C000001814

Martindale

The complete drug reference

Thirty-second edition

Edited by

Kathleen Parfitt

BSc, FRPharmS

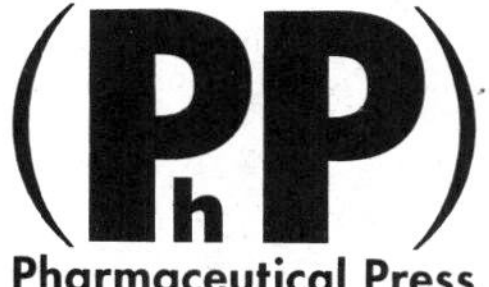

Published by the Pharmaceutical Press
1 Lambeth High Street, London SEI 7JN, UK

First edition of *Martindale: The Extra Pharmacopoeia* was published in 1883. *Squire's Companion* was incorporated in the twenty-third edition in 1952.

Thirty-second edition published 1999

© 1999 Pharmaceutical Press

Printed in the United States of America by World Color Book Services, Taunton, Massachusetts

ISBN 0 85369 429 X

ISSN 0263-5364

All rights reserved. No part of this publication may be reproduced, stored in a retrieval system, or transmitted in any form or by any means, without the prior written permission of the copyright holder.

The publisher makes no representation, express or implied, with regard to the accuracy of the information contained in this book and cannot accept any legal responsibility or liability for any errors or omissions that may be made.

A catalogue record for this book is available from the British Library

Preface

Over the years Marti has become much more than the name 'pharmacopoeia' implid so for this new edition the subtitle 'Extra Pharmacopoeia' has beplaced by 'The Complete Drug Reference'. Martindale is now pued every three years. It is also available electronically on CD arMartindale Online.

The aim of Martincis to provide practising pharmacists and physicians with unbiasealuated information on drugs and medicines used throughout the wı It therefore has to develop as the body of knowledge on existing c grows, new drugs emerge, new preparations are launched, old prepons abandoned, reformulated, or redefined, and the information neof those practising pharmacy and medicine continue to evolve. We ltried to ensure that the new edition continues to meet these needs.

All the drug monograjrom the last edition have been revised, more than 300 having been ded and more than 250 added, and organised into chapters that reflectuses of the drugs being described. One of the new features of this ecn is the creation of an Interactions section within drug monographsnake the information more accessible both in the book and electronly. A new Bronchodilators chapter draws together drugs that we'ormerly described in the Antimuscarinics, Prophylactic Anti-asthrAgents, Sympathomimetics, and Xanthines chapters and includes ıase treatment reviews for Asthma and for Chronic Obstructive Puhary Disease.

The disease treatmentriews, 644 in all and generally located in the chapter introductions, ḥ also been thoroughly revised in order to reflect current trends aprovide key references. Cross-references to these reviews appear in monographs of the drugs cited; the reviews can also be accessed via general index. It is hoped that these reviews will be of use to readers o want an overview of a particular disease and its drug treatment and vprovide a useful starting point for those who want to pursue particulaspects further.

The information on prietary preparations, an important feature of Martindale, has been uped and presented more concisely.

Martindale is based cpublished information and more than 30 000 selected references are :luded. Our aim is to evaluate the literature, covering important stucs, guidelines, and useful reviews and placing them in context. Multintre studies, meta-analyses, and systematic reviews are playing a gwing and important role in the study of drug treatment, and their findgs and conclusions are considered in many of our chapters. However, ere is also a place for the anecdotal report and the small study, and inrmation from such sources is included where appropriate.

The sheer bulk of Mandale was making it rather unwieldy to use and strenuous editorial efforhave been made this time to reduce the size of the book without sacrifing content.

Martindale is not a bok of standards. Inclusion of a substance or a preparation is not to be cnsidered as a recommendation for use, nor does it confer any status on tl substance or preparation. While considerable efforts have been made tcheck the material in Martindale, the publisher cannot accept any respoibility for errors and omissions. Also the reader is assumed to posses the necessary knowledge to interpret the information that Martincle provides.

Arrangement

Part 1 (pages 1–1539 contains 4336 monographs arranged in 51 chapters. These chaptersgenerally bring together monographs on drugs and groups of drugs thathave similar uses or actions. The introductions of those chapters that decribe drugs used in the management of disease contain disease treatmnt reviews—descriptions of those diseases together with reviews of the choice of treatments.

Part 2 (pages 1541–1646) consists of a series of 827 short monographs arranged in the alphabetical order of their main titles. It includes monographs on some new drugs, on drugs not easily classified, on herbals, and on drugs no longer used clinically but still of interest. There are also monographs on toxic substances, the effects of which may require drug therapy.

Part 3 (pages 1647–2057) contains proprietary preparations from a range of countries. For this edition we have covered Australia, Austria, Belgium, Canada, France, Germany, Ireland, Italy, the Netherlands, Norway, South Africa, Spain, Sweden, Switzerland, UK, and USA. We have also included some proprietary preparations from Japan. The information provided includes the proprietary name, the manufacturer or distributor, the active ingredients with cross-references to the drug monographs, and a summary of the indications as given by the manufacturer.

Indexes

Directory of Manufacturers. In Martindale the names of manufacturers and distributors are abbreviated. Their full names are given in this directory together with the full address if it is available. This directory contains some 5400 entries.

General Index. To make fullest use of the contents of Martindale the general index should always be consulted. The exhaustive index includes entries for drugs (approved names, synonyms, and chemical names), preparations, pharmacological and therapeutic groups, and clinical uses (disease treatment reviews). As in previous editions, the index is arranged alphabetically 'word-by-word' rather than 'letter-by-letter'. The index indicates the column in which the relevant entry appears as well as the page.

Nomenclature

Martindale Identity Numbers. Each monograph title is followed by an identity number in brackets which consists of a maximum of 6 figures followed by a check character. These numbers are used in our computer manipulation and their purpose is to identify monographs in Martindale.

Titles and Synonyms. The title of each monograph is in English, with preference being given to British Approved Names (BAN), United States Adopted Names (USAN), and International Nonproprietary Names (INN). These 3 authorities are shown where appropriate. A European Directive (92/27/EEC) requiring the use of Recommended International Nonproprietary Names (rINNs) in the labelling of medicinal products throughout member states of the European Community had not been implemented in the UK at the time of going to press. However, we have acknowledged the move towards replacing BAN by rINN by giving more prominence to INN names. Names given as synonyms include commonly used abbreviated names; Latin versions of *Ph. Eur.* titles; English, American, and Latin synonyms; names used in other languages when these may not be readily identifiable; manufacturers' code numbers; and chemical names. In some approved names it is now general policy to use 'f' for 'ph' in sulpha, 't' for 'th', and 'i' for 'y'; for this reason entries in alphabetical lists and indexes should be sought in alternative spellings if the expected spellings are not found. A table of contracted names for ions and groups used in approved names and titles is given on page xi.

CAS Registry Numbers. Chemical Abstracts Service (CAS) registry numbers are provided, where available, for each monograph substance to help readers refer to other information systems. Numbers for various forms of the monograph substance are listed with the variation in form given in parentheses.

Atomic and Molecular Weights

Atomic weights are based on the table of Atomic Weights as revised in 1995 by the Commission on Atomic Weights and Isotopic Abundance, International Union of Pure and Applied Chemistry and based on the ^{12}C scale (see page xii). Molecular weights are given corrected to one place of decimals or to four significant figures for relative weights of less than 100.

Pharmacopoeias

The selected pharmacopoeias in which each substance appears are listed. Current copies of the pharmacopoeias and their addenda should be consulted for confirmation and for details of standards.

The pharmacopoeias covered include: Austrian, Belgian, *British, British Veterinary,* Chinese, *European, French, German*, International, Italian, *Japanese,* Netherlands, *Polish,* Portuguese, *Swiss,* and *United States* (including the *Formulary*). Those *italicised* in the above list either appeared as new editions or were revised by supplements since the last edition of Martindale, and have been examined for this 32nd edition.

The abbreviations for these pharmacopoeias are included in the list of abbreviations used in Martindale, see page ix which also includes details of the edition and/or supplement(s) consulted.

Several countries are parties to the Convention on the Elaboration of a European Pharmacopoeia. This means that they must adopt the standards of the European Pharmacopoeia. These countries are currently Austria, Belgium, Bosnia-Herzegovina, Croatia, Cyprus, Czech Republic, Denmark, Finland, France, Germany, Greece, Iceland, Ireland, Italy, Luxembourg, the Netherlands, Norway, Portugal, Slovakia, Slovenia, Spain, Sweden, Switzerland, Turkey, the United Kingdom of Great Britain and Northern Ireland, and the Former Yugoslav Republic of Macedonia. Hence the European Pharmacopoeia is cited in the drug monograph lists of pharmacopoeias rather than these individual national pharmacopoeias.

Official preparations, mainly from the current British and US Pharmacopoeias, are listed at the end of drug monographs.

Pharmaceutical Information

Information on the chemical and physical properties of each substance is given when it is likely to be of use or interest, but only when it is certain that it applies to the form of substance being described in the monograph.

PERCENTAGE STRENGTHS. Unless otherwise stated, solutions of solids in liquids are expressed as percentage w/v, of liquids in liquids as percentage v/v, and of gases in liquids as percentage w/w.

SOLUBILITY. The figures given for solubility in each monograph have generally been obtained from the major pharmacopoeias in which the substance is described, but should not be considered absolute. Unless otherwise indicated in the text, the figures are for solubility at temperatures between 15° and 25°. The information usually relates to w/v solubilities but in some cases is v/v if the monograph substance itself is a liquid. Where solubilities are given in words, the following terms describe the indicated solubility ranges:

solubility	
very soluble	1 in less than 1
freely soluble	1 in 1 to 1 in 10
soluble	1 in 10 to 1 in 30
sparingly soluble	1 in 30 to 1 in 100
slightly soluble	1 in 100 to 1 in 1000
very slightly soluble	1 in 1000 to 1 in 10 000
practically insoluble	1 in more than 10 000

STORAGE. Substances and preparations should be stored under conditions which prevent contamination and diminish deterioration, and the conditions of storage given in the text indicate the precautions recommended in specific cases. Where authorities differ, we have included the most stringent storage requirement. The term 'a cool place' is generally used to describe a place in which the temperature is between 8° and 15°. In general, the storage conditions apply to the monograph substance and not its solutions or preparations.

TEMPERATURE. Temperatures are expressed in degrees Celsius (centigrade) unless otherwise indicated.

Pharmacological and Therapeuınformation

Information on adverse effects, treatmentverse effects, precautions (including contra-indications), interactioıarmacokinetics, and uses and administration of each substance is ɪed by concise statements and these may be elaborated and expanɑy referenced reviews and abstracts from papers and other publicatiхhis edition contains about 11 300 such abstracts or reviews base information in an ever widening range of publications.

Much information has been found in ːes such as World Health Organization publications, government re and legislation, and other official and standard publications. Manurers' literature has been considered in the light of other available ination.

The risks of administering drugs in pregy are well known and the general principle is to give a drug only whe benefit to the individual mother outweighs the risk to the fetus. W there is a clear risk it is noted under the Precautions or Adverse Ef heading but safety should not be inferred from the absence of a statet for any drug.

Doses

Doses are described under the Uses and Anistration heading with as much detail as is necessary and availablenless otherwise stated the doses represent the average range of quties which are generally regarded as suitable for adults when adistered by mouth. More information on doses and drug administon may be given in the abstracts or reviews. Unless otherwise speci, glucose injection is 5% w/v and sodium chloride injection is 0.9%.

When doses for children are expressed arange of quantities within specified age limits, the lower dose applies æ lower age and the higher dose at the higher age.

Acknowledgements

The Editor would like to acknowledge invaluable advice and assistance so willingly provided by AB Pral. Thanks are also due to DN Bateman, PR Jackson, T Pullar, LE Rany, M Summerhayes, and WW Yeo for reading and commenting on drs of this edition.

The Editor is grateful to the many organiions that have helped in providing information, including the World alth Organization and the British Pharmacopoeia Commission.

Martindale staff have been able to call free on the expertise of other members of the Royal Pharmaceutical Soci's staff. In particular the Editor is grateful to JEF Reynolds, DK Mehtaıd the editorial staff of the British National Formulary, and the staff of library and information department. Thanks are due to M Davis and ELaughton for work on the Preparations database and for other editial tasks, and also to SL Jefferson and RL Stock who contributed this edition.

The contents of this 32nd edition were ɪnned, written, checked, indexed, keyed, proofed, and processed by ıe Martindale staff. The Editor is pleased to acknowledge the skills d commitment of all the Martindale staff and to record her gratitude: Claire Ryan for clerical assistance and, towards the end of the producon cycle, to Evelyn Doh, Pauline Lloyd, and Maria Robinson for a subantial amount of keying; to the Staff Editors Alison Brayfield, Catherir Cadart, Kathleen Eager, Sue Funnell, Prakash Gotecha, Sue Handy, Rhda Lee, Julie McGlashan, Gail Neathercoat, and Keith Riley; to the Asistant Editors Paul Blake and Anne Parsons; and to the Senior AssistantEditor Sean Sweetman.

London January 1999

Abbreviations

For abbreviations of the names of manufacturers or their distributors, see Directory of Manufacturers, p.2059.

≈—approximately equals.
ACE—angiotensin-converting enzyme.
agg.—aggregate (in botanical names), including 2 or more species which resemble each other closely.
AIDS—acquired immunodeficiency syndrome.
a.m.—ante meridiem, 'before noon'.
ARC—AIDS-related complex.
Aust.—Austria.
Aust. P.—Austrian Pharmacopoeia 1990 (Österreichisches Arzneibuch) including Addenda 1990 and 1991.
Austral.—Australia.
BAN—British Approved Name.
BANM—British Approved Name Modified.
Belg. P.—Belgian Pharmacopoeia 1980 (Pharmacopée Belge, Sixième Edition) and Supplements to 1988.
BMA—British Medical Association.
BNF—British National Formulary.
b.p.—boiling point.
BP—British Pharmacopoeia. Unless otherwise specified, BP references are to the 1998 edition including Amendments No. 1.
BP (Vet)—British Pharmacopoeia (Veterinary) 1998 and Amendments No. 1.
BPC—British Pharmaceutical Codex.
Br.—British.
BUN—Blood-urea-nitrogen.
°C—degrees Celsius (centigrade). Unless otherwise indicated in the text, temperatures are expressed in this thermometric scale.
C.—*Campylobacter*, *Candida*, *Chlamydia*, or *Corynebacterium*.
Canad.—Canada.
CAPD—continuous ambulatory peritoneal dialysis.
CAS—Chemical Abstracts Service.
CCPD—continuous cycle peritoneal dialysis.
CDC—Centers for Disease Control (USA).
Chin. P.—Chinese Pharmacopoeia 1990.
CI—Colour Index.
CNS—central nervous system.
cP—centipoise(s).
CPMP—Committee on Proprietary Medicinal Products of the European Union.
CRM—the former Committee on the Review of Medicines (UK).
CSF—cerebrospinal fluid.
CSM—Committee on Safety of Medicines (UK).
cSt—centistokes.
D & C—designation applied in USA to dyes permitted for use in drugs and cosmetics.
d.c.—direct current.
DHSS—the former Department of Health and Social Security (UK).
DNA—deoxyribonucleic acid.
DOE—Department of the Environment (UK).
DoH—Department of Health (UK).
DPF—Dental Practitioners' Formulary (UK).
DTF—Drug Tariff Formulary.
ECG—electrocardiogram.
ECT—electroconvulsive therapy.
Ecuad.—Ecuador.
ed.—editor(s) *or* edited by *or* edition.
EEC—European Economic Community, now the European Union.
EEG—electro-encephalogram.
e.g.—*exempli gratia* 'for example'.
ENL—erythema nodosum leprosum.
ENT—ear, nose, and throat.
ESR—erythrocyte sedimentation rate.
ESRD—end-stage renal disease.
et al.—*et alii*, 'and others': for three or more co-authors or co-workers.
EU—European Union.
Eur. P.—see Ph. Eur.
Ext. D & C—designation applied in USA to dyes permitted for use in external drug and cosmetic preparations.
°F—degrees Fahrenheit.
FAC—Food Additives and Contaminants Committee of the Ministry of Agriculture, Fisheries and Food (UK).
FAO—Food and Agriculture Organization of the United Nations.
FAO/WHO—Food and Agriculture Organization of the United Nations *and the* World Health Organization.
FDA—Food and Drug Administration of USA.
FdAC—Food Advisory Committee of the Ministry of Agriculture, Fisheries and Food (UK).
FD & C—designation applied in USA to dyes permitted for use in foods, drugs, and cosmetics.
FEV_1—forced expiratory volume in 1 second.
FIP—Fédération Internationale Pharmaceutique.
f.p.—freezing point.
FPA—Family Planning Association (UK).
Fr.—France.
Fr. P.—French Pharmacopoeia 1982 (Pharmacopée Francaise, Xe Edition) and Supplements 1 to 13.
g—gram(s).
Ger.—Germany.
Ger. P.— German Pharmacopoeia (Deutsches Arzneibuch, 1998).
GFR—glomerular filtration rate.
Hb— haemoglobin.
Hib—*Haemophilus influenzae* type b.
HIV—human immunodeficiency virus.
HLA—human lymphocyte antigens.
HLB—hydrophilic-lipophilic balance.
HSE—Health and Safety Executive (UK).
Hung.—Hungary.
IARC—International Agency for Research on Cancer.
ibid.—*ibidem*, 'in the same place (journal or book)'.
idem—'the same': used for the same authors and titles.
i.e.—*id est*, 'that is'.
Ig—immunoglobulin.
INN—International Nonproprietary Name.
Int. P.—International Pharmacopoeia 3rd ed., Volume 1, 1979; Volume 2, 1981; Volume 3, 1988; and Volume 4, 1994.
IPCS—International Programme on Chemical Safety.
IQ—intelligence quotient.
IR—infra-red.
Irl.—Ireland.
ISO—International Organization for Standardization.
It. P.—Italian Pharmacopoeia 1985 (Farmacopea Ufficiale della Repubblica Italiana, Edizione Nona) and Supplements 1 to 3.
Ital.—Italy.
iu—international unit(s).
IUD—intra-uterine device.
IUPAC—International Union of Pure and Applied Chemistry.

J—joule(s).
Jpn—Japan.
Jpn P.—The Pharmacopoeia of Japan, 13th ed., 1996.
K—kelvin.
kcal—kilocalorie(s).
kg—kilogram(s).
kJ—kilojoule(s).
Kor.—Korea.
lb—pound(s) avoirdupois.
LD_{50}—a dose lethal to 50% of the specified animals or micro-organisms.
Lf—limit flocculation.
m—metre(s).
m^2—square metre(s).
m^3—cubic metre(s).
M—molar.
MAFF—Ministry of Agriculture, Fisheries and Food (UK).
MAOI—monoamine oxidase inhibitor.
max.—maximum.
MBC—minimum bactericidal concentration.
MCA—Medicines Control Agency (UK).
mEq—milliequivalent(s).
mg—milligram(s).
MIC—minimum inhibitory concentration.
min—minute.
min.—minimum.
MJ—megajoule(s).
mL—millilitre(s).
mm—millimetre(s).
mm^2—square millimetre(s).
mm^3—cubic millimetre(s).
mmHg—millimetre(s) of mercury.
mmol—millimole.
mol—mole.
mol. wt—molecular weight.
Mon.—Monaco.
mosmol—milliosmole.
m.p.—melting point.
MRC—Medical Research Council (UK).
μg—microgram(s).
μL—microlitre(s).
μm—micrometre(s).
NCTC—National Collection of Type Cultures (Central Public Health Laboratory, London, England).
Neth.—The Netherlands.
Neth. P.—Netherlands Pharmacopoeia 1983 (Nederlandse Farmacopee, Negende Uitgave) and Supplements to 1993.
ng—nanogram(s).
NIH—National Institutes of Health (USA).
nm—nanometre(s).
Norw.—Norway.
NSAID—nonsteroidal anti-inflammatory drug.
OP—over proof.
o/w—oil-in-water.
P—probability.
Pa—pascal(s).
PBI—protein-bound iodine.
pCO_2—plasma partial pressure (concentration) of carbon dioxide.
p_aCO_2—arterial plasma partial pressure (concentration) of carbon dioxide.
pg—picogram(s).
pH—the negative logarithm of the hydrogen ion concentration.
Ph. Eur.—European Pharmacopoeia, 3rd ed., 1997 and Supplements 1998 and 1999.
Pharm. Soc. Lab. Rep.—Royal Pharmaceutical Society's Laboratory Report.
PHLS—Public Health Laboratory Service (UK).
pINN—Proposed International Nonproprietary Name.
pINNM—Proposed International Nonproprietary Name Modified.
pK_a—the negative logarithm of the dissociation constant.
p.m.—*post meridiem*, 'afternoon'.
pO_2—plasma partial pressure (concentration) of oxygen.
p_aO_2—arterial plasma partial pressure (concentration) of oxygen.
Pol.—Poland.
Pol. P.—Polish Pharmacopoeia (Farmakopea Polska) 5th ed., Volume 1, 1990; Volume 2, 1993; Supplement 1, 1995; Volume 3, 1996.
Port.—Portugal.
Port. P.—Portuguese Pharmacopoeia 1986 (Farmacopoeia Portuguesa V) and Supplements to 1991.
ppm—parts per million.
PSGB—The Pharmaceutical Society of Great Britain. Now the Royal Pharmaceutical Society of Great Britain.
q.s.—*quantum sufficit*, 'as much as suffices'.
q.v.—*quod vide*, 'which see'.
RCGP—Royal College of General Practitioners (UK).
RIMA—reversible inhibitor of monoamine oxidase type A.
rINN—Recommended International Nonproprietary Name.
rINNM—Recommended International Nonproprietary Name Modified.
RNA—ribonucleic acid.
RPSGB—The Royal Pharmaceutical Society of Great Britain.
S. Afr.—South Africa.
SGOT—serum glutamic oxaloacetic transaminase (serum aspartate aminotransferase *now preferred*).
SGPT—serum glutamic pyruvic transaminase (serum alanine aminotransferase *now preferred*).
SI—Statutory Instrument *or* Système International d'Unités (International System of Units).
SLE—systemic lupus erythematosus.
sp.—species (plural spp.).
sp. gr.—specific gravity.
SSRI—selective serotonin reuptake inhibitor.
St—stokes.
subsp.—subspecies.
suppl—supplement(s).
Swed.—Sweden.
Swiss P.—Swiss Pharmacopoeia 1997 (Pharmacopoea Helvetica, 8e édition, Edition Française) and Supplement 1998.
Switz.—Switzerland.
Thai.—Thailand.
TPN—total parenteral nutrition.
UK—United Kingdom.
UNICEF—United Nations Children's Fund.
UP—under proof.
US and **USA**—United States of America.
USAN—United States Adopted Name.
USNF—The United States 'National Formulary 18', 1995, and Supplements 1 to 9.
USP—The United States Pharmacopeia 23, 1995, and Supplements 1 to 9.
UV—ultraviolet.
var.—variety.
vol.—volume(s).
v/v—volume in volume.
v/w—volume in weight.
WHO—World Health Organization.
w/o—water-in-oil.
wt—weight.
wt per mL—weight per millilitre.
w/v—weight in volume.
w/w—weight in weight.

Contracted Names for Ions and Groups

Contracted Name	Chemical Name
acetonide	isopropylidene ether of a dihydric alcohol
aceturate	*N*-acetylglycinate
acistrate	2′-acetate (ester) and stearate (salt)
acoxil	acetoxymethyl
amsonate	4,4′-diaminostilbene-2,2′-disulphonate
anisatil	2-(4-methoxyphenyl)-2-oxoethyl
axetil	1-acetoxyethyl
besylate (besilate)	benzenesulphonate
bezomil	(benzoyloxy)methyl
buciclate	*trans*-4-butylcyclohexanecarboxylate
bunapsilate	3,7-di-*tert*-butylnaphthalene-1,5-disulphonate
buteprate	17-(1-oxobutoxy) (ester) and 21-(1-oxopropoxy) (ester)
camsylate (camsilate)	camphor-10-sulphonate
caproate	hexanoate
carbesilate	4-carboxybenzenesulphonate
cilexetil	(*RS*)-1-{[(cyclohexyloxy)carbonyl]oxy}ethyl
closylate (closilate)	4-chlorobenzenesulphonate
crobefate	(±)-(*E*)-6-hydroxy-4′-methoxy-3-(*p*-methoxybenzylidene)flavone phosphate ion (2−)
cromacate	[(6-hydroxy-4-methyl-2-oxo-2*H*-chromen-7-yl)oxy]acetate
cromesilate	6,7-dihydroxycoumarin-4-methanesulphonate
cyclotate (ciclotate)	4-methylbicyclo[2.2.2]oct-2-ene-l-carboxylate
cypionate (cipionate)	3-cyclopentylpropionate
deanil	2-dimethylaminoethyl
dibudinate	2,6-di-*tert*-butylnaphthalene-1,5-disulphonate
dibunate	2,6-di-*tert*-butyl-l-naphthalenesulphonate
digolil	2-(2-hydroxyethoxy)ethyl
diolamine	diethanolamine
dipivoxil	(2,2-dimethyl-1-oxopropoxy)methyl or (pivaloyloxy)methyl (=pivoxil)
dofosfate	octadecyl hydrogen phosphate
edamine	ethylenediamine
edetate	ethylenediamine-*NNN′N′*-tetra-acetate
edisylate (edisilate)	ethane-1,2-disulphonate
embonate	4,4′-methylenebis(3-hydroxy-2-naphthoate) (=pamoate)
enanthate (enantate)	heptanoate
epolamine	1-pyrrolidineethanol
erbumine	*tert*-butylamine
estolate	propionate dodecyl sulphate
esylate (esilate)	ethanesulphonate
etabonate	(ethoxycarbonyl)oxy (=ethyl carbonate)
farnesil	(2*E*,6*E*)-3,7,11-trimethyl-2,6,10-dodecatrienyl
fendizoate	2-[(2′-hydroxy-4-biphenylyl)carbonyl]benzoate
fostedate	tetradecyl hydrogen phosphate
gluceptate	glucoheptonate
hybenzate (hibenzate)	2-(4-hydroxybenzoyl)benzoate
hyclate	monohydrochloride hemi-ethanolate hemihydrate
isethionate (isetionate)	2-hydroxyethanesulphonate
lauryl sulphate (laurilsulfate)	dodecyl sulphate
megallate	3,4,5-trimethoxybenzoate
meglumine	*N*-methylglucamine
mesylate (mesilate)	methanesulphonate
metembonate	4,4′-methylenebis(3-methoxy-2-naphthoate)
mofetil	2-(morpholino)ethyl
napadisylate (napadisilate)	naphthalene-1,5-disulphonate
napsylate (napsilate)	naphthalene-2-sulphonate
olamine	ethanolamine
oxoglurate	2-oxoglutarate
pamoate	4,4′-methylenebis(3-hydroxy-2-naphthoate) (=embonate)
pendetide	N^6-{*N*-[2-({2-[bis(carboxymethyl)amino]-ethyl}(carboxymethyl)amino)ethyl]-*N*-(carboxymethyl)glycyl}-N^2-(*N*-glycyl-L-tyrosyl)-L-lysine
pentexil	1-hydroxyethyl pivalate
phenpropionate	3-phenylpropionate
pivalate	trimethylacetate
pivoxetil	1-(2-methoxy-2-methylpropionyloxy)ethyl
pivoxil	(2,2-dimethyl-1-oxopropoxy)methyl or (pivaloyloxy)methyl (=dipivoxil)
polistirex	sulphonated styrene-divinylbenzene copolymer complex
proxetil	1-[(isopropoxycarbonyl)oxy]ethyl
steaglate	stearoyloxyacetate
suleptanate	sodium 7-[methyl(2-sulphonatomethyl)carbamoyl]heptanoyl
tebutate	*tert*-butylacetate
tenoate	2-thiophenecarboxylate
teprosilate	3-(theophyllin-7-yl)propanesulphonate
theoclate (teoclate)	8-chlorotheophyllinate
tofesilate	2-(theophyllin-7-yl)ethanesulphonate
tosylate (tosilate)	toluene-4-sulphonate
triclofenate	2,4,5-trichlorophenolate
triflutate	trifluoroacetate
trolamine	triethanolamine
troxundate	3,6,9-trioxaundecanoate
xinafoate	1-hydroxy-2-naphthoate

Atomic Weights of the Elements— $^{12}C=12$

Atomic Number	Name	Symbol	Atomic Weight
89	Actinium	Ac	*
13	Aluminium	Al	26.981538
95	Americium	Am	*
51	Antimony	Sb	121.760
18	Argon	Ar	39.948
33	Arsenic	As	74.92160
85	Astatine	At	*
56	Barium	Ba	137.327
97	Berkelium	Bk	*
4	Beryllium	Be	9.012182
83	Bismuth	Bi	208.98038
5	Boron	B	10.811
35	Bromine	Br	79.904
48	Cadmium	Cd	112.411
55	Caesium	Cs	132.90545
20	Calcium	Ca	40.078
98	Californium	Cf	*
6	Carbon	C	12.0107
58	Cerium	Ce	140.116
17	Chlorine	Cl	35.4527
24	Chromium	Cr	51.9961
27	Cobalt	Co	58.933200
29	Copper	Cu	63.546
96	Curium	Cm	*
66	Dysprosium	Dy	162.50
99	Einsteinium	Es	*
68	Erbium	Er	167.26
63	Europium	Eu	151.964
100	Fermium	Fm	*
9	Fluorine	F	18.9984032
87	Francium	Fr	*
64	Gadolinium	Gd	157.25
31	Gallium	Ga	69.723
32	Germanium	Ge	72.61
79	Gold	Au	196.96655
72	Hafnium	Hf	178.49
2	Helium	He	4.002602
67	Holmium	Ho	164.93032
1	Hydrogen	H	1.00794
49	Indium	In	114.818
53	Iodine	I	126.90447
77	Iridium	Ir	192.217
26	Iron	Fe	55.845
36	Krypton	Kr	83.80
57	Lanthanum	La	138.9055
103	Lawrencium	Lr	*
82	Lead	Pb	207.2
3	‡Lithium	Li	6.941
71	Lutetium	Lu	174.967
12	Magnesium	Mg	24.3050
25	Manganese	Mn	54.938049
101	Mendelevium	Md	*
80	Mercury	Hg	200.59
42	Molybdenum	Mo	95.94
60	Neodymium	Nd	144.24
10	Neon	Ne	20.1797
93	Neptunium	Np	*
28	Nickel	Ni	58.6934
41	Niobium	Nb	92.90638
7	Nitrogen	N	14.00674
102	Nobelium	No	*
76	Osmium	Os	190.23
8	Oxygen	O	15.9994
46	Palladium	Pd	106.42
15	Phosphorus	P	30.973761
78	Platinum	Pt	195.078
94	Plutonium	Pu	*
84	Polonium	Po	*
19	Potassium	K	39.0983
59	Praseodymium	Pr	140.90765
61	Promethium	Pm	*
91	†Protactinium	Pa	231.03588
88	Radium	Ra	*
86	Radon	Rn	*
75	Rhenium	Re	186.207
45	Rhodium	Rh	102.90550
37	Rubidium	Rb	85.4678
44	Ruthenium	Ru	101.07
62	Samarium	Sm	150.36
21	Scandium	Sc	44.955910
34	Selenium	Se	78.96
14	Silicon	Si	28.0855
47	Silver	Ag	107.8682
11	Sodium	Na	22.989770
38	Strontium	Sr	87.62
16	Sulphur	S	32.066
73	Tantalum	Ta	180.9479
43	Technetium	Tc	*
52	Tellurium	Te	127.60
65	Terbium	Tb	158.92534
81	Thallium	Tl	204.3833
90	†Thorium	Th	232.0381
69	Thulium	Tm	168.93421
50	Tin	Sn	118.710
22	Titanium	Ti	47.867
74	Tungsten	W	183.84
109	Unnilennium	Une	*
106	Unnilhexium	Unh	*
108	Unniloctium	Uno	*
105	Unnilpentium	Unp	*
104	Unnilquadium	Unq	*
107	Unnilseptium	Uns	*
110	Ununnilium	Uun	*
111	Unununium	Uuu	*
92	†Uranium	U	238.0289
23	Vanadium	V	50.9415
54	Xenon	Xe	131.29
70	Ytterbium	Yb	173.04
39	Yttrium	Y	88.90585
30	Zinc	Zn	65.39
40	Zirconium	Zr	91.224

Elements marked (*) have no stable nuclides and IUPAC states "there is no general agreement on which of the isotopes of the radioactive elements is, or is likely to be judged 'important' and various criteria such as 'longest half-life', 'production in quantity', 'used commercially', etc., have been applied in the Commission's choice." However, atomic weights are given for radioactive elements marked (†) as they do have a characteristic terrestrial isotopic composition. Commercially available lithium (‡) materials have atomic weights ranging from 6.94 to 6.99; if a more accurate value is required, it must be determined for the specific material.

Part 1

Monographs on Drugs and Ancillary Substances

Analgesics Anti-inflammatory Drugs and Antipyretics

The compounds described in this chapter are used mainly in the relief of pain, inflammation and, sometimes, fever. They can be grouped broadly into one of the categories briefly described below.

Gold compounds

Gold compounds are used mainly for their anti-inflammatory effect in active progressive rheumatoid arthritis and progressive juvenile chronic arthritis; they may also be beneficial in psoriatic arthritis. The mechanism of action of gold compounds in rheumatic disorders is as yet unknown.

For further discussion of the actions and uses of gold compounds, see Sodium Aurothiomalate, p.83.

Nonsteroidal Anti-inflammatory Drugs

Nonsteroidal anti-inflammatory drugs (NSAIDs) are a group of unrelated organic acids that have analgesic, anti-inflammatory, and antipyretic properties. NSAIDs are inhibitors of the enzyme cyclo-oxygenase, which results in the direct inhibition of the biosynthesis of prostaglandins and thromboxanes from arachidonic acid (see p.1411 and p.704). There are 2 forms of cyclo-oxygenase, COX-1, which is the constitutive form of the enzyme, and COX-2, which is the form induced in the presence of inflammation. Inhibition of COX-2 is therefore thought to be responsible for at least some of the analgesic, anti-inflammatory, and antipyretic properties of NSAIDs whereas inhibition of COX-1 is thought to produce some of their toxic effects, particularly those on the gastro-intestinal tract. Most of the NSAIDs currently available for clinical use inhibit both COX-1 and COX-2.

Aspirin (see under Salicylates, below) is also considered to be an NSAID, but it irreversibly acetylates cyclo-oxygenase whereas other NSAIDs compete with arachidonic acid at the active site of cyclo-oxygenase.

NSAIDs are used for the relief of mild to moderate pain, minor febrile conditions, and for acute and chronic inflammatory disorders such as osteoarthritis, rheumatoid arthritis, juvenile chronic arthritis, and ankylosing spondylitis. Indomethacin and some other NSAIDs are used to close patent ductus arteriosus in premature neonates. Some NSAIDs are applied topically for the relief of muscular and rheumatic pain, and some are used in ophthalmic preparations for ocular inflammatory disorders.

For further discussion of the actions and uses of NSAIDs, see p.63.

Opioid Analgesics

Opioid analgesics include the opium alkaloids morphine and codeine and their derivatives as well as synthetic substances with agonist, partial agonist, or mixed agonist-antagonist activity at opioid receptors. The term opiate analgesics refers only to those opioids derived from opium, or their semisynthetic congeners. The term narcotic analgesic has legal connotations and is no longer used pharmacologically or clinically.

The majority of opioids are used as analgesics, and morphine is the standard against which all other opioid analgesics are compared. Weak opioids such as codeine or dextropropoxyphene are used in the treatment of moderate to severe pain, and are often combined with non-opioid analgesics such as aspirin, other NSAIDs, or paracetamol. Strong opioids such as morphine are used in severe acute and chronic pain, including cancer pain. Some opioids such as codeine, morphine, and diamorphine are also used as antitussives, although the latter two are usually reserved for use in terminal lung disease. Some opioid analgesics such as fentanyl and its congeners are used mainly as adjuncts to anaesthesia; some of these may also be used in higher doses as the sole anaesthetic drug. Opioids with these uses are described in this chapter.

Opioids such as dextromethorphan and pholcodine that are used exclusively as antitussives are discussed under Cough, p.1052. Opioids such as diphenoxylate and loperamide that are used exclusively in the treatment of diarrhoea are discussed under Gastro-intestinal Drugs, p.1167.

Opioids can produce physical dependence and withdrawal symptoms on sudden discontinuation. They are also subject to abuse.

For further discussion of the actions and uses of Opioid Analgesics, see p.67.

Para-aminophenol derivatives

Paracetamol is the principal para-aminophenol derivative in use. Acetanilide (p.12) and phenacetin (p.78) were formerly used but have generally been replaced by safer analgesics. Propacetamol (p.81) is hydrolysed to paracetamol in the plasma.

Paracetamol has analgesic and antipyretic properties and weak anti-inflammatory activity. The mechanism of analgesic action remains to be fully elucidated, but may be due to inhibition of prostaglandin synthesis both centrally and peripherally. Paracetamol is used for the relief of mild to moderate pain and minor febrile conditions.

Benorylate (p.21) is an ester of aspirin and paracetamol with similar uses as the individual components.

For further discussion of the actions and uses of paracetamol, see p.72.

Salicylates

Aspirin and other salicylates are NSAIDs (see above) and have analgesic, anti-inflammatory, and antipyretic properties. They are inhibitors of the enzyme cyclo-oxygenase, which results in the direct inhibition of the biosynthesis of prostaglandins and thromboxanes from arachidonic acid (see p.1411 and p.704). Salicylates are used for the relief of mild to moderate pain, minor febrile conditions, and for acute and chronic inflammatory disorders such as osteoarthritis, rheumatoid arthritis, juvenile chronic arthritis, and ankylosing spondylitis. Some salicylates are applied topically in rubefacient preparations for the relief of muscular and rheumatic pain. Aspirin also inhibits platelet aggregation and is used in cardiovascular disorders. Non-acetylated salicylates do not have antiplatelet activity.

Benorylate (p.21) is an ester of aspirin and paracetamol with similar uses as the individual components.

For further discussion of the actions and uses of salicylates, see Aspirin, p.16.

Fever and hyperthermia

The hypothalamus is the centre of the thermoregulatory system and is responsible for maintaining the body temperature at a set point (known as the set-point temperature) which is normally 37°. Mechanisms which produce or conserve body heat include passive heat absorption from the environment, peripheral vasoconstriction, and thermogenic processes such as metabolic reactions and shivering. Heat loss is achieved mainly through sweating and peripheral vasodilatation. Body temperature may be elevated by a number of causes and it is important to distinguish between these as the appropriate treatment may vary according to the mechanisms of the temperature increase.

Fever (pyrexia) is defined as an increase in body temperature due to an elevated thermoregulatory set-point temperature. Common causes of fever include infections, inflammatory disorders, neoplastic disease, and some drug treatment. The term hyperthermia (hyperpyrexia) has been used when the set point is not altered, but there is a disturbance of thermoregulatory control. This may be due to injury to the hypothalamus, defective heat loss as occurs in dehydration, or excessive heat production following strenuous activities or as a reaction to certain drugs such as anaesthetics (malignant hyperthermia) or antipsychotics (neuroleptic malignant syndrome).

Treatment of fever. Whenever possible the underlying cause of the fever should be identified and treated first.[1] Apart from pregnant women or patients who are already dehydrated or malnourished or those with cardiac, respiratory, or neurological diseases, body temperatures up to 41° are relatively harmless.[1] It is not clear if there is any value in treating fever at lower temperatures. Antipyretics have been given to febrile children but studies have shown that such treatment did not necessarily improve their comfort[2] and might even prolong any infection.[3] It has also been suggested[4] that in severe infection the use of antipyretics might increase mortality. It has been noted[4] that the WHO recommend that in developing countries antipyretics should not be given routinely to children with fever; they should be reserved for those with severe discomfort or high fever. In the UK, antipyretic therapy is recommended to treat post-immunisation fever developing after some vaccines.[5] However, if the fever persists after the second dose of antipyretic medical advice should be sought. Antipyretics have also been given as prophylaxis against febrile convulsions, especially in those with a previous history of such seizures or in those with epilepsy. However, antipyretic therapy does not appear to prevent recurrence of febrile convulsions (p.338).[1,6,7] There is also little to support the use of antipyretics for prophylaxis of post-immunisation fever although some suggest offering it to infants at higher risk of seizures receiving diphtheria-tetanus-pertussis or polio immunisation.[5]

Methods for reducing body temperature in fever include the use of antipyretics and/or physical means. Dissipation of body heat may be aided by removing excess clothing or bedding, maintaining a cool environment, and avoiding movement. Maintaining an adequate fluid intake is important. Fanning and tepid sponging are often employed although opinion on their value varies.[1,6,8] Cold baths should not be used as they may actually increase body temperature by inducing vasoconstriction. One study has suggested that antipyretics may be more effective than physical methods for reducing fever in children but the best response was obtained using an antipyretic with tepid sponging.[8] Antipyretics used include paracetamol, salicylates such as aspirin and some other NSAIDs. In fever they appear to promote the return of the set-point temperature to normal by inhibiting central synthesis and release of prostaglandins that mediate the effect of endogenous pyrogens in the hypothalamus. They cannot lower the body temperature below normal and are ineffective against raised body temperature not associated with fever. Some NSAIDs such as indomethacin and naproxen may be of value both for the differential diagnosis and the management of neoplastic fever as they appear to be more effective in reducing this type of fever than against fever associated with infections.

Paracetamol is usually the antipyretic of choice in infants and children; salicylates are generally contra-indicated in these patients because of the possible link between their use and the development of Reye's syndrome. Ibuprofen appears to be as effective as paracetamol[9] and may be of use when an alternative is required,[10] but there is still relatively little experience of its use and safety in infants and children.

Treatment of hyperthermia. Hyperthermia may produce body temperatures greater than 41°. It can result from heat stroke which may be an extreme form of exertional hyperthermia or may occur when there is an underlying thermoregulation defect, usually in sedentary, elderly subjects. Other causes include drug-induced hyperthermia and thyrotoxic crisis. Hyperthermia can also be induced by a number of drugs either during normal usage or following overdosage. Hyperthermia associated with anaesthesia is discussed under malignant hyperthermia (p.1314). Hyperthermia associated with antipsychotics is discussed under neuroleptic malignant syndrome (p.651). Some drugs that can cause hyperthermia in overdosage include antimuscarinics, salicylates, amphetamines, MAOIs, and cocaine. As with fever, the underlying causes should be identified and treated with appropriate supportive care. These high temperatures are life-threatening and should be lowered immediately. One of the most rapid and effective means of cooling is to immerse the patient in very cold water but core temperature should be monitored to avoid inducing hypothermia.[11] Some consider evaporative cooling methods to be more efficient.[12] Intravenous or intraperitoneal administration of cool fluids, gastric lavage or enemas with ice water have also been used.[11,13] Antipyretics are ineffective since the high temperatures are a result of thermoregulatory failure.

When hyperthermia is associated with muscle rigidity and fulminant hypermetabolism of skeletal muscle, as in the neuroleptic malignant syndrome and malignant hyperthermia, temperature reductions may be obtained using the muscle relaxant dantrolene. There is also anecdotal evidence that dantrolene may produce beneficial effects for the treatment of similar symptoms resulting from poisoning with various agents but the manufacturers have warned physicians that they should not regard dantrolene as an effective treatment for all types of hyperthermia and rigidity accompanying poisoning. In severe cases of hyperthermia when neuromuscular hyperactivity may also impair ventilation a neuromuscular blocker has been used, although suxamethonium is best avoided as it can itself precipitate malignant hyperthermia. Although experience in a small number of patients suggests that dantrolene can hasten cooling in patients with heat stroke when used with conventional cooling methods there is no evidence that it affects outcome.[14]

1. Drwal-Klein LA, Phelps SJ. Antipyretic therapy in the febrile child. *Clin Pharm* 1992; **11:** 1005–21.
2. Kramer MS, *et al.* Risks and benefits of paracetamol antipyresis in young children with fever of presumed viral origin. *Lancet* 1991; **337:** 591–4.
3. Doran TF, *et al.* Acetaminophen: more harm than good for chickenpox? *J Pediatr* 1989; **114:** 1045–8.
4. Shann F. Antipyretics in severe sepsis. *Lancet* 1995; **345:** 338.
5. Anonymous. Prophylactic paracetamol with childhood immunisation? *Drug Ther Bull* 1990; **28:** 73–4.
6. Joint Working Group of the Research Unit of the Royal College of Physicians and the British Paediatric Association. Guidelines for the management of convulsions with fever. *Br Med J* 1991; **303:** 634–6.
7. Uhari M, *et al.* Effect of acetaminophen and of low intermittent doses of diazepam on prevention of recurrences of febrile seizures. *J Pediatr* 1995; **126:** 991–5.
8. Kinmonth A-L, *et al.* Management of feverish children at home. *Br Med J* 1992; **305:** 1134–6.
9. McIntyre J, Hull D. Comparing efficacy and tolerability of ibuprofen and paracetamol in fever. *Arch Dis Child* 1996; **74:** 164–7.
10. Anonymous. Junifen suspension—ibuprofen for febrile children. *Drug Ther Bull* 1991; **29:** 11–12.
11. Simon HB. Hyperthermia. *N Engl J Med* 1993; **329:** 483–7.
12. Slovis CM. Hyperthermia. *N Engl J Med* 1994; **330:** 218–19.
13. Duthie DJR. Heated-related illness. *Lancet* 1998; **352:** 1329–30.
14. Channa AB, *et al.* Is dantrolene effective in heat stroke patients? *Crit Care Med* 1990; **18:** 290–2.

Musculoskeletal and joint disorders

The **rheumatic disorders** are a wide range of painful disorders affecting primarily the joints and related structures of the musculoskeletal system, but there may also be widespread involvement of other systems. The term arthritis is used when the disease is largely confined to the joints. Some of the most common forms of arthritis are discussed in this section and these include rheumatoid arthritis, osteoarthritis, juvenile chronic arthritis, and the spondyloarthropathies such as ankylosing spondylitis. Other conditions that are associated with arthritis and which are discussed elsewhere include gout (p.390) and systemic lupus erythematosus (p.1029).

The names **soft-tissue rheumatism** (see below) and non-articular rheumatism, have been used to describe a number of painful conditions associated with disease of the structures that surround a joint. For a discussion of the management of **low back pain**, see below.

Juvenile chronic arthritis. Juvenile chronic arthritis is a term used to describe a clinically heterogeneous group of idiopathic arthritides occurring in children under 16 years of age.

Methods of treatment are generally the same as for rheumatoid arthritis in adults (see below), although for some drugs there is limited experience of their use in children. Juvenile chronic arthritis is one of the limited number of indications for the use of aspirin in children.

References.

1. Rose CD, Doughty RA. Pharmacological management of juvenile rheumatoid arthritis. *Drugs* 1992; **43:** 849–63.
2. Giannini EH, Cassidy JT. Methotrexate in juvenile rheumatoid arthritis: do the benefits outweigh the risks? *Drug Safety* 1993; **9:** 325–39.
3. Kalla AA, *et al.* A risk-benefit assessment of slow-acting antirheumatic drugs in rheumatoid arthritis. *Drug Safety* 1994; **11:** 21–36.
4. Southwood TR. Arthritis in children. In: Snaith ML, ed. *ABC of rheumatology.* London: BMJ Publishing Group, 1996: 52–6.
5. Malleson PN. Management of childhood arthritis. Part 2: chronic arthritis. *Arch Dis Child* 1997; **76:** 541–4.
6. Woo P, Wedderburn LR. Juvenile chronic arthritis. *Lancet* 1998; **351:** 969–73. Correction. *ibid.*; 1292.

Osteoarthritis. Osteoarthritis is a diverse collection of diseases also known as osteoarthrosis, degenerative joint disease, or joint failure. It is characterised by progressive disintegration of articular cartilage, usually accompanied by new bone formation at joint margins and beneath the involved cartilage. There may be synovial inflammation, particularly in advanced disease, but it is different in nature to that seen with rheumatoid arthritis and is usually only a minor component of the disease. Osteoarthritis may be a sequel to trauma, inflammation, or metabolic disorders, but usually the underlying origin is not apparent.

Although there have been claims based largely on *animal* studies that various drugs are chondroprotective, there is no evidence from controlled studies in humans that any treatment is disease-modifying. Management is therefore aimed at relief of pain and maintenance of joint function.

Physical methods of treatment include physiotherapy, heat and cold therapy, exercises, splinting, and weight reduction in the obese. Acupuncture and transcutaneous electrical nerve stimulation (TENS) are also used in the management of osteoarthritis.

A non-opioid analgesic such as paracetamol is usually tried first for the relief of pain. An NSAID may be tried when paracetamol is ineffective or when there is a significant inflammatory component but there is the risk of adverse effects with prolonged use of NSAIDs, especially in the elderly. There has also been concern that NSAIDs such as indomethacin may accelerate osteoarthritis. When the use of NSAIDs is considered essential misoprostol is sometimes administered concurrently in an attempt to reduce gastro-intestinal adverse effects such as peptic ulceration and haemorrhage. Weak opioids such as codeine or dihydrocodeine are sometimes used in combination with paracetamol if the pain is unresponsive to paracetamol alone. Topical analgesics such as NSAIDs or capsaicin, or rubefacients may provide slight relief of pain but their role, if any, is unclear. Systemic corticosteroids have no place in the management of osteoarthritis. Intra-articular or peri-articular injections of corticosteroids are somewhat controversial but may be of help in some patients with localised inflammation, although if used they should only be given infrequently and as adjunctive therapy.

Surgery, including joint replacement, is of great benefit to patients with severe osteoarthritis that cannot be effectively managed by physical or medical therapy.

References.

1. Ghosh P. Nonsteroidal anti-inflammatory drugs and chondroprotection: a review of the evidence. *Drugs* 1993; **46:** 834–46.
2. Puett DW, Griffin MR. Published trials of nonmedicinal and noninvasive therapies for hip and knee osteoarthritis. *Ann Intern Med* 1994; **121:** 133–40.
3. Brandt KD. Toward pharmacologic modification of joint damage in osteoarthritis. *Ann Intern Med* 1995; **122:** 874–5.
4. Jones A, Doherty M. Osteoarthritis. In: Snaith ML, ed. *ABC of rheumatology.* London: BMJ Publishing Group, 1996: 28–31.
5. Wollheim FA. Current pharmacological treatment of osteoarthritis. *Drugs* 1996; **52** (suppl 3): 27–38.
6. Anonymous. What can be done about osteoarthritis? *Drug Ther Bull* 1996; **34:** 33–5.
7. Creamer P, Hochberg MC. Osteoarthritis. *Lancet* 1997; **350:** 503–9.
8. Eccles M, *et al.* North of England evidence based guideline development project: summary guideline for non-steroidal anti-inflammatory drugs versus basic analgesia in treating the pain of degenerative arthritis. *Br Med J* 1998; **317:** 526–30.

Rheumatoid arthritis. Rheumatoid arthritis is a common chronic systemic inflammatory disease that predominantly affects the synovial joints and results in progressive diability and increased mortality. Early rheumatoid arthritis is characterised primarily by inflammation of the synovium; as the disease progresses the patient suffers destruction of cartilage and bone. Extra-articular features commonly include general malaise, fatigue, weight loss, fever, and anaemia. Features associated with more severe forms of the disease include vasculitis, pericarditis, pleurisy, pleural effusion, pulmonary interstitial fibrosis, peripheral neuropathies, subcutaneous and pulmonary nodules, scleritis, and Sjögren's syndrome. Palindromic rheumatism is characterised by repeated episodes of arthritis and periarthritis without fever; the joints appear normal between attacks.

The cause of rheumatoid arthritis is probably multifactorial. There may well be an immunological component because about 80% of patients with rheumatoid arthritis have raised serum concentrations of rheumatoid factors, which are antibodies directed against immunoglobulin G (IgG). However, these antibodies are also found in other diseases and their role is unclear in the pathogenesis of rheumatoid arthritis. Another hypothesis proposes that rheumatoid arthritis may be the result of some infectious agent. Whatever the initial trigger, evidence is accumulating that release of cytokines such as tumour necrosis factor alpha (TNF-α) and interleukins (IL-1 and IL-6) following activation of T-lymphocytes by unknown antigens and macrophages maintain the chronic systemic and synovial inflammation characteristic in rheumatoid arthritis.

The incidence of rheumatoid arthritis is initially higher in women than in men but equalises in later life, and it has been suggested that androgens may have some sort of protective effect.

The severity and course of the disease varies greatly between patients. Disease activity usually fluctuates during the first few months and it is difficult to predict the course of the disease at this stage. Some patients will have a mild disease and may only experience brief attacks with little or no disease progression. However, the vast majority of patients will have intermittent relapses and remissions with an overall pattern of slowly progressive joint destruction and deformity. A few patients may have very severe and rapidly progressive disease.

Since there is no curative treatment for rheumatoid arthritis, management is aimed at alleviating pain and improving or maintaining joint function. This is accomplished through physiotherapy as well as the use of drugs. In some cases surgery may be required.

The choice of drugs for relief of pain depends upon the severity of symptoms. In mild cases an analgesic such as paracetamol may be all that is required but most patients need the additional anti-inflammatory effect provided by an NSAID. Although there is little apparent difference between the various NSAIDs in terms of anti-inflammatory activity, patient responses vary widely. When starting an NSAID the dose should be gradually increased to the recommended maximum over one to two weeks; if the response is inadequate after a total of about four weeks, or if adverse effects are intolerable, other NSAIDs should be tried. Misoprostol is sometimes administered with NSAIDs in an attempt to reduce gastro-intestinal adverse effects such as peptic ulceration and haemorrhage. Topical analgesics such as

NSAIDs or capsaicin, or rubefacients may provide slight relief of pain but their role, if any, is unclear.

Although NSAIDs provide symptomatic relief they do not affect the release of cytokines in conventional doses and therefore do not suppress the rate of cartilage erosion or alter the course of the disease. Because of the risks of toxicity the use of disease modifying antirheumatic drugs (DMARDs) (also referred to as second-line drugs) had conventionally been delayed until there was overt evidence of progressive disease but it is now clear that irreversible joint damage commonly occurs early in the disease and many rheumatologists now add a DMARD shortly after rheumatoid arthritis has been diagnosed in order to try and arrest or slow this deterioration.[1] There is some evidence from controlled studies[2,3] to indicate that early aggressive treatment can improve prognosis, at least in the short-term, but whether it should be given to all patients with very early disease remains to be determined.[4] It is also unclear whether early use of DMARDs will reduce long-term disability[1] but a recent multicentre study[5] has indicated their potential; data from 2888 patients with rheumatoid arthritis followed up for an average of 9 years, indicated that consistent use of DMARDs is associated with an improvement in long-term functional outcomes,[5] compared with patients who had used such drugs inconsistently.

DMARDs are a diverse group with different structures and probably different modes of action; they include the antimalarials (chloroquine, hydroxychloroquine), sulphasalazine, gold compounds (auranofin, sodium aurothiomalate), penicillamine, methotrexate, azathioprine, cyclophosphamide, and cyclosporin. It is thought that the mechanism of action of most of the DMARDs may involve blockade of the release or activity of cytokines to some degree, although other mechanisms may also be involved; current hypotheses on the modes of action of some have been discussed.[6] DMARDs have been referred to as slow-acting antirheumatic drugs as, unlike the NSAIDs, any therapeutic effect may not be apparent for 4 to 6 months. If, however, the response is inadequate after at least 6 months of therapy another DMARD should be tried.

The long-term use of DMARDs is limited by toxicity and loss of efficacy. Many patients do not continue to take a particular drug for more than one or two years. Discontinuation of therapy in a patient who has shown improvement may initiate a relapse. However, drug withdrawal may be considered by some clinicians for patients in complete remission, although evidence for the benefit of either continuing or discontinuing DMARDs in such patients is lacking.[7] In a randomised, placebo-controlled study[8] of stopping DMARDs in rheumatoid arthritis, the risk of synovitis was doubled in patients who discontinued active therapy. In the authors' opinion, DMARDs should be continued in patients with a good response as the risk of adverse effects during long-term therapy was observed to be low. However, since 62% of the placebo group went for a full year without experiencing a rheumatoid flare, it may be reasonable for some patients to consider stopping treatment. In a further study[9] in patients who had discontinued DMARDs, restarting therapy with the same antirheumatic drug when the disease flared up again was effective in most cases.

As adverse reactions with DMARDs frequently occur and may be life threatening, all patients require careful monitoring to avoid severe toxicity.[10,11] Patients who relapse during treatment with one DMARD may gain benefit when a different one is substituted. Treatment with more than one DMARD in various regimens is being tried but there is little available evidence to assess benefit.[1] A meta-analysis[12] of 5 different combinations of DMARDs found that although efficacy might be greater than single DMARDs, toxicity was also increased. However some combinations have produced favourable results.

There is little agreement on which DMARD should be used first and their selection is largely based on individual experience and preference. At present, data from comparative studies are insufficient to allow more than a crude ranking of the DMARDs with regard to efficacy and toxicity, but a number of reviews and analyses have been published to aid the rational selection of these drugs in rheumatoid arthritis.[1,13-23] Some meta-analyses[13,15] of generally short-term comparative studies suggest that methotrexate, intramuscular gold (sodium aurothiomalate), sulphasalazine, and penicillamine are more or less equivalent in efficacy, while the antimalarials and oral gold (auranofin) appear to be somewhat less effective. Intramuscular gold exhibited the highest toxicity while the antimalarials and oral gold had relatively low toxicity rates.[13] Another meta-analysis[14] considered that antimalarials and methotrexate had the best ratio of toxicity to efficacy.

Intramuscular gold has long been used for the treatment of rheumatoid arthritis and is often the standard against which the efficacy of other treatments is measured. Although it is still extensively prescribed, its toxicity and poor long-term efficacy has led to renewed debate over its place in antirheumatic therapy.[24,25] Oral gold is less toxic but is also much less effective. Early enthusiasm for penicillamine has also been somewhat curtailed by a high incidence of adverse effects. The antimalarials are less effective than most other DMARDs but as they are generally less toxic and better tolerated they may be preferred in patients with milder forms of disease. Although sulphasalazine was originally introduced for the treatment of rheumatoid arthritis, results of early studies were unfavourable and it subsequently found its main use in the treatment of inflammatory bowel disease. However, re-investigation many years later demonstrated its efficacy and is now often one of the DMARDs of first choice.[1,23] Immunosuppressants have also been used in rheumatoid arthritis but there are concerns over long-term toxicity. However, methotrexate can improve disease activity when given once weekly in low doses that are too small to produce systemic immunosuppression and when used in this manner adverse effects occur commonly but are usually mild. In a recent long-term study[26] almost two-thirds of patients were still taking methotrexate after 5 years. The risk of hepatotoxicity remains a concern, but many rheumatologists[1,19,20] consider methotrexate to be a first choice DMARD. Improvement generally begins earlier with methotrexate than with other DMARDs. Concomitant use of folic acid or folinic acid is recommended by some as this can reduce the toxicity of methotrexate without reducing efficacy,[27,28] but the timing of administration may be important. The use of other immunosuppressants is more debatable but azathioprine and cyclophosphamide are still used in some patients with severe disease who have failed to respond to other drugs, especially in those with extra-articular manifestations such as vasculitis. Cyclosporin has also been shown to be effective in rheumatoid arthritis but, because of concern over nephrotoxicity, it is considered that it is best reserved for refractory disease; the use of low-dose regimens may help to minimise adverse effects. The microemulsion formulation of cyclosporin possesses a more predictable and improved absorption profile compared with the conventional oral formulation, and may enable lower doses to be used for a good clinical response.[29]

The use of corticosteroids in rheumatoid arthritis is controversial. Although systemic corticosteroids can suppress the symptoms of the disease, their usefulness is limited by adverse effects. They are usually reserved for use in patients with severe rapidly progressing disease that has failed to respond to other antirheumatics or when there are severe extra-articular effects. Systemic corticosteroids have also been used temporarily to control disease activity during initiation of DMARDs. In spite of problems with the adverse effects of corticosteroids it has been suggested that, in line with current thinking on the earlier use of more aggressive therapy for the control of inflammation, early use of short-term corticosteroids might also be appropriate.[30] Although corticosteroids are associated with bone loss,[31] this appears to be dose-related[32] and, at low doses, the benefits of corticosteroid therapy on inflammation and mobility might result in a reduced loss of bone in patients with rheumatoid arthritis. There is some evidence[49] to suggest that the rate of joint destruction may be substantially reduced by corticosteroids in low doses (such as prednisolone 7.5 mg daily) in patients with moderate to severe rheumatoid arthritis of less than 2 years duration; the corticosteroid should be gradually discontinued after 2 to 4 years to avoid possible long-term adverse effects. It is imperative that reduction in joint destruction should be distinguished from mere symptomatic improvement, which, at low corticosteroid doses, lasts only for 6 to 12 months. Intra-articular injections of corticosteroids may be used when there are acute flares affecting one or a few individual joints but they should be given infrequently.

A wide range of other drugs has been tried in rheumatoid arthritis,[16,21,33,34] but for most there is little clearcut evidence of efficacy. Studies[35,36] indicate that minocycline can produce modest beneficial effects in patients with rheumatoid arthritis, but the clinical significance of these improvements has been questioned[37] and it remains to be determined what role, if any, minocycline would have in the management of rheumatoid arthritis. Testosterone has produced clinical improvement in male and postmenopausal female patients. Much research has been conducted into using immunomodulators and immunotherapy. Interferons have produced results similar to conventional DMARDs but the need for repeated injections is a drawback. Other drugs that have been tried[38-40] include amiprilose, leflunomide, mycophenolate mofetil, zileuton, oral desensitisation with collagen, and immunoglobulins. Interest in the possible role of cytokines in the pathogenesis of rheumatoid arthritis has led to studies of various inhibitors of TNF-α such as tumour necrosis factor antibodies (e.g. infliximab), soluble tumour necrosis factor receptor (etanercept), and tumour necrosis factor receptor fusion protein, as well as interleukin antagonists.[41,42] A CD4 antibody (IDEC-CE9.1) and matrix metalloprotease inhibitors have also been studied. Other methods of treatment that are under investigation include gene therapy and autologous bone marrow transplantation. A rheumatoid arthritis vaccine is also in clinical trials. Some studies suggest that addition of fish oils and/or evening primrose oil to standard antirheumatic therapy might help to reduce pain and joint swelling.

Findings that significant skeletal bone loss occurs early in the disease have raised the question of the need for general measures to prevent osteoporosis in patients with rheumatoid arthritis.[30] Some[30] consider the use of oestrogen therapy in postmenopausal women with rheumatoid arthritis to be appropriate but to date the overall effect of such treatment is unclear.[43-45] The use of bisphosphonates such as disodium pamidronate is being studied.[46]

The treatment of rheumatoid arthritis during pregnancy presents its own problems; the rational selection of suitable drugs has been discussed in a number of reviews.[47,48]

1. Anonymous. Modifying disease in rheumatoid arthritis. *Drug Ther Bull* 1998; **36:** 3–6.
2. van der Heide A, *et al.* The effectiveness of early treatment with "second-line" antirheumatic drugs: a randomized, controlled trial. *Ann Intern Med* 1996; **124:** 699–707.
3. Egsmose C, *et al.* Patients with rheumatoid arthritis benefit from early 2nd line therapy: 5 year followup of a prospective double blind placebo controlled study. *J Rheumatol* 1995; **22:** 2208–13.
4. Wollheim FA. Disease modifying drugs in rheumatoid arthritis. *Br Med J* 1997; **314:** 766–7.
5. Fries JF, *et al.* Reduction in long-term disability in patients with rheumatoid arthritis by disease-modifying antirheumatic drug-based treatment strategies. *Arthritis Rheum* 1996; **39:** 616–22.
6. Choy E, Kingsley G. How do second-line agents work? *Br Med Bull* 1995; **51:** 472–92.
7. Gómez-Reino JJ. Long-term therapy for rheumatoid arthritis. *Lancet* 1996; **347:** 343–4.
8. ten Wolde S, *et al.* Randomised placebo-controlled study of stopping second-line drugs in rheumatoid arthritis. *Lancet* 1996; **347:** 347–52.
9. ten Wolde S, *et al.* Effect of resumption of second line drugs in patients with rheumatoid arthritis that flared up after treatment discontinuation. *Ann Rheum Dis* 1997; **56:** 235–9.
10. Wijnands MJH, van Riel PLCM. Management of adverse effects of disease-modifying antirheumatic drugs. *Drug Safety* 1995; **13:** 219–27.
11. Lehmann T, *et al.* Toxicity of antirheumatic drugs. *Med J Aust* 1997; **116:** 378–83.
12. Felson DT, *et al.* The efficacy and toxicity of combination therapy in rheumatoid arthritis: a meta-analysis. *Arthritis Rheum* 1994; **37:** 1487–91.
13. Felson DT, *et al.* The comparative efficacy and toxicity of second-line drugs in rheumatoid arthritis. *Arthritis Rheum* 1990; **33:** 1449–61.
14. Felson DT, *et al.* Use of short-term efficacy/toxicity tradeoffs to select second-line drugs in rheumatoid arthritis: a metaanalysis of published clinical trials. *Arthritis Rheum* 1992; **35:** 1117–25.
15. Capell HA, *et al.* Second line (disease modifying) treatment in rheumatoid arthritis: which drug for which patient? *Ann Rheum Dis* 1993; **52:** 423–8.
16. Brooks PM. Clinical management of rheumatoid arthritis. *Lancet* 1993; **341:** 286–90.
17. Porter DR, Sturrock RD. Medical management of rheumatoid arthritis. *Br Med J* 1993; **307:** 425–8.
18. Kalla AA, *et al.* A risk-benefit assessment of slow-acting antirheumatic drugs in rheumatoid arthritis. *Drug Safety* 1994; **11:** 21–36.
19. Cash JM, Klippel JH. Second-line drug therapy for rheumatoid arthritis. *N Engl J Med* 1994; **330:** 1368–75.

20. Anonymous. Drugs for rheumatoid arthritis. *Med Lett Drugs Ther* 1994; **36:** 101–106.
21. Luqmani R, *et al.* Clinical pharmacology and modification of autoimmunity and inflammation in rheumatoid disease. *Drugs* 1994; **47:** 259–85.
22. Akil M, Amos RS. Rheumatoid arthritis: treatment. In: Snaith ML, ed. *ABC of rheumatology.* London: BMJ Publishing Group, 1996: 44–7.
23. Jackson CG, Williams HJ. Disease-modifying antirheumatic drugs: using their clinical pharmacological effects as a guide to their selection. *Drugs* 1998; **56:** 337–44.
24. Anonymous. Gold therapy in rheumatoid arthritis. *Lancet* 1991; **338:** 19–20.
25. Pincus T, Wolfe F. Treatment of rheumatoid arthritis: challenges to traditional paradigms. *Ann Intern Med* 1991; **115:** 825–7.
26. Weinblatt ME, *et al.* Methotrexate in rheumatoid arthritis: a five-year prospective multicenter study. *Arthritis Rheum* 1994; **37:** 1492–8.
27. Shiroky JB, *et al.* Low-dose methotrexate with leucovorin (folinic acid) in the management of rheumatoid arthritis: results of a multicenter randomized, double-blind, placebo-controlled trial. *Arthritis Rheum* 1993; **36:** 795–803.
28. Morgan SL, *et al.* Supplementation with folic acid during methotrexate therapy for rheumatoid arthritis: a double-blind, placebo-controlled trial. *Ann Intern Med* 1994; **121:** 833–41.
29. Tugwell P. International consensus recommendations on cyclosporin use in rheumatoid arthritis. *Drugs* 1995; **50:** 48–56.
30. Sambrook PN. Osteoporosis in rheumatoid arthritis: what is the role of antirheumatic therapy? *Lancet* 1994; **344:** 3–4.
31. Laan RFJM, *et al.* Low-dose prednisone induces rapid reversible axial bone loss in patients with rheumatoid arthritis: a randomized, controlled study. *Ann Intern Med* 1993; **119:** 963–8.
32. Saag KG, *et al.* Low dose long-term corticosteroid therapy in rheumatoid arthritis: an analysis of serious adverse events. *Am J Med* 1994; **96:** 115–23.
33. Capell HA, Brzeski M. Slow drugs: slow progress? Use of slow acting antirheumatic drugs (SAARDs) in rheumatoid arthritis. *Ann Rheum Dis* 1992; **51:** 424–9.
34. Miller-Blair DJ, Robbins DL. Rheumatoid arthritis: new science, new treatment. *Geriatrics* 1993; **48:** 28–38.
35. Kloppenburg M, *et al.* Minocycline in active rheumatoid arthritis. *Arthritis Rheum* 1994; **37:** 629–36.
36. Tilley BC, *et al.* Minocycline in rheumatoid arthritis: a 48-week, double-blind, placebo-controlled trial. *Ann Intern Med* 1995; **122:** 81–9.
37. McKendry RJR. Is rheumatoid arthritis caused by an infection? *Lancet* 1995; **345:** 1319–20.
38. Panush RS, Arend WP. Rheumatology. *JAMA* 1997; **277:** 1899–1900.
39. Choy EHS, Scott DL. Drug treatment of rheumatic diseases in the 1990s: achievements and future developments. *Drugs* 1997; **53:** 337–48.
40. Schiff M. Emerging treatments for rheumatoid arthritis. *Am J Med* 1997; **102** (suppl 1A): 11S–15S.
41. Buckley CD. Treatment of rheumatoid arthritis. *Br Med J* 1997; **315:** 236–8.
42. Koopman WJ, Moreland LW. Rheumatoid arthritis: anticytokine therapies on the horizon. *Ann Intern Med* 1998; **128:** 231–3.
43. van den Brink, *et al.* Adjuvant oestrogen therapy does not improve disease activity in postmenopausal patients with rheumatoid arthritis. *Ann Rheum Dis* 1993; **52:** 862–5.
44. MacDonald AG, *et al.* Effects of hormone replacement therapy in rheumatoid arthritis: a double blind placebo-controlled study. *Ann Rheum Dis* 1994; **53:** 54–7.
45. Hall GM, *et al.* A randomised controlled trial of the effect of hormone replacement therapy on disease activity in postmenopausal rheumatoid arthritis. *Ann Rheum Dis* 1994; **53:** 112–16.
46. Eggelmeijer F, *et al.* Increased bone mass with pamidronate treatment in rheumatoid arthritis: results of a three-year randomized, double-blind trial. *Arthritis Rheum* 1996; **39:** 396–402.
47. Witter FR. Clinical pharmacokinetics in the treatment of rheumatoid arthritis in pregnancy. *Clin Pharmacokinet* 1993; **25:** 444–9.
48. Østensen M. Optimisation of antirheumatic drug treatment in pregnancy. *Clin Pharmacokinet* 1994; **27:** 486–503.
49. Kirwan JR. The Arthritis and Rheumatism Council Low-dose Glucocorticoid Study Group. The effect of glucocorticoids on joint destruction in rheumatoid arthritis. *N Engl J Med* 1995; **333:** 142–6.

Soft-tissue rheumatism. Soft-tissue rheumatism includes a number of conditions such as fibromyalgia (fibrositis, muscular rheumatism, myofascial pain), humeral epicondylitis (e.g. tennis or golfer's elbow), frozen shoulder, Tietze's syndrome, fascitis, tendinitis, tenosynovitis, bursitis (e.g. housemaid's knee), and sprains and strains. It has a variety of causes and may be associated with overuse, trauma, infection, or systemic inflammatory diseases. Inflamed or displaced tissue may impinge on nearby nerves and produce compression neuropathies such as carpal tunnel syndrome. Soft-tissue rheumatic conditions are usually benign and can remit spontaneously. The management of some of these conditions has been reviewed.[1-6,11] Most will respond to selective rest of the affected region and splinting where appropriate. Gentle exercise, massage, application of heat, cold, or rubefacients can also be of benefit. Many soft tissue lesions respond to local injection of a corticosteroid given with a local anaesthetic.[7] Short-term use of oral NSAIDs may help to relieve pain and reduce inflammation of soft-tissue trauma. Topical formulations of NSAIDs have been used but although they are more effective than placebo for pain relief their role, if any, is unclear. Capsaicin has also been tried as a topical analgesic.

Pyridoxine has been suggested as a treatment option for carpal tunnel syndrome but there is significant controversy surrounding its efficacy[8] and high doses of pyridoxine given for prolonged periods have been associated with sensory neuropathy. There have been anecdotal reports of beneficial responses of carpal tunnel syndrome to hormone replacement therapy.[9,10]

1. Dawson DM. Entrapment neuropathies of the upper extremities. *N Engl J Med* 1993; **329:** 2013–18.
2. Campbell P, Lawton JO. Heel pain: diagnosis and management. *Br Med J* 1994; **52:** 380–5.
3. Barry M, Jenner JR. Pain in the neck, shoulder, and arm. In: Snaith ML, ed. *ABC of rheumatology.* London: BMJ Publishing Group, 1996: 6–9.
4. Shipley M. Pain in the hand and wrist. In: Snaith ML, ed. *ABC of rheumatology.* London: BMJ Publishing Group, 1996: 1–5.
5. Muhammed N, *et al.* Peripheral nerve entrapment syndromes: diagnosis and management. *Br J Hosp Med* 1995; **53:** 141–6.
6. Reveille JD. Soft-tissue rheumatism: diagnosis and treatment. *Am J Med* 1997; **102** (suppl 1A): 23S–29S.
7. Caldwell JR. Intra-articular corticosteroids. *Drugs* 1996; **52:** 507–14.
8. Copeland DA, Stoukides CA. Pyridoxine in carpel tunnel syndrome. *Ann Pharmacother* 1994; **28:** 1042–4.
9. Confino-Cohen R, *et al.* Response of carpal tunnel syndrome to hormone replacement therapy. *Br Med J* 1991; **303:** 1514.
10. Hall GM, *et al.* Carpal tunnel syndrome and hormone replacement therapy. *Br Med J* 1992; **304:** 382.
11. Doherty M, Jones A. Fibromyalgia syndrome. In: Snaith ML, ed. *ABC of rheumatology.* London: BMJ Publishing Group, 1996: 24–7.

Spondyloarthropathies. The spondyloarthropathies are a group of seronegative arthritides which include ankylosing spondylitis, psoriatic arthritis, arthritis associated with inflammatory bowel disorders (enteropathic arthritis), and arthritis associated with infection as in reactive arthritis (aseptic arthritis).

Ankylosing spondylitis is characterised by arthritis of the spine and sacroiliac joints and sometimes there is also asymmetrical peripheral involvement. Males under 40 years of age are predominantly affected. The aim of management of the disease is to reduce pain and stiffness and to prevent spine and joint deformity, which is accomplished using a combination of active physical therapy and drug therapy. Exercises are used to strengthen muscles and to maintain a good posture and range of movement in joints. NSAIDs are used to relieve pain and inflammation, thus allowing the exercises to be performed. Some patients may require concomitant treatment with other non-opioid analgesics such as paracetamol for additional pain control. Indomethacin has been considered by some to be the NSAID of choice, although individual patient tolerance and preference often dictate the final choice of drug. Misoprostol is sometimes administered with NSAIDs in an attempt to reduce gastro-intestinal adverse effects such as peptic ulceration and haemorrhage. Phenylbutazone is sometimes used when other drugs are unsuitable but it should be noted that the use of phenylbutazone in the UK has been limited to hospital rheumatology departments because of the risk of occasional serious adverse effects. Systemic corticosteroids are rarely indicated but intra-articular injections of corticosteroids may be beneficial when one or two peripheral joints are severely affected. Although NSAIDs reduce inflammation in ankylosing spondylitis they do not influence the progression of the disease. Sulphasalazine, which has proven efficacy in ankylosing spondylitis (mainly in patients with peripheral involvement), may help to control severe or refractory disease; the efficacy of other second-line or disease modifying antirheumatic drugs used in rheumatoid arthritis (see above) remains to be demonstrated.

Psoriatic arthritis (or psoriatic arthropathy) is an inflammatory seronegative arthritis occurring in patients with psoriasis. In some patients the spine may be involved when the condition may be indistinguishable from ankylosing spondylitis. Less frequently some patients have a form of symmetrical arthritis resembling rheumatoid arthritis (see above). The psoriasis (p.1075) and the arthritis usually require separate treatment. Treatment of the arthritis is initially as for ankylosing spondylitis with NSAIDs and physical therapy. If these methods fail treatment with a disease modifying antirheumatic drug should be instituted. Gold compounds have been tried. Immunosuppressants such as azathioprine or methotrexate may be useful for severe or progressive cases but potential liver toxicity may limit the long-term use of methotrexate in some patients. Sulphasalazine has also been tried in some patients. Chloroquine and hydroxychloroquine should be avoided since they may precipitate skin reactions (see p.428). Systemic corticosteroids have little or no place in the management of psoriatic arthritis.

Reactive arthritis is characterised by sterile synovitis following 1 to 4 weeks after an infection most commonly of the gastro-intestinal or genito-urinary tract. Extra-articular features involving the skin, eyes, or genito-urinary tract may or may not be present. Reactive arthritis is also a feature of Reiter's syndrome. Reactive arthritis is treated with physical therapy and NSAIDs and, if indicated, intra-articular injections of corticosteroids; the role of antibacterials is less certain (see under Bone and Joint Infections, p.117).

References.

1. Gran JT, Husby G. Ankylosing spondylitis: current drug treatment. *Drugs* 1992; **44:** 585–603.
2. Svenungsson B. Reactive arthritis. *Br Med J* 1994; **308:** 671–2.
3. Keat A. Spondyloarthropathies. In: Snaith ML, ed. *ABC of rheumatology.* London: BMJ Publishing Group, 1996: 48–51.
4. Toussirot E, Wendling D. Current guidelines for the drug treatment of ankylosing spondylitis. *Drugs* 1998; **56:** 225–40.

Still's disease. Still's disease is characterised by a high fever, polyarthritis, and an evanescent pink macular rash that is most prominent during bouts of fever; patients are seronegative for rheumatoid factor. Onset is usually in children under 5 years of age, but can occur in adults. Treatment is usually with aspirin or other NSAIDs or corticosteroids.

The name Still's disease has been used rather inconsistently to describe some types of juvenile chronic arthritis (see above).

References.

1. Watts RA, Scott DGI. Rashes and vasculitis. In: Snaith ML, ed. *ABC of rheumatology.* London: BMJ Publishing Group, 1996: 69–73.
2. Evans RH. Pyrexia of unknown origin. *Br Med J* 1997; **314:** 583–6.

Pain

Pain is not only associated with physical suffering or hurting but has an emotional or mental component, hence its definition by the International Association for the Study of Pain as 'an unpleasant sensory and emotional experience associated with actual or potential tissue damage, or described in terms of such damage.' The emotional as well as the physical aspects need to be considered during treatment.

Under normal circumstances pain is the result of stimulation of peripheral receptors which transmit impulses through pain pathways to the brain. Pain receptors or nociceptors are of two basic types: mechanoheat and polymodal receptors. Mechanoheat receptors have a high stimulation threshold and respond to intense or potentially damaging noxious stimuli. These receptors are associated with rapidly conducting thinly myelinated Aδ fibres and their stimulation produces rapid sharp localised pain that serves to activate withdrawal reflexes. The other type of receptors are referred to as polymodal nociceptors as they respond to mechanical, thermal, or chemical insults. These receptors are also activated by cellular components that are released following tissue damage. Their impulses are transmitted slowly along unmyelinated C type fibres and produce dull, aching, and poorly localised pain with a slower onset.

Nerve fibres from nociceptors terminate in the dorsal root of the spinal cord before transmission by ascending pathways to the brain. There have been many theories on the processing of pain signals at the spinal level but the 'gate theory' proposed by Melzack and Wall is one of the best known. This theory postulates that the transmission of impulses, arriving from different receptors, to the brain is modulated by a gate mechanism in the substantia gelatinosa. Stimulation of small fibres opens the gate and facilitates transmission whereas stimulation of large fibres, which normally carry non-painful sensory input can close the gate and inhibit transmission. Transmission also appears to be modulated by several other mechanisms which can influence the sensitivity of the gate. Inhibitory control over the gate is produced by descending fibres from the brain which in turn are influenced by input from all parts of the body and by input from the cortex so that cognitive processes such as past experience can influence the perception of pain. When output through the gate exceeds a critical level transmission to the brain occurs to produce withdrawal reflexes, autonomic responses, and the sensation of pain. Feedback from this response system acts further to modulate the gate control system.

Pain associated with tissue damage results in increased sensitivity of the sensory system so that pain can occur in the absence of a clear stimulus. There may be a reduction in the pain threshold (*allodynia*) resulting in an exaggerated response (*hyperalgesia*) or a prolonged effect (*hyperpathia*). The effect of stimulation of high threshold nociceptors is usually transient but inflammatory mediators such as bradykinin, histamine, serotonin, and prostaglandins produced in response to tissue damage can produce peripheral sensitisation so that these receptors respond to low intensity or innocuous stimuli. Due to this increased activity central sensitisation also occurs. Neurones in the dorsal horn undergo prolonged alterations in their response properties so that they respond to input from fibres which do not normally evoke pain such as low threshold Aβ fibres which are activated by tactile stimuli.

Pain is often classified as being acute or chronic in nature although some forms of pain regarded as being chronic may consist of intermittent attacks of pain followed by relatively long pain-free periods. **Acute pain** is associated with trauma or disease and usually has a well defined location, character, and timing. It is accompanied by symptoms of autonomic hyperactivity such as tachycardia, hypertension, sweating, and mydriasis. Pain lasting more than a few months is usually regarded as being **chronic pain** and generally presents a different clinical picture. It is not necessarily readily associated with trauma or disease and its localisation, character, and timing are more vague than with acute pain. Furthermore, as the autonomic nervous system adapts, the signs of autonomic hyperactivity associated with acute pain disappear. However, patients with chronic pain experience physical, psychological, social, and functional deterioration. These demoralising factors contribute towards exacerbation of pain and must be considered during its treatment.

From an aetiological perspective, pain may be considered as being psychogenic or as being associated with an underlying disease or trauma. Psychogenic pain may rarely be delusional (only responding to psychiatric treatment) or may be due to psychologically induced chronic physiological changes. Patients with the latter type of psychogenic pain may develop chronic illness behaviour patterns, tend to respond poorly to conventional analgesics, and need behavioural therapy.

Physiologically, pain may be divided into nociceptive pain and neurogenic pain. *Nociceptive pain* follows activation of nociceptors by noxious stimuli as described above but is not associated with injury to peripheral nerves or the CNS. It may be somatic or visceral in nature, depending on which peripheral receptors or nerves are involved. Somatic pain is usually well localised and may be described as deeply located, sharp or dull, nagging, stabbing, throbbing, or pressure-like. Visceral pain is generally less localised and more diffuse than somatic pain and may be referred to remote areas of the body. Depending on the structure involved it is variously described as deeply located, aching, nagging, cramping, or pressing and may be accompanied by nausea and vomiting. Nociceptive pain usually responds to treatment with conventional analgesics.

The terms *neurogenic* or *neuropathic pain* are often used interchangeably to describe pain resulting from damage or dysfunction of peripheral nerves/receptors or of the central nervous system. The term neurogenic pain covers sympathetically maintained pains including causalgia and reflex sympathetic dystrophy, and painful conditions such as postherpetic and trigeminal neuralgia, and diabetic neuropathy. Pain associated with central nervous tissue, such as in central post-stroke pain (the thalamic syndrome) is referred to as central pain. The clinical signs of neurogenic pain can vary greatly. Some of the more common features include heightened pain sensitivity and sensations of superficial burning or stabbing (lancinating) pain. The pain may be associated with areas of sensory deficit or some form of autonomic instability. Neurogenic pain responds poorly to conventional analgesics and can be difficult to treat.

References.

1. International Association for the Study of Pain. Classification of chronic pain: descriptions of chronic pain syndromes and definitions of pain terms. *Pain* 1986; (suppl 3): S1–S225.
2. Melzack R, Wall PD. Pain mechanisms: a new theory. *Science* 1965; **150:** 971–9.
3. Markenson JA. Mechanisms of chronic pain. *Am J Med* 1996; **101** (suppl 1A): 6S–18S.

General management of pain. There are several approaches to the management of pain, and combining approaches can result in an additive or greatly enhanced effect.

Early treatment is important as unrelieved pain can have profound psychological effects on the patient, and acute pain that is poorly managed initially can degenerate into chronic pain, which may prove to be much more difficult to treat. It is important to assess and treat the mental and emotional aspects of the pain as well as its physical aspects. Although drug therapy is the mainstay of pain treatment the addition of psychological, behavioural, or physical methods can enhance analgesia.

The transmission of pain impulses to the brain can be inhibited at a number of levels. Pain may be managed at a peripheral level as in the use of ice packs or NSAIDs to inhibit local responses to trauma and prevent stimulation of nociceptors. Techniques such as nerve blocks or cryoanalgesia can be used to inhibit peripheral transmission of pain. Intervention of pain processing at the spinal level can be accomplished using stimulation techniques or spinal injections of opioids, local anaesthetics, or other drugs. Analgesics such as the opioids can alter central processing of pain impulses.

The WHO has devised a regimen for the use of analgesics in the treatment of chronic cancer pain and this has been used by some authorities as the basis for a graded clinical approach in the treatment of both acute and chronic pain. In the WHO regimen drugs are selected from an analgesic ladder which starts with the use of a non-opioid analgesic alone. If pain is not controlled a weak opioid may be added. If this is not effective the weak opioid is replaced by a strong opioid and the non-opioid analgesic may be withdrawn. Some pain, such as neurogenic pain, incident bone pain, and some forms of visceral pain, respond poorly or not at all to opioid analgesics given in tolerable doses and at each stage, the analgesic therapy may be supplemented by the use of co-analgesics or other pharmacological or nonpharmacological adjuvant treatment to enhance analgesia and limit side-effects. The WHO ladder is described in more detail under Cancer Pain (see below).

Other methods of pain control that may be tried either alone or in combination with analgesics include physical methods such as physiotherapy, nervous system stimulation methods, and surgery. Physiotherapy can be an important part of pain management and may include massage and the application of heat and cold in many forms.

A number of stimulation techniques exist for the management of pain of which acupuncture and transcutaneous electrical nerve stimulation (TENS) are the most widely used. The rationale behind the use of TENS, in which the peripheral nerves supplying the painful area are stimulated by applying a low-intensity, high frequency electrical current across the skin, lies in the 'gate theory' of pain (see Pain, above). It is suggested that stimulation of large rapidly conducting myelinated nerves which normally transmit low-threshold tactile input closes the gate to transmission of pain through the spinal column by slow conducting unmyelinated nerves. However, other mechanisms may also contribute to the effect of TENS. In acupuncture, stimulation is achieved by insertion of small needles into specific acupuncture points. Heat or a small electrical pulsed current is sometimes applied to the needles to enhance the effect. There is much conflicting data on its mode of action. It may in part be explained by the 'gate theory', but opioidergic mechanisms are also involved as endogenous opioid peptides are produced and its effects can be reversed with the antagonist naloxone.

References.

1. Justins D. Modern approaches to pain management. *Prescribers' J* 1993; **33:** 221–6.
2. Justins D. Non-malignant chronic pain. *Prescribers' J* 1993; **33:** 259–66.
3. Lewis KS, *et al.* Effect of analgesic treatment on the physiological consequences of acute pain. *Am J Hosp Pharm* 1994; **51:** 1539–54.
4. Justins DM. Chronic pain management. *Br J Hosp Med* 1994; **52:** 12–16.
5. Reidenberg MM, Portenoy RK. The need for an open mind about the treatment of chronic nonmalignant pain. *Clin Pharmacol Ther* 1994; **55:** 367–9.
6. American Pain Society Quality of Care Committee. Quality improvement guidelines for the treatment of acute pain and cancer pain. *JAMA* 1995; **274:** 1874–80.
7. Anonymous. Pain: under-recognized and undertreated? *WHO Drug Inf* 1996; **10:** 36–8.
8. Gloth FM. Concerns with chronic analgesic therapy in elderly patients. *Am J Med* 1996; **101** (suppl 1A): 19S–24S.
9. Katz WA. Approach to the management of nonmalignant pain. *Am J Med* 1996; **101** (suppl 1A): 54S–63S.
10. McQuay H, *et al.* Treating acute pain in hospital. *Br Med J* 1997; **314:** 1531–5.
11. American Academy of Pain Medicine and the American Pain Society. The use of opioids for the treatment of chronic pain: a consensus statement. *Clin J Pain* 1997; **13:** 6–8.

Analgesics and analgesic adjuvants. Described below are drugs or groups of drugs used in the treatment of pain, including non-opioid and opioid analgesics and some drugs used as adjuvant analgesics.

Non-opioid analgesics. Paracetamol and aspirin and other NSAIDs are the first choice for treating mild or moderate pain and are used in moderate or severe pain to potentiate the effects of opioids. They are suitable for use in acute or chronic pain. Aspirin and other NSAIDs are thought to act by inhibiting cyclo-oxygenase and preventing prostaglandin formation; it is uncertain how paracetamol acts. NSAIDs are particularly effective in bone pain of malignant origin and pain due to inflammation. Aspirin and paracetamol are of similar potency in most types of pain but paracetamol only has a weak anti-inflammatory effect. Dependence and tolerance are not a problem with non-opioid analgesics but as the dose is increased, their efficacy reaches a ceiling. Most NSAIDs have a greater analgesic effect than aspirin or paracetamol in single doses but it has not been established whether this is true when used repeatedly in chronic pain. Adverse effects can limit the use of non-opioid analgesics. Aspirin and other NSAIDs inhibit blood platelet function, adversely affect the gastro-intestinal tract, and can precipitate hypersensitivity reactions including asthma. Paracetamol does not have the haematological or gastro-intestinal adverse effects of aspirin but large doses can produce severe or sometimes fatal hepatotoxicity; patients with cachexia or those with existing liver disease may be more susceptible.

Weak opioid analgesics. Codeine is traditionally the weak opioid analgesic of choice; alternatives include dextropropoxyphene and dihydrocodeine. Weak opioids are often given with non-opioid analgesics for the treatment of moderate or moderate to severe opioid-sensitive pain. Combinations of codeine with paracetamol produce a small but significant increase in analgesia compared with paracetamol alone and might be appropriate for occasional pain relief, but the incidence of adverse effects increases with repeated use. Combinations of dextropropoxyphene with paracetamol are no more effective than paracetamol alone for acute pain; efficacy in chronic pain is unclear and adverse effects may become troublesome.

Strong opioid analgesics. Strong opioids are mainly used in the treatment of severe acute non-malignant pain and cancer pain (see below). Their use in chronic non-malignant pain is somewhat controversial because of fears of psychological dependence and respiratory depression. However, in practice such problems rarely occur and those fears should not prevent patients being given effective analgesic therapy. Respiratory depression induced by opioids is generally a short-lived phenomenon that usually occurs in opioid-naive patients and is antagonised by pain. Although physical dependence can occur with continued use of opioids, withdrawal symptoms may be avoided by gradually tapering doses when the opioid is discontinued. The risk of psychological dependence and addictive behaviour is low when opioids are used to treat pain. Strong opioids include full agonists such as morphine, diamorphine, hydromorphone, methadone, pethidine, oxycodone, levorphanol, fentanyl, and alfentanil; partial agonists such as buprenorphine; and mixed agonist-antagonists such as pentazocine, butorphanol, nalbuphine, and dezocine. However, the use of opioids in the latter two groups can be compromised by their propensity to precipitate withdrawal symptoms in opioid-dependent individuals.

Morphine is the strong opioid of choice. The oral route is the most desirable route of administration and is appropriate for the control of acute and chronic pain in many patients. Morphine is well absorbed when given orally and has a short half-life so that administration of an immediate-release oral preparation offers a flexible means of dosage titration. Once initial pain relief is achieved, administration of modified-release morphine tablets every 12 hours may be more convenient for maintenance of analgesia in chronic pain, but this does reduce dosage flexibility and extra doses of immediate-release oral morphine may be required for breakthrough or incident bone pain. Other routes such as intramuscular or intravenous injection for emergency pain control or intermittent infusion for patient-controlled analgesia may be used. Alternative routes should also be used where there would be problems with oral administration as in patients with persistent vomiting or at risk of vomiting, or with dysphagia, malabsorption, delayed gastric emptying, or intestinal obstruction.

Occasionally an alternative to morphine may be useful. Methadone, levorphanol, or oxycodone have a longer duration of action than morphine, but it should be noted that methadone and levorphanol, which have long half-lives, may accumulate and therefore should not be used long term because of progressive CNS depression. A rapid onset of action is provided by pethidine, alfentanil, and fentanyl, and dextromoramide is useful if a short action is needed. Diamorphine may be preferred to morphine when the parenteral route has to be used because the volume of solution to be injected is less with diamorphine than with morphine.

Troublesome adverse effects of opioids include sedation, nausea, vomiting, constipation, and, most seriously, respiratory depression. Tolerance generally develops to all of these effects except constipation, which should be prevented by regular use of laxatives. If tolerance to the analgesic effects of a particular opioid necessitates a dose increase which produces unacceptable side-effects, then another opioid may be tried since cross-tolerance is not complete.

Antidepressants. Subantidepressant doses of tricyclic antidepressants are considered to be useful in chronic neurogenic pain of the burning, dysaesthetic type such as postherpetic neuralgia and diabetic neuropathy; shooting pain has also been reported to respond to tricyclics. The primary role of antidepressants in the management of chronic pain is for patients whose pain is refractory to conventional analgesics or for whom the adverse effects of treatment are intolerable. They may be used in addition to conventional analgesics, and are particularly useful in the treatment of cancer pain of mixed aetiology. There is little evidence for an analgesic effect of antidepressants in acute pain but musculoskeletal pain has sometimes responded to tricyclic antidepressants. Amitriptyline has also been found to be useful for the prophylaxis of various headaches including migraine (p.443). Amitriptyline is usually the tricyclic that is selected for the treatment of chronic neurogenic pain, but other tricyclics have also been tried; the tetracyclic antidepressant mianserin and the selective serotonin reuptake inhibitors, fluoxetine and paroxetine have also been used but there is no evidence that these newer antidepressants have greater analgesic efficacy than the tricyclics.

Antiepileptics have membrane-stabilising properties that have been found useful in the relief of neurogenic pain especially when there is a stabbing (lancinating) element, as in trigeminal neuralgia; there have also been reports of efficacy in the treatment of diabetic neuropathy and for migraine prophylaxis (p.443). Side-effects are a problem with antiepileptics. Carbamazepine appears to be the antiepileptic most frequently used for neurogenic pain. Other drugs with membrane stabilising properties have also been used. **Antiarrhythmics** such as mexiletine and flecainide are reputed to be more effective than antiepileptics in neurogenic pain, but must be used with extreme caution in patients with cardiac disorders. Intravenous administration of lignocaine is potentially dangerous but has been useful in a limited number of patients with chronic pain syndromes such as adiposis dolorosa (Dercum's disease), neuralgic disorders, and diabetic neuropathy.

Corticosteroids have produced improvement, often substantial, in neurogenic pain, including pain caused by nerve compression or infiltration and sympathetically maintained pain. They are also of use in patients with cancer to relieve headache caused by raised intracranial pressure and for refractory pain caused by bone metastases. Corticosteroids also have added benefits of increasing well-being and appetite. Dexamethasone, methylprednisolone, and prednisolone have been used for pain management, sometimes in the form of long-acting depot injections administered locally with or without a local anaesthetic. The exact mechanism of action of corticosteroids in analgesia is not clear but may involve relief of pressure on nervous tissue by reduction of inflammation and oedema.

The use of **antipsychotics**, such as the phenothiazines, as adjuvant analgesics is controversial and apart from methotrimeprazine there is little convincing evidence that they produce useful analgesia. Methotrimeprazine is sometimes used as an adjunct in palliative care for the management of pain and associated restlessness, distress, or vomiting.

Hydroxyzine provides additional analgesia when used with opioids and has a useful antiemetic effect; it has been used in postoperative pain and chronic cancer pain.

Caffeine has been used with the aim of enhancing the effects of non-opioid and opioid analgesics but is of debatable benefit. There are similar doubts about whether caffeine enhances the effect of ergotamine in the treatment of migraine (p.446). In addition to doubts about caffeine enhancing the analgesic effect, it can add to gastro-intestinal adverse effects and in large doses can itself cause headache.

Muscle relaxants. Benzodiazepines and other muscle relaxants such as baclofen or dantrolene are useful for relieving muscle spasm (p.1303) in acute pain or cancer pain. Baclofen has been reported to be effective in the treatment of rectal or vesical tenesmus and in neurogenic pain states. Spasmolytics such as hyoscine may be useful in conjunction with analgesics in the treatment of visceral cancer pain due to the distension of hollow organs.

Bone modulating drugs such as calcitonin and bisphosphonates may be useful in cancer pain arising from bone metastases (see below) but have a slow onset of action and are second choice to NSAIDs. Bisphosphonates may cause an initial transient increase in bone pain.

Miscellaneous drugs. Following the discovery that epidural or intrathecal injection of opioids can produce effective analgesia many other drugs have been tried by these routes, either alone or with opioids or local anaesthetics, but their role, if any, in the management of pain remains to be determined. Some of these drugs, such as clonidine and ketamine, also appear to have analgesic properties when given by other routes.

See below under Some Analgesic Techniques for discussions of the use of inhalational analgesics, nerve blocks, patient-controlled analgesia, and rubefacients and topical analgesics.

References.

1. Pon D, Hart LL. IV lidocaine as an analgesic. *DICP Ann Pharmacother* 1989; **23:** 602–4.
2. American Pain Society. Principles of analgesic use in the treatment of acute pain and chronic cancer pain, 2nd edition. *Clin Pharm* 1990; **9:** 601–11.
3. Bushnell TG, Justins DM. Choosing the right analgesic: a guide to selection. *Drugs* 1993; **46:** 394–408.
4. Rummans TA. Nonopioid agents for treatment of acute and subacute pain. *Mayo Clin Proc* 1994; **69:** 481–90.
5. Patt RB, *et al.* The neuroleptics as adjuvant analgesics. *J Pain Symptom Manage* 1994; **9:** 446–53.
6. Sawynok J. Pharmacological rationale for the clinical use of caffeine. *Drugs* 1995; **49:** 37–50.
7. McQuay H, *et al.* Anticonvulsant drugs for management of pain: a systematic review. *Br Med J* 1995; **311:** 1047–52.
8. McQuay HJ, *et al.* A systematic review of antidepressants in neuropathic pain. *Pain* 1996; **68:** 217–27.
9. McQuay HJ, Moore RA. Antidepressants and chronic pain: effective analgesia in neuropathic pain and other syndromes. *Br Med J* 1997; **314:** 763–4.
10. Anonymous. Drugs for pain. *Med Lett Drugs Ther* 1998; **40:** 79–84.

Some analgesic techniques. INHALATIONAL ANALGESICS. Some inhalational anaesthetics are used in subanaesthetic doses for their analgesic effect.

Nitrous oxide with oxygen is used to provide analgesia and sedation during dental procedures. A mixture of nitrous oxide 50% v/v and oxygen 50% v/v can provide good analgesia without loss of consciousness and is suitable for self-administration. It is used for short procedures such as dressing changes,[1,2] for pain relief during childbirth,[3] in the management of postoperative pain,[1] as an aid to postoperative physiotherapy, and for acute pain in emergency situations such as in ambulances. Continuous inhalation of nitrous oxide-oxygen has been tried for periods longer than 24 hours in the management of pain in terminal cancer.[4] However, such a practice is not usually otherwise recommended[1] as it may result in megaloblastic bone-marrow changes. Isoflurane and enflurane are sometimes used alone in subanaesthetic doses to provide analgesia in obstetrics and other painful procedures although some workers have been unable to confirm an analgesic effect with subanaesthetic doses.

Methoxyflurane at concentrations of 0.3 to 0.8% v/v has been used for analgesia in dentistry and childbirth but daily use is not recommended because of its nephrotoxic potential.

Trichloroethylene in concentrations of 0.35 to 0.5% v/v has been used in some countries to provide analgesia for obstetrics, emergency management of trauma, and other acutely painful procedures.

1. Hull CJ. Control of pain in the perioperative period. *Br Med Bull* 1988; **44:** 341–56.
2. Gaukroger PB. Pediatric analgesia: which drug, which dose? *Drugs* 1991; **41:** 52–9.
3. Brownridge P. Treatment options for the relief of pain during childbirth. *Drugs* 1991; **41:** 69–80.
4. Fosburg MT, Crone RK. Nitrous oxide analgesia for refractory pain in the terminally ill. *JAMA* 1983; **250:** 511–13.

NERVE BLOCKS. Nerve blocks produce analgesia by interrupting the nervous transmission of pain signals either by temporary inhibition of conduction or by destruction of the nerve. Nerve blocks may be used in the management of acute or chronic pain associated with a well defined anatomical site, especially when the pain is unresponsive to or not adequately controlled by conventional therapy. Nerve blocks are either used alone or with analgesics in an attempt to enhance analgesia and reduce side-effects. The route of administration and method employed depend on the site to be blocked but may include peripheral nerve block, autonomic nerve blocks such as sympathetic nerve blocks and coeliac plexus block, and central nerve blocks such as epidural (including caudal) and spinal block. Local anaesthetics are used when a temporary effect is required. For a longer duration more destructive blocks using neurolytic agents such as phenol or alcohol or freezing of the nerve (cryoanalgesia) may be used, but even with these, the effects may last no more than a few months. Furthermore, neurolytic solutions produce variable and non-selective neural damage with poor correlation between pain relief and histological damage and some consider the risk of complications to outweigh the benefits obtained.[1]

The use of nerve blocks in the management of cancer has declined following the refinement of the use of conventional analgesics. In light of the risks and limited duration of effect, some consider that the value of such techniques may be limited to patients with a life expectancy of 3 months or less[2] and the main benefit of nerve blocks in cancer is to produce maximum pain relief rapidly. However, others support the view that chemical and thermal neurolysis can provide long-term control of severe cancer pain without a substantial incidence of adverse effects.[3] Neurolytic blocks may be of particular value in cancer pain syndromes involving the viscera or the torso, but are rarely applicable in the management of extremity pain.[4] Neurogenic pain is rarely helped by somatic neural block and may even be aggravated,[1] but block of the splanchnic nerves or coeliac plexus with alcohol or phenol is reputed to be effective in relieving severe intractable pain caused by cancer of the pancreas, stomach, small intestine, gallbladder, or other abdominal viscera, especially when the cancer has not spread to the parietal peritoneum.[5] Similar neurolytic blocks preceded by a local anaesthetic have also been used in patients with severe intractable pain of chronic pancreatitis, postcholecystectomy syndrome, or other chronic abdominal visceral diseases unrelieved by medical or surgical therapy.

Central nerve blocks using local anaesthetics with or without opioids are used for the management of acute pain such as labour pain during childbirth and postoperative pain; they are also sometimes used for cancer pain.[1,6]

Sympathetic nerve blocks using repeated injections of local anaesthetics or neurolytic agents have been used for sympathetically maintained pain. Intravenous regional sympathetic block is an alternative when a single limb is involved;[1] guanethidine is one of the drugs that has been used.[7]

Injections of local anaesthetics with or without corticosteroids are often used for blocks of localised painful joints. Nerve blocks are also used to block localised painful trigger areas[8] such as postoperative or post-traumatic neuroma formation and for focal muscle pain.

1. Hanks GW, Justins DM. Cancer pain: management. *Lancet* 1992; **339:** 1031–6.
2. WHO. Cancer pain relief and palliative care: report of a WHO expert committee. *WHO Tech Rep Ser 804*, 1990.
3. American Society of Anesthesiologists Task Force on Pain Management, Cancer Pain Section. Practice guidelines for cancer pain management. *Anesthesiology* 1996; **84:** 1243–7.
4. Marshall KA. Managing cancer pain: basic principles and invasive treatments. *Mayo Clin Proc* 1996; **71:** 472–7.
5. Bonica JJ. Management of pain with regional analgesia. *Postgrad Med J* 1984; **60:** 897–904.
6. Hunt R, Massolino J. Spinal bupivacaine for the pain of cancer. *Med J Aust* 1989; **150:** 350.
7. Hannington-Kiff JG. Relief of causalgia in limbs by regional intravenous guanethidine. *Br Med J* 1979; **2:** 367–8.
8. Foley KM. The treatment of cancer pain. *N Engl J Med* 1985; **313:** 84–95.

PATIENT-CONTROLLED ANALGESIA. Patient-controlled analgesia involves the use of automated delivery systems that enable patients to administer doses of an analgesic to themselves on demand. Doses of opioids are usually given intravenously, their frequency being controlled by each patient within the safety limits of the delivery system.

Patient-controlled analgesia has proved popular with patients and nursing staff and has been used successfully by children as young as 5 years of age[1,2] and by the elderly.[3] It is useful for the control of pain from a variety of causes including postoperative pain.[4,5] Nitrous oxide in oxygen has a long history of effective use in patient-controlled analgesia during childbirth; patient-controlled opioid analgesia may not be suitable for such pain.[6]

The safety and efficacy of patient-controlled opioid analgesia largely depends on the availability of adequately trained staff and reliable pumps designed to minimise the possibility of programming errors or tampering by patients or visitors. There have been isolated reports of patients receiving very large doses through deliberate operation of the system by relatives,[7] electrical interference,[8] or incorrect use by the patient or staff.[9,10]

In the simplest type of patient-controlled analgesia the patient is able to self-administer a fixed bolus dose on demand; further doses are not then permitted until a pre-programmed lockout interval has expired. Bolus doses are adjusted to prevent overdosage but maintain analgesic blood concentrations. Variable-dose patient-controlled analgesia has also been tried in which the patient selects one of several doses, although this method offered no advantage over fixed-dose systems in one study.[11] Some devices allow the dose to be administered as a short infusion to reduce adverse effects associated with high peak concentrations of opioids. In another commonly used method, sometimes described as patient-augmented analgesia, the patient is given a continuous background infusion which is supplemented by self-administered bolus doses. However, with this method patients may receive more opioids without any improvement in analgesia;[12,13] they may also experience more adverse effects such as nausea and vomiting, respiratory depression, drowsiness, and pruritus,[13,14] although this may depend on the size of the dose used for the background infusion.[15] It remains to be seen if there is any advantage with the more sophisticated devices that can be programmed to adjust the background infusion according to the frequency of the bolus demands.

Many opioids have been tried for patient-controlled analgesia. Morphine or pethidine are the most commonly used opioids but oxymorphone or hydromorphone may be useful alternatives. Also consideration should be given to the risks from the accumulation of the pethidine metabolite, norpethidine. The agonist-antagonist nalbuphine may also be a useful alternative because of its ceiling effect on respiratory depression. The use of buprenorphine and methadone may be limited by their long half-lives, while the action of drugs such as fentanyl and its analogues may be too short.

Most experience has been with the intravenous route, but the intramuscular, subcutaneous, epidural, and intrathecal routes have also been used. Epidural or intrathecal administration may allow the use of smaller doses but the development of respiratory depression can be delayed when using the epidural route; a greater degree of patient monitoring may be required when using either of these routes.[16] Epidural administration of bupivacaine with an opioid analgesic such as fentanyl has been tried for use in patient-controlled analgesia, and may allow reduced opioid doses, although whether this confers any clinical benefit is questionable.[17]

Other routes are also being investigated.

1. Berde CB, *et al.* Patient-controlled analgesia in children and adolescents: a randomized, prospective comparison with intramuscular administration of morphine for postoperative analgesia. *J Pediatr* 1991; **118:** 460–6.
2. Irwin M, *et al.* Evaluation of a disposable patient-controlled analgesia device in children. *Br J Anaesth* 1992; **68:** 411–13.
3. Egbert AM, *et al.* Randomized trial of postoperative patient-controlled analgesia vs intramuscular narcotics in frail elderly men. *Arch Intern Med* 1990; **150:** 1897–1903.
4. Mitchell RWD, Smith G. The control of acute postoperative pain. *Br J Anaesth* 1989; **63:** 147–58.
5. Rowbotham DJ. The development and safe use of patient-controlled analgesia. *Br J Anaesth* 1992; **68:** 331–2.
6. McIntosh DG, Rayburn WF. Patient-controlled analgesia in obstetrics and gynecology. *Obstet Gynecol* 1991; **78:** 1129–35.
7. Lam FY. Patient-controlled analgesia by proxy. *Br J Anaesth* 1993; **70:** 113.
8. Notcutt WG, *et al.* Overdose of opioid from patient-controlled analgesia pumps. *Br J Anaesth* 1992; **69:** 95–7.
9. Farmer M, Harper NJN. Unexpected problems with patient controlled analgesia. *Br Med J* 1992; **304:** 574.
10. Johnson T, Daugherty M. Oversedation with patient controlled analgesia. *Anaesthesia* 1992; **47:** 81–2.
11. Love DR, *et al.* A comparison of variable-dose patient-controlled analgesia with fixed-dose patient-controlled analgesia. *Anesth Analg* 1996; **83:** 1060–4.
12. Parker RK, *et al.* Patient-controlled analgesia: does a concurrent opioid infusion improve pain management after surgery? *JAMA* 1991; **266:** 1947–52.
13. Doyle E, *et al.* Comparison of patient-controlled analgesia with and without a background infusion after lower abdominal surgery in children. *Br J Anaesth* 1993; **71:** 670–3.
14. Smythe MA, *et al.* Patient-controlled analgesia versus patient-controlled analgesia plus continuous infusion after hip replacement surgery. *Ann Pharmacother* 1996; **30:** 224–7.
15. Doyle E, *et al.* Patient-controlled analgesia with low dose background infusions after lower abdominal surgery in children. *Br J Anaesth* 1993; **71:** 818–22.
16. Hill HF, Mather LE. Patient-controlled analgesia: pharmacokinetic and therapeutic considerations. *Clin Pharmacokinet* 1993; **24:** 124–40.
17. Cooper DW, *et al.* Patient-controlled extradural analgesia with bupivacaine, fentanyl, or a mixture of both, after Caesarean section. *Br J Anaesth* 1996; **76:** 611–15.

RUBEFACIENTS AND TOPICAL ANALGESICS. Rubefacients or counter-irritants can relieve superficial or deep-seated pain probably by producing counter stimulation, which according to the 'gate theory' of pain (see Pain, above) helps to inhibit the transmission of pain signals. Their topical application produces hyperaemia or irritation of the skin and they are used alone or as an adjunct to massage in the management of a variety of painful musculoskeletal conditions. Some are also traditionally used in preparations for the symptomatic relief of minor peripheral vascular disorders such as chilblains. Substances commonly used in rubefacient preparations include nicotinate and salicylate compounds, essential oils, capsicum, solutions of ammonia, camphor, and nonivamide. Capsaicin, which is one of the active ingredients of capsicum, is used alone as a topical analgesic in a range of painful conditions, including neurogenic pain and rheumatic disorders. It appears to produce its analgesic effect partly through depletion of substance P, one of the neurotransmitters in pain pathways.[1,2] The effect of capsaicin does not rely on vasodilatation in the skin and it is therefore not considered to be a traditional counter-irritant but has been included in rubefacient preparations for the relief of muscular and rheumatic pain.

Application of heat to the skin can also help to relieve pain and melted hard paraffin has been used in wax baths as an adjunct to physiotherapy for painful joints and sprains. Warm kaolin poultices have also been used as a means of applying heat for pain relief.

Some NSAIDs have been used topically in the treatment of soft-tissue injuries and inflammatory musculoskeletal conditions, although this route does not necessarily avoid the adverse effects of systemic treatment. There is some evidence[3] to suggest that topical NSAIDs might be more effective than placebo but without comparative studies against other forms of treatment some[4] consider that their therapeutic role is unclear.

Other agents used as topical analgesics include compounds such as ethyl chloride and the halogenated hydrocarbon propellants; their evaporation produces an intense cold that numbs the tissues.

Local anaesthetics are sometimes included in topical preparations used for the relief of painful skin and musculoskeletal disorders.

1. Clarke IMC. Peppering pain, *Lancet* 1993; **342:** 1130.
2. Fusco BM, Giacovazzo M. Peppers and pain: the promise of capsaicin. *Drugs* 1997; **53:** 909–14.
3. Moore RA, *et al.* Quantitive systematic review of topically applied non-steroidal anti-inflammatory drugs. *Br Med J* 1998; **316:** 333–8.
4. Duerden M, *et al.* Topical NSAIDs are better than placebo. *Br Med J* 1998; **317:** 280–1.

Pain in infants and children. Pain has often been undertreated in infants and children because of fears of respiratory depression, cardiovascular collapse, depressed levels of consciousness, and addiction with potent analgesics. Assessment of pain is also a problem in children of all ages and it is not that long since it was widely believed that neonates were incapable of feeling pain.

Most **neonates** requiring analgesia and receiving respiratory support can be managed with an infusion of morphine, although the infusion rate may need to be adjusted before they are completely weaned from mechanical ventilation. In neonates who are breathing spontaneously there is a substantial risk of respiratory depression with powerful opioid analgesics. Morphine sulphate has been used in such neonates but should be limited to those under intensive care, as for example after major surgery. For mention of the provision of analgesia in neonates in intensive care see Intensive Care under Sedation, p.638. Fentanyl citrate and codeine phosphate have also been used in neonates. Experience with the newer partial opioid agonists such as buprenorphine, nalbuphine, and meptazinol is limited. Sucrose solutions have been shown to reduce physiologic and behavioural indicators of stress and pain in neonates undergoing painful procedures although there had been some doubt expressed over whether this indicates effective analgesia.

In **infants and children** opioids are still the mainstay of analgesia for moderate to severe pain and morphine is the standard against which the others are compared. Techniques of continuous intravenous infusion with or without initial loading doses have become popular for postoperative pain relief, but titration of the infusion rate is necessary to achieve a balance between analgesia and respiratory depression. Subcutaneous infusions of morphine have also been used, mostly for the relief of terminal cancer pain in children. Intramuscular injections can provide excellent analgesia but are painful and therefore probably only suitable for short-term use. Other opioid analgesics used in infants and children have included codeine, buprenorphine, fentanyl, meptazinol, nalbuphine, papaveretum, and pethidine. Patient-controlled analgesia using morphine has been tried in children (see above).

Morphine has been given to children by the epidural route; experience with the intrathecal route is more limited.

Other methods of opioid drug delivery of possible value in paediatric analgesia include transmucosal, nasal, and transdermal administration.

Lytic cocktails (see p.77) consisting of chlorpromazine, pethidine, and/or promethazine have been administered parenterally for sedation and analgesia in paediatric patients, but some authorities have recommended that alternatives should be considered.

Local anaesthetics do not have the side-effects associated with opioid analgesics and are of particular value in neonates and children. They are especially suitable for the management of acute pain in day-care situations. Single injections given by the epidural route are often used to provide analgesia during and after surgery. Continuous epidural infusions of local anaesthetics have also been used. However, simpler techniques such as wound infiltration or peripheral nerve blocks can also provide effective analgesia for some procedures and are free of the problems of lower limb weakness or urinary retention associated with caudal blocks. Surface anaesthesia provided by application of eutectic creams (see p.1296) containing lignocaine with prilocaine to intact skin may be sufficient for some minor painful procedures in children, although use in those under 1 year of age is not recommended.

Non-opioid analgesics are used in children, either alone for minor pain or as an adjunct to opioid analgesics in severe pain; they are often given by the rectal route. Paracetamol is frequently the drug first employed but it lacks any anti-inflammatory effect. The use of aspirin in children is greatly limited because of its association with Reye's syndrome. Other NSAIDs are useful for pain associated with inflammation but, like aspirin, can produce severe gastro-intestinal side-effects.

Cancer pain in children may be treated using the analgesic ladder scheme described under Cancer Pain (see below).

References.

1. Lloyd-Thomas AR. Pain management in paediatric patients. *Br J Anaesth* 1990; **64:** 85–104.
2. Commission on the provision of surgical services. *Report of the working party on pain after surgery.* London: Royal College of Surgeons of England and College of Anaesthetists, 1990.
3. Schecter NL, *et al.* Report of the consensus conference on the management of pain in childhood cancer. *Pediatrics* 1990; **86:** 813–34.
4. Gaukroger PB. Paediatric analgesia: which drug? which dose? *Drugs* 1991; **41:** 52–9.
5. Bhatt-Mehta V, Rosen DA. Management of acute pain in children. *Clin Pharm* 1991; **10:** 667–85.
6. Selbst SM. Analgesia in children: why is it underused in emergency departments? *Drug Safety* 1992; **7:** 8–13.
7. Burrows FA, Berde CB. Optimal pain relief in infants and children. *Br Med J* 1993; **307:** 815–16.
8. Anonymous. Treating moderate and severe pain in infants. *Drug Ther Bull* 1994; **32:** 21–4.
9. Anonymous. Managing acute pain in children. *Drug Ther Bull* 1995; **33:** 41–4 and 79.
10. Anonymous. Managing chronic pain in children. *Drug Ther Bull* 1995; **33:** 52–5.
11. Bhatt-Mehta V. Current guidelines for the treatment of acute pain in children. *Drugs* 1996; **51:** 760–76.
12. Ball AJ, Ferguson S. Analgesia and analgesic drugs in paediatrics. *Br J Hosp Med* 1996; **55:** 586–90.
13. Anderson BJ, *et al.* Size, myths and the clinical pharmacokinetics of analgesia in paediatric patients. *Clin Pharmacokinet* 1997; **33:** 313–27.

Specific pain states

Cancer pain. The pain cancer patients experience may be acute, chronic, or intermittent and is often complex in nature. The pain may result from the disease itself as a result of tumour involvement of the viscera and extension into soft tissues, tumour-induced nerve compression and injury, or raised intracranial pressure, or bone metastases. Many patients will have more than one type of pain. Pain may also arise as a result of side-effects of treatment, or from a concurrent disease, and may be exacerbated by emotional or mental changes. There may also be exacerbations due to movement (incident pain) or worsening of cancer.

Pain relief involves the treatment of the cause of the pain as well as treatment of the pain itself, together with explanation, reassurance, and supportive care to improve any mental and social complicating factors. The mainstay of cancer pain management is drug treatment with non-opioid or opioid analgesics, or both together, plus adjuvant analgesics if necessary. Most cancer pain is opioid sensitive but a small proportion of patients (about 10 to 20%) may experience pain that responds poorly or not at all to opioid analgesics given at tolerable doses. Such types of pain can be difficult to treat and examples include neurogenic pain resulting from nerve destruction or compression, incident bone pain, pancreatic pain, and muscle spasm.

In the management of cancer pain the aim is to achieve adequate continuous pain relief with the minimum of side-effects and this calls for regular monitoring of the treatment. Unmanageable adverse effects of one analgesic may be eliminated by changing to another. The non-opioids aspirin and other NSAIDS are associated with gastropathy and bleeding complications, and paracetamol in high doses is hepatotoxic. Opioids can induce nausea and vomiting, and constipation can be a difficult problem to control. Any sedation should be assessed, for while it may be useful in the management of acute pain, it is undesirable in patients with chronic pain. Although tolerance, physical dependence, and withdrawal symptoms can occur with continued use of opioids, this does not prevent their effective use for cancer pain. Withdrawal symptoms may be avoided by gradually tapering doses on discontinuing a drug. Psychological dependence and addictive behaviour do not occur when opioids are used in cancer patients, so fears of their development should not restrict use of these analgesics. Also, respiratory depression is not a problem; indeed opioid-sensitive pain appears to protect against it, although it may occur if the source of opioid-sensitive pain is removed (e.g. by surgery) without adequate reduction in opioid dosage.

Guidelines for the relief of cancer pain, published by WHO in 1986[1] and revised in 1996,[2] are widely endorsed by specialists in pain relief and the care of the terminally ill.[3-18] Patients should be assessed individually and, wherever possible, treatment should be given by mouth. It should be given regularly and the treatment should follow the accepted three-step 'analgesic ladder'.[1,2] This approach is often described as **treatment 'by mouth, by the clock, and by the ladder'**. Regular dosage rather than treatment as required aims to prevent pain re-emerging and to minimise the expectation of pain. The analgesic ladder consists of 3 stages, treatment beginning at step 1 and progressing to step 3 if pain increases; it can be used for children as well as adults. The stages are as follows:

1. a non-opioid analgesic such as aspirin, other NSAIDs, or paracetamol; an adjuvant (see below) may also be given if necessary to tackle specific pain or associated symptoms
2. a weak opioid analgesic such as codeine or dihydrocodeine plus a non-opioid analgesic; an adjuvant may also be given
3. a strong opioid analgesic, preferably oral morphine; a non-opioid analgesic may also be given, as may an adjuvant.

Non-opioids and weak opioids have a ceiling effect above which increasing the dose does not increase analgesic efficacy. Using analgesics with different pharmacological actions together can produce additive or synergistic increases in analgesia but only one analgesic from each of the 3 groups should be used at the same time.

Adjuvant drugs that may be necessary at any stage include antidepressants, antiepileptics, and class I antiarrhythmics for neurogenic pain, corticosteroids for nerve compression and headache resulting from raised intracranial pressure, and muscle relaxants for muscle spasm. Radiotherapy and radioisotopes such as strontium-89 may be of use when the bone pain of metastases is unresponsive to NSAIDs alone. Bone modulating drugs such as calcitonin and bisphosphonates may be of additional benefit but have a slow onset of action and bisphosphonates may cause an initial transient increase in pain. Corticosteroids have been used as an alternative to NSAIDs in refractory bone pain but long-term use should be avoided. Nerve blocks with local anaesthetics or neurolytic solutions may benefit a few patients, in particular those with sympathetically maintained pain or specific localised pain (see above). Physiotherapy and relaxation techniques may be useful for painful muscle spasm. Adjuvant therapy should be fully explored before moving on to the next 'rung' of the treatment ladder or increasing the dosage of an opioid analgesic. For further details of analgesic adjuvants, see above.

The **strong opioid** of choice is morphine given by mouth as a solution or tablets every 4 hours or as modified-release formulations every 12 to 24 hours. There are no 'standard' doses; they have ranged from 2.5 to over 2500 mg of morphine sulphate every 4 hours, although most patients need far less than 100 mg every 4 hours. The oral solution or standard tablets should be used for breakthrough pain in patients receiving modified-release preparations.

Alternative opioids if morphine is not tolerated have included standardised opium, hydromorphone, levorphanol, oxycodone, or tramadol. Methadone and pethidine have also been used but are of limited value because of the risk of accumulation of methadone and a toxic metabolite of pethidine and the relatively short duration of action of pethidine. Accumulation is also a risk with levorphanol. 'Brompton Cocktail' mixtures or elixirs, which contained diamorphine or morphine and cocaine with or without chlorpromazine, are now obsolete.

Although the oral route is generally preferred, other routes, such as rectal administration, may be necessary if, for example, there is intractable vomiting, inability to swallow, or unconsciousness. When injections become necessary a continuous subcutaneous infusion may be preferable to repeated subcutaneous or intramuscular injections. In the UK diamorphine hydrochloride is often preferred to morphine sulphate for parenteral administration because it is more soluble and allows a smaller dose volume; hydromorphone hydrochloride is an alternative to diamorphine. Morphine has also been given intravenously by bolus injection or infusion.

Epidural or intrathecal administration of opioids, either by injection or infusion, has been used when conventional routes have failed. Some advocate the use of these routes because smaller doses may produce analgesia equivalent to that of larger doses given by mouth or parenterally, although there has been little conclusive evidence for a lower incidence of side-effects or a better quality of analgesia.

Other routes of administration that have been investigated include buccal, sublingual, and nebulised routes, but these are not recommended for morphine because there is no current evidence of clinical advantage over conventional routes.[15] However, buprenorphine is administered sublingually and may be a useful alternative in patients with dysphagia, although experience of long-term use in cancer pain is limited. Fentanyl can be administered via a transdermal system that provides continuous and controlled delivery for 72 hours.

Automated delivery systems for self-administration of parenteral analgesics (patient-controlled analgesia) have been used for administration of opioid analgesics (see above).

1. WHO. *Cancer pain relief.* Geneva: WHO, 1986.
2. WHO. *Cancer pain relief.* 2nd ed. Geneva: WHO, 1996.
3. Hillier R. Control of pain in terminal cancer. *Br Med Bull* 1990; **46:** 279–91.
4. American Pain Society. Principles of analgesic use in the treatment of acute pain and chronic cancer pain, 2nd edition. *Clin Pharm* 1990; **9:** 601–11.
5. WHO. Cancer pain relief and palliative care: report of a WHO expert committee. *WHO Tech Rep Ser 804* 1990.
6. Schechter NL, *et al.* Report of the consensus conference on the management of pain in childhood cancer. *Pediatrics* 1990; **86:** 813–34.
7. Hanks GW, Justins DM. Cancer pain: management. *Lancet* 1992; **339:** 1031–6.
8. Davis CL, Hardy JR. Palliative care. *Br Med J* 1994; **308:** 1359–62.
9. Hammack JE, Loprinzi CL. Use of orally administered opioids for cancer-related pain. *Mayo Clin Proc* 1994; **69:** 384–90.
10. Lamer TJ. Treatment of cancer-related pain: when orally administered medications fail. *Mayo Clin Proc* 1994; **69:** 473–80.
11. US Agency for Health Care Policy and Research. Management of cancer pain: adults. *Am J Hosp Pharm* 1994; **51:** 1643–56.
12. American Society of Anesthesiologists Task Force on Pain Management, Cancer Pain Section. Practice guidelines for cancer pain management. *Anesthesiology* 1996; **84:** 1243–57.
13. Marshall KA. Managing cancer pain: basic principles and invasive treatments. *Mayo Clin Proc* 1996; **71:** 472–7.
14. Levy MH. Pharmacologic treatment of cancer pain. *N Engl J Med* 1996; **335:** 1124–32.
15. Expert Working Group of the European Association for Palliative Care. Morphine in cancer pain: modes of administration. *Br Med J* 1996; **312:** 823–6.
16. Thürlimann B, de Stoutz ND. Causes and treatment of bone pain of malignant origin. *Drugs* 1996; **51:** 383–98.
17. O'Neill B, Fallon M. ABC of palliative care. Principles of palliative care and pain control. *Br Med J* 1997; **315:** 801–4.
18. Sykes J, *et al.* ABC of palliative care. Difficult pain problems. *Br Med J* 1997; **315:** 867–9.

Central pain. Central pain is a neurogenic pain arising from lesions of the CNS. Pain following a cerebrovascular accident has been referred to as thalamic syndrome but is now commonly known as central post-stroke pain and may arise not only from classical stroke but also from surgery or trauma to the head. The pain, which has been described as burning, stabbing, and aching, may be mild to intolerable and occurs spontaneously or in response to a mild stimulus.

As for other types of neurogenic pain, opioid analgesics are ineffective and management of central post-stroke pain involves the use of antidepressants and antiepileptics.[1-3] Early peripheral sympathetic blockade may produce temporary relief in some cases. Mexiletine may be of use in patients with refractory pain;[4] lignocaine may also be of use to relieve acute painful crises.[5] Transcutaneous electrical nerve stimulation (TENS) may occasionally be of help but some advocate brain or spinal cord stimulation. Surgical treatment generally gives disappointing results.

1. Bowsher D. Neurogenic pain syndromes and their management. *Br Med Bull* 1991; **47:** 644–66.
2. Illis LS. Central pain. *Br Med J* 1990; **300:** 1284–6.
3. Bowsher D. Cerebrovascular disease: sensory consequences of stroke. *Lancet* 1993; **341:** 156.
4. Awerbuch GI, Sandyk R. Mexiletine for thalamic pain syndrome. *Int J Neurosci* 1990; **55:** 129–33.
5. Edmondson EA, *et al.* Systemic lidocaine therapy for post-stroke pain. *South Med J* 1993; **86:** 1093–6.

Colic pain. Biliary colic is associated with gallstones (p.1642) or other biliary disorders that result in obstruction of the bile ducts. Morphine may relieve the accompanying pain, but as it can also produce spasm of the sphincter of Oddi it can raise intrabiliary pressure and exacerbate the pain. It is therefore usually recommended that morphine and its derivatives should either be avoided in patients with biliary disorders or that they should be given with an antispasmodic. Opioid analgesics such as pethidine or phenazocine, which have less smooth muscle activity than morphine, may be more suitable. Prostaglandins have also been implicated in the aetiology of biliary colic and NSAIDs such as diclofenac,[1,2] indomethacin, ketoprofen,[3] and lysine aspirin[3] have been successfully used to relieve the pain of biliary colic. Other drugs that have been tried for their action on biliary smooth muscle and the sphincter of Oddi include antimuscarinics.

Ureteral obstruction, such as in the formation and passage of renal calculi (see p.888), produces painful **renal** or **ureteral colic**. The acute pain of renal or ureteral colic may be relieved using opioid analgesics such as pethidine that have a minimal effect on smooth muscle. NSAIDs may also be of use as it is believed that the pain may be partially mediated by prostaglandins. Diclofenac sodium given intramuscularly[4-6] or rectally[7] appears to be of similar efficacy to pethidine. Antimuscarinics have also been used.

1. Grossi E, *et al.* Different pharmacological approaches to the treatment of acute biliary colic. *Curr Ther Res* 1986; **40:** 876–82.
2. Lundstam S, *et al.* Diclofenac compared with a narcotic analgesic in the treatment of biliary pain. *Curr Ther Res* 1987; **42:** 395–9.
3. Magrini M, *et al.* Successful treatment of biliary colic with intravenous ketoprofen or lysine acetylsalicylate. *Curr Med Res Opin* 1985; **9:** 454–60.
4. Hetherington JW, Philp NH. Diclofenac sodium versus pethidine in acute renal colic. *Br Med J* 1986; **292:** 237–8.
5. Sanahuja J, *et al.* Intramuscular diclofenac sodium versus intravenous Baralgin in the treatment of renal colic. *DICP Ann Pharmacother* 1990; **24:** 361–4.
6. Collaborative Group of the Spanish Society of Clinical Pharmacology. Comparative study of the efficacy of dipyrone, diclofenac sodium and pethidine in acute renal colic. *Eur J Clin Pharmacol* 1991; **40:** 543–6.
7. Thompson JF, *et al.* Rectal diclofenac compared with pethidine injection in acute renal colic. *Br Med J* 1989; **299:** 1140–1.

Diabetic neuropathy. Sensory polyneuropathy, a complication of diabetes mellitus, is the commonest of the neuropathies producing neurogenic pain. The pain is mainly experienced as a burning sensation, sometimes accompanied by shooting, or aching pain. Painful neuropathy benefits from optimal diabetic control[1] (see p.315). Non-opioid analgesics such as aspirin or other NSAIDs, or paracetamol may be tried, although neurogenic pain is often resistant to conventional analgesics, and the treatment of painful diabetic neuropathy is generally as for postherpetic neuralgia[2] (see below). Relief may be obtained using tricyclic antidepressants[3-5] with or without a phenothiazine. Selective serotonin reuptake inhibitors have been tried but studies[5-7] suggest that they are ineffective or less effective than tricyclic antidepressants. Antiepileptics can be used to control any shooting or stabbing components of the pain. Antiarrhythmics such as lignocaine[8] given intravenously or mexiletine[9,10] given orally have been shown to be effective against some components of the pain and may be worth trying in unresponsive patients. Topical application of capsaicin may relieve pain in some patients.[11,12]

1. Fedele D, Giugliano D. Peripheral diabetic neuropathy: current recommendations and future prospects for its prevention and management. *Drugs* 1997; **54:** 414–21.
2. Bowsher D. Neurogenic pain syndromes and their management. *Br Med Bull* 1991; **47:** 644–66.
3. Kvinesdal B, *et al.* Imipramine treatment of painful diabetic neuropathy. *JAMA* 1984; **251:** 1727–30.
4. Max MB, *et al.* Amitriptyline relieves diabetic neuropathy pain in patients with normal or depressed mood. *Neurology* 1987; **37:** 589–96.
5. Max MB, *et al.* Effects of desipramine, amitriptyline, and fluoxetine on pain in diabetic neuropathy. *N Engl J Med* 1992; **326:** 1250–6.
6. Sindrup SH, *et al.* The selective serotonin reuptake inhibitor citalopram relieves the symptoms of diabetic neuropathy. *Clin Pharmacol Ther* 1992; **52:** 547–52.
7. Sindrup SH, *et al.* The selective serotonin reuptake inhibitor paroxetine is effective in the treatment of diabetic neuropathy symptoms. *Pain* 1990; **42:** 135–44.
8. Kastrup J, *et al.* Treatment of chronic painful diabetic neuropathy with intravenous lidocaine infusion. *Br Med J* 1986; **292:** 173.
9. Dejgård A, *et al.* Mexiletine for treatment of chronic painful diabetic neuropathy. *Lancet* 1988; **i:** 9–11.
10. Stracke H, *et al.* Mexiletine in the treatment of diabetic neuropathy. *Diabetes Care* 1992; **15:** 1550–5.
11. Capsaicin Study Group. Treatment of painful diabetic neuropathy with topical capsaicin: a multicenter, double-blind vehicle-controlled study. *Arch Intern Med* 1991; **151:** 2225–9.
12. Biesbroeck R, *et al.* A double-blind comparison of topical capsaicin and oral amitriptyline in painful diabetic neuropathy. *Adv Therapy* 1995; **12:** 111–20.

Dysmenorrhoea. Dysmenorrhoea is painful menstruation and can be classified as primary or secondary. In the more common primary form discomfort and pain arise from uterine contractions produced by release of prostaglandins from the endometrium in the luteal phase of the menstrual cycle. For this reason, drugs that inhibit ovulation or prostaglandin production are often effective treatments.[1] NSAIDs inhibit cyclo-oxygenase (prostaglandin synthetase) and are usually the drugs of first choice. Those most commonly used have included aspirin, diflunisal, flurbiprofen, ibuprofen, indomethacin, ketoprofen, mefenamic acid, naproxen, and piroxicam. Theoretically, mefenamic acid has the advantage of inhibiting both the synthesis and the peripheral action of prostaglandins, but clinical studies have not consistently shown fenamates to be more effective than other cyclo-oxygenase inhibitors. NSAIDs are taken at the onset of discomfort and continued for a few days while symptoms persist.

Patients who fail to respond to NSAIDs may benefit from the use of progestogens either alone for part of the cycle or more usually together with oestrogens in the form of oral contraceptive preparations.

Antispasmodic drugs such as hyoscine butylbromide are included in some preparations promoted for the relief of spasm associated with dysmenorrhoea.

Secondary dysmenorrhoea is pain associated with various other disorders such as endometriosis, and treatment should first be aimed at the underlying cause.

1. Shapiro SS. Treatment of dysmenorrhoea and premenstrual syndrome with non-steroidal anti-inflammatory drugs. *Drugs* 1988; **36:** 475–90.

Headache. Aspirin and other NSAIDs, or paracetamol are often tried first for the symptomatic treatment of various types of headache including migraine (p.443) and tension-type headache (p.444). An NSAID given at the onset of symptoms may successfully treat an acute attack of migraine. NSAIDs may also be effective for the prophylaxis of migraine, although they are not considered first-line treatment.

Weak opioid analgesics such as codeine are sometimes included in oral compound analgesic preparations used in the initial treatment of migraine or tension-type headache, but are best avoided, especially in patients who experience frequent attacks.

Labour pain. It is important to assess the adverse effects, on both the mother and the fetus, when selecting any method for the management of labour pain. Measures such as relaxation, hydrotherapy, transcutaneous electrical nerve stimulation (TENS), and acupuncture are sometimes used, but additional or alternative pharmacological methods of analgesia are requested by the majority of women in labour.[1]

Opioid analgesics have been administered systemically in the management of labour pain for many years, although they do not appear to provide adequate analgesia in most patients at a tolerable dosage. Pethidine tends to be the most commonly used drug. Unfortunately, like all opioids, it can cross the placenta and produce respiratory depression in the fetus and, when given by intramuscular injection, the onset of action can be unpredictable. Intravenous administration by intermittent doses or continuous infusion or patient-controlled intravenous analgesia has been tried in an attempt to improve pain control, but such techniques are thus far not considered superior to epidural blocks (see below) and do not appear to be widely used.[1]

The inhalational anaesthetic **nitrous oxide**, given with oxygen, is suitable for self-administration and is commonly used to relieve labour pain. It is relatively safe and can produce substantial analgesia in most patients. Other inhalational analgesics are also sometimes used (see above).

Epidural analgesia with a local anaesthetic can provide effective pain relief during labour. The caudal route was once widely employed for epidural analgesia but it has now largely been superseded by the lumbar route. Although epidural analgesia has been associated with an increased risk of prolonged labour, forceps delivery, and caesarean section,[2] and may not improve maternal experience of childbirth, it is still considered to be beneficial to both mother and baby, particularly in high-risk cases.[1,3] However, it does require management by suitably experienced staff and the availability of resuscitation facilities to avoid maternal complications. It has been suggested[4,5] that since a request for epidural analgesia is more likely to be made by women experiencing slow, complicated, painful labour, it is difficult to quantify the effect of the epidural itself on the outcome of labour, and exactly how it may modify labour remains unclear. In the mother epidural analgesia prevents many of the adverse physiological responses associated with the stress of pain and general anaesthesia. Neonates appear to do better after maternal epidural block than after non-epidural opioid analgesics or general anaesthesia, and the incidence of neonatal mortality may be lower, particularly in low birth-weight neonates.[3]

Epidural block has few contra-indications. In the absence of coagulopathy it may be of particular value in pre-eclampsia as it produces beneficial haemodynamic changes.[3] Serious adverse events are rare and usually arise from administration errors.[1,3] However, profound hypotension can occur as a result of sympathetic block.[6] Other effects may include diminished patient awareness of uterine contractions and of giving birth, sensations of weakness, numbness and paraesthesia of the lower limbs, impaired mobility, bladder distension, and pyrexia or uncontrollable shivering.[1,3] Many of these effects are associated with motor block and can be reduced by using doses of local anaesthetic lower than those required for surgery. Epidural analgesia can also prolong the second stage of labour and the use of oxytocin may be required.[3] Further details of the adverse effects and precautions for epidural block can be found under Central Block on p.1281 and p.1283 respectively. Occasionally epidural administration of local anaesthetics does not produce adequate analgesia due to patchy or incomplete block.[6]

Bupivacaine is one of the local anaesthetics most commonly used in epidural analgesia.

Opioid analgesics have been administered epidurally but are not particularly effective for labour pain when used alone.[6,7] Adequate analgesia is usually only obtained with doses that are associated with nausea, sedation, and disorientation.[1] Severe pruritus can also be a problem with some opioids such as morphine. Delayed respiratory depression is also a potential hazard, but may be less of a problem with drugs such as pethidine or fentanyl.[1,6] Epidural opioids are considered to be most useful when given in combination with epidural local anaesthetics. The addition of small doses of opioid analgesics to bupivacaine provides additional pain relief and reduces the amount of local anaesthetic required as well as the degree of motor block.[6,7] The addition of an opioid can also control epidural-induced shivering.[7] Several opioids have been tried epidurally with bupivacaine but it has not yet been determined which is the most suitable for pain relief during labour; favourable results have been obtained with drugs such as fentanyl or sufentanil. The use of drugs such as clonidine with local anaesthetics or opioids is also being studied.

Once the initial block is established additional analgesia can be provided through a catheter by intermittent 'top-up' doses or by a continuous epidural infusion;[1,8] a combination of the two methods forms the basis of some types of patient-controlled epidural analgesia,[8,9] but there is some concern that the safety of such patient-controlled epidural anaesthesia remains largely untested.[10]

A spinal block given before the epidural block reduces the degree of motor block associated with epidural analgesia and allows the patient to be ambulatory during labour.[9,11-14] Combined **spinal-epidural analgesia** provides the rapid onset of spinal block and the flexibility of continuous epidural block.[4,8]

Although there is renewed interest in the use of **spinal blocks** in labour[9] they do not appear to have been widely used alone for the relief of labour pain and it is considered[4] that no single drug or combination of drugs by this route reliably provides adequate analgesia for the duration of labour. The use of spinal blocks in obstetrics has been more commonly associated with anaesthesia and management of postoperative pain in caesarean section.[1] Spinal blocks with local anaesthetics have a greater tendency to produce hypotension and headache than epidural blocks, and this appears to be particularly so in pregnant patients.[15] Although spinal block using opioids may control labour pain, some consider that they are unsuitable for use alone because they also produce a greater incidence of adverse effects in pregnant patients.[15] Further details of the adverse effects and precautions for spinal block can be found under Central Block on p.1281 and p.1283 respectively.

The technique of paracervical local anaesthetic block has been largely abandoned in labour pain[1] because of the high incidence of fetal arrhythmias, acidosis, and asphyxia and isolated reports of fetal death.

1. Brownridge P. Treatment options for the relief of pain during childbirth. *Drugs* 1991; **41:** 69–80.
2. Thorp JA, *et al.* The effect of intrapartum epidural analgesia on nulliparous labor: a randomized, controlled, prospective trial. *Am J Obstet Gynecol* 1993; **169:** 851–8.
3. Reynolds F. Epidural analgesia in obstetrics. *Br Med J* 1989; **299:** 751–2.
4. Eberle RL, Norris MC. Labour analgesia: a risk-benefit analysis. *Drug Safety* 1996; **14:** 239–51.
5. McGrady EM. Extradural analgesia: does it affect progress and outcome in labour? *Br J Anaesth* 1997; **78:** 115–17.
6. Anonymous. Pain relief in labour: old drugs, new route. *Lancet* 1991; **337:** 1446–7.
7. Reynolds F. Extradural opioids in labour. *Br J Anaesth* 1989; **63:** 251–3.
8. Collis RE. Regional analgesia in labour: a new look. *Hosp Med* 1998; **59:** 388–92.
9. Kan RE, Hughes SC. Recent developments in analgesia during labour. *Drugs* 1995; **50:** 417–22.
10. Bogod D. Advances in epidural analgesia for labour: progress versus prudence. *Lancet* 1995; **345:** 1129–30.
11. Collis RE, *et al.* Combined spinal epidural analgesia with ability to walk throughout labour. *Lancet* 1993; **341:** 767–8. Correction *ibid.*; 1038.
12. Camann W, Abouleish A. Spinal epidural analgesia and walking throughout labour. *Lancet* 1993; **341:** 1095.
13. Collis RE, *et al.* Randomised comparison of combined spinal-epidural and standard epidural analgesia in labour. *Lancet* 1995; **345:** 1413–16.
14. Nageotte MP, *et al.* Epidural analgesia compared with combined spinal-epidural analgesia during labor in nulliparous women. *N Engl J Med* 1997; **337:** 1715–19.
15. Kestin IG. Spinal anaesthesia in obstetrics. *Br J Anaesth* 1991; **66:** 596–607.

Low back pain. Low back pain (sometimes referred to by the lay term lumbago), is an extremely common complaint in the industrialised world but only a small percentage of patients suffer from a recognised organic disease. The most frequent identifiable causes include mechanical or degenerative damage (e.g. disc disease), inflammatory diseases, infections, malignant neoplasms, and bone diseases (e.g. osteoporosis, osteomalacia, Paget's disease). Of these, disc disease appears to be the most common major disorder seen in back pain clinics. In patients with a herniated or prolapsed disc, the rupture of one of the fibrocartilagenous intervertebral discs can exert pressure on spinal nerves and produce a condition characterised by severe and often acute pain radiating from the back along the distribution of the nerves affected. In lumbar disc herniation the sciatic nerve may be involved and patients experience pain (sciatica), usually in one leg along the typical distribution of the nerve.

Treatment for acute back pain should be given early to prevent the condition becoming chronic. For simple back pain in the absence of nerve root symptoms or signs of serious spinal pathology paracetamol should be tried in the first instance, but if this fails to give relief then an NSAID should be substituted. If neither of these drugs controls the pain adequately, paracetamol may be combined with a weak opioid; strong opioid analgesics should be avoided if possible. Analgesics should be given regularly rather than when required. A short course of a muscle relaxant such as diazepam or baclofen may also be considered. Unless patients are in great pain or unable to stand or walk, bed rest is no longer recommended for simple back pain as it promotes chronicity. Even when necessary, bed rest should be limited to up to 3 days. Early physical activity, even if it causes some discomfort, should be encouraged since this improves the rate of recovery. Specific exercises do not appear to be useful for acute back pain but manipulation may be considered during the first weeks after onset.

As opposed to simple back pain, restriction of activity and bed rest may be justified in the treatment of sciatica. Epidural injections of corticosteroids with or without local anaesthetics, using either the caudal or lumbar route, may facilitate recovery. Manipulation should not be used for patients with evidence of nerve root entrapment as it may exacerbate the lesion. Surgery is indicated in patients with herniated disc if conservative treatment fails or if there is severe nerve compression. Dissolution of the disc by injection of enzymes (chemonucleosis) such as chymopapain or collagenase appears to be an effective alternative to surgery, but anaphylactic reactions may occasionally occur.

The prevalence of chronic or recurrent back problems is high, and in the majority of cases, the source of the pain cannot be identified; for many patients, chronic pain is not the same as acute back pain lasting longer and treatment is difficult. Surgery may be indicated for disc disease (see above) or spondylosis. Local injections of corticosteroids, sclerosant injections into ligaments, or cryotherapy to facet joints have all been tried but the success rate of these procedures is low. Rehabilitation programmes combining physical and psychological approaches to managing back pain are alternative options available. Transcutaneous electrical nerve stimulation (TENS), acupuncture, and neurolytic nerve blocks are other methods that have been tried for intractable chronic back pain.

References.

1. Bush K. Lower back pain and sciatica: how best to manage them. *Br J Hosp Med* 1994; **51:** 216–22.
2. Royal College of General Practitioners. *Clinical guidelines for the management of acute low back pain: low back pain evidence review.* London: Royal College of General Practitioners, 1996.
3. Jayson MIV. Back pain. *Br Med J* 1996; **313:** 355–8.
4. Jenner JR, Barry M. Low back pain. In: Snaith ML, ed. *ABC of rheumatology.* London: BMJ Publishing Group, 1996: 10–13.
5. Deyo RA. Acute low back pain: a new paradigm for management. *Br Med J* 1996; **313:** 1343–4.
6. Jayson MIV. Why does acute back pain become chronic? *Br Med J* 1997; **314:** 1639–40.
7. van Tulder MW, *et al.* Conservative treatment of acute and chronic nonspecific low back pain: a systematic review of randomized controlled trials of the most common interventions. *Spine* 1997; **22:** 2128–56.

Myocardial infarction pain. The severe pain of acute myocardial infarction is located in the retrosternal area with radiation to the arms, neck, jaw, and epigastrium. Pain relief is of benefit not only in its own right but also because pain may cause adverse haemodynamic effects such as increases in blood pressure, heart rate, and stroke volume. Although early treatment of the myocardial infarction (p.791) may relieve pain dramatically, opioid analgesics are the first-line treatment for pain and should be given intravenously as soon as possible, that is before hospital admission, to patients with suspected infarction. Opioids can also help to reduce anxiety. An inhaled mixture of nitrous oxide and oxygen has sometimes been used to provide pain relief before arrival in hospital; sublingual glyceryl trinitrate or an alternative fast-acting nitrate may also be given.

Diamorphine or morphine given by slow intravenous injection have generally been the opioids of choice, partly because of a more advantageous haemodynamic profile, but pethidine has also been used. The intramuscular route should only be used if venous access is unobtainable since it is relatively ineffective in shocked patients, complicates the enzymatic assessment of the infarction, and may result in large haematomas when patients are given thrombolytics. Alternative analgesics include nalbuphine or buprenorphine, although the latter may not produce pain relief as quickly as diamorphine. Pentazocine's cardiovascular effects make it unsuitable for use during or after myocardial infarction.

References.

1. Herlitz J. Analgesia in myocardial infarction. *Drugs* 1989; **37:** 939–44.
2. Wyllie HR, Dunn FG. Pre-hospital opiate and aspirin administration in patients with suspected myocardial infarction. *Br Med J* 1994; **308:** 760–1.
3. Weston CFM, *et al.* Guidelines for the early management of patients with myocardial infarction. *Br Med J* 1994; **308:** 767–71.

Neurogenic pain syndromes. The definition and characteristics of neurogenic pain are described under Pain, above. Treatment can be difficult since neurogenic pain responds poorly to conventional analgesics.[1] The painful disorders characterised by neurogenic pain (either as the predominant form of pain or as one component of the overall pain) discussed in this section are Central Pain, Diabetic Neuropathy, Phantom Limb Pain, Postherpetic Neuralgia, Sympathetic Pain Syndromes such as reflex sympathetic dystrophy and causalgia, and Trigeminal Neuralgia.

1. Bowsher D. Neurogenic pain syndromes and their management. *Br Med Bull* 1991; **47:** 644–66.

Orofacial pain. Orofacial pain may arise from a wide range of disorders so its effective management depends very much on the correct identification and treatment of any underlying cause, which may include dental disease, cluster headache (p.443), migraine (p.443), trigeminal neuralgia (see below), sinusitis (p.142), ear disease such as otitis media (p.134), giant cell arteritis (p.1021), aneurysms, and neoplasms. However, a large number of patients have a type of facial pain of unknown cause which is typically exacerbated by stress and can develop into a chronic debilitating disorder. Many patients with such idiopathic facial pain respond to non-opioid analgesics, explanation, and reassurance. Antidepressants such as the tricyclics are often of value. Treatment should be continued for several months if pain recurrence on withdrawal is to be avoided. Psychological treatments can also be helpful. Botulinum A toxin has been tried for the relief of facial pain associated with some disorders of the orofacial muscles.

References.

1. Feinmann C, Peatfield R. Orofacial neuralgia: diagnosis and treatment guidelines. *Drugs* 1993; **46:** 263–8.
2. Hunter S. The management of "psychogenic" orofacial pain. *Br Med J* 1992; **304:** 329–30.

Pancreatic pain. Pain in pancreatitis (p.1613) can be severe and may require the administration of opioid analgesics. Unfortunately, morphine and its derivatives can produce spasm of the sphincter of Oddi, so if one of these opioids is used it should be given with an antispasmodic. Pethidine has a minimal effect on smooth muscle and may be given intravenously for pain relief in acute pancreatitis; phenazocine is another suitable opioid analgesic.

Concerns over the long-term use of opioids in non-malignant pain should not prevent the patient being given effective analgesia which may be achieved by following the general principles recommended by the WHO for treatment of cancer pain (see above). Mild attacks of pain may be treated using non-opioid analgesics with or without antispasmodics such as antimuscarinics. Patients experiencing inadequate pain relief may progress to weak opioids and then if necessary to stronger opioids. Analgesics should be given before meals to help to alleviate the postprandial exacerbation of pain. Administration should be on a regular basis and doses titrated for each patient. Pancreatic extracts are probably worth trying but if the pain is not eased they should be withdrawn and reserved for those with symptomatic malabsorption. Coeliac plexus block has been used for the relief of severe intractable pain in some patients with chronic pancreatitis; it has also been used similarly in patients with cancer of the pancreas. However, the benefits of such a block are unclear.

References.

1. Trewby PN. Chronic pancreatitis. *Prescribers' J* 1991; **31:** 111–17.
2. Mergener K, Baillie J. Chronic pancreatitis. *Lancet* 1997; **350:** 1379–85.

Phantom limb pain. Phantom limb pain is associated with an amputated limb and is more common when there has been severe pre-amputation pain. It is frequently a mixture of neurogenic and other types of pain. Management may be difficult[1,2] but in a survey of war veteran amputees, for those who took any form of treatment for phantom limb pain, conventional analgesics such as NSAIDs or paracetamol with or without opioid analgesics were reported as being satisfactory.[2] Transcutaneous electrical nerve stimulation (TENS) was another method used by some and considered to be at least as effective as other therapies. Tricyclic antidepressants and antiepileptics may be of help for the neurogenic components of the pain[1,3] and some relief may be obtained with sympathetic blocks.[1] From a review[4] of studies investigating the effect of regional anaesthesia in preventing phantom limb pain in patients undergoing lower-limb amputation it appeared that epidural blockade started before and continuing for the duration of surgery or for several days after amputation conferred more protection from long-term pain than blockade commenced late intra-operatively or postoperatively. However, a recent randomised, double-blind, controlled trial[5] failed to demonstrate any beneficial effect of pre-emptive analgesia using epidural blockade in such patients.

1. Stannard CF. Phantom limb pain. *Br J Hosp Med* 1993; **50:** 583–7.
2. Wartan SW, *et al.* Phantom pain and sensation among British veteran amputees. *Br J Anaesth* 1997; **78:** 652–9.
3. Ward A, *et al.* Phantom limb pain—a pain beyond reach? *Hosp Pharm* 1998; **5:** 241–6.
4. Katz J. Prevention of phantom limb pain by regional anaesthesia. *Lancet* 1997; **349:** 519–20.
5. Nikolajsen L, *et al.* Randomised trial of epidural bupivacaine and morphine in prevention of stump and phantom pain in lower-limb amputation. *Lancet* 1997; **350:** 1353–7.

Postherpetic neuralgia. About 10% of patients who have had acute herpes zoster still experience pain one or more months after the rash has healed. The elderly are the most susceptible. The pain of postherpetic neuralgia is neurogenic resulting from peripheral nerve injury, and typically follows a dermatomal distribution commonly affecting the head, neck, and limbs. Some have described the pain as burning, others as aching. The affected area is extremely sensitive to any stimuli; even the pressure of clothing can produce unbearable pain. Spontaneous remission of postherpetic neuralgia occurs in many patients within a few months. In a small percentage of patients the pain can last for several years.

Postherpetic neuralgia is difficult to treat. The ideal approach would be to prevent the neuralgia from developing by treatment given when the acute zoster develops. Antivirals and other drugs such as corticosteroids and local and regional anaesthesia have been tried but without noted success in preventing postherpetic neuralgia, although some drugs may reduce the duration. Treatment is therefore based on managing the neuralgia once it develops.

The value of conventional analgesics is limited because of the neurogenic character of the pain and treatment relies on the tricyclic antidepressants which appear to help some patients. Antiepileptics have been used, but their value in postherpetic neuralgia is unclear, though they may help in those with sharp pain. However, their adverse effects make them unsuitable in the elderly. Nerve blocks and surgical techniques may provide temporary pain relief, but results have generally been disappointing. Transcutaneous electrical nerve stimulation (TENS) may be effective in some patients. Topical application of capsaicin may produce some benefit. Topical preparations of aspirin, indomethacin, or local anaesthetics are considered to have shown some promise.

References.

1. Anonymous. Postherpetic neuralgia. *Lancet* 1990; **336:** 537–8.
2. Robertson DRC, George CF. Treatment of post herpetic neuralgia in the elderly. *Br Med Bull* 1990; **46:** 113–123
3. Bowsher D. Neurogenic pain syndromes and their management. *Br Med Bull* 1991; **47:** 644–66.
4. Lee JJ, Gauci CAG. Postherpetic neuralgia: current concepts and management. *Br J Hosp Med* 1994; **52:** 565–70.
5. Kost RG, Straus SE. Postherpetic neuralgia—pathogenesis, treatment, and prevention. *N Engl J Med* 1996; **335:** 32–42.

Postoperative pain. Pain is not a necessary or unavoidable consequence of surgery and, if unrelieved, can increase morbidity. Unfortunately pain relief following surgery has often been inadequate, and it is now recognised that the traditional approach of giving an opioid analgesic such as morphine in fixed intramuscular doses as required to control pain is no longer valid. Pain control should be adjusted for each patient and each situation, and if treatment can be given safely to prevent postoperative pain, so much the better.

Pure opioid agonists, in particular morphine, are still the mainstay of management of postoperative pain, although the opioid may only be part of treatment. Differences between pure agonists are largely pharmacokinetic and drugs such as fentanyl, diamorphine, or pethidine have been used when a faster onset of action is required. Pure opioid agonists can control most postoperative pain but the desired degree of analgesia has to be balanced against adverse effects such as nausea, vomiting, and respiratory depression. Partial opioid agonists or mixed agonist-antagonists such as buprenorphine, pentazocine, nalbuphine, butorphanol, and meptazinol are less likely to produce respiratory depression, but as they have a weaker analgesic action than morphine, their use for postoperative pain is limited.

Although the intramuscular administration of opioids is simple, it is also painful and can produce widely fluctuating plasma concentrations with the risk of respiratory depression. Patients are also dependent on nursing staff to administer the injections regularly if adequate analgesia is to be maintained. Unfortunately, alternative methods of opioid administration are limited. The oral route is not suitable for opioids in the immediate postoperative period but may be convenient later on when gastro-intestinal function has recovered. Opioid analgesics have also been given by the rectal, subcutaneous, sublingual, buccal, transdermal and intranasal routes in the treatment of postoperative pain, but, because of unreliable absorption and/or slow onset of action, these routes are, like the oral route, not ideal immediately following surgery.

The intravenous route is widely used; an effective means of providing opioid-induced analgesia in the immediate postoperative period is to administer a variable rate intravenous infusion with an initial bolus dose plus subsequent top-up boluses if necessary. Patient-controlled analgesia (see above) has proved popular with patients and nursing staff.

Opioids injected via the epidural or intrathecal routes provide excellent analgesia. Insertion of a catheter during surgery makes it easier to give subsequent continuous infusion or 'on-demand' bolus injections. Morphine is the opioid analgesic most commonly used, but opioids such as fentanyl that are more lipid soluble may be preferable when the injection is given epidurally. Although the doses used are relatively small, there is a high incidence of nausea, vomiting, urinary retention, pruritus, and respiratory depression. This last effect may be delayed, so close monitoring of respiratory function is necessary.

The lack of sedative effects with NSAIDs makes them of particular value in the management of acute pain after day-case surgery, but they are usually considered to be unsuitable as sole analgesics immediately after major surgery. They can, however, be used effectively with other drugs, and it is now apparent that concomitant administration of an NSAID with an opioid enables the dose of the opioid to be reduced without loss of analgesic effect. However, the risk of gastric ulceration, impaired coagulation, and reduced renal function may limit the use of NSAIDs in some patients. Diclofenac, flurbiprofen, ketoprofen, and ketorolac are among the NSAIDs used for postoperative pain. Diclofenac, ketoprofen, and ketorolac may be given by injection.

Nerve blocks with local anaesthetics carried out during surgery often produce profound analgesia in the immediate postoperative period. However, effects are only temporary and repeated administration may be impractical. Local infiltration of anaesthetic at the site of operation is a simple method of preventing postoperative wound pain. Central nerve blocks obtained with epidural or intrathecal administration of local anaesthetics produce excellent analgesia and use of a long-acting drug such as bupivacaine can produce prolonged pain relief. Insertion of a catheter during the operation allows subsequent administration by infusion or bolus injection. Hypotension is a potentially serious problem with central nerve blocks and necessitates constant monitoring of blood pressure. Administration of mixtures of opioids and local anaesthetics epidurally or intrathecally has permitted good postoperative analgesia to be obtained in some situations using relatively smaller doses of each drug. A wide range of other drugs such as clonidine have also been tried by these routes either alone or with opioids or local anaesthetics, but their role, if any, remains to be determined.

Pre-operative use of analgesics or local anaesthetics (pre-emptive analgesia) may also reduce postoperative pain.

References.

1. Commission on the provision of surgical services. *Report of the working party on pain after surgery.* London: Royal College of Surgeons of England and College of Anaesthetists, 1990.
2. Anonymous. Managing postoperative pain. *Drug Ther Bull* 1993; **31:** 11–12.
3. Nuutinen LS, *et al.* A risk-benefit appraisal of injectable NSAIDs in the management of postoperative pain. *Drug Safety* 1993; **9:** 380–93.
4. Howard R. Preoperative and postoperative pain control. *Arch Dis Child* 1993; **69:** 699–703.
5. Katz J. Preop analgesia for postop pain. *Lancet* 1993; **342:** 65–6.
6. Kehlet H. Postoperative pain relief—what is the issue? *Br J Anaesth* 1994; **72:** 375–8.
7. Leith S, *et al.* Extradural infusion analgesia for postoperative pain relief. *Br J Anaesth* 1994; **73:** 552–8.
8. Chrubasik S, Chrubasik J. Selection of the optimum opioid for extradural administration in the treatment of postoperative pain. *Br J Anaesth* 1995; **74:** 121–2.
9. Cashman J, McAnulty G. Nonsteroidal anti-inflammatory drugs in perisurgical pain management: mechanisms of action and rationale for optimum use. *Drugs* 1995; **49:** 51–70.
10. American Society of Anesthesiologists Task Force on Pain Management, Acute Pain Section. Practice guidelines for acute pain management in the perioperative setting. *Anesthesiology* 1995; **82:** 1071–81.
11. McQuay HJ. Pre-emptive analgesia: a systematic review of clinical studies. *Ann Med* 1995; **27:** 249–56.
12. Raja SN. Is an ounce of preoperative local anesthetic better than a pound of postoperative analgesic? *Reg Anesth* 1996; **21:** 277–80.
13. Follin SL, Charland SL. Acute pain management: operative or medical procedures and trauma. *Ann Pharmacother* 1997; **31:** 1068–76.

Sickle-cell crisis. The management of pain of sickle-cell crisis (p.703) is similar to that of other forms of acute pain. The pain of mild crises may be controlled using analgesics such as NSAIDs or weak opioid analgesics.[1,2] Crises severe enough to necessitate hospital admission usually require the use of stronger opioid analgesics but NSAIDs may be useful as an adjunct for bone pain. Inhalation of a mixture of nitrous oxide and oxygen may be a useful analgesic during transfer to hospital.[3] Partial agonist and antagonist opioids such as buprenorphine or pentazocine are not recommended to treat acute pain before transfer to hospital.[3] Some patients appear to prefer pethidine to morphine but many workers[1,2,4] avoid its use if possible as control of pain may be inadequate and doses of pethidine commonly used to manage crises may lead to accumulation of its neuroexcitatory metabolite norpethidine and precipitate seizures (see also p.76). Diamorphine has been used as an alternative to morphine. As the dose of opioid required to control the pain can vary considerably, not only during each episode but also from one episode to another and between individual patients patient-controlled analgesia (see above) may be of help to manage the pain once initial pain relief has been obtained with loading doses of parenteral opioids;[2,5] opioids used have included morphine and fentanyl. The use of continuous epidural analgesia with local anaesthetics alone or in combination with opioids has been tried. A randomised trial[6] of morphine for the management of severe painful sickle-cell crises in children showed that oral modified-release morphine was a safe and effective alternative to continuous intravenous morphine.

A recent double-blind study appeared to indicate that high doses of methylprednisolone might shorten the duration of painful crises but there was a suggestion that there might be a rebound phenomenon with treated patients more likely to experience further crises soon after discharge.[7]

1. Davies SC, Oni L. Management of patients with sickle cell disease. *Br Med J* 1997; **315:** 656–60.
2. Vijay V, *et al.* The anaesthetist's role in acute sickle cell crisis. *Br J Anaesth* 1998; **80:** 820–8.
3. Report of a working party of the Standing Medical Advisory Committee on sickle cell, thalassaemia and other haemoglobinopathies. London: HMSO, 1993.
4. Pryle BJ, *et al.* Toxicity of norpethidine in sickle cell crisis. *Br Med J* 1992; **304:** 1478–9.
5. Grundy R, *et al.* Practical management of pain in sickling disorders. *Arch Dis Child* 1993; **69:** 256–9.
6. Jacobson SJ, *et al.* Randomised trial of oral morphine for painful episodes of sickle-cell disease in children. *Lancet* 1997; **350:** 1358–61.
7. Griffin TC, *et al.* High-dose intravenous methylprednisolone therapy for pain in children and adolescents with sickle cell disease. *N Engl J Med* 1994; **330:** 733–7.

Sympathetic pain syndromes. Reflex sympathetic dystrophy and causalgia are neurogenic pain syndromes, with apparent involvement of the sympathetic nervous system.

Reflex sympathetic dystrophy (also referred to as complex regional pain syndrome type I, algodystrophy, Sudeck's atrophy, post-traumatic osteoporosis, or shoulder-hand syndrome) is a severely painful syndrome of the limbs. Patients with reflex sympathetic dystrophy who respond to a sympatholytic procedure (see below) have been described as having 'sympathetically maintained pain' while those who do not as having 'sympathetic-independent pain'. Reflex sympathetic dystrophy is usually precipitated by injury or follows lack of use of the affected limb. There may be accompanying autonomic hyperactivity and trophic changes of skin and bone. **Causalgia** (complex regional pain syndrome type II) may be regarded as a specific type of reflex sympathetic dystrophy which follows damage to a peripheral nerve. The pain is continuous, diffuse, and burning, and is easily exacerbated. Its onset can be within days or weeks of an initial injury.

Management of reflex sympathetic dystrophy involves trying to restore normal function by treating the causative injury and easing the acute pain, followed by sympathetic nerve block with a local anaesthetic and aggressive physiotherapy as it is important that the patient starts using the affected limb again. Neurolytic nerve block with phenol has also been tried. Intravenous regional sympathetic block with the adrenergic blocking drug guanethidine is used, although opinions as to its efficacy vary.

Stimulation techniques such as transcutaneous electrical nerve stimulation (TENS) have been employed in some patients. Alpha blockers such as phenoxybenzamine or high doses of corticosteroids might produce some improvement. In refractory patients it might be worth trying antidepressants, antiepileptics, and other drugs used in the general treatment of neurogenic pain (see under Postherpetic Neuralgia, above). Application of the topical analgesic capsaicin has also been tried for reflex sympathetic dystrophy. Preliminary data from small numbers of patients suggest that bisphosphonates may be beneficial in controlling pain in some patients with reflex sympathetic dystrophy.

References.

1. Charlton JE. Management of sympathetic pain. *Br Med Bull* 1991; **47:** 601–18.
2. Bowsher D. Neurogenic pain syndromes and their management. *Br Med Bull* 1991; **47:** 644–66.
3. Yasuda JM, Schroeder DJ. Guanethidine for reflex sympathetic dystrophy. *Ann Pharmacother* 1994; **28:** 338–41.
4. Schott GD. An unsympathetic view of pain. *Lancet* 1995; **345:** 634–6.
5. Murray P, Atkinson R. Reflex sympathetic dystrophy. *Br J Hosp Med* 1995; **53:** 35–40.
6. Paice E. Reflex sympathetic dystrophy. *Br Med J* 1995; **310:** 1645–8.
7. Lloyd-Thomas AR, Lauder G. Reflex sympathetic dystrophy in children. *Br Med J* 1995; **310:** 1648–9.
8. Jadad AR, *et al.* Intravenous regional sympathetic blockade for pain relief in reflex sympathetic dystrophy: a systematic review and a randomized, double-blind crossover study. *J Pain Symptom Manage* 1995; **10:** 13–20.
9. Schott GD. Interrupting the sympathetic outflow in causalgia and reflex sympathetic dystrophy: a futile procedure for many patients. *Br Med J* 1998; **316:** 792.
10. Schott GD. Bisphosphonates for pain relief in reflex sympathetic dystrophy? *Lancet* 1997; **350:** 1117. Correction. *ibid.* 1998; **351:** 682.

Trigeminal neuralgia. Trigeminal neuralgia (tic douloureux) is a neurogenic pain characterised by sudden, brief, sharp, agonising, episodic pain in the distribution of one or more branches of the fifth cranial nerve. There may be several episodes (lasting several seconds or minutes) a day over a number of weeks, followed by a pain-free interval which may last for weeks or years. Trigeminal neuralgia generally has a 'trigger zone' in which even a very light stimulus such as a draught of air produces pain. In some cases firm pressure applied around but not to the zone itself may help to relieve pain. Trigeminal neuralgia may be idiopathic or may be secondary to nerve compression (such as that caused by a tumour), facial injury, or multiple sclerosis.

Carbamazepine is the drug of first choice for the management of trigeminal neuralgia and initially may produce satisfactory pain relief in 70% or more of patients. However, increasingly larger doses may be required. Also side-effects can be troublesome. If pain relief is inadequate then the addition of phenytoin may help; baclofen has also been added to carbamazepine therapy. These drugs may also be used alone or together in patients intolerant of carbamazepine. Other antiepileptics such as sodium valproate and clonazepam have also been used in carbamazepine-intolerant patients; oxcarbazepine is another possible alternative.

In many patients drug therapy eventually fails to control the pain or produces unacceptable side-effects and invasive procedures become necessary. One method frequently used is the selective destruction of pain bearing nerve fibres with radiofrequency thermocoagulation; instillation of glycerol has also been used to achieve the same effect but the efficacy and safety of the procedure is debatable. Microvascular decompression of the trigeminal nerve root has also been used in intractable cases.

References.

1. Sweet WH. The treatment of trigeminal neuralgia (tic douloureux). *N Engl J Med* 1986; **315:** 174–7.
2. Zakrzewska JM. Medical management of trigeminal neuralgia. *Br Dent J* 1990; **168:** 399–401.
3. Bowsher D. Neurogenic pain syndromes and their management. *Br Med Bull* 1991; **47:** 644–66.
4. Green MW, Selman JE. Review article: the medical management of trigeminal neuralgia. *Headache* 1991; **31:** 588–92.

Aceclofenac (2545-k)

Aceclofenac *(BAN, rINN).*

Aceclofenacum. [*o*-(2,6-Dichloroanilino)phenyl]acetate glycolic acid ester; 2-(2,6-Dichloroanalino)phenylacetoxyacetic acid.

$C_{16}H_{13}Cl_2NO_4$ = 354.2.

CAS — 89796-99-6.

Pharmacopoeias. In *Eur.* (see p.viii).

A white or almost white, crystalline powder. Practically **insoluble** in water; soluble in alcohol and in methyl alcohol; freely soluble in acetone and in dimethylformamide. **Protect** from light.

Adverse Effects

As for NSAIDs in general, p.63.

Hypersensitivity. Leukocytoclastic vasculitis, a type III hypersensitivity reaction, with lung haemoptysis has been reported in a patient following therapy with aceclofenac.[1]

1. Epelde F, Boada L. Leukocytoclastic vasculitis and hemoptysis after treatment with aceclofenac. *Ann Pharmacother* 1995; **29:** 1168.

Precautions

As for NSAIDs in general, p.65.

Aceclofenac should be avoided in patients with moderate to severe renal impairment.

Interactions

For interactions associated with NSAIDs, see p.65.

Pharmacokinetics

Aceclofenac is well absorbed from the gastro-intestinal tract; peak plasma concentrations are reached 1 to 3 hours after an oral dose. Aceclofenac is more than 99% bound to plasma proteins. The plasma-elimination half-life is approximately 4 hours. About two-thirds of a dose is excreted in the urine, mainly as hydroxymetabolites.

Uses and Administration

Aceclofenac, a phenylacetic acid derivative, is an NSAID (see p.65) related to diclofenac (p.32). It is used in the management of osteoarthritis, rheumatoid arthritis, and ankylosing spondylitis.

The usual dose of aceclofenac is 100 mg given twice daily by mouth. The initial dose should be reduced to 100 mg daily in patients with hepatic impairment.

Preparations

Proprietary Preparations (details are given in Part 3)
Belg.: Biofenac; ***Irl.:*** Airtal; ***Spain:*** Airtal; Airtal Difucrem; Falcol; Gerbin; Sanein; ***Swed.:*** Barcan; ***UK:*** Preservex.

Acemetacin (12308-x)

Acemetacin *(BAN, rINN).*

Bay-f-4975; TVX-1322. *O*-[(1-*p*-Chlorobenzoyl-5-methoxy-2-methylindol-3-yl)acetyl]glycolic acid.

$C_{21}H_{18}ClNO_6$ = 415.8.

CAS — 53164-05-9.

Acemetacin, a glycolic acid ester of indomethacin (p.45), is an NSAID (p.63). Its pharmacological activity is due to both acemetacin and its major metabolite indomethacin (p.45). Acemetacin is used in rheumatoid arthritis, osteoarthritis, and low back pain, and for postoperative pain and inflammation. Usual daily doses are 120 to 180 mg by mouth in divided doses. Acemetacin is eliminated by both hepatic and renal routes and pharmacokinetics are not affected by moderate renal or hepatic impairment and appear to be unchanged in the elderly.

References.

1. Jones RW, *et al.* Comparative pharmacokinetics of acemetacin in young subjects and elderly patients. *Br J Clin Pharmacol* 1991; **31:** 543–5.

Preparations

Proprietary Preparations (details are given in Part 3)
Aust.: Rheutrop; ***Belg.:*** Altren†; ***Ger.:*** Peran; Rantudil; ***Ital.:*** Acemix; Solart; ***Spain:*** Espledol; Oldan; ***Switz.:*** Tilur; ***UK:*** Emflex.

Acetanilide (2603-e)

Antifebrin. *N*-Phenylacetamide.

C_8H_9NO = 135.2.

CAS — 103-84-4.

Pharmacopoeias. In *Fr.*

Acetanilide, a para-aminophenol derivative related to paracetamol (p.72), has analgesic and antipyretic properties. It was replaced by safer analgesics.

Preparations

Proprietary Preparations (details are given in Part 3)
Multi-ingredient: ***Fr.:*** Gripponyl†.

Actarit (13756-g)

Actarit *(rINN).*

(*p*-Acetamidophenyl)acetic acid.

$C_{10}H_{11}NO_3$ = 193.2.

CAS — 18699-02-0.

Actarit is reported to be an immunomodulator. It is used in the treatment of rheumatoid arthritis.

References.

1. Nobunaga M. Long term administration study of a new DMARD actarit on rheumatoid arthritis. *Rinsho Iyaku* 1994; **10:** 947–62.

Preparations

Proprietary Preparations (details are given in Part 3)
Jpn: Mover.

Alclofenac (2605-y)

Alclofenac *(BAN, USAN, rINN).*

W-7320. (4-Allyloxy-3-chlorophenyl)acetic acid.

$C_{11}H_{11}ClO_3$ = 226.7.

CAS — 22131-79-9.

Alclofenac, a phenylacetic acid derivative related to diclofenac (p.31), is an NSAID (p.63). It was used in musculoskeletal and joint disorders but following reports of toxicity, especially skin reactions, it was generally withdrawn from the market. It was also used as the aminoethanol derivative.

Preparations

Proprietary Preparations (details are given in Part 3)
Belg.: Mervan†; ***Switz.:*** Mervan†.

Alfentanil Hydrochloride (12339-b)

Alfentanil Hydrochloride *(BANM, USAN, rINNM).*

Alfentanili Hydrochloridum; R-39209. *N*-{1-[2-(4-Ethyl-5-oxo-2-tetrazolin-1-yl)ethyl]-4-(methoxymethyl)-4-piperidyl}propionanilide hydrochloride.

$C_{21}H_{32}N_6O_3,HCl$ = 453.0.

CAS — 71195-58-9 (alfentanil); 69049-06-5 (anhydrous alfentanil hydrochloride); 70879-28-6 (alfentanil hydrochloride, monohydrate).

Pharmacopoeias. In *Eur.* (see p.viii) and *US.*

A white or almost white powder. Alfentanil hydrochloride 109 µg is approximately equivalent to 100 µg of alfentanil.

Freely **soluble** to soluble in water; freely soluble in alcohol, in chloroform, and in methyl alcohol; sparingly soluble in acetone. **Protect** from light.

CAUTION. *Avoid contact with the skin and the inhalation of particles of alfentanil hydrochloride.*

Dependence and Withdrawal

As for Opioid Analgesics, p.67.

Adverse Effects and Treatment

As for Opioid Analgesics in general, p.68, and for Fentanyl, p.38.

Effects on the cardiovascular system. A report of 2 cases of sinus arrest during intubation following administration of alfentanil 30 µg per kg body-weight.[1] For further reference to the cardiovascular effects of alfentanil, see under Anaesthesia in Uses and Administration, below.

1. Maryniak JK, Bishop VA. Sinus arrest after alfentanil. *Br J Anaesth* 1987; **59:** 390–1.

Effects on mental function. Like fentanyl, alfentanil 7.5 or 15 µg per kg body-weight intravenously had no effect on memory in healthy subjects.[1] In another study impairment of memory for new facts did occur 2 hours after operation in patients anaesthetised with alfentanil 7.5 µg per kg, but not in those given fentanyl;[2] methohexitone might have contributed to the impairment.

1. Scamman FL, *et al.* Ventilatory and mental effects of alfentanil and fentanyl. *Acta Anaesthesiol Scand* 1984; **28:** 63–7.
2. Kennedy DJ, Ogg TW. Alfentanil and memory function: a comparison with fentanyl for day case termination of pregnancy. *Anaesthesia* 1985; **40:** 537–40.

Effects on the respiratory system. Alfentanil, like other opioid agonists, causes dose-related respiratory depression; it is significant with doses of more than 1000 µg. Recovery has been reported to be faster after alfentanil than after fentanyl (see p.38),[1,2] possibly reflecting the shorter elimination half-life of alfentanil. Even so, accumulation of alfentanil is possible with large doses over a prolonged period. Profound analgesia is accompanied by marked respiratory depression which may persist or recur postoperatively.

After an initial rapid recovery from anaesthesia, 2 patients suffered sudden respiratory arrest about an hour after the end of alfentanil infusion;[3] both responded to treatment with naloxone. Close monitoring of respiration in the initial postoperative period was recommended and this was reinforced by the manufacturers;[4] factors such as hyperventilation and the use of opioid premedication might enhance or prolong the respiratory depressant effects of alfentanil.

1. Andrews CJH, *et al.* Ventilatory effects during and after continuous infusion of fentanyl or alfentanil. *Br J Anaesth* 1983; **55:** 211S–16S.
2. Scamman FL, *et al.* Ventilatory and mental effects of alfentanil and fentanyl. *Acta Anaesthesiol Scand* 1984; **28:** 63–7.
3. Sebel PS, *et al.* Respiratory depression after alfentanil infusion. *Br Med J* 1984; **289:** 1581–2.
4. Waldron HA, Cookson RF. Respiratory depression after alfentanil infusion. *Br Med J* 1985; **290:** 319.

Precautions

As for Opioid Analgesics in general, p.68.

Elderly. Scott and Stanski[1] found that elderly patients had increased brain sensitivity to alfentanil as demonstrated by

EEG changes and lower doses might be indicated in older patients for pharmacodynamic rather than pharmacokinetic reasons. See also under Pharmacokinetics, below.

1. Scott JC, Stanski DR. Decreased fentanyl and alfentanil dose requirements with age: a simultaneous pharmacokinetic and pharmacodynamic evaluation. *J Pharmacol Exp Ther* 1987; **240:** 159–66.

Inflammatory bowel disease. Patients with Crohn's disease required higher doses of alfentanil than control patients[1] although there were no differences in alfentanil pharmacokinetics between the 2 groups of patients.

1. Gesink-van der Veer BJ, *et al.* Influence of Crohn's disease on the pharmacokinetics and pharmacodynamics of alfentanil. *Br J Anaesth* 1993; **71:** 827–34.

Neonates. Alfentanil given to preterm infants undergoing paralysis and mechanical ventilation for respiratory distress syndrome resulted in a rapid and significant fall in heart rate and blood pressure emphasising that proper evaluation of the pharmacological and clinical effects was necessary.[1]

1. Marlow N, *et al.* Hazards of analgesia for newborn infants. *Arch Dis Child* 1988; **63:** 1293.

Pregnancy. The manufacturers contra-indicate the use of alfentanil in labour or before clamping of the cord during caesarean section because of its placental transfer and risk of neonatal respiratory depression.

Interactions

For interactions associated with opioid analgesics, see p.69.

Drugs that depress the heart or increase vagal tone, such as beta blockers and anaesthetic drugs, may predispose patients given alfentanil to develop bradycardia and hypotension. Concomitant administration of alfentanil and non-vagolytic muscle relaxants may produce bradycardia and possibly asystole.

The metabolism of alfentanil is inhibited by ketoconazole resulting in a risk of prolonged or delayed respiratory depression. A similar effect has been reported with fluconazole.

Antibacterials. The elimination half-life of alfentanil was increased and clearance decreased when given after a 7-day course of *erythromycin* by mouth in healthy subjects.[1] Other hepatic enzyme inhibitors and drugs interfering with hepatic blood flow might also affect the clearance of alfentanil.

1. Bartkowski RR, *et al.* Inhibition of alfentanil metabolism by erythromycin. *Clin Pharmacol Ther* 1989; **46:** 99–102.

Antifungals. Administration of alfentanil one hour after intravenous or oral *fluconazole* decreased the clearance of alfentanil by 60 and 55% respectively and increased the mean half-life of alfentanil from 1.5 hours to 2.7 and 2.5 hours respectively.[1]

1. Palkama VJ, *et al.* The effect of intravenous and oral fluconazole on the pharmacokinetics and pharmacodynamics of intravenous alfentanil. *Anesth Analg* 1998; **87:** 190–4.

Pharmacokinetics

After parenteral administration alfentanil hydrochloride has a rapid onset and short duration of action. Alfentanil is highly protein bound (about 90%) and has a small volume of distribution. Its terminal elimination half-life is about 1 to 2 hours. It is metabolised in the liver by oxidative *N*- and *O*-dealkylation to inactive metabolites which are excreted in the urine. Alfentanil can cross the blood-brain barrier. It also crosses the placenta and has been detected in colostrum.

Alfentanil is less lipid-soluble than fentanyl, but more so than morphine. It is highly bound to plasma protein, principally to α_1-acid glycoprotein. Decreased lipid solubility can be expected to limit penetration of the blood-brain barrier when compared with fentanyl, but the majority of unbound alfentanil is unionised and can rapidly gain access to the CNS. It has a smaller volume of distribution than fentanyl. The elimination half-life of alfentanil is shorter than that of fentanyl. The manufacturers have given values for a three-compartment pharmacokinetic model with a distribution half-life of 0.4 to 3.1 minutes, a redistribution half-life of 4.6 to 21.6 minutes, and a terminal elimination half-life of 64.1 to 129.3 minutes following single bolus injections of 50 or 125 μg per kg body-weight. Accumulation is less likely than with fentanyl, but can occur following repeated or continuous administration especially in patients with reduced clearance. The mean elimination half-life reported is usually about 90 minutes, but this is reduced in children and increased in the elderly, in hepatic impairment, in the obese, and during cardiopulmonary bypass (see below).

Reviews of the pharmacokinetics of alfentanil.

1. Hull CJ. The pharmacokinetics of alfentanil in man. *Br J Anaesth* 1983; **55:** 157S–64S.
2. Mather LE. Clinical pharmacokinetics of fentanyl and its newer derivatives. *Clin Pharmacokinet* 1983; **8:** 422–46.
3. Davis PJ, Cook DR. Clinical pharmacokinetics of the newer intravenous anaesthetic agents. *Clin Pharmacokinet* 1986; **11:** 18–35.
4. Bodenham A, Park GR. Alfentanil infusions in patients requiring intensive care. *Clin Pharmacokinet* 1988; **15:** 216–26.
5. Scholz J, *et al.* Clinical pharmacokinetics of alfentanil, fentanyl and sufentanil. *Clin Pharmacokinet* 1996; **31:** 275–92.

Administration. CONTINUOUS INTRAVENOUS INFUSION. The limited number of detailed studies of alfentanil by continuous intravenous infusion[1-3] have found pharmacokinetic parameters to be similar to those after a single bolus injection, but with some conflicting results; they have generally involved only small numbers of patients.

Van Beem *et al.*[4] used a dosage regimen recommended for surgery under general anaesthesia in 29 patients undergoing orthopaedic surgery. After an initial bolus intravenous injection of alfentanil 50 μg per kg body-weight, an intravenous infusion of 1 μg per kg per minute was started immediately and continued for 44 to 445 minutes; a second bolus injection of 50 μg per kg was given immediately before incision and an additional bolus injection of 1 mg given if necessary. The time course of the plasma-alfentanil concentration fitted a two-compartmental model in 26 patients. Terminal half-lives varied widely from 56 to 226 minutes (mean 106 minutes), the highest values being mainly in patients over 60 years. There was no significant correlation between pharmacokinetic parameters and the duration of the infusion or the total dose. Plasma clearance and volumes of distribution did not correlate significantly with body-weight although steady-state volume of distribution was enlarged with increasing age. The mean estimated steady-state concentration was 293 ng per mL (range 147 to 636 ng per mL).

1. Fragen RJ, *et al.* Pharmacokinetics of the infusion of alfentanil in man. *Br J Anaesth* 1983; **55:** 1077–81.
2. Shafer A, *et al.* Pharmacokinetics and pharmacodynamics of alfentanil infusions during general anesthesia. *Anesth Analg* 1986; **65:** 1021–8.
3. Reitz JA, *et al.* The pharmacokinetics of alfentanil in gynecologic surgical patients. *J Clin Pharmacol* 1986; **26:** 60–4.
4. van Beem H, *et al.* Pharmacokinetics of alfentanil during and after a fixed rate infusion. *Br J Anaesth* 1989; **62:** 610–15.

INTRAMUSCULAR. See under Administration in the Elderly, below.

Administration in patients with burns. The volume of distribution and total clearance of alfentanil were reduced and its elimination half-life prolonged in patients with burns.[1] This was due, in part, to raised concentrations of α_1-acid glycoprotein leading to increased protein binding.

1. Macfie AG, *et al.* Disposition of alfentanil in burns patients. *Br J Anaesth* 1992; **69:** 447–50.

Administration during cardiopulmonary bypass. The elimination half-life of alfentanil increased from 72 minutes before bypass to 195 minutes afterwards in 5 patients undergoing cardiopulmonary bypass.[1] This was attributed to an increase in volume of distribution, based in part on a dilution-induced decrease in plasma protein binding. Others[2,3] found that on starting cardiopulmonary bypass total serum concentrations of alfentanil were halved, mainly because of dilution of α_1-acid glycoprotein and an increase in unbound alfentanil.

1. Hug CC, *et al.* Alfentanil pharmacokinetics in patients before and after cardiopulmonary bypass. *Anesth Analg* 1983; **62:** 266.
2. Kumar K, *et al.* The effect of cardiopulmonary bypass on plasma protein binding of alfentanil. *Eur J Clin Pharmacol* 1988; **35:** 47–52.
3. Hynynen M, *et al.* Plasma concentration and protein binding of alfentanil during high-dose infusion for cardiac surgery. *Br J Anaesth* 1994; **72:** 571–6.

Administration in children. Alfentanil has been shown to have a shorter elimination half-life (about 40 minutes) and a smaller volume of distribution in children than in adults.[1] See also under Administration in Hepatic Impairment, below.

1. Meistelman C, *et al.* A comparison of alfentanil pharmacokinetics in children and adults. *Anesthesiology* 1987; **66:** 13–16.

Administration in the elderly. Plasma clearance of alfentanil following 50 μg per kg body-weight as a single intravenous dose was reduced in elderly patients aged more than 65 years when compared with that in healthy young adults.[1] Mean elimination half-life was 137 minutes in the elderly and 83 minutes in the young adults. Volumes of distribution were similar and Helmers *et al.*[1] considered that reduced clearance might be due to decreased hepatic metabolism in the elderly. In a study in male patients Scott and Stanski[2] found the terminal elimination half-life of alfentanil to increase with age, although clearance was not significantly affected. In patients given alfentanil 1 μg per kg per minute by continuous intravenous infusion during orthopaedic surgery,[3] terminal half-life increased linearly with age in those older than 40 years and steady-state volume of distribution was enlarged with increasing age; clearance did not correlate significantly with age and was thought to be more variable during a continuous infusion in long-term surgery than after a single bolus injection. Lemmens *et al.*[4] reported that the effects of age on alfentanil pharmacokinetics were dependent on gender. In their study total plasma clearance decreased and terminal half-life increased with increasing age in women, but not in men. It has been suggested that this effect in women may be more dependent on menopausal status than on age.[5]

In a study[6] in elderly patients plasma concentrations of alfentanil were greater and the maximum concentration occurred earlier when alfentanil was injected into the deltoid muscle compared with injection into the gluteal muscle.

1. Helmers H, *et al.* Alfentanil kinetics in the elderly. *Clin Pharmacol Ther* 1984; **36:** 239–43.
2. Scott JC, Stanski DR. Decreased fentanyl and alfentanil dose requirements with age: a simultaneous pharmacokinetic and pharmacodynamic evaluation. *J Pharmacol Exp Ther* 1987; **240:** 159–66.
3. van Beem H, *et al.* Pharmacokinetics of alfentanil during and after a fixed rate infusion. *Br J Anaesth* 1989; **62:** 610–15.
4. Lemmens HJM, *et al.* Influence of age on the pharmacokinetics of alfentanil: gender dependence. *Clin Pharmacokinet* 1990; **19:** 416–22.
5. Rubio A, Cox C. Sex, age and alfentanil pharmacokinetics. *Clin Pharmacokinet* 1991; **21:** 81.
6. Virkkilä M, *et al.* Pharmacokinetics and effects of im alfentanil as premedication for day-case ophthalmic surgery in elderly patients. *Br J Anaesth* 1993; **71:** 507–11.

Administration in hepatic impairment. Total plasma clearance and protein binding of alfentanil were decreased in patients with alcoholic cirrhosis when compared with control subjects. Elimination half-life was prolonged from 90 to 219 minutes in the cirrhotic patients following a single intravenous dose of 50 μg per kg body-weight and was attributed in part to alterations in binding sites of α_1-acid glycoprotein.[1] There might be different effects on alfentanil disposition in patients with non-alcoholic cirrhosis or other liver disorders.[2] The pharmacokinetics of alfentanil were apparently not affected in children with cholestatic hepatic disease whereas clearance was reduced postoperatively in 3 patients who had undergone liver transplantation.[3]

1. Ferrier C, *et al.* Alfentanil pharmacokinetics in patients with cirrhosis. *Anesthesiology* 1985; **62:** 480–4.
2. Bower S, *et al.* Effects of different hepatic pathologies on disposition of alfentanil in anaesthetized patients. *Br J Anaesth* 1992; **68:** 462–5.
3. Davis PJ, *et al.* Effects of cholestatic hepatic disease and chronic renal failure on alfentanil pharmacokinetics in children. *Anesth Analg* 1989; **68:** 579–83.

Administration in obesity. Bentley *et al.*[1] reported the pharmacokinetics of alfentanil to be altered in obesity. Elimination half-life was 172 minutes in 6 obese patients compared with 92 minutes in 7 who were not obese. Plasma clearance of alfentanil was also decreased, although Maitre *et al.*[2] found that obesity had no effect on clearance, but it did have a direct relationship with the volume of the central compartment.

1. Bentley JB, *et al.* Obesity and alfentanil pharmacokinetics. *Anesth Analg* 1983; **62:** 251.
2. Maitre PO, *et al.* Population pharmacokinetics of alfentanil: the average dose-plasma concentration relationship and interindividual variability in patients. *Anesthesiology* 1987; **66:** 3–12.

Administration in renal impairment. The pharmacokinetics of alfentanil were not affected significantly in adults[1] or children[2] with chronic renal failure. In another study[3] increased volume of distribution of alfentanil at steady-state was associated with decreased plasma protein binding in patients with chronic renal failure.

1. Van Peer A, *et al.* Alfentanil kinetics in renal insufficiency. *Eur J Clin Pharmacol* 1986; **30:** 245–7.
2. Davis PJ, *et al.* Effects of cholestatic hepatic disease and chronic renal failure on alfentanil pharmacokinetics in children. *Anesth Analg* 1989; **68:** 579–83.
3. Chauvin M, *et al.* Pharmacokinetics of alfentanil in chronic renal failure. *Anesth Analg* 1987; **66:** 53–6.

Uses and Administration

Alfentanil is a short-acting opioid (p.69) related to fentanyl (p.39).

Alfentanil is used in surgical procedures as an analgesic and adjunct to general anaesthetics or as a primary anaesthetic. It is also used as an analgesic and respiratory depressant in the management of mechanically ventilated patients under intensive care.

Alfentanil is administered intravenously as the hydrochloride. Doses are expressed in terms of alfentanil base. A peak effect may be seen within 1.5 to 2 minutes of an injection and analgesia can be expected to last for up to 10 minutes; dose supplements are therefore required if it is to be used for more prolonged surgical procedures. It may be given by continuous intravenous infusion in ventilated patients.

The dosage of alfentanil employed depends on whether the patient has spontaneous respiration or assisted ventilation and on the expected duration of anaesthesia. When used as an adjunct in the *maintenance of general anaesthesia* the recommended initial dose in the UK in adults with spontaneous respiration is up to 500 μg given slowly over about 30 seconds; supplementary doses of 250 μg may be given. Ventilated adults and children may be given 30 to 50 μg per kg body-weight with supplements of 15 μg per kg. When given by infusion to ventilated adults and children there is an initial loading dose of 50 to 100 μg per kg given as a bolus or by infusion over 10 minutes, and this is followed by infusion at a rate of 0.5 to 1.0 μg per kg per minute. Typical doses that have been used in the USA are as follows: for procedures lasting less than 30 minutes in adults with spontaneous respiration or assisted ventilation is 8 to 20 μg per kg body-weight followed by supplementary doses of 3 to 5 μg per kg every 5 to 20 minutes or an infusion of 0.5 to 1.0 μg per kg per minute. When the expected duration of anaesthesia is longer than 30 minutes, the initial dose for adults with assisted ventilation is 20 to 75 μg per kg followed by supplementary doses of 5 to 15 μg per kg or an infusion of 0.5 to 3.0 μg per kg per minute. If alfentanil has been given in anaesthetic doses (see below) for the induction of anaesthesia infusion rates may need to be reduced by 30 to 50% during the first hour of maintenance. Maintenance infusions of alfentanil should be discontinued 10 to 30 minutes before the anticipated end of surgery.

The dose for the *induction of anaesthesia* in patients with assisted ventilation undergoing procedures of at least 45 minutes is 130 to 245 μg per kg followed by an inhalation anaesthetic or maintenance doses of alfentanil of 0.5 to 1.5 μg per kg per minute.

In intensive care ventilated adults may be given alfentanil initially at an infusion rate of 2 mg per hour or a loading dose of 5 mg may be given in divided doses over 10 minutes or more slowly if hypotension or bradycardia occur. Thereafter a suitable rate of infusion should be determined for each patient (rates of 0.5 to 10 mg per hour have been used); patients should be carefully monitored and the duration of treatment should not generally exceed 4 days. During continuous infusion additional bolus injections of 0.5 to 1.0 mg may be given if required to provide analgesia for short painful procedures that may be carried out in intensive care.

Doses are adjusted according to the needs of the patient. Children may require higher or more frequent doses than adults, whereas the elderly or debilitated patients may require lower or less frequent doses.

Reviews.

1. Larijani GE, Goldberg ME. Alfentanil hydrochloride: a new short-acting narcotic analgesic for surgical procedures. *Clin Pharm* 1987; **6:** 275–82.
2. Clotz MA, Nahata MC. Clinical uses of fentanyl, sufentanil, and alfentanil. *Clin Pharm* 1991; **10:** 581–93.

Administration. Alfentanil is usually administered by intravenous injection or infusion, but has also been given intramuscularly[1,2] or epidurally (see under Labour Pain and under Postoperative Pain, below).

1. Arendt-Nielsen L, *et al.* Analgesic efficacy of im alfentanil. *Br J Anaesth* 1990; **65:** 164–8.
2. Virkkilä M, *et al.* Pharmacokinetics and effects of im alfentanil as premedication for day-case ophthalmic surgery in elderly patients. *Br J Anaesth* 1993; **71:** 507–11.

Anaesthesia. Alfentanil, like fentanyl (p.40), appears to produce fewer circulatory changes than morphine and may be preferred for anaesthetic use, especially in cardiovascular surgery.

De Lange *et al.*[1] noted that continuous infusions of alfentanil produced greater cardiovascular stability than frequent intravenous bolus injections in coronary artery bypass patients. Nauta *et al.*[2] showed that anaesthetic induction with alfentanil by rapid infusion resulted in little change in cardiovascular dynamics and a speedy recovery. In a study of haemodynamic responses to anaesthesia and surgery, induction with alfentanil 125 μg per kg body-weight, fentanyl 75 μg per kg, or sufentanil 15 μg per kg all provided satisfactory anaesthesia in patients undergoing heart valve replacement.[3] Alfentanil is generally considered to have a shorter duration of action than fentanyl and has been associated with a more rapid recovery from anaesthesia by some workers,[4] but not by others.[5-7] Psychomotor function has taken several hours to return to normal after alfentanil anaesthesia despite rapid immediate recovery.[8] Similar cardiovascular stability[9] and attenuation of the hormonal response to stress[10] have been achieved with alfentanil and fentanyl, but the effects of alfentanil were of shorter duration. Crawford *et al.*[11] found that alfentanil 10 μg per kg or 40 μg per kg prevented any increase in heart rate or blood pressure after tracheal intubation and was associated with decreased plasma-noradrenaline concentrations. Profound hypotension and bradycardia occurred with the higher dose. Others[12] gave alfentanil 75 μg per kg immediately before induction of anaesthesia without causing clinically significant hypotension or bradycardia although cardiovascular and catecholamine responses to tracheal intubation were totally obtunded; this was possibly because of the concomitant use of suxamethonium and an antimuscarinic. However, 4 of the 10 patients given alfentanil 75 μg per kg[12] developed chest wall rigidity and a smaller dose such as 30 μg per kg might be preferable. Alfentanil has been used successfully in conjunction with propofol to facilitate intubation without using a neuromuscular blocking drug in adults[13,14] and in children;[15,16] doses used in adults for nasotracheal intubation have been alfentanil 10 or 20 μg per kg and propofol 2.5 mg per kg.[13,14]

For *ophthalmic anaesthesia* alfentanil 10 μg per kg was considered by some to be a reasonable alternative to fentanyl 2.5 μg per kg;[17] both blood pressure and heart rate fell by the same extent with either drug whereas the fall in intra-ocular pressure was significantly greater and quicker with alfentanil. Others[18] reported either drug to satisfactorily reduce intra-ocular pressure and the haemodynamic responses associated with intubation prior to ophthalmic surgery.

For a discussion of the drugs used to facilitate intubation and of opioids such as alfentanil used to control the pressor response and the rise of intra-ocular pressure associated with intubation, see under Anaesthesia, p.1302.

Total intravenous anaesthesia using alfentanil together with propofol has been successful in adults[7,19-21] and children.[22]

For reference to a study indicating that pretreatment with alfentanil can reduce the pain associated with injection of the anaesthetic drug propofol, see p.1230.

1. De Lange S, *et al.* Alfentanil-oxygen anesthesia: comparison of continuous infusion and frequent bolus techniques for coronary artery surgery. *Anesthesiology* 1981; **55:** A42.
2. Nauta J, *et al.* Anesthetic induction with alfentanil: a new short-acting narcotic analgesic. *Anesth Analg* 1982; **61:** 267–72.
3. Bovill JG, *et al.* Comparison of fentanyl, sufentanil, and alfentanil anesthesia in patients undergoing valvular heart surgery. *Anesth Analg* 1984; **63:** 1081–6.
4. Kay B, Venkataraman P. Recovery after fentanyl and alfentanil in anaesthesia for minor surgery. *Br J Anaesth* 1983; **55:** 169S–71S.
5. Cooper GM, *et al.* Effect of alfentanil and fentanyl on recovery from brief anaesthesia. *Br J Anaesth* 1983; **55:** 179S–82S
6. Brown EM, *et al.* Fentanyl/alfentanil for pelvic laparoscopy. *Can Anaesth Soc J* 1984; **31:** 251–4.
7. Jenstrup M, *et al.* Total iv anaesthesia with propofol-alfentanil or propofol-fentanyl. *Br J Anaesth* 1990; **64:** 717–22.
8. Moss E, *et al.* Comparison of recovery after halothane or alfentanil anaesthesia for minor surgery. *Br J Anaesth* 1987; **59:** 970–7.
9. Rucquoi M, Camu F. Cardiovascular responses to large doses of alfentanil and fentanyl. *Br J Anaesth* 1983; **55:** 223S–30S.
10. Hynynen M, *et al.* Continuous infusion of fentanyl or alfentanil for coronary artery surgery: effects on plasma cortisol concentration, β-endorphin immunoreactivity and arginine vasopressin. *Br J Anaesth* 1986; **58:** 1260–6.
11. Crawford DC, *et al.* Effects of alfentanil on the pressor and catecholamine responses to tracheal intubation. *Br J Anaesth* 1987; **59:** 707–12.
12. Scheinin B, *et al.* Alfentanil obtunds the cardiovascular and sympathoadrenal responses to suxamethonium-facilitated laryngoscopy and intubation. *Br J Anaesth* 1989; **62:** 385–92.
13. Alcock R, *et al.* Comparison of alfentanil with suxamethonium in facilitating nasotracheal intubation in day-case anaesthesia. *Br J Anaesth* 1993; **70:** 34–7.
14. Coghlan SFE. *et al.* Use of alfentanil with propofol for nasotracheal intubation without neuromuscular block. *Br J Anaesth* 1993; **70:** 89–91.
15. Steyn MP, *et al.* Tracheal intubation without neuromuscular block in children. *Br J Anaesth* 1994; **72:** 403–6.
16. McConaghy P, Bunting HE. Assessment of intubating conditions in children after induction with propofol and varying doses of alfentanil. *Br J Anaesth* 1994; **73:** 596–9.
17. Mostafa SM, *et al.* Comparison of effects of fentanyl and alfentanil on intra-ocular pressure. *Anaesthesia* 1986; **41:** 493–8.
18. Sweeney J, *et al.* Modification by fentanyl and alfentanil of the intraocular pressure response to suxamethonium and tracheal intubation. *Br J Anaesth* 1989; **63:** 688–91.
19. Reyneke CJ, *et al.* Alfentanil and propofol infusions for surgery in the burned patient. *Br J Anaesth* 1989; **63:** 418–22.
20. Taylor IN, *et al.* Pharmacodynamic stability of a mixture of propofol and alfentanil. *Br J Anaesth* 1992; **69:** 168–71.
21. Sandin R. Propofol and alfentanil mixture. *Br J Anaesth* 1993; **70:** 382–3.
22. Browne BL, *et al.* Propofol and alfentanil in children: infusion technique and dose requirement for total iv anaesthesia. *Br J Anaesth* 1992; **69:** 570–6.

CAESAREAN SECTION. The manufacturers contra-indicate the use of alfentanil before clamping the cord during caesarean section because of the risk of respiratory depression in the neonate. Study of alfentanil 30 μg per kg body-weight in women undergoing caesarean section was abandoned by Leuwer *et al.*[1] after massive respiratory depression had occurred in 4 of 5 neonates. However, alfentanil has been used successfully to minimise haemodynamic responses to intubation and surgery in patients with severe cardiovascular disorders undergoing caesarean section.[2,3] A baby delivered following the successful use of alfentanil 35 μg per kg in a mother with severe aortic stenosis[2] was apnoeic and unresponsive with poor muscle tone; it responded rapidly to naloxone. Alfentanil 10 μg per kg immediately before induction attenuated the cardiovascular response to intubation in patients with severe pregnancy-induced hypertension[3] and was considered a suitable alternative to fentanyl 2.5 μg per kg; no effect on neonatal mortality could be attributed to anaesthetic technique. However, it has been suggested that the use of smaller doses of alfentanil of 7.5 μg per kg with magnesium sulphate 30 mg per kg may provide better cardiovascular control.[4]

1. Leuwer M, *et al.* Pharmacokinetics and pharmacodynamics of an equipotent fentanyl and alfentanil dose in mother and infant during caesarean section. *Br J Anaesth* 1990; **64:** 398P–9P.
2. Redfern N, *et al.* Alfentanil for caesarean section complicated by severe aortic stenosis: a case report. *Br J Anaesth* 1987; **59:** 1309–12.
3. Rout CC, Rocke DA. Effects of alfentanil and fentanyl on induction of anaesthesia in patients with severe pregnancy-induced hypertension. *Br J Anaesth* 1990; **65:** 468–74.
4. Ashton WB, *et al.* Attenuation of the pressor response to tracheal intubation by magnesium sulphate with and without alfentanil in hypertensive proteinuric patients undergoing caesarean section. *Br J Anaesth* 1991; **67:** 741–7.

PHAEOCHROMOCYTOMA. Alfentanil does not release histamine and may be the opioid of choice in the anaesthetic management of patients with phaeochromocytoma.[1] It has a very rapid onset of action, good vasodilating properties, and a relatively short elimination half-life. These patients are often very somnolent for the first 48 hours after surgery and postoperative opioid dosage requirements may be less than expected. Alfentanil infusion continued into the postoperative period allows careful titration of dosage.

1. Hull CJ. Phaeochromocytoma: diagnosis, preoperative preparation and anaesthetic management. *Br J Anaesth* 1986; **58:** 1453–68.

Pain. LABOUR PAIN. The manufacturers contra-indicate the use of alfentanil in labour because of its placental transfer and the risk of neonatal respiratory depression.

Administration of alfentanil 30 μg per kg body-weight per hour by continuous epidural infusion, with supplementary epidural bolus doses of 30 μg per kg as necessary, provided unsatisfactory pain relief during labour and there was evidence of neonatal hypotonia.[1]

1. Heytens L, *et al.* Extradural analgesia during labour using alfentanil. *Br J Anaesth* 1987; **59:** 331–7.

POSTOPERATIVE PAIN. Epidural alfentanil may be a better choice than epidural fentanyl in the relief of postoperative pain.[1]

Chrubasik *et al.*[2] found that continuous on-demand epidural infusions of alfentanil 200 μg per hour or fentanyl 20 μg per hour provided comparable analgesia to morphine 200 μg per hour in the early postoperative period; alfentanil (16 minutes) and fentanyl (13 minutes) had the advantage of more rapid onset of analgesia than morphine (44 minutes). However, some considered that there was no overall advantage of epidural over intravenous administration in patients receiving alfentanil either as patient-controlled analgesia[3] or as a continuous infusion.[4]

1. Morgan M. The rational use of intrathecal and extradural opioids. *Br J Anaesth* 1989; **63:** 165–88.
2. Chrubasik J, *et al.* Relative analgesic potency of epidural fentanyl, alfentanil, and morphine in treatment of postoperative pain. *Anesthesiology* 1988; **68:** 929–33.
3. Chauvin M, *et al.* Equivalence of postoperative analgesia with patient-controlled intravenous or epidural alfentanil. *Anesth Analg* 1993; **76:** 1251–8.
4. van den Nieuwenhuyzen MCO, *et al.* Epidural vs intravenous infusion of alfentanil in the management of postoperative pain following laparotomies. *Acta Anaesthesiol Scand* 1996; **40:** 1112–18.

Preparations

USP 23: Alfentanil Injection.

Proprietary Preparations (details are given in Part 3)

Aust.: Rapifen; ***Austral.:*** Rapifen; ***Belg.:*** Rapifen; ***Canad.:*** Alfenta; ***Fr.:*** Rapifen; ***Ger.:*** Rapifen; ***Irl.:*** Rapifen; ***Ital.:*** Fentalim; ***Neth.:*** Rapifen; ***Norw.:*** Rapifen; ***S.Afr.:*** Rapifen; ***Spain:*** Fanaxal; Limifen; ***Swed.:*** Rapifen; ***Switz.:*** Rapifen; ***UK:*** Rapifen; ***USA:*** Alfenta.

Alminoprofen (16021-j)

Alminoprofen *(rINN)*.

4-[(2-Methylallyl)amino]hydratropic acid.

$C_{13}H_{17}NO_2$ = 219.3.

CAS — 39718-89-3.

Alminoprofen, a propionic acid derivative related to ibuprofen (p.44), is an NSAID (p.63). It has been used in inflammatory and rheumatic disorders in doses of up to 900 mg daily by mouth.

Preparations

Proprietary Preparations (details are given in Part 3)
Fr.: Minalfene.

Aloxiprin (2607-z)

Aloxiprin *(BAN, rINN)*.

CAS — 9014-67-9.

Pharmacopoeias. In *Br.*

A polymeric condensation product of aluminium oxide and aspirin. A fine white or slightly pink, odourless or almost odourless, powder. It contains 7.5 to 8.5% of aluminium and 79.0 to 87.4% of total salicylates. Aloxiprin 600 mg is approximately equivalent to 500 mg of aspirin. Practically **insoluble** in water, in alcohol, and in ether; slightly soluble in chloroform.

Adverse Effects, Treatment, and Precautions

As for Aspirin, p.16.

Aloxiprin, like aspirin, should not generally be given to children under the age of 12 years because of the risk of Reye's syndrome.

Interactions

For interactions associated with salicylates, see Aspirin, p.17.

Pharmacokinetics

Aloxiprin is hydrolysed in the gastro-intestinal tract to salicylate, the rate of breakdown being low in the acid conditions of the stomach and greater at the higher pH values of the intestine.

Uses and Administration

Aloxiprin, a polymeric condensation product of aluminium oxide and aspirin, has actions similar to those of aspirin (p.18) and has been used as an analgesic and anti-inflammatory in musculoskeletal and joint disorders. A usual dose was 600 mg to 1.2 g three times daily by mouth. Aloxiprin should be taken 30 minutes before food.

Aloxiprin has also been used in the treatment and prevention of thrombo-embolic disorders.

Preparations

BP 1998: Aloxiprin Tablets.

Proprietary Preparations (details are given in Part 3)
Aust.: Palaprin; ***Irl.:*** Palaprin†; ***Switz.:*** Lyman†; Rumatral†; Thrombace; Tiatral†.

Multi-ingredient: ***Austral.:*** Migran-eze†; Perpain†; Rheumat-Eze†; ***UK:*** Askit.

Alphaprodine Hydrochloride (6203-b)

Alphaprodine Hydrochloride *(BANM, rINNM)*.

Nu-1196. (±)-1,3-Dimethyl-4-phenyl-4-piperidyl propionate hydrochloride.

$C_{16}H_{23}NO_2,HCl$ = 297.8.

CAS — 77-20-3 (alphaprodine); 14405-05-1 (alphaprodine hydrochloride); 561-78-4 (alphaprodine hydrochloride, ±).

Alphaprodine hydrochloride is an opioid analgesic (p.67) chemically related to and with an action resembling that of pethidine (p.76), but more rapid in onset and of shorter duration. It was formerly used in obstetrics, as pre-operative medication, for minor surgical procedures, and for dental procedures.

References.

1. Fuller HD. Cyanosis of the hands following the use of alphaprodine in dental anaesthesia. *Can Anaesth Soc J* 1986; **33:** 213–15.

Aluminium Aspirin (2608-c)

Aluminum Acetylsalicylate; Aluminum Aspirin; Aspirin Aluminium. Bis(2-acetoxybenzoato-*O'*)hydroxyaluminium.

$C_{18}H_{15}AlO_9$ = 402.3.

CAS — 23413-80-1.

Pharmacopoeias. In *Jpn.*

Aluminium aspirin is a salicylic acid derivative (see Aspirin, p.16) that has been given by mouth in the management of fever, pain, and musculoskeletal and joint disorders.

Preparations

Proprietary Preparations (details are given in Part 3)
Ital.: Alupir†.

Multi-ingredient: ***Aust.:*** Kratofin; ***Ger.:*** Deskoval N†; ***S.Afr.:*** Analgen-SA; ***Spain:*** Meridol.

Amfenac Sodium (12354-m)

Amfenac Sodium *(BANM, USAN, rINNM)*.

AHR-5850; AHR-5850D. Sodium (2-amino-3-benzoylphenyl)acetate monohydrate.

$C_{15}H_{12}NNaO_3,H_2O$ = 295.3.

CAS — 51579-82-9 (amfenac); 61618-27-7 (amfenac sodium).

Amfenac sodium, an arylacetic derivative, is an NSAID (p.63) that has been used for the relief of pain and inflammation.

Preparations

Proprietary Preparations (details are given in Part 3)
Jpn: Fenazox†.

Amidopyrine (2609-k)

Aminophenazone *(rINN)*; Amidazofen; Amidopyrine-Pyramidon; Aminopyrine; Dimethylaminoantipyrine; Dimethylaminophenazone. 4-Dimethylamino-1,5-dimethyl-2-phenyl-4-pyrazolin-3-one.

$C_{13}H_{17}N_3O$ = 231.3.

CAS — 58-15-1.

Pharmacopoeias. In *Aust., It.,* and *Port.*

Amidopyrine, a pyrazolone derivative, is an NSAID (p.63), but the risk of agranulocytosis is sufficiently great to render it unsuitable for use. Onset of agranulocytosis may be sudden and unpredictable. Amidopyrine has been used in the form of a variety of salts or complexes including topically as the salicylate.

Precautions. CARCINOGENICITY. Some[1] consider that amidopyrine should be regarded as a potential carcinogen because it reacted readily with nitrous acid to form dimethylnitrosamine. The reaction was catalysed by thiocyanate present in the saliva particularly in smokers.

1. Boyland E, Walker SA. Catalysis of the reaction of aminopyrine and nitrite by thiocyanate. *Arzneimittelforschung* 1974; **24:** 1181–4.

PORPHYRIA. Amidopyrine has been associated with clinical exacerbations of porphyria and is considered unsafe in porphyric patients.[1]

1. Moore MR, McColl KEL. *Porphyria: drug lists.* Glasgow: Porphyria Research Unit, University of Glasgow, 1991.

Preparations

Proprietary Preparations (details are given in Part 3)
Ital.: Farmidone†; Ftalazone†; Fugantil†; Malivan†; Piroreumal†; Rosetin†; Termidon†; Tiomidone†.

Multi-ingredient: ***Belg.:*** Do-Do†; ***Ital.:*** Clormetadone†; Flexipyrin†; Hibersulfan†; Nevrazon†; Novodone†; Reused†; Temoxa†; Tiopirin†; Virdex; ***Switz.:*** Clinit†; Thermocutan.

Aminopropylone (14142-q)

Aminopropylon. *N*-(2,3-Dihydro-1,5-dimethyl-3-oxo-2-phenyl-1*H*-pyrazol-4-yl)-2-(dimethylamino)propanamide.

$C_{16}H_{22}N_4O_2$ = 302.4.

CAS — 3690-04-8.

Aminopropylone is an NSAID (p.63) used in topical preparations, usually in a concentration of 5% with a heparinoid, for the local treatment of pain and inflammatory conditions. The hydrochloride has been used similarly.

Preparations

Proprietary Preparations (details are given in Part 3)

Multi-ingredient: ***Ital.:*** Artrocur; Lisiflen†; Vessiflex.

Ammonium Salicylate (12370-m)

$C_7H_9NO_3$ = 155.2.

CAS — 528-94-9.

Ammonium salicylate is a salicylic acid derivative used topically in rubefacient preparations similarly to methyl salicylate (p.55) for the relief of pain in musculoskeletal and joint disorders.

Preparations

Proprietary Preparations (details are given in Part 3)

Multi-ingredient: ***Austral.:*** Radian-B; ***Irl.:*** Radian-B; ***UK:*** Aspellin; Radian-B.

Ampiroxicam (2484-x)

Ampiroxicam *(BAN, rINN)*.

CP-65703. 4-[1-(Ethoxycarbonyloxy)ethoxy]-2-methyl-N^2-pyridyl-2*H*-1,2-benzothiazine-3-carboxamide 1,1-dioxide.

$C_{20}H_{21}N_3O_7S$ = 447.5.

CAS — 99464-64-9.

Ampiroxicam is an NSAID (p.63) that is reported to be metabolised to piroxicam (p.80).

Amtolmetin Guacil (15445-q)

Amtolmetin Guacil *(rINN)*.

MED-15; ST-679. *N*-[(1-Methyl-5-*p*-toluoylpyrrol-2-yl)acetyl]glycine *o*-methoxyphenyl.

$C_{24}H_{24}N_2O_5$ = 420.5.

CAS — 87344-06-7.

Amtolmetin guacil is an NSAID (p.63). It is an ester prodrug of tolmetin (p.89) used in painful and inflammatory disorders. It is given by mouth in daily doses of 600 to 1200 mg.

Preparations

Proprietary Preparations (details are given in Part 3)
Ital.: Artromed; Eufans.

Amyl Salicylate (16508-j)

Isoamyl Salicylate; Isopentyl Salicylate. 3-Methylbutyl 2-hydroxybenzoate.

$C_{12}H_{16}O_3$ = 208.3.

CAS — 87-20-7.

Pharmacopoeias. In *Fr.*

Amyl salicylate is a salicylic acid derivative used topically in rubefacient preparations similarly to methyl salicylate (p.55) for its analgesic and anti-inflammatory actions. It has also been used in perfumery.

Preparations

Proprietary Preparations (details are given in Part 3)

Multi-ingredient: ***Belg.:*** Revocyl†; ***Fr.:*** Baume Aroma; Baume Dalet; Baume Saint-Bernard; Sedartryl; ***Spain:*** Balsamo Analgesic Karmel; Linimento Klari.

Anileridine (6204-v)

Anileridine *(BAN, rINN)*.

Ethyl 1-(4-aminophenethyl)-4-phenylpiperidine-4-carboxylate.

$C_{22}H_{28}N_2O_2$ = 352.5.

CAS — 144-14-9.

Pharmacopoeias. In *US.*

A white to yellowish-white, odourless or almost odourless, crystalline powder. When exposed to light and air it oxidises and darkens in colour. There are 2 crystalline forms, melting at about 80° and about 89° respectively.

Very slightly **soluble** in water; soluble 1 in 2 of alcohol and 1 in 1 of chloroform; soluble in ether but solutions may be turbid. **Store** in airtight containers. Protect from light.

Anileridine Hydrochloride (6205-g)

Anileridine Hydrochloride *(BANM, rINNM)*.

$C_{22}H_{28}N_2O_2,2HCl$ = 425.4.

CAS — 126-12-5.

Pharmacopoeias. In *US.*

A white or almost white odourless crystalline powder. Anileridine hydrochloride 30 mg is approximately equivalent to 25 mg of anileridine. **Soluble** 1 in 5 of water and 1 in 80 of alcohol; practically insoluble in chloroform and in ether. A 5% solution in water has a pH of 2.5 to 3.0. **Store** in airtight containers. Protect from light.

Anileridine Phosphate (6206-q)

Anileridine Phosphate *(BANM, rINNM)*.

$C_{22}H_{28}N_2O_2,H_3PO_4$ = 450.5.

CAS — 4268-37-5.

Anileridine phosphate 32 mg is approximately equivalent to 25 mg of anileridine.

Anileridine, a phenylpiperidine derivative, is an opioid analgesic (p.67) chemically related to and with actions resembling those of pethidine (p.76). It is used in the management of moderate to severe pain, including labour pain, and as an adjunct to anaesthesia. Anileridine is used as the hydrochloride and phosphate with doses expressed as anileridine base.

The usual dose of anileridine by mouth is 25 to 50 mg every 6 hours given as the hydrochloride.

The usual subcutaneous or intramuscular dose of anileridine for pain is 25 to 50 mg every 4 to 6 hours given as the phosphate, although for severe pain single doses of 75 to 100 mg may be given. The total daily dosage should not exceed 200 mg.

As an adjunct to anaesthesia, 50 to 100 mg of anileridine (as the phosphate) is added to 500 mL of glucose injection (5%) and the equivalent of 5 to 10 mg of anileridine is given by slow intravenous injection followed by slow intravenous infusion of the solution at the rate of about 600 μg of anileridine per minute.

Preparations

USP 23: Anileridine Hydrochloride Tablets; Anileridine Injection.

Proprietary Preparations (details are given in Part 3)
Canad.: Leritine.

Aspirin (2601-s)

Aspirin *(BAN).*

Acetylsal. Acid; Acetylsalicylic Acid; Acidum Acetylsalicylicum; Polopiryna; Salicylic Acid Acetate. *O*-Acetylsalicylic acid; 2-Acetoxybenzoic acid.

$C_9H_8O_4$ = 180.2.

CAS — 50-78-2.

NOTE. The use of the name Aspirin is limited; in some countries it is a trade-mark.
Compounded preparations of aspirin and codeine phosphate in the proportions, by weight, 50 parts to 1 part have the British Approved Name Co-codaprin.
Compounded preparations of aspirin and codeine phosphate in USP 23 may be represented by the name Co-codaprin.

Pharmacopoeias. In *Chin., Eur.* (see p.viii), *Int., Jpn, Pol.,* and *US.*

Colourless or white crystals or white crystalline powder; odourless or almost odourless. **Solubilities** 1 in 300 of water, 1 in 5 of alcohol, 1 in 17 of chloroform, and 1 in 10 to 15 of ether. **Store** in airtight containers. Aspirin is stable in dry air, but gradually hydrolyses in contact with moisture to acetic and salicylic acids.

Adverse Effects and Treatment

The adverse effects of NSAIDs in general are described on p.63.

The most common adverse effects occurring with therapeutic doses of aspirin are gastro-intestinal disturbances such as nausea, dyspepsia, and vomiting. Gastro-intestinal symptoms may be minimised by giving aspirin with food. Irritation of the gastric mucosa with erosion, ulceration, haematemesis, and melaena may occur. Histamine H_2-receptor antagonists, proton-pump inhibitors, and prostaglandin analogues such as misoprostol have been used in the management of aspirin-induced mucosal damage (see under Peptic Ulcer Disease, p.1174). Slight blood loss, which is often asymptomatic, may occur in about 70% of patients; it is not usually of clinical significance but may, in a few patients cause iron-deficiency anaemia during long-term therapy. Such occult blood loss is not affected by administration of aspirin with food but may be reduced by use of enteric-coated or other modified-release tablets or the use of histamine H_2-receptor antagonists or high doses of antacids. Major upper gastro-intestinal bleeding occurs rarely.

Some persons, especially those with asthma, chronic urticaria, or chronic rhinitis, exhibit notable sensitivity to aspirin which may provoke various reactions including urticaria and other skin eruptions, angioedema, rhinitis, and severe, even fatal, paroxysmal bronchospasm and dyspnoea. Persons sensitive to aspirin often exhibit cross-sensitivity to other NSAIDs. See under Hypersensitivity, below for additional details.

Aspirin increases the bleeding time, decreases platelet adhesiveness, and, in large doses, may cause hypoprothrombinaemia. It may cause other blood disorders, including thrombocytopenia.

Aspirin and other salicylates may cause hepatotoxicity, particularly in patients with juvenile chronic arthritis or other connective tissue disorders.

In children the use of aspirin has been implicated in some cases of Reye's syndrome, thus leading to severe restrictions on the indications for aspirin therapy in children. For further details see under Reye's Syndrome, below.

Aspirin given rectally may cause local irritation; anorectal stenosis has been reported.

Mild chronic salicylate intoxication, or salicylism, usually occurs only after repeated administration of large doses. Salicylism can also occur following excessive topical application of salicylates. Symptoms include dizziness, tinnitus, deafness, sweating, nausea and vomiting, headache, and mental confusion, and may be controlled by reducing the dosage. Symptoms of more severe intoxication or of acute poisoning following overdosage include hyperventilation, fever, restlessness, ketosis, and respiratory alkalosis and metabolic acidosis. Depression of the central nervous system may lead to coma; cardiovascular collapse and respiratory failure may also occur. In children drowsiness and metabolic acidosis commonly occur; hypoglycaemia may be severe.

In acute salicylate overdosage by mouth the stomach should be emptied by lavage. Repeated doses of activated charcoal may be given by mouth with the aim not only of preventing absorption of any salicylate remaining in the stomach but also of aiding elimination of any that has been absorbed. Fluid and electrolyte management is the mainstay of treatment with the immediate aim being correction of acidosis, hyperpyrexia, hypokalaemia, and dehydration. Alkaline diuresis, haemodialysis, or haemoperfusion are effective methods of removing salicylate from the plasma.

Measurement of plasma-salicylate concentration can be useful in assessing the severity of an overdose. However, the severity of the overdosage could be underestimated if outcome is based on early plasma concentrations as absorption of aspirin can be delayed due to reduced gastric emptying, formation of concretions in the stomach, or as a result of ingestion of enteric-coated preparations. In order to ensure that peak plasma concentrations of salicylate are measured it has been suggested that for overdosage with non-enteric coated preparations of aspirin, measurements should commence not less than 6 hours after ingestion and should be repeated until a decline in plasma concentration has been observed. Patients who overdose with enteric preparations require continual monitoring of plasma concentrations.

References to salicylate toxicity and its management.

1. Notarianni L. A reassessment of the treatment of salicylate poisoning. *Drug Safety* 1992; **7:** 292–303.
2. Woods D, *et al.* Acute toxicity of drugs: salicylates. *Pharm J* 1993; **250:** 576–8.
3. Collee GG, Hanson GC. The management of acute poisoning. *Br J Anaesth* 1993; **70:** 562–73.
4. Watson JE, Tagupa ET. Suicide attempt by means of aspirin enema. *Ann Pharmacother* 1994; **28:** 467–9.

Effects on the blood. In addition to its beneficial effects on platelets aspirin can cause adverse blood effects. An indication of this toxicity is given by an early reference[1] to reports submitted to the UK Committee on Safety of Medicines (CSM). There were 787 reports of adverse reactions to aspirin reported to the CSM between June 1964 and January 1973. These included 95 reports of blood disorders (17 fatal) including thrombocytopenia (26; 2 fatal), aplastic anaemia (13; 7 fatal), and agranulocytosis or pancytopenia (10; 2 fatal). Aspirin has also been associated with haemolytic anaemia in patients with glucose-6-phosphate dehydrogenase deficiency.[2]

1. Cuthbert MF. Adverse reactions to non-steroidal antirheumatic drugs. *Curr Med Res Opin* 1974; **2:** 600–9.
2. Magee P, Beeley L. Drug-induced blood dyscrasias. *Pharm J* 1991; **246:** 396–7.

Effects on blood pressure. For reference to the effects of aspirin on blood pressure compared with other NSAIDs, see p.63.

Effects on the gastro-intestinal tract. Clinical and epidemiological evidence suggests that aspirin produces dose-related gastro-intestinal toxicity[1,2] that is sometimes, but rarely, fatal.[2] Studies[3,4] indicate that even doses of 300 mg daily or less carry a risk of peptic ulcer bleeding. Preliminary studies suggest that very small doses of aspirin can produce prophylactic benefits in cardiovascular disease without the risk of gastro-intestinal toxicity, but further study is required.[5] There appears to be no convincing evidence that the risk of major gastro-intestinal bleeding associated with a 75-mg dose is reduced by using enteric-coated or modified-release formulations rather than soluble aspirin.[6] All known NSAIDs have the potential for causing acute damage to the gastric mucosa (see p.64), and comparative studies of acute gastric mucosal damage caused by such drugs consistently associate aspirin with the most severe lesions.[1]

1. Graham DY, Smith JL. Aspirin and the stomach. *Ann Intern Med* 1986; **104:** 390–8.
2. Roderick PJ, *et al.* The gastrointestinal toxicity of aspirin: an overview of randomised controlled trials. *Br J Clin Pharmacol* 1993; **35:** 219–26.
3. Silagy CA, *et al.* Adverse effects of low-dose aspirin in a healthy elderly population. *Clin Pharmacol Ther* 1993; **54:** 84–9.
4. Weil J, *et al.* Prophylactic aspirin and risk of peptic ulcer bleeding. *Br Med J* 1995; **310:** 827–30.
5. Lee M, *et al.* Dose effects of aspirin on gastric prostaglandins and stomach mucosal injury. *Ann Intern Med* 1994; **120:** 184–9.
6. Anonymous. Which prophylactic aspirin? *Drug Ther Bull* 1997; **35:** 7–8.

Effects on hearing. Studies have indicated that tinnitus develops at serum-salicylate concentrations above 200 μg per mL.[1] However, results from one study[2] demonstrated considerable intersubject variation in the response of the human ear to a particular serum-salicylate concentration and tinnitus may occur at lower plasma-salicylate concentrations. Patients with pre-existing hearing loss may not experience tinnitus despite serum-salicylate concentrations of 311 to 677 μg per mL.[1] Day and co-workers[2] demonstrated a graded increase in intensity of hearing loss and tinnitus with increasing salicylate dose and plasma concentration. For example at an average total plasma-salicylate concentration of 110 μg per mL, the hearing loss at any given frequency was about 12 decibels; such a deficit may be relevant to patients with pre-existing hearing impairment.[2]

1. Mongan E, *et al.* Tinnitus as an indication of therapeutic serum salicylate levels. *JAMA* 1973; **226:** 142–5.
2. Day RO, *et al.* Concentration-response relationships for salicylate-induced ototoxicity in normal volunteers. *Br J Clin Pharmacol* 1989; **28:** 695–702.

Effects on the heart. Salicylate poisoning may result in cardiovascular collapse but details of such cases have not been widely reported. Berk and Andersen[1] described 2 patients with salicylate intoxication who developed asystole following the intravenous administration of diazepam. They suggested that diazepam-induced respiratory depression affected the acid-base balance so that the concentration of non-ionised membrane-penetrating fraction of salicylate was increased.

1. Berk WA, Andersen JC. Salicylate-associated asystole: report of two cases. *Am J Med* 1989; **86:** 505–6.

Effects on the kidneys. Although abuse of combined analgesic preparations containing aspirin has been implicated in the development of analgesic nephropathy, kidney damage associated with the therapeutic use of aspirin alone appears to be comparatively rare. Many studies have failed to find an increased risk of renal damage in patients taking aspirin.[1-8]

1. New Zealand Rheumatism Association Study. Aspirin and the kidney. *Br Med J* 1974; **1:** 593–6.
2. Walker BR, *et al.* Aspirin and renal function. *N Engl J Med* 1977; **297:** 1405.
3. Akyol SM, *et al.* Renal function after prolonged consumption of aspirin. *Br Med J* 1982; **284:** 631–2.
4. Bonney SL, *et al.* Renal safety of two analgesics used over the counter: ibuprofen and aspirin. *Clin Pharmacol Ther* 1986; **40:** 373–7.
5. Sandler DP, *et al.* Analgesic use and chronic renal disease. *N Engl J Med* 1989; **320:** 1238–43.
6. Pommer W, *et al.* Regular analgesic intake and the risk of end-stage renal failure. *Am J Nephrol* 1989; **9:** 403–12.
7. Dubach UC, *et al.* An epidemiologic study of abuse of analgesic drugs: effects of phenacetin and salicylate on mortality and cardiovascular morbidity (1968 to 1987). *N Engl J Med* 1991; **324:** 155–60.
8. Perneger TV, *et al.* Risk of kidney failure associated with the use of acetaminophen, aspirin, and nonsteroidal antiinflammatory drugs. *N Engl J Med* 1994; **331:** 1675–9.

Effects on the liver. Aspirin-induced hepatic injury is generally mild and manifests as a mild to moderate elevation in aminotransferase values; however, there is a risk of severe liver injury.[1] One review[2] reported an increase in aminotransferase values in 59 of 439 patients given aspirin; the increase was considered to be probably related to aspirin in 23 of the 59 patients. Hepatotoxicity appears to be correlated with serum-salicylate concentrations greater than 150 μg per mL and with active rheumatoid disease. Aspirin-induced liver injury is usually reversible on discontinuing the drug.[2]

See also under Reye's Syndrome, below.

1. Lewis JH. Hepatic toxicity of nonsteroidal anti-inflammatory drugs. *Clin Pharm* 1984; **3:** 128–38.
2. Freeland GR, *et al.* Hepatic safety of two analgesics used over the counter: ibuprofen and aspirin. *Clin Pharmacol Ther* 1988; **43:** 473–9.

Hypersensitivity. An examination of published literature[1] to estimate the rate of sensitivity reactions to aspirin and cross-sensitivity to other analgesics found that the main clinical feature of patients who have aspirin hypersensitivity included middle-age, female sex, diagnoses of asthma or rhinitis, a personal or family history of atopy, and a history of nasal polyps. The occurrence of aspirin sensitivity in patients with asthma and nasal polyps had been referred to in some reports as the 'aspirin triad'. Other sensitivities often found concomitantly included allergy to food dyes such as tartrazine and to other drugs such as other NSAIDs. The response to individual NSAIDs is believed to be closely linked to the extent to which they inhibit prostaglandin synthesis.[2,3] There may be a dose threshold below which no detectable symptoms occur and patients who may be tolerant of regular low-dose aspirin may develop symptoms when they take larger doses.[3] Some[3] use a formal challenge with a 300-mg dose of aspirin by mouth to confirm a diagnosis of NSAID sensitivity but others[4] consider this to be a dangerous technique and use inhalation of lysine aspirin which they consider to be a safer and more predictable alternative.

1. Kwoh CK, Feinstein AR. Rates of sensitivity reactions to aspirin: problems in interpreting the data. *Clin Pharmacol Ther* 1986; **40:** 494–505.
2. Power I. Aspirin-induced asthma. *Br J Anaesth* 1993; **71:** 619–21.
3. Frew A. Selected side-effects: 13. non-steroidal anti-inflammatory drugs and asthma. *Prescribers' J* 1994; **34:** 74–7.
4. Davies BH. NSAIDs and asthma. *Prescribers' J* 1994; **34:** 163–4.

DESENSITISATION. Successful desensitisation has been achieved using various oral aspirin challenge protocols.[1,2] Incremental doses of aspirin (starting at 30 mg) are given until an allergic response is obtained; aspirin is readministered at the dose that caused the response and again incremental doses are given until finally a 650-mg dose is tolerated. After desensitisation, an interruption of continuous aspirin administration results in the reappearance of sensitivity.

1. Asad SI, *et al.* Effect of aspirin in "aspirin sensitive" patients. *Br Med J* 1984; **288:** 745–8.
2. Stevenson DD. Desensitization of aspirin-sensitive asthmatics: a therapeutic alternative? *J Asthma* 1983; **20:** 31–8.

Hypoglycaemia. A review of the literature[1] on drug-induced hypoglycaemia has highlighted the fact that overdosage with salicylates can produce hypoglycaemia in children. Although it is recognised[1,2] that therapeutic doses of salicylates in adults can lower blood-glucose concentrations in diabetic and non-diabetic subjects alike, opinion on the clinical significance of this effect varies. Salicylates have been implicated in a few cases of hypoglycaemia in adults[1] and some[2] suggest that patients with renal impairment or those receiving large doses, such as in the treatment of rheumatoid arthritis, may be at risk. Hypoglycaemia has been reported in one patient with renal failure following excessive application of a topical preparation containing salicylic acid.[3]

1. Seltzer HS. Drug-induced hypoglycemia: a review of 1418 cases. *Endocrinol Metab Clin North Am* 1989; **18:** 163–83.
2. Pandit MK, *et al.* Drug-induced disorders of glucose tolerance. *Ann Intern Med* 1993; **118:** 529–39.
3. Raschke R, *et al.* Refractory hypoglycemia secondary to topical salicylate intoxication. *Arch Intern Med* 1991; **151:** 591–3.

Reye's syndrome. Reye's syndrome is a disorder occurring almost exclusively in children and is characterised by acute encephalopathy and fatty degeneration of the liver. Many factors may be involved in its aetiology but it typically occurs after a viral infection such as chickenpox or influenza and may be precipitated by a chemical trigger. Several large studies, as well as individual case reports, have found an association between Reye's syndrome and the prior ingestion of aspirin.[1-4] The evidence for other salicylates could not be adequately evaluated.[3] Although the role of aspirin and possibly other salicylates in the pathogenesis of Reye's syndrome remains to be determined, the use of aspirin and other acetylated salicylates as analgesics or antipyretics for children under the age of 12 years is generally not recommended. Some authorities also extend this precaution to non-acetylated salicylates. Most authorities consider one of the few acceptable indications remaining for the use of aspirin in children to be juvenile chronic arthritis. One group of workers[5] who re-examined some of the original studies suggested that there might also be a link between Reye's syndrome and the use of antiemetics, phenothiazines, and some other antihistamines, but their conclusions have been criticised.[6]

1. Waldman RJ, *et al.* Aspirin as a risk factor in Reye's syndrome. *JAMA* 1982; **247:** 3089–94.
2. Halpin TJ, *et al.* Reye's syndrome and medication use. *JAMA* 1982; **248:** 687–91.
3. Hurwitz ES, *et al.* Public health service study of Reye's syndrome and medications: report of the main study. *JAMA* 1987; **257:** 1905–11.
4. Hall SM, *et al.* Preadmission antipyretics in Reye's syndrome. *Arch Dis Child* 1988; **63:** 857–66.
5. Casteels-Van Daele M, Eggermont E. Reye's syndrome. *Br Med J* 1994; **308:** 919–20.
6. Hall SM. Reye's syndrome. *Br Med J* 1994; **309:** 411.

Precautions

The precautions of NSAIDs in general are described on p.65.

Aspirin should be cautiously employed, if at all, in patients prone to dyspepsia or known to have a lesion of the gastric mucosa. It should not be administered to patients with haemophilia or other haemorrhagic disorders, or to patients with gout since low doses increase urate concentrations.

Aspirin should be used with caution in patients with asthma or allergic disorders. It should not be given to patients with a history of sensitivity reactions to aspirin or other NSAIDs, which includes those in whom attacks of asthma, angioedema, urticaria, or rhinitis have been precipitated by aspirin or any other NSAID (for further details of risk factors see Hypersensitivity under Adverse Effects, above).

Caution is necessary when renal or hepatic function is impaired; aspirin should be avoided in severe renal or hepatic impairment. Aspirin should be used cautiously in dehydrated patients and in the presence of uncontrolled hypertension.

High doses may precipitate acute haemolytic anaemia in patients with glucose 6-phosphate dehydrogenase deficiency. Aspirin may interfere with insulin and glucagon control in diabetics (see Hypoglycaemia under Adverse Effects, above).

The use of aspirin in children under the age of 12 years is extremely limited because of the risk of Reye's syndrome (see under Adverse Effects, above, and under Uses and Administration, below).

Although low-dose aspirin might be used in some pregnant patients, analgesic doses of aspirin should not be used at term as it may be associated with prolongation of labour and with maternal and neonatal bleeding. High doses may cause closure of fetal ductus arteriosus before birth and possibly persistent pulmonary hypertension in the newborn (see under Pregnancy, below); kernicterus may occur in jaundiced neonates. Mothers who are breast feeding their infants should not take aspirin.

Continuous prolonged use of aspirin should be avoided in the elderly because of the risk of gastro-intestinal bleeding.

Aspirin should be discontinued several days before scheduled surgical procedures (see below).

Pregnancy. The potential adverse effects of aspirin when used during pregnancy have been reviewed.[1] Salicylates readily cross the placenta and have been shown to be teratogenic in *animals*. Although some studies and anecdotal reports have implicated aspirin in the formation of congenital abnormalities, most large studies[2-4] have failed to find any significant risk or evidence of teratogenicity. Analysis of data collected by the Slone Epidemiology Unit Birth Defects Study suggests that use of aspirin during the early months of pregnancy, when the fetal heart is developing, is not associated with an increased risk of cardiac defects.[5] The ability of aspirin, however, to alter platelet function may be a potential risk. There have been a few reports of haemorrhagic disorders in infants whose mothers had consumed aspirin during pregnancy[6] and of salicylate-associated haemorrhagic complications in mothers.[7] However, no clinically significant adverse effects on maternal or neonatal bleeding or on fetal ductus flow were reported in 6 controlled studies which evaluated low-dose aspirin (less than 325 mg daily) in pregnancy-induced hypertension.[8] It appeared that the degree of cyclo-oxygenase inhibition produced by aspirin was unlikely to be great enough to cause premature closure of the ductus arteriosus or to affect the pulmonary blood vessels.[1] However, in some studies in patients considered to have high-risk pregnancies the risk of abruptio placentae[9] or consequent perinatal death[10] was increased by maternal administration of aspirin. For reference to a possible association between aspirin and other NSAIDs and persistent pulmonary hypertension of the newborn, see under NSAIDs, p.65.

Although aspirin has the potential to inhibit uterine contractions of labour it was considered that intermittent or low dose aspirin therapy was unlikely to inhibit cyclo-oxygenase for long enough to prolong pregnancy or labour.[1]

1. de Swiet M, Fryers G. The use of aspirin in pregnancy. *J Obstet Gynaecol* 1990; **10:** 467–82.
2. Slone D, *et al.* Aspirin and congenital malformations. *Lancet* 1976; **1:** 1373–5.
3. Shapiro S, *et al.* Perinatal mortality and birth-weight in relation to aspirin taken during pregnancy. *Lancet* 1976; **i:** 1375–6.
4. Winship KA, *et al.* Maternal drug histories and central nervous system anomalies. *Arch Dis Child* 1984; **59:** 1052–60.
5. Werler MM, *et al.* The relation of aspirin use during the first trimester of pregnancy to congenital cardiac defects. *N Engl J Med* 1989; **321:** 1639–42.
6. Bleyer WA, Breckenridge RT. Studies on the detection of adverse drug reactions in the newborn II: the effects of prenatal aspirin on newborn hemostasis. *JAMA* 1970; **213:** 2049–53.
7. Collins E, Turner G. Maternal effects of regular salicylate ingestion in pregnancy. *Lancet* 1975; **ii:** 335–7.
8. Imperiale TF, Petrulis AS. A meta-analysis of low-dose aspirin for the prevention of pregnancy-induced hypertensive disease. *JAMA* 1991; **266:** 261–4.
9. Sibai BM, *et al.* Prevention of preeclampsia with low-dose aspirin in healthy, nulliparous pregnant women. *N Engl J Med* 1993; **329:** 1213–18.
10. Hamid R, *et al.* Low dose aspirin in women with raised maternal serum alpha-fetoprotein and abnormal Doppler waveform patterns from the uteroplacental circulation. *Br J Obstet Gynaecol* 1994; **101:** 481–4.

Surgical procedures. Aspirin prolongs bleeding time, mainly by inhibiting platelet aggregation. This effect is irreversible and new platelets must be released into the circulation before bleeding time can return to normal. Therefore aspirin therapy should be discontinued several days before surgical procedures. In some clinical situations, aspirin may have been given shortly before a surgical procedure. When emergency coronary bypass surgery is required following myocardial infarction, most patients would have received aspirin as part of the initial treatment for infarction. Perioperative bleeding, transfusion requirements, and surgical re-exploration rates may be increased when aspirin is given.[1] Administration of desmopressin acetate may reduce the risk of perioperative bleeding (see under Haemorrhagic Disorders, p.1246).

Aspirin is sometimes given during the second and third trimester for the prevention of pregnancy-induced hypertensive disease (see under Hypertension, p.788). Studies indicate that when given in a dose of 325 mg daily or less, clinically significant effects on maternal or neonatal bleeding do not occur.[2] Some have suggested that aspirin therapy may increase the risk of formation of extradural haematoma thus making epidural anaesthesia inadvisable[3] but a recent study[4] found that low-dose aspirin during pregnancy did not increase the risk of bleeding complications during epidural anaesthesia.

Patients on low-dose aspirin, in whom tourniquets are used for nerve blocks or other procedures, may be at increased risk of developing purpuric rash.[5]

It has been suggested that in patients undergoing dermatological surgery, aspirin need only be stopped before surgery in those patients with a prolonged bleeding time, whereas patients with a normal bleeding time could continue therapy.[6]

1. Goldman S, *et al.* Improvement in early saphenous vein graft patency after coronary artery bypass surgery with antiplatelet therapy: results of a Veterans Administration Cooperative Study. *Circulation* 1988; **77:** 1324–32.
2. Imperiale TF, Petrulis AS. A meta-analysis of low-dose aspirin for the prevention of pregnancy-induced hypertensive disease. *JAMA* 1991; **266:** 260–4.
3. Macdonald R. Aspirin and extradural blocks. *Br J Anaesth* 1991; **66:** 1–3.
4. Sibai BM, *et al.* Low-dose aspirin in nulliparous women: safety of continuous epidural block and correlation between bleeding time and maternal-neonatal bleeding complications. *Am J Obstet Gynecol* 1995; **172:** 1553–7.
5. Runcie CJ, *et al.* Aspirin and intravenous regional blocks. *Br J Hosp Med* 1990; **43:** 229–30.
6. Lawrence C, *et al.* Effect of aspirin and nonsteroidal antiinflammatory drug therapy on bleeding complications in dermatologic surgical patients. *J Am Acad Dermatol* 1994; **31:** 988–92.

Interactions

The interactions of NSAIDs in general are described on p.65.

Some of the effects of aspirin on the gastro-intestinal tract are enhanced by alcohol. Concurrent administration of aspirin and dipyridamole may result in an increase in peak plasma-salicylate concentration and area under the curve. Administration of drugs such as metoclopramide in patients with migraine headache results in earlier absorption of aspirin and higher peak plasma-salicylate concentrations. Metoprolol may increase peak plasma-salicylate concentrations. Salicylate intoxication has occurred in patients on high-dose salicylate regimens and carbonic anhydrase inhibitors. Serum-salicylate concentrations may be reduced by concurrent administration of corticosteroids. This interaction is likely to be important in patients receiving high-dose long-term salicylate treatment. Conversely, salicylate toxicity may occur if corticosteroids are withdrawn. Also the risk of gastro-intestinal bleeding and ulceration associated with aspirin is increased when used with corticosteroids. Antacids and adsorbents may increase the excretion of aspirin in alkaline urine. Administration of gold compounds with aspirin may exacerbate aspirin-induced liver damage. Aspirin may enhance the activity of coumarin anticoagulants, sulphonylurea hypoglycaemic drugs, methotrexate, phenytoin, and valproic acid. Aspirin diminishes the effects of uricosurics such as probenecid and sulphinpyrazone. The concomitant use of aspirin and other NSAIDs should be avoided because of the increased risk of adverse effects. Aspirin may decrease the plasma concentration of some other NSAIDs, for example, fenbufen, indomethacin, and piroxicam. The manufacturer of mifepristone advises that aspirin or NSAIDs should be avoided for 8 to 12 days after mifepristone use because of a theoretical risk that these prostaglandin synthetase inhibitors may alter the efficacy of mifepristone.

A review[1] of potential drug interactions related to aspirin.

1. Miners JO. Drug interactions involving aspirin (acetylsalicylic acid) and salicylic acid. *Clin Pharmacokinet* 1989; **17:** 327–44.

ACE inhibitors. For a discussion of aspirin and other NSAIDs reducing the activity of ACE inhibitors, see p.808.

Antifungals. Plasma-salicylate concentrations in an 8-year-old child receiving long-term aspirin therapy for rheumatic heart disease were markedly reduced when treatment with griseofulvin was started.[1] It was suggested that griseofulvin might interfere with absorption of aspirin.

1. Phillips KR, *et al.* Griseofulvin significantly decreases serum salicylate concentrations. *Pediatr Infect Dis J* 1993; **12:** 350–2.

Calcium-channel blockers. The antiplatelet effects of aspirin and calcium-channel blockers may be increased when they are used together; there have been isolated reports[1,2] of disturbed haemostasis including abnormal bruising, prolonged bleeding times and ecchymosis in patients taking aspirin and verapamil concurrently.

1. Ring ME, *et al.* Clinically significant antiplatelet effects of calcium-channel blockers. *J Clin Pharmacol* 1986; **26:** 719–20.
2. Verzino E, *et al.* Verapamil-aspirin interaction. *Ann Pharmacother* 1994; **28:** 536–7.

General anaesthetics. For the effect of aspirin on thiopentone anaesthesia, see p.1233.

Spironolactone. For the effect of aspirin in patients taking spironolactone, see p.947.

Pharmacokinetics

Aspirin and other salicylates are absorbed rapidly from the gastro-intestinal tract but absorption following rectal administration is less reliable than after oral administration. Aspirin and other salicylates can also be absorbed through the skin.

Following oral administration, absorption of non-ionised aspirin occurs in the stomach and intestine. Some aspirin is hydrolysed to salicylate in the gut wall. After absorption aspirin is rapidly converted to salicylate but during the first 20 minutes following oral administration, aspirin is the predominant form of the drug in the plasma. Aspirin is 80 to 90% bound to plasma proteins and is widely distributed; its volume of distribution is reported to be 170 mL per kg body-weight in adults. As plasma-drug concentrations increase, the binding sites on the proteins become saturated and the volume of distribution increases. Both aspirin and salicylate have pharmacological activity; only aspirin has an anti-platelet effect. Salicylate is extensively bound to plasma proteins and is rapidly distributed to all body parts. Salicylate appears in breast milk and crosses the placenta.

Salicylate is mainly eliminated by hepatic metabolism; the metabolites include salicyluric acid, salicyl phenolic glucuronide, salicylic acyl glucuronide, gentisic acid, and gentisuric acid. The formation of the major metabolites, salicyluric acid and salicyl phenolic glucuronide is easily saturated and follows Michaelis-Menten kinetics; the other metabolic routes are first-order processes. As a result, steady-state plasma-salicylate concentrations increase disproportionately with dose. Following a 325-mg aspirin dose, elimination is a first-order process and the plasma-salicylate half-life is about 2 to 3 hours; at high aspirin doses, the half-life increases to 15 to 30 hours. Salicylate is also excreted unchanged in the urine; the amount excreted by this route increases with increasing dose and also depends on urinary pH, about 30% of a dose being excreted in alkaline urine compared with 2% of a dose in acidic urine. Renal excretion involves glomerular filtration, active renal tubular secretion, and passive tubular reabsorption.

Salicylate is removed by haemodialysis.

References.

1. Needs CJ, Brooks PM. Clinical pharmacokinetics of the salicylates. *Clin Pharmacokinet* 1985; **10:** 164–77.

Uses and Administration

Aspirin is a salicylate NSAID (p.65). Aspirin and other salicylates have analgesic, anti-inflammatory, and antipyretic properties; they act as inhibitors of the enzyme cyclo-oxygenase, which results in the direct inhibition of the biosynthesis of prostaglandins and thromboxanes from arachidonic acid (see p.1411 and p.704). Aspirin also inhibits platelet aggregation; non-acetylated salicylates do not.

Aspirin is used for the relief of mild to moderate pain such as headache, dysmenorrhoea, myalgias, and dental pain. It is also used in the management of pain and inflammation in acute and chronic rheumatic disorders such as rheumatoid arthritis, juvenile chronic arthritis, osteoarthritis, and ankylosing spondylitis. In the treatment of minor febrile conditions, such as colds or influenza, aspirin is of value for the reduction of temperature and relief of the headache and the joint and muscle pains.

Aspirin is also used for its antiplatelet activity in the initial treatment of cardiovascular disorders such as angina pectoris and myocardial infarction and for the prevention of cardiovascular events in a variety of conditions or procedures for patients at risk. For further details see under Antiplatelet Therapy, below.

Aspirin is usually taken by mouth. Gastric irritation may be reduced by taking doses after food. Various dosage forms are available including plain uncoated tablets, buffered tablets, dispersible tablets, enteric-coated tablets, and modified-release tablets. In some instances aspirin may be administered rectally by suppository.

The usual dose of aspirin by mouth as an analgesic and antipyretic is 0.3 to 0.9 g, which may be repeated every 4 to 6 hours according to clinical needs, to a maximum of 4 g daily. The dose of suppositories is 0.6 to 0.9 g every 4 hours to a maximum of 3.6 g daily.

Plasma-salicylate concentrations of 150 to 300 μg per mL are required for optimal anti-inflammatory activity but may produce tinnitus; more serious adverse effects occur at concentrations above 300 μg per mL. Doses need to be adjusted individually to achieve optimum concentrations. Generally doses of about 4 to 8 g daily in divided doses are used for acute rheumatic disorders such as rheumatoid arthritis or osteoarthritis. Doses of up to 5.4 g daily in divided doses may be sufficient in chronic conditions.

Indications for aspirin therapy in children are extremely limited because of the risk of Reye's syndrome (see under Adverse Effects, above), and include juvenile chronic arthritis and Still's disease. Suggested doses for children are 80 to 100 mg per kg body-weight daily in 5 or 6 divided doses with up to 130 mg per kg daily used in acute exacerbations if necessary.

Sodium aspirin has also been used for the treatment of pain and fever.

Antiplatelet therapy. Aspirin's antiplatelet activity has led to its use or investigation in a variety of disorders.[1-4] It is used as part of the initial treatment of unstable angina (p.780) and is given in the early treatment of myocardial infarction (p.791); it may also be of some benefit in the initial treatment of acute ischaemic stroke (p.799). It is of value for the secondary prevention of cardiovascular events in patients with stable or unstable angina or those with acute or prior myocardial infarction. Similarly, aspirin reduces the risk of future serious vascular events, including stroke, in patients who have already suffered an ischaemic stroke or transient ischaemic attack and is of use in the long-term management of atrial fibrillation (see under Cardiac Arrhythmias, p.782) for the prevention of stroke in patients with contra-indications to warfarin or if there are no other risk factors for stroke. The value of aspirin for primary prevention of angina, myocardial infarction, and stroke is unclear but it might be of benefit in patients at high risk of occlusive vascular disease. Although aspirin may prevent venous thrombo-embolism (p.802) following surgery other treatments have been preferred. However, it is recommended for use in preventing thrombotic complications associated with procedures such as angioplasty and coronary bypass grafting (see under Reperfusion and Revascularisation Procedures, p.797). Aspirin is often given as an adjunct to patients with peripheral arterial thrombo-embolism (p.794) to prevent propagation of the clot and also to prevent post-operative complications. It may have some effect in delaying disease progression in patients with peripheral arterial disease (p.794) but a recent analysis[5] concluded that there was probably insufficient evidence to support its prophylactic use in patients with intermittent claudication and no additional cardiovascular risk factors. Similarly, the benefit of aspirin for prevention of cardiovascular events in patients with diabetes mellitus (see under Diabetic Complications, p.315) and who have no other cardiovascular risk factors remains to be determined. The value of adding aspirin to anticoagulants for the prophylaxis of thrombo-embolism in patients with artificial heart valves (see p.801) is also unclear. Aspirin's range of activities, including its antiplatelet activity, is put to use in the treatment of Kawasaki disease (see below). It is also used to treat thrombotic symptoms associated with antiphospholipid syndrome, such as occurs in patients with systemic lupus erythematosus (p.1029), and has been recommended for prophylactic use in pregnant patients with antiphospholipid antibodies who are at risk of fetal loss. Aspirin has also been tried in pregnancy-induced hypertension (see under Hypertension, p.788) for the prevention of pre-eclampsia and intra-uterine growth retardation but it appears that its use may be justified only in women at high risk.

Aspirin is an inhibitor of the enzyme cyclo-oxygenase, the reaction being considered to be due to an irreversible acetylation process. In blood platelets such enzyme inhibition prevents the synthesis of thromboxane A_2, a compound which is a vasoconstrictor, causes platelet aggregation and is thus potentially thrombotic. In blood vessel walls the enzyme inhibition prevents the synthesis of prostacyclin, which is a vasodilator, has anti-aggregating properties and is thus potentially anti-thrombotic. Aspirin therefore appears to have paradoxical biological effects. The duration of these effects, however, may be somewhat different with the effects on the vascular tissue generally being shorter lived than the effects on the platelets (although the animal species studied, the type of blood vessel employed, and the prevailing experimental conditions may alter the results). The differing duration of effects may be explained by the fact that vascular cells regain the ability to regenerate prostacyclin in a few hours but platelets are unable to re-synthesise cyclo-oxygenase thus resulting in no new thromboxane A_2 being produced until, after about 24 hours, more platelets are released by the bone marrow; as platelet activity in bone marrow may also be affected by aspirin it is generally considered that aspirin need not be given more frequently than once daily for inhibition of platelet aggregation to occur. The inhibitory effect on thromboxane is rapid and unrelated to serum concentrations of aspirin, this probably being due to inactivation of cyclo-oxygenase in platelets in the presystemic circulation. Since the effect is unrelated to systemic bioavailability controlled-release and dermal delivery preparations which do not achieve high systemic concentrations of aspirin are being developed to limit extra-platelet effects of aspirin. Inhibition is cumulative on repeat administration and it has been estimated that a daily dose of 20 to 50 mg will result in virtually complete suppression of platelet thromboxane synthesis within a few days. Large doses can produce maximum suppression almost instantaneously.

Several pharmacological studies have attempted to find a dose of aspirin that would inhibit synthesis of platelet thromboxane A_2 while sparing the effect on prostacyclin production[6-8] but it has been pointed out[4] that in patients with vascular disease accompanying or caused by endothelial dysfunction, such as in atherosclerosis, a selective sparing of vascular prostacyclin production may not be obtained at any effective antiplatelet dose. However, Hirsh *et al.*[9] have suggested that the clinical relevance of inhibiting the synthesis of prostacyclin has been exaggerated. Experimental evidence indicates that aspirin is thrombogenic only at extremely high doses (200 mg per kg body-weight), far exceeding the minimum dose required to inhibit prostacyclin production. Also aspirin is clinically effective as an antithrombotic drug at doses that inhibit the synthesis of prostacyclin. Further support for the lack of importance of inhibition of prostacyclin synthesis comes from epidemiological studies in patients with arthritis given large doses of aspirin and patients with congenital cyclo-oxygenase deficiency; neither of these groups of patients have experienced an excess of thrombotic episodes.

In the series of meta-analyses conducted by the Antiplatelet Trialists' Collaboration[10-12] doses of 75 to 325 mg were the most commonly tested; doses in this range appeared to be equally effective for their antiplatelet effect; larger doses did not appear to be superior and caused more gastro-intestinal adverse effects. Whether lower doses offer the same efficacy with reduced gastro-intestinal toxicity remains to be determined (see Effects on the Gastro-intestinal Tract, above). A more recent analysis[5] concluded that a dose of 75 mg daily should be effective for secondary prophylaxis of vascular events although for patients with suspected or proven myocardial infarction a suitable dose may be 150 mg daily for the first month followed by 75 mg thereafter. Because doses in the order of 75 mg daily take a few days to exert a full antiplatelet effect treatment should be initiated with a loading dose such as 150 to 300 mg if immediate suppression is desirable as in the initial treatment of acute myocardial infarction and unstable angina. Aspirin should be chewed or dispersed in water; chewing a tablet of aspirin ensures that some buccal absorption occurs.

1. Patrono C. Aspirin as an antiplatelet drug. *N Engl J Med* 1994; **330:** 1287–94.
2. Lutomski DM, *et al.* Pharmacokinetic optimisation of the treatment of embolic disorders. *Clin Pharmacokinet* 1995; **28:** 67–92.
3. Catella-Lawson F, Fitzgerald GA. Long term aspirin in the prevention of cardiovascular disorders: recent developments and variations on a theme. *Drug Safety* 1995; **13:** 69–75.
4. Schrör K. Antiplatelet drugs: a comparative review. *Drugs* 1995; **50:** 7–28.
5. Eccles M, *et al.* North of England evidence based guideline development project: guideline on the use of aspirin as secondary prophylaxis for vascular disease in primary care. *Br Med J* 1998; **316:** 1303–9.
6. Patrignani P, *et al.* Selective cumulative inhibition of platelet thromboxane production by low-dose aspirin in healthy subjects. *J Clin Invest* 1982; **69:** 1366–72.
7. Weksler BB, *et al.* Differential inhibition by aspirin of vascular and platelet prostaglandin synthesis in atherosclerotic patients. *N Engl J Med* 1983; **308:** 800–5.
8. McLeod LJ, *et al.* The effects of different doses of some acetylsalicylic acid formulations on platelet function and bleeding times in healthy subjects. *Scand J Haematol* 1986; **36:** 379–84.
9. Hirsh J, *et al.* Aspirin and other platelet active drugs: relationship among dose, effectiveness, and side effects. *Chest* 1989; **95** (suppl 2): 12S–18S.
10. Antiplatelet Trialists' Collaboration. Collaborative overview of randomised trials of antiplatelet therapy—I: prevention of death, myocardial infarction, and stroke by prolonged antiplatelet therapy in various categories of patients. *Br Med J* 1994; **308:** 81–106. Correction. *ibid.*: 1540.
11. Antiplatelet Trialists' Collaboration. Collaborative overview of randomised trials of antiplatelet therapy—II: maintenance of vascular graft or arterial patency by antiplatelet therapy. *Br Med J* 1994; **308:** 159–68.
12. Antiplatelet Trialists' Collaboration. Collaborative overview of randomised trials of antiplatelet therapy—III: reduction in venous thrombosis and pulmonary embolism by antiplatelet prophylaxis among surgical and medical patients. *Br Med J* 1994; **308:** 235–46.

Behçet's syndrome. For reference to a recommendation that aspirin may be used with colchicine to prevent acute exacerbations of Behçet's syndrome, see p.1018.

Cataract. It has been suggested that some anti-inflammatory drugs might have beneficial effects against cataract formation but evidence to support or disprove the hypothesis that aspirin has a protective effect against cataract formation is considered inconclusive.[1,2] One study in the US in over 22 000 males concluded that low-dose aspirin (325 mg on alternate days) for 5 years was unlikely to have a major effect on cataract formation but that a slightly decreased risk for cataract extraction could not be excluded.[3] In a later study[4] in the UK ophthalmic examination of over 1800 patients who were receiving 300 to 1200 mg of aspirin daily for transient ischaemic attacks failed to confirm any protective effect.

1. Cheng H. Aspirin and cataract. *Br J Ophthalmol* 1992; **76:** 257–8.
2. Anonymous. Preventing cataract. *Lancet* 1992; **340:** 883–4.
3. Seddon JM, *et al.* Low dose aspirin and risks of cataract in a randomised trial of US physicians. *Arch Ophthalmol* 1991; **109:** 252–5.
4. UK-TIA Study Group. Does aspirin affect the rate of cataract formation? Cross-sectional results during a randomised double-blind placebo controlled trial to prevent serious vascular events. *Br J Ophthalmol* 1992; **76:** 259–61.

Dysmenorrhoea. The pain of dysmenorrhoea (p.9) arises from uterine contractions produced by release of prostaglandins from the endometrium in the luteal phase of the menstrual cycle. Drugs such as aspirin and other NSAIDs that inhibit prostaglandin production through inhibition of cyclo-oxygenase are effective drugs in the treatment of dysmenorrhoea.

Fever. Methods for controlling fever (see p.1) include the use of antipyretics and/or physical cooling methods. Paracetamol, salicylates such as aspirin and some other NSAIDs are the main antipyretics used. However, salicylates are generally contra-indicated in infants and children because of the possible link between their use and the development of Reye's syndrome (see under Adverse Effects, above).

Headache. An NSAID such as aspirin is often tried first for the symptomatic treatment of various types of headache including migraine (see p.443) and tension-type headache (see p.444). Aspirin given at the onset of symptoms can successfully treat an acute attack of migraine. However, absorption may be poor due to gastric stasis which is commonly present in migraine. For this reason dispersible and effervescent preparations and compound preparations containing drugs such as metoclopramide which relieve gastric stasis have been advocated. NSAIDs may also be effective prophylactic drugs for migraine, although propranolol or pizotifen are generally preferred.

References.

1. Tfelt-Hansen P, Olesen J. Effervescent metoclopramide and aspirin (Migravess) versus effervescent aspirin or placebo for migraine attacks: a double-blind study. *Cephalalgia* 1984; **4:** 107–11.
2. Buring JE, *et al.* Low-dose aspirin for migraine prophylaxis. *JAMA* 1990; **264:** 1711–13.
3. The Oral Sumatriptan and Aspirin plus Metoclopramide Comparative Study Group. A study to compare oral sumatriptan with oral aspirin plus oral metoclopramide in the acute treatment of migraine. *Eur Neurol* 1992; **32:** 177–84.
4. Tfelt-Hansen P, *et al.* The effectiveness of combined oral lysine acetylsalicylate and metoclopramide compared with oral sumatriptan for migraine. *Lancet* 1995; **346:** 923–6.

Kawasaki disease. Aspirin has been given in regimens with normal immunoglobulins to children with Kawasaki disease (p.1524) because of its anti-inflammatory, antipyretic, and antiplatelet activity.[1-5]

The optimum dose and duration of treatment with aspirin is not yet established but the usual practice is to use an anti-inflammatory regimen until the fever has settled and then convert to an antithrombotic regimen. Usual initial doses used have ranged from 30 to 120 mg per kg body-weight daily. Some clinicians recommend administration of aspirin in a dose of 80 to 100 mg per kg daily in 4 divided doses until the patient is afebrile or for the first 14 days after the onset of symptoms. Once fever and signs of inflammatory disease resolve, the aspirin dose is reduced to 3 to 5 mg per kg daily as a single dose for its antiplatelet effect. Aspirin may be discontinued 6 to 8 weeks after the onset of illness but is usually continued for at least one year if coronary abnormalities are present and is continued indefinitely if coronary aneurysms persist.

It has been noted[6] that aspirin has never been demonstrated in a prospective study to reduce the prevalence of coronary artery abnormalities in children with Kawasaki disease and recent studies[3,5] indicate that the incidence of such abnormalities following treatment was similar for regimens using high or low doses of aspirin. In view of the potential risks and lack of obvious cardiac benefits of high-dose aspirin some[6] consider that an argument could be made for use of a low dose such as 3 to 5 mg per kg daily to prevent thrombosis, with other drugs such as paracetamol or ibuprofen being added for fever control or severe arthritis.

1. Dajani AS, *et al.* Diagnosis and therapy of Kawasaki disease in children. *Circulation* 1993; **87:** 1776–80.
2. Dajani AS, *et al.* Guidelines for long-term management of patients with Kawasaki disease: report from the Committee on Rheumatic Fever, Endocarditis, and Kawasaki Disease, Council on Cardiovascular Disease in the Young, American Heart Association. *Circulation* 1994; **89:** 916–22.
3. Durongpisitkul K, *et al.* The prevention of coronary artery aneurysm in Kawasaki disease: a meta-analysis on the efficacy of aspirin and immunoglobulin treatment. *Pediatrics* 1995; **96:** 1057–61.
4. Samuel J, O'Sullivan J. Kawasaki disease. *Br J Hosp Med* 1996; **55:** 9–14.
5. Terai M, Shulman ST. Prevalence of coronary artery abnormalities in Kawasaki disease is highly dependent on gamma globulin dose but independent of salicylate dose. *J Pediatr* 1997; **131:** 888–93.
6. Newburger JW. Treatment of Kawasaki disease. *Lancet* 1996; **347:** 1128.

Leg ulcers. A 4-month placebo controlled study[1] in 20 patients suggested that aspirin 300 mg daily aided healing of chronic venous leg ulcers; the mechanism of action was unclear.[2] However, the validity of the findings has been challenged.[3] The management of leg ulcers is discussed on p.1076.

1. Layton AM, *et al.* Randomised trial of oral aspirin for chronic venous leg ulcers. *Lancet* 1994; **344:** 164–5.
2. Ibbotson SH, *et al.* The effect of aspirin on haemostatic activity in the treatment of chronic venous leg ulceration. *Br J Dermatol* 1995; **132:** 422–6.
3. Ruckley CV, Prescott RJ. Treatment of chronic leg ulcers. *Lancet* 1994; **344:** 1512–13.

Malignant neoplasms. For references to studies suggesting that regular use of aspirin and other NSAIDs may reduce the risk of developing malignant neoplasms of the gastro-intestinal tract, see under NSAIDs, p.66.

Pain. Aspirin and other salicylates are used in the management of mild to moderate pain (p.4). Aspirin is of similar analgesic efficacy to paracetamol but possesses greater anti-inflammatory activity. Salicylate compounds are commonly used in rubefacient preparations for topical application (see p.7). Aspirin may also be used as an adjunct to opioids in the management of severe pain such as cancer pain (p.8). Aspirin was once widely used in the treatment of rheumatoid arthritis (p.2) but has been superseded by other NSAIDs that are better tolerated. Paracetamol is the preferred choice of non-opioid analgesic for pain in infants and children (p.7) because of the association of aspirin with Reye's syndrome in this age group (see under Adverse Effects, above). However, juvenile chronic arthritis (p.2) and Still's disease (p.4) are among the limited number of indications for the use of aspirin in children.

Dependence and tolerance are not a problem with non-opioid analgesics such as aspirin, but there is a ceiling of efficacy, above which increasing the dose has no further therapeutic effect.

Polycythaemia vera. Aspirin in low doses has been used to provide symptomatic relief for erythromelalgia in patients with polycythaemia vera (p.495).

Preparations

BP 1998: Aspirin and Caffeine Tablets; Aspirin Tablets; Co-codaprin Tablets; Dispersible Aspirin Tablets; Dispersible Co-codaprin Tablets; Effervescent Soluble Aspirin Tablets;
USP 23: Acetaminophen and Aspirin Tablets; Acetaminophen, Aspirin, and Caffeine Capsules; Acetaminophen, Aspirin, and Caffeine Tablets; Aspirin and Codeine Phosphate Tablets; Aspirin Capsules; Aspirin Delayed-release Capsules; Aspirin Delayed-release Tablets; Aspirin Effervescent Tablets for Oral Solution; Aspirin Extended-release Tablets; Aspirin Suppositories; Aspirin Tablets; Aspirin, Alumina, and Magnesia Tablets; Aspirin, Alumina, and Magnesium Oxide Tablets; Aspirin, Caffeine, and Dihydrocodeine Bitartrate Capsules; Aspirin, Codeine Phosphate, Alumina, and Magnesia Tablets; Aspirin, Codeine Phosphate, and Caffeine Capsules; Aspirin, Codeine Phosphate, and Caffeine Tablets; Buffered Aspirin Tablets; Butalbital and Aspirin Tablets; Butalbital, Aspirin, and Caffeine Capsules; Butalbital, Aspirin, and Caffeine Tablets; Butalbital, Aspirin, Caffeine, and Codeine Phosphate Capsules; Carisoprodol and Aspirin Tablets; Carisoprodol, Aspirin, and Codeine Phosphate Tablets; Oxycodone and Aspirin Tablets; Pentazocine Hydrochloride and Aspirin Tablets; Propoxyphene Hydrochloride, Aspirin, and Caffeine Capsules; Propoxyphene Napsylate and Aspirin Tablets.

Proprietary Preparations (details are given in Part 3)
Aust.: Acimetten; Algobene; Aspiricor; Aspro; ASS; Colfarit; Corsalbene; Thrombo ASS; ***Austral.:*** Aspro; Astrix; Bex; Bufferin†; Cardiprin; Cartia; Disprin; Disprin Direct; Ecotrin; Solprin; Spren; SRA†; Vincent's Powders; Winsprin†; ***Belg.:*** Acenterine; Asaflow; Asarid; Aspirine; Aspro; Catalgix; Dispril; Dolean†; Rhodine; Rhonal; ***Canad.:*** Asaphen; Aspergum; Aspirin Plus Stomach Guard; Bufferin; Coryphen; Ecotrin†; Entrophen; Headache Tablets; Novasen; ***Fr.:*** Actispirine†; Aspro; Catalgine; Claragine; Juvepirine; Rhonal; Sargepirine; ***Ger.:*** Acesal; Acesal Calcium; Acetylin; Apernyl†; Aspalox†; Aspro; ASS; Bonakiddi†; Bonfal†; Colfarit†; Contradol†; Contrheuma†; Gepan†; Godamed; Hermes ASS; HerzASS; Melabon†; Micristin; Miniasal; monobeltin†; Protectin-OPT†; Sanocapt†; Santasal N; Spalt; Temagin ASS†; Togal ASS; ***Irl.:*** Ascriptin; Aspro; Caprin; Claradin†; Clonteric; Disprin; Lowasa; Nu-Seals; Resprin; ***Ital.:*** Acesal; Apernyl†; Ascriptin; Aspergum†; Aspiglicina; Aspirina; Aspirina 03; Aspirina 05; Aspirinetta; Aspro; Bufferin; Cardioaspirin; Cemirit; Domupirina†; Dreimal†; Endydol†; Kilios; Kynosina†; Rectosalyl†; ***Neth.:*** Aspro; Rhonal†; ***Norw.:*** Albyl-E; Bamycor; Dispril; Globentyl; Globoid; Novid; ***S.Afr.:*** ASAtard; Aspro; Disprin; Ecotrin; ***Spain:*** AAS; Adiro; Algho; Asboi†; Aspidolce†; Aspinfantil; Aspirina; Aspro; Biontop†; Bioplak; Calmantina; Dulcipirina†; Helver Sal; Mejoral Infantil; Okal Infantil; Orravina; Rhonal; Saspryl; Tromalyt; Upsalgina; ***Swed.:*** Acetard†; Albyl minor; Asaferm†; Asalite†; Bamycor; Bamyl; Dispril; Magnecyl; Reumyl†; Trombyl; ***Switz.:*** Aspro; Colfarit†; Demoprin nouvelle formule; Dolean pH 8†; Enterosarine†; Rhonal†; Tiatral 100 SR; Togal ASS; ***UK:*** Angettes; Aspro; Beechams Lemon Tablets; Caprin; Disprin; Disprin Direct; Enprin; Fynnon Calcium Aspirin; Nu-Seals; Phensic Soluble†; Platet†; PostMI; ***USA:*** 8-Hour Bayer Timed-Release; Adprin-B; Arthritis Foundation Pain Reliever; Arthritis Pain Formula; Arthritis Pain Tablets; ASA†; Ascriptin; Aspergum; Asprimox; Bayer Low Adult Strength; Bufferin; Buffex; Cama Arthritis Pain Reliever; Easprin; Ecotrin; Empirin; Extra Strength Bayer Plus; Extra Strength Tri-Buffered Bufferin†; Genprin; Halfprin; Heartline; Magnaprin; Norwich Extra Strength; Regular Strength Bayer; St. Joseph Adult Chewable; ZORprin.

Multi-ingredient: numerous preparations are listed in Part 3.

Auranofin (5293-j)

Auranofin *(BAN, USAN, rINN).*

SKF-39162; SKF-D-39162. (1-Thio-β-D-glucopyranosato)(triethylphosphine)gold 2,3,4,6-tetra-acetate.

$C_{20}H_{34}AuO_9PS$ = 678.5.

CAS — 34031-32-8.

Auranofin has a gold content of about 29%.

Adverse Effects and Treatment

The most common adverse effects of auranofin involve the gastro-intestinal tract with nausea, abdominal pain, and sometimes vomiting, but most often diarrhoea which can affect up to 50% of patients and may be severe enough to cause patients to withdraw from treatment. Other adverse effects are similar to those experienced with sodium aurothiomalate (p.83), although they appear to be less troublesome in that fewer patients have been reported to discontinue treatment with auranofin than with injectable gold. As with other gold salts, treatment of adverse effects is generally symptomatic (see p.84). A bulking agent such as bran or modifying the diet to increase bulk or a temporary reduction in dosage may help the diarrhoea.

Reviews.

1. Tozman ECS, Gottlieb NL. Adverse reactions with oral and parenteral gold preparations. *Med Toxicol* 1987; **2:** 177–89.

Effects on the gastro-intestinal tract. Diarrhoea and abdominal pain are frequent adverse effects in patients taking auranofin. The mechanism of gastro-intestinal toxicity has not been established but may be associated with a reversible defect in intestinal permeability.[1] Colitis and eosinophilia have been reported in a patient taking auranofin.[2]

1. Behrens R, *et al.* Investigation of auranofin-induced diarrhoea. *Gut* 1986; **27:** 59–65.
2. Michet CJ, *et al.* Auranofin-associated colitis and eosinophilia. *Mayo Clin Proc* 1987; **62:** 142–4.

Effects on the kidneys. In a retrospective review[1] of 1283 patients who had received auranofin for treatment of rheumatoid arthritis 41 were found to have developed proteinuria. Treatment of proteinuria in the majority of patients consisted of discontinuing auranofin therapy. Long-term follow-up of 36 patients indicated that proteinuria had resolved in 31 patients within 2 years and in 29 patients within 1 year. Seven of 8 patients later rechallenged with auranofin had no relapses. In a further review of 2 comparative double-blind studies using gold compounds in the treatment of rheumatoid arthritis, proteinuria was found to have developed in 27% (23 of 85) of patients treated with sodium aurothiomalate, in 17% (42 of 247) of those treated with auranofin, and in 17% (36 of 210) of those receiving placebo. All patients were receiving NSAIDs.

1. Katz WA, *et al.* Proteinuria in gold-treated rheumatoid arthritis. *Ann Intern Med* 1984; **101:** 176–9.

Precautions

As for Sodium Aurothiomalate, p.84. Urine and blood tests should be carried out monthly. Auranofin should be administered with caution to patients with inflammatory bowel disease.

Interactions

As for Sodium Aurothiomalate, p.84.

Pharmacokinetics

Auranofin is incompletely absorbed from the gastro-intestinal tract, only about 25% of the gold being absorbed. Gold from auranofin is bound to plasma proteins as well as to red blood cells. After 2 to 3 months of treatment the steady-state serum concentration of gold is reported to be about 0.5 μg per mL. The average terminal plasma half-life of gold at steady state is about 26 days while the biological half-life is 81 days. Tissue retention and total gold accumulation in the body are less than with intramuscular gold. Gold from auranofin penetrates into synovial fluid.

Most of a dose of auranofin appears in the faeces due to its poor absorption. About 60% of the absorbed gold from auranofin is excreted in the urine and the remainder in the faeces.

Reviews.

1. Blocka KLN, *et al.* Clinical pharmacokinetics of oral and injectable gold compounds. *Clin Pharmacokinet* 1986; **11:** 133–43.

Uses and Administration

Auranofin has similar actions and uses to those of sodium aurothiomalate (p.84). It is given by mouth in progressive rheumatoid arthritis (p.2); such oral treatment is less toxic than intramuscular gold but is also much less effective. The usual initial dose of auranofin is 6 mg daily either as a single dose or in two divided doses. Treatment should be continued for at least 6 months to assess the response; the dose may be increased after 6 months, if the response is inadequate, to 3 mg three times daily. If the response is still inadequate after 3 months at this dosage, then treatment should be discontinued.

Asthma. Auranofin is not usually used in the management of asthma (p.745) but studies[1] indicate that it can have a corticosteroid-sparing effect.

1. Bernstein IL, *et al.* A placebo-controlled multicenter study of auranofin in the treatment of patients with corticosteroid-dependent asthma. *J Allergy Clin Immunol* 1996; **98;** 317–24.

Lupus. Since the introduction of less toxic drugs gold salts are now rarely used in the treatment of systemic lupus erythematosus (p.1029), however, there have been anecdotal reports suggesting that auranofin may still be of use in patients with discoid lupus erythematosus[1] or cutaneous lupus erythematosus[2] refractory to conventional treatment.

1. Dalziel K, *et al.* Treatment of chronic discoid lupus erythematosus with an oral gold compound (auranofin). *Br J Dermatol* 1986; **115:** 211–16.
2. Farrell AM, Bunker CB. Oral gold therapy in cutaneous lupus erythematosus (revisited). *Br J Dermatol* 1996; **135** (suppl 47): 41.

Psoriasis. Although efficacy for topical auranofin in the treatment of plaque-type psoriasis (p.1075) has been demonstrated in a placebo-controlled study,[1] the high incidence of adverse skin reactions, such as contact dermatitis, was thought to outweigh any benefit.

1. Helm KF, *et al.* Topical auranofin ointment for the treatment of plaque psoriasis. *J Am Acad Dermatol* 1995; **33:** 517–19.

Preparations

Proprietary Preparations (details are given in Part 3)
Aust.: Ridaura; ***Austral.:*** Ridaura; ***Belg.:*** Ridaura; ***Canad.:*** Ridaura; ***Fr.:*** Ridauran; ***Ger.:*** Ridaura; ***Irl.:*** Ridaura; ***Ital.:*** Crisofin†; Ridaura; ***Neth.:*** Ridaura; ***Norw.:*** Ridaura; ***S.Afr.:*** Ridaura; ***Spain:*** Crisinor; Ridaura; ***Swed.:*** Ridaura; ***Switz.:*** Ridaura; ***UK:*** Ridaura; ***USA:*** Ridaura.

Aurothioglucose (5294-z)

1-Aurothio-D-glucopyranose; (D-Glucosylthio)gold; Gold Thioglucose. (1-Thio-D-glucopyranosato)gold.

$C_6H_{11}AuO_5S = 392.2.$

CAS — 12192-57-3.

Pharmacopoeias. In US.

A yellow odourless or almost odourless powder. Freely **soluble** in water; practically insoluble in alcohol, acetone, chloroform, and ether. It is stabilised by the addition of a small amount of sodium acetate. A 1% solution in water has a pH of about 6.3. Aqueous solutions are unstable on long standing. **Store** in airtight containers. Protect from light.

Aurothioglucose has a gold content of about 50%.

Adverse Effects, Treatment, and Precautions

As for Sodium Aurothiomalate, p.83.

Interactions

As for Sodium Aurothiomalate, p.84.

Pharmacokinetics

As for Sodium Aurothiomalate, p.84; absorption is slower and more irregular.

Uses and Administration

Aurothioglucose has similar actions and uses to those of sodium aurothiomalate (p.84). It is used in the treatment of rheumatoid arthritis (p.2) and juvenile chronic arthritis (p.2). Aurothioglucose is administered intramuscularly as a suspension in oil in arthritic disorders in an initial weekly dose of 10 mg increasing gradually to 50 mg weekly. Therapy is continued at weekly intervals until a total dose of 0.8 to 1 g has been given; if improvement has occurred at this stage with no signs of toxicity 50 mg may then be given at intervals of 3 or 4 weeks. Children, 6 to 12 years, may be given one-quarter the adult dose, to a maximum of 25 mg per dose.

Preparations

USP 23: Aurothioglucose Injectable Suspension.

Proprietary Preparations (details are given in Part 3)
Austral.: Gold-50; ***Canad.:*** Solganal; ***Ger.:*** Aureotan; ***Neth.:*** Auromyose; ***USA:*** Solganal.

Aurotioprol (12407-d)

Sodium 3-aurothio-2-hydroxypropane-1-sulphonate.

$C_3H_6AuNaO_4S_2 = 390.2.$

CAS — 27279-43-2.

Aurotioprol has a gold content of about 50%.

Aurotioprol is a gold compound with similar actions and uses to those of sodium aurothiomalate (p.83). It is given by intramuscular injection for the treatment of rheumatoid arthritis (p.2). The initial dose is 25 mg weekly, increased to 50 to 100 mg weekly, until a total dose of 1.2 to 1.5 g has been given. This may be followed by a dose of 50 to 100 mg intramuscularly every month.

Preparations

Proprietary Preparations (details are given in Part 3)
Belg.: Allochrysine; ***Fr.:*** Allochrysine.

Azapropazone (2610-w)

Azapropazone *(BAN, rINN).*

AHR-3018; Apazone *(USAN)*; Mi85; NSC-102824. 5-Dimethylamino-9-methyl-2-propylpyrazolo[1,2-*a*][1,2,4]benzotriazine-1,3(2*H*)-dione.

$C_{16}H_{20}N_4O_2 = 300.4.$

CAS — 13539-59-8.

Pharmacopoeias. In Br.

A white to pale yellow, crystalline powder. Very slightly **soluble** in water and in chloroform; soluble in alcohol; dissolves in solutions of alkali hydroxides.

Adverse Effects

As for NSAIDs in general, p.63.

Some adverse effects appear to be more common with azapropazone than with other NSAIDs. Analysis of spontaneous reporting of adverse reactions to the UK Committee on Safety of Medicines revealed that azapropazone had been associated with the highest risk of gastro-intestinal reactions compared with 6 other NSAIDs, as well as with a relatively high frequency of renal, hepatic, allergic, and haematological reactions.[1]

1. Committee on Safety of Medicines/Medicines Control Agency. *Current Problems* 1994; **20:** 9–11.

Effects on the blood. The Committee on Safety of Medicines (CSM) in the UK had received 6 reports of Coombs positive haemolytic anaemia associated with azapropazone between January 1984 and March 1985 and the manufacturers 6 reports of auto-immune haemolysis over 10 years.[1] One group of workers[2] who reported haemolytic anaemia and reversible pulmonary infiltration, suggestive of an allergic or immune reaction, in 3 patients noted that since 1976 the CSM had received 18 reports of haemolytic anaemia and 11 reports of allergic alveolitis, pulmonary fibrosis, or fibrosing alveolitis. Fatal haemolytic anaemia has subsequently been reported in one patient.[3]

1. Chan-Lam D, *et al.* Red cell antibodies and autoimmune haemolysis after treatment with azapropazone. *Br Med J* 1986; **293:** 1474.
2. Albazzaz MK, *et al.* Alveolitis and haemolytic anaemia induced by azapropazone. *Br Med J* 1986; **293:** 1537–8.
3. Montgomery RD, Babb RG. Alveolitis and haemolytic anaemia induced by azapropazone. *Br Med J* 1987; **294:** 375.

Effects on the gastro-intestinal tract. In a review[1] of the relative safety of 7 oral NSAIDs, the UK Committee on Safety of Medicines commented that azapropazone was associated with the highest risk of gastro-intestinal reactions in both epidemiological studies and an analysis of spontaneous reporting of adverse reactions. Although it appeared that some patients over 60 years of age had received doses exceeding those recommended for this age group it was considered that even when this was taken into account a marked difference remained between gastro-intestinal reactions for azapropazone compared with other NSAIDs. The Committee recommended that azapropazone should be restricted for use in rheumatoid arthritis, ankylosing spondylitis and acute gout and only when other NSAIDs have been ineffective. Its use in patients with a history of peptic ulceration was contra-indicated. It was also recommended that when used in patients over 60 years of age for rheumatoid arthritis or ankylosing spondylitis the dose should be restricted to a maximum of 600 mg daily.

1. Committee on Safety of Medicines/Medicines Control Agency. *Current Problems* 1994; **20:** 9–11.

Effects on the kidneys. Acute interstitial nephritis (one patient)[1] and reversible non-oliguric renal failure (one patient)[2] have been reported during treatment with azapropazone.

1. Sipilä R, *et al.* Acute renal failure during azapropazone therapy. *Mayo Clin Proc* 1983; **58:** 209–10.
2. Goldstein AJ, Grech P. Reversible non-oliguric renal failure during treatment with low dose azapropazone. *Br Med J* 1986; **293:** 698.

Effects on the liver. Hepatitis and erythema multiforme developed in one patient 2 to 3 weeks after starting azapropazone for osteoarthritis.[1]

1. Lo TCN, Dymock IW. Azapropazone induced hepatitis. *Br Med J* 1988; **297:** 1614.

Effects on the lungs. See under Effects on the Blood, above.

Effects on the skin. Of 917 reports of adverse reactions associated with azapropazone forwarded to the WHO Collaborating Centre for International Drug Monitoring[1] before September 1984, 190 (21%) were of photosensitivity. Of 154 reports of photosensitivity evaluated a causal relationship to use of azapropazone was considered certain in 6, probable in 138, and possible in 10. In May 1994 the Committee on Safety of Medicines in the UK stated[2] that since 1976 they had received 464 reports of photosensitivity reactions associated with azapropazone and commented that, when corrected for prescription volume, reporting of this reaction was 50 times greater than with other commonly prescribed NSAIDs. They recommended that patients should be advised to avoid direct exposure to sunlight or to use sunblock preparations.

1. Olsson S, *et al.* Photosensitivity during treatment with azapropazone. *Br Med J* 1985; **291:** 939.
2. Committee on Safety of Medicines/Medicines Control Agency. Photosensitivity associated with azapropazone (Rheumox). *Current Problems* 1994; **20:** 6.

Precautions

As for NSAIDs in general, p.65. Azapropazone is also contra-indicated in patients with a history or evidence of peptic ulceration, inflammatory bowel disorders, or blood disorders. Reduced doses should be given to elderly patients and patients with renal impairment; its use should be avoided in patients with severe renal impairment. Its use should also be avoided in breast-feeding mothers.

Patients should be advised to avoid direct exposure to sunlight or to use sunblock preparations.

Porphyria. Azapropazone was considered to be unsafe in patients with acute porphyria because it has been shown to be porphyrinogenic in *animal* or *in-vitro* systems.[1]

1. Moore MR, McColl KEL. *Porphyria: drug lists.* Glasgow: Porphyria Research Unit, University of Glasgow, 1991.

Interactions

For interactions associated with NSAIDs, see p.65.

Pharmacokinetics

Azapropazone is absorbed from the gastro-intestinal tract and peak plasma concentrations are reached about 4 hours after administration. It is highly protein bound. A half-life of 12 to 24 hours has been reported. Azapropazone is excreted in the urine as unchanged drug (about 65%), 8-hydroxyazapropazone, and glucuronide or sulphate metabolites. Very small amounts are excreted in breast milk.

References.

1. Bald R, *et al.* Excretion of azapropazone in human breast milk. *Eur J Clin Pharmacol* 1990; **39:** 271–3.

Uses and Administration

Azapropazone is an NSAID (see p.65), structurally related to phenylbutazone (p.79). It also has uricosuric properties. Because azapropazone appears to be associated with a higher incidence of adverse effects than with some other NSAIDs its use in the UK is restricted to the treatment of rheumatoid arthritis, ankylosing spondylitis, and acute gout in patients for whom other NSAIDs have been ineffective.

For the treatment of rheumatoid arthritis or ankylosing spondylitis the usual dose in the UK is 1.2 g daily in 2 or 4 divided doses by mouth. Patients over 60 years of age or those with reduced renal function may be given 300 mg twice daily but azapropazone should be avoided in patients with severe renal impairment.

Usually uricosuric drugs should not be given during an acute attack of gout as they may prolong its duration, but azapropazone appears to be suitable for the treatment of acute gout. In acute gout 1.8 g may be given daily in divided doses until the attack is resolving (usually by the fourth day), then reduced to 1.2 g daily until symptoms have disappeared. An adequate fluid intake should be maintained. If symptoms persist appropriate alternative treatment (see p.390) should be considered. For elderly patients and those with reduced renal function, as long as they have a creatinine clearance of 60 mL or more per minute, the dose is 1.8 g daily in divided doses for the first 24 hours followed by 1.2 g daily. This should be reduced as soon as possible to a maximum of 600 mg daily.

Azapropazone has been given intravenously in some countries.

Preparations

BP 1998: Azapropazone Capsules; Azapropazone Tablets.

Proprietary Preparations (details are given in Part 3)
Aust.: Prolixan; ***Ger.:*** Prolixan†; Tolyprin; ***Irl.:*** Rheumox; ***Neth.:*** Prolixan; ***S.Afr.:*** Rheumox†; ***Swed.:*** Prolixana; ***Switz.:*** Prolixan; ***UK:*** Rheumox.

Multi-ingredient: ***Aust.:*** Algo-Prolixan; Myo-Prolixan†; ***Ger.:*** Dolo-Prolixan†; ***Switz.:*** Dolo-Prolixan.

Bendazac (2614-j)

Bendazac *(BAN, USAN, rINN).*

AF-983; Bindazac. (1-Benzyl-1*H*-indazol-3-yloxy)acetic acid.

$C_{16}H_{14}N_2O_3$ = 282.3.
CAS — 20187-55-7.

Bendazac Lysine (16536-a)

Bendazac Lysine *(BANM, rINNM).*

AF-1934. L-Lysine-(1-benzyl-1*H*-indazol-3-yloxy)acetic acid.

$C_{22}H_{28}N_4O_5$ = 428.5.
CAS — 81919-14-4.

Bendazac is an NSAID (p.63) structurally related to indomethacin (p.45). It has been used topically in preparations containing 1 and 3% for the treatment of various inflammatory skin disorders.

Bendazac lysine has been used in the management of cataract, 2 drops of a 0.5% solution being instilled three times daily. It has also been given by mouth for similar purposes.

References.

1. Balfour JA, Clissold SP. Bendazac lysine: a review of its pharmacological properties and therapeutic potential in the management of cataracts. *Drugs* 1990; **39:** 575–96.

Preparations

Proprietary Preparations (details are given in Part 3)
Aust.: Versus; ***Ital.:*** Bendalina; Versus; ***Spain:*** Bendalina†.

Benorylate (2611-e)

Benorylate *(BAN).*

Benorilate *(rINN)*; FAW-76; Fenasprate; Win-11450. 4-Acetamidophenyl *O*-acetylsalicylate.

$C_{17}H_{15}NO_5$ = 313.3.
CAS — 5003-48-5.

Pharmacopoeias. In *Br.*

A white or almost white, odourless or almost odourless, crystalline powder. Practically **insoluble** in water; sparingly soluble in alcohol and in methyl alcohol; soluble in acetone and in chloroform.

Adverse Effects, Treatment, and Precautions

As for Aspirin, p.16, and Paracetamol, p.72.

Benorylate may cause nausea, indigestion, heartburn, and constipation; drowsiness, diarrhoea, and skin rashes have also been reported. Some patients have experienced dizziness, tinnitus, and deafness associated with high blood-salicylate concentrations.

Benorylate, like aspirin (see p.17), should not generally be given to children under the age of 12 years because of the risk of Reye's syndrome.

When an overdose of benorylate is suspected, it has been suggested that plasma concentrations of both salicylate and paracetamol should be measured since a normal plasma-paracetamol concentration cannot necessarily be assumed from a normal plasma-salicylate measurement.

References.

1. Aylward M. Toxicity of benorylate. *Br Med J* 1973; **2:** 118.
2. Symon DNK, *et al.* Fatal paracetamol poisoning from benorylate therapy in child with cystic fibrosis. *Lancet* 1982; **ii:** 1153–4.

Interactions

For the interactions associated with aspirin, see p.17, and for those associated with paracetamol, see p.74.

Pharmacokinetics

Benorylate is slowly absorbed virtually unchanged from the gastro-intestinal tract. Following absorption, benorylate is rapidly metabolised to salicylate and paracetamol. It is excreted mainly as metabolites of salicylic acid and paracetamol in the urine.

Uses and Administration

Benorylate is an aspirin-paracetamol ester with analgesic, anti-inflammatory, and antipyretic properties. It is used in the treatment of mild to moderate pain (p.4) and fever (p.1). It is also used in osteoarthritis (p.2), rheumatoid arthritis (p.2), and soft-tissue rheumatism (p.4). Benorylate is given by mouth, preferably after food, in doses of 2 g twice daily for mild to moderate pain and fever. Doses for osteoarthritis, quiescent rheumatoid arthritis, and soft-tissue rheumatism are up to 6 g daily in divided doses. In active rheumatoid arthritis 4 g twice daily may be required. In elderly patients reduced doses of 2 g twice daily or possibly 2 g in the morning and 4 g at night should be given; a maximum daily dose of 6 g should not be exceeded.

Preparations

BP 1998: Benorilate Oral Suspension; Benorilate Tablets.

Proprietary Preparations (details are given in Part 3)
Belg.: Benortan†; Duvium; ***Fr.:*** Longalgic; Salipran; ***Ger.:*** Benortan†; ***Irl.:*** Benoral; ***Ital.:*** Bentum†; ***Neth.:*** Benortan†; ***Spain:*** Doline; Vetedol; ***Switz.:*** Benortan†; Duvium; ***UK:*** Benoral.

Benoxaprofen (2612-l)

Benoxaprofen *(BAN, USAN, rINN).*

Compound 90459; LRCL-3794. 2-[2-(4-Chlorophenyl)benzoxazol-5-yl]propionic acid.

$C_{16}H_{12}ClNO_3$ = 301.7.
CAS — 51234-28-7.

Benoxaprofen is an NSAID (p.63) structurally related to ibuprofen (p.44). It was formerly given by mouth in rheumatoid arthritis and osteoarthritis but because of reports of adverse reactions and fatalities the manufacturers halted worldwide marketing in the early 1980s, of the preparation known as Opren. Side-effects that have occurred with benoxaprofen include skin disorders, notably photosensitivity reactions but also erythema multiforme and the Stevens-Johnson syndrome, onycholysis and other nail disorders, gastro-intestinal disturbances including peptic ulceration and bleeding, blood disorders such as thrombocytopenia, cholestatic jaundice and other liver or biliary disorders, and renal failure.

Benzydamine Hydrochloride

(2613-y)

Benzydamine Hydrochloride *(BANM, USAN, rINNM).*

AF-864; Benzindamine Hydrochloride. 3-(1-Benzyl-1*H*-indazol-3-yloxy)-*NN*-dimethylpropylamine hydrochloride.

$C_{19}H_{23}N_3O,HCl$ = 345.9.

CAS — 642-72-8 (benzydamine); 132-69-4 (benzydamine hydrochloride).

Pharmacopoeias. In *Br.* and *Pol.*

A white crystalline powder. Very **soluble** in water; freely soluble in alcohol and in chloroform; practically insoluble in ether. A 10% solution in water has a pH of 4.0 to 5.5.

Adverse Effects

Following topical application to the skin local reactions such as erythema or rash may occur and photosensitivity has been reported. Following use as mouth and throat preparations, numbness or stinging sensations of the oral mucosa have been reported.

Effects on the kidneys. A 57-year-old woman who had used 400 g of a topical cream containing benzydamine hydrochloride 3% over a period of 4 months was found to have raised plasma concentrations of creatinine and urea consistent with a substantial reduction in glomerular filtration rate.[1]

1. O'Callaghan CA, *et al.* Renal disease and use of topical non-steroidal anti-inflammatory drugs. *Br Med J* 1994; **308:** 110–11.

Uses and Administration

Benzydamine hydrochloride is an NSAID (p.65). It is used topically on the skin in concentrations of 3 to 5% in painful musculoskeletal and soft-tissue disorders. Benzydamine hydrochloride is also used as a mouthwash or spray in concentrations of 0.15% for the relief of inflammatory conditions of the mouth and throat. It has also been given by mouth, rectally, or by intramuscular or intravenous injection for the relief of painful and inflammatory conditions, and as a solution for vaginal irrigation.

Benzydamine salicylate (benzasal) has been used topically on the skin as a 6% cream or spray.

Mouth disorders. Results of a randomised placebo-controlled study in patients undergoing radiotherapy for oropharyngeal cancer indicated that benzydamine as an oral rinse was effective in reducing the area and severity of mucositis.[1] Benzydamine has been used locally for the management of mouth ulcers (p.1172) although one study[2] found it no more useful than placebo.

1. Epstein JB, *et al.* Prevention of oral mucositis in radiation therapy: a controlled study with benzydamine hydrochloride rinse. *Int J Radiat Oncol Biol Phys* 1989; **16:** 1571–5.
2. Matthews RW, *et al.* Clinical evaluation of benzydamine, chlorhexidine, and placebo mouthwashes in the management of recurrent aphthous stomatitis. *Oral Surg Oral Med Oral Pathol* 1987; **63:** 189–91.

Preparations

BP 1998: Benzydamine Cream; Benzydamine Mouthwash; Benzydamine Oromucosal Spray.

Proprietary Preparations (details are given in Part 3)
Aust.: Tantum; ***Austral.:*** Difflam; Difflam Anti-inflammatory Solution; Difflam Anti-inflammatory Throat Spray; ***Canad.:*** Sun-Benz; Tantum; ***Fr.:*** Opalgyne; ***Ger.:*** Tantum Verde; ***Irl.:*** Difflam; ***Ital.:*** Afloben; Benzirin; Flogaton†; Ginesal; Multum; Saniflor Dentifricio; Saniflor Vena; Tantum; Verax; ***Neth.:*** Tantum†; ***S.Afr.:*** Andolex; Tantum†; ***Spain:*** Fulgium; Rosalgin; Tantum; Tantum Verde; ***Swed.:*** Andolex; ***Switz.:*** Bucco-Tantum; Rhino-Tantum†; Tantum†; ***UK:*** Difflam.

Multi-ingredient: ***Austral.:*** Difflam Anti-inflammatory Antiseptic Mouth Gel; Difflam Anti-Inflammatory Cough Lozenges; Difflam Anti-inflammatory Lozenges; Difflam Dental†; Difflam-C; ***Fr.:*** Hexo-Imotryl; ***Ital.:*** Algolisina; Leucorsan; Linea F; ***S.Afr.:*** Andolex-C; ***Spain:*** Bristaciclina Dental; Dolosarto; Etermol Antitusivo; Maxilase Antibiotica†; Mentamida; Prosturol; Sinus†; Tantum; Tantum Ciclina; Vinciseptil Otico.

Benzyl Nicotinate (9212-g)

Benzyl pyridine-3-carboxylate.

$C_{13}H_{11}NO_2$ = 213.2.

CAS — 94-44-0.

Pharmacopoeias. In *Ger.*

Benzyl nicotinate is used in topical preparations as a rubefacient.

Preparations

Proprietary Preparations (details are given in Part 3)

Ger.: Dermotherma N†; Kausalpunkt N†; Pykaryl T; Rheubalmin Bad Nico; Rubriment.

Multi-ingredient: ***Aust.:*** Ambenat; Bayolin; Derivon; Expectal-Balsam; Forapin; Igitur-antirheumatische; Igitur-Rheumafluid†; Menthoneurin; Mobilisin plus; Pelvichthol; Pilowal†; Rheumex; Rubizon-Rheumagel; Rubriment; Thermo-Rheumon; Thrombophob; Tifenso; ***Austral.:*** Pergalen†; ***Belg.:*** Bayoline†; Forapin; Thrombophob†; ***Fr.:*** Bayoline†; Lumbalgine; Pergalen†; ***Ger.:*** ABC Warme-Salbe; ABC-Bad†; Akrotherm; Algonerg†; Amasin†; Ambene N; Arthrodestal N; Auroanalin; Bartelin nico; Bayolin†; Brachialin percutan N; Brachont; Camphopin; Capsamol; Caye Balsam; Contrheuma; Cor-Select; Cuxaflex N; Cuxaflex Thermo; Cycloarthrin†; Dolo-Exhirud†; Dolo-Menthoneurin Cre-Sa; Dolo-Rubriment; Dolorgiet; DoloVisano Salbe; Emasex-N; Etrat Sportsalbe†; Expectal Balsam†; exrheudon OPT; Fibraflex N†; Fibraflex-W-Creme N†; Fibraflex†; Flexocutan N†; Forapin E; Glutisal-buton-Salbe†; Glutisal†; Heilit; Hot Thermo; Hyperiagil†; Ichtho-Himbin†; Intradermi Fluid N; Judolor†; K_5 "spezial"†; Keptan S†; Lomazell forte N; Marament Balsam W; Mediment†; Menthoneurin-Vollbad N; mikanil N; Mussera†; Myalgol N; Mydalgan†; Nitro-Praecordin N; Ortholan mit Salicylester; Ostochont; Pelvichthol N; Percutase N; Pergalen†; Pernionin; Pernionin Teil-Bad N; Pernionin Voll-Bad N; Phardol 10†; Phardol N Balsam†; Phardol Rheuma; Phlogont-Thermal; Praecordin S; Reumaless; Rheu-Do†; Rheubalmin; Rheubalmin Thermo; Rheuma Bad; Rheuma Liquidum; rheuma-loges N Balsam†; Rheuma-Salbe; Rheuma-Salbe Lichtenstein; rheumamed†; Rheumasalbe; Rheumasan N; Rheumasan†; Rheumasit; Rheumex†; Rheumyl N†; Rheumyl†; Riker Sport†; Rosarthron forte; Rubriment; Rubriment-N; Salhumin Gel N; Salirheuman†; Segmentocut Thermo; Spolera therm†; stadasan Thermo†; Tachynerg N; Terbintil†; Thermo Mobilisin; thermo-loges; Thermo-Menthoneurin; Thermo-Menthoneurin Bad; Thermo-Rheumon; Thermosan†; Thermosenex; Turgostad†; Vehiculan NF†; Venothromb†; Warme-Gel; Zuk Thermo; ***Irl.:*** Bayolin†; ***Ital.:*** Lasoreuma; Salonpas; Sloan; ***Neth.:*** Menthoneurin; Sloan's balsem; ***S.Afr.:*** Forapin†; Thrombophob; ***Swed.:*** Remysal N†; ***Switz.:*** Artragel; Assan-Thermo; Brachialin†; Demotherm Pommade contre le rhumatisme; Dolo Demotherm; Forapin; Histalgane; Incutin; Marament-N; Neo-Liniment†; Roliwol S; Thermocutan; ***UK:*** Bayolin†; Salonair.

Bezitramide (6208-s)

Bezitramide *(BAN, rINN).*

R-4845. 4-[4-(2,3-Dihydro-2-oxo-3-propionyl-1*H*-benzimidazol-1-yl)piperidino]-2,2-diphenylbutyronitrile.

$C_{31}H_{32}N_4O_2$ = 492.6.

CAS — 15301-48-1.

Bezitramide is an opioid analgesic (p.67) which has been given by mouth in daily doses of 5 to 15 mg in the treatment of severe pain. Its action is slow in onset, but prolonged.

References.

1. Meijer DKF, *et al.* Pharmacokinetics of the oral narcotic analgesic bezitramide and preliminary observations on its effect on experimentally induced pain. *Eur J Clin Pharmacol* 1984; **27:** 615–18.

Preparations

Proprietary Preparations (details are given in Part 3)

Belg.: Burgodin; ***Neth.:*** Burgodin†.

Bornyl Salicylate (11271-z)

Borneol Salicylate. 2-Hydroxybenzoic acid 1,7,7-trimethylbicyclo[2.2.1]hept-2-yl ester.

$C_{17}H_{22}O_3$ = 274.4.

CAS — 560-88-3.

Bornyl salicylate is a salicylic acid derivative that is used topically in rubefacient preparations similarly to methyl salicylate (p.55) for the relief of pain in musculoskeletal and joint disorders.

Preparations

Proprietary Preparations (details are given in Part 3)

Multi-ingredient: ***Aust.:*** Forapin; ***Belg.:*** Forapin; ***Ger.:*** Contrheuma-Gel forte N; Forapin E; Terbintil†; ***S.Afr.:*** Forapin†; ***Switz.:*** Acidodermil; Forapin; Hygiodermil; Sedodermil.

Bromfenac Sodium (2896-k)

Bromfenac Sodium *(USAN, rINNM).*

AHR-10282; AHR-10282B. Sodium [2-amino-3-(*p*-bromobenzoyl)phenyl]acetate sesquihydrate.

$C_{15}H_{11}BrNNaO_3,1\frac{1}{2}H_2O$ = 383.2.

CAS — 91714-94-2 (bromfenac); 91714-93-1 (bromfenac sodium); 120638-55-3 (bromfenac sodium).

Bromfenac sodium, a phenylacetic acid derivative related to diclofenac (p.31), is an NSAID (p.63). It was withdrawn from the market following reports of severe and sometimes fatal hepatic failure.

Preparations

Proprietary Preparations (details are given in Part 3)

USA: Duract†.

Bufexamac (2618-a)

Bufexamac *(BAN, rINN).*

Bufexamacum. 2-(4-Butoxyphenyl)acetohydroxamic acid.

$C_{12}H_{17}NO_3$ = 223.3.

CAS — 2438-72-4.

Pharmacopoeias. In *Eur.* (see p.viii) and *Jpn.*

A white or almost white, crystalline powder. Practically **insoluble** in water; soluble in dimethylformamide; slightly soluble in ethyl acetate and in methyl alcohol. **Protect** from light.

Bufexamac is an NSAID (p.63) that is applied topically in concentrations of 5% in various skin disorders. Stinging and burning may occur after application; hypersensitivity reactions have been reported.

Preparations

Proprietary Preparations (details are given in Part 3)

Aust.: Bufexan; Droxaryl; Flogocid†; Parfenac; ***Austral.:*** Paraderm; ***Belg.:*** Bufexine; Droxaryl; ***Canad.:*** Norfemac; ***Fr.:*** Bufal; Calmaderm; Parfenac; ***Ger.:*** Allergipuran N; Bufederm; duradermal; Ekzemase; Jomax; Logomed Ekzem-Salbe; Malipuran; Parfenac; Windol; ***Ital.:*** Parfenal; Viafen; ***Neth.:*** Droxaryl†; Parfenac; ***S.Afr.:*** Parfenac; ***Switz.:*** Flogocid; Parfenac; ***UK:*** Parfenac†.

Multi-ingredient: ***Austral.:*** Fungo; Paraderm Plus; ***Belg.:*** Flogocid; ***Ger.:*** Bufeproct; Haemomac; Logomed Hamorrhoiden; Mastu S; Proctoparf; ***Switz.:*** Flogocid NN.

Bumadizone Calcium (2619-t)

Bumadizone Calcium *(rINNM).*

Calcium 2-(1,2-diphenylhydrazinocarbonyl)hexanoate hemihydrate.

$(C_{19}H_{21}N_2O_3)_2Ca,\frac{1}{2}H_2O$ = 699.8.

CAS — 3583-64-0 (bumadizone); 34461-73-9 (bumadizone calcium).

Bumadizone calcium is an NSAID (p.63) that is reported to be metabolised to phenylbutazone (p.79) and oxyphenbutazone (p.72). Its use was limited by the risk of agranulocytosis and other haematological adverse effects.

Preparations

Proprietary Preparations (details are given in Part 3)

Ger.: Rheumatol†; ***S.Afr.:*** Eumotol†.

Buprenorphine (19995-d)

Buprenorphine *(BAN).*

Buprenorphinum; RX-6029-M. (6*R*,7*R*,14*S*)-17-Cyclopropylmethyl-7,8-dihydro-7-[(1*S*)-1-hydroxy-1,2,2-trimethylpropyl]-6-*O*-methyl-6,14-ethano-17-normorphine; (2*S*)-2-[(−)-(5*R*,6*R*,7*R*,14*S*)-9a-Cyclopropylmethyl-4,5-epoxy-3-hydroxy-6-methoxy-6,14-ethanomorphinan-7-yl]-3,3-dimethylbutan-2-ol.

$C_{29}H_{41}NO_4$ = 467.6.

CAS — 52485-79-7.

Pharmacopoeias. In *Eur.* (see p.viii).

A white or almost white crystalline powder. Very slightly **soluble** in water; freely soluble in acetone; soluble in methyl alcohol; slightly soluble in cyclohexane. It dissolves in dilute solutions of acids. **Protect** from light.

Buprenorphine Hydrochloride (6209-w)

Buprenorphine Hydrochloride *(BANM, USAN, rINNM).*

Buprenorphini Hydrochloridum; CL-112302; NIH-8805; UM-952.

$C_{29}H_{41}NO_4,HCl$ = 504.1.

CAS — 53152-21-9.

Pharmacopoeias. In *Eur.* (see p.viii) and *US.*

A white or almost white crystalline powder. Buprenorphine hydrochloride 107.8 μg is approximately equivalent to 100 μg of buprenorphine. Sparingly **soluble** in water; soluble in alcohol; freely soluble in methyl alcohol; practically insoluble in cyclohexane. A 1% solution in water has a pH between 4.0 and 6.0. **Store** in airtight containers. Protect from light.

Dependence and Withdrawal

As for Opioid Analgesics, p.67.

Buprenorphine may have a lower potential for producing dependence than pure agonists such as morphine. However, it has been subject to abuse. Abrupt withdrawal of buprenorphine is said to produce only a mild abstinence syndrome.

Adverse Effects and Treatment

As for Opioid Analgesics in general, p.68.

Treatment of adverse effects is similar to that for other opioid analgesics (p.68). The effects of buprenorphine are not readily reversed by naloxone (see under Effects on the Respiratory System, below); doxapram may be of some benefit.

Adverse effects reported following administration of buprenorphine injection in 8187 patients were, nausea (8.8%), vomiting (7.4%), drowsiness (4.3%), sleeping (1.9%), dizziness (1.2%), sweating (0.98%), headache (0.55%), confusion (0.53%), lightheadedness (0.38%), blurred vision (0.28%), euphoria (0.27%), dry mouth (0.11%), depression (0.09%), and hallucinations (0.09%).[1] Some studies have reported nausea, vomiting, and dizziness to be more troublesome with buprenorphine than with morphine.[2,3]

In a trial of *sublingual* buprenorphine 50 of 141 cancer patients withdrew because of side-effects, especially dizziness, nausea, vomiting, and drowsiness; constipation was not reported.[4] One woman developed a painless ulcer on the upper surface of her tongue after she had put sublingual buprenorphine tablets on rather than under her tongue.[5]

Shock occurred in 2 patients 2 hours after receiving *epidural* buprenorphine 300 μg;[6] treatment with naloxone was unsuccessful but symptoms disappeared spontaneously after 2 to 3 hours.

1. Harcus AW, *et al.* Methodology of monitored release of a new preparation: buprenorphine. *Br Med J* 1979; **2:** 163–5.
2. Sear JW, *et al.* Buprenorphine for postoperative analgesia. *Br J Anaesth* 1979; **51:** 71.
3. Kjaer M, *et al.* A comparative study of intramuscular buprenorphine and morphine in the treatment of chronic pain of malignant origin. *Br J Clin Pharmacol* 1982; **13:** 487–92.
4. Robbie DS. A trial of sublingual buprenorphine in cancer pain. *Br J Clin Pharmacol* 1979; **7** (suppl 3): 315S–17S.
5. Lockhart SP, Baron JH. Tongue ulceration after lingual buprenorphine. *Br Med J* 1984; **288:** 1346.
6. Christensen FR, Andersen LW. Adverse reaction to extradural buprenorphine. *Br J Anaesth* 1982; **54:** 476.

Effects on mental function. Psychotomimetic effects have been relatively uncommon with buprenorphine. Harcus *et al.*[1] reported hallucinations in only 7 of 8147 patients (0.09%) given buprenorphine by injection. There have been reports of hallucinations following sublingual buprenorphine in 1 patient[2] and following epidural injection in 5 patients.[3]

1. Harcus AW, *et al.* Methodology of monitored release of a new preparation: buprenorphine. *Br Med J* 1979; **2:** 163–5.
2. Paraskevaides EC. Near fatal auditory hallucinations after buprenorphine. *Br Med J* 1988; **296:** 214.
3. MacEvilly M, O'Carroll C. Hallucinations after epidural buprenorphine. *Br Med J* 1989; **298:** 928–9.

Effects on the respiratory system. There have been varying reports on the occurrence of respiratory depression in association with buprenorphine. It might be subject to a 'ceiling effect' in that respiratory depression does not necessarily increase proportionately with dose. However, high doses of 30 or 40 μg per kg body-weight given as sole intravenous analgesic in balanced anaesthesia have been associated with significant and severe respiratory depression.[1]

Respiratory depression may be delayed in onset and more prolonged than that seen with morphine and is not readily reversed by naloxone, possibly because buprenorphine is very firmly bound to opioid receptors. A study of sublingual buprenorphine for postoperative pain relief was abandoned when 3 of the first 16 patients showed signs of late-onset respiratory depression after the second dose of buprenorphine; the respiratory depression did not respond to naloxone.[2] Successful reversal has been demonstrated in healthy subjects with buprenorphine-induced respiratory depression given large doses of naloxone 5 or 10 mg, but not with 1 mg; reversal was gradual in onset and decreased the duration of the normally prolonged respiratory depression.[3] The respiratory depressant and analgesic effects of buprenorphine were decreased by the *concomitant* administration of naloxone.[4]

1. Schmidt JF, *et al.* Postoperative pain relief with naloxone: severe respiratory depression and pain after high dose buprenorphine. *Anaesthesia* 1985; **40:** 583–6.
2. Thörn S-E, *et al.* Prolonged respiratory depression caused by sublingual buprenorphine. *Lancet* 1988; **i:** 179–80.
3. Gal TJ. Naloxone reversal of buprenorphine-induced respiratory depression. *Clin Pharmacol Ther* 1989; **45:** 66–71.
4. Lehmann KA, *et al.* Influence of naloxone on the postoperative analgesic and respiratory effects of buprenorphine. *Eur J Clin Pharmacol* 1988; **34:** 343–52.

Precautions

As for Opioid Analgesics in general, p.68.

Buprenorphine has opioid antagonist actions and may precipitate withdrawal symptoms if given to patients physically dependent on opioids.

Respiratory depression, if it occurs, is relatively slow in onset and of prolonged duration; it may not be readily reversed by naloxone.

There is a risk that, with partial opioid agonists such as buprenorphine, their antagonistic effects might impair more effective analgesic therapy. This appeared to happen in 2 cancer patients both of whom were given sublingual buprenorphine that was later substituted by morphine.[1] Conventional doses of morphine were inadequate and in one patient raising the dose of morphine proved fatal.

1. Overweg-van Kints J, Stricker BHC. Falende pijnbestrijding tijdens sublinguaal gebruik van buprenorfine. *Ned Tijdschr Geneeskd* 1987; **131:** 1973–4.

Abuse. See under Dependence and Withdrawal, above.

Breast feeding. Some authorities consider that the amount of buprenorphine distributed into breast milk is probably too small to be harmful to a breast-fed infant. From a study[1] of one breast-feeding mother who was receiving buprenorphine 4 mg daily it was estimated that at the age of 4 weeks the total amount ingested by the infant during a 24-hour period was 3.28 μg for buprenorphine and 0.33 μg for norbuprenorphine.

1. Marquet P, *et al.* Buprenorphine withdrawal syndrome in a newborn. *Clin Pharmacol Ther* 1997; **62:** 569–71.

Pregnancy and the neonate. An infant born to a mother who was being treated with buprenorphine 4 mg daily for diamorphine addiction suffered a minor withdrawal syndrome 2 days after birth.[1] The infant rapidly recovered without any treatment. No further signs of withdrawal occurred when breast feeding was abruptly stopped at the age of 8 weeks.

1. Marquet P, *et al.* Buprenorphine withdrawal syndrome in a newborn. *Clin Pharmacol Ther* 1997; **62:** 569–71.

Interactions

For interactions associated with opioid analgesics, see p.69.

Pharmacokinetics

Following intramuscular injection, buprenorphine rapidly reaches peak plasma concentrations. Absorption also takes place through the buccal mucosa following sublingual administration. Buprenorphine is about 96% bound to plasma proteins. Plasma elimination half-lives have ranged from 1.2 to 7.2 hours; there is a lack of correlation between plasma concentrations and analgesic activity. Some is metabolised in the liver to *N*-dealkylbuprenorphine (norbuprenorphine) and conjugated metabolites, but buprenorphine is excreted predominantly unchanged in the faeces; there is some evidence for enterohepatic recirculation. Metabolites are excreted in the urine, but very little unchanged drug. Buprenorphine is subject to considerable first-pass metabolism following oral administration. Small amounts of buprenorphine are distributed into breast milk.

Administration. BUCCAL ROUTE. Absorption of sublingual buprenorphine is relatively slow. In a 10-hour study[1] plasma concentrations following 400 or 800 μg sublingually peaked at about 200 minutes (range 90 to 360 minutes) and buprenorphine was still detected in plasma at the end of the study. Systemic availability was about 55% (range 16 to 94%) and absorption was more or less complete 5 hours after a dose. However, the authors of a subsequent study[2] considered that this was an overestimation, possibly due to methodological flaws. The later study results indicated that the bioavailability of sublingual buprenorphine is about 30% and that sublingual holding times between 3 and 5 minutes are bioequivalent.

1. Bullingham RES, *et al.* Sublingual buprenorphine used postoperatively: ten hour plasma drug concentration analysis. *Br J Clin Pharmacol* 1982; **13:** 665–73.
2. Mendelson J, *et al.* Bioavailability of sublingual buprenorphine. *J Clin Pharmacol* 1997; **37:** 31–7.

Administration in children. The terminal elimination half-life of buprenorphine was only about 1 hour in small children aged about 4 to 7 years given 3 μg per kg body-weight intravenously as premedication, but could not be estimated reliably because of the rapid decline in plasma-buprenorphine concentrations.[1] Clearance values did however appear higher than in adults; steady-state volume of distribution was similar. Premature neonates (gestational age 27 to 32 weeks) given a similar dose followed by an infusion of 0.72 μg per kg per hour had a considerably lower clearance rate and had a mean elimination half-life of 20 hours.[2] Although this dosing regimen appeared to be safe, sedation was judged to be inadequate in 4 of the 12 neonates studied. It was suggested that as buprenorphine given by infusion might not produce consistent sedation and analgesia in premature neonates, it could not be recommended for use in neonatal care.

1. Olkkola KT, *et al.* Pharmacokinetics of intravenous buprenorphine in children. *Br J Clin Pharmacol* 1989; **28:** 202–4.
2. Barrett DA, *et al.* The pharmacokinetics and physiological effect of buprenorphine infusion in premature neonates. *Br J Clin Pharmacol* 1993; **36:** 215–19.

Administration in renal impairment. Buprenorphine clearance appears to occur mainly by hepatic extraction and metabolism and would not be expected to be related to renal function, whereas metabolites are excreted in urine. Buprenorphine kinetics were similar in a study in anaesthetised healthy patients and those with renal impairment, with a mean elimination half-life of 398 and 239 minutes respectively.[1] Plasma concentrations of the metabolites norbuprenorphine and buprenorphine-3-glucuronide were increased about 4 times and 15 times respectively in patients with renal impairment,[1] but significant pharmacological activity was unlikely since norbuprenorphine has little analgesic activity compared with the parent compound and buprenorphine-3-glucuronide has none.

1. Hand CW, *et al.* Buprenorphine disposition in patients with renal impairment: single and continuous dosing, with special reference to metabolites. *Br J Anaesth* 1990; **64:** 276–82.

Uses and Administration

Buprenorphine is an opioid analgesic (p.69) classified as a partial opioid agonist. It is used for the relief of moderate to severe pain and as an adjunct to anaesthesia. Buprenorphine is also used in the treatment of opioid dependence.

Buprenorphine has a relatively slow onset but prolonged duration of action. Following intramuscular injection analgesia is apparent within 30 minutes and lasts up to 6 hours. A slower more prolonged response is achieved following sublingual administration.

Buprenorphine is used as the hydrochloride but doses are expressed in terms of the equivalent amount of the base. The dose by intramuscular or slow intravenous injection for moderate to severe pain is 300 to 600 μg repeated every 6 to 8 hours as required. Children over 6 months may be given 3 to 6 μg per kg body-weight by injection every 6 to 8 hours; up to 9 μg per kg may be given if required in refractory cases.

Doses of 200 to 400 μg are given sublingually every 6 to 8 hours. Suggested sublingual doses for children over 6 months are: 16 to 25 kg body-weight, 100 μg; 25 to 37.5 kg, 100 to 200 μg; and 37.5 to 50 kg, 200 to 300 μg.

When used in balanced anaesthesia 300 μg may be given intramuscularly or 400 μg sublingually for premedication; 300 to 450 μg may be given intravenously as a perioperative analgesic supplement.

Buprenorphine is generally described as a mixed agonist-antagonist acting mainly as a partial agonist at μ opioid receptors, with some antagonist activity at κ receptors. It has also been shown to bind at μ, δ, and κ opioid binding sites and to have high affinity for the μ and δ receptor and lesser affinity for the κ receptor.[1] Buprenorphine, like fentanyl, has high lipid solubility, but has a lower intrinsic activity than fentanyl. Differences between buprenorphine and pure μ opioid agonists such as fentanyl, including relatively slow onset of action, prolonged duration of action, resistance to antagonism by naloxone, and lack of correlation between plasma concentrations and analgesic effects, have been explained by differences in the way buprenorphine binds to opioid receptors. In a study *in vitro* buprenorphine had slow rates of association and dissociation from the opioid receptor when compared with fentanyl.[2]

1. Bovill JG. Which potent opioid? Important criteria for selection. *Drugs* 1987; **33:** 520–30.
2. Boas RA, Villiger JW. Clinical actions of fentanyl and buprenorphine: the significance of receptor binding. *Br J Anaesth* 1985; **57:** 192–6.

Anaesthesia. Buprenorphine may be used for premedication and as an adjunct to anaesthesia. It has also been used after anaesthesia with fentanyl and in one study[1] buprenorphine antagonised the respiratory rate depression following fentanyl as effectively as naloxone.

1. Boysen K, *et al.* Buprenorphine antagonism of ventilatory depression following fentanyl anaesthesia. *Acta Anaesthesiol Scand* 1988; **32:** 490–2.

Opioid dependence. Buprenorphine is used in the treatment of opioid dependence (p.67). It has shown promise in the treatment and detoxification of diamorphine addicts since it suppresses craving for diamorphine and there is only a mild abstinence syndrome when buprenorphine is abruptly withdrawn.[1-3] In a comparative study sublingual buprenorphine 2 mg daily was acceptable and as effective as oral methadone 30 mg daily in the detoxification of diamorphine addicts.[4] Higher sublingual doses of buprenorphine or different routes of administration may be necessary in practice. In other studies sublingual buprenorphine 8 mg daily was as effective as oral methadone 60 mg daily[5] but less effective than oral methadone 80 mg daily.[6] Fudala *et al.*[7] considered daily doses of 8 mg sublingually to be preferable to 8 mg every other day, although alternate-day dosing could be tolerated.

In some countries buprenorphine is available in combination with naloxone for the treatment of opioid dependence.

1. WHO. WHO expert committee on drug dependence: twenty-fifth report. *WHO Tech Rep Ser 775* 1989.
2. Guthrie SK. Pharmacologic interventions for the treatment of opioid dependence and withdrawal. *DICP Ann Pharmacother* 1990; **24:** 721–34.
3. O'Connor PG, *et al.* Three methods of opioid detoxification in a primary care setting: a randomized trial. *Ann Intern Med* 1997; **127:** 526–30.
4. Bickel WK, *et al.* A clinical trial of buprenorphine: comparison with methadone in the detoxification of heroin addicts. *Clin Pharmacol Ther* 1988; **43:** 72–8.
5. Johnson RE, *et al.* A controlled trial of buprenorphine treatment for opioid dependence. *JAMA* 1992; **267:** 2750–5.
6. Ling W, *et al.* A controlled trial comparing buprenorphine and methadone maintenance in opioid dependence. *Arch Gen Psychiatry* 1996; **53:** 401–407.
7. Fudala PJ, *et al.* Use of buprenorphine in the treatment of opioid addiction: II physiologic and behavioural effects of daily and alternate-day administration and abrupt withdrawal. *Clin Pharmacol Ther* 1990; **47:** 525–34.

Pain. ACUTE PAIN. Buprenorphine can be given intramuscularly, intravenously, or sublingually for the control of *postoperative* pain although the intravenous route may be preferred for acute pain relief. The epidural route has also been used.[1-3] Patient-controlled analgesia with intravenous[4] and intramuscular[5] buprenorphine has been effective although its long half-life may limit such use.

Buprenorphine had no adverse cardiovascular effects when given intravenously after open-heart surgery,[6] suggesting that it was a suitable analgesic for patients with unstable circulation. It was also considered suitable for the relief of pain in *myocardial infarction*.[7]

1. Murphy DF, MacEvilly M. Pain relief with epidural buprenorphine after spinal fusion: a comparison with intramuscular morphine. *Acta Anaesthesiol Scand* 1984; **28:** 144–6.
2. Bilsback P, *et al.* Efficacy of the extradural administration of lofentanil, buprenorphine or saline in the management of postoperative pain. *Br J Anaesth* 1985; **57:** 943–8.
3. Gundersen RY, *et al.* Postoperative pain relief with high-dose epidural buprenorphine: a double-blind study. *Acta Anaesthesiol Scand* 1986; **30:** 664–7.
4. Gibbs JM, *et al.* Patient administration of iv buprenorphine for postoperative pain relief using the 'Cardiff' demand analgesia apparatus. *Br J Anaesth* 1982; **54:** 279–84.
5. Harmer M, *et al.* Intramuscular on demand analgesia: double blind controlled trial of pethidine, buprenorphine, morphine, and meptazinol. *Br Med J* 1983; **286:** 680–2.
6. Rosenfeldt FL, *et al.* Haemodynamic effects of buprenorphine after heart surgery. *Br Med J* 1978; **2:** 1602–3.
7. Hayes MJ, *et al.* Randomised trial comparing buprenorphine and diamorphine for chest pain in suspected myocardial infarction. *Br Med J* 1979; **2:** 300–2.

CHRONIC PAIN. Sublingual buprenorphine has been used successfully in the control of cancer pain although in one study[1] 50 of 141 patients withdrew because of side-effects, especially dizziness, nausea, vomiting, and drowsiness; constipation was not reported. Following single intramuscular doses of buprenorphine 300 μg or morphine 10 mg in cancer patients with moderate to severe chronic pain there was no difference in peak analgesic effects or the time to reach these effects; buprenorphine had a significantly longer duration of action, but dizziness, nausea, and vomiting were more of a problem.[2] In another study intramuscular buprenorphine had a similar duration of effect to intramuscular morphine; pain relief was more delayed with sublingual buprenorphine but lasted longer.[3] However, Hull[4] did not recommend buprenorphine in advanced cancer because of its partial morphine antagonist properties (see also under Precautions, above).

1. Robbie DS. A trial of sublingual buprenorphine in cancer pain. *Br J Clin Pharmacol* 1979; **7:** 315S–17S.
2. Kjaer M, *et al.* A comparative study of intramuscular buprenorphine and morphine in the treatment of chronic pain of malignant origin. *Br J Clin Pharmacol* 1982; **13:** 487–92.
3. Wallenstein SL, *et al.* Crossover trials in clinical analgesic assays: studies of buprenorphine and morphine. *Pharmacotherapy* 1986; **6:** 228–35.
4. Hull FM. The management of pain in advanced cancer. *J Clin Pharm Ther* 1990; **15:** 303–6.

Preparations

Proprietary Preparations (details are given in Part 3)
Aust.: Temgesic; ***Austral.:*** Temgesic; ***Belg.:*** Temgesic; ***Fr.:*** Subutex; Temgesic; ***Ger.:*** Temgesic; ***Irl.:*** Temgesic; ***Ital.:*** Finibron†; Temgesic; ***Neth.:*** Temgesic; ***Norw.:*** Temgesic; ***S.Afr.:*** Temgesic; ***Spain:*** Buprex; Prefin; ***Swed.:*** Temgesic; ***Switz.:*** Temgesic; ***UK:*** Temgesic; ***USA:*** Buprenex.

Butibufen Sodium (12475-l)

Butibufen Sodium *(rINNM)*.

FF-106 (butibufen). Sodium 2-(4-isobutylphenyl)butyrate.

$C_{14}H_{19}NaO_2$ = 242.3.

CAS — 55837-18-8 (butibufen); 60682-24-8 (butibufen sodium).

Butibufen sodium is an NSAID (p.63) that has been used by mouth in inflammatory and rheumatic disorders.

Preparations

Proprietary Preparations (details are given in Part 3)
Spain: Mijal.

Butorphanol Tartrate (6210-m)

Butorphanol Tartrate *(BANM, USAN, rINNM)*.

levo-BC-2627 (butorphanol). (−)-17-(Cyclobutylmethyl)morphinan-3,14-diol hydrogen tartrate.

$C_{21}H_{29}NO_2,C_4H_6O_6$ = 477.5.

CAS — 42408-82-2 (butorphanol); 58786-99-5 (butorphanol tartrate).

Pharmacopoeias. In *US.*

A white powder. Sparingly **soluble** in water; slightly soluble in methyl alcohol; insoluble in alcohol, in chloroform, in ether, in ethyl acetate, and in hexane; soluble in dilute acids. A solution in water is slightly acidic. **Store** in airtight containers.

Dependence and Withdrawal

As for Opioid Analgesics, p.67.

Butorphanol may have a lower potential for producing dependence than pure agonists such as morphine. However, it has been subject to abuse. Abrupt discontinuation of chronic butorphanol administration has produced a less severe withdrawal syndrome than with morphine.

Adverse Effects and Treatment

As for Opioid Analgesics in general, p.68, and for Pentazocine, p.75.

Headache, and feelings of floating may also occur. Hallucinations and other psychotomimetic effects are rare and have been reported less frequently than with pentazocine. In addition insomnia and nasal congestion may occur frequently when butorphanol is given intranasally.

Because butorphanol has opioid agonist and antagonist activity, naloxone is the recommended antagonist for the treatment of overdosage.

Effects on the respiratory system. Butorphanol 2 mg produces a similar degree of respiratory depression to morphine 10 mg, but a ceiling effect is apparent with higher doses of butorphanol.[1] It has been reported to be a less potent respiratory depressant than fentanyl,[2] but more potent than nalbuphine.[3]

1. Nagashima H, *et al.* Respiratory and circulatory effects of intravenous butorphanol and morphine. *Clin Pharmacol Ther* 1976; **19:** 738–45.
2. Dryden GE. Voluntary respiratory effects of butorphanol and fentanyl following barbiturate induction: a double-blind study. *J Clin Pharmacol* 1986; **26:** 203–7.
3. Zucker JR, *et al.* Respiratory effects of nalbuphine and butorphanol in anesthetized patients. *Anesth Analg* 1987; **66:** 879–81.

Precautions

As for Opioid Analgesics in general, p.68.

Although cardiovascular effects may be less than with pentazocine, butorphanol should generally be avoided after myocardial infarction.

Butorphanol may precipitate withdrawal symptoms if given to patients physically dependent on opioids. The dosage regimen of butorphanol may need to be adjusted in the elderly and in patients with hepatic or renal impairment.

Abuse. There has been a report of fibrous myopathy associated with chronic intramuscular abuse of butorphanol.[1]

1. Wagner JM, Cohen S. Fibrous myopathy from butorphanol injections. *J Rheumatol* 1991; **18:** 1934–5.

Pregnancy. Two instances of sinusoidal fetal heart rate pattern were noted out of 188 consecutive cases of butorphanol administration in active-phase labour.[1]

1. Welt SI. Sinusoidal fetal heart rate and butorphanol administration. *Am J Obstet Gynecol* 1985; **152:** 362–3.

Interactions

For interactions associated with opioid analgesics, see p.69.

Pharmacokinetics

Butorphanol is absorbed from the gastro-intestinal tract but it undergoes extensive first-pass metabolism. Peak plasma concentrations occur 0.5 to 1 hour after intramuscular and nasal administration and 1 to 1.5 hours after oral administration. Butorphanol has a plasma elimination half-life of about 3 hours. About 80% is bound to plasma proteins.

Butorphanol is extensively metabolised in the liver through hydroxylation, *N*-dealkylation, and conjugation, only 5% being excreted unchanged. Excretion is mainly in the urine; about 11 to 14% of a parenteral dose is excreted in the bile. It crosses the placenta and is distributed into breast milk.

References.

1. Shyu WC, *et al.* Multiple-dose phase I study of transnasal butorphanol. *Clin Pharmacol Ther* 1993; **54:** 34–41.
2. Shyu WC, *et al.* The absolute bioavailability of transnasal butorphanol in patients experiencing rhinitis. *Eur J Clin Pharmacol* 1993; **45:** 559–62.
3. Shyu WC, *et al.* The effects of age and sex on the systemic availability and pharmacokinetics of transnasal butorphanol. *Eur J Clin Pharmacol* 1994; **47:** 57–60.

Uses and Administration

Butorphanol tartrate, a phenanthrene derivative, is an opioid analgesic (p.69) pharmacologically similar to pentazocine (p.75). Butorphanol is used for the relief of moderate to severe pain and as an adjunct to anaesthesia. Onset of analgesia is reported within 10 to 15 minutes of intramuscular injection and may last for 3 to 4 hours. With intranasal administration, onset of action is also within 10 to 15 minutes but duration of action is longer and can be up to 5 hours.

For the relief of moderate to severe pain, butorphanol tartrate is given in doses of 1 to 4 mg by intramuscular injection or in doses of 0.5 to 2 mg by intravenous injection every 3 to 4 hours. It may also been given as a nasal spray, in usual doses of 1 mg (1 spray in 1 nostril), repeated after 60 to 90 minutes, if necessary. This sequence may be repeated after 3 to 4 hours as needed. An initial dose of 2 mg (1 spray in each nostril) may be given for severe pain, but should not be repeated until 3 to 4 hours later.

For premedication 2 mg may be given intramuscularly 60 to 90 minutes before surgery. For use in balanced anaesthesia a usual dose is 2 mg given intravenously shortly before induction followed by 0.5 to 1 mg intravenously in increments during anaesthesia.

The dosage of butorphanol may need to be adjusted in the elderly and in patients with hepatic or renal impairment. When given by injection the initial dose for pain should be half the usual initial adult dose. Subsequent doses should be determined by the patient's response; a dosage interval of 6 to 8 hours has been recommended. For nasal administration the initial dose should be limited to 1 mg followed by 1 mg after 90 to 120 minutes if necessary; subsequent doses if required should generally be given at intervals of not less than 6 hours.

References.

1. Atkinson BD, *et al.* Double-blind comparison of intravenous butorphanol (Stadol) and fentanyl (Sublimaze) for analgesia during labor. *Am J Obstet Gynecol* 1994; **171:** 993–8.
2. Gillis JC, *et al.* Transnasal butorphanol: a review of its pharmacodynamic and pharmacokinetic properties, and therapeutic potential in acute pain management. *Drugs* 1995; **50:** 157–75.

Headache. Butorphanol has been advocated for use as a nasal spray in the treatment of migraine, but its place in therapy, if any, remains to be established.

References.

1. Freitag FG. The acute treatment of migraine with transnasal butorphanol (TNB). *Headache Q* 1993; **4** (suppl 3): 22–8.
2. Hoffert MJ, *et al.* Transnasal butorphanol in the treatment of acute migraine. *Headache* 1995; **35:** 65–9.

Pruritus. Preliminary results from a small study[1] of 6 patients with severe opioid-induced pruritus unresponsive to diphenhydramine indicated that intranasal butorphanol 2 mg administered every 4 to 6 hours may be an effective treatment.

1. Dunteman E, *et al.* Transnasal butorphanol for the treatment of opioid-induced pruritus unresponsive to antihistamines. *J Pain Symptom Manage* 1996; **12:** 255–60.

Preparations

USP 23: Butorphanol Tartrate Injection.

Proprietary Preparations (details are given in Part 3)
Canad.: Stadol; ***Spain:*** Verstadol; ***USA:*** Stadol.

Capsaicin (9679-a)

(*E*)-8-Methyl-*N*-vanillylnon-6-enamide.

$C_{18}H_{27}NO_3$ = 305.4.

CAS — 404-86-4.

NOTE. Do not confuse capsaicin with capsicin (p.1559) which is capsicum oleoresin.

Pharmacopoeias. In *US.*

The active principle of the dried ripe fruits of *Capsicum* spp.

An off-white powder. Melting range 57° to 66°. Practically **insoluble** in cold water; soluble in alcohol and in chloroform; slightly soluble in carbon disulphide. **Store** in a cool place in airtight containers. Protect from light.

CAUTION. *Capsaicin should be handled with care. Particles should not be inhaled nor come into contact with any part of the body.*

Adverse Effects

A warm, stinging, or burning sensation may be experienced at the site of application; this usually disappears after a few days of use but may persist longer if applications are less frequent than recommended (see Uses and Administration, below). Coughing, sneezing, or respiratory irritation may occur if dried cream residue is inhaled.

Precautions

Contact with eyes and broken or irritated skin should be avoided. The hands should be washed after application of the cream, unless the hands are the treated areas, in which case, they should be washed 30 minutes after application. If bandages are used to cover treated areas they should not be wound too tightly. Thick applications of the cream should be avoided.

Uses and Administration

Capsaicin is used as a topical analgesic in painful conditions such as postherpetic neuralgia after the lesions have healed, diabetic neuropathy, osteoarthritis, and rheumatoid arthritis. The use of topical analgesics is discussed on p.7. For adults and children over 2 years of age capsaicin is usually applied sparingly 3 or 4 times daily as a 0.025% or 0.075% cream. A more concentrated cream containing 0.25% capsaicin is available in some countries for adults and children over 12 years of age, and is applied sparingly twice a day. Capsaicin cream should be rubbed well into the skin until little or no residue is left on the surface. Therapeutic response may not be evident for 1 to 2 weeks for arthritic disorders, or 2 to 4 weeks for neuralgias (or even longer if the head or neck are involved). The UK manufacturer recommends that for the management of painful diabetic neuropathy, capsaicin should only be used under specialist supervision and that treatment should be reviewed after the first 8 weeks and regularly re-evaluated thereafter. Although not a counter-irritant itself, capsaicin has been included in rubefacient preparations for the relief of muscular and rheumatic pain.

Action. The analgesic effect following topical application of capsaicin is attributed to its ability to deplete the neuropeptide substance P from local sensory C-type nerve fibres.[1-5] Its action in depleting substance P, after repeated applications, serves to reduce the transmission of pain impulses to the CNS. Since effect of capsaicin does not rely on vasodilatation in the skin it is therefore not considered to be a traditional counter-irritant.

1. Rumsfield JA, West DP. Topical capsaicin in dermatologic and peripheral pain disorders. *DICP Ann Pharmacother* 1991; **25:** 381–7.
2. Cordell GA, Araujo OE. Capsaicin: identification, nomenclature, and pharmacotherapy. *Ann Pharmacother* 1993; **27:** 330–6.
3. Winter J, *et al.* Capsaicin and pain mechanisms. *Br J Anaesth* 1995; **75:** 157–68.
4. Del Bianco E, *et al.* The effects of repeated dermal application of capsaicin to the human skin on pain and vasodilatation induced by intradermal injection of acid and hypertonic solutions. *Br J Clin Pharmacol* 1996; **41:** 1–60.
5. Fusco BM, Giacovazzo M. Peppers and pain: the promise of capsaicin. *Drugs* 1997; **53:** 909–14.

Cluster headache. Prevention of occurrence of attacks of cluster headache (p.443) using repeated applications of capsaicin to the nasal mucosa has been reported.[1]

1. Fusco BM, *et al.* Preventative effect of repeated nasal applications of capsaicin in cluster headache. *Pain* 1994; **59:** 321–5.

Micturition disorders. Intravesical capsaicin has been tried for painful bladder disorders and to treat bladder detrusor hyperreflexia.[1,2] Instillation into the ureter has also been tried in the management of the loin pain/haematuria syndrome.[3]

For a discussion of the more usual management of urinary incontinence, see p.454.

1. Nitti VW. Intravesical capsaicin for treatment of neurogenic bladder. *Lancet* 1994; **343:** 1448.
2. Lazzeri M, *et al.* Intravesical capsaicin for treatment of severe bladder pain: a randomized placebo controlled study. *J Urol (Baltimore)* 1996; **156:** 947–52.
3. Bultitude MI. Capsaicin in treatment of loin pain/haematuria syndrome. *Lancet* 1995; **345:** 921–2.

Neurogenic pain. Capsaicin has been tried topically in various types of pain that may be mediated by the neurotransmitter, substance P, including neurogenic pain, which does not generally respond to conventional systemic analgesics. Topical capsaicin is used in the management of diabetic neuropathy (p.9) and postherpetic neuralgia (p.10), but while a meta-analysis[1] of randomised, double-blind, placebo-controlled studies and later studies[2] suggested that it is effective in painful diabetic neuropathy the evidence for efficacy in postherpetic neuralgia was considered[1] to be less convincing. Other types of neurogenic pain that capsaicin has been tried in include reflex sympathetic dystrophy[3] (p.11), postmastectomy neuroma,[4,5] and stump pain.[6]

1. Zhang WY, Li Wan Po A. The effectiveness of topically applied capsaicin. *Eur J Clin Pharmacol* 1994; **46:** 517–22.
2. Biesbroeck R, *et al.* A double-blind comparison of topical capsaicin and oral amitriptyline in painful diabetic neuropathy. *Adv Therapy* 1995; **12:** 111–20.
3. Cheshire WP, Snyder CR. Treatment of reflex sympathetic dystrophy with topical capsaicin: case report. *Pain* 1990; **42:** 307–11.
4. Watson CPN, Evans RJ. The postmastectomy pain syndrome and topical capsaicin: a randomized trial. *Pain* 1992; **51:** 375–9.

5. Dini D, *et al.* Treatment of the post-mastectomy pain syndrome with topical capsaicin. *Pain* 1993; **54:** 223–6.
6. Rayner HC, *et al.* Relief of local stump pain by capsaicin cream. *Lancet* 1989; **ii:** 1276–7.

Pruritus. Substance P is a possible mediator of itch sensations and capsaicin has been tried in pruritus (p.1075) associated with various diseases and haemodialysis.[1-4] It has also been used to provide relief from pruritus induced by hetastarch[5] and for the itch and pain associated with PUVA therapy.[6,7]

1. Breneman DL, *et al.* Topical capsaicin for treatment of hemodialysis-related pruritus. *J Am Acad Dermatol* 1992; **26:** 91–4.
2. Leibsohn E. Treatment of notalgia paresthetica with capsaicin. *Cutis* 1992; **49:** 335–6.
3. Fölster-Holst R, Brasch J. Effect of topically applied capsaicin on pruritus in patients with atopic dermatitis. *J Dermatol Treat* 1996; **7:** 13–15.
4. Hautmann G, *et al.* Aquagenic pruritus, PUVA and capsaicin treatments. *Br J Dermatol* 1994; **131:** 920–1.
5. Szeimies R-M, *et al.* Successful treatment of hydroxyethyl starch-induced pruritus with topical capsaicin. *Br J Dermatol* 1994; **131:** 380–2.
6. Burrows NP, Norris PG. Treatment of PUVA-induced skin pain with capsaicin. *Br J Dermatol* 1994; **131:** 584–5.
7. Kirby B, Rogers S. Treatment of PUVA itch with capsaicin. *Br J Dermatol* 1997; **137:** 152.

Psoriasis. Since substance P has been implicated in the pathophysiology of several inflammatory dermatological processes, capsaicin has been tried in a number of skin disorders including psoriasis.[1,2]

The usual management of psoriasis is discussed on p.1075.

1. Bernstein JE, *et al.* Effects of topically applied capsaicin on moderate and severe psoriasis vulgaris. *J Am Acad Dermatol* 1986; **15:** 504–7.
2. Ellis CN, *et al.* A double-blind evaluation of topical capsaicin in pruritic psoriasis. *J Am Acad Dermatol* 1993; **29:** 438–42.

Rheumatic disorders. Topical capsaicin is used for the temporary relief of the pain of arthritis. From the results of a meta-analysis[1] of randomised, double-blind placebo-controlled studies and later studies[2] it appears that capsaicin is effective in easing the pain of osteoarthritis (p.2) but its role, if any, is unclear; published evidence[3] for efficacy in rheumatoid arthritis (p.2) appears to be limited. Capsaicin may be a useful therapy for pain associated with primary fibromyalgia,[4] which responds poorly to conventional treatment.

1. Zhang WY, Li Wan Po A. The effectiveness of topically applied capsaicin. *Eur J Clin Pharmacol* 1994; **46:** 517–22.
2. Altman RD, *et al.* Capsaicin cream 0.025% as monotherapy for osteoarthritis: a double-blind study. *Semin Arthritis Rheum* 1994; **23** (suppl 3): 25–33.
3. Deal CL, *et al.* Treatment of arthritis with topical capsaicin: a double-blind trial. *Clin Ther* 1991; **13:** 383–95.
4. McCarty DJ, *et al.* Treatment of pain due to fibromyalgia with topical capsaicin: a pilot study. *Semin Arthritis Rheum* 1994; **23** (suppl 3): 41–7.

Preparations

Proprietary Preparations (details are given in Part 3)
Aust.: Capsiplast; ***Austral.:*** Capsig†; Zostrix; ***Canad.:*** Axsain; Capzasin-P; Zostrix; ***Irl.:*** Axsain; ***Spain:*** Capsidol; Gelcen; Katrum; Priltam; ***Swed.:*** Capsina; ***UK:*** Axsain; ***USA:*** Capsin; Capzasin-P; Dolorac; No Pain-HP; R-Gel; Zostrix.

Multi-ingredient: ***Aust.:*** Rubizon-Rheumagel; ***Canad.:*** Arthricare Odor Free; Heet; Methacin; Midalgan; ***Fr.:*** Capsic; ***Ger.:*** Capsamol; Rheumaliment†; Thermazet†; ***Irl.:*** Algipan; Radian-B; ***Ital.:*** Disalgil; ***Neth.:*** Cremes Tegen Spierpijn†; ***UK:*** Zacin; ***USA:*** Arthricare Odor Free; Heet; Menthacin; Pain Doctor; Pain X; Ziks.

Carbaspirin Calcium (2620-l)

Carbaspirin Calcium *(USAN)*.

Carbasalate Calcium *(rINN)*; Calcium Acetylsalicylate Carbamide; Calcium Carbaspirin; Carbasalatum Calcicum; Carbasalatum Calcium.

$C_{19}H_{18}CaN_2O_9$ = 458.4.

CAS — 5749-67-7.

Pharmacopoeias. In *Eur.* (see p.viii).

A 1:1 complex of calcium acetylsalicylate and urea. A white crystalline powder. It contains 99 to 101% of an equimolecular compound of calcium di[2-(acetyloxy)benzoate] and urea, calculated with reference to the anhydrous substance. Freely **soluble** in water and in dimethylformamide; practically insoluble in acetone and in anhydrous methyl alcohol. **Store** in airtight containers.

Adverse Effects, Treatment, and Precautions

As for Aspirin, p.16.

Carbaspirin calcium, like aspirin, should not generally be given to children under the age of 12 years because of the risk of Reye's syndrome.

Interactions

For interactions associated with aspirin, see p.17.

Uses and Administration

Carbaspirin calcium is metabolised to aspirin following absorption; it thus has the actions of aspirin (p.18). Carbaspirin calcium is given in doses equivalent to 250 mg to 1 g of aspirin (maximum 4 g daily) for pain or fever and in doses equivalent to 0.5 to 2 g of aspirin every 4 hours (maximum 6 g daily) for rheumatic disorders. Carbaspirin calcium has also been used in the management of thrombo-embolic disorders.

Preparations

Proprietary Preparations (details are given in Part 3)
Aust.: Iromin; ***Belg.:*** Solupsa; ***Fr.:*** Solupsan; ***Irl.:*** Ascal†; ***Neth.:*** Ascal; ***Spain:*** Ascal 38; ***Switz.:*** Alcacyl; Iromin†.

Multi-ingredient: ***Aust.:*** Irocopar cC; Irocophan; Iromin Chinin C; ***Fr.:*** Cephalgan; ***Switz.:*** Alca-C; Alcacyl-B_1†; Calonat; Irocopar†.

Carfentanil Citrate (18911-a)

Carfentanil Citrate *(USAN, rINNM)*.

R-33799. Methyl 1-phenethyl-4-(*N*-phenylpropionamido)isonipecotate citrate.

$C_{24}H_{30}N_2O_3,C_6H_8O_7$ = 586.6.

CAS — 59708-52-0 (carfentanil); 61380-27-6 (carfentanil citrate).

Carfentanil citrate is an opioid analgesic related to fentanyl (p.38). It has been used in veterinary medicine.

Celecoxib (3624-n)

Celecoxib *(pINN)*.

SC-58635. *p*-[5-*p*-Tolyl-3-(trifluoromethyl)pyrazol-1-yl]benzenesulfonamide.

$C_{17}H_{14}F_3N_3O_2S$ = 381.4.

CAS — 169590-42-5.

Celecoxib is an NSAID (p.63) reported to be a selective inhibitor of cyclo-oxygenase-2 (COX-2). It is used in the treatment of rheumatoid arthritis and osteoarthritis.

Choline Magnesium Trisalicylate (2624-c)

CAS — 64425-90-7.

Adverse Effects, Treatment, and Precautions

As for Aspirin, p.16.

The use of aspirin and other acetylated salicylates is generally not recommended for children under the age of 12 years because of the risk of Reye's syndrome, unless specifically indicated. Some authorities also extend this precaution to non-acetylated salicylates.

Effects on the liver. References.

1. Cersosimo RJ, Matthews SJ. Hepatotoxicity associated with choline magnesium trisalicylate: case report and review of salicylate-induced hepatotoxicity. *Drug Intell Clin Pharm* 1987; **21:** 621–5.

Interactions

For interactions associated with salicylates, see Aspirin, p.17.

Uses and Administration

Choline magnesium trisalicylate is a combination of the salicylic acid derivatives choline salicylate (p.25) and magnesium salicylate (p.51). It has analgesic, anti-inflammatory, and antipyretic actions similar to those of aspirin (p.18). Following oral administration, choline magnesium trisalicylate dissociates and the salicylate moiety is rapidly absorbed. Each unit dose of 500 mg of salicylate is provided by approximately 293 mg of choline salicylate with 362 mg of magnesium salicylate (anhydrous). Choline magnesium trisalicylate is used in osteoarthritis, rheumatoid arthritis, and other arthritides in doses equivalent to 1 or 1.5 g of salicylate twice daily by mouth; doses may also be given as a single daily dose if required. A dose of 750 mg given three times daily may be more suitable for elderly patients. Choline magnesium trisalicylate is also used in the general management of other forms of pain and for fever.

Preparations

Proprietary Preparations (details are given in Part 3)
Canad.: Trilisate; ***Irl.:*** Trilisate†; ***UK:*** Trilisate†; ***USA:*** Tricosal; Trilisate.

Choline Salicylate (2625-k)

Choline Salicylate *(BAN, USAN, rINN)*.

(2-Hydroxyethyl)trimethylammonium salicylate.

$C_{12}H_{19}NO_4$ = 241.3.

CAS — 2016-36-6.

Pharmacopoeias. Br. includes Choline Salicylate Solution.

Choline salicylate 1 g is approximately equivalent to 750 mg of aspirin. Choline Salicylate Solution (BP 1998) is an aqueous solution containing 47.5 to 52.5% of choline salicylate. It is a clear colourless liquid. It may contain a suitable antimicrobial preservative.

Uses and Administration

Choline salicylate is a salicylic acid derivative (see Aspirin, p.16) used in the treatment of pain and fever, and in the management of rheumatic disorders. It is given by mouth in doses of 435 to 870 mg every four hours as necessary for pain and fever, and in doses of 4.8 to 7.2 g daily in divided doses for rheumatic disorders.

Choline salicylate is also used as a local analgesic. Solutions containing up to 20% choline salicylate are used in ear disorders such as the relief of pain in otitis media and externa but are considered to be of doubtful value; they are also used to soften ear wax as an aid to removal (see p.1190). An 8.7% gel is used for lesions of the mouth (p.1172). Choline salicylate is also applied topically in a rubefacient preparation in a concentration of 3.9% for the relief of muscular and rheumatic pain.

Choline salicylate is also given in the form of choline magnesium trisalicylate (see p.25).

Adverse effects. There has been a report[1] of a 21-month-old boy who developed salicylate poisoning after his mother had rubbed the contents of 3 tubes of 'Bonjela' teething ointment (containing a total of 2.61 g of choline salicylate) on his gums over 48 hours.

1. Paynter AS, Alexander FW. Salicylate intoxication caused by teething ointment. *Lancet* 1979; **ii:** 1132.

Preparations

BP 1998: Choline Salicylate Dental Gel; Choline Salicylate Ear Drops.

Proprietary Preparations (details are given in Part 3)
Austral.: Applicaine; Ora-Sed Jel†; ***Belg.:*** Teejel; ***Canad.:*** Teejel; ***Ger.:*** Audax; Rheumavincin†; ***Irl.:*** Audax; Teejel; ***S.Afr.:*** Audax†; ***UK:*** Audax; Dinnefords Teejel; ***USA:*** Arthropan.

Multi-ingredient: ***Aust.:*** Mundisal; Tifenso; ***Austral.:*** Bonjela; Seda-Gel; ***Belg.:*** Givalex; ***Fr.:*** Givalex; Pansoral; ***Ger.:*** Givalex; Mundisal; ***Irl.:*** Bonjela; ***Spain:*** Aldo Otico; Paidoterin Descongestivo†; ***Switz.:*** Mundisal; Pansoral; ***UK:*** Bonjela; Earex Plus.

Cinchophen (2627-t)

Cinchophen *(BAN, rINN)*.

Acifenokinolin; Phenylcinchoninic Acid; Quinophan. 2-Phenylquinoline-4-carboxylic acid.

$C_{16}H_{11}NO_2$ = 249.3.

CAS — 132-60-5.

Cinchophen and its derivatives were formerly used in the treatment of gout but were associated with severe and unpredictable hepatotoxicity.

Cinmetacin (12572-y)

Cinmetacin *(rINN)*.

(1-Cinnamoyl-5-methoxy-2-methylindol-3-yl)acetic acid.

$C_{21}H_{19}NO_4$ = 349.4.

CAS — 20168-99-4.

Cinmetacin is an NSAID (p.63) that has been given by mouth or by rectal suppository in musculoskeletal and joint disorders.

Preparations

Proprietary Preparations (details are given in Part 3)
Spain: Cetanovo†.

Clofexamide (12585-a)

Clofexamide *(rINN)*.

ANP-246. 2-(4-Chlorophenoxy)-*N*-(2-diethylaminoethyl)acetamide.

$C_{14}H_{21}ClN_2O_2$ = 284.8.

CAS — 1223-36-5.

Clofexamide has been used topically as the hydrochloride in preparations for musculoskeletal, joint, and soft-tissue disorders.

Preparations

Proprietary Preparations (details are given in Part 3)
Multi-ingredient: ***Fr.:*** Perclusone.

Clofezone (2628-x)

Clofezone *(rINN)*.

ANP-3260. An equimolar combination of clofexamide and phenylbutazone.

$C_{14}H_{21}ClN_2O_2.C_{19}H_{20}N_2O_2.2H_2O$ = 629.2.

CAS — 60104-29-2.

Clofezone, a combination molecule containing clofexamide (p.25) and phenylbutazone (p.79), has been used topically in preparations for musculoskeletal, joint, and soft-tissue disorders.

Preparations

Proprietary Preparations (details are given in Part 3)
Multi-ingredient: ***Fr.:*** Perclusone.

Clonixin (2630-j)

Clonixin (*USAN, rINN*).

CBA-93626; Sch-10304. 2-(3-Chloro-o-toluidino)nicotinic acid.

$C_{13}H_{11}ClN_2O_2$ = 262.7.

CAS — 17737-65-4.

Clonixin is an NSAID (p.63). It has been used as the lysine salt in doses of up to 250 mg four times daily by mouth for the relief of pain. Clonixin has also been given as the lysine salt by intramuscular or intravenous injection and as a rectal suppository.

References.

1. Eberhardt R, *et al.* Analgesic efficacy and tolerability of lysine-clonixinate versus ibuprofen in patients with gonarthrosis. *Curr Ther Res* 1995; **56:** 573–80.

Preparations

Proprietary Preparations (details are given in Part 3)
Spain: Dolalgial.

Cloracetadol (14174-z)

Cloracetadol (*rINN*).

N-[4-(2,2,2-Trichloro-1-hydroxyethoxy)phenyl]acetamide.

$C_{10}H_{10}Cl_3NO_3$ = 298.5.

CAS — 15687-05-5.

Cloracetadol is reported to have analgesic, antipyretic, and anti-inflammatory properties.

Preparations

Proprietary Preparations (details are given in Part 3)
Multi-ingredient: ***Ital.:*** Pisol†.

Codeine (6211-b)

Codeine (*BAN*).

Codeinum; Methylmorphine; Metilmorfina; Morphine Methyl Ether. 7,8-Didehydro-4,5-epoxy-3-methoxy-17-methylmorphinan-6-ol monohydrate.

$C_{18}H_{21}NO_3,H_2O$ = 317.4.

CAS — 76-57-3 (anhydrous codeine); 6059-47-8 (codeine monohydrate).

Pharmacopoeias. In *Eur.* (see p.viii), *Int.*, and *US.*

Codeine is obtained from opium or made by methylating morphine. It occurs as colourless or white crystals or white crystalline powder. M.p. 155° to 159°. It effloresces slowly in dry air.

Slightly **soluble** (1 in 120) of water and soluble in boiling water; soluble 1 in 2 of alcohol, 1 in 0.5 of chloroform, and 1 in 50 of ether. A 0.5% solution in water has a pH of more than 9. **Store** in airtight containers. Protect from light.

Codeine Hydrochloride (6212-v)

Codeine Hydrochloride (*BANM*).

$C_{18}H_{21}NO_3,HCl,2H_2O$ = 371.9.

CAS — 1422-07-7 (anhydrous codeine hydrochloride).

Pharmacopoeias. In *Aust., Br.*, and *Swiss.*

Small colourless crystals or a white crystalline powder. **Soluble** in water; slightly soluble in alcohol; practically insoluble in chloroform and in ether. **Protect** from light.

Codeine Phosphate (6213-g)

Codeine Phosphate (*BANM*).

Codeine Phosphate Hemihydrate; Codeini Phosphas; Codeini Phosphas Hemihydricus; Codeinii Phosphas; Methylmorphine Phosphate.

$C_{18}H_{21}NO_3,H_3PO_4,\frac{1}{2}H_2O$ = 406.4.

CAS — 52-28-8 (anhydrous codeine phosphate); 41444-62-6 (codeine phosphate hemihydrate); 5913-76-8 (codeine phosphate sesquihydrate).

NOTE. Compounded preparations of codeine phosphate and aspirin in the proportions 1 part to 50 parts by weight, respectively, have the British Approved Name Co-codaprin.

Compounded preparations of codeine phosphate and paracetamol have the British Approved Name Co-codamol; proportions are expressed as *x/y*, with *x* and *y* being the amount in mg of codeine phosphate and paracetamol, respectively.

Compounded preparations of paracetamol (acetaminophen) and codeine phosphate in USP 23 may be represented by the name Co-codAPAP and preparations of aspirin and codeine phosphate in USP 23 by the name Co-codaprin.

Pharmacopoeias. In *Chin., Eur.* (see p.viii), *Int., Jpn, Pol.*, and *US.*

Chin. specifies $1\frac{1}{2}H_2O$. *Int.* permits $1\frac{1}{2}H_2O$ or $\frac{1}{2}H_2O$.

Eur. also has a monograph for Codeine Phosphate Sesquihydrate ($C_{18}H_{21}NO_3,H_3PO_4,1\frac{1}{2}H_2O$ = 424.4).

The hemihydrate and the sesquihydrate occur as small odourless, colourless or white crystals or a white crystalline powder. Ph. Eur. **solubilities** for the hemihydrate or sesquihydrate are: freely soluble in water; slightly soluble in alcohol; practically insoluble in ether. USP solubilities for the hemihydrate are: soluble 1 in 2.5 of water and 1 in 0.5 of water at 80°; soluble 1 in 325 of alcohol and 1 in 125 of boiling alcohol. A 4% solution in water has a pH of 4.0 to 5.0. **Store** in airtight containers. Protect from light.

Incompatibility. Acetylation of codeine phosphate by aspirin has occurred in solid dosage forms containing the two drugs, even at a low moisture level.[1] *Animal* work suggested that the analgesic activity of codeine was not affected by acetylation.[2]

1. Galante RN, *et al.* Solid-state acetylation of codeine phosphate by aspirin. *J Pharm Sci* 1979; **68:** 1494–8.
2. Buckett WR, *et al.* The analgesic properties of some 14-substituted derivatives of codeine and codeinone. *J Pharm Pharmacol* 1964; **16:** 174–82.

Codeine Sulphate (6214-q)

Codeine Sulphate (*BANM*).

Codeine Sulfate.

$(C_{18}H_{21}NO_3)_2,H_2SO_4,3H_2O$ = 750.9.

CAS — 1420-53-7 (anhydrous codeine sulphate); 6854-40-6 (codeine sulphate trihydrate).

Pharmacopoeias. In *US.*

White crystals, usually needle-like, or white crystalline powder. **Soluble** 1 in 30 of water, 1 in 6.5 of water at 80°, and 1 in 1300 of alcohol; insoluble in chloroform and in ether. **Store** in airtight containers. Protect from light.

Stability. Codeine sulphate solutions appear to be intrinsically more stable than codeine phosphate solutions.[1]

1. Powell MF. Enhanced stability of codeine sulfate: effect of pH, buffer, and temperature on the degradation of codeine in aqueous solution. *J Pharm Sci* 1986; **75:** 901–3.

Dependence and Withdrawal

As for Opioid Analgesics, p.67. Codeine is subject to abuse (see under Precautions, below), but produces less euphoria and sedation than morphine.

Neonatal opioid dependence. Some of the symptoms characteristic of the neonatal abstinence syndrome were seen in a neonate whose mother had taken about 90 mg of codeine daily during the last 2 months of pregnancy.[1]

1. Khan K, Chang J. Neonatal abstinence syndrome due to codeine. *Arch Dis Child* 1997; **76:** F59–F60.

Adverse Effects and Treatment

As for Opioid Analgesics in general, p.68.

In therapeutic doses codeine is much less liable than morphine to produce adverse effects, although constipation may be troublesome with long-term use. Following large doses of codeine, excitement and convulsions may occur.

Codeine, like morphine, has a dose-related histamine-releasing effect. Anaphylactic reactions following intravenous administration have been reported, rarely.

Effects on mental function. Central effects of codeine phosphate appeared to be limited, but dose-related, in subjects given 30, 60, or 90 mg; visuo-motor coordination was altered with doses of 60 and 90 mg and dynamic visual acuity with 90 mg.[1] Drowsiness reported by 3 subjects receiving 90 mg of codeine phosphate could not be linked with impaired performance whereas nausea in 3 could.

1. Bradley CM, Nicholson AN. Effects of a μ-opioid receptor agonist (codeine phosphate) on visuo-motor coordination and dynamic visual acuity in man. *Br J Clin Pharmacol* 1986; **22:** 507–12.

Effects on the pancreas. A 26-year-old woman developed acute pancreatitis on 2 separate occasions a few hours after taking a single, 40-mg dose of codeine.[1] There was no history of alcohol consumption and her recovery was uneventful.

1. Hastier P, *et al.* Pancreatitis induced by codeine: a case report with positive rechallenge. *Gut* 1997; **41:** 705–6.

Effects on the skin. Pruritus and burning erythemato-vesicular plaques that developed in a patient in response to oral codeine were attributed to a fixed drug eruption.[1]

1. Gonzalo-Garijo MA, Revenga-Arranz F. Fixed drug eruption due to codeine. *Br J Dermatol* 1996; **135:** 498–9.

Overdosage. Acute codeine intoxication in 430 children, due to accidental ingestion of antitussive preparations, was analysed by von Mühlendahl *et al.*[1] The children were nearly all between 1 and 6 years old. Symptoms in decreasing order of frequency included somnolence, rash, miosis, vomiting, itching, ataxia, and swelling of the skin. Respiratory failure occurred in 8 children and 2 died; all 8 had taken 5 mg or more per kg body-weight. Infants are at special risk and there have been reports of fatality[2] or near fatality[3] following inappropriate treatment in 3-month-old infants given mixtures containing codeine.

Opioid toxicity, in addition to severe salicylate toxicity, has occurred in adults following overdoses of aspirin and codeine tablets.[4]

1. von Mühlendahl KE, *et al.* Codeine intoxication in childhood. *Lancet* 1976; **ii:** 303–5.
2. Ivey HH, Kattwinkel J. Danger of Actifed-C. *Pediatrics* 1976; **57:** 164–5.
3. Wilkes TCR, *et al.* Apnoea in a 3-month-old baby prescribed compound linctus containing codeine. *Lancet* 1981; **i:** 1166–7.
4. Leslie PJ, *et al.* Opiate toxicity after self poisoning with aspirin and codeine. *Br Med J* 1986; **292:** 96.

Precautions

As for Opioid Analgesics in general, p.68.

Abuse. Although the risk of dependence on codeine is low with normal use,[1] it is the subject of deliberate abuse. In the UK linctuses containing codeine are particularly liable to abuse. Reports in the literature include the use in New Zealand of codeine-containing preparations to produce demethylated products known as "Homebake" containing variable amounts of morphine;[2] and abuse of co-codaprin tablets for their codeine content.[3-5]

1. Rowden AM, Lopez JR. Codeine addiction. *DICP Ann Pharmacother* 1989; **23:** 475–7.
2. Shaw JP. Drug misuse in New Zealand. *Pharm J* 1987; **238:** 607.
3. Sakol MS, Stark CR. Codeine abuse. *Lancet* 1989; **ii:** 1282.
4. Paterson JR, *et al.* Codeine abuse from co-codaprin. *Lancet* 1990; **335:** 224.
5. Sakol MS, Stark CR. Codeine abuse from co-codaprin. *Lancet* 1990; **335:** 224.

Children. See under Overdosage, above, and under Uses and Administration, below.

Driving. Codeine phosphate 50 mg alone and in combination with alcohol had a deleterious effect on driving skills in a simulated driving test.[1]

1. Linnoila M, Häkkinen S. Effects of diazepam and codeine, alone and in combination with alcohol, on simulated driving. *Clin Pharmacol Ther* 1974; **15:** 368–73.

Interactions

For interactions associated with opioid analgesics, see p.69.

For reference to a suggestion that quinidine can inhibit the analgesic effect of codeine, see under Metabolism in Pharmacokinetics, below.

Pharmacokinetics

Codeine and its salts are absorbed from the gastro-intestinal tract. Rectal absorption of codeine phosphate has been reported. Ingestion of codeine phosphate produces peak plasma-codeine concentrations in about one hour. Codeine is metabolised by *O*- and *N*-demethylation in the liver to morphine, norcodeine, and other metabolites including normorphine and hydrocodone. Codeine and its metabolites are excreted almost entirely by the kidney, mainly as conjugates with glucuronic acid.

The plasma half-life has been reported to be between 3 and 4 hours after administration by mouth or intramuscular injection.

References.

1. Ebbighausen WOR, *et al.* Mass fragmentographic detection of normorphine in urine of man after codeine intake. *J Pharm Sci* 1973; **62:** 146–8.
2. Bechtel WD, Sinterhauf K. Plasma level and renal excretion of [³H] codeine phosphate in man and in the dog. *Arzneimittelforschung* 1978; **28:** 308–11.
3. Cone EJ, *et al.* Comparative metabolism of codeine in man, rat, dog, guinea-pig and rabbit: identification of four new metabolites. *J Pharm Pharmacol* 1979; **31:** 314–17.
4. Rogers JF, *et al.* Codeine disposition in smokers and nonsmokers. *Clin Pharmacol Ther* 1982; **32:** 218–27.
5. Moolenaar F, *et al.* Rectal versus oral absorption of codeine phosphate in man. *Biopharm Drug Dispos* 1983; **4:** 195–9.
6. Posey BL, Kimble SN. High-performance liquid chromatographic study of codeine, norcodeine and morphine as indicators of codeine ingestion. *J Anal Toxicol* 1984; **8:** 68–74.

Administration. In a comparative study[1] codeine had an oral/intramuscular analgesic relative potency ratio of 6:10. This was high compared with that of morphine and was attributed to protection from rapid first-pass metabolism rather than more efficient absorption following oral administration.

1. Beaver WT, *et al.* Analgesic studies of codeine and oxycodone in patients with cancer I: comparisons of oral with intramuscular codeine and of oral with intramuscular oxycodone. *J Pharmacol Exp Ther* 1978; **207:** 92–100.

Metabolism. The analgesic effect of codeine may be partly due to its metabolite morphine and it has been suggested that its efficacy may be impaired in patients who are poor metabolisers of codeine[1-3] or in those who are also receiving drugs such as quinidine which impair its metabolism.[1] However, Quiding *et al.*[4] found that patients unable to demethylate codeine to produce detectable plasma concentrations of morphine obtained a similar analgesic effect to patients with detectable plasma morphine concentrations. A study[5] involving infants aged 6 to 10 months has indicated that children were capable of demethylating codeine to morphine at the age of 6 months although glucuronidation of the morphine appeared to be impaired when compared with older children.

1. Desmeules J, *et al.* Impact of environmental and genetic factors on codeine analgesia. *Eur J Clin Pharmacol* 1991; **41:** 23–6.
2. Chen ZR, *et al.* Disposition and metabolism of codeine after single and chronic doses in one poor and seven extensive metabolisers. *Br J Clin Pharmacol* 1991; **31:** 381–90.
3. Sindrup SH, *et al.* Codeine increases pain thresholds to copper vapor laser stimuli in extensive but not poor metabolizers of sparteine. *Clin Pharmacol Ther* 1991; **49:** 686–93.
4. Quiding H, *et al.* Analgesic effect and plasma concentrations of codeine and morphine after two dose levels of codeine following oral surgery. *Eur J Clin Pharmacol* 1993; **44:** 319–23.
5. Quiding H, *et al.* Infants and young children metabolise codeine to morphine: a study after single and repeated rectal administration. *Br J Clin Pharmacol* 1992; **33:** 45–9.

Uses and Administration

Codeine, a phenanthrene derivative, is an opioid analgesic (p.69). It is much less potent as an analgesic than morphine and has relatively mild sedative effects.

Codeine or its salts, especially the phosphate, are administered by mouth in the form of linctuses for the relief of cough, and as tablets for the relief of mild to moderate pain, often in association with a non-opioid analgesic. Codeine phosphate with aspirin or paracetamol is sometimes known as co-codaprin or co-codamol (Co-codAPAP), respectively (see NOTE, above). The phosphate is also given by injection, usually by the intramuscular or subcutaneous route, for the relief of pain; the intravenous route has also been used in adults.

Doses are similar by mouth or by injection.

For the relief of pain codeine phosphate may be given in doses of 30 to 60 mg every 4 hours to a maximum of 240 mg daily. Children aged 1 to 12 years may be given 500 µg per kg body-weight 4 to 6 times daily.

To allay unproductive cough codeine phosphate may be given in doses of 15 to 30 mg three to four times a day. Children aged 5 to 12 years may be given 7.5 to 15 mg three to four times a day and those aged 1 to 5 years, 3 mg three to four times a day (but see below).

Codeine is also used as tablets or in mixtures for the symptomatic relief of acute diarrhoea in adult doses of 30 mg given 3 to 4 times daily.

Other codeine salts used include the hydrochloride, sulphate, acephyllinate, camsylate, and hydrobromide. Codeine polistirex (a codeine and sulphonated diethenylbenzene-ethenylbenzene copolymer complex) is used in modified-release preparations.

A meta-analysis[1] comparing paracetamol-codeine combinations versus paracetamol alone concluded that in single dose studies addition of codeine to paracetamol produced a comparatively small but statistically significant increase in analgesic effect; multidose studies showed an increased incidence of side-effects with the combination.

1. de Craen AJM, *et al.* Analgesic efficacy and safety of paracetamol-codeine combinations versus paracetamol alone: a systematic review. *Br Med J* 1996; **313:** 321–5.

Administration in children. Dosage recommendations for codeine in the treatment of pain or cough are generally restricted to those over 1 year of age. However, Lloyd-Thomas[1] considered codeine to be an effective analgesic in neonates and children. With a single dose of codeine phosphate 1 mg per kg body-weight by mouth or by intramuscular injection there was a relatively small risk of respiratory depression in neonates, but significant respiratory depression has occurred with multiple doses and patients should be observed closely.[1] Case reports of adverse reactions such as vasodilatation, severe hypotension, and apnoea in infants and children after intravenous administration of codeine have precluded its use by this route in children of all ages.[2]

Antimotility drugs such as codeine should not be used in infants and young children with acute diarrhoea[3,4] and in chronic diarrhoea codeine has been restricted to those over 4 to 5 years old.

Cough suppressants containing codeine or similar opioids are generally not recommended for administration to children and should be avoided in those under 1 year of age.

1. Lloyd-Thomas AR. Pain management in paediatric patients. *Br J Anaesth* 1990; **64:** 85–104.
2. Marsh DF, *et al.* Opioid systems and the newborn. *Br J Anaesth* 1997; **79:** 787–95.
3. Anonymous. Drugs in the management of acute diarrhoea in infants and young children. *Bull WHO* 1989; **67:** 94–6.
4. Cimolai N, Carter JE. Antimotility agents for paediatric use. *Lancet* 1990; **336:** 874.

Preparations

BP 1998: Co-codamol Tablets; Co-codaprin Tablets; Codeine Linctus; Codeine Phosphate Oral Solution; Codeine Phosphate Tablets; Dispersible Co-codaprin Tablets; Paediatric Codeine Linctus;
USP 23: Acetaminophen and Codeine Phosphate Capsules; Acetaminophen and Codeine Phosphate Oral Solution; Acetaminophen and Codeine Phosphate Oral Suspension; Acetaminophen and Codeine Phosphate Tablets; Aspirin and Codeine Phosphate Tablets; Aspirin, Codeine Phosphate, Alumina, and Magnesia Tablets; Aspirin, Codeine Phosphate, and Caffeine Capsules; Aspirin, Codeine Phosphate, and Caffeine Tablets; Butalbital, Aspirin, Caffeine, and Codeine Phosphate Capsules; Carisoprodol, Aspirin, and Codeine Phosphate Tablets; Codeine Phosphate Injection; Codeine Phosphate Tablets; Codeine Sulfate Tablets; Guaifenesin and Codeine Phosphate Syrup; Terpin Hydrate and Codeine Elixir.

Proprietary Preparations (details are given in Part 3)
Aust.: Codipertussin; Tricodein; ***Austral.:*** Actacode; Codate†; Codelix†; Codlin†; ***Belg.:*** Bronchodine; Codocalyptol; Glottyl; Pectocalmine Gommes†; ***Fr.:*** Neo-Codion; Paderyl; Pectoral Edulcor; ***Ger.:*** Bronchicum Mono Codein; Bronchoforton Kodeinsaft†; codi OPT; Codicaps mono; Codicept†; Codicompren; Codiforton; Codipertussin†; Codipront mono; Contrapect infant N†; Contrapect†; Dicton; Neo-Codion NN; Optipect Kodein; Tricodein; Tryasol; Tussamag Codeintropfen; Tussipect mono†; Tussoretard SN; ***Irl.:*** Codant; Diarrest; ***Neth.:*** Rami Hoeststroop voor Kinderen†; ***S.Afr.:*** Xeramax; ***Spain:*** Bisoltus; Codeisan; Histaverin; Perduretas Codeina; Solcodein†; ***Switz.:*** Tricodein; ***UK:*** Evacode; Galcodine.

Multi-ingredient: numerous preparations are listed in Part 3.

Cymene (2631-z)

p-Cymene; *p*-Cymol. 4-Isopropyl-1-methylbenzene; 4-Isopropyltoluene.

$C_{10}H_{14}$ = 134.2.
CAS — 25155-15-1; 99-87-6 (p-cymene).

Cymene has been used as a topical local analgesic for the relief of pain in rheumatic conditions.

Preparations

Proprietary Preparations (details are given in Part 3)
Spain: Dolcymene†.

Multi-ingredient: ***Fr.:*** Neuriplege.

Devil's Claw Root (3082-w)

Harpagophyti Radix; Harpagophyton; Harpagophytum; Harpagophytum Procumbens; Teufelskrallenwurzel.

Pharmacopoeias. In *Eur.* (see p.viii).

The cut and dried tuberous, secondary roots of *Harpagophytum procumbens* (Pedaliaceae). Greyish-brown to dark brown with a bitter taste. Contains not less than 1.2% harpagoside ($C_{24}H_{30}O_{11}$=494.5). **Protect** from light.

Devil's claw root is used in herbal remedies for musculoskeletal and joint disorders.

Preparations

Proprietary Preparations (details are given in Part 3)
Fr.: Algophytum; Harpadol; Lyophytum†; ***Ger.:*** Arthrosetten H; Arthrotabs; Defencid; Dolo-Arthrodynat; Dolo-Arthrosetten H; Doloteffin; Harpagoforte Asmedic; Jucurba N; Kai Fu†; Rheuma-Sern; Rheuma-Tee†; Rheuma-Teufelskralle HarpagoMega; Salus; ***Ital.:*** Artigel†; ***Spain:*** Fitokey Harpagophytum†; Harpagofito Orto; Hartiosen.

Multi-ingredient: ***Austral.:*** Arthritic Pain Herbal Formula 1; Devils Claw Plus; Green Lipped Mussel†; Harpagophytum Complex; Herbal Arthritis Formula; Lifesystem Herbal Formula 1 Arthritic Aid; Lifesystem Herbal Formula 12 Willowbark; Prost-1; Willowbark Plus Herbal Formula 11; ***Fr.:*** Actisane Douleurs Articulaires; Arkophytum; Artrosan; ***Ital.:*** Artoxan; ***UK:*** Arthrotone.

Dextromoramide (6215-p)

Dextromoramide *(BAN, pINN).*

Dextrodiphenopyrine; *d*-Moramid; Pyrrolamidol. (+)-1-(3-Methyl-4-morpholino-2,2-diphenylbutyryl)pyrrolidine.

$C_{25}H_{32}N_2O_2$ = 392.5.
CAS — 357-56-2.

Dextromoramide Tartrate (6216-s)

Dextromoramide Tartrate *(BANM, pINNM).*

Bitartrate de Dextromoramide; Dextromoramide Acid Tartrate; Dextromoramide Hydrogen Tartrate; Dextromoramidi Tartras; Tartarato de Dextromoramida.

$C_{25}H_{32}N_2O_2,C_4H_6O_6$ = 542.6.
CAS — 2922-44-3.

Pharmacopoeias. In *Eur.* (see p.viii).

A white crystalline or amorphous powder. Dextromoramide tartrate 6.9 mg is approximately equivalent to 5 mg of dextromoramide. **Soluble** in water; sparingly soluble in alcohol; very slightly soluble in ether. A 1% solution in water has a pH of 3.0 to 4.0.

Dependence and Withdrawal, Adverse Effects, Treatment, and Precautions

As for Opioid Analgesics, p.67. Dextromoramide is subject to abuse. It is reported to be less sedating than morphine.

Interactions

For interactions associated with opioid analgesics, see p.69.

Uses and Administration

Dextromoramide is an opioid analgesic (p.69) structurally related to methadone (p.54) and is used in the treatment of severe pain. It is not recommended for use in obstetric analgesia because of an increased risk of neonatal depression.

Dextromoramide is given as the tartrate by mouth or by rectum. It has also been given by subcutaneous or intramuscular injection and similar analgesic effects have been claimed for the same dose whether given by mouth or by injection. The analgesic effect begins after about 20 to 30 minutes, but its duration of action is only about 2 to 3 hours.

The usual dose is the equivalent of dextromoramide 5 mg by mouth increased if necessary up to 20 mg. Dextromoramide is given by injection in doses of 5 mg.

Dextromoramide is also given rectally as suppositories containing the equivalent of 10 mg.

An initial dose equivalent to not more than 80 µg per kg body-weight has been suggested by the manufacturers for use in children.

Preparations

BP 1998: Dextromoramide Injection; Dextromoramide Tablets.

Proprietary Preparations (details are given in Part 3)
Austral.: Palfium; ***Belg.:*** Palfium; ***Fr.:*** Palfium; ***Irl.:*** Palfium; ***Ital.:*** Narcolo†; ***Neth.:*** Palfium; ***UK:*** Palfium.

Dextropropoxyphene (13408-s)

Dextropropoxyphene *(BAN, pINN).*

Propoxyphene. (+)-(1*S*,2*R*)-1-Benzyl-3-dimethylamino-2-methyl-1-phenylpropyl propionate.

$C_{22}H_{29}NO_2$ = 339.5.
CAS — 469-62-5.

Dextropropoxyphene Hydrochloride (6217-w)

Dextropropoxyphene Hydrochloride *(BANM, pINNM).*

Cloridrato de Dextropropoxifeno; Dextropropoxypheni Hydrochloridum; Propoxyphene Hydrochloride *(USAN).*

$C_{22}H_{29}NO_2,HCl$ = 375.9.
CAS — 1639-60-7.

NOTE. Compounded preparations of dextropropoxyphene hydrochloride and paracetamol in the proportions 1 part to 10 parts by weight, respectively, have the British Approved Name Co-proxamol.

Pharmacopoeias. In *Eur.* (see p.viii) and *US.*

A white or almost white odourless crystalline powder. Ph. Eur. **solubilities** are: very soluble in water; freely soluble in alcohol, practically insoluble in ether. USP solubilities are: freely soluble in water; soluble in alcohol, in acetone, and in chloroform; practically insoluble in ether. **Store** in airtight containers and protect from light.

Dextropropoxyphene Napsylate (6218-e)

Dextropropoxyphene Napsylate *(BANM).*

Dextropropoxyphene Napsilate *(pINNM)*; Propoxyphene Napsylate *(USAN).* Dextropropoxyphene naphthalene-2-sulphonate monohydrate.

$C_{22}H_{29}NO_2,C_{10}H_8O_3S,H_2O$ = 565.7.
CAS — 17140-78-2 (anhydrous dextropropoxyphene napsylate); 26570-10-5 (dextropropoxyphene napsylate monohydrate).

NOTE. Compounded preparations of dextropropoxyphene (propoxyphene) napsylate and paracetamol (acetaminophen) in USP 23 may be represented by the name Co-proxAPAP.

Pharmacopoeias. In *Br.* and *US.*

An odourless or almost odourless white powder. Dextropropoxyphene napsylate 100 mg is approximately equivalent to 66 mg of dextropropoxyphene hydrochloride. Practically **insoluble** in water; soluble 1 in 15 of alcohol and 1 in 10 of chloroform; soluble in acetone and in methyl alcohol. **Store** in airtight containers.

Dependence and Withdrawal

As for Opioid Analgesics, p.67. Dextropropoxyphene has been subject to abuse (see under Precautions, below).

Reports of dextropropoxyphene dependence and its treatment.

1. Wall R, *et al.* Addiction to Distalgesic (dextropropoxyphene). *Br Med J* 1980; **280:** 1213–14.
2. D'Abadie NB, Lenton JD. Propoxyphene dependence: problems in management. *South Med J* 1984; **77:** 299–301.

Adverse Effects

As for Opioid Analgesics in general, p.68. In the recommended dosage the adverse effects of dextropropoxyphene are less marked than those of morphine. Gastro-intestinal effects, dizziness, and drowsiness are the most common. Liver impairment has been reported.

There are a disturbing number of fatalities from either accidental or intentional overdosage with dextropropoxyphene. Many reports emphasise the rapidity with which death ensues; death within an hour of overdosage is considered by some not to be uncommon and can occur within 15 minutes. Overdosage is often complicated by patients also taking alcohol and using mixed preparations such as dextropropoxyphene with paracetamol or aspirin.

Symptoms of overdosage are similar to those of opioid poisoning in general, but in addition patients may experience psychotic reactions. There may be cardiac conduction abnormalities and arrhythmias.

Dextropropoxyphene injections are painful and have had a very destructive effect on soft tissues and veins when dextropropoxyphene has been abused in this way.

Anorectal reactions have followed the prolonged use of suppositories containing dextropropoxyphene; the reactions appear to be dose dependent.

Effects on the blood. A 12-year history of haemolysis and subsequent significant haemolytic anaemia in an elderly woman[1] was associated with chronic, periodic, and occasionally excessive intake of co-proxamol.

1. Fulton JD, McGonigal G. Steroid responsive haemolytic anaemia due to dextropropoxyphene paracetamol combination. *J R Soc Med* 1989; **82:** 228.

Effects on the ears. A report of complete nerve deafness associated with chronic abuse of co-proxamol was made to the UK Committee on Safety of Medicines.[1] The Committee had received 2 other reports of permanent hearing loss attributed to co-proxamol abuse; transient hearing loss had also been reported in 2 patients taking usual doses; 7 further reports described tinnitus.

1. Ramsay BC. Complete nerve deafness after abuse of co-proxamol. *Lancet* 1991; **338:** 446–7.

Effects on the liver. There have been occasional reports of jaundice in patients taking dextropropoxyphene without paracetamol. Many of the 49 suspected hepatic reactions with dextropropoxyphene reported to the UK Committee on Safety of Medicines by 1985[1] had involved dextropropoxyphene in association with paracetamol; clinical features including malaise, jaundice, raised serum transaminases, and sometimes fever, were however generally characteristic of dextropropoxyphene alone. Relapsing jaundice mimicking biliary disease was attributable to the dextropropoxyphene component of co-proxamol in 3 patients,[2] whereas there was no abnormality of liver function in 11 patients on long-term co-proxamol analgesia.[3]

1. Committee on Safety of Medicines. Hepatotoxicity with dextropropoxyphene. *Current Problems 17* 1986.
2. Bassendine MF, *et al.* Dextropropoxyphene induced hepatotoxicity mimicking biliary tract disease. *Gut* 1986; **27:** 444–9.
3. Hutchinson DR, *et al.* Liver function in patients on long-term paracetamol (co-proxamol) analgesia. *J Pharm Pharmacol* 1986; **38:** 242–3.

Hypoglycaemia. References to a hypoglycaemic effect of dextropropoxyphene.[1,2]

1. Wiederholt IC, *et al.* Recurrent episodes of hypoglycemia induced by propoxyphene. *Neurology* 1967; **17:** 703–4.
2. Almirall J, *et al.* Propoxyphene-induced hypoglycemia in a patient with chronic renal failure. *Nephron* 1989; **53:** 273–5.

Overdosage. There have been several reviews or retrospective studies of acute self-poisoning with dextropropoxyphene.[1-3] At a symposium on the safety and efficacy of dextropropoxyphene[4] many of the participants dealt with the problems of dextropropoxyphene overdosage, often in conjunction with paracetamol and sometimes with alcohol. Profound and even fatal CNS depression can develop rapidly as a result of the dextropropoxyphene content and in many cases death has occurred within an hour.[5] The quantity likely to be fatal is small. Whittington[6] suggested that 15 tablets or less of co-proxamol could lead to death and this is close to the figure of 20 tablets suggested by Young and Lawson.[7] A number of papers reviewed the cases of poisoning in different countries; one of these on poisoning in the USA[8] demonstrated that the incidence of dextropropoxyphene-associated deaths reached a peak in 1977 and has been falling since then at a rate that is not matched by a decline in prescribing. Also Finkle[8] could not demonstrate a connection between the metabolite nordextropropoxyphene and the fatalities. However, nordextropropoxyphene, like dextropropoxyphene, is considered to have local anaesthetic activity and Henry and Cassidy[9] implicated membrane stabilising activity as a major factor responsible for the severe cardiac depressant effect of dextropropoxyphene.

1. Young RJ. Dextropropoxyphene overdosage: pharmacological considerations and clinical management. *Drugs* 1983; **26:** 70–9.
2. Madsen PS, *et al.* Acute propoxyphene self-poisoning in 222 consecutive patients. *Acta Anaesthesiol Scand* 1984; **28:** 661–5.
3. Segest E. Poisoning with dextropropoxyphene in Denmark. *Hum Toxicol* 1987; **6:** 203–7.
4. Bowen D, *et al.* (ed). Distalgesic; safety and efficacy. *Hum Toxicol* 1984; **3** (suppl): 1S–238S.
5. Proudfoot AT. Clinical features and management of Distalgesic overdose. *Hum Toxicol* 1984; **3** (suppl): 85S–94S.
6. Whittington RM. Dextropropoxyphene deaths: coroner's report. *Hum Toxicol* 1984; **3** (suppl): 175S–85S.
7. Young RJ, Lawson AAH. Distalgesic poisoning—cause for concern. *Br Med J* 1980; **280:** 1045–7.
8. Finkle BS. Self-poisoning with dextropropoxyphene and dextropropoxyphene compounds: the USA experience. *Hum Toxicol* 1984; **3** (suppl): 115S–34S.
9. Henry JA, Cassidy SL. Membrane stabilising activity: a major cause of fatal poisoning. *Lancet* 1986; **i:** 1414–17.

Treatment of Adverse Effects

As for Opioid Analgesics in general, p.68.

Rapid treatment of overdosage with naloxone and assisted respiration is essential. Cardiac effects may not be reversed by naloxone. Gastric lavage and administration of activated charcoal may be of value but dialysis is of little use.

Convulsions may require control with an anticonvulsant, bearing in mind that the CNS depressant effects of dextropropoxyphene might be exacerbated (see also under Interactions, below). Stimulants should not be used because of the risk of inducing convulsions.

Patients taking overdoses of dextropropoxyphene with paracetamol will also require treatment for paracetamol poisoning (p.72). Mixtures of dextropropoxyphene and aspirin may be involved; the treatment of aspirin poisoning is described on p.16.

Reviews.

1. Proudfoot AT. Clinical features and management of Distalgesic overdose. *Hum Toxicol* 1984; **3** (suppl): 85S–94S.

Precautions

As for Opioid Analgesics in general, p.68.

Abuse. There have been reports of the abuse of dextropropoxyphene,[1] and Lader[2] considered that the ready availability of dextropropoxyphene made it liable to abuse although it was a relatively weak opioid analgesic. However, Finkle[3] thought there was no evidence that dextropropoxyphene was frequently associated with abuse, and Turner[4] concluded that, although there was abuse potential, it was of relatively low importance in terms of the community as a whole.

A severe withdrawal syndrome has been reported[5] in one elderly patient who covertly consumed a daily dose of dextropropoxyphene of 1 to 3 g for at least 12 months. The patient was treated by a gradually decreasing dosage schedule of dextropropoxyphene over 9 weeks.

1. Tennant FS. Complications of propoxyphene abuse. *Arch Intern Med* 1973; **132:** 191–4.
2. Lader M. Abuse of weak opioid analgesics. *Hum Toxicol* 1984; **3** (suppl): 229S–36S.
3. Finkle BS. Self-poisoning with dextropropoxyphene and dextropropoxyphene compounds: the USA experience. *Hum Toxicol* 1984; **3** (suppl): 115S–34S.
4. Turner P. Final remarks. *Hum Toxicol* 1984; **3** (suppl): 237S–8S.
5. Hedenmalm K. A case of severe withdrawal syndrome due to dextropropoxyphene. *Ann Intern Med* 1995; **123:** 473.

Breast feeding. See under Pharmacokinetics, below.

Porphyria. Dextropropoxyphene has been associated with clinical exacerbations of porphyria and is considered unsafe in porphyric patients.[1]

1. Moore MR, McColl KEL. *Porphyria: drug lists.* Glasgow: Porphyria Research Unit, University of Glasgow, 1991.

Interactions

For interactions associated with opioid analgesics, see p.69.

Plasma concentrations of dextropropoxyphene are increased by ritonavir, with a resultant risk of toxicity; concomitant administration should be avoided.

CNS depressants, including alcohol, may contribute to the hazards of dextropropoxyphene. The convulsant action of high doses of dextropropoxyphene may be enhanced by CNS stimulants.

Dextropropoxyphene interacts with several other drugs through inhibition of liver metabolism. Drugs reported to be affected include antidepressants, benzodiazepines, beta blockers, carbamazepine (see p.341), phenobarbitone (see p.351), phenytoin (see p.354), and warfarin.

Antimuscarinics. A suggested interaction between *orphenadrine* and dextropropoxyphene has been questioned (see p.465).

Pharmacokinetics

Dextropropoxyphene is readily absorbed from the gastro-intestinal tract, the napsylate tending to be more slowly absorbed than the hydrochloride, but both are subject to considerable first-pass metabolism. Peak plasma concentrations occur about 1 to 2 hours after ingestion. It is rapidly distributed and concentrated in the liver, lungs, and brain. About 80% of dextropropoxyphene and its metabolites are reported to be bound to plasma proteins. Dextropropoxyphene crosses the placenta. It has been detected in breast milk but some authorities consider that the amount is too small to be harmful to a breast-fed infant.

Dextropropoxyphene is *N*-demethylated to nordextropropoxyphene (norpropoxyphene), in the liver. It is excreted in the urine mainly as metabolites. It is now recognised that dextropropoxyphene and nordextropropoxyphene have prolonged elimination half-lives; values of 6 to 12 hours and 30 to 36 hours, respectively, have been reported. Accumulation of dextropropoxyphene and its metabolites may occur with repeated doses and nordextropropoxyphene may contribute to the toxicity seen with overdosage.

Reviews.

1. Pearson RM. Pharmacokinetics of propoxyphene. *Hum Toxicol* 1984; **3** (suppl): 37S–40S.

Administration in the elderly. The elimination half-lives of dextropropoxyphene and its metabolite nordextropropoxyphene were prolonged in healthy elderly subjects when compared with young controls.[1] After multiple dosing median half-lives of dextropropoxyphene and nordextropropoxyphene were 36.8 and 41.8 hours respectively in the elderly compared with 22.0 and 22.1 hours in the young subjects. In this study[1] there was a strong correlation between half-life of nordextropropoxyphene and estimated creatinine clearance.

1. Flanagan RJ, *et al.* Pharmacokinetics of dextropropoxyphene and nordextropropoxyphene in young and elderly volunteers after single and multiple dextropropoxyphene dosage. *Br J Clin Pharmacol* 1989; **28:** 463–9.

Administration in hepatic impairment. Plasma concentrations of dextropropoxyphene were higher in patients with cirrhosis given the drug than in healthy controls whereas concentrations of nordextropropoxyphene were lower.[1]

1. Giacomini KM, *et al.* Propoxyphene and norpropoxyphene plasma concentrations after oral propoxyphene in cirrhotic patients with and without surgically constructed portacaval shunt. *Clin Pharmacol Ther* 1980; **28:** 417–24.

Administration in renal impairment. Higher and more persistent plasma concentrations of dextropropoxyphene and nordextropropoxyphene in anephric patients when compared with healthy subjects[1] were attributed to decreased first-pass metabolism of dextropropoxyphene and decreased renal excretion of nordextropropoxyphene in the anephric patients.

1. Gibson TP, *et al.* Propoxyphene and norpropoxyphene plasma concentrations in the anephric patient. *Clin Pharmacol Ther* 1980; **27:** 665–70.

Uses and Administration

Dextropropoxyphene is an opioid analgesic (p.69) structurally related to methadone (p.54). It has mild analgesic activity and is administered by mouth as the hydrochloride or napsylate to alleviate mild to moderate pain. Unlike the laevo-isomer (levopropoxyphene, p.1063), dextropropoxyphene has little antitussive activity.

Dextropropoxyphene is mainly used in conjunction with other analgesics with anti-inflammatory and antipyretic effects, such as aspirin and paracetamol. In the UK the usual dose is 65 mg of dextropropoxyphene hydrochloride or 100 mg of the napsylate given three or four times daily. In the USA similar doses are given every 4 hours up to a maximum total daily dose of 390 mg of the hydrochloride and 600 mg of the napsylate. Compounded preparations of dextropropoxyphene hydrochloride (1 part) and paracetamol (10 parts) have the British Approved Name co-proxamol; a usual strength of this combination is dextropropoxyphene hydrochloride 32.5 mg with paracetamol 325 mg. Compounded preparations of dextropropoxyphene napsylate and paracetamol may be known in the USA as co-proxAPAP.

In a detailed review of the analgesic effectiveness of dextropropoxyphene, Beaver[1] observed that, with respect to single oral doses, the weight of evidence pointed to the recommended doses of dextropropoxyphene being no more and probably less effective than usual doses of paracetamol, aspirin, or other NSAIDs. However, the comparative effectiveness may vary substantially depending on the cause of the pain. When it comes to comparative studies involving combinations of dextropropoxyphene with other analgesics, findings are even less clear-cut; there are studies showing some benefit from such a combination and others showing no benefit. The effectiveness of co-proxamol (dextropropoxyphene with paracetamol) has long been a matter of controversy yet despite this a recent survey[2] conducted in 30 UK teaching hospitals found that co-proxamol was the most widely used paracetamol-containing analgesic. It was suggested that the popularity of co-proxamol was purely down to prescribing habits passed on to new medical staff, rather than hard evidence regarding efficacy. This view has been refuted by Sykes *et al.*[3] who say that a large number of studies have demonstrated clear analgesic effects for dextropropoxyphene. However, any assumption that the combination was widely used because it was more effective than paracetamol alone was not supported by a systematic overview of single dose studies by Li Wan Po and Zhang.[4] They concluded that while co-proxamol was indeed an effective analgesic it was no better than paracetamol alone. While the evidence from this and other systematic reviews indicate that co-proxamol should be replaced by paracetamol alone for acute pain the position for chronic use is considered to be not so clear.[5]

1. Beaver WT. Analgesic efficacy of dextropropoxyphene and dextropropoxyphene-containing combinations: a review. *Hum Toxicol* 1984; **3** (suppl): 191S–220S.
2. Haigh S. 12 Years on: co-proxamol revisited. *Lancet* 1996; **347:** 1840–1. Correction. *ibid.*; **348:** 346.
3. Sykes JV, *et al.* Coproxamol revisited. *Lancet* 1996; **348:** 408.
4. Li Wan Po A, Zhang WY. Systematic overview of co-proxamol to assess analgesic effects of addition of dextropropoxyphene to paracetamol. *Br Med J* 1997; **315:** 1565–71. Correction *ibid.* 1998; **316:** 116 and 656.
5. Anonymous. Co-proxamol or paracetamol for acute pain? *Drug Ther Bull* 1998; **36:** 80.

Preparations

BP 1998: Co-proxamol Tablets; Dextropropoxyphene Capsules; ***USP 23:*** Propoxyphene Hydrochloride and Acetaminophen Tablets; Propoxyphene Hydrochloride Capsules; Propoxyphene Hydrochloride, Aspirin, and Caffeine Capsules; Propoxyphene Napsylate and Acetaminophen Tablets; Propoxyphene Napsylate and Aspirin Tablets; Propoxyphene Napsylate Oral Suspension; Propoxyphene Napsylate Tablets.

Proprietary Preparations (details are given in Part 3)

Austral.: Doloxene; ***Belg.:*** Depronal; ***Canad.:*** 642; Darvon-N; Novo-Propoxyn; ***Fr.:*** Antalvic; ***Ger.:*** Develin; Dolo-Neurotrat†; ***Irl.:*** Doloxene; ***Ital.:*** Liberen; ***Neth.:*** Depronal; ***S.Afr.:*** Doloxene; Doxypol†; ***Spain:*** Darvon; Deprancol; ***Swed.:*** Dexofen; Dolotard; Doloxene; ***Switz.:*** Depronal; ***UK:*** Doloxene; ***USA:*** Darvon; Darvon-N; Dolene; PP-Cap.

Multi-ingredient: ***Aust.:*** Algo-Prolixan; APA; Contraforte; Sigmalin B_6 forte; Ultrapyrin†; ***Austral.:*** Capadex; Di-Gesic; Doloxene Co†; Paradex; ***Belg.:*** Distalgic; Yamalen New; Yamalen†; ***Canad.:*** 692; Darvon-N Compound†; Darvon-N with ASA†; ***Fr.:*** Di-Antalvic; Propofan; ***Ger.:*** Dolo-Prolixan†; Rosimon-Neu†; Ultrapyrin†; ***Irl.:*** Cosalgesic; Distalgesic; Doloxene Compound; ***Ital.:*** Femidol†; ***Norw.:*** Aporex; ***S.Afr.:*** Distalgesic; Doloxene Co; Doxyfene; Lentogesic; Synap; ***Swed.:*** Dexodon; Distalgesic; Doleron; Paraflex comp.; ***Switz.:*** Distalgesic; Dolo-Prolixan; ***UK:*** Cosalgesic; Distalgesic; Doloxene Compound†; ***USA:*** Darvocet-N; Darvon Compound; E-Lor†; Genagesic; PC-Cap; Propacet; Proxy†; Wygesic.

Dezocine (12637-j)

Dezocine *(USAN, rINN).*

Wy-16225. (−)-13β-Amino-5,6,7,8,9,10,11α,12-octahydro-5α-methyl-5,11-methanobenzocyclodecen-3-ol.

$C_{16}H_{23}NO$ = 245.4.

CAS — 53648-55-8.

Dependence and Withdrawal

As for Opioid Analgesics, p.67.

According to a WHO expert committee[1] the potential for physical dependence on dezocine was low in *animals* and had not been studied in humans. Assessment of the morphine-like subjective and miotic effects of dezocine indicated that it had the potential to be abused, but suggested that its abuse potential was less than that of morphine.[2] In 1989, in the absence of reports of actual abuse of dezocine, WHO[1] rated its likelihood as moderate and considered that international control was not warranted.

1. WHO. WHO expert committee on drug dependence: twenty-fifth report. *WHO Tech Rep Ser 775* 1989.
2. Jasinski DR, Preston KL. Assessment of dezocine for morphine-like subjective effects and miosis. *Clin Pharmacol Ther* 1985; **38:** 544–8.

Adverse Effects and Treatment

As for Opioid Analgesics in general, p.68.

Because dezocine has opioid agonist and antagonist activity, naloxone is the recommended antagonist for the treatment of overdose.

In a preliminary study pronounced dizziness occurred in most patients given single intravenous doses of dezocine 5 to 20 mg.[1]

1. Oosterlinck W, Verbaeys A. Preliminary clinical experience with dezocine, a new potent analgesic. *Curr Med Res Opin* 1980; **6:** 472–4.

Effects on mental function. At high doses symptoms suggestive of psychotomimetic effects were more frequent after dezocine than after morphine,[1] but a WHO expert committee[2] considered that, although dezocine produced miosis and other opioid effects such as euphoria, there was no evidence for the dysphoric sedative and hallucinogenic effects seen with pentazocine.

1. Romagnoli A, Keats AS. Ceiling respiratory depression by dezocine. *Clin Pharmacol Ther* 1984; **35:** 367–73.
2. WHO. WHO expert committee on drug dependence: twenty-fifth report. *WHO Tech Rep Ser 775* 1989.

Effects on the respiratory system. Respiratory depression following intravenous administration of dezocine or morphine 10 mg per 70 kg body-weight was similar although dezocine was associated with a more rapid onset and a brief higher peak activity;[1] unlike morphine a ceiling effect for respiratory depression occurred at a cumulative dose of 30 mg of dezocine per 70 kg. In patients undergoing cardiac catheterisation relatively low intravenous doses of dezocine or morphine (0.125 mg per kg) had no clinically important haemodynamic or respiratory effects.[2]

1. Romagnoli A, Keats AS. Ceiling respiratory depression by dezocine. *Clin Pharmacol Ther* 1984; **35:** 367–73.
2. Rothbard RL, *et al.* Hemodynamic and respiratory effects of dezocine, ciramadol, and morphine. *Clin Pharmacol Ther* 1985; **38:** 84–8.

Precautions

As for Opioid Analgesics in general, p.68.

Dezocine may precipitate withdrawal symptoms if given to patients who are physically dependent on opioids (see below).

Opioid-dependent subjects maintained on oral methadone in a daily dose of 30 mg were challenged with different doses of intramuscular dezocine ranging from 7.5 to 60 mg.[1] Dezocine produced primarily antagonist-like effects and precipitated a withdrawal syndrome which was not directly dose-related in magnitude. The greatest withdrawal effects were seen in the mid-dose range and the least with the higher doses. These results suggest that lower doses of dezocine should have a relatively low abuse liability in opioid-dependent patients.

1. Strain EC, *et al.* Opioid antagonist effects of dezocine in opioid-dependent humans. *Clin Pharmacol Ther* 1996; **60:** 206–17.

Interactions

For interactions associated with opioid analgesics, see p.69.

Pharmacokinetics

Dezocine is readily absorbed following intramuscular administration. It appears to be metabolised in the liver and excreted mainly as the glucuronide conjugate in the urine.

In pharmacokinetic studies in healthy subjects dezocine displayed the characteristics of a drug with very extensive distribution, high clearance, and short half-life.[1] It was rapidly and almost completely absorbed after intramuscular or subcutaneous administration. Following a 10 mg dose a mean peak serum concentration of 18.9 ng per mL was achieved 0.57 hour after intramuscular administration and a peak of 11.1 ng per mL was achieved 1.2 hours after subcutaneous administration. Mean elimination half-lives were similar regardless of the route of injection: in one study they were 2.4 or 2.2 hours respectively after intravenous or intramuscular administration and, in another, they were 2.7 or 2.5 hours after intravenous or subcutaneous administration.

1. Locniskar A, *et al.* Pharmacokinetics of dezocine, a new analgesic: effect of dose and route of administration. *Eur J Clin Pharmacol* 1986; **30:** 121–3.

Uses and Administration

Dezocine is an opioid analgesic (p.69). It is structurally related to pentazocine (p.75) and, likewise, has mixed opioid agonist/antagonist actions. Dezocine is used for the relief of moderate to severe pain and is given by injection. The usual intramuscular dose is 10 mg, repeated every 3 to 6 hours as necessary; doses ranging from 5 to 20 mg may be given according to requirements. The intravenous dose is 2.5 to 10 mg repeated every 2 to 4 hours with the usual initial dose being 5 mg. The manufacturers suggest a maximum total daily dose of 120 mg.

References.

1. O'Brien JJ, Benfield P. Dezocine: a preliminary review of its pharmacodynamic and pharmacokinetic properties, and therapeutic efficacy. *Drugs* 1989; **38:** 226–48.

Preparations

Proprietary Preparations (details are given in Part 3)

USA: Dalgan.

Diacerein (1729-k)

Diacerein *(rINN).*

Diacerhein; Diacetylrhein; Rhein Diacetate; SF-277. 9,10-Dihydro-4,5-dihydroxy-9,10-dioxo-2-anthroic acid diacetate.

$C_{19}H_{12}O_8$ = 368.3.

CAS — 13739-02-1.

Diacerein is an anthraquinone derivative that has been used in osteoarthritis (p.2) in doses of 50 to 100 mg daily by mouth. Its active metabolite, rhein, a constituent of rhubarb (p.1212) is reported to act as an interleukin-1 inhibitor. Diarrhoea is a common side-effect with diacerein.

References.

1. Debord P, *et al.* Influence of renal function on the pharmacokinetics of diacerein after a single oral dose. *Eur J Drug Metab Pharmacokinet* 1994; **19:** 13–19.
2. Spencer CM, Wilde MI. Diacerein. *Drugs* 1997; **53:** 98–106.

Preparations

Proprietary Preparations (details are given in Part 3)

Fr.: Art; ***Ital.:*** Artrodar; Benedar†; Diadar†; Fisiodar.

Diamorphine Hydrochloride (6219-l)

Diamorphine Hydrochloride *(BANM).*

Diacetylmorphine Hydrochloride; Heroin Hydrochloride. 4,5-Epoxy-17-methylmorphinan-3,6-diyl diacetate hydrochloride monohydrate.

$C_{21}H_{23}NO_5,HCl,H_2O$ = 423.9.

CAS — 561-27-3 (diamorphine); 1502-95-0 (diamorphine hydrochloride).

Pharmacopoeias. In Br.

A white or almost white crystalline powder, odourless when freshly prepared but develops an odour of acetic acid on storage. Freely **soluble** in water and in chloroform; soluble in alcohol; practically insoluble in ether. **Protect** from light.

Incompatibility. Diamorphine hydrochloride is incompatible with mineral acids and alkalis and with chlorocresol.[1]

Cyclizine may precipitate from mixtures with diamorphine hydrochloride at concentrations of cyclizine greater than 10 mg per mL, in the presence of sodium chloride, or as the concentration of diamorphine relative to cyclizine increases; mixtures of diamorphine and cyclizine are also liable to precipitate after 24 hours.

Mixtures of diamorphine and haloperidol are liable to precipitate after 24 hours if the haloperidol concentration is above 2 mg per mL. Under some conditions mixtures of metoclopramide and diamorphine may become discoloured and should be discarded.

1. McEwan JS, Macmorran GH. The compatibility of some bactericides. *Pharm J* 1947; **158:** 260–2.

Stability. Diamorphine is relatively unstable in aqueous solution and is hydrolysed to 6-*O*-monoacetylmorphine and then morphine to a significant extent at room temperature; 3-*O*-mono-acetylmorphine is only occasionally detected. The rate of decomposition is at a minimum at about pH 4.[1,2]

Cooper *et al.*[3] studied the stability of aqueous solutions of diamorphine in chloroform water and concluded that such solutions should be used within 3 weeks of preparation when stored at room temperature. Twycross[4] commented that the degradation products of diamorphine were not devoid of analgesic activity. Using a more sensitive analytical method Beaumont[5] reported that although the pH range of maximum stability of diamorphine in aqueous solution was 3.8 to 4.4, the addition of buffers reduced stability. Simple unbuffered chloroform water gave maximum stability, the shelf-life of such a solution being 4 weeks at room temperature.

The BP recommends that solutions for injection be prepared immediately before use by dissolving Diamorphine Hydrochloride for Injection in Water for Injections. This may pose a problem with solutions for subcutaneous infusion when concentrated solutions may remain in infusion pump reservoirs for some time.[6] Investigation of 9 concentrations of diamorphine stored at 4 different temperatures for 8 weeks[7] revealed instability under conditions of concentration, time, and temperature prevalent during subcutaneous infusion. Degradation of diamorphine occurred at all concentrations (0.98 to 250 mg per mL) at temperatures of 4° and above; the effect of temperature was significant at 21° and 37°. The percentage fall in diamorphine concentration was directly related to initial concentration and was accompanied by a corresponding increase in 6-*O*-monoacetylmorphine and, to a lesser extent, morphine; other possible breakdown products such as 3-*O*-monoacetylmorphine were not present in detectable quantities. Diamorphine degradation was associated with a fall in pH and the development of a strong acetic acid-like odour. Precipitation and a white turbidity was seen in solutions of 15.6 mg per mL and above after incubation for 2 weeks at 21° and 37°. Omar *et al.*[7] noted that solutions for infusion are generally freshly prepared and used within 24 hours, but advised that signs of precipitation should be watched for, especially when using longer-term infusions and high concentrations of diamorphine.

In another stability study[8] diamorphine hydrochloride in concentrations of both 1 and 20 mg per mL in sodium chloride 0.9% was stable for a minimum of 15 days at room temperature (23° to 25°) and 4° when stored in a PVC container. In one type of disposable infusion device (Infusor) similar solutions were stable for 15 days even at 31°. In another infusion device (Intermate 200) diamorphine was stable for a minimum of 15 days at both concentrations and all temperatures except for the 1 mg per mL solution kept at 31° when stability was only maintained for a minimum of 2 days. When stored in glass syringes both strengths of diamorphine hydrochloride were stable for 15 days at 4° and at room temperature the 1 mg per mL solution was stable for a minimum of 7 days and the 20 mg per mL solution was stable for a minimum of 12 days. There were no substantial changes in physical appearance or pH.

1. Davey EA, Murray JB. Hydrolysis of diamorphine in aqueous solutions. *Pharm J* 1969; **203:** 737.
2. Davey EA, Murray JB. Determination of diamorphine in the presence of its degradation products using gas liquid chromatography. *Pharm J* 1971; **207:** 167.
3. Cooper H, *et al.* Stability of diamorphine in chloroform water mixture. *Pharm J* 1981; **226:** 682–3.
4. Twycross RG. Stability of diamorphine in chloroform water. *Pharm J* 1981; **227:** 218.
5. Beaumont IM. Stability of diamorphine in chloroform water. *Pharm J* 1981; **227:** 41.
6. Jones VA, *et al.* Diamorphine stability in aqueous solution for subcutaneous infusion. *Br J Clin Pharmacol* 1987; **23:** 651P.
7. Omar OA, *et al.* Diamorphine stability in aqueous solution for subcutaneous infusion. *J Pharm Pharmacol* 1989; **41:** 275–7.
8. Kleinberg ML, *et al.* Stability of heroin hydrochloride in infusion devices and containers for intravenous administration. *Am J Hosp Pharm* 1990; **47:** 377–81.

Dependence and Withdrawal

As for Opioid Analgesics, p.67. Diamorphine is subject to abuse (see under Adverse Effects, Treatment, and Precautions, below).

Diamorphine is used for substitution therapy in the management of opioid dependence (see under Uses and Administration, below).

Adverse Effects, Treatment, and Precautions

As for Opioid Analgesics in general, p.68.

Pulmonary oedema after overdosage is a common cause of fatalities among diamorphine addicts. Nausea and hypotension are claimed to be less common than with morphine.

There are many reports of adverse effects associated with the abuse of diamorphine, usually obtained illicitly in an adulterated form.

Abuse. Most of the reports of adverse effects with diamorphine involve its abuse. In addition to the central effects, there are effects caused by the administration methods and by the adulterants.[1] Thus in many instances it is difficult to identify the factor causing the toxicity. Most body systems are involved including the immune system,[2] kidneys,[3] liver,[4] respiratory system,[5,6] and the nervous system.[7-10] Other aspects of the illicit use of diamorphine include fatal overdose[11] and smuggling by swallowing packages of drug[12] or other methods of internal bodily concealment.

1. Hendrickse RG, *et al.* Aflatoxins and heroin. *Br Med J* 1989; **299:** 492–3.
2. Husby G, *et al.* Smooth muscle antibody in heroin addicts. *Ann Intern Med* 1975; **83:** 801–5.
3. Cunningham EE, *et al.* Heroin-associated nephropathy. *JAMA* 1983; **250:** 2935–6.
4. Weller IVD, *et al.* Clinical, biochemical, serological, histological and ultrastructural features of liver disease in drug abusers. *Gut* 1984; **25:** 417–23.
5. Anderson K. Bronchospasm and intravenous street heroin. *Lancet* 1986; **i:** 1208.
6. Hughes S, Calverley PMA. Heroin inhalation and asthma. *Br Med J* 1988; **297:** 1511–12.
7. Sempere AP, *et al.* Spongiform leucoencephalopathy after inhaling heroin. *Lancet* 1991; **338:** 320.
8. Roulet Perez E, *et al.* Toxic leucoencephalopathy after heroin ingestion in a 2½-year-old child. *Lancet* 1992; **340:** 729.
9. Zuckerman GB. Neurologic complications following intranasal administration of heroin in an adolescent. *Ann Pharmacother* 1996; **30:** 778–81.
10. Kriegstein AR, *et al.* Heroin inhalation and progressive spongiform leukoencephalopathy. *N Engl J Med* 1997; **336:** 589–90.
11. Kintz P, *et al.* Toxicological data after heroin overdose. *Hum Toxicol* 1989; **8:** 487–9.
12. Stewart A, *et al.* Body packing—a case report and review of the literature. *Postgrad Med J* 1990; **66:** 659–61.

Administration. Although generally free from complications, sterile abscess formation was reported in 2 patients with advanced cancer receiving diamorphine by continuous subcutaneous infusions.[1]

1. Hoskin PJ, *et al.* Sterile abscess formation by continuous subcutaneous infusion of diamorphine. *Br Med J* 1988; **296:** 1605.

EPIDURAL ROUTE. Acute dysphoric reactions have been reported after the use of epidural diamorphine.[1]

1. Holder KJ, Morgan BM. Dysphoria after extradural diamorphine. *Br J Anaesth* 1994; **72:** 728.

Breast feeding. See under Opioid Dependence in Uses and Administration, below.

Phaeochromocytoma. Diamorphine can liberate endogenous histamine which may in turn stimulate release of catecholamines. Its use provoked hypertension and tachycardia in a patient with phaeochromocytoma.[1]

1. Chaturvedi NC, *et al.* Diamorphine-induced attack of paroxysmal hypertension in phaeochromocytoma. *Br Med J* 1974; **2:** 538.

Pregnancy and the neonate. Some references to diamorphine dependence in pregnant women and the effects on the fetus and neonate.

1. Fricker HS, Segal S. Narcotic addiction, pregnancy, and the newborn. *Am J Dis Child* 1978; **132:** 360–6.
2. Ostrea EM, Chavez CJ. Perinatal problems (excluding neonatal withdrawal) in maternal drug addiction: a study of 830 cases. *J Pediatr* 1979; **94:** 292–5.
3. Lifschitz MH, *et al.* Fetal and postnatal growth of children born to narcotic-dependent women. *J Pediatr* 1983; **102:** 686–91.
4. Klenka HM. Babies born in a district general hospital to mothers taking heroin. *Br Med J* 1986; **293:** 745–6.
5. Gregg JEM, *et al.* Inhaling heroin during pregnancy: effects on the baby. *Br Med J* 1988; **296:** 754.
6. Little BB, *et al.* Maternal and fetal effects of heroin addiction during pregnancy. *J Reprod Med* 1990; **35:** 159–62.

Interactions

For interactions associated with opioid analgesics, see p.69.

Pharmacokinetics

Diamorphine hydrochloride is well absorbed from the gastro-intestinal tract and following subcutaneous or intramuscular injection. Following injection it is rapidly converted to the active metabolite 6-*O*-monoacetylmorphine (6-acetylmorphine) in the blood and then to morphine. Orally administered diamorphine is subject to extensive first-pass metabolism to morphine; neither diamorphine nor 6-acetylmorphine have been detected in the blood following administration of diamorphine by this route. Both diamorphine and 6-acetylmorphine readily cross the blood-brain barrier. Morphine glucuronides are the main excretion products in the urine.

Reviews and studies of the pharmacokinetics of diamorphine.

1. Boerner U, *et al.* The metabolism of morphine and heroin in man. *Drug Metab Rev* 1975; **4:** 39–73.
2. Inturrisi CE, *et al.* The pharmacokinetics of heroin in patients with chronic pain. *N Engl J Med* 1984; **310:** 1213–17.
3. Moore RA, *et al.* Opiate metabolism and excretion. *Baillieres Clin Anaesthesiol* 1987; **1:** 829–58.
4. Barrett DA, *et al.* Morphine kinetics after diamorphine infusion in premature neonates. *Br J Clin Pharmacol* 1991; **32:** 31–7.

Administration. Diamorphine is much more lipid-soluble and has a more rapid onset and shorter duration of action than morphine. Although deacetylation to morphine occurs rapidly in the blood it occurs only slowly in the cerebrospinal fluid following intraspinal injection of diamorphine.[1] After intrathecal injection diamorphine was removed from spinal fluid much more rapidly than morphine.[2] Peak plasma concentrations of morphine following epidural diamorphine injection were significantly higher and were achieved significantly faster than after epidural injection of morphine.[3]

1. Morgan M. The rational use of intrathecal and extradural opioids. *Br J Anaesth* 1989; **63:** 165–88.
2. Moore A, *et al.* Spinal fluid kinetics of morphine and heroin. *Clin Pharmacol Ther* 1984; **35:** 40–5.
3. Watson J, *et al.* Plasma morphine concentrations and analgesic effects of lumbar extradural morphine and heroin. *Anesth Analg* 1984; **63:** 629–34.

Administration in children. Loading doses of diamorphine of either 50 μg per kg body-weight or 200 μg per kg were given as an infusion over 30 minutes to 19 ventilated neonates followed by a continuous infusion of 15 μg per kg per hour, and the pharmacokinetics of the products of diamorphine metabolism (morphine, morphine-6-glucuronide, and morphine-3-glucuronide) studied.[1] Although the overall elimination of morphine was reduced compared with adults, the relative contributions of the various metabolic routes of morphine remained similar between neonates and adults. Data from this study did not indicate any advantage for the higher loading dose (see also under Uses and Administration, below).

1. Barrett DA, *et al.* Morphine, morphine-6-glucuronide and morphine-3-glucuronide pharmacokinetics in newborn infants receiving diamorphine infusions. *Br J Clin Pharmacol* 1996; **41:** 531–7.

Uses and Administration

Diamorphine hydrochloride is an opioid analgesic (p.69). It is an acetylated morphine derivative and is a more potent opioid analgesic than morphine (p.58). Diamorphine is used for the relief of severe pain especially in terminal illnesses. It is also used similarly to morphine for the relief of dyspnoea due to pulmonary oedema resulting from left ventricular failure. Diamorphine has a powerful cough suppressant effect and has been given as Diamorphine Linctus (BPC 1973) to control cough associated with terminal lung cancer although morphine is now preferred.

In the treatment of acute pain standard doses of diamorphine hydrochloride by subcutaneous or intramuscular injection are 5 to 10 mg every 4 hours. Doses equivalent to a quarter to one half of the corresponding intramuscular dose have been used for slow intravenous injection. For the pain of myocardial infarction diamorphine hydrochloride is given in doses of 5 mg by slow intravenous injection at a rate of 1 mg per minute with a further dose of 2.5 to 5 mg if required; doses may be reduced by half for elderly or frail patients. Doses of 2.5 to 5 mg have been given intravenously at the same rate for acute pulmonary oedema. For chronic pain 5 to 10 mg may be given by mouth or by subcutaneous or intramuscular injection every 4 hours; the dose may be increased according to needs. Diamorphine hydrochloride may also be administered by continuous subcutaneous infusion or intraspinally. For the treatment of cough in terminal disease, doses of diamorphine hydrochloride 1.5 to 6 mg every 4 hours may be given.

Because of its abuse potential diamorphine is carefully controlled and in many countries it is not available for clinical use; by dose adjustment morphine can provide equivalent analgesia. There has been much debate regarding the relative merits of analgesia with diamorphine or morphine. Many now regard oral morphine to be the strong opioid analgesic of choice although diamorphine hydrochloride may be preferred for administration by injection because it is more soluble in water thus allowing the use of smaller dose volumes. Diamorphine hydrochloride may also be preferred to morphine salts for intraspinal administration because it is more lipid-soluble.

As a guide to relative potency diamorphine hydrochloride 5 mg intramuscularly is approximately equivalent to 10 mg by mouth which in turn is approximately equivalent to morphine sulphate 15 mg by mouth.

Administration in children. In a study of the effects of diamorphine in 34 premature infants (gestational age 26 to 40 weeks), a loading dose of 50 μg per kg body-weight given as an intravenous infusion over 30 minutes followed by a continuous infusion at a rate of 15 μg per kg per hour was considered to be safe and resulted in plasma concentrations of morphine comparable with those that usually produce adequate analgesia in children and adults; the duration of the infusion ranged from 14 to 149 hours.[1] Small but significant reductions in heart rate and mean blood pressure were noted but these were not associated with any clinical deterioration. The fall in respiration rate reflected the desired intention to encourage synchronisation of the infants' breathing with the ventilator.[1] The authors concluded that intravenous diamorphine could be given safely to neonates and would provide adequate analgesia. A later study[2] indicated that the use of a 200 µg per kg loading dose conferred no benefit over a 50 µg per kg dose and might produce undesirable physiological effects. Continuous intravenous infusions of 7 µg per kg per hour have been used in neonates not requiring ventilation.[3]

The subcutaneous route appeared to be as effective and safe as the intravenous route for administration of diamorphine infusions in children for postoperative pain relief following elective abdominal surgery.[4] The dose of diamorphine used in both groups of children was 1 mg per kg body-weight administered at a rate of 20 µg per kg per hour.

1. Elias-Jones AC, *et al.* Diamorphine infusion in the preterm neonate. *Arch Dis Child* 1991; **66:** 1155–7.
2. Barker DP, *et al.* Randomised, double blind trial of two loading dose regimens of diamorphine in ventilated newborn infants. *Arch Dis Child* 1995; **73:** F22–F26.
3. Blanchard S. Analgesic use in neonatal necrotising enterocolitis. *Pharm J* 1992; **248:** 52.
4. Semple D, *et al.* Comparison of iv and sc diamorphine infusions for the treatment of acute pain in children. *Br J Anaesth* 1996; **76:** 310–12.

Opioid dependence. Many opiate misusers have expressed a preference for withdrawal using diamorphine rather than methadone. In a comparative study stabilisation was achieved using either diamorphine or methadone 1 mg per mL oral solutions;[1] patients could not identify which they had been given. Whenever signs of physical withdrawal were observed 10 mL of either solution was given and the total amount over the first 24 hours taken as the patient's daily requirement. The mean dose of diamorphine required for stabilisation was 55 mg compared with 36 mg for methadone. Some centres have administered diamorphine in the form of reefers.

Breast feeding has been used to treat diamorphine dependence in the offspring of dependent mothers but this is no longer considered to be the best method and some authorities recommend that breast feeding should be stopped.

1. Ghodse AH, *et al.* Comparison of oral preparations of heroin and methadone to stabilise opiate misusers as inpatients. *Br Med J* 1990; **300:** 719–20.

Pain. ACUTE PAIN. Rapid pain relief may be obtained with the intravenous injection of diamorphine. Other routes include the intraspinal route for which diamorphine is well suited because of its lipid solubility and pharmacokinetics. Epidural doses of diamorphine have ranged from 0.5 to 10 mg.[1] Macrae *et al.*[2] found diamorphine 5 mg produced rapid analgesia whether given intramuscularly (in 1 mL of 0.9% sodium chloride) or epidurally (in 10 mL of 0.9% sodium chloride) for pain following caesarean section, but analgesia was significantly more prolonged and more intense following epidural injection; itching was reported by 50% of patients undergoing epidural analgesia. Continuous epidural infusion of diamorphine 0.5 mg per hour in 15 mL of 0.125% bupivacaine provided postoperative analgesia superior to that with either drug alone in patients undergoing major abdominal gynaecological surgery.[3] Continuous epidural infusion of diamorphine 0.4 to 0.6 mg per hour in 0.15% bupivacaine produced analgesia superior to that with either epidural bolus injection of diamorphine 3.6 mg in 9 mL of 0.9% saline or patient-controlled intravenous administration of diamorphine at a maximum rate of 1 mg per 5 minutes in patients undergoing total abdominal hysterectomy.[4] However, more patients receiving the continuous epidural infusion were hypoxaemic than in the other 2 groups. Diamorphine 5 mg in 8 mL of 0.9% sodium chloride produced comparable analgesia to 8 mL of 0.375% bupivacaine when given epidurally during labour but the duration was longer with diamorphine; addition of adrenaline appeared to improve the quality and duration of analgesia with diamorphine.[5] The addition of diamorphine 5 mg to 10 mL of 0.25% bupivacaine also enhanced pain relief when given epidurally in the first stage of labour.[6] In a similar study addition of diamorphine to bupivacaine produced a high incidence of pruritus and drowsiness.[7]

Diamorphine has also been given intrathecally for postoperative analgesia and should be effective at lower doses than with the epidural route because of greater CSF concentrations. Reay *et al.*[8] reported that diamorphine 0.25 or 0.5 mg administered intrathecally with bupivacaine spinal anaesthesia both provided greater postoperative analgesia than bupivacaine alone, but the incidence of adverse effects, especially nausea, vomiting, and urinary retention, was still high with either dose and they could not recommend the routine use of this technique. Intrathecal administration of diamorphine with bupivacaine has also been used for analgesia during labour.[9]

1. Morgan M. The rational use of intrathecal and extradural opioids. *Br J Anaesth* 1989; **63:** 165–88.
2. Macrae DJ, *et al.* Double-blind comparison of the efficacy of extradural diamorphine, extradural phenoperidine and im diamorphine following caesarean section. *Br J Anaesth* 1987; **59:** 354–9.
3. Lee A, *et al.* Postoperative analgesia by continuous extradural infusion of bupivacaine and diamorphine. *Br J Anaesth* 1988; **60:** 845–50.
4. Madej TH, *et al.* Hypoxaemia and pain relief after lower abdominal surgery: comparison of extradural and patient-controlled analgesia. *Br J Anaesth* 1992; **69:** 554–7.
5. Keenan GMA, *et al.* Extradural diamorphine with adrenaline in labour: comparison with diamorphine and bupivacaine. *Br J Anaesth* 1991; **66:** 242–6.
6. McGrady EM, *et al.* Epidural diamorphine and bupivacaine in labour. *Anaesthesia* 1989; **44:** 400–3.
7. Bailey CR, *et al.* Diamorphine-bupivacaine mixture compared with plain bupivacaine for analgesia. *Br J Anaesth* 1994; **72:** 58–61.
8. Reay BA, *et al.* Low-dose intrathecal diamorphine analgesia following major orthopaedic surgery. *Br J Anaesth* 1989; **62:** 248–52.
9. Kestin IG, *et al.* Analgesia for labour and delivery using incremental diamorphine and bupivacaine via a 32-gauge intrathecal catheter. *Br J Anaesth* 1992; **68:** 244–7.

CHRONIC PAIN. Patients with chronic opioid-sensitive pain are often treated with diamorphine given by continuous subcutaneous infusion using a small battery-operated syringe driver. The following technique was described by Dover.[1] Diamorphine hydrochloride 1 g can be dissolved in 1.6 mL of water to give a solution with a volume of 2.4 mL (415 mg per mL), but the maximum suggested concentration is 250 mg per mL. If the analgesic requirement is not known the following protocol is recommended:

(1) Start injections every 4 hours of 2.5 or 5 mg diamorphine, or if the patient has a already been taking opioids, a dose that is equivalent to the last dose.

(2) If this is unsatisfactory increase this dose in 50% increments until the patient reports even a little pain relief.

(3) Calculate the 24-hour requirement by multiplying by six, and start the infusion at this level.

(4) Increase the 24-hour dosage in the pump by 50% increments until the pain is controlled. Note that requirements may vary from less than 20 mg to more than 5 g per 24 hours.

When starting an infusion it is important not to allow any breakthrough pain. This may be achieved either by starting the infusion more than 2 hours before the previous oral dose wears off or by giving a loading dose injection of the 4-hourly requirement.

Although generally free from complications, sterile abscess formation was reported in 2 patients with advanced cancer receiving diamorphine by continuous subcutaneous infusions.[2]

The intraventricular route was used successfully in 2 patients with intractable cancer pain.[3]

1. Dover SB. Syringe driver in terminal care. *Br Med J* 1987; **294:** 553–5.
2. Hoskin PJ, *et al.* Sterile abscess formation by continuous subcutaneous infusion of diamorphine. *Br Med J* 1988; **296:** 1605.
3. Reeve WG, Todd JG. Intraventricular diamorphine via an Ommaya shunt for intractable cancer pain. *Br J Anaesth* 1990; **65:** 544–7.

Preparations

BP 1998: Diamorphine Injection;
BPC 1973: Diamorphine Linctus.

Proprietary Preparations (details are given in Part 3)
UK: Diagesil.

Diclofenac (13409-w)

Diclofenac *(BAN, rINN).*
[2-(2,6-Dichloroanilino)phenyl]acetic acid.
$C_{14}H_{11}Cl_2NO_2$ = 296.1.
CAS — 15307-86-5.

Diclofenac Diethylamine (11328-c)

Diclofenac Diethylamine *(BANM).*
$C_{18}H_{22}Cl_2N_2O_2$ = 369.3.
CAS — 78213-16-8.

Diclofenac Potassium (15163-x)

Diclofenac Potassium *(BANM, USAN, rINNM).*
CGP-45840B. Potassium [*o*-(2,6-dichloroanilino)phenyl]acetate.
$C_{14}H_{10}Cl_2KNO_2$ = 334.2.
CAS — 15307-81-0.

Diclofenac Sodium (2632-c)

Diclofenac Sodium *(BANM, USAN, rINNM).*
Diclofenacum Natricum; Diclophenac Sodium; GP-45840.
Sodium [2-(2,6-dichloroanilino)phenyl]acetate.
$C_{14}H_{10}Cl_2NNaO_2$ = 318.1.
CAS — 15307-79-6.

NOTE. DICL is a code approved by the BP for use on single unit doses of eye drops containing diclofenac sodium where the individual container may be too small to bear all the appropriate labelling information.

Pharmacopoeias. In *Eur.* (see p.viii), *Jpn*, and *US.*

A white to slightly yellowish hygroscopic crystalline powder. Sparingly **soluble** in water; soluble in alcohol; slightly soluble in acetone; practically insoluble in ether; freely soluble in methyl alcohol. The pH of a 1% solution in water is between 7.0 and 8.5. **Store** in airtight container. Protect from light.

Adverse Effects

As for NSAIDs in general, p.63.

There may be pain and, occasionally, tissue damage at the site of injection when diclofenac is given intramuscularly. Diclofenac suppositories may cause local irritation. Transient burning and stinging may occur with diclofenac ophthalmic solution.

A review of worldwide clinical studies with diclofenac[1] has reported the incidence of drug-associated adverse effects to be about 12%; about 16% of patients who experienced adverse effects discontinued treatment (a figure corresponding to about 2% of the entire patient sample). The most frequently reported adverse effects were gastro-intestinal and were reported in 7.6% of patients. CNS-related adverse effects were reported in 0.7% of patients and allergy or local reactions in 0.4%. This and other reviews[2] have shown that adverse effects associated with diclofenac are usually mild and transient and appear to be unrelated to the dose of drug given.

1. Willkens RF. Worldwide clinical safety experience with diclofenac. *Semin Arthritis Rheum* 1985; **15** (suppl 1): 105–10.
2. Small RE. Diclofenac sodium. *Clin Pharm* 1989; **8:** 545–8.

Effects on the blood. Results of a large survey undertaken to assess the relation between agranulocytosis, aplastic anaemia, and drug exposure indicated that diclofenac was significantly associated with aplastic anaemia, providing an estimated tenfold increase in risk.[1] There are reports of other haematological abnormalities including haemolytic anaemia,[2] thrombocytopenia,[3-5] neutropenia,[5] and agranulocytosis[6] occurring in patients given diclofenac.

Localised spontaneous bleeding,[7,8] bruising,[9,10] inhibition of platelet aggregation,[7,8] and prolonged bleeding time[10] have been reported.

1. The International Agranulocytosis and Aplastic Anemia Study. Risks of agranulocytosis and aplastic anemia: a first report of their relation to drug use with special reference to analgesics. *JAMA* 1986; **256:** 1749–57.
2. López A, *et al.* Autoimmune hemolytic anemia induced by diclofenac. *Ann Pharmacother* 1995; **29:** 787.
3. Kramer MR, *et al.* Severe reversible autoimmune haemolytic anaemia and thrombocytopenia associated with diclofenac therapy. *Scand J Haematol* 1986; **36:** 118–20.
4. George S, Rahi AHS. Thrombocytopenia associated with diclofenac therapy. *Am J Health-Syst Pharm* 1995; **52:** 420–1.
5. Kim HL, Kovacs MJ. Diclofenac-associated thrombocytopenia and neutropenia. *Ann Pharmacother* 1995; **29:** 713–15.
6. Colomina P, Garcia S. Agranulocytosis caused by diclofenac. *DICP Ann Pharmacother* 1989; **23:** 507.
7. Michalevicz R, Seligsohn U. Clinical bleeding due to diclofenac (Voltaren). *Arthritis Rheum* 1982; **25:** 599.
8. Price AJ, Obeid D. Spontaneous non-gastrointestinal bleeding associated with diclofenac. *Lancet* 1989; **ii:** 1520.
9. Parapia L, Cox JA. Spontaneous platelet aggregation after diclofenac treatment. *Br Med J* 1984; **288:** 368.
10. Khazan U, *et al.* Diclofenac sodium and bruising. *Ann Intern Med* 1990; **112:** 472–3.

Effects on electrolytes. There have been case reports of diclofenac being associated with the development of symptoms resembling the syndrome of inappropriate antidiuretic hormone secretion in elderly women.[1,2] Also the UK Committee on Safety of Medicines had received a report of fatal hyponatraemia in another elderly woman.[2]

1. Petersson I, *et al.* Water intoxication associated with non-steroidal anti-inflammatory drug therapy. *Acta Med Scand* 1987; **221:** 221–3.
2. Cheung NT, *et al.* Syndrome of inappropriate secretion of antidiuretic hormone induced by diclofenac. *Br Med J* 1993; **306:** 186.

Effects on the eyes. A patient who had been taking diclofenac for several years and had increasingly complained of dry, gritty eyes noticed that eye irritation disappeared within 3 days when diclofenac had to be discontinued because of gastro-intestinal effects.[1]

1. Reid ALA, Henderson R. Diclofenac and dry, irritable eyes. *Med J Aust* 1994; **160:** 308.

Effects on the gastro-intestinal tract. The most frequent adverse effects reported in patients given diclofenac are gastro-intestinal in nature. Typical reactions include epigastric pain, nausea, vomiting, and diarrhoea. Rarely peptic ulcer and gastro-intestinal bleeding have occurred. Diclofenac has also been implicated as the causative agent in colonic ulceration,[1] small bowel perforation,[2] and pseudomembranous colitis.[3] Rectal administration of diclofenac suppositories may cause local reactions such as itching, burning, or exacerbation of haemorrhoids.

1. Carson J, *et al.* Colonic ulceration and bleeding during diclofenac therapy. *N Engl J Med* 1990; **323:** 135.
2. Deakin M, *et al.* Small bowel perforation associated with an excessive dose of slow release diclofenac sodium. *Br Med J* 1988; **297:** 488–9.
3. Gentric A, Pennec YL. Diclofenac-induced pseudomembranous colitis. *Lancet* 1992; **340:** 126–7.

Effects on the kidneys. Renal papillary necrosis[1] and nephrotic syndrome[2-4] have been reported in patients taking diclofenac. See also under Effects on Electrolytes, above.

1. Scott SJ, *et al.* Renal papillary necrosis associated with diclofenac sodium. *Br Med J* 1986; **292:** 1050.
2. Beun GDM, *et al.* Isolated minimal change nephropathy associated with diclofenac. *Br Med J* 1987; **295:** 182–3.
3. Yinnon AM, *et al.* Nephrotic syndrome associated with diclofenac sodium. *Br Med J* 1987; **295:** 556.
4. Tattersall J, *et al.* Membranous nephropathy associated with diclofenac. *Postgrad Med J* 1992; **68:** 392–3.

Effects on the liver. Elevations of serum aminotransferase activity and clinical hepatitis,[1-6] including fatal fulminant hepatitis[2,5] have occurred in patients taking diclofenac. There has also been a case report of hepato-renal damage attributed to diclofenac.[7] Analysis[8] of 180 of the cases of diclofenac-associated hepatic injury received by the FDA between November 1988 and June 1991 suggested an increased risk of hepatotoxicity in female patients and those taking diclofenac for osteoarthritis. Hepatotoxicity had been detected within 6 months of starting diclofenac in 85% of the patients. The biochemical pattern of injury was hepatocellular or mixed hepatocellular in 66% of patients and cholestatic injury was found in 8% of patients. Signs of hypersensitivity were uncommon and it was considered that the mechanism of hepatic injury was likely to be a metabolic idiosyncratic reaction rather than due to intrinsic toxicity of diclofenac.

1. Dunk AA, *et al.* Diclofenac hepatitis. *Br Med J* 1982; **284:** 1605–6.
2. Breen EG, *et al.* Fatal hepatitis associated with diclofenac. *Gut* 1986; **27:** 1390–3.
3. Schapira D, *et al.* Diclofenac-induced hepatotoxicity. *Postgrad Med J* 1986; **62:** 63–5.
4. Ryley NG, *et al.* Diclofenac associated hepatitis. *Gut* 1989; **30:** A708.
5. Helfgott SM, *et al.* Diclofenac-associated hepatotoxicity. *JAMA* 1990; **264:** 2660–2.
6. Purcell P, *et al.* Diclofenac hepatitis. *Gut* 1991; **32:** 1381–5.
7. Diggory P, *et al.* Renal and hepatic impairment in association with diclofenac administration. *Postgrad Med J* 1989; **64:** 507–8.
8. Banks AT, *et al.* Diclofenac-associated hepatotoxicity: analysis of 180 cases reported to the Food and Drug Administration as adverse reactions. *Hepatology* 1995; **22:** 820–7.

Effects on the skin. Self-limiting skin reactions such as rash or pruritus may occur in patients given diclofenac. More serious skin reactions attributed to diclofenac include bullous dermatitis[1] and erythema multiforme.[2] Local irritation and necrosis has occurred on intramuscular injection of diclofenac.[3,4]

1. Gabrielsen TØ, *et al.* Drug-induced bullous dermatosis with linear IgA deposits along the basement membrane. *Acta Derm Venereol (Stockh)* 1981; **61:** 439–41.
2. Morris BAP, Remtulla SS. Erythema multiforme major following use of diclofenac. *Can Med Assoc J* 1985; **133:** 665.
3. Stricker BHC, van Kasteren BJ. Diclofenac-induced isolated myonecrosis and the Nicolau syndrome. *Ann Intern Med* 1992; **117:** 1058.
4. Pillans PI, O'Connor N. Tissue necrosis and necrotising fasciitis after intramuscular administration of diclofenac. *Ann Pharmacother* 1995; **29:** 264–6.

Hypersensitivity. Aspirin-sensitive asthmatic patients have developed reactions (rhinorrhoea, tightness of chest, wheezing, dyspnoea) when challenged with diclofenac in doses of 10 to 25 mg[1] and the CSM in the UK have received a report of one aspirin-sensitive patient who died from acute asthma 4 hours after a single 25-mg dose of diclofenac.[2]

Anaphylactic shock has been reported.[3]

1. Szczeklik A, *et al.* Asthmatic attacks induced in aspirin-sensitive patients by diclofenac and naproxen. *Br Med J* 1977; **2:** 231–2.
2. Committee on Safety of Medicines/Medicines Control Agency. Avoid all NSAIDs in aspirin-sensitive patients. *Current Problems* 1993; **19:** 8.
3. Dux S, *et al.* Anaphylactic shock induced by diclofenac. *Br Med J* 1983; **286:** 1861.

Precautions

As for NSAIDs in general, p.65.

The manufacturers recommend that ophthalmic preparations containing diclofenac should not be used by patients who wear soft contact lenses.

Administration of intravenous diclofenac is contra-indicated in patients with moderate or severe renal impairment, hypovolaemia, or dehydration; in patients with a history of haemorrhagic diathesis, cerebrovascular bleeding (including suspected), or asthma; and in patients undergoing surgery with a high risk of haemorrhage.

Breast feeding. See under Pharmacokinetics, below.

Porphyria. Diclofenac sodium has been associated with clinical exacerbations of porphyria and is considered unsafe in porphyric patients.[1]

1. Moore MR, McColl KEL. *Porphyria: drug lists.* Glasgow: Porphyria Research Unit, University of Glasgow, 1991.

Interactions

For interactions associated with NSAIDs, see p.65.

Diclofenac should not be administered intravenously to patients already receiving other NSAIDs, or anticoagulants including low-dose heparin.

Deterioration in renal function has been attributed to the concomitant use of diclofenac with *triamterene*[1] or with *cyclosporin*.[2] The area under the concentration-time curve for diclofenac was doubled in the presence of cyclosporin[3] and the manufacturer of cyclosporin recommends that the dosage of diclofenac should be reduced by about a half when diclofenac is used with cyclosporin.

One group of workers[4] has found that the area under the curve for diclofenac was reduced by 20% when it was administered as a single 100-mg daily dose in the form of a modified-release preparation to subjects receiving *misoprostol* 800 µg daily. Concomitant administration was also associated with an increase in the incidence and severity of gastro-intestinal effects. Studies by the manufacturer[5] had failed to find any significant pharmacokinetic interactions between diclofenac and misoprostol when administered in a formulation containing diclofenac 50 mg and misoprostol 200 µg. A similar reduction in the area under the curve for diclofenac has been reported[6] following administration of diclofenac after pretreatment with *sucralfate*.

Cholestyramine appears substantially to reduce the bioavailability of diclofenac when the two drugs are given together;[7] *colestipol* produces a similar but smaller effect.

The manufacturer of acetylcholine chloride ophthalmic preparations has stated that there have been reports that *acetylcholine* and *carbachol* have been ineffective when used in patients treated with topical (ophthalmic) NSAIDs.

1. Härkönen M, Ekblom-Kullberg S. Reversible deterioration of renal function after diclofenac in patient receiving triamterene. *Br Med J* 1986; **293:** 698–9.
2. Branthwaite JP, Nicholls A. Cyclosporin and diclofenac interaction in rheumatoid arthritis. *Lancet* 1991; **337:** 252.
3. Kovarik JM, *et al.* Cyclosporine and nonsteroidal antiinflammatory drugs: exploring potential drug interactions and their implications for the treatment of rheumatoid arthritis. *J Clin Pharmacol* 1997; **37:** 336–43.
4. Dammann HG, *et al.* Differential effects of misoprostol and ranitidine on the pharmacokinetics of diclofenac and gastrointestinal symptoms. *Br J Clin Pharmacol* 1993; **36:** 345–9.
5. Karim A. Pharmacokinetics of diclofenac and misoprostol when administered alone or as a combination product. *Drugs* 1993; **45** (suppl 1): 7–14.
6. Pedrazzoli J, *et al.* Short-term sucralfate administration alters potassium diclofenac absorption in healthy male volunteers. *Br J Clin Pharmacol* 1997; **43:** 104–108.
7. Al-balla SR, *et al.* The effects of cholestyramine and colestipol on the absorption of diclofenac in man. *Int J Clin Pharmacol Ther* 1994; **32:** 441–5.

Pharmacokinetics

Diclofenac is rapidly absorbed when given as an oral solution, rectal suppository, or by intramuscular injection. It is absorbed more slowly when given as enteric-coated tablets, especially when this dosage form is given with food. Although orally-administered diclofenac is almost completely absorbed, it is subject to first-pass metabolism so that about 50% of the drug reaches the systemic circulation in the unchanged form. Diclofenac is also absorbed percutaneously. At therapeutic concentrations it is more than 99% bound to plasma proteins. Diclofenac penetrates synovial fluid where concentrations may persist even when plasma concentrations fall; diclofenac is distributed into breast milk but the amount is considered by some authorities to be too small to be harmful to a breast-fed infant. The terminal plasma half-life is about 1 to 2 hours. Diclofenac is metabolised to 4′-hydroxydiclofenac, 5-hydroxydiclofenac, 3′-hydroxydiclofenac and 4′,5-dihydroxydiclofenac. It is then excreted in the form of glucuronide and sulphate conjugates, mainly in the urine (about 65%) but also in the bile (about 35%).

References.

1. Fowler PD, *et al.* Plasma and synovial fluid concentrations of diclofenac sodium and its major hydroxylated metabolites during long-term treatment of rheumatoid arthritis. *Eur J Clin Pharmacol* 1983; **25:** 389–94.
2. Maggi CA, *et al.* Comparative bioavailability of diclofenac hydroxyethylpyrrolidine vs diclofenac sodium in man. *Eur J Clin Pharmacol* 1990; **38:** 207–8.
3. Davies NM, Anderson KE. Clinical pharmacokinetics of diclofenac: therapeutic insights and pitfalls. *Clin Pharmacokinet* 1997; **33:** 184–213.

Uses and Administration

Diclofenac, a phenylacetic acid derivative, is an NSAID (p.65). It is used mainly as the sodium salt for the relief of pain and inflammation in various conditions: musculoskeletal and joint disorders such as rheumatoid arthritis, osteoarthritis, and ankylosing spondylitis; peri-articular disorders such as bursitis and tendinitis; soft-tissue disorders such as sprains and strains; and other painful conditions such as renal colic, acute gout, dysmenorrhoea, and following some surgical procedures. It has also been used in some countries for the management of fever.

The maximum total daily dose of diclofenac sodium by any route is 150 mg. The usual dose by mouth or rectally is 75 to 150 mg daily in divided doses. Modified-release preparations of diclofenac sodium are available for oral use. Diclofenac has also been given in equivalent doses by mouth as the free acid in dispersible preparations for short-term treatment up to 3 months long. Diclofenac sodium may also be given by deep intramuscular injection into the gluteal muscle in a dose of 75 mg once daily or, if required in severe conditions, 75 mg twice daily. Diclofenac sodium may also be given as a continuous or intermittent intravenous infusion in glucose 5% or sodium chloride 0.9% (both previously buffered with sodium bicarbonate). For the treatment of postoperative pain a dose of 75 mg may be given over 30 to 120 minutes. The dose may be repeated if necessary after 4 to 6 hours. To prevent postoperative pain, 25 to 50 mg diclofenac sodium may be given after surgery over 15 to 60 minutes followed by 5 mg per hour. The maximum period recommended for parenteral use is 2 days. Diclofenac sodium is also used intramuscularly in renal colic in a dose of 75 mg repeated once after 30 minutes if necessary. In children 1 to 12 years old the dose by mouth or rectally for juvenile chronic arthritis is 1 to 3 mg per kg body-weight daily in divided doses.

Diclofenac sodium is also used as a 0.1% **ophthalmic solution** for the prevention of intra-operative miosis during cataract extraction, for the treatment of postoperative inflammation following cataract extraction, and for pain in corneal epithelial defects following photorefractive keratectomy. For the prevention of miosis, one drop is instilled in the appropriate eye 4 times during the 2 hours before surgery and for the treatment of postoperative inflammation, one drop is instilled 4 times daily for up to 28 days starting 24 hours after surgery. For the control of post-photorefractive keratectomy pain, one drop is instilled twice in the hour before surgery, then one drop twice at 5-minute intervals immediately after the procedure, and then one drop every 2 to 5 hours during the waking hours for up to 24 hours.

Diclofenac diethylamine is used **topically** as a gel containing the equivalent of 1% of diclofenac sodium for the local symptomatic relief of pain and inflammation; it is applied to the affected site 3 to 4 times daily; treatment should be reviewed after 14 days or after 28 days if used for osteoarthritis. Diclofenac epolamine (diclofenac hydroxyethylpyrrolidine; DHEP) is also used topically.

Diclofenac has also been given by mouth as the potassium salt. Diclofenac is available in combination with misoprostol (see p.1419) for patients at risk of NSAID-induced peptic ulceration.

Reviews.

1. Todd PA, Sorkin EM. Diclofenac sodium: a reappraisal of its pharmacodynamic and pharmacokinetic properties, and therapeutic efficacy. *Drugs* 1988; **35:** 244–85.
2. Small RE. Diclofenac sodium. *Clin Pharm* 1989; **8:** 545–8.

Administration. TOPICAL. Some references to the use of plasters providing sustained topical release of diclofenac epolamine.

1. Galeazzi M, Marcolongo R. A placebo-controlled study of the efficacy and tolerability of a nonsteroidal anti-inflammatory drug, DHEP plaster, in inflammatory peri- and extra-articular rheumatological diseases. *Drugs Exp Clin Res* 1993; **19:** 107–15.
2. Dreiser RL, Tisne-Camus M. DHEP plasters as a topical treatment of knee osteoarthritis—a double-blind placebo-controlled study. *Drugs Exp Clin Res* 1993; **19:** 117–23.

Actinic keratoses. Although topical application of a preparation containing diclofenac 3% in a 2.5% hyaluronic acid gel has been reported[1] to have been effective when tried in the treatment of actinic keratoses (p.492) a randomised double-blind study[2] indicated that this preparation was not significantly more effective than the use of the hyaluronic acid gel alone.

1. Rivers JK, McLean DI. An open study to assess the efficacy and safety of topical 3% diclofenac in a 2.5% hyaluronic acid gel for the treatment of actinic keratoses. *Arch Dermatol* 1997; **133:** 1239–42.
2. McEwan LE, Smith JG. Topical diclofenac/hyaluronic acid gel in the treatment of solar keratoses. *Australas J Dermatol* 1997; **38:** 187–9.

Preparations

BP 1998: Diclofenac Tablets; Slow Diclofenac Tablets;
USP 23: Diclofenac Sodium Delayed-release Tablets.

Proprietary Preparations (details are given in Part 3)
Aust.: Algefit; Dedolor; Deflamat; Diclobene; Diclomelan; Diclosyl; Fenaren; Magluphen†; Naclof†; Tratul; Voltaren; ***Austral.:*** Arthrotec; Diclohexal; Fenac; Voltaren; Voltaren Ophtha; ***Belg.:*** Cataflam; Polyflam†; Voltaren; ***Canad.:*** Arthrotec; Novo-Difenac; Nu-Diclo; Voltaren; Voltaren Ophtha; ***Fr.:*** Flector; Voldal; Voltarene; Xenid; ***Ger.:*** Allvoran; Arthotec; Arthrex; Arthrex Duo; Benfofen; Delphinac; Diclac; Diclo; Diclo-OPT†; Diclo-Puren; Diclo-saar; Diclo-Spondyril†; Diclo-Tablinen; Diclo-Wolff; Dicloberl†; Diclofenbeta; Diclomerck; Diclophlogont; Diclorektal; Dignofenac†; Dolgit-Diclo; dolobasan†; DoloVisano Diclo†; duravolten; Effekton; Jenafenac; Lexobene; Monoflam; Myogit; Rewodina; Rheumasan D†; Sigafenac; Silino†; Toryxil; Voltaren; Voltaren Ophtha; ***Irl.:*** Arthrotec; Cataflam; Diclac; Diclo; Diclomel; Difene; Vologen; Voltarol; ***Ital.:*** Artrotec; Cataflam; Dealgic; Deflamat; Diclocular; Dicloftil; Dicloreum; Fenadol; Flector; Flogofenac; Forgenac; Misofenac; Novapirina; Ribex Flu; Voltaren; ***Neth.:*** Arthrotec; Cataflam; Naclof; Voltaren; ***Norw.:*** Arthrotec; Naclof†; Voltaren; ***S.Afr.:*** Anfenax†; Arcanafenac; Arthrotec; Brovaflamp†; Cataflam; Cliniflam†; Diclofam; Difenac; Flexagen; Fortfen; Infla-Ban; Naclof; Panamor; Pharmaflam†; Sodiclo; Veltex; Voltaren; ***Spain:*** Di Retard; Dolotren; Liberalgium; Luase; Voltaren; Voltaren Emulgel; ***Swed.:*** Arthrotec; Naclof†; Voltaren; Voltaren T; ***Switz.:*** Arthrotec; diclo-basan; Diclosifar; Ecofenac; Flector; Grofenac; Inflamac; Olfen; Primofenac; Rheufenac; Rhumalgan†; Vifenac; Voltarene; Voltarene Emulgel; Voltarene Ophtha; Voltarene Rapide; ***UK:*** Arthrotec; Dicloflex; Diclomax Retard; Diclotard; Diclovol; Diclozip; Digenac; Flamatak; Flamrase; Flexotard; Isclofen; Lofensaid; Motifene; Rhumalgan; Slofenac; Valenac†; Volraman; Volsaid; Voltarol; Voltarol Ophtha; ***USA:*** Arthrotec; Cataflam; Voltaren.

Multi-ingredient: ***Aust.:*** Dolo-Neurobion; Neodolpasse; Neurofenac; ***Ger.:*** B-Voltaren†; Combaren; Neuro-Effekton†; Neurofenac†; ***Ital.:*** Voltamicin; ***Spain:*** Coneurase†; Dolo Nervobion; ***Switz.:*** Voltamicin; ***UK:*** Dexomon.

Diethylamine Salicylate (2633-k)

$C_{11}H_{17}NO_3 = 211.3.$
CAS — 4419-92-5.
Pharmacopoeias. In *Br.*

White or almost white, odourless or almost odourless crystals. Very **soluble** in water; freely soluble in alcohol and in chloroform. **Protect** from light. Avoid contact with iron or iron salts.

Diethylamine salicylate is a salicylic acid derivative used topically in rubefacient preparations similarly to methyl salicylate (p.55) for rheumatic and muscular pain.

Preparations

BP 1998: Diethylamine Salicylate Cream.

Proprietary Preparations (details are given in Part 3)
Aust.: Algesal; Rheumagel†; ***Belg.:*** Algesal; ***Canad.:*** Algesal; Physiogesic; ***Fr.:*** Algesal†; ***Ital.:*** Algesal; Algoflex Same; ***Neth.:*** Algesal; ***Norw.:*** Algesal; ***Spain:*** Algoderm; Artrogota; ***Swed.:*** Algesal; ***UK:*** Algesal; Lloyd's Cream.

Multi-ingredient: ***Aust.:*** Derivon; Dolo-Menthoneurin; Igitur-antirheumatische; Igitur-Rheumafluid†; Kalisyl; Latesyl; Pasta rubra salicylata; Reparil; Rheugesal; Thermal; ***Austral.:*** Rubesal; ***Belg.:*** Algesal; Reparil; ***Fr.:*** Algesal Suractive; Reparil; Traumalgyl; ***Ger.:*** ABC Warme-Salbe; Algesal; Algesalona; Arthro-Menthoneurin†; Bartelin N; Bartelin nico; Brachialin percutan N; Contrheuma V + T Bad N; Dolo-Menthoneurin; Doloneuro; Fibraflex†; Reparil-Gel N; Rheubalmin; Rheuma Bad; Rheumasan Bad; Rheumex†; Rheumichthol Bad; Rheumyl N†; Rheumyl†; Spolera therm†; ***Ital.:*** Aspercreme; Cloristamina†; Reparil; Sedalpan; Via Mal Trauma Gel; ***Neth.:*** Algesal Forte; ***Norw.:*** Thermal; ***S.Afr.:*** Analgen†; Reparil; ***Spain:*** Algesal; Doctomitil; Dolmitin; Fepari; Radio Salil; ***Swed.:*** Remysal N†; ***Switz.:*** Algesal; Algesalona; Brachialin†; Dolo-Menthoneurin†; Proctalgen; Reparil; Reparil N; Roliwol B; ***UK:*** Fiery Jack.

Diethylsalicylamide (13411-b)

N,N-Diethyl-2-hydroxybenzamide.
$C_{11}H_{15}NO_2 = 193.2.$
CAS — 19311-91-2.

Diethylsalicylamide is a salicylic acid derivative (see Aspirin, p.16) that has been used in the treatment of pain and fever.

Preparations

Proprietary Preparations (details are given in Part 3)
Multi-ingredient: ***Fr.:*** Sedarene†.

Difenpiramide (12650-e)

Diphenpyramide; Z-876. *N*-(2-Pyridyl)-2-(biphenyl-4-yl)acetamide.
$C_{19}H_{16}N_2O = 288.3.$
CAS — 51484-40-3.

Difenpiramide is an NSAID (p.63) that has been used in musculoskeletal, joint, and soft-tissue disorders.

Preparations

Proprietary Preparations (details are given in Part 3)
Ital.: Difenax†.

Diflunisal (2635-t)

Diflunisal *(BAN, USAN, rINN).*
Diflunisalum; MK-647. 5-(2,4-Difluorophenyl)salicylic acid.
$C_{13}H_8F_2O_3 = 250.2.$
CAS — 22494-42-4.
Pharmacopoeias. In *Eur.* (see p.viii) and *US.*

A white to off-white, practically odourless, crystalline powder. **Solubilities** are: practically insoluble in water; freely soluble to soluble in alcohol; freely soluble in methyl alcohol; soluble in acetone, in ether, and in ethyl acetate; slightly soluble in chloroform, in carbon tetrachloride, and in dichloromethane; practically insoluble in petroleum spirit; dissolves in dilute solutions of alkali hydroxides. **Protect** from light.

Adverse Effects and Treatment

As for NSAIDs in general, p.63. The commonest side-effects occurring with diflunisal are gastro-intestinal disturbances, headache, and rash. Peptic ulceration and gastro-intestinal bleeding have been reported. Dizziness, drowsiness, insomnia, and tinnitus may also occur.

Effects on the blood. Haematological adverse effects associated with diflunisal therapy appear to be infrequent. Thrombocytopenia associated with diflunisal-induced peripheral platelet destruction has been reported in a patient with rheumatoid arthritis.[1] Heinz-body haemolytic anaemia has also been reported, see under Hypersensitivity, below.

1. Bobrove AM. Diflunisal-associated thrombocytopenia in a patient with rheumatoid arthritis. *Arthritis Rheum* 1988; **31:** 148–9.

Effects on the kidneys. There has been a report[1] of acute interstitial nephritis, presenting as acute oliguric renal failure, erythroderma, and eosinophilia following the use of diflunisal.

1. Chan LK, *et al.* Acute interstitial nephritis and erythroderma associated with diflunisal. *Br Med J* 1980; **280:** 84–5.

Effects on the skin. Reports of Stevens-Johnson syndrome associated with diflunisal.[1,2] See also under Hypersensitivity, below.

1. Hunter JA, *et al.* Diflunisal and Stevens-Johnson syndrome. *Br Med J* 1978; **2:** 1088.
2. Grom JA, *et al.* Diflunisal-induced erythema multiforme major. *Hosp Formul* 1986; **21:** 353–4.

Hypersensitivity. Three cases of hypersensitivity to diflunisal in which the main clinical features were fever, elevated liver enzyme values, erythroderma, and eosinophilia, have been reported.[1] Heinz-body haemolytic anaemia occurred in one of the patients.

1. Cook DJ, *et al.* Three cases of diflunisal hypersensitivity. *Can Med Assoc J* 1988; **138:** 1029–30.

Overdosage. Diflunisal poisoning has sometimes been fatal.[1,2] A dose of 15 g has been reported to have caused death when no other drugs were involved but a dose of 7.5 g has also been fatal when taken with other drugs. The treatment of a diflunisal overdose should involve gastric lavage and supportive care; the benefit of forced diuresis has not been established.[1]

1. Court H, Volans GN. Poisoning after overdose with non-steroidal anti-inflammatory drugs. *Adverse Drug React Acute Poisoning Rev* 1984; **3:** 1–21.
2. Levine B, *et al.* Diflunisal related fatality: a case report. *Forensic Sci Int* 1987; **35:** 45–50.

Precautions

As for NSAIDs in general, p.65. Diflunisal may need to be given in reduced dosage in patients with renal impairment and should not be given when renal impairment is severe.

Interactions

For interactions associated with NSAIDs, see p.65.

Aspirin may produce a small decrease in the plasma concentration of diflunisal. Diflunisal has been reported to increase the plasma concentrations of indomethacin and paracetamol; the concomitant administration of diflunisal and indomethacin has been associated with fatal gastro-intestinal haemorrhage and therefore the combination should not be used. Antacids may reduce the absorption of diflunisal.

Benzodiazepines. For the effect of diflunisal on plasma concentrations of *oxazepam,* see p.663.

Probenecid. Average steady state plasma concentrations of diflunisal were increased by 65% when it was administered with probenecid.[1] This was due mainly to reduced formation of the phenolic and acyl glucuronides. However, plasma concentrations of these glucuronides and the sulphate conjugate were also increased even more because probenecid also reduced their renal clearance.

1. Macdonald JI, *et al.* Effect of probenecid on the formation and elimination kinetics of the sulphate and glucuronide conjugates of diflunisal. *Eur J Clin Pharmacol* 1995; **47:** 519–23.

Pharmacokinetics

Diflunisal is well absorbed from the gastro-intestinal tract and peak plasma concentrations occur about 2 to 3 hours after ingestion of a single dose. It is extensively bound (more than 99%) to plasma protein and has an plasma half-life of about 8 to 12 hours. Diflunisal exhibits non-linear pharmacokinetics so that doubling the dose produces a greater than doubling of drug accumulation. Due to the long half-life and non-linear kinetics, several days are required to reach steady-state serum concentrations following multiple dosing. The time to steady-state concentrations can be reduced by giving an initial loading dose. Concentrations of diflunisal in synovial fluid reach about 70% of those in plasma. Diflunisal is excreted in the urine mainly as glucuronide conjugates. Some biliary recycling may also occur. Diflunisal is distributed into breast milk with concentrations reported to be about 2 to 7% of those in plasma.

References.

1. Loewen GR, *et al.* Effect of dose on the glucuronidation and sulphation kinetics of diflunisal in man: single dose studies. *Br J Clin Pharmacol* 1988; **26:** 31–9.
2. Eriksson L-O, *et al.* Influence of renal failure, rheumatoid arthritis and old age on the pharmacokinetics of diflunisal. *Eur J Clin Pharmacol* 1989; **36:** 165–74.
3. Verbeeck RK, *et al.* The effect of multiple dosage on the kinetics of glucuronidation and sulphation of diflunisal in man. *Br J Clin Pharmacol* 1990; **29:** 381–9.
4. Nuernberg B, *et al.* Pharmacokinetics of diflunisal in patients. *Clin Pharmacokinet* 1991; **20:** 81–9.
5. Macdonald JI, *et al.* Sex-difference and the effects of smoking and oral contraceptive steroids on the kinetics of diflunisal. *Eur J Clin Pharmacol* 1990; **38:** 175–9.

Uses and Administration

Diflunisal is a salicylic acid derivative (see Aspirin, p.18) but it is not hydrolysed to salicylate and its clinical effects are considered to resemble more closely those of propionic acid derivative NSAIDs (p.65). Diflunisal is used in the acute or long-term management of mild to moderate pain, pain and inflammation associated with osteoarthritis and rheumatoid arthritis, and symptoms of primary dysmenorrhoea. The usual initial dose for pain relief is 1000 mg followed by a maintenance dose of 500 mg every 12 hours. In some patients 250 mg every 8 to 12 hours may be sufficient but some may require 500 mg every 8 hours. Maintenance doses greater than 1500 mg daily are not recommended. The usual dose for arthritis is 500 to 1000 mg daily; this dose may be given as a single dose or as 2 divided doses.

Diflunisal may need to be given in reduced dosage in patients with renal impairment and should not be given when renal impairment is severe.

Diflunisal arginine has been used similarly given by mouth or by intramuscular or intravenous injection.

Preparations

BP 1998: Diflunisal Tablets;
USP 23: Diflunisal Tablets.

Proprietary Preparations (details are given in Part 3)
Aust.: Fluniget; ***Austral.:*** Dolobid; ***Belg.:*** Biartac; Diflusal; ***Canad.:*** Dolobid; ***Fr.:*** Dolobis; ***Ger.:*** Fluniget; ***Irl.:*** Dolobid; ***Ital.:*** Adomal†; Aflogos; Artrodol; Citidol†; Difludol; Diflunil†; Diflusan†; Dolisal†; Dolobid; Fluodonil; Flustar†; Nalgisa†; Noaldol†; Reuflos†; ***Neth.:*** Dolocid; ***Norw.:*** Diflonid; Donobid; ***S.Afr.:*** Dolobid; ***Spain:*** Dolobid; Ilacen†; ***Swed.:*** Diflonid†; Donobid; ***Switz.:*** Unisal; ***UK:*** Dolobid; ***USA:*** Dolobid.

Dihydrocodeine Phosphate (6221-g)

Dihydrocodeine Phosphate *(BANM, rINNM).*
Hydrocodeine Phosphate.
$C_{18}H_{23}NO_3,H_3PO_4$ = 399.4.
CAS — 24204-13-5.
Pharmacopoeias. In *Jpn.*

Dihydrocodeine Tartrate (6222-q)

Dihydrocodeine Tartrate *(BANM, rINNM).*
Dihydrocodeine Acid Tartrate; Dihydrocodeine Bitartrate; Drocode Bitartrate; Hydrocodeine Bitartrate. 4,5-Epoxy-3-methoxy-17-methylmorphinan-6-ol hydrogen tartrate.
$C_{18}H_{23}NO_3,C_4H_6O_6$ = 451.5.
CAS — 125-28-0 (dihydrocodeine); 5965-13-9 (dihydrocodeine tartrate).

NOTE. Compounded preparations of dihydrocodeine tartrate and paracetamol in the proportions 1 part to 50 parts by weight, respectively, have the British Approved Name Co-dydramol.

Pharmacopoeias. In *Aust., Br., Ger., Pol.,* and *US.*

Odourless, or almost odourless, colourless crystals or white crystalline powder. Freely **soluble** in water; sparingly soluble in alcohol; practically insoluble in ether. A 10% solution in water has a pH of 3.2 to 4.2. **Store** in airtight containers. Protect from light.

Dependence and Withdrawal

As for Opioid Analgesics, p.67. Dihydrocodeine has been subject to abuse (see under Precautions, below).

Adverse Effects and Treatment

As for Opioid Analgesics in general, p.68; side-effects from dihydrocodeine are less pronounced than those from morphine.

For reference to increased postoperative pain associated with the use of dihydrocodeine, see under Pain in Uses and Administration, below.

Overdosage. A 29-year-old man who had taken 2.1 g of dihydrocodeine had biochemical evidence of acute renal and hepatic impairment when admitted 13 hours after the overdose.[1] Severe life-threatening respiratory depression subsequently developed 36 hours after the overdose and only responded to treatment with naloxone after large doses (a total of 46.6 mg of naloxone) over a long period (106 hours). Commenting on this report some questioned the evidence for hepatic impairment and considered that the raised liver enzyme values were of muscular origin as a result of rhabdomyolysis.[2-4] Rhabdomyolysis might also have contributed to renal failure.

An anaphylactoid reaction following an overdose of an unspecified number of dihydrocodeine tablets[5] appeared to respond to intravenous naloxone.

1. Redfern N. Dihydrocodeine overdose treated with naloxone infusion. *Br Med J* 1983; **287:** 751–2.
2. Buckley BM, Vale JA. Dihydrocodeine overdose treated with naloxone infusion. *Br Med J* 1983; **287:** 1547.
3. Blain PG, Lane RJM. Dihydrocodeine overdose treated with naloxone infusion. *Br Med J* 1983; **287:** 1547.
4. Wen P. Dihydrocodeine overdose treated with naloxone infusion. *Br Med J* 1983; **287:** 1548.
5. Panos MZ, *et al.* Use of naloxone in opioid-induced anaphylactoid reaction. *Br J Anaesth* 1988; **61:** 371.

Precautions

As for Opioid Analgesics in general, p.68.

Abuse. Dihydrocodeine has been reported to be widely abused by opiate addicts.[1-3]

1. Swadi H, *et al.* Misuse of dihydrocodeine tartrate (DF 118) among opiate addicts. *Br Med J* 1990; **300:** 1313.
2. Robertson JR, *et al.* Misuse of dihydrocodeine tartrate (DF 118) among opiate addicts. *Br Med J* 1990; **301:** 119.
3. Strang J, *et al.* Misuse of dihydrocodeine tartrate (DF 118) among opiate addicts. *Br Med J* 1990; **301:** 119.

Elderly. Despite some impaired renal function an elderly group of patients[1] appeared to handle dihydrocodeine similarly to healthy young subjects. There was marked variability in all measurements and on the basis of this study no clear conclusions on guidelines for dosage in elderly patients could be drawn. However, the recommendation that small doses be given initially with subsequent doses according to response was endorsed.

1. Davis KN, *et al.* The effect of ageing on the pharmacokinetics of dihydrocodeine. *Eur J Clin Pharmacol* 1989; **37:** 375–9.

Renal impairment. Caution is necessary when giving dihydrocodeine to patients with severe renal impairment. Severe narcosis occurred in a patient with anuria and on maintenance haemodialysis after she had received dihydrocodeine by mouth for 4 days.[1] She responded to treatment with naloxone. See also under Pharmacokinetics, below.

1. Barnes JN, Goodwin FJ. Dihydrocodeine narcosis in renal failure. *Br Med J* 1983; **286:** 438–9.

Interactions

For interactions associated with opioid analgesics, see p.69.

Pharmacokinetics

The pharmacokinetics of dihydrocodeine may be similar to those of codeine (p.26).

There have been few pharmacokinetic studies of dihydrocodeine. In one study[1] peak plasma concentrations of dihydrocodeine were achieved 1.6 and 1.8 hours after an oral dose of 30 and 60 mg, respectively; elimination half-lives varied between about 3.5 and 4.5 hours. The rate of absorption was independent of dose and oral bioavailability was only about 20%, possibly because of substantial first-pass metabolism in the gut wall or liver.

1. Rowell FJ, *et al.* Pharmacokinetics of intravenous and oral dihydrocodeine and its acid metabolites. *Eur J Clin Pharmacol* 1983; **25:** 419–24.

Administration in renal impairment. The pharmacokinetics of dihydrocodeine tartrate, given by mouth as a single 60-mg dose, were affected in 9 patients with chronic renal failure treated with haemodialysis when compared with 9 healthy subjects.[1] Time to peak plasma concentration in those with renal failure was 3 hours compared with 1 hour in healthy subjects; the area under the plasma concentration/time curve was greater in those with renal failure; and after 24 hours dihydrocodeine was still detectable in the plasma of all renal failure patients, but in only 3 of the healthy subjects.

1. Barnes JN, *et al.* Dihydrocodeine in renal failure: further evidence for an important role of the kidney in the handling of opioid drugs. *Br Med J* 1985; **290:** 740–2.

Uses and Administration

Dihydrocodeine is an opioid analgesic (p.69). It is related to codeine (p.27) and has similar analgesic activity. Dihydrocodeine is used for the relief of moderate to severe pain and has also been used as a cough suppressant.

For analgesia the usual dose of dihydrocodeine tartrate by mouth is 30 mg after food every 4 to 6 hours. For severe pain 40 to 80 mg may be given three times daily. Children over 4 years of age may be given 0.5 to 1 mg per kg body-weight every 4 to 6 hours. Modified-release preparations are available for twice daily administration in adults with chronic severe pain.

Dihydrocodeine tartrate may also be given by deep subcutaneous or intramuscular injection in doses of up to 50 mg every 4 to 6 hours. Doses equivalent to those used orally may be given to children over 4 years of age.

As a cough suppressant dihydrocodeine tartrate may be given by mouth in doses of 10 mg every 4 to 6 hours. Children over 4 years of age have been given 200 μg per kg every 4 to 6 hours.

Dihydrocodeine tartrate (1 part) and paracetamol (50 parts) in combination, have been given the British Approved Name co-dydramol; a usual strength of this combination is dihydrocodeine tartrate 10 mg with paracetamol 500 mg. The usual dose of dihydrocodeine tartrate when given in this manner is 10 to 20 mg every 4 to 6 hours to a total daily maximum dose of 80 mg. Alternative compounded preparations of dihydrocodeine with non-opioid analgesics are also available; dosage and strength varies with formulations.

Dihydrocodeine phosphate has also been used. Other salts of dihydrocodeine used, mainly for their antitussive effects, include the hydrochloride and the thiocyanate. Dihydrocodeine polistirex has been used in modified-release preparations.

Dyspnoea. Johnson *et al.*[1] reported some benefit with dihydrocodeine in normocapnic patients severely disabled by breathlessness due to chronic airflow obstruction. A dose of 15 mg was taken 30 minutes before exercise up to three times a day.

1. Johnson MA, *et al.* Dihydrocodeine for breathlessness in 'pink puffers'. *Br Med J* 1983; **286:** 675–7.

Pain. Dihydrocodeine is used in the management of moderate to severe pain. However, Seymour *et al.*[1] have reported the phenomenon of dose-related increased postoperative pain in patients given 25 or 50 mg dihydrocodeine tartrate intravenously following dental surgery. Henry[2] proposed that dihydrocodeine might act as an antagonist in situations where acute pain was accompanied by high opioid activity. Dihydrocodeine continues to be prescribed for dental pain, although other analgesics such as ibuprofen[3] might be more effective.

1. Seymour RA, *et al.* Dihydrocodeine-induced hyperalgesia in postoperative dental pain. *Lancet* 1982; **i:** 1425–6.
2. Henry JA. Dihydrocodeine increases dental pain. *Lancet* 1982; **ii:** 223.
3. Frame JW, *et al.* A comparison of ibuprofen and dihydrocodeine in relieving pain following wisdom teeth removal. *Br Dent J* 1989; **166:** 121–4.

Preparations

BP 1998: Co-dydramol Tablets; Dihydrocodeine Injection; Dihydrocodeine Oral Solution; Dihydrocodeine Tablets;
USP 23: Aspirin, Caffeine, and Dihydrocodeine Bitartrate Capsules.

Proprietary Preparations (details are given in Part 3)
Aust.: Codidol; Paracodin; ***Austral.:*** Paracodin; Rikodeine; ***Belg.:*** Codicontin; Paracodine; ***Fr.:*** Dicodin; ***Ger.:*** DHC; Paracodin; Paracodin N; Paracodin retard†; Remedacen; Tiamon Mono; ***Irl.:*** DF 118; DHC Continus; Hydol; Paracodin; ***Ital.:*** Paracodina; ***S.Afr.:*** DF 118; Paracodin; ***Spain:*** Contugesic; Paracodina; Tosidrin; ***Switz.:*** Codicontin; Hydrocodeinon; Paracodin; ***UK:*** DF 118; DHC Continus.

Multi-ingredient: ***Aust.:*** Paracodin; ***Austral.:*** Codox; Senetuss†; Tuscodin†; ***Belg.:*** Paracodine; ***Ger.:*** Antitussivum Burger; Makatussin forte†; Makatussin Tropfen forte; Monacant†; Monapax mit Dihydrocodein†; Paracodin retard; Priatan†; ***Irl.:*** Paramol; ***Ital.:*** Cardiazol-Paracodina; ***Spain:*** Traquivan; ***Switz.:*** Escotussin; Makatussin forte; Neo Makatussin N; Paracodin retard; Pulmocure†; ***UK:*** Galake; Paramol; Remedeine; ***USA:*** DHC Plus; Synalgos-DC; Triaprin-DC†; Vanex Grape.

Dipipanone Hydrochloride (6224-s)

Dipipanone Hydrochloride *(BANM, rINNM).*
Phenylpiperone Hydrochloride; Piperidyl Methadone Hydrochloride; Piperidylamidone Hydrochloride. (±)-4,4-Diphenyl-6-piperidinoheptan-3-one hydrochloride monohydrate.
$C_{24}H_{31}NO,HCl,H_2O$ = 404.0.
CAS — 467-83-4 (dipipanone); 856-87-1 (dipipanone hydrochloride).
Pharmacopoeias. In *Br.*

An odourless or almost odourless, white, crystalline powder. Sparingly **soluble** in water; freely soluble in alcohol and in acetone; practically insoluble in ether. A 2.5% solution in water has a pH of 4.0 to 6.0.

Dipipanone hydrochloride is an opioid analgesic (p.67) structurally related to methadone (p.53). Used alone it is reported to be less sedating than morphine. It is used in the treatment of moderate or severe pain.

Dipipanone hydrochloride is usually administered with cyclizine hydrochloride in order to reduce the incidence of nausea and vomiting, but the use of opioid preparations containing an antiemetic is not recommended for the management of chronic pain as an antiemetic is usually only required for the first few days of treatment. The usual dose of dipipanone hydrochloride given by mouth is 10 mg, repeated every 6 hours. The dose may be increased if necessary in increments of 5 mg; it is seldom necessary to exceed a dose of 30 mg. Following administration by mouth the effect begins within an hour and lasts about 4 to 6 hours.

Preparations of dipipanone hydrochloride with cyclizine hydrochloride are subject to abuse.

Preparations

BP 1998: Dipipanone and Cyclizine Tablets.

Proprietary Preparations (details are given in Part 3)

Multi-ingredient: ***Irl.:*** Diconal; ***S.Afr.:*** Wellconal; ***UK:*** Diconal.

Diproqualone (16607-k)

Diproqualone (*rINN*).

3-(2,3-Dihydroxypropyl)-2-methyl-4(3*H*)-quinazolinone.

$C_{12}H_{14}N_2O_3$ = 234.3.

CAS — 36518-02-2.

Diproqualone is an analgesic that has been used as the camsylate in doses of 600 to 1200 mg daily in divided doses by mouth.

Preparations

Proprietary Preparations (details are given in Part 3)

Multi-ingredient: *Switz.:* Algopriv.

Dipyrone (2638-f)

Dipyrone (*BAN, USAN*).

Metamizole Sodium (*pINN*); Aminopyrine-sulphonate Sodium; Analginum; Metamizole; Metamizolum Natricum; Methampyrone; Natrium Novaminsulfonicum; Noramidazophenum; Noraminophenazonum; Novamidazofen; NSC-73205; Sodium Noramidopyrine Methanesulphonate; Sulpyrine. Sodium *N*-(2,3-dimethyl-5-oxo-1-phenyl-3-pyrazolin-4-yl)-*N*-methylaminomethanesulphonate monohydrate.

$C_{13}H_{16}N_3NaO_4S,H_2O$ = 351.4.

CAS — 68-89-3 (anhydrous dipyrone); 5907-38-0 (dipyrone monohydrate).

NOTE. Dipyrone is referred to in some countries by the colloquial name 'Mexican aspirin'.

Pharmacopoeias. In *Chin., Eur.* (see p.viii), *Jpn,* and *Pol.*

A white or almost white crystalline powder. Very **soluble** in water; soluble in alcohol. **Protect** from light.

Adverse Effects and Precautions

Administration of dipyrone is associated with an increased risk of agranulocytosis and with shock.

Effects on the blood. Data collected from 8 population groups in Europe and Israel by the International Agranulocytosis and Aplastic Anemia Study[1] revealed that there was a significant regional variability in the rate-ratio estimate for agranulocytosis and dipyrone (0.9 in Budapest to 33.3 in Barcelona). Although a large relative increase in risk between agranulocytosis and use of dipyrone was found, the incidence was less than some previous reports had suggested.

1. The International Agranulocytosis and Aplastic Anemia Study. Risks of agranulocytosis and aplastic anemia: a first report of their relation to drug use with special reference to analgesics. *JAMA* 1986; **256:** 1749–57.

Effects on the skin. Dipyrone has been considered responsible for a case of drug-induced toxic epidermal necrolysis.[1]

1. Roujeau J-C, *et al.* Sjögren-like syndrome after drug-induced toxic epidermal necrolysis. *Lancet* 1985; **i:** 609–11.

Hypersensitivity. Cross-sensitivity between aspirin and dipyrone occurred in one patient.[1] Dipyrone produced an exacerbation of dyspnoea, cyanosis, and respiratory arrest.

1. Bartoli E, *et al.* Drug-induced asthma. *Lancet* 1976; **i:** 1357.

Porphyria. Dipyrone has been associated with clinical exacerbations of porphyria and is considered unsafe in porphyric patients.[1]

1. Moore MR, McColl KEL. *Porphyria: drug lists.* Glasgow: Porphyria Research Unit, University of Glasgow, 1991.

Pharmacokinetics

Following oral administration dipyrone is rapidly hydrolysed in gastric juice to the active metabolite 4-methyl-amino-antipyrine which after absorption undergoes metabolism to 4-formyl-amino-antipyrine and other metabolites. Dipyrone is also rapidly undetectable in plasma following intravenous administration. None of the metabolites of dipyrone are extensively bound to plasma proteins. Most of a dose is excreted in the urine as metabolites. Dipyrone metabolites are also distributed into breast milk.

References.

1. Heinemeyer G, *et al.* The kinetics of metamizol and its metabolites in critical-care patients with acute renal dysfunction. *Eur J Clin Pharmacol* 1993; **45:** 445–50.
2. Levy M, *et al.* Clinical pharmacokinetics of dipyrone and its metabolites. *Clin Pharmacokinet* 1995; **28:** 216–34.
3. Zylber-Katz E, *et al.* Dipyrone metabolism in liver disease. *Clin Pharmacol Ther* 1995; **58:** 198–209.

Uses and Administration

Dipyrone, an NSAID (p.65), is the sodium sulphonate of amidopyrine (p.15) and has similar properties. Because of the risk of serious adverse effects its use is justified only in severe pain where no alternative is available or suitable. Dipyrone has been given by mouth in doses of 0.5 to 4 g daily in divided doses. It has also been given by intramuscular or intravenous injection and rectally as a suppository.

A magnesium cogener of dipyrone, metamizole magnesium has been used similarly to dipyrone as has the calcium cogener metamizole calcium.

Preparations

Proprietary Preparations (details are given in Part 3)
Aust.: Inalgon Neu; Novalgin; Spasmo Inalgon Neu; *Belg.:* Novalgine; *Fr.:* Novalgine†; Pyrethane; *Ger.:* Analgin; Analgit; Baralgin; Berlosin; Neuro-Brachont N†; Neuro-Fortamin S†; Norgesic N†; Novalgin; *Ital.:* Novalgina; Trisalgina; *Neth.:* Novalgin; *Spain:* Adolkin; Afebrin; Dolemicin; Dolo Buscopan†; Huberdor†; Lasain; Neo Melubrina; Nolotil; Optalgin; Pirenil Rectal†; *Swed.:* Novalgin; *Switz.:* Minalgin; Novalgine.

Multi-ingredient: *Aust.:* Baralgin†; Buscopan Compositum; Dolpasse†; Nealgon†; Spasmium comp; *Belg.:* Baralgin†; Buscopan Compositum; Visceralgine Compositum; *Fr.:* Algo-Buscopan†; Avafortan; Baralgine†; Cefaline-Pyrazole; Optalidon a la Noramidopyrine; Salgydal a la noramidopyrine; Visceralgine Forte; *Ger.:* Duo-Norgesic N†; Neuro-Fortamin†; Spondylon†; *Hung.:* Quarelin; *Ital.:* Artrocur†; Baralgina†; Buscopan Compositum; Condol†; Eblimon†; Sistalgin Compositum†; Soma Complex; Spasmamide Composta†; *S.Afr.:* Baralgan†; Buscopan Compositum; Norifortan; Scopex Co†; *Spain:* Baralgin†; Buscapina Compositum; Nolotil Compositum; Syntaverin†; Vapin Complex; *Switz.:* Baralgine†; Buscopan Compositum†; Dolo-Neurobion†; Influbene†; Panax†; Rectopyrine†.

Droxicam (2737-h)

Droxicam (*rINN*).

5-Methyl-3-(2-pyridyl)-2*H*,5*H*-1,3-oxazino[5,6-*c*]-[1,2]benzothiazine-2,4(3*H*)-dione 6,6-dioxide.

$C_{16}H_{11}N_3O_5S$ = 357.3.

CAS — 90101-16-9.

Droxicam is an NSAID (p.63) reported to act as a prodrug for piroxicam (p.80). It has been given by mouth for pain and inflammation associated with musculoskeletal, joint, and soft-tissue disorders but marketing was suspended in December 1994 because it was associated with adverse liver effects.

Effects on the liver. Up to October 1993 the Spanish National System of Pharmacovigilance had received 82 spontaneous reports of hepatic damage associated with droxicam[1] and in December 1994 the European Union Committee for Proprietary Medicinal Products recommended that marketing authorisation for droxicam should be suspended pending further studies. An industry sponsored study[1] (submitted in December 1994) of 8910 patients who had taken droxicam identified one patient whose hepatic damage was considered to be attributable to droxicam, a figure comparable with the base-line estimate observed for NSAIDs in general (see p.65).

1. García-Rodríguez LA, *et al.* Acute liver injury and droxicam use in the region of Friuli-Venezia Giulia. *Br J Clin Pharmacol* 1995; **40:** 103–6.

Preparations

Proprietary Preparations (details are given in Part 3)
Ital.: Dobenam†; Droxar†; *Spain:* Drogelon†; Ferpan†; Ombolan†; Pensatron†.

Eltenac (2797-j)

Eltenac (*rINN*).

4-(2,6-Dichloroanilino)-3-thiopheneacetic acid.

$C_{12}H_9Cl_2NO_2S$ = 302.2.

CAS — 72895-88-6.

Eltenac is an NSAID (p.63) used in veterinary medicine.

Enadoline Hydrochloride (17326-c)

Enadoline Hydrochloride (*USAN, rINNM*).

CI-977. *N*-Methyl-*N*-[(5*R*,7*S*,8*S*)-7-(1-pyrrolidinyl)-1-oxaspiro[4.5]dec-8-yl]-4-benzofuranacetamide monohydrochloride.

$C_{24}H_{32}N_2O_3,HCl$ = 433.0.

CAS — 124378-77-4 (enadoline); 124439-07-2 (enadoline hydrochloride).

Enadoline hydrochloride is an opioid analgesic (p.67) reported to have selective κ agonist activity. It is under investigation for the treatment of severe pain and severe head injury.

References.

1. Reece PA, *et al.* Diuretic effects, pharmacokinetics, and safety of a new centrally acting kappa-opioid agonist (CI-977) in humans. *J Clin Pharmacol* 1994; **34:** 1126–32.
2. Pande AC, *et al.* Analgesic efficacy of enadoline versus placebo or morphine in postsurgical pain. *Clin Neuropharmacol* 1996; **19:** 451–6.

Enoxolone (1608-p)

Enoxolone (*BAN, rINN*).

Glycyrrhetic Acid; Glycyrrhetinic Acid. 3β-Hydroxy-11-oxo-olean-12-en-30-oic acid.

$C_{30}H_{46}O_4$ = 470.7.

CAS — 471-53-4.

Enoxolone is a complex triterpene prepared from glycyrrhizinic acid, a constituent of liquorice. Enoxolone is used locally in preparations for the treatment of non-infective inflammatory disorders of the skin, mouth, throat, and rectum.

Derivatives of enoxolone, including its aluminium salt (p.1191), acetoxolone (p.1176), and carbenoxolone (p.1182) are used in the treatment of peptic ulcer disease and other gastro-intestinal disorders.

Enoxolone is a potent inhibitor of the enzyme 11β-hydroxysteroid dehydrogenase which inactivates cortisol and concomitant application of enoxolone with hydrocortisone has been shown in *animal* studies to potentiate the activity of hydrocortisone in skin.[1] Whether this also increases the systemic absorption and toxicity of hydrocortisone remains to be determined.[2]

1. Teelucksingh S, *et al.* Potentiation of hydrocortisone activity in skin by glycyrrhetinic acid. *Lancet* 1990; **335:** 1060–3.
2. Greaves MW. Potentiation of hydrocortisone activity in skin by glycerrhetinic acid. *Lancet* 1990; **336:** 876.

Preparations

Proprietary Preparations (details are given in Part 3)
Fr.: P.O. 12.

Multi-ingredient: *Fr.:* Anolan†; Arthrodont; Hexalyse; Lelong Irritations; Pyreflor; Sedorrhoide; Valda Mal de Gorge†; Valda Septol; *Ital.:* Acnesan; Antalgola Plus†; Eudent con Glysan; Katosilver; Lenipasta; Lenirose; Neo-Stomygen; Pastiglie Valda; Sterox†; Valda F3; Viderm; *Spain:* Angi†; Angileptol; Anginovag; Pentalmicina; Roberfarin.

Epirizole (2640-c)

Epirizole (*USAN, pINN*).

DA-398; Mepirizole. 4-Methoxy-2-(5-methoxy-3-methylpyrazol-1-yl)-6-methylpyrimidine.

$C_{11}H_{14}N_4O_2$ = 234.3.

CAS — 18694-40-1.

Pharmacopoeias. In *Jpn.*

Epirizole is an NSAID (p.63) that has been used by mouth.

Preparations

Proprietary Preparations (details are given in Part 3)
Jpn: Mebron.

Eptazocine Hydrobromide (12698-b)

Eptazocine Hydrobromide (*rINNM*).

ST-2121. (−)-(1*S*,6*S*)-2,3,4,5,6,7-Hexahydro-1,4-dimethyl-1,6-methano-1*H*-4-benzazonin-10-ol hydrobromide.

$C_{15}H_{21}NO,HBr$ = 312.2.

CAS — 72522-13-5 (eptazocine); 72150-17-5 (eptazocine hydrobromide).

Eptazocine hydrobromide is reported to be an opioid analgesic (p.67) with mixed opioid agonist and antagonist actions.

Preparations

Proprietary Preparations (details are given in Part 3)
Jpn: Sedapain†.

Etenzamide (2641-k)

Etenzamide (*BAN*).

Ethenzamide (*rINN*); Aethoxybenzamidum; Ethoxybenzamide; Ethylsalicylamide; HP-209. 2-Ethoxybenzamide.

$C_9H_{11}NO_2$ = 165.2.

CAS — 938-73-8.

Pharmacopoeias. In *Aust.* and *Jpn.*

Etenzamide is a salicylic acid derivative (see Aspirin, p.16). It has been given in doses of up to 4 g daily in divided doses by mouth.

Preparations

Proprietary Preparations (details are given in Part 3)
Belg.: Simil NF; *Fr.:* Trancalgyl†; *Ger.:* Euffekt†.

Multi-ingredient: *Aust.:* Coldadolin; Dolmix†; Helopyrin; Neuro-European; Nisicur; Seltoc; Ultrapyrin†; *Fr.:* Cephyl; *Ger.:* Antifohnon-N; Antipanin N†; Ascorbin-Chinin-Dragees Michallik†; Doregrippin S†; ergo sanol spezial†; ergo sanol†; Eu-Med S†; Glutisal; Kolton grippale N; Neopyrin-N†; Octadon†; Optipyrin S†; Prostatin N†; Temagin†; Toximer†; Ultrapyrin†; *Ital.:* Etocil Caffeina†; Etocil Pirina†; *Switz.:* Algopriv; Ergosanol; Ergosanol a la cafeine; Ergosanol special; Ergosanol special a la cafeine; Melabon†; Melaforte†; Nicaphlogyl; Seranex sans codeine.

Etersalate (3553-h)

Etersalate (*rINN*).

Eterilate; Eterylate; Etherylate. 2-(4-Acetamidophenoxy)ethyl salicylate, acetate (ester).

$C_{19}H_{19}NO_6$ = 357.4.

CAS — 62992-61-4.

Etersalate is a salicylic acid derivative (see Aspirin, p.16) that was used in the treatment of pain, fever, and in rheumatic disorders and for its antiplatelet action.

Preparations

Proprietary Preparations (details are given in Part 3)
Spain: Daital†.

Ethoheptazine Citrate (6225-w)

Ethoheptazine Citrate *(BANM, rINNM).*

Wy-401. Ethyl 1-methyl-4-phenylperhydroazepine-4-carboxylate dihydrogen citrate.

$C_{16}H_{23}NO_2,C_6H_8O_7$ = 453.5.

CAS — 77-15-6 (ethoheptazine); 6700-56-7 (ethoheptazine citrate); 2085-42-9 ((±)-ethoheptazine citrate).

Ethoheptazine citrate is an opioid analgesic (p.67) structurally related to pethidine (p.76). It is employed as an analgesic in the short-term treatment of mild to moderate pain, usually in conjunction with other compounds such as aspirin and meprobamate. The usual dose is 75 to 150 mg three or four times daily.

Preparations

Proprietary Preparations (details are given in Part 3)

Multi-ingredient: ***Canad.:*** Equagesic; ***Irl.:*** Equagesic†; ***S.Afr.:*** Equagesic; ***UK:*** Equagesic.

Ethyl Nicotinate (9231-s)

$C_8H_9NO_2$ = 151.2.

CAS — 614-18-6.

Ethyl nicotinate is used in topical preparations as a rubefacient.

Preparations

Proprietary Preparations (details are given in Part 3)
Aust.: Mucotherm.

Multi-ingredient: ***Aust.:*** Thermal; ***Belg.:*** Algex†; Transvane†; ***Ger.:*** Striatridin; ***Irl.:*** Transvasin; ***Ital.:*** Linimento Bertelli†; ***Norw.:*** Thermal; ***Swed.:*** Transvasin; ***Switz.:*** Baume Esco Forte; Sloan Baume; Thermocutan; ***UK:*** PR Heat Spray; Transvasin.

Ethyl Salicylate (12707-l)

Ethyl 2-hydroxybenzoate.

$C_9H_{10}O_3$ = 166.2.

CAS — 118-61-6.

Ethyl salicylate is a salicylic acid derivative that has been used similarly to methyl salicylate (p.55) in concentrations of up to 5% in topical rubefacient preparations for the relief of pain in musculoskeletal, joint, and soft-tissue disorders.

Preparations

Proprietary Preparations (details are given in Part 3)

Multi-ingredient: ***Austral.:*** Deep Heat; Radian-B; ***Belg.:*** Rado-Salil; ***Ger.:*** Contrheuma-Gel forte N; Terbintil†; ***Ital.:*** Remy; ***Switz.:*** Alginex†; ***UK:*** Aspellin; Deep Heat Spray; Dubam; Ralgex.

Ethylmorphine Hydrochloride (6226-e)

Ethylmorphine Hydrochloride *(BANM).*

Aethylmorphinae Hydrochloridum; Aethylmorphini Hydrochloridum; Chlorhydrate de Codéthyline; Cloridrato de Etilmorfina; Ethylmorphini Hydrochloridum; Ethylmorphinium Chloride. 3-*O*-Ethylmorphine hydrochloride dihydrate; 7,8-Didehydro-4,5-epoxy-3-ethoxy-17-methylmorphinan-6-ol hydrochloride dihydrate.

$C_{19}H_{23}NO_3,HCl,2H_2O$ = 385.9.

CAS — 76-58-4 (ethylmorphine); 125-30-4 (ethylmorphine hydrochloride).

Pharmacopoeias. In *Chin., Eur.* (see p.viii), *Jpn,* and *Pol.*

A white or almost white crystalline powder. **Soluble** in water and in alcohol; practically insoluble in ether. A 2% solution in water has a pH of 4.3 to 5.7. **Protect** from light.

Ethylmorphine hydrochloride is an opioid analgesic (p.67) and has properties similar to those of codeine (p.26). It is used mainly as a cough suppressant. It has also been used for its analgesic and antidiarrhoeal properties and has been given in eye drops as a lymphagogue.

Ethylmorphine free base and the camphorate and camsylate have also been used.

References

1. Aasmundstad TA, *et al.* Biotransformation and pharmacokinetics of ethylmorphine after a single oral dose. *Br J Clin Pharmacol* 1995; **39:** 611–20.

Preparations

Proprietary Preparations (details are given in Part 3)
Belg.: Codethyline; ***Fr.:*** Trachyl; ***UK:*** Collins Elixir.

Multi-ingredient: ***Aust.:*** Modiscop; ***Belg.:*** Neo-Codion; Solucamphre; Theralene Pectoral; Tux; ***Fr.:*** Bronpax; Camphodionyl; Curibronches†; Doudol†; Ephydion; Eubispasme Codethyline; Humex; Marrubene Codethyline; Ozothine; Pecto 6†; Peter's Sirop; Polery; Pulmosodyl; Pulmospir†; Quintopan Adult; Sedophon; Sirop Pectoral adulte; Sirop Pectoral enfant; Theralene Pectoral†; Thiosedal; Tussipax; Tussipax a l'Euquinine; Vegetoserum; ***Ger.:*** Expectorans Solucampher†; Neo-Codion N†; Neo-Codion†; Noviform-Aethylmorphin†; ***Ital.:*** Codetilina-Eucaliptolo He; Mindol-Merck; Pantosse†; ***Norw.:*** Cosylan; Solvipect comp; Sterk hostesirup; ***Spain:*** Cidantos†; Demusin; Diptol Antihist†; Eucalyptospirine; Neodemusin†; Sedalmerck; Super Koki†; ***Swed.:*** Cocillana-Etyfin; Cosylan; Lepheton; ***Switz.:*** Ipeca; Neo-Codion Adultes†; Neo-Codion Enfants†; Neo-Codion†; Phol-Tux; Saintbois nouvelle formule; Sano Tuss; Solucamphre.

Etodolac (12717-j)

Etodolac *(BAN, USAN, rINN).*

AY-24236; Etodolic Acid. 1,8-Diethyl-1,3,4,9-tetrahydropyrano[3,4-*b*]indol-1-ylacetic acid.

$C_{17}H_{21}NO_3$ = 287.4.

CAS — 41340-25-4.

Pharmacopoeias. In *Br.*

A white or almost white crystalline powder. Practically **insoluble** in water; freely soluble in alcohol.

Adverse Effects and Precautions

As for NSAIDs in general, p.63.

The presence of phenolic metabolites of etodolac in the urine may give rise to a false-positive reaction for bilirubin.

Effects on the blood. A report[1] of a patient who had agranulocytosis associated with the use of etodolac.

1. Cramer RL, *et al.* Agranulocytosis associated with etodolac. *Ann Pharmacother* 1994; **28:** 458–60.

Effects on the gastro-intestinal tract. Etodolac may produce less gastric toxicity than naproxen.[1,2]

1. Taha AS, *et al.* Effect of repeated therapeutic doses of naproxen and etodolac on gastric and duodenal mucosal prostaglandins (PGs) in rheumatoid arthritis (RA). *Gut* 1989; **30:** A751.
2. Bianchi Porro G, *et al.* A double-blind gastroscopic evaluation of the effects of etodolac and naproxen on the gastrointestinal mucosa of rheumatic patients. *J Intern Med* 1991; **229:** 5–8.

Interactions

For interactions associated with NSAIDs, see p.65.

Pharmacokinetics

Etodolac is a chiral compound given as the racemate. Peak plasma concentrations of the active (S)-enantiomer and of the inactive (R)-enantiomer are usually obtained within about 2 hours of administration by mouth but plasma concentrations of the (R)-enantiomer have been reported to greatly exceed those of the (S)-enantiomer. Both enantiomers are highly bound to plasma protein. Both enantiomers are distributed to the synovial fluid, although the difference in their concentrations may not be as marked as the difference in plasma concentrations. The plasma half-life of total etodolac has been reported to be about 7 hours; excretion is predominantly in the urine mainly as hydroxylated metabolites and glucuronide conjugates; some may be excreted in the bile.

References.

1. Brocks DR, *et al.* Stereoselective disposition of etodolac enantiomers in synovial fluid. *J Clin Pharmacol* 1991; **31:** 741–6.
2. Brocks DR, *et al.* The stereoselective pharmacokinetics of etodolac in young and elderly subjects, and after cholecystectomy. *J Clin Pharmacol* 1992; **32:** 982–9.
3. Brocks DR, Jamali F. Etodolac clinical pharmacokinetics. *Clin Pharmacokinet* 1994; **26:** 259–74.

Uses and Administration

Etodolac, a pyrano-indoleacetic acid derivative, is an NSAID (p.65). It is used for rheumatoid arthritis and osteoarthritis and for the treatment of acute pain.

For the treatment of rheumatoid arthritis and osteoarthritis, the recommended dosage of etodolac in the UK is 400 to 600 mg daily given in single or divided doses. In the USA the recommended dose is initially 600 to 1000 mg daily in divided doses adjusted according to response to a maximum of 1200 mg daily. Modified-release preparations are available for once daily administration in the treatment of rheumatoid arthritis or osteoarthritis.

For the treatment of acute pain, the recommended dose is 200 to 400 mg every 6 to 8 hours to a usual maximum of 1000 mg daily although some patients have been given up to 1200 mg daily.

Preparations

BP 1998: Etodolac Capsules; Etodolac Tablets.

Proprietary Preparations (details are given in Part 3)
Aust.: Lodine†; ***Canad.:*** Ultradol; ***Fr.:*** Lodine; ***Ital.:*** Edolan†; Lodine; Zedolac†; ***Switz.:*** Lodine; ***UK:*** Lodine; ***USA:*** Lodine.

Etofenamate (2644-x)

Etofenamate *(BAN, USAN, rINN).*

B-577; Bay-d-1107; TV-485; TVX-485; WHR-5020. 2-(2-Hydroxyethoxy)ethyl *N*-(ααα-trifluoro-*m*-tolyl)anthranilate.

$C_{18}H_{18}F_3NO_4$ = 369.3.

CAS — 30544-47-9.

Etofenamate is an NSAID (p.63) that has been applied topically in a concentration of 5 or 10% for the relief of pain and inflammation associated with musculoskeletal, joint, and soft-tissue disorders. It has also been given by deep intramuscular injection in single doses of 1 g.

Preparations

Proprietary Preparations (details are given in Part 3)
Aust.: Rheumon; Traumon; ***Belg.:*** Flexium; ***Ger.:*** Algesalona E; Rheuma-Gel; Rheumon; Traumon; ***Ital.:*** Bayro; ***Spain:*** Afrolate; Deiron†; Flogoprofen; Zenavan; ***Switz.:*** Etofen; Rheumon; Traumalix.

Multi-ingredient: ***Aust.:*** Thermo-Rheumon; ***Ger.:*** Thermo-Rheumon.

Etorphine Hydrochloride (6227-l)

Etorphine Hydrochloride *(BANM, rINNM).*

M-99; 19-Propylorvinol Hydrochloride. (6*R*, 7*R*, 14*R*)-7,8-Dihydro-7-(1*R*-1-hydroxy-1-methylbutyl)-6-*O*-methyl-6,14α-ethenomorphine hydrochloride; (2*R*)-2-[(−)-(5*R*, 6*R*, 7*R*, 14*R*)-4,5-Epoxy-3-hydroxy-6-methoxy-9a-methyl-6,14-ethenomorphinan-7-yl]pentan-2-ol hydrochloride.

$C_{25}H_{33}NO_4,HCl$ = 448.0.

CAS — 14521-96-1 (etorphine); 13764-49-3 (etorphine hydrochloride).

Pharmacopoeias. In *BP(Vet).*

A white or almost white microcrystalline powder. Sparingly **soluble** in water and in alcohol; very slightly soluble in chloroform; practically insoluble in ether. A 2% solution in water has a pH of 4.0 to 5.5. **Protect** from light.

CAUTION. *Etorphine hydrochloride is extremely potent and extraordinary care should be taken in any procedure in which it is used. Any spillage on the skin should be washed off at once. In the case of accidental injection or absorption through broken skin or mucous membrane, a reversing agent should be injected immediately.*

Dependence and Withdrawal

As for Opioid Analgesics, p.67.

Adverse Effects and Treatment

As for Opioid Analgesics in general, p.68.

Etorphine hydrochloride is highly potent and rapid acting; minute amounts can exert serious effects leading to coma. It may be absorbed through skin and mucous membranes. It is thus advisable to inject an antagonist immediately following contamination of skin or mucous membranes with preparations containing etorphine hydrochloride and to wash the affected areas copiously. Accidental injection or needle scratch should also be treated immediately by injecting an antagonist. Naloxone is preferred as the antagonist in medical treatment. However, veterinary preparations of etorphine are supplied with a preparation containing diprenorphine hydrochloride (Revivon) and this should be used for immediate first-aid antagonism if naloxone is not available.

Uses and Administration

Etorphine hydrochloride is a highly potent opioid analgesic (p.69) used for reversible neuroleptanalgesia in veterinary medicine. For a description of neuroleptanalgesia, see under Anaesthetic Techniques on p.1220. It is given with acepromazine maleate or methotrimeprazine (Immobilon) to restrain animals and prior to minor veterinary surgery. The duration of action of etorphine is up to about 45 to 90 minutes depending on the species but it may be longer in man, especially if the large animal preparation is involved.

Famprofazone (2645-r)

Famprofazone *(BAN, rINN)*.

4-Isopropyl-2-methyl-3-[methyl(α-methylphenethyl)aminomethyl]-1-phenyl-3-pyrazolin-5-one.

$C_{24}H_{31}N_3O = 377.5$.

CAS — 22881-35-2.

Famprofazone has analgesic and antipyretic properties and has been given by mouth, usually in conjunction with other analgesics.

Preparations

Proprietary Preparations (details are given in Part 3)
Multi-ingredient: ***Ger.:*** Gewodin.

Felbinac (2491-t)

Felbinac *(BAN, USAN, rINN)*.

CL-83544; LJC-10141. Biphenyl-4-ylacetic acid.

$C_{14}H_{12}O_2 = 212.2$.

CAS — 5728-52-9.

Adverse Effects and Precautions

Mild local reactions such as erythema, dermatitis, and pruritus have occurred in patients using felbinac topically. Bronchospasm or wheeziness has also been reported.

Felbinac preparations should be avoided in patients with a history of hypersensitivity reactions to aspirin or other NSAIDs.

The UK Committee on Safety of Medicines had received 49 reports of adverse reactions associated with felbinac by October 1989, about 11 months after it was released on the UK market.[1] Bronchospasm or wheeziness was reported in 8 patients using felbinac gel. Four of these patients had a history of asthma of whom 3 were reported to have had a similar reaction to aspirin or other NSAIDs. Other reported reactions included skin rashes (17 cases), local application site reactions (7), and dyspepsia (6).

1. Committee on Safety of Medicines. Felbinac (Traxam) and bronchospasm. *Current Problems 27* 1989.

Uses and Administration

Felbinac, an active metabolite of fenbufen (p.37), is an NSAID (p.65). It is used topically in the symptomatic treatment of soft-tissue injuries when it is applied as a 3% gel or a 3.17% foam to unbroken skin over affected areas 2 to 4 times daily. The total daily dose of gel or foam should not exceed 25 g regardless of the size or number of affected areas. Therapy should be reviewed after 14 days.

Diisopropanolamine felbinac has been used similarly.

References.

1. Hosie GAC. The topical NSAID, felbinac, versus oral ibuprofen: a comparison of efficacy in the treatment of acute lower back injury. *Br J Clin Res* 1993; **4:** 5–17.

Preparations

Proprietary Preparations (details are given in Part 3)
Aust.: Target; ***Belg.:*** Flexfree; ***Ger.:*** Dolinac; Target; ***Irl.:*** Traxam; ***Ital.:*** Dolinac; Traxam; ***Jpn:*** Napageln; ***S.Afr.:*** Dolinac; ***Switz.:*** Target; ***UK:*** Traxam.

Fenbufen (2646-f)

Fenbufen *(BAN, USAN, rINN)*.

CL-82204; Fenbufenum. 4-(Biphenyl-4-yl)-4-oxobutyric acid.

$C_{16}H_{14}O_3 = 254.3$.

CAS — 36330-85-5.

Pharmacopoeias. In *Eur.* (see p.viii) and *Jpn.*

A white fine crystalline powder. Very slightly **soluble** in water; slightly soluble in alcohol, in acetone, and in dichloromethane.

Adverse Effects and Precautions

As for NSAIDs in general, p.63, although the commonest side-effects of fenbufen are skin rashes. Disorders such as erythema multiforme and Stevens-Johnson syndrome have also been reported. A small number of patients who develop rash may go on to develop a severe illness characterised by a pulmonary eosinophilia or an allergic alveolitis. Treatment with fenbufen should be discontinued immediately if a rash appears.

Effects on the blood. Haemolytic anaemia[1] and aplastic anaemia[2] have been reported in patients receiving fenbufen.

1. Martland T, Stone WD. Haemolytic anaemia associated with fenbufen. *Br Med J* 1988; **297:** 921.
2. Andrews R, Russell N. Aplastic anaemia associated with a non-steroidal anti-inflammatory drug: relapse after exposure to another such drug. *Br Med J* 1990; **301:** 38.

Effects on the lungs. In January 1989 the UK Committee on Safety of Medicines reported that it had received 7 reports of a suspected association between rash and an allergic interstitial lung disorder in patients receiving fenbufen.[1] In 5 patients, the lung disorder was diagnosed as pulmonary eosinophilia; in the 2 other patients the pulmonary component of the reaction was described as allergic alveolitis. Several of these reactions have been reported in the literature.[2,3]

1. Committee on Safety of Medicines. Fenbufen, rash and pulmonary eosinophilia. *Current Problems 24* 1989.
2. Swinburn CR. Alveolitis and haemolytic anaemia induced by azapropazone. *Br Med J* 1987; **294:** 375.
3. Burton GH. Rash and pulmonary eosinophilia associated with fenbufen. *Br Med J* 1990; **300:** 82–3.

Effects on the skin. In September 1988 the UK Committee on Safety of Medicines reported[1] that it was still receiving large numbers of reports of adverse reactions to fenbufen when such reports were expected to have declined. Fenbufen was the most commonly reported suspect drug in 1986 and 1987. At the time of the report more than 6000 such reports had been received, 80% concerning mucocutaneous reactions and most involving a generalised florid erythematous rash, often with pruritus. There were 178 reports of erythema multiforme, 30 of Stevens-Johnson syndrome, and 2 fatalities.

1. Committee on Safety of Medicines. Fenbufen and mucocutaneous reactions. *Current Problems 23* 1988.

Hypersensitivity. See under Effects on the Lungs (above).

Interactions

For interactions associated with NSAIDs, see p.65.

Concomitant administration of fenbufen and aspirin may result in decreased serum concentrations of fenbufen and its metabolites.

Pharmacokinetics

Fenbufen is absorbed from the gastro-intestinal tract and peak plasma concentrations are reached in about 70 minutes. Fenbufen is over 99% bound to plasma proteins. It is metabolised in the liver to active metabolites. Fenbufen and its metabolites are reported to have plasma half-lives of about 10 hours and are mainly eliminated as conjugates in the urine.

Uses and Administration

Fenbufen, a propionic acid derivative, is an NSAID (p.65). It is given by mouth for the relief of pain and inflammation associated with musculoskeletal and joint disorders such as rheumatoid arthritis, osteoarthritis, and ankylosing spondylitis in doses of 900 mg daily by mouth; the dose may be either 450 mg in the morning and evening or 300 mg in the morning with 600 mg in the evening.

Preparations

BP 1998: Fenbufen Capsules; Fenbufen Tablets.

Proprietary Preparations (details are given in Part 3)
Aust.: Lederfen; ***Fr.:*** Cinopal; ***Ger.:*** Lederfen†; ***Irl.:*** Lederfen; ***Ital.:*** Cinopal; ***S.Afr.:*** Cinopal; ***Spain:*** Cincopal; ***UK:*** Lederfen.

Fenoprofen Calcium (2649-h)

Fenoprofen Calcium *(BANM, USAN, pINNM)*.

69323; 53858 (acid); Lilly-61169 (sodium salt). Calcium (±)-2-(3-phenoxyphenyl)propionate dihydrate.

$(C_{15}H_{13}O_3)_2Ca,2H_2O = 558.6$.

CAS — 31879-05-7 (fenoprofen); 34597-40-5 (anhydrous fenoprofen calcium); 53746-45-5 (fenoprofen calcium dihydrate).

Pharmacopoeias. In *Br.* and *US.*

A white or almost white odourless or almost odourless crystalline powder. Fenoprofen calcium (dihydrate) 1.1 g is approximately equivalent to 1 g of fenoprofen. BP **solubilities** are: slightly soluble in water and in chloroform; soluble in alcohol. USP solubilities are: slightly soluble in water and in methyl alcohol; practically insoluble in chloroform. **Store** in airtight containers.

Adverse Effects

As for NSAIDs in general, p.63. Dysuria, cystitis, haematuria, interstitial nephritis, and renal failure have been reported with fenoprofen. Nephrotic syndrome, which may be preceded by fever, rash, arthralgia, oliguria, azotaemia, and anuria, has also occurred. Upper respiratory infection and nasopharyngitis have been reported. There have been reports of severe hepatic reactions, including jaundice and fatal hepatitis.

Effects on the blood. Haematological adverse effects including agranulocytosis,[1] aplastic anaemia,[2] and thrombocytopenia[3,4] have been reported in patients taking fenoprofen; the manufacturers also report haemolytic anaemia.

1. Simon SD, Kosmin M. Fenoprofen and agranulocytosis. *N Engl J Med* 1978; **299:** 490.
2. Ashraf M, *et al.* Aplastic anaemia associated with fenoprofen. *Br Med J* 1982; 284: 1301–2.
3. Simpson RE, *et al.* Acute thrombocytopenia associated with fenoprofen. *N Engl J Med* 1978; **298:** 629–30.
4. Katz ME, Wang P. Fenoprofen-associated thrombocytopenia. *Ann Intern Med* 1980; **92:** 262.

Effects on the kidneys. References to reversible renal failure and nephrotic syndrome in patients taking fenoprofen.[1-4]

1. Brezin JH, *et al.* Reversible renal failure and nephrotic syndrome associated with nonsteroidal anti-inflammatory drugs. *N Engl J Med* 1979; **301:** 1271–3.
2. Curt GA, *et al.* Reversible rapidly progressive renal failure with nephrotic syndrome due to fenoprofen calcium. *Ann Intern Med* 1980; **92:** 72–3.
3. Handa SP. Renal effects of fenoprofen. *Ann Intern Med* 1980; **93:** 508–9.
4. Lorch J, *et al.* Renal effects of fenoprofen. *Ann Intern Med* 1980; **93:** 509.

Effects on the liver. Cholestatic jaundice and hepatitis developed in a 68-year-old woman after treatment with fenoprofen 600 mg four times daily for 7 weeks. Subsequent administration of naproxen and indomethacin did not result in hepatotoxicity.[1] However, there has been a report of cross-hepatotoxicity between fenoprofen and naproxen in one patient.[2]

1. Stennett DJ, *et al.* Fenoprofen-induced hepatotoxicity. *Am J Hosp Pharm* 1978; **35:** 901.
2. Andrejak M, *et al.* Cross hepatotoxicity between non-steroidal anti-inflammatory drugs. *Br Med J* 1987; **295:** 180–1.

Effects on the skin. Toxic epidermal necrolysis was associated with fenoprofen in 2 patients.[1]

1. Stotts JS, *et al.* Fenoprofen-induced toxic epidermal necrolysis. *J Am Acad Dermatol* 1988; **18:** 755–7.

Precautions

As for NSAIDs in general, p.65.

Interactions

For interactions associated with NSAIDs, see p.65.

Aspirin is reported to reduce plasma concentrations of fenoprofen.

Phenobarbitone might increase the rate of metabolism of fenoprofen.[1]

1. Helleberg L, *et al.* A pharmacokinetic interaction in man between phenobarbitone and fenoprofen, a new anti-inflammatory agent. *Br J Clin Pharmacol* 1974; **1:** 371–4.

Pharmacokinetics

Fenoprofen is readily absorbed from the gastro-intestinal tract; bioavailability is about 85% but food and milk may reduce the rate and extent of absorption. Peak plasma concentrations occur 1 to 2 hours after a dose. The plasma half-life is about 3 hours. Fenoprofen is 99% bound to plasma proteins. About 90% of a dose is excreted in the urine in 24 hours, chiefly as the glucuronide and the glucuronide of hydroxylated fenoprofen. Small amounts have been distributed into breast milk.

Uses and Administration

Fenoprofen, a propionic acid derivative, is an NSAID (p.65). It is used as the calcium salt in the management of mild to moderate pain and for the relief of pain and inflammation associated with disorders such as osteoarthritis, rheumatoid arthritis, and ankylosing spondylitis. A usual dose is the equivalent of 200 to 600 mg of fenoprofen three or four times daily. It has been recommended that the total daily dose should not exceed 3 to 3.2 g.

Preparations

BP 1998: Fenoprofen Tablets;
USP 23: Fenoprofen Calcium Capsules; Fenoprofen Calcium Tablets.

Proprietary Preparations (details are given in Part 3)
Aust.: Nalfon; ***Belg.:*** Fepron†; ***Canad.:*** Nalfon; ***Fr.:*** Nalgesic; ***Irl.:*** Fenopron; Progesic†; ***Ital.:*** Fepron; ***Neth.:*** Fepron†; ***S.Afr.:*** Fenopron; ***UK:*** Fenopron; Progesic†; ***USA:*** Nalfon.

Fentanyl (12127-z)

Fentanyl *(BAN, rINN)*.

Fentanylum. *N*-(1-Phenethyl-4-piperidyl) propionanilide.

$C_{22}H_{28}N_2O = 336.5$.

CAS — 437-38-7.

Pharmacopoeias. In *Eur.* (see p.viii).

A white or almost white polymorphic powder. Practically **insoluble** in water; freely soluble in alcohol and in methyl alcohol. **Protect** from light.

Fentanyl Citrate (6228-y)

Fentanyl Citrate *(BANM, USAN, rINNM)*.

Fentanyli Citras; McN-JR-4263-49; Phentanyl Citrate; R-4263.

N-(1-Phenethyl-4-piperidyl)propionanilide dihydrogen citrate.

$C_{22}H_{28}N_2O,C_6H_8O_7 = 528.6$.

CAS — 990-73-8.

Pharmacopoeias. In *Chin., Eur.* (see p.viii), *Jpn, Pol.,* and *US*.

White granules, a white crystalline powder, or a white or almost white powder. Fentanyl citrate 157 μg is approximately equivalent to 100 μg of fentanyl. Sparingly **soluble** to soluble in water; sparingly soluble in alcohol; slightly soluble in chloroform; soluble to freely soluble in methyl alcohol. **Protect** from light.

CAUTION. *Avoid contact with skin and the inhalation of particles of fentanyl citrate.*

Incompatibility. Fentanyl citrate is incompatible with thiopentone sodium and methohexitone sodium.

A thick white precipitate formed in the intravenous tubing when fentanyl citrate with droperidol was given shortly after nafcillin sodium. There was no precipitate when fentanyl citrate alone was mixed with nafcillin sodium.[1]

Fentanyl citrate underwent rapid and extensive loss when admixed with fluorouracil in polyvinyl chloride (PVC) containers.[2] The loss was due to sorption of fentanyl to the PVC containers as a result of the alkaline pH of the admixture, and presumably could occur from admixture of fentanyl citrate with any sufficiently alkaline drug.

See also under Stability, below.

1. Jeglum EL, *et al.* Nafcillin sodium incompatibility with acidic solutions. *Am J Hosp Pharm* 1981; **38:** 462, 464.
2. Xu QA, *et al.* Rapid loss of fentanyl citrate admixed with fluorouracil in polyvinyl chloride containers. *Ann Pharmacother* 1997; **31:** 297–302.

Stability. In a 48-hour study fentanyl citrate was stable when stored at room temperature under usual light conditions in glass or polyvinyl chloride containers of 5% glucose or 0.9% sodium chloride solution;[1] the concentration of fentanyl delivered by a patient-controlled system was relatively constant throughout a 30-hour study period. Fentanyl citrate injection diluted to 20 μg per mL with 0.9% sodium chloride was stable for 30 days at 3° or 23° in polyvinyl chloride reservoirs for portable infusion pumps.[2] An admixture of fentanyl citrate and bupivacaine in 0.9% sodium chloride[3] appeared compatible and stable when stored for up to 30 days at 3° or 23° in a portable infusion pump. In another study[4] the stability of solutions containing fentanyl, bupivacaine, and adrenaline, alone and in combination was studied over a period of 56 days when stored at various temperatures in the light or in the dark in polyvinyl chloride (PVC) bags. Both fentanyl and bupivacaine were adsorbed from solution onto the PVC for the first 3 days but thereafter concentrations of these agents remained relatively stable; freezing appeared to slow the concentration change for bupivacaine but not for fentanyl. Solutions containing adrenaline became more acidic during the study as the adrenaline progressively deteriorated but this was greatly reduced by freezing. Autoclaving produced a further reduction in the concentration of all agents. There was no sign of precipitation from any of the solutions studied. Fentanyl is potentially unstable in PVC containers when admixed with alkaline drugs (see under Incompatibility, above).

1. Kowalski SR, Gourlay GK. Stability of fentanyl citrate in glass and plastic containers and in a patient-controlled delivery system. *Am J Hosp Pharm* 1990; **47:** 1584–7.
2. Allen LV, *et al.* Stability of fentanyl citrate in 0.9% sodium chloride solution in portable infusion pumps. *Am J Hosp Pharm* 1990; **47:** 1572–4.
3. Tu Y-H, *et al.* Stability of fentanyl citrate and bupivacaine hydrochloride in portable pump reservoirs. *Am J Hosp Pharm* 1990; **47:** 2037–40.
4. Dawson PJ, *et al.* Stability of fentanyl, bupivacaine and adrenaline solutions for extradural infusion. *Br J Anaesth* 1992; **68:** 414–17.

Dependence and Withdrawal

As for Opioid Analgesics, p.67. Fentanyl and illicitly manufactured analogues are subject to abuse (see under Precautions, below).

Movement disorders, extreme irritability, and symptoms characteristic of opioid abstinence syndrome have been reported in children after withdrawal of prolonged fentanyl infusions.[1] One group of workers reported that plasma concentrations required to produce satisfactory sedation increased steadily in neonates receiving continuous infusions suggesting the development of tolerance to the sedating effects of fentanyl.[2]

1. Lane JC, *et al.* Movement disorder after withdrawal of fentanyl infusion. *J Pediatr* 1991; **119:** 649–51.
2. Arnold JH, *et al.* Changes in the pharmacodynamic response to fentanyl in neonates during continuous infusion. *J Pediatr* 1991; **119:** 639–43.

Adverse Effects and Treatment

As for Opioid Analgesics in general, p.68.

Respiratory depression which occurs especially with high doses of fentanyl responds to naloxone (see also under Effects on the Respiratory System, below). Atropine may be used to block the vagal effects of fentanyl such as bradycardia. Unlike morphine, fentanyl is reported not to cause significant histamine release. Transient hypotension may follow intravenous administration. Muscle rigidity may occur and may require administration of neuromuscular blockers.

Local reactions such as rash, erythema, and itching have been reported with the transdermal patches.

Effects on the cardiovascular system. For a reference to the effects of fentanyl on histamine release compared with some other opioids, see under Pethidine, p.76.

Effects on mental function. Fentanyl had some dose-related effects on mental function and motor activity in healthy subjects,[1] but immediate and delayed recall were not affected. See also under Alfentanil (p.12).

There has been an isolated report[2] of acute toxic delirium in a 14-year-old boy treated with transdermal fentanyl.

1. Scamman FL, *et al.* Ventilatory and mental effects of alfentanil and fentanyl. *Acta Anaesthesiol Scand* 1984; **28:** 63–7.
2. Kuzma PJ, *et al.* Acute toxic delirium: a uncommon reaction to transdermal fentanyl. *Anesthesiology* 1995; **83:** 869–71.

Effects on the nervous system. There have been reports of seizures with low and high doses of fentanyl or sufentanil.[1] There was, however, no EEG evidence of cortical seizure activity in a patient who had seizure-like muscle movements during a fentanyl infusion;[2] the muscle movements might have been due to myoclonus produced by depression of higher CNS inhibitory centres or to a pronounced form of opioid-induced muscle rigidity.

For a report of encephalopathy associated with prolonged use of fentanyl and midazolam in infants in intensive care, see under Encephalopathy in the Adverse Effects of Diazepam, p.662.

1. Zaccara G, *et al.* Clinical features, pathogenesis and management of drug-induced seizures. *Drug Safety* 1990; **5:** 109–51.
2. Scott JC, Sarnquist FH. Seizure-like movements during a fentanyl infusion with absence of seizure activity in a simultaneous EEG recording. *Anesthesiology* 1985; **62:** 812–14.

Effects on the respiratory system. Fentanyl, like other opioid agonists, causes dose-related respiratory depression; it is significant with intravenous fentanyl doses of more than 200 μg and may be more prolonged than analgesia. Anaesthesia with fentanyl may result in either prolonged or delayed respiratory depression postoperatively.[1] If present at the end of operation it should be reversed by an opioid antagonist such as naloxone; alternatively a respiratory stimulant such as doxapram that does not reverse analgesia has been given. Buprenorphine has also been tried for the reversal of respiratory depression induced by fentanyl (see Anaesthesia, p.23). Because of the risk of delayed respiratory depression patients should continue to be monitored postoperatively until spontaneous breathing has been re-established. Severe respiratory depression in a 14-month-old child following intravenous sedation with fentanyl and midazolam has highlighted the necessity for careful monitoring when administering respiratory depressants concurrently.[2]

Rigidity of the respiratory muscles (chest wall rigidity) may occur during fentanyl anaesthesia. The effects can be minimised by using a slow intravenous injection but administration of a neuromuscular blocker may be required to allow artificial ventilation; rigidity has been reversed postoperatively by naloxone. Sanford *et al.* reported[3] that similar muscle rigidity induced by alfentanil could be attenuated by pretreatment with a benzodiazepine whereas small doses of neuromuscular blockers appeared to be ineffective.

The risk of respiratory depression associated with epidural administration of fentanyl, a highly lipid-soluble opioid, has been considered relatively small and only slight ventilatory depression was noted[4] following a dose of 50 μg. However, profound delayed respiratory depression has been reported in 2 women 100 minutes[5] and 80 minutes[6] respectively after fentanyl 100 μg had been administered epidurally for caesarean section. No adverse effects on neonatal respiration or neurobehaviour were detected in a study[7] of neonates of mothers given epidural infusions of bupivacaine and fentanyl during labour.

Respiratory depression is also a risk with topically applied fentanyl preparations. Severe hypoventilation with some fatalities has occurred in patients receiving fentanyl through a transdermal patch for minor painful conditions.[8]

1. Bennett MRD, Adams AP. Postoperative respiratory complications of opiates. *Clin Anaesthesiol* 1983; **1:** 41–56.
2. Yaster M, *et al.* Midazolam-fentanyl intravenous sedation in children: case report of respiratory arrest. *Pediatrics* 1990; **86:** 463–7.
3. Sanford TJ, *et al.* Pretreatment with sedative-hypnotics, but not with nondepolarizing muscle relaxants, attenuates alfentanil-induced muscle rigidity. *J Clin Anesth* 1994; **6:** 473–80.
4. Morisot P, *et al.* Ventilatory response to carbon dioxide during extradural anaesthesia with lignocaine and fentanyl. *Br J Anaesth* 1989; **63:** 97–102.
5. Brockway MS, *et al.* Profound respiratory depression after extradural fentanyl. *Br J Anaesth* 1990; **64:** 243–5.
6. Wang CY. Respiratory depression after extradural fentanyl. *Br J Anaesth* 1992; **69:** 544.
7. Porter J, *et al.* Effect of epidural fentanyl on neonatal respiration. *Anesthesiology* 1998; **89:** 79–85.
8. *FDC Reports Pink Sheet* 1994; January 24: 12.

Effects on the skin. Report of one patient[1] who developed a macular rash covering the whole body, except for the face and scalp, while using transdermal fentanyl patches.

1. Stoukides CA, Stegman M. Diffuse rash associated with transdermal fentanyl. *Clin Pharm* 1992; **11:** 222.

Precautions

As for Opioid Analgesics in general, p.68.

Caution is advised in patients with myasthenia gravis; the effects of muscular rigidity on respiration may be particularly pronounced in these patients.

Absorption of fentanyl from transdermal patches may be increased as the temperature rises and patients should therefore avoid exposing the patch to external heat; similarly, patients with fever may require monitoring because of increased absorption. It may take 17 hours or longer for plasma concentrations of fentanyl to decrease by 50% after removal of a patch; patients who have experienced side-effects should be monitored for up to 24 hours and those requiring replacement opioid therapy should initially receive low doses increased gradually thereafter.

Acute opioid withdrawal syndrome has been seen in cancer patients switched from modified-release oral morphine to transdermal fentanyl despite adequate analgesia being maintained.[1]

1. Anonymous. Opiate withdrawal with transdermal fentanyl. *Pharm J* 1995; **255:** 680.

Abuse. Several synthetic analogues of fentanyl, so-called 'designer drugs' have been manufactured illicitly for recreational use, particularly in the USA. They are highly potent and respiratory depression and death may occur very rapidly.[1] The 'fentanyls' have been smoked or snorted as well as injected intravenously.

Fentanyl analogues identified by WHO[2,3] as being subject to street abuse or likely to be abused include: alpha-methylfentanyl (also known as 'China white' or 'synthetic heroin'), 3-methylfentanyl, acetyl-alpha-methylfentanyl, alpha-methylthiofentanyl, para-fluorofentanyl, beta-hydroxyfentanyl, beta-hydroxy-3-methylfentanyl, thiofentanyl, and 3-methylthiofentanyl.

Fentanyl itself is also subject to illicit use. It is chemically unrelated to morphine and therefore not reactive to screening tests for opioids. It has therefore been recommended[4] that fentanyl should be tested for specifically in cases with suspended opioid misuse.

Used fentanyl transdermal patches may contain significant amounts of fentanyl[5] and have been subject to abuse. The manufacturers advise that used patches should be folded firmly in half, adhesive side inwards to conceal the release membrane, and disposed of safely.

1. Buchanan JF, Brown CR. 'Designer drugs': a problem in clinical toxicology. *Med Toxicol* 1988; **3:** 1–17.
2. WHO. WHO expert committee on drug dependence: twenty-fourth report. *WHO Tech Rep Ser 761* 1988.
3. WHO. WHO expert committee on drug dependence: twenty-sixth report. *WHO Tech Rep Ser 787* 1989.
4. Berens AIL, *et al.* Illicit fentanyl in Europe. *Lancet* 1996; **347:** 1334–5.
5. Marquardt KA, *et al.* Fentanyl remaining in a transdermal system following three days of continuous use. *Ann Pharmacother* 1995; **29:** 969–71.

Administration. Fentanyl is much more lipid-soluble than morphine and after standard single intravenous doses has a rapid onset and short duration of action. However, fentanyl is rapidly redistributed in the body and has a longer elimination half-life than morphine (see Pharmacokinetics, below). Hence with high or repeated doses fentanyl becomes a relatively long-acting drug and to avoid accumulation patients should be monitored and doses adjusted accordingly.

Repeated intra-operative doses of fentanyl should be given with care, since not only may the respiratory depression persist into the postoperative period but it may become apparent for the first time postoperatively when the patient is away from immediate nursing attention.

Interactions

For interactions associated with opioid analgesics, see p.69.

Benzodiazepines. For the effects of concomitant use of opioids such as fentanyl with benzodiazepines, see under Analgesics in the Interactions of Diazepam, p.663.

Propofol. For reference to the effect that concomitant administration of fentanyl has on blood concentrations of propofol, see p.1230.

Pharmacokinetics

After parenteral administration fentanyl citrate has a rapid onset and short duration of action. It is metabolised in the liver by *N*-dealkylation and hydroxylation. Metabolites and some unchanged drug are excreted mainly in the urine. The short duration of action is probably due to rapid redistribution into the tissues rather than metabolism and excretion. An elimination half-life of about 4 hours reflects slower release from tissue depots. About 80% has been reported to be bound to plasma proteins. Fentanyl appears in the cerebrospinal fluid. It crosses the placenta and small amounts have been detected in breast milk.

In reviewing pharmacokinetic studies of fentanyl Mather[1] attributed marked differences in results to differences in assay methods. Moore *et al.*[2] also emphasised the need for sensitive assay methods because the potency of fentanyl meant the use of small doses. Terminal half-lives ranging from 2 to 7 hours have been reported in healthy subjects and surgical patients. However, the duration of action of fentanyl after a single intravenous dose of up to 100 μg may be only 30 to 60 minutes as a result of rapid redistribution into the tissues. The manufacturers have given values for a three-compartment pharmacokinetic model with a distribution time of 1.7 minutes, a redistribution time of 13 minutes, and a terminal elimination half-life of 219 minutes. Administration of repeated or large doses may result in accumulation and a more prolonged action.

The clinical significance of secondary peak plasma-fentanyl concentrations and the possible role of entero-systemic recirculation[3] has been controversial, but Moore *et al.*[2] considered that irregular decay curves were not unlikely for lipophilic compounds such as fentanyl, especially in patients undergoing operations and subject to large changes in blood flow. Unexpectedly high plasma-fentanyl concentrations in a patient following epidural administration were thought to be a result of aortic clamping and might reflect the effect of changes in blood flow.[4]

The main metabolites of fentanyl excreted in the urine have been identified as 4-*N*-(*N*-propionylanilino) piperidine and 4-*N*-(*N*-hydroxypropionylanilino) piperidine; 1-(2-phenethyl)-4-*N*-(*N*-hydroxypropionylanilino) piperidine is a minor metabolite.[5] According to Moore *et al.*[2] fentanyl has no active or toxic metabolites.

1. Mather LE. Clinical pharmacokinetics of fentanyl and its newer derivatives. *Clin Pharmacokinet* 1983; **8:** 422–46.
2. Moore RA, *et al.* Opiate metabolism and excretion. *Baillieres Clin Anaesthesiol* 1987; **1:** 829–58.
3. Bennett MRD, Adams AP. Postoperative respiratory complications of opiates. *Clin Anaesthesiol* 1983; **1:** 41–56.
4. Bullingham RES, *et al.* Unexpectedly high plasma fentanyl levels after epidural use. *Lancet* 1980; **i:** 1361–2.
5. Goromaru T, *et al.* Identification and quantitative determination of fentanyl metabolites in patients by gas chromatography-mass spectrometry. *Anesthesiology* 1984; **61:** 73–7.

Administration. Some references to the pharmacokinetics of fentanyl following constant rate intravenous infusion,[1] transdermal application,[2-5] use of the oral transmucosal route,[6] intranasal administration,[7] and subcutaneous infusion.[8]

1. Duthie DJR, *et al.* Pharmacokinetics of fentanyl during constant rate iv infusion for the relief of pain after surgery. *Br J Anaesth* 1986; **58:** 950–6.
2. Sebel PS, *et al.* Transdermal absorption of fentanyl and sufentanil in man. *Eur J Clin Pharmacol* 1987; **32:** 529–31.
3. Ridout G, *et al.* Pharmacokinetic considerations in the use of newer transdermal formulations. *Clin Pharmacokinet* 1988; **15:** 114–31.
4. Duthie DJR, *et al.* Plasma fentanyl concentrations during transdermal delivery of fentanyl to surgical patients. *Br J Anaesth* 1988; **60:** 614–18.
5. Plezia PM, *et al.* Transdermal fentanyl: pharmacokinetics and preliminary clinical evaluation. *Pharmacotherapy* 1989; **9:** 2–9.
6. Streisand JB, *et al.* Absorption and bioavailability of oral transmucosal fentanyl citrate. *Anesthesiology* 1991; **75:** 223–9.
7. Walter SH, *et al.* Pharmacokinetics of intranasal fentanyl. *Br J Anaesth* 1993; **70** (suppl 1): 108.
8. Miller RS, *et al.* Plasma concentrations of fentanyl with subcutaneous infusion in palliative care patients. *Br J Clin Pharmacol* 1995; **40:** 553–6.

Administration during cardiopulmonary bypass. The pharmacokinetics of fentanyl during cardiopulmonary bypass.[1,2] In general, studies indicate that serum concentrations of fentanyl decrease initially and then remain stable during the bypass procedure. The fall in concentrations has been attributed to haemodilution although adsorption to the bypass apparatus has also been demonstrated.

1. Buylaert WA, *et al.* Cardiopulmonary bypass and the pharmacokinetics of drugs: an update. *Clin Pharmacokinet* 1989; **17:** 10–26.
2. Gedney JA, Ghosh S. Pharmacokinetics of analgesics, sedatives and anaesthetic agents during cardiopulmonary bypass. *Br J Anaesth* 1995; **75:** 344–51.

Administration in the elderly. Bentley *et al.*[1] reported the elimination half-life of fentanyl to be increased from 265 minutes in patients with a mean age of 36 years to 945 minutes in those with a mean age of 67 years. Scott and Stanski[2] were critical of the relatively short sampling time used and in contrast to Bentley *et al.* they found that major fentanyl pharmacokinetic parameters did not correlate with age. However, elderly patients had increased brain sensitivity to fentanyl, as demonstrated by EEG changes[2] and lower doses might be indicated in older patients for pharmacodynamic rather than pharmacokinetic reasons.

1. Bentley JB, *et al.* Age and fentanyl pharmacokinetics. *Anesth Analg* 1982; **61:** 968–71.
2. Scott JC, Stanski DR. Decreased fentanyl and alfentanil dose requirements with age: a simultaneous pharmacokinetic and pharmacodynamic evaluation. *J Pharmacol Exp Ther* 1987; **240:** 159–66.

Administration in hepatic impairment. The pharmacokinetics of fentanyl were not affected significantly in surgical patients with cirrhosis of the liver.[1] Moore *et al.*[2] considered that fentanyl had not been associated with clinical problems when given to patients with liver dysfunction.

1. Haberer JP, *et al.* Fentanyl pharmacokinetics in anaesthetized patients with cirrhosis. *Br J Anaesth* 1982; **54:** 1267–70.
2. Moore RA, *et al.* Opiate metabolism and excretion. *Baillieres Clin Anaesthesiol* 1987; **1:** 829–58.

Administration in infants and children. The disposition of intravenous fentanyl 10 to 50 μg per kg body-weight in 14 neonates undergoing various major surgical procedures was highly variable.[1] The mean elimination half-life of 317 minutes and other pharmacokinetic parameters including volume of distribution and total body clearance were greater than reported in adults, but both pharmacodynamic and pharmacokinetic mechanisms appeared responsible for the very prolonged respiratory depression that can occur in neonates after fentanyl anaesthesia. In 9 premature neonates given fentanyl 30 μg per kg intravenously for induction of anaesthesia[2] the elimination half-life ranged from 6 to 32 hours, but cautious interpretation was advised because of the method of calculation.

1. Koehntop DE, *et al.* Pharmacokinetics of fentanyl in neonates. *Anesth Analg* 1986; **65:** 227–32.
2. Collins C, *et al.* Fentanyl pharmacokinetics and hemodynamic effects in preterm infants during ligation of patent ductus arteriosus. *Anesth Analg* 1985; **64:** 1078–80.

Administration in renal impairment. Clearance of fentanyl from plasma was reported to be enhanced in surgical patients with end-stage renal disease,[1] although clearance was reduced and elimination half-life increased in patients with renal failure undergoing transplantation,[2] possibly because of the influence of uraemia on metabolism in the liver. Nevertheless, Moore *et al.*[2] noted that fentanyl had no active or toxic metabolites and had not been associated with clinical problems when given to patients with renal dysfunction.

1. Corall IM, *et al.* Plasma concentrations of fentanyl in normal surgical patients and those with severe renal and hepatic disease. *Br J Anaesth* 1980; **52:** 101P.
2. Moore RA, *et al.* Opiate metabolism and excretion. *Baillieres Clin Anaesthesiol* 1987; **1:** 829–58.

Uses and Administration

Fentanyl, a phenylpiperidine derivative, is a potent opioid analgesic (p.69) chemically related to pethidine (p.77) and is primarily a μ-opioid agonist.

Fentanyl is used as an analgesic, an adjunct to general anaesthetics, and as an anaesthetic for induction and maintenance. It is also used as a respiratory depressant in the management of mechanically ventilated patients under intensive care. When used with an antipsychotic such as droperidol it can induce a state of neuroleptanalgesia in which the patient is calm and indifferent to his surroundings and is able to cooperate with the surgeon.

Fentanyl is usually administered by intramuscular or intravenous injection as the citrate or in transdermal patches as the base. It has also been given by epidural injection or by the transmucosal route as the citrate. Doses are expressed in terms of the base.

It is more lipid soluble than morphine and following an intravenous injection of 100 μg the effects of fentanyl begin almost immediately, although maximum analgesia and respiratory depression may not occur for several minutes; the average duration of action is 30 to 60 minutes although analgesia may only last for 10 to 20 minutes in an unpremedicated adult. Increasing the dose to 50 μg per kg body-weight can give pain relief for 4 to 6 hours.

For premedication 50 to 100 μg of fentanyl may be given intramuscularly 30 to 60 minutes before the induction of anaesthesia. As an adjunct to general anaesthesia, fentanyl is usually given by intravenous injection. Dosage recommendations show a wide range depending on the technique. Patients with spontaneous respiration may be given 50 to 200 μg of fentanyl as an initial dose with supplements of 50 μg. In the USA it is recommended that doses above 2 μg per kg body-weight should be used in conjunction with assisted ventilation. Significant respiratory depression follows doses of more than 200 μg. Patients whose ventilation is assisted may be given 300 to 3500 μg (up to 50 μg per kg) as an initial dose with supplements of 100 to 200 μg or higher depending on the patient's response. High doses have been reported to moderate or attenuate the response to surgical stress (see under Anaesthesia, below).

Reduced doses are used in the elderly.

In the UK recommended initial doses for use as an adjunct to general anaesthesia for children above 2 years of age range from 3 to 5 μg per kg intravenously for those with spontaneous respiration; supplements of 1 μg per kg may be given. When ventilation is assisted, the initial recommended dose is 15 μg per kg, with supplements of 1 to 3 μg per kg. In the USA doses as low as 2 to 3 μg per kg are employed in children between the ages of 2 and 12 years. See also under Administration in Infants and Children, below.

Similar doses to those used for premedication may also be given by intramuscular injection postoperatively, and by intramuscular or slow intravenous injection as an adjunct to regional anaesthesia.

For the treatment of intractable chronic pain in adults when opioid analgesia is indicated transdermal patches delivering amounts of fentanyl ranging from 25 to 100 μg per hour are available. Doses should be individually titrated for each patient according to previous opioid usage. Initial dosages should not exceed 25 μg per hour in opioid-naive patients. During transfer to treatment with fentanyl patches previous opioid analgesic therapy should be phased out gradually in order to allow for the gradual increase in plasma-fentanyl concentrations. Patches should be replaced every 72 hours with the new patch being applied to a different site; use of the same area of the skin should be avoided for several days. More than one patch may be applied at the same time if doses greater than 100 μg per hour are required; additional or alternative analgesic therapy should be considered if doses greater than 300 μg per hour are required. Elderly or debilitated patients should be observed carefully for signs of toxicity and the dose reduced if necessary. Fentanyl patches are not appropriate for acute or postoperative pain.

A lozenge-on-a-stick lollipop dosage form of fentanyl citrate for transmucosal delivery has been used as a premedicant and analgesic in anaesthesia. Lozenges containing the equivalent of 100, 200, 300, or 400 μg of fentanyl base are available. Adults may receive up to a maximum of 5 μg per kg (2.5 to 5 μg per kg in the elderly); children weighing more than

10 kg may receive up to 15 μg per kg. The maximum dose for adults and children, regardless of weight, is 400 μg. Patients receiving the lozenges require constant supervision, including monitoring of respiratory function.

References.

1. Clotz MA, Nahata MC. Clinical uses of fentanyl, sufentanil, and alfentanil. *Clin Pharm* 1991; **10:** 581–93.

Administration. INTRANASAL ROUTE. Studies[1,2] indicating that intranasal administration of fentanyl is as effective as intravenous administration for postoperative pain management and that it can be used in a patient-controlled analgesia system.

1. Striebel HW, *et al.* Intranasal fentanyl titration for postoperative pain management in an unselected population. *Anaesthesia* 1993; **48:** 753–7.
2. Striebel HW, *et al.* Patient-controlled intranasal analgesia: a method for noninvasive postoperative pain management. *Anesth Analg* 1996; **83:** 548–51.

TRANSDERMAL ROUTE. The manufacturers state that the use of transdermal fentanyl is contra-indicated in the management of acute or postoperative pain because the problems of dose titration in the short term increase the possibility of development of significant respiratory depression (see also under Adverse Effects, above).

For patients who have been receiving a strong opioid analgesic for chronic intractable pain the initial dose of the fentanyl patch should be based on the previous 24-hour opioid requirement. Use of a patch providing 25 μg of fentanyl per hour is approximately equivalent to oral administration of 90 mg of morphine sulphate daily.

References.

1. Jeal W, Benfield P. Transdermal fentanyl: a review of its pharmacological properties and therapeutic efficacy in pain control. *Drugs* 1997; **53:** 109–38.

TRANSMUCOSAL ROUTE. A lozenge-on-a-stick lollipop dosage form of fentanyl for transmucosal administration appears to be effective for sedation and analgesia before anaesthesia or painful procedures in children[1,2] and in adults.[3] The formulation is also under investigation for breakthrough cancer pain in opioid-tolerant patients. It has been noted[4] that this route of administration can cause all the adverse effects of parenteral opioids; nausea and vomiting are common and potentially lethal respiratory depression can occur.

1. Nelson PS, *et al.* Comparison of oral transmucosal fentanyl citrate and an oral solution of meperidine, diazepam, and atropine for premedication in children. *Anesthesiology* 1989; **70:** 616–21.
2. Schechter NL, *et al.* The use of oral transmucosal fentanyl citrate for painful procedures in children. *Pediatrics* 1995; **95:** 335–9.
3. Macaluso AD, *et al.* Oral transmucosal fentanyl citrate for premedication in adults. *Anesth Analg* 1996; **82:** 158–61.
4. Anonymous. Oral transmucosal fentanyl citrate. *Med Lett Drugs Ther* 1994; **36:** 24–5.

Administration in infants and children. Robinson and Gregory[1] reported satisfactory anaesthesia with high-dose fentanyl citrate (30 to 50 μg per kg body-weight) in premature infants when used as sole anaesthetic, in conjunction with pancuronium, for ligation of patent ductus arteriosus; cardiovascular stability was maintained throughout the procedure. However, Friesen and Henry[2] found significant hypotension in preterm infants given either fentanyl 20 μg per kg, isoflurane, halothane, or ketamine; systolic arterial pressure was best maintained with the ketamine technique. Anand *et al.*[3] reported that the surgical stress response in preterm babies was abolished by the addition of fentanyl 10 μg per kg intravenously to the anaesthetic regimen of nitrous oxide and tubocurarine. Dose responses of fentanyl in neonatal anaesthesia have been discussed by Yaster.[4] For sedation and analgesia during intensive care an infusion rate of 2 to 4 μg per kg per hour has been useful and associated with cardiovascular stability.[5] Although the use of fentanyl for prolonged sedation of infants and children during ventilatory support is reported to be widespread there is a lack of evidence of its safety and efficacy for this use.[6] In one double-blind placebo-controlled study[7] investigating the use of a continuous fentanyl infusion for 5 days in premature neonates receiving mechanical ventilation for respiratory distress syndrome, it was noted that although fentanyl was effective in reducing physiological indicators of pain and stress, there was an increased need for ventilatory support associated with the use of fentanyl compared with placebo. Fentanyl was infused initially in a dose of 5 μg per kg over 20 minutes, and thereafter in a decreasing dosage schedule over 120 hours from a rate of 2 μg per kg per hour to 0.5 μg per kg per hour. The authors pointed out that the results of this study could not assess the effects of fentanyl on long-term outcome and a larger multi-centre study was required. There have also been reports of possible tolerance and withdrawal symptoms associated with prolonged administration of fentanyl (see under Dependence and Withdrawal, above).

See also under Transmucosal Route, above and Postoperative Pain, below.

1. Robinson S, Gregory GA. Fentanyl-air-oxygen anesthesia for ligation of patent ductus arteriosus in preterm infants. *Anesth Analg* 1981; **60:** 331–4.
2. Friesen RH, Henry DB. Cardiovascular changes in preterm neonates receiving isoflurane, halothane, fentanyl, and ketamine. *Anesthesiology* 1986; **64:** 238–42.
3. Anand KJS, *et al.* Randomised trial of fentanyl anaesthesia in preterm babies undergoing surgery: effects on the stress response. *Lancet* 1987; **i:** 243–8.
4. Yaster M. The dose response of fentanyl in neonatal anesthesia. *Anesthesiology* 1987; **66:** 433–5.
5. Lloyd-Thomas AR. Pain management in paediatric patients. *Br J Anaesth* 1990; **64:** 85–104.
6. Kauffman RE. Fentanyl, fads, and folly: who will adopt the therapeutic orphans? *J Pediatr* 1991; **119:** 588–9.
7. Orsini AJ, *et al.* Routine use of fentanyl infusions for pain and stress reduction in infants with respiratory distress syndrome. *J Pediatr* 1996; **129:** 140–5.

Anaesthesia. Fentanyl and its newer congeners alfentanil and sufentanil are shorter-acting than morphine and appear to produce fewer circulatory changes; they may be preferred for use as supplements during anaesthesia with inhalational or intravenous drugs.

In a comparative study of opioid supplements to nitrous oxide anaesthesia fentanyl and sufentanil were equally preferable to morphine or pethidine in terms of haemodynamic changes to stress and rates of recovery.[1] For further comparisons between fentanyl and its congeners, see under alfentanil (p.14) and under sufentanil (p.86). The cardiovascular stress response to intubation was attenuated by the use of fentanyl 3 μg per kg body-weight intravenously as an adjunct to thiopentone induction in elderly patients,[2] and fentanyl 2.5 μg per kg or alfentanil 10 μg per kg decreased intra-ocular pressure and reduced the haemodynamic responses associated with intubation when given at induction to adults undergoing ophthalmic operations[3] or women with severe pregnancy-induced hypertension undergoing caesarean section.[4] For a discussion of the use of opioids such as fentanyl to attenuate these responses to intubation, see under Anaesthesia, p.1302.

High doses of fentanyl are used in an attempt to reduce the cardiovascular, endocrine, and metabolic changes that may accompany surgery. When attenuation of surgical stress is especially important, for example in cardiac surgery, intravenous fentanyl 50 to 100 μg per kg in conjunction with oxygen and a neuromuscular blocker, and sometimes up to 150 μg per kg may be used for general anaesthesia.

Attenuation of metabolic and endocrine responses has been achieved with high-dose fentanyl (at least 50 μg per kg) given before the onset of surgery,[5] but appeared to have little effect on established responses when given after the start of surgery.[6] Supplementation with fentanyl 15 μg per kg at induction of anaesthesia with nitrous oxide-oxygen suppressed β-endorphin, ACTH, growth hormone, cortisol, and glucose response to pelvic surgery.[7]

Stanley and Webster[8] found that fentanyl up to 50 μg per kg as sole anaesthetic produced minimal changes in cardiovascular dynamics in patients undergoing mitral valvular replacement, although Wynands *et al.*[9] were unable to confirm stable haemodynamics using a loading dose of 75 μg per kg, sometimes followed by an infusion of 0.75 μg per kg per minute up to a total dose of about 160 μg per kg. Induction of anaesthesia with an intravenous bolus of fentanyl 100 μg per kg prevented the increased plasma-catecholamine concentrations associated with perioperative stress and attenuated circulatory responses in patients undergoing cholecystectomy when compared with those who underwent a balanced technique of anaesthesia with fentanyl 5 μg per kg at induction followed by continuous infusion of 3 μg per kg per hour.[10] Total intravenous anaesthesia with fentanyl and propofol has been successful.[11]

For the use of fentanyl for anaesthesia in neonates and children, see under Administration in Infants and Children, above.

Neuroleptanalgesia. An injection of short-acting fentanyl 50 μg per mL with the longer-acting antipsychotic droperidol 2.5 mg per mL is available and has been used for neuroleptanalgesia, premedication, and as an adjunct to anaesthesia. However, such a fixed-ratio combination has been criticised as irrational and having the potential to cause distressing and possibly lethal adverse effects.[12]

1. Ghoneim MM, *et al.* Comparison of four opioid analgesics as supplements to nitrous oxide anaesthesia. *Anesth Analg* 1984; **63:** 405–12.
2. Chung F, Evans D. Low-dose fentanyl: haemodynamic response during induction and intubation in geriatric patients. *Can Anaesth Soc J* 1985; **32:** 622–8.
3. Sweeney J, *et al.* Modification by fentanyl and alfentanil of the intraocular pressure response to suxamethonium and tracheal intubation. *Br J Anaesth* 1989; **63:** 688–91.
4. Rout CC, Rocke DA. Effects of alfentanil and fentanyl on induction of anaesthesia in patients with severe pregnancy-induced hypertension. *Br J Anaesth* 1990; **65:** 468–74.
5. Hall, GM. Fentanyl and the metabolic response to surgery. *Br J Anaesth* 1980; **52:** 561–2.
6. Bent JM, *et al.* Effects of high-dose fentanyl anaesthesia on the established metabolic and endocrine response to surgery. *Anaesthesia* 1984; **39:** 19–23.
7. Lacoumenta S, *et al.* Fentanyl and the β-endorphin, ACTH and glucoregulatory hormonal response to surgery. *Br J Anaesth* 1987; **59:** 713–20.
8. Stanley TH, Webster LR. Anesthetic requirements and cardiovascular effects of fentanyl-oxygen and fentanyl-diazepam-oxygen anesthesia in man. *Anesth Analg* 1978; **57:** 411–16.
9. Wynands JE, *et al.* Blood pressure response and plasma fentanyl concentrations during high- and very high-dose fentanyl anesthesia for coronary artery surgery. *Anesth Analg* 1983; **62:** 661–5.
10. Klingstedt C, *et al.* High- and low-dose fentanyl anesthesia: circulatory and plasma catecholamine responses during cholecystectomy. *Br J Anaesth* 1987; **59:** 184–8.
11. Jenstrup M, *et al.* Total iv anaesthesia with propofol-alfentanil or propofol-fentanyl. *Br J Anaesth* 1990; **64:** 717–22.
12. Anonymous. Innovar: a follow-up. *Med Lett Drugs Ther* 1981; **23:** 74–5.

PHAEOCHROMOCYTOMA. Unlike morphine and some other opioids, fentanyl and alfentanil do not release histamine and may be used safely in the anaesthetic management of patients with phaeochromocytoma.[1] Alfentanil may be the opioid of choice.

1. Hull CJ. Phaeochromocytoma: diagnosis, preoperative preparation and anaesthetic management. *Br J Anaesth* 1986; **58:** 1453–68.

POSTOPERATIVE SHIVERING. As pethidine appears to be effective in the treatment of postoperative shivering a number of other opioids including fentanyl have also been tried but not all opioids are necessarily effective. Fentanyl was reported to be effective in one study.[1]

1. Alfonsi P, *et al.* Fentanyl, as pethidine, inhibits post anaesthesia shivering. *Br J Anaesth* 1993; **70** (suppl 1): 38.

Intensive care. Despite the short duration of action of fentanyl after single doses, rapid redistribution in the body results in an elimination half-life longer than that of morphine. Consequently fentanyl is not a short-acting drug when used for analgesia in intensive care, and Aitkenhead[1] considered that it offered little advantage over morphine.

See also under Administration in Infants and Children, above.

1. Aitkenhead AR. Analgesia and sedation in intensive care. *Br J Anaesth* 1989; **63:** 196–206.

Pain. LABOUR PAIN. Fentanyl has been reported to be an effective analgesic during active labour. An intravenous dose of 50 or 100 μg was given every hour on request to a mean cumulative dose of 140 μg (range 50 to 600 μg). Temporary analgesia and mild sedation were apparent in each treated woman when compared with controls. Onset of analgesia was within 5 minutes of a dose and was sustained for about 45 minutes.[1] In a non-blinded comparative study[2] equivalent analgesia was obtained during early and late labour with intravenous fentanyl 50 to 100 μg every hour or pethidine 25 to 50 mg every 2 to 3 hours; there were fewer maternal and immediate neonatal side-effects with fentanyl.

Opioids have also been given epidurally in labour and, although fentanyl is unreliable when used alone,[3] it does enhance the epidural analgesia achieved with the local anaesthetic bupivacaine when given as a bolus epidural injection[4] or by continuous epidural infusion[5] and may increase overall maternal satisfaction with labour.[6] Lirzin *et al.*[4] reported increased duration of pain relief when fentanyl 80 μg was added to epidural 0.25% bupivacaine. Jones *et al.*[5] demonstrated beneficial results with continuous epidural analgesia. They compared a loading dose of 0.5% bupivacaine 6 mL and fentanyl 100 μg epidurally followed by epidural infusion of 0.08% bupivacaine 15 mL per hour plus fentanyl 37.5 μg per hour, with bupivacaine alone. However, they subsequently reported profound respiratory depression 100 minutes after the use of bupivacaine and fentanyl epidural analgesia and strongly advised that patients be observed continuously for 2 to 3 hours after such treatment.[7] Excellent analgesia has been reported with low-dose bupivacaine and fentanyl by continuous epidural infusion,[8,9] and Reynolds[10] agreed with Herman *et al.*[11] that local anaesthetic-opioid combinations might be the way ahead. The reduction in the minimum local analgesic concentration of epidural bupivacaine for labour pain increased with increasing dose of fentanyl added to bupivacaine.[12] However, the incidence of pruritus increased significantly with fentanyl in a dose of 4 μg per mL and therefore the optimum dose of fentanyl may be 3 μg per mL for bupivacaine-sparing epidural analgesia during labour.

1. Rayburn W, *et al.* Fentanyl citrate analgesia during labor. *Am J Obstet Gynecol* 1989; **161:** 202–6.
2. Rayburn WF, *et al.* Randomized comparison of meperidine and fentanyl during labor. *Obstet Gynecol* 1989; **74:** 604–6.
3. Reynolds F. Extradural opioids in labour. *Br J Anaesth* 1989; **63:** 251–3.
4. Lirzin JD, *et al.* Controlled trial of extradural bupivacaine with fentanyl, morphine or placebo for pain relief in labour. *Br J Anaesth* 1989; **62:** 641–4.
5. Jones G, *et al.* Comparison of bupivacaine and bupivacaine with fentanyl in continuous extradural analgesia during labour. *Br J Anaesth* 1989; **63:** 254–9.
6. Murphy JD, *et al.* Bupivacaine versus bupivacaine plus fentanyl for epidural analgesia: effect on maternal satisfaction. *Br Med J* 1991; **302:** 564–7.
7. McClure JH, Jones G. Comparison of bupivacaine and bupivacaine with fentanyl in continuous extradural analgesia during labour. *Br J Anaesth* 1989; **63:** 637–40.

8. Chestnut DH, *et al.* Continuous infusion epidural analgesia during labor: a randomized, double-blind comparison of 0.0625% bupivacaine/0.0002% fentanyl versus 0.125% bupivacaine. *Anesthesiology* 1988; **68:** 754–9.
9. Chestnut DH, *et al.* Continuous epidural infusion of bupivacaine-fentanyl during the second stage of labor. *Anesthesiology* 1989; **71:** A841.
10. Reynolds F. Extradural opioids in labour. *Br J Anaesth* 1990; **64:** 529.
11. Herman NL, *et al.* Extradural opioids in labour. *Br J Anaesth* 1990; **64:** 528–9.
12. Lyons G, *et al.* Extradural pain relief in labour: bupivacaine sparing by extradural fentanyl is dose dependent. *Br J Anaesth* 1997; **78:** 493–7.

POSTOPERATIVE PAIN. Small intravenous bolus doses of opioid analgesic may be injected immediately after surgery for postoperative analgesia and faster acting opioids such as fentanyl may be preferable to morphine.[1] Fentanyl has also been given by epidural injection in doses of 100 or 200 μg or by continuous epidural infusion in doses of 20 to 80 μg per hour; patient-controlled systems have been used.[2]

Epidural fentanyl or sufentanil provided effective postoperative analgesia following caesarean section with comparable adverse effect profiles.[3] The suggested optimal dose of fentanyl was 100 μg. For references comparing epidural fentanyl with alfentanil, see under Postoperative Pain in Uses and Administration of Alfentanil, p.14. In reviewing postoperative pain management Lutz and Lamer[4] considered epidural opioids to provide superior analgesia to systemically administered opioids. Fentanyl may be administered through a lumbar epidural catheter that is often inserted immediately postoperatively. After an initial loading dose of 1 to 1.5 μg per kg body-weight of fentanyl, infusion at the rate of 0.7 to 2 μg per kg per hour is begun and continued for about 48 hours on average. Some prefer to use intermittent injection.

Combined opioid and local anaesthetic epidural infusions have also proved effective, for example fentanyl 1 μg per mL with bupivacaine 0.1%; both could be infused at lower rates than either drug alone. Although a study[5] comparing bupivacaine-fentanyl combinations with each drug alone for epidural analgesia following caesarean section confirmed an additive analgesic effect for the combination, there was no demonstrable clinical benefit compared with fentanyl alone in this patient group who expect early mobilisation. However, the combination may be of greater benefit in patients for whom early ambulation is not routine.

Fentanyl has also been given by epidural injection to children for postoperative analgesia.[6]

Fentanyl has been tried by intrathecal injection for postoperative pain.[7]

1. Mitchell RWD, Smith G. The control of acute postoperative pain. *Br J Anaesth* 1989; **63:** 147–58.
2. Morgan M. The rational use of intrathecal and extradural opioids. *Br J Anaesth* 1989; **63:** 165–88.
3. Grass JA, *et al.* A randomized, double-blind, dose-response comparison of epidural fentanyl versus sufentanil analgesia after cesarean section. *Anesth Analg* 1997; **85:** 365–71.
4. Lutz LJ, Lamer TJ. Management of postoperative pain: review of current techniques and methods. *Mayo Clin Proc* 1990; **65:** 584–96.
5. Cooper DW, *et al.* Patient-controlled extradural analgesia with bupivacaine, fentanyl, or a mixture of both, after caesarean section. *Br J Anaesth* 1996; **76:** 611–15.
6. Lejus C, *et al.* Postoperative extradural analgesia in children: comparison of morphine with fentanyl. *Br J Anaesth* 1994; **72:** 156–9.
7. Sudarshan G, *et al.* Intrathecal fentanyl for post-thoracotomy pain. *Br J Anaesth* 1995; **75:** 19–22.

Preparations

USP 23: Fentanyl Citrate Injection.

Proprietary Preparations (details are given in Part 3)
Aust.: Durogesic; ***Austral.:*** Sublimaze; ***Canad.:*** Duragesic; Sublimaze; ***Ger.:*** Durogesic; ***Irl.:*** Durogesic; Sublimaze; ***Ital.:*** Durogesic; Fentanest; ***Neth.:*** Durogesic; ***Norw.:*** Durogesic; Leptanal; ***S.Afr.:*** Durogesic; Sublimaze; Tanyl; ***Spain:*** Fentanest; ***Swed.:*** Durogesic; Leptanal; ***UK:*** Durogesic; Sublimaze; ***USA:*** Duragesic; Sublimaze.

Multi-ingredient: ***Aust.:*** Thalamonal; ***Austral.:*** Marcain plus Fentanyl; ***Belg.:*** Thalamonal; ***Canad.:*** Innovar†; ***Ger.:*** Thalamonal; ***Ital.:*** Leptofen; ***Neth.:*** Thalamonal; ***Swed.:*** Leptanal comp†; ***Switz.:*** Thalamonal†; ***UK:*** Thalamonal†; ***USA:*** Innovar.

Fentiazac (12747-x)

Fentiazac *(BAN, USAN, rINN).*

BR-700; Wy-21894. [4-(4-Chlorophenyl)-2-phenylthiazol-5-yl]acetic acid.

$C_{17}H_{12}ClNO_2S$ = 329.8.

CAS — 18046-21-4.

Fentiazac is an NSAID (p.63) that has been used for the relief of pain and inflammation associated with musculoskeletal, joint, peri-articular, and soft-tissue disorders. It has also been used in the treatment of fever. Fentiazac has been given in usual doses of 100 to 200 mg once or twice daily by mouth. Fentiazac has also been applied topically as a 5% cream and has been given rectally as the calcium salt.

Preparations

Proprietary Preparations (details are given in Part 3)
Aust.: Norvedan; ***Fr.:*** Fentac†; ***Ital.:*** Domureuma†; Flogene; Norvedan†; O-Flam; ***Spain:*** Dermisone Fentiazaco†; Donorest; Riscalon.

Fepradinol (3788-r)

Fepradinol *(rINN).*

(±)-α-{[(2-Hydroxy-1,1-dimethylethyl)amino]methyl}benzyl alcohol.

$C_{12}H_{19}NO_2$ = 209.3.

CAS — 63075-47-8.

Fepradinol is an NSAID (p.63) that has been used topically in a concentration of 6% for the relief of pain and inflammation. The hydrochloride has been used similarly.

Preparations

Proprietary Preparations (details are given in Part 3)
Spain: Dalgen; Flexidol.

Feprazone (2650-a)

Feprazone *(BAN, rINN).*

DA-2370; Phenylprenazone; Prenazone. 4-(3-Methylbut-2-enyl)-1,2-diphenylpyrazolidine-3,5-dione.

$C_{20}H_{20}N_2O_2$ = 320.4.

CAS — 30748-29-9 (feprazone); 57148-60-4 (feprazone piperazine salt 1 : 1).

Adverse Effects and Precautions

As for NSAIDs in general, p.63.

Effects on the blood. Thrombocytopenia and immune-complex-mediated haemolytic anaemia were associated with feprazone in a 21-year-old student.[1]

1. Bell PM, Humphrey CA. Thrombocytopenia and haemolytic anaemia due to feprazone. *Br Med J* 1982; **284:** 17.

Effects on the skin. Report[1] of a 9-year-old girl who had localised dermographism in areas of hyperpigmented skin that had resulted from a fixed drug reaction to feprazone.

1. Pellicano R, *et al.* Localized dermographism at the site of a fixed drug eruption. *Br J Dermatol* 1995; **132:** 156–8.

Pharmacokinetics

Feprazone is absorbed from the gastro-intestinal tract with peak plasma concentrations occurring 4 to 6 hours after ingestion. It has a plasma half-life of about 24 hours.

Uses and Administration

Feprazone, a phenylbutazone (p.79) derivative, is an NSAID (p.65). It has been used in mild to moderate pain, fever, and inflammation associated with musculoskeletal and joint disorders in initial doses of up to 600 mg daily in divided doses by mouth; maintenance doses of up to 400 mg daily have been given. Feprazone has also been given rectally and used topically as a 5% cream.

Pinazone, the piperazine salt of feprazone, has been used similarly.

Preparations

Proprietary Preparations (details are given in Part 3)
Aust.: Zepelin; ***Ital.:*** Zepelin; ***Spain:*** Brotazona; Cocresol†; Rangozona†; Represil†; Reuflodol.

Multi-ingredient: ***Ital.:*** Fepramol†; Solvelin†.

Floctafenine (2651-t)

Floctafenine *(BAN, USAN, rINN).*

R-4318; RU-15750. 2,3-Dihydroxypropyl *N*-(8-trifluoromethyl-4-quinolyl)anthranilate.

$C_{20}H_{17}F_3N_2O_4$ = 406.4.

CAS — 23779-99-9.

Pharmacopoeias. In *Jpn.*

Adverse Effects and Precautions

As for NSAIDs in general, p.63. Anaphylactic shock has been reported in patients given floctafenine; anaphylactic reactions may be preceded by minor allergic manifestations, therefore floctafenine should be discontinued in any patient who develops signs suggestive of allergy (such as pruritus or urticaria). Reactions may also involve the liver. Floctafenine may cross-react with glafenine (p.42) and should not be given to patients who have experienced glafenine-associated reactions.

Porphyria. Floctafenine was considered to be unsafe in patients with acute porphyria because it has been shown to be porphyrinogenic in *animals* or *in vitro* systems.[1]

1. Moore MR, McColl KEL. *Porphyria: drug lists* Glasgow: Porphyria Research Unit, University of Glasgow, 1991.

Interactions

For interactions associated with NSAIDs, see p.65.

Pharmacokinetics

Floctafenine is absorbed from the gastro-intestinal tract; peak plasma concentrations are obtained 1 to 2 hours after ingestion. Its plasma half-life is about 8 hours. It is metabolised in the liver to floctafenic acid. It is excreted mainly as glucuronide conjugates in the urine and bile.

Uses and Administration

Floctafenine, an anthranilic acid derivative related to glafenine (p.42), is an NSAID (p.65) used in doses of up to 1.2 g daily, in divided doses, by mouth for the short-term relief of pain.

Preparations

Proprietary Preparations (details are given in Part 3)
Belg.: Idarac; ***Canad.:*** Idarac; ***Fr.:*** Idarac; ***Irl.:*** Idarac; ***Ital.:*** Idarac; ***Neth.:*** Idalon; ***Spain:*** Idarac.

Flufenamic Acid (2652-x)

Flufenamic Acid *(BAN, USAN, rINN).*

CI-440; CN-27554; INF-1837; NSC-82699. *N*-(ααα-Trifluoro-*m*-tolyl)anthranilic acid.

$C_{14}H_{10}F_3NO_2$ = 281.2.

CAS — 530-78-9.

Adverse Effects and Precautions

As for NSAIDs in general, p.63.

Effects on the gastro-intestinal tract. Acute proctocolitis associated with oral flufenamic acid in one patient.[1]

1. Ravi S, *et al.* Colitis caused by non-steroidal anti-inflammatory drugs. *Postgrad Med J* 1986; **62:** 773–6.

Porphyria. Flufenamic acid has been associated with acute attacks of porphyria and is considered unsafe in patients with acute porphyria.[1]

1. Moore MR, McColl KEL. *Porphyria: drug lists.* Glasgow: Porphyria Research Unit, University of Glasgow, 1991.

Uses and Administration

Flufenamic acid, an anthranilic acid derivative related to mefenamic acid (p.52), is an NSAID (p.65). Flufenamic acid is mainly used topically in a concentration of 2.5 to 3.5% for the relief of pain and inflammation associated with musculoskeletal, joint, and soft-tissue disorders. It has also been given by mouth.

Preparations

Proprietary Preparations (details are given in Part 3)
Ger.: Dignodolin; Rheuma Lindofluid; Sastridex†.

Multi-ingredient: ***Aust.:*** Mobilisin; Mobilisin plus; Rheugesal; ***Belg.:*** Mobilisin; ***Ger.:*** Algesalona; Flexocutan N†; Mobilisin; Thermo Mobilisin; ***Ital.:*** Mobilisin; ***S.Afr.:*** Flexilat†; ***Spain:*** Movilisin; ***Switz.:*** Algesalona; Assan; Assan-Thermo; Mobilisin.

Flunixin Meglumine (16811-r)

Flunixin Meglumine *(BANM, USAN, rINNM).*

Sch-14714 (flunixin). 2-{[2-Methyl-3-(trifluoromemthyl)phenyl]amino}-3-pyridinecarboxylic acid compounded with 1-deoxy-1-(methylamino)-D-glucitol (1:1); 2-(α^3,α^3,α^3-Trifluoro-2,3,-xylidino)nicotinic acid compounded with 1-deoxy-1-(methylamino)-D-glucitol (1:1).

$C_{14}H_{11}F_3N_2O_2.C_7H_{17}NO_5$ = 491.5.

CAS — 38677-85-9 (flunixin); 42461-84-7 (flunixin meglumine).

Pharmacopoeias. In *BP(vet).* Also in *US* for veterinary use only.

A white to almost white crystalline powder. **Soluble** to freely soluble in water, in alcohol, and in methyl alcohol. A 5% solution in water has a pH of 7.0 to 9.0. **Store** in airtight containers at a temperature not exceeding 25°.

Flunixin meglumine is an NSAID (p.63) used in veterinary medicine for relief of pain and inflammation in acute and chronic disorders and as adjunctive therapy in the treatment of endotoxic or septic shock and mastitis.

Flunoxaprofen (16812-f)

Flunoxaprofen *(rINN).*

RV-12424. (+)-2-(*p*-Fluorophenyl)-α-methyl-5-benzoxazoleacetic acid.

$C_{16}H_{12}FNO_3$ = 285.3.

CAS — 66934-18-7.

Flunoxaprofen, a propionic acid derivative, is an NSAID (p.63) that has been given for the relief of painful and inflammatory conditions by mouth, as a rectal suppository, and as a 5% topical gel. It has also been used as a vaginal irrigation.

Preparations

Proprietary Preparations (details are given in Part 3)
Ital.: Priaxim.

Flupirtine Maleate (18644-z)

Flupirtine Maleate *(BANM, USAN, rINNM)*.

D-9998; W-2964M. Ethyl 2-amino-6-(4-fluorobenzylamino)-3-pyridylcarbamate maleate.

$C_{15}H_{17}FN_4O_2.C_4H_4O_4$ = 420.4.

CAS — 56995-20-1 (flupirtine); 75507-68-5 (flupirtine maleate).

Flupirtine maleate is an analgesic that has been given for the relief of pain (p.4) in usual doses of 100 mg three or four times daily by mouth or in doses of 150 mg three or four times daily as a rectal suppository; daily doses of up to 600 mg by mouth or 900 mg rectally have been used where necessary.

References.

1. Friedel HA, Fitton A. Flupirtine: a review of its pharmacological properties, and therapeutic efficacy in pain states. *Drugs* 1993; **45:** 548–69.

Preparations

Proprietary Preparations (details are given in Part 3)
Ger.: Katadolon; Trancopal Dolo.

Flurbiprofen (2653-r)

Flurbiprofen *(BAN, USAN, rINN)*.

BTS-18322; U-27182. 2-(2-Fluorobiphenyl-4-yl)propionic acid.

$C_{15}H_{13}FO_2$ = 244.3.

CAS — 5104-49-4.

Pharmacopoeias. In *Br., Fr., Jpn,* and *US.*

A white or almost white crystalline powder. Practically **insoluble** in water; freely soluble in alcohol, in acetone, in chloroform, in ether, and in methyl alcohol; soluble in acetonitrile; dissolves in aqueous solutions of alkali hydroxides and carbonates. **Store** in airtight containers.

Flurbiprofen Sodium (11385-h)

Flurbiprofen Sodium *(BANM, rINNM)*.

Sodium (±)-2-(2-fluoro-4-biphenylyl)propionate dihydrate.

$C_{15}H_{12}FNaO_2,2H_2O$ = 302.3.

CAS — 56767-76-1.

Pharmacopoeias. In *Br.* and *US.*

A white to creamy-white, crystalline powder. Sparingly **soluble** in water; soluble in alcohol; practically insoluble in dichloromethane.

Adverse Effects

As for NSAIDs in general, p.63.

Minor symptoms of ocular irritation including transient burning and stinging have been reported following the instillation of flurbiprofen sodium eye drops; there may be increased bleeding from ocular surgery and wound healing may be delayed. Local irritation may occur following rectal administration of flurbiprofen.

Reports from the manufacturers on the range and incidence of the side-effects of flurbiprofen.[1,2]

1. Sheldrake FE, *et al.* A long-term assessment of flurbiprofen. *Curr Med Res Opin* 1977; **5:** 106–16.
2. Brooks CD, *et al.* Clinical safety of flurbiprofen. *J Clin Pharmacol* 1990; **30:** 342–51.

Effects on the CNS. A severe symmetrical parkinsonian syndrome developed in a 52-year-old man who had taken flurbiprofen 50 mg 3 times daily for 7 days.[1]

1. Enevoldson TP, *et al.* Acute parkinsonism associated with flurbiprofen. *Br Med J* 1990; **300:** 540–1.

Effects on the kidneys. Renal papillary necrosis has been described in one patient associated with the use of flurbiprofen for many years.[1] Acute flank pain and reversible renal dysfunction, similar to that seen with suprofen (see p.88) has been reported in 2 patients treated with flurbiprofen.[2,3]

1. Nafría EC, *et al.* Renal papillary necrosis induced by flurbiprofen. *DICP Ann Pharmacother* 1991; **25:** 870–1.
2. Kaufhold J, *et al.* Flurbiprofen-associated tubulointerstitial nephritis. *Am J Nephrol* 1991; **11:** 144–6.
3. McIntire SC, *et al.* Acute flank pain and reversible renal dysfunction associated with nonsteroidal anti-inflammatory drug use. *Pediatrics* 1993; **92:** 459–60.

Effects on the liver. A case of cholestatic jaundice probably due to flurbiprofen has been reported.[1]

1. Kotowski KE, Grayson MF. Side effects of non-steroidal anti-inflammatory drugs. *Br Med J* 1982; **285:** 377.

Effects on the skin. Cutaneous vasculitis apparently due to flurbiprofen occurred in a 59-year-old woman with long-standing rheumatoid arthritis.[1]

1. Wei N. Flurbiprofen and cutaneous vasculitis. *Ann Intern Med* 1990; **112:** 550–1.

Precautions

As for NSAIDs in general, p.65.

Flurbiprofen sodium eye drops should not be used in patients with active epithelial herpes simplex keratitis. Patients with a history of herpes simplex keratitis should be monitored closely when undergoing treatment with flurbiprofen sodium eye drops.

Breast feeding. See under Pharmacokinetics, below.

Interactions

For interactions associated with NSAIDs, see p.65.

The manufacturer of acetylcholine chloride ophthalmic preparations has stated that there have been reports that acetylcholine and carbachol have been ineffective when used in patients treated with topical (ophthalmic) NSAIDs.

Pharmacokinetics

Flurbiprofen is readily absorbed from the gastro-intestinal tract with peak plasma concentrations occurring about 1 to 2 hours after ingestion. It is about 99% bound to plasma proteins and has a plasma half-life of about 3 to 6 hours. It is metabolised mainly by hydroxylation and conjugation in the liver and excreted in urine. Flurbiprofen is distributed into breast milk in amounts considered by some authorities to be too small to be harmful to a breast-fed infant.

Flurbiprofen is a chiral compound given as the racemate and the above pharmacokinetic characteristics refer to the racemic mixture. Allowance may have to be made for the different activities of the enantiomers.

References.

1. Aarons L, *et al.* Plasma and synovial fluid kinetics of flurbiprofen in rheumatoid arthritis. *Br J Clin Pharmacol* 1986; **21:** 155–63.
2. Smith IJ, *et al.* Flurbiprofen in post-partum women: plasma and breast milk disposition. *J Clin Pharmacol* 1989; **29:** 174–84.
3. Kean WF, *et al.* The pharmacokinetics of flurbiprofen in younger and elderly patients with rheumatoid arthritis. *J Clin Pharmacol* 1992; **32:** 41–8.
4. Davies NM. Clinical pharmacokinetics of flurbiprofen and its enantiomers. *Clin Pharmacokinet* 1995; **28:** 100–14.

Uses and Administration

Flurbiprofen, a propionic acid derivative, is an NSAID (p.65). It is used in musculoskeletal and joint disorders such as ankylosing spondylitis, osteoarthritis, and rheumatoid arthritis, in soft-tissue disorders such as sprains and strains, for postoperative pain, and in mild to moderate pain including dysmenorrhoea and migraine. Flurbiprofen sodium is used in eye drops to inhibit intra-operative miosis and to control postoperative inflammation of the anterior segment of the eye.

Flurbiprofen is given in usual doses of 150 to 200 mg daily by mouth in divided doses, increased to 300 mg daily in acute or severe conditions if necessary. A modified-release preparation for once daily administration is also available. Patients with dysmenorrhoea may be given an initial dose of 100 mg followed by 50 to 100 mg every four to six hours to a maximum total daily dose of 300 mg. Doses given rectally as suppositories are similar to those given by mouth.

To inhibit intra-operative miosis during ocular surgery one drop of flurbiprofen sodium 0.03% is instilled into the eye every 30 minutes beginning 2 hours before surgery and ending not less than 30 minutes before surgery. To control postoperative inflammation the same dosage regimen is used before ocular surgery followed 24 hours after surgery by the instillation of one drop four times daily for one to three weeks. Flurbiprofen sodium eye drops have also been used in the topical treatment of cystoid macular oedema.

Flurbiprofen axetil has been given in some countries by intravenous injection for severe pain.

Preparations

BP 1998: Flurbiprofen Eye Drops; Flurbiprofen Tablets;
USP 23: Flurbiprofen Sodium Ophthalmic Solution; Flurbiprofen Tablets.

Proprietary Preparations (details are given in Part 3)
Aust.: Froben; Ocuflur; ***Austral.:*** Ocufen; ***Belg.:*** Froben; Ocuflur; ***Canad.:*** Ansaid; Froben; Novo-Flurprofen; Ocufen; ***Fr.:*** Cebutid; Ocufen; ***Ger.:*** Froben; Ocuflur; ***Irl.:*** Fenomel; Froben; Ocufen; ***Ital.:*** Froben; Ocufen; Transact Lat; ***Mon.:*** Antadys; ***Neth.:*** Froben; ***S.Afr.:*** Froben; Ocufen; Trans Act$_{LAT}$; ***Spain:*** Froben; Neo Artrol; Ocuflur; Tulip; ***Switz.:*** Froben; Ocuflur; ***UK:*** Froben; Ocufen; ***USA:*** Ansaid; Ocufen.

Fosfosal (15322-t)

Fosfosal *(rINN)*.

UR-1521. 2-Phosphono-oxybenzoic acid.

$C_7H_7O_6P$ = 218.1.

CAS — 6064-83-1.

Fosfosal is a salicylic acid derivative (see Aspirin, p.16). It has been given in usual doses of 1.2 g up to three times daily by mouth for the treatment of pain.

Preparations

Proprietary Preparations (details are given in Part 3)
Spain: Aydolid; Disdolen; Protalgia.

Multi-ingredient: ***Spain:*** Aydolid Codeina; Disdolen Codeina.

Furprofen (19751-m)

4-(2-Furanylcarbonyl)-α-methylbenzeneacetic acid.

$C_{14}H_{12}O_4$ = 244.2.

CAS — 66318-17-0.

Furprofen, a propionic acid derivative, is an NSAID (p.63) that has been given by mouth in doses of 200 to 400 mg daily for the relief of pain.

Preparations

Proprietary Preparations (details are given in Part 3)
Ital.: Dolex.

Glafenine (2654-f)

Glafenine *(rINN)*.

Glaphenine. 2,3-Dihydroxypropyl *N*-(7-chloro-4-quinolyl)anthranilate.

$C_{19}H_{17}ClN_2O_4$ = 372.8.

CAS — 3820-67-5.

Pharmacopoeias. In *Fr.*

Adverse Effects and Precautions

Glafenine is a common cause of anaphylaxis. There may be hepatotoxicity (which may be fatal), nephrotoxicity, and gastro-intestinal disturbances. It should be discontinued at the first sign of any allergic reaction.

Glafenine may cross-react with floctafenine and should not be given to patients who have experienced adverse reactions to floctafenine.

Patients taking glafenine should drink plenty of fluids to reduce the risk of crystallisation in the urinary tract.

Uses and Administration

Glafenine, an anthranilic acid derivative, is an NSAID (p.65) that was used for the relief of all types of pain. However, its high incidence of anaphylactic reactions has led to its withdrawal from the market in most countries. Glafenine hydrochloride was also used.

Preparations

Proprietary Preparations (details are given in Part 3)
Ital.: Glifan†; ***Switz.:*** Glifanan†.

Glucametacin (2655-d)

Glucametacin *(rINN)*.

2-{2-[1-(4-Chlorobenzoyl)-5-methoxy-2-methylindol-3-yl]acetamido}-2-deoxy-D-glucose.

$C_{25}H_{27}ClN_2O_8$ = 518.9.

CAS — 52443-21-7.

Glucametacin, a derivative of indomethacin (p.45), is an NSAID (p.63) that was given by mouth in musculoskeletal, joint, peri-articular, and soft-tissue disorders.

Preparations

Proprietary Preparations (details are given in Part 3)
Ital.: Teoremac†; ***Spain:*** Euminex†.

Glycol Salicylate (2656-n)

Ethylene Glycol Monosalicylate; Hydroxyethylis Salicylas. 2-Hydroxyethyl salicylate.

$C_9H_{10}O_4$ = 182.2.

CAS — 87-28-5.

Pharmacopoeias. In *Eur.* (see p.viii).

An oily, colourless or almost colourless liquid. Sparingly **soluble** in water; freely soluble in alcohol; very soluble in acetone, in ether, and in dichloromethane. **Protect** from light.

Glycol salicylate is a salicylic acid derivative used similarly to methyl salicylate (p.55) in topical rubefacient preparations in concentrations of 5 to 15% for the relief of muscular and rheumatic pain.

Preparations

Proprietary Preparations (details are given in Part 3)
Ger.: Dolo-Arthrosenex N; Kytta; Lumbinon; Norgesic†; Phardol Mono; Phlogont; Phlogont Rheuma; Rheu-Do mite†; Rheubalmin N; Rheunerton†; Spolera forte†; Traumasenex; Zuk Rheuma.

Multi-ingredient: ***Aust.:*** Ambenat; Bayolin; Dolex; Etrat; Igitur-Rheumafluid†; Menthoneurin; Mobilisin; Mobilisin plus; Moviflex; Rheumex; Rubizon-Rheumagel; Rubriment; Venosin; Venostasin†; ***Austral.:*** Deep Heat; Euky Bear Limberub†; ***Belg.:*** Algipan; Bayoline†; Mobilisin; Percutalgine; Rado-Salil; ***Canad.:*** Midalgan; ***Fr.:*** Algipan†; Bayoline†; Lao-Dal; Lumbalgine; Percutalgine; ***Ger.:*** Algonerg†; Ambene N; Arthrodestal N; Auroanalin; Bayolin†; Brachont; Caye Balsam; Contrheuma; Contrheuma flussig†; Contrheuma V + T Bad N; Cuxaflex N; Cuxaflex Thermo; Cycloarthrin†; Dolo Mobilat; Dolo-Exhirud†; Dolo-Menthoneurin CreSa; Dolo-Rubriment; Doloneuro; Dolorgiet; DoloVisano Salbe; Enelbin-Salbe forte†; Essaven Sportgel; Etrat Sportgel; exrheudon OPT; Fibraflex N†; Fibraflex-W-Creme N†; Fibraflex†; Flexocutan N†; Heilit Rheuma-Bad N-Kombi†; Hot Thermo; Hyperiagil†; Infrotto Ultra; Infrotto†; Keptan S†; Li-iL Rheuma-Bad; Makinil†; Mediment†; Menthoneurin-Salbe; Menthoneurin-Vollbad N; Midysalb; mikanil N; Mobilisin; Myalgol N; Mydalgan†; Ortholan mit Salicylester; Ostochont; Percutase N; Phardol 10†; Phardol N Balsam†; Phardol Rheuma; Phlogont-Thermal; Pinofit†; Probaphen†; Pumilen-Balsam†; Rheu-Do†; Rheubalmin Thermo; Rheuma Bad; Rheuma Liquidum; Rheuma-Salbe; Rheuma-Salbe Lichtenstein; Rheumichthol Bad; Riker Sport†; Rubriment-N; Salhumin Gel N; Salirheuman†; Segmentocut Thermo; Sportino Akut; stadasan Thermo†; Thermo-Menthoneurin; Thermo-Menthoneurin Bad; Thermosenex; Thrombo-Enelbin N†; Trauma-Puren; Vehiculan NF†; Venoplant; Venostasin; Vertebralon N†; Warme-Gel; Zuk Thermo; ***Irl.:*** Algipan; Bayolin†; Cremalgin†; ***Ital.:*** Balsamo Sifcamina; Disalgil; Lasoreuma; Mobilisin; Salonpas; Sloan; Thermogene†; ***Neth.:*** Cremes Tegen Spierpijn†; Menthoneurin; Sloan's balsem; ***S.Afr.:*** Flexilat†; ***Spain:*** Movilisin; Percutalin; ***Switz.:*** Artragel; Assan; Assan-Thermo; Contugel†; Demotherm Pommade contre le rhumatisme; Dolo Demotherm; Dolo-Arthrosenex; Dolo-Veniten; Dolorex; Dolorex Neo; Histalgane; Histalgane mite; Incutin; Methylan†; Midalgan; Mobilisin; Moviflex; Nicagel†; Prelloran; Radalgin; Roliwol B; Roliwol S; Spolera "plus"†; Sportusal; Sportusal Spray sine heparino; Venostasin comp†; ***UK:*** Algipan; Bayolin†; Cremalgin; Deep Heat Spray; Dubam; Fiery Jack; Ralgex; Ralgex (low-odour); Ralgex Freeze Spray; Salonair.

Gold Keratinate (12797-q)

Aurothiopolypeptide.

CAS — 9078-78-8.

A gold compound stated to contain 13% of Au.

Gold keratinate has similar actions and uses to those of sodium aurothiomalate (p.83). It was given by intramuscular injection for the treatment of arthritic disorders.

Preparations

Proprietary Preparations (details are given in Part 3)
Ger.: Auro-Detoxin†.

Hexyl Nicotinate (9240-w)

n-Hexyl nicotinate.

$C_{12}H_{17}NO_2$ = 207.3.

CAS — 23597-82-2.

Hexyl nicotinate is used in topical preparations as a rubefacient.

Preparations

Proprietary Preparations (details are given in Part 3)
Multi-ingredient: ***Belg.:*** Transvane†; ***Irl.:*** Transvasin; ***Swed.:*** Transvasin; ***UK:*** Transvasin.

Hydrocodone Hydrochloride (6229-j)

Hydrocodone Hydrochloride *(BANM, rINNM).*

$C_{18}H_{21}NO_3,HCl,2\frac{1}{2}H_2O$ = 380.9.

CAS — 25968-91-6 (anhydrous hydrocodone hydrochloride).

Hydrocodone Tartrate (6231-p)

Hydrocodone Tartrate *(BANM, rINNM).*

Dihydrocodeinone Acid Tartrate; Hydrocodone Acid Tartrate; Hydrocodone Bitartrate *(USAN)*; Hydrocodoni Bitartras; Hydrocone Bitartrate. 6-Deoxy-3-*O*-methyl-6-oxomorphine hydrogen tartrate hemipentahydrate; (−)-(5*R*)-4,5-Epoxy-3-methoxy-9a-methylmorphinan-6-one hydrogen tartrate hemipentahydrate.

$C_{18}H_{21}NO_3,C_4H_6O_6,2\frac{1}{2}H_2O$ = 494.5.

CAS — 125-29-1 (hydrocodone); 143-71-5 (anhydrous hydrocodone tartrate); 34195-34-1 (hydrocodone tartrate hemipentahydrate).

NOTE. Compounded preparations of hydrocodone tartrate (bitartrate) and paracetamol (acetaminophen) in USP 23 may be represented by the name Co-hycodAPAP.

Pharmacopoeias. In *Aust., Belg., Ger., Swiss,* and *US.*

Fine, white crystals or crystalline powder. **Soluble** in water; slightly soluble in alcohol; insoluble in chloroform and in ether. A 2% solution in water has a pH of 3.2 to 3.8. **Store** in airtight containers. Protect from light.

Hydrocodone, a phenanthrene derivative, is an opioid analgesic (p.67) related to codeine (p.26) and has similar actions, but is more potent on a weight for weight basis. Hydromorphone is one of the metabolites of hydrocodone.

Hydrocodone is used chiefly as the tartrate for the relief of irritant cough, though it has no particular advantage over codeine. It is also used for the relief of moderate to moderately severe pain. Hydrocodone tartrate with paracetamol is sometimes known as co-hycodAPAP.

Hydrocodone tartrate is taken by mouth in doses of 5 to 10 mg every 4 to 6 hours.

Hydrocodone hydrochloride is given by injection. The polistirex (a hydrocodone and sulphonated diethenylbenzene-ethenylbenzene copolymer complex) is used in modified-release preparations.

Hydrocodone has also been used in the treatment of dyspnoea.

Preparations

USP 23: Hydrocodone Bitartrate and Acetaminophen Tablets; Hydrocodone Bitartrate Tablets.

Proprietary Preparations (details are given in Part 3)
Belg.: Biocodone; ***Canad.:*** Hycodan; Robidone; ***Ger.:*** Dicodid; ***Norw.:*** Hydrokon†; ***Switz.:*** Dicodid.

Multi-ingredient: ***Austral.:*** Hycomine; ***Canad.:*** Caldomine-DH; Calmydone; Coristex-DH; Coristine-DH; Dimetane Expectorant-DC; Hycomine; Mercodol with Decapryn; Novahistex DH; Novahistex DH Expectorant; Novahistine DH; Triaminic Expectorant DH; Tussaminic DH; ***USA:*** Alor; Amacodone; Anaplex HD; Anexsia; Atuss EX; Atuss G; Atuss HD; Azdone†; Bancap HC; Ceta Plus; Chlorgest-HD†; Co-Gesic; Co-Tuss V; Codamine; Codan†; Codiclear DH; Codimal DH; Cophene XP; Damason-P; Deconamine CX; Dolacet; Donatussin DC; Duocet; Duratuss HD; ED Tuss HC; ED-TLC; Endagen-HD; Endal-HD; Endal-HD Plus; Entuss Expectorant; Entuss Pediatric†; Entuss-D; Entuss-D Jr; H-Tuss-D; Histinex HC; Histinex PV; Histussin D; Histussin HC; Hy-Phen; Hyco-Pap; HycoClear Tuss; Hycodan; Hycomine; Hycomine Compound; Hycomine Pediatric; Hycotuss Expectorant; Hydrocet; Hydrocodone CP; Hydrocodone GF; Hydrocodone HD; Hydrocodone PA; Hydrogesic; Hydromet; Hydromine†; Hydropane; Hydrophene DH; Iodal; Iotussin HC; Kwelcof; Lorcet; Lortab; Lortab ASA; Marcof; Margesic H; Medipain†; Nasatuss; Norcet†; Norco; Oncet; P-V-Tussin; Panacet; Panasal; Pancof-HC; Para-Hist HD; Pneumotussin HC; Protuss; Protuss-D; Rolatuss with Hydrocodone; Ru-Tuss with Hydrocodone; S-T Forte; S-T Forte 2; SRC Expectorant; Stagesic; Statuss Green; T-Gesic; Triaminic Expectorant DH; Tussafed HC; Tussafin Expectorant; Tussanil DH; Tussend; Tussgen; Tussigon; Tussionex Pennkinetic; Tyrodone; Unituss HC; Vanex Expectorant; Vanex-HD; Vetuss HC; Vicodin; Vicodin Tuss; Vicoprofen; Zydone.

Hydromorphone Hydrochloride (6233-w)

Hydromorphone Hydrochloride *(BANM, rINNM).*

Dihydromorphinone Hydrochloride. 6-Deoxy-7,8-dihydro-6-oxomorphine hydrochloride; (−)-(5*R*)-4,5-Epoxy-3-hydroxy-9a-methylmorphinan-6-one hydrochloride.

$C_{17}H_{19}NO_3,HCl$ = 321.8.

CAS — 466-99-9 (hydromorphone); 71-68-1 (hydromorphone hydrochloride).

Pharmacopoeias. In *Aust., Ger.,* and *US.*

A fine white or almost white odourless crystalline powder. **Soluble** 1 in 3 of water; sparingly soluble in alcohol; practically insoluble in ether. **Store** in airtight containers. Protect from light.

Incompatibility. Colour change from pale yellow to light green occurred when solutions of minocycline hydrochloride or tetracycline hydrochloride were mixed with hydromorphone hydrochloride in 5% glucose injection.[1] Mixtures of hydromorphone hydrochloride and dexamethasone sodium phosphate exhibited concentration-dependent incompatibility.[2] White cloudiness, haziness, or precipitation developed 4 hours after mixing thiopentone sodium and hydromorphone hydrochloride.[3]

Stability of mixtures of fluorouracil and hydromorphone hydrochloride in 0.9% sodium chloride or 5% glucose was dependent on the concentration of fluorouracil present.[4] Hydromorphone hydrochloride 0.5 mg per mL with fluorouracil 1 mg per mL was stable for at least 7 days at 32° and for at least 35 days at 23°, 4°, or −20°. When the concentration of fluorouracil was increased to 16 mg per mL, hydromorphone was noted to decompose incurring unacceptable losses after 3 days at 32° or after 7 days at 23°, but was stable for at least 35 days at 4° or −20°.

1. Nieves-Cordero AL, *et al.* Compatibility of narcotic analgesic solutions with various antibiotics during simulated Y-site injection. *Am J Hosp Pharm* 1985; **42:** 1108–9.
2. Walker SE, *et al.* Compatibility of dexamethasone sodium phosphate with hydromorphone hydrochloride or diphenhydramine hydrochloride. *Am J Hosp Pharm* 1991; **48:** 2161–6.
3. Chiu MF, Schwartz ML. Visual compatibility of injectable drugs used in the intensive care unit. *Am J Health-Syst Pharm* 1997; **54:** 64–5.
4. Xu QA, *et al.* Stability and compatibility of fluorouracil with morphine sulfate and hydromorphone hydrochloride. *Ann Pharmacother* 1996; **30:** 756–61.

Dependence and Withdrawal

As for Opioid Analgesics, p.67.

Adverse Effects, Treatment, and Precautions

As for Opioid Analgesics in general, p.68.

Interactions

For interactions associated with opioid analgesics, see p.69.

Pharmacokinetics

Hydromorphone hydrochloride is rapidly but incompletely absorbed from the gastro-intestinal tract following oral administration. A plasma elimination half-life of about 2.5 hours has been reported after oral or intravenous administration. Hydromorphone appears to be widely distributed in the tissues and it crosses the placenta. It is metabolised in the liver and excreted in the urine mainly as conjugated hydromorphone, dihydroisomorphine, and dihydromorphine.

References.

1. Vallner JJ, *et al.* Pharmacokinetics and bioavailability of hydromorphone following intravenous and oral administration to human subjects. *J Clin Pharmacol* 1981; **21:** 152–6.

Uses and Administration

Hydromorphone hydrochloride, a phenanthrene derivative, is an opioid analgesic (p.69). It is related to morphine (p.58) but with a greater analgesic potency. It is a useful alternative to morphine sulphate for subcutaneous administration since its greater solubility in water allows a smaller dose volume. Following injection onset of action usually occurs within 15 minutes and analgesia is reported to last for about 3 to 5 hours; after oral administration onset of analgesia is usually within 30 minutes.

Hydromorphone hydrochloride is used for the relief of moderate to severe pain. It is administered by subcutaneous or intramuscular injection in initial doses of 1 to 2 mg every 4 to 6 hours as necessary. It may also be given by slow intravenous injection or by intravenous or subcutaneous infusion, with doses adjusted according to individual requirements. Higher parenteral doses may be given to opioid-tolerant patients using a highly concentrated solution containing 10 mg per mL that allows smaller dose volumes. In the UK, doses of hydromorphone hydrochloride by mouth are 1.3 to 2.6 mg every 4 hours. In the USA doses of 2 mg may be given by mouth every 4 to 6 hours; doses may be increased to 4 mg or more for severe pain. Modified-release formulations of hydromorphone hydrochloride are available for twice-daily administration. By rectum, the usual dose is 3 mg every 6 to 8 hours.

Hydromorphone hydrochloride is given, as a syrup, in doses of 1 mg repeated every 3 to 4 hours for the relief of non-productive cough.

References.

1. Urquhart ML, *et al.* Patient-controlled analgesia: a comparison of intravenous versus subcutaneous hydromorphone. *Anesthesiology* 1988; **69:** 428–32.
2. Bruera E, *et al.* Patient-controlled subcutaneous hydromorphone versus continuous subcutaneous infusion for the treatment of cancer pain. *J Natl Cancer Inst* 1988; **80:** 1152–4.
3. Moulin DE, *et al.* Comparison of continuous subcutaneous and intravenous hydromorphone infusions for management of cancer pain. *Lancet* 1991; **337:** 465–8.

Preparations

USP 23: Hydromorphone Hydrochloride Injection; Hydromorphone Hydrochloride Tablets.

Proprietary Preparations (details are given in Part 3)

Canad.: Dilaudid; Hydromorph; ***Ger.:*** Dilaudid; ***Irl.:*** Dilaudid†; Palladone; ***UK:*** Palladone; ***USA:*** Dilaudid; HydroStat IR.

Multi-ingredient: ***Ger.:*** Dilaudid-Atropin; ***Swed.:*** Dilaudid-Atropin; ***Switz.:*** Dilaudid-Atropin; ***USA:*** Dilaudid Cough.

Ibuprofen (2657-h)

Ibuprofen *(BAN, USAN, rINN)*.

Ibuprofeno; Ibuprofenum; RD-13621; U-18573. 2-(4-Isobutylphenyl)propionic acid.

$C_{13}H_{18}O_2$ = 206.3.

CAS — 15687-27-1.

Pharmacopoeias. In *Chin., Eur.* (see p.viii), *Int., Jpn, Pol.,* and *US.*

A white or almost white crystalline powder or colourless crystals with a slight characteristic odour. Practically **insoluble** in water; very soluble in alcohol and in chloroform; freely to very soluble in acetone and in methyl alcohol; freely soluble in ether and in dichloromethane; slightly soluble in ethyl acetate; it dissolves in dilute aqueous solutions of alkali hydroxides and carbonates. **Store** in airtight containers.

Adverse Effects, Treatment, and Precautions

As for NSAIDs in general, p.63. Ibuprofen may be better tolerated than other NSAIDs.

Symptoms of nausea, vomiting, and tinnitus have been reported after ibuprofen overdosage. More serious toxicity is uncommon, but gastric emptying followed by supportive measures is recommended if the quantity ingested within the previous 2 hours exceeds 100 mg per kg body-weight.

An analysis[1] of the outcome of treatment of 83 915 children found that the risk of hospitalisation for gastro-intestinal bleeding, renal failure, or anaphylaxis was no greater in children given ibuprofen than in those given paracetamol.

1. Lesko SM, Mitchell AA. An assessment of the safety of pediatric ibuprofen. *JAMA* 1995; **273:** 929–33.

Breast feeding. The amount of ibuprofen distributed into breast milk is considered by some authorities to be too small to be harmful to a breast-fed infant although some manufacturers recommend that breast feeding should be avoided during ibuprofen treatment, including topical application. A recent study[1] estimated that a breast-fed infant would ingest about 0.0008% of the maternal dose.

1. Walter K, Dilger C. Ibuprofen in human milk. *Br J Clin Pharmacol* 1997; **44:** 211–12.

Effects on the blood. Blood disorders including agranulocytosis, aplastic anaemia,[1] pure white-cell aplasia,[2] and thrombocytopenia[3] have been reported in patients taking ibuprofen. Fatal haemolytic anaemia occurred in a man taking ibuprofen and oxazepam.[4]

1. Gryfe CI, Rubenzahl S. Agranulocytosis and aplastic anemia possibly due to ibuprofen. *Can Med Assoc J* 1976; **114:** 877.
2. Mamus SW, *et al.* Ibuprofen-associated pure white-cell aplasia. *N Engl J Med* 1986; **314:** 624–5.
3. Jain S. Ibuprofen-induced thrombocytopenia. *Br J Clin Pract* 1994; **48:** 51.
4. Guidry JB, *et al.* Fatal autoimmune hemolytic anemia associated with ibuprofen. *JAMA* 1979; **242:** 68–9.

Effects on the CNS. Aseptic meningitis has occurred in patients taking NSAIDs. A review[1] of NSAID-related CNS adverse effects summarised 23 literature reports of NSAID-associated aseptic meningitis; 17 reports involved ibuprofen, 4 sulindac, 1 naproxen, and 1 tolmetin. Of the 23 reports, 11 involved patients with a diagnosis of systemic lupus erythematosus. Typically the reaction is seen in patients who have just recommenced NSAID treatment after a gap in their treatment. Within a few hours of restarting the NSAID the patient experiences fever, headache, and a stiff neck; abdominal pain may be present. The patient may become lethargic and eventually comatose. Symptoms resolve if the NSAID is stopped. It is believed to be a hypersensitivity reaction but there does not appear to be cross-reactivity between NSAIDs. More recently, a 56-year-old man with rheumatoid arthritis developed symptoms of aseptic meningitis 2 hours after ingesting ibuprofen.[2] The authors believed this to be the first reported case of ibuprofen-induced aseptic meningitis in a patient with rheumatoid arthritis.

1. Hoppmann RA, *et al.* Central nervous system side effects of nonsteroidal anti-inflammatory drugs: aseptic meningitis, psychosis, and cognitive dysfunction. *Arch Intern Med* 1991; **151:** 1309–13.
2. Horn AC, Jarrett SW. Ibuprofen-induced aseptic meningitis in rheumatoid arthritis. *Ann Pharmacother* 1997; **31:** 1009–11.

Effects on electrolytes. A patient with pre-existing renal disease developed severe hyponatraemia and symptoms of severe water intoxication after receiving ibuprofen.[1] All symptoms resolved on discontinuation of ibuprofen.

1. Blum M, Aviram A. Ibuprofen induced hyponatraemia. *Rheumatol Rehabil* 1980; **19:** 258–9.

Effects on the eyes. Reversible amblyopia has been reported in patients receiving ibuprofen.[1,2] For reference to effects on the optic nerve associated with ibuprofen, see p.64.

1. Collum LMT, Bowen DI. Ocular side-effects of ibuprofen. *Br J Ophthalmol* 1971; **55:** 472–7.
2. Palmer CAL. Toxic amblyopia from ibuprofen. *Br Med J* 1972; **3:** 765.

Effects on the gastro-intestinal tract. Ibuprofen and other NSAIDs can cause dyspepsia, nausea and vomiting, gastro-intestinal bleeding, and peptic ulcers and perforation. Colitis and its exacerbation have occurred.[1,2]

1. Ravi S, *et al.* Colitis caused by non-steroidal anti-inflammatory drugs. *Postgrad Med J* 1986; **62:** 773–6.
2. Clements D, *et al.* Colitis associated with ibuprofen. *Br Med J* 1990; **301:** 987.

Effects on the kidneys. Reports of adverse renal effects with ibuprofen include an increase in serum creatinine concentration,[1] acute renal failure,[2-5] and nephrotic syndrome.[6] Cystitis, haematuria, and interstitial nephritis may occur. Acute flank pain and reversible renal dysfunction, similar to that seen with suprofen (p.88), has been reported in some patients treated with ibuprofen.[7,8] See also under Effects on Electrolytes, above.

1. Whelton A, *et al.* Renal effects of ibuprofen, piroxicam, and sulindac in patients with asymptomatic renal failure: a prospective, randomized, crossover comparison. *Ann Intern Med* 1990; **112:** 568–76.
2. Brandstetter RD, Mar DD. Reversible oliguric renal failure associated with ibuprofen treatment. *Br Med J* 1978; **2:** 1194–5.
3. Kimberly RP, *et al.* Apparent acute renal failure associated with therapeutic aspirin and ibuprofen administration. *Arthritis Rheum* 1979; **22:** 281–5.
4. Spierto RJ, *et al.* Acute renal failure associated with the use of over-the-counter ibuprofen. *Ann Pharmacother* 1992; **26:** 714.
5. Fernando AHN, *et al.* Renal failure after topical use of NSAIDs. *Br Med J* 1994; **308:** 533.
6. Justiniani FR. Over-the-counter ibuprofen and nephrotic syndrome. *Ann Intern Med* 1986; **105:** 303.
7. McIntire SC, *et al.* Acute flank pain and reversible renal dysfunction associated with nonsteroidal anti-inflammatory drug use. *Pediatrics* 1993; **92:** 459–60.
8. Wattad A, *et al.* A unique complication of nonsteroidal anti-inflammatory drug use. *Pediatrics* 1994; **93:** 693.

Effects on the skin. Skin rashes may occur during hypersensitivity reactions. Serious dermatological problems in the category of erythema multiforme bullosum, including the Stevens-Johnson syndrome, as well as toxic epidermal necrolysis have been reported in patients taking ibuprofen.[1]

1. Sternlieb P, Robinson RM. Side effects of ibuprofen. *Ann Intern Med* 1980; **92:** 570.

Hypersensitivity. A fatal asthma attack occurred in a 65-year-old-woman, with adult-onset asthma, 30 minutes after ingestion of ibuprofen 800 mg.[1]

For other hypersensitivity reactions or possible reactions see also under Effects on the CNS and under Effects on the Skin, above.

1. Ayres JG, *et al.* Asthma death due to ibuprofen. *Lancet* 1987; **i:** 1082.

Meningitis. For reports of aseptic meningitis following administration of ibuprofen, see under Effects on the CNS, above.

Overdosage. There has been a review[1] of cases of ibuprofen overdose reported to the National Poisons Information Service of the UK in the 2 years following its introduction as an 'over-the-counter' medication. Although there was a substantial increase in the number of cases reported, no concurrent increase in severity of poisoning was demonstrated and in only 1 of 203 cases was ibuprofen thought to have caused serious problems. It was concluded that ibuprofen appeared to be much less toxic in acute overdose than either aspirin or paracetamol. However, subsequent reports illustrate the complexity of major overdosage with ibuprofen. A syndrome of coma, hyperkalaemia with cardiac arrhythmias, metabolic acidosis, pyrexia, and respiratory and renal failure was reported[2] in a 17-year-old man following major overdosage with ibuprofen and minor overdosage with doxepin. Hyperkalaemia was not evident until 14 hours after hospital admission and was thought to be due to a combination of potassium replacement for initial hypokalaemia, acidosis, muscle damage, and ibuprofen-induced renal failure. A 6-year-old child developed shock, coma, and metabolic acidosis following ingestion of a dose of ibuprofen equivalent to 300 mg per kg body-weight.[3] Treatment consisting of intubation, mechanical ventilation, fluid resuscitation, gastric lavage, and activated charcoal proved successful. In another report,[4] in which a 21-month-old child had ingested the equivalent of 500 mg per kg of ibuprofen, the presenting symptoms were acute renal failure with severe metabolic acidosis. The child developed tonic-clonic seizures 46 hours after ingestion, with significant hypocalcaemia and hypomagnesaemia, which may have been exacerbated by the administration of sodium polystyrene sulphonate and frusemide. The seizures which could not be controlled with diazepam, phenytoin, and phenobarbitone ceased following correction of electrolyte balance.

1. Perry SJ, *et al.* Ibuprofen overdose: the first two years of over–the–counter sales. *Hum Toxicol* 1987; **6:** 173–8.
2. Menzies DG, *et al.* Fulminant hyperkalaemia and multiple complications following ibuprofen overdose. *Med Toxicol Adverse Drug Exp* 1989; **4:** 468–71.
3. Zuckerman GB, Uy CC. Shock, metabolic acidosis, and coma following ibuprofen overdose in a child. *Ann Pharmacother* 1995; **29:** 869–71.
4. Al-Harbi NN, *et al.* Hypocalcemia and hypomagnesemia after ibuprofen overdose. *Ann Pharmacother* 1997; **31:** 432–4.

Interactions

For interactions associated with NSAIDs, see p.65.

Moclobemide enhances the effects of ibuprofen.

Lipid regulating drugs. For a report of rhabdomyolysis and renal failure attributed to an interaction between ibuprofen and *ciprofibrate*, see p.1270.

Pharmacokinetics

Ibuprofen is absorbed from the gastro-intestinal tract and peak plasma concentrations occur about 1 to 2 hours after ingestion. Ibuprofen is also absorbed following rectal administration. There is some absorption following topical application to the skin. For example, one manufacturer reports that percutaneous absorption from one topical dose form is about 5% of that obtained following administration of an oral dose form. Ibuprofen is 90 to 99% bound to plasma proteins and has a plasma half-life of about 2 hours. It is rapidly excreted in the urine mainly as metabolites and their conjugates. About 1% is excreted in urine as unchanged ibuprofen and about 14% as conjugated ibuprofen. There appears to be little if any distribution into breast milk.

The above figures refer to racemic ibuprofen. However, ibuprofen's disposition is stereoselective and there is some metabolic conversion of the inactive R(−)-enantiomer to the active S(+)-enantiomer (dexibuprofen).

References.

1. Davies NM. Clinical pharmacokinetics of ibuprofen: the first 30 years. *Clin Pharmacokinet* 1998; **34:** 101–54.

Uses and Administration

Ibuprofen, a propionic acid derivative, is an NSAID (p.65). Its anti-inflammatory properties may be weaker than those of some other NSAIDs.

Ibuprofen is used in the management of mild to moderate pain and inflammation in conditions such as dysmenorrhoea, headache including migraine, postoperative pain, dental pain, musculoskeletal and joint disorders such as ankylosing spondylitis, osteoarthritis, and rheumatoid arthritis including juvenile chronic arthritis, peri-articular disorders such as bursitis and tenosynovitis, and soft-tissue disorders such as sprains and strains. It is also used to reduce fever.

Ibuprofen has also been used as an alternative to indomethacin in the treatment of patent ductus arteriosus.

The usual dose by mouth for painful conditions in adults is 1.2 to 1.8 g daily in divided doses although maintenance doses of 0.6 to 1.2 g daily may be effective in some patients. If necessary the dose may be increased; in the UK the maximum recommended dose is 2.4 g daily whereas in the USA it is 3.2 g daily. Modified-release preparations of ibuprofen are available for once- or twice daily dosing, although actual dosages vary with different preparations. Patients with rheumatoid arthritis generally require higher doses of ibuprofen than those with osteoarthritis. The recommended dose for fever reduction in adults is 200 to 400 mg every 4 to 6 hours to a maximum of 1.2 g daily.

In the UK the usual dose by mouth for the treatment of pain or fever in children is 20 to 30 mg per kg body-weight daily in divided doses. Alternatively, total daily doses to be given in divided doses may be expressed in terms of age and are: 6 to 12 months, 150 mg; 1 to 2 years, 150 to 200 mg; 3 to 7 years, 300 to 400 mg; and 8 to 12 years, 600 to 800 mg. Up to 40 mg per kg may be given daily in juvenile chronic arthritis if necessary. Ibuprofen is not generally recommended for children weighing less than 7 kg and some manufacturers suggest a maximum daily dose of 500 mg in those weighing less than 30 kg.

In the USA, suggested doses for children are: for fever, 5 to 10 mg per kg (depending on the severity of the fever) and for pain, 10 mg per kg; doses may be given every 6 to 8 hours up to a maximum daily dose of 40 mg per kg. A usual daily dose in the USA for juvenile chronic arthritis in children aged 6 months to 12 years is up to 40 mg per kg.

Ibuprofen is also applied topically as a 5% cream, gel, or spray solution.

Ibuprofen is usually given as the base but various salts, esters, and other complexes are also used. These include lysine and sodium salts, guaiacol and pyridoxine esters, and aminoethanol, isobutanolammonium, and meglumine derivatives.

Ibuprofen is usually administered as a racemic mixture but preparations containing only the S(+)-isomer (dexibuprofen) are available in some countries.

Cystic fibrosis. In patients with cystic fibrosis (see p.119), the inflammatory response to chronic pulmonary infection with *Pseudomonas* organisms contributes to lung destruction. Ibuprofen has shown beneficial anti-inflammatory effects in an *animal* model of chronic endobronchial *Pseudomonas* infections and is therefore being studied in patients with cystic fibrosis[1,2] in the hope of providing a safer alternative to corticosteroids to reduce pulmonary inflammation. A study[3] in patients with cystic fibrosis and mild lung disease, indicated that ibuprofen given in high doses for four years slowed the progression of the lung disease without serious adverse effects. Initial doses were in the region of 20 to 30 mg per kg bodyweight to a maximum of 1600 mg but were then adjusted individually to achieve peak plasma concentrations of 50 to 100 μg per mL.

1. Konstan MW, *et al.* Ibuprofen in children with cystic fibrosis: pharmacokinetics and adverse effects. *J Pediatr* 1991; **118:** 956–64.
2. Davis PB. Cystic fibrosis from bench to bedside. *N Engl J Med* 1991; **325:** 575–7.
3. Konstan MW, *et al.* Effect of high-dose ibuprofen in patients with cystic fibrosis. *N Engl J Med* 1995; **332:** 848–54.

Patent ductus arteriosus. For a suggestion that ibuprofen might be a better choice than indomethacin for the treatment of patent ductus arteriosus, see under Indomethacin on p.47.

Preparations

BP 1998: Ibuprofen Cream; Ibuprofen Gel; Ibuprofen Oral Suspension; Ibuprofen Tablets;
USP 23: Ibuprofen and Pseudoephedrine Hydrochloride Tablets; Ibuprofen Oral Suspension; Ibuprofen Tablets.

Proprietary Preparations (details are given in Part 3)
Aust.: Avallone; Brufen; Dismenol neu; Dolgit; Dolibu; Dolofort; Doloren; Duafen; Ibudol; Ibugel; Ibupron; Iburem; Ibutop; Imbun; Junifen†; Kratalgin; Nurofen; Seractil; Tabcin; Urem†; ***Austral.:*** ACT-3; Actiprofen; Brufen; Codral Period Pain†; Ibu-Cream†; Nurofen; Rafen; Tri-Profen; ***Belg.:*** Brufen; Bufedon; Dolgit†; Dolofin†; Exidol†; Ibu-Slow; Ibutop; Inabrin; Junifen; Malafene; Motrin; Nurofen; ***Canad.:*** Actiprofen; Advil; Medipren†; Motrin; Novo-Profen; ***Fr.:*** Advil; Algifene; Analgyl†; Brufen; Dolgit; Ergix; Fenalgic†; Gelufene; Ibutop; Nureflex; Nurofen; Oralfene; Tiburon; ***Ger.:*** Aktren; Anco; Brufen; Cesra; Contraneural; Dentigoa; Dignoflex; Dimidon†; Dismenol N; Dolgit; Dolo neos; Dolo-Dolgit†; Dolo-Puren; Dolormin; dura-Ibu; duraibuprofen; Dysdolen†; Esprenit; Exneural; Fibraflex†; Gynofug; Ibol†; Ibu; ibu-Attritin†; Ibu-Vivimed; Ibubest; Ibubeta; Ibuflam; Ibufug; Ibuhexal; Ibumerck; Ibuphlogont; Ibuprof; Ibutad; Ibutop; Imbun; Jenaprofen; Kontagripp Mono; Logomed Schmerz; Mensoton; Mobilat; Novogent; Optalidon; Opturem; Parsal; Pfeil; Schmerz-Dolgit; Seclodin; stadasan†; Tabalon; Tempil; Togal N; Trauma-Dolgit; Trombufen†; Urem; ***Irl.:*** Actiprofen; Advil; Brufen; Bufigen; Cunil; Ibugel; Melfen; Nurofen; Proflex; ***Ital.:*** Aciril; Algofen; Antalgil; Arfen; Artrene†; Asepsal; Benflogin; Brufen; Brufort; Calmine; Cibalgina Due Fast; Dolocyl; Faspic; Flubenil; Focus†; Gineflor; Ginenorm; Inabrin†; Kos; Moment; Neo-Mindol; Nurofen; Prontalgin†; ***Neth.:*** Advil; Brufen; Femapirin†; Ibosure†; Ibumetin†; Nerofen†; Nurofen; Zafen; ***Norw.:*** Brufen; Ibumetin; Ibux; ***S.Afr.:*** Abbifen†; Adfen; Antiflam; Betagesic; Betaprofen; Brufen; Brugesic; Clinofen†; Dynofen; Ibopain; Ibufarm†; Ibuleve; Ibumed; Inza; Magnatex; Nurofen; Ranfen; Rofen; Solufen†; ***Spain:*** Actifen†; Actimidol; Aldospray Analgesico; Algiasdin; Algisan; Altior; Cusialgil†; Dalsy; Doctril; Dolocyl; Dorival; Ediluna; Espidifen; Evasprin†; Faspic; Femaprim; Femidol; Ibenon; Incefal†; Isdol; Kalma; Leonal; Librofem†; Liderfeme†; Lisi-Budol†; Medipren†; Narfen; Neobrufen; Noalgil; Nurofen; Pocyl; Sadefen; Sedaspray†; Solufena; Spidifen†; Todalgil; ***Swed.:*** Brufen; Duobrus; Ibumetin; Ipren; Nurofen; ***Switz.:*** Algifor; Antalgit†; Brufen; Bufeno; Dismenol N; Dolgit; Dolocyl; Dologel; Ecoprofen; Ibufen-L; Ibugel; Ibulgan†; Ibumed; Iproben; Iprogel; Irfen; Motrin; Neo-Helvagit†; Nurofen; Optifen; Panax N; Redufen; Serviprofen; Solufen; Spedifen; ***UK:*** Advil; Anadin Ibuprofen†; Apsifen; Arthrofen; Brufen; Cuprofen; Ebufac; Femafen†; Fenbid; Galprofen; Ibrufhalal; Ibufac; Ibugel; Ibular; Ibuleve; Ibumed†; Ibumousse; Ibuspray; Ibutop Cuprofen; Ibutop Ralgex; Inoven; Isisfen; Junifen; Librofem; Lidifen; Migrafen; Motrin; Novaprin; Nurofen; Nurofen Advance; Pacifene; Phor Pain; Proflex; Relcofen; Rimafen; ***USA:*** Aches-N-Pain†; Advil; Arthritis Foundation Ibuprofen†; Bayer Select Pain Relief Formula; Cramp End†; Dynafed IB; Excedrin IB†; Genpril; Haltran; Ibifon; Ibu; Ibu-Tab†; Ibuprin; Ibuprohm; Medipren†; Menadol; Midol IB; Motrin; Nuprin; PediaProfen; Rufen†; Saleto-200; Trendar†.

Multi-ingredient: ***Canad.:*** Advil Cold & Sinus; Dayquil Sinus with Pain Relief; Dristan Sinus; ***Fr.:*** Rhinadvil; Rhinureflex; Vicks Rhume; ***Irl.:*** Advil Cold & Flu; Codafen Continus; ***S.Afr.:*** Advil CS; Lotem; Mypaid; Myprodol; Nurofen Cold & Flu; ***Spain:*** Nurogrip; Salvarina; ***Swed.:*** Ardinex; ***Switz.:*** Ibufen-L; ***UK:*** Advil Cold & Sinus; Codafen Continus; Deep Relief; Lemsip Power +; Nurofen Cold & Flu; Nurofen Plus; Solpaflex; Vicks Action; ***USA:*** Advil Cold & Sinus; Dimetapp Sinus Caplets; Dristan Sinus; Motrin IB Sinus; Sine-Aid IB; Vicoprofen.

Ibuproxam (12841-a)

Ibuproxam *(rINN)*.
4-Isobutylhydratropohydroxamic acid.
$C_{13}H_{19}NO_2 = 221.3$.
CAS — 53648-05-8.

Ibuproxam is an NSAID (p.63) that has been used in musculoskeletal, joint, and soft-tissue disorders by mouth or as a rectal suppository and has also been applied topically.

Preparations

Proprietary Preparations (details are given in Part 3)
Ital.: Deflogon†; Ibudros; ***Spain:*** Nialen; ***Switz.:*** Ibudros†.

Imidazole Salicylate (16848-e)

Imidazole Salicylate *(rINN)*.
Imidazole compounded with salicylic acid.
$C_{10}H_{10}N_2O_3 = 206.2$.
CAS — 36364-49-5.

Imidazole salicylate is a salicylic acid derivative (see Aspirin, p.16) that has been used in the treatment of fever and inflammatory respiratory-tract and otorhinolaryngeal disorders. Imidazole salicylate has been given in doses of up to 2.25 g daily in divided doses by mouth. It has also been given as a rectal suppository and has been applied topically as a 5% gel for the relief of muscular and rheumatic pain.

Preparations

Proprietary Preparations (details are given in Part 3)
Ital.: Flogozen; Fluenzen; Selezen.

Indomethacin (2658-m)

Indomethacin *(BAN, USAN)*.
Indometacin *(rINN)*; Indometacinum. [1-(4-Chlorobenzoyl)-5-methoxy-2-methylindol-3-yl]acetic acid.
$C_{19}H_{16}ClNO_4 = 357.8$.
CAS — 53-86-1.
Pharmacopoeias. In *Chin., Eur.* (see p.viii), *Int., Jpn,* and *US.*

A white to yellow-tan, odourless or almost odourless, crystalline powder. It exhibits polymorphism. Practically **insoluble** in water; soluble 1 in 50 of alcohol, 1 in 30 of chloroform, and 1 in 40 of ether. **Protect** from light. Indomethacin is unstable in alkaline solution.

Indomethacin Sodium (19343-w)

Indomethacin Sodium *(BANM, USAN)*.
Indometacin Sodium *(rINNM)*; Indomethacin Sodium Trihydrate. Sodium 1-(4-chlorobenzoyl)-5-methoxy-2-methylindole-3-acetate, trihydrate.
$C_{19}H_{15}ClNNaO_4,3H_2O = 433.8$.
CAS — 74252-25-8.
Pharmacopoeias. In *US.*

Protect from light.

Incompatibility. Indomethacin sodium injection is reconstituted with preservative-free sodium chloride for injection or water for injection. Preparations containing glucose should not be used; reconstitution at a pH below 6 may cause precipitation of indomethacin. Visual incompatibility has been reported between indomethacin sodium injection and tolazoline hydrochloride,[1] 7.5 and 10% glucose injection, calcium gluconate, dobutamine, dopamine, cimetidine,[2] gentamicin sulphate, and tobramycin sulphate.[3] A pH below 6 may account for the visual incompatibility of indomethacin sodium and several of these drugs.

1. Marquardt ED. Visual compatibility of tolazoline hydrochloride with various medications during simulated Y-site injection. *Am J Hosp Pharm* 1990; **47:** 1802–3.
2. Ishisaka DY, *et al.* Visual compatibility of indomethacin sodium trihydrate with drugs given to neonates by continuous infusion. *Am J Hosp Pharm* 1991; **48:** 2442–3.
3. Thompson DF, Heflin NR. Incompatibility of injectable indomethacin with gentamicin sulfate or tobramycin sulfate. *Am J Hosp Pharm* 1992; **49:** 836–8.

Stability. A reconstituted solution of indomethacin sodium 500 μg per mL was stable for 14 days when stored at 2° to 6° in either the manufacturer's original glass vial or in a polypropylene syringe.[1]

1. Walker SE, *et al.* Stability of reconstituted indomethacin sodium trihydrate in original vials and polypropylene syringes. *Am J Health-Syst Pharm* 1998; **55:** 154–8.

Adverse Effects

Adverse effects are more frequent with indomethacin than with many other NSAIDs (see p.63), the most common being gastro-intestinal disturbances, headache, dizziness, and lightheadedness. Gastro-intestinal perforation, ulceration, and bleeding may also occur; rarely, intestinal strictures have been reported. Other adverse effects include depression, drowsiness, tinnitus, confusion, insomnia, psychiatric disturbances, syncope, convulsions, coma, peripheral neuropathy, blurred vision, corneal deposits, and other ocular effects, oedema and weight gain, hypertension, haematuria, skin rashes, pruritus, urticaria, stomatitis, alopecia, and hypersensitivity reactions. Leucopenia, purpura, thrombocytopenia, aplastic anaemia, haemolytic anaemia, agranulocytosis, epistaxis, hyperglycaemia, hyperkalaemia, and vaginal bleeding have been reported. There have also been reports of hepatitis, jaundice, and renal failure. Hypersensitivity reactions may also occur in aspirin-sensitive patients. Rectal irritation has been reported occasionally in patients who have received indomethacin suppositories.

Adverse effects associated with the use of indomethacin in premature **neonates** also include haemorrhagic, renal, gastro-intestinal, metabolic, and coagulation disorders; pulmonary hypertension, intracranial bleeding, fluid retention, and exacerbation of infection may also occur.

Effects on the blood. There were 1261 reports of adverse reactions to indomethacin reported to the UK Committee on Safety of Medicines between June 1964 and January 1973. These included 157 reports of blood disorders (25 fatal) including thrombocytopenia (35; 5 fatal), aplastic anaemia (17; no fatalities), and agranulocytosis or leucopenia (21; 3 fatal).[1] Subsequently, the First Report from the International Agranulocytosis and Aplastic Anemia Study confirmed a significant relationship between the use of indomethacin and agranulocytosis and aplastic anaemia.[2]

Although use of indomethacin in 20 women being treated for premature labour did not affect maternal prothrombin or activated partial thromboplastin time, maternal bleeding time during therapy was increased.[3] However, no cases of neonatal intraventricular haemorrhage or maternal postpartum haemorrhage were seen.

1. Cuthbert MF. Adverse reactions to non-steroidal antirheumatic drugs. *Curr Med Res Opin* 1974; **2:** 600–10.
2. The International Agranulocytosis and Aplastic Anemia Study. Risks of agranulocytosis and aplastic anemia: a first report of their relation to drug use with special reference to analgesics. *JAMA* 1986; **256:** 1749–57.
3. Lunt CC, *et al.* The effect of indomethacin tocolysis on maternal coagulation status. *Obstet Gynecol* 1994; **84:** 820–2.

Effects on cerebral blood flow. See under Patent Ductus Arteriosus in Uses and Administration, below.

Effects on electrolytes. Hyporeninaemia, hypoaldosteronism, and hyperkalaemia have been associated with administration of indomethacin.[1-5] See also under Effects on the Kidneys, below.

1. Zimran A, *et al.* Incidence of hyperkalaemia induced by indomethacin in a hospital population. *Br Med J* 1985; **291:** 107–8.
2. Tan SY, *et al.* Indomethacin-induced prostaglandin inhibition with hyperkalemia: a reversible cause of hyporeninemic hypoaldosteronism. *Ann Intern Med* 1979; **90:** 783–5.
3. MacCarthy EP, *et al.* Indomethacin-induced hyperkalaemia. *Med J Aust* 1979; **1:** 550.
4. Beroniade V, *et al.* Indomethacin-induced inhibition of prostaglandin with hyperkalemia. *Ann Intern Med* 1979; **91:** 499–500.
5. Findling JW, *et al.* Indomethacin-induced hyperkalemia in three patients with gouty arthritis. *JAMA* 1980; **244:** 1127–8.

Effects on the eyes. Severe and irreversible retinopathy, presumably due to long-term ingestion of high doses of indomethacin occurred in a 33-year-old man.[1] A summary of previous literature reports of indomethacin-induced ocular effects indicated that indomethacin was retinotoxic, although to what degree was uncertain. For reference to effects on the optic nerve associated with indomethacin, see p.64.

1. Graham CM, Blach RK. Indomethacin retinopathy: case report and review. *Br J Ophthalmol* 1988; **72:** 434–8.

Effects on the gastro-intestinal tract. Nausea, vomiting, dyspepsia, gastro-intestinal lesions, and serious reactions including gastro-intestinal bleeding, ulceration, and perforation have occurred in patients receiving indomethacin. Although it is well established that NSAIDs can produce adverse effects on the upper gastro-intestinal tract, indomethacin and other NSAIDs can also affect the large intestines.[1]

Between January 1965 and 1985 the Committee on Safety of Medicines in the UK had recorded 12 cases of intestinal perforation (7 deaths), 5 cases of intestinal ulceration (1 death), and 2 cases of intestinal ulceration and perforation (no deaths).[2]

Intestinal perforation has been observed in **neonates** following enteral administration of indomethacin.[3] However, intravenous administration appears to be associated with a lower incidence of adverse effects.[4] Of 2482 preterm neonates given indomethacin intravenously 146 were reported as having experienced adverse effects.[4] Half of the reports (73) were rated as being possibly, probably, or definitely related to the drug treatment by the reporting physician. There were 18 reports of gastro-intestinal bleeding and 13 reports of necrotising enterocolitis.

1. Oren R, Ligumsky M. Indomethacin-induced colonic ulceration and bleeding. *Ann Pharmacother* 1994; **28:** 883–5.
2. Stewart JT, *et al.* Anti-inflammatory drugs and bowel perforations and haemorrhage. *Br Med J* 1985; **290:** 787–8.
3. Alpan G, *et al.* Localized intestinal perforations after enteral administration of indomethacin in premature infants. *J Pediatr* 1985; **106:** 277–81.
4. Walters M. Tolerance of intravenous indomethacin treatment for premature infants with patent ductus arteriosus. *Br Med J* 1988; **297:** 773–4.

Effects on the joints. For references to concern that NSAIDs such as indomethacin may accelerate the rate of cartilage destruction in patients with osteoarthritis, see under NSAIDs, p.64.

Effects on the kidneys. Acute renal failure,[1-3] nephrotic syndrome,[4] and renal papillary necrosis[5] have been reported in patients given indomethacin. There have been suggestions that misoprostol might reduce the risk of indomethacin-induced renal toxicity.[6,7]

Renal dysfunction has also occurred in **neonates** given indomethacin intravenously for patent ductus arteriosus. Of 2482 neonates treated in the UK between 1980 and 1988, indomethacin-associated adverse effects reported to the manufacturer[8] included renal failure or shutdown (10 neonates), fall in urea concentration (12), hyponatraemia (16), and increase in creatinine concentration (5). The renal impairment was not usually sustained or serious, but in neonates with pre-existing renal impairment, indomethacin therapy may lead to serious deterioration. Autopsy of 6 neonates who had had prolonged exposure to indomethacin *in utero* and had died of persistent anuria showed cystic dilatation of the superficial nephrons, ischaemia of the inner renal cortex, and interstitial fibrosis.[9]

1. Walshe JJ, Venuto RC. Acute oliguric renal failure induced by indomethacin: possible mechanism. *Ann Intern Med* 1979; **91:** 47–9.
2. Bernheim JL, Korzets Z. Indomethacin-induced renal failure. *Ann Intern Med* 1979; **91:** 792.
3. Chan X. Fatal renal failure due to indomethacin. *Lancet* 1987; **ii:** 340.
4. Boiskin I, *et al.* Indomethacin and the nephrotic syndrome. *Ann Intern Med* 1987; **106:** 776–7.
5. Mitchell H, *et al.* Indomethacin-induced renal papillary necrosis in juvenile chronic arthritis. *Lancet* 1982; **ii:** 558–9.
6. Weir MR, *et al.* Minimization of indomethacin-induced reduction in renal function by misoprostol. *J Clin Pharmacol* 1991; **31:** 729–35.
7. Wong F, *et al.* The effect of misoprostol on indomethacin-induced renal dysfunction in well-compensated cirrhosis. *J Hepatol* 1995; **23:** 1–7.
8. Walters M. Tolerance of intravenous indomethacin treatment for premature infants with patent ductus arteriosus. *Br Med J* 1988; **297:** 773–4.
9. van der Heijden BJ, *et al.* Persistent anuria, neonatal death, and renal microcystic lesions after prenatal exposure to indomethacin. *Am J Obstet Gynecol* 1994; **171:** 617–23.

Effects on the liver. Cholestasis occurred in a 52-year-old woman several days after starting indomethacin;[1] liver function values returned to normal once indomethacin was discontinued.

1. Cappell MS, *et al.* Indomethacin-associated cholestasis. *J Clin Gastroenterol* 1988; **10:** 445–7.

Hypersensitivity. Hypersensitivity reactions including acute asthma have been reported following the use of indomethacin suppositories,[1] eye drops,[2] or capsules[3] by patients who were aspirin-sensitive or had a history of asthma.

1. Timperman J. A fatal asthmatic attack following administration of an indomethacin suppository. *J Forensic Med* 1971; **18:** 30–2.
2. Sheehan GJ, *et al.* Acute asthma attack due to ophthalmic indomethacin. *Ann Intern Med* 1989; **111:** 337–8.
3. Johnson NM, *et al.* Indomethacin-induced asthma in aspirin-sensitive patients. *Br Med J* 1977; **2:** 1291.

Precautions

As for NSAIDs in general, p.65.

Indomethacin should be administered with caution to patients with epilepsy, parkinsonism, or psychiatric disorders. Dizziness may affect the performance of skilled tasks such as driving. Patients on long-term indomethacin therapy should be examined regularly for adverse effects, and some authorities particularly recommend periodic blood and ophthalmic examinations. Rectal administration should be avoided in patients with proctitis and haemorrhoids.

In addition indomethacin should not be given to **neonates** with untreated infection, with significantly impaired renal function, or with necrotising enterocolitis. Infants who are bleeding (especially gastro-intestinal bleeding or intracranial haemorrhage) or who have thrombocytopenia or coagulation defects should not be given indomethacin and those receiving indomethacin should be monitored during treatment for signs of bleeding. Electrolytes and renal function should also be monitored and if anuria or marked oliguria is evident at the time of a scheduled second or third dose, administration should be delayed until renal function has returned to normal.

False-negative results in the dexamethasone suppression test have been reported in patients taking indomethacin.

Breast feeding. Convulsions in a one-week old breast-fed infant appeared to be associated with ingestion of indomethacin by the mother;[1] the child had normal motor and mental development at the age of 1 year and seizures had not recurred. Indomethacin has been detected in breast milk, but some workers[2] consider that the amount is so small that it should not constitute a contra-indication to breast feeding.

1. Eeg-Olofsson O, *et al.* Convulsions in a breast-fed infant after maternal indomethacin. *Lancet* 1978; **ii:** 215.
2. Beaulac-Baillargeon L, Allard G. Distribution of indomethacin in human milk and estimation of its milk to plasma ratio in vitro. *Br J Clin Pharmacol* 1993; **36:** 413–16.

Elderly. Following a study[1] of the pharmacokinetics of indomethacin in the elderly it was suggested that the maintenance dose of indomethacin in elderly patients should be reduced by 25%. The total clearance of indomethacin in elderly subjects had been reduced when compared with that in young subjects; this was thought to be due to reduced hepatic metabolism in the elderly.

1. Oberbauer R, *et al.* Pharmacokinetics of indomethacin in the elderly. *Clin Pharmacokinet* 1993; **24:** 428–34.

Pregnancy. See under Premature Labour in Uses and Administration, below.

Interactions

For interactions associated with NSAIDs, see p.65.

Concurrent administration of anti-inflammatory doses of aspirin decreases indomethacin blood concentrations by about 20%. Administration of diflunisal with indomethacin decreases the renal clearance and increases plasma concentrations of indomethacin. Combined use of diflunisal and indomethacin has resulted in fatal gastro-intestinal haemorrhage; therefore, these drugs should not be used concurrently. Plasma concentrations of indomethacin are likely to be increased in patients receiving probenecid.

Concomitant administration of indomethacin has been reported to increase plasma concentrations of *aminoglycoside antibiotics*, increase the bioavailability of *tiludronate*, and to enhance the effect of *desmopressin*.

The manufacturer of acetylcholine chloride ophthalmic preparations has stated that there have been reports that *acetylcholine* and *carbachol* have been ineffective when used in patients treated with topical (ophthalmic) NSAIDs.

Antipsychotics. A report[1] of severe drowsiness and confusion in patients given *haloperidol* with indomethacin.

1. Bird HA, *et al.* Drowsiness due to haloperidol/indomethacin in combination. *Lancet* 1983; **i:** 830–1.

Pharmacokinetics

Indomethacin is readily absorbed from the gastro-intestinal tract in adults; peak plasma concentrations are reached about 2 hours after a dose. Absorption may be slowed by food or by aluminium or magnesium containing antacids. In premature neonates, absorption of oral indomethacin is poor and incomplete. The bioavailability of rectal suppositories in adults has been reported to be comparable with or slightly less than the bioavailability with oral dosage forms.

Indomethacin is about 99% bound to plasma proteins. It is distributed into synovial fluid, the CNS, and placenta. Low concentrations have been distributed into breast milk. The terminal plasma half-life has been reported to range from 2.6 to 11.2 hours in adults. The terminal half-life in neonates has been reported to be between 15 and 30 hours. Indomethacin is metabolised in the liver to its glucuronide conjugate and to desmethylindomethacin, desbenzoylindomethacin, desmethyl-desbenzoylindomethacin, and to their glucuronides. Some indomethacin undergoes N-deacylation. Indomethacin and its conjugates undergo enterohepatic circulation. Excretion of indomethacin and its metabolites is predominantly in the urine with lesser amounts appearing in the faeces.

References.

1. Moise KJ, *et al.* Placental transfer of indomethacin in the human pregnancy. *Am J Obstet Gynecol* 1990; **162:** 549–54.
2. Lebedevs TH, *et al.* Excretion of indomethacin in breast milk. *Br J Clin Pharmacol* 1991; **32:** 751–4.
3. Wiest DB, *et al.* Population pharmacokinetics of intravenous indomethacin in neonates with symptomatic patent ductus arteriosus. *Clin Pharmacol Ther* 1991; **49:** 550–7.
4. Beaulac-Baillargeon L, Allard G. Distribution of indomethacin in human milk and estimation of its milk to plasma ratio in vitro. *Br J Clin Pharmacol* 1993; **36:** 413–16.

Uses and Administration

Indomethacin, an indole acetic acid derivative, is an NSAID (p.65).

It is used in musculoskeletal and joint disorders including ankylosing spondylitis, osteoarthritis, rheumatoid arthritis, and acute gout, and in peri-articular disorders such as bursitis and tendinitis. It may also be used in inflammation, pain, and oedema following orthopaedic procedures, in mild to moderate pain in conditions such as dysmenorrhoea, and it has been used as an adjunct to opioids in the management of postoperative pain, and in the treatment of fever. Indomethacin is also used as the sodium salt to close patent ductus arteriosus in premature infants (see below).

The usual initial dose by mouth in chronic musculoskeletal and joint disorders is 25 mg two or three times daily increased, if required, by 25 to 50 mg daily at weekly intervals to 150 to 200 mg daily. To alleviate night pain and morning stiffness, 100 mg of the total daily dose may be administered by mouth, or rectally as a suppository, on retiring. Alternatively, the total daily dose may be administered by rectum as 100 mg in the morning and at night. The total daily combined dose by mouth and by rectum should not exceed 200 mg. In acute gout the daily dose is 150 to 200 mg in divided doses until all symptoms and signs subside; in dysmenorrhoea up to 75 mg daily has been suggested.

Modified-release preparations of indomethacin are available for administration once or twice daily.

Indomethacin has been used topically as 0.5 or 1% eye drops to prevent miosis during cataract surgery and to prevent cystoid macular oedema; the usual dose is one drop instilled 4 times daily (beginning on the day before surgery, where relevant).

When used to close patent ductus arteriosus in premature infants indomethacin sodium is given as a short course of therapy of three intravenous injections given at 12- to 24-hour intervals; each injection should be given over 5 to 10 seconds. Indomethacin sodium injection is reconstituted with preservative-free sodium chloride for injection or water for injection; glucose solutions should not be used. The dose of indomethacin sodium (expressed as indomethacin) depends upon the age of the neonate and the following doses have been suggested based upon the age at the first dose: less than 48 hours old, 200 μg per kg body-weight initially followed by two further doses of 100 μg per kg each; 2 to 7 days old, three doses of 200 μg per kg each; over 7 days old, 200 μg per kg initially followed by two further doses of 250 μg per kg each. If, 48 hours after this course of therapy the ductus remains open or re-opens a second course of therapy may be employed, but if this produces no response surgery may be necessary.

Meglumine indomethacin and a lipid soluble ester of indomethacin, indomethacin farnesil ($C_{34}H_{40}ClNO_4$=562.1), have also been used for painful and inflammatory conditions. A complex of indomethacin and L-arginine, known as indoarginine, has been used in pain, inflammation, and febrile conditions.

Bartter's syndrome. The treatment of Bartter's syndrome can often be difficult (see p.1150). Blocking the kinin-prostaglandin axis with a cyclo-oxygenase inhibitor such as indomethacin improves hypokalaemia and other clinical features (including growth retardation) in children with the syndrome.[1-3]

1. Littlewood JM, *et al.* Treatment of childhood Bartter's syndrome with indomethacin. *Lancet* 1976; **ii:** 795.
2. Seidel C, *et al.* Pre-pubertal growth in the hyperprostaglandin E syndrome. *Pediatr Nephrol* 1995; **9:** 723–8.
3. Craig JC, Falk MC. Indomethacin for renal impairment in neonatal Bartter's syndrome. *Lancet* 1996; **347:** 550.

Diabetes insipidus. In nephrogenic diabetes insipidus (p.1237) the treatment is mainly with water replacement in conjunction with thiazide diuretics and restricted sodium intake but a variety of other drugs have also been tried. Indomethacin and other prostaglandin synthetase inhibitors have been reported to decrease urine volume in all types of this disorder.

References.

1. Rosen GH, *et al.* Indomethacin for nephrogenic diabetes insipidus in a four-week-old infant. *Clin Pharm* 1986; **5:** 254–6.
2. Libber S, *et al.* Treatment of nephrogenic diabetes insipidus with prostaglandin synthesis inhibitors. *J Pediatr* 1986; **108:** 305–11.
3. Allen HM, *et al.* Indomethacin in the treatment of lithium-induced nephrogenic diabetes insipidus. *Arch Intern Med* 1989; **149:** 1123–6.
4. Martinez EJ, *et al.* Lithium-induced nephrogenic diabetes insipidus treated with indomethacin. *South Med J* 1993; **86:** 971–3.

Malignant neoplasms. Some NSAIDs such as indomethacin may be of value both for the differential diagnosis and the management of neoplastic fever as they appear to be more effective in reducing this type of fever than against fever associated with infections.[1] Indomethacin has also been tried for the treatment of fever and flu-like symptoms associated with interleukin-2 therapy although there has been concern over exacerbation of renal toxicity (see p.542). It has been suggested that indomethacin might also possess some antineoplastic activity.[2]

1. Engervall P, *et al.* Antipyretic effect of indomethacin in malignant lymphoma. *Acta Med Scand* 1986; **219:** 501–5.
2. Mertens WC, *et al.* Effect of indomethacin plus ranitidine in advanced melanoma patients on high-dose interleukin-2. *Lancet* 1992; **340:** 397–8.

Neonatal intraventricular haemorrhage. Indomethacin is one of a number of drugs that have been tried prophylactically to prevent the development of intraventricular haemorrhage in neonates at risk (see p.709). Several mechanisms have been proposed for its possible action including reduction of cerebral flow as a result of vasoconstriction, reduction of oxygen free-radical damage, and accelerated maturation of blood vessels around the ventricles. Early studies[1-3] of the use of indomethacin for prevention of intraventricular haemorrhage produced conflicting results. A more recent large multicentre study[4] suggested that indomethacin can reduce the incidence and severity of intraventricular haemorrhage, especially for the more severe forms, but it has been noted[5] that there was an unusually large number of neonates with severe intraventricular haemorrhage in the control group. Neonates who received indomethacin were given a dose of 100 µg per kg body-weight intravenously at 6 to 12 hours after delivery and then every 24 hours for 2 additional doses. A concern with the use of indomethacin is the possibility that it may produce cerebral ischaemia due to its vasoconstrictor action and therefore increase the risk of developmental handicaps. A review[6] of studies of prophylactic indomethacin concluded that more studies of possible adverse effects and long-term outcome are needed before indomethacin can be recommended for routine use. However, follow-up[7] at 3 years of age of the infants included in the multicentre study reported no adverse effects on cognitive or motor development.

Another study[8] has indicated that indomethacin does not prevent the progression of existing low grade intraventricular haemorrhage.

1. Ment LR, *et al.* Randomized indomethacin trial for prevention of intraventricular hemorrhage in very low birth weight infants. *J Pediatr* 1985; **107:** 937–43.
2. Rennie JM, *et al.* Early administration of indomethacin to preterm infants. *Arch Dis Child* 1986; **61:** 233–8.
3. Bada HS, *et al.* Indomethacin reduces the risks of severe intraventricular hemorrhage. *J Pediatr* 1989; **115:** 631–7.
4. Ment LR, *et al.* Low-dose indomethacin and prevention of intraventricular hemorrhage: a multicenter randomized trial. *Pediatrics* 1994; **93:** 543–50.
5. Volpe JJ. Brain injury caused by intraventricular hemorrhage: is indomethacin the silver bullet for prevention? *Pediatrics* 1994; **93:** 673–7.
6. Fowlie PW. Prophylactic indomethacin: systematic review and meta-analysis. *Arch Dis Child* 1996; **74:** F81–F87.
7. Ment LR, *et al.* Neurodevelopmental outcome at 36 months' corrected age of preterm infants in the multicenter indomethacin intraventricular hemorrhage prevention trial. *Pediatrics* 1996; **98:** 714–18.
8. Ment LR, *et al.* Low-dose indomethacin therapy and extension of intraventricular hemorrhage: a multicenter randomized trial. *J Pediatr* 1994; **124:** 951–5.

Patent ductus arteriosus. The ductus arteriosus is a vascular channel present in the fetal circulation that connects the pulmonary artery and the descending aorta. After birth, various mechanisms, including a fall in prostaglandin concentration, trigger closure of the ductus arteriosus and the output from the right ventricle is thus channelled completely into the pulmonary circulation. In some infants the ductus arteriosus fails to close, a condition known as persistent patent ductus arteriosus, and in such infants the pulmonary circulation is reduced as blood is diverted into the descending aorta. This condition may be found in infants with congenital heart defects when it may be an isolated lesion or part of a more complex cardiac abnormality. More commonly it occurs in premature neonates, especially those with respiratory distress syndrome. In some infants a patent ductus arteriosus is necessary for maintaining some oxygenation of the blood, for example in infants with pulmonary artery atresia or transposition of the great arteries. These infants require treatment with a prostaglandin such as alprostadil or dinoprostone to maintain patency of the ductus arteriosus until surgery can be performed to correct the malformation.

Not all infants with patent ductus arteriosus require treatment. Some infants may be asymptomatic or have only slight clinical symptoms and no immediate intervention is required. In many cases spontaneous closure will occur after several months, or if closure does not occur surgical ligation may be performed if clinical symptoms persist. Infants with haemodynamically significant ductus arteriosus, signs of heart failure, and who require ventilation should undergo treatment.

Initial management of persistent patent ductus arteriosus involves fluid restriction, diuretics, correction of anaemia, and support of respiration. If this fails to control symptoms after 24 to 48 hours then indomethacin is generally given to promote closure of the ductus.[1-4] Some workers[5] advocate treatment with indomethacin as soon as symptoms become apparent rather than delaying treatment until signs of congestive failure develop. Early treatment may significantly reduce the morbidities arising from a persistent patent ductus arteriosus. Chlorothiazide and frusemide are common diuretics used. There has been concern that frusemide may promote delayed ductus closure in infants with respiratory distress syndrome,[2,6] although the concurrent use of frusemide does not seem to inhibit closure during treatment with indomethacin[7] and may reduce adverse renal effects of indomethacin.[7,8] Indomethacin probably leads to closure of the ductus through inhibition of prostaglandin synthesis. It is usually given intravenously as the sodium salt. The current practice is to give 3 doses at intervals of usually 12 to 24 hours with the amount depending on the age of the neonate. Indomethacin has been given by mouth where the injection is unavailable, but absorption of oral indomethacin is poor and incomplete in premature neonates. A second course of injections may be given 48 hours after the first course if the ductus remains open or has re-opened. Should that fail (which may be the case in 25% of infants treated[1,9]) then surgery is required.

Several studies have investigated whether prolonged maintenance therapy would result in more effective closure of the patent ductus arteriosus and thereby decrease the recurrence rate. One study[10] demonstrated a decreased need for surgical closure and reduced recurrences in neonates treated with standard intravenous indomethacin therapy followed by maintenance therapy (intravenous indomethacin 200 µg per kg body-weight per day for an additional 5 days) compared with infants treated with standard indomethacin therapy. Similar beneficial findings were reported[11] in infants given prolonged low-dose indomethacin therapy (100 µg per kg per day for 6 days) compared with infants given standard indomethacin therapy. An additional benefit was a lower incidence of adverse effects; fewer infants experienced a rise in serum creatinine or urea concentrations. Prophylactic administration of indomethacin has been found to be of benefit,[5,12,13] but more data are needed on the incidence of possible adverse effects and neurodevelopmental outcomes before routine use of this strategy can be recommended.[13] Although prophylactic therapy reduces the chance of developing a symptomatic patent ductus arteriosus, there does not appear to be any additional advantage in reducing the risk of some morbidities in comparison with early symptomatic treatment.[5]

Ibuprofen also appears to be effective in closing a patent ductus arteriosus,[14-17] and it has been suggested that ibuprofen might be a better choice than indomethacin as, unlike indomethacin, it does not have adverse effects on renal and cerebral haemodynamics and oxygenation.[14,15,17] However, some workers[18] found that when indomethacin was given by continuous intravenous infusion, rather than by rapid injection, the usual fall in cerebral blood flow velocity was avoided.

1. Silove ED. Pharmacological manipulation of the ductus arteriosus. *Arch Dis Child* 1986; **61:** 827–9.
2. Bhatt V, Nahata MC. Pharmacologic management of patent ductus arteriosus. *Clin Pharm* 1989; **8:** 17–33.
3. Barst RJ, Gersony WM. The pharmacological treatment of patent ductus arteriosus: a review of the evidence. *Drugs* 1989; **38:** 249–66.
4. Archer N. Patent ductus arteriosus in the newborn. *Arch Dis Child* 1993; **69:** 529–32.
5. Clyman RI. Recommendations for the postnatal use of indomethacin: an analysis of four separate treatment strategies. *J Pediatr* 1996; **128:** 601–7.
6. Anonymous. Delayed closure of the ductus. *Lancet* 1983; **ii:** 436.
7. Yeh TF, *et al.* Furosemide prevents the renal side effects of indomethacin therapy in premature infants with patent ductus arteriosus. *J Pediatr* 1982; **101:** 433–7.
8. Nahata MC, *et al.* Furosemide can prevent decline in urine output in infants receiving indomethacin for patent ductus closure: a multidose study. *Infusion* 1988; **12:** 11–12 and 15.
9. Gersony WM, *et al.* Effects of indomethacin in premature infants with patent ductus arteriosus: results of a national collaborative study. *J Pediatr* 1983; **102:** 895–906.
10. Hammerman C, Aramburo MJ. Prolonged indomethacin therapy for the prevention of recurrences of patent ductus arteriosus. *J Pediatr* 1990; **117:** 771–6.
11. Rennie JM, Cooke RWI. Prolonged low dose indomethacin for persistent ductus arteriosus of prematurity. *Arch Dis Child* 1991; **66:** 55–8.
12. Couser RJ, *et al.* Prophylactic indomethacin therapy in the first twenty-four hours of life for the prevention of patent ductus arteriosus in preterm infants treated prophylactically with surfactant in the delivery room. *J Pediatr* 1996; **128:** 631–7.
13. Fowlie PW. Prophylactic indomethacin: systematic review and meta-analysis. *Arch Dis Child* 1996; **74:** F81–F87.
14. Patel J, *et al.* Ibuprofen treatment of patent ductus arteriosus. *Lancet* 1995; **346:** 255.
15. Van Overmeire B, *et al.* Treatment of patent ductus arteriosus with ibuprofen. *Arch Dis Child* 1997; **76:** F179–F184.
16. Varvarigou A, *et al.* Early ibuprofen administration to prevent patent ductus arteriosus in premature newborn infants. *JAMA* 1996; **275:** 539–44.
17. Mosca F, *et al.* Comparative evaluation of the effects of indomethacin and ibuprofen on cerebral perfusion and oxygenation in preterm infants with patent ductus arteriosus. *J Pediatr* 1997; **131:** 549–54.
18. Hammerman C, *et al.* Continuous versus multiple rapid infusions of indomethacin: effects on cerebral blood flow velocity. *Pediatrics* 1995; **95:** 244–8.

Polyhydramnios. Reports[1,2] of the beneficial effects of indomethacin in the management of polyhydramnios (an excessive accumulation of amniotic fluid).

1. Kirshon B, *et al.* Indomethacin therapy in the treatment of symptomatic polyhydramnios. *Obstet Gynecol* 1990; **75:** 202–5.
2. Ash K, *et al.* TRAP sequence—successful outcome with indomethacin treatment. *Obstet Gynecol* 1990; **76:** 960–2.

Premature labour. The most common approach to postponing premature labour (p.760) with drugs is with a selective beta agonist. However, as prostaglandins have a role in uterine contraction and cervical ripening and dilatation, prostaglandin synthetase inhibitors such as indomethacin have also been used. Comparative studies[1,2] have demonstrated that indomethacin and ritodrine are equally effective in inhibiting uterine contractions and delaying delivery in patients in preterm labour who have intact membranes and in whom the gestational age is less than or equal to 34 weeks. In one study[2] an initial oral loading dose of indomethacin 50 mg was given, followed by 25 to 50 mg orally every 4 hours until contractions stopped and then by a maintenance dose of 25 mg every 4 to 6 hours. In the other comparative study[1] indomethacin was given as a 100-mg rectal suppository followed by 25 mg orally every 4 hours for 48 hours; if regular uterine contractions persisted 1 to 2 hours after the initial suppository, an additional 100-mg suppository was given before beginning oral therapy. Terbutaline was given for maintenance therapy.

Unfortunately indomethacin can adversely affect the fetus and whether the risk is increased the earlier it is used in gestation is not clear. One study, for example, indicated an increased risk at or before 30 weeks' gestation[3] while another did not.[1] Reported adverse effects include: transient constriction of the ductus arteriosus,[4,5] pulmonary hypertension,[2] bronchopulmonary dysplasia,[6] reduced volume of amniotic fluid (oligohydramnios)[2,5] and possible renal damage.[7] As a result of the risks associated with indomethacin it is generally reserved as a second-line tocolytic or for combination with an intravenous tocolytic[8] when an additive effect is required at very early gestation.

1. Morales WJ, *et al.* Efficacy and safety of indomethacin versus ritodrine in the management of preterm labor: a randomized study. *Obstet Gynecol* 1989; **74:** 567–72.
2. Besinger RE, *et al.* Randomized comparative trial of indomethacin and ritodrine for the long-term treatment of preterm labor. *Am J Obstet Gynecol* 1991; **164:** 981–8.
3. Norton ME, *et al.* Neonatal complications after the administration of indomethacin for preterm labor. *N Engl J Med* 1993; **329:** 1602–7.

4. Moise KJ, *et al.* Indomethacin in the treatment of premature labor: effects on the fetal ductus arteriosus. *N Engl J Med* 1988; **319:** 327–31.
5. Hallak M, *et al.* Indomethacin for preterm labor: fetal toxicity in a dizygotic twin gestation. *Obstet Gynecol* 1991; **78:** 911–13.
6. Eronen M, *et al.* Increased incidence of bronchopulmonary dysplasia after antenatal administration of indomethacin to prevent preterm labor. *J Pediatr* 1994; **124:** 782–8.
7. van der Heijden BJ, *et al.* Persistent anuria, neonatal death, and renal microcystic lesions after prenatal exposure to indomethacin. *Am J Obstet Gynecol* 1994; **171:** 617–23.
8. Johnson P. Suppression of preterm labour: current concepts. *Drugs* 1993; **45:** 684–92.

Preparations

BP 1998: Indometacin Capsules; Indometacin Suppositories;
USP 23: Indomethacin Capsules; Indomethacin Extended-release Capsules; Indomethacin for Injection; Indomethacin Oral Suspension; Indomethacin Suppositories.

Proprietary Preparations (details are given in Part 3)
Aust.: Flexidin; Gaurit; Indocid; Indocollyre; Indohexal; Indomelan; Indoptol; Liometacen; Luiflex; Ralicid; ***Austral.:*** Arthrexin; Hicin; Indocid; Indocid PDA; Indomed; Indoptol; Indospray; ***Belg.:*** Dolcidium†; Indocid; Indoptol; Luiflex; ***Canad.:*** Indocid; Indocid PDA; Indocollyre; Indotec; Novo-Methacin; Nu-Indo; Rhodacine; ***Fr.:*** Ainscrid; Chrono-Indocid; Indocid; Indocollyre; ***Ger.:*** Amuno; Amuno M†; Chibro-Amuno 3; Confortid; durametacin†; Elmetacin; Indo; Indo Top; Indo-paed; Indo-Phlogont; Indo-Tablinen; Indocontin; Indomet-ratiopharm; Indomisal; Indorektal; Inflam; Jenacin; Mobilat; Rheubalmin Indo; Sigadoc; Vonum†; ***Irl.:*** Cidomel; Flexin Continus; Idomed; Imbrilon; Indocid; Indocid PDA; Indomod; ***Ital.:*** Boutycin†; Cidalgon†; Imet; Indocid; Indocollirio; Indom Collirio; Indoxen; Liometacen; Metacen; Peralgon†; ***Jpn:*** Infree; Inteban†; ***Neth.:*** Dolazol†; Dometin†; Indocid; Indocid PDA; Indoptol; ***Norw.:*** Confortid; Indocid; ***S.Afr.:*** Acuflex; Aflamin; Arthrexin; Articulen; Betacin; Dynametcin†; Elmetacin; Famethacin; Flamaret; Flamecid; Indocid; Indoflam†; Indoflex†; Indomed†; Indotal†; Mediflex; Methabid†; Methamax; Methocaps; Nisaid-25; Restameth-SR; Rumitard†; ***Spain:*** Aliviosin; Artrinovo; Butidil†; Flogoter; Inacid; Indo Framan; Indocaf; Indoftol; Indolgina; Indonilo; Mederreumol; Neo Decabutin; Reumo; Reusin; ***Swed.:*** Confortid; Indomee; ***Switz.:*** Bonidon; Confortid†; Elmetacin; Helvecin; Indo-Mepha; Indocid; Indophtal; Indoptic; Servimeta†; ***UK:*** Artracin; Flexin Continus; Imbrilon; Indocid; Indocid PDA; Indolar SR; Indomax; Indomod; Indotard; Maximet SR; Mobilan†; Pardelprin; Rheumacin; Rimacid; Slo-Indo; ***USA:*** Indochron; Indocin.

Multi-ingredient: ***Aust.:*** Vonum; ***Ger.:*** Inflam; Vonum cutan†; ***Ital.:*** Difmetre; Solitacina†; ***Spain:*** Artri; Artrivia Prednisolona†; Betartrinovo; Combiflexona†; Fiacin; Indosolona†; Ramatocina†; ***Switz.:*** Ralur.

Isamfazone (5131-t)

Isamfazone *(rINN)*.

Pir-353. (−)-*N*-Methyl-*N*-(α-methylphenethyl)-6-oxo-3-phenyl-1(6*H*)-pyridazineacetamide.

$C_{22}H_{23}N_3O_2$ = 361.4.

CAS — 55902-02-8.

Isamfazone is an NSAID (p.63) that was used for the symptomatic treatment of musculoskeletal, joint, and peri-articular disorders and to reduce fever.

Preparations

Proprietary Preparations (details are given in Part 3)

Multi-ingredient: ***Spain:*** Combiflexona†; Frenespan†.

Isonixin (12870-d)

Isonixin *(rINN)*.

2-Hydroxy-*N*-(2,6-dimethylphenyl)nicotinamide.

$C_{14}H_{14}N_2O_2$ = 242.3.

CAS — 57021-61-1.

Isonixin is an NSAID (p.63) that has been used in the management of pain and inflammation associated with musculoskeletal and joint disorders. Isonixin has been used in doses of 400 mg two to four times daily by mouth or by rectal suppository. It has also been applied topically as a 2.5% cream.

Preparations

Proprietary Preparations (details are given in Part 3)
Spain: Nixyn.

Multi-ingredient: ***Spain:*** Nixyn.

Kebuzone (2661-r)

Kebuzone *(pINN)*.

Ketophenylbutazone. 4-(3-Oxobutyl)-1,2-diphenylpyrazolidine-3,5-dione.

$C_{19}H_{18}N_2O_3$ = 322.4.

CAS — 853-34-9.

Kebuzone, a phenylbutazone derivative, is an NSAID (p.63). It has been used in musculoskeletal, joint, and soft-tissue disorders in doses of up to 1.5 g daily in divided doses by mouth. Kebuzone has also been given as the sodium salt by intramuscular injection in doses equivalent to 1 g of base.

Porphyria. Kebuzone was considered to be unsafe in patients with acute porphyria because it has been shown to be porphyrinogenic in *animals* or *in-vitro* systems.[1]

1. Moore MR, McColl KEL. *Porphyria: drug lists.* Glasgow: Porphyria Research Unit, University of Glasgow, 1991.

Preparations

Proprietary Preparations (details are given in Part 3)
Aust.: Ketazon; ***Ger.:*** Ketazon; ***Ital.:*** Chetopir†.

Multi-ingredient: ***Aust.:*** Rheumesser.

Ketobemidone (6234-e)

Ketobemidone *(BAN, rINN)*.

Cetobemidone. 1-(4-*m*-Hydroxyphenyl-1-methyl-4-piperidyl)propan-1-one.

$C_{15}H_{21}NO_2$ = 247.3.

CAS — 469-79-4.

Ketobemidone is an opioid analgesic (p.67). It has been given as the hydrochloride by mouth, by injection, or rectally, sometimes with an antispasmodic; the usual dose has been 5 to 10 mg.

References.

1. Anderson P, *et al.* Clinical pharmacokinetics of ketobemidone: its bioavailability after rectal administration. *Eur J Clin Pharmacol* 1981; **19:** 217–23.

Preparations

Proprietary Preparations (details are given in Part 3)
Norw.: Ketorax; ***Swed.:*** Ketodur; Ketogan Novum.

Multi-ingredient: ***Norw.:*** Ketogan; ***Swed.:*** Ketogan.

Ketoprofen (2662-f)

Ketoprofen *(BAN, USAN, rINN)*.

Ketoprofenum; RP-19583. *(RS)*-2-(3-Benzoylphenyl)propionic acid.

$C_{16}H_{14}O_3$ = 254.3.

CAS — 22071-15-4 (ketoprofen); 57469-78-0 (ketoprofen lysine); 57495-14-4 (ketoprofen sodium); 22161-81-5 (dexketoprofen).

Pharmacopoeias. In *Eur.* (see p.viii), *Jpn*, and *US.*

A white or almost white, crystalline powder. M.p. 92° to 97°. Practically **insoluble** in water; freely soluble in alcohol, in acetone, and in dichloromethane. **Store** in airtight containers.

Adverse Effects and Precautions

As for NSAIDs in general, p.63.

When ketoprofen is administered intramuscularly there may be pain at the injection site and occasionally tissue damage. Ketoprofen suppositories may cause local irritation.

Effects on the pancreas. A report of pancreatitis associated with ketoprofen.[1]

1. Cobb TK, Pierce JR. Acute pancreatitis associated with ketoprofen. *South Med J* 1992; **85:** 430–1.

Hypersensitivity. Life-threatening asthma, urticaria, and angioedema developed in 2 aspirin-sensitive patients after taking ketoprofen 50 mg by mouth.[1] Cardiac and respiratory arrest occurred in an asthmatic patient shortly after taking ketoprofen.[2]

There has been a report[3] of delayed skin hypersensitivity in a patient who used a topical gel containing ketoprofen. The reaction recurred on rechallenge to ketoprofen gel but not to a similar gel containing diclofenac. The authors of the report noted that the UK Committee on Safety of Medicines had received 15 reports of skin reactions to ketoprofen gel, including two each of dermatitis and urticaria.

1. Frith P, *et al.* Life-threatening asthma, urticaria, and angiœdema after ketoprofen. *Lancet* 1978; **ii:** 847–8.
2. Schreuder G. Ketoprofen: possible idiosyncratic acute bronchospasm. *Med J Aust* 1990; **152:** 332–3.
3. Oh VMS. Ketoprofen gel and delayed hypersensitivity dermatitis. *Br Med J* 1994; **309:** 512.

Myasthenia gravis. There has been a brief report[1] of a single dose of ketoprofen 50 mg by mouth precipitating a cholinergic crisis in a patient with well-controlled myasthenia gravis. The patient had previously noted a similar but milder reaction with aspirin, but not with paracetamol.

1. McDowell IFW, McConnell JB. Cholinergic crisis in myasthenia gravis precipitated by ketoprofen. *Br Med J* 1985; **291:** 1094.

Photosensitivity. Ketoprofen has been reported to cause photosensitivity reactions.[1]

1. Anonymous. Drugs that cause photosensitivity. *Med Lett Drugs Ther* 1986; **28:** 51–2.

Renal impairment. The elimination half-life and unbound plasma concentrations of the *(S)*-enantiomer of ketoprofen are increased in patients with impaired renal function;[1] this appears to be principally attributable to impaired renal clearance of the acyl-glucuronide conjugates in a stereoselective fashion, with subsequent hydrolysis of the unstable conjugate back to the aglycone producing increased plasma-ketoprofen concentrations.[2] It has been suggested[2] that dosage adjustments are indicated only for patients with moderately severe renal failure (creatinine clearance of less than 20 mL per minute).

1. Hayball PJ, *et al.* The influence of renal function on the enantioselective pharmacokinetics and pharmacodynamics of ketoprofen in patients with rheumatoid arthritis. *Br J Clin Pharmacol* 1993; **36:** 185–93.
2. Skeith KJ, *et al.* The influence of renal function on the pharmacokinetics of unchanged and acyl-glucuroconjugated ketoprofen enantiomers after 50 and 100 mg racemic ketoprofen. *Br J Clin Pharmacol* 1996; **42:** 163–9.

Interactions

For interactions associated with NSAIDs, see p.65. Probenecid delays the excretion of ketoprofen and decreases its extent of protein binding resulting in increased plasma-ketoprofen concentrations.

Pharmacokinetics

Ketoprofen is readily absorbed from the gastro-intestinal tract; peak plasma concentrations occur about 0.5 to 2 hours after a dose. When ketoprofen is given with food, the bioavailability is not altered but the rate of absorption is slowed. Ketoprofen is well absorbed from the intramuscular and rectal routes; only a small amount of ketoprofen is absorbed following topical application. Ketoprofen is 99% bound to plasma proteins and substantial concentrations of drug are found in the synovial fluid. The elimination half-life in plasma is about 1.5 to 4 hours. Ketoprofen is metabolised mainly by conjugation with glucuronic acid, and is excreted mainly in the urine.

Ketoprofen possesses a chiral centre. It is usually given as the racemate but its pharmacological actions appear to be due largely to the *(S)*-enantiomer, dexketoprofen. The pharmacokinetics of ketoprofen appear to exhibit little stereoselectivity (but see under Renal Impairment, above).

References.

1. Debruyne D, *et al.* Clinical pharmacokinetics of ketoprofen after single intravenous administration as a bolus or infusion. *Clin Pharmacokinet* 1987; **12:** 214–21.
2. Flouvat B, *et al.* Pharmacokinetics of ketoprofen in man after repeated percutaneous administration. *Arzneimittelforschung* 1989; **39:** 812–15.
3. Jamali F, Brocks DR. Clinical pharmacokinetics of ketoprofen and its enantiomers. *Clin Pharmacokinet* 1990; **19:** 197–217.
4. Geisslinger G, *et al.* Pharmacokinetics of ketoprofen enantiomers after different doses of the racemate. *Br J Clin Pharmacol* 1995; **40;** 73–5.

Uses and Administration

Ketoprofen, a propionic acid derivative, is an NSAID (p.65). Its anti-inflammatory properties may be weaker than those of some other NSAIDs.

Ketoprofen is used in musculoskeletal and joint disorders such as ankylosing spondylitis, osteoarthritis, and rheumatoid arthritis, and in peri-articular disorders such as bursitis and tendinitis. It is also used in dysmenorrhoea, postoperative pain, in painful and inflammatory conditions such as acute gout or soft-tissue disorders, and to reduce fever.

In the treatment of rheumatic disorders a usual daily dose of ketoprofen by mouth is 100 to 200 mg in 2 to 4 divided doses; modified-release formulations taken once daily may also be used. In the USA some manufacturers suggest an initial oral doses of 75 mg three times daily or 50 mg four times daily increased as needed to a maximum of 300 mg daily in divided doses. Ketoprofen may also be administered rectally as suppositories in a usual dose of 100 mg at night. The total daily combined dose by mouth and by rectum should not exceed 200 mg. The dose by mouth for the treatment of other painful conditions including dysmenorrhoea is 25 to 50 mg every 6 to 8 hours.

Ketoprofen may be given by deep intramuscular injection into the gluteal muscle for acute exacerbations of musculoskeletal, joint, peri-articular and soft-tissue disorders and in the management of pain following orthopaedic surgery. Doses of 50 to 100 mg may be given every 4 hours, up to a maximum dose of 200 mg in 24 hours for up to 3 days. Ketoprofen is also applied as a 2.5% gel 2 to 4 times daily for up to 7 days for local pain relief.

Ketoprofen has also been used as the lysine and as the sodium salt.

Ketoprofen is usually administered as a racemic mixture but preparations containing only the S(+)-isomer (dexketoprofen) are available in some countries.

Reviews.

1. Mauleón D, *et al.* Preclinical and clinical development of dexketoprofen. *Drugs* 1996; **52:** 24–46.

Preparations

BP 1998: Ketoprofen Capsules.

Proprietary Preparations (details are given in Part 3)
Aust.: Actron; Keprodol; Profenid; Toprek; ***Austral.:*** Orudis; Oruvail; ***Belg.:*** Birofenid; Fastum; Rofenid; Toprek; ***Canad.:*** Apo-Keto; Novo-Keto; Orafen; Orudis; Oruvail; Rhodis; Rhovail; ***Fr.:*** Bi-Profenid; Ketum; Profenid; Topfena; Toprec; ***Ger.:*** Alrheumun; europan†; Gabrilen; Orudis; Spondylon; ***Irl.:*** Alrheumat†; Orudis; Orugesic; Oruvail; ***Ital.:*** Artrosilene; Dexal†; Fastum; Flexen; Iso-K†; Kefenid†; Ketalgin†; Ketartrium; Keto†; Ketodol; Ketofen; Meprofen; Oki; Orudis; Profenil†; Reuprofen; Salient†; Sinketol; Toprek; Zepelindue; ***Neth.:*** Orudis; Oscorel; ***Norw.:*** Orudis; ***S.Afr.:*** Fastum; Ketoflam; Myproflam; Orucote; Orudis†; Oruject; Oruvail; ***Spain:*** Arcental; Extraplus; Fastum; Ketosolan; Orudis; Reumoquin; ***Swed.:*** Orudis; Prodon; ***Switz.:*** Fastum; Orudis; Profenid†; ***UK:*** Alrheumat†; Fenoket; Jomethid; Ketil; Ketocid; Ketovail†; Ketozip; Larafen; Orudis; Oruvail; Powergel; Solpaflex; ***USA:*** Actron; Orudis; Oruvail.

Ketorolac Trometamol (16867-j)

Ketorolac Trometamol *(BANM, rINNM).*

Ketorolac Tromethamine *(USAN)*; RS-37619-00-31-3. (±)-5-Benzoyl-2,3-dihydro-1*H*-pyrrolizine-1-carboxylic acid compound with 2-amino-2-(hydroxymethyl)-1,3-propanediol (1 : 1).

$C_{19}H_{24}N_2O_6$ = 376.4.

CAS — 74103-06-3 (ketorolac); 74103-07-4 (ketorolac trometamol).

Pharmacopoeias. In US.

A white to off-white, crystalline powder. Freely **soluble** in water and in methyl alcohol; slightly soluble in alcohol and in tetrahydrofuran; practically insoluble in acetone, in acetonitrile, in butyl alcohol, in dichloromethane, in dioxan, in ethyl acetate, in hexane, and in toluene. A 1% solution in water has a pH between 5.7 and 6.7. **Store** in airtight containers and protect from light.

Adverse Effects

As for NSAIDs in general, p.63.

Concern over the high incidence of reported adverse effects with ketorolac trometamol has led to its withdrawal from the market in some countries while in others its permitted dosage and maximum duration of treatment has been reduced. Adverse effects reported include gastro-intestinal disturbances including gastro-intestinal bleeding (especially in the elderly), perforation, and peptic ulceration. Hypersensitivity reactions such as anaphylaxis, rash, bronchospasm, laryngeal oedema, and hypotension have also occurred. Other adverse effects reported include drowsiness, dizziness, headache, mental and sensory changes, sweating, dry mouth, thirst, fever, convulsions, myalgia, aseptic meningitis, hypertension, dyspnoea, pulmonary oedema, bradycardia, fluid retention, increases in blood urea and creatinine, acute renal failure, hyponatraemia, hyperkalaemia, urinary frequency or retention, nephrotic syndrome, flank pain with or without haematuria, purpura, thrombocytopenia, epistaxis, inhibition of platelet aggregation, increased bleeding time, postoperative wound haemorrhage, haematoma, flushing or pallor, and pancreatitis. Severe skin reactions including Stevens-Johnson syndrome and Lyell's syndrome have been reported. Liver function changes may occur; hepatitis and liver failure have been reported. There may be pain at the site of injection.

Adverse effects reported with ketorolac are mainly those common to all NSAIDs with gastro-intestinal reactions being the most frequent followed by haematological, renal, hypersensitivity, and then neurological reactions. Since the launch of ketorolac in 1990, 97 reactions with a fatal outcome have been reported worldwide.[1] The causes of death were as follows: gastro-intestinal bleeding or perforation (47 cases); renal impairment or insufficiency (20); anaphylaxis or asthma (7); haemorrhagic reactions (4); and unexplained or miscellaneous causes (19). Concern over the safety of ketorolac has led to adverse reactions being monitored closely and to the implementation of restrictions on dose and duration of treatment (see under Uses and Administration, below). A postmarketing surveillance study,[2] led by Dr B Strom for the US manufacturer, has examined the risks of parenteral ketorolac in 9 900 patients who received 10 272 courses of ketorolac. Gastro-intestinal bleeding and operative site bleeding were expected to be the major risks of ketorolac, and were the major foci of this study. The results of the study indicated a dose-response relationship with average daily ketorolac dose for both gastro-intestinal bleeding and operative site bleeding, and an association with duration of therapy beyond 5 days for gastro-intestinal bleeding. The risk of serious gastro-intestinal bleeding and operative site bleeding was higher for elderly patients [the manufacturer recommends that the elderly should not receive daily doses greater than 60 mg]. Although the overall associations between ketorolac use and both gastro-intestinal bleeding and operative site bleeding are small, the risk becomes clinically important as doses increase, in elderly patients, and, for gastro-intestinal bleeding only, when used for longer than 5 days. The US manufacturer has consequently emphasised that ketorolac is a potent NSAID and is indicated only for the short-term management of moderate to severe pain and not for minor or chronic painful conditions; its administration carries many risks and related adverse effects can be serious especially when used inappropriately. After examining data from the Strom study the EU Committee for Proprietary Medicinal Products adopted the opinion that ketorolac had a narrow therapeutic margin but that it was indicated for the short-term management of moderate to severe acute postoperative pain.

Further references to ketorolac's adverse effects are given below.[3-11]

1. Committee on Safety of Medicines/Medicines Control Agency. Ketorolac: new restrictions on dose and duration of treatment. *Current Problems* 1993; **19:** 5–6.
2. Strom BL, *et al.* Parenteral ketorolac and risk of gastrointestinal and operative site bleeding: a postmarketing surveillance study. *JAMA* 1996; **275:** 376–82.
3. Rotenberg FA, Giannini VS. Hyperkalemia associated with ketorolac. *Ann Pharmacother* 1992; **26:** 778–9.
4. Boras-Uber LA, Brackett NC. Ketorolac-induced acute renal failure. *Am J Med* 1992; **92:** 450–2. Correction *ibid.*; **93:** 117.
5. Schoch PH, *et al.* Acute renal failure in an elderly woman following intramuscular ketorolac administration. *Ann Pharmacother* 1992; **26:** 1233–6.
6. Goetz CM, *et al.* Anaphylactoid reaction following ketorolac tromethamine administration. *Ann Pharmacother* 1992; **26:** 1237–8.
7. Randi ML, *et al.* Haemolytic uraemic syndrome during treatment with ketorolac trometamol. *Br Med J* 1993; **306:** 186.
8. Fong J, Gora ML. Reversible renal insufficiency following ketorolac therapy. *Ann Pharmacother* 1993; **27:** 510–12.
9. Corelli RL, Gericke KR. Renal insufficiency associated with intramuscular administration of ketorolac tromethamine. *Ann Pharmacother* 1993; **27:** 1055–7.
10. Buck ML, Norwood VF. Ketorolac-induced acute renal failure in a previously healthy adolescent. *Pediatrics* 1996; **98:** 294–6.
11. Feldman HI, *et al.* Parenteral ketorolac: the risk for acute renal failure. *Ann Intern Med* 1997; **126:** 193–9.

Precautions

As for NSAIDs in general, p.65.

In light of the concern over the toxicity of ketorolac it has been recommended that ketorolac should not be used during pregnancy or labour and that it should not be given to mothers who are breast feeding.

Ketorolac is contra-indicated in patients with a history of hypersensitivity to aspirin or other NSAIDs, a history of asthma, nasal polyps, bronchospasm, or angioedema, a history of peptic ulceration or gastro-intestinal bleeding, in patients with moderate or severe renal impairment, and in those with hypovolaemia or dehydration. The dose of ketorolac should be reduced in the elderly and in patients weighing less than 50 kg. It is recommended that patients with mild renal impairment should receive a reduced dose of ketorolac and undergo close monitoring of renal function. Ketorolac should be used with caution in heart failure, hepatic impairment and other conditions leading to reduction in blood volume or in renal blood flow. Ketorolac should be withdrawn if clinical symptoms of liver disease develop. Ketorolac should not be given to patients with coagulation or haemorrhagic disorders or those with confirmed or suspected cerebrovascular bleeding. It is contra-indicated as a prophylactic analgesic before surgery and for intraoperative use; it should not be given postoperatively to those who have undergone procedures with a high risk of haemorrhage.

Dizziness may affect the performance of skilled tasks such as driving.

Interactions

For interactions associated with NSAIDs, see p.65.

Ketorolac should not be given to patients already receiving anticoagulants or to those who will require prophylactic anticoagulant therapy, including low-dose heparin. The risk of ketorolac-associated bleeding is increased by other NSAIDs or aspirin and by oxpentifylline and concomitant use should be avoided. Probenecid increases the half-life and plasma concentrations of ketorolac and the two drugs should not be given together.

The manufacturer of acetylcholine chloride ophthalmic preparations has stated that there have been reports that acetylcholine and carbachol have been ineffective when used in patients treated with topical (ophthalmic) NSAIDs.

Pharmacokinetics

Ketorolac trometamol is absorbed following intramuscular or oral administration. At physiological pH ketorolac trometamol dissociates to form an anionic ketorolac molecule which is less hydrophilic than the trometamol salt. The peak plasma concentration of ketorolac is reached within about 30 to 60 minutes; absorption following intramuscular administration may be slower than that following oral administration in some individuals. Ketorolac is over 99% bound to plasma protein. It does not readily penetrate the blood-brain barrier. Ketorolac crosses the placenta and small amounts of drug are distributed into breast milk. The terminal plasma half-life is about 4 to 6 hours, but is about 6 to 7 hours in the elderly and 9 to 10 hours in patients with renal dysfunction. The major metabolic pathway is glucuronic acid conjugation; there is some *para*-hydroxylation. About 90% of a dose is excreted in urine as unchanged drug and conjugated and hydroxylated metabolites, the remainder is excreted in the faeces.

References.

1. Jung D, *et al.* Pharmacokinetics of ketorolac tromethamine in humans after intravenous, intramuscular and oral administration. *Eur J Clin Pharmacol* 1988; **35:** 423–5.
2. Wischnik A, *et al.* The excretion of ketorolac tromethamine into breast milk after multiple oral dosing. *Eur J Clin Pharmacol* 1989; **36:** 521–4.
3. Buckley M M-T, Brogden RN. Ketorolac: a review of its pharmacodynamic and pharmacokinetic properties, and therapeutic potential. *Drugs* 1990; **39:** 86–109.
4. Resman-Targoff BH. Ketorolac: a parenteral nonsteroidal anti-inflammatory drug. *DICP Ann Pharmacother* 1990; **24:** 1098–1104.
5. Jallad NS, *et al.* Pharmacokinetics of single-dose oral and intramuscular ketorolac tromethamine in the young and elderly. *J Clin Pharmacol* 1990; **30:** 76–81.
6. Olkkola KT, Maunuksela E-L. The pharmacokinetics of postoperative intravenous ketorolac tromethamine in children. *Br J Clin Pharmacol* 1991; **31:** 182–4.
7. Hayball PJ, *et al.* The pharmacokinetics of ketorolac enantiomers following intramuscular administration of the racemate. *Br J Clin Pharmacol* 1994; **37:** 75–8.
8. Brocks DR, Jamali F. Clinical pharmacokinetics of ketorolac tromethamine. *Clin Pharmacokinet* 1992; **23:** 415–27.

Uses and Administration

Ketorolac, a pyrrolizine carboxylic acid derivative structurally related to indomethacin (p.46), is an NSAID (p.65). It is used principally as an analgesic.

Ketorolac is used intramuscularly, intravenously, or orally as the trometamol salt in the short-term management of moderate to severe postoperative pain. However, it should be noted that because of concerns over the high incidence of reported adverse effects with ketorolac its dosage and maximum duration of use are restricted. In the UK the recommended initial dose by the parenteral route is 10 mg of ketorolac trometamol followed by 10 to 30 mg every 4 to 6 hours as required, although ketorolac may be given as often as every 2 hours in the initial postoperative period if required. The total maximum daily dose is 90 mg (60 mg in the elderly, patients with mild renal impairment, and in those weighing less than 50 kg). Intravenous injections should be administered over at least 15 seconds. The recommended maximum duration for parenteral therapy is 2 days and patients should be transferred to oral therapy as soon as possible. During transfer from parenteral to oral therapy the combined daily dose on the day of converting for all forms of ketorolac trometamol should not exceed 90 mg (60 mg in the elderly, patients with mild renal impairment, and in those weighing less than 50 kg) of which no more than 40 mg should be given orally. The recommended oral dose in the UK is 10 mg every 4 to 6 hours (every 6 to 8 hours in the elderly) to a maximum of 40 mg daily for a maximum duration of 7 days. In the USA it is recommended that the maximum combined duration of use of parenteral and oral ketorolac should not exceed 5 days.

Ketorolac trometamol is also used as 0.5% eye drops to relieve ocular itching associated with seasonal allergic conjunctivitis. Ketorolac trometamol eye drops 0.5% have also been used for the topical treatment of cystoid macular oedema and for the prevention and reduction of inflammation associated with ocular surgery.

Reviews.

1. Gillis JC, Brogden RN. Ketorolac: a reappraisal of its pharmacodynamic and pharmacokinetic properties and therapeutic use in pain management. *Drugs* 1997; **53:** 139–88.

Preparations

USP 23: Ketorolac Tromethamine Injection; Ketorolac Tromethamine Tablets.

Proprietary Preparations (details are given in Part 3)
Austral.: Toradol; ***Belg.:*** Aculare; Taradyl; ***Canad.:*** Acular; Toradol; ***Fr.:*** Tora-Dol†; ***Ger.:*** Acular; ***Irl.:*** Acular; ***Ital.:*** Acular; Lixidol; Tora-Dol; ***Neth.:*** Acular†; ***Norw.:*** Toradol; ***S.Afr.:*** Acular; Tora-Dol; ***Spain:*** Droal; Tonum; Toradol; ***Swed.:*** Toradol; ***Switz.:*** Tora-Dol; ***UK:*** Acular; Toradol; ***USA:*** Acular; Toradol.

Lefetamine Hydrochloride (19403-g)

Lefetamine Hydrochloride *(rINNM).*

(−)-*N*,*N*-Dimethyl-1,2-diphenylethylamine hydrochloride.

$C_{16}H_{19}N,HCl$ = 261.8.

CAS — 7262-75-1 (lefetamine); 14148-99-3 (lefetamine hydrochloride).

Lefetamine hydrochloride has analgesic properties and has been given by mouth, by rectal suppository, and by intramuscular or subcutaneous injection.

Preparations

Proprietary Preparations (details are given in Part 3)
Ital.: Santenol.

Levomethadone Hydrochloride (9871-a)

Levomethadone Hydrochloride *(rINNM).*

(−)-Methadone Hydrochloride. (−)-6-Dimethylamino-4,4-diphenylheptan-3-one hydrochloride.

$C_{21}H_{27}NO,HCl$ = 345.9.

CAS — 125-58-6 (levomethadone); 5967-73-7 (levomethadone hydrochloride).

Levomethadone is an opioid analgesic (p.67). It is the active isomer of racemic methadone (p.53) and is used similarly as the hydrochloride in the treatment of severe pain.

References.

1. Olsen GD, *et al.* Clinical effects and pharmacokinetics of racemic methadone and its optical isomers. *Clin Pharmacol Ther* 1977; **21:** 147–57.

Preparations

Proprietary Preparations (details are given in Part 3)
Ger.: L-Polamidon.

Levomethadyl Acetate (6235-l)

Levomethadyl Acetate *(USAN).*

Levacetylmethadol *(rINN)*; *l*-α-Acetylmethadol; LAAM; LAM; *l*-Methadyl Acetate. (−)-4-Dimethylamino-1-ethyl-2,2-diphenylpentyl acetate.

$C_{23}H_{31}NO_2$ = 353.5.

CAS — 1477-40-3 (levomethadyl); 34433-66-4 (levomethadyl acetate); 43033-72-3 (levomethadyl acetate hydrochloride).

NOTE. Levomethadyl Acetate Hydrochloride is *USAN.*

Dependence and Withdrawal, Adverse Effects, Treatment, and Precautions

As for Opioid Analgesics in general, p.67.

As it may take 2 to 3 days before the effects of levomethadyl acetate become apparent after intravenous injection its potential for abuse is considered to be very low.

Interactions

For interactions associated with opioid analgesics, see p.69.

Pharmacokinetics

Levomethadyl acetate is absorbed from the gastro-intestinal tract. It has a slow onset and long duration of action. It is metabolised to compounds which have morphine-like activity and a long half-life. The metabolites *l*-α-noracetylmethadol and *l*-α-dinoracetylmethadol have been identified in plasma while methadol and normethadol have been identified in urine.

References.

1. Kaiko RF, Inturrisi CE. Disposition of acetylmethadol in relation to pharmacologic action. *Clin Pharmacol Ther* 1975; **18:** 96–103.
2. Henderson GL, *et al.* Plasma l-α-acetylmethadol (LAAM) after acute and chronic administration. *Clin Pharmacol Ther* 1977; **21:** 16–25.

Uses and Administration

Levomethadyl acetate, a diphenylheptane derivative, is an opioid analgesic (p.69). It is a derivative of methadone (p.54) and has been used similarly in the management of opioid dependence. The longer duration of action of levomethadyl acetate allows intermittent administration and it is given as the hydrochloride by mouth three times a week or on alternate days as maintenance treatment. However, it has a slow onset of action and supplements of other short-acting opiates or a non-opioid withdrawal suppressant may be required to prevent withdrawal symptoms during the first three days of treatment.

Initial doses range from 20 to 40 mg with increments of 5 to 10 mg being given at 48- or 72-hour intervals until an acceptable maintenance dose is achieved which should generally not exceed 140 mg.

References.

1. Eissenberg T, *et al.* Dose-related efficacy of levomethadyl acetate for treatment of opioid dependence: a randomized clinical trial. *JAMA* 1997; **277:** 1945–51.

Preparations

Proprietary Preparations (details are given in Part 3)
USA: ORLAAM.

Levorphanol Tartrate (6236-y)

Levorphanol Tartrate *(BANM, rINNM).*

Levorphan Tartrate; Levorphanol Bitartrate; Methorphinan Tartrate. (−)-9a-Methylmorphinan-3-ol hydrogen tartrate dihydrate.

$C_{17}H_{23}NO,C_4H_6O_6,2H_2O$ = 443.5.

CAS — 77-07-6 (levorphanol); 125-72-4 (levorphanol tartrate, anhydrous); 5985-38-6 (levorphanol tartrate dihydrate).

Pharmacopoeias. In *It.* and *US.*

Practically white odourless crystalline powder. **Soluble** 1 in 50 of water and 1 in 120 of alcohol; insoluble in chloroform and in ether.

Levorphanol tartrate, a phenanthrene derivative, is a potent opioid analgesic (p.67) used in the management of moderate to severe pain and for premedication. The analgesic effect usually begins about 10 to 60 minutes after oral administration and lasts up to about 8 hours.

In the management of pain a usual initial dose of levorphanol tartrate by mouth is 2 mg repeated in 6 to 8 hours if necessary. The maximum initial daily dose in non-opioid tolerant patients should not exceed 12 mg.

Levorphanol tartrate may be given by intramuscular or subcutaneous injection in initial doses of 1 to 2 mg, repeated in 6 to 8 hours if necessary. Levorphanol tartrate may also be given by slow intravenous injection in an initial dose of up to 1 mg in divided doses, repeated in 3 to 6 hours if necessary. The maximum initial daily dose by the parenteral route in non-opioid tolerant patients should not exceed 8 mg.

For premedication, a usual dose is 1 to 2 mg by intramuscular or subcutaneous injection given 60 to 90 minutes before surgery.

Elderly or debilitated patients may require lower doses.

Preparations

USP 23: Levorphanol Tartrate Injection; Levorphanol Tartrate Tablets.

Proprietary Preparations (details are given in Part 3)
Canad.: Levo-Dromoran†; ***USA:*** Levo-Dromoran.

Lithium Salicylate (2663-d)

$C_7H_5LiO_3$ = 144.1.

CAS — 552-38-5.

Lithium salicylate is a salicylic acid derivative (see Aspirin, p.16) that has been used in rheumatic disorders, but its use cannot be recommended because of the pharmacological effect of the lithium ion.

Preparations

Proprietary Preparations (details are given in Part 3)
Multi-ingredient: ***Fr.:*** Antigoutteux Rezall.

Lonazolac Calcium (11435-t)

Lonazolac Calcium *(rINNM).*

Calcium 3-(4-chlorophenyl)-1-phenylpyrazol-4-ylacetate.

$C_{34}H_{24}CaCl_2N_4O_4$ = 663.6.

CAS — 53808-88-1 (lonazolac); 75821-71-5 (lonazolac calcium).

Lonazolac calcium is an NSAID (p.63). It has been used in pain, inflammation, and musculoskeletal and joint disorders in usual doses of up to 600 mg daily, in divided doses, by mouth. Suppositories have also been employed in doses of 400 mg twice daily.

Preparations

Proprietary Preparations (details are given in Part 3)
Aust.: Irritren; ***Belg.:*** Irritren†; ***Ger.:*** Argun; arthro akut; Irritren; ***Switz.:*** Irritren†.

Lornoxicam (6486-p)

Lornoxicam *(BAN, USAN, rINN).*

Chlorotenoxicam; Chlortenoxicam; CTX; Ro-13-9297. 6-Chloro-4-hydroxy-2-methyl-*N*-2-pyridyl-2*H*-thieno[2,3-e][1,2]-thiazine-3-carboxamide 1,1-dioxide.

$C_{13}H_{10}ClN_3O_4S_2$ = 371.8.

CAS — 70374-39-9.

Lornoxicam is an NSAID (p.63). It has been used in pain, inflammation, and musculoskeletal and joint disorders in usual doses of 8 to 16 mg daily, in divided doses.

References.

1. Balfour JA, *et al.* Lornoxicam: a review of its pharmacology and therapeutic potential in the management of painful and inflammatory conditions. *Drugs* 1996; **51:** 639–57.
2. Skjodt NM, Davies NM. Clinical pharmacokinetics of lornoxicam: a short half-life oxicam. *Clin Pharmacokinet* 1998; **34:** 421–8.

Preparations

Proprietary Preparations (details are given in Part 3)
Swed.: Xefo.

Loxoprofen Sodium (11675-l)

Loxoprofen Sodium *(rINNM).*

CS-600 (loxoprofen). Sodium (±)-*p*-[(2-oxocyclopentyl)methyl]hydratropate dihydrate.

$C_{15}H_{17}O_3Na,2H_2O$ = 304.3.

CAS — 68767-14-6 (loxoprofen); 80382-23-6 (loxoprofen sodium dihydrate).

Pharmacopoeias. In *Jpn.*

Loxoprofen sodium is an NSAID (p.63) given by mouth for the management of pain and inflammation associated with musculoskeletal and joint disorders or operative procedures.

Preparations

Proprietary Preparations (details are given in Part 3)
Jpn: Loxonin.

Lysine Aspirin (9560-m)

Aspirin DL-Lysine; Lysine Acetylsalicylate; DL-Lysine Acetylsalicylate.

$C_{15}H_{22}N_2O_6$ = 326.3.

CAS — 62952-06-1.

Pharmacopoeias. In *Fr.*

Lysine aspirin 900 mg is approximately equivalent to 500 mg of aspirin.

Adverse Effects, Treatment, and Precautions

As for Aspirin, p.16. Shock has been reported in patients given lysine aspirin by injection.

Lysine aspirin, like aspirin, should not generally be given to children under the age of 12 years because of the risk of Reye's syndrome.

Interactions

For interactions associated with aspirin, see p.17.

Uses and Administration

Lysine aspirin has analgesic, anti-inflammatory, and antipyretic actions similar to those of aspirin (see p.18). Following administration, lysine aspirin dissociates into lysine and aspirin; aspirin is then hydrolysed to salicylic acid. Lysine aspirin is used in the treatment of pain, fever, and rheumatic disorders. It is given by mouth in doses equivalent to 0.5 to 1 g of aspirin, repeated every 4 hours as needed up to a maximum of 3 g of aspirin daily (2 g daily in the elderly) for pain and fever. The dose for rheumatic disorders is 4 to 6 g of aspirin daily in 3 or 4 divided doses. Lysine aspirin is also given intramuscularly or intravenously in similar doses; the maximum daily parenteral dose is 4 g of aspirin for very severe pain and 6 g of aspirin for rheumatic disorders.

Lysine aspirin is also used in combination with metoclopramide in the treatment of migraine.

Lysine aspirin has also been used in the management of thrombo-embolic disorders.

References.

1. Tfelt-Hansen P, *et al.* The effectiveness of combined oral lysine acetylsalicylate and metoclopramide compared with oral sumatriptan for migraine. *Lancet* 1995; **346:** 923–6.

For a suggestion that lysine aspirin might be more suitable than aspirin for the diagnosis of sensitivity to NSAIDs, see under Hypersensitivity on p.16.

Preparations

Proprietary Preparations (details are given in Part 3)
Belg.: Aspegic; Cardegic; ***Fr.:*** Aspegic; Kardegic; ***Ger.:*** Aspisol; ***Ital.:*** Aspegic; Aspidol; Cardirene; Flectadol; Quinton†; Tomasl†; ***Jpn:*** Venopirin†; ***Neth.:*** Aspegic; ***Spain:*** ASL; Aspegic; Inyesprin; Lysinotol; Solusprin; ***Switz.:*** Alcacyl instant; Aspegic; Kardegic; ***UK:*** Laboprin†.

Multi-ingredient: ***Belg.:*** Migpriv; ***Fr.:*** Migpriv; ***Neth.:*** Migrafin; ***Spain:*** Dolo Coneurase†; Fluxal; Neurodif; Neurogobens.

Magnesium Salicylate (2664-n)

$C_{14}H_{10}MgO_6,4H_2O$ = 370.6.
CAS — 18917-89-0 (anhydrous magnesium salicylate); 18917-95-8 (magnesium salicylate tetrahydrate).
Pharmacopoeias. In US.

White, odourless, efflorescent, crystalline powder. Anhydrous magnesium salicylate 1 g is approximately equivalent to 1.2 g of aspirin. **Soluble** in water and in alcohol; freely soluble in methyl alcohol; slightly soluble in ether. **Store** in airtight containers.

Adverse Effects, Treatment, and Precautions

As for Aspirin, p.16.

The use of aspirin and other acetylated salicylates is generally not recommended for children under the age of 12 years because of the risk of Reye's syndrome, unless specifically indicated. Some authorities also extend this precaution to non-acetylated salicylates such as magnesium salicylate.

There is an additional caution in renal impairment because of the risk of hypermagnesaemia.

Interactions

For interactions associated with salicylates, see Aspirin, p.17.

Uses and Administration

Magnesium salicylate has analgesic, anti-inflammatory, and antipyretic actions similar to those of aspirin (see p.18). It is used in the treatment of pain and fever and in the management of inflammatory conditions such as osteoarthritis, rheumatoid arthritis, and other arthritides. Usual doses of magnesium salicylate, expressed in terms of anhydrous magnesium salicylate, are 300 to 600 mg by mouth every 4 hours for pain or fever. A total daily dose of 3.5 g should not be exceeded. A dose of 545 mg to 1.2 g given 3 to 4 times daily is used for arthritic disorders.

Preparations

USP 23: Magnesium Salicylate Tablets.

Proprietary Preparations (details are given in Part 3)
Canad.: Back-Ese M; Doans Backache Pills; Herbogesic; ***USA:*** Backache Maximum Strength Relief; Bayer Select Maximum Strength Backache; Doans; Magan; Mobidin; Momentum Muscular Backache Formula; Nuprin Backache.

Multi-ingredient: ***USA:*** Extra Strength Doans PM; Magsal; Maximum Strength Arthriten; Mobigesic; Myogesic.

Meclofenamate Sodium (2665-h)

Meclofenamate Sodium *(BANM, USAN, rINNM).*
$C_{14}H_{10}Cl_2NNaO_2,H_2O$ = 336.1.
CAS — 6385-02-0.
Pharmacopoeias. In US. BP(Vet) includes Meclofenamic Acid.

A white to creamy white, odourless to almost odourless, crystalline powder. Freely **soluble** in water, the solution sometimes being somewhat turbid due to partial hydrolysis and absorption of carbon dioxide; soluble in methyl alcohol; slightly soluble in chloroform; practically insoluble in ether. **Store** in airtight containers. Protect from light.

Adverse Effects and Precautions

As for NSAIDs in general, p.63.

The commonest adverse effect in 2500 patients who received meclofenamate sodium in double-blind or long-term studies was gastro-intestinal disturbance.[1] Diarrhoea occurred in 11.2% of patients in double-blind studies and 32.8% of patients in long-term studies (up to 3 years). Ulcers were detected in 22 patients during therapy and skin rashes occurred in 4% of patients. Transient increases in serum aminotransferases and BUN occurred in some patients.

1. Preston SN. Safety of sodium meclofenamate (Meclomen™). *Curr Ther Res* 1978; **23** (suppl 4S): S107–12.

Effects on the blood. Case reports of agranulocytosis[1] and thrombocytopenia[2] associated with meclofenamate therapy.

1. Wishner AJ, Milburn PB. Meclofenamate sodium-induced agranulocytosis and suppression of erythropoiesis. *J Am Acad Dermatol* 1985; **13:** 1052–3.
2. Rodriguez J. Thrombocytopenia associated with meclofenamate. *Drug Intell Clin Pharm* 1981; **15:** 999.

Interactions

For interactions associated with NSAIDs, see p.65.

Pharmacokinetics

Meclofenamate sodium is readily absorbed when given by mouth. Peak plasma concentrations occur about 0.5 to 1 hour after ingestion. Meclofenamate is over 99% bound to plasma proteins. The plasma elimination half-life of meclofenamate sodium is about 2 to 4 hours. It is metabolised by oxidation, hydroxylation, dehalogenation, and conjugation with glucuronic acid and excreted in urine mainly as glucuronide conjugates of the metabolites. About 20 to 30% is recovered in the faeces. One of the metabolites, a 3-hydroxymethyl compound, is reported to be active.

References.

1. Koup JR, *et al.* A single and multiple dose pharmacokinetic and metabolism study of meclofenamate sodium. *Biopharm Drug Dispos* 1990; **11:** 1–15.

Uses and Administration

Meclofenamate sodium, an anthranilic acid derivative similar to mefenamic acid (p.52), is an NSAID (p.65). It is given by mouth in musculoskeletal and joint disorders such as osteoarthritis and rheumatoid arthritis, in mild to moderate pain, and in dysmenorrhoea and menorrhagia.

Doses of meclofenamate sodium are expressed in terms of the equivalent amount of meclofenamic acid. In arthritic conditions it is given in doses of 200 to 400 mg daily; daily doses are usually given in 3 to 4 divided doses. For relief of mild to moderate pain doses are 50 to 100 mg every 4 to 6 hours; the daily dose should not exceed 400 mg. The dose in the treatment of dysmenorrhoea and menorrhagia is 100 mg three times daily for up to 6 days during menstruation.

Meclofenamic acid has been given as a rectal suppository, and is also used in veterinary medicine.

Preparations

USP 23: Meclofenamate Sodium Capsules.

Proprietary Preparations (details are given in Part 3)
Aust.: Meclomen; ***Ital.:*** Lenidolor; Meclodol; Meclomen†; Movens; ***S.Afr.:*** Meclomen; ***Spain:*** Meclomen; ***Switz.:*** Meclomen†; ***USA:*** Meclodium†; Meclomen†.

Mefenamic Acid (2666-m)

Mefenamic Acid *(BAN, USAN, rINN).*
Acidum Mefenamicum; CI-473; CN-35355; INF-3355. *N*-(2,3-Xylyl)anthranilic acid.
$C_{15}H_{15}NO_2$ = 241.3.
CAS — 61-68-7.
Pharmacopoeias. In *Eur.* (see p.viii), *Jpn, Pol.,* and *US.*

A white to almost white, microcrystalline powder. Practically **insoluble** in water; slightly soluble in alcohol, in dichloromethane, and in methyl alcohol; sparingly soluble in chloroform; soluble in solutions of alkali hydroxides. **Store** in airtight containers. Protect from light.

Adverse Effects

As for NSAIDs in general, p.63. Diarrhoea and rashes may occur and necessitate discontinuation of treatment. Other effects reported include drowsiness, thrombocytopenia, occasionally haemolytic anaemia, and rarely aplastic anaemia. Convulsions are a prominent feature of overdosage with mefenamic acid.

Effects on the blood. References to haematological reactions in patients taking mefenamic acid including haemolytic anaemia,[1] leucopenia,[2] neutropenia,[3] and agranulocytosis.[4]

1. Scott GL, *et al.* Autoimmune haemolytic anaemia and mefenamic acid therapy. *Br Med J* 1968; **3:** 534–5.
2. Burns A, Young RE. Mefenamic acid induced leucopenia in the elderly. *Lancet* 1984; **ii:** 46.
3. Handa SI, Freestone S. Mefenamic acid-induced neutropenia and renal failure in elderly females with hypothyroidism. *Postgrad Med J* 1990; **66:** 557–9.
4. Muroi K, *et al.* Treatment of drug-induced agranulocytosis with granulocyte-colony stimulating factor. *Lancet* 1989; **ii:** 55.

Effects on the gastro-intestinal tract. Reversible steatorrhoea has occurred[1] and mefenamic acid may provoke colitis in patients without a past history of this condition.[2]

1. Marks JS, Gleeson MH. Steatorrhoea complicating therapy with mefenamic acid. *Br Med J* 1975; **4:** 442.
2. Ravi S, *et al.* Colitis caused by non-steroidal anti-inflammatory drugs. *Postgrad Med J* 1986; **62:** 773–6.

Effects on the kidneys. Mefenamic acid has been reported to produce nephrotoxic effects. Of special concern are reports of the development of nonoliguric renal failure in elderly patients who had experienced diarrhoea and vomiting while taking mefenamic acid and had continued to take the drug. It is normally recommended that mefenamic acid be discontinued in the event of diarrhoea and it was suggested that in these patients the gastro-intestinal toxicity had led to fluid and electrolyte depletion, thus predisposing these patients to mefenamic acid's nephrotoxicity.[1] A recent report[2] of nonoliguric renal failure in elderly patients given mefenamic acid for musculoskeletal pain serves as a reminder of this adverse effect.

1. Taha A, *et al.* Non-oliguric renal failure during treatment with mefenamic acid in elderly patients: a continuing problem. *Br Med J* 1985; **291:** 661–2.
2. Grant DJ, MacConnachie AM. Mefenamic acid is more dangerous than most. *Br Med J* 1995; **311:** 392.

Effects on the pancreas. A report of pancreatitis associated with mefenamic acid.[1]

1. van Walraven AA, *et al.* Pancreatitis caused by mefenamic acid. *Can Med Assoc J* 1982; **126:** 894.

Effects on the skin. Bullous pemphigoid, together with haemolytic anaemia and diarrhoea,[1] and fixed drug eruptions[2,3] have been associated with the use of mefenamic acid. Additionally, Stevens-Johnson syndrome, together with cholestatic hepatitis and haemolytic anaemia, in one patient has been attributed to mefenamic acid therapy.[4] It is generally recommended that mefenamic acid should be withdrawn if skin reactions develop.

1. Shepherd AN, *et al.* Mefenamic acid-induced bullous pemphigoid. *Postgrad Med J* 1986; **62:** 67–8.
2. Wilson CL, Otter A. Fixed drug eruption associated with mefenamic acid. *Br Med J* 1986; **293:** 1243.
3. Long CC, *et al.* Fixed drug eruption to mefenamic acid: a report of three cases. *Br J Dermatol* 1992; **126:** 409–11.
4. Chan JCN, *et al.* A case of Stevens-Johnson syndrome, cholestatic hepatitis and haemolytic anaemia associated with use of mefenamic acid. *Drug Safety* 1991; **6:** 230–4.

Overdosage. Mefenamic acid overdose has been associated with CNS toxicity, especially with convulsions.[1] Coma[2,3] has also been reported.

1. Court H, Volans GN. Poisoning after overdose with non-steroidal anti-inflammatory drugs. *Adverse Drug React Acute Poisoning Rev* 1984; **3:** 1–21.
2. Gössinger H, *et al.* Coma in mefenamic acid poisoning. *Lancet* 1982; **ii:** 384.
3. Hendrickse MT. Mefenamic acid overdose mimicking brainstem stroke. *Lancet* 1988; **ii:** 1019.

Precautions

As for NSAIDs in general, p.65. In addition mefenamic acid is contra-indicated in patients with inflammatory bowel disease. Patients who develop diarrhoea or rash while receiving mefenamic acid should discontinue therapy. Some consider that blood counts and liver function should be monitored during long-term therapy.

Mefenamic acid may give a false positive in tests for the presence of bile in the urine.

Porphyria. Mefenamic acid was considered to be unsafe in patients with acute porphyria although there is conflicting experimental evidence of porphyrinogenicity.[1]

1. Moore MR, McColl KEL. *Porphyria: drug lists.* Glasgow: Porphyria Research Unit, University of Glasgow, 1991.

Interactions

For interactions associated with NSAIDs, see p.65.

Pharmacokinetics

Mefenamic acid is absorbed from the gastro-intestinal tract. Peak plasma concentrations occur about 2 to 4 hours after ingestion. The plasma elimination half-life is reported to be 2 to 4 hours. Mefenamic acid is extensively bound to plasma proteins. Small amounts have been detected in breast milk. Over 50% of a dose may be recovered in the urine, as unchanged drug or conjugates of mefenamic acid and its metabolites.

Uses and Administration

Mefenamic acid, an anthranilic acid derivative, is an NSAID (p.65), although its anti-inflammatory properties are considered to be minor.

It is used in mild to moderate pain including headache, dental pain, postoperative and postpartum pain, and dysmenorrhoea, in musculoskeletal and joint disorders such as osteoarthritis and rheumatoid arthritis, in menorrhagia, and in children with fever and juvenile chronic arthritis. The usual dose by mouth is up to 500 mg three times daily. A suggested dose for children over 6 months of age is 25 mg per kg body-weight daily in divided doses. In the US where mefenamic acid is only licensed for the treatment of acute pain in adults it is recommended that it should not be given for longer than 7 days at a time, but in the UK this restriction is only applied to children unless they are receiving mefenamic acid for juvenile chronic arthritis.

Preparations

BP 1998: Mefenamic Acid Capsules;
USP 23: Mefenamic Acid Capsules.

Proprietary Preparations (details are given in Part 3)
Aust.: Parkemed; ***Austral.:*** Mefic; Ponstan; ***Canad.:*** Ponstan; ***Fr.:*** Ponstyl; ***Ger.:*** Parkemed; Ponalar; ***Irl.:*** Mefac; Pinalgesic; Ponalgic; Ponmel; Ponstan; ***Ital.:*** Lysalgo; Parke-Med†; ***S.Afr.:*** Clinstan†; Fenamin; Mefalgic; Ponac; Ponstan; Ponstel; ***Spain:*** Coslan; ***Switz.:*** Ecopan†; Mefenacide; Ponstan; ***UK:*** Contraflam; Dysman; Meflam; Opustan; Ponstan; ***USA:*** Ponstel.

Meloxicam (2751-d)

Meloxicam *(BAN, rINN).*

UH-AC-62. 4-Hydroxy-2-methyl-*N*-(5-methyl-2-thiazolyl)-2*H*-1,2-benzothiazine-3-carboxamide 1,1-dioxide.

$C_{14}H_{13}N_3O_4S_2$ = 351.4.

CAS — 71125-38-7.

Adverse Effects

As for NSAIDs in general, p.63.

Between September 1996, when meloxicam was first marketed in the UK, and mid June 1998 the UK Committee on Safety of Medicines had received a total of 773 reports of 1339 suspected adverse reactions for meloxicam.[1] Of all the reactions 41% were gastro-intestinal and of these 18% involved gastro-intestinal perforation, ulceration and/or bleeding; the mean age of the patients involved had been 64 years. Although most patients recovered after withdrawal of meloxicam and/or treatment, 5 had died. A total of 193 reactions involved the skin, the most common being pruritus, rash, and urticaria. There were also reports of angioedema (25), photosensitivity (12), and bullous dermatoses, including erythema multiforme and Stevens Johnson syndrome (5). No patients died from skin reactions and most recovered after meloxicam was withdrawn. Other frequently reported reactions were neurological (mostly headache), cardiovascular (oedema and palpitations), dizziness, flushing, and fatigue.

It has been proposed that selective inhibitors of cyclo-oxygenase-2, such as meloxicam, might produce fewer adverse effects than other NSAIDs but there appears to be no convincing evidence that the risk of severe gastro-intestinal events is lower with meloxicam than with other NSAIDs at equi-effective doses.[2]

1. Committee on Safety of Medicines/Medicines Control Agency. Meloxicam (Mobic): gastrointestinal and skin reactions. *Current Problems* 1998; **24:** 13.
2. Anonymous. Meloxicam—a safer NSAID? *Drug Ther Bull* 1998; **36:** 62–4.

Precautions

As for NSAIDs in general, p.65.

Meloxicam should be avoided in patients with renal failure unless receiving dialysis, in severe hepatic failure, and in bleeding disorders. Rectal administration should be avoided in patients with a history of proctitis, haemorrhoids, or rectal bleeding.

Renal impairment. The pharmacokinetics of meloxicam were not substantially altered in patients with a creatinine clearance of 41 to 60 mL per minute compared with those with normal renal function.[1] In those with a creatinine clearance of 20 to 40 mL per minute, total plasma-meloxicam concentrations were lower but meloxicam free fractions were higher. Such free meloxicam concentrations were similar to the other groups. On the basis of these results, it was suggested that it was not necessary to reduce meloxicam doses in patients with a creatinine clearance greater than 20 mL per minute.

1. Boulton-Jones JM, *et al.* Meloxicam pharmacokinetics in renal impairment. *Br J Clin Pharmacol* 1997; **43:** 35–40.

Interactions

For interactions associated with NSAIDs, see p.65.

There may be an increased risk of bleeding during concomitant use of meloxicam and oxpentifylline.

Pharmacokinetics

Meloxicam is well absorbed following oral administration. It is 99% bound to plasma proteins. Meloxicam has a plasma-elimination half-life of approximately 20 hours. It is extensively metabolised mainly by oxidation and excreted in similar amounts in the urine and in the faeces; less than 3% of a dose is excreted unchanged. The volume of distribution is increased in severe renal failure.

References.

1. Narjes H, *et al.* Pharmacokinetics and tolerability of meloxicam after i.m. administration. *Br J Clin Pharmacol* 1996; **41:** 135–9.
2. Türck D, *et al.* Clinical pharmacokinetics of meloxicam. *Arzneimittelforschung* 1997; **47:** 253–8.

Administration in renal impairment. For reference to the pharmacokinetics of meloxicam in renal impairment, see under Precautions, above.

Uses and Administration

Meloxicam, an oxicam derivative, is an NSAID (p.65). It is reported to be a selective inhibitor of cyclo-oxygenase-2 (COX-2). Meloxicam is used in the management of rheumatoid arthritis, for the short-term symptomatic treatment of acute exacerbations of osteoarthritis, and for the symptomatic treatment of ankylosing spondylitis.

In the treatment of rheumatoid arthritis, meloxicam is given by mouth in a usual dose of 15 mg daily as a single dose. In the treatment of acute exacerbations of osteoarthritis the usual daily dose of meloxicam by mouth is 7.5 mg, increased if necessary to a maximum of 15 mg daily given as a single dose. Doses of 15 mg daily, by mouth, are used in the treatment of ankylosing spondylitis.

A dose of 7.5 mg daily is recommended for long-term treatment in the elderly. The recommended maximum daily dose in dialysis patients is 7.5 mg.

Meloxicam may be given by rectal suppository in doses similar to those used orally.

Preparations

Proprietary Preparations (details are given in Part 3)
Aust.: Mobic; Movalis; ***Belg.:*** Mobic; ***Fr.:*** Mobic; ***Ger.:*** Mobec; ***Irl.:*** Mobic; ***Ital.:*** Mobic; ***Neth.:*** Movicox; ***S.Afr.:*** Mobic; ***Spain:*** Movalis; Parocin; Uticox; ***Swed.:*** Mobic; ***Switz.:*** Mobicox; ***UK:*** Mobic.

Meptazinol Hydrochloride (12932-r)

Meptazinol Hydrochloride *(BANM, USAN, rINNM).*

IL-22811 (meptazinol); WY-22811 (meptazinol). 3-(3-Ethyl-1-methylperhydroazepin-3-yl)phenol hydrochloride.

$C_{15}H_{23}NO,HCl$ = 269.8.

CAS — 54340-58-8 (meptazinol); 59263-76-2 (meptazinol hydrochloride); 34154-59-1 (±-meptazinol hydrochloride).

Pharmacopoeias. In Br.

A white or almost white powder. Meptazinol hydrochloride 115.6 mg is approximately equivalent to 100 mg of meptazinol. Very **soluble** in water; freely soluble in alcohol; very soluble in methyl alcohol; very slightly soluble in acetone; dissolves in dilute solutions of alkali hydroxides.

Dependence and Withdrawal

As for Opioid Analgesics, p.67.

In assessing the dependence potential of meptazinol, a WHO expert committee[1] noted that abrupt discontinuation of chronic meptazinol administration precipitated only slight withdrawal signs in *animals* and that meptazinol did not suppress opioid withdrawal signs and symptoms in humans dependent on morphine. Abuse had not been reported. They considered that the likelihood of abuse was moderate and that international control was not warranted in 1989.

1. WHO. WHO expert committee on drug dependence: twenty-fifth report. *WHO Tech Rep Ser 775* 1989.

Adverse Effects, Treatment, and Precautions

As for Opioid Analgesics in general, p.68.

Meptazinol is claimed to have a low incidence of respiratory depression. The incidence of psychotomimetic effects such as hallucinations has been reported to be low. As meptazinol possesses antagonist as well as agonist properties, naloxone is the recommended antagonist for the treatment of overdosage.

Meptazinol has the potential to precipitate withdrawal symptoms if given to patients who are physically dependent on opioids.

Effects on the respiratory system. Meptazinol is said to have a relatively low potential for respiratory depression and in healthy subjects was reported to produce substantially less respiratory depression than morphine or pentazocine at usual analgesic doses.[1] Respiratory depression does occur in anaesthetised patients. A profound reduction in minute volume was observed after the start of surgery in healthy adults following meptazinol 100 mg intravenously.[2] When compared with pethidine in anaesthetised patients meptazinol 1 mg per kg body-weight intravenously produced less respiratory depression than pethidine 1 mg per kg, but more than pethidine 0.5 mg per kg.[3] Ventilatory depressant effects were similar in another study,[4] although a second injection produced a further decrease in ventilation only with pethidine. Compensatory mechanisms may come into play following repeated doses of meptazinol but Lee and Drummond[4] considered that intravenous administration of meptazinol during anaesthesia should be viewed with as much caution as with any other opioid. In a comparison with morphine[5] similar effects on ventilation were seen with meptazinol by intravenous infusion postoperatively when patients were monitored continuously. In another postoperative study[6] respiratory rate fell following meptazinol or morphine, although their effects on central regulation of respiration differed; CO_2 sensitivity seemed to be impaired by morphine but not meptazinol.

Respiratory arrest occurred after an overdose of 50 meptazinol 200-mg tablets and a quarter of a bottle of whisky.[7] Full recovery eventually followed supportive measures although spontaneous respiration was not re-established by naloxone intravenously to a cumulative total dose of 10 mg.

1. Jordan C, *et al.* A comparison of the respiratory effects of meptazinol, pentazocine and morphine. *Br J Anaesth* 1979; **51:** 497–502.
2. Hardy PAJ. Meptazinol and respiratory depression. *Lancet* 1983; **ii:** 576.
3. Wilkinson DJ, *et al.* Meptazinol— a cause of respiratory depression in general anaesthesia. *Br J Anaesth* 1985; **57:** 1077–84.
4. Lee A, Drummond GB. Ventilatory effects of meptazinol and pethidine in anaesthetised patients. *Br J Anaesth* 1987; **59:** 1127–33.
5. Frater RAS, *et al.* Analgesia-induced respiratory depression: comparison of meptazinol and morphine in the postoperative period. *Br J Anaesth* 1989; **63:** 260–5.
6. Verborgh C, Camu F. Post-surgical pain relief with zero-order intravenous infusions of meptazinol and morphine: a double-blind placebo-controlled evaluation of their effects on ventilation. *Eur J Clin Pharmacol* 1990; **38:** 437–42.
7. Davison AG, *et al.* Meptazinol overdose producing near fatal respiratory depression. *Hum Toxicol* 1987; **6:** 331.

Hepatic impairment. See under Pharmacokinetics, below.

Interactions

For interactions associated with opioid analgesics, see p.69.

Pharmacokinetics

Following oral administration of meptazinol peak plasma concentrations have been achieved within 0.5 to 2 hours, but bioavailability is low since it undergoes extensive first-pass metabolism. Systemic availability is improved after rectal administration. Peak plasma concentrations have been achieved 30 minutes after rectal or intramuscular administration. Plasma protein binding has averaged only about 27%. Elimination half-lives of about 2 hours have been reported. Meptazinol is extensively metabolised in the liver and is excreted mainly in the urine as the glucuronide conjugate. Less than 10% of a dose has been recovered from the faeces. Meptazinol crosses the placenta.

References.

1. Franklin RA, *et al.* Studies on the metabolism of meptazinol, a new analgesic drug. *Br J Clin Pharmacol* 1976; **3:** 497–502.
2. Franklin RA, *et al.* Studies on the absorption and disposition of meptazinol following rectal administration. *Br J Clin Pharmacol* 1977; **4:** 163–7.
3. Davies G, *et al.* Pharmacokinetics of meptazinol in man following repeated intramuscular administration. *Eur J Clin Pharmacol* 1982; **23:** 535–8.
4. Norbury HM, *et al.* Pharmacokinetics of the new analgesic, meptazinol, after oral and intravenous administration to volunteers. *Eur J Clin Pharmacol* 1983; **25:** 77–80.
5. Murray GR, *et al.* The systemic availability of meptazinol in man after oral and rectal doses. *Eur J Clin Pharmacol* 1989; **36:** 279–82.

Administration in the elderly. A lower clearance and longer elimination half-life has been reported for meptazinol in elderly patients, but dosage reduction was not considered warranted on pharmacokinetic grounds. Mean half-lives in elderly and young subjects were 3.39 and 1.94 hours respectively following single oral doses[1] and 2.93 and 2.06 hours respectively following intravenous administration.[2]

1. Norbury HM, *et al.* Pharmacokinetics of meptazinol after single and multiple oral administration to elderly patients. *Eur J Clin Pharmacol* 1984; **27:** 223–6.
2. Murray GR, *et al.* Pharmacokinetics of meptazinol after parenteral administration in the elderly. *Eur J Clin Pharmacol* 1987; **31:** 733–6.

Administration in hepatic impairment. Oral bioavailability of meptazinol appeared to be enhanced in patients with liver disease. Mean peak plasma concentrations of 184 ng per mL, 131 ng per mL, and 53 ng per mL were measured in cirrhotic patients, patients with non-cirrhotic liver disease, and patients with normal liver function, respectively, after a single oral dose of meptazinol, although there was no evidence of accumulation after chronic dosing.[1] There were no significant differences in plasma clearance after an intravenous dose. Reduced oral doses of meptazinol might be advisable in cirrhotic patients.

1. Birnie GG, *et al.* Enhanced oral bioavailability of meptazinol in cirrhosis. *Gut* 1987; **28:** 248–54.

Pregnancy and the neonate. In women given an intramuscular injection of 100 to 150 mg during labour, meptazinol was found to cross the placenta readily but was rapidly eliminated from the neonate.[1] This contrasted with pethidine which was known to be excreted very slowly from neonates. As in the adult, elimination of meptazinol by the neonate appeared to take place mainly by conjugation with glucuronic acid.[2] A half-life of 3.4 hours, similar to that in adults, has been reported in the neonate,[3] in contrast to 22.7 hours for pethidine in neonates.

Disposition of meptazinol appears not to be significantly affected by pregnancy. Mean half-lives of 1.36 and 1.68 hours were reported in pregnant and non-pregnant women, respectively,[4] compared with 2.06 hours in men.

1. Franklin RA, *et al.* Preliminary studies on the disposition of meptazinol in the neonate. *Br J Clin Pharmacol* 1981; **12:** 88–90.
2. Dowell PS, *et al.* Routes of meptazinol conjugation in the neonate. *Br J Clin Pharmacol* 1982; **14:** 748–9.
3. Jackson MBA, Robson PJ. Preliminary clinical and pharmacokinetic experiences in the newborn when meptazinol is compared with pethidine as an obstetric analgesic. *Postgrad Med J* 1983; **59** (suppl 1): 47–51.
4. Murray GR, *et al.* The disposition of meptazinol after single and multiple intravenous administration to pregnant and non-pregnant women. *Eur J Clin Pharmacol* 1989; **36:** 273–7.

Uses and Administration

Meptazinol is an opioid agonist-antagonist with partial opioid agonist activity at the μ_1 opioid receptor (see p.69); it also has cholinergic activity. Meptazinol is used in the treatment of moderate to severe pain. It has a shorter duration of action than morphine. Meptazinol may also be used as an adjunct for analgesia during surgery.

Meptazinol is given by mouth as the base or by intramuscular or intravenous injection as the hydrochloride but doses are expressed in terms of the base. The intramuscular dose is the equivalent of 75 to 100 mg of meptazinol given every 2 to 4 hours; for obstetric pain a dose of 2 mg per kg body-weight (100 to 150 mg) may be used.

Meptazinol hydrochloride may also be given by slow intravenous injection in doses equivalent to 50 to 100 mg of meptazinol every 2 to 4 hours.

For the short-term treatment of moderate pain meptazinol may be given by mouth in a dose of 200 mg every 3 to 6 hours.

References.

1. Holmes B, Ward A. Meptazinol: a review of its pharmacodynamic and pharmacokinetic properties and therapeutic efficacy. *Drugs* 1985; **30:** 285–312.

Administration. EPIDURAL ROUTE. Epidural administration of meptazinol 90 mg for postoperative pain was reported to be superior to intramuscular administration of 90 mg.[1] Others[2,3] tried epidural meptazinol for analgesia after caesarean section, but discouraged its use. In one study[2] a 30-mg dose was ineffective with an unacceptable incidence of adverse effects and in the other[3] a 60-mg dose was ineffective because of its short duration of action.

The manufacturers in the UK state that the injectable formulation is not suitable for epidural or intrathecal use.

1. Verborgh C, *et al.* Meptazinol for postoperative pain relief in man: comparison of extradural and im administration. *Br J Anaesth* 1987; **59:** 1134–9.
2. Francis RI, Lockhart AS. Epidural meptazinol. *Anaesthesia* 1986; **41:** 88–9.
3. Birks RJS, Marsh DRG. Epidural meptazinol. *Anaesthesia* 1986; **41:** 883.

Administration in children. Experience with meptazinol in children has been limited; Ridley *et al.*[1] reported 1 mg per kg body-weight intramuscularly to be as effective as pethidine for post-tonsillectomy pain.

1. Ridley SA, *et al.* Meptazinol versus pethidine for post-operative pain relief in children. *Anaesthesia* 1986; **41:** 263–7.

Preparations

BP 1998: Meptazinol Injection; Meptazinol Tablets.

Proprietary Preparations (details are given in Part 3)
Aust.: Meptidol; ***Ger.:*** Meptid; ***Irl.:*** Meptid; ***UK:*** Meptid.

Methadone Hydrochloride (6237-j)

Methadone Hydrochloride *(BANM, pINNM).*

Amidine Hydrochloride; Amidone Hydrochloride; (±)-Methadone Hydrochloride; Methadoni Hydrochloridum; Phenadone. (±)-6-Dimethylamino-4,4-diphenylheptan-3-one hydrochloride.

$C_{21}H_{27}NO,HCl = 345.9.$

CAS — 76-99-3 (methadone); 297-88-1 (methadone, ±); 1095-90-5 (methadone hydrochloride); 125-56-4 (methadone hydrochloride, ±).

Pharmacopoeias. In *Chin., Eur.* (see p.viii), and *US.*

Odourless colourless crystals or white crystalline powder. **Soluble** in water; freely soluble in alcohol and in chloroform; practically insoluble in ether and in glycerol. A 1% solution has a pH of 4.5 to 6.5. **Store** in airtight containers. Protect from light.

Incompatibility. Physical incompatibility as judged by loss of clarity was reported when an intravenous solution of methadone hydrochloride was mixed with those of aminophylline, ammonium chloride, amylobarbitone sodium, chlorothiazide sodium, heparin sodium, methicillin sodium, nitrofurantoin sodium, novobiocin sodium, pentobarbitone sodium, phenobarbitone sodium, phenytoin sodium, quinalbarbitone sodium, sodium bicarbonate, sodium iodide, sulphadiazine sodium, sulphafurazole diethanolamine, or thiopentone sodium.[1]

There appears to be adequate evidence that stable solutions containing methadone hydrochloride and hydroxybenzoate esters can be formulated but the risk of precipitation exists if syrup preserved with hydroxybenzoates is used to extemporaneously prepare a methadone mixture 1 mg per mL to the DTF formula.[2] An oral formulation of methadone hydrochloride 5 mg per mL containing methyl hydroxybenzoate 0.1% as preservative rather than chloroform has been reported stable for at least 4 months at room temperature.[3]

1. Patel JA, Phillips GL. A guide to physical compatibility of intravenous drug admixtures. *Am J Hosp Pharm* 1966; **23:** 409–11.
2. *PSGB Lab Report P/80/1* 1980.
3. Ching MS, *et al.* Stability of methadone mixture with methyl hydroxybenzoate as a preservative. *Aust J Hosp Pharm* 1989; **19:** 159–61.

Dependence and Withdrawal

As for Opioid Analgesics, p.67. Methadone withdrawal symptoms are similar to, but more prolonged, than those produced by morphine or diamorphine. They develop more slowly and do not usually appear until 24 to 48 hours after the last dose.

Methadone is used for substitution therapy in the management of opioid dependence (see under Uses and Administration, below).

Adverse Effects and Treatment

As for Opioid Analgesics in general, p.68.

Methadone is subject to accumulation in the body and has a more prolonged effect than morphine. It may have a relatively greater respiratory depressant effect than morphine and, although reported to be less sedating, repeated administration of methadone may result in marked sedation. After gross overdosage symptoms are similar to those of morphine poisoning. Pulmonary oedema after overdosage is a common cause of fatalities among addicts.

Methadone causes pain at injection sites; subcutaneous injection causes local tissue irritation and induration.

Commenting on the risk of using methadone for opioid withdrawal Harding-Pink[1] pointed out that most cases of methadone poisoning occurred in persons not on maintenance and were often children or family members of maintenance patients. Methadone is highly toxic to anyone who is not tolerant to opioids; 50 to 100 mg can be life-threatening in non-tolerant adults and 10 mg can be fatal in a young child.

1. Harding-Pink D. Opioid toxicity: methadone: one person's maintenance dose is another's poison. *Lancet* 1993; **341:** 665–6.

Effects on the endocrine system. Hypoadrenalism has been demonstrated in chronic methadone addicts. Findings consistent with deficient ACTH production and subsequent secondary hypoadrenalism were reported by Dackis *et al.*[1] whereas Pullan *et al.*[2] found evidence of methadone-induced primary adrenal cortical hypofunction.

1. Dackis CA, *et al.* Methadone induced hypoadrenalism. *Lancet* 1982; **ii:** 1167.
2. Pullan PT, *et al.* Methadone-induced hypoadrenalism. *Lancet* 1983; **i:** 714.

Effects on the nervous system. Choreic movements in a patient on long-term methadone maintenance treatment for diamorphine addiction disappeared when methadone was discontinued.[1]

1. Wasserman S, Yahr MD. Choreic movements induced by the use of methadone. *Arch Neurol* 1980; **37:** 727–8.

Effects on sexual function. Sexual performance was impaired in 29 male diamorphine addicts receiving methadone maintenance therapy.[1] The function of secondary sex organs was markedly suppressed when compared with untreated diamorphine addicts or controls and serum-testosterone concentrations were 43% lower in those on methadone.

1. Cicero TJ, *et al.* Function of the male sex organs in heroin and methadone users. *N Engl J Med* 1975; **292:** 882–7.

Precautions

As for Opioid Analgesics in general, p.68.

Administration. Methadone has a long half-life and accumulation may occur with repeated doses, especially in elderly or debilitated patients.[1] An 81-year-old woman given methadone 5 mg three times a day by mouth for 2 days became deeply unconscious but awoke immediately when given naloxone 400 μg intravenously.[2]

Sudden death in 10 diamorphine addicts occurred between 2 and 6 days after starting a methadone maintenance programme.[3] The mean prescribed dose of methadone at the time of death had been about 60 mg. There was evidence of chronic persistent hepatitis in all cases and liver disease could have reduced methadone clearance resulting in higher than expected blood concentrations. Liver function tests and urine testing for the presence of drugs prior to entry into methadone maintenance programmes and lower starting doses might decrease the likelihood of such deaths. Wu and Henry[4] noted that, like dextropropoxyphene, methadone has membrane stabilising activity and can block nerve conduction. They suggested that the sudden deaths were mainly due to accumulation of methadone over several days resulting in complications such as cardiac arrhythmias or cardiovascular collapse.

For the effects of hepatic impairment and renal impairment on the disposition of methadone, see under Pharmacokinetics, below.

1. Twycross RG. A comparison of diamorphine-with-cocaine and methadone. *Br J Clin Pharmacol* 1977; **4:** 691–3.
2. Symonds P. Methadone and the elderly. *Br Med J* 1977; **i:** 512.
3. Drummer OH, *et al.* Deaths of heroin addicts starting on a methadone maintenance programme. *Lancet* 1990; **335:** 108.
4. Wu C, Henry JA. Deaths of heroin addicts starting on methadone maintenance. *Lancet* 1990; **335:** 424.

Breast feeding. Methadone is distributed into breast milk and death of the 5-week-old infant of a mother on methadone maintenance was attributed to methadone received via his mother's milk.[1] Others have suggested that the amount of methadone in breast milk was unlikely to have any pharmacological effect on the infant.[2,3]

1. Smialek JE, *et al.* Methadone deaths in children. *JAMA* 1977; **238:** 2516–17.
2. Anonymous. Methadone in breast milk. *Med Lett Drugs Ther* 1979; **21:** 52.
3. Wojnar-Horton RE, *et al.* Methadone distribution and excretion into breast milk of clients in a methadone maintenance programme. *Br J Clin Pharmacol* 1997; **44:** 543–7.

Pregnancy and the neonate. Methadone is not recommended for use in labour because its prolonged duration of action increases the risk of neonatal respiratory depression.

Neonatal withdrawal syndrome and low birth-weight are immediate problems in the infants born to women receiving methadone for the management of opioid addiction; increased still-birth rates have also been noted.[1-3] Rosen and Johnson[2] studied the first 18 months of life of children born to methadone-maintained mothers. In the neonatal period moderate to severe opioid abstinence syndrome occurred in 75% of infants, as well as reduced head circumference and raised systolic blood pressure. At follow-up over 18 months these children had a higher incidence of otitis media, of reduced head circumference, and of abnormal eye findings when compared with drug-free controls. Neurobehavioural abnormalities and lower scores on mental and motor developmental indices were thought to be possible predictors of later learning and behavioural problems. Lifschitz *et al.*[4] could discern no specific effect of methadone or diamorphine on intrauterine and postnatal growth.

1. Blinick G, *et al.* Methadone maintenance, pregnancy, and progeny. *JAMA* 1973; **225:** 477–9.
2. Rosen TS, Johnson HL. Children of methadone-maintained mothers: follow-up to 18 months of age. *J Pediatr* 1982; **101:** 192–6.
3. Kalter H, Warkany J. Congenital malformations. *N Engl J Med* 1983; **308:** 491–7.
4. Lifschitz MH, *et al.* Fetal and postnatal growth of children born to narcotic-dependent women. *J Pediatr* 1983; **102:** 686–91.

Interactions

For interactions associated with opioid analgesics, see p.69.

Methadone is metabolised in the liver to inactive metabolites by the mixed-function oxidase system and thus interactions are likely with enzyme inducers. Withdrawal symptoms have been reported in patients maintained on methadone when they were given *phenobarbitone*,[1] *phenytoin*,[2,3] or *rifampicin*.[4-6] Furthermore, *histamine H_2 antagonists* such as cimetidine (see p.69) and *selective serotonin reuptake inhibitors* such as fluoxetine[7] and fluvoxamine[7,8] may enhance the effects of some opioid analgesics; such interactions may lead to methadone toxicity. Concomitant administration of methadone and *fluconazole* has been reported[9] to result in increased serum concentrations of methadone although the authors of the study considered that for patients being treated for opioid dependence the interaction was unlikely to require adjustment of the methadone dose. Drugs that *acidify* or *alkalinise* the urine may have an effect on methadone pharmacokinetics since body clearance is increased at acidic pH and decreased at alkaline pH.[10]

Methadone possibly increases plasma concentrations of *zidovudine* (see p.631).

1. Liu S-J, Wang RIH. Case report of barbiturate-induced enhancement of methadone metabolism and withdrawal syndrome. *Am J Psychiatry* 1984; **141:** 1287–8.
2. Finelli PF. Phenytoin and methadone tolerance. *N Engl J Med* 1976; **294:** 227.
3. Tong TG, *et al.* Phenytoin-induced methadone withdrawal. *Ann Intern Med* 1981; **94:** 349–51.
4. Kreek MJ, *et al.* Rifampin-induced methadone withdrawal. *N Engl J Med* 1976; **294:** 1104–6.
5. Bending MR, Skacel PO. Rifampicin and methadone withdrawal. *Lancet* 1977; **i:** 1211.
6. Raistrick D, *et al.* Methadone maintenance and tuberculosis treatment. *Br Med J* 1996; **313:** 925–6.
7. Eap CB, *et al.* Fluvoxamine and fluoxetine do not interact in the same way with the metabolism of the enantiomers of methadone. *J Clin Psychopharmacol* 1997; **17:** 113–17.
8. Bertschy G, *et al.* Probable metabolic interaction between methadone and fluvoxamine in addict patients. *Ther Drug Monit* 1994; **16:** 42–5.
9. Cobb MN, *et al.* The effect of fluconazole on the clinical pharmacokinetics of methadone. *Clin Pharmacol Ther* 1998; **63:** 655–62.
10. Nilsson M-I, *et al.* Effect of urinary pH on the disposition of methadone in man. *Eur J Clin Pharmacol* 1982; **22:** 337–42.

Pharmacokinetics

Methadone hydrochloride is readily absorbed from the gastro-intestinal tract and following subcutaneous or intramuscular injection. It is widely distributed in the tissues, diffuses across the placenta, and is distributed into breast milk. It is extensively protein bound. Methadone is metabolised in the liver, mainly by *N*-demethylation and cyclisation, and the metabolites are excreted in the bile and urine. It has a prolonged half-life and is subject to accumulation.

In reviews of the pharmacokinetics of methadone[1,2] particular reference has been made to its long elimination half-life, accumulation following repeated doses, and wide interindividual variations.

Methadone is rapidly absorbed after administration by mouth and has high oral bioavailability. Peak plasma concentrations have been reported 1 to 5 hours after oral administration of a single dose in tablet form. It undergoes considerable tissue distribution and protein binding is reported to be 60 to 90% with α_1-acid glycoprotein being the main binding protein in plasma. Metabolism to the major metabolite 2-ethylidine-1,5-dimethyl-3,3-diphenylpyrrolidine and the minor metabolite 2-ethyl-3,3-diphenyl-5-methylpyrrolidine, both of them inactive, occurs in the liver. These metabolites are excreted in the faeces and urine together with unchanged methadone. Other metabolites, including methadol and normethadol, have also been described. The liver may also serve as a major storage site of unchanged methadone which is taken up, bound nonspecifically by the liver, and released again mainly unchanged. Urinary excretion of methadone is pH-dependent, the lower the pH the greater the clearance.

In addition to marked interindividual variations there are differences in the pharmacokinetics of methadone following single or multiple doses. Elimination half-lives vary considerably (a range of 15 to 60 hours has been quoted) and may be much longer than the 18 hours reported following a single dose. Careful adjustment of dosage is necessary with repeated administration.

Most studies have been in addicts. Plasma concentrations have been found to vary widely during methadone maintenance therapy with large differences between patients and wide fluctuations in individual patients. Interindividual variations in kinetics have also been seen in cancer patients.

1. Säwe J. High-dose morphine and methadone in cancer patients: clinical pharmacokinetic considerations of oral treatment. *Clin Pharmacokinet* 1986; **11:** 87–106.
2. Moore RA, *et al.* Opiate metabolism and excretion. *Baillieres Clin Anaesthesiol* 1987; **1:** 829–58.

Administration. Methadone is considerably more lipid-soluble than morphine. A study of plasma concentrations and analgesia following their intramuscular injection indicated that more rapid and greater relief of pain might be achieved if lipid-soluble opioid analgesics were injected into the deltoid rather than the gluteal muscle; there was no significant difference in absorption of morphine from the two sites.[1]

Other routes of administration investigated in pharmacokinetic studies include continuous intravenous infusion[2] and continuous epidural infusion.[3]

1. Grabinski PY, *et al.* Plasma levels and analgesia following deltoid and gluteal injections of methadone and morphine. *J Clin Pharmacol* 1983; **23:** 48–55.
2. Denson DD, *et al.* Pharmacokinetics of continuous intravenous infusion of methadone in the early post-burn period. *J Clin Pharmacol* 1990; **30:** 70–5.
3. Shir Y, *et al.* Plasma concentrations of methadone during postoperative patient-controlled extradural analgesia. *Br J Anaesth* 1990; **65:** 204–9.

Administration in hepatic impairment. Overall Moore *et al.*[1] considered that hepatic dysfunction did not unduly disrupt methadone metabolism and Novick *et al.*[2] suggested that maintenance dosage of methadone need not be changed in stable chronic liver disease, although abrupt changes in hepatic status might result in substantial alterations in methadone disposition requiring dosage adjustments.

In a study of patients on methadone maintenance therapy[2] apparent terminal half-life of methadone was prolonged from a mean of 18.8 hours in those with healthy livers to 35.5 hours in patients with severe chronic liver disease. However plasma concentrations were not increased in such patients, possibly because the storage capacity of the liver was decreased.

1. Moore RA, *et al.* Opiate metabolism and excretion. *Baillieres Clin Anaesthesiol* 1987; **1:** 829–58.
2. Novick DM, *et al.* Methadone disposition in patients with chronic liver disease. *Clin Pharmacol Ther* 1981; **30:** 353–62.

Administration in renal impairment. The urinary excretion of methadone was reduced in renal failure,[1] but plasma concentrations were within the usual range and faecal excretion accounted for the majority of the dose. Very little methadone was removed by peritoneal dialysis or haemodialysis.

1. Kreek MJ, *et al.* Methadone use in patients with chronic renal disease. *Drug Alcohol Depend* 1980; **5:** 197–205.

Pregnancy. Plasma concentrations of methadone were reduced in methadone-maintained pregnant women, probably due to enhanced metabolism.[1] It was suggested that the dose of methadone might need to be increased in such patients.

1. Pond SM, *et al.* Altered methadone pharmacokinetics in methadone-maintained pregnant women. *J Pharmacol Exp Ther* 1985; **233:** 1–6.

Uses and Administration

Methadone hydrochloride, a diphenylheptane derivative, is an opioid analgesic (p.69) that is primarily a μ opioid agonist. Single doses of methadone have a less marked sedative action than single doses of morphine. Methadone is a racemic mixture and levomethadone (p.50) is the active isomer. Methadone hydrochloride is used in the treatment of severe pain; it may be of use for those patients who experience excitation or exacerbation of pain with morphine. It is also used in the management of opioid dependence. Methadone has a depressant action on the cough centre and has been used as a cough suppressant in terminal illness, although some authorities discourage this use because of the risks of accumulation.

The analgesic effect of methadone begins about 10 to 20 minutes after parenteral injection and about 30 to 60 minutes after administration by mouth, the effect of a single dose usually lasting about 4 hours. As accumulation occurs following repeated doses, the effects become more prolonged.

The analgesic dose of methadone hydrochloride ranges from 2.5 to 10 mg given at intervals of 3 to 8 hours depending on the pain. A commonly used range is 5 to 10 mg every 6 to 8 hours initially, adjusted according to response. To avoid the risk of accumulation and opioid overdosage it is recommended that in prolonged use methadone should not be administered more than twice daily. It may be given by mouth or by subcutaneous or intramuscular injection; if repeated injections are required the intramuscular route is preferred to the subcutaneous.

Methadone hydrochloride is used as part of the treatment of dependence on opioids, although prolonged use of methadone itself may result in dependence. In the treatment of opioid withdrawal, or detoxification, methadone is given initially in doses sufficient to suppress withdrawal symptoms. A mixture containing 1 mg per mL of methadone hydrochloride is used in the UK for opioid dependent persons. A dose of 10 to 20 mg of methadone hydrochloride by mouth may be given initially and increased as necessary by 10 to 20 mg daily until there are no signs of withdrawal or intoxication. After stabilisation, which can often be achieved with a daily dose of 40 to 60 mg, the dose of methadone is gradually decreased until total withdrawal is achieved. Similar doses may also be given by subcutaneous or intramuscular injection. Some treatment schedules for opioid dependence involve prolonged maintenance therapy with methadone where the daily dose is adjusted carefully for the individual; there have been reports of some patients receiving 120 mg or more daily.

For the control of intractable cough associated with terminal lung cancer, methadone hydrochloride is usually given in the form of a linctus in a dose of 1 to 2 mg every 4 to 6 hours, but reduced to twice daily on prolonged use.

Levomethadone is used similarly in the treatment of severe pain.

References.

1. Olsen GD, *et al.* Clinical effects and pharmacokinetics of racemic methadone and its optical isomers. *Clin Pharmacol Ther* 1977; **21:** 147–57.

Administration. Although duration of action following single doses of methadone is similar to that with morphine it increases considerably with multiple dosing of methadone because of the long elimination half-life (see Pharmacokinetics, above). The minimum effective dose of methadone can be difficult to titrate for the individual patient. A fixed 10-mg oral dose with a flexible patient-controlled dosage interval has been used in patients with chronic cancer pain.[1] Dosage not more frequently than every 4 hours during the first 3 to 5 days, followed by a fixed dose every 8 to 12 hours depending on the patient's requirements, was advised.

A suggested dose for patients who need to switch from oral morphine to methadone because of poor pain control is one tenth of the total daily dose of morphine, but not greater than 100 mg given at intervals determined by the patient and not more frequently than every 3 hours.[2]

When switching from oral to parenteral administration Säwe[3] suggests that the dose of methadone should be halved and adjusted thereafter as necessary.

Apart from subcutaneous or intramuscular injection methadone has also been given intravenously or intraspinally. Evidence of the prolonged effect of methadone was demonstrated when a single intravenous bolus dose of 20 mg resulted in postoperative analgesia lasting about 25 hours.[4] Methadone has also been tried intravenously in children to prevent postoperative pain; a dose of 200 μg per kg bodyweight was given perioperatively followed postoperatively by 50 μg per kg every 10 minutes until the patient was both comfortable and adequately alert.[5] An initial 2-hour loading intravenous infusion of methadone 100 to 200 μg per kg bodyweight per hour to provide rapid analgesia followed by infusion at a lower maintenance rate of 10 to 20 μg per kg per hour for continuous pain relief has been used in burn patients.[6] Epidural methadone has been used successfully in doses of up to 5 mg for analgesia in association with bupivacaine.[7,8]

1. Säwe J, *et al.* Patient-controlled dose regimen of methadone for chronic cancer pain. *Br Med J* 1981; **282:** 771–3.
2. Morley JS, *et al.* Methadone in pain uncontrolled by morphine. *Lancet* 1993; **342:** 1243.
3. Säwe J. High-dose morphine and methadone in cancer patients: clinical pharmacokinetic considerations of oral treatment. *Clin Pharmacokinet* 1986; **11:** 87–106.
4. Gourlay GK, *et al.* Methadone produces prolonged postoperative analgesia. *Br Med J* 1982; **284:** 630–1.
5. Berde CB, *et al.* Comparison of morphine and methadone for prevention of postoperative pain in 3- to 7-year-old children. *J Pediatr* 1991; **119:** 136–41.

6. Denson DD, *et al.* Pharmacokinetics of continuous intravenous infusion of methadone in the early post-burn period. *J Clin Pharmacol* 1990; **30:** 70–5.
7. Drenger B, *et al.* Extradural bupivacaine and methadone for extracorporeal shock-wave lithotripsy. *Br J Anaesth* 1989; **62:** 82–6.
8. Martin CS, *et al.* Extradural methadone and bupivacaine in labour. *Br J Anaesth* 1990; **65:** 330–2.

Opioid dependence. The treatment of opioid dependence is discussed on p.67. The following formula is not official but is that formerly listed in the Drug Tariff Formulary for Methadone Mixture 1 mg per mL. The preparation is 2.5 times the strength of Methadone Linctus (BP 1998) and is intended only for drug-dependent persons.

Methadone Mixture 1 mg/mL

methadone hydrochloride 10 mg

Green S and Tartrazine Solution (BP 1980) 0.02 mL

Compound Tartrazine Solution (BP 1980) 0.08 mL

syrup, unpreserved 5 mL

chloroform water, double-strength to 10 mL.

Some commercially available forms of methadone mixture 1 mg per mL employ a preservative system based on hydroxybenzoate esters rather than chloroform; however, syrup preserved with hydroxybenzoate esters may be unsuitable for extemporaneous dispensing (see under Incompatibility, above).

References.

1. Ghodse AH, *et al.* Comparison of oral preparations of heroin and methadone to stabilise opiate misusers as inpatients. *Br Med J* 1990; **300:** 719–20.
2. Wolff K, *et al.* Measuring compliance in methadone maintenance patients: use of a pharmacologic indicator to "estimate" methadone plasma levels. *Clin Pharmacol Ther* 1991; **50:** 199–207.
3. Wilson P, *et al.* Methadone maintenance in general practice: patients, workload, and outcomes. *Br Med J* 1994; **309:** 641–4.
4. Farrell M, *et al.* Methadone maintenance treatment in opiate dependence: a review. *Br Med J* 1994; **309:** 997–1001.

Preparations

BP 1998: Methadone Injection; Methadone Linctus; Methadone Tablets;
USP 23: Methadone Hydrochloride Injection; Methadone Hydrochloride Oral Concentrate; Methadone Hydrochloride Oral Solution; Methadone Hydrochloride Tablets.

Proprietary Preparations (details are given in Part 3)
Aust.: Heptadon; ***Austral.:*** Physeptone; ***Irl.:*** Physeptone; ***Ital.:*** Eptadone; ***Neth.:*** Symoron; ***S.Afr.:*** Physeptone; ***Spain:*** Metasedin; Sedo; ***Switz.:*** Ketalgine; ***UK:*** Martindale Methadone Mixture DTF; Methadose; Methex; Physeptone; ***USA:*** Dolophine; Methadose.

Methyl Butetisalicylate (12947-v)

Methyl Diethylacetylsalicylate. Methyl *O*-(2-ethylbutyryl)salicylate.

$C_{14}H_{18}O_4$ = 250.3.

Methyl butetisalicylate is a salicylic acid derivative that has been used similarly to methyl salicylate (p.55) as a 30% rubefacient cream for the relief of musculoskeletal, joint, and soft-tissue pain.

Preparations

Proprietary Preparations (details are given in Part 3)
Fr.: Doloderm; ***Ital.:*** Doloderm.

Methyl Gentisate (14229-j)

2,5-Dihydroxybenzoic acid methyl ester.

$C_8H_8O_4$ = 168.1.
CAS — 2150-46-1.

Methyl gentisate has been used topically for the relief of musculoskeletal and joint pain.

Preparations

Proprietary Preparations (details are given in Part 3)
Multi-ingredient: ***Ital.:*** Reumacort.

Methyl Nicotinate (9253-z)

Methyl Nicotinate *(USAN).*
Methyl pyridine-3-carboxylate.

$C_7H_7NO_2$ = 137.1.
CAS — 93-60-7.

Pharmacopoeias. In *Br.*

White or almost white crystals or crystalline powder with a characteristic odour; m.p. 40° to 42°. Very **soluble** in water, in alcohol, and in chloroform; freely soluble in ether.

Methyl nicotinate is used in topical preparations as a rubefacient.

Preparations

Proprietary Preparations (details are given in Part 3)
Austral.: Vas†; ***UK:*** Vitathone†.

Multi-ingredient: ***Aust.:*** Berggeist; Forapin; ***Austral.:*** Deep Heat; ***Belg.:*** Algipan; Decontractyl; Percutalgine; ***Canad.:*** Arthricare Odor Free; Arthricare Triple Medicated; Decontractyl; Midalgan; ***Fr.:*** Algipan†; Capsic; Carudol; Decontractyl; Lumirelax†; Sedartryl; ***Ger.:*** Arthro-Menthoneurin†; Cobed†; Contrheuma flussig†; Contrheuma-Gel forte N; Doloneuro; Forapin E; Kytta-Balsam f; Menthoneurin-Vollbad N; Midysalb; Mydalgan†; Pernionin; Pernionin Teil-Bad N; Pernionin Voll-Bad N; RH 50 percutan†; Rheumasan N; Spondylon; Symphytum Ro-Plex (Rowo-777)†; Terbintil†; Thermo-Menthoneurin Bad; ***Irl.:*** Algipan; Cremalgin†; ***Ital.:*** Aspercreme; Balsamo Sifcamina; Cloristamina†; Difmedol†; Relaxar; Sedalpan; ***Neth.:*** Cremes Tegen Spierpijn†; ***Spain:*** Balsamo Midalgan; Doctofril Antiinflamat; Doctomitil; Percutalin; Radio Salil; ***Switz.:*** Baume Kytta†; Forapin†; Kytta Baume; Methylan†; Midalgan; Nicagel†; Radalgin; Roliwol; ***UK:*** Algipan; Cremalgin; Deep Heat Spray; Dubam; Fiery Jack; Ralgex; Ralgex (low-odour); Red Oil; ***USA:*** Arthricare Odor Free; Arthricare Triple Medicated; Musterole.

Methyl Salicylate (2667-b)

Methyl Sal.; Methylis Salicylas. Methyl 2-hydroxybenzoate.

$C_8H_8O_3$ = 152.1.
CAS — 119-36-8.

Pharmacopoeias. In *Eur.* (see p.viii), *Jpn,* and *Pol.* Also in *USNF,* which allows in addition to synthetic methyl salicylate, that obtained from the leaves of *Gaultheria procumbens* (Ericaceae) and the bark of *Betula lenta* (Betulaceae). The source of the methyl salicylate must be indicated on the label.

A colourless or pale yellow or reddish liquid with a strong persistent characteristic aromatic odour.

Very slightly to slightly **soluble** in water; soluble 1 in 7 of alcohol (70%); miscible with alcohol, with fixed oils, and with volatile oils. **Store** in airtight containers. Protect from light. Certain plastic containers, such as those made from polystyrene, are unsuitable for liniments or ointments containing methyl salicylate.

NOTE. The BP directs that methyl salicylate be dispensed or supplied when Oil of Wintergreen, Wintergreen, or Wintergreen Oil is prescribed or demanded, unless it is ascertained that Methyl Salicylate Liniment (BP 1998) is required. Wintergreen Oil has also been known as Sweet Birch Oil.

Adverse Effects, Treatment, and Precautions

Salicylate intoxication can occur following ingestion or topical application of methyl salicylate (see Adverse Effects of Aspirin, p.16).

Ingestion of methyl salicylate poses the threat of severe, rapid-onset salicylate poisoning because of its liquid concentrated form and lipid solubility.[1] It is readily absorbed from the gastro-intestinal tract and most is rapidly hydrolysed to free salicylate. The symptoms, which may appear within 2 hours of ingestion, are similar to those of salicylate poisoning in general (see Adverse Effects of Aspirin, p.16), although methyl salicylate is expected to be more toxic because of its lipid solubility. There have been reports of fatalities following ingestion of as little as 4 mL in a child and 6 mL in an adult, although the adult lethal dose is estimated to be 30 mL.[1] Topical Chinese herbal medicinal oils may contain methyl salicylate in variable amounts, and salicylate poisoning has been reported in a woman who had attempted suicide by taking such a preparation, Red Flower Oil.[2] The authors also noted that some patients took small amounts of this preparation orally in an attempt to enhance its analgesic effects.

Like other salicylates, methyl salicylate may be absorbed through intact skin.[1] Percutaneous absorption is enhanced by exercise, heat, occlusion, or disruption of the integrity of the skin. The amount absorbed will also be increased by application to large areas of skin. Results from a study in healthy subjects demonstrated that a considerable amount of salicylic acid may be absorbed through the skin after topical application of products containing methyl salicylate.[3] Both the rate and extent of absorption increase after repeated application; the bioavailability of the ointment preparation used in the study increased from 15% after the second dose to 22% after the third to eighth dose. The authors recommend that topical analgesic preparations containing methyl salicylate or other salicylates should be used with caution in patients at increased risk of developing salicylate adverse effects (see Precautions of Aspirin, p.17). Results from another study[4] demonstrating high tissue to plasma ratios following topical application of a methyl salicylate formulation suggest that direct penetration and not recirculation in the blood is responsible for the salicylate concentrations found. The results also demonstrated that methyl salicylate is extensively metabolised to salicylic acid in the dermal and subcutaneous tissues following topical administration.

1. Chan TYK. Potential dangers from topical preparations containing methyl salicylate. *Hum Exp Toxicol* 1996; **15:** 747–50.
2. Chan TH, *et al.* Severe salicylate poisoning associated with the intake of Chinese medicinal oil ('Red Flower Oil'). *Aust N Z J Med* 1995; **25:** 57.
3. Morra P, *et al.* Serum concentrations of salicylic acid following topical applied salicylate derivatives. *Ann Pharmacother* 1996; **30:** 935–40.
4. Cross SE, *et al.* Is there tissue penetration after application of topical salicylate formulations? *Lancet* 1997; **350:** 636.

Interactions

Absorption of methyl salicylate through the skin can occur following excessive topical application, and interactions would be expected to be as for other salicylates (see Interactions of Aspirin, p.17).

Anticoagulants. Potentiation of warfarin anticoagulation has been reported[1,2] following topical application of methyl salicylate preparations.

1. Littleton F. Warfarin and topical salicylates. *JAMA* 1990; **263:** 2888.
2. Tam LS, *et al.* Warfarin interactions with Chinese traditional medicines: danshen and methyl salicylate medicated oil. *Aust N Z J Med* 1995; **25:** 258.

Uses and Administration

Methyl salicylate is a salicylic acid derivative that is irritant to the skin and is used topically in rubefacient preparations for the relief of pain in musculoskeletal, joint, and soft-tissue disorders. It is also used for minor peripheral vascular disorders such as chilblains and as an ingredient in inhalations for the symptomatic relief of upper respiratory-tract disorders.

Preparations

BP 1998: Kaolin Poultice; Methyl Salicylate Liniment; Methyl Salicylate Ointment; Surgical Spirit.

Proprietary Preparations (details are given in Part 3)
Austral.: Linsal; ***Ger.:*** Phlogont Rheuma; Rheumabad N†; Rheumax; ***S.Afr.:*** Thermo-Rub; ***USA:*** Argesic; Exocaine; Gordogesic.

Multi-ingredient: ***Aust.:*** Aciforin; Carl Baders Divinal; DDD; Derivon; Diphlogen; Embrocation; Leukona-Rheuma-Bad; Mayfit akut; Mayfit chronisch; Medizinalbad†; Neo-Phlogicid; Onycho Phytex; Pasta rubra salicylata; Phytex; Red Point†; Tineafax; Trafuril†; Traumasalbe; ***Austral.:*** Alcusal Sport; Analgesic Balm†; Analgesic Rub†; Biosal; Bosisto's Eucalyptus Rub; Cremor Menthol†; Deep Heat; Dencorub; Dencorub Extra Strength; Methyl Salicylate Compound Liniment; Methyl Salicylate Ointment Compound; Metsal; Metsal AR Heat Rub; Metsal Heat Rub; Painguard†; PC Arthri-Spray; Phytex†; Quelfas A†; Radian-B; Solarub†; Vicks Inhaler; ***Belg.:*** Baume Dalet; Iodex MS†; Mitosyl; Pelarol†; Rado-Salil; Reflexspray; ***Canad.:*** Absorbine Analgesic; Alsirub; Analgesic Balm; Analgesic Rub (NCP)†; Antiphlogistine Rub A-535; Arthricare Triple Medicated; Artritol; Baume Analgesique; Baume Analgesique Medicamente; Ben-Gay Original; Ben-Gay Ultra; Buckley's White Rub; Buckleys Pain Relief; Cal Mo Dol; Calmomusc; Carboseptol; Carmatis; Corn Salve; Deep Heating; Heet; Inarub; Infraline; Instant Rub; Kiro Rub; Medicated Analgesic Cream; Nasal Jelly; Pain Buster; Penetrating Rub; Physio-Rub; Pommade au The des Bois; Rheumalan; Rheumatisme; SJ Liniment; Therapeutic Soothing Ice; Thermo Rub; Thunas Salve for Rheumatic Pains; ***Fr.:*** Baume Bengue; Baume Disalgyl†; Capsic; Disalgyl; Eutalgic; Inongan; Kamol; Lao-Dal; ***Ger.:*** Brachialin percutan N; Camphopin; Clinit N†; Cuxaflex N; Dalet-Balsam; DDD; Dermalid†; Dolorsan-Balsam; Finalgon N Schmerzpflaster; Heilit; Heilit Rheuma-Olbad; Hewedolor; Hoemarin Rheuma; Hoevenol; Kneipp Rheuma Bad; Leukona-Rheuma-Bad N; Li-iL Rheuma-Bad; Marament Balsam W; Onymyken S†; Pernionin; Pernionin N; Pernionin Teil-Bad N; Psoriasis-Salbe M; Reumaless; Rheubalmin Bad; Rheuma-Pasc N; Rheumaliment†; Rosarthron forte; Salus Nieren-Blasen-Tee Nr.23; Salus Rheuma-Tee Krautertee Nr. 12; Schupps Heilkrauter Rheumabad; Segmentocut†; Trauma-Salbe Rodler 301 N; Vipracutan†; Vipratox; ***Irl.:*** Bengue's Balsam; Listerine; Monphytol; Phytex; Radian-B; ***Ital.:*** Balsamo Italstadium; Kindian†; Linimento Bertelli†; Neo Eubalsamina†; Salonpas; Soluzione Composta Alcoolica Saponosa di Coaltar; Vegetallumina; Vicks Inalante; ***Neth.:*** Sloan's liniment†; Tijgerolie†; ***S.Afr.:*** Chisi; Counterpain; Docrub; Radian; Warm-Up; ***Spain:*** Aerospray Analgesico†; Antiseptico Dent Donner†; Arnicon; Artrodesmol Extra; Balsamo Midalgan; Bartal†; Bellacanfor†; Buco Regis; Carbocaina; Dolokey; Elixir Dental Formahina†; Embrocacion Gras; Halogedol; Inhalador; Lapiz Termo Compositum†; Liderflex; Linimento Naion; Linimento Sloan; Masagil; Mentobox†; Mostazola†; Nixyn; Odontocromil c Sulfamida; Piorlis; Pomada Balsamica; Pomada Revulsiva; Porosan†; Radio Salil; Reflex; Regal; Termosan; Vicks Inhalador; ***Swed.:*** Sloan's liniment†; Trafuril†; ***Switz.:*** Antiphlogistine; Baby Liberol; Baume Esco; Baume Esco Forte; Brachialin†; Carmol "blanche"†; Carmol "thermogene"†; Carmol†; Decongestine†; Embropax; Emplatre Croix D; Fortalis; Huile analgesique "Polar-Bar"; Incutin; Kernosan Huile de Massage; Liberol; Marament-N; Massorax; Neo-Decongestine†; Neo-Liniment†; Olbas; Pasta boli; Phlogantine†; Pirom; Roliwol; Sedasept; Sloan Baume; Sloan Liniment; Vicks Inhaler N; ***UK:*** 9 Rubbing Oils; Aezodent; Antiseptic Foot Balm; Aspellin; Balmosa; Bengue's Balsam; Chymol Emollient Balm; DDD; Deep Heat Massage; Deep Heat Maximum Strength; Deep Heat Rub; Deep Heat Spray; Dermacreme; Dubam; Eftab; Germolene; Gonne Balm; Kleer Cream; Listerine Antiseptic Mouthwash; Massage Balm Arnica; Menthol and Wintergreen Heat Product†; Mentholatum Balm†; Mentholatum Nasal Inhaler; Monphytol; Nasal Inhaler; Olbas; Phytex; PR Heat Spray; Psorin; Radian-B; Ralgex; Salonair; TCP; Vapour Rub; Vicks Inhaler; ***USA:*** Analgesic Balm; Arthricare Triple Medicated; Arthritis Hot Creme; Astring-O-Sol; Banalg; Ben-Gay; Ben-Gay Ultra; Betuline; Cool-Mint Listerine; Deep Heating Lotion; Deep Heating Rub; Deep-Down Rub; Dermal-Rub; Dermolin; Flex-all 454; FreshBurst Listerine; Gordobalm; Heet; Icy Hot; Improved Analgesic; infraRUB; Iodex with Methyl Salicylate; Ivy-Chex; Listerine; Massengill; Maximum Strength Flexall 454; Methagual; Methalgen; Minit-Rub; Muscle Rub; Musterole; Musterole Extra; Pain Bust-R II; Pain Doctor; Panalgesic; Panalgesic Gold; Paralgesic; Phylorinol; Soltice; Sports Spray†; Thera-gesic; Ziks.

Mofebutazone (2670-f)

Mofebutazone *(rINN)*.

Monobutazone; Monophenylbutazone. 4-Butyl-1-phenylpyrazolidine-3,5-dione.

$C_{13}H_{16}N_2O_2$ = 232.3.

CAS — 2210-63-1.

Mofebutazone, a derivative of phenylbutazone (p.79), is an NSAID (p.63). It has been used in the management of musculoskeletal and joint disorders. Mofebutazone has been given by mouth, by rectal suppository, and by intramuscular injection of the sodium salt.

Preparations

Proprietary Preparations (details are given in Part 3)
Ger.: Diadin M; Mofesal; Mofesal N.

Multi-ingredient: *Aust.:* Clinit; *Ger.:* Algonerg†; Clinit N†; Glutisal-buton-Salbe†; Vasotonin forte; *Switz.:* Clinit†.

Mofezolac (5515-l)

Mofezolac *(rINN)*.

3,4-bis(*p*-Methoxyphenyl)-5-isoxazoleacetic acid.

$C_{19}H_{17}NO_5$ = 339.3.

CAS — 78967-07-4.

Mofezolac is an NSAID (p.63).

Morazone Hydrochloride (2671-d)

Morazone Hydrochloride *(BANM, rINNM)*.

1,5-Dimethyl-4-(3-methyl-2-phenylmorpholinomethyl)-2-phenyl-4-pyrazolin-3-one hydrochloride.

$C_{23}H_{27}N_3O_2,HCl$ = 413.9.

CAS — 6536-18-1 (morazone); 50321-35-2 (morazone hydrochloride).

Morazone hydrochloride, a pyrazolone derivative, is an NSAID (p.63). It was used, usually in conjunction with other analgesics, by mouth and has also been given by subcutaneous or intramuscular injection.

Preparations

Proprietary Preparations (details are given in Part 3)

Multi-ingredient: *Ger.:* Rosimon-Neu†.

Morniflumate (3845-j)

Morniflumate *(USAN, rINN)*.

UP-164. 2-Morpholinoethyl 2-(α,α,α-trifluoro-*m*-toluidino)nicotinate.

$C_{19}H_{20}F_3N_3O_3$ = 395.4.

CAS — 65847-85-0.

Morniflumate, the morpholinoethyl ester of niflumic acid (p.63), is an NSAID (p.63). It has been used in inflammatory conditions in doses of 700 mg given twice daily by mouth, or rectally as suppositories.

Preparations

Proprietary Preparations (details are given in Part 3)
Fr.: Nifluril; *Ital.:* Flomax; Morniflu; Niflam; *Spain:* Actol†; Niflactol; *Switz.:* Nifluril.

Morphine (6239-c)

Morphine *(BAN)*.

7,8-Didehydro-4,5-epoxy-17-methylmorphinan-3,6-diol.

$C_{17}H_{19}NO_3$ = 285.3.

CAS — 57-27-2 (anhydrous morphine); 6009-81-0 (morphine monohydrate).

Morphine is the chief alkaloid of opium which is the dried or partially dried latex from the capsules of *Papaver somniferum*. It may more commonly be obtained now from the whole plant which is harvested as Poppy straw; a concentrate of poppy straw is known as CPS.

Morphine Hydrochloride (6241-w)

Morphine Hydrochloride *(BANM)*.

Morphini Hydrochloridum; Morphinii Chloridum; Morphinum Chloratum.

$C_{17}H_{19}NO_3,HCl,3H_2O$ = 375.8.

CAS — 52-26-6 (anhydrous morphine hydrochloride); 6055-06-7 (morphine hydrochloride trihydrate).

Pharmacopoeias. In *Chin., Eur.* (see p.viii), *Int., Jpn,* and *Pol.*

Colourless, silky needles, cubical masses or a white or almost white, crystalline powder. It is efflorescent in a dry atmosphere. **Soluble** in water and in glycerol; slightly soluble in alcohol; practically insoluble in ether. **Store** in airtight containers. Protect from light.

Incompatibility. See under Morphine Sulphate, below.

Morphine Sulphate (6242-e)

Morphine Sulphate *(BANM)*.

Morphine Sulfate; Morphini Sulfas.

$(C_{17}H_{19}NO_3)_2,H_2SO_4,5H_2O$ = 758.8.

CAS — 64-31-3 (anhydrous morphine sulphate); 6211-15-0 (morphine sulphate pentahydrate).

Pharmacopoeias. In *Eur.* (see p.viii), *Int.,* and *US.*

Odourless, white or almost white, acicular crystals, cubical masses, or crystalline powder. When exposed to air it gradually loses water of hydration. It darkens on prolonged exposure to light. Ph. Eur. **solubilities** are: soluble in water; very slightly soluble in alcohol; practically insoluble in toluene. USP solubilities are: soluble 1 in 16 of water and 1 in 1 of water at 80°; soluble 1 in 570 of alcohol and 1 in 240 of alcohol at 60°; insoluble in chloroform and in ether. **Store** in airtight containers. Protect from light.

Incompatibility. Morphine salts are sensitive to changes in pH and morphine is liable to be precipitated out of solution in an alkaline environment. Compounds incompatible with morphine salts include aminophylline and sodium salts of barbiturates and phenytoin. Other incompatibilities, sometimes attributed to particular formulations, have included:

- aciclovir sodium—precipitate noted two hours after admixture with morphine sulphate solution;[1]
- chlorpromazine hydrochloride injection—precipitation was considered to be due to chlorocresol present in the morphine sulphate injection;[2]
- doxorubicin—addition of morphine sulphate 1 mg per mL to doxorubicin hydrochloride liposomal injection 0.4 mg per mL in dextrose 5% resulted in turbidity changes;[3]
- fluorouracil—immediate precipitate formed after admixture of fluorouracil 1 or 16 mg per mL with morphine sulphate 1 mg per mL in dextrose 5% or sodium chloride 0.9%;[4]
- frusemide—precipitate noted one hour after admixture with morphine sulphate solution;[1]
- heparin sodium—incompatibility has been reported from straightforward additive studies.[5] A more recent study[6] indicated that morphine sulphate and heparin sodium were only incompatible at morphine sulphate concentrations greater than 5 mg per mL and that this incompatibility could be prevented by using 0.9% sodium chloride solution as the admixture diluent rather than water;
- pethidine hydrochloride—incompatibility has been noted following admixture with morphine sulphate;[5,7]
- prochlorperazine edisylate—immediate precipitation was attributed to phenol in the morphine sulphate injection formulation;[8,9]
- promethazine hydrochloride—cloudiness was reported to develop when 12.5 mg of promethazine hydrochloride was drawn into a syringe containing morphine sulphate 8 mg.[10] Others[7] have noted no incompatibility;
- tetracyclines—colour change from pale yellow to light green occurred when solutions of minocycline hydrochloride or tetracycline hydrochloride were mixed with morphine sulphate in 5% glucose injection.[11]

1. Pugh CB, *et al.* Visual compatibility of morphine sulphate and meperidine hydrochloride with other injectable drugs during simulated Y-site injection. *Am J Hosp Pharm* 1991; **48:** 123–5.
2. Crapper JB. Mixing chlorpromazine and morphine. *Br Med J* 1975; **i:** 33.
3. Trissel LA, *et al.* Compatibility of doxorubicin hydrochloride liposome injection with selected other drugs during simulated Y-site administration. *Am J Health-Syst Pharm* 1997; **54:** 2703–13.
4. Xu QA, *et al.* Stability and compatibility of fluorouracil with morphine sulfate and hydromorphone hydrochloride. *Ann Pharmacother* 1996; **30:** 756–61.
5. Patel JA, Phillips GL. A guide to physical compatibility of intravenous drug admixtures. *Am J Hosp Pharm* 1966; **23:** 409–11.
6. Baker DE, *et al.* Compatibility of heparin sodium and morphine sulfate. *Am J Hosp Pharm* 1985; **42:** 1352–5.
7. Parker WA. Physical compatibilities of preanesthetic medications. *Can J Hosp Pharm* 1976; **29:** 91–2.
8. Stevenson JG, Patriarca C. Incompatibility of morphine sulfate and prochlorperazine edisylate in syringes. *Am J Hosp Pharm* 1985; **42:** 2651.
9. Zuber DEL. Compatibility of morphine sulfate injection and prochlorperazine edisylate injection. *Am J Hosp Pharm* 1987; **44:** 67.
10. Fleischer NM. Promethazine hydrochloride—morphine sulfate incompatibility. *Am J Hosp Pharm* 1973; **30:** 665.
11. Nieves-Cordero AL, *et al.* Compatibility of narcotic analgesic solutions with various antibiotics during simulated Y-site injection. *Am J Hosp Pharm* 1985; **42:** 1108–9.

Stability. Solutions of morphine sulphate for intravenous infusion appear to be relatively stable. In one study[1] 0.04 mg per mL and 0.4 mg per mL solutions retained more than 90% of their initial concentration of morphine sulphate when stored at 4° or 23° for 7 days, whether or not they were protected from light. Solutions prepared from commercially available injection or from powder, in 0.9% sodium chloride or 5% glucose, and stored in polyvinyl chloride bags or glass bottles were equally stable. In a further study[2] 10 mg per mL or 5 mg per mL solutions of morphine sulphate in glucose or sodium chloride and stored in portable infusion pump cassettes retained more than 95% of their initial concentration when kept at 23° for 30 days. A 0.9% solution of sodium chloride containing morphine sulphate 2 mg per mL was stable for 6 weeks when stored in polypropylene syringes at ambient temperatures in the light or dark but a similar solution which also contained 0.1% sodium metabisulphite lost 15% of its potency during the same period.[3] Stability of such a solution with or without sodium metabisulphite was considered to be unacceptable when stored in glass syringes in the dark.[4]

1. Vecchio M, *et al.* The stability of morphine intravenous infusion solutions. *Can J Hosp Pharm* 1988; **41:** 5–9, 43.
2. Walker SE, *et al.* Hydromorphone and morphine stability in portable infusion pump cassettes and minibags. *Can J Hosp Pharm* 1988; **41:** 177–82.
3. Grassby PF. The stability of morphine sulphate in 0.9 per cent sodium chloride stored in plastic syringes. *Pharm J* 1991; **248:** HS24–HS25.
4. Grassby PF, Hutchings L. Factors affecting the physical and chemical stability of morphine sulphate solutions stored in syringes. *Int J Pharm Pract* 1993; **2:** 39–43.

References to the stability of morphine in Kaolin and Morphine Mixture (BP).

1. Helliwell K, Game P. Stability of morphine in kaolin and morphine mixture BP. *Pharm J* 1981; **227:** 128–9.
2. Helliwell K, Jennings P. Kaolin and morphine mixture BP: effects of containers on the stability of morphine. *Pharm J* 1984; **232:** 682.

Morphine Tartrate (6243-l)

Morphine Tartrate *(BANM)*.

$(C_{17}H_{19}NO_3)_2,C_4H_6O_6,3H_2O$ = 774.8.

CAS — 302-31-8 (anhydrous morphine tartrate); 6032-59-3 (morphine tartrate trihydrate).

Incompatibility. See under Morphine Sulphate, above.

Dependence and Withdrawal

As for Opioid Analgesics, p.67.

Dependence associated with morphine and closely related μ-agonists appears to result in more severe withdrawal symptoms than that associated with κ-receptor agonists. With morphine, withdrawal symptoms usually begin within a few hours, reach a peak within 36 to 72 hours, and then gradually subside.

Adverse Effects and Treatment

As for Opioid Analgesics in general, p.68.

Effects on the cardiovascular system. For a reference to the effects of morphine on histamine release compared with some other opioids, see under Pethidine, p.76.

Effects on the muscles. There has been a report of severe rectovaginal spasms in one patient following intrathecal administration of morphine.[1] The spasms were successfully controlled with midazolam.

1. Littrell RA, *et al.* Muscle spasms associated with intrathecal morphine therapy: treatment with midazolam. *Clin Pharm* 1992; **11:** 57–9.

Effects on the nervous system. Myoclonus has been reported in patients with advanced malignant disease receiving high doses of morphine.[1] It was unrelated to plasma-morphine concentrations and was attributed in part to the concurrent use of other drugs including antidepressants, antipsychotics, and NSAIDs. Quinn[2] questioned the diagnosis of myoclonus and the role of morphine. McQuay[3] also criticised the importance attached to myoclonus by Potter *et al.*[1] and considered it probably the least common and least important of all the side-effects of morphine.

Glare *et al.*[4] have reported myoclonus in 2 cancer patients with renal impairment on high stable doses of morphine; the metabolite normorphine, found in the plasma of both patients, might have been responsible.

It has been reported that myoclonus induced by morphine may be successfully controlled using a benzodiazepine such as midazolam.[5]

1. Potter JM, *et al.* Myoclonus associated with treatment with high doses of morphine: the role of supplemental drugs. *Br Med J* 1989; **299:** 150–3.
2. Quinn N. Myoclonus associated with high doses of morphine. *Br Med J* 1989; **299:** 683–4.
3. McQuay HJ, *et al.* Myoclonus associated with high doses of morphine. *Br Med J* 1989; **299:** 684.
4. Glare PA, *et al.* Normorphine, a neurotoxic metabolite? *Lancet* 1990; **335:** 725–6.
5. Holdsworth MT, *et al.* Continuous midazolam infusion for the management of morphine-induced myoclonus. *Ann Pharmacother* 1995; **29:** 25–9.

Precautions

As for Opioid Analgesics in general, p.68.

Biliary-tract disorders. See under Precautions of Opioid Analgesics, p.68.

Hepatic impairment. In view of its hepatic metabolism, caution is generally advised when giving morphine to patients with impaired liver function (but see under Pharmacokinetics, below). Some advise that administration should be avoided or the dose reduced because of the risk of precipitating a coma. Twycross and Lack[1] considered that moderate hepatic insufficiency does not affect morphine metabolism whereas severe hepatic failure may.

The mean elimination half-life of morphine in 12 patients with cirrhosis was almost twice that in 10 healthy subjects after administration of a modified-release oral morphine preparation (MST-Continus) and peak serum concentrations were almost three times as high.[2] Patients with cirrhosis exhibited a greater degree of sedation but none developed encephalopathy. It was recommended that the dose for modified-release preparations should be reduced and the frequency of administration prolonged for patients with cirrhosis.

1. Twycross RG, Lack SA. *Oral morphine in advanced cancer*. 2nd ed. Beaconsfield: Beaconsfield Publishers, 1989.
2. Kotb HIM, *et al.* Pharmacokinetics of controlled release morphine (MST) in patients with liver cirrhosis. *Br J Anaesth* 1997; **79:** 804–6.

Neonates. Preterm neonates who had been randomly allocated to receive morphine to aid mechanical ventilation showed no difference in IQ, motor impairment, or behaviour compared with similar neonates who received non-opioid treatment when assessed at 5 to 6 years of age.[1]

1. MacGregor R, *et al.* Outcome at 5-6 years of prematurely born children who received morphine as neonates. *Arch Dis Child* 1998; **79:** F40–F43.

Phaeochromocytoma. Morphine and some other opioids can induce the release of endogenous histamine and thereby stimulate catecholamine release making them unsuitable for use in patients with phaeochromocytoma. For further details, see p.69.

Renal impairment. Severe and prolonged respiratory depression has occurred in patients with renal impairment given morphine. Osborne *et al.*[1] attributed toxicity in 3 such patients to the accumulation of the active metabolite morphine-6-glucuronide. Hasselström *et al.*[2] found plasma concentrations of this metabolite to be ten times higher than normal in a 7-year-old girl with haemolytic uraemic syndrome given morphine intravenously although the half-life of morphine was also prolonged. Calleja *et al.*[3] reported plasma concentrations of morphine-6-glucuronide to be persistently increased 19 days after stopping morphine by intravenous infusion in a 17-year-old girl with normal renal function. They suggested that alterations in bowel flora following antibiotic therapy or inhibition of morphine-3-glucuronide glucuronidation by lorazepam might be responsible. Osborne *et al.*[4] have also reported that accumulation of morphine can occur in renal failure, although to a lesser extent than accumulation of metabolites (see also under Pharmacokinetics, below).

1. Osborne RJ, *et al.* Morphine intoxication in renal failure: the role of morphine-6-glucuronide. *Br Med J* 1986; **292:** 1548–9.
2. Hasselström J, *et al.* Long lasting respiratory depression induced by morphine-6-glucuronide? *Br J Clin Pharmacol* 1989; **27:** 515–18.
3. Calleja MA, *et al.* Persistently increased morphine-6-glucuronide concentrations. *Br J Anaesth* 1990; **64:** 649.
4. Osborne R, *et al.* The pharmacokinetics of morphine and morphine glucuronides in kidney failure. *Clin Pharmacol Ther* 1993; **54:** 158–67.

Interactions

For interactions associated with opioid analgesics, see p.69.

For references to myoclonus associated with morphine and the concurrent use of other drugs, see Effects on the Nervous System under Adverse Effects, above.

Benzodiazepines. An additive sedative effect is to be expected between opioid analgesics and benzodiazepines and has been reported with morphine and midazolam.[1]

For reference to a suggestion that lorazepam may inhibit morphine-3-glucuronide glucuronidation, see Renal Impairment under Precautions, above.

1. Tverskoy M, *et al.* Midazolam-morphine sedative interaction in patients. *Anesth Analg* 1989; **68:** 282–5.

Cisapride. Plasma concentrations of morphine have been increased following concomitant oral administration with cisapride.[1]

1. Rowbotham DJ, *et al.* Effect of cisapride on morphine absorption after oral administration of sustained-release morphine. *Br J Anaesth* 1991; **67:** 421–5.

Histamine H_2 antagonists. See under Opioid Analgesics, p.69.

Local Anaesthetics. Prior use of epidural chloroprocaine has been reported[1] to reduce the duration of epidural morphine analgesia.

1. Eisenach JC, *et al.* Effect of prior anesthetic solution on epidural morphine analgesia. *Anesth Analg* 1991; **73:** 119–23.

Metoclopramide. Reports on the effects of metoclopramide on morphine have included an increased rate of onset and degree of sedation when metoclopramide was given by mouth with modified-release morphine[1] and antagonism of the effects of morphine on gastric emptying by intravenous metoclopramide.[2]

1. Manara AR, *et al.* The effect of metoclopramide on the absorption of oral controlled release morphine. *Br J Clin Pharmacol* 1988; **25:** 518–21.
2. McNeill MJ, *et al.* Effect of iv metoclopramide on gastric emptying after opioid premedication. *Br J Anaesth* 1990; **64:** 450–2.

Tricyclic antidepressants. Both clomipramine and amitriptyline significantly increased the plasma availability of morphine when given to cancer patients taking oral morphine solution.[1] It was noted however that the potentiation of the analgesic effects of morphine by these drugs might not be confined to increased bioavailability of morphine; the dose of tricyclic to use with morphine in the treatment of cancer pain should be decided by clinical evaluation rather than by pharmacokinetic data.

1. Ventafridda V, *et al.* Antidepressants increase bioavailability of morphine in cancer patients. *Lancet* 1987; **i:** 1204.

Pharmacokinetics

Morphine salts are well absorbed from the gastrointestinal tract but have poor oral bioavailability since they undergo extensive first-pass metabolism in the liver and gut. After subcutaneous or intramuscular injection morphine is readily absorbed into the blood. The majority of a dose of morphine is conjugated with glucuronic acid in the liver and gut to produce morphine-3-glucuronide and morphine-6-glucuronide. The latter is considered to contribute to the analgesic effect of morphine, especially when repeated doses are given by mouth. Morphine-3-glucuronide on the other hand may antagonise the analgesic action of morphine and morphine-6-glucuronide and it has been suggested that it might be responsible for the paradoxical pain observed in some patients given morphine. Other active metabolites include normorphine, codeine, and morphine ethereal sulphate. Enterohepatic circulation probably occurs. Morphine is distributed throughout the body but mainly in the kidneys, liver, lungs, and spleen, with lower concentrations in the brain and muscles. Morphine crosses the blood-brain barrier less readily than more lipid-soluble opioids such as diamorphine, but it has been detected in the cerebrospinal fluid as have its highly polar metabolites morphine-3-glucuronide and morphine-6-glucuronide. Morphine diffuses across the placenta and traces also appear in breast milk and sweat. About 35% is protein bound. Mean plasma elimination half-lives of 1.7 hours for morphine and 2.4 to 6.7 hours for morphine-3-glucuronide have been reported.

Up to 10% of a dose of morphine may eventually be excreted, as conjugates, through the bile into the faeces. The remainder is excreted in the urine, mainly as conjugates. About 90% of total morphine is excreted in 24 hours with traces in urine for 48 hours or more.

Much has been published on the metabolism and disposition of morphine and its relevance to the clinical use of morphine, in particular the analgesic effect of repeated oral doses and the relative potency of oral to parenteral doses. There has been uncertainty as to the contributions in man of first-pass metabolism in the liver and gut, the possible role of renal metabolism, the analgesic activity and clinical importance of the metabolite morphine-6-glucuronide, and enterohepatic circulation. There has also been interest in the effects of the metabolite morphine-3-glucuronide.

A major role for the kidney rather than the liver in the metabolism of morphine was proposed by McQuay and Moore[1,2] in 1984. Around that time Hanks and Aherne[3] considered that the liver, gut wall, and kidney might all be important, but later they and others[4,5] rejected the kidney as a major site of morphine metabolism and considered the liver and possibly the gut to have a predominant role. In 1987 Moore *et al.*[6] noted that, although morphine conjugation was generally assumed to occur primarily in the liver, the evidence was not compelling, yet neither the intestines nor the kidney seemed likely sites for extrahepatic metabolism.

Hanks *et al.*[4] sought to explain the more favourable oral to parenteral potency ratio of 1:2 or 1:3 associated with repeated dosage of morphine as opposed to single-dose ratios of 1:6 or 1:8. They concluded that the increased analgesic efficacy of repeated oral doses of morphine when compared with a single oral dose might be due to the active metabolite morphine-6-glucuronide making a significant contribution to the overall analgesic effect; they also maintained that enterohepatic circulation of morphine might be a contributory factor. McQuay *et al.*[7] considered there was no convincing evidence that repeated doses were more effective than single doses. Hanks *et al.*[8] re-affirmed their belief that there was a difference between the results with single or repeated doses of morphine; they considered the likeliest explanation to be the analgesic contribution of morphine-6-glucuronide with enterohepatic circulation of morphine and its metabolites probably being of secondary importance.[9]

Osborne *et al.*[10] have demonstrated the analgesic activity of morphine-6-glucuronide when given to cancer patients and Paul *et al.*[11] have reported *animal* work implying that morphine-6-glucuronide acts through the same receptor mechanisms as morphine. In a small study in 3 cancer patients Hanna *et al.*[12] found that morphine-6-glucuronide administered intrathecally had greater analgesic activity than intrathecal morphine and persisted for longer in the lumbar cerebrospinal fluid; morphine-6-glucuronide was not detected in CSF following the intrathecal administration of morphine. It now seems accepted that morphine-6-glucuronide makes a major contribution to the analgesic activity of morphine.[13-15] Preliminary studies also suggest that morphine-6-glucuronide may cause less toxicity than morphine.[16]

The pharmacokinetics of morphine-6-glucuronide have been investigated by Hanna *et al.*[17] They found the terminal half-life of about 2 hours for injected morphine-6-glucuronide to be similar to that for morphine or morphine-6-glucuronide resulting from morphine metabolism; volume of distribution and clearance rate were significantly smaller for injected morphine-6-glucuronide than for morphine.

Morphine-3-glucuronide is also a major metabolite of morphine. Findings in *animals* indicate that this metabolite may antagonise the analgesic action of morphine and morphine-6-glucuronide.[18] It has also been suggested that abnormal metabolism of morphine to produce morphine-3-glucuronide but no morphine-6-glucuronide may explain the unexpected lack of pain relief or even the worsening of pain in some patients given morphine.[19,20]

1. McQuay H, Moore A. Metabolism of narcotics. *Br Med J* 1984; **288:** 237.
2. Moore A, *et al.* Morphine kinetics during and after renal transplantation. *Clin Pharmacol Ther* 1984; **35:** 641–5.
3. Hanks GW, Aherne GW. Morphine metabolism: does the renal hypothesis hold water? *Lancet* 1985; **i:** 221–2.
4. Hanks GW, *et al.* Explanation for potency of repeated oral doses of morphine? *Lancet* 1987; **ii:** 723–5.
5. Bodenham A, *et al.* Extrahepatic morphine metabolism in man during the anhepatic phase of orthotopic liver transplantation. *Br J Anaesth* 1989; **63:** 380–4.
6. Moore RA, *et al.* Opiate metabolism and excretion. *Baillieres Clin Anaesthesiol* 1987; **1:** 829–58.
7. McQuay HJ, *et al.* Potency of oral morphine. *Lancet* 1987; **ii:** 1458–9.
8. Hanks GW, *et al.* Enterohepatic circulation of morphine. *Lancet* 1988; **i:** 469.
9. Hanks GW, Wand PJ. Enterohepatic circulation of opioid drugs: is it clinically relevant in the treatment of cancer patients? *Clin Pharmacokinet* 1989; **17:** 65–8.
10. Osborne R, *et al.* Analgesic activity of morphine-6-glucuronide. *Lancet* 1988; **i:** 828.
11. Paul D, *et al.* Pharmacological characterization of morphine-6β-glucuronide, a very potent morphine metabolite. *J Pharmacol Exp Ther* 1989; **251:** 477–83.
12. Hanna MH, *et al.* Analgesic efficacy and CSF pharmacokinetics of intrathecal morphine-6-glucuronide: comparison with morphine. *Br J Anaesth* 1990; **64:** 547–50.
13. Osborne R, *et al.* Morphine and metabolite behavior after different routes of morphine administration: demonstration of the importance of the active metabolite morphine-6-glucuronide. *Clin Pharmacol Ther* 1990; **47:** 12–19.
14. McQuay HJ, *et al.* Oral morphine in cancer pain: influences on morphine and metabolite concentration. *Clin Pharmacol Ther* 1990; **48:** 236–44.
15. Portenoy RK, *et al.* The metabolite morphine-6-glucuronide contributes to the analgesia produced by morphine infusion in patients with pain and normal renal function. *Clin Pharmacol Ther* 1992; **51:** 422–31.
16. Thompson PI, *et al.* Respiratory depression following morphine and morphine-6-glucuronide in normal subjects. *Br J Clin Pharmacol* 1995; **40:** 145–52.
17. Hanna MH, *et al.* Disposition of morphine-6-glucuronide and morphine in healthy volunteers. *Br J Anaesth* 1991; **66:** 103–7.
18. Smith MT, *et al.* Morphine-3-glucuronide—a potent antagonist of morphine analgesia. *Life Sci* 1990; **47:** 579–85.
19. Morley JS, *et al.* Paradoxical pain. *Lancet* 1992; **340:** 1045.
20. Morley JS, *et al.* Methadone in pain uncontrolled by morphine. *Lancet* 1993; **342:** 1243.

Administration. There have been many studies on the pharmacokinetics of morphine following administration by various routes and methods. They include administration by the buccal route (see below), modified-release oral preparations,[1,2] the rectal route,[3,4] the pulmonary route,[5,6] continuous subcutaneous compared with intravenous infusion,[7] and the intraspinal route.[8-12]

Morgan[13] discussed briefly the pharmacokinetic aspects of opioids given by epidural and intrathecal injection. Slow dural transfer of morphine and its prolonged presence in the cerebrospinal fluid appeared to correlate with its slow onset and long duration of action by these routes. More lipid-soluble opioids, such as diamorphine and pethidine, entered and left the CSF more rapidly than morphine.

Osborne *et al.*[14] studied the pharmacokinetics of morphine administered by 5 different routes—intravenous bolus injection and oral, sublingual, buccal, and modified-release buccal tablets—with particular reference to morphine-6-glucuronide, the active metabolite. This metabolite occurred in large quantities after intravenous administration and plasma concentrations rapidly exceeded those of morphine. Following oral administration morphine-6-glucuronide and morphine-3-glucuronide were present in quantities similar to those seen after intravenous morphine; morphine concentrations in plasma were very low and the mean morphine-6-glucuronide to morphine area under the curve ratio was 9.7 to 1. There was delayed absorption with attenuation and delay of peak morphine and metabolite plasma concentrations following sublingual or buccal administration.

Babul and Darke[15] found that, compared with oral administration, concentrations of morphine were higher and those of its glucuronides lower when morphine was given rectally suggesting avoidance of first-pass metabolism.

1. Pinnock CA, *et al.* Absorption of controlled release morphine sulphate in the immediate postoperative period. *Br J Anaesth* 1986; **58:** 868–71.
2. Savarese JJ, *et al.* Steady-state pharmacokinetics of controlled release oral morphine sulphate in healthy subjects. *Clin Pharmacokinet* 1986; **11:** 505–10.
3. Moolenaar F, *et al.* Drastic improvement in the rectal absorption profile of morphine in man. *Eur J Clin Pharmacol* 1985; **29:** 119–21.
4. Cole L, *et al.* Further development of a morphine hydrogel suppository. *Br J Clin Pharmacol* 1990; **30:** 781–6.
5. Ward ME, *et al.* Morphine pharmacokinetics after pulmonary administration from a novel aerosol delivery system. *Clin Pharmacol Ther* 1997; **62:** 596–609.
6. Masood AR, Thomas SHL. Systemic absorption of nebulized morphine compared with oral morphine in healthy subjects. *Br J Clin Pharmacol* 1996; **41:** 250–2.
7. Waldmann CS, *et al.* Serum morphine levels: a comparison between continuous subcutaneous infusion and continuous intravenous infusion in postoperative patients. *Anaesthesia* 1984; **39:** 768–71.
8. Gustafsson LL, *et al.* Disposition of morphine in cerebrospinal fluid after epidural administration. *Lancet* 1982; **i:** 796.
9. Moore A, *et al.* Spinal fluid kinetics of morphine and heroin. *Clin Pharmacol Ther* 1984; **35:** 40–5.
10. Max MB, *et al.* Epidural and intrathecal opiates: cerebrospinal fluid and plasma profiles in patients with chronic cancer pain. *Clin Pharmacol Ther* 1985; **38:** 631–41.
11. Nordberg G, *et al.* Extradural morphine: influence of adrenaline admixture. *Br J Anaesth* 1986; **58:** 598–604.
12. Ionescu TI, *et al.* The pharmacokinetics of intradural morphine in major abdominal surgery. *Clin Pharmacokinet* 1988; **14:** 178–86.
13. Morgan M. The rational use of intrathecal and extradural opioids. *Br J Anaesth* 1989; **63:** 165–88.
14. Osborne R, *et al.* Morphine and metabolite behavior after different routes of morphine administration: demonstration of the importance of the active metabolite morphine-6-glucuronide. *Clin Pharmacol Ther* 1990; **47:** 12–19.
15. Babul N, Darke AC. Disposition of morphine and its glucuronide metabolites after oral and rectal administration: evidence of route specificity. *Clin Pharmacol Ther* 1993; **54:** 286–92.

BUCCAL ROUTE. Conflicting results from studies on buccal administration of morphine may reflect differences in formulation[1] and hence absorption. Bell *et al.*[2] reported equivalent analgesia with buccal and intramuscular morphine although Fisher *et al.*[3] found marked interindividual variability with mean peak serum concentrations of morphine some eight times lower after a buccal tablet than after an intramuscular injection and occurring a mean of 4 hours later. Morphine sulphate in aqueous solution has been reported to be moderately well absorbed from the buccal mucosa.[4] Absolute bioavailability for morphine was estimated to be 23.8% after an oral solution, 22.4% after a modified-release oral tablet (MST Continus), and 20.2% after a modified-release buccal tablet, with maximum plasma-morphine concentrations at 45 minutes, 2.5 hours, and 6 hours respectively; mean ratios of area under the plasma concentration-time curve for morphine-6-glucuronide to morphine in plasma were 11:1 after buccal and oral morphine compared with 2:1 for intravenous morphine.[5] There was considerable inter-subject variation in plasma concentrations of the morphine metabolites, morphine-3-glucuronide and morphine-6-glucuronide, following buccal administration of morphine as a modified-release formulation[6] and lack of pain relief was subsequently reported with this buccal formulation.[7] Poor absorption of morphine from modified-release buccal tablets when compared with intramuscular injection was also reported by Simpson *et al.*;[8] bitterness of the tablets, leading to their premature removal, and poor dissolution may have contributed.

1. Calvey TN, Williams NE. Pharmacokinetics of buccal morphine. *Br J Anaesth* 1990; **64:** 256.
2. Bell MDD, *et al.* Buccal morphine—a new route for analgesia? *Lancet* 1985; **i:** 71–3.
3. Fisher AP, *et al.* Serum morphine concentrations after buccal and intramuscular morphine administration. *Br J Clin Pharmacol* 1987; **24:** 685–7.
4. Al-Sayed-Omar O, *et al.* Influence of pH on the buccal absorption of morphine sulphate and its major metabolite, morphine-3-glucuronide. *J Pharm Pharmacol* 1987; **39:** 934–5.
5. Hoskin PJ, *et al.* The bioavailability and pharmacokinetics of morphine after intravenous, oral and buccal administration in healthy volunteers. *Br J Clin Pharmacol* 1989; **27:** 499–505.
6. Manara AR, *et al.* Pharmacokinetics of morphine following administration by the buccal route. *Br J Anaesth* 1989; **62:** 498–502.
7. Manara AR, *et al.* Analgesic efficacy of perioperative buccal morphine. *Br J Anaesth* 1990; **64:** 551–5.
8. Simpson KH, *et al.* An investigation of premedication with morphine given by the buccal or intramuscular route. *Br J Clin Pharmacol* 1989; **27:** 377–80.

Administration in the elderly. The pharmacokinetics of morphine were compared in 7 elderly (60 to 69 years) and 13 young subjects, all of them healthy, following a single intravenous injection of morphine sulphate 10 mg per 70 kg bodyweight.[1] Although the terminal rate of drug disappearance from plasma was faster in the elderly group, apparent volume of distribution at steady state was about half that of the young group and plasma clearance was reduced.

1. Owen JA, *et al.* Age-related morphine kinetics. *Clin Pharmacol Ther* 1983; **34:** 364–8.

Administration in hepatic impairment. The liver is a major site of morphine metabolism and therefore impaired liver function could be expected to affect elimination. There is some evidence that in cirrhosis glucuronidation might be relatively spared compared with other metabolic processes and that some extrahepatic metabolism may occur. Several studies have served to illustrate these points; hepatic extraction of morphine was impaired in cirrhotic patients, but less than expected;[1] morphine metabolism was minimal during the anhepatic phase of liver transplantation, but increased markedly when the new liver was reperfused;[2] morphine metabolism was virtually complete following liver transplantation with only 4.5% unchanged morphine being excreted in the urine 24 hours after administration;[3] morphine elimination was reduced when hepatic blood flow was impaired.[4]

1. Crotty B, *et al.* Hepatic extraction of morphine is impaired in cirrhosis. *Eur J Clin Pharmacol* 1989; **36:** 501–6.
2. Bodenham A, *et al.* Extrahepatic morphine metabolism in man during the anhepatic phase of orthotopic liver transplantation. *Br J Anaesth* 1989; **63:** 380–4.
3. Shelly MP, *et al.* Pharmacokinetics of morphine in patients following orthotopic liver transplantation. *Br J Anaesth* 1989; **63:** 375–9.
4. Manara AR, *et al.* Morphine elimination and liver blood flow: a study in patients undergoing distal splenorenal shunt. *Br J Hosp Med* 1989; **42:** 148 (abstract).

Administration in infants and children. The pharmacokinetics of morphine in children are similar to those in adults;[1-3] in each case an elimination half-life of about 2 hours has been reported following intravenous administration of morphine. Pharmacokinetic differences have however been observed in neonates given morphine by intravenous infusion. An elimination half-life of 13.9 ± 6.4 hours was reported in 8 neonates aged 1 to 30 days.[4] In another study 7 neonates aged 1 to 4 days had a mean elimination half-life of 6.81 hours compared with 3.91 hours in 4 infants aged 17 to 65 days; clearance of morphine was also significantly reduced in the newborn group.[5] The metabolism of morphine in 12 children aged 1 to 16 years was compared with that in 9 premature infants aged 2 to 12 days.[6] As expected, plasma clearance was lower in the neonates than in the children, probably due to a reduction in the metabolism of morphine in the neonates, as well as to immature renal function. Morphine-3-glucuronide and morphine-6-glucuronide were however detected in plasma or urine from children and neonates indicating that preterm infants can metabolise morphine by glucuronidation, although capacity to do so was enhanced after the neonatal period. However, Hartley *et al.*[7] have reported that while morphine-3-glucuronide could be measured in plasma samples from premature neonates obtained at 2 hours and 24 hours morphine-6-glucuronide could only be measured in samples obtained at 24 hours. Also in another study of 16 acutely ill infants of less than 32 weeks gestational age 6 did not conjugate morphine at all and eliminated it in the urine unchanged.[8] The pharmacokinetics of morphine were very variable in preterm and term neonates given a single intravenous dose in the first week of life;[9] nearly 80% of morphine remained unbound. The 10 preterm infants with a gestational age of up to 30 weeks had a mean elimination half-life of 10.0 hours compared with 6.7 hours in 3 term neonates.

1. Dahlström B, *et al.* Morphine kinetics in children. *Clin Pharmacol Ther* 1979; **26:** 354–65.
2. Stanski DR, *et al.* Kinetics of high-dose intravenous morphine in cardiac surgery patients. *Clin Pharmacol Ther* 1976; **19:** 752–6.
3. Olkkola KT, *et al.* Clinical pharmacokinetics and pharmacodynamics of opioid analgesics in infants and children. *Clin Pharmacokinet* 1995; **5:** 385–404.
4. Koren G, *et al.* Postoperative morphine infusion in newborn infants: assessment of disposition characteristics and safety. *J Pediatr* 1985; **107:** 963–7.
5. Lynn AM, Slattery JT. Morphine pharmacokinetics in early infancy. *Anesthesiology* 1987; **66:** 136–9.
6. Choonara IA, *et al.* Morphine metabolism in children. *Br J Clin Pharmacol* 1989; **28:** 599–604.
7. Hartley R, *et al.* Pharmacokinetics of morphine infusion in premature neonates. *Arch Dis Child* 1993; **69:** 55–8.
8. Bhat R, *et al.* Morphine metabolism in acutely ill preterm newborn infants. *J Pediatr* 1992; **120:** 795–9.
9. Bhat R, *et al.* Pharmacokinetics of a single dose of morphine in preterm infants during the first week of life. *J Pediatr* 1990; **117:** 477–81.

Administration in renal impairment. Only a small amount of morphine is excreted unchanged in the urine. There are conflicting reports of morphine accumulation; some for,[1,2] others against.[3-5] It does seem clear though that morphine metabolites accumulate in patients with renal impairment;[5-9] the half-life of the active metabolite morphine-6-glucuronide was reported to be prolonged and its clearance reduced when morphine-6-glucuronide was administered to patients with renal impairment.[10] Opioid intoxication[11] and a prolonged opioid effect[12] in patients with renal failure has been associated with morphine-6-glucuronide (see also under Precautions, above).

1. Ball M, *et al.* Renal failure and the use of morphine in intensive care. *Lancet* 1985; **i:** 784–6.
2. Osborne R, *et al.* The pharmacokinetics of morphine and morphine glucuronides in kidney failure. *Clin Pharmacol Ther* 1993; **54:** 158–67.
3. Säwe J, *et al.* Kinetics of morphine in patients with renal failure. *Lancet* 1985; **ii:** 211.
4. Woolner DF, *et al.* Renal failure does not impair the metabolism of morphine. *Br J Clin Pharmacol* 1986; **22:** 55–9.
5. Chauvin M, *et al.* Morphine pharmacokinetics in renal failure. *Anesthesiology* 1987; **66:** 327–31.
6. Säwe J, Odar-Cederlöf I. Kinetics of morphine in patients with renal failure. *Eur J Clin Pharmacol* 1987; **32:** 377–82.
7. Wolff J, *et al.* Influence of renal function on the elimination of morphine and morphine glucuronides. *Eur J Clin Pharmacol* 1988; **34:** 353–7.
8. Sear JW, *et al.* Studies on morphine disposition: influence of renal failure on the kinetics of morphine and its metabolites. *Br J Anaesth* 1989; **62:** 28–32.
9. Peterson GM, *et al.* Plasma levels of morphine and morphine glucuronides in the treatment of cancer pain: relationship to renal function and route of administration. *Eur J Clin Pharmacol* 1990; **38:** 121–4.
10. Hanna MH, *et al.* Morphine-6-glucuronide disposition in renal impairment. *Br J Anaesth* 1993; **70:** 511–14.
11. Osborne RJ, *et al.* Morphine intoxication in renal failure: the role of morphine-6-glucuronide. *Br Med J* 1986; **292:** 1548–9.
12. Bodd E, *et al.* Morphine-6-glucuronide might mediate the prolonged opioid effect of morphine in acute renal failure. *Hum Exp Toxicol* 1990; **9:** 317–21.

Uses and Administration

Morphine, a phenanthrene derivative and the principal alkaloid of opium, is an opioid analgesic (p.69) with agonist activity mainly at μ opioid receptors and perhaps at κ and δ receptors. It acts mainly on the CNS and smooth muscle. Although morphine is predominantly a CNS depressant it has some central stimulant actions which result in nausea and vomiting and miosis. Morphine generally increases smooth muscle tone, especially the sphincters of the gastro-intestinal and biliary tracts.

Morphine may produce both physical and psychological dependence (see p.67) and should therefore be used with discrimination. Tolerance may also develop.

Morphine is used for the relief of moderate to severe pain, especially in pain associated with cancer, myocardial infarction, and surgery. In addition to relieving pain, morphine also alleviates the anxiety associated with severe pain and it is useful as a hypnotic where sleeplessness is due to pain.

Morphine reduces intestinal motility but its role, if any, in the symptomatic treatment of diarrhoea is very limited. It also relieves dyspnoea associated with various conditions, including that due to pulmonary oedema resulting from left ventricular failure. It is an effective cough suppressant, but codeine is usually preferred as there is less risk of dependence; morphine may however be necessary to control intractable cough associated with terminal lung cancer. Morphine has been used pre-operatively as an adjunct to anaesthesia for pain relief and to allay anxiety. It has also been used in high doses as a general anaesthetic in specialised procedures.

Administration and dosage. Morphine is usually administered as the sulphate, although the hydrochloride and the tartrate are used in similar doses. Routes of administration include the oral, subcutaneous, intramuscular, intravenous, intraspinal, and rectal routes. Subcutaneous injections are considered not suitable for oedematous patients. Parenteral doses may be intermittent injections or continuous or intermittent infusions adjusted according to individual analgesic requirements.

Doses should generally be reduced in the elderly or debilitated or in patients with hepatic or renal impairment (see also under Precautions, above).

Doses by mouth for pain are usually in the range of 5 to 20 mg every 4 hours and may be given as an aqueous solution of the hydrochloride or sulphate, or as tablets; with modified-release preparations the 24-hour dose may be given as a single dose or in 2 divided doses. As with the other routes, high oral doses may be required for effective analgesia, especially in palliative care.

Morphine is sometimes administered rectally generally as suppositories in doses of 10 to 30 mg every 4 hours.

The usual dose by subcutaneous or intramuscular injection is 10 mg every 4 hours but may range from 5 to 20 mg. Children up to 1 month of age may be given 150 μg per kg body-weight every 4 hours; those aged 1 to 12 months, 200 μg per kg; 1 to 5 years, 2.5 to 5 mg; 6 to 12 years, 5 to 10 mg. See also under Administration in Infants and Children, below.

Doses of up to 15 mg have been given by slow intravenous injection, sometimes as a loading dose for continuous or patient-controlled infusion. For continuous intravenous administration maintenance doses have generally ranged from 0.8 to 80 mg per hour, although some patients have required and been given much higher doses. Similar doses have been given by continuous subcutaneous infusion.

For myocardial infarction 10 mg may be given by intravenous injection at a rate of 2 mg per minute followed by a further 5 to 10 mg if necessary; half this dose should be used in elderly or debilitated patients.

Intraspinal doses are in the region of 5 mg for an initial epidural injection; if pain relief is unsatisfactory after one hour, further doses of 1 to 2 mg may be given up to a total dose of 10 mg per 24 hours. The recommended initial dose for continuous epidural infusion is 2 to 4 mg per 24 hours increased if necessary by 1 to 2 mg. Intrathecal administration of morphine and its salts has tended to be less common than epidural administration. Doses of 0.2 to 1 mg have been injected intrathecally on a single occasion.

In acute pulmonary oedema 5 to 10 mg may be given by intravenous injection at a rate of 2 mg per minute.

For the control of intractable cough associated with terminal lung cancer, morphine hydrochloride oral solution is given in an initial dose of 5 mg every 4 hours.

Administration. CONTINUOUS INFUSION. Both acute and chronic pain have been controlled satisfactorily by continuous intravenous or subcutaneous infusions of morphine sulphate[1-3] but diamorphine hydrochloride or hydromorphone hydrochloride may be preferred for subcutaneous infusion because their greater solubility in water allows a smaller dose volume. Continuous subcutaneous infusions may be preferred to continuous intravenous infusions.[4] Although one group of workers[5] found continuous subcutaneous infusion to be less effective then epidural administration for relief of postoperative pain, it was still considered to provide simple and relatively effective analgesia with a low rate of adverse effects.

See also under Patient-controlled Analgesia, below.

1. Waldmann CS, *et al.* Serum morphine levels: a comparison between continuous subcutaneous infusion and continuous intravenous infusion in postoperative patients. *Anaesthesia* 1984; **39:** 768–71.
2. Goudie TA, *et al.* Continuous subcutaneous infusion of morphine for postoperative pain relief. *Anaesthesia* 1985; **40:** 1086–92.
3. Stuart GJ, *et al.* Continuous intravenous morphine infusions for terminal pain control: a retrospective review. *Drug Intell Clin Pharm* 1986; **20:** 968–72.
4. Drexel H. Long-term continuous subcutaneous and intravenous opioid infusions. *Lancet* 1991; **337:** 979.
5. Hindsholm KB, *et al.* Continuous subcutaneous infusion of morphine—an alternative to extradural morphine for postoperative pain relief. *Br J Anaesth* 1993; **71;** 580–2.

INTRA-ARTICULAR ROUTE. Intra-articular injection of morphine into the knee at the end of arthroscopy has been reported to provide some degree of postoperative pain relief;[1,2] such pain relief may be more pronounced than that produced by the same dose given intravenously.[1] The effect appears to be due to the action of morphine on peripheral opioid receptors.[3] However, there have been conflicting results on whether addition of morphine to intra-articular bupivacaine improves analgesia.[4,5] Doses of morphine reported to have been injected intra-articularly have ranged from 1 to 5 mg.

1. Stein C, *et al.* Analgesic effect of intra-articular morphine after arthroscopic knee surgery. *N Engl J Med* 1991; **325:** 1123–6.
2. Joshi GP, *et al.* Intra-articular morphine for pain relief after anterior cruciate ligament repair. *Br J Anaesth* 1993; **70:** 87–8.
3. Stein C, *et al.* Local analgesic effect of endogenous opioid peptides. *Lancet* 1993; **342:** 321–4.
4. Laurent SC, *et al.* Addition of morphine to intra-articular bupivacaine does not improve analgesia after day-case arthroscopy. *Br J Anaesth* 1994; **72:** 170–3.
5. Heine MF, *et al.* Intra-articular morphine after arthroscopic knee operation. *Br J Anaesth* 1994; **73:** 413–15.

INTRASPINAL ROUTE. Morphine is given epidurally and intrathecally to relieve both acute and chronic pain. However, reviews on the role of spinal opioids have generally concluded that they should be reserved for pain not controlled by more conventional methods of administration.[1-3] When converting from more conventional routes of administration McQuay[3] suggested that 1% of the total daily dose could be tried as the daily intrathecal dose and 10% as the epidural dose.

Intrathecal morphine may be delivered continuously via an implanted programmable infusion pump for the long-term management of chronic non-malignant and cancer pain.

See also under Patient-controlled Analgesia, below.

1. Anonymous. Spinal opiates revisited. *Lancet* 1986; **i:** 655–6.
2. Gustafsson LL, Wiesenfeld-Hallin Z. Spinal opioid analgesia: a critical update. *Drugs* 1988; **35:** 597–603.
3. McQuay HJ. Opioids in chronic pain. *Br J Anaesth* 1989; **63:** 213–26.

PATIENT-CONTROLLED ANALGESIA. Morphine is one of the most frequently used opioid analgesics for patient-controlled analgesia (see p.7). Most experience has been with the intravenous route, but the intramuscular, subcutaneous, oral, pulmonary, and epidural[1] routes have also been used. Reasonable initial settings recommended for intravenous administration have been a demand dose of 1 mg of morphine sulphate (or its equivalent) and a lockout interval of 5 to 10 minutes.[2]

1. Sjöström S, *et al.* Patient-controlled analgesia with extradural morphine or pethidine. *Br J Anaesth* 1988; **60:** 358–66.
2. Anonymous. Patient-controlled analgesia. *Med Lett Drugs Ther* 1989; **31:** 104.

PULMONARY ROUTE. For reference to the use of nebulised morphine see under Dyspnoea, below.

Administration in infants and children. The management of pain in infants and children is discussed on p.7. Morphine is widely used[1] and may be given to *neonates* who require analgesia as a result of surgery, invasive procedures, or intensive care. They do however have enhanced susceptibility to the respiratory depression associated with opioids although those already receiving respiratory support are at less risk. Allowance also has to be made for morphine's altered pharmacokinetics in this group (see above). Most neonates receiving respiratory support can be managed with an infusion of morphine 10 μg per kg body-weight per hour; the dose should not exceed 15 μg per kg per hour. In neonates who are breathing spontaneously there is a substantial risk of respiratory depression with powerful opioid analgesics such as morphine, and its administration to such neonates should be limited to those under intensive care, as after major surgery. Morphine 5 to 7 μg per kg per hour by intravenous infusion allows adequate analgesia without respiratory depression, but the infusion rate should be titrated against response. Suggested infusion rates range from 5 to 15 μg per kg per hour. Bolus injections should be avoided. The use of opioids for sedation and analgesia in neonates in intensive care is mentioned on p.638; morphine is considered to be a more rational choice than fentanyl in such a setting where long-term infusions are required.

In *infants and children* opioids are still the mainstay of analgesia and morphine is the standard against which the others are compared. Techniques of continuous intravenous infusion have become popular for postoperative pain relief. From the age of 5 to 6 months morphine metabolism appears to conform to an adult pattern; in younger infants the regimens for neonates (see above) should be followed. Titration of infusion rate against patient response minimises the risks and most have found 10 to 30 μg per kg per hour to be satisfactory with minimal respiratory depression; if required a loading dose of morphine 100 to 200 μg per kg may be given initially with bolus top-up doses of 50 to 100 μg per kg every 4 hours. Subcutaneous infusions of morphine 30 to 60 μg per kg per hour have been used for the relief of terminal cancer pain in children, but for postoperative analgesia the dose needed should be similar to that for intravenous infusion. An intramuscular injection of morphine 100 to 200 μg per kg provides excellent short-term analgesia. Patient-controlled analgesia using morphine has been tried in children as young as 5 years of age.

Some spinal doses of morphine in children are as follows: caudal epidural block, 100 μg per kg; thoracic or lumbar epidural block, 50 μg per kg. Intrathecal doses of 20 or 30 μg per kg have provided satisfactory postoperative pain relief, but respiratory depression occurred in 10 to 25% respectively.

Guidelines[2] for the control of pain associated with *major trauma* in children recommend that after resuscitation a bolus dose of 25 μg per kg body-weight of morphine should be given intravenously with further doses of 10 μg per kg at intervals of 10 minutes titrated against the patient's response. However, it should be noted that opioid analgesics should not be given to patients with appreciable head injuries whose conscious level is depressed or fluctuating.

1. Lloyd-Thomas AR. Pain management in paediatric patients. *Br J Anaesth* 1990; **64:** 85–104.
2. Lloyd-Thomas AR, Anderson I. Paediatric trauma: secondary survey. *Br Med J* 1990; **301:** 433–7.

Cancer pain. The starting dose of morphine in cancer pain depends on the type of analgesic previously taken; 5 to 10 mg every 4 hours is enough to replace a non-opioid or a weaker opioid analgesic whereas 10 to 20 mg or more may be necessary to replace an opioid of equivalent strength to morphine. Doses should be increased gradually until the lowest effective analgesic dose is reached, taking into account any 'rescue' doses that have been administered to relieve breakthrough pain. There are no 'standard' doses; they have ranged from 2.5 to over 2500 mg of morphine sulphate every 4 hours, although most patients need far less than 100 mg every 4 hours. For patients on 4-hourly regimens, a double dose may be taken at bedtime to avoid waking up in the night. The initial dose of a modified-release preparation is 10 to 20 mg every 12 hours if replacing paracetamol or no previous analgesic, but 20 to 30 mg every 12 hours if replacing a weaker opioid. The dose and not the frequency of administration should be altered if required; some formulations allow administration once every 24 hours. Immediate-release formulations should be used to manage breakthrough pain during dose titration of modified-release preparations. Some argue that dose titration should always be carried out with immediate-release preparations, only transferring to modified-release formulations once the optimum analgesic dose has been achieved.

References.

1. Expert Working Group of the European Association for Palliative Care. Morphine in cancer pain: modes of administration. *Br Med J* 1996; **312:** 823–6.

Dyspnoea. In the treatment of dyspnoea, doses of morphine tend to be smaller than those used for pain relief. Morphine hydrochloride or sulphate may be given as an oral solution in carefully titrated doses, starting at a dose of 5 mg every 4 hours; as little as 2.5 mg every 4 hours may be sufficient for opioid-naive patients.[1] In acute pulmonary oedema, 5 to 10 mg may be given by slow intravenous injection. In irreversible malignant chest disease a test dose of 5 mg by mouth should be repeated every 4 hours with 5 to 10 mg at bedtime; if necessary the dose may be increased gradually up to 15 to 20 mg every 4 hours. If the patient is already receiving morphine for pain a 50% increase in dose may be tried.[2] Patients have also obtained relief from subcutaneous injection.[3]

Although one group of workers[4] reported that a low dose of nebulised morphine (mean dose 1.7 mg) improved exercise endurance in patients with dyspnoea due to advanced chronic lung disease, several subsequent studies[5-7] have failed to obtain significant improvements with doses up to 40 mg. It is considered that current evidence does not support the use of nebulised morphine for breathlessness.[1] Furthermore, bronchospasm, particularly at high doses can be a problem and there is no consensus on the optimal dose, schedule of administration, or method of dose titration.

1. Davis CL. ABC of palliative care: breathlessness, cough, and other respiratory problems. *Br Med J* 1997; **315:** 931–4.
2. Twycross RG, Lack SA. *Oral morphine in advanced cancer.* 2nd ed. Beaconsfield: Beaconsfield Publishers, 1989.
3. Bruera E, *et al.* Subcutaneous morphine for dyspnea in cancer patients. *Ann Intern Med* 1993; **119:** 906–7.
4. Young IH, *et al.* Effect of low dose nebulised morphine on exercise endurance in patients with chronic lung disease. *Thorax* 1989; **44:** 387–90.
5. Beauford W, *et al.* Effects of nebulized morphine sulfate on the exercise tolerance of the ventilatory limited COPD patients. *Chest* 1993; **104:** 175–8.
6. Noseda A, *et al.* Disabling dyspnoea in patients with advanced disease: lack of effect of nebulized morphine. *Eur Respir J* 1997; **10:** 1079–83.
7. Jankelson D, *et al.* Lack of effect of high doses of inhaled morphine on exercise endurance in chronic obstructive pulmonary disease. *Eur Respir J* 1997; **10:** 2270–4.

Intensive care. When used to provide analgesia for patients in intensive care, morphine has a relatively slow onset of action, but longer term rather than rapid-onset analgesia can be achieved by a loading dose of 10 to 15 mg, in adults, followed by an infusion of 2 to 3 mg per hour; the dose must be individually titrated.

Preparations

BP 1998: Chloroform and Morphine Tincture *(Chlorodyne)*; Morphine and Atropine Injection; Morphine Sulphate Injection; Morphine Suppositories; Morphine Tablets;
USP 23: Morphine Sulfate Injection.

Proprietary Preparations (details are given in Part 3)
Aust.: Kapanol; Morapid; Mundidol; Oramorph; Vendal; ***Austral.:*** Anamorph; Kapanol; MS Contin; Ordine; ***Belg.:*** MS Contin; Stellaphine†; Stellorphine; ***Canad.:*** Epimorph†; Kadian; M-Eslon; Morphitec; MOS; MS Contin; MSIR; Oramorph; Statex; ***Fr.:*** Moscontin; Skenan; ***Ger.:*** Capros; M-long; MSI; MSR; MST; Sevredol; ***Irl.:*** Morstel; MST Continus; MXL; Oramorph; Sevredol; ***Ital.:*** MS Contin; Oblioser†; Relipain†; Skenan; ***Neth.:*** Kapanol; MS Contin; Noceptin; Sevredol; Skenan; ***Norw.:*** Dolcontin; Kapanol; ***S.Afr.:*** MST Continus; SRM-Rhotard; ***Spain:*** Morfina Miro†; Morfina Serra; MST Continus; Oblioser; Sevredol; ***Swed.:*** Dolcontin; Loceptin; Maxidon; Oramorph; ***Switz.:*** MST Continus;

Sevredol; ***UK:*** Morcap; MST Continus; MXL; Oramorph; Sevredol; SRM-Rhotard†; Zomorph; ***USA:*** Astramorph PF; Duramorph; Infumorph; Kadian; MS Contin; MS/L; MS/S; MSIR; OMS Concentrate; Oramorph; RMS; Roxanol.

Multi-ingredient: ***Aust.:*** Modiscop; ***Austral.:*** Morphalgin; Morthat†; ***Belg.:*** Spasma; ***Irl.:*** Cyclimorph; Diocalm; ***Ital.:*** Cardiostenol; ***S.Afr.:*** Chloropect; Collodyne; Cyclimorph; Diastat†; Enterodyne; Pectrolyte; ***Swed.:*** Spasmofen; ***UK:*** Collis Browne's; Cyclimorph; Diocalm Dual Action; Enterosan; Nepenthe†; Opazimes.

Morpholine Salicylate (9591-w)

2-Hydroxybenzoic acid compounded with morpholine (1 : 1).

$C_{11}H_{15}NO_4$ = 225.2.

CAS — 147-90-0.

Morpholine salicylate is a salicylic acid derivative (see Aspirin, p.16) that has been used by mouth or topically for musculoskeletal disorders.

Preparations

Proprietary Preparations (details are given in Part 3)
Fr.: Pyradol†; Retarcyl†; ***Ital.:*** Deposal†.

Nabumetone (12990-p)

Nabumetone *(BAN, USAN, rINN).*

BRL-14777; Nabumetonum. 4-(6-Methoxy-2-naphthyl)butan-2-one.

$C_{15}H_{16}O_2$ = 228.3.

CAS — 42924-53-8.

Pharmacopoeias. In *Eur.* (see p.viii).

A white or almost white crystalline powder. Practically **insoluble** in water; freely soluble in acetone; slightly soluble in methyl alcohol. **Protect** from light.

Adverse Effects and Precautions

As for NSAIDs in general, p.63.

Effects on the gastro-intestinal tract. Like other NSAIDs nabumetone can produce adverse effects on the gastro-intestinal tract, although some studies have produced favourable comparisons with ibuprofen[1] or naproxen.[2]

1. Roth SH, *et al.* A controlled study comparing the effects of nabumetone, ibuprofen, and ibuprofen plus misoprostol on the upper gastrointestinal tract mucosa. *Arch Intern Med* 1993; **153:** 2565–71.
2. Roth SH, *et al.* A longterm endoscopic evaluation of patients with arthritis treated with nabumetone vs naproxen. *J Rheumatol* 1994; **21:** 1118–23.

Effects on the lungs. Pulmonary fibrosis developed in a 68-year-old woman receiving nabumetone 1500 mg; symptoms appeared after 2 weeks of therapy and worsened during the next 6 weeks.[1] There was rapid resolution on withdrawal of nabumetone and treatment with oral corticosteroids.

1. Morice A, *et al.* Pulmonary fibrosis associated with nabumetone. *Postgrad Med J* 1991; **67:** 1021–2.

Effects on the skin. Pseudoporphyria characterised by blistering on the neck and hands developed in a 36-year-old woman taking nabumetone and auranofin for rheumatoid arthritis.[1] Stopping auranofin had no effect on the blistering which only resolved once nabumetone was withdrawn. The authors of the report stated that the UK Committee on Safety of Medicines had received 3 additional reports of pseudoporphyria suspected to be caused by nabumetone.

1. Varma S, Lanigan SW. Pseudoporphyria caused by nabumetone. *Br J Dermatol* 1998; **138:** 549–50.

Interactions

For interactions associated with NSAIDs, see p.65.

Pharmacokinetics

Although nabumetone is well absorbed from the gastro-intestinal tract plasma concentrations following oral administration are too small to be measured as it undergoes rapid and extensive first-pass metabolism in the liver to the principal active compound 6-methoxy-2-naphthylacetic acid (6-MNA) and other inactive metabolites. 6-MNA is more than 99% bound to plasma proteins. 6-MNA diffuses into synovial fluid. There is considerable interindividual variation in the plasma elimination half-life of 6-MNA, especially in the elderly; some reported mean values at steady state include 22 to about 27 hours for young adults and about 25 and 34 hours in elderly patients. 6-MNA eventually undergoes further metabolism by *O*-methylation and conjugation. About 80% of a dose is excreted in the urine as inactive or conjugated metabolites and less than 1% as unchanged 6-MNA.

References.

1. Brier ME, *et al.* Population pharmacokinetics of the active metabolite of nabumetone in renal dysfunction. *Clin Pharmacol Ther* 1995; **57:** 622–7.
2. Davies NM. Clinical pharmacokinetics of nabumetone: the dawn of selective cyclo-oxygenase-2 inhibition? *Clin Pharmacokinet* 1997; **33:** 403–16.

Uses and Administration

Nabumetone is a non-active prodrug whose major metabolite is an NSAID (p.65) structurally similar to naproxen (p.62). It is used for the relief of pain and inflammation associated with osteoarthritis and rheumatoid arthritis in a usual dose of 1 g by mouth taken as a single dose in the evening; if necessary 0.5 to 1 g may be given additionally in the morning. It has been recommended that a dose of 1 g daily should not be exceeded in elderly patients and that 500 mg daily may be satisfactory in some cases.

References.

1. Anonymous. Nabumetone—a new NSAID. *Med Lett Drugs Ther* 1992; **34:** 38–40.
2. Friedel HA, *et al.* Nabumetone: a reappraisal of its pharmacology and therapeutic use in rheumatic diseases. *Drugs* 1993; **45:** 131–56.
3. Proceedings of a symposium: continuing developments with nabumetone: an investigators' update. *Am J Med* 1993; 95 (suppl 2A): 1S–45S.
4. Dahl SL. Nabumetone: a "nonacidic" nonsteroidal antiinflammatory drug. *Ann Pharmacother* 1993; **27:** 456–63.

Preparations

BP 1998: Nabumetone Oral Suspension; Nabumetone Tablets.

Proprietary Preparations (details are given in Part 3)
Belg.: Relifex†; ***Canad.:*** Relafen; ***Ger.:*** Arthaxan; ***Irl.:*** Relifex; ***Ital.:*** Artaxan; Nabuser; Relifex†; ***Neth.:*** Mebutan; ***Norw.:*** Relifex; ***S.Afr.:*** Relifen; Relisan; Relitone; ***Spain:*** Dolsinal; Listran; Relif; ***Swed.:*** Relifex; ***Switz.:*** Balmox; ***UK:*** Relifex; ***USA:*** Relafen.

Nalbuphine Hydrochloride (6244-y)

Nalbuphine Hydrochloride *(BANM, USAN, rINNM).*

EN-2234A. 17-Cyclobutylmethyl-7,8-dihydro-14-hydroxy-17-normorphine hydrochloride; (−)-(5R,6S,14S)-9a-Cyclobutylmethyl-4,5-epoxymorphinan-3,6,14-triol hydrochloride.

$C_{21}H_{27}NO_4$,HCl = 393.9.

CAS — 20594-83-6 (nalbuphine); 23277-43-2 (nalbuphine hydrochloride).

Incompatibility has been reported between injections of nalbuphine hydrochloride and nafcillin sodium,[1] diazepam,[2] pentobarbitone sodium,[2] or thiethylperazine maleate.[2]

1. Jeglum EL, *et al.* Nafcillin sodium incompatibility with acidic solutions. *Am J Hosp Pharm* 1981; **38:** 462–4.
2. Jump WG, *et al.* Compatibility of nalbuphine hydrochloride with other preoperative medications. *Am J Hosp Pharm* 1982; **39:** 841–3.

Dependence and Withdrawal

As for Opioid Analgesics, p.67.

A WHO expert committee considered in 1989 that the likelihood of nalbuphine abuse was low to moderate and was not great enough to warrant international control.[1] Abuse had been reported infrequently and the withdrawal syndrome produced when naloxone was given after continuous nalbuphine administration was less severe than that in morphine dependence.

1. WHO. WHO expert committee on drug dependence: twenty-fifth report. *WHO Tech Rep Ser 775* 1989.

Adverse Effects and Treatment

As for Opioid Analgesics in general, p.68.

Headache may occur. Nausea and vomiting occur less than with other opioids. Hallucinations and other psychotomimetic effects are rare and have been reported much less frequently than with pentazocine.

Because nalbuphine has opioid agonist and antagonist activity, naloxone is the recommended antagonist for the treatment of overdose.

Effects on the respiratory system. Nalbuphine produces similar respiratory depression to morphine at equianalgesic doses, but there is a ceiling effect with nalbuphine and, unlike morphine, respiratory depression does not increase appreciably with higher doses.[1] In a cumulative-dose study[2] a plateau effect was seen with nalbuphine above a total dose of 30 mg per 70 kg body-weight intravenously. Pugh *et al.*[3] noted similar ventilatory depression with single intravenous doses of nalbuphine of 15, 30, or 60 mg per 70 kg; naloxone failed to reverse the depression at the highest dose.

1. Klepper ID, *et al.* Respiratory function following nalbuphine and morphine in anaesthetized man. *Br J Anaesth* 1986; **58:** 625–9.
2. Romagnoli A, Keats AS. Ceiling effect for respiratory depression by nalbuphine. *Clin Pharmacol Ther* 1980; **27:** 478–85.
3. Pugh GC, *et al.* Effect of nalbuphine hydrochloride on the ventilatory and occlusion pressure responses to carbon dioxide in volunteers. *Br J Anaesth* 1989; **62:** 601–9.

Precautions

As for Opioid Analgesics in general, p.68.

Nalbuphine may precipitate withdrawal symptoms if given to patients physically dependent on opioids.

The dose of nalbuphine should be reduced in patients with hepatic or renal impairment.

Pregnancy. When used for analgesia during labour greater placental transfer and more sedation in mothers and their infants has been demonstrated with nalbuphine than with pethidine.[1] There have also been reports of bradycardia and respiratory depression in neonates whose mothers received nalbuphine during labour.[2,3] It was considered that nalbuphine should be given with caution during labour, especially by the intravenous route. Guillonneau *et al.*[2] recommended subcutaneous administration and advised that nalbuphine should not be given around the expected time of delivery.

Further references on the transplacental transfer of nalbuphine are given under Pharmacokinetics, below.

1. Wilson CM, *et al.* Transplacental gradient of pethidine and nalbuphine in labour. *Br J Clin Pharmacol* 1986; **21:** 571P–2P.
2. Guillonneau M, *et al.* Perinatal adverse effects of nalbuphine given during parturition. *Lancet* 1990; **335:** 1588.
3. Sgro C, *et al.* Perinatal adverse effects of nalbuphine given during labour. *Lancet* 1990; **336:** 1070.

Interactions

For interactions associated with opioid analgesics, see p.69.

Pharmacokinetics

Following intramuscular injection nalbuphine has been reported to produce peak plasma concentrations after 30 minutes. It is metabolised in the liver and is excreted predominantly in the faeces as unchanged drug and conjugates. About 7% of a dose has been reported to be excreted in the urine as unchanged drug, its conjugates, and metabolites.

Nalbuphine crosses the placenta.

There appears to be considerable first-pass metabolism of nalbuphine following its administration by mouth.

The plasma elimination half-life of nalbuphine has generally been cited as about 5 hours. Aitkenhead *et al.*[1] reported a mean half-life of 222 minutes (range 111-460 minutes) following intravenous administration in healthy subjects; clearance was high and likely to be affected by changes in hepatic blood flow. In anaesthetised patients given nalbuphine intravenously clearance was lower and a mean half-life of 135.5 minutes (range 69.8 to 262.7 minutes) was reported.[2]

Bioavailability of an oral nalbuphine preparation in healthy subjects was only 11.8% (range 6.1 to 20.1%), half-life was about 279 minutes, and time to peak plasma concentration about 47 minutes.[1] Kay *et al.*[3] gave an oral preparation of nalbuphine postoperatively and reported a half-life of about 242 minutes and peak plasma concentrations at about 107 minutes.

Jaillon *et al.*[4] concluded from a comparison of the intravenous pharmacokinetics of nalbuphine in children aged 1½ to 8½ years, young healthy adults, and patients over 65 years of age that the dose and rate of administration of nalbuphine would probably need to be increased for children and reduced in the elderly; the children had received a dose of nalbuphine hydrochloride of 200 μg per kg body-weight and the adults 10 mg. Systemic clearance of nalbuphine following intravenous administration decreased significantly with age. The mean elimination half-life of nalbuphine was 0.9 hours in the children, 2 hours in the young adults, and 2.3 hours in the elderly. Following administration of a 30-mg dose by mouth the mean elimination half-life was 10.6 hours in the young adults and 6.5 hours in the elderly. However, mean peak serum concentrations of nalbuphine were much higher in the elderly than in the young adults and this probably reflected the difference in absolute bioavailability between the two groups, 46% in the elderly as compared with 12% in the young adults.

1. Aitkenhead AR, *et al.* The pharmacokinetics of oral and intravenous nalbuphine in healthy volunteers. *Br J Clin Pharmacol* 1988; **25:** 264–8.
2. Sear JW, *et al.* Disposition of nalbuphine in patients undergoing general anaesthesia. *Br J Anaesth* 1987; **59:** 572–5.
3. Kay B, *et al.* Pharmacokinetics of oral nalbuphine in postoperative patients. *Br J Anaesth* 1987; **59:** 1327P.
4. Jaillon P, *et al.* Pharmacokinetics of nalbuphine in infants, young healthy volunteers, and elderly patients. *Clin Pharmacol Ther* 1989; **46:** 226–33.

Pregnancy. References.

1. Wilson CM, *et al.* Transplacental gradient of pethidine and nalbuphine in labour. *Br J Clin Pharmacol* 1986; **21:** 571P–2P.
2. Dadabhoy ZP, *et al.* Transplacental transfer of nalbuphine in patients undergoing cesarean section: a pilot study. *Acta Anaesthesiol Ital* 1988; **39:** 227–32.
3. Nicolle E, *et al.* Therapeutic monitoring of nalbuphine: transplacental transfer and estimated pharmacokinetics in the neonate. *Eur J Clin Pharmacol* 1996; **49:** 485–9.

Uses and Administration

Nalbuphine hydrochloride, a phenanthrene derivative, is an opioid analgesic (p.69). It has mixed opioid agonist-antagonist activity. It is used for the relief of moderate to severe pain, including that associated with myocardial infarction, and as an adjunct to anaesthesia. Nalbuphine hydrochloride is reported to act within 15 minutes of subcutaneous or intramuscular injection or within 2 to 3 minutes of intravenous injection and generally to produce analgesia for 3 to 6 hours. It is given subcutaneously, intramuscularly, or intravenously.

The dose of nalbuphine hydrochloride for pain relief is 10 to 20 mg every 3 to 6 hours as required. Doses of 10 to 30 mg have been given by slow intravenous injection in myocardial infarction; a second dose of 20 mg may be given after 30 minutes if necessary. Children may be given up to 300 μg per kg bodyweight initially, repeated once or twice as necessary.

Premedication has been carried out using doses of 100 to 200 μg per kg. As an adjunct to anaesthesia a usual dose is 0.3 to 1.0 mg per kg body-weight given intravenously over 10 to 15 minutes at induction; in the USA doses of up to 3 mg per kg have been used. Maintenance doses of 250 to 500 μg per kg are given at half-hourly intervals.

Nalbuphine is generally described as a mixed agonist-antagonist acting mainly as an agonist at κ opioid receptors and as an antagonist or partial agonist at μ receptors. It has shown antagonist activity similar to that seen with naloxone in opioid-dependent subjects.[1] Nalbuphine is structurally related to naloxone and oxymorphone. Pharmacologically nalbuphine is qualitatively similar to pentazocine, but nalbuphine is a more potent antagonist at μ opioid receptors, is less likely to produce psychotomimetic effects such as hallucinations, and is reported to produce no significant cardiovascular effects in patients with ischaemic heart disease. It differs from pure μ agonists such as morphine in that its analgesic, sedative, and respiratory depressant actions are subject to a 'ceiling' effect and may not increase proportionately with dose.

1. Preston KL, *et al.* Antagonist effects of nalbuphine in opioid-dependent human volunteers. *J Pharmacol Exp Ther* 1989; **248:** 929–37.

Pain. ACUTE PAIN. Although nalbuphine has the possible advantage of a 'ceiling' effect for respiratory depression this effect may also be applicable to analgesia. When nalbuphine was used for *postoperative* pain relief following abdominal surgery Pugh and Drummond[1] reported an apparent reversal of analgesic effect at high doses. In comparative studies of pain relief following various types of surgery nalbuphine has been reported to be inferior to morphine following hip replacement,[2] but of longer duration and with fewer complications than pethidine.[3] Nalbuphine has been administered postoperatively in patient-controlled analgesia and has been found as effective as pethidine[4] or morphine.[5] Because of its μ-opioid antagonist properties nalbuphine has been used to reverse the side-effects of μ agonists without reducing analgesia[6] although increased pain has sometimes been reported.

Labour. McAteer *et al.*[7] reported that nalbuphine given intravenously in a patient-controlled device was preferred to pethidine given similarly for labour pain, whereas Wilson *et al.*[8] found no advantage with intramuscular nalbuphine over pethidine for labour pain. More recently, severe respiratory depression has been reported in neonates following the use of nalbuphine; subcutaneous administration and avoidance of the expected delivery time was advised (see Pregnancy under Precautions, above).

1. Pugh GC, Drummond GB. A dose-response study with nalbuphine hydrochloride for pain in patients after upper abdominal surgery. *Br J Anaesth* 1987; **59:** 1356–63.
2. Fee JPH, *et al.* Analgesia after hip replacement surgery: comparison of nalbuphine with morphine. *Br J Anaesth* 1989; **63:** 756–8.
3. Brock-Utne JG, *et al.* A comparison of nalbuphine and pethidine for postoperative pain relief after orthopaedic surgery. *S Afr Med J* 1985; **68:** 391–3.
4. Sprigge JS, Otton PE. Nalbuphine versus meperidine for postoperative analgesia: a double-blind comparison using the patient controlled analgesic technique. *Can Anaesth Soc J* 1983; **30:** 517–21.
5. Christiansen S. Nalbuphine in patient-controlled analgesia: a comparison with morphine. *Curr Ther Res* 1987; **41:** 933–45.
6. Chalmers PC, *et al.* Double-blind comparison of intravenous nalbuphine and placebo in the amelioration of side-effects of epidural narcotics. *Pain Clin* 1988; **2:** 49–56.
7. McAteer EJ, *et al.* Patient controlled analgesia in labour: a comparison of nalbuphine and pethidine. *Br J Anaesth* 1986; **58:** 122P.
8. Wilson CM, *et al.* A double-blind comparison of intramuscular pethidine and nalbuphine in labour. *Anaesthesia* 1986; **41:** 1207–13.

CHRONIC PAIN. Using subcutaneous administration Stambaugh[1] found nalbuphine to provide equivalent analgesia to morphine in chronic cancer pain and with fewer complications, but McQuay[2] noted that a ceiling of analgesic efficacy (equivalent to morphine 30 mg) appeared to restrict the value of nalbuphine in chronic pain.

1. Stambaugh JE. Evaluation of nalbuphine: efficacy and safety in the management of chronic pain associated with advanced malignancy. *Curr Ther Res* 1982; **31:** 393–401.
2. McQuay HJ. Opioids in chronic pain. *Br J Anaesth* 1989; **63:** 213–26.

Preparations

Proprietary Preparations (details are given in Part 3)
Aust.: Nubain; ***Canad.:*** Nubain; ***Fr.:*** Nubain; ***Ger.:*** Nubain; ***S.Afr.:*** Nubain; ***Switz.:*** Nubain; ***UK:*** Nubain; ***USA:*** Nubain.

Naproxen (2672-n)

Naproxen *(BAN, USAN, rINN).*

Naproxenum; RS-3540. (+)-2-(6-Methoxy-2-naphthyl)propionic acid.

$C_{14}H_{14}O_3$ = 230.3.

CAS — 22204-53-1.

Pharmacopoeias. In *Chin., Eur.* (see p.viii), *Jpn,* and *US.*

A white or off-white, almost odourless, crystalline powder. Practically **insoluble** in water; soluble in alcohol and in methyl alcohol; freely soluble in chloroform and in dehydrated alcohol; sparingly soluble in ether. **Store** in airtight containers. Protect from light.

Naproxen Sodium (2673-h)

Naproxen Sodium *(BANM, USAN, rINNM).*

RS-3650.

$C_{14}H_{13}NaO_3$ = 252.2.

CAS — 26159-34-2.

Pharmacopoeias. In *US.*

A white to creamy-white crystalline powder. Each 550 mg of naproxen sodium is approximately equivalent to 500 mg of naproxen. **Soluble** in water and methyl alcohol; sparingly soluble in alcohol; very slightly soluble in acetone; practically insoluble in chloroform and in toluene. **Store** in airtight containers.

Adverse Effects

As for NSAIDs in general, p.63.

Administration of suppositories containing naproxen may cause rectal irritation and occasional bleeding.

Effects on the blood. Haematological adverse effects reported in patients receiving naproxen include haemolytic anaemia,[1,2] aplastic anaemia,[3] and agranulocytosis.[4]

1. Hughes JA, Sudell W. Hemolytic anemia associated with naproxen. *Arthritis Rheum* 1983; **26:** 1054.
2. Lo TCN, Martin MA. Autoimmune haemolytic anaemia associated with naproxen suppositories. *Br Med J* 1986; **292:** 1430.
3. McNeil P, *et al.* Naproxen-associated aplastic anaemia. *Med J Aust* 1986; **145:** 53–4.
4. Nygard N, Starkebaum G. Naproxen and agranulocytosis. *JAMA* 1987; **257:** 1732.

Effects on the CNS. Aseptic meningitis has been associated with naproxen therapy.[1] Details of one patient who suffered recurrent attacks are provided by Weksler and Lehany.[1]

There has been a report[2] of a patient with Parkinson's disease whose symptoms had previously been well-controlled but who deteriorated when she was given naproxen. She improved on withdrawal of naproxen and the effect was confirmed by rechallenge. It was noted that the UK Committee on Safety of Medicines had records of one case of parkinsonism associated with a combined preparation of naproxen and misoprostol and 12 other reports of tremor or ataxia precipitated by naproxen.

1. Weksler BB, Lehany AM. Naproxen-induced recurrent aseptic meningitis. *DICP Ann Pharmacother* 1991; **25:** 1183–4.
2. Shaunak S, *et al.* Exacerbation of idiopathic Parkinson's disease by naproxen. *Br Med J* 1995; **311:** 422.

Effects on the eyes. Keratopathy, characterised by whorl-like corneal opacities, occurred in a woman receiving naproxen; complete regression occurred after discontinuation of naproxen.[1] There has also been a report of exacerbation of glaucoma in a 65-year-old woman given naproxen.[2]

For reference to effects on the optic nerve associated with naproxen, see p.64.

1. Szmyd L, Perry HD. Keratopathy associated with the use of naproxen. *Am J Ophthalmol* 1985; **99:** 598.
2. Fincham JE. Exacerbation of glaucoma in an elderly female taking naproxen sodium: a case report. *J Geriatr Drug Ther* 1989; **3:** 139–43.

Effects on the gastro-intestinal tract. Gastro-intestinal adverse effects are among the most frequently reported during short- and long-term treatment with naproxen. Acute proctocolitis associated with the use of naproxen has been reported[1] in one patient. Oesophageal ulceration reported in 7 patients[2] may have arisen due to incorrect consumption (such as taking the dosage without fluids or lying down after administration) but other causes could not be dismissed.

1. Ravi S, *et al.* Colitis caused by non-steroidal anti-inflammatory drugs. *Postgrad Med J* 1986; **62:** 773–6.
2. Kahn LH, *et al.* Over-the-counter naproxen sodium and esophageal injury. *Ann Intern Med* 1997; **126:** 1006.

Effects on the kidneys. Acute renal failure,[1] renal papillary necrosis,[2] interstitial nephritis,[3] and hyperkalaemia[1] have been reported in patients receiving naproxen. As with other NSAIDs, renal adverse effects occur more frequently in patients with certain risk factors such as volume depletion, diuretic therapy, heart failure, and pre-existing renal dysfunction.[1]

1. Todd PA, Clissold SP. Naproxen: a reappraisal of its pharmacology, and therapeutic use in rheumatic diseases and pain states. *Drugs* 1990; **40:** 91–137.
2. Caruana RJ, Semble EL. Renal papillary necrosis due to naproxen. *J Rheumatol* 1984; **11:** 90–1.
3. Quigley MR, *et al.* Concurrent naproxen- and penicillamine-induced renal disease in rheumatoid arthritis. *Arthritis Rheum* 1982; **25:** 1016–19.

Effects on the liver. There have been a few reports[1,2] of moderate to severe jaundice attributed to naproxen.

1. Victorino RMM, *et al.* Jaundice associated with naproxen. *Postgrad Med J* 1980; **56:** 368–70.
2. Andrejak M, *et al.* Cross hepatotoxicity between non-steroidal anti-inflammatory drugs. *Br Med J* 1987; **295:** 180–1.

Effects on the lungs. See under Hypersensitivity, below.

Effects on the salivary glands. For reference to salivary gland swelling associated with naproxen therapy, see under Hypersensitivity, below.

Effects on the skin. Cutaneous reactions reported in patients receiving naproxen include erythema nodosum,[1] lichen planus,[2] and toxic pustular skin eruption.[3]

Photodermatitis, characterised by vesicle formation or increased skin fragility on sun-exposed skin, has been reported in adults[4-6] and children.[7,8]

Relapse of subacute cutaneous lupus erythematosus has been reported in one patient to be possibly associated with the administration of naproxen.[9]

For reference to facial scars of unknown origin developing in children receiving NSAIDs, and in particular naproxen, see under NSAIDs, p.65.

1. Grattan CEH, Kennedy CTC. Naproxen induced erythema nodosum. *Br Med J* 1984; **288:** 114.
2. Heymann WR, *et al.* Naproxen-induced lichen planus. *J Am Acad Dermatol* 1984; **10:** 299–301.
3. Page SR, Grattan CEH. Pustular reaction to naproxen with cholestatic jaundice. *Br Med J* 1986; **293:** 510.
4. Howard AM, *et al.* Pseudoporphyria due to naproxen. *Lancet* 1985; **i:** 819–20.
5. Rivers JK, Barnetson RS. Naproxen-induced bullous photodermatitis. *Med J Aust* 1989; **151:** 167–8.
6. Levy ML, *et al.* Naproxen-induced pseudoporphyria: a distinctive photodermatitis. *J Pediatr* 1990; **117:** 660–4.
7. Parodi A, *et al.* Possible naproxen-induced relapse of subacute cutaneous lupus erythematosus. *JAMA* 1992; **268:** 51–2.
8. Lang BA, Finlayson LA. Naproxen-induced pseudoporphyria in patients with juvenile rheumatoid arthritis. *J Pediatr* 1994; **124:** 639–42.
9. Cox NH, Wilkinson DS. Dermatitis artefacta as the presenting feature of auto-erythrocyte sensitization syndrome and naproxen-induced pseudoporphyria in a single patient. *Br J Dermatol* 1992; **126:** 86–9.

Hypersensitivity. All of 11 aspirin-sensitive asthmatic patients developed reactions (rhinorrhoea, tightness of chest, wheezing, dyspnoea) after taking naproxen in doses of 40 to 80 mg.[1] Hypersensitivity to individual NSAIDs is believed to be closely linked to the extent to which these drugs inhibit prostaglandin (see under Aspirin, p.16). There may therefore be a dose threshold below which no detectable symptoms occur. Such an effect has been reported[2] in a patient previously stabilised on naproxen for about one year who had a hypersensitivity reaction following a dosage increase.

A hypersensitivity reaction characterised by pulmonary infiltrates with eosinophilia[3,4] has been reported in patients taking naproxen. There has also been a report of a generalised hypersensitivity reaction with acute eosinophilic colitis in a 57-year-old woman treated with naproxen for osteoarthritis.[5]

Bilateral swelling of the major salivary glands, a generalised rash, and eosinophilia suggestive of a hypersensitivity response has been reported in a patient following use of naproxen.[6]

1. Szczeklik A, *et al.* Asthmatic attacks induced in aspirin-sensitive patients by diclofenac and naproxen. *Br Med J* 1977; **2:** 231–2.
2. Briscoe-Dwyer L, Etzel JV. Dyspnea and periorbital edema following an increase in naproxen dose. *Ann Pharmacother* 1994; **28:** 1110.
3. Nader DA, Schillaci RF. Pulmonary infiltrates with eosinophilia due to naproxen. *Chest* 1983; **83:** 280–2.
4. Buscaglia AJ, *et al.* Pulmonary infiltrates associated with naproxen. *JAMA* 1984; **251:** 65–6.
5. Bridges AJ, *et al.* Acute eosinophilic colitis and hypersensitivity reaction associated with naproxen therapy. *Am J Med* 1990; **89:** 526–7.
6. Knulst AC, *et al.* Salivary gland swelling following naproxen therapy. *Br J Dermatol* 1995; **133:** 647–9.

Precautions

As for NSAIDs in general, p.65.

Breast feeding. The amount of naproxen distributed into breast milk is considered by some authorities to be too small to be harmful to a breast-fed infant although some manufacturers recommend that breast feeding should be avoided during naproxen therapy. In a study[1] of one breast-fed infant only 0.26% of the mother's dose was recovered from the infant.

1. Jamali F, Stevens DRS. Naproxen excretion in milk and its uptake by the infant. *Drug Intell Clin Pharm* 1983; **17:** 910–11.

Parkinsonism. For a report of a patient whose symptoms of Parkinson's disease were exacerbated by naproxen, see under Effects on the CNS in Adverse Effects, above.

Interactions

For interactions associated with NSAIDs, see p.65.

The excretion of naproxen is delayed by probenecid resulting in raised plasma concentrations of naproxen.

Antiepileptics. For the effect of naproxen on the protein binding of valproic acid, see p.363.

Pharmacokinetics

Naproxen and naproxen sodium are readily absorbed from the gastro-intestinal tract. Peak plasma concentrations are attained about 1 to 2 hours after ingestion of naproxen sodium and in about 2 to 4 hours after ingestion of naproxen. Food reduces the rate but not the extent of absorption. Naproxen and naproxen sodium are also well absorbed following rectal administration but absorption is slower compared with the oral route. At therapeutic concentrations naproxen is more than 99% bound to plasma proteins. Plasma concentrations of naproxen increase proportionally with dose up to about 500 mg daily; at higher doses there is an increase in clearance caused by saturation of plasma proteins. Naproxen diffuses into synovial fluid; it crosses the placenta and is distributed into breast milk in small amounts. Naproxen has a plasma elimination half-life of about 13 hours. Approximately 95% of a dose is excreted in urine as naproxen and 6-*O*-desmethylnaproxen and their conjugates. Less than 5% of a dose has been recovered in the faeces.

References.

1. Bruno R, *et al.* Naproxen kinetics in synovial fluid of patients with osteoarthritis. *Br J Clin Pharmacol* 1988; **26:** 41–4.
2. Bertin P, *et al.* Sodium naproxen: concentration and effect on inflammatory response mediators in human rheumatoid synovial fluid. *Eur J Clin Pharmacol* 1994; **46:** 3–7.
3. Davies NM, Anderson KE. Clinical pharmacokinetics of naproxen. *Clin Pharmacokinet* 1997; **32:** 268–93.

Uses and Administration

Naproxen, a propionic acid derivative, is an NSAID (p.65).

Naproxen is used in musculoskeletal and joint disorders such as ankylosing spondylitis, osteoarthritis, and rheumatoid arthritis including juvenile chronic arthritis. It is also used in dysmenorrhoea, headache including migraine, postoperative pain, soft-tissue disorders, acute gout, and to reduce fever. Naproxen is usually given by mouth as the free acid or as the sodium salt.

In the treatment of rheumatic disorders, the usual dose of naproxen or naproxen sodium is the equivalent of 500 mg to 1 g of naproxen daily either as a single dose or in 2 divided doses. A dose of 10 mg per kg body-weight daily of naproxen in 2 divided doses has been used in children over 5 years of age with juvenile chronic arthritis.

In other painful conditions such as dysmenorrhoea and acute musculoskeletal disorders the usual initial dose is the equivalent of 500 mg of naproxen followed by 250 mg every 6 to 8 hours, up to a maximum daily dose of 1250 mg after the first day.

In acute gout an initial dose equivalent to 750 mg of naproxen followed by 250 mg every 8 hours is used.

Modified-release preparations are available in some countries for once daily administration.

For the treatment of migraine, the equivalent of 750 mg of naproxen can be given at the first symptom of an impending attack and, if necessary, this may be followed after at least half an hour by further doses of 250 to 500 mg throughout the day to a total maximum daily dose of 1250 mg. See below for a suggested dose for the prophylaxis of migraine.

Rectal administration of naproxen in doses of 500 mg once or twice daily is sometimes employed.

Naproxen has also been used as the piperazine, aminobutanol, and lysine salts and as naproxen cetrimonium. Naproxen is available in combination with misoprostol (p.1419) for patients at risk of NSAID-induced peptic ulceration.

Reviews.

1. Todd PA, Clissold SP. Naproxen: a reappraisal of its pharmacology, and therapeutic use in rheumatic diseases and pain states. *Drugs* 1990; **40:** 91–137.

Headache. An NSAID such as naproxen is among the drugs tried first for the symptomatic treatment of various types of headache including migraine (p.443) and tension-type headache (p.444). An NSAID given at the onset of symptoms can successfully treat an acute attack of migraine.[1] NSAIDs also appear to be effective for the prophylaxis of migraine, although propranolol or pizotifen are generally preferred. Studies have indicated that naproxen sodium 550 mg given twice daily may be useful for reducing the number of attacks suffered.[2-5]

1. Treves TA, *et al.* Naproxen sodium versus ergotamine tartrate in the treatment of acute migraine attacks. *Headache* 1992; **32:** 280–2.
2. Sargent J, *et al.* A comparison of naproxen sodium to propranolol hydrochloride and a placebo control for the prophylaxis of migraine headache. *Headache* 1985; **25:** 320–4.
3. Welch KMA, *et al.* Successful migraine prophylaxis with naproxen sodium. *Neurology* 1985; **35:** 1304–10.
4. Sances G, *et al.* Naproxen sodium in menstrual migraine prophylaxis: a double-blind placebo controlled study. *Headache* 1990; **30:** 705–9.
5. Bellavance AJ, Meloche JP. A comparative study of naproxen sodium, pizotyline and placebo in migraine prophylaxis. *Headache* 1990; **30:** 710–15.

Malignant neoplasms. Some NSAIDs such as naproxen may be of value both for the differential diagnosis and the management of neoplastic fever[1,2] as they appear to be more effective in reducing this type of fever than against fever associated with infections.

1. Chang JC, Gross HM. Neoplastic fever responds to the treatment of an adequate dose of naproxen. *J Clin Oncol* 1985; **3:** 552–8.
2. Azeemuddin SK, *et al.* The effect of naproxen on fever in children with malignancies. *Cancer* 1987; **59:** 1966–8.

Preparations

BP 1998: Naproxen Oral Suspension; Naproxen Suppositories; Naproxen Tablets;
USP 23: Naproxen Oral Suspension; Naproxen Sodium Tablets; Naproxen Tablets.

Proprietary Preparations (details are given in Part 3)
Aust.: Miranax; Naprobene; Nycopren; Proxen; Xenopan; ***Austral.:*** Anaprox; Inza; Naprogesic; Naprosyn; Naxen†; Proxen; Synflex†; ***Belg.:*** Apra-Gel; Apranax; Diparene†; Naprosyne; Nycopren†; ***Canad.:*** Apo-Napro-Na; Naprosyn; Naxen; Novo-Naprox; Nu-Naprox; Roche; Synflex; ***Fr.:*** Apranax; Naprosyne; ***Ger.:*** Apranax; Dysmenalgit; Malexin; Napro-Dorsch†; Proxen; ***Irl.:*** Genoxen; Gerinap; Napmel; Naprex; Naprosyn; Synflex; ***Ital.:*** Alganil†; Aperdan; Artroxen; Axer; Floginax; Flogogin; Floxalin; Gibinap; Gibixen; Gynestrel; Laser; Leniartril; Naprium†; Naprius; Naprodol; Naprorex; Naprosyn; Natrioxen; Neo Eblimon; Nitens; Numidan; Piproxen; Praxenol†; Prexan; Primeral; Proxine; Synalgo; Synflex; Ticoflex; Xenar; ***Neth.:*** Aleve; Femex; Naprocoat; Naprosyne; Naprovite; Nycopren; ***Norw.:*** Alpoxen; Ledox; Napren; Naprosyn; ***S.Afr.:*** Acusprain; Clinosyn†; Nafasol; Napflam†; Naprel; Naproscript†; Naprosyn; Naxen; Pranoxen; Proxen; Synflex; Traumox; ***Spain:*** Aliviomas; Antalgin; Denaxpren; Ilagane; Lundiran; Naprokes; Naprosyn; Naproval; Proxen; Rofanten†; ***Swed.:*** Alpoxen; Miranax; Naprelan†; Naprosyn; Pronaxen; ***Switz.:*** Apranax; Naprolag†; Naprosyn; Nycopren; Proxen; Servinaprox; ***UK:*** Arthrosin; Arthroxen; Condrotec; Laraflex; Napratec; Naprosyn; Nycopren; Pranoxen Continus†; Prosaid; Rheuflex†; Rimoxyn; Synflex; Timpron; Valrox†; ***USA:*** Aleve; Anaprox; Naprelan; Naprosyn.

Multi-ingredient: ***Ital.:*** Flogogin.

Narceine (14234-e)

6-({6-[2-(Dimethylamino)ethyl]-2-methoxy-3,4-(methylenedioxy)phenyl}acetyl)-o-veratric acid; 6-({6-[2-(Dimethylamino)ethyl]-4-methoxy-1,3-benzodioxol-5-yl}acetyl)-2,3-dimethoxybenzoic acid.

$C_{23}H_{27}NO_8$ = 445.5.
CAS — 131-28-2.

Narceine is an opioid analgesic (p.67) that was used in cough preparations for its antitussive action; the phosphate was used similarly.

Preparations

Proprietary Preparations (details are given in Part 3)
Multi-ingredient: ***Ital.:*** Paneraj†.

Nefopam Hydrochloride (2674-m)

Nefopam Hydrochloride *(BANM, USAN, rINNM).*

Benzoxazocine; Fenazoxine; R-738. 3,4,5,6-Tetrahydro-5-methyl-1-phenyl-1*H*-2,5-benzoxazocine hydrochloride.

$C_{17}H_{19}NO,HCl$ = 289.8.

CAS — 13669-70-0 (nefopam); 23327-57-3 (nefopam hydrochloride).

Adverse Effects and Treatment

Side-effects occurring with nefopam include nausea, vomiting, sweating, drowsiness, insomnia, urinary retention, lightheadedness, nervousness, mental confusion, blurred vision, headache, dry mouth, and tachycardia. Euphoria, hallucinations, and convulsions have occasionally been reported, as has temporary pink discoloration of the urine. Symptoms of overdosage have included CNS and cardiovascular toxicity.

Effects on the urinary tract. In January 1989, the UK Committee on Safety of Medicines[1] reported that it had received 53 reports in which nefopam was associated with the development of urinary retention or symptoms of hesitancy, poor stream, or dribbling. In one case there was a history of prostatism.

1. Committee on Safety of Medicines. Nefopam hydrochloride (Acupan). *Current Problems 24* 1989.

Overdosage. A report[1] of a fatal overdose of nefopam, and details of 9 patients who recovered with routine supportive treatment.

1. Piercy DM, *et al.* Death due to overdose of nefopam. *Br Med J* 1981; **283:** 1508–9.

Precautions

Nefopam is contra-indicated in patients with a history of convulsive disorders. It should be used with caution in the elderly and in patients with glaucoma, urinary retention, or impaired hepatic or renal function.

Interactions

It has been recommended that nefopam should not be given to patients receiving MAOIs and should be used cautiously in those receiving tricyclic antidepressants. The adverse effects of nefopam may be additive to those of other drugs with antimuscarinic or sympathomimetic activity.

Pharmacokinetics

Nefopam is absorbed from the gastro-intestinal tract. Peak plasma concentrations occur 1 to 3 hours after administration by mouth and about 1.5 hours after intramuscular injection. About 73% is bound to plasma proteins. Nefopam is distributed into breast milk. It has an elimination half-life of about 4 hours. It is extensively metabolised and excreted mainly in urine, in which less than 5% of a dose is excreted unchanged. About 8% of a dose is excreted via the faeces.

Distribution into breast milk. Studies in 5 healthy nursing mothers given nefopam for post-episiotomy pain indicated that nefopam was present in human milk in an equivalent concentration to that in plasma.[1] It was calculated that on a body-weight basis a breast-fed infant would receive less than 3% of the maternal dose.

1. Liu DTY, *et al.* Nefopam excretion in human milk. *Br J Clin Pharmacol* 1987; **23:** 99–101.

Uses and Administration

Nefopam hydrochloride is a non-opioid analgesic considered to act centrally, although its mechanism of action is unclear. It also has some antimuscarinic and sympathomimetic actions. Nefopam hydrochloride is used for the relief of moderate acute and chronic pain. The usual dose range by mouth is 30 to 90 mg three times daily; the suggested initial doses are 60 mg three times daily but 30 mg three times daily in elderly patients. Nefopam hydrochloride may also be given in doses of 20 mg by intramuscular injection, repeated every 6 hours if necessary; it is recommended that the patient should always be lying down when receiving the injection and should remain so for 15 to 20 minutes afterwards; it has also been given by slow intravenous injection.

References.

1. Heel RC, *et al*. Nefopam: a review of its pharmacological properties and therapeutic efficacy. *Drugs* 1980; **19:** 249–67.

Preparations

Proprietary Preparations (details are given in Part 3)
Belg.: Acupan; ***Fr.:*** Acupan; ***Ger.:*** Ajan; Silentan; ***Irl.:*** Acupan; ***Ital.:*** Acupan†; Nefadol; Nefam; Oxadol; ***S.Afr.:*** Acupan†; ***Spain:*** Acupan; ***Switz.:*** Acupan; ***UK:*** Acupan.

Nicoboxil (9216-w)

Nicoboxil *(rINN)*.

Butoxyethyl Nicotinate. 2-Butoxyethyl nicotinate.

$C_{12}H_{17}NO_3$ = 223.3.

CAS — 13912-80-6.

Nicoboxil is a nicotinate used in topical preparations as a rubefacient. It is also included in some topical preparations used for the treatment of acne vulgaris.

Preparations

Proprietary Preparations (details are given in Part 3)
Multi-ingredient: ***Aust.:*** Finalgon; ***Austral.:*** Finalgon; ***Canad.:*** Actinac; Finalgon; ***Ger.:*** Finalgon; Ortholan†; ***Irl.:*** Actinac; ***Ital.:*** Anti-Acne; ***Spain:*** Finalgon; ***UK:*** Actinac.

Nicomorphine Hydrochloride (13012-l)

Nicomorphine Hydrochloride *(BANM, rINNM)*.

3,6-Di-O-nicotinoylmorphine hydrochloride; (−)-(5R,6S)-4,5-Epoxy-9a-methylmorphin-7-en-3,6-diyl dinicotinate hydrochloride.

$C_{29}H_{25}N_3O_5,HCl$ = 532.0.

CAS — 639-48-5 (nicomorphine); 12040-41-4 (nicomorphine hydrochloride); 35055-78-8 (nicomorphine xHCl).

Nicomorphine hydrochloride is an opioid analgesic (p.67) used in the treatment of pain. It is given by mouth in initial doses of 5 to 10 mg daily or by intramuscular, slow intravenous, or subcutaneous injection in usual doses of 10 to 20 mg; it may also be given rectally.

References.

1. Koopman-Kimenai PM, *et al*. Pharmacokinetics of intramuscular nicomorphine and its metabolites in man. *Eur J Clin Pharmacol* 1991; **41:** 375–8.

Preparations

Proprietary Preparations (details are given in Part 3)
Aust.: Vilan; ***Neth.:*** Vilan; ***Switz.:*** Vilan.

Nifenazone (2676-v)

Nifenazone *(BAN, rINN)*.

N-(2,3-Dimethyl-5-oxo-1-phenyl-3-pyrazolin-4-yl)nicotinamide.

$C_{17}H_{16}N_4O_2$ = 308.3.

CAS — 2139-47-1.

Nifenazone is an NSAID (p.63) that has been used in musculoskeletal and joint disorders given by mouth or rectally.

Preparations

Proprietary Preparations (details are given in Part 3)
Ger.: Nicopyron†; ***Ital.:*** Algotrex†; Neopiran†; Reumatosil; Supermidone†; ***Spain:*** Thylin†.
Multi-ingredient: ***Ital.:*** Teknadone†.

Niflumic Acid (2677-g)

Niflumic Acid *(rINN)*.

UP-83. 2-(ααα-Trifluoro-m-toluidino)nicotinic acid.

$C_{13}H_9F_3N_2O_2$ = 282.2.

CAS — 4394-00-7.

Pharmacopoeias. In *Fr.*

Adverse Effects and Precautions

As for NSAIDs in general, p.63. Fluoride-associated osteosis has been reported with prolonged use. Niflumic acid should be discontinued if hypersensitivity skin reactions appear.

Uses and Administration

Niflumic acid, a nicotinic acid derivative, is an NSAID (p.65). It has been used in inflammatory and musculoskeletal and joint disorders in usual doses of about 250 mg three times daily by mouth; up to 1500 mg daily has been used in severe disorders. It has also been used topically as a 3% cream or ointment or 2.5% gel. The morpholinoethyl ester morniflumate (p.56) has similar uses.

Niflumic acid glycinamide has been used topically in inflammatory mouth disorders.

Preparations

Proprietary Preparations (details are given in Part 3)
Aust.: Actol; ***Belg.:*** Niflugel; Nifluril; ***Fr.:*** Flunir; Niflugel; Nifluril; ***Ger.:*** Actol; ***Ital.:*** Niflam; ***Spain:*** Actol†; Niflactol Topico; ***Switz.:*** Niflugel; Nifluril.
Multi-ingredient: ***Fr.:*** Nifluril.

Nimesulide (13017-k)

Nimesulide *(BAN, rINN)*.

R-805. 4′-Nitro-2′-phenoxymethanesulphonanilide.

$C_{13}H_{12}N_2O_5S$ = 308.3.

CAS — 51803-78-2.

Nimesulide is an NSAID (p.63) reported to be a selective inhibitor of cyclo-oxygenase-2 (COX-2). It has been given in doses of up to 200 mg twice daily by mouth or rectally for inflammatory conditions, fever, and pain. Nimesulide betadex (nimesulide betacyclodextrin complex) has been used similarly.

References.

1. Bennett A, *et al*. Nimesulide: a multifactorial therapeutic approach to the inflammatory process? a 7-year clinical experiences. *Drugs* 1993; **46:** (suppl 1): 1–283.
2. Davis R, Brogden RN. Nimesulide: an update of its pharmacodynamic and pharmacokinetic properties, and therapeutic efficacy. *Drugs* 1994; **48:** 431–54.
3. Senna GE, *et al*. Nimesulide in the treatment of patients intolerant of aspirin and other NSAIDs. *Drugs* 1996; **14:** 94–103.
4. Vizzardi M, *et al*. Nimesulide beta cyclodextrin (nimesulide-betadex) versus nimesulide in the treatment of pain after arthroscopic surgery. *Curr Ther Res* 1998; **59:** 162–71.

Adverse effects. Although *thrombocytopenia* is a common feature in patients infected with HIV one group of workers considered that thrombocytopenia in one of their patients was related to the use of nimesulide.[1]

There has been a report[2] of a patient who developed *fulminant hepatic failure* after treatment with nimesulide.

1. Pasticci MB, *et al*. Nimesulide, thrombocytopenic purpura, and human immunodeficiency virus (HIV) infection. *Ann Intern Med* 1990; **112:** 233–4.
2. McCormick PA, *et al*. COX 2 inhibitor and fulminant hepatic failure. *Lancet* 1999; **353:** 40–1.

Premature labour. Nimesulide has been tried as an alternative to indomethacin to delay labour in a patient with a history of preterm delivery.[1] Nimesulide was given from 16 to 34 weeks of gestation and a successful delivery started 6 days after withdrawal. There appeared to be no adverse effect on fetal renal function or the ductus arteriosus. The authors suggested that fetal prostaglandin synthesis might be mainly mediated through cyclo-oxygenase-1 and that a relatively selective cyclo-oxygenase-2 inhibitor such as nimesulide might produce fewer adverse effects on the fetus than other non-selective NSAIDs.

1. Sawdy R, *et al*. Use of a cyclo-oxygenase type-2-selective non-steroidal anti-inflammatory agent to prevent preterm delivery. *Lancet* 1997; **350:** 265–6.

Preparations

Proprietary Preparations (details are given in Part 3)
Belg.: Mesulid; ***Irl.:*** Aulin; ***Ital.:*** Algolider; Aulin; Eudolene; Fansidol; Flolid; Laidor; Ledoren; Mesid; Mesulid; MF 110; Nide; Nidol; Nimedex; Nimesulene; Nims; Nisal; Remov; Resulin; Sulide; Teonim; ***Spain:*** Antifloxil; Guaxan; ***Switz.:*** Aulin; Nisulid.

Nonivamide (9265-t)

Nonivamide *(rINN)*.

Nonylvanillamide. N-Vanillylnonamide; N-[(4-Hydroxy-3-methoxyphenyl)methyl]nonanamide.

$C_{17}H_{27}NO_3$ = 293.4.

CAS — 2444-46-4.

NOTE. Use of the term 'synthetic capsaicin' to describe nonivamide has arisen from the use of nonivamide as an adulterant for capsaicin and capsicum oleoresin.

Nonivamide is used in topical preparations as a rubefacient.

Preparations

Proprietary Preparations (details are given in Part 3)
Ger.: ABC Warme-Pflaster Sensitive.
Multi-ingredient: ***Aust.:*** Finalgon; Forapin; Rubriment; ***Austral.:*** Bansuk†; Finalgon; ***Belg.:*** Forapin; ***Canad.:*** Finalgon; ***Ger.:*** ABC Warme-Salbe; Akrotherm; Clinit N†; Elacur NO†; Enelbin-Salbe forte†; Finalgon; Histajodol N; Infrotto Ultra; Lomazell forte N; Mydalgan†; Ortholan†; Ostochont; Rheuma Liquidum; Rheumasalbe; Rheumasan†; Rubriment; Salirheuman†; Thermosan†; Vertebralon N†; ***S.Afr.:*** Forapin†; ***Spain:*** Finalgon; ***Switz.:*** Forapin; Histalgane; Radalgin; Roliwol S; Thermocutan.

Nonsteroidal Anti-inflammatory Drugs (2600-p)

NSAIDs.

Adverse Effects and Treatment

The commonest side-effects occurring during therapy with NSAIDs are generally gastro-intestinal disturbances, such as gastro-intestinal discomfort, nausea, and diarrhoea; these are usually mild and reversible but in some patients peptic ulcer and severe gastro-intestinal bleeding may occur. It has been proposed that the gastro-intestinal effects of NSAIDs are due to inhibition of cyclo-oxygenase-1 (COX-1) but whether use of an NSAID which is a highly selective inhibitor of COX-2 improves gastro-intestinal tolerance remains unproven.

CNS-related side-effects include headache, vertigo, dizziness, nervousness, tinnitus, depression, drowsiness, and insomnia. Hypersensitivity reactions may occur occasionally and include fever, angioedema, bronchospasm, and rashes. Hepatotoxicity and aseptic meningitis, which occur rarely, may also be hypersensitivity reactions. Some patients may experience visual disturbances.

Haematological adverse effects of NSAIDs include anaemias, thrombocytopenia, neutropenia, eosinophilia, and agranulocytosis. Unlike aspirin, inhibition of platelet aggregation is reversible with other NSAIDs.

Some NSAIDs have been associated with nephrotoxicity such as interstitial nephritis and nephrotic syndrome; renal failure may be provoked by NSAIDs especially in patients with pre-existing renal impairment. Haematuria has also occurred. Fluid retention may occur, rarely precipitating congestive heart failure in elderly patients. Long-term use or abuse of analgesics, including NSAIDs, has been associated with nephropathy. Other adverse effects include photosensitivity. Alveolitis, pulmonary eosinophilia, pancreatitis, Stevens-Johnson syndrome, and toxic epidermal necrolysis are other rare adverse effects. Induction or exacerbation of colitis has also been reported.

Further details concerning the adverse effects of the individual NSAIDs may be found under their respective monographs.

The relative toxicity of NSAIDs is a continuing subject of debate.[1] Attempts have been made to rank these drugs according to their toxicity on various body systems.[2] For further details see below under individual headings.

1. Skeith KJ, *et al*. Differences in NSAID tolerability profiles: fact or fiction? *Drug Safety* 1994; **10:** 183–95.
2. Committee on Safety of Medicines/Medicines Control Agency. Relative safety of oral non-aspirin NSAIDs. *Current Problems* 1994; **20:** 9–11.

Effects on the blood. The UK Committee on Safety of Medicines recently provided data on the reports it had received between July 1963 and January 1993 on agranulocytosis and neutropenia.[1] Several groups of drugs were commonly implicated, among them NSAIDs for which there were 133 reports of agranulocytosis (45 fatal) and 187 of neutropenia (15 fatal). The most frequently implicated NSAID was phenylbutazone with 74 reports of agranulocytosis (39 fatal) and 40 of neutropenia (4 fatal).

1. Committee on Safety of Medicines/Medicines Control Agency. Drug-induced neutropenia and agranulocytosis. *Current Problems* 1993; **19:** 10–11.

Effects on blood pressure. A meta-analysis[1] of 50 randomised trials studying the effects of NSAIDs on blood pressure in a total of 771 patients found that NSAIDs had elevated mean supine blood pressure by 5 mmHg. Piroxicam, indomethacin, and ibuprofen had produced the greatest increase but the effect was only found to be statistically significant for piroxicam. Aspirin, sulindac, and flurbiprofen produced the smallest elevation in blood pressure while the effect of tiaprofenic acid, diclofenac, and naproxen was intermediate. The increase was more marked in studies in which patients had received antihypertensive therapy than in those where such treatment had not been used. NSAIDs had antagonised all antihypertensive therapy but the effect had been greater against beta blockers and vasodilators than against diuretics. An earlier meta-analysis of intervention studies had produced similar results.[2] Of the 1324 patients who had received NSAIDs, increases in mean arterial pressure were greatest in hypertensive patients who had taken either indomethacin, naproxen, or piroxicam, although results were only significant for indomethacin and naproxen. Sulindac and aspirin had minimal effects on mean arterial pressure.

It has been suggested that the use of NSAIDs in the elderly may increase the risk of the need for antihypertensive therapy.[3] A study[3] of 9411 patients aged 65 years or older who had just started treatment with antihypertensives found that 41% had used NSAIDs in the previous year compared with 26% of 9629 control patients not being treated with antihypertensive therapy.

1. Johnson AG, *et al.* Do nonsteroidal anti-inflammatory drugs affect blood pressure? *Ann Intern Med* 1994; **121:** 289–300.
2. Pope JE, *et al.* A meta-analysis of the effects of nonsteroidal anti-inflammatory drugs on blood pressure. *Arch Intern Med* 1993; **153:** 477–84.
3. Gurwitz JH, *et al.* Initiation of antihypertensive treatment during nonsteroidal anti-inflammatory drug therapy. *JAMA* 1994; **272:** 781–6.

Effects on the CNS. A literature review[1] revealed that headache, hearing loss, and tinnitus are the most frequent CNS adverse effects in patients taking NSAIDs. Aseptic meningitis has occurred rarely in patients using naproxen, sulindac, or tolmetin, but the most common reports are in patients with systemic lupus erythematosus who were receiving ibuprofen. Reports of psychosis appear to be rare and have involved indomethacin or sulindac, but in the reviewers' experience it is probably under-reported and is typically seen in elderly patients given indomethacin. The role of NSAIDs in the development of cognitive decline in the elderly is unclear: they have been associated with memory impairment and attention deficits in elderly patients;[1,2] however some authors have also reported that long-term NSAID use may reduce the rate of cognitive decline[3] or the risk of developing Alzheimer's disease.[4]

1. Hoppmann RA, *et al.* Central nervous system side effects of nonsteroidal anti-inflammatory drugs: aseptic meningitis, psychosis, and cognitive dysfunction. *Arch Intern Med* 1991; **151:** 1309–13.
2. Saag KG, *et al.* Nonsteroidal antiinflammatory drugs and cognitive decline in the elderly. *J Rheumatol* 1995; **22:** 2142–7.
3. Rozzini R, *et al.* Protective effect of chronic NSAID use on cognitive decline in older persons. *J Am Geriatr Soc* 1996; **44:** 1025–9.
4. Stewart WF, *et al.* Risk of Alzheimer's disease and duration of NSAID use. *Neurology* 1997; **48:** 626–32.

Effects on electrolytes. See under Effects on the Kidneys, below.

Effects on the eyes. Ocular effects such as blurred vision occur rarely in patients taking NSAIDs. Other more serious effects on the eyes associated with NSAIDs also appear to be rare. In the USA the National Registry of Drug-Induced Ocular Side Effects analysed 144 reports they received of possible adverse optic nerve reactions associated with the use of NSAIDs.[1] Of the 24 cases of papilloedema with or without pseudotumour cerebri more than half were associated with propionic acid derivatives, but it was considered that the data indicated that, on rare occasions, most NSAIDs could cause this effect; the number of reports for individual drugs was: ibuprofen (7 reports), indomethacin (5), naproxen (5), meclofenamate (3), diflunisal (1), ketoprofen (1), sulindac (1), and tolmetin (1). Almost two-thirds of the 120 cases of optic or retrobulbar neuritis were also associated with propionic acid derivatives; the number of reports for individual drugs was: ibuprofen (43), naproxen (17), indomethacin (9), benoxaprofen (8), phenylbutazone (8), piroxicam (8), zomepirac (7), sulindac (6), fenoprofen (5), oxyphenbutazone (3), meclofenamate (2), tolmetin (2), diflunisal (1), and ketoprofen (1).

1. Fraunfelder FT, *et al.* Possible optic nerve side effects associated with nonsteroidal anti-inflammatory drugs. *J Toxicol Cutan Ocul Toxicol* 1994; **13:** 311–16.

Effects on the gastro-intestinal tract. NSAIDs can cause clinically important damage of the gastro-intestinal tract. The complex mechanisms involved are not fully understood,[1-11] although there is considerable interest in the role of cyclo-oxygenase-1 (COX-1) inhibition in gastro-intestinal toxicity and in the development of potentially less toxic selective COX-2 inhibitors.[12] The gastric mucosa is damaged both by local and systemic effects of NSAIDs.[13] The local effect is pH-dependent and varies between individual drugs. The systemic effect is pH-independent, can occur with any route of administration, and is less drug specific; it is this effect that is thought to involve COX-1 inhibition.

NSAIDs may increase the incidence of bleeding in the upper gastro-intestinal tract and of perforation, but serious complications are relatively infrequent. Although the effects of NSAIDs on the upper gastro-intestinal tract are well recognised they have also been associated with damage to the distal small intestine and colon.[14-20] Risk factors continue to be studied and so far the most important patient-related factors for upper gastro-intestinal toxicity are old age, a history of peptic ulcers or bleeding of the gastro-intestinal tract, and concomitant use of corticosteroids. A pilot study has also suggested that NSAIDs can produce a high degree of gastro-intestinal toxicity in children.[21] Whether infection with *Helicobacter pylori* affects the risk for NSAID-induced peptic ulcers is unclear.[22] Duration of therapy is not thought to influence the risk for serious events; a recent cohort study[23] has found that the risk of gastro-intestinal bleeding or perforation with NSAIDs is constant throughout treatment.

Several studies[24-26] have been conducted on the relative toxicity of oral NSAIDs on the upper gastro-intestinal tract and various rankings of these drugs have been discussed.[27-29] The UK Committee on Safety of Medicines (CSM)[29] examined 10 epidemiological studies for 7 oral non-aspirin NSAIDs and also examined the spontaneous reports they had received of gastro-intestinal effects associated with NSAIDs. The CSM concluded that azapropazone was associated with the highest risk of gastro-intestinal reactions and ibuprofen with the lowest risk. Piroxicam, ketoprofen, indomethacin, naproxen, and diclofenac had an intermediate risk; it was considered that the risk for piroxicam might be higher than for the other NSAIDs with intermediate toxicity. In a systematic review[30] of controlled epidemiological studies that found a relation between NSAID use and hospital admission for gastric haemorrhage or perforation, the low risk of serious gastric toxicity with ibuprofen appeared to be attributable mainly to the low doses used clinically; higher doses of ibuprofen are associated with a similar risk as other NSAIDs. For reference to an association between aspirin and the most severe gastric lesions compared with other NSAIDs, see p.16.

There has been concern that topical use of NSAIDs may also be associated with gastro-intestinal toxicity but a case-controlled study[31] concluded that topical administration was not associated with significant upper gastro-intestinal bleeding or perforation.

Apart from the selection of an NSAID with a lower risk for gastro-intestinal toxicity, other methods used for the prevention or treatment of NSAID-induced gastropathy are discussed under the treatment of peptic ulcer disease on p.1174.

1. Kendall MJ, Horton RC. Clinical pharmacology and therapeutics. *Postgrad Med J* 1990; **66:** 166–85.
2. Hawkey CJ. Non-steroidal anti-inflammatory drugs and peptic ulcers. *Br Med J* 1990; **300:** 278–84.
3. Holvoet J, *et al.* Relation of upper gastrointestinal bleeding to non-steroidal anti-inflammatory drugs and aspirin: a case-control study. *Gut* 1991; **32:** 730–4.
4. Griffin MR, *et al.* Nonsteroidal anti-inflammatory drug use and increased risk for peptic ulcer disease in elderly persons. *Ann Intern Med* 1991; **114:** 257–63.
5. Kuwayama H, *et al.* Gastroduodenal mucosal injury by nonsteroidal anti-inflammatory drugs. *Drug Invest* 1990; **2** (suppl 1): 22–6.
6. Schoen RT, Vender RJ. Mechanisms of nonsteroidal anti-inflammatory drug-induced gastric damage. *Am J Med* 1989; **86:** 449–58.
7. Szabo S, *et al.* Non-steroidal anti-inflammatory drug-induced gastropathy: mechanisms and management. *Med Toxicol Adverse Drug Exp* 1989; **4:** 77–94.
8. Soll AH. UCLA Conference. Nonsteroidal anti-inflammatory drugs and peptic ulcer disease. *Ann Intern Med* 1991; **114:** 307–19.
9. Gabriel SE, *et al.* Risk for serious gastrointestinal complications related to use of nonsteroidal anti-inflammatory drugs. *Ann Intern Med* 1991; **115:** 787–96.
10. Hayllar J, *et al.* Gastroprotection and nonsteroidal anti-inflammatory drugs (NSAIDs): rationale and clinical implications. *Drug Safety* 1992; **7:** 86–105.
11. Willett LR, *et al.* Epidemiology of gastrointestinal damage associated with nonsteroidal anti-inflammatory drugs. *Drug Safety* 1994; **10:** 170–81.
12. Hayllar J, Bjarnason I. NSAIDs, Cox-2 inhibitors, and the gut. *Lancet* 1995; **346:** 521–2.
13. Bjorkman DJ. Nonsteroidal anti-inflammatory drug-induced gastrointestinal injury. *Am J Med* 1996; **101** (suppl 1A): 25S–32S.
14. Riddell RH, *et al.* Non-steroidal anti-inflammatory drugs as a possible cause of collagenous colitis: a case-control study. *Gut* 1992; **33:** 683–6.
15. Gibson GR, *et al.* Colitis induced by nonsteroidal anti-inflammatory drugs: report of four cases and review of the literature. *Arch Intern Med* 1992; **152:** 625–32.
16. Allison MC, *et al.* Gastrointestinal damage associated with the use of nonsteroidal antiinflammatory drugs. *N Engl J Med* 1992; **327:** 749–54.
17. Gleeson M, *et al.* Colitis associated with non-steroidal anti-inflammatory drugs. *Lancet* 1994; **344:** 1028.
18. Kwo PY, Tremaine WJ. Nonsteroidal anti-inflammatory drug-induced enteropathy: case discussion and review of the literature. *Mayo Clin Proc* 1995; **70:** 55–61.
19. Gleeson MH, *et al.* Non-steroidal anti-inflammatory drugs, salicylates, and colitis. *Lancet* 1996; **347:** 904–5.
20. Evans JMM, *et al.* Non-steroidal anti-inflammatory drugs are associated with emergency admission to hospital for colitis due to inflammatory bowel disease. *Gut* 1997; **40:** 619–22.
21. Mulberg AE, *et al.* Identification of nonsteroidal antiinflammatory drug-induced gastroduodenal injury in children with juvenile rheumatoid arthritis. *J Pediatr* 1993; **122:** 647–9.
22. Marshall B. NSAIDs and Helicobacter pylori: therapeutic options. *Lancet* 1998; **352:** 1001–3.
23. MacDonald TM, *et al.* Association of upper gastrointestinal toxicity of non-steroidal anti-inflammatory drugs with continued exposure: cohort study. *Br Med J* 1997; **315:** 1333–7.
24. Kaufman DW, *et al.* Nonsteroidal anti-inflammatory drug use in relation to major upper gastrointestinal bleeding. *Clin Pharmacol Ther* 1993; **53:** 485–94.
25. García Rodríguez LA, Jick H. Risk of upper gastrointestinal bleeding and perforation associated with individual non-steroidal anti-inflammatory drugs. *Lancet* 1994; **343:** 769–72.
26. Langman MJS, *et al.* Risks of bleeding peptic ulcer associated with individual non-steroidal anti-inflammatory drugs. *Lancet* 1994; **343:** 1075–8.
27. Bateman DN. NSAIDs: time to re-evaluate gut toxicity. *Lancet* 1994; **343:** 1051–2.
28. Smith CC, *et al.* NSAIDs and gut toxicity. *Lancet* 1994; **344:** 56–7.
29. Committee on Safety of Medicines/Medicines Control Agency. Relative safety of oral non-aspirin NSAIDs. *Current Problems* 1994; **20:** 9–11.
30. Henry D, *et al.* Variability in risk of gastrointestinal complications with individual non-steroidal anti-inflammatory drugs: results of a collaborative meta-analysis. *Br Med J* 1996; **312:** 1563–6.
31. Evans JMM, *et al.* Topical non-steroidal anti-inflammatory drugs and admission to hospital for upper gastrointestinal bleeding and perforation: a record linkage case-control study. *Br Med J* 1995; **311:** 22–6.

Effects on the joints. There is concern that NSAIDs such as indomethacin may accelerate the rate of cartilage destruction in patients with osteoarthritis.[1,2]

1. Rashad S, *et al.* Effect of non-steroidal anti-inflammatory drugs on the course of osteoarthritis. *Lancet* 1989; **ii:** 519–22.
2. Huskisson EC, *et al.* Effects of antiinflammatory drugs on the progression of osteoarthritis of the knee. *J Rheumatol* 1995; **22:** 1941–6.

Effects on the kidneys. NSAIDs can produce a number of different renal disorders following systemic or topical administration,[1] some of which are due to their inhibition of prostaglandin synthesis.[2,3] Under normal conditions prostaglandins appear to have little effect on renal homoeostasis but in the presence of renal vasoconstriction their vasodilator action increases renal blood flow and thereby helps to maintain renal function.[4,5] Patients whose renal function is being maintained by prostaglandins are therefore at risk from NSAIDs. Such patients include those with impaired circulation, the elderly, those on diuretics, and those with heart failure or renal vascular disease.[2,4] Other risk factors for renal impairment with NSAIDs include dehydration, cirrhosis, surgery, sepsis,[6] and a history of gout or hyperuricaemia.[6,7] The half-life of an NSAID may be a more important determinant of the risk of developing functional renal impairment than the ingested dose.[7]

ACE inhibitors can also produce renal impairment and combined use with NSAIDs should be undertaken with great care. Prostaglandin inhibition may also lead to salt and water retention particularly when there is pre-existing hypertension or sodium depletion.[4] NSAIDs, therefore, tend to counteract the action of diuretics and antihypertensives.[2,4] There have been isolated reports of severe hyponatraemia and other symptoms resembling the syndrome of inappropriate antidiuretic hormone secretion in patients taking NSAIDs.[8,9]

Potassium homoeostasis is less dependent on prostaglandins and hyperkalaemia occurs infrequently with NSAIDs.[3] It is more likely to occur in patients with specific risk factors such as those receiving potassium supplements or potassium-sparing diuretics.[3] Indomethacin appears to be the main NSAID implicated (see also p.45).

NSAIDs may cause acute interstitial nephritis, perhaps involving an allergic response,[2,3] and it may progress to interstitial fibrosis or papillary necrosis.[3,10]

Analgesic abuse or prolonged excessive use can produce nephropathy, a condition characterised by renal papillary necrosis and chronic interstitial nephritis, and, eventually, renal failure.[11] Phenacetin, a para-aminophenol derivative, has long been recognised as being one of the main drugs responsible for analgesic nephropathy,[12,13] but nephropathy has also been associated with the long-term use of NSAIDs and paracetamol without phenacetin.[14]

1. O'Callaghan CA, *et al.* Renal disease and use of topical non-steroidal anti-inflammatory drugs. *Br Med J* 1994; **308:** 110–11.
2. Kendall MJ, Horton RC. Clinical pharmacology and therapeutics. *Postgrad Med J* 1990; **66:** 166–85.
3. Whelton A, Hamilton CW. Nonsteroidal anti-inflammatory drugs: effects on kidney function. *J Clin Pharmacol* 1991; **31:** 588–98.
4. Harris K. The role of prostaglandins in the control of renal function. *Br J Anaesth* 1992; **69;** 233–5.
5. Kenny GNC. Potential renal, haematological and allergic adverse effects associated with nonsteroidal anti-inflammatory drugs. *Drugs* 1992; **44** (suppl 5): 31–7.
6. MacDonald TM. Selected side-effects: 14. non-steroidal anti-inflammatory drugs and renal damage. *Prescribers' J* 1994; **34:** 77–80.
7. Henry D, *et al.* Consumption of non-steroidal anti-inflammatory drugs and the development of functional renal impairment in elderly subjects: results of a case-control study. *Br J Clin Pharmacol* 1997; **44:** 85–90.
8. Petersson I, *et al.* Water intoxication associated with non-steroidal anti-inflammatory drug therapy. *Acta Med Scand* 1987; **221:** 221–3.
9. Cheung NT, *et al.* Syndrome of inappropriate secretion of antidiuretic hormone induced by diclofenac. *Br Med J* 1993; **306:** 186.
10. Sandler DP, *et al.* Nonsteroidal anti-inflammatory drugs and the risk for chronic renal disease. *Ann Intern Med* 1991; **115:** 165–72.
11. De Broe ME, Elseviers MM. Analgesic nephropathy. *N Engl J Med* 1998; **338:** 446–52.
12. Sandler DP, *et al.* Analgesic use and chronic renal disease. *N Engl J Med* 1989; **320:** 1238–43.
13. Dubach UC, *et al.* An epidemiologic study of abuse of analgesic drugs: effects of phenacetin and salicylate on mortality and cardiovascular morbidity (1968 to 1987). *N Engl J Med* 1991; **324:** 155–60.
14. Perneger TV, *et al.* Risk of kidney failure associated with the use of acetaminophen, aspirin, and nonsteroidal antiinflammatory drugs. *N Engl J Med* 1994; **331:** 1675–9.

Effects on the liver. A retrospective study involving over 220 000 adults who were either using, or had used, NSAIDs identified a small excess risk of serious, acute non-infectious liver injury; in current users there was a twofold increase in risk and there was a predominance of the cholestatic type of liver injury among such patients. Nonetheless, admissions to hospital for liver injury had been rare.[1] In a review[2] of cohort and case-control studies describing an association between NSAIDs and liver disease, the strongest evidence emerged for sulindac. There were also a significant number of reports of hepatotoxicity on rechallenge with diclofenac. Evidence of hepatotoxicity for other NSAIDs was weak, although the risk appeared to be high when they were used with other hepatotoxic drugs. However, the overall incidence of liver disease with NSAIDs was very low.

1. García Rodríguez LA, *et al.* The role of non-steroidal anti-inflammatory drugs in acute liver injury. *Br Med J* 1992; **305:** 865–8. Correction. *ibid.*: 920.
2. Manoukian AV, Carson JL. Nonsteroidal anti-inflammatory drug-induced hepatic disorders. *Drug Safety* 1996; **15:** 64–71.

Effects on the lungs. Adverse pulmonary effects such as pneumonitis, alveolitis, pulmonary infiltrates, and pulmonary fibrosis, often suggestive of an allergic or immune reaction, have been reported with a number of NSAIDs. For references, see under individual monographs.

Effects on the pancreas. A review[1] of drug-induced pancreatitis considered that sulindac was amongst the drugs for which a definite association with pancreatitis had been established. There had been isolated reports of pancreatitis with ketoprofen, mefenamic acid, and piroxicam but any association was considered to be questionable. For further references see under individual monographs.

1. Underwood TW, Frye CB. Drug-induced pancreatitis. *Clin Pharm* 1993; **12:** 440–8.

Effects on the skin. The diverse cutaneous reactions to NSAIDs have been reviewed.[1] Of 250 children attending a rheumatology clinic 34 (13.6%) were found to have 4 or more facial scars of unknown origin.[2] This number of scars was found in 22.2% of the 116 children who had received naproxen and in 9.2% of the 87 who had received other NSAIDs. Children affected were more likely to have light skin and blue or green eyes. It was not known whether this was a form of phototoxic reaction but pseudoporphyria-like eruptions associated with NSAIDs, and naproxen in particular (see p.61), have been reported.

See also under Hypersensitivity, below.

1. Bigby M, Stern R. Cutaneous reactions to nonsteroidal anti-inflammatory drugs. *J Am Acad Dermatol* 1985; **12:** 866–76.
2. Wallace CA, *et al.* Increased risk of facial scars in children taking nonsteroidal antiinflammatory drugs. *J Pediatr* 1994; **125:** 819–22.

Hypersensitivity. NSAIDs have produced a wide range of hypersensitivity reactions in susceptible individuals; the most common include skin rashes, urticaria, rhinitis, angioedema, bronchoconstriction, and anaphylactic shock. Hypersensitivity to NSAIDs appears to occur more frequently in patients with asthma or allergic disorders but other risk factors have been identified (for further details see under Aspirin, p.16). The occurrence of aspirin sensitivity in patients with asthma and nasal polyps has been referred to as the 'aspirin triad'. There is considerable cross-reactivity between aspirin and other NSAIDs and it is generally recommended that patients who have had a hypersensitivity reaction to aspirin or any other NSAID should avoid all NSAIDs. For references to hypersensitivity reactions associated with NSAIDs, see under individual monographs.

Overdosage. The clinical signs and symptoms following acute overdosage of NSAIDs and methods of treatment have been reviewed.[1] In general, symptoms of NSAID poisoning are mild, and usually include nausea and vomiting, headache, drowsiness, blurred vision, and dizziness. There have been isolated case reports of more serious toxicity, including seizures, hypotension, apnoea, coma, and renal failure, although usually after ingestion of substantial quantities. Seizures are a particular problem with mefenamic acid overdosage.

Treatment of NSAID overdosage is entirely supportive. Gastric lavage and activated charcoal may be of benefit within 1 hour of ingestion. Multiple doses of activated charcoal may be useful in enhancing elimination of NSAIDs with long half-lives such as piroxicam and sulindac. Forced diuresis, haemodialysis, or haemoperfusion are unlikely to be of benefit for NSAID overdosage, although haemodialysis may be required if oliguric renal failure develops.

1. Smolinske SC, *et al.* Toxic effects of nonsteroidal anti-inflammatory drugs in overdose: an overview of recent evidence on clinical effects and dose-response relationships. *Drug Safety* 1990; **5:** 252–74.

Precautions

NSAIDs should not be given to patients with peptic ulceration and should be used with caution in patients with a history of such disorders. To reduce the risk of gastro-intestinal effects, the drug may be taken with or after food or milk. Antacids, histamine H_2-receptor antagonists, omeprazole, sucralfate, or misoprostol may be used for a similar purpose (see under Peptic Ulcer Disease, p.1174). However, food, milk, and such measures may reduce the rate and extent of drug absorption. Some authorities recommend that NSAIDs associated with the lowest risk of gastro-intestinal toxicity (see Effects on the Gastro-intestinal Tract, under Adverse Effects, above) should be tried first in the lowest recommended dose, and not more than one NSAID should be used at a time.

NSAIDs should be used with caution in patients with infections, since symptoms such as fever and inflammation may be masked, and also used with caution in patients with asthma or allergic disorders. NSAIDs are contra-indicated in patients with a history of hypersensitivity reactions to aspirin or other NSAIDs, including those in whom attacks of asthma, angioedema, urticaria, or rhinitis have been precipitated by aspirin or any other NSAID.

Other general precautions to be observed include administration to patients with haemorrhagic disorders, hypertension, and impaired renal, hepatic, or cardiac function. Patients undergoing therapy with some NSAIDs may need to be monitored for the development of blood, kidney, liver, or eye disorders. NSAIDs should be used with caution in the elderly and may need to be given in reduced doses.

Regular use of NSAIDs during the 3rd trimester of pregnancy may result in closure of fetal ductus arteriosus *in utero*, and possibly in persistent pulmonary hypertension of the newborn. The onset of labour may be delayed and its duration increased.

Some NSAIDs can interfere with thyroid function tests by lowering serum-thyroid hormone concentrations.

Further details concerning the precautions of the individual NSAIDs may be found under their respective monographs.

Pregnancy. Results from a case-control interview study[1] suggest that prenatal ingestion of aspirin or other NSAIDs may be implicated in persistent pulmonary hypertension of the newborn. The authors suggest that these drugs may be responsible for gestational structural or functional alterations of the pulmonary vasculature. However, they interpret their results with caution and also suggest that the primary cause may be the underlying disorder for which the NSAIDs or aspirin were ingested. They were unable to pinpoint in which trimester the drugs may have their proposed action, and conclude that further evaluation is necessary.

1. Van Marter LJ, *et al.* Persistent pulmonary hypertension of the newborn and smoking and aspirin and nonsteroidal antiinflammatory drug consumption during pregnancy. *Pediatrics* 1996; **97:** 658–63.

Interactions

Notable interactions involving NSAIDs include enhancement of the effects of oral anticoagulants (especially by azapropazone and phenylbutazone) and increased plasma concentrations of lithium, methotrexate, and cardiac glycosides. The risk of nephrotoxicity may be increased if given with ACE inhibitors, cyclosporin, tacrolimus, or diuretics. Effects on renal function may lead to reduced excretion of some drugs. There may also be an increased risk of hyperkalaemia with ACE inhibitors and potassium-sparing diuretics. The antihypertensive effects of some antihypertensives including ACE inhibitors, beta blockers, and diuretics may be reduced. Convulsions may occur due to an interaction with quinolones. NSAIDs may enhance the effects of phenytoin and sulphonylurea antidiabetics. The effects of NSAIDs might be enhanced by use with moclobemide. The concomitant use of more than one NSAID (including aspirin) should be avoided because of the increased risk of adverse effects. The risk of gastro-intestinal bleeding and ulceration associated with NSAIDs is increased when used with corticosteroids or, possibly, alcohol, bisphosphonates, or oxpentifylline. There may be an increased risk of haemotoxicity during concomitant use of zidovudine and NSAIDs; blood counts 1 to 2 weeks after starting use together are recommended. The manufacturer of mifepristone advises that NSAIDs or aspirin should be avoided for 8 to 12 days after mifepristone use because of a theoretical risk that these prostaglandin synthetase inhibitors may alter the efficacy of mifepristone.

Further details concerning the interactions of the individual NSAIDs may be found under their respective monographs.

References.

1. Brouwers JRBJ, de Smet PAGM. Pharmacokinetic-pharmacodynamic drug interactions with nonsteroidal anti-inflammatory drugs. *Clin Pharmacokinet* 1994; **27:** 462–85.
2. Bishnoi A, *et al.* Effect of commonly prescribed nonsteroidal anti-inflammatory drugs on thyroid hormone measurements. *Am J Med* 1994; **96:** 235–8.

Antihypertensives. For reference to the relative effects of NSAIDs in antagonising different types of antihypertensive drugs, see Effects on Blood Pressure under Adverse Effects, above.

Pharmacokinetics

Details of the pharmacokinetics of individual NSAIDs may be found under their respective monographs.

General reviews.

1. Woodhouse KW, Wynne H. The pharmacokinetics of non-steroidal anti-inflammatory drugs in the elderly. *Clin Pharmacokinet* 1987; **12:** 111–22.
2. Walson PD, Mortensen ME. Pharmacokinetics of common analgesics, anti-inflammatories and antipyretics in children. *Clin Pharmacokinet* 1989; **17** (suppl 1): 116–37.
3. Netter P, *et al.* Recent findings on the pharmacokinetics of non-steroidal anti-inflammatory drugs in synovial fluid. *Clin Pharmacokinet* 1989; **17:** 145–62.
4. Lapicque F, *et al.* Protein binding and stereoselectivity of non-steroidal anti-inflammatory drugs. *Clin Pharmacokinet* 1993; **25:** 115–25.
5. Simkin PA, *et al.* Articular pharmacokinetics of protein-bound antirheumatic agents. *Clin Pharmacokinet* 1993; **25:** 342–50.

Uses and Administration

Many of the effects of NSAIDs appear to be due to their inhibitory action on cyclo-oxygenases which are involved in the biosynthesis of prostaglandins and thromboxanes from arachidonic acid (see p.1411 and p.704). Prostaglandins have an important role in the production of pain, inflammation, and fever, and NSAIDs therefore find their main use as analgesics, anti-inflammatories, and antipyretics. Administered as single doses or in short-term intermittent therapy they provide adequate analgesia to relieve mild to moderate pain. However, it may take up to three weeks of use before their anti-inflammatory effects become evident. The combined analgesic and anti-inflammatory effects of NSAIDs make them particularly useful for the symptomatic relief of painful and/or inflammatory conditions including rheumatic disorders such as rheumatoid arthritis, osteoarthritis, and the spondyloarthropathies, and also in peri-articular disorders, and soft-tissue rheumatism. NSAIDs, but not aspirin or other salicylates, are also used to treat acute gouty arthritis.

Administration of NSAIDs is usually by mouth, with or after food, although some such as diclofenac, ketoprofen, ketorolac, piroxicam, and tenoxicam can be given by intramuscular injection; ketorolac and tenoxicam can also be given by intravenous injection. Some NSAIDs are applied topically.

Several NSAIDs are used in ophthalmic preparations for the inhibition of intra-operative miosis, control of postoperative ocular inflammation, and prevention of cystoid macular oedema.

Although there have been many studies comparing the efficacy of one NSAID with one or several others there has been no wide-ranging comparison between all NSAIDs to allow them to be ranked in order of efficacy. Generally, it is felt that there is little difference in anti-inflammatory activity between the various NSAIDs and choice is largely empirical. Responses of individual patients varies widely. Thus, if a patient fails to respond to one NSAID, another drug may be successful. However, it has been recommended that NSAIDs associated with a low risk of gastro-intestinal toxicity (see above) should generally be preferred and the lowest effective dose used.

Action. It has been proposed that NSAIDs act through inhibition of cyclo-oxygenase-1 (COX-1) and cyclo-oxygenase-2 (COX-2) and that inhibition of COX-1 is associated with adverse gastro-intestinal effects while inhibition of COX-2 is associated with anti-inflammatory activity.[1-6] Hence the interest in NSAIDs that are selective inhibitors of COX-2; meloxicam and nimesulide are two such drugs. COX-2 inhibitors may also have a potential use in other diseases in which COX-2 might be implicated.[4] Even if COX-2 inhibitors are associated with a reduced incidence of gastric toxicity, any potential drawbacks of prolonged COX-2 inhibition at other locations are as yet unknown.[4,5]

There is increasing evidence that NSAIDs may also have a central mechanism of action that augments the peripheral mechanism.[6]

Many NSAIDs possess centres of chirality within their molecular structure, with different chiral forms (enantiomers) having different degrees of pharmacological activity.[7,8] For example, indomethacin, its analogues, and some arylpropionic acids are chiral drugs with the S(+) enantiomer in most cases showing the dominant pharmacological activity. However, the ratio of S/R activity varies between drugs and between animal species. NSAIDs are generally administered clinically as the racemate with only a few currently being given as the (S)-enantiomer. The chirality of a drug may have subtle effects on its toxicity and interactions, and it may be more desirable to administer a drug as its active enantiomer.[8]

See individual monographs for references relating to the stereoselective pharmacokinetics of some NSAIDs.

1. Hayllar J, Bjarnason I. NSAIDs, Cox-2 inhibition, and the gut. *Lancet* 1995; **346:** 521–2.
2. Bennett A, Tavares IA. NSAIDs, Cox-2 inhibitors, and the gut. *Lancet* 1995; **346:** 1105.
3. Vane JR. NSAIDs, Cox-2 inhibitors, and the gut. *Lancet* 1995; **346:** 1105–6.
4. Jouzeau J-Y, *et al.* Cyclo-oxygenase isoenzymes: how recent findings affect thinking about nonsteroidal anti-inflammatory drugs. *Drugs* 1997; **53:** 563–82.
5. Richardson C, Emery P. The clinical implications of inhibition of the inducible form of cyclo-oxygenase. *Drug Safety* 1996; **15:** 249–60.
6. Cashman JN. The mechanisms of action of NSAIDs in analgesia. *Drugs* 1996; **52** (suppl 5): 13–23.
7. Kean WF, *et al.* Chirality in antirheumatic drugs. *Lancet* 1991; **338:** 1565–8.
8. Hayball PJ. Chirality and nonsteroidal anti-inflammatory drugs. *Drugs* 1996; **52** (suppl 5): 47–58.

Colic pain. Prostaglandins have been implicated in the aetiology of biliary colic (see Colic Pain, p.8), and some NSAIDs such as diclofenac, indomethacin, and ketoprofen have been used to relieve such pain.

Ectopic ossification. The use of NSAIDs appears to be a promising alternative to inhibition of mineralisation with etidronate in the prevention of ectopic ossification (p.730) after surgery or trauma.

References.

1. Schmidt SA, *et al.* The use of indomethacin to prevent the formation of heterotopic bone after total hip replacement: a randomized, double-blind clinical trial. *J Bone Joint Surg (Am)* 1988; **70A:** 834–8.
2. Pagnani MJ, *et al.* Effect of aspirin on heterotopic ossification after total hip arthroplasty in men who have osteoarthrosis. *J Bone Joint Surg (Am)* 1991; **73A:** 924–9.
3. Knelles D, *et al.* Prevention of heterotopic ossification after total hip replacement: a prospective, randomised study using acetylsalicylic acid, indomethacin and fractional or single-dose irradiation. *J Bone Joint Surg (Br)* 1997; **79B:** 596–602.

Eye disorders. Miosis resistant to conventional mydriatics often develops during ocular surgery, possibly due to release of prostaglandins and other substances associated with trauma. NSAIDs, which are prostaglandin synthetase inhibitors, are therefore used prophylactically as eye drops before ocular surgery to ameliorate intra-operative miosis but there has been some doubt that the effect they produce is of clinical significance. Those commonly used include diclofenac, indomethacin, flurbiprofen, and suprofen. These drugs do not possess intrinsic mydriatic properties. The use of conventional mydriatics is discussed on p.454.

Some NSAIDs are used topically or systemically in a number of inflammatory ocular disorders, including those following ocular surgery (see below). They are used as alternatives to corticosteroids in the management of postoperative ocular inflammation and alone or with corticosteroids to prevent or relieve cystoid macular oedema, a complication following some types of ocular surgery. However, their role in the treatment of macular oedema associated with uveitis (p.1030) is less clear. NSAIDs are also used in the treatment of scleritis (see p.1029).

Some references to the use of NSAIDs in ophthalmology are given below.

1. Flach AJ. Cyclo-oxygenase inhibitors in ophthalmology. *Surv Ophthalmol* 1992; **36:** 259–84.
2. Koay P. The emerging roles of topical non-steroidal anti-inflammatory agents in ophthalmology. *Br J Ophthalmol* 1996; **80:** 480–5.

POSTOPERATIVE INFLAMMATORY OCULAR DISORDERS. Corticosteroids are used topically for the control of **postoperative ocular inflammation** but caution is required as they can delay wound healing and mask postoperative infection. They should only be used for short periods as they can cause glaucoma in susceptible individuals. NSAIDs are also used topically in the management of postoperative ocular inflammation,[1-4] although there is some doubt over efficacy. However, in one study[5] eye drops containing diclofenac sodium were found to be more effective than those containing prednisolone sodium phosphate in reducing the increase in blood-aqueous humour leakage after cataract surgery. In another study[6] diclofenac appeared to be as effective as betamethasone in controlling postoperative inflammation following strabismus surgery.

Cystoid macular oedema is a complication following cataract or retinal detachment surgery which arises from a disturbance of the blood-retinal barrier. A number of NSAIDs,[7-9] including diclofenac, flurbiprofen, indomethacin, and ketorolac are used topically with or without corticosteroids to prevent or relieve cystoid macular oedema. NSAIDs such as indomethacin are also used systemically in the management of cystoid macular oedema.

1. Pappas HR, *et al.* Topical indomethacin therapy before argon laser trabeculoplasty. *Am J Ophthalmol* 1985; **99:** 571–5.
2. Weinreb RN, *et al.* Flurbiprofen pretreatment in argon laser trabeculoplasty for primary open-angle glaucoma. *Arch Ophthalmol* 1984; **102:** 1629–32.
3. Bizzotto MF, *et al.* Efficacy of flurbiprofen versus placebo on postoperative course following cataract extraction. *Drugs Exp Clin Res* 1984; **10:** 421–5.
4. Sabiston DW, Robinson IG. An evaluation of the anti-inflammatory effect of flurbiprofen after cataract extraction. *Br J Ophthalmol* 1987; **71:** 418–21.
5. Kraff MC, *et al.* Inhibition of blood-aqueous humor barrier breakdown with diclofenac: a fluorophotometric study. *Arch Ophthalmol* 1990; **108:** 380–3.
6. Wright M, *et al.* Comparison of the efficacy of diclofenac and betamethasone following strabismus surgery. *Br J Ophthalmol* 1997; **81:** 299–301.
7. Jampol LM. Pharmacologic therapy of aphakic and pseudophakic cystoid macular edema. *Ophthalmology* 1985; **92:** 807–10.
8. Flach AJ, *et al.* Effectiveness of ketorolac tromethamine 0.5% ophthalmic solution for chronic aphakic and pseudophakic cystoid macular edema. *Am J Ophthalmol* 1987; **103:** 479–86.
9. Jampol LM, *et al.* Nonsteroidal anti-inflammatory drugs and cataract surgery. *Arch Ophthalmol* 1994; **112:** 891–4.

Fever. Methods for controlling fever (p.1) include the use of antipyretics and/or physical cooling methods. Paracetamol, salicylates and some other NSAIDs are the main antipyretics used. Paracetamol is usually the antipyretic of choice in infants and children; salicylates are generally contra-indicated in these patients because of the possible link between their use and the development of Reye's syndrome (see under Adverse Effects of Aspirin, p.17). Ibuprofen appears to be an effective alternative to paracetamol but there is relatively little experience of its use and safety in infants and children.

Gout. NSAIDs are the drugs usually used first for the treatment of acute attacks of gout (p.390). Since the treatment of chronic gout can lead to the mobilisation of urate crystals from established tophi to produce acute attacks, NSAIDs may also be used for the prophylaxis of acute gout during the first few months of antihyperuricaemic therapy.

Headache. An NSAID is often tried first for the symptomatic treatment of various types of headache including migraine (p.443) and tension-type headache (p.444). An NSAID given at the onset of symptoms can successfully treat an acute attack of migraine. NSAIDs may also be effective prophylactic drugs for migraine, although propranolol or pizotifen are generally preferred. Chronic paroxysmal hemicrania, a rare variant of cluster headache (p.443), responds to indomethacin.

Kidney disorders. Although NSAIDs can produce adverse effects on the kidney (see above) they may have a role in the management of some types of glomerular kidney disease (p.1021). They may be of use for the control of proteinuria due to nephrotic syndrome except when there is overt renal failure.

Malignant neoplasms. Results of a study by the American Cancer Society[1] have suggested that regular use of aspirin may reduce the risk of developing fatal cancer of the oesophagus, stomach, colon, or rectum. Death rates due to other gastro-intestinal cancers did not appear to be affected. Although a number of other studies[2-5] appear to support the reduced risk of colorectal cancer in regular users of aspirin or other NSAIDs, it is considered[6-9] that further studies are still required before any firm conclusions can be made. Also a recent study[10] found no evidence of an association between the use of aspirin and the incidence of colorectal cancer although the authors suggest that these results may be explained by the short treatment period and the low dose of aspirin used. It has also been pointed out[6-8] that long-term use of aspirin may itself be associated with an increased risk of certain other diseases, including cancer of the urinary-tract.

Treatment with sulindac has been found to be of benefit in patients with familiar adenomatous polyposis (p.87).

For a discussion of the treatment and prophylaxis of malignant neoplasms of the gastro-intestinal tract, see p.487.

1. Thun MJ, *et al.* Aspirin use and the risk of fatal cancer. *Cancer Res* 1993; **53:** 1322–7.
2. Rosenberg L, *et al.* A hypothesis: nonsteroidal anti-inflammatory drugs reduce the incidence of large-bowel cancer. *J Natl Cancer Inst* 1991; **83:** 355–8.
3. Logan RFA, *et al.* Effect of aspirin and non-steroidal anti-inflammatory drugs on colorectal adenomas: case-control study of subjects participating in the Nottingham faecal occult blood screening programme. *Br Med J* 1993; **307:** 285–9.
4. Giovannucci E, *et al.* Aspirin use and the risk for colorectal cancer and adenoma in male health professionals. *Ann Intern Med* 1994; **121:** 241–6.
5. Giovannucci E, *et al.* Aspirin and the risk of colorectal cancer in women. *N Engl J Med* 1995; **333:** 609–14.
6. Paganini-Hill A. Aspirin and colorectal cancer. *Br Med J* 1993; **307:** 278–9.
7. Farmer KC, *et al.* Aspirin and non-steroidal anti-inflammatory drugs in the chemoprevention of colorectal cancer. *Med J Aust* 1993; **159:** 649–50.
8. Garewal HS. Aspirin in the prevention of colorectal cancer. *Ann Intern Med* 1994; **121:** 303–4.
9. Koutsos MI, *et al.* Can nonsteroidal anti-inflammatory drugs be recommended to prevent colon cancer in high risk elderly patients? *Drugs Aging* 1995; **6:** 421–5.
10. Stürmer T, *et al.* Aspirin use and colorectal cancer: post-trial follow-up data from the Physicians' Health Study. *Ann Intern Med* 1998; **128:** 713–20.

Menstrual disorders. NSAIDs have been used or tried in a number of disorders associated with menstruation.

Drug therapy is the treatment of choice for idiopathic menorrhagia (p.1461). Menorrhagia is thought to be associated with abnormalities of prostaglandin production, and treatment with NSAIDs such as ibuprofen, mefenamic acid, or naproxen is often employed. When administered during menstruation, such drugs reduce uterine blood loss by an average of 30% in women with menorrhagia. There does not appear to be any evidence to suggest that any one NSAID is more effective than any other.

NSAIDs are also used for dysmenorrhoea (p.9). The pain of dysmenorrhoea arises from uterine contractions produced by release of prostaglandins from the endometrium in the luteal phase of the menstrual cycle. Drugs that inhibit ovulation or prostaglandin production are often effective treatments and NSAIDs are usually the drugs of first choice. Mefenamic acid may have a theoretical advantage over other NSAIDs in being able to inhibit both the synthesis and the peripheral action of prostaglandins, but clinical studies have not shown fenemates to be more effective.

Migraine. See under Headache, above.

Orthostatic hypotension. Fludrocortisone is usually the first drug tried in the treatment of orthostatic hypotension (p.1040) when nonpharmacological treatment has failed. NSAIDs such as flurbiprofen, ibuprofen, or indomethacin may be used alone or added to treatment if the response is inadequate.

Pain. NSAIDs have a similar analgesic effect to aspirin and paracetamol in single doses but in regular full dosage, they have both a lasting analgesic and an anti-inflammatory effect. NSAIDs are used in the management of mild to moderate pain (p.4) and are of particular value in pain due to inflammation. NSAIDs may also be used as an adjunct to opioids in the management of severe pain such as cancer pain (p.8) and are particularly effective in bone pain of malignant origin. NSAIDs may be used in the treatment of acute low back pain (p.10) if paracetamol fails to provide adequate pain relief. Short-term use of oral NSAIDs may help to relieve pain and reduce inflammation of soft-tissue rheumatism (p.4); topical formulations of some NSAIDs are also used but their therapeutic role, if any, is unclear. NSAIDs provide symptomatic relief for rheumatic disorders such as rheumatoid arthritis (p.2) and spondyloarthropathies (p.4), but they do not alter the course of the disease and additional antirheumatic drugs may need to be given to prevent irreversible joint damage. NSAIDs may also be used as an alternative to paracetamol for osteoarthritis (p.2). NSAIDs may be of benefit for inflammatory pain in infants and children (p.7), although paracetamol is generally the preferred non-opioid analgesic in this age group. NSAIDs may be used for postoperative pain (p.11), and are of particular value following day-case surgery because of their lack of sedative effects. They are not usually considered to be strong enough as the sole analgesic following major surgery, but may be used with stronger analgesics and may allow dosage reduction of concomitant opioids. The pain of mild sickle-cell crises (p.11) may be controlled by analgesics such as NSAIDs or weak opioids; NSAIDs may be used with strong opioids for severe crises.

Dependence and tolerance are not a problem with non-opioid analgesics such as NSAIDs, but there is a ceiling of efficacy, above which increasing the dose has no further therapeutic effect.

Urinary incontinence. Prostaglandin synthetase inhibitors, such as flurbiprofen and indomethacin, have been studied in the management of urge incontinence (p.454) because of their weak effect on detrusor instability but their therapeutic value has not been established.

Opioid Analgesics (6200-n)

Dependence and Withdrawal

Drug dependence of the opioid type is a state arising from repeated administration of an opioid; it is characterised by an overwhelming need to continue taking the drug or one with similar properties, by a tendency to increase the dose owing to the development of tolerance, and by psychological and physical dependence on the drug. Cross-tolerance and cross-dependence can be expected between opioids acting at the same receptors. Opioid analgesics, in particular diamorphine, are abused for their euphoriant effects and dependence develops rapidly with regular use. Dependence as a result of legitimate therapeutic use is much less of a problem.

Abrupt withdrawal of opioids from persons physically dependent on them precipitates a withdrawal syndrome, the severity of which depends on the individual, the drug used, the size and frequency of the dose, and the duration of drug use. Withdrawal symptoms may also follow the administration of an opioid antagonist such as naloxone or an agonist/antagonist such as pentazocine to opioid-dependent persons. Neonatal opioid dependence may occur in the offspring of opioid-dependent mothers and these infants may suffer withdrawal symptoms at birth.

Opioid analgesics can be classified according to the receptors at which they act (see under Uses and Administration, below) and withdrawal syndromes are characteristic for a receptor type. Dependence associated with morphine and closely related μ-agonists appears to result in more severe withdrawal symptoms than that associated with κ-receptor agonists. Onset and duration of withdrawal symptoms also vary according to the duration of action of the specific drug. With morphine and diamorphine *withdrawal symptoms* usually begin within a few hours, reach a peak within 36 to 72 hours, and then gradually subside; they develop more slowly with methadone. Withdrawal symptoms include yawning, mydriasis, lachrymation, rhinorrhoea, sneezing, muscle tremor, weakness, sweating, anxiety, irritability, disturbed sleep or insomnia, restlessness, anorexia, nausea, vomiting, loss of weight, diarrhoea, dehydration, leucocytosis, bone pain, abdominal and muscle cramps, gooseflesh, vasomotor disturbances, and increases in heart rate, respiratory rate, blood pressure, and temperature. Some physiological values may not return to normal for several months following the acute withdrawal syndrome.

Withdrawal symptoms may be terminated by a suitable dose of the original or a related opioid. Tolerance diminishes rapidly after withdrawal so that a previously tolerated dose may prove fatal.

For a discussion of the treatment of opioid dependence and neonatal opioid dependence, see below.

Diagnosis of dependence. Naloxone (p.987) and other opioid antagonists have been used to diagnose opioid dependence. Detection of opioids in hair[1] has been used in the assessment of addicts.

1. Strang J, *et al.* Hair analysis for drugs of abuse. *Lancet* 1990; **335:** 740.

Treatment of opioid dependence. The treatment of opioid dependence has been the subject of a number of reviews and discussions.[1-6]

Planned withdrawal (**detoxification**) may be effected slowly or rapidly. Opioids, themselves, have a long history of use in the management of opioid dependence; the usual method in many countries is to replace the drug of dependence with methadone given as a liquid oral preparation, and then gradually withdraw the methadone if possible. Methadone is considered to be particularly suitable for withdrawal therapy because it can be given orally and its long half-life allows once daily administration. Liquid oral preparations are usually preferred. Oral diamorphine has been used similarly to methadone; reefers containing diamorphine have also been used in some centres. Dihydrocodeine tablets have been used successfully. A more recent introduction is levomethadyl acetate which appears to have similar properties to methadone. Its extremely long half-life allows maintenance to be achieved with administration three times weekly. Buprenorphine given sublingually has also shown promise in the treatment of opioid dependence.

Iatrogenic opioid dependence may occur in patients receiving μ-agonists such as morphine, fentanyl, or pethidine for the management of acute pain or in an intensive care setting for more than 5 to 10 days. Methadone has been used successfully to manage opioid withdrawal in adult intensive care patients.[7] However, some[8] avoid using methadone to manage withdrawal in children because of the stigma of its associations with managing withdrawal in drug addicts. In physically dependent but non-addicted patients, gradual weaning using the same opioid that was used therapeutically is preferred where possible, although in some cases, it may be necessary to change to a different opioid because of ease of administration, duration of action, and ability to taper the dose; virtually any opioid can be used.[8]

Other drugs used in the management of opioid withdrawal include alpha$_2$-adrenoceptor agonists such as clonidine and opioid antagonists such as naltrexone and naloxone. Clonidine may help to suppress symptoms of opioid withdrawal, such as anxiety, insomnia, and muscle aches. It appears to be more effective when used in the control of symptoms following abrupt withdrawal than when used during gradual withdrawal of methadone. Hypotension may limit its usefulness in some patients. The clonidine analogue lofexidine may produce similar results to those obtained with clonidine and appears to be less sedating and hypotensive.

Naltrexone and naloxone block the euphoriant effects of opioids although their use in detoxification as monotherapy is limited by unacceptable opioid withdrawal effects. Naltrexone may be used with clonidine and some workers have reported that withdrawal can be achieved within a few days using combined therapy.[9,10] Moreover, naloxone and naltrexone are being used in the relatively new technique of rapid or ultra rapid opioid detoxification.[11,12] Detoxification with, in most cases, naloxone or naltrexone is achieved while the patient is heavily sedated or under general anaesthesia and hence unaware of any unpleasant withdrawal symptoms. However, although rapid, with detoxification within 24 hours, and with a high initial success rate, the technique itself is not without risks and it does not obviate the need for maintenance treatment (see below).

Concomitant counselling and other psychosocial services have been shown to be important in the outcome of withdrawal therapy.[13] Detoxification alone does not ensure long-term abstinence.

A number of other drugs may be of use as adjuncts in the management of withdrawal symptoms. Diphenoxylate with atropine may be used for the control of diarrhoea. Promethazine has been used for its antiemetic and sedative actions. Beta blockers such as propranolol may be of use for patients with pronounced somatic anxiety symptoms. A short course of thioridazine may also be suitable for anxiety. Benzodiazepines or chlormethiazole can be given to relieve anxiety and associated insomnia but only short courses should be used in order to minimise the risk of dependence and abuse.

Long-term **maintenance** treatment (stabilisation treatment) with an opioid is sometimes used, in conjunction with psychosocial support, to enable the patient to acquire some form of social stability. Methadone is most commonly used; the use of diamorphine although feasible[14] is controversial[15] and is advocated by only a few individual centres. The use of methadone for maintenance has been reviewed.[16] Naltrexone can be effective in maintaining abstinence in opioid addicts following detoxification, especially after rapid or ultra rapid detoxification. It is considered that naltrexone would probably be of most use in highly motivated addicts with good sociological and psychological support to discourage impulsive use of opioids.[1,17,18]

The problems associated with the management of the **pregnant** patient with opioid dependence have been discussed by Gerada *et al.*[19] and the management of neonatal opioid dependence is discussed in detail below. The aim should be to stabilise the patient first using methadone since acute withdrawal can result in fetal death. Drug withdrawal is best done slowly during the second trimester. It has been suggested that if patients present during the final trimester and cannot be detoxified, maintenance with diamorphine might be preferable to the use of methadone as it might produce less severe withdrawal symptoms in the neonate.[20]

1. Herridge P, Gold MS. Pharmacological adjuncts in the treatment of opioid and cocaine addicts. *J Psychoactive Drugs* 1988; **20:** 233–42.
2. Guthrie SK. Pharmacologic interventions for the treatment of opioid dependence and withdrawal. *DICP Ann Pharmacother* 1990; **24:** 721–34.
3. DOH. *Drug misuse and dependence: guidelines on clinical management.* London: HMSO, 1991.
4. Wodak A. Managing illicit drug use: a practical guide. *Drugs* 1994; **47:** 446–57.
5. Mattick RP, Hall W. Are detoxification programmes effective? *Lancet* 1996; **347:** 97–100.
6. Seivewright NA, Greenwood J. What is important in drug misuse treatment? *Lancet* 1996; **347:** 373–6.
7. Böhrer H, *et al.* Methadone treatment of opioid withdrawal in intensive care patients. *Lancet* 1993; **341:** 636–7.
8. Yaster M, *et al.* The management of opioid and benzodiazepine dependence in infants, children, and adolescents. *Pediatrics* 1996; **98:** 135–40.
9. Charney DS, *et al.* The combined use of clonidine and naltrexone as a rapid, safe, and effective treatment of abrupt withdrawal from methadone. *Am J Psychiatry* 1986; **143:** 831–7.
10. Brewer C, *et al.* Opioid withdrawal and naltrexone induction in 48-72 hours with minimal drop-out, using a modification of the naltrexone-clonidine technique. *Br J Psychiatry* 1988; **153:** 340–3.
11. Justins D. Rapid opioid detoxification under anaesthesia. *Hosp Med* 1998; **59:** 180.
12. Cook TM, Collins PD. Rapid opioid detoxification under anaesthesia. *Hosp Med* 1998; **59:** 245–7.
13. McLellan AT, *et al.* The effects of psychosocial services in substance abuse treatment. *JAMA* 1993; **269:** 1953–9.
14. Perneger TV, *et al.* Randomised trial of heroin maintenance programme for addicts who fail in conventional drug treatments. *Br Med J* 1998; **317:** 13–18.
15. Farrell M, Hall W. The Swiss heroin trials: testing alternative approaches. *Br Med J* 1998; **316:** 639.
16. Farrell M, *et al.* Methadone maintenance treatment in opiate dependence: a review. *Br Med J* 1994; **309:** 997–1001.
17. Ginzburg HM, MacDonald MG. The role of naltrexone in the management of drug abuse. *Med Toxicol* 1987; **2:** 83–92.
18. Gonzalez JP, Brogden RN. Naltrexone: a review of its pharmacodynamic and pharmacokinetic properties and therapeutic efficacy in the management of opioid dependence. *Drugs* 1988; **35:** 192–213.
19. Gerada C, *et al.* Management of the pregnant opiate user. *Br J Hosp Med* 1990; **43:** 138–41.
20. Thomas CS, Osborn M. Inhaling heroin during pregnancy. *Br Med J* 1988; **296:** 1672.

NEONATAL OPIOID DEPENDENCE. Infants born to opioid-dependent mothers may suffer withdrawal symptoms including CNS hyperirritability, gastro-intestinal dysfunction, respiratory distress, and vague autonomic symptoms including yawning, sneezing, mottling, and fever.[1] Onset of symptoms is partly dependent on the drug abused and varies from shortly after birth to 2 weeks of age, although most symptoms appear within 72 hours. Some symptoms may persist for 3 months or more. Breast feeding has been used to treat opioid dependence in the offspring of dependent mothers but this is no longer considered to be the best method and some authorities recommend that breast feeding should be stopped. Finnegan[1] considered that, in general, the safest methods for treating the infant included the use of titrated doses of either paregoric (a preparation in the USP containing opium) or phenobarbitone.

The American Academy of Pediatrics[2] in considering neonatal drug withdrawal in general recommended that treatment of the neonate should be primarily supportive and considered that many infants manifesting drug withdrawal symptoms could be managed in this way. They advised adoption of abstinence scoring methods to judge the need for drug therapy. Drugs that have been used for opioid withdrawal include paregoric, diluted tincture of opium, morphine, methadone, diazepam, chlorpromazine, phenobarbitone, and clonidine. Naloxone should not routinely be given to infants of opioid-dependent mothers because of the risk of seizures with abrupt opioid withdrawal. The Committee[2] made no hard and fast recommendations but considered that, when appropriate, specific drug therapy should be used for treatment of withdrawal symptoms. Thus for opioid withdrawal, tincture of opium is the preferred drug.

Kandall *et al.*[3] compared paregoric with phenobarbitone and concluded that paregoric was the treatment of choice for the neonatal abstinence syndrome that included opioid withdrawal. Calabrese and Gulledge[4] considered that paregoric, phenobarbitone, chlorpromazine, or diazepam could be used with comparable efficacy to treat neonatal opioid withdrawal symptoms as they emerge. Rivers,[5] however, noted that chlorpromazine has tended to be the preferred treatment in the UK. Other UK workers have reported the use of phenobarbitone, chloral hydrate, and chlorpromazine either singly or in combination;[6,7] Gregg *et al.*[8] recommended treatment with pure aqueous morphine sulphate by mouth.

1. Finnegan LP. Outcome of children born to women dependent upon narcotics. *Adv Alcohol Subst Abuse* 1982; **1:** 55–101.
2. American Academy of Pediatrics, Committee on Drugs. Neonatal drug withdrawal. *Pediatrics* 1998; **101:** 1079–88. Correction. *ibid.*; **102:** 660 [dosage error].
3. Kandall SR, *et al.* Opiate v CNS depressant therapy in neonatal drug abstinence syndrome. *Am J Dis Child* 1983; **137:** 378–82.
4. Calabrese JR, Gulledge AD. The neonatal narcotic abstinence syndrome: a brief review. *Can J Psychiatry* 1985; **30:** 623–6.
5. Rivers RPA. Neonatal opiate withdrawal. *Arch Dis Child* 1986; **61:** 1236–9.
6. Klenka HM. Babies born in a district general hospital to mothers taking heroin. *Br Med J* 1986; **293:** 745–6.
7. Alroomi LG, *et al.* Maternal narcotic abuse and the newborn. *Arch Dis Child* 1988; **63:** 81–3.
8. Gregg JEM, *et al.* Maternal narcotic abuse and the newborn. *Arch Dis Child* 1988; **63:** 684.

Adverse Effects

In normal doses the commonest side-effects of opioid analgesics are nausea, vomiting, constipation, drowsiness, and confusion; tolerance to these side-effects generally develops with long-term use, but not to constipation. Micturition may be difficult and there may be ureteric or biliary spasm; there is also an antidiuretic effect. Dry mouth, dizziness, sweating, facial flushing, headache, vertigo, bradycardia, tachycardia, palpitations, orthostatic hypotension, hypothermia, restlessness, changes of mood, decreased libido or potency, hallucinations, and miosis also occur. These effects tend to occur more commonly in ambulant patients than in those at rest in bed and in those without severe pain. Raised intracranial pressure occurs in some patients. Muscle rigidity has been reported following high doses. The euphoric activity of opioids has led to their abuse. For a discussion of opioid dependence, see above.

Larger doses of opioids produce respiratory depression and hypotension, with circulatory failure and deepening coma. Convulsions may occur, especially in infants and children. Rhabdomyolysis progressing to renal failure has been reported in overdosage. Death may occur from respiratory failure. Toxic doses of specific opioids vary considerably with the individual and regular users may tolerate large doses. The triad of coma, pinpoint pupils, and respiratory depression is considered indicative of opioid overdosage; dilatation of the pupils occurs as hypoxia develops. Pulmonary oedema after overdosage is a common cause of fatalities among opioid addicts.

Morphine and some other opioids have a dose-related histamine-releasing effect which may be responsible in part for reactions such as urticaria and pruritus as well as hypotension and flushing. Contact dermatitis has been reported and pain and irritation may occur on injection. Anaphylactic reactions following intravenous injection have been reported rarely.

Apart from analgesia, pharmacological effects of opioid analgesics include CNS depression with respiratory depression, cough suppression, and sedation, and effects on smooth muscle including reduced gastro-intestinal motility. The adverse effects associated with individual opioid analgesics may reflect to some extent their activity at specific opioid receptors (for a description of the different opioid receptors and associated activity, see Uses and Administration, below) or may result from a direct toxic effect.[1,2] Some adverse effects of pure opioid agonists, such as the respiratory depressant effect of morphine, are dose-related, whereas agonist/antagonists such as buprenorphine, butorphanol, and nalbuphine exhibit a 'ceiling effect' as the dose increases. Tolerance develops to some side-effects, e.g. nausea and vomiting, but not to others, such as constipation.

The type and extent of side-effects experienced in practice may also be influenced by the circumstances of use, that is, whether or not opioid-sensitive pain is present, whether the opioid analgesic is being given for the control of chronic severe pain or acute pain, and on the route of administration. In reviewing the use of opioids in *chronic pain* McQuay[3] commented that, despite worries to the contrary, respiratory depression and dependence liability are not generally a problem when appropriate doses are used to treat opioid-sensitive pain. In fact the presence of opioid-sensitive pain appears to protect against the respiratory depressant effect, although it may occur if the source of opioid-sensitive pain is removed (e.g. by surgery) without adequate reduction in opioid dosage. The side-effects of opioid analgesics when used in advanced cancer have been put into context by Twycross and Lack.[4] They consider constipation to be the most troublesome adverse effect and state that significant respiratory depression is rarely seen, if used as they suggest, since pain antagonises the central depressant effects of morphine.

In the context of *acute postoperative pain* opioid-induced respiratory depression is of concern whereas short-term postoperative use is unlikely to cause dependence (although see under Treatment of Opioid Dependence, above for references to iatrogenic physical dependence).[5] It was hoped that administration of opioids by the *spinal route* would result in fewer side-effects, especially respiratory depression. In postoperative pain relief with spinal opioids, the incidence of side-effects is said to be low when patients are properly monitored.[6] However, Morgan[7] has reported pruritus, nausea and vomiting, and urinary retention to be common and respiratory depression to occur; more seriously the appearance of respiratory depression could be considerably delayed. Morgan[7] considered all opioid analgesics to have the propensity to produce respiratory depression when given spinally, although it appeared more common with morphine. Delayed respiratory depression has been attributed to the poor lipid solubility of morphine, but does occur after other opioids. Some have considered that despite earlier worries, potentially fatal late respiratory depression was as rare with the spinal route as postoperative respiratory depression with the conventional route.[8,9] Disputes regarding the frequency of respiratory depression associated with even conventional methods of administration of opioid analgesics might be due to the methods used for measuring respiratory effects. Wheatley *et al.*[10] found continuous pulse oximetry a more sensitive index of respiratory depression than simply measuring the frequency of ventilation. When spinal routes of administration are compared, the incidence of ventilatory depression has been reported to be higher following intrathecal than epidural administration of morphine.[11]

1. Duthie DJR, Nimmo WS. Adverse effects of opioid analgesic drugs. *Br J Anaesth* 1987; **59:** 61–77.
2. Schug SA, *et al.* Adverse effects of systemic opioid analgesics. *Drug Safety* 1992; **7:** 200–13.
3. McQuay HJ. Opioids in chronic pain. *Br J Anaesth* 1989; **63:** 213–26.
4. Twycross RG, Lack SA. *Oral morphine in advanced cancer.* 2nd ed. Beaconsfield: Beaconsfield Publishers, 1989.
5. Mitchell RWD, Smith G. The control of acute postoperative pain. *Br J Anaesth* 1989; **63:** 147–58.
6. Lutz LJ, Lamer TJ. Management of postoperative pain: review of current techniques and methods. *Mayo Clin Proc* 1990; **65:** 584–96.
7. Morgan M. The rational use of intrathecal and extradural opioids. *Br J Anaesth* 1989; **63:** 165–88.
8. Anonymous. Spinal opiates revisited. *Lancet* 1986; **i:** 655–6.
9. McQuay HJ. Spinal opiates. *Br J Hosp Med* 1987; **37:** 354–5.
10. Wheatley RG, *et al.* Postoperative hypoxaemia: comparison of extradural, i.m. and patient-controlled opioid analgesia. *Br J Anaesth* 1990; **64:** 267–75.
11. Gustafsson LL, *et al.* Adverse effects of extradural and intrathecal opiates: report of a nationwide survey in Sweden. *Br J Anaesth* 1982; **54:** 479–85.

Effects on the biliary tract and liver. Serum concentrations of amylase and hydroxybutyric acid dehydrogenase may be raised after administration of opioids due to spasm of the sphincter of Oddi.[1] Serum-aspartate aminotransferase (SGOT) and serum-alanine aminotransferase (SGPT) concentrations can be raised by opioids and they could induce an increase in serum-lactic dehydrogenase concentration of hepatic origin by increasing intrabiliary pressure.[1]

1. Clark F. Drugs and enzymes. *Adverse Drug React Bull* 1977; (Oct.): 232–5.

Effects on the cardiovascular system. For reference to histamine release and cardiovascular effects following the intravenous administration of some opioids see under Pethidine, p.76.

Effects on the endocrine system. Endogenous opioid peptides may have a role in the regulation of endocrine function. Morphine, as well as endorphin and enkephalins, has been found to stimulate prolactin release[1] and synthetic analogues of morphine are reported to have similar properties. Opioids such as morphine are also part of a large group of drugs implicated in causing hyperglycaemia.[2]

1. Hell K, Wernze H. Drug-induced changes in prolactin secretion: clinical implications. *Med Toxicol* 1988; **3:** 463–98.
2. O'Byrne S, Feely J. Effects of drugs on glucose tolerance in non-insulin-dependent diabetics (part II). *Drugs* 1990; **40:** 203–19.

Treatment of Adverse Effects

In acute poisoning by an opioid taken by mouth the stomach should be emptied. A laxative may be given to aid peristalsis.

Intensive supportive therapy may be required to correct respiratory failure and shock. In addition, the specific antagonist naloxone is used to counteract very rapidly the severe respiratory depression and coma produced by excessive doses of opioid analgesics (see p.987). Since naloxone has a shorter duration of action than many opioids patients who have already responded should be kept under close observation for signs of relapse and repeated injections given according to the respiratory rate and depth of coma. Alternatively, in situations where one of the longer acting opioids is known or suspected to be the cause of symptoms a continuous intravenous infusion of naloxone, adjusted according to response, may be used.

The use of opioid antagonists such as naloxone in persons physically dependent on opioids may induce withdrawal symptoms.

References.

1. Henry J, Volans G. ABC of poisoning. Analgesics: opioids. *Br Med J* 1984; **289:** 990–3.

Constipation. For reference to the use of naloxone to relieve opioid-induced constipation without compromising analgesic control in patients receiving long-term therapy with opioids, see under Reversal of Opioid Effects in the Uses and Administration of Naloxone, p.987.

Precautions

Opioid analgesics are generally contra-indicated in respiratory depression and obstructive airways disease. One exception is the use of some opioids such as morphine in some forms of dyspnoea (see below). They are also contra-indicated or should be used with great caution in acute alcoholism, convulsive disorders, head injuries, and conditions in which intracranial pressure is raised. They should not be given to comatose patients.

Opioid analgesics should be given with caution or in reduced doses to patients with hypothyroidism, adrenocortical insufficiency, asthma, impaired kidney or liver function, prostatic hyperplasia, hypotension, shock, inflammatory or obstructive bowel disorders, or myasthenia gravis.

Discontinuation of therapy with opioid analgesics should be carried out gradually in patients who may have developed physical dependence, to avoid precipitating withdrawal symptoms (see Dependence, above).

Opioid analgesics should be given with great care to infants, especially neonates. Their administration during labour may cause respiratory depression in the newborn infant. Babies born to opioid-dependent mothers may suffer withdrawal symptoms (see under Neonatal Opioid Dependence, above).

Dosage should be reduced in elderly or debilitated patients.

Opioid analgesics with some antagonist activity, such as buprenorphine, butorphanol, nalbuphine, or pentazocine, may precipitate withdrawal symptoms in physically dependent patients who have recently used pure agonists such as morphine.

Drowsiness may affect the ability to perform skilled tasks; those so affected should not drive or operate machinery.

Asthma. Opioids are usually contra-indicated in asthma,[1] however Barnes and Chung[2] considered that they were safe in controlled asthma, but should be avoided during acute exacerbations.

1. Gorchein A. Difficult asthma. *Br Med J* 1989; **299:** 1031.
2. Barnes PJ, Chung KF. Difficult asthma. *Br Med J* 1989; **299:** 1031–2.

Biliary-tract disorders. It is usually recommended that opioids such as morphine should either be avoided in patients with biliary disorders or that they should be given with an antispasmodic. Morphine can cause an increase in intrabiliary pressure as a result of effects on the sphincter of Oddi[1] and might therefore be expected to exacerbate rather than relieve pain in patients with biliary colic (p.8) or other biliary-tract disorders. Biliary-type pain has also been induced in patients given morphine after cholecystectomy.[2]

Hahn *et al.*[3] found morphine to cause the most marked delay in gallbladder emptying when compared with pethidine, pentazocine, or butorphanol in healthy subjects; they considered this confirmation that morphine should be avoided in biliary disorders and also considered that the other opioid analgesics could be used until something better is available. Vieira *et al.*[4] found that fentanyl and sufentanil do not constrict the common bile duct like morphine and therefore may be suitable for perioperative pain control in patients in whom spasm of the common bile duct is undesirable.

1. Helm JF, *et al.* Effects of morphine on the human sphincter of Oddi. *Gut* 1988; **29:** 1402–7.
2. Roberts-Thomson IC, *et al.* Sympathetic activation: a mechanism for morphine induced pain and rises in liver enzymes after cholecystectomy? *Gut* 1990; **31:** 217–21.
3. Hahn M, *et al.* The effect of four narcotics on cholecystokinin octapeptide stimulated gall bladder contraction. *Aliment Pharmacol Ther* 1988; **2:** 129–34.

4. Vieira ZEG, *et al.* Evaluation of fentanyl and sufentanil on the diameter of the common bile duct by ultrasonography in man: a double blind, placebo controlled study. *Int J Clin Pharmacol Ther* 1994; **32:** 274–7.

Hepatic impairment. Although some patients with hepatic dysfunction have been reported to be particularly sensitive to opioids, many patients with liver impairment have been reported to tolerate opioids normally.[1]

1. Hanks GW, Aherne GW. Morphine metabolism: does the renal hypothesis hold water? *Lancet* 1985; **i:** 221–2.

Infants and children. There is some evidence to suggest that children under 6 months of age are more sensitive to opioids; neonates in particular may be more sensitive to respiratory depression with morphine than adults. Pharmacokinetic differences may contribute to this increased sensitivity. Nevertheless morphine is probably the drug of choice for postoperative analgesia (p.59).

References.

1. Choonara IA. Pain relief. *Arch Dis Child* 1989; **64:** 1101–2.
2. Marsh DF, *et al.* Opioid systems and the newborn. *Br J Anaesth* 1997; **79:** 787–95.

Phaeochromocytoma. Morphine and some other opioids can induce the release of endogenous histamine and thereby stimulate catecholamine release. Both diamorphine[1] and pethidine[2] have been reported to cause hypertension when given to patients with phaeochromocytoma and histamine-releasing opioids should be avoided in such patients. Alfentanil, like fentanyl, does not release histamine and may be the opioid of choice in the anaesthetic management of patients with phaeochromocytoma.[3]

1. Chaturvedi NC, *et al.* Diamorphine-induced attack of paroxysmal hypertension in phaeochromocytoma. *Br Med J* 1974; **2:** 538.
2. Lawrence CA. Pethidine-induced hypertension in phaeochromocytoma. *Br Med J* 1978; **1:** 149–50.
3. Hull CJ. Phaeochromocytoma: diagnosis, preoperative preparation and anaesthetic management. *Br J Anaesth* 1986; **58:** 1453–68.

Interactions

As serious and sometimes fatal reactions have occurred following administration of pethidine to patients receiving MAOIs (including moclobemide), pethidine and related drugs are contra-indicated in patients taking MAOIs or within 14 days of stopping such treatment; other opioid analgesics should be avoided or given with extreme caution (for further details, see p.305). Life-threatening reactions have also been reported when selegiline, a selective inhibitor of monoamine oxidase type B, has been given with pethidine. The depressant effects of opioid analgesics are enhanced by other CNS depressants such as alcohol, anaesthetics, anxiolytics, hypnotics, tricyclic antidepressants, and antipsychotics. Cyclizine may counteract the haemodynamic benefits of opioids. Cimetidine inhibits the metabolism of some opioids, especially pethidine.

The actions of opioids may in turn affect the activities of other compounds. For instance, their gastro-intestinal effects may delay absorption as with mexiletine or may be counteractive as with cisapride, metoclopramide, or domperidone. Opioid premedicants such as papaveretum have been reported to reduce serum concentrations of ciprofloxacin when given concomitantly.

Antivirals. Ritonavir and possibly other HIV-protease inhibitors may increase the area under the curve of some opioids. The increases expected for dextropropoxyphene or pethidine were considered by the manufacturer of ritonavir to be large enough to recommend that these opioids should not be used with ritonavir. Other opioids predicted to have large or moderate increases included alfentanil, fentanyl, hydrocodone, methadone, oxycodone, and tramadol and it was recommended that monitoring of drug concentrations and/or adverse effects were required when used with ritonavir. It was considered that ritonavir might possibly reduce the area under the curve of codeine, hydromorphone, or morphine.

Histamine H_2 antagonists. Histamine H_2 antagonists may enhance the effects of some opioid analgesics. Cimetidine was reported to alter the clearance and volume of distribution of pethidine[1] whereas ranitidine did not.[2] Morphine has been considered less likely to interact with cimetidine than other opioids such as pethidine because of differences in metabolism. However, although cimetidine did not affect the disposition of morphine in one study in healthy subjects[3] there have been isolated reports of possible interactions between morphine and H_2 antagonists including apnoea, confusion, and muscle twitching associated with concomitant cimetidine and morphine[4] and confusion associated with concomitant ranitidine and morphine.[5] There has also been a report[6] of a patient receiving regular analgesia with methadone by mouth and morphine subcutaneously who required treatment with naloxone after becoming unresponsive 6 days after ulcer prophylaxis with cimetidine had been started.

1. Guay DRP, *et al.* Cimetidine alters pethidine disposition in man. *Br J Clin Pharmacol* 1984; **18:** 907–14.
2. Guay DRP, *et al.* Ranitidine does not alter pethidine disposition in man. *Br J Clin Pharmacol* 1985; **20:** 55–9.
3. Mojaverian P, *et al.* Cimetidine does not alter morphine disposition in man. *Br J Clin Pharmacol* 1982; **14:** 809–13.
4. Fine A, Churchill DN. Potentially lethal interaction of cimetidine and morphine. *Can Med Assoc J* 1981; **124:** 1434, 1436.
5. Martinez-Abad M, *et al.* Ranitidine-induced confusion with concomitant morphine. *Drug Intell Clin Pharm* 1988; **22:** 914–15.
6. Sorkin EM, Ogawa GS. Cimetidine potentiation of narcotic action. *Drug Intell Clin Pharm* 1983; **17:** 60–1.

Uses and Administration

Pharmacologically the opioid analgesics are broadly similar; qualitative and quantitative differences may be dependent on their interaction with **opioid receptors**. There are several types of opioid receptor and they are distributed in distinct patterns through the central and peripheral nervous systems. The three main types in the CNS were originally designated μ (mu), κ (kappa), and δ (delta) although they have recently been reclassified as OP_3, OP_2, and OP_1 respectively. Activities attributed to the stimulation of these receptors have been as follows:

μ—analgesia (mainly at supraspinal sites), respiratory depression, miosis, reduced gastro-intestinal motility, and euphoria; μ_1 (supraspinal analgesia) and μ_2 (respiratory depression and gastro-intestinal activity) subtypes have been postulated;

κ—analgesia (mainly in the spinal cord); less intense miosis and respiratory depression, dysphoria and psychotomimetic effects;

δ—less certain in man, but probably analgesia; selective for enkephalins.

Other receptors include σ (sigma) and ε (epsilon) receptors. The psychotomimetic effects of agonist-antagonists such as pentazocine that are poorly antagonised by naloxone have been thought by some to be mediated by σ receptors.

Opioids act at one or more of these receptors as full agonists, partial agonists, or antagonists. Morphine and similar opioid agonists (sometimes called μ agonists) are considered to act primarily at μ and perhaps at κ and δ receptors. Opioid agonist-antagonists such as pentazocine appear to act as κ agonists and μ antagonists whereas buprenorphine is a partial agonist at μ receptors with some antagonist activity at κ receptors. The opioid antagonist naloxone acts at μ, κ, and δ receptors.

In addition to differing affinities for particular receptors the degree of activation once bound also differs. The full agonist morphine produces maximum activation at the μ receptor and its effects increase with dose, whereas partial agonists and agonist-antagonists may demonstrate a 'ceiling effect' in that above a certain level their effects do not increase proportionately with dose.

Other differences between opioid analgesics may relate to their lipid solubility and pharmacokinetics; speed of onset and duration of action may influence the choice of analgesic.

Opioid analgesics are sometimes classified as weak opioids or strong opioids. **Weak opioids** include codeine, dextropropoxyphene, and dihydrocodeine and are used, often with non-opioid analgesics, in the treatment of moderate or moderate to severe pain. **Strong opioids** are used in severe acute and chronic pain. The principal strong opioid is morphine. Others include: buprenorphine, diamorphine, fentanyl, methadone, pentazocine, and pethidine.

Morphine is the strong opioid of choice. It is absorbed when given orally and has a short half-life so that administration of an immediate-release oral preparation offers a flexible means of dosage titration. Once initial pain relief is achieved, administration of a modified-release morphine preparation once or twice daily may be more convenient for maintenance of analgesia in chronic pain, but this does reduce dosage flexibility and extra doses of immediate-release oral morphine may be required for breakthrough or incident pain.

Occasionally an alternative to morphine may be useful. Methadone, levorphanol, or oxycodone have a longer duration of action than morphine, but it should be noted that methadone and levorphanol, which have long half-lives, may accumulate and therefore should not be used long-term because of progressive CNS depression. A rapid onset of action is provided by pethidine, alfentanil, and fentanyl, and dextromoramide is useful if a short action is needed. Diamorphine may be preferred to morphine when an opioid has to be given by injection since the volume of solution to be injected is less with diamorphine than with morphine.

The oral route is the most desirable route of administration for opioid analgesics and is appropriate for the control of acute and chronic pain in many patients. Other routes are used though, such as intramuscular or intravenous injection for emergency pain control, intermittent infusion for patient-controlled analgesia, or continuous subcutaneous infusion for patients with advanced cancer. Rectal or transdermal administration is also possible with a few opioids. Alternative routes are also of use where there would be problems with oral administration as in patients with persistent vomiting or at risk of vomiting, with dysphagia, malabsorption, delayed gastric emptying, intestinal obstruction, severe weakness, or in a coma.

In addition to being used for the relief of pain opioids are used in anaesthesia for premedication, induction, or maintenance. In balanced anaesthesia they are used in conjunction with an anaesthetic and a neuromuscular blocker. When used with a compound such as droperidol they can produce a state of mild sedation with analgesia called neuroleptanalgesia.

Some opioids are used for analgesia, sedation, and suppression of respiration in the management of mechanically ventilated patients under intensive care (p.638).

Codeine is used for the suppression of cough; for intractable cough in terminal illness morphine may be used.

Opioids may relieve some forms of dyspnoea; morphine and diamorphine are probably the most commonly used, but dihydrocodeine and hydrocodone have also been tried.

Methadone is used in the treatment of opioid dependence (see above) and buprenorphine and levomethadyl acetate have also shown promise.

Opioid analgesics possess some of the properties of naturally occurring or **endogenous opioid peptides.** Endogenous peptides include the enkephalins, endorphins, and dynorphins; their polypeptide precursors may also be precursors for non-opioid peptides. Pro-enkephalin is the precursor of met- and leu-enkephalin; pro-opiomelanocortin is the precursor of beta-endorphin, beta-lipotrophin, melanocyte-stimulating hormone, and corticotrophin; and prodynorphin is the precursor of dynorphins and neoendorphins. Endogenous opioid peptides are widely distributed in the CNS with specific groups of peptides in other parts of the body. They appear to function as neurotransmitters, modulators of neurotransmission, or neurohormones. Their presence in the hypothalamus suggests a role in the regulation of endocrine function. Opioids have been shown to stimulate the release of some pituitary hormones, including prolactin and growth hormone, and to inhibit the release of others, including corticotrophin.

References.

1. Cherny NI. Opioid analgesics: comparative features and prescribing guidelines. *Drugs* 1996; **51:** 713–37.
2. Upton RN, *et al.* Pharmacokinetic optimisation of opioid treatment in acute pain therapy. *Clin Pharmacokinet* 1997; **33:** 225–44.

Action. Some references to opioid receptors.

1. Pleuvry BJ. Opioid receptors and their ligands: natural and unnatural. *Br J Anaesth* 1991; **66:** 370–80.
2. Pleuvry BJ. Opioid receptors and awareness of the Greek alphabet. *Br J Hosp Med* 1992; **48:** 678–81.
3. Atcheson R, Lambert DG. Update on opioid receptors. *Br J Anaesth* 1994; **73:** 132–4.
4. Dhawan BN, *et al.* International Union of Pharmacology. XII. Classification of opioid receptors. *Pharmacol Rev* 1996; **48:** 567–86.
5. Lambert DG. Recent advances in opioid pharmacology. *Br J Anaesth* 1998; **81:** 1–2.

Administration in infants and children. The management of pain in neonates, infants, and children is discussed on p.7. Opioids are widely used.[1,2] Neonates can be treated with strong opioids such as morphine if receiving respiratory support. Care is necessary because of the neonate's enhanced susceptibility to the respiratory depressant effects of opioids. Allowance also needs to be made for the altered pharmacokinetics of opioids in this group. The use of opioids for sedation and analgesia in neonates in intensive care is mentioned on p.638.

Older infants and children can be treated effectively with morphine or other opioid analgesics and from the age of 5 or 6 months morphine metabolism follows the course seen in adults.

1. Lloyd-Thomas AR. Pain management in paediatric patients. *Br J Anaesth* 1990; **64:** 85–104.
2. Bhatt-Mehta V. Current guidelines for the treatment of acute pain in children. *Drugs* 1996; **51:** 760–76.

Anaesthesia. Opioid analgesics have been given intravenously as supplements during general anaesthesia with inhalational or intravenous drugs. They have also been widely used before surgery to reduce anxiety, smooth induction of anaesthesia, reduce overall anaesthetic requirements, and provide postoperative pain relief. Very high doses of morphine have been infused intravenously to produce anaesthesia for cardiac surgery, but shorter acting drugs such as fentanyl and related opioids are generally used now; some may prefer agonist-antagonist opioids. Sedation and respiratory depression may be prolonged necessitating assisted ventilation; reversal of these effects can be achieved by opioid antagonists such as naloxone. For a discussion of the various drugs used to achieve and maintain conditions suitable for surgery, including the use of opioids in the induction and maintenance of anaesthesia, see p.1220. Opioid analgesics, most commonly fentanyl, have been used with a neuroleptic to induce a state known as neuroleptanalgesia in which the patient is calm and indifferent to the surroundings yet is responsive to commands. For a brief discussion of neuroleptanalgesia and similar anaesthetic techniques, see p.1220.

POSTOPERATIVE SHIVERING. Pethidine appears to be effective in the treatment of postoperative shivering (see p.1219) but not all opioids are necessarily effective.

PREMEDICATION. Opioids, including morphine and its derivatives, papaveretum, and pethidine, have been widely used before surgery to reduce anxiety, smooth induction of anaesthesia, reduce overall anaesthetic requirements, and provide postoperative pain relief. Some now consider that the routine use of opioids is largely traditional and in view of the high incidence of side-effects advocate restriction to patients already in pain or who will experience pain before induction of anaesthesia. For a discussion of the drugs used to achieve and maintain conditions suitable for surgery, including the use of opioids for premedication, see under Anaesthesia on p.1220.

Cough. Opioids are used to suppress cough (p.1052). Pholcodine (p.1068) and dextromethorphan (p.1057) are the most commonly used opioids, although both lack any intrinsic analgesic activity. Of the analgesic opioids, codeine is the most widely used as a cough suppressant. However, these opioids are seldom sufficiently potent to be effective in severe cough. Morphine and diamorphine are used for the relief of intractable cough in terminal illness, although morphine is now preferred. Methadone has also been used but should be avoided as it has a long duration of action and tends to accumulate. Cough suppressants containing codeine or similar opioids are not recommended for administration to children, and should be avoided in those under 1 year of age.

Diarrhoea. Oral rehydration therapy, which is the treatment of choice for acute diarrhoea (p.1168), prevents dehydration, but it does not necessarily shorten the duration of the diarrhoea. Therefore opioids such as codeine have been used for their antimotility action as adjuncts in the management of acute diarrhoea. However, the WHO considers that such antidiarrhoeal drug therapy is of limited value, may delay the expulsion of causative organisms, and should never be given to children. Furthermore opioids should not be used in conditions where inhibition of peristalsis should be avoided, where abdominal distension develops, or in diarrhoeal conditions such as severe ulcerative colitis or antibiotic-associated colitis.

Dyspnoea. Dyspnoea has been defined as a subjective feeling of abnormally uncomfortable, difficult, or laboured breathing. It is associated with respiratory, cardiovascular, metabolic, and haematological disorders or other diseases which interfere with oxygenation of the blood. Dyspnoea is best relieved by treatment of the underlying disorder: the treatment of dyspnoea associated with asthma and chronic obstructive pulmonary disease is discussed on p.745 and p.747 respectively. However, many patients may remain symptomatic.

Oxygen may reduce dyspnoea in some patients even if dyspnoea is not related to hypoxia. Also a flow of air directed across the face by a fan can be effective.

Diazepam has been tried in the treatment of dyspnoea (particularly in the 'pink and puffing' patient) in the belief that reduction of an elevated respiratory drive may alleviate respiratory distress.[1] Benefits observed in some patients have not, however, been confirmed. The hazards of the administration of benzodiazepines to patients with any form of respiratory depression or pulmonary insufficiency should be remembered (see Precautions for Diazepam, p.663). However, benzodiazepines may be helpful in patients with advanced cancer who have rapid shallow respiration, especially when this is associated with anxiety.[2,3] Diazepam, lorazepam, and midazolam are benzodiazepines that have been tried in such patients. Methotrimeprazine is occasionally used as an alternative.

Opioids may relieve some forms of dyspnoea[1,3] especially that due to acute left ventricular failure, pulmonary oedema, and malignant chest disease. The cause of dyspnoea should be established since the use of opioids is generally not advised, or only with extreme caution, in patients with obstructive airways disease whose dyspnoea may be relieved by other means. Morphine and diamorphine are probably the most commonly used opioids in dyspnoea but dihydrocodeine, hydrocodone, and oxymorphone have also been tried.

Nebulised morphine had been reported to improve exercise endurance in some patients with dyspnoea due to advanced chronic lung disease but current evidence does not support its use.[3]

In patients with advanced cancer and intractable dyspnoea unresponsive to the above measures, chlorpromazine may be useful to relieve air hunger and sedate dying patients who have unrelieved distress;[2] midazolam may be used as an alternative. Promethazine has also been used. High doses of a corticosteroid such as dexamethasone may help to relieve dyspnoea in patients with airways obstruction due to a tumour by reducing oedema around the tumour.

1. Tobin MJ. Dyspnea: pathophysiologic basis, clinical presentation, and management. *Arch Intern Med* 1990; **150:** 1604–13.
2. Walsh D. Dyspnoea in advanced cancer. *Lancet* 1993; **342:** 450–1.
3. Davis CL. ABC of palliative care: breathlessness, cough, and other respiratory problems. *Br Med J* 1997; **315:** 931–4.

Pain. Opioid analgesics are used for the relief of acute and chronic pain (p.4). Not every type of pain responds; neurogenic pain, for example, is not alleviated by opioid therapy. Those types of acute pain that may respond include pain associated with intensive care, labour (p.9), myocardial infarction (p.10), and sickle-cell crisis (p.11). Postoperative pain also responds (p.11). Colic pain responds to opioid therapy (p.8), but some opioids such as morphine also stimulate smooth muscle and may exacerbate such pain; when morphine has been employed, it has been with an antispasmodic. The paediatric use of opioid analgesics to relieve pain is discussed under Administration in Infants and Children, above.

Cancer pain is the most common form of chronic pain treated with opioid analgesics (see p.8). Other forms include pancreatic pain (p.10), although, as with colic, opioids such as morphine that can stimulate smooth muscle may exacerbate the pain.

Sometimes pain that should respond to morphine may not respond and may even worsen. An excess of the metabolite morphine-3-glucuronide may be the cause (see p.57).

Opioids are sometimes used with local anaesthetics to produce central nerve blocks (p.6) for the management of acute pain and for cancer pain.

Many opioids have been tried for patient-controlled analgesia (p.7); morphine and pethidine are the most commonly used but oxymorphone or hydromorphone may be useful alternatives.

There has been recent interest in the local analgesic effects of opioids.[1,2]

1. Thompson DF, Pierce DR. Local analgesia with opioid drugs. *Ann Pharmacother* 1995; **29:** 189–90.
2. Stein C. The control of pain in peripheral tissue by opioids. *N Engl J Med* 1995; **332:** 1685–90.

HEADACHE. Weak opioid analgesics such as codeine are sometimes included in oral compound analgesic preparations used in the initial treatment of migraine (see p.443) or tension-type headache (see p.444), but are best avoided, especially in patients who experience frequent attacks.

Sedation. In addition to their analgesic action opioids have been used in a variety of procedures for their sedative properties. Mention of this use of opioids can be found in the discussions of anaesthesia (p.1220), endoscopy (p.638), and intensive care (p.638).

Tetanus. Opioid analgesics can be used to provide analgesia and additional sedation in patients undergoing treatment for tetanus. Morphine has also been given to control the sympathetic overactivity in such patients.[1] For discussions of the overall treatment of tetanus, see p.145 and p.1304.

1. Rocke DA, *et al.* Morphine in tetanus—the management of sympathetic nervous system overactivity. *S Afr Med J* 1986; **70:** 666–8.

Opium (6246-z)

Gum Opium; Opium Crudum; Raw Opium.

Pharmacopoeias. In *Chin., Eur.* (see p.viii), and *US.*

Aust., Chin., Ger., It., Neth., and *US* also include a monograph for Prepared Opium. *Jpn* includes only Prepared Opium. *Jpn* also includes a diluted opium powder containing 1% of anhydrous morphine.

Opium is the air-dried latex obtained by incision from the unripe capsules of *Papaver somniferum* (Papaveraceae). It has a characteristic odour, a blackish-brown colour, and a bitter taste. The Ph. Eur. specifies that it should contain not less than 10% of anhydrous morphine, not less than 2% of anhydrous codeine, and not more than 3% of anhydrous thebaine; the USP specifies not less than 9.5% of anhydrous morphine. Opium contains a variable mixture of other alkaloids including noscapine and papaverine.

The exuded latex is dried and manipulated to form cakes of uniform composition, variously shaped according to the country of origin, and known in commerce as Turkish, Indian, or European opium.

Protect from light.

NOTE. The Ph. Eur. states that Opium is intended only as the starting material for the manufacture of galenical preparations and is not dispensed as such.

Prepared Opium (Opium Titratum; Powdered Opium; Pulvis Opii; Standardised Opium Powder) is opium, dried, powdered, and adjusted in strength. The BP 1988 included a similar preparation containing 9.5 to 10.5% of anhydrous morphine.

The USP specifies that it should contain 10.0 to 10.5% of anhydrous morphine and allows any of its diluents for powdered extracts with the exception of starch.

Dependence and Withdrawal, Adverse Effects, Treatment, and Precautions

As for Opioid Analgesics in general, p.67.

Reports of squill-associated cardiac toxicity resulting from the abuse of opiate squill linctus (Gee's linctus).[1,2]

1. Thurston D, Taylor K. Gee's linctus. *Pharm J* 1984; **233:** 63.
2. Smith W, *et al.* Wenckebach's phenomenon induced by cough linctus. *Br Med J* 1986; **292:** 868.

Interactions

For interactions associated with opioid analgesics, see p.69.

Uses and Administration

Opium has the properties of opioid analgesics (p.69). Its analgesic and sedative actions are due mainly to its content of morphine (p.58). It acts less rapidly than morphine since opium appears to be more slowly absorbed; the relaxing action of the papaverine and noscapine on intestinal muscle makes it more constipating than morphine.

Opium is used as prepared opium, as Opium Tincture (BP 1998) or (USP 23), or as Camphorated Opium Tincture (BP 1998) or Paregoric (USP 23) in various oral preparations. These have included Opiate Squill Linctus (BP 1998) (Gee's linctus) for cough.

Paregoric (USP 23) has been advocated in the USA for the treatment of neonatal opioid dependence.

Preparations

BP 1998: Camphorated Opium Tincture *(Paregoric)*; Concentrated Camphorated Opium Tincture; Opium Tincture *(Laudanum)*;
USP 23: Opium Tincture; Paregoric.

Proprietary Preparations (details are given in Part 3)

Multi-ingredient: ***Canad.:*** Diban; Donnagel-PG; ***Fr.:*** Colchimax; Eubispasme Codethyline; Lamaline; Paregorique; Pectipar†; Pectospir†; Pectovox†; Premidan Adult†; Tuberol†; ***Spain:*** Cunticina Adultos†; Digestovital; Kolotanino†; Salvacolina; Tanagel; ***Switz.:*** Bromocod N; Pectocalmine; ***UK:*** Nepenthe†; ***USA:*** B & O Supprettes No. 15A; B & O Supprettes No. 16A; Donnagel-PG†; Parepectolin.

Hydrochlorides of Mixed Opium Alkaloids

(15940-f)

Alkaloidorum Opii Hydrochloridum; Extractum Concentratum Opii; Omnoponum; Opialum; Opium Concentratum.

Pharmacopoeias. Preparations of the hydrochlorides of mixed opium alkaloids are included in *Jpn.*

Papaveretum (6250-e)

Papaveretum *(BAN).*

A mixture of 253 parts of morphine hydrochloride, 23 parts of papaverine hydrochloride, and 20 parts of codeine hydrochloride.

CAS — 8002-76-4.

NOTE. Do not confuse papaveretum with papaverine (p.1614).

Pharmacopoeias. In *Br.*

Papaveretum (BP 1998) contains 80.0 to 88.4% of anhydrous morphine hydrochloride, 8.3 to 9.2% of papaverine hydrochloride, and 6.6 to 7.4% of anhydrous codeine hydrochloride.

15.4 mg of Papaveretum (BP 1998) contains the equivalent of approximately 10 mg of the major component, anhydrous morphine.

A white or almost white crystalline powder. **Soluble** in water, sparingly soluble in alcohol. A 1.5% solution in water has a pH of 3.7 to 4.7. **Protect** from light.

Dependence and Withdrawal, Adverse Effects, Treatment, and Precautions

As for Opioid Analgesics in general, p.67.

Papaveretum has been confused with papaverine (p.1614) and in one such case[1] a patient became unconscious after self-injection of papaveretum in mistake for papaverine.

1. Robinson LQ, Stephenson TP. Self injection treatment for impotence. *Br Med J* 1989; **299:** 1568.

Interactions

For interactions associated with opioid analgesics, see p.69.

Uses and Administration

Hydrochlorides of mixed opium alkaloids have the properties of opioid analgesics (p.69). In the UK, papaveretum formerly contained the hydrochlorides of morphine, codeine, noscapine, and papaverine. However, because of concern over the potential genotoxicity of noscapine (p.1065) UK preparations containing papaveretum were reformulated to exclude the noscapine component and the name papaveretum was redefined in the BP 1993 to reflect this change of formulation. It is possible that in other countries the term papaveretum is still being used to describe a mixture containing noscapine.

Mixtures of opium alkaloids such as papaveretum have the analgesic and sedative properties of morphine (p.58) and are used in the treatment of moderate to severe pain and for pre-operative sedation.

In adults papaveretum is generally administered by subcutaneous or intramuscular injection in doses of 7.7 to 15.4 mg every 4 hours. The initial dose in the elderly should not exceed 7.7 mg. Papaveretum may also be given intravenously in doses of one-quarter to one-half the corresponding subcutaneous or intramuscular dose.

Infants aged up to 1 month may be given 115.5 μg per kg body-weight and infants aged up to 1 year, 115.5 to 154 μg per kg. Children aged 1 to 12 years may be given 154 to 231 μg per kg.

For pre-operative medication papaveretum is given intramuscularly or subcutaneously sometimes in conjunction with hyoscine hydrobromide.

Papaveretum has also been given by mouth with aspirin for the management of moderate to severe pain.

Preparations

BP 1998: Papaveretum Injection.

Proprietary Preparations (details are given in Part 3)
Canad.: Pantopon†; ***S.Afr.:*** Omnopon; ***Switz.:*** Escopon†; ***UK:*** Omnopon†; ***USA:*** Pantopon.

Multi-ingredient: ***Switz.:*** Spasmosol; ***UK:*** Aspav.

Oxametacin (13052-x)

Oxametacin *(rINN).*

Oxamethacin. 1-(4-Chlorobenzoyl)-5-methoxy-2-methylindole-3-acetohydroxamic acid.

$C_{19}H_{17}ClN_2O_4$ = 372.8.

CAS — 27035-30-9.

Oxametacin, an indomethacin (p.45) derivative, is an NSAID (p.63). It has been used in musculoskeletal and joint disorders given by mouth or rectally.

Preparations

Proprietary Preparations (details are given in Part 3)
Ital.: Restid†; ***Spain:*** Restid†.

Oxaprozin (13055-d)

Oxaprozin *(BAN, USAN, rINN).*

Wy-21743. 3-(4,5-Diphenyloxazol-2-yl)propionic acid.

$C_{18}H_{15}NO_3$ = 293.3.

CAS — 21256-18-8.

Pharmacopoeias. In *Jpn.*

Adverse Effects and Precautions

As for NSAIDs in general, p.63.

Diagnosis and testing. False-positive results for testing of benzodiazepines in urine have been reported in patients taking oxaprozin.[1] The manufacturer[2] has commented that the interaction occurs with some immunoassay tests and that thin-layer chromatography can successfully discriminate between benzodiazepines and oxaprozin. False-positive results for a fluorescence polarisation immunoassay for phenytoin have also been reported in patients receiving oxaprozin.[3]

1. Pulini M. False-positive benzodiazepine urine test due to oxaprozin. *JAMA* 1995; **273:** 1905.
2. Raphan H, Adams MH. False-positive benzodiazepine urine test due to oxaprozin. *JAMA* 1995; **273:** 1905–6.
3. Patel T, *et al.* Assay interaction between oxaprozin and phenytoin. *Ann Pharmacother* 1997; **31:** 254.

Effects on the liver. A report[1] of fatal fulminant hepatitis in a 56-year-old woman who had received 600 to 1200 mg of oxaprozin daily for about 6 weeks.

1. Purdum PP, *et al.* Oxaprozin-induced fulminant hepatitis. *Ann Pharmacother* 1994; **28:** 1159–61.

Interactions

For interactions associated with NSAIDs, see p.65.

Pharmacokinetics

Oxaprozin is slowly but extensively absorbed from the gastro-intestinal tract and is highly bound to plasma proteins. At steady state, which may take several days to achieve, the accumulation half-life is about 25 hours after a 600-mg dose and 21 hours after a 1200-mg dose. Oxaprozin is metabolised mainly in the liver by microsomal oxidation and conjugation with glucuronic acid to form inactive metabolites which are excreted in the urine and faeces.

References.

1. Karim A. Inverse nonlinear pharmacokinetics of total and protein unbound drug (oxaprozin): clinical and pharmacokinetic implications. *J Clin Pharmacol* 1996; **36:** 985–97.
2. Karim A, *et al.* Oxaprozin and piroxicam, nonsteroidal antiinflammatory drugs with long half-lives: effect of protein-binding differences on steady-state pharmacokinetics. *J Clin Pharmacol* 1997; **37:** 267–78.

Uses and Administration

Oxaprozin, a propionic acid derivative, is an NSAID (p.65). It is used in the treatment of osteoarthritis and rheumatoid arthritis in a usual dose of 1200 mg given once daily by mouth, although in osteoarthritis patients with low body-weight or mild disease may respond to an initial dose of 600 mg daily. The recommended maximum daily dose is 1800 mg or 26 mg per kg body-weight, whichever is the lower.

References.

1. Miller LG. Oxaprozin: a once-daily nonsteroidal anti-inflammatory drug. *Clin Pharm* 1992; **11:** 591–603.
2. Anonymous. Oxaprozin for arthritis. *Med Lett Drugs Ther* 1993; **35:** 15–16.

Preparations

Proprietary Preparations (details are given in Part 3)
S.Afr.: Deflam; ***USA:*** Daypro.

Oxycodone Hydrochloride (6248-k)

Oxycodone Hydrochloride *(BANM, USAN, rINNM).*

7,8-Dihydro-14-hydroxycodeinone hydrochloride; Dihydrone Hydrochloride; NSC-19043 (oxycodone); Oxycone Hydrochloride; Thecodine. 6-Deoxy-7,8-dihydro-14-hydroxy-3-*O*-methyl-6-oxomorphine hydrochloride; (−)-(5*R*,6*S*,14*S*)-4,5-Epoxy-14-hydroxy-3-methoxy-9a-methylmorphinan-6-one hydrochloride.

$C_{18}H_{21}NO_4,HCl$ = 351.8.

CAS — 76-42-6 (oxycodone); 124-90-3 (oxycodone hydrochloride).

NOTE. Compounded preparations of oxycodone and paracetamol (acetaminophen) in USP 23 may be represented by the name Co-oxycodAPAP.

Pharmacopoeias. In *Aust., Belg., Fr., Jpn,* and *US* (some specify the trihydrate).

White to off-white, odourless, hygroscopic crystals or powder. **Soluble** in water; slightly soluble in alcohol. **Store** in airtight containers.

Oxycodone Terephthalate (18469-c)

4,5α-Epoxy-14-hydroxy-3-methoxy-17-methylmorphinan-6-one 1,4-benzenedicarboxylate (2:1) salt.

$(C_{18}H_{21}NO_4)_2.C_8H_6O_4$ = 796.9.

CAS — 64336-55-6.

Pharmacopoeias. In *US.*

Store in airtight containers.

Dependence and Withdrawal, Adverse Effects, Treatment, and Precautions

As for Opioid Analgesics in general, p.67.

Effects on the respiratory system. References to respiratory depression occurring in children given oxycodone.

1. Olkkola KT, *et al.* Pharmacokinetics and ventilatory effects of intravenous oxycodone in postoperative children. *Br J Clin Pharmacol* 1994; **38:** 71–6.
2. Kalso E. Pharmacokinetics and ventilatory effects of intravenous oxycodone in postoperative children. *Br J Clin Pharmacol* 1995; **39:** 214.

Hepatic impairment. The clearance and elimination of oxycodone were shown to be prolonged in 6 female patients with end-stage liver cirrhosis awaiting liver transplantations.[1] Significant ventilatory depression was also observed. Pharmacokinetic values after successful transplantation were similar to those previously reported for healthy adults. It was recommended that, when administering oxycodone to patients with end-stage liver disease, the dosing frequency should be reduced and the dose lowered.

1. Tallgren M, *et al.* Pharmacokinetics and ventilatory effects of oxycodone before and after liver transplantation. *Clin Pharmacol Ther* 1997; **61:** 655–61.

Porphyria. Oxycodone was considered to be unsafe in patients with acute porphyria because it has been shown to be porphyrinogenic in *animals* or *in vitro* systems.[1]

1. Moore MR, McColl KEL. *Porphyria: drug lists.* Glasgow: Porphyria Research Unit, University of Glasgow, 1991.

Interactions

For interactions associated with opioid analgesics, see p.69.

Pharmacokinetics

Oxycodone is absorbed from the gastro-intestinal tract. It is metabolised to noroxycodone and, to a lesser extent, oxymorphone (p.72). Both metabolites undergo glucuronidation and are excreted with unchanged drug in urine. The elimination half-life of oxycodone is reported to be 2 to 3 hours.

References.

1. Pöyhiä R, *et al.* The pharmacokinetics of oxycodone after intravenous injection in adults. *Br J Clin Pharmacol* 1991; **32:** 516–18.
2. Leow KP, *et al.* Single-dose and steady-state pharmacokinetics and pharmacodynamics of oxycodone in patients with cancer. *Clin Pharmacol Ther* 1992; **52:** 487–95.
3. Olkkola KT, *et al.* Pharmacokinetics and ventilatory effects of intravenous oxycodone in postoperative children. *Br J Clin Pharmacol* 1994; **38:** 71–6.
4. Mandema JW, *et al.* Characterization and validation of a pharmacokinetic model for controlled-release oxycodone. *Br J Clin Pharmacol* 1996; **42:** 747–56.
5. Kaiko RF, *et al.* Pharmacokinetic-pharmacodynamic relationships of controlled-release oxycodone. *Clin Pharmacol Ther* 1996; **59:** 52–61.

Uses and Administration

Oxycodone, a phenanthrene derivative, is an opioid analgesic (p.69). Oxycodone hydrochloride is given by mouth for the relief of moderate to moderately severe pain in a dose of 5 mg every 6 hours. Combined preparations containing oxycodone hydrochloride and aspirin or paracetamol are also used. Some preparations with paracetamol may be known as co-oxycodAPAP. Higher doses of oxycodone have been used for the control of severe pain. Oxycodone hydrochloride may also be given by mouth as a modified-release preparation every 12 hours.

Oxycodone has been given rectally every 6 to 8 hours in suppositories containing 30 mg of oxycodone (as the pectinate) or 10 to 40 mg of oxycodone hydrochloride.

Oxycodone terephthalate is also used by mouth.

References.

1. Kalso E, Vainio A. Morphine and oxycodone hydrochloride in the management of cancer pain. *Clin Pharmacol Ther* 1990; **47:** 639–46.
2. Sunshine A, *et al.* Analgesic efficacy of controlled-release oxycodone in postoperative pain. *J Clin Pharmacol* 1996; **36:** 595–603.

Preparations

USP 23: Oxycodone and Acetaminophen Capsules; Oxycodone and Acetaminophen Tablets; Oxycodone and Aspirin Tablets; Oxycodone Hydrochloride Oral Solution; Oxycodone Hydrochloride Tablets.

Proprietary Preparations (details are given in Part 3)
Austral.: Endone; Proladone; ***Canad.:*** Oxycontin; Supeudol; ***Fr.:*** Eubine; ***USA:*** Oxycontin; OxyIR; Roxicodone.

Multi-ingredient: ***Austral.:*** Percodan†; ***Canad.:*** Endocet; Endodan; Oxycocet; Oxycodan; Percocet; Percodan; Roxicet; ***USA:*** Percocet; Percodan; Roxicet; Roxilox; Roxiprin; Tylox.

Oxymorphone Hydrochloride (6249-a)

Oxymorphone Hydrochloride *(BANM, rINNM).*

7,8-Dihydro-14-hydroxymorphinone hydrochloride; Oximorphone Hydrochloride. 6-Deoxy-7,8-dihydro-14-hydroxy-6-oxomorphine hydrochloride; (−)-(5*R*,6*S*,14*S*)-4,5-Epoxy-3,14-dihydroxy-9a-methylmorphinan-6-one hydrochloride.

$C_{17}H_{19}NO_4,HCl = 337.8.$

CAS — 76-41-5 (oxymorphone); 357-07-3 (oxymorphone hydrochloride).

Pharmacopoeias. In *US.*

A white or slightly off-white odourless powder, darkening on exposure to light. **Soluble** 1 in 4 of water, 1 in 100 of alcohol, and 1 in 25 of methyl alcohol; very slightly soluble in chloroform and in ether. **Store** in airtight containers. Protect from light.

Oxymorphone hydrochloride, a phenanthrene derivative, is an opioid analgesic (p.67) with actions and uses similar to those of morphine (p.56), apart from a lack of cough suppressant activity. Oxymorphone is used in the treatment of moderate to severe pain, including pain in obstetrics, and is reported to provide analgesia for 3 to 6 hours. It may also be used as an adjunct to anaesthesia and to relieve dyspnoea due to pulmonary oedema resulting from left ventricular failure.

Oxymorphone hydrochloride is given in initial doses of 1 to 1.5 mg, repeated every 4 to 6 hours as necessary, by intramuscular or subcutaneous injection; 500 µg may be given by intravenous injection. The usual dose for analgesia during labour is 0.5 to 1 mg intramuscularly.

Oxymorphone hydrochloride is given rectally in a suppository in a dose of 5 mg every 4 to 6 hours.

Pain. Oxymorphone hydrochloride has been reported to be a suitable alternative to morphine or pethidine for patient-controlled analgesia after caesarean section.[1,2] A loading dose of 1 mg has been given intravenously in four divided doses at 15-minute intervals to produce initial analgesia. Patients have then self-administered bolus doses of up to 300 µg as required with an 8-minute lockout interval between doses.

1. Sinatra RS, Harrison DM. Oxymorphone in patient-controlled analgesia. *Clin Pharm* 1989; **8:** 541, 544.
2. Sinatra RS, *et al.* A comparison of morphine, meperidine, and oxymorphone as utilised in patient-controlled analgesia following cesarean delivery. *Anesthesiology* 1989; **70:** 585–90.

Preparations

USP 23: Oxymorphone Hydrochloride Injection; Oxymorphone Hydrochloride Suppositories.

Proprietary Preparations (details are given in Part 3)
Canad.: Numorphan; ***USA:*** Numorphan.

Oxyphenbutazone (2678-q)

Oxyphenbutazone *(BAN, rINN).*

G-27202; Hydroxyphenylbutazone; Oxifenbutazona; Oxyphenbutazonum. 4-Butyl-1-(4-hydroxyphenyl)-2-phenylpyrazolidine-3,5-dione monohydrate.

$C_{19}H_{20}N_2O_3,H_2O = 342.4.$

CAS — 129-20-4 (anhydrous oxyphenbutazone); 7081-38-1 (oxyphenbutazone monohydrate).

Pharmacopoeias. In *Eur.* (see p.viii) and *US.*

A white to yellowish-white, odourless, crystalline powder. Practically **insoluble** in water; soluble 1 in 1.5 of alcohol, 1 in 4 of chloroform, and 1 in 15 of ether; freely soluble in acetone; it dissolves in dilute solutions of alkali hydroxides. **Store** in airtight containers. Protect from light.

Adverse Effects and Precautions

As for Phenylbutazone, p.79. Adverse effects on the blood may be more frequent with oxyphenbutazone than with phenylbutazone.

Porphyria. Oxyphenbutazone has been associated with clinical exacerbations of porphyria and is considered unsafe in porphyric patients.[1]

1. Moore MR, McColl KEL. *Porphyria: drug lists.* Glasgow: Porphyria Research Unit, University of Glasgow, 1991.

Interactions

For interactions associated with NSAIDs, see p.65.

Uses and Administration

Oxyphenbutazone, a metabolite of phenylbutazone (p.79), is an NSAID (p.63). It has been applied topically to the eye as an anti-inflammatory ointment (usually 10%) in conditions such as episcleritis. Oxyphenbutazone was used systemically in disorders such as ankylosing spondylitis, osteoarthritis, and rheumatoid arthritis but such use is no longer considered justified owing to the risk of severe haematological adverse effects. The piperazine salt has also been used.

Preparations

BP 1998: Oxyphenbutazone Eye Ointment;
USP 23: Oxyphenbutazone Tablets.

Proprietary Preparations (details are given in Part 3)
Aust.: Tanderil; ***Ger.:*** Californit†; Phlogont†; Tanderil†; ***Irl.:*** Tanderil†; ***S.Afr.:*** Otone†; ***Spain:*** Diflamil; ***Switz.:*** Tanderil†; ***UK:*** Tanderil†.

Multi-ingredient: ***Ger.:*** Dolo-Phlogase†; Mindaril†; Phlogase†; ***Irl.:*** Tanderil Chloramphenicol†; ***Ital.:*** Difmedol†; ***Switz.:*** Mindaril†.

Paracetamol (2679-p)

Paracetamol *(BAN, rINN).*

Acetaminophen; *N*-Acetyl-*p*-aminophenol; Paracetamolum. 4′-Hydroxyacetanilide; *N*-(4-Hydroxyphenyl)acetamide.

$C_8H_9NO_2 = 151.2.$

CAS — 103-90-2.

NOTE. Compounded preparations containing paracetamol have been given the following British Approved Names:
Co-codamol, codeine phosphate and paracetamol, the proportions being expressed in the form *x*/*y* where *x* and *y* are the strengths in milligrams of codeine phosphate and paracetamol respectively;
Co-dydramol, dihydrocodeine tartrate and paracetamol in the proportions, by weight, 1 part to 50 parts respectively;
Co-methiamol, DL-methionine and paracetamol, the proportions being expressed in the form *x*/*y* where *x* and *y* are the strengths in milligrams of DL-methionine and paracetamol respectively;
Co-proxamol, dextropropoxyphene hydrochloride and paracetamol in the proportions, by weight, 1 part to 10 parts respectively.
Compounded preparations containing paracetamol (acetaminophen) in USP 23 may be represented by the following names:
Co-bucafAPAP for butalbital, paracetamol, and caffeine;
Co-codAPAP for paracetamol and codeine phosphate;
Co-hycodAPAP for hydrocodone bitartrate and paracetamol;
Co-oxycodAPAP for oxycodone and paracetamol; and
Co-proxAPAP for dextropropoxyphene napsylate (propoxyphene napsylate) and paracetamol.

Pharmacopoeias. In *Chin., Eur.* (see p.viii), *Int., Jpn, Pol.,* and *US.*

A white odourless crystalline powder. Sparingly **soluble** in water; soluble 1 in 20 of boiling water, 1 in 10 of alcohol, and 1 in 15 of 1*N* sodium hydroxide; very slightly soluble in dichloromethane and in ether. **Store** in airtight containers. Protect from light.

Adverse Effects and Treatment

Side-effects of paracetamol are rare and usually mild, although haematological reactions including thrombocytopenia, leucopenia, pancytopenia, neutropenia, and agranulocytosis have been reported. Skin rashes, and other hypersensitivity reactions occur occasionally.

Overdosage with paracetamol can result in severe liver damage and sometimes acute renal tubular necrosis. Prompt treatment with acetylcysteine or methionine is essential and is discussed under Overdosage, below.

Effects on the kidneys. For reference to evidence that abuse or prolonged excessive use of analgesics, including paracetamol, can produce nephropathy, see under NSAIDs, p.64.

See also under Overdosage, below.

Effects on the pancreas. A review of drug-induced pancreatitis reported that pancreatitis associated with paracetamol had only occurred in patients taking more than recommended doses and even then it had been a rare reaction.[1]

1. Underwood TW, Frye CB. Drug-induced pancreatitis. *Clin Pharm* 1993; **12:** 440–8.

Hypersensitivity. Reactions, characterised by urticaria, dyspnoea, and hypotension, have occurred following the administration of paracetamol to adults[1,2] and children.[3] Angioedema has also been reported.[4] Fixed drug eruptions, confirmed by rechallenge, have been described.[5-7]

1. Stricker BHC, *et al.* Acute hypersensitivity reactions to paracetamol. *Br Med J* 1985; **291:** 938–9.
2. Van Diem L, Grilliat JP. Anaphylactic shock induced by paracetamol. *Eur J Clin Pharmacol* 1990; **38:** 389–90.
3. Ellis M, *et al.* Immediate adverse reactions to acetaminophen in children: evaluation of histamine release and spirometry. *J Pediatr* 1989; **114:** 654–6.
4. Idoko JA, *et al.* Angioneurotic oedema following ingestion of paracetamol. *Trans R Soc Trop Med Hyg* 1986; **80:** 175.
5. Thomas RHM, Munro DD. Fixed drug eruption due to paracetamol. *Br J Dermatol* 1986; **115:** 357–9.
6. Cohen HA, *et al.* Fixed drug eruption caused by acetaminophen. *Ann Pharmacother* 1992; **26:** 1596–7.
7. Harris A, Burge SM. Vasculitis in a fixed drug eruption due to paracetamol. *Br J Dermatol* 1995; **133:** 790–1.

Overdosage. Acute overdosage with paracetamol, whether accidental or deliberate, is relatively common. The consequences can be extremely serious because of the narrow margin between therapeutic and toxic doses. Ingestion of as little as 10 to 15 g of paracetamol by adults may cause severe hepatocellular necrosis and, less often, renal tubular necrosis.

Early features of overdosage such as nausea and vomiting usually settle within 24 hours; other early symptoms may include lethargy and sweating. Abdominal pain may be the first indication of liver damage, which is not usually apparent for 24 to 48 hours and sometimes may be delayed for up to 4 to 6 days after ingestion. Liver damage is generally at a maximum 72 to 96 hours after ingestion. Hepatic failure, encephalopathy, coma, and death may result. Complications of hepatic failure, include acidosis, cerebral oedema, haemorrhage, hypoglycaemia, hypotension, infection, and renal failure. An increasing prothrombin time is a reliable indicator of deteriorating liver function and it is recommended by some that the prothrombin time should be measured regularly. Measurement of serum concentrations of aspartate aminotransferase and alanine aminotransferase is also considered to be of value.[27] Patients receiving enzyme-inducing drugs or those with a history of alcohol abuse are at special risk of hepatic damage, as may be patients suffering from malnutrition such as those with anorexia or AIDS. It has also been suggested that fasting may predispose to hepatotoxicity.[1]

Acute renal failure with acute tubular necrosis may develop, even in the absence of severe liver damage. Other non-hepatic symptoms that have been reported following paracetamol overdosage include myocardial abnormalities and pancreatitis.

Toxicity following overdosage with paracetamol has been attributed to the production of a minor but highly reactive metabolite, *N*-acetyl-*p*-benzoquinoneimine (NABQI) by mixed function oxidase enzymes in the liver and kidney. The amount of NABQI produced after normal doses of paracetamol is usually completely detoxified by conjugation with glutathione and excreted as mercaptopurine and cysteine conjugates. However, following paracetamol overdosage, tissue stores of glutathione become depleted, allowing NABQI to accumulate and bind to sulfhydryl groups within hepatocytes causing cell damage. Substances capable of replenishing depleted stores of glutathione, such as acetylcysteine or methionine, are thus used as antidotes in paracetamol overdosage. Acetylcysteine may also be involved in the repair of damaged tissue.

Treatment of paracetamol overdosage. The management of paracetamol overdosage as practised in the UK and US has been the subject of several reviews.[2-11]

Prompt treatment is essential, even when there are no obvious symptoms, and all patients should be admitted to hospital. Gastric lavage should be carried out especially if the overdose was taken within the previous 2 hours; full supportive measures should also be instituted. Some centres give activated charcoal to reduce gastro-intestinal absorption, especially in cases of multiple drug overdosage. However, if acetylcysteine or methionine is to be administered by mouth the charcoal is best cleared from the stomach to prevent it reducing the absorption of the antidote.

In order to assess the risk of liver damage, the plasma-paracetamol concentration should be determined as soon as possible, but not within 4 hours of ingestion, to ensure that peak concentrations are recorded. The patient's plasma-paracetamol concentration is compared against a standard nomogram reference line on a plot of plasma-paracetamol concentration against hours after ingestion. A semi-logarithmic plot or a linear plot may be used, see Figure 1 (p.73) and Figure 2 (p.73). Generally, antidote treatment is required if the patient's plasma-paracetamol concentration is higher than this line. Plasma-paracetamol measured more than 16 hours after ingestion are not reliable indicators of hepatic toxicity. Furthermore, the nomogram may not be suitable for use when patients have taken modified-release preparations of paracetamol.[12,13] Some suggestions for modified strategies for the use of the Rumack-Matthew nomogram in the face of overdosage with modified-release preparations have been made.[14-16]

Antidote treatment should be started as soon as possible after suspected paracetamol ingestion and should not be delayed while awaiting the results of plasma assays. Once the results become available, treatment may be stopped if the initial concentration is below the nomogram reference line. However, if the initial concentration is above the reference line, the full course of antidote must be administered and should not be discontinued when subsequent plasma concentrations fall below the reference line. Patients receiving enzyme-inducing drugs such as carbamazepine, phenytoin, phenobarbitone, rifampicin, or those with malnutrition or a history of alcohol abuse should receive an antidote if their plasma-paracetamol concentrations are up to 50% below the standard reference line.

Figure 1. A semi-logarithmic plot of plasma-paracetamol concentration against hours after ingestion.

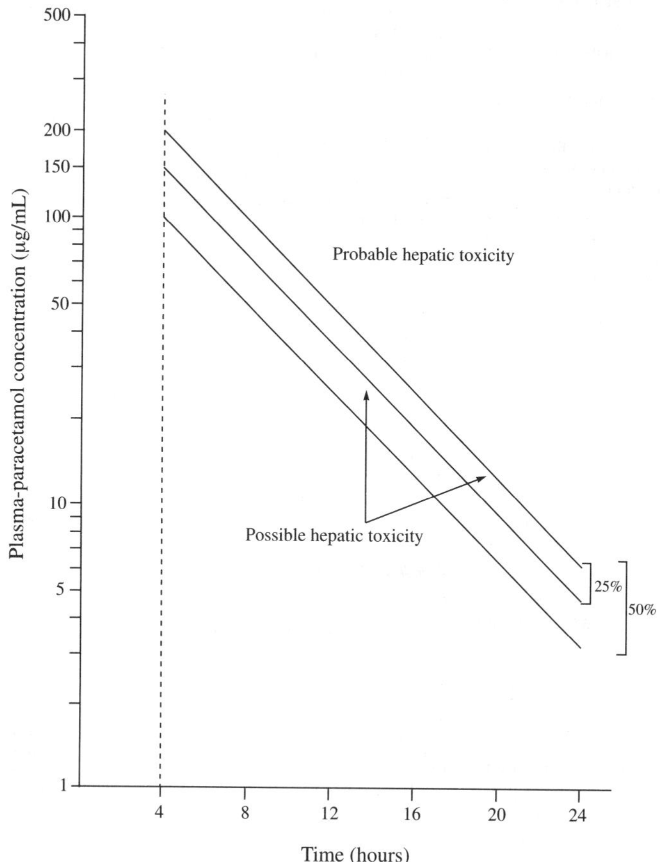

Adapted from Rumack BH, Matthew HJ. Acetaminophen poisoning and toxicity. *Pediatrics* 1975; **55:** 871–6.

Notes for the use of this chart:
1. The time coordinates refer to time after ingestion.
2. Plasma-paracetamol concentrations drawn before 4 hours may not represent peak concentrations.
3. The graph should be used only in relation to a single acute ingestion.
4. The solid line 25% below the standard nomogram is included to allow for possible errors in plasma assays and estimated time from ingestion of an overdose.
5. The solid line 50% below the standard nomogram is to assess the possible hepatic toxicity in patients receiving enzyme-inducing drugs or with malnutrition or a history of alcohol abuse.

Figure 2. A linear plot of plasma-paracetamol concentration against hours after ingestion.

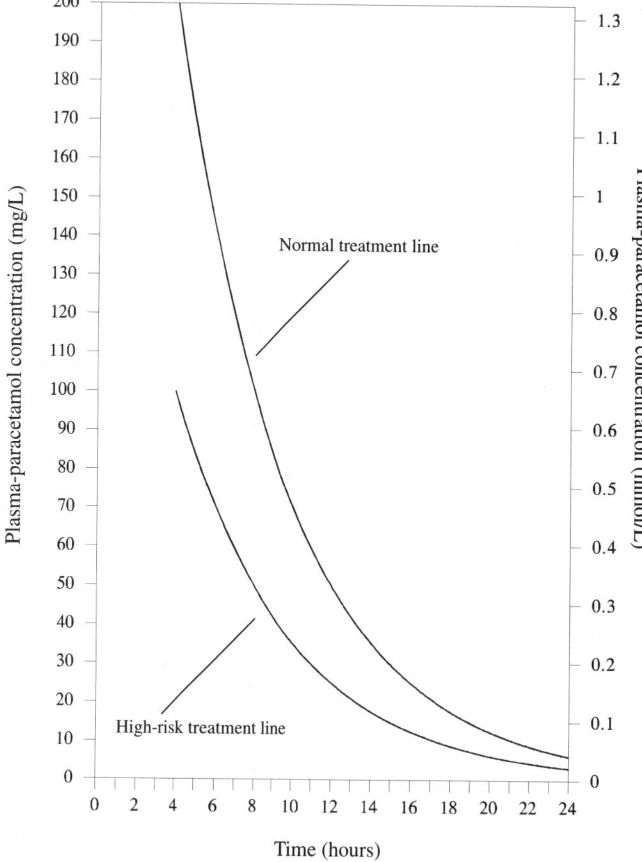

Courtesy of P A Routledge.

Notes for the use of this chart:
1. The time coordinates refer to time after ingestion.
2. Plasma-paracetamol concentrations drawn before 4 hours may not represent peak concentrations.
3. The graph should be used only in relation to a single acute ingestion.
4. Patients whose plasma-paracetamol concentrations are above the normal treatment line should be treated.
5. Patients on enzyme-inducing drugs or with malnutrition or a history of alcohol abuse should be treated if their plasma-paracetamol concentrations are above the high-risk treatment line.

Choice of antidote. Acetylcysteine (p.1052) is usually the antidote of choice but there is some variance over the route of administration used. Although intravenous administration has been associated with anaphylactic reactions it is the preferred route in the UK because of concerns over the effects of vomiting and activated charcoal on oral absorption. Nausea and vomiting are amongst the most common early symptoms of paracetamol overdosage and may be exacerbated by the extremely disagreeable taste and odour of oral acetylcysteine. However, oral administration is the usual route of choice in the USA and experience there suggests that it is effective and that the outcome of treatment is not adversely affected by the use of activated charcoal.

An alternative in the UK is methionine (p.984) by mouth, which is cheaper and easier to administer than intravenous acetylcysteine. It may also be used in the UK in situations where a patient cannot be transferred to hospital provided it is given within 10 to 12 hours of the overdose. Methionine absorption is impaired if activated charcoal has been administered or in patients who are vomiting.

Acetylcysteine is most effective when administered during the first 8 hours following ingestion of the overdose and the effect diminishes progressively thereafter. It used to be believed that starting treatment more than 15 hours after overdosage was of no benefit and might possibly aggravate the risk of hepatic encephalopathy. However, late administration has now been shown to be safe,[17] and studies of patients treated up to 36 hours after ingestion suggest that beneficial results may be obtained up to and possibly beyond 24 hours.[18,19] Furthermore, administration of intravenous acetylcysteine to patients who had already developed fulminant hepatic failure has been shown to reduce morbidity and mortality.[20]

In the UK, an initial dose of 150 mg per kg body-weight of acetylcysteine in 200 mL of glucose 5% is given intravenously over 15 minutes, followed by an intravenous infusion of 50 mg per kg in 500 mL of glucose 5% over the next 4 hours and then 100 mg per kg in one litre over the next 16 hours. The volume of intravenous fluids should be modified for children. If an anaphylactoid reaction develops, the infusion should be stopped and an antihistamine administered; it may be possible to continue the acetylcysteine infusion at a slower rate. In the USA, acetylcysteine is given by mouth in an initial dose of 140 mg per kg as a 5% solution followed by 70 mg per kg every 4 hours for an additional 17 doses. Some[21] have suggested using a larger loading dose of acetylcysteine when it is given orally with activated charcoal whereas others[22] have found that the efficacy of acetylcysteine is not adversely affected by prior administration of activated charcoal and consider that increasing the acetylcysteine dose appears to be unwarranted.

Methionine is an alternative to acetylcysteine and, likewise, is most effective when given as early as possible following paracetamol overdosage. However, it is not as effective in late presentation[5,23-25] and the incidence and severity of hepatic damage is greater if treatment with methionine is started more than 10 hours after ingestion; it may also precipitate hepatic encephalopathy.[5]

The usual dose of methionine is 2.5 g by mouth every 4 hours for 4 doses starting less than 10 to 12 hours after ingestion of the paracetamol. It has also been given intravenously. The literature relating to the use of methionine in paracetamol poisoning is, in general, imprecise as to the form of methionine used. In the UK, the doses quoted above refer to DL-methionine. Preparations containing both methionine and paracetamol (co-methiamol) have been formulated for use in situations where overdosage may occur. However, the issue of whether methionine should be routinely added to paracetamol preparations is contentious for medical and ethical reasons.

Histamine H_2-receptor antagonists. It has been suggested that since cimetidine blocks the hepatic cytochrome P450 mixed function oxidase system, it might be of use as an adjunct to acetylcysteine for patients whose production of the toxic metabolite of paracetamol is increased due to enzyme induction. Although there have been several anecdotal reports claiming benefit for cimetidine in patients with paracetamol poisoning, there is no current evidence to support these claims.[11,26]

Liver transplantation may be considered as a last recourse in some patients.

1. Whitcomb DC, *et al.* Association of acetaminophen hepatotoxicity with fasting and ethanol use. *JAMA* 1994; **272:** 1845–50.
2. Keays R, Williams R. Paracetamol poisoning and liver failure. *Prescribers' J* 1989; **29:** 155–62.
3. Scott DK, Vale JA. Paracetamol poisoning. *Pharm J* 1990; **245:** 95–7.
4. Lewis RK, Paloucek FP. Assessment and treatment of acetaminophen overdose. *Clin Pharm* 1991; **10:** 765–74.

5. Janes J, Routledge PA. Recent developments in the management of paracetamol (acetaminophen) poisoning. *Drug Safety* 1992; **7:** 170–7.
6. Bray GP. Liver failure induced by paracetamol. *Br Med J* 1993; **306:** 157–8.
7. Ferner R. Paracetamol poisoning—an update. *Prescribers' J* 1993; **33:** 45–50.
8. Collee GG, Hanson GC. The Management of acute poisoning *Br J Anaesth* 1993; **70:** 562–73.
9. Makin AJ, *et al.* Management of severe cases of paracetamol overdosage. *Br J Hosp Med* 1994; **52:** 210–13.
10. Vale JA, Proudfoot AT. Paracetamol (acetaminophen) poisoning. *Lancet* 1995; **346:** 547–52.
11. Prescott LF. Paracetamol overdose. In: *Paracetamol (acetaminophen): a critical bibliographic review.* London: Taylor & Francis, 1996: 401–73.
12. Graudins A, *et al.* Overdose of extended-release acetaminophen. *N Engl J Med* 1995; **333:** 196.
13. Vassallo S, *et al.* Use of the Rumack-Matthew nomogram in cases of extended-release acetaminophen toxicity. *Ann Intern Med* 1996; **125:** 940.
14. Temple AR, Mrazik TJ. Move on extended-release acetaminophen. *N Engl J Med* 1995; **333:** 1508.
15. Graudins A, *et al.* Move on extended-release acetaminophen. *N Engl J Med* 1995; **333:** 1508–9.
16. Cetasuk EW, *et al.* Extended-release acetaminophen overdose. *JAMA* 1996; **275:** 686.
17. Parker D, *et al.* Safety of late acetylcysteine treatment in paracetamol poisoning. *Hum Exp Toxicol* 1990; **9:** 25–7.
18. Smilkstein MJ, *et al.* Efficacy of oral N-acetylcysteine in the treatment of acetaminophen overdose: analysis of the National Multicenter Study (1976 to 1985). *N Engl J Med* 1988; **319:** 1557–62.
19. Harrison PM, *et al.* Improved outcome of paracetamol-induced fulminant hepatic failure by late administration of acetylcysteine. *Lancet* 1990; **335:** 1572–3.
20. Keays R, *et al.* Intravenous acetylcysteine in paracetamol induced fulminant hepatic failure: a prospective controlled trial. *Br Med J* 1991; **303:** 1026–9.
21. Chamberlain JM, *et al.* Use of activated charcoal in a simulated poisoning with acetaminophen: a new loading dose for N-acetylcysteine? *Ann Emerg Med* 1993; **22:** 1398–1402.
22. Spiller HA, *et al.* A prospective evaluation of the effect of activated charcoal before oral N-acetylcysteine in acetaminophen overdose. *Ann Emerg Med* 1994; **23:** 519–23.
23. Vale JA, *et al.* Intravenous N-acetylcysteine: the treatment of choice in paracetamol poisoning? *Br Med J* 1979; **2:** 1435–6.
24. Vale JA, *et al.* Treatment of acetaminophen poisoning: the use of oral methionine. *Arch Intern Med* 1981; **141:** 394–6.
25. Tee LGB, *et al.* N-Acetylcysteine for paracetamol overdose. *Lancet* 1986; **i:** 331–2.
26. Kaufenberg AJ, Shepherd MF. Role of cimetidine in the treatment of acetaminophen poisoning. *Am J Health-Syst Pharm* 1998; **55:** 1516–19.
27. Routledge P, *et al.* Paracetamol (acetaminophen) poisoning. *Br Med J* 1998; **317:** 1609–10.

Precautions

Paracetamol should be given with care to patients with impaired kidney or liver function. It should also be given with care to patients with alcohol dependence.

Breast feeding. The amount of paracetamol distributed into breast milk is considered by some authorities to be too small to be harmful to a breast-fed infant. Pharmacokinetic studies in 12 nursing mothers given a single dose of paracetamol showed that peak paracetamol concentrations in breast milk of 10 to 15 μg per mL were achieved in 1 to 2 hours. Plasma concentrations were determined in 2 mothers; a breast milk/plasma ratio of about 1 was reported.[1] Similar findings were reported from another study.[2]

1. Berlin CM, *et al.* Disposition of acetaminophen in milk, saliva, and plasma of lactating women. *Pediatr Pharmacol* 1980; **1:** 135–41.
2. Hurden EL, *et al.* Excretion of paracetamol in human breast milk. *Arch Dis Child* 1980; **55:** 969–72.

Renal impairment. Caution is recommended when giving paracetamol to patients with renal impairment. Plasma concentrations of paracetamol and its glucuronide and sulphate conjugates are increased in patients with moderate renal failure and in patients on dialysis.[1-3] It has been suggested that paracetamol itself may be regenerated from these metabolites.[1,2] There are conflicting data on whether the conjugates of paracetamol accumulate in patients with renal impairment receiving multiple doses.[2,3]

1. Prescott LF, *et al.* Paracetamol disposition and metabolite kinetics in patients with chronic renal failure. *Eur J Clin Pharmacol* 1989; **36:** 291–7.
2. Martin U, *et al.* The disposition of paracetamol and the accumulation of its glucuronide and sulphate conjugates during multiple dosing in patients with chronic renal failure. *Eur J Clin Pharmacol* 1991; **41:** 43–6.
3. Martin U, *et al.* The disposition of paracetamol and its conjugates during multiple dosing in patients with end-stage renal failure maintained on haemodialysis. *Eur J Clin Pharmacol* 1993; **45:** 141–5.

Interactions

The risk of paracetamol toxicity may be increased in patients receiving other potentially hepatotoxic drugs or drugs that induce liver microsomal enzymes. The absorption of paracetamol may be accelerated by drugs such as metoclopramide. Excretion may be affected and plasma concentrations altered when administered with probenecid. Cholestyramine reduces the absorption of paracetamol if given within one hour of paracetamol administration.

Antibacterials. For the effects of paracetamol on chloramphenicol, see p.183.

Anticoagulants. For the effects of paracetamol on oral anticoagulants, see under Warfarin, p.966.

Antiepileptics. For the effects of paracetamol on lamotrigine, see p.348.

Antivirals. For reports of adverse effects of the liver associated with concomitant use of paracetamol and antiviral drugs, see under Interferons, p.617 and Zidovudine, p.631.

Probenecid. Pretreatment with probenecid can decrease paracetamol clearance and increase its plasma half-life.[1] Although urinary excretion of the sulphate and glucuronide conjugates of paracetamol are reduced, that of paracetamol is unchanged.

1. Kamali F. The effect of probenecid on paracetamol metabolism and pharmacokinetics. *Eur J Clin Pharmacol* 1993; **45:** 551–3.

Pharmacokinetics

Paracetamol is readily absorbed from the gastro-intestinal tract with peak plasma concentrations occurring about 10 to 60 minutes after oral administration. Paracetamol is distributed into most body tissues. It crosses the placenta and is present in breast milk. Plasma-protein binding is negligible at usual therapeutic concentrations but increases with increasing concentrations. The elimination half-life of paracetamol varies from about 1 to 3 hours.

Paracetamol is metabolised predominantly in the liver and excreted in the urine mainly as the glucuronide and sulphate conjugates. Less than 5% is excreted as unchanged paracetamol. A minor hydroxylated metabolite (*N*-acetyl-*p*-benzoquinoneimine) which is usually produced in very small amounts by mixed-function oxidases in the liver and kidney and which is usually detoxified by conjugation with glutathione may accumulate following paracetamol overdosage and cause tissue damage.

Absorption. The absorption of paracetamol was slow and incomplete in vegetarian subjects compared with non-vegetarian subjects.[1]

1. Prescott LF, *et al.* Impaired absorption of paracetamol in vegetarians. *Br J Clin Pharmacol* 1993; **36:** 237–40.

Uses and Administration

Paracetamol, a para-aminophenol derivative, has analgesic and antipyretic properties and weak anti-inflammatory activity. Paracetamol is given by mouth or as a rectal suppository for mild to moderate pain and for fever (p.1). Paracetamol is often the analgesic or antipyretic of choice especially in patients in whom salicylates or other NSAIDs are contra-indicated. Such patients include asthmatics or those with a history of peptic ulcer, or children in whom salicylates are contra-indicated because of the risk of Reye's syndrome.

The usual adult dose by mouth is 0.5 to 1 g every 4 to 6 hours up to a maximum of 4 g daily. Usual doses in children are: under 3 months, 10 mg per kg body-weight (reduce to 5 mg per kg if jaundiced); 3 months to 1 year, 60 to 120 mg; 1 to 5 years, 120 to 250 mg; 6 to 12 years, 250 to 500 mg. These doses may be given every 4 to 6 hours when necessary up to a maximum of 4 doses in 24 hours. For post-immunisation pyrexia, a dose of 60 mg has been recommended for children 2 to 3 months of age. A second dose may be given after four to six hours; if the pyrexia persists after that dose, the parent should seek medical advice.

Rectal doses for adults and children over 12 years of age are 0.5 to 1 g. Rectal doses in younger children are: 1 to 5 years, 125 to 250 mg; 6 to 12 years, 250 to 500 mg. Doses may be administered up to 4 times daily.

References.

1. Prescott LF. *Paracetamol (acetaminophen): a critical bibliographic review.* London: Taylor & Francis, 1996.

Headache. Non-opioid analgesics such as paracetamol, aspirin, and other NSAIDs are often tried first for the symptomatic treatment of various types of headache including migraine (see p.443) and tension-type headache (see p.444). These drugs given at the onset of symptoms can successfully treat an acute attack of migraine. However, absorption may be poor due to gastric stasis which is commonly present in migraine. For this reason dispersible and effervescent preparations and compound preparations containing drugs such as metoclopramide which relieve gastric stasis have been advocated.

Pain. Paracetamol is used in the management of mild to moderate pain (p.4). It is of similar potency to aspirin, but with weak anti-inflammatory activity. Paracetamol may also be used as an adjunct to opioids in the management of severe pain such as cancer pain (p.8). Paracetamol is the preferred choice for pain in infants and children (p.7) because of the association of aspirin with Reye's syndrome in this age group (see p.17). In the treatment of rheumatic disorders, a weak anti-inflammatory effect limits the role of paracetamol. However, it may be of benefit for simple pain control in rheumatoid arthritis (p.2) and ankylosing spondylitis (see under Spondyloarthropathies, p.4), although these patients usually require the additional anti-inflammatory effects provided by NSAIDs. Synovial inflammation is usually only a minor component of osteoarthritis (p.2), and paracetamol is generally recommended as first choice of treatment before NSAIDs are tried. Paracetamol is useful for the relief of acute low back pain (p.10).

Dependence and tolerance are not a problem with non-opioid analgesics such as paracetamol, but there is a ceiling of efficacy, above which increasing the dose has no further therapeutic effect.

Preparations

BP 1998: Co-codamol Tablets; Co-dydramol Tablets; Co-proxamol Tablets; Dispersible Paracetamol Tablets; Paediatric Paracetamol Oral Solution; Paracetamol Oral Suspension; Paracetamol Tablets; Soluble Paracetamol Tablets;

USP 23: Acetaminophen and Aspirin Tablets; Acetaminophen and Caffeine Capsules; Acetaminophen and Caffeine Tablets; Acetaminophen and Codeine Phosphate Capsules; Acetaminophen and Codeine Phosphate Oral Solution; Acetaminophen and Codeine Phosphate Oral Suspension; Acetaminophen and Codeine Phosphate Tablets; Acetaminophen and Diphenhydramine Citrate Tablets; Acetaminophen and Pseudoephedrine Hydrochloride Tablets; Acetaminophen Capsules; Acetaminophen for Effervescent Oral Solution; Acetaminophen Oral Solution; Acetaminophen Oral Suspension; Acetaminophen Suppositories; Acetaminophen Tablets; Acetaminophen, Aspirin, and Caffeine Capsules; Acetaminophen, Aspirin, and Caffeine Tablets; Acetaminophen, Dextromethorphan Hydrobromide, Doxylamine Succinate, and Pseudoephedrine Hydrochloride Oral Solution; Acetaminophen, Diphenhydramine Hydrochloride, and Pseudoephedrine Hydrochloride Tablets; Butalbital, Acetaminophen, and Caffeine Capsules; Butalbital, Acetaminophen, and Caffeine Tablets; Hydrocodone Bitartrate and Acetaminophen Tablets; Isometheptene Mucate, Dichloralphenazone, and Acetaminophen Capsules; Oxycodone and Acetaminophen Capsules; Oxycodone and Acetaminophen Tablets; Propoxyphene Hydrochloride and Acetaminophen Tablets; Propoxyphene Napsylate and Acetaminophen Tablets.

Proprietary Preparations (details are given in Part 3)

Aust.: Apacet†; Duaneo; Enelfa†; Kratofin simplex; Mexalen; Momentum; Parakapton; Peinfort†; Tylenol; ***Austral.:*** Ceetamol†; Dymadon; Junior Disprol†; Lemsip; Ordov Febrigesic; Panacete†; Panadol; Panamax; Paralgin; Parasin†; Paraspen†; Setamol; Tempra; Tylenol; ***Belg.:*** Curpol; Dafalgan; Dolprone; Efferalgan; Lemgrip; Lonarid Mono; Neuridon; Panadol; Pe-Tam; Perdolan Mono; Sanicopyrine; Supadol Mono†; Tempra; ***Canad.:*** 222 AF; Abenol; Acetab; AF Anacin; Alsiphene; Anacin-3†; Artritol; Atasol; Cephanol; Headarest†; Novo-Gesic; Pain Aid Free; Panadol; Pediatrix; Robigesic; Rounox; Tantaphen; Tempra; Tylenol; ***Fr.:*** Aferadol; Claradol; Dafalgan; Doliprane; Dolko; Dolotec; Efferalgan; Geluprane; Gynospasmine; Malgis†; Oralgan; Panadol; Paralyoc; ***Ger.:*** Anaflon†; Anti-Algos; Ben-u-ron; Captin; Contac Erkaltungs-Trunk; Dignocetamol†; Dolarist†; Dolofugin†; Doloreduct; Dolorfug†; Dorocoff-Paracetamol; duracetamol; Enelfa; Eu-Med Schmerzzapfschen†; Fensum; Finiweh; Freka-cetamol†; Grippostad; Larylin Heissgetrank gegen Schmerzen und Fieber; Logomed Schmerz- /Fieber; Lonarid Mono†; Mandrogripp; Mogil†; Momentum Analgetikum; Mono Praecimed; Mono-Tri-medil†; NeoCitran; NilnOcen; Octadon N†; Paedialgon; Pyromed S; Sinpro junior†; Sinpro-N†; Togal; Treupel mono; Verlapyrin N†; Vivimed; ***Irl.:*** Calpol; Cetamol†; Disprol; Hedex†; Panadol; Paralief; Paralink; Parasol†; Suotex†; Tylenol; ***Ital.:*** Acetamol; Calpol†; Efferalgan; Neo-Fepramol; Panadol; Puernol; Sanipirina†; Tachipirina; ***Neth.:*** Daro†; Darocet†; Hedex†; Kinder Finimal; Momentum; Panadol; Sinaspril-Paracetamol; ***Norw.:*** Alvedon; Panodil; Paracet; Pinex; ***S.Afr.:*** Antalgic; Arcanagesic; Brunomol; Calpol; Cetapon†; Compu-Pain†; Dolorol; Doxypol†; Dynadol; Empaped; Ennagesic†; Entalgic; Farmacetamol; Fevamol; Lyteca†; Maxadol-P; Medpramol; Napamol; Pacimol; Painamol; Pamol; Panado; Prolief; Pyradol; Pyragesic†; Setamol†; Temol; Tylenol; Winpain; Xeramax; ***Spain:*** Acertol; Actron; Akindol; Alginina†; Analter; Antidol; Apiretal; Aspac; Asplin; Auxidor†; Calmanticold; Cupanol; Desfebre†; Dolgesic; Dolostop; Drazin†; Duorol; Efferalgan; Febranine; Febrectal Simple; Gelocatil; Hedex†; Melabon Infantil; Nofedol; Panadol; Panrectal†; Pediapirin; Pirinasol; Prontina†; Sinmol; Stopain†; Temperal; Termalgin; Tylenol; Zatinol; Zolben; ***Swed.:*** Alvedon; Curadon; Lemsip; Panodil; Reliv; ***Switz.:*** Acetalgine; Bebesan N†; Ben-u-ron; Comprimes analgesiques no 534; Contre-Douleurs P; Dafalgan; Democyl; Demogripal; Dolprone; Fortalidon P; Influbene N; Malex N†; Neo-Treupine†; Nina; Ortensan; Panadol; Spalt N; Stellacyl nouvelle formule†; Treupel N; Treuphadol; Tylenol; Zolben; ***UK:*** Alvedon; Anadin Paracetamol; Aspro Paraclear†; Calpol; Disprol; Elkamol; Fanalgic; Fennings Children's Powders; Hedex; Infadrops; Medinol; Miradol; Pain Relief Syrup for Children; Paldesic; Panadol; Panaleve; Paracets; Paraclear; Paramin; Placidex; Salzone; Tixymol; Tramil; ***USA:*** Acephen; Aceta; AlbaTemp; Alka-Seltzer Advanced Formula†; Apacet; Apap; Arthritis Foundation Pain Reliever, Aspirin Free†; Arthritis Pain Formula Aspirin Free; Aspirin Free Anacin; Aspirin Free Pain Relief; Bromo Seltzer; Childrens Dynafed Jr; Childrens Mapap; Dapa; Dolanex; Dorcol Children's Fever & Pain Reducer; Extra Strength Datril†; Extra Strength Dynafed EX; Feverall; Genapap; Genebs; Halenol; Liquiprin; Mapap; Maranox; Meda; Myapap; Neopap; Oraphen-PD; Panadol; Panex; Phenaphen†; Redutemp; Ridenol; Silapap; Snaplets-FR; St. Joseph Aspirin-Free for Children; Suppap; Tapanol; Tempra; Tylenol; Uni-Ace.

Multi-ingredient: numerous preparations are listed in Part 3.

Parsalmide (13084-v)

Parsalmide *(rINN)*.

54106-CB; MY-41-6. 5-Amino-*N*-butyl-*O*-(prop-2-ynyl)salicylamide; 5-Amino-*N*-butyl-2-(prop-2-ynyloxy)benzamide.

$C_{14}H_{18}N_2O_2$ = 246.3.

CAS — 30653-83-9.

Parsalmide is an NSAID (p.63) that was given by mouth or rectally for the relief of painful and inflammatory conditions.

Preparations

Proprietary Preparations (details are given in Part 3)

Ital.: Sinovial†.

Pentamorphone (10368-c)

Pentamorphone *(USAN, rINN)*.

A-4492; RX-77989. 7,8-Didehydro-4,5α-epoxy-3-hydroxy-17-methyl-14-(pentylamino)morphinan-6-one.

$C_{22}H_{28}N_2O_3$ = 368.5.

CAS — 68616-83-1.

Pentamorphone is a synthetic opioid that has been studied as an analgesic.

References.

1. Wong HY, *et al.* Pentamorphone for management of postoperative pain. *Anesth Analg* 1991; **72:** 656–60.
2. Kelly WB, *et al.* A comparison of pentamorphone and fentanyl in balanced anaesthesia during general surgery. *Can J Anaesth* 1994; **41:** 703–9.

Pentazocine (6251-l)

Pentazocine *(BAN, USAN, rINN)*.

NIH-7958; NSC-107430; Win-20228. (2*R**,6*R**,11*R**)-1,2,3,4,5,6-Hexahydro-6,11-dimethyl-3-(3-methylbut-2-enyl)-2,6-methano-3-benzazocin-8-ol.

$C_{19}H_{27}NO$ = 285.4.

CAS — 359-83-1.

Pharmacopoeias. In *Br., It., Jpn,* and *US.*

A white or creamy-white powder. Pentazocine 100 mg is approximately equivalent to 112.8 mg of pentazocine hydrochloride or 131.6 mg of pentazocine lactate.

Soluble 1 in more than 1000 of water, 1 in 11 of alcohol, 1 in 2 of chloroform, and 1 in 42 of ether; soluble in acetone; sparingly soluble in ethyl acetate. **Store** in airtight containers. Protect from light.

Pentazocine Hydrochloride (6252-y)

Pentazocine Hydrochloride *(BANM, USAN, rINNM)*.

$C_{19}H_{27}NO,HCl$ = 321.9.

CAS — 2276-52-0; 64024-15-3.

Pharmacopoeias. In *Br., It.,* and *US.*

A white or pale cream crystalline powder. **Soluble** 1 in 30 of water, 1 in 20 of alcohol, 1 in 4 of chloroform; practically insoluble in ether; very slightly soluble in acetone. A 1% solution in water has a pH of 4.0 to 6.0. **Store** in airtight containers. Protect from light.

Pentazocine Lactate (6253-j)

Pentazocine Lactate *(BANM, USAN, rINNM)*.

$C_{19}H_{27}NO,C_3H_6O_3$ = 375.5.

CAS — 17146-95-1.

Pharmacopoeias. In *Br.*

A white to pale cream powder. Sparingly **soluble** in water, in alcohol, and in chloroform; freely soluble in methyl alcohol. Dissolves in aqueous solution of alkali hydroxides. A 1% solution in water has a pH of 5.5 to 6.5.

Incompatibility. Commercial injections of pentazocine lactate are reported to be incompatible with soluble barbiturates and other alkaline substances including sodium bicarbonate. Diazepam and chlordiazepoxide have also been reported to be incompatible, as have glycopyrronium bromide[1] and nafcillin sodium.[2]

1. Ingallinera TS, *et al.* Compatibility of glycopyrrolate injection with commonly used infusion solutions and additives. *Am J Hosp Pharm* 1979; **36:** 508–10.
2. Jeglum EL, *et al.* Nafcillin sodium incompatibility with acidic solutions. *Am J Hosp Pharm* 1981; **38:** 462, 464.

Dependence and Withdrawal

As for Opioid Analgesics, p.67. Pentazocine is subject to abuse.

Pentazocine does produce physical dependence, but withdrawal symptoms are substantially less severe than with morphine. It does not typically produce drug-seeking behaviour of the same degree or intensity as morphine or other prototypic μ agonists, nor does it substitute for morphine in dependent subjects.[1] Pentazocine injection has been abused,[2] but street abuse, especially in the USA, has more often involved the intravenous use of crushed tablets of pentazocine and tripelennamine ('T's and Blues').[3-5] A decreased incidence of pentazocine abuse in the USA appeared to coincide with the introduction of oral tablets incorporating naloxone,[1] the rationale being that naloxone antagonises the effect of pentazocine if illicitly injected, but has no effect when taken by mouth. Some continued to abuse the new pentazocine/naloxone formulation;[6] intravenous abuse in one woman, who was unaware of the reformulation, resulted in opioid withdrawal symptoms and severe hypertension.[7] A 1989 report from the WHO committee[1] rated the likelihood of abuse of pentazocine as moderate, based on its pharmacological profile, dependence potential, and actual abuse. The committee considered that it should continue to be scheduled as a psychotropic substance rather than a narcotic drug.

1. WHO. WHO expert committee on drug dependence: twenty-fifth report. *WHO Tech Rep Ser 775* 1989.
2. Hunter R, Ingram IM. Intravenous pentazocine abuse by a nurse. *Lancet* 1983; **ii:** 227.
3. Poklis A, Whyatt PL. Current trends in the abuse of pentazocine and tripelennamine: the metropolitan St. Louis experience. *J Forensic Sci* 1980; **25:** 72–8.
4. Senay EC. Clinical experience with T's and B's. *Drug Alcohol Depend* 1985; **14:** 305–11.
5. Jackson C, *et al.* Fatal intracranial hemorrhage associated with phenylpropanolamine, pentazocine, and tripelennamine overdose. *J Emerg Med* 1985; **3:** 127–32.
6. Reed DA, Schnoll SH. Abuse of pentazocine-naloxone combination. *JAMA* 1986; **256:** 2562–4.
7. Reinhart S, Barrett SM. An acute hypertensive response after intravenous use of a new pentazocine formulation. *Ann Emerg Med* 1985; **14:** 591–3.

Adverse Effects

As for Opioid Analgesics in general, p.68.

Pentazocine may cause hallucinations and other psychotomimetic effects such as nightmares and thought disturbances. High doses may result in hypertension and tachycardia; increased aortic and pulmonary artery pressure with an increase in cardiac work has followed intravenous administration in patients with myocardial infarction. As with morphine respiratory depression occurs, but pentazocine is said to have a 'ceiling' effect in that the depth of respiratory depression does not increase proportionately with higher doses.

Rare adverse effects with pentazocine have included agranulocytosis and toxic epidermal necrolysis.

Pentazocine injections may be painful. Local tissue damage may occur at injection sites particularly after subcutaneous injection or multiple doses; there have been reports of muscle fibrosis associated with intramuscular injections.

Effects on the blood. There have been reports of agranulocytosis associated with pentazocine.[1-3]

1. Marks A, Abramson N. Pentazocine and agranulocytosis. *Ann Intern Med* 1980; **92:** 433.
2. Haibach H, *et al.* Pentazocine-induced agranulocytosis. *Can Med Assoc J* 1984; **130:** 1165–6.
3. Sheehan M, *et al.* Pentazocine-induced agranulocytosis. *Can Med Assoc J* 1985; **132:** 1401.

Effects on the CNS. A report of oculogyric crisis associated with the use of pentazocine.[1]

1. Burstein AH, Fullerton T. Oculogyric crisis possibly related to pentazocine. *Ann Pharmacother* 1993; **27:** 874–6.

Effects on the skin. Toxic epidermal necrolysis in a 62-year-old man was attributed to pentazocine;[1] he had taken 50 to 75 mg every 4 hours for 8 days. His severe uraemia was attributed to fluid loss through the skin.

1. Hunter JAA, Davison AM. Toxic epidermal necrolysis associated with pentazocine therapy and severe reversible renal failure. *Br J Dermatol* 1973; **88:** 287–90.

Treatment of Adverse Effects

As for Opioid Analgesics in general, p.68. Because pentazocine has opioid agonist and antagonist activity, naloxone is the recommended antagonist for the treatment of overdosage.

Precautions

As for Opioid Analgesics in general, p.68.

Pentazocine has weak opioid antagonist actions and may precipitate withdrawal symptoms if given to patients who are physically dependent on opioids. It should generally be avoided after myocardial infarction and in patients with heart failure or arterial or pulmonary hypertension.

When frequent injections are needed, pentazocine should be given intramuscularly rather than subcutaneously and the injection sites should be varied.

Abuse. See under Dependence and Withdrawal, above.

Porphyria. Pentazocine has been associated with acute attacks of porphyria and is considered unsafe in patients with acute porphyria.[1]

1. Moore MR, McColl KEL. *Porphyria: drug lists.* Glasgow: Porphyria Research Unit, University of Glasgow, 1991.

Interactions

For interactions associated with opioid analgesics, see p.69.

Tobacco smoking. Evidence that smokers metabolised about 40% more pentazocine than non-smokers, although there was large inter-subject variation;[1] tobacco smoking might induce liver enzymes responsible for drug oxidation.[1]

1. Vaughan DP, *et al.* The influence of smoking on the inter-subject variation in pentazocine elimination. *Br J Clin Pharmacol* 1976; **3:** 279–83.

Pharmacokinetics

Pentazocine is absorbed from the gastro-intestinal tract; following administration by mouth, peak plasma concentrations are reached in 1 to 3 hours and the half-life is reported to be about 4 hours. After intramuscular injection, peak plasma concentrations are reached in 15 minutes to 1 hour. About 60% has been reported to be bound to plasma protein. Pentazocine undergoes extensive first-pass metabolism in the liver; oral bioavailability is low with only about half of a dose reaching the systemic circulation. Metabolites and a small amount of unchanged drug are excreted in the urine. It diffuses across the placenta.

References.

1. Ehrnebo M, *et al.* Pentazocine binding to blood cells and plasma proteins. *Clin Pharmacol Ther* 1974; **16:** 424–9.
2. Ehrnebo M, *et al.* Bioavailability and first-pass metabolism of oral pentazocine in man. *Clin Pharmacol Ther* 1977; **22:** 888–92.
3. Bullingham RES, *et al.* Clinical pharmacokinetics of narcotic agonist-antagonist drugs. *Clin Pharmacokinet* 1983; **8:** 332–43.

Administration in hepatic impairment. Clearance of pentazocine was significantly reduced and terminal half-life and oral bioavailability increased in cirrhotic patients when compared with healthy subjects.[1]

1. Neal EA, *et al.* Enhanced bioavailability and decreased clearance of analgesics in patients with cirrhosis. *Gastroenterology* 1979; **77:** 96–102.

Uses and Administration

Pentazocine, a benzomorphan derivative, is an opioid analgesic (p.69) that has mixed opioid agonist/antagonist actions. Agonist activity is thought to be predominantly at κ opioid receptors (with possibly some σ receptor activity); it acts as a weak antagonist or partial agonist at μ receptors. Pentazocine is used for the relief of moderate to severe pain. It may also be used for pre-operative sedation and as an adjunct to anaesthesia. Its analgesic effect declines more rapidly than that of morphine.

Pentazocine is administered by mouth as the hydrochloride. A usual dose is 25 to 100 mg of pentazocine hydrochloride every 3 to 4 hours after food. Children aged 6 to 12 years may be given 25 mg every 3 to 4 hours.

Pentazocine is also administered by subcutaneous, intramuscular, and intravenous injection as the lactate. The usual dose is the equivalent of pentazocine 30 to 60 mg every 3 to 4 hours; it should not be necessary to exceed 360 mg daily. Also if frequent injections are needed, the intramuscular route should be used rather than the subcutaneous route, and the injection sites should be varied. In the USA single intravenous doses of not more than 30 mg are advised. For children over 1 year, the maximum single dose should not exceed 1 mg per kg body-weight subcutaneously or intramuscularly, or 500 μg per kg intravenously.

Pentazocine is also given rectally as the lactate in suppositories usually in a dose of the equivalent of pentazocine 50 mg up to 4 times daily.

As a deterrent to abuse a combined oral preparation of pentazocine hydrochloride and naloxone hydrochloride is available in some countries.

Preparations

BP 1998: Pentazocine Capsules; Pentazocine Injection; Pentazocine Suppositories; Pentazocine Tablets;

USP 23: Pentazocine and Naloxone Hydrochlorides Tablets; Pentazocine Hydrochloride and Aspirin Tablets; Pentazocine Hydrochloride Tablets; Pentazocine Lactate Injection.

Proprietary Preparations (details are given in Part 3)

Aust.: Fortral; ***Austral.:*** Fortral; ***Belg.:*** Fortal; ***Canad.:*** Talwin; ***Fr.:*** Fortal; ***Ger.:*** Fortral; ***Irl.:*** Fortral; ***Ital.:*** Liticon†; Pentafen; Pentalgina; Talwin; Talwin-Tab; ***Neth.:*** Fortral; ***Norw.:*** Fortralin;

S.Afr.: Opsronim; Sosenol; ***Spain:*** Sosegon; ***Swed.:*** Fortalgesic; ***Switz.:*** Fortalgesic; ***UK:*** Fortral†; ***USA:*** Talwin; Talwin NX.

Multi-ingredient: ***Irl.:*** Fortagesic; ***USA:*** Emergent-Ez; Talacen; Talwin Compound.

Pethidine Hydrochloride (6254-z)

Pethidine Hydrochloride *(BANM, rINNM).*

Meperidine Hydrochloride; Pethidini Hydrochloridum. Ethyl 1-methyl-4-phenylpiperidine-4-carboxylate hydrochloride.

$C_{15}H_{21}NO_2,HCl = 283.8.$

CAS — 57-42-1 (pethidine); 50-13-5 (pethidine hydrochloride).

Pharmacopoeias. In *Chin., Eur.* (see p.viii), *Int., Jpn, Pol.,* and *US.*

A fine white odourless crystalline powder.

Ph. Eur. **solubilities:** very soluble in water; freely soluble in alcohol; practically insoluble in ether. USP solubilities: very soluble in water; soluble in alcohol; sparingly soluble in ether. A 5% solution has a pH of about 5. **Store** in airtight containers. Protect from light.

Incompatibility. Solutions of pethidine hydrochloride are acidic. They are incompatible with barbiturate salts and loss of clarity was also observed in an early additive study[1] with other drugs including aminophylline, heparin sodium, methicillin sodium, morphine sulphate, nitrofurantoin sodium, phenytoin sodium, sodium iodide, sulphadiazine sodium, and sulphafurazole diethanolamine. Colour change from pale yellow to light green occurred when solutions of minocycline hydrochloride or tetracycline hydrochloride were mixed with pethidine hydrochloride in 5% glucose injection.[2] In the same study an immediate precipitate occurred on admixture with cefoperazone sodium or mezlocillin sodium; with nafcillin sodium an immediate cloudy appearance cleared on agitation. Incompatibility has also been observed between pethidine hydrochloride and aciclovir sodium, imipenem, frusemide,[3] liposomal doxorubicin hydrochloride,[4] and idarubicin.[5] Solutions of cefazolin sodium[6] and pethidine hydrochloride mixed in 5% glucose injection turned light yellow after 5 days storage at 25°; the admixture was stable for at least 20 days at 4°.

1. Patel JA, Phillips GL. A guide to physical compatibility of intravenous drug admixtures. *Am J Hosp Pharm* 1966; **23:** 409–11.
2. Nieves-Cordero AL, *et al.* Compatibility of narcotic analgesic solutions with various antibiotics during simulated Y-site injection. *Am J Hosp Pharm* 1985; **42:** 1108–9.
3. Pugh CB, *et al.* Visual compatibility of morphine sulfate and meperidine hydrochloride with other injectable drugs during simulated Y-site injection. *Am J Hosp Pharm* 1991; **48:** 123–5.
4. Trissel LA, *et al.* Compatibility of doxorubicin hydrochloride liposome injection with selected other drugs during simulated Y-site administration. *Am J Health-Syst Pharm* 1997; **54:** 2708–13.
5. Turowski RC, Durthaler JM. Visual compatibility of idarubicin hydrochloride with selected drugs during simulated Y-site injection. *Am J Hosp Pharm* 1991; **48:** 2181–4.
6. Lee DKT, *et al.* Stability of cefazolin sodium and meperidine hydrochloride. *Am J Health-Syst Pharm* 1996; **53:** 1608–10.

Stability. Pethidine hydrochloride injection 100 mg per mL was stable for at least 24 hours at room temperature when diluted to a concentration of 300 mg per litre in glucose 5% and 4% and in sodium chloride injection (0.9%) and sodium chloride injection (0.9%) diluted 1 in 5.[1]

Accelerated stability studies using elevated temperatures and humidities to simulate tropical conditions classified pethidine hydrochloride as a 'less stable drug substance'.[2] It was suggested that during quality assurance of preparations containing pethidine hydrochloride particular attention should be paid to their stability.

1. Rudd L, Simpson P. Pethidine stability in intravenous solutions. *Med J Aust* 1978; **2:** 34.
2. WHO. WHO expert committee on specifications for pharmaceutical preparations: thirty-first report. *WHO Tech Rep Ser 790* 1990.

Dependence and Withdrawal

As for Opioid Analgesics, p.67. Doses of pethidine as large as 3 or 4 g daily have been taken by addicts. As tolerance to the CNS stimulant and antimuscarinic effects is not complete with these very large doses, muscle twitching, tremor, mental confusion, dilated pupils, and sometimes convulsions may be present.

Withdrawal symptoms appear more rapidly than with morphine and are of shorter duration.

For the abuse of pethidine analogues, see under Precautions, below.

Adverse Effects and Treatment

As for Opioid Analgesics in general, p.68.

The effects on smooth muscle may be relatively less intense than with morphine and constipation occurs less frequently. After overdosage, symptoms are generally similar to those of morphine poisoning. However, stimulation of the CNS and convulsions may also occur, especially in tolerant individuals or following toxic doses by mouth; these have been attributed mainly to the metabolite norpethidine. Local reactions often follow injection of pethidine; general hypersensitivity reactions occur rarely. The intravenous administration of pethidine may result in increased heart rate.

The incidence of adverse effects in hospitalised patients receiving pethidine was monitored by the Boston Collaborative Drug Surveillance Program.[1] Following pethidine by mouth adverse reactions were reported in 16 of 366 patients and mainly involved the gastro-intestinal tract. Following pethidine by injection 102 of 3268 patients had adverse effects, the central nervous system being involved in 38.

1. Miller RR, Jick H. Clinical effects of meperidine in hospitalized medical patients. *J Clin Pharmacol* 1978; **18:** 180–9.

Effects on the cardiovascular system. Histamine release was more frequent after pethidine than after morphine, fentanyl, or sufentanil administered intravenously for the induction of anaesthesia.[1] Increased plasma-histamine concentrations occurred in 5 of 16 patients given pethidine in a mean dose of 4.3 mg per kg body-weight and were generally accompanied by hypotension, tachycardia, erythema, and increased plasma-adrenaline concentrations. Only 1 of 10 given morphine and none of those receiving fentanyl or sufentanil showed evidence of histamine release. All of the histamine releasers were young women.

1. Flacke JW, *et al.* Histamine release by four narcotics: a double-blind study in humans. *Anesth Analg* 1987; **66:** 723–30.

Effects on the nervous system. CNS excitatory effects of pethidine such as tremors, muscle twitches, and convulsions have been associated with toxic doses and have been attributed to the metabolite norpethidine. Accumulation of norpethidine may occur if large doses of pethidine are repeated at short intervals and is especially likely when renal function is impaired.[1-10]

1. Kaiko RF, *et al.* Central nervous system excitatory effects of meperidine in cancer patients. *Ann Neurol* 1983; **13:** 180–5.
2. Lieberman AN, Goldstein M. Reversible parkinsonism related to meperidine. *N Engl J Med* 1985; **312:** 509.
3. Mauro VF, *et al.* Meperidine-induced seizure in a patient without renal dysfunction or sickle cell anemia. *Clin Pharm* 1986; **5:** 837–9.
4. Morisy L, Platt D. Hazards of high-dose meperidine. *JAMA* 1986; **255:** 467–8.
5. Armstrong PJ, Bersten A. Normeperidine toxicity. *Anesth Analg* 1986; **65:** 536–8.
6. Eisendrath SJ, *et al.* Meperidine-induced delirium. *Am J Psychiatry* 1987; **144:** 1062–5.
7. Kyff JV, Rice TL. Meperidine-associated seizures in a child. *Clin Pharm* 1990; **9:** 337–8.
8. Pryle BJ, *et al.* Toxicity of norpethidine in sickle cell crisis. *Br Med J* 1992; **304:** 1478–9.
9. Hagmeyer KO, *et al.* Meperidine-related seizures associated with patient-controlled analgesia pumps. *Ann Pharmacother* 1993; **27:** 29–32.
10. Stone PA, *et al.* Norpethidine toxicity and patient controlled analgesia. *Br J Anaesth* 1993; **71:** 738–40.

Precautions

As for Opioid Analgesics in general, p.68.

It should also be given cautiously to patients with supraventricular tachycardia or with a history of convulsive disorders.

Abuse. A synthetic analogue of pethidine, MPPP (1-methyl-4-phenyl-4-propionoxypiperidine), manufactured illicitly for recreational use, achieved notoriety when it was accidentally contaminated with MPTP (1-methyl-4-phenyl-1,2,3,6-tetrahydropyridine) leading to an epidemic of parkinsonism among intravenous drug abusers.[1] The World Health Organization has also identified another analogue, PEPAP (1-phenylethyl-4-phenyl-4-acetoxypiperidine) as being liable to abuse.[2]

1. Buchanan JF, Brown CR. 'Designer drugs': a problem in clinical toxicology. *Med Toxicol* 1988; **3:** 1–17.
2. WHO. WHO expert committee on drug dependence: twenty-fourth report. *WHO Tech Rep Ser 761* 1988.

Elderly. Pethidine had a slower elimination rate in elderly compared with young patients and a reduction in total daily dose might be necessary in elderly patients receiving repeated doses of pethidine.[1] Another study concluded that age-related changes in disposition were not sufficient to warrant modification of pethidine dosage regimens.[2]

1. Holmberg L, *et al.* Comparative disposition of pethidine and norpethidine in old and young patients. *Eur J Clin Pharmacol* 1982; **22:** 175–9.
2. Herman RJ, *et al.* Effects of age on meperidine disposition. *Clin Pharmacol Ther* 1985; **37:** 19–24.

Phaeochromocytoma. Pethidine provoked episodes of hypertension in a patient with phaeochromocytoma; the effect was suppressed by labetalol.[1] Like other histamine-releasing opioids, pethidine should be used with caution in such patients.

1. Lawrence CA. Pethidine-induced hypertension in phaeochromocytoma. *Br Med J* 1978; **1:** 149–50.

Pregnancy and the neonate. Pethidine is widely used for analgesia during labour. It rapidly crosses the placenta and like other opioid analgesics may cause respiratory depression in the neonate although this may be less than with morphine. Respiratory depression varies according to the timing and size of the maternal dose.

Fetal depression was not apparent when delivery occurred within 1 hour of pethidine administration, but was present in 6 of 24 infants delivered 1 to 3 hours after injection and in all of 5 infants delivered 3 to 6 hours after injection.[1] Cooper *et al.*[2] noted higher blood concentrations of pethidine in infants delivered within 1 hour of a single dose of pethidine 150 mg intramuscularly when compared with those born following administration 1 to 4 hours before delivery. The role of pethidine metabolites is not certain, but relatively little of a dose might have been metabolised by the mother within 1 hour. Hogg *et al.*[3] reported that neonates appeared able to metabolise pethidine although probably more slowly than adults. They also showed that the amounts of pethidine and norpethidine excreted by the neonate increased significantly with the maternal dose-delivery interval for intervals of up to 5 hours and considered that most of the placentally transferred pethidine should be excreted by the third day. Elimination of pethidine took up to 6 days in the neonates studied by Cooper *et al.*[2] In another study,[4] depressed neonatal responses persisted for the first 2 days of life; depression was dose-related being greatest with the highest dose of pethidine (75 to 150 mg within 4 hours of delivery).

Further references on the transplacental transfer of pethidine can be found under Pregnancy in Pharmacokinetics, below.

Neither psychological nor physical effects were found in 5-year-old children of mothers who had received pethidine during labour.[5] Neonatal behaviour does not appear to have been affected significantly by pethidine, although it has been acknowledged that the relationship between maternal analgesia in labour and subsequent infant behaviour is by no means simple.[6] The results of early studies which suggested an excess of cases of cancer in children whose mothers received pethidine during labour have been refuted by a more recent and larger study.[7]

1. Morrison JC, *et al.* Metabolites of meperidine related to fetal depression. *Am J Obstet Gynecol* 1973; **115:** 1132–7.
2. Cooper LV, *et al.* Elimination of pethidine and bupivacaine in the newborn. *Arch Dis Child* 1977; **52:** 638–41.
3. Hogg MIJ, *et al.* Urinary excretion and metabolism of pethidine and norpethidine in the newborn. *Br J Anaesth* 1977; **49:** 891–9.
4. Hodgkinson R, *et al.* Double-blind comparison of the neurobehaviour of neonates following the administration of different doses of meperidine to the mother. *Can Anaesth Soc J* 1978; **25:** 405–11.
5. Buck C. Drugs in pregnancy. *Can Med Assoc J* 1975; **112:** 1285.
6. Anonymous. To measure life. *Lancet* 1981; **ii:** 291–2.
7. Golding J, *et al.* Childhood cancer, intramuscular vitamin K, and pethidine given during labour. *Br Med J* 1992; **305:** 341–6.

Renal impairment. Caution is necessary when pethidine is given to patients with renal impairment. Evidence of CNS excitation, including seizures and twitches, in 2 patients with renal insufficiency receiving multiple doses of pethidine was attributed to accumulation of the metabolite norpethidine; they both had high norpethidine : pethidine plasma concentration ratios.[1]

See also under Pharmacokinetics, below.

1. Szeto HH, *et al.* Accumulation of normeperidine, an active metabolite of meperidine, in patients with renal failure or cancer. *Ann Intern Med* 1977; **86:** 738–41.

Interactions

For interactions associated with opioid analgesics, see p.69.

Very severe reactions, including coma, severe respiratory depression, cyanosis, and hypotension have occurred in patients receiving MAOIs (including moclobemide) and given pethidine. There are also reports of hyperexcitability, convulsions, tachycardia, hyperpyrexia, and hypertension. Pethidine should not be given to patients receiving MAOIs or within 14 days of their discontinuation. Concurrent administration of pethidine and phenothiazines has produced severe hypotensive episodes and may prolong the respiratory depression due to pethidine.

Plasma concentrations of pethidine are increased by ritonavir, with a resultant risk of toxicity; concomitant administration should be avoided.

Barbiturates. Opioid analgesics and barbiturates can be expected to have additive CNS depressant effects. Prolonged sedation with pethidine in the presence of phenobarbitone has also been attributed to induction of *N*-demethylation of pethidine, resulting in the enhanced formation of the potentially neurotoxic metabolite norpethidine.[1,2]

1. Stambaugh JE, *et al.* A potentially toxic drug interaction between pethidine (meperidine) and phenobarbitone. *Lancet* 1977; **i:** 398–9.
2. Stambaugh JE, *et al.* The effect of phenobarbital on the metabolism of meperidine in normal volunteers. *J Clin Pharmacol* 1978; **18:** 482–90.

Histamine H_2 Antagonists. Cimetidine reduced the clearance and volume of distribution of pethidine in healthy subjects,[1] whereas ranitidine did not.[2]

1. Guay DRP, *et al.* Cimetidine alters pethidine disposition in man. *Br J Clin Pharmacol* 1984; **18:** 907–14.
2. Guay DRP, *et al.* Ranitidine does not alter pethidine disposition in man. *Br J Clin Pharmacol* 1985; **20:** 55–9.

MAOIs. Some of the most serious interactions involving pethidine have been with non-selective MAOIs and have been manifest as enhanced depressant effects or hyperexcitability (see above). However, a life-threatening interaction has also been reported between pethidine and selegiline, a selective monoamine oxidase type B inhibitor.[1] Also, symptoms suggestive of a mild serotonin syndrome developed in a 73-year-old woman taking moclobemide (a reversible inhibitor of monoamine oxidase), nortriptyline, and lithium after she was given pethidine intravenously.[2]

1. Zornberg GL, *et al.* Severe adverse interaction between pethidine and selegiline. *Lancet* 1991; **337:** 246. Correction. *ibid.*; 440.
2. Gillman PK. Possible serotonin syndrome with moclobemide and pethidine. *Med J Aust* 1995; **162:** 554.

Phenothiazines. Prochlorperazine prolonged the respiratory depressant effect of pethidine in healthy subjects.[1] Enhanced CNS depression and hypotension were reported when healthy subjects were given chlorpromazine in addition to pethidine; there was evidence of increased *N*-demethylation of pethidine.[2]

1. Steen SN, Yates M. Effects of benzquinamide and prochlorperazine, separately and combined with meperidine, on the human respiratory center. *Clin Pharmacol Ther* 1972; **13:** 153.
2. Stambaugh JE, Wainer IW. Drug interaction: meperidine and chlorpromazine, a toxic combination. *J Clin Pharmacol* 1981; **21:** 140–6.

Phenytoin. The hepatic metabolism of pethidine appears to be enhanced by phenytoin. Concomitant administration resulted in reduced half-life and bioavailability in healthy subjects; blood concentrations of norpethidine were increased.[1]

1. Pond SM, Kretschzmar KM. Effect of phenytoin on meperidine clearance and normeperidine formation. *Clin Pharmacol Ther* 1981; **30:** 680–6.

Pharmacokinetics

Pethidine hydrochloride is absorbed from the gastro-intestinal tract, but only about 50% of the drug reaches the systemic circulation because of first-pass metabolism. Absorption following intramuscular injection is variable. Peak plasma concentrations have been reported 1 to 2 hours after oral administration. It is about 60 to 80% bound to plasma proteins.

Pethidine is metabolised in the liver by hydrolysis to pethidinic acid (meperidinic acid) or demethylation to norpethidine (normeperidine) and hydrolysis to norpethidinic acid (normeperidinic acid), followed by partial conjugation with glucuronic acid. Norpethidine is pharmacologically active and its accumulation may result in toxicity. Pethidine is reported to have a plasma elimination half-life of about 3 to 6 hours in healthy subjects; the metabolite norpethidine is eliminated more slowly, with a half-life reported to be up to about 20 hours. Both pethidine and norpethidine appear in the cerebrospinal fluid. At the usual values of urinary pH or if the urine is alkaline, only a small amount of pethidine is excreted unchanged; urinary excretion of pethidine and norpethidine is enhanced by acidification of the urine. Pethidine crosses the placenta and is distributed into breast milk.

Reviews of the pharmacokinetics of pethidine.

1. Edwards DJ, *et al.* Clinical pharmacokinetics of pethidine: 1982. *Clin Pharmacokinet* 1982; **7:** 421–33.
2. Moore RA, *et al.* Opiate metabolism and excretion. *Baillieres Clin Anaesthesiol* 1987; **1:** 829–58.

Administration. The elimination half-life of pethidine was prolonged and plasma clearance decreased when given perioperatively compared with postoperatively.[1]

During labour the pharmacokinetics of pethidine may depend on the method of administration. In a comparison of intramuscular injection at different sites, absorption of pethidine from the gluteus muscle was impaired and the deltoid muscle was preferred.[2]

No statistically significant differences were found in pharmacokinetic parameters for deltoid and gluteal intramuscular injections in elderly postoperative patients.[3] However, substantial interpatient variability was noted for both sites, and the authors suggested that more rapid and predictable routes such as intravenous injection may be more appropriate for postoperative use in the elderly.

1. Tamsen A, *et al.* Patient-controlled analgesic therapy, part 1: pharmacokinetics of pethidine in the per- and postoperative periods. *Clin Pharmacokinet* 1982; **7:** 149–63.
2. Lazebnik N, *et al.* Intravenous, deltoid, or gluteus administration of meperidine during labor? *Am J Obstet Gynecol* 1989; **160:** 1184–9.
3. Erstad BL, *et al.* Site-specific pharmacokinetics and pharmacodynamics of intramuscular meperidine in elderly postoperative patients. *Ann Pharmacother* 1997; **31:** 23–8.

Administration in hepatic impairment. The terminal half-life of pethidine was prolonged to about 7 hours in cirrhotic patients compared with 3 hours in healthy subjects and was attributed to impairment of the drug-metabolising activity of the liver.[1] Another study concluded that although impaired hepatic metabolism might confer relative protection from norpethidine toxicity in patients with cirrhosis, there might be an increased risk of cumulative toxicity because of slow elimination of the metabolite.[2]

1. Klotz U, *et al.* The effect of cirrhosis on the disposition and elimination of meperidine in man. *Clin Pharmacol Ther* 1974; **16:** 667–75.
2. Pond SM, *et al.* Presystemic metabolism of meperidine to normeperidine in normal and cirrhotic subjects. *Clin Pharmacol Ther* 1981; **30:** 183–8.

Administration in renal impairment. Plasma protein binding of pethidine was reported to be decreased in renal disease and ranged from 58.2% in healthy subjects to 31.8% in anuric patients.[1] The same workers also reported impaired elimination of pethidine in patients with renal dysfunction.[2]

See also under Precautions, above.

1. Chan K, *et al.* Plasma protein binding of pethidine in patients with renal disease. *J Pharm Pharmacol* 1983; **35:** 94P.
2. Chan K, *et al.* The influence of renal dysfunction on the disposition of pethidine in man. *Br J Clin Pharmacol* 1984; **17:** 198P.

Pregnancy. Some references to the pharmacokinetics of pethidine during labour are given below.

1. Tomson G, *et al.* Maternal kinetics and transplacental passage of pethidine during labour. *Br J Clin Pharmacol* 1982; **13:** 653–9.
2. Kuhnert BR, *et al.* Disposition of meperidine and normeperidine following multiple doses during labor: I mother. *Am J Obstet Gynecol* 1985; **151:** 406–9.
3. Kuhnert BR, *et al.* Disposition of meperidine and normeperidine following multiple doses during labor: II fetus and neonate. *Am J Obstet Gynecol* 1985; **151:** 410–15.

Uses and Administration

Pethidine hydrochloride, a phenylpiperidine derivative, is a synthetic opioid analgesic (p.69) that acts mainly as a μ opioid agonist. Pethidine is used for the relief of most types of moderate to severe acute pain including the pain of labour. It is more lipid soluble than morphine and has a less potent and shorter lasting analgesic effect; analgesia usually lasts for 2 to 4 hours. Its short duration of action and accumulation of its potentially neurotoxic metabolite norpethidine on repeated administration make it unsuitable for the management of chronic pain. Pethidine has a weaker action on smooth muscle than morphine and its lower potential to increase biliary pressure makes it suitable when opioid analgesics are required to manage pain associated with biliary colic and pancreatitis. It is also used as pre-operative medication and as an adjunct to anaesthesia. It has been given with phenothiazines such as promethazine to achieve basal narcosis. Pethidine has little effect on cough or on diarrhoea.

For the relief of pain, pethidine hydrochloride is given in doses of 50 to 150 mg by mouth every 4 hours. It may also be given by intramuscular or subcutaneous injection in doses of 25 to 100 mg and by slow intravenous injection in doses of 25 to 50 mg repeated after 4 hours. For postoperative pain the subcutaneous or intramuscular doses may be given every 2 to 3 hours if necessary. In children, doses of 0.5 to 2 mg per kg body-weight may be given by mouth or by intramuscular injection.

In obstetric analgesia 50 to 100 mg may be given by intramuscular or subcutaneous injection as soon as contractions occur at regular intervals. This dose may be repeated after 1 to 3 hours if necessary up to a maximum of 400 mg in 24 hours.

For pre-operative medication 25 to 100 mg may be given intramuscularly or subcutaneously about 1 hour before operation; children may be given 0.5 to 2 mg per kg. As an adjunct to nitrous oxide-oxygen anaesthesia 10 to 25 mg may be given by slow intravenous injection.

Administration. In addition to conventional routes of administration pethidine has been given epidurally[1-4] and intrathecally.[5] It has also been given intravenously[6,7] and intranasally[8] by patient-controlled analgesia. However, some consider that the use of pethidine should be avoided in patient-controlled analgesia because of the increased risk of norpethidine-induced seizures[9] (see also under Effects on the Nervous System, above).

1. Perriss BW. Epidural pethidine in labour: a study of dose requirements. *Anaesthesia* 1980; **35:** 380–2.
2. Husemeyer RP, *et al.* A study of pethidine kinetics and analgesia in women in labour following intravenous, intramuscular and epidural administration. *Br J Clin Pharmacol* 1982; **13:** 171–6.
3. Perriss BW, *et al.* Analgesia following extradural and im pethidine in post-caesarean section patients. *Br J Anaesth* 1990; **64:** 355–7.
4. Blythe JG, *et al.* Continuous postoperative epidural analgesia for gynecologic oncology patients. *Gynecol Oncol* 1990; **37:** 307–10.
5. Acalovschi I, *et al.* Saddle block with pethidine for perineal operations. *Br J Anaesth* 1986; **58:** 1012–16.
6. Tamsen A, *et al.* Patient-controlled analgesic therapy, part II: individual analgesic demand and analgesic plasma concentrations of pethidine in postoperative pain. *Clin Pharmacokinet* 1982; **7:** 164–75.
7. Rayburn W, *et al.* Intravenous meperidine during labor: a randomized comparison between nursing- and patient-controlled administration. *Obstet Gynecol* 1989; **74:** 702–6.
8. Striebel WH, *et al.* Intranasal meperidine titration for postoperative pain relief. *Anesth Analg* 1993; **76:** 1047–51.
9. Hagmeyer KO, *et al.* Meperidine-related seizures associated with patient-controlled analgesia pumps. *Ann Pharmacother* 1993; **27:** 29–32.

Eclampsia and pre-eclampsia. See Lytic Cocktails under Sedation, below.

Pain. Pethidine may be preferred to morphine when rapid control of acute pain is required. It is widely used in obstetrics to control the pain of labour and for postoperative pain relief following caesarean section or other surgical procedures.

In a study of patients with intractable pain the minimum effective analgesic blood concentration ranged from 100 to 820 ng per mL (median 250 ng per mL) in 15 of 16; the remaining patient failed to obtain analgesia with pethidine. Additional measures were considered necessary[1] if the minimum effective concentration exceeded 400 ng per mL.

Pethidine has traditionally been given by intermittent intramuscular injection in the treatment of acute pain, but inconsistent pain relief can be expected because of fluctuating blood-pethidine concentrations;[2] continuous intravenous infusion might be more effective for acute pain. For reference to various routes of administration, see Administration, above.

1. Mather LE, Glynn CJ. The minimum effective analgesic blood concentration of pethidine in patients with intractable pain. *Br J Clin Pharmacol* 1982; **14:** 385–90.
2. Edwards DJ, *et al.* Clinical pharmacokinetics of pethidine: 1982. *Clin Pharmacokinet* 1982; **7:** 421–33.

SICKLE-CELL CRISIS. Concern has been expressed over the continued use of pethidine for analgesia in painful crises in sickle-cell disease. Control of pain may be inadequate and doses commonly used to manage crises may lead to accumulation of the neuroexcitatory metabolite of pethidine and precipitate seizures.[1,2] See also under Effects on the Nervous System, above.

1. Pryle BJ, *et al.* Toxicity of norpethidine in sickle cell crisis. *Br Med J* 1992; **304:** 1478–9.
2. Harrison JFM, *et al.* Pethidine in sickle cell crisis. *Br Med J* 1992; **305:** 182.

Sedation. Some references to the use of pethidine for endoscopy are given below.

1. Chokhavatia S, *et al.* Sedation and analgesia for gastrointestinal endoscopy. *Am J Gastroenterol* 1993; **88:** 393–6.
2. Bahal-O'Mara N, *et al.* Sedation with meperidine and midazolam in pediatric patients undergoing endoscopy. *Eur J Clin Pharmacol* 1994; **47:** 319–23.

LYTIC COCKTAILS. Lytic cocktails consisting of chlorpromazine, pethidine, and/or promethazine have been given intravenously in some countries for the management of pre-eclampsia and imminent eclampsia.[1] However, the use of phenothiazines is generally not recommended late in pregnancy. The more usual treatment of pre-eclampsia and eclampsia is primarily aimed at reducing hypertension (see Hypertension in Pregnancy, under Hypertension, p.788); the management of eclampsia, which is the convulsive phase, is discussed on p.338.

Lytic cocktails have also been used for sedation and analgesia in paediatric patients, generally by the intramuscular route, although intravenous injections have also been used. However, there is a high rate of therapeutic failure as well as serious adverse effects with such combinations, and the American Academy of Pediatrics[2] has recommended that alternative sedatives and analgesics should be considered; guidelines have been drawn up should it be appropriate to use a lytic cocktail. Lytic cocktails are not the most appropriate means of sedation for short procedures since patients must be monitored for approximately one hour before the procedure while the drugs take effect, and for even longer during the recovery period.[3]

1. WHO. The hypertensive disorders of pregnancy. *WHO Tech Rep Ser 758* 1987.
2. American Academy of Pediatrics Committee on Drugs. Reappraisal of Lytic cocktail/Demerol, Phenergan, and Thorazine (DPT) for the sedation of children. *Pediatrics* 1995; **95:** 598–602.
3. Barst SM, *et al.* A comparison of propofol and Demerol-Phenergan-Thorazine for brief, minor, painful procedures in a pediatric hematology-oncology clinic. *Int J Pediatr Hematol/Oncol* 1995; **1:** 587–91.

Shivering. For reference to the use of pethidine in the management of shivering associated with anaesthesia, see under Adverse Effects of General Anaesthetics, p.1219. Pethidine has also been used to treat amphotericin-induced shaking chills.[1]

1. Burks LC, *et al.* Meperidine for the treatment of shaking chills and fever. *Arch Intern Med* 1980; **140:** 483–4.

Preparations

BP 1998: Pethidine Injection; Pethidine Tablets;
USP 23: Meperidine Hydrochloride Injection; Meperidine Hydrochloride Syrup; Meperidine Hydrochloride Tablets.

Proprietary Preparations (details are given in Part 3)
Aust.: Alodan; ***Belg.:*** Dolantine; ***Canad.:*** Demerol; ***Fr.:*** Dolosal; ***Ger.:*** Dolantin; ***Spain:*** Dolantina; ***Switz.:*** Centralgine; Dolantine†; ***USA:*** Demerol.

Multi-ingredient: ***Austral.:*** Marcain plus Pethidine; ***Canad.:*** Pamergan†; ***Ger.:*** Psyquil compositum†; ***Spain:*** Petigan Miro†; ***UK:*** Pamergan P100; ***USA:*** Atropine and Demerol; Mepergan.

Phenacetin (2681-h)

Phenacetin *(rINN).*

Aceto-*p*-phenetidide; Acetophenetidin; Acetylphenetidin; Fenacetina; Paracetophenetidin; Phenacetinum. *p*-Acetophenetidide; 4′-Ethoxyacetanilide; *N*-(4-Ethoxyphenyl)acetamide.

$C_{10}H_{13}NO_2$ = 179.2.

CAS — 62-44-2.

Pharmacopoeias. In *Eur.* (see p.viii), *Jpn,* and *Pol.*

A fine, white, crystalline powder or white, glistening, crystalline scales. Very slightly **soluble** in water, soluble in alcohol, and slightly soluble in ether.

Adverse Effects

Phenacetin may cause methaemoglobinaemia, sulphaemoglobinaemia, and haemolytic anaemia.

Prolonged administration of large doses of analgesic mixtures containing phenacetin has been associated with the development of renal papillary necrosis (see p.64) and transitional-cell carcinoma of the renal pelvis.

Uses and Administration

Phenacetin, a para-aminophenol derivative, has analgesic and antipyretic properties. It was usually given with aspirin, caffeine, or codeine but is now little used because of adverse haematological effects and nephrotoxicity.

Preparations

Proprietary Preparations (details are given in Part 3)
Multi-ingredient: ***Fr.:*** Gripponyl†; Hemagene Tailleur; Polypirine.

Phenazocine Hydrobromide (6256-k)

Phenazocine Hydrobromide *(BANM, rINNM).*

1,2,3,4,5,6-Hexahydro-6,11-dimethyl-3-phenethyl-2,6-methano-3-benzazocin-8-ol hydrobromide hemihydrate.

$C_{22}H_{27}NO,HBr,\frac{1}{2}H_2O$ = 411.4.

CAS — 127-35-5 (phenazocine); 1239-04-9 (anhydrous phenazocine hydrobromide).

Phenazocine hydrobromide is an opioid analgesic (p.67). It is considered to be less sedating than morphine. It also has a weaker action on smooth muscle than morphine and its lower potential to increase biliary pressure makes it suitable when opioid analgesics are required to manage pain associated with biliary colic and pancreatitis.

Phenazocine hydrobromide may be given for the relief of severe pain. It acts within 20 minutes after administration by mouth and the analgesic effect may last up to 6 hours. The usual oral or sublingual dose is 5 mg every 4 to 6 hours, though single doses of up to 20 mg may be given.

Preparations

Proprietary Preparations (details are given in Part 3)
UK: Narphen.

Phenazone (2684-v)

Phenazone *(BAN, rINN).*

Analgésine; Antipyrin; Antipyrine; Azophenum; Fenazona; Phenazonum. 1,5-Dimethyl-2-phenyl-4-pyrazolin-3-one.

$C_{11}H_{12}N_2O$ = 188.2.

CAS — 60-80-0.

Pharmacopoeias. In *Eur.* (see p.viii), *Jpn,* and *US.*

Colourless, odourless crystals or white or almost white crystalline powder. Very **soluble** in water and in dichloromethane; freely soluble to very soluble in alcohol; freely soluble in chloroform; sparingly soluble in ether. Solutions in water are neutral to litmus. **Store** in airtight containers and protect from light.

Phenazone and Caffeine Citrate (2683-b)

Antipyrino-Coffeinum Citricum; Migrenin.

Pharmacopoeias. In *Aust.* and *Jpn.*

A powder usually containing phenazone 90%, caffeine 9%, and citric acid monohydrate 1%.

Phenazone Salicylate (2682-m)

Antipyrin Salicylate; Salipyrin.

$C_{11}H_{12}N_2O,C_7H_6O_3$ = 326.3.

CAS — 520-07-0.

Pharmacopoeias. In *Aust.* and *Fr.*

Adverse Effects and Precautions

Phenazone is liable to give rise to skin eruptions and in susceptible individuals even small doses may have this effect. Hypersensitivity reactions and nephrotoxicity have been reported. Large doses by mouth may cause nausea, drowsiness, coma, and convulsions.

Effects on the blood. Phenazone had been shown to cause haemolytic anaemia in certain individuals with a deficiency of glucose-6-phosphate dehydrogenase.[1] Episodes of agranulocytosis were reported[2] in 6 women using a cream containing phenazone; all recovered on withdrawal.

1. Prankerd TAJ. Hemolytic effects of drugs and chemical agents. *Clin Pharmacol Ther* 1963; **4:** 334–50.
2. Delannoy A, Schmit J-C. Agranulocytosis after cutaneous contact with phenazone. *Eur J Haematol* 1993; **50:** 124.

Effects on the kidneys. Phenazone is considered nephrotoxic but only limited clinical information on phenazone is available because it has been mainly used in association with phenacetin.[1]

1. Prescott LF. Analgesic nephropathy: a reassessment of the role of phenacetin and other analgesics. *Drugs* 1982; **23:** 75–149.

Effects on the skin. In a summary[1] of 77 cases of fixed drug eruption phenazone derivatives were considered to be the causative agent in 9 of the 14 cases that were severe generalised reactions.

1. Stubb S, *et al.* Fixed drug eruptions: 77 cases from 1981 to 1985. *Br J Dermatol* 1989; **120:** 583.

Hypersensitivity. Immediate allergic reactions to phenazone have been reported.[1,2] In one patient leucopenia was detected 8 weeks later.[1]

1. Kadar D, Kalow W. Acute and latent leukopenic reaction to antipyrine. *Clin Pharmacol Ther* 1980; **28:** 820–22.
2. McCrea JB, *et al.* Allergic reaction to antipyrine, a marker of hepatic enzyme activity. *DICP Ann Pharmacother* 1989; **23:** 38–40.

Porphyria. Phenazone was considered to be unsafe in patients with acute porphyria because it has been shown to be porphyrinogenic in *animals* or *in vitro* systems.[1]

1. Moore MR, McColl KEL. *Porphyria: drug lists.* Glasgow: Porphyria Research Unit, University of Glasgow, 1991.

Interactions

Phenazone affects the metabolism of some other drugs and its metabolism is affected by other drugs that increase or reduce the activity of liver enzymes.

Pharmacokinetics

Phenazone is absorbed from the gastro-intestinal tract and peak plasma concentrations are obtained within 1 to 2 hours of ingestion. It is distributed throughout the body fluids with concentrations in the saliva and breast milk reaching about the same levels as those in plasma. Less than 10% is bound to plasma proteins and it has an elimination half-life of about 12 hours. Phenazone is metabolised in the liver to 3 major metabolites 3-hydroxymethylphenazone, 4-hydroxyphenazone, and norphenazone. Phenazone, 3-hydroxymethylphenazone, and glucuronidated metabolites are all excreted in the urine. A small portion may be eliminated via the bile.

Uses and Administration

Phenazone is an NSAID (p.65) and has been given by mouth; phenazone and caffeine citrate and phenazone salicylate have similarly been given by mouth as analgesics.

Solutions containing about 5% of phenazone have been used topically as ear drops in disorders such as acute otitis media (but see below).

Phenazone is used as a test for the effect of other drugs or the effect of a disease state on the activity of drug-metabolising enzymes in the liver.

Diagnosis and testing. A review[1] of normal plasma-phenazone pharmacokinetics, urinary metabolite disposition, and total body clearances of phenazone in the presence of cirrhosis, fatty liver, hepatitis, and cholestatis.

1. St Peter JV, Awni WM. Quantifying hepatic function in the presence of liver disease with phenazone (antipyrine) and its metabolites. *Clin Pharmacokinet* 1991; **20:** 50–65.

Otitis media. There seems to be no justification[1] for the inclusion of phenazone in local preparations used in treating acute otitis media (p.134). It is presumably included in such preparations because it is believed to have a local anti-inflammatory, and therefore, analgesic action. It would, however, seem unlikely that phenazone would have any action on the skin of the intact tympanic membrane and, therefore, on the pain which is due primarily to the stretching and distention of the membrane.

In general, no topical treatment is considered effective in acute otitis media.

1. Carlin WV. Is there any justification for using phenazone in a local application prescribed for the treatment of acute otitis media? *Br Med J* 1987; **294:** 1333.

Preparations

USP 23: Antipyrine and Benzocaine Otic Solution; Antipyrine, Benzocaine, and Phenylephrine Hydrochloride Otic Solution.

Proprietary Preparations (details are given in Part 3)
Austral.: Erasol; ***Ger.:*** Aequiton-P; Eu-Med; Migrane-Kranit mono; Spondylon N†; ***Irl.:*** Tropex; ***S.Afr.:*** Aurone; Oto-Phen; ***Swed.:*** Spalt N.

Multi-ingredient: ***Aust.:*** Asthma Efeum†; Asthma-Frenon; Bellasthman; Coffo Selt; Otalgan; Spalt; ***Austral.:*** Auralgan; ***Belg.:*** Otalgan; Otocalmine; Ouate Hemostatique; Parmentier; Tympalgine; ***Canad.:*** Auralgan; ***Fr.:*** Brulex; HEC; Hyalurectal†; Migralgine; Otipax; Ovules Sedo-Hemostatiques du Docteur Jouve; Theinol; ***Ger.:*** Coffeemed N; Cor-Neo-Nervacit-S†; Cosavil†; Efisalin N†; Eu-Med SC†; Felsol Neo; Furacin-Otalgicum†; Ilvico†; Kephalosan†; Migranex†; Migranin; Otalgan; Otodolor; Par-Isalon†; Sanalgutt-S†; Spondylon N†; Spondylon S†; Titralgan†; ***Irl.:*** Auraltone†; ***Ital.:*** Emocicatrol†; Mentalgina†; Otalgan; Otomidone; Otopax; ***Norw.:*** Antineuralgica; Codalgin; Fanalgin; ***S.Afr.:*** Atrofed†; Auralgicin; Aurasept; Aurone Forte; Covancaine; Ilvico; Otised; Oto-Phen Forte; Universal Earache Drops; ***Spain:*** AB FE; Crema Antisolar Evanesce†; Epistaxol; Hemostatico Antisep Asen; Oftalmo†; Otalgan; Otosedol; Otosmo†; Pomada Heridas; Quimpedor; Tabletas Quimpe; Timpanalgesic†; ***Swed.:*** Doleron; Koffazon; ***Switz.:*** Otalgan; Otipax; Otosan; Otothricinol; Radolor†; Seranex sans codeine; Spasmosol†; Spedralgin sans codeine; Spirogel; ***USA:*** Allergen; Analgesic Otic Solution; Aurafair Otic†; Auralgan; Auroto; Benzotic; Otocalm; Tympagesic.

Phenazopyridine Hydrochloride (2685-g)

Phenazopyridine Hydrochloride *(BANM, USAN, rINNM).*

Chloridrato de Fenazopiridina; NC-150; NSC-1879; W-1655. 3-Phenylazopyridine-2,6-diyldiamine hydrochloride.

$C_{11}H_{11}N_5,HCl$ = 249.7.

CAS — 94-78-0 (phenazopyridine); 136-40-3 (phenazopyridine hydrochloride).

Pharmacopoeias. In *Pol.* and *US.*

A light or dark red to dark violet crystalline powder, odourless or with a slight odour.

Soluble 1 in 300 of cold water, 1 in 20 of boiling water, 1 in 59 of alcohol, 1 in 331 of chloroform, and 1 in 100 of glycerol; very slightly soluble in ether. **Store** in airtight containers.

REMOVAL OF STAINS. Phenazopyridine stains may be removed from fabric by soaking in a solution of sodium dithionite 0.25%.

Adverse Effects

Phenazopyridine hydrochloride has caused gastro-intestinal side-effects, headache, and rashes. Hepatotoxicity, haemolytic anaemia, methaemoglobinaemia, and acute renal failure have also been reported, generally associated with overdosage or with therapeutic doses in patients with impaired renal function. Crystal deposits of phenazopyridine have formed in the urinary tract.

Abnormal coloration of body tissues or fluids may occur. Staining of contact lenses has occurred.

Effects on the CNS. Aseptic meningitis, characterised by distinct episodes of fever and confusion, in a patient was associated with the administration of phenazopyridine.[1]

1. Herlihy TE. Phenazopyridine and aseptic meningitis. *Ann Intern Med* 1987; **106:** 172–3.

Precautions

Phenazopyridine hydrochloride is contra-indicated in patients with impaired renal function or severe hepatitis or those with glucose-6-phosphate dehydrogenase deficiency. Treatment should be discontinued if the skin or sclerae become discoloured. Phenazopyridine may interfere with urinalysis based on colour reactions or spectrometry.

Pharmacokinetics

Phenazopyridine hydrochloride is absorbed from the gastro-intestinal tract. It is excreted mainly in the urine; up to 65% may be excreted as unchanged phenazopyridine and 18% as paracetamol.

Uses and Administration

Phenazopyridine is an azo dye that exerts an analgesic effect on the mucosa of the urinary tract and is used to provide symptomatic relief of pain and irritability in conditions such as cystitis and prostatitis (see under Urinary-tract Infections, p.149), and urethritis (p.149). It is given by mouth as the hydrochloride in usual doses of 200 mg three times daily after food. If given in conjunction with an antibacterial for the treatment of urinary-tract infections it is recommended that phenazopyridine hydrochloride should be given for not more than 2 days. During administration the urine is tinged either orange or red and underclothes are apt to be stained.

Urinary-tract infections. There is currently no well-substantiated role for phenazopyridine in the treatment of urinary-tract infections and its adverse effects are potentially serious.[1]

1. Zelenitsky SA, Zhanel GG. Phenazopyridine in urinary tract infections. *Ann Pharmacother* 1996; **30:** 866–8.

Preparations

USP 23: Oxytetracycline and Phenazopyridine Hydrochlorides and Sulfamethizole Capsules; Phenazopyridine Hydrochloride Tablets.

Proprietary Preparations (details are given in Part 3)
Belg.: Uropyrine; ***Canad.:*** Phenazo; Pyridium; ***Fr.:*** Pyridium†; ***Ger.:*** Pyridium†; Spasmosan†; ***S.Afr.:*** Azodine; Pyridium; ***USA:*** Azo-Standard; Baridium; Eridium†; Geridium†; Phenazodine†; Prodium; Pyridiate; Pyridium; Uro-Trac; Urodine†; Urogesic.

Multi-ingredient: ***Aust.:*** Gastrotest; ***Canad.:*** Azo Gantrisin†; ***Ger.:*** Spasmo Nierofu†; Spasmo-Urolcear†; Urospasmon; ***S.Afr.:*** Azo-Mandelamine†; ***Spain:*** Furantoina Sedante†; Micturol Sedante; Urogobens Antiespasmo; ***Switz.:*** Urospasmon†; ***USA:*** Azo Gantanol†; Azo Gantrisin†; Pyridium Plus†; Urobiotic-250†.

Phenicarbazide (2689-w)

Phenicarbazide *(rINN).*

Phenylsemicarbazide. 1-Phenylsemicarbazide.

$C_7H_9N_3O = 151.2$.

CAS — 103-03-7.

Phenicarbazide has analgesic properties. It has been given by mouth.

Preparations

Proprietary Preparations (details are given in Part 3)
Multi-ingredient: ***Fr.:*** Polypirine.

Phenoperidine Hydrochloride (6257-a)

Phenoperidine Hydrochloride *(BANM, rINNM).*

R-1406. Ethyl 1-(3-hydroxy-3-phenylpropyl)-4-phenylpiperidine-4-carboxylate hydrochloride.

$C_{23}H_{29}NO_3,HCl = 403.9$.

CAS — 562-26-5 (phenoperidine); 3627-49-4 (phenoperidine hydrochloride).

Incompatible with propanidid and solutions of methohexitone sodium and thiopentone sodium.

Dependence and Withdrawal, Adverse Effects, Treatment, and Precautions

As for Opioid Analgesics in general, p.67 and Pethidine, p.76.

Muscular rigidity may require treatment with neuromuscular blockers. Some cases of jaundice have been reported.

Hepatic impairment. Phenoperidine is metabolised in the liver and caution is generally advised in patients with liver disease. However, a pharmacokinetic study[1] indicated that dosage modification might not be necessary when hepatic function was only slightly or moderately impaired.

1. Isherwood CN, *et al.* Elimination of phenoperidine in liver disease. *Br J Anaesth* 1984; **56:** 843–7.

Interactions

For interactions associated with opioid analgesics, see p.69.

Pharmacokinetics

Although normally given by injection, there is some absorption of phenoperidine from the gastro-intestinal tract. It is extensively metabolised in the liver to pethidine and norpethidine, which are mainly excreted in the urine.

References.

1. Milne L, *et al.* Plasma concentration and metabolism of phenoperidine in man. *Br J Anaesth* 1980; **52:** 537–40.
2. Isherwood CN, *et al.* Elimination of phenoperidine in liver disease. *Br J Anaesth* 1984; **56:** 843–7.
3. Fischler M, *et al.* Pharmacokinetics of phenoperidine in anaesthetized patients undergoing general surgery. *Br J Anaesth* 1985; **57:** 872–6.
4. Fischler M, *et al.* Pharmacokinetics of phenoperidine in patients undergoing cardiopulmonary bypass. *Br J Anaesth* 1985; **57:** 877–82.
5. Milne LA, *et al.* Effect of urine pH on the elimination of phenoperidine. *Br J Clin Pharmacol* 1983; **16:** 101–3.

Uses and Administration

Phenoperidine hydrochloride is an opioid analgesic (p.69) related to pethidine (p.77). It is usually given by intravenous injection.

Phenoperidine hydrochloride produces surgical analgesia and has also been used with an antipsychotic such as droperidol, to induce neuroleptanalgesia. Phenoperidine has also been used as an analgesic and respiratory depressant in patients requiring long-term assisted ventilation in intensive care.

In anaesthesia in which spontaneous respiration is maintained, an average initial intravenous dose of phenoperidine hydrochloride for adults is up to 1 mg; supplements of 500 μg may be given every 40 to 60 minutes. Significant respiratory depression follows doses of more than 1 mg. In anaesthesia with assisted ventilation, the initial dose is 2 to 5 mg with supplementary doses of 1 mg.

Similar doses have been given by intramuscular injection in intensive care.

Preparations

Proprietary Preparations (details are given in Part 3)
Austral.: Operidine; ***Fr.:*** R 1406; ***Swed.:*** Lealgin; ***UK:*** Operidine†.

Phenylbutazone (2686-q)

Phenylbutazone *(BAN, rINN).*

Butadione; Fenilbutazona; Phenylbutazonum. 4-Butyl-1,2-diphenylpyrazolidine-3,5-dione.

$C_{19}H_{20}N_2O_2 = 308.4$.

CAS — 50-33-9 (phenylbutazone); 129-18-0 (phenylbutazone sodium); 4985-25-5 (phenylbutazone piperazine).

Pharmacopoeias. In *Chin., Eur.* (see p.viii), *Jpn, Pol.,* and *US.*

A white or off-white, odourless, crystalline powder. Ph. Eur. **solubilities** are: practically insoluble in water; sparingly soluble in alcohol; soluble in ether; it dissolves in alkaline solutions. USP solubilities are: very slightly soluble in water; soluble in alcohol; freely soluble in acetone and in ether. **Store** in airtight containers. Protect from light.

Adverse Effects

Nausea, vomiting, epigastric distress, diarrhoea, oedema due to salt retention, skin rashes, dizziness, drowsiness, headache, and blurred vision may occur. More serious reactions include gastric irritation with ulceration and gastro-intestinal bleeding, ulcerative stomatitis, hepatitis, jaundice, haematuria, nephritis, renal failure, pancreatitis, ocular toxicity, and goitre. Phenylbutazone may precipitate heart failure and may also cause an acute pulmonary syndrome with dyspnoea and fever. Salivary gland enlargement, hypersensitivity reactions including asthma, and severe generalised reactions including lymphadenopathy, erythema multiforme, Stevens-Johnson syndrome, toxic epidermal necrolysis, and exfoliative dermatitis have been reported.

The most serious adverse effects of phenylbutazone are related to bone-marrow depression and include agranulocytosis and aplastic anaemia. Leucopenia, pancytopenia, haemolytic anaemia, and thrombocytopenia may also occur. These adverse haematological reactions have resulted in the indications for use of phenylbutazone being restricted (see under Uses and Administration, below). Blood disorders may develop soon after starting treatment or may occur suddenly after prolonged treatment, and regular haematological monitoring should be carried out as discussed under Precautions, below.

The adverse effects of NSAIDs in general are described on p.63.

Effects on the blood. Both phenylbutazone[1-3] and oxyphenbutazone[1,3] are well known for their adverse effects on the blood and especially for fatal agranulocytosis and aplastic anaemia. Some indication of the extent of this toxicity can be obtained from the records of the UK Committee on Safety of Medicines[4] which showed that between July 1963 and January 1993 it had received 74 reports of agranulocytosis (39 fatal) associated with phenylbutazone and 40 reports of neutropenia (4 fatal). Up-to-date figures were not provided on oxyphenbutazone, but it is considered to be more toxic to the bone marrow than phenylbutazone.[1]

1. Anonymous. Phenylbutazone and oxyphenbutazone: time to call a halt. *Drug Ther Bull* 1984; **22:** 5–6.
2. Böttiger LE, Westerholm B. Drug-induced blood dyscrasias in Sweden. *Br Med J* 1973; **3:** 339–43.
3. The International Agranulocytosis and Aplastic Anemia Study. Risks of agranulocytosis and aplastic anemia: a first report of their relation to drug use with special reference to analgesics. *JAMA* 1986; **256:** 1749–57.
4. Committee on Safety of Medicines/Medicines Control Agency. Drug-induced neutropenia and agranulocytosis. *Current Problems* 1993; **19:** 10–11.

Precautions

Phenylbutazone is contra-indicated in patients with blood disorders or active gastro-intestinal disorders such as peptic ulcer or inflammatory bowel disease and also in patients with a history of any such disorders. It is also contra-indicated in patients with cardiovascular, pulmonary, or thyroid disease, in those with severe impairment of hepatic or renal function, and in those with a history of hypersensitivity to aspirin or other NSAIDs. It is also contra-indicated in patients with salivary gland disorders or Sjögren's syndrome. It may aggravate systemic lupus erythematosus.

Blood-cell counts should be performed before and regularly during therapy in patients receiving the drug for more than 1 week but should not be relied upon to predict dysplasia; monitoring of hepatic and renal function is also recommended. Patients should be told to discontinue the drug at the first signs of toxic effects and to report at once the appearance of symptoms such as fever, sore throat, stomatitis, skin rashes, bruising, and weight gain or oedema. Treatment should also be withdrawn if symptoms of the acute pulmonary syndrome including dyspnoea and fever develop.

It should be used with caution in elderly patients who may require reduced doses. Courses of treatment should be kept as short as possible. Dizziness or drowsiness may affect the performance of skilled tasks such as driving.

The precautions to be taken with NSAIDs in general are described on p.65.

Porphyria. Oxyphenbutazone, a metabolite of phenylbutazone, has been associated with clinical exacerbations of porphyria and is considered unsafe in porphyric patients.[1] Phenylbutazone is also considered to be unsafe although there is conflicting experimental evidence on porphyrinogenicity.

1. Moore MR, McColl KEL. *Porphyria: drug lists.* Glasgow: Porphyria Research Unit, University of Glasgow, 1991.

Interactions

For interactions associated with NSAIDs, see p.65. Additionally the elimination half-life of phenylbutazone is reduced in patients pretreated with drugs that increase liver microsomal enzyme activity. Concurrent administration of methylphenidate or anabolic steroids and phenylbutazone may increase the serum concentration of the metabolite oxyphenbutazone. Cholestyramine reduces the absorption of phenylbutazone.

A report[1] in 2 patients of side-effects including headaches, dizziness, ambulatory instability, tingles, and transient diplopia suggesting a potentiation of neurological adverse effects attributed to concomitant administration of phenylbutazone and misoprostol.

1. Jacquemier JM, *et al.* Neurosensory adverse effects after phenylbutazone and misoprostol combined treatment. *Lancet* 1989; **ii:** 1283.

Pharmacokinetics

Phenylbutazone is readily absorbed from the gastro-intestinal tract with peak plasma concentrations occurring about 2 hours after ingestion. It is also readily absorbed when administered rectally. Phenylbutazone is widely distributed throughout body fluids and tissues; it diffuses into the synovial fluid, crosses the placenta, and small amounts enter the CNS and breast milk. It is 98% bound to plasma proteins. It is extensively metabolised in the liver by oxidation and by conjugation with glucuronic acid. Oxyphenbutazone, γ-hydroxyphenbutazone, and *p*,γ-dihydroxyphenylbutazone are formed by oxidation but only small amounts appear in urine, the remainder being further metabolised. It is mainly excreted in the urine as metabolites although about a quarter of a dose may be excreted in the faeces. The plasma elimination half-life is about 70 hours but it is subject to large interindividual variations.

Uses and Administration

Phenylbutazone, a pyrazolone derivative, is an NSAID (p.65). However, because of its toxicity it is not employed as a general analgesic or antipyretic. Although phenylbutazone is effective in almost all musculoskeletal and joint disorders including ankylosing spondylitis, acute gout, osteoarthritis, and rheumatoid arthritis, it should only be used in acute conditions where less toxic drugs have failed. In the UK the use of phenylbutazone is restricted to the hospital treatment of ankylosing spondylitis unresponsive to other drugs.

In the UK the recommended initial dose is 200 mg given by mouth two to three times daily for 2 days; thereafter the dose is reduced to the minimum effective amount, which is usually 200 to 300 mg daily given in divided doses. Treatment should be given for the shortest period possible.

Elderly patients may require reduced doses.

In some countries phenylbutazone has also been given as a rectal suppository and applied topically for musculoskeletal pain and in soft-tissue injury. It has also been given intramuscularly as the sodium salt. Other salts of phenylbutazone that have been used in musculoskeletal, joint, and soft-tissue disorders include the calcium, megallate, and piperazine salts.

Preparations

USP 23: Phenylbutazone Capsules; Phenylbutazone Tablets.

Proprietary Preparations (details are given in Part 3)
Aust.: Butazolidin; ***Austral.:*** Butazolidin; ***Belg.:*** Butazolidin; ***Canad.:*** Alka Butazolidin†; Butazolidin†; Novo-Butazone; ***Fr.:*** Butazolidine; ***Ger.:*** Ambene; Butazolidin; Demoplas; exrheudon OPT; ***Irl.:*** Butacote†; Butazolidin†; ***Ital.:*** Butazina†; Butazolidina†; Carudol†; Kadol; Ticinil Calcico†; Ticinil†; ***Neth.:*** Butazolidin; ***S.Afr.:*** Butrex†; Inflazone; Scriptozone†; ***Spain:*** Butadiona†; Butazolidina; Carudol; ***Swed.:*** Butazolidin†; ***Switz.:*** Butadion; Butazolidine; Butazolidine Alca†; ***UK:*** Butacote; Butazone; ***USA:*** Butazolidin†; Cotylbutazone†.

Multi-ingredient: ***Aust.:*** Ambene; Ambene N; Delta-Tomanol; ***Fr.:*** Alpha-Kadol†; Carudol; Dermiclone†; Dextrarine Phenylbutazone; Penetradol†; Traumalgyl; ***Ger.:*** Ambene Comp; Glutisalbuton†; Neuro-Demoplas†; ***Ital.:*** Lisabutina†; ***Spain:*** Artrodesmol Extra; Doctofril Antiinflamat; ***Switz.:*** Butaparin; Carudol; Hepabuzone.

Phenyramidol Hydrochloride (2690-m)

Phenyramidol Hydrochloride *(BANM, USAN).*

Fenyramidol Hydrochloride *(rINNM)*; IN-511; MJ-505; NSC-17777. 1-Phenyl-2-(2-pyridylamino)ethanol hydrochloride; α-(2-Pyridylaminomethyl)benzyl alcohol hydrochloride.

$C_{13}H_{14}N_2O,HCl = 250.7.$

CAS — 553-69-5 (phenyramidol); 326-43-2 (phenyramidol hydrochloride).

Phenyramidol hydrochloride has analgesic and skeletal muscle relaxant properties and was used by mouth in the treatment of muscular pain and stiffness. It may enhance the effects of coumarin anticoagulants (p.966) and of phenytoin (p.354).

Preparations

Proprietary Preparations (details are given in Part 3)
Ger.: Cabral†; ***Ital.:*** Anabloc†; Analexin†.

Picenadol Hydrochloride (19658-g)

Picenadol Hydrochloride *(USAN, rINNM).*

LY-150720; LY-136595((−)-isomer); LY-136596((+)-isomer). (±)-*trans*-*m*-(1,3-Dimethyl-4-propyl-4-piperidyl)phenol hydrochloride.

$C_{16}H_{25}NO,HCl = 283.8.$

CAS — 79201-85-7 (picenadol); 74685-16-8 (picenadol hydrochloride).

Picenadol hydrochloride is an opioid analgesic (p.67) with mixed agonist-antagonist properties. The (+)-isomer is reported to have opioid agonist activity and the (−)-isomer antagonist activity. It has been studied for its analgesic efficacy following oral or intramuscular administration.

References.

1. Brunelle RL, *et al.* Analgesic effect of picenadol, codeine, and placebo in patients with postoperative pain. *Clin Pharmacol Ther* 1988; **43:** 663–7.
2. Goldstein DJ, *et al.* Picenadol in a large multicenter dental pain study. *Pharmacotherapy* 1994; **14:** 54–9.

Picolamine Salicylate (9592-e)

NOTE. Picolamine is *rINN.*

Picolamine salicylate is a salicylic acid derivative that has been used similarly to methyl salicylate (p.55) in concentrations of 10% in topical rubefacient preparations for the treatment of musculoskeletal, joint, peri-articular, and soft-tissue disorders.

Preparations

Proprietary Preparations (details are given in Part 3)
Fr.: Reflex; ***Spain:*** Algiospray.

Piketoprofen (19662-h)

Piketoprofen *(rINN).*

m-Benzoyl-*N*-(4-methyl-2-pyridyl)hydratropamide.

$C_{22}H_{20}N_2O_2 = 344.4.$

CAS — 60576-13-8.

Piketoprofen is an NSAID (p.63) that has been used topically as the hydrochloride in concentrations of about 2% in musculoskeletal, joint, peri-articular, and soft-tissue disorders.

Preparations

Proprietary Preparations (details are given in Part 3)
Spain: Calmatel; Triparsean.

Piritramide (6259-x)

Piritramide *(BAN, rINN).*

Pirinitramide; R-3365. 1-(3-Cyano-3,3-diphenylpropyl)-4-piperidinopiperidine-4-carboxamide.

$C_{27}H_{34}N_4O = 430.6.$

CAS — 302-41-0.

Piritramide is an opioid analgesic (p.67).

It is used for the management of severe pain including post-operative pain, for premedication, and to provide analgesia during anaesthesia. It is given by intramuscular, subcutaneous, or slow intravenous injection as the tartrate in doses equivalent of up to about 30 mg of the base.

Porphyria. Piritramide was considered to be unsafe in patients with acute porphyria because it has been shown to be porphyrinogenic in *animals* or *in vitro* systems.[1]

1. Moore MR, McColl KEL. *Porphyria: drug lists.* Glasgow: Porphyria Research Unit, University of Glasgow, 1991.

Preparations

Proprietary Preparations (details are given in Part 3)
Aust.: Dipidolor; ***Belg.:*** Dipidolor; ***Ger.:*** Dipidolor; ***Neth.:*** Dipidolor; ***Swed.:*** Piridolan†.

Piroxicam (2692-v)

Piroxicam *(BAN, USAN, rINN).*

CP-16171; Piroxicamum. 4-Hydroxy-2-methyl-*N*-(2-pyridyl)-2*H*-1,2-benzothiazine-3-carboxamide 1,1-dioxide.

$C_{15}H_{13}N_3O_4S = 331.3.$

CAS — 36322-90-4.

Pharmacopoeias. In *Eur.* (see p.viii) and *US.*

An off-white to light tan or light yellow, odourless crystalline powder. It is polymorphic and forms a monohydrate that is yellow. Ph. Eur. **solubilities** are: practically insoluble in water; sparingly soluble in alcohol; soluble in dichloromethane. USP solubilities are: very slightly soluble in water, in dilute acids, and in most organic solvents; slightly soluble in alcohol and in aqueous alkaline solutions. **Store** in airtight containers. Protect from light.

Adverse Effects

As for NSAIDs in general, p.63.

Local irritation and occasionally bleeding may occur with piroxicam suppositories and there may be pain and occasionally tissue damage at the injection site on intramuscular administration.

A report[1] of the adverse reactions associated with piroxicam received by the Medicines Safety Centre in South Africa during 1981-86 including two reactions, paraesthesia and hair loss, not previously recorded in the literature.

1. Gerber D. Adverse reactions of piroxicam. *Drug Intell Clin Pharm* 1987; **21:** 707–10.

Effects on the blood. Decreases in haemoglobin and haematocrit not associated with obvious gastro-intestinal bleeding, have occurred in patients taking piroxicam. Thrombocytopenia, thrombocytopenic purpura,[1] and aplastic anaemia[2] have been described in patients on piroxicam.

1. Bjørnstad H, Vik Ø. Thrombocytopenic purpura associated with piroxicam. *Br J Clin Pract* 1986; **40:** 42.
2. Lee SH, *et al.* Aplastic anaemia associated with piroxicam. *Lancet* 1982; **i:** 1186.

Effects on electrolytes. Reversible hyperkalaemic hyperchloraemic acidosis has been reported[1,2] in patients receiving piroxicam. Severe hyponatraemia and symptoms resembling the syndrome of inappropriate antidiuretic hormone secretion have also been associated with piroxicam.[3]

See also under Effects on the Kidneys, below.

1. Grossman LA, Moss S. Piroxicam and hyperkalemic acidosis. *Ann Intern Med* 1983; **99:** 282.
2. Miller KP, *et al.* Severe hyperkalemia during piroxicam therapy. *Arch Intern Med* 1984; **144:** 2414–15.
3. Petersson I, *et al.* Water intoxication associated with non-steroidal anti-inflammatory drug therapy. *Acta Med Scand* 1987; **221:** 221–3.

Effects on the kidneys. Acute nephropathy with characteristic features of Henoch-Schönlein purpura,[1] acute renal failure,[2] uraemia with hyperkalaemia, and acute interstitial nephritis[3] have been associated with systemic administration of piroxicam. Nephrotic syndrome and interstitial nephritis has been reported in a patient following topical application of piroxicam gel.[4]

1. Goebel KM, Mueller-Brodmann W. Reversible overt nephropathy with Henoch-Schönlein purpura due to piroxicam. *Br Med J* 1982; **284:** 311–12.
2. Frais MA, *et al.* Piroxicam-induced renal failure and hyperkalemia. *Ann Intern Med* 1983; **99:** 129–30.
3. Mitnick PD, Klein WJ. Piroxicam-induced renal disease. *Arch Intern Med* 1984; **144:** 63–4.
4. O'Callaghan CA, *et al.* Renal disease and use of topical non-steroidal anti-inflammatory drugs. *Br Med J* 1994; **308:** 110–11.

Effects on the liver. Necrosis of the liver has been associated with piroxicam. Details have been supplied on 3 patients,[1,2] of whom 2 died.

1. Lee SM, *et al.* Subacute hepatic necrosis induced by piroxicam. *Br Med J* 1986; **293:** 540–1.
2. Paterson D, *et al.* Piroxicam induced submassive necrosis of the liver. *Gut* 1992; **33;** 1436–8.

Effects on the pancreas. A report[1] of pancreatitis associated with piroxicam.

1. Haye OL. Piroxicam and pancreatitis. *Ann Intern Med* 1986; **104:** 895.

Effects on the skin. As with other NSAIDs, rash has occurred in patients taking piroxicam. Phototoxic reactions have been described.[1] Serious skin reactions attributed to piroxicam therapy include toxic epidermal necrolysis[2] and pemphigus vulgaris.[3]

1. Stern RS. Phototoxic reactions to piroxicam and other nonsteroidal antiinflammatory agents. *N Engl J Med* 1983; **309:** 186–7.
2. Chosidow O, *et al.* Intestinal involvement in drug-induced toxic epidermal necrolysis. *Lancet* 1991; **337:** 928.
3. Martin RL, *et al.* Fatal pemphigus vulgaris in a patient taking piroxicam. *N Engl J Med* 1983; **309:** 795–6.

Overdosage. Details of 16 patients who were considered to have taken an overdosage of piroxicam alone were reported[1] to the National Poisons Information Service of the UK. Thirteen patients (including 5 children) experienced no symptoms after doses estimated to be up to 300 to 400 mg; 2 patients complained of dizziness and blurred vision after 200 to 300 mg; the last patient who claimed to have taken 600 mg presented in coma, regained consciousness within one hour, and had recovered fully within 24 hours.

1. Court H, Volans GN. Poisoning after overdose with non-steroidal anti-inflammatory drugs. *Adverse Drug React Acute Poisoning Rev* 1984; **3:** 1–21.

Precautions

As for NSAIDs in general, p.65.

Breast feeding. See under Pharmacokinetics, below.

Porphyria. Piroxicam has been associated with clinical exacerbations of porphyria and is considered unsafe in porphyric patients.[1]

1. Moore MR, McColl KEL. *Porphyria: drug lists.* Glasgow: Porphyria Research Unit, University of Glasgow, 1991.

Interactions

For interactions associated with NSAIDs, see p.65.

Concurrent administration of aspirin results in decreased plasma concentrations of piroxicam to about 80% of normal. Concomitant administration of piroxicam and ritonavir may result in increased plasma concentrations of piroxicam and carries an increased risk of toxicity; use together should be avoided.

Pharmacokinetics

Piroxicam is well absorbed from the gastro-intestinal tract; peak plasma concentrations are reached 3 to 5 hours after an oral dose. Piroxicam is also absorbed to some degree following topical application. Piroxicam is 99% bound to plasma proteins. It has been detected in breast milk in concentrations of 1 to 3% of those in maternal plasma, but such amounts are considered by some authorities to be too small to be harmful to a breast-fed infant. Piroxicam has a long plasma elimination half-life of approximately 50 hours. It is metabolised in the liver by hydroxylation and conjugation with glucuronic acid and excreted predominantly in the urine with smaller amounts in the faeces. Enterohepatic recycling occurs. Less than 5% of the dose is excreted unchanged in the urine.

References.

1. Østensen M. Piroxicam in human breast milk. *Eur J Clin Pharmacol* 1983; **25:** 829–30.
2. Richardson CJ, *et al.* Piroxicam and 5′-hydroxypiroxicam kinetics following multiple dose administration of piroxicam. *Eur J Clin Pharmacol* 1987; **32:** 89–91.
3. Doogan DP. Topical non-steroidal anti-inflammatory drugs. *Lancet* 1989; **ii:** 1270–1.
4. Mäkelä A-L, *et al.* Steady state pharmacokinetics of piroxicam in children with rheumatic diseases. *Eur J Clin Pharmacol* 1991; **41:** 79–81 (higher clearance and shorter half-life in children).
5. Rudy AC, *et al.* The pharmacokinetics of piroxicam in elderly persons with and without renal impairment. *Br J Clin Pharmacol* 1994; **37:** 1–5.

6. Deroubaix X, *et al.* Oral bioavailability of CHF1194, an inclusion complex of piroxicam and β-cyclodextrin, in healthy subjects under single dose and steady-state conditions. *Eur J Clin Pharmacol* 1995; **47:** 531–6.

7. Karim A, *et al.* Oxaprozin and piroxicam, nonsteroidal antiinflammatory drugs with long half-lives: effect of protein-binding differences on steady-state pharmacokinetics. *J Clin Pharmacol* 1997; **37:** 267–78.

Uses and Administration

Piroxicam, an oxicam derivative, is an NSAID (p.65). It is used in musculoskeletal and joint disorders such as ankylosing spondylitis, osteoarthritis, rheumatoid arthritis including juvenile chronic arthritis, in soft-tissue disorders, and in acute gout.

In rheumatic disorders a usual initial dose of piroxicam by mouth is 20 mg daily as a single dose. Daily maintenance doses may vary between 10 and 30 mg given in single or divided doses; administration of doses in excess of 20 mg daily for more than a few days is associated with an increased risk of gastro-intestinal adverse effects. Because of the long half-life, steady-state concentrations are not reached for 7 to 12 days. In acute musculoskeletal conditions an initial dose of 40 mg daily may be given for 2 days followed by 20 mg daily for 1 to 2 weeks. Piroxicam is also used in acute gout, the usual dose being 40 mg daily for 5 to 7 days. Piroxicam is given in similar doses as a rectal suppository or on a short-term basis by intramuscular injection.

Piroxicam is also used in the local treatment of a variety of painful or inflammatory conditions as a topical gel in a concentration of 0.5% applied three or four times daily; treatment should be reviewed after 4 weeks. Piroxicam has been used in some countries as a 1% cream and as eye drops in a concentration of 0.5%.

Piroxicam may also be used in children aged 6 years or over with juvenile chronic arthritis. The usual dose by mouth is 5 mg daily in those weighing less than 15 kg, 10 mg daily in those weighing 16 to 25 kg, 15 mg daily in those weighing 26 to 45 kg, and 20 mg daily in those weighing 46 kg or over.

Piroxicam betadex (piroxicam beta cyclodextrin complex) is used in some preparations for painful and inflammatory disorders; such a complex may have a more rapid onset of therapeutic effect due to its enhanced solubility but at present there is little evidence to support the manufacturer's claim that it has improved gastro-intestinal tolerability. Other piroxicam salts or compounds that have also been used include piroxicam cinnamate (cinnoxicam), piroxicam choline, and piroxicam pivalate.

Reviews.

1. Lee CR, Balfour JA. Piroxicam-β-cylodextrin: a review of its pharmacodynamic and pharmacokinetic properties, and therapeutic potential in rheumatic diseases and pain states. *Drugs* 1994; **48:** 907–29.

Preparations

BP 1998: Piroxicam Capsules; Piroxicam Gel;
USP 23: Piroxicam Capsules.

Proprietary Preparations (details are given in Part 3)

Aust.: Brexin; Felden; Pirocam; ***Austral.:*** Candyl; Feldene; Fensaid; Mobilis; Pirox; Rosig; ***Belg.:*** Brexine; Feldene; ***Canad.:*** Feldene; Novo-Pirocam; Nu-Pirox; ***Fr.:*** Brexin; Cycladol; Feldene; Geldene; Inflaced; Olcam; ***Ger.:*** Brexidol; durapirox; Fasax; Felden; Flexase; Jenapirox; Piro-Phlogont; Piro-Puren; Pirobeta; Piroflam; Pirorheum; Pirorheuma; Pirox; Pirox-Spondyril†; Piroximerck; Pra-Brexidol; Rheumitin; ***Irl.:*** Feldene; Geroxicam; Pericam; ***Ital.:*** Antiflog; Artroxicam; Brexin; Bruxicam; Cicladol; Cicladol L†; Ciclafast; Clevian; Dexicam; Feldene; Flodol; Flogobene; Lampoflex; Nirox; Piroftal; Pivaloxicam; Polipirox; Reucam; Reudene; Reumagil; Riacen; Roxene; Roxenil; Roxiden; Roxim†; Sinartrol; Unicam†; Zacam; Zelis; Zen; Zunden; ***Neth.:*** Brexine; Feldene; ***Norw.:*** Brexidol; Felden; Pirox; Tetram; ***S.Afr.:*** Brexecam; Feldene; Pixicam; Pyrocaps; Rheugesic; Roxicam; Xycam; ***Spain:*** Artragil; Brexinil; Cycladol; Dekamega; Doblexan; Feldene; Improntal; Salcacam; Salvacam; Sasulen; Vitaxicam; ***Swed.:*** Brexidol; Felden; ***Switz.:*** Felden; Pirocam; Pirosol; ***UK:*** Feldene; Flamatrol; Larapam; Piroflam; Pirozip; ***USA:*** Feldene.

Pranoprofen (3847-c)

Pranoprofen *(rINN).*

α-Methyl-5*H*-[1]-benzopyrano[2,3-*b*]pyridine-7-acetic acid.

$C_{15}H_{13}NO_3$ = 255.3.

CAS — 52549-17-4.

Pharmacopoeias. In *Jpn.*

Pranoprofen, a propionic acid derivative, is an NSAID (p.63). It has been given in doses of 75 mg three times daily by mouth for the treatment of pain, inflammation, and fever. Pranoprofen has also been used as eye drops in a concentration of 0.1% for ocular inflammation.

References.

1. Notivol R, *et al.* Treatment of chronic nonbacterial conjunctivitis with a cyclo-oxygenase inhibitor or a corticosteroid. *Am J Ophthalmol* 1994; **117:** 651–6.

Preparations

Proprietary Preparations (details are given in Part 3)
Belg.: Pranox; ***Jpn:*** Niflan; ***Spain:*** Oftalar.

Proglumetacin Maleate (13174-q)

Proglumetacin Maleate *(BANM, rINNM).*

CR-604; Protacine Maleate. 3-{4-[2-(1-*p*-Chlorobenzoyl-5-methoxy-2-methylindol-3-ylacetoxy)ethyl]piperazin-1-yl}propyl 4-benzamido-*N*,*N*-dipropylglutaramate dimaleate.

$C_{46}H_{58}ClN_5O_8,2C_4H_4O_4$ = 1076.6.

CAS — 57132-53-3 (proglumetacin); 59209-40-4 (proglumetacin maleate).

Proglumetacin maleate, an indoleacetic acid derivative related to indomethacin (p.45), is an NSAID (p.63). It has been used in musculoskeletal and joint disorders in doses of up to 450 mg daily, in divided doses, by mouth.

References.

1. Appelboom T, Franchimont P. Proglumetacin versus indometacin in rheumatoid arthritis: a double-blind multicenter study. *Adv Therapy* 1994; **11:** 228–34.

2. Martens M. Double-blind randomized comparison of proglumetacin and naproxen sodium in the treatment of patients with ankle sprains. *Curr Ther Res* 1995; **56:** 639–48.

Preparations

Proprietary Preparations (details are given in Part 3)
Aust.: Protaxon; ***Belg.:*** Tolindol; ***Ger.:*** Protaxon; ***Ital.:*** Afloxan; Proxil; ***Spain:*** Prodamox; Protaxil.

Propacetamol Hydrochloride (13537-a)

Propacetamol Hydrochloride *(rINNM).*

Propacetamoli Hydrochloridum. The hydrochloride of *N*,*N*-diethylglycine ester with paracetamol.

$C_{14}H_{20}N_2O_3,HCl$ = 300.8.

CAS — 66532-85-2 (propacetamol).

Pharmacopoeias. In *Eur.* (see p.viii).

A white or almost white crystalline powder. Freely **soluble** in water; slightly soluble in dehydrated alcohol; practically insoluble in acetone. **Protect** from moisture.

Propacetamol, a para-aminophenol derivative, is hydrolysed to paracetamol (p.72) in the plasma. It has been given as the hydrochloride intramuscularly or intravenously in doses of 1 to 2 g for the treatment of pain (p.4) and fever (p.1).

A report[1] of occupational contact dermatitis in 3 nurses arising from the preparation of injections of propacetamol.

1. Barband A, *et al.* Occupational allergy to propacetamol. *Lancet* 1995; **346:** 902.

Preparations

Proprietary Preparations (details are given in Part 3)
Belg.: Pro-Dafalgan; ***Fr.:*** Pro-Dafalgan; ***Ital.:*** Pro-Efferalgan; ***Switz.:*** Pro-Dafalgan.

Propiram Fumarate (2695-p)

Propiram Fumarate *(BANM, USAN, rINNM).*

Bay-4503; FBA-4503. *N*-(1-Methyl-2-piperidinoethyl)-*N*-(2-pyridyl)propionamide hydrogen fumarate.

$C_{16}H_{25}N_3O,C_4H_4O_4$ = 391.5.

CAS — 15686-91-6 (propiram); 13717-04-9 (propiram fumarate).

Propiram fumarate is an agonist-antagonist opioid analgesic (p.67) classified as a partial agonist at μ opioid receptors. It has been given by mouth for the relief of moderate to severe pain.

References.

1. Goa KL, Brogden RN. Propiram: a review of its pharmacodynamic and pharmacokinetic properties, and clinical use as an analgesic. *Drugs* 1993; **46:** 428–45.

Propyl Nicotinate (19727-m)

$C_9H_{11}NO_2$ = 165.2.

Propyl nicotinate is used in topical preparations as a rubefacient.

Preparations

Proprietary Preparations (details are given in Part 3)
Ger.: Elacur; Nicodan; Nicodan N†.
Multi-ingredient: ***Ger.:*** Elacur NO†.

Propyphenazone (2696-s)

Propyphenazone *(BAN, rINN).*

Isopropylantipyrine; Isopropylantipyrinum; Isopropylphenazone; Propifenazona; Propyphenazonum. 4-Isopropyl-2,3-dimethyl-1-phenyl-3-pyrazolin-5-one.

$C_{14}H_{18}N_2O$ = 230.3.

CAS — 479-92-5.

Pharmacopoeias. In *Eur.* (see p.viii) and *Jpn.*

A white or slightly yellowish crystalline powder. Slightly **soluble** in water; freely soluble in alcohol and in dichloromethane; soluble in ether. **Protect** from light.

Propyphenazone, a pyrazolone derivative related to phenazone (p.78), has analgesic and antipyretic properties. It has been given by mouth and as a rectal suppository in the treatment of pain and fever. There have been some reports of severe hypersensitivity reactions in patients receiving propyphenazone.

Porphyria. Propyphenazone has been associated with clinical exacerbations of porphyria and is considered unsafe in porphyric patients.[1]

1. Moore MR, McColl KEL. *Porphyria: drug lists.* Glasgow: Porphyria Research Unit, University of Glasgow, 1991.

Preparations

Proprietary Preparations (details are given in Part 3)
Aust.: Dim-Antos; ***Belg.:*** Cibalgine†; ***Ger.:*** Arantil P†; Demex; Eufibron; Hewedolor propy†; Isoprochin P; ***Ital.:*** Causyth†; Cibalgina†; Pireuma; ***Spain:*** Budirol†; Cibalgina.

Multi-ingredient: ***Aust.:*** Adolorin; Adoluron CC; APA; Asthma; Asticol; Avamigran; Cedanon; Coldagrippin; Contraforte; Contralorin; Eu-Med; Gewadal; Influvidon; Melabon; Migradon; Montamed; Neokratin; Nervan; Neuro-Europan; Normensan; Rapidol; Sanalgit†; Saridon; Spasmoplus; Tonopan; Toximer; Vivimed; ***Belg.:*** Migraine-Kranit Nova; Migraine-Kranit†; Neuridon Forte; Optalidon; Saridon; Spasmo-Cibalgine; Spasmoplus; ***Fr.:*** Polypirine; ***Ger.:*** Agevis†; Ariven SN†; Avamigran N; Cibalen†; Clinit N†; Commotional S†; Copyrkal N†; Dolo-Phlogase†; Ergo-Kranit; Eu-Med SC†; Eudorlin†; Fomagrippin N; Fortalidon S†; Gentil†; Gewodin; Grippostad†; Ichtho-Bellol compositum S; Ichthospasmin N†; Kephalosan†; Mandrorhinon†; Migrane-Kranit N; Migranex spezial N†; Migratan S; Neuro-Demoplas†; Neuro-Spondyril S†; Norgesic N; Novo Petrin; Optalidon N; Optalidon special Noc; Ozabran N†; Saridon; Spasmo-Cibalgin compositum S; Spasmo-Cibalgin S; Temagin†; Tispol S; Titretta; Titretta analgica B†; Titretta analgica†; Verla-3†; ***Ital.:*** Alfazina; Azerodol; Caffalgina; Cistalgan; Etocil Pirina†; Exit†; Fargepirina†; Flexidone; Flexipyrin†; Influrem; Influvit; Megal†; Micranet; Mindol-Merck; Neo-Optalidon; Odontalgico Dr. Knapp con Vit. B1; Omniadol; Optalidon; Ozopulmin Antipiretico†; Ribelfan; Saridon; Saridon senza Caffeina†; Sedol; Spasmo-Cibalgina; Spasmoplus; Uniplus; Upsa Plus; Veramon; Vitialgin; Xival†; ***Neth.:*** Daro Hoofdpijnpoeders; Sanalgin; Saridon; ***S.Afr.:*** Ilvico; ***Spain:*** Abdominol; Bronquimar; Calmoplex; Cibalgina Compuesta; Dolodens; Espasmo Cibalgina†; Fenalgin; Flexagil; Hubergrip; Leodin†; Lotanal†; Megral†; Melabon; Meloka; Optalidon; Quimpedor; Rectolmin Antiterm†; Saridon; Sedalmerck; Sedatermin†; Spasmalfher†; Sulmetin Papaver; Sulmetin Papaverina; Supra Leodin†; Tabletas Quimpe; Tonopan; ***Switz.:*** Angifebrine; Barbamin; Caposan; Cerebrol; Comprimes analgesiques "S"; Dialgine forte N; Dismenol†; Dolopyrine; Dolostop; Epizon†; Escalgin sans codeine; Escoflex Compositum†; Escogripp sans codeine; Escogripp†; Febracyl; Fortalidon sans codeine†; Fortalidon†; Gewodine; Gubamine; Kafa; Melabon†; Melaforte†; Nicaphlogyl; Novidol; Quadronal†; Radolor†; Sanalgin; Saridon; Seranex sans codeine; Sinedal; Siniphen; Sonotryl; Spasmanodine†; Spasmo-Barbamin; Spasmo-Barbamine compositum; Spasmo-Cibalgin; Spasmo-Cibalgin comp; Spasmosol†; Spedralgin sans codeine; Tonopan.

Proquazone (13180-v)

Proquazone *(BAN, USAN, rINN).*

43-715; RU-43-715-n. 1-Isopropyl-7-methyl-4-phenylquinazolin-2(1*H*)-one.

$C_{18}H_{18}N_2O$ = 278.3.

CAS — 22760-18-5.

Proquazone is an NSAID (p.63). It is given by mouth in musculoskeletal and joint disorders in usual doses of 600 to 900 mg daily in divided doses; up to 1.2 g daily may be given for up to 7 days if necessary. It may also be given by rectal suppository.

References.

1. Clissold SP, Beresford R. Proquazone: a review of its pharmacodynamic and pharmacokinetic properties, and therapeutic efficacy in rheumatic diseases and pain states. *Drugs* 1987; **33:** 478–50.

Preparations

Proprietary Preparations (details are given in Part 3)
Aust.: Biarison; ***Switz.:*** Biarison†.

Protizinic Acid (2697-w)

Protizinic Acid *(rINN)*.
2-(7-Methoxy-10-methylphenothiazin-2-yl)propionic acid.
$C_{17}H_{17}NO_3S$ = 315.4.
CAS — 13799-03-6.

Protizinic acid is an NSAID (p.63) that has been used in musculoskeletal and joint disorders.

Ramifenazone (2660-x)

Ramifenazone *(rINN)*.
Isopropylaminophenazone; Isopyrin. 4-Isopropylamino-2,3-dimethyl-1-phenyl-3-pyrazolin-5-one.
$C_{14}H_{19}N_3O$ = 245.3.
CAS — 3615-24-5.

NOTE. The name Isopyrin has also been applied to isoniazid.

Ramifenazone is an NSAID (p.63) that has been used in preparations for painful and inflammatory conditions. The hydrochloride salt was given by mouth and the salicylate applied topically.

Preparations

Proprietary Preparations (details are given in Part 3)
Multi-ingredient: ***Aust.:*** Delta-Tomanol.

Remifentanil Hydrochloride

(13662-d)

Remifentanil Hydrochloride *(BANM, USAN, rINNM)*.
GI-87084B. 4-Carboxyl-4-(*N*-phenylpropionamido)-1-piperidine propionic acid dimethyl ester monohydrate.
$C_{20}H_{28}N_2O_5,HCl$ = 412.9.
CAS — 132539-07-2.

Remifentanil hydrochloride 1.1 mg is approximately equivalent to 1 mg of remifentanil.

Incompatibility. The manufacturers state that remifentanil hydrochloride should not be mixed with lactated Ringer's injection with or without 5% glucose injection. It should not be mixed in the same solution for intravenous administration as propofol or blood products. Incompatibilities have been reported between chlorpromazine hydrochloride 2 mg per mL and remifentanil 25 µg per mL (as the hydrochloride) in 5% glucose and cefoperazone sodium 40 mg per mL or amphotericin 0.6 mg/mL and remifentanil 250 µg per mL (as the hydrochloride) in 5% glucose.[1]

1. Trissel LA, *et al.* Compatibility of remifentanil hydrochloride with selected drugs during simulated Y-site administration. *Am J Health-Syst Pharm* 1997; **54:** 2192–6.

Dependence and Withdrawal

As for Opioid Analgesics, p.67.

Adverse Effects and Treatment

As for Opioid Analgesics in general, p.68 and for Fentanyl, p.38.

Precautions

As for Opioid Analgesics in general, p.68.

Initial doses should be reduced in elderly patients.

Administration. Remifentanil hydrochloride injections containing glycine should not be given by the epidural or intrathecal routes.

Hepatic impairment. Although the pharmacokinetics of remifentanil are not changed in patients with severe hepatic impairment, such patients may be more sensitive to the respiratory depressant effects and should be monitored with doses titrated to individual requirements.

Renal impairment. The pharmacokinetics of remifentanil are not changed in patients with severe renal impairment (a creatinine clearance of less than 10 mL per minute) and the manufacturers have stated that the carboxylic acid metabolite is unlikely to accumulate to clinically active concentrations in such patients following remifentanil infusions of up to 2 µg per kg per minute for up to 12 hours. Dosage adjustments relative to that used in other patients are considered to be unnecessary.

Interactions

For interactions associated with opioid analgesics, see p.69.

Pharmacokinetics

Following parenteral administration remifentanil hydrochloride has a rapid onset and short duration of action. Its effective biological half-life is about 3 to 10 minutes and is independent of dose. Remifentanil is about 70% bound to plasma proteins, principally to α_1-acid glycoprotein. It is hydrolysed by non-specific esterases in blood and tissues to an essentially inactive carboxylic acid metabolite. Approximately 95% of a dose of remifentanil is excreted in the urine as the metabolite.

The manufacturers of remifentanil have given values for a three-compartment pharmacokinetic model with a rapid distribution half-life of 1 minute, a slower distribution half-life of 6 minutes, and a terminal elimination half-life of 10 to 20 minutes.

References to the pharmacokinetics of remifentanil are given below.

1. Egan TD. Remifentanil pharmacokinetics and pharmacodynamics: a preliminary appraisal. *Clin Pharmacokinet* 1995; **29:** 80–94.

Uses and Administration

Remifentanil, an anilidopiperidine derivative, is an opioid analgesic (p.69) related to fentanyl (p.39). It is a short-acting µ-receptor opioid agonist used for analgesia during induction and/or maintenance of general anaesthesia. It is also used to provide analgesia into the immediate postoperative period. Remifentanil is administered intravenously as the hydrochloride, usually by infusion. Its onset of action is within 1 minute and the duration of action is 5 to 10 minutes. Doses are expressed in terms of remifentanil base. Initial doses in elderly patients should be half the recommended adult doses and then titrated to individual requirements.

When used to provide analgesia during induction of anaesthesia an intravenous infusion is given in doses of 0.5 to 1.0 µg per kg body-weight per minute. An additional initial intravenous bolus of 1 µg per kg may be administered over 30 to 60 seconds if the patient is to be intubated less than 8 minutes after the start of the infusion.

For provision of analgesia during maintenance of anaesthesia in ventilated patients, infusion doses range from 0.05 to 2.0 µg per kg per minute depending on the anaesthetic drug employed and adjusted according to patient response. Supplemental intravenous boluses of 0.5 to 1 µg per kg may be given every 2 to 5 minutes in response to light anaesthesia or intense surgical stress. The infusion dosage in spontaneous respiration is initially 0.04 µg per kg per minute adjusted according to response within a usual range of 0.025 to 0.1 µg per kg per minute. Bolus doses are not recommended during spontaneous ventilation.

For continuation of analgesia into the immediate postoperative period doses by intravenous infusion range from 0.025 to 0.2 µg per kg per minute; supplemental intravenous bolus doses are not recommended during the postoperative period.

Remifentanil may also be used as the analgesic component of local or regional anaesthesia with or without benzodiazepine sedation.

Remifentanil has a very rapid offset of action and no residual opioid action remains 5 to 10 minutes after discontinuation of an infusion. Consideration should therefore be given to provision of alternative analgesics administered in sufficient time before discontinuation of remifentanil to provide continuous and more prolonged postoperative pain relief when appropriate.

References and reviews.

1. Bacon R, *et al.* Early extubation after open-heart surgery with total intravenous anaesthetic technique. *Lancet* 1995; **345:** 133–4.
2. Duthie DJR, *et al.* Remifentanil and coronary artery surgery. *Lancet* 1995; **345:** 649–50.
3. Patel SS, Spencer CM. Remifentanil. *Drugs* 1996; **52:** 417–27.
4. Duthie DJR. Remifentanil and tramadol. *Br J Anaesth* 1998; **81:** 51–7.

Preparations

Proprietary Preparations (details are given in Part 3)
Fr.: Ultiva; ***Ger.:*** Ultiva; ***Ital.:*** Ultiva; ***Neth.:*** Ultiva; ***UK:*** Ultiva; ***USA:*** Ultiva.

Salacetamide (11612-x)

Salacetamide *(rINN)*.
L-749. *N*-Acetylsalicylamide.
$C_9H_9NO_3$ = 179.2.
CAS — 487-48-9.

Salacetamide is a salicylic acid derivative (see Aspirin, p.16) that was used in the relief of pain and fever.

Preparations

Proprietary Preparations (details are given in Part 3)
Multi-ingredient: ***Ger.:*** Eu-Med SC†; Octadon†.

Salamidacetic Acid (2622-j)

Carbamoylphenoxyacetic acid; Salicylamide *O*-acetic acid. (2-Carbamoylphenoxy)acetic acid.
$C_9H_9NO_4$ = 195.2.
CAS — 25395-22-6 (salamidacetic acid); 3785-32-8 (sodium salamidacetate).

Salamidacetic acid is a salicylic acid derivative (see Aspirin, p.16) that has also been used as the sodium and diethylamine salts for the treatment of musculoskeletal and joint disorders.

Preparations

Proprietary Preparations (details are given in Part 3)
Aust.: Akistin†; ***Ger.:*** Clinit N; ***Ital.:*** Neosalid†.

Multi-ingredient: ***Aust.:*** Ambene; Rheumesser; ***Ger.:*** Arbid†; Caye Balsam; Flexurat; Glutisal-buton-Salbe†; Hewedolor B†; Hewedolor forte; Mussera†; Rhinoinfant†.

Salicylamide (2700-l)

Salicylamide *(BAN, rINN)*.
2-Hydroxybenzamide.
$C_7H_7NO_2$ = 137.1.
CAS — 65-45-2.
Pharmacopoeias. In *Aust.*, *Pol.*, and *US.*

A white practically odourless crystalline powder. Slightly **soluble** in water and in chloroform; soluble in alcohol and in propylene glycol; freely soluble in ether and in solutions of alkalis.

Salicylamide is a salicylic acid derivative (see Aspirin, p.16) but is not hydrolysed to salicylate; it is almost completely metabolised to inactive metabolites during absorption and on first pass through the liver. It is given in doses of 325 to 650 mg or more by mouth, usually with other analgesics, three or four times daily for pain and fever. Salicylamide is also applied topically in rubefacient preparations in concentrations of about 5% for the relief of muscular and rheumatic pain.

Preparations

Proprietary Preparations (details are given in Part 3)
Aust.: Isosal; ***Ital.:*** Sinedol†; Urtosal†.

Multi-ingredient: ***Aust.:*** Influvidon; Isosal; Rilfit†; Rubriment; Sigmalin B_6; Sigmalin B_6 forte; Sigmalin B_6 ohne Coffein; Spalt; ***Belg.:*** Antigrip†; Intralgin†; Myalgesic; Percutalgine; ***Canad.:*** Achrocidin†; ***Fr.:*** Percutalgine; ***Ger.:*** ABC-Bad†; Anti.opt†; Antigrippalin†; Arbid†; Chinavit†; Coffalon; Gentarol N†; Gentil†; Glutisal; Glutisal-buton†; Glutisal†; Grippostad†; Kontagripp-RR†; Kontagripp†; Melabon N†; Ortholan†; Poikicin†; Refagan N†; Rheumadrag†; Romigal N†; Rosimon-Neu†; Salistoperm; Siguran N†; Spasmo-Gentarol N†; Spondylon S†; Treupel-N†; ***Ital.:*** Anticorizza; Azerodol; Exit†; Refagan†; ***S.Afr.:*** Ascold; Colcaps; Flutex; Histamed Co; Ilvico; Intralgin†; ***Spain:*** Boncicol†; Coricidin; Doloana; Fiorinal Codeina†; Fiorinal†; Hubergrip; Nefrolit†; Percutalin; Pridio; Prontal†; Rinomicine; Rinomicine Activada; Tuscalman†; Yendol; ***Switz.:*** Comba-Gripp; Demogripp†; Escalgin sans codeine; Escogripp sans codeine; Escogripp†; Grippalgine N; No Grip; Novidol; Osa; Siniphen; ***UK:*** Intralgin; ***USA:*** Anodynos; BC; Lobac; Presalin; Rhinogesic; Rid-a-Pain with Codeine; S-A-C; Saleto; Saleto-D; Salocol; Salphenyl; Tri-Pain; Triaprin-DC†.

Salix (11536-n)

Salicis Cortex; Willow Bark.
Pharmacopoeias. In *Ger.*

Salix consists of the dried bark of *Salix alba* and other species of *Salix* (Salicaceae), notably *S. fragilis*, *S. purpurea*, and *S. pentandra*. It contains variable amounts of tannin and also of salicin ($C_{13}H_{18}O_7$ = 286.3) which has antipyretic and analgesic actions similar to those of aspirin. Salix has been used in a variety of herbal remedies for painful and inflammatory conditions and for fever. It was once used as a bitter.

Preparations

Proprietary Preparations (details are given in Part 3)
Aust.: Biogelat Erkaltungs & Grippe; ***Canad.:*** Saliton; ***Ger.:*** Rheumakaps; Rheumatab Salicis; Schmerzetten†; Tamanybonsan.

Multi-ingredient: ***Aust.:*** Digestodoron; Grippefloran; Kneipp Grippe-Tee; ***Austral.:*** Arthritic Pain Herbal Formula 1; Harpagophytum Complex; Lifesystem Herbal Formula 1 Arthritic Aid; Lifesystem Herbal Formula 12 Willowbark; Prost-1; Salagesic; Willowbark Plus Herbal Formula 11; ***Canad.:*** Arthrisan; ***Fr.:*** Arkophytum; Canteine Bouteille†; Digestodoron; Mediflor Tisane Circulation du Sang No 12; Passinevryl†; Santane A_4; ***Ger.:*** entero sanol†; Grippe-Tee Stada†; Hevert-Erkaltungs-Tee; Hevert-Gicht-Rheuma-Tee comp; Kneipp Rheuma Tee N; Knufinke Blasen- und Nieren-Tee Uro-K†; Nephrubin; Passiorin†; Rheumex†; ***Ital.:*** Depurativo; Donalg; Fluend; Passiflorine; Tauma; ***Spain:*** Passiflorine; ***Switz.:*** Dragees antirhumatismales fortes; Dragees contre les maux de tete; Phytomed Rhino; Tisane antirhumatismale; Tisane antirhumatismale "H"†; Valverde contre les douleurs†; ***UK:*** Digestodoron; Herbal Pain Relief; Ligvites.

Salol (9315-y)

Phenyl salicylate.

$C_{13}H_{10}O_3$ = 214.2.

CAS — 118-55-8.

Pharmacopoeias. In *Aust.* and *Pol.*

Salol is a salicylic acid derivative (see Aspirin, p.16). It was formerly used as an intestinal antiseptic, but effective doses were toxic owing to the liberation of phenol. It is used in oral preparations containing hexamine for the treatment of lower urinary-tract infections.

Salol has been used topically as a sunscreen.

Preparations

Proprietary Preparations (details are given in Part 3)
Austral.: Aussie Tan Sunstick.

Multi-ingredient: ***Aust.:*** Carl Baders Divinal; ***Austral.:*** Lip-Sed†; ***Canad.:*** Franzbranns; ***Fr.:*** Borostyrol; Saprol†; ***Ger.:*** Parodontal F5 med; Urodil N†; ***Swed.:*** Munvatten†; ***Switz.:*** Borostyrol N; Dermophil Indien; ***USA:*** Atrosept; Dolsed; Prosed/DS; Trac Tabs 2X; UAA; Uridon Modified; Urimar-T; Urised; Urogesic Blue.

Salsalate (2702-j)

Salsalate *(BAN, USAN, rINN).*

NSC-49171; Salicyl Salicylate; Salicylosalicylic Acid; Salicylsalicylic Acid; Salysal; Sasapyrine. *O*-(2-Hydroxybenzoyl)salicylic acid.

$C_{14}H_{10}O_5$ = 258.2.

CAS — 552-94-3.

Pharmacopoeias. In *US.*

Store in airtight containers.

Adverse Effects, Treatment, and Precautions

As for Aspirin, p.16.

The use of aspirin and other acetylated salicylates is generally not recommended for children under the age of 12 years because of the risk of Reye's syndrome, unless specifically indicated. Some authorities also extend this precaution to non-acetylated salicylates such as salsalate.

Salsalate has been reported to interfere with thyroid function tests.

Effects on the gastro-intestinal tract. Salsalate is associated with less faecal blood loss than aspirin and has been reported to cause fewer gastric lesions than piroxicam.[1] However, small-bowel ulcerations were reported in a patient when salsalate was added to a regimen of ranitidine and metoclopramide which had been prescribed for duodenal ulcer.[2]

1. Porro GB, *et al.* Salsalate in the treatment of rheumatoid arthritis: a double-blind clinical and gastroscopic trial versus piroxicam: II—endoscopic evaluation. *J Int Med Res* 1989; **17:** 320–3.
2. Souza Lima MA. Ulcers of the small bowel associated with stomach-bypassing salicylates. *Arch Intern Med* 1985; **145:** 1139.

Effects on the kidneys. Minimal-change nephrotic syndrome has been associated with salsalate in one patient.[1]

1. Vallès M, Tovar JL. Salsalate and minimal-change nephrotic syndrome. *Ann Intern Med* 1987; **107:** 116.

Interactions

For interactions associated with salicylates, see Aspirin, p.17.

Pharmacokinetics

Salsalate is insoluble in acidic gastric fluids but is soluble in the small intestine. One molecule of salsalate is hydrolysed to 2 molecules of salicylic acid; hydrolysis occurs both in the small intestine and following absorption of the parent compound. Additional details on the pharmacokinetics of salicylic acid are provided in aspirin (see p.18). Not all of the absorbed salsalate is hydrolysed and about 13% of salsalate is excreted as glucuronide conjugates in the urine; thus, the amount of salicylic acid available from salsalate is less than that from aspirin when the two drugs are given in equimolar equivalents of salicylic acid.

Uses and Administration

Salsalate is a salicylic acid derivative that has analgesic, anti-inflammatory, and antipyretic actions similar to those of aspirin (see p.18). It is used for pain and fever and also in inflammatory disorders such as osteoarthritis and rheumatoid arthritis. A usual dose is up to 3 g daily given by mouth in divided doses with food.

Preparations

USP 23: Salsalate Capsules; Salsalate Tablets.

Proprietary Preparations (details are given in Part 3)
Canad.: Disalcid; ***Ger.:*** Disalgesic†; ***Spain:*** Atisuril†; Umbradol; ***UK:*** Disalcid†; ***USA:*** Amigesic; Argesic-SA; Artha-G; Disalcid; Marthritic; Mono-Gesic; Salflex; Salsitab.

Sarracenia Purpurea (18472-e)

Pitcher Plant.

The roots and leaves of *Sarracenia purpurea* (Sarraceniaceae) have been used in the form of an aqueous distillate, administered by local injection, for neuromuscular or neuralgic pain.

Preparations

Proprietary Preparations (details are given in Part 3)
USA: Sarapin†.

Sodium Aurothiomalate (5296-k)

Sodium Aurothiomalate *(rINN).*

Gold Sodium Thiomalate; Sodium Aurothiosuccinate.

CAS — 12244-57-4 (xNa, anhydrous); 39377-38-3 (2Na monohydrate).

Pharmacopoeias. In *Br., Jpn,* and *US.*

The BP description is a fine, pale yellow, hygroscopic powder with a slight odour. It consists mainly of the disodium salt of (aurothio)succinic acid ($C_4H_3AuNa_2O_4S$ = 390.1) and has a gold content of 44.5 to 46.0% calculated on the dried material. Very **soluble** in water. A 10% solution in water has a pH of 6.0 to 7.0.

The USP defines a mixture of the monosodium and disodium salts of gold thiomalic acid[(aurothio)succinic acid] ($C_4H_4AuNaO_4S$ = 368.1 and $C_4H_3AuNa_2O_4S$ = 390.1) that has a gold content of 44.8 to 49.6%, and 49.0 to 52.5% calculated on the dried glycerol-free material. A 10% solution in water has a pH of 5.8 to 6.5.

Store in airtight containers. Protect from light.

Adverse Effects

Reports show a wide range for the incidence of adverse effects of sodium aurothiomalate. However, authorities consider that with careful treatment about one-third of patients will experience adverse effects. It is also considered that about 5% of patients will experience severe adverse effects and that some of the effects will be fatal. The most common effects involve the skin and mucous membranes with pruritus (an early sign of intolerance) and stomatitis (often with a metallic taste) being the most prominent. Rashes with pruritus often occur after 2 to 6 months of intramuscular treatment and may necessitate discontinuation of therapy. Other reactions affecting the skin and mucous membranes include erythema, maculopapular eruptions, erythema multiforme, urticaria, eczema, seborrhoeic dermatitis, lichenoid eruptions, alopecia, exfoliative dermatitis, glossitis, pharyngitis, vaginitis, photosensitivity reactions, and irreversible pigmentation (chrysiasis).

Toxic effects on the blood include eosinophilia, thrombocytopenia, leucopenia, agranulocytosis, and aplastic anaemia.

Effects on the kidneys include mild transient proteinuria which may lead to heavy proteinuria, haematuria, and nephrosis.

Other effects reported include pulmonary fibrosis, toxic hepatitis, cholestatic jaundice, peripheral neuritis, encephalitis, psychoses, fever, and gastro-intestinal disorders including enterocolitis. Gold deposits may occur in the eyes. Vasomotor or nitritoid reactions, with weakness, flushing, palpitations, and dyspnoea, may occur following injection of sodium aurothiomalate. Local irritation may also follow injection.

Sometimes there is an initial exacerbation of the arthritic condition.

A number of the adverse effects of gold have an immunogenic component.

Reviews.

1. Tozman ECS, Gottlieb NL. Adverse reactions with oral and parenteral gold preparations. *Med Toxicol* 1987; **2:** 177–89.

Effects on the blood. Blood disorders such as leucopenia, granulocytopenia, and thrombocytopenia have occurred in patients receiving gold therapy. Eosinophilia has been reported to be the most frequent haematological abnormality.[1] It is estimated that thrombocytopenia develops in 1 to 3% of patients receiving gold salts.[2]

Fatal consumption coagulopathy occurred in 4 children following the second injection of sodium aurothioglucose or sodium aurothiomalate.[3]

1. Foster RT. Eosinophilia—a marker of gold toxicity. *Can J Hosp Pharm* 1985; **85:** 150–1.
2. Coblyn JS, *et al.* Gold-induced thrombocytopenia: a clinical and immunogenetic study of twenty-three patients. *Ann Intern Med* 1981; **95:** 178–81.
3. Jacobs JC, *et al.* Consumption coagulopathy after gold therapy for JRA. *J Pediatr* 1984; **105:** 674–5.

Effects on the cardiovascular system. Vasomotor or nitritoid reactions associated with administration of gold compounds are usually transient and self-limiting and although they may be mild there have been isolated reports of associated complications such as myocardial infarction, stroke, transient ischaemic attack, and transient monocular visual loss.[1] Most reactions have been associated with sodium aurothiomalate (a reported incidence of 4.7%) but they have also occurred with auranofin and sodium aurothioglucose. Tachyphylaxis usually occurs to the reactions and most patients are able to continue treatment but paradoxically in some the severity increases with repeated doses; 2.8% of patients receiving sodium aurothiomalate may require a change of treatment due to recurrent reactions. Transfer to sodium aurothioglucose may be an option in patients who derive significant benefit from gold injections but it is important firstly to distinguish such reactions from true anaphylactic reactions to gold.

1. Ho M, Pullar T. Vasomotor reactions with gold. *Br J Rheumatol* 1997; **36:** 154–6.

Effects on the gastro-intestinal tract. A case report of enterocolitis due to sodium aurothiomalate has been published[1] and 27 other cases associated with gold therapy reviewed.

1. Jackson CW, *et al.* Gold induced enterocolitis. *Gut* 1986; **27:** 452–56.

Effects on the immune system. Details of a patient who developed an immune deficiency syndrome that was attributed to gold therapy with sodium aurothiomalate.[1]

1. Haskard DO, Macfarlane D. Adult acquired combined immune deficiency in a patient with rheumatoid arthritis on gold. *J R Soc Med* 1988; **81:** 548–9.

Effects on the kidneys. Proteinuria developed in 21 patients while receiving a standard regimen of sodium aurothiomalate.[1] The severity of the proteinuria varied greatly and in 11 it increased for 4 months after treatment was stopped. Eight patients were considered to have developed the nephrotic syndrome. The median duration of proteinuria was 11 months, resolving in all 21 patients when treatment was withdrawn; at 24 months 3 patients were still experiencing proteinuria and it was not until 39 months that all were free of the condition. Renal biopsy indicated several types of kidney damage.

See under Auranofin (p.20) for a comparative incidence of proteinuria in patients receiving sodium aurothiomalate or auranofin.

1. Hall CL, *et al.* The natural course of gold nephropathy: long term study of 21 patients. *Br Med J* 1987; **295:** 745–8.

Effects on the liver. Some reports of hepatotoxicity with sodium aurothiomalate.[1,2]

1. Favreau M, *et al.* Hepatic toxicity associated with gold therapy. *Ann Intern Med* 1977; **87:** 717–19.
2. Edelman J, *et al.* Liver dysfunction associated with gold therapy for rheumatoid arthritis. *J Rheumatol* 1983; **10:** 510–11.

Effects on the lungs. 'Gold lung' is the term used to describe symptoms of dyspnoea on exertion, weakness, dry cough, and malaise developing some weeks or months after starting gold treatment. Pulmonary insufficiency may eventually develop. The pulmonary lesions usually subside on withdrawal of gold therapy, although persistent symptoms have been reported. Nonbacterial thrombotic endocarditis associated with gold-induced pulmonary disease has also been reported.[1] This was considered to be a manifestation of gold-induced immune complex deposition.

1. Kollef MH, *et al.* Nonbacterial thrombotic endocarditis associated with gold induced pulmonary disease. *Ann Intern Med* 1988; **108:** 903–4.

Effects on the nervous system. Reports of sodium aurothiomalate adversely affecting the nervous system.[1-5]

1. Dick DJ, Raman D. The Guillain-Barre syndrome following gold therapy. *Scand J Rheumatol* 1982; **11:** 119–20.
2. Schlumpf U, *et al.* Neurologic complications induced by gold treatment. *Arthritis Rheum* 1983; **26:** 825–31 (Guillain-Barré syndrome and neuropathy with myokymia).
3. Cerinic MM, *et al.* Gold polyneuropathy in juvenile rheumatoid arthritis. *Br Med J* 1985; **290:** 1042.
4. Cohen M, *et al.* Acute disseminated encephalomyelitis as a complication of treatment with gold. *Br Med J* 1985; **290:** 1179–80.
5. Dubowitz MN, *et al.* Gold-induced neuroencephalopathy responding to dimercaprol. *Lancet* 1991; **337:** 850–1.

Effects on the skin. Chrysiasis is a distinctive pigmentation that develops in light-exposed skin of patients receiving parenteral gold salts. In a study[1] of 31 patients with chrysiasis who were receiving intramuscular sodium aurothiomalate for rheumatoid arthritis, it was noted that visible changes developed above a threshold equivalent to 20 mg per kg bodyweight gold content. The severity of the pigmentation depended upon cumulative dose. Focal aggregates of gold are deposited in the reticular and papillary dermis with no obvious increase in melanin. The pigmentation is permanent but benign, although the cosmetic effects may cause some patients distress. Prevention of chrysiasis is difficult but avoidance of exposure to sunlight may be helpful.

1. Smith RW, *et al.* Chrysiasis revisited: a clinical and pathological study. *Br J Dermatol* 1995; **133:** 671–8.

Hypersensitivity. Many adverse effects associated with gold treatment have an immunological basis. Small amounts of nickel have been detected in sodium aurothiomalate injection[1] and in sodium aurothioglucose injection[2] and it has been suggested that gold therapy may exacerbate or induce hypersensitivity to nickel.[1-3]

1. Choy EHS, *et al.* Nickel contamination of gold salts: link with gold-induced skin rash. *Br J Rheumatol* 1997; **36:** 1054–8.
2. Wijnands MJH, *et al.* Chrysotherapy provoking exacerbation of contact hypersensitivity to nickel. *Lancet* 1990; **335:** 867–8.
3. Fulton RA, *et al.* Another hazard of gold therapy? *Ann Rheum Dis* 1982; **41:** 100–1.

Pancreatitis. It was suggested that pancreatitis reported in a woman receiving gold injections and in a woman on oral gold therapy may have been due to a hypersensitivity reaction.[1]

1. Eisemann AD, *et al.* Pancreatitis and gold treatment of rheumatoid arthritis. *Ann Intern Med* 1989; **111:** 860–1.

Treatment of Adverse Effects

The treatment of the adverse effects of gold is usually symptomatic and most effects resolve when gold therapy is withdrawn. In severe cases a chelating agent such as dimercaprol (p.979) may be employed.

Precautions

Gold therapy is contra-indicated in exfoliative dermatitis, systemic lupus erythematosus, necrotising enterocolitis, and pulmonary fibrosis. It should be used with caution in patients with renal or hepatic impairment and in the elderly but is contra-indicated in severe renal or hepatic disorders. Patients with a history of haematological disorders or who have previously shown toxicity to heavy metals should not be given gold salts, nor should any severely debilitated patient.

It is recommended that diabetes mellitus and heart failure should be adequately controlled in any patient before gold is given. Patients with a history of urticaria, eczema, or colitis should be treated with caution. Patients with a poor sulphoxidation state may be more susceptible to adverse effects of sodium aurothiomalate.

It is generally recommended that gold salts should not be given to pregnant patients or to patients who are breast feeding.

Concurrent administration of gold salts with other therapy capable of inducing blood disorders should be undertaken with caution, if at all.

Due to the possibility of vasomotor reactions, patients should remain recumbent for about 10 minutes after each injection.

The urine should be tested for albumin before each injection and the blood should be examined for signs of depressed haemopoiesis. Patients should be warned to report the appearance of sore throat or tongue, metallic taste, pruritus, rash, buccal ulceration, easy bruising, purpura, epistaxis, bleeding gums, menorrhagia, pyrexia, indigestion, diarrhoea, or unexplained malaise. Effects such as eosinophilia, proteinuria, pruritus, and rash arising during gold treatment should be allowed to resolve before therapy is continued.

Annual chest X-rays should be carried out.

Breast feeding. Gold has been detected in breast milk[1,2] and found bound to the red blood cells of breast-fed babies.[2] In a report[1] of one breast-fed infant it was calculated that the weight-adjusted dose of gold received by the infant exceeded that received by the mother although the infant exhibited no ill-effects during 100 days of breast feeding and developed normally thereafter. Nonetheless, because of the relatively high exposure it was recommended that breast-fed infants should be closely monitored.

1. Bennett PN, *et al.* Use of sodium aurothiomalate during lactation. *Br J Clin Pharmacol* 1990; **29:** 777–9.
2. Needs CJ, Brooks PM. Antirheumatic medication during lactation. *Br J Rheumatol* 1985; **24:** 291–7.

Porphyria. Gold compounds are considered to be unsafe in porphyric patients.[1]

1. Moore MR, McColl KEL. *Porphyria: drug lists.* Glasgow: Porphyria Research Unit, University of Glasgow, 1991.

Pregnancy. Although there have been a number of healthy neonates born after *in-utero* exposure to gold compounds[1,2] *animal* studies and one report[1] of malformation in a child born to a woman treated with sodium aurothiomalate led to a suggestion that gold might possibly have teratogenic effects.

1. Rogers JG, *et al.* Possible teratogenic effects of gold. *Aust Paediatr J* 1980; **16:** 194–5.
2. Bennett PN, *et al.* Use of sodium aurothiomalate during lactation. *Br J Clin Pharmacol* 1990; **29:** 777–9.

Interactions

There is an increased risk of toxicity when gold compounds are administered concurrently with other nephrotoxic, hepatotoxic, or myelosuppressive drugs. Concurrent use of gold compounds with penicillamine may increase the risk of haematologic or renal adverse reactions.

For a discussion on the effects of previous therapy with gold salts affecting penicillamine toxicity, see under penicillamine (p.990).

Pharmacokinetics

Sodium aurothiomalate is absorbed readily after intramuscular injection and 85 to 95% becomes bound to plasma proteins. With doses of 50 mg weekly a steady-state serum concentration of gold of about 3 to 5 μg per mL is reached in 5 to 8 weeks. It is widely distributed to body tissues and fluids, including synovial fluid, and accumulates in the body.

The serum half-life of gold is about 5 or 6 days but this increases after successive doses and after a course of treatment, gold may be found in the urine for up to 1 year or more owing to its presence in deep body compartments. Sodium aurothiomalate is mainly excreted in the urine, with smaller amounts in the faeces.

Gold has been detected in the fetus following administration of sodium aurothiomalate to the mother. Gold is distributed into breast milk.

Reviews.

1. Blocka KLN, *et al.* Clinical pharmacokinetics of oral and injectable gold compounds. *Clin Pharmacokinet* 1986; **11:** 133–43.
2. Tett SE. Clinical pharmacokinetics of slow-acting antirheumatic drugs. *Clin Pharmacokinet* 1993; **25:** 392–407.

Uses and Administration

Sodium aurothiomalate and other gold salts are used mainly for their anti-inflammatory effect in active progressive rheumatoid arthritis and progressive juvenile chronic arthritis; they may also be beneficial in psoriatic arthritis. They are generally reserved for use as second-line drugs in patients whose symptoms are unresponsive to or inadequately controlled by NSAIDs alone.

Sodium aurothiomalate therapy should only be undertaken where facilities are available to carry out the tests specified under Precautions, above.

Sodium aurothiomalate is given by deep intramuscular injection; the area should be gently massaged and, due to the possibility of vasomotor reactions, the patient should remain recumbent for 10 minutes and kept under close observation for 30 minutes after each injection. Initially 10 mg is given in the first week to test the patient's tolerance. If satisfactory, this is followed by doses of 25 to 50 mg at weekly intervals until signs of remission occur, when the dosage interval is increased to 2 weeks until full remission occurs; the dosage interval is then further increased gradually to every 4 to 6 weeks and treatment may be continued for up to 5 years after remission. Improvement may not be seen until a total dose of 300 to 500 mg has been administered. If no major improvement has been observed after a total of 1 g has been given (excluding the test dose) therapy should be discontinued; alternatively in the absence of toxicity, 100 mg may be given weekly for 6 weeks; should there be no response at this dose other forms of therapy should be tried. In patients who relapse while receiving maintenance therapy, the interval between doses should be reduced to one week and should not be increased again until control has been obtained but if no response is obtained within 2 months, alternative treatment should be used. It is important to avoid complete relapse since a second course of gold therapy is not usually effective.

For children with progressive juvenile chronic arthritis the suggested initial weekly dose is 1 mg per kg body-weight to a maximum of 50 mg weekly (a suitable test dose is one-tenth to one-fifth of the calculated initial weekly dose for 2 to 3 weeks). With full remission, the dosage interval may be increased to 4 weeks. If no improvement has occurred after 20 weeks, the dose could be raised slightly or another antirheumatic drug tried.

NSAIDs may be continued when sodium aurothiomalate therapy is initiated.

Other gold compounds that have been used include auranofin (p.19), aurothioglucose (p.20), aurotioprol (p.20), gold keratinate (p.43), and sodium aurothiosulphate (p.85).

Pemphigus and pemphigoid. Corticosteroids are the main treatment for blistering in pemphigus and pemphigoid (see p.1075). Systemic gold therapy has been used in combination with corticosteroids to permit a reduction in corticosteroid dosage. However, it has been suggested that evidence for the steroid-sparing effect is lacking and that gold therapy should be reserved for patients who cannot tolerate corticosteroids or in whom they are contra-indicated.[1]

1. Bystryn J-C, Steinman NM. The adjuvant therapy of pemphigus: an update. *Arch Dermatol* 1996; **132:** 203–12.

Rheumatic disorders. Gold compounds are among the disease modifying antirheumatic drugs (DMARDs) that may be used in the treatment of rheumatoid arthritis (p.2) and juvenile chronic arthritis (p.2). There is little agreement on which of the various DMARDs should be tried first and their selection is largely based on individual experience and preference. Despite its toxicity intramuscular gold has long been used for the treatment of rheumatoid arthritis and is often the standard against which the efficacy of other treatments is measured. Oral gold is less toxic but is also much less effective. Gold compounds may also be of benefit in psoriatic arthritis (see under Spondyloarthropathies, p.4).

References.

1. Epstein WV, *et al.* Effect of parenterally administered gold therapy on the course of adult rheumatoid arthritis. *Ann Intern Med* 1991; **114:** 437–44.
2. Anonymous. Gold therapy in rheumatoid arthritis. *Lancet* 1991; **338:** 19–20.
3. Klinkhoff AV, Teufel A. How low can you go? Use of very low dosage of gold in patients with mucocutaneous reactions. *J Rheumatol* 1995; **22:** 1657–9.

Preparations

BP 1998: Sodium Aurothiomalate Injection;
USP 23: Gold Sodium Thiomalate Injection.

Proprietary Preparations (details are given in Part 3)

Aust.: Tauredon; ***Austral.:*** Myocrisin; ***Canad.:*** Myochrysine; ***Ger.:*** Tauredon; ***Irl.:*** Myocrisin; ***Norw.:*** Myocrisin; ***S.Afr.:*** Myocrisin; ***Spain:*** Miocrin; ***Swed.:*** Myocrisin; ***Switz.:*** Tauredon; ***UK:*** Myocrisin; ***USA:*** Aurolate; Myochrysine†.

Sodium Aurothiosulphate (5297-a)

Sodium Aurotiosulfate *(rINN)*; Gold Sodium Thiosulphate; Sodium Dithiosulfatoaurate.

$Na_3Au(S_2O_3)_2,2H_2O$ = 526.2.

CAS — 10233-88-2 (anhydrous sodium aurothiosulphate); 10210-36-3 (sodium aurothiosulphate dihydrate).

Sodium aurothiosulphate has a gold content of about 37%.

Sodium aurothiosulphate has similar actions and uses to those of sodium aurothiomalate (p.83). It has been given by intramuscular injection.

Preparations

Proprietary Preparations (details are given in Part 3)
Ital.: Fosfocrisolo.

Sodium Gentisate (2704-c)

Sodium Gentisate *(rINN)*.

Gentisato Sodico; Natrii Gentisas. Sodium 2,5-dihydroxybenzoate dihydrate.

$C_7H_5NaO_4,2H_2O$ = 212.1.

CAS — 490-79-9 (gentisic acid); 4955-90-2 (anhydrous sodium gentisate).

Pharmacopoeias. In *Fr.*

Sodium gentisate was used in the treatment of musculoskeletal and joint disorders.

Preparations

Proprietary Preparations (details are given in Part 3)
Multi-ingredient: ***Ger.:*** Rheumadrag†.

Sodium Salicylate (2705-k)

Natrii Salicylas. Sodium 2-hydroxybenzoate.

$C_7H_5NaO_3$ = 160.1.

CAS — 54-21-7.

Pharmacopoeias. In *Eur.* (see p.viii), *Int.*, *Jpn*, *Pol.*, and *US.*

Colourless small crystals, shiny flakes, or white or faintly pink amorphous or microcrystalline powder, odourless or with a faint characteristic odour.

Sodium salicylate 1 g is approximately equivalent to 1.1 g of aspirin.

Freely **soluble** in water; sparingly soluble in alcohol; freely soluble in glycerol; very soluble in boiling water and in boiling alcohol; practically insoluble in ether. Concentrated aqueous solutions are liable to deposit crystals of the hexahydrate on standing. A freshly prepared 10% solution in water is neutral or acid to litmus. **Store** in airtight containers. Protect from light.

Adverse Effects, Treatment, and Precautions

As for Aspirin, p.16.

When sodium salicylate is used in the treatment of rheumatic fever its high sodium content may cause problems in patients with cardiac complications.

The use of aspirin and other acetylated salicylates is generally not recommended for children under the age of 12 years because of the risk of Reye's syndrome, unless specifically indicated. Some authorities also extend this precaution to non-acetylated salicylates such as sodium salicylate.

Effects on the eyes. Retinal haemorrhages were reported in a 60-year-old woman taking sodium salicylate 6 g daily by mouth for 2 months and in a 10-year-old girl taking sodium salicylate, 4 g daily by mouth, for 40 days.[1] In both cases the haemorrhages were gradually resolved after the treatment was stopped.

1. Mortada A, Abboud I. Retinal haemorrhages after prolonged use of salicylates. *Br J Ophthalmol* 1973; **57:** 199–200.

Interactions

For interactions associated with salicylates, see Aspirin, p.17.

Uses and Administration

Sodium salicylate is a salicylic acid derivative that has analgesic, anti-inflammatory, and antipyretic actions similar to those of aspirin (p.18). It is used in the treatment of pain, fever, and in rheumatic disorders such as osteoarthritis and rheumatoid arthritis. The usual oral dose of sodium salicylate for pain or fever is 325 to 650 mg every four hours as required. The oral dose for rheumatic disorders is 3.6 to 5.4 g daily in divided doses. Sodium salicylate has also been used in the symptomatic treatment of rheumatic fever but its high sodium content may cause problems in patients with cardiac complications.

Sodium salicylate has also been given by intravenous infusion.

References.

1. Seymour RA, *et al.* The efficacy and pharmacokinetics of sodium salicylate in post-operative dental pain. *Br J Clin Pharmacol* 1984; **17:** 161–3.

Preparations

USP 23: Sodium Salicylate Tablets.

Proprietary Preparations (details are given in Part 3)
Canad.: Dodds; Saliject†; ***UK:*** Fennings Mixture†; Jackson's Febrifuge.

Multi-ingredient: ***Austral.:*** Drixine Cough Suppressant†; ***Belg.:*** Baseler Haussalbe; ***Canad.:*** Plax; Thunas Tab for Menstrual Pain; ***Fr.:*** Aromabyl; Bain de Bouche Bancaud†; Glyco-Thymoline; Theinol; ***Ger.:*** Anastil†; Fangyol-Med-Bad†; Gelonida NA; Ilvico†; Kolton grippale N†; Monacant†; Salimar-Bad L; Uriginex†; ***Ital.:*** Creosolactol Bambini†; Reused†; Salicilato Attivato Ana†; ***S.Afr.:*** Colphen; Ilvico; ***UK:*** Doans†; TCP; ***USA:*** Cystex; Pabalate; Scot-Tussin Original 5-Action; Tussirex.

Sodium Thiosalicylate (16988-d)

$C_7H_5O_2NaS$ = 176.2.

Sodium thiosalicylate is a salicylic acid derivative (see Aspirin, p.16) used in the treatment of musculoskeletal disorders, osteoarthritis, rheumatic fever, and acute gout. It is used in usual doses of 50 to 150 mg intramuscularly.

Preparations

Proprietary Preparations (details are given in Part 3)
USA: Pirosal; Rexolate; Thiocyl.

Spiradoline Mesylate (963-t)

Spiradoline Mesylate *(USAN)*.

Spiradoline Mesilate *(rINNM)*; U-62066E. (±)-2-(3,4-Dichlorophenyl)-*N*-methyl-*N*-[(5R*,7S*,8S*)-7-(1-pyrrolidinyl)-1-oxaspiro[4.5]dec-8-yl]acetamide methanesulphonate.

$C_{22}H_{30}Cl_2N_2O_2,CH_4O_3S$ = 521.5.

CAS — 87151-85-7 (spiradoline); 87173-97-5 (spiradoline mesylate).

Spiradoline mesylate is an opioid analgesic (p.67) under investigation. It has high affinity for κ opioid receptors but adverse mental effects may limit its use.

Sufentanil Citrate (13274-e)

Sufentanil Citrate *(BANM, USAN, rINNM)*.

R-33800; R-30730 (sufentanil); Sufentanili Citras. *N*-{4-(Methoxymethyl)-1-[2-(2-thienyl)ethyl]-4-piperidyl}propionanilide citrate.

$C_{22}H_{30}N_2O_2S,C_6H_8O_7$ = 578.7.

CAS — 56030-54-7 (sufentanil); 60561-17-3 (sufentanil citrate).

Pharmacopoeias. In *Eur.* (see p.viii) and *US.*

A white or almost white powder. **Soluble** in water; soluble to sparingly soluble in alcohol; sparingly soluble in acetone and in chloroform; freely soluble in methyl alcohol. Sufentanil citrate 15 μg is approximately equivalent to 10 μg of sufentanil. **Protect** from light.

CAUTION. *Avoid contact with skin and the inhalation of particles of sufentanil citrate.*

Dependence and Withdrawal

As for Opioid Analgesics, p.67.

Adverse Effects, Treatment, and Precautions

As for Opioid Analgesics in general, p.68 and Fentanyl, p.38.

Administration in the elderly. The pharmacokinetics of sufentanil in elderly patients have been variable in different studies, but Monk *et al.*[1] considered that there had been no evidence overall for differences between the elderly and younger adults. Nevertheless, as with fentanyl the manufacturer advises reduced initial doses in the elderly.

1. Monk JP, *et al.* Sufentanil: a review of its pharmacological properties and therapeutic use. *Drugs* 1988; **36:** 286–313.

Administration in obesity. The elimination half-life and volume of distribution of sufentanil were increased in obese subjects.[1] The manufacturers recommend that for obese patients more than 20% above ideal body-weight the dosage of sufentanil should be determined on the basis of the patients' lean body-weight.

1. Schwartz AE, *et al.* Pharmacokinetics of sufentanil in the obese. *Anesthesiology* 1986; **65** (suppl 3A): A562.

Breast feeding. Concentrations of sufentanil were similar in colostrum and serum in 7 women given sufentanil by continuous epidural infusion during the first postoperative day following caesarean section. In the light of its poor oral availability such an amount was not considered to be a hazard to the breast-feeding infant, and a maternal dose of 5 μg per hour epidurally was considered to be safe for such infants.[1]

1. Ausseur A, *et al.* Continuous epidural infusion of sufentanil after caesarean section: concentration in breast milk. *Br J Anaesth* 1994; **72** (suppl 1): 106.

Effects on the cardiovascular system. For a reference to the effects of sufentanil on histamine release compared with some other opioids, see under Pethidine, p.76.

Effects on the nervous system. There have been reports of tonic-clonic movements or seizures in a few patients receiving sufentanil.[1] There was no evidence of cortical seizure activity in one patient whose EEG was recorded,[2] suggesting that the observed myoclonus was not a convulsion or seizure.

1. Zaccara G, *et al.* Clinical features, pathogenesis and management of drug-induced seizures. *Drug Safety* 1990; **5:** 109–51.
2. Bowdle TA. Myoclonus following sufentanil without EEG seizure activity. *Anesthesiology* 1987; **67:** 593–5.

Effects on the respiratory system. Sufentanil, like other opioid agonists, causes dose-related respiratory depression. There have been reports of significant respiratory depression associated with chest wall rigidity in the early postoperative period after anaesthesia with sufentanil.[1,2]

1. Goldberg M, *et al.* Postoperative rigidity following sufentanil administration. *Anesthesiology* 1985; **63:** 199–201.
2. Chang J, Fish KJ. Acute respiratory arrest and rigidity after anesthesia with sufentanil: a case report. *Anesthesiology* 1985; **63:** 710–11.

Interactions

For interactions associated with opioid analgesics, see p.69.

Benzodiazepines. For the effects of concomitant use of opioids such as sufentanil with benzodiazepines, see under Analgesics in the Interactions of Diazepam, p.663.

Pharmacokinetics

Following parenteral administration sufentanil citrate has a rapid onset and short duration of action. The terminal elimination half-life of sufentanil is about 2.5 hours. It is extensively bound to plasma proteins (about 90%). It is metabolised in the liver and small intestine by *N*-dealkylation and *O*-demethylation and the metabolites are excreted in the urine.

Some reviews of the pharmacokinetics of sufentanil.

1. Mather LE. Clinical pharmacokinetics of fentanyl and its newer derivatives. *Clin Pharmacokinet* 1983; **8:** 422–46.
2. Davis PJ, Cook DR. Clinical pharmacokinetics of the newer intravenous anaesthetic agents. *Clin Pharmacokinet* 1986; **11:** 18–35.
3. Monk JP, *et al.* Sufentanil: a review of its pharmacological properties and therapeutic use. *Drugs* 1988; **36:** 286–313.
4. Scholz J, *et al.* Clinical pharmacokinetics of alfentanil, fentanyl and sufentanil: an update. *Clin Pharmacokinet* 1996; **31:** 275–92.

Sufentanil is very lipid-soluble. Like alfentanil it is highly bound to plasma protein, principally to α_1-acid glycoprotein. The elimination half-life lies between that of alfentanil and fentanyl. The manufacturers of sufentanil have given values for a three-compartment pharmacokinetic model with a distribution half-life of 1.4 minutes, a redistribution half-life of 17.1 minutes, and an elimination half-life of 164 minutes. Accumulation may be relatively limited when compared with fentanyl. In practice the pharmacokinetics of sufentanil may vary according to the age and condition of the patient and the procedures undertaken. For example, the elimination half-life of sufentanil has been reported to be longer in patients undergoing cardiac surgery (595 minutes),[1] in hyperventilated patients (232 minutes),[2] and in those undergoing abdominal aortic surgery (more than 12 hours).[3]

1. Howie MB, *et al.* Serum concentrations of sufentanil and fentanyl in the post-operative course in cardiac surgery patients. *Anesthesiology* 1984; **61:** A131.
2. Schwartz AE, *et al.* Pharmacokinetics of sufentanil in neurosurgical patients undergoing hyperventilation. *Br J Anaesth* 1989; **63:** 385–8.
3. Hudson RJ, *et al.* Pharmacokinetics of sufentanil in patients undergoing abdominal aortic surgery. *Anesthesiology* 1989; **70:** 426–31.

Administration. References to the pharmacokinetics of sufentanil administered epidurally,[1] intrathecally,[1] and transdermally.[2]

1. Ionescu TI, *et al.* Pharmacokinetic study of extradural and intrathecal sufentanil anaesthesia for major surgery. *Br J Anaesth* 1991; **66:** 458–64.
2. Sebel PS, *et al.* Transdermal absorption of fentanyl and sufentanil in man. *Eur J Clin Pharmacol* 1987; **32:** 529–31.

Administration in hepatic impairment. Because of the efficient hepatic extraction and clearance of sufentanil[1] liver dysfunction might be expected to affect its pharmacokinetics.

1. Schedewie H, *et al.* Sufentanil and fentanyl hepatic extraction rate and clearance in obese patients undergoing gastroplasty. *Clin Pharmacol Ther* 1988; **43:** 132.

Administration in infants and children. Age-related differences in the pharmacokinetics of sufentanil in paediatric patients undergoing cardiovascular surgery were noted by Greeley *et al.*[1] Neonates (up to 1 month old) had a significantly lower plasma clearance rate and greater elimination half-life than infants (1 month to 2 years), children, and adolescents. Davis *et al.*[2] found that infants and small children (1 month to 3 years) with cardiac disease had higher clearance rates and shorter elimination half-lives than reported for adults.

1. Greeley WJ, *et al.* Sufentanil pharmacokinetics in pediatric cardiovascular patients. *Anesth Analg* 1987; **66:** 1067–72.
2. Davis PJ, *et al.* Pharmacodynamics and pharmacokinetics of high-dose sufentanil in infants and children undergoing cardiac surgery. *Anesth Analg* 1987; **66:** 203–8.

Administration in renal impairment. Sear[1] found the pharmacokinetics of sufentanil to be unaffected in patients with chronic renal failure, although Wiggum *et al.*[2] reported elevated plasma concentrations of sufentanil in one such patient.

1. Sear JW. Sufentanil disposition in patients undergoing renal transplantation: influence of choice of kinetic model. *Br J Anaesth* 1989; **63:** 60–7.
2. Wiggum DC, *et al.* Postoperative respiratory depression and elevated sufentanil levels in a patient with chronic renal failure. *Anesthesiology* 1985; **63:** 708–10.

Uses and Administration

Sufentanil, a phenylpiperidine derivative, is an opioid analgesic (p.69) related to fentanyl (p.39). It is highly lipid-soluble and more potent than fentanyl. Sufentanil is used as an analgesic adjunct in anaesthesia and as a primary anaesthetic drug in procedures requiring assisted ventilation. It has a rapid onset and recovery is considered to be more rapid than with fentanyl.

Sufentanil is administered intravenously as the citrate either by slow injection or as an infusion. Lower initial doses are advised in the elderly and debilitated patients. For obese patients more than 20% above ideal body-weight the dosage of sufentanil should be determined on the basis of the patients' lean body-weight. In all patients supplementary maintenance doses should be according to individual response and length of procedure. Doses are expressed in terms of sufentanil base. Doses of up to 8 µg of sufentanil per kg body-weight produce profound analgesia. Doses of 8 µg or more per kg produce a deep level of anaesthesia but are associated with prolonged respiratory depression and assisted ventilation may be required in the postoperative period.

When used as an analgesic adjunct to anaesthesia with nitrous oxide and oxygen for surgical procedures lasting up to 8 hours, the total dosage should not exceed 1 µg per kg per hour. It is customary to give up to 75% of the dose before intubation followed as necessary during surgery by additional injections of 10 to 50 µg or by a suitable continuous or intermittent infusion administered so that the total hourly dose is not exceeded. Thus, for an operation lasting 1 to 2 hours the total dose would be 1 to 2 µg per kg with 0.75 to 1.5 µg per kg being given before intubation.

When used as the primary anaesthetic drug in major surgery doses of 8 to 30 µg per kg are employed with 100% oxygen; doses of 25 to 30 µg per kg block sympathetic response including catecholamine release and are indicated in procedures such as cardiovascular surgery or neurosurgery. Anaesthesia may be maintained by additional injections of 0.5 to 10 µg per kg or by a suitable continuous or intermittent infusion administered so that the total dosage for the procedure does not exceed 30 µg per kg.

All the above doses relate to the use of sufentanil in adults; experience of paediatric use is more limited. Children undergoing cardiovascular surgery may be given sufentanil, with 100% oxygen, in an initial dose of 10 to 25 µg per kg with maintenance doses of up to 25 to 50 µg.

Sufentanil has also been given epidurally for the relief of pain (see below). Recommended doses for labour and delivery are 10 to 15 µg administered epidurally with 10 mL bupivacaine 0.125% with or without adrenaline; the dose may be repeated twice at not less than one-hour intervals until delivery.

General reviews of sufentanil.

1. Monk JP, *et al.* Sufentanil: a review of its pharmacological properties and therapeutic use. *Drugs* 1988; **36:** 286–313.
2. Clotz MA, Nahata MC. Clinical uses of fentanyl, sufentanil, and alfentanil. *Clin Pharm* 1991; **10:** 581–93.

Administration. Sufentanil is usually administered intravenously, but the epidural route is also used (see below). Intranasal administration (see under Anaesthesia and under Sedation, below) or intrathecal administration (see below) have also been tried.

EPIDURAL. In a laboratory assessment of epidural sufentanil in healthy subjects,[1] a dose of 50 µg produced analgesia for 2 to 3 hours; analgesia was intensified and prolonged and respiratory and other side-effects, especially drowsiness, were reduced by the addition of adrenaline. Epidural sufentanil or fentanyl provided effective postoperative analgesia following caesarean section with comparable adverse effect profiles.[2] Sufentanil doses of 20 and 30 µg showed equivalent efficacy and provided greater analgesia for a longer duration than a dose of 10 µg. Addition of sufentanil to the local anaesthetic bupivacaine has improved the quality of epidural analgesia.[3] Effective analgesia has been achieved in children with epidural sufentanil.[4]

Epidural administration of sufentanil has been tried for patient-controlled analgesia but appeared to have little advantage over patient-controlled analgesia using morphine given intravenously.[5]

1. Klepper ID, *et al.* Analgesic and respiratory effects of extradural sufentanil in volunteers and the influence of adrenaline as an adjuvant. *Br J Anaesth* 1987; **59:** 1147–56.
2. Grass JA, *et al.* A randomized, double-blind, dose-response comparison of epidural fentanyl versus sufentanil analgesia after cesarean section. *Anesth Analg* 1997; **85:** 365–71.
3. Reynolds F. Extradural opioids in labour. *Br J Anaesth* 1989; **63:** 251–3.
4. Benlabed M, *et al.* Analgesia and ventilatory response to CO_2 following epidural sufentanil in children. *Anesthesiology* 1987; **67:** 948–51.
5. Grass JA, *et al.* Patient-controlled analgesia after cesarean delivery: epidural sufentanil versus intravenous morphine. *Reg Anesth* 1994; **19:** 90–7.

INTRATHECAL. Sufentanil has been given by the intrathecal route for labour pain. There was no significant difference in terms of effects on fetal heart rate when intrathecal sufentanil was compared with epidural bupivacaine,[1] although the authors suggested that fetal heart rate should be monitored carefully when either drug is used. A combination of sufentanil, bupivacaine, and adrenaline administered intrathecally provided excellent analgesia during labour and had a more rapid onset, a longer duration of action, and reduced local anaesthetic requirements compared with epidural administration.[2] Intrathecal sufentanil and bupivacaine provided shorter duration of analgesia when administered during the advanced stages of labour compared with early labour.[3]

1. Nielsen PE, *et al.* Fetal heart rate changes after intrathecal sufentanil or epidural bupivacaine for labor analgesia: incidence and clinical significance. *Anesth Analg* 1996; **83:** 742–6.
2. Kartawiadi SL, *et al.* Spinal analgesia during labor with low-dose bupivacaine, sufentanil, and epinephrine: a comparison with epidural analgesia. *Reg Anesth* 1996; **21:** 191–6.
3. Viscomi CM, *et al.* Duration of intrathecal labor analgesia: early versus advanced labor. *Anesth Analg* 1997; **84:** 1108–12.

Anaesthesia. Sufentanil, like fentanyl (p.40), appears to produce fewer circulatory changes than morphine and may be preferred for anaesthetic use, especially in cardiovascular surgery.

In a comparative study fentanyl and sufentanil were equally preferable to morphine or pethidine as adjuncts to nitrous oxide anaesthesia in terms of haemodynamic changes to stress and rates of recovery.[1] Flacke *et al.*[2] compared these same 4 drugs and found sufentanil to be the most satisfactory, especially in terms of the haemodynamic and autonomic stability achieved. Sufentanil also compared favourably with fentanyl when used for the induction and maintenance of anaesthesia for coronary artery bypass surgery[3] and when given in lower doses by continuous infusion for outpatient anaesthesia.[4]

Sufentanil anaesthesia for major surgery has been assessed in a multicentre study;[5] to prevent the majority of adverse reactions pre-operative assessment of the patient's circulatory volume, concomitant administration of muscle relaxants, ready availability of vagolytic agents, and a cumulative dose of no more than 1 µg per kg body-weight per hour, were recommended.

Premedication with sufentanil administered intranasally has been tried in children[6,7] and in adults.[8]

Neuroleptanalgesia. Sufentanil is one of the opioids that have been used with a neuroleptic to produce neuroleptanalgesia.

1. Ghoneim MM, *et al.* Comparison of four opioid analgesics as supplements to nitrous oxide anesthesia. *Anesth Analg* 1984; **63:** 405–12.
2. Flacke JW, *et al.* Comparison of morphine, meperidine, fentanyl, and sufentanil in balanced anesthesia: a double-blind study. *Anesth Analg* 1985; **64:** 897–910.
3. Mathews HML, *et al.* Comparison of fentanyl and sufentanil anaesthesia for patients undergoing coronary artery bypass grafting. *Br J Anaesth* 1987; **59:** 939–40P.
4. Phitayakorn P, *et al.* Comparison of continuous sufentanil and fentanyl infusions for outpatient anaesthesia. *Can J Anaesth* 1987; **34:** 242–5.
5. Murkin JM. Sufentanil anaesthesia for major surgery: the multicentre Canadian clinical trial. *Can J Anaesth* 1989; **36:** 343–9.
6. Henderson JM, *et al.* Pre-induction of anesthesia in pediatric patients with nasally administered sufentanil. *Anesthesiology* 1988; **68:** 671–5.
7. Zedie N, *et al.* Comparison of intranasal midazolam and sufentanil premedication in pediatric outpatients. *Clin Pharmacol Ther* 1996; **59:** 341–8.
8. Helmers JHJH, *et al.* Comparison of intravenous and intranasal sufentanil absorption and sedation. *Can J Anaesth* 1989; **36:** 494–7.

Pain. For the use of sufentanil in the management of pain, see under Epidural and Intrathecal Administration, above.

Sedation. Some references to the use of sufentanil for sedation are given below. See also under Anaesthesia, above.

1. Bates BA, *et al.* A comparison of intranasal sufentanil and midazolam to intramuscular meperidine, promethazine, and chlorpromazine for conscious sedation in children. *Ann Emerg Med* 1994; **24:** 646–51.
2. Lefrant JY, *et al.* Sufentanil short duration infusion for postoperative sedation in critically ill patients. *Br J Anaesth* 1995; **74** (suppl 1): 114.

Preparations

USP 23: Sufentanil Citrate Injection.

Proprietary Preparations (details are given in Part 3)
Aust.: Sufenta; ***Belg.:*** Sufenta; ***Canad.:*** Sufenta; ***Fr.:*** Sufenta; ***Ger.:*** Sufenta; ***Ital.:*** Fentatienil; ***Neth.:*** Sufenta; ***Norw.:*** Sufenta; ***S.Afr.:*** Sufenta; ***Swed.:*** Sufenta; ***Switz.:*** Sufenta; ***USA:*** Sufenta.

Sulindac (2706-a)

Sulindac *(BAN, USAN, rINN).*

MK-231; Sulindacum. (*Z*)-[5-Fluoro-2-methyl-1-(4-methylsulphinylbenzylidene)inden-3-yl]acetic acid.

$C_{20}H_{17}FO_3S$ = 356.4.

CAS — 38194-50-2.

Pharmacopoeias. In Eur. (see p.viii) and US.

A yellow, odourless or almost odourless, polymorphic, crystalline powder. Ph. Eur. **solubilities** are: very slightly soluble in water and in ether; sparingly soluble in alcohol; soluble in dichloromethane; dissolves in dilute solutions of alkali hydroxides. USP solubilities are: practically insoluble in water and in petroleum spirit; slightly soluble in alcohol, in acetone, in chloroform, and in methyl alcohol; very slightly soluble in isopropyl alcohol and in ethyl acetate. **Protect** from light.

Adverse Effects

As for NSAIDs in general, p.63, and for Indomethacin, p.45. Urine discoloration has occasionally been reported with sulindac.

Sulindac metabolites have been reported as major or minor components in renal stones.

A report of 4 patients and a short review of 8 previously reported cases of serious adverse reactions to sulindac;[1] reactions included fever and skin, liver, CNS, lymph node, bone-marrow, and lung involvement.

1. Park GD, *et al.* Serious adverse reactions associated with sulindac. *Arch Intern Med* 1982; **142:** 1292–4.

Effects on the blood. Agranulocytosis,[1] thrombocytopenia,[2] haemolytic anaemia,[3] and aplastic anaemia[4] have been reported in patients taking sulindac.

1. Romeril KR, *et al.* Sulindac induced agranulocytosis and bone marrow culture. *Lancet* 1981; **ii:** 523.
2. Karachalios GN, Parigorakis JG. Thrombocytopenia and sulindac. *Ann Intern Med* 1986; **104:** 128.
3. Johnson FP, *et al.* Immune hemolytic anemia associated with sulindac. *Arch Intern Med* 1985; **145:** 1515–16.
4. Andrews R, Russell N. Aplastic anaemia associated with a non-steroidal anti-inflammatory drug: relapse after exposure to another such drug. *Br Med J* 1990; **301:** 38.

Effects on the CNS. Acute deterioration of parkinsonism occurred in a patient following the introduction of sulindac therapy.[1]

See also under Hypersensitivity, below.

1. Sandyk R, Gillman MA. Acute exacerbation of Parkinson's disease with sulindac. *Ann Neurol* 1985; **17:** 104–5.

Effects on the endocrine system. Reversible gynaecomastia associated with sulindac therapy has been reported in one patient.[1] There has also been a report[2] of reversible hypothyroidism in an elderly patient taking sulindac.

1. Kapoor A. Reversible gynecomastia associated with sulindac therapy. *JAMA* 1983; **250:** 2284–5.
2. Iyer RP, Duckett GK. Reversible secondary hypothyroidism induced by sulindac. *Br Med J* 1985; **290:** 1788.

Effects on the gallbladder. A "sludge" composed of crystalline metabolites of sulindac has been found in the common bile duct during surgery for biliary obstruction in patients who had been taking sulindac.[1]

1. Anonymous. Rare complication with sulindac. *FDA Drug Bull* 1989; **19:** 4.

Effects on the kidneys. Sulindac-induced renal impairment, interstitial nephritis, and nephrotic syndrome have been reported.[1]

The ability of NSAIDs to inhibit renal prostaglandin synthesis is an important factor in the development of renal toxicity. Generally, inhibition of prostaglandin synthesis has no significant effect on renal blood flow or glomerular filtration rate. However, patients with reduced renal perfusion have increased dependence on prostaglandin synthesis for renal haemodynamic function. In these patients, inhibition of prostaglandin synthesis can produce deleterious effects on renal blood flow and glomerular filtration rate. It has been suggested that sulindac, as a prodrug, may not inhibit renal prostaglandin synthesis in therapeutic doses. However, this potentially important therapeutic advantage has not been uniformly observed in short-term studies in patients with renal dysfunction.[2-4]

There have been reports of renal stones consisting of between 10 and 90% of sulindac metabolites developing in patients treated with sulindac.[5]

1. Whelton A, *et al.* Sulindac and renal impairment. *JAMA* 1983; **249:** 2892.
2. Klassen DK, *et al.* Sulindac kinetics and effects on renal function and prostaglandin excretion in renal insufficiency. *J Clin Pharmacol* 1989; **29:** 1037–42.
3. Eriksson L-O, *et al.* Effects of sulindac and naproxen on prostaglandin excretion in patients with impaired renal function and rheumatoid arthritis. *Am J Med* 1990; **89:** 313–21.
4. Whelton A, *et al.* Renal effects of ibuprofen, piroxicam, and sulindac in patients with asymptomatic renal failure. *Ann Intern Med* 1990; **112:** 568–76.
5. Anonymous. Rare complication with sulindac. *FDA Drug Bull* 1989; **19:** 4.

Effects on the liver. Hepatotoxicity reported in patients receiving sulindac includes hepatocellular injury and cholestatic jaundice.[1,2] Symptoms of hypersensitivity including rash, fever, or eosinophilia have been reported in 35 to 55% of patients with sulindac-induced liver damage;[2] in these patients the liver damage occurred usually within 4 to 8 weeks of beginning sulindac therapy. For reference to a report citing the strongest evidence for an association of sulindac with liver disease compared with other NSAIDs, see under NSAIDs, p.65.

See also under Effects on the Skin, below.

1. Gallanosa AG, Spyker DA. Sulindac hepatotoxicity: a case report and review. *Clin Toxicol* 1985; **23:** 205–38.
2. Tarazi EM, *et al.* Sulindac-associated hepatic injury: analysis of 91 cases reported to the Food and Drug Administration. *Gastroenterology* 1993; **104:** 569–74.

Effects on the lungs. For reference to pneumonitis associated with sulindac therapy, see under Hypersensitivity, below.

Effects on the pancreas. Reports[1-4] of pancreatitis associated with sulindac therapy.

1. Goldstein J, *et al.* Sulindac associated with pancreatitis. *Ann Intern Med* 1980; **93:** 151.
2. Siefkin AD. Sulindac and pancreatitis. *Ann Intern Med* 1980; **93:** 932–3.
3. Lilly EL. Pancreatitis after administration of sulindac. *JAMA* 1981; **246:** 2680.
4. Memon AN. Pancreatitis and sulindac. *Ann Intern Med* 1982; **97:** 139.

Effects on the skin. Toxic epidermal necrolysis has occurred in patients taking sulindac.[1] In one patient toxic hepatitis and the Stevens-Johnson/toxic epidermal necrolysis syndrome resulted in death.[2]

An unusual pernio-like reaction affecting the toes and confirmed by rechallenge has also been reported.[3]

Sulindac has also been reported to cause photosensitivity reactions.[4]

1. Small RE, Garnett WR. Sulindac-induced toxic epidermal necrolysis. *Clin Pharm* 1988; **7:** 766–71.
2. Klein SM, Khan MA. Hepatitis, toxic epidermal necrolysis and pancreatitis in association with sulindac therapy. *J Rheumatol* 1983; **10:** 512–13.
3. Reinertsen LJ. Unusual pernio-like reaction to sulindac. *Arthritis Rheum* 1981; **24:** 1215.
4. Anonymous. Drugs that cause photosensitivity. *Med Lett Drugs Ther* 1986; **28:** 51–2.

Hypersensitivity. Hypersensitivity reactions to sulindac include pneumonitis,[1,2] generalised lymphadenopathy,[3] aseptic meningitis,[4] and anaphylactoid reaction.[5]

See also under Effects on the Liver and under Effects on the Skin, above.

1. Smith FE, Lindberg PJ. Life-threatening hypersensitivity to sulindac. *JAMA* 1980; **244:** 269–70.
2. Fein M. Sulindac and pneumonitis. *Ann Intern Med* 1981; **95:** 245.
3. Sprung DJ. Sulindac causing a hypersensitivity reaction with peripheral and mediastinal lymphadenopathy. *Ann Intern Med* 1982; **97:** 564.
4. Fordham von Reyn C. Recurrent aseptic meningitis due to sulindac. *Ann Intern Med* 1983; **99:** 343–4.
5. Hyson CP, Kazakoff MA. A severe multisystem reaction to sulindac. *Arch Intern Med* 1991; **151:** 387–8.

Precautions

As for NSAIDs in general, p.65.

Sulindac metabolites have been reported as major or minor components in renal stones. It should therefore be used with caution in patients with a history of renal stones and such patients should be kept well hydrated while receiving sulindac.

The dose of sulindac may need to be reduced in patients with liver or renal function impairment.

Interactions

For interactions associated with NSAIDs, see p.65.

Dimethyl sulphoxide reduces plasma concentrations of the active metabolite of sulindac and concomitant administration of the two drugs has also resulted in peripheral neuropathy. Diflunisal and aspirin are reported to reduce the plasma concentration of the active metabolite of sulindac. Unlike other NSAIDs, sulindac is reported not to reduce the antihypertensive effects of drugs such as thiazide diuretics, but nevertheless the manufacturers recommend that blood pressure be closely monitored in patients taking antihypertensives and sulindac together.

Pharmacokinetics

Sulindac is absorbed from the gastro-intestinal tract. It is metabolised by reversible reduction to the sulphide metabolite, which appears to be the biologically active form, and by irreversible oxidation to the sulphone metabolite. Peak plasma concentrations of the sulphide metabolite are achieved in about 2 hours. The mean elimination half-life of sulindac is about 7 to 8 hours and of the sulphide metabolite about 16 to 18 hours. Sulindac and its metabolites are highly bound to plasma protein. About 50% is excreted in the urine mainly as the sulphone metabolite and its glucuronide conjugate, with smaller amounts of sulindac and its glucuronide conjugate. Sulindac and its metabolites are also excreted in bile and undergo extensive enterohepatic circulation.

References.

1. Davies NM, Watson MS. Clinical pharmacokinetics of sulindac: a dynamic old drug. *Clin Pharmacokinet* 1997; **32:** 437–59.

Uses and Administration

Sulindac is an NSAID (p.65). It is structurally related to indomethacin (p.46); its biological activity appears to be due to its sulphide metabolite. Sulindac is used in musculoskeletal and joint disorders such as ankylosing spondylitis, osteoarthritis, and rheumatoid arthritis, and also in the short-term management of acute gout and peri-articular conditions such as bursitis and tendinitis. It is also used to reduce fever.

A usual dose of sulindac by mouth is initially 150 or 200 mg twice daily reduced according to response. The maximum recommended daily dose is 400 mg. The UK manufacturers recommend that the treatment of peri-articular disorders should be limited to 7 to 10 days; for acute gout, 7 days of therapy is usually adequate. The dose may need to be reduced in patients with liver or renal function impairment.

Sulindac sodium has been given by rectal suppository in doses of 200 to 400 mg daily.

Gastro-intestinal disorders. In placebo-controlled studies[1,2] sulindac 150 to 200 mg twice daily for 6 to 9 months has reduced the number and size of polyps in patients with familial adenomatous polyposis but the effect may be incomplete and in one study[2] only polyps less than 2 mm in size regressed. The size and number of polyps has been reported[1] to increase on discontinuation of treatment and long-term therapy is therefore being studied. However, some workers[3] have observed diminution of sulindac's effectiveness with long-term treatment although others[4] have reported that they have managed recurrences by adjustment of the maintenance dosage used; it appeared that there were individual variations in sensitivity to sulindac with respect to prevention of polyps recurrence although 200 mg daily appeared to be an average maintenance dose needed.[4] Whether sulindac prevents malignant degeneration is unknown but there has been a report[5] of a patient who developed rectal cancer during long-term therapy for familial adenomatous polyposis. Some[1] consider that sulindac is unlikely to replace surgery as primary therapy for familial adenomatous polyposis.

Sulindac has also been reported to have produced beneficial effects in a patient with duodenal polyps associated with Gardner's syndrome[6] but a placebo-controlled study has suggested that it may not be effective against sporadic type colonic polyps.[7]

For a discussion of evidence suggesting that regular use of NSAIDs may protect against various types of malignant neoplasms of the gastro-intestinal tract, see under Malignant Neoplasms in NSAIDs, p.66.

1. Giardiello FM, *et al.* Treatment of colonic and rectal adenomas with sulindac in familial adenomatous polyposis. *N Engl J Med* 1993; **328:** 1313–16.
2. Debinski HS, *et al.* Effect of sulindac on small polyps in familial adenomatous polyposis. *Lancet* 1995; **345:** 855–6.
3. Tonelli F, Valanzano R. Sulindac in familial adenomatous polyposis. *Lancet* 1993; **342:** 1120.
4. Labayle D, *et al.* Sulindac in familial adenomatous polyposis. *Lancet* 1994; **343:** 417–18.
5. Thorson AG, *et al.* Rectal cancer in FAP patient after sulindac. *Lancet* 1994; **343:** 180.
6. Parker AL, *et al.* Disappearance of duodenal polyps in Gardner's syndrome with sulindac therapy. *Am J Gastroenterol* 1993; **88:** 93–4.
7. Ladenheim J, *et al.* Effect of sulindac on sporadic colonic polyps. *Gastroenterology* 1995; **108:** 1083–7.

Premature labour. The most common approach to postponing premature labour (p.760) with drugs is with a selective beta agonist. However, as prostaglandins have a role in uterine contraction and cervical ripening and dilatation, prostaglandin synthetase inhibitors such as indomethacin have also been used. Sulindac has also been tried[1,2] as an alternative to indomethacin as it appears to have little placental transfer and may therefore have fewer fetal side-effects.[1]

1. Carlan SJ, *et al.* Randomized comparative trial of indomethacin and sulindac for the treatment of refractory preterm labor. *Obstet Gynecol* 1992; **79:** 223–8.
2. Carlan SJ, *et al.* Outpatient oral sulindac to prevent recurrence of preterm labor. *Obstet Gynecol* 1995; **85:** 769–74.

Preparations

BP 1998: Sulindac Tablets;
USP 23: Sulindac Tablets.

Proprietary Preparations (details are given in Part 3)
Aust.: Clinoril; ***Austral.:*** Aclin; Clinoril; Clusinol; Saldac; ***Belg.:*** Clinoril; ***Canad.:*** Apo-Sulin; Clinoril; Novo-Sundac; ***Fr.:*** Arthrocine; ***Irl.:*** Clinoril; ***Ital.:*** Aflodac; Algocetil; Citireuma; Clinoril; Clisundac†; Lyndac; Reumyl†; Sudac†; Sulartrene; Sulen; Sulic; Sulinol; Sulreuma†; ***Neth.:*** Clinoril; ***Norw.:*** Clinoril; ***S.Afr.:*** Clinoril; R-Flex; ***Spain:*** Sulindal; ***Swed.:*** Clinoril; ***Switz.:*** Clinoril; ***UK:*** Clinoril; ***USA:*** Clinoril.

Superoxide Dismutase (992-n)

SOD.

A group of water-soluble protein congeners widely distributed in nature which catalyse the conversion of superoxide radicals to peroxide. Several different forms exist, which vary in their metal content; forms containing copper or copper and zinc are common.

Orgotein (13043-t)

Orgotein *(BAN, USAN, rINN).*

Bovine Superoxide Dismutase; Ormetein.

CAS — 9016-01-7.

A superoxide dismutase produced from beef liver as Cu-Zn mixed chelate. Mol. wt about 33 000 with a compact conformation maintained by about 4 gram-atoms of chelated divalent metal.

Pegorgotein (17849-x)

Pegorgotein *(USAN, rINN).*

PEG-SOD; Win-22118.

CAS — 155773-57-2.

A superoxide dismutase conjugated with polyethylene glycol to prolong its duration of action.

Sudismase (5782-p)

Sudismase *(rINN).*

CAS — 110294-55-8.

A human *N*-acetylsuperoxide dismutase produced by recombinant DNA technology and containing a copper and zinc prosthetic group.

Adverse Effects

Anaphylaxis and other hypersensitivity reactions, sometimes fatal, have been reported with orgotein. Local reactions and pain may occur at the site of injection of orgotein.

Pharmacokinetics

References.

1. Tsao C, *et al.* Pharmacokinetics of recombinant human superoxide dismutase in healthy volunteers. *Clin Pharmacol Ther* 1991; **50:** 713–20.
2. Uematsu T, *et al.* Pharmacokinetics and safety of intravenous recombinant human superoxide dismutase (NK341) in healthy subjects. *Int J Clin Pharmacol Ther* 1994; **32:** 638–41.
3. Jadot G, *et al.* Clinical pharmacokinetics and delivery of bovine superoxide dismutase. *Clin Pharmacokinet* 1995; **28:** 17–25.
4. Rosenfeld WN, *et al.* Safety and pharmacokinetics of recombinant human superoxide dismutase administered intrathecally to premature neonates with respiratory distress syndrome. *Pediatrics* 1996; **97:** 811–17.
5. Davis JM, *et al.* Safety and pharmacokinetics of multiple doses of recombinant human CuZn superoxide dismutase administered intrathecally to premature neonates with respiratory distress syndrome. *Pediatrics* 1997; **100:** 24–30.

Uses and Administration

Superoxide dismutases have anti-inflammatory properties. Orgotein, a bovine derived superoxide dismutase, has been given by local injection, into the joints for degenerative joint disorders, but hypersensitivity reactions have limited its use. It has also been tried for the amelioration of side-effects from radiotherapy. Forms of human superoxide dismutase derived by recombinant DNA technology have been developed.

Superoxide dismutases are also under investigation for their free-radical scavenging properties in a variety of conditions including the prevention of bronchopulmonary dysplasia in neonates.

Head injury. Pegorgotein was found[1] to be little more effective than placebo in improving neurological outcome or reducing mortality in patients with severe head injury.

1. Young B, *et al.* Effects of pegorgotein on neurologic outcome of patients with severe head injury: a multicenter, randomized controlled trial. *JAMA* 1996; **276:** 538–43.

Motor neurone disease. A small percentage of patients with familial amyotrophic lateral sclerosis (see Motor Neurone Disease, p.1625) have been shown to have a mutation in the gene encoding for the enzyme copper-zinc superoxide dismutase but there has been no consensus as to whether patients with this mutation should be given superoxide dismutase supplements.[1]

1. Orrell RW, deBelleroche JS. Superoxide dismutase and ALS. *Lancet* 1994; **344:** 1651–2.

Neonatal respiratory distress syndrome. A preliminary double-blind placebo-controlled study[1] in 45 neonates with severe respiratory distress syndrome showed that orgotein 0.25 mg per kg body-weight every 12 hours by subcutaneous injection was helpful in reducing the severity of bronchopulmonary dysplasia. For discussions on the more usual drugs used in the management of bronchopulmonary dysplasia and neonatal respiratory distress syndrome see p.1018 and p.1025.

1. Rosenfeld W, *et al.* Prevention of bronchopulmonary dysplasia by administration of bovine superoxide dismutase in preterm infants with respiratory distress syndrome. *J Pediatr* 1984; **105:** 781–5.

Radiotherapy. Although some studies[1,2] indicate that orgotein can ameliorate the side-effects of radiotherapy for bladder tumours one study[3] was terminated prematurely because of unacceptable hypersensitivity reactions and apparent inefficacy.

1. Edsmyr F, *et al.* Orgotein efficacy in ameliorating side effects due to radiation therapy I: double-blind, placebo-controlled trial in patients with bladder tumors. *Curr Ther Res* 1976; **19:** 198–211.
2. Sanchiz F, *et al.* Prevention of radioinduced cystitis by orgotein: a randomized study. *Anticancer Res* 1996; **16:** 2025–8.
3. Nielsen OS, *et al.* Orgotein in radiation treatment of bladder cancer: a report on allergic reactions and lack of radioprotective effect. *Acta Oncol* 1987; **26:** 101–4.

Preparations

Proprietary Preparations (details are given in Part 3)
Aust.: Peroxinorm†; ***Ger.:*** Peroxinorm†; ***Ital.:*** Artrolasi†; Interceptor†; Orgo-M†; Oxinorm†; Serosod†; ***Spain:*** Ontosein; Peroxinorm†.

Suprofen (13292-y)

Suprofen *(BAN, USAN, rINN).*

R-25061; Sutoprofen. 2-[4-(2-Thenoyl)phenyl]propionic acid.

$C_{14}H_{12}O_3S$ = 260.3.

CAS — 40828-46-4.

Pharmacopoeias. In US.

A white to off-white, odourless or almost odourless, powder. Sparingly **soluble** in water.

Adverse Effects and Precautions

Ocular administration of suprofen may cause local reactions including discomfort, itching, redness, iritis, pain, chemosis, photophobia, and rarely punctate epithelial staining. Hypersensitivity may occur. Suprofen eye drops should not be used in patients with active herpes simplex keratitis.

Adverse renal reactions following oral administration have ended its use as an oral NSAID.

A clinical syndrome of flank pain and acute renal failure associated with oral suprofen has been reported;[1] the syndrome is unlike other nephrotoxic syndromes related to NSAIDs.

1. Hart D, *et al.* Suprofen-related nephrotoxicity: a distinct clinical syndrome. *Ann Intern Med* 1987; **106:** 235–8.

Interactions

The manufacturer of acetylcholine chloride ophthalmic preparations has stated that there have been reports that acetylcholine and carbachol have been ineffective when used in patients treated with topical (ophthalmic) NSAIDs.

Uses and Administration

Suprofen is an NSAID (p.65). Suprofen is used to inhibit the miosis that may occur during ocular surgery and is administered as 1% eye drops. On the day of surgery, 2 drops are instilled into the conjunctival sac 3 hours, 2 hours, and then 1 hour before surgery. Two drops may be instilled into the conjunctival sac every 4 hours during the day before surgery. It was formerly given by mouth in mild to moderate pain and in osteoarthritis and rheumatoid arthritis but, following reports of adverse renal reactions, marketing of the oral dose form was suspended worldwide.

Preparations

USP 23: Suprofen Ophthalmic Solution.

Proprietary Preparations (details are given in Part 3)
USA: Profenal.

Suxibuzone (2707-t)

Suxibuzone *(rINN).*

4-Butyl-4-hydroxymethyl-1,2-diphenylpyrazolidine-3,5-dione hydrogen succinate (ester).

$C_{24}H_{26}N_2O_6$ = 438.5.

CAS — 27470-51-5.

Suxibuzone, a derivative of phenylbutazone (p.79), is an NSAID (p.63) that has been applied topically at a concentration of about 7% in musculoskeletal and joint disorders. Concern over safety and toxicity has led to its withdrawal from the market in many countries.

Preparations

Proprietary Preparations (details are given in Part 3)
Spain: Danilon; ***Switz.:*** Flamilon†.

Multi-ingredient: ***Spain:*** Lapiz Termo Compositum†.

Tenidap Sodium (4865-m)

Tenidap Sodium *(BANM, USAN, rINNM).*

CP-66248 (tenidap); CP-66248-2 (tenidap sodium); CP-66248-02 (tenidap sodium). (*Z*)-5-Chloro-3-(α-hydroxy-2-thenylidene)-2-oxoindoline-1-carboxamide sodium.

$C_{14}H_8ClN_2NaO_3S$ = 342.7.

CAS — 120210-48-2 (tenidap); 119784-94-0 (tenidap sodium).

Tenidap is an NSAID (p.63) that also acts as a cytokine modulator. It has been studied in the treatment of rheumatoid arthritis and osteoarthritis but because of concern over its potential effect on bone mineral density its development for these indications was abandoned.

Tenoxicam (13305-h)

Tenoxicam *(BAN, USAN, rINN).*

Ro-12-0068; Ro-12-0068/000; Tenoxicamum. 4-Hydroxy-2-methyl-*N*-(2-pyridyl)-2*H*-thieno[2,3-e][1,2]thiazine-3-carboxamide 1,1-dioxide.

$C_{13}H_{11}N_3O_4S_2$ = 337.4.

CAS — 59804-37-4.

Pharmacopoeias. In Eur. (see p.viii).

A yellow, polymorphic, crystalline powder. Practically **insoluble** in water; very slightly soluble in alcohol; sparingly soluble in dichloromethane; it dissolves in solutions of acids and alkalis. **Protect** from light.

Adverse Effects and Precautions

As for NSAIDs in general, p.63.

Adverse effects associated with tenoxicam have been reviewed.[1] The majority of adverse effects relate to the gastro-intestinal tract (11.4%), nervous system (2.8%), or skin (2.5%).

1. Todd PA, Clissold SP. Tenoxicam: an update of its pharmacology and therapeutic efficacy in rheumatic diseases. *Drugs* 1991; **41:** 625–46.

Effects on the kidney. A review[1] of the effects of tenoxicam on renal function concluded that tenoxicam could be given at normal recommended doses to elderly patients or those with mild to moderate renal impairment who were not at high risk of renal failure or receiving potentially nephrotoxic therapy. Data from the manufacturer's database[1] on 67 063 patients, including 17 005 over 65 years of age, who had received tenoxicam indicated that there had been 45 adverse events relating to urinary system function. The prevalence of adverse events was similar in elderly and non-elderly patients, the most common effects being dysuria and renal pain. Seven of the events had been described as severe.

1. Heintz RCA. Tenoxicam and renal function. *Drug Safety* 1995; **12:** 110–19.

Effects on the liver. A report[1] of acute hepatitis associated with the use of tenoxicam.

1. Sungur C, *et al.* Acute hepatitis caused by tenoxicam. *Ann Pharmacother* 1994; **28:** 1309.

Effects on the skin. A report of three cases of toxic epidermal necrolysis (Lyell's syndrome) associated with tenoxicam.[1]

See also above.

1. Chosidow O, *et al.* Toxidermies sévères au ténoxicam (Tilcotil®). *Ann Dermatol Venereol* 1991; **118:** 903–4.

Interactions

For interactions associated with NSAIDs, see p.65.

Pharmacokinetics

Tenoxicam is well absorbed following oral administration; peak plasma concentrations occur within about 2 hours in fasting subjects; this may be delayed to about 6 hours when tenoxicam is given with food but the extent of absorption is not affected. Tenoxicam is over 98.5% protein bound and penetrates synovial fluid. The plasma elimination half-life is about 60 to 75 hours; with daily administration, steady-state concentrations are reached within 10 to 15 days. Tenoxicam is completely metabolised to inactive metabolites which are excreted mainly in the urine; there is some biliary excretion of glucuronide conjugates of the metabolites.

References.

1. Nilsen OG. Clinical pharmacokinetics of tenoxicam. *Clin Pharmacokinet* 1994; **26:** 16–43.
2. Guentert TW, *et al.* Relative bioavailability of oral dosage forms of tenoxicam. *Arzneimittelforschung* 1994; **44:** 1051–4.

Uses and Administration

Tenoxicam, a piroxicam (p.81) analogue, is an NSAID (p.65). It is used in the symptomatic management of osteoarthritis and rheumatoid arthritis and also in the short-term management of soft-tissue injury. Tenoxicam is given by mouth as a single daily dose usually of 20 mg. In acute musculoskeletal disorders treatment for up to 7 days is usually sufficient but in severe cases it may be given for up to a maximum of 14 days. Doses similar to those given by mouth have been given by intramuscular or intravenous injection for initial treatment for 1 to 2 days. Tenoxicam has also been given by rectal suppository.

References.

1. Todd PA, Clissold SP. Tenoxicam: an update of its pharmacology and therapeutic efficacy in rheumatic diseases. *Drugs* 1991; **41:** 625–46.

Preparations

Proprietary Preparations (details are given in Part 3)
Aust.: Liman; Tilcotil; ***Austral.:*** Tilcotil; ***Belg.:*** Tilcotil; ***Canad.:*** Mobiflex; ***Fr.:*** Tilcotil; ***Ger.:*** Liman; Tilcotil; ***Irl.:*** Mobiflex; ***Ital.:*** Dolmen; Rexalgan; Tilcotil; ***Neth.:*** Tilcotil; ***S.Afr.:*** Tilcotil; ***Spain:*** Artriunic; Reutenox; Tilcotil; ***Swed.:*** Alganex; ***Switz.:*** Tilcotil; ***UK:*** Mobiflex.

Tetrydamine (3915-l)

Tetrydamine *(USAN).*

Tetridamine *(rINN)*; POLI-67. 4,5,6,7-Tetrahydro-2-methyl-3-(methylamino)-2*H*-indazole.

$C_9H_{15}N_3$ = 165.2.

CAS — 17289-49-5.

Tetrydamine is an NSAID (p.63) that has been used as the maleate as a douche in the treatment of vaginitis.

Preparations

Proprietary Preparations (details are given in Part 3)
Spain: Fomene; Tesos.

Thurfyl Salicylate (2708-x)

Tetrahydrofurfuryl salicylate.

$C_{12}H_{14}O_4$ = 222.2.

CAS — 2217-35-8.

Thurfyl salicylate is a salicylic acid derivative that has been used similarly to methyl salicylate (p.55) in topical rubefacient preparations at concentrations of up to 14% for musculoskeletal, joint, peri-articular, and soft-tissue disorders.

Preparations

Proprietary Preparations (details are given in Part 3)
Multi-ingredient: ***Belg.:*** Transvane†; ***Irl.:*** Transvasin; ***Swed.:*** Transvasin; ***UK:*** Transvasin.

Tiaprofenic Acid (2709-r)

Tiaprofenic Acid *(BAN, rINN)*.

Acidum Tiaprofenicum; FC-3001; RU-15060. 2-(5-Benzoyl-2-thienyl)propionic acid.

$C_{14}H_{12}O_3S = 260.3$.

CAS — 33005-95-7.

Pharmacopoeias. In *Eur.* (see p.viii).

A white or almost white, crystalline powder. Practically **insoluble** in water; freely soluble in alcohol, in acetone, and in dichloromethane. **Protect** from light.

Adverse Effects and Precautions

As for NSAIDs in general, p.63.

Tiaprofenic acid may cause cystitis, bladder irritation, and other urinary-tract symptoms (see below). It should not be given to patients with active urinary-tract disorders or prostatic disease or a history of recurrent urinary-tract disorders. It should be stopped immediately if urinary-tract symptoms occur and urinalysis and urine culture performed.

Breast feeding. See under Pharmacokinetics, below.

Effects on the urinary tract. Cystitis and bladder irritation have been associated with the use of tiaprofenic acid.[1-6] In August 1994 the UK Committee on Safety of Medicines (CSM) stated[4] that since the introduction of tiaprofenic acid in the UK in 1982 they had received 69 reports of cystitis and 32 other reports of urinary-tract symptoms associated with tiaprofenic acid including frequency, dysuria, and haematuria whereas only 8 cases of cystitis had been reported for all other NSAIDs combined. Analysis of spontaneous reports received by WHO[7] confirmed that cystitis was more commonly associated with tiaprofenic acid than with other NSAIDs. The Australian Adverse Drug Reaction Advisory Committee had received similar reports.[3] Since the 1994 warning, the CSM[8] had received reports of a further 74 cases of cystitis, but the majority of these had occurred before the warning was issued. The duration of treatment in patients affected had varied considerably. Most patients recovered when tiaprofenic acid was withdrawn.

The CSM recommended that tiaprofenic acid should not be given to patients with pre-existing urinary-tract disorders and that it should be stopped in patients who develop urinary-tract symptoms. Patients should be advised that if they develop symptoms such as urinary frequency, nocturia, urgency, or pain on urination, or have blood in their urine they should stop taking tiaprofenic acid and consult their doctor.

1. Ahmed M, Davison OW. Severe cystitis associated with tiaprofenic acid. *Br Med J* 1991; **303:** 1376.
2. O'Neill GFA. Tiaprofenic acid as a cause of non-bacterial cystitis. *Med J Aust* 1994; **160:** 123–5.
3. Australian Adverse Drug Reactions Advisory Committee. Update on tiaprofenic acid and urinary symptoms. *Aust Adverse Drug React Bull* 1994; **13:** 6.
4. Committee on Safety of Medicines/Medicines Control Agency. Severe cystitis with tiaprofenic acid (Surgam). *Current Problems* 1994; **20:** 11.
5. Harrison WJ, *et al.* Adverse reactions to tiaprofenic acid mimicking interstitial cystitis. *Br Med J* 1994; **309:** 574.
6. Mayall FG, *et al.* Cystitis and ureteric obstruction in patients taking tiaprofenic acid. *Br Med J* 1994: **309:** 599.
7. The ADR Signals Analysis Project (ASAP) Team. How does cystitis affect a comparative risk profile of tiaprofenic acid with other non-steroidal antiinflammatory drugs? An international study based on spontaneous reports and drug usage data. *Pharmacol Toxicol* 1997; **80:** 211–17.
8. Crawford MLA, *et al.* Severe cystitis associated with tiaprofenic acid. *Br J Urol* 1997; **79:** 578–84.

Interactions

For interactions associated with NSAIDs, see p.65.

Pharmacokinetics

Tiaprofenic acid is absorbed from the gastro-intestinal tract with peak plasma concentrations being reached within about 1.5 hours after oral administration. It has a short elimination half-life of about 2 hours and is highly bound to plasma proteins (about 98%). Excretion of tiaprofenic acid and its metabolites is mainly in the urine in the form of acyl glucuronides; some is excreted in the bile. Tiaprofenic acid is distributed into breast milk in amounts considered to be too small to be harmful to a breast-fed infant.

References.

1. Davies NM. Clinical pharmacokinetics of tiaprofenic acid and its enantiomers. *Clin Pharmacokinet* 1996; **31:** 331–47.

Uses and Administration

Tiaprofenic acid, a propionic acid derivative, is an NSAID (p.65). It is used for the relief of pain and inflammation in musculoskeletal and joint disorders such as ankylosing spondylitis, osteoarthritis, and rheumatoid arthritis, in peri-articular disorders such as fibrositis and capsulitis, and in soft-tissue disorders such as sprains and strains. The usual dose by mouth is 600 mg daily given in 2 or 3 divided doses or once daily as a modified-release preparation. Tiaprofenic acid may be given rectally when the dose by suppository is 300 mg twice daily. It has also been given intramuscularly as the trometamol salt in acute conditions.

References.

1. Plosker GL, Wagstaff AJ. Tiaprofenic acid: a reappraisal of its pharmacological properties and use in the management of rheumatic diseases. *Drugs* 1995; **50:** 1050–75.

Preparations

Proprietary Preparations (details are given in Part 3)
Austral.: Surgam; ***Belg.:*** Artiflam; Surgam; ***Canad.:*** Albert Tiafen; Surgam; ***Fr.:*** Surgam; ***Ger.:*** Lindotab; Surgam; ***Irl.:*** Surgam; ***Ital.:*** Artroreuma; Suralgan; Surgamyl; Tiaprorex; ***Neth.:*** Surgam; ***S.Afr.:*** Surgam; ***Spain:*** Derilate; Surgamic; ***Switz.:*** Surgam; ***UK:*** Surgam.

Tiaramide Hydrochloride (2710-j)

Tiaramide Hydrochloride *(BANM, USAN, rINNM)*.

NTA-194; Tiaperamide Hydrochloride. 5-Chloro-3-{2-[4-(2-hydroxyethyl)piperazin-1-yl]-2-oxoethyl}benzothiazolin-2-one hydrochloride.

$C_{15}H_{18}ClN_3O_3S,HCl = 392.3$.

CAS — 32527-55-2 (tiaramide); 35941-71-0 (tiaramide hydrochloride).

Pharmacopoeias. In *Jpn.*

Tiaramide hydrochloride is an NSAID (p.63) that has been given by mouth for the relief of pain and inflammation.

Preparations

Proprietary Preparations (details are given in Part 3)
Jpn: Solantal.

Tilidate Hydrochloride (6262-z)

Tilidate Hydrochloride *(BANM)*.

Tilidine Hydrochloride *(USAN, pINNM)*; Gö 1261-C; W-5759A. (±)-Ethyl *trans*-2-dimethylamino-1-phenylcyclohex-3-ene-1-carboxylate hydrochloride hemihydrate.

$C_{17}H_{23}NO_2,HCl,\frac{1}{2}H_2O = 318.8$.

CAS — 20380-58-9 (tilidate); 27107-79-5 (anhydrous tilidate hydrochloride); 24357-97-9 (anhydrous +-trans-tilidate hydrochloride).

Dependence and Withdrawal, Adverse Effects, Treatment, and Precautions

As for Opioid Analgesics in general, p.67.

Porphyria. Tilidate has been associated with clinical exacerbations of porphyria and is considered unsafe in porphyric patients.[1]

1. Moore MR, McColl KEL. *Porphyria: drug lists.* Glasgow: Porphyria Research Unit, University of Glasgow, 1991.

Interactions

For interactions associated with opioid analgesics, see p.69.

Pharmacokinetics

Tilidate is absorbed from the gastro-intestinal tract. It is metabolised and excreted in the urine mainly as metabolites nortilidate (nortilidine) and bisnortilidate (bisnortilidine). Nortilidate is responsible for the analgesic activity of tilidate.

References.

1. Vollmer K-O, *et al.* Pharmacokinetics of tilidine and metabolites in man. *Arzneimittelforschung* 1989; **39:** 1283–8.

Uses and Administration

Tilidate hydrochloride is an opioid analgesic (p.69). It is used in the control of moderate to severe pain.

Tilidate hydrochloride may be given by intravenous, intramuscular, or subcutaneous injection in doses of up to 400 mg daily; usual doses as a suppository are 75 mg four times daily, or by mouth 50 mg four times daily. As a deterrent to abuse a combined oral preparation of tilidate hydrochloride with naloxone hydrochloride is available in some countries.

Preparations

Proprietary Preparations (details are given in Part 3)
Belg.: Valoron; Valtran; ***Ger.:*** Tilidalor; Valoron N; ***S.Afr.:*** Valoron; ***Spain:*** Tilitrate; ***Switz.:*** Valoron.

Tinoridine Hydrochloride (2711-z)

Tinoridine Hydrochloride *(rINNM)*.

Tienoridine Hydrochloride; Y-3642 (tinoridine). Ethyl 2-amino-6-benzyl-4,5,6,7-tetrahydrothieno[2,3-c]pyridine-3-carboxylate hydrochloride.

$C_{17}H_{20}N_2O_2S,HCl = 352.9$.

CAS — 24237-54-5 (tinoridine); 25913-34-2 (tinoridine hydrochloride).

Tinoridine hydrochloride is an NSAID (p.63) that has been given by mouth for pain and inflammation.

Preparations

Proprietary Preparations (details are given in Part 3)
Jpn: Nonflamin.

Tolfenamic Acid (2712-c)

Tolfenamic Acid *(BAN, rINN)*.

N-(3-Chloro-*o*-tolyl)anthranilic acid.

$C_{14}H_{12}ClNO_2 = 261.7$.

CAS — 13710-19-5.

Adverse Effects and Precautions

As for NSAIDs in general, p.63. Dysuria, most commonly in males, probably due to local irritation of the urethra by a metabolite, has also been reported. Tremor, euphoria, and fatigue have also occurred.

Effects on the lungs. Pulmonary infiltration has been associated with tolfenamic acid treatment in 6 patients.[1]

1. Strömberg C, *et al.* Pulmonary infiltrations induced by tolfenamic acid. *Lancet* 1987; **ii:** 685.

Interactions

For interactions associated with NSAIDs, see p.65.

Pharmacokinetics

Tolfenamic acid is readily absorbed from the gastro-intestinal tract. Time to peak plasma concentrations depends on the formulation; peak plasma concentrations are reached about 60 to 90 minutes after administration of the tablets, but take about 2 hours to be reached when using the capsules. Tolfenamic acid is about 99% bound to plasma proteins. The plasma half-life is about 2 hours. Tolfenamic acid is metabolised in the liver; the metabolites and unchanged drug are conjugated with glucuronic acid. About 90% of an ingested dose is excreted in the urine and the remainder in the faeces.

Uses and Administration

Tolfenamic acid, an anthranilic acid derivative related to mefenamic acid (p.52), is an NSAID (p.65). In the treatment of acute attacks of migraine tolfenamic acid is given in a usual dose of 200 mg when the first symptoms appear; if a satisfactory response is not obtained this dose may be repeated once after 1 to 2 hours if using the tablets, or 2 to 3 hours if using the capsules. Tolfenamic acid has also been given for the relief of mild to moderate pain in disorders such as dysmenorrhoea, rheumatoid arthritis, or osteoarthritis in doses of 100 to 200 mg three times daily by mouth.

Preparations

Proprietary Preparations (details are given in Part 3)
Aust.: Clotam; ***Neth.:*** Rociclyn; ***Switz.:*** Clotam; ***UK:*** Clotam.

Tolmetin Sodium (2713-k)

Tolmetin Sodium *(BANM, USAN, rINNM)*.

McN-2559-21-98; McN-2559 (tolmetin). Sodium (1-methyl-5-*p*-toluoylpyrrol-2-yl)acetate dihydrate.

$C_{15}H_{14}NNaO_3,2H_2O = 315.3$.

CAS — 26171-23-3 (tolmetin); 35711-34-3 (anhydrous tolmetin sodium); 64490-92-2 (tolmetin sodium dihydrate).

Pharmacopoeias. In *US.*

A light yellow to light orange crystalline powder. Freely **soluble** in water and in methyl alcohol; slightly soluble in alcohol; very slightly soluble in chloroform.

Adverse Effects and Precautions

As for NSAIDs in general, p.63.

Effects on the blood. Case reports of agranulocytosis[1] and thrombocytopenia[2] associated with tolmetin.

1. Sakai J, Joseph MW. Tolmetin and agranulocytosis. *N Engl J Med* 1978; **298:** 1203.
2. Lockhart JM. Tolmetin-induced thrombocytopenia. *Arthritis Rheum* 1982; **25:** 1144–5.

Effects on the CNS. See under Hypersensitivity, below.

Effects on the gastro-intestinal tract. Erosive oesophagitis has been reported[1] in an 11-year-old child following ingestion of a dose of tolmetin while lying down and without drinking any water.

1. Palop V, *et al.* Tolmetin-induced esophageal ulceration. *Ann Pharmacother* 1997; **31:** 929.

Effects on the kidneys. Interstitial nephritis[1] and nephrotic syndrome[2,3] have been reported in patients given tolmetin.

1. Katz SM, *et al.* Tolmetin: association with reversible renal failure and acute interstitial nephritis. *JAMA* 1981; **246:** 243–5.
2. Chatterjee GP. Nephrotic syndrome induced by tolmetin. *JAMA* 1981; **246:** 1589.
3. Tietjen DP. Recurrence and specificity of nephrotic syndrome due to tolmetin. *Am J Med* 1989; **87:** 354–5.

Hypersensitivity. Anaphylactic shock,[1] urticaria and angioedema,[2] and aseptic meningitis[3] are among the hypersensitivity reactions reported in patients taking tolmetin.

1. Rossi AC, Knapp DE. Tolmetin-induced anaphylactoid reactions. *N Engl J Med* 1982; **307:** 499–500.

2. Ponte CD, Wisman R. Tolmetin-induced urticaria/angioedema. *Drug Intell Clin Pharm* 1985; **19:** 479–80.
3. Ruppert GB, Barth WF. Tolmetin-induced aseptic meningitis. *JAMA* 1981; **245:** 67–8.

Interactions

For interactions associated with NSAIDs, see p.65.

Pharmacokinetics

Tolmetin is almost completely absorbed from the gastro-intestinal tract and peak plasma concentrations are attained about 30 to 60 minutes after ingestion. It is extensively bound to plasma proteins (over 99%) and has a biphasic plasma half-life of about 1 to 2 hours and 5 hours respectively. Tolmetin penetrates synovial fluid and very small amounts are distributed into breast milk. It is excreted in the urine as an inactive dicarboxylic acid metabolite and its glucuronide and as tolmetin glucuronide with small amounts of unchanged drug.

Uses and Administration

Tolmetin sodium is an NSAID (p.65). It is used in musculoskeletal and joint disorders such as ankylosing spondylitis, osteoarthritis, and rheumatoid arthritis, including juvenile chronic arthritis, and in peri-articular disorders such as fibrositis and bursitis. The usual initial dose is the equivalent of 400 mg of tolmetin three times daily by mouth; maintenance doses of 600 to 1800 mg daily in divided doses have been used. In juvenile chronic arthritis it is given in usual initial doses equivalent to 20 mg of tolmetin per kg body-weight daily in divided doses; maintenance doses of 15 to 30 mg per kg daily have been used. The maximum daily dose of tolmetin recommended for adults and children is 30 mg per kg up to a maximum total of 1800 mg.

Tolmetin has been used as the free acid in similar doses rectally, and has been applied as a 5% topical gel.

Preparations

USP 23: Tolmetin Sodium Capsules; Tolmetin Sodium Tablets.

Proprietary Preparations (details are given in Part 3)
Aust.: Tolectin; ***Belg.:*** Tolectin; ***Canad.:*** Tolectin; ***Ger.:*** Tolectin†; ***Irl.:*** Tolectin; ***Ital.:*** Reutol†; Tolectin; ***Neth.:*** Tolectin; ***S.Afr.:*** Tolectin; ***Spain:*** Artrocaptin; ***Switz.:*** Tolectin; ***UK:*** Tolectin†; ***USA:*** Tolectin.

Tramadol Hydrochloride (6263-c)

Tramadol Hydrochloride *(BANM, USAN, rINNM).*

CG-315; CG-315E; U-26225A. (±)-*trans*-2-Dimethylaminomethyl-1-(3-methoxyphenyl)cyclohexanol hydrochloride.

$C_{16}H_{25}NO_2$,HCl = 299.8.

CAS — 27203-92-5 (tramadol); 22204-88-2 (tramadol hydrochloride); 36282-47-0 (tramadol hydrochloride).

Dependence and Withdrawal

As for Opioid Analgesics, p.67. Tramadol may have lower potential for producing dependence than morphine.

References.

1. Richter W, *et al.* Clinical investigation on the development of dependence during oral therapy with tramadol. *Arzneimittelforschung* 1985; **35:** 1742–4.

The UK Committee on Safety of Medicines[1] commented in October 1996 that since June 1994 they have received reports of drug dependence in 5 patients and withdrawal symptoms associated with tramadol in 28 patients, which corresponded to a reporting rate of about 1 in 6000. Doses in excess of the recommended maximum of 400 mg daily had been taken by 5 of the patients. The duration of treatment before onset of these effects ranged from 10 to 409 days (average 3 months). Withdrawal symptoms reported were typically those of opioid withdrawal in general.

1. Committee on Safety of Medicines/Medicines Control Agency. Tramadol—(Zydol, Tramake and Zamadol). *Current Problems* 1996; **22:** 11.

Adverse Effects and Treatment

As for Opioid Analgesics in general, p.68. Tramadol may produce fewer typical opioid adverse effects such as less respiratory depression and less constipation.

In addition to hypotension, hypertension has occasionally been reported. Anaphylaxis, hallucinations, and confusion have also been reported.

Effects on the CNS. The UK Committee on Safety of Medicines (CSM)[1] commented in February 1995 that since June 1994 they had received reports of 15 patients who had experienced confusion and/or hallucinations while taking tramadol. The majority of the reactions developed 1 to 7 days after starting treatment and resolved rapidly on withdrawal in most patients. It was noted that psychiatric reactions comprised about 10% of all reactions reported with tramadol. In a later comment[2] in October 1996, the CSM noted that 27 reports of convulsion and one of worsening epilepsy had been received, which corresponded to a reporting rate of about 1 in 7000. Of the 5 patients receiving intravenous tramadol, 2 had been given doses well in excess of those recommended (equivalent to 1.45 and 4.0 g daily). Of the patients receiving oral tramadol, the majority were taking other drugs, including tricyclic antidepressants (TCAs) and selective serotonin reuptake inhibitors (SSRIs). A similar pattern was reported by the Food and Drug Administration[3] in the USA: of 124 cases of seizure reported from March 1995 to July 1996, 30 suggested doses taken in excess of the recommended 400 mg or at shorter time intervals than those recommended, and in 72 cases drugs with the potential to lower the seizure threshold, including SSRIs and TCAs, had been taken.

A debilitating CNS-mediated reaction to an initial dose of tramadol has been described in a patient.[4] Symptoms, which lasted approximately 4 hours, included ataxia, dilatation of the pupils, numbness in all limbs, tremulousness, and dysphoria. Although the exact mechanism of the reaction is not known, based on phenotyping results, it was suspected that since the patient was an extensive metaboliser with very high activity of the cytochrome P450 isozyme CYP2D6, high concentrations of the active *O*-desmethyl metabolite were the cause. The patient recovered with no sequelae.

1. Committee on Safety of Medicines/Medicines Control Agency. Tramadol (Zydol)—psychiatric reactions. *Current Problems* 1995; **21:** 2.
2. Committee on Safety of Medicines/Medicines Control Agency. Tramadol—(Zydol, Tramake and Zamadol). *Current Problems* 1996; **22:** 11.
3. Kahn LH, *et al.* Seizures reported with tramadol. *JAMA* 1997; **278:** 1661.
4. Gleason PP, *et al.* Debilitating reaction following the initial dose of tramadol. *Ann Pharmacother* 1997; **31:** 1150–2.

Effects on the respiratory system. Respiratory depression has been reported after tramadol infusion anaesthesia,[1] although in a postoperative study[2] tramadol had no significant respiratory depressant effect when equianalgesic doses of morphine, pentazocine, pethidine, piritramide, and tramadol were compared.

1. Paravicini D, *et al.* Tramadol-infusionsanaesthesie mit substitution von enfluran und differenten lachgaskonzentrationen. *Anaesthesist* 1985; **34:** 20–7.
2. Fechner R, *et al.* Clinical investigations on the effect of morphine, pentazocine, pethidine, piritramide and tramadol on respiration. *Anasth Intensivmed* 1985; **26:** 126–32.

Precautions

As for Opioid Analgesics in general, p.68.

The dosage interval should be increased to 12 hours in patients with renal or liver impairment. Tramadol should not be used if there is severe renal impairment. Removal by haemodialysis is reported to be very slow.

Tramadol should be used with care in patients with a history of epilepsy or those susceptible to seizures. See also Effects on the CNS under Adverse Effects, above.

Anaesthesia. The manufacturers warn against using tramadol during very light planes of general anaesthesia because of possible intra-operative awareness, although it may be used intra-operatively provided anaesthesia is maintained by the continuous administration of a potent volatile anaesthetic. Intra-operative awareness was reported in 65% of a group of 20 patients when used to provide analgesia during light general anaesthesia with nitrous oxide and intermittent enflurane.[1] However, in a study by Coetzee *et al.*[2] in 51 patients given tramadol during stable light continuous isoflurane-nitrous oxide anaesthesia there was no clinically significant lightening of anaesthesia. Budd[3] had commented that during extensive use of tramadol intra-operatively over several years, there had not been any incidence of recall in any patient treated at their clinic.

1. Lehmann KA, *et al.* Zur bedeutung von Tramadol als intraoperativem analgetikum: eine randomisierte doppelblindstudie im vergleich zu placebo. *Der Anaesthetist* 1985; **34:** 11–19.
2. Coetzee JF, *et al.* Effect of tramadol on depth of anaesthesia. *Br J Anaesth* 1996; **76:** 415–18.
3. Budd K. Tramadol. *Br J Anaesth* 1995; **75:** 500.

Interactions

For interactions associated with opioid analgesics, see p.69.

Carbamazepine is reported to diminish the analgesic activity of tramadol by reducing serum concentrations.

The risk of seizures is increased if tramadol is administered concomitantly with other drugs that have the potential to lower the seizure threshold. See also under Effects on the CNS under Adverse Effects, above.

Tramadol inhibits reuptake of noradrenaline and serotonin and enhances serotonin release and there is the possibility that it may interact with other drugs that enhance monoaminergic neurotransmission including lithium, tricyclic antidepressants, and selective serotonin reuptake inhibitors; it should not be given to patients receiving MAOIs or within 14 days of their discontinuation.

Metabolism of tramadol is mediated by the cytochrome P450 isozyme CYP2D6. Concomitant administration with specific inhibitors of this enzyme, such as *quinidine*, may increase concentrations of tramadol and lower concentrations of its active metabolite but the clinical consequences of this effect are unclear.

Anticoagulants. Tramadol was reported to have potentiated the anticoagulant effect of *phenprocoumon* in 2 patients,[1] and of *warfarin* in 1 patient.[2] However, a randomised, double-blind, placebo-controlled study[3] in 19 patients failed to find evidence of an interaction between phenprocoumon and tramadol.

1. Madsen H, *et al.* Interaction between tramadol and phenprocoumon. *Lancet* 1997; **350:** 637.
2. Scher ML, *et al.* Potential interaction between tramadol and warfarin. *Ann Pharmacother* 1997; **31:** 646–7.
3. Boeijina JK, *et al.* Is there interaction between tramadol and phenprocoumon? *Lancet* 1997; **350:** 1552.

Antidepressants. For reference to a possible case of serotonin syndrome associated with concomitant administration of tramadol and *sertraline*, see under Fluoxetine, p.287.

Pharmacokinetics

Tramadol is readily absorbed following oral administration but is subject to first-pass metabolism. Tramadol is metabolised by *N*- and *O*-demethylation and glucuronidation or sulphation in the liver. The metabolite *O*-desmethyltramadol is pharmacologically active. Tramadol is excreted mainly in the urine predominantly as metabolites. Tramadol is widely distributed, crosses the placenta, and appears in small amounts in breast milk. The elimination half-life following oral administration is about 6 hours.

Production of the active metabolite *O*-desmethyltramadol is dependent on the cytochrome P450 isozyme CYP2D6, which exhibits genetic polymorphism.[1] For a reference to a debilitating CNS-mediated reaction in a patient who was an extensive metaboliser with high CYP2D6 activity, see under Effects on the CNS in Adverse Effects, above.

1. Poulsen L, *et al.* The hypoalgesic effect of tramadol in relation to CYP2D6. *Clin Pharmacol Ther* 1996; **60:** 636–44.

Uses and Administration

Tramadol hydrochloride is an opioid analgesic (p.69). It also has noradrenergic and serotonergic properties that may contribute to its analgesic activity. Tramadol is used for moderate to severe pain.

Tramadol hydrochloride is given by mouth, by the intramuscular, subcutaneous, or intravenous route, or by suppository. Usual doses by mouth are 50 to 100 mg every 4 to 6 hours. Tramadol hydrochloride may also be given orally as a modified-release preparation twice daily. The total daily dosage by mouth should not exceed 400 mg.

A dose of 50 to 100 mg may be given every 4 to 6 hours by intramuscular injection, intravenous injection over 2 to 3 minutes, or by intravenous infusion. For the treatment of postoperative pain, the initial dose is 100 mg followed by 50 mg every 10 to 20 minutes if necessary to a total maximum (including the initial dose) of 250 mg in the first hour. Thereafter, doses are 50 to 100 mg every 4 to 6 hours up to a total daily dose of 600 mg.

Rectal doses by suppository are 100 mg up to 4 times a day.

References.

1. Anonymous. Tramadol—a new analgesic. *Drug Ther Bull* 1994; **32:** 85–6. Correction. *ibid.*: 96.
2. Radbruch L, *et al.* A risk-benefit assessment of tramadol in the management of pain. *Drug Safety* 1996; **15:** 8–29.
3. Williams HJ. Tramadol hydrochloride: something new in oral analgesic therapy. *Curr Ther Res* 1997; **58:** 215–26.
4. Lewis KS, Han NH. Tramadol: a new centrally acting analgesic. *Am J Health-Syst Pharm* 1997; **54:** 643–52.
5. Duthie DJR. Remifentanil and tramadol. *Br J Anaesth* 1998; **81:** 51–7.

Preparations

Proprietary Preparations (details are given in Part 3)
Aust.: Nobligan; Tramal; ***Belg.:*** Contramal; Dolzam; ***Fr.:*** Topalgic; ***Ger.:*** Amadol; Tradol; Trama; Trama-Dorsch; Tramabeta; Tramadolor; Tramadura; Tramagetic; Tramagit; Tramal; Tramamerck; Tramedphano; ***Irl.:*** Tramake; Zydol; ***Ital.:*** Contramal; Fortradol; ***Neth.:*** Theradol; Tramagetic; Tramal; ***S.Afr.:*** Tramal; ***Spain:*** Adolonta; Tralgiol; ***Swed.:*** Nobligan; Tiparol; Tradolan; ***Switz.:*** Tramadolor; Tramal; ***UK:*** Tramake; Zamadol; Zydol; ***USA:*** Ultram.

Multi-ingredient: ***Ger.:*** Tramundin.

Trefentanil (16797-c)

Trefentanil *(rINN).*

N-{1-[2-(4-Ethyl-5-oxo-Δ^2-tetrazolin-1-yl)ethyl]-4-phenyl-4-piperidyl}-2′-fluoropropionanilide.

$C_{25}H_{31}FN_6O_2$ = 466.6.

CAS — 120656-74-8 (trefentanil); 120656-93-1 (trefentanil hydrochloride).

NOTE. Trefentanil Hydrochloride is *USAN.*

Trefentanil is an opioid analgesic (p.67) reported to have a shorter duration of action than alfentanil (p.12).

References.

1. Cambareri JJ, *et al.* A-3665, a new short-acting opioid: a comparison with alfentanil. *Anesth Analg* 1993; **76:** 812–16.
2. Lemmens HJM, *et al.* Pharmacokinetic-pharmacodynamic modeling in drug development: application to the investigational opioid trefentanil. *Clin Pharmacol Ther* 1994; **56:** 261–71.

Triethanolamine Salicylate (9593-l)

Trolamine Salicylate (*pINNM*).

Triethanolamine salicylate is a salicylic acid derivative used similarly to methyl salicylate (p.55) in topical rubefacient preparations in a concentration of 10 to 15% for the relief of muscular and rheumatic pain. It has also been used as a sunscreen.

In contrast to methyl salicylate, which undergoes considerable absorption and produces high subcutaneous and dermal concentrations of salicylic acid after application to intact skin, concentrations of salicylic acid after topical application of triethanolamine salicylate were substantially lower in tissue[1] and undetectable in serum.[2]

1. Cross SE, *et al.* Is there tissue penetration after application of topical salicylate formulations? *Lancet* 1997; **350:** 636.
2. Morra P, *et al.* Serum concentrations of salicylic acid following topically applied salicylate derivatives. *Ann Pharmacother* 1996; **30:** 935–40.

Preparations

Proprietary Preparations (details are given in Part 3)
Austral.: Dencorub Arthritis; Metsal AR Analgesic; ***Canad.:*** Antiphlogistine Rub A-535 No Odour; Aspercreme; Ben-Gay No Odor; Miosal; Myoflex; Royflex; Sportscreme†; ***Spain:*** Bexidermil; Topicrem; ***USA:*** Analgesia Creme; Aspercreme; Coppertone Tan Magnifier; Exocaine Odor Free†; Mobisyl; Myoflex; Pro-gesic; Sportscreme; Tropical Blend Tan Magnifier.

Multi-ingredient: ***Austral.:*** Metsal Analgesic; ***Canad.:*** Ease Pain Away; Myoflex Ice Plus.

Ufenamate (3654-q)

Ufenamate (*rINN*).

Butyl Flufenamate. Butyl *N*-(α,α,α-trifluoro-*m*-tolyl)anthranilate.

$C_{18}H_{18}F_3NO_2$ = 337.3.
CAS — 67330-25-0.

Ufenamate is an NSAID (p.63) used as a 5% cream or ointment in inflammatory skin disorders.

Preparations

Proprietary Preparations (details are given in Part 3)
Jpn: Fenazol.

Viminol Hydroxybenzoate (2715-t)

Viminol Hydroxybenzoate (*rINNM*).

Diviminol Hydroxybenzoate; Z-424 (viminol). 1-[1-(2-Chlorobenzyl)pyrrol-2-yl]-2-(di-*sec*-butyl)aminoethanol 4-hydroxybenzoate.

$C_{21}H_{31}ClN_2O,C_7H_6O_3$ = 501.1.
CAS — 21363-18-8 (viminol); 21466-60-4; 23784-10-3 (both viminol hydroxybenzoate).

Viminol hydroxybenzoate has analgesic and antipyretic properties. It has been given in doses equivalent to up to 400 mg of viminol daily, in divided doses, by mouth.

Preparations

Proprietary Preparations (details are given in Part 3)
Ital.: Dividol.

Zaltoprofen (3052-b)

Zaltoprofen (*rINN*).

CN-100. (±)-10,11-Dihydro-α-methyl-10-oxodibenzo[*b,f*]thiepin-2-acetic acid.

$C_{17}H_{14}O_3S$ = 298.4.
CAS — 89482-00-8.

Zaltoprofen is an NSAID (p.63) which has been given by mouth for musculoskeletal and joint disorders.

References.

1. Ishizaki T, *et al.* Pharmacokinetic profile of a new nonsteroidal anti-inflammatory agent, CN-100, in humans. *Drug Invest* 1991; **3:** 1–7.

Ziconotide (20097-h)

Ziconotide (*rINN*).

SNX-111. L-Cysteinyl-L-lysylglycyl-L-lysylglycl-L-alanyl-L-lysyl-L-cysteinyl-L-seryl-L-arginyl-L-leucyl-L-methionyl-L-tyrosyl-L-α-aspartyl-L-cysteinyl-L-cysteinyl-L-threonylglycyl-L-seryl-L-cysteinyl-L-arginyl-L-serylglycyl-L-lysyl-L-cysteinamide cyclic(1→16),(8→20),(15→25)-tris(disulfide).

$C_{102}H_{172}N_{36}O_{32}S_7$ = 2639.1.

Ziconotide is a peptide derived from sea snails. It is reported to be a neurone-specific calcium antagonist and is being studied in the management of various types of pain, including neurogenic pain, and in other conditions such as head trauma.

Anthelmintics

This chapter describes the important helminth or worm infections that occur in man (see Table 1) and the anthelmintics used to treat them.

Choice of Anthelmintic

Helminth infections are among the most common infections in man, affecting a large proportion of the world's population, mainly in tropical regions. In developing countries they pose a large threat to public health, and contribute to the prevalence of malnutrition, anaemia, eosinophilia, and pneumonia. Helminth infections causing severe morbidity include lymphatic filariasis (a cause of elephantiasis), onchocerciasis (river blindness), and schistosomiasis. These infections can affect the majority of populations in endemic areas with major economic and social consequences. WHO are making strenuous efforts to control a number of these infections in endemic areas. Control of these infections in both individuals and populations depends not only on the use of chemotherapeutic agents but also on preventing transmission by advice on food preparation and hygiene, the provision of adequate sanitation and sewage treatment (especially where sewage is used as fertiliser), the provision of safe potable water supplies, and effective vector control.

The worms that cause infection in man generally fall either into the phylum Platyhelminthes, which includes the cestodes or tapeworms and the trematodes or flukes, or into the phylum Nematoda which includes the nematodes or roundworms.

The **cestodes** (flatworms, segmented worms, or tapeworms) cause infection in man in most parts of the world. Man may be the definitive host and harbour the adult worm in the intestine or an intermediate host carrying the larval form. With the exception of *Hymenolepis nana* the adult worms do not usually multiply within the same host. However, larval forms may be produced and, as with infection or ingestion of these forms, systemic infection may develop. Cestode infections include:

- cysticercosis
- diphyllobothriasis
- echinococcosis
- hymenolepiasis
- taeniasis.

The **nematodes**, or roundworms, represent a large group of worms some of which are capable of producing infections in man. In many cases man is the primary (definitive) host but human infections caused by parasites for which animals are the primary hosts also occur. Nematodes do not generally multiply in man; strongyloidiasis is an exception as reinfection can occur without environmental re-exposure. Nematode infections are most common in warm, moist climates but some species of nematode can tolerate cool or arid conditions and infective forms can persist in the environment for long periods. An understanding of the life cycle of the infective species is necessary for diagnostic tests to be made at appropriate times, usually to coincide with the infective stage of the cycle and for the choice of appropriate control measures.

The nematode infections can be divided into filarial infections, intestinal infections, and tissue infections.

Filarial nematodes are endemic in large areas of the tropics and produce considerable morbidity. The adult worms may live for several years releasing large numbers of motile embryos known as microfilariae into the blood or skin, depending on the species. Transmission is usually by biting insects which form the intermediate host. In some endemic areas multiple infections with filarial nematodes are common. Filarial nematode infections include:

- loiasis
- lymphatic filariasis
- mansonella infections
- onchocerciasis.

Intestinal nematode infections (roundworms) are very common especially in developing countries in the tropics and subtropics. Children are particularly at risk and these infections contribute to morbidity through malnutrition, vitamin deficiencies, diarrhoea, anaemia, and pneumonia. Poor sanitation and sewage disposal perpetuate infections with soil-borne nematodes. Several different worm infections may often be endemic in the same part of the world, resulting in mixed infections. When that occurs broad spectrum anthelmintics may be used to reduce the overall infection burden in the population (see under Ascariasis, below). Intestinal nematode infections include:

- angiostrongyliasis
- ascariasis
- capillariasis
- enterobiasis
- hookworm infections
- strongyloidiasis
- trichostrongyliasis
- trichuriasis.

The *tissue nematodes* represent a miscellaneous group causing a variety of pathological conditions in man. In cutaneous larva migrans and toxocariasis the nematodes have a primary animal host and the human disease is caused by infection with infective larvae which do not subsequently mature in man. Trichinosis and gnathostomiasis affect a number of carnivorous animals and man is an incidental host. Syngamosis is primarily an infection of domestic fowl and wild birds although infection in man has been reported rarely. In dracunculiasis man is the primary (definitive) host. Although these diseases are not generally fatal they cause a considerable degree of morbidity and treatment is complicated by the lack of effective, non-toxic systemic anthelmintics. Tissue nematode infections include:

- angiostrongyliasis
- cutaneous larva migrans
- dracunculiasis
- gnathostomiasis
- syngamosis
- toxocariasis
- trichinosis.

Trematode (or fluke) infections are caused by parasitic worms of the class Trematoda. There are 4 categories of fluke which are pathogenic in man; the blood flukes *Schistosoma* spp., the intestinal flukes *Fasciolopsis, Heterophyes, Metagonimus,* and *Nanophyetus* spp., the liver flukes *Clonorchis, Fasciola,* and *Opisthorchis* spp., and the lung flukes *Paragonimus* spp. Symptoms are usually only seen in heavy infections and commonly include fever, pain, and eosinophilia. Trematode infections include:

- intestinal fluke infections
- liver fluke infections
- lung fluke infections
- schistosomiasis.

Ancylostomiasis

See under Hookworm Infections, below. Larvae of *Ancylostoma* spp. are also a cause of cutaneous larva migrans (see below).

Angiostrongyliasis

Two forms of angiostrongyliasis are recognised and both are due to accidental infection with species of the animal nematode *Angiostrongylus.*

Infection with the larvae of the rat lungworm *A. cantonensis* causes an eosinophilic meningoencephalitis. Transmission follows ingestion of raw or undercooked snails or crustaceans or contaminated vegetables. The disease is generally self-limiting. Treatment with mebendazole has been suggested but severe host reaction to the dying larvae may result.

Intestinal infection with *A. costaricensis* can cause eosinophilic gastro-enteritis. It most commonly occurs in children following ingestion of vegetables contaminated by infected slugs. Surgical resection of the affected bowel may be necessary but treatment with mebendazole or thiabendazole has been suggested.

Ascariasis

Ascariasis is an infection caused by *Ascaris lumbricoides*, the common roundworm or giant roundworm. The term roundworm is also applied to nematodes in general. It is usually an infection of the small intestine but on rare occasions there may be severe ectopic infections. It is commonly found in the tropics and especially in rural areas. Eggs are excreted in the faeces and can remain viable in moist soil for several years. On ingestion of mature eggs the larvae hatch and penetrate the intestinal wall. They migrate in the blood stream via the liver to the lungs where they enter the alveoli. The larvae then move up the bronchial tree and are swallowed. The mature adult develops in the intestines, and it has been estimated that a gravid female is produced about 2 months after infection. The life span of the adult worm is 1 to 2 years. Ascariasis may be asymptomatic. When symptoms of intestinal infection do occur they include anorexia, abdominal pain, and diarrhoea; nutritional deficiency may result. The pulmonary stage may cause pneumonitis and bronchospasm often accompanied by eosinophilia. Heavy infections can cause intestinal or biliary obstruction. Migration of the worm from the small intestine can produce ectopic infection of the urinary-genital tract, lungs, liver, or heart. Such infections are rare but serious.

Children are at greatest risk of *Ascaris* infection and one study[1] has suggested that child-targeted treatment can be more cost-effective in reducing disease cases than programmes of mass chemotherapy in areas where infection is endemic.

Table 1. Helminths: classification and diseases.

Group	Helminth	Common Name	Clinical infection
Cestodes (tapeworms)	*Diphyllobothrium latum*	broad fish tapeworm	diphyllobothriasis
	Echinococcus spp.		echinococcosis (hydatid disease)
	Hymenolepis nana	dwarf tapeworm	hymenolepiasis
	*Taenia saginata**	beef tapeworm	taeniasis
	*Taenia solium**	pork tapeworm	cysticercosis (larval form), taeniasis (adult worm)
Nematodes (filarial)	*Brugia malayi*		lymphatic filariasis (Malayan, brugian)
	Brugia timori		lymphatic filariasis (Timorian, brugian)
	Loa loa	eye-worm	loiasis
	Mansonella spp.		Mansonella infections
	Onchocerca volvulus		onchocerciasis (river blindness)
	Wuchereria bancrofti		lymphatic filariasis (bancroftian)
Nematodes (intestinal)	*Ancylostoma duodenale*	Old World hookworm	ancylostomiasis
	Angiostrongylus costaricensis		angiostrongyliasis
	Necator americanus	New World hookworm	necatoriasis
	*Ascaris lumbricoides**	common roundworm, giant roundworm	ascariasis
	Capillaria philippinensis		capillariasis
	*Enterobius vermicularis**	threadworm, pinworm	enterobiasis
	Strongyloides stercoralis	sometimes called threadworm in USA	strongyloidiasis
	Trichostrongylus spp.		trichostrongyliasis
	*Trichuris trichiura**	whipworm	trichuriasis
Nematodes (tissue)	*Ancylostoma* spp.	dog/cat hookworm	cutaneous larva migrans (creeping eruption)
	Angiostrongylus cantonensis		angiostrongyliasis
	Dracunculus medinensis	guinea-worm	dracunculiasis (dracontiasis)
	Gnathostoma spinigerum		gnathostomiasis
	Syngamus spp.	gapeworm	syngamosis
	Toxocara spp.*		toxocariasis (visceral larva migrans, ocular larva migrans)
	*Trichinella spiralis**		trichinosis (trichinellosis)
Trematodes (flukes)	*Clonorchis sinensis*	Chinese liver fluke	clonorchiasis
	Fasciola hepatica	liver fluke	fascioliasis
	Fasciolopsis buski	intestinal fluke	fasciolopsiasis
	Heterophyes heterophyes	intestinal fluke	heterophyiasis
	Metagonimus yokogawi	intestinal fluke	metagonimiasis
	Nanophyetus salmincola	intestinal fluke	nanophyetiasis
	Opisthorchis spp.	liver fluke	opisthorchiasis
	Paragonimus spp.	oriental lung fluke	paragonimiasis
	Schistosoma spp.	blood fluke	schistosomiasis

NOTE: Infections due to worms marked with an asterisk may occur in temperate climates. Infections due to other worms are generally limited to tropical or localised areas, but may occur in travellers who have visited those areas.

Treatment is with a benzimidazole carbamate derivative such as albendazole or mebendazole with both drugs being equally highly effective. Pyrantel embonate is an alternative. Such broad-spectrum therapy can be useful if the patient is suffering from a mixed intestinal nematode infection. Drugs such as thiabendazole with little or no activity against *Ascaris* should be avoided for the initial treatment of mixed infections since they may stimulate the worm to migrate to a different body site. Other anthelmintics effective in ascariasis include levamisole and piperazine salts.

1. Guyatt HL, *et al.* Control of Ascaris infection by chemotherapy: which is the most cost-effective option? *Trans R Soc Trop Med Hyg* 1995; **89:** 16–20.

Capillariasis

Capillariasis is caused by infection with *Capillaria philippinensis,* a nematode endemic in the Philippines and southern Thailand. Infection in man is through eating raw or undercooked freshwater fish containing infective larvae. The larvae mature in the intestines and the adults produce both eggs and infective larvae so that auto-infection occurs and heavy infections can result. Symptoms are mostly gastro-intestinal, with abdominal pain, vomiting, and severe prolonged diarrhoea leading to cachexia and muscle wasting. The infection has a mortality rate of between 20 and 30% if untreated. Prolonged treatment with mebendazole or, alternatively, albendazole, is necessary.

Clonorchiasis

See under Liver Fluke Infections, below.

Cutaneous larva migrans

Cutaneous larva migrans (creeping eruption) occurs when man becomes infected with the larvae of animal hookworms, usually *Ancylostoma braziliense* or *A. caninum*, hookworms of cats and dogs. Other hookworms may also be involved or may cause other infections (see Hookworm Infections, below). The larvae penetrate the skin and then migrate causing characteristic trails in the skin. This migration can persist for several months and can be a source of intense pruritus. Occasionally larvae migrate to the lungs causing eosinophilia and pulmonary symptoms. Thiabendazole given by mouth or applied topically is the standard treatment although albendazole and ivermectin are possible alternatives.

Infection with *Gnathostoma spinigerum* or *Strongyloides stercoralis* can also cause cutaneous larva migrans (see Gnathostomiasis and Strongyloidiasis, below). Ocular and visceral larva migrans are features of toxocariasis (see below).

References.

1. Rodilla F, *et al.* Current treatment recommendations for cutaneous larva migrans. *Ann Pharmacother* 1994; **28:** 672–3.

Cysticercosis

Cysticercosis is a systemic infection caused by the larval form (cysticercus) of *Taenia solium.* Infection is acquired through ingestion of eggs in contaminated food or water, or directly from individuals harbouring the adult worm. The eggs hatch in the intestine and the larvae spread systemically to almost any body tissue. Invasion of the brain is known as neurocysticercosis and is a common cause of epilepsy in endemic areas. The most effective treatment for neurocysticercosis has been debated.[1] In the absence of large randomised studies, opinion have been divided over whether cysticidal drugs should be given routinely in neurocysticercosis or reserved for selected patients.[1] Some have suggested that they might be associated with long-term sequelae,[2] and have reiterated that the ideal solution is prevention by ensuring adequate sanitation and sewage treatment and thorough cooking of meat that may be contaminated. When anthelmintics are considered necessary, praziquantel is used to treat neurocysticercosis and is usually given with a corticosteroid to prevent an inflammatory response to dead and dying larvae. Albendazole is an alternative treatment that some consider to be preferable; a corticosteroid or antihistamine is also administered to counter any inflammatory reaction. In some cases surgical removal of cysts may be the preferred treatment.

Infection with the adult worm of *T. solium* is discussed under Taeniasis, below.

1. Anonymous. Cerebral cysticercosis: what can be expected of cysticidal drugs? *WHO Drug Inf* 1995; **9:** 135–8.
2. Carpio A, *et al.* Is the course of neurocysticercosis modified by treatment with antihelminthic agents? *Arch Intern Med* 1995; **155:** 1982–8.

Diphyllobothriasis

Diphyllobothriasis is an intestinal infection with the fish tapeworm *Diphyllobothrium latum* and other *Diphyllobothrium* spp. and is acquired in man through ingestion of raw, infected, freshwater fish. The infection is rarely symptomatic. However, because the adult worm competes for vitamin B_{12}, some patients may develop megaloblastic anaemia with its associated neurological symptoms. Concentrations of other vitamins may also be reduced. Treatment is with a single dose of praziquantel. Niclosamide is an alternative. Vitamin supplements should also be given to correct any deficiencies.

Dracunculiasis

Dracunculiasis (dracontiasis, guinea-worm infection) is caused by infection with the nematode *Dracunculus medinensis*. It has been endemic in parts of Africa and Asia but is increasingly coming under control and the hope is that it will soon be eradicated. The disease is transmitted through drinking water containing larvae that develop in freshwater crustaceans. The larvae penetrate the intestinal mucosa and mature in connective tissue. The adult female migrates to the subcutaneous tissues normally of the legs after about 1 year. Ulceration of the overlying skin releases larvae which are ingested by the crustacean host to complete the life cycle. The first symptom is the lesion caused by the emerging worm, although a generalised hypersensitivity reaction may also occur. Secondary infection is a common complication.

The most effective method of controlling dracunculiasis is by provision of safe drinking water. The WHO eradication campaign is based on health education, and the provision of safe water by measures including water treatment with pesticides such as temefos and encouraging the use of domestic filters.

There is no effective direct drug therapy against any stage in man. The traditional treatment is removal of the adult worm by gentle traction sometimes over several weeks. Metronidazole or thiabendazole may provide symptomatic benefit in the management of dracunculiasis although they have no direct anthelmintic effect. They are thought to act by weakening the anchorage of the worms within the subcutaneous tissues, thus allowing them to be removed more quickly.

Echinococcosis

Echinococcosis, or hydatid disease, in man is infection with the larval stage of *Echinococcus granulosus* or *E. multilocularis*. These two species cause distinct forms of the disease known as cystic echinococcosis and alveolar echinococcosis respectively. Various animals are involved in the transmission of the disease, man becoming infected through ingestion of eggs from contaminated faeces. The eggs hatch in the intestine and the embryos penetrate the intestinal wall and invade body organs, usually the liver. The embryo develops into a cyst which slowly increases in size and may remain intact for many years. Symptomatic infection usually only occurs when the cyst is large enough to cause obstruction or to compress adjacent structures, or if rupture occurs. Where possible, surgical removal of the intact cyst is the first line of treatment.

In **cystic echinococcosis**, drugs may be given locally or systemically before surgery to kill infective larvae within the cyst and reduce the risk of further infection. They are also given postoperatively if a cyst ruptures during surgery. Local injection of larvicidal agents such as alcohol, cetrimide, and hypertonic saline have been used. Chemotherapy is also used as an adjunct. The preferred drug for associated systemic treatment is albendazole. Mebendazole may be used, although some have suggested it is not as effective as albendazole. Praziquantel has also been reported to be effective. Albendazole, mebendazole, or praziquantel may also be used when surgery is not possible. Albendazole may be a suitable alternative to surgery as initial treatment in uncomplicated cases and administration with cimetidine may increase its effectiveness.

A further option when surgery is not possible is the PAIR (puncture/aspiration/injection/re-aspiration) procedure which consists of ultrasound-guided cyst puncture followed by aspiration of the cyst fluid, local injection of alcohol or hypertonic saline into the cyst, and re-aspiration of the cyst contents. Concomitant chemotherapy is recommended.

E. multilocularis infection (**alveolar echinococcosis**) is more invasive and is characterised by a tumour-like infiltrative growth; it usually requires both surgery and long-term treatment with a benzimidazole such as albendazole although some patients have improved on albendazole alone.

References.

1. WHO Informal Working Group on Echinococcosis. Guidelines for treatment of cystic and alveolar echinococcosis in humans. *Bull WHO* 1996; **74:** 231–42.
2. Kumar A, Chattopadhyay TK. Management of hydatid disease of the liver. *Postgrad Med J* 1992; **68:** 853–6.
3. Wen H, *et al.* Diagnosis and treatment of human hydatidosis. *Br J Clin Pharmacol* 1993; **35:** 565–74.

Enterobiasis

Enterobiasis is an infection with *Enterobius vermicularis* (pinworm, threadworm). It is one of the few intestinal nematodes which is common in temperate climates and is particularly common in young children. Like trichuriasis (see below) it is an infection of the large intestine and transmission follows ingestion or inhalation of mature eggs. The larvae mature in the gut in about 2 months. The eggs are not released into the gut contents but the mature female migrates to the anus at night and lays its eggs on the perianal and perineal skin. The eggs become infective within 6 hours. Diagnosis is based on detecting eggs around the anus. The most common symptom is perianal itching but many infections are asymptomatic. Rarely ectopic disease such as appendicitis or salpingitis may occur. The adult worm has a life span of about 6 weeks and, if reinfection can be prevented, the infection is self-limiting. While additional hygiene measures can prevent reinfection, treatment of the whole family with an anthelmintic should remain the main therapeutic response; more than one course may be required.

Treatment is with a benzimidazole carbamate derivative such as albendazole or mebendazole or with pyrantel embonate. Such broad-spectrum therapy can be useful if the patient is suffering from a mixed intestinal nematode infection. Other anthelmintics used in enterobiasis include piperazine, or viprynium embonate.

Fascioliasis

See under Liver Fluke Infections, below.

Fasciolopsiasis

See under Intestinal Fluke Infections, below.

Gnathostomiasis

Gnathostomiasis is an infection with, in most cases, the larval form of the nematode *Gnathostoma spinigerum*, although other *Gnathostoma* spp. have been identified. *G. spinigerum* inhabits the stomach of cats and dogs. Eggs shed in their faeces are ingested by freshwater crustaceans and hatch into larvae which are ingested by fish or other animals; man acquires the infection by consumption of the raw or undercooked flesh of these secondary hosts. Once ingested the larva penetrates the gut wall and migrates via the liver to a wide variety of other tissues including skin, eyes, and CNS. Rarely, dermal infiltration may result in cutaneous larva migrans (see above).

The preferred treatment of gnathostomiasis is surgical removal of the gnathostome but this is rarely possible. Albendazole has been reported to be effective.

Heterophyiasis

See under Intestinal Fluke Infections, below.

Hookworm infections

Infections with the hookworms *Ancylostoma duodenale* (ancylostomiasis) and *Necator americanus* (necatoriasis) are a major cause of iron-deficiency anaemia in large areas of the tropics and sub-tropics, especially in rural communities. Eggs deposited in warm moist soil hatch into larvae which develop further into the infective form. Infection is normally by penetration through the skin although it may be by ingestion. The larvae migrate to the lungs from where they are swallowed and mature to the adult form in the small intestine. Eggs appear in the faeces about 6 to 8 weeks after infection and the adult worm may live for several years. *A. duodenale* larvae are capable of remaining dormant in the tissues, only maturing to the adult when climatic conditions are favourable. Symptoms correspond to the stage of infection. Visitors to endemic areas may develop intense pruritus, erythema, and a papulovesicular eruption at the site of infection known as ground itch. Migration through the lungs during the first infection may cause pneumonitis and bronchospasm with accompanying eosinophilia. The main symptoms of intestinal infection are iron-deficiency anaemia and severe hypoalbuminaemia. In addition, abdominal pain, diarrhoea, and weight loss may occur.

Treatment is usually with a benzimidazole carbamate derivative such as mebendazole or albendazole, and such broad-spectrum therapy can also be useful if the patient is suffering from a mixed intestinal nematode infection. Other anthelmintics used in hookworm include levamisole or pyrantel embonate, but these may be less effective against *N. americanus* than against *A. duodenale*. Iron-deficiency anaemia caused by hookworm infections responds rapidly to oral iron therapy; folic acid supplements may be necessary in some patients. Mass treatment programmes may be necessary in endemic areas to reduce the overall burden of infection.[1-3]

There is some evidence to suggest[4] that human infection with animal hookworms, some of which were previously thought to cause only cutaneous larva migrans (see above), may also occasionally cause enteric infections characterised by eosinophilia.

1. Nahmias J, *et al.* Evaluation of albendazole, pyrantel, bephenium, pyrantel-praziquantel, and pyrantel-bephenium for single-dose mass treatment of necatoriasis. *Ann Trop Med Parasitol* 1989; **83:** 625–9.
2. Bradley M, *et al.* The epidemiology and control of hookworm infection in the Burma Valley area of Zimbabwe. *Trans R Soc Trop Med Hyg* 1993; **87:** 145–7.
3. Krepel HP, *et al.* Treatment of mixed Oesophagostomum and hookworm infection: effect of albendazole, pyrantel pamoate, levamisole and thiabendazole. *Trans R Soc Trop Med Hyg* 1993; **87:** 87–9.
4. Schad GA. Hookworms: pets to humans. *Ann Intern Med* 1994; **120:** 434–5.

Hymenolepiasis

Hymenolepiasis is an infection of the intestine with *Hymenolepis nana*, or dwarf tapeworm. Infection is acquired through ingestion of eggs in contaminated food or water or on hands and can be passed directly from person to person. It is more common in children. Clinical symptoms occur in heavy infections and include diarrhoea and abdominal pain. Treatment is with a single dose of praziquantel or a 7 day course of niclosamide.

Intestinal fluke infections

The intestinal fluke infections **fasciolopsiasis**, **heterophyiasis**, **metagonimiasis**, and **nanophyetiasis** are caused by *Fasciolopsis buski*, *Heterophyes heterophyes* and some other *Heterophyes* spp., *Metagonimus yokogawai*, and *Nanophyetus salmincola* respectively. Fasciolopsiasis, heterophyiasis, and metagonimiasis are endemic in the Far East and Southeast Asia, with heterophyiasis also being common in the Middle East. Nanophyetiasis has occurred increasingly in the Pacific northwest of the USA. Fasciolopsiasis is caused by the ingestion of infected plants, while undercooked or raw infected fish are the sources of *H. heterophyes*, *M. yokogawai*, and *N. salmincola* infections.

Fasciolopsiasis is usually asymptomatic, but heavy infections can cause diarrhoea, abdominal pain, and, rarely, intestinal obstruction and an allergic oedematous reaction. Metagonimiasis is also generally asymptomatic but may cause mild diarrhoea, while pain and mucous diarrhoea are common in heterophyiasis. Similar gastro-intestinal symptoms occur with eosinophilia in nanophyetiasis. Eggs of *M. yokogawai* and *H. heterophyes* may rarely penetrate the bowel wall and enter the bloodstream to be deposited in various organs, leading to serious complications such as cardiac failure or fatal embolism in the heart or brain.

Treatment of intestinal fluke infections is with praziquantel.[1]

1. WHO. Control of foodborne trematode infections. *WHO Tech Rep Ser 849* 1995.

Liver fluke infections

Fasciola hepatica, *Opisthorchis viverrini*, *O. felineus*, and *Clonorchis sinensis* are liver flukes transmitted by the ingestion of infected aquatic plants, grasses or water (*F. hepatica*), or raw or undercooked fish (*Opisthorchis* spp., *C. sinensis*). **Fascioliasis** is primarily a disease of sheep and cattle and human infections occur where these animals are raised, whereas **clonorchiasis** and **opisthorchiasis** are seen mainly in Southeast Asia and eastern Europe.

Fascioliasis in the acute phase is usually characterised by fever, gastro-intestinal symptoms, pain due to liver enlargement, and marked eosinophilia, but these symptoms decline as the worms enter their final habitat in the bile ducts. Acute symptoms occur rarely with clonorchiasis and opisthorchiasis and infections tend to be asymptomatic for many years. Adult flukes live in the bile ducts and symptoms of biliary-tract obstruction appear after repeated or heavy infections with liver flukes. Cholangiocarcinoma (bile duct cancer) is now generally accepted to be associated with liver fluke infection although its exact pathogenesis is unclear.

Praziquantel is used for the treatment of most liver fluke infections.[1] Bithionol is more effective than praziquantel in fascioliasis and is the preferred treatment, although triclabendazole may become the treatment of choice;[1] dehydroemetine has also been used.

Praziquantel remains the treatment of choice for clonorchiasis and opisthorchiasis.[1]

1. WHO. Control of foodborne trematode infections. *WHO Tech Rep Ser 849* 1995.

Loiasis

Loiasis is an infection with the filarial nematode *Loa loa* which occurs in areas of Central and West Africa. It is transmitted by the biting tabanid fly *Chrysops*. The infective larvae mature to adult worms which migrate through subcutaneous tissues and occasionally the subconjunctiva. Symptoms include pruritus, swelling, and pain, with occasional subcutaneous swellings, often on the arms or legs, that are characteristic of the disease. Passage of a worm through the subconjunctiva produces intense conjunctivitis. Eosinophilia may be severe, especially in visitors from non-endemic areas. Other complications include renal disease, endomyocardial fibrosis, encephalopathy, and peripheral neuropathy.

Treatment is with diethylcarbamazine which is effective against the microfilariae, larval forms, and a proportion of adult worms. In some cases, treatment has been associated with acute encephalitis, particularly in patients with heavy microfilaraemia. It has been assumed that this may be related to blockage of capillaries in the brain and meninges and for this reason small doses of diethylcarbamazine are given initially in combination with a corticosteroid and antihistamine, gradually increasing to full therapeutic doses over several days. However this does not eliminate the risk of encephalitis entirely and the role of the microfilariae in this syndrome has been questioned. Some consider that ivermectin could be useful but, as with diethylcarbamazine, there is concern over its potential neurotoxic effects in patients with heavy microfilaraemia.

Diethylcarbamazine is also used for prophylaxis but it has been suggested that it should be reserved for subjects at high risk of exposure. Vector control is regarded as impractical and methods aimed at reducing contact with the vector such as window screens and protective clothing are recommended.

Lung fluke infections

The lung fluke infection **paragonimiasis** is caused by *Paragonimus* spp., commonly *P. westermani*, with human infections occurring in Asia, Africa, and Central or South America. The disease is transmitted by the ingestion of raw infected freshwater crabs or crayfish, or from infected drinking water.

The flukes mature in the lungs where they cause local necrosis, haemorrhage, inflammation, and fibrosis. Symptoms of paragonimiasis include fever, pain, and chest complaints, but the majority of light to moderate infections are asymptomatic. The worms may also develop at other sites, particularly the brain where they can cause epilepsy, symptoms of cerebral tumours, or cerebral embolism, which may be fatal.

Treatment is with praziquantel or bithionol. Triclabendazole has been studied.

Lymphatic filariasis

Lymphatic filariasis arises from infection with *Wuchereria bancrofti* (bancroftian filariasis), *Brugia malayi*, or *B. timori* (both known as brugian filariasis and as Malayan and Timorian filariasis respectively). It occurs in tropical and subtropical regions. Larval forms are transmitted by mosquitos. The larvae penetrate the lymphatic system where they mature to adult worms that may live for many years. Infective microfilariae are produced within 3 to 6 months and enter the peripheral blood stream, from where they are ingested by further mosquito vectors in which new larvae develop.

Lymphatic filariasis may be asymptomatic but both acute and chronic symptoms also occur. Inflammatory reactions to immature and adult worms in the lymphatic system produce episodic adenolymphangitis with fever. In men bancroftian filariasis characteristically presents as epididymo-orchitis. Abscesses may occasionally occur, particularly with brugian filariasis. Chronic lymphadenopathy is frequently seen. The main clinical features in chronic bancroftian filariasis are hydrocele, lymphoedema, elephantiasis, and chyluria. Chronic brugian filariasis typically causes lymphoedema and elephantiasis in the limb below the knee or elbow. Tropical pulmonary eosinophilia is a clinical variant of filarial disease, particularly *W. bancrofti* infection. The symptoms include cough, wheezing, and eosinophilia. If untreated the condition can progress to chronic interstitial fibrosis.

There is no entirely satisfactory treatment of lymphatic filariasis. Diethylcarbamazine kills microfilariae and a proportion of immature and adult worms and is widely used for both treatment and prophylaxis. Treatment can precipitate severe immunological reactions to the dead and dying worms. Large hydroceles and elephantiasis are generally not reversible and usually require surgical intervention.[1] However, treatment with coumarins may reduce the lymphoedema and so lead to improvement.[2,3] There has also been a suggestion that elephantiasis may be linked to local secondary bacterial or fungal infections, and that simple measures such as regular washing could also produce improvement.[4] Tropical pulmonary eosinophilia responds to diethylcarbamazine but about 20% of patients may relapse and require re-treatment.[1] Diethylcarbamazine is also used in the mass control of filariasis in all subjects in an endemic area (for further details, see p.100).

Ivermectin, which is also effective against microfilariae, has produced promising results in several studies and may become an alternative or adjunct to diethylcarbamazine (see p.102).

In recent studies, albendazole combined with diethylcarbamazine or ivermectin has shown promise.

Control measures aimed at reducing the intensity of transmission include educating local communities on the use of insecticidal sprays and impregnated bed nets, and the use of mass chemotherapy treatment. Effective vector control is considered to be too expensive in most endemic areas.

1. WHO. Lymphatic filariasis: the disease and its control: fifth report of the WHO expert committee on filariasis. *WHO Tech Rep Ser 821* 1992.
2. Casley-Smith JR, *et al*. Treatment of filarial lymphoedema and elephantiasis with 5,6-benzo-α-pyrone (coumarin). *Br Med J* 1993; **307:** 1037–41.
3. Anonymous. Coumarins: symptomatic relief of filarial lymphoedema. *WHO Drug Inf* 1993; **7:** 177–8.
4. McGregor A. Washing off elephantiasis. *Lancet* 1994; **344:** 121.

Mansonella infections

Infections with the filarial nematodes *Mansonella perstans, M. ozzardi*, and *M. streptocerca* are generally asymptomatic but a variety of symptoms including malaise, fever, joint pain, and meningeal symptoms have been described. Infection is transmitted by biting midges and flies. Treatment with diethylcarbamazine may be effective depending on the infecting species. Mebendazole may be effective alone or in combination with levamisole in *M. perstans*. Ivermectin has been suggested for *M. ozzardi* infections and may be the drug of choice for *M. streptocerca*.

Metagonimiasis

See under Intestinal Fluke Infections, above.

Nanophyetiasis

See under Intestinal Fluke Infections, above.

Necatoriasis

See under Hookworm Infections, above.

Onchocerciasis

Onchocerciasis (river blindness) is caused by infection with the filarial nematode *Onchocerca volvulus*. It is endemic in large areas of Africa and areas of Central or South America. It is particularly prevalent near fast flowing rivers, the breeding ground of the blackfly which is the vector of this parasite. Following infection, the larvae mature into adults in fibrous nodules, usually in the subcutaneous tissue. The adults release large numbers of microfilariae which are responsible for the major symptoms of the disease in the skin and the eye. Symptoms of skin involvement range from an intensely pruritic erythematous rash to chronic skin changes and severe pendulous lymphoedema. Microfilariae in the eye are a major cause of blindness in endemic areas.

Onchocerciasis is controlled with ivermectin.[1-3] Ivermectin rapidly eliminates microfilariae from the skin and more gradually from the eye.[3] It does not eliminate the adult worms although it suppresses release of microfilariae for several cycles.

Ivermectin is donated without charge by *Merck Sharp & Dohme* through the Mectizan Expert Committee (MEC) for human use in community-wide mass treatment programmes in all countries in which onchocerciasis is endemic, where it is given once a year to all but pregnant women, breast-feeding mothers of recently born babies, children weighing less than 15 kg, and those unable to walk or otherwise seriously ill.[4] Control of the disease in endemic areas thus relies upon the administration of ivermectin once or twice a year and this should be combined with vector control.[2] For further details, see under Ivermectin, p.102.

Before the introduction of ivermectin, diethylcarbamazine citrate was the usual treatment for onchocerciasis, but it is no longer recommended by WHO.[2,3] The major limitations to its use are the severe allergic reaction (the Mazzotti reaction) associated with its microfilaricidal action, aggravation of existing ocular lesions or precipitation of new ones, and the need to give repeated courses of treatment for continued suppression of the disease.[3]

Suramin has also been used in the treatment of onchocerciasis and is effective against adult worms.[2,3] However, its use is restricted because of its toxicity.

Amocarzine has also been evaluated in onchocerciasis.[3]

1. Van Laethen Y, Lopes C. Treatment of onchocerciasis. *Drugs* 1996; **52:** 861–9.
2. *WHO model prescribing information: drugs used in parasitic diseases*. 2nd ed. Geneva: WHO, 1995.
3. WHO. Onchocerciasis and its control: report of a WHO expert committee on onchocerciasis control. *WHO Tech Rep Ser 852* 1995.
4. Pond B. Distribution of ivermectin by health workers. *Lancet* 1990; **335:** 1539.

Opisthorchiasis

See under Liver Fluke Infections, above.

Paragonimiasis

See under Lung Fluke Infections, above.

Schistosomiasis

Schistosomiasis is a parasitic infection caused by *Schistosoma* spp., largely *S. mansoni, S. japonicum,* and *S. haematobium*, and to a lesser extent *S. intercalatum* and *S. mekongi*. The disease is seen mainly in Africa, Asia, South America, and the Caribbean, where it is a hazard to individuals exposed to fresh water containing the intermediate host, infected freshwater snails.

Free-swimming cercariae are released from the snail and penetrate human skin causing a pruritic papular rash in sensitised individuals (swimmer's itch). Parasites mature in the lungs and liver within about 6 weeks, then migrate to the blood vessels, the bladder, or intestines. Mature female worms produce eggs which are excreted in urine or stools, or become lodged in tissues, and immunological reactions to these eggs results in disease. The acute reaction to egg deposition has been termed Katayama fever, a self-limiting but sometimes fatal illness resembling serum sickness and most frequently seen in *S. japonicum* infection. The chronic phase of infection is often asymptomatic for many years but usually results in granuloma formation and fibrosis in tissues where eggs are deposited, such as the liver, lungs, intestines, or urinary tract, the site depending on the infecting species.

Praziquantel is used for the treatment of chronic schistosomiasis and is effective against all species of schistosomes. Metriphonate and oxamniquine are alternatives that may be used against *S. haematobium* and *S. mansoni* respectively.

Niclosamide is used as a molluscicide for the treatment of water in schistosomiasis control programmes. Copper sulphate or sodium pentachlorophenate have also been used but to a lesser extent.

Schistosomiasis vaccines are in development.

References.

1. WHO. The control of schistosomiasis: second report of the WHO expert committee. *WHO Tech Rep Ser 830* 1993.

Strongyloidiasis

Strongyloidiasis is an infection of the small intestine caused by *Strongyloides stercoralis*, known as threadworm in the USA. It generally occurs in the tropics and subtropics and can also occur in some areas of South and East Europe, Japan, and the USA. In contrast with other intestinal nematodes, the eggs of *S. stercoralis* hatch before leaving the gastro-intestinal tract, and can cause autoinfection, particularly in immunocompromised patients. Larvae reaching the soil can either mature into free-living adults or remain in an infective larval stage. Infective larvae cause infection by penetrating the skin. The larvae migrate to the lungs, move up the bronchial tree to be swallowed, and finally penetrate the mucosa of the small intestine where they mature. Eggs are deposited about 28 days after initial infection.

Infection may be asymptomatic, but commonly patients have symptoms relating to the stages of infection. Penetration of larvae through the skin causes intense pruritus and an erythematous rash. The rash may follow the course of migration and is one of the causes of cutaneous larva migrans (see above). An inflammatory response to migration through the lungs may be seen and this may include pneumonitis and bronchospasm. In heavy infections, which are most common in immunocompromised patients as a result of autoinfection, massive pulmonary invasion may occur resulting in fatal alveolar haemorrhage. Abdominal symptoms include colicky pain, diarrhoea, and vomiting, leading to nutritional deficiencies and weight loss. Eosinophilia may also be present. Disseminated disease may occur in immunocompromised patients including severe pulmonary and abdominal symptoms, shock, encephalopathy, meningitis, and Gram-negative septicaemia. Since strongyloidiasis is commonly fatal in these patients, vulnerable patients from endemic areas should be screened regularly and treated promptly at the first sign of infection.

Ivermectin is effective for the treatment of strongyloidiasis and is considered by some authorities to be the drug of choice. Thiabendazole was widely used and still is in some countries. Albendazole is more effective and better tolerated than thiabendazole. Mebendazole has also been suggested but it must be administered for longer periods than albendazole since it has only a limited effect on migrating larvae. These broad-spectrum anthelmintics (thiabendazole excepted) are also useful if the patient is suffering from a mixed intestinal nematode infection.

Syngamosis

Syngamosis, or gapeworm infection, is caused by *Syngamus* spp. and is primarily an infection of domestic fowl and wild birds and mammals, although infection in man has been reported rarely. Man may become infected by eating foods contaminated with infective larvae which penetrate the intestinal wall and migrate to the lungs where they mature into adult worms. The major symptom is a cough due to irritation of the bronchi and increased mucus production. The infection may be confused with asthma. Thiabendazole and mebendazole have been used successfully to treat the infection in man.

Taeniasis

Taeniasis is an infection of the intestine with beef tapeworm, *Taenia saginata*, or pork tapeworm, *T. solium*, acquired through ingestion of raw or undercooked meat that is contaminated. The larval form of *T. solium* can cause systemic infection, cysticercosis (see above).

Infection with the adult worm usually produces symptoms only when the worm reaches a size that can cause obstruction or related problems. Segments of the worm containing eggs may be excreted in the faeces so maintaining the cycle of reproduction. Treatment is with a single dose of praziquantel, which has the advantage of also being active, in higher doses, against the larval form of *T. solium*. Niclosamide is also effective but is only active against adult worms.

Toxocariasis

Toxocariasis is infection with the larval form of *Toxocara canis* and less commonly *T. cati*. The adult worms live in the intestines of dogs and cats respectively and man becomes infected when eggs excreted in animal faeces are ingested. Once ingested the eggs hatch and the larvae migrate from the intestine to other organs most commonly the liver, lung, and eye. Most infections are asymptomatic but two clinical syndromes, ocular larva migrans and visceral larva migrans, can occur, usually in children.

Ocular larva migrans occurs when larvae invade the eye causing a granuloma which may impair vision and can cause blindness. There is no specific treatment.[1] Anthelmintics such as albendazole or thiabendazole, corticosteroids, ocular surgery and laser photocoagulation have been employed but assessment of their efficacy is difficult because of the variable natural course of the disease.

The clinical symptoms of visceral larva migrans depend upon the organs involved but commonly include cough, fever, wheezing, and hepatomegaly. Encephalitis and seizures may occur and there is usually an eosinophilia. Acute infection normally resolves without treatment.[2] However, severe or prolonged infections may be treated with diethylcarbamazine citrate. Albendazole, mebendazole and thiabendazole have also been used.

1. Shields JA. Ocular toxocariasis: a review. *Surv Ophthalmol* 1984; **28:** 361–81.
2. Gillespie SH. Human toxocariasis. *Commun Dis Rep* 1993; **3:** R140–R143.

Trichinosis

Trichinosis (trichinellosis) is an infection caused by *Trichinella spiralis*. Man becomes infected through ingestion of raw or undercooked meat, usually pork, which contains infective larvae. The larvae mature into adult worms in the small intestine and the mature female deposits larvae which migrate in the blood to skeletal muscle and sometimes to the myocardium. Symptoms usually occur only in heavy infections. Invasion of the intestines by the maturing adult worms can cause diarrhoea, abdominal pain, and vomiting followed about a week later by hypersensitivity reactions to the migrating larvae. These may include eosinophilia, fever, muscle pain, periorbital oedema and more rarely encephalitis, myocarditis, or pneumonia which may be fatal.

All patients with confirmed or suspected infection should be treated to prevent the continued production of larvae. Mebendazole is considered to be the anthelmintic of choice in some countries. Albendazole, flubendazole, thiabendazole, or pyrantel embonate may also be effective. A corticosteroid should be given for severe hypersensitivity reactions.

Trichostrongyliasis

Trichostrongyliasis is an infection of the small intestine caused by *Trichostrongylus* spp. including *T. colubriformis*. It is normally a parasite of herbivores but infections in man have been found. *Trichostrongylus* spp. have a similar life cycle to *Ancylostoma duodenale* (see Hookworm Infections, above). Pyrantel embonate, albendazole, or mebendazole are recommended for the treatment of trichostrongyliasis.

Trichuriasis

Trichuriasis is an infection of the large intestine with *Trichuris trichiura*, sometimes known as whipworm. Distribution is worldwide but most infections occur in the tropics and subtropics. Eggs are excreted in the faeces and can remain viable in the soil for extended periods. Under optimum conditions the eggs become infective in about 2 to 4 weeks. Following ingestion, larvae are released from the eggs and develop within the wall of the small intestine for about 3 to 10 days before migrating to the lumen of the large intestine where they remain attached to the mucosal lining. Eggs are detectable in the faeces about 1 to 3 months after infection. Trichuriasis is often asymptomatic but heavy infection can result in anaemia, diarrhoea, and rectal prolapse.

Treatment is with a benzimidazole carbamate derivative such as albendazole or mebendazole and such broad-spectrum therapy can be useful if the patient is suffering from a mixed intestinal nematode infection.

Abamectin (2774-q)

Abamectin *(USAN, rINN)*.

MK-0936. A mixture of abamectin component B_{1a} and abamectin component B_{1b}.

CAS — 65195-55-3 (component B_{1a}); 65195-56-4 (component B_{1b}).

Abamectin is an avermectin anthelmintic used in veterinary medicine for nematode infections. It is also used as a systemic veterinary ectoparasiticide.

Albendazole (752-p)

Albendazole *(BAN, USAN, rINN)*.

SKF-62979. Methyl 5-propylthio-1*H*-benzimidazol-2-ylcarbamate.

$C_{12}H_{15}N_3O_2S$ = 265.3.

CAS — 54965-21-8.

Pharmacopoeias. In *Chin.* and *US.*

A white to faintly yellowish powder. Practically **insoluble** in water and in alcohol; very slightly soluble in ether and in dichloromethane; freely soluble in anhydrous formic acid.

Adverse Effects and Precautions

As for Mebendazole, p.104.

Albendazole is teratogenic in *animals* (see Pregnancy and Breast Feeding, below).

Although generally well-tolerated, the following adverse reactions were reported in the first phase of WHO-coordinated studies[1] involving 30 patients given *high-dose* therapy with albendazole for the treatment of cystic echinococcosis [hydatid disease]: raised serum-transaminase levels (2 patients); reduced leucocyte counts (1); gastro-intestinal symptoms (1); allergic conditions (1); and loss of hair (1). Treatment was stopped in a further patient with alveolar echinococcosis because of depressed bone-marrow activity. In the second phase of these studies[2] 109 patients were given albendazole and 20 experienced adverse effects; similar findings were reported with mebendazole. The range of effects with albendazole was: elevation of transaminases (5 patients); abdominal pain and other gastro-intestinal symptoms (7); severe headache (4); loss of hair (2); leucopenia (2); fever and fatigue (1); thrombocytopenia (1); and urticaria and itching (1). Albendazole had to be withdrawn in 5 patients because of adverse effects, although in 3 the withdrawal was only temporary.

Albendazole should only be used in the treatment of echinococcosis if there is constant medical supervision with regular monitoring of serum-transaminase concentrations and of leucocyte and platelet counts. Patients with liver damage should be treated with reduced doses of benzimidazole carbamates, if at all.[2]

1. Davis A, *et al.* Multicentre clinical trials of benzimidazolecarbamates in human echinococcosis. *Bull WHO* 1986; **64:** 383–8.
2. Davis A, *et al.* Multicentre clinical trials of benzimidazolecarbamates in human cystic echinococcosis (phase 2). *Bull WHO* 1989; **67:** 503–8.

Effects on growth. A multiple-dose regimen of albendazole in children with asymptomatic trichuriasis has been reported to be associated with impaired growth in those with low levels of infection.[1] However it was considered that this should not deter the use of single doses in mass treatment programmes.[2]

1. Forrester JE, *et al.* Randomised trial of albendazole and pyrantel in symptomless trichuriasis in children. *Lancet* 1998; **352:** 1103–8.
2. Winstanley P. Albendazole for mass treatment of asymptomatic trichuris infections. *Lancet* 1998; **352:** 1080–1.

Effects on the liver. In a series of 40 patients given albendazole for echinococcosis, 7 developed abnormalities in liver function tests during therapy.[1] Six had a hepatocellular type of abnormality attributable to albendazole; the seventh had cholestatic jaundice which was probably not due to albendazole.

1. Morris DL, Smith PG. Albendazole in hydatid disease—hepatocellular toxicity. *Trans R Soc Trop Med Hyg* 1987; **81:** 343–4.

Pregnancy and breast feeding. Albendazole is teratogenic in some *animal* species and the UK manufacturers have stated that it is contra-indicated in pregnant women or in women thought to be pregnant. They also advise that women of childbearing age should take effective precautions, with non-hormonal contraceptive measures, against conception during and within one month of completing treatment with albendazole. In the USA the manufacturers, while not recommending albendazole for pregnant patients, have stated that if it is used in pregnancy, then such use should only be where the potential benefit justifies the risk to the fetus; this is in accord with albendazole being classified in FDA pregnancy category C.

It is not known whether albendazole or its metabolites are distributed into breast milk.

Interactions

Plasma concentrations of the active metabolite of albendazole (albendazole sulphoxide) were reported to be raised by approximately 50% in a study in 8 patients receiving concomitant *dexamethasone*.[1]

The plasma concentration of albendazole sulphoxide has also been increased by concomitant administration of *praziquantel*,[2] although the practical consequences of this were considered uncertain. Concentrations of albendazole sulphoxide have also been found to be raised in bile and hydatid cyst fluid by administration of albendazole with *cimetidine*, which may increase its effectiveness in the treatment of echinococcosis.[3]

1. Jung H, *et al.* Dexamethasone increases plasma levels of albendazole. *J Neurol* 1990; **237:** 279–80.
2. Homeida M, *et al.* Pharmacokinetic interaction between praziquantel and albendazole in Sudanese men. *Ann Trop Med Parasitol* 1994; **88:** 551–9.
3. Wen H, *et al.* Initial observation on albendazole in combination with cimetidine for the treatment of human cystic echinococcosis. *Ann Trop Med Parasitol* 1994; **88:** 49–52.

Pharmacokinetics

Albendazole is poorly absorbed from the gastro-intestinal tract, but rapidly undergoes extensive first-pass metabolism. The principal metabolite albendazole sulphoxide has anthelmintic activity and a plasma half-life of about 8.5 hours. Albendazole sulphoxide is widely distributed throughout the body including into the bile and cerebrospinal fluid. It is approximately 70% bound to plasma protein.

Albendazole sulphoxide is eliminated in the bile; only a small amount appears to be excreted in the urine.

References.

1. Marriner SE, *et al.* Pharmacokinetics of albendazole in man. *Eur J Clin Pharmacol* 1986; **30:** 705–8.
2. Jung H, *et al.* Clinical pharmacokinetics of albendazole in patients with brain cysticercosis. *J Clin Pharmacol* 1992; **32:** 28–31.
3. Steiger U, *et al.* Albendazole treatment of echinococcosis in humans: effects on microsomal metabolism and drug tolerance. *Clin Pharmacol Ther* 1990; **47:** 347–53.
4. Morris DL, *et al.* Penetration of albendazole sulphoxide into hydatid cysts. *Gut* 1987; **28:** 75–80.

Uses and Administration

Albendazole is a benzimidazole carbamate anthelmintic structurally related to mebendazole (p.104) and with similar activity. Albendazole is used in the treatment of the cestode infections cysticercosis and echinococcosis (hydatid disease) in relatively high doses. In some countries it is used in the treatment of single and mixed intestinal nematode infections including ascariasis, enterobiasis, hookworm, strongyloidiasis, and trichuriasis. It may also be used in the treatment of capillariasis, gnathostomiasis, and trichostrongyliasis. Albendazole may be effective in the treatment of the tissue nematode infections cutaneous larva migrans, toxocariasis, and trichinosis and in combination with other anthelmintics in the treatment of the filarial nematode infection lymphatic filariasis. For discussions of these infections and their treatment, see under Choice of Anthelmintic (p.92). See also below.

In the treatment of **echinococcosis**, albendazole is given by mouth with meals in a dose of 400 mg twice daily for 28 days for patients weighing over 60 kg. A dose of 15 mg per kg body-weight daily in two divided doses (to a maximum total daily dose of 800 mg) has been suggested for patients weighing less than 60 kg. For cystic echinococcosis the 28-day course may be repeated after 14 days without treatment to a total of 3 treatment cycles. For alveolar echinococcosis, cycles of 28 days of treatment followed by 14 days without treatment may need to continue for months or years.

In the treatment of **neurocysticercosis**, albendazole 400 mg twice daily for patients weighing over 60 kg (or 15 mg per kg daily in two divided doses to a maximum total daily dose of 800 mg in those weighing less than 60 kg) is given for 8 to 30 days.

Albendazole is given by mouth, usually as a single dose, in the treatment of single or mixed **intestinal nematode infections**. The usual dose for adults and children aged 2 years or over with ascariasis, enterobiasis, hookworm infections, or trichuriasis is 400 mg as a single dose. In enterobiasis the dose may be repeated in 1 to 2 weeks. Some authorities suggest that the dose in children with enterobiasis is 100 mg. In strongyloidiasis, 400 mg is given daily for 3 consecutive days; this may be repeated after 3 weeks if necessary.

Albendazole has also been used to treat children with **giardiasis** (p.575); suggested doses are 400 mg daily for 5 days.

Ascariasis. Albendazole is used as an alternative to mebendazole in the treatment of ascariasis (see p.92). Both drugs are equally highly effective with a cure rate greater than 98% reported for albendazole in one study.[1]

1. Albonico M, *et al.* A randomized controlled trial comparing mebendazole and albendazole against Ascaris, Trichuris and hookworm infections. *Trans R Soc Trop Med Hyg* 1994; **88:** 585–9.

Capillariasis. Albendazole in a dose of 400 mg daily for 10 days has been suggested[1] as an alternative to mebendazole for the treatment of capillariasis (p.93).

1. Anonymous. Drugs for parasitic infections. *Med Lett Drugs Ther* 1998; **40:** 1–12.

Cutaneous larva migrans. Albendazole has been reported to be effective in the treatment of cutaneous larva migrans[1-3] and may be an alternative to standard treatment with thiabendazole (p.93). Albendazole, generally in a dose of 400 mg daily for three[1] or five[2] days, has alleviated the discomfort of cutaneous larva migrans. A single dose of 400 mg also appears to be effective.[3]

1. Jones SK, *et al.* Oral albendazole for the treatment of cutaneous larva migrans. *Br J Dermatol* 1990; **122:** 99–101.
2. Sanguigni S, *et al.* Albendazole in the therapy of cutaneous larva migrans. *Trans R Soc Trop Med Hyg* 1990; **84:** 831.
3. Oriheula AR, Torres JR. Single dose of albendazole in the treatment of cutaneous larva migrans. *Arch Dermatol* 1990; **126:** 398–9.

Cysticercosis. Albendazole is used in the treatment of neurocysticercosis (p.93) as an alternative to praziquantel;[1,2] some consider albendazole to be preferable.[3-5] Albendazole has also been reported to be effective in extra-ocular cysticercosis.[6]

1. Sotelo J, *et al.* Short course of albendazole therapy for neurocysticercosis. *Arch Neurol* 1988; **45:** 1130–3.
2. Botero D, *et al.* Short course albendazole treatment for neurocysticercosis in Columbia. *Trans R Soc Trop Med Hyg* 1993; **87:** 576–7.
3. Cruz M, *et al.* Albendazole versus praziquantel in the treatment of cerebral cysticercosis: clinical evaluation. *Trans R Soc Trop Med Hyg* 1991; **85:** 244–7.
4. Takayanagui OM, Jardim E. Therapy for neurocysticercosis: comparison between albendazole and praziquantel. *Arch Neurol* 1992; **49:** 290–4.
5. Mehta SS, *et al.* Albendazole versus praziquantel for neurocysticercosis. *Am J Health-Syst Pharm* 1998; **55:** 598–600.
6. Sihota R, Honavar SG. Oral albendazole in the management of extraocular cysticercosis. *Br J Ophthalmol* 1994; **78:** 621–3.

Echinococcosis. Albendazole is used in the treatment of echinococcosis (p.94) as an adjunct to, or instead of, surgery. It is generally preferred to mebendazole.

References.

1. Horton RJ. Chemotherapy of Echinococcus infection in man with albendazole. *Trans R Soc Trop Med Hyg* 1989; **83:** 97–102.
2. Davis A, *et al.* Multicentre clinical trials of benzimidazolecarbamates in human cystic echinococcosis (phase 2). *Bull WHO* 1989; **67:** 503–8.
3. Todorov T, *et al.* Factors influencing the response to chemotherapy in human cystic echinococcosis. *Bull WHO* 1992; **70:** 347–58.
4. Teggi A, *et al.* Therapy of human hydatid disease with mebendazole and albendazole. *Antimicrob Agents Chemother* 1993; **37:** 1679–84.
5. Gil-Grande LA, *et al.* Randomised controlled trial of efficacy of albendazole in intra-abdominal hydatid disease. *Lancet* 1993; **342:** 1269–72.
6. Liu Y-H, *et al.* Computer tomography of liver in alveolar echinococcosis treated with albendazole. *Trans R Soc Trop Med Hyg* 1993; **87:** 319–21.
7. Wen H, *et al.* Initial observation on albendazole in combination with cimetidine for the treatment of human cystic echinococcosis. *Ann Trop Med Parasitol* 1994; **88:** 49–52.

Gnathostomiasis. Albendazole has been reported to be effective in the treatment of gnathostomiasis (p.94). Doses of 400 mg once or twice daily have been given for 2 or 3 weeks.[1-3]

1. Kraivichian P, *et al.* Albendazole for the treatment of human gnathostomiasis. *Trans R Soc Trop Med Hyg* 1992; **86:** 418–21.
2. Suntharasamai P, *et al.* Albendazole stimulates outward migration of Gnathostoma spinigerum to the dermis in man. *Southeast Asian J Trop Med Public Health* 1992; **23:** 716–22.
3. Anonymous. Drugs for parasitic infections. *Med Lett Drugs Ther* 1998; **40:** 1–12.

Hookworm infections. Hookworm infections are commonly treated with benzimidazole carbamates such as albendazole (see p.94). Albendazole, in a single 400 mg dose, produced an 84% cure rate and an 82% reduction in egg count in patients not cured in 77 patients with light necatoriasis (*Necator americanus* infection).[1] In another study,[2] although the cure rate was only 56.8% following a single 400 mg dose of albendazole this was superior to treatment with mebendazole which had a cure rate of 22.4%.

1. Nahmias J, *et al.* Evaluation of albendazole, pyrantel, bephenium, pyrantel-praziquantel and pyrantel-bephenium for single-dose mass treatment of necatoriasis. *Ann Trop Med Parasitol* 1989; **83:** 625–9.
2. Albonico M, *et al.* A randomized controlled trial comparing mebendazole and albendazole against Ascaris, Trichuris and hookworm infections. *Trans R Soc Trop Med Hyg* 1994; **88:** 585–9.

Lymphatic filariasis. Albendazole is not generally used in the treatment of lymphatic filariasis (see p.95). However, recent studies have suggested that albendazole in combination with ivermectin may be more effective than either drug alone for reduction of microfilaraemia in bancroftian filariasis.[1,2] Similarly, albendazole combined with diethylcarbamazine has shown promise.[2]

1. Addiss DG, *et al.* Randomised placebo-controlled comparison of ivermectin and albendazole alone and in combination for Wuchereria bancrofti microfilaraemia in Haitian children. *Lancet* 1997; **350:** 480–4. Correction. *ibid.*; 1036.
2. Ismail MM, *et al.* Efficacy of single dose combinations of albendazole, ivermectin and diethylcarbamazine for the treatment of bancroftian filariasis. *Trans R Soc Trop Med Hyg* 1998; **92:** 94–7.

Microsporidiosis. Albendazole has been tried in the treatment of microsporidiosis,[1-5] a protozoal infection increasingly seen in patients with AIDS (see p.576). Albendazole is also employed empirically in the treatment of HIV-associated diarrhoea (p.601).

1. Blanshard C, *et al.* Treatment of intestinal microsporidiosis with albendazole in patients with AIDS. *AIDS* 1992; **6:** 311–13.
2. Dieterich DT, *et al.* Treatment with albendazole for intestinal disease due to Enterocytozoon bieneusi in patients with AIDS. *J Infect Dis* 1994; **169:** 178–82.
3. Franzen C, *et al.* Intestinal microsporidiosis with Septata intestinalis in a patient with AIDS—response to albendazole. *J Infect* 1995; **31:** 237–9.
4. Dore GJ, *et al.* Disseminated microsporidiosis due to Septata intestinalis in nine patients infected with the human immunodeficiency virus: response to therapy with albendazole. *Clin Infect Dis* 1995; **21:** 70–6.
5. Molina J-M, *et al.* Albendazole for treatment and prophylaxis of microsporidiosis due Encephalitozoon intestinalis in patients with AIDS: a randomized double-blind controlled trial. *J Infect Dis* 1998; **177:** 1373–7.

Strongyloidiasis. Albendazole is generally preferred to thiabendazole or mebendazole in the treatment of strongyloidiasis (p.95) although some authorities now consider ivermectin to be the drug of choice.

References.

1. Rossignol JF, Maisonneuve H. Albendazole: placebo-controlled study in 870 patients with intestinal helminthiasis. *Trans R Soc Trop Med Hyg* 1983; **77:** 707–11.
2. Chanthavanich P, *et al.* Repeated doses of albendazole against strongyloidiasis in Thai children. *Southeast Asian J Trop Med Public Health* 1989; **20:** 221–6.
3. Mojon M, Nielsen PB. Treatment of Strongyloides stercoralis with albendazole: a cure rate of 86 per cent. *Zentralbl Bakteriol Mikrobiol Hyg [A]* 1987; **263:** 619–24.
4. Archibald LK, *et al.* Albendazole is effective treatment for chronic strongyloidiasis. *Q J Med* 1993; **86:** 191–5.

Toxocariasis. Albendazole is one of the drugs that might be used for the treatment of toxocariasis (see p.96) and in one small study[1] albendazole produced improvement similar to that achieved with thiabendazole but with fewer problems.

1. Stürchler D, *et al.* Thiabendazole vs albendazole in treatment of toxocariasis: a clinical trial. *Ann Trop Med Parasitol* 1989; **83:** 473–8.

Trichinosis. Albendazole may be effective in the treatment of trichinosis (p.96). Andrews *et al.*[1] described the use of albendazole to treat a patient infected with *Trichinella pseudospiralis.* A retrospective study in 44 patients with trichinosis comparing albendazole treatment with thiabendazole found that, while the two drugs were of comparable efficacy, albendazole was the better tolerated.[2]

1. Andrews JRH, *et al.* Trichinella pseudospiralis in humans: description of a case and its treatment. *Trans R Soc Trop Med Hyg* 1994; **88:** 200–3.
2. Cabié A, *et al.* Albendazole versus thiabendazole as therapy for trichinosis: a retrospective study. *Clin Infect Dis* 1996; **22:** 1033–5.

Trichostrongyliasis. Albendazole in a single dose of 400 mg has been suggested[1] as an alternative to pyrantel embonate or mebendazole in the treatment of trichostrongyliasis (p.96).

1. Anonymous. Drugs for parasitic infections. *Med Lett Drugs Ther* 1998; **40:** 1–12.

Trichuriasis. Albendazole is used in the treatment of trichuriasis (p.96). It is normally given in a single dose and is often used in mixed intestinal nematode infections.[1] However, it has been reported[1-3] that in groups of children with mixed intestinal worm infections single doses of albendazole are ineffective in eliminating *Trichuris trichiura* and multiple doses are required to produce worthwhile reductions in egg production. Treatment for 3 days has been suggested for heavy infection[4] (for a suggestion that such regimens may be associated with impaired growth in less heavily infected children, see Effects on Growth under Adverse Effects, above).

1. Hall A, Anwar KS. Albendazole and infections with Trichuris trichiura and Giardia intestinalis. *Southeast Asian J Trop Med Public Health* 1991; **22:** 84–7.
2. Hall A, Nahar Q. Albendazole and infections with Ascaris lumbricoides and Trichuris trichiura in children in Bangladesh. *Trans R Soc Trop Med Hyg* 1994; **88:** 110–12.
3. Albonico M, *et al.* A randomized controlled trial comparing mebendazole and albendazole against Ascaris, Trichuris and hookworm infections. *Trans R Soc Trop Med Hyg* 1994; **88:** 585–9.
4. Anonymous. Drugs for parasitic infections. *Med Lett Drugs Ther* 1998; **40:** 1–12.

Preparations

USP 23: Albendazole Tablets.

Proprietary Preparations (details are given in Part 3)
Aust.: Eskazole; ***Austral.:*** Eskazole; Zentel; ***Fr.:*** Zentel; ***Ger.:*** Eskazole; ***Ital.:*** Zentel; ***Neth.:*** Eskazole; ***S.Afr.:*** Paranthil; Zentel; ***Spain:*** Eskazole; ***Switz.:*** Zentel; ***UK:*** Eskazole; ***USA:*** Albenza.

Amocarzine (18938-g)

Amocarzine (*rINN*).

CGP-6140. 4-Methyl-4′-(*p*-nitroanilino)thio-1-piperazinecarboxanilide.

$C_{18}H_{21}N_5O_2S$ = 371.5.

CAS — 36590-19-9.

NOTE. Amocarzine has sometimes been referred to as thiocarbamazine.

Amocarzine is an antifilarial anthelmintic, derived from amoscanate, which is active against the adult worms of *Onchocerca volvulus.* It is under investigation for the oral treatment of onchocerciasis (p.95).

References.

1. Soula G, *et al.* Activity of thiocarbamazine in patients dually infected with schistosoma and onchocerca volvulus. *Lancet* 1989; **i:** 726. [See NOTE on nomenclature of amocarzine, above].
2. Lecaillon JB, *et al.* Pharmacokinetics of CGP 6140 (amocarzine) after oral administration of single 100-1600 mg doses to patients with onchocerciasis. *Br J Clin Pharmacol* 1990; **30:** 625–8.
3. Lecaillon JB, *et al.* The influence of food on the pharmacokinetics of CGP 6140 (amocarzine) after oral administration of a 1200 mg single dose to patients with onchocerciasis. *Br J Clin Pharmacol* 1990; **30:** 629–33.
4. Poltera AA, *et al.* Onchocercacidal effects of amocarzine (CGP 6140) in Latin America. *Lancet* 1991; **337:** 583–4.
5. Cooper PJ, *et al.* Onchocerciasis in Ecuador: evolution of chorioretinopathy after amocarzine treatment. *Br J Ophthalmol* 1996; **80:** 337–42.

Amoscanate (12371-b)

Amoscanate *(rINN).*

C-9333-Go/CGP-4540; GO-9333; Nithiocyamine. 4-*p*-Nitroanilinophenyl isothiocyanate.

$C_{13}H_9N_3O_2S$ = 271.3.

CAS — 26328-53-0.

Amoscanate is an isothiocyanate anthelmintic which has been tried in the treatment of hookworm infections. In China it has been used against schistosomiasis due to *Schistosoma japonicum.*

Trivalent Antimony Compounds (14110-f)

Antimony Potassium Tartrate (755-e)

Antim. Pot. Tart.; Brechweinstein; Kalii Stibyli Tartras; Potassium Antimonyltartrate; Stibii et Kalii Tartras; Tartar Emetic; Tartarus Stibiatus. Dipotassium bis{μ-[2,3-dihydroxybutanedioato(4-)-O^1,O^2:O^3,O^4]}-diantimonate(2-) trihydrate; Dipotassium bis[μ-tartrato(4-)]diantimonate(2-) trihydrate.

$C_8H_4K_2O_{12}Sb_2,3H_2O$ = 667.9.

CAS — 11071-15-1 (anhydrous antimony potassium tartrate); 28300-74-5 (antimony potassium tartrate trihydrate).

Pharmacopoeias. In *Fr., It.,* and *US.* In some pharmacopoeias the monograph substance is described as $C_4H_4KO_7Sb,½H_2O$ (= 333.9).

Odourless, colourless, transparent crystals or white powder. The crystals effloresce on exposure to air and do not readily rehydrate even when exposed to high humidity.

Soluble 1 in 12 of water, 1 in 3 of boiling water, and 1 in 15 of glycerol; practically insoluble in alcohol. Solutions in water are acid to litmus.

Incompatible with acids and alkalis, salts of heavy metals, albumin, soap, and tannins.

Antimony Sodium Tartrate (756-l)

Antim. Sod. Tart.; Sodium Antimonyltartrate; Stibium Natrium Tartaricum. Disodium bis{μ-[2,3-dihydroxybutanedioato(4-)-O^1,O^2:O^3,O^4]}diantimonate(2-); Disodium bis{μ-[L-(+)-tartrato(4-)]}diantimonate(2-).

$C_8H_4Na_2O_{12}Sb_2$ = 581.6.

CAS — 34521-09-0.

Pharmacopoeias. In *Int.* (as $C_4H_4NaO_7Sb$ = 308.8) and *US.*

Odourless, colourless, transparent crystals or white powder. The crystals effloresce on exposure to air.

Freely **soluble** in water; practically insoluble in alcohol. **Incompatible** with acids and alkalis, salts of heavy metals, albumin, soap, and tannins.

Stibocaptate (810-h)

Stibocaptate *(BAN).*

Sodium Stibocaptate *(rINN)*; Antimony Sodium Dimercaptosuccinate; Ro-4-1544/6; Sb-58; TWSb/6. Antimony sodium *meso*-2,3-dimercaptosuccinate. The formula varies from $C_{12}H_{11}NaO_{12}S_6Sb_2$ = 806.1 to $C_{12}H_6Na_6O_{12}S_6Sb_2$ = 916.0.

CAS — 3064-61-7 ($C_{12}H_6Na_6O_{12}S_6Sb_2$).

Stibophen (811-m)

Estibofeno; Fouadin; Stibophenum. Bis[4,5-dihydroxybenzene-1,3-disulphonato(4–)-O^4,O^5]antimonate(5–) pentasodium heptahydrate.

$C_{12}H_4Na_5O_{16}S_4Sb,7H_2O$ = 895.2.

CAS — 15489-16-4 (stibophen heptahydrate).

Pharmacopoeias. In *It.*

Adverse Effects and Treatment

Trivalent antimony compounds are more toxic than pentavalent antimonials such as sodium stibogluconate, possibly because they are excreted much more slowly. The most serious adverse effects are on the heart and liver. There are invariably ECG changes during treatment, but hypotension, bradycardia, and cardiac arrhythmias are more serious. Sudden death or cardiovascular collapse may occur at any time. Elevated liver enzyme values are common; liver damage with hepatic failure and death is most likely in patients with pre-existing hepatic disease.

Adverse effects immediately after intravenous administration of trivalent antimonials, in particular the tartrates, have included coughing, chest pain, pain in the arms, vomiting, abdominal pain, fainting, and collapse, especially after rapid injection. Extravasation during injection is extremely painful because of tissue damage. An anaphylactoid reaction characterised by an urticarial rash, husky voice, and collapse has been reported after the sixth or seventh intravenous injection of a course of treatment.

Numerous less immediate adverse effects have occurred including gastro-intestinal disturbances, muscular and joint pains, arthritis, pneumonia, dyspnoea, headache, dizziness, weakness, pruritus, skin rashes, facial oedema, fever, haemolytic anaemia, and kidney damage.

Large doses of antimony compounds taken by mouth have an emetic action. Continuous treatment with small doses of antimony may give rise to symptoms of subacute poisoning similar to those of chronic arsenical poisoning.

Treatment of severe poisoning with antimony compounds is similar to that for arsenic poisoning (see p.1551); dimercaprol may be of benefit.

References.

1. Stemmer KL. Pharmacology and toxicology of heavy metals: antimony. *Pharmacol Ther* 1976; **1:** 157–60.

Precautions

Trivalent antimony therapy has generally been superseded by less toxic treatment. It is contra-indicated in the presence of lung, heart, liver, and kidney disease. Intravenous injections should be administered very slowly and stopped if coughing, vomiting, or substernal pain occurs; extravasation should be avoided.

Some antimony compounds such as the tartrates cause severe pain and tissue necrosis and should not be given by intramuscular or subcutaneous injection.

In the event of trivalent antimony compounds being used then patients with glucose-6-phosphate dehydrogenase deficiency should be excluded. WHO lists stibophen[1] among the anthelmintics to be avoided in patients with this deficiency.

1. WHO. Glucose-6-phosphate dehydrogenase deficiency. *Bull WHO* 1989; **67:** 601–11.

Pharmacokinetics

Antimony compounds are poorly absorbed from the gastro-intestinal tract.

They are slowly excreted, mainly in the urine, following parenteral administration. Antimony accumulates in the body during treatment and persists for several months afterwards. Trivalent antimony has a greater affinity for cell proteins than for plasma proteins.

Uses and Administration

Trivalent antimony compounds were used in the treatment of the protozoal infection leishmaniasis until the advent of the less toxic pentavalent compounds. They continued to be used in the treatment of schistosomiasis, but have now been superseded by less toxic and more easily administered drugs such as praziquantel.

Antimony sodium tartrate was formerly used as an emetic and expectorant.

Preparations

Proprietary Preparations (details are given in Part 3)
Ital.: Formix†.

Multi-ingredient: ***Fr.:*** Montavon; ***Neth.:*** Rami Hoeststroop†.

Areca (758-j)

Areca Nuts; Arecae Semen; Arekasame; Betel Nuts; Noix d'Arec.

Pharmacopoeias. In *Jpn.*

Areca consists of the dried ripe seeds of *Areca catechu* (Palmae) containing the alkaloid arecoline. It was formerly used in the treatment of tapeworm infection. Arecoline has been used in veterinary medicine as a purgative and taenifuge.

Areca has sialogogue properties and is used in eastern countries as a masticatory. It is also chewed in conjunction with calcium hydroxide for its mild intoxicant and euphoriant properties. An increased incidence of oral leucoplakia and oral carcinoma has been reported in persons in the habit of chewing areca (betel nuts).

General references.

1. Arjungi KN. Areca nut: a review. *Arzneimittelforschung* 1976; **26:** 951–6.

Carcinogenicity. Ashby *et al.*[1] suggested that increased oral cancer associated with the chewing of 'quids' composed of areca, lime, and, occasionally, tobacco leaf, might be associated with the arecaidine content. However, Burton-Bradley[2] pointed out that there was no direct evidence that areca causes oral cancer and that other agents may be implicated. There does appear to be evidence of a link between the chewing of similar areca nut products and the development of oral submucous fibrosis,[3,4] a premalignant condition.

1. Ashby J, *et al.* Betel nuts, arecaidine, and oral cancer. *Lancet* 1979; **i:** 112.
2. Burton-Bradley BG. Is "betel chewing" carcinogenic? *Lancet* 1979; **ii:** 903.
3. Murlidhar V, Upmanyu G. Tobacco chewing, oral submucous fibrosis, and anaesthetic risk. *Lancet* 1996; **347:** 1840.
4. Babu S, *et al.* Oral fibrosis among teenagers chewing tobacco, areca nut, and Pan masala. *Lancet* 1996; **348:** 692.

Effects on the lungs. Evidence suggesting that there is an association between betel-nut chewing and bronchoconstriction in asthmatic patients.[1,2]

1. Taylor RFH, *et al.* Betel-nut chewing and asthma. *Lancet* 1992; **339:** 1134–6.
2. Kiyingi KS. Betel nut chewing and asthma. *Lancet* 1992; **340:** 59–60.

Effects on the nervous system. CNS symptoms in 2 patients were due to withdrawal from betel-nut chewing, a custom almost universal among people living under traditional conditions in Papua New Guinea and other Asian and Melanesian countries.[1] Syndromes associated with the practice range from habituation to addiction and psychosis. Severe extrapyramidal symptoms in 2 chronic schizophrenic patients have been reported[2] following chewing of betel nuts.

1. Wiesner DM. Betel-nut withdrawal. *Med J Aust* 1987; **146:** 453.
2. Deahl MP. Psychostimulant properties of betel nuts. *Br Med J* 1987; **294:** 841.

Ascaridole (761-s)

Ascaridol. 1-Isopropyl-4-methyl-2,3-dioxabicyclo[2.2.2]oct-5-ene.

$C_{10}H_{16}O_2$ = 168.2.

CAS — 512-85-6.

The active principle of chenopodium oil. It is an unstable liquid which is liable to explode when heated or when treated with organic acids.

Ascaridole has the same actions as chenopodium oil (see below).

Bephenium Hydroxynaphthoate (762-w)

Bephenium Hydroxynaphthoate *(BAN, rINN).*

Naphthammonum. Benzyldimethyl(2-phenoxyethyl)ammonium 3-hydroxy-2-naphthoate.

$C_{28}H_{29}NO_4$ = 443.5.

CAS — 7181-73-9 (bephenium); 3818-50-6 (bephenium hydroxynaphthoate).

Pharmacopoeias. In *Int.*

Bephenium hydroxynaphthoate is an anthelmintic formerly used in the treatment of hookworm infections due to *Ancylostoma duodenale.*

Preparations

Proprietary Preparations (details are given in Part 3)
Irl.: Alcopar†; ***UK:*** Alcopar†.

Betanaphthol (763-e)

β-Naftol; Naphthol. Naphth-2-ol.

$C_{10}H_8O$ = 144.2.

CAS — 135-19-3.

Pharmacopoeias. In *Aust., Pol.,* and *Swiss.*

Betanaphthol was formerly used as an anthelmintic in hookworm and tapeworm infections, but it has been superseded by less toxic and more efficient drugs.

Betanaphthol has a potent parasiticidal effect and was used as an ointment in the treatment of scabies, ringworm, and other skin diseases.

Betanaphthyl benzoate was used similarly.

Preparations

Proprietary Preparations (details are given in Part 3)

Multi-ingredient: ***Aust.:*** Salvyl; ***Fr.:*** Carbonaphtine Pectinee†; Intesticarbine†; ***Ital.:*** Tioderma†; ***Spain:*** Salva Infantes.

Bithionol (2210-k)

Bithionol *(BAN, rINN).*

Bitionol. 2,2′-Thiobis(4,6-dichlorophenol).

$C_{12}H_6Cl_4O_2S$ = 356.1.

CAS — 97-18-7.

Pharmacopoeias. Fr. includes bithionol oxide for veterinary use.

Adverse Effects

Adverse effects in patients taking bithionol by mouth include anorexia, nausea, vomiting, abdominal discomfort, diarrhoea, salivation, dizziness, headache, and skin rashes.

Photosensitivity reactions have occurred in persons using soap containing bithionol. Cross-sensitisation with other halogenated disinfectants has also occurred.

Uses and Administration

Bithionol is a chlorinated bis-phenol with bactericidal and anthelmintic properties. It is active against most trematodes (flukes). Bithionol is used in preference to praziquantel in fascioliasis (p.94) and is also used in paragonimiasis as an alternative to praziquantel (p.95). It has been given in a dose of 30 to 50 mg per kg body-weight by mouth on alternate days for 10 to 15 doses. WHO recommends a regimen of 30 mg per kg body-weight daily for 5 days to treat fascioliasis.

Bithionol is no longer used topically as a bactericide because of photosensitivity reactions.

References.

1. Singh TS, *et al.* Pulmonary paragonimiasis: clinical features, diagnosis and treatment of 39 cases in Manipur. *Trans R Soc Trop Med Hyg* 1986; **80:** 967–71.
2. Farid Z, *et al.* Treatment of acute toxaemic fascioliasis. *Trans R Soc Trop Med Hyg* 1988; **82:** 299.
3. Farag HF, *et al.* Bithionol (Bitin) treatment in established fascioliasis in Egyptians. *J Trop Med Hyg* 1988; **91:** 240–4.

Chenopodium Oil (768-c)

Aetheroleum Chenopodii; Esencia de Quenopodio Vermífuga; Oil of American Wormseed; Wurmsamenöl.

CAS — 8006-99-3.

Pharmacopoeias. In *It.*

Distilled with steam from the fresh flowering and fruiting plants, excluding roots, of *Chenopodium ambrosioides* var. *anthelminticum.* It contains ascaridole.

CAUTION. *Chenopodium oil may explode when heated.*

Chenopodium oil was formerly used as an anthelmintic for the expulsion of roundworms (*Ascaris*) and hookworms. It is toxic and has caused numerous fatalities.

The use of chenopodium herb as a flavouring agent is not recommended.

Clorsulon (18980-p)

Clorsulon *(BAN, USAN, rINN).*

MK-401. 4-Amino-6-(trichlorovinyl)benzene-1,3-disulphonamide.

$C_8H_8Cl_3N_3O_4S_2$ = 380.7.

CAS — 60200-06-8.

Pharmacopoeias. In *US.*

A white to off-white powder. Slightly **soluble** in water; freely soluble in methyl alcohol and in acetonitrile; very slightly soluble in dichloromethane.

Clorsulon is a veterinary anthelmintic used in the treatment of liver fluke infections.

Closantel (1984-s)

Closantel *(BAN, USAN, rINN).*

R-31520 (closantel); R-34828 (closantel sodium). 5′-Chloro-4′-(4-chloro-α-cyanobenzyl)-3,5-di-iodosalicyl-*o*-toluidide.

$C_{22}H_{14}Cl_2I_2N_2O_2$ = 663.1.

CAS — 57808-65-8 (closantel); 61438-64-0 (closantel sodium).

Closantel is a veterinary anthelmintic used in the treatment of liver fluke infections.

Loss of eyesight was reported in 11 women who received closantel (Flukiver) in mistake for a gynaecological product.[1] Sight was restored after closantel administration was stopped but incapacitating eye pain remained. Closantel had been provided as part of a charitable drug donation without adequate product information.

1. 't Hoen E, *et al.* Harmful human use of donated veterinary drug. *Lancet* 1993; **342:** 308–9.

Diamphenethide (12639-c)

Diamphenethide *(BAN).*

Diamfenetide *(rINN)*; Diamfenetidum. β,β′-Oxybis(aceto-*p*-phenetidide).

$C_{20}H_{24}N_2O_5$ = 372.4.

CAS — 36141-82-9.

Diamphenethide is a veterinary anthelmintic that has been used for the control of fascioliasis in sheep.

Dichlorophen (771-e)

Dichlorophen *(BAN, rINN).*

Di-phenthane-70; G-4. 2,2′-Methylenebis(4-chlorophenol).

$C_{13}H_{10}Cl_2O_2$ = 269.1.

CAS — 97-23-4.

Pharmacopoeias. In *Aust., Br.,* and *Fr.*

A white or slightly cream-coloured powder with a not more than slightly phenolic odour. Practically **insoluble** in water; freely soluble in alcohol; very soluble in ether.

Dichlorophen is an anthelmintic that was used in the treatment of infection by tapeworms but has been superseded by praziquantel or niclosamide.

Dichlorophen also has antifungal and antibacterial activity and has been used topically in the treatment of fungal infections and as a germicide in soaps and cosmetics.

Preparations

BP 1998: Dichlorophen Tablets.

Proprietary Preparations (details are given in Part 3)
S.Afr.: Anthiphen†.

Multi-ingredient: ***Ger.:*** Fissan-Brustwarzensalbe†; Ovis†; ***S.Afr.:*** Mycota; ***Switz.:*** Balsafissan†; ***UK:*** Germolene; Mycota.

Diethylcarbamazine Citrate (772-l)

Diethylcarbamazine Citrate *(BANM, rINNM).*

Diethylcarbam. Cit.; Diethylcarbamazine Acid Citrate; Diethylcarbamazini Citras; Ditrazini Citras; RP-3799. *NN*-Diethyl-4-methylpiperazine-1-carboxamide dihydrogen citrate.

$C_{10}H_{21}N_3O,C_6H_8O_7$ = 391.4.

CAS — 90-89-1 (diethylcarbamazine); 1642-54-2 (diethylcarbamazine citrate).

Pharmacopoeias. In *Chin., Eur.* (see p.viii), *Int., Jpn,* and *US.*

A white, crystalline, slightly hygroscopic powder, odourless or with a slight odour. M.p. about 136° to 138° with decomposition. Very **soluble** in water; soluble or sparingly soluble in alcohol; practically insoluble in acetone, in chloroform, and in ether. **Store** in airtight containers. Solutions should be protected from light.

Adverse Effects

Adverse effects directly attributable to diethylcarbamazine include nausea and vomiting. Headache, dizziness, and drowsiness may occur.

Hypersensitivity reactions arise from the death of the microfilariae. These can be serious, especially in onchocerciasis where there may also be sight-threatening ocular toxicity; fatalities have been reported. Encephalitis may be exacerbated in patients with loiasis and fatalities have occurred.

Reactions occurring during diethylcarbamazine treatment of lymphatic filariasis are basically of 2 types: pharmacological dose-dependent responses and a response of the infected host to the destruction and death of parasites.[1] Reactions of the first type include weakness, dizziness, lethargy, anorexia, and nausea. They begin within 1 to 2 hours of taking diethylcarbamazine, and persist for a few hours. Reactions of the second type are less likely to occur and less severe in bancroftian than in brugian filariasis. They may be systemic or local, both with and without fever. Systemic reactions may occur a few hours after the first oral dose of diethylcarbamazine and generally do not last for more than 3 days. They include headache, aches in other parts of the body, joint pain, dizziness, anorexia, malaise, transient haematuria, allergic reactions, vomiting, and sometimes attacks of bronchial asthma in asthmatic patients. Fever and systemic reactions are positively associated with microfilaraemia. Systemic reactions are reduced if diethylcarbamazine is given in spaced doses or in repeated small doses. They eventually cease spontaneously and interruption of treatment is rarely necessary; symptomatic treatment with antipyretics or analgesics may be helpful. Local reactions tend to occur later in the course of treatment and last longer; they also disappear spontaneously and interruption of treatment is not necessary. Local reactions include lymphadenitis, abscess, ulceration, and transient lymphoedema; funiculitis and epididymitis may also occur in bancroftian filariasis.

In most patients with onchocerciasis the microfilaricidal activity of diethylcarbamazine leads to a series of events with dermal, ocular, and systemic components, known as the Mazzotti reaction, within minutes to hours after its administration.[2] Clinical manifestations can be severe, dangerous, and debilitating and WHO no longer recommends the use of diethylcarbamazine in onchocerciasis. Systemic reactions include increased itching, rash, headache, aching muscles, joint pain, painful swollen and tender lymph nodes, fever, tachycardia and hypotension, and vertigo. Most patients experience eye discomfort in the first few hours after diethylcarbamazine treatment. Punctate keratitis can develop as can optic neuritis and visual field loss.

It has been suggested that the release of interleukin-6 may be implicated in diethylcarbamazine's adverse effects in patients with lymphatic filariasis.[3]

1. WHO. Lymphatic filariasis: the disease and its control: fifth report of the WHO expert committee on filariasis. *WHO Tech Rep Ser 821* 1992.
2. WHO. WHO expert committee on onchocerciasis: third report. *WHO Tech Rep Ser 752* 1987.
3. Yazdanbakhsh M, *et al.* Serum interleukin-6 levels and adverse reactions to diethylcarbamazine in lymphatic filariasis. *J Infect Dis* 1992; **166:** 453–4.

Precautions

Treatment with diethylcarbamazine should be closely supervised since hypersensitivity reactions are common and may be severe, especially in patients with onchocerciasis or loiasis. Patients with onchocerciasis should be monitored for eye changes. (The use of diethylcarbamazine to treat onchocerciasis is no longer recommended.)

Infants, pregnant women, the elderly, and the debilitated, especially those with cardiac or renal disease, are normally excluded when diethylcarbamazine is used in mass treatment schedules.

The use of diethylcarbamazine 2 mg per kg body-weight as a provocative day test for the detection of microfilariae of nocturnally periodic *Wuchereria bancrofti* in the blood, was not suitable in the presence of onchocerciasis or loiasis.[1]

1. McMahon JE, *et al.* Tanzania filariasis project: a provocative day test with diethylcarbamazine for the detection of microfilariae of nocturnally periodic Wuchereria bancrofti in the blood. *Bull WHO* 1979; **57:** 759–65.

Pregnancy. *Animal* studies[1] suggest that the uterine hypermotility induced by diethylcarbamazine is mediated via prostaglandin synthesis; this might explain the mechanism of the abortifacient action previously reported.[2]

1. Joseph CA, Dixon PAF. Possible prostaglandin-mediated effect of diethylcarbamazine on rat uterine contractility. *J Pharm Pharmacol* 1984; **36:** 281–2.
2. Subbu VSV, Biswas AR. Ecbolic effect of diethyl carbamazine. *Indian J Med Res* 1971; **59:** 646–7.

Renal impairment. For a study on the effects of renal impairment on the pharmacokinetics of diethylcarbamazine, see under Pharmacokinetics, below.

Pharmacokinetics

Diethylcarbamazine citrate is readily absorbed from the gastro-intestinal tract and also through the skin and conjunctiva. It is widely distributed in tissues and is excreted in the urine unchanged and as the *N*-oxide metabolite. Urinary excretion and hence plasma half-life is dependent on urinary pH.

A pharmacokinetic study in 6 patients with onchocerciasis[1] indicating that diethylcarbamazine is absorbed quickly and almost completely from the gastro-intestinal tract and is eliminated largely as unchanged drug in urine with relatively small amounts being excreted as the *N*-oxide metabolite. Following a single radioactively labelled dose of diethylcarbamazine citrate 0.5 mg per kg body-weight, administered by mouth as an aqueous solution, peak plasma concentrations of 100 to 150 ng per mL were achieved in 1 to 2 hours, followed by a sharp decline, then a marked secondary rise 3 to 6 hours after dosing followed by a steady decline. The half-life ranged from 9 to 13 hours. Urinary excretion of diethylcarbamazine and diethylcarbamazine *N*-oxide was complete within 96 hours; between 4 and 5% of the dose was recovered in the faeces. Disposition kinetics were similar in 5 healthy subjects given a single 50-mg tablet of diethylcarbamazine citrate. Peak plasma concentrations were initially 80 to 200 ng per mL, with a secondary rise 3 to 9 hours after dosing, the terminal half-life ranged from 5 to 13 hours, and urinary excretion of unchanged diethylcarbamazine and the *N*-oxide was complete within 48 hours.

When an alkaline urinary pH was maintained the elimination half-life of diethylcarbamazine and the area under the plasma concentration versus time curve were significantly increased compared with values when an acidic urinary pH was maintained.[2] However, alkalinisation of the urine in an attempt to decrease the dose of diethylcarbamazine in onchocerciasis was unlikely to be of practical value.[3]

1. Edwards G, *et al.* Diethylcarbamazine disposition in patients with onchocerciasis. *Clin Pharmacol Ther* 1981; **30:** 551–7.
2. Edwards G, *et al.* The effect of variations in urinary pH on the pharmacokinetics of diethylcarbamazine. *Br J Clin Pharmacol* 1981; **12:** 807–12.
3. Awadzi K, *et al.* The effect of moderate urine alkalinisation on low dose diethylcarbamazine therapy in patients with onchocerciasis. *Br J Clin Pharmacol* 1986; **21:** 669–76.

Renal impairment. Results in patients with chronic renal impairment and healthy subjects, given a single 50-mg dose of diethylcarbamazine citrate by mouth, indicating that the plasma half-life of diethylcarbamazine is prolonged and its 24-hour urinary excretion considerably reduced in those with moderate and severe degrees of renal impairment.[1] Mean plasma half-lives in 7 patients with severe renal impairment (creatinine clearance less than 25 mL per minute), 5 patients with moderate renal impairment (creatinine clearance between 25 and 60 mL per minute), and 4 healthy subjects were 15.1, 7.7, and 2.7 hours, respectively. The patient with the longest plasma half-life of 32 hours did not have the poorest renal function, but it was considered likely that the abnormally slow elimination of diethylcarbamazine was due to the high urine pH (7) resulting from sodium bicarbonate therapy. A further patient with a half-life longer than expected also had a less acidic urine.

1. Adjepon-Yamoah KK, *et al.* The effect of renal disease on the pharmacokinetics of diethylcarbamazine in man. *Br J Clin Pharmacol* 1982; **13:** 829–34.

Uses and Administration

Diethylcarbamazine citrate is an anthelmintic used in the treatment of lymphatic filariasis due to *Wuchereria bancrofti* (bancroftian filariasis), *Brugia malayi*, or *B. timori* (both known as brugian filariasis and as Malayan and Timorian filariasis respectively). It is also used in loiasis due to *Loa loa*. It was used in onchocerciasis due to *Onchocerca volvulus* before ivermectin became available. Diethylcarbamazine is active against both the microfilariae and adult worms of *W. bancrofti*, *B. malayi*, and *Loa loa*, but only against the microfilariae of *O. volvulus*. It has been tried in *Mansonella* infections and may be most effective against *M. streptocerca*. Diethylcarbamazine is also used in the treatment of toxocariasis (visceral larva migrans). For discussions of these infections and their treatment, see under Choice of Anthelmintic, p.92. See also below.

Diethylcarbamazine citrate is usually administered by mouth as tablets.

In the treatment of filarial infections due to *W. bancrofti, B. malayi, B. timori*, and *Loa loa* the manufacturer recommends 6 mg per kg body-weight daily in 3 divided doses for 3 weeks, given in an initial dosage of 1 mg per kg daily, gradually increased to 6 mg per kg daily over 3 days then maintained for 3 weeks, to reduce the incidence and severity of hypersensitivity reactions due to the destruction of microfilariae. However, in bancroftian filariasis WHO recommends 6 mg per kg daily for 12 days, and in brugian filariasis a dose of 3 to 6 mg per kg daily for 6 to 12 days. In the treatment of loiasis, WHO recommends a dose of 1 mg per kg as a single dose initially, doubled on two successive days and then adjusted to 2 to 3 mg per kg three times daily for a further 18 days. A corticosteroid may be given concurrently in the treatment of filarial infections. Similar doses are given for 3 weeks in the treatment of toxocariasis.

In the prophylaxis of bancroftian filariasis a dose of 50 mg monthly has been recommended and in the prophylaxis of loiasis a dose of 300 mg weekly.

In areas where lymphatic filariasis is endemic, mass treatment campaigns can reduce the intensity of transmission and incidence of disease. Diethylcarbamazine has been used in the form of medicated salt in some countries to control lymphatic filariasis.

Administration. Diethylcarbamazine was first used as the chloride, but is now produced as the dihydrogen citrate which contains only half its weight as base. In reporting doses it is therefore important to indicate whether they refer to a specific salt or to the base; unless otherwise stated, it can generally be assumed that the dose refers to the citrate.[1]

1. WHO. Lymphatic filariasis: fourth report of the WHO expert committee on filariasis. *WHO Tech Rep Ser 702* 1984.

Loiasis. Diethylcarbamazine is the main drug used in the management of loiasis (p.94).

References.

1. Nutman TB, *et al.* Loa loa infection in temporary residents of endemic regions: recognition of a hyperresponsive syndrome with characteristic clinical manifestations. *J Infect Dis* 1986; **154:** 10–18.
2. Nutman TB, *et al.* Diethylcarbamazine prophylaxis for human loiasis: results of a double-blind study. *N Engl J Med* 1988; **319:** 752–6.
3. Nutman TB, Ottesen EA. Diethylcarbamazine and human loiasis. *N Engl J Med* 1989; **320:** 320.

Lymphatic filariasis. Diethylcarbamazine citrate is the main drug used in the treatment of lymphatic filariasis (p.95). In endemic areas where more than 5% of the population is infected, mass treatment of the entire population (excluding neonates, pregnant women, and debilitated individuals) can reduce the intensity of transmission and the incidence of disease. However, compliance may be a problem with the usual multidose treatment regimens. Administering the doses at weekly intervals was shown to improve compliance and efficacy.[1] Single doses of 6 mg per kg body-weight clear microfilariae from the blood more slowly than the conventional multiple-dose regimens, but microfilaraemia after 12 months has been shown to be comparable with either regimen for both bancroftian and brugian filariasis.[2,3] Studies have shown that single doses of 3 or 6 mg per kg body-weight repeated at intervals of 6 or 12 months can maintain microfilaraemia at low levels.[4,5] In a study comparing a single dose every 6 months, a low dose every month, and the use of medicated cooking salt with the standard regimen, all three alternative regimens were superior to the standard regimen and the use of medicated salt or low monthly doses were the most effective.[6,7] The effectiveness of medicated salt has been confirmed by other investigators.[8,9] Combination of diethylcarbamazine with ivermectin has been reported to be more effective than either drug alone.[10-12] Diethylcarbamazine with albendazole has also shown promise.[13]

Diethylcarbamazine has also been used diagnostically. Detecting microfilariae in lymphatic filariasis can be difficult because of their nocturnal periodicity. Small doses of diethylcarbamazine can stimulate the microfilariae thus aiding their detection in the daytime in blood specimens.[14] For cautions against using such a test in patients with loiasis or onchocerciasis, see Precautions, above. Also it has been suggested that measurements on finger-prick blood samples may not be as accurate as those carried out on samples of venous blood.[15]

1. Eberhard ML, *et al.* Effectiveness of spaced doses of diethylcarbamazine citrate for the control of bancroftian filariasis. *Trop Med Parasitol* 1989; **40:** 111–13.
2. Andrade LD, *et al.* Comparative efficacy of three different diethylcarbamazine regimens in lymphatic filariasis. *Trans R Soc Trop Med Hyg* 1995; **89:** 319–21.
3. Hakim SL, *et al.* Single-dose diethylcarbamazine in the control of periodic brugian filariasis in Peninsular Malaysia. *Trans R Soc Trop Med Hyg* 1995; **89:** 686–9.
4. Kimura E, *et al.* Long-term efficacy of single-dose mass treatment with diethylcarbamazine citrate against diurnally subperiodic Wuchereria bancrofti: eight years' experience in Samoa. *Bull WHO* 1992; **70:** 769–76.
5. Meyrowitsch DW, *et al.* Mass diethylcarbamazine chemotherapy for control of bancroftian filariasis: comparative efficacy of standard treatment and two semi-annual single-dose treatments. *Trans R Soc Trop Med Hyg* 1996; **90:** 69–73.
6. Meyrowitsch DW, *et al.* Mass DEC chemotherapy for control of bancroftian filariasis: comparative efficacy of four strategies two years after start of treatment. *Trans R Soc Trop Med Hyg* 1996; **90:** 423–8.
7. Meyrowitsch DW, Simonsen PE. Long-term effect of mass diethylcarbamazine chemotherapy on bancroftian filariasis: results at four years after start of treatment. *Trans R Soc Trop Med Hyg* 1998; **92:** 98–103.
8. Liu J, *et al.* Mass treatment of filariasis using DEC-medicated salt. *J Trop Med Hyg* 1992; **95:** 132–5.
9. Reddy GS, Venkateswaralu N. Mass administration of DEC-medicated salt for filariasis control in the endemic population of Karaikal, South India: implementation and impact assessment. *Bull WHO* 1996; **74:** 85–90.
10. Glaziou P, *et al.* Double-blind controlled trial of a single dose of the combination ivermectin 400 μg/kg plus diethylcarbamazine 6 mg/kg for the treatment of bancroftian filariasis: results at six months. *Trans R Soc Trop Med Hyg* 1994; **88:** 707–8.
11. Moulia-Pelat JP, *et al.* Advantages of an annual single dose of ivermectin 400 μg/kg plus diethylcarbamazine for community treatment of bancroftian filariasis. *Trans R Soc Trop Med Hyg* 1995; **89:** 682–5.
12. Bockarie MJ, *et al.* Randomised community-based trial of annual single-dose diethylcarbamazine with or without ivermectin against Wuchereria bancrofti infection in human beings and mosquitoes. *Lancet* 1998; **351:** 162–8.
13. Ismail MM, *et al.* Efficacy of single dose combinations of albendazole, ivermectin and diethylcarbamazine for the treatment of bancroftian filariasis. *Trans R Soc Trop Med Hyg* 1998; **92:** 94–7.
14. Sabry M. A quantitative analysis of the diagnostic value of diethylcarbamazine provocation in endemic Wuchereria bancrofti infection. *Trans R Soc Trop Med Hyg* 1988; **82:** 117–21.
15. Eberhard ML, *et al.* Persistence of microfilaremia in bancroftian filariasis after diethylcarbamazine citrate therapy. *Trop Med Parasitol* 1988; **39:** 128–30.

Preparations

USP 23: Diethylcarbamazine Citrate Tablets.

Proprietary Preparations (details are given in Part 3)

Austral.: Hetrazan; ***Canad.:*** Hetrazan; ***Fr.:*** Notezine†; ***Ger.:*** Hetrazan†; ***Spain:*** Filarcidan†; ***UK:*** Hetrazan.

Doramectin (14635-v)

Doramectin *(BAN, USAN, rINN).*

UK-67994.

CAS — 117704-25-3.

Doramectin is an avermectin anthelmintic used in veterinary medicine for nematode infections. It is also used as a systemic veterinary ectoparasiticide.

Embelia (777-k)

Vidang.

CAS — 550-24-3 (embelic acid).

The dried fruits of *Embelia ribes* and *E. robusta* (= *E. tsjeriamcottam*) (Myrsinaceae), containing about 2.5% of embelic acid (embelin).

Embelia has been used in India and other eastern countries for the expulsion of tapeworms.

Eprinomectin (19088-e)

Eprinomectin *(USAN, rINN).*

Eprinomectina; Eprinomectine; MK-397. A mixture of eprinomectin component B_{1a} and eprinomectin component B_{1b}.

CAS — 159628-36-1 (eprinomectin); 123997-26-2 (eprinomectin); 133305-88-1 (component B_{1a}); 133305-89-2 (component B_{1b}).

Eprinomectin is an avermectin anthelmintic used in veterinary medicine for nematode infections. It is also used as a systemic veterinary ectoparasiticide.

Febantel (12729-a)

Febantel *(BAN, USAN, rINN).*

Bay-h-5757; BAY-Vh-5757. 2′-[2,3-Bis(methoxycarbonyl)guanidino]-5′-phenylthio-2-methoxyacetanilide; Dimethyl {2-[2-(2-methoxyacetamido)-4-(phenylthio)phenyl]imidocarbonyl}dicarbamate.

$C_{20}H_{22}N_4O_6S$ = 446.5.

CAS — 58306-30-2.

Febantel is a veterinary anthelmintic used in the treatment of nematode infections of the gastro-intestinal tract and lungs and in tapeworm infections.

Fenbendazole (778-a)

Fenbendazole *(BAN, USAN, rINN).*

Hoe-881V. Methyl 5-phenylthio-1*H*-benzimidazol-2-ylcarbamate.

$C_{15}H_{13}N_3O_2S$ = 299.3.

CAS — 43210-67-9.

Pharmacopoeias. In Eur. (see p.viii).

A white or almost white powder. Practically **insoluble** in water; very slightly soluble in methyl alcohol; sparingly soluble in dimethylformamide. **Protect** from light.

Fenbendazole is a benzimidazole anthelmintic structurally related to mebendazole (see p.104). It is used in veterinary practice.

Flubendazole (12756-r)

Flubendazole *(BAN, USAN, rINN).*

Fluoromebendazole; R-17889. Methyl 5-(4-fluorobenzoyl)-1*H*-benzimidazol-2-ylcarbamate.

$C_{16}H_{12}FN_3O_3$ = 313.3.

CAS — 31430-15-6.

Flubendazole, a benzimidazole carbamate anthelmintic, is an analogue of mebendazole (p.104) and has similar actions and uses.

For the treatment of enterobiasis in adults and children, flubendazole 100 mg is given by mouth as a single dose, repeated if necessary after 2 to 3 weeks. For ascariasis, hookworm infections, and trichuriasis 100 mg is given twice daily for 3 days. For discussions of these infections and their treatment, see under Choice of Anthelmintic, p.92.

References.

1. Feldmeier H, *et al.* Flubendazole versus mebendazole in intestinal helminthic infections. *Acta Trop (Basel)* 1982; **39:** 185–9.
2. Kan SP. The anthelmintic effects of flubendazole on Trichuris trichiura and Ascaris lumbricoides. *Trans R Soc Trop Med Hyg* 1983; **77:** 668–70.
3. Dominguez-Vazquez A, *et al.* Comparison of flubendazole and diethylcarbamazine in treatment of onchocerciasis. *Lancet* 1983; **i:** 139–43.
4. Tellez-Giron E, *et al.* Treatment of neurocysticercosis with flubendazole. *Am J Trop Med Hyg* 1984; **33:** 627–31.
5. Nocera T, *et al.* Value of flubendazole in the treatment of scabies. *Eur J Dermatol* 1996; **6:** 154–5.

Preparations

Proprietary Preparations (details are given in Part 3)
Fr.: Fluvermal; *Spain:* Flicum.

Haloxon (12815-c)

Haloxon *(BAN, rINN).*

Bis(2-chloroethyl) 3-chloro-4-methylcoumarin-7-yl phosphate.

$C_{14}H_{14}Cl_3O_6P = 415.6.$

CAS — 321-55-1.

Pharmacopoeias. In *BP(Vet).*

A white or almost white, odourless or almost odourless powder. M.p. 88° to 93°. Practically **insoluble** in water; freely soluble in alcohol, in acetone, and in chloroform.

Haloxon is an organophosphorus compound used as an anthelmintic in veterinary medicine.

For a description of the toxic effects of organophosphorus compounds and the treatment of acute poisoning, see organophosphorus insecticides (p.1408).

Hexachloroparaxylene (781-y)

Chloxyle; Hetol; Hexachloroparaxylol. 1,4-Bis(trichloromethyl)benzene.

$C_8H_4Cl_6 = 312.8.$

CAS — 68-36-0.

Hexachloroparaxylene has been used in China and the former USSR as an anthelmintic, principally to treat the liver fluke infections clonorchiasis and opisthorchiasis, but other treatment is preferred.

Adverse effects reported with hexachloroparaxylene have included gastro-intestinal disturbances, cardiac arrhythmias, nephrotoxicity, and haemolysis.

Hycanthone Mesylate (783-z)

Hycanthone Mesilate *(rINNM)*; Hydroxylucanthone Methanesulphonate; NSC-134434 (hycanthone); Win-24933 (hycanthone). 1-(2-Diethylaminoethylamino)-4-hydroxymethylthioxanthen-9-one methanesulphonate.

$C_{20}H_{24}N_2O_2S,CH_3SO_3H = 452.6.$

CAS — 3105-97-3 (hycanthone); 23255-93-8 (hycanthone mesylate).

NOTE. Hycanthone is *USAN.*

Hycanthone has been used as a schistosomicide in the individual or mass treatment of infection with *Schistosoma haematobium* and *S. mansoni.*

Owing to its toxicity and concern about possible carcinogenicity, mutagenicity, and teratogenicity, hycanthone has been replaced by other drugs such as praziquantel.

Ivermectin (12874-b)

Ivermectin *(BAN, USAN, rINN).*

CAS — 70288-86-7 (ivermectin); 70161-11-4 (component B_{1a}); 70209-81-3 (component B_{1b}).

Pharmacopoeias. In *Eur.* (see p.viii).

A mixture of ivermectin component H_2B_{1a} (5-*O*-demethyl-22,23-dihydroavermectin A_{1a}; $C_{48}H_{74}O_{14} = 875.1$) and ivermectin component H_2B_{1b} (25-(1-methylethyl)-5-*O*-demethyl-25-de(1-methylpropyl)-22,23-dihydroavermectin A_{1a}; $C_{47}H_{72}O_{14} = 861.1$). It contains not less than 90% of component H_2B_{1a} and not less than 95% of components H_2B_{1a} and H_2B_{1b} together, calculated with reference to the anhydrous substance.

A white or yellowish-white, hygroscopic, crystalline powder. Practically **insoluble** in water; soluble in alcohol; freely soluble in dichloromethane. **Store** in airtight containers.

Adverse Effects and Precautions

The adverse effects reported with ivermectin are generally consistent with a mild Mazzotti reaction arising from its effect on the microfilariae. They include fever, pruritus, arthralgia, myalgia, asthenia, postural hypotension, tachycardia, oedema, lymphadenopathy, gastro-intestinal symptoms, sore throat, cough, and headache. The effects tend to be transient and if treatment is required they respond to analgesics and antihistamines.

Ivermectin may cause mild ocular irritation. Somnolence, transient eosinophilia, and raised liver enzyme values have also been reported.

There is some distribution into breast milk (see Breast Feeding, below). Administration of ivermectin is not recommended during pregnancy. Mass treatment is generally withheld from pregnant women (see Pregnancy, below), children under 15 kg body-weight, and the seriously ill.

Some studies have shown quite a high incidence of adverse effects with ivermectin and have associated the effects with the severity of infection.[1-3] However, in none of these studies were the reactions considered to be life-threatening and only symptomatic treatment was required. The severity, incidence, and duration of adverse reactions was reported to be reduced after repeated annual administration.[4] When larger groups of patients were considered in the Onchocerciasis Control Programme (OCP) in West Africa a much lower incidence of adverse reactions was observed in patients given ivermectin for the first time[5] and when treatment was repeated a year later that incidence was reduced even further. The results from several trials in this programme[6] show 93 severe reactions in 50 929 patients (1.83%), most of the reactions being postural hypotension or dizziness (53). A more recent study[7] has found 22 severe reactions in 17 877 patients treated for onchocerciasis in an area also endemic for *Loa loa* infection, and demonstrated a relationship to heavy *L. loa* microfilaraemia. It was suggested that ivermectin should be used with caution for mass onchocerciasis treatment programmes in areas where loiasis and onchocerciasis co-exist.

Some supervision is considered necessary after administration of ivermectin;[2,6] the OCP recommendation[6] is for resident nurses to monitor patients for a period of 36 hours after treatment, whatever the level of endemicity. However, the incidence of adverse reactions reported after repeated doses appears to be lower than after the first dose and the need for supervision on re-treatment has been questioned.[8]

Neurotoxicity observed in some breeds of *dogs* has not been seen in *cattle* or *horses*[9] nor was it reported in man in the above studies. Another potential concern was the prolongation of prothrombin times observed by Homeida *et al.*[10] in 28 patients given ivermectin, but others have not confirmed this effect[11] or observed any bleeding disorders.[12]

There has been some concern over the use of ivermectin to treat scabies in elderly patients following a report suggesting a possible link to an increased incidence of death among a cohort of 47 patients.[13] It has, however, been argued that no such association has been seen in other populations of elderly patients and that the statistical methods used by the original authors were deficient.[14-16] There was no evidence of an increase in death rate associated with ivermectin in a community-based trial in Papua New Guinea of diethylcarbamazine with or without ivermectin for lymphatic filariasis.[17]

1. Kumaraswami V, *et al.* Ivermectin for the treatment of Wuchereria bancrofti filariasis: efficacy and adverse reactions. *JAMA* 1988; **259:** 3150–3.
2. Rothova A, *et al.* Side-effects of ivermectin in treatment of onchocerciasis. *Lancet* 1989; **i:** 1439–41.
3. Zea-Flores R, *et al.* Adverse reactions after community treatment of onchocerciasis with ivermectin in Guatemala. *Trans R Soc Trop Med Hyg* 1992; **86:** 663–6.
4. Burnham GM. Adverse reactions to ivermectin treatment for onchocerciasis: results of a placebo-controlled, double-blind trial in Malawi. *Trans R Soc Trop Med Hyg* 1993; **87:** 313–17.
5. De Sole G, *et al.* Lack of adverse reactions in ivermectin treatment of onchocerciasis. *Lancet* 1990; **335:** 1106–7.
6. De Sole G, *et al.* Adverse reactions after large-scale treatment of onchocerciasis with ivermectin: combined results from eight community trials. *Bull WHO* 1989; **67:** 707–19.
7. Gardon J, *et al.* Serious reactions after mass treatment of onchocerciasis with ivermectin in an area endemic for Loa loa infection. *Lancet* 1997; **350:** 18–22.
8. Whitworth JAG, *et al.* A community trial of ivermectin for onchocerciasis in Sierra Leone: adverse reactions after the first five treatment rounds. *Trans R Soc Trop Med Hyg* 1991; **85:** 501–5.
9. WHO. WHO expert committee on onchocerciasis: third report. *WHO Tech Rep Ser 752* 1987.
10. Homeida MMA, *et al.* Prolongation of prothrombin time with ivermectin. *Lancet* 1988; **i:** 1346–7.
11. Richards FO, *et al.* Ivermectin and prothrombin time. *Lancet* 1989; **i;** 1139–40.
12. Pacque MC, *et al.* Ivermectin and prothrombin time. *Lancet* 1989; **i:** 1140.
13. Barkwell R, Shields S. Deaths associated with ivermectin treatment of scabies. *Lancet* 1997; **349:** 1144–5.
14. Diazgranados JA, Costa JL. Deaths after ivermectin treatment. *Lancet* 1997; **349:** 1698.
15. Reintjes R, Hoek C. Deaths associated with ivermectin for scabies. *Lancet* 1997; **350:** 215.
16. Coyne PE, Addiss DG. Deaths associated with ivermectin for scabies. *Lancet* 1997; **350:** 215–16.
17. Alexander NDE, *et al.* Absence of ivermectin-associated excess deaths. *Trans R Soc Trop Med Hyg* 1998; **92:** 342.

Breast feeding. The distribution of ivermectin into breast milk has limited its use in breast-feeding mothers. Ogbuokiri *et al.*[1] measured ivermectin concentrations in the milk of 4 healthy lactating women who had been given a standard dose of ivermectin; the mean concentration in breast milk was 14.13 ng per mL. These workers felt that in view of this low concentration the precaution of excluding lactating mothers from ivermectin mass treatment programmes should be reconsidered. Some authorities have recommended that ivermectin should not be given to mothers who are breast feeding until the infant is at least one week old.

1. Ogbuokiri JE, *et al.* Ivermectin levels in human breast milk. *Eur J Clin Pharmacol* 1994; **46:** 89–90.

Pregnancy. It is recommended that pregnant women should be excluded from mass treatment schedules with ivermectin. While women who are known to be pregnant can be excluded, it is recognised that women not yet diagnosed as pregnant or unwilling to admit their pregnancy have been treated. Pacqué *et al.*[1] assessed 203 pregnancy outcomes to women who had received ivermectin during pregnancy mostly during the first 12 weeks. They found that the rates of major congenital malformation, miscarriage, and still-birth associated with ivermectin were similar to those in untreated mothers. Chippaux *et al.*[2] studied another 110 women also inadvertently given ivermectin during pregnancy and observed a similar lack of adverse effect on pregnancy outcome. They considered that the precaution of avoiding the administration of ivermectin to women notifying a pregnancy should be adequate.

1. Pacqué M, *et al.* Pregnancy outcome after inadvertent ivermectin treatment during community-based distribution. *Lancet* 1990; **336:** 1486–9.
2. Chippaux J-P, *et al.* Absence of any adverse effect of inadvertent ivermectin treatment during pregnancy. *Trans R Soc Trop Med Hyg* 1993; **87:** 318.

Pharmacokinetics

Ivermectin is absorbed from the gastro-intestinal tract following oral administration with peak plasma concentrations being obtained after approximately 4 hours. Ivermectin is reported to be approximately 93% bound to plasma proteins and has a plasma elimination half-life of about 12 hours. It undergoes metabolism and is excreted largely as metabolites over a period of about 2 weeks, chiefly in the faeces, with less than 1% appearing in the urine and less than 2% in breast milk (see also Breast Feeding, above).

Uses and Administration

Ivermectin is a semisynthetic derivative of one of the avermectins, a group of macrocyclic lactones produced by *Streptomyces avermitilis.*

It has a microfilaricidal action in onchocerciasis and reduces the microfilarial load without the toxicity seen with diethylcarbamazine. Ivermectin also has a microfilaricidal action in lymphatic filariasis and has been used in its treatment. Ivermectin is also active in some other worm infections. It is used in the treatment of strongyloidiasis and has been tried in some *Mansonella* infections. For details of these infections and their treatment, see under Choice of Anthelmintic, p.92. See also below.

A single dose of 3 to 12 mg based roughly on 150 μg per kg body-weight by mouth for patients weighing more than 15 kg and over 5 years of age is given annually or every 6 months in the treatment of onchocerciasis. This schedule has been adopted in the mass treatment of subjects in infected areas. No food should be taken for 2 hours before or after the dose.

Ivermectin 200 μg per kg as a single dose, or daily on two consecutive days, is suggested for the treatment of strongyloidiasis.

Reviews.

1. Ottesen EA, Campbell WC. Ivermectin in human medicine. *J Antimicrob Chemother* 1994; **34:** 195–203.

Cutaneous larva migrans. There are some reports[1,2] of ivermectin being effective in the treatment of cutaneous larva migrans (p.93).

1. Caumes E, *et al.* Efficacy of ivermectin in the therapy of cutaneous larva migrans. *Arch Dermatol* 1992; **128:** 994–5.
2. Caumes E, *et al.* A randomized trial of ivermectin versus albendazole for the treatment of cutaneous larva migrans. *Am J Trop Med Hyg* 1993; **49:** 641–4.

Epilepsy. An improvement in seizure control was noted in 34 of 91 patients with epilepsy (p.335) who received ivermectin for onchocerciasis.[1] The seizures might have been provoked by microfilariae in the CNS and improvement could be connected with its microfilaricidal effect. Another explanation might lie in ivermectin's GABA agonist activity.[2]

1. Kipp W, *et al.* Improvement in seizures after ivermectin. *Lancet* 1992; **340:** 789–90.
2. Costa JL, Diazgranados JA. Ivermectin for spasticity in spinal-cord injury. *Lancet* 1994; **343:** 739.

Intestinal nematode infections. Ivermectin activity has been observed in man against *Ascaris lumbricoides*, *Strongyloides stercoralis*, and *Trichuris trichiura*.[1] Roundworm expulsion has been reported as a 'side-effect' of ivermectin when used in community-based treatment of onchocerciasis.[2] When a controlled study was carried out,[3] single doses of 150 or 200 μg of ivermectin per kg body-weight produced cure rates of 94% in strongyloidiasis (see below) and above 67% in ascariasis, trichuriasis, and enterobiasis. Although some activity has been observed against *Necator americanus*,[1] cure rates for hookworm were considered unsatisfactory.[3] Whitworth *et al.*[4] have reported that they observed no activity against *Trichuris* contrary to other observations.

1. Freedman DO, *et al.* The efficacy of ivermectin in the chemotherapy of gastrointestinal helminthiasis in humans. *J Infect Dis* 1989; **159:** 1151–3.
2. Whitworth JAG, *et al.* Community-based treatment with ivermectin. *Lancet* 1988; **ii:** 97–8.
3. Naquira C, *et al.* Ivermectin for human strongyloidiasis and other intestinal helminths. *Am J Trop Med Hyg* 1989; **40:** 304–9.
4. Whitworth JAG, *et al.* A field study of the effect of ivermectin on intestinal helminths in man. *Trans R Soc Trop Med Hyg* 1991; **85:** 232–4.

Loiasis. There is evidence of reduced microfilaraemia following ivermectin treatment[1-4,7] in patients with loiasis (p.94), but concern over its potential for neurotoxicity in patients with a high microfilarial burden.[5,6]

1. Martin-Prevel Y, *et al.* Reduction of microfilaraemia with single high-dose of ivermectin in loiasis. *Lancet* 1993; 342: 442.
2. Ranque S, *et al.* Decreased prevalence and intensity of Loa loa infection in a community treated with ivermectin every three months for two years. *Trans R Soc Trop Med Hyg* 1996; **90:** 429–30.
3. Duong TH, *et al.* Reduced Loa loa microfilaria count ten to twelve months after a single dose of ivermectin. *Trans R Soc Trop Med Hyg* 1997; **91:** 592–3.
4. Gardon J, *et al.* Marked decrease in Loa loa microfilaraemia six and twelve months after a single dose of ivermectin. *Trans R Soc Trop Med Hyg* 1997; **91:** 593–4.
5. Anonymous. Encephalitis following treatment of loiasis. *WHO Drug Inf* 1991; **5:** 113–14.
6. Gardon J, *et al.* Serious reactions after mass treatment of onchocerciasis with ivermectin in an area endemic for Loa loa infection. *Lancet* 1997; **350:** 18–22.
7. Chippaux J-P, *et al.* Impact of repeated large scale ivermectin treatments on the transmission of Loa loa. *Trans R Soc Trop Med Hyg* 1998; **92:** 454–8.

Lymphatic filariasis. Ivermectin has produced promising results in several studies in the treatment of lymphatic filariasis (p.95) and may become an alternative or adjunct to diethylcarbamazine if a suitable treatment schedule can be found. Ivermectin is effective against the microfilariae of lymphatic filariasis and it has been suggested that in high doses it may have some activity against the adult worm.[1,2] Single doses of ivermectin, usually of 100 μg per kg body-weight, have been shown to eliminate microfilariae more rapidly than a course of diethylcarbamazine, but the effect is less sustained.[3-6] However, a sustained effect can be obtained by giving ivermectin regularly, for example every 6 months[2,7] or by giving a larger dose at less frequent intervals. A single dose of 200 μg per kg has produced a response that has lasted for up to 2 years.[1] A dose of 400 μg per kg has also produced a sustained response.[2,8] Another suggested approach is to treat the patient with a single dose of ivermectin plus diethylcarbamazine;[9] this combination has been successful in annual treatment campaign.[10-12] Ivermectin in combination with albendazole may also be effective.[12,13]

1. Eberhard ML, *et al.* Long-term suppression of microfilaraemia following ivermectin treatment. *Trans R Soc Trop Med Hyg* 1992; **86:** 287–8.
2. Moulia-Pelat JP, *et al.* Ivermectin 400 μg/kg: long-term suppression of microfilariae in Bancroftian filariasis. *Trans R Soc Trop Med Hyg* 1994; **88:** 107–9.
3. Sabry M, *et al.* A placebo-controlled double-blind trial for the treatment of bancroftian filariasis with ivermectin or diethylcarbamazine. *Trans R Soc Trop Med Hyg* 1991; **85:** 640–3.
4. Cartel J-L, *et al.* Single versus repeated doses of ivermectin and diethylcarbamazine for the treatment of Wuchereria bancrofti var pacifica microfilaremia: results at 12 months of a double-blind study. *Trop Med Parasitol* 1991; **42:** 335–8.
5. Zheng H, *et al.* Efficacy of ivermectin for control of microfilaremia recurring after treatment with diethylcarbamazine I: clinical and parasitologic observations. *Am J Trop Med Hyg* 1991; **45:** 168–74.
6. Dreyer G, *et al.* Treatment of bancroftian filariasis in Recife, Brazil: a two-year comparative study of the efficacy of single treatments with ivermectin or diethylcarbamazine. *Trans R Soc Trop Med Hyg* 1995; **89:** 98–102.
7. Nguyen NL, *et al.* Control of bancroftian filariasis is an endemic area of Polynesia by ivermectin 400 μg/kg. *Trans R Soc Trop Med Hyg* 1996; **90:** 689–91.
8. Nguyen NL, *et al.* Advantages of ivermectin at a single dose of 400 μg/kg compared with 100 μg/kg for community treatment of lymphatic filariasis in Polynesia. *Trans R Soc Trop Med Hyg* 1994; **88:** 461–4.
9. Glaziou P, *et al.* Double-blind controlled trial of a single dose of the combination ivermectin 400 μg/kg plus diethylcarbamazine 6 mg/kg for the treatment of bancroftian filariasis: results at six months. *Trans R Soc Trop Med Hyg* 1994; **88:** 707–8.
10. Moulia-Pelat JP, *et al.* Advantages of an annual single dose of ivermectin 400 μg/kg plus diethylcarbamazine for community treatment of bancroftian filariasis. *Trans R Soc Trop Med Hyg* 1995; **89:** 682–5.
11. Bockarie MJ, *et al.* Randomised community-based trial of annual single-dose diethylcarbamazine with or without ivermectin against Wuchereria bancrofti infection in human beings and mosquitoes. *Lancet* 1998; **351:** 162–8.
12. Ismail MM, *et al.* Efficacy of single dose combinations of albendazole, ivermectin and diethylcarbamazine for the treatment of bancroftian filariasis. *Trans R Soc Trop Med Hyg* 1998; **92:** 94–7.
13. Addiss DG, *et al.* Randomised placebo-controlled comparison of ivermectin and albendazole alone and in combination for Wuchereria bancrofti microfilaraemia in Haitian children. *Lancet* 1997; **350:** 480–4. Correction. *ibid.*; 1036.

Mansonella infections. The response of *Mansonella* infections (p.95) to ivermectin depends on the species. It may be effective against *Mansonella ozzardi*, but studies in *M. perstans* infection have not shown ivermectin to produce a substantial reduction in microfilaraemia.[1,2] A good response to ivermectin has been reported in patients infected with *M. streptocerca*.[3]

1. Schulz-Key H, *et al.* Efficacy of ivermectin in the treatment of concomitant Mansonella perstans infections in onchocerciasis patients. *Trans R Soc Trop Med Hyg* 1993; **87:** 227–9.
2. Van den Enden E, *et al.* Treatment failure of a single high dose of ivermectin for Mansonella perstans filariasis. *Trans R Soc Trop Med Hyg* 1993; **87:** 90.
3. Fischer P, *et al.* Treatment of human Mansonella streptocerca infection with ivermectin. *Trop Med Int Hlth* 1997; **2:** 191–9.

Onchocerciasis. Ivermectin has a microfilaricidal action against *Onchocerca volvulus* and is the main drug used in the control of onchocerciasis (p.95). A single dose rapidly eliminates microfilariae from the skin and gradually eliminates them from the cornea and anterior chamber of the eye.[1] Ivermectin does not eliminate the adult worms but does suppress the release of microfilariae from the adult worm for several cycles which accounts for its prolonged activity. Its action against *O. volvulus* has been attributed to a GABA-agonist effect. Studies have also indicated that ivermectin inhibits the transmission of microfilariae by reducing their uptake from man by the insect vector.[2-5]

Ivermectin is donated without charge by *Merck Sharp & Dohme* through the Mectizan Expert Committee (MEC) for human use in community-wide mass treatment programmes in all countries in which onchocerciasis is endemic, where it is given once a year to all but pregnant women, breast-feeding mothers of recently born babies, children weighing less than 15 kg, and those unable to walk or otherwise seriously ill.[6] Several studies have confirmed the long-term safety and efficacy of such programmes.[7-11]

The ocular microfilarial load can be safely reduced by ivermectin[1,12] and early lesions of the anterior segment of the eye have improved.[12] A reduction in the incidence[13] and progression[14] of optic nerve damage has also been reported but the effect on posterior segment disease is less certain.[15] Improvements in skin lesions have been reported.[16] Administration every 6 months produces a more rapid reduction of microfilariae than administration every year,[17] but it is difficult to tell whether any long-term advantages outweigh the disadvantages of more frequent administration. In non-endemic areas, repeated doses may be necessary to reduce recurrence; a study in the UK found that patients given three doses at monthly intervals had fewer relapses at 6 months than patients who received a single dose, but relapses were nevertheless seen in 50% of patients at 12 months.[18] Others have suggested that treatment may need to be repeated every 4 to 6 months.[19]

1. Newland HS, *et al.* Effect of single-dose ivermectin therapy on human Onchocerca volvulus infection with onchocercal ocular involvement. *Br J Ophthalmol* 1988; **72:** 561–9.
2. Taylor HR, *et al.* Impact of mass treatment of onchocerciasis with ivermectin on the transmission of infection. *Science* 1990; **250:** 116–18.
3. Trpis M, *et al.* Effect of mass treatment of a human population with ivermectin on transmission of Onchocerca volvulus by Simulium yahense in Liberia, West Africa. *Am J Trop Med Hyg* 1990; **42:** 148–56.
4. Chavasse DC, *et al.* Low level ivermectin coverage and the transmission of onchocerciasis. *Trans R Soc Trop Med Hyg* 1995; **89:** 534–7.
5. Boussinesq M, *et al.* Onchocerca volvulus: striking decrease in transmission in the Vina valley (Cameroon) after eight annual large scale ivermectin treatments. *Trans R Soc Trop Med Hyg* 1997; **91:** 82–6.
6. Pond B. Distribution of ivermectin by health workers. *Lancet* 1990; **335:** 1539.
7. De Sole G, *et al.* Adverse reactions after large-scale treatment of onchocerciasis with ivermectin: combined results from eight community trials. *Bull WHO* 1989; **67:** 707–19.
8. Pacqué M, *et al.* Safety of and compliance with community-based ivermectin therapy. *Lancet* 1990; **335:** 1377–80.
9. Pacqué M, *et al.* Community-based treatment of onchocerciasis with ivermectin: safety, efficacy, and acceptability of yearly treatment. *J Infect Dis* 1991; **163:** 381–5.
10. Steel C, *et al.* Immunologic responses to repeated ivermectin treatment in patients with onchocerciasis. *J Infect Dis* 1991; **164:** 581–7.
11. Whitworth JAG, *et al.* A community trial of ivermectin for onchocerciasis in Sierra Leone: clinical and parasitological responses to four doses given at six-monthly interval. *Trans R Soc Trop Med Hyg* 1992; **86:** 277–80.
12. Dadzie KY, *et al.* Changes in ocular onchocerciasis after two rounds of community-based ivermectin treatment in a holo-endemic onchocerciasis focus. *Trans R Soc Trop Med Hyg* 1991; **85:** 267–71.
13. Abiose A, *et al.* Reduction in incidence of optic nerve disease with annual ivermectin to control onchocerciasis. *Lancet* 1993; **341:** 130–4.
14. Cousens SN, *et al.* Impact of annual dosing with ivermectin on progression of onchocercal visual field loss. *Bull WHO* 1997; **75:** 229–36.
15. Whitworth JAG, *et al.* Effects of repeated doses of ivermectin on ocular onchocerciasis: community-based trial in Sierra Lione. *Lancet* 1991; **338:** 1100–1103.
16. Pacqué M, *et al.* Improvements in severe onchocercal skin disease after a single dose of ivermectin. *Am J Med* 1991; **90:** 590–4.
17. Greene BM, *et al.* A comparison of 6-, 12-, and 24-monthly dosing with ivermectin for treatment of onchocerciasis. *J Infect Dis* 1991; **163:** 376–80.
18. Churchill DR, *et al.* A trial of a three-dose regimen of ivermectin for the treatment of patients with onchocerciasis in the UK. *Trans R Soc Trop Med Hyg* 1994; **88:** 242.
19. Greene BM. Modern medicine versus an ancient scourge: progress toward control of onchocerciasis. *J Infect Dis* 1992; **166:** 15–21.

Scabies and pediculosis. Scabies is usually treated with a topically applied acaricide (p.1401). However, a single oral dose of ivermectin has been reported to be effective.[1,2] In a study of 11 patients with uncomplicated scabies, a single oral dose of ivermectin 200 μg per kg body-weight was effective in curing infection after 4 weeks. In a group of 11 patients, also infected with the human immunodeficiency virus, scabies was cured in 8 patients after 2 weeks.[1] Two of the remaining 3 patients received a second dose of ivermectin which cured the scabies infection by the fourth week. Crusted (Norwegian) scabies has also been reported to be effectively treated by a single oral dose of 12 mg of ivermectin in addition to topical application of 3% salicylic acid ointment in 2 patients; the treatment was effective in under one week.[2]

Ivermectin has also been investigated as a possible treatment for pediculosis, although again, topically applied insecticides are the usual method of control (see p.1401). A study *in vitro* and in *animals* showed that ivermectin killed nymphs and females of the human body louse (*Pediculus humanus humanus*). Ivermectin was known to be effective against other louse species that infect a range of *animals*.[3]

1. Meinking TL, *et al.* The treatment of scabies with ivermectin. *N Engl J Med* 1995; **333:** 26–30.
2. Aubin F, Humbert P. Ivermectin for crusted (Norwegian) scabies. *N Engl J Med* 1995; **332:** 612.
3. Mumcuoglu KY, *et al.* Systemic activity of ivermectin on the human body louse (Anoplura: Pediculidae). *J Med Entomol* 1990; **27:** 72–5.

Strongyloidiasis. Ivermectin is effective in the treatment of strongyloidiasis (p.95) and is considered by some authorities to be the drug of choice.

References.

1. Naquira C, *et al.* Ivermectin for human strongyloidiasis and other intestinal helminths. *Am J Trop Med Hyg* 1989; **40:** 304–9.
2. Wijesundera M de S, Sanmuganathan PS. Ivermectin therapy in chronic strongyloidiasis. *Trans R Soc Trop Med Hyg* 1992; **86:** 291.
3. Lyagoubi M, *et al.* Chronic persistent strongyloidiasis cured by ivermectin. *Trans R Soc Trop Med Hyg* 1992; **86:** 541.
4. Datry A, *et al.* Treatment of Strongyloides stercoralis infection with ivermectin compared with albendazole: results of an open study of 60 cases. *Trans R Soc Trop Med Hyg* 1994; **88:** 344–5.
5. Gann PH, *et al.* A randomized trial of single- and two-dose ivermectin versus thiabendazole for treatment of strongyloidiasis. *J Infect Dis* 1994; **169:** 1076–9.

Preparations

Proprietary Preparations (details are given in Part 3)
Austral.: Stromectol; ***Fr.:*** Mectizan; ***USA:*** Mectizan; Stromectol.

Levamisole Hydrochloride (788-x)

Levamisole Hydrochloride *(BANM, USAN, rINNM).*

Cloridrato de Levamizol; ICI-59623; Levamisoli Hydrochloridum; NSC-177023; R-12564; RP-20605; *l*-Tetramisole Hydrochloride; *l*-Tetramisole Hydrochloride. (−)-(S)-2,3,5,6-Tetrahydro-6-phenylimidazo[2,1-*b*]thiazole hydrochloride.

$C_{11}H_{12}N_2S,HCl = 240.8.$

CAS — 14769-73-4 (levamisole); 16595-80-5 (levamisole hydrochloride).

Pharmacopoeias. In *Chin., Eur.* (see p.viii), and *US.*

A white to almost white crystalline powder. Levamisole hydrochloride 1.18 g is approximately equivalent to 1 g of levamisole. Freely **soluble** in water; soluble in alcohol; practically insoluble in ether; slightly soluble in dichloromethane. A 5% solution has a pH of 3.0 to 4.5. **Protect** from light.

Adverse Effects

When given in single doses for the treatment of ascariasis or other worm infections, levamisole is generally well tolerated and side-effects are usually limited to nausea, vomiting, diarrhoea, abdominal pain, dizziness, and headache.

When levamisole is used as an immunostimulant and given for longer periods, adverse effects are more frequent and diverse and, in common with other immunomodulators, may sometimes result from exacerbation of the primary underlying disease. Adverse effects associated especially with the more prolonged administration of levamisole have included: hypersensitivity reactions such as fever, an influenza-like syndrome, arthralgia, muscle pain, skin rashes, and cutaneous vasculitis; central nervous system effects including headache, insomnia, dizziness, and convulsions; haematological abnormalities such as agranulocytosis, leucopenia, and thrombocytopenia; and gastro-intestinal disturbances, including an abnormal taste in the mouth.

A review from the manufacturers of 46 controlled studies in which 2635 cancer patients received adjuvant levamisole treatment.[1] Most patients received levamisole on 3 consecutive days every 2 weeks (1102 patients) or on 2 consecutive days every week (1156 patients), usually in a daily dose of 150 mg. Levamisole can cause several side-effects, such as skin rash, nausea, vomiting, and a metallic or bitter taste in the mouth, which although troublesome are relatively trivial and may regress during therapy or disappear on cessation of therapy. A total of 38 patients developed agranulocytosis and of these 36 had received weekly treatment. Several contracted possible life-threatening infections and 2 died of septic shock.

1. Amery WK, Butterworth BS. Review/commentary: the dosage regimen of levamisole in cancer: is it related to efficacy and safety? *Int J Immunopharmacol* 1983; **5:** 1–9.

Effects on the endocrine system. Rechallenge confirmed that levamisole was responsible for inappropriate antidiuretic hormone syndrome in a patient receiving levamisole with fluorouracil.[1]

1. Tweedy CR, *et al.* Levamisole-induced syndrome of inappropriate antidiuretic hormone. *N Engl J Med* 1992; **326:** 1164.

Effects on the liver. Elevated aspartate aminotransferase concentrations in 2 of 11 patients given levamisole for recurrent pyoderma suggested liver toxicity, a very rarely occurring side-effect.[1] More recently, liver enzyme concentrations were reported to be raised in a 14-year-old boy treated with levamisole for minimal change nephrotic syndrome.[2]

1. Papageorgiou P, *et al.* Levamisole in chronic pyoderma. *J Clin Lab Immunol* 1982; **8:** 121–7.
2. Bulugahapitiya DTD. Liver toxicity in a nephrotic patient treated with levamisole. *Arch Dis Child* 1997; **76:** 289.

Effects on the nervous system. Reports[1,2] of inflammatory leucoencephalopathy were associated with the use of fluorouracil and levamisole in 4 patients being treated for adenocarcinoma of the colon. Active demyelination was demonstrated in 2 patients.[1] Clinical improvement occurred when chemotherapy was stopped; three patients were treated with corticosteroids.[1] A similar syndrome has been reported in a patient with a history of hepatitis C who received levamisole alone.[3]

1. Hook CC, *et al.* Multifocal inflammatory leukoencephalopathy with 5-fluorouracil and levamisole. *Ann Neurol* 1992; **31:** 262–7.
2. Kimmel DW, Schutt AJ. Multifocal leukoencephalopathy: occurrence during 5-fluorouracil and levamisole therapy and resolution after discontinuation of chemotherapy. *Mayo Clin Proc* 1993; **68:** 363–5.
3. Lucia P, *et al.* Multifocal leucoencephalopathy induced by levamisole. *Lancet* 1996; **348:** 1450.

Precautions

The use of levamisole should be avoided in patients with pre-existing blood disorders. Patients receiving levamisole in combination with fluorouracil should undergo appropriate monitoring of haematological and hepatic function.

Agranulocytosis. The presence of HLA B27 in seropositive rheumatoid arthritis is an important predisposing factor to the development of agranulocytosis during treatment with levamisole; it is recommended that the use of levamisole in this group should be avoided.[1]

1. Mielants H, Veys EM. A study of the hematological side effects of levamisole in rheumatoid arthritis with recommendations. *J Rheumatol* 1978; **5** (suppl 4): 77–83.

Sjögren's syndrome. The appearance of side-effects in 9 of 10 patients with rheumatoid arthritis and Sjögren's syndrome while being treated with levamisole led to abandonment of the study.[1] Levamisole should be given with caution, if at all, to patients with Sjögren's syndrome.

1. Balint G, *et al.* Sjögren's syndrome: a contraindication to levamisole treatment? *Br Med J* 1977; **2:** 1386–7.

Interactions

The US manufacturer reports that levamisole can produce a disulfiram-like reaction with alcohol.

Increased plasma-phenytoin concentrations have been observed in patients taking phenytoin with levamisole and fluorouracil (see under Phenytoin, p.356). For an increase in warfarin's activity when given with levamisole and fluorouracil, see p.969.

Pharmacokinetics

Levamisole is rapidly absorbed from the gastro-intestinal tract. Maximum plasma concentrations are attained within 1.5 to 4 hours. It is extensively metabolised in the liver. The plasma half-life for levamisole is 3 to 4 hours and for the metabolites is 16 hours. It is excreted mainly in the urine as metabolites and a small proportion in the faeces. About 70% of the administered dose is excreted in the urine over 3 days, with about 5% as unchanged levamisole.

Some studies of the pharmacokinetics of levamisole.[1,2]

1. Kouassi E, *et al.* Novel assay and pharmacokinetics of levamisole and p-hydroxylevamisole in human plasma and urine. *Biopharm Drug Dispos* 1986; **7:** 71–89.
2. Luyckx M, *et al.* Pharmacokinetics of levamisole in healthy subjects and cancer patients. *Eur J Drug Metab Pharmacokinet* 1982; **7:** 247–54.

Uses and Administration

Levamisole hydrochloride is the active laevo-isomer of tetramisole hydrochloride. It is used as an anthelmintic and as an adjuvant in malignant disease. It has also been tried in several conditions where its stimulant effect on the depressed immune response might be useful.

Levamisole is active against intestinal nematode worms and appears to act by paralysing susceptible worms which are subsequently eliminated from the intestines. In particular, levamisole is effective in the treatment of ascariasis (p.92). It is also used in hookworm infections (p.94).

Doses of levamisole hydrochloride are expressed in terms of the equivalent amount of levamisole. The usual dose in ascariasis is 150 mg of levamisole by mouth as a single dose; children have been given 3 mg per kg body-weight as a single dose. For the hookworm infection ancylostomiasis or for mixed ascariasis-hookworm infections, 300 mg is given over 1 or 2 days; children have been given 6 mg per kg over 1 to 2 days. Another dose schedule widely used for ascariasis and hookworm infections in both adults and children is 2.5 mg per kg as a single dose, repeated after 7 days in cases of severe hookworm infection.

Levamisole affects the immune response. The term 'immunostimulant' has often been used; it is appropriate only in so far as restoration of a depressed response is concerned; stimulation above normal levels does not seem to occur. Levamisole influences host defences by modulating cell-mediated immune responses; it restores depressed T-cell functions. Levamisole has been tried in a wide variety of disorders involving the immune response, including bacterial and viral infections and rheumatic disorders, although in these conditions results have not been encouraging.

It is also used as an adjunct in patients with malignant disease, although it is not clear that any response is due to levamisole's action on the immune system. Recurrences of adenocarcinoma of the colon inhibited by adjuvant treatment with levamisole and fluorouracil following resection of tumours with regional lymph node involvement. A suggested dose is levamisole 50 mg by mouth every 8 hours for 3 days starting 7 to 30 days after surgery and this treatment course is repeated every 14 days. Fluorouracil is administered concurrently, but not starting until 21 to 34 days after surgery (i.e. if the first course of levamisole is given within 20 days of surgery, fluorouracil therapy is started with the second course of levamisole).

Reviews.

1. Janssen PAJ. The levamisole story. *Prog Drug Res* 1976; **20:** 347–83.
2. Renoux G. The general immunopharmacology of levamisole. *Drugs* 1980; **20:** 89–99.
3. Amery WKP, Bruynseels JPJM. Levamisole, the story and the lessons. *Int J Immunopharmacol* 1992; **14:** 481–6.

Behçet's syndrome. Levamisole is one of the many drugs that have been tried in the treatment of Behçet's syndrome although it is not one of the preferred treatments (see p.1018). There have been reports of individual patients with Behçet's syndrome improving on levamisole treatment.[1]

See also under Mouth Ulceration, below.

1. Lavery HA, Pinkerton JHM. Successful treatment of Behcet's syndrome with levamisole., *Br J Dermatol* 1985; **113:** 372–3.

Malignant neoplasms. Levamisole has been tried in the adjuvant treatment of various malignant neoplasms[1,2] with conflicting results. Attention has concentrated on its use in adenocarcinoma of the colon as a result of a study that indicated that it might be beneficial if given together with fluorouracil shortly after surgery.[3] Further investigation demonstrated that adjuvant treatment with both compounds could reduce the incidence of recurrence and, at least within the 3.5 years of the study, increase survival.[4] Follow-up for a median of 6.5 years confirmed these results.[5] This benefit was demonstrated in patients with resectable adenocarcinoma of the colon where there was regional lymph node involvement (stage C). Patients with tumours classified as stage B_2 where invasion extended to serosa or pericolonic fat were also studied,[4] but more time needed to pass before the results could be interpreted. The treatment of colon cancer is discussed on p.487 where the US recommendation is given that patients with stage C colon cancer should receive adjuvant fluorouracil and levamisole therapy.

How levamisole exerts its effect is unclear. Its effect on the immune system may not necessarily be involved.[4] Also it is ineffective when given alone to patients with stage C disease.[4-6]

1. Spreafico F. Use of levamisole in cancer patients. *Drugs* 1980; **20:** 105–16.
2. Amery WK, Butterworth BS. Review/commentary: the dosage regimen of levamisole in cancer: is it related to efficacy and safety? *Int J Immunopharmacol* 1983; **5:** 1–9.
3. Laurie JA, *et al.* Surgical adjuvant therapy of large-bowel carcinoma: an evaluation of levamisole and the combination of levamisole and fluorouracil: the North Central Cancer Treatment Group and the Mayo Clinic. *J Clin Oncol* 1989; **7:** 1447–56.
4. Moertel CG, *et al.* Levamisole and fluorouracil for adjuvant therapy of resected colon carcinoma. *N Engl J Med* 1990; **322:** 352–8.
5. Moertel CG, *et al.* Fluorouracil plus levamisole as effective adjuvant therapy after resection of stage III colon carcinoma: a final report. *Ann Intern Med* 1995; **122:** 321–6.
6. Chlebowski RT, *et al.* Long-term survival following levamisole or placebo adjuvant treatment of colorectal cancer: a Western Cancer Study Group trial. *Oncology* 1988; **45:** 141–3.

Mansonella infections. Levamisole is one of the drugs that has been suggested for the treatment of *Mansonella* infections (p.95). It has been given with mebendazole and there have been reports[1,2] of patients responding.

1. Maertens K, Wery M. Effect of mebendazole and levamisole on Onchocerca volvulus and Dipetalonema perstans. *Trans R Soc Trop Med Hyg* 1975; **69:** 359–60.
2. Bernberg HC, *et al.* The combined treatment with levamisole and mebendazole for a perstans-like filarial infection in Rhodesia. *Trans R Soc Trop Med Hyg* 1979; **73:** 233–4.

Mouth ulceration. Levamisole might be beneficial in severe mouth ulceration (p.1172) but is limited by its adverse effects. In reviewing levamisole in recurrent aphthous stomatitis, Miller[1] observed that beneficial results have been reported with levamisole in open studies, but results of double-blind studies have been conflicting. Nevertheless Miller reported that there have been patients with severe recurrent aphthous stomatitis refractory to all other modes of treatment who have responded to levamisole. Dosage has been with 150 mg daily in divided doses given for 3 days at the first sign of ulceration, followed by 11 days without treatment, repeated as necessary.

1. Miller MF. Use of levamisole in recurrent aphthous stomatitis. *Drugs* 1980; **20:** 131–6.

Renal disorders. In a randomised double-blind study, children with frequently relapsing corticosteroid-sensitive and corticosteroid-dependent nephrotic syndrome were given placebo or levamisole 2.5 mg per kg body-weight on alternate days and steroid therapy was gradually withdrawn.[1] Of 31 children being treated with levamisole 14 were still in remission 112 days after the start of the study compared with 4 of 30 receiving placebo. For a discussion of the treatment of glomerular kidney disorders, including the nephrotic syndrome, see p.1021.

1. British Association for Paediatric Nephrology. Levamisole for corticosteroid-dependent nephrotic syndrome in childhood. *Lancet* 1991; **337:** 1555–7.

Vitiligo. Pasridia and Khera[1] have reported that levamisole can halt the progression of vitiligo (hypopigmentation). In their study, 34 out of 36 patients with limited slow-spreading disease responded to treatment within 2 to 4 months. Patients received 150 mg of oral levamisole daily on 2 consecutive days each week. Patients who were additionally treated with topical fluocinolone or clobetasol had higher rates of repigmentation.

The more usual treatment of vitiligo is discussed under Pigmentation Disorders, p.1075.

1. Pasricha JS, Khera V. Effect of prolonged treatment with levamisole on vitiligo with limited and slow-spreading disease. *Int J Dermatol* 1994; **33:** 584–7.

Preparations

USP 23: Levamisole Hydrochloride Tablets.

Proprietary Preparations (details are given in Part 3)
Austral.: Ergamisol; ***Belg.:*** Ergamisol; ***Canad.:*** Ergamisol; ***Fr.:*** Solaskil; ***Ger.:*** Ergamisol; ***Irl.:*** Ketrax; ***Ital.:*** Ergamisol; Immunol†; ***Neth.:*** Ergamisol; ***S.Afr.:*** Ergamisol; ***UK:*** Ketrax; ***USA:*** Ergamisol.

Male Fern (790-j)

Aspidium; Farnwurzel; Felce Maschio; Feto Macho; Filix Mas; Fougère Mâle; Helecho Macho; Rhizoma Filicis Maris.

The rhizome, frond-bases, and apical bud of *Dryopteris filix-mas* agg. (Polypodiaceae), collected late in the autumn, divested of the roots and dead portions and carefully dried, retaining the internal green colour. It contains not less than 1.5% of filicin. During storage the green colour of the interior gradually disappears, often after a lapse of 6 months, and such material is unfit for medicinal use. The BPC 1973 extract should be **stored** in airtight containers, protected from light.

Filicin is the mixture of ether-soluble substances obtained from male fern. Its activity is chiefly due to flavaspidic acid, a phloroglucinol derivative.

Male fern has anthelmintic properties and was formerly administered as male fern extract (aspidium oleoresin) for the expulsion of tapeworms. However, male fern is highly toxic and has been superseded by other drugs.

Adverse effects include headache, nausea and vomiting, severe abdominal cramp, diarrhoea, dyspnoea, albuminuria, hyperbilirubinaemia, dizziness, tremors, convulsions, visual disturbances including blindness (possibly permanent), stimulation of uterine muscle, coma, respiratory failure, bradycardia, and cardiac failure. Fatalities have occurred.

Preparations

Proprietary Preparations (details are given in Part 3)

Multi-ingredient: ***Aust.:*** Digestodoron; ***Fr.:*** Digestodoron; ***Ger.:*** Discmigon; ***UK:*** Digestodoron.

Mebendazole (791-z)

Mebendazole *(BAN, USAN, rINN)*.

Mebendazolum; R-17635. Methyl 5-benzoyl-1*H*-benzimidazol-2-ylcarbamate.

$C_{16}H_{13}N_3O_3$ = 295.3.

CAS — 31431-39-7.

Pharmacopoeias. In *Chin., Eur.* (see p.viii), *Int., Pol.,* and *US.*

A white to slightly yellow almost odourless powder. Practically **insoluble** in water, in alcohol, in chloroform, in dichloromethane, in ether, and in dilute mineral acids; freely soluble in formic acid. **Protect** from light.

Adverse Effects

Since mebendazole is poorly absorbed from the gastro-intestinal tract at the usual therapeutic doses, side-effects have generally been restricted to gastro-intestinal disturbances, such as transient abdominal pain and diarrhoea, and have tended to occur in patients being treated for heavy intestinal infection. Headache and dizziness have been reported. Adverse effects have been reported more frequently with the high doses tried in echinococcosis and have included allergic reactions, raised liver enzyme values, alopecia, and bone marrow depression.

In the first phase[1] of WHO-coordinated multicentre studies on the treatment of echinococcosis (hydatid disease) involving *Echinococcus granulosus* or *E. multilocularis*, the most frequent adverse effects in the 139 patients given *high-dose* mebendazole generally for 3 months were reduced leucocyte count (25), gastro-intestinal symptoms (22), and raised serum-transaminase values (22). Other adverse effects were allergic conditions such as fever and skin reactions (4), CNS symptoms including headache (6), and loss of hair (7). Seven patients stopped treatment because of side-effects.

The second phase of studies[2] compared albendazole with mebendazole in more prolonged high-dosage schedules for cystic *E. granulosus* infection. Adverse effects were similar to those reported with the first phase. However, in the first phase the allergic consequences of the 14 ruptured lung cysts and the 4 ruptured liver cysts that occurred with mebendazole were not reported. In the second phase 2 patients suffered anaphylactic shock as a result of rupture of a lung cyst and a cyst in the abdominal cavity. These 2 patients were withdrawn from mebendazole treatment as were another 4 patients as a consequence of their adverse reactions, although in 3 the withdrawal was only temporary.

Although albendazole is preferred to mebendazole in the treatment of echinococcosis, if either agent is used, then there should be constant medical supervision with regular monitoring of serum-transaminase concentrations and of leucocyte and platelet counts. Patients with liver damage should be treated with reduced doses of benzimidazole carbamates, if at all.[2]

1. Davis A, *et al.* Multicentre clinical trials of benzimidazolecarbamates in human echinococcosis. *Bull WHO* 1986; **64:** 383–8.
2. Davis A, *et al.* Multicentre clinical trials of benzimidazolecarbamates in human cystic echinococcosis (phase 2). *Bull WHO* 1989; **67:** 503–8.

Overdosage. Respiratory arrest and tachyarrhythmia associated with continuous convulsions were reported[1] in an 8-week- old infant following accidental poisoning with mebendazole. Treatment by exchange transfusion and anticonvulsants was successful.

1. el Kalla S, Menon NS. Mebendazole poisoning in infancy. *Ann Trop Paediatr* 1990; **10:** 313–14.

Precautions

Mebendazole is teratogenic in *rats* (see Pregnancy and Breast Feeding, below).

Patients receiving high doses of mebendazole, such as those with echinococcosis, should be supervised closely with blood counts and liver function being monitored.

Monitoring drug concentrations. In a retrospective analysis of patients who had received high doses of mebendazole for echinococcosis,[1] no relationship was found between dose and plasma concentration of mebendazole and considerable intra- and interindividual variation in plasma concentrations was observed, emphasising the need for repeated monitoring. Several patients appeared to have what were considered to be subtherapeutic plasma concentrations.

1. Luder PJ, *et al.* Treatment of hydatid disease with high oral doses of mebendazole: long-term follow-up of plasma mebendazole levels and drug interactions. *Eur J Clin Pharmacol* 1986; **31:** 443–8.

Pregnancy and breast feeding. Mebendazole is teratogenic in *rats* and the manufacturers in the UK have stated that it is contra-indicated in pregnant women, including those who are thought to be or may be pregnant. In the USA the manufacturers, while not recommending mebendazole for pregnant patients, have stated that if it is used in pregnancy, especially during the first trimester, then such use should only be where the potential benefit justifies the risk to the fetus; this is in accord with mebendazole being classified in FDA pregnancy category C. They noted that where they had evidence of mebendazole being used by pregnant women, including those in their first trimester, then the incidence of malformations and spontaneous abortions was no greater than that observed in the general population.

It is not known whether distribution into breast milk occurs.

Interactions

The concomitant administration of *phenytoin* or *carbamazepine* has been reported to lower plasma-mebendazole concentrations in patients receiving high doses for echinococcosis, presumably as a result of enzyme induction; *valproate* had no such effect.[1] Plasma concentrations of mebendazole have been raised when the enzyme inhibitor *cimetidine* has been given concomitantly, and there has been a report of this effect resulting in the resolution of previously unresponsive hepatic hydatid cysts.[2]

1. Luder PJ, *et al.* Treatment of hydatid disease with high oral doses of mebendazole: long-term follow-up of plasma mebendazole levels and drug interactions. *Eur J Clin Pharmacol* 1986; **31:** 443–8.
2. Bekhti A, Pirotte J. Cimetidine increases serum mebendazole concentrations: implications for treatment of hepatic hydatid cysts. *Br J Clin Pharmacol* 1987; **24:** 390–2.

Pharmacokinetics

Mebendazole is poorly absorbed from the gastro-intestinal tract and undergoes extensive first-pass elimination, being metabolised in the liver, eliminated in the bile as unchanged drug and metabolites, and excreted in the faeces. Only about 2% of a dose is excreted unchanged or as metabolites in the urine. Mebendazole is highly protein bound.

Bioavailability. It has been suggested[1] that the poor bioavailability of mebendazole observed at therapeutic dose levels is due to a combination of high first-pass elimination and the very low solubility of the compound. Modification of the dose form rather than administration of large doses may be a more rational method of increasing plasma concentrations in the treatment of extra-intestinal infections.[1]

1. Dawson M, *et al.* The pharmacokinetics and bioavailability of a tracer dose of [^{3}H]-mebendazole in man. *Br J Clin Pharmacol* 1985; **19:** 79–86.

Uses and Administration

Mebendazole, a benzimidazole carbamate derivative, is an anthelmintic with activity against most nematodes and some other worms; activity against some larval stages and ova has also been demonstrated. Mebendazole's anthelmintic activity is considered to be dependent on the inhibition or destruction of cytoplasmic microtubules in the worm's intestinal or absorptive cells. Inhibition of glucose uptake and depletion of glycogen stores follow as do other inhibitory effects leading to death of the worm within several days.

Mebendazole, being poorly absorbed from the gastro-intestinal tract, is used principally in the treatment of the intestinal nematode infections ascariasis (roundworm infection), enterobiasis (pinworm or threadworm infections), hookworm infections (ancylostomiasis and necatoriasis), and trichuriasis (whipworm infection); it is useful in mixed infections. During treatment with mebendazole, migration of worms with expulsion through the mouth and nose has occurred in some patients heavily infected with *Ascaris*. Mebendazole is also used in the treatment of capillariasis and trichostrongyliasis and has been used in strongyloidiasis. Other nematode infections which may respond to mebendazole are infection with the filarial nematode *Mansonella perstans*, the tissue infections toxocariasis and trichinosis, and infections with the primary animal parasites *Angiostrongylus spp*. Mebendazole has also been tried in high doses in the treatment of echinococcosis (hydatid disease). For discussions of these infections and their treatment, see under Choice of Anthelmintic, p.92. See also below.

Mebendazole is given by mouth. The usual dose for adults and children aged over 2 years with enterobiasis is 100 mg as a single dose, repeated if necessary after 2 to 3 weeks; for ascariasis, hookworm infections, and trichuriasis the usual dose is 100 mg twice daily for 3 days, although a single dose of 500 mg may be effective.

Angiostrongyliasis. Mebendazole has been used for the treatment of angiostrongyliasis (p.92). A suggested dose for infections with *Angiostrongylus cantonensis* is 100 mg twice daily for 5 days. For those due to *A. costaricensis* a higher dose of 200 to 400 mg three times daily for 10 days has been suggested.[1]

1. Anonymous. Drugs for parasitic infections. *Med Lett Drugs Ther* 1998; **40:** 1–12.

Capillariasis. Mebendazole in a dose of 200 mg twice daily for 20 days has been suggested[1] for the treatment of capillariasis (p.93).

1. Anonymous. Drugs for parasitic infections. *Med Lett Drugs Ther* 1998; **40:** 1–12.

Echinococcosis. Mebendazole has been used in echinococcosis,[1-6] but albendazole is generally preferred (see p.94). The usual dose of mebendazole in cystic echinococcosis is 40 to 50 mg per kg body-weight daily for at least 3 to 6 months.[7] A similar dose is used as an adjuvant to surgery. For alveolar echinococcosis, the dose is adjusted after 4 weeks to produce a plasma concentration of at least 250 nmol per litre (74 ng per mL), although adults should not receive more than 6g daily. Treatment is continued for at least 2 years following radical surgery, or indefinitely in inoperable cases.

1. Ammann RW, *et al.* Recurrence rate after discontinuation of long-term mebendazole therapy in alveolar echinococcosis (preliminary results). *Am J Trop Med Hyg* 1990; **43:** 506–15.
2. Messaritakis J, *et al.* High mebendazole doses in pulmonary and hepatic hydatid disease. *Arch Dis Child* 1991; **66:** 532–3.
3. Teggi A, *et al.* Therapy of human hydatid disease with mebendazole and albendazole. *Antimicrob Agents Chemother* 1993; **37:** 1679–84.
4. Göçmen A, *et al.* Treatment of hydatid disease in childhood with mebendazole. *Eur Respir J* 1993; **6:** 253–7.
5. Ammann RW, *et al.* Effect of chemotherapy on the larval mass and the long-term course of alveolar echinococcosis. *Hepatology* 1994; **19:** 735–42.
6. Erdinçler P, *et al.* The role of mebendazole in the surgical treatment of central nervous system hydatid disease. *Br J Neurosurg* 1997; **11:** 116–20.

7. WHO Informal Working Group on Echinococcosis. Guidelines for treatment of cystic and alveolar echinococcosis in humans. *Bull WHO* 1996; **74:** 231–42.

Giardiasis. Some patients with giardiasis (p.575) are reported to have responded to mebendazole.[1] However, when mebendazole was compared with metronidazole in a controlled study of patients with giardiasis, the response to mebendazole was not encouraging with a dose of 600 mg given in 3 divided doses over one day.[2] Another report[3] was also not encouraging although it suggested mebendazole might be more effective in children.

1. Al-Waili NS, *et al.* Therapeutic use of mebendazole in giardial infections. *Trans R Soc Trop Med Hyg* 1988; **82:** 438.
2. Gascón J, *et al.* Failure of mebendazole treatment in Giardia lamblia infection. *Trans R Soc Trop Med Hyg* 1989; **83:** 647.
3. Gascón J, *et al.* Mebendazole and metronidazole in giardial infections. *Trans R Soc Trop Med Hyg* 1990; **84:** 694.

Mansonella infections. Mebendazole is one of the drugs that has been suggested for the treatment of infections with *Mansonella perstans* (p.95). Some patients have responded to mebendazole with levamisole[1,2] or to mebendazole alone.[3]

1. Maertens K, Wery M. Effect of mebendazole and levamisole on Onchocerca volvulus and Dipetalonema perstans. *Trans R Soc Trop Med Hyg* 1975; **69:** 359–60.
2. Bernberg HC, *et al.* The combined treatment with levamisole and mebendazole for a perstans-like filarial infection in Rhodesia. *Trans R Soc Trop Med Hyg* 1979; **73:** 233–4.
3. Wahlgren M, Frolov I. Treatment of Dipetalonema perstans infections with mebendazole. *Trans R Soc Trop Med Hyg* 1983; **77:** 422–3.

Strongyloidiasis. Mebendazole has been used for the treatment of strongyloidiasis (p.95), but needs to be given for longer periods than albendazole to control auto-infection, so that of the two benzimidazole carbamates, albendazole is preferred.[1-3]

1. Wilson KH, Kauffman CA. Persistent Strongyloides stercoralis in a blind loop of the bowel: successful treatment with mebendazole. *Arch Intern Med* 1983; **143:** 357–8.
2. Mravak S, *et al.* Treatment of strongyloidiasis with mebendazole. *Acta Trop (Basel)* 1983; **40:** 93–4.
3. Pelletier LL, Baker CB. Treatment failures following mebendazole therapy for chronic strongyloidiasis. *J Infect Dis* 1987; **156:** 532–3.

Syngamosis. Mebendazole has been used successfully[1] to treat syngamosis (p.96).

1. Timmons RF, *et al.* Infection of the respiratory tract with Mammomanogamus (Syngamus) laryngeus: a new case in Largo, Florida, and a summary of previously reported cases. *Am Rev Respir Dis* 1983; **128:** 566–9.

Toxocariasis. Mebendazole has been used in the treatment of toxocariasis (p.96). Magnaval and Charlet[1] reported that mebendazole produced similar improvement to that obtained with thiabendazole but with a lower incidence of adverse effects.

1. Magnaval JF, Charlet JP. Efficacité comparée du thiabendazole et du mébendazole dans le traitement de la toxocarose. *Therapie* 1987; **42:** 541–4.

Trichinosis. Mebendazole is used for the treatment of trichinosis and is considered the anthelmintic of choice in some countries (see p.96).

References.

1. Levin ML. Treatment of trichinosis with mebendazole. *Am J Trop Med Hyg* 1983; **32:** 980–3.

Preparations

USP 23: Mebendazole Tablets.

Proprietary Preparations (details are given in Part 3)
Aust.: Pantelmin; ***Austral.:*** Sqworm; Vermox; ***Belg.:*** Vermox; ***Canad.:*** Vermox; ***Ger.:*** Surfont; Vermox; ***Irl.:*** Vermox; ***Ital.:*** Vermox; ***Neth.:*** Madicure; Vermox; ***Norw.:*** Vermox; ***S.Afr.:*** Anthex; Cipex; D-Worm; Vermox; Wormgo; ***Spain:*** Bantenol; Lomper; Mebendan; Oxitover; Sufil; Sulfil†; ***Swed.:*** Vermox; ***Switz.:*** Vermicidin†; Vermox; ***UK:*** Ovex; Pripsen; Vermox; ***USA:*** Vermox.

Metriphonate (3594-e)

Metriphonate *(BAN).*

Metrifonate *(rINN)*; Bayer-L-1359; DETF; Metrifonatum; Trichlorfon *(USAN)*; Trichlorphon. Dimethyl 2,2,2-trichloro-1-hydroxyethylphosphonate.

$C_4H_8Cl_3O_4P$ = 257.4.

CAS — 52-68-6.

Pharmacopoeias. In *Eur.* (see p.viii), *Int.*, and *US.*

A white crystalline powder. M.p. about 78° with decomposition. Freely **soluble** in water, in alcohol, in acetone, in chloroform, and in ether; very soluble in dichloromethane; very slightly soluble in hexane and in pentane. Decomposed by alkali. **Store** at a temperature not exceeding 25°. Protect from light.

CAUTION. *Metriphonate is very toxic when inhaled, swallowed, or spilled on the skin. It can be removed from the skin by washing with soap and water. Contaminated material should be immersed in a 2% aqueous solution of sodium hydroxide for several hours.*

Adverse Effects, Treatment, and Precautions

Metriphonate is generally well tolerated, but may cause nausea, vomiting, abdominal pain, diarrhoea, headache, dizziness, and weakness.

It is an organophosphorus compound and because of its anticholinesterase properties depresses plasma-cholinesterase concentrations. Atropine has been used to relieve cholinergic side-effects without affecting metriphonate's activity against *Schistosoma haematobium.* Patients treated with metriphonate should not be given depolarising muscle relaxants such as suxamethonium for at least 48 hours. The administration of metriphonate should be avoided in those recently exposed to insecticides or other agricultural chemicals with anticholinesterase activity.

For a description of the toxic effects of organophosphorus compounds and the treatment of acute poisoning, see under organophosphorus insecticides (p.1408).

Metriphonate depresses cholinesterase activity and there has been the occasional report of severe cholinergic adverse effects.[1] However, it does not usually give rise to troublesome effects at doses normally employed, even though there may temporarily be almost complete inhibition of plasma cholinesterase and considerable inhibition of erythrocyte cholinesterase[2] (but see also under Alzheimer's Disease, below).

The environmental aspects of metriphonate usage have been considered by WHO.[3]

1. Jamnadas VP, Thomas JEP. Metriphonate and organophosphate poisoning. *Cent Afr J Med* 1979; **25:** 130.
2. Pleština R, *et al.* Effect of metrifonate on blood cholinesterases in children during the treatment of schistosomiasis. *Bull WHO* 1972; **46:** 747–59.
3. Trichlorfon. *Environmental Health Criteria 132.* Geneva: WHO, 1992.

Pregnancy. WHO reported[1] that metriphonate had not shown embryotoxicity or teratogenicity. Despite these negative findings WHO did not recommend the administration of metriphonate to pregnant patients unless immediate intervention was essential. There has been a report of an infant born with massive hydrocephalus and a large meningomyelocele whose mother had been treated twice during the second month of her pregnancy with metriphonate[2] and a possible link between congenital abnormalities and the use of metriphonate to eradicate fish parasites.[3]

1. WHO. The control of schistosomiasis: second report of the WHO expert committee. *WHO Tech Rep Ser 830* 1993.
2. Monson MH, Alexander K. Metrifonate in pregnancy. *Trans R Soc Trop Med Hyg* 1984; **78:** 565.
3. Czeizel AE, *et al.* Environmental trichlorfon and cluster of congenital abnormalities. *Lancet* 1993; **341:** 539–42.

Pharmacokinetics

Metriphonate is absorbed following oral administration and some is converted to dichlorvos which is considered to be the active moiety. Plasma concentrations of dichlorvos are about 1% of those of metriphonate with peak concentrations of both substances occurring within 2 hours. Excretion is via the kidney, mainly as glucuronides.

References.

1. Nordgren I, *et al.* Plasma levels of metrifonate and dichlorvos during treatment of schistosomiasis with Bilarcil. *Am J Trop Med Hyg* 1980; **29:** 426–30.
2. Nordgren I, *et al.* Levels of metrifonate and dichlorvos in plasma and erythrocytes during treatment of schistosomiasis with Bilarcil. *Acta Pharmacol Toxicol* 1981; **49** (suppl V): 79–86.
3. Pettigrew LC, *et al.* Pharmacokinetics, pharmacodynamics, and safety of metrifonate in patients with Alzheimer's disease. *J Clin Pharmacol* 1998; **38:** 236–45.

Uses and Administration

Metriphonate is an organophosphorus compound and is converted in the body to the active metabolite dichlorvos (p.1404), an anticholinesterase.

Metriphonate has anthelmintic activity against *Schistosoma haematobium* and is given by mouth as an alternative to praziquantel in the treatment of schistosomiasis due to *S. haematobium.* It is usually given in three doses of 7.5 to 10 mg of metriphonate per kg body-weight at intervals of 2 weeks.

Metriphonate has also been used as an insecticide and as a parasiticide in fish and domestic animals.

Alzheimer's disease. Metriphonate, like a number of other cholinesterase inhibitors has been tried in the treatment of Alzheimer's disease (p.1386). Studies[1,2] have indicated that it can produce modest benefits. However, clinical studies are reported to have been halted following reports of muscle weakness, sometimes requiring respiratory support.

1. Becker RE, *et al.* Effects of metrifonate on cognitive decline in Alzheimer disease: a double-blind, placebo-controlled, 6-month study. *Alzheimer Dis Assoc Disord* 1998; **12:** 54–7.
2. Morris JC, *et al.* Metrifonate benefits cognitive, behavioral, and global function in patients with Alzheimer's disease. *Neurology* 1998; **50:** 1222–30.

Schistosomiasis. While praziquantel is now the main treatment for schistosomiasis (p.95), metriphonate is an alternative for infection due to *Schistosoma haematobium.*

Metriphonate owes its activity against *S. haematobium* to its metabolite dichlorvos which is a cholinesterase inhibitor; it is not active against other *Schistosoma* spp. The standard dose in the treatment of *S. haematobium* infection is 7.5 to 10 mg per kg body-weight given on 3 occasions at intervals of 2 weeks.[1] Cure rates with this schedule in schistosomiasis control programmes range from 40 to more than 80%, with a reduction of more than 80% in egg counts among those not cured. A comparison with praziquantel showed little difference in response between either drug.[2] However, metriphonate's dosage schedule of 3 doses at intervals of 2 weeks has caused problems of patient compliance.[3] Other dosage schedules have been tried. In one group of trials, the cure rate at 6 months following treatment with 1, 2, or 3 doses was 28, 65, and 84% respectively. Another study showed that 5 mg per kg given three times in one day produced similar results to a standard dosage schedule.[4]

1. WHO. WHO model prescribing information: drugs used in parasitic diseases. Geneva: WHO, 1995.
2. King CH, *et al.* Chemotherapy-based control of schistosomiasis haematobia. I. Metrifonate versus praziquantel in control of intensity and prevalence of infection. *Am J Trop Med Hyg* 1988; **39:** 295–305.
3. Aden Abdi Y, Gustafsson LL. Poor patient compliance reduces the efficacy of metrifonate treatment of Schistosoma haematobium in Somalia. *Eur J Clin Pharmacol* 1989; **36:** 161–4.
4. Aden Abdi Y, Gustafsson LL. Field trial of the efficacy of a simplified and standard metrifonate treatments of Schistosoma haematobium. *Eur J Clin Pharmacol* 1989; **37:** 371–4.

Preparations

Proprietary Preparations (details are given in Part 3)
Ger.: Bilarcil†.

Morantel Tartrate (12977-e)

Morantel Tartrate *(BANM, USAN, pINNM).*

CP-12009-18; UK-2964-18. *(E)*-1,4,5,6-Tetrahydro-1-methyl-2-[2-(3-methyl-2-thienyl)vinyl]pyrimidine hydrogen tartrate.

$C_{12}H_{16}N_2S,C_4H_6O_6$ = 370.4.

CAS — 20574-50-9 (morantel); 26155-31-7 (morantel tartrate).

Morantel is an analogue of pyrantel. The tartrate is used as a veterinary anthelmintic in the treatment of gastro-intestinal roundworms.

Moxidectin (11024-d)

Moxidectin *(BAN, USAN, rINN).*

CL-301423. (6*R*,15*S*)-5-*O*-Demethyl-28-deoxy-25-[(*E*)-1,3-dimethylbut-1-enyl]-6,28-epoxy-23-oxomilbemycin B (*E*)-23-*O*-methyloxime.

$C_{37}H_{53}NO_8$ = 639.8.

CAS — 113507-06-5.

Moxidectin is a milbemycin anthelmintic used in veterinary medicine. It is also used as a systemic veterinary ectoparasiticide.

Netobimin (2190-g)

Netobimin *(BAN, USAN, rINN).*

Sch-32481. 2-{3-Methoxycarbonyl-2-[2-nitro-5-(propylthio)phenyl]guanidino}ethanesulphonic acid.

$C_{14}H_{20}N_4O_7S_2$ = 420.5.

CAS — 88255-01-0.

Netobimin is an anthelmintic used in veterinary medicine.

Niclosamide (793-k)

Niclosamide *(BAN, USAN, rINN).*

Anhydrous Niclosamide; Bay-2353; Niclosamida Anidra; Niclosamidum Anhydricum; Phenasale. 2′,5-Dichloro-4′-nitrosalicylanilide; 5-Chloro-*N*-(2-chloro-4-nitrophenyl)-2-hydroxybenzamide.

$C_{13}H_8Cl_2N_2O_4$ = 327.1.

CAS — 50-65-7.

Pharmacopoeias. In *Chin., Eur.* (see p.viii), *Int.*, and *Pol.*
Int. permits the anhydrous substance or the monohydrate.

Yellowish-white to yellowish, fine crystals. Practically **insoluble** in water; slightly soluble in dehydrated alcohol; sparingly soluble in acetone. **Store** in airtight containers. Protect from light.

Niclosamide Monohydrate (15873-b)

Niclosamide Monohydrate *(BANM)*.

Niclosamida Mono-hidratada; Niclosamidum Monohydricum.

$C_{13}H_8Cl_2N_2O_4,H_2O = 345.1.$

Pharmacopoeias. In *Eur.* (see p.viii).
Int. permits the monohydrate or the anhydrous substance under the title Niclosamide.

Yellowish, fine crystals. Practically **insoluble** in water; slightly soluble in dehydrated alcohol; sparingly soluble in acetone. **Protect** from light.

Adverse Effects

Gastro-intestinal disturbances may occur occasionally with niclosamide. Lightheadedness and pruritus have been reported less frequently.

Pharmacokinetics

Niclosamide is not significantly absorbed from the gastro-intestinal tract.

Uses and Administration

Niclosamide is an anthelmintic which is active against most tapeworms, including the beef tapeworm (*Taenia saginata*), the pork tapeworm (*T. solium*), the fish tapeworm (*Diphyllobothrium latum*), the dwarf tapeworm (*Hymenolepis nana*), and the dog tapeworm (*Dipylidium caninum*). For discussions of the treatment of tapeworm infections see Diphyllobothriasis p.93, Hymenolepiasis p.94, and Taeniasis p.96. Its activity against these worms appears to be due to inhibition of mitochondrial oxidative phosphorylation; anaerobic ATP production is also affected.

Niclosamide is administered in tablets, which must be chewed thoroughly before swallowing and washed down with water.

For infections with pork tapeworm a single 2-g dose is given after a light breakfast. Niclosamide is not active against the larval form (cysticerci) and although the risk of inducing cysticercosis appears to be theoretical, a laxative is given about 2 hours after the dose to expel the killed worms and minimise the possibility of the migration of ova of *T. solium* into the stomach; also an antiemetic may be given before treatment.

For infections with beef or fish tapeworms the 2-g dose of niclosamide may be divided, with 1 g taken after breakfast and 1 g an hour later.

In dwarf-tapeworm infections an initial dose of 2 g is given on the first day followed by 1 g daily for 6 days.

Children aged 2 to 6 years are given half the above doses and those under 2 years of age are given one-quarter the above doses.

Unless expulsion of the worm is aided by a laxative, portions are voided in a partially digested form after treatment with niclosamide; the scolex is rarely identifiable.

Niclosamide is used as a molluscicide for the treatment of water in schistosomiasis control programmes (see p.95).

Preparations

BP 1998: Niclosamide Tablets.

Proprietary Preparations (details are given in Part 3)
Austral.: Yomesan†; ***Belg.:*** Yomesan; ***Fr.:*** Tredemine; ***Ger.:*** Yomesan; ***Ital.:*** Yomesan; ***Neth.:*** Yomesan; ***S.Afr.:*** Yomesan; ***Swed.:*** Yomesan; ***Switz.:*** Yomesane†; ***UK:*** Yomesan; ***USA:*** Niclocide†.

Niridazole (794-a)

Niridazole *(BAN, USAN, rINN)*.

BA-32644; NSC-136947. 1-(5-Nitrothiazol-2-yl)imidazolidin-2-one.

$C_6H_6N_4O_3S = 214.2.$

CAS — 61-57-4.

Pharmacopoeias. In *Fr., Int.*, and *It.*

Adverse Effects

Common side-effects with niridazole include anorexia, nausea, vomiting, diarrhoea, abdominal pain, abnormal taste, dizziness, and headache.

Less frequent, but more serious, are effects on the CNS including insomnia, anxiety, agitation, confusion, hallucinations, and convulsions; they have occurred especially in patients with impaired liver function such as those with severe hepato-intestinal schistosomiasis.

Hypersensitivity reactions have been reported and may be associated with destruction of parasites; they have included skin rashes, fever, and peripheral eosinophilia.

Other adverse effects reported occasionally with niridazole include ECG abnormalities. Impaired spermatogenesis has been reported and it has been shown in *animal* and *in-vitro* studies to have carcinogenic, mutagenic, and embryotoxic effects.

Haemolysis may occur in persons with a deficiency of glucose-6-phosphate dehydrogenase. The urine may be coloured a deep brown because of the presence of niridazole metabolites.

References.

1. Urman HK, *et al.* Carcinogenic effects of niridazole. *Cancer Lett* 1975; **1:** 69–74.
2. El-Beheiry AH, *et al.* Niridazole and fertility in bilharzial men. *Arch Androl* 1982; **8:** 297–300.
3. Abdu-Aguye I, Sambo-Donga L. Influence of dosing interval and in-patient versus out-patient status on incidence of side-effects of niridazole. *Hum Toxicol* 1986; **5:** 275–8.

Uses and Administration

Niridazole is a nitrothiazole derivative that has been given in the treatment of schistosomiasis, but it has been superseded by other drugs.

Preparations

Proprietary Preparations (details are given in Part 3)
Switz.: Ambilhar†.

Nitroscanate (13027-t)

Nitroscanate *(BAN, USAN, rINN)*.

CGA-23654. 4-(4-Nitrophenoxy)phenyl isothiocyanate.

$C_{13}H_8N_2O_3S = 272.3.$

CAS — 19881-18-6.

Nitroscanate is an isothiocyanate anthelmintic used in veterinary practice.

Nitroxynil (13029-r)

Nitroxynil *(BAN)*.

Nitroxinil *(rINN)*. 4-Hydroxy-3-iodo-5-nitrobenzonitrile.

$C_7H_3IN_2O_3 = 290.0.$

CAS — 1689-89-0 (nitroxynil); 27917-82-4 (nitroxynil eglumine).

Pharmacopoeias. In *BP(Vet)*. Also in *Fr.* for veterinary use.

A yellow to yellowish brown powder. Practically **insoluble** in water; slightly soluble in alcohol; sparingly soluble in ether; it dissolves in solutions of alkali hydroxides. **Protect** from light.

Nitroxynil is a veterinary anthelmintic used in the treatment of fascioliasis and some gastro-intestinal roundworms in cattle and sheep. It is also used to treat gapeworm infection (syngamosis) in game birds.

Oxamniquine (795-t)

Oxamniquine *(BAN, USAN, rINN)*.

UK-4271. 1,2,3,4-Tetrahydro-2-isopropylaminomethyl-7-nitro-6-quinolylmethanol.

$C_{14}H_{21}N_3O_3 = 279.3.$

CAS — 21738-42-1.

Pharmacopoeias. In *Fr., Int.*, and *US.*

A yellow-orange crystalline solid. Sparingly **soluble** in water; soluble in acetone, chloroform, and methyl alcohol. A 1% suspension has a pH of 8.0 to 10.0.

Adverse Effects

Oxamniquine caused severe pain at the injection site when administered intramuscularly and is no longer given by this route.

It is generally well tolerated following administration by mouth, although dizziness with or without drowsiness occurs in at least a third of patients, beginning up to 3 hours after a dose and usually lasting for up to 6 hours. Other common side-effects include headache and gastro-intestinal effects such as nausea, vomiting, and diarrhoea.

Allergic-type reactions including urticaria, pruritic skin rashes, and fever may occur. Liver enzyme values have been raised transiently in some patients. Epileptiform convulsions have been reported, especially in patients with a history of convulsive disorders. Hallucinations and excitement have occurred rarely.

A reddish discoloration of urine, probably due to a metabolite of oxamniquine, has been reported.

Effects on body temperature. Although a modest post-treatment rise in temperature has been reported occasionally from several areas, fever is not a common side-effect of oxamniquine, except in Egypt where it appears to be characteristic. The cause is not known. Increased immune complexes and excretion of antigens occurred in only half the cases, there is no evidence that Egyptian patients metabolise the drug differently to produce a pyrogenic metabolite, and the effect has not been seen in other areas where a similar high-dose regimen is used.[1]

1. Foster R. A review of clinical experience with oxamniquine. *Trans R Soc Trop Med Hyg* 1987; **81:** 55–9.

Effects on the nervous system. In 37 patients with *Schistosoma mansoni* infection treated successfully with oxamniquine,[1] dizziness and drowsiness were most common but the only significant adverse effect was the development of EEG abnormalities in 6 of 34 patients whose pre-treatment EEG was normal. Of the 3 patients with pre-existing EEG abnormalities one suffered a grand mal seizure during therapy as previously reported,[2] one did not suffer seizures, and the third received phenytoin prophylaxis during oxamniquine therapy. It was considered prudent to administer anticonvulsant drugs prior to initiating oxamniquine therapy in patients with a history of seizure disorder. Since completion of this study a patient with no history of seizures suffered a grand mal seizure 2 hours after each of the second and third doses of oxamniquine.

The main neuropsychiatric side-effects seen in 180 Brazilian patients with *Schistosoma mansoni* infection treated with single oral doses of oxamniquine were: drowsiness (50.6%), dizziness (41.1%), headache (16.1%), temporary amnesia (2.2%), behavioural disturbances (1.7%), chills (1.1%), and seizures (1.1%).[3] An EEG was performed before and after treatment in 20 patients; there were alterations in 3 but they were not associated with neuropsychiatric changes.

1. Krajden S, *et al.* Safety and toxicity of oxamniquine in the treatment of Schistosoma mansoni infections, with particular reference to electroencephalographic abnormalities. *Am J Trop Med Hyg* 1983; **32:** 1344–6.
2. Keystone JS. Seizures and electroencephalograph changes associated with oxamniquine therapy. *Am J Trop Med Hyg* 1978; **27:** 360–2.
3. de Carvalho SA, *et al.* Neurotoxicidade do oxamniquine no tratamento da infeção humana pelo Schistosoma mansoni. *Rev Inst Med Trop S Paulo* 1985; **27:** 132–42.

Precautions

Oxamniquine should be used with caution in epileptics or patients with a history of epilepsy. Patients should be warned that oxamniquine can cause dizziness or drowsiness and if affected they should not drive or operate machinery.

Pharmacokinetics

Oxamniquine is readily absorbed following administration by mouth. Peak plasma concentrations are achieved 1 to 3 hours after a dose and the plasma half-life is 1 to 2.5 hours.

It is extensively metabolised to inactive metabolites, principally the 6-carboxy derivative, which are excreted in the urine. About 70% of a dose of oxamniquine is excreted as the 6-carboxy metabolite within 12 hours of administration; traces of 2-carboxy metabolite have also been detected in the urine.

Daneshmend and Homeida studied the pharmacokinetics of oxamniquine in Sudanese subjects,[1] including 9 patients with advanced hepatosplenic schistosomiasis and 5 controls, following a single 1-g oral dose. In the 9 patients peak plasma concentrations ranged from 300 to 2252 ng per mL (mean, 1267 ng per mL) 1 to 3 hours after the dose compared with 1205 to 2619 ng per mL (mean, 1983 ng per mL) after 1 to 2 hours in the 5 healthy subjects. Mean plasma half-lives for patients and controls were 151.2 and 111.0 minutes, respectively. There were no significant differences in time to reach peak concentration or plasma half-lives. It seemed that elimination of oxamniquine may be non-linear and, although the mean peak plasma concentration was 36% lower in patients than in controls, the higher dosage requirements noted in Sudanese patients were unlikely to be due to lower plasma concentrations. There was no correlation between severity of the disease and pharmacokinetic values.

1. Daneshmend TK, Homeida MA. Oxamniquine pharmacokinetics in hepatosplenic schistosomiasis in the Sudan. *J Antimicrob Chemother* 1987; **19:** 87–93.

Uses and Administration

Oxamniquine is an anthelmintic used in the treatment of schistosomiasis caused by *Schistosoma mansoni*, but not by other *Schistosoma* spp. It causes worms to shift from the mesenteric veins to the liver where the male worms are retained; the female worms return to the mesentery, but can no longer release eggs. Resistance may occur.

Oxamniquine is given by mouth, preferably after food, in the treatment of schistosomiasis due to *S. mansoni*. Dosage depends on the geographical origin of the infection and total doses range from 15 mg per kg body-weight given as a single dose to 60 mg per kg given over 2 to 3 days. A single dose should not exceed 20 mg per kg.

Schistosomiasis. Oxamniquine is an alternative to praziquantel for the treatment of schistosomiasis (p.95) due to *Schistosoma mansoni*,[1] although resistance has occurred particularly in South America.[2]

The dose ranges between a single dose of 15 mg per kg body-weight and 60 mg per kg given over 2 or 3 days.[1,2] Doses in the low range have been used effectively in South America, the Caribbean, and West Africa while patients in Egypt, South Africa, and Zimbabwe require doses at the top end of the range; intermediate doses may be effective in other parts of Africa.[2]

After the appropriate therapeutic dose of oxamniquine, cure rates of at least 60%, and often more than 90%, can be expected. Egg excretion in those not cured will be reduced by over 80%, and usually by over 90%, one year after treatment.[2]

1. WHO. The control of schistosomiasis: second report of the WHO expert committee. *WHO Tech Rep Ser 830* 1993.
2. WHO. The control of schistosomiasis: report of a WHO expert committee. *WHO Tech Rep Ser 728* 1985.

Preparations

USP 23: Oxamniquine Capsules.

Proprietary Preparations (details are given in Part 3)
Fr.: Vansil†; *UK:* Vansil†; *USA:* Vansil.

Oxantel Embonate (796-x)

Oxantel Embonate *(BANM, rINNM)*.

CP-14445-16; Oxantel Pamoate *(USAN)*. (*E*)-3-[2-(1,4,5,6-Tetrahydro-1-methylpyrimidin-2-yl)vinyl]phenol 4,4′-methylenebis(3-hydroxy-2-naphthoate).

$C_{13}H_{16}N_2O,C_{23}H_{16}O_6$ = 604.6.

CAS — 36531-26-7 (oxantel); 68813-55-8 (oxantel embonate); 42408-84-4 (oxantel embonate).

Oxantel embonate is an analogue of pyrantel embonate formerly used in the treatment of trichuriasis.

Oxfendazole (13060-x)

Oxfendazole *(BAN, USAN, rINN)*.

RS-8858. Methyl 5-phenylsulphinyl-1*H*-benzimidazol-2-ylcarbamate.

$C_{15}H_{13}N_3O_3S$ = 315.3.

CAS — 53716-50-0.

Pharmacopoeias. In *BP(Vet)*. Also in *Fr.* for veterinary use.

A white or almost white powder with a slight characteristic odour. Practically **insoluble** in water; slightly soluble in acetone, in chloroform, in ether, and in methyl alcohol. **Protect** from light.

Oxfendazole is a benzimidazole anthelmintic structurally related to mebendazole (see p.104). It is used in veterinary practice.

Oxibendazole (13062-f)

Oxibendazole *(BAN, USAN, rINN)*.

SKF-30310. Methyl 5-propoxy-1*H*-benzimidazol-2-ylcarbamate.

$C_{12}H_{15}N_3O_3$ = 249.3.

CAS — 20559-55-1.

Oxibendazole is a benzimidazole anthelmintic structurally related to mebendazole (see p.104). It is used in veterinary practice.

Oxyclozanide (13071-d)

Oxyclozanide *(BAN, rINN)*.

ICI-46683. 3,3′,5,5′,6-Pentachloro-2′-hydroxysalicylanilide.

$C_{13}H_6Cl_5NO_3$ = 401.5.

CAS — 2277-92-1.

Pharmacopoeias. In *BP(Vet)*.

A pale cream or cream-coloured, odourless or almost odourless powder. Very slightly **soluble** in water; soluble in alcohol; freely soluble in acetone; slightly soluble in chloroform.

Oxyclozanide is a veterinary anthelmintic used in the control of fascioliasis in cattle and sheep.

Piperazine (13973-z)

$C_4H_{10}N_2$ = 86.14.

CAS — 110-85-0.

Pharmacopoeias. In *US*.

White to off-white lumps or flakes with an ammoniacal odour. M.p. 109° to 113°. Piperazine 44.4 mg is approximately equivalent to 100 mg of piperazine hydrate.

Soluble in water and in alcohol; practically insoluble in ether. **Store** in airtight containers. Protect from light.

Piperazine Adipate (799-d)

Piperaz. Adip.; Piperazini Adipas; Piperazinum Adipicum.

$C_4H_{10}N_2,C_6H_{10}O_4$ = 232.3.

CAS — 142-88-1.

Pharmacopoeias. In *Eur.* (see p.viii), *Int.*, and *Jpn*.

A white crystalline powder. Piperazine adipate 120 mg is approximately equivalent to 100 mg of piperazine hydrate. **Soluble** in water; practically insoluble in alcohol.

Piperazine Citrate (801-n)

Hydrous Tripiperazine Dicitrate; Piperazini Citras.

$(C_4H_{10}N_2)_3,2C_6H_8O_7,xH_2O$ = 642.7 (anhydrous substance).

CAS — 144-29-6 (anhydrous piperazine citrate); 41372-10-5 (piperazine citrate hydrate).

Pharmacopoeias. In *Chin.*, *Eur.* (see p.viii), *Int.*, and *US*.

A white, odourless or almost odourless, crystalline or granular powder. It contains a variable amount of water. Piperazine citrate 125 mg is approximately equivalent to 100 mg of piperazine hydrate; if calculations are based on anhydrous piperazine citrate, then 110 mg is approximately equivalent to 100 mg of piperazine hydrate.

Soluble in water; practically insoluble in alcohol and in ether. A 10% solution in water has a pH of about 5.

A decrease in the content of piperazine [as citrate] in syrups on storage was attributed to interaction with fructose and glucose formed by hydrolysis of sucrose.[1] A syrup prepared with sorbitol lost no potency when stored at 25° for 14 months.

1. Nielsen A, Reimer P. The stability of piperazine in syrup. *Arch Pharm Chemi (Sci)* 1975; **3:** 73–8.

Piperazine Hydrate (802-h)

Piperazini Hydras; Piperazinum Hydricum. Piperazine hexahydrate.

$C_4H_{10}N_2,6H_2O$ = 194.2.

CAS — 142-63-2.

Pharmacopoeias. In *Eur.* (see p.viii).

Colourless deliquescent crystals. M.p. about 43°.

The dosage of the salts of piperazine is usually expressed in terms of piperazine hydrate; 100 mg of piperazine hydrate is approximately equivalent to 44.4 mg of piperazine, to 120 mg of piperazine adipate, to 125 mg of piperazine citrate, and to 104 mg of piperazine phosphate.

Freely **soluble** in water and in alcohol; very slightly soluble in ether. A 5% solution in water has a pH of 10.5 to 12.0. **Store** in airtight containers. Protect from light.

Piperazine Phosphate (803-m)

Piperazini Phosphas.

$C_4H_{10}N_2,H_3PO_4,H_2O$ = 202.1.

CAS — 14538-56-8 (anhydrous piperazine phosphate); 18534-18-4 (piperazine phosphate monohydrate).

Pharmacopoeias. In *Br.*, *Chin.*, and *Jpn*.

A white odourless or almost odourless crystalline powder. Piperazine phosphate 104 mg is approximately equivalent to 100 mg of piperazine hydrate. Sparingly **soluble** in water; practically insoluble in alcohol. A 1% solution in water has a pH of 6.0 to 6.5.

Adverse Effects

Serious adverse effects are rare with piperazine and are generally evidence of overdosage or impaired excretion. Nausea, vomiting, diarrhoea, abdominal pain, headache, skin rashes, and urticaria occasionally occur. Severe neurotoxicity and EEG abnormalities have been reported with symptoms including somnolence, dizziness, nystagmus, muscular incoordination and weakness, ataxia, paraesthesia, myoclonic contractions, choreiform movements, tremor, convulsions, and loss of reflexes.

Transient visual disturbances such as blurred vision have occurred occasionally and there were reports of cataract formation after treatment with piperazine although they do not appear to have been substantiated.

Hypersensitivity reactions such as bronchospasm, Stevens-Johnson syndrome, and angioedema have occurred in some individuals.

Piperazine has been taken off the market in some European countries because of general concern about its safety.[1] A study carried out in Sweden on 2 healthy subjects had indicated that mononitrosation of piperazine can occur in the stomach to produce the potential carcinogen *N*-mononitrosopiperazine; the more potent *N,N*-dinitrosopiperazine was not found.[2] However, the disease risk to man from such *N*-nitroso compounds has been questioned[3] and certainly reports of tumours associated with the use of piperazine have not been traced. Also in the UK the Committee on Review of Medicines (CRM) concluded on reviewing piperazine that the incidence of serious adverse effects was low and that, with appropriate pack warnings, piperazine products could remain as medicines available to the public through pharmacies.[1]

1. Anonymous. Data sheet changes for piperazine in pregnancy. *Pharm J* 1988; **240:** 367.
2. Bellander BTD, *et al.* Nitrosation of piperazine in the stomach. *Lancet* 1981; **ii:** 372.
3. Tannenbaum SR. N-nitroso compounds: a perspective on human exposure. *Lancet* 1983; **i:** 629–32.

Effects on the blood. A 4-year-old African boy with glucose-6-phosphate dehydrogenase deficiency developed haemolytic anaemia.[1] No cause for the haemolysis was found except that 2 days previously he had taken Pripsen (piperazine and senna). Severe thrombocytopenia with epistaxis and haemoptysis which developed in a 61-year-old man after piperazine self-medication was probably the result of sensitisation to piperazine 15 years earlier.[2]

1. Buchanan N, *et al.* G-6-PD deficiency and piperazine. *Br Med J* 1971; **2:** 110.
2. Cork MJ, *et al.* Pruritus ani, piperazine, and thrombocytopenia. *Br Med J* 1990; **301:** 1398.

Effects on the liver. A reaction resembling viral hepatitis occurred on 2 occasions in a 25-year-old woman after the administration of piperazine; it appeared to be a hypersensitivity reaction.[1]

1. Hamlyn AN, *et al.* Piperazine hepatitis. *Gastroenterology* 1976; **70:** 1144–7.

Hypersensitivity. There has been a report[1] of a patient experiencing a serum-sickness-like illness associated with piperazine and this was followed by a delayed hypersensitivity vasculitis.

See also Effects on the Blood and Effects on the Liver, above.

1. Balzan M, Cacciottolo JM. Hypersensitivity vasculitis associated with piperazine therapy. *Br J Dermatol* 1994; **131:** 133–4.

Precautions

Piperazine is contra-indicated in patients with epilepsy or severe renal impairment and should be given with care to patients with neurological disturbances or impaired renal function. It should also be avoided or given with extreme caution in patients with hepatic impairment.

Breast feeding. The UK manufacturers (of Pripsen) report that piperazine is distributed into breast milk. Mothers should be advised to take a dose after breast feeding then not to breast feed for 8 hours during which period milk should be expressed and discarded at the regular feeding times.

Pregnancy. It has been reported that piperazine is teratogenic in *rabbits* and that there have been isolated reports of fetal malformations following clinical use, though no causal relationship has been established. Two infants with malformations have been described briefly:[1] one had bilateral hare lip, cleft palate, and anophthalmia; the other had an abnormality of one foot. Both mothers had taken Pripsen (piperazine with senna). The UK manufacturers of Pripsen advise against use in pregnancy, especially during the first trimester, unless immediate treatment with piperazine is essential.

1. Leach FN. Management of threadworm infestation during pregnancy. *Arch Dis Child* 1990; **65:** 399–400.

Interactions

The anthelmintic effects of piperazine and pyrantel may be antagonised when the two compounds are used together. The possibility that piperazine may enhance the adverse effects of phenothiazines such as chlorpromazine is discussed on p.654.

Pharmacokinetics

Piperazine is readily absorbed from the gastro-intestinal tract and is almost completely excreted in the urine within 24 hours, partly as metabolites. The rate at which different individuals excrete piperazine has been reported to vary widely.

References.

1. Hanna S, Tang A. Human urinary excretion of piperazine citrate from syrup formulations. *J Pharm Sci* 1973; **62:** 2024–5.
2. Bellander BTD, *et al.* Nitrosation of piperazine in the stomach. *Lancet* 1981; **ii:** 372.
3. Fletcher-KA, *et al.* Urinary piperazine excretion in healthy Caucasians. *Ann Trop Med Parasitol* 1982; **76:** 77–82.

Uses and Administration

Piperazine is an anthelmintic effective against the intestinal nematodes *Ascaris lumbricoides* (roundworm) and *Enterobius vermicularis* (pinworm, threadworm) though other anthelmintics are usually preferred (see the discussions on the treatment of ascariasis and enterobiasis on p.92 and p.94). In roundworms piperazine produces a neuromuscular block leading to a flaccid muscle paralysis in susceptible worms which are then easily dislodged from their position by the movement of the gut and are expelled in the faeces.

Piperazine is usually administered as the citrate or phosphate, but the adipate may also be used. Dosage is generally stated in terms of the hexahydrate, piperazine hydrate.

For the treatment of roundworm infection in adults and children over 12 years of age, a single dose equivalent to 4.5 g of piperazine hydrate is given by mouth. Children aged 9 to 12 years may given the equivalent of 3.75 g, those aged 6 to 8 years the equivalent of 3 g, those aged 4 to 5 years the equivalent of 2.25 g, and those aged 1 to 3 years the equivalent of 1.5 g. Children under 1 year should receive piperazine on medical advice only; a dose of 120 mg per kg body-weight has been suggested. The dose is repeated after 14 days.

For elimination of threadworms, treatment is generally given for 7 days. Adults and children over 12 years of age are given the equivalent of 2.25 g of the hydrate once daily, children aged 7 to 12 years the equivalent of 1.5 g daily, those aged 4 to 6 years the equivalent of 1.125 g daily, and those aged 1 to 3 years the equivalent of 750 mg daily. Children under 1 year should receive piperazine on medical advice only; a dose of 45 to 75 mg per kg has been suggested. A second course after a 7-day interval may be required.

Another schedule that is employed for a preparation of piperazine with senna is a single dose of 4 g of the phosphate for adults and children over 6 years of age, repeated after 14 days for threadworm infections, or repeated monthly if necessary for up to 3 months to treat and prevent reinfection with roundworms.

Preparations

BP 1998: Piperazine Citrate Elixir; Piperazine Phosphate Tablets; ***USP 23:*** Piperazine Citrate Syrup; Piperazine Citrate Tablets.

Proprietary Preparations (details are given in Part 3)

Aust.: Tasnon; ***Canad.:*** Entacyl; Veriga; Verimex; Versol; ***Fr.:*** Antelmina; Nematorazine†; Solucamphre; ***Irl.:*** Citrazine; ***Ital.:*** Citropiperazina; Uvilon†; ***S.Afr.:*** Ascarient†; Pip-A-Ray†; Pipralen; Piprine; Wormelix†; ***Spain:*** Ceforcal†; Mimedran; Vermi; ***UK:*** Ectodyne; Expelix†; Pripsen; Worm; Wormex.

Multi-ingredient: ***Belg.:*** Solucamphre; ***Fr.:*** Carudol; Uraseptine Rogier†; Uromil; Vermifuge; ***Irl.:*** Antepar†; Pripsen; ***Spain:*** Thioderazine B1†; ***Switz.:*** Carudol; ***UK:*** Pripsen.

Pomegranate Bark (804-b)

Granado; Granati Cortex; Granatrinde; Granatum; Grenadier; Melograno; Pomegranate; Pomegranate Root Bark; Romeira.

Pharmacopoeias. In *Chin.* which specifies Pomegranate Rind.

The dried bark of the stem and root of *Punica granatum* (Punicaceae) containing about 0.4 to 0.9% of alkaloids. Pomegranate Rind, the dried pericarp separated from the fruit of the pomegranate, contains gallotannic acid but no alkaloids.

Pomegranate bark has been used for the expulsion of tapeworms.

Praziquantel (13161-h)

Praziquantel *(BAN, USAN, rINN)*.

EMBAY-8440; Praziquantelum. 2-Cyclohexylcarbonyl-1,2,3,6,7,11b-hexahydropyrazino[2,1-*a*]isoquinolin-4-one.

$C_{19}H_{24}N_2O_2$ = 312.4.

CAS — 55268-74-1.

Pharmacopoeias. In *Chin., Eur.* (see p.viii), *Int.*, and *US.*

White or practically white crystalline powder; odourless or with a faint characteristic odour. Very slightly **soluble** in water; freely soluble in alcohol, in chloroform, and in dichloromethane. **Protect** from light.

Adverse Effects

Side-effects with praziquantel may be common but they are usually mild and transient. Headache, diarrhoea, dizziness, drowsiness, malaise, abdominal discomfort, nausea, and vomiting have been reported most frequently. Hypersensitivity reactions such as fever, urticaria, pruritic skin rashes, and eosinophilia may occur; they may be due to death of the infecting parasites. Raised liver enzyme values have been reported rarely.

Most patients with neurocysticercosis who are given praziquantel suffer adverse nervous system effects, including headache, hyperthermia, seizures, and intracranial hypertension, which are thought to result from an inflammatory response to dead and dying parasites in the CNS. The concomitant administration of corticosteroids is advised in such patients.

Effects on the gastro-intestinal tract. Colicky abdominal pain and bloody diarrhoea occurred in a small community in Zaire shortly after treatment for *Schistosoma mansoni* infection with single doses of praziquantel 40 mg per kg body-weight by mouth.[1] A similar syndrome has been reported in some patients with *Schistosoma japonicum* infection given praziquantel.[2] The abdominal pain occurring in these patients was very different from the mild abdominal discomfort much more commonly reported with praziquantel therapy.

1. Polderman AM, *et al.* Side effects of praziquantel in the treatment of Schistosoma mansoni in Maniema, Zaire. *Trans R Soc Trop Med Hyg* 1984; **78:** 752–4.
2. Watt G, *et al.* Bloody diarrhoea after praziquantel therapy. *Trans R Soc Trop Med Hyg* 1986; **80:** 345–6.

Effects on the nervous system. Adverse nervous system effects are common in patients with neurocysticercosis given praziquantel. Neurological symptoms have also been reported[1] with the much lower doses of praziquantel used in the treatment of taeniasis in a patient with undiagnosed neurocysticercosis.

1. Flisser A, *et al.* Neurological symptoms in occult neurocysticercosis after single taenicidal dose of praziquantel. *Lancet* 1993; **342:** 748.

Precautions

Praziquantel should not be used in patients with ocular cysticercosis because of the risk of severe eye damage resulting from destruction of the parasite.

Patients should be warned that praziquantel may cause dizziness or drowsiness and if affected they should not drive or operate machinery during or for 24 hours after treatment.

Praziquantel is distributed into breast milk and mothers should not breast feed during or for 72 hours after treatment.

Interactions

Some workers have proposed the use of *dexamethasone* to prevent the inflammatory response due to destroyed cysticerci in praziquantel treatment of cysticercosis.[1] However, since dexamethasone has been reported approximately to halve plasma concentrations of praziquantel,[2] it has been suggested that it be reserved for the short-term treatment of praziquantel-induced intracranial hypertension.[1]

Carbamazepine,[3] *phenytoin*,[3] and *chloroquine*[4] have also been reported to reduce the bioavailability of praziquantel while *cimetidine* has been reported to increase praziquantel bioavailability.[5,6]

For reference to plasma concentrations of the active metabolite of *albendazole* being increased by concomitant administration of praziquantel, see p.96.

1. Del Brutto OH, Sotelo J. Neurocysticercosis: an update. *Rev Infect Dis* 1988; **10:** 1075–87.
2. Vazquez ML, *et al.* Plasma levels of praziquantel decrease when dexamethasone is given simultaneously. *Neurology* 1987; **37:** 1561–2.
3. Quinn DI, Day RO. Drug interactions of clinical importance: an updated guide. *Drug Safety* 1995; **12:** 393–452.
4. Masimirembwa CM, *et al.* The effect of chloroquine on the pharmacokinetics and metabolism of praziquantel in rats and in humans. *Biopharm Drug Dispos* 1994; **15:** 33–43.
5. Metwally A, *et al.* Effect of cimetidine, bicarbonate and glucose on the bioavailability of different formulations of praziquantel. *Arzneimittelforschung* 1995; **45:** 516–18.
6. Jung H, *et al.* Pharmacokinetic study of praziquantel administered alone and in combination with cimetidine in a single-day therapeutic regimen. *Antimicrob Agents Chemother* 1997; **41:** 1256–9.

Pharmacokinetics

Praziquantel is rapidly absorbed after administration by mouth, even when taken with a meal; more than 80% of a dose is reported to be absorbed. Peak plasma concentrations are achieved 1 to 3 hours after a dose, but there is a pronounced first-pass effect and praziquantel undergoes rapid and extensive metabolism in the liver being hydroxylated to metabolites that are thought to be inactive. It is distributed to the CSF. The plasma elimination half-life of praziquantel is 1 to 1.5 hours and that of the metabolites about 4 hours.

It is excreted in the urine, mainly as metabolites, about 80% of the dose being eliminated within 4 days and more than 90% of this in the first 24 hours.

Praziquantel is distributed into breast milk.

References to the pharmacokinetics of praziquantel.

1. Leopold G, *et al.* Clinical pharmacology in normal volunteers of praziquantel, a new drug against schistosomes and cestodes: an example of a complex study covering both tolerance and pharmacokinetics. *Eur J Clin Pharmacol* 1978; **14:** 281–91.
2. Bühring KU, *et al.* Metabolism of praziquantel in man. *Eur J Drug Metab Pharmacokinet* 1978; **3:** 179–90.
3. Patzschke K, *et al.* Serum concentrations and renal excretion in humans after oral administration of praziquantel—results of three determination methods. *Eur J Drug Metab Pharmacokinet* 1979; **3:** 149–56.
4. Mandour M El M, *et al.* Pharmacokinetics of praziquantel in healthy volunteers and patients with schistosomiasis. *Trans R Soc Trop Med Hyg* 1990; **84:** 389–93.

Uses and Administration

Praziquantel is an anthelmintic with a broad spectrum of activity against trematodes (flukes) including all species of *Schistosoma* pathogenic to man and cestodes (tapeworms). It is used in the treatment of cysticercosis, diphyllobothriasis, hymenolepiasis, schistosomiasis, taeniasis, and intestinal, liver, and lung fluke infections. For discussions of these infections and their treatment, see under Choice of Anthelmintic, p.92. See also below.

Praziquantel is administered by mouth with food.

In the treatment of schistosomiasis in adults and children it is given on one day as three doses of 20 mg per kg body-weight at intervals of 4 to 6 hours or it is given as a single dose of 40 mg per kg.

Doses in adults and children in the liver fluke infections clonorchiasis and opisthorchiasis are 25 mg per kg three times daily for one or two days or a single dose of 40 mg per kg. Similar doses may be used in lung fluke and intestinal fluke infections.

Single doses of 5 to 25 mg per kg are used in adults and children in tapeworm infections.

Praziquantel is used in the treatment of neurocysticercosis in a dose of 50 mg per kg daily in 3 divided doses for 15 days. A corticosteroid should be given concomitantly to reduce the severity of adverse effects.

Reviews.

1. Pearson RD, Guerrant RL. Praziquantel: a major advance in anthelmintic therapy. *Ann Intern Med* 1983; **99:** 195–8. Correction. *ibid.*; 574.
2. King CH, Mahmoud AAF. Drugs five years later: praziquantel. *Ann Intern Med* 1989; **110:** 290–6.

Cysticercosis. Praziquantel is used in the treatment of neurocysticercosis (p.93) although albendazole may be more effective.

References.

1. Sotelo J, *et al.* Therapy of parenchymal brain cysticercosis with praziquantel. *N Engl J Med* 1984; **310:** 1001–7.
2. Del Brutto OH, Sotelo J. Neurocysticercosis: an update. *Rev Infect Dis* 1988; **10:** 1075–87.
3. Crimmins D, *et al.* Neurocysticercosis: an under-recognized cause of neurological problems. *Med J Aust* 1990; **152:** 434–8.
4. Moodley M, Moosa A. Treatment of neurocysticercosis: is praziquantel the new hope? *Lancet* 1989; **i:** 262–3.
5. Sotelo J. Praziquantel for neurocysticercosis. *Lancet* 1989; **i:** 897.
6. Sotelo J, *et al.* Praziquantel for cysticercosis of the brain parenchyma. *N Engl J Med* 1984; **311:** 734.
7. Ciferri F. Delayed CSF reaction to praziquantel. *Lancet* 1988; **i:** 642–3.
8. Takayanagui JM, Jardim E. Therapy for neurocysticercosis: comparison between albendazole and praziquantel. *Arch Neurol* 1992; **49:** 290–4.
9. Mehta SS, *et al.* Albendazole versus praziquantel for neurocysticercosis. *Am J Health-Syst Pharm* 1998; **55:** 598–600.

Echinococcosis. Praziquantel may be used as an adjunct to surgery in echinococcosis (p.94). Praziquantel has been reported to possess a scolicidal effect against *Echinococcus granulosus in vitro*[1] and there has been a report of the successful treatment of disseminated peritoneal hydatid disease with praziquantel and surgery.[2] In this case praziquantel was effective against the small cysts; 2 large cysts were removed surgically, one before praziquantel was started. However, activity in 9 other patients given praziquantel was disappointing.[3]

1. Morris DL, *et al.* Protoscolicidal effect of praziquantel— in vitro and electron microscopical studies on Echinococcus granulosus. *J Antimicrob Chemother* 1986; **18:** 687–91.
2. Henriksen T-H, *et al.* Treatment of disseminated peritoneal hydatid disease with praziquantel. *Lancet* 1989; **i:** 272.
3. Piens MA, *et al.* Praziquantel dans l'hydatidose humaine: évaluation par traitement médical pré-opératoire. *Bull Soc Pathol Exot Filiales* 1989; **82:** 503–12.

Intestinal fluke infections. Praziquantel is used in the treatment of the intestinal fluke infections fasciolopsiasis, heterophyiasis, metagonimiasis, and nanophyetiasis (see p.94). It is given in a usual recommended dose of 25 mg per kg body-weight three times daily for one day. However, single doses of 15 mg per kg, 25 mg per kg, or 40 mg per kg all yielded a cure rate of 100% in a study in 72 primary school children in Thailand who were harbouring *Fasciolopsis buski* suggesting that a single dose of 15 mg per kg at bedtime might be tried.[1] Nine patients infected with the trematode *Nanophyetus salmincola* were treated with praziquantel 20 mg per kg body-weight three times daily for one day and were negative for eggs in their stools 2 to 12 weeks later.[2]

1. Harinasuta T, *et al.* Efficacy of praziquantel on fasciolopsiasis. *Arzneimittelforschung* 1984; **34:** 1214–15.
2. Fritsche TR, *et al.* Praziquantel for treatment of human Nanophyetus salmincola (Troglotrema salmincola) infection. *J Infect Dis* 1989; **160:** 896–9.

Liver fluke infections. Praziquantel is used in the treatment of clonorchiasis and opisthorchiasis, and has also been used in the treatment of fascioliasis although in this latter infection bithionol or triclabendazole are preferred (see p.94).

Various studies have shown praziquantel to be effective in clonorchiasis[1-4] and opisthorchiasis,[5,6] although one study in opisthorchiasis[7] showed that re-infection was common despite praziquantel therapy, particularly in those with heavy initial infection. Recently a study in Thailand[8] confirmed that mass treatment for opisthorchiasis with a single dose of praziquantel was beneficial, although it was suggested that ideally treatment should be given twice a year.

While praziquantel is not the drug of choice for fascioliasis, there has been a report[9] of successful treatment of a patient with severe fascioliasis. Subsequent studies[10-12] have, however, shown praziquantel to be of little benefit.

1. Soh C-J. Clonorchis sinensis: experimental and clinical studies with praziquantel in Korea. *Arzneimittelforschung* 1984; **34:** 1156–9.
2. Chen C-Y, Hsieh W-C. Clonorchis sinensis: epidemiology in Taiwan and clinical experience with praziquantel. *Arzneimittelforschung* 1984; **34:** 1160–2.
3. Kuang Q-H, *et al.* Clonorchiasis: treatment with praziquantel in 50 cases. *Arzneimittelforschung* 1984; **34:** 1162–3.
4. Lee S-H. Large scale treatment of clonorchis sinensis infections with praziquantel under field conditions. *Arzneimittelforschung* 1984; **34:** 1227–8.
5. Bunnag D, *et al.* Opisthorchis viverrini: clinical experience with praziquantel in hospital for tropical diseases. *Arzneimittelforschung* 1984; **34:** 1173–4.
6. Ambroise-Thomas P, *et al.* Therapeutic results in opisthorchiasis with praziquantel in a reinfection-free environment in France. *Arzneimittelforschung* 1984; **34:** 1177–9.
7. Upatham ES, *et al.* Rate of re-infection by Opisthorchis viverrini in an endemic northeast Thai community after chemotherapy. *Int J Parasitol* 1988; **18:** 643–9.
8. Pungpak S, *et al.* Opisthorchis viverrini infection in Thailand: studies on the morbidity of the infection and resolution following praziquantel treatment. *Am J Trop Med Hyg* 1997; **56:** 311–14.
9. Schiappacasse RH, *et al.* Successful treatment of severe infection with Fasciola hepatica with praziquantel. *J Infect Dis* 1985; **152:** 1339–40.
10. Farag HF, *et al.* A short note on praziquantel in human fascioliasis. *J Trop Med Hyg* 1986; **89:** 79–80.
11. Farid Z, *et al.* Treatment of acute toxaemic fascioliasis. *Trans R Soc Trop Med Hyg* 1988; **82:** 299.
12. Farid Z, *et al.* Unsuccessful use of praziquantel to treat acute fascioliasis in children. *J Infect Dis* 1986; **154:** 920–1.

Lung fluke infections. Praziquantel is used in the treatment of the lung fluke infection paragonimiasis (p.95).

References.

1. Vanijanonta S, *et al.* Paragonimus heterotremus and other Paragonimus spp. in Thailand: pathogenesis clinic and treatment. *Arzneimittelforschung* 1984; **34:** 1186–8.
2. Pachucki CT, *et al.* American paragonimiasis treated with praziquantel. *N Engl J Med* 1984; **311:** 582–3.

Protozoal infections. During a study of the efficacy of praziquantel in tapeworm infections it was noted that praziquantel also had a significant effect against the protozoans *Entamoeba histolytica* and *Giardia duodenalis*.[1] For a discussion of the more conventional antiprotozoal drugs used in these infections, see p.573 and p.575.

1. Flisser A, *et al.* Effect of praziquantel on protozoan parasites. *Lancet* 1995; **345:** 316–17.

Schistosomiasis. Praziquantel is the main drug that is used in the treatment of schistosomiasis (p.95). It is effective against all species of schistosomes.[1] The manufacturers recommend a dose of 20 mg per kg body-weight given three times in one day for all schistosomal infections. WHO[1] recommends a single dose of 40 mg per kg. WHO considers[1] that in the field such treatment will produce a cure rate of 60 to 90% with a reduction in egg count in those not cured of 90 to 95%. Good as such results are, a single dose or one day's sole treatment should not be considered as all that is required to achieve a permanent cure or prevent reinfection, and any treatment plan should be reassessed after 6 or 12 months.[2,3] Such an approach with annual screening and targeted chemotherapy is now accepted as providing, at least in some endemic areas, successful protection for children against intense infection and consequent hepatic disease.[3]

Several studies indicate that doses lower than those recommended above might be effective and in some control programmes 20 mg per kg might be enough for *S. haematobium*[4-6] or 30 mg per kg for *S. mansoni*.[4] It remains to be seen if such low doses lead to problems of resistance as has been suggested with oxamniquine.[7] However, refractory infections have been reported. A 4-day treatment course was needed to produce a complete cure in one patient who relapsed twice following standard one-day treatment regimens.[8] Hepatic impairment, specifically hepatic fibrosis, is a feature of some schistosomal infections and patients with such liver involvement have benefited from treatment with praziquantel.[3,9]

1. WHO. The control of schistosomiasis: second report of the WHO expert committee. *WHO Tech Rep Ser 830* 1993.
2. Anonymous. The chemotherapy of schistosomiasis control. *Bull WHO* 1986; **64:** 23–5.
3. Anonymous. Mass treatment of schistosomiasis with praziquantel. *WHO Drug Inf* 1988; **2:** 184–5.
4. Taylor P, *et al.* Efficacy of low doses of praziquantel for Schistosoma mansoni and S. haematobium. *J Trop Med Hyg* 1988; **91:** 13–17.
5. King CH, *et al.* Dose-finding study for praziquantel therapy of Schistosoma haematobium in Coast Province, Kenya. *Am J Trop Med Hyg* 1989; **40:** 507–13.
6. Hatz C, *et al.* Ultrasound scanning for detecting morbidity due to Schistosoma haematobium and its resolution following treatment with different doses of praziquantel. *Trans R Soc Trop Med Hyg* 1990; **84:** 84–8.
7. Coles GC, *et al.* Tolerance of Kenyan Schistosoma mansoni to oxamniquine. *Trans R Soc Trop Med Hyg* 1987; **81:** 782–5.
8. Murray-Smith SQ, *et al.* A case of refractory schistosomiasis. *Med J Aust* 1996; **165:** 458.
9. Zwingenberger K, *et al.* Praziquantel in the treatment of hepatosplenic schistosomiasis: biochemical disease markers indicate deceleration of fibrogenesis and diminution of portal flow obstruction. *Trans R Soc Trop Med Hyg* 1990; **84:** 252–6.

Taeniasis. Praziquantel is used in the treatment of taeniasis (p.96). It has been studied in the mass control of taeniasis when a single dose of 5 mg per kg body-weight was used.[1]

Praziquantel is also effective against the larval form of *Taenia solium* and is used to treat neurocysticercosis (see above).

1. Cruz M, *et al.* Operational studies on the control of Taenia solium taeniasis/cysticercosis in Ecuador. *Bull WHO* 1989; **67:** 401–7

Preparations

USP 23: Praziquantel Tablets.

Proprietary Preparations (details are given in Part 3)

Austral.: Biltricide; ***Fr.:*** Biltricide; ***Ger.:*** Biltricide; Cesol; Cysticide; ***Neth.:*** Biltricide; ***S.Afr.:*** Biltricide; Cysticide; ***USA:*** Biltricide.

Pyrantel Embonate (805-v)

Pyrantel Embonate *(BANM, rINNM).*

CP-10423-16; Pirantel Pamoate; Pyrantel Pamoate *(USAN).* 1,4,5,6-Tetrahydro-1-methyl-2-[(*E*)-2-(2-thienyl)vinyl]pyrimidine 4,4′-methylenebis(3-hydroxy-2-naphthoate).

$C_{11}H_{14}N_2S,C_{23}H_{16}O_6 = 594.7.$

CAS — 15686-83-6 (pyrantel); 22204-24-6 (pyrantel embonate).

Pharmacopoeias. In *Chin., Int., Jpn, Pol.,* and *US.*

A yellow to tan-coloured solid. Pyrantel embonate 2.9 g is approximately equivalent to 1 g of pyrantel. Practically **insoluble** in water and in methyl alcohol; soluble in dimethyl sulphoxide; slightly soluble in dimethylformamide. **Protect** from light.

Adverse Effects and Precautions

The adverse effects of pyrantel embonate are generally mild and transient. The most frequent are gastro-intestinal effects such as nausea and vomiting, anorexia, abdominal pain, and diarrhoea. Other adverse effects reported include headache, dizziness, drowsiness, insomnia, skin rashes, and elevated liver enzyme values.

Pyrantel embonate should be used with caution in patients with impaired liver function.

Interactions

The anthelmintic effects of both pyrantel and piperazine may be antagonised when the two compounds are used together.

Pharmacokinetics

Only a small proportion of a dose of pyrantel embonate is absorbed from the gastro-intestinal tract. Up to about 7% is excreted as unchanged drug and metabolites in the urine but over half of the dose is excreted unchanged in the faeces.

Uses and Administration

Pyrantel embonate is an anthelmintic effective against intestinal nematodes including roundworms (*Ascaris lumbricoides*), threadworms (*Enterobius vermicularis*), and *Trichostrongylus* spp., the tissue nematode *Trichinella spiralis*, and hookworms, although it is possibly less effective against *Necator americanus* hookworms than against *Ancylostoma duodenale*. Pyrantel is not effective against whipworm (*Trichuris trichiura*). Pyrantel embonate is one of the anthelmintics that may be used in the treatment of infections with these worms, as discussed under Choice of Anthelmintic, p.92. It appears to act by paralysing susceptible worms which are then dislodged by peristaltic activity.

Single or mixed infections due to susceptible worms in adults and children may be treated with a single oral dose equivalent to 10 mg of pyrantel per kg body-weight. Ascariasis occurring alone may only require 5 mg per kg; a single dose of 2.5 mg per kg has been used in mass treatment programmes. In necatoriasis, 10 mg per kg daily for 3 days or 20 mg per kg daily for 2 days may be necessary. The response in enterobiasis may be improved by repeating the 10 mg per kg dose after 2 to 4 weeks. In trichinosis a dose of 10 mg per kg daily for 5 days has been suggested.

Preparations

USP 23: Pyrantel Pamoate Oral Suspension.

Proprietary Preparations (details are given in Part 3)
Aust.: Combantrin; ***Austral.:*** Anthel; Combantrin; Early Bird; ***Canad.:*** Combantrin; Jaa Pyral; ***Fr.:*** Combantrin; Helmintox; ***Ger.:*** Helmex; ***Ital.:*** Combantrin; ***S.Afr.:*** Combantrin; ***Spain:*** Lombriareu; Trilombrin; ***Switz.:*** Cobantril; ***UK:*** Combantrin†; ***USA:*** Antiminth; Pin-Rid; Pin-X; Reese's Pinworm.

Rafoxanide (13206-f)

Rafoxanide *(BAN, USAN, rINN).*

MK-990. 3′-Chloro-4′-(4-chlorophenoxy)-3,5-di-iodosalicylanilide.

$C_{19}H_{11}Cl_2I_2NO_3$ = 626.0.

CAS — 22662-39-1.

Rafoxanide is an anthelmintic used for the treatment of fascioliasis in sheep and cattle.

Santonin (807-q)

Santoninum. (3S,3aS,5aS,9bS)-3a,5,5a,9b-Tetrahydro-3,5a,9-trimethylnaphtho[1,2-*b*]furan-2,8(3*H*,4*H*)-dione.

$C_{15}H_{18}O_3$ = 246.3.

CAS — 481-06-1.

Pharmacopoeias. In *Jpn.*

A crystalline lactone obtained from the dried unexpanded flowerheads of *Artemisia cina* (santonica, wormwood) and other species of *Artemisia* (Compositae).

Santonin was formerly used as an anthelmintic in the treatment of roundworm (*Ascaris*) infection, but has been superseded by other less toxic anthelmintics.

It is used as a flavouring agent in food.

Tetramisole Hydrochloride (814-g)

Tetramisole Hydrochloride *(BANM, USAN, rINNM).*

ICI-50627; McN-JR-8299-11; R-8299. (±)-2,3,5,6-Tetrahydro-6-phenylimidazo[2,1-*b*]thiazole hydrochloride.

$C_{11}H_{12}N_2S,HCl$ = 240.8.

CAS — 5036-02-2 (tetramisole); 5086-74-8 (tetramisole hydrochloride).

Pharmacopoeias. In *Fr.* for veterinary use.

Tetramisole hydrochloride is an anthelmintic used in veterinary practice for the control of nematode infections. It is a racemic mixture and the laevo-isomer, levamisole hydrochloride (p.102), accounts for most of its activity.

Thiabendazole (816-p)

Thiabendazole *(BAN, USAN).*

Tiabendazole *(rINN)*; E233; MK-360; Tiabendazolum. 2-(Thiazol-4-yl)-1*H*-benzimidazole.

$C_{10}H_7N_3S$ = 201.2.

CAS — 148-79-8.

Pharmacopoeias. In *Chin., Eur.* (see p.viii), *Int.*, and *US.*

A white or almost white, odourless or almost odourless, crystalline powder. Practically **insoluble** in water; slightly soluble in alcohol, in acetone, and in dichloromethane; slightly or very slightly soluble in ether; very slightly soluble in chloroform; it dissolves in dilute mineral acids. **Protect** from light.

Adverse Effects

Dizziness and gastro-intestinal disturbances, especially anorexia, nausea, and vomiting, are common during treatment with thiabendazole. Other adverse effects occurring occasionally include pruritus, skin rashes, headache, fatigue, drowsiness, drying of mucous membranes, hyperglycaemia, disturbance of vision including colour vision, leucopenia, tinnitus, effects on the liver including cholestasis and parenchymal damage, enuresis, crystalluria, and bradycardia and hypotension. There have also been reports of erythema multiforme, fatal Stevens-Johnson syndrome, toxic epidermal necrolysis, convulsions, and effects on mental state.

Fever, chills, angioedema, and lymphadenopathy have been reported, but may represent allergic response to dead parasites rather than to thiabendazole.

The urine of some patients taking thiabendazole may have a characteristic odour similar to that following the ingestion of asparagus; it is attributed to the presence of a thiabendazole metabolite.

Effects on the liver. Dry mouth with swollen parotid and salivary glands suggestive of the sicca complex preceded the development of cholestatic jaundice in a 17-year-old boy given thiabendazole.[1]

1. Davidson RN, *et al.* Intrahepatic cholestasis after thiabendazole. *Trans R Soc Trop Med Hyg* 1988; **82:** 620.

Hypersensitivity. Severe erythema multiforme developed in a patient 16 days after a course of thiabendazole.[1] Many of the lesions encircled pre-existing melanocytic naevi.

1. Humphreys F, Cox NH. Thiabendazole-induced erythema multiforme with lesions around melanocytic naevi. *Br J Dermatol* 1988; **118:** 855–6.

Precautions

Thiabendazole is teratogenic in *mice*. It should be used with caution in patients with hepatic or renal impairment. Thiabendazole causes drowsiness in some patients and those affected should not drive or operate machinery.

Thiabendazole should not be used in mixed worm infections involving *Ascaris lumbricoides* as it can cause these roundworms to migrate; live roundworms have emerged through the mouth or nose.

Renal impairment. Thiabendazole and its 5-hydroxy metabolite did not accumulate in an anephric patient on haemodialysis and haemoperfusion and receiving treatment for severe strongyloidiasis.[1] However, the potentially toxic conjugated glucuronide and sulphate metabolites did accumulate. The clearance of all 3 metabolites was poor by haemodialysis; haemoperfusion was much more efficient, although for rapid removal the haemoperfusion columns should be changed every hour.

1. Bauer L, *et al.* The pharmacokinetics of thiabendazole and its metabolites in an anephric patient undergoing hemodialysis and hemoperfusion. *J Clin Pharmacol* 1982; **22:** 276–80.

Interactions

Theophylline. For the effect of thiabendazole on serum concentrations of theophylline, see p.770.

Pharmacokinetics

Thiabendazole is readily absorbed from the gastro-intestinal tract and reaches peak concentrations in the plasma after 1 to 2 hours. It is metabolised to 5-hydroxythiabendazole and excreted principally in the urine as glucuronide or sulphate conjugates; about 90% is recovered in the urine within 48 hours of ingestion, but only 5% in the faeces. Absorption may occur from preparations applied to the skin or eyes.

References.

1. Tocco DJ, *et al.* Absorption, metabolism, and excretion of thiabendazole in man and laboratory animals. *Toxicol Appl Pharmacol* 1966; **9:** 31–9.

Uses and Administration

Thiabendazole, a benzimidazole derivative, is an anthelmintic with activity against most nematode worms; activity against some larval stages and ova has also been demonstrated. The mode of action is not certain, but thiabendazole may inhibit the fumarate-reductase system of worms thereby interfering with their source of energy.

Thiabendazole is used in the treatment of cutaneous larva migrans, dracunculiasis (guinea worm infection), and toxocariasis. It may also be used in the treatment of strongyloidiasis, and can provide symptomatic relief during the larval invasion stage of trichinosis. Thiabendazole is also active against some intestinal nematodes, but should not be used as primary therapy; the treatment of mixed infections including ascariasis is not recommended since thiabendazole may cause the worms to migrate to other body organs causing serious complications. For discussions of the treatment of the above infections see under Choice of Anthelmintic, p.92. See also below.

Thiabendazole is given by mouth, with meals, usually in a dose of 25 mg per kg body-weight twice daily for 2 or more days, the duration depending on the type of infection; the daily dose should not exceed 3 g. For those unable to tolerate 2 doses daily, 25 mg per kg may be given after the largest meal on day 1 and repeated 24 hours later after a similar meal on day 2. For mass treatment, a single dose of 50 mg per kg after the evening meal is suggested although the incidence of adverse effects may be higher than with 2 doses of 25 mg per kg.

In cutaneous larva migrans, 25 mg per kg may be given twice daily for 2 days, repeated after 2 days if necessary; topical treatment with a 10 to 15% suspension intended for oral use has also been advocated as an alternative or adjunct to oral treatment.

In dracunculiasis, 25 to 50 mg per kg may be given twice daily for one day; in massive infection a further 50 mg per kg may be given after 5 to 8 days. Alternatively 25 to 37.5 mg per kg may be given twice daily for 3 days.

In strongyloidiasis, 25 mg per kg may be given twice daily for 2 days or 50 mg per kg as a single dose; when the infection is disseminated treatment for at least 5 days may be necessary.

In trichinosis, 25 mg per kg may be given twice daily for 2 to 4 successive days.

In toxocariasis, 25 mg per kg may be given twice daily for 7 days.

Thiabendazole also has some antifungal activity. It is used as a fungicidal preservative for certain foods.

Angiostrongyliasis. Thiabendazole has been suggested as an alternative to mebendazole for the treatment of infections with *Angiostrongylus costaricensis* (see p.92), although the high dose of 25 mg per kg body-weight three times a day for 3 days considered necessary is likely to be toxic and may have to be decreased.[1]

1. Anonymous. Drugs for parasitic infections. *Med Lett Drugs Ther* 1998; **40:** 1–12.

Dracunculiasis. Thiabendazole[1,2] may be used for symptomatic treatment of dracunculiasis (p.93), although it has no direct anthelmintic effect. It is used to facilitate removal of the worm from subcutaneous tissues.

1. Muller R. Guinea worm disease: epidemiology, control, and treatment. *Bull WHO* 1979; **57:** 683–9.
2. Kale OO, *et al.* Controlled comparative trial of thiabendazole and metronidazole in the treatment of dracontiasis. *Ann Trop Med Parasitol* 1983; **77:** 151–7.

Fungal infections. Thiabendazole[1] has been reported to be of some success in the treatment of chromoblastomycosis which is discussed on p.368.

1. Ollé-Goig JE, Domingo J. A case of chromomycosis treated with thiabendazole. *Trans R Soc Trop Med Hyg* 1983; **77:** 773–4.

Strongyloidiasis. Thiabendazole may be used in the treatment of strongyloidiasis, but albendazole or ivermectin are generally preferred (see p.95).

References.

1. Grove DI. Treatment of strongyloidiasis with thiabendazole: an analysis of toxicity and effectiveness. *Trans R Soc Trop Med Hyg* 1982; **76:** 114–18.
2. Barnish G, Barker J. An intervention study using thiabendazole suspension against strongyloides fuelleborni-like infections in Papua New Guinea. *Trans R Soc Trop Med Hyg* 1987; **81:** 60–3.

Syngamosis. Thiabendazole has been used successfully[1,2] to treat syngamosis when it has occurred in man (see p.96).

1. Grell GAC, *et al.* Syngamus in a West Indian. *Br Med J* 1978; **2:** 1464.
2. Leers W-D, *et al.* Syngamosis, an unusual case of asthma: the first reported case in Canada. *Can Med Assoc J* 1985; **132:** 269–70.

Preparations

BP 1998: Tiabendazole Tablets;
USP 23: Thiabendazole Oral Suspension; Thiabendazole Tablets.

Proprietary Preparations (details are given in Part 3)
Austral.: Mintezol; ***Canad.:*** Mintezol; ***Irl.:*** Mintezol; ***S.Afr.:*** Mintezol†; ***Spain:*** Triasox; ***UK:*** Mintezol; ***USA:*** Mintezol.

Thiacetarsamide (19922-g)

p-[Bis(carboxymethylmercapto)arsino]benzamide; 4-Carbamylphenyl bis[carboxymethylthio]arsenite.

$C_{11}H_{12}AsNO_5S_2$ = 377.3.

CAS — 531-72-6.

Pharmacopoeias. In *US.*

Thiacetarsamide is an anthelmintic used in veterinary medicine.

Thiophanate (13328-s)

Thiophanate *(BAN)*.

4,4′-o-Phenylenebis(ethyl 3-thioallophanate).

$C_{14}H_{18}N_4O_4S_2$ = 370.4.

CAS — 23564-06-9.

Thiophanate is an anthelmintic used in veterinary practice for the control of nematode infections.

Triclabendazole (3230-g)

Triclabendazole *(BAN, rINN)*.

5-Chloro-6-(2,3-dichlorophenoxy)-2-(methylthio)benzimidazole.

$C_{14}H_9Cl_3N_2OS$ = 359.7.

CAS — 68786-66-3.

Triclabendazole is a benzimidazole anthelmintic used in veterinary practice and with a potential role in the treatment of human fascioliasis. Triclabendazole is also under investigation for the treatment of human paragonimiasis.

Liver fluke infections. Although bithionol or praziquantel are currently used to treat fascioliasis (p.94), WHO[1] anticipated that triclabendazole would become the drug of choice. A possible dosage schedule was two doses of 5 mg per kg bodyweight given after meals, with an interval of 6 to 8 hours between the two doses.[1] In a study from Chile, 19 of 24 patients with chronic hepatic fascioliasis were treated successfully with a single dose of triclabendazole 10 mg per kg after an overnight fast.[2]

1. WHO. Control of foodborne trematode infections. *WHO Tech Rep Ser 849* 1995.
2. Apt W, *et al.* Treatment of human chronic fascioliasis with triclabendazole: drug efficacy and serologic response. *Am J Trop Med Hyg* 1995; **52:** 532–5.

Lung fluke infections. Encouraging results were reported from a pilot study of triclabendazole[1] in the treatment of paragonimiasis (p.95).

1. Ripert C, *et al.* Therapeutic effect of triclabendazole in patients with paragonimiasis in Cameroon: a pilot study. *Trans R Soc Trop Med Hyg* 1992; **86:** 417.

Viprynium Embonate (819-e)

Viprynium Embonate *(BAN)*.

Pyrvinium Embonate; Pyrvinium Pamoate; Viprynium Pamoate. Bis{6-dimethylamino-2-[2-(2,5-dimethyl-1-phenylpyrrol-3-yl)vinyl]-1-methylquinolinium} 4,4′-methylenebis(3-hydroxy-2-naphthoate).

$C_{52}H_{56}N_6,C_{23}H_{14}O_6$ = 1151.4.

CAS — 3546-41-6.

NOTE. Pyrvinium Chloride is *rINN.*

Pharmacopoeias. In *US.*

A bright orange or orange-red to almost black crystalline powder. Viprynium embonate 7.5 mg is approximately equivalent to 5 mg of viprynium.

Practically **insoluble** in water and in ether; very slightly soluble in methyl alcohol; slightly soluble in chloroform and in methoxyethanol; freely soluble in glacial acetic acid. **Store** in airtight containers. Protect from light.

Adverse Effects

Viprynium occasionally causes nausea, vomiting, and diarrhoea. Hypersensitivity reactions and photosensitivity have been reported.

Viprynium stains the stools bright red and may stain clothing if vomiting occurs.

Pharmacokinetics

Viprynium embonate is not significantly absorbed from the gastro-intestinal tract.

Uses and Administration

Viprynium embonate is an effective anthelmintic in the treatment of enterobiasis (p.94), but has generally been superseded by other drugs such as albendazole, mebendazole, flubendazole, or pyrantel embonate.

It has been administered by mouth in a single dose equivalent to 5 mg of viprynium per kg body-weight, repeated after 2 to 3 weeks if necessary.

Preparations

USP 23: Pyrvinium Pamoate Oral Suspension; Pyrvinium Pamoate Tablets.

Proprietary Preparations (details are given in Part 3)

Aust.: Molevac; ***Belg.:*** Vanquin†; ***Canad.:*** Vanquin; ***Fr.:*** Povanyl; ***Ger.:*** Molevac; Pyrcon; ***Ital.:*** Vanquin; ***Norw.:*** Vanquin; ***Spain:*** Pamoxan; ***Swed.:*** Vanquin; ***Switz.:*** Molevac.

Antibacterials

In this chapter are antimicrobial agents used principally in the treatment and prophylaxis of bacterial infections. They include antibiotics, sulphonamides, quinolones, and antimycobacterial agents; in practice the term 'antibiotics' often encompasses all of these agents. Antibacterial agents described elsewhere include metronidazole (p.585) which, as well as being an antiprotozoal agent, is used in the treatment of anaerobic bacterial infections. Immunological approaches to the treatment and prophylaxis of bacterial infections are discussed under Vaccines Immunoglobulins and Antisera, p.1500.

In addition, disinfectants and preservatives (p.1097) are used to kill or inhibit the growth of micro-organisms.

Drug Groups

Although antibiotics and other antibacterials are a very diverse class of compounds they are often classified and discussed in groups. They may be classified according to their mode of action or spectrum of antimicrobial activity, but generally those with similar chemical structures are grouped together.

Aminoglycosides

The aminoglycosides are a closely-related group of bactericidal antibiotics derived from bacteria of the order Actinomycetales or, more specifically, the genus *Streptomyces* (framycetin, kanamycin, neomycin, paromomycin, streptomycin, and tobramycin) and the genus *Micromonospora* (gentamicin and sissomicin). They are polycationic compounds that contain an aminocyclitol, usually 2-deoxystreptamine, or streptidine in streptomycin and related compounds, with cyclic amino-sugars attached by glycosidic linkages. Therefore, they have also been termed aminoglycosidic aminocyclitols. The sulphate salts are generally used.

The aminoglycosides have broadly similar toxicological features. Ototoxicity is a major limitation to their use; streptomycin and gentamicin are generally considered to be more toxic to the vestibular branch of the eighth cranial nerve and neomycin and kanamycin to be more toxic to the auditory branch. Other adverse effects common to the group include nephrotoxicity, neuromuscular blocking activity, and allergy, including cross-reactivity.

The pharmacokinetics of the aminoglycosides are very similar. Little is absorbed from the gastro-intestinal tract but they are generally well-distributed in the body after parenteral administration although penetration into the CSF is poor. They are excreted unchanged in the urine by glomerular filtration.

The aminoglycosides have a similar antimicrobial spectrum and appear to act by interfering with bacterial protein synthesis, possibly by binding irreversibly to the 30S and to some extent the 50S portions of the bacterial ribosome. The manner in which they bring about cell death is not fully understood. They are most active against Gram-negative rods. *Staphylococcus aureus* is susceptible to the aminoglycosides but otherwise most Gram-positive bacteria, and also anaerobic bacteria, are naturally resistant. They show enhanced activity with penicillins against some enterococci and streptococci. Bacterial resistance to streptomycin may occur by mutation whereas with the other aminoglycosides it is usually associated with the plasmid-mediated production of inactivating enzymes which are capable of phosphorylation, acetylation, or adenylation. The aminoglycosides have a postantibiotic effect, that is antibacterial activity persisting after concentrations have dropped below minimum inhibitory concentrations.

Streptomycin was the first aminoglycoside to become available commercially and was isolated from a strain of *Streptomyces griseus* in 1944. Its use is now restricted mainly to the treatment of tuberculosis when it is always administered in association with other antituberculous drugs because of the rapid development of resistance. *Dihydrostreptomycin*, a reduction product of streptomycin, is only rarely used because of its toxicity. The *neomycin* complex of antibiotics were the next to be isolated; neomycin itself is mainly a mixture of the B and C isomers and neomycin B is considered to be identical with *framycetin*. Because of their toxicity they are not given systemically. The related compound *paromomycin* also has antiprotozoal and anthelmintic properties and may be used in the treatment of intestinal amoebiasis, cestode infections, cryptosporidiosis, and leishmaniasis. *Kanamycin* is less toxic than neomycin and can be used systemically. However, it is not active against *Pseudomonas aeruginosa* and has generally been replaced by gentamicin and other newer aminoglycosides, although it has been used in penicillin-resistant gonorrhoea.

Gentamicin was isolated from *Micromonospora purpurea* in 1963 and, being active against *Ps. aeruginosa* and *Serratia marcescens*, is widely used in the treatment of life-threatening infections. *Tobramycin* is one of several components of the nebramycin complex of aminoglycosides produced by *Streptomyces tenebrarius*. It has an antimicrobial spectrum very similar to that of gentamicin and is reported to be more active against *Ps. aeruginosa*. *Amikacin*, a semisynthetic derivative of kanamycin, has a side-chain rendering it less susceptible to inactivating enzymes. It has a spectrum of activity like that of gentamicin but Gram-negative bacteria resistant to gentamicin, tobramycin, and kanamycin are often sensitive. *Sissomicin* is closely related structurally to gentamicin, and *netilmicin* is the *N*-ethyl derivative of sissomicin. Netilmicin may be active against some gentamicin-resistant strains of bacteria although not to the same extent as amikacin. Other aminoglycosides include *isepamicin and micronomicin*.

Because of their potential toxicity and antimicrobial spectrum, aminoglycosides should in general only be used for the treatment of serious infections. Doses must be carefully regulated to maintain plasma concentrations within the therapeutic range but avoiding accumulation, especially in patients with renal impairment. Neomycin and framycetin, which are considered too toxic to be given parenterally, have been given by mouth to suppress the intestinal flora. The topical use of neomycin and gentamicin has been associated with allergic reactions and the emergence of resistant bacteria. Gentamicin or tobramycin are the drugs of choice in the treatment of life-threatening infections due to aminoglycoside-sensitive organisms and are often used in association with other antibacterials. With the continuing emergence of resistant strains, amikacin and netilmicin should be reserved for severe infections resistant to gentamicin and the other aminoglycosides.

Antimycobacterials

The antimycobacterials are a miscellaneous group of antibacterials whose spectrum of activity includes *Mycobacterium* spp. and which are used in the treatment of tuberculosis, leprosy, and other mycobacterial infections. They include the rifamycins, also known as ansamycins or rifomycins, a group of antibiotics isolated from a strain of *Amycolatopsis mediterranei* (*Nocardia mediterranei*; *Streptomyces mediterranei*). Rifamycins described in this chapter include *rifamycin sodium*, a rifamycin rarely used as it has been superseded by more effective drugs, and a newer rifamycin, *rifaximin*. The main antibiotic in this group, *rifampicin*, is a mainstay of regimens for the treatment of tuberculosis and leprosy, and is increasingly being used for other infections. The related drug *rifabutin* is also used in mycobacterial disease, especially opportunistic mycobacterial infections due to *Mycobacterium avium* complex (MAC).

Another drug widely used for tuberculosis is *isoniazid*, a derivative of isonicotinic acid; it is invariably used in combination with other drugs to avoid or delay emergence of resistance. *Pyrazinamide*, a nicotinamide derivative, is also an important component of combination regimens for tuberculosis, while *ethambutol* and the aminoglycoside *streptomycin* may be added where resistance to first-line drugs is likely. The thiosemicarbazone derivative *thiacetazone* is now less widely used in tuberculosis because of its toxicity and because more effective drugs are available, but is sometimes employed in developing countries. Other drugs that have been used to treat tuberculosis include *aminosalicylic acid* and its salts, *capreomycin*, and *cycloserine*.

The sulphones have been employed since the 1940s in the treatment of leprosy, but the only one widely used now is *dapsone*, an important component of multidrug regimens. Its action is thought to involve inhibition of folate metabolism, similarly to the sulphonamides, and dapsone is also used in the prophylactic treatment of malaria and in *Pneumocystis carinii* pneumonia. Also important in the treatment of leprosy is the phenazine dye *clofazimine*, which has a role in the treatment of type 2 lepra reactions as well and has been used in other mycobacterial infections. The thioamides *ethionamide* and *prothionamide* have been used in the treatment of leprosy and tuberculosis, but have generally been replaced by less toxic drugs, for example, by *ofloxacin* or *minocycline* in alternative antileprotic regimens.

Cephalosporins and related Beta Lactams

The cephalosporins or cephem antibiotics are semisynthetic antibiotics derived from cephalosporin C a natural antibiotic produced by the mould *Cephalosporium acremonium*. The active nucleus, 7-aminocephalosporanic acid, is very closely related to the penicillin nucleus, 6-aminopenicillanic acid, and consists of a beta-lactam ring fused with a 6-membered dihydrothiazine ring and having an acetoxymethyl group at position 3. Cephalosporin C has a side-chain at position 7 derived from D-α-aminoadipic acid. Chemical modification of positions 3 and 7 has resulted in a series of drugs with different characteristics. Substitution at the 7-amino group tends to affect antibacterial action whereas at position 3 it may have more of an effect on pharmacokinetic properties.

The cephalosporins are bactericidal and, similarly to the penicillins, they act by inhibiting synthesis of the bacterial cell wall. The most widely used system of classification of cephalosporins is by generations and is based on the general features of their antibacterial activity, but may depend to some extent on when they were introduced. Succeeding generations generally have increasing activity against Gram-negative bacteria. *Cephalothin* was one of the first cephalosporins to become available and is representative of the **first-generation** cephalosporins. It has good activity against a wide spectrum of Gram-positive bacteria including penicillinase-producing, but not methicillin-resistant, staphylococci; enterococci are, however, resistant. Its activity against Gram-negative bacteria is modest. Cephalothin is not absorbed from the gastro-intestinal tract and must be administered parenterally although intramuscular administration is painful. Cephalothin has generally been replaced by *cephazolin* or *cephradine*. *Cephaloridine* is now rarely used because of its nephrotoxicity. Cephradine is absorbed from the gastro-intestinal tract and can be administered both by mouth and by injection. *Cefroxadine* (the oxymethyl derivative of cephradine), *cefadroxil*, *cefatrizine*, *cephalexin* and its pivaloyloxymethyl ester *pivcephalexin* are all administered by mouth. All of these drugs have a very similar spectrum of antimicrobial activity to cephalothin. *Cefaclor* is also given by mouth. It has similar activity to cephalothin against Gram-positive cocci, but because of its greater activity against Gram-negative bacteria, particularly *Haemophilus influenzae*, it is often classified as a second-generation drug. *Cefprozil* is an oral cephalosporin with a longer half-life than cefaclor.

Cephamandole was the first available **second-generation** cephalosporin. It has similar or slightly less activity than cephalothin against Gram-positive bacteria, but greater stability to hydrolysis by beta-lactamases produced by Gram-negative bacteria and enhanced activity against many of the Enterobacteriaceae and *Haemophilus influenzae*. *Cefuroxime* has a similar spectrum of activity to cephamandole although it is even more resistant to hydrolysis by beta-lactamases. *Cefuroxime axetil*, the acetoxyethyl ester of cefuroxime, is administered by mouth. Other drugs classified as second-generation cephalosporins and administered parenterally include *cefonicid*, *ceforanide*, and *cefotiam*; these all have spectra of activity similar to cephamandole. Cephamycins (see below) are also classified with second-generation cephalosporins.

The **third-generation** cephalosporins, sometimes referred to as **extended-spectrum** cephalosporins are even more stable to hydrolysis by beta-lactamases than cephamandole and cefuroxime. Compared with the earlier generations of cephalosporins they have a wider spectrum and greater potency of activity against Gram-negative organisms including most clinically important Enterobacteriaceae. Their activity against Gram-positive organisms is said to be less than that of the first-generation drugs, but they are very active against streptococci. *Cefotaxime* was the first of this group to become available and it has relatively modest activity against *Pseudomonas aeruginosa*. *Cefmenoxime*, *cefodizime*, *ceftizoxime*, and *ceftriaxone* are all very similar to cefotaxime in their antimicrobial activity. These drugs are all administered parenterally and differ mainly in their pharmacokinetic characteristics. *Cefixime* is a third-generation cephalosporin given by mouth; others include *cefdinir*, *cefetamet pivoxil*, *cefpodoxime proxetil*, and *ceftibuten*. *Latamoxef* is an **oxacephalosporin** which differs from the true cephalosporins in that the S atom of the 7-aminocephalosporanic acid nucleus is replaced by an O atom. It differs from cefotaxime mainly in its enhanced activity against *Bacteroides fragilis*. *Ceftazidime* is typical of a group of parenteral third-generation cephalosporins with enhanced activity against *Ps. aeruginosa*. *Cefoperazone* is similar in its activity to ceftazidime. *Cefpiramide* is structurally related to cefoperazone and has comparable activity. Although *cefsulodin* is classified as a third-generation cephalosporin its activity against Gram-negative bacteria is confined to *Ps. aeruginosa*. The newer cephalosporins *cefepime* and *cefpirome* have been described by some as **fourth-generation** because of their broad spectrum of activity.

The semisynthetic **cephamycins** are chemical modifications of cephamycin C, a beta-lactam antibiotic produced naturally by *Streptomyces* spp. They differ from the cephalosporins by the addition of a 7-α-methoxy group to the 7-aminocephalosporanic acid nucleus. Steric hindrance by this methoxy group is considered to be responsible for their greater stability to beta-lactamases. For practical purposes they are generally classified with the second-generation cephalosporins, but are more active against anaerobic bacteria, especially *Bacteroides fragilis*. *Cefoxitin* was one of the first cephamycins available; *cefmetazole* and *cefotetan* have been introduced more recently. Others include *cefbuperazone* and *cefminox*. All these cephamycins must be administered by the parenteral route.

Imipenem was the first of the **carbapenem** group of antibiotics to become available; it is the *N*-formimidoyl derivative of thienamycin which is produced by *Streptomyces cattleya*. It is bactericidal, and, similarly to the cephalosporins, acts by inhibiting synthesis of the bacterial cell wall. It has a very broad spectrum of antimicrobial activity including Gram-positive and Gram-negative aerobic and anaerobic organisms; it has good activity against both *Ps. aeruginosa* and *B. fragilis*. Imipenem is administered parenterally in association with cilastatin, a dehydropeptidase I inhibitor which inhibits the renal metabolism of imipenem. A newer carbapenem, *meropenem*, is relatively stable to renal dehydropeptidase.

The **monobactams** were first identified as monocyclic beta-lactams isolated from bacteria; they are now produced synthetically. *Aztreonam* was the first commercially available monobactam. It too is bactericidal with a similar action on bacterial cell-wall synthesis to the cephalosporins. Its antimicrobial activity, however, differs from imipenem and the newer cephalosporins in that it is restricted to Gram-negative aerobic organisms. It has good activity against *Ps. aeruginosa*. Aztreonam is administered by the parenteral route. Other monobactams include *carumonam*.

Carbacephems are structurally related to the cephalosporins, but the S atom of the 7-aminocephalosporanic acid nucleus is replaced by a methylene group. *Loracarbef* is an oral carbacephem.

Chloramphenicols

Chloramphenicol is an antibiotic which was first isolated from cultures of *Streptomyces venezuelae* in 1947 but is now produced synthetically. It has a relatively simple structure and is a derivative of dichloroacetic acid with a nitrobenzene moiety. Chloramphenicol was the first broad-spectrum antibiotic to be discovered; it acts by interfering with bacterial protein synthesis and is mainly bacteriostatic. Its range of activity is similar to that of tetracycline and includes Gram-positive and Gram-negative bacteria, rickettsias, and chlamydias. The sensitivity of *Salmonella typhi, Haemophilus influenzae*, and *Bacteroides fragilis* to chloramphenicol have provided the principal indications for its use.

After one or two years' use chloramphenicol was found to have a serious and sometimes fatal depressant effect on the bone marrow. The 'grey syndrome', another potentially fatal adverse effect, was reported later in newborn infants. As a result of this toxicity the use of chloramphenicol has been restricted in many countries; it should only be given when there is no suitable alternative and never for minor infections.

Chloramphenicol is active when given by mouth and, unlike most other antibacterials, it diffuses into the CSF even when the meninges are not inflamed. The majority of a dose is inactivated in the liver, only a small proportion appearing unchanged in the urine.

Chloramphenicol is used for typhoid fever in many countries although resistance is sometimes a problem. For *Haemophilus influenzae* infections, especially meningitis, the emergence of ampicillin-resistant strains led to a reappraisal of the use of chloramphenicol. Some workers have considered that ampicillin and chloramphenicol should both be given to patients with meningitis until the sensitivity of the infecting organisms is known; however, the newer third-generation cephalosporins have challenged this use. It is now used as an alternative to cephalosporins in *H. influenzae* meningitis. Chloramphenicol is also effective against many anaerobic bacteria and may be valuable in such conditions as cerebral abscess where anaerobes such as *Bacteroides fragilis* are often involved, although metronidazole may be preferred.

Chloramphenicol sodium succinate is used parenterally and the palmitate, which is almost tasteless, is given in oral suspensions. Ophthalmic preparations of chloramphenicol are used widely in some countries for a variety of infections.

Thiamphenicol is a semisynthetic derivative of chloramphenicol in which the nitro group on the benzene ring has been replaced by a methylsulphonyl group, resulting, in general, in a loss of activity *in vitro*. It has been claimed that thiamphenicol is less toxic than chloramphenicol and there have been fewer reports of aplastic anaemia but reversible bone-marrow depression may occur more frequently. Unlike chloramphenicol, thiamphenicol is not metabolised in the liver to any extent and is excreted largely unchanged in the urine. It has been used similarly to chloramphenicol in some countries.

Azidamfenicol is another analogue of chloramphenicol that has been used topically in the treatment of eye and skin infections.

Glycopeptides

Vancomycin has a glycopeptide structure; it acts by interfering with bacterial cell wall synthesis and is very active against Gram-positive cocci. Intravenous vancomycin is reserved for the treatment of severe staphylococcal infections and for the treatment and prophylaxis of endocarditis when other antibacterials cannot be used either because of patient sensitivity or bacterial resistance. It is the treatment of choice for infections caused by methicillin-resistant staphylococci. Vancomycin hydrochloride is poorly absorbed when taken by mouth; it is used in the treatment of pseudomembranous colitis. *Teicoplanin* is a glycopeptide with similar properties to vancomycin, but a longer duration of action. It can be given intramuscularly as well as intravenously. *Ramoplanin* is under investigation, especially for topical use in skin infections.

Lincosamides

Lincomycin is an antibiotic produced by a strain of *Streptomyces lincolnensis* and was first described in 1962; *clindamycin* is the 7-chloro-7-deoxy derivative of lincomycin.

Although not related structurally to erythromycin and the other macrolide antibiotics, the lincosamides have similar antimicrobial activity and act at the same site on the bacterial ribosome to suppress protein synthesis.

The lincosamides are bacteriostatic or bactericidal depending on the concentration and are active mainly against Gram-positive bacteria, and against *Bacteroides* spp. They also appear to have some antiprotozoal activity. Clindamycin and lincomycin have qualitatively similar activity but clindamycin is more active than lincomycin *in vitro*. Cross-resistance occurs between the lincosamide, streptogramin, and macrolide groups of antibiotics.

The lincosamides have been used, like erythromycin, as an alternative to penicillin but reports of the occurrence of severe and sometimes fatal pseudomembranous colitis in association with lincomycin and clindamycin have led to the recommendation that they should only be used when there is no suitable alternative.

Both lincomycin and clindamycin can be given orally and parenterally but clindamycin is much better absorbed from the gastro-intestinal tract and less affected by the presence of food in the stomach. They both penetrate well into bone and have been used successfully in osteomyelitis. They have also been used topically in the treatment of acne vulgaris.

The main indication for the use of lincosamides is now in the treatment of severe anaerobic infections although metronidazole (p.587) or some beta lactams may be a more suitable choice in such infections; clindamycin also has a role in the prophylaxis of endocarditis in penicillin-allergic patients. It has been used, usually with other antiprotozoals, in babesiosis, chloroquine-resistant malaria, and toxoplasmosis.

Macrolides

The macrolides are a large group of antibiotics mainly derived from *Streptomyces* spp. and having a common macrocyclic lactone ring to which one or more sugars are attached. They are all weak bases and only slightly soluble in water. Their properties are very similar and in general they have low toxicity and the same spectrum of antimicrobial activity with cross-resistance between individual members of the group. The macrolides are bacteriostatic or bactericidal, depending on the concentration and the type of micro-organism, and are thought to interfere with bacterial protein synthesis. Their antimicrobial spectrum is similar to that of benzylpenicillin but they are also active against such organisms as *Legionella pneumophila*, *Mycoplasma pneumoniae*, and some rickettsias and chlamydias.

Erythromycin was discovered in 1952 and is the only macrolide to be used widely. It is destroyed by gastric acid and must therefore be given as enteric-coated formulations or as one of its more stable salts or esters such as the stearate or ethyl succinate. Hepatotoxicity has been reported after the administration of erythromycin, most commonly as the estolate. Erythromycin lactobionate or gluceptate may be given intravenously. Cardiac arrhythmias have been reported occasionally after intravenous administration. Erythromycin is used as an alternative to penicillin in many infections, especially in patients who are allergic to penicillin, and, similarly to tetracycline, in the treatment of infections due to *Mycoplasma pneumoniae* and *Chlamydia trachomatis*, and in acne vulgaris. It is also used in the treatment of infections caused by *Legionella pneumophila*.

The other macrolides include *spiramycin* which has been used extensively in Europe and has also been used in the treatment and prophylaxis of toxoplasmosis and may be useful in the treatment of cryptosporidiosis.

Oleandomycin has been used orally and parenterally as the phosphate. Its ester, *triacetyloleandomycin*, is better absorbed from the gastro-intestinal tract but, like erythromycin estolate, has proved hepatotoxic. *Josamycin, kitasamycin, midecamycin*, and *rokitamycin* have been used in Europe and/or Japan.

More recent macrolides include *azithromycin, clarithromycin, dirithromycin*, and *roxithromycin*. These drugs all appear to have essentially similar properties to erythromycin although they may differ in their pharmacokinetics. Clarithromycin and, to a lesser extent, azithromycin are more active than erythromycin against opportunistic mycobacteria such as *Mycobacterium avium* complex. Clarithromycin is also used in the treatment of leprosy and in regimens for the eradication of *Helicobacter pylori* in peptic ulcer disease. Both azithromycin and clarithromycin have activity against protozoa including *Toxoplasma gondii*.

Flurithromycin is among other macrolides investigated.

Tylosin is a macrolide used in veterinary medicine.

The **streptogramin** group of antibiotics are also derived from *Streptomyces* spp. and include *pristinamycin* and *virginiamycin*. They consist of two components, which act synergistically and they are therefore also known as synergistins. One of the components is structurally related to the macrolides, and they have a similar spectrum of antimicrobial activity to erythromycin. Semisynthetic derivatives such as RP-56500 (quinupristin/dalfopristin) may be useful in the treatment of infections with multi-drug resistant organisms including methicillin-resistant *Staphylococcus aureus* and vancomycin-resistant enterococci.

Cross-resistance is often observed between the macrolides, lincosamides, and streptogramins.

Penicillins

Penicillin was the first antibiotic to be used therapeutically and was originally obtained, as a mixture of penicillins known as F, G, X, and K, from the mould *Penicillium notatum*. Better yields were achieved using *P. chrysogenum* and benzylpenicillin (penicillin G) was selectively produced by adding the precursor phenylacetic acid to the fermentation medium. The term 'penicillin' is now used generically for the entire group of natural and semisynthetic penicillins. Penicillins are still widely used; they are generally well tolerated, apart from hypersensitivity reactions, and are usually bactericidal by virtue of their inhibitory action on the synthesis of the bacterial cell wall.

They all have the same ring structure and are monobasic acids which readily form salts and esters; 6-aminopenicillanic acid, the penicillin nucleus, consists of a fused thiazolidine ring and a beta-lactam ring with an amino group at the 6-position.

The earlier or so-called 'natural' penicillins were produced by adding different side-chain precursors to fermentations of the *Penicillium* mould; *benzylpenicillin*, with a phenylacetamido side-chain at the 6-position, and *phenoxymethylpenicillin* (penicillin V), with a phenoxyacetamido side-chain, were 2 of the first and are still widely used. Benzylpenicillin can be considered the parent compound of the penicillins and is active mainly against Gram-positive bacteria and *Neisseria* spp. It is inactivated by penicillinase-producing bacteria and because of its instability in gastric acid it is usually injected. Long-acting preparations include *procaine penicillin* and *benzathine penicillin* which slowly release benzylpenicillin after injection. Phenoxymethylpenicillin is acid-stable and therefore given by mouth but it is also inactivated by penicillinase. It is generally used for relatively mild infections.

When no side-chain precursor is added to the fermentation medium 6-aminopenicillanic acid itself is obtained. A range of penicillins has been synthesised from 6-aminopenicillanic acid by substitution at the 6-amino position in an effort to improve on the instability of benzylpenicillin to gastric acid and penicillinases, to widen its antimicrobial spectrum, and to reduce its rapid rate of renal excretion. Two phenoxypenicillins in which the side-chain is α-phenoxypropionamido (*phenethicillin*) or α-phenoxybutyramido (*propicillin*) are more stable to acid than benzylpenicillin but offer no advantage over phenoxymethylpenicillin.

Methicillin has a 2,6-dimethoxybenzamido group at the 6-position and was the first penicillin found to be resistant to destruction by staphylococcal penicillinase. However, it is not acid-resistant and has to be injected. The isoxazolyl penicillins, *cloxacillin, dicloxacillin, flucloxacillin*, and *oxacillin*, are resistant to penicillinase and gastric acid. They have very similar chemical structures and differ mainly in their absorption characteristics. *Nafcillin* is a similar penicillinase-resistant antibiotic but is irregularly absorbed when taken by mouth.

Ampicillin has a D(−)-α-aminophenylacetamido side-chain and a broader spectrum of activity than benzylpenicillin; although generally less active against Gram-positive bacteria, some Gram-negative organisms including *Escherichia coli, Haemophilus influenzae*, and *Salmonella* spp. are sensitive although resistance is being reported increasingly. *Pseudomonas* spp. are not sensitive. Ampicillin is acid-stable and can be given by mouth but is destroyed by penicillinase. *Amoxycillin*, with a D(−)-α-aminohydroxyphenylacetamido side-chain, only differs from ampicillin by the addition of a hydroxyl group, but is better absorbed from the gastro-intestinal tract. A number of prodrugs including *bacampicillin, hetacillin, metampicillin*, and *pivampicillin* are also said to be better absorbed and are hydrolysed to ampicillin *in vivo*.

Carbenicillin, with an α-carboxyphenylacetamido side-chain, has marked activity against *Pseudomonas aeruginosa* and some *Proteus* spp. but otherwise is generally less active than ampicillin. It has to be given by injection and large doses are required. *Carfecillin* and *carindacillin* are the phenyl and indanyl esters of carbenicillin respectively and are hydrolysed to carbenicillin *in vivo* when taken by mouth. *Sulbenicillin* has an α-phenylsulphoacetamido side-chain and *ticarcillin* an α-carboxythienylacetamido side-chain and both have similar activity to carbenicillin; ticarcillin is more active against *Ps. aeruginosa*. The ureidopenicillins *azlocillin* and *mezlocillin*, and the closely related drug *piperacillin* are more active than carbenicillin against *Ps. aeruginosa* and have a wider range of activity against Gram-negative bacteria.

Temocillin, a 6-α-methoxy derivative of ticarcillin, is resistant to many beta-lactamases and is active against most Gram-negative aerobic bacteria, but not *Ps. aeruginosa*.

Mecillinam is a penicillanic acid derivative with a substituted amidino group in the 6-position. Unlike the 6-aminopenicillanic acid derivatives it is active mainly against Gram-negative bacteria, although *Ps. aeruginosa*, and *Bacteroides* spp. are considered resistant. Mecillinam is not active orally and is given by mouth as *pivmecillinam* which is hydrolysed to mecillinam on absorption.

The beta-lactamase inhibitors *clavulanic acid*, *sulbactam*, and *tazobactam* are used to extend the antimicrobial range of certain beta-lactam antibiotics.

Quinolones

The quinolonecarboxylic acids, carboxyquinolones, or 4-quinolones are a group of synthetic antibacterials structurally related to nalidixic acid. The term 4-quinolone has been used as a generic name for the common 4-oxo-1,4-dihydroquinoline skeleton. Under this system nalidixic acid, a naphthyridene derivative, is an 8-aza-4-quinolone, cinoxacin, a cinnoline derivative, is a 2-aza-4-quinolone, and pipemidic and piromidic acids, pyrido-pyrimidine derivatives, are 6,8-diaza-4-quinolones.

Nalidixic acid is active against Gram-negative bacteria but has little activity against *Pseudomonas* and Gram-positive organisms. Because bactericidal concentrations can only be achieved in urine its use has generally been limited to the treatment of urinary-tract infections.

Modification of the structure of nalidixic acid has produced related antibacterials such as *oxolinic acid, cinoxacin*, and *acrosoxacin*. Although some of these have a greater activity *in vitro* against Gram-negative organisms and activity against some Gram-positive organisms, none has been considered to represent a significant clinical advance over nalidixic acid; acrosoxacin is only used in the treatment of gonorrhoea. Addition of a piperazinyl radical at position 7, as in *pipemidic acid*, appears to confer some activity against *Pseudomonas*. *Flumequine* was the first fluorinated 4-quinolone to be synthesised, but has no piperazinyl group. Addition of the 7-piperazinyl group and a fluorine atom at position 6 has produced a group of fluorinated piperazinyl quinolones or fluoroquinolones with a broader spectrum of activity than nalidixic acid and pharmacokinetic properties more suitable for the treatment of systemic infections. They include *ciprofloxacin, enoxacin, fleroxacin, grepafloxacin, levofloxacin, lomefloxacin, nadifloxacin, norfloxacin, ofloxacin, pefloxacin, rufloxacin, sparfloxacin*, and *trovafloxacin*. *Danofloxacin, enrofloxacin*, and *marbofloxacin* are used in veterinary practice. Development of *difloxacin* for human use was suspended because of the high incidence of adverse effects, but it is used in veterinary practice. *Temafloxacin* was withdrawn worldwide because of toxicity.

The fluoroquinolones are very active against aerobic Gram-negative bacilli and cocci including the Enterobacteriaceae, *Haemophilus influenzae*, *Moraxella (Branhamella) catarrhalis*, and *Neisseria gonorrhoeae* and are also active against *Pseudomonas aeruginosa*. They are generally less active against Gram-positive organisms such as staphylococci and much less active against streptococci such as *Streptococcus pneumoniae*, although some fluoroquinolones have now been developed with increased activity against these organisms. They also have activity against mycobacteria, mycoplasmas, rickettsias, and *Plasmodium falciparum*. Some, for example ofloxacin, have useful activity against *Chlamydia trachomatis*. Activity against anaerobic bacteria is generally poor. There is concern that the emergence of resistant strains of organisms may limit the usefulness of fluoroquinolones in future.

One disadvantage of all the quinolone antibacterials is that they are generally not recommended for use in children, adolescents, and pregnant and breast feeding women because of their propensity to cause joint erosions in immature *animals*.

Sulphonamides and Diaminopyrimidines

The sulphonamides are analogues of *p*-aminobenzoic acid. The first sulphonamide of clinical importance was *Prontosil*, an azo dye which is metabolised *in vivo* to *sulphanilamide*. It was synthesised in Germany in 1932. Many sulphonamides have since been synthesised; they differ only slightly in their antimicrobial activity, but vary in their pharmacokinetic properties. The sulphonamides have been classified according to their rate of excretion as short-, medium- or intermediate-, long-, and ultra-long-acting. The **short-acting** sulphonamides are excreted in the urine in high concentrations and have therefore been of particular use in the treatment of urinary-tract infections. The solubility in urine of earlier short-acting sulphonamides, such as *sulphapyridine*, and their acetyl metabolites is low and hence crystalluria has been reported frequently. Of the short-acting sulphonamides most commonly used, *sulphadiazine* also has low solubility in urine whereas *sulphadimidine* and *sulphafurazole* and their acetyl conjugates are very soluble. Three short-acting sulphonamides (triple sulphonamides) have been given together to reduce the risk of crystalluria, as the constituent sulphonamides can co-exist in solution in urine without affecting each other's solubility. Preparations of mixed sulphonamides have, however, generally been replaced by the more soluble sulphonamides. The **medium-acting** sulphonamides such as *sulphamethoxazole*, the **long-acting** sulphonamides such as *sulphadimethoxine, sulphamethoxydiazine*, and *sulphamethoxypyridazine*, and the **ultra-long-acting** sulphonamides such as *sulfadoxine* and *sulfametopyrazine* do not attain such high concentrations in the urine and rarely cause crystalluria. Sulphonamides which are slowly excreted from the body do appear, however, to have been more commonly implicated in the development of reactions such as the Stevens-Johnson syndrome.

The sulphonamides are usually bacteriostatic, and interfere with folic acid synthesis of susceptible organisms; their broad spectrum of antimicrobial activity has, however, been limited by the development of resistance. The clinical use of sulphonamides has therefore been greatly reduced; in general they are indicated only in the treatment of urinary-tract infections and a few other disorders such as nocardiosis. Sulphonamides such as *sulphaguanidine, succinylsulphathiazole*, and *phthalylsulphathiazole* are poorly absorbed from the gastro-intestinal tract and have been used for the treatment of gastro-intestinal infections although they are now rarely indicated. *Silver sulphadiazine* and *mafenide acetate* are applied topically for their antibacterial action in patients with burns. *Sulphasalazine* (p.1215) a conjugate of 5-aminosalicylic acid (mesalazine) and sulphapyridine is used in the treatment of inflammatory bowel diseases and in rheumatoid arthritis.

Groups of drugs structurally related to the sulphonamides include the thiazides and carbonic anhydrase inhibitors (p.778) which are used for their diuretic activity, and the sulphonylureas (p.331) which are used for their hypoglycaemic activity.

Trimethoprim is a diaminopyrimidine which also inhibits folic acid synthesis but at a different stage in the metabolic pathway to that inhibited by the sulphonamides. It has a similar spectrum of antimicrobial activity to sulphonamides and often demonstrates synergy *in vitro* with these drugs. Trimethoprim was initially available only in combination with sulphonamides, most commonly with sulphamethoxazole as co-trimoxazole. It is now used alone particularly in the treatment of infections of the urinary and respiratory tracts. Analogues of trimethoprim include *baquiloprim, brodimoprim, ormetoprim*, and *tetroxoprim*.

Co-trimoxazole generally replaced sulphonamides alone in the treatment of systemic infections, although its use has also been restricted in some countries and trimethoprim may be preferred. Co-trimoxazole is however indicated for *Pneumocystis carinii* pneumonia and may be useful in protozoal infections such as toxoplasmosis. Other sulphonamides which have been used in combination with trimethoprim include sulphadiazine (see *co-trimazine*), sulfametopyrazine, sulfametrole, sulphamethoxypyridazine, and sulphamoxole (see *co-trifamole*). Sulphadiazine has been used in combination with tetroxoprim (see *co-tetroxazine*).

Sulphonamides have also been used in association with the diaminopyrimidine, pyrimethamine (p.436) in the treatment or prophylaxis of some protozoal infections. Commonly used combinations are sulfadoxine and pyrimethamine for malaria, and sulphadiazine and pyrimethamine for the treatment of toxoplasmosis.

Tetracyclines

The tetracyclines are a group of antibiotics, originally derived from certain *Streptomyces* spp., having the same tetracyclic nucleus, naphthacene, and similar properties. Unlike the penicillins and aminoglycosides they are usually bacteriostatic at the concentrations achieved in the body but act similarly to the aminoglycosides by interfering with protein synthesis in susceptible organisms.

Tetracyclines all have a broad spectrum of activity which includes Gram-positive and Gram-negative bacteria, chlamydias, rickettsias, mycoplasmas, spirochaetes, some mycobacteria, and some protozoa, but the emergence of resistant strains and the development of other antimicrobials has often reduced their value. Adverse effects have also restricted their usefulness. Gastro-intestinal disturbances are common and other important toxic effects include deposition in bones and teeth, precluding their use in pregnancy and young children; anti-anabolic effects, especially in patients with renal impairment; fatty changes in the liver; and photosensitivity, especially with demeclocycline. Allergic reactions are relatively uncommon. Because of these adverse effects tetracyclines should be avoided in pregnant women, children, and, apart from doxycycline and minocycline, patients with renal impairment.

The first tetracycline to be introduced was *chlortetracycline* in 1948 and, like chloramphenicol which was discovered about the same time, it was found to have a broad spectrum of activity and to be active by mouth unlike benzylpenicillin or streptomycin, the only other antibiotics then in use. The discovery of chlortetracycline was followed closely by that of *oxytetracycline* and then *tetracycline*, a reduction product of chlortetracycline which may be produced semisynthetically. All 3 have very similar properties although chlortetracycline is less well absorbed, and oxytetracycline may cause less staining of teeth. *Demeclocycline*, demethylated chlortetracycline, has a longer half-life than tetracycline. However, phototoxic reactions have been reported most frequently with demeclocycline. It has been used with some success in patients with the syndrome of inappropriate secretion of antidiuretic hormone.

The 4 tetracyclines mentioned so far (chlortetracycline, oxytetracycline, tetracycline, and demeclocycline) are all natural products that have been isolated from *Streptomyces* spp. The more recent tetracyclines, methacycline, doxycycline, and minocycline are semisynthetic derivatives. *Methacycline*, like demeclocycline, has a longer half-life than tetracycline and has been given twice daily. *Doxycycline* and *minocycline*, 2 more recent semisynthetic tetracycline derivatives, are both more active *in vitro* than tetracycline against many species. More importantly, minocycline is active against some tetracycline-resistant bacteria including strains of staphylococci. Both are well absorbed and, unlike the other tetracyclines, absorption is not significantly affected by the presence of food. They can be given in lower doses than the older members of the group and, having long half-lives, doxycycline is usually given once daily and minocycline twice daily. Also, they do not accumulate significantly in patients with renal impairment and can, therefore, be given to such patients. Both doxycycline and minocycline are more lipid-soluble than the other tetracyclines and they penetrate well into tissues. The use of minocycline may, however, be limited by its vestibular side-effects.

Because of the emergence of resistant organisms and the discovery of drugs with narrower antimicrobial spectra, tetracyclines are not generally the antibiotics of choice in Gram-positive or Gram-negative infections. However they have a place in the treatment of chlamydial infections, rickettsial infections such as typhus and the spotted fevers, mycoplasmal infections such as atypical pneumonia, and pelvic inflammatory disease, Lyme disease, brucellosis, tularaemia, plague, cholera, periodontal disease, and acne. The tetracyclines have also been useful in the treatment of penicillin-allergic patients suffering from venereal diseases, anthrax, actinomycosis, bronchitis, and leptospirosis. Minocycline may sometimes be used in multidrug regimens for leprosy.

Miscellaneous Antibacterials

Spectinomycin is an aminocyclitol antibacterial with some similarities to streptomycin although it is not an aminoglycoside. Spectinomycin is active against a wide range of bacteria but its clinical use is restricted to the treatment of chancroid and gonorrhoea. Trospectomycin, a water-soluble derivative, has been investigated.

Mupirocin is an antibacterial produced by *Pseudomonas fluorescens* with activity against most strains of staphylococci and streptococci and also some Gram-negative bacteria. It is applied topically.

Fosfomycin is a derivative of phosphonic acid; it is active against a range of Gram-positive and Gram-negative bacteria and is administered by mouth or parenterally.

The fusidane antibacterial *fusidic acid* is derived from *Fusidium coccineum* and has narrow spectrum of antibacterial activity, but it is very active against *Staphylococcus aureus* and has been used both topically and systemically in the treatment of staphylococcal infections. Resistance develops readily and it is often given in conjunction with other antibacterials.

The polymyxins are basic antibacterials produced by the growth of different strains of *Bacillus polymyxa* (*B. aerosporus*). *Polymyxin B* and *colistin* have been used clinically, but their systemic use has been more or less abandoned because of their toxicity, notably to the kidneys and nervous system. They are not absorbed when taken by mouth and have therefore been given in gastro-intestinal infections for their bactericidal activity against Gram-negative bacteria. They continue to be widely used as components of topical preparations.

Bacitracin, gramicidin, and *tyrothricin* are polypeptide antibacterials also produced by certain strains of *Bacillus* spp. but they are active against Gram-positive bacteria. Like the polymyxins, they are toxic when used systemically and are therefore mainly used topically.

The halogenated hydroxyquinoline *clioquinol* has antibacterial, antifungal, and antiprotozoal activity. It was formerly used in gastro-intestinal infections including amoebiasis but is of little value and can produce severe neurotoxicity. It is now mainly used locally for superficial infections of the skin and external ear. Topical application to extensive areas of skin can result in significant systemic absorption, especially if an occlusive dressing is used. *Chlorquinaldol* and *halquinol* are used similarly.

Urinary antimicrobials such as *nitrofurantoin*, and also *hexamine* which has generally been given as the hippurate or mandelate, may be used in the treatment and prophylaxis of infections of the lower urinary tract. They are concentrated in the urine, but do not usually achieve antimicrobial concentrations in the blood.

Choice of Antibacterial

Ideally, antibacterial treatment of infections should be chosen after the infecting organisms have been identified and the results of sensitivity tests are known. In practice, empirical treatment is often necessary initially, bearing in mind local patterns of infection and resistance. Other factors such as site of infection and tissue penetration are also important in deciding which antibacterial to give.

The prophylactic use of antibacterials is restricted mainly to patients undergoing some types of surgery. Other groups requiring infection prophylaxis include patients at special risk of developing endocarditis and those who have had rheumatic fever, who are splenectomised, or who are immunocompromised.

Abscess, abdominal

See under Abscess, Liver and under Peritonitis below.

Abscess, brain

Brain abscesses can result from otitis media, sinusitis, trauma, or dental sepsis, or they may be metastatic secondary to, for example, lung abscesses. Treatment entails surgical removal of pus and high doses of antibacterials. Ideally the choice of antibacterial depends on the infecting organisms and penetration by the antibacterial into brain tissue and abscess pus. Until organisms can be cultured empirical treatment should be given.

The site and origin of the brain abscess is a guide to the likely organisms; infections are often mixed and usually involve anaerobes. A report[1] from the UK noted that benzylpenicillin with metronidazole is appropriate against the *Streptococcus milleri* and anaerobes commonly found in frontal abscesses secondary to paranasal sinusitis; chloramphenicol or ampicillin or, more often, a third-generation cephalosporin with metronidazole and an aminoglycoside are used for temporal lobe and cerebellar abscesses which are often otogenic and may contain enterobacteria (usually *Proteus* spp.) with mixtures of anaerobes; and high-dose flucloxacillin with fusidic acid or rifampicin can be given for abscesses secondary to trauma, in which *Staphylococcus aureus* should be suspected (vancomycin is an alternative if allergy or bacterial resistance is a problem). Maximum doses of beta-lactams are advocated to ensure adequate penetration into the brain abscess.

Opportunistic infections in immunocompromised patients may present as brain abscesses.

1. Donald FE. Treatment of brain abscess. *J Antimicrob Chemother* 1990; **25:** 310–12.

Abscess, liver

Bacteria commonly responsible for pyogenic liver abscesses include Enterobacteriaceae, especially *Escherichia coli*; anaerobes, especially *Bacteroides fragilis*; and *Streptococcus milleri* (these can be microaerophilic). As elsewhere in the abdomen (see under Peritonitis, below), infections are often mixed. Treatment involves aspiration or drainage of pus and the administration of high doses of antibacterials. Broad-spectrum empirical therapy should be started immediately; more specific therapy may be possible when the results of cultures following diagnostic percutaneous aspiration of the abscess are known. Antibacterial therapy has been successful without surgical intervention. Gentamicin with clindamycin have been commonly used[1,2] but various combinations of other antibacterials, including cefoxitin, chloramphenicol, carboxypenicillins, third-generation cephalosporins, and metronidazole, might be appropriate.[2] However, intravenous antibacterial treatment without surgical intervention was not consistently successful,[3] although this might have been due to inadequate treatment against enteric anaerobes, especially *B. fragilis*.[2]

For the treatment of amoebic liver abscess, see under Amoebiasis in Antiprotozoals, p.573.

1. Herbert DA, *et al.* Pyogenic liver abscesses: successful non-surgical therapy. *Lancet* 1982; **i:** 134–6.
2. Herbert DA, *et al.* Medical management of pyogenic liver abscesses. *Lancet* 1985; **i:** 1384.
3. McCorkell SJ, Niles NL. Pyogenic liver abscesses: another look at medical management. *Lancet* 1985; **i:** 803–6.

Abscess, lung

Lung abscesses are often secondary to aspiration pneumonia and are discussed under Pneumonia, below. The organisms involved are commonly anaerobic bacteria.

Actinomycosis

Actinomycosis is mainly caused by the oral commensal *Actinomyces israelii*, a Gram-positive anaerobic or microaerophilic bacterium. Other species sometimes responsible include *A. meyeri*, *A. naeslundii*, and *A. viscosus*. One of the commonest forms has been cervicofacial actinomycosis, generally associated with poor oral hygiene and dental procedures.[1] Other forms include abdominal,[2] pulmonary, and disseminated actinomycosis; pelvic actinomycosis is associated with the use of intra-uterine contraceptive devices.

The antibacterial of choice is benzylpenicillin intravenously in high doses for several weeks, followed by oral penicillin (e.g. phenoxymethylpenicillin) for several months.[1,2] Strains relatively resistant to benzylpenicillin have proved sensitive to amoxycillin.[3] Tetracycline is an alternative in patients allergic to penicillin. Other alternatives include erythromycin or clindamycin. In one patient, actinomycosis resistant to conventional treatment responded to a prolonged course of ciprofloxacin.[4]

1. Anonymous. Essential drugs: systemic mycoses. *WHO Drug Inf* 1991; **5:** 129–36.
2. Stringer MD, Cameron AEP. Abdominal actinomycosis: a forgotten disease? *Br J Hosp Med* 1987; **38:** 125–7.
3. Martin MV. The use of oral amoxycillin for the treatment of actinomycosis: a clinical and in vitro study. *Br Dent J* 1984; **156:** 252–4.
4. Macfarlane DJ, *et al.* Treatment of recalcitrant actinomycosis with ciprofloxacin. *J Infect* 1993; **27:** 177–80.

Anaerobic bacterial infections

Anaerobic bacteria predominate in the normal microbial flora of man and are a common cause of infections, especially those arising from the gastro-intestinal tract, upper respiratory tract, skin, or vagina. Common anaerobic pathogens are *Bacteroides*, *Prevotella* (formerly non-fragilis *Bacteroides*), *Fusobacterium*, *Clostridium*, *Peptostreptococcus*, and *Actinomyces* spp. Apart from single species infections such as tetanus, gas gangrene, pseudomembranous colitis, and actinomycosis, most anaerobic infections are of mixed aetiology. Abscesses are often a feature. Infections include: brain abscess; acute necrotising gingivitis and other periodontal infections; chronic otitis media and chronic sinusitis; aspiration pneumonia and lung abscess; peritonitis and intra-abdominal abscess; bacterial vaginosis and pelvic inflammatory disease; cellulitis, ulcers, bite and other wound infections.[1] Sensitivity testing *in vitro* is often impractical and treatment for non-species-specific infections is usually empirical. Benzylpenicillin was traditionally considered the antibacterial of choice when *B. fragilis* was unlikely (infections above the diaphragm) although resistance is increasingly a problem. Antibacterials with activity against the *B. fragilis* group and other anaerobic pathogens include metronidazole and other 5-nitroimidazole derivatives, chloramphenicol, clindamycin, cefoxitin, antipseudomonal penicillins, imipenem-cilastatin, and combinations of a beta-lactam and beta-lactamase inhibitor.[2]

Clinical isolates of anaerobic bacteria in the USA[3] have shown increasing resistance of the *B. fragilis* group (including *B. distasonis*, *B. fragilis*, *B. ovatus*, *B. thetaiotaomicron*, and *B. vulgatus*) to clindamycin, continuing penicillin resistance in non-fragilis *Bacteroides* spp. (now reclassified as *Prevotella* spp. and including the type species *P. melaninogenica*), and rare beta-lactamase-mediated resistance of *Fusobacterium* to penicillin. Resistance of some *Clostridium* spp. to penicillin and clindamycin had declined, but no changes were noted for *Cl. perfringens*.

The *B. fragilis* group are the most frequently isolated anaerobic bacteria in clinical infections and all members of the group may be pathogenic.[4] Most strains produce beta lactamase and thus are resistant to penicillins and cephalosporins although there is varied susceptibility within the group.[5] In an ongoing USA survey of susceptibility patterns[6] the most active drugs *in vitro* against *B. fragilis* group strains were imipenem, metronidazole, and chloramphenicol; resistance to cefoxitin, clindamycin, and piperacillin was not widespread and combinations of beta-lactamase inhibitors with penicillins or cephalosporins (e.g. ampicillin or cefoperazone with sulbactam; ticarcillin with clavulanate) were also very active. Others have reported similar results.[5] On the basis of activity *in vitro* in another study[7] metronidazole, imipenem, ticarcillin with clavulanate, cefoxitin, and amoxycillin with clavulanate were considered suitable for the treatment of *B. fragilis* group infections. A clinical isolate of *B. fragilis*, simultaneously resistant to metronidazole, amoxycillin with clavulanate, and imipenem, was reported in the UK;[8] treatment with clindamycin was successful on this occasion.

1. Styrt B, Gorbach SL. Recent developments in the understanding of the pathogenesis and treatment of anaerobic infections (first of two parts). *N Engl J Med* 1989; **321:** 240–6.
2. Styrt B, Gorbach SL. Recent developments in the understanding of the pathogenesis and treatment of anaerobic infections (second of two parts). *N Engl J Med* 1989; **321:** 298–302.
3. Musial CE, Rosenblatt JE. Antimicrobial susceptibilities of anaerobic bacteria isolated at the Mayo Clinic during 1982 through 1987: comparison with results from 1977 through 1981. *Mayo Clin Proc* 1989; **64:** 392–9.
4. Brook I. The clinical importance of all members of the Bacteroides fragilis group. *J Antimicrob Chemother* 1990; **25:** 473–4.
5. Cuchural GJ, *et al.* Comparative activities of newer β-lactam agents against members of the Bacteroides fragilis group. *Antimicrob Agents Chemother* 1990; **34:** 479–80.
6. Cornick NA, *et al.* The antimicrobial susceptibility patterns of the Bacteroides fragilis group in the United States, 1987. *J Antimicrob Chemother* 1990; **25:** 1011–19.
7. Jacobs MR, *et al.* β-Lactamase production, β-lactam sensitivity and resistance to synergy with clavulanate of 737 Bacteroides fragilis group organisms from thirty-three US centres. *J Antimicrob Chemother* 1990; **26:** 361–70.
8. Turner P, *et al.* Simultaneous resistance to metronidazole, co-amoxiclav, and imipenem in clinical isolate of Bacteroides fragilis. *Lancet* 1995; **345:** 1275–7.

Anthrax

Anthrax is a zoonotic disease caused by *Bacillus anthracis*, a spore-forming Gram-positive aerobe. It is rare in western countries. The commonest type is cutaneous anthrax; pulmonary, gastro-intestinal, and meningitic anthrax can also occur and in these types the prognosis is poor.

Benzylpenicillin is the antibacterial of choice[1,2] although some resistant strains of *B. anthracis* have been reported. Knudson[1] cited the following treatment regimens: for mild uncomplicated cutaneous anthrax, phenoxymethylpenicillin potassium 7.5 mg per kg bodyweight by mouth every 6 hours for 5 to 7 days; for more extensive cutaneous disease, procaine penicillin 10 mg per kg intramuscularly every 12 hours for 5 to 7 days; for pulmonary, intestinal, and meningeal anthrax, immediate treatment with benzylpenicillin by continuous intravenous infusion, 50 mg per kg in the first hour followed by 200 mg per kg every 24 hours. Once septicaemia has developed a fatal outcome is likely due to toxin release and Knudson[1] advised the use of anthrax antitoxin, if available, in conjunction with antibacterials. Benzylpenicillin 10 mg per kg intramuscularly every 12 hours for 5 to 7 days has been used prophylactically if contaminated meat has been ingested or if *B. anthracis* has been inadvertently injected beneath the skin. Vaccine is available for active immunisation against anthrax. Combined penicillin and vaccine prophylaxis has been used for pulmonary anthrax prophylaxis.[1]

A tetracycline or erythromycin may be used in patients unable to take penicillin.[2,3]

1. Knudson GB. Treatment of anthrax in man: history and current concepts. *Milit Med* 1986; **151:** 71–7.
2. Anonymous. The choice of antibacterial drugs. *Med Lett Drugs Ther* 1998; **40:** 33–42.
3. Anonymous. Anthrax: memorandum from a WHO meeting. *Bull WHO* 1996; **74:** 465–70.

Antibiotic-associated colitis

See under Gastro-enteritis, below.

Arthritis, bacterial

See under Bone and Joint Infections, below.

Bacillary angiomatosis

See under Cat Scratch Disease, below.

Bacterial vaginosis

Bacterial vaginosis (anaerobic vaginosis; nonspecific vaginitis) is a common and often distressing vaginal condition associated with a fishy-smelling vaginal discharge and an abnormal vaginal flora. The abnormal flora comprises *Gardnerella vaginalis* and *Bacteroides* and *Mobiluncus* spp.[1] It is not generally considered to be exclusively a sexually transmitted disease. An association has been reported between bacterial vaginosis and premature births of low-weight infants, and treatment early in the second trimester of pregnancy is advised.[2,3]

Usual treatment is with metronidazole or clindamycin either by mouth or intravaginally;[3-5] the duration is usually 5 or 7 days depending on the drug and preparation used although single oral doses of metronidazole have been employed. However, relapse is common after any of these treatment regimens.[2]

1. Blackwell A. Anaerobic vaginosis: therapeutic and epidemiological aspects. *J Antimicrob Chemother* 1984; **14:** 445–8.
2. Hay PE. Therapy of bacterial vaginosis. *J Antimicrob Chemother* 1998; **41:** 6–9.
3. Anonymous. Management of bacterial vaginosis. *Drug Ther Bull* 1998; **36:** 33–5.
4. WHO. *WHO model prescribing information: drugs used in sexually transmitted diseases and HIV infection.* Geneva: WHO, 1995.
5. Centers for Disease Control. 1998 Guidelines for treatment of sexually transmitted diseases. *MMWR* 1998; **47** (RR-1): 70–4.

Biliary-tract infections

Infections of the biliary tract are usually associated with obstructive and inflammatory conditions such as cholecystitis and cholangitis. Complications can include gangrene, hepatic or intraperitoneal abscesses, peritonitis, and septicaemia. The organisms involved are typically gut flora including Gram-negative aerobes such as *Escherichia coli* and *Klebsiella* spp. and anaerobes including *Bacteroides fragilis*.

Treatment of uncomplicated acute cholecystitis is usually conservative. Antibacterials including cephalosporins, tetracyclines, or broad-spectrum penicillins are commonly given, although some have questioned that use.[1] For more severe infections including suppurative cholangitis, prompt treatment with appropriate antibacterial drugs is necessary. Since biliary obstruction prevents adequate concentrations of many antibacterials being achieved in the bile, the main aim of treatment is to control bacteraemia. Antibacterials used, often in combination, include cephalosporins, aminoglycosides, ampicillin (or amoxycillin), piperacillin, fluoroquinolones, metronidazole, clindamycin, and imipenem.[2,3] In most cases of obstruction, definitive treatment depends on restoring drainage of bile by surgical or medical treatment of gallstones (p.1642).

Antibacterial prophylaxis is commonly employed in biliary surgery (see Surgical Infection, below) to prevent acute cholangitis and wound infections. Cephalosporins are often used for this purpose.[2]

Antibacterials may also have a role as maintenance therapy in recurrent cholangitis.

1. Bouchier IAD. Gallstones. *Br Med J* 1990; **300:** 592–7.
2. van den Hazel SJ, *et al.* Role of antibiotics in the treatment and prevention of acute and recurrent cholangitis. *Clin Infect Dis* 1994; **19:** 279–86.
3. Peña C, Gudiol F. Cholecystitis and cholangitis: spectrum of bacteria and role of antibiotics. *Dig Surg* 1996; **13:** 317–20.

Bites and stings

Wound infections following cat or dog bites are often due to the Gram-negative aerobe *Pasteurella multocida*. The treatment of choice for *P. multocida* is benzylpenicillin and it should be given for infections evident within 24 hours of a bite;[1] tetracycline is an alternative in patients allergic to penicillin. The fluoroquinolone ciprofloxacin has been used successfully to treat *P. multocida* cellulitis associated with a cat bite.[2]

In addition to *P. multocida*, other bacteria involved in cat or dog bite wound infections include *Staphylococcus, Streptococcus, Bacteroides,* and *Fusobacterium* spp. and their presence will influence the choice of treatment. For example, a penicillinase-resistant penicillin may be necessary if *Staph. aureus* is present. Also, combinations of antibacterials may be necessary in patients allergic to penicillin since tetracycline, the alternative suggested against *P. multocida* infection, has only limited activity against aerobic Gram-positive cocci. Amoxycillin with clavulanic acid is reported to be effective against most wound pathogens.[3]

More unusual organisms include *Capnocytophaga canimorsus* (formerly called dysgonic fermenter type 2 or DF-2) which has been associated in particular with dog bites, but also with cat bites. It is an opportunistic pathogen especially hazardous to immunocompromised patients including splenectomised patients; the best treatment is benzylpenicillin,[4] amoxycillin-clavulanic acid, or erythromycin.[5] Reports of severe *C. canimorsus* infection following dog bites,[6,7] including fatal septicaemia in an otherwise healthy man, have highlighted the importance of early antibacterial treatment and debridement.

See also under Cat Scratch Disease (below).

If necessary prophylaxis or treatment for rabies (p.1531) should be instituted.

Among the more unusual infections acquired from animals is seal finger, caused by an as yet unidentified organism and treated with tetracycline.[8] The Gram-negative bacilli *Spirillum minus* (or *minor*) and *Streptobacillus moniliformis* are both causes of rat-bite fever. In each case the treatment of choice is benzylpenicillin;[9] a tetracycline or streptomycin are alternatives.

Envenomation following bites and stings by snakes, scorpions, spiders, and some marine animals is usually treated symptomatically and with specific antivenoms and antisera (see for example Box Jellyfish Sting, p.1516, Scorpion Stings, p.1533, Snake Bites, p.1534, Spider Bites, p.1534, and Stone Fish Venom Antisera, p.1535).

1. Elliot DL, *et al.* Pet-associated illness. *N Engl J Med* 1985; **313:** 985–95.
2. Richards CAL, Emmanuel FXS. Treatment of Pasteurella multocida cellulitis with ciprofloxacin. *J Infect* 1992; **24:** 216–17.
3. Goldstein EJC. Bite wounds and infections. *Clin Infect Dis* 1992; **14:** 633–8.
4. McCarthy M, Zumla A. DF-2 infection. *Br Med J* 1988; **297:** 1355–6.
5. Morgan MS, Cruickshank JG. Prevention of postsplenectomy sepsis. *Lancet* 1993; **341:** 700–1.
6. Gallen IW, Ispahani P. Fulminant Capnocytophaga canimorsus (DF-2) septicaemia. *Lancet* 1991; **337:** 308.
7. Kristensen KS, *et al.* Capnocytophaga canimorsus infection after dog-bite. *Lancet* 1991; **337:** 849.
8. Beck B, Smith TG. Seal finger: an unsolved medical problem in Canada. *Can Med Assoc J* 1976; **115:** 105–9.
9. Anonymous. The choice of antibacterial drugs. *Med Lett Drugs Ther* 1998; **40:** 33–42.

Bone and joint infections

In *bacterial arthritis* (septic arthritis) joints may be infected via the blood with a variety of organisms including staphylococci, streptococci, enterococci, Enterobacteriaceae, *Pseudomonas aeruginosa*, and anaerobes although the commonest is probably *Staphylococcus aureus*. *Haemophilus influenzae* is a common cause in young children as is *Neisseria gonorrhoeae* in sexually active young adults. In addition to gonococcal arthritis other specific types of bacterial arthritis include Lyme disease, and meningococcal, salmonellal, and tuberculous arthritis (see under the appropriate disease for further details).

With the exception of *N. gonorrhoeae*, infecting organisms in *osteomyelitis* (infection of bone) are similar to those in bacterial arthritis.[1-11]

In *reactive arthritis* (aseptic arthritis) joint inflammation follows infection elsewhere in the body. It is generally secondary to sexually transmitted infections, especially chlamydial infections, or to enteric infections. Reactive arthritis in association with urethritis or cervicitis, or both, is termed Reiter's syndrome.

Empirical treatment regimens for bacterial arthritis or osteomyelitis usually include antistaphylococcal antibacterials such as flucloxacillin, nafcillin, clindamycin, and fusidic acid; children under 5 years may be given amoxycillin or cefuroxime because of the likelihood of *H. influenzae* infection. Treatment is generally initiated with high doses given intravenously and may need to continue for 6 weeks in acute bacterial arthritis or osteomyelitis. Chronic disease may require longer term treatment although the oral route may be used after initial parenteral therapy.

Oral ciprofloxacin[12,13] or ofloxacin[14] have been used successfully in the treatment of osteomyelitis due to susceptible organisms, but the value of fluoroquinolones against Gram-positive bacteria is controversial and there appears to be increasing resistance to them among methicillin-resistant *Staph. aureus* and coagulase-negative staphylococci.[15]

For reference to infection prophylaxis in orthopaedic patients, see under Surgical Infection, below.

Reactive arthritis is treated with anti-inflammatories; the role of antibacterials is less certain. Results in arthritis associated with chlamydial infections have been more promising than in that triggered by enteric infections.[16] Long-term treatment with a tetracycline in addition to an NSAID has been reported to shorten the duration of reactive arthritis resulting from *Chlamydia trachomatis* infection.[17]

For mention of the use of tetracyclines, usually minocycline, in the treatment of *rheumatoid arthritis*, see under Musculoskeletal and Joint Disorders, p.261.

1. Goldenberg DL, Reed JI. Bacterial arthritis. *N Engl J Med* 1985; **312:** 764–71.
2. Dickie AS. Current concepts in the management of infections in bones and joints. *Drugs* 1986; **32:** 458–75.
3. Anonymous. Bacterial arthritis. *Lancet* 1986; **ii:** 721–2.
4. Sexton DJ, McDonald M. Osteomyelitis: approaching the 1990s. *Med J Aust* 1990; **153:** 91–6.
5. Dirschl DR, Almekinders LC. Osteomyelitis: common causes and treatment recommendations. *Drugs* 1993; **45:** 29–43.
6. Haas DW, McAndrew MP. Bacterial osteomyelitis in adults: evolving considerations in diagnosis and treatment. *Am J Med* 1996; **101:** 550–61.
7. Hamed KA, *et al.* Pharmacokinetic optimisation of the treatment of septic arthritis. *Clin Pharmacokinet* 1996; **31:** 156–63.
8. Cimmino MA. Recognition and management of bacterial arthritis. *Drugs* 1997; **54:** 50–60.
9. Lew DP, Waldvogel FA. Osteomyelitis. *N Engl J Med* 1997; **336:** 999–1007.
10. Mader JT, *et al.* A practical guide to the diagnosis and management of bone and joint infections. *Drugs* 1997; **54:** 253–64.
11. Goldenberg DL. Septic arthritis. *Lancet* 1998; **351:** 197–202.
12. Gentry LO, Rodriguez GG. Oral ciprofloxacin compared with parenteral antibiotics in the treatment of osteomyelitis. *Antimicrob Agents Chemother* 1990; **34:** 40–3.
13. Dan M, *et al.* Oral ciprofloxacin treatment of Pseudomonas aeruginosa osteomyelitis. *Antimicrob Agents Chemother* 1990; **34:** 849–52.
14. Gentry LO, Rodriguez-Gomez G. Ofloxacin versus parenteral therapy for chronic osteomyelitis. *Antimicrob Agents Chemother* 1991; **35:** 538–41.
15. Cruciani M, Bassetti D. The fluoroquinolones as treatment for infections caused by Gram-positive bacteria. *J Antimicrob Chemother* 1994; **33:** 403–17.

16. Svenungsson B. Reactive arthritis. *Br Med J* 1994; **308:** 671–2.
17. Lauhio A. Reactive arthritis: consider combination treatment. *Br Med J* 1994; **308:** 1302–3.

Botulism

For a discussion of botulism and its management, see p.1506.

Bronchitis

Bronchitis may be defined as inflammation of the bronchi and is associated with excessive sputum production and cough. The bronchi of healthy people are said to be nearly always sterile whereas the upper respiratory tract is often colonised with commensal bacteria including *Streptococcus pneumoniae* and *Haemophilus influenzae*.

Acute bronchitis in previously healthy subjects is commonly associated with viral respiratory infections such as colds and influenza. There may sometimes be secondary bacterial infection that responds to antibacterial therapy as for acute exacerbations of chronic bronchitis (see below). *Acute bronchiolitis* occurs in infants as a result mainly of viral infection and antibacterials are not given routinely (see Respiratory Syncytial Virus Infection, p.602).

Chronic bronchitis and emphysema often occur together and have been termed chronic obstructive pulmonary disease (chronic obstructive airways disease). Acute exacerbations of chronic bronchitis may be viral in origin, but bacteria are often present in purulent sputum, the commonest being *Str. pneumoniae* and *H. influenzae*; *Moraxella (Branhamella) catarrhalis* is increasingly reported.

The value of antibacterial treatment in both acute bronchitis and acute exacerbation of chronic disease has been controversial and difficult to assess.[1-5] Following a comparison of broad-spectrum antibacterial (amoxycillin, co-trimoxazole, or doxycycline) with placebo, Anthonisen *et al.*[6] considered that antibacterials were justified in exacerbations of chronic obstructive pulmonary disease characterised by increased dyspnoea, sputum production, and sputum purulence. A meta-analysis of randomised studies indicated a small improvement due to therapy in patients with exacerbations of disease.[7] If antibacterials are given it is common practice to give a 7- to 10-day oral course of a broad-spectrum drug such as amoxycillin with or without clavulanic acid, ampicillin, an oral cephalosporin such as cefaclor or cefuroxime axetil, co-trimoxazole, erythromycin or a newer macrolide such as azithromycin or clarithromycin, tetracycline, or trimethoprim (preferred to co-trimoxazole in the UK), the choice depending on local patterns of resistance. Long-term prophylaxis in patients with frequent exacerbations is controversial.

Bronchitis associated with *Chlamydia pneumoniae* (formerly TWAR strain of *C. psittaci*) and responding to tetracycline or erythromycin has also been reported.[8]

The symptomatic relief of chronic bronchitis is discussed under Chronic Obstructive Pulmonary Disease on p.747.

1. Gonzales R, Sande M. What will it take to stop physicians from prescribing antibiotics in acute bronchitis? *Lancet* 1995; **345:** 665–6.
2. Hahn DL. Antibiotics in acute bronchitis. *Lancet* 1995; **345:** 1244–5.
3. Anonymous. Antibiotics for exacerbations of chronic bronchitis? *Lancet* 1987; **ii:** 23–4.
4. Staley H, *et al.* Is an objective assessment of antibiotic therapy in exacerbations of chronic bronchitis possible? *J Antimicrob Chemother* 1993; **31:** 193–7.
5. O'Brien KL, *et al.* Cough illness/bronchitis—principles of judicious use of antimicrobial agents. *Pediatrics* 1998; **101** (suppl): 178–81.
6. Anthonisen NR, *et al.* Antibiotic therapy in exacerbations of chronic obstructive pulmonary disease. *Ann Intern Med* 1987; **106:** 196–204.
7. Saint S, *et al.* Antibiotics in chronic obstructive pulmonary disease exacerbations: a meta-analysis. *JAMA* 1995; **273:** 957–60.
8. Grayston JT, *et al.* A new respiratory tract pathogen: Chlamydia pneumoniae strain TWAR. *J Infect Dis* 1990; **161:** 618–25.

Brucellosis

Brucellosis (formerly known as undulant fever) is caused by *Brucella* spp., aerobic Gram-negative bacteria found primarily in animals and transmitted to humans. The principal species affecting man are *Brucella abortus*, from cattle; *B. melitensis*, from sheep, goats, camels, and sometimes cattle; and *B. suis* from pigs. Brucellosis has often been associated with consumption of unpasteurised milk or its products and although rare or controlled in countries such as the UK it remains a problem in many areas, including the Mediterranean region and Middle East. Rarely, human infection can result from exposure to live veterinary vaccines.[1]

Treatment of brucellosis has been with rifampicin plus doxycycline, but some now prefer doxycycline plus streptomycin. The regimen recommended by WHO is rifampicin 600 to 900 mg with doxycycline 200 mg both given daily in the morning as a single dose for at least 6 weeks.[2] Administration of doxycycline and rifampicin for 30 days was found by some workers[3] to result in higher relapse rates than those for the regimen of tetracycline and streptomycin previously recommended by WHO. However, in a multinational comparative study of 143 patients with acute brucellosis,[4] a 45-day regimen of rifampicin and doxycycline was comparable with a regimen of doxycycline 200 mg daily with a meal for 45 days and streptomycin 1 g intramuscularly daily for 21 days; a third regimen of tetracycline 500 mg 4 times daily for 21 days and streptomycin 1 g intramuscularly daily for 14 days was associated with a 41% failure rate and could not be recommended. Doxycycline for 6 weeks and streptomycin for the first 2 weeks also proved effective in a Spanish study[5] and was considered preferable to doxycycline and rifampicin. An overview of studies also indicated that doxycycline plus streptomycin was associated with lower relapse rates than rifampicin plus doxycycline and the former was recommended as the preferred combination.[6] An interaction between rifampicin and doxycycline, in which concentrations of doxycycline were reduced when the two were given together,[7] might explain the reduced efficacy of this combination. A suggested regimen in non-pregnant adults is thus doxycycline 200 mg daily for 6 weeks together with streptomycin 1 g daily for 2 to 3 weeks.[8]

Resistance to rifampicin has emerged following therapy despite administration with doxycycline.[9]

Rifampicin with co-trimoxazole was effective in the treatment of **children**[10] although the authors of a multicentre study in Kuwaiti children[11] considered that rifampicin should be reserved for complicated brucellosis because of the risk of serious adverse effects and development of resistance in areas endemic for tuberculosis. They recommended oxytetracycline or doxycycline for 3 weeks with gentamicin intramuscularly for the first 5 days in children over 8 years old, co-trimoxazole being given instead of a tetracycline in younger children. Co-trimoxazole has also been used alone to treat brucellosis but relapse has been found to be common.[2]

For the treatment of brucellosis during **pregnancy** WHO recommends rifampicin as the drug of choice and that co-trimoxazole or tetracycline should only be given if rifampicin is unavailable; streptomycin is contra-indicated.[2]

In the treatment of **neurobrucellosis** the length of therapy appears to be of critical importance; relapses may occur after treatment lasting only 2 to 3 weeks and a regimen of tetracycline 2 g daily and rifampicin 600 to 900 mg daily given for 8 to 12 weeks supplemented with streptomycin 1 g daily for 6 weeks has consequently been recommended by some.[12] There have also been reports of the successful use of similar triple therapy in the treatment of endocarditis due to *Brucella melitensis*.[13]

A vaccine is available in some countries for active immunisation of individuals at high risk of contracting brucellosis.

1. Blasco JM, Díaz R. Brucella melitensis Rev-1 vaccine as a cause of human brucellosis. *Lancet* 1993; **342:** 805.
2. FAO/WHO. Joint FAO/WHO expert committee on brucellosis: sixth report. *WHO Tech Rep Ser 740* 1986.
3. Ariza J, *et al.* Comparative trial of rifampin-doxycycline versus tetracycline-streptomycin in the therapy of human brucellosis. *Antimicrob Agents Chemother* 1985; **28:** 548–51.
4. Acocella G, *et al.* Comparison of three different regimens in the treatment of acute brucellosis: a multicenter multinational study. *J Antimicrob Chemother* 1989; **23:** 433–9. Correction *ibid.*; **24:** 629.
5. Cisneros JM, *et al.* Multicenter prospective study of treatment of Brucella melitensis brucellosis with doxycycline for 6 weeks plus streptomycin for 2 weeks. *Antimicrob Agents Chemother* 1990; **34:** 881–3.
6. Solera J, *et al.* Recognition and optimum treatment of brucellosis. *Drugs* 1997; **53:** 245–56.
7. Colmenero JD, *et al.* Possible implications of doxycycline-rifampin interaction for treatment of brucellosis. *Antimicrob Agents Chemother* 1994; **38:** 2798–2802.
8. Friedland JS. Brucellosis. *Prescribers' J* 1993; **33:** 24–8.
9. De Rautlin de la Roy YM, *et al.* Rifampicin resistance in a strain of Brucella melitensis after treatment with doxycycline and rifampicin. *J Antimicrob Chemother* 1986; **18:** 648–9.
10. Llorens-Terol J, Busquets RM. Brucellosis treated with rifampicin. *Arch Dis Child* 1980; **55:** 486–8.
11. Lubani MM, *et al.* A multicenter therapeutic study of 1100 children with brucellosis. *Pediatr Infect Dis* 1989; **8:** 75–8.
12. Shakir RA. Neurobrucellosis. *Postgrad Med J* 1986; **62:** 1077–9.
13. Farid Z, Trabolsi B. Successful treatment of two cases of brucella endocarditis with rifampicin. *Br Med J* 1985; **291:** 110.

Campylobacter enteritis

See under Gastro-enteritis, below.

Cat scratch disease

Cat scratch disease usually occurs after a cat scratch or bite. The condition is characterised by regional lymphadenopathy and is often self-limiting, but may be disseminated in immunocompromised patients. With uncertainty over aetiology there has been no specific antibacterial therapy, but there are reports of successful treatment with gentamicin[1] or co-trimoxazole[2] in children and with ciprofloxacin[3] in adults.

In the 1980s a Gram-negative bacillus presumed to be responsible for cat scratch disease was isolated[4,5] and subsequently named *Afipia felis*.[6] However, it now appears that *Bartonella henselae* (formerly *Rochalimaea henselae*) is the main cause of cat scratch disease[6-8] and that *A. felis* causes few, if any, cases, although there is some evidence that both organisms might have a joint role.[9] Bacillary angiomatosis, in which both *B. henselae* and *B. quintana*[10] (the causative organism of trench fever) have been implicated, may represent a disseminated form of cat scratch disease occurring predominantly in HIV-infected patients. However, in contrast to the response seen in cat scratch disease, the disseminated disease in immunocompromised patients has not responded to ciprofloxacin,[11,12] but has responded to treatment with doxycycline[11-14] or erythromycin.[11] Care is required in patients with AIDS since the lesions of bacillary angiomatosis closely resemble those of Kaposi's sarcoma, and if the diagnosis is missed life-saving antibacterial therapy may not be given.[15]

1. Bogue CW, *et al.* Antibiotic therapy for cat-scratch disease? *JAMA* 1989; **262:** 813–16.
2. Collipp PJ. Cat-scratch disease therapy. *Am J Dis Child* 1989; **143:** 1261.
3. Holley HP. Successful treatment of cat-scratch disease with ciprofloxacin. *JAMA* 1991; **265:** 1563–5.
4. Wear DJ, *et al.* Cat scratch disease: a bacterial infection. *Science* 1983; **221:** 1403–5.
5. English CK, *et al.* Cat-scratch disease: isolation and culture of the bacterial agent. *JAMA* 1988; **259:** 1347–52.
6. Birtles RJ, *et al.* Cat scratch disease and bacillary angiomatosis: aetiological agents and the link with AIDS. *Commun Dis Rep* 1993; **3:** R107–R110.
7. Relman DA, *et al.* The agent of bacillary angiomatosis: an approach to the identification of uncultured pathogens. *N Engl J Med* 1990; **323:** 1573–80.
8. Flexman JP, *et al.* Bartonella henselae is a causative agent of cat scratch disease in Australia. *J Infect* 1995; **31:** 241–5.
9. Alkan S, *et al.* Dual role for Afipia felis and Rochalimaea henselae in cat-scratch disease. *Lancet* 1995; **345:** 385.
10. Koehler JE, *et al.* Isolation of Rochalimaea species from cutaneous and osseous lesions of bacillary angiomatosis. *N Engl J Med* 1992; **327:** 1625–31.
11. Tappero JW, Koehler JE. Cat-scratch disease and bacillary angiomatosis. *JAMA* 1991; **266:** 1938–9.
12. Tucker RM, *et al.* Cat-scratch disease and bacillary angiomatosis. *JAMA* 1991; **266:** 1939.
13. Kemper CA, *et al.* Visceral bacillary epithelioid angiomatosis: possible manifestations of disseminated cat scratch disease in the immunocompromised host: a report of two cases. *Am J Med* 1990; **89:** 216–22.
14. Mui BSK, *et al.* Response of HIV-associated disseminated cat scratch disease to treatment with doxycycline. *Am J Med* 1990; **89:** 229–31.
15. Taylor AG, *et al.* Cat-scratch, Kaposi's sarcoma, and bacillary angiomatosis. *Lancet* 1993; **342:** 686.

Cellulitis

See under Skin Infections, below.

Cervicitis

Gonorrhoea in women occurs predominantly as cervicitis, but mucopurulent cervicitis is frequently caused by sexually transmitted *Chlamydia trachomatis*. The two infections often occur together and should be treated concurrently. Guidelines for treatment are given under Gonorrhoea, and Chlamydial Infections, below.

Chancroid

Chancroid is one of the classical sexually transmitted diseases and is caused by the Gram-negative bacterium *Haemophilus ducreyi*. It occurs worldwide, but is endemic in parts of Africa and South East Asia where it is a frequent cause of genital ulceration and a risk factor in the transmission of HIV. Chancroid has also become an important sexually transmitted disease in the USA.[1]

The treatment of choice for chancroid in most endemic areas has been a multidose course of erythromycin or co-trimoxazole[2] although single-dose treatment regimens might be preferable if compliance is a problem. Treatment failure may be more common in patients also infected with HIV, especially with single-dose regimens.[1]

Specific regimens have been provided by the Centers for Disease Control (CDC) in the USA and by the WHO. CDC has recommended[1] either erythromycin 500 mg four times daily by mouth for 7 days; or a single intramuscular injection of ceftriaxone 250 mg; or a single oral dose of azithromycin 1 g; or ciprofloxacin 500 mg twice daily by mouth for 3 days. WHO has recommended[3] erythromycin 500 mg three times daily by mouth for 7 days, alternatives being a single intramuscular injection of ceftriaxone 250 mg, a single oral dose of ciprofloxacin 500 mg, or a single intramuscular injection of spectinomycin 2 g. Co-trimoxazole 960 mg twice daily by mouth for 7 days has also been used in some countries. High failure rates have been reported with ceftriaxone,[4] and its future usefulness may be limited.

Sexual partners of patients with chancroid should also be treated.

1. Centers for Disease Control. 1998 Guidelines for treatment of sexually transmitted diseases. *MMWR* 1998; **47** (RR-1): 18–20.
2. Dangor Y, *et al.* Treatment of chancroid. *Antimicrob Agents Chemother* 1990; **34:** 1308–11.
3. WHO. *WHO model prescribing information: drugs used in sexually transmitted diseases and HIV infection.* Geneva: WHO, 1995.
4. Tyndall M, *et al.* Ceftriaxone no longer predictably cures chancroid in Kenya. *J Infect Dis* 1993; **167:** 469–71.

Chlamydial infections

The species *Chlamydia pneumoniae*, *C. psittaci*, and *C. trachomatis* are all pathogens in man and are generally sensitive to tetracyclines or erythromycin. *C. pneumoniae* is a respiratory pathogen formerly called TWAR (Taiwan acute respiratory) agent and considered then to be a strain of *C. psittaci*; it was first described as a cause of community-acquired pneumonia (see Pneumonia, below), but has since been associated with a wide variety of clinical presentations and has been implicated in the pathogenesis of ischaemic heart disease. *C. psittaci* is transmitted to man from birds and causes psittacosis which also affects the lungs (see Psittacosis, below).

Chlamydia trachomatis infections. *C. trachomatis* causes a wide range of diseases. Many are sexually transmitted and the spectrum is similar to that with *Neisseria gonorrhoeae* (see Gonorrhoea, below); infections with the two organisms often occur concurrently. Pregnant women infected with *C. trachomatis* may be at risk of premature rupture of membranes and preterm labour (see Premature Labour, below). They may also infect their offspring to cause ophthalmia neonatorum (see Neonatal Conjunctivitis, below) or pneumonia (below).

Guidelines for the treatment of uncomplicated urethral, endocervical, or rectal infections with *C. trachomatis* from the WHO[1] recommend a 7-day oral course of doxycycline or tetracycline; alternatives are erythromycin or a sulphonamide. The Centers for Disease Control in the USA[2] recommend either doxycycline for 7 days or a single oral dose of azithromycin; alternatives are 7-day courses of ofloxacin or of erythromycin. Sexual partners of those infected with *C. trachomatis* should be tested and treated.[1,2] Pregnant women should be given erythromycin[1,2] or amoxycillin[2] to eradicate *C. trachomatis* infection and prevent perinatal transmission. Azithromycin is a further alternative.[2]

For further reference to sexually transmitted *C. trachomatis* infections, see under the headings Epididymitis, Pelvic Inflammatory Disease, and Urethritis (all below).

Specific serotypes of *C. trachomatis* are responsible for another sexually transmitted disease, lymphogranuloma venereum (see Lymphogranuloma Venereum, below).

Reactive arthritis (see Bone and Joint Infections, above) may be secondary to chlamydial infections.

Other *C. trachomatis* infections that are not sexually transmitted include trachoma and inclusion conjunctivitis in adults (see Trachoma, below).

1. WHO. *WHO model prescribing information: drugs used in sexually transmitted diseases and HIV infection.* Geneva: WHO, 1995.
2. Centers for Disease Control. 1998 Guidelines for treatment of sexually transmitted diseases. *MMWR* 1998; **47** (RR-1): 53–9.

Cholera and other vibrio infections

See under Gastro-enteritis, below.

Cystic fibrosis

Cystic fibrosis is a genetic disorder associated with the production of abnormally viscous mucus. This results in blocked ducts in many organs, but most importantly in the lungs and pancreas. The underlying defect is mutation in the gene which codes for cystic fibrosis transmembrane conductance regulator (CFTR), a protein which functions as a chloride channel.[1] Mutation results in defective ion transport with reduced chloride ion secretion and accelerated sodium ion absorption, and related changes in the composition and properties of mucin secreted. Now that patients with cystic fibrosis usually survive into adulthood, it is increasingly seen to be a multisystem disease. However, the main clinical manifestations are still pulmonary disease, with recurrent bacterial infections and the production of copious viscous sputum, and malabsorption due to pancreatic insufficiency. Other complications include male infertility and liver disease. There is increased salt loss in sweat.

Various diagnostic methods are available[2,3] and clinical diagnosis of cystic fibrosis may be confirmed by establishing that chloride concentrations in sweat are raised, using the pilocarpine sweat test (see *Martindale*, 29th ed. p.1335). Nowadays identification of gene mutation is possible and should ideally be used for further confirmation of the diagnosis.

Decreases in the morbidity of patients with cystic fibrosis and improved survival are largely due to the management of pulmonary disease with antibacterials and physiotherapy and to nutritional management. Several reviews have discussed both established and experimental treatments.[4-11]

Pulmonary disease is the major cause of mortality. Cystic fibrosis is an underlying cause of bronchiectasis (chronic dilatation of the bronchi) as a result of excessive secretion of mucus and recurrent infections. Cough and excessive production of sputum are characteristic of cystic fibrosis and the lungs are generally colonised with bacterial pathogens, especially mucoid strains of *Pseudomonas aeruginosa*. Pseudomonal pulmonary infection is the major cause of morbidity and mortality in cystic fibrosis. Monitoring of bacterial pathogens in the sputum, including their sensitivity, is necessary for rational treatment.[12] Apart from *Ps. aeruginosa*, *Staphylococcus aureus* is often present and may be the predominant pathogen in infants. *Burkholderia cepacia* (formerly *Pseudomonas cepacia*), said to be virtually nonpathogenic in healthy subjects, is being increasingly isolated in cystic fibrosis patients and cross-infection is causing widespread concern.[13] In a proportion who acquire it *B. cepacia* has been associated with rapid deterioration and death.[14] Other bacteria isolated include *Haemophilus influenzae* and atypical *Mycobacteria* spp.

Some intervene early and give antibacterials prophylactically as soon as cystic fibrosis has been diagnosed, that is before there is necessarily any evidence of infection. In one study, infants given continuous treatment with oral flucloxacillin once cystic fibrosis had been picked up by neonatal screening had fewer hospital admissions, lower rates of *Staph. aureus* isolation, and less morbidity than those given antibacterials episodically only when indicated clinically.[15]

Once present, eradication of *Ps. aeruginosa* is difficult and not permanent. Acute exacerbations of pulmonary infection are treated with antipseudomonal antibacterials administered intravenously, usually an aminoglycoside (e.g. tobramycin) with a penicillin (e.g. ticarcillin) or a third-generation cephalosporin (e.g. ceftazidime); ceftazidime has also been given alone. High doses are necessary because of the poor penetration of these antipseudomonal antibacterials into the site of infection and their increased renal clearance in patients with cystic fibrosis, as well as the difficulties of penetrating mucoid strains of *Ps. aeruginosa*.[16] Alternatively, ciprofloxacin can be given by mouth; it has been widely used successfully for short-term treatment although it is not generally recommended in infants and children. There is uncertainty over the value of long-term prophylaxis and its attendant risks, including the development of bacterial resistance. Some treat acute exacerbations as they occur whereas others give regular intermittent courses of intravenous antipseudomonal antibacterials. For example, in some units[12] a 10- to 14-day course is given intravenously every 3 months to any patient with cystic fibrosis in whom *Ps. aeruginosa* has been recovered from the sputum more than once or twice, regardless of symptoms. The intravenous antibacterials can often be given safely at home.[17] Inhaled antibacterials including gentamicin with carbenicillin,[18] tobramycin alone[19] and with ticarcillin,[20] or colistin[21] have also been used in patients chronically infected with *Ps. aeruginosa*, and interest in this route of administration is likely to increase,[22] especially with improvements in nebuliser systems and techniques.[23] In one study,[24] chronic colonisation was prevented by giving ciprofloxacin and inhalations of colistin for 3 weeks whenever *Ps. aeruginosa* was isolated from routine sputum cultures. Active immunisation with a *Pseudomonas aeruginosa* vaccine or passive immunisation with antibodies against *Ps. aeruginosa* are under investigation.

Infection with *B. cepacia* is difficult to treat because the majority of antipseudomonal antibacterials are not effective. Co-trimoxazole has been suggested for *B. cepacia* infections[25] and temocillin has shown promise,[26] but David[12] considered the best hope was to stop antipseudomonal treatment so that *B. cepacia* might be replaced by *Ps. aeruginosa*. Firm guidance about the risks and consequences of colonisation has been difficult to give since attitudes to *B. cepacia* are evolving rapidly.[13] Transmission of *B. cepacia* in cystic fibrosis patients appears to be mainly by social contact,[27,28] although some have reported otherwise.[29]

Antistaphylococcal antibacterials such as flucloxacillin may be used for *Staph. aureus* infection, but eradication from the sputum is very difficult.[12,30] Fusidic acid has been given in combination with an antistaphylococcal penicillin.[31]

After isolation of *H. influenzae* from the sputum some prefer to treat immediately with amoxycillin rather than wait for new symptoms to appear.[12]

The effects of cystic fibrosis in the lungs are complex and treatment of infections may not halt the progression of lung destruction. Many other interventions have been tried. Dornase alfa (recombinant human deoxyribonuclease; rhDNase) is administered by aerosol inhalation and reduces the viscosity of the sputum by breaking down the large quantities of DNA released by degenerating inflammatory cells. The use of dornase alfa has been associated with some improvement in lung function and it might be a useful adjunct to bronchial drainage, although it is unclear whether it prevents the development of progressive lung damage (see p.1059). Mucolytics such as acetylcysteine are generally not considered to be effective in cystic fibrosis.[32,33]

Other interventions tried with some evidence of benefit include management of the inflammatory response in the lungs with corticosteroids[34] (by mouth[35] or by inhalation,[36] although a randomised controlled study[37] with inhaled corticosteroid failed to demonstrate benefit) or with the NSAID ibuprofen.[38] Alpha$_1$-proteinase inhibitor, the main inhibitor of neutrophil elastase in the lung has also been investigated[39] as has oxpentifylline,[40] a drug with anticytokine activity. A preliminary study[41] suggested that administration of eicosapentaenoic acid could reduce sputum production by modifying the production of leukotriene B_4, a possible mediator of the inflammatory response.

Bronchodilators may be useful in selected patients but are not used routinely. Both beta$_2$-adrenoceptor stimulants such as salbutamol[42] and antimuscarinics such as ipratropium have been used.[43]

Experimental treatment aimed at modifying the pulmonary disease process includes ion transport therapy involving the administration of aerosolised drugs which either inhibit sodium ion absorption across airway epithelia, for example the sodium channel blocker amiloride,[44,45] or induce chloride ion secretion, for example the triphosphate nucleotides adenosine triphosphate (ATP) and uridine triphosphate (UTP).

In patients with severe lung disease, oxygen therapy may give some relief of symptoms but its effect on mortality and morbidity is uncertain.[46] At present the only available treatment for patients with end stage pulmonary disease is lung transplantation.

Nutritional management of cystic fibrosis should ensure adequate calorie intake from a balanced diet in order to counteract malabsorption due to pancreatic insufficiency and the increased metabolic requirements of patients with cystic fibrosis.[47,48] Supplements of the fat-soluble vitamins A, D, and E, and sometimes vitamin K may be necessary. Pancreatic enzymes, as pancreatin or pancrelipase, are taken before or with each meal or snack. Inactivation of pancreatic enzymes by gastric acid can be decreased by the use of histamine H_2-antagonists such as cimetidine[49] or a proton pump inhibitor such as omeprazole.[50]

Somatic **gene therapy** represents the nearest approach to a cure for cystic fibrosis. It aims to introduce the normal CFTR gene sequence into cells of affected tissue. Most effort has been directed at gene delivery to the lungs using adenovirus vectors or liposomes, but results have been variable.[51-53] For a discussion of the general principles of gene therapy, see p.1583.

1. Koch C, Høiby N. Pathogenesis of cystic fibrosis. *Lancet* 1993; **341:** 1065–9.
2. Stern RC. The diagnosis of cystic fibrosis. *N Engl J Med* 1997; **336:** 487–91.
3. Wallis C. Diagnosing cystic fibrosis: blood, sweat, and tears. *Arch Dis Child* 1997; **76:** 85–91.
4. Alton E, *et al.* New treatments for cystic fibrosis. *Br Med Bull* 1992; **48:** 785–804.
5. Fiel SB. Clinical management of pulmonary disease in cystic fibrosis. *Lancet* 1993; **341:** 1070–4.
6. Tizzano EF, Buchwald M. Recent advances in cystic fibrosis research. *J Pediatr* 1993; **122:** 985–8.
7. Wallace CS, *et al.* Pharmacologic management of cystic fibrosis. *Clin Pharm* 1993; **12:** 657–74.
8. Webb AK, David TJ. Clinical management of children and adults with cystic fibrosis. *Br Med J* 1994; **308:** 459–62.
9. Anonymous. Therapeutic approaches to cystic fibrosis: memorandum from a joint WHO/ICF(M)A meeting. *Bull WHO* 1994; **72:** 341–52.
10. Ramsey BW. Management of pulmonary disease in patients with cystic fibrosis. *N Engl J Med* 1996; **335:** 179–88.
11. Rosenstein BJ, Zeitlin PL. Cystic fibrosis. *Lancet* 1998; **351:** 277–82.
12. David TJ. Cystic fibrosis. *Arch Dis Child* 1990; **65:** 152–7.
13. Anonymous. Pseudomonas cepacia—more than a harmless commensal? *Lancet* 1992; **339:** 1385–6.
14. Walters S, Smith EG. Pseudomonas cepacia in cystic fibrosis: transmissibility and its implications. *Lancet* 1993; **342:** 3–4.
15. Beardsmore CS, *et al.* Pulmonary function in infants with cystic fibrosis: the effect of antibiotic treatment. *Arch Dis Child* 1994; **71:** 133–7.
16. Anonymous. Antibiotic dosage in cystic fibrosis. *Lancet* 1985; **i:** 1020–1.
17. Gilbert J, *et al.* Home intravenous antibiotic treatment in cystic fibrosis. *Arch Dis Child* 1988; **63:** 512–17.
18. Hodson ME, *et al.* Aerosol carbenicillin and gentamicin treatment of Pseudomonas aeruginosa infection in patients with cystic fibrosis. *Lancet* 1981; **ii:** 1137–9.
19. Ramsey BW, *et al.* Efficacy of aerosolized tobramycin in patients with cystic fibrosis. *N Engl J Med* 1993; **328:** 1740–6.
20. Wall MA, *et al.* Inhaled antibiotics in cystic fibrosis. *Lancet* 1983; **i:** 1325.
21. Jensen T, *et al.* Colistin inhalation therapy in cystic fibrosis patients with chronic Pseudomonas aeruginosa lung infection. *J Antimicrob Chemother* 1987; **19:** 831–8.
22. Littlewood JM, *et al.* Aerosol antibiotic treatment in cystic fibrosis. *Arch Dis Child* 1993; **68:** 788–92.
23. Hung JCC, *et al.* Evaluation of two commercial jet nebulisers and three compressors for the nebulisation of antibiotics. *Arch Dis Child* 1994; **71:** 335–8.
24. Valerius NH, *et al.* Prevention of chronic Pseudomonas aeruginosa colonisation in cystic fibrosis by early treatment. *Lancet* 1991; **338:** 725–6.
25. Anonymous. The choice of antibacterial drugs. *Med Lett Drugs Ther* 1998; **40:** 33–42.
26. Taylor RFH, *et al.* Temocillin and cystic fibrosis: outcome of intravenous administration in patients infected with Pseudomonas cepacia. *J Antimicrob Chemother* 1992; **29:** 341–4.
27. Govan JRW, *et al.* Evidence for transmission of Pseudomonas cepacia by social contact in cystic fibrosis. *Lancet* 1993; **342:** 15–19.
28. Mahenthiralingam E, *et al.* Burkholderia cepacia in cystic fibrosis. *N Engl J Med* 1995; **332:** 819.
29. Steinbach S, *et al.* Transmissibility of Pseudomonas cepacia infection in clinic patients and lung-transplant recipients with cystic fibrosis. *N Engl J Med* 1994; **331:** 981–7.
30. Littlewood JM. An overview of the management of cystic fibrosis. *J R Soc Med* 1986; **79** (suppl 12): 55–63.
31. Jensen T, *et al.* Clinical experiences with fusidic acid in cystic fibrosis patients. *J Antimicrob Chemother* 1990; **25** (suppl B): 45–52.
32. Stafanger G, *et al.* The clinical effect and the effect on the ciliary motility of oral N-acetylcysteine in patients with cystic fibrosis and primary ciliary dyskinesia. *Eur Respir J* 1988; **1:** 161–7.
33. Ratjen F, *et al.* A double-blind placebo controlled trial with oral ambroxol and N-acetylcysteine for mucolytic treatment in cystic fibrosis. *Eur J Pediatr* 1985; **144:** 374–8.
34. Price JF, Greally P. Corticosteroid treatment in cystic fibrosis. *Arch Dis Child* 1993; **68:** 719–21.
35. Eigen H, *et al.* A multicenter study of alternate-day prednisone therapy in patients with cystic fibrosis. *J Pediatr* 1995; **126:** 515–23.
36. Van Haren EHJ, *et al.* The effects of the inhaled corticosteroid budesonide on lung function and bronchial hyperresponsiveness in adult patients with cystic fibrosis. *Respir Med* 1995; **89:** 209–14.
37. Balfour-Lynn IM, *et al.* Randomised controlled trial of inhaled corticosteroids (fluticasone propionate) in cystic fibrosis. *Arch Dis Child* 1997; **77:** 124–30.
38. Konstan MW, *et al.* Effect of high-dose ibuprofen in patients with cystic fibrosis. *N Engl J Med* 1995; **332:** 848–54.
39. McElvaney NG, *et al.* Aerosol α-1-antitrypsin treatment for cystic fibrosis. *Lancet* 1991; **337:** 392–4.
40. Aronoff SC, *et al.* Effects of pentoxifylline on sputum neutrophil elastase and pulmonary function in patients with cystic fibrosis: preliminary observations. *J Pediatr* 1994; **125:** 992–7.
41. Lawrence R, Sorrell T. Eicosapentaenoic acid in cystic fibrosis: evidence of a pathogenetic role for leukotriene B_4. *Lancet* 1993; **342:** 465–9.
42. Eggleston P, *et al.* A controlled trial of long-term bronchodilator therapy in cystic fibrosis. *Chest* 1991; **99:** 1088–92.
43. Weintraub SJ, Eschenbacher WL. The inhaled bronchodilators ipratropium bromide and metaproterenol in adults with CF. *Chest* 1989; **95:** 861–4.
44. Knowles MR, *et al.* A pilot study of aerosolized amiloride for the treatment of lung disease in cystic fibrosis. *N Engl J Med* 1990; **322:** 1189–94.
45. Bowler IM, *et al.* Nebulised amiloride in respiratory exacerbations of cystic fibrosis: a randomised controlled trial. *Arch Dis Child* 1995; **73:** 427–30.
46. Zinman R, *et al.* Nocturnal home oxygen in the treatment of hypoxemic cystic fibrosis patients. *J Pediatr* 1989; **114:** 368–77.
47. Bowler IM, *et al.* Resting energy expenditure and substrate oxidation rates in cystic fibrosis. *Arch Dis Child* 1993; **68:** 754–9.
48. Green MR, *et al.* Nutritional management of the infant with cystic fibrosis. *Arch Dis Child* 1995; **72:** 452–6.
49. Perry RS, Gallagher J. Management of maldigestion associated with pancreatic insufficiency. *Clin Pharm* 1985; **4:** 161–9.
50. Heijerman HG, *et al.* Omeprazole enhances the efficacy of pancreatin (Pancrease) in cystic fibrosis. *Ann Intern Med* 1991; **114:** 200–1.
51. Colledge WH, Evans MJ. Cystic fibrosis gene therapy. *Br Med Bull* 1995; **51:** 82–90.
52. Coutelle C. Gene therapy approaches for cystic fibrosis. *Biologicals* 1995; **23:** 21–5.
53. Southern KW. Gene therapy for cystic fibrosis: current issues. *Br J Hosp Med* 1996; **55:** 495–9.

Diarrhoea, infective

See under Gastro-enteritis, below.

Diphtheria

Diphtheria is caused by infection, usually of the upper respiratory tract or the skin, with the Gram-positive aerobe *Corynebacterium diphtheriae*. It is distributed worldwide and despite the effectiveness of immunisation (see Diphtheria Vaccines, p.1507), diphtheria is still common in parts of the world, including the tropics. Although the risk to travellers is said to be low, diphtheria should be considered in patients returning from tropical countries with a sore throat.[1] Russia and other republics of the former USSR have experienced an epidemic.[2]

The most serious manifestations of infection are due to exotoxin produced by toxigenic strains and thus treatment is primarily with diphtheria antitoxin. Erythromycin or benzylpenicillin are also given to eliminate *C. diphtheriae*, thereby terminating toxin production and preventing the spread of infection to contacts. Close contacts of primary cases of diphtheria may be given a 7-day prophylactic course of erythromycin by mouth, in addition to boosters or primary immunisation with diphtheria vaccine. Non-toxigenic *C. diphtheriae* is the most common isolate in clinical cases in the UK[3] and generally causes a less severe form of the disease; it does, however, have the potential to cause invasive disease in some patients.[4]

Asymptomatic carriers may harbour non-toxigenic strains of *C. diphtheriae* that can be converted to toxigenic strains. A single intramuscular injection of benzathine penicillin has been less effective than oral erythromycin, but may be used if compliance is uncertain;[5] clindamycin for 7 days by mouth has also eliminated the carrier state,[5] but erythromycin remains the drug of choice. Bacteriological follow-up should be carried out 2 weeks after completing treatment to be certain *C. diphtheriae* has been eradicated from carriers.[6]

1. Anonymous. Toxigenic Corynebacterium diphtheriae associated with the Haj. *Commun Dis Rep* 1991; **1:** 143.
2. Hardy IRB, *et al.* Current situation and control strategies for resurgence of diphtheria in newly independent states of the former Soviet Union. *Lancet* 1996; **347:** 1739–44.
3. Begg N, Balraj V. Diphtheria: are we ready for it? *Arch Dis Child* 1995; **73:** 568–72.
4. Efstratiou A, *et al.* Non-toxigenic Corynebacterium diphtheriae var gravis in England. *Lancet* 1993; **341:** 1592–3.
5. McCloskey RV, *et al.* Treatment of diphtheria carriers: benzathine penicillin, erythromycin, and clindamycin. *Ann Intern Med* 1974; **81:** 788–91.
6. Miller LW, *et al.* Diphtheria carriers and the effect of erythromycin therapy. *Antimicrob Agents Chemother* 1974; **6:** 166–9.

Ear infections

See under Otitis Externa, and Otitis Media, below.

Ehrlichiosis

Infections with rickettsia-like bacteria of the *Ehrlichia* genus are rare and at one time the only species isolated from humans was *E. sennetsu*, the cause of Sennetsu fever in Japan. *E. canis* is responsible for a tick-borne disease in *dogs* and a closely related species, *E. chaffeensis*, causes human ehrlichiosis.[1] A granulocytic *Ehrlichia* species closely related to *E. phagocytophila* and *E. equi* appears to be responsible for cases of human granulocytic ehrlichiosis in parts of the USA[1,2] and probably in Europe.[3] A large proportion of infections occur after a tick bite. As with other rickettsial infections, treatment is with a tetracycline;[1,2,4] chloramphenicol has been used as an alternative.[4] Antibiotic susceptibility testing has suggested that rifamycins and quinolones, particularly trovafloxacin, are promising alternatives in the granulocytic form of infections.[5]

1. Dumler JS, Bakken JS. Ehrlichial diseases of humans: emerging tick-borne infections. *Clin Infect Dis* 1995; **20:** 1102–10.
2. Bakken JS, *et al.* Clinical and laboratory characteristics of human granulocytic ehrlichiosis. *JAMA* 1996; **275:** 199–205.
3. Brouqui P, *et al.* Human granulocytic ehrlichiosis in Europe. *Lancet* 1995; **346:** 782–3.
4. Schaffner W, Standaert SM. Ehrlichiosis—in pursuit of an emerging infection. *N Engl J Med* 1996; **334:** 262–3.
5. Klein MB, *et al.* Antibiotic susceptibility of the newly cultivated agent of human granulocytic ehrlichiosis: promising activity of quinolones and rifamycins. *Antimicrob Agents Chemother* 1997; **41:** 76–9.

Endocarditis

Infective endocarditis is caused by infection of the endocardium following invasion of the blood stream by bacteria or fungi and particularly affects the heart valves. Infection may follow an acute or subacute course depending in part on the organisms responsible. Virtually any organism can cause endocarditis but streptococci, enterococci, and staphylococci continue to be major culprits. The commonest bacteria responsible are the alpha haemolytic streptococci originating mainly from the mouth and throat; they have been called viridans streptococci or even '*Streptococcus viridans*' (although this is not a true species) and include *Str. mitis*, *Str. mutans*, *Str. oralis*, *Str. salivarius*, and *Str. sanguis*. Other streptococci originate in the gut and include *Str. bovis*. Enterococci (faecal streptococci) also originate in the gut and include *Enterococcus faecalis* and to a lesser extent *E. faecium*. Endocarditis due to all these bacteria is commonly subacute or insidious. Acute endocarditis is often due to *Staphylococcus aureus*, a common cause in intravenous drug abusers, but may also be caused by coagulase-negative staphylococci, particularly *Staph. lugdunensis*. *Staph. epidermidis* is often responsible for prosthetic valve infection. Gram-negative bacteria such as the Enterobacteriaceae, *Pseudomonas* spp., and the HACEK group of slow-growing organisms (*Haemophilus*, *Actinobacillus*, *Cardiobacterium*, *Eikenella*, *Kingella*); the rickettsia *Coxiella burnetii* (the cause of Q fever, below); and fungi such as *Candida* and *Aspergillus* are less common causes of endocarditis.

There are consensus recommendations for the treatment and prophylaxis of endocarditis.

Endocarditis treatment. Guidelines for the treatment of streptococcal, enterococcal, and staphylococcal endocarditis were produced by the British Society for Antimicrobial Chemotherapy in 1998[1] and, with the addition of HACEK endocarditis, by the American Heart Association in 1995.[2] Although these guidelines are broadly accepted there may be differing views on detail including choice of antibacterial, route of administration, and duration of treatment. Treatment depends on identification of the infecting organisms and their sensitivity to antibacterials. Blood should therefore be taken for culture before treatment is started; MICs should be measured. *Empirical treatment* with benzylpenicillin plus gentamicin may then be given until the laboratory results are known; vancomycin should be given instead of benzylpenicillin if staphylococcal infection is likely.[1] There is synergy between penicillin and aminoglycosides against streptococci. Viridans streptococci are generally much more sensitive to penicillin than enterococci and gentamicin may sometimes be stopped once the laboratory results are known.

Briefly, the 1998 **UK** guidelines[1] are as follows.

- STREPTOCOCCAL ENDOCARDITIS.

  For *penicillin-sensitive streptococci* (viridans streptococci and *Str. bovis* with a benzylpenicillin MIC of 0.1 μg or less per mL): intravenous bolus injections of benzylpenicillin 1.2 g every 4 hours and gentamicin 80 mg twice daily both given for 2 weeks.

  For *streptococci less sensitive to penicillin* (viridans streptococci and *Str. bovis* with a benzylpenicillin MIC of more than 0.1 μg per mL): benzylpenicillin and gentamicin as above, but both given for 4 weeks.

  For *streptococci in penicillin-allergic patients*: initially either vancomycin 1 g intravenously twice daily or teicoplanin 400 mg intravenously every 12 hours for three doses and then a maintenance dose of 400 mg daily; either drug should be given for 4 weeks, together with gentamicin as above for the first 2 weeks.

- ENTEROCOCCAL ENDOCARDITIS.

  For *gentamicin-sensitive or low-level resistant enterococci* (MIC less than 100 μg per mL): intravenous bolus injections of ampicillin or amoxycillin 2 g every 4 hours and gentamicin 80 mg twice daily, both given for 4 weeks.

  For *gentamicin highly-resistant enterococci* (MIC at least 2000 μg per mL): ampicillin or amoxycillin as above, but for a minimum of 6 weeks; streptomycin may also be given if sensitivity can be demonstrated.

  For *enterococci in penicillin-allergic patients*: as for streptococci in penicillin-allergic patients above, except that gentamicin should be given for all 4 weeks of treatment.

- STAPHYLOCOCCAL ENDOCARDITIS.

  For *penicillin-sensitive staphylococci*: intravenous bolus injections of benzylpenicillin 1.2 g every 4 hours for four weeks plus gentamicin 80 to 120 mg every 8 hours for the first week.

  For *staphylococci resistant to penicillins generally but sensitive to methicillin/flucloxacillin*: intravenous bolus injections of flucloxacillin 2 g every 4 hours for 4 weeks plus gentamicin as for penicillin-sensitive staphylococci.

  For *staphylococci resistant to methicillin/flucloxacillin* and in *penicillin-allergic patients*: vancomycin 1 g intravenously twice daily for 4 weeks plus gentamicin as for penicillin-sensitive staphylococci.

  In difficult cases of endocarditis due to coagulase-negative staphylococci or *Staph. aureus*, rifampicin may occasionally be added to therapy, usually with vancomycin.

The 1995 **USA** guidelines[2] are as follows.

- STREPTOCOCCAL AND ENTEROCOCCAL ENDOCARDITIS.

  For *penicillin-sensitive streptococci* (viridans streptococci and *Str. bovis* with a benzylpenicillin MIC of 0.1 μg or less per mL): there are 3 alternative regimens, namely benzylpenicillin alone for 4 weeks; ceftriaxone alone for 4 weeks; or benzylpenicillin with gentamicin, each for 2 weeks only. Streptomycin has been used as an alternative to gentamicin but gentamicin is now preferred. Doses are: intravenous benzylpenicillin 7.2 to 10.8 g daily by continuous infusion or in 6 divided doses; intravenous or intramuscular ceftriaxone 2 g once daily; intramuscular or intravenous gentamicin 1 mg per kg body-weight every 8 hours.

  For *relatively resistant streptococci* (viridans streptococci and *Str. bovis* with a benzylpenicillin MIC greater than 0.1 μg per mL but less than 0.5 μg per mL): intravenous benzylpenicillin 10.8 g daily by continuous infusion or in 6 divided doses for 4 weeks with gentamicin as above for 2 weeks.

  For *more resistant bacteria* (enterococci or viridans streptococci with a benzylpenicillin MIC of 0.5 μg or more per mL): there are three alternative regimens, namely intravenous benzylpenicillin 10.8 to 18.0 g daily by continuous infusion or in 6 divided doses with gentamicin as above; or intravenous ampicillin 12.0 g daily by continuous infusion or in 6 divided doses again with gentamicin as above; or intravenous vancomycin 30 mg per kg daily in two divided doses, the total daily dose not exceeding 2 g, again with gentamicin as above. Both drugs in each regimen should be given for 4 to 6 weeks. Streptomycin has again been used as an alternative to gentamicin but gentamicin is now preferred. Resistance is, however, emerging among enterococcal strains to vancomycin and to gentamicin and streptomycin as well as to the penicillins. Where resistance to vancomycin is modest, teicoplanin is suggested as an alternative. Some patients with multiply-resistant enterococcal infection whose treatment fails may need to be considered for surgical intervention.

  For *streptococci and enterococci in penicillin-allergic patients or those allergic to other beta-lactams*: intravenous vancomycin 30 mg per kg daily in two divided doses for 4 weeks, the total daily dose not exceeding 2 g. For more resistant bacteria vancomycin should be given with gentamicin as above, both for 4 to 6 weeks.

- STAPHYLOCOCCAL ENDOCARDITIS.

  For *methicillin-susceptible staphylococci* in the *absence of prosthetic material*: intravenous nafcillin or oxacillin 2 g every 4 hours for 4 to 6 weeks with or without gentamicin 1 mg per kg intramuscularly or intravenously every 8 hours for 3 to 5 days. For *methicillin-resistant* staphylococci, intravenous vancomycin 30 mg per kg daily in 2 divided doses is given for 4 to 6 weeks, the total daily dose not exceeding 2 g.

  For *methicillin-susceptible staphylococci in the presence of prosthetic material*: intravenous nafcillin or oxacillin 2 g every 4 hours with oral rifampicin 300 mg every 8 hours for 6 weeks or more and gentamicin as above for the initial 2 weeks. For methicillin-resistant staphylococci, nafcillin or oxacillin are replaced by intravenous vancomycin 30 mg per kg daily in 2 or 4 divided doses for 6 weeks or more, the total daily dose not exceeding 2 g.

  For *methicillin-susceptible staphylococci in penicillin-allergic patients or those allergic to other beta-lactams* in the *absence of prosthetic material*, intravenous cephazolin 2 g every 8 hours for 4 to 6 weeks or other first-generation cephalosporin (except in immediate-type hypersensitivity) with or without gentamicin as above for 3 to 5 days. Alternatively intravenous vancomycin 30 mg per kg daily in 2 divided doses is given for 4 to 6 weeks, the total daily dose not exceeding 2 g. In the *presence of prosthetic material*, such patients receive the regimen described above but with nafcillin or oxacillin replaced by vancomycin or a first-generation cephalosporin.

- HACEK ENDOCARDITIS.

  Traditionally the HACEK group of organisms have been susceptible to ampicillin, but recently resistant strains have been identified and monotherapy with ampicillin is no longer recommended. Preferred treatment is therefore with intramuscular or intravenous ceftriaxone 2 g once daily for 4 weeks, although cefotaxime or other third-generation cephalosporin may be substituted. Alternatively, intravenous ampicillin 12 g daily by continuous infusion or in 6 divided doses with intramuscular or intravenous gentamicin 1 mg per kg every 8 hours may be given, both for 4 weeks. Therapy should be extended to 6 weeks for prosthetic valve endocarditis.

Endocarditis prophylaxis. Patients at risk of developing endocarditis, including those with valvular heart disease, prosthetic valves, or other cardiac abnormalities and those with a history of endocarditis or rheumatic fever, should be given antibacterials prophylactically when about to undergo dental operations, tonsillectomy, or other procedures liable to lead to bacteraemia. Antibacterials should be administered so that adequate blood and tissue concentrations are achieved throughout the procedure. They are generally given as a single dose before the procedure, sometimes repeated about 6 hours later; the oral route is used if possible. A penicillin such as amoxycillin, with or without an aminoglycoside such as gentamicin, is used, reflecting the bacteria usually responsible (see above). Clindamycin, vancomycin, or teicoplanin are used in penicillin-allergic patients. UK and USA guidelines for prophylaxis are similar. Recommendations from the British Society for Antimicrobial Chemotherapy were published in 1982[3] and amended in 1986,[4] 1990,[5] 1992,[6] and 1997.[7] Updated recommendations from the American Heart Association were also published in 1997.[8]

UK guidelines are as follows.

- DENTAL PROCEDURES.

  Prior application of chlorhexidine or other suitable antiseptic to the gingival margins may reduce the severity of any bacteraemia.

  Under local or no anaesthesia (including patients with a prosthetic valve, but not in those who have endocarditis): amoxycillin or clindamycin by mouth. Amoxycillin is preferred provided that patients are not penicillin-allergic and have not received penicillin more than once in the previous month. Doses are: amoxycillin 3 g or clindamycin 600 mg as a single oral dose 1 hour before the procedure.

  Under general anaesthesia: amoxycillin in one of 3 regimens, namely: amoxycillin 1 g intravenously just before induction then 0.5 g by mouth 6 hours later; or 3 g by mouth 4 hours before anaesthesia and repeated once as soon as possible after the operation; or amoxycillin 3 g with probenecid 1 g both by mouth 4 hours before the operation. Those who are allergic to penicillin or have received it more than once in the previous month should be referred to hospital.

  In special-risk patients referred to hospital (i.e. those who are to have a general anaesthetic and have prosthetic heart valves or are unable to receive penicillin because of allergy or receipt of penicillin more than once in the previous month; those who have previously had endocarditis): amoxycillin plus gentamicin or vancomycin plus gentamicin. When penicillin *can* be given: amoxycillin 1 g and gentamicin 120 mg both intravenously just before induction and amoxycillin 0.5 g by mouth 6 hours later. When penicillin *cannot* be used: vancomycin 1 g by slow intravenous infusion over at least 100 minutes followed by gentamicin 120 mg intravenously just before induction or 15 minutes before the surgical procedure. Intravenous teicoplanin 400 mg just before induction or 15 minutes before the procedure may be substituted for vancomycin. A second alternative is clindamycin 300 mg intravenously over at least 10 minutes just before induction or 15 minutes before the surgical procedure followed 6 hours later by 150 mg by mouth or by intravenous infusion over at least 10 minutes.

- UPPER RESPIRATORY TRACT PROCEDURES.

  As for dental procedures (above), but the postoperative antibacterial may need to be given parenterally if swallowing is painful.

- GENITO-URINARY PROCEDURES.

  As for dental procedures in special-risk patients (above), but not clindamycin. If there is urinary infection prophylaxis should also be effective against these infecting organisms.

- GASTRO-INTESTINAL, OBSTETRIC, AND GYNAECOLOGICAL PROCEDURES.

  Prophylaxis is only necessary in patients with prosthetic valves or those who have previously had endocarditis and then as for dental procedures in special-risk patients (above), but not clindamycin.

USA guidelines[8] are as follows.

- DENTAL, ORAL, RESPIRATORY-TRACT, OR OESOPHAGEAL PROCEDURES.

  Standard oral regimen: amoxycillin 2 g an hour beforehand.

  Patients unable to take oral antibacterials: ampicillin 2 g intravenously or intramuscularly up to 30 minutes before the procedure.

  Penicillin-allergic patients: clindamycin 600 mg by mouth an hour beforehand, or cephalexin or cefadroxil 2 g by mouth an hour beforehand, or azithromycin or clarithromycin 500 mg by mouth an hour beforehand.

  Penicillin-allergic patients unable to take oral antibacterials: clindamycin 600 mg intravenously or cephazolin 1 g intravenously or intramuscularly up to 30 minutes before the procedure.

- GENITO-URINARY AND GASTRO-INTESTINAL (EXCLUDING OESOPHAGEAL) PROCEDURES.

  Moderate-risk patients: amoxycillin 2 g by mouth an hour beforehand, or ampicillin 2 g intravenously or intramuscularly up to 30 minutes before the procedure.

Moderate-risk patients who are penicillin-allergic: vancomycin 1 g intravenously over 1 to 2 hours, with completion of the infusion up to 30 minutes before the procedure.

High-risk patients: ampicillin 2 g plus gentamicin 1.5 mg per kg (up to a maximum total of 120 mg) intravenously or intramuscularly up to 30 minutes before the procedure, followed 6 hours later by ampicillin 1 g intravenously or intramuscularly or by amoxycillin 1 g by mouth.

High-risk patients who are penicillin-allergic: vancomycin 1 g intravenously over 1 to 2 hours plus gentamicin 1.5 mg per kg (up to 120 mg) intravenously or intramuscularly, with completion of the infusion and injection up to 30 minutes before the procedure.

1. Working Party of the British Society for Antimicrobial Chemotherapy. Antibiotic treatment of streptococcal, enterococcal, and staphylococcal endocarditis. *Heart* 1998; **79:** 207–10.
2. Wilson WR, *et al.* Antibiotic treatment of adults with infective endocarditis due to streptococci, enterococci, staphylococci, and HACEK microorganisms. *JAMA* 1995; **274:** 1706–13.
3. Working Party of the British Society for Antimicrobial Chemotherapy. The antibiotic prophylaxis of infective endocarditis. *Lancet* 1982; **ii:** 1323–6.
4. Simmons NA, *et al.* Prophylaxis of infective endocarditis. *Lancet* 1986; **i:** 1267.
5. Endocarditis Working Party of the British Society for Antimicrobial Chemotherapy. Antibiotic prophylaxis of infective endocarditis. *Lancet* 1990; **335:** 88–9.
6. Simmons NA, *et al.* Antibiotic prophylaxis and infective endocarditis. *Lancet* 1992; **339:** 1292–3.
7. Littler WA, *et al.* Changes in recommendations about amoxycillin prophylaxis for prevention of endocarditis. *Lancet* 1997; **350:** 1100.
8. Dajani AS, *et al.* Prevention of bacterial endocarditis: recommendations by the American Heart Association. *JAMA* 1997; **277:** 1794–1801.

Endometritis

Endometritis (or endomyometritis) is a uterine infection that may be a part of pelvic inflammatory disease (below) or may be a postoperative complication of caesarean section.

Antibacterial prophylaxis may be given at caesarean section after cord clamping to prevent postpartum endometritis as well as wound infection. In the UK 1 to 3 parenteral doses of a beta lactam after delivery has been recommended.[1] USA surgical prophylaxis guidelines have suggested an intravenous dose of cephazolin in high-risk patients;[2] ampicillin is an alternative.[3] Other antibacterials used have included cefotetan or cefoxitin.[4] However, postpartum infection has sometimes occurred despite prophylaxis.

Early postpartum endometritis has a polymicrobial aetiology. In one study the most common organisms isolated included *Gardnerella vaginalis*, *Peptococcus* spp., *Bacteroides* spp., *Staphylococcus epidermidis*, group B streptococci, and *Ureaplasma urealyticum*.[5] *Chlamydia trachomatis* has been implicated more often in late postpartum endometritis, but a wide variety of microorganisms may also be responsible including genital mycoplasmas and, to a lesser extent, facultative and anaerobic bacteria.[6]

In the USA, standard empirical therapy for postpartum endometritis has been a short course of intravenous antibacterials, often clindamycin with gentamicin, given until the patient has been afebrile and asymptomatic for 24 to 48 hours and followed by a course of oral treatment, often with amoxycillin. However, several studies have indicated that oral therapy is not necessary after successful intravenous therapy.[7-9]

1. Pollock AV. Surgical prophylaxis—the emerging picture. *Lancet* 1988; **i:** 225–30.
2. Anonymous. Antimicrobial prophylaxis in surgery. *Med Lett Drugs Ther* 1997; **39:** 97–102.
3. Glick M, Guglielmo BJ. Antibiotic prophylaxis in cesarean section. *DICP Ann Pharmacother* 1990; **24:** 841–6.
4. Watts DH, *et al.* Upper genital tract isolates at delivery as predictors of post-cesarean infections among women receiving antibiotic prophylaxis. *Obstet Gynecol* 1991; **77:** 287–92.
5. Rosene K, *et al.* Polymicrobial early postpartum endometritis with facultative and anaerobic bacteria, genital mycoplasmas, and Chlamydia trachomatis: treatment with piperacillin or cefoxitin. *J Infect Dis* 1986; **153:** 1028–37.
6. Hoyme UB, *et al.* Microbiology and treatment of late postpartum endometritis. *Obstet Gynecol* 1986; **68:** 226–32.
7. Hager WD, *et al.* Efficacy or oral antibiotics following parenteral antibiotics for serious infections in obstetrics and gynecology. *Obstet Gynecol* 1989; **73:** 326–9.
8. Morales WJ, *et al.* Short course of antibiotic therapy in treatment of postpartum endomyometritis. *Am J Obstet Gynecol* 1989; **161:** 568–72.
9. Dinsmoor MJ, *et al.* A randomized, double-blind, placebo-controlled trial of oral antibiotic therapy following intravenous antibiotic therapy for postpartum endometritis. *Obstet Gynecol* 1991; **77:** 60–2.

Enterococcal infections

Enterococcal infections are causing increasing concern, particularly with the emergence of drug-resistant strains.[1-7] Enterococci, principally *Enterococcus faecalis* (formerly *Streptococcus faecalis*) but also *E. faecium* and *E. avium*, can cause a variety of infections including those of the biliary tract and urinary tract, endocarditis, and peritonitis. Since they are frequently present in the gut flora they are a common cause of nosocomial infections. Enterococci are resistant to cephalosporins, tetracyclines, macrolides, and chloramphenicol. The emergence of resistance to gentamicin, penicillins, and the glycopeptide antimicrobials vancomycin and teicoplanin has compromised the previously standard treatment for enterococcal infections of a penicillin or glycopeptide with gentamicin. There can be no general recommendations for treatment at present and the choice of antibacterial should be made according to locally prevailing patterns of resistance and antibacterial sensitivity tests. Because of the lack of effective antibacterials emphasis has been placed on measures to prevent the spread of vancomycin-resistant enterococci. Guidelines have been published by the USA Hospital Infection Control Practices Advisory Committee,[8] and it has been suggested that they could be adapted for use by other countries.[9]

1. Moellering RC. The enterococcus: a classic example of the impact of antimicrobial resistance on therapeutic options. *J Antimicrob Chemother* 1991; **28:** 1–12.
2. Eliopoulos GM. Increasing problems in the therapy of enterococcal infections. *Eur J Clin Microbiol Infect Dis* 1993; **12:** 409–12.
3. Tailor SAN, *et al.* Enterococcus, an emerging pathogen. *Ann Pharmacother* 1993; **27:** 1231–42.
4. Johnson AP. The pathogenicity of enterococci. *J Antimicrob Chemother* 1994; **33:** 1083–9.
5. Spera RV, Farber VF. Multidrug-resistant Enterococcus faecium: an untreatable nosocomial pathogen. *Drugs* 1994; **48:** 678–88.
6. Morris JG, *et al.* Enterococci resistant to multiple antimicrobial agents, including vancomycin. *Ann Intern Med* 1995; **123:** 250–9.
7. Landman D, Quale JM. Management of infections due to resistant enterococci: a review of therapeutic options. *J Antimicrob Chemother* 1997; **40:** 161–70.
8. Hospital Infection Control Practices Advisory Committee (HICPAC). Recommendations for preventing the spread of vancomycin resistance. *MMWR* 1995; **44** (RR-12): 1–13.
9. Fraise AP. The treatment and control of vancomycin resistant enterococci. *J Antimicrob Chemother* 1996; **38:** 753–6.

Epididymitis

Epididymitis is often associated with urethritis and in young men occurs most commonly as a complication of sexually transmitted infection with *Neisseria gonorrhoeae* and especially *Chlamydia trachomatis*, but may occur in homosexual males as a result of infection with enteric organisms, particularly *Escherichia coli*. For chlamydial epididymitis WHO[1] recommends a 7-day oral course of tetracycline hydrochloride 500 mg four times daily or doxycycline 100 mg twice daily; for those unable to tolerate tetracycline they advise a 7-day course of erythromycin 500 mg four times daily. Unless it can be excluded, patients should also be treated concurrently for gonorrhoea (below). In the USA, the Centers for Disease Control[2] recommends empirical treatment for epididymitis likely to have been caused by gonococcal or chlamydial infection with a single intramuscular dose of ceftriaxone 250 mg together with doxycycline 100 mg twice daily by mouth for 10 days; if the cause is thought to be an enteric organism ofloxacin 300 mg twice daily by mouth for 10 days is recommended.

In men over 35 years and in children epididymitis is usually secondary to urinary-tract infection with *Pseudomonas aeruginosa* and other Gram-negative bacilli and is not sexually transmitted.

1. WHO. *WHO model prescribing information: drugs used in sexually transmitted diseases and HIV infection*. Geneva: WHO, 1995.
2. Centers for Disease Control. 1998 Guidelines for treatment of sexually transmitted diseases. *MMWR* 1998; **47** (RR-1): 86–8.

Epiglottitis

In acute epiglottitis rapid swelling of the epiglottis and surrounding soft tissues results in sudden airway obstruction which can be fatal. It is often due to bacteraemic infection with *Haemophilus influenzae* type b and has occurred primarily in young children. However, the incidence has decreased in this age group since the introduction of haemophilus influenzae vaccine.[1] Acute epiglottitis also occurs in adults.[1]

Treatment and prophylaxis is similar to that for Haemophilus influenzae meningitis (see under Meningitis, below). Immediate management includes the maintenance of an adequate airway and the intravenous administration of antibacterials active against *H. influenzae* type b. Chloramphenicol has been the drug of choice, but third-generation cephalosporins such as cefotaxime and ceftriaxone are increasingly used.[2] Prophylaxis with rifampicin may be given to index cases and contacts.

1. Frantz TD, *et al.* Acute epiglottitis in adults: analysis of 129 cases. *JAMA* 1994; **272:** 1358–60.
2. Sawyer SM, *et al.* Successful treatment of epiglottitis with two doses of ceftriaxone. *Arch Dis Child* 1994; **70:** 129–32.

Escherichia coli enteritis

See under Gastro-enteritis, below.

Eye infections

During 1980 in a UK hospital, investigation of the microbial flora of patients with acute bacterial infection of the external eye, including acute bacterial conjunctivitis, corneal ulceration, blepharitis, dacryocystitis, and discharging sockets revealed that *Staphylococcus aureus*, *Streptococcus pneumoniae*, and *Haemophilus influenzae* were the main pathogens.[1] A similar study in the USA[2] in children with acute conjunctivitis found *Moraxella catarrhalis* in addition, and probable viral infections in 16%. *Staph. aureus* was predominantly isolated from control subjects. In the UK study, all pathogens isolated were sensitive to chloramphenicol which remained the most effective topical antibacterial with the least overall resistance of 6%; tetracycline was the next most effective. Gentamicin was the drug of choice for infections due to *Pseudomonas aeruginosa* and coliform bacilli.[1] Chloramphenicol eye drops are very widely used in patients with red eyes although untreated simple bacterial conjunctivitis is a self-limiting condition that resolves within about 2 weeks.[3] However, there is debate concerning this use of chloramphenicol—see Ocular Use, under Precautions of Chloramphenicol, p.183. Other antibacterials used topically in eye preparations include sulphacetamide, trimethoprim with polymyxin B, fluoroquinolones such as ciprofloxacin and ofloxacin with a spectrum of activity similar to that of the aminoglycosides gentamicin or tobramycin, neomycin, and fusidic acid which is active against staphylococci.

Subconjunctival injections or systemic treatment may be necessary in serious infections.

Infective endophthalmitis (infection inside the eye) generally follows accidental or surgical trauma to the eye and should be treated aggressively according to the causative organisms. The commonest source of infection is the patient's own bacterial flora; *Staphylococcus epidermidis* is reported to be the infective organism in about 40% of cases, while other Gram-positive organisms are responsible for about a further 30% of cases.[4,5] *Bacillus cereus* has emerged as a particularly virulent cause of endophthalmitis.[6] Gram-negative bacteria such as *Pseudomonas aeruginosa* and *Proteus* spp. are common, while a few cases are due to fungal infections.[5,7] Treatment is still controversial. Fisch[4] reported that most patients received parenteral antibacterials in addition to intra-ocular administration, but Hughes and Hill[5] state that the systemic route is of limited value. In addition, a US National Eye Institute-sponsored study[8] investigating the use of immediate postoperative vitrectomy with or without systemic antibacterial therapy concluded that additional therapy provided no advantage over vitrectomy alone for postoperative endophthalmitis. Direct injection into the vitreous appears to be the most favoured route, in combination with subconjunctival and topical therapy. The antibacterials commonly used have included aminoglycosides (such as amikacin or gentamicin) in combination with either vancomycin[5,7,8] or a cephalosporin.[7] Empirical use of aminoglycosides has, however, been questioned because of their possible retinal toxicity.[9] Vancomycin with ceftazidine[10,11] or vancomycin alone[10] (if tests show absence of Gram-negative infection) have been suggested as alternatives. The fluoroquinolones and carbapenems may also be useful but experience with these drugs is limited.[7] Infections with *Staph. epidermidis* are reported to respond more favourably than infections with other organisms.[4,5,7] The choice of treatment for *B. cereus* endophthalmitis has been based on *in-vitro* studies; active antibacterials have included gentamicin with vancomycin or clindamycin.[6]

Gonococcal conjunctivitis is mentioned under Gonorrhoea (below) and chlamydial conjunctivitis (inclusion conjunctivitis) under Trachoma (below). Chlamydial and gonococcal eye infections in neonates are discussed under Neonatal Conjunctivitis (below). For a discussion of *Acanthamoeba* keratitis in contact lens wearers see p.573. For a discussion of fungal eye infections and their treatment, see p.369.

1. Seal DV, *et al.* Aetiology and treatment of acute bacterial infection of the external eye. *Br J Ophthalmol* 1982; **66:** 357–60.
2. Weiss A, *et al.* Acute conjunctivitis in childhood. *J Pediatr* 1993; **122:** 10–14.
3. Buckley SA. Survey of patients taking topical medication at their first presentation to eye casualty. *Br Med J* 1990; **300:** 1497–8.
4. Fisch A, *et al.* Epidemiology of infective endophthalmitis in France. *Lancet* 1991; **338:** 1373–6.
5. Hughes DS, Hill RJ. Infectious endophthalmitis after cataract surgery. *Br J Ophthalmol* 1994; **78:** 227–32.
6. David DB, *et al.* Bacillus cereus endophthalmitis. *Br J Ophthalmol* 1994; **78:** 577–80.
7. Hassan IJ. Endophthalmitis—problems, progress and prospects. *J Antimicrob Chemother* 1994; **33:** 383–6.
8. Endophthalmitis Vitrectomy Study Group. Results of the Endophthalmitis Vitrectomy Study. *Arch Ophthalmol* 1995; **113:** 1479–96.
9. Campochiaro PA, Lim JI. Aminoglycoside toxicity in the treatment of endophthalmitis. *Arch Ophthalmol* 1994; **112:** 48–53.
10. Donahue SP, *et al.* Empiric treatment of endophthalmitis: are aminoglycosides necessary? *Arch Ophthalmol* 1994; **112:** 45–7.
11. Aaberg TM, *et al.* Intraocular ceftazidime as an alternative to the aminoglycosides in the treatment of endophthalmitis. *Arch Ophthalmol* 1994; **112:** 18–19.

Gas gangrene

Clostridium spp. are anaerobic Gram-positive bacteria some of which cause gas gangrene with muscle necrosis and systemic toxicity as a result of toxin formation. *Cl. perfringens* is the species most frequently responsible. Gas gangrene is usually associated with traumatic or surgical wounds. Treatment is primarily by surgical debridement of all necrotic muscle and the administration of large doses of benzylpenicillin. Alternative antibacterials have included clindamycin, metronidazole, imipenem, a tetracycline, or chloramphenicol. Hyperbaric oxygen is used as an adjunct to surgical debridement. Gas-gangrene antitoxins (p.1511) are rarely used nowadays.

Benzylpenicillin is also recommended as prophylaxis against gas gangrene in patients undergoing high amputations of lower limbs or following major trauma; metronidazole is an alternative in patients allergic to penicillin.

Gastro-enteritis

Diarrhoea is a symptom of simple gastro-enteritis and of most intestinal infections. It is a major problem in developing countries, but is common worldwide. Although viruses are often responsible, the severest forms of infectious diarrhoea are generally those due to bacteria. Common bacterial pathogens include *Campylobacter jejuni*, *Escherichia coli*, *Salmonella enteritidis*, *Shigella* spp., *Vibrio cholerae*, and *Yersinia enterocolitica*. Intestinal protozoa also cause diarrhoea and are of increasing importance in AIDS-associated diarrhoea. For discussions of viral and protozoal gastro-enteritis and their treatment, see p.595 and p.574 respectively. In acute diarrhoea of any aetiology the priority is to maintain hydration by prevention or treatment of fluid and electrolyte depletion, especially in infants and the elderly. Oral rehydration therapy is discussed under Diarrhoea on p.1168.

The treatment of bacterial diarrhoea has been reviewed.[1-6] Antibacterial therapy is usually unnecessary in mild and self-limiting gastro-enteritis, but invasive organisms may cause systemic illness. Empirical antimicrobial therapy is not generally recommended[5] but may be considered in high-risk adult patients (such as the elderly, those with certain pre-existing medical conditions, and those with severe dysenteric symptoms). Some individual commentators,[6] however, believe this approach to be unnecessarily cautious. Antibacterial therapy is justified when some specific infections are confirmed (see below for further details).

'Food poisoning' is generally a self-limiting form of gastro-enteritis although serious outbreaks of food-borne illness have been associated with bacteria such as *Salmonella enteritidis*. Other common food-poisoning organisms include *Listeria monocytogenes*, *Campylobacter* spp, *Yersinia enterocolitica*, *Vibrio parahaemolyticus*, and *E. coli*. An enterotoxin is responsible for food poisoning associated with *Staphylococcus aureus*, *Clostridium* spp., and *Bacillus* spp.[7,8]

In **infants and children** oral rehydration therapy is universally recognised as initial treatment of acute diarrhoea, but has been underutilised in both developed and developing countries.[9,10] Antibacterials have little place in management in most cases and their inappropriate use has contributed to a high prevalence of antibiotic resistance in commensal bacteria.[9] WHO[10,11] has stipulated that antibacterials should only be used in children with acute diarrhoea when there is dysentery or suspected cholera; *Shigella* is the most important cause of dysentery in young children. Giardiasis and amoebiasis should also be treated. WHO emphasised[10] that oral preparations containing streptomycin or dihydrostreptomycin, neomycin, halogenated hydroxyquinolones, or nonabsorbable sulphonamides (sulphaguanidine, succinylsulphathiazole, phthalylsulphathiazole) should not be used. For reference to the treatment of enteropathogenic *E. coli* (EPEC) diarrhoea in infants, see under Escherichia coli Enteritis, below.

HIV-associated diarrhoea. As discussed on p.601, diarrhoea is common in HIV infection and AIDS and causative organisms may be bacterial, protozoal, or viral.[12,13] The most common bacterial cause is the *Mycobacterium avium* complex; others include *Campylobacter*, *Salmonella*, and *Shigella* spp. Supportive care and appropriate conventional antibacterial therapy may be adequate, as described under Opportunistic Mycobacterial Infections on p.133 and under the specific infections, below.

Travellers' diarrhoea. Acute diarrhoea associated with travel occurs worldwide. The most common bacterial pathogen is enterotoxigenic *E. coli*, although enteroadherent *E. coli* is also sometimes associated with travellers' diarrhoea. Other bacteria include *Campylobacter jejuni*, *Salmonella* and *Shigella* spp., *Vibrio cholerae*, and non-cholera vibrios such as *V. parahaemolyticus*. Viruses and the protozoa *Giardia intestinalis*, *Entamoeba histolytica*, and *Cryptosporidium* may also be responsible. Published recommendations for the management of travellers' diarrhoea are similar in principle but differ in detail.[14-18] Clinical features depend on the pathogen responsible and treatment varies according to severity and duration of diarrhoea. Onset of diarrhoea is generally delayed with *Giardia* and *Entamoeba* because of the incubation period. Diarrhoea is often mild and self-limiting and increased fluid intake or, oral rehydration therapy is all that will be required. Symptomatic treatment with antimotility drugs such as loperamide may be of benefit in mild to moderate diarrhoea. Bismuth salicylate may be used to reduce the frequency of diarrhoea. Although antimicrobial therapy is not indicated in most cases of infective diarrhoea, empirical treatment with a fluoroquinolone has been effective for moderate to severe attacks. Co-trimoxazole has also been used, but there is a risk of severe skin reactions and bone-marrow depression and increasing bacterial resistance is causing concern. When the infecting bacteria are known, for example, *Campylobacter*, *Salmonella*, or *Shigella* spp., the specific therapy described below may be necessary.

The risk of developing travellers' diarrhoea can be reduced by avoiding possibly contaminated foods as embodied in the advice to 'cook it, boil it, peel it, or forget it'. A number of prophylactic drug regimens have been suggested, including bismuth salicylate and various antibacterials, usually a fluoroquinolone or co-trimoxazole. Recently a single dose of ciprofloxacin was reported to be successful in professional soldiers.[19] However, routine antimicrobial prophylaxis is not generally recommended because of the danger of drug reactions, supra-infections, and increasing bacterial resistance and should probably be reserved for those at special risk. Many authorities prefer early treatment, including self-medication, with clear instructions on when medical help should be sought.

1. Gorbach SL. Bacterial diarrhoea and its treatment. *Lancet* 1987; **ii:** 1378–82.
2. Anonymous. Quinolones in acute non-travellers' diarrhoea. *Lancet* 1990; **336:** 282.
3. Guerrant RL, Bobak DA. Bacterial and protozoal gastroenteritis. *N Engl J Med* 1991; **325:** 327–40.
4. Watson AJM. Diarrhoea. *Br Med J* 1992; **304:** 1302–4.
5. Farthing M, *et al.* The management of infective gastroenteritis in adults: a consensus statement by an expert panel convened by the British Society for the Study of Infection. *J Infect* 1996; **33:** 143–52.
6. Gorbach SL. Treating diarrhoea. *Br Med J* 1997; **314:** 1776–7.
7. Waites WM, Arbuthnott JP. Foodborne illness: an overview. *Lancet* 1990; **336:** 722–5.
8. Roberts D. Sources of infection: food. *Lancet* 1990; **336:** 859–61.
9. Walker-Smith JA. Underutilisation of oral rehydration in the treatment of gastroenteritis. *Drugs* 1988; **36** (suppl 4): 61–4.
10. WHO. *The rational use of drugs in the management of acute diarrhoea in children.* Geneva: WHO, 1990.
11. WHO. *The management and prevention of diarrhoea: practical guidelines.* 3rd ed. Geneva: WHO, 1993.
12. Dupont HL, Marshall GD. HIV-associated diarrhoea and wasting. *Lancet* 1995; **346:** 352–6.
13. Sharpstone D, Gazzard B. Gastrointestinal manifestations of HIV infection. *Lancet* 1996; **348:** 379–83.
14. Cartwright RY. Travellers' diarrhoea. *Br Med Bull* 1993; **49:** 348–62.
15. Nathwani D, Wood MJ. The management of travellers' diarrhoea. *J Antimicrob Chemother* 1993; **31:** 623–6.
16. DuPont HL, Ericsson CD. Prevention and treatment of traveler's diarrhea. *N Engl J Med* 1993; **328:** 1821–7.
17. Farthing MJG. Travellers' diarrhoea. *Br Med J* 1993; **306:** 1425–6.
18. Anonymous. Advice for travelers. *Med Lett Drugs Ther* 1998; **40:** 47–50.
19. Salam I, *et al.* Randomised trial of single-dose ciprofloxacin for travellers' diarrhoea. *Lancet* 1994; **344:** 1537–9.

Antibiotic-associated colitis. Colonisation of the colon with *Clostridium difficile*, a toxin-producing Gram-positive anaerobe, is the most common identifiable cause of antibiotic-associated diarrhoea and pseudomembranous colitis. It has been associated with the use of most antibacterials, but particularly with clindamycin, lincomycin, ampicillin, amoxycillin, ciprofloxacin, and cephalosporins. The diarrhoea may be mild and self-limiting or debilitating and persistent. Although the diarrhoea generally resolves within a few days of discontinuation of the offending drug together with fluid and electrolyte replacement, early specific antibacterial therapy should be given to patients with severe illness characterised by high fever, marked abdominal pain, and marked leucocytosis and to elderly, toxic, or debilitated patients, or those unresponsive to supportive therapy.[1,2] Antidiarrhoeal drugs should be avoided since they may aggravate the condition and may occasionally increase the possibly of toxic megacolon.[1]

Vancomycin or metronidazole are widely used.[1,2] Metronidazole tends to be the drug of first choice for patients with mild to moderate symptoms with vancomycin being used in those who do not respond to metronidazole, in those who are severely immunocompromised, and in those with severe illness.[1,2] This view is also endorsed by expert bodies in the USA whose aim is to provide guidelines for preventing the spread of vancomycin resistance.[3] Metronidazole can be given orally or intravenously as appropriate. Vancomycin is only given orally; it should not be given intravenously since it does not give rise to adequate concentrations of the drug in the bowel lumen.[1] Absorption of vancomycin after enteral administration is usually minimal, although significant serum concentrations have been detected in a few patients.[4,5] *Cl. difficile*, including organisms isolated from patients who have had recurrences of colitis after treatment with vancomycin, are generally highly susceptible to vancomycin.[6,7] Response to vancomycin is usually good unless treatment has been delayed until the patient is moribund, or has ileus, toxic megacolon, or a colonic perforation. The severity of the diarrhoea often decreases within 48 to 72 hours, but cessation may take a week or more. Relapses are quite common,[8] but usually respond to re-treatment with vancomycin or metronidazole.[1]

Other drugs that appear to be effective in the treatment of antibiotic-associated colitis include teicoplanin,[9-11] fusidic acid,[11,12] and bacitracin,[13] although experience with their use remains limited.

The anion-exchange resins cholestyramine and colestipol hydrochloride have been shown to bind the *Cl. difficile* toxin *in vitro*, and cholestyramine has been used to treat pseudomembranous colitis.[14] The use of vancomycin together with cholestyramine has been suggested,[15] but the value of the combination is uncertain.

Oral immunoglobulin A, given in combination with vancomycin, was effective in controlling severe diarrhoea in a child who had not responded to other therapies.[16] Normal immunoglobulin given intravenously was also effective when added to vancomycin and metronidazole therapy in two elderly patients unresponsive to antibacterials alone.[17]

Treatment aimed at recolonising the gut with non-pathogenic organisms has included administration of lactic-acid-producing organisms such as *Lactobacillus*,[18] and the yeasts *Saccharomyces boulardii*,[19,20] and *S. cerevisiae*.[21]

In patients with antibiotic-associated diarrhoea, but not colitis or *Cl. difficile* colonisation, a role for intestinal overgrowth of *Candida* spp.[22] or a reduction in enteric anaerobes has been suggested.

1. Tabaqchali S, Jumaa P. Diagnosis and management of Clostridium difficile infection. *Br Med J* 1995; **310:** 1375–80.
2. Fekety R, Shah AB. Diagnosis and treatment of Clostridium difficile colitis. *JAMA* 1993; **269:** 71–5.
3. Hospital Infection Control Practices Advisory Committee (HICPAC). Recommendations for preventing the spread of vancomycin resistance. *MMWR* 1994; **44** (RR-12): 1–13.
4. Bryan CS, White WL. Safety of oral vancomycin in functionally anephric patients. *Antimicrob Agents Chemother* 1978; **14:** 634–5.
5. Pasic M, *et al.* Systemic absorption after local intracolonic vancomycin in pseudomembranous colitis. *Lancet* 1993; **342:** 443.
6. Dzink J, Bartlett JG. In vitro susceptibility of Clostridium difficile isolates from patients with antibiotic-associated diarrhea or colitis. *Antimicrob Agents Chemother* 1980; **17:** 695–8.
7. Levett PN. Time-dependent killing of Clostridium difficile by metronidazole and vancomycin. *J Antimicrob Chemother* 1991; **27:** 55–62.
8. Walters BAJ, *et al.* Relapse of antibiotic associated colitis: endogenous persistence of Clostridium difficile during vancomycin therapy. *Gut* 1983; **24:** 206–12.
9. de Lalla F, *et al.* Treatment of Clostridium difficile-associated disease with teicoplanin. *Antimicrob Agents Chemother* 1989; **33:** 1125–7.
10. de Lalla F, *et al.* Prospective study of oral teicoplanin versus oral vancomycin for therapy of pseudomembranous colitis and Clostridium difficile-associated diarrhea. *Antimicrob Agents Chemother* 1992; **36:** 2192–6.
11. Wenisch C, *et al.* Comparison of vancomycin, teicoplanin, metronidazole, and fusidic acid for the treatment of Clostridium difficile-associated diarrhea. *Clin Infect Dis* 1996; **22:** 813–18.
12. Cronberg S, *et al.* Fusidic acid for the treatment of antibiotic-associated colitis induced by Clostridium difficile. *Infection* 1984; **12:** 276–9.
13. Dudley MN, *et al.* Oral bacitracin vs vancomycin therapy for Clostridium difficile-induced diarrhea: a randomized double-blind trial. *Arch Intern Med* 1986; **146:** 1101–4.
14. Pruksananonda P, Powell KR. Multiple relapses of Clostridium difficile-associated diarrhea responding to an extended course of cholestyramine. *Pediatr Infect Dis J* 1989; **8:** 175–8.
15. Shwed JA, Rodvold KA. Anion-exchange resins and oral vancomycin in pseudomembranous colitis. *DICP Ann Pharmacother* 1989; **23:** 70–1.
16. Tjellström B, *et al.* Oral immunoglobulin A supplement in treatment of Clostridium difficile enteritis. *Lancet* 1993; **341;** 701–2.
17. Salcedo J, *et al.* Intravenous immunoglobulin therapy for severe Clostridium difficile colitis. *Gut* 1997; **41:** 366–70.
18. Gorbach SL, *et al.* Successful treatment of relapsing Clostridium difficile colitis with Lactobacillus GG. *Lancet* 1987; **ii:** 1519.
19. Surawicz CM, *et al.* Prevention of antibiotic-associated diarrhea by Saccharomyces boulardii: a prospective study. *Gastroenterology* 1989; **96:** 981–8.
20. McFarland LV, *et al.* A randomized placebo-controlled trial of Saccharomyces boulardii in combination with standard antibiotics for Clostridium difficile disease. *JAMA* 1994; **271:** 1913–18.
21. Schellenberg D, *et al.* Treatment of Clostridium difficile diarrhoea with brewer's yeast. *Lancet* 1994; **343:** 171–2.
22. Danna PL, *et al.* Role of candida in pathogenesis of antibiotic-associated diarrhoea in elderly inpatients. *Lancet* 1991; **337:** 511–14.

Campylobacter enteritis. *Campylobacter jejuni* is a major cause of acute diarrhoea. *C. coli* is less common and *C. upsaliensis* has been identified only recently as a probable enteropathogen.[1] Food is a common source of infection and Skirrow[2] has reviewed *Campylobacter* enteritis as a foodborne illness. In the UK, several sources are responsible[3] including contaminated food and water and one important source is from doorstep deliveries of foil-topped bottled milk that have been pecked by birds.[3-5]

Erythromycin or ciprofloxacin are of benefit[6] in severely affected patients, but the infection is usually self-limiting and fluid and electrolyte replacement is generally sufficient. A tetracycline may be an alternative antimicrobial.[6] Treatment with erythromycin can eradicate the organism from the faeces,[7-9] but may not reduce the duration of symptoms unless treatment is started early in the course of the disease.[7-9] Some strains of *Campylobacter* are resistant to erythromycin,[10] and resistance is also an increasing problem with ciprofloxacin.[11] Multiple drug resistance has been reported.[12] Treatment with oral immunoglobulin A had beneficial effects in 1 patient.[13]

Severe systemic infections with *C. fetus* require parenteral therapy with imipenem or gentamicin,[6] depending on susceptibility. Other alternatives include third-generation cephalosporins or chloramphenicol.

There is some evidence of an association between *C. jejuni* infection and the Guillain-Barré syndrome.[14]

1. Goossens H, *et al.* Is "Campylobacter upsaliensis" an unrecognised cause of human diarrhoea? *Lancet* 1990; **335:** 584–6.
2. Skirrow MB. Foodborne illness: Campylobacter. *Lancet* 1990; **336:** 921–3.
3. Pebody RG, *et al.* Outbreaks of campylobacter infection: rare events for a common pathogen. *Commun Dis Rep* 1997; **7:** R33–R37.
4. Phillips CA. Bird attacks on milk bottles and campylobacter infection. *Lancet* 1995; **346:** 386.
5. Stuart J, *et al.* Outbreak of campylobacter enteritis in a residential school associated with bird pecked bottle tops. *Commun Dis Rep* 1997; **7:** R38–R40.
6. Anonymous. The choice of antibacterial drugs. *Med Lett Drugs Ther* 1998; **40:** 33–42.
7. Anders BJ, *et al.* Double-blind placebo controlled trial of erythromycin for treatment of campylobacter enteritis. *Lancet* 1982; **i:** 131–2.
8. Mandal BK, *et al.* Double-blind placebo-controlled trial of erythromycin in the treatment of clinical campylobacter infection. *J Antimicrob Chemother* 1984; **13:** 619–23.
9. Williams D, *et al.* Early treatment of Campylobacter jejuni enteritis. *Antimicrob Agents Chemother* 1989; **33:** 248–50.
10. Taylor DN, *et al.* Erythromycin-resistant campylobacter infections in Thailand. *Antimicrob Agents Chemother* 1987; **31:** 438–42.
11. Piddock LJV. Quinolone resistance and Campylobacter spp. *J Antimicrob Chemother* 1995; **36:** 891–8.
12. Winstanley TG, *et al.* Multiple antibiotic resistance in a strain of Campylobacter jejuni acquired in Jordan. *J Antimicrob Chemother* 1993; **31:** 178–9.
13. Hammerström V, *et al.* Oral immunoglobulin treatment in Campylobacter jejuni enteritis. *Lancet* 1993; **341:** 1036.
14. Rees JH, *et al.* Campylobacter jejuni infection and Guillain-Barré syndrome. *N Engl J Med* 1995; **333:** 1374–9.

Cholera and other vibrio infections. Cholera results from infection with the enterotoxin-producing Gram-negative bacillus *Vibrio cholerae* which causes acute secretory diarrhoea. It can be associated with two serogroups of *V. cholerae*, O1 and O139. Serogroup O1 can then be divided into two biotypes (classical and El Tor) and each of these has three serotypes (Inaba, Ogawa, and Hikojima). The seventh pandemic began in 1961 in South East Asia and reached South America in January 1991.[1-6] This pandemic is caused by *V. cholerae* O1 biotype El Tor. It is the longest pandemic recorded this century and shows no sign of abating. In late 1992 and 1993 epidemic cholera caused by *V. cholerae* O139 was reported in India and Bangladesh and subsequently identified in Thailand and other Asian countries. *V. cholerae* O139 became the dominant strain in India in less than 2 months and some workers declared it responsible for the eighth cholera pandemic.[2] However, there is some evidence that by 1994 it was abating and that by 1996 O1 was again the prevalent type in India and Bangladesh. There appears to be no cross-immunity between O1 and the O139 serogroup.

Individuals can reduce the risk of contracting cholera by avoiding possibly contaminated foodstuffs, good personal hygiene, and boiling or otherwise disinfecting drinking water. Methods of preventing or containing cholera epidemics include ensuring a safe water supply, providing good sanitation, and promoting safe handling and preparation of foods; mass chemoprophylaxis, vaccination, and travel and trade restrictions are not effective[7] although newer vaccines are showing more promise.

The majority of cases of vibrio gastro-enteritis are mild to moderate and generally require no therapy other than fluid and electrolyte replacement with an appropriate oral rehydration solution (see Diarrhoea, p.1168). Patients with severe gastro-enteritis, dehydration, and shock should receive vigorous fluid replacement, preferably intravenously.[8] Antimicrobial therapy has been shown to decrease the duration and volume of diarrhoea in cholera and may also decrease the duration of other vibrio diarrhoeas.[9] Tetracycline, chloramphenicol, and erythromycin were all effective in the treatment of O1 cholera according to an early WHO report.[10] More recently WHO[7] recommended a single dose of doxycycline as the treatment of choice for adults except pregnant women. Tetracycline, co-trimoxazole, furazolidone, erythromycin, and chloramphenicol are alternatives, with furazolidone being preferred for pregnant women and co-trimoxazole for children. Recommendations from the USA for adults specify a tetracycline as the first choice with co-trimoxazole or a fluoroquinolone such as ciprofloxacin as alternatives.[11] A recent study has suggested that single-dose ciprofloxacin might be preferred to doxycycline, particularly in areas of tetracycline resistance.[12] The O139 strain is reported to be sensitive to ciprofloxacin,[13] erythromycin,[13] and tetracyclines,[2] but resistant to co-trimoxazole.[2] There has also been some resistance to furazolidone.[2] Multiple drug resistance may be a problem; differing sensitivity and resistance patterns have been reported for the 2 biotypes classical and El Tor *V. cholerae*.[14] The outbreak strain in Rwandan refugees was resistant to tetracycline, doxycycline, co-trimoxazole, chloramphenicol, and ampicillin.[2]

Mass chemoprophylaxis is not recommended but may be justified for household contacts,[1,10] especially those at high risk because of age or pregnancy.[1] The type of cholera vaccines traditionally available are not very effective although some promising results have been reported with the use of oral vaccines in areas where cholera is endemic.

Marine or halophilic *Vibrio* spp. known to cause gastro-enteritis include *V. parahaemolyticus* which is responsible for food poisoning from raw or undercooked seafood especially in Japan.[15,16] Another halophilic sp., *V. vulnificus*, is increasingly associated with wound infection and septicaemia.[15] On the basis of *in-vitro* sensitivity testing[17] and anecdotal clinical experience, empirical therapy with aminoglycosides, ceftazidime, imipenem, or ciprofloxacin should all be effective.[18]

1. Anonymous. Cholera. *Commun Dis Rep* 1991; **1:** R48–50.
2. Crowcroft NS. Cholera: current epidemiology. *Commun Dis Rep* 1994; **4:** R157–64.
3. Swerdlow SL, Ries AA. Vibrio cholerae non-O1—the eighth pandemic? *Lancet* 1993; **342:** 382–3.
4. Mahon BE, *et al.* Reported cholera in the United States, 1992-1994: a reflection of global changes in cholera epidemiology. *JAMA* 1996; **276:** 307–12.
5. Seas C, Gotuzzo E. Cholera: overview of epidemiologic, therapeutic, and preventive issues learned from recent epidemics. *Int J Infect Dis* 1996; **1:** 37–46.
6. Sánchez JL, Taylor DN. Cholera. *Lancet* 1997; **349:** 1825–30.
7. WHO. *Guidelines for cholera control.* Geneva: WHO, 1993.
8. Morris JG, Black RE. Cholera and other vibrioses in the United States. *N Engl J Med* 1985; **312:** 343–50.
9. Blake PA. Vibrios on the half shell: what the walrus and the carpenter didn't know. *Ann Intern Med* 1983; **99:** 558–9.
10. WHO. WHO expert committee on cholera: second report. *WHO Tech Rep Ser 352* 1967.
11. Anonymous. The choice of antibacterial drugs. *Med Lett Drugs Ther* 1998; **40:** 33–42.
12. Khan WA, *et al.* Randomised controlled comparison of single-dose ciprofloxacin and doxycycline for cholera caused by Vibrio cholerae O1 or O139. *Lancet* 1996; **348:** 296–300.
13. Dhar U, *et al.* Clinical features, antimicrobial susceptibility and toxin production in Vibrio cholerae O139 infection: comparison with V. cholerae O1 infection. *Trans R Soc Trop Med Hyg* 1996; **90:** 402–5.
14. Siddique AK, *et al.* Simultaneous outbreaks of contrasting drug resistant classic and El Tor Vibrio cholerae O1 in Bangladesh. *Lancet* 1989; **ii:** 396.
15. Anonymous. Shuck your oysters with care. *Lancet* 1990; **336:** 215–16.
16. Doyle MP. Foodborne illness: pathogenic Escherichia coli, Yersinia enterocolitica, and Vibrio parahaemolyticus. *Lancet* 1990; **336:** 1111–15.
17. French GL, *et al.* Antimicrobial susceptibilities of halophilic vibrios. *J Antimicrob Chemother* 1989; **24:** 183–94.
18. French GL. Antibiotics for marine vibrios. *Lancet* 1990; **336:** 568–9.

Escherichia coli enteritis. *Escherichia coli* is a normal intestinal commensal and member of the Gram-negative family of bacteria the Enterobacteriaceae. Pathogenic strains causing distinct syndromes of diarrhoeal disease and also associated with foodborne illness include: enteropathogenic *E. coli* (EPEC)—an important cause of infantile diarrhoea in many developing countries; enteroinvasive *E. coli* (EIEC)—producing an invasive type of diarrhoea resembling that of *Shigella* dysentery; enterotoxigenic *E. coli* (ETEC)—an important cause of travellers' diarrhoea (see above); and enterohaemorrhagic *E. coli* (EHEC)—associated with haemorrhagic colitis, haemolytic uraemic syndrome, and thrombotic thrombocytopenic purpura.[1] Enteroadherent *E. coli* (EAEC) is a cause of chronic diarrhoea in young children.[2]

Although these organisms are generally sensitive to a wide range of antibacterials only special categories of *E. coli* diarrhoea should be treated.[2]

Neonates with severe EPEC diarrhoea have been given oral non-absorbable antibacterials such as neomycin or gentamicin although in older children or adults this diarrhoea is said by some to be self-limiting.[2] However, Hill *et al.*[3] noted improvement with antibacterials beyond the neonatal period; they subsequently reported EPEC infection to be a common treatable cause of life-threatening *chronic* diarrhoea in infancy and suggested that it was frequently associated with travel to a developing country.[4] Symptoms could become persistent and life-threatening in previously healthy infants, requiring intravenous rehydration and parenteral antibacterials such as gentamicin and penicillin.[4]

Verotoxin-producing strains of EHEC, in particular serotype O157, have been associated with bloody diarrhoea, haemorrhagic colitis, and haemolytic uraemic syndrome in the UK[5] and the USA,[6,7] especially in young children. Cases have generally been linked with the consumption of foods derived from cattle, although there have been outbreaks in the USA[8] associated with the consumption of alfalfa sprouts. *E. coli* O157 has also been reported as a cause of epidemic haemorrhagic colitis in Africa, where it may be difficult to distinguish from shigellosis.[9,10] Antibacterial treatment was of no evident benefit, but a retrospective study reported from Canada[11] indicated that treatment with ampicillin, amoxycillin, or co-trimoxazole might be of value. A later view,[12] however, expressed uncertainty as to whether antibacterial treatment influences the course of enterohaemorrhagic *E. coli* infection and the development of haemolytic-uraemic syndrome or thrombotic thrombocytopenic purpura; the non-antibacterial treatment of these two latter complications is discussed in Plasma, under Thrombotic Microangiopathies, p.726.

1. Doyle MP. Pathogenic Escherichia coli, Yersinia enterocolitica, and Vibrio parahaemolyticus. *Lancet* 1990; **336:** 1111–15.
2. Gorbach SL. Bacterial diarrhoea and its treatment. *Lancet* 1987; **ii:** 1378–82.
3. Hill SM, *et al.* Antibiotics for Escherichia coli gastroenteritis. *Lancet* 1988; **i:** 771–2.
4. Hill SM, *et al.* Enteropathogenic Escherichia coli and life threatening chronic diarrhoea. *Gut* 1991; **32:** 154–8.
5. PHLS Working Group on Vero cytotoxin producing Escherichia coli (VTEC). Interim guidelines for the control of infections with Vero cytotoxin producing Escherichia coli (VTEC). *Commun Dis Rep* 1995; **5:** R77–81.
6. MacDonald KL, Osterholm MT. The emergence of Escherichia coli O157:H7 infection in the United States: the changing epidemiology of food borne disease. *JAMA* 1993; **269:** 2264–6.
7. Bell BP, *et al.* A multistate outbreak of Escherichia coli O157:H7-associated bloody diarrhea and hemolytic uremic syndrome from hamburgers: the Washington experience. *JAMA* 1994; **272:** 1349–53.
8. Centers for Disease Control. Outbreaks of Escherichia coli O157: H7 infection associated with eating alfalfa sprouts—Michigan and Virginia, June-July 1997. *MMWR* 1997; **46:** 741–4.
9. Isaäcson M, *et al.* Haemorrhagic colitis epidemic in Africa. *Lancet* 1993; **341:** 961.
10. Paquet C, *et al.* Aetiology of haemorrhagic colitis epidemic in Africa. *Lancet* 1993; **342:** 175.
11. Cimolai N, *et al.* Antibiotics for Escherichia coli O157:H7 enteritis? *J Antimicrob Chemother* 1989; **23:** 807–8.
12. Farthing M, *et al.* The management of infective gastroenteritis in adults: a consensus statement by an expert panel convened by the British Society for the Study of Infection. *J Infect* 1996; **33:** 143–52.

Necrotising enterocolitis. Necrotising enterocolitis in the newborn is thought to result from hypoxia or ischaemic injury to the intestinal mucosa with subsequent infection. Bacteria implicated in the disease include *Pseudomonas*, *Escherichia coli*, *Klebsiella*, *Salmonella* spp., and *Clostridium* spp. Treatment involves suspension of oral feeding, intravenous fluid therapy, and surgical excision of the affected gut. References to the use of oral vancomycin for the treatment[1] of neonatal necrotising enterocolitis indicate that it may be of benefit. In a comparison of intravenous regimens to treat the condition it was reported that ampicillin with gentamicin appeared as effective as vancomycin with cefotaxime in neonates over 2200 g birth-weight, but in smaller neonates results were better with vancomycin and cefotaxime.[2]

Necrotising enteritis in older children and adults, known as pigbel, has been attributed to toxins produced by *Clostridium perfringens*. Both sporadic and epidemic forms are predominantly seen in the highlands of Papua New Guinea, but sporadic cases have been reported elsewhere. Treatment is supportive with surgical intervention where necessary. A vaccine is available for prophylaxis.

1. Han VKM. An outbreak of Clostridium difficile necrotizing enterocolitis: a case for oral vancomycin therapy? *Pediatrics* 1983; **71:** 935–41.
2. Scheifele DW, *et al.* Comparison of two antibiotic regimens for neonatal necrotizing enterocolitis. *J Antimicrob Chemother* 1987; **20:** 421–9.

Salmonella enteritis. *Salmonella* spp. are Gram-negative bacteria belonging to the Enterobacteriaceae family. They can be divided into those causing enteric fever, namely *S. typhi* and *S. paratyphi*, where infection is systemic although affecting the gastro-intestinal tract (see under Typhoid and Paratyphoid Fever, below) and non-typhoid *Salmonella*, including *S. enteritidis* and *S. typhimurium* which cause acute gastro-enteritis usually through food poisoning. There are numerous *Salmonella* serotypes identified with food poisoning and they have often been named according to the place where they were first isolated. The increase in salmonellosis in Great Britain has been almost entirely due to *S. enteritidis*[1] and this reflects an increase internationally.[2] Non-typhoid *Salmonella* spp. can cause invasive salmonellosis which may be manifest as septicaemia or localised infections such as meningitis or osteomyelitis.

Uncomplicated non-typhoid Salmonella enteritis is usually managed by fluid and electrolyte replacement. Attempts to eradicate the carrier state with antibacterial therapy (for example fluoroquinolones) appear to have been unsuccessful so far[3] and routine use is not recommended.[4] Patients with underlying debility or evidence of invasive salmonellosis should be given antibacterial therapy. Amoxycillin, ampicillin, or co-trimoxazole have been suggested[5,6] as have trimethoprim, cefotaxime,[6] ceftriaxone,[6] a fluoroquinolone[6] such as ciprofloxacin,[7] or chloramphenicol.[6] However, there is concern over the emergence of resistant strains, particularly to the fluoroquinolones.[8,9] Multiresistant R-type strains of *S. typhimurium* DT 104 have also been reported.[10-12]

1. Baird-Parker AC. Foodborne salmonellosis. *Lancet* 1990; **336:** 1231–5.
2. Rodrigue DC, *et al.* International increase in Salmonella enteritidis: a new pandemic? *Epidemiol Infect* 1990; **105:** 21–7.
3. Nagler JM, *et al.* Salmonella gastroenteritis: longterm follow-up of an outbreak after treatment with norfloxacin or co-trimoxazole. *J Antimicrob Chemother* 1994; **34:** 291–4.
4. Farthing M. The management of infective gastroenteritis in adults: a consensus statement by an expert panel convened by the British Society for the Study of Infection. *J Infect* 1996; **33:** 143–52.
5. Gorbach SL. Bacterial diarrhoea and its treatment. *Lancet* 1987; **ii:** 1378–82.
6. Anonymous. The choice of antibacterial drugs. *Med Lett Drugs Ther* 1998; **40:** 33–42.
7. Leigh DA. The treatment of a large outbreak of acute bacterial gastroenteritis with ciprofloxacin. *J Antimicrob Chemother* 1992; **30:** 733–5.
8. Wilcox MH, Spencer RC. Quinolones and salmonella gastroenteritis. *J Antimicrob Chemother* 1992; **30:** 221–8.
9. Frost JA, *et al.* Increasing ciprofloxacin resistance in salmonellas in England and Wales 1991-1994. *J Antimicrob Chemother* 1996; **37:** 85–91.
10. Threlfall EJ, *et al.* Increasing spectrum of resistance in multiresistant Salmonella typhimurium. *Lancet* 1996; **347:** 1053–4.
11. Anonymous. Multidrug-resistant Salmonella serotype typhimurium—United States, 1996. *JAMA* 1996; **277:** 1513.
12. Anonymous. Emergence of multidrug-resistant salmonella. *WHO Drug Inf* 1997; **11:** 21.

Shigellosis. Shigellosis (bacillary dysentery) is an enteric infection caused by the *Shigella* spp. *S. dysenteriae*, *S. flexneri*, *S. boydii*, or *S. sonnei*. They are Gram-negative bacteria belonging to the Enterobacteriaceae and are able to invade the colon. Depending on the species involved, the disease ranges from mild self-limiting secretory diarrhoea to severe colitis and dysentery with blood and mucus in the stools. *S. dysenteriae* is the most common in the developing world and causes the most severe disease. In developed countries *S. flexneri* and *S. sonnei* are more common. Some *S. flexneri* can cause severe colitis and toxic dilatation of the colon has been reported in travellers.[1] *S. sonnei* is the least pathogenic of the species.

As with any form of diarrhoea rehydration is the key to treatment. Antibacterial therapy may be with ampicillin (amoxycillin appears to be less effective), co-trimoxazole (or trimethoprim), nalidixic acid, or fluoroquinolones such as ciprofloxacin, but will depend on the prevailing resistance patterns (see below) and the severity of the disease. Bacterial resistance is common and some consider that antibacterials should be restricted to the most severe cases, particularly those due to *S. dysenteriae*;[2] in the UK, the Public Health Laboratory Services (PHLS) Working Group has concluded that therapy is seldom indicated for *S. sonnei* infections.[3] WHO[4] have advised that children with *Shigella* dysentery should be given antimicrobial therapy and recommended co-trimoxazole as treatment of choice with nalidixic acid or ampicillin as alternatives; they have noted that resistance to ampicillin is frequent.[5]

The rapid development of resistance and the emergence of multiresistant strains of *Shigella*, particularly in developing countries, has led to some changes in treatment recommendations.[5] In 1992, Bennish and Salam[6] considered that in developing countries nalidixic acid had become the preferred drug unless ampicillin or co-trimoxazole were known to be effective in the region. For *S. dysenteriae* it might be necessary to use pivmecillinam. They concluded that the fluoroquinolones should continue to be reserved for infections resistant to nalidixic acid or pivmecillinam.[6] Reduced susceptibility to fluoroquinolones of some strains of *S. sonnei* has been reported from Japan.[7] Fluoroquinolones are generally not used in children although a study[8] in Bangladesh has used ciprofloxacin in children with shigellosis and found it to be of similar efficacy to pivmecillinam. In studies from Israel, the third-generation cephalosporins ceftriaxone[9] or cefixime[10] were more effective than ampicillin or co-trimoxazole, respectively, in children with shigellosis. Other studies in adults in Bangladesh found cefixime to be ineffective compared with pivmecillinam[11] and azithromycin to be effective, although slightly less so, than ciprofloxacin.[12]

Oral shigella vaccines are under investigation for prophylaxis.

1. Wilson APR, *et al.* Toxic dilatation of the colon in shigellosis. *Br Med J* 1990; **301:** 1325–6.
2. Kaya IS, *et al.* Danger of antibiotic resistance in shigellosis. *Lancet* 1990; **336:** 186.
3. PHLS Working Group on the control of Shigella sonnei infection. Revised guidelines for the control of Shigella sonnei infection and other infective diarrhoeas. *Commun Dis Rep* 1993; **3:** R69–70.
4. WHO. *The rational use of drugs in the management of acute diarrhoea in children.* Geneva: WHO, 1990.
5. WHO. *The management and prevention of diarrhoea: practical guidelines.* 3rd ed. Geneva: WHO, 1993.
6. Bennish ML, Salam MA. Rethinking options for the treatment of shigellosis. *J Antimicrob Chemother* 1992; **30:** 243–7.
7. Horiuchi S, *et al.* Reduced susceptibilities of Shigella sonnei strains isolated from patients with dysentery to fluoroquinolones. *Antimicrob Agents Chemother* 1993; **37:** 2486–9.
8. Salam MA, *et al.* Randomised comparison of ciprofloxacin suspension and pivmecillinam for childhood shigellosis. *Lancet* 1998; **352:** 522–7.
9. Varsano I, *et al.* Comparative efficacy of ceftriaxone and ampicillin for treatment of severe shigellosis in children. *J Pediatr* 1991; **118:** 627–32.
10. Ashkenazi S, *et al.* A randomized, double-blind study comparing cefixime and trimethoprim-sulfamethoxazole in the treatment of childhood shigellosis. *J Pediatr* 1993; **123:** 817–21.
11. Salam MA, *et al.* Treatment of shigellosis: IV. Cefixime is ineffective in shigellosis in adults. *Ann Intern Med* 1995; **123:** 505–8.
12. Khan WA, *et al.* Treatment of shigellosis: V. Comparison of azithromycin and ciprofloxacin. *Ann Intern Med* 1997; **126:** 697–703.

Yersinia enteritis. *Yersinia enterocolitica* is a Gram-negative bacteria of the Enterobacteriaceae family and the species most commonly responsible for yersiniosis. The predominant form of infection is an enteric illness with or without mesenteric adenitis[1] although clinical manifestations can range from self-limited enterocolitis to potentially fatal systemic infection and post-infection complications can include erythema nodosum and reactive arthritis.[2] *Y. enterocolitica* is a recognised food-borne pathogen[3] and in some temperate countries rivals *Salmonella* and exceeds *Shigella* as a cause of acute gastro-enteritis; pigs are a major reservoir. Increased susceptibility to *Yersinia* infection has occurred in patients with iron overload treated with desferrioxamine and this is discussed further on p.976.

Isolates of *Y. enterocolitica* are reported to be susceptible to co-trimoxazole, aminoglycosides, chloramphenicol, tetracycline, third-generation cephalosporins, and quinolones *in vitro*.[1,2] As with any form of diarrhoea rehydration is the key to treatment and most forms of mild uncomplicated enteritis do not require antibacterial treatment. When necessary, Hoogkamp-Korstanje[1] considered drugs with good intracellular activity such as trimethoprim, co-trimoxazole, tetracycline, chloramphenicol, or fluoroquinolones to be the treatment of choice. In the absence of controlled comparative studies Cover and Aber[2] recommended doxycycline or co-trimoxazole for complicated gastro-intestinal and focal extra-intestinal infections or doxycycline and an aminoglycoside empirically in bacteraemia. Co-trimoxazole as first choice or alternatively a fluoroquinolone, an aminoglycoside, cefotaxime, or ceftizoxime have also been recommended.[4] One patient with chronic *Yersinia* infection who responded well to tetracycline or co-trimoxazole, but relapsed on withdrawal, has been treated successfully with ciprofloxacin.[5]

1. Hoogkamp-Korstanje JAA. Antibiotics in Yersinia enterocolitica infections. *J Antimicrob Chemother* 1987; **20:** 123–31.
2. Cover TL, Aber RC. Yersinia enterocolitica. *N Engl J Med* 1989; **321:** 16–24.
3. Doyle MP. Pathogenic Escherichia coli, Yersinia enterocolitica, and Vibrio parahaemolyticus. *Lancet* 1990; **336:** 1111–15.
4. Anonymous. The choice of antibacterial drugs. *Med Lett Drugs Ther* 1998; **40:** 33–42.
5. Read RC, Barry RE. Relapsing yersinia infection. *Br Med J* 1990; **300:** 1694.

Gonorrhoea

Gonorrhoea is a sexually transmitted disease caused by infection of mucosa with *Neisseria gonorrhoeae* (gonococcus), a Gram-negative bacterium. It occurs predominantly as urethritis in men and cervicitis in women and also as pharyngitis, proctitis, or conjunctivitis. Complications of gonococcal infections include pelvic inflammatory disease (below) in women and epididymitis (above) in men. Disseminated gonococcal infection results from gonococcal bacteraemia and may lead to septic arthritis, an arthritis-dermatitis syndrome (not to be confused with Reiter's disease which has been associated with non-gonococcal or nonspecific urethritis), and more rarely with conditions such as endocarditis or meningitis. Gonorrhoea in pregnant women may cause neonatal gonococcal conjunctivitis (ophthalmia neonatorum).

Infection with *Chlamydia trachomatis* (see under Chlamydial Infections, above) often occurs along with gonorrhoea and should be treated concomitantly.

N. gonorrhoeae used to be sensitive to penicillins and tetracyclines but in some areas, including the USA, this is no longer the case. Gonococcal resistance includes plasmid-mediated penicillin resistance, due to penicillinase-producing *N. gonorrhoeae* (PPNG); high-level plasmid-mediated tetracycline resistance (TRNG); and chromosomally mediated resistance (CMRNG), not due to beta-lactamase production, including resistance to penicillin, tetracycline, cefoxitin, or spectinomycin.[1,2]

The prevalence of gonococcal resistance has required changes in treatment recommendations.

In 1986, WHO[3] recommended penicillins or tetracyclines for areas where gonococcal resistance was low; cephalosporins or spectinomycin where resistance had reduced the efficacy of drugs such as benzylpenicillin, tetracycline, and co-trimoxazole; or kanamycin, thiamphenicol, or co-trimoxazole, drugs that might be cheaper and more widely available than cephalosporins or spectinomycin, although geographically their efficacy varied considerably. In the 1991 report from WHO,[4] penicillins, tetracyclines, and other older drugs were no longer included in the regimens recommended for most areas. The 1995 WHO recommendations state resistance to penicillins is so widespread that they are rarely regarded as useful.[5]

In the USA the wide distribution of antimicrobial-resistant *N. gonorrhoeae*, as documented by the Gonococcal Isolate Surveillance Project,[2] has also necessitated revised treatment guidelines. In 1998 the Centers for Disease Control (CDC)[6] recommended single-dose ceftriaxone, cefixime, ciprofloxacin, or ofloxacin as the treatment of choice for uncomplicated gonorrhoea, rather than penicillin or tetracycline, plus either single-dose azithromycin or a 7-day course of doxycycline for chlamydial infection that commonly co-exists with gonorrhoea.

However, in Britain[7] the incidence of penicillinase-producing *N. gonorrhoeae* has remained relatively low, despite their rapid spread in some parts of the world (especially Africa and South East Asia), although increasing penicillin resistance is reported in some areas.[8] A single oral dose of ampicillin or amoxycillin together with probenecid may often be effective for uncomplicated gonorrhoea acquired locally. Fluoroquinolones or spectinomycin are alternatives. If gonorrhoea has been acquired overseas a fluoroquinolone, a cephalosporin, or spectinomycin should be used.

Of concern are the increasing number of reports of resistance to newer antigonococcal drugs such as the fluoroquinolones from the UK,[9] the western Pacific region,[10] Canada,[11] and the USA.[12,13]

Recommended *treatment regimens* from WHO in 1995[5] and CDC in 1998[6] are as follows. Where appropriate, sexual partners should be tested and treated.

UNCOMPLICATED GONOCOCCAL INFECTIONS IN ADULTS.

1. WHO (for anogenital infections): a single dose of ceftriaxone 250 mg intramuscularly; or ciprofloxacin 500 mg (or an equivalent fluoroquinolone) by mouth; or spectinomycin 2 g intramuscularly. An oral cephalosporin such as cefixime 400 mg may also be used.

Alternatives that may be useful in some countries, depending on the prevalence of resistance: kanamycin 2 g intramuscularly as a single dose; or thiamphenicol 2.5 g by mouth once daily for 2 days; or co-trimoxazole 4.8 g once daily by mouth for three days.

For pharyngeal infections, treatment with either ceftriaxone or co-trimoxazole is recommended.

2. CDC (for uncomplicated infections in general): a single intramuscular dose of ceftriaxone 125 mg or single oral doses of cefixime 400 mg, ciprofloxacin 500 mg, or ofloxacin 400 mg. Other cephalosporins or fluoroquinolones may be substituted. Spectinomycin 2 g as a single intramuscular dose is an alternative in patients who cannot tolerate cephalosporins or fluoroquinolones. For pharyngeal infections they recommend ceftriaxone, ciprofloxacin, or ofloxacin. In each case CDC advocates concomitant treatment for presumptive chlamydial infections with either azithromycin 1 g orally as a single dose or doxycycline 100 mg twice daily for 7 days.

CDC recommends a cephalosporin or spectinomycin for pregnant women with gonorrhoea, and erythromycin or amoxycillin for chlamydial infection.

GONOCOCCAL EYE INFECTIONS IN ADULTS.

WHO[5] recommends a single dose of ceftriaxone 250 mg intramuscularly, or spectinomycin 2 g intramuscularly, or ciprofloxacin 500 mg by mouth together with frequent irrigation of the infected eye with saline. Kanamycin 2 g intramuscularly is another alternative. CDC[6] recommends a single dose of ceftriaxone 1 g intramuscularly together with irrigation of the infected eye with saline.

DISSEMINATED GONOCOCCAL INFECTIONS IN ADULTS.

WHO[5] recommends ceftriaxone 1 g intramuscularly or intravenously once daily or spectinomycin 2 g intramuscularly twice daily for 7 days. Another third-generation cephalosporin may be substituted if neither of these drugs is available. The following regimens are recommended by CDC:[6] initially ceftriaxone 1 g intramuscularly or intravenously every 24 hours, ceftizoxime 1 g intravenously every 8 hours, or cefotaxime 1 g intravenously every 8 hours. Ciprofloxacin 500 mg intravenously every 12 hours, ofloxacin 400 mg intravenously every 12 hours, or spectinomycin 2 g intramuscularly every 12 hours may be substituted in patients allergic to beta-lactams. Once improvement has been established for 24 to 48 hours oral therapy with cefixime 400 mg, ciprofloxacin 500 mg, or ofloxacin 400 mg, all twice daily may be substituted for the remainder of the 1-week treatment period. For gonococcal *meningitis* and *endocarditis* CDC advises ceftriaxone 1 to 2 g intravenously every 12 hours initially. Treatment for meningitis should continue for 10 to 14 days and for endocarditis for at least 4 weeks.

GONOCOCCAL INFECTIONS IN INFANTS AND CHILDREN.

Infants born to mothers with gonorrhoea are at high risk of infection and require prophylactic treatment. WHO[5] recommends a single intramuscular injection of ceftriaxone 50 mg per kg body-weight (maximum 125 mg), or spectinomycin 25 mg per kg (maximum 75 mg), or kanamycin 25 mg per kg (maximum 75 mg) if ceftriaxone is not available. CDC[6] suggests a single injection of ceftriaxone 25 to 50 mg per kg (maximum 125 mg). For those infants with disseminated gonococcal infection (sepsis, arthritis, meningitis) they[6] recommend a 7-day course of ceftriaxone or cefotaxime, extended to 10 to 14 days if meningitis is present. The prevention and treatment of neonatal gonococcal conjunctivitis is discussed under Neonatal Conjunctivitis, below.

The treatment recommended by CDC[6] for *children* with gonococcal infections, most commonly due to sexual abuse in pre-adolescents, is as for adults in those weighing 45 kg or more. Under a body-weight of 45 kg CDC recommends a single intramuscular dose of ceftriaxone 125 mg or spectinomycin 40 mg per kg (maximum 2 g) for those with uncomplicated infections; for disseminated infection they recommend an intramuscular or intravenous dose of ceftriaxone 50 mg per kg (maximum 1 g) once daily for 7 days, extended to 10 to 14 days and a maximum dose of 2 g in those weighing more than 45 kg.

1. Judson FN. Management of antibiotic-resistant Neisseria gonorrhoeae. *Ann Intern Med* 1989; **110:** 5–7.
2. Schwarcz SK, *et al.* National surveillance of antimicrobial resistance in Neisseria gonorrhoeae. *JAMA* 1990; **264:** 1413–17.
3. WHO. WHO expert committee on venereal diseases and treponematoses: sixth report. *WHO Tech Rep Ser 736* 1986: 118–23.
4. WHO. Management of patients with sexually transmitted diseases. *WHO Tech Rep Ser 810* 1991: 84–6.
5. WHO. *WHO model prescribing information: drugs used in sexually transmitted diseases and HIV infection.* Geneva: WHO, 1995.
6. Centers for Disease Control. 1998 Guidelines for treatment of sexually transmitted diseases. *MMWR* 1998; **47** (RR-1): 59–69.
7. Bignell C. The eradication of gonorrhoea. *Br Med J* 1994; **309:** 1103–4.
8. Lewis DA, *et al.* A one-year survey of Neisseria gonorrhoeae isolated from patients attending an east London genitourinary medicine clinic: antibiotic susceptibility patterns and patients' characteristics. *Genitourin Med* 1995; **71:** 13–17.
9. Gransden WR, *et al.* Decreased susceptibility of Neisseria gonorrhoeae to ciprofloxacin. *Lancet* 1990; **335:** 51. Correction. *ibid.*; 302.
10. Tapsall JW. Surveillance of antibiotic resistance in Neisseria gonorrhoeae and implications for the therapy of gonorrhoea. *Int J STD AIDS* 1995; **6:** 233–6.
11. Yeung KH, Dillon JR. Norfloxacin resistant Neisseria gonorrhoeae in North America. *Lancet* 1990; **336:** 759.
12. Gordon SM, *et al.* The emergence of Neisseria gonorrhoeae with decreased susceptibility to ciprofloxacin in Cleveland, Ohio: epidemiology and risk factors. *Ann Intern Med* 1996; **125:** 465–70.
13. Knapp JS, *et al.* Emerging in vitro resistance to quinolones in penicillinase-producing Neisseria gonorrhoeae strains in Hawaii. *Antimicrob Agents Chemother* 1994; **38:** 2200–3.

Granuloma inguinale

Granuloma inguinale or donovanosis is caused by the Gram-negative bacterium *Calymmatobacterium granulomatis* and occurs most commonly in the tropics and subtropics, especially Papua New Guinea and India. It is characterised by genital ulcers and is generally considered to be a sexually transmitted disease.

WHO[1] recommends co-trimoxazole 960 mg twice daily by mouth for 14 days as treatment of choice. Alternative drugs they suggest for patients not responding to co-trimoxazole include tetracycline, chloramphenicol, and gentamicin. Streptomycin is no longer recommended because of its toxicity and the need to reserve it for tuberculosis. In the USA the Centers for Disease Control and Prevention[2] recommend treatment with co-trimoxazole 960 mg twice daily or doxycycline 100 mg twice daily, both for a minimum of 3 weeks, with ciprofloxacin 750 mg twice daily or erythromycin 500 mg four times daily also for 3 weeks as alternatives. The addition of an aminoglycoside may be considered if lesions do not respond during the first few days of treatment.

1. WHO. *WHO model prescribing information: drugs used in sexually transmitted diseases and HIV infection.* Geneva: WHO, 1995.
2. Centers for Disease Control. 1998 Guidelines for treatment of sexually transmitted diseases. *MMWR* 1998; **47** (RR-1): 26–7.

Haemophilus influenzae infections

Haemophilus influenzae is a Gram-negative bacterium that colonises the upper respiratory tract in the majority of healthy people. Most are carriers of non-encapsulated strains, but a small proportion carry *H. influenzae* type b, the commonest encapsulated strain. Serious invasive infections have usually been caused by type b strains and have occurred mainly in young children. They include the bacteraemic diseases meningitis, pneumonia, epiglottitis, cellulitis, and arthritis. Non-encapsulated strains commonly cause otitis media, sinusitis, and conjunctivitis and infect patients with chronic bronchitis. However, they too can cause invasive infections such as pneumonia, septicaemia, and meningitis[1] and, with the introduction of *H. influenzae* type b vaccines, non-encapsulated strains may be responsible for a greater proportion of invasive *H. influenzae* disease.

For further details of these infections and their management see under the specific disease side-headings.

Ampicillin and chloramphenicol have been the antibacterials of choice against *H. influenzae*, but increasing resistance, especially to ampicillin, should be borne in mind; there have been several reports of multiresistant strains.[2-5] Injectable cephalosporins are popular alternatives for multiresistant type b organisms although there is controversy over their effectiveness against fully sensitive strains when compared with ampicillin or chloramphenicol or both; experience has been favourable with cefotaxime and ceftriaxone, but there is argument over the efficacy of cefuroxime.[6]

For serious *H. influenzae* infections cefotaxime, ceftriaxone, or chloramphenicol are currently preferred. For less serious infections, ampicillin, amoxycillin (with or without clavulanic acid), oral second- or third-generation cephalosporins, co-trimoxazole (or trimethoprim in the UK), tetracyclines, and the macrolides azithromycin and clarithromycin are suggested alternatives.

In the UK, secondary prophylaxis with rifampicin is given following *H. influenzae* type b meningitis (see below). A vaccine against *H. influenzae* type b is available and vaccination is included in the infant immunisation schedules in some countries including the UK and USA.

1. Falla TJ, *et al.* Population-based study of non-typable Haemophilus influenzae invasive disease in children and neonates. *Lancet* 1993; **341:** 851–4.
2. Sturm AW, *et al.* Outbreak of multiresistant non-encapsulated Haemophilus influenzae infections in a pulmonary rehabilitation centre. *Lancet* 1990; **335:** 214–16.
3. Brightman CAJ, *et al.* Family outbreak of chloramphenicol-ampicillin resistant Haemophilus influenzae type b disease. *Lancet* 1990; **335:** 351–2.
4. Barclay K, *et al.* Multiresistant Haemophilus influenzae. *Lancet* 1990; **335:** 549.
5. Scott GM, *et al.* Outbreaks of multiresistant Haemophilus influenzae infection. *Lancet* 1990; **335:** 925.
6. Powell M. Chemotherapy for infections caused by Haemophilus influenzae: current problems and future prospects. *J Antimicrob Chemother* 1991; **27:** 3–7.

Helicobacter pylori infections

Antibacterial therapy is used to eradicate *Helicobacter pylori* infection in peptic ulcer disease (p.1174) and MALT lymphoma (p.484).

Infections in immunocompromised patients

Patients with a defective immune system are at special risk of infection. Primary immune deficiency is rare, whereas secondary deficiency is more common: immunosuppressive therapy, cancer and its treatment, HIV infection, and splenectomy may all cause neutropenia and impaired humoral and cellular immunity in varying degrees. The risk of infection is linked to the duration and severity of neutropenia.

Infectious diseases are a major cause of morbidity and mortality in patients with AIDS (see HIV-associated Infections, p.600). Some are due to common pathogens, but others are opportunistic and are caused by normally avirulent commensals. Children with HIV infection appear to be at special risk of serious bacterial infections with common encapsulated bacteria. For further reference to some bacterial infections associated with AIDS, see under Gastro-enteritis (above), Opportunistic Mycobacterial Infections (below), and Tuberculosis (below). Fungal, protozoal, and viral infections which can affect immunocompromised patients are discussed under Infections in Immunocompromised Patients, p.369, p.575, and p.601, respectively. Secondary and opportunistic infections in patients with HIV infection are discussed under HIV-associated Infections, p.600.

Common causative organisms of unexplained fever in neutropenic patients include the Gram-negative bacteria *Pseudomonas aeruginosa, Escherichia coli,* and *Klebsiella* spp. and the Gram-positive bacteria staphylococci, streptococci, enterococci, and *Corynebacterium* spp. Gram-negative organisms have generally been responsible for most immediate life-threatening infections, but with the wider use of selective gut decontamination and of central venous catheters the spectrum of bacteria has changed and Gram-positive infections are occurring more frequently;[1,2] chemotherapy-induced mucositis and the prophylactic use of quinolones may also contribute to the increased prevalence of Gram-positive infections.[3] In neutropenic cancer patients Gram-positive bacteria, including staphylococci and viridans streptococci, appear to have become the predominant infecting organisms. Other bacteria implicated include the Gram-negative organism *Stenotrophomonas maltophilia (Xanthomonas maltophilia, Pseudomonas maltophilia).*[4]

TREATMENT. Onset of fever in neutropenic patients is indicative of serious infection which may progress to septicaemia and death and empirical antibacterial therapy should be started immediately.

The severity of infections depends on the level and duration of neutropenia, and factors such as severe mucositis or prolonged vascular access have a bearing on the likely infecting organisms. It is consequently difficult to produce a standard regimen for empirical treatment of infections in neutropenic patients. In addition the choice of empirical therapy needs to be adapted depending on changing patterns of infecting organisms and the emergence of drug resistant pathogens.[5,6] While a combination of an aminoglycoside and a beta lactam has been commonly used, monotherapy is becoming increasingly popular.

Monotherapy with ceftazidime has been shown to be as effective as combination therapy, even in severely neutropenic patients,[7,8] although activity against Gram-positive infections may be inadequate. Carbapenems (imipenem/cilastatin or meropenem) have activity against both Gram-positive and Gram-negative organisms and provide an alternative monotherapy. The monobactams, which have little activity against Gram-positive organisms, are a less suitable choice. The fluoroquinolones have been studied but results are conflicting.[9-11]

Combination therapy usually includes an aminoglycoside (amikacin, gentamicin, or netilmicin) with an antipseudomonal cephalosporin or penicillin. Other combinations studied in an attempt to avoid aminoglycoside-related toxicity and the need for monitoring blood concentrations include combinations of two or more beta lactams[12] and the monobactam aztreonam with flucloxacillin.[13] However, there are concerns over both the activity and possible selection of resistant organisms with some of these regimens.[14] Withdrawal of the aminoglycoside when the patient stabilises or improves is less effective than continuing with the complete regimen.[15] Vancomycin or teicoplanin have been used in the initial regimen in centres with a high incidence of methicillin-resistant *Staphylococcus* spp.,[16] but have not been shown to produce additional benefits elsewhere.[17] They are more often used as adjuncts if there is evidence of Gram-positive infection. The emergence of vancomycin-resistant strains of *Enterococcus* spp. and *Staphylococcus* spp. means that empirical use of vancomycin should probably be discouraged.[18]

The optimum duration of therapy is still controversial.[14] Antibacterial treatment can be discontinued after 5 to 7 days in patients in whom both the infection and the neutropenia resolve. In patients with continuing neutropenia, prolonged antibacterial use can predispose to fungal superinfections, but re-infection is a potential hazard if the drugs are stopped. Antibacterial treatment can probably be stopped after 10 days in such patients[14] or 5 to 7 days after the fever resolves[19] provided that the patients are subsequently closely monitored and suitable prophylaxis is continued.

An ongoing series of studies by the International Antimicrobial Therapy Cooperative Group of the European Organisation for Research and Treatment of Cancer has attempted to assess the efficacy of a range of therapeutic and prophylactic strategies[6] and the Infectious Diseases Society of America is publishing a series of guidelines.[19]

The routine use of colony-stimulating factors as an adjunct to antibacterial treatment is not generally recommended[19] but may be indicated in neutropenic patients at high risk of serious infections or infection-related complications; examples include some patients with malignant neoplasms[20] and those with persistent severe neutropenia and infections that are not responsive to antibacterials alone.[19]

PROPHYLAXIS. Most infections in immunosuppressed patients are caused by organisms from their own alimentary tract and in cancer patients, for example, may follow chemotherapy-induced mucosal damage to the tract. Despite the efficacy of antibacterial prophylaxis in nonfebrile patients likely to be neutropenic, the Infectious Diseases Society of America[19] discourages routine use; reasons include toxicity of the antibacterial, potential fungal overgrowth, and problems of bacterial resistance (see below). Most experience with prophylaxis has been in patients with leukaemia. Possible prophylactic regimens included selective decontamination of the alimentary tract using oral nonabsorbable antibacterials such as gentamicin, nystatin, vancomycin, framycetin, polymyxin B, and colistin or oral absorbable drugs such as co-trimoxazole or the fluoroquinolones (see also under Intensive Care, below).

Complete elimination of gastro-intestinal flora using neomycin, polymyxin B, cephaloridine, and amphotericin was more successful than selective decontamination at reducing the incidence of graft-versus-host disease and severe infections in children undergoing bone-marrow transplantation.[21] Recently, prophylaxis with fluoroquinolones has been commonly used although, general, prophylaxis with these drugs has resulted in reduction in Gram-negative but not in Gram-positive infections in immunocompromised patients.[3,22] In response to the increasing incidence of Gram-positive infections in these patients, combination prophylaxis with fluoroquinolones and phenoxymethylpenicillin[23] or rifampicin[24] has been tried. Nevertheless, concern about the emergence of resistant organisms has led to the recommendation that routine prophylaxis should be avoided.[19]

Immunocompromised patients may benefit from appropriate immunisation against common infections, although precautions relating to the administration of live vaccines in such patients should be observed (p.1501).

The duration and severity of neutropenia can be reduced by the use granulocyte or granulocyte-macrophage colony-stimulating factors, and this may be a useful adjunct in infection control in selected patients.[20]

For further reference to prophylaxis in high-risk patients, see under Intensive Care, below.

1. Anonymous. Surveillance cultures in neutropenia. *Lancet* 1989; **i:** 1238–9.
2. Oppenheim BA. The changing pattern of infection in neutropenic patients. *J Antimicrob Chemother* 1998; **41** (suppl D): 7–11.
3. Meunier F. Prevention of infections in neutropenic patients with pefloxacin. *J Antimicrob Chemother* 1990; **26** (suppl B): 69–73.
4. Kerr KG, *et al.* Pseudomonas maltophilia infections in neutropenic patients and the use of imipenem. *Postgrad Med J* 1990; **66:** 1090.
5. Klastersky J. Science and pragmatism in the treatment and prevention of neutropenic infection. *J Antimicrob Chemother* 1998; **41** (suppl D): 13–24.
6. Viscoli C. The evolution of the empirical management of fever and neutropenia in cancer patients. *J Antimicrob Chemother* 1998; **41** (suppl D): 65–80.
7. Pizzo PA, *et al.* A randomized trial comparing ceftazidime alone with combination antibiotic therapy in cancer patients with fever and neutropenia. *N Engl J Med* 1986; **315:** 552–8.
8. De Pauw BE, *et al.* Ceftazidime compared with piperacillin and tobramycin for the empiric treatment of fever in neutropenic patients with cancer: a multicenter randomized trial. *Ann Intern Med* 1994; **120:** 834–44.
9. Meunier F, *et al.* Prospective randomized evaluation of ciprofloxacin versus piperacillin plus amikacin for empiric antibiotic therapy of febrile granulocytopenic cancer patients with lymphomas and solid tumours. *Antimicrob Agents Chemother* 1991; **35:** 873–8.
10. Johnson PRE, *et al.* A randomized trial of high-dose ciprofloxacin versus azlocillin and netilmicin in the empirical therapy of febrile neutropenic patients. *J Antimicrob Chemother* 1992; **30:** 203–14.
11. Malik IA, *et al.* Randomised comparison of oral ofloxacin alone with combination of parenteral antibiotics in neutropenic febrile patients. *Lancet* 1992; **339:** 1092–6. [N.B. Correction to ofloxacin dosage (it should be 400 mg twice daily) in *Lancet* 1992; **340:** 128].
12. Winston DJ, *et al.* Beta-lactam antibiotic therapy in febrile granulocytopenic patients: a randomized trial comparing cefoperazone plus piperacillin, ceftazidime plus piperacillin, and imipenem alone. *Ann Intern Med* 1991; **115:** 849–59.
13. Heney D, *et al.* Aztreonam therapy in children with febrile neutropenia: a randomized trial of aztreonam plus flucloxacillin versus piperacillin plus gentamicin. *J Antimicrob Chemother* 1991; **28:** 117–29.
14. Boogaerts MA. Anti-infective strategies in neutropenia. *J Antimicrob Chemother* 1995; **36** (suppl A): 167–78.
15. EORTC International Antimicrobial Therapy Cooperative Group. Ceftazidime combined with a short or long course of amikacin for empirical therapy of gram-negative bacteremia in cancer patients with granulocytopenia. *N Engl J Med* 1987; **317:** 1692–8.
16. Menichetti F, *et al.* Effects of teicoplanin and those of vancomycin in initial empirical antibiotic regimen for febrile, neutropenic patients with hematological malignancies. *Antimicrob Agents Chemother* 1994; **38:** 2041–6.
17. European Organization for Research and Treatment of Cancer (EORTC) International Antimicrobial Therapy Cooperative Group and the National Cancer Institute of Canada—Clinical Trials Group. Vancomycin added to empirical combination antibiotic therapy for fever in granulocytopenic cancer patients. *J Infect Dis* 1991; **163:** 951–8.
18. Centers for Disease Control. Hospital Infection Control Practices Advisory Committee (HICPAC). Recommendations for preventing the spread of vancomycin resistance. *MMWR* 1995; **44** (RR-12): 1–13.
19. Hughes WT, *et al.* 1997 Guidelines for the use of antimicrobial agents in neutropenic patients with unexplained fever. *Clin Infect Dis* 1997; **25:** 551–73.
20. American Society of Clinical Oncology. Recommendations for the use of hematopoietic colony-stimulating factors: evidence-based, clinical practice guidelines. *J Clin Oncol* 1994; **12:** 2471–2508.
21. Vossen JM, *et al.* Prevention of infection and graft-versus-host disease by suppression of intestinal microflora in children treated with allogeneic bone marrow transplantation. *Eur J Clin Microbiol Infect Dis* 1990; **9:** 14–23.
22. Engels EA, *et al.* Efficacy of quinolone prophylaxis in neutropenic cancer patients: a meta-analysis. *J Clin Oncol* 1998; **16:** 1179–87.

23. International Antimicrobial Therapy Cooperative Group of the European Organization for Research and Treatment of Cancer (EORTC). Reduction of fever and streptococcal bacteremia in granulocytopenic patients with cancer: a trial of oral penicillin V or placebo combined with pefloxacin. *JAMA* 1994; **272:** 1183–9.
24. Bow EJ, *et al.* Quinolone-based antibacterial chemoprophylaxis in neutropenic patients: effect of augmented gram-positive activity on infectious morbidity. *Ann Intern Med* 1996; **125:** 183–90.

Intensive care

Similarly to immunocompromised patients (above), those in intensive care units are often very susceptible to endogenous infections, especially respiratory and urinary-tract infections, arising from gastro-intestinal colonisation by aerobic Gram-negative bacilli acquired in hospital. Selective digestive tract decontamination (SDD) using oral non-absorbable antibacterial regimens and selective parenteral and enteral antisepsis regimens (SPEAR) incorporating selective decontamination together with systemic antibacterial prophylaxis have been used in an attempt to prevent colonisation and infection in these high-risk patients although its effectiveness is debated.

Selective decontamination is achieved by elimination of aerobic, potentially pathogenic, organisms from throat and intestines while preserving the indigenous, mostly anaerobic, flora.[1] Regimens commonly include two or three non-absorbable or poorly absorbed antibacterial drugs, for example colistin, neomycin, norfloxacin, or polymyxin, in combination with an antifungal, usually amphotericin. The drugs are usually applied topically to the oropharyngeal mucosa in addition to oral or intragastric administration, although local application to the oropharynx alone is also reported to be effective.[2,3] A parenteral third-generation cephalosporin, usually cefotaxime, may be given for a few days until oral medication takes effect.[4,5] Strict adherence to the protocol is reported to be necessary for maximum efficacy[6] and constant monitoring for the emergence of antimicrobial resistance is considered essential[5,6] although so far this has rarely been seen in practice.[6,7] However, most regimens have little or no activity against potential Gram-positive pathogens such as *Enterococcus* spp., and so their use may increase the risk for colonisation and infection with these organisms.[8] There is particular concern over the emergence of vancomycin-resistant strains.

Despite numerous clinical studies, many of which have shown a reduction in potential Gram-negative pathogens[4,5,9] and in the incidence of respiratory-tract infections,[2,3] it has been difficult to demonstrate that SDD or SPEAR reduces mortality[10-13] although a meta-analysis[14] of randomised controlled trials concluded that a combination of a systemic and topical antibacterial could be beneficial. It has been suggested[15] that equivalent infection control could be achieved more economically by emphasis on high standards of hygiene and avoidance of histamine H_2-receptor antagonists, which could allow overgrowth of potentially pathogenic bacteria as a result of the change in gastric pH.

Another potential source of infection in intensive care is from the use of **intravascular catheters**. The organisms implicated most frequently have been coagulase-negative staphylococci.[16] Prevention and control of infection depend on good aseptic technique and care of the insertion site, and also catheter design.[16,17] Catheters should be removed as soon as possible (often after 48 to 72 hours for peripheral lines) and any infections treated promptly with antibacterials; vancomycin or teicoplanin are appropriate for empirical treatment so long as resistance is not a problem.[16] The effectiveness of antibacterial prophylaxis has not been fully tested, although there are some favourable early studies.[18] Topical antiseptics and antibacterials have produced promising results.[16] Antibacterials could also prove useful in reducing or eliminating colonisation of the catheter lumen[19] and catheters coated with antibacterials[20] or heparin[21] are under investigation. Randomised clinical studies have shown that the use of catheters coated with minocycline and rifampicin[22] or with antiseptics (p.1098) can reduce the risk of systemic infections.

The importance of maintaining high standards of infection control, including handwashing, in intensive care units has been reinforced by the increasing incidence of nosocomial infections that are difficult to treat such as vancomycin-resistant enterococci and *Acinetobacter*. In one such outbreak due to *A. baumannii* some strains were resistant to imipenem and all other antibacterials except polymyxin B and sulbactam.[23] Intensive infection control measures and irrigation of all open wounds with polymyxin B solution were used to eliminate infection and colonisation.

1. van Saene HKF, Stoutenbeek CP. Selective decontamination. *J Antimicrob Chemother* 1987; **20:** 462–5.
2. Rodriguez-Roldan JM, *et al.* Prevention of nosocomial lung infection in ventilated patients: use of an antimicrobial pharyngeal nonabsorbable paste. *Crit Care Med* 1990; **18:** 1239–42.
3. Pugin J, *et al.* Oropharyngeal decontamination decreases incidence of ventilator-associated pneumonia: a randomized, placebo-controlled, double-blind clinical trial. *JAMA* 1991; **265:** 2704–10.
4. Ledingham IM, *et al.* Triple regimen of selective decontamination of the digestive tract, systemic cefotaxime, and microbiological surveillance for prevention of acquired infection in intensive care. *Lancet* 1988; **i:** 785–90.
5. Tetteroo GWM, *et al.* Selective decontamination to reduce gram-negative colonisation and infections after oesophageal resection. *Lancet* 1990; **335:** 704–7.
6. Tetteroo GWM, *et al.* Bacteriology of selective decontamination: efficacy and rebound colonisation. *J Antimicrob Chemother* 1994; **34:** 139–48.
7. van Saene HKF, *et al.* Cefotaxime combined with selective decontamination in long term intensive care unit patients: virtual absence of emergence of resistance. *Drugs* 1988; **35** (suppl 2): 29–34.
8. Bontes MJM, *et al.* Colonization and infection with Enterococcus faecalis in intensive care units: the role of antimicrobial agents. *Antimicrob Agents Chemother* 1995; **39:** 2783–6.
9. Aerdts SJA, *et al.* Prevention of bacterial colonization of the respiratory tract and stomach of mechanically ventilated patients by a novel regimen of selective decontamination in combination with initial systemic cefotaxime. *J Antimicrob Chemother* 1990; **26** (suppl A): 59–76.
10. Loirat P, *et al.* Selective digestive decontamination in intensive care unit patients. *Intensive Care Med* 1992; **18:** 182–8.
11. Vandenbroucke-Grauls CMJE, Vandenbroucke JP. Effect of selective decontamination of the digestive tract on respiratory tract infections and mortality in the intensive care unit. *Lancet* 1991; **338:** 859–62.
12. van Saene HKF, *et al.* Selective decontamination of the digestive tract in the intensive care unit: current status and future prospects. *Crit Care Med* 1992; **20:** 691–703.
13. Selective Decontamination of the Digestive Tract Trialists' Collaborative Group. Meta-analysis of randomised controlled trials of selective decontamination of the digestive tract. *Br Med J* 1993; **307:** 525–32.
14. Liberati A, *et al.* Antibiotic prophylaxis in adult patients treated in intensive care units. Acute Respiratory Infections Module of the Cochrane Database of Systematic Reviews (updated 1 December 1997). Available in the Cochrane Library; Issue 1. Oxford: Update Software; 1998.
15. Atkinson SW, Bihari DJ. Selective decontamination of the gut. *Br Med J* 1993; **306:** 286–7.
16. Elliott TSJ. Line-associated bacteraemias. *Commun Dis Rep* 1993; **3:** R91–R96.
17. Raad I. Intravascular-catheter-related infections. *Lancet* 1998; **351:** 893–8.
18. Spafford PS, *et al.* Prevention of central venous catheter-related coagulase-negative staphylococcal sepsis in neonates. *J Pediatr* 1994; **125:** 259–63.
19. Yassien M, *et al.* Modulation of biofilms of Pseudomonas aeruginosa by quinolones. *Antimicrob Agents Chemother* 1995; **39:** 2262–8.
20. Raad I, *et al.* Antibiotics and prevention of microbial colonization of catheters. *Antimicrob Agents Chemother* 1995; **39:** 2397–2400.
21. Appelgren P, *et al.* Does surface heparinisation reduce bacterial colonisation of central venous catheters? *Lancet* 1995; **345:** 130.
22. Raad I, *et al.* Central venous catheters coated with minocycline and rifampin for the prevention of catheter-related colonization and bloodstream infections: a randomized, double-blind trial. *Ann Intern Med* 1997; **127:** 267–74.
23. Go ES, *et al.* Clinical and molecular epidemiology of acinetobacter infections sensitive only to polymyxin B and sulbactam. *Lancet* 1994; **344:** 1329–32.

Legionnaires' disease

Legionnaires' disease is a legionella pneumonia caused by the Gram-negative bacterium *Legionella pneumophila*. Serious outbreaks have been associated with infected air-conditioning systems or water supplies. Pontiac fever is a milder, usually self-limiting, influenza-like illness also caused by *L. pneumophila* as well as by other *Legionella* spp. Legionellosis has been suggested as a broad term to cover pneumonic and non-pneumonic clinical syndromes caused by any *Legionella* spp.; other species include *L. bozemanii, L. micdadei* (Pittsburgh pneumonia agent), and *L. wadsworthii*.

Erythromycin is the usual treatment for *Legionella* infections; azithromycin or clarithromycin may be acceptable alternatives.[1,2] Fluoroquinolones are alternatives to the macrolides.[2] Rifampicin may be given in addition especially in severe or deteriorating illness or in immunocompromised patients.[1,2]

1. Roig J, *et al.* Treatment of legionnaires' disease: current recommendations. *Drugs* 1993; **46:** 63–79.
2. Stout JE, Yu VL. Legionellosis. *N Engl J Med* 1997; **337:** 682–7.

Leprosy

Leprosy (Hansen's disease) is a chronic disease caused by *Mycobacterium leprae*; it affects the peripheral nervous system, the skin, and some other tissues. It is transmitted from person-to-person when bacilli are shed from the nose and skin lesions of infected patients, but most individuals are naturally immune, and symptoms are suppressed. Clinical leprosy may be regarded as a consequence of deficient cell-mediated immunity in susceptible individuals. For the purpose of grouping patients for chemotherapy, leprosy may be classified as multibacillary or paucibacillary.

Multibacillary leprosy occurs when cellular immunity is largely deficient, and includes the sub-groups lepromatous (LL), borderline lepromatous (BL), and mid-borderline leprosy (BB) as well as any other types giving a positive skin smear for acid-fast bacilli. Generally the lepromin test (p.1596) is negative. Paucibacillary leprosy results when cellular immunity is only partially deficient, and includes the sub-groups borderline tuberculoid (BT), tuberculoid (TT), and indeterminate leprosy (I) when the skin smear is negative. Generally the lepromin test is positive.

Reactive episodes may be seen in leprosy patients undergoing treatment; they are known as *lepra reactions* and unless treated may lead to deformity and disability. Most reactions belong to one of two main types. *Type 1* lepra reactions or reversal reactions are delayed hypersensitivity reactions (type IV hypersensitivity) and respond to analgesics and corticosteroids. *Type 2* lepra reactions, also known as erythema nodosum leprosum (ENL), represent a humoral antibody response (type III hypersensitivity) to dead bacteria. Drugs used in mild type 2 lepra reactions include analgesics, chloroquine, and stibophen. Drug treatment of severe type 2 lepra reactions consists of corticosteroids, thalidomide, or clofazimine.[1] Antileprotic drug therapy is generally continued during lepra reactions.

Dapsone given on its own was for a long time the mainstay of leprosy treatment. However, the emergence of resistance to dapsone and to other antileprotics led to the use of multidrug therapy regimens consisting of 2 or 3 drugs with dapsone, rifampicin, and clofazimine being the standard ones. Newer alternatives include clarithromycin, minocycline, and ofloxacin. Ethionamide or prothionamide have been used in place of clofazimine in light-skinned patients, but are no longer recommended because of their severe hepatotoxicity.

The most widely used multidrug regimens are those recommended by WHO[2] and in these the choice of drugs and length of treatment are based on the patient's bacillary load. Patients were originally classified as having multibacillary or paucibacillary leprosy according to the degree of skin-smear positivity. However, the lack of facilities for bacteriological examination of skin smears has led to classification increasingly being made on clinical grounds. WHO now classifies patients with more than 5 skin lesions as multibacillary, and those with less than 5 skin lesions as paucibacillary. It further classifies patients with only one skin lesion as having paucibacillary single-lesion leprosy.

MULTIBACILLARY LEPROSY.

The standard regimen recommended by WHO for multibacillary leprosy[2] is rifampicin 600 mg and clofazimine 300 mg both given once a month under supervision together with clofazimine 50 mg and dapsone 100 mg both daily in self-administered doses. Treatment is continued for 2 years.[2] Since patient compliance has been considered essential for successful treatment, the monthly rifampicin and clofazimine doses are given under supervision and dapsone ingestion can be verified by a urine spot test. However, WHO now recommends that delivery systems should be more flexible to adapt to individual circumstances since cure rates have been high even when regimens are not strictly adhered to.[2] In addition, shorter treatment schedules of about 12 months are being investigated[2] although there is some concern that even the standard 2-year regimen may not be sufficient (see below under Relapse). Two studies[3-5] of a 1-year regimen of rifampicin (6 or 12 months), ethionamide, and dapsone or clofazimine demonstrated good clinical results, but an unacceptable incidence of hepatotoxicity. An 8-month regimen, comprising daily supervised treatment with rifampicin, ethionamide, dapsone, and clofazimine for 8 weeks, followed by unsupervised daily ethionamide, dapsone, and clofazimine for 6 months also proved effective.[6] The problems of hepatotoxicity may be reduced by newer drugs such as the fluoroquinolones ofloxacin and pefloxacin, the macrolide clarithromycin, and the tetracycline minocycline.[7] In particular, there is great interest in the combination of ofloxacin with rifampicin, which may offer the possibility of a much shorter (1-month) treatment regimen.[2] In the meantime, WHO[2] recommends the following alternative 2-year treatment regimens utilising these newer drugs when the standard regimen cannot be used, either because of rifampicin resistance or toxicity or because of refusal to accept clofazimine due to the skin pigmentation it causes. When rifampicin cannot be given clofazimine 50 mg daily together with ofloxacin 400 mg and minocycline 100 mg for the first 6 months is recommended, then continuing for a further 18 months with clofazimine together with minocycline or ofloxacin. When clofazimine cannot be given ofloxacin 400 mg daily or minocycline 100 mg daily may be substituted in the standard regimen.[8] Alternatively, rifampicin 600 mg, ofloxacin 400 mg, and minocycline 100 mg could be administered once a month for 24 months.[2]

Immunotherapy with *Mycobacterium w* vaccine in addition to standard multidrug treatment has also been shown to reduce treatment time in initial studies[9-11] although a small increase in the incidence of type 1 lepra reactions has been observed.[12]

PAUCIBACILLARY LEPROSY.

The WHO recommended regimen[2] for paucibacillary leprosy is rifampicin 600 mg once monthly under supervision and dapsone 100 mg daily, self-administered. Treatment is continued for 6 months. If there are severe toxic effects with dapsone it should be stopped and clofazimine substituted.[8] The WHO considers that a single dose of rifampicin 600 mg, ofloxacin 400 mg and minocycline 100 mg given in combination is a suitable alternative for patients with single lesion paucibacillary leprosy,[2] although some[13] have reservations about the clinical study[14] comparing this regimen with the standard 6-month treatment. Short-course regimens that have been shown to be effective in the treatment of paucibacillary leprosy include: rifampicin 900 mg weekly for 8 weeks; rifampicin 900 mg weekly for 12 weeks; and rifampicin 600 mg in association with dapsone 100 mg, each given daily for 6 days.[15] However, the time to achieve cure may be unacceptably long in a substantial minority of paucibacillary patients treated with current short-course regimens.[16] Treatment with rifampicin 600 mg daily and ofloxacin 400 mg daily for one month is under investigation for both paucibacillary and multibacillary leprosy.[8]

RELAPSE.

Relapse following a recommended course of multidrug therapy for multibacillary or paucibacillary leprosy can occur and WHO recommends re-treatment with the original regimen.[2] Although the relapse rate following multidrug therapy for multibacillary leprosy generally appears to be low,[2,17] there has been concern at the set duration of treatments for both multibacillary[18,19] and paucibacillary[20] leprosy now recommended by WHO rather than continuing treatment until skin smears are negative. Long-term follow-up suggests that patients with a high initial bacterial load may be at increased risk of relapse, and may require closer surveillance following completion of treatment.[21]

PREGNANCY.

Pregnant and breast feeding leprosy patients experience clinical deterioration and in general antileprotic therapy is continued in such patients.

PROPHYLAXIS.

Leprosy is spread from person to person, so household contacts may be at risk. Administration of dapsone prophylaxis to some household contacts[22,23] may prevent disease in this high-risk group. WHO[2] suggests that contacts of newly diagnosed cases should be examined for evidence of leprosy and then advised how to watch for early signs of the disease; prophylaxis with rifampicin or other antileprotics is not recommended in leprosy control programmes. BCG vaccine appears to be protective. Vaccines specifically against leprosy are under investigation.

ELIMINATION.

The multidrug therapy regimens recommended by WHO have been widely implemented in recent years. Their success led to the World Health Assembly setting a goal in 1991 of elimination of leprosy as a public health problem by the year 2000: that is reducing the prevalence to less than 1 case per 10 000 population in endemic areas. However, reducing the prevalence to this level is likely to become increasingly difficult as programmes are extended to remote areas, and there is still a need for rehabilitation programmes for those disabled by the disease.

1. Lockwood DNJ. The management of erythema nodosum leprosum: current and future options. *Lepr Rev* 1996; **67:** 253–9.
2. WHO. WHO expert committee on leprosy. *WHO Tech Rep Ser 874* 1998.
3. Pattyn SR, *et al.* Combined regimens of one year duration in the treatment of multibacillary leprosy—I. Combined regimens with rifampicin administered during one year. *Lepr Rev* 1989; **60:** 109–17.
4. Pattyn SR, *et al.* Combined regimens of one year duration in the treatment of multibacillary leprosy—II. Combined regimens with rifampicin administered during 6 months. *Lepr Rev* 1989; **60:** 118–23.
5. Pattyn SR, *et al.* Status of the multibacillary leprosy patients treated with combined regimens of 1 year duration, after a mean follow-up of more than 5 years. *Lepr Rev* 1991; **62:** 337–9.
6. Pattyn SR, *et al.* Ambulatory treatment of multibacillary leprosy with a regimen of 8 months duration. *Lepr Rev* 1992; **63:** 36–40.
7. Noordeen SK, Hombach JM. Leprosy. In: *WHO. Tropical disease research: progress 1991-1992.* Eleventh programme report of the UNDP/World Bank/WHO special programme for Research and Training in Tropical Diseases (TDR). Geneva: WHO, 1993.
8. WHO. Chemotherapy of leprosy. *WHO Tech Rep Ser 847* 1994.
9. Zaheer SA, *et al.* Combined multidrug and Mycobacterium w vaccine therapy in patients with multibacillary leprosy. *J Infect Dis* 1993; **167:** 401–10.
10. Zaheer SA, *et al.* Addition of immunotherapy with Mycobacterium w vaccine to multi-drug therapy benefits multibacillary leprosy patients. *Vaccine* 1995; **13:** 1102–10.
11. Katoch K, *et al.* Treatment of bacilliferous BL/LL cases with combined chemotherapy and immunotherapy. *Int J Lepr* 1995; **63:** 202–12.
12. Kar HK, *et al.* Reversal reaction in multibacillary leprosy patients following MDT with and without immunotherapy with a candidate for an antileprosy vaccine, Mycobacterium w. *Lepr Rev* 1993; **64:** 219–26.
13. Lockwood DNJ. Rifampicin/minocycline and ofloxacin (ROM) for single lesions—what is the evidence? *Lepr Rev.* 1997; **68:** 299–300.
14. Single-lesion Multicentre Trial Group. Efficacy of single-dose multidrug therapy for the treatment of single-lesion paucibacillary leprosy. *Lepr Rev* 1997; **68:** 341–9.
15. Pattyn SR, *et al.* Evaluation of five treatment regimens, using either dapsone monotherapy or several doses of rifampicin in the treatment of paucibacillary leprosy. *Lepr Rev* 1990; **61:** 151–6.
16. Pattyn SR, *et al.* Eight years of follow-up of paucibacillary patients treated with short-course regimens. *Lepr Rev* 1992; **63:** 80–2.
17. World Health Organisation Leprosy Unit. Risk of relapse in leprosy. *Indian J Lepr* 1995; **67:** 13–26.
18. Jakeman P. Risk of relapse in multibacillary leprosy. *Lancet* 1995; **345:** 4–5.
19. Waters MFR. Relapse following various types of multidrug therapy in multibacillary leprosy. *Lepr Rev* 1995; **66:** 1–9. Correction. *ibid.*; 192.
20. Kar PK, *et al.* A clinicopathological study of multidrug therapy in borderline tuberculoid leprosy. *J Indian Med Assoc* 1994; **92:** 336–7.
21. Desikan KV. The risk of relapse after multidrug therapy in leprosy. *Lepr Rev* 1997; **68:** 114–16.
22. Filice GA, Fraser DW. Management of household contacts of leprosy patients. *Ann Intern Med* 1978; **88:** 538–42.
23. Dayal R, Bharadwaj VP. Prevention and early detection of leprosy in children. *J Trop Pediatr* 1995; **41:** 132–8.

Leptospirosis

Leptospirosis is an infectious disease caused by serovars of the spirochaete *Leptospira interrogans*, the commonest in the UK being *L. hardjo* and *L. icterohaemorrhagiae*.[1] *Leptospira* are widely distributed in wild and domestic animals, including cattle. Rats are a common source of infection in man and transmission is often by contact with water or soil contaminated with infected urine. In England and Wales there were 299 confirmed cases of leptospirosis during 1985–9;[1] the main occupational group at risk was farmers and agricultural workers. The data were insufficient to confirm whether recreational water users such as canoeists were at increased risk, but outbreaks among such groups have been reported elsewhere.[2] The majority of symptomatic patients have no more than a mild influenza-like illness, although a small proportion develop Weil's disease with haemorrhagic complications and severe liver and kidney failure.

The use of antibacterials is controversial since many recover without treatment. However, when leptospirosis is suspected treatment within 4 to 7 days has been recommended to prevent complications.[3,4] The intravenous administration of either benzylpenicillin 900 mg, ampicillin 1 g, or erythromycin 500 mg every 6 hours, or the oral administration of amoxycillin 500 mg every 8 hours or doxycycline 100 mg twice daily has been suggested;[4] treatment is continued for 7 days. Benzylpenicillin has been given intravenously in higher doses for severe leptospirosis; 7.2 to 9.6 g daily for 5 days followed by 1.44 g daily for a further 5 days has been advocated.[5] However, intravenous doses of 900 mg every 6 hours for 7 days have proved successful even when given late in the course of illness.[6] In severe infections, supportive therapy with analgesics and antiemetics may be required. Renal function should be monitored and dialysis instigated if necessary, and blood products may be necessary to control haemorrhagic complications.[3]

Doxycycline has reduced the incidence of leptospirosis when given prophylactically to USA soldiers in Panama.[7] Leptospirosis vaccines are available in some countries.

1. Ferguson IR. Leptospirosis update. *Br Med J* 1991; **302** 128–9.
2. Centers for Disease Control. Outbreak of leptospirosis among white-water rafters—Costa Rica, 1996. *MMWR* 1997; **46:** 577–9.
3. Ferguson I. Uncommon infections I: leptospirosis. *Prescribers' J* 1991; **31:** 185–9.
4. Ferguson IR. Leptospirosis surveillance: 1990-1992. *Commun Dis Rep* 1993; **3:** R47–R48.
5. Anonymous. Leptospira outbreak in cattle and man. *J R Coll Gen Pract* 1985; **35:** 36.
6. Watt G, *et al.* Placebo-controlled trial of intravenous penicillin for severe and late leptospirosis. *Lancet* 1988; **i:** 433–5.
7. Takafuji ET, *et al.* An efficacy trial of doxycycline chemoprophylaxis against leptospirosis. *N Engl J Med* 1984; **310:** 497–500.

Listeriosis

Listeriosis is caused by *Listeria monocytogenes*, a Gram-positive bacterium widespread in the environment and capable of growing at low temperatures. Increased awareness of *L. monocytogenes* as a human pathogen has followed recent epidemics of listeriosis associated with the consumption of contaminated food products including soft cheeses, coleslaw, and pasteurised milk. *L. monocytogenes* has since been detected in many types of food, especially uncooked hot dogs, undercooked chicken, and pâté.[1] A comprehensive review of listeriosis from the Centers for Disease Control[2] in the USA acknowledged that it is a relatively rare infection and that despite epidemics of infection associated with identified food products it typically occurs sporadically and the source of infection is usually not certain. Infection occurs primarily in pregnant women, neonates, the elderly, and immunocompromised patients. Clinical manifestations vary. Pregnant women may have relatively mild flu-like symptoms, but infection may result in spontaneous abortion, fetal death, or perinatal sepsis or meningitis in the neonate. Non-perinatal listeriosis may cause sepsis but commonly presents as meningitis. Endocarditis has occurred in patients with cardiac lesions. Focal infections following initial bacteraemia occur mainly in immunocompromised patients.

The treatment of choice is generally ampicillin with gentamicin,[2,3] although some have advocated ampicillin alone;[4] synergy has been reported *in vitro*. Ampicillin or amoxycillin alone may be used in pregnant women.[5] In penicillin-allergic patients co-trimoxazole, erythromycin, and tetracycline are alternatives,[2] but the choice of treatment in these patients is more difficult. Gentamicin with chloramphenicol or with vancomycin has been used and rifampicin has been effective experimentally;[3] erythromycin plus gentamicin has been successful.[6] *In-vitro* testing of various antimicrobial combinations showed those containing gentamicin to be most effective at killing *L. monocytogenes* and those containing rifampicin to be least effective.[7] A strain of *L. monocytogenes* with plasmid-mediated resistance to chloramphenicol, erythromycin, streptomycin, and tetracycline has been reported from France,[8] but such multiresistance had not then emerged in the UK.[9] However, according to MacGowan,[3] tetracycline should not be used to treat listeriosis in the UK because of bacterial resistance.

Further details specifically concerning neonatal listerial meningitis and its treatment can be found under Meningitis, below.

1. Jones D. Foodborne listeriosis. *Lancet* 1990; **336:** 1171–4.
2. Gellin BG, Broome CV. Listeriosis. *JAMA* 1989; **261:** 1313–20.
3. MacGowan AP. Listeriosis—the therapeutic options. *J Antimicrob Chemother* 1990; **26:** 721–2.
4. Kessler SL, Dajani AS. Listeria meningitis in infants and children. *Pediatr Infect Dis J* 1990; **9:** 61–3.

5. Wilkinson P. Uncommon infections 2: listeriosis. *Prescribers' J* 1992; **32:** 26–31.
6. MacGowan AP, *et al.* Maternal listeriosis in pregnancy without fetal or neonatal infection. *J Infect* 1991; **22:** 53–7.
7. MacGowan AP, *et al.* In-vitro synergy testing of nine antimicrobial combinations against Listeria monocytogenes. *J Antimicrob Chemother* 1990; **25:** 561–6.
8. Poyart-Salmeron C, *et al.* Transferable plasmid-mediated antibiotic resistance in Listeria monocytogenes. *Lancet* 1990; **335:** 1422–6.
9. MacGowan AP, *et al.* Antibiotic resistance of Listeria monocytogenes. *Lancet* 1990; **336:** 513–14.

Lyme disease

Lyme disease is a seasonal infectious disease caused by the spirochaete *Borrelia burgdorferi* and transmitted primarily by *Ixodes* ticks. It was first recognised in the 1970s in Lyme, Connecticut,[1] but when the spirochaete responsible was later identified, Lyme disease was found to occur worldwide with regional variations. Lyme disease is a multisystem disease[2] that principally affects the skin, nervous system, heart, and joints, and can be divided into 3 stages. In the early stage a characteristic skin lesion, erythema migrans, may be accompanied by flu-like or meningitis-like symptoms. This may be followed weeks or months later by signs of disseminated infection including neurological and cardiac abnormalities and even years later by chronic arthritis and the late skin manifestation acrodermatitis chronica atrophicans, both signs of persistent infection.

Appropriate treatment should prove curative, especially in the early stages. Current recommendations for treatment[2-6] give oral doxycycline (or tetracycline) or amoxycillin as the antibacterials of choice for **early stage** Lyme disease and mild neurological and cardiac symptoms. Alternatives include oral cephalosporins such as cefuroxime or azithromycin. In pregnant women or young children amoxycillin (or phenoxymethylpenicillin) may be used or erythromycin in those allergic to penicillin, although erythromycin has been associated with a high failure rate. In general duration of treatment ranges from 10 to 21 days, but depends on individual response.

Intravenous ceftriaxone, cefotaxime, or benzylpenicillin are recommended for **late stage** Lyme disease including meningitis, serious cardiac symptoms, and arthritis; doxycycline or amoxycillin by mouth for 30 days have also been used in Lyme arthritis.

Preventive measures against Lyme disease include the use of tick repellents and physical protection.[7] After tick bites empirical treatment with doxycycline may be warranted in endemic areas where the probability of infection is high,[8] but generally the risk of infection is low,[9] particularly if the tick is removed promptly. The risk of infection may be greater if the tick has fed to repletion.[10] Most guidelines do not support the use of empirical antibacterial therapy following tick bites, and the cost-effectiveness of parenteral therapy in those with positive serological test results and nonspecific symptoms has been questioned.[11,12] Lyme disease vaccines are under investigation.

1. Steere AC. Lyme disease. *N Engl J Med* 1989; **321:** 586–96.
2. Sigal LH, ed. A symposium: National Clinical Conference on Lyme Disease. *Am J Med* 1995; **98** (suppl 4A): 1S–84S.
3. American Academy of Pediatrics Committee on Infectious Diseases. Treatment of Lyme borreliosis. *Pediatrics* 1991; **88:** 176–9.
4. Cryan B, Wright DJM. Lyme disease in paediatrics. *Arch Dis Child* 1991; **66:** 1359–63.
5. Weber K, Pfister H-W. Clinical management of Lyme borreliosis. *Lancet* 1994; **343:** 1017–20.
6. O'Connell S. Lyme disease in the United Kingdom. *Br Med J* 1995; **310:** 303–8.
7. Couch P, Johnson CE. Prevention of Lyme disease. *Am J Hosp Pharm* 1992; **49:** 1164–73.
8. Magid D, *et al.* Prevention of Lyme disease after tick bites: a cost-effectiveness analysis. *N Engl J Med* 1992; **327:** 534–41.
9. Shapiro ED, *et al.* A controlled trial of antimicrobial prophylaxis for Lyme disease after deer-tick bites. *N Engl J Med* 1992; **327:** 1769–73.
10. Matuschka F-R, Spielman A. Risk of infection from and treatment of tick bite. *Lancet* 1993; **342:** 529–30.
11. Lightfoot RW, *et al.* Empiric parenteral antibiotic treatment of patients with fibromyalgia and fatigue and a positive serologic result for lyme disease: a cost-effectiveness analysis. *Ann Intern Med* 1993; **119:** 503–9.
12. Luft BJ, *et al.* Appropriateness of parenteral antibiotic treatment for patients with presumed Lyme disease: a joint statement of the American College of Rheumatology and the Council of the Infectious Diseases Society of America. *Ann Intern Med* 1993; **119:** 518.

Lymphogranuloma venereum

Lymphogranuloma venereum or chlamydial lymphogranuloma is caused by infection with certain serotypes of *Chlamydia trachomatis* and is endemic in tropical areas, but may also occur in the developed world. It is a sexually transmitted disease and in the early phase may cause genital ulceration although the commonest clinical manifestation is inguinal lymphadenopathy. There is multisystem involvement and late complications, including those related to fibrosis and abnormal lymphatic drainage, may require surgery.

The antimicrobial treatment of choice is with a tetracycline given by mouth. WHO[1] have recommended treatment for 2 weeks or more with doxycycline or tetracycline; possible alternatives are erythromycin, sulphadiazine, or other sulphonamides. In the USA the Centers for Disease Control[2] recommend treatment for 3 weeks with doxycycline or alternatively with erythromycin.

1. WHO. *WHO model prescribing information: drugs used in sexually transmitted diseases and HIV infection.* Geneva: WHO, 1995.
2. Centers for Disease Control. 1998 Guidelines for treatment of sexually transmitted diseases. *MMWR* 1998; **47** (RR-1): 27–8.

Melioidosis. Melioidosis is caused by the Gram-negative aerobic bacterium *Burkholderia pseudomallei* (*Pseudomonas pseudomallei*), and has been found mainly in south-east Asia and northern Australia. Its true incidence and distribution may be much wider than originally thought;[1] diagnosis is difficult because of the broad spectrum of clinical manifestations. Pulmonary melioidosis is probably the commonest form and has been treated with doxycycline for 3 to 6 months.[2] Chronic or subacute non-bacteraemic melioidosis has also been treated long term with tetracycline or co-trimoxazole.[2]

Septicaemic melioidosis is an important cause of death in Thailand. Because *B. pseudomallei* is intrinsically resistant to many antibacterials, including aminoglycosides and the early beta lactams, it is unresponsive to many empirical regimens for septicaemia.[1] Until recently treatment has been based on anecdotal regimens, but in a study from Thailand[3] intravenous ceftazidime halved the mortality of severe melioidosis when compared with conventional parenteral treatment with high doses of chloramphenicol intravenously, doxycycline, and co-trimoxazole. As a result ceftazidime came to be considered the treatment of choice for septicaemic melioidosis.[1] Parenteral treatment for a minimum of 7 days is followed by oral maintenance therapy with amoxycillin-clavulanic acid or the conventional regimen (chloramphenicol, doxycycline, and co-trimoxazole);[3] amoxycillin-clavulanic acid has shown promise[3] and appears to be a safe alternative to the conventional regimen for the oral treatment of melioidosis.[4] However, resistance to ceftazidime and amoxycillin-clavulanic acid has been reported,[5] emphasising the importance of careful monitoring for the emergence of resistance during treatment. Ceftazidime plus co-trimoxazole, both given intravenously, has been advocated by some for severe melioidosis, especially in patients with septicaemia.[6] Imipenem is more active *in vitro* against *B. pseudomallei* than ceftazidime[7] and has been suggested as an alternative.[8]

B. pseudomallei has the potential for prolonged latency as demonstrated by a Vietnam war veteran who presented with melioidosis of the bone 18 years after exposure to the organism.[9] He was treated with ceftriaxone intravenously for 8 weeks followed by oral ciprofloxacin.

1. Dance DAB. Pseudomonas pseudomallei: danger in the paddy fields. *Trans R Soc Trop Med Hyg* 1991; **85:** 1–3.
2. Guard RW, *et al.* Melioidosis in far north Queensland: a clinical and epidemiological review of twenty cases. *Am J Trop Med Hyg* 1984; **33:** 467–73.
3. White NJ, *et al.* Halving of mortality of severe melioidosis by ceftazidime. *Lancet* 1989; **ii:** 697–701.
4. Rajchanuvong A, *et al.* A prospective comparison of co-amoxiclav and the combination of chloramphenicol, doxycycline, and co-trimoxazole for the oral maintenance treatment of melioidosis. *Trans R Soc Trop Med Hyg* 1995; **89:** 546–9.
5. Dance DAB, *et al.* Development of resistance to ceftazidime and co-amoxiclav in Pseudomonas pseudomallei. *J Antimicrob Chemother* 1991; **28:** 321–4.
6. Sookpranee M, *et al.* Multicenter prospective randomized trial comparing ceftazidime plus co-trimoxazole with chloramphenicol plus doxycycline and co-trimoxazole for treatment of severe melioidosis. *Antimicrob Agents Chemother* 1992; **36:** 158–62.
7. Dance DAB, *et al.* The antimicrobial susceptibility of Pseudomonas pseudomallei; emergence of resistance in vitro and during treatment. *J Antimicrob Chemother* 1989; **24:** 295–309.
8. Anonymous. The choice of antibacterial drugs. *Med Lett Drugs Ther* 1998; **40:** 33–42.
9. Koponen MA, *et al.* Melioidosis: forgotten but not gone. *Arch Intern Med* 1991; **151:** 605–8.

Meningitis

Initiation of bacterial meningitis involves colonisation of the nasopharynx by the bacterial pathogen, invasion into the bloodstream (bacteraemia), survival in the bloodstream (enhanced in encapsulated bacteria), invasion of the meninges, bacterial replication, and subarachnoid-space inflammation.[1,2] The bacteria most often responsible for meningitis are *Streptococcus pneumoniae* (pneumococci), *Haemophilus influenzae*, and *Neisseria meningitidis* (meningococci). Other causes include *Listeria monocytogenes*, Gram-negative enteric bacilli, and *Pseudomonas aeruginosa*. *H. influenzae* is more common in infants and young children whereas in neonates *Escherichia coli* and group B streptococci are the most frequent causes. Overall *H. influenzae* meningitis has appeared to be more common in the USA than in the UK but, as elsewhere, its incidence has decreased following the introduction of immunisation with *H. influenzae* type b vaccine.

Choice of treatment. Doctors in the UK are advised[3] to give emergency treatment with parenteral benzylpenicillin to all suspected cases of meningitis before transfer to hospital (see also under Meningococcal Meningitis, below). Subsequent treatment depends on identification of the infecting organism and its susceptibility to antibacterials. Other factors affecting choice of antibacterial include penetration into the CSF and bactericidal activity once there. Once in hospital, penicillin and chloramphenicol have been the mainstays of treatment in adults and children and may be given **empirically** until the results of culture and susceptibility tests are known, but third-generation cephalosporins are increasingly preferred because of resistance. In the UK in 1989, Finch[4] recommended empirical treatment with chloramphenicol (ampicillin is often given as well, but the combination is of no proven benefit and there is increasing ampicillin resistance among *H. influenzae*) or with cefuroxime or cefotaxime. Authors working in the USA,[2,5] have advised the following empirical treatments: cefotaxime or ceftriaxone, with the addition of ampicillin in patients less than 3 months of age or over 50 years, in whom Listeria meningitis is more prevalent. They have also recommended addition of vancomycin to any empirical regimen when highly penicillin-resistant or cephalosporin-resistant pneumococcal meningitis is suspected. Vancomycin with ceftazidime is recommended in patients with recent head trauma, neurosurgery or CSF shunts.[5] Immunocompromised patients should receive ampicillin with ceftazidime.[5] Penicillin-allergic patients can be given chloramphenicol but it may not be effective against Gram-negative enteric bacilli or resistant pneumococci. There have been treatment failures with cefuroxime in *H. influenzae* meningitis[6] and, in comparative studies,[7,8] ceftriaxone has generally been superior to cefuroxime in children with bacterial meningitis; ceftriaxone and cefotaxime appear to have comparable efficacy.[9] Encouraging preliminary results have been obtained with meropenem as an alternative to cephalosporins for empirical treatment.[10,11]

The chosen antibacterials are generally given intravenously in relatively high doses. Treatment regimens should be reconsidered as soon as microbiological information is available. Management of the commonest forms of bacterial meningitis is discussed below.

Neonatal meningitis is uncommon but remains a life-threatening emergency often associated with bacteraemia and shock. Group B streptococci and *E. coli* are the commonest pathogens, *L. monocytogenes* is the third most common cause in the UK, and *Staphylococcus epidermidis* may be responsible for meningitis after invasive neurosurgery.[12] Empirical treatment with ampicillin or chloramphenicol together with gentamicin has been widely used, but extended-spectrum cephalosporins such as cefotaxime or ceftazidime are often preferred, plus ampicillin if *L. monocytogenes* is suspected.[4] USA authors[2] have advised that for neonates up to 4 weeks of age, ampicillin plus cefotaxime or ampicillin plus an aminoglycoside should be given; vancomycin should also be added when highly penicillin-resistant or cephalosporin-resistant pneumococcal meningitis is suspected. In preterm, low-birth-weight neonates, vancomycin should be given with ceftazidime because of the higher risk of nosocomial infection with staphylococci or Gram-negative bacilli.[5] A committee of the American Academy of Pediatrics[13] has recommended that, once the infecting organism is known, benzylpenicillin or ampicillin be given for group B streptococci and ampicillin for *L. monocytogenes*, both for 14 days; treatment of Gram-negative enteric infection should be based on susceptibility tests and continued for at least 3 weeks.

In the UK Gandy and Rennie[12] advocated an aggressive approach to the treatment of neonatal meningitis with cefotaxime, penicillin, and gentamicin initially then, once the organisms were known, cefotaxime for *E. coli* and ceftazidime for *Pseudomonas*. Gentamicin was continued mainly to treat the associated septicaemia. They supported the use of intraventricular gentamicin but considered intrathecal administration via the lumbar route to be ineffective. The necessity for gentamicin and its intraventricular administration were both severely criticised;[14,15] Heyderman and Levin[16] considered that, since the only studies to date had demonstrated a poorer outcome with intraventricular aminoglycosides, they should not be advocated. For other organisms Gandy and Rennie[12] suggested penicillin plus gentamicin for 3 weeks for group B streptococci, ampicillin or penicillin with gentamicin for *L. monocytogenes*, and systemic antibiotics with intraventricular vancomycin for *Staph. epidermidis* infection of ventriculoperitoneal shunts.

In **infants** immediately beyond the neonatal period (1 to 3 months of age) infecting organisms may be as for neonates or children older than 3 months (*N. meningitidis, Str. pneumoniae*, or *H. influenzae*) and initial treatment with ampicillin together with cefotaxime has been recommended in the UK.[17] Authors from the USA,[2,5] have advised ampicillin with either cefotaxime or ceftriaxone for infants aged 4 to 12 weeks; vancomycin should also be added when highly penicillin-resistant or cephalosporin-resistant pneumococcal meningitis is suspected.[2] For **older infants and children** the UK authors[17] have recommended cefotaxime or ceftriaxone in preference to benzylpenicillin or ampicillin together with chloramphenicol. Opinion in the USA[2] is that ampicillin may or may not be given with the cephalosporin.

Adjunctive treatment. Mortality and morbidity, including deafness in children, remain high in meningitis despite increasingly effective antibacterials. As well as microbial virulence the host response to infection is important. Endotoxins and other microbial products, resulting from bacterial lysis following antibacterial treatment, are able to provoke an inflammatory response by triggering the release of cytokines including interleukin-1 and tumour necrosis factor. There is thus a possible role for anti-inflammatory drugs in the treatment of bacterial meningitis.[18,19] The role of corticosteroids has been the subject of considerable debate.[2,5,20-24] Some have suggested they may have a role in certain circumstances. There has been support for the use of dexamethasone in preventing deafness in children associated with *H. influenzae* type b meningitis[2,22-24] although the decreasing incidence of this type of meningitis since the introduction of immunisation casts further doubt on the value of such treatment. Additionally, some authors[2,5] have advocated dexamethasone use in bacterial meningitis in high-risk patients or in those with severe mental impairment, cerebral oedema, or very high intracranial pressure. However, the general view does appear to be against[2,5,20-24] *routine* adjunctive use, whether in children or adults.

GRAM-NEGATIVE ENTERIC AND PSEUDOMONAL MENINGITIS. Meningitis due to Gram-negative enteric bacteria occurs especially in neonates (see above), the elderly, and the immunocompromised and as a complication of neurosurgery. Treatment is generally with a third-generation cephalosporin such as cefotaxime; gentamicin or another suitable aminoglycoside may sometimes be given as well. For meningitis caused by *Pseudomonas aeruginosa* ceftazidime plus an aminoglycoside is used.[2,4,5] Intraventricular administration of an aminoglycoside has sometimes been judged necessary, but see under Neonatal Meningitis, above.

HAEMOPHILUS INFLUENZAE MENINGITIS. This is mainly a disease of preschool children and was nearly always caused by encapsulated type b strains of *H. influenzae* acquired from close contact, but the incidence has decreased as a result of immunisation. A third-generation cephalosporin such as cefotaxime or ceftriaxone is the treatment of choice;[2,4,5] there have been treatment failures with cefuroxime.[6] Chloramphenicol is an alternative. Ampicillin is less useful now because of resistance, but can be given for beta-lactamase-negative strains. Treatment for a minimum of 7 to 10 days after fever has subsided may be necessary.[4,25]

Prophylaxis. Since treatment does not eliminate nasopharyngeal carriage of *H. influenzae* type b, rifampicin should be given to index cases in the usual prophylactic dose for 4 days before discharge from hospital. Secondary cases should be prevented by giving rifampicin for 4 days to household and classroom contacts.[26]

For active immunisation of children against *H. influenzae* type b, see under Haemophilus Influenzae Vaccines, p.1511.

LISTERIA MENINGITIS. See above under Neonatal Meningitis. See also under Listeriosis, above.

MENINGOCOCCAL MENINGITIS. Benzylpenicillin is the treatment of choice for meningitis caused by *N. meningitidis*,[2,4,5] probably the commonest form of meningococcal infection (see under Meningococcal Infections, below), although reduced sensitivity has been reported in some strains[27-29] and has resulted in treatment failure;[30] high doses of benzylpenicillin are recommended. Alternatives are third-generation cephalosporins such as cefotaxime or ceftriaxone.[1,2,4,5,31] Parenteral benzylpenicillin is given, preferably intravenously, before transfer to hospital if meningococcal infection seems likely.[3,32-36] Duration of treatment is empirical but since *N. meningitidis* is rapidly cleared from the CSF and relapse is uncommon, treatment is generally continued for 5 days after resolution of fever and signs of meningitis;[4] a 7-day course is generally effective.[33]

Prophylaxis. Penicillin may not eliminate the carrier state and therefore rifampicin should be given for 2 days prior to hospital discharge, in the usual prophylactic dose. Secondary cases of meningococcal infection should be prevented by giving prophylactic treatment to close contacts of the index case, especially members of the same household who have had close prolonged contact with the case.[3,37] Rifampicin given for 2 days is the prophylactic of choice for the prevention of secondary cases.[3,37] Alternatives to rifampicin include a single oral dose of ciprofloxacin or an intramuscular dose of ceftriaxone.[3,37]

Where possible, vaccination should be performed in those contacts who have received prophylaxis.[3,37] Vaccines are available against group A and C meningococci or against groups A, C, Y, and W135 meningococci, and are under investigation against group B.

PNEUMOCOCCAL MENINGITIS. Meningitis due to *Str. pneumoniae* is most common in adults and infants, but can occur at any age. It is said to be the most serious form of meningitis with mortality exceeding 20%.[4] Benzylpenicillin or phenoxymethylpenicillin have been treatments of choice although strains with reduced sensitivity to penicillins are increasingly reported (see under Pneumonia, below) and a third-generation cephalosporin such as cefotaxime or ceftriaxone is often the initial treatment of choice; benzylpenicillin may be substituted if the organism is subsequently shown to be sensitive to it. Treatment should generally continue for 7 to 10 days after fever subsides,[4] with some clinicians preferring a minimum of 10 days.[25] Pneumococcal strains resistant to cephalosporins have recently emerged and vancomycin is recommended with or without rifampicin in addition to cefotaxime or ceftriaxone where such pneumococci are prevalent.[2,5] However, one difficulty is that third-generation cephalosporins may not be available in developing countries; chloramphenicol may still prove useful in those countries with a high incidence of bacterial meningitis,[38,39] but treatment failures have been reported with chloramphenicol in penicillin-resistant pneumococcal meningitis.[40]

Prophylaxis. A pneumococcal vaccine is available, but its effectiveness in preventing meningitis has not been established.

1. Tunkel AR, *et al.* Bacterial meningitis: recent advances in pathophysiology and treatment. *Ann Intern Med* 1990; **112:** 610–23.
2. Tunkel AR, Scheld WM. Acute bacterial meningitis. *Lancet* 1995; **346:** 1675–80.
3. PHLS Meningococcal Infections Working Group and Public Health Medicine Environmental Group. Control of meningococcal disease: guidance for consultants in communicable disease control. *Commun Dis Rep* 1995; **5:** R189–R195.
4. Finch R. Bacterial meningitis. *Prescribers' J* 1989; **29:** 2–11.
5. Quagliarello VJ, Scheld WM. Treatment of bacterial meningitis. *N Engl J Med* 1997; **336:** 708–16.
6. Arditi M, *et al.* Cefuroxime treatment failure and Haemophilus influenzae meningitis: case report and review of literature. *Pediatrics* 1989; **84:** 132–5.
7. Lebel MH, *et al.* Comparative efficacy of ceftriaxone and cefuroxime for treatment of bacterial meningitis. *J Pediatr* 1989; **114:** 1049–54.
8. Schaad UB, *et al.* A comparison of ceftriaxone and cefuroxime for the treatment of bacterial meningitis in children. *N Engl J Med* 1990; **322:** 141–7.
9. Peltola H, *et al.* Randomised comparison of chloramphenicol, ampicillin, cefotaxime, and ceftriaxone for childhood bacterial meningitis. *Lancet* 1989; **i:** 1281–7.
10. Schmutzhard E, *et al.* A randomised comparison of meropenem with cefotaxime or ceftriaxone for the treatment of bacterial meningitis in adults. *J Antimicrob Chemother* 1995; **36** (suppl A): 85–97.
11. Klugman KP, *et al.* Randomized comparison of meropenem with cefotaxime for treatment of bacterial meningitis. *Antimicrob Agents Chemother* 1995; **39:** 1140–6.
12. Gandy G, Rennie J. Antibiotic treatment of suspected neonatal meningitis. *Arch Dis Child* 1990; **65:** 1–2.
13. American Academy of Pediatrics Committee on Infectious Diseases. Treatment of bacterial meningitis. *Pediatrics* 1988; **81:** 904–7. [See also Savarino SJ, *et al. Pediatrics* 1989; **83:** 632–3 and McCracken GH, *ibid.*, 633 (correction; cefotaxime should *not* be used for pseudomonal meningitis).]
14. Short A. Antibiotic treatment of suspected neonatal meningitis. *Arch Dis Child* 1990; **65:** 810.
15. Tarlow MJ. Antibiotic treatment of suspected neonatal meningitis. *Arch Dis Child* 1990; **65:** 810.
16. Heyderman RS, Levin M. Antibiotic treatment of suspected neonatal meningitis. *Arch Dis Child* 1991; **66:** 170.
17. Klein NJ, *et al.* Antibiotic choices for meningitis beyond the neonatal period. *Arch Dis Child* 1992; **67:** 157–9.
18. Anonymous. Steroids and meningitis. *Lancet* 1989; **ii:** 1307–8.
19. Finch RG, Mandragos C. Corticosteroids in bacterial meningitis. *Br Med J* 1991; **302:** 607–8.
20. Harvey DR, Stevens JP. What is the role of corticosteroids in meningitis? *Drugs* 1995; **50:** 945–50.
21. Townsend GC, Scheld WM. The use of corticosteroids in the management of bacterial meningitis in adults. *J Antimicrob Chemother* 1996; **37:** 1051–61.
22. McIntyre PB, *et al.* Dexamethasone as adjunctive therapy in bacterial meningitis: a meta-analysis of randomized clinical trials since 1988. *JAMA* 1997; **278:** 925–31.
23. American Academy of Pediatrics Committee on Infectious Diseases. Dexamethasone therapy for bacterial meningitis in infants and children. *Pediatrics* 1990; **86:** 130–3.
24. The Meningitis Working Party of the British Paediatric Immunology and Infectious Diseases Group. Should we use dexamethasone in meningitis? *Arch Dis Child* 1992; **67:** 1398–1401.
25. O'Neill P. Meningitis: how long to treat bacterial meningitis. *Lancet* 1993; **341:** 530. Correction. *ibid.*: 642.
26. Cartwright KAV, *et al.* Chemoprophylaxis for Haemophilus influenzae type b. *Br Med J* 1991; **302:** 546–7.
27. Jones DM, Sutcliffe EM. Meningococci with reduced susceptibility to penicillin. *Lancet* 1990; **335:** 863–4.
28. Saez Nieto JA, *et al.* Meningococci moderately resistant to penicillin. *Lancet* 1990; **336:** 54.
29. Riley G, *et al.* Penicillin resistance in Neisseria meningitidis. *N Engl J Med* 1991; **324:** 997.
30. Turner PC, *et al.* Treatment failure in meningococcal meningitis. *Lancet* 1990; **335:** 732–3.
31. Klein NJ, *et al.* Management of meningococcal infections. *Br J Hosp Med* 1993; **50:** 42–9.
32. Welsby PD, Golledge CL. Meningococcal meningitis. *Br Med J* 1990; **300:** 1150–1.
33. Begg N. Reducing mortality from meningococcal disease. *Br Med J* 1992; **305:** 133–4.
34. Strang JR, Pugh EJ. Meningococcal infections: reducing the case fatality rate by giving penicillin before admission to hospital. *Br Med J* 1992; **305:** 141–3.
35. Cartwright K, *et al.* Early treatment with parenteral penicillin in meningococcal disease. *Br Med J* 1992; **305:** 143–7.
36. Cartwright K, *et al.* Initial management of suspected meningococcal infection: parenteral benzylpenicillin is vital. *Br Med J* 1994; **309:** 1160–1.
37. American Academy of Pediatrics, Canadian Paediatric Society. Meningococcal disease prevention and control strategies for practice-based physicians. *Pediatrics* 1996; **97:** 404–11.
38. Pécoul B, *et al.* Long-acting chloramphenicol versus intravenous ampicillin for treatment of bacterial meningitis. *Lancet* 1991; **338:** 862–6.
39. Kumar P, Verma IC. Antibiotic therapy for bacterial meningitis in children in developing countries. *Bull WHO* 1993; **71:** 183–8.
40. Friedland IR, Klugman KP. Failure of chloramphenicol therapy in penicillin-resistant pneumococcal meningitis. *Lancet* 1992; **339:** 405–8.

Meningococcal infections

The meningococcus *Neisseria meningitidis* is a Gram-negative bacterium classified into several serotypes including groups A, B, and C. It occurs worldwide and can cause endemic and epidemic infection. Group A is mainly responsible for epidemics in the developing world. In the USA most infections have been caused by group B or group C meningococci; the relative importance of group C has been increasing in North America. Group B has been the most prevalent in the UK and Europe although there has been some increase in group C infections. Infections have occurred predominantly in young children under 5 years, but there has been an increased incidence in teenagers and young adults in recent UK outbreaks. Meningococcal disease has traditionally been associated with poverty and overcrowding; the only established risk factor is close contact with an index case, hence the importance of prophylaxis. Clinical infection is preceded by asymptomatic nasopharyngeal carriage of meningococci and spread of infection is usually via respiratory droplets from asymptomatic carriers. Bacteraemia is probably the primary event in all forms of meningococcal disease; clinical manifestations range from mild sore throat or transient fever to fulminant disease. A vasculitic rash (petechiae or purpura) is often associated with meningococcal infection. Meningococcal infection most commonly manifests as septicaemia, which can be rapidly fatal, particularly if fulminating, with mortality ranging from 15% up to 80% in severe forms, or as meningococcal meningitis, in which the infection is confined to the CNS and is associated with mortality rates of 5% or less. Meningococcal meningitis may also occur in conjunction with meningococcal septicaemia. Less usual forms of metastatic meningococcal infection include polyarthritis, pericarditis, pneumonitis, and genito-urinary-tract infections.

Despite some uncertainty as to whether patients with suspected meningococcal septicaemia rather than meningitis would benefit from early penicillin treatment, it is still generally recommended for all patients with suspected meningococcal disease. Thus, when meningococcal infection seems likely benzylpenicillin should be given parenterally, preferably intravenously, before transfer to hospital. For details of the treatment and prophylaxis of meningococcal infections, see Meningococcal Meningitis, under Meningitis, above.

References.

1. Peltola H. Early meningococcal disease: advising the public and the profession. *Lancet* 1993; **342:** 509–10.
2. Klein NJ, *et al.* Management of meningococcal infections. *Br J Hosp Med* 1993; **50:** 42–9.
3. PHLS Meningococcal Infections Working Group and Public Health Medicine Environmental Group. Control of meningococcal disease: guidance for consultants in communicable disease control. *Commun Dis Rep* 1995; **5:** R189–R195.
4. American Academy of Pediatrics and Canadian Paediatric Society. Meningococcal disease prevention and control strategies for practice-based physicians. *Pediatrics* 1996; **97:** 404–11.

Mouth infections

Infections of the mouth include those of dental origin such as dental caries, abscesses, gingivitis, and periodontal infections, and those without a dental origin. Infections arising in the nasal cavity, middle ear, oropharynx, and paranasal sinuses can also affect the oral cavity. This discussion deals mainly with infections of dental origin.

The organisms most often encountered in oral infections are viridans streptococci, a variety of anaerobes, and facultative streptococci.[1] Over the years the emphasis has shifted from treatment to prevention of oral diseases.[2]

Dental caries is caused by the erosion of tooth enamel due to acid produced by bacteria (usually *Streptococcus mutans*) in plaque. Fluoride in various forms is used in dental caries prophylaxis, where it may promote remineralisation or reduce acid production by plaque bacteria.[2] Sugar-free chewing gum can help prevent caries by stimulating the production of saliva.[3] Dental caries vaccines have also been investigated.

The term periodontal disease encompasses specific conditions affecting the gingiva and the supporting connective tissue and alveolar bone.[4] Gingivitis is thought to be caused by a nonspecific bacterial plaque flora that gradually changes from predominantly Gram-positive to more Gram-negative. Gingivitis may or may not develop into periodontitis, but periodontitis is always preceded by gingivitis. Periodontitis is associated with a Gram-negative anaerobic microflora. Most gingivitis and periodontitis can be prevented and treated by adequate oral hygiene and plaque removal using mechanical means such as toothbrushes. Mechanical removal of calculus is necessary where the build up is significant. Antiseptics may also help to reduce plaque accumulation and several including cetylpyridinium chloride[5] and chlorhexidine[6,7] have been used.

Penicillin has continued to be an effective drug in combating oral pathogens, and erythromycin or metronidazole to be alternatives. In one study,[8] strict anaerobes isolated from dentoalveolar abscesses were generally susceptible to benzylpenicillin, amoxycillin, erythromycin, clindamycin, and metronidazole; all facultative anaerobes were resistant to metronidazole, but most were susceptible to the other antibacterial agents. Fusiform bacteria and spirochaetes have been linked with acute necrotising ulcerative gingivitis (also called Vincent's infection or trench mouth);[9] systemic metronidazole is often the treatment of choice. Tinidazole has also been used. Tetracyclines or metronidazole have been used for chronic periodontal disease.[10] Antibacterials and antiseptics delivered locally to the periodontal pocket may be of value.

1. Guralnick W. Odontogenic infections. *Br Dent J* 1984; **156:** 440–7.
2. WHO. Recent advances in oral health: report of a WHO expert committee. *WHO Tech Rep Ser 826* 1992.
3. Edgar WM. Sugar substitutes, chewing gum and dental caries—a review. *Br Dent J* 1998; **184:** 29–32.
4. Williams RC. Periodontal disease. *N Engl J Med* 1990; **322:** 373–82.
5. Ashley FP, *et al.* The effect of a 0.1% cetylpyridinium chloride mouthrinse on plaque and gingivitis in adult subjects. *Br Dent J* 1984; **157:** 191–6.
6. Brecx M, *et al.* Efficacy of Listerine, Meridol and chlorhexidine mouthrinses on plaque, gingivitis and plaque bacteria vitality. *J Clin Periodontol* 1990; **17:** 292–7.
7. de la Rosa M, *et al.* The use of chlorhexidine in the management of gingivitis in children. *J Periodontol* 1988; **59:** 387–9.
8. Lewis MAO, *et al.* Antibiotic susceptibilities of bacteria isolated from acute dentoalveolar abscesses. *J Antimicrob Chemother* 1989; **23:** 69–77.
9. Johnson BD, Engel D. Acute necrotizing ulcerative gingivitis: a review of diagnosis, etiology and treatment. *J Periodontol* 1986; **57:** 141–50.
10. Watts TLP. Periodontitis for medical practitioners. *Br Med J* 1998; **316:** 993–6.

Mycetoma

Mycetoma is a localised chronic infection seen especially in the tropics and subtropics and involving subcutaneous tissue, bone, and skin. It has been termed Madura foot when affecting the sole of the foot. Mycetomas caused by fungi (p.369) such as *Madurella mycetomatis* are called eumycetomas and those caused by the filamentous bacteria, actinomycetes, are called actinomycetomas. *Nocardia brasiliensis* is the commonest actinomycete responsible; others include *Actinomadura madurae*, *A. pelletieri*, and *Streptomyces somaliensis*. For details of systemic infections caused by *Nocardia* spp., see under Nocardiosis, below.

Various treatment regimens for actinomycetomas have been tried. Mahgoub[1] found co-trimoxazole with streptomycin or dapsone with streptomycin to be the most effective although *Streptomyces somaliensis* infection did not always respond. Two further regimens, sulfadoxine with pyrimethamine and streptomycin or rifampicin with streptomycin, were suitable for second-line therapy.[1] Cures were achieved after treatment for 4 to 24 months.[1] In a study of antibacterial activity *in vitro* against strains of *Streptomyces somaliensis* isolated from mycetoma patients, rifampicin was the most effective followed by erythromycin, tobramycin, fusidic acid, and streptomycin in decreasing order of activity; all strains were resistant to trimethoprim.[2] The successful use of hyperbaric oxygen in addition to co-trimoxazole[3] or of amoxycillin-clavulanic acid[4] in the treatment of *N. brasiliensis* actinomycetoma previously resistant to conventional therapy has been described.

1. Mahgoub ES. Medical management of mycetoma. *Bull WHO* 1976; **54:** 303–10.
2. Nasher MA, *et al.* In vitro studies of antibiotic sensitivities of Streptomyces somaliensis—a cause of human actinomycetoma. *Trans R Soc Trop Med Hyg* 1989; **83:** 265–8.
3. Walker RM, *et al.* Beneficial effects of hyperbaric oxygen therapy in Nocardia brasiliensis soft-tissue infection. *Med J Aust* 1991; **155:** 122–3.
4. Gomez A, *et al.* Amoxicillin and clavulanic acid in the treatment of actinomycetoma. *Int J Dermatol* 1993; **32:** 218–20.

Necrotising enterocolitis

See under Gastro-enteritis, above.

Necrotising fasciitis

Necrotising fasciitis is a severe soft-tissue infection resulting in necrosis of the subcutaneous tissue and adjacent fascia together with severe systemic illness. It may be caused by a mixture of aerobic and anaerobic organisms, but can be due to group A streptococci or staphylococci alone and may be associated with a toxic shock syndrome (below).

Treatment involving radical surgical excision of the affected tissues may be avoided in some patients treated with large doses of appropriate antibacterials.[1] For streptococcal necrotising fasciitis high-dose benzylpenicillin should be used; clindamycin may be added in severe cases.[2] Erythromycin should be avoided because of the risk of resistance.[2] Staphylococcal infections are treated with a penicillinase-resistant penicillin, cephazolin, or vancomycin (for resistant strains).[1] Since diagnosis can be difficult, it may be advisable to treat as for a mixed infection with antibacterials active against anaerobes (e.g. clindamycin) and also an aminoglycoside or third-generation cephalosporin against Gram-negative rods initially, in addition to benzylpenicillin.[3] A broad-spectrum penicillin-beta-lactamase-inhibitor combination or imipenem-cilastatin may also be used.[1] Hyperbaric oxygen therapy has also been beneficial although prospective controlled studies are lacking.[4]

1. Gorbach SL. IDCP guidelines: necrotizing skin and soft tissue infections. Part I: necrotizing fasciitis. *Infect Dis Clin Pract* 1996; **5:** 406–11.
2. Anonymous. Invasive group A streptococcal infections in Gloucestershire. *Commun Dis Rep* 1994; **4:** 97.
3. Chelsom J, *et al.* Necrotising fasciitis due to group A streptococci in western Norway: incidence and clinical features. *Lancet* 1994; **344:** 1111–15.
4. Leach RM, *et al.* Hyperbaric oxygen therapy. *Br Med J* 1998; **317:** 1140–3.

Neonatal conjunctivitis

Conjunctivitis of the newborn, also known as ophthalmia neonatorum, is defined as any conjunctivitis with discharge occurring during the first 28 days of life.[1] That due to *Neisseria gonorrhoeae* is the most serious; it usually appears by the third day after birth, can rapidly result in blindness, and systemic infections, especially severe septicaemia, may occur. *Chlamydia trachomatis* is another major cause of neonatal conjunctivitis; it characteristically occurs 5 to 14 days after birth and is less threatening to sight than gonococcal infection, but may also infect the nasopharynx and may cause pneumonia. Chlamydial conjunctivitis is more common than gonococcal conjunctivitis in developed countries. Both these organisms are sexually transmitted and the infants of mothers with such genital-tract infections are infected during their passage through the birth canal. Other less serious bacterial causes of neonatal conjunctivitis include *Staphylococcus aureus*, *Streptococcus pneumoniae*, *Haemophilus* spp., and *Pseudomonas* spp.; they are often hospital-acquired.[1]

The management of gonococcal and chlamydial neonatal conjunctivitis varies from country to country depending on the prevalence of gonorrhoea and *C. trachomatis* infection and on bacterial resistance.

PROPHYLAXIS. The ideal method of prophylaxis is to treat the infected mother during pregnancy, but this is not always possible. Where the risk of *gonococcal infection* is high, ocular prophylaxis at birth is particularly important because of the rapid onset of conjunctivitis and its potential seriousness and is preferable to early diagnosis and treatment of the neonate.[2] Cleansing of the neonate's eyes immediately after birth followed by the topical application of either tetracycline 1% eye ointment, erythromycin 0.5% or 1% eye ointment, or silver nitrate 1% eye drops is advised[3,4] and is sometimes required by law.[3] Silver nitrate[1] is active against all strains of *N. gonorrhoeae* regardless of their susceptibility to antibacterials; it is inexpensive and widely available, but may cause chemical conjunctivitis and has been ineffective in preventing chlamydial conjunctivitis (see below). Tetracycline has been reported to be as effective as silver nitrate in protecting against gonococcal conjunctivitis caused by multiresistant strains[5] and WHO now lists it as the drug of choice.[4]

The value of prophylaxis against *chlamydial neonatal conjunctivitis* is less certain. Tetracycline ointment has been reported to be less effective in preventing chlamydial infection than gonococcal infection[5] and erythromycin ointment has also been unreliable.[6] Silver nitrate is generally considered ineffective,[1] despite an unexpected reduction in the incidence of chlamydial conjunctivitis in one study.[5] Screening and treatment of pregnant women for *C. trachomatis* infection may be a more effective method of control than ocular prophylaxis.[5,7] This approach also tackles the more serious problem of chlamydial pneumonia.[8]

Neonatal conjunctivitis continues to cause blindness, especially in developing countries. Povidone-iodine is less expensive and perhaps more readily available in such countries than silver nitrate or erythromycin. In a study in Kenya involving more than 3000 infants[9] a 2.5% ophthalmic solution of povidone-iodine appeared to be a more effective prophylactic than either a 1% ophthalmic solution of silver nitrate or erythromycin 0.5% eye ointment. In particular there were fewer cases of chlamydial conjunctivitis with povidone-iodine.

TREATMENT. *Gonococcal neonatal conjunctivitis* must be treated systemically. WHO[4] have recommended ceftriaxone 50 mg per kg. body-weight by intramuscular injection as a single dose (to a maximum of 125 mg) or, if ceftriaxone is not available, spectinomycin 25 mg per kg (to a maximum of 75 mg) or kanamycin 25 mg per kg (to a maximum of 75 mg) by intramuscular injection as a single dose. When systemic treatment is not available tetracycline 1% eye ointment should be applied to both eyes every hour until the infant can be transferred to a facility offering systemic treatment. Where the prevalence of penicillin-resistant gonococci is less than 1%, benzylpenicillin 60 mg per kg daily intravenously or intramuscularly in divided doses for 7 days might be given.[10] WHO formerly advised that systemic therapy should be accompanied by hourly conjunctival irrigation and by application of a topical antibacterial preparation such as tetracycline or erythromycin eye ointment until the discharge was eliminated.[1,10]

The CDC[3] recommends a single intravenous or intramuscular injection of ceftriaxone 25 to 50 mg per kg (up to 125 mg) when there is no evidence of disseminated infection.

See also under Gonorrhoea (above) for the treatment of infants exposed to gonorrhoea at birth or with established gonococcal infection at any site.

For *nongonococcal neonatal conjunctivitis* WHO[4] and CDC[3] recommend erythromycin 50 mg per kg daily in divided doses by mouth for 10 to 14 days. There is no indication that topical therapy is of additional benefit.[3,10]

1. WHO. *Conjunctivitis of the newborn: prevention and treatment at the primary health care level.* Geneva: WHO, 1986.
2. Laga M, *et al.* Epidemiology and control of gonococcal ophthalmia neonatorum. *Bull WHO* 1989; **67:** 471–8.
3. Centers for Disease Control. 1998 Guidelines for treatment of sexually transmitted diseases. *MMWR* 1998; **47** (RR-1): 56–7, 65–6, 69.
4. WHO. *WHO model prescribing information: drugs used in sexually transmitted infections and HIV infection.* Geneva: WHO, 1995.
5. Laga M, *et al.* Prophylaxis of gonococcal and chlamydial ophthalmia neonatorum: a comparison of silver nitrate and tetracycline. *N Engl J Med* 1988; **318:** 653–7.
6. Black-Payne C, *et al.* Failure of erythromycin ointment for post natal ocular prophylaxis of chlamydial conjunctivitis. *Pediatr Infect Dis J* 1989; **8:** 491–5.
7. Hammerschlag MR, *et al.* Efficacy of neonatal ocular prophylaxis for the prevention of chlamydial and gonococcal conjunctivitis. *N Engl J Med* 1989; **320:** 769–72.
8. Schachter J. Why we need a program for the control of Chlamydia trachomatis. *N Engl J Med* 1989; **320:** 802–4.
9. Isenberg SJ, *et al.* A controlled trial of povidone-iodine as prophylaxis against ophthalmia neonatorum. *N Engl J Med* 1995; **332:** 562–6.
10. WHO. WHO expert committee on venereal diseases and treponematoses: sixth report. *WHO Tech Rep Ser 736* 1986: 125.

Nocardiosis

Nocardia spp. are Gram-positive aerobic branching bacteria that cause systemic or localised infection. The principal pathogenic species in man is *N. asteroides*; others include *N. brasiliensis, N. pseudobrasiliensis,* and *N. caviae*. Localised chronic infection or actinomycetoma is described under Mycetoma (above). Systemic nocardiosis is primarily a lung infection and often involves abscess formation; it occurs especially in immunocompromised patients and may be disseminated with abscesses in the brain and subcutaneous tissues.

The treatment of choice has been a sulphonamide such as sulphadiazine or, more recently, co-trimoxazole,[1-4] although a study *in vitro* indicated that the fixed ratio of trimethoprim:sulphamethoxazole in co-trimoxazole might contain too little trimethoprim for optimal activity.[5] Sulphafurazole[6] has been used successfully.

Various other antibacterials are active *in vitro* against *N. asteroides* and in one study imipenem, amikacin, and minocycline were the most effective overall, with ciprofloxacin the most active fluoroquinolone tested and ceftriaxone and cefpirome the most active cephalosporins.[7] The susceptibility patterns of other *Nocardia* spp. may differ. Synergy against *N. asteroides* has been demonstrated *in vitro* between imipenem or amikacin and trimethoprim:sulphamethoxazole (1:20);[8] imipenem and cefotaxime;[8] ampicillin and erythromycin;[9] amikacin and cefuroxime;[10] amikacin and co-trimoxazole;[10] and amikacin and amoxycillin with clavulanic acid.[10]

There have been reports of the effective treatment of nocardiosis with amikacin,[10,11] minocycline,[12,13] or ciprofloxacin with doxycycline.[14]

Treatment needs to be prolonged and may continue for 6 to 12 months.

1. Abdi EA, *et al.* Nocardia infection in splenectomized patients: case reports and a review of the literature. *Postgrad Med J* 1987; **63:** 455–8.
2. Smego RA, *et al.* Treatment of systemic nocardiosis. *Lancet* 1987; **i:** 456.
3. Filice GA. Treatment of nocardiosis. *Lancet* 1987; **i:** 1261–2.
4. Varghese GK, *et al.* Nocardia brasiliensis meningitis. *Postgrad Med J* 1992; **68:** 986.
5. Bennett JE, Jennings AE. Factors influencing susceptibility of Nocardia species to trimethoprim-sulfamethoxazole. *Antimicrob Agents Chemother* 1978; **13:** 624–7.
6. Poland GA, *et al.* Nocardia asteroides pericarditis: report of a case and review of the literature. *Mayo Clin Proc* 1990; **65:** 819–24.
7. Gombert ME, *et al.* Susceptibility of Nocardia asteroides to new quinolones and β-lactams. *Antimicrob Agents Chemother* 1987; **31:** 2013–14.
8. Gombert ME, Aulicino TM. Synergism of imipenem and amikacin in combination with other antibiotics against Nocardia asteroides. *Antimicrob Agents Chemother* 1983; **24:** 810–11.
9. Finland M, *et al.* Synergistic action of ampicillin and erythromycin against Nocardia asteroides: effect of time of incubation. *Antimicrob Agents Chemother* 1974; **5:** 344–53.
10. Goldstein FW, *et al.* Amikacin-containing regimens for treatment of nocardiosis in immunocompromized patients. *Eur J Clin Microbiol* 1987; **6:** 198–200.
11. Meier B, *et al.* Successful treatment of a pancreatic Nocardia asteroides abscess with amikacin and surgical drainage. *Antimicrob Agents Chemother* 1986; **29:** 150–1.
12. Petersen EA, *et al.* Minocycline treatment of pulmonary nocardiosis. *JAMA* 1983; **250:** 930–2.
13. Naka W, *et al.* Unusually located lymphocutaneous nocardiosis caused by Nocardia brasiliensis. *Br J Dermatol* 1995; **132:** 609–13.
14. Bath PMW, *et al.* Treatment of multiple subcutaneous Nocardia asteroides abscesses with ciprofloxacin and doxycycline. *Postgrad Med J* 1989; **65:** 190–1.

Obstetric disorders

See under: Endometritis (the prophylaxis and treatment of postpartum endometritis, a complication of caesarean section), above; Premature Labour, below; and Urinary-Tract Infections in Pregnancy, below. See also Neonatal Conjunctivitis, above, and Perinatal Streptococcal Infections, below.

Opportunistic mycobacterial infections

Environmental mycobacteria are widespread, and a number of species other than those responsible for leprosy and tuberculosis are facultative parasites capable of producing disease in man. These organisms, which have been referred to as atypical, nontuberculous, tuberculoid, opportunistic, or MOTT mycobacteria (mycobacteria other than tuberculous), are rarely, if ever, transmitted from person to person but are acquired from the environment. The diseases produced include localised skin and soft tissue lesions, pulmonary infections, and lymphadenitis, but disseminated infections may develop rapidly in immunocompromised patients such as those with AIDS and now represent one of the most common opportunistic bacterial infections in patients with advanced AIDS.

Localised lesions, invariably following inoculation, are most commonly due to the slow-growing species *Mycobacterium marinum* ('swimming pool' or 'fish-tank' granuloma), *M. ulcerans* (Buruli ulcer), and the fast-growing species *M. chelonae* (*M. chelonei*), *M. abscessus* (formerly *M. chelonae* subspecies), and *M. fortuitum*. Ulcerated lesions due to *M. haemophilum* have been described mainly in immunocompromised patients.

Pulmonary disease, which is clinically indistinguishable from pulmonary tuberculosis, has most frequently been attributed to the *M. avium* complex (MAC; *M. avium-intracellulare* complex; MAIC), *M. kansasii*, and to a lesser extent *M. xenopi*; less common causes include *M. chelonae*, *M. malmoense*, *M. scrofulaceum*, *M. simiae*, and *M. szulgai*.

Lymphadenitis, which is usually self-limiting and occurs particularly in children under 5 years of age, may be caused by many species but the great majority of cases are due to the related *M. avium* complex and *M. scrofulaceum* (sometimes collectively known as the MAIS complex).

Dissemination of opportunistic mycobacterial infections may occur rapidly in patients with depressed cellular immunity. The majority of cases have been attributed to the *M. avium* complex; species implicated more recently include *M. celatum* and *M. genavense*.

The course of treatment depends on the site and nature of infection. Response to chemotherapy is often difficult to predict as *in vitro* sensitivity of the organisms may not reflect the response obtained *in vivo*. Clinical improvements may still be achieved despite resistance *in vitro* to the individual drugs used in a regimen and selection of drugs is often on the basis of the best activity *in vitro*.[1-3] Most assessments of treatment have been based on retrospective surveys of empirical therapy and anecdotal reports.

Surgical resection remains valuable in localised disease,[3] either alone or in combination with chemotherapy, although the risk of spreading infection to deeper tissues[4] should be borne in mind.

MYCOBACTERIUM AVIUM COMPLEX (MAC).

Infections with *Mycobacterium avium* complex are traditionally regarded as difficult to treat, and prolonged therapy with a multi-drug regimen is usually required.[3] In patients with AIDS, lifelong therapy may be necessary. The optimum treatment regimen has yet to be determined. Before the introduction of the newer macrolides, clarithromycin and azithromycin, most regimens comprised ethambutol, rifampicin, and ciprofloxacin, sometimes with the addition of clofazimine.[5,6] Amikacin was added for severe infections or at the beginning of therapy. Isoniazid has been used occasionally,[3,7-9] but is omitted from most regimens currently in use. In the USA, its inclusion is actively discouraged[10] and in Australia it is added only if concurrent infection with *M. tuberculosis* is suspected.[11] Rifabutin has been shown to be effective[8,12] and has now largely replaced rifampicin in regimens for the treatment of MAC infections. A dose-ranging study of clarithromycin[13] confirmed its efficacy against MAC but, not surprisingly, resistance emerged in a large proportion of patients who continued to receive clarithromycin monotherapy, reinforcing the necessity for it to be given as part of combination therapy.[14] Cross-resistance with azithromycin has also been reported.[15] Synergy has been demonstrated between clarithromycin and many of the drugs used in MAC.[16] Currently the most common combination of drugs in use is clarithromycin (or azithromycin) plus ethambutol and rifabutin.[10,11,17-21] Clofazimine is commonly included either as a fourth drug or as an alternative to clarithromycin, and ciprofloxacin is a possible alternative third or fourth drug. Amikacin or streptomycin is added when parenteral therapy is necessary.

Other drugs tried in the management of MAC infection in small numbers of patients include interferons[22-24] and corticosteroids.[25]

Prophylaxis. Chemoprophylaxis is used to reduce the incidence of disseminated MAC disease in patients with advanced HIV infection. There appears to be a tendency to delay starting prophylaxis until later in the disease process; in 1993 the National Institutes of Health (NIH) in the USA recommended[10] starting at a blood CD4+ count of less than 100 per mm^3 but in 1995 commentators[26] considered that there was little advantage starting above a blood CD4+ count of 75 per mm^3, and the 1997 guidelines[27] from the US Public Health Service and the Infectious Diseases Society of America (USPHS/IDSA) recommend starting prophylaxis at a CD4+ count of 50 per mm^3.

Azithromycin,[28,29] clarithromycin,[30] and rifabutin[31] have been shown to be effective given as monotherapy. Combination therapy with azithromycin and rifabutin was more effective than either drug alone[28] but was less well tolerated. In the USA, azithromycin or clarithromycin are preferred to rifabutin for prophylaxis.[27]

Although prophylaxis is not considered necessary in immunocompetent individuals, vaccination with BCG has been found incidentally to provide protection against MAC infection in children.[32,33]

OTHER OPPORTUNISTIC MYCOBACTERIA.

In pulmonary and systemic disease due to *M. kansasii* rifampicin and ethambutol have been used for 9 to 15 months,[34,35] although a research committee of the British Thoracic Society concluded that treatment for up to 24 months may be necessary in immunocompromised patients.[36] Since the relapse rate following this regimen was similar to that seen in patients who had previously received isoniazid as part of standard therapy for presumed tuberculosis, the authors concluded that there was no advantage in adding isoniazid to therapy for *M. kansasii*.[36] Nevertheless, and despite reports of resistance to isoniazid *in vitro*,[36,37] several studies have supported prolonged treatment with isoniazid in combination with rifampicin and ethambutol.[37-39] This regimen incorporating isoniazid is recommended by the American Thoracic Society,[21] and should be continued for 18 months with at least 12 months of negative sputum cultures. Other antimycobacterial drug regimens have been used, but inclusion of rifampicin in a multidrug regimen improves therapeutic outcome.[40] Treatment regimens used for *M. xenopi* also include ethambutol and rifampicin with[41,42] or without[34] isoniazid, and regimens including ciprofloxacin.[43]

Imipenem,[44] doxycycline, erythromycin, amikacin with or without cefoxitin,[45] and clarithromycin[46] have been used for *M. chelonae* infections. Treatment of localised infection may be surgical; antibacterial treatment is not always necessary. Similarly, treatment of localised *M. fortuitum* infection may be surgical.[45] Amikacin with or without cefoxitin has been used for disseminated disease[45] and amikacin has been applied topically for mycobacterial keratitis.[47] Ciprofloxacin in association with cefoxitin has been used successfully for soft tissue abscess following surgical drainage and curettage.[48] Another fluoroquinolone ofloxacin has been used successfully in patients with pulmonary infection,[44] or surgical wound infection.[49]

For *M. marinum* infections (swimming-pool granuloma or fish-tank granuloma) rifampicin and ethambutol,[50] rifampicin and isoniazid, minocycline and co-trimoxazole,[4] clarithromycin and rifabutin,[51] or monotherapy with clarithromycin, minocycline, doxycycline, or co-trimoxazole[21] have been used.

Surgical treatment and intensive antibacterial regimens have been used for *M. scrofulaceum* infections,[41] while Buruli ulcer, due to *M. ulcerans*, which is difficult to treat, requires surgery,[2,41] often major; antimycobacterials have been used but results with rifampicin and clofazimine have often been clinically disappointing.[2] Phenytoin, applied locally, was reported to induce healing in 3 patients with Buruli ulcer.[52] *M. haemophilum* infection in a patient with rheumatoid arthritis and ulcerated nodules on his legs responded to treatment with rifampicin, ciprofloxacin, and clarithromycin.[53]

Treatment of disseminated *M. genavense* infection in HIV-infected patients has been similar to that for MAC infection.[54] The strain of *M. celatum* isolated from one patient had a susceptibility pattern halfway between that of MAC and *M. tuberculosis*; symptomatic improvement was achieved with a regimen of isoniazid, rifampicin, and ethambutol.[55]

1. Grange JM, Yates MD. Infections caused by opportunist mycobacteria: a review. *J R Soc Med* 1986; **79:** 226–9.
2. Grange JM. Environmental mycobacteria and human disease. *Lepr Rev* 1991; **62:** 353–61.
3. WHO. *WHO model prescribing information: drugs used in mycobacterial diseases*. Geneva: WHO, 1991.
4. Gray SF, *et al.* Fish tank granuloma. *Br Med J* 1990; **300:** 1069–70.
5. Chiu J, *et al.* Treatment of disseminated Mycobacterium avium complex infection in AIDS with amikacin, ethambutol, rifampin, and ciprofloxacin. *Ann Intern Med* 1990; **113:** 358–61.
6. Kemper CA, *et al.* Treatment of Mycobacterium avium complex bacteremia in AIDS with a four-drug oral regimen: rifampin, ethambutol, clofazimine, and ciprofloxacin. *Ann Intern Med* 1992; **116:** 466–72.
7. Agins BD, *et al.* Effect of combined therapy with ansamycin, clofazimine, ethambutol and isoniazid for Mycobacterium avium infection in patients with AIDS. *J Infect Dis* 1989; **159:** 784–7.
8. Hoy J, *et al.* Quadruple-drug therapy for Mycobacterium avium-intracellular bacteremia in AIDS patients. *J Infect Dis* 1990; **161:** 801–5.
9. Reddy MV, *et al.* In vitro and in vivo synergistic effect of isoniazid with streptomycin and clofazimine against Mycobacterium avium complex (MAC). *Tubercle Lung Dis* 1994; **75:** 208–12.
10. Masur H, and the Public Health Service Task Force on Prophylaxis and Therapy for Mycobacterium avium Complex. Recommendations on prophylaxis and therapy for disseminated Mycobacterium avium complex disease in patients infected with the human immunodeficiency virus. *N Engl J Med* 1993; **329:** 898–904.
11. Hoy JF, *et al.* HIV and non-tuberculous mycobacterial infection. *Med J Aust* 1996; **164:** 543–5.
12. Dautzenberg B, *et al.* Early bactericidal activity of rifabutin versus that of placebo in treatment of disseminated Mycobacterium avium complex bacteremia in AIDS patients. *Antimicrob Agents Chemother* 1996; **40:** 1722–5.
13. Chaisson RE, *et al.* Clarithromycin therapy for bacteremic Mycobacterium avium complex disease: a randomized, double-blind, dose-ranging study in patients with AIDS. *Ann Intern Med* 1994; **121:** 905–11.
14. Goldberger M, Masur H. Clarithromycin therapy for Mycobacterium avium complex disease in patients with AIDS: potential and problems. *Ann Intern Med* 1994: **121:** 974–6.
15. Heifets L, *et al.* Mycobacterium avium strains resistant to clarithromycin and azithromycin. *Antimicrob Agents Chemother* 1993; **37:** 2364–70.
16. Piersimoni C, *et al.* Activity of seven antimicrobial agents, alone and in combination, against AIDS-associated isolates of Mycobacterium avium complex. *J Antimicrob Chemother* 1995; **36:** 497–502.
17. Anonymous. Drugs for AIDS and associated infections. *Med Lett Drugs Ther* 1995; **37:** 87–94.
18. Miller R. HIV-associated respiratory disease. *Lancet* 1996; **348:** 307–12.
19. Sharpstone D, Gazzard B. Gastrointestinal manifestations of HIV infection. *Lancet* 1996; **348:** 379–83.
20. Shafran SD, *et al.* A comparison of two regimens for the treatment of Mycobacterium avium complex bacteremia in AIDS: rifabutin, ethambutol, and clarithromycin versus rifampin, ethambutol, clofazimine, and ciprofloxacin. *N Engl J Med* 1996; **335:** 377–83.
21. American Thoracic Society. Diagnosis and treatment of disease caused by nontuberculous mycobacteria. *Am J Respir Crit Care Med* 1997; **156:** S1–S25.
22. Squires KE, *et al.* Interferon-γ and Mycobacterium avium-intracellulare infection. *J Infect Dis* 1989; **159:** 599–600.
23. Holland SM, *et al.* Treatment of refractory disseminated nontuberculous mycobacterial infection with interferon gamma. *N Engl J Med* 1994; **330:** 1348–55.
24. Maziarz RT, *et al.* Reversal of infection with Mycobacterium avium intracellulare by treatment with alpha-interferon in a patients with hairy cell leukaemia. *Ann Intern Med* 1988; **109:** 292–4.
25. Wormser GP, *et al.* Low-dose dexamethasone as adjunctive therapy for disseminated Mycobacterium avium complex infections in AIDS patients. *Antimicrob Agents Chemother* 1994; **38:** 2215–17.
26. Ostroff SM, *et al.* Preventing disseminated Mycobacterium avium complex disease in patients infected with human immunodeficiency virus. *Clin Infect Dis* 1995; **21** (suppl 1): S72–S76.
27. Centers for Disease Control. 1997 USPHS/IDSA guidelines for the prevention of opportunistic infections in persons infected with human immunodeficiency virus. *MMWR* 1997; **46** (RR-12): 12–13.
28. Havlir DV, *et al.* Prophylaxis against disseminated Mycobacterium avium complex with weekly azithromycin, daily rifabutin, or both. *N Engl J Med* 1996; **335:** 392–8.
29. Oldfield EC, *et al.* Once weekly azithromycin therapy for prevention of Mycobacterium avium complex infection in patients with AIDS: a randomized, double-blind, placebo-controlled multicenter trial. *Clin Infect Dis* 1998; **26:** 611–19.
30. Pierce M, *et al.* A randomized trial of clarithromycin as prophylaxis against disseminated Mycobacterium avium complex infection in patients with advanced acquired immunodeficiency syndrome. *N Engl J Med* 1996; **335:** 384–91.
31. Nightingale SD, *et al.* Two controlled trials of rifabutin prophylaxis against Mycobacterium avium complex infection in AIDS. *N Engl J Med* 1993; **329:** 828–33.
32. Trnka L, *et al.* Six years' experience with the discontinuation of BCG vaccination 4: protective effect of BCG vaccination against the Mycobacterium avium intracellulare complex. *Tubercle Lung Dis* 1994; **75:** 348–52.
33. Romanus V, *et al.* Atypical mycobacteria in extrapulmonary disease among children: incidence in Sweden from 1969 to 1990, related to changing BCG-vaccination coverage. *Tubercle Lung Dis* 1995; **76:** 300–10.
34. Campbell IA. Pulmonary disease due to opportunistic mycobacteria. *Saudi Med J* 1990; **11:** 89–91.
35. Banks J, *et al.* Pulmonary infection with Mycobacterium kansasii in Wales, 1970-9: review of treatment and response. *Thorax* 1983; **38:** 271–4.
36. Jenkins PA, *et al.* Mycobacterium kansasii pulmonary infection: a prospective study of the results of nine months of treatment with rifampicin and ethambutol. *Thorax* 1994; **49:** 442–5.
37. Evans SA, *et al.* Pulmonary Mycobacterium kansasii infection: comparison of the clinical features, treatment and outcome with pulmonary tuberculosis. *Thorax* 1996; **51:** 1248–52.
38. Levine B, Chaisson RE. Mycobacterium kansasii: a cause of treatable pulmonary disease associated with advanced human immunodeficiency virus (HIV) infection. *Ann Intern Med* 1991; **114:** 861–8.
39. Sauret J, *et al.* Treatment of pulmonary disease caused by Mycobacterium kansasii: results of 18 vs 12 months' chemotherapy. *Tubercle Lung Dis* 1995; **76:** 104–8.
40. Schraufnagel DE, *et al.* Short-course chemotherapy for mycobacteriosis kansasii? *Can Med Assoc J* 1984; **130:** 34–8.
41. Bailey WC. Treatment of atypical mycobacterial disease. *Chest* 1983; **84:** 625–8.
42. Prosser AJ. Spinal infection with Mycobacterium xenopi. *Tubercle* 1986; **67:** 229–32.
43. Kahana LM, Spino M. Ciprofloxacin in patients with mycobacterial infections: experience in 15 patients. *DICP Ann Pharmacother* 1991; **25:** 919–24.
44. Yew WW, *et al.* Ofloxacin and imipenem in the treatment of Mycobacterium fortuitum and Mycobacterium chelonae lung infections. *Tubercle* 1990; **71:** 131–3.
45. Wallace RJ, *et al.* Treatment of nonpulmonary infections due to Mycobacterium fortuitum and Mycobacterium chelonei on the basis of in vitro susceptibilities. *J Infect Dis* 1985; **152:** 500–14.
46. Wallace RJ, *et al.* Clinical trial of clarithromycin for cutaneous (disseminated) infection due to Mycobacterium chelonae. *Ann Intern Med* 1993; **119:** 482–60.
47. Huang SCM, *et al.* Non-tuberculous mycobacterial keratitis: a study of 22 cases. *Br J Ophthalmol* 1996; **80:** 962–8.
48. Westmoreland D, *et al.* Case report: soft tissue abscess caused by Mycobacterium fortuitum. *J Infect Dis* 1990; **20:** 223–5.
49. Yew WW, *et al.* Ofloxacin therapy of Mycobacterium fortuitum infection: further experience. *J Antimicrob Chemother* 1990; **25:** 880–1.
50. Donta ST, *et al.* Therapy of Mycobacterium marinum infections: use of tetracyclines vs rifampin. *Arch Intern Med* 1986; **146:** 902–4.
51. Laing RBS, *et al.* New antimicrobials against Mycobacterium marinum infection. *Br J Dermatol* 1994; **131:** 914.
52. Adjei O, *et al.* Phenytoin in the treatment of Buruli ulcer. *Trans R Soc Trop Med Hyg* 1998; **92:** 108–9.
53. Darling TN, *et al.* Treatment of Mycobacterium haemophilum infection with an antibiotic regimen including clarithromycin. *Br J Dermatol* 1994; **131:** 376–9.
54. Pechère M, *et al.* Clinical and epidemiologic features of infection with Mycobacterium genavense. *Arch Intern Med* 1995; **155:** 400–4.
55. Piersimoni C, *et al.* Disseminated infection due to Mycobacterium celatum in patient with AIDS. *Lancet* 1994; **344:** 332.

Osteomyelitis

See under Bone and Joint Infections, above.

Otitis externa

Otitis externa or inflammation of the skin of the external auditory canal may be due to infection with bacteria, viruses, or fungi or secondary to skin disorders such as eczema, although more than one factor is often responsible for chronic disease. Treatment includes thorough cleansing and the use of appropriate antibacterial ear drops, often containing a corticosteroid as well, even though some have doubted the value of topical antibacterials. (Note that the UK Committee on Safety of Medicines has warned that ear drops containing aminoglycosides, such as gentamicin, neomycin, or framycetin, or polymyxins should not be used when the ear drum is perforated because of the risk of ototoxicity.[1]) Systemic antibacterials may be necessary in severe cases of otitis externa.

The various types of otitis externa and their management have been described by Keene.[2] Briefly, for a *boil or furuncle* in the ear canal a ribbon gauze wick soaked in ichthammol in glycerol ear drops or magnesium sulphate paste may be inserted to reduce the swelling; alternatively dexamethasone, framycetin, and gramicidin ear drops may be used. Systemic treatment with flucloxacillin should be given if staphylococcal infection is likely.[2] In *acute diffuse otitis externa* (*swimmer's ear*) *Staphylococcus aureus* and *Pseudomonas* spp. are often present. Treatment includes instillation of ear drops such as dexamethasone, framycetin, and gramicidin or gentamicin and hydrocortisone, using a wick if it proves difficult.[2] In a report from Germany, topical gentamicin was generally successful and oral fluoroquinolones were effective in most cases not responding to topical treatment.[3] *'Malignant' otitis externa*, due to fulminating infection especially with *Pseudomonas*, is uncommon but can occur in, for example, elderly diabetics. Topical antibacterials are not effective and systemic treatment with antipseudomonal drugs such as gentamicin or ceftazidime, together with metronidazole if anaerobes are present, is essential.[2] Oral ciprofloxacin given for 6 or more weeks has been used successfully in infection due predominantly to *Ps. aeruginosa*[4,5] and some have considered that fluoroquinolones, in particular ciprofloxacin, may become the antibacterials of choice in malignant otitis externa.[6] However, resistance to ciprofloxacin has been reported.[7] In *eczematous otitis externa* gentamicin with hydrocortisone ear drops can be used if infection is suspected.[2]

1. Committee on Safety of Medicines. Preparations used in the topical treatment of otitis externa. *Current Problems 5* 1981.
2. Keene M. Otitis externa. *Prescribers' J* 1990; **30:** 229–35.
3. Elies W. Local chemotherapy of selected bacterial infections of the ear. *J Antimicrob Chemother* 1990; **26:** 303–5.
4. Hickey SA, *et al.* Treating malignant otitis with oral ciprofloxacin. *Br Med J* 1989; **299:** 550–1.
5. Lang R, *et al.* Successful treatment of malignant external otitis with oral ciprofloxacin: report of experience with 23 patients. *J Infect Dis* 1990; **161:** 537–40.
6. Giamarellou H. Malignant otitis externa: the therapeutic evolution of a lethal infection. *J Antimicrob Chemother* 1992; **30:** 745–51.
7. Cooper MA, *et al.* Ciprofloxacin resistance developing during treatment of malignant otitis externa. *J Antimicrob Chemother* 1993; **32:** 163–4.

Otitis media

Otitis media or inflammation of the middle ear can be acute or chronic, serous (with effusion; secretory) or suppurative. Reviews[1,2] illustrate the continuing confusion over terminology and differences in management, despite the fact that otitis media is one of the most frequent childhood illnesses seen in general practice. Diagnosis can be difficult[3] and according to Glover[1] can only be achieved by viewing the tympanic membrane (ear drum) or by the presence of a discharge. He classified otitis media as *acute serous otitis media*, secondary to Eustachian tube dysfunction and characterised by discomfort; *acute suppurative otitis media*, due to bacterial or viral infection, with pain ranging from mild earache to severe pain and a red ear drum bulging from an acute purulent effusion that may rupture with purulent discharge; *chronic serous otitis media*, or the 'glue ear' syndrome, characterised by deafness; and *chronic suppurative otitis media*, associated with perforation and/or cholesteatoma and characterised by discharge and deafness. There may be some overlap in the use of these terms. According to Shah,[4] *serous otitis media* (also termed secretory or non-suppurative otitis media, otitis media with effusion, and 'glue ear') is the commonest middle ear disorder in children; the fluid present may be serous, mucoid, mucopurulent, or of mixed variety; there are no acute symptoms and signs of inflammation; and the fluid is often sterile. He acknowledged the close relationship between acute otitis media and serous otitis media in young children. Others[5] have considered terms such as acute suppurative or acute serous otitis to be unhelpful since the diagnosis could not be made in practice, and preferred the use of acute otitis media.

ACUTE OTITIS MEDIA is seen especially in young children and is often due to bacterial or viral infections (frequently both), sometimes associated with upper respiratory-tract infection, although infecting organisms are not always identified. The commonest bacterial pathogens are *Streptococcus pneumoniae*, followed by *Haemophilus influenzae*, with *Moraxella (Branhamella) catarrhalis*[6] an increasingly important cause. Treatment aims to relieve symptoms, avoid complications, and prevent relapse, recurrence, and progression to the chronic state.[1] Sometimes an analgesic such as paracetamol may be all that is required as long as frequent inspection is possible. However, it is common practice to prescribe a systemic antibacterial as well as an analgesic,[7] although the need for routine antibacterial treatment is increasingly being questioned.[3,5,8,9] Ear drops containing antibacterials, corticosteroids, or local anaesthetics are not effective, neither are topical and systemic decongestants, antihistamines, and mucolytics.[1] Systemic antibacterial treatment aims to speed resolution and prevent complications. However, while clinical studies have shown only modest benefits from routine administration of antibacterials[10-12] and experience from countries where antibacterials are not given routinely for acute otitis media suggests that there is no consequent increase in complications,[9,12] some clinicians argue that the routine use of antibacterials is clinically justifiable.[13-16] Amoxycillin is often the drug of choice; alternatives include erythromycin with or without a sulphonamide such as sulphafurazole, or an oral cephalosporin such as cefaclor, cefixime, or cefuroxime axetil. Co-trimoxazole is used in come countries but it is not generally recommended in the UK. Amoxycillin with clavulanic acid may be given when beta-lactamase-resistant strains of *H. influenzae* or *M. catarrhalis* are prevalent. Penicillin-resistant strains of *Str. pneumoniae* have been reported in children with otitis media[17] and are reported to be increasingly prevalent.[18] However, many penicillin-resistant strains remain sensitive to amoxycillin, although the situation will need continued evaluation.[18,19] Duration of therapy has varied from 5 to 10 or more days; some have claimed that shorter courses are effective[20,21] and in one study[22] amoxycillin for 3 days appeared to be as effective as for 10 days. However, short courses should probably not be used in children under 2 years of age[16,20] or in others at high risk of treatment failure.[20] Longer treatment for 20 days has not been found to be more efficacious than 10 days.[23]

Antibacterial prophylaxis has been tried in children at high risk including those with *recurrent acute otitis media*,[24] but it remains controversial.[1] In the UK, it is suggested that prophylaxis with trimethoprim or erythromycin may be tried during the winter. In the USA amoxycillin or sulphafurazole has been recommended for prophylaxis.[25] The use of xylitol chewing gum, which inhibits the growth of *Str. pneumoniae*, has been reported to reduce the incidence of acute otitis media.[26]

SEROUS OTITIS MEDIA (otitis media with effusion) is common in children and may be associated with recurrent upper respiratory-tract infection. Many are asymptomatic, the fluid is usually sterile, and the condition can resolve spontaneously.[4] Optimal treatment is controversial.[2] Careful assessment and follow-up without medication is the conservative approach, but according to Shah[4] a broad-spectrum antibacterial such as amoxycillin for 5 to 10 days should be tried in young children with serous otitis media following an infection. Those at special risk such as children with cleft palate should be referred to a specialist. In the USA, Bluestone[25] has recommended amoxycillin as first-line therapy. However, a meta-analysis has suggested that, although a short course of antibacterials might clear the effusion in the short term, the effect is not sustained.[27] Recent US guidelines for managing otitis media with effusion in young children[28] state that most cases resolve spontaneously, although they noted that in the previously mentioned meta-analysis of controlled studies[27] there was a 14% increase in the resolution rate with antibacterial treatment; a typical course lasted for 10 days. They considered management options for uncomplicated otitis media with effusion in an otherwise healthy child of 1 to 3 years to be either observation or antibacterial therapy; adverse effects and the possible development of bacterial resistance should be borne in mind.[28] Corticosteroids, antihistamines, and decongestants were not recommended.[28] Nevertheless, Berman[29] states that the use of corticosteroids in combination with antibacterials should still be considered a treatment option.

CHRONIC OTITIS MEDIA can include recurrent episodes of acute infection, chronic suppurative otitis media, and prolonged serous otitis media. There have been various definitions of *chronic suppurative otitis media*. Glover[1] has divided it into 2 types associated with deafness and/or discharge. In one (tubo-tympanic disease) there is typically perforation of the ear drum, deafness, and a profuse mucoid discharge associated with upper respiratory-tract infection, the commonest infecting organisms being *Str. pneumoniae*, *Staph. aureus*, and *H. influenzae*. In the other (attico-antral disease) there may be cholesteatoma with bone involvement and the commonest infecting organisms are *Pseudomonas aeruginosa* and *Proteus* spp. Treatment of chronic suppurative otitis media is controversial. Although the value of systemic antibacterials has been debated,[1] in the UK they are recommended for use during acute exacerbations. The mainstay of treatment is thorough cleansing. Local treatment with corticosteroids or astringents as in otitis externa (above) may be beneficial, particularly with infections of mastoid cavities. Antibacterial ear drops are suggested when perforation of the ear drum is present. The UK Committee on Safety of Medicines has warned of the dangers of ototoxicity when ear drops containing aminoglycosides or polymyxins are used in the presence of a perforated ear drum in patients with otitis externa, but specialists consider that untreated chronic suppurative otitis media is more likely to result in deafness than is the use of these ear drops.[1] In *Pseudomonas* infection ear drops like gentamicin and hydrocortisone are frequently used.[1] Local application of the fluoroquinolones ciprofloxacin or ofloxacin[14] has shown promise and may prove a safer alternative than these ear drops.[30]

In the USA initial oral therapy with amoxycillin-clavulanic acid, cefaclor, or erythromycin-sulphafurazole has been advocated for chronic suppurative otitis media,[31] but even so ear drops continue to be popular.[2] In a study from Israel[32] intravenous mezlocillin or ceftazidime together with daily suction and debridement, but no topical antibacterial therapy, was reported to be successful in treating children with chronic suppurative otitis media without cholesteatoma; *Ps. aeruginosa* had been present in most cultures and other organisms included Gram-negative enteric bacilli, *Staph. aureus*, and *H. influenzae*. Anaerobic organisms have also been implicated frequently.[33] A community-based study in Kenya found that oral amoxycillin and topical antibacterial and corticosteroid drops given in addition to regular cleansing was more effective than either cleansing alone or no treatment.[34]

1. Glover GW. Otitis media. *Prescribers' J* 1990; **30:** 218–24.
2. Lisby-Sutch SM, *et al.* Therapy of otitis media. *Clin Pharm* 1990; **9:** 15–34.
3. Froom J, *et al.* Diagnosis and antibiotic treatment of acute otitis media: report from International Primary Care Network. *Br Med J* 1990; **300:** 582–6.
4. Shah NS. Serous otitis media. *Prescribers' J* 1990; **30:** 225–8.
5. Bollag U, Bollag-Albrecht E. Recommendations derived from practice audit for the treatment of acute otitis media. *Lancet* 1991; **338:** 96–9.
6. Marchant CD. Spectrum of disease due to Branhamella catarrhalis in children with particular reference to acute otitis media. *Am J Med* 1990; **88** (suppl 5A): 15S–19S.
7. Anonymous. Management of acute otitis media and glue ear. *Drug Ther Bull* 1995; **33:** 12–15.
8. Browning GG. Childhood otalgia: acute otitis media 1. *Br Med J* 1990; **300:** 1005–6.
9. Majeed A, Harris T. Acute otitis media in children. *Br Med J* 1997; **315:** 321–2.
10. Rosenfeld RM, *et al.* Clinical efficacy of antimicrobial drugs for acute otitis media: metaanalysis of 5400 children from thirty-three randomized trials. *J Pediatr* 1994; **124:** 355–67.
11. Del Mar C, *et al.* Are antibiotics indicated as initial treatment for children with acute otitis media? A meta-analysis. *Br Med J* 1997; **314:** 1526–9.
12. Froom J, *et al.* Antimicrobials for acute otitis media? A review from the International Primary Care Network. *Br Med J* 1997; **315:** 98–102.
13. Carlin SA, *et al.* Host factors and the early therapeutic response in acute otitis media. *J Pediatr* 1991; **118:** 178–83.
14. Burke P, *et al.* Acute red ear in children: controlled trial of non-antibiotic treatment in general practice. *Br Med J* 1991; **303:** 558–62.
15. Dowell SF, *et al.* Otitis media—principles of judicious use of antimicrobial agents. *Pediatrics* 1998; **101** (suppl): 165–71.
16. Paradise JL. Short-course antimicrobial treatment for acute otitis media: not best for infants and young children. *JAMA* 1997; **278:** 1640–2.
17. Klugman KP. Management of antibiotic-resistant pneumococcal infections. *J Antimicrob Chemother* 1994; **34:** 191–3.
18. Klugman KP. Epidemiology, control and treatment of multiresistant pneumococci. *Drugs* 1996; **52** (suppl 2): 42–6.
19. Pelton SI. New concepts in the pathophysiology and management of middle ear disease in childhood. *Drugs* 1996; **52** (suppl 2): 62–7.
20. Pichichero ME. Changing the treatment paradigm for acute otitis media in children. *JAMA* 1998; **279:** 1748–50.
21. Kozyrskj AL, *et al.* Treatment of acute otitis media with a shortened course of antibiotics: a meta-analysis. *JAMA* 1998; **279:** 1736–42.
22. Chaput de Saintonge DM, *et al.* Trial of three-day and ten-day courses of amoxycillin in otitis media. *Br Med J* 1982; **284:** 1078–81.
23. Mandel EM, *et al.* Efficacy of 20- versus 10-day antimicrobial treatment for acute otitis media. *Pediatrics* 1995; **96:** 5–13.
24. Paradise JL. Antimicrobial drugs and surgical procedures in the prevention of otitis media. *Pediatr Infect Dis J* 1989; **8** (suppl 1): S35–7.
25. Bluestone CD. Management of otitis media in infants and children: current role of old and new antimicrobial agents. *Pediatr Infect Dis J* 1988; **7:** S129–36.
26. Uhari M, *et al.* Xylitol chewing gum in prevention of acute otitis media: double blind randomised trial. *Br Med J* 1996; **313:** 1180–4.
27. Williams RL, *et al.* Use of antibiotics in preventing recurrent acute otitis media and in treating otitis media with effusion: a meta-analytic attempt to resolve the brouhaha. *JAMA* 1993; **270:** 1344–51.
28. The Otitis Media Guideline Panel. Managing otitis media with effusion in young children. *Pediatrics* 1994; **94:** 766–73.
29. Berman S. Otitis media in children. *N Engl J Med* 1995; **332:** 1560–5.
30. Elies W. Local chemotherapy of selected bacterial infections of the ear. *J Antimicrob Chemother* 1990; **26:** 303–5.
31. Nelson JD. Chronic suppurative otitis media. *Pediatr Infect Dis J* 1988; **7:** 446–8.
32. Fliss DM, *et al.* Medical management of chronic suppurative otitis media without cholesteatoma in children. *J Pediatr* 1990; **116:** 991–6.
33. Wintermeyer SM, Nahata MC. Chronic suppurative otitis media. *Ann Pharmacother* 1994; **28:** 1089–99.
34. Smith AW, *et al.* Randomised controlled trial of treatment of chronic suppurative otitis media Kenyan schoolchildren *Lancet* 1996; **348:** 1128–33.

Pancreatitis

The overall management of pancreatitis is discussed on p.1613. Although the value of prophylactic antibacterials in acute pancreatitis is not proven, early treatment with cefuroxime markedly reduced mortality in a study of patients with acute necrotising pancreatitis[1] and a retrospective study[2] reported a reduction in the incidence, but not in the time of onset, of infection in those receiving prophylactic therapy.

1. Sainio V, *et al.* Early antibiotic treatment in acute necrotising pancreatitis. *Lancet* 1995; **346:** 663–7.
2. Ho HS, Frey CF. The role of antibiotic prophylaxis in severe acute pancreatitis. *Arch Surg* 1997; **132:** 487–93.

Pelvic inflammatory disease

Pelvic inflammatory disease is a broad term for infectious disorders of the upper genital tract in women and may include endometritis, salpingitis, tubo-ovarian abscess, and pelvic peritonitis. It is generally due to ascending infection through the cervix and uterus to the fallopian tubes, resulting in salpingitis, and from there may extend to the ovaries and peritoneum. Long-term complications include infertility and ectopic pregnancy. Pelvic inflammatory disease has become more common and has been the subject of several reviews.[1-3] The use of intra-uterine contraceptive devices might increase the likelihood of pelvic inflammatory disease although the risk may have been overstated;[1] it appears to be greatest during the first 20 days after insertion of the device.[4]

The majority of these infections are probably sexually transmitted and at one time were mainly due to *Neisseria gonorrhoeae*, but *Chlamydia trachomatis* is increasingly responsible and may be the commonest cause of pelvic inflammatory disease in some areas. Other organisms that have been isolated include *Mycoplasma hominis*; *Ureaplasma urealyticum*; anaerobes such as

Bacteroides, *Peptococcus*, and *Peptostreptococcus* spp.; Gram-negative enteric aerobes such as *Escherichia coli*; and Gram-positive aerobes such as group B streptococci. Some of these organisms occur in the abnormal vaginal flora associated with bacterial vaginosis (above). Thus, the aetiology of pelvic inflammatory disease appears to be polymicrobial; some think that primary infection with *N. gonorrhoeae* or *C. trachomatis*, or both, allows opportunistic infection with aerobic and anaerobic bacteria.[1]

Treatment regimens are of necessity broad spectrum and empirical and should include antibacterials active against the major pathogens. Many consider that treatment should be started in hospital so that drugs can be given parenterally. For inpatients WHO[5] has recommended doxycycline intravenously or by mouth plus ceftriaxone intramuscularly or an oral regimen of ciprofloxacin, doxycycline, and metronidazole. Both regimens should be continued for at least 4 days, or for at least 48 hours after clinical improvement, followed by doxycycline by mouth for 10 to 14 days. For outpatients a single-dose treatment for uncomplicated gonorrhoea such as ceftriaxone intramuscularly is suggested[5] (see Gonorrhoea, above) together with metronidazole and either doxycycline or tetracycline by mouth for 10 days. Further examples of suitable treatment regimens have been provided by the Centers for Disease Control in the USA.[6] For parenteral administration cefoxitin or cefotetan may be given intravenously together with doxycycline orally or intravenously (regimen A) or clindamycin intravenously together with gentamicin intramuscularly or intravenously (regimen B), in each case continued for 24 hours after substantial clinical improvement has occurred and then followed by doxycycline by mouth to complete a total of 14 days' treatment. In regimen A, clindamycin or metronidazole may be added to doxycycline for continued therapy in patients with tubo-ovarian abscesses. In regimen B continuation may be with oral clindamycin rather than doxycycline. For oral treatment ofloxacin plus metronidazole by mouth for 14 days may be employed. Alternatively, a single intramuscular dose of cefoxitin plus probenecid by mouth, or of ceftriaxone or equivalent cephalosporin, together with doxycycline by mouth for 14 days may be used.

In the UK metronidazole plus doxycycline (or erythromycin) is suggested for patients with pelvic inflammatory disease, although gonorrhoea should also be treated if present; a cephalosporin such as cefotaxime plus doxycycline may be necessary in patients who are severely ill.

1. Pearce JM. Pelvic inflammatory disease. *Br Med J* 1990; **300:** 1090–1.
2. Dodson MG. Optimum therapy for acute pelvic inflammatory disease. *Drugs* 1990; **39:** 511–22.
3. McCormack WM. Pelvic inflammatory disease. *N Engl J Med* 1994; **330:** 115–19.
4. Farley TMM, *et al.* Intrauterine devices and pelvic inflammatory disease: an international perspective. *Lancet* 1992; **339:** 785–8.
5. WHO. *WHO model prescribing information: drugs used in sexually transmitted disease and HIV infection.* Geneva: WHO, 1995.
6. Centers for Disease Control. 1998 Guidelines for treatment of sexually transmitted diseases. *MMWR* 1998; **47** (RR-1): 79–86.

Peptic ulcer disease

The Gram-negative bacterium *Helicobacter pylori* (formerly *Campylobacter pylori*) is involved in the aetiology of gastritis and peptic ulceration and treatment regimens to eradicate the organism have been devised. For a discussion of peptic ulcer disease and its treatment, including antibacterial therapy, see p.1174.

Perinatal streptococcal infections

Group B streptococci are a major cause of perinatal infections, often leading to neonatal pneumonia or septicaemia, sometimes with meningitis, although the incidence varies in different parts of the world. Infections are acquired through maternal genital carriage during pregnancy. *Prevention* of group B streptococcal infection in infants may be achieved by giving appropriate antibacterials to the mother during labour.[1,2] Ideally maternal carriers of group B streptococci would be identified during pregnancy, but this may not be practical. Factors that increase the risk of acquiring neonatal infection include premature labour, prolonged rupture of membranes, maternal fever, a previous child with neonatal group B streptococcal infection, and multiple pregnancy and they will influence the decision of whether or not to give intrapartum antibacterial prophylaxis to the mother. A penicillin is the preferred drug. Guidelines in the USA[1,3] allow prophylactic strategies based either on prenatal screening or on risk factor analysis. They have recommended ampicillin or benzylpenicillin given intravenously during labour, or alternatively clindamycin or erythromycin in women allergic to penicillin. However, these policies have their critics.[4,5] In other parts of the world, including Europe, the incidence of neonatal streptococcal infections is much lower and the US model for prophylaxis may not be appropriate.[6,7]

Another strategy suggested for areas with a high incidence of neonatal group B streptococcal disease (above 1.5 per 1000 live births) is administration of a single dose of penicillin to all neonates at birth.[8]

As mentioned under Premature Labour, below, the elimination of group B streptococci in pregnant women might also reduce the risk of premature labour.

Streptococcus group B vaccines are under investigation for administration to pregnant women to prevent neonatal infection.

1. Centers for Disease Control. Prevention of prenatal group B streptococcal disease: a public health perspective *MMWR* 1996; **45** (RR-7): 1–24.
2. van Oppen C, Feldman R. Antibiotic prophylaxis of neonatal group B streptococcal infections. *Br Med J* 1993; **301:** 411–12.
3. American Academy of Pediatrics, Committee on Infectious Diseases and Committee on Fetus and Newborn. Revised guidelines for prevention of early-onset group B streptococcal (GBS) infection. *Pediatrics* 1997; **99:** 489–96.
4. Benitz WE. The neonatal group B streptococcal debate. *Pediatrics* 1998; **101:** 494–5.
5. Ledger WJ. CDC guidelines for the prevention of perinatal group B streptococcal disease: are they appropriate? *Infect Dis Clin Pract* 1998; **7:** 188–93.
6. Simpson AJA, Heard SR. Group B Streptococcus. *Lancet* 1995; **346:** 700.
7. Jakobi P, *et al.* New CDC guidelines for prevention of perinatal group B streptococcal disease. *Lancet* 1996; **348:** 969.
8. Siegel JD, Cushion NB. Prevention of early-onset group B streptococcal disease: another look at single-dose penicillin at birth. *Obstet Gynecol* 1996; **87:** 692–8.

Peritonitis

Intra-abdominal infections include peritonitis, which may be complicated by intraperitoneal abscesses, and abscesses of the intra-abdominal viscera such as those of the liver (see under Abscess, Liver, above), pancreas, and spleen. Infective peritonitis may be primary or secondary or may be a complication of continuous ambulatory peritoneal dialysis (CAPD).

Primary peritonitis. In primary or spontaneous bacterial peritonitis there is no specific focus of infection and it occurs most often as a complication of ascites. Infecting bacteria include *Escherichia coli*, other Enterobacteriaceae, and streptococci. Initial treatment has been with broad-spectrum chemotherapy such as ampicillin plus an aminoglycoside, but third-generation cephalosporins such as cefotaxime are considered by some to be the treatment of choice.[1] Other alternatives include other broad-spectrum penicillins, carbapenems, and combinations of penicillins or cephalosporins with beta-lactamase inhibitors.[2] Ofloxacin by mouth has been reported to be as effective as intravenous cefotaxime in one study in uncomplicated infections.[3] In another study the administration of oral norfloxacin for selective intestinal decontamination appeared to prevent spontaneous bacterial peritonitis in cirrhotic patients with low levels of ascitic fluid protein[4] and prophylaxis with norfloxacin has been recommended to decrease the recurrence of spontaneous bacterial peritonitis.[1] Co-trimoxazole has also been reported to be an effective prophylactic.[5]

Secondary peritonitis. Secondary peritonitis is associated with perforation of the gastro-intestinal tract, conditions such as appendicitis and diverticulitis, and contamination at surgery. Infections are generally mixed and originate from the gastro-intestinal tract. Bacteria responsible include *E. coli* and other Enterobacteriaceae; anaerobes, especially *Bacteroides fragilis*; enterococci; and sometimes *Pseudomonas aeruginosa*. Broad-spectrum antibacterial therapy is therefore necessary, at least until the infecting organisms are known, and a combination of 2 or 3 drugs is often given. The intravenous route is generally preferred. An aminoglycoside such as gentamicin or a cephalosporin plus metronidazole or clindamycin has often been used, but many other regimens have been tried. However, the emergence of organisms resistant to third-generation cephalosporins and of isolates of *B. fragilis* resistant to clindamycin may favour the use of aminoglycosides, fluoroquinolones, or carbapenems with metronidazole in susceptible patients.[2] Secondary intraperitoneal abscesses occur as complications of disorders such as appendicitis; they should be drained[6] and antibacterials similar to those for secondary peritonitis should be given. For reference to the prevention of postoperative infection, see under Surgical Infection, below.

CAPD peritonitis. Peritonitis is the main complication of CAPD, a technique widely used in end-stage renal failure, and has been the subject of detailed reviews.[7,8] Unlike secondary peritonitis, above, a single infecting organism is often responsible. A working party of the British Society for Antimicrobial Chemotherapy (BSAC)[9] noted that the commonest source of infection is contamination when the dialysis bag or transfer set is changed; others include catheters, bacteraemia, upper respiratory-tract secretions, and, possibly, organisms that have passed through the gut wall or from the fallopian tubes. *Staphylococcus epidermidis* causes about half the episodes of confirmed peritonitis and many other organisms causing peritonitis in CAPD such as alpha-haemolytic streptococci, 'diphtheroids', and *Staph. aureus* are also skin bacteria. The Enterobacteriaceae and *Pseudomonas aeruginosa* together account for almost a fifth of the infecting organisms. BSAC[9] recommend that CAPD-associated peritonitis should be treated promptly with antibacterials given by the intraperitoneal route, rather than orally or intravenously, since precise therapeutic and non-toxic concentrations can be delivered to the site of infection; with many antibacterials adequate serum concentrations are achieved within a few hours of intraperitoneal administration. CAPD should be continued as usual with antibacterials added to the dialysis fluid. In the severely ill patient, an intravenous or intraperitoneal loading dose may be given to ensure prompt therapeutic concentrations. There is a possibility that antibacterial activity might be reduced by the peritoneal dialysate,[10] but pharmacokinetic considerations appear to favour the peritoneal route.[11]

Initial **empirical treatment** of CAPD peritonitis must be effective against both Gram-positive and Gram-negative pathogens. BSAC[9] recommended a combination of vancomycin and an aminoglycoside such as gentamicin, netilmicin, or tobramycin. Once the pathogen and its sensitivity are known, either vancomycin or the aminoglycoside should be discontinued. Intermittent dosing with vancomycin and gentamicin has been tried, but experience is limited.[8] As an alternative to the above regimen cefuroxime or ceftazidime may be used.[9] In order to avoid indiscriminate use of vancomycin and thus reduce the emergence of resistant organisms empirical treatment with a first-generation cephalosporin such as cephazolin together with an aminoglycoside may be used or alternatively the cephalosporin in this combination may be replaced with nafcillin, clindamycin, vancomycin, or ciprofloxacin in order of preference.[12] The optimum length of treatment remains controversial but the working party[9] recommend continuation for at least 5 days after resolution of clinical signs and symptoms and clearing of the effluent; usually a total of 7 to 10 days is adequate. Others consider a minimum of 10 days of treatment to be necessary,[8] or at least 21 days in patients with *Staph. aureus* or Gram-negative infections.[12]

For peritonitis due to *Ps. aeruginosa*, BSAC recommend a combination of an antipseudomonal penicillin such as azlocillin or ticarcillin and an aminoglycoside; ceftazidime is an alternative but this too should be combined with an aminoglycoside. Failure to respond promptly is an indication for early catheter removal. Flucloxacillin or vancomycin are recommended[9] for *Staph. aureus* infections, ampicillin or vancomycin for *Enterococcus faecalis* infections, and vancomycin for diphtheroids. If bowel perforation is likely metronidazole may be given along with vancomycin and an aminoglycoside.[8]

Long-term antibacterial **prophylaxis** is not advised by BSAC,[9] but dramatic reductions in peritonitis rates have been achieved with programmes based on stringent aseptic wound care and on minimising contact of the CAPD system with household water.[13]

Williams and Coles[14] have highlighted the importance of staphylococci as a cause of peritonitis in CAPD and have discussed the possible role of rifampicin in combination therapy for persistent or recurrent peritonitis and in the treatment of biofilm and catheter-related infections. Urokinase has been used in conjunction with rifampicin in relapsing peritonitis and may facilitate penetration of rifampicin into the catheter biofilm,[8] although the importance of biofilm in peritonitis is uncertain.[14] Suppression of nasal carriage of *Staph. aureus* with rifampicin[12,14] or mupirocin[12] might reduce the risk of catheter exit-site infection.

Other antibacterials used successfully in the treatment of CAPD-peritonitis include intraperitoneal ciprofloxacin.[15-17] The oral route would offer advantages and ciprofloxacin by mouth has shown promise[18] although resistance may be a problem.[19] Teicoplanin has been used instead of vancomycin.[20]

1. Gilbert JA, Kamath PS. Spontaneous bacterial peritonitis: an update. *Mayo Clin Proc* 1995; **70:** 365–70.
2. Johnson CC, *et al.* Peritonitis: update on pathophysiology, clinical manifestations, and management. *Clin Infect Dis* 1997; **24:** 1035–47.
3. Navasa M *et al.* Randomized comparative study of oral ofloxacin versus intravenous cefotaxime in spontaneous bacterial peritonitis. *Gastroenterology* 1996; **111:** 1011–17.
4. Soriano G, *et al.* Selective intestinal decontamination prevents spontaneous bacterial peritonitis. *Gastroenterology* 1991; **100:** 477–81.
5. Singh N, *et al.* Trimethoprim-sulfamethoxazole for the prevention of spontaneous bacterial peritonitis in cirrhosis: a randomized trial. *Ann Intern Med* 1995; **122:** 595–8.
6. Anonymous. Percutaneous drainage of the abdominal abscess. *Lancet* 1982; **i:** 889–90.
7. Horton MW, *et al.* Treatment of peritonitis in patients undergoing continuous ambulatory peritoneal dialysis. *Clin Pharm* 1990; **9:** 102–18.
8. Mawhinney WM, *et al.* Development and treatment of peritonitis in continuous ambulatory peritoneal dialysis. *Int J Pharm Pract* 1991; **1:** 10–18.
9. Working Party of the British Society for Antimicrobial Chemotherapy. Diagnosis and management of peritonitis in continuous ambulatory peritoneal dialysis. *Lancet* 1987; **i:** 845–9.
10. Craddock CF. CAPD peritonitis. *Lancet* 1987; **i:** 1320–1.
11. Keller E, *et al.* Drug therapy in patients undergoing continuous ambulatory peritoneal dialysis: clinical pharmacokinetic considerations. *Clin Pharmacokinet* 1990; **18:** 104–17.
12. Keane WF, *et al.* Peritoneal dialysis-related peritonitis treatment recommendations: 1996 update. *Perit Dial Int* 1996; **16:** 557–73.
13. Ludlam H, *et al.* Prevention of peritonitis in continuous ambulatory peritoneal dialysis. *Lancet* 1990; **335:** 1161.
14. Williams JD, Coles GA. Gram-positive infections related to CAPD. *J Antimicrob Chemother* 1991; **27** (suppl B): 31–5.
15. Ludlam HA, *et al.* Intraperitoneal ciprofloxacin for the treatment of peritonitis in patients receiving continuous ambulatory peritoneal dialysis (CAPD). *J Antimicrob Chemother* 1990; **25:** 843–51.
16. Ludlam H, *et al.* Short course ciprofloxacin therapy for CAPD peritonitis. *J Antimicrob Chemother* 1990; **26:** 162–4.
17. Dryden MS, *et al.* Low dose intraperitoneal ciprofloxacin for the treatment of peritonitis in patients receiving continuous ambulatory peritoneal dialysis (CAPD). *J Antimicrob Chemother* 1991; **28:** 131–9.
18. Fleming LW, *et al.* Oral ciprofloxacin in the treatment of peritonitis in patients on continuous ambulatory peritoneal dialysis. *J Antimicrob Chemother* 1990; **25:** 441–8.
19. Wilcox MH, Finch RG. Ciprofloxacin and CAPD peritonitis. *J Antimicrob Chemother* 1990; **26:** 447–8.
20. Neville LO, *et al.* Efficacy and safety of teicoplanin in Gram-positive peritonitis in patients on peritoneal dialysis. *J Antimicrob Chemother* 1988; **21** (suppl A): 123–31.

Pertussis

Pertussis or whooping cough is caused by infection with the respiratory pathogen *Bordetella pertussis*, a Gram-negative aerobic bacterium. The related species *B. parapertussis* causes a similar but generally milder illness. Pertussis is very infectious and occurs most frequently in children, but may be more common in adults than once thought.[1,2] The incidence of pertussis has been greatly reduced by the active immunisation of infants (see under Pertussis Vaccines, p.1526) and effective prevention by the adequate uptake of vaccine remains the ultimate objective. Reporting on a resurgence of pertussis in the USA in 1993, thought to be due in part to failure of whole-cell pertussis vaccine, Christie *et al.*[3] considered that, in addition to an accelerated schedule of vaccination, prompt use of erythromycin for treatment and prophylaxis may help to contain epidemics.

Erythromycin is the antibacterial of choice at any stage of the disease. Once infection has occurred erythromycin is thought to render the patient non-infectious by eliminating nasopharyngeal carriage of *B. pertussis*. Such treatment is unlikely to affect the clinical course of pertussis because diagnosis is difficult until the paroxysmal stage, by which time the bacteria have already damaged the respiratory tract and released their toxins.[4] Erythromycin is also given prophylactically to close contacts. Erythromycin 50 mg per kg body-weight daily for 14 days, whether for treatment or prophylaxis, has been recommended,[5] and the estolate ester was favoured in order to achieve maximum blood concentrations. However, a 7-day course of erythromycin estolate was reported to be as effective as a 14-day course for treatment.[6] Courses of azithromycin for 5 days or clarithromycin for 7 days were also effective.[7] Decreased transmission and severity of the disease has been seen in adults and adolescents in a confined setting, when erythromycin (as base or ethyl succinate) was used for treatment, and prophylaxis in those exposed, and especially when started within 14 days of the first case being identified.[8] Erythromycin prophylaxis was also effective in a family setting, especially if started before the occurrence of the first secondary case.[9]

Strains of *B. pertussis* resistant to erythromycin have been reported in the USA, but do not appear to be widespread.[10] Co-trimoxazole has been suggested as an alternative to erythromycin for both treatment and prophylaxis.[10]

1. Mortimer EA. Pertussis and its prevention: a family affair. *J Infect Dis* 1990; **161:** 473–9.
2. Wright SW, *et al.* Pertussis infection in adults with persistent cough. *JAMA* 1995; **273:** 1044–6.
3. Christie CDC, *et al.* The 1993 epidemic of pertussis in Cincinnati: resurgence of disease in a highly immunized population of children. *N Engl J Med* 1994; **331:** 16–21.
4. Moxon ER, Rappuoli R. Modern vaccines: Haemophilus influenzae infections and whooping cough. *Lancet* 1990; **335:** 1324–9.
5. Bass JW. Pertussis: current status of prevention and treatment. *Pediatr Infect Dis* 1985; **4:** 614–19.
6. Halperin SA, *et al.* Seven days of erythromycin estolate is as effective as fourteen days for the treatment of Bordetella pertussis infections. *Pediatrics* 1997; **100:** 65–71.
7. Aoyama T, *et al.* Efficacy of short-term treatment of pertussis with clarithromycin and azithromycin. *J Pediatr* 1996; **129:** 761–4.
8. Steketee RW, *et al.* Evidence for a high attack rate and efficacy of erythromycin prophylaxis in a pertussis outbreak in a facility for the developmentally disabled. *J Infect Dis* 1988; **157:** 434–40.
9. De Serres G, *et al.* Field effectiveness of erythromycin prophylaxis to prevent pertussis within families. *Pediatr Infect Dis J* 1995; **14:** 969–75.
10. Centers for Disease Control. Erythromycin-resistant Bordetella pertussis—Yuma County, Arizona, May-October 1994. *MMWR* 1994; **43:** 807–10.

Pharyngitis

Pharyngitis and tonsillitis are upper respiratory-tract infections with similar causes and occur especially in children. Acute pharyngitis is an inflammatory syndrome of the oropharynx that may include the tonsils whereas tonsillitis is strictly speaking a more localised infection. The commonest causes are viral and 'sore throat' is often a symptom of the common cold as well as influenza and infectious mononucleosis. For further details of these viral infections, see under Choice of Antiviral, p.595.

The most important bacterial cause of acute pharyngitis and tonsillitis is the group A beta-haemolytic streptococcus, *Streptococcus pyogenes*. An erythrogenic toxin-producing strain causes pharyngitis and tonsillitis in scarlet fever.

In view of the prevalence of a viral cause, opinions have differed over whether and when to treat pharyngitis with antimicrobial drugs. Some have advocated waiting until a definite diagnosis of *Str. pyogenes* infection is made, but others treat immediately if streptococcal pharyngitis is suspected because of the risk of longer term complications such as rheumatic fever and the need to eradicate *Str. pyogenes* from the throat.[1-3] The incidence of rheumatic fever has been low for many years in developed countries, but recently there has been evidence of a resurgence in the USA. Thus, in addition to shortening the illness and interrupting transmission, the antibacterial treatment of streptococcal pharyngitis also serves as primary prevention of rheumatic fever (see below). However, in countries in which the incidence of rheumatic fever remains low the routine administration of antibacterials for the management of sore throats is discouraged.[4,5]

Penicillin is the standard treatment for streptococcal pharyngitis or tonsillitis, generally as phenoxymethylpenicillin by mouth for 10 days; benzylpenicillin may be given by injection initially. A single intramuscular injection of benzathine penicillin is perhaps the treatment of choice, especially if compliance with a 10-day course of oral penicillin is unlikely, and is advocated by WHO and the American Heart Association for the primary prevention of rheumatic fever (see under Rheumatic Fever, below), but the injection may not be available in some countries. Ampicillin should probably be avoided because of the risk of maculopapular rash if the patient proves to have infectious mononucleosis.[6] Erythromycin or another macrolide may be given to penicillin-allergic patients, except where there is evidence of significant resistance, as in Japan[7] and Finland;[8] it may also be a better choice than penicillin if there is a likelihood of infection with *Arcanobacterium (Corynebacterium) haemolyticum* (see below). Oral cephalosporins are another alternative.

Despite the general effectiveness of penicillin a trend of increasing numbers of relapses and recurrent infections has been noted.[9] Some treatment failures have been attributed to poor patient compliance with a 10-day course of penicillin and attempts to overcome this have included giving fewer daily doses or shortening the length of treatment. Twice-daily doses of phenoxymethylpenicillin 250 mg were reported to be as effective as doses three times daily,[10] but a single daily dose of 750 mg was not.[11] Courses of phenoxymethylpenicillin shorter than 10 days have not proved effective.[12,13] There is some evidence that shorter courses may be possible with some alternative antibacterials. Studies have shown 5-day course of erythromycin[14] or cefotiam hexetil,[15] 3-day[16] or 5-day[17] courses of azithromycin, and a 4-day course of cefuroxime axetil[18] to be as effective as a 10-day course of phenoxymethylpenicillin.

In addition to poor compliance, treatment failures with penicillin, leading to recurrent infection, might be explained by the presence of beta-lactamase-producing oropharyngeal bacteria that are able to protect *Str. pyogenes* against penicillin.[19] Antibacterials less susceptible to beta lactamase have been effective, sometimes more so than phenoxymethylpenicillin. They include the oral cephalosporins cefaclor,[20] cefuroxime axetil,[21] cefixime,[22] cefprozil,[23] and cefadroxil[24] and the combined preparation amoxycillin with clavulanic acid[25,26] (like ampicillin, amoxycillin should perhaps be avoided because of the risk of maculopapular rash if the patient turns out to have infectious mononucleosis). Clindamycin has eradicated *Str. pyogenes* and beta-lactamase-producing bacteria in children of 12 years and under with recurrent tonsillitis, but might be less effective in older patients.[27] It was also effective where penicillin and erythromycin had failed in an outbreak of streptococcal pharyngitis.[28]

Pharyngeal carriage of *Str. pyogenes* is common, especially in primary school children and thus its presence does not necessarily reflect acute infection. Eradication may be beneficial in selected cases and has been achieved by a single intramuscular injection of benzathine penicillin together with a 4-day course of oral rifampicin;[29] a 10-day course of oral clindamycin has also been effective.[30] In order to ensure that outbreaks of *Str. pyogenes* are prevented in closely confined populations, some have recommended prophylactic antibacterials for *all* members of these populations, without exception.[31]

Other bacterial causes of pharyngitis include *Arcanobacterium (Corynebacterium) haemolyticum, Chlamydia pneumoniae, Corynebacterium diphtheriae* (see under Diphtheria, above), *Neisseria gonorrhoeae* (see under Gonorrhoea, above), group C beta-haemolytic streptococci, and anaerobic bacteria.

A. haemolyticum is thought to be an important cause of pharyngitis in adolescents and young adults; there is often an accompanying scarlatiniform rash. It has been reported to respond to a single injection of benzathine penicillin or a 10-day course of erythromycin by mouth, but not to phenoxymethylpenicillin.[32]

Pharyngitis is often associated with infection with *Chlamydia pneumoniae* (formerly known as the TWAR strain of *C. psittaci*). Tetracycline or erythromycin are effective antibacterials.[33]

1. Anonymous. Bacterial pharyngitis. *Lancet* 1987; **i:** 1241–2.
2. Marcovitch H. Sore throats. *Arch Dis Child* 1990; **65:** 249–50.
3. Lang SDR, Singh K. The sore throat: when to investigate and when to prescribe. *Drugs* 1990; **40:** 854–62.
4. Little P, *et al.* Reattendance and complications in a randomised trial of prescribing strategies for sore throat: the medicalising effect of prescribing antibiotics. *Br Med J* 1997; **315:** 350–2.
5. Del Mar CB, Glasziou PP. Antibiotics for the symptoms and complications of sore throat (Cochrane Review). Available in the Cochrane Library; Issue 3. Oxford: Update Software; 1998.
6. Green AD. Treatment of choice for childhood tonsillitis. *Br Med J* 1986; **293:** 1030.

7. Maruyama S, *et al.* Sensitivity of group A streptococci to antibiotics: prevalence of resistance to erythromycin in Japan. *Am J Dis Child* 1979; **133:** 1143–5.
8. Seppälä H, *et al.* Resistance to erythromycin in group A streptococci. *N Engl J Med* 1992; **326:** 292–7.
9. Dillon HC. Streptococcal pharyngitis in the 1980s. *Pediatr Infect Dis J* 1987; **6:** 123–30.
10. Gerber MA, *et al.* Twice-daily penicillin in the treatment of streptococcal pharyngitis. *Am J Dis Child* 1985; **139:** 1145–8.
11. Gerber MA, *et al.* Failure of once-daily penicillin V therapy for streptococcal pharyngitis. *Am J Dis Child* 1989; **143:** 153–5.
12. Gerber MA, *et al.* Five vs ten days of penicillin V therapy for streptococcal pharyngitis. *Am J Dis Child* 1987; **141:** 224–7.
13. Strömberg A, *et al.* Five versus ten days treatment of group A streptococcal pharyngotonsillitis: a randomized controlled clinical trial with phenoxymethylpenicillin and cefadroxil. *Scand J Infect Dis* 1988; **20:** 37–46.
14. Adam D, *et al.* Five days of erythromycin estolate versus ten days of penicillin V in the treatment of group A streptococcal tonsillopharyngitis in children. *Eur J Clin Microbiol Infect Dis* 1996; **15:** 712–17.
15. Carbon C, *et al.* A double-blind randomized trial comparing the efficacy and safety of a 5-day course of cefotiam hexetil with that of a 10-day course of penicillin V in adult patients with pharyngitis caused by group A β-haemolytic streptococci. *J Antimicrob Chemother* 1995; **35:** 843–54.
16. O'Doherty B, *et al.* Azithromycin versus penicillin V in the treatment of paediatric patients with acute streptococcal pharyngitis/tonsillitis. *Eur J Clin Microbiol Infect Dis* 1996; **15:** 718–24.
17. Hooton TM. A comparison of azithromycin and penicillin V for the treatment of streptococcal pharyngitis. *Am J Med* 1991; **91**(3A): 23S–26S.
18. Aujard Y, *et al.* Comparative efficacy and safety of four-day cefuroxime axetil and ten-day penicillin treatment of group A beta-hemolytic streptococcal pharyngitis in children. *Pediatr Infect Dis J* 1995; **14:** 295–300.
19. Brook I. The role of β-lactamase-producing bacteria in the persistence of streptococcal tonsillar infection. *Rev Infect Dis* 1984; **6:** 601–7.
20. Stillerman M. Comparison of oral cephalosporins with penicillin therapy for group A streptococcal pharyngitis. *Pediatr Infect Dis* 1986; **5:** 649–54.
21. Gooch WM, *et al.* Efficacy of cefuroxime axetil suspension compared with that of penicillin V suspension in children with group A streptococcal pharyngitis. *Antimicrob Agents Chemother* 1993; **37:** 159–63.
22. Kiani R, *et al.* Comparative, multicenter studies of cefixime and amoxicillin in the treatment of respiratory tract infections. *Am J Med* 1988; **85** (suppl 3A): 6–13.
23. Milatovic D, *et al.* Cefprozil versus penicillin V in treatment of streptococcal tonsillopharyngitis. *Antimicrob Agents Chemother* 1993; **37:** 1620–3.
24. Milatovic D, Knauer J. Cefadroxil versus penicillin in the treatment of streptococcal tonsillopharyngitis. *Eur J Clin Microbiol Infect Dis* 1989; **8:** 282–8.
25. Brook I. Treatment of patients with acute recurrent tonsillitis due to group A β-haemolytic streptococci: a prospective randomized study comparing penicillin and amoxycillin/clavulanate potassium. *J Antimicrob Chemother* 1989; **24:** 227–33.
26. Dykhuizen RS, *et al.* Phenoxymethyl penicillin versus co-amoxiclav in the treatment of acute streptococcal pharyngitis, and the role of β-lactamase activity in saliva. *J Antimicrob Chemother* 1996; **37:** 133–8.
27. Foote PA, Brook I. Penicillin and clindamycin therapy in recurrent tonsillitis: effect of microbial flora. *Arch Otolaryngol Head Neck Surg* 1989; **115:** 856–9.
28. Raz R, *et al.* Clindamycin in the treatment of an outbreak of streptococcal pharyngitis in a kibbutz due to beta-lactamase producing organisms. *J Chemother* 1990; **2:** 182–4.
29. Tanz RR, *et al.* Penicillin plus rifampin eradicates pharyngeal carriage of group A streptococci. *J Pediatr* 1985; **106:** 876–80.
30. Tanz RR, *et al.* Clindamycin treatment of chronic pharyngeal carriage of group A streptococci. *J Pediatr* 1991; **119:** 123–8.
31. Gray GC, *et al.* Hyperendemic Streptococcus pyogenes infection despite prophylaxis with penicillin G benzathine. *N Engl J Med* 1991; **325:** 92–7.
32. Miller RA, *et al.* Corynebacterium hemolyticum as a cause of pharyngitis and scarlatiniform rash in young adults. *Ann Intern Med* 1986; **105:** 867–72.
33. Grayston JT, *et al.* A new respiratory tract pathogen: Chlamydia pneumoniae strain TWAR. *J Infect Dis* 1990; **161:** 618–25.

Pinta

See under Syphilis, below.

Plague

Plague is caused by the Gram-negative bacillus *Yersinia pestis* (*Yersinia pseudotuberculosis* subsp. *pestis*) and is usually transmitted to man via rodents and their infected fleas. It has occurred as worldwide pandemics, for example, the Black Death in Europe in the Middle Ages. In the 1980s the largest numbers of cases reported were in Tanzania, Vietnam, Brazil, and Peru.[1] Plague may take several forms of which bubonic plague is the most common; others include pneumonic, septicaemic, and meningitic plague. Treatment with streptomycin, tetracycline, or chloramphenicol is highly effective in all forms if recognised early.[2] Many consider streptomycin to be the antibacterial of choice,[1] but the possibility of a 'Herxheimer' type reaction resulting from the bactericidal effect of streptomycin has prompted some to prefer tetracycline or to use lower doses of streptomycin together with tetracycline. Chloramphenicol has been preferred in meningitic plague because it crosses the blood-brain barrier.

Commenting on the plague epidemic that occurred in India in 1994, workers from US Centers for Disease Control[3] also noted that streptomycin continues to be the drug of choice for treating plague, that tetracycline and gentamicin are alternatives, and that chloramphenicol is preferred for plague meningitis. They considered that prophylaxis should be given to those who have had face-to-face contact or who have occupied a closed space with someone who has pneumonic plague. For prophylaxis, tetracycline can be given to adults and older children or sulphonamides to children of 8 years or less; chloramphenicol is also effective.[3]

Infection with a strain of *Y. pestis* resistant to all the drugs usually effective against plague identified in a patient from Madagascar[4] responded to treatment with co-trimoxazole and streptomycin.

A vaccine is available for active immunisation.

1. Butler T. The black death past and present 1: plague in the 1980s. *Trans R Soc Trop Med Hyg* 1989; **83:** 458–60.
2. Public Health Laboratory Service Communicable Disease Surveillance Centre. Plague. *Br Med J* 1983; **287:** 118–19.
3. Campbell GL, Hughes JM. Plague in India: a new warning from an old nemesis. *Ann Intern Med* 1995; **122:** 151–3.
4. Galimand M, *et al.* Multidrug resistance in Yersinia pestis mediated by a transferable plasmid. *N Engl J Med* 1997; **337:** 677–80.

Pneumonia

Pneumonia, or inflammation of the lungs with consolidation, is mostly due to bacterial or viral infection, but may be caused by fungi in immunocompromised patients or by the aspiration of chemical irritants. Interstitial pneumonitis is a common complication in cancer patients and has also been associated with certain drugs, for example amiodarone, bleomycin, and nitrofurantoin; sometimes a hypersensitivity reaction has been suspected.

The aetiology of infective pneumonia, and therefore the choice of treatment, differs according to whether it is community-acquired or hospital-acquired (nosocomial) and whether the patient was previously healthy, has chronic lung disease or other debilitating condition, is very young or very old, is immunocompromised, or has pneumonia as a result of aspiration.

Community-acquired pneumonia. In community-acquired pneumonia[1-4,43] the commonest pathogen in previously healthy subjects is *Streptococcus pneumoniae* (pneumococcus). Onset of pneumococcal pneumonia can be very rapid and treatment should be started promptly. *Str. pneumoniae* has usually been considered sensitive to the penicillins benzylpenicillin, amoxycillin, or ampicillin; to cephalosporins; to erythromycin; or to co-trimoxazole, but a 1991 review of resistance patterns in Europe[5] concluded that *Str. pneumoniae* no longer had predictable antibacterial susceptibility. The problem of resistant pneumococci on a worldwide basis has been noted in a recent review[6] and such resistance is a major concern in the USA,[7,8] highlighting the need for a more effective pneumococcal vaccine. Penicillin-resistant strains, some with high levels of resistance have been reported in various countries, especially Spain.[9-12] Penicillin-resistant *Str. pneumoniae* is also being increasingly identified in Australia.[13] In a survey between 1986 and 1989 of 61 centres in the UK all strains of *Str. pneumoniae* tested were sensitive to penicillin,[14] but localised pockets of resistance have been reported[15] and there appears to be a general trend in the UK of increases in the incidence of pneumococci resistant to, or with reduced susceptibility to, penicillin and other antibacterials commonly used for treatment.[16] However, the routine use of penicillin for community-acquired pneumonia may still be reasonable in many countries and, indeed, the latest study in Spain[12] noted that, although there were increased levels of resistance to penicillins and to cephalosporins, this had not been associated with increased mortality so that these antibacterials remained the drugs of choice. Erythromycin or macrolide resistance has also been reported in some countries,[17-19] especially in France where macrolide consumption is relatively high.[5] In the 1986–9 UK survey[14] 99% of strains were susceptible to erythromycin, although there was increased reporting of resistant strains in the 1992 review.[16] Resistance to co-trimoxazole and chloramphenicol has been noted in Pakistan.[20]

Mycoplasma pneumoniae is also an important cause of community-acquired pneumonia. Epidemics occur about every 4 years and the one underway in Europe in 1991 would probably have been responsible for up to 20% of all community-acquired pneumonia during 1992.[21] Erythromycin or tetracycline are the antibacterials of choice against *M. pneumoniae*; erythromycin is usually recommended when mycoplasmal pneumonia is suspected.[21,22] The wisdom of giving erythromycin alone for initial treatment of community-acquired pneumonia has been questioned[23] since even during *M. pneumoniae* epidemics pneumococci remain the commonest cause and, although they are usually sensitive to erythromycin, resistance has increasingly, albeit rarely,[14] been reported.[17-19] Giving erythromycin together with a penicillin has therefore been suggested,[21] although as noted above penicillin-resistant pneumococci have also been reported.

Other bacteria that may be responsible for community-acquired pneumonia include *Staphylococcus aureus*, which usually occurs as a secondary bacterial infection following influenza and is associated with high mortality; *Haemophilus influenzae* and, more recently, *Moraxella (Branhamella) catarrhalis*[24] especially in patients with chronic lung disease; *Legionella pneumophila* (see Legionnaires' Disease, above); *Chlamydia psittaci* (see Psittacosis, below); *Chlamydia pneumoniae* (formerly known as the TWAR strain of *Chlamydia psittaci*);[25] and *Coxiella burnetii* (see Q fever, below). Gram-negative bacilli rarely cause pneumonia in the community, especially in previously healthy patients. Anaerobic bacteria are associated with aspiration pneumonia. Viruses are the commonest pathogens in young children.

Guidelines for the initial *empirical* treatment of community-acquired pneumonia in the UK[22] and in the USA[26] have been published by the British and the American Thoracic Societies respectively. In the UK[22] treatment is usually with benzylpenicillin, ampicillin, or amoxycillin. Erythromycin is an alternative in penicillin-allergic patients and should also be given during epidemics of mycoplasmal pneumonia and when *Legionella* is suspected. Second- or third-generation cephalosporins such as cefuroxime or cefotaxime are other alternatives to penicillin treatment.[22] An antistaphylococcal penicillin such as flucloxacillin should be added to treatment during influenza epidemics. Severe pneumonia of unknown aetiology may be treated by a combination of erythromycin and a second- or third-generation cephalosporin; an alternative regimen is ampicillin with flucloxacillin and erythromycin.[22] In the USA,[26] the preferred treatment in outpatients with uncomplicated disease and under 60 years of age is erythromycin (or azithromycin or clarithromycin if the patients are intolerant to erythromycin or if they are smokers when *H. influenzae* may also be a consideration). Tetracycline is an alternative if there is macrolide allergy or intolerance. Outpatients who are over 60 years of age or who have co-existing disease should be given a second-generation cephalosporin, or co-trimoxazole, or a combination of a beta-lactam and a beta-lactamase inhibitor, the latter option being also with a macrolide if *Legionella* infection is a concern; rifampicin may be added for hospitalised patients if there is confirmed *Legionella* infection.[26] For severe pneumonia in hospitalised patients a macrolide is given (again with rifampicin if appropriate); in addition, an aminoglycoside and a third-generation cephalosporin with antipseudomonal activity are employed or other antipseudomonal drugs such as imipenem/cilastatin or ciprofloxacin may be used.[26] Local patterns of resistance should be borne in mind (see, e.g. pneumococci, above). Definitive treatment recommendations for pneumonia due to penicillin-resistant pneumococci are lacking;[16] high-dose penicillin therapy may be adequate for strains with intermediate resistance.[12,27] Penicillin-resistant *H. influenzae* may be a problem in some areas. Many isolates of *Moraxella (Branhamella) catarrhalis* produce beta lactamase and are resistant to penicillins, but patients have responded to amoxycillin with clavulanic acid (co-amoxiclav), cefotaxime, or co-trimoxazole.[24] An aminoglycoside has been added to initial therapy in patients at special risk of Gram-negative bacillary pneumonia, including those with chronic lung disease, alcoholism, diabetes, heart failure, and chronic debility.[28] Atypical pneumonias such as those caused by *Chlamydia* or *Coxiella burnetii* may be treated with erythromycin or tetracycline; azithromycin and clarithromycin are possible alternatives for *C. pneumoniae* infections.[29]

In *children* pneumonia is caused by a wider spectrum of organisms than in adults.[30] Pneumonia in neonates is usually due to organisms acquired from the mother's genital tract, especially group B streptococci, *Escherichia coli*, and *Klebsiella pneumoniae*; initial treatment with gentamicin and benzylpenicillin or ampicillin has been suggested. For prophylaxis against group B streptococci in neonates, see under Perinatal Streptococcal Infections, above. In the USA, *Chlamydia trachomatis* is said to be the commonest cause in infants up to 3 months of age;[30] erythromycin is the treatment of choice or, alternatively, sulphafurazole.[31] Viruses, especially respiratory syncytial virus, are the commonest pathogens in infants and children up to 4 years of age and, as in adults, pneumococci are the commonest bacterial pathogens.[30] Although the pathogens are often not identified all children with pneumonia should be given antibacterials because of the possibility of bacterial infection.[30] Benzylpenicillin or ampicillin is effective, but severely ill infants should be given flucloxacillin and an aminoglycoside as well; erythromycin is used to treat chlamydial and mycoplasmal infection.[30] In developing countries acute lower respiratory-tract infection is a major cause of childhood mortality, especially in children under 5 years. Most die from pneumonia due to *Str. pneumoniae* or *H. influenzae*. In guidance from WHO[32] for the management of these infections in small hospitals, both organisms were considered to be sensitive usually to benzylpenicillin, ampicillin, amoxycillin, co-trimoxazole, and chloramphenicol and these drugs were included in protocols for the treatment of pneumonia, according to severity. However, in a study from Pakistan[20] the majority of isolates of *Str. pneumoniae* were resistant or had decreased susceptibility to at least one antibacterial, especially co-trimoxazole (62%) (recommended by WHO[32] as an alternative to procaine penicillin, amoxycillin, or ampicillin) and chloramphenicol (39%) (recommended by WHO[32] for very severe pneumonia). Even so, community-based treatment of pneumonia with a standard course of oral co-trimoxazole was of benefit in Nepalese[33] and Indian[34] infants. For children with only mild acute respiratory infections the WHO recommendation to provide supportive care without antibacterials[32] has been endorsed by an Indonesian study in which ampicillin was of no benefit.[35]

Hospital-acquired pneumonia. Most reports on hospital-acquired or nosocomial pneumonia have been from the USA.[1] Aerobic Gram-negative bacilli such as *Pseudomonas* and *Klebsiella* are the dominant cause and two or more pathogens are often found. *Staph. aureus* and *Legionella* spp. may also cause a substantial amount of nosocomial pneumonia.[1] Broad-spectrum antibacterial therapy is essential initially with, for example, a third-generation cephalosporin such as cefotaxime or ceftazidime or an antipseudomonal penicillin together with an aminoglycoside. Monotherapy with monobactams, cephalosporins, or imipenem has also been used.[36] In one study,[37] intravenous ciprofloxacin was as effective as ceftazidime, but treatment failures with ciprofloxacin included persisting *Staph. aureus* and streptococcal infections. Nosocomial pneumonia is especially likely in immunocompromised or neutropenic patients. Prophylactic measures in ventilated patients are those mentioned under Intensive Care, above.

Immunocompromised patients. Immunosuppressed patients are at special risk of pneumonia. In addition to the bacteria mentioned above they are susceptible to opportunistic infections with *Mycobacterium tuberculosis* (see under Tuberculosis, below); viruses such as *Cytomegalovirus*; and fungi, in particular *Pneumocystis carinii*, are also causes of pneumonia in these patients.

Interstitial pneumonitis is a common complication in cancer patients. It may sometimes be drug-related, but diagnosis of the cause is difficult. Early empirical treatment with erythromycin and co-trimoxazole, active against *Legionella*, *Mycoplasma*, and *Pneumocystis carinii*, has been advocated,[38] although individualised patient-directed care may be preferable.[39]

Aspiration pneumonia. Aspiration of organisms present in the upper respiratory tract into the lungs, often as a result of loss of consciousness or difficulty in swallowing, can cause aspiration pneumonia. When community-acquired the organisms responsible are predominantly anaerobes, but in hospital-acquired aspiration pneumonia Gram-negative bacilli and *Staph. aureus* are also found.[1] Anaerobic pulmonary infections have been reviewed by Bartlett.[40] Confusion has arisen over the term 'aspiration pneumonia' because it has also been applied more generally to aspiration, for example, of gastric acid (Mendelson's syndrome), resulting in chemical pneumonitis and not associated with bacterial infection. *Lung abscess* generally characterises late-stage aspiration pneumonia involving anaerobic bacteria. The aetiology is rarely established, but specific anaerobic bacteria involved include *Peptostreptococcus*, *Prevotella melaninogenica* (*Bacteroides melaninogenicus*), and *Fusobacterium nucleatum*. Nearly all patients with anaerobic pulmonary infections are treated empirically. Benzylpenicillin used to be considered the treatment of choice, but this is less certain now because of increasing resistance in anaerobes, often due to beta-lactamase production, and because of a study demonstrating the superiority of clindamycin.[41] Another study has reinforced the value of clindamycin in the presence of penicillin-resistant *Prevotella melaninogenica*.[42] Responses to metronidazole alone have been poor. Antibacterial regimens advocated include benzylpenicillin intravenously (despite its apparent inferiority to clindamycin); clindamycin orally or intravenously; or an aminopenicillin such as amoxycillin or ampicillin with metronidazole, each given intravenously or by mouth.[22,40] Most patients with lung abscess receive parenteral therapy until they become afebrile and show clinical improvement; oral therapy may then continue for weeks or months if necessary. Most of the available information relates to lung abscess but is probably applicable to aspiration pneumonia without abscess as well.

1. Macfarlane JT. Treatment of lower respiratory infections. *Lancet* 1987; **ii:** 1446–9.
2. Innes JA. Community acquired pneumonia. *Br Med J* 1987; **295:** 1083–4.
3. Anonymous. Antibiotics for community-acquired pneumonia in adults. *Drug Ther Bull* 1988; **26:** 13–16.
4. Bartlett JG, Mundy LM. Community-acquired pneumonia. *N Engl J Med* 1995; **333:** 1618–24.
5. Baquero F, *et al.* A review of antibiotic resistance patterns of Streptococcus pneumoniae in Europe. *J Antimicrob Chemother* 1991; **28** (suppl C): 31–8.
6. Friedland IR, McCracken GH. Management of infections caused by antibiotic-resistant Streptococcus pneumoniae. *N Engl J Med* 1994; **331:** 377–82.
7. Breiman RF, *et al.* Emergence of drug-resistant pneumococcal infections in the United States. *JAMA* 1994; **271:** 1831–5.
8. Hofmann J, *et al.* The prevalence of drug-resistant Streptococcus pneumoniae in Atlanta. *N Engl J Med* 1995; **333:** 481–6.
9. Anonymous. Penicillin-resistant pneumococci. *Lancet* 1988; **i:** 1142–3.
10. Casal J, *et al.* Increase in resistance to penicillin in pneumococci in Spain. *Lancet* 1989; **i:** 735.
11. Klugman KP, Koornhof HJ. Worldwide increase in pneumococcal antibiotic resistance. *Lancet* 1989: **ii:** 444.
12. Pallares R, *et al.* Resistance to penicillin and cephalosporin and mortality from severe pneumococcal pneumonia in Barcelona, Spain. *N Engl J Med* 1995; **333:** 474–80. Correction. *ibid.*; 1655.
13. Collignon PJ, Bell JM. Drug-resistant Streptococcus pneumoniae: the beginning of the end for many antibiotics? *Med J Aust* 1996: **164:** 64–7.
14. Spencer RC, *et al.* A three year survey of clinical isolates in the United Kingdom and their antimicrobial susceptibility. *J Antimicrob Chemother* 1990; **26:** 435–46.
15. Ridgway EJ, Allen KD. Penicillin resistance in pneumococci. *J Antimicrob Chemother* 1991; **27:** 251–2.
16. George RC, *et al.* Antibiotic-resistant pneumococci in the United Kingdom. *Commun Dis Rep* 1992; **2:** R37–R43.
17. Eykyn SJ. Pneumococcaemia caused by erythromycin-resistant Streptococcus pneumoniae type 14. *Lancet* 1988; **ii:** 1086.
18. Verhaegen J, *et al.* Erythromycin-resistant Streptococcus pneumoniae. *Lancet* 1988; **ii:** 1432–3.
19. Warren RE, *et al.* Erythromycin-resistant Streptococcus pneumoniae. *Lancet* 1988; **ii:** 1433. Correction. *ibid.* 1989; **i:** 58.
20. Mastro TD, *et al.* Antimicrobial resistance of pneumococci in children with acute lower respiratory tract infection in Pakistan. *Lancet* 1991; **337:** 156–9.
21. Anonymous. Mycoplasma pneumoniae. *Lancet* 1991; **337:** 651–2.
22. The British Thoracic Society. Guidelines for the management of community-acquired pneumonia in adults admitted to hospital. *Br J Hosp Med* 1993; **49:** 346–50.
23. Davies AJ, Jolley A. Community-acquired pneumonia. *Lancet* 1991; **337:** 1101.
24. Wright PW, *et al.* A descriptive study of 42 cases of Branhamella catarrhalis pneumonia. *Am J Med* 1990; **88** (suppl 5A): 2S–8S.
25. Grayston JT, *et al.* A new respiratory tract pathogen: Chlamydia pneumoniae strain TWAR. *J Infect Dis* 1990; **161:** 618–25.
26. American Thoracic Society. Guidelines for the initial management of adults with community-acquired pneumonia: diagnosis, assessment of severity, and initial antimicrobial therapy. *Am Rev Respir Dis* 1993; **148:** 1418–26.
27. Klugman KP. Pneumococcal resistance to antibiotics. *Clin Microbiol Rev* 1990; **3:** 171–96.
28. McGehee JL, *et al.* Treatment of pneumonia in patients at risk of infection with Gram-negative bacilli. *Am J Med* 1988; **84:** 597–602.
29. Hammerschlag MR. Antimicrobial susceptibility and therapy of infections caused by Chlamydia pneumoniae. *Antimicrob Agents Chemother* 1994; **38:** 1873–8.
30. Anonymous. Pneumonia in childhood. *Lancet* 1988; **i:** 741–3.
31. Anonymous. Drugs for sexually transmitted diseases. *Med Lett Drugs Ther* 1995; **37:** 117–22.
32. WHO. *Respiratory infections in children: management in small hospitals*. Geneva: WHO, 1988.
33. Pandey MR, *et al.* Reduction in total under-five mortality in western Nepal through community-based antimicrobial treatment of pneumonia. *Lancet* 1991; **338:** 993–7.
34. Bang AT, *et al.* Pneumonia in neonates: can it be managed in the community? *Arch Dis Child* 1993; **68:** 550–6.
35. Sutrisna B, *et al.* Randomised, controlled trial of effectiveness of ampicillin in mild acute respiratory infections in Indonesian children. *Lancet* 1991; **338:** 471–4.
36. LaForce FM. Systemic antimicrobial therapy of nosocomial pneumonia: monotherapy versus combination therapy. *Eur J Clin Microbiol Infect Dis* 1989; **8:** 61–8.
37. Rapp RP, *et al.* Intravenous ciprofloxacin versus ceftazidime for treatment of nosocomial pneumonia and urinary tract infection. *Clin Pharm* 1991; **10:** 49–55.
38. Browne MJ, *et al.* A randomized trial of open lung biopsy versus empiric antimicrobial therapy in cancer patients with diffuse pulmonary infiltrates. *J Clin Oncol* 1990; **8:** 222–9.
39. Bustamante CI, Wade JC. Treatment of interstitial pneumonia in cancer patients: is empiric antibiotic therapy the answer? *J Clin Oncol* 1990; **8:** 200–2.
40. Bartlett JG. Treatment of anaerobic pulmonary infections. *J Antimicrob Chemother* 1989; **24:** 836–40.
41. Levison ME, *et al.* Clindamycin compared with penicillin for the treatment of anaerobic lung abscess. *Ann Intern Med* 1983; **98:** 466–71.
42. Gudiol F, *et al.* Clindamycin vs penicillin for anaerobic lung infections: high rate of penicillin failures associated with penicillin-resistant Bacteroides melaninogenicus. *Arch Intern Med* 1990; **150:** 2525–9.
43. Brown PD, Lerner SA. Community-acquired pneumonia. *Lancet* 1998; **352:** 1295–1302.

Pregnancy and the neonate

For infections associated specifically with pregnancy, see under Endometritis (above), Perinatal Streptococcal Infections (above), and Premature Labour (below).

Premature labour

There is evidence of an association between premature rupture of membranes, maternal genito-urinary infection, and preterm labour. Various bacteria have been implicated, including group B streptococci, *Chlamydia trachomatis* (above), and those associated with bacterial vaginosis (above) and adjunctive antibacterial treatment is under evaluation.

In one study penicillin reduced the incidence of preterm labour when given to pregnant women with group B streptococci in their urine, vagina, and cervix.[1] Premature labour also increases the risk of neonates acquiring group B streptococcal infection from their mothers and intrapartum antibacterials may be employed to reduce this risk—see Perinatal Streptococcal Infections, above. In other studies, erythromycin appeared to reduce the risk of premature rupture of membranes in pregnant women with *C. trachomatis* infection.[2,3]

Antibacterial treatment after premature rupture of membranes might also be beneficial. A meta-analysis[4] of randomised, controlled trials involving women with premature rupture of membranes before 37 weeks' gestation concluded that systemic antibacterial therapy reduced the incidence of delivery within one week and reduced chorioamnionitis and postpartum infection. A reduction in neonatal sepsis and intraventricular haemorrhage was also reported in this[4] and another meta-analysis.[5] Antibacterials used have included ampicillin, mezlocillin, piperacillin, erythromycin, ceftizoxime and cephalexin. A further meta-analysis[6] of studies in women with premature labour but *without* premature rupture of membranes found that the potential benefit of antibacterials in terms of reduced neonatal infection was outweighed by an apparent increased risk of neonatal mortality.

1. Thomsen AC, *et al.* Antibiotic elimination of group-B streptococci in urine in prevention of preterm labour. *Lancet* 1987; **i:** 591–3.
2. Cohen I, *et al.* Improved pregnancy outcome following successful treatment of chlamydial infection. *JAMA* 1990; **263:** 3160–3.
3. McGregor JA, *et al.* Cervicovaginal microflora and pregnancy outcome: results of a double-blind, placebo-controlled trial of erythromycin treatment. *Am J Obstet Gynecol* 1990; **163:** 1580–91.
4. Mercer BM, Arheart KL. Antimicrobial therapy in expectant management of preterm premature rupture of the membranes. *Lancet* 1995; **346:** 1271–9. Correction. *ibid.* 1996; **347:** 410.
5. Egarter C, *et al.* Antibiotic treatment in preterm premature rupture of membranes and neonatal morbidity: a metaanalysis. *Am J Obstet Gynecol* 1996; **174:** 589–97.
6. Egarter C, *et al.* Adjunctive antibiotic treatment in preterm labor and neonatal morbidity: a meta-analysis. *Obstet Gynecol* 1996; **88:** 303–9.

Proctitis

The treatment of rectal infections caused by *Neisseria gonorrhoeae* and *Chlamydia trachomatis* is discussed under Gonorrhoea and Chlamydial Infections, above.

Ceftriaxone 125 mg intramuscularly together with doxycycline 100 mg twice daily by mouth for 7 days is recommended by the Centers for Disease Control in the USA[1] for empirical treatment of sexually transmitted proctitis and should be effective against *N. gonorrhoeae* and *C. trachomatis*.

Proctitis may also be associated with herpes simplex infections (p.597).

1. Centers for Disease Control. 1998 Guidelines for treatment of sexually transmitted diseases. *MMWR* 1998; **47** (RR-1): 104–5.

Prostatitis

See under Urinary-tract Infections, below.

Psittacosis

The causative organism of psittacosis is *Chlamydia psittaci*. It is usually transmitted to humans by direct or indirect contact with infected birds and the primary site of infection is the lung.[1] Transmission between humans is common with what was formerly thought to be the TWAR strain of *C. psittaci*,[2] but is now known to be a different species, *C. pneumoniae*,[3] that also causes pneumonia. The clinical presentation of psittacosis can vary widely from a mild 'flu-like' illness to a fulminating toxic state with multiple organ involvement.[1] Most patients will have a cough, although this is not always prominent. Tetracyclines are the treatment of choice[1,4] and early therapy may be life-saving; a 21-day course has been recommended since relapses have occurred after shorter periods.[1] An alternative is chloramphenicol.[4] Erythromycin or a similar macrolide have also been used successfully.[5,6]

1. Macfarlane JT, Macrae AD. Psittacosis. *Br Med Bull* 1983; **39:** 163–7.
2. Anonymous. TWAR—Chlamydia in a new guise? *Lancet* 1988; **i:** 974–5.
3. Grayston JT, *et al.* A new respiratory tract pathogen: Chlamydia pneumoniae strain TWAR. *J Infect Dis* 1990; **161:** 618–25.
4. Anonymous. The choice of antibacterial drugs. *Med Lett Drugs Ther* 1998; **40:** 33–42.
5. Morrison WM, *et al.* An outbreak of psittacosis. *J Infect* 1991; **22:** 71–5.
6. Chang KP, Veitch PC. Fever, haematuria, proteinuria, and a parrot. *Lancet* 1997; **350:** 1674.

Q fever

Q fever (or query fever) is a rickettsial infection (below) caused by *Coxiella burnetii*. It is a zoonosis occurring worldwide and is transmitted to humans from domestic animals such as cattle and sheep, mainly by inhalation of infected dust. Acute infection generally presents as a febrile influenza-like illness that may progress to pneumonia. Endocarditis is the most frequent manifestation of chronic infection and the most serious form of Q fever; infection may be difficult to eradicate and prolonged treatment is generally required. There is also evidence in patients who have not experienced cardiac involvement of long-term sequelae including lethargy and fatigue.

A tetracycline such as doxycycline has been the treatment of choice for Q fever; alternatively chloramphenicol has been used. Erythromycin may be adequate for Q fever pneumonia,[1] at least in mild cases;[2] results with erythromycin were favourable in a retrospective review.[3] However, Q fever pneumonia may often resolve without treatment and the role of antibacterial therapy is not clear.[4]

Q fever endocarditis is more difficult to treat. Raoult[5] described tetracycline as the mainstay of treatment, although it fails to eradicate *C. burnetii* when used alone and various combinations of antibacterials have been tried. A study *in vitro*[6] showed that isolates of *C. burnetii* associated with chronic infection were less sensitive to antibacterials than those from acute Q fever, but that fluoroquinolones alone or with rifampicin might be of value. Long-term treatment with doxycycline plus rifampicin[7] or with ciprofloxacin alone[8] has been successful in individual patients with endocarditis, whereas pefloxacin alone[9] was not. Following a retrospective comparison of doxycycline alone or with rifampicin, fluoroquinolones (ofloxacin or pefloxacin), or co-trimoxazole, Levy *et al.*[10] recommended treatment for at least 3 years with doxycycline plus a fluoroquinolone; doxycycline plus rifampicin also appeared effective, but in most cases rifampicin had been stopped after a few months because of interactions with anticoagulant often prescribed at the same time. Raoult[5] also concluded that no current treatment eradicated Q fever endocarditis within 2 years and, like Levy *et al.*,[10] recommended that it be treated with doxycycline together with a fluoroquinolone for a minimum of 3 years. Other regimens that have been investigated have included chloroquine plus doxycycline.[5]

A vaccine is available in some countries for use in occupational groups who regularly handle potentially infected animal tissues.

1. D'Angelo LJ, Hetherington R. Q fever treated with erythromycin. *Br Med J* 1979; **2:** 305–6.
2. Marrie TJ, *et al.* Q fever pneumonia associated with exposure to wild rabbits. *Lancet* 1986; **i:** 427–9.
3. Pérez-del-Molino A, *et al.* Erythromycin and the treatment of Coxiella burnetii pneumonia. *J Antimicrob Chemother* 1991; **28:** 455–9.
4. Lieberman D, *et al.* Q-fever pneumonia in the Negev region of Israel: a review of 20 patients hospitalised over a period of one year. *J Infect* 1995; **30:** 135–40.
5. Raoult D. Treatment of Q fever. *Antimicrob Agents Chemother* 1993; **37:** 1733–6.
6. Yeaman MR, *et al.* Antibiotic susceptibilities of two Coxiella burnetii isolates implicated in distinct clinical syndromes. *Antimicrob Agents Chemother* 1989; **33:** 1052–7.
7. Brecker SJD, Eykyn SJ. Q-fever endocarditis twenty-five years on. *Lancet* 1989; **ii:** 684–5.
8. Yebra M, *et al.* Ciprofloxacin in a case of Q fever endocarditis. *N Engl J Med* 1990; **323:** 614.
9. Cacoub P, *et al.* Q-fever endocarditis and treatment with the fluoroquinolones. *Arch Intern Med* 1991; **151:** 816, 818.
10. Levy PY, *et al.* Comparison of different antibiotic regimens for therapy of 32 cases of Q fever endocarditis. *Antimicrob Agents Chemother* 1991; **35:** 533–7.

Relapsing fever

Relapsing fever is caused by spirochaetes of the *Borrelia* genus that are transmitted to humans by body lice or ornithodoros ticks. *B. recurrentis* causes louse-borne relapsing fever and can occur widely, but is endemic especially in Ethiopia. Many species of *Borrelia* may cause tick-borne relapsing fever.

The treatment of choice for infection due to *B. recurrentis* is a tetracycline; benzylpenicillin is an alternative.[1] Therapy with single oral doses of tetracycline,[2,3] erythromycin,[2,3] or chloramphenicol[3] has been effective. Antibacterial treatment often causes a Jarisch-Herxheimer reaction characterised by rigor, fever and hypotension which may be fatal.[2,4] Therapies used in an attempt to prevent this reaction include paracetamol and corticosteroids.[2,4] Recently the use of antibodies against tumour necrosis factor α has shown promise.[5]

Tick-borne relapsing fever is milder than the louse-borne variety, but has been treated similarly.

1. Anonymous. The choice of antibacterial drugs. *Med Lett Drugs Ther* 1998; **40:** 33–42.
2. Butler T, *et al.* Borrelia recurrentis infection: single-dose antibiotic regimens and management of the Jarisch-Herxheimer reaction. *J Infect Dis* 1978; **137:** 573–7.
3. Perine PL, Teklu B. Antibiotic treatment of louse-borne relapsing fever in Ethiopia: a report of 377 cases. *Am J Trop Med Hyg* 1983; **32:** 1096–1100.
4. Butler T. Relapsing fever: new lessons about antibiotic action. *Ann Intern Med* 1985; **102:** 397–9.
5. Fekade D, *et al.* Prevention of Jarisch-Herxheimer reactions by treatment with antibodies against tumor necrosis factor α. *N Engl J Med* 1996; **335:** 311–15.

Respiratory-tract infections

Principal community-acquired bacterial pathogens in the respiratory tract continue to be *Streptococcus pneumoniae* and *Haemophilus influenzae*,[1] although *Moraxella (Branhamella) catarrhalis*[2-4] is increasingly important in some areas. Other respiratory pathogens include *Chlamydia pneumoniae* (formerly TWAR strain of *C. psittaci*), *Legionella pneumophila,* and *Mycoplasma pneumoniae*. *Streptococcus pyogenes* is the predominant cause of pharyngitis. *Staphylococcus aureus* and aerobic Gram-negative bacilli such as *Pseudomonas aeruginosa* and *Klebsiella* spp. may be responsible for hospital-acquired (nosocomial) infections.

Community-acquired lower respiratory-tract infections are very common and are traditionally considered to be viral in origin, but Macfarlane and Colleagues[5] reported that bacterial pathogens similar to those causing pneumonia were commonly isolated from patients with these milder respiratory infections; even so about one quarter of patients failed to respond satisfactorily to empirical antibacterial treatment.

Broad-spectrum antibacterials such as a penicillin or erythromycin may be necessary in some cases of uncomplicated upper or lower respiratory-tract infection. First line empirical treatment with a fluoroquinolone should be avoided because of poor activity against streptococci.[6,7] In respiratory-tract infections complicating chronic obstructive pulmonary disease, amoxycillin has been recommended for first-line treatment.[8] If a further course is necessary, drugs with activity against penicillin-resistant *H. influenzae* and *M. catarrhalis* should probably be given, such as amoxycillin with clavulanic acid, a fluoroquinolone (bearing in mind that they are not very active against *Str. pneumoniae*), or a second-generation cephalosporin.

For details on infections of the upper respiratory tract, see under Epiglottitis (p.122), Pharyngitis (p.137), and Sinusitis (p.142); see also Otitis Media (p.134). For infections of the lower respiratory tract, see under Bronchitis (p.118), Cystic Fibrosis (p.119), and Pneumonia (p.138); those with a specific cause include Legionnaires' Disease (p.128), Nocardiosis (p.133), Pertussis (p.137), and Tuberculosis (p.146).

1. Finch RG. Epidemiological features and chemotherapy of community-acquired respiratory tract infections. *J Antimicrob Chemother* 1990; **26** (suppl E): 53–61.
2. Davies BI, Maesen FPV. Treatment of Branhamella catarrhalis infections. *J Antimicrob Chemother* 1990; **25:** 1–4.
3. Wallace RJ, *et al.* Antibiotic susceptibilities and drug resistance in Moraxella (Branhamella) catarrhalis. *Am J Med* 1990; **88** (suppl 5A): 46S–50S.
4. Murphy TF. Branhamella catarrhalis: epidemiological and clinical aspects of a human respiratory tract pathogen. *Thorax* 1998; **53:** 124–8.
5. Macfarlane JT, *et al.* Prospective study of aetiology and outcome of adult lower-respiratory-tract infections in the community. *Lancet* 1993; **341:** 511–14.
6. Körner RJ, *et al.* Dangers of oral fluoroquinolone treatment in community acquired upper respiratory tract infections. *Br Med J* 1994; **308:** 191–2.
7. Hosker HSR, *et al.* Management of community acquired lower respiratory tract infection. *Br Med J* 1994; **308:** 701–5.
8. Hosker H, *et al.* Antibiotics in chronic obstructive pulmonary disease. *Br Med J* 1994; **308:** 871–2.

Rheumatic fever

Acute rheumatic fever occurs especially in children aged 6 to 15 years as a consequence of upper respiratory-tract infections, such as pharyngitis or tonsillitis, with rheumatogenic strains of the group A beta-haemolytic streptococcus *Streptococcus pyogenes*. The pathogenesis of rheumatic fever is not known, but an immune mechanism may be involved. There may be a latent period of 1 to 5 weeks after the initial infection, before clinical manifestations of rheumatic fever appear. The major ones are arthritis, carditis, chorea, erythema marginatum, and subcutaneous nodules. Those affecting the heart are the most serious and are a major cause of cardiovascular death in children and young adults in developing countries. Rheumatic fever has been associated with poverty and overcrowding and has declined dramatically in developed countries, but is still a major problem in the developing world. However, in the 1980s there was evidence of a resurgence in the USA with outbreaks of rheumatic fever reported in middle-class children[1] and military recruits.[2] Increased pathogenicity of *Str. pyogenes* serotypes might have contributed to this resurgence.[3]

Similar guidelines for the primary and secondary prevention of rheumatic fever have been published by WHO[4] and the American Heart Association (AHA).[5] Rheumatic fever can usually be prevented by *primary prophylaxis*, that is, by the prompt treatment of streptococcal upper respiratory-tract infection with eradication of group A streptococci from the throat. Penicillin is the drug of choice, either as a single intramuscular injection of benzathine penicillin or as a course of phenoxymethylpenicillin by mouth for 10 days. An injection containing benzathine penicillin and procaine penicillin has been used in children.[5] Erythromycin may be given to patients allergic to penicillin. Other macrolides or oral cephalosporins may also be used. For further details on the treatment of streptococcal sore throat, see under Pharyngitis, above. Treatment failure is more common after oral antibacterials and in the USA most of these patients are streptococcal carriers.[5] Treatment of chronic carriers is not usually necessary, but eradication of pharyngeal carriage has been achieved by an injection of benzathine penicillin plus rifampicin by mouth for 4 days;[6] a 10-day course of oral clindamycin has also been effective.[7] Broad-based primary prophylaxis in communities rather than individuals is controversial and requires careful planning, but, for example, penicillin prophylaxis did control an epidemic of acute tonsillitis associated with *Str. pyogenes* in a junior detention centre.[8] However, a study in military recruits demonstrated that *Str. pyogenes* infection could not be prevented in closely confined communities unless all individuals in the population received prophylaxis.[9]

If acute rheumatic fever occurs, a full therapeutic course of penicillin should be given initially, as for primary prevention, to eradicate group A streptococci.[5] Treatment then comprises bed rest and anti-inflammatory drugs, usually corticosteroids or salicylates, in an attempt to prevent valvular scarring. However, it is unclear whether anti-inflammatory treatment has any influence on such long-term sequelae.[10] *Secondary prevention* is then continued with prolonged antibacterial prophylaxis because of the high risk of recurrent attacks of rheumatic fever following subsequent streptococcal upper respiratory-tract infections. Again, penicillin is the preferred antibacterial, the usual recommendation being an intramuscular injection of benzathine penicillin every 4 weeks, although injections every 3 weeks may be warranted where the risk of recurrence is high.[4,5] This advice has been influenced by reports of high recurrence rates with the monthly regimen in such situations.[11] A 12-year study in Taiwan[12] confirmed that prophylaxis with benzathine penicillin injections every 3 weeks is more effective than injections every 4 weeks and it was recommended that the 3-week regimen should be used in adults and children with a recent episode of rheumatic fever, especially in developing countries where exposure to streptococci is still intense. In addition, pharmacokinetic studies have indicated relatively low serum concentrations of penicillin in the fourth week after an intramuscular injection of benzathine penicillin,[13,14] despite the successful use of monthly injections in most patients. Alternatively, oral prophylaxis with phenoxymethylpenicillin or sulphadiazine may be given; erythromycin is suggested for the rare patient who is allergic to penicillin and sulphonamides. Sulphonamides should *not* be used for primary prevention because they do not eradicate the streptococci. The duration of secondary prophylaxis depends on the individual patient, but in those who have not had rheumatic carditis it should generally continue for a minimum of 5 years after the last attack of rheumatic fever, and at least until the age of 18 or early 20s.[5] A study from Chile supported this view.[15] Those who have had rheumatic carditis but without residual valvular disease should perhaps receive prophylaxis for 10 years[5] or at least until the age of 25 years.[4] For those with carditis and persistent valvular disease, prophylaxis should continue at least until the age of 40 years, or sometimes for life.[5] Fears of serious allergic reactions associated with long-term benzathine penicillin prophylaxis appear to be unfounded.[16]

Household contacts of rheumatic fever patients who themselves have positive streptococcal cultures should be treated.[5]

Patients with rheumatic valvular heart disease as a result of rheumatic fever are at risk of developing infective endocarditis and should receive additional appropriate short-term antibacterial prophylaxis when undergoing dental and some surgical procedures (see Endocarditis, above).

1. Veasy LG, *et al.* Resurgence of acute rheumatic fever in the intermountain area of the United States. *N Engl J Med* 1987; **316:** 421–7.
2. Wallace MR, *et al.* The return of acute rheumatic fever in young adults. *JAMA* 1989; **262:** 2557–61.
3. Schwartz B, *et al.* Changing epidemiology of group A streptococcal infection in the USA. *Lancet* 1990; **336:** 1167–71.
4. WHO. Rheumatic fever and rheumatic heart disease. *WHO Tech Rep Ser 764* 1988.
5. Dajani A, *et al.* Treatment of acute streptococcal pharyngitis and prevention of rheumatic fever: a statement for health professionals. *Pediatrics* 1995; **96:** 758–64.
6. Tanz RR, *et al.* Penicillin plus rifampin eradicates pharyngeal carriage of group A streptococci. *J Pediatr* 1985; **106:** 876–80.
7. Tanz RR, *et al.* Clindamycin treatment of chronic pharyngeal carriage of group A streptococci. *J Pediatr* 1991; **119:** 123–8.
8. Colling A, *et al.* Minimum amount of penicillin prophylaxis required to control Streptococcus pyogenes epidemic in closed community. *Br Med J* 1982; **285:** 95–6.
9. Gray GC, *et al.* Hyperendemic Streptococcus pyogenes infection despite prophylaxis with penicillin G benzathine. *N Engl J Med* 1991; **325:** 92–7.
10. Stollerman GH. Rheumatic fever. *Lancet* 1997; **349:** 935–42.
11. Ayoub EM. Prophylaxis in patients with rheumatic fever: every three or every four weeks? *J Pediatr* 1989; **115:** 89–91.
12. Lue H-C, *et al.* Long-term outcome of patients with rheumatic fever receiving benzathine penicillin G prophylaxis every three weeks versus every four weeks. *J Pediatr* 1994; **125:** 812–16.
13. Kaplan EL, *et al.* Pharmacokinetics of benzathine penicillin G: serum levels during the 28 days after intramuscular injection of 1,200,000 units. *J Pediatr* 1989; **115:** 146–50.
14. Meira ZMA, *et al.* Evaluation of secondary prophylactic schemes, based on benzathine penicillin G, for rheumatic fever in children. *J Pediatr* 1993; **123:** 156–8.
15. Berrios X, *et al.* Discontinuing rheumatic fever prophylaxis in selected adolescents and young adults: a prospective study. *Ann Intern Med* 1993; **118:** 401–6. Correction. *ibid.*; **119:** 173.
16. International Rheumatic Fever Study Group. Allergic reactions to long-term benzathine penicillin prophylaxis for rheumatic fever. *Lancet* 1991; **337:** 1308–10.

Rickettsial infections

Bacteria of the Rickettsiaceae family that infect man include *Rickettsia* spp. (see under Spotted Fevers and under Typhus, below) and *Coxiella burnetii* (see under Q fever, above). *Ehrlichia* spp. (see under Ehrlichiosis, above), are rickettsia-like bacteria. *Bartonella quintana* (formerly *Rochalimaea quintana*) (see under Trench Fever, below) is no longer classified as a rickettsia. The treatment of choice for rickettsial infections is usually a tetracycline or chloramphenicol;[1,2] a fluoroquinolone such as ciprofloxacin has also been used.[2]

1. WHO Working Group on Rickettsial Diseases. Rickettsioses: a continuing disease problem. *Bull WHO* 1982; **60:** 157–64.
2. Raoult D, Drancourt M. Antimicrobial therapy of rickettsial diseases. *Antimicrob Agents Chemother* 1991; **35:** 2457–62.

Salmonella enteritis

See under Gastro-enteritis, above.

Salpingitis

See under Pelvic Inflammatory Disease, above.

Septicaemia

Traditionally, transient bacteraemia (the presence of bacteria in the blood) has been regarded as a fairly common condition which does not usually cause complications, whereas uncontrolled bacteraemia leads to septicaemia with serious symptoms such as fever and shock. This distinction has not always been adhered to in published sources and the terms have sometimes been used interchangeably. Added to this, the identification of the cascade of inflammatory mediators involved and the realisation that what had been called 'sepsis' could arise in the absence of infection have prompted reassessment of the terminology used both in the UK and in the USA.[1] In the UK, Lynne and Cohen[2] considered that the term 'septicaemia' should no longer be used since it does not distinguish between mild and severe disease. They preferred the term 'sepsis syndrome' for patients with a generalised systemic response together with evidence of organ dysfunction and 'septic shock' to describe patients who also have hypotension not due to hypovolaemia or cardiac causes. The American College of Chest Physicians and Society of Critical Care Medicine has proposed the following series of definitions to cover the spectrum of syndromes resulting from this inflammatory response:[1,3]

- **systemic inflammatory response syndrome** (SIRS), the systemic inflammatory response to infection or various other severe clinical insults including pancreatitis, ischaemia, trauma, and haemorrhagic shock
- **sepsis**, the SIRS caused specifically by infection
- **severe sepsis**, sepsis associated with organ dysfunction, perfusion abnormalities (such as lactic acidosis, oliguria, or an acute alteration in mental status), or hypotension
- **septic shock**, sepsis with hypotension, despite adequate fluid resuscitation, together with perfusion abnormalities
- **multiple organ dysfunction syndrome** (MODS), the presence of altered organ function in an acutely ill patient such that homoeostasis cannot be maintained without intervention; it may be a cause as well as a consequence of SIRS.

Septicaemia can be caused by a wide range of bacteria.[4] **Community-acquired** primary septicaemia arises spontaneously and is often associated with a specific infectious disease, such as meningococcal septicaemia with meningococcal meningitis (above) or streptococcal septicaemia with pneumonia (above). *Streptococcus pneumoniae* and *Haemophilus influenzae* are common causes of primary septicaemia in children (although this pattern is changing in countries where immunisation against *H. influenzae* type b is routine); Gram-negative rods and group B streptococci are commonest in neonates. **Hospital-acquired** septicaemia is often iatrogenic and may occur as a complication of surgery or indwelling catheters[5,6] or may be associated with neutropenia in cancer patients (see under Infections in Immunocompromised Patients, above). It is often associated with acute respiratory distress syndrome (p.1017).

Whatever the cause, septicaemia requires prompt treatment without waiting for the results of laboratory tests. Choice of antibacterial depends on the probable source of infection. For example, urinary-tract infection is likely to be associated with Gram-negative septicaemia due to *Escherichia coli*; abdominal sepsis with Gram-negative septicaemia due to mixed infection with *E. coli*, enterococci, and anaerobic bacteria; and skin sepsis, bacterial arthritis, acute osteomyelitis, and cardiovascular shunts with Gram-positive septicaemia due to staphylococci. The antibacterials used should also reflect current patterns of bacterial resistance in the community or hospital. *Empirical treatment* has often been initiated with a penicillin and an aminoglycoside, metronidazole being added if anaerobic infection is suspected. In the UK recommended treatment is with either a broad-spectrum penicillin plus an aminoglycoside, or a third-generation cephalosporin alone, or meropenem alone, or imipenem-cilastatin alone for initial empirical therapy. Metronidazole may be added if anaerobic organisms are suspected, and flucloxacillin or vancomycin if Gram-positive organisms are suspected. USA guidelines[7] recommend either a third- or fourth-generation cephalosporin (cefotaxime, ceftizoxime, ceftriaxone, or cefepime), or ticarcillin-clavulanic acid, or piperacillin-tazobactam, or imipenem-cilastatin, or meropenem, each with an aminoglycoside (gentamicin, tobramycin, or amikacin) for the initial treatment of life-threatening sepsis in adults. When there is some information on which to base choice of treatment, but before the infecting organisms are definitely known, they have suggested the following treatment:

- suspected bacterial endocarditis—gentamicin with vancomycin
- suspected methicillin-resistant staphylococci—vancomycin, with or without gentamicin and/or rifampicin
- intra-abdominal or pelvic infections likely to involve anaerobes—ticarcillin-clavulanic acid, ampicillin-sulbactam, piperacillin-tazobactam, imipenem-cilastatin, meropenem, cefoxitin, or cefotetan, each with or without an aminoglycoside, or alternatively metronidazole or clindamycin with an aminoglycoside, or possibly trovafloxacin
- suspected biliary-tract infection—piperacillin or mezlocillin plus metronidazole, piperacillin-tazobactam, or ampicillin-sulbactam, each with or without an aminoglycoside.

Once the infecting organisms have been identified, choice of treatment will again depend on their sensitivity and current patterns of resistance in the community or hospital. Specific types of septicaemia studied and reviewed in the literature include that due to Gram-negative bacteria in general,[8,9] *Pseudomonas aeruginosa,*[10] *Serratia* spp.,[11] staphylococci,[12] *Streptococcus pyogenes,*[13] *Str. pneumoniae,*[14] and enterococci.[15] For comments on the consequences of emerging multidrug-resistant strains of enterococci and staphylococci, see Enterococcal Infections, above, and Staphylococcal Infections, below.

In addition to antimicrobial therapy, patients with septic shock[16-18] require rigorous supportive measures (p.798).

Septicaemia is generally most lethal in the very old and the very young.

Neonatal septicaemia may be divided into **early-onset**, which is acquired from the mother's genital tract and manifests itself during the first few days after birth, and **late-onset** which may be nosocomially acquired. Bacteria commonly causing early-onset sepsis include enterococci, *E. coli, H. influenzae, Listeria monocytogenes,* and streptococci. Some of these organisms may also produce meningitis in the neonate (above). Empirical treatment for both early- and late-onset sepsis is based on similar principles to those in other patients, giving consideration to local patterns of infection and resistance and to the suitability of individual antibacterials for this age group. However, early-onset sepsis is usually best controlled by prenatal treatment of the mother or by perinatal prophylaxis. Prophylaxis for group B streptococcal infections is discussed under Perinatal Streptococcal Infections, above. While vancomycin has been shown to prevent infections with coagulase-negative staphylococci,[19] widespread prophylactic use of this drug is not recommended.[20] Intravenous administration of normal immunoglobulin has been tried for the prevention of septicaemia in preterm neonates with variable results (p.1525).

Treatment failure despite apparently adequate anti-infective therapy might be due in part to a continuing inflammatory process and attempts to modify this are under investigation. Endotoxin, a lipopolysaccharide associated with the cell membrane of Gram-negative bacteria, is an important mediator in the septic syndrome. Endotoxin release may occur spontaneously or during antibacterial therapy.[21] When in the circulation it stimulates the release of endogenous mediators such as interleukin-1, interleukin-6, tumour necrosis factor alpha, and other cytokines.[22] These in turn induce a cascade of secondary inflammatory mediators resulting eventually in endothelial damage and severe haemodynamic and metabolic derangements. It is now understood that a similar inflammatory response also occurs following non-infective insults. However, adjunctive therapy with endotoxin antibodies, anticytokines such as anakinra and tumour necrosis factor antibodies, soluble tumour necrosis factor receptor, bactericidal permeability increasing protein, nitric oxide synthase inhibitors, guanylate cyclase inhibitors such as methylene blue, and platelet-activating factor antagonists have generally produced disappointing results.[23,24] Recent theories suggest that a more complex interplay of pro- and anti-inflammatory responses may be involved in the pathophysiology of SIRS and MODS and this may explain the failure of these predominantly anti-inflammatory treatment modalities.[25]

1. Bone RC. Why new definitions of sepsis and organ failure are needed. *Am J Med* 1993; **95:** 348–50.
2. Lynn WA, Cohen J. Management of septic shock. *J Infect* 1995; **30:** 207–12.
3. American College of Chest Physicians/Society of Critical Care Medicine Consensus Conference Committee. Definitions for sepsis and organ failure and guidelines for the use of innovative therapies in sepsis. *Crit Care Med* 1992; **20:** 864–74.
4. Eykyn SJ, *et al.* The causative organisms of septicaemia and their epidemiology. *J Antimicrob Chemother* 1990; **25** (suppl C): 41–58.
5. Dickinson GM, Bisno AL. Infections associated with indwelling devices: concepts of pathogenesis; infections associated with intravascular devices. *Antimicrob Agents Chemother* 1989; **33:** 597–601.
6. Dickinson GM, Bisno AL. Infections associated with indwelling devices: infections related to extravascular devices. *Antimicrob Agents Chemother* 1989; **33:** 602–7.
7. Anonymous. The choice of antibacterial drugs. *Med Lett Drugs Ther* 1998; **40:** 33–42.
8. Dudley MN. Overview of gram-negative sepsis. *Am J Hosp Pharm* 1990; **47** (suppl 3): 53–60.
9. DiPiro JT. Pathophysiology and treatment of gram-negative sepsis. *Am J Hosp Pharm* 1990; **47** (suppl 3): S6–S10.
10. Hilf M, *et al.* Antibiotic therapy for Pseudomonas aeruginosa bacteremia: outcome correlations in a prospective study of 200 patients. *Am J Med* 1989; **87:** 540–6.
11. Saito H, *et al.* Serratia bacteremia: review of 118 cases. *Rev Infect Dis* 1989; **11:** 912–20.
12. Eykyn SJ. Staphylococcal sepsis: the changing pattern of disease and therapy. *Lancet* 1988; **i:** 100–4.
13. Anonymous. Invasive streptococci. *Lancet* 1989; **ii:** 1255.
14. Davies AJ, Kumaratne DS. The continuing problem of pneumococcal infection. *J Antimicrob Chemother* 1988; **21:** 387–91.
15. Montecalvo MA, *et al.* Outbreak of vancomycin-, ampicillin-, and aminoglycoside-resistant Enterococcus faecium bacteremia in an adult oncology unit. *Antimicrob Agents Chemother* 1994; **38:** 1363–7.
16. Glauser MP, *et al.* Septic shock: pathogenesis. *Lancet* 1991; **338:** 732–6.
17. Cohen J, Glauser MP. Septic shock: treatment. *Lancet* 1991; **338:** 736–9.
18. Astiz ME, Rackow EC. Septic shock. *Lancet* 1998; **351:** 1501–5.
19. Kacica MA, *et al.* Prevention of gram-positive sepsis in neonates weighing less than 1500 grams. *J Pediatr* 1994; **125:** 253–8.
20. Barefield ES, Philips JB. Vancomycin prophylaxis for coagulase-negative staphylococcal bacteremia. *J Pediatr* 1994; **125:** 230–2.
21. Prins JM. Clinical relevance of antibiotic-induced endotoxin release. *Antimicrob Agents Chemother* 1994; **38:** 1211–18.
22. Blackwell TS, Christman JW. Sepsis and cytokines: current status. *Br J Anaesth* 1996; **77:** 110–17.
23. Verhoef J, *et al.* Issues in the adjunct therapy of severe sepsis. *J Antimicrob Chemother* 1996; **38:** 167–82.
24. Opal SM, Yu RL. Antiendotoxin strategies for the prevention and treatment of septic shock: new approaches and future directions. *Drugs* 1998; **55:** 497–508.
25. Bone RC. Immunologic dissonance: a continuing evolution in our understanding of the systemic inflammatory response syndrome (SIRS) and the multiple organ dysfunction syndrome (MODS). *Ann Intern Med* 1996; **125:** 680–7.

Sexually transmitted diseases

The sexually transmitted diseases, formerly termed venereal diseases, are defined as a group of communicable diseases that are transferred mainly by sexual contact. More than 20 pathogens are known to be transmitted sexually. They include the bacteria *Haemophilus ducreyi* (see Chancroid, p.118), *Neisseria gonorrhoeae* (see Gonorrhoea, p.126), *Treponema pallidum* (see Syphilis, p.145), *Calymmatobacterium granulomatis* (see Granuloma Inguinale, p.126), *Chlamydia trachomatis* (see Lymphogranuloma Venereum, p.130 and Chlamydial Infections, p.119), and mycoplasmas including *Ureaplasma urealyticum.*

Clinical syndromes associated with sexually transmitted diseases include urethritis (p.149) and epididymitis (p.122) in men; cervicitis (p.118), pelvic inflammatory disease (p.135), and bacterial vaginosis (p.117) in women; and proctitis (p.140). Perinatal transmission of sexually transmitted pathogens from the mother can result in neonatal conjunctivitis (p.132) or pneumonia (p.138).

For discussions of some viral sexually transmitted diseases, see under HIV Infection and AIDS (p.599), Hepatitis (p.595), and Herpesvirus Infections (p.596) in Antivirals. Trichomoniasis is discussed in Antiprotozoals, p.577.

General guidelines for the management of sexually transmitted diseases are published,[1,2] and the epidemiology of sexually transmitted diseases and implications for travellers has been reviewed.[3]

1. WHO. *WHO model prescribing information: drugs used in sexually transmitted diseases and HIV infection:* Geneva: WHO, 1995.
2. Centers for Disease Control. 1998 Guidelines for treatment of sexually transmitted diseases. *MMWR* 1998 **47** (RR-1): 1–116.
3. Mulhall BP. Sexually transmissible diseases and travel. *Br Med Bull* 1993; **49:** 394–411.

Shigellosis

See under Gastro-enteritis, above.

Sickle-cell disease

For prophylaxis against pneumococcal infection in sickle-cell disease, see under Spleen Disorders, below.

Sinusitis

Sinusitis or inflammation of the paranasal sinuses is more common in adults than children. It can be caused by viral, bacterial, or fungal infection or may be secondary to other disorders such as allergy. Serious complications include bacterial meningitis and brain abscess.

Acute sinusitis often results from viral upper respiratory-tract infections. Similarly to acute otitis media the most frequent bacterial pathogens are *Streptococcus pneumoniae* and unencapsulated *Haemophilus influenzae*, with *Moraxella (Branhamella) catarrhalis* increasingly important in children. Other bacterial causes, especially in adults, include mixed anaerobic bacteria (usually associated with dental disease and more frequent in chronic sinusitis), *Staphylococcus aureus, Streptococcus pyogenes*, and Gram-negative bacteria including Enterobacteriaceae and *Pseudomonas aeruginosa* (in nosocomial sinusitis). About 5% of primary sinusitis in young adults has been associated with *Chlamydia pneumoniae.*

Acute sinusitis may resolve spontaneously, and a study failed to show any clinical benefit from antibacterial treatment of acute maxillary sinusitis.[1] When antibacterials are considered necessary treatment should be given for an adequate length of time, usually 2 weeks.[2,3] Topical decongestants may also be used to promote drainage and ventilation.[2,3] The choice of antibacterial is similar to that for acute otitis media (above). Effective antibacterials include amoxycillin with or without clavulanic acid, co-trimoxazole, cefuroxime, erythromycin, and azithromycin;[2] the emergence of penicillin-resistant strains of *H. influenzae, M. catarrhalis*, and *Str. pneumoniae* is causing concern.[4] Patients with evidence of severe infections may require intravenous therapy with vancomycin and ceftriaxone or cefotaxime initially.[4] Tetracycline or erythromycin are the most effective antibacterials against *Chlamydia pneumoniae.*[5]

Failure to treat acute sinusitis which does not resolve spontaneously can result in chronic sinusitis or occasionally in complications such as brain abscess or meningitis. Exacerbations of chronic sinusitis are treated as for acute infection. Management of chronic sinusitis is based on reducing obstruction of the sinus cavity using antihistamines, decongestants, anti-inflammatory drugs (including corticosteroids), and saline washes as appropriate.[2,6,7] The usefulness of antibacterials is more contentious,[6] although some clinicians advocate prolonged courses as part of initial treatment.[2,7] Surgical intervention may be necessary if medical treatment fails. The treatment of the non-infective aspects of rhinitis is discussed on p.400.

1. van Buchem FL, *et al.* Primary-care-based randomised placebo-controlled trial of antibiotic treatment in acute maxillary sinusitis. *Lancet* 1997; **349:** 683–7.
2. Evans KL. Diagnosis and management of sinusitis. *Br Med J* 1994; **309:** 1415–22.
3. Evans KL. Recognition and management of sinusitis. *Drugs* 1998. **56:** 59–71.
4. Gwaltney JM. Acute community-acquired sinusitis. *Clin Infect Dis* 1996; **23:** 1209–25.
5. Grayston JT, *et al.* A new respiratory tract pathogen: Chlamydia pneumoniae strain TWAR. *J Infect Dis* 1990; **161:** 618–25.
6. Rowe-Jones J, Mackay I. Management of sinusitis: sinusitis and rhinitis, or rhinosinusitis? *Br Med J* 1995; **310:** 670.
7. Wald ER. Chronic sinusitis in children. *J Pediatr* 1995; **127:** 339–47.

Skin infections

Bacterial infections of the skin and soft-tissue include the pyodermas, namely impetigo, erysipelas, cellulitis, folliculitis, furunculosis, and ecthyma gangrenosum; necrotising soft-tissue infections (see also under Necrotising Fasciitis, above); infections of bites and stings (see above); ulcerating skin infections; infected burns; and toxin-mediated bacterial disease such as staphylococcal scalded skin syndrome.[1] Common causes are *Staphylococcus aureus* and *Streptococcus pyogenes*. For specific cutaneous infections, e.g. anthrax, see under the appropriate side-heading. Acne and rosacea, skin disorders of less certain aetiology but treated with antibacterials are discussed on p.1072 and p.1076, respectively.

Topical antibacterials and antiseptics may be useful for the treatment of superficial skin infections, but antibacterials should only be used short term because of the risks of bacterial resistance and contact allergy.[2] Antibacterials of value systemically, like gentamicin and fusidic acid, are better not used topically.[2] Systemic toxicity is also a possibility, for example the topical use of neomycin in patients with extensive skin damage may result in deafness.

Phenoxymethylpenicillin (or benzylpenicillin if parenteral therapy is required) remains the treatment of choice for systemic therapy of streptococcal infections.[3] Erythromycin may be used in patients unable to tolerate penicillin, but there are reports of increasing resistance. Failure of penicillin to control aggressive streptococcal infections may be due to the presence of a high bacterial load, and in this situation clindamycin may be more effective.[3] A penicillinase-resistant penicillin such as flucloxacillin is required for staphylococcal infections, or erythromycin as an alternative for those unable to tolerate penicillins.

Impetigo is the most superficial skin infection and is especially contagious. In the UK it is usually caused by *Staph. aureus*, but in West Indian and Asian immigrants *Str. pyogenes* is more likely; the two may co-exist.[1] Phenoxymethylpenicillin or erythromycin is still generally the oral treatment of choice for non-bullous streptococcal impetigo,[4] but treatment with an antistaphylococcal antibacterial should be considered in patients who fail to respond.[3,5] Where the pathogen is *Staph. aureus* (bullous impetigo) flucloxacillin is indicated as initial treatment; erythromycin is a suitable alternative in penicillin-allergic patients.[1] Cephalexin has also been effective.[6] Topical antibacterials are widely used but resistance has been encountered with tetracyclines, gentamicin, and fusidic acid;[1] mupirocin has proved topically effective against both streptococci and staphylococci[7] including methicillin-resistant *Staph. aureus*, but again resistant strains have been reported.[1]

Erysipelas is a rapidly spreading infection of the skin complicated by lymphatic involvement and is largely caused by *Str. pyogenes* and other beta-haemolytic streptococci although *Staph. aureus* occasionally produce a similar picture. Penicillin is usually indicated, but staphylococcal erysipelas should be treated with a penicillinase-resistant penicillin; erythromycin is an acceptable alternative in penicillin-hypersensitive patients.[1]

Cellulitis is a more deep-seated spreading infection largely caused by *Str. pyogenes* or *Staph. aureus*. Clinical differentiation of the cause is often difficult, so antibacterial treatment should be active against both organisms.[3] The principles of treatment are similar to those for erysipelas although parenteral therapy is needed more often. *Haemophilus influenzae* is an occasional cause of localised cellulitis and as resistance to ampicillin or chloramphenicol may be a problem, cefuroxime may be preferable.[1] Puncture wounds of the foot may result in cellulitis due to *Pseudomonas aeruginosa* infection which usually responds to ciprofloxacin.[5] Prophylactic treatment has sometimes been recommended in patients with recurrent erysipelas or cellulitis; in one study prolonged low-dose therapy with erythromycin was effective.[8]

Folliculitis and **furunculosis** are usually due to *Staph. aureus*. Antibacterials are required only in the presence of systemic symptoms or spreading cellulitis; less severe infections usually respond to the application of moist heat. The drug of choice is an antistaphylococcal penicillin such as flucloxacillin or erythromycin for penicillin-allergic patients.[1] Recurrent furunculosis can be serious in at-risk patients such as those undergoing dialysis. Attempts to reduce the nasal carriage of staphylococci have included the use of short-course rifampicin or long-term low-dose clindamycin.[9] Nasal creams containing chlorhexidine and neomycin or mupirocin are also used to eliminate nasal carriage of staphylococci.

Ecthyma gangrenosum usually affects severely immunocompromised patients and is generally caused by *Ps. aeruginosa*. Treatment should be with an aminoglycoside together with an antipseudomonal beta lactam such as azlocillin or ceftazidime.[1]

Ulceration of the skin may result from localised infection, as for example in necrotising infections, or may be secondary to pressure, vascular disease, or neuropathy. An antibacterial is indicated when there is definite evidence of tissue sepsis and those used have included an antistaphylococcal penicillin such as flucloxacillin with metronidazole or clindamycin when anaerobes are present, and gentamicin, ceftazidime, or ciprofloxacin for Gram-negative enteric organisms and *Ps. aeruginosa*.[1] In the case of secondary ulcers such as pressure sores[10] and leg ulcers,[11] prevention is the key to management. Antiseptics can be applied topically, but may impair wound healing. In general antibacterials are not recommended for topical use.[10,11] Metronidazole as a topical solution[12] or by mouth[13] has been used successfully to treat foul-smelling anaerobically infected pressure sores and leg ulcers, although the evidence for oral use in this condition was criticised.[14]

Burns become colonised by skin staphylococci including *Staph. aureus*, but infection may also arise from gut or upper respiratory tract flora, especially *Ps. aeruginosa*. Sepsis remains the major fatal complication. Prophylactic and especially topical antibacterials encourage resistance and may be toxic. Silver sulphadiazine cream has a broad spectrum and is especially active against Gram-negative bacteria although resistance can occur; mafenide acetate is also used. An essential element of management is removal of devitalised tissue, preferably before it has been heavily colonised. Infections with *Str. pyogenes* or *Staph. aureus* require aggressive treatment: for streptococcal infection penicillin is usually given with flucloxacillin to cover other colonising organisms that may be beta-lactamase producers; for staphylococcal infection a penicillinase-resistant penicillin is used; and for *Ps. aeruginosa* infection an aminoglycoside plus an antipseudomonal beta-lactam is used.[1]

Staphylococcal scalded skin syndrome is a toxin-mediated exfoliative dermatitis. Fluid and protein losses should be corrected and antistaphylococcal drugs such as flucloxacillin should be prescribed to eliminate the primary focus of infection.

Diabetic skin infections. Foot infections are a major problem in diabetic patients. They are polymicrobial and therapy to cover common pathogens should be used until the results of cultures are known. The following empirical treatment has been suggested.[15] For mild infections: oral treatment with amoxycillin/clavulanic acid or alternatively clindamycin, cephalexin, or cefuroxime axetil; for moderate infections: parenteral treatment with ticarcillin/clavulanic acid or ampicillin/sulbactam or alternatively clindamycin, cefoxitin, cefotetan, or cefotaxime; for severe infections: imipenem/cilastatin, aztreonam with clindamycin, or ciprofloxacin or ofloxacin with clindamycin.

Fungating tumours may produce a smell similar to that associated with anaerobic infection, suggesting colonisation of the tumour with anaerobes. Topical metronidazole has been applied to fungating tumours and other severe skin lesions to control offensive odour, supplemented by metronidazole irrigation for cleansing large or deep cavities.[16,17]

1. Finch R. Skin and soft-tissue infections. *Lancet* 1988; **i:** 164–8.
2. Anonymous. Topical antibiotics and antiseptics for the skin. *Drug Ther Bull* 1987; **25:** 97–9.
3. Bisno AL, Stevens DL. Streptococcal infections of skin and soft tissues. *N Engl J Med* 1996; **334:** 240–5.
4. Feder HM, *et al.* Is penicillin still the drug of choice for non-bullous impetigo? *Lancet* 1991; **338:** 803–5.
5. Failla DM, Pankey GA. Optimum outpatient therapy of skin and skin structure infections. *Drugs* 1994; **48:** 172–8.
6. Demidovich CW, *et al.* Impetigo: Current etiology and comparison of penicillin, erythromycin and cephalexin therapies. *Am J Dis Child* 1990; **144:** 1313–15.
7. Carruthers R. Prescribing antibiotics for impetigo. *Drugs* 1988; **36:** 364–9.
8. Kremer M, *et al.* Long-term antimicrobial therapy in the prevention of recurrent soft-tissue infections. *J Infect* 1991; **22:** 37–40.
9. Anonymous. Recurrent staphylococcal skin infections. *Lancet* 1988; **ii:** 1346–7.
10. Anonymous. Treatment of pressure ulcers. *Med Lett Drugs Ther* 1990; **32:** 17–18.
11. Gilliland EL, Wolfe JHN. Leg ulcers. *Br Med J* 1991; **303:** 776–9.
12. Jones PH, *et al.* Treatment of anaerobically infected pressure sores with topical metronidazole. *Lancet* 1978; **i:** 214.
13. Baker PG, Haig G. Metronidazole in the treatment of chronic pressure sores and ulcers: a comparison with standard treatments in general practice. *Practitioner* 1981; **225:** 569–73.
14. Anonymous. Does metronidazole help leg ulcers and pressure sores? *Drug Ther Bull* 1982; **20:** 9–10.
15. Joseph WS. Treatment of lower extremity infections in diabetics. *Drugs* 1991; **42:** 984–96.
16. Allwood MC, *et al.* Metronidazole topical gel. *Pharm J* 1986; **236:** 158.
17. Anonymous. Management of smelly tumours. *Lancet* 1990; **335:** 141–2.

Spleen disorders

Splenectomised patients and those with hyposplenism associated with, for example, sickle-cell disease have impaired immunity and like other immunocompromised patients (above) are at increased risk of infection. Children are at special risk. Pneumococci (*Streptococcus pneumoniae*) are the commonest infecting bacteria and may cause severe overwhelming infection that is rapid in onset and sometimes fatal. Hence, prophylaxis with an oral penicillin such as phenoxymethylpenicillin is advocated. Pneumococcal vaccine is also used; the newer ones may be more effective than earlier vaccines. Other organisms implicated include *Neisseria meningitidis*, *Haemophilus influenzae*, and *Escherichia coli* in splenectomised patients and *Salmonella* in children with sickle-cell disease. More unusual organisms include *Capnocytophaga canimorsus* (formerly called DF-2) which may cause opportunistic infections in splenectomised patients following animal bites. There may also be an increased risk of falciparum malaria and babesiosis.

SPLENECTOMISED PATIENTS. Guidelines for prophylaxis based on published evidence and expert opinion have been published in the UK.[1] Immunisation with polyvalent pneumococcal vaccine is recommended for all asplenic patients and those with functional hyposplenism. *Haemophilus influenzae* (Hib) vaccine is recommended for all patients who have not previously received this vaccine. Meningococcal immunisation is not routinely recommended since the vaccine currently available does not protect against the group B strain of *N. meningitidis* causing most infections in the UK. However, it is recommended for patients travelling to destinations where group A and C strains are more prevalent. Influenza vaccination may be beneficial. Lifelong prophylaxis with a suitable antibacterial should be offered. Phenoxymethylpenicillin is usually given, but amoxycillin may be preferred, particularly in adults, as it is better absorbed following oral administration and has a broader spectrum of activity. Erythromycin is a suitable alternative in those unable to tolerate penicillins. On a practical level, compliance with lifelong prophylaxis is difficult, but is particularly important in patients with underlying immunodeficiency, in children up to the age of 16 years, and for the first two years after splenectomy. Patients should keep a supply of a suitable antibacterial for immediate administration should symptoms of infection occur, and be instructed to seek medical advice urgently.

SICKLE-CELL DISEASE. Children with sickle-cell disease are particularly susceptible to severe pneumococcal infection which may be manifest as septicaemia, meningitis, or pneumonia.

Penicillin prophylaxis is usually combined with early administration of a polyvalent pneumococcal vaccine. However, despite the introduction of the 23-valent vaccine, there is little evidence that it produces substantial protection in children under 2 years of age. The value of prophylaxis with oral penicillin was demonstrated by Gaston *et al.*[2] Phenoxymethylpenicillin 125 mg twice daily is effective in young children but amoxycillin may be preferred in adults since it is better absorbed and has a broader spectrum.[1] There is evidence to suggest that, in children who have received pneumococcal immunisation, there is no benefit in continuing penicillin prophylaxis beyond the age of 5 years[3] although indefinite prophylaxis has been recommended for those who have had a previous pneumococcal septic event.[4] Fears that prolonged prophylaxis could encourage the emergence of resistant pneumococci have not been substantiated.[5] Neonatal screening for sickle-cell disease is advocated, but compliance with regular penicillin prophylaxis may be poor and effective follow-up is necessary if the full benefit of such screening is to be achieved.[6,7] Nevertheless, availability of penicillin in the home, even if not taken regularly, means that it can be readily used if febrile illness occurs.[2,6] If children with sickle-cell disease develop a febrile illness they are generally treated in hospital with intravenous antibacterials, although outpatient management may often be possible.[8]

1. Working Party of the British Committee for Standards in Haematology Clinical Haematology Task Force. Guidelines for the prevention and treatment of infection in patients with an absent or dysfunctional spleen. *Br Med J* 1996; **312:** 430–4.
2. Gaston MH, *et al.* Prophylaxis with oral penicillin in children with sickle cell anemia: a randomized trial. *N Engl J Med* 1986; **314:** 1593–9.
3. Falletta JM, *et al.* Discontinuing penicillin prophylaxis in children with sickle cell anemia. *J Pediatr* 1995; **127:** 685–90.
4. Hongeng S, *et al.* Recurrent Streptococcus pneumoniae sepsis in children with sickle cell disease. *J Pediatr* 1997; **130:** 814–16. Correction. *ibid.*; **131:** 232.
5. Norris CF, *et al.* Pneumococcal colonization in children with sickle cell disease. *J Pediatr* 1996; **129:** 821–7.
6. Milne RIG. Assessment of care of children with sickle cell disease: implications for neonatal screening programmes. *Br Med J* 1990; **300:** 371–4.
7. Cummins D, *et al.* Penicillin prophylaxis in children with sickle cell disease in Brent. *Br Med J* 1991; **302:** 989–90.
8. Willimas JA, *et al.* A randomized study of outpatient treatment with ceftriaxone for selected febrile children with sickle cell disease. *N Engl J Med* 1993; **329:** 472–6.

Spotted fevers

Rickettsial infections of the spotted fever group are transmitted to man by ticks and have also been called tick typhus. They include Rocky Mountain spotted fever, due to *Rickettsia rickettsii* and occurring especially in the USA; boutonneuse or Mediterranean spotted fever, due to *R. conorii* and occurring in Mediterranean countries including the Middle East, Africa, and India; Queensland tick typhus, due to *R. australis* and occurring in Australia; north Asian tick typhus, due to *R. sibirica* and occurring in Siberia and Mongolia; and oriental spotted fever, due to *R. japonica* and occurring in Japan. Rickettsialpox, due to *R. akari*, is transmitted from mice by mites and occurs in the USA, Russia, and Africa.

Spotted fevers are recognised increasingly as a cause of febrile illness associated usually but not always with a purpuric rash and are becoming an important cause of imported fevers in non-endemic areas.[1] Rocky Mountain spotted fever has been one of the most severe of these fevers, but others are potentially serious. A tetracycline, often doxycycline, or chloramphenicol is the treatment of choice for all the spotted fevers. In Rocky Mountain spotted fever tetracycline 25 to 50 mg per kg body-weight daily or chloramphenicol 50 to 75 mg per kg daily for 7 to 10 days markedly reduced mortality.[1] Because tetracyclines are generally contra-indicated in young children, chloramphenicol has been recommended in the USA for children with Rocky Mountain spotted fever under the age of 9, but some still prefer to use tetracycline;[2] as demonstrated in Mediterranean spotted fever, shorter courses of tetracycline might be effective.[3] Relapses have occurred in patients with Mediterranean spotted fever treated with chloramphenicol.[4] Other alternatives to tetracycline used in Mediterranean spotted fever have included erythromycin[5] and ciprofloxacin.[6] Erythromycin was effective, but less so than tetracycline, in children with Mediterranean spotted fever.[5] Short 2-day courses of ciprofloxacin or doxycycline were curative in adults whose disease was not severe, although there was a more rapid response to doxycycline.[6]

Rickettsialpox can be mistaken for chickenpox. However, it will respond to tetracycline although patients have generally recovered without treatment.[7]

1. Anonymous. Bitten, hot, and mostly spotty. *Lancet* 1991; **337:** 143–4.
2. Abramson JS, Givner LB. Should tetracycline be contraindicated for therapy of presumed Rocky Mountain spotted fever in children less than 9 years of age? *Pediatrics* 1990; **86:** 123–4.
3. Yagupsky P. Tetracycline for Rocky Mountain spotted fever. *Pediatrics* 1991; **87:** 124.
4. Shaked Y, *et al.* Relapse of rickettsial Mediterranean spotted fever and murine typhus after treatment with chloramphenicol. *J Infect* 1989; **18:** 35–7.
5. Muñoz-Espin T, *et al.* Erythromycin versus tetracycline for treatment of Mediterranean spotted fever. *Arch Dis Child* 1986; **61:** 1027–9.
6. Gudiol F, *et al.* Randomized double-blind evaluation of ciprofloxacin and doxycycline for Mediterranean spotted fever. *Antimicrob Agents Chemother* 1989; **33:** 987–8.
7. Kass EM, *et al.* Rickettsialpox in a New York City hospital, 1980 to 1989. *N Engl J Med* 1994; **331:** 1612–17.

Staphylococcal infections

Staphylococci are Gram-positive bacteria pathogenic to man. Species may be differentiated by various methods including the coagulase test. Those species of clinical importance are *Staphylococcus aureus*, which is usually coagulase-positive, and *Staph. epidermidis* and *Staph. saprophyticus*, which are coagulase-negative.

Staph. aureus colonises the skin and mucous membranes naturally and many people, including neonates, may be staphylococcal carriers from time to time. Localised *Staph. aureus* infections may follow surgery or trauma and commonly result in abscess formation. Staphylococcal skin infections include impetigo and furunculosis. Conditions associated with staphylococcal extracellular toxin production include staphylococcal scalded skin syndrome, toxic shock syndrome, and staphylococcal food poisoning. Staphylococcal septicaemia is usually a consequence of local infection and may sometimes be associated with intravascular or intraperitoneal catheters or with intravenous drug abuse. Septicaemia often results in staphylococcal endocarditis. Other possible complications of septicaemia are pneumonia and bone and joint infections, although in these cases aspiration or local trauma, respectively, may be the cause.

Staph. epidermidis is also a natural inhabitant of skin and mucous membranes and an increasingly important nosocomial pathogen. Many infections are hospital-acquired and are often associated with indwelling catheters. There has been an increased incidence of bacteraemia due to *Staph. epidermidis* in neonatal units.

Staph. saprophyticus is a common cause of urinary-tract infections in young women.

Staphylococci were sensitive to benzylpenicillin when it was first introduced, but the majority of strains are now resistant as a result of penicillinase production. Methicillin and other penicillinase-resistant penicillins such as flucloxacillin were developed because of their activity against these resistant staphylococci. However, methicillin-resistant staphylococci soon emerged. Both coagulase-negative staphylococci and *Staph. aureus* resistant to methicillin are generally resistant to all beta-lactams and often exhibit multiple resistance to other antibacterials (see Methicillin, p.225). More studies have been published on methicillin-resistant *Staph. aureus* (MRSA) than methicillin-resistant coagulase-negative staphylococci, but both types are a serious problem in hospitals around the world. Resistant strains may be endemic to a single hospital or may be epidemic causing outbreaks of infection at more than one hospital. Colonisation of hospital staff and patients with methicillin-resistant staphylococci is an important factor in the spread of these infections. Current trends are towards health care at home rather than in hospital and there are reports suggesting that MRSA is becoming more prevalent in the community.[1-3,8]

Revised guidelines for the control of MRSA in hospital were produced by a combined working party of the British Society for Antimicrobial Chemotherapy, the Hospital Infection Society, and the Infection Control Nurses Association in 1998.[4] They advise prompt isolation of infected or colonised patients, screening of patients and staff in contact with such patients, the use of protective clothing and handwashing with an antiseptic detergent or alcoholic rub; and the use by all patients of an antiseptic detergent for washing and bathing. For eradication of nasal carriage they recommend mupirocin nasal ointment or, if the strain is mupirocin-resistant, chlorhexidine and neomycin cream. Eradication at other colonised sites is more difficult: antiseptic detergents may be used for skin and hair washing; mupirocin in a macrogol basis for small infected skin lesions, but not for burns or large raw areas; hexachlorophane dusting powder for axillae and groins; and systemic rifampicin with fusidic acid or ciprofloxacin for throat or sputum colonisation if absolutely necessary.[4] For the treatment of severe infections due to MRSA they recommend vancomycin or teicoplanin, possibly combined with rifampicin, as the treatment of choice. Similarly recommendations have been made in a consensus review published in the USA.[5]

Although ciprofloxacin may be used the emergence of widespread resistance in methicillin-sensitive and methicillin-resistant *Staph. aureus* limits its usefulness (see p.187). Combination therapy may be helpful. Rifampicin is highly active against MRSA, but it must always be used in combination with another drug to prevent the emergence of resistance. Combinations of rifampicin with gentamicin, vancomycin, co-trimoxazole, fusidic acid, quinolones, or novobiocin have been tried.

There has been concern over isolated reports from around the world of resistance or reduced susceptibility to vancomycin,[6] and in response the Centers for Disease Control in the USA produced interim guidelines.[7]

Staphylococcal vaccines have been used for the prophylaxis and treatment of staphylococcal infections.

For the management of staphylococcal infections in general, see under the specific disease headings.

1. Rosenberg J. Methicillin-resistant Staphylococcus aureus (MRSA) in the community: who's watching? *Lancet* 1995; **346:** 132–3.
2. Herold BC, *et al.* Community-acquired methicillin-resistant Staphylococcus aureus in children with no identified predisposing risk. *JAMA* 1998; **279:** 593–8.
3. Collignon P, *et al.* Community-acquired meticillin-resistant Staphylococcus aureus in Australia. *Lancet* 1998; **352:** 145–6.
4. Combined Working Party of the British Society for Antimicrobial Chemotherapy, the Hospital Infection Society and the Infection Control Nurses Association. Revised guidelines for the control of methicillin-resistant Staphylococcus aureus infection in hospitals. *J Hosp Infect* 1998; **39:** 253–90.
5. Mulligan ME, *et al.* Methicillin-resistant Staphylococcus aureus: a consensus review of the microbiology, pathogenesis, and epidemiology with implications for prevention and management. *Am J Med* 1993; **94:** 313–28.
6. CDC. Update: Staphylococcus aureus with reduced susceptibility to vancomycin—United States, 1997. *MMWR* 1997; **46:** 813–15.
7. CDC. Interim guidelines for prevention and control of staphylococcal infection associated with reduced susceptibility to vancomycin. *MMWR* 1997; **46:** 626–8, 635.
8. Lowy FD. Staphylococcus aureus infections. *N Engl J Med* 1998; **339:** 520–32.

Surgical infection

Infection is an important cause of postoperative surgical morbidity and mortality. The value of infection *prophylaxis* is well established in certain types of surgery, especially abdominal surgery and where prostheses are implanted, although recommendations as to the choice of antibacterial and the route, timing, and duration of administration may vary. Keighley[1] has listed the major problems in surgical infection as: wound infection, which may be trivial or deep-seated; intra-abdominal, subphrenic, or pelvic abscesses; septicaemia; gas gangrene; and infected foreign bodies, including prostheses. The risk of postoperative infection is closely linked to the degree of contamination at operation. Categories of contamination include clean, clean-contaminated (potentially contaminated), contaminated, and dirty operations.[1] Clean operations exclude those involving the gastro-intestinal, urinary, or respiratory tracts. Clean-contaminated operations include those where the gastro-intestinal or respiratory tracts are opened, but there is no apparent contamination. Contaminated operations include those where there is acute inflammation or spillage from a hollow viscus. Dirty operations include those where there is pus, gangrene, or a perforated viscus. In addition, surgery to repair compound fractures and lacerations due to animal or human bites is considered 'dirty'. The use of antibacterials for the management of dirty surgery is considered to be therapeutic rather than prophylactic and should continue for several days postoperatively.[2]

Guidelines for the *treatment* of intra-abdominal infections have been produced in the USA by the Surgical Infection Society.[3]

ANTIMICROBIAL PROPHYLAXIS. Strictly speaking the term 'prophylaxis' should be confined to elective procedures with no evidence of sepsis at the time of operation. If possible any pre-existing infections should be treated before admission for surgery. For prophylaxis it is customary to give antibacterials systemically as a single pre-operative dose whereas more prolonged administration is necessary when they are given therapeutically.

Contaminating organisms. The choice of prophylactic antibacterial will be influenced by the likely contaminants for a particular surgical procedure. For example, Keighley[1] cites *Escherichia coli* and other Enterobacteriaceae as important pathogens in appendicectomy, gastro-oesophageal, biliary, and colorectal surgery; *Bacteroides* spp. in appendicectomy and colorectal surgery; *Clostridium perfringens* in gastro-oesophageal, biliary, and colorectal surgery; *Enterococcus faecalis* in gastro-oesophageal and biliary surgery; and staphylococci in gastro-oesophageal surgery. Staphylococci are also likely pathogens in cardiovascular, orthopaedic, and head and neck surgery;[2] *Staphylococcus aureus* infection may complicate 'clean' operations despite prophylaxis[4] and has been shown to be a common cause of sepsis in elective colorectal surgery.[5]

Route of administration. Systemic administration, usually by the intravenous route, is generally preferred. The chosen antibacterial is usually given as a single dose intravenously just before operation at the induction of anaesthesia. The pharmacokinetic properties should be such that adequate serum concentrations are maintained throughout the surgical procedure.[1] Additional doses may be necessary when surgery is prolonged, when there is massive blood loss, or when an antibacterial with a short half-life is used.[2] More controversial routes have included topical or intra-incisional administration and peritoneal lavage. Oral administration of non-absorbable antibacterials to suppress the intestinal flora was traditionally used before large bowel surgery and neomycin with erythromycin is still given for this purpose in the USA. For reference to selective digestive tract decontamination (SDD), see under Intensive Care, above. Other means of administration include bone cement and chains of beads for implantation, both containing gentamicin and used prophylactically in orthopaedic surgery.[6,7]

Choice of antibacterial. The most commonly used antibacterials are cephalosporins, aminoglycosides, and metronidazole. Cephazolin is commonly used in the USA.[2] Cefoxitin or cefotetan have greater activity against bowel anaerobes and may be preferred for colorectal surgery. Clindamycin is also indicated for some procedures.[2] If methicillin-resistant staphylococci are likely wound pathogens, prophylaxis with vancomycin may be necessary but it should not be used routinely since this may encourage the emergence of vancomycin-resistant enterococci.

The necessity for antibacterial prophylaxis in minimally invasive procedures such as laparoscopy and endoscopy is often not clear.[8]

Certain categories of patient continue to be at long-term risk of infection after surgery and include splenectomised patients who have impaired immunity and are at risk of pneumococcal and other infections (see under Spleen Disorders, above). Patients at special risk of endocarditis require prophylaxis when undergoing dental and some surgical procedures (see Endocarditis, above). Some have advocated similar prophylaxis in patients with joint prostheses undergoing dental treatment,[9] but a working party for the British Society for Antimicrobial Chemotherapy considers such prophylaxis to be unjustified.[10]

1. Keighley MRB. Infection: prophylaxis. *Br Med Bull* 1988; **44:** 374–402.
2. Anonymous. Antimicrobial prophylaxis in surgery. *Med Lett Drugs Ther* 1997; **39:** 97–102.
3. Bohnen JMA, *et al.* Guidelines for clinical care: anti-infective agents for intra-abdominal infection: a Surgical Infection Society policy statement. *Arch Surg* 1992; **127:** 83–9.

4. Kernodle DS, *et al.* Failure of cephalosporins to prevent Staphylococcus aureus surgical wound infections. *JAMA* 1990; **263:** 961–6.
5. Morris DL, *et al.* A comparison of aztreonam/metronidazole and cefotaxime/metronidazole in elective colorectal surgery: antimicrobial prophylaxis must include Gram-positive cover. *J Antimicrob Chemother* 1990; **25:** 673–8.
6. Henry SL, Galloway KP. Local antibacterial therapy for the management of orthopaedic infections: pharmacokinetic considerations. *Clin Pharmacokinet* 1995; **29:** 36–45.
7. Wininger DA, Fass RJ. Antibiotic-impregnated cement and beads for orthopedic infections. *Antimicrob Agents Chemother* 1996; **40:** 2675–9.
8. Wilson APR. Antibiotic prophylaxis and infection control measures in minimally invasive surgery. *J Antimicrob Chemother* 1995; **36:** 1–5.
9. Grant A, Hoddinott C. Joint replacement, dental surgery, and antibiotic prophylaxis. *Br Med J* 1992; **304:** 959.
10. Simmons NA, *et al.* Case against antibiotic prophylaxis for dental treatment of patients with joint prostheses. *Lancet* 1992; **339:** 301.

Syphilis

Syphilis is a sexually transmitted disease caused by the spirochaete *Treponema pallidum* and occurs worldwide. Non-venereal treponematoses occurring principally in the tropics include endemic syphilis or bejel, also caused by *T. pallidum*; pinta, caused by *T. carateum*; and yaws, caused by *T. pertenue*.

Syphilis may be acquired or congenital (see below) and in each case has early and late stages. In acquired sexually transmitted disease the *early* stage includes primary and secondary syphilis and early latent infection, defined as of not more than 2 years' duration by WHO[1,2] or of less than 1 year's duration by the Centers for Disease Control (CDC) in the USA.[3] (Latent infection is when serological tests are positive, but the patient is asymptomatic.) *Late* stage disease includes late latent infection and all late clinical stages. Some term all these late clinical stages tertiary syphilis whereas others use tertiary for benign gummatous syphilis and quaternary for the more serious complications of cardiovascular syphilis and neurosyphilis.[4] The term *neurosyphilis* has generally been applied to late-stage symptomatic neurological disease, although it is recognised that CNS invasion by *T. pallidum* is common in early syphilis and that CNS involvement may occur at any stage.

The incidence of syphilis fell dramatically after the introduction of penicillin and *T. pallidum* remains sensitive to it. There has, however, been a resurgence of syphilis,[5] linked in part with HIV infection. In HIV-infected patients syphilis appears more virulent and neurosyphilis occurs more quickly in these immunocompromised patients. Like other diseases causing genital ulcers, syphilis is a risk factor for HIV infection.

The treatment of choice for both early and late syphilis is still penicillin and long-acting injections are generally used. WHO guidelines[2] recommend either benzathine penicillin or procaine penicillin. The preferred penicillin in the UK is procaine penicillin[6] whereas benzathine penicillin is preferred in the USA.[3] Treatment for late syphilis is less well-established than that for early disease and is usually for longer. Benzylpenicillin may be preferred for neurosyphilis and congenital syphilis. For a summary of WHO and CDC treatment guidelines, see below.

Penetration of penicillin into the CNS is poor following the intramuscular injection of benzathine penicillin. Since *T. pallidum* may be present in the CNS in early disease and in view of the recent resurgence of syphilis in parts of the USA and its rapid progression, including the early development of neurological disease in patients with concomitant HIV infection, the efficacy of benzathine penicillin has been questioned.[7-9] In 1998 CDC[3] recommended no change in therapy for primary, secondary, or late latent syphilis in HIV-infected patients; early latent syphilis in HIV-infected patients should be treated as for primary and secondary syphilis. Others[9] have considered that higher total doses of benzathine penicillin, as for late disease, must be given to HIV-infected patients even with early syphilis to reduce the likelihood of a relapse to neurosyphilis and perhaps to control lesions. Likewise, a lower incidence of neurosyphilis in HIV-infected patients reported from Europe has been attributed by some to the 3 injections of benzathine penicillin used in Holland,[10] or 10 to 14 days of procaine penicillin in the UK,[11] as opposed to the single dose of benzathine penicillin used to treat early syphilis in the USA. Relapses have been reported in some HIV-infected patients in the USA despite the adoption of high multiple-dose regimens in all stages of syphilis.[12] However, the high doses of benzylpenicillin recommended by CDC for the treatment of neurosyphilis (see below) were not consistently effective in patients with HIV infection and symptomatic neurosyphilis.[13]

Patients *allergic to penicillin* have been given tetracycline or erythromycin although their efficacy is less well established.

A Jarisch-Herxheimer reaction may occur after the first dose of antibacterial, especially in patients with early syphilis, and some advocate corticosteroid cover.[4]

Congenital syphilis may result from transplacental infection at any stage of pregnancy and any stage of maternal syphilis. There has been a dramatic increase in its incidence in the USA and renewed concern about the efficacy of treatment with benzathine penicillin.[14] Both WHO[1,2] and CDC[3] prefer a course of benzylpenicillin or procaine penicillin rather than benzathine penicillin for infants with congenital syphilis.

Recommended *treatment regimens* for acquired and congenital syphilis from WHO in 1995[2] and CDC in 1998[3] are as follows. Sexual partners should be examined and treated.

EARLY SYPHILIS.

1. WHO: benzathine penicillin 1.8 g (2.4 million units) intramuscularly in a single session, usually given as 2 injections at separate sites, or procaine penicillin 1.2 g (1.2 million units) intramuscularly daily for 10 days. WHO note that some recommend longer regimens for secondary and latent syphilis and give benzathine penicillin weekly for 3 consecutive weeks or procaine penicillin daily for 2 weeks.

Alternatives for non-pregnant penicillin-allergic patients: doxycycline 100 mg by mouth twice daily for 15 days or tetracycline hydrochloride 500 mg by mouth 4 times daily for 15 days. Pregnant women allergic to penicillin may be given erythromycin 500 mg by mouth 4 times daily for 15 days (but see below).

2. CDC: Benzathine penicillin 1.8 g intramuscularly in a single dose. Alternatives for penicillin-allergic patients: doxycycline 100 mg twice daily, or tetracycline 500 mg four times daily, each by mouth for 2 weeks. A further though less effective alternative is erythromycin 500 mg four times daily, by mouth for 2 weeks; ceftriaxone may also be considered.

LATE SYPHILIS.

1. WHO: procaine penicillin 1.2 g intramuscularly daily for 3 weeks or benzathine penicillin 1.8 g intramuscularly once weekly for 3 consecutive weeks. For those with neurosyphilis: benzylpenicillin 2.4 g (4 million units) intravenously every 4 hours for 2 weeks, or, if compliance can be ensured, procaine penicillin 1.2 g intramuscularly daily plus probenecid 500 mg orally 4 times daily for 2 weeks.

2. CDC: benzathine penicillin 1.8 g intramuscularly weekly for 3 consecutive weeks. Alternatives: doxycycline or tetracycline by mouth for 4 weeks. For those with neurosyphilis: benzylpenicillin 1.8 to 2.4 g (3 to 4 million units) intravenously every 4 hours for 10 to 14 days or, if outpatient compliance can be ensured, procaine penicillin 2.4 g (2.4 million units) intramuscularly daily together with probenecid 500 mg by mouth 4 times daily, both for 10 to 14 days.

SYPHILIS IN PREGNANCY.

Penicillin as under early and late syphilis together with close surveillance. CDC[3] note that some recommend a second dose of benzathine penicillin a week after the initial dose for patients with early syphilis. According to CDC[3] pregnant patients who are allergic to penicillin should be given penicillin, after desensitisation if necessary, since the alternatives, tetracyclines, are contra-indicated during pregnancy and erythromycin cannot be relied on to cure an infected fetus. WHO, on the other hand, advise against desensitisation in a primary care setting and suggest that erythromycin, although inferior, should be given in these circumstances. The mother should be re-treated with tetracyclines after delivery, and the infant assessed and treated.

CONGENITAL SYPHILIS.

1. WHO: for early congenital syphilis in infants up to 2 years of age and having abnormal CSF: benzylpenicillin 30 mg per kg body-weight (50 000 units per kg) intramuscularly or intravenously daily in 2 divided doses for 10 days or procaine penicillin 50 mg per kg (50 000 units per kg) intramuscularly daily in a single dose for 10 days. For infants with normal CSF: benzathine penicillin 37.5 mg per kg (50 000 units per kg) intramuscularly as a single-session treatment (although some treat all as if the CSF were abnormal). Children older than 2 years: benzylpenicillin 120 to 180 mg per kg (200 000 to 300 000 units per kg) to a maximum of 1.44 g (2.4 million units) intravenously daily in divided doses for 2 weeks.

2. CDC: Benzylpenicillin 30 mg per kg intravenously every 12 hours for the first 7 days of life and every 8 hours thereafter for a total of 10 days or procaine penicillin 50 mg per kg intramuscularly daily for 10 days. Infants at risk of congenital syphilis but without clinical evidence of infection may be given a single intramuscular injection of benzathine penicillin 37.5 mg per kg. Older infants and children thought to have congenital syphilis or neurological involvement should be given benzylpenicillin 30 mg per kg every 4 to 6 hours for 10 days.

NON-VENEREAL TREPONEMATOSES.

When the prevalence of endemic syphilis (bejel), pinta, or yaws is 10% or more WHO[1] recommend mass treatment of the entire population with a single intramuscular injection of benzathine penicillin 900 mg (1.2 million units) or half this dose in children under 10 years.

1. WHO. WHO expert committee on venereal diseases and treponematoses: sixth report. *WHO Tech Rep Ser 736* 1986: 126–39.
2. WHO. *WHO model prescribing information: drugs used in sexually transmitted diseases and HIV infection.* Geneva: WHO, 1995.
3. Centers for Disease Control. 1998 Guidelines for treatment of sexually transmitted diseases. *MMWR* 1998; **47** (RR-1): 28–46.
4. Thin RN. Treatment of venereal syphilis. *J Antimicrob Chemother* 1989; **24:** 481–3.
5. Rolfs RT, Nakashima AK. Epidemiology of primary and secondary syphilis in the United States, 1981 through 1989. *JAMA* 1990; **264:** 1432–7.
6. Anderson J, *et al.* Primary and secondary syphilis, 20 years' experience 3: diagnosis, treatment, and follow up. *Genitourin Med* 1989; **65:** 239–43.
7. Musher DM. How much penicillin cures early syphilis? *Ann Intern Med* 1988; **109:** 849–51.
8. Lukehart SA, *et al.* Invasion of the central nervous system by Treponema pallidum: implications for diagnosis and treatment. *Ann Intern Med* 1988; **109:** 855–62.
9. Musher DM, *et al.* Effect of human immunodeficiency virus (HIV) infection on the course of syphilis and on the response to treatment. *Ann Intern Med* 1990; **113:** 872–81.
10. Esselink R, *et al.* Low frequency of neurosyphilis in HIV-infected individuals. *Lancet* 1993; **341:** 571.
11. O'Farrell N, Thin RN. Neurosyphilis and HIV. *Lancet* 1993; **341:** 1224.
12. Malone JL, *et al.* Syphilis and neurosyphilis in a human immunodeficiency virus type-1 seropositive population: evidence for frequent serologic relapse after therapy. *Am J Med* 1995; **99:** 55–63.
13. Gordon SM, *et al.* The response of symptomatic neurosyphilis to high-dose intravenous penicillin G in patients with human immunodeficiency virus infection. *N Engl J Med* 1994; **331:** 1469–73.
14. Ikeda MK, Janson HB. Evaluation and treatment of congenital syphilis. *J Pediatr* 1990; **117:** 843–52.

Tetanus

Clostridium tetani is a Gram-positive anaerobic spore-forming bacillus present in soil and faeces. The toxin it produces, tetanospasmin, causes tetanus or lockjaw, with uncontrolled muscle spasm. Tetanus can be prevented by active immunisation with tetanus vaccine or passive immunisation with tetanus immunoglobulin. Nowadays it occurs predominantly in developing countries and especially in neonates. In developed countries immunity may be relatively low in the elderly.

In addition to the control of muscle spasm with drugs such as diazepam (see p.1304 for the symptomatic treatment of tetanus), treatment includes the use of tetanus immunoglobulin to neutralise any circulating toxin and the administration of benzylpenicillin. A tetracycline[1] or metronidazole[2] have been suggested as possible alternatives to benzylpenicillin and some now consider metronidazole to be preferable to benzylpenicillin.[3]

In rural developing countries where tetanus is common and active immunisation little practised, pre-operative metronidazole or penicillin might be used for patients undergoing emergency operations who have not been immunised against tetanus; the duration of antibacterial cover depends on the contamination risk.[4]

1. Anonymous. The choice of antibacterial drugs. *Med Lett Drugs Ther* 1998; **40:** 33–42.
2. Ahmadsyah I, Salim A. Treatment of tetanus: an open study to compare the efficacy of procaine penicillin and metronidazole. *Br Med J* 1985; **291:** 648–50.

3. Sanford JP. Tetanus—forgotten but not gone. *N Engl J Med* 1995; **332:** 812–13.
4. Anonymous. Postoperative tetanus. *Lancet* 1984; **ii:** 964–5.

Tonsillitis

See under Pharyngitis, above.

Toxic shock syndrome

Toxic shock syndrome is an acute febrile illness associated with multisystem failure and caused by a toxin, usually toxic shock syndrome toxin-1 (TSST-1), produced by *Staphylococcus aureus*.[1,2] Bacteraemia has been reported to be absent in most cases.[3] In the early 1980s toxic shock syndrome was reported predominantly in menstruating women using high-absorbency tampons, but it is now appreciated that foci of staphylococcal infection such as surgical wounds, burns, abscesses, and sinuses are often responsible.[1,2] Treatment of the acute phase requires prevention of further production or absorption of toxin by local measures such as removal of tampons or packing, wound debridement, or drainage of abscesses; elimination of the toxin-producing bacteria by antistaphylococcal antibacterials given intravenously initially; fluid replacement; and sometimes corticosteroids.[1,2] Todd[1] recommended continuing antibacterial treatment for 10 days during the convalescent phase to reduce the risk of recurrence.

More recently group A beta-haemolytic streptococci (*Streptococcus pyogenes*) have been associated with a similar toxin-related syndrome.[4,5] Benzylpenicillin is the treatment of choice[6] but, since it may be difficult to exclude staphylococcal toxic shock syndrome, an antistaphylococcal drug such as flucloxacillin should also be given.[6] Clinical improvement has been reported in a patient after administration of intravenous normal immunoglobulins.[7]

Toxic shock syndromes may be associated with necrotising fasciitis (see above).

1. Todd JK. Therapy of toxic shock syndrome. *Drugs* 1990; **39:** 856–61.
2. Williams GR. The toxic shock syndrome. *Br Med J* 1990; **300:** 960.
3. Eykyn SJ. Staphylococcal sepsis: the changing pattern of disease and therapy. *Lancet* 1988; **i:** 100–4.
4. Cone LA, *et al.* Clinical and bacteriologic observations of a toxic shock-like syndrome due to Streptococcus pyogenes. *N Engl J Med* 1987; **317:** 146–9.
5. Stevens DL, *et al.* Severe group A streptococcal infections associated with a toxic shock-like syndrome and scarlet fever toxin A. *N Engl J Med* 1989; **321:** 1–7.
6. Sanderson P. Do streptococci cause toxic shock? *Br Med J* 1990; **301:** 1006–7.
7. Barry W, *et al.* Intravenous immunoglobulin therapy for toxic shock syndrome. *JAMA* 1992; **267:** 3315–16.

Trachoma

Trachoma results from chronic eye infection with certain *Chlamydia trachomatis* serotypes and is endemic in parts of Africa, the Middle East, and India where it is an important cause of blindness. It is not a sexually transmitted disease, but is associated with poverty, poor sanitation, and poor personal hygiene. The reservoir is chronic eye infection and transmission may be via fingers, fomites, and flies. Inclusion conjunctivitis in infants (see under Neonatal Conjunctivitis, above) and in adults is associated with sexually transmitted genital *C. trachomatis* infection and can progress to trachoma when there is persistent or recurrent eye infection.

Guidelines for trachoma control published by WHO in 1981 outlined topical or oral treatment with a tetracycline or alternatively with erythromycin or a sulphonamide.[1] Topical chemotherapy for trachoma must be intensive and prolonged, 6 weeks being the minimum recommended duration for continuous intensive treatment with tetracycline 1% ophthalmic ointment. With less frequent applications, the duration of treatment must be prolonged and may need to be extended to months or even years. The recommended intermittent treatment schedule consists of applications of tetracycline twice daily for 5 consecutive days or once daily for 10 days, each month and for 6 months each year, to be repeated as necessary. Short courses with topical tetracyclines can be used for the control of bacterial infections during seasonal epidemics of conjunctivitis and may have to be repeated annually. Oral therapy with tetracycline or doxycycline for 3 to 4 weeks has also been effective for selective treatment in well monitored programmes. Erythromycin and related macrolides administered by mouth or topically to the eye have been of benefit in trachoma, but have been less widely used. Topical therapy with sulphonamides appears only partially effective; adequate treatment with oral sulphonamides requires full therapeutic doses for approximately 2 to 3 weeks and may be associated with adverse reactions.

A single oral dose of azithromycin has been reported to produce a similar rate of resolution to conventional treatment with topical tetracycline for 6 weeks.[2] In the USA, some[3] recommend azithromycin as the treatment of choice for trachoma, with combined oral and topical treatment with either a tetracycline or a sulphonamide as an alternative.

The view has been expressed that in endemic areas the provision of clean water, regular face washing, and the use of tetracycline eye ointment by those infected might eradicate trachoma.[4]

A vaccine against *C. trachomatis* is also under investigation.[5]

1. Dawson CR, *et al. Guide to trachoma control.* Geneva: WHO, 1981.
2. Bailey RL, *et al.* Randomised controlled trial of single-dose azithromycin in treatment of trachoma. *Lancet* 1993; **342:** 453–6.
3. Anonymous. The choice of antibacterial drugs. *Med Lett Drugs Ther* 1998; **40:** 33–42.
4. Potter AR. Avoidable blindness. *Br Med J* 1991; **302:** 922–3.
5. Coghlan A. Shapely vaccine targets chlamydia. *New Scientist* 1996; **152:** 18.

Trench fever

Trench fever is a louse-borne bacterial infection so named because of its prevalence among soldiers in the First World War. It is caused by *Bartonella quintana* (formerly *Rochalimaea quintana*) which was until recently classified as a rickettsia. *B. quintana* and *B. henselae* have also been implicated in bacillary angiomatosis, especially in immunocompromised patients, and *B. henselae* is considered to be a cause of cat scratch disease (above).

Reports from France[1] and the USA[2] of *B. quintana* bacteraemia, sometimes with endocarditis, in the urban poor prompted the suggestion that trench fever has returned.[3] A typical case of trench fever in Marseilles has been described[4] and might herald an increasing incidence as a result of migration from endemic areas, poverty, and louse infestation.

Treatment of trench fever has usually been with a tetracycline such as doxycycline or with erythromycin. Other antibacterials, for example ceftriaxone, were also used in cases of bacteraemia,[2] but there was limited follow-up and clear recommendations could not be given. Similarly, optimal therapy for *Bartonella* endocarditis has not been identified; however, it has been suggested that the usual treatment for blood culture-negative endocarditis (a penicillin plus an aminoglycoside) should be effective.[5]

1. Drancourt M, *et al.* Bartonella (Rochalimaea) quintana endocarditis in three homeless men. *N Engl J Med* 1995; **332:** 419–23.
2. Spach DH, *et al.* Bartonella (Rochalimaea) quintana bacteremia in inner-city patients with chronic alcoholism. *N Engl J Med* 1995; **332:** 424–8.
3. Relman DA. Has trench fever returned? *N Engl J Med* 1995; **332:** 463–4.
4. Stein A, Raoult D. Return of trench fever. *Lancet* 1995; **345:** 450–1.
5. Raoult D, *et al.* Diagnosis of 22 new cases of Bartonella endocarditis. *Ann Intern Med* 1996; **125:** 646–52. Correction. *ibid.* 1997; **127:** 249.

Tuberculosis

Tuberculosis is a chronic infectious disease caused primarily by *Mycobacterium tuberculosis* or sometimes *M. bovis*; the closely related form *M. africanum* has occasionally been implicated as a cause of human tuberculosis. Infection is usually due to inhalation of infected droplet nuclei, and the lung is generally the first organ affected, but the primary infection is usually asymptomatic.

In the majority of subjects infection and concomitant inflammatory reactions resolve once acquired immunity develops and any surviving organisms become dormant, but in a few patients, particularly in young children or immunocompromised patients, there may be a progression to active primary disease. Dormant organisms may also become reactivated in some patients to produce disease, particularly following changes in immune status. Hypersensitivity reactions to mycobacterial proteins may cause extensive tissue damage, and virtually any organ of the body can be involved.

During recent years there has been an increase in the incidence of tuberculosis, particularly among the urban poor, and also in association with the spread of HIV infection. WHO declared tuberculosis a global emergency in 1993. Particularly worrying is the increase in multidrug-resistant strains and poor compliance with drug treatment is seen as a contributory factor. In the USA, there has been emphasis on improving compliance with drug therapy and monitoring responses to limit the further spread of multidrug-resistant disease.[1,2] Direct supervision of treatment has been shown to be effective in both urban and rural settings,[3-6] and attempts have been made to simplify drug regimens to facilitate this, including the use of intermittent therapy and combination preparations.[7] The feasibility of implantable dosage forms is also being investigated.[8] A decrease in reported cases of tuberculosis in New York City from 1992 through 1994 has been attributed mainly to better rates of treatment completion and expanded use of directly observed therapy.[9]

WHO applies the term DOTS to its tuberculosis control strategy; it has also been used as an acronym for directly observed treatment, short-course.

Treatment. The introduction of rifampicin, with its rapid bactericidal activity, in the 1970s allowed the development of short-course chemotherapy for the treatment of tuberculosis. Treatment regimens formerly relied on oral daily isoniazid and thiacetazone for periods of 12 to 18 months supplemented by parenteral streptomycin for the first 2 months. Reasons for the high failure rate commonly encountered with such regimens included poor compliance, failure of streptomycin to suppress active disease during the initial treatment phase, and toxicity of the drugs used. Modern short-course therapy involves an initial phase (2 months) using a combination of drugs to produce rapid killing of the bacilli, with the majority of patients having no organisms detectable in sputum smears after 2 months, and a continuation phase of 4 to 6 months using fewer drugs with the aim of eliminating any remaining organisms and thus preventing recurrence.

FIRST-LINE DRUGS. First-choice **antituberculous drugs**, often referred to as primary or 'first-line' drugs include isoniazid, rifampicin, pyrazinamide, ethambutol, and streptomycin. Thiacetazone has also been regarded as a first-line drug in developing countries but WHO recommends that ethambutol be substituted in patients with HIV infection whenever possible since this patient group is at high risk of severe and sometimes fatal skin reactions with thiacetazone. In fact, current WHO recommended treatment regimens do not include thiacetazone. However, the suggestion that thiacetazone should be dropped for routine treatment[10,11] in general has proved controversial.[12,13] The short-course regimens recommended by WHO[14] combine drugs with potent bactericidal activity (isoniazid, rifampicin), with sterilising activity against semi-dormant bacilli (rifampicin, pyrazinamide) with the ability to suppress drug-resistant mutants (isoniazid, rifampicin), and which may be administered 2 or 3 times weekly (isoniazid, rifampicin, pyrazinamide, streptomycin, ethambutol).

WHO recommends treatment regimens based on disease characteristics.[14,15] To ensure compliance, WHO considers direct observation of therapy to be essential during the initial phase and desirable in patients receiving rifampicin during the continuation phase.[14,15]

For newly diagnosed patients with active pulmonary tuberculosis and patients with severe tuberculosis at any site the following regimens are recommended: for the initial phase, isoniazid, rifampicin, and pyrazinamide plus either streptomycin or ethambutol daily for 2 months; then for the continuation phase either isoniazid plus rifampicin daily (or 3 times each week for both drugs for intermittent therapy) for a further 4 months or isoniazid plus ethambutol daily for a further 6 months. (Ethambutol and streptomycin are omitted from the initial phase in some national guidelines for patient groups in whom the risk of drug resistance is small.)

For re-treatment after relapse, treatment failure, or default patients should receive isoniazid, rifampicin, pyrazinamide, and ethambutol daily for 3 months, supplemented with streptomycin daily for the first 2 months as directly observed therapy (initial phase) then, if the sputum is smear-negative, isoniazid, rifampicin, and ethambutol daily (or 3 times each week for all drugs) for a further 5 months (continuation phase).

For patients with smear-negative pulmonary tuberculosis and patients with less severe infections at other sites the preferred regimen is isoniazid, rifamycin, and pyrazinamide daily for 2 months (initial phase) then either isoniazid and ethambutol daily for 6 months or isoniazid and rifampicin daily (or 3 times each week for both drugs) for 4 months (continuation phase).

The choice of regimen depends on local patterns of drug resistance and the availability of drugs and medical supervision, and are embodied in national treatment protocols in many countries including the UK[16] and USA.[17,18] Recently there has been increased awareness of the potential hepatotoxicity of first-line drugs such as isoniazid, rifampicin, and pyrazinamide. Pyrazinamide is generally regarded as producing the most severe form of hepatotoxicity of the three, and further details covering this and special precautions for its use in patients with liver disorders are given in the drug monograph (p.241). WHO and UK guidelines recommend interrupting drug therapy if liver dysfunction occurs, and cautiously re-introducing the same drugs (including pyrazinamide) on resolution.[14,19] Patients in whom complete cessation of therapy is hazardous may be given streptomycin and ethambutol until hepatic function recovers.

SECOND-LINE DRUGS. Other drugs used in the treatment of tuberculosis, such as the aminosalicylates, capreomycin, cycloserine, ethionamide, prothionamide, and kanamycin are considered to be secondary drugs and have been used if resistance or toxicity to the 'first-line' drugs develops during therapy, but are generally less effective and/or more toxic. The increasing problem of tuberculosis resistant to conventional first-line drugs has also led to increased interest in the development of new agents, and in various drugs such as the fluoroquinolones and the rifamycin derivative rifabutin.

RESISTANCE. The incidence of drug-resistant strains of *Mycobacterium tuberculosis* has increased steadily over recent years in many countries, including the USA.[20,21] Isoniazid resistance is most common but multidrug-resistant strains have also occurred, often in HIV-infected individuals, resulting in disease which is very difficult to treat and often fatal. Such resistance is considered to result from poor management of tuberculosis control[22] and administration of tuberculosis treatment under direct observation has reduced the rates of primary drug resistance, acquired drug resistance, and relapse in the USA.[3,9] In the UK[23] rates of multidrug-resistant tuberculosis remained lower than those in the USA, but are rising. The first reported outbreak of hospital-acquired multidrug-resistant tuberculosis in England and Wales has occurred on an HIV unit.[24]

In areas with a high rate of initial drug resistance, ethambutol or streptomycin is added during the initial phase;[14,15] drug selection may be re-evaluated once sensitivity results are available. As discussed above, patients who relapse after an initial treatment course are generally given a second prolonged and directly observed treatment course with first-line drugs. Patients who relapse following the WHO standard re-treatment regimen or who are otherwise suspected of having multidrug-resistant tuberculosis should receive at least three drugs which the patient has not already received and which do not share cross-resistance to drugs received previously; these should be given under direct observation for at least 3 months followed by a continuation phase of at least 18 months with at least 2 of the drugs. WHO recommends inclusion of an injectable aminoglycoside (amikacin, capreomycin, or kanamycin) and pyrazinamide, even if the patient has previously received it, in the initial phase.[25] Cross-resistance exists between fluoroquinolones, between cycloserine and terizidone, and between thiacetazone and prothionamide or ethionamide.[25] Cross-resistance between rifampicin and rifabutin is also commonly observed. There appears to be no cross-resistance between fluoroquinolones and other antituberculous drugs, but fluoroquinolone-resistant tuberculosis can emerge rapidly as a result of inadequate or inappropriate treatment.[26] Cross-resistance patterns among aminoglycosides are complex.[25]

CHILDREN. Children and infants can be treated with similar regimens to adults.[16-18] Ethambutol is not usually given to young children because of difficulty in detecting ocular toxicity.

PREGNANCY AND THE NEONATE. Tuberculosis during pregnancy poses a serious risk to the fetus and neonate if not detected early and treated properly in the mother.[27] Pregnant patients with clinical tuberculosis are treated similarly to non-pregnant patients, although streptomycin, other aminoglycosides, and capreomycin should be avoided because they can cause ototoxicity in the fetus. Ethionamide and prothionamide are also best avoided.[16] The American Thoracic Society and CDC[18] have also advised against the routine use of pyrazinamide because the risk of teratogenicity had not been determined. Consequently, since the standard 6-month regimen includes pyrazinamide, they recommend a minimum of 9 months of therapy preferably with isoniazid, rifampicin, and ethambutol initially. However, others have used pyrazinamide in pregnancy.[27] Also in the USA, pregnant women who react positively to a tuberculin skin test, but who have a normal chest X-ray, may be offered immediate prophylaxis with isoniazid (see Preventive Therapy, below) if they have risk factors for tuberculosis; those without risk factors are referred for prophylaxis after delivery.[27] Following two reports of isoniazid-related hepatitis deaths in the postpartum period, some delay prophylaxis with isoniazid until 3 to 6 months post partum.[27]

The neonate of a mother with current tuberculosis should receive isoniazid for 3 months (UK)[16] or 6 months (USA)[18] then the infant should be re-evaluated. BCG vaccination is recommended by some authorities when isoniazid is stopped.[14,16]

HIV INFECTION. Patients with HIV infection are particularly prone to active tubercular disease, both pulmonary and extrapulmonary. Studies suggest that such patients respond well to conventional regimens,[28] although malabsorption of antimycobacterials may occur[29] and has been associated with acquired drug resistance,[30] and mortality is higher than in HIV-negative patients.[14] Also, there may be an increased incidence of adverse reactions to antimycobacterials in HIV-positive individuals,[28] particularly to thiacetazone.[31] WHO recommend that ethambutol should be used in place of both thiacetazone and streptomycin in patients with HIV infection.[14] Most regimens suggested for treating tuberculosis in patients with HIV infection are versions of standard short-course therapy with rifampicin, isoniazid, ethambutol, and pyrazinamide (see above), and most commentators emphasise the importance of directly observed therapy to ensure compliance.[32] It has been suggested that these regimens should be adopted for treatment of all patients regardless of HIV status thus avoiding the necessity to test for HIV before starting treatment,[10,11] but this may not be practical in some developing countries.[12,13] In the USA, treatment is recommended for a minimum of 9 months.[17]

Drug-resistant tuberculosis is a problem,[33,34] with up to 90% of cases of drug-resistant disease in the USA occurring in HIV-infected persons:[33] regimens must be modified as in non-HIV-infected patients. Multiple drug-resistant tuberculosis can be rapidly fatal in patients with HIV infection and early, effective treatment is essential, and should continue for 18-24 months after smears become negative.[35]

Prolonged or lifetime prophylaxis with isoniazid has been given to patients with HIV infection following the completion of tuberculosis treatment in the UK.[36] Preventive therapy is also used in some countries to prevent first episodes of active disease (see below).

ADJUNCTIVE THERAPY. Injection of suspensions of killed *Mycobacterium vaccae* has been shown to improve immune responsiveness in patients with pulmonary tuberculosis,[37] and such **immunotherapy** may be a beneficial addition to chemotherapy.[38-40]

The use of **corticosteroids** in uncomplicated pulmonary tuberculosis should be avoided but they have a role in selected patients with severe pulmonary and severe extrapulmonary disease, and for patients with severe hypersensitivity reactions to antituberculous drugs.[14,41,42] They should never be given to patients with active disease without protective chemotherapy cover and they must be used with caution in patients with dormant disease in whom they may reactivate disease. For further details on the possible role of corticosteroids as an adjunct to antituberculous therapy, see p.1030.

Preventive Therapy (Chemoprophylaxis). Chemoprophylaxis is intended to prevent the occurrence of acute tuberculosis in patients with asymptomatic tuberculous infection (that is, those with a positive tuberculin skin test but no evidence of active disease), and in susceptible contacts, and to curb its spread through the community.

Chemoprophylaxis is not recommended routinely in developing countries and the primary objective as elsewhere should be to treat active tuberculosis.[14] Chemoprophylaxis is generally with isoniazid for 6 to 12 months. It is more widely used in the USA than in the UK and other countries where vaccination with BCG vaccine (p.1505) is employed. Rifampicin, and occasionally ethambutol may be used if the likelihood of drug resistance is high.[18]

The American Thoracic Society and the Centers for Disease Control[18] have issued detailed recommendations for prophylactic treatment of tuberculosis. Prophylaxis with isoniazid for 6 to 12 months is generally recommended for the following categories of patients who exhibit a positive tuberculin skin test:

1) Household members and other close associates of newly diagnosed potentially infectious tuberculosis patients.

2) Persons whose skin tests have become positive within the past 2 years.

3) Patients in special clinical situations such as those with diabetes mellitus, Hodgkin's disease, leukaemia, end-stage renal failure, or those receiving prolonged corticosteroid or immunosuppressive therapy, or intravenous drug abusers, or those with substantial rapid weight loss or chronic undernutrition.

In addition, chemoprophylaxis may be offered to persons with negative skin tests in certain high-risk situations.

Prophylaxis is also recommended for persons infected with HIV who react positively to tuberculin but have no evidence of disease. HIV-positive patients should not receive BCG vaccine because of the risk of disseminated infection.[43]

For reference to prophylaxis in pregnant women and the neonate, see above.

The British Thoracic Society's Joint Tuberculosis Committee advises that chemoprophylaxis may be given to some contacts with strongly positive tuberculin Heaf test reactions, but without clinical or radiological evidence of tuberculous disease.[44] They recommend that chemoprophylaxis should be given to contacts under 16 years old who have not had BCG vaccination and have positive tuberculin reactions and should be considered in children who have received BCG vaccination and who have a strongly positive tuberculin reaction. Also, children under 2 years old who are close contacts of cases with positive sputum smears and who have not had BCG vaccination should be given chemoprophylaxis whatever their tuberculin status.[16]

The resurgence of tuberculosis has increased the risk of nosocomial infection in patients and health care workers and has prompted guidance on preventing its transmission in health care settings.[44]

HIV INFECTION. Since HIV infection increases both the individual's susceptibility to primary infection with *M. tuberculosis* and to progression to active tuberculosis in individuals with existing *M. tuberculosis* infection, effective tuberculosis control is particularly important in this population. BCG immunisation is not recommended in individuals with HIV infection since there is a risk of disseminated infection. Chemoprophylaxis has been shown to reduce the incidence of tuberculosis when given to persons with HIV infection, particularly in those with a positive tuberculin reaction.[45] Current practice is to give chemoprophylaxis to individuals identified as being at greatest risk of tuberculosis. In 1994, IUAT and WHO[47] supported prophylaxis with isoniazid for 6 to 12 months in HIV-infected individuals with a positive tuberculin test, once active tuberculosis had been excluded. Further research was necessary before, for example, the merits of life-long or extended preventive therapy in areas of high tuberculosis transmission or the role of prophylaxis in anergic individuals could be assessed. In the USA, chemoprophylaxis is also offered to HIV-infected persons with negative tuberculin tests who are considered to be at high risk of contracting the infection.[18,48]

In developing countries with a high prevalence of tuberculosis, the difficulties in providing preventive chemotherapy to all HIV-infected individuals at risk may be overwhelming.[46] WHO has suggested that preventive chemotherapy may be restricted to selected at-risk groups such as health-care workers and selected individuals.[14]

1. Bellin E. Failure of tuberculosis control: a prescription for change. *JAMA* 1994; **271:** 708–9.
2. Bloch AB, *et al.* Nationwide survey of drug-resistant tuberculosis in the United States. *JAMA* 1994; **271:** 665–71.
3. Weis SE, *et al.* The effect of directly observed therapy on the rates of drug resistance and relapse in tuberculosis. *N Engl J Med* 1994; **330:** 1179–84.
4. Wilkinson D. High-compliance tuberculosis treatment programme in a rural community. *Lancet* 1994; **343:** 647–8.
5. Bayer R, Wilkinson D. Directly observed therapy for tuberculosis: history of an idea. *Lancet* 1995; **345:** 1545–8. Correction. *ibid.*; **346:** 322.
6. China Tuberculosis Control Collaboration. Results of directly observed-therapy in 112 842 Chinese patients with smear-positive tuberculosis. *Lancet* 1996; **347:** 358–62.
7. Moulding T, *et al.* Fixed-dose combinations of antituberculous medications to prevent drug resistance. *Ann Intern Med* 1995; **122:** 951–4.
8. Gangadharam PRJ, *et al.* Experimental chemotherapy of tuberculosis using single dose treatment with isoniazid in biodegradable polymers. *J Antimicrob Chemother* 1994; **33:** 265–71.
9. Frieden TR, *et al.* Tuberculosis in New York City—turning the tide. *N Engl J Med* 1995; **333:** 229–33.
10. Nunn P. Thiacetazone should not be used routinely—or primum non nocere. *Tubercle Lung Dis* 1995; **76** (suppl 2): 3.
11. Elliott AM, Foster SD. Thiacetazone: time to call a halt? *Tubercle Lung Dis* 1996; **77:** 27–9.
12. Rieder HL. Controversies in tuberculosis control: thioacetazone may be used routinely—pro. *Tubercle Lung Dis* 1995; **76** (suppl 2): 3.
13. van Gorkom J, Kibuga DK. Cost-effectiveness and total costs of three alternative strategies for the prevention and management of severe skin reactions attributable to thiacetazone in the treatment of human immunodeficiency virus positive patients with tuberculosis in Kenya. *Tubercle Lung Dis* 1996; **77:** 30–6.
14. WHO. *TB/HIV: A clinical manual.* Geneva: WHO, 1996.
15. WHO. *Treatment of tuberculosis: guidelines for national programmes.* Geneva: WHO, 1997.
16. Joint Tuberculosis Committee of the British Thoracic Society. Chemotherapy and management of tuberculosis in the United Kingdom: recommendations 1998. *Thorax* 1998; **53:** 536–48.
17. Centers for Disease Control. Initial therapy for tuberculosis in the era of multidrug resistance: recommendations of the Advisory Council for the Elimination of Tuberculosis. *MMWR* 1993; **42:** 1–8.
18. American Thoracic Society and the Centers for Disease Control. Treatment of tuberculosis and tuberculosis infection in adults and children. *Am J Respir Crit Care Med* 1994; **149:** 1359–74.
19. Ormerod LP, *et al.* Hepatotoxicity of antituberculosis drugs. *Thorax* 1996; **51:** 111–13.
20. Iseman MD. Treatment of multidrug-resistant tuberculosis. *N Engl J Med* 1993; **329:** 784–91.
21. Pablos-Mendez A, *et al.* Global surveillance for antituberculosis-drug resistance, 1994-1997. *N Engl J Med* 1998; **338:** 1641–9. Correction. *ibid.*; **339:** 139.
22. Nunn P, Felten M. Surveillance of resistance to antituberculosis drugs in developing countries. *Tubercle Lung Dis* 1994; **75:** 163–7.
23. Bennett DE, *et al.* Drug resistant tuberculosis in England and Wales, 1993-1995. *Thorax* 1996; **51** (suppl 3): A8.
24. Anonymous. Outbreak of hospital acquired multidrug resistant tuberculosis. *Commun Dis Rep* 1995; **5:** 161.
25. WHO. *Guidelines for the management of drug-resistant tuberculosis.* Geneva: WHO, 1997.
26. Sullivan EA, *et al.* Emergence of fluoroquinolone-resistant tuberculosis in New York City. *Lancet* 1995; **345:** 1148–50.
27. Davidson PT. Managing tuberculosis during pregnancy. *Lancet* 1995; **346:** 199–200.
28. Small PM, *et al.* Treatment of tuberculosis in patients with advanced human immunodeficiency virus infection. *N Engl J Med* 1991; **324:** 289–94.
29. Peloquin CA, *et al.* Malabsorption of antimycobacterial medications. *N Engl J Med* 1993; **329:** 1122–3.
30. Patel KB, *et al.* Drug malabsorption and resistant tuberculosis in HIV-infected patients. *N Engl J Med* 1995; **332:** 336–7.
31. Nunn P, *et al.* Cutaneous hypersensitivity reactions due to thiacetazone in HIV-1 seropositive patients treated for tuberculosis. *Lancet* 1991; **337:** 627–30.
32. De Cock KM, Wilkinson D. Tuberculosis control in resource-poor countries: alternative approaches in the era of HIV. *Lancet* 1995; **346:** 675–7.
33. Snider DE, Roper WL. The new tuberculosis. *N Engl J Med* 1992; **326:** 703–5.
34. Edlin BR, *et al.* An outbreak of multidrug-resistant tuberculosis among hospitalized patients with the acquired immunodeficiency syndrome. *N Engl J Med* 1992; **326:** 1514–21.
35. Drobniewski F. Is death inevitable with multiresistant TB plus HIV infection? *Lancet* 1997; **349:** 71–2.
36. Subcommittee of the Joint Tuberculosis Committee of the British Thoracic Society. Guidelines on the management of tuberculosis and HIV infection in the United Kingdom. *Br Med J* 1992; **304:** 1231–3.
37. Bahr GM, *et al.* Improved immunotherapy for pulmonary tuberculosis with Mycobacterium vaccae. *Tubercle* 1990; **71:** 259–66.
38. Etemadi A, *et al.* Immunotherapy for drug-resistant tuberculosis. *Lancet* 1992; **340:** 1360–1.
39. Stanford JL, Grange JM. New concepts for the control of tuberculosis in the twenty first century. *J R Coll Physicians Lond* 1993; **27:** 218–23.
40. Prior JG, *et al.* Immunotherapy with Mycobacterium vaccae combined with second line chemotherapy in drug-resistant abdominal tuberculosis. *J Infect* 1995; **31:** 59–61.
41. Horne NW, ed. *Modern drug treatment of tuberculosis.* 7th ed. London: The Chest, Heart and Stroke Association, 1990.
42. Alzeer AH, FitzGerald JM. Corticosteroids and tuberculosis: risks and use as adjunct therapy. *Tubercle Lung Dis* 1993; **74:** 6–11.
43. Centers for Disease Control. 1997 USPHS/IDSA guidelines for the prevention of opportunistic infections in persons infected with human immunodeficiency virus. *MMWR* 1997; **46** (RR-12): 10–12.
44. Joint Tuberculosis Committee of the British Thoracic Society. Control and prevention of tuberculosis in the United Kingdom: Code of Practice 1994. *Thorax* 1994; **49:** 1193–1200.
45. Wilkinson D, *et al.* Effect of preventive treatment for tuberculosis in adults infected with HIV: systematic review of randomised placebo controlled trials. *Br Med J* 1998; **317:** 625–9.
46. De Cock KM, *et al.* Preventive therapy for tuberculosis in HIV-infected persons: international recommendations, research, and practice. *Lancet* 1995; **345:** 833–6.
47. International Union Against Tuberculosis and Lung Disease (IUATLD) and the Global Programme on AIDS and the Tuberculosis Programme of the World Health Organization (WHO). Tuberculosis preventive therapy in HIV-infected individuals: a joint statement. *Tubercle Lung Dis* 1994; **75:** 96–8.
48. Kaplan JE, *et al.* USPHS/IDSA guidelines for the prevention of opportunistic infections in persons infected with human immunodeficiency virus: an overview. *Clin Infect Dis* 1995; **21** (suppl 1): S12–S31.

Tularaemia

Tularaemia is caused by the Gram-negative bacillus *Francisella tularensis* which primarily affects rodents and rabbits but may be transmitted to man, usually by handling infected animals or carcasses, or by the bites of insect vectors. It may take several forms, the most common of which is the ulceroglandular form, characterised by rash and ulceration at the site of inoculation accompanied by fever and lymphadenopathy; other forms include the typhoidal and pneumonic forms, which have a higher mortality rate.

Streptomycin is considered the antibacterial of choice in severe disease,[1,2] although gentamicin may be an alternative in patients who cannot tolerate streptomycin.[2] Tetracycline or chloramphenicol may be given by mouth; clinical relapses are more frequent than with the aminoglycosides,[2,3] although relapsed disease will respond to a further course. Some patients have also responded to high-dose intravenous erythromycin.[4]

Because of the difficulty in obtaining streptomycin in the USA, the literature on alternative drugs for the treatment of tularaemia was reviewed.[5] On the basis of this review it was concluded that:

- gentamicin is an acceptable alternative to streptomycin and should be considered the alternative antibacterial of choice for serious cases of nonmeningitic tularaemia
- tetracycline might be a reasonable alternative to gentamicin and could be given by mouth in less severely ill patients, but there is a relatively high relapse rate with tetracycline
- chloramphenicol should be considered when tularaemic meningitis is suspected—like tetracycline it is associated with a relatively high relapse rate, but has the advantage over both aminoglycosides and tetracycline of good penetration of the CNS
- imipenem-cilastatin (1 case) and the fluoroquinolones ciprofloxacin and norfloxacin (6 cases) have shown promise, but further studies are needed before they can be recommended.

A tularaemia vaccine is available in some countries for active immunisation against the disease.

1. Corwin WC, Stubbs SP. Further studies on tularemia in the Ozarks: review of forty-four cases during a three-year period. *JAMA* 1952; **149:** 343–5.
2. Evans ME, *et al.* Tularemia: a 30-year experience with 88 cases. *Medicine (Baltimore)* 1985; **64:** 251–69.
3. Ford-Jones L, *et al.* "Muskrat fever": two outbreaks of tularemia near Montreal. *Can Med Assoc J* 1982; **127:** 298–9.
4. Westerman EL, McDonald J. Tularemia pneumonia mimicking Legionnaires' disease: isolation of organism on CYE agar and successful treatment with erythromycin. *South Med J* 1983; **76:** 1169–70.
5. Enderlin G, *et al.* Streptomycin and alternative agents for the treatment of tularemia: review of the literature. *Clin Infect Dis* 1994; **19:** 42–7.

Typhoid and paratyphoid fever

Typhoid and paratyphoid fever are systemic infections caused respectively by *Salmonella typhi* and *S. paratyphi* A, B, or C, Gram-negative bacteria belonging to the Enterobacteriaceae family. They are sometimes termed collectively 'enteric fever' but, although infection follows invasion of the intestinal mucosa and reinfection of the intestines subsequently occurs, dissemination in the blood leads to more widespread systemic effects. Typhoid and paratyphoid are endemic in many countries and, in most, typhoid is more common. In the UK most cases are contracted abroad; in the period 1981-90 the majority of those in England and Wales with typhoid and paratyphoid A fever had been infected in the Indian subcontinent whereas the majority of paratyphoid B fever had been picked up in Mediterranean and Middle East countries.[1]

Treatment of typhoid fever has generally been with chloramphenicol or alternatively amoxycillin, ampicillin, or co-trimoxazole. However, there has been a spread of strains of *S. typhi* resistant to chloramphenicol, ampicillin, amoxycillin, trimethoprim, and co-trimoxazole,[2-8] especially in the Indian subcontinent, in the Middle East, and possibly in South and South-East Asia. Fluoroquinolones such as ciprofloxacin or third-generation cephalosporins such as cefotaxime, ceftriaxone, and cefoperazone are effective for typhoid fever due to multiresistant strains, with fluoroquinolones generally the more effective.[9] Reporting from the Central Public Health Laboratory on the incidence of chloramphenicol-resistant strains of *S. typhi* in the UK in 1991, Rowe *et al.*[10] recommended that treatment with ciprofloxacin should be considered, especially when patients have come from areas endemic for these resistant strains. In 1994, the recommendation to use ciprofloxacin for initial treatment of enteric fever in the UK still stood.[11] However, the increasing incidence of ciprofloxacin resistance in multiresistant *S. typhi* has been noted in both developing and developed countries.[12,13] Fluoroquinolones are generally contra-indicated in children and in pregnant women because of potential toxicity, but there is evidence of the successful use of ciprofloxacin or ofloxacin in multiresistant infection in children[14-16] and some have recommended their use in these patients.[9] Similarly, ciprofloxacin was effective in the second and third trimester of pregnancy[17,18] and some have suggested that it could be used in pregnancy if the organism was resistant to amoxycillin or ampicillin.[17]

On recovery, typhoid patients may continue to excrete *S. typhi* in the faeces or urine for several weeks. Unlike these convalescent carriers, chronic carriers may excrete *S. typhi* for years without any symptoms; eradication is difficult and prolonged courses of treatment are necessary. An increased risk of biliary-tract and bile-related cancers has been associated with chronic carriage of *S. typhi*, and the importance of eradication has been emphasised.[19] Typhoid vaccines are used for the prevention of typhoid fever.

Paratyphoid fever is less common and generally milder than typhoid fever. Treatment is similar.

1. Anonymous. Enteric fever England and Wales 1981-90. *Commun Dis Rep* 1991; **1:** 72.
2. Rowe B, *et al.* Spread of multiresistant Salmonella typhi. *Lancet* 1990; **336:** 1065.
3. Mikhail IA, *et al.* Antibiotic-multiresistant Salmonella typhi in Egypt. *Trans R Soc Trop Med Hyg* 1989; **83:** 120.
4. Anand AC, *et al.* Epidemic multiresistant enteric fever in eastern India. *Lancet* 1990; **335:** 352.
5. Jesudasan MV, John TJ. Multiresistant Salmonella typhi in India. *Lancet* 1990; **336:** 252.
6. Gupta BL, *et al.* Multiresistant Salmonella typhi in India. *Lancet* 1990; **336:** 252.
7. Wallace M, Yousif AA. Spread of multiresistant Salmonella typhi. *Lancet* 1990; **336:** 1065–6.
8. Mandal BK. Treatment of multiresistant typhoid fever. *Lancet* 1990; **336:** 1383.
9. White NJ, *et al.* Fluoroquinolone antibiotics in children with multidrug resistant typhoid. *Lancet* 1996; **348:** 547.
10. Rowe B, *et al.* Ciprofloxacin and typhoid fever. *Lancet* 1992; **339:** 740.
11. Brown NM, *et al.* Ciprofloxacin resistance in Salmonella paratyphi A. *J Antimicrob Chemother* 1994; **33:** 1258–9.
12. Rowe B, *et al.* Ciprofloxacin-resistant Salmonella typhi in the UK. *Lancet* 1995; **346:** 1302.
13. Mitchell DH. Ciprofloxacin-resistant Salmonella typhi: an emerging problem. *Med J Aust* 1997; **167:** 172.
14. Cheesbrough JS, *et al.* Quinolones in children with invasive salmonellosis. *Lancet* 1991; **338:** 127.
15. Dutta P, *et al.* Ciprofloxacin for treatment of severe typhoid fever in children. *Antimicrob Agents Chemother* 1993; **37:** 1197–9.
16. Vinh H, *et al.* Two or three days of ofloxacin treatment for uncomplicated multidrug-resistant typhoid fever in children. *Antimicrob Agents Chemother* 1996; **40:** 958–61.
17. Leung D, *et al.* Treatment of typhoid in pregnancy. *Lancet* 1995; **346:** 648.
18. Koul PA, *et al.* Ciprofloxacin for multiresistant enteric fever in pregnancy. *Lancet* 1995; **346:** 307–8.
19. Caygill CPJ, *et al.* Cancer mortality in chronic typhoid and paratyphoid carriers. *Lancet* 1994; **343:** 83–4.

Typhus

Rickettsial infections or fevers of the typhus group are transmitted to man by various insect vectors. Louse-borne or epidemic typhus, due to *Rickettsia prowazekii*, and flea-borne or murine typhus, due to the closely related *R. typhi* (formerly called *R. mooseri*), have occurred worldwide. Scrub typhus is due to *Orientia tsutsugamushi* (formerly *R. tsutsugamushi*) transmitted by mites and occurs mainly in Asia, Australia, and the Pacific Islands.

Tetracycline, often doxycycline, or chloramphenicol is the treatment of choice for these infections although strains of *O. tsutsugamushi* resistant to doxycycline and chloramphenicol have been reported in Thailand.[1] There is some evidence that ciprofloxacin may prove effective.[2] Prophylaxis for scrub typhus with doxycycline has shown promise when started before exposure to infection.[3] Typhus vaccines are available for active immunisation against louse-borne typhus.

1. Watt G, *et al.* Scrub typhus infections poorly responsive to antibiotics in northern Thailand. *Lancet* 1996; **348:** 86–9.
2. Eaton M, *et al.* Ciprofloxacin treatment of typhus. *JAMA* 1989; **262:** 772–3.
3. Twartz JC, *et al.* Doxycycline prophylaxis for human scrub typhus. *J Infect Dis* 1982; **146:** 811–18.

Urethritis

Infective urethritis is a sexually transmitted disease seen most frequently in men. One of the commonest causes is *Neisseria gonorrhoeae*. Nongonococcal urethritis or nonspecific urethritis may be due to *Chlamydia trachomatis* in up to 50% of cases and *Ureaplasma urealyticum* (formerly T-strain mycoplasma) in up to 40%, but often the cause is unknown. Other organisms implicated have included *Mycoplasma genitalium*. Gonococcal and chlamydial infections frequently occur together and, since specific therapy for gonorrhoea is often not effective against *C. trachomatis*, treatment for the two infections should be given concomitantly otherwise postgonococcal urethritis due to *C. trachomatis* may follow the cure of gonorrhoea. The treatment of chlamydial urethritis is discussed under Chlamydial Infections (above) and that for gonococcal urethritis under Gonorrhoea (above).

For nonchlamydial nongonococcal urethritis the Centers for Disease Control in the USA[1] recommend a single 1-g dose of azithromycin by mouth or a 7-day course of doxycycline 100 mg twice daily. Alternative regimens are erythromycin 500 mg four times daily or ofloxacin 300 mg twice daily, in each case for 7 days.[1] Persistent or recurrent nongonococcal urethritis should be treated with a single oral 2-g dose of metronidazole plus oral erythromycin 500 mg four times daily for 7 days.[1]

1. Centers for Disease Control. 1998 Guidelines for treatment of sexually transmitted diseases. *MMWR* 1998; **47** (RR-1): 49–52.

Urinary-tract infections

Infections of the urinary tract are especially common in women. They are frequently due to enteric bacteria, in particular *Escherichia coli*, although a common cause in young women is *Staphylococcus saprophyticus*, a coagulase-negative staphylococcus. Other urinary pathogens include *Staph. epidermidis*, enterococci, and *Pseudomonas* spp. An arbitrary definition of urinary-tract infection has been significant bacteriuria with 10^5 or more colony forming units per mL of a midstream urine specimen; some also consider lower counts to be indicative of infection. Most urinary-tract infections are isolated uncomplicated infections of the lower urinary tract. Recurrent infections may be due to relapse, or more often, re-infection and are more serious. Patients with complicated urinary-tract infections associated with urinary-tract abnormalities or diseases such as diabetes mellitus may be at risk of kidney damage.

Infections of the lower urinary tract in *women* generally present as cystitis (inflammation of the bladder) and symptoms include dysuria, frequency, and urgency together with pyuria and significant bacteriuria; the urethral syndrome is similar, but there is no significant bacteriuria. In the upper urinary tract acute pyelonephritis may occur as a complication of cystitis or, more rarely may result from septicaemia. Asymptomatic bacteriuria may progress to acute pyelonephritis in *pregnant women* and should therefore be treated.

Urinary-tract infections in *men* are less common and are often associated with abnormalities of the genito-urinary tract such as prostatic hyperplasia. Acute bacterial prostatitis is usually caused by organisms similar to those responsible for cystitis in women. Chronic bacterial prostatitis is difficult to treat; the antibacterials used must be able to penetrate into the prostatic fluid. For other genito-urinary infections in men, see under Epididymitis and under Urethritis, above.

In preschool *children*, especially girls, asymptomatic bacteriuria together with vesicoureteric reflux can result in renal scarring and should be treated; the use of prophylactic antibacterials is complex and controversial. Long-term follow-up of girls who have had asymptomatic bacteriuria suggests that new kidney damage does not occur after 4 years of age, but highlights the importance of diagnosis and treatment in younger children.

The significance of asymptomatic bacteriuria in *old age* is disputed, but most consider treatment to be unnecessary.

Infections associated with *indwelling bladder catheters* occur in both men and women and probably account for the majority of hospital-acquired urinary-tract infections.

Treatment. Antibacterials used to treat urinary-tract infections need to be excreted in adequate concentrations in the urine. For *acute uncomplicated infections* oral amoxycillin, ampicillin, co-trimoxazole, nalidixic acid, nitrofurantoin, or trimethoprim (preferred to co-trimoxazole in the UK) have been given although the choice will depend on local patterns of bacterial resistance; *E. coli* resistant to ampicillin and amoxycillin is widespread. Alternatives when resistance is prevalent include amoxycillin with clavulanic acid, oral cephalosporins, fluoroquinolones such as ciprofloxacin, or fosfomycin. In pregnant women, nitrofurantoin or a beta lactam can be used. Standard treatment schedules have been for 5 to 7 days; 3-day or single-dose regimens can also be effective and may be preferred in women. Urinary alkalinising agents such as potassium citrate and sodium citrate have been given by mouth to relieve the pain of cystitis caused by lower urinary-tract infections. Recurrent infections may require long-term low-dose antibacterial prophylaxis.

Acute pyelonephritis may require broad-spectrum parenteral treatment initially with, for example, aztreonam, ceftazidime, cefuroxime, ciprofloxacin, or gentamicin.

Chronic bacterial prostatitis may require treatment for several weeks with trimethoprim, erythromycin, or a fluoroquinolone.

Catheter-related bladder infections may sometimes respond to localised treatment with bladder washouts containing chlorhexidine.

References.

1. Brumfitt W. Progress in understanding urinary infections. *J Antimicrob Chemother* 1991; **27:** 9–22.
2. Wilkie ME, *et al.* Diagnosis and management of urinary tract infection in adults. *Br Med J* 1992; **305:** 1137–41.
3. Stamm WE, Hooton TM. Management of urinary tract infections in adults. *N Engl J Med* 1993; **329:** 1328–34.
4. Grüneberg RN. Changes in urinary pathogens and their antibiotic sensitivities, 1971–1992. *J Antimicrob Chemother* 1994; **33** (suppl A): 1–8.
5. Thomson KS, *et al.* USA resistance patterns among UTI pathogens. *J Antimicrob Chemother* 1994; **33** (suppl A): 9–15.
6. Kunin CM. Chemoprophylaxis and suppressive therapy in the management of urinary tract infections. *J Antimicrob Chemother* 1994; **33** (suppl A): 51–62.
7. Reeves DS. A perspective on the safety of antibacterials used to treat urinary tract infections. *J Antimicrob Chemother* 1994; **33** (suppl A): 111–20.
8. Brumfitt W, Hamilton-Miller JMT. Consensus viewpoint on management of urinary infections. *J Antimicrob Chemother* 1994; **33** (suppl A): 147–53.
9. Maskell R. Management of recurrent urinary tract infections in adults. *Prescribers' J* 1995; **35:** 1–11.
10. Ronald A, Sanche SE. Antimicrobial management of urinary tract infections. *Curr Opin Infect Dis* 1995; **8:** 420–3.
11. Nicolle LE. A practical guide to the management of complicated urinary tract infection. *Drugs* 1997; **53:** 583–92.

CATHETER RELATED. References.

1. Anonymous. Catheter-acquired urinary tract infection. *Lancet* 1991; **338:** 857–8.
2. Harding GKM, *et al.* How long should catheter-acquired urinary tract infection in women be treated: a randomized controlled study. *Ann Intern Med* 1991; **114:** 713–19.
3. van der Wall E, *et al.* Prophylactic ciprofloxacin for catheter-associated urinary-tract infection. *Lancet* 1992; **339:** 946–51.

ELDERLY. References.

1. Morgan MG, *et al.* Treatment of urinary infection in the elderly. *Infection* 1990; **18:** 326–31.
2. Abrutyn E, *et al.* Does asymptomatic bacteriuria predict mortality and does antimicrobial treatment reduce mortality in elderly ambulatory women? *Ann Intern Med* 1994; **120:** 827–33. Correction. *ibid.*; **121:** 901.
3. Nicolle LE. Urinary tract infection in the elderly. *J Antimicrob Chemother* 1994; **33** (suppl A): 99–109.
4. Ouslander JG, *et al.* Does eradicating bacteriuria affect the severity of chronic urinary incontinence in nursing home residents? *Ann Intern Med* 1995; **122:** 749–54.
5. Abrutyn E, *et al.* Does treatment of asymptomatic bacteriuria in older ambulatory women reduce subsequent symptoms of urinary tract infection? *J Am Geriatr Soc* 1996; **44:** 293–5.

INFANTS AND CHILDREN. References.

1. Verrier Jones K. Antimicrobial treatment for urinary tract infections. *Arch Dis Child* 1990; **65:** 327–30.
2. White RHR. Management of urinary tract infection and vesicoureteric reflux in children: 1. *Br Med J* 1990; **300:** 1391–2.
3. Working Group of the Research Unit, Royal College of Physicians. Guidelines for the management of acute urinary tract infection in childhood. *J R Coll Physicians Lond* 1991; **25:** 36–42.
4. Smellie JM, *et al.* Retrospective study of children with renal scarring associated with reflux and urinary infection. *Br Med J* 1994; **308:** 1193–6.
5. Ansari BM, *et al.* Urinary tract infection in children: part 1: epidemiology, natural history, diagnosis and management. *J Infect* 1995; **30:** 3–6.
6. Watson AR. Urinary tract infection in early childhood. *J Antimicrob Chemother* 1994; **34** (suppl A): 53–60. Correction. *ibid.* 1995; **35:** 561.
7. Gordon I. Vesico-ureteric reflux, urinary-tract infection, and renal damage in children. *Lancet* 1995; **346:** 489–90.
8. Anonymous. The management of urinary tract infection in children. *Drug Ther Bull* 1997; **35:** 65–9.

MEN. References.

1. Lipsky BA. Urinary tract infections in men: epidemiology, pathophysiology, diagnosis, and treatment. *Ann Intern Med* 1989; **110:** 138–50.
2. Leigh DA. Prostatitis—an increasing clinical problem for diagnosis and management. *J Antimicrob Chemother* 1993; **32** (suppl A): 1–9.

PREGNANCY. References.

1. Tan JS, File TM. Treatment of bacteriuria in pregnancy. *Drugs* 1992; **44:** 972–80.
2. Vercaigne LM, Zhanel GG. Recommended treatment for urinary tract infection in pregnancy. *Ann Pharmacother* 1994; **28:** 248–51.
3. Bint AJ, Hill D. Bacteriuria of pregnancy—an update on significance, diagnosis and management. *J Antimicrob Chemother* 1994; **33** (suppl A): 93–7.

WOMEN. References.

1. Johnson JR, Stamm WE. Urinary tract infections in women: diagnosis and treatment. *Ann Intern Med* 1989; **111:** 906–17.
2. Brumfitt W, Hamilton-Miller JMT. Prophylactic antibiotics for recurrent urinary tract infections. *J Antimicrob Chemother* 1990; **25:** 505–12.
3. Hamilton-Miller JMT. The urethral syndrome and its management. *J Antimicrob Chemother* 1994; **33** (suppl A): 63–73.
4. Kunin CM. Urinary tract infections in females. *Clin Infect Dis* 1994; **18:** 1–12.
5. Anonymous. Managing urinary tract infection in women. *Drug Ther Bull* 1998; **36:** 30–2.

Whipple's disease

Whipple's disease is a rare chronic systemic infection associated with a bacillus recently identified as *Tropheryma whippelii*.[1] It was once considered to be a disease predominantly involving the small intestine and resulting in malabsorption, but may affect virtually all organs. There is probably central nervous system involvement in all patients with Whipple's disease, although it may only be evident in 10 to 20%.[2] Before the use of antibacterial therapy the disease was invariably fatal. The treatment generally recommended is benzylpenicillin (sometimes given as procaine penicillin) and streptomycin parenterally for two weeks, followed by co-trimoxazole orally for one year.[2-5] Such long-term treatment with co-trimoxazole, a drug that crosses the blood-brain barrier, is advisable because of the relatively high frequency and seriousness of CNS relapse. These relapses respond less well to antibacterial treatment;[3] chloramphenicol has been used in those not responding to the above regimen and one patient with CNS relapse improved on ceftriaxone given intravenously.[6] A patient intolerant of co-trimoxazole was given phenoxymethylpenicillin and probenecid after the initial 14-day course of benzylpenicillin and streptomycin.[7] There has also been a report of benefit in a penicillin-allergic patient treated with erythromycin.[8]

1. Relman DA, *et al.* Identification of the uncultured bacillus of Whipple's disease. *N Engl J Med* 1992; **327:** 293–301.
2. Dobbins WO. Whipple's disease. *Mayo Clin Proc* 1988; **63:** 623–4.
3. Keinath RD, *et al.* Antibiotic treatment and relapse in Whipple's disease: long-term follow-up of 88 patients. *Gastroenterology* 1985; **88:** 1867–73.
4. Fleming JL, *et al.* Whipple's disease: clinical, biochemical, and histopathologic features and assessment of treatment in 29 patients. *Mayo Clin Proc* 1988; **63:** 539–51.

5. Singer R. Diagnosis and treatment of Whipple's disease. *Drugs* 1998; **55:** 699–704.
6. Adler CH, Galetta SL. Oculo-facial-skeletal myorhythmia in Whipple disease: treatment with ceftriaxone. *Ann Intern Med* 1990; **112:** 467–9.
7. Rickman LS, *et al.* Brief report: uveitis caused by Tropheryma whippelii (Whipple's bacillus). *N Engl J Med* 1995; **332:** 363–6.
8. Bowles KM, *et al.* A 35-year-old with swollen knees who had recurrent fever and pericarditis, then diarrhoea before getting better. *Lancet* 1996; **348:** 1356.

Yaws

See under Syphilis, above.

Yersinia enteritis

See under Gastro-enteritis, above.

Acediasulfone Sodium (8231-n)

Acediasulfone Sodium *(rINN).*

Sodium Diaphenylsulphonacetate. *N-p*-Sulphanilylphenylglycine sodium.

$C_{14}H_{13}N_2NaO_4S$ = 328.3.

CAS — 127-60-6.

Acediasulfone sodium is reported to have antibacterial properties and is used topically in the treatment of local infections of the ear.

Preparations

Proprietary Preparations (details are given in Part 3)

Multi-ingredient: ***Aust.:*** Ciloprin cum Anaesthetico; ***Swed.:*** Ciloprin; ***Switz.:*** Ciloprine ca.

Aconiazide (1947-b)

Aconiazide *(rINN).*

α-Isonicotinylhydrazone *o*-tolyloxyacetic acid.

$C_{15}H_{13}N_3O_4$ = 299.3.

CAS — 13410-86-1.

Aconiazide is an antituberculous drug under investigation.

Acrosoxacin (12323-t)

Acrosoxacin *(BAN).*

Rosoxacin *(USAN, rINN)*; Win-35213. 1-Ethyl-1,4-dihydro-4-oxo-7-(4-pyridyl)quinoline-3-carboxylic acid.

$C_{17}H_{14}N_2O_3$ = 294.3.

CAS — 40034-42-2.

Adverse Effects and Precautions

As for Nalidixic Acid, p.228.

Dizziness, drowsiness, and visual disturbances may occur relatively frequently and patients should be advised not to drive or operate machinery if affected.

Uses and Administration

Acrosoxacin is a 4-quinolone antibacterial with actions similar to those of nalidixic acid. It is active against *Neisseria gonorrhoeae* and is given by mouth in the treatment of gonorrhoea (p.126) as a single dose of 300 mg, preferably on an empty stomach.

Preparations

Proprietary Preparations (details are given in Part 3)

Fr.: Eracine; ***Ger.:*** Winuron†; ***Irl.:*** Eradacin†; ***Ital.:*** Rosacin†; ***Spain:*** Eradacil†; ***UK:*** Eradacin†.

Alatrofloxacin Mesylate (5383-c)

Alatrofloxacin Mesylate *(USAN).*

Alatrofloxacin Mesilate *(rINNM)*; CP-116517-27. 7-{(1*R*,5*S*,6*s*)-6-[(*S*)-2-((*S*)-2-Aminopropionamido)propionamido]-3-azabicyclo[3.1.0]hex-3-yl}-1-(2,4-difluorophenyl)-6-fluoro-1,4-dihydro-4-oxo-1,8-naphthyridine-3-carboxylic acid monomethanesulphonate.

$C_{26}H_{25}F_3N_6O_5,CH_3SO_3H$ = 654.6.

CAS — 157182-32-6 (alatrofloxacin); 157605-25-9 (alatrofloxacin mesylate).

Alatrofloxacin is a prodrug of the fluoroquinolone antibacterial trovafloxacin (p.267) and is used intravenously as the mesylate in the treatment of susceptible infections. Details of doses are given under trovafloxacin.

Preparations

Proprietary Preparations (details are given in Part 3)

USA: Trovan.

Amifloxacin (14126-q)

Amifloxacin *(BAN, USAN, rINN).*

Win-49375; Win-49375-3 (amifloxacin mesylate). 6-Fluoro-1,4-dihydro-1-methylamino-4-oxo-7-(4-methylpiperazin)-1-ylquinoline-3-carboxylic acid; 6-Fluoro-1,4-dihydro-1-(methylamino)-7-(4-methyl-1-piperazinyl)-4-oxo-3-quinolinecarboxylic acid.

$C_{16}H_{19}FN_4O_3$ = 334.3.

CAS — 86393-37-5 (amifloxacin); 88036-80-0 (amifloxacin mesylate).

Amifloxacin is a fluoroquinolone antibacterial.

Amikacin (184-z)

Amikacin *(BAN, rINN).*

Amicacina; Amikacinum. 6-*O*-(3-Amino-3-deoxy-α-D-glucopyranosyl)-4-*O*-(6-amino-6-deoxy-α-D-glucopyranosyl)-*N*[1]-[(2*S*)-4-amino-2-hydroxybutyryl]-2-deoxystreptamine.

$C_{22}H_{43}N_5O_{13}$ = 585.6.

CAS — 37517-28-5.

Pharmacopoeias. In *Eur.* (see p.viii), *Int.*, *Pol.*, and *US.*

A semisynthetic derivative of kanamycin A. A white or almost white crystalline powder. Sparingly **soluble** in water; practically insoluble in alcohol and in acetone; slightly soluble in methyl alcohol. A 1% solution in water has a pH of 9.5 to 11.5. **Store** in airtight containers.

Amikacin Sulphate (3-k)

Amikacin Sulphate *(BANM, rINNM).*

Amikacin Sulfate *(USAN)*; Amikacini Sulfas; BB-K8.

$C_{22}H_{43}N_5O_{13},2H_2SO_4$ = 781.8.

CAS — 39831-55-5.

Pharmacopoeias. In *Chin.*, *Eur.* (see p.viii), *Int.*, *Jpn*, *Pol.*, and *US.*

A white or almost white crystalline powder. 1.3 g of monograph substance is approximately equivalent to 1 g of amikacin. Ph. Eur. states that it contains not less than 72.3% and not more than the equivalent of 76.8% of amikacin, calculated with reference to the dried substance. The pH of a 1% solution is between 2.0 and 4.0. The USP permits amikacin sulphate having a molar ratio of amikacin to H_2SO_4 of either 1:2 or 1:1.8. The pH of a 1% solution is between 2.0 and 4.0 and between 6.0 and 7.3 respectively. It loses not more than 13.0% of its weight on drying.

Freely **soluble** in water; practically insoluble in alcohol and in acetone. Solutions may darken from colourless to pale yellow but this does not indicate a loss of potency. **Store** in airtight containers.

Incompatibilities. For discussion of the incompatibility of aminoglycosides, including amikacin, with beta lactams, see under Gentamicin Sulphate, p.212. Amikacin is also reported to be incompatible with various other drugs. However, reports are contradictory in many cases, and other factors, such as the strength and composition of the vehicles used, may play a role.

Adverse Effects, Treatment, and Precautions

As for Gentamicin Sulphate, p.212. Peak plasma concentrations of amikacin greater than 30 to 35 μg per mL or trough concentrations greater than 5 to 10 μg per mL should be avoided. Amikacin affects auditory (cochlear) function to a greater extent than gentamicin.

Interactions

As for Gentamicin Sulphate, p.213.

Antimicrobial Action

As for Gentamicin Sulphate, p.213. It is active against a similar range of organisms although it is also reported to have some activity against *Nocardia asteroides*, *Mycobacterium tuberculosis*, and some atypical mycobacterial strains. MICs of amikacin for the most sensitive organisms range from about 0.1 to 8 μg per mL or more, which are generally higher than those for gentamicin; however higher doses than for gentamicin can be tolerated, permitting peak serum concentrations up to about 30 to 35 μg per mL. Amikacin is not degraded by many of the common enzymes often responsible for acquired aminoglycoside resistance. In consequence, cross-resistance with gentamicin and other aminoglycosides is infrequent and amikacin may be effective against strains resistant to other aminoglycosides. However, resistant strains of Gram-negative bacteria and staphylococci have been reported, and some authorities feel that its use should be restricted to infections resistant to other aminoglycosides, although reports differ as to the extent and speed of the development of amikacin resistance where it has been widely used.

References.

1. Ho YII, *et al.* In-vitro activities of aminoglycoside-aminocyclitols against mycobacteria. *J Antimicrob Chemother* 1997; **40:** 27–32.

Pharmacokinetics

As for Gentamicin Sulphate, p.213.

After intramuscular injection of amikacin sulphate peak plasma concentrations equivalent to about 20 μg of amikacin per mL are achieved one hour after a 500-mg dose, reducing to about 2 μg per mL 10 hours after injection. A plasma concentration of 38 μg per mL has been reported after the intravenous infusion of 500 mg over 30 minutes, reduced to 18 μg per mL one hour later. Amikacin has been detected in body tissues and fluids after injection; it crosses the placenta but does not readily penetrate into the CSF, although substantial penetration of the blood-brain barrier has been reported in children with meningitis.

A plasma half-life of about 2 to 3 hours has been reported in patients with normal renal function. Most of a dose is excreted by glomerular filtration in the urine within 24 hours.

References.

1. Vanhaeverbeek M, *et al.* Pharmacokinetics of once-daily amikacin in elderly patients. *J Antimicrob Chemother* 1993; **31:** 185–7.
2. Gaillard J-L, *et al.* Cerebrospinal fluid penetration of amikacin in children with community-acquired bacterial meningitis. *Antimicrob Agents Chemother* 1995; **39:** 253–5.
3. Bressolle F, *et al.* Population pharmacokinetics of amikacin in critically ill patients. *Antimicrob Agents Chemother* 1996; **40:** 1682–9.
4. Canis F, *et al.* Pharmacokinetics and bronchial diffusion of single daily dose amikacin in cystic fibrosis patients. *J Antimicrob Chemother* 1997; **39:** 431–3.
5. Tod M, *et al.* Population pharmacokinetic study of amikacin administered once or twice daily to febrile, severely neutropenic adults. *Antimicrob Agents Chemother* 1998; **42:** 849–56.

Uses and Administration

Amikacin is a semisynthetic aminoglycoside antibiotic derived from kanamycin and is used similarly to gentamicin (p.214) in the treatment of severe Gram-negative and other infections. It is given as the sulphate, and is generally reserved for the treatment of severe infections caused by susceptible bacteria that are resistant to gentamicin and tobramycin. Amikacin has also been given with antimycobacterials in the treatment of opportunistic mycobacterial infections (p.133). As with gentamicin, amikacin may be used with penicillins and with cephalosporins; the injections should be given at separate sites.

Doses of amikacin sulphate are expressed in terms of amikacin base. A suggested dose for adults and children is the equivalent of 15 mg of amikacin per kg body-weight daily in equally divided doses every 8 or 12 hours by intramuscular injection. It has been suggested that in life-threatening infections, the dose may be increased in adults up to a maximum of 500 mg every 8 hours. A dose of 7.5 mg per kg daily in two divided doses (equivalent to 250 mg twice daily in adults) has been suggested for the treatment of uncomplicated urinary-tract infections. The same doses may be given by slow intravenous injection over 2 to 3 minutes or by intravenous infusion. In adults, 500 mg in 100 to 200 mL of diluent has been infused over 30 to 60 minutes; proportionately less fluid should be given to children.

A suggested dosage regimen in neonates is the equivalent of 10 mg of amikacin per kg as a loading dose, followed by 15 mg per kg daily in two divided doses. If given by intravenous infusion an infusion period of 1 to 2 hours is recommended. It has been suggested that doses may need to be adjusted in preterm neonates: one suggested regimen is 10 mg per kg initially, then 7.5 mg per kg every 18 to 24 hours thereafter.

Treatment should preferably not continue for longer than 7 to 10 days, and in consequence the total dose given to adults should not exceed 15 g. Peak plasma concentrations greater than 30 to 35 μg per mL or trough plasma concentrations greater than 5 to 10 μg per mL should be avoided. It is recommended that dosage should be adjusted in all patients according to plasma-amikacin concentrations, and this is particularly important where factors such as age, renal impairment, or dose may predispose to toxicity, or where there is a risk of subtherapeutic concentrations. For discussion of the methods of calculating aminoglycoside dosage requirements, see p.214. As with some other aminoglycosides, there are preliminary results suggesting that equivalent efficacy can be obtained from once-daily dosage with amikacin without increasing toxicity, but such dosage regimens are not yet established.

A 0.25% solution has been instilled into body cavities in adults.

A liposomal formulation of amikacin is under investigation.

Preparations

USP 23: Amikacin Sulfate Injection.

Proprietary Preparations (details are given in Part 3)
Aust.: Biklin; ***Austral.:*** Amikin; ***Belg.:*** Amukin; ***Canad.:*** Amikin; ***Fr.:*** Amiklin; ***Ger.:*** Biklin; ***Irl.:*** Amikin; ***Ital.:*** Amicasil; Amikan; BB-K8; Chemacin; Dramigel; Likacin; Lukadin; Migracin; Mikavir; Pierami; Sifamic; ***Neth.:*** Amukin; ***S.Afr.:*** Amikin; Kacinth; ***Spain:*** Biclin; Kanbine; ***Swed.:*** Biklin; ***Switz.:*** Amikine; ***UK:*** Amikin; ***USA:*** Amikin.

Aminosalicylic Acid (7551-s)

4-Aminosalicylic Acid; Aminosalylum; Para-aminosalicylic Acid; PAS; Pasalicylum. 4-Amino-2-hydroxybenzoic acid.

$C_7H_7NO_3$ = 153.1.

CAS — 65-49-6.

NOTE. Distinguish from 5-aminosalicylic acid (Mesalazine, p.1199).

Pharmacopoeias. In *Aust.* and *US.*

A white or almost white, bulky powder which darkens on exposure to air and light; it is odourless or has a slight acetous odour.

Slightly **soluble** in water and ether; soluble in alcohol. A saturated solution in water has a pH of 3.0 to 3.7.

Aqueous solutions are unstable. The USP directs that a solution must not be used if it is darker in colour than a freshly prepared solution. **Store** at a temperature not exceeding 30° in airtight containers. Protect from light.

Calcium Aminosalicylate (7552-w)

Aminosalicylate calcium; Calcii Para-aminosalicylas; Calcium PAS. Calcium 4-amino-2-hydroxybenzoate trihydrate.

$(C_7H_6NO_3)_2Ca,3H_2O$ = 398.4.

CAS — 133-15-3 (anhydrous calcium aminosalicylate).

Pharmacopoeias. In *Aust;* and in *Jpn* ($7H_2O$).

Calcium aminosalicylate 1.3 g is approximately equivalent to 1 g of aminosalicylic acid.

Sodium Aminosalicylate (7571-y)

Aminosalicylate Sodium; Aminosalylnatrium; Natrii Aminosalicylas; Natrii Para-aminosalicylas; Pasalicylum Solubile; Sodium Para-aminosalicylate; Sodium PAS. Sodium 4-amino-2-hydroxybenzoate dihydrate.

$C_7H_6NNaO_3,2H_2O$ = 211.1.

CAS — 133-10-8 (anhydrous sodium aminosalicylate); 6018-19-5 (sodium aminosalicylate dihydrate).

Pharmacopoeias. In *Aust., Chin., It., Pol., Swiss,* and *US.*

White to cream-coloured practically odourless crystalline powder. Sodium aminosalicylate 1.38 g is approximately equivalent to 1 g of aminosalicylic acid. **Soluble** 1 in 2 of water; sparingly soluble in alcohol; very slightly soluble in chloroform and in ether. A 2% solution in water has a pH of 6.5 to 8.5.

Aqueous solutions are unstable and should be freshly prepared. The USP directs that solutions should be prepared within 24 hours of administration and that a solution must not be used if it is darker in colour than a freshly prepared solution. **Store** at a temperature not exceeding 40° in airtight containers. Protect from light.

Solutions of sodium aminosalicylate in sorbitol or syrup degraded more quickly to *m*-aminophenol than those in glycerol or propylene glycol.[1] Colour developed in all solutions but was not found to be an accurate indicator of decomposition of sodium aminosalicylate as it reflected only oxidation of *m*-aminophenol.

1. Blake MI, *et al.* Effect of vehicle on the stability of sodium aminosalicylate in liquid dosage forms. *Am J Hosp Pharm* 1973; **30:** 441–3.

Adverse Effects and Treatment

Aminosalicylic acid and its salts may cause the side-effects of salicylates (see Aspirin, p.16).

Gastro-intestinal side-effects are common and include nausea, vomiting, and diarrhoea; they may be reduced by giving doses with food or in association with an antacid but occasionally may be severe enough that therapy has to be withdrawn. Alteration of gastro-intestinal function may lead to malabsorption of vitamin B_{12}, folate, and lipids. Salts of aminosalicylic acid may be better tolerated than the acid. Tolerance in children is better than in adults.

Hypersensitivity reactions have been reported in 5 to 10% of adults, usually during the first few weeks of treatment, and include fever, skin rashes, less commonly, arthralgia, lymphadenopathy, hepatosplenomegaly, and rarely, a syndrome resembling infectious mononucleosis. Other adverse effects which have been attributed to a hypersensitivity reaction to aminosalicylate include jaundice and encephalitis. Blood disorders reported include haemolytic anaemia in patients with glucose-6-phosphate dehydrogenase deficiency, agranulocytosis, eosinophilia, leucopenia, and thrombocytopenia. Psychosis may occasionally occur. Prolonged treatment may induce goitre and hypothyroidism. Crystalluria may occur.

Effects on the liver. Drug-induced hepatitis occurred in 0.32% of 7492 patients receiving antituberculous drugs; aminosalicylic acid was the most common cause.[1]

1. Rossouw JE, Saunders SJ. Hepatic complications of antituberculous therapy. *Q J Med* 1975; **44:** 1–16.

Precautions

Aminosalicylic acid and its salts should be administered with great care to patients with impaired renal or hepatic function and in patients with gastric ulcer. They should be used with caution in patients with glucose-6-dehydrogenase deficiency. The sodium salt should be administered with caution to patients with heart failure.

Aminosalicylates interfere with tests for glycosuria using copper reagents and for urobilinogen using Erhlich's reagent.

Pregnancy and breast feeding. The use of aminosalicylic acid or its salts is not recommended in pregnant patients due to gastro-intestinal intolerance.[1] In addition, the literature suggests that first-trimester exposure may be associated with congenital defects.[2]

Small amounts of aminosalicylic acid are present in breast milk. A maximum concentration of 1.1 μg per mL has been reported in a lactating woman 3 hours after administration of a 4 g dose of aminosalicylic acid.[3]

1. Snider D. Pregnancy and tuberculosis. *Chest* 1984; **86:** 10S–13S.
2. Briggs GG, *et al. Drugs in pregnancy and lactation.* 4th ed. Baltimore: Williams and Wilkins, 1994: 33a
3. Holdiness MR. Antituberculosis drugs and breast feeding. *Arch Intern Med* 1984; **144:** 1988.

Interactions

The adverse effects of aminosalicylates and salicylates may be additive. Probenecid may also increase toxicity by delaying renal excretion and enhancing plasma concentrations of aminosalicylate. The activity of aminosalicylic acid may be antagonised by ester-type local anaesthetics such as procaine.

Antimicrobial Action

Aminosalicylic acid is bacteriostatic and is active only against mycobacteria. It has a relatively weak action compared with other antituberculous drugs but most strains of *Mycobacterium tuberculosis* have been reported to be inhibited by 1 μg per mL. Resistance develops quickly if aminosalicylic acid is used alone.

Pharmacokinetics

When given by mouth, aminosalicylic acid and its salts are readily absorbed, and peak plasma concentrations occur after about 1 to 4 hours.

Aminosalicylate diffuses widely through body tissues and fluids, although diffusion into the CSF occurs only if the meninges are inflamed. Some aminosalicylate is bound to plasma proteins.

Aminosalicylate is metabolised in the intestine and liver primarily by acetylation. Urinary excretion is rapid, and 80% or more of a dose is excreted within 24 hours; 50% or more of the dose is excreted as the acetylated metabolite. The half-life of aminosalicylic acid is approximately 1 hour.

Aminosalicylate is distributed into breast milk (see under Precautions above, for more details).

Uses and Administration

Aminosalicylic acid and its salts are given by mouth in the treatment of tuberculosis (p.146) when other more potent drugs cannot be used. They should always be given with other antituberculous drugs.

Aminosalicylic acid may be given, often as the sodium salt, in a daily dose of 10 to 12 g in 2 or 3 divided doses for adults and 150 to 300 mg per kg body-weight in 3 or 4 divided doses for children.

A wide range of dosage forms has been used in an attempt to overcome the bulk and exceedingly unpleasant taste of the aminosalicylates. The salts appear to be better tolerated than the free acid and solutions in iced water prepared immediately before use may be less unpleasant to take.

Administration in renal impairment. Most clinicians recommend that aminosalicylic acid should be avoided in patients with renal impairment.[1] An increase in plasma clearance of aminosalicylic acid (attributed to increased hepatic metabolism) has been noted in patients with renal impairment, so attempting to give aminosalicylate in reduced doses to such patients may lead to subtherapeutic serum concentrations.[2]

1. Appel GB, Neu HC. The nephrotoxicity of antimicrobial agents (first of three parts). *N Engl J Med* 1977; **296:** 663–70.
2. Holdiness MR. Clinical pharmacokinetics of the antituberculosis drugs. *Clin Pharmacokinet* 1984; **9:** 511–44.

Diagnosis and testing. Aminosalicylic acid has been used in a test for pancreatic function.[1,2]

1. Hoek FJ, *et al.* Improved specificity of the PABA test with p-aminosalicylic acid (PAS). *Gut* 1987; **28:** 468–73.
2. Puntis JWL, *et al.* Simplified oral pancreatic function test. *Arch Dis Child* 1988; **63:** 780–4.

Inflammatory bowel disease. Together with corticosteroids, derivatives of 5-aminosalicylic acid are one of the mainstays of the treatment of inflammatory bowel disease (p.1171). However, aminosalicylic acid (4-aminosalicylic acid) has also been investigated, and promising results have been reported with enemas in ulcerative colitis.[1-4]

1. Campieri M, *et al.* 4-Aminosalicylic acid (4-ASA) and 5-aminosalicylic acid (5-ASA) in topical treatment of ulcerative colitis patients. *Gastroenterology* 1984; **86:** 1039.
2. Ginsberg AL, *et al.* Treatment of left-sided ulcerative colitis with 4-aminosalicylic acid enemas: a double-blind, placebo-controlled trial. *Ann Intern Med* 1988; **108:** 195–9.
3. Sharma MP, Duphare HV. 4-Aminosalicylic acid enemas for ulcerative colitis. *Lancet* 1989; **i:** 450.
4. O'Donnell LJD, *et al.* Double blind, controlled trial of 4-aminosalicylic acid and prednisolone enemas in distal ulcerative colitis. *Gut* 1992; **33:** 947–9.

Preparations

USP 23: Aminosalicylate Sodium Tablets; Aminosalicylic Acid Tablets.

Proprietary Preparations (details are given in Part 3)
Canad.: Nemasol; ***Ger.:*** Pas-Fatol N; ***Ital.:*** Eupasal Sodico†; Salf-Pas; ***Swed.:*** Na-PAS†; ***Switz.:*** Perfusion de PAS; ***USA:*** Paser.

Amoxycillin (4-a)

Amoxycillin *(BAN).*

Amoxicillin *(rINN).* (6*R*)-6-[α-D-(4-Hydroxyphenyl)glycylamino]penicillanic acid.

$C_{16}H_{19}N_3O_5S$ = 365.4.

CAS — 26787-78-0.

Amoxycillin Sodium (5-t)

Amoxycillin Sodium *(BANM).*

Amoxicillin Sodium *(rINNM)*; Amoxicilina Sódica; Amoxicillinum Natricum.

$C_{16}H_{18}N_3NaO_5S$ = 387.4.

CAS — 34642-77-8.

Pharmacopoeias. In *Eur.* (see p.viii) and *Pol.*

A white or almost white very hygroscopic powder. 1.06 g of monograph substance is approximately equivalent to 1 g of amoxycillin. Each g of monograph substance represents about 2.6 mmol of sodium. Very **soluble** in water; sparingly soluble in dehydrated alcohol; very slightly soluble in acetone. A 10% solution in water has a pH of 8.0 to 10.0.

Store in airtight containers.

References.

1. Cook B, *et al.* The stability of amoxycillin sodium in intravenous infusion fluids. *J Clin Hosp Pharm* 1982; **7:** 245–50.
2. Ashwin J, *et al.* Stability and administration of intravenous Augmentin. *Pharm J* 1987; **238:** 116–18.
3. McDonald C, *et al.* The stability of amoxycillin sodium in normal saline and glucose (5%) solutions in the liquid and frozen states. *J Clin Pharm Ther* 1989; **14:** 45–52.

Amoxycillin Trihydrate (6-x)

Amoxycillin Trihydrate *(BANM).*

Amoxicillin Trihydrate *(rINNM)*; Amoxicillin *(USAN)*; Amoxicillinum Trihydricum; BRL-2333.

$C_{16}H_{19}N_3O_5S,3H_2O$ = 419.5.

CAS — 61336-70-7.

NOTE. Compounded preparations of amoxycillin (as the trihydrate or as the sodium salt) and clavulanic acid (as potassium clavulanate) have the British Approved Name Co-amoxiclav; the proportions are expressed in the form *x/y*, where *x* and *y* are the strengths in milligrams of amoxycillin and clavulanic acid respectively.

Compounded preparations of amoxycillin (amoxicillin) (as the trihydrate) and potassium clavulanate (clavulanate potassium) in USP 23 may be represented by the name Co-amoxiclav.

Pharmacopoeias. In *Chin., Eur.* (see p.viii), *Jpn, Pol.*, and *US.*

A white or almost white crystalline powder. 1.15 g of monograph substance is approximately equivalent to 1 g of amoxycillin. Slightly **soluble** in water, in methyl alcohol, and in alcohol; practically insoluble in carbon tetrachloride, chloroform, ether, and fixed oils. It dissolves in dilute solutions of acids and of alkali hydroxides. A 0.2% solution in water has a pH of 3.5 to 6.0. **Store** in airtight containers.

Adverse Effects and Precautions

As for Ampicillin, p.153.

The incidence of diarrhoea is less with amoxycillin than ampicillin.

Hepatitis and cholestatic jaundice have been reported with the combination amoxycillin with clavulanic acid; the clavulanic acid component has been implicated. Erythema multiforme (including the Stevens-Johnson syndrome), toxic epidermal necrolysis, and exfoliative dermatitis have also been attributed occasionally to amoxycillin with clavulanic acid.

Effects on the liver. Hepatitis and cholestatic jaundice associated with the combination amoxycillin with clavulanic acid (co-amoxiclav) have been reported[1-4] and by 1993 the UK Committee on Safety of Medicines (CSM) had received 138 reports of hepato-biliary disorders, 3 of which were fatal.[5] They warned that, although usually reversible, the reaction often occurred after stopping therapy with a delay of up to 6 weeks. It appeared that the clavulanic acid was probably responsible. Retrospective analysis of cases reported in Australia[6] and a cohort study in the UK[7] found increasing age and prolonged treatment to be major risk factors for jaundice following co-amoxiclav; male sex is also a risk factor. By 1997 the CSM considered that cholestatic jaundice occurred with a frequency of about 1 in 6000 adult patients and that the risk of acute liver injury was about six times greater with co-amoxiclav than with amoxycillin alone. Therefore it now recommends that co-amoxiclav should be reserved for bacterial infections likely to be caused by amoxycillin resistant strains, and that treatment should not usually exceed 14 days.[8]

1. Stricker BHC, *et al.* Cholestatic hepatitis due to antibacterial combination of amoxicillin and clavulanic acid (Augmentin). *Dig Dis Sci* 1989; **34:** 1576–80.
2. Wong FS, *et al.* Augmentin-induced jaundice. *Med J Aust* 1991; **154:** 698–701.
3. Larrey D, *et al.* Hepatitis associated with amoxycillin-clavulanic acid combination report of 15 cases. *Gut* 1992; **33:** 368–71.
4. Hebbard GS, *et al.* Augmentin-induced jaundice with a fatal outcome. *Med J Aust* 1992; **156:** 285–6.
5. Committee on Safety of Medicines/Medicines Control Agency. Cholestatic jaundice with co-amoxiclav. *Current Problems* 1993; **19:** 2.
6. Thomson JA, *et al.* Risk factors for the development of amoxycillin-clavulanic acid associated jaundice. *Med J Aust* 1995; **162:** 638–40.
7. Rodríguez LAG, *et al.* Risk of acute liver injury associated with the combination of amoxicillin and clavulanic acid. *Arch Intern Med* 1996; **156:** 1327–32.
8. Committee on Safety of Medicines/Medicines Control Agency. Revised indications for co-amoxiclav (Augmentin). *Current Problems* 1997; **23:** 8.

Interactions

As for Benzylpenicillin, p.160.

Antimicrobial Action

As for Ampicillin, p.153.

Amoxycillin has been reported to be more active *in vitro* than ampicillin against *Enterococcus faecalis, Helicobacter pylori,* and *Salmonella* spp. but less active against *Shigella* spp.

It is inactivated by beta lactamases and complete cross-resistance has been reported between amoxycillin and ampicillin. The spectrum of activity of amoxycillin may be extended by the concomitant use of a beta-lactamase inhibitor such as clavulanic acid (p.190). As well as reversing resistance to amoxycillin in beta-lactamase-producing strains of species otherwise sensitive, clavulanic acid has also been reported to enhance the activity of amoxycillin against several species not generally considered sensitive. These have included *Bacteroides, Legionella,* and *Nocardia* spp. and *Burkholderia (Pseudomonas) pseudomallei.* However, *Ps. aeruginosa, Serratia marcescens,* and many other Gram-negative bacteria remain resistant. Transferable resistance has been reported in *H. pylori.*

Pharmacokinetics

Amoxycillin is resistant to inactivation by gastric acid. It is more rapidly and more completely absorbed than ampicillin when given by mouth. Peak plasma-amoxycillin concentrations of about 5 μg per mL have been observed 1 to 2 hours after a dose of 250 mg, with detectable amounts present for up to 8 hours. Doubling the dose can double the concentration. The presence of food in the stomach does not appear to diminish the total amount absorbed.

Amoxycillin is given by injection as the sodium salt and, in general, similar concentrations are achieved with intramuscular as with oral administration.

About 20% is bound to plasma proteins in the circulation and plasma half-lives of 1 to 1.5 hours have been reported. The half-life may be longer in neonates and the elderly; in renal failure the half-life may be 7 to 20 hours. Amoxycillin is widely distributed at varying concentrations in body tissues and fluids. It crosses the placenta; small amounts are distributed into breast milk. Little amoxycillin passes into the CSF unless the meninges are inflamed.

Amoxycillin is metabolised to a limited extent to penicilloic acid which is excreted in the urine. About 60% of an oral dose of amoxycillin is excreted unchanged in the urine in 6 hours by glomerular filtration and tubular secretion. Urinary concentrations above 300 μg per mL have been reported after a dose of 250 mg. Probenecid retards renal excretion. Amoxycillin is removed by haemodialysis. High concentrations have been reported in bile; some may be excreted in the faeces.

Amoxycillin with clavulanic acid. The pharmacokinetics of amoxycillin and clavulanic acid (p.190) are broadly similar and neither appears to affect the other to any great extent.

References.

1. Adam D, *et al.* Pharmacokinetics of amoxicillin and clavulanic acid administered alone and in combination. *Antimicrob Agents Chemother* 1982; **22:** 353–7.
2. Davies BE, *et al.* Pharmacokinetics of amoxycillin and clavulanic acid in haemodialysis patients following intravenous administration of Augmentin. *Br J Clin Pharmacol* 1988; **26:** 385–90.
3. Gould IM, *et al.* Amoxycillin/clavulanic acid levels in lower respiratory secretions. *J Antimicrob Chemother* 1988; **22:** 88–90.
4. Grange JD, *et al.* Pharmacokinetics of amoxycillin/clavulanic acid in serum and ascitic fluid in cirrhotic patients. *J Antimicrob Chemother* 1989; **23:** 605–11.
5. Jones AE, *et al.* Pharmacokinetics of intravenous amoxycillin and potassium clavulanate in seriously ill children. *J Antimicrob Chemother* 1990; **25:** 269–74.
6. Huisman-de Boer JJ, *et al.* Amoxicillin pharmacokinetics in preterm infants with gestational ages of less than 32 weeks. *Antimicrob Agents Chemother* 1995; **39:** 431–4.
7. Charles BG, *et al.* Population pharmacokinetics of intravenous amoxicillin in very low birth weight infants. *J Pharm Sci* 1997; **86:** 1288–92.

Uses and Administration

Amoxycillin is the 4-hydroxy analogue of ampicillin (p.154) and is used in a similar variety of susceptible infections. These include actinomycosis, biliary-tract infections, bronchitis, endocarditis (particularly for prophylaxis), gastro-enteritis (including salmonella enteritis, but not shigellosis), gonorrhoea, Lyme disease, mouth infections, otitis media, pneumonia, spleen disorders (pneumococcal infection prophylaxis), typhoid and paratyphoid fever, and urinary-tract infections. The beta-lactamase inhibitor clavulanic acid (p.190) widens amoxycillin's antimicrobial spectrum and a combined preparation (co-amoxiclav) can be used when resistance to amoxycillin is prevalent, for example in respiratory-tract infections due to *Haemophilus influenzae* or *Moraxella (Branhamella) catarrhalis,* in the empirical treatment of animal bites, or in infections such as chancroid and melioidosis. For details of these infections and their treatment, see under Choice of Antibacterial, p.116.

It is given as part of treatment regimens to eradicate *Helicobacter pylori* infection in patients with peptic ulcer disease (p.1174).

Administration and dosage. Amoxycillin is given by mouth as the trihydrate and by injection as the sodium salt. Doses are expressed in terms of the equivalent amount of amoxycillin.

The usual oral dose is amoxycillin 250 to 500 mg every 8 hours. Children up to 10 years of age may be given 125 to 250 mg every 8 hours; under 20 kg body-weight a dose of 20 to 40 mg per kg daily has been suggested.

Higher oral doses of amoxycillin, either as a single dose or in short courses, are used in some conditions. For example, amoxycillin is given as a single dose of 3 g, with probenecid 1 g, in the treatment of uncomplicated gonorrhoea in areas where gonococci remain sensitive. A dose of 3 g repeated once after 8 or 10 to 12 hours may be used for dental abscesses or uncomplicated acute urinary-tract infections, respectively. For the prophylaxis of endocarditis in susceptible patients amoxycillin 2 or 3 g is given about 1 hour before dental procedures under local or no anaesthesia. A high-dose regimen of amoxycillin 3 g twice daily may be used in patients with severe or recurrent infections of the respiratory tract. If necessary, children aged 3 to 10 years with otitis media may be given 750 mg twice daily for 2 days. For the eradication of *H. pylori,* amoxycillin is given in combination with either metronidazole or clarithromycin and a bismuth compound or an antisecretory drug; doses of amoxycillin have been 1.5 to 2.25 g daily in 2 to 4 divided doses.

Amoxycillin is administered by intramuscular or slow intravenous injection in doses of 500 mg every 8 hours. In severe infections 1 g of amoxycillin may be given every 6 hours by slow intravenous injection over 3 to 4 minutes or by infusion over 30 to 60 minutes. Children up to 10 years of age may be given 50 to 100 mg per kg body-weight daily by injection in divided doses.

Doses should be reduced in severe renal impairment.

Amoxycillin with clavulanic acid. Amoxycillin in combination with clavulanic acid (co-amoxiclav) is administered by mouth in a ratio of amoxycillin (as the trihydrate) 2, 4, or 7 parts to 1 part of clavulanic acid (as the potassium salt), or intravenously in a ratio of 5 parts of amoxycillin (as the sodium salt) to 1 part of clavulanic acid (as the potassium salt). Doses of the combination, calculated on amoxycillin content, are similar to those for amoxycillin alone.

References.

1. Speller DCE, *et al.*, eds. Clavulanate/β-lactam antibiotics: further experience. *J Antimicrob Chemother* 1989; **24** (suppl B): 1–226.
2. Todd PA, Benfield P. Amoxicillin/clavulanic acid: an update of its antibacterial activity, pharmacokinetic properties and therapeutic use. *Drugs* 1990; **39:** 264–307.

Preparations

BP 1998: Amoxicillin Capsules; Amoxicillin Injection; Amoxicillin Oral Suspension; Co-amoxiclav Tablets;
USP 23: Amoxicillin and Clavulanate Potassium for Oral Suspension; Amoxicillin and Clavulanate Potassium Tablets; Amoxicillin Capsules; Amoxicillin for Oral Suspension; Amoxicillin Tablets.

Proprietary Preparations (details are given in Part 3)
Aust.: Amoxid; Amoxilan; Clamoxyl; Gonoform; Ospamox; Supramox; ***Austral.:*** Alphamox; Amoxil; Ampexin; Bgramin; Cilamox; Fisamox; Ibiamox†; Moxacin; ***Belg.:*** Amoxi†; Amoxycaps†; Amoxypen†; Clamoxyl; Clavucid; Flemoxin; Hiconcil; Moxaline†; Novabritine; ***Canad.:*** Amoxil; Novamoxin; Nu-Amoxi; ***Fr.:*** A-Gram; Amodex; Amophar; Bactox; Bristamox; Clamoxyl; Flemoxine; Gramidil; Hiconcil; Zamocilline; ***Ger.:*** Amagesan; Amc-Puren; Amoxi; amoxi-basan†; Amoxi-Diolan; Amoxi-Hefa; Amoxi-Tablinen; Amoxi-Wolff; Amoxibeta; Amoxibiocin†; Amoxihexal; Amoxillat; Amoximerck; Amoxypen; Clamoxyl; Cuxacillin; Dignoamoxicillin†; dura AX; Flui-Amoxicillin; Glassatan†; Infectomox; Jephoxin; Padiamox†; Sigamopen; Ulcolind Amoxi; ***Irl.:*** Almodan; Amoxil; Clonamox; Galenamox; Geramox; Hiconcil†; Oramox; Pinamox; Roxillin; ***Ital.:*** Alfamox; AM 73†; Amoflux; Amox; Amoxibiotic†; Amox-

illin; Amoxina; Amoxipen; Aspenil†; Bradimox; Cabermox†; Dodemox; Helimox; Ibiamox; Isimoxin; Majorpen†; Mopen; Neo-Ampiplus; Neotetranase; Pamocil; Piramox†; Simoxil; Simplamox†; Sintopen; Velamox; Zamocillin†; Zimox; ***Neth.:*** Clamoxyl; Flemoxin; ***Norw.:*** Amimox; Amoxillin; Imacillin; ***S.Afr.:*** Acucil; Amocillin; Amoxil; Amoxyfizz; AMX†; Arcanacillin†; Betamox; C-Mox; Ibiamox†; Ipcamox; Maxcil; Moxan; Moxymax; Moxypen; Norimox†; Penmox; Pharmoxin†; Polymox†; Promoxil; Ranmoxy; Rocillin; Saltermox; Spectramox; Ultramox; Unimox; Xeracil; Xillin†; Zoxil; ***Spain:*** Actimoxi; Agerpen; Amitron; Amoflamisan; Amox; Amoxaren; Amoxi Gobens; Amoxibacter; Amoxidel; Amoximedical; Amoxipen†; Apamox; Ardine; Bimoxi†; Bioxidona; Blenox; Bolchipen; Borbalan; Brondix; Cidanamox†; Clamoxyl; Co Amoxin; Dacala†; Damoxicil; Dobriciclin; Edoxil; Eupen; Halitol; Hosboral; Inexbron; Mediamox†; Metifarma; Morgenxil; Moxipin†; Novagcilina; Precopen; Raudopen; Recefril†; Reloxyl; Remisan; Riotapen; Salvapen; Suamoxil; Superpeni; Tolodina; ***Swed.:*** Amimox; Amoxiferm†; Bristamox; Flemoxin; Imacillin; ***Switz.:*** amoxi-basan; Amoxi-Mepha; Amoximex; Antiotic; Azilline; Clamoxyl; Flemoxin; Helvamox; Penimox; Pharmamox†; Rivoxicillin; Servamox; Sigamopen†; Spectroxyl; Supramox; ***UK:*** Almodan; Amix; Amopen; Amoram; Amoxil; Amoxymed†; Amrit; Flemoxin†; Galenamox; Rimoxallin; ***USA:*** Amoxil; Biomox†; Polymox†; Trimox; Wymox.

Multi-ingredient: ***Aust.:*** Augmentin; Clavamox; Helicocin; ***Austral.:*** Augmentin; Clamoxyl; Clavulin; Losec Helicopak; ***Belg.:*** Augmentin; ***Canad.:*** Clavulin; ***Fr.:*** Augmentin; Ciblor; ***Ger.:*** Augmentan; Flanamox; ***Irl.:*** Augmentin; ***Ital.:*** Augmentin; Clavulin; Dicil†; Duplamox Mucolitico†; Duplamox†; Flanamox†; Moxacin†; Moxiprim†; Neoduplamox; Stacillin†; Velamox D†; ***Neth.:*** Augmentin; ***Norw.:*** Bremide; ***S.Afr.:*** Augmentin; Flumox; Hiconcil-NS; Macropen; Megapen; Suprapen; ***Spain:*** Agerpen Mucolitico; Amo Resan; Amoxi Gobens Mucol; Amoxidel Bronquial; Amoxtiol; Amoxyplus; Amoxyvinco Mucolitico; Ardine Bronquial; Augmentine; Bigpen; Bimoxi Mucolitico†; Bisolvon Amoxycilina; Brisantin†; Brolimine Antibiotico†; Bronco Tonic N F; Bronconovag; Bronquium Amoxicilina; Broxamox†; Burmicin; Cilinvita Bronquial†; Clamoxyl Mucolitico; Clavepen; Clavius†; Clavucid; Clavumox; Combitorax; Damoxicil Mucolitico; Duonasa; Edoxil Mucolitico; Eupeclanic; Eupen Bronquial; Flubiotic; Hortemox†; Hosboral Bronquial; Inexbron Mucolitico; Inmupen; Kelsopen; Metifarma Mucolit; Moxipin Mucolitico†; Neumobronquial†; Pangamox; Precopen Mucolitico; Prosbis†; Pulmo Borbalan; Reloxyl Mucolitico; Remisan Mucolitico; Salvapen Mucolitico; Sinus†; Sobrepin Amoxi†; Superpeni Mucolitico; Ultramoxil†; ***Swed.:*** Spektramox; ***Switz.:*** Augmentin; ***UK:*** Augmentin; Augmentin-Duo; ***USA:*** Augmentin; Prevpac.

Amphomycin (7-r)

Amphomycin *(BAN, USAN)*.

Amfomycin *(pINN)*.

CAS — 1402-82-0.

A polypeptide antibiotic produced by the growth of *Streptomyces canus*.

Amphomycin has an antibacterial action against Gram-positive bacteria, and has been applied topically as the calcium salt in combination with other drugs in the treatment of skin infections.

Preparations

Proprietary Preparations (details are given in Part 3)

Multi-ingredient: ***Aust.:*** Ecomytrin; Ecomytrin-Hydrocortison; ***Norw.:*** Ecomytrin-Hydrocortison†; ***Spain:*** Ecomitrin†; ***Swed.:*** Ecomytrin-Hydrocortison†; Ecomytrin†; ***Switz.:*** Ecomytrin-Hydrocortison†.

Ampicillin (8-f)

Ampicillin *(BAN, USAN, rINN)*.

Aminobenzylpenicillin; Ampicillinum; Ampicillinum Anhydricum; Anhydrous Ampicillin; AY-6108; BRL-1341; NSC-528986; P-50. (6*R*)-6-(α-D-Phenylglycylamino)penicillanic acid.

$C_{16}H_{19}N_3O_4S$ = 349.4.

CAS — 69-53-4.

NOTE. Compounded preparations of equal parts by weight of ampicillin and flucloxacillin have the British Approved Name Co-fluampicil.

Pharmacopoeias. In *Eur.* (see p.viii), *Jpn*, and *Pol.*
Int. and *US* permit anhydrous or the trihydrate.

A white, crystalline powder. Sparingly to slightly **soluble** in water; slightly soluble in methyl alcohol; practically insoluble in alcohol, acetone, carbon tetrachloride, chloroform, ether, and fixed oils. It dissolves in dilute solutions of acids and of alkali hydroxides. A 0.25% solution in water has a pH of 3.5 to 5.5 and a 1% solution in water has a pH of 3.5 to 6.0. **Store** at a temperature not exceeding 30° in airtight containers.

Ampicillin Sodium (9-d)

Ampicillin Sodium *(BANM, USAN, rINNM)*.

Aminobenzylpenicillin Sodium; Ampicillinnatrium; Ampicillinum Natricum.

$C_{16}H_{18}N_3NaO_4S$ = 371.4.

CAS — 69-52-3.

Pharmacopoeias. In *Chin.*, *Eur.* (see p.viii), *Int.*, *Jpn*, *Pol.*, and *US.*

A white hygroscopic powder. 1.06 g of monograph substance is approximately equivalent to 1 g of ampicillin. Each g of monograph substance represents about 2.7 mmol of sodium.

Freely **soluble** in water; sparingly soluble in acetone; practically insoluble in ether, in liquid paraffin, and in fixed oils. A 10% solution in water has a pH of 8 to 10. **Store** in airtight containers.

The **stability** of solutions of ampicillin sodium is dependent on many factors including concentration, pH, temperature, and the nature of the vehicle. Stability decreases in the presence of glucose, fructose, invert sugar, dextrans, hetastarch, sodium bicarbonate, and lactate. It is recommended that reconstituted solutions of ampicillin sodium for injection should be administered immediately after preparation, and should not be frozen. Solutions for infusion are stable for varying periods and details are given in the manufacturers' literature.

Incompatibility. The incompatibility of ampicillin sodium and aminoglycosides is well established. Incompatibilities have also been reported with a wide range of other drugs, including other antibacterials, and appear to be more pronounced at higher concentrations and in solutions also containing glucose.

References.

1. Lynn B. The stability and administration of intravenous penicillins. *Br J Intraven Ther* 1981; **2**(Mar): 22–39.

Ampicillin Trihydrate (10-c)

Ampicillin Trihydrate *(BANM, rINNM)*.

Ampicillin; Ampicillinum Trihydricum.

$C_{16}H_{19}N_3O_4S,3H_2O$ = 403.5.

CAS — 7177-48-2.

Pharmacopoeias. In *Eur.* (see p.viii) and *Pol.* In *Jpn* under the title Ampicillin. *Int.* and *US* permit anhydrous or the trihydrate under the title Ampicillin.

A white crystalline powder. 1.15 g of monograph substance is approximately equivalent to 1 g of ampicillin. Slightly **soluble** in water and in methyl alcohol; practically insoluble in alcohol, in chloroform, in ether, and in fixed oils. It dissolves in dilute solutions of acids and of alkali hydroxides. A 0.25% solution in water has a pH of 3.5 to 5.5. **Store** at a temperature not exceeding 30° in airtight containers.

Adverse Effects

As for Benzylpenicillin p.159. Skin rashes are among the most common side-effects and are generally either urticarial or maculopapular; the urticarial reactions are typical of penicillin hypersensitivity while the erythematous maculopapular eruptions are characteristic of ampicillin and amoxycillin and often appear more than 7 days after commencing treatment. Such rashes may be due to hypersensitivity to the beta-lactam moiety or to the amino group in the side chain, or to a toxic reaction. The occurrence of a maculopapular rash during ampicillin administration does not necessarily preclude the subsequent administration of other penicillins. Since in practice it may be difficult to distinguish between hypersensitive and toxic responses, skin testing for hypersensitivity may be advisable before another penicillin is used in patients who have had ampicillin rashes. Most patients with infectious mononucleosis develop a maculopapular rash when treated with ampicillin, and patients with other lymphoid disorders such as lymphatic leukaemia and possibly HIV infection also appear to be at higher risk. More serious skin reactions may occur and erythema multiforme associated with ampicillin has occasionally been reported.

Gastro-intestinal adverse effects particularly diarrhoea and also nausea and vomiting occur quite frequently, usually following administration by mouth. Pseudomembranous colitis has also been reported.

Precautions

As for Benzylpenicillin p.160.

Ampicillin should be discontinued if a skin rash occurs. It should preferably not be given to patients with infectious mononucleosis since they are especially susceptible to ampicillin-induced skin rashes; patients with lymphatic leukaemia or possibly HIV infection may also be at increased risk of developing skin rashes.

Myasthenia gravis. The symptoms of a woman with myasthenia gravis were exacerbated when she was given ampicillin.[1]

1. Argov Z, *et al.* Ampicillin may aggravate clinical and experimental myasthenia gravis. *Arch Neurol* 1986; **43**: 255–6.

Interactions

As for Benzylpenicillin, p.160.

Allopurinol. An increased frequency of skin rashes has been reported in patients receiving ampicillin or amoxycillin together with allopurinol, compared with those receiving antibacterial alone,[1] but this could not be confirmed in a subsequent study.[2]

1. Jick H, Porter JB. Potentiation of ampicillin skin reactions by allopurinol or hyperuricemia. *J Clin Pharmacol* 1981; **21**: 456–8.
2. Hoigné R, *et al.* Occurrence of exanthems in relation to aminopenicillin preparations and allopurinol. *N Engl J Med* 1987; **316**: 1217.

Chloroquine. The absorption of ampicillin has been reduced in healthy subjects by chloroquine taken concomitantly.[1]

1. Ali HM. Reduced ampicillin bioavailability following oral coadministration with chloroquine. *J Antimicrob Chemother* 1985; **15**: 781–4.

Antimicrobial Action

Ampicillin is a beta-lactam antibiotic. It is bactericidal and has a similar mode of action to that of benzylpenicillin (p.160), but as an aminopenicillin with an amino group side chain attached to the basic penicillin structure ampicillin is better able to penetrate the outer membrane of some Gram-negative bacteria and has a broader spectrum of activity.

Spectrum of activity. (See also Resistance, below). It resembles benzylpenicillin in its action against Gram-positive organisms, including *Streptococcus pneumoniae,* and other streptococci but, apart perhaps from *Enterococcus faecalis,* it is slightly less potent than benzylpenicillin. *Listeria monocytogenes* is highly sensitive. The Gram-negative cocci *Moraxella (Branhamella) catarrhalis, Neisseria gonorrhoeae,* and *N. meningitidis* are sensitive. Ampicillin is more active than benzylpenicillin against some Gram-negative bacilli including *Haemophilus influenzae* and Enterobacteriaceae such as *Escherichia coli, Proteus mirabilis, Salmonella* and *Shigella* spp. It is inactive against *Pseudomonas aeruginosa*. Ampicillin also has activity similar to benzylpenicillin against other organisms including many anaerobes and *Actinomyces* spp.

Minimum inhibitory concentrations for sensitive Gram-positive organisms have been reported to range from 0.02 to 1.5 μg per mL and for Gram-negative organisms from 0.03 to 3 μg per mL.

Activity with other antimicrobials. There is synergy against some beta-lactamase-producing organisms between ampicillin and beta-lactamase inhibitors such as clavulanic acid or sulbactam, and also penicillinase-stable drugs such as cloxacillin or flucloxacillin. Synergy has also been demonstrated between ampicillin and aminoglycosides against a range of organisms, including enterococci. Variable effects including synergy, antagonism, or indifference have been reported between ampicillin and other beta-lactams, bacteriostatic drugs such as chloramphenicol, and rifampicin.

Resistance. Like benzylpenicillin, ampicillin is inactivated by beta lactamases although other mechanisms may be responsible for resistance in some species. There are geographical variations in the incidence of resistance, but most staphylococci and many strains of *E. coli, H. influenzae*, *M. catarrhalis*, *N. gonorrhoeae*, and *Salmonella* and *Shigella* spp. are resistant.

Pharmacokinetics

Ampicillin is relatively stable in the acid gastric secretion and is moderately well absorbed from the gastro-intestinal tract after oral administration. Food can interfere with the absorption of ampicillin so doses should preferably be taken at least 30 minutes before meals. Peak concentrations in plasma are attained in about 1 to 2 hours and following a dose of 500 mg by mouth are reported to range from 2 to 6 μg per mL.

Ampicillin is given by injection as the sodium salt and following the intramuscular administration of 500 mg peak plasma concentrations occur within about 1 hour and are reported to range from 7 to 14 μg per mL.

Ampicillin is widely distributed and therapeutic concentrations can be achieved in ascitic, pleural, and joint fluids. It crosses the placenta into the fetal circulation and small amounts are distributed into breast milk. There is little diffusion into the CSF except when the meninges are inflamed. About 20% is bound to plasma proteins and the plasma half-life is about 1 to 1.5 hours, but this may be increased in neonates and the elderly; in renal impairment half-lives of 7 to 20 hours have been reported.

Ampicillin is metabolised to some extent to penicilloic acid which is excreted in the urine.

Renal clearance of ampicillin occurs partly by glomerular filtration and partly by tubular secretion; it is retarded by the concomitant administration of probenecid. About 20 to 40% of an orally administered dose may be excreted unchanged in the urine in 6 hours; urinary concentrations have ranged from 0.25 to 1 mg per mL following a dose of 500 mg. Following parenteral administration about 60 to 80% is excreted in the urine within 6 hours. Ampicillin is removed by haemodialysis. High concentrations are reached in bile; it undergoes enterohepatic recycling and some is excreted in the faeces.

Ampicillin with sulbactam. The pharmacokinetics of ampicillin and sulbactam are broadly similar and neither appears to affect the other to any great extent.

References.

1. Wright N, Wise R. The elimination of sulbactam alone and combined with ampicillin in patients with renal dysfunction. *J Antimicrob Chemother* 1983; **11:** 583–7.
2. Rho JP, *et al.* Single-dose pharmacokinetics of intravenous ampicillin plus sulbactam in healthy elderly and young adult subjects. *J Antimicrob Chemother* 1989; **24:** 573–80.
3. Valcke YJ, *et al.* Penetration of ampicillin and sulbactam in the lower airways during respiratory infections. *Antimicrob Agents Chemother* 1990; **34:** 958–62.
4. Meyers BR, *et al.* Pharmacokinetics of ampicillin-sulbactam in healthy elderly and young volunteers. *Antimicrob Agents Chemother* 1991; **35:** 2098–2101.
5. Wildfeuer A, *et al.* Pharmacokinetics of ampicillin and sulbactam in patients undergoing heart surgery. *Antimicrob Agents Chemother* 1991; **35:** 1772–6.

Uses and Administration

Ampicillin is used in the treatment of a variety of infections due to susceptible organisms (see Antimicrobial Action, above). They include biliary-tract infections, bronchitis, endocarditis, gastro-enteritis (including salmonella enteritis and shigellosis), gonorrhoea, listeriosis, meningitis, otitis media, perinatal streptococcal infections (intrapartum prophylaxis against group B streptococci), peritonitis, pneumonia, septicaemia, typhoid and paratyphoid fever, and urinary-tract infections. Resistance to ampicillin is increasingly a problem in some infections, for example, gonorrhoea, pneumococcal infections, respiratory-tract infections due to *Haemophilus influenzae* or *Moraxella (Branhamella) catarrhalis*, salmonella infections, shigellosis, and infections due to *Escherichia coli*. For details of these infections and their treatment, see under Choice of Antibacterial, p.116. If beta-lactamase-producing organisms are present, ampicillin can be administered with a beta-lactamase inhibitor such as sulbactam (see below) or a penicillinase-resistant drug such as cloxacillin or flucloxacillin. It may also be administered in association with an aminoglycoside to increase the spectrum of organisms covered; it is advisable to administer the injections separately.

Administration and dosage. The dosage of ampicillin will depend on the severity of the disease, the age of the patient, and renal function; the dose should be reduced in severe renal impairment. Ampicillin is usually administered by mouth as the trihydrate and by injection as the sodium salt. Doses are expressed in terms of the equivalent amount of ampicillin. The usual dose by mouth is 0.25 to 1 g of ampicillin every 6 hours. It is recommended that ampicillin be taken at least 30 minutes before or 2 hours after food. Children may be given half the adult dose.

For urinary-tract infections, ampicillin 500 mg is given every 8 hours.

For typhoid and paratyphoid where *Salmonella typhi* strains remain sensitive to ampicillin, a dose of 1 to 2 g every 6 hours for two weeks is suggested for acute infections, and for 4 to 12 weeks in carriers.

Ampicillin 2 or 3.5 g administered, in association with probenecid 1 g, as a single dose by mouth, has been used in the treatment of uncomplicated gonorrhoea, in areas where gonococci remain sensitive.

Ampicillin is administered by injection in usual doses of 500 mg every 4 to 6 hours intramuscularly, or it may be given by slow intravenous injection over 3 to 5 minutes or by infusion. Higher parenteral doses of 1 to 2 g given intravenously over 10 to 15 minutes every 3 to 6 hours (maximum 14 g daily) have been suggested for serious infections such as meningitis. Children may be given half the adult dose. For infants and children with meningitis, doses of 150 to 200 mg per kg daily in divided doses have been suggested. A suggested dose, given to the mother, for intrapartum prophylaxis against group B streptococcal infection in the neonate is ampicillin 2 g by intravenous injection initially then 1 g every 4 hours until delivery.

Ampicillin may also be administered by other routes usually as a supplement to systemic therapy. Intraperitoneal or intrapleural injections are given in a dose of ampicillin 500 mg daily dissolved in 5 to 10 mL of water. For intra-articular injection, ampicillin 500 mg daily is given dissolved in up to 5 mL of water or a solution of procaine hydrochloride 0.5%.

Ampicillin benzathine has also been administered by intramuscular injection.

Ampicillin with sulbactam. The sodium salts of ampicillin and sulbactam (p.250) may be given intramuscularly or intravenously in the treatment of infections due to beta-lactamase-producing organisms. Doses are expressed in terms of the equivalent amounts of ampicillin and sulbactam; available injections contain ampicillin and sulbactam in the ratio 2:1, respectively. The usual dose is ampicillin 1 g with sulbactam 0.5 g every 6 hours; doses may be doubled in severe infections.

For oral administration sultamicillin (p.257), a mutual prodrug of ampicillin and sulbactam, may be used.

Ampicillin may be administered in combination with other antibacterials, including cloxacillin and flucloxacillin (known as co-fluampicil), to produce a wider spectrum of activity.

Preparations

BP 1998: Ampicillin Capsules; Ampicillin Injection; Ampicillin Oral Suspension; Co-fluampicil Capsules; Co-fluampicil Oral Suspension;
USP 23: Ampicillin and Probenecid Capsules; Ampicillin and Probenecid for Oral Suspension; Ampicillin and Sulbactam for Injection; Ampicillin Capsules; Ampicillin for Injectable Suspension; Ampicillin for Injection; Ampicillin for Oral Suspension; Ampicillin Tablets.

Proprietary Preparations (details are given in Part 3)
Aust.: Binotal; Doktacillin; Penglobe; Standacillin; ***Austral.:*** Alphacin; Austrapen; Penbritin†; ***Belg.:*** Penbritin; Pentrexyl; ***Canad.:*** Ampicin; Nu-Ampi; Penbritin; ***Fr.:*** Peniclinet†; Prototapen†; Totapen; ***Ger.:*** Amblosin†; Ampensaar†; Ampi-Tablinen†; Ampicillat†; Binotal; duraampicillin; Jenampin; Pen-Bristol†; Penstabil†; ***Irl.:*** Amfipen; Clonamp; Novapen; Penbritin; Pentrexyl†; Vidopen; ***Ital.:*** Ampen†; Ampi-Zoja†; Ampilan†; Ampilisa; Ampilux; Ampiplus Simplex; Ampisint†; Amplipenyl†; Amplital; Amplizer; Citicil; Gramcillina†; Ibimicyn; Lampocillina; Penampil†; Pentrexyl; Platocillina; Principen†; Radiocillina†; Sesquicillina†; Totalciclina†; ***Jpn:*** Herpen; ***Neth.:*** Amfipen†; Pentrexyl; ***Norw.:*** Doktacillin; Pentrexyl; ***S.Afr.:*** Ampi-Rol; Ampicyn†; Ampimax; Ampipen; Ampisalt; Be-Ampicil; Co-Cillin; Dyna-Ampcil; Excillin; Hexacillin; M-P-Cil†; Penbritin; Penrite; Pentrex†; Petercillin; Ranamp; Spectracil; Statcillin†; ***Spain:*** Ampiplus; Antibiopen; Britapen; Ciarbiot; Electopen; Gobemicina; Nuvapen; Sintecilina†; Togram†; Ultrabion†; ***Swed.:*** Doktacillin; Pentrexyl; ***Switz.:*** Arcocillin†; Cimexillin†; Servicillin†; ***UK:*** Amfipen; Flu-Amp; Magnapen; Penbritin; Rimacillin; Vidopen; ***USA:*** D-Amp†; Marcillin; Omnipen; Omnipen-N; Polycillin-N†; Polycillin-PRB†; Polycillin†; Principen; Principen with Probenecid†; Totacillin; Totacillin-N†.

Multi-ingredient: ***Aust.:*** Totocillin†; Unasyn; ***Austral.:*** Ampicyn; ***Fr.:*** Unacim; ***Ger.:*** Broncho-Binotal†; Totocillin†; Unacid; ***Irl.:*** Ampiclox; ***Ital.:*** Ampiplus; Amplium; Bethacil; Diamplicil; Duplexcillina; Duplexil; Infectrin; Loricin; Sobrepin Antibiotico†; Unasyn; ***S.Afr.:*** Ampiclox; Apen; Cloxam; Megamox; Pentrex-F†; ***Spain:*** Alongamicina Balsa; Alongamicina†; Ampiciliber Bronquial†; Ampiorus Balsamico†; Bacimex†; Bactosone Retard; Bactosone†; Bio Espectrum; Bisolvon Ampicil Retard†; Bisolvon Ampicilina†; Brixilon†; Bronco Pensusan; Broncobacter†; Broncotyfen†; Combitorax Ampicilina†; Complexobiotico Bals†; Electopen Balsam Retard; Electopen Balsam†; Electopen Retard; Espectral; Espectral Balsamico; Espectrosira; Etro; Etro Balsamico; Exapenil Mucolitico†; Galotam; Gobemicina Retard; Hispamicina Retard; Maxicilina; Miliken Mucol Med Retard; Miliken Mucol Retard; Miliken Mucolitico; Mucorex Ampicilina; Neo Penprobal†; Nuvapen Mucolitico Retard†; Nuvapen Retard†; Pectosan Ampicilina; Pectox Ampicilina; Penisintex Bronquial; Pulminflamatoria; Pulmospin; Pulmosterin Retard; Resan Mucolitico; Resan Retard; Resisten Retard; Retarpen; Retarpen Balsamico; Retarpen Mucolitico; Sinus†; Ultrabion; Ultrabion Balsamico; Ultrapenil; Unasyn; ***Switz.:*** Pencloxin†; ***UK:*** Ampiclox†; Dicapen†; Flu-Amp; Magnapen; ***USA:*** Unasyn.

Apramycin Sulphate (15966-s)

Apramycin Sulphate *(BANM, rINNM).*

47657 (apramycin); EL-857 (apramycin); EL-857/820 (apramycin); Nebramycin Factor 2 (apramycin). 4-*O*-[(2*R*,3*R*,4a*S*,6*R*,7*S*,8*R*,8a*R*)-3-Amino-6-(4-amino-4-deoxy-α-D-glucopyranosyloxy)-8-hydroxy-7-methylaminoperhydropyrano[3,2-*b*]pyran-2-yl]-2-deoxystreptamine sulphate.

$C_{21}H_{41}N_5O_{11},2\frac{1}{2}H_2SO_4$ = 784.8.
CAS — 37321-09-8 (apramycin); 41194-16-5 (apramycin sulphate).

NOTE. Apramycin is *USAN.*

Pharmacopoeias. In *BP(Vet).*

The sulphate of an antibiotic produced by *Streptomyces tenebrarius* or by other means.

A light brown hygroscopic powder or granules. Freely **soluble** in water; practically insoluble in alcohol, in methyl alcohol, in acetone, and in ether. **Store** at a temperature not exceeding 25°.

Apramycin is an aminoglycoside antibiotic used as the sulphate in veterinary practice.

Arbekacin Sulphate (19281-l)

Arbekacin Sulphate *(rINNM).*

ABK (arbekacin); AHB-DBK (arbekacin); HABA-Dibekacin (arbekacin). *O*-3-Amino-3-deoxy-α-D-glucopyranosyl-(1→4)-*O*-[2,6-diamino-2,3,4,6-tetradeoxy-α-D-*erythro*-hexopyranosyl-(1→6)]-*N'*-[(2*S*)-4-amino-2-hydroxybutyryl]-2-deoxy-L-streptamine sulphate.

$C_{22}H_{44}N_6O_{10},xH_2S0_4$ = 552.6 (arbekacin).
CAS — 51025-85-5 (arbekacin).

Arbekacin is an aminoglycoside derived from dibekacin and has general properties similar to those of gentamicin (p.212). It is used as the sulphate in the treatment of serious infections due to methicillin-resistant *Staphylococcus aureus* and is given intramuscularly in doses of 150 to 200 mg daily in 2 divided doses. The same dose may also be given by intravenous infusion over 0.5 to 2 hours. Dosage should be adjusted based on serum-arbekacin concentration monitoring.

Preparations

Proprietary Preparations (details are given in Part 3)
Jpn: Habekacin.

Arsanilic Acid (12394-e)

Arsanilic Acid *(BAN, rINN).*

Aminarsonic Acid; AS-101. *p*-Aminobenzenearsonic acid; 4-Aminophenylarsonic acid.

$C_6H_8AsNO_3$ = 217.1.
CAS — 98-50-0.

NOTE. The code AS-101 has been used for an immunomodulator under investigation in the treatment of AIDS.

Pharmacopoeias. In *US* for veterinary use only.

A white to off-white crystalline powder. **Soluble** in hot water and in amyl alcohol; slightly soluble in cold water, in alcohol, and in acetic acid; practically insoluble in acetone, in chloroform, and in ether. Soluble in solutions of alkali carbonates; sparingly soluble in concentrated mineral acids; practically insoluble in dilute mineral acids.

Sodium Arsanilate (13241-h)

Sodium Arsanilate (*BANM, rINNM*).

Sodium Aminarsonate; Sodium Anilarsonate. Sodium 4-aminophenylarsonate.

$C_6H_7AsNNaO_3$ = 239.0.

CAS — 127-85-5.

Pharmacopoeias. *Fr.* includes the anhydrous substance and the trihydrate.

Arsanilic acid and sodium arsanilate are used in veterinary medicine for the prophylaxis and treatment of enteric infections in pigs and also as growth-promoting agents.

Aspoxicillin (1960-n)

Aspoxicillin (*rINN*).

TA-058. (2*S*,5*R*,6*R*)-6-{(2*R*)-2-[(2*R*)-2-Amino-3-(methylcarbamoyl)propionamido]-2-(*p*-hydroxyphenyl)acetamido}-3,3-dimethyl-7-oxo-4-thia-1-azabicyclo[3.2.0]-heptane-2-carboxylic acid.

$C_{21}H_{27}N_5O_7S$ = 493.5.

CAS — 63358-49-6.

Aspoxicillin is a ureidopenicillin given intravenously in the treatment of susceptible infections.

Preparations

Proprietary Preparations (details are given in Part 3)
Jpn: Doyle.

Astromicin Sulphate (12404-x)

Astromicin Sulphate (*pINNM*).

Abbott-44747; Astromicin Sulfate (*USAN*); Fortimicin A Sulphate; KW-1070. 4-Amino-1-(2-amino-*N*-methylacetamido)-1,4-dideoxy-3-*O*-(2,6-diamino-2,3,4,6,7-pentadeoxy-β-L-*lyxo*-heptopyranosyl)-6-*O*-methyl-L-*chiro*-inositol sulphate.

$C_{17}H_{35}N_5O_6,2H_2SO_4$ = 601.6.

CAS — 55779-06-1 (astromicin); 72275-67-3 (astromicin sulphate); 66768-12-5 (xH_2SO_4).

Pharmacopoeias. In *Jpn*.

An antibiotic produced by *Micromonospora* spp.

Astromicin is an aminoglycoside with actions and uses similar to those of gentamicin (p.212). It is used as the sulphate and administered intramuscularly, or by slow intravenous injection over 0.5 to 1 hour, in a usual dosage equivalent to 400 mg of astromicin daily in 2 divided doses. Dosage should be adjusted based on serum-astromicin concentration monitoring.

Preparations

Proprietary Preparations (details are given in Part 3)
Jpn: Fortimicin.

Avilamycin (3342-j)

Avilamycin (*BAN, USAN*).

LY-048740.

$C_{61}H_{88}Cl_2O_{32}$ (avilamycin A) = 1404.2.

CAS — 11051-71-1 (avilamycin); 69787-79-7 (avilamycin A); 69787-80-0 (avilamycin C).

Avilamycin is an antibacterial used in veterinary medicine as a production enhancer.

Avoparcin (11-k)

Avoparcin (*BAN, USAN, rINN*).

Compound 254.

CAS — 37332-99-3.

A glycopeptide antibiotic produced by *Amycolatopsis coloradensis* (*Streptomyces candidus*) or by any other means.

Avoparcin is a glycopeptide antibiotic that has been incorporated into animal feedstuffs to promote growth.

There is evidence of cross-resistance between avoparcin and vancomycin.[1] Suggestions that vancomycin-resistant organisms could enter the human population from the food chain as a result of the use of avoparcin as a growth promoter in animals[2,3] have been disputed by the manufacturers of avoparcin.[4,5]

The use of avoparcin as a growth promoter in animals has been banned in the European Union.

1. Klare I, *et al.* vanA-mediated high-level glycopeptide resistance in Enterococcus faecium from animal husbandry. *FEMS Microbiol Lett* 1995; **125:** 165–72.
2. Howarth F, Poulter D. Vancomycin resistance: time to ban avoparcin? *Lancet* 1996; **347:** 1047.
3. Wise R. Avoparcin and animal feedstuff. *Lancet* 1996; **347:** 1835.
4. Mudd A. Vancomycin resistance and avoparcin. *Lancet* 1996; **347:** 1412.
5. Mudd AJ. Is it time to ban all antibiotics as animal growth-promoting agents? *Lancet* 1996; **348:** 1454–5.

Azidamfenicol (12-a)

Azidamfenicol (*BAN, rINN*).

Azidamphenicol; Azidoamphenicol; Bayer 52910. 2-Azido-*N*-[(α*R*,β*R*)-β-hydroxy-α-hydroxymethyl-4-nitrophenethyl]acetamide.

$C_{11}H_{13}N_5O_5$ = 295.3.

CAS — 13838-08-9.

Azidamfenicol is an antibiotic that is related structurally to chloramphenicol (p.182). It has been used as 1% eye drops or eye ointment in the treatment of bacterial eye infections.

Preparations

Proprietary Preparations (details are given in Part 3)
Ger.: Berlicetin-Augentropfen; Posifenicol; Thilocanfol.

Azidocillin (13-t)

Azidocillin (*BAN, rINN*).

Azidobenzylpenicillin; BRL-2534; SPC-297D. (6*R*)-6-(D-2-Azido-2-phenylacetamido)penicillanic acid.

$C_{16}H_{17}N_5O_4S$ = 375.4.

CAS — 17243-38-8.

Azidocillin is a semisynthetic penicillin with actions and uses similar to those of phenoxymethylpenicillin (p.236). It is given by mouth as the sodium salt in doses of 750 mg twice daily in the treatment of susceptible infections. The potassium salt has also been used.

Preparations

Proprietary Preparations (details are given in Part 3)
Aust.: Longatren; ***Ger.:*** Syncillin; ***Ital.:*** Longatren†.

Azithromycin (3467-b)

Azithromycin (*BAN, USAN, rINN*).

CP-62993; XZ-450. (2*R*,3*S*,4*R*,5*R*,8*R*,10*R*,11*R*,12*S*,13*S*,14*R*)-13-(2,6-Dideoxy-3-*C*-3-*O*-dimethyl-α-L-*ribo*hexopyranosyloxy)-2-ethyl-3,4,10-trihydroxy-3,5,6,8,10,12,14-heptamethyl-11-(3,4,6-trideoxy-3-dimethylamino-β-D-*xylo*hexopyranosyloxy)-1-oxa-6-azacyclopentadecan-15-one dihydrate; 9-Deoxo-9a-aza-9a-methyl-9a-homoerythromycin A dihydrate.

$C_{38}H_{72}N_2O_{12},2H_2O$ = 785.0.

CAS — 83905-01-5 (anhydrous azithromycin); 117772-70-0 (azithromycin dihydrate).

Pharmacopoeias. In *US*.

A 0.2% solution in methyl alcohol (50%) has a pH of 9.0 to 11.0. **Store** in airtight containers.

Adverse Effects and Precautions

As for Erythromycin, p.204. Gastro-intestinal disturbances are the most frequent adverse effect but are usually mild and less frequent than with erythromycin. Transient elevations of liver enzyme values have been reported and, rarely, cholestatic jaundice. Rashes, headache, and dizziness may occur. Transient alternations in neutrophil counts have been seen in patients receiving azithromycin. The manufacturers suggest that azithromycin should not be used in patients with hepatic impairment.

Effects on the ears. Reversible sensorineural hearing loss was reported in 3 patients who received azithromycin 500 mg daily together with clofazimine and ethambutol for the treatment of disseminated *Mycobacterium avium* complex infection.[1]

1. Wallace MR, *et al.* Ototoxicity with azithromycin. *Lancet* 1994; **343:** 241.

Effects on fluid and electrolyte homoeostasis. The syndrome of inappropriate antidiuretic hormone (SIADH) secretion was associated with azithromycin treatment in 1 patient.[1,2]

1. Cadle RM, *et al.* Symptomatic syndrome of inappropriate antidiuretic hormone secretion associated with azithromycin. *Ann Pharmacother* 1997; **31:** 1308–10.
2. Kintzel PE. Correction: symptomatic syndrome of inappropriate antidiuretic hormone secretion associated with azithromycin. *Ann Pharmacother* 1998; **32:** 388.

Effects on the kidneys. Acute interstitial nephritis leading to irreversible renal failure has been reported in a patient who received azithromycin for 9 days.[1]

1. Mansoor GA, *et al.* Azithromycin-induced acute interstitial nephritis. *Ann Intern Med* 1993; **119:** 636–7.

Eosinophilia. A syndrome characterised by eosinophilia, arthralgia, fever, and rash was associated in one patient with administration of azithromycin or roxithromycin on separate occasions.[1] The original authors believed the condition represented the Churg-Strauss syndrome although this was disputed in correspondence[2] and attributed to the eosinophilia-myalgia syndrome.

1. Hübner C, *et al.* Macrolide-induced Churg-Strauss syndrome in a patient with atopy. *Lancet* 1997; **350:** 563.
2. Kränke B, Aberer W. Macrolide-induced Churg-Strauss syndrome in patient with atopy. *Lancet* 1997; **350:** 1551–2.

Interactions

For a discussion of drug interactions with macrolide antibacterials, see Erythromycin, p.205.

Increased rifabutin toxicity has been reported in patients receiving azithromycin and rifabutin.

Antimicrobial Action

As for Erythromycin, p.205. It is less active than erythromycin against streptococci and staphylococci, but has greater activity than erythromycin *in vitro* against some Gram-negative pathogens such as *Haemophilus influenzae* and *Moraxella (Branhamella) catarrhalis*, as well as having activity against some of the Enterobacteriaceae such as *Escherichia coli* and *Salmonella* and *Shigella* spp. Azithromycin is also more active than erythromycin against *Chlamydia trachomatis* and some opportunistic mycobacteria, including *Mycobacterium avium* complex. It has activity against the protozoa *Toxoplasma gondii* and *Plasmodium falciparum*.

References.

1. Hamilton-Miller JMT. In-vitro activities of 14-, 15- and 16-membered macrolides against Gram-positive cocci. *J Antimicrob Chemother* 1992; **29:** 141–7.
2. Gordillo ME, *et al.* In vitro activity of azithromycin against bacterial enteric pathogens. *Antimicrob Agents Chemother* 1993; **37:** 1203–5.
3. Agacfidan A, *et al.* In vitro activity of azithromycin (CP-62,993) against Chlamydia trachomatis and Chlamydia pneumoniae. *Antimicrob Agents Chemother* 1993; **37:** 1746–8.

Resistance. The pattern of resistance to azithromycin is similar to that seen with clarithromycin (p.189).

Pharmacokinetics

Following oral administration about 40% of a dose of azithromycin is bioavailable. Absorption from the capsule formulation, but not the tablet formulation, is reduced by food. Peak plasma concentrations are achieved 2 to 3 hours after a dose, but azithromycin is extensively distributed to the tissues, and tissue concentrations subsequently remain much higher than those in the blood; in contrast to most other antibacterials, plasma concentrations are therefore of little value as a guide to efficacy. High concentrations are taken up into white blood cells. There is little diffusion into the CSF when the meninges are not inflamed. Small amounts of azithromycin are demethylated in the liver, and it is excreted in bile as unchanged drug and metabolites. About 6% of an oral dose (representing about 20% of the amount in the systemic circulation) is excreted in the urine. The terminal elimination half-life is probably in excess of 40 hours.

Reviews and references.

1. Lalak NJ, Morris DL. Azithromycin clinical pharmacokinetics. *Clin Pharmacokinet* 1993; **25:** 370–4.
2. Nahata MC, *et al.* Pharmacokinetics of azithromycin in pediatric patients after oral administration of multiple doses of suspension. *Antimicrob Agents Chemother* 1993; **37:** 314–16.
3. Luke DR, *et al.* Safety, toleration, and pharmacokinetics of intravenous azithromycin. *Antimicrob Agents Chemother* 1996; **40:** 2577–81.
4. Rapp RP. Pharmacokinetics and pharmacodynamics of intravenous and oral azithromycin: enhanced tissue activity and minimal drug interactions. *Ann Pharmacother* 1998; **32:** 785–93.

Uses and Administration

Azithromycin is a nitrogen-containing macrolide or azalide with actions and uses similar to those of erythromycin (p.206).

Azithromycin may also be used as a component of regimens in the treatment of *Mycobacterium avium* complex (MAC) infections (see under Opportunistic

Mycobacterial Infections, p.133) and may be used as an alternative to rifabutin for prophylaxis. It has been tried in protozoal infections including toxoplasmosis (p.576).

It is given by mouth as the dihydrate; doses are calculated in terms of the base. The capsule formulation should be given at least an hour before, or 2 hours after, meals.

The usual dose for uncomplicated genital infections due to *Chlamydia trachomatis* is the equivalent of 1 g of azithromycin as a single dose. A single dose of 2 g may be given for uncomplicated gonorrhoea. For other infections due to susceptible organisms including otitis media, respiratory-tract infections, and skin infections the dose is 500 mg as a single dose daily for 3 or more days. Alternatively, an initial dose of 500 mg may be followed by 250 mg daily for a further 4 days. For prophylaxis of disseminated MAC infections, azithromycin 1.2 g may be given once weekly. In children, the dose suggested in the UK is 10 mg per kg body-weight once daily for 3 days. In the USA, the dose recommended for children for pneumonia or otitis media is 10 mg per kg on the first day then 5 mg per kg daily for a further 4 days, and the dose for pharyngitis or tonsillitis is 12 mg per kg once daily for 5 days.

Azithromycin dihydrate may also be given initially by intravenous infusion in doses equivalent to 500 mg of azithromycin as a single daily dose in the treatment of community acquired pneumonia and pelvic inflammatory disease.

Reviews.

1. Peters DH, *et al.* Azithromycin: a review of its antimicrobial activity, pharmacokinetic properties and clinical efficacy. *Drugs* 1992; **44:** 750–99.

Inflammatory bowel disease. Azithromycin, in combination with rifabutin, has been studied in the treatment of Crohn's disease (see Inflammatory Bowel Disease, p.1171). The rationale for this use is based on the putative involvement of *Mycobacterium paratuberculosis* as a causative factor for the disease.

Preparations

USP 23: Azithromycin Capsules; Azithromycin for Oral Suspension.

Proprietary Preparations (details are given in Part 3)
Aust.: Zithromax; ***Austral.:*** Zithromax; ***Belg.:*** Zitromax; ***Canad.:*** Zithromax; ***Fr.:*** Zithromax; ***Ger.:*** Zithromax; ***Irl.:*** Zithromax; ***Ital.:*** Azitrocin; Ribotrex; Trozocina; Zitromax; ***Neth.:*** Zithromax; ***Norw.:*** Azitromax; ***S.Afr.:*** Zithromax; ***Spain:*** Goxil; Toraseptol; Vinzam; Zentavion; Zitromax; ***Swed.:*** Azitromax; ***Switz.:*** Zithromax; ***UK:*** Zithromax; ***USA:*** Zithromax.

Azlocillin Sodium (14-x)

Azlocillin Sodium *(BANM, rINNM).*

BAY-e-6905. Sodium (6*R*)-6-[D-2-(2-oxoimidazolidine-1-carboxamido)-2-phenylacetamido]penicillanate.

$C_{20}H_{22}N_5NaO_6S$ = 483.5.

CAS — 37091-66-0 (azlocillin); 37091-65-9 (azlocillin sodium).

NOTE. Azlocillin is *USAN*.

Pharmacopoeias. In *Br., Pol.,* and *US.*

A white to pale yellow hygroscopic powder. 1.05 g of monograph substance is approximately equivalent to 1 g of azlocillin. Each g of monograph substance represents about 2.1 mmol of sodium. **Soluble** in water; very soluble in methyl alcohol; practically insoluble in acetone, in chloroform, and in ether. A 10% solution in water has a pH of 6 to 8. **Store** in airtight containers at a temperature not exceeding 25°.

Incompatibility has been reported with aminoglycosides, ciprofloxacin, metronidazole, and tetracyclines.

Adverse Effects and Precautions

As for Carbenicillin Sodium, p.162.

As azlocillin sodium has a lower sodium content than carbenicillin sodium, hypernatraemia and hypokalaemia are less likely to occur. Prolongation of bleeding time has been less frequent and less severe than with carbenicillin.

Hypouricaemia. Reports of transient asymptomatic decreases in serum-uric acid concentrations during treatment with azlocillin.[1,2]

1. Faris HM, Potts DW. Azlocillin and serum uric acid. *Ann Intern Med* 1983; **98:** 414.
2. Ernst JA, Sy ER. Effect of azlocillin on uric acid levels in serum. *Antimicrob Agents Chemother* 1983; **24:** 609–10.

Interactions

As for Benzylpenicillin, p.160.

For the effect of azlocillin on the clearance of *cefotaxime*, and a report of neurotoxicity, see p.168. For reference to azlocillin affecting the disposition of *ciprofloxacin*, see p.187.

See also above for incompatibilities.

Antimicrobial Action

Azlocillin has an antimicrobial action similar to that of piperacillin (p.237). Its activity *in vitro* against Enterobacteriaceae is generally less than that of mezlocillin or piperacillin, but it has comparable activity to piperacillin against *Pseudomonas aeruginosa*.

Pharmacokinetics

Azlocillin is not absorbed from the gastro-intestinal tract to any significant extent. It is reported to have nonlinear dose-dependent pharmacokinetics. Doubling of an intravenous dose results in more than double the plasma concentration. Between 20 and 46% of azlocillin in the circulation is bound to plasma proteins. The plasma half-life is usually about 1 hour, but longer in neonates; in patients with renal impairment half-lives of 2 to 6 hours have been reported.

Azlocillin is widely distributed in body tissues and fluids. It crosses the placenta into the fetal circulation and small amounts are distributed into breast milk. There is little diffusion into the CSF except when the meninges are inflamed.

Azlocillin is reported to be metabolised to a limited extent. About 50 to 70% of a dose is excreted unchanged in the urine by glomerular filtration and tubular secretion within 24 hours of administration, so that high urinary concentrations are achieved. Azlocillin is partly excreted in the bile where it is also found in high concentrations.

Plasma concentrations are enhanced if probenecid is administered concomitantly.

Azlocillin is removed by haemodialysis.

Uses and Administration

Azlocillin is a ureidopenicillin and, like piperacillin (p.238), is used primarily for the treatment of infections caused by *Pseudomonas aeruginosa*. It has been used particularly for septicaemia, and infections of the respiratory and urinary tracts, and also for peritonitis; for details of these infections see under Choice of Antibacterial, p.116. Azlocillin is commonly administered in association with an aminoglycoside; however they should be administered separately as they have been shown to be incompatible.

Administration and dosage. Azlocillin is administered intravenously as the sodium salt. Doses are expressed in terms of the equivalent amount of azlocillin. A 10% solution in a suitable diluent is given by slow injection for doses of 2 g or less; higher doses should be infused over 20 to 30 minutes.

The usual dose is 5 g every 8 hours for life-threatening infections or 2 g every 8 hours for less severe infections and urinary-tract infections.

The following doses may be used for children: premature infants, 50 mg per kg body-weight twice daily; neonates less than 7 days old, 100 mg per kg twice daily; infants between 7 days and 1 year, 100 mg per kg three times daily; children up to 14 years, 75 mg per kg three times daily.

The interval between doses may need to be increased in moderate to severe renal impairment; additional dosage reductions may be needed in patients with both renal and hepatic impairment.

Preparations

BP 1998: Azlocillin Injection;
USP 23: Azlocillin for Injection.

Proprietary Preparations (details are given in Part 3)
Aust.: Securopen; ***Austral.:*** Securopen†; ***Ger.:*** Securopen; ***Irl.:*** Securopen; ***Ital.:*** Securopen; ***Norw.:*** Securopen; ***UK:*** Securopen.

Aztreonam (13266-e)

Aztreonam *(BAN, USAN, rINN).*

Azthreonam; SQ-26776. (*Z*)-2-{2-Aminothiazol-4-yl-[(2*S*,3*S*)-2-methyl-4-oxo-1-sulphoazetidin-3-ylcarbamoyl]methyleneamino-oxy}-2-methylpropionic acid.

$C_{13}H_{17}N_5O_8S_2$ = 435.4.

CAS — 78110-38-0.

Pharmacopoeias. In *US.*

A white crystalline powder. Slightly **soluble** in methyl alcohol; very slightly soluble in dehydrated alcohol; practically insoluble in ethyl acetate, in chloroform, and in toluene; soluble in dimethylformamide and in dimethyl sulphoxide. **Store** in airtight containers.

Aztreonam has been reported to be **incompatible** with metronidazole, nafcillin, and vancomycin.

References.

1. Bell RG, *et al.* Stability of intravenous admixtures of aztreonam and cefoxitin, gentamicin, metronidazole, or tobramycin. *Am J Hosp Pharm* 1986; **43:** 1444–53.
2. Riley CM, Lipford LC. Interaction of aztreonam with nafcillin in intravenous admixtures. *Am J Hosp Pharm* 1986; **43:** 2221–4.
3. Belliveau PP, *et al.* Stability of aztreonam and ampicillin sodium-sulbactam sodium in 0.9% sodium chloride injection. *Am J Hosp Pharm* 1994; **51:** 901–4.
4. Trissel LA, Martinez JF. Compatibility of aztreonam with selected drugs during simulated Y-site administration. *Am J Health-Syst Pharm* 1995; **52:** 1086–90.
5. Trissel LA, *et al.* Compatibility and stability of aztreonam and vancomycin hydrochloride. *Am J Health-Syst Pharm* 1995; **52:** 2560–4.

Adverse Effects

The adverse effects of aztreonam are similar to those of other beta-lactams (see Benzylpenicillin, p.159, and Cephalothin, p.179). Hypersensitivity reactions, including skin rashes, urticaria, eosinophilia, and rarely anaphylaxis, may occur in patients receiving aztreonam, although it has been reported to be only weakly immunogenic (see also under Precautions, below). Gastro-intestinal effects include diarrhoea, nausea, vomiting, and an abnormal taste.

Phlebitis or thrombophlebitis has been reported after the intravenous administration of aztreonam, and pain or swelling after intramuscular injection.

Administration of aztreonam may result in the overgrowth of non-susceptible organisms, including Gram-positive cocci. Pseudomembranous colitis may develop.

Other adverse effects that have been reported with aztreonam include jaundice and hepatitis, increases in liver enzymes, and prolongation of prothrombin and partial thromboplastin times.

Effects on the skin. References.

1. McDonald BJ, *et al.* Toxic epidermal necrolysis possibly linked to aztreonam in bone marrow transplant patients. *Ann Pharmacother* 1992; **26:** 34–5.

Precautions

Aztreonam should not be given to patients who are hypersensitive to it and should be administered with caution to those known to be hypersensitive to other beta-lactams although the incidence of cross-sensitivity appears to be low (but see below).

It should be used with caution in patients with renal or hepatic impairment.

Aztreonam is said to show little cross-reactivity with other beta-lactams,[1,2] but there have been isolated reports of immediate hypersensitivity to aztreonam in patients with a history of hypersensitivity to penicillin.[3,4]

1. Saxon A, *et al.* Lack of cross-reactivity between aztreonam, a monobactam antibiotic, and penicillin in penicillin-allergic subjects. *J Infect Dis* 1984; **149:** 16–22.
2. Adkinson NF. Immunogenicity and cross-allergenicity of aztreonam. *Am J Med* 1990; **88** (suppl 3C): 12S–15S.
3. Alvarez JS, *et al.* Immediate hypersensitivity to aztreonam. *Lancet* 1990; **335:** 1094.
4. Hantson P, *et al.* Immediate hypersensitivity to aztreonam and imipenem. *Br Med J* 1991; **302:** 294–5.

Interactions

Caution is recommended in patients receiving aztreonam and oral anticoagulant therapy because of the possibility of increased prothrombin time.

Antimicrobial Action

Aztreonam is bactericidal and acts similarly to the penicillins by inhibiting synthesis of the bacterial cell wall; it has a high affinity for the penicillin-binding protein 3 (PBP-3) of Gram-negative bacteria. The activity of aztreonam is restricted to Gram-negative aerobic organisms, including beta-lactamase-producing strains, with poor or no activity against Gram-positive aerobes or anaerobic organisms. It is active against most Enterobacteriaceae including *Escherichia coli*, *Klebsiella*, *Proteus*, *Providencia*, *Salmonella*, *Serratia*, *Shigella*, and *Yersinia* spp. Most of these organisms are inhibited *in vitro* by a concentration of aztreonam of 4 μg or less per mL. Some strains of *Enterobacter* and *Citrobacter* spp. are resistant. Aztreonam is active against *Pseudomonas aeruginosa* with MICs of 16 μg or less per mL. Most strains of other *Pseudomonas* spp. are insensitive. Aztreonam has good activity against *Haemophilus influenzae* and *Neisseria* spp.; most strains are inhibited by concentrations of 0.5 μg or less per mL.

Synergy has been reported *in vitro* between aztreonam and aminoglycosides against *Ps. aeruginosa* and some *Enterobacteriaceae*.

Aztreonam is stable to hydrolysis by many beta-lactamases and appears to be a poor inducer of beta-lactamase production. Acquired resistance has occasionally been reported.

References.

1. Parry MF. Aztreonam susceptibility testing: a retrospective analysis. *Am J Med* 1990; **88** (suppl 3C): 7S–11S.

Pharmacokinetics

Aztreonam is poorly absorbed from the gastro-intestinal tract and is therefore administered parenterally. Absorption after intramuscular injection is good; peak plasma concentrations of about 46 μg per mL have been achieved within one hour of a 1-g dose. Aztreonam has a plasma half-life of approximately 1.7 hours. The half-life may be prolonged in neonates, in renal impairment, and to some extent in patients with hepatic impairment. About 56% in the circulation is bound to plasma proteins. It is widely distributed in body tissues and fluids, including bile. Diffusion into the CSF is poor unless the meninges are inflamed. It crosses the placenta and enters the fetal circulation; small amounts are distributed into breast milk.

Aztreonam is not extensively metabolised. The principal metabolite, SQ-26992, is inactive and is formed by opening of the beta-lactam ring; it has a much longer half-life than the parent compound. Aztreonam is excreted predominantly in the urine, by renal tubular secretion and glomerular filtration; about 60 to 70% of a dose appears within 8 hours as unchanged drug with only small quantities of metabolites. Only small amounts of unchanged drug and metabolites are excreted in the faeces.

Aztreonam is removed by haemodialysis and to a lesser extent by peritoneal dialysis.

Reviews.

1. Mattie H. Clinical pharmacokinetics of aztreonam: an update. *Clin Pharmacokinet* 1994; **26:** 99–106.

Uses and Administration

Aztreonam is a monobactam or monocyclic beta-lactam antibiotic used parenterally as an alternative to aminoglycosides or third-generation cephalosporins for the treatment of infections caused by susceptible Gram-negative aerobic organisms. These have included bone and joint infections, gonorrhoea, intra-abdominal and pelvic infections, lower respiratory-tract infections including pseudomonal infections in patients with cystic fibrosis, meningitis, septicaemia, skin and soft tissue infections, and urinary-tract infections. For details of these infections and their treatment, see under Choice of Antibacterial, p.116. To broaden the spectrum of activity for empirical treatment of infections, aztreonam should be used in conjunction with other antibacterials. Concurrent use of an aminoglycoside may be of benefit in serious *Pseudomonas aeruginosa* infections.

Aztreonam is usually administered parenterally by deep intramuscular injection, by slow intravenous injection over 3 to 5 minutes, or by intravenous infusion over 20 to 60 minutes. It is given in doses ranging from 1 to 8 g daily, administered in divided doses every 6 to 12 hours, according to the severity of the infection. Single doses over 1 g should be administered by the intravenous route. A single intramuscular dose of 1 g has been recommended for the treatment of gonorrhoea or cystitis.

Infants older than one week and children may be given aztreonam 30 mg per kg body-weight every 6 or 8 hours. For severe infections, children of 2 years or older may be given 50 mg per kg every 6 or 8 hours; a total daily dose of 8 g should not be exceeded.

Dosage should be reduced in moderate to severe renal impairment. The manufacturers have recommended that patients with renal impairment be given a usual initial dose followed by a maintenance dose adjusted according to their creatinine clearance: those with a clearance of 10 to 30 mL per minute, half the initial dose; those with a clearance of less than 10 mL per minute, one-quarter of the initial dose. They suggest that a supplementary dose of one-eighth of the initial dose be given to patients on haemodialysis after each dialysis session.

General references.

1. Brogden RN, Heel RC. Aztreonam: a review of its antibacterial activity, pharmacokinetic properties and therapeutic use. *Drugs* 1986; **31:** 96–130.
2. Neu HC. ed. Aztreonam's role in the treatment of Gram-negative infections. *Am J Med* 1990; **88** (suppl 3C): 1S–43S.

Clinical studies with aztreonam.

1. Smith G, *et al.* The use of aztreonam in serious Gram-negative infections. *J Antimicrob Chemother* 1988; **21:** 233–41.
2. DeMaria A, *et al.* Randomized clinical trial of aztreonam and aminoglycoside antibiotics in the treatment of serious infections caused by Gram-negative bacilli. *Antimicrob Agents Chemother* 1989; **33:** 1137–43.
3. DuPont HL, *et al.* Oral aztreonam, a poorly absorbed yet effective therapy for bacterial diarrhoea in US travellers to Mexico. *JAMA* 1992; **267:** 1932–5.

Preparations

USP 23: Aztreonam for Injection; Aztreonam Injection.

Proprietary Preparations (details are given in Part 3)
Aust.: Azactam; ***Austral.:*** Azactam; ***Belg.:*** Azactam; ***Fr.:*** Azactam; ***Ger.:*** Azactam; ***Irl.:*** Azactam; ***Ital.:*** Azactam; Primbactam; ***Jpn:*** Azactam; ***Neth.:*** Azactam; ***Norw.:*** Azactam; ***Spain:*** Azactam; Urobactam; ***Swed.:*** Azactam; ***Switz.:*** Azactam; ***UK:*** Azactam; ***USA:*** Azactam.

Bacampicillin Hydrochloride (15-r)

Bacampicillin Hydrochloride *(BANM, USAN, rINNM)*.

Ampicillin Ethoxycarbonyloxyethyl Hydrochloride; Bacampicillini Hydrochloridum; Carampicillin; EPC-272. 1-(Ethoxycarbonyloxy)ethyl (6*R*)-6-(α-D-phenylglycylamino)penicillanate hydrochloride.

$C_{21}H_{27}N_3O_7S,HCl = 502.0.$

CAS — 50972-17-3 (bacampicillin); 37661-08-8 (bacampicillin hydrochloride).

Pharmacopoeias. In *Eur.* (see p.viii), *Jpn*, and *US*.

A white or practically white hygroscopic powder or granules. 1.44 g of monograph substance is approximately equivalent to 1 g of ampicillin. **Soluble** in water and in dichloromethane; freely soluble in alcohol and in chloroform; very slightly soluble in ether. A 2% solution in water has a pH of 3.0 to 4.5. **Store** at a temperature not exceeding 25° in airtight containers.

Adverse Effects and Precautions

As for Ampicillin, p.153. Diarrhoea has been reported to occur less frequently with bacampicillin.

Interactions

As for Benzylpenicillin, p.160.

Antimicrobial Action

Bacampicillin has the antimicrobial action of ampicillin *in vivo* (p.153). It possesses no intrinsic activity and needs to be hydrolysed to ampicillin.

Pharmacokinetics

Bacampicillin is more rapidly and completely absorbed from the gastro-intestinal tract than ampicillin, to which it is hydrolysed in the intestinal wall and plasma. Peak plasma-ampicillin concentrations occur about 30 to 60 minutes after administration by mouth, and are approximately twice those after an equivalent dose of ampicillin. The absorption of bacampicillin from tablets does not appear to be affected by the presence of food in the stomach. About 75% of a dose is excreted in the urine as ampicillin within 8 hours.

Uses and Administration

Bacampicillin has actions and uses similar to those of ampicillin (p.154) to which it is rapidly hydrolysed after administration. It is given as the hydrochloride in doses of 400 to 800 mg two or three times daily by mouth; children over 5 years of age have been given 200 mg three times daily.

In uncomplicated gonorrhoea a single dose of bacampicillin hydrochloride 1.6 g together with probenecid 1 g may be given in areas where gonococci remain sensitive.

Preparations

USP 23: Bacampicillin Hydrochloride for Oral Suspension; Bacampicillin Hydrochloride Tablets.

Proprietary Preparations (details are given in Part 3)
Aust.: Penglobe; ***Belg.:*** Bacampicin; Bacocil; Penglobe; ***Canad.:*** Penglobe; ***Fr.:*** Bacampicine; Penglobe; ***Ger.:*** Ambacamp; Penglobe; ***Irl.:*** Ambaxin†; ***Ital.:*** Albaxin†; Amplibac†; Bacacil; Penglobe; ***Neth.:*** Penglobe†; ***Spain:*** Ambaxino; Penglobe; Velbacil; ***Swed.:*** Penglobe; ***Switz.:*** Bacacil†; Bacampicin; ***UK:*** Ambaxin†; ***USA:*** Spectrobid.

Bacitracin (17-d)

Bacitracin *(BAN, rINN)*.

Bacitracinum.

CAS — 1405-87-4.

Pharmacopoeias. In *Chin.*, *Eur.* (see p.viii), *Int.*, *Pol.*, and *US*.

The Ph. Eur. states that bacitracin consists of one or more of the antimicrobial polypeptides produced by certain strains of *Bacillus licheniformis* and by *B. subtilis* var. *Tracy*. The USP states that it is a polypeptide produced by the growth of an organism of the *licheniformis* group of *Bacillus subtilis*.

It is a white to pale buff hygroscopic powder, odourless or with a slight odour. The Ph. Eur. specifies a potency of not less than 60 units per mg calculated on the dried substance, and the USP a potency of not less than 40 units per mg. Freely **soluble** in water; freely soluble or soluble in alcohol; soluble in methyl alcohol, and in glacial acetic acid, the solution in the organic solvents usually showing some insoluble residue; practically insoluble in acetone, in chloroform, and in ether. A 1% solution has a pH of 6 to 7.

Bacitracin is precipitated from solutions and inactivated by salts of many of the heavy metals. Solutions in water deteriorate rapidly at room temperature. **Store** at a temperature of 8° to 15° in airtight containers.

Bacitracin Zinc (16-f)

Bacitracin Zinc *(BANM, rINNM)*.

Bacitracins Zinc Complex; Bacitracinum Zincum; Zinc Bacitracin.

CAS — 1405-89-6.

Pharmacopoeias. In *Eur.* (see p.viii), *Int.*, *Pol.*, and *US*.

The zinc complex of bacitracin.

A white or pale yellowish-grey or tan hygroscopic powder, odourless or with a slight odour. Slightly or sparingly **soluble** in water; slightly soluble in alcohol; very slightly soluble in ether. A saturated solution in water has a pH of 6.0 to 7.5. **Store** in a cool place in airtight containers.

Incompatibility. Bacitracin was slowly inactivated in bases containing stearyl alcohol, cholesterol, polyoxyethylene derivatives, and sodium lauryl sulphate, and was rapidly inactivated in bases containing water, macrogols, propylene glycol, glycerol, cetylpyridinium chloride, benzalkonium chloride, ichthammol, phenol, and tannic acid.[1]

1. Plaxco JM, Husa WJ. The effect of various substances on the antibacterial activity of bacitracin in ointments. *J Am Pharm Assoc (Sci)* 1956; **45:** 141–5.

Stability. Bacitracin zinc was more stable than bacitracin and could be stored for 18 months at temperatures up to 40° without appreciable loss. Lozenges of bacitracin zinc and ointments and tablets containing bacitracin zinc with neomycin were more stable than the corresponding bacitracin preparations. Bacitracin zinc was less bitter than bacitracin and the taste was more readily disguised.[1]

1. Gross HM, *et al.* Zinc bacitracin in pharmaceutical preparations. *Drug Cosmet Ind* 1954; **75:** 612–13.

Units

The second International Standard Preparation (1964) of bacitracin zinc contains 74 units per mg.

Adverse Effects

When administered systemically bacitracin may produce severe nephrotoxicity. Nausea and vomiting may occur, as well as pain at the site of injection. Hypersensitivity reactions, including rashes and anaphylaxis, have occurred with both systemic, and more rarely with topical, administration.

Interactions

Additive nephrotoxicity would be anticipated if bacitracin is given systemically with other nephrotoxic drugs. Bacitracin is reported to enhance the neuromuscular blocking action of other drugs.

Antimicrobial Action

Bacitracin interferes with bacterial cell wall synthesis by blocking the function of the lipid carrier molecule that transfers cell wall subunits across the cell membrane. It is active against many Gram-positive bacteria including staphylococci, streptococci (particularly group A streptococci), and clostridia. It is also active against *Actinomyces*, *Treponema pallidum*, and some Gram-negative species such as *Neisseria* and *Haemophilus influenzae*, although most Gram-negative organisms are resistant.

Acquired bacterial resistance to bacitracin rarely occurs, but resistant strains of staphylococci have been detected.

Pharmacokinetics

Bacitracin is not appreciably absorbed from the gastro-intestinal tract. When administered by intramuscular injection it is rapidly absorbed; doses of 200 to 300 units per kg body-weight every 6 hours produce plasma concentrations of up to 2 units per mL. About 10 to 40% of a single injected dose is excreted in the urine within 24 hours. Bacitracin readily diffuses into the pleural and ascitic fluids but little passes into the CSF. Absorption is reported to be negligible following topical application but may occur after peritoneal lavage.

Uses and Administration

Bacitracin and bacitracin zinc are applied topically often in conjunction with other antibacterials such as neomycin and polymyxin B, and sometimes with corticosteroids, in the treatment of local infections due to susceptible organisms. Absorption from open wounds and from the bladder or peritoneal cavity may lead to adverse effects although the dose-limiting toxicity of combined preparations is considered to be due to neomycin.

Bacitracin has been given by mouth in the treatment of antibiotic-associated colitis due to *Clostridium difficile*. Parenteral administration is usually avoided because of toxicity but bacitracin has been given intramuscularly.

Preparations

BP 1998: Polymyxin and Bacitracin Eye Ointment;
USP 23: Bacitracin and Polymyxin B Sulfate Topical Aerosol; Bacitracin for Injection; Bacitracin Ointment; Bacitracin Ophthalmic Ointment; Bacitracin Zinc and Polymyxin B Sulfate Ointment; Bacitracin Zinc and Polymyxin B Sulfate Ophthalmic Ointment; Bacitracin Zinc Ointment; Neomycin and Polymyxin B Sulfates and Bacitracin Ointment; Neomycin and Polymyxin B Sulfates and Bacitracin Ophthalmic Ointment; Neomycin and Polymyxin B Sulfates and Bacitracin Zinc Ointment; Neomycin and Polymyxin B Sulfates and Bacitracin Zinc Ophthalmic Ointment; Neomycin and Polymyxin B Sulfates, Bacitracin Zinc, and Hydrocortisone Acetate Ophthalmic Ointment; Neomycin and Polymyxin B Sulfates, Bacitracin Zinc, and Hydrocortisone Ointment; Neomycin and Polymyxin B Sulfates, Bacitracin Zinc, and Hydrocortisone Ophthalmic Ointment; Neomycin and Polymyxin B Sulfates, Bacitracin Zinc, and Lidocaine Ointment; Neomycin and Polymyxin B Sulfates, Bacitracin, and Hydrocortisone Acetate Ointment; Neomycin and Polymyxin B Sulfates, Bacitracin, and Hydrocortisone Acetate Ophthalmic Ointment; Neomycin and Polymyxin B Sulfates, Bacitracin, and Lidocaine Ointment; Neomycin Sulfate and Bacitracin Ointment; Neomycin Sulfate and Bacitracin Zinc Ointment; Polymyxin B Sulfate and Bacitracin Zinc Topical Aerosol; Polymyxin B Sulfate and Bacitracin Zinc Topical Powder.

Proprietary Preparations (details are given in Part 3)
Aust.: Rhinocillin B; ***Canad.:*** Baciguent; Bacitin; ***USA:*** Ak-Tracin; Baci-IM; Baciguent.

Multi-ingredient: ***Aust.:*** Baneocin; Cicatrex; Eucillin; Nebacetin; Polybactrin; Riker Antibiotic-Spray; ***Austral.:*** Cicatrin; Myci-tracin†; Nemdyn; Neosporin; Spersin†; ***Belg.:*** Nebacetine†; Neobacitracine; Rikosol†; ***Canad.:*** Antibiotic Ointment; Antibiotique Onguent; Baciguent Plus Pain Reliever; Bacimyxin; Bioderm; Cicatrin; Cortisporin; Emercreme No 4; Lanabiotic; Neo Bace; Neosporin; Neotopic; Optimyxin; Ozonol Antibiotic Plus; Polycidin; Polyderm; Polysporin; Polysporin Triple Antibiotic; Polytopic; Polytracin; ***Fr.:*** Bacicoline; Bacteomycine; Collunovar; Lysopaine; Maxilase-Bacitracine; Oropivalone Bacitracine; Pimafucort†; ***Ger.:*** Anginomycin; Batrax; Bivacyn; Cicatrex; Medicrucin-blau†; Medicrucin-gelb N†; Nebacetin; Neobac; Neotracin; Polybactrin†; Polyspectran; Polyspectran HC; Polyspectran OS†; Prednitracin; Tonsilase†; ***Irl.:*** Biotrin†; Cicatrin; Polybactrin; Polybactrin Soluble†; Polyfax; ***Ital.:*** Bimixin; Cicatrene; Enterostop; Orobicin; Prednigamma†; ***Neth.:*** Bacicoline-B; Nebacetin†; Polyspectran B†; ***Norw.:*** Bacimycin; ***S.Afr.:*** Cicatrin; Nebacetin†; Neosporin; Polysporin; ***Spain:*** Alantomicina; Alantomicina Complex; Bacisporin; Banedif; Bio Hubber Fuerte; Dermisone Tri Antibiotic; Dermo Hubber; Indertal†; Infalina†; Linitul Antibiotico; Lizipaina; Neo Bacitrin; Neo Bacitrin Hidrocortis; Oxidermiol Enzima; Phonal; Pomada Antibiotica; Puodermina Hidrocor†; Rinobanedif; Tricin†; Tulgrasum Antibiotico; Tyroneomicin; Tyropenicilin R†; ***Swed.:*** Nebacetin†; ***Switz.:*** Bacimycine; Baneopol; Batramycine; Cicatrex; Lysopaine; Nebacetin†; Neosporin-B†; Neotracin; Oro-Pivalone; Polybactrin Soluble†; Polybactrin†; Prednitracin; ***UK:*** Cicatrin; Polybactrin†; Polyfax; Tri-Cicatrin†; Tribiotic†; ***USA:*** Ak-Poly-Bac; Ak-Spore; Alba-3; Aquaphor Antibiotic; Bactine First Aid Antibiotic Plus Anesthetic; Betadine First Aid Antibiotics + Moisturizer; Betadine Plus First Aid Antibiotics & Pain Reliever; Campho-Phenique Antibiotic Plus Pain Reliever Ointment; Clomycin; Coracin; Cortisporin; Lanabiotic; Medi-Quik†; Mycitracin; Mycitracin Plus; Neocin; Neomixin; Neosporin; Neosporin Plus; Neotal; Neotricin HC; Neotricin†; Ocutricin; Polycin-B; Polysporin; Septa; Spectrocin Plus; Topisporin†; Tribiotic Plus; Triple Antibiotic.

Balofloxacin (17613-d)

Balofloxacin *(rINN)*.

Q-35. (±)-1-Cyclopropyl-6-fluoro-1,4-dihydro-8-methoxy-7-[3-(methylamino)piperidino]-4-oxo-3-quinolinecarboxylic acid.

$C_{20}H_{24}FN_3O_4$ = 389.4.

CAS — 127294-70-6.

Balofloxacin is a fluoroquinolone antibacterial.

Bambermycin (12416-n)

Bambermycin *(BAN, pINN)*.

Bambermycins *(USAN)*; Flavophospholipol.

CAS — 11015-37-5.

An antibiotic complex containing mainly moenomycin A and moenomycin C and which may be obtained from cultures of *Streptomyces bambergiensis* or by other means.

Bambermycin is used as a growth promotor in pigs, poultry, and cattle.

Baquiloprim (2485-r)

Baquiloprim *(BAN, rINN)*.

138OU. 5-(8-Dimethylamino-7-methyl-5-quinolylmethyl)pyrimidin-2,4-diyldiamine.

$C_{17}H_{20}N_6$ = 308.4.

CAS — 102280-35-3.

Baquiloprim is a diaminopyrimidine antibacterial used in veterinary medicine in combination with sulphadimethoxine or sulphadimidine.

Bekanamycin Sulphate (18-n)

Bekanamycin Sulphate *(rINNM)*.

Aminodeoxykanamycin Sulphate; Bekanamycini Sulfas; Kanamycin B Sulphate; KDM; NK-1006. 6-*O*-(3-Amino-3-deoxy-α-D-glucopyranosyl)-2-deoxy-4-*O*-(2,6-diamino-2,6-dideoxy-α-D-glucopyranosyl)-D-streptamine sulphate.

$C_{18}H_{37}N_5O_{10},2.5H_2SO_4$ = 728.7.

CAS — 4696-76-8 (bekanamycin); 70550-99-1 (bekanamycin sulphate).

Pharmacopoeias. In *Jpn.*

1.5 g of monograph substance is approximately equivalent to 1 g of bekanamycin.

Bekanamycin is an aminoglycoside and is a congener of kanamycin. It has actions and uses similar to those of gentamicin (p.212). It has been given as the sulphate intramuscularly in usual doses of 400 to 600 mg daily, in divided doses; it has also been given topically and by mouth. It is reported to be more toxic than kanamycin.

Preparations

Proprietary Preparations (details are given in Part 3)
Ital.: Kanendos; Stereocidin†; ***Jpn:*** Kanendomycin.

Multi-ingredient: ***Ital.:*** Micomplex†; Situalin Antibiotico; Viscloben Antibiotico; Visumetazone Antibiotico; Visumicina.

Benethamine Penicillin (19-h)

Benethamine Penicillin *(BAN, rINN)*.

Benzyl(phenethyl)ammonium (6*R*)-6-(2-phenylacetamido)penicillanate.

$C_{15}H_{17}N,C_{16}H_{18}N_2O_4S$ = 545.7.

CAS — 751-84-8.

Pharmacopoeias. In *Br.*

A white crystalline powder. Benethamine penicillin 950 mg is approximately equivalent to 600 mg of benzylpenicillin (1 million units).

Very slightly **soluble** in water; slightly soluble in alcohol; sparingly soluble in acetone and in chloroform. **Store** at a temperature not exceeding 30° in airtight containers.

Benethamine penicillin is a poorly soluble derivative of benzylpenicillin (p.159) with similar actions and uses, although it is not recommended for chronic, severe, or deep-seated infections. After deep intramuscular injection it forms a depot from which it is slowly absorbed and hydrolysed to benzylpenicillin. Benethamine penicillin is usually given in conjunction with benzylpenicillin sodium and procaine penicillin to produce both an immediate and a prolonged effect; overall, the effect lasts for 2 to 3 days.

Preparations

Proprietary Preparations (details are given in Part 3)

Multi-ingredient: ***Fr.:*** Biclinocilline.

Benzathine Penicillin (20-a)

Benzathine Penicillin *(BAN)*.

Benzathine Benzylpenicillin *(rINN)*; Benzathini Benzylpenicillinum; Benzethacil; Benzilpenicillina Benzatinica; Benzylpenicillinum Benzathinum; Penicillin G Benzathine; Penzaethinum G. *NN'*-Dibenzylethylenediammonium bis[(6*R*)-6-(2-phenylacetamido)penicillanate].

$C_{16}H_{20}N_2(C_{16}H_{18}N_2O_4S)_2$ = 909.1.

CAS — 1538-09-6 (anhydrous benzathine penicillin); 5928-83-6 (benzathine penicillin monohydrate); 41372-02-5 (benzathine penicillin tetrahydrate).

Pharmacopoeias. In *Chin.*, *Eur.* (see p.viii), *Int.*, *Pol.*, and *US* (as the tetrahydrate).

A white powder. Benzathine penicillin 900 mg is approximately equivalent to 720 mg of benzylpenicillin (1.2 million units).

Very slightly **soluble** in water; slightly soluble in alcohol; freely soluble in dimethylformamide and in formamide; practically insoluble in ether. The pH of a 0.05% solution of the tetrahydrate in equal quantities of water and dehydrated alcohol is 4.0 to 6.5. **Store** at a temperature not exceeding 30° in airtight containers.

Adverse Effects and Precautions

As for Benzylpenicillin, p.159.

Non-allergic (embolic-toxic) reactions similar to those reported after administration of procaine penicillin, p.240, have been reported rarely with benzathine penicillin.

Benzathine penicillin should not be injected intravascularly since ischaemic reactions may occur.

Interactions

As for Benzylpenicillin, p.160.

Pharmacokinetics

When benzathine penicillin is given by intramuscular injection, it forms a depot from which it is slowly released and hydrolysed to benzylpenicillin. Peak plasma concentrations are produced in about 24 hours and are lower than those following an equivalent dose of benzylpenicillin potassium or sodium. However, depending on the dose, benzylpenicillin is usually detectable in plasma for up to 4 weeks (but see below).

Distribution into the CSF is reported to be poor.

Due to the slow absorption from the site of injection, benzylpenicillin has been detected in the urine for up to 12 weeks after a single dose.

Benzathine penicillin is relatively stable in the presence of gastric juice, but absorption from the gastro-intestinal tract is variable. Plasma concentrations of benzylpenicillin achieved following an oral dose are lower than those from the same dose of a soluble penicillin; peak concentrations are also produced less rapidly, but may persist for longer.

Plasma concentrations. Benzathine penicillin has been given every 4 weeks for secondary prophylaxis against rheumatic fever, although some advocate administration every 3 weeks to ensure adequate plasma concentrations of benzylpenicillin. Typical concentrations achieved after a single intramuscular injection of benzathine penicillin 900 mg have been cited as about 0.1, 0.02, and 0.002 μg per mL on days 1, 14, and 32 respectively. In one study[1] adequate concentrations (defined as 0.02 μg or more per mL) were seen in more than 80% of serum samples at 3 weeks, but in only 36% at 4 weeks. In a further study,[2] in which single doses of 900 mg, 1.35 g and 1.8 g were compared, it appeared that doses higher than the 900-mg dose of benzathine penicillin usually recommended might prolong the duration of protective plasma concentrations of benzylpenicillin (defined as above 0.025 μg per mL) and improve the efficacy of dosing every 4 weeks for prophylaxis against rheumatic fever.

1. Kaplan EL, *et al.* Pharmacokinetics of benzathine penicillin G: serum levels during the 28 days after intramuscular injection of 1 200 000 units. *J Pediatr* 1989; **115:** 146–50.
2. Currie BJ, *et al.* Penicillin concentrations after increased doses of benzathine penicillin G for prevention of secondary rheumatic fever. *Antimicrob Agents Chemother* 1994; **38:** 1203–4.

Pregnancy. The pharmacokinetics of benzathine penicillin appear to be altered in late pregnancy. Of 10 healthy pregnant women given benzathine penicillin 1.8 g intramuscularly before caesarean section, only 4 achieved adequate serum concentrations of benzylpenicillin (for syphilis, at least 0.018 μg per mL) for 7 days.[1]

1. Nathan L, *et al.* Penicillin levels following the administration of benzathine penicillin G in pregnancy. *Obstet Gynecol* 1993; **82:** 338–42.

Uses and Administration

Benzathine penicillin has the same antimicrobial action as benzylpenicillin (p.160) to which it is hydrolysed gradually following deep intramuscular injection. This results in a prolonged effect, but because of the relatively low blood concentrations of benzylpenicillin produced, its use should be restricted to micro-organisms that are highly susceptible to benzylpenicillin. In acute infections, and when bacteraemia is present, the initial treatment should be with benzylpenicillin by injection.

Infections treated with benzathine penicillin include diphtheria (asymptomatic carriers), pharyngitis (*Streptococcus pyogenes; Arcanobacterium (Corynebacterium) haemolyticum*), rheumatic fever (primary and secondary prophylaxis), and syphilis (including non-venereal treponematoses). For details of these infections and their treatment, see under Choice of Antibacterial, p.116.

Administration and dosage. Benzathine penicillin is administered by deep intramuscular injection, sometimes in association with procaine penicillin. It has been given by mouth for mild infections, although phenoxymethylpenicillin is usually preferred.

For early syphilis, a single dose of benzathine penicillin 1.8 g by deep intramuscular injection is given, usually as 2 injections at separate sites. In late syphilis, 1.8 g is given at weekly intervals for 3 consecutive weeks. Benzathine penicillin is not usually recommended for the treatment of neurosyphilis because of reports of inadequate penetration into the CSF. Infants up to 2 years of age may be given a single intramuscular dose of 37.5 mg per kg body-weight for the treatment of congenital syphilis provided there is no evidence of infection in the CSF.

For the treatment of other treponemal infections, such as yaws, pinta, and endemic syphilis (bejel), a single intramuscular dose of benzathine penicillin 900 mg is given, or 450 mg in children.

For streptococcal pharyngitis and the primary prevention of rheumatic fever the adult dose is a single intramuscular injection of 900 mg; children under 30 kg body-weight may be given 450 to 675 mg. To prevent recurrences of acute rheumatic fever 900 mg is given intramuscularly every 3 or 4 weeks; a dose of 450 mg has been recommended for children under 30 kg body-weight.

Preparations

USP 23: Penicillin G Benzathine and Penicillin G Procaine Injectable Suspension; Penicillin G Benzathine Injectable Suspension; Penicillin G Benzathine Oral Suspension; Penicillin G Benzathine Tablets; Sterile Penicillin G Benzathine.

Proprietary Preparations (details are given in Part 3)
Aust.: Retarpen; ***Austral.:*** Bicillin L-A; ***Belg.:*** Penadur; ***Canad.:*** Bicillin L-A; Megacillin; ***Fr.:*** Extencilline; ***Ger.:*** Pendysin; ***Irl.:*** Penidural†; ***Ital.:*** Diaminocillina; Wycillina; ***Neth.:*** Penidural; ***S.Afr.:*** Bicillin L-A; Penilente LA; ***Spain:*** Benzetacil; Cepacilina; Peniroger Retard†; Provipen Benzatina†; ***Switz.:*** Penadur†; Stabicilline†; ***UK:*** Penidural†; ***USA:*** Bicillin L-A; Permapen.

Multi-ingredient: ***Aust.:*** Retarpen compositum; ***Austral.:*** Bicillin All Purpose†; ***Canad.:*** Bicillin A-P; ***Ger.:*** Depotpen†; Retacillin; Tardocillin; ***Ital.:*** Tri-Wycillina; ***Neth.:*** Penidural D/F; ***S.Afr.:*** Penilente Forte; Ultracillin; ***Spain:*** Benzetacil Compuesta; Cepacilina; Davurmicin†; Neocepacilina; Penilevel Retard; Provipen†; ***Switz.:*** Penadur 6-3-3†; ***USA:*** Bicillin C-R.

Benzathine Phenoxymethylpenicillin (21-t)

Penicillin V Benzathine (*USAN*); Phenoxymethylpenicillini Dibenzylaethylendiaminum. *N,N'*-Dibenzylethylenediammonium bis[(6*R*)-6-(2-phenoxyacetamido)penicillanate].

$(C_{16}H_{18}N_2O_5S)_2,C_{16}H_{20}N_2$ = 941.1.

CAS — 5928-84-7 (anhydrous benzathine phenoxymethylpenicillin); 63690-57-3 (benzathine phenoxymethylpenicillin tetrahydrate).

Pharmacopoeias. In *Aust.* and *US.*

An almost white powder with a characteristic odour. Benzathine phenoxymethylpenicillin 1.3 g is approximately equivalent to 1 g of phenoxymethylpenicillin. **Soluble** 1 in 3200 of water, 1 in 330 of alcohol, 1 in 42 of chloroform, 1 in 910 of ether, and 1 in 37 of acetone. A 3% suspension in water has a pH of 4.0 to 6.5. **Store** in airtight containers.

Benzathine phenoxymethylpenicillin has actions and uses similar to those of phenoxymethylpenicillin (p.236) and is administered as an oral suspension in the treatment of susceptible mild to moderate infections. Doses are expressed in terms of phenoxymethylpenicillin.

Preparations

USP 23: Penicillin V Benzathine Oral Suspension.

Proprietary Preparations (details are given in Part 3)
Aust.: Ospen; Pen-Os; Star-Pen; ***Austral.:*** Abbocillin-V; Cilicaine V; ***Belg.:*** Oracilline; ***Canad.:*** Pen-Vee; PVF; ***Fr.:*** Oracilline; ***Ger.:*** InfectoBicillin; Ospen†; ***Spain:*** Benoral; ***Switz.:*** Ospen; Phenocillin.

Benzylpenicillin (181-l)

Benzylpenicillin (*BAN, rINN*).

Crystalline Penicillin G; Penicillin; Penicillin G. (2*S*,5*R*,6*R*)-3,3-Dimethyl-7-oxo-6-(2-phenylacetamido)-4-thia-1-azabicyclo[3.2.0]heptane-2-carboxylic acid; (6*R*)-6-(2-Phenylacetamido)penicillanic acid.

$C_{16}H_{18}N_2O_4S$ = 334.4.

CAS — 61-33-6.

The name benzylpenicillin is commonly used to describe either benzylpenicillin potassium or benzylpenicillin sodium as these are the forms in which benzylpenicillin is used.

In *Martindale*, benzylpenicillin means either the potassium or sodium salt.

Benzylpenicillin Potassium (182-y)

Benzylpenicillin Potassium (*BANM, rINNM*).

Benzylpenicillinum Kalicum; Penicillin G Potassium.

$C_{16}H_{17}KN_2O_4S$ = 372.5.

CAS — 113-98-4.

Pharmacopoeias. In *Chin., Eur.* (see p.viii), *Int., Jpn, Pol.,* and *US.*

The potassium salt of 6-phenylacetamidopenicillanic acid, an antimicrobial acid produced by growing certain strains of *Penicillium notatum* or related organisms or obtained by any other means.

A white or almost white crystalline powder. Each g of monograph substance represents about 2.7 mmol of potassium. Very **soluble** in water; sparingly soluble in alcohol; practically insoluble in fixed oils and in liquid paraffin. A 10% solution in water has a pH of 5.5 to 7.5 and a 6% solution has a pH of 5.0 to 7.5. **Store** in airtight containers.

Stability and **incompatibility**, as for Benzylpenicillin Sodium, below.

Benzylpenicillin Sodium (22-x)

Benzylpenicillin Sodium (*BANM, rINNM*).

Benzylpenicillinum Natricum; Penicillin G Sodium.

$C_{16}H_{17}N_2NaO_4S$ = 356.4.

CAS — 69-57-8.

Pharmacopoeias. In *Chin., Eur.* (see p.viii), *Int., Pol.,* and *US.*

The sodium salt of 6-phenylacetamidopenicillanic acid, an antimicrobial acid produced by growing certain strains of *Penicillium notatum* or related organisms or obtained by any other means.

A white or almost white crystalline powder. Each g of monograph substance represents about 2.8 mmol of sodium. Very **soluble** in water; practically insoluble in fixed oils and in liquid paraffin. A 10% solution in water has a pH of 5.5 to 7.5 and a 6% solution has a pH of 5.0 to 7.5. **Store** in airtight containers.

Stability. Benzylpenicillin sodium or potassium is hydrolysed in aqueous solutions by degradation of the β-lactam ring and hydrolysis is accelerated by increased temperature or alkaline conditions; inactivation also occurs under acid conditions. Degradation products include penillic, penicillenic, and penicilloic acids which lower the pH and cause a progressive increase in the rate of deterioration; *N*-formylpenicillamine and very small amounts of penicillamine have also been detected. Degradation is minimal at about pH 6.8 and deterioration of benzylpenicillin in solution may be retarded by using a citrate buffer. Dilute solutions are more stable than concentrated ones.

Incompatibility. Benzylpenicillin has been reported to be incompatible with metal ions and some rubber products. Its stability may be affected by ionic and nonionic surfactants, oxidising and reducing agents, alcohols, glycerol, glycols, macrogols and other hydroxy compounds, some paraffins and bases, some preservatives for example chlorocresol or thiomersal, carbohydrate solutions in an alkaline pH, fat emulsions, blood and blood products, and viscosity modifiers. Benzylpenicillin is incompatible with a wide range of acidic and basic drugs (see Stability, above) and with a number of other antimicrobials, including amphotericin, some cephalosporins, and vancomycin. Benzylpenicillin and aminoglycosides are mutually incompatible and injections should be administered at separate sites.

References.

1. Lynn B. The stability and administration of intravenous penicillins. *Br J Intraven Ther* 1981; **2** (Mar): 22–39.
2. Bird AE, *et al.* N-Formylpenicillamine and penicillamine as degradation products of penicillins in solution. *J Pharm Pharmacol* 1986; **38:** 913–17.

Units

The second International Standard Preparation (1952) of benzylpenicillin sodium contained 1670 units of penicillin per mg but was discontinued in 1968 since penicillin can now be characterised completely by chemical tests. Despite this, doses of benzylpenicillin are still expressed in units in some countries.

Benzylpenicillin potassium 600 mg or benzylpenicillin sodium 600 mg have generally been considered to be approximately equivalent to 1 million units (1 mega unit).

Adverse Effects

The most common adverse effects of benzylpenicillin are hypersensitivity reactions, especially skin rashes; anaphylaxis occasionally occurs and has sometimes been fatal. Other adverse effects have generally been associated with large intravenous doses of benzylpenicillin; patients with impaired renal function are also at increased risk. These adverse effects include haemolytic anaemia and neutropenia, both of which might have some immunological basis; prolongation of bleeding time and defective platelet function; convulsions and other signs of CNS toxicity (encephalopathy has followed intrathecal administration and can be fatal); and electrolyte disturbances because of the administration of large amounts of potassium or sodium when benzylpenicillin potassium or sodium, respectively, are administered.

Hepatitis and cholestatic jaundice have been reported rarely with some penicillins, notably penicillinase-resistant penicillins such as flucloxacillin and oxacillin, and also combinations of amoxycillin or ticarcillin with clavulanic acid.

Nephropathy and interstitial nephritis, which may have some immunological basis, has been especially associated with methicillin, but may be produced by other penicillins.

Some patients with syphilis and other spirochaete infections may experience a Jarisch-Herxheimer reaction shortly after starting treatment with penicillin, which is probably due to the release of endotoxins from the killed treponemes and should not be mistaken for a hypersensitivity reaction. Symptoms include fever, chills, headache, and reactions at the site of the lesions. The reaction can be dangerous in cardiovascular syphilis or where there is a serious risk of increased local damage such as with optic atrophy.

Gastro-intestinal effects like diarrhoea and nausea are the most common adverse effects following oral administration of benzylpenicillin; a sore mouth or tongue or a black hairy tongue have occasionally been reported. Pseudomembranous colitis has been associated with the use of most antibiotics; of the penicillins, ampicillin or amoxycillin have been implicated most frequently (see Antibiotic-associated Colitis, p.123).

Hypersensitivity. The overall incidence of allergic reactions to penicillin has been reported to vary from about 1 to 10% although some patients may have been incorrectly labelled 'allergic to penicillin'. Anaphylactic reactions occur in about 0.05% of patients, usually after parenteral administration but they have also been reported after taking penicillin by mouth.

Hypersensitivity to penicillin gives rise to a wide variety of clinical syndromes. Immediate reactions include anaphylaxis, angioedema, urticaria, and some maculopapular rashes. Late reactions may include serum sickness-like reactions and haemolytic anaemia. Reactions are considered to be due mainly to breakdown products (produced *in vitro* before administration) or metabolites of penicillin, and possibly penicillin itself, acting as haptens which when combined with proteins and other macromolecules produce potential antigens. As the hypersensitivity is related to the basic penicillin structure, patients who are genuinely allergic to benzylpenicillin must be assumed to be allergic to all penicillins; sensitised patients may also react to the cephalosporins and other beta-lactam antibiotics. For comment on crossreactivity with penicillamine, see under Penicillamine, Precautions, p.990.

Tests for hypersensitivity may be used to determine those patients most likely to develop serious allergic reactions to penicillins. Skin tests are used to evaluate the current risk of immediate or accelerated IgE-mediated reactions, the most serious being anaphylaxis. Both the major and minor determinants of penicillin hypersensitivity should be used; the major determinant is available as penicilloyl-polylysine (p.1616) and a minor-determinant mixture consisting of benzylpenicillin and its derivatives, including penicilloic acid and benzylpenicilloylamine can be used, although if this is not available a solution of benzylpenicillin may be substituted. Adrenaline should be available in case an anaphylactic reaction develops. The results of skin tests are unreliable if a significant time has elapsed before beginning therapy. A number of *in-vitro* tests including the radioallergosorbent test (RAST) have been developed.

Desensitisation may be attempted in patients allergic to penicillin when treatment with penicillin is considered essential. It involves the administration of very small doses of penicillin given at relatively short intervals of 15 minutes or more, and gradually increased to therapeutic concentrations. However, desensitisation may be hazardous and should only be carried out if the patient can be monitored continuously and adrenaline and resuscitation equipment are immediately available. Desensitisation should be regarded as temporary, and allergic reactions may recur during the next exposure to penicillin.

Neutropenia. Neutropenia has been widely reported in patients receiving high doses of beta-lactams and an incidence of from 5 to more than 15% has been reported in patients treated for 10 days or more. Warning signs include fever, rash, and eosinophilia. Monitoring of the leucocyte count is recommended during long-term treatment with high doses. Some have proposed a direct toxic effect whereas others have postulated an immune mechanism.

References to hypersensitivity reactions associated with penicillins.

1. Sullivan TJ, *et al.* Skin testing to detect penicillin allergy. *J Allergy Clin Immunol* 1981; **68:** 171–80.
2. Beeley L. Allergy to penicillin. *Br Med J* 1984; **288:** 511–12.
3. Holgate ST. Penicillin allergy: how to diagnose and when to treat. *Br Med J* 1988; **296:** 1213–14.
4. Anonymous. Penicillin allergy in childhood. *Lancet* 1989; **i:** 420.
5. Surtees SJ, *et al.* Allergy to penicillin: fable or fact? *Br Med J* 1991; **302:** 1051–2. [With comments from several authors—*Br Med J* 1991; **302:** 1462–3.]
6. Lin RY. A perspective on penicillin allergy. *Arch Intern Med* 1992; **152:** 930–7.
7. Anonymous. Penicillin allergy. *Drug Ther Bull* 1996; **34:** 87–8.

References to neutropenia associated with penicillins.

1. Anonymous. Antibiotic-induced neutropenia. *Lancet* 1985; **ii:** 814.
2. Neftel KA, *et al.* Inhibition of granulopoiesis in vivo and in vitro by β-lactam antibiotics. *J Infect Dis* 1985; **152:** 90–8.
3. Olaison L, Alestig K. A prospective study of neutropenia induced by high doses of β-lactam antibiotics. *J Antimicrob Chemother* 1990; **25:** 449–53.

References to CNS effects associated with penicillins.

1. Schliamser SE, *et al.* Neurotoxicity of β-lactam antibiotics: predisposing factors and pathogenesis. *J Antimicrob Chemother* 1991; **27:** 405–25.

Precautions

Patients known to be hypersensitive to penicillins should be given an antibacterial of another class. However, sensitised patients may also react to the cephalosporins and other beta-lactams. Desensitisation may be necessary if treatment with a penicillin is essential (see Adverse Effects, above). Penicillins should be given with caution to patients with a history of allergy, especially to drugs.

Care is necessary if very high doses of penicillins are given, especially if renal function is poor, because of the risk of neurotoxicity. The intrathecal route should be avoided. Care is also necessary if large doses of the potassium or sodium salts are given to patients with impaired renal function or heart failure, and high doses of benzylpenicillin potassium should be used with caution in patients receiving potassium-containing drugs or potassium-sparing diuretics. Renal and haematological status should be monitored during prolonged and high-dose therapy. Because of the Jarisch-Herxheimer reaction, care is also necessary when treating patients with spirochaete infections, particularly syphilis.

Contact with penicillin should be avoided since skin sensitisation may occur.

Penicillin therapy changes the normal bacterial flora and can lead to supra-infection with penicillin-resistant organisms including *Pseudomonas* or *Candida*, particularly with prolonged use.

Penicillins may interfere with some diagnostic tests such as those for urinary glucose using copper sulphate, direct antiglobulin (Coombs') tests, and some tests for urinary or serum proteins. Penicillins may interfere with tests that use bacteria, for example the Guthrie test for phenylketonuria using *Bacillus subtilis* organisms.

Interactions

Probenecid prolongs the half-life of benzylpenicillin by competing with it for renal tubular secretion and may be used therapeutically for this purpose. Benzylpenicillin may also interact with bacteriostatic antibacterials such as chloramphenicol, and tetracyclines (see under Antimicrobial Action, below) and may be incompatible *in vitro* with other drugs including a number of other antibacterials (see above).

The possibility of a prolonged bleeding time following oral treatment with a broad-spectrum drug like ampicillin should be borne in mind in patients receiving anticoagulants.

For the effect of penicillins on *methotrexate*, see p.549 and for the effect on *oral contraceptives*, see p.1433.

Antimicrobial Action

Benzylpenicillin is a beta-lactam antibiotic and has a bactericidal action against Gram-positive bacteria, Gram-negative cocci, some other Gram-negative bacteria, spirochaetes, and actinomycetes.

Mechanism of action. It exerts its killing action on growing and dividing bacteria by inhibiting bacterial cell-wall synthesis, although the mechanisms involved are still not precisely understood. Bacterial cell walls are held rigid and protected against osmotic rupture by peptidoglycan. Benzylpenicillin inhibits the final cross-linking stage of peptidoglycan production by binding to and inactivating transpeptidases, penicillin-binding proteins on the inner surface of the bacterial cell membrane. However, it is now realised that other earlier stages in cell-wall synthesis can also be inhibited. Other mechanisms involved include bacterial lysis by the inactivation of endogenous inhibitors of bacterial autolysins.

Its action is inhibited by penicillinase and other beta-lactamases that are produced during the growth of certain micro-organisms.

Many Gram-negative organisms are intrinsically resistant by virtue of the inability of benzylpenicillin to penetrate their outer membranes. Intrinsic resistance can also be due to structural differences in the target penicillin-binding proteins. See under Resistance, below, for reference to acquired resistance.

Spectrum of activity. The following pathogenic organisms are usually sensitive to benzylpenicillin:

Gram-positive aerobes and anaerobes including *Bacillus anthracis, Clostridium perfringens, Cl. tetani, Corynebacterium diphtheriae, Erysipelothrix rhusiopathiae, Listeria monocytogenes, Peptostreptococcus* spp., non-beta-lactamase-producing staphylococci, and streptococci including *Streptococcus agalactiae* (group B), *Str. pneumoniae* (pneumococci), *Str. pyogenes* (group A), and some viridans streptococci; enterococci are relatively insensitive.

Gram-negative cocci including *Neisseria meningitidis* (meningococci) and *Neisseria gonorrhoeae* (gonococci).

Gram-negative bacilli including *Pasteurella multocida, Streptobacillus moniliformis*, and *Spirillum minus* (or *minor*); most Gram-negative bacilli, including *Pseudomonas* spp. and Enterobacteriaceae, are insensitive although some strains of *Proteus mirabilis* and *Escherichia coli* may be inhibited by high concentrations of benzylpenicillin.

Gram-negative anaerobes including *Prevotella* (non-fragilis *Bacteroides*) and *Fusobacterium* spp.

Other organisms including *Actinomyces* and the spirochaetes, *Borrelia, Leptospira*, and *Treponema* spp.

Mycobacteria, fungi, mycoplasmas, and rickettsias are not sensitive.

Minimum inhibitory concentrations (MICs) of benzylpenicillin for the most sensitive organisms (gonococci, meningococci, non-beta-lactamase-producing staphylococci, and streptococci) have been reported to range from 0.005 to 0.05 µg per mL; the maximum bactericidal effect is at concentrations about 4 times the MIC.

Activity with other antimicrobials. Benzylpenicillin may exhibit synergy with other antimicrobials particularly the aminoglycosides and such combinations have been used against enterococci and other relatively insensitive bacteria. Its activity may be enhanced by clavulanic acid and other beta-lactamase inhibitors, and both enhancement and antagonism have been demonstrated for beta-lactam combinations. Antagonism has been reported to occur with some bacteriostatic drugs, such as chloramphenicol, that interfere with active bacterial growth necessary for benzylpenicillin to achieve its effect.

Resistance. Susceptible Gram-positive bacteria acquire resistance to beta-lactams mainly through the induction of beta-lactamases, including penicillinases. These enzymes are liberated extracellularly and hydrolyse the beta-lactam ring. This resistance is usually plasmid-mediated and can be transferred from one bacterium to another. Gram-negative bacteria produce beta-lactamases within their cell membranes which may be chromosomally or plasmid-mediated; all Gram-negative species probably contain small amounts of beta-lactamases. Resistance in Gram-negative species may also be due to changes in their outer membrane resulting in the failure of beta-lactams to reach their target penicillin-binding proteins. Changes in the binding characteristics of penicillin-binding proteins may also result in resistance in Gram-positive and Gram-negative bacteria.

Most strains of *Staphylococcus aureus* are now resistant to benzylpenicillin. *Streptococcus pneumoniae* with reduced susceptibility or complete resistance to benzylpenicillin have increasingly been reported. Strains of *Neisseria meningitidis* with reduced sensitivity to benzylpenicillin have been identified. Penicillinase-producing *Neisseria gonorrhoeae* are widespread; reduced sensitivity of gonococci to benzylpenicillin may also result from alterations in penicillin-binding proteins. Resistant strains of other species usually sensitive to benzylpenicillin have emerged among *Bacillus anthracis* and *Corynebacterium diphtheriae*. Most strains of *Haemophilus influenzae* and *Moraxella (Branhamella) catarrhalis* are now resistant.

Some organisms, usually Gram-positive cocci such as staphylococci or streptococci, may develop tolerance and are inhibited but not killed by benzylpenicillin; in such cases the minimum bactericidal concentration (MBC) is much greater than the minimum inhibitory concentration (MIC).

Pharmacokinetics

Benzylpenicillin rapidly appears in the blood following intramuscular injection of water-soluble salts, and maximum concentrations are usually reached in 15 to 30 minutes; peak plasma concentrations of about 12 μg per mL have been reported after single doses of 600 mg.

When given by mouth, benzylpenicillin is inactivated fairly rapidly by gastric acid and only up to about 30% is absorbed, mainly from the duodenum; maximum plasma-penicillin concentrations usually occur in about an hour. In order to attain plasma-penicillin concentrations after oral administration similar to those following intramuscular injection, up to 5 times as much benzylpenicillin may be necessary. Absorption varies greatly in different individuals and is better in patients with reduced gastric acid production including neonates and the elderly. Food decreases the absorption of benzylpenicillin and oral doses are best given at least half an hour before or 2 to 3 hours after a meal.

Benzylpenicillin is widely distributed at varying concentrations in body tissues and fluids. It appears in pleural, pericardial, peritoneal, and synovial fluids but in the absence of inflammation diffuses only to a small extent into abscess cavities, avascular areas, the eye, the middle ear, and the CSF. Inflamed tissue is, however, more readily penetrated and, for example, in meningitis higher concentrations of benzylpenicillin are achieved in the CSF. Active transport out of the CSF is reduced by probenecid. In patients with uraemia other organic acids may accumulate in the CSF and compete with benzylpenicillin for active transport; toxic concentrations of benzylpenicillin sufficient to cause convulsions can result.

Benzylpenicillin diffuses across the placenta into the fetal circulation, and small amounts appear in breast milk.

The plasma half-life is about 30 minutes although it may be longer in neonates and the elderly because of incomplete renal function. In renal impairment the half-life may be increased to about 10 hours. Approximately 60% is reported to be bound to plasma protein.

Benzylpenicillin is metabolised to a limited extent and the penicilloic acid derivative has been recovered in the urine. Benzylpenicillin is rapidly excreted in the urine, principally by tubular secretion and about 20% of a dose given by mouth appears unchanged in the urine; about 60 to 90% of a dose of aqueous benzylpenicillin given intramuscularly appears in the urine mainly within the first hour. Significant concentrations are achieved in bile, but in patients with normal renal function only small amounts are excreted via the bile. Benzylpenicillin is removed by haemodialysis.

Renal tubular secretion is inhibited by probenecid (p.395), which is sometimes given to increase plasma-penicillin concentrations.

Uses and Administration

Benzylpenicillin is used in the treatment of a variety of infections due to susceptible organisms (see Antimicrobial Action, above). They include abscess, actinomycosis, anthrax, bites and stings, diphtheria, endocarditis, gas gangrene, leptospirosis, Lyme disease, meningitis, meningococcal infections, necrotising enterocolitis, necrotising fasciitis, neonatal conjunctivitis (if gonococci are sensitive), perinatal streptococcal infections (intrapartum prophylaxis against group B streptococci), pharyngitis (or tonsillitis), pneumonia, skin infections, surgical infection (prophylaxis in first trimester abortion in women at high risk for pelvic infection), syphilis (neurosyphilis and congenital syphilis), tetanus, toxic shock syndrome, and Whipple's disease. For details of these infections and their treatment, see under Choice of Antibacterial, p.116.

Administration and dosage. Benzylpenicillin is usually administered intramuscularly or intravenously. For some indications benzathine penicillin (p.158) or procaine penicillin (p.240), which provide a prolonged effect, are preferred; they are given intramuscularly. Benzylpenicillin is sometimes given by mouth for infections of moderate severity, but one of the acid-resistant penicillins such as phenoxymethylpenicillin (p.236) is preferable.

Benzylpenicillin is available as the potassium or sodium salt. The dose of benzylpenicillin should be sufficient to achieve an optimum bactericidal concentration in the blood as rapidly as possible; concentrations may be increased by concurrent administration of probenecid (p.395). In some countries, doses are still expressed in units (see above).

For some infections doses of 0.6 to 2.4 g of benzylpenicillin daily in 2 to 4 divided doses by intramuscular or slow intravenous injection or intravenous infusion may be adequate, but higher doses given intravenously, often by infusion, are more usual for severe infections. For example, in streptococcal endocarditis benzylpenicillin 7.2 g daily (1.2 g every 4 hours) intravenously, usually with an aminoglycoside, has been recommended; doses of 18 g or more daily are not unusual for less sensitive streptococci and enterococci. In meningococcal and pneumococcal meningitis benzylpenicillin 9.6 to 14.4 g daily (2.4 g every 4 to 6 hours) intravenously has been recommended; up to 18 g daily has sometimes been suggested for meningococcal meningitis. Such high doses may need to be reduced in patients with renal impairment.

High doses should be administered slowly to avoid irritation of the CNS and electrolyte imbalance, and a rate of not more than 300 mg per minute has been recommended for intravenous doses above 1.2 g.

Infants and children from 1 month to 12 years may be given 100 mg per kg daily in 4 divided doses; infants aged 1 to 4 weeks, 75 mg per kg daily in 3 divided doses; and neonates 50 mg per kg daily in 2 divided doses.

As in adults, higher paediatric doses may be necessary in severe infections. A dose of 180 to 300 mg per kg daily given intravenously in 4 to 6 divided doses has been recommended for meningitis in infants and children from 1 month to 12 years of age; infants aged 1 to 4 weeks may be given 150 mg per kg daily in 3 divided doses; neonates up to 7 days old may be given 100 mg per kg daily in 2 divided doses.

In patients with suspected meningococcal infection an intravenous or intramuscular injection of benzylpenicillin should be given before transfer to hospital. Suggested doses are: adults and children aged 10 years or more, 1.2 g; children aged 1 to 9 years, 600 mg; children under 1 year, 300 mg.

A suggested dose for intrapartum prophylaxis against group B streptococcal infection is benzylpenicillin 3 g initially then 1.5 g every 4 hours until delivery.

Other routes. For subconjunctival injection, 300 or 600 mg of benzylpenicillin may be dissolved in 0.5 to 1.0 mL of water, or another suitable solvent such as lignocaine 2% with or without adrenaline 1 in 100 000.

Benzylpenicillin is sometimes given by mouth in adult doses of 125 to 312 mg three or four times daily, administered on an empty stomach.

Intrathecal injections are no longer recommended.

Preparations

BP 1998: Benzylpenicillin Injection; Fortified Procaine Benzylpenicillin Injection;
USP 23: Penicillin G Potassium Capsules; Penicillin G Potassium for Injection; Penicillin G Potassium for Oral Solution; Penicillin G Potassium Injection; Penicillin G Potassium Tablets; Penicillin G Potassium Tablets for Oral Solution; Penicillin G Sodium for Injection.

Proprietary Preparations (details are given in Part 3)
Austral.: Benpen; Crystapen†; ***Canad.:*** Crystapen; Megacillin; Novo-Pen-G; ***Irl.:*** Crystapen; ***S.Afr.:*** Benzatec; Novopen; ***Spain:*** Cilina†; Cilipen†; Coliriocilina; Pekamin; Penibiot; Penibiot Lidocaina; Penilevel; Peniroger; Sodiopen; Unicilina; ***UK:*** Crystapen; ***USA:*** Pentids†; Pfizerpen.

Multi-ingredient: ***Aust.:*** Antipen; Fortepen; Ophcillin N; Retarpen compositum; ***Austral.:*** Bicillin All Purpose†; ***Belg.:*** Combicilline†; ***Canad.:*** Bicillin A-P; ***Fr.:*** Biclinocilline; Bipenicilline†; Gomenol-Syner-Penicilline; ***Ger.:*** Bipensaar; Hydracillin; Jenacillin A; Megacillin forte†; Retacillin; ***Ital.:*** Tri-Wycillina; ***Neth.:*** Bicilline; Penidural D/F; ***S.Afr.:*** Penilente Forte; Ultracillin; ***Spain:*** Anapen; Aquicilina D A; Benzetacil Compuesta; Broncosolvente EP†; Cepacilina; Cilina 400†; Davurmicin†; Neocepacilina; Neopenyl; Neumobiot; Penibiot Retard†; Penilevel Retard; Peniroger Procain†; Provipen†; Tyropenicilin R†; ***Switz.:*** Penadur 6-3-3†; ***UK:*** Bicillin.

Betamipron (15257-m)

Betamipron *(rINN)*.

N-Benzoyl-β-alanine; CS-443. 3-Benzamidopropionic acid.

$C_{10}H_{11}NO_3$ = 193.2.

CAS — 3440-28-6.

Betamipron is a renal protectant used in combination with the carbapenem antibiotic panipenem to reduce its adverse renal effects.

Preparations

Proprietary Preparations (details are given in Part 3)

Multi-ingredient: ***Jpn:*** Carbenin.

Biapenem (13919-s)

Biapenem (*USAN, rINN*).

CL-186815; L-627; LJC-10627. 6-{[(4R,5S,6S)-2-Carboxy-6-[(1R)-1-hydroxyethyl]-4-methyl-7-oxo-1-azabicyclo[3.2.0]hept-2-en-3-yl]thio}-6,7-dihydro-5H-pyrazolo[1,2-*a*]-s-triazol-4-ium hydroxide, inner salt.

$C_{15}H_{18}N_4O_4S$ = 350.4.

CAS — 120410-24-4.

Biapenem is a carbapenem beta-lactam antibiotic similar to imipenem (p.216). Like meropenem (p.224) it is reported to be more stable to renal dehydropeptidase I than imipenem.

References.

1. Hikida M, *et al.* Low neurotoxicity of LJC 10,627, a novel 1β-methyl carbapenem antibiotic: inhibition of γ-aminobutyric acid$_A$, benzodiazepine, and glycine receptor binding in relation to lack of central nervous system toxicity in rats. *Antimicrob Agents Chemother* 1993; **37:** 199–202.
2. Malanoski GJ, *et al.* In vitro activity of biapenem against clinical isolates of Gram-positive and Gram-negative bacteria. *Antimicrob Agents Chemother* 1993; **37:** 2009–16.
3. Aldridge KE, *et al.* In vitro activity of biapenem (L-627), a new carbapenem, against anaerobes. *Antimicrob Agents Chemother* 1994; **38:** 889–93.
4. Yeo S-F, Livermore DM. Comparative in-vitro activity of biapenem and other carbapenems against Haemophilus influenzae isolates with known resistance mechanisms to ampicillin. *J Antimicrob Chemother* 1994; **33:** 861–5.
5. Chen HY, Livermore DM. In-vitro activity of biapenem, compared with imipenem and meropenem, against Pseudomonas aeruginosa strains and mutants with known resistance mechanisms. *J Antimicrob Chemother* 1994; **33:** 949–58.
6. Piddock LJV, Jin YF. Activity of biapenem (LJC 10627) against 51 imipenem-resistant bacteria and selection and characterisation of biapenem-resistant mutants. *J Antimicrob Chemother* 1995; **36:** 845–50.
7. Koeppe P, *et al.* Biapenem pharmacokinetics in healthy volunteers and in patients with impaired renal function. *Arzneimittelforschung* 1997; **47:** 1250–6.
8. Kozawa O, *et al.* Pharmacokinetics and safety of a new parenteral carbapenem antibiotic, biapenem (L-627), in elderly subjects. *Antimicrob Agents Chemother* 1998; **42:** 1433–6.

Brodimoprim (16546-x)

Brodimoprim (*rINN*).

2,4-Diamino-5-(4-bromo-3,5-dimethoxybenzyl)pyrimidine.

$C_{13}H_{15}BrN_4O_2$ = 339.2.

CAS — 56518-41-3.

Brodimoprim is closely related structurally to trimethoprim (p.265) and is used in the treatment of infections of the respiratory tract and ear.

General references.

1. Braunsteiner AR, Finsinger F. Brodimoprim: therapeutic efficacy and safety in the treatment of bacterial infections. *J Chemother* 1993; **5:** 507–11.

The mean terminal half-life of brodimoprim in serum after administration of a single 400-mg dose by mouth to 8 healthy subjects was 25.9 hours.[1]

1. Kalager T, *et al.* Pharmacokinetics of brodimoprim in serum and skin blister fluid. *Chemotherapy* 1985; **31:** 405–9.

Preparations

Proprietary Preparations (details are given in Part 3)
Ital.: Hyprim; Unitrim.

Calcium Sulphaloxate (4901-j)

Calcium Sulphaloxate (*BANM*).

Calcium Sulfaloxate (*rINNM*). Calcium 4′-[(hydroxymethylcarbamoyl)sulphamoyl]phthalanilate pentahydrate.

$(C_{16}H_{14}N_3O_7S)_2Ca,5H_2O$ = 914.9.

CAS — 14376-16-0 (sulphaloxic acid); 59672-20-7 (calcium sulphaloxate).

Calcium sulphaloxate is a sulphonamide with properties similar to those of sulphamethoxazole (p.254). It is poorly absorbed, about 95% remaining in the intestine, and has been given for its antibacterial action in the gastro-intestinal tract.

Preparations

Proprietary Preparations (details are given in Part 3)
Ger.: Intestin-Euvernil N†.

Capreomycin Sulphate (7554-l)

Capreomycin Sulphate (*BANM, rINNM*).

34977; Capreomycin Sulfate (*USAN*); Capromycin Sulphate.

CAS — 11003-38-6 (capreomycin); 1405-37-4 (capreomycin sulphate).

Pharmacopoeias. In *Br., Chin.,* and *US.*

A mixture of the sulphates of the polypeptide antimicrobial substances produced by certain strains of *Streptomyces capreolus* and containing not less than 90% of capreomycin I. The BP specifies that it contains not less than 700 units per mg.

Capreomycin I consists of capreomycin IA ($C_{25}H_{44}N_{14}O_8$=668.7) and capreomycin IB ($C_{25}H_{44}N_{14}O_7$=652.7) which predominates. Capreomycin II which makes up about 10% of the mixture consists of capreomycin IIA and capreomycin IIB.

A white or almost white solid or amorphous powder. Very **soluble** in water; practically insoluble in alcohol, chloroform, ether, and most other organic solvents. A 3% solution in water has a pH of 4.5 to 7.5. **Store** at a temperature not exceeding 15° in airtight containers.

Adverse Effects

The effects of capreomycin on the kidney and eighth cranial nerve are similar to those of aminoglycosides such as gentamicin (p.212). Nitrogen retention, renal tubular dysfunction, and progressive renal damage may occur. Hypokalaemia has been reported. Vertigo, tinnitus, and occasionally hearing loss may also occur and are sometimes irreversible. Abnormalities in liver function have been reported when capreomycin has been administered with other antituberculous drugs. Hypersensitivity reactions including urticaria, maculopapular rashes, and sometimes fever have been reported. Leucocytosis and leucopenia have also been observed. Eosinophilia commonly occurs with capreomycin. Capreomycin also has a neuromuscular blocking action. There may be pain, induration, and excessive bleeding at the site of intramuscular injection; sterile abscesses may also form.

Precautions

Capreomycin should be given with care and in reduced dosage to patients with impaired renal function. Care is also essential in patients with signs of eighth cranial nerve damage. It is advisable to monitor renal and auditory function and serum-potassium concentrations in patients before and during therapy.

Interactions

Care should be taken when capreomycin is used with other drugs that have neuromuscular blocking activity. It should not be administered with other drugs that are ototoxic or nephrotoxic.

Antimicrobial Action

Capreomycin is bacteriostatic against various mycobacteria. An MIC of 10 μg per mL has been reported for *Mycobacterium tuberculosis*, though this varies greatly with the media used. Resistance develops readily if capreomycin is used alone. It shows cross-resistance with kanamycin and neomycin.

References.

1. Ho YII, *et al.* In-vitro activities of aminoglycoside-aminocyclitols against mycobacteria. *J Antimicrob Chemother* 1997; **40:** 27–32.

Pharmacokinetics

Capreomycin is poorly absorbed from the gastro-intestinal tract. A dose of 1 g administered intramuscularly has been reported to give a peak serum concentration of about 30 μg per mL after 1 or 2 hours. About 50% of a dose is excreted unchanged in the urine by glomerular filtration within 12 hours.

Uses and Administration

Capreomycin is used in the treatment of tuberculosis (p.146) as part of a multidrug regimen when resistance to or toxicity from primary drugs has developed.

Capreomycin is administered as the sulphate by deep intramuscular injection. The usual adult dose is the equivalent of 1 g of capreomycin base (maximum 20 mg per kg bodyweight) given daily for 2 to 4 months, then two or three times a week for the remainder of therapy. Experience in children is limited.

As with aminoglycosides, the dose of capreomycin in patients with reduced renal function must be adjusted based on creatinine clearance; the desired steady-state serum capreomycin level is 10 μg per mL.

Preparations

BP 1998: Capreomycin Injection;
USP 23: Capreomycin for Injection.

Proprietary Preparations (details are given in Part 3)
Aust.: Capastat; ***Austral.:*** Capastat; ***Canad.:*** Capastat; ***Ger.:*** Ogostal†; ***Spain:*** Capastat; ***UK:*** Capastat; ***USA:*** Capastat.

Carbadox (12522-m)

Carbadox (*BAN, USAN, pINN*).

GS-6244. Methyl 3-quinoxalin-2-ylmethylenecarbazate 1,4-dioxide.

$C_{11}H_{10}N_4O_4$ = 262.2.

CAS — 6804-07-5.

Carbadox is an antibacterial that has been used in veterinary practice for treating swine dysentery and enteritis and for promoting growth. However, its use has been prohibited in the UK following reports of carcinogenicity.

Carbenicillin Sodium (24-f)

Carbenicillin Sodium (*BANM, rINNM*).

BRL-2064; Carbenicillin Disodium (*USAN*); Carbenicillinum Natricum; α-Carboxybenzylpenicillin Sodium; CP-15-639-2; GS-3159 (carbenicillin potassium); NSC-111071. The disodium salt of (6R)-6-(2-carboxy-2-phenylacetamido)penicillanic acid.

$C_{17}H_{16}N_2Na_2O_6S$ = 422.4.

CAS — 4697-36-3 (carbenicillin); 4800-94-6 (carbenicillin disodium); 17230-86-3 (carbenicillin potassium).

Pharmacopoeias. In *Eur.* (see p.viii), *Jpn, Pol.,* and *US.*

A white or slightly yellowish, hygroscopic powder. 1.1 g of monograph substance is approximately equivalent to 1 g of carbenicillin. Each g of monograph substance represents about 4.7 mmol of sodium. Freely **soluble** in water; soluble in alcohol and in methyl alcohol; practically insoluble in chloroform and in ether. A 1% solution in water has a pH of 6.5 to 8.0. A 5% solution in water has a pH of 5.5 to 7.5. **Store** at a temperature between 2° and 8° in airtight containers. Protect from light.

Carbenicillin sodium has been reported to be **incompatible** with aminoglycosides, tetracyclines, and a number of other drugs including antimicrobials.

Adverse Effects

As for Benzylpenicillin, p.159.

Pain at the injection site and phlebitis may occur. Electrolyte disturbances, particularly hypokalaemia or hypernatraemia, may follow the administration of large doses of carbenicillin sodium.

A dose-dependent coagulation defect has been reported, especially in patients with renal failure. Carbenicillin appears to interfere with platelet function thereby prolonging bleeding time; purpura and haemorrhage from mucous membranes and elsewhere may result.

Precautions

As for Benzylpenicillin, p.160.

Carbenicillin sodium should be given with caution to patients on a restricted sodium diet.

Carbenicillin sodium and other antipseudomonal penicillins have been shown to be incompatible with gentamicin and some other aminoglycosides *in vitro* and they should therefore be administered separately.

See above for other possible incompatibilities.

Interactions

As for Benzylpenicillin, p.160.

Antimicrobial Action

Carbenicillin has a bactericidal mode of action similar to that of benzylpenicillin, but with an extended spectrum of activity against Gram-negative bacteria. The most important feature of carbenicillin is its activity against *Pseudomonas aeruginosa*, although high concentrations are generally necessary. Activity against *Ps. aeruginosa* and some other organisms can be enhanced by gentamicin and other aminoglycosides. Carbenicillin is also active against *Proteus*, including indole-positive spp. such as *Pr. vulgaris*. It is comparable with ampicillin against other Gram-negative bacteria. Sensitive organisms include some Enterobacteriaceae, for example *Escherichia coli* and *Enterobacter* spp.; *Haemophilus influenzae*; and *Neisseria* spp. *Klebsiella* spp. are usually insensitive. Its activity against Gram-positive bacteria is less than that of benzylpenicillin. Anaerobic organisms are generally susceptible to carbenicillin, but for *Bacteroides fragilis* high concentrations are required.

Minimum inhibitory concentrations (MICs) of carbenicillin against bacteria considered susceptible range from about 0.1 to 32 μg per mL. Against *Ps. aeruginosa* an MIC of 16 to 32 μg per mL has been cited, but much higher concentrations may be necessary; isolates have been considered by some to be resistant when the MIC exceeds 128 μg per mL.

Resistance. Carbenicillin is inactivated by penicillinases and some other beta-lactamases, although it is more stable to the chromosomally-mediated beta-lactamases produced by some Gram-negative organisms including *Ps. aeruginosa* and some *Proteus* spp. Resistance to carbenicillin may develop in *Ps. aeruginosa* during treatment with carbenicillin or other beta-lactams. This resistance may be intrinsic where there are changes in cell wall permeability or penicillin-binding proteins or it may be due to plasmid-mediated beta-lactamase production that may be transferred to and from certain strains of Enterobacteriaceae.

There may be cross-resistance between carbenicillin and other antipseudomonal penicillins.

Outbreaks of pseudomonal resistance to carbenicillin have been associated with extensive use in, for example, hospital burns units.

Pharmacokinetics

Carbenicillin is not absorbed from the gastro-intestinal tract and has therefore been given either intramuscularly or intravenously.

The half-life of carbenicillin is reported to be about 1 to 1.5 hours; it is increased in patients with renal impairment, especially if there is hepatic impairment, and also in neonates. Half-lives of 10 to 20 hours have been reported in severe renal impairment. Clearance is enhanced in patients with cystic fibrosis. Carbenicillin is approximately 50% bound to plasma proteins. Distribution of carbenicillin in the body is similar to that of other penicillins. Small amounts have been detected in breast milk. There is little diffusion into the CSF except when the meninges are inflamed.

Relatively high concentrations have been reported in bile, but carbenicillin is excreted principally by renal tubular secretion and glomerular filtration.

Administration of probenecid increases and prolongs the plasma concentrations of carbenicillin.

Carbenicillin is removed by haemodialysis and, to some extent, by peritoneal dialysis.

Uses and Administration

Carbenicillin is a carboxypenicillin that has been given by injection as the disodium salt, often in conjunction with gentamicin, in the treatment of infections due to *Pseudomonas aeruginosa*; however, other antipseudomonal penicillins such as ticarcillin (p.263) or piperacillin (p.237) are now preferred. It has also been given to treat serious infections due to non-penicillinase-producing strains of *Proteus* spp.

Esters of carbenicillin such as carfecillin (p.163) and carindacillin (p.163), have been given by mouth in the treatment of urinary-tract infections.

Preparations

BP 1998: Carbenicillin Injection;
USP 23: Carbenicillin for Injection.

Proprietary Preparations (details are given in Part 3)
Austral.: Carbapen†; ***Canad.:*** Pyopen†; ***Ital.:*** Geopen; ***Spain:*** Geopen; ***UK:*** Pyopen†.

Carfecillin Sodium (25-d)

Carfecillin Sodium *(BANM, pINNM).*

BRL-3475; Carbenicillin Phenyl Sodium *(USAN)*. Sodium (6*R*)-6-(2-phenoxycarbonyl-2-phenylacetamido)penicillanate.

$C_{23}H_{21}N_2NaO_6S$ = 476.5.

CAS — 27025-49-6 (carfecillin); 21649-57-0 (carfecillin sodium).

Carfecillin is the phenyl ester of carbenicillin (p.162) to which it is hydrolysed following absorption from the gastro-intestinal tract. Its use is restricted to the treatment of urinary-tract infections due to *Pseudomonas* spp. and other sensitive bacteria including *Proteus* spp.

Preparations

Proprietary Preparations (details are given in Part 3)
Ital.: Urocarf.

Carindacillin Sodium (26-n)

Carindacillin Sodium *(BANM, pINNM).*

Carbenicillin Indanyl Sodium *(USAN)*; CP-15464-2. Sodium (6*R*)-6-[2-(indan-5-yloxycarbonyl)-2-phenylacetamido]penicillanate.

$C_{26}H_{25}N_2NaO_6S$ = 516.5.

CAS — 35531-88-5 (carindacillin); 26605-69-6 (carindacillin sodium).

Pharmacopoeias. In *US.*

A white to off-white powder. **Soluble** in water and alcohol. A 10% solution in water has a pH of 5 to 8. 1.4 g of monograph substance is approximately equivalent to 1 g of carbenicillin. Each g of monograph substance represents about 1.9 mmol of sodium. **Store** in airtight containers.

Carindacillin is the indanyl ester of carbenicillin (p.162) to which it is hydrolysed following absorption from the gastro-intestinal tract. Its use is restricted to the treatment of urinary-tract infections due to *Pseudomonas* spp. and other sensitive bacteria including *Proteus* spp.

It is given by mouth as carindacillin sodium. Usual doses, expressed in terms of carbenicillin, are 382 to 764 mg four times daily.

Preparations

USP 23: Carbenicillin Indanyl Sodium Tablets.

Proprietary Preparations (details are given in Part 3)
Canad.: Geopen†; ***Ger.:*** Carindapen†; ***USA:*** Geocillin.

Carumonam Sodium (18916-d)

Carumonam Sodium *(BANM, USAN, rINNM).*

AMA-1080 (carumonam); Ro-17-2301 (carumonam); Ro-17-2301/006 (carumonam sodium). (*Z*)-(2-Aminothiazol-4-yl){[(2*S*,3*S*)-2-carbamoyloxymethyl-4-oxo-1-sulphoazetidin-3-yl]carbamoyl}methyleneamino-oxyacetic acid, disodium salt.

$C_{12}H_{12}N_6Na_2O_{10}S_2$ = 510.4.

CAS — 87638-04-8 (carumonam); 86832-68-0 (carumonam sodium).

Carumonam sodium is a monobactam antibiotic with a spectrum of antimicrobial action *in vitro* similar to that of aztreonam (p.157). It is given by intramuscular or intravenous injection in a usual dose of 1 to 2 g daily in two divided doses.

Clinical experience with carumonam.

1. Hoepelman AIM, *et al.* Carumonam (Ro-17-2301; AMA-1080) compared with gentamicin for treatment of complicated urinary tract infections. *Antimicrob Agents Chemother* 1988; **32:** 473–6.

Preparations

Proprietary Preparations (details are given in Part 3)
Jpn: Amasulin.

Cefaclor (27-h)

Cefaclor *(BAN, USAN, pINN).*

Cefaclorum; Compound 99638. (7*R*)-3-Chloro-7-(α-D-phenylglycylamino)-3-cephem-4-carboxylic acid monohydrate.

$C_{15}H_{14}ClN_3O_4S,H_2O$ = 385.8.

CAS — 53994-73-3 (anhydrous cefaclor); 70356-03-5 (cefaclor monohydrate).

Pharmacopoeias. In *Eur.* (see p.viii) and *US. Jpn* includes the anhydrous substance.

A white to off-white, or slightly yellow, crystalline powder. 1.05 g of monograph substance is approximately equivalent to 1 g of anhydrous cefaclor. Slightly **soluble** in water; practically insoluble in methyl alcohol, in chloroform, and in dichloromethane. A 2.5% aqueous suspension has a pH of 3.0 to 4.5. **Store** in airtight containers.

Adverse Effects and Precautions

As for Cephalexin, p.178.

Hypersensitivity. Serum-sickness-like reactions may be more common with cefaclor than several other oral antibacterials[1] especially in young children who have received a number of courses of cefaclor;[2] typical features included skin reactions and arthralgia. A relatively high incidence of anaphylactic reactions has been reported from Japan.[3]

There has been a report of myocarditis that developed as a hypersensitivity reaction to cefaclor in a 12-year-old child.[4]

1. McCue JD. Delayed detection of serum sickness caused by oral antimicrobials. *Adv Therapy* 1990; **7:** 22–7.
2. Vial T, *et al.* Cefaclor-associated serum sickness-like disease: eight cases and review of the literature. *Ann Pharmacother* 1992; **26:** 910–14.
3. Hama R, Mori K. High incidence of anaphylactic reactions to cefaclor. *Lancet* 1988; **i:** 1331.
4. Beghetti M, *et al.* Hypersensitivity myocarditis caused by an allergic reaction to cefaclor. *J Pediatr* 1998; **132:** 172–3.

The UK manufacturer recommends that prothrombin time should be monitored in patients receiving cefaclor and warfarin following rare reports of increased prothrombin times. It is not known whether this interaction is related to the vitamin K-related hypoprothrombinaemia observed with some cephalosporins (see Cephamandole, p.180), but cefaclor does not contain the side chain usually implicated in this reaction.

Interactions

As for Cephalexin, p.178.

Antimicrobial Action

Cefaclor is bactericidal and has antimicrobial activity similar to that of cephalexin (p.178) but is reported to be more active against Gram-negative bacteria including *Escherichia coli, Klebsiella pneumoniae, Neisseria gonorrhoeae,* and *Proteus mirabilis,* and especially against *Haemophilus influenzae*. It is active against some beta-lactamase-producing strains of *H. influenzae*. It may be less resistant to staphylococcal penicillinase than cephalexin or cephradine and a marked inoculum effect has been reported *in vitro*.

Pharmacokinetics

Cefaclor is well absorbed from the gastro-intestinal tract but plasma concentrations are slightly lower than those achieved with cephalexin or cephradine. Doses of 250, 500, and 1000 mg by mouth produce peak plasma concentrations of about 6, 13, and 23 μg per mL respectively at 0.5 to 1 hour. The presence of food may delay the absorption of cefaclor, but the total amount absorbed is unchanged. A plasma half-life of 0.5 to 1 hour has been reported; it may be slightly prolonged in patients with renal impairment. About 25% is bound to plasma proteins.

Cefaclor appears to be widely distributed in the body; it crosses the placenta and low concentrations have been detected in breast milk. It is rapidly excreted by the kidneys; up to 85% of a dose appears unchanged in the urine within 8 hours, the greater part within 2 hours. High concentrations of cefaclor are achieved in the urine within 8 hours of a dose; peak concentrations of 600, 900, and 1900 μg per mL have been reported after doses of 250, 500, and 1000 mg respectively. Probenecid delays excretion. Some cefaclor is removed by haemodialysis.

References.

1. Wise R. The pharmacokinetics of the oral cephalosporins—a review. *J Antimicrob Chemother* 1990; **26** (suppl E): 13–20.

Uses and Administration

Cefaclor is a cephalosporin antibiotic administered by mouth similarly to cephalexin in the treatment of susceptible infections including upper and lower respiratory-tract infections, skin infections, and urinary-tract infections. Some classify cefaclor as a second-generation cephalosporin and its greater activity against *Haemophilus influenzae* makes it more suitable than cephalexin for the treatment of infections such as otitis media. For details of these infections and their treatment, see under Choice of Antibacterial, p.116.

Cefaclor is given as the monohydrate. Doses are expressed in terms of the equivalent amount of anhydrous cefaclor. The usual adult dose is 250 to 500 mg every 8 hours; up to 4 g daily has been given. A suggested dose for children over 1 month of age is 20 mg per kg body-weight daily in three divided doses, increased if necessary to 40 mg per kg daily, but not exceeding a total daily dose of 1 g. A common dosage regimen is: children over 5 years, 250 mg three times daily; 1 to 5 years, 125 mg three times daily; under 1 year, 62.5 mg three times daily.

Preparations

USP 23: Cefaclor Capsules; Cefaclor for Oral Suspension.

Proprietary Preparations (details are given in Part 3)
Aust.: Ceclor; ***Austral.:*** Ceclor; Keflor; ***Belg.:*** Ceclor; ***Canad.:*** Ceclor; ***Fr.:*** Alfatil; ***Ger.:*** Cec; Ceclorbeta; Cef-Diolan; Cefa-Wolff; Cefabiocin†; Cefallone; Infectocef; Panoral; Sigacefal; ***Irl.:*** Distaclor; ***Ital.:*** Panacef; ***Neth.:*** Ceclor; ***S.Afr.:*** Cec; Ceclor; Kloclor; Vercef; ***Spain:*** Ceclor; ***Swed.:*** Kefolor; ***Switz.:*** Ceclor; ***UK:*** Distaclor; Keftid; ***USA:*** Ceclor.

Multi-ingredient: ***Ger.:*** Muco Panoral.

Cefadroxil (28-m)

Cefadroxil *(BAN, USAN, pINN).*

BL-S578; Cefadroxilum; Cephadroxil; MJF-11567-3. (7*R*)-7-(α-D-4-Hydroxyphenylglycylamino)-3-methyl-3-cephem-4-carboxylic acid monohydrate.

$C_{16}H_{17}N_3O_5S,H_2O$ = 381.4.

CAS — 50370-12-2 (anhydrous cefadroxil); 119922-85-9 (cefadroxil hemihydrate); 66592-87-8 (cefadroxil monohydrate).

Pharmacopoeias. In *Chin., Eur.* (see p.viii), and *US. Jpn* includes the anhydrous substance.

A white to off-white crystalline powder. Slightly **soluble** in water; practically insoluble or very slightly soluble in alcohol; practically insoluble in chloroform and in ether. A 5% suspension in water has a pH of 4 to 6. **Store** in airtight containers at a temperature not exceeding 30°. Protect from light.

Adverse Effects and Precautions

As for Cephalexin, p.178.

Interactions

As for Cephalexin, p.178.

Antimicrobial Action

As for Cephalexin, p.178.

Pharmacokinetics

Cefadroxil is well absorbed from the gastro-intestinal tract. After doses of 500 mg and 1 g by mouth, peak plasma concentrations of about 16 and 30 μg per mL respectively are obtained after 1.5 to 2 hours. Although peak concentrations are similar to those of cephalexin, plasma concentrations are more sustained. Administration with food does not appear to affect the absorption of cefadroxil. About 20% of cefadroxil in the circulation is reported to be bound to plasma proteins. The plasma half-life of cefadroxil is about 1.5 hours and is prolonged in patients with impaired renal function.

Cefadroxil is widely distributed to body tissues and fluids. It crosses the placenta and appears in breast milk.

More than 90% of a dose of cefadroxil may be excreted unchanged in the urine within 24 hours by glomerular filtration and tubular secretion; peak urinary concentrations of greater than 1 mg per mL have been reported after a dose of 500 mg. Cefadroxil is removed by haemodialysis.

References.

1. Tanrisever B, Santella PJ. Cefadroxil: a review of its antibacterial, pharmacokinetic and therapeutic properties in comparison with cephalexin and cephradine. *Drugs* 1986; **32** (suppl 3): 1–16.
2. Wise R. The pharmacokinetics of the oral cephalosporins—a review. *J Antimicrob Chemother* 1990; **26** (suppl E): 13–20.
3. Garrigues TM, *et al.* Dose-dependent absorption and elimination of cefadroxil in man. *Eur J Clin Pharmacol* 1991; **41**: 179–83.

Uses and Administration

Cefadroxil is a first-generation cephalosporin antibiotic that is the para-hydroxy derivative of cephalexin (p.178), and is used similarly in the treatment of mild to moderate susceptible infections. It is administered by mouth, and doses are expressed in terms of the anhydrous substance. Usually, 1 to 2 g is given daily as a single dose or in 2 divided doses. The following doses have been suggested for children: 500 mg twice daily for those over 6 years of age, 250 mg twice daily for children aged 1 to 6 years, and 25 mg per kg body-weight daily in divided doses for infants under 1 year.

Doses should be reduced in patients with impaired renal function.

Preparations

USP 23: Cefadroxil Capsules; Cefadroxil for Oral Suspension; Cefadroxil Tablets.

Proprietary Preparations (details are given in Part 3)
Aust.: Biodroxil; Duracef; ***Belg.:*** Duracef; Moxacef; ***Canad.:*** Duricef; ***Fr.:*** Oracefal; ***Ger.:*** Bidocef; Cedrox; Gruncef; ***Irl.:*** Ultracef; ***Ital.:*** Cefadril; Ceoxil; Cephos; Crenodyn; Droxicef†; Ibidroxil†; Kefroxil†; Oradroxil; ***Jpn:*** Sedral; ***Neth.:*** Moxacef†; ***S.Afr.:*** Cefadrox; Cipadur; Dacef; Duracef; ***Spain:*** Cefroxil†; Duracef; ***Swed.:*** Cefamox; ***Switz.:*** Duracef; ***UK:*** Baxan; ***USA:*** Duricef; Ultracef†.

Cefapirin Sodium (29-b)

Cefapirin Sodium *(BANM, pINNM).*

BL-P-1322; Cephapirin Sodium *(USAN).* Sodium (7*R*)-7-[2-(4-pyridylthio)acetamido]cephalosporanate; Sodium (7*R*)-3-acetoxymethyl-7-[2-(4-pyridylthio)acetamido]-3-cephem-4-carboxylate.

$C_{17}H_{16}N_3NaO_6S_2$ = 445.4.

CAS — 21593-23-7 (cefapirin); 24356-60-3 (cefapirin sodium).

Pharmacopoeias. In *It., Jpn,* and *US.*

US also includes Cephapirin Benzathine for veterinary use.

A white to off-white crystalline powder. 1.05 g of monograph substance is approximately equivalent to 1 g of cefapirin. Each g of monograph substance represents about 2.2 mmol of sodium. Very **soluble** in water; practically insoluble in most organic solvents. A 1% solution in water has a pH of 6.5 to 8.5. **Store** in airtight containers.

Cefapirin is a first-generation cephalosporin antibiotic with actions and uses very similar to those of cephalothin (p.179). It is used as the sodium salt and the usual adult dose is the equivalent of 0.5 to 1 g of cefapirin every 4 to 6 hours by intramuscular injection or intravenously. In severe infections up to 12 g daily may be given, preferably intravenously.

Reduced doses may be necessary in patients with impaired renal function.

Preparations

USP 23: Cephapirin for Injection.

Proprietary Preparations (details are given in Part 3)
Fr.: Cefaloject; ***Ital.:*** Piricef†; ***Spain:*** Brisfirina; ***USA:*** Cefadyl†.

Multi-ingredient: ***Spain:*** Brisfirina Balsamica.

Cefatrizine (30-x)

Cefatrizine *(BAN, USAN, pINN).*

BL-S640; SKF-60771; S-640P. (7*R*)-7-(α-D-4-Hydroxyphenylglycylamino)-3-(1*H*-1,2,3-triazol-4-ylthiomethyl)-3-cephem-4-carboxylic acid.

$C_{18}H_{18}N_6O_5S_2$ = 462.5.

CAS — 51627-14-6.

Pharmacopoeias. *Jpn* includes Propylene Glycol Cefatrizine.

Cefatrizine is a cephalosporin antibiotic with actions and uses similar to those of cephalexin (p.178), although it might be more active *in vitro*. It is given by mouth, as a compound with propylene glycol, in usual doses equivalent to 500 mg twice daily of cefatrizine.

Preparations

Proprietary Preparations (details are given in Part 3)
Belg.: Cefaperos; ***Fr.:*** Cefaperos; ***Ital.:*** Biotrixina; Cefatrix; Cefotrizin; Cetrazil; Cetrinox; Faretrizin; Ipatrizina; Kefoxina; Ketrizin; Lampotrix†; Latocef; Miracef; Novacef; Orotrix; Tamyl; Tricef; Trixidine; Trixilan; Trizina; Zanitrin†; Zinaf; Zitrix; ***Jpn:*** Cepticol.

Cefazedone Sodium (15311-c)

Cefazedone Sodium *(BANM, rINNM).*

EMD-30087. Sodium (7*R*)-7-[2-(3,5-dichloro-4-oxo-1-pyridyl)acetamido]-3-(5-methyl-1,3,4-thiadiazol-2-ylthiomethyl)-3-cephem-4-carboxylate.

$C_{18}H_{14}Cl_2N_5NaO_5S_3$ = 570.4.

CAS — 56187-47-4 (cefazedone); 63521-15-3 (cefazedone sodium).

1.1 g of monograph substance is approximately equivalent to 1 g of cefazedone. Each g of monograph substance represents about 1.75 mmol of sodium.

Cefazedone is a cephalosporin antibiotic. It has been administered intravenously as the sodium salt in a dose of up to the equivalent of cefazedone 6 g daily in two or three divided doses.

Preparations

Proprietary Preparations (details are given in Part 3)
Ger.: Refosporin†.

Cefbuperazone Sodium (16565-d)

Cefbuperazone Sodium *(rINNM).*

BMY-25182; T-1982 (both cefbuperazone). Sodium 7-[(2*R*,3*S*)-2-(4-ethyl-2,3-dioxopiperazin-1-ylcarboxamido)-3-hydroxybutyramido]-7-methoxy-3-(1-methyl-1*H*-tetrazol-5-ylthiomethyl)-3-cephem-4-carboxylate.

$C_{22}H_{28}N_9NaO_9S_2$ = 649.6.

CAS — 76610-84-9 (cefbuperazone).

NOTE. Cefbuperazone is *USAN.*

Pharmacopoeias. In *Jpn.*

Cefbuperazone is a cephamycin antibiotic similar to cefoxitin (p.170) and is given by injection as the sodium salt. Its spectrum of activity includes Enterobacteriaceae, but more especially anaerobic bacteria such as *Bacteroides fragilis*. Cefbuperazone does not appear to be active against cefoxitin-resistant strains of *B. fragilis*.

Cefbuperazone has an *N*-methylthiotetrazole side-chain. For adverse effects and drug interactions associated with the presence of this side-chain, see under Cephamandole, p.180.

References.

1. Prabhala RH, *et al.* In vitro activity of cefbuperazone, a new cephamycin, against anaerobic bacteria. *Antimicrob Agents Chemother* 1985; **27**: 640–2.
2. Wexler H, *et al.* In vitro activity of cefbuperazone against anaerobic bacteria. *Antimicrob Agents Chemother* 1985; **27**: 674–6.
3. Del Bene VE, *et al.* In vitro activity of cefbuperazone compared with that of other new β-lactam agents against anaerobic Gram-negative bacilli and contribution of β-lactamase to resistance. *Antimicrob Agents Chemother* 1985; **27**: 817–20.
4. Dias MBS, *et al.* In vitro activity of cefbuperazone against Bacteroides spp. *Antimicrob Agents Chemother* 1985; **27**: 968–70.
5. Tanaka H, *et al.* Biliary penetration of cefbuperazone in the presence and absence of obstructive jaundice. *J Antimicrob Chemother* 1987; **20**: 417–20.

Cefcanel Daloxate (6465-m)

Cefcanel Daloxate *(rINN).*

2,3-Dihydroxy-2-butenyl (6*R*,7*R*)-7-[(*R*)-mandelamido]-3-{[(5-methyl-1,3,4-thiadiazol-2-yl)thio]methyl}-8-oxo-5-thia-1-azabicyclo[4.2.0]oct-2-ene-2-carboxylate, cyclic 2,3-carbonate, ester with L-alanine.

$C_{19}H_{18}N_4O_5S_3.C_8H_9NO_4$ = 661.7.

CAS — 41952-52-7 (cefcanel); 97275-40-6 (cefcanel daloxate).

Cefcanel is a cephalosporin antibiotic that has been investigated by mouth as the daloxate.

References.

1. Chin NX, *et al.* In vitro activity of cefcanel versus other oral cephalosporins. *Eur J Clin Microbiol Infect Dis* 1991; **10**: 676–82.
2. Nicolle LE, *et al.* Comparison of three days' therapy with cefcanel or amoxicillin for the treatment of acute uncomplicated urinary tract infection. *Scand J Infect Dis* 1993; **25**: 631–7.
3. Edwall B, *et al.* Pharmacokinetics of oral cefcanel daloxate hydrochloride in healthy volunteers and patients with various degrees of impaired renal function. *J Antimicrob Chemother* 1994; **33**: 281–8.
4. Köhler W, Schenk P. Cephalosporinbehandlung der sinusitis maxillaris. *Laryngorhinootologie* 1995; **74**: 355–60.

Cefcapene (17075-y)

Cefcapene *(rINN).*

(6*R*,7*R*)-7-[(*Z*)-2-(2-Amino-4-thiazolyl)-2-pentenamido]-3-(hydroxymethyl)-8-oxo-5-thia-1-azabicyclo[4.2.0]oct-2-ene-2-carboxylic acid carbamate.

$C_{17}H_{19}N_5O_6S_2$ = 453.5.

CAS — 135889-00-8.

Cefcapene is an oral cephalosporin antibacterial under investigation as the pivaloyloxymethyl ester, cefcapene pivoxil.

Cefdinir (10948-y)

Cefdinir *(BAN, USAN, rINN).*

CI-983; FK-482. (−)-(6*R*,7*R*)-7-[2-(2-Amino-4-thiazolyl)glyoxylamido]-8-oxo-3-vinyl-5-thia-1-azabicyclo[4.2.0]oct-2-ene-2-carboxylic acid, 7^2-(*Z*)-oxime; 7-{(2-Amino-1,3-thiazol-4-yl)-2-[(*Z*)-hydroxyimino]acetamido}-3-vinylcephem-4-carboxylic acid.

$C_{14}H_{13}N_5O_5S_2$ = 395.4.

CAS — 91832-40-5.

Cefdinir is a third-generation oral cephalosporin antibiotic similar to cefixime (p.165). It is reported to be much more active *in vitro* than cefixime against *Staphylococcus aureus* and *Enterococcus faecalis*, but is less active against some Enterobacteriaceae. It is given by mouth in a usual dose of 600 mg daily as a single dose or in two divided doses. Children may be given 14 mg per kg body-weight daily up to a maximum of 600 mg. Doses should be reduced in patients with renal impairment (with a creatinine clearance of less than 30 mL per minute) to 300 mg once daily.

References.

1. Neu HC, *et al.* Comparative in vitro activity and β-lactamase stability of FK-482, a new oral cephalosporin. *Antimicrob Agents Chemother* 1989; **33**: 1795–1800.
2. Wise R, *et al.* The in-vitro activity of cefdinir (FK-482), a new oral cephalosporin. *J Antimicrob Chemother* 1991; **28**: 239–48.
3. Perea EJ, Iglesias MCG. Comparative in-vitro activity of cefdinir against multiresistant Haemophilus influenzae. *J Antimicrob Chemother* 1994; **34**: 161–4.
4. Marchese A, *et al.* Antistaphylococcal activity of cefdinir, a new oral third-generation cephalosporin, alone and in combination with other antibiotics, at supra- and sub-MIC levels. *J Antimicrob Chemother* 1995; **35**: 53–66.
5. Cook PJ, *et al.* Distribution of cefdinir, a third generation cephalosporin antibiotic, in serum and pulmonary compartments. *J Antimicrob Chemother* 1996; **37**: 331–9.

Preparations

Proprietary Preparations (details are given in Part 3)
Jpn: Cefzon; ***USA:*** Omnicef.

Cefditoren (15883-g)

Cefditoren *(rINN).*

(+)-(6*R*,7*R*)-7-[2-(2-Amino-4-thiazolyl)glyoxylamido]-3-[(*Z*)-2-(4-methyl-5-thiazolyl)vinyl]-8-oxo-5-thia-1-azabicyclo[4.2.0]oct-2-ene-2-carboxylic acid 7^2-(*Z*)-(*O*-methyloxime).

$C_{19}H_{18}N_6O_5S_3$ = 506.6.

CAS — 104145-95-1.

Cefditoren is a cephalosporin antibiotic with a broad spectrum of activity. It is given by mouth as the pivaloyloxymethyl ester, cefditoren pivoxil.

For reference to carnitine deficiency occurring after the administration of some pivaloyloxymethyl esters, see Pivampicillin, p.238.

Preparations

Proprietary Preparations (details are given in Part 3)
Jpn: Meiact.

Cefepime Hydrochloride (17329-t)

Cefepime Hydrochloride *(BANM, USAN, rINNM).*

BMY-28142 (cefepime). {6R-[6α,7β(Z)]}-1-[(7-{[(2-Amino-4-thiazolyl)-(methoxyimino)acetyl]amino}-2-carboxy-8-oxo-5-thia-1-azabicyclo[4.2.0]oct-2-en-3-yl)methyl]-1-methylpyrrolidinium chloride monohydrochloride monohydrate; 7-{(2-Amino-1,3-thiazol-4-yl)-2-[(Z)-methoxyimino]acetamido}-3-(1-methylpyrrolidiniomethyl)-3-cephem-4-carboxylate hydrochloride.

$C_{19}H_{25}ClN_6O_5S_2,HCl,H_2O = 571.5.$

CAS — 88040-23-7 (cefepime); 123171-59-5 (cefepime hydrochloride monohydrate).

Adverse Effects and Precautions

As for Cephalothin Sodium, p.179.

References.

1. Neu HC. Safety of cefepime: a new extended-spectrum parenteral cephalosporin. *Am J Med* 1996; **100** (suppl 6A): 68S–75S.

Antimicrobial Action

Cefepime is a fourth-generation cephalosporin antibiotic and is active against a wide range of Gram-positive and Gram-negative aerobic organisms. Against Gram-positive cocci, its activity is similar to that of cefotaxime (p.168) and includes staphylococci (but not methicillin-resistant *Staphylococcus aureus*) and streptococci. Against Enterobacteriaceae, it has a broader spectrum of activity than other cephalosporins, including activity against organisms producing chromosomally mediated beta-lactamases such as *Enterobacter* spp. and *Proteus vulgaris*. Against *Pseudomonas aeruginosa*, it has similar or slightly less activity than ceftazidime (p.174), although it may be active against some strains resistant to ceftazidime.

References.

1. Neu HC, *et al.* The activity of BMY 28142, a new broad spectrum β-lactamase stable cephalosporin. *J Antimicrob Chemother* 1986; **17:** 441–52.
2. Watanabe N, *et al.* Comparative in-vitro activities of newer cephalosporins cefclidin, cefepime, and cefpirome against ceftazidime- or imipenem-resistant Pseudomonas aeruginosa. *J Antimicrob Chemother* 1992; **30:** 633–41.
3. Thornsberry C, *et al.* In-vitro activity of cefepime and other antimicrobials: survey of European isolates. *J Antimicrob Chemother* 1993; **32** (suppl B): 31–53.
4. Kessler RE, Fung-Tomc J. Susceptibility of bacterial isolates to β-lactam antibiotics from US clinical trials over a 5-year period. *Am J Med* 1996; **100** (suppl 6A): 13S–19S.
5. Palmer SM, *et al.* Bactericidal killing activities of cefepime, ceftazidime, cefotaxime, and ceftriaxone against Staphylococcus aureus and β-lactamase-producing strains of Enterobacter aerogenes and Klebsiella pneumoniae in an in vitro infection model. *Antimicrob Agents Chemother* 1995; **39:** 1764–71.

Pharmacokinetics

Cefepime is administered by injection as the hydrochloride. It is rapidly and almost completely absorbed following intramuscular injection and mean peak plasma concentrations of about 14 and 30 μg per mL have been reported about 1.5 hours after doses of 0.5 and 1.0 g respectively. Within 30 minutes of intravenous administration of similar doses, peak plasma concentrations of about 40 and 80 μg per mL are achieved. The plasma half-life of cefepime is approximately 2 hours and is prolonged in patients with renal impairment. About 20% of cefepime is bound to plasma proteins.

Cefepime is widely distributed in body tissues and fluids. High concentrations are achieved in bile. Low concentrations have been detected in breast milk.

Cefepime is eliminated principally by the kidneys and about 85% of a dose is recovered unchanged in the urine. Cefepime is substantially removed by haemodialysis.

References.

1. Okamoto MP, *et al.* Cefepime clinical pharmacokinetics. *Clin Pharmacokinet* 1993; **25:** 88–102.
2. Rybak M. The pharmacokinetic profile of a new generation of parenteral cephalosporin. *Am J Med* 1996; **100** (suppl 6A): 39S–44S.
3. Reed MD, *et al.* Pharmacokinetics of intravenously and intramuscularly administered cefepime in infants and children. *Antimicrob Agents Chemother* 1997; **41:** 1783–7.

Uses and Administration

Cefepime is a fourth-generation cephalosporin antibiotic used in the treatment of infections due to susceptible organisms. They include infections of the urinary tract, respiratory tract, and skin. For details of these infections and their treatment, see under Choice of Antibacterial, p.116.

Cefepime is given as the hydrochloride by deep intramuscular injection, or intravenously by slow injection over 3 to 5 minutes or by infusion over at least 30 minutes. Doses are expressed in terms of the equivalent amount of cefepime. The usual dose is 1 to 2 g daily in two divided doses for mild to moderate infections, increased to 4 g daily in severe infections, although up to 6 g daily in three divided doses has been given.

Dosage should be reduced in renal impairment. The manufacturers recommend a normal initial loading dose followed by suitable maintenance doses according to creatinine clearance and the severity of the infection: creatinine clearance 30 to 60 mL per minute, 0.5 to 2 g every 24 hours; 11 to 29 mL per minute, 0.5 to 1 g every 24 hours; and 10 mL per minute or less, 0.25 to 0.5 g every 24 hours. Patients undergoing haemodialysis should be given a repeat dose after each dialysis session, while those undergoing continuous ambulatory peritoneal dialysis should receive normal recommended doses at intervals of 48 hours.

Reviews.

1. Various. Cefepime: a β-lactamase-stable extended-spectrum cephalosporin. *J Antimicrob Chemother* 1993; **32** (suppl B): 1–214.
2. Barradell LB, Bryson HM. Cefepime: a review of its antibacterial activity, pharmacokinetic properties and therapeutic use. *Drugs* 1994; **47:** 471–505.
3. Okamoto MP, *et al.* Cefepime: a new fourth-generation cephalosporin. *Am J Hosp Pharm* 1994; **51:** 463–77.
4. Wynd MA, Paladins JA. Cefepime: a fourth-generation parenteral cephalosporin. *Ann Pharmacother* 1996; **30:** 1414–24.

Preparations

Proprietary Preparations (details are given in Part 3)
Aust.: Maxipime; ***Austral.:*** Maxipime; ***Belg.:*** Maxipime; ***Canad.:*** Maxipime; ***Fr.:*** Axepim; ***Ger.:*** Maxipime; ***Ital.:*** Cepim; Cepimex; Maxipime; ***Neth.:*** Maxipime; ***S.Afr.:*** Maxipime; ***Spain:*** Maxipime; ***Swed.:*** Maxipime; ***Switz.:*** Maxipime; ***USA:*** Maxipime.

Cefetamet (3412-l)

Cefetamet *(USAN, rINN).*

LY-097964; Ro-15-8074; Ro-15-8075 (cefetamet pivoxil). (Z)-7-[2-(2-Aminothiazol-4-yl)-2-methoxyiminoacetamido]-3-methyl-3-cephem-4-carboxylic acid.

$C_{14}H_{15}N_5O_5S_2 = 397.4.$

CAS — 65052-63-3 (cefetamet); 65243-33-6 (cefetamet pivoxil).

Cefetamet is a third-generation cephalosporin antibiotic similar to cefixime (below). It is given by mouth as the hydrochloride of the pivaloyloxymethyl ester, cefetamet pivoxil hydrochloride, which is hydrolysed to cefetamet *in vivo*. The usual dose is 500 mg twice daily.

For reference to carnitine deficiency occurring after the administration of some pivaloyloxymethyl esters, see Pivampicillin, p.238.

Reviews.

1. Bryson HM, Brogden RN. Cefetamet pivoxil: a review of its antibacterial activity, pharmacokinetic properties and therapeutic use. *Drugs* 1993; **45:** 589–621.
2. Blouin RA, Stoeckel K. Cefetamet pivoxil clinical pharmacokinetics. *Clin Pharmacokinet* 1993; **25:** 172–88.

Preparations

Proprietary Preparations (details are given in Part 3)
Aust.: Globocef; ***Ger.:*** Globocef; ***Ital.:*** Globocef; ***Switz.:*** Globocef.

Cefixime (12006-g)

Cefixime *(BAN, USAN, rINN).*

Cefiximum; CL-284635; FK-027; FR-17027. (Z)-7-[2-(2-Aminothiazol-4-yl)-2-(carboxymethoxyimino)acetamido]-3-vinyl-3-cephem-4-carboxylic acid trihydrate.

$C_{16}H_{15}N_5O_7S_2,3H_2O = 507.5.$

CAS — 79350-37-1.

Pharmacopoeias. In *Eur.* (see p.viii) and *US.*

A white or almost white to light yellow, slightly hygroscopic, crystalline powder. 1.12 g of monograph substance is approximately equivalent to 1 g of anhydrous cefixime. Slightly **soluble** to practically insoluble in water; slightly soluble in alcohol; sparingly soluble in dehydrated alcohol; freely soluble in methyl alcohol; soluble in glycerol and in propylene glycol; sparingly soluble in acetone; very slightly soluble in 70% sorbitol and in octanol; practically insoluble in ether, in ethyl acetate, and in hexane. A 5% suspension in water has a pH of 2.6 to 4.1. **Store** at a temperature not exceeding 30° in airtight containers. Protect from light.

Adverse Effects and Precautions

As for Cephalothin Sodium, p.179.

The most frequently reported adverse effects of cefixime are gastro-intestinal disturbances, especially diarrhoea. Cefixime should be discontinued if diarrhoea is severe.

Although cefixime does not have the *N*-methylthiotetrazole side chain usually associated with hypoprothrombinaemia (see Cephamandole, p.180), increases in prothrombin times have occurred in a few patients.

Antibiotic-associated colitis. For reports of diarrhoea and pseudomembranous colitis associated with cefixime, see Cephalothin, p.179.

Interactions

Care should be exercised in patients receiving anticoagulants and cefixime concomitantly due to the possibility that cefixime may increase prothrombin times (see above).

Antimicrobial Action

Cefixime is a bactericidal antibiotic and is stable to hydrolysis by many beta-lactamases. It has a mode of action and spectrum of activity similar to that of the third-generation cephalosporin cefotaxime (p.168), but some Enterobacteriaceae are less susceptible to cefixime. *Haemophilus influenzae*, *Moraxella (Branhamella) catarrhalis*, and *Neisseria gonorrhoeae* are sensitive, including penicillinase-producing strains. Of the Gram-positive bacteria, streptococci are sensitive to cefixime but staphylococci, enterococci, and *Listeria* spp. are not.

Enterobacter spp., *Pseudomonas aeruginosa*, and *Bacteroides* spp. are resistant to cefixime.

References.

1. Barry AL, Jones RN. Cefixime: spectrum of antibacterial activity against 16 016 clinical isolates. *Pediatr Infect Dis J* 1987; **6:** 954–7.
2. Neu HC. In vitro activity of a new broad spectrum, beta-lactamase-stable oral cephalosporin, cefixime. *Pediatr Infect Dis J* 1987; **6:** 958–62.
3. Stone JW, *et al.* Cefixime, in-vitro activity, pharmacokinetics and tissue penetration. *J Antimicrob Chemother* 1989; **23:** 221–8.

Pharmacokinetics

Only 40 to 50% of an oral dose of cefixime is absorbed from the gastro-intestinal tract, whether taken before or after meals, although the rate of absorption may be decreased in the presence of food. Cefixime is better absorbed from oral suspension than from tablets. Absorption is fairly slow. Peak plasma concentrations of 2 to 3 μg per mL and 3.7 to 4.6 μg per mL have been reported between 2 and 6 hours after single doses of 200 and 400 mg, respectively. The plasma half-life is usually about 3 to 4 hours and may be prolonged when there is renal impairment. About 65% of cefixime in the circulation is bound to plasma proteins.

Information on the distribution of cefixime in body tissues and fluids is limited. It crosses the placenta.

Relatively high concentrations may be achieved in bile and urine. About 20% of an oral dose (or 50% of an absorbed dose) is excreted unchanged in the urine within 24 hours. Up to 60% may be eliminated by nonrenal mechanisms; there is no evidence of metabolism but some is probably excreted into the faeces from bile. It is not substantially removed by dialysis.

References.

1. Brittain DC, *et al.* The pharmacokinetic and bactericidal characteristics of oral cefixime. *Clin Pharmacol Ther* 1985; **38:** 590–4.
2. Guay DRP, *et al.* Pharmacokinetics of cefixime (CL-284,635; FK027) in healthy subjects and patients with renal insufficiency. *Antimicrob Agents Chemother* 1986; **30:** 485–90.
3. Faulkner RD, *et al.* Pharmacokinetics of cefixime in the young and elderly. *J Antimicrob Chemother* 1988; **21:** 787–94.
4. Stone JW, *et al.* Cefixime, in-vitro activity, pharmacokinetics and tissue penetration. *J Antimicrob Chemother* 1989; **23:** 221–8.
5. Westphal JF, *et al.* Biliary excretion of cefixime: assessment in patients provided with T-tube drainage. *Antimicrob Agents Chemother* 1993; **37:** 1488–91.
6. Somekh E, *et al.* Penetration and bactericidal activity of cefixime in synovial fluid. *Antimicrob Agents Chemother* 1996; **40:** 1198–1200.

Uses and Administration

Cefixime is generally classified as a third-generation cephalosporin antibiotic and is given by mouth in the treatment of susceptible infections, (see Antimicrobial Action, above), including gonorrhoea, otitis media, pharyngitis, lower respiratory-tract infections such as bronchitis, and urinary-tract infections. For details of these infections and their treatment, see under Choice of Antibacterial, p.116.

Cefixime is available as the trihydrate and doses are expressed in terms of anhydrous cefixime. It is given by mouth in adult doses of 200 to 400 mg daily as a single dose or in two divided doses. Children under 50 kg body-weight may be given 8 mg per kg daily as an oral suspension, again as a single dose or in two divided doses.

Doses should be reduced in patients with moderate to severe renal impairment. A dose of 200 mg daily should not be exceeded in patients with a creatinine clearance of less than 20 mL per minute.

For uncomplicated gonorrhoea, a single oral dose of 400 mg is given.

General references.

1. Brogden RN, Campoli-Richards DM. Cefixime: a review of its antibacterial activity, pharmacokinetic properties and therapeutic potential. *Drugs* 1989; **38:** 524–50.
2. Leggett NJ, *et al.* Cefixime. *DICP Ann Pharmacother* 1990; **24:** 489–95.
3. Adam D, Wallace RJ, eds. Symposium on cefixime. *Drugs* 1991; **42** (suppl 4): 1–32.
4. Markham A, Brogden RN. Cefixime: a review of its therapeutic efficacy in lower respiratory tract infections. *Drugs* 1995; **49:** 1007–22.

Preparations

USP 23: Cefixime for Oral Suspension; Cefixime Tablets.

Proprietary Preparations (details are given in Part 3)
Aust.: Aerocef; Tricef; ***Canad.:*** Suprax; ***Fr.:*** Oroken; ***Ger.:*** Cephoral; Suprax; Uro-Cephoral; ***Irl.:*** Suprax; ***Ital.:*** Cefixoral; Suprax; Unixime; ***Jpn:*** Cefspan; ***Neth.:*** Fixim; ***S.Afr.:*** Fixime; ***Spain:*** Denvar; Necopen; ***Swed.:*** Tricef; ***Switz.:*** Cephoral; ***UK:*** Suprax; ***USA:*** Suprax.

Cefluprenam (17616-m)

Cefluprenam *(rINN)*.

(−)-{(*E*)-3-[(6*R*,7*R*)-7-[2-(5-Amino-1,2,4-thiadiazol-3-yl)glyoxylamido]-2-carboxy-8-oxo-5-thia-1-azabicyclo[4.2.0]oct-2-en-3-yl]allyl}(carbamoylmethyl)ethylmethylammonium hydroxide, inner salt, 7[2]-(*Z*)-[*O*-(fluoromethyl)oxime].

$C_{20}H_{25}FN_8O_6S_2$ = 556.6.

CAS — 116853-25-9.

Cefluprenam is a cephalosporin antibacterial. It has been tried in the treatment of susceptible infections.

Cefmenoxime Hydrochloride (15312-k)

Cefmenoxime Hydrochloride *(USAN, rINNM)*.

Abbott-50192; Cefmenoxime Hemihydrochloride; SCE-1365 (cefmenoxime). (*Z*)-(7*R*)-7-[2-(2-Aminothiazol-4-yl)-2-methoxyiminoacetamido]-3-[(1-methyl-1*H*-tetrazol-5-yl)thiomethyl]-3-cephem-4-carboxylic acid hydrochloride.

$(C_{16}H_{17}N_9O_5S_3)_2$,HCl = 1059.6.

CAS — 65085-01-0 (cefmenoxime); 75738-58-8 (cefmenoxime hydrochloride).

Pharmacopoeias. In *Jpn* and *US*.

White to light orange-yellow crystals or crystalline powder. Very slightly **soluble** in water; freely soluble in formamide; slightly soluble in methyl alcohol; practically insoluble in dehydrated alcohol and in ether. **Store** in airtight containers.

Cefmenoxime is a third-generation cephalosporin antibiotic with actions and uses similar to those of cefotaxime (p.168). It is administered as the hydrochloride by intramuscular injection, or intravenously by injection or infusion in the treatment of susceptible infections. Doses are expressed in terms of the equivalent amount of cefmenoxime. The usual dose is 1 to 4 g daily in 2 to 4 divided doses, although up to 9 g daily has been given in severe infections. Children have been given 40 to 80 mg per kg body-weight daily in 2 to 4 divided doses; higher doses have been used in severe infections. Neonates have been given 40 to 60 mg per kg in 2 or 3 divided doses.

Like cephamandole (p.180), cefmenoxime has an *N*-methylthiotetrazole side-chain and coagulopathy and a disulfiram-like interaction with alcohol have been reported rarely.

References.

1. Campoli-Richards DM, Todd PA. Cefmenoxime: a review of its antibacterial activity, pharmacokinetic properties and therapeutic use. *Drugs* 1987; **34:** 188–221.
2. Evers J, *et al.* Elimination of cefmenoxime during continuous haemofiltration. *Eur J Clin Pharmacol* 1993; **44** (suppl 1): S31–S32.

Preparations

USP 23: Cefmenoxime for Injection.

Proprietary Preparations (details are given in Part 3)
Aust.: Tacef; ***Ger.:*** Tacef; ***Jpn:*** Bestcall.

Cefmetazole (17134-p)

Cefmetazole *(USAN, rINN)*.

U-72791. (6*R*,7*S*)-7-{2-[(Cyanomethyl)thio]acetamido}-7-methoxy-3-{[(1-methyl-1*H*-tetrazol-5-yl)thio]methyl}-8-oxo-5-thia-1-azabicyclo-[4.2.0]oct-2-ene-2-carboxylic acid.

$C_{15}H_{17}N_7O_5S_3$ = 471.5.

CAS — 56796-20-4.

Pharmacopoeias. In *US*.

Cefmetazole Sodium (12540-v)

Cefmetazole Sodium *(USAN, rINNM)*.

CS-1170; SKF-83088; U-72791A.

$C_{15}H_{16}N_7NaO_5S_3$ = 493.5.

CAS — 56796-39-5.

Pharmacopoeias. In *Jpn* and *US*.

1.05 g of cefmetazole sodium is approximately equivalent to 1 g of cefmetazole. Each g of monograph substance represents about 2 mmol of sodium.

Very **soluble** in water and in methyl alcohol; soluble in acetone; practically insoluble in chloroform. A 10% solution in water has a pH of 4.2 to 6.2. **Store** in airtight containers.

Adverse Effects and Precautions

As for Cephalothin Sodium, p.179.

Cefmetazole contains an *N*-methylthiotetrazole side-chain and like cephamandole (p.180) has the potential to cause hypoprothrombinaemia and bleeding.

Effects on the blood. References.

1. Breen GA, St Peter WL. Hypoprothrombinemia associated with cefmetazole. *Ann Pharmacother* 1997; **31:** 180–3.

Interactions

As for Cephamandole, p.180.

Antimicrobial Action

Cefmetazole is a cephamycin antibiotic with a similar spectrum of antibacterial activity to that of cefoxitin (p.170), including the anaerobe *Bacteroides fragilis*.

References.

1. Cornick NA, *et al.* Activity of cefmetazole against anaerobic bacteria. *Antimicrob Agents Chemother* 1987; **31**: 2010–12.

Pharmacokinetics

Following cefmetazole 2 g intravenously every 6 hours, as the sodium salt, peak and trough plasma concentrations of 138 and 6 μg per mL have been achieved. Cefmetazole is 65 to 85% bound to plasma proteins, depending on the plasma concentration. A plasma half-life of about 1.1 to 1.5 hours has been reported; it is prolonged in patients with renal impairment. There is limited information on the distribution of cefmetazole. Small amounts have been detected in breast milk. Relatively high concentrations have been achieved in bile.

The majority of a dose is excreted unchanged in the urine resulting in high concentrations; up to 85% of a dose has been recovered within 12 hours. Cefmetazole is partly excreted by renal tubular secretion and probenecid prolongs elimination.

Cefmetazole is removed to some extent by haemodialysis.

References.

1. Ito MK, *et al.* Intraoperative serum, bile, and gallbladder-wall concentrations of cefmetazole in patients undergoing cholecystectomy. *Clin Pharm* 1988; **7:** 467–8.
2. Ko H, *et al.* Pharmacokinetics of intravenously administered cefmetazole and cefoxitin and effects of probenecid on cefmetazole elimination. *Antimicrob Agents Chemother* 1989; **33:** 356–61.
3. Ko H, *et al.* Pharmacokinetics of single-dose cefmetazole following intramuscular administration of cefmetazole sodium to healthy male volunteers. *Antimicrob Agents Chemother* 1989; **33:** 508–12.
4. Tan JS, *et al.* Pharmacokinetics of intravenous cefmetazole with emphasis on comparison between predicted theoretical levels in tissue and actual skin window fluid levels. *Antimicrob Agents Chemother* 1989; **33:** 924–7.
5. Halstenson CE, *et al.* Disposition of cefmetazole in healthy volunteers and patients with impaired renal function. *Antimicrob Agents Chemother* 1990; **34:** 519–23.
6. Borin MT, *et al.* Pharmacokinetics and dose proportionality of cefmetazole in healthy young and elderly volunteers. *Antimicrob Agents Chemother* 1990; **34:** 1944–8.

Uses and Administration

Cefmetazole is a cephamycin antibiotic generally classified with the second-generation cephalosporins and used similarly to cefoxitin (p.171) in the treatment and prophylaxis of anaerobic and mixed bacterial infections, especially intra-abdominal and pelvic infections. It may also be used in the treatment of gonorrhoea. For details of these infections and their treatment, see under Choice of Antibacterial, p.116.

It is administered intravenously as the sodium salt by infusion over 10 to 60 minutes or by slow injection over 3 to 5 minutes. Cefmetazole sodium is also administered intramuscularly in some countries. Doses are expressed in terms of the equivalent amount of cefmetazole.

The usual adult dose is 2 g intravenously every 6 to 12 hours. The interval between doses should be 12, 16, or 24 hours in patients with mild, moderate, or severe renal impairment, respectively; patients with virtually no renal function may be given cefmetazole every 48 hours, after haemodialysis.

For uncomplicated gonorrhoea the usual dose is 1 g as a single intramuscular injection, together with probenecid 1 g by mouth.

For surgical infection prophylaxis, a single dose of 1 or 2 g may be given intravenously 30 to 90 minutes before surgery and repeated if necessary after 8 and 16 hours. At caesarean section a single 2-g dose may be given intravenously to the mother after the umbilical cord is clamped; alternatively a 1-g dose may be given and repeated after 8 and 16 hours.

References.

1. Finch R, *et al.* eds. Cefmetazole: a clinical appraisal. *J Antimicrob Chemother* 1989; **23** (suppl D): 1–142.

Preparations

USP 23: Cefmetazole for Injection; Cefmetazole Injection.

Proprietary Preparations (details are given in Part 3)
Ital.: Cefadel; Decacef; Metacaf; Metafar; Metasal; Metazol; ***Jpn:*** Cefmetazon; ***Spain:*** Cemetol; ***USA:*** Zefazone.

Cefminox Sodium (18922-r)

Cefminox Sodium *(pINNM)*.

MT-141. Sodium 7-{2-[(*S*)-2-amino-2-carboxyethyl]thioacetamido}-7-methoxy-3-(1-methyl-1*H*-tetrazol-5-ylthiomethyl)-3-cephem-4-carboxylate.

$C_{16}H_{20}N_7NaO_7S_3$ = 541.6.

CAS — 75481-73-1 (cefminox).

Cefminox sodium is a cephamycin antibiotic similar to cefoxitin sodium (p.170).

Cefminox has an *N*-methylthiotetrazole side-chain. For adverse effects and drug interactions associated with the presence of this side-chain, see under Cephamandole, p.180.

References.

1. Watanabe S, Omoto S. Pharmacology of cefminox, a new bactericidal cephamycin. *Drugs Exp Clin Res* 1990; **16:** 461–7.
2. Soriano F, *et al.* Comparative susceptibility of cefminox and cefoxitin to β-lactamases of Bacteroides spp. *J Antimicrob Chemother* 1991; **28:** 55–60.
3. Aguilar L, *et al.* Cefminox: correlation between in-vitro susceptibility and pharmacokinetics and serum bactericidal activity in healthy volunteers. *J Antimicrob Chemother* 1994; **33:** 91–101.
4. Hoellman DB, *et al.* In vitro activities of cefminox against anaerobic bacteria compared with those of nine other compounds. *Antimicrob Agents Chemother* 1998; **42:** 495–501.

Preparations

Proprietary Preparations (details are given in Part 3)
Jpn: Meicelin; ***Spain:*** Alteporina; Tencef.

Cefodizime Sodium (18923-f)

Cefodizime Sodium *(BANM, rINNM)*.

HR-221; S-771221B; THR-221; TRH-221. The disodium salt of (*Z*)-7-[2-(2-Aminothiazol-4-yl)-2-methoxyiminoacetamido]-3-(5-carboxymethyl-4-methylthiazol-2-ylthiomethyl)-3-cephem-4-carboxylic acid.

$C_{20}H_{18}N_6Na_2O_7S_4$ = 628.6.

CAS — 69739-16-8 (cefodizime); 86329-79-5 (cefodizime sodium).

1.08 g of monograph substance is approximately equivalent to 1 g of cefodizime. Each g of monograph substance represents about 3.2 mmol of sodium.

Adverse Effects and Precautions

As for Cefotaxime Sodium, p.168.

Interactions

Probenecid reduces the renal clearance of cefodizime.

Antimicrobial Action

Cefodizime has similar antimicrobial activity to that of cefotaxime (p.168) although cefodizime has no active metabolite. It has variable activity against *Citrobacter* spp., and *Pseudomonas aeruginosa* and *Bacteroides fragilis* are generally resistant.

Pharmacokinetics

Cefodizime is administered by injection as the sodium salt. Intramuscular administration of 1 g cefodizime produces peak plasma concentrations of about 60 to 75 μg per mL at about 1 to 1.5 hours. Immediately after intravenous administration of 1 or 2 g cefodizime mean peak plasma concentrations of 215 and 394 μg per mL, respectively, have been achieved. Cefodizime is about 80% bound to plasma proteins and is widely distributed into body tissues and fluids. It crosses the placenta and small amounts have been detected in breast milk. Plasma elimination is reported to be triphasic with a terminal elimination half-life of about 4 hours. The half-life is prolonged by renal impairment.

The majority of a dose is excreted unchanged in the urine; up to 80% of a dose has been recovered within 24 hours. Cefodizime is mainly excreted by glomerular filtration with some tubular secretion. Probenecid delays excretion. Cefodizime is removed by dialysis.

References.

1. Conte JE. Pharmacokinetics of cefodizime in volunteers with normal or impaired renal function. *J Clin Pharmacol* 1994; **34:** 1066–70.
2. Lenfant B, *et al.* Pharmacokinetics of cefodizime following single doses of 0.5, 1.0, 2.0, and 3.0 grams administered intravenously to healthy volunteers. *Antimicrob Agents Chemother* 1995; **39:** 2037–41.
3. Scaglione F, *et al.* Pharmacokinetic study of cefodizime and ceftriaxone in sera and bones of patients undergoing hip arthroplasty. *Antimicrob Agents Chemother* 1997; **41:** 2292–4.

Uses and Administration

Cefodizime is a third-generation cephalosporin antibiotic with uses similar to those of cefotaxime (p.169).

Cefodizime is administered as the disodium salt by intramuscular injection or intravenously by injection or infusion in the treatment of susceptible infections. Doses are expressed in terms of the equivalent amount of cefodizime. The usual adult dose is 1 g every 12 hours for urinary-tract infections and lower respiratory-tract infections; alternatively, a single daily dose of 2 g may be given in urinary-tract infections. Single doses over 1 g should be given intravenously. Doses should be reduced in renal impairment.

References.

1. Finch RG, *et al.*, eds. Cefodizime: a third generation cephalosporin with immunomodulating properties. *J Antimicrob Chemother* 1990; **26** (suppl C): 1–134.
2. Barradell LB, Brogden RN. Cefodizime: a review of its antibacterial activity, pharmacokinetic properties and therapeutic use. *Drugs* 1992; **44:** 800–834.

Preparations

Proprietary Preparations (details are given in Part 3)
Aust.: Timecef; ***Ger.:*** Modivid†; ***Irl.:*** Modivid; ***Ital.:*** Diezime; Modivid; Timecef; ***UK:*** Timecef.

Cefonicid Sodium (16566-n)

Cefonicid Sodium *(BANM, USAN, rINNM)*.

SKF-D-75073-Z_2; SKF-D-75073-Z (cefonicid monosodium). The disodium salt of 7-[(R)-mandelamido]-3-(1-sulphomethyl-1*H*-tetrazol-5-ylthiomethyl)-3-cephem-4-carboxylic acid.

$C_{18}H_{16}N_6Na_2O_8S_3$ = 586.5.

CAS — 61270-58-4 (cefonicid); 61270-78-8 (cefonicid disodium); 71420-79-6 (cefonicid monosodium).

Pharmacopoeias. In US.

1.08 g of monograph substance is approximately equivalent to 1 g of cefonicid. Each g of monograph substance represents about 3.4 mmol of sodium.

Freely **soluble** in water, in sodium chloride 0.9%, and in glucose 5%; very slightly soluble in dehydrated alcohol; soluble in methyl alcohol. A 5% solution in water has a pH of 3.5 to 6.5. **Store** in airtight containers.

Adverse Effects and Precautions

As for Cephalothin Sodium, p.179.

Cefonicid contains a substituted *N*-methylthiotetrazole side-chain, a structure associated with hypoprothrombinaemia (see Cephamandole, p.180).

Effects on the blood. References.

1. Riancho JA, *et al.* Life-threatening bleeding in a patient treated with cefonicid. *Ann Intern Med* 1995; **123:** 472–3.

Interactions

As for Cephamandole, p.180.

Antimicrobial Action

Cefonicid sodium has an antimicrobial action and pattern of resistance similar to that of cephamandole (p.180), although it is generally less active against Gram-positive cocci.

Pharmacokinetics

Cefonicid is administered parenterally as the sodium salt. After intramuscular administration of a dose of 1 g peak plasma concentrations ranging from 67 to 126 μg per mL have been achieved after 1 to 2 hours. More than 90% of cefonicid in the circulation is bound to plasma proteins. Cefonicid has a plasma half-life of approximately 4.5 hours, which is prolonged in patients with renal impairment.

Therapeutic concentrations of cefonicid have been reported in a wide range of body tissues and fluids.

Up to 99% of a dose of cefonicid is excreted unchanged in the urine within 24 hours. The excretion of cefonicid is decreased by the concomitant administration of probenecid.

References.

1. Trang JM, *et al.* Effect of age and renal function on cefonicid pharmacokinetics. *Antimicrob Agents Chemother* 1989; **33:** 142–6.
2. Furlanut M, *et al.* Pharmacokinetics of cefonicid in children. *Eur J Clin Pharmacol* 1989; **36:** 79–82.
3. Benson JM, *et al.* In vitro protein binding of cefonicid and cefuroxime in adult and neonatal sera. *Antimicrob Agents Chemother* 1993; **37:** 1343–7.

Uses and Administration

Cefonicid is a second-generation cephalosporin antibiotic used similarly to cephamandole in the treatment of susceptible infections and for surgical infection prophylaxis.

It is administered at the sodium salt by deep intramuscular injection, or intravenously by slow injection over 3 to 5 minutes or by infusion. Doses are expressed in terms of the equivalent amount of cefonicid. The usual dose is cefonicid 1 g once daily. For uncomplicated urinary-tract infections a dose of 0.5 g once daily is recommended; up to 2 g once daily has been given in severe infections. More than 1 g should not be injected intramuscularly into a single site.

For patients with impaired renal function a loading dose of 7.5 mg per kg body-weight is recommended followed by reduced maintenance doses according to the creatinine clearance and the severity of the infection. A dose supplement is not required following dialysis.

For surgical infection prophylaxis, a single dose of 1 g given one hour prior to surgical incision is usually sufficient, but may be administered daily for a further 2 days in prosthetic arthroplasty or open-heart surgery.

References.

1. Saltiel E, Brogden RN. Cefonicid: a review of its antibacterial activity, pharmacological properties and therapeutic use. *Drugs* 1986; **32:** 222–59.

Preparations

USP 23: Cefonicid for Injection.

Proprietary Preparations (details are given in Part 3)
Belg.: Monocid; ***Ital.:*** Biocil; Cefodie; Cefosporin; Chefir; Delsacid; Fonicef; Ipacid; Lisa; Modiem; Monobios; Monocid; Parecid; Praticef; Sintocef; Unicef; Unicid; ***Spain:*** Monocid; Unidie; ***USA:*** Monocid.

Cefoperazone Sodium (187-a)

Cefoperazone Sodium *(BANM, USAN, rINNM)*.

CP-52640-2; CP-52640 (anhydrous cefoperazone); CP-52640-3 (cefoperazone dihydrate); T-1551 (cefoperazone or sodium salt). Sodium (7*R*)-7-[(*R*)-2-(4-ethyl-2,3-dioxopiperazin-1-ylcarboxamido)-2-(4-hydroxyphenyl)acetamido]-3-[(1-methyl-1*H*-tetrazol-5-yl)thiomethyl]-3-cephem-4-carboxylate.

$C_{25}H_{26}N_9NaO_8S_2$ = 667.7.

CAS — 62893-19-0 (cefoperazone); 62893-20-3 (cefoperazone sodium).

Pharmacopoeias. In *Chin., Jpn, Pol.,* and *US.*

1.03 g of monograph substance is approximately equivalent to 1 g of cefoperazone. Each g of monograph substance represents about 1.5 mmol of sodium.

A white to pale buff crystalline powder. Freely **soluble** in water and in methyl alcohol; slightly soluble in dehydrated alcohol; practically insoluble in acetone, in ethyl acetate, and in ether.

A 25% solution in water has a pH of 4.5 to 6.5. **Store** in airtight containers.

Incompatibility. As with most beta-lactams, admixture of cefoperazone sodium with aminoglycosides is not recommended because of the potential for inactivation of either drug.

There have been reports of incompatibility with other drugs including diltiazem,[1] pentamidine,[2] perphenazine,[3] pethidine,[4] and promethazine.[5]

1. Gayed AA, *et al.* Visual compatibility of diltiazem injection with various diluents and medications during simulated Y-site injection. *Am J Health-Syst Pharm* 1995; **52:** 516–20.
2. Lewis JD, El-Gendy A. Cephalosporin-pentamidine isethionate incompatibilities. *Am J Health-Syst Pharm* 1996; **53:** 1461–2.
3. Gasca M, *et al.* Visual compatibility of perphenazine with various antimicrobials during simulated Y-site injection. *Am J Hosp Pharm* 1987; **44:** 574–5.
4. Nieves-Cordero AL, *et al.* Compatibility of narcotic analgesic solutions with various antibiotics during simulated Y-site injection. *Am J Hosp Pharm* 1985; **42:** 1108–9.
5. Scott SM. Incompatibility of cefoperazone and promethazine. *Am J Hosp Pharm* 1990; **47:** 519.

Adverse Effects and Precautions

As for Cephalothin Sodium, p.179.

Like cefotaxime (p.168), cefoperazone has the potential for colonisation and superinfection with resistant organisms. Changes in bowel flora may be more marked than with cefotaxime because of the greater biliary excretion of cefoperazone; diarrhoea may occur more often.

Cefoperazone contains an *N*-methylthiotetrazole side-chain, a structure associated with hypoprothrombinaemia (see Cephamandole, p.180). Hypoprothrombinaemia has been reported in patients treated with cefoperazone and has rarely been associated with bleeding episodes. Prothrombin time should be monitored in patients at risk of hypoprothrombinaemia and vitamin K administered if necessary.

Interactions

As for Cephamandole, p.180.

Antimicrobial Action

Cefoperazone has antimicrobial activity similar to that of ceftazidime (p.174), although it is slightly less active against some Enterobacteriaceae. It has good activity against *Pseudomonas aeruginosa*, but is less active than ceftazidime.

Cefoperazone is more susceptible than cefotaxime to hydrolysis by certain beta-lactamases.

Activity, particularly against Enterobacteriaceae and *Bacteroides* spp. has been enhanced in the presence of the beta-lactamase inhibitor sulbactam; resistant *Ps. aeruginosa* are not sensitive to the combination.

References.

1. Fass RJ, *et al.* In vitro activities of cefoperazone and sulbactam singly and in combination against cefoperazone-resistant members of the family Enterobacteriaceae and nonfermenters. *Antimicrob Agents Chemother* 1990; **34:** 2256–9.
2. Clark RB, *et al.* Multicentre study on antibiotic susceptibilities of anaerobic bacteria to cefoperazone-sulbactam and other antimicrobial agents. *J Antimicrob Chemother* 1992; **29:** 57–67.

Pharmacokinetics

Cefoperazone is administered parenterally as the sodium salt. After intramuscular administration of doses equivalent to cefoperazone 1 or 2 g, peak plasma concentrations of 65 and 97 μg per mL have been reported after 1 to 2 hours. The plasma half-life of cefoperazone is about 2 hours, but may be prolonged in neonates and in patients with hepatic or biliary-tract disease. Cefoperazone is 82 to 93% bound to plasma proteins, depending on the concentration.

Cefoperazone is widely distributed in body tissues and fluids, although penetration into the CSF is generally poor. It crosses the placenta, and low concentrations have been detected in breast milk.

Cefoperazone is excreted principally in the bile where it rapidly achieves high concentrations. Urinary excretion is primarily by glomerular filtration. Up to 30% of a dose is excreted unchanged in the urine within 12 to 24 hours; this proportion may be increased in patients with hepatic or biliary disease. Cefoperazone A, a degradation product less active than cefoperazone, has been found only rarely *in vivo*.

References to the pharmacokinetics of cefoperazone with sulbactam.

1. Reitberg DP, *et al.* Multiple-dose pharmacokinetics and toleration of intravenously administered cefoperazone and sulbactam when given as single agents or in combination. *Antimicrob Agents Chemother* 1988; **32:** 42–6.
2. Johnson CA, *et al.* Pharmacokinetics and pharmacodynamics of cefoperazone-sulbactam in patients on continuous ambulatory peritoneal dialysis. *Antimicrob Agents Chemother* 1988; **32:** 51–6.
3. Rho JP, *et al.* Effect of impaired renal function on the pharmacokinetics of coadministered cefoperazone and sulbactam. *J Antimicrob Chemother* 1992; **29:** 701–9.
4. Danziger LH, *et al.* Steady-state pharmacokinetics of cefoperazone and sulbactam in patients with acute appendicitis. *Ann Pharmacother* 1994; **28:** 703–7.

Uses and Administration

Cefoperazone is a third-generation cephalosporin antibiotic used similarly to ceftazidime (p.174) in the treatment of susceptible infections, especially those due to *Pseudomonas* spp. It is not recommended for the treatment of meningitis because of poor penetration into the CSF.

Cefoperazone is administered as the sodium salt by deep intramuscular injection or intravenously by intermittent or continuous infusion. Doses are expressed in terms of the equivalent amount of cefoperazone. The usual dose for adults is 2 to 4 g daily in two divided doses. In severe infections, up to 12 g daily in two to four divided doses may be given. In general, the dose should not exceed 4 g daily in patients with liver disease or biliary obstruction or 2 g daily in those with both liver and kidney impairment; if higher doses are used plasma concentrations of cefoperazone should be monitored. If cefoperazone is given in association with an aminoglycoside, the drugs should be administered separately. Cefoperazone is also given with the beta-lactamase inhibitor sulbactam.

Preparations

USP 23: Cefoperazone for Injection; Cefoperazone Injection.

Proprietary Preparations (details are given in Part 3)
Aust.: Cefobid; ***Canad.:*** Cefobid†; ***Fr.:*** Cefobis; ***Ger.:*** Cefobis; ***Ital.:*** Bioperazone; Cefazone; Cefobid†; Cefogram; Cefoneg; Cefoper; Cefosint; Dardum; Farecef; Ipazone; Kefazon; Mediper†; Novobiocyl; Perocef; Prontokef; Tomabef; Zoncef; ***Spain:*** Cefobid; ***Switz.:*** Cefobis†; ***USA:*** Cefobid.

Multi-ingredient: ***Aust.:*** Sulperazon†.

Ceforanide (12541-g)

Ceforanide *(BAN, USAN, rINN).*

BL-S786. 7-[2-(α-Amino-*o*-tolyl)acetamido]-3-(1-carboxymethyl-1*H*-tetrazol-5-ylthiomethyl)-3-cephem-4-carboxylic acid.

$C_{20}H_{21}N_7O_6S_2$ = 519.6.

CAS — 60925-61-3.

Pharmacopoeias. In *US.*

A 5% suspension in water has a pH of 2.5 to 4.5. **Store** in airtight containers.

Ceforanide is a second-generation cephalosporin antibiotic with actions and uses similar to those of cephamandole (p.180), although it is reported to be less active *in vitro* against some bacteria, including staphylococci and *Haemophilus influenzae*. It is used in the treatment of susceptible infections and for surgical infection prophylaxis.

It is given as the lysine salt but doses are expressed in terms of the equivalent amount of ceforanide. It has been administered by deep intramuscular injection, or intravenously by slow injection over 3 to 5 minutes or by infusion, in doses of 1 to 2 g every 12 hours. A suggested dose in children has been 20 mg per kg body-weight daily in two divided doses. For surgical infection prophylaxis a dose of 1 to 2 g intravenously one hour prior to surgical incision has been recommended for adults.

Ceforanide contains a substituted *N*-methylthiotetrazole side-chain, a structure associated with hypoprothrombinaemia and alcohol intolerance (see Cephamandole, p.180). Probenecid does not affect the renal excretion of ceforanide.

References.

1. Campoli-Richards DM, *et al.* Ceforanide: a review of its antibacterial activity, pharmacokinetic properties and clinical efficacy. *Drugs* 1987; **34:** 411–37.

Preparations

USP 23: Ceforanide for Injection.

Proprietary Preparations (details are given in Part 3)
Belg.: Precef.

Cefoselis (17617-b)

Cefoselis *(rINN).*

(−)-5-Amino-2-({(6*R*,7*R*)-7-[2-(2-amino-4-thiazolyl)glyoxylamido]-2-carboxy-8-oxo-5-thia-1-azabicyclo[4.2.0]oct-2-en-3-yl}methyl)-1-(2-hydroxyethyl)pyrazolium hydroxide, inner salt, 7^2-(*Z*)-(*O*-methyloxime).

$C_{19}H_{22}N_8O_6S_2$ = 522.6.

CAS — 122841-10-5.

Cefoselis is a cephalosporin antibacterial used in the treatment of susceptible bacterial infections.

Cefotaxime Sodium (32-f)

Cefotaxime Sodium *(BANM, USAN, rINNM).*

Cefotaximum Natricum; CTX; HR-756; RU-24756. Sodium (7*R*)-7-[(*Z*)-2-(2-aminothiazol-4-yl)-2-(methoxyimino)acetamido]cephalosporanate; Sodium (7*R*)-3-acetoxymethyl-7-[(*Z*)-2-(2-aminothiazol-4-yl)-2-(methoxyimino)acetamido]-3-cephem-4-carboxylate.

$C_{16}H_{16}N_5NaO_7S_2$ = 477.4.

CAS — 63527-52-6 (cefotaxime); 64485-93-4 (cefotaxime sodium).

Pharmacopoeias. In *Chin., Eur.* (see p.viii), *Jpn, Pol.,* and *US.*

A white or off-white to pale yellow, hygroscopic, crystalline powder. 1.05 g of monograph substance is approximately equivalent to 1 g of cefotaxime. Each g of monograph substance represents about 2.09 mmol of sodium.

Freely **soluble** to very soluble in water; sparingly soluble in methyl alcohol; practically insoluble in ether and in other organic solvents. A 10% solution has a pH of between 4.5 and 6.5. **Store** in airtight containers at a temperature not exceeding 30°. Protect from light.

Incompatibility. Cefotaxime sodium has been reported to be incompatible with alkaline solutions such as sodium bicarbonate. The manufacturers recommend that it should be administered separately from aminoglycosides.

Adverse Effects and Precautions

As for Cephalothin Sodium, p.179. Arrhythmias have been associated with rapid bolus infusion through a central venous catheter in a few cases.

The broad-spectrum third-generation cephalosporins have the potential for colonisation and superinfection with resistant organisms such as *Pseudomonas aeruginosa*, *Enterobacter* spp., *Candida*, and enterococci, at various sites in the body, although the incidence has generally been low with cefotaxime. Changes in bowel flora are a predisposing factor and have been more marked with cefoperazone and ceftriaxone, possibly because of their greater biliary excretion. Pseudomembranous colitis, associated with *Clostridium difficile* infection, may occasionally be seen with any of the third-generation cephalosporins.

Reviews on adverse effects associated with third-generation cephalosporins.

1. Neu HC. Third generation cephalosporins: safety profiles after 10 years of clinical use. *J Clin Pharmacol* 1990; **30:** 396–403.
2. Fekety FR. Safety of parenteral third-generation cephalosporins. *Am J Med* 1990; **88** (suppl 4A): 38S–44S.

Antibiotic-associated colitis. It has been suggested[1] that cefotaxime is associated with an increased risk of *Clostridium difficile* diarrhoea in elderly patients; however, the manufacturer[2] has disputed this, arguing that cefotaxime compares favourably with alternative third-generation cephalosporins.

1. Impallomeni M, *et al.* Increased risk of diarrhoea caused by Clostridium difficile in elderly patients receiving cefotaxime. *Br Med J* 1995; **311:** 1345–6.
2. Rothschild E, *et al.* Risk of diarrhoea due to Clostridium difficile during cefotaxime treatment. *Br Med J* 1996; **312:** 778.

Interactions

As for many cephalosporins, probenecid reduces the renal clearance of cefotaxime, resulting in higher and prolonged plasma concentrations of cefotaxime and its desacetyl metabolite.

The total body clearance of cefotaxime has been reduced in patients with normal and reduced renal function by the concomitant administration of the ureidopenicillins azlocillin[1] or mezlocillin.[2] Doses of cefotaxime may need to be reduced if either of these penicillins is being given. Encephalopathy with focal motor status and generalised convulsions have been reported in a patient with renal failure given cefotaxime and high doses of azlocillin.[3]

1. Kampf D, *et al.* Kinetic interactions between azlocillin, cefotaxime, and cefotaxime metabolites in normal and impaired renal function. *Clin Pharmacol Ther* 1984; **35:** 214–20.
2. Rodondi LC, *et al.* Influence of coadministration on the pharmacokinetics of mezlocillin and cefotaxime in healthy volunteers and in patients with renal failure. *Clin Pharmacol Ther* 1989; **45:** 527–34.
3. Wroe SJ, *et al.* Focal motor status epilepticus following treatment with azlocillin and cefotaxime. *Med Toxicol* 1987; **2:** 233–4.

Antimicrobial Action

Cefotaxime is a third-generation cephalosporin antibiotic. It has a bactericidal action similar to cephamandole, but a broader spectrum of activity. It is highly stable to hydrolysis by most beta-lactamases and has greater activity against Gram-negative bacteria than first- or second-generation cephalosporins. Although cefotaxime is generally considered to have slightly less activity than first-generation cephalosporins against Gram-positive bacteria, many streptococci are very sensitive to it.

Desacetylcefotaxime is an active metabolite of cefotaxime and there may be additive or synergistic effects against some species.

Minimum inhibitory concentrations (MICs) of cefotaxime for susceptible organisms have been reported to range from about 0.03 to 16 μg per mL. An MIC of 8 μg or less per mL has been taken to indicate susceptibility and 64 μg or more per mL, resistance. Many studies express activity in terms of MIC_{90}, the concentration at which 90% of organisms are inhibited. MICs are generally close to minimum bactericidal concentrations (MBCs) although tolerance has been reported.

Spectrum of activity. Among Gram-negative bacteria cefotaxime is active *in vitro* against many Enterobacteriaceae including *Citrobacter* and *Enterobacter* spp., *Escherichia coli, Klebsiella* spp., both indole-positive and indole-negative *Proteus, Providencia, Salmonella, Serratia, Shigella,* and *Yersinia* spp. Other susceptible Gram-negative bacteria, including penicillin-resistant strains, are *Haemophilus influenzae, Moraxella (Branhamella) catarrhalis, Neisseria gonorrhoeae,* and *N. meningitidis. Brucella melitensis* is also reported to be sensitive. For many of these Gram-negative bacteria the MIC is under 1 μg per mL and often much less. Some strains of *Pseudomonas* spp. are moderately susceptible to cefotaxime, but most are resistant. Desacetylcefotaxime is active against many of these Gram-negative bacteria, but not against *Pseudomonas* spp.

Among Gram-positive bacteria cefotaxime is active against staphylococci and streptococci. *Staphylococcus aureus,* including penicillinase-producing strains but not methicillin-resistant *Staph. aureus,* is sensitive with an MIC_{90} of about 2 to 4 μg per mL, reduced in the presence of desacetylcefotaxime. *Staph. epidermidis* is sensitive with an MIC_{90} of about 8 μg per mL, but penicillinase-producing strains are resistant. *Streptococcus agalactiae* (group B streptococci), *Str. pneumoniae,* and *Str. pyogenes* (group A streptococci) are all very sensitive (MIC_{90} 0.1 μg or less per mL) although truly penicillin-resistant pneumococci are apparently not sensitive. Enterococci and *Listeria monocytogenes* are resistant.

Cefotaxime is active against some anaerobic bacteria. *Bacteroides fragilis* may be moderately sensitive, but many strains are resistant; synergy has been demonstrated with desacetylcefotaxime *in vitro. Clostridium perfringens* is sensitive, but most *Cl. difficile* are resistant.

Other organisms sensitive to cefotaxime include the spirochaete *Borrelia burgdorferi* and the causative organism of chancroid, *Haemophilus ducreyi.*

Activity with other antimicrobials. In addition to possible synergy or additive effects with desacetylcefotaxime, the activity of cefotaxime may be enhanced by aminoglycosides such as gentamicin; synergy has been demonstrated *in vitro* against Gram-negative bacteria including *Pseudomonas aeruginosa.* There have also been reports of enhanced activity *in vitro* with other antibacterials including fosfomycin and ciprofloxacin and variable results with penicillins.

Resistance may develop during treatment with cefotaxime due to derepression of chromosomally-mediated beta-lactamases, and has been reported particularly in *Enterobacter* spp., with multiresistant strains emerging during treatment. This type of resistance has also developed in other bacteria including *Citrobacter, Serratia,* and *Pseudomonas* spp. Another mechanism of cefotaxime resistance is the development of plasma-mediated, extended-spectrum beta-lactamases, and this has occurred in *Klebsiella* spp. and also other Enterobacteriaceae. Resistance in *Str. pneumoniae* is due to the production of altered penicillin-binding proteins.

References to the antimicrobial activity of cefotaxime and other third-generation cephalosporins, including the problem of bacterial resistance.

1. Neu HC. Pathophysiologic basis for the use of third-generation cephalosporins. *Am J Med* 1990; **88** (suppl 4A): 3S–11S.
2. Chow JW, *et al.* Enterobacter bacteremia: clinical features and emergence of antibiotic resistance during therapy. *Ann Intern Med* 1991; **115:** 585–90.
3. Sanders CC. New β-lactams: new problems for the internist. *Ann Intern Med* 1991; **115:** 650–1.
4. Thomson KS, *et al.* High-level resistance to cefotaxime and ceftazidime in Klebsiella pneumoniae isolates from Cleveland, Ohio. *Antimicrob Agents Chemother* 1991; **35:** 1001–3.
5. Piddock LJV, *et al.* Prevalence and mechanism of resistance to 'third-generation' cephalosporins in clinically relevant isolates of Enterobacteriaceae from 43 hospitals in the UK, 1990-1991. *J Antimicrob Chemother* 1997; **39:** 177–87.

Pharmacokinetics

Cefotaxime is administered by injection as the sodium salt. It is rapidly absorbed after intramuscular injection and mean peak plasma concentrations of about 12 and 20 μg per mL have been reported 30 minutes after 0.5 and 1 g of cefotaxime, respectively. Immediately after the intravenous injection of 0.5, 1, or 2 g of cefotaxime mean peak plasma concentrations of 38, 102, and 215 μg per mL, respectively, have been achieved with concentrations ranging from about 1 to 3 μg per mL after 4 hours. The plasma half-life of cefotaxime is about one hour and that of the active metabolite desacetylcefotaxime is about 1.5 hours; half-lives are increased in neonates and in patients with severe renal impairment, especially those of the metabolite, and a reduction in dosage may be necessary. The effects of liver disease on clearance of cefotaxime and its metabolite have been variable, but in general dosage adjustment has not been considered necessary. About 40% of cefotaxime in the circulation is reported to be bound to plasma proteins.

Cefotaxime and desacetylcefotaxime are widely distributed in body tissues and fluids; therapeutic concentrations are achieved in the CSF particularly when the meninges are inflamed. It crosses the placenta and low concentrations have been detected in breast milk.

Following partial metabolism in the liver to desacetylcefotaxime and inactive metabolites, elimination is mainly by the kidneys and about 40 to 60% of a dose has been recovered unchanged in the urine within 24 hours; a further 20% is excreted as the desacetyl metabolite. Probenecid competes for renal tubular secretion with cefotaxime resulting in higher and prolonged plasma concentrations of cefotaxime and its desacetyl metabolite. Cefotaxime and its metabolites are removed by haemodialysis.

Relatively high concentrations of cefotaxime and desacetylcefotaxime are achieved in bile and about 20% of a dose has been recovered in the faeces.

N.B. Reported pharmacokinetic values may relate to cefotaxime plus its active metabolite, desacetylcefotaxime, when microbiological assays have been used.

References to the pharmacokinetics of cefotaxime.

1. Asmar BI, *et al.* Cefotaxime diffusion into the cerebrospinal fluid of children with meningitis. *Antimicrob Agents Chemother* 1985; **28:** 138–40.
2. Fick RB, *et al.* Penetration of cefotaxime into respiratory secretions. *Antimicrob Agents Chemother* 1987; **31:** 815–17.
3. Kearns GL, *et al.* Cefotaxime and desacetylcefotaxime pharmacokinetics in very low birth weight neonates. *J Pediatr* 1989; **114:** 461–7.
4. Sjölin J, *et al.* Penetration of cefotaxime and desacetylcefotaxime into brain abscesses in humans. *Antimicrob Agents Chemother* 1991; **35:** 2606–10.
5. Nau R, *et al.* Passage of cefotaxime and ceftriaxone into cerebrospinal fluid of patients with uninflamed meninges. *Antimicrob Agents Chemother* 1993; **37:** 1518–24.

References to the pharmacokinetics of cefotaxime in liver disease.

1. Höffken G, *et al.* Pharmacokinetics of cefotaxime and desacetyl-cefotaxime in cirrhosis of the liver. *Chemotherapy* 1984; **30:** 7–17.
2. Graninger W, *et al.* Cefotaxime and desacetyl-cefotaxime blood levels in hepatic dysfunction. *J Antimicrob Chemother* 1984; **14** (suppl B): 143–6.
3. Hary L, *et al.* The pharmacokinetics of ceftriaxone and cefotaxime in cirrhotic patients with ascites. *Eur J Clin Pharmacol* 1989; **36:** 613–16.
4. Ko RJ, *et al.* Pharmacokinetics of cefotaxime and desacetylcefotaxime in patients with liver disease. *Antimicrob Agents Chemother* 1991; **35:** 1376–80.

References to the pharmacokinetics of cefotaxime in renal impairment.

1. Matzke GR, *et al.* Cefotaxime and desacetyl cefotaxime kinetics in renal impairment. *Clin Pharmacol Ther* 1985; **38:** 31–6.
2. Paap CM, *et al.* Pharmacokinetics of cefotaxime and its active metabolite in children with renal dysfunction. *Antimicrob Agents Chemother* 1991; **35:** 1879–83.
3. Paap CM, *et al.* Cefotaxime and metabolite disposition in two pediatric continuous ambulatory peritoneal dialysis patients. *Ann Pharmacother* 1992; **26:** 341–3.
4. Paap CM, Nahata MC. The relation between type of renal disease and renal drug clearance in children. *Eur J Clin Pharmacol* 1993; **44:** 195–7.

Uses and Administration

Cefotaxime is a third-generation cephalosporin antibiotic used in the treatment of infections due to susceptible organisms (see Antimicrobial Action, above), especially serious and life-threatening infections. They include brain abscess, endocarditis, gonorrhoea, intensive care (selective parenteral and enteral antisepsis regimens), Lyme disease, meningitis, peritonitis (primary or spontaneous), pneumonia, septicaemia, surgical infection (prophylaxis), and typhoid fever. For details of these infections and their treatment, see under Choice of Antibacterial, p.116.

Administration and dosage. Cefotaxime is given as the sodium salt by deep intramuscular injection or intravenously by slow injection over 3 to 5 minutes or by infusion over 20 to 60 minutes. Doses are expressed in terms of the equivalent amount of cefotaxime. It is usually given in doses of 2 to 6 g daily in 2 to 4 divided doses. In severe infections up to 12 g may be given daily by the intravenous route in up to 6 divided doses; pseudomonal infections usually require more than 6 g daily, but a cephalosporin with greater antipseudomonal activity, such as ceftazidime, is preferable. Children may be given 100 to 150 mg of cefotaxime per kg body-weight (50 mg per kg for neonates) daily in 2 to 4 divided doses, increased to 200 mg per kg (150 to 200 mg per kg for neonates) daily if necessary. Doses of cefotaxime should be reduced in severe renal impairment; after an initial loading dose of 1 g, halving the dose while maintaining the usual frequency of dosing has been suggested.

In the treatment of gonorrhoea a single 1-g dose of cefotaxime is given.

For surgical infection prophylaxis, 1 g is administered 30 to 90 minutes before surgery. At caesarean section 1 g is given intravenously to the mother as soon as the umbilical cord is clamped and two further doses intramuscularly or intravenously 6 and 12 hours later.

Cefotaxime may be administered in association with an aminoglycoside as synergy may occur against some Gram-negative organisms, but the drugs should be administered separately. It has sometimes been used with another beta-lactam to broaden the spectrum of activity. Cefotaxime has also been used in association with metronidazole in the treatment of mixed aerobic-anaerobic infections.

General references to third-generation cephalosporins.

1. Neu HC, *et al.,* eds. Third-generation cephalosporins: a decade of progress in the treatment of severe infections. *Am J Med* 1990; **88** (suppl 4A): 1S–45S.

General references to cefotaxime.

1. Todd PA, Brogden RN. Cefotaxime: an update of its pharmacology and therapeutic use. *Drugs* 1990; **40:** 608–51.
2. Gentry LO. Cefotaxime and prophylaxis: new approaches with a proven agent. *Am J Med* 1990; **88** (suppl 4A): 32S–37S.
3. Davies A, Speller DCE, eds. Cefotaxime—recent clinical investigations. *J Antimicrob Chemother* 1990; **26** (suppl A): 1-83.
4. Brogden RN, Spencer CM. Cefotaxime: a reappraisal of its antibacterial activity and pharmacokinetic properties, and a review of its therapeutic efficacy when administered twice daily for the treatment of mild to moderate infections. *Drugs* 1997; **53:** 483–510.

Preparations

BP 1998: Cefotaxime Injection;
USP 23: Cefotaxime for Injection; Cefotaxime Injection.

Proprietary Preparations (details are given in Part 3)
Aust.: Claforan; ***Austral.:*** Claforan; ***Belg.:*** Claforan; ***Canad.:*** Claforan; ***Fr.:*** Claforan; ***Ger.:*** Claforan; ***Irl.:*** Claforan; ***Ital.:*** Claforan; Zariviz; ***Neth.:*** Claforan; ***Norw.:*** Claforan; ***S.Afr.:*** Claforan; ***Spain:*** Cefacron; Claforan; Primafen; ***Swed.:*** Claforan; ***Switz.:*** Claforan; ***UK:*** Claforan; ***USA:*** Claforan.

Cefotetan Disodium (15313-a)

Cefotetan Disodium *(BANM, USAN, rINNM)*.

ICI-156834; YM-09330 (both cefotetan or disodium salt). (7S)-7-[(4-Carbamoylcarboxymethylene-1,3-dithietan-2-yl)carboxamido]-7-methoxy-3-[(1-methyl-1*H*-tetrazol-5-yl)thiomethyl]-3-cephem-4-carboxylic acid, disodium salt.

$C_{17}H_{15}N_7Na_2O_8S_4$ = 619.6.

CAS — 69712-56-7 (cefotetan); 74356-00-6 (cefotetan disodium).

Pharmacopoeias. US includes Cefotetan and Cefotetan Disodium. Jpn includes Cefotetan.

1.08 g of cefotetan disodium is approximately equivalent to 1 g of cefotetan. A 10% solution in water has a pH of 4.0 to 6.5. Each g of monograph substance represents about 3.2 mmol of sodium.

Store in airtight containers.

There may be **incompatibility** with aminoglycosides. Precipitation has been reported with promethazine hydrochloride.

References.

1. Das Gupta V, *et al.* Chemical stability of cefotetan disodium in 5% dextrose and 0.9% sodium chloride injections. *J Clin Pharm Ther* 1990; **15:** 109–14.
2. Erickinson SH, Ulici D. Incompatibility of cefotetan disodium and promethazine hydrochloride. *Am J Health-Syst Pharm* 1995; **52:** 1347.

Adverse Effects and Precautions

As for Cephalothin Sodium, p.179.

Cefotetan contains an *N*-methylthiotetrazole side-chain and like cephamandole (p.180) has the potential to cause hypoprothrombinaemia and bleeding.

Cefotetan, especially at high doses, may interfere with the Jaffé method of measuring creatinine concentrations to produce falsely elevated values; this should be borne in mind when measuring renal function.

Effects on the blood. Haemolytic anaemia occurred following cefotetan treatment in a patient on two occasions.[1] On the second occasion, haemolysis was accompanied by acute renal failure. The mechanism of the reaction was thought to be due to immune complex formation.

1. Wagner BKJ, *et al.* Cefotetan disodium-induced hemolytic anemia. *Ann Pharmacother* 1992; **26:** 199–200.

Interactions

As for Cephamandole, p.180.

Antimicrobial Action

Cefotetan is a cephamycin antibiotic with a mode of action and spectrum of activity similar to that of cefoxitin (p.170). It is generally much more active *in vitro* than cefoxitin against the Gram-negative Enterobacteriaceae, but has similar activity against *Bacteroides fragilis* and may be less active against some other *Bacteroides* spp.

References.

1. Wexler HM, Finegold SM. In vitro activity of cefotetan compared with that of other antimicrobial agents against anaerobic bacteria. *Antimicrob Agents Chemother* 1988; **32:** 601–4.

Pharmacokinetics

After intramuscular injection of cefotetan, peak plasma concentrations of about 70 μg per mL at 1 hour and 90 μg per mL at 3 hours have been reported after doses of 1 and 2 g, respectively. The plasma half-life of cefotetan is usually in the range of 3.0 to 4.6 hours and is prolonged in patients with renal impairment. About 88% of cefotetan in the circulation may be bound to plasma proteins, depending on the plasma concentration.

Cefotetan is widely distributed in body tissues and fluids. It crosses the placenta and low concentrations have been detected in breast milk. High concentrations are achieved in bile.

Cefotetan is excreted in the urine, primarily by glomerular filtration, as unchanged drug; 50 to 80% of a dose has been recovered in the urine in 24 hours and high concentrations are achieved. Small amounts of the tautomeric form of cefotetan have been detected in both plasma and urine.

Biliary excretion of cefotetan probably accounts for nonrenal clearance.

Some cefotetan is removed by dialysis.

References.

1. Owen AWMC, *et al.* The pharmacokinetics of cefotetan excretion in the unobstructed biliary tree. *J Antimicrob Chemother* 1983; **11** (suppl A): 217–21.
2. Smith BR, *et al.* Cefotetan pharmacokinetics in volunteers with various degrees of renal function. *Antimicrob Agents Chemother* 1986; **29:** 887–93.
3. Browning MJ, *et al.* Pharmacokinetics of cefotetan in patients with end-stage renal failure on maintenance dialysis. *J Antimicrob Chemother* 1986; **18:** 103–6.
4. Carver PL, *et al.* Pharmacokinetics and pharmacodynamics of total and unbound cefoxitin and cefotetan in healthy volunteers. *J Antimicrob Chemother* 1989; **23:** 99–106.
5. Zimmerman J, *et al.* Absolute bioavailability and noncompartmental analysis of intravenous and intramuscular Cefotan (cefotetan) in normal volunteers. *J Clin Pharmacol* 1989; **29:** 151–7.
6. Martin C, *et al.* Clinical pharmacokinetics of cefotetan. *Clin Pharmacokinet* 1994; **26:** 248–58.

Uses and Administration

Cefotetan is a cephamycin antibiotic generally classified with the second-generation cephalosporins and used similarly to cefoxitin (p.171) in the treatment and prophylaxis of anaerobic and mixed bacterial infections, especially intra-abdominal and pelvic infections.

It is administered as the disodium salt by deep intramuscular injection or intravenously by slow injection over 3 to 5 minutes or by infusion. Doses are expressed in terms of the equivalent amount of cefotetan. The usual dose for adults is 1 or 2 g every 12 hours. For the treatment of life-threatening infections, 3 g every 12 hours may be given intravenously. Dosage should be reduced in patients with severely impaired renal function. Those with a creatinine clearance of 10 to 30 mL per minute may be given the usual dose every 24 hours and those with a creatinine clearance of less than 10 mL per minute, every 48 hours.

For infection prophylaxis during surgical procedures an intravenous dose of 1 or 2 g is administered 30 to 60 minutes before surgery or, in caesarean section, as soon as the umbilical cord is clamped.

References.

1. DiPiro JT, May JR. Use of cephalosporins with enhanced antianaerobic activity for treatment and prevention of anaerobic and mixed infections. *Clin Pharm* 1988; **7:** 285–302.

Preparations

USP 23: Cefotetan for Injection; Cefotetan Injection.

Proprietary Preparations (details are given in Part 3)
Aust.: Ceftenon; ***Austral.:*** Apatef; ***Belg.:*** Apacef; ***Canad.:*** Cefotan; ***Fr.:*** Apacef; ***Ger.:*** Apatef†; ***Ital.:*** Apatef; Cepan†; Darvilen†; ***Jpn:*** Yamatetan; ***USA:*** Cefotan.

Cefotiam Hydrochloride (12542-q)

Cefotiam Hydrochloride *(BANM, USAN, rINNM)*.

Abbott-48999; CGP-14221E (cefotiam or hydrochloride); SCE-963. 7-[2-(2-Amino-1,3-thiazol-4-yl)acetamido]-3-[1-(2-dimethylaminoethyl)-1*H*-tetrazol-5-ylthiomethyl]-3-cephem-4-carboxylic acid dihydrochloride.

$C_{18}H_{23}N_9O_4S_3$,2HCl = 598.6.

CAS — 61622-34-2 (cefotiam); 66309-69-1 (cefotiam hydrochloride).

Pharmacopoeias. In Jpn and US.

1.14 g of monograph substance is approximately equivalent to 1 g of cefotiam.

Store in airtight containers.

Cefotiam is a cephalosporin antibiotic with actions and uses similar to those of cephamandole (p.180). It is administered intravenously or intramuscularly as the hydrochloride in doses equivalent to up to 6 g of cefotiam daily in divided doses, according to the severity of the infection.

Cefotiam hexetil hydrochloride, a prodrug of cefotiam, is given by mouth in doses equivalent to 200 to 400 mg of cefotiam twice daily.

References.

1. Brogard JM, *et al.* Clinical pharmacokinetics of cefotiam. *Clin Pharmacokinet* 1989; **17:** 163–74.

Preparations

USP 23: Cefotiam for Injection.

Proprietary Preparations (details are given in Part 3)
Aust.: Spizef; ***Belg.:*** Pansporine†; ***Fr.:*** Taketiam; Texodil; ***Ger.:*** Spizef; ***Ital.:*** Sporidyn†; ***Jpn:*** Pansporin; ***Switz.:*** Halospor†.

Cefoxitin Sodium (33-d)

Cefoxitin Sodium *(BANM, USAN, rINNM)*.

Cefoxitinum Natricum; L-620388; MK-306. Sodium 3-carbamoyloxymethyl-7-methoxy-7-(2-thienylacetamido)-3-cephem-4-carboxylate.

$C_{16}H_{16}N_3NaO_7S_2$ = 449.4.

CAS — 35607-66-0 (cefoxitin); 33564-30-6 (cefoxitin sodium).

Pharmacopoeias. In Eur. (see p.viii), Jpn, Pol., and US.

1.05 g of cefoxitin sodium is approximately equivalent to 1 g of cefoxitin. Each g of monograph substance represents about 2.2 mmol of sodium. A white or almost white hygroscopic powder. Very **soluble** in water; slightly soluble in acetone; sparingly soluble in alcohol and in dimethylformamide; soluble in methyl alcohol; practically insoluble in chloroform and in ether. **Store** in airtight containers at a temperature not exceeding 8°.

Adverse Effects and Precautions

As for Cephalothin Sodium, p.179.

Cefoxitin may interfere with the Jaffé method of measuring creatinine concentrations to produce falsely high values; this should be borne in mind when measuring renal function.

Effects on the gastro-intestinal tract. Marked changes in anaerobic, facultative, and aerobic faecal flora have been noted with cefoxitin.[1]

1. Mulligan ME, *et al.* Alterations in human fecal flora, including ingrowth of Clostridium difficile, related to cefoxitin therapy. *Antimicrob Agents Chemother* 1984; **26:** 343–6.

Interactions

Probenecid reduces the renal clearance of cefoxitin.

Antimicrobial Action

Cefoxitin is a cephamycin antibiotic which, like the other beta-lactams, is bactericidal and is considered to act through the inhibition of bacterial cell wall synthesis.

It has a similar spectrum of activity to cephamandole (p.180) but is more active against anaerobic bacteria, especially *Bacteroides fragilis*.

Cefoxitin can induce the production of beta-lactamases by some bacteria, and combinations of cefoxitin with other beta-lactams have been shown to be antagonistic *in vitro*.

Cefoxitin itself is considered to be resistant to a wide range of beta-lactamases, including those produced by *Bacteroides* spp. However, acquired resistance to cefoxitin has been reported in *B. fragilis* (see Anaerobic Bacterial Infections, p.116) and has been attributed to beta-lactamase as well as to alterations in penicillin-binding proteins or to outer membrane proteins; there may be cross-resistance to other antibacterials.

References.

1. Cuchural GJ, *et al.* Transfer of β-lactamase-associated cefoxitin resistance in Bacteroides fragilis. *Antimicrob Agents Chemother* 1986; **29:** 918–20.
2. Piddock LJV, Wise R. Cefoxitin resistance in Bacteroides species: evidence indicating two mechanisms causing decreased susceptibility. *J Antimicrob Chemother* 1987; **19:** 161–70.
3. Brogan O, *et al.* Bacteroides fragilis resistant to metronidazole, clindamycin and cefoxitin. *J Antimicrob Chemother* 1989; **23:** 660–2.
4. Wexler HM, Halebian S. Alterations to the penicillin-binding proteins in the Bacteroides fragilis group: a mechanism for non-β-lactamase mediated cefoxitin resistance. *J Antimicrob Chemother* 1990; **26:** 7–20.
5. Cherubin CE, Applemen MD. Susceptibility of cefoxitin-resistant isolates of bacteroides to other agents including β-lactamase inhibitor/β-lactam combinations. *J Antimicrob Chemother* 1993; **32:** 168–70.

Pharmacokinetics

Cefoxitin is not absorbed from the gastro-intestinal tract; it is given parenterally as the sodium salt. After 1 g by intramuscular injection a peak plasma concentration of up to 30 μg per mL at 20 to 30 minutes has been reported whereas concentrations of 125, 72, and 25 μg per mL have been achieved after the intravenous injection of 1 g over 3, 30, and 120 minutes respectively. Cefoxitin is about 70% bound to plasma proteins. It has a plasma half-life of 45 to 60 minutes which is prolonged in renal impairment. Cefoxitin is widely distributed in the body but there is normally little penetration into the CSF, even when the meninges are inflamed. It crosses the placenta and has been detected in breast milk. Relatively high concentrations are achieved in bile.

The majority of a dose is excreted unchanged by the kidneys, up to about 2% being metabolised to descarbamylcefoxitin which is virtually inactive. Cefoxitin is excreted in the urine by glomerular filtration and tubular secretion and about 85% of a dose is recovered within 6 hours; probenecid slows this excretion. After an intramuscular dose of 1 g, peak concentrations in the urine are usually greater than 3 mg per mL.

Cefoxitin is removed by haemodialysis.

References.

1. Feldman WE, *et al.* Penetration of cefoxitin into cerebrospinal fluid of infants and children with bacterial meningitis. *Antimicrob Agents Chemother* 1982; **21:** 468–71.
2. Hansbrough JF, Clark JE. Concentrations of cefoxitin in gall-bladder bile of cholecystectomy patients. *Antimicrob Agents Chemother* 1982; **22:** 709–10.

Uses and Administration

Cefoxitin is a cephamycin antibiotic which differs structurally from the cephalosporins by the addition of a 7-α-methoxy group to the 7-β-aminocephalosporanic acid nucleus.

It is generally classified with the second-generation cephalosporins and can be used similarly to cephamandole for the treatment of susceptible infections. However, because of its activity against *Bacteroides fragilis* and other anaerobic bacteria, it is used principally in the treatment and prophylaxis of anaerobic and mixed bacterial infections, especially intra-abdominal and pelvic infections. Indications include endometritis (prophylaxis at caesarean section), pelvic inflammatory disease, and surgical infection (prophylaxis). It may also be used in the treatment of gonorrhoea and urinary-tract infections. For details of these infections and their treatment, see under Choice of Antibacterial, p.116.

Administration and dosage. Cefoxitin is administered as the sodium salt by deep intramuscular injection, by slow intravenous injection over 3 to 5 minutes, or by intermittent or continuous intravenous infusion.

Doses are expressed in terms of the equivalent amount of cefoxitin. The usual adult dose is 1 or 2 g every 8 hours although it may be given more frequently (every 4 or 6 hours). In severe infections up to 12 g daily has been recommended. Children and neonates may be given 20 to 40 mg per kg bodyweight every 12 hours for neonates up to 1 week old, every 8 hours for those aged 1 to 4 weeks, and every 6 to 8 hours for older infants and children; in severe infections, up to 200 mg per kg daily may be given, to a maximum of 12 g daily.

In renal impairment, dosage should be reduced according to the creatinine-clearance rate. In adults, after an initial loading dose of 1 to 2 g, suggested maintenance doses are: creatinine clearance of 30 to 50 mL per minute, 1 to 2 g every 8 to 12 hours; 10 to 29 mL per minute, 1 to 2 g every 12 to 24 hours; 5 to 9 mL per minute, 0.5 to 1 g every 12 to 24 hours; and below 5 mL per minute, 0.5 to 1 g every 24 to 48 hours. The loading dose should be repeated after each haemodialysis.

For the treatment of uncomplicated urinary-tract infections, cefoxitin 1 g twice daily has been given intramuscularly. For the treatment of uncomplicated gonorrhoea, a single dose of 2 g intramuscularly has been given in association with probenecid 1 g by mouth.

For surgical infection prophylaxis, the usual dose is cefoxitin 2 g intramuscularly or intravenously 30 to 60 minutes prior to the procedure and then every 6 hours, not usually for more than 24 hours. Infants and children undergoing surgical procedures can be given doses of 30 to 40 mg per kg body-weight, at the same time intervals as adults; neonates may also be given 30 to 40 mg per kg, but at intervals of 8 to 12 hours.

At caesarean section a single 2-g dose may be given intravenously to the mother as soon as the umbilical cord is clamped. Some consider a 3-dose regimen, with further 2-g doses 4 and 8 hours after the initial dose, to be more effective in preventing complications such as endometritis than a single dose.

Reviews.

1. DiPiro JT, May JR. Use of cephalosporins with enhanced anti-anaerobic activity for treatment and prevention of anaerobic and mixed infections. *Clin Pharm* 1988; **7:** 285–302.
2. Goodwin CS. Cefoxitin 20 years on: is it still useful? *Rev Med Microbiol* 1995; **6:** 146–53.

Preparations

BP 1998: Cefoxitin Injection;
USP 23: Cefoxitin for Injection; Cefoxitin Injection.

Proprietary Preparations (details are given in Part 3)
Aust.: Mefoxitin; ***Austral.:*** Mefoxin; ***Belg.:*** Mefoxin; ***Canad.:*** Mefoxin; ***Fr.:*** Mefoxin; ***Ger.:*** Mefoxitin; ***Irl.:*** Mefoxin; ***Ital.:*** Betacef; Cefociclin; Mefoxin; Stovaren†; Tifox; ***Neth.:*** Mefoxin; ***Norw.:*** Mefoxitin; ***S.Afr.:*** Mefoxin; ***Spain:*** Cefaxicina; Mefoxitin; ***Swed.:*** Mefoxitin; ***Switz.:*** Mefoxitin; ***UK:*** Mefoxin; ***USA:*** Mefoxin.

Cefozopran (15884-q)

Cefozopran *(rINN)*.

SCE-2787. (−)-1-{[(6*R*,7*R*)-7-[2-(5-Amino-1,2,4-thiadiazol-3-yl)glyoxylamido]-2-carboxy-8-oxo-5-thia-1-azabicyclo[4.2.0]oct-2-en-3-yl]methyl}-1*H*-imidazo[1,2-*b*]pyridazin-4-ium hydroxide inner salt, 7^2-(*Z*)-(*O*-methyloxime).

$C_{19}H_{17}N_9O_5S_2$ = 515.5.

CAS — 113359-04-9.

Cefozopran is a cephalosporin antibiotic administered parenterally as the hydrochloride.

References.

1. Iwahi T, *et al.* In vitro and in vivo activities of SCE-2787, a new parenteral cephalosporin with a broad antibacterial spectrum. *Antimicrob Agents Chemother* 1992; **36:** 1358–66.
2. Paulfeuerborn W, *et al.* Comparative pharmacokinetics and serum bactericidal activities of SCE-2787 and ceftazidime. *Antimicrob Agents Chemother* 1993; **37:** 1835–41.

Cefpimizole Sodium (16567-h)

Cefpimizole Sodium *(USAN, rINNM)*.

AC-1370 (cefpimizole); U-63196 (cefpimizole); U-63196E. Sodium (1-{4-carboxy-7-[(*R*)-2-(5-carboxyimidazol-4-ylcarboxamido)-2-phenylacetamido]-3-cephem-3-ylmethyl}-4-pyridinio)ethylsulphate.

$C_{28}H_{25}N_6NaO_{10}S_2$ = 692.7.

CAS — 84880-03-5 (cefpimizole); 85287-61-2 (cefpimizole sodium).

Cefpimizole sodium is a cephalosporin antibiotic that has been administered parenterally. It has been classified as a third-generation cephalosporin with antipseudomonal activity, but it is generally less active than cefotaxime or ceftazidime.

Preparations

Proprietary Preparations (details are given in Part 3)
Jpn: Renilan†.

Cefpiramide (14940-j)

Cefpiramide *(USAN, rINN)*.

SM-1652; WY-44635. (7*R*)-7-[(*R*)-2-(4-Hydroxy-6-methylnicotinamido)-2-(4-hydroxyphenyl)acetamido]-3-(1-methyl-1*H*-tetrazol-5-ylthiomethyl)-3-cephem-4-carboxylic acid.

$C_{25}H_{24}N_8O_7S_2$ = 612.6.

CAS — 70797-11-4.

Pharmacopoeias. In *US.*

Store in airtight containers.

A 5% suspension in water has a pH of 3.0 to 5.0.

Cefpiramide Sodium (16569-b)

Cefpiramide Sodium *(USAN, rINNM)*.

$C_{25}H_{23}N_8NaO_7S_2$ = 634.6.

CAS — 74849-93-7.

Pharmacopoeias. In *Jpn.*

1.04 g of monograph substance is approximately equivalent to 1 g of cefpiramide. Each g of monograph substance represents about 1.6 mmol of sodium.

Cefpiramide is a third-generation cephalosporin antibiotic related to cefoperazone (p.167) and with similar activity against *Pseudomonas aeruginosa*, but possibly less active against Enterobacteriaceae. Cefpiramide is also active against staphylococci and streptococci and marginal activity against enterococci *in vitro* has been reported. Cefpiramide contains an *N*-methylthiotetrazole side-chain, a structure associated with hypoprothrombinaemia (see Cephamandole, p.180), alcohol intolerance, and potentiation of anticoagulants.

It is given by intravenous injection or infusion as the sodium salt in the treatment of susceptible infections. A usual adult dose is 1 to 2 g daily in two divided doses.

Pharmacokinetic characteristics include a relatively long plasma half-life of about 4.5 hours, extensive plasma protein binding, and high biliary excretion.

References to the antibacterial activity of cefpiramide.

1. Barry AL, *et al.* Cefpiramide: comparative in-vitro activity and β-lactamase stability. *J Antimicrob Chemother* 1985; **16:** 315–25.
2. Quentin C, *et al.* Comparative in vitro activity of cefpiramide, a new parenteral cephalosporin. *Eur J Clin Microbiol Infect Dis* 1988; **7:** 544–9.

References to the pharmacokinetics of cefpiramide.

1. Nakagawa K, *et al.* Pharmacokinetics of cefpiramide (SM-1652) in humans. *Antimicrob Agents Chemother* 1984; **25:** 221–5.
2. Conte JE. Pharmacokinetics of cefpiramide in volunteers with normal or impaired renal function. *Antimicrob Agents Chemother* 1987; **31:** 1585–8.
3. Brogard JM, *et al.* High hepatic excretion in humans of cefpiramide, a new cephalosporin. *Antimicrob Agents Chemother* 1988; **32:** 1360–4.
4. Demotes-Mainard F, *et al.* Pharmacokinetics and protein binding of cefpiramide in patients with alcoholic cirrhosis. *Clin Pharmacol Ther* 1991; **49:** 263–9.
5. Demotes-Mainard F, *et al.* Cefpiramide kinetics and plasma protein binding in cholestasis. *Br J Clin Pharmacol* 1994; **37:** 295–7.

Preparations

USP 23: Cefpiramide for Injection.

Proprietary Preparations (details are given in Part 3)
Jpn: Sepatren.

Cefpirome Sulphate (18924-d)

Cefpirome Sulphate *(BANM, rINNM)*.

Cefpirome Sulfate *(USAN)*; HR-810 (cefpirome or cefpirome sulphate). (*Z*)-7-[2-(2-Aminothiazol-4-yl)-2-methoxyiminoacetamido]-3-(1-pyrindiniomethyl)-3-cephem-4-carboxylate sulphate.

$C_{22}H_{22}N_6O_5S_2,H_2SO_4$ = 612.7.

CAS — 84957-29-9 (cefpirome); 98753-19-6 (cefpirome sulphate).

Adverse Effects and Precautions

As for Cephalothin, p.179. Cefpirome is reported to interfere with the Jaffé method of measuring creatinine concentrations to determine renal function.

References.

1. Rubinstein E, *et al.* A review of the adverse events profile of cefpirome. *Drug Safety* 1993; **9:** 340–5.

Interactions

Probenecid reduces the renal clearance of cefpirome.

Antimicrobial Action

Cefpirome is a fourth-generation cephalosporin antibiotic that is stable to a wide range of beta-lactamases. It has a spectrum of activity similar to that of the third-generation cephalosporin cefotaxime (p.168), but it appears to be more active *in vitro* against staphylococci, some enterococci, some Enterobacteriaceae, and *Pseudomonas aeruginosa*. Cefpirome may be less active than ceftazidime (p.174) against *Ps. aeruginosa*.

References to the antibacterial action of cefpirome *in vitro*.

1. Wise R, *et al.* The antimicrobial activity of cefpirome, a new cephalosporin. *J Antimicrob Chemother* 1985; **15:** 449–56.
2. Jones RN, Fuchs PC. Activity of cefepime (BMY-28142) and cefpirome (HR-810) against Gram-negative bacilli resistant to cefotaxime or ceftazidime. *J Antimicrob Chemother* 1989; **23:** 163–5.
3. Eng RHK, *et al.* In-vitro and in-vivo activity of cefpirome (HR-810) against methicillin-susceptible and -resistant Staphylococcus aureus and Streptococcus faecalis. *J Antimicrob Chemother* 1989; **23:** 373–81.
4. Schäfer V, *et al.* In-vitro activity of cefpirome against isolates from patients with urinary tract, lower respiratory tract and wound infections. *J Antimicrob Chemother* 1992; **29** (suppl A): 7–12.
5. Cheng AFB, *et al.* The antimicrobial activity and β-lactamase stability of cefpirome, a new fourth-generation cephalosporin in comparison with other agents. *J Antimicrob Chemother* 1993; **31:** 699–709.

6. Piérard D, *et al.* Comparative in-vitro activity of cefpirome against isolates from intensive care and haematology/oncology units. *J Antimicrob Chemother* 1998; **41:** 443–50.

Pharmacokinetics

Cefpirome is administered by injection as the sulphate. Mean peak serum concentrations of 80 to 90 μg per mL are attained after a single intravenous 1-g dose. The elimination half-life is about 2 hours and is prolonged in patients with renal impairment. Cefpirome is less than 10% bound to plasma proteins.

Cefpirome is widely distributed into body tissues and fluids. It is mainly excreted by the kidneys and 80 to 90% of a dose is recovered unchanged in the urine. Significant amounts are removed by haemodialysis.

References.

1. Kavi J, *et al.* Pharmacokinetics and tissue penetration of cefpirome, a new cephalosporin. *J Antimicrob Chemother* 1988; **22:** 911–16.
2. Saxby MF, *et al.* Penetration of cefpirome in prostatic tissue. *J Antimicrob Chemother* 1990; **25:** 488–90.
3. Baldwin DR, *et al.* The penetration of cefpirome into the potential sites of pulmonary infection. *J Antimicrob Chemother* 1991; **28:** 79–86.
4. Wilcox MH, *et al.* Relationship between cefpirome clearance, serum creatinine, weight and age in patients treated for infection. *J Antimicrob Chemother* 1991; **28:** 291–9.
5. Nakayama I, *et al.* Single- and multiple-dose pharmacokinetics of intravenous cefpirome (HR-810) to healthy volunteers. *J Clin Pharmacol* 1992; **32:** 256–66.
6. Veys N, *et al.* Single-dose pharmacokinetics of cefpirome in patients receiving hemodialysis and in patients treated by continuous ambulatory peritoneal dialysis. *Clin Pharmacol Ther* 1993; **54:** 395–401.
7. Strenkoski LC, Nix DE. Cefpirome clinical pharmacokinetics. *Clin Pharmacokinet* 1993; **25:** 263–73.
8. Nahata MC, *et al.* Pharmacokinetics of cefpirome in pediatric patients. *Antimicrob Agents Chemother* 1995; **39:** 2348–9.
9. Friedland IR, *et al.* Concentrations of cefpirome in cerebrospinal fluid of children with bacterial meningitis after a single intravenous dose. *Antimicrob Agents Chemother* 1998; **42:** 199–201.

Uses and Administration

Cefpirome is a fourth-generation cephalosporin antibiotic used in the treatment of infections due to susceptible organisms. They include infections of the urinary tract, respiratory tract, and skin, and also septicaemia and infections in immunocompromised patients. For details of these infections and their treatment, see under Choice of Antibacterial, p.116.

Cefpirome is given by intravenous injection over 3 to 5 minutes or infusion over 20 to 30 minutes as the sulphate in doses of 1 or 2 g every 12 hours.

Dosage should be reduced in renal impairment. The manufacturers recommend a loading dose of 1 or 2 g depending on the severity of infection, followed by suitable maintenance doses according to creatinine clearance and severity of infection: creatinine clearance 20 to 50 mL per minute, 0.5 or 1 g twice daily; 5 to 20 mL per minute, 0.5 or 1 g once daily; 5 mL per minute or less (in haemodialysis patients), 0.5 or 1 g once daily plus a half-dose after each dialysis session.

References.

1. Brown EM, *et al.* eds. Cefpirome: a novel extended spectrum cephalosporin. *J Antimicrob Chemother* 1992; **29** (suppl A): 1–104.
2. Wiseman LR, Lamb HM. Cefpirome: a review of its antibacterial activity, pharmacokinetic properties and clinical efficacy in the treatment of severe nosocomial infections and febrile neutropenia. *Drugs* 1997; **54:** 117–40.

Preparations

Proprietary Preparations (details are given in Part 3)
Aust.: Cedixen; Cefrom; ***Austral.:*** Cefrom; ***Belg.:*** Cefrom; ***Fr.:*** Cefrom; ***Neth.:*** Cefrom; ***Swed.:*** Cefrom; ***Switz.:*** Cefrom; ***UK:*** Cefrom.

Cefpodoxime Proxetil (1990-q)

Cefpodoxime Proxetil *(BANM, USAN, rINNM).*

CS-807; U-76252. The 1-[(isopropoxycarbonyl)oxy]ethyl ester of (*Z*)-7-[2-(2-amino-1,3-thiazol-4-yl)-2-methoxyiminoacetamido]-3-methoxymethyl-3-cephem-4-carboxylic acid.

$C_{21}H_{27}N_5O_9S_2$ = 557.6.

CAS — 80210-62-4 (cefpodoxime); 87239-81-4 (cefpodoxime proxetil).

1.3 g of cefpodoxime proxetil is approximately equivalent to 1 g of cefpodoxime.

Adverse Effects and Precautions

As for Cephalothin Sodium, p.179.

The most frequently reported adverse effects of cefpodoxime are gastro-intestinal disturbances, especially diarrhoea.

Interactions

Absorption of cefpodoxime is decreased by concurrent ingestion of antacids or histamine H_2-receptor antagonists. Probenecid reduces the renal excretion of cefpodoxime.

Antimicrobial Action

As for Cefixime, p.165. Cefpodoxime also has some activity against *Staphylococcus aureus*, and may be more active than cefixime against penicillin-resistant strains of *Streptococcus pneumoniae*.

References.

1. Valentini S, *et al.* In-vitro evaluation of cefpodoxime. *J Antimicrob Chemother* 1994; **33:** 495–508.

Pharmacokinetics

Cefpodoxime proxetil is de-esterified in the intestinal epithelium following oral administration, to release active cefpodoxime in the bloodstream. Bioavailability is about 50% in fasting subjects and may be increased in the presence of food. Absorption is decreased in conditions of low gastric acidity. Plasma concentrations of about 1.5, 2.5, and 4.0 μg per mL have been achieved 2 to 3 hours after oral doses of 100, 200, and 400 mg cefpodoxime respectively. About 20 to 30% of cefpodoxime is bound to plasma proteins. The plasma half-life is about 2 to 3 hours and is prolonged in patients with impaired renal function.

Cefpodoxime reaches therapeutic concentrations in the respiratory and genito-urinary tracts and bile. It has been detected in low concentrations in breast milk.

Cefpodoxime is excreted unchanged in the urine. It is removed by dialysis.

Pharmacokinetics of cefpodoxime.

1. Hughes GS, *et al.* Effects of gastric pH and food on the pharmacokinetics of a new oral cephalosporin, cefpodoxime proxetil. *Clin Pharmacol Ther* 1989; **46:** 674–85.
2. O'Neill P, *et al.* Pharmacokinetics and inflammatory fluid penetration of cefpodoxime proxetil in volunteers. *Antimicrob Agents Chemother* 1990; **34:** 232–4.
3. Borin MT, *et al.* Pharmacokinetics of cefpodoxime in plasma and skin blister fluid following oral dosing of cefpodoxime proxetil. *Antimicrob Agents Chemother* 1990; **34:** 1094–9.
4. Borin MT, *et al.* Pharmacokinetic and tolerance studies of cefpodoxime after single- and multiple-dose oral administration of cefpodoxime proxetil. *J Clin Pharmacol* 1991; **31:** 1137–45.
5. Peter JVS, *et al.* Disposition of cefpodoxime proxetil in healthy volunteers and patients with impaired renal function. *Antimicrob Agents Chemother* 1992; **36:** 126–31.
6. Muller-Serieys C, *et al.* Penetration of cefpodoxime proxetil in lung parenchyma and epithelial lining fluid of non-infected patients. *Antimicrob Agents Chemother* 1992; **36:** 2099–2103.
7. Borin MT, *et al.* Disposition of cefpodoxime proxetil in hemodialysis patients. *J Clin Pharmacol* 1992; **32:** 1038–44.
8. Johnson CA, *et al.* Pharmacokinetics and ex vivo susceptibility of cefpodoxime proxetil in patients receiving continuous ambulatory peritoneal dialysis. *Antimicrob Agents Chemother* 1993; **37:** 2650–5.
9. Borin MT, *et al.* Pharmacokinetics of cefpodoxime proxetil in healthy young and elderly volunteers. *J Clin Pharmacol* 1994; **34:** 774–81.
10. Borin MT, Forbes KK. Effect of food on absorption of cefpodoxime proxetil oral suspension in adults. *Antimicrob Agents Chemother* 1995; **39:** 273–5.
11. Takasugi N, *et al.* Penetration of cefpodoxime into uterine and vaginal secretions from postpartum women after a single oral dose of cefpodoxime proxetil. *Antimicrob Agents Chemother* 1996; **40:** 1832–4.

Uses and Administration

Cefpodoxime is a third-generation cephalosporin antibiotic used similarly to cefixime (p.166) in the treatment of susceptible infections. It is given by mouth as the proxetil ester which is hydrolysed on absorption to cefpodoxime. Doses are expressed in terms of the equivalent amount of cefpodoxime. Absorption may be enhanced if cefpodoxime proxetil is administered with food. The usual adult dose is 100 to 200 mg every 12 hours for respiratory-tract and urinary-tract infections. A dose of 200 or 400 mg every 12 hours may be given for skin infections. In children doses of 8 to 10 mg per kg body-weight daily may be given as a single dose or in two divided doses, up to a maximum of 200 mg daily for respiratory-tract infections or 400 mg daily for otitis media.

The interval between doses should be extended in patients with severe renal impairment (creatinine clearance of less than about 40 mL per minute).

For uncomplicated gonorrhoea, a single dose of 200 mg may be given.

References.

1. Moore EP, *et al.*, eds. Cefpodoxime proxetil: a third-generation oral cephalosporin. *J Antimicrob Chemother* 1990; **26** (suppl E): 1–101.
2. Adam D, *et al.*, eds. Cefpodoxime proxetil: a new third generation oral cephalosporin. *Drugs* 1991; **42** (suppl 3): 1–66.
3. Frampton JE, *et al.* Cefpodoxime proxetil: a review of its antibacterial activity, pharmacokinetic properties and therapeutic potential. *Drugs* 1992; **44:** 889–917.
4. Chocas EC, *et al.* Cefpodoxime proxetil: a new, broad-spectrum, oral cephalosporin. *Ann Pharmacother* 1993; **27:** 1369–77.

Preparations

Proprietary Preparations (details are given in Part 3)
Aust.: Biocef; Otreon; ***Austral.:*** Orelox; ***Fr.:*** Cefodox†; Orelox; ***Ger.:*** Orelox; Podomexef; ***Irl.:*** Cefodox; ***Ital.:*** Cefodox; Orelox; Otreon; ***Jpn:*** Banan; ***Neth.:*** Orelox; ***S.Afr.:*** Orelox; ***Spain:*** Orelox; Otreon; ***Swed.:*** Orelox; ***Switz.:*** Orelox; Podomexef; ***UK:*** Orelox; ***USA:*** Vantin.

Cefprozil (9390-n)

Cefprozil *(BAN, USAN, rINN).*

BMY-28100-03-800; BMY-28100 (*cis* isomer); BMY-28167 (*trans* isomer). (6*R*,7*R*)-7-[(*R*)-2-Amino-2-(*p*-hydroxyphenyl)acetamido]-8-oxo-3-(1-propenyl)-5-thia-1-azabicyclo[4.2.0]oct-2-ene-2-carboxylic acid monohydrate; 7-(D-4-Hydroxyphenylglycylamino)-3-[(*E*)prop-1-enyl]cephem-4-carboxylic acid monohydrate.

$C_{18}H_{19}N_3O_5S,H_2O$ = 407.4.

CAS — 92665-29-7 (anhydrous cefprozil); 121123-17-9 (cefprozil monohydrate).

Pharmacopoeias. In US.

1.05 g of monograph substance is approximately equivalent to 1 g of anhydrous cefprozil. A 0.5% solution in water has a pH of 3.5 to 6.5. **Store** in airtight containers.

Adverse Effects and Precautions

As for Cephalexin, p.178.

Hypersensitivity. Serum sickness-like reactions were reported in 4 patients, 3 of them children, given cefprozil.[1] Such reactions have been associated with cefaclor (p.163), but whether they represent a class-related hypersensitivity reaction is not yet clear.

1. Lowery N, *et al.* Serum sickness-like reactions associated with cefprozil therapy. *J Pediatr* 1994; **125:** 325–8.

Interactions

As for Cephalexin, p.178.

Antimicrobial Action

Cefprozil is bactericidal and has antimicrobial activity similar to that of cefaclor (p.163).

References.

1. Leitner F, *et al.* BMY-28100, a new oral cephalosporin. *Antimicrob Agents Chemother* 1987; **31:** 238–43.
2. Chin N-X, Neu HC. Comparative antibacterial activity of a new oral cephalosporin, BMY-28100. *Antimicrob Agents Chemother* 1987; **31:** 480–3.
3. Scribner RK, *et al.* In vitro activity of BMY-28100 against common isolates from pediatric infections. *Antimicrob Agents Chemother* 1987; **31:** 630–1.
4. Eliopoulos GM, *et al.* In vitro activity of BMY-28100, a new oral cephalosporin. *Antimicrob Agents Chemother* 1987; **31:** 653–6.
5. Arguedas AG, *et al.* In-vitro activity of cefprozil (BMY-28100) and loracarbef (LY-163892) against pathogens obtained from middle ear fluid. *J Antimicrob Chemother* 1991; **27:** 311–18.

Pharmacokinetics

Cefprozil is well absorbed from the gastro-intestinal tract with a reported bioavailability of 90 to 95%. Doses of 250, 500, and 1000 mg by mouth produce peak plasma concentrations of 6, 10, and 18 μg per mL respectively at 1 to 2 hours. The presence of food is reported to have little or no effect on the absorption of cefprozil. A plasma half-life of 1 to 1.4 hours has been reported; it is increased in patients with impaired renal function, up to about 6 hours in those with end-stage renal failure. Approximately 35 to 45% of cefprozil is bound to plasma proteins.

Cefprozil is widely distributed in the body tissues. Concentrations of cefprozil in tonsillar and adenoidal tissue are reported to be about 40 to 50% of those in plasma, and less than 0.3% of a 1000-mg dose has been recovered in breast milk in 24 hours. About 60% of a dose is excreted unchanged in the urine in the first 8 hours by glomerular filtration and tubular secretion. High concentrations of cefprozil are achieved in the urine; concentrations of 700, 1000, and 2900 μg per mL have been reported within 4 hours of doses of 250, 500, and 1000 mg respectively. Some cefprozil is removed by haemodialysis.

References.

1. Nye K, *et al.* Pharmacokinetics and tissue penetration of cefprozil. *J Antimicrob Chemother* 1990; **25:** 831–5.
2. Barbhaiya RH, *et al.* Comparison of cefprozil and cefaclor pharmacokinetics and tissue penetration. *Antimicrob Agents Chemother* 1990; **34:** 1204–9.
3. Barbhaiya RH, *et al.* Comparison of the effects of food on the pharmacokinetics of cefprozil and cefaclor. *Antimicrob Agents Chemother* 1990; **34:** 1210–13.
4. Sáez-Llorens X, *et al.* Pharmacokinetics of cefprozil in infants and children. *Antimicrob Agents Chemother* 1990; **34:** 2152–5.
5. Shyu WC, *et al.* Pharmacokinetics of cefprozil in healthy subjects and patients with renal impairment. *J Clin Pharmacol* 1991; **31:** 362–71.
6. Shyu WC, *et al.* Pharmacokinetics of cefprozil in healthy subjects and patients with hepatic impairment. *J Clin Pharmacol* 1991; **31:** 372–6.
7. Lode H, *et al.* Multiple-dose pharmacokinetics of cefprozil and its impact on intestinal flora of volunteers. *Antimicrob Agents Chemother* 1992; **36:** 144–9.
8. Shyu WC, *et al.* Oral absolute bioavailability and intravenous dose-proportionality of cefprozil in humans. *J Clin Pharmacol* 1992; **32:** 798–803.
9. Shyu WC, *et al.* Penetration of cefprozil into tonsillar and adenoidal tissues. *Antimicrob Agents Chemother* 1993; **37:** 1080–3.
10. Shyu WC, *et al.* Penetration of cefprozil into middle ear fluid of patients with otitis media. *Antimicrob Agents Chemother* 1994; **38:** 2210–12.

Uses and Administration

Cefprozil is an oral cephalosporin antibiotic consisting of *cis* and *trans* isomers in a ratio of about 90:10. It is used similarly to cefaclor (p.163) in the treatment of susceptible infections, including upper and lower respiratory-tract infections and skin and soft tissue infections, and should probably be classified as a second-generation cephalosporin.

Cefprozil is given as the monohydrate. Doses are expressed in terms of the equivalent amount of anhydrous cefprozil. The usual adult dose is 250 or 500 mg twice daily or 500 mg once daily. A suggested dose for children is 7.5 or 15 mg per kg bodyweight every twelve hours. Doses may be reduced in patients with impaired renal function; half the standard dose has been suggested for patients with a creatinine clearance of less than 30 mL per minute.

Reviews.

1. Wiseman LR, Benfield P. Cefprozil: a review of its antibacterial activity, pharmacokinetic properties, and therapeutic potential. *Drugs* 1993; **45:** 295–317.
2. Barriere SL. Review of in vitro activity, pharmacokinetic characteristics, safety, and clinical efficacy of cefprozil, a new oral cephalosporin. *Ann Pharmacother* 1993; **27:** 1082–9.

Preparations

USP 23: Cefprozil for Oral Suspension; Cefprozil Tablets.

Proprietary Preparations (details are given in Part 3)
Canad.: Cefzil; ***S.Afr.:*** Prozef; ***Spain:*** Arzimol; Brisoral; ***UK:*** Cefzil; ***USA:*** Cefzil.

Cefquinome (6466-b)

Cefquinome *(BAN, rINN).*

HR111V. (Z)-7-[2-(2-Amino-1,3-thiazol-4-yl)-2-(methoxyimino)acetamido]-3-(5,6,7,8-tetrahydroquinoliniomethyl)-3-cephem-4-carboxylate.

$C_{23}H_{24}N_6O_5S_2$ = 528.6.

CAS — 84957-30-2 (cefquinome); 123766-80-3 (cefquinome sulphate).

NOTE. Cefquinome Sulfate is *USAN.*

Cefquinome is a fourth-generation cephalosporin antibacterial used in veterinary medicine.

Cefroxadine (12543-p)

Cefroxadine *(USAN, rINN).*

CGP-9000. (7R)-[D-2-Amino-2-(cyclohexa-1,4-dienyl)acetamido]-3-methoxy-3-cephem-4-carboxylic acid.

$C_{16}H_{19}N_3O_5S$ = 365.4.

CAS — 51762-05-1.

Pharmacopoeias. Jpn includes the dihydrate.

Cefroxadine is a cephalosporin antibiotic with actions and uses similar to those of cephalexin (p.178). It has been given by mouth in doses of 0.5 to 2 g daily in divided doses.

References.

1. Scaglione F, *et al.* Cefroxadine in the treatment of children affected by respiratory and ENT diseases: a multicentre study involving 1072 in-patients. *Drugs Exp Clin Res* 1989; **15:** 71–6.

Preparations

Proprietary Preparations (details are given in Part 3)
Ital.: Oraspor†.

Cefsulodin Sodium (12544-s)

Cefsulodin Sodium *(BANM, USAN, rINNM).*

Abbott-46811; CGP-7174E; SCE-129; Sulcephalosporin Sodium. Sodium 3-(4-carbamoylpyridiniomethyl)-7-[(2R)-2-phenyl-2-sulphoacetamido]-3-cephem-4-carboxylate.

$C_{22}H_{19}N_4NaO_8S_2$ = 554.5.

CAS — 62587-73-9 (cefsulodin); 52152-93-9 (cefsulodin sodium).

Pharmacopoeias. In *Jpn.*

1.04 g of monograph substance is approximately equivalent to 1 g of cefsulodin. Each g of monograph substance represents about 1.8 mmol of sodium.

Adverse Effects and Precautions

As for Cephalothin Sodium, p.179.

Antimicrobial Action

Cefsulodin is a bactericidal antibiotic with activity against *Pseudomonas aeruginosa* as great as that of ceftazidime (p.174), but no significant activity against other Gram-negative bacteria. Gram-positive bacteria and anaerobes are not very susceptible. Its activity against *Ps. aeruginosa* may be enhanced by aminoglycosides.

Cefsulodin is stable to hydrolysis by many beta-lactamases, but emergence of resistant *Ps. aeruginosa* has been reported during treatment with cefsulodin.

Pharmacokinetics

Cefsulodin is administered parenterally as the sodium salt. It has a plasma half-life of approximately 1.6 hours, prolonged in renal impairment. Up to 30% of cefsulodin in the circulation is bound to plasma proteins. Therapeutic concentrations have been reported in a wide range of body tissues and fluids. The major route of excretion of cefsulodin is via the urine, mainly by glomerular filtration. Clearance may be enhanced in cystic fibrosis, although there have been conflicting reports.

References.

1. Granneman GR, *et al.* Cefsulodin kinetics in healthy subjects after intramuscular and intravenous injection. *Clin Pharmacol Ther* 1982; **31:** 95–103.
2. Reed MD, *et al.* Single-dose pharmacokinetics of cefsulodin in patients with cystic fibrosis. *Antimicrob Agents Chemother* 1984; **25:** 579–81.
3. Hedman A, *et al.* Increased renal clearance of cefsulodin due to higher glomerular filtration rate in cystic fibrosis. *Clin Pharmacokinet* 1990; **18:** 168–75.

Uses and Administration

Cefsulodin is a third-generation cephalosporin antibiotic with a narrow spectrum of activity that has been used similarly to ceftazidime (below) for the treatment of infections caused by susceptible strains of *Pseudomonas aeruginosa.*

It is administered as the sodium salt by intramuscular injection, or intravenously by slow injection or by infusion. Doses are expressed in terms of the equivalent amount of cefsulodin. The usual dose for adults is 1 to 4 g daily in two to four divided doses; in severe infections daily doses of 6 g or more may be required. Children may be given doses of 20 to 50 mg per kg body-weight daily; up to 100 mg per kg daily has been given in severe infections.

Patients with renal impairment should be given cefsulodin sodium in a usual loading dose; subsequent doses should be reduced or the dosage interval prolonged.

References.

1. Smith BR. Cefsulodin and ceftazidime, two antipseudomonal cephalosporins. *Clin Pharm* 1984; **3:** 373–85.
2. Wright DB. Cefsulodin. *Drug Intell Clin Pharm* 1986; **20:** 845–9.

Preparations

Proprietary Preparations (details are given in Part 3)
Aust.: Monaspor; Pseudocef; ***Fr.:*** Pyocefal; ***Ger.:*** Pseudocef; ***Jpn:*** Takesulin; ***Neth.:*** Monaspor†; ***UK:*** Monaspor†.

Ceftazidime (12545-w)

Ceftazidime *(BAN, USAN, rINN).*

GR-20263; LY-139381. (Z)-(7R)-7-[2-(2-Aminothiazol-4-yl)-2-(1-carboxy-1-methylethoxyimino)acetamido]-3-(1-pyridiniomethyl)-3-cephem-4-carboxylate pentahydrate.

$C_{22}H_{22}N_6O_7S_2,5H_2O$ = 636.7.

CAS — 72558-82-8 (anhydrous ceftazidime); 78439-06-2 (ceftazidime pentahydrate).

Pharmacopoeias. In *Pol.* and *US.*

A white to cream coloured crystalline powder. Ceftazidime pentahydrate 1.16 g is approximately equivalent to 1 g of anhydrous ceftazidime. Slightly **soluble** in water; practically insoluble in alcohol; soluble in dimethyl sulphoxide; slightly soluble in dimethylformamide and in methyl alcohol; practically insoluble in acetone, in chloroform, in dioxan, in ether, in ethyl acetate, and in toluene; soluble in alkali. A 0.5% solution in water has a pH of 3 to 4. **Store** in airtight containers.

Ceftazidime for injection is available as a dry powder containing ceftazidime together with sodium carbonate. When reconstituted ceftazidime sodium is formed with the evolution of carbon dioxide. An alternative formulation, ceftazidime with arginine, appears to overcome the problems associated with effervescence.[1] In some countries a frozen injection containing ceftazidime sodium is also used.

1. Stiles ML, *et al.* Gas production of three brands of ceftazidime. *Am J Hosp Pharm* 1991; **48:** 1727–9.

Incompatibility. It has been reported that ceftazidime does not cause decreased activity when incubated in solution with *gentamicin*[1] or *tobramycin*[2] at 37°, or when mixed with tobramycin in serum.[3] Ceftazidime and tobramycin[4] were also stable for up to 16 hours at room temperature when combined in a dextrose-containing dialysis solution, and for a further 8 hours at 37°. However the manufacturers recommend that ceftazidime, like most other beta-lactams, should not be mixed with an aminoglycoside in the same giving set or syringe because of the potential for inactivation of either drug.

Ceftazidime is generally considered to be compatible with *metronidazole*, but degradation of ceftazidime has been reported.[5] Precipitation has occurred with *vancomycin*,[6] although in one study[7] ceftazidime and/or vancomycin were stable in a dextrose-containing peritoneal dialysis solution when kept for 6 days in a refrigerator or 48 to 72 hours at room temperature. Ceftazidime and *teicoplanin*[8] were stable in combination in a peritoneal dialysis solution at 37° for 8 hours when it had been stored at 4°, but not when previously stored at 25°. Ceftazidime was not stable when mixed in solution with *aminophylline*.[9] There was some evidence of possible incompatibility with *pentamidine*.[10]

1. Elliott TSJ, *et al.* Stability of gentamicin in combination with selected new β-lactam antibiotics. *J Antimicrob Chemother* 1984; **14:** 668–9.
2. Elliott TSJ, *et al.* Stability of tobramycin in combination with selected new β-lactam antibiotics. *J Antimicrob Chemother* 1986; **17:** 680–1.
3. Pennell AT, *et al.* Effect of ceftazidime, cefotaxime, and cefoperazone on serum tobramycin concentrations. *Am J Hosp Pharm* 1991; **48:** 520–2.
4. Mason NA, *et al.* Stability of ceftazidime and tobramycin sulfate in peritoneal dialysis solution. *Am J Hosp Pharm* 1992; **49:** 1139–42.
5. Messerschmidt W. Pharmazeutische kompatibilität von ceftazidim und metronidazol. *Pharm Ztg* 1990; **135:** 36–8.
6. Cairns CJ, Robertson J. Incompatibility of ceftazidime and vancomycin. *Pharm J* 1987; **238:** 577.
7. Vaughan LM, Poon CY. Stability of ceftazidime and vancomycin alone and in combination in heparinized and non-heparinized peritoneal dialysis solution. *Ann Pharmacother* 1994; **28:** 572–6
8. Manduru M. *et al.* Stability of ceftazidime sodium and teicoplanin sodium in a peritoneal dialysis solution. *Am J Health-Syst Pharm* 1996; **53:** 2731–4.
9. Pleasants RA, *et al.* Compatibility of ceftazidime and aminophylline admixtures for different methods of intravenous infusion. *Ann Pharmacother* 1992; **26:** 1221–6.
10. Lewis JD. El-Gendy A. Cephalosporin-pentamidine isethionate incompatibilities. *Am J Health-Syst Pharm* 1996; **53:** 1462–3.

Stability. References.

1. Richardson BL, *et al.* The pharmacy of ceftazidime. *J Antimicrob Chemother* 1981; **8** (suppl B): 233–6.
2. Brown AF, *et al.* Freeze thaw stability of ceftazidime. *Br J Parenter Ther* 1985; **6:** 43, 45, 50.
3. Walker SE, Dranitsaris G. Ceftazidime stability in normal saline and dextrose in water. *Can J Hosp Pharm* 1988; **41:** 65–6, 69–71.
4. Wade CS, *et al.* Stability of ceftazidime and amino acids in parenteral nutrient solutions. *Am J Hosp Pharm* 1991; **48:** 1515–19.
5. Stiles ML, *et al.* Stability of ceftazidime (with arginine) and of cefuroxime sodium in infusion-pump reservoirs. *Am J Hosp Pharm* 1992; **49:** 2761–4.
6. Stewart JT, *et al.* Stability of ceftazidime in plastic syringes and glass vials under various storage conditions. *Am J Hosp Pharm* 1992; **49:** 2765–8.
7. Nahata MC, *et al.* Stability of ceftazidime (with arginine) stored in plastic syringes at three temperatures. *Am J Hosp Pharm* 1992; **49:** 2954–6.
8. Bednar DA, *et al.* Stability of ceftazidime (with arginine) in an elastomeric infusion device. *Am J Health-Syst Pharm* 1995; **52:** 1912–14.

9. van Doorne H, *et al.* Ceftazidime degradation rates for predicting stability in a portable infusion-pump reservoir. *Am J Health-Syst Pharm* 1996; **53:** 1302–5.
10. Stendal TL, *et al.* Drug stability and pyridine generation in ceftazidime injection stored in an elastomeric infusion device. *Am J Health-Syst Pharm* 1998; **55:** 683–5.

Adverse Effects and Precautions

As for Cephalothin Sodium, p.179.

Like cefotaxime (p.168), ceftazidime has the potential for colonisation and superinfection with resistant organisms. The risk of superinfection with, for example, *Staphylococcus aureus* may be higher than with cefotaxime, since ceftazidime is less active against staphylococci.

Effects on the blood. References.

1. Hui CH, Chan LC. Agranulocytosis associated with cephalosporin. *Br Med J* 1993; **307:** 484.

Effects on the nervous system. References.

1. Al-Zahawi MF, *et al.* Hallucinations in association with ceftazidime. *Br Med J* 1988; **297:** 858.
2. Jackson GD, Berkovic SL. Ceftazidime encephalopathy: absence status and toxic hallucinations. *J Neurol Neurosurg Psychiatry* 1992; **55:** 33–4.

Effects on the skin. References.

1. Vinks SATMM, *et al.* Photosensitivity due to ambulatory intravenous ceftazidime in cystic fibrosis patient. *Lancet* 1993; **341:** 1221–2.

Interactions

Unlike many other cephalosporins, probenecid has little effect on the renal clearance of ceftazidime.

References.

1. Verhagen CA, *et al.* The renal clearance of cefuroxime and ceftazidime and the effect of probenecid on their tubular excretion. *Br J Clin Pharmacol* 1994; **37:** 193–7.

Antimicrobial Action

Ceftazidime has a bactericidal action and broad spectrum of activity similar to that of cefotaxime (p.168), but increased activity against *Pseudomonas* spp.; it is less active against staphylococci and streptococci. Unlike cefotaxime it has no active metabolite.

Ceftazidime is highly stable to hydrolysis by most beta-lactamases. It is active *in vitro* against many Gram-negative bacteria including *Pseudomonas aeruginosa*, *Burkholderia (Pseudomonas) pseudomallei*, and Enterobacteriaceae including *Citrobacter* and *Enterobacter* spp., *Escherichia coli*, *Klebsiella* spp., both indole-positive and indole-negative *Proteus*, *Providencia*, *Salmonella*, *Serratia*, and *Shigella* spp. and *Yersinia enterocolitica*. Other susceptible Gram-negative bacteria include *Haemophilus influenzae*, *Moraxella (Branhamella) catarrhalis*, and *Neisseria* spp. Among Gram-positive bacteria it is active against some staphylococci and streptococci, but methicillin-resistant staphylococci, enterococci, and *Listeria monocytogenes* are generally resistant. Ceftazidime is active against some anaerobes, although most strains of *Bacteroides fragilis* and *Clostridium difficile* are resistant.

Minimum inhibitory concentrations (MICs) of 8 μg or less per mL have been taken to indicate susceptibility to ceftazidime and MICs of 32 μg or more per mL, resistance. An MIC of about 4 μg per mL has been reported for *Ps. aeruginosa*.

The activity of ceftazidime against *Pseudomonas aeruginosa* and some Enterobacteriaceae may be enhanced by aminoglycosides. Antagonism has been reported *in vitro* between ceftazidime and chloramphenicol.

Resistance. As with cefotaxime, resistance may develop during treatment due to the derepression of chromosomally mediated beta-lactamases. It has been noted particularly in *Pseudomonas* spp. and in Enterobacteriaceae including *Citrobacter*, *Enterobacter* spp. and *Proteus vulgaris*. Resistance may also occur due to the production of plasmid-mediated extended-spectrum beta-lactamases, particularly in *Klebsiella* spp. and *E. coli*.

Pharmacokinetics

Ceftazidime is administered by injection as the sodium salt or in solution with arginine. Mean peak plasma concentrations of 17 and 39 μg per mL have been reported approximately one hour after intramuscular administration of 0.5 and 1 g of ceftazidime, respectively. Five minutes after intravenous bolus injections of 0.5, 1, and 2 g of ceftazidime, mean plasma concentrations of 45, 90, and 170 μg per mL, respectively, have been reported. The plasma half-life of ceftazidime is about 2 hours, but this is prolonged in patients with renal impairment and in neonates. Clearance may be enhanced in patients with cystic fibrosis. It is about 10% bound to plasma proteins.

Ceftazidime is widely distributed in body tissues and fluids; therapeutic concentrations are achieved in the CSF when the meninges are inflamed. It crosses the placenta and is distributed into breast milk.

Ceftazidime is passively excreted in bile, although only a small proportion is eliminated by this route. It is mainly excreted by the kidneys, almost exclusively by glomerular filtration; probenecid has little effect on the excretion. About 80 to 90% of a dose is recovered unchanged in the urine within 24 hours. It is removed by haemodialysis and peritoneal dialysis.

Studies of the pharmacokinetics of ceftazidime.

a. General.

1. Mouton JW, *et al.* Pharmacokinetics of ceftazidime in serum and suction blister fluid during continuous and intermittent infusions in healthy volunteers. *Antimicrob Agents Chemother* 1990; **34:** 2307–11.
2. Bressolle F, *et al.* Endotracheal and aerosol administrations of ceftazidime in patients with nosocomial pneumonia: pharmacokinetics and absolute bioavailability. *Antimicrob Agents Chemother* 1992; **36:** 1404–11.

b. Biliary excretion.

1. Bouza E, *et al.* Comparison of ceftazidime concentrations in bile and serum. *Antimicrob Agents Chemother* 1983; **24:** 104–6.
2. Leung JWC, *et al.* The effect of obstruction on the biliary excretion of cefoperazone and ceftazidime. *J Antimicrob Chemother* 1990; **25:** 399–406.

c. CNS distribution.

1. Modai J, *et al.* Penetration of ceftazidime into cerebrospinal fluid of patients with bacterial meningitis. *Antimicrob Agents Chemother* 1983; **24:** 126–8.
2. Fong IW, Tomkins KB. Penetration of ceftazidime into the cerebrospinal fluid of patients with and without evidence of meningeal inflammation. *Antimicrob Agents Chemother* 1984; **26:** 115–16.
3. Green HT, *et al.* Penetration of ceftazidime into intracranial abscess. *J Antimicrob Chemother* 1989; **24:** 431–6.
4. Nau R, *et al.* Cerebrospinal fluid ceftazidime kinetics in patients with external ventriculostomies. *Antimicrob Agents Chemother* 1996; **40:** 763–6.

d. Other distribution.

1. O'Donoghue MAT, *et al.* Ceftazidime in middle ear fluid. *J Antimicrob Chemother* 1989; **23:** 664–6.
2. Langer M, *et al.* Penetration of ceftazidime into bronchial secretions in critically ill patients. *J Antimicrob Chemother* 1991; **28:** 925–32.

e. Pharmacokinetics in cystic fibrosis.

1. Leeder JS, *et al.* Ceftazidime disposition in acute and stable cystic fibrosis. *Clin Pharmacol Ther* 1984; **36:** 355–62.
2. Hedman A, *et al.* Influence of the glomerular filtration rate on renal clearance of ceftazidime in cystic fibrosis. *Clin Pharmacokinet* 1988; **15:** 57–65.

f. Pharmacokinetics in premature neonates.

1. van den Anker JN, *et al.* Ceftazidime pharmacokinetics in preterm infants: effects of renal function and gestational age. *Clin Pharmacol Ther* 1995; **58:** 650–9.
2. van den Anker JN, *et al.* Ceftazidime pharmacokinetics in preterm infants: effect of postnatal age and postnatal exposure to indomethacin. *Br J Clin Pharmacol* 1995; **40:** 439–43.
3. van den Anker JN, *et al.* Once-daily versus twice-daily administration of ceftazidime in the preterm infant. *Antimicrob Agents Chemother* 1995; **39:** 2048–50.

g. Pharmacokinetics in the elderly.

1. LeBel M, *et al.* Pharmacokinetics of ceftazidime in elderly volunteers. *Antimicrob Agents Chemother* 1985; **28:** 713–15.
2. Higbee MD, *et al.* Pharmacokinetics of ceftazidime in elderly patients. *Clin Pharm* 1989; **8:** 59–62.
3. Sirgo MA, Norris S. Ceftazidime in the elderly: appropriateness of twice-daily dosing. *DICP Ann Pharmacother* 1991; **25:** 284–8.

h. Pharmacokinetics in hepatic impairment.

1. El Touny M, *et al.* Pharmacokinetics of ceftazidime in patients with liver cirrhosis and ascites. *J Antimicrob Chemother* 1991; **28:** 95–100.

i. Pharmacokinetics in renal impairment.

1. Welage LS, *et al.* Pharmacokinetics of ceftazidime in patients with renal insufficiency. *Antimicrob Agents Chemother* 1984; **25:** 201–4.
2. Leroy A, *et al.* Pharmacokinetics of ceftazidime in normal and uremic subjects. *Antimicrob Agents Chemother* 1984; **25:** 638–42.
3. Ackerman BH, *et al.* Effect of decreased renal function on the pharmacokinetics of ceftazidime. *Antimicrob Agents Chemother* 1984; **25:** 785–6.
4. Lin N-S, *et al.* Single- and multiple-dose pharmacokinetics of ceftazidime in infected patients with varying degrees of renal function. *J Clin Pharmacol* 1989; **29:** 331–7.
5. Kinowski J-M, *et al.* Multiple-dose pharmacokinetics of amikacin and ceftazidime in critically ill patients with septic multiple-organ failure during intermittent hemofiltration. *Antimicrob Agents Chemother* 1993; **37:** 464–73.
6. Demotes-Mainard F, *et al.* Pharmacokinetics of intravenous and intraperitoneal ceftazidime in chronic ambulatory peritoneal dialysis. *J Clin Pharmacol* 1993; **33:** 475–9.

Uses and Administration

Ceftazidime is a third-generation cephalosporin antibiotic with enhanced activity against *Pseudomonas aeruginosa*. It is used in the treatment of susceptible infections (see Antimicrobial Action, above), especially those due to *Pseudomonas* spp. They include biliary-tract infections, bone and joint infections, cystic fibrosis (respiratory-tract infections), endophthalmitis, infections in immunocompromised patients (neutropenic patients), melioidosis, meningitis, peritonitis, pneumonia, upper respiratory-tract infections, septicaemia, skin infections (including burns, ecthyma gangrenosum, and ulceration), surgical infections (prophylaxis), and urinary-tract infections. For details of these infections and their treatment, see under Choice of Antibacterial, p.116.

Administration and dosage. Ceftazidime is available as the pentahydrate but it is formulated with sodium carbonate, to form the sodium salt in solution, or with arginine. Doses are expressed in terms of anhydrous ceftazidime. It is administered by deep intramuscular injection, slow intravenous injection over 3 to 5 minutes, or intravenous infusion over up to 30 minutes. The usual dose for adults ranges from 1 to 6 g daily in divided doses every 8 or 12 hours. The higher doses are used in severe infections especially in immunocompromised patients. In adults with cystic fibrosis who have pseudomonal lung infections, high doses of 90 to 150 mg per kg bodyweight daily in 3 divided doses are used; up to 9 g daily has been given to adults with normal renal function. Single doses of more than 1 g should be given intravenously.

Children are usually given ceftazidime 30 to 100 mg per kg daily in 2 or 3 divided doses, but in severely ill children up to 150 mg per kg daily to a maximum of 6 g daily may be given in 3 divided doses. Neonates and infants up to 2 months old have been given 25 to 60 mg per kg daily in 2 divided doses.

In the elderly the dose should generally not exceed 3 g daily.

In patients with impaired renal function the dosage of ceftazidime may need to be reduced. Following a loading dose of 1 g, maintenance doses are based on the creatinine clearance. Suggested maintenance doses are: creatinine clearance 31 to 50 mL per minute, 1 g every 12 hours; 16 to 30 mL per minute, 1 g every 24 hours; 6 to 15 mL per minute, 0.5 g every 24 hours; and less than 5 mL per minute, 0.5 g every 48 hours. In severe infections these doses may need to be increased by 50%. In these patients ceftazidime trough serum concentrations should not exceed 40 μg per mL. In patients undergoing peritoneal dialysis a loading dose of 1 g may be given followed by 500 mg every 24 hours; ceftazidime sodium may also be added to the dialysis fluid, usually 125 to 250 mg of ceftazidime for 2 litres of dialysis fluid. In patients on haemodialysis a loading dose of 1 g is given and should be repeated after each dialysis period.

For surgical infection prophylaxis in patients undergoing prostatic surgery, a dose of 1 g may be given at induction of anaesthesia and repeated if necessary when the catheter is removed.

Ceftazidime can be used in association with an aminoglycoside, another beta-lactam such as piperacillin, or vancomycin in patients with severe neutropenia, or, if infection with *Bacteroides fragilis* is suspected, in association with an antibiotic such as clindamycin or metronidazole. The drugs should generally be administered separately.

References.

1. Rains CP, *et al.* Ceftazidime: an update of its antibacterial activity, pharmacokinetic properties and therapeutic efficacy. *Drugs* 1995; **49:** 577–617.

Preparations

USP 23: Ceftazidime for Injection; Ceftazidime Injection.

Proprietary Preparations (details are given in Part 3)
Aust.: Fortum; Kefazim; ***Austral.:*** Fortum; ***Belg.:*** Glazidim; Kefadim; ***Canad.:*** Ceptaz; Fortaz; Tazidime; ***Fr.:*** Fortum; ***Ger.:*** Fortum; ***Irl.:*** Fortum; ***Ital.:*** Ceftim; Glazidim; Panzid†; Spectrum; Starcef; ***Neth.:*** Fortum; ***Norw.:*** Fortum; ***S.Afr.:*** Fortum; Kefzim; ***Spain:*** Fortam; Kefamin; Potendal; ***Swed.:*** Fortum; ***Switz.:*** Fortam; ***UK:*** Fortum; Kefadim; ***USA:*** Ceptaz; Fortaz; Tazicef; Tazidime.

Ceftezole Sodium (34-n)

Ceftezole Sodium *(rINNM).*

Sodium (7*R*)-7-[2-(1*H*-tetrazol-1-yl)acetamido]-3-(1,3,4-thiadiazol-2-ylthiomethyl)-3-cephem-4-carboxylate.

$C_{13}H_{11}N_8NaO_4S_3$ = 462.5.

CAS — 26973-24-0 (ceftezole); 41136-22-5 (ceftezole sodium).

Ceftezole is a cephalosporin antibiotic with properties similar to those of cephalothin (p.179). It may be administered as the sodium salt by the intramuscular route.

Preparations

Proprietary Preparations (details are given in Part 3)
Ital.: Alomen.

Ceftibuten (1793-h)

Ceftibuten *(BAN, USAN, rINN).*

7432-S; Sch-39720. 7-[2-(2-Amino-1,3-thiazol-4-yl)-4-carboxyisocrotonamide]-3-cephem-4-carboxylic acid.

$C_{15}H_{14}N_4O_6S_2$ = 410.4.

CAS — 97519-39-6.

Adverse Effects and Precautions

As for Cephalothin Sodium, p.179.

The most frequently reported adverse effects of ceftibuten are gastro-intestinal disturbances, especially diarrhoea, and headache.

Antimicrobial Action

As for Cefixime, p.165. It is less active *in vitro* against *Streptococcus pneumoniae.*

References.

1. Shawar R, *et al.* Comparative in vitro activity of ceftibuten (Sch-39720) against bacterial enteropathogens. *Antimicrob Agents Chemother* 1989; **33:** 781–4.
2. Bragman SGL, Casewell MW. The in-vitro activity of ceftibuten against 475 clinical isolates of Gram-negative bacilli, compared with cefuroxime and cefadroxil. *J Antimicrob Chemother* 1990; **25:** 221–6.
3. Wise R, *et al.* Ceftibuten—in-vitro activity against respiratory pathogens, β-lactamase stability and mechanism of action. *J Antimicrob Chemother* 1990; **26:** 209–13.

Pharmacokinetics

Ceftibuten is rapidly absorbed from the gastro-intestinal tract following oral administration, although the rate and extent of absorption are some what decreased by the presence of food. Peak plasma concentrations of about 17.0 μg per mL are attained about 2 hours after a 400-mg dose. The plasma half-life of ceftibuten is about 2.0 to 2.3 hours and is prolonged in patients with renal impairment. Ceftibuten is 60 to 77% bound to plasma proteins.

Ceftibuten distributes into middle-ear fluid and bronchial secretions. About 10% of a dose is converted to the *trans*-isomer, which has about one-eighth of the activity of the *cis*-isomer. Ceftibuten is excreted mainly in the urine and also in the faeces. Significant amounts are removed by haemodialysis.

References.

1. Wise R, *et al.* Pharmacokinetics and tissue penetration of ceftibuten. *Antimicrob Agents Chemother* 1990; **34:** 1053–5.
2. Kearns GL, *et al.* Single-dose pharmacokinetics of ceftibuten (SCH-39720) in infants and children. *Antimicrob Agents Chemother* 1991; **35:** 2078–84.
3. Kelloway JS, *et al.* Pharmacokinetics of ceftibuten-cis and its trans metabolite in healthy volunteers and in patients with chronic renal insufficiency. *Antimicrob Agents Chemother* 1991; **35:** 2267–74.
4. Kearns GL, Young RA. Ceftibuten pharmacokinetics and pharmacodynamics: focus on paediatric use. *Clin Pharmacokinet* 1994; **26:** 169–89.
5. Lin C, *et al.* Multiple-dose pharmacokinetics of ceftibuten in healthy volunteers. *Antimicrob Agents Chemother* 1995; **39:** 356–8.
6. Lin C, *et al.* Pharmacokinetics and dose proportionality of ceftibuten in men. *Antimicrob Agents Chemother* 1995; **39:** 359–61.
7. Lin C, *et al.* Penetration of ceftibuten into middle ear fluid *Antimicrob Agents Chemother* 1996; **40:** 1394–6.

Uses and Administration

Ceftibuten is an oral third-generation cephalosporin antibiotic used similarly to cefixime (p.166) in the treatment of urinary-tract and respiratory-tract infections. It is given by mouth as the dihydrate, but doses are expressed in terms of anhydrous ceftibuten. The usual adult dose is 400 mg once daily. Children over 6 months of age and weighing 45 kg or less may be given 9 mg per kg body-weight daily as a single dose.

Doses should be reduced in patients with moderate to severe renal impairment (creatinine clearance below 50 mL per minute).

Reviews.

1. Wiseman LR, Balfour JA. Ceftibuten: review of its antibacterial activity, pharmacokinetic properties and clinical efficacy. *Drugs* 1994; **47:** 784–808.
2. Nelson JD, McCracken GH (eds). Ceftibuten: a new orally active cephalosporin for pediatric infections. *Pediatr Infect Dis J* 1995; **14** (suppl): S76–S133.
3. Guay DRP. Ceftibuten: a new expanded-spectrum oral cephalosporin. *Ann Pharmacother* 1997; **31:** 1022–33.

Preparations

Proprietary Preparations (details are given in Part 3)
Aust.: Caedex; ***Ger.:*** Keimax; ***Irl.:*** Cedax; ***Ital.:*** Cedax; Isocef; ***Jpn:*** Seftem; ***Neth.:*** Cedax; ***S.Afr.:*** Cedax; ***Spain:*** Biocef; Cedax; Cepifran; ***Swed.:*** Cedax; ***Switz.:*** Cedax; ***UK:*** Cedax; ***USA:*** Cedax.

Ceftiofur Sodium (3853-j)

Ceftiofur Sodium *(BANM, USAN).*

CM-31-916; CM-31916 (ceftiofur); U-64279A (ceftiofur hydrochloride); U-64279-E. Sodium (6*R*,7*R*)-7-[2-(2-Amino-4-thiazolyl)-glyoxylamido]-3-mercaptomethyl-8-oxo-5-thia-1-azabicyclo[4.2.0]oct-2-ene-2-carboxylate, 7²-(*Z*)-(*O*-methyloxime), 2-furoate (ester).

$C_{19}H_{16}N_5NaO_7S_3$ = 545.5.

CAS — 80370-57-6 (ceftiofur); 103980-44-5 (ceftiofur hydrochloride); 104010-37-9 (ceftiofur sodium);.

Ceftiofur sodium is a cephalosporin antibiotic used in veterinary practice.

Ceftizoxime Sodium (12546-e)

Ceftizoxime Sodium *(BANM, USAN, rINNM).*

FK-749; FR-13749; SKF-88373-Z. Sodium (*Z*)-7-[2-(2-amino-thiazol-4-yl)-2-methoxyiminoacetamido]-3-cephem-4-carboxylate.

$C_{13}H_{12}N_5NaO_5S_2$ = 405.4.

CAS — 68401-81-0 (ceftizoxime); 68401-82-1 (ceftizoxime sodium).

Pharmacopoeias. In *Jpn* and *US.*

A white to pale yellow crystalline powder. 1.06 g of monograph substance is approximately equivalent to 1 g of ceftizoxime. Each g of monograph substance represents about 2.5 mmol of sodium. Freely **soluble** in water. A 10% solution in water has a pH of 6 to 8. **Store** in airtight containers.

References.

1. Lesko AB, *et al.* Ceftizoxime stability in iv solutions. *DICP Ann Pharmacother* 1989; **23:** 615–18.

Adverse Effects and Precautions

As for Cefotaxime Sodium, p.168.

Interactions

Probenecid reduces the renal clearance of ceftizoxime.

Antimicrobial Action

As for Cefotaxime Sodium, p.168, although ceftizoxime has no active metabolite.

Pharmacokinetics

After intramuscular injection of 0.5 and 1 g of ceftizoxime, mean peak plasma concentrations of about 14 and 39 μg per mL respectively have been reported after 1 hour. The plasma half-life of ceftizoxime is about 1.7 hours and is prolonged in neonates and in renal impairment. Only 30% of ceftizoxime in the circulation is bound to plasma proteins.

Ceftizoxime is widely distributed in body tissues and fluids; therapeutic concentrations are achieved in the CSF when the meninges are inflamed. It crosses the placenta and low concentrations have been detected in breast milk.

Nearly all of a dose is excreted unchanged in the urine within 24 hours of administration, thus achieving high urinary concentrations. Ceftizoxime is excreted by tubular secretion as well as glomerular filtration and the concomitant administration of probenecid results in higher and more prolonged plasma concentrations. Some ceftizoxime is removed by dialysis.

References.

1. Jordan NS, *et al.* Comparative pharmacokinetics of ceftizoxime and cefotaxime in healthy volunteers. *Curr Ther Res* 1986; **40:** 133–40.
2. Vallée F, LeBel M. Comparative study of pharmacokinetics and serum bactericidal activity of ceftizoxime and cefotaxime. *Antimicrob Agents Chemother* 1991; **35:** 2057–64.
3. Fujii R. Investigation of half-life and clinical effects of ceftizoxime in premature and newborn infants. *Drug Invest* 1990; **2:** 143–9.
4. Reed MD, *et al.* Ceftizoxime disposition in neonates and infants during the first six months of life. *DICP Ann Pharmacother* 1991; **25:** 344–7.
5. Guglielmo BJ, *et al.* Pharmacokinetics and pharmacodynamics of ceftizoxime in abscess fluid. *J Antimicrob Chemother* 1997; **39:** 437–8.

Uses and Administration

Ceftizoxime is a third-generation cephalosporin antibiotic used similarly to cefotaxime (p.169) for the treatment of susceptible infections.

It is administered as the sodium salt by deep intramuscular injection, or intravenously as a slow injection over 3 to 5 minutes or as a continuous or intermittent infusion. If 2 g of ceftizoxime is injected intramuscularly the dose should be divided between sites.

Doses are expressed in terms of the equivalent amount of ceftizoxime. It is usually given in a dose of 1 to 2 g every 8 to 12 hours. In severe or life-threatening infections 2 to 3 g every 8 hours may be given, although doses of up to 12 g daily have been used. Children over 3 months of age may be given 30 to 60 mg per kg body-weight daily in 2 to 4 divided doses; this may be increased to 100 to 150 mg per kg daily in severe infections.

For the treatment of urinary-tract infections, a dose of 0.5 to 1 g every 12 hours has been used. A single intramuscular dose of 1 g has been given in uncomplicated gonorrhoea.

Doses should be modified in patients with impaired renal function. The manufacturers have suggested the following dosage schedule after a loading dose of 0.5 to 1 g: according to the severity of infection, 0.5 to 1.5 g every 8 hours for those with mild renal impairment (creatinine clearance 50 to 79 mL per minute); 0.25 to 1 g every 12 hours in moderate to severe impairment (creatinine clearance 5 to 49 mL per minute); and 0.25 to 0.5 g every 24 hours or 0.5 to 1 g every 48 hours, after dialysis, for those with a creatinine clearance of less than 5 mL per minute.

References.

1. Richards DM, Heel RC. Ceftizoxime: a review of its antibacterial activity, pharmacokinetic properties and therapeutic use. *Drugs* 1985; **29:** 281–329.

Preparations

USP 23: Ceftizoxime for Injection; Ceftizoxime Injection.

Proprietary Preparations (details are given in Part 3)
Aust.: Cefizox; ***Canad.:*** Cefizox; ***Fr.:*** Cefizox; ***Ger.:*** Ceftix; ***Irl.:*** Cefizox; ***Ital.:*** Eposerin; ***Jpn:*** Epocelin; ***Neth.:*** Cefizox; ***Spain:*** Cefizox; Epocelin; ***UK:*** Cefizox†; ***USA:*** Cefizox.

Ceftriaxone Sodium (12547-l)

Ceftriaxone Sodium *(BANM, USAN, rINNM)*.

Ceftriaxonum Natricum; Ro-13-9904; Ro-13-9904/000 (ceftriaxone). (*Z*)-7-[2-(2-Aminothiazol-4-yl)-2-methoxyiminoacetamido]-3-[(2,5-dihydro-6-hydroxy-2-methyl-5-oxo-1,2,4-triazin-3-yl)thiomethyl]-3-cephem-4-carboxylic acid, disodium salt, sesquaterhydrate.

$C_{18}H_{16}N_8Na_2O_7S_3,3\frac{1}{2}H_2O = 661.6$.

CAS — 73384-59-5 (ceftriaxone); 74578-69-1 (ceftriaxone sodium, anhydrous); 104376-79-6 (ceftriaxone sodium sesquaterhydrate).

Pharmacopoeias. In Eur. (see p.viii), *Pol.*, and *US.*

An almost white to yellowish, slightly hygroscopic, crystalline powder. 1.19 g of monograph substance is approximately equivalent to 1 g of ceftriaxone. Each g of monograph substance represents about 3.0 mmol of sodium.

Freely or very **soluble** in water; very slightly soluble in alcohol and dehydrated alcohol; sparingly soluble in methyl alcohol.

A 10% solution in water has a pH of 6 to 8. **Store** in airtight containers at a temperature not exceeding 30°. Protect from light.

Incompatibility. The UK manufacturer warns of incompatibility if ceftriaxone sodium is mixed with calcium-containing solutions or with aminoglycosides, fluconazole, labetalol, vancomycin, or amsacrine. Published reports of incompatibility have included that between ceftriaxone and vancomycin[1] or pentamidine.[2]

1. Pritts D, Hancock D. Incompatibility of ceftriaxone with vancomycin. *Am J Hosp Pharm* 1991; **48:** 77.
2. Lewis JD, El-Gendy A. Cephalosporin-pentamidine isethionate incompatibilities. *Am J Health-Syst Pharm* 1996; **53:** 1461–2.

Stability. References.

1. Nahata MC. Stability of ceftriaxone sodium in peritoneal dialysis solutions. *DICP Ann Pharmacother* 1991; **25:** 741–2.
2. Canton E, Esteban MJ. Stability of ceftriaxone solution. *J Antimicrob Chemother* 1992; **30:** 397–8.
3. Bailey LC, *et al.* Stability of ceftriaxone sodium in injectable solutions stored frozen in syringes. *Am J Hosp Pharm* 1994; **51:** 2159–61.
4. Plumridge RJ *et al.* Stability of ceftriaxone sodium in polypropylene syringes at −20, 4, and 20°C. *Am J Health-Syst Pharm* 1996; **53:** 2320–3.

Adverse Effects and Precautions

As for Cefotaxime Sodium, p.168.

Changes in bowel flora may be more marked than with cefotaxime because of the greater biliary excretion of ceftriaxone; diarrhoea may occur more often, especially in children. Biliary sludge or pseudolithiasis due to a precipitate of calcium ceftriaxone has been seen occasionally in patients receiving ceftriaxone. Similarly, deposition of the calcium salt has occurred rarely in the urine. Ceftriaxone is highly protein-bound and is able to displace bilirubin from albumin binding sites, causing hyperbilirubinaemia; its use should be avoided in jaundiced neonates.

Neutropenia has been reported with most cephalosporins; a complex mechanism has been attributed to that associated with ceftriaxone. There have been rare reports of fatal haemolysis associated with ceftriaxone.

Ceftriaxone has an *N*-methylthiotriazine ring rather than the *N*-methylthiotetrazole side-chain seen in cephalosporins such as cephamandole (p.180), but might still have the potential to cause hypoprothrombinaemia.

Administration in neonates. References to the displacement of bilirubin by ceftriaxone in neonates.

1. Gulian J-M, *et al.* Bilirubin displacement by ceftriaxone in neonates: evaluation by determination of 'free' bilirubin and erythrocyte-bound bilirubin. *J Antimicrob Chemother* 1987; **19:** 823–9.
2. Fink S, *et al.* Ceftriaxone effect on bilirubin-albumin binding. *Pediatrics* 1987; **80:** 873–5.

Effects on the biliary tract. Using abdominal ultrasonography, biliary sludge or pseudolithiasis was found in about 40% of severely ill children being treated with high doses of ceftriaxone[1] and was later reported in adults.[2,3] The sludge has been identified as a calcium salt of ceftriaxone.[4] Patients are often asymptomatic and the sludge usually dissolves once ceftriaxone is discontinued. Gallstones with ceftriaxone as a major component have been identified in a patient given long-term high-dose treatment.[5] Similarly, a bile-duct stone composed of ceftriaxone occurred with high-dose ceftriaxone in a child.[6]

In another report, intractable hiccups were associated with ceftriaxone-related pseudolithiasis in a 10-year-old boy.[7]

1. Schaad UB, *et al.* Reversible ceftriaxone-associated biliary pseudolithiasis in children. *Lancet* 1988; **ii:** 1411–13.
2. Pigrau C, *et al.* Ceftriaxone-associated biliary pseudolithiasis in adults. *Lancet* 1989; **ii:** 165.
3. Heim-Duthoy KL, *et al.* Apparent biliary pseudolithiasis during ceftriaxone therapy. *Antimicrob Agents Chemother* 1990; **34:** 1146–9.
4. Park HZ, *et al.* Ceftriaxone-associated gallbladder sludge: identification of calcium-ceftriaxone salt as a major component of gallbladder precipitate. *Gastroenterology* 1991; **100:** 1665–70.
5. Lopez AJ, *et al.* Ceftriaxone-induced cholelithiasis. *Ann Intern Med* 1991; **115:** 712–14.
6. Robertson FM, *et al.* Ceftriaxone choledocholithiasis. *Pediatrics* 1996; **98:** 133–5.
7. Bonioli E, *et al.* Pseudolithiasis and intractable hiccups in a boy receiving ceftriaxone. *N Engl J Med* 1994; **331:** 1532.

Effects on the blood. References.

1. Haubenstock A, *et al.* Hypoprothrombinaemic bleeding associated with ceftriaxone. *Lancet* 1983; **i:** 1215–16.
2. Rey D, *et al.* Ceftriaxone-induced granulopenia related to a peculiar mechanism of granulopoiesis inhibition. *Am J Med* 1989; **87:** 591–2.
3. Bernini JC, *et al.* Fatal hemolysis induced by ceftriaxone in a child with sickle cell anemia. *J Pediatr* 1995; **126:** 813–15.
4. Lascari AD, Amyot K. Fatal hemolysis caused by ceftriaxone. *J Pediatr* 1995; **126:** 816–17.
5. Scimeca PG, *et al.* Hemolysis after treatment with ceftriaxone. *J Pediatr* 1996; **128:** 163.

Effects on the gastro-intestinal tract. References.

1. Nahata MC, Miller MA. Diarrhoea associated with ceftriaxone and its implications in paediatric patients. *J Clin Pharm Ther* 1989; **14:** 305–7.
2. Samonis G, *et al.* Prospective evaluation of effects of broad-spectrum antibiotics on gastrointestinal yeast colonization of humans. *Antimicrob Agents Chemother* 1993; **37:** 51–3.

Effects on the pancreas. References.

1. Zimmermann AE, *et al.* Ceftriaxone-induced acute pancreatitis. *Ann Pharmacother* 1993; **27:** 36–7.

Interactions

Ceftriaxone has an *N*-methylthiotriazine side-chain and may have the potential to increase the effects of anticoagulants and to cause a disulfiram-like reaction with alcohol, as may cephalosporins with the related *N*-methylthiotetrazole side chain (see Cephamandole, p.180).

Unlike many cephalosporins, probenecid does not affect the renal excretion of ceftriaxone.

Antimicrobial Action

As for Cefotaxime Sodium, p.168, although ceftriaxone has no active metabolite.

References.

1. Goldstein FW, *et al.* Resistance to ceftriaxone and other β-lactams in bacteria isolated in the community. *Antimicrob Agents Chemother* 1995; **39:** 2516–19.

Pharmacokinetics

Ceftriaxone demonstrates nonlinear dose-dependent pharmacokinetics because of its protein binding; about 85 to 95% is bound to plasma protein depending on the plasma concentration of ceftriaxone.

Mean peak plasma concentrations of about 40 and 80 μg per mL have been reported 2 hours after intramuscular injection of 0.5 and 1 g of ceftriaxone respectively. The plasma half-life of ceftriaxone is not dependent on the dose and varies between 6 and 9 hours; it may be prolonged in neonates. The half-life does not change appreciably in patients with moderate renal impairment, but it may be prolonged in severe renal impairment especially when there is also hepatic impairment.

Ceftriaxone is widely distributed in body tissues and fluids. It crosses both inflamed and non-inflamed meninges, generally achieving therapeutic concentrations in the CSF. It crosses the placenta and low concentrations have been detected in breast milk. High concentrations are achieved in bile.

About 40 to 65% of a dose of ceftriaxone is excreted unchanged in the urine, principally by glomerular filtration; the remainder is excreted in the bile and is ultimately found in the faeces as unchanged drug and microbiologically inactive compounds.

Reviews.

1. Hayton WL, Stoeckel K. Age-associated changes in ceftriaxone pharmacokinetics. *Clin Pharmacokinet* 1986; **11:** 76–86.
2. Yuk JH, *et al.* Clinical pharmacokinetics of ceftriaxone. *Clin Pharmacokinet* 1989; **17:** 223–35.

Some studies of the pharmacokinetics of ceftriaxone.

a. Distribution into the CNS.

1. Latif R, Dajani AS. Ceftriaxone diffusion into cerebrospinal fluid of children with meningitis. *Antimicrob Agents Chemother* 1983; **23:** 46–8.
2. Chandrasekar PH, *et al.* Diffusion of ceftriaxone into the cerebrospinal fluid of adults. *J Antimicrob Chemother* 1984; **14:** 427–30.
3. Lucht F, *et al.* The penetration of ceftriaxone into human brain tissue. *J Antimicrob Chemother* 1990; **26:** 81–6.
4. Nau R, *et al.* Passage of cefotaxime and ceftriaxone into cerebrospinal fluid of patients with uninflamed meninges. *Antimicrob Agents Chemother* 1993; **37:** 1518–24.
5. Gaillard J-L, *et al.* Concentrations of ceftriaxone in cerebrospinal fluid of children with meningitis receiving dexamethasone therapy. *Antimicrob Agents Chemother* 1994; **38:** 1209–10.

b. Pharmacokinetics in hepatobiliary disease.

1. Stoeckel K, *et al.* Single-dose ceftriaxone kinetics in liver insufficiency. *Clin Pharmacol Ther* 1984; **36:** 500–9.
2. Hary L, *et al.* The pharmacokinetics of ceftriaxone and cefotaxime in cirrhotic patients with ascites. *Eur J Clin Pharmacol* 1989; **36:** 613–16.
3. Toth A, *et al.* Pharmacokinetics of ceftriaxone in liver-transplant recipients. *J Clin Pharmacol* 1991; **31:** 722–8.
4. Van Delden OM, *et al.* Biliary excretion of ceftriaxone into non-stagnant and stagnant bile. *J Antimicrob Chemother* 1994; **33:** 193–4.

c. Pharmacokinetics in renal impairment.

The pharmacokinetics of ceftriaxone are not markedly altered in mild to moderate renal impairment,[1] but the half-life can be prolonged in severe or end-stage renal disease.[1-4] Ceftriaxone is generally not removed by peritoneal dialysis[4] or by haemodialysis[1-3] although Garcia and colleagues[5] have reported a decrease in half-life during haemodialysis. In many patients no alteration in dosage is necessary, but some individuals have reduced non-renal clearance despite apparently normal hepatic function.[2,3] It is advisable to monitor plasma ceftriaxone in patients with severe renal impairment and unknown non-renal clearance.

1. Patel IH, *et al.* Ceftriaxone pharmacokinetics in patients with various degrees of renal impairment. *Antimicrob Agents Chemother* 1984; **25:** 438–42.
2. Stoeckel K, *et al.* Single-dose ceftriaxone kinetics in functionally anephric patients. *Clin Pharmacol Ther* 1983; **33:** 633–41.
3. Cohen D, *et al.* Pharmacokinetics of ceftriaxone in patients with renal failure and in those undergoing hemodialysis. *Antimicrob Agents Chemother* 1983; **24:** 529–32.
4. Ti T-Y, *et al.* Kinetic disposition of intravenous ceftriaxone in normal subjects and patients with renal failure on hemodialysis or peritoneal dialysis. *Antimicrob Agents Chemother* 1984; **25:** 83–7.
5. Garcia RL, *et al.* Single-dose pharmacokinetics of ceftriaxone in patients with end-stage renal disease and hemodialysis. *Chemotherapy* 1988; **34:** 261–6.

d. Pharmacokinetics in surgery.

1. Jungbluth GL, *et al.* Ceftriaxone disposition in open-heart surgery patients. *Antimicrob Agents Chemother* 1989; **33:** 850–6.
2. Martin C, *et al.* Pharmacokinetics and tissue penetration of a single dose of ceftriaxone (1,000 milligrams intravenously) for antibiotic prophylaxis in thoracic surgery. *Antimicrob Agents Chemother* 1992; **36:** 2804–7.
3. Martin C, *et al.* Concentrations of prophylacic [sic] ceftriaxone in abdominal tissues during pancreatic surgery. *J Antimicrob Chemother* 1997; **40:** 445–8.
4. Scaglione F, *et al.* Pharmacokinetic study of cefodizime and ceftriaxone in sera and bones of patients undergoing hip arthroplasty. *Antimicrob Agents Chemother* 1997; **41:** 2292–4.

e. Pharmacokinetics in pregnancy and lactation.

1. Bourget P, *et al.* Pharmacokinetics and protein binding of ceftriaxone during pregnancy. *Antimicrob Agents Chemother* 1993; **37:** 54–9.
2. Bourget P, *et al.* Ceftriaxone distribution and protein binding between maternal blood and milk postpartum. *Ann Pharmacother* 1993; **27:** 294–7.

Uses and Administration

Ceftriaxone is a third-generation cephalosporin antibiotic used similarly to cefotaxime for the treatment of susceptible infections. They include chancroid, endocarditis, gastro-enteritis (invasive salmonellosis; shigellosis), gonorrhoea, Lyme disease, meningitis (including meningococcal meningitis prophylaxis), septicaemia, surgical infection (prophylaxis), syphilis, typhoid fever, and Whipple's disease. For details of these infections and their treatment, see under Choice of Antibacterial, p.116.

Administration and dosage. Ceftriaxone is administered as the sodium salt by slow intravenous injection over 2 to 4 minutes, by intermittent intravenous infusion over at least 30 minutes, or by deep intramuscular injection. If more than 1 g is to be injected intramuscularly then the dose should be divided between more than one site. Doses are expressed in terms of the equivalent amount of ceftriaxone. It is usually given to adults in a dose of 1 to 2 g daily as a single dose or in two divided doses; in severe infections up to 4 g daily may be given. Suggested doses for infants and children are 20 to 50 mg per kg body-weight once daily; for severe infections up to 80 mg per kg daily may be given. In neonates, the maximum dose should not exceed 50 mg per kg; intravenous doses in neonates should be given over 60 minutes. Doses above 50 mg per kg should be administered by intravenous infusion only.

A single intramuscular dose of 250 mg is recommended for the treatment of uncomplicated gonorrhoea in adults.

For surgical infection prophylaxis in adults, a single dose of 1 g may be administered 0.5 to 2 hours prior to surgery; a 2-g dose is suggested before colorectal surgery.

For the prevention of secondary cases of meningococcal meningitis a single intramuscular dose of 250 mg has been suggested for adults and 125 mg for children.

A reduction in dosage may be necessary in patients with severe renal impairment and in those with both impaired renal and hepatic function; plasma concentrations should be monitored in such patients.

References.

1. Brogden RN, Ward A. Ceftriaxone: a reappraisal of its antibacterial activity and pharmacokinetic properties, and an update on its therapeutic use with particular reference to once-daily administration. *Drugs* 1988; **35:** 604–45.

Preparations

BP 1998: Ceftriaxone Injection;
USP 23: Ceftriaxone for Injection; Ceftriaxone Injection.

Proprietary Preparations (details are given in Part 3)
Aust.: Rocephin; ***Austral.:*** Rocephin; ***Belg.:*** Rocephine; ***Canad.:*** Rocephin; ***Fr.:*** Rocephine; ***Ger.:*** Rocephin; ***Irl.:*** Rocephin; ***Ital.:*** Rocefin; ***Neth.:*** Rocephin; ***Norw.:*** Rocephalin; ***S.Afr.:*** Rocephin; ***Spain:*** Hosbocin†; Rocefalin; ***Swed.:*** Rocephalin; ***Switz.:*** Rocephine; ***UK:*** Rocephin; ***USA:*** Rocephin.

Cefuroxime (15872-m)

Cefuroxime *(BAN, USAN, rINN).*
640/359. (*Z*)-3-Carbamoyloxymethyl-7-[2-(2-furyl)-2-methoxyiminoacetamido]-3-cephem-4-carboxylic acid.
$C_{16}H_{16}N_4O_8S$ = 424.4.
CAS — 55268-75-2.

Cefuroxime Axetil (16570-x)

Cefuroxime Axetil *(BANM, USAN, rINNM).*
CCI-15641.
$C_{20}H_{22}N_4O_{10}S$ = 510.5.
CAS — 64544-07-6.
Pharmacopoeias. In *Eur.* (see p.viii), *Pol.,* and *US.*

A white or almost white amorphous powder. 1.20 g of cefuroxime axetil is approximately equivalent to 1 g of cefuroxime. Slightly **soluble** in water, in alcohol, in dehydrated alcohol, and in ether; soluble in acetone, in chloroform, in ethyl acetate, and in methyl alcohol.
Store in airtight containers. Protect from light.

Cefuroxime Sodium (35-h)

Cefuroxime Sodium *(BANM, rINNM).*
Cefuroximum Natricum.
$C_{16}H_{15}N_4NaO_8S$ = 446.4.
CAS — 56238-63-2.
Pharmacopoeias. In *Eur.* (see p.viii), *Jpn, Pol.,* and *US.*

1.05 g of cefuroxime sodium is approximately equivalent to 1 g of cefuroxime. Each g of monograph substance represents about 2.2 mmol of sodium.

A white or almost white or faintly yellow, slightly hygroscopic powder. Ph. Eur. **solubilities** are: freely soluble in water, very slightly soluble in alcohol; practically insoluble in ether. The USP has: soluble in water, sparingly soluble in alcohol; insoluble in acetone, in chloroform, in ether, in ethyl acetate, and in toluene. Ph. Eur. states that a 1% solution in water has a pH of 5.5 to 8.5 and the USP that a 10% solution in water has a pH of 6.0 to 8.5.
Store in airtight containers at a temperature not exceeding 25°.

Cefuroxime sodium may be **incompatible** with aminoglycosides.

References.

1. Barnes AR. Chemical stabilities of cefuroxime sodium and metronidazole in an admixture for intravenous infusion. *J Clin Pharm Ther* 1990; **15:** 187–96.
2. Stiles ML, *et al.* Stability of ceftazidime (with arginine) and of cefuroxime sodium in infusion-pump reservoirs. *Am J Hosp Pharm* 1992; **49:** 2761–4.
3. Hebron B, Scott H. Shelf life of cefuroxime eye-drops when dispensed in artificial tear preparations. *Int J Pharm Pract* 1993; **2:** 163–7.

Adverse Effects and Precautions

As for Cephalothin Sodium, p.179.

Gastro-intestinal disturbances, including diarrhoea, nausea, and vomiting, have occurred in some patients receiving cefuroxime axetil. There have been rare reports of erythema multiforme, including the Stevens-Johnson syndrome, and toxic epidermal necrolysis.

Antibiotic-associated colitis. For reports of pseudomembranous colitis associated with cefuroxime axetil, see Cephalothin, p.179.

Interactions

Probenecid reduces the renal clearance of cefuroxime.

Antimicrobial Action

Cefuroxime is bactericidal and has a similar spectrum of antimicrobial action, and pattern of resistance, to that of cephamandole (p.180). It is more resistant to hydrolysis by beta-lactamases than cephamandole, and therefore may be more active against beta-lactamase-producing strains of, for example, *Haemophilus influenzae* and *Neisseria gonorrhoeae.* However, treatment failures have occurred in patients with *H. influenzae* meningitis given cefuroxime and might be associated with a relatively high minimum bactericidal concentration (MBC) when compared with the minimum inhibitory concentration (MIC) or with a significant inoculum effect. Reduced affinity of penicillin-binding proteins for cefuroxime has also been reported responsible for resistance in a beta-lactamase-negative strain of *H. influenzae.*

References.

1. Arditi M, *et al.* Cefuroxime treatment failure and Haemophilus influenzae meningitis: case report and review of literature. *Pediatrics* 1989; **84:** 132–5.
2. Mendelman PM, *et al.* Cefuroxime treatment failure of nontypable Haemophilus influenzae meningitis associated with alteration of penicillin-binding proteins. *J Infect Dis* 1990; **162:** 1118–23.
3. Brown NM, *et al.* Cefuroxime resistance in Haemophilus influenzae. *Lancet* 1992; **340:** 552.

Pharmacokinetics

Cefuroxime axetil is absorbed from the gastro-intestinal tract and is rapidly hydrolysed in the intestinal mucosa and blood to cefuroxime. Absorption was erratic from the tablets originally marketed; an improved formulation was introduced in 1987. The absorption of cefuroxime axetil is enhanced in the presence of food. Peak plasma concentrations are reported about 2 to 3 hours after an oral dose. The sodium salt is given by intramuscular or intravenous injection. Peak plasma concentrations of about 27 μg per mL have been achieved 45 minutes after an intramuscular dose of 750 mg with measurable amounts present 8 hours after a dose. Up to 50% of cefuroxime in the circulation is bound to plasma proteins. The plasma half-life is about 70 minutes and is prolonged in patients with renal impairment and in neonates.

Cefuroxime is widely distributed in the body including pleural fluid, sputum, bone, synovial fluid, and aqueous humour, but only achieves therapeutic concentrations in the CSF when the meninges are inflamed. It crosses the placenta and has been detected in breast milk.

Cefuroxime is excreted unchanged, by glomerular filtration and renal tubular secretion, and high concentrations are achieved in the urine. Following injection, most of a dose of cefuroxime is excreted within 24 hours, the majority within 6 hours. Probenecid competes for renal tubular secretion with cefuroxime resulting in higher and more prolonged plasma concentrations of cefuroxime. Small amounts of cefuroxime are excreted in bile.

Plasma concentrations are reduced by dialysis.

References to the pharmacokinetics of cefuroxime.

1. Lang CC, *et al.* Bioavailability of cefuroxime axetil: comparison of standard and abbreviated methods. *J Antimicrob Chemother* 1990; **25:** 645–50.
2. Winter J, Dhillon P. Penetration of cefuroxime into bronchial mucosa following oral administration of cefuroxime axetil. *J Antimicrob Chemother* 1991; **27:** 556–8.
3. Ridgway E, *et al.* The pharmacokinetics of cefuroxime axetil in the sick elderly patient. *J Antimicrob Chemother* 1991; **27:** 663–8.
4. Powell DA, *et al.* Pharmacokinetics of cefuroxime axetil suspension in infants and children. *Antimicrob Agents Chemother* 1991; **35:** 2042–5.
5. Konishi K, *et al.* Pharmacokinetics of cefuroxime axetil in patients with normal and impaired renal function. *J Antimicrob Chemother* 1993; **31:** 413–20.
6. Kossman T, *et al.* Penetration of cefuroxime into the cerebrospinal fluid of patients with traumatic brain injury. *J Antimicrob Chemother* 1996; **37:** 161–7.
7. Jenkins CDG, *et al.* Comparative intraocular penetration of topical and injected cefuroxime. *Br J Ophthalmol* 1996; **80:** 685–8.
8. Stoeckel K, *et al.* Penetration of cefetamet pivoxil and cefuroxime axetil into the maxillary sinus mucosa at steady state. *Antimicrob Agents Chemother* 1996; **40:** 780–3.

Uses and Administration

Cefuroxime is a second-generation cephalosporin antibiotic used in the treatment of susceptible infections (see Antimicrobial Action, above). These have included bone and joint infections, bronchitis (and other lower respiratory-tract infections), gonorrhoea, meningitis (although treatment failures have been reported in *H. influenzae* meningitis, see p.130), otitis media, peritonitis, pharyngitis, sinusitis, skin infections (including soft-tissue infections), surgical infection (prophylaxis), and urinary-tract infections. For details of all these infections and their treatment, see under Choice of Antibacterial, p.116.

Administration and dosage. Cefuroxime is administered by mouth as the acetoxyethyl ester, cefuroxime axetil, in the form of tablets or suspension or by injection as the sodium salt. Absorption from the gastro-intestinal tract is enhanced if cefuroxime axetil is given after food. Cefuroxime sodium may be given by deep intramuscular injection, by slow intravenous injection over 3 to 5 minutes, or by intravenous infusion. Doses of cefuroxime axetil and cefuroxime sodium are expressed in terms of the equivalent amount of cefuroxime.

Usual oral doses are 125 mg twice daily for uncomplicated urinary-tract infections and 250 to 500 mg twice daily for respiratory-tract infections. A suggested dose for children more than 3 months of age is 125 mg twice daily or 10 mg per kg body-weight twice daily to a maximum of 250 mg daily. Children over 2 years of age with otitis media may be given 250 mg twice daily or 15 mg per kg twice daily to a maximum of 500 mg daily.

By injection the usual dose is 750 mg of cefuroxime every 8 hours but in more severe infections 1.5 g may be given intravenously every 8 or 6 hours. Infants and children can be given 30 to 60 mg per kg body-weight daily, increased to 100 mg per kg daily if necessary, given in 3 or 4 divided doses. Neonates may be given similar total daily doses but administered in 2 or 3 divided doses.

Parenteral doses may need to be reduced in renal impairment. The manufacturers suggest that the usual adult dose of 750 mg should only be given twice daily when the creatinine clearance is between 10 and 20 mL per minute and once daily when it is below 10 mL per minute. Patients undergoing haemodialysis should receive an additional 750-mg dose following each dialysis; those undergoing continuous peritoneal dialysis may be given 750 mg twice daily.

For the treatment of meningitis due to sensitive strains of bacteria, cefuroxime is administered intravenously in doses of 3 g every 8 hours. Infants and children are given 200 to 240 mg per kg daily intravenously in 3 or 4 divided doses, which may be decreased to 100 mg per kg daily after 3 days or when there is clinical improvement. For neonates, a dose of 100 mg per kg daily, decreased to 50 mg per kg daily when indicated, has been recommended.

In the treatment of gonorrhoea a single dose of 1.5 g by intramuscular injection, divided between 2 injection sites, has been suggested. A single 1-g oral dose of cefuroxime has been given for uncomplicated gonorrhoea. In each case an oral dose of probenecid 1 g may be administered in conjunction with cefuroxime.

For surgical infection prophylaxis the usual dose is 1.5 g of cefuroxime intravenously prior to the procedure; this may be supplemented by 750 mg intravenously or intramuscularly every 8 hours for up to 24 to 48 hours depending upon the procedure. For total joint replacement 1.5 g of cefuroxime powder may be mixed with the methylmethacrylate cement.

References.

1. Perry CM, Brogden RN. Cefuroxime axetil: a review of its antibacterial activity, pharmacokinetic properties and therapeutic efficacy. *Drugs* 1996; **52:** 125–58.

Preparations

BP 1998: Cefuroxime Axetil Tablets; Cefuroxime Injection;
USP 23: Cefuroxime Axetil Tablets; Cefuroxime for Injection; Cefuroxime Injection.

Proprietary Preparations (details are given in Part 3)
Aust.: Curocef; Zinnat; ***Belg.:*** Kefurox; Zinacef; Zinnat; ***Canad.:*** Ceftin; Kefurox; Zinacef; ***Fr.:*** Cepazine; Zinnat; ***Ger.:*** Elobact; Zinacef; Zinnat; ***Irl.:*** Zinacef; Zinnat; ***Ital.:*** Biociclin; Biofurex; Bioxima; Cefamar; Cefoprim; Cefumax; Cefur; Cefurex; Cefurin; Colifossim; Curoxim; Deltacef; Duxima; Gibicef; Ipacef; Itorex; Kefox; Kesint; Lafurex; Lamposporin†; Medoxim; Oraxim; Polixima; Supero; Tilexim; Ultroxim†; Zinnat; Zoref; ***Neth.:*** Zinacef; Zinnat; ***Norw.:*** Lifurox; Zinacef; ***S.Afr.:*** Zinacef; Zinnat; ***Spain:*** Curoxima; Nivador; Selan; Zinnat; ***Swed.:*** Axacef; Lifurox; Zinacef; Zinnat; ***Switz.:*** Zinacef; Zinat; ***UK:*** Zinacef; Zinnat; ***USA:*** Ceftin; Kefurox; Zinacef.

Cefuzonam (2900-x)

Cefuzonam *(rINN).*

Cefuzoname. (*Z*)-7-[2-(2-Aminothiazol-4-yl)-2-methoxyiminoacetamido]-3-(1,2,3-thiadiazol-5-ylthiomethyl)-3-cephem-4-carboxylic acid.

$C_{16}H_{15}N_7O_5S_4$ = 513.6.
CAS — 82219-78-1.

Cefuzonam is a cephalosporin antibiotic; it has been administered by intravenous injection or infusion as the sodium salt. Concern has been expressed over reports of severe skin reactions associated with its use.

Preparations

Proprietary Preparations (details are given in Part 3)
Jpn: Cosmosin†.

Cephacetrile Sodium (36-m)

Cephacetrile Sodium *(USAN).*

Cefacetrile Sodium *(BANM, pINNM);* BA-36278A. Sodium (7*R*)-7-(2-cyanoacetamido)cephalosporanate; Sodium (7*R*)-3-acetoxymethyl-7-(2-cyanoacetamido)-3-cephem-4-carboxylate.

$C_{13}H_{12}N_3NaO_6S$ = 361.3.
CAS — 10206-21-0 (cephacetrile); 23239-41-0 (cephacetrile sodium).

Cephacetrile is a cephalosporin antibiotic with actions and uses similar to those of cephalothin (p.179). It has been given parenterally as the sodium salt.

Preparations

Proprietary Preparations (details are given in Part 3)
Ital.: Celospor†; ***Switz.:*** Celospor†.

Cephalexin (37-b)

Cephalexin *(BAN, USAN).*

Cefalexin *(pINN);* 66873; Cefalexinum. (7*R*)-3-Methyl-7-(α-D-phenylglycylamino)-3-cephem-4-carboxylic acid monohydrate.

$C_{16}H_{17}N_3O_4S,H_2O$ = 365.4.
CAS — 15686-71-2 (anhydrous cephalexin); 23325-78-2 (cephalexin monohydrate).

Pharmacopoeias. In *Chin., Eur.* (see p.viii), *Jpn, Pol.,* and *US. It.* also includes Cephalexin Sodium.

A white or almost white crystalline powder. 1.05 g of monograph substance is approximately equivalent to 1 g of anhydrous cephalexin. **Soluble** 1 in about 100 of water; practically insoluble in alcohol, in chloroform, and in ether. A 0.5% solution in water has a pH of 4.0 to 5.5 and a 5% suspension in water has a pH of 3.0 to 5.5. **Store** at a temperature not exceeding 30° in airtight containers. Protect from light.

Cephalexin Hydrochloride (9391-h)

Cephalexin Hydrochloride *(BANM, USAN).*

Cefalexin Hydrochloride *(pINNM);* LY-061188.

$C_{16}H_{17}N_3O_4S,HCl,H_2O$ = 401.9.
CAS — 105879-42-3.

Pharmacopoeias. In *US.*

A white to off-white crystalline powder. 1.16 g of monograph substance is approximately equivalent to 1 g of anhydrous cephalexin. **Soluble** 1 in 100 of water, acetone, acetonitrile, alcohol, dimethylformamide, and methyl alcohol; practically insoluble in chloroform, in ether, in ethyl acetate, and in isopropyl alcohol. A 1% solution in water has a pH of 1.5 to 3.0. **Store** in airtight containers.

Adverse Effects and Precautions

As for Cephalothin Sodium, p.179.

The most common adverse effects of cephalexin and other oral cephalosporins are generally gastro-intestinal disturbances and hypersensitivity reactions. Pseudomembranous colitis has been reported.

References.

1. Dave J, *et al.* Cephalexin induced toxic epidermal necrolysis. *J Antimicrob Chemother* 1991; **28:** 477–8.
2. Baran R, Perrin C. Fixed-drug eruption presenting as an acute paronychia. *Br J Dermatol* 1991; **125:** 592–5.
3. Clark RF. Crystalluria following cephalexin overdose. *Pediatrics* 1992; **89:** 672–4.
4. Murray KM, Camp MS. Cephalexin-induced Stevens-Johnson syndrome. *Ann Pharmacother* 1992; **26:** 1230–3.

Interactions

The renal excretion of cephalexin, and many other cephalosporins, is delayed by probenecid.

Hormonal contraceptives. There have been isolated reports of cephalexin decreasing the efficacy of oestrogen-containing oral contraceptives.[1] For a discussion of decreased efficacy of oral contraceptives and the need for additional contraceptive methods in patients taking broad-spectrum antibacterials, see under Hormonal Contraceptives, p.1433.

1. Friedman M, *et al.* Cephalexin and Microgynon-30 do not go well together. *J Obstet Gynaecol* 1982; **2:** 195–6.

Antimicrobial Action

As for Cephalothin Sodium, p.179, although cephalexin is generally less potent. Some strains of Gram-negative bacteria may be inhibited only by the high concentrations achievable in the urinary tract. *Haemophilus influenzae* shows varying sensitivity to cephalexin.

Pharmacokinetics

Cephalexin is almost completely absorbed from the gastro-intestinal tract and produces a peak plasma concentration of about 18 μg per mL one hour after a 500-mg oral dose; doubling the dose doubles the peak concentration. If cephalexin is taken with food, absorption may be delayed, but the total amount absorbed is not appreciably altered. Up to 15% of a dose is bound to plasma proteins. The plasma half-life is about 1 hour; it increases with reduced renal function.

Cephalexin is widely distributed in the body but does not enter the CSF in significant quantities. It crosses the placenta and small quantities are found in breast milk. Cephalexin is not metabolised. About 80% or more of a dose is excreted unchanged in the urine in the first 6 hours by glomerular filtration and tubular secretion; urinary concentrations greater than 1 mg per mL have been achieved after a dose of 500 mg. Probenecid delays urinary excretion. Therapeutically effective concentrations may be found in the bile and some may be excreted by this route.

Cephalexin is removed by haemodialysis and peritoneal dialysis.

References.

1. Wise R. The pharmacokinetics of the oral cephalosporins—a review. *J Antimicrob Chemother* 1990; **26** (suppl E): 13–20.

Uses and Administration

Cephalexin is a first-generation cephalosporin antibacterial. It is administered by mouth for the treatment of susceptible infections including those of the respiratory and urinary tracts and of the skin (see under Choice of Antibacterial, p.116). For severe infections treatment with parenteral cephalosporins is to be preferred.

Cephalexin is given as the monohydrate or hydrochloride. Doses are expressed in terms of the equivalent amount of anhydrous cephalexin.

The usual dose for adults is 1 to 2 g daily given in divided doses at 6-, 8-, or 12-hourly intervals; in severe or deep-seated infections the dose can be increased to up to 6 g daily but when high doses are required the use of a parenteral cephalosporin should be considered. Children may be given 25 to 100 mg per kg body-weight daily in divided doses to a maximum of 4 g daily.

For the prophylaxis of recurrent urinary-tract infection, cephalexin may be given in a dose of 125 mg at night.

Doses may need to be reduced in severe renal impairment.

Cephalexin sodium or cephalexin lysine are available in some countries for parenteral use.

Preparations

BP 1998: Cefalexin Capsules; Cefalexin Oral Suspension; Cefalexin Tablets;
USP 23: Cephalexin Capsules; Cephalexin for Oral Suspension; Cephalexin Tablets.

Proprietary Preparations (details are given in Part 3)
Aust.: Cepexin; Cephalobene; Keflex; Ospexin; Sanaxin; ***Austral.:*** Ceporex†; Ibilex; Keflex; ***Belg.:*** Ceporex; Keforal; ***Canad.:*** Keflex; Novo-Lexin; Nu-Cephalex; ***Fr.:*** Cefacet; Ceporexine; Keforal; ***Ger.:*** Cephalex; Ceporexin; Oracef; ***Irl.:*** Ceporex; Kefexin; Keflex; ***Ital.:*** Abiocef†; Cefadros†; Cepo†; Ceporex; Coliceflor†; Domucef†; Ibilex†; Keforal; Lafarin; Latoral†; Lorexina†; Sintolexyn†; Zetacef-lis†; Zetacef†; ***Neth.:*** Ceporex†; Keforal; ***Norw.:*** Keflex; ***S.Afr.:*** Betacef; Ceporex†; Cerexin; Fexin; Keflex; Lenocef; Ranceph; ***Spain:*** Bioscefal; Cefadina†; Cefalexgobens; Cefalorex†; Cefamiso; Cefibacter†; Ciliceft†; Defaxina; Efemida; Karilexina; Kefloridina; Lexibiotico; Lexincef; Sporol†; Sulquipen; Torlasporin; Ultralexin†; Valesporin†; ***Swed.:*** Keflex; ***Switz.:*** Ceporex†; Keflex; Servispor; ***UK:*** Ceporex; Keflex; Kiflone; ***USA:*** Biocef; Cefanex; Keflet†; Keflex; Keftab; Zartan†.

Multi-ingredient: ***Ital.:*** Focet†; Fosfolexin†; Kufaprim†; ***Spain:*** Kefloridina Mucolitico; Prindex Mucolitico†.

Cephalonium (39-g)

Cephalonium *(BAN).*

Cefalonium *(pINN);* 41071; Carbamoylcefaloridine. (7*R*)-3-(4-Carbamoyl-1-pyridiniomethyl)-7-[2-(2-thienyl)acetamido]-3-cephem-4-carboxylate.

$C_{20}H_{18}N_4O_5S_2$ = 458.5.
CAS — 5575-21-3.

Pharmacopoeias. In *BP(Vet).*

A white or almost white crystalline powder. Very slightly **soluble** in water and in methyl alcohol; soluble in dimethyl sulphoxide; practically insoluble in alcohol, in dichloromethane, and in ether. It dissolves in dilute acids and in alkaline solutions. **Store** at temperature not exceeding 30°. Protect from light.

Cephalonium is a cephalosporin antibacterial used in veterinary practice.

Cephaloridine (40-f)

Cephaloridine *(BAN, USAN).*

Cefaloridine *(pINN)*; 40602; Cefaloridinum. (7*R*)-3-(1-Pyridiniomethyl)-7-[(2-thienyl)acetamido]-3-cephem-4-carboxylate.

$C_{19}H_{17}N_3O_4S_2$ = 415.5.

CAS — 50-59-9.

Pharmacopoeias. In *Aust., Belg., Fr., It., Jpn, Neth.,* and *Port.*

Cephaloridine was one of the first cephalosporin antibacterials to be available clinically. It has properties similar to those of cephalothin (below), but is more nephrotoxic and is seldom used now.

It has usually been administered intramuscularly in doses of 0.5 to 1 g two or three times daily.

Preparations

Proprietary Preparations (details are given in Part 3)
Belg.: Cepalorin†; ***Fr.:*** Ceporine†; ***Ital.:*** Ceporin†; Dinasint†; Faredina†; Floridin†; Keflodin†; Latorex†; Lauridin†.

Cephalothin Sodium (41-d)

Cephalothin Sodium *(BANM, USAN).*

Cefalotin Sodium *(pINNM)*; 38253; Cefalotinum Natricum; Sodium Cephalothin. Sodium (7*R*)-7-[2-(2-thienyl)acetamido]cephalosporanate; Sodium (7*R*)-3-acetoxymethyl-7-[2-(2-thienyl)acetamido]-3-cephem-4-carboxylate.

$C_{16}H_{15}N_2NaO_6S_2$ = 418.4.

CAS — 153-61-7 (cephalothin); 58-71-9 (cephalothin sodium).

Pharmacopoeias. In *Chin., Eur.* (see p.viii), *Jpn, Pol.,* and *US.*

A white to off-white, almost odourless, crystalline powder. 1.06 g of monograph substance is approximately equivalent to 1 g of cephalothin. Each g of monograph substance represents 2.39 mmol of sodium.

Freely **soluble** in water; slightly soluble in dehydrated alcohol; freely soluble in 0.9% sodium chloride solution and in glucose solutions; practically insoluble in ether, and most other organic solvents. A 10 or 25% solution in water has a pH of 4.5 to 7.0. **Store** at a temperature not exceeding 30° in airtight containers. Protect from light.

Cephalothin sodium has been reported to be **incompatible** with aminoglycosides and with many other drugs. Precipitation may occur in solutions with a pH of less than 5.

Adverse Effects

The adverse effects associated with cephalothin and other cephalosporins are broadly similar to those described for penicillins (see Benzylpenicillin, p.159). The most common are hypersensitivity reactions, including skin rashes, urticaria, eosinophilia, fever, reactions resembling serum sickness, and anaphylaxis.

There may be a positive response to the Coombs' test although haemolytic anaemia rarely occurs. Neutropenia and thrombocytopenia have occasionally been reported. Agranulocytosis has been associated rarely with some cephalosporins. Bleeding complications related to hypoprothrombinaemia and/or platelet dysfunction have occurred especially with cephalosporins and cephamycins having a methylthiotetrazole side-chain, including cephamandole, cefbuperazone, cefmenoxime, cefmetazole, cefonicid, cefoperazone, ceforanide, cefotetan, cefpiramide, and latamoxef. The presence of a methylthiadiazolethiol side-chain, as in cephazolin, or a methylthiotriazine ring, as in ceftriaxone, might also be associated with such bleeding disorders.

Nephrotoxicity has been reported with cephalothin although it is less toxic than cephaloridine. Acute renal tubular necrosis has followed excessive dosage and has also been associated with its use in older patients or those with pre-existing renal impairment, or with the concomitant administration of nephrotoxic drugs such as aminoglycosides. Acute interstitial nephritis is also a possibility as a manifestation of hypersensitivity.

Transient increases in liver enzyme values have been reported. Hepatitis and cholestatic jaundice have occurred rarely with some cephalosporins.

Convulsions and other signs of CNS toxicity have been associated with high doses, especially in patients with severe renal impairment.

Gastro-intestinal adverse effects such as nausea, vomiting, and diarrhoea have been reported rarely. Prolonged use may result in overgrowth of non-susceptible organisms and, as with other broad-spectrum antibiotics, pseudomembranous colitis may develop (see also below).

There may be pain at the injection site following intramuscular administration, and thrombophlebitis has occurred following intravenous infusion of cephalosporins. Cephalothin appears to be more likely to cause such local reactions than other cephalosporins.

Antibiotic-associated colitis. Pseudomembranous colitis has been associated with the use of most antibiotics, including the cephalosporins. The newer broad-spectrum cephalosporins have also been implicated[1-3] and in the UK the Committee on Safety of Medicines (CSM)[4] has warned of the dangers of pseudomembranous colitis with the newer, as well as the older, oral cephalosporins. In addition to 33 reports of pseudomembranous colitis associated with cephalexin, cephradine, cefadroxil, and cefaclor, 6 of which proved fatal, they had received 12 reports of probable or confirmed cases with cefuroxime axetil and 15 with cefixime, one of them fatal. In clinical trials of cefuroxime axetil and cefixime, diarrhoea and pseudomembranous colitis appeared to be dose-related and therefore the CSM recommended that higher doses should be reserved for severe infections. In any event they advised that treatment should be discontinued if symptoms suggestive of pseudomembranous colitis arise.

For further discussion of the management of this condition, see p.123.

1. de Lalla F, *et al.* Third generation cephalosporins as a risk factor for Clostridium difficile-associated disease: a four-year survey in a general hospital. *J Antimicrob Chemother* 1989; **23:** 623–31.
2. Golledge CL, *et al.* Extended spectrum cephalosporins and Clostridium difficile. *J Antimicrob Chemother* 1989; **23:** 929–31.
3. Freiman JP, *et al.* Pseudomembranous colitis associated with single-dose cephalosporin prophylaxis. *JAMA* 1989; **262:** 902.
4. Committee on Safety of Medicines. Pseudomembranous (antibiotic-associated) colitis and diarrhoea with cephalosporins. *Current Problems 32* 1991.

Effects on the kidneys. References.

1. Zhanel GG. Cephalosporin-induced nephrotoxicity: does it exist? *DICP Ann Pharmacother* 1990; **24:** 262–5.

Precautions

Cephalothin should not be given to patients who are hypersensitive to it or to other cephalosporins. About 10% of penicillin-sensitive patients may also be allergic to cephalosporins although the true incidence is uncertain; great care should be taken if cephalothin is to be given to such patients. Care is also necessary in patients with known histories of allergy.

Cephalothin should be given with caution to patients with renal impairment; a dosage reduction may be necessary. Renal and haematological status should be monitored especially during prolonged and high-dose therapy. Cephalothin and some other cephalosporins and cephamycins (ceforanide, cefotetan, cefoxitin, and cefpirome) may interfere with the Jaffé method of measuring creatinine concentrations and may produce falsely high values; this should be borne in mind when measuring renal function. Positive results to the direct Coombs' test have been found during treatment with cephalothin and these can interfere with blood cross-matching. The urine of patients being treated with cephalothin may give false-positive reactions for glucose using copper-reduction reactions.

Interactions

The concomitant use of a nephrotoxic drug such as the aminoglycoside gentamicin may increase the risk of kidney damage with cephalothin. There is also some evidence for enhanced nephrotoxicity with a loop diuretic like frusemide, but this is less certain than with frusemide and cephaloridine. Similarly to the penicillins, the renal excretion of cephalothin and many other cephalosporins is inhibited by probenecid. There may be antagonism between cephalothin and bacteriostatic antibacterials.

Antimicrobial Action

Cephalothin is a beta-lactam antibiotic. It is bactericidal and acts similarly to benzylpenicillin (p.160) by inhibiting synthesis of the bacterial cell wall. It is most active against Gram-positive cocci, and has moderate activity against some Gram-negative bacilli.

Sensitive Gram-positive cocci include both penicillinase- and non-penicillinase-producing staphylococci, although methicillin-resistant staphylococci are usually resistant; most streptococci are also sensitive, but not penicillin-resistant *Streptococcus pneumoniae;* enterococci are usually resistant. Some Gram-positive anaerobes are also sensitive. Cephalothin is usually inactive against *Listeria monocytogenes.*

Among Gram-negative bacteria cephalothin has activity against some Enterobacteriaceae including strains of *Escherichia coli, Klebsiella pneumoniae, Proteus mirabilis, Salmonella,* and *Shigella* spp., but not against *Enterobacter,* indole-positive *Proteus,* or *Serratia* spp. It is also active against *Haemophilus influenzae, Moraxella (Branhamella) catarrhalis,* and *Neisseria* spp. *Bacteroides fragilis* and *Pseudomonas aeruginosa* are not sensitive, neither are mycobacteria, mycoplasma, and fungi.

The minimum inhibitory concentrations of cephalothin for susceptible Gram-positive cocci range from about 0.1 to 1 μg per mL; for the majority of susceptible Gram-negative bacteria concentrations of 1 to 16 μg or more per mL are usually required.

Resistance of bacteria to cephalothin may be due to several mechanisms: the drug may be prevented from reaching its site of action, for example in some Gram-negative organisms the cell wall may be a potential barrier; the target penicillin-binding proteins may be altered so that cephalothin cannot bind with these proteins; or, most importantly, the organism may produce beta-lactamases (cephalosporinases). Cephalothin is relatively resistant to hydrolysis by staphylococcal beta-lactamase, but is inactivated by a variety of beta-lactamases produced by Gram-negative organisms; resistance of Gram-negative organisms often depends on more than one factor. Resistance can be chromosomally or plasmid-mediated and may sometimes be inducible by cephalosporins.

Certain strains of bacteria may be inhibited but not killed by cephalosporins or penicillins and in such cases the minimum bactericidal concentration (MBC) is much greater than the minimum inhibitory concentration (MIC); this is known as tolerance.

As well as with other cephalosporins, some cross-resistance may occur between cephalothin and the penicillinase-resistant penicillins.

Pharmacokinetics

Cephalothin is poorly absorbed from the gastro-intestinal tract. After intramuscular injection peak plasma concentrations of about 10 and 20 μg per mL are achieved within 30 minutes of doses of 0.5 and 1 g, respectively. A concentration of 30 μg per mL has been reported 15 minutes after the intravenous injection of a 1-g dose; a range of 14 to 20 μg per mL has been achieved by the continuous intravenous infusion of 500 mg per hour.

Cephalothin is widely distributed in body tissues and fluids except the brain and CSF where the concentrations achieved are low and unpredictable. It crosses the placenta into the fetal circulation and low concentrations have been detected in breast milk. The plasma half-life varies from about 30 to 50 minutes, but may be longer in patients with renal impairment, especially that of the metabolite. About 70% of cephalothin in the circulation is bound to plasma proteins.

Approximately 20 to 30% of cephalothin is rapidly deacetylated in the liver and about 60 to 70% of a dose is excreted in the urine by the renal tubules within 6 hours as cephalothin and the relatively inactive metabolite, desacetylcephalothin. High urine concentrations of 0.8 and 2.5 mg per mL have been observed following intramuscular doses of 0.5 and 1 g, respectively. Probenecid blocks the renal excretion of cephalothin. A very small amount is excreted in bile.

Uses and Administration

Cephalothin is a first-generation cephalosporin antibiotic that has been used in the treatment of infections due to susceptible bacteria, particularly staphylococci, but has generally been replaced by cephazolin or cephradine; these in turn are being replaced by newer cephalosporins.

Cephalothin is given as the sodium salt by slow intravenous injection over 3 to 5 minutes or by intermittent or continuous infusion. It may be given intramuscularly but this route is painful. Doses are expressed in terms of the equivalent amount of cephalothin. The usual dose has been 0.5 to 1 g of cephalothin every 4 to 6 hours; up to 12 g daily has been given in severe infections.

Reduced doses are recommended if cephalothin has to be given to patients with impaired renal function.

Preparations

USP 23: Cephalothin for Injection; Cephalothin Injection.

Proprietary Preparations (details are given in Part 3)
Aust.: Keflin; ***Austral.:*** Keflin Neutral; ***Belg.:*** Keflin†; ***Canad.:*** Ceporacin; Keflin; ***Fr.:*** Keflin; ***Ger.:*** Cepovenin†; ***Irl.:*** Keflin†; ***Ital.:*** Keflin; ***Neth.:*** Ceporacin†; Keflin; ***Norw.:*** Keflin; ***S.Afr.:*** Keflin; ***Spain:*** Keflin; ***Swed.:*** Keflin; ***Switz.:*** Keflin N†; ***USA:*** Keflin†.

Cephamandole (42-n)

Cephamandole *(BAN)*.

Cefamandole *(USAN, rINN)*; 83405; Compound 83405. (7*R*)-7-D-Mandelamido-3-(1-methyl-1*H*-tetrazol-5-ylthiomethyl)-3-cephem-4-carboxylic acid; {6*R*-[6α,7β(*R**)]}-7-[(hydroxyphenylacetyl)amino]-3-{[(1-methyl-1*H*-tetrazol-5-yl)thio]methyl}-8-oxo-5-thia-1-azabicyclo[4.2.0]oct-2-ene-2-carboxylic acid.

$C_{18}H_{18}N_6O_5S_2$ = 462.5.

CAS — 34444-01-4.

Cephamandole Nafate (18358-s)

Cephamandole Nafate *(BAN)*.

Cefamandole Nafate *(USAN, rINNM)*; 106223. Sodium (7*R*)-7-[(2*R*)-2-formyloxy-2-phenylacetamido]-3-(1-methyl-1*H*-tetrazol-5-ylthiomethyl)-3-cephem-4-carboxylate.

$C_{19}H_{17}N_6NaO_6S_2$ = 512.5.

CAS — 42540-40-9.

Pharmacopoeias. In *Pol.* and *US.*

A white, odourless, crystalline solid. 1.11 g of monograph substance is approximately equivalent to 1 g of cephamandole activity and represents 2.2 mmol of sodium.

Soluble in water and in methyl alcohol; practically insoluble in ether, in chloroform, and in cyclohexane. A 10% solution in water has a pH of 3.5 to 7.0. **Store** in airtight containers.

Cephamandole nafate has been reported to be **incompatible** with aminoglycosides and with metronidazole. Formulations of cephamandole nafate available for injection contain sodium carbonate and are incompatible with solutions containing calcium or magnesium salts. When reconstituted with water the sodium carbonate rapidly hydrolyses about 30% of the ester to cephamandole sodium; during storage of the reconstituted solution at room temperature carbon dioxide is produced.

References.

1. Frable RA, *et al.* Stability of cefamandole nafate injection with parenteral solutions and additives. *Am J Hosp Pharm* 1982; **39:** 622–7. Correction. *ibid.*; 1479.

Cephamandole Sodium (43-h)

Cephamandole Sodium *(BANM)*.

Cefamandole Sodium *(rINNM)*.

$C_{18}H_{17}N_6NaO_5S_2$ = 484.5.

CAS — 30034-03-8.

Pharmacopoeias. In *Jpn* and *US.*

A white to light yellowish-white odourless crystalline powder. 1.05 g of monograph substance is approximately equivalent to 1 g of cephamandole and represents 2.2 mmol of sodium. Freely **soluble** in water and in dimethylformamide; soluble in methyl alcohol; slightly soluble in dehydrated alcohol; and very slightly soluble in acetone. A 10% solution in water has a pH of 3.5 to 7.0.

Adverse Effects and Precautions

As for Cephalothin Sodium, p.179.

Cephamandole has an *N*-methylthiotetrazole side-chain and may cause bleeding as a result of hypoprothrombinaemia which is usually reversible with administration of vitamin K. An alteration in intestinal flora was once thought responsible for this vitamin K-associated hypoprothrombinaemia, but interference with prothrombin synthesis now seems more likely.

Effects on the blood. References.

1. Lipsky JJ. Antibiotic-associated hypoprothrombinaemia. *J Antimicrob Chemother* 1988; **21:** 281–300.
2. Shearer MJ, *et al.* Mechanism of cephalosporin-induced hypoprothrombinemia: relation to cephalosporin side chain, vitamin K metabolism, and vitamin K status. *J Clin Pharmacol* 1988; **28:** 88–95.
3. Welage LS, *et al.* Comparative evaluation of the pharmacokinetics of N-methylthiotetrazole following administration of cefoperazone, cefotetan, and cefmetazole. *Antimicrob Agents Chemother* 1990; **34:** 2369–74.

Interactions

A disulfiram-like interaction with alcohol may occur and has been attributed to the *N*-methylthiotetrazole side-chain of cephamandole. Patients receiving cephamandole should therefore avoid alcohol during, and for at least several days after, treatment. Interactions are also possible with preparations containing significant amounts of alcohol.

Cephamandole, and other cephalosporins containing an *N*-methylthiotetrazole side-chain, may enhance the hypoprothrombinaemic response to anticoagulants as discussed under Warfarin (p.966).

Probenecid reduces the renal clearance of cephamandole and many other cephalosporins.

References.

1. Portier H, *et al.* Interaction between cephalosporins and alcohol. *Lancet* 1980; **ii:** 263.
2. Drummer S, *et al.* Antabuse-like effect of β-lactam antibiotics. *N Engl J Med* 1980; **303:** 1417–18.

Antimicrobial Action

Cephamandole is bactericidal and acts similarly to cephalothin, but has a broader spectrum of activity. It generally has similar or less activity against Gram-positive staphylococci and streptococci, but is resistant to some beta-lactamases produced by Gram-negative bacteria. It is more active than cephalothin against many of the Enterobacteriaceae including some strains of *Enterobacter, Escherichia coli, Klebsiella, Salmonella*, and indole-positive *Proteus* spp. However, resistance to cephamandole and other beta-lactams has emerged in some species, notably *Enterobacter*, during treatment with cephamandole. Cephamandole is very active *in vitro* against *Haemophilus influenzae* although an inoculum effect has been reported for beta-lactamase-producing strains. Like cephalothin, most strains of *Bacteroides fragilis* are resistant to cephamandole, as are *Pseudomonas* spp.

The minimum inhibitory concentrations of cephamandole for susceptible Gram-positive bacteria have been reported to range from about 0.1 to 2.0 µg per mL; for most susceptible Gram-negative bacteria concentrations of 0.5 to 8.0 µg per mL are usually required.

References.

1. Sabath LD. Reappraisal of the antistaphylococcal activities of first-generation (narrow-spectrum) and second-generation (expanded-spectrum) cephalosporins. *Antimicrob Agents Chemother* 1989; **33:** 407–11.

Pharmacokinetics

Cephamandole is poorly absorbed from the gastro-intestinal tract. It is given intramuscularly or intravenously, usually as the nafate which is rapidly hydrolysed to release cephamandole *in vivo*. Peak plasma concentrations for cephamandole of about 13 and 25 µg per mL have been achieved 0.5 to 2 hours after intramuscular doses of 0.5 and 1 g respectively; concentrations are very low after 6 hours. About 70% is bound to plasma proteins. The plasma half-life varies from about 0.5 to 1.2 hours depending on the route of injection; it is prolonged in patients with renal impairment.

Cephamandole is widely distributed in body tissues and fluids including bone, joint fluid, and pleural fluid; it diffuses into the CSF when the meninges are inflamed, but concentrations are unpredictable. Cephamandole has also been detected in breast milk. It is rapidly excreted unchanged by glomerular filtration and renal tubular secretion; about 80% of a dose is excreted within 6 hours and high urinary concentrations are achieved. Probenecid competes for renal tubular secretion with cephamandole resulting in higher and prolonged plasma concentrations of cephamandole. Therapeutic concentrations of cephamandole are achieved in bile.

It is removed by haemodialysis to some extent.

Uses and Administration

Cephamandole is a second-generation cephalosporin antibiotic used in the treatment of infections due to susceptible bacteria (see Antimicrobial Action, above) and for surgical infection prophylaxis.

It is given principally as cephamandole nafate (the sodium salt of cephamandole formyl ester). Doses are expressed in terms of the equivalent amount of cephamandole. It is administered by deep intramuscular injection, by slow intravenous injection over 3 to 5 minutes, or by intermittent or continuous infusion in doses of 0.5 to 2 g every 4 to 8 hours depending on the severity of the infection. Children over 1 month of age may be given 50 to 100 mg per kg body-weight daily in divided doses; 150 mg per kg daily may be given in severe infections, but this dose should not be exceeded.

Doses should be reduced for patients with impaired renal function. After an initial dose of 1 to 2 g the following maintenance doses have been recommended: for patients with a creatinine clearance of 50 to 80 mL per minute, 0.75 to 2 g every 6 hours; 25 to 50 mL per minute, 0.75 to 2 g every 8 hours; 10 to 25 mL per minute, 0.5 to 1.25 g every 8 hours; 2 to 10 mL per minute, 0.5 to 1 g every 12 hours; and less than 2 mL per minute, 0.25 to 0.75 g every 12 hours.

If the addition of an aminoglycoside to cephamandole therapy is necessary, then they should be administered separately.

For surgical infection prophylaxis a dose of 1 or 2 g intravenously or intramuscularly one-half to one hour before surgical incision, followed by 1 or 2 g every 6 hours for 24 to 48 hours, is recommended. For patients undergoing procedures involving implantation of prosthetic devices, cephamandole should be continued for up to 72 hours.

Preparations

USP 23: Cefamandole Nafate for Injection; Cefamandole Sodium for Injection; Sterile Cefamandole Sodium.

Proprietary Preparations (details are given in Part 3)

Aust.: Mandokef; ***Austral.:*** Mandol; ***Belg.:*** Mandol; ***Canad.:*** Mandol; ***Fr.:*** Kefandol; ***Ger.:*** Mandokef; ***Irl.:*** Kefadol; ***Ital.:*** Bergacef†; Cedol; Cefam; Cefamen†; Cefaseptolo†; Cefiran; Cemado; Fado†; Ibiman†; Lampomandol; Mancef; Mandokef; Mandolsan; Neocefal; Pavecef†; Septomandolo; ***Neth.:*** Mandol; ***S.Afr.:*** Mandokef; ***Spain:*** Mandokef; ***Switz.:*** Mandokef; ***UK:*** Kefadol; ***USA:*** Mandol†.

Cephazolin (18366-s)

Cephazolin *(BAN)*.

Cefazolin *(pINN)*. 3-[(5-Methyl-1,3,4-thiadiazol-2-yl)thiomethyl]-7-(tetrazol-1-ylacetamido)-3-cephem-4-carboxylic acid.

$C_{14}H_{14}N_8O_4S_3$ = 454.5.

CAS — 25953-19-9.

Pharmacopoeias. In *US.*

A white to slightly off-white odourless crystalline powder. Slightly **soluble** in water, in alcohol, and in methyl alcohol; soluble in dimethylformamide and in pyridine; sparingly soluble in acetone; very slightly soluble in ethyl acetate, in isopropyl alcohol, and in methyl isobutyl ketone; practically insoluble in chloroform, in dichloromethane, and in ether. **Store** in airtight containers.

Cephazolin Sodium (44-m)

Cephazolin Sodium *(BANM)*.

Cefazolin Sodium *(USAN, pINNM)*; 46083; Cefazolinum Natricum; SKF-41558.

$C_{14}H_{13}N_8NaO_4S_3$ = 476.5.

CAS — 27164-46-1.

Pharmacopoeias. In *Chin., Eur.* (see p.viii), *Jpn,* and *US.*

A white to off-white almost odourless, very hygroscopic, crystalline powder. 1.05 g of monograph substance is approximately equivalent to 1 g of cephazolin. Each g of monograph substance represents about 2.1 mmol of sodium.

Freely **soluble** in water, in sodium chloride 0.9% solution, and in glucose solutions; very slightly soluble in alcohol; practically insoluble in ether and in chloroform. A 10% solution in water has a pH of 4.0 to 6.0. **Store** at a temperature not exceeding 30° in airtight containers. Protect from light.

Cephazolin sodium has been reported to be **incompatible** with aminoglycosides and many other drugs. When the pH of a solution exceeds 8.5 there may be hydrolysis and when it is below 4.5 insoluble cephazolin may be precipitated.

Stability. References.

1. Nahata MC, Ahalt PA. Stability of cefazolin sodium in peritoneal dialysis solutions. *Am J Hosp Pharm* 1991; **48:** 291–2.

Adverse Effects and Precautions

As for Cephalothin Sodium, p.179. Similarly to cephalosporins with a *N*-methylthiotetrazole side-chain, cephazolin has been associated with causing hypoprothrombinaemia (see Cephamandole, p.180).

Effects on the nervous system. References.

1. Manzella JP, *et al.* CNS toxicity associated with intraventricular injection of cefazolin: report of three cases. *J Neurosurg* 1988; **68:** 970–1.
2. Martin ES, *et al.* Seizures after intraventricular cefazolin administration. *Clin Pharm* 1992; **11:** 104–5.

Interactions

Cephazolin contains a methylthiadiazolethiol side-chain and, similarly to cephalosporins containing the related *N*-methylthiotetrazole side-chain (see Cephamandole, p.180), may cause a disulfiram-like reaction with alcohol, and possibly enhance the effects of warfarin.

The renal excretion of cephazolin and many other cephalosporins is delayed by probenecid.

Antimicrobial Action

As for Cephalothin Sodium, p.179, although cephazolin is more sensitive to staphylococcal beta-lactamase.

The minimum inhibitory concentrations of cephazolin for susceptible Gram-positive cocci range from about 0.1 to 1 μg per mL; for the majority of susceptible Gram-negative bacteria concentrations of greater than 1 μg per mL are required.

Pharmacokinetics

Cephazolin is poorly absorbed from the gastro-intestinal tract and is given by intramuscular or intravenous injection. Following a dose of 500 mg given intramuscularly, peak plasma concentrations of 30 μg or more per mL are obtained after 1 to 2 hours. About 85% of cephazolin in the circulation is bound to plasma proteins. The plasma half-life of cephazolin is about 1.8 hours, and is increased in patients with renal impairment. Cephazolin diffuses into bone and into ascitic, pleural, and synovial fluid but not appreciably into the CSF. It crosses the placenta into the fetal circulation; only low concentrations are detected in breast milk.

Cephazolin is excreted unchanged in the urine, mainly by glomerular filtration with some renal tubular secretion, at least 80% of a dose given intramuscularly being excreted within 24 hours. Peak urine concentrations of more than 1 and 4 mg per mL have been reported after intramuscular doses of 0.5 and 1 g respectively. Probenecid delays excretion. Cephazolin is removed to some extent by haemodialysis.

High biliary concentrations have been reported, although the amount excreted by this route is small.

Uses and Administration

Cephazolin is a first-generation cephalosporin antibiotic used in the treatment of a variety of infections due to susceptible organisms, including biliary-tract infections, endocarditis (staphylococcal), and peritonitis (associated with continuous ambulatory peritoneal dialysis). It is also used for surgical infection prophylaxis, including prophylaxis of endometritis at caesarean section. For details of these infections, and their treatment, see under Choice of Antibacterial, p.116.

Administration and dosage. Cephazolin is given as the sodium salt by deep intramuscular injection, by slow intravenous injection over 3 to 5 minutes, or by intravenous infusion. Doses are expressed in terms of the equivalent amount of cephazolin. The usual adult dose is 0.5 to 1 g every 6 to 12 hours. The usual maximum daily dose is 6 g, although up to 12 g has been used in severe life-threatening infections. Children over 1 month may be given 25 to 50 mg per kg body-weight daily in three or four divided doses, increased in severe infections to a maximum of 100 mg per kg daily.

For the prophylaxis of infection during surgery, a 1 g dose is given half to one hour prior to the operation, followed by 0.5 to 1 g during surgery for lengthy procedures. A dose of 0.5 to 1 g is given every 6 to 8 hours postoperatively for 24 hours, or up to 5 days in certain cases.

Dosage should be reduced in patients with renal impairment and various modifications have been recommended. The manufacturers suggest the following for adults following a loading dose: creatinine clearance 55 mL or more per minute, usual doses; creatinine clearance 35 to 54 mL per minute, usual doses but at intervals of at least 8 hours; creatinine clearance 11 to 34 mL per minute, half the usual dose every 12 hours; creatinine clearance 10 mL or less per minute, half the usual dose every 18 to 24 hours.

Other routes of administration used for cephazolin sodium include intraperitoneal administration in peritoneal dialysis solutions and intra-ocular injections.

In some countries a modified-release intramuscular formulation of cephazolin sodium together with the less soluble dibenzylamine salt of cephazolin, in the ratio of 1:4, has been used.

Preparations

BP 1998: Cefazolin Injection;
USP 23: Cefazolin for Injection; Cefazolin Injection.

Proprietary Preparations (details are given in Part 3)

Aust.: Gramaxin†; Kefzol; Zolicef; ***Austral.:*** Cefamezin; Kefzol; ***Belg.:*** Cefacidal; Kefzol; ***Canad.:*** Ancef; Kefzol; ***Fr.:*** Cefacidal; Kefzol; ***Ger.:*** Baktozil†; Basocef; Elzogram; Gramaxin; ***Irl.:*** Kefzol†; ***Ital.:*** Acef; Biazolina; Bor-Cefazol†; Cefabiozim; Cefamezin; Cefazil; Cefazina†; Cromezin; Firmacef; Lampocef†; Recef; Sicef; Totacef; Zolin; Zolisint; ***Jpn:*** Cefamezin; ***Neth.:*** Cefacidal; Kefzol; ***S.Afr.:*** Cefacidal; Izacef; Kefzol; Ranzol; ***Spain:*** Areuzolin; Brizolina; Camil†; Caricef; Cefa Resan; Cefabiot; Cefacene; Cefadrex; Cefakes; Cefamezin; Cefamusel; Dacovo†; Fazoplex; Filoklin; Gencefal; Intrazolina; Karidina; Kefol; Kurgan; Neofazol; Tasep; Zolival; ***Switz.:*** Kefzol; Servicef; ***UK:*** Kefzol; ***USA:*** Ancef; Kefzol; Zolicef.

Multi-ingredient: ***Spain:*** Daren†; Tecfazolina.

Cephradine (45-b)

Cephradine *(BAN, USAN)*.

Cefradine *(rINN)*; Cefradinum; SKF-D-39304; SQ-11436; SQ-22022 (cephradine dihydrate). (7*R*)-7-(α-D-Cyclohexa-1,4-dienylglycylamino)-3-methyl-3-cephem-4-carboxylic acid.

$C_{16}H_{19}N_3O_4S$ = 349.4.

CAS — 38821-53-3 (anhydrous cephradine); 31828-50-9 (non-stoichiometric cephradine hydrate); 58456-86-3 (cephradine dihydrate).

Pharmacopoeias. In *Eur.* (see p.viii), *Jpn, Pol.,* and *US* which allows the anhydrous form, the monohydrate, or the dihydrate.

A white to slightly yellow, hygroscopic crystalline powder. Sparingly **soluble** in water; practically insoluble or very slightly soluble in alcohol and in chloroform; practically insoluble in ether. A 1% solution in water has a pH of 3.5 to 6.0. Commercially available injections contain sodium carbonate or arginine as neutralisers.

Store at a temperature not exceeding 30° in airtight containers. Protect from light.

Injections containing sodium carbonate are **incompatible** with solutions such as compound sodium lactate injection which contain calcium salts.

References.

1. Wang Y-C J, Monkhouse DC. Solution stability of cephradine neutralized with arginine or sodium bicarbonate. *Am J Hosp Pharm* 1983; **40:** 432.
2. Mehta AC, *et al.* Chemical stability of cephradine injection solutions. *Intensive Therapy Clin Monit* 1988; **9:** 195–6.

Adverse Effects and Precautions

As for Cephalexin, p.178. Intramuscular injections of cephradine can be painful and thrombophlebitis has occurred following intravenous injection.

Interactions

As for Cephalexin, p.178.

Antimicrobial Action

As for Cephalexin, p.178.

Pharmacokinetics

Cephradine is rapidly and almost completely absorbed from the gastro-intestinal tract. Doses of 250, 500, and 1000 mg given by mouth have produced peak plasma concentrations of about 9, 17, and 24 μg per mL respectively at 1 hour and are similar to those achieved with cephalexin. Absorption is delayed by the presence of food although the total amount absorbed is not appreciably altered. Following intramuscular injection peak plasma concentrations of about 6 and 14 μg per mL have been obtained within 1 to 2 hours of doses of 500 mg and 1 g respectively.

Only about 6 to 20% is reported to be bound to plasma proteins. A plasma half-life of about 1 hour has been reported; this is prolonged in patients with renal impairment. Cephradine is widely distributed to body tissues and fluids, but does not enter the CSF in significant quantities. Therapeutic concentrations may be found in the bile. It crosses the placenta into the fetal circulation and is distributed in small amounts into breast milk.

Cephradine is excreted unchanged in the urine by glomerular filtration and tubular secretion, over 90% of an oral dose or 60 to 80% of an intramuscular dose being recovered within 6 hours. Peak urinary concentrations of about 3 mg per mL have been achieved after a 500-mg dose by mouth. Probenecid delays excretion.

Cephradine is removed by haemodialysis and peritoneal dialysis.

References.

1. Wise R. The pharmacokinetics of the oral cephalosporins—a review. *J Antimicrob Chemother* 1990; **26** (suppl E): 13–20.
2. Schwinghammer TL, *et al.* Pharmacokinetics of cephradine administered intravenously and orally to young and elderly subjects. *J Clin Pharmacol* 1990; **30:** 893–9.

Uses and Administration

Cephradine is a first-generation cephalosporin antibiotic administered by mouth similarly to cephalexin (p.178) and by the parenteral route similarly to cephazolin (p.181) in the treatment of susceptible infections and in the prophylaxis of infections during surgical procedures.

Cephradine is given by mouth in doses of 1 to 2 g daily in two to four divided doses; up to 4 g daily may be given by this route. In severe infections it should be given parenterally, by deep intramuscular injection or intravenously by slow injection over 3 to 5 minutes or by infusion, in doses of 2 to 4 g daily in four divided doses; up to 8 g daily may be given by the parenteral route. The usual daily dose by mouth for children is 25 to 50 mg per kg body-weight; by injection 50 to 100 mg per kg daily may be given, increasing to 300 mg per kg daily in severe infections.

For surgical infection prophylaxis, 1 to 2 g may be given pre-operatively by the intramuscular or intravenous route; subsequent parenteral or oral doses are given as appropriate.

Dosage should be reduced in patients with renal impairment.

Preparations

BP 1998: Cefradine Capsules;
USP 23: Cephradine Capsules; Cephradine for Injection; Cephradine for Oral Suspension; Cephradine Tablets.

Proprietary Preparations (details are given in Part 3)
Aust.: Sefril; ***Belg.:*** Velosef; ***Canad.:*** Velosef†; ***Fr.:*** Doncef; Kelsef; Zadyl; Zeefra; ***Ger.:*** Sefril†; ***Irl.:*** Velosef; ***Ital.:*** Cefamid†; Cefrabiotic; Cefrasol†; Celex†; Cesporan†; Citicef; Ecosporina; Lenzacef†; Lisacef; Samedrin†; Velocef†; ***Neth.:*** Maxisporin; Velosef; ***S.Afr.:*** Bactocef; Cefril; ***Spain:*** Cefral†; Septacef; Velocef; ***Switz.:*** Sefril†; ***UK:*** Nicef; Velosef; ***USA:*** Velosef.

Chloramphenicol (49-p)

Chloramphenicol *(BAN, rINN).*

Chloramphenicolum; Chloranfenicol; Cloranfenicol; Kloramfenikol; Laevomycetinum. 2,2-Dichloro-*N*-[(αR,βR)-β-hydroxy-α-hydroxymethyl-4-nitrophenethyl]acetamide.

$C_{11}H_{12}Cl_2N_2O_5$ = 323.1.

CAS — 56-75-7.

NOTE. CPL is a code approved by the BP for use on single unit doses of eye drops containing chloramphenicol where the individual container may be too small to bear all the appropriate labelling information.

Pharmacopoeias. In *Chin., Eur.* (see p.viii), *Int., Jpn, Pol.,* and *US.*

An antimicrobial substance produced by the growth of certain strains of *Streptomyces venezuelae*, but now mainly prepared synthetically.

A white to greyish-white or yellowish-white, fine crystalline powder or fine crystals, needles, or elongated plates. **Soluble** 1 in 400 of water; freely soluble in alcohol, in propylene glycol, in acetone, and in ethyl acetate; slightly soluble in ether. A 2.5% suspension in water has a pH of 4.5 to 7.5. **Store** in airtight containers. Protect from light.

Solubility. Both urea[1] and benzalkonium chloride[2] have been reported to improve the solubility of chloramphenicol in water; the latter combination reportedly showed synergistic activity *in vitro* against *Pseudomonas aeruginosa.*[2]

1. Goldberg AH, *et al.* Increasing dissolution rates and gastrointestinal absorption of drugs via solid solutions and eutectic mixtures IV: chloramphenicol-urea system. *J Pharm Sci* 1966; **55:** 581–3.
2. Yousef RT, Ghobashy AA. Solubilization of chloramphenicol by benzalkonium chloride and study of their combined activity against Pseudomonas aeruginosa. *Acta Pharm Suec* 1968; **5:** 385–92.

Stability. Chloramphenicol is reported to be stable in aqueous solution over a wide pH range,[1] although stability can be improved with suitable buffering: one study reported a loss of about 50% from unbuffered aqueous solutions on storage for 290 days at 20° to 22°, whereas the loss from solutions buffered to pH 7.4 with borax was only 14%.[2] Loss of chloramphenicol (by hydrolysis) is increased by heating: about 4% is lost from aqueous solution on heating at 100° for 30 minutes, and 10% at 115° for about 30 minutes.[3] Heating at 98° to 100° for 30 minutes has been suggested for sterilisation of eye drops and it was calculated that no more than 10% potency would be lost in drops sterilised in this manner and stored for 4 months at 20° or 2 years at 4°.[3] However aqueous solutions must be protected from light since photochemical decomposition occurs,[4,5] with yellowing of the solution and development of an acid pH.[4]

The stability of chloramphenicol in ointment bases has also been investigated:[6] it was found to be more stable in oil-in-water emulsion bases than water-in-oil bases, and stability was better in bases containing wool fat than those with cetyl alcohol.

1. Higuchi T, *et al.* The kinetics of degradation of chloramphenicol in solution II: over-all disappearance rate from buffered solutions. *J Am Pharm Assoc (Sci)* 1954; **43:** 129–34.
2. Brunzell A. Determination of the hydrolytic decomposition of chloramphenicol in water-containing preparations. *Svensk Farm Tidskr* 1957; **6:** 129–38.
3. Heward M, *et al.* Stability to heat and subsequent storage of chloramphenicol eye-drops BPC. *Pharm J* 1970; **204:** 386–7.
4. Shih IK. Photodegradation products of chloramphenicol in aqueous solution. *J Pharm Sci* 1971; **60:** 1889–90.
5. de Vries H, *et al.* Photochemical decomposition of chloramphenicol in a 0.25% eyedrop and in a therapeutic intraocular concentration. *Int J Pharmaceutics* 1984; **20:** 265–71.
6. Attia MA, *et al.* Stability of chlortetracycline hydrochloride and chloramphenicol in some ophthalmic ointment bases. *Pharmazie* 1985; **40:** 629–31.

Chloramphenicol Palmitate (48-q)

Chloramphenicol Palmitate *(BANM, rINNM).*

Chloramphenicol α-Palmitate; Chloramphenicoli Palmitas; Palmitylchloramphenicol.

$C_{27}H_{42}Cl_2N_2O_6$ = 561.5.

CAS — 530-43-8.

Pharmacopoeias. In *Chin., Eur.* (see p.viii), *Int.,* and *US.*

A fine, white or almost white, unctuous, crystalline powder. M.p. 87° to 95°. 1.7 g of monograph substance is approximately equivalent to 1 g of chloramphenicol.

Practically **insoluble** in water; sparingly soluble in alcohol; freely soluble in acetone and in chloroform; soluble in ether; very slightly soluble in hexane. **Store** in airtight containers. Protect from light.

Chloramphenicol palmitate occurs in several polymorphic forms and the thermodynamically stable form (polymorph A) has low bioavailability following oral administration.

Polymorphism. Chloramphenicol palmitate exists in 3 crystalline and one amorphous polymorphic forms. Peak blood concentrations of chloramphenicol are much higher after administration of polymorph B, or the amorphous form, than after equivalent doses of polymorph A.[1,2] The polymorph B is metastable but is reported to demonstrate good stability at room temperature; polymorph C is unstable and is readily converted to the A form at elevated temperatures.[3]

1. Aguiar AJ, *et al.* Effect of polymorphism on the absorption of chloramphenicol from chloramphenicol palmitate. *J Pharm Sci* 1967; **56:** 847–51.
2. Banerjee S, *et al.* Serum levels of chloramphenicol in children, rhesus monkeys, and cats after administration of chloramphenicol palmitate suspension. *J Pharm Sci* 1971; **60:** 153–5.
3. Borka L. The stability of chloramphenicol palmitate polymorphs: solid and solution phase transformations. *Acta Pharm Suec* 1971; **8:** 365–72.

Stability. Chloramphenicol palmitate suspension in a syrup basis became curdled and discoloured after storage in a rigid amber polyvinyl chloride bottle for 2 years, but kept well when stored in amber glass bottles for the same period.[1]

1. Shah RC, *et al.* Suitability of rigid polyvinyl chloride bottles for liquid oral products. *Pharm J* 1978; **221:** 58–9.

Chloramphenicol Sodium Succinate (46-v)

Chloramphenicol Sodium Succinate *(BANM, rINNM).*

Chloramphenicol α-Sodium Succinate; Chloramphenicoli Natrii Succinas. Sodium (2*R*,3*R*)-2-(2,2-dichloroacetamido)-3-hydroxy-3-(4-nitrophenyl)propyl succinate.

$C_{15}H_{15}Cl_2N_2NaO_8$ = 445.2.

CAS — 982-57-0.

Pharmacopoeias. In *Eur.* (see p.viii) and *US. Chin.* includes Chloramphenicol Hydrogen Succinate.

A white or yellowish-white hygroscopic powder. 1.4 g of monograph substance is approximately equivalent to 1 g of chloramphenicol. Each g of monograph substance represents about 2.2 mmol of sodium.

Very **soluble** in water; freely soluble in alcohol; practically insoluble in ether. A 25% solution in water has a pH of 6.4 to 7.0. **Store** in airtight containers. Protect from light.

Incompatibilities. Incompatibility or loss of activity has been reported between chloramphenicol and a wide variety of other substances. Other factors, especially, drug concentration, may play a part and many interactions are chiefly seen with concentrated solutions.

Adverse Effects

Chloramphenicol may cause serious and sometimes fatal adverse effects. Some of its toxicity is thought to be due to effects on mitochondrial protein synthesis. The most serious adverse effect of chloramphenicol is its depression of the bone marrow, which can take 2 different forms. The first is a fairly common dose-related reversible depression occurring usually when plasma-chloramphenicol concentrations exceed 25 μg per mL and is characterised by morphological changes in the bone marrow, decreased iron utilisation, reticulocytopenia, anaemia, leucopenia, and thrombocytopenia. This effect may be due to inhibition of protein synthesis in the mitochondria of bone marrow cells.

The second and apparently unrelated form of bone-marrow toxicity is severe irreversible aplastic anaemia. This is fairly rare, with a suggested incidence of about 1:20 000 to 1:50 000, although the incidence varies throughout the world, and is not considered to be dose-related. The aplasia usually develops after a latent period of weeks or even months and has been suggested to be the result of a nitrated benzene radical produced *in vivo*. It is considered that victims may have some genetic or biochemical predisposition but there is no way of identifying susceptible patients. Although the majority of cases have followed oral administration aplasia has also occurred after intravenous and topical (eye drops) dosage of chloramphenicol. Survival is most likely in those with early onset aplasia but they may subsequently develop acute non-lymphoblastic leukaemia.

A toxic manifestation—'the grey syndrome'—characterised by abdominal distension, vomiting, ashen colour, hypothermia, progressive pallid cyanosis, irregular respiration, and circulatory collapse followed by death in a few hours or days, has occurred in premature and other newborn infants receiving large doses of chloramphenicol. The syndrome is associated with high plasma concentrations of chloramphenicol, due to reduced capacity for glucuronidation and decreased glomerular filtration in children of this age, leading to drug accumulation. Recovery is usually complete if the drug is withdrawn early enough after onset, but up to 40% of infants with the full-blown syndrome may die. The syndrome has also been reported in infants born to mothers given chloramphenicol in late pregnancy. A similar syndrome has been reported in adults and older children given very high doses.

Prolonged oral administration of chloramphenicol may induce bleeding, either by bone-marrow depression or by reducing the intestinal flora with consequent inhibition of vitamin K synthesis. Haemolytic anaemia has occurred in some patients with the Mediterranean form of glucose 6-phosphate dehydrogenase deficiency, but is rare in patients with milder forms of the deficiency.

Peripheral as well as optic neuritis has been reported in patients receiving chloramphenicol, usually over prolonged periods. Although ocular symptoms are often reversible if treatment is withdrawn early, permanent visual impairment or blindness has occurred.

Other neurological symptoms have included encephalopathy with confusion and delirium, mental depression, and headache. Ototoxicity has also occurred, especially after the use of ear drops.

Hypersensitivity reactions including rashes, fever, and angioedema may occur especially after topical use; anaphylaxis has occurred but is rare. Jarisch-Herxheimer-like reactions may also occur. Gastrointestinal symptoms including nausea, vomiting, and diarrhoea can follow oral administration. Disturbances of the oral and intestinal flora may cause stomatitis, glossitis, and rectal irritation. Patients may experience an intensely bitter taste following rapid intravenous administration of chloramphenicol sodium succinate.

A review[1] of the toxicity of chloramphenicol, including the potential role of the *p*-nitro group in producing aplastic anaemia. Derivatives such as thiamphenicol, which lack this grouping are not associated with increased incidence of aplastic anaemia.

1. Yunis AA. Chloramphenicol: relation of structure to activity and toxicity. *Ann Rev Pharmacol Toxicol* 1988; **28:** 83–100.

Overdosage. Charcoal haemoperfusion was found to be far superior to exchange transfusion in the removal of chloramphenicol from blood, although it did not prevent death in a 7-week-old infant with the grey baby syndrome following a dosage error.[1]

1. Freundlich M, *et al.* Management of chloramphenicol intoxication in infancy by charcoal hemoperfusion. *J Pediatr* 1983; **103:** 485–7.

Precautions

Chloramphenicol is contra-indicated in patients with a history of hypersensitivity or toxic reaction to the drug. It should never be given systemically for minor infections or for prophylaxis. Repeated courses and prolonged treatment should be avoided and it should not be used in patients with pre-existing bone-marrow depression or blood dyscrasias. Routine periodic blood examinations are advisable in all patients, but will not warn of aplastic anaemia.

Concomitant administration of chloramphenicol with other drugs liable to depress bone-marrow function should be avoided.

Reduced doses should be given to patients with impaired liver function. Excessive blood concentrations may also occur following administration of usual doses to patients with severe renal impairment and in premature and full-term neonates who have immature metabolic processes. Monitoring of plasma-chloramphenicol concentrations may be desirable in patients with risk factors. A suggested range for peak plasma concentrations is 10 to 25 µg per mL and 5 to 15 µg per mL for trough concentrations.

Because of the risk of the 'grey syndrome' newborn infants should never be given chloramphenicol systemically, unless it may be life-saving and there is no alternative treatment. The use of chloramphenicol is probably best avoided during pregnancy, particularly in the last trimester, and in nursing mothers since chloramphenicol given to the mother is distributed into breast milk.

Chloramphenicol may interfere with the development of immunity and it should not be given during active immunisation.

Ocular use. Ocular chloramphenicol is widely used in Britain for the treatment of superficial eye infections. In view of the potential for serious toxicity, such as aplastic anaemia, following systemic absorption some, particularly in the USA, have advised that its ocular use should be restricted to situations where there is no alternative treatment.[1] However, apart from patients with a personal or family history of blood dyscrasias, the use, particularly of short courses, was defended by several specialists in the UK,[2-4] and the arguments have been the subject of several reviews.[5-7] Prospective case-control studies should help to clarify the risk,[8] and one such involving 145 patients with aplastic anaemia and 1226 controls found that only 3 of the patients had been exposed to ocular chloramphenicol and calculated that the absolute risk was no more than 0.5 cases per million treatment courses.[9]

1. Doona M, Walsh JB. Use of chloramphenicol as topical eye medication: time to cry halt? *Br Med J* 1995; **310:** 1217–18.
2. Mulla RJ, *et al.* Is it time to stop using chloramphenicol on the eye: fears are based on only six cases. *Br Med J* 1995; **311:** 450.
3. Buckley RJK, *et al.* Is it time to stop using chloramphenicol on the eye: safe in patients with no history of blood dyscrasia. *Br Med J* 1995; **311:** 450.
4. Hall AV, *et al.* Is it time to stop using chloramphenicol on the eye: risk is low in short courses. *Br Med J* 1995; **311:** 450–1.
5. McGhee CNJ, Anastas CN. Widespread ocular use of topical chloramphenicol: is there justifiable concern regarding idiosyncratic aplastic anaemia? *Br J Ophthalmol* 1996; **80:** 182–4.
6. Rayner SA, Buckley RJ. Ocular chloramphenicol and aplastic anaemia: is there a link? *Drug Safety* 1996; **14:** 273–6.
7. Titcomb L. Ophthalmic chloramphenicol and blood dyscrasias: a review. *Pharm J* 1997; **258:** 28–35.
8. Gordon-Smith EC, *et al.* Is it time to stop using chloramphenicol on the eye: prospective study of aplastic anaemia should give definitive answer. *Br Med J* 1995; **311:** 451.
9. Laporte J-R, *et al.* Possible association between ocular chloramphenicol and aplastic anaemia—the absolute risk is very low. *Br J Clin Pharmacol* 1998; **46:** 181–4.

Porphyria. Chloramphenicol has been associated with acute attacks of porphyria and is considered unsafe in patients with acute porphyria.[1]

1. Moore MR, McColl KEL. *Porphyria: drug lists.* Glasgow: Porphyria Research Unit, University of Glasgow, 1991.

Interactions

Chloramphenicol is inactivated in the liver and may, therefore, interact with drugs that are metabolised by hepatic microsomal enzymes. For example, chloramphenicol enhances the effects of coumarin anticoagulants such as dicoumarol and warfarin sodium, some hypoglycaemics such as chlorpropamide and tolbutamide, and antiepileptics such as phenytoin, and may reduce the metabolism of cyclophosphamide to its active form. Conversely the metabolism of chloramphenicol may be increased by inducers of hepatic enzymes such as phenobarbitone or rifampicin. Contradictory results have been reported with paracetamol and phenytoin.

Chloramphenicol may decrease the effects of iron and vitamin B_{12} in anaemic patients and impair the action of oral contraceptives.

For the effects of chloramphenicol on the activity of other antibacterials, see under Antimicrobial Action, below.

Antiepileptics. For reference to the effects of chloramphenicol on phenobarbitone and phenytoin, see p.351 and p.354, respectively. While serum concentrations of chloramphenicol are usually reduced by the hepatic enzyme induction that occurs with phenobarbitone,[1,2] when given with phenytoin elevated and potentially toxic serum-chloramphenicol concentrations have resulted,[2] apparently due to competition for binding sites, although increased metabolism may alternatively lead to decreased serum-chloramphenicol concentrations.

1. Bloxham RA, *et al.* Chloramphenicol and phenobarbitone—a drug interaction. *Arch Dis Child* 1979: **54:** 76–7.
2. Krasinski K, *et al.* Pharmacologic interactions among chloramphenicol, phenytoin and phenobarbital. *Pediatr Infect Dis* 1982; **1:** 232–5.

Cimetidine. Fatal aplastic anaemia of rapid onset has occurred in 2 patients who received intravenous chloramphenicol and cimetidine concomitantly.[1,2] As there is usually a latent period of 2 weeks to 12 months before aplastic anaemia develops following chloramphenicol therapy it is plausible that an additive or synergistic effect may have occurred between the 2 drugs to cause bone-marrow toxicity.

1. Farber BF, Brody JP. Rapid development of aplastic anemia after intravenous chloramphenicol and cimetidine therapy. *South Med J* 1981; **74:** 1257–8.
2. West BC, *et al.* Aplastic anemia associated with parenteral chloramphenicol: review of 10 cases, including the second case of possible increased risk with cimetidine. *Rev Infect Dis* 1988; **10:** 1048–51.

Cyclophosphamide. For the effect of chloramphenicol on cyclophosphamide, see p.517.

Oral contraceptives. For the suggestion that chloramphenicol may reduce the efficacy of oral contraceptives, see Hormonal Contraceptives, p.1433.

Paracetamol. Contradictory results have been reported in patients receiving both chloramphenicol and paracetamol. Buchanan and Moodley[1] reported an increase in chloramphenicol half-life from 3.25 to 15 hours when intravenous paracetamol was given to 6 patients in intensive care 2 hours after intravenous chloramphenicol. In contrast, Spika and colleagues,[2] in a study in 5 children found that the half-life of intravenous chloramphenicol was reduced from 3 to 1.2 hours, concomitant with an increase in clearance, when oral paracetamol was given 30 minutes beforehand. Furthermore, Kearns and colleagues,[3] in a study in 26 children found no evidence of altered disposition when oral paracetamol was given to patients receiving intravenous chloramphenicol, and Stein and colleagues[4] found no significant change in chloramphenicol pharmacokinetics in 5 patients given oral chloramphenicol and paracetamol.

1. Buchanan N, Moodley GP. Interaction between chloramphenicol and paracetamol. *Br Med J* 1979; **2:** 307–8.
2. Spika JS, *et al.* Interaction between chloramphenicol and acetaminophen. *Arch Dis Child* 1986; **61:** 1121–4.
3. Kearns GL, *et al.* Absence of a pharmacokinetic interaction between chloramphenicol and acetaminophen in children. *J Pediatr* 1985; **107:** 134–9.
4. Stein CM, *et al.* Lack of effect of paracetamol on the pharmacokinetics of chloramphenicol. *Br J Clin Pharmacol* 1989; **27:** 262–4.

Preservatives. For a report of interaction between sulphite antoxidants and chloramphenicol, see p.1126.

Antimicrobial Action

Chloramphenicol is a bacteriostatic antibiotic with a broad spectrum of action against both Gram-positive and Gram-negative bacteria, as well as some other organisms.

Mechanism of action. Chloramphenicol is thought to enter sensitive cells by an active transport process. Within the cell it binds to the 50S subunit of the bacterial ribosome at a site adjacent to the site of action of the macrolides and clindamycin, and inhibits bacterial protein synthesis by preventing attachment of aminoacyl transfer RNA to its acceptor site on the ribosome, thus preventing peptide bond formation by peptidyl transferase. The block in protein synthesis results in a primarily bacteriostatic action, although it may be bactericidal to some organisms, including *Haemophilus influenzae*, *Neisseria meningitidis*, and *Streptococcus pneumoniae*, at concentrations about 2 to 4 times the inhibitory concentration.

Spectrum of activity. Chloramphenicol has activity against many types of bacteria although in most cases there are less toxic alternatives available. The following pathogens are usually susceptible (but see also Resistance, below).

Gram-positive cocci including staphylococci such as *Staph. epidermidis* and some strains of *Staph. aureus*, and streptococci such as *Str. pneumoniae*, *Str. pyogenes*, and the viridans streptococci. Methicillin-resistant staphylococci and *Enterococcus faecalis* are considered to be resistant.

Other Gram-positive species including *Bacillus anthracis*, *Corynebacterium diphtheriae*, and anaerobes such as *Peptococcus* and *Peptostreptococcus* spp.

Gram-negative cocci such as *Neisseria meningitidis* and *N. gonorrhoeae* are usually highly sensitive, as are *Haemophilus influenzae* and a variety of other Gram-negative bacteria including *Brucella abortus*, *Campylobacter* spp., *Legionella pneumophila, Pasteurella*, and *Vibrio* spp. The Enterobacteriaceae vary in their susceptibility, and many strains have shown acquired resistance, but *Escherichia coli*, and strains of *Klebsiella* spp., *Proteus mirabilis*, *Salmonella*, *Shigella*, and *Yersinia* spp. have been reported to be susceptible. Many strains of *Enterobacter*, indole positive *Proteus*, and *Serratia* spp. are resistant, or at best moderately susceptible. *Pseudomonas aeruginosa* is invariably resistant although *Burkholderia* (formerly *Pseudomonas*) spp. may be susceptible.

Some Gram-negative anaerobes are susceptible, or moderately so, including *Bacteroides fragilis*, *Veillonella*, and *Fusobacterium* spp.

Other susceptible organisms include *Actinomyces* spp., *Leptospira* spp., spirochaetes such as *Treponema pallidum*, chlamydias, mycoplasmas, and rickettsias. *Nocardia* spp. are resistant. Chloramphenicol is ineffective against fungi, protozoa, and viruses.

Minimum inhibitory concentrations (MICs) for the most sensitive organisms such as *Haemophilus influenzae* or *Neisseria* spp. range from about 0.25 to 2 µg per mL, but organisms with MICs of up to about 12 µg per mL are generally considered susceptible.

Activity with other antimicrobials. As with other bacteriostatic antimicrobials the possibility exists of an antagonistic effect if chloramphenicol is given with a bactericidal drug, and some antagonism has been demonstrated *in vitro* between chloramphenicol and various beta lactams and aminoglycosides but the clinical significance of most of these interactions is usually held to be doubtful. Because of the adjacency of their binding sites on the ribosome chloramphenicol may competitively inhibit the effects of macrolides or lincosamides such as clindamycin.

Resistance. Acquired resistance has been widely reported, although the prevalence of resistance has tended to decline where use of the drug has become less frequent. The most commonly seen form of resistance has been the production of an acetyltransferase that inactivates the drug. Such resistance is usually plasmid-mediated and may be associated with resistance to other drugs such as the tetracyclines. Other mechanisms that may reduce sensitivity to chloramphenicol include reduced permeability or uptake, and ribosomal mutation.

The actual incidence of resistance varies considerably in different countries and different centres. Epidemics of chloramphenicol-resistant *Salmonella* and *Shigella* spp. have occurred in the past, and although the prevalence of resistance in *Salmonella* spp. has been reported to be negligible except in parts of South or South-east Asia, resistant salmonellal infections acquired in these regions are increasingly being seen elsewhere. Resistance among *Haemophilus* and *Neisseria* spp. occurs, and the latter may be problematic in developing countries, although it does not yet seem to be widespread. However, resistant strains of enterococci and pneumococci are reported to be relatively common in some areas, and over 50% of staphylococcal strains have been reported to show resistance in some hospitals.

Pharmacokinetics

Chloramphenicol is readily absorbed when given by mouth. Blood concentrations of 10 μg per mL or more may be reached about 1 or 2 hours after a single dose of 1 g by mouth and blood concentrations of about 18.5 μg per mL have been reported after multiple 1-g doses. Chloramphenicol palmitate is hydrolysed to chloramphenicol in the gastro-intestinal tract prior to absorption, and the sodium succinate, which is given parenterally, is probably hydrolysed to free drug mainly in the liver, lungs, and kidneys; such hydrolysis may be incomplete in infants and neonates contributing to the variable pharmacokinetics in this age group. Chloramphenicol sodium succinate is, even in adults, only partially and variably hydrolysed so that blood concentrations of chloramphenicol obtained after parenteral administration of the sodium succinate are often lower than those obtained after administration of chloramphenicol by mouth, with up to 30% of a dose excreted unchanged in the urine before hydrolysis can take place.

Chloramphenicol is widely distributed in body tissues and fluids; it enters the CSF, giving concentrations of about 50% of those existing in the blood even in the absence of meningitis; it diffuses across the placenta into the fetal circulation, into breast milk, and into the aqueous and vitreous humours of the eye. It also enters the aqueous humour following topical application. Up to about 60% in the circulation is bound to plasma protein. The half-life of chloramphenicol has been reported to range from 1.5 to 4 hours; the half-life is prolonged in patients with severe liver impairment and is also much longer in neonates. Renal impairment has relatively little effect on the half-life of the active drug, due to its extensive metabolism, but may lead to accumulation of the inactive metabolites.

Chloramphenicol is excreted mainly in the urine but only 5 to 10% of an oral dose appears unchanged; the remainder is inactivated in the liver, mostly by conjugation with glucuronic acid. About 3% is excreted in the bile. However, most is reabsorbed and only about 1%, mainly in the inactive form, is excreted in the faeces.

The absorption, metabolism, and excretion of chloramphenicol are subject to considerable interindividual variation, especially in infants and children, making monitoring of plasma concentrations necessary to determine pharmacokinetics in a given patient.

Uses and Administration

The liability of chloramphenicol to provoke life-threatening adverse effects, particularly bone-marrow aplasia, has severely limited its clinical usefulness, although it is still widely used in some countries. It should never be given systemically for minor infections and regular blood counts are usually advisable during treatment. The third-generation cephalosporins are now favoured for many of the former indications of chloramphenicol. There are consequently few unambiguous indications for the use of chloramphenicol. It has been used in severe typhoid and other salmonellal infections, although it does not eliminate the carrier state. Chloramphenicol is an alternative to a third-generation cephalosporin in the treatment of bacterial meningitis, both empirically and against sensitive organisms such as *Haemophilus influenzae*. It has been used in the treatment of severe anaerobic infections, particularly in brain abscesses, and in infections below the diaphragm where *Bacteroides fragilis* is often implicated; however, other drugs are usually preferred. Although the tetracyclines remain the treatment of choice in rickettsial infections such as typhus and the spotted fevers, chloramphenicol is also used as an alternative where the tetracyclines cannot be given.

Other bacterial infections in which chloramphenicol may be used as an alternative to other drugs include anthrax, severe systemic infections with *Campylobacter fetus*, ehrlichiosis, severe gastro-enteritis, gas gangrene, granuloma inguinale, severe *Haemophilus influenzae* infections other than meningitis (for example in epiglottitis), listeriosis, severe melioidosis, plague (especially if meningitis develops), psittacosis, tularaemia (especially when meningitis is suspected), and Whipple's disease. For details of these infections and their treatment, see under Choice of Antibacterial, p.116.

Chloramphenicol is extensively used in the topical treatment of ear and, in particular, eye infections, despite the fact that many of these are mild and self-limiting. It is also used topically in the treatment of skin infections.

When given by mouth, chloramphenicol is usually administered in capsules or as a suspension of chloramphenicol palmitate. When oral administration is not feasible water-soluble chloramphenicol sodium succinate may be given intravenously, but oral therapy should be substituted as soon as possible; an intravenous dose should be injected over at least one minute. Administration by intramuscular injection is controversial because of doubts whether absorption is adequate. In some countries chloramphenicol has been given rectally as suppositories.

Doses are expressed in terms of chloramphenicol base and are similar whether administered by mouth or intravenously. For adults and children the usual dose is 50 mg per kg body-weight daily in divided doses every 6 hours; up to 100 mg per kg daily may be given in meningitis or severe infections due to moderately resistant organisms, although these higher doses should be reduced as soon as possible. To minimise the risk of relapse it has been recommended that treatment should be continued after the patient's temperature has returned to normal for a further 4 days in rickettsial diseases and for 8 to 10 days in typhoid fever.

Where there is no alternative to the use of chloramphenicol, premature and full-term neonates may be given daily doses of 25 mg per kg body-weight and full-term infants over the age of 2 weeks may be given up to 50 mg per kg daily, in 4 divided doses. Monitoring of plasma concentrations is essential to avoid toxicity.

In patients with impaired hepatic function or severe renal impairment the dose of chloramphenicol may need to be reduced because of decreased metabolism or excretion.

In the treatment of eye infections chloramphenicol is usually applied as a 0.5% solution or as a 1% ointment.

Chloramphenicol has also been used in the form of various other derivatives including the arginine succinate, the cinnamate, the glycinate, the glycinate sulphate, the palmitoylglycolate, the pantothenate, the steaglate, the stearate, and the hydrogen succinate.

Administration. INTRAMUSCULAR ADMINISTRATION. When parenteral administration of chloramphenicol is necessary the intravenous route is generally preferred although the intramuscular route has been advocated. Shann and others[1] reported adequate serum concentrations after intramuscular injection, contrary to the widely held belief that chloramphenicol sodium succinate is poorly absorbed by this route, and claimed that pain on injection was minimal. Following a study in children with bacterial meningitis[2] they suggested treatment with intramuscular chloramphenicol for 2 or 3 days, followed by oral therapy. However, Coulthard and Lamb[3] found that children describe intramuscular chloramphenicol as amongst the worst treatments they ever receive, and certainly much worse than the insertion of intravenous cannulae.

1. Shann F, *et al.* Absorption of chloramphenicol sodium succinate after intramuscular administration in children. *N Engl J Med* 1985; **313:** 410–14.
2. Shann F, *et al.* Chloramphenicol alone versus chloramphenicol plus penicillin for bacterial meningitis in children. *Lancet* 1985; **ii** 681–3.
3. Coulthard MG, Lamb WH. Antibiotics: intramuscular or intravenous? *Lancet* 1985; **ii:** 1015.

Preparations

BP 1998: Chloramphenicol Capsules; Chloramphenicol Ear Drops; Chloramphenicol Eye Drops; Chloramphenicol Eye Ointment; Chloramphenicol Sodium Succinate Injection;
USP 23: Chloramphenicol and Hydrocortisone Acetate for Ophthalmic Suspension; Chloramphenicol and Polymyxin B Sulfate Ophthalmic Ointment; Chloramphenicol and Prednisolone Ophthalmic Ointment; Chloramphenicol Capsules; Chloramphenicol Cream; Chloramphenicol for Ophthalmic Solution; Chloramphenicol Ophthalmic Ointment; Chloramphenicol Ophthalmic Solution; Chloramphenicol Otic Solution; Chloramphenicol Palmitate Oral Suspension; Chloramphenicol Sodium Succinate for Injection; Chloramphenicol, Polymyxin B Sulfate, and Hydrocortisone Acetate Ophthalmic Ointment.

Proprietary Preparations (details are given in Part 3)

Aust.: Biophenicol; Halomycetin; Kemicetin; Oleomycetin; ***Austral.:*** Chloromycetin; Chloroptic†; Chlorsig; ***Belg.:*** Chloromycetin†; Fenicol†; Isopto Fenicol†; Kemicetina; ***Canad.:*** Chloromycetin; Chloroptic; Diochloram; Novo-Chlorocap; Optho-Chloram; Pentamycetin; Sopamycetin†; ***Fr.:*** Cebenicol; Tifomycine†; ***Ger.:*** Aquamycetin; Berlicetin; Chloramsaar N; Chloroptic†; Dispaphenicol†; Oleomycetin; Paraxin; Posifenicol C; Thilocanfol C; ***Irl.:*** Chloromycetin; Chloroptic; Sno Phenicol†; ***Ital.:*** Chemicetina; Chloromycetin; Cloramfen; Micoclorina†; Micodry†; Mycetin; Sificetina; Vitamfenicolo; ***Neth.:*** Globenicol; ***S.Afr.:*** Chloramex; Chlorcol; Chloromycetin; Chloroptic; Chlorphen; Fenicol; Lennacol†; Spersanicol; Troymycetin†; ***Spain:*** Chemicetina; Chloromycetin; Cloramplast†; Cloranfe; Cloranfenic; Clorofenicina†; Isopto Fenicol; Normofenicol; Plastodermo†; ***Swed.:*** Chloromycetin; Isopto Fenicol; ***Switz.:*** Chloromycetin; Septicol; Serviclofen†; Spersanicol; Suismycetin†; ***UK:*** Chloromycetin; Kemicetine; Sno Phenicol; ***USA:*** Ak-Chlor; Chloromycetin; Chloroptic.

Multi-ingredient: ***Aust.:*** Cortison Kemicetin; Oleomycetin-Prednison; ***Austral.:*** Chlorocort; Chloromyxin†; ***Belg.:*** De Icol; Viscocort; ***Canad.:*** Actinac; Elase-Chloromycetin; Ophthocort; Pentamycetin-HC; Sopamycetin/HC†; ***Fr.:*** Cebedexacol; ***Ger.:*** Amindan†; Aquapred; Berlicetin-Ohrentropfen; Biofenicol-N†; Corti-Flexiole; Dexa-Biofenicol-N†; Fibrolan mit Chloromycetin†; Ichthoseptal; Iruxol; Mindaril†; Oleomycetin-Prednison; Pima Biciron†; Positex†; Spersadex Comp; Spersadexolin; Spersidu C†; ***Irl.:*** Actinac; Iruxol†; Tanderil Chloramphenicol†; ***Ital.:*** Antibioptal; Aurizone†; Betabioptal; Chemyterral†; Colbiocin; Corti-Fluoral; Cortison Chemicetina; Cosmiciclina; Dexoline; Eubetal Antibiotico; Fluorobioptal; Geomix†; Idracemi; Iruxol; Otomicetina; Vasofen; Vitecaf; Xantervit Antibiotico; ***Norw.:*** Spersadex med kloramfenikol; ***S.Afr.:*** Chloramex H†; Corti-Flexiole†; Covomycin; Covomycin-D; Covotop; Spersacet C; Spersadex Comp; Spersadexoline; ***Spain:*** Amidrin Bio†; Blefarida; Clo Zinc; Clor Hemi; Cortison Chemicet Topica; Cortison Chemicetina†; Cortivel; Dermisone Epitelizante†; Dexa Fenic; Dexafenicol; Dexam Constric; Dorsec†; Epitelizante; Fluo Fenic; Ginesona†; Hidroc Cloranf; Icol; Medricol; Medrivas Antib; Otosedol Biotico; Parkelase Chloromycetin; Pomada Llorens Sulfaclor†; Predni Azuleno; Ultralan†; ***Swed.:*** Chloromycetin Hydrocortison†; ***Switz.:*** Bacicoline†; Cortiphenol H†; Herpidu Chloramphenicol†; Mindaril†; Septicortin; Spersacet C; Spersadex Comp; Spersadexoline; Spersanicol vitamine†; ***UK:*** Actinac; Chloromycetin Hydrocortisone; ***USA:*** Chloromycetin Hydrocortisone; Elase-Chloromycetin; Ophthocort†.

Chlorquinaldol (1601-n)

Chlorquinaldol *(BAN, rINN)*.

5,7-Dichloro-2-methylquinolin-8-ol.

$C_{10}H_7Cl_2NO$ = 228.1.

CAS — 72-80-0.

Pharmacopoeias. In *Pol.*

Chlorquinaldol is a halogenated hydroxyquinoline with properties similar to those of clioquinol (p.193). It is mainly applied topically in infected skin conditions and in vaginal infections.

Preparations

Proprietary Preparations (details are given in Part 3)
Austral.: Steroxin†; ***Fr.:*** Gynotherax†; ***Switz.:*** Sterosan†.

Multi-ingredient: ***Aust.:*** Neriquinol; Ultraquinol; ***Fr.:*** Nerisone C; ***Ger.:*** Dignoquine†; Nerisona C; Proctospre; Sirinal†; Tyrosirinal†; Vobaderm Plus†; ***Irl.:*** Locoid C; ***Ital.:*** Eczecur†; Impetex; Nerisona C; Proctocort†; ***Mon.:*** Colposeptine; ***Norw.:*** Cortikinol†; Locoidol; ***S.Afr.:*** Locoid C†; ***Spain:*** Amplidermis; Claral Plus; Colposeptina†; Lidobama Plus†; Quinortar; Temetex Compositum†; ***Swed.:*** Sterosan-Hydrocortisone†; ***Switz.:*** Candio E†; Lidazon; Proctospre; Sano-Angin†; Temetex C†; ***UK:*** Locoid C.

Chlortetracycline (50-n)

Chlortetracycline *(BAN, rINN)*.

(4*S*,4a*S*,5a*S*,6*S*,12a*S*)-7-Chloro-4-dimethylamino-1,4,4a,5,5a,6,11,12a-octahydro-3,6,10,12,12a-pentahydroxy-6-methyl-1,11-dioxonaphthacene-2-carboxamide; 7-Chlorotetracycline.

$C_{22}H_{23}ClN_2O_8$ = 478.9.

CAS — 57-62-5.

Chlortetracycline Hydrochloride (52-m)

Chlortetracycline Hydrochloride *(BANM, rINNM)*.

Chlortetracyclini Hydrochloridum.

$C_{22}H_{23}ClN_2O_8$,HCl = 515.3.

CAS — 64-72-2.

NOTE. Aureomycin and aureomycin hydrochloride were used as nonproprietary names for chlortetracycline hydrochloride; these names are now used in some countries as proprietary names.

Pharmacopoeias. In *Chin., Eur.* (see p.viii), *Int., Pol.,* and *US.*

US also includes Chlortetracycline Bisulfate for veterinary use.

An antimicrobial substance produced by the growth of certain strains of *Streptomyces aureofaciens* or by any other means.

Yellow odourless crystalline powder. **Soluble** 1 in 75 of water and 1 in 560 of alcohol; soluble in solutions of alkali hydroxides and carbonates; practically insoluble in acetone, chloroform, dioxan, and ether. A 1% solution in water has a pH of 2.3 to 3.3. **Store** in airtight containers. Protect from light.

Incompatibilities. Preparations of chlortetracycline have an acid pH and incompatibility may reasonably be expected with alkaline preparations or drugs unstable at low pH.

Adverse Effects and Precautions

As for Tetracycline Hydrochloride, p.259.

Interactions

As for Tetracycline Hydrochloride, p.260.

Antimicrobial Action

As for Tetracycline Hydrochloride, p.260. It is somewhat less active against many Gram-negative organisms.

Pharmacokinetics

As for Tetracycline Hydrochloride, p.260.

Chlortetracycline is poorly absorbed from the gastro-intestinal tract compared with other tetracyclines. It is reported to be rapidly inactivated in the body with a half-life of about 6 hours and is largely eliminated by biliary excretion. About 45% of a dose is protein bound. Only a small amount is excreted in the urine and although it is not recommended in patients with renal impairment accumulation would not be likely despite an increase in half-life to 7 to 11 hours.

Uses and Administration

Chlortetracycline is a tetracycline derivative with uses similar to those of tetracycline (p.261).

It is given by mouth as the hydrochloride in a usual dose of 250 to 500 mg four times daily, preferably one hour before, or 2 hours after, meals. However, it is more often used topically as a 1% ophthalmic ointment and as a 3% cream or ointment for application to the skin.

Mouth ulceration. In a double-blind placebo-controlled study[1] involving 57 patients with recurrent aphthous ulcers (p.1172) chlortetracycline 250 mg in 10 mL of water used as a mouth rinse for one minute 4 times daily for 4 consecutive days and repeated if necessary after a rinse-free period of one week, was found to be an effective local treatment. See also under Tetracycline (p.261).

1. Henricsson V, Axéll T. Treatment of recurrent aphthous ulcers with Aureomycin mouth rinse or Zendium dentifrice. *Acta Odontol Scand* 1985; **43:** 47–52.

Preparations

BP 1998: Chlortetracycline Eye Ointment; Chlortetracycline Ointment;
USP 23: Chlortetracycline Hydrochloride Capsules; Chlortetracycline Hydrochloride Ointment; Chlortetracycline Hydrochloride Ophthalmic Ointment.

Proprietary Preparations (details are given in Part 3)
Aust.: Aureomycin; ***Austral.:*** Aureomycin; ***Belg.:*** Aureomycin; Aureomycine; ***Canad.:*** Aureomycin; ***Fr.:*** Aureomycine; ***Ger.:*** Aureomycin; ***Irl.:*** Aureomycin; ***Ital.:*** Aureomicina; ***Neth.:*** Aureomycin; ***Norw.:*** Aureomycin; ***S.Afr.:*** Aureomycin; ***Spain:*** Aureomicina; Dermosa Aureomicina; ***Swed.:*** Aureomycin; ***Switz.:*** Aureomycin; ***UK:*** Aureomycin; ***USA:*** Aureomycin†.

Multi-ingredient: ***Aust.:*** Aureocort; ***Canad.:*** Aureocort†; ***Ger.:*** Aureodelf; Aureomycin N; ***Irl.:*** Aureocort; Deteclo; ***Ital.:*** Aureocort; Aureomix; ***S.Afr.:*** Tritet; ***Spain:*** Antiblefarica; Poliantib; ***UK:*** Aureocort; Deteclo.

Ciclacillin (63-g)

Ciclacillin *(BAN, rINN)*.

Cyclacillin *(USAN)*; Wy-4508. (6*R*)-6-(1-Aminocyclohexanecarboxamido)penicillanic acid.

$C_{15}H_{23}N_3O_4S$ = 341.4.

CAS — 3485-14-1.

Pharmacopoeias. In *Jpn* and *US.*

A 1% solution in water has a pH of 4.0 to 6.5. **Store** in airtight containers.

Ciclacillin is an aminopenicillin with properties similar to those of ampicillin (p.153), although it is generally less active *in vitro*. It has been given in doses of 250 to 500 mg four times daily by mouth.

Preparations

USP 23: Cyclacillin for Oral Suspension; Cyclacillin Tablets.

Proprietary Preparations (details are given in Part 3)
Belg.: Wypicil†.

Cilastatin Sodium (16578-v)

Cilastatin Sodium *(BANM, USAN, rINNM)*.

MK-791. (*Z*)-(*S*)-6-Carboxy-6-[(*S*)-2,2-dimethylcyclopropanecarboxamido]hex-5-enyl-L-cysteine, monosodium salt.

$C_{16}H_{25}N_2NaO_5S$ = 380.4.

CAS — 82009-34-5 (cilastatin); 81129-83-1 (cilastatin sodium).

Pharmacopoeias. In *US.*

A white to tan powder. **Soluble** in water and in methyl alcohol. A 1% solution in water has a pH of 6.5 to 7.5. **Store** at a temperature less than 8°.

Cilastatin sodium is an inhibitor of dehydropeptidase I, an enzyme found in the brush border of the renal tubules. It is administered concurrently with the antibiotic imipenem (p.216) to prevent its renal metabolism to microbiologically inactive and potentially nephrotoxic products. This increases the concentrations of imipenem achieved in the urine and protects against any nephrotoxic effects, which were seen with high doses of imipenem given experimentally to *animals*.

Cilastatin has no antibacterial activity itself, and does not affect the antibacterial activity of imipenem.

Preparations

USP 23: Imipenem and Cilastatin for Injectable Suspension; Imipenem and Cilastatin for Injection.

Proprietary Preparations (details are given in Part 3)

Multi-ingredient: ***Aust.:*** Zienam; ***Austral.:*** Primaxin; ***Belg.:*** Tienam; ***Canad.:*** Primaxin; ***Fr.:*** Tienam; ***Ger.:*** Zienam; ***Ital.:*** Imipem; Tenacid; Tienam; ***Neth.:*** Tienam; ***Norw.:*** Tienam; ***S.Afr.:*** Tienam; ***Spain:*** Tienam; ***Swed.:*** Tienam; ***Switz.:*** Tienam; ***UK:*** Primaxin; ***USA:*** Primaxin.

Cinoxacin (5655-n)

Cinoxacin *(BAN, USAN, rINN)*.

64716; Azolinic Acid; Compound 64716. 1-Ethyl-1,4-dihydro-4-oxo-1,3-dioxolo[4,5-*g*]cinnoline-3-carboxylic acid.

$C_{12}H_{10}N_2O_5$ = 262.2.

CAS — 28657-80-9.

Pharmacopoeias. In *US.*

White to yellowish-white, odourless crystalline solid. Practically **insoluble** in water and in most common organic solvents; soluble in alkaline solution. **Store** in airtight containers.

Adverse Effects and Precautions

As for Nalidixic Acid, p.228.

Cinoxacin is not recommended in patients with severe renal impairment, and the dosage should be reduced in those with mild to moderate renal impairment.

References.

1. Stricker BHC, *et al.* Anaphylactic reactions to cinoxacin. *Br Med J* 1988; **297:** 1434–5.

Interactions

As for Nalidixic Acid, p.228.

Antimicrobial Action

As for Nalidixic Acid, p.228. Cross-resistance with nalidixic acid has been shown.

Pharmacokinetics

Cinoxacin is rapidly and almost completely absorbed following administration by mouth. Peak serum concentrations of about 15 μg per mL have been obtained 1 to 3 hours after a 500-mg dose. The plasma half-life is about 1 to 1.5 hours. Cinoxacin has been reported to be more than 60% bound to plasma proteins.

Cinoxacin appears to be metabolised in the liver and is excreted via the kidney. Over 95% of a dose appears in the urine within 24 hours, over half as unaltered drug and the remainder as inactive metabolites. Mean urinary concentrations of about 300 μg per mL have been achieved during the first 4 hours after administration of a 500-mg dose by mouth. Urinary excretion is reduced by probenecid and in patients with renal impairment.

Uses and Administration

Cinoxacin is a 4-quinolone antibacterial with actions and uses similar to those of nalidixic acid (p.229). In the treatment of urinary-tract infections the usual adult dose is 500 mg twice daily by mouth for 7 to 14 days; for prophylaxis a single dose of 500 mg daily at bedtime may be given. Dosage should be reduced in mild to moderate renal impairment; cinoxacin is not recommended in patients with severe renal impairment.

References.

1. Sisca TS, *et al.* Cinoxacin: a review of its pharmacological properties and therapeutic efficacy in the treatment of urinary tract infections. *Drugs* 1983; **25:** 544–69.

Preparations

USP 23: Cinoxacin Capsules.

Proprietary Preparations (details are given in Part 3)
Aust.: Cinobac; ***Belg.:*** Cinobac; ***Ger.:*** Cinobactin; ***Ital.:*** Cinobac; Nossacin; Noxigram; Uroc; Uronorm; Uroxacin; ***Neth.:*** Cinobac†; ***S.Afr.:*** Cinobactin; ***Swed.:*** Cinobactin†; ***UK:*** Cinobac; ***USA:*** Cinobac.

Ciprofloxacin (16850-v)

Ciprofloxacin *(BAN, USAN, rINN)*.

Bay-q-3939; Ciprofloxacinum. 1-Cyclopropyl-6-fluoro-1,4-dihydro-4-oxo-7-piperazin-1-ylquinoline-3-carboxylic acid.

$C_{17}H_{18}FN_3O_3$ = 331.3.

CAS — 85721-33-1.

Pharmacopoeias. In *Eur.* (see p.viii) and *US.*

A pale yellow, crystalline powder. Practically **insoluble** in water; very slightly soluble in dehydrated alcohol and in dichloromethane; soluble in dilute acetic acid. **Store** in airtight containers. Protect from light.

Ciprofloxacin Hydrochloride (11305-s)

Ciprofloxacin Hydrochloride *(BANM, USAN, rINNM)*.

Bay-o-9867; Ciprofloxacini Hydrochloridum. Ciprofloxacin hydrochloride monohydrate.

$C_{17}H_{18}FN_3O_3$,HCl,H_2O = 385.8.

CAS — 86483-48-9 (anhydrous ciprofloxacin hydrochloride); 86393-32-0 (ciprofloxacin hydrochloride monohydrate).

Pharmacopoeias. In *Eur.* (see p.viii), *Pol.,* and *US.*

Faintly yellowish to light yellow crystals or crystalline powder. 291.1 mg is approximately equivalent to 250 mg of ciprofloxacin. Sparingly **soluble** to soluble in water; slightly soluble in acetic acid and in methyl alcohol; very slightly soluble in dehydrated alcohol; practically insoluble in acetone, in acetonitrile, in dichloromethane, in ethyl acetate, and in hexane. A 2.5% solution in water has a pH of 3.0 to 4.5. **Store** in airtight containers. Protect from light.

Ciprofloxacin Lactate (11306-w)

Ciprofloxacin Lactate *(BANM, rINNM)*.

$C_{17}H_{18}FN_3O_3$,$C_3H_6O_3$ = 421.4.

CAS — 97867-33-9.

127 mg is approximately equivalent to 100 mg of ciprofloxacin.

Incompatibility. Ciprofloxacin infusion is stated by the manufacturers to have a pH of 3.9 to 4.5 and to be incompatible with injections chemically or physically unstable at this pH range. Incompatibility has been reported between ciprofloxacin and a range of drugs including some other antibacterials.[1-4]

1. Lyall D, Blythe J. Ciprofloxacin lactate infusion. *Pharm J* 1987; **238:** 290.
2. Jim LK. Physical and chemical compatibility of intravenous ciprofloxacin with other drugs. *Ann Pharmacother* 1993; **27:** 704–7.

3. Janknegt R, *et al.* Quinolones and penicillins incompatibility. *DICP Ann Pharmacother* 1989; **23:** 91–2.
4. Goodwin SD, *et al.* Compatibility of ciprofloxacin injection with selected drugs and solutions. *Am J Hosp Pharm* 1991; **48:** 2166–71.

Adverse Effects

Ciprofloxacin is generally well tolerated. The range of adverse effects associated with ciprofloxacin and the other fluoroquinolone antibacterials is broadly similar to that with earlier quinolones such as nalidixic acid (p.228). They most often involve the gastro-intestinal tract, CNS, or skin.

Gastro-intestinal disturbances include nausea, vomiting, diarrhoea, abdominal pain, and dyspepsia and are the most frequent adverse effects. Pseudomembranous colitis has been reported rarely.

Headache, dizziness, and restlessness are among the commonest effects on the CNS. Others include tremor, drowsiness, insomnia, nightmares, and visual and other sensory disturbances and, more rarely, hallucinations, psychotic reactions, depression, and convulsions. Paraesthesia and peripheral neuropathy have occurred occasionally.

In addition to rash and pruritus, hypersensitivity-type reactions affecting the skin have included, rarely, vasculitis, erythema multiforme, Stevens-Johnson syndrome, and toxic epidermal necrolysis. Photosensitivity has occurred, and may be more frequent with some newer fluoroquinolones such as lomefloxacin and sparfloxacin. Anaphylaxis has been reported. As with other quinolone antibacterials reversible arthralgia has sometimes occurred and joint erosions have been documented in immature *animals*. Tendon damage has been reported.

Other adverse effects reported with ciprofloxacin include transient increases in serum creatinine or blood urea nitrogen and, occasionally, acute renal failure secondary to interstitial nephritis; crystalluria; elevated liver enzyme values, jaundice, and hepatitis; haematological disturbances including eosinophilia, leucopenia, thrombocytopenia and, very rarely, haemolytic anaemia or agranulocytosis; myalgia; gynaecomastia; and cardiovascular effects including tachycardia.

As with other antibacterials superinfection with organisms not very susceptible to ciprofloxacin is possible. Such organisms include *Candida*, *Clostridium difficile*, and *Streptococcus pneumoniae*.

Pain and irritation may occur at the site of injection accompanied rarely by phlebitis or thrombophlebitis.

General reviews of the adverse effects of fluoroquinolone antibacterials.

1. Stahlmann R. Safety profile of the quinolones. *J Antimicrob Chemother* 1990; **26** (suppl D): 31–44.
2. Paton JH, Reeves DS. Adverse reactions to the fluoroquinolones. *Adverse Drug React Bull* 1992; (April): 575–8.
3. Domagala JM. Structure-activity and structure-side-effect relationships for the quinolone antibacterials. *J Antimicrob Chemother* 1994; **33:** 685–706.
4. Rubinstein E, *et al.* The use of fluoroquinolones in neutropenic patients—analysis of adverse effects. *J Antimicrob Chemother* 1994; **34:** 7–19.
5. Ball P, Tillotson G. Tolerability of fluoroquinolone antibiotics: past, present and future. *Drug Safety* 1995; **13:** 343–58.

Reviews and surveys of the adverse effects of ciprofloxacin.

1. Arcieri GM, *et al.* Safety of intravenous ciprofloxacin: a review. *Am J Med* 1989; **87** (suppl 5A): 92S–97S.
2. Schacht P, *et al.* Safety of oral ciprofloxacin: an update based on clinical trial results. *Am J Med* 1989; **87** (suppl 5A): 98S–102S.
3. Kennedy N, *et al.* Safety profile of ciprofloxacin during long-term therapy for pulmonary tuberculosis. *J Antimicrob Chemother* 1993; **32:** 897–902.

Effects on the blood. Haematological disturbances including eosinophilia, leucopenia, thrombocytopenia, and, very rarely, haemolytic anaemia have been reported with ciprofloxacin. In addition, transient reductions in factor VIII and von Willebrand's factor leading to bleeding in 2 patients receiving ciprofloxacin has been reported.[1]

1. Castaman G, Rodeghiero F. Acquired transitory von Willebrand syndrome with ciprofloxacin. *Lancet* 1994; **343:** 492.

Effects on the gastro-intestinal tract. Reports of pseudomembranous colitis or superinfection with *Clostridium difficile* associated with ciprofloxacin and other fluoroquinolones.

1. Dan M, Samra Z. Clostridium difficile colitis associated with ofloxacin therapy. *Am J Med* 1989; **87:** 479.
2. Cain DB, O'Connor ME. Pseudomembranous colitis associated with ciprofloxacin. *Lancet* 1990; **336:** 946.
3. Bates CJ, *et al.* Ciprofloxacin and Clostridium difficile infection. *Lancet* 1990; **336:** 1193.
4. Low N, Harries A. Ciprofloxacin and pseudomembranous colitis. *Lancet* 1990; **336:** 1510.
5. Hillman RJ, *et al.* Ciprofloxacin as a cause of Clostridium difficile-associated diarrhoea in an HIV antibody-positive patient. *J Infect* 1990; **21:** 205–7.
6. Golledge CL, *et al.* Ciprofloxacin and Clostridium difficile-associated diarrhoea. *J Antimicrob Chemother* 1992; **30:** 141–7.
7. McFarland LV, *et al.* Ciprofloxacin-associated Clostridium difficile disease. *Lancet* 1995; **346:** 977–8.

Effects on the kidneys. References to renal toxicity associated with ciprofloxacin and other fluoroquinolones.

1. Rippelmeyer DJ, Synhavsky A. Ciprofloxacin and allergic interstitial nephritis. *Ann Intern Med* 1988; **109:** 170.
2. Ying LS, Johnson CA. Ciprofloxacin-induced interstitial nephritis. *Clin Pharm* 1989; **8:** 518–21.
3. Rastogi S, *et al.* Allergic nephropathy associated with ciprofloxacin. *Mayo Clin Proc* 1990; **65:** 987–9.
4. Allon M, *et al.* Acute renal failure due to ciprofloxacin. *Arch Intern Med* 1990; **150:** 2187–9.
5. George MJ, *et al.* Acute renal failure after an overdose of ciprofloxacin. *Arch Intern Med* 1991; **151:** 620.
6. Simpson J, *et al.* Typhoid fever, ciprofloxacin, and renal failure. *Arch Dis Child* 1991; **66:** 1083–4.
7. Yew WW, *et al.* Ciprofloxacin-induced renal dysfunction in patients with mycobacterial lung infections. *Tubercle Lung Dis* 1995; **76:** 173–5.
8. Hestin D, *et al.* Norfloxacin-induced nephrotic syndrome. *Lancet* 1995; **345:** 732–3.

Effects on the liver. References to hepatotoxicity associated with ciprofloxacin and other fluoroquinolones.

1. Grassmick BK, *et al.* Fulminant hepatic failure possibly related to ciprofloxacin. *Ann Pharmacother* 1992; **26:** 636–9.
2. Sherman O, Beizer JL. Possible ciprofloxacin-induced acute cholestatic jaundice. *Ann Pharmacother* 1994; **28:** 1162–4.
3. Villeneuve J-P, *et al.* Suspected ciprofloxacin-induced hepatotoxicity. *Ann Pharmacother* 1995; **29:** 257–9.
4. Jones SE, Smith RH. Quinolones may induce hepatitis. *Br Med J* 1997; **314:** 869.

Effects on the musculoskeletal system. Reversible arthralgia has sometimes occurred with the fluoroquinolone antibacterials;[1] joint erosions have been documented in immature *animals*. In one case report, treatment with pefloxacin might have contributed to the destructive arthropathy that occurred in a 17-year-old youth.[2]

More recently there have been reports of tendinitis and tendon rupture associated with fluoroquinolones.[3-6] By July 1995 the UK Committee on Safety of Medicines (CSM) had received 21 reports of tendon damage, often of the Achilles tendon, associated with these antibacterials—11 with ciprofloxacin and 10 with ofloxacin.[6] The risk of tendon damage might be increased by the concomitant use of corticosteroids and appeared more common with increasing age.[6] The CSM warned that at the first sign of pain or inflammation the quinolone should be discontinued and the affected limb rested until the tendon symptoms had resolved.[6] Similar warnings have been issued in other countries.

1. Alfaham M, *et al.* Arthropathy in a patient with cystic fibrosis taking ciprofloxacin. *Br Med J* 1987; **295:** 699.
2. Chevalier X, *et al.* A case of destructive polyarthropathy in a 17-year-old youth following pefloxacin treatment. *Drug Safety* 1992; **7:** 310–14.
3. Huston KA. Achilles tendinitis and tendon rupture due to fluoroquinolone antibiotics. *N Engl J Med* 1994; **331:** 748.
4. Szarfman A, *et al.* More on fluoroquinolone antibiotics and tendon rupture. *N Engl J Med* 1995; **332:** 193.
5. Carrasco JM, *et al.* Tendinitis associated with ciprofloxacin. *Ann Pharmacother* 1997; **31:** 120.
6. Committee on Safety of Medicines/Medicines Control Agency. Tendon damage associated with quinolone antibiotics. *Current Problems* 1995; **21:** 8.

Effects on the nervous system. By 1991 the UK Committee on Safety of Medicines had received 26 reports of convulsions associated with ciprofloxacin, 1 with norfloxacin, and 1 with ofloxacin.[1] They noted that convulsions could occur both in patients with epilepsy and in those with no previous history of convulsions.

Other recent reports of CNS toxicity associated with ciprofloxacin have included eosinophilic meningitis,[2] delirium,[3] and acute psychoses.[4,5] Peripheral neuropathy,[6] dysaesthesia,[7] catatonia,[8] sleep disturbances,[9] hemiparesis,[10] and tinnitus[11] have also been reported.

There has also been a report of a Tourette-like syndrome associated with ofloxacin.[12]

1. Committee on Safety of Medicines. Convulsions due to quinolone antimicrobial agents. *Current Problems 32* 1991.
2. Asperilla MO, *et al.* Eosinophilic meningitis associated with ciprofloxacin. *Am J Med* 1989; **87:** 589–90.
3. Jay GT, Fitzgerald JM. Ciprofloxacin-induced delirium. *Ann Pharmacother* 1997; **31:** 252.
4. McCue JD, Zandt JR. Acute psychoses associated with the use of ciprofloxacin and trimethoprim-sulfamethoxazole. *Am J Med* 1991; **90:** 528–9.
5. Reeves RR. Ciprofloxacin-induced psychosis. *Ann Pharmacother* 1992; **26:** 930–1.
6. Aoun M, *et al.* Peripheral neuropathy associated with fluoroquinolones. *Lancet* 1992; **340:** 127.
7. Zehnder D, *et al.* Painful dysaesthesia with ciprofloxacin. *Br Med J* 1995; **311:** 1204.
8. Akhtar S, Ahmad H. Ciprofloxacin-induced catatonia. *J Clin Psychiatry* 1993; **54:** 115–16.
9. Upton C. Sleep disturbance in children treated with ofloxacin. *Br Med J* 1994; **309:** 1411.
10. Rosolen A, *et al.* Acute hemiparesis associated with ciprofloxacin. *Br Med J* 1994; **309:** 1411.
11. Paul J, Brown NM. Tinnitus and ciprofloxacin. *Br Med J* 1995; **311:** 232.
12. Thomas RJ, Reagan DR. Association of a Tourette-like syndrome with ofloxacin. *Ann Pharmacother* 1996; **30:** 138–41.

Hypersensitivity. Hypersensitivity and skin reactions have been associated with ciprofloxacin and other fluoroquinolones. Reports have included anaphylaxis (which has been fatal),[1-4] serum sickness,[5] toxic epidermal necrolysis,[6-8] laryngeal oedema,[9] and vasculitis.[10-12] Fatal vasculitis has been reported with ofloxacin.[13]

1. Davis H, *et al.* Anaphylactoid reactions reported after treatment with ciprofloxacin. *Ann Intern Med* 1989; **111:** 1041–3.
2. Peters B, Pinching AJ. Fatal anaphylaxis associated with ciprofloxacin in a patient with AIDS related complex. *Br Med J* 1989; **298:** 605.
3. Wurtz RM, *et al.* Anaphylactoid drug reactions to ciprofloxacin and rifampicin in HIV-infected patients. *Lancet* 1989; **i:** 955–6.
4. Assouad M, *et al.* Anaphylactoid reactions to ciprofloxacin. *Ann Intern Med* 1995; **122:** 396–7.
5. Slama TG. Serum sickness-like illness associated with ciprofloxacin. *Antimicrob Agents Chemother* 1990; **34:** 904–5.
6. Tham TCK, *et al.* Possible association between toxic epidermal necrolysis and ciprofloxacin. *Lancet* 1991; **338:** 522.
7. Moshfeghi M, Mandler HD. Ciprofloxacin-induced toxic epidermal necrolysis. *Ann Pharmacother* 1993; **27:** 1467–9.
8. Yerasi AB, Oertel MD. Ciprofloxacin-induced toxic epidermal necrolysis. *Ann Pharmacother* 1996; **30:** 297.
9. Baciewicz AM, *et al.* Laryngeal edema related to ciprofloxacin therapy. *Ann Pharmacother* 1992; **26:** 1456.
10. Choe U, *et al.* Ciprofloxacin-induced vasculitis. *N Engl J Med* 1989; **320:** 257–8.
11. Stubbings J, *et al.* Cutaneous vasculitis due to ciprofloxacin. *Br Med J* 1992; **305:** 29.
12. Drago F, *et al.* Henoch-Schönlein purpura induced by fluoroquinolones. *Br J Dermatol* 1994; **131:** 448.
13. Pace JL, Gatt P. Fatal vasculitis associated with ofloxacin. *Br Med J* 1989; **299:** 658.

Superinfection. Reports of superinfection with *Streptococcus pneumoniae*.[1-3] For references to superinfection with *Clostridium difficile* and associated pseudomembranous colitis, see under Effects on the Gastro-intestinal Tract, above.

1. Righter J. Pneumococcal meningitis during intravenous ciprofloxacin therapy. *Am J Med* 1990; **88:** 548.
2. Gordon JJ, Kauffman CA. Superinfection with Streptococcus pneumoniae during therapy with ciprofloxacin. *Am J Med* 1990; **89:** 383–4.
3. Lee BL, *et al.* Infectious complications with respiratory pathogens despite ciprofloxacin therapy. *N Engl J Med* 1991; **325:** 520–1.

Precautions

Ciprofloxacin should be used with caution in patients with epilepsy or a history of CNS disorders. Since ciprofloxacin and related fluoroquinolones have, like nalidixic acid, been shown to cause degenerative changes in weight-bearing joints of young *animals*, it has been suggested that these compounds should not be used in children, adolescents, pregnant women, or breast-feeding mothers. Tendon damage may occur rarely with fluoroquinolones (see above) and treatment should be discontinued if patients experience tendon pain, inflammation, or rupture.

Care is necessary in patients with impaired hepatic or renal function, glucose-6-phosphate dehydrogenase deficiency, or myasthenia gravis. An adequate fluid intake should be maintained during treatment with ciprofloxacin and excessive alkalinity of the urine avoided because of the risk of crystalluria. Exposure to strong sunlight or sunlamps should also be avoided. The ability to drive or operate machinery may be impaired by ciprofloxacin, especially when alcohol is also taken.

Administration in children. Since ciprofloxacin and other fluoroquinolones can cause degenerative changes in weight-bearing joints of young *animals* they should only be used in children and adolescents where their use may be justified if the benefits outweigh the risks.[1,2]

1. Schaad UB, *et al.* Use of fluoroquinolones in pediatrics: consensus report of an International Society of Chemotherapy commission. *Pediatr Infect Dis J* 1995; **14:** 1–9.
2. Green SDR. Indications and restrictions of fluoroquinolone use in children. *Br J Hosp Med* 1996; **56:** 420–3.

Exposure to ultraviolet light. Loss of antibacterial activity has been reported following irradiation of ciprofloxacin solutions by ultraviolet light.[1] In addition to the possible hazard of photosensitivity reactions, a reduction in both cutaneous and circulating levels of ciprofloxacin was predicted in patients exposed to sunlight through window glass or longer wavelength ultraviolet (UVA) radiation from sunbeds.[1]

1. Phillips G, *et al.* The loss of antibiotic activity of ciprofloxacin by photodegradation. *J Antimicrob Chemother* 1990; **26:** 783–9.

Interference with diagnostic tests. Ciprofloxacin did not interfere with determination of urinary-glucose concentrations carried out with Clinitest, Diastix, or Tes-Tape,[1] but pseudoglycosuria, a false-positive reaction for glucose in urine, has been reported with BM-Test-7 in elderly patients given ciprofloxacin for urinary-tract infections.[2]

1. Tartaglione TA, Flint NB. Effect of imipenem-cilastatin and ciprofloxacin on tests for glycosuria. *Am J Hosp Pharm* 1985; **42:** 602–5.
2. Drysdale L, *et al.* Pseudoglycosuria and ciprofloxacin. *Lancet* 1988; **ii:** 961.

Myasthenia gravis. Caution is advised in patients with myasthenia gravis given fluoroquinolones, following reports of the possible exacerbation of symptoms in one patient[1] and unmasking of subclinical myasthenia gravis in another[2] by ciprofloxacin. Exacerbation of myasthenia gravis has also been reported with norfloxacin.[3]

1. Moore B, *et al.* Possible exacerbation of myasthenia gravis by ciprofloxacin. *Lancet* 1988; **i:** 882.
2. Mumford CJ, Ginsberg L. Ciprofloxacin and myasthenia gravis. *Br Med J* 1990; **301:** 818.
3. Rauser EH, *et al.* Exacerbation of myasthenia gravis by norfloxacin. *DICP Ann Pharmacother* 1990; **24:** 207–8.

Interactions

The range of drug interactions reported with ciprofloxacin and other fluoroquinolones continues to grow. Fluoroquinolones are known to inhibit hepatic drug metabolism and may interfere with the clearance of drugs metabolised by the liver such as theophylline. On the other hand, cations like aluminium, magnesium, or iron reduce the absorption of ciprofloxacin and related drugs when given concomitantly.

For physical or chemical incompatibilities with ciprofloxacin, see above.

ANALGESICS. Concurrent administration of *fenbufen* with quinolones may increase the incidence of quinolone CNS adverse effects. Reviews[1,2] have noted that 7 cases of convulsions associated with the use of fenbufen and enoxacin have been reported to the Japanese regulatory authorities. The UK Committee on Safety of Medicines has recognised that convulsions may occur due to an interaction between the quinolones and NSAIDs; by 1991, 3 such interactions had been reported to them.[3] Adverse neurological effects have also been reported in a patient receiving *naproxen* and chloroquine when ciprofloxacin was administered, which abated when the antirheumatic drugs were withdrawn.[4]

Ciprofloxacin also interacts with *opioid analgesics*; peak serum concentrations of ciprofloxacin given by mouth pre-operatively were significantly reduced when intramuscular *papaveretum* was injected concomitantly.[5] The manufacturers recommend that opioids should not be administered peri-operatively to patients receiving ciprofloxacin.

ANTACIDS AND METAL IONS. The absorption of ciprofloxacin and other fluoroquinolones is reduced by *antacids* containing *aluminium* or *magnesium* and also by *calcium, iron,* and *zinc* salts.[6] *Sucralfate* releases aluminium ions in the stomach and thereby reduces the absorption of ciprofloxacin[7,8] and other fluoroquinolones, including norfloxacin[9] and ofloxacin. In addition, concomitant administration of antacids or oral iron preparations might antagonise the antibacterial activity of fluoroquinolone within the gut lumen.[10] *Dairy products* with a high calcium content might also interfere with the absorption of fluoroquinolones.[11-13] *Enteral feeds*, which contain cations, have also been found to reduce absorption of ciprofloxacin.[14] A reduction in ciprofloxacin bioavailability has also been reported following concomitant administration of *chewable tablets* of didanosine which contain aluminium and magnesium ion buffering agents.[15]

ANTIBACTERIALS. The simultaneous administration of parenteral ciprofloxacin and *azlocillin* has resulted in higher and more prolonged serum concentrations of ciprofloxacin.[16]

ANTICOAGULANTS. For reports of ciprofloxacin and other quinolones enhancing the effect of oral anticoagulants, see under Warfarin, p.966.

ANTINEOPLASTICS AND IMMUNOSUPPRESSANTS. Absorption of oral ciprofloxacin appears to be reduced after cytotoxic chemotherapy.[17] There has been a report of enhanced nephrotoxicity in a patient who received ciprofloxacin and *cyclosporin*,[18] although a review[19] found no correlation between concurrent treatment and alterations in pharmacokinetics or pharmacodynamics.

ANTIVIRALS. Both ciprofloxacin and *foscarnet* can cause convulsions and two patients developed generalised tonic-clonic seizures while receiving the drugs concurrently.[20]

ANXIOLYTICS. For an isolated report of increased blood concentrations of *midazolam* associated with the concomitant administration of ciprofloxacin, see under Diazepam, p.663.

HISTAMINE H_2-ANTAGONISTS. *Cimetidine* has been reported to reduce the clearance of pefloxacin[21] and *ranitidine* given intravenously has reduced the bioavailability of oral enoxacin.[22]

PHENYTOIN. For conflicting reports of the effect of ciprofloxacin on serum-*phenytoin* concentrations, see p.354.

PROBENECID. The urinary excretion of ciprofloxacin and some other fluoroquinolones is reduced by the concomitant administration of probenecid; plasma concentrations are not necessarily increased.

XANTHINES. Ciprofloxacin and other fluoroquinolones (to a greater or lesser extent) decrease the clearance of *theophylline* (p.768) and *caffeine* (p.750) from the body. Seizures have occurred in patients given ciprofloxacin and theophylline concomitantly and in one such report[23] serum-theophylline concentrations were normal. Fluoroquinolones can be neurotoxic in their own right (see Adverse Effects, above).

1. Janknegt R. Drug interactions with quinolones. *J Antimicrob Chemother* 1990; **26** (suppl D): 7–29.
2. Christ W. Central nervous system toxicity of quinolones: human and animal findings. *J Antimicrob Chemother* 1990; **26** (suppl B): 219–25.
3. Committee on Safety of Medicines. Convulsions due to quinolone antimicrobial agents. *Current Problems 32* 1991.
4. Rollof J, Vinge E. Neurologic adverse effects during concomitant treatment with ciprofloxacin, NSAIDs, and chloroquine: possible drug interaction. *Ann Pharmacother* 1993; **27:** 1058–9.
5. Morran C, *et al.* Brief report: pharmacokinetics of orally administered ciprofloxacin in abdominal surgery. *Am J Med* 1989; **87** (suppl 5A): 86S–88S.
6. Lomaestro BM, Bailie GR. Absorption interactions with fluoroquinolones: 1995 update. *Drug Safety* 1995; **12:** 314–33.
7. Garrelts JC, *et al.* Sucralfate significantly reduces ciprofloxacin concentrations in serum. *Antimicrob Agents Chemother* 1990; **34:** 931–3.
8. Van Slooten AD, *et al.* Combined use of ciprofloxacin and sucralfate. *DICP Ann Pharmacother* 1991; **25:** 578–82.
9. Parpia SH, *et al.* Sucralfate reduces the gastrointestinal absorption of norfloxacin. *Antimicrob Agents Chemother* 1989; **33:** 99–102.
10. Lewin CS, Smith JT. 4-Quinolones and multivalent ions. *J Antimicrob Chemother* 1990; **26:** 149.
11. Neuvonen PJ, *et al.* Interference of dairy products with the absorption of ciprofloxacin. *Clin Pharmacol Ther* 1991; **50:** 498–502.
12. Kivistö KT, *et al.* Inhibition of norfloxacin absorption by dairy products. *Antimicrob Agents Chemother* 1992; **36:** 489–91.
13. Neuvonen PJ, Kivistö KT. Milk and yoghurt do not impair the absorption of ofloxacin. *Br J Clin Pharmacol* 1992; **33:** 346–8.
14. Healy DP, *et al.* Ciprofloxacin absorption is impaired in patients given enteral feedings orally and via gastrostomy and jejunostomy tubes. *Antimicrob Agents Chemother* 1996; **40:** 6–10.
15. Sahai J, *et al.* Cations in the didanosine tablet reduce ciprofloxacin bioavailability. *Clin Pharmacol Ther* 1993; **53:** 292–7.
16. Barriere SL, *et al.* Alteration in the pharmacokinetic disposition of ciprofloxacin by simultaneous administration of azlocillin. *Antimicrob Agents Chemother* 1990; **34:** 823–6.
17. Johnson EJ, *et al.* Reduced absorption of oral ciprofloxacin after chemotherapy for haematological malignancy. *J Antimicrob Chemother* 1990; **25:** 837–42.
18. Elston RA, Taylor J. Possible interaction of ciprofloxacin with cyclosporin A. *J Antimicrob Chemother* 1988; **21:** 679–80.
19. Hoey LL, Lake KD. Does ciprofloxacin interact with cyclosporine? *Ann Pharmacother* 1994; **28:** 93–6.
20. Fan-Havard P, *et al.* Concurrent use of foscarnet and ciprofloxacin may increase the propensity for seizures. *Ann Pharmacother* 1994; **28:** 869–72.
21. Sörgel F, *et al.* Effects of cimetidine on the pharmacokinetics of pefloxacin in healthy volunteers. *Rev Infect Dis* 1988; **10** (suppl 1): S137.
22. Grasela TH, *et al.* Inhibition of enoxacin absorption by antacids or ranitidine. *Antimicrob Agents Chemother* 1989; **33:** 615–17.
23. Bader MB. Role of ciprofloxacin in fatal seizures. *Chest* 1992; **101:** 883–4.

Antimicrobial Action

Ciprofloxacin is bactericidal and acts by inhibiting the A subunit of DNA gyrase (topoisomerase) which is essential in the reproduction of bacterial DNA. It has a broader spectrum of activity and is more potent *in vitro* than the non-fluorinated quinolone nalidixic acid. Activity may be reduced in acid media.

Spectrum of activity (see also Resistance, below). Among Gram-negative aerobic bacteria ciprofloxacin is active *in vitro* against Enterobacteriaceae including *Escherichia coli* and *Citrobacter, Enterobacter, Klebsiella, Proteus, Providencia, Salmonella, Serratia, Shigella,* and *Yersinia* spp; the MIC_{90} for most of these is reported to be 1 μg or less per mL. It is also active against *Pseudomonas aeruginosa* (MIC_{90} about 2 μg per mL), but less so against other *Pseudomonas* spp. *Haemophilus ducreyi, H. influenzae, Moraxella (Branhamella) catarrhalis, Neisseria gonorrhoeae,* and *N. meningitidis* are all very sensitive, including beta-lactamase-producing strains of *H. influenzae, M. catarrhalis,* and *N. gonorrhoeae.* Other Gram-negative aerobic bacteria reported to be sensitive to ciprofloxacin have included *Acinetobacter* spp., *Campylobacter* spp., *Gardnerella vaginalis, Helicobacter pylori, Legionella* spp., *Pasteurella multocida,* and *Vibrio* spp. Variable activity has been reported against *Brucella melitensis.*

Among Gram-positive aerobic bacteria ciprofloxacin is active against staphylococci including penicillinase-producing andnonproducing strains (MIC_{90} 1 μg or less per mL) and against some methicillin-resistant strains. Streptococci, in particular *Streptococcus pneumoniae*, and enterococci are less susceptible. Other Gram-positive bacteria sensitive to ciprofloxacin *in vitro* are *Corynebacterium* spp. and *Listeria monocytogenes.*

Most anaerobic bacteria, including *Bacteroides fragilis* and *Clostridium difficile*, are resistant to ciprofloxacin although some other *Bacteroides* and *Clostridium* spp. may be susceptible.

Ciprofloxacin has some activity against mycobacteria, mycoplasmas, rickettsias, and the protozoan *Plasmodium falciparum. Chlamydia trachomatis* is not very susceptible and *Nocardia asteroides* and *Ureaplasma urealyticum* are usually considered to be resistant. The spirochaete *Treponema pallidum* and fungi are also resistant.

Activity with other antimicrobial agents. There have been some reports of enhanced activity *in vitro* when ciprofloxacin has been used with other antimicrobials such as azlocillin against *Staphylococcus aureus* and *Pseudomonas aeruginosa*, imipenem against *Ps. aeruginosa*, and cefotaxime or clindamycin against anaerobic bacteria.

Acquired resistance. Resistant strains, particularly of *Staph. aureus* (including methicillin-resistant strains) and *Ps. aeruginosa* have emerged during treatment with ciprofloxacin (see below for reports of other resistant bacteria). There is complete cross-resistance between ciprofloxacin and the other fluoroquinolones, but not between ciprofloxacin and nalidixic acid. Like nalidixic acid, resistance to ciprofloxacin appears, so far, to be chromosomally rather than plasmid-mediated.

Resistance. Acquired resistance to ciprofloxacin and other fluoroquinolones has occurred most frequently in staphylococci[1-3] and *Pseudomonas aeruginosa*;[4] cross-resistance to unrelated antibacterials has been described in *Ps. aeruginosa.*[5] Resistance has also been reported in *Campylobacter* spp. initially linked with the widespread veterinary use of quinolones[6,7] and subsequently becoming more clinically important;[8,9] similarly there have been reports of increasing quinolone resistance in both non-typhoid *Salmonella* spp.[10] as well as *S. typhi*[11-13] and *S. paratyphi.*[14] Resistance to fluoroquinolones has also been reported in other Enterobacteriaceae including *Escherichia coli,*[15,16] *Serratia marcescens,*[17] *Shigella sonnei,*[18] and *Haemophilus influenzae.*[19,20] Decreased susceptibility of *Neisseria gonorrhoeae* has been described[21,22] and resistant strains have now been reported.[23] Mutational resistance has developed in mycobacteria following monotherapy with ciprofloxacin.[24] Fluoroquinolone-resistant strains of *Mycobacterium tuberculosis* have been isolated from patients with tuberculosis.[25]

Excretion of ciprofloxacin in sweat has been suggested to be a contributory factor in the development of resistance to *Staphylococcus epidermidis* and possibly other skin-dwelling bacteria.[26]

1. Oppenheim BA, *et al.* Outbreak of coagulase negative staphylococcus highly resistant to ciprofloxacin in a leukaemia unit. *Br Med J* 1989; **299:** 294–7.
2. Blumberg HM, *et al.* Rapid development of ciprofloxacin resistance in methicillin-susceptible andresistant Staphylococcus aureus. *J Infect Dis* 1991; **163:** 1279–85.
3. Trucksis M, *et al.* Emerging resistance to fluoroquinolones in staphylococci: an alert. *Ann Intern Med* 1991; **114:** 424–6.
4. Acar JF, Francoual S. The clinical problems of bacterial resistance to the new quinolones. *J Antimicrob Chemother* 1990; **26** (suppl B): 207–13.
5. Aubert G, *et al.* Emergence of quinolone-imipenem cross-resistance in Pseudomonas aeruginosa after fluoroquinolone therapy. *J Antimicrob Chemother* 1992; **29:** 307–12.
6. Endtz HP, *et al.* Quinolone resistance in campylobacter isolated from man and poultry following the introduction of fluoroquinolones in veterinary medicine. *J Antimicrob Chemother* 1991; **27:** 199–208.
7. Bowler I, Day D. Emerging quinolone resistance in campylobacters. *Lancet* 1992; **340:** 245.
8. Segreti J, *et al.* High-level quinolone resistance in clinical isolates of Campylobacter jejuni. *J Infect Dis* 1992; **165:** 667–70.

9. McIntyre M, Lyons M. Resistance to ciprofloxacin in Campylobacter spp. *Lancet* 1993; **341:** 188.
10. Frost JA, *et al.* Increasing ciprofloxacin resistance in salmonellas in England and Wales 1991-1994. *J Antimicrob Chemother* 1996; **37:** 85–91.
11. Rowe B, *et al.* Ciprofloxacin-resistant Salmonella typhi in the UK. *Lancet* 1995; **346:** 1302.
12. Mitchell DH. Ciprofloxacin-resistant Salmonella typhi: an emerging problem. *Med J Aust* 1997; **167:** 172.
13. Murdoch DA, *et al.* Epidemic ciprofloxacin-resistant Salmonella typhi in Tajikistan. *Lancet* 1998; **351:** 339.
14. Bhutta ZA. Quinolone-resistant Salmonella paratyphi B meningitis in a newborn: a case report. *J Infect* 1997; **35:** 308–10.
15. Aguiar JM, *et al.* The emergence of highly fluoroquinolone-resistant Escherichia coli in community-acquired urinary tract infections. *J Antimicrob Chemother* 1992; **29:** 349–50.
16. Threlfall EJ, *et al.* High-level resistance to ciprofloxacin in Escherichia coli. *Lancet* 1997; **349:** 403.
17. Fujimaki K, *et al.* Quinolone resistance in clinical isolate of Serratia marcescens. *Antimicrob Agents Chemother* 1989; **33:** 785–7.
18. Horiuchi S, *et al.* Reduced susceptibilities of Shigella sonnei strains isolated from patients with dysentery to fluoroquinolones. *Antimicrob Agents Chemother* 1993; **37:** 2486–9.
19. Barriere SL, Hindler JA. Ciprofloxacin-resistant Haemophilus influenzae infection in a patient with chronic lung disease. *Ann Pharmacother* 1993; **27:** 309–10.
20. Gould IM, *et al.* Quinolone resistant Haemophilus influenzae. *J Antimicrob Chemother* 1994; **33:** 187–8.
21. Jephcott AE, Turner A. Ciprofloxacin resistance in gonococci. *Lancet* 1990; **335:** 165.
22. Gordon SM, *et al.* The emergence of Neisseria gonorrhoeae with decreased susceptibility to ciprofloxacin in Cleveland, Ohio: epidemiology and risk factors. *Ann Intern Med* 1996; **125:** 465–70.
23. Kam K, *et al.* Quinolone-resistant Neisseria gonorrhoeae in Hong Kong. *Sex Transm Dis* 1996; **23:** 103–8.
24. Wallace RJ, *et al.* Activities of ciprofloxacin and ofloxacin against rapidly growing mycobacterial with demonstration of acquired resistance following single-drug therapy. *Antimicrob Agents Chemother* 1990; **34:** 65–70.
25. Sullivan EA, *et al.* Emergence of fluoroquinolone-resistant tuberculosis in New York City. *Lancet* 1995; **345:** 1148–50.
26. Høiby N, *et al.* Excretion of ciprofloxacin in sweat and multiresistant Staphylococcus epidermidis. *Lancet* 1997; **349:** 167–9.

Pharmacokinetics

Ciprofloxacin is rapidly and well absorbed from the gastro-intestinal tract. Oral bioavailability is approximately 70% and a peak plasma concentration of about 2.5 μg per mL is achieved 1 to 2 hours after a dose of 500 mg by mouth. Absorption may be delayed by the presence of food, but is not substantially affected overall. The plasma half-life is about 3.5 to 4.5 hours and there is evidence of modest accumulation. Half-life may be prolonged in severe renal failure—a value of 8 hours has been reported in end-stage renal disease—and to some extent in the elderly. There is limited information on the effect of liver dysfunction; in one study the half-life of ciprofloxacin was slightly prolonged in patients with severe cirrhosis of the liver. With one or two exceptions, most studies have shown the pharmacokinetics of ciprofloxacin to be not markedly affected by cystic fibrosis.

Plasma protein binding ranges from 20 to 40%. Ciprofloxacin is widely distributed in the body and tissue penetration is generally good. It appears in the CSF, but concentrations are only about 10% of those in plasma when the meninges are not inflamed. Ciprofloxacin crosses the placenta and is distributed into breast milk. High concentrations are achieved in bile.

Ciprofloxacin is eliminated principally by urinary excretion, but non-renal clearance may account for about a third of elimination and includes hepatic metabolism, biliary excretion, and possibly transluminal secretion across the intestinal mucosa. At least 4 active metabolites have been identified. Oxociprofloxacin appears to be the major urinary metabolite and sulphociprofloxacin the primary faecal metabolite. Urinary excretion is by active tubular secretion as well as glomerular filtration and is reduced by probenecid; it is virtually complete within 24 hours. About 40 to 50% of an oral dose is excreted unchanged in the urine and about 15% as metabolites. Up to 70% of a parenteral dose may be excreted unchanged within 24 hours and 10% as metabolites. Faecal excretion over 5 days has accounted for 20 to 35% of an oral dose and 15% of an intravenous dose.

Only small amounts of ciprofloxacin are removed by haemodialysis or peritoneal dialysis.

Comparative pharmacokinetics of the fluoroquinolones.

1. Neuman M. Clinical pharmacokinetics of the newer antibacterial 4-quinolones. *Clin Pharmacokinet* 1988; **14:** 96–121.

Reviews of the pharmacokinetics of ciprofloxacin.

1. Vance-Bryan K, *et al.* Clinical pharmacokinetics of ciprofloxacin. *Clin Pharmacokinet* 1990; **19:** 434–61.

Studies on the distribution of ciprofloxacin.

1. Sweeney G, *et al.* Penetration of ciprofloxacin into the aqueous humour of the uninflamed human eye after oral administration. *J Antimicrob Chemother* 1990; **26:** 99–105.
2. Cover DL, Mueller BA. Ciprofloxacin penetration into human breast milk: a case report. *DICP Ann Pharmacother* 1990; **24:** 703–4.
3. Nau R, *et al.* Penetration of ciprofloxacin into the cerebrospinal fluid of patients with uninflamed meninges. *J Antimicrob Chemother* 1990; **25:** 965–73.
4. Trautmann M, *et al.* Penetration of ciprofloxacin into the spinal fluid in patients with viral and bacterial meningitis. *Arzneimittelforschung* 1990; **40:** 611–13.
5. Mertes PM, *et al.* Penetration of ciprofloxacin into heart valves, myocardium, mediastinal fat, and sternal bone marrow in humans. *Antimicrob Agents Chemother* 1990; **34:** 398–401.
6. Darouiche R, *et al.* Levels of rifampin and ciprofloxacin in nasal secretions: correlation with MIC_{90} and eradication of nasopharyngeal carriage of bacteria. *J Infect Dis* 1990; **162:** 1124–7.
7. Jacobs F, *et al.* Penetration of ciprofloxacin into human pleural fluid. *Antimicrob Agents Chemother* 1990; **34:** 934–6.
8. Fabre D, *et al.* Steady-state pharmacokinetics of ciprofloxacin in plasma from patients with nosocomial pneumonia: penetration of the bronchial mucosa. *Antimicrob Agents Chemother* 1991; **35:** 2521–5.
9. Dan M, *et al.* Distribution of ciprofloxacin in ascitic fluid following administration of a single oral dose of 750 milligrams. *Antimicrob Agents Chemother* 1992; **36:** 677–8.
10. Dan M, *et al.* The penetration of ciprofloxacin into bronchial mucosa, lung parenchyma, and pleural tissue after intravenous administration. *Eur J Clin Pharmacol* 1993; **44:** 101–2.
11. Decré D, Bergogne-Bérézin E. Pharmacokinetics of quinolones with special reference to the respiratory tree. *J Antimicrob Chemother* 1993; **31:** 331–43.
12. Catchpole C, *et al.* The comparative pharmacokinetics and tissue penetration of single-dose ciprofloxacin 400 mg iv and 750 mg po. *J Antimicrob Chemother* 1994; **33:** 103–10.
13. Leeming JP, *et al.* Ocular penetration of topical ciprofloxacin and norfloxacin drops and their effect upon eyelid flora. *Br J Ophthalmol* 1994; **78:** 546–8.
14. Edmiston CE, *et al.* Penetration of ciprofloxacin and fleroxacin into biliary tract. *Antimicrob Agents Chemother* 1996; **40:** 787–8.

Pharmacokinetics of ciprofloxacin in patients with cystic fibrosis.

1. LeBel M, *et al.* Pharmacokinetics and pharmacodynamics of ciprofloxacin in cystic fibrosis patients. *Antimicrob Agents Chemother* 1986; **30:** 260–6.
2. Davis RL, *et al.* Pharmacokinetics of ciprofloxacin in cystic fibrosis. *Antimicrob Agents Chemother* 1987; **31:** 915–19.
3. Steen HJ, *et al.* Clinical and pharmacokinetic aspects of ciprofloxacin in the treatment of acute exacerbations of pseudomonas infection in cystic fibrosis patients. *J Antimicrob Chemother* 1989; **24:** 787–95.
4. Christensson BA, *et al.* Increased oral bioavailability of ciprofloxacin in cystic fibrosis patients. *Antimicrob Agents Chemother* 1992; **36:** 2512–17.
5. Schaefer HG, *et al.* Pharmacokinetics of ciprofloxacin in pediatric cystic fibrosis patients. *Antimicrob Agents Chemother* 1996; **40:** 29–34.

Pharmacokinetics of ciprofloxacin in the elderly.

1. LeBel M, *et al.* Pharmacokinetics of ciprofloxacin in elderly subjects. *Pharmacotherapy* 1986; **6:** 87–91.
2. Kees F, *et al.* Pharmacokinetics of ciprofloxacin in elderly patients. *Arzneimittelforschung* 1989; **39:** 524–7.
3. Ljungberg B, Nilsson-Ehle I. Pharmacokinetics of ciprofloxacin in the elderly: increased oral bioavailability and reduced renal clearance. *Eur J Clin Microbiol Infect Dis* 1989; **8:** 515–20.
4. Shah A, *et al.* Pharmacokinetics of high-dose intravenous ciprofloxacin in young and elderly and in male and female subjects. *Antimicrob Agents Chemother* 1995; **39:** 1003–6.

Pharmacokinetics of ciprofloxacin in liver impairment.

1. Esposito S, *et al.* Pharmacokinetics of ciprofloxacin in impaired liver function. *Int J Clin Pharmacol Res* 1989; **9:** 37–41.

Pharmacokinetics of ciprofloxacin in renal impairment.

1. Roberts DE, Williams JD. Ciprofloxacin in renal failure. *J Antimicrob Chemother* 1989; **23:** 820–3.
2. Dharmasena D, *et al.* Pharmacokinetics of intraperitoneal ciprofloxacin in patients on CAPD. *J Antimicrob Chemother* 1989; **23:** 253–9.
3. Plaisance KI, *et al.* Effect of renal function on the bioavailability of ciprofloxacin. *Antimicrob Agents Chemother* 1990; **34:** 1031–4.
4. MacGowan AP, *et al.* Serum ciprofloxacin concentrations in patients with severe sepsis being treated with ciprofloxacin 200 mg iv bd irrespective of renal function. *J Antimicrob Chemother* 1994; **33:** 1051–4.
5. Shah A, *et al.* Pharmacokinetics of intravenous ciprofloxacin in normal and renally impaired subjects. *J Antimicrob Chemother* 1996; **38:** 103–16.

Pharmacokinetics of ciprofloxacin in seriously ill patients.

1. Forrest A, *et al.* Development of a population pharmacokinetic model and optimal sampling strategies for intravenous ciprofloxacin. *Antimicrob Agents Chemother* 1993; **37:** 1065–72.
2. Forrest A, *et al.* Pharmacodynamics of intravenous ciprofloxacin in seriously ill patients. *Antimicrob Agents Chemother* 1993; **37:** 1073–81.
3. Cohn SM, *et al.* Enteric absorption of ciprofloxacin during the immediate postoperative period. *J Antimicrob Chemother* 1995; **36:** 717–21.
4. Garrelts JC, *et al.* Ciprofloxacin pharmacokinetics in burn patients. *Antimicrob Agents Chemother* 1996; **40:** 1153–6.
5. Owens RC, *et al.* Oral bioavailability and pharmacokinetics of ciprofloxacin in patients with AIDS. *Antimicrob Agents Chemother* 1997; **41:** 1508–11.

Uses and Administration

Ciprofloxacin is a fluorinated 4-quinolone or fluoroquinolone antibacterial with a wider spectrum of activity than nalidixic acid (see Antimicrobial Action, above) and more favourable pharmacokinetics for use in systemic infections. It has been used in the treatment of a wide range of infections including biliary-tract infections, infected bites and stings (animal bites), bone and joint infections, brucellosis, cat scratch disease, chancroid, exacerbations of cystic fibrosis, gastro-enteritis (including travellers' diarrhoea and campylobacter enteritis, cholera, salmonella enteritis, and shigellosis), gonorrhoea, infections in immunocompromised patients (neutropenia), legionnaires' disease, meningitis (meningococcal meningitis prophylaxis), otitis externa, otitis media, peritonitis, Q fever, lower respiratory-tract infections (including pseudomonal infections in cystic fibrosis, but excluding infections due to *Streptococcus pneumoniae* such as pneumococcal pneumonia), septicaemia, skin infections (including soft-tissue infections), spotted fevers, surgical infection prophylaxis, typhoid and paratyphoid fever, typhus, and urinary-tract infections. Fluoroquinolones such as ciprofloxacin and ofloxacin have been tried in the treatment of opportunistic mycobacterial infections and tuberculosis; ofloxacin may be used in the treatment of leprosy. Fluoroquinolones such as ciprofloxacin and ofloxacin are used topically in the treatment of eye infections. For details of all these infections and their treatment, see under Choice of Antibacterial, p.116.

Administration and dosage. Ciprofloxacin is given by mouth as the hydrochloride or by intravenous infusion over 30 to 60 minutes as a solution of the lactate in a concentration of 1 to 2 mg per mL. Eye drops of ciprofloxacin hydrochloride are available in some countries.

The usual adult oral dose of ciprofloxacin ranges from 250 to 750 mg twice daily depending on the severity and nature of the infection. The usual intravenous dose is 100 to 400 mg twice daily. A dose of 100 mg twice daily by mouth is recommended in women with acute uncomplicated cystitis. Single oral doses of 250 or 500 mg are used for the treatment of gonorrhoea, depending upon patterns of resistance. A single oral dose of 500 mg is suggested for meningococcal meningitis prophylaxis. A single oral dose of 750 mg is suggested for surgical infection prophylaxis, given 60 to 90 minutes before the procedure.

For acute exacerbations of cystic fibrosis associated with *Pseudomonas aeruginosa* infection ciprofloxacin may be given to adolescents and children aged 5 years or more in a dose of 20 mg per kg by mouth twice daily, up to a maximum of 750 mg twice daily. Alternatively a recommended dose of 10 mg per kg may be given by intravenous infusion over 60 minutes three times daily, to a maximum of 400 mg three times daily.

Ciprofloxacin is not generally recommended for other uses in children and adolescents (see Precautions, above) but, if considered essential, doses of 5 to 15 mg per kg body-weight twice daily by mouth or 4 to 8 mg per kg twice daily intravenously have been suggested.

Doses should be reduced in patients with severe renal impairment. Halving the dose has been suggested when the creatinine clearance is less than 20 mL per minute or alternatively the dosage interval may be increased; ideally plasma concentrations of ciprofloxacin should be monitored.

General references to fluoroquinolone antibacterials.

1. Hooper DC, Wolfson JS. Fluoroquinolone antimicrobial agents. *N Engl J Med* 1991; **324:** 384–94.
2. von Rosenstiel N, Adam D. Quinolone antibacterials: an update of their pharmacology and therapeutic use. *Drugs* 1994; **47:** 872–901.
3. Balfour JA, Goa KL, eds. Proceedings of the 5th International symposium on new quinolones. *Drugs* 1995; **49** (suppl 2): 1–505.

General references to ciprofloxacin.

1. Campoli-Richards DM, *et al.* Ciprofloxacin: a review of its antibacterial activity, pharmacokinetic properties and therapeutic use. *Drugs* 1998; **35:** 373–447.
2. Neu HC, ed. Ciprofloxacin: major advances in intravenous and oral quinolone therapy. *Am J Med* 1989; **87** (suppl 5A): 1S–287S.
3. Brown EM, *et al.*, eds. Ciprofloxacin—defining its role today. *J Antimicrob Chemother* 1990; **26** (suppl F): 1–193.
4. Davis R, *et al.* Ciprofloxacin: an updated review of its pharmacology, therapeutic efficacy and tolerability. *Drugs* 1996; **51:** 1019–74.

Administration. Although the usual maximum doses of ciprofloxacin are 750 mg orally or 400 mg intravenously twice daily, higher doses have been used. Notably, the US manufacturer recommends an intravenous dose of 400 mg three times daily in severe infections other than those of the urinary tract.

In a study in patients with suspected shigellosis, a single oral dose of ciprofloxacin 1 g or 1 g daily for 2 days was as effective as the conventional dose of 500 mg twice daily for 5 days except in patients infected with *Shigella dysenteriae* type 1.[1] A single oral dose of ciprofloxacin 500 mg appeared to be effective when given early for the empirical treatment of travellers' diarrhoea.[2] A patient with a renal cyst infection unresponsive to conventional antibacterial therapy improved on ciprofloxacin 600 mg intravenously twice daily for 7 days followed by oral therapy without evidence of toxicity.[3]

1. Bennish ML, *et al.* Treatment of shigellosis III: comparison of one- or two-dose ciprofloxacin with standard 5-day therapy: a randomized, blinded trial. *Ann Intern Med* 1992; **117:** 727–34.
2. Salam I, *et al.* Randomised trial of single-dose ciprofloxacin for travellers' diarrhoea. *Lancet* 1994; **344:** 1537–9.
3. Rossi SJ, *et al.* High-dose ciprofloxacin in the treatment of a renal cyst infection. *Ann Pharmacother* 1993; **27:** 38–9.

Inflammatory bowel disease. As discussed on p.1171 ciprofloxacin has gained some favour in the management of inflammatory bowel disease, largely on an empirical basis since controlled studies are lacking. Ciprofloxacin has been given in combination with metronidazole to treat active Crohn's disease.[1]

1. Prantera C, *et al.* An antibiotic regimen for the treatment of active Crohn's disease: a randomized, controlled clinical trial of metronidazole plus ciprofloxacin. *Am J Gastroenterol* 1996; **91:** 328–32.

Preparations

BP 1998: Ciprofloxacin Intravenous Infusion; Ciprofloxacin Tablets;
USP 23: Ciprofloxacin Injection; Ciprofloxacin Ophthalmic Solution; Ciprofloxacin Tablets.

Proprietary Preparations (details are given in Part 3)
Aust.: Ciloxan; Ciproxin; ***Austral.:*** Ciloxan; Ciproxin; ***Belg.:*** Ciloxan; Ciproxine; ***Canad.:*** Ciloxan; Cipro; ***Fr.:*** Ciflox; Uniflox; ***Ger.:*** Ciloxan; Ciprobay; ***Irl.:*** Ciproxin; ***Ital.:*** Cifloxt†; Ciproxin; Flociprin; ***Neth.:*** Ciproxin; ***Norw.:*** Cilox; Ciproxin; ***S.Afr.:*** Ciloxan; Ciprobay; ***Spain:*** Baycip; Belmacina; Catex; Ceprimax; Cetraxal; Cipobacter; Ciprok; Cunesin; Estecina; Globuce; Huberdoxina; Inkamil; Oftaciclox; Piprol; Plenolyt; Quipro; Rigoran; Sepcen; Septocipro; Tam; Velmonit; ***Swed.:*** Ciloxan; Ciproxin; ***Switz.:*** Ciloxan; Ciproxine; ***UK:*** Ciloxan; Ciproxin; ***USA:*** Ciloxan; Cipro.

Multi-ingredient: ***USA:*** Cipro HC Otic.

Clarithromycin (1891-b)

Clarithromycin *(BAN, USAN, rINN).*

A-56268; Abbott-56268; TE-031.

(2*R*,3*S*,4*S*,5*R*,6*R*,8*R*,10*R*,11*R*,12*S*,13*R*)-3-(2,6-Dideoxy-3-*C*,3*O*-dimethyl-α-L-*ribo*-hexopyranosyloxy)-11,12-dihydroxy-6-methoxy-2,4,6,8,10,12-hexamethyl-9-oxo-5-(3,4,6-trideoxy-3-dimethylamino-β-D-*xylo*-hexopyranosyloxy)pentadecan-13-olide; 6-*O*-Methylerythromycin.

$C_{38}H_{69}NO_{13}$ = 748.0.

CAS — 81103-11-9.

Pharmacopoeias. In US.

A 0.2% suspension in methyl alcohol (5%) has a pH of 7.5 to 10.0. **Store** in airtight containers.

Adverse Effects and Precautions

As for Erythromycin, p.204. Gastro-intestinal disturbances are the most frequent adverse effect but are usually mild and less frequent than with erythromycin. Taste disturbances, stomatitis, glossitis, and tooth discoloration have occurred. Transient elevations of liver enzyme values, cholestatic jaundice, and hepatitis have been reported. Headache and rashes from mild skin eruptions to, rarely, Stevens-Johnson syndrome have occurred. There have also been reports of transient CNS effects such as anxiety, dizziness, insomnia, hallucinations, and confusion. Other adverse effects include hypoglycaemia and thrombocytopenia.

Intravenous administration may cause phlebitis and pain at the injection site.

Caution is required in patients with impaired renal or hepatic function. It should not be used during pregnancy if possible: high doses have been associated with embryotoxicity in *animal* studies.

Effects on the blood. Single cases of thrombocytopenia[1] and thrombocytopenic purpura[2] associated with clarithromycin administration have been reported.

1. Price TA, Tuazon CU. Clarithromycin-induced thrombocytopenia. *Clin Infect Dis* 1992; **15:** 563–4.
2. Oteo JA, *et al.* Clarithromycin-induced thrombocytopenic purpura. *Clin Infect Dis* 1994; **19:** 1170–1.

Effects on the eyes. Corneal opacities, reversible on discontinuation of treatment, were reported in a patient receiving clarithromycin as part of a regimen for disseminated *Mycobacterium avium* complex infection.[1]

1. Dorrell L, *et al.* Toxicity of clarithromycin in the treatment of Mycobacterium avium complex infection in a patient with AIDS. *J Antimicrob Chemother* 1994; **34:** 605–6.

Effects on the gastro-intestinal tract. Pseudomembranous colitis associated with *Clostridium difficile* developed in a child receiving clarithromycin.[1]

1. Braegger CP, Nadal D. Clarithromycin and pseudomembranous enterocolitis. *Lancet* 1994; **343:** 241–2.

Effects on the heart. QT prolongation and torsade de pointes was associated with clarithromycin administration in 2 patients.[1] Impaired renal function in 1 patient and impaired hepatic function and organic heart disease in both could have increased their susceptibility to this adverse effect.

1. Lee KL, *et al.* QT prolongation and torsades de pointes associated with clarithromycin. *Am J Med* 1998; **104:** 395–6.

Effects on the pancreas. A case of pancreatitis was reported in a patient receiving clarithromycin.[1]

1. Liviu L, *et al.* Pancreatitis induced by clarithromycin. *Ann Intern Med* 1996; **125:** 701.

Effects on the skin. In addition to skin rashes and other hypersensitivity reactions which occasionally occur in patients receiving macrolides, leukocytoclastic vasculitis has been reported in a patient receiving clarithromycin.[1]

1. Gavura SR, Nusinowitz S. Leukocytoclastic vasculitis associated with clarithromycin. *Ann Pharmacother* 1998; **32:** 543–5.

Fever. Fever associated with clarithromycin was reported in one patient.[1]

1. Kadayifci A, *et al.* Clarithromycin-induced fever in a patient with Helicobacter pylori gastritis. *Ann Pharmacother* 1997; **31:** 788.

Interactions

For a discussion of drug interactions with macrolide antibacterials, see Erythromycin, p.205.

Increased rifabutin toxicity has been reported in patients receiving clarithromycin and rifabutin (p.242) and there has been a report of delirium following concurrent use with fluoxetine (p.286).

Antiretroviral drugs. In a study of healthy subjects[1] concurrent administration of the HIV-protease inhibitor *ritonavir* inhibited the metabolism of clarithromycin, producing elevated plasma concentrations and a prolonged half-life. The metabolism of ritonavir was not affected significantly. It has been suggested that other HIV-protease inhibitors, and also *delavirdine*, may have a similar effect on clarithromycin.

Decreased concentrations of *zidovudine* (p.631) have been reported in patients also taking clarithromycin and the manufacturer recommends that doses of the two drugs should be separated by 1 to 2 hours.

1. Ouell et D, *et al.* Assessment of the pharmacokinetic interaction between ritonavir and clarithromycin. *Clin Pharmacol Ther* 1996; **59:** 143.

Cimetidine. Although a study in healthy subjects suggested that some pharmacokinetic parameters of clarithromycin are altered by concurrent cimetidine administration,[1] the clinical significance of such changes are unknown.

1. Amsden GW, *et al.* Oral cimetidine prolongs clarithromycin absorption. *Antimicrob Agents Chemother* 1998; **42:** 1578–80.

Omeprazole. In a study in healthy subjects, increased concentrations of clarithromycin and its active metabolite were observed in gastric tissue and mucus and, to a lesser extent, in plasma during concomitant administration of omeprazole.[1] In addition, administration of clarithromycin with omeprazole resulted in higher and more prolonged plasma concentrations of omeprazole. The investigators suggest that this interaction could account for the synergistic action observed with this combination when used for eradication of *Helicobacter pylori*. However, the manufacturers of clarithromycin have noted that no dosage alteration to either drug is necessary.

1. Gustavson LE, *et al.* Effect of omeprazole on concentrations of clarithromycin in plasma and gastric tissue at steady state. *Antimicrob Agents Chemother* 1995; **39:** 2078–83.

Antimicrobial Action

As for Erythromycin, p.205. It is reported to be more active than erythromycin against susceptible streptococci and staphylococci *in vitro*, as well as against some other species including *Moraxella (Branhamella) catarrhalis, Legionella* spp., *Chlamydia trachomatis* and *Ureaplasma urealyticum*. MICs are usually 2- to 4-fold lower than for erythromycin. Clarithromycin is reported to be more active than erythromycin or azithromycin against some mycobacteria, including *Mycobacterium avium* complex, and against *M. leprae.* It is reported to have some *in vitro* activity against the protozoan *Toxoplasma gondii,* and may have some activity against cryptosporidia. The major metabolite, 14-hydroxyclarithromycin, is also active, and may enhance the activity of clarithromycin *in vivo*, notably against *Haemophilus influenzae*.

Activity with other antimicrobials. Clarithromycin has been reported to enhance the activity of a number of antimycobacterials including ethambutol, isoniazid, pyrazinamide, and rifampicin against *Mycobacterium tuberculosis*.[1,2]

1. Cavalieri SJ, *et al.* Synergistic activities of clarithromycin and antituberculous drugs against multi-drug-resistant Mycobacterium tuberculosis. *Antimicrob Agents Chemother* 1995; **39:** 1542–5.
2. Mor N, Esfandiari A. Synergistic activities of clarithromycin and pyrazinamide against Mycobacterium tuberculosis in human macrophages. *Antimicrob Agents Chemother* 1997; **41:** 2035–6.

Resistance. Erythromycin-resistant isolates of *Streptococcus pneumoniae* are commonly cross-resistant to clarithromycin.[1] The incidence of resistance to clarithromycin and other macrolides is higher among penicillin-resistant strains than among penicillin-sensitive strains.[2] Clarithromycin-resistant isolates of *Helicobacter pylori* are also emerging.[3,4] Genetic mutations responsible for clarithromycin resistance have been identified in *H. pylori*[5] and in *Mycobacterium* spp.[6,7] Since resistance develops rapidly in *Mycobacterium avium* during clarithromycin monotherapy, combination therapy is usually recommended. However, resistance to clarithromycin in an AIDS patient with systemic *Mycobacterium avium* complex infection, despite combined treatment with clofazimine, has been described.[8]

1. Lonks JR, Medeiros AA. High rate of erythromycin and clarithromycin resistance among Streptococcus pneumoniae isolates from blood cultures from Providence, RI. *Antimicrob Agents Chemother* 1993; **37:** 1742–5.
2. Barry AL, *et al.* Macrolide resistance among Streptococcus pneumoniae and Streptococcus pyogenes isolates from out-patients in the USA. *J Antimicrob Chemother* 1997; **40:** 139–40.
3. López-Brea M, *et al.* Evolution of resistance to metronidazole and clarithromycin in Helicobacter pylori clinical isolates from Spain. *J Antimicrob Chemother* 1997; **40:** 279–81.
4. Hultén K, *et al.* Macrolide resistance in Helicobacter pylori: mechanism and stability in strains from clarithromycin-treated patients. *Antimicrob Agents Chemother* 1997; **41:** 2550–3.
5. Versalovic J, *et al.* Mutations in 23S rRNA are associated with clarithromycin resistance in Helicobacter pylori. *Antimicrob Agents Chemother* 1996; **40:** 477–80.
6. Nash KA, Inderlied CB. Genetic basis of macrolide resistance in Mycobacterium avium isolated from patients with disseminated disease. *Antimicrob Agents Chemother* 1995; **39:** 2625–30.
7. Wallace RJ, *et al.* Genetic basis for clarithromycin resistance among isolates of Mycobacterium chelonae and Mycobacterium abscessus. *Antimicrob Agents Chemother* 1996; **40:** 1676–81.
8. De Wit S, *et al.* Acquired resistance to clarithromycin as combined therapy in Mycobacterium avium intracellulare infection. *Lancet* 1993; **341:** 53–4.

Pharmacokinetics

Clarithromycin is rapidly absorbed from the gastro-intestinal tract following oral administration, and undergoes first-pass metabolism; the bioavailability of the parent drug is about 55%. The extent of absorption is relatively unaffected by the presence of food. Peak concentrations of clarithromycin and its principal active metabolite 14-hydroxyclarithromycin are reported to be about 0.6 and 0.7 μg per mL respectively following a single 250-mg dose by mouth; at steady-state the same dose given every 12 hours as tablets produces peak concentrations of clarithromycin of about 1 μg per mL. The same dose given as a suspension produces a steady-state plasma concentration of about 2 μg per mL.

The pharmacokinetics of clarithromycin are non-linear and dose dependent; high doses may produce disproportionate increases in peak concentration of the parent drug, due to saturation of the metabolic pathways.

The drug and its principal metabolite are widely distributed, and tissue concentrations exceed those in serum, in part because of intracellular uptake. Clarithromycin has been detected in breast milk. It is extensively metabolised in the liver, and excreted in faeces via the bile. Substantial amounts are excreted in urine; at steady-state about 20% and 30% respectively of a 250-mg or 500-mg dose is excreted in this way, as unchanged drug. 14-Hydroxyclarithromycin as well as other metabolites are also excreted in the urine accounting for 10 to 15% of the dose. The terminal half-life of clarithromycin is reportedly about 3 to 4 hours in patients receiving 250-mg doses twice daily, and about 5 to 7 hours in those receiving 500 mg twice daily. The half-life is prolonged in renal impairment.

References.

1. Chu S-y, *et al.* Clarithromycin pharmacokinetics in healthy young and elderly volunteers. *J Clin Pharmacol* 1992; **32:** 1045–9.
2. Gan VN, *et al.* Pharmacokinetics of a clarithromycin suspension in infants and children. *Antimicrob Agents Chemother* 1992; **36:** 2478–80.
3. Chu S-y, *et al.* Effect of moderate or severe hepatic impairment on clarithromycin pharmacokinetics. *J Clin Pharmacol* 1993; **33:** 480–5.
4. Chu S-y, *et al.* Single- and multiple-dose pharmacokinetics of clarithromycin, a new macrolide antibacterial. *J Clin Pharmacol* 1993; **33:** 719–26.
5. Fraschini F, *et al.* Clarithromycin clinical pharmacokinetics. *Clin Pharmacokinet* 1993; **25:** 189–204.

Uses and Administration

Clarithromycin is a macrolide derived from erythromycin with similar actions and uses (p.206). It is given in the treatment of respiratory-tract infections (including otitis media) and in skin and soft-tissue infections. Clarithromycin is also used in the treatment of leprosy and for prophylaxis and treatment of opportunistic mycobacterial infections. For details of all these infections and their treatment, see under Choice of Antibacterial, p.116.

Clarithromycin may be given to eradicate *Helicobacter pylori* in treatment regimens for peptic ulcer disease (p.1174). It has been tried in protozoal infections, including toxoplasmosis (p.576).

Clarithromycin is given by mouth or by intravenous infusion. Usual doses in adults are 250 mg twice daily by mouth, increased to 500 mg twice daily if necessary in severe infection. A course is usually for 7 to 14 days. Children may be given 7.5 mg per kg body-weight twice daily for 5 to 10 days.

The usual intravenous dose is 500 mg twice daily, given as an intravenous infusion over 60 minutes using a solution containing about 0.2% of clarithromycin. Intravenous treatment may continue for 2 to 5 days, but should be changed to clarithromycin by mouth when possible. In patients with severe renal impairment (creatinine clearance of less than 30 mL per minute) dosage may need to be halved.

For disseminated infection due to *Mycobacterium avium* complex, clarithromycin may be given in a dose of 500 mg twice daily by mouth, in conjunction with other antimycobacterials. For leprosy, clarithromycin 500 mg daily by mouth has been given as part of an alternative multidrug therapy regimen (p.128).

For the eradication of *H. pylori* associated with peptic ulcer disease, clarithromycin is given in combination with a proton pump inhibitor or a histamine H_2-receptor antagonist and sometimes also another antibacterial. Suggested regimens include 7-day triple therapy with clarithromycin 250 mg or 500 mg twice daily plus omeprazole and either a nitroimidazole or amoxycillin, and 14-day dual therapy with clarithromycin 250 mg four times daily or 500 mg three times daily plus ranitidine bismutrex.

Reviews.

1. Peters DH, Clissold SP. Clarithromycin: a review of its antimicrobial activity, pharmacokinetic properties and therapeutic potential. *Drugs* 1992; **44:** 117–64.
2. Barradell LB, *et al.* Clarithromycin: a review of its pharmacological properties and therapeutic use in Mycobacterium avium-intracellulare complex infection in patients with acquired immune deficiency syndrome. *Drugs* 1993; **46:** 289–312.
3. Williams JD, Sefton AM. Comparison of macrolide antibiotics *J Antimicrob Chemother* 1993; **31** (suppl C): 11–26.
4. Markham A, McTavish D. Clarithromycin and omeprazole: as Helicobacter pylori eradication therapy in patients with H. pylori-associated gastric disorders. *Drugs* 1996; **51:** 161–78.

Inflammatory bowel disease. Clarithromycin, in combination with rifabutin, has been studied in the treatment of Crohn's disease (see Inflammatory Bowel Disease, p.1171). The rationale for this use is based on the putative involvement of *Mycobacterium paratuberculosis* as a causative factor for the disease.

Preparations

USP 23: Clarithromycin for Oral Suspension; Clarithromycin Tablets.

Proprietary Preparations (details are given in Part 3)
Aust.: Klacid; Maclar; ***Austral.:*** Klacid; ***Belg.:*** Biclar; ***Canad.:*** Biaxin; ***Fr.:*** Naxy; Zeclar; ***Ger.:*** Biaxin HP; Cyllind; Klacid; Mavid; ***Irl.:*** Klacid; ***Ital.:*** Klacid; Macladin; Veclam; ***Neth.:*** Klacid; ***Norw.:*** Klacid; ***S.Afr.:*** Klacid; ***Spain:*** Bremon; Klacid; Kofron; ***Swed.:*** Klacid; ***Switz.:*** Klacid; Klaciped; ***UK:*** Klaricid; ***USA:*** Biaxin.

Multi-ingredient: *USA:* Prevpac.

Clavulanic Acid (18258-v)

Clavulanic Acid *(BAN, rINN).*

BRL-14151; MM-14151. *(Z)*-(2*R*,5*R*)-3-(2-Hydroxyethylidene)-7-oxo-4-oxa-1-azabicyclo[3.2.0]heptane-2-carboxylic acid.

$C_8H_9NO_5$ = 199.2.

CAS — 58001-44-8 (clavulanic acid); 57943-81-4 (sodium clavulanate).

Potassium Clavulanate (153-p)

Potassium Clavulanate *(BANM, rINNM).*

BRL-14151K; Clavulanate Potassium *(USAN)*; Kalii Clavulanas.

$C_8H_8KNO_5$ = 237.3.

CAS — 61177-45-5.

NOTE. Compounded preparations of amoxycillin (as the trihydrate or as the sodium salt) and clavulanic acid (as potassium clavulanate) have the British Approved Name Co-amoxiclav; the proportions are expressed in the form *x/y*, where *x* and *y* are the strengths in milligrams of amoxycillin and clavulanic acid respectively.

Compounded preparations of amoxycillin (amoxicillin) (as the trihydrate) and potassium clavulanate (clavulanate potassium) in USP 23 may be represented by the name Co-amoxiclav.

Pharmacopoeias. In *Eur.* (see p.viii), *Jpn, Pol.,* and *US.*

A white to off-white hygroscopic, crystalline powder. 1.19 g of potassium clavulanate is approximately equivalent to 1 g of clavulanic acid. Freely **soluble** in water; slightly soluble in alcohol; very slightly soluble in acetone; soluble in methyl alcohol with decomposition. A 1% solution in water has a pH of 5.5 to 8.0. **Stability** in aqueous solution is not good, but is optimal at pH 6.0 to 6.3. **Store** in airtight containers.

Clavulanic acid is produced by cultures of *Streptomyces clavuligerus*. It has a beta-lactam structure resembling that of the penicillin nucleus except that the fused thiazolidine ring of the penicillins is replaced by an oxazolidine ring. In general, clavulanic acid has only weak antibacterial activity. It is a potent progressive inhibitor of plasmid-mediated and some chromosomal beta-lactamases produced by Gram-negative bacteria including *Haemophilus ducreyi, H. influenzae, Neisseria gonorrhoeae, Moraxella (Branhamella) catarrhalis, Bacteroides fragilis,* and some Enterobacteriaceae. It is also an inhibitor of the beta-lactamases produced by *Staphylococcus aureus*. Clavulanic acid can permeate bacterial cell walls and can therefore inactivate both extracellular enzymes and those that are bound to the cell. Its mode of action depends on the particular enzyme inhibited, but it generally acts as a competitive, and often irreversible, inhibitor. Clavulanic acid consequently enhances the activity of penicillin and cephalosporin antibacterials against many resistant strains of bacteria. However, it is generally less effective against chromosomally mediated type 1 beta-lactamases; therefore, many *Citrobacter, Enterobacter, Morganella,* and *Serratia* spp., and *Pseudomonas aeruginosa* remain resistant. Some plasmid-mediated extended-spectrum beta-lactamases in *Klebsiella pneumoniae*, some other Enterobacteriaceae, and *Ps. aeruginosa* are also not inhibited by beta-lactamase inhibitors.

It is given as potassium clavulanate by mouth and injection in combination with amoxycillin (co-amoxiclav) (p.151), and by injection in combination with ticarcillin (p.263).

Administration of clavulanate with penicillins has been associated with the development of cholestatic jaundice and hepatitis (see Amoxycillin, Adverse Effects, p.152) and therefore the use of co-amoxiclav has declined (see below).

Because of the risk of cholestatic jaundice co-amoxiclav is not a treatment of choice for common bacterial infections. In the UK, the Committee on Safety of Medicines[1] recommends that it should be reserved for bacterial infections likely to be caused by amoxycillin resistant beta-lactamase producing strains and that treatment should not usually exceed 14 days. It may be considered in the following main indications:

- sinusitis, otitis media, recurrent tonsillitis
- acute exacerbations of chronic bronchitis
- bronchopneumonia
- urinary-tract infections, especially when recurrent or complicated, but not prostatitis
- septic abortion, pelvic or puerperal sepsis, and intra-abdominal sepsis
- cellulitis, animal bites, and severe dental abscess with spreading cellulitis.

1. Committee on Safety of Medicines/Medicines Control Agency. Revised indications for co-amoxiclav (Augmentin). *Current Problems* 1997; **23:** 8.

Antimicrobial Action. General references.

1. Payne DJ, *et al.* Comparative activities of clavulanic acid, sulbactam and tazobactam against clinically important β-lactamases. *Antimicrob Agents Chemother* 1994; **38:** 767–72.
2. Nicolas-Chanoine MH. Inhibitor-resistant β-lactamases. *J Antimicrob Chemother* 1997; **40:** 1–3.

Pharmacokinetics. The pharmacokinetics of clavulanic acid are similar to those of amoxycillin and ticarcillin with which it is administered. The following pharmacokinetic properties have been reported: peak concentrations of about 2 to 4 μg per mL one to two hours after administration of 125 mg by mouth; up to 30% bound to plasma proteins; half-life of approximately 1 hour; and variable urinary excretion of unchanged drug of up to 60% of the total dose within 6 hours of oral administration. The excretion of clavulanic acid is not significantly affected by the administration of probenecid, suggesting that it is cleared predominantly by glomerular filtration. It may be metabolised more extensively than amoxycillin. Clearance of clavulanic acid decreases with decreasing renal function, but not to the same extent as for amoxycillin. Clavulanic acid is removed by haemodialysis.

References.

1. Watson ID, *et al.* Clinical pharmacokinetics of enzyme inhibitors in antimicrobial chemotherapy. *Clin Pharmacokinet* 1988; **15:** 133–64.

Preparations

BP 1998: Co-amoxiclav Tablets;
USP 23: Amoxicillin and Clavulanate Potassium for Oral Suspension; Amoxicillin and Clavulanate Potassium Tablets; Ticarcillin and Clavulanic Acid for Injection; Ticarcillin and Clavulanic Acid Injection.

Proprietary Preparations (details are given in Part 3)
Belg.: Clavucid.

Multi-ingredient: ***Aust.:*** Augmentin; Clavamox; Timenten; ***Austral.:*** Augmentin; Clamoxyl; Clavulin; Timentin; ***Belg.:*** Augmentin; Timentin; ***Canad.:*** Clavulin; Timentin; ***Fr.:*** Augmentin; Ciblor; Claventin; ***Ger.:*** Augmentan; Betabactyl; ***Irl.:*** Augmentin; Timentin; ***Ital.:*** Augmentin; Clavucar; Clavulin; Neoduplamox; Stacillin†; Timentin; ***Neth.:*** Augmentin; Timentin; ***Norw.:*** Bremide; ***S.Afr.:*** Augmentin; ***Spain:*** Amoxyplus; Augmentine; Bigpen; Burmicin; Clavepen; Clavius†; Clavucid; Clavumox; Duonasa; Eupeclanic; Inmupen; Kelsopen; Pangamox; Ultramoxil†; ***Swed.:*** Spektramox; ***Switz.:*** Augmentin; Timenten; ***UK:*** Augmentin; Augmentin-Duo; Timentin; ***USA:*** Augmentin; Timentin.

Clemizole Penicillin (53-b)

Clemizole Penicillin (*BAN, rINN*).

Clemizole Benzylpenicillin; Penicillin G Clemizole. 1-[1-(4-Chlorobenzyl)benzimidazol-2-ylmethyl]pyrrolidinium (6*R*)-6-(2-phenylacetamido)penicillanate.

$C_{16}H_{18}N_2O_4S,C_{19}H_{20}ClN_3$ = 660.2.

CAS — 6011-39-8.

Clemizole penicillin is a long-acting preparation of benzylpenicillin (p.159) with similar properties and uses.

Preparations

Proprietary Preparations (details are given in Part 3)
Aust.: Clemipen; ***Ger.:*** Megacillin for Injection†; ***Switz.:*** Megacilline.

Multi-ingredient: ***Aust.:*** Antipen; ***Ger.:*** Megacillin forte†; ***Spain:*** Anapen; Neopenyl.

Clinafloxacin Hydrochloride (15475-y)

Clinafloxacin Hydrochloride (*USAN, rINNM*).

CI-960 (clinafloxacin); PD-127391.

$C_{17}H_{17}ClFN_3O_3,HCl$ = 402.2.

CAS — 105956-97-6 (clinafloxacin); 105956-99-8 (clinafloxacin hydrochloride).

NOTE. (±)-7-(3-Amino-1-pyrrolidinyl)-8-chloro-1-cyclopropyl-6-fluoro-1,4-dihydro-4-oxo-3-quinolinecarboxylic acid hydrochloride

Clinafloxacin is a fluoroquinolone antibacterial.

References.

1. Bron NJ, *et al.* The tolerance and pharmacokinetics of clinafloxacin (CI-960) in healthy subjects. *J Antimicrob Chemother* 1996; **38:** 1023–9.
2. Wise R, *et al.* Pharmacokinetics and inflammatory fluid penetration of clinafloxacin. *Antimicrob Agents Chemother* 1998; **42:** 428–30.
3. Ednie LM, *et al.* Comparative activities of clinafloxacin against Gram-positive and -negative bacteria. *Antimicrob Agents Chemother* 1998; **42:** 1269–73.
4. Fuchs PC, *et al.* In vitro activities of clinafloxacin against contemporary clinical bacterial isolates from 10 North American centers. *Antimicrob Agents Chemother* 1998; **42:** 1274–7.

Clindamycin Hydrochloride (55-g)

Clindamycin Hydrochloride (*BANM, rINNM*).

Chlorodeoxylincomycin Hydrochloride; (7*S*)-Chloro-7-deoxylincomycin Hydrochloride; Clindamycini Hydrochloridum; U-21251 (clindamycin). Methyl 6-amino-7-chloro-6,7,8-trideoxy-*N*-[(2*S*,4*R*)-1-methyl-4-propylprolyl]-1-thio-L-*threo*-D-*galacto*-octopyranoside hydrochloride.

$C_{18}H_{33}ClN_2O_5S,HCl$ = 461.4.

CAS — 18323-44-9 (clindamycin); 21462-39-5 (anhydrous clindamycin hydrochloride); 58207-19-5 (clindamycin hydrochloride monohydrate).

NOTE. Clindamycin is *USAN*.
The name Clinimycin, which was formerly used for clindamycin, has also been used for a preparation of oxytetracycline.

Pharmacopoeias. In *Chin., Eur.* (see p.viii), *Pol.,* and *US.*

A white or almost white crystalline powder, odourless or with a faint mercaptan-like odour. It contains a variable quantity of water. 1.13 g of monograph substance is approximately equivalent to 1 g of clindamycin. Ph. Eur. **solubilities** are: very soluble in water; slightly soluble in alcohol. USP solubilities are: freely soluble in water, dimethylformamide, and methyl alcohol; soluble in alcohol; practically insoluble in acetone. A 10% solution in water has a pH of 3.0 to 5.5. **Store** at a temperature not exceeding 30° in airtight containers.

Clindamycin Palmitate Hydrochloride (54-v)

Clindamycin Palmitate Hydrochloride (*BANM, USAN, rINNM*).

U-25179E. Clindamycin 2-palmitate hydrochloride.

$C_{34}H_{63}ClN_2O_6S,HCl$ = 699.9.

CAS — 36688-78-5 (clindamycin palmitate); 25507-04-4 (clindamycin palmitate hydrochloride).

Pharmacopoeias. In *US.*

A white to off-white amorphous powder with a characteristic odour. 1.6 g of monograph substance is approximately equivalent to 1 g of clindamycin. **Soluble** 1 in 3 of alcohol and 1 in 9 of ethyl acetate; freely soluble in water, in chloroform, and in ether; very soluble in dimethylformamide. A 1% solution in water has a pH of 2.8 to 3.8. **Store** in airtight containers.

Clindamycin Phosphate (56-q)

Clindamycin Phosphate (*BANM, USAN, rINNM*).

Clindamycini Phosphas; U-28508. Clindamycin 2-(dihydrogen phosphate).

$C_{18}H_{34}ClN_2O_8PS$ = 505.0.

CAS — 24729-96-2.

Pharmacopoeias. In *Eur.* (see p.viii), *Jpn,* and *US.*

A white to off-white, odourless or almost odourless, hygroscopic, crystalline powder. 1.2 g of monograph substance is approximately equivalent to 1 g of clindamycin. **Soluble** 1 in 2.5 of water; slightly soluble in dehydrated alcohol; very slightly soluble in acetone and in alcohol; practically insoluble in chloroform, in dichloromethane, and in ether. A 1% solution in water has a pH of 3.5 to 4.5. **Store** at a temperature not exceeding 30° in airtight containers.

Incompatibilities. Solutions of clindamycin salts have an acid pH and incompatibility may reasonably be expected with alkaline preparations, or with drugs unstable at low pH. Clindamycin phosphate is incompatible with natural rubber closures.

Stability. Oesterling[1] reported that in buffered aqueous solution, clindamycin showed maximum stability at pH 3 to 5; after storage for 2 years at 25° not more than 10% degradation would occur in the pH range 1 to 6.5. At pH 0.4 to 4 hydrolysis of clindamycin to 1-dethiomethyl-1-hydroxyclindamycin and methyl mercaptan occurred; at pH 5 to 10 lincomycin was formed. Clindamycin phosphate, which was less bitter than the hydrochloride, was most stable in solution at pH 3.5 to 6.5.[2]

Clindamycin 15 mg per mL (as the phosphate salt) in sterile water for injections was stable for the full study period of 91 days when protected from light and stored at either 4° or 22°.[3]

1. Oesterling TO. Aqueous stability of clindamycin. *J Pharm Sci* 1970; **59:** 63–7.
2. Oesterling TO, Rowe EL. Hydrolysis of lincomycin-2-phosphate and clindamycin-2-phosphate. *J Pharm Sci* 1970; **59:** 175–9.
3. Nahata MC, *et al.* Stability of cimetidine hydrochloride and of clindamycin phosphate in water for injection stored in glass vials at two temperatures. *Am J Hosp Pharm* 1993; **50:** 2559–61.

Adverse Effects

Clindamycin is reported to produce diarrhoea in about 2 to 20% of patients after systemic administration; in some patients severe antibiotic-associated or pseudomembranous colitis may develop, and has proved fatal. The syndrome, which may develop during therapy or for up to several weeks after it, appears to be due to toxins produced by *Clostridium* spp., most notably *C. difficile.* It has been reported to be more frequent in women and in elderly patients, and may also occur rarely after topical administration. Other gastro-intestinal effects reported with clindamycin include nausea, vomiting, abdominal pain or cramps, and unpleasant or metallic taste after high intravenous doses.

Hypersensitivity reactions, including skin rashes in up to 10% of patents, urticaria, and very rarely anaphylaxis, have occurred. Other adverse effects include transient leucopenia or occasionally agranulocytosis, eosinophilia, thrombocytopenia, erythema multiforme, polyarthritis, and abnormalities of liver function tests; in some cases overt jaundice and hepatic damage have been reported. Although local irritation is stated to be rare, intramuscular injection has led to sterile abscess, and thrombophlebitis may occur after intravenous administration. Some parenteral formulations contain benzyl alcohol which may cause fatal 'gasping syndrome' in neonates.

Topical application may be associated with local irritation and contact dermatitis; sufficient clindamycin may be absorbed to produce systemic effects. Cervicitis, vaginitis, or vulvovaginal irritation has been reported with intravaginal use; a small amount of systemic absorption also occurs.

Effects on the cardiovascular system. Cardiac arrest occurred in a 50-year-old woman after rapid injection of 600 mg of undiluted clindamycin phosphate into a central intravenous line. Further injections were given over 30 minutes without cardiovascular complications.[1]

1. Aucoin P, *et al.* Clindamycin-induced cardiac arrest. *South Med J* 1982; **75:** 768.

Effects on the gastro-intestinal tract. References to antibiotic-associated colitis and the role of clindamycin.

1. Tedesco FJ, *et al.* Clindamycin-associated colitis: a prospective study. *Ann Intern Med* 1974; **81:** 429–33.
2. Robertson MB, *et al.* Incidence of antibiotic-related diarrhoea and pseudomembranous colitis: a prospective study of lincomycin, clindamycin and ampicillin. *Med J Aust* 1977; **1:** 243–6.
3. Committee on Safety of Medicines. Antibiotic induced colitis. *Adverse Reactions Series 17* 1979.
4. Borriello SP, Larson HE. Antibiotic and pseudomembranous colitis. *J Antimicrob Chemother* 1981; **7** (suppl A): 53–62.
5. Milstone EB, *et al.* Pseudomembranous colitis after topical application of clindamycin. *Arch Dermatol* 1981; **117:** 154–5.
6. Parry MF, Rha C-K. Pseudomembranous colitis caused by topical clindamycin phosphate. *Arch Dermatol* 1986; **122:** 583–4.
7. Young GP, *et al.* Antibiotic-associated colitis caused by Clostridium difficile: relapse and risk factors. *Med J Aust* 1986; **144:** 303–6.

Effects on the lymphatic system. Lymphadenitis was associated with clindamycin administration in one patient.[1]

1. Southern PM. Lymphadenitis associated with the administration of clindamycin. *Am J Med* 1997; **103:** 164–5.

Effects on the skin. A report of toxic epidermal necrolysis associated with clindamycin.[1]

1. Paquet P, *et al.* Toxic epidermal necrolysis following clindamycin treatment. *Br J Dermatol* 1995; **132:** 665–6.

Treatment of Adverse Effects

Clindamycin should be withdrawn immediately if significant diarrhoea or colitis occurs. Metronidazole or vancomycin may be used to treat antibiotic-associated pseudomembranous colitis. For further details, see under Gastro-enteritis, p.123.

Precautions

Clindamycin should not be given to patients hypersensitive to it or to the closely-related drug lincomycin. It should be used with caution in patients with gastro-intestinal disease, particularly those with a history of colitis. Clindamycin should be withdrawn immediately if significant diarrhoea or colitis occurs. Elderly and female patients may be more likely to experience severe diarrhoea or pseudomembranous colitis. Caution has also been advised in atopic patients, and in those with hepatic or renal impairment who may require dosage adjustment. Periodic tests of liver and kidney function and blood counts have been recommended in patients receiving prolonged therapy, and in infants. Clindamycin is distributed into breast milk and breast feeding should be avoided during therapy.

AIDS. Clindamycin was poorly tolerated by patients with AIDS in a study of its use for prophylaxis of toxoplasmic encephalitis (but see also below). Despite the use of relatively low doses of clindamycin (300 mg twice daily) 23 of 52 patients reported adverse effects that necessitated temporary or permanent withdrawal of the drug, the most frequent adverse reactions being diarrhoea and skin rash. The clindamycin arm of the study had to be terminated prematurely.[1]

1. Jacobson MA, *et al.* Toxicity of clindamycin as prophylaxis for AIDS-associated toxoplasmic encephalitis. *Lancet* 1992; **339:** 333–4.

Interactions

Clindamycin may enhance the effect of drugs with neuromuscular blocking activity (p.1306) and there is a potential danger of respiratory depression. Additive respiratory depressant effects may also occur with opioids. Clindamycin may antagonise the activity of parasympathomimetics. For reports of synergistic and antagonistic antimicrobial activity with other antibacterials, see Antimicrobial Action, below.

Adsorbents. In 16 healthy subjects given clindamycin alone and with a kaolin-pectin suspension it was found that the suspension had no effect on the extent of clindamycin absorption but did markedly reduce the absorption rate.[1]

1. Albert KS, *et al.* Pharmacokinetic evaluation of a drug interaction between kaolin-pectin and clindamycin. *J Pharm Sci* 1978; **67:** 1579–82.

Antimicrobial Action

Clindamycin is a lincosamide antibiotic with a primarily bacteriostatic action against Gram-positive aerobes and a wide range of anaerobic bacteria.

Mechanism of action. Lincosamides such as clindamycin bind to the 50S subunit of the bacterial ribosome, similarly to macrolides such as erythromycin (p.205), and inhibit the early stages of protein synthesis. The action of clindamycin is predominantly bacteriostatic although high concentrations may be slowly bactericidal against sensitive strains.

Spectrum of activity. Clindamycin is active against most aerobic Gram-positive bacteria including streptococci, staphylococci, *Bacillus anthracis,* and

Corynebacterium diphtheriae; enterococci, however, are generally resistant.

Clindamycin has good activity against a wide range of anaerobic bacteria. Susceptible Gram-positive anaerobes include *Eubacterium, Propionibacterium, Peptococcus*, and *Peptostreptococcus* spp., and many strains of *Clostridium perfringens* and *Cl. tetani*. Among Gram-negative anaerobes susceptible to clindamycin are *Fusobacterium* spp. (although *F. varium* is usually resistant), *Veillonella*, and *Bacteroides* spp. including the *B. fragilis* group.

Apart from *Mycoplasma hominis*, clindamycin is generally less active than erythromycin against *Mycoplasma* spp. Several *Actinomyces* spp. and *Nocardia asteroides* are reported to be susceptible.

Most Gram-negative aerobic bacteria, including the Enterobacteriaceae, are resistant to clindamycin; unlike erythromycin, *Neisseria gonorrhoeae, N. meningitidis, and Haemophilus influenzae* are generally resistant to clindamycin.

Fungi, yeasts, and viruses are also resistant; however, clindamycin has been reported to have some antiprotozoal activity against *Toxoplasma gondii* and *Plasmodium* spp.

Minimum inhibitory concentrations (MICs) of clindamycin have been reported to be as low as 0.002 μg per mL for the most sensitive strains of *Streptococcus pneumoniae* but MICs for sensitive streptococci, staphylococci, and anaerobes such as *Bacteroides fragilis* or *Fusobacterium* spp. are usually in the range 0.01 to 0.5 μg per mL. Organisms with MICs up to about 1.6 μg per mL are considered sensitive, and those with MICs between about 1.6 and 4.8 μg per mL of moderate sensitivity.

Activity with other antimicrobials. Synergistic activity has been reported between clindamycin and ceftazidime or metronidazole, and also with ciprofloxacin against some anaerobes. However, there is some evidence that clindamycin inhibits the bactericidal activity of the aminoglycosides, although conflicting reports have suggested variable degrees of synergy against anaerobic organisms. Because of the adjacency of their binding sites on the ribosome, clindamycin may competitively inhibit the effects of macrolides or chloramphenicol. Clindamycin has been reported to diminish the activity of ampicillin *in vitro* against *Staph. aureus*. It is reported to enhance the activity of primaquine against *Pneumocystis carinii*.

Resistance. Most Gram-negative aerobes, such as the Enterobacteriaceae, are intrinsically resistant to clindamycin, but acquired resistance also occurs in normally-sensitive strains. The mechanisms of resistance are the same as those for erythromycin, namely methylation of the ribosomal binding site, chromosomal mutation of the ribosomal protein, and in a few staphylococcal isolates enzymic inactivation by a plasmid-mediated adenyltransferase. Methylation of the ribosome leads to cross-resistance between the lincosamides and macrolides and streptogramins (the MLS_B phenotype); this type of resistance is usually plasmid mediated and inducible. Complete cross-resistance exists between clindamycin and lincomycin.

The incidence of resistance varies with the organism and the geographical location; it is more frequent in organisms that are also erythromycin resistant, and many strains of methicillin-resistant *Staphylococcus aureus* are also resistant to clindamycin. In some countries and institutions there is evidence of an increase in resistance amongst the *Bacteroides fragilis* group to 25% of strains or more.

Action. References suggesting that clindamycin may reduce microbial adherence and enhance phagocytosis by its effects on bacterial slime (glycocalyx).

1. Veringa EM, *et al.* Enhancement of opsonophagocytosis of Bacteroides spp by clindamycin in subinhibitory concentrations. *J Antimicrob Chemother* 1981; **23:** 577–87.
2. Veringa EM, *et al.* The role of glycocalyx in surface phagocytosis of Bacteroides spp. in the presence and absence of clindamycin. *J Antimicrob Chemother* 1989; **23:** 711–20.
3. Khardori N, *et al.* Effect of subinhibitory concentrations of clindamycin and trospectomycin on the adherence of Staphylococcus epidermidis in an in vitro model of vascular catheter colonization. *J Infect Dis* 1991; **164:** 108–13.

References suggesting that the antibacterial effects of clindamycin may be independent of plasma concentrations.

1. Xue IB, *et al.* Variation in postantibiotic effect of clindamycin against clinical isolates of Staphylococcus aureus and implications for dosing of patients with osteomyelitis. *Antimicrob Agents Chemother* 1996; **40:** 1403–7.
2. Klepser ME, *et al.* Bactericidal activity of low-dose clindamycin administered at 8- and 12-hour intervals against Staphylococcus aureus, Streptococcus pneumoniae, and Bacteroides fragilis. *Antimicrob Agents Chemother* 1997; **41:** 630–5.

Activity against protozoa and fungi. References.

1. Lewis C. Antiplasmodial activity of 7-halogenated lincomycins. *J Parasitol* 1968; **54:** 169–70.
2. Araujo FG, Remington JS. Effect of clindamycin on acute and chronic toxoplasmosis in mice. *Antimicrob Agents Chemother* 1874; **5:** 647–51.
3. Mack DG, McLeod R. New micromethod to study the effect of antimicrobial agents on Toxoplasma gondii: comparison of sulfadoxine and sulfadiazine individually and in combination with pyrimethamine and study of clindamycin, metronidazole, and cyclosporin A. *Antimicrob Agents Chemother* 1984; **26:** 26–30.
4. Queener SF, *et al.* Activity of clindamycin with primaquine against Pneumocystis carinii in vitro and in vivo. *Antimicrob Agents Chemother* 1988; **32:** 807–13.
5. Blais J, *et al.* Effect of clindamycin on intracellular replication, protein synthesis, and infectivity of Toxoplasma gondii. *Antimicrob Agents Chemother* 1993; **37:** 2571–7.
6. Fichera ME, *et al.* In vitro assays elucidate peculiar kinetics of clindamycin action against Toxoplasma gondii. *Antimicrob Agents Chemother* 1995; **39:** 1530–7.

Activity with other antimicrobials. References to antimicrobial synergy and antagonism between clindamycin and other antimicrobials.

1. Meers PD. Bacteroides infections. *Lancet* 1973; **ii:** 573.
2. Busch DF, *et al.* Activity of combinations of antimicrobial agents against Bacteroides fragilis. *J Infect Dis* 1976; **133:** 321–8.
3. Sanders CC, *et al.* Effects of clindamycin on derepression of β-lactamases in Gram-negative bacteria. *J Antimicrob Chemother* 1983; **12** (suppl C): 97–104.
4. Brook I, *et al.* Synergism between penicillin, clindamycin, or metronidazole and gentamicin against species of the Bacteroides melaninogenicus and Bacteroides fragilis groups. *Antimicrob Agents Chemother* 1984; **25:** 71–7.
5. George WL. In vitro antibacterial activity of the combination of clindamycin and ceftazidime. *Antimicrob Agents Chemother* 1984; **25:** 657–8.
6. Brook I, Walker RI. Interaction between penicillin, clindamycin or metronidazole and gentamicin against species of clostridia and anaerobic and facultatively anaerobic Gram-positive cocci. *J Antimicrob Chemother* 1984; **15:** 31–7.
7. Whiting JL, *et al.* Interactions of ciprofloxacin with clindamycin, metronidazole, cefoxitin, cefotaxime, and mezlocillin against Gram-positive and Gram-negative anaerobic bacteria. *Antimicrob Agents Chemother* 1987; **31:** 1379–82.
8. Arditi M, Yogev R. In vitro interaction between rifampin and clindamycin against pathogenic coagulase-negative staphylococci. *Antimicrob Agents Chemother* 1989; **33:** 245–7.

Resistance. Although there is usually cross-resistance between clindamycin and macrolides (see above) a resistance pattern has recently been identified that results in resistance to macrolides while retaining susceptibility to clindamycin.[1]

1. Sutcliffe J, *et al.* Streptococcus pneumoniae and Streptococcus pyogenes resistant to macrolides but sensitive to clindamycin: a common resistance pattern mediated by an efflux system. *Antimicrob Agents Chemother* 1996; **40:** 1817–24.

Pharmacokinetics

About 90% of a dose of clindamycin hydrochloride is absorbed from the gastro-intestinal tract; concentrations of 2 to 3 μg per mL occur within 1 hour after a 150-mg dose of clindamycin, with average concentrations of about 0.7 μg per mL after 6 hours. After doses of 300 and 600 mg peak plasma concentrations of 4 and 8 μg per mL, respectively, have been reported. Absorption is not significantly diminished by food in the stomach but the rate of absorption may be reduced. Clindamycin palmitate hydrochloride is rapidly hydrolysed following oral administration to provide free clindamycin.

Following parenteral administration the biologically inactive clindamycin phosphate is also hydrolysed to clindamycin. When the equivalent of 300 mg of clindamycin is injected intramuscularly a mean peak plasma concentration of 6 μg per mL is achieved within 3 hours; 600 mg gives a peak concentration of 9 μg per mL. In children, peak concentrations may be reached within one hour. When the same doses are infused intravenously peak concentrations of 7 and 10 μg per mL are achieved by the end of infusion.

Small amounts of clindamycin may be absorbed from topical application to the skin; bioavailability from topical preparations of the hydrochloride and phosphate (the former in an extemporaneous formulation) has been reported to be about 7.5% and 2% respectively.

About 5% of an intravaginal dose may be absorbed systemically.

Clindamycin is widely distributed in body fluids and tissues including bone but it does not reach the CSF in significant concentrations. It diffuses across the placenta into the fetal circulation and has been reported to appear in breast milk. High concentrations occur in bile. It accumulates in leucocytes and macrophages. Over 90% of clindamycin in the circulation is bound to plasma proteins. The half-life is 2 to 3 hours, although this may be prolonged in pre-term neonates and patients with severe renal impairment.

Clindamycin undergoes metabolism, presumably in the liver, to the active *N*-demethyl and sulphoxide metabolites, and also some inactive metabolites. About 10% of a dose is excreted in the urine as active drug or metabolites and about 4% in the faeces; the remainder is excreted as inactive metabolites. Excretion is slow, and takes place over several days. It is not effectively removed from the blood by dialysis.

AIDS patients. Clindamycin was reported to have higher bioavailability, lower plasma clearance, and a lower volume of distribution in patients with AIDS than in healthy volunteers.[1] This may partly be explained by increased binding to plasma proteins.[2]

1. Gatti G, *et al.* Comparative study of bioavailabilities and pharmacokinetics of clindamycin in healthy volunteers and patients with AIDS. *Antimicrob Agents Chemother* 1993; **37:** 1137–43.
2. Flaherty JF, *et al.* Protein binding of clindamycin in sera of patients with AIDS. *Antimicrob Agents Chemother* 1996; **40:** 1134–8.

Uses and Administration

Clindamycin is a lincosamide antibiotic which is a chlorinated derivative of lincomycin. It is a primarily bacteriostatic antibacterial used chiefly in the treatment of serious anaerobic infections, notably due to *Bacteroides fragilis*, and in some staphylococcal and streptococcal infections. However, because of its potential for causing pseudomembranous colitis (see Adverse Effects, above) it is usually used only when alternative drugs are unsuitable. Amongst the conditions that it may be used to treat are liver abscess, actinomycosis, staphylococcal bone and joint infections, the carrier state of diphtheria, gas gangrene, various gynaecological infections including bacterial vaginosis, endometritis, and pelvic inflammatory disease (the latter two in combination with an aminoglycoside), necrotising fasciitis, secondary peritonitis, streptococcal pharyngitis (usually to treat the carrier state), pneumonia (especially lung abscess), septicaemia, and skin infections involving heavy colonisation with streptococci or anaerobes. It is used in the prophylaxis of endocarditis in penicillin-allergic patients, in the prevention of perinatal streptococcal infections, and in combination with other drugs for the prophylaxis of surgical infection. For details of these bacterial infections and their treatment, see under Choice of Antibacterial, p.116.

Clindamycin is also applied topically in the treatment of acne (p.1072).

Clindamycin also has some antiprotozoal actions, and has been used, usually in combination with other antiprotozoals, in various infections (see below) including babesiosis, malaria, and toxoplasmosis; it may also be used in combination with primaquine in the treatment of *Pneumocystis carinii* pneumonia.

Clindamycin is given by mouth as capsules containing the hydrochloride or as oral liquid preparations containing the palmitate hydrochloride. The capsules should be taken with a glass of water. Doses are expressed in terms of the equivalent amount of clindamycin.

The usual dose by mouth is the equivalent of 150 to 300 mg of clindamycin every 6 hours; in severe infections the dose may be increased to 450 mg every 6 hours. Children may be given 3 to 6 mg per kg body-weight every 6 hours; those under one-year-old or weighing 10 kg or less should receive at least 37.5 mg every 8 hours.

For prophylaxis in patients at risk of developing endocarditis and who cannot be given a penicillin, an oral dose of clindamycin 600 mg given one hour before procedures such as dental extractions, under local or no anaesthesia, has been suggested. For patients at special risk undergoing dental procedures involving general anaesthesia, an intravenous dose of clindamycin 300 mg given over at least 10 minutes, at induction or 15 minutes before the procedure, followed 6 hours later by oral or intravenous clindamycin 150 mg has been suggested.

Clindamycin is given parenterally as the phosphate. It is given by intramuscular injection, or by intermittent or continuous intravenous infusion, as a solution usually diluted to not more than 6 mg per mL, although some authorities allow up to 18 mg per mL; the rate of infusion should be not more than 30 mg per minute. Not more than 1.2 g should be administered as a single one-hour infusion, and not more than 600 mg should be given as a single intramuscular injection.

The usual parenteral dose is the equivalent of 0.6 to 2.7 g of clindamycin daily in divided doses; up to 4.8 g daily has been given intravenously in very severe infections. Children over the age of 1 month may be given the equivalent of 15 to 40 mg per kg body-weight daily in divided doses; in severe infections they should receive a total dose of not less than 300 mg of clindamycin daily. Neonates have been given 15 to 20 mg per kg daily.

Topical formulations containing 1% of clindamycin phosphate are used for the treatment of acne. The hydrochloride may be applied similarly, but systemic absorption may be greater (see Pharmacokinetics, above).

A 2% cream containing clindamycin phosphate is used for the treatment of bacterial vaginosis, the equivalent of about 100 mg clindamycin being given intravaginally at night for 3 to 7 days.

Administration. A number of studies have suggested that a parenteral regimen of clindamycin 600 mg three times daily is as effective as giving the same dose four times daily,[1] or as giving 900 mg three times daily.[2,3]

1. Buchwald D, *et al.* Effect of hospitalwide change in clindamycin dosing schedule on clinical outcome. *Rev Infect Dis* 1989; **11:** 619–24.
2. Chin A, *et al.* Cost analysis of two clindamycin dosing regimens. *DICP Ann Pharmacother* 1989; **23:** 980–3.
3. Chatwani A, *et al.* Clindamycin dosage scheduling for acute pelvic infection. *Am J Obstet Gynecol* 1990; **163:** 240.

Babesiosis. Clindamycin, 1.2 g twice daily intravenously or 600 mg three times daily by mouth, in association with quinine, 650 mg three times daily by mouth, has been recommended in the USA for the treatment of babesiosis (p.574) caused by *Babesia microti*.[1] Children could be given clindamycin 20 to 40 mg per kg body-weight daily and quinine 25 mg per kg daily, both by mouth in 3 divided doses.[1] Treatment is continued for 7 days. However, WHO, while noting that the combination was reported to be successful in the few patients requiring specific treatment, stated that further confirmation of its effectiveness was required.[2]

1. Anonymous. Drugs for parasitic infections. *Med Lett Drugs Ther* 1998; **40:** 1–12.
2. WHO. WHO model prescribing information—drugs used in parasitic diseases. Geneva: WHO, 1995.

Malaria. Clindamycin 900 mg three times daily for 5 days plus quinine sulphate 650 mg three times daily for 3 to 7 days, both given by mouth, is one of the suggested treatments[1] for chloroquine-resistant falciparum malaria (p.422). Parenteral clindamycin plus quinine has also been tried in severe falciparum malaria.[2]

1. Anonymous. Drugs for parasitic infections. *Med Lett Drugs Ther* 1998; **40:** 1–12.
2. Kremsner PG, *et al.* Quinine plus clindamycin improves chemotherapy of severe malaria in children. *Antimicrob Agents Chemother* 1995; **39:** 1603–5.

Pneumocystis carinii pneumonia. Clindamycin may be used with primaquine as an alternative to co-trimoxazole for the treatment of *Pneumocystis carinii* pneumonia in patients with AIDS (p.370). A suggested dose[1] is clindamycin 600 mg intravenously, or 300 to 450 mg by mouth, every 6 hours with primaquine 30 mg by mouth daily, for 21 days. Clindamycin with primaquine is not normally recommended for prophylaxis although there are reports of it being tried.[2]

1. Anonymous. Drugs for parasitic infections. *Med Lett Drugs Ther* 1998; **40:** 1–12.
2. Kay R, DuBois RE. Clindamycin/primaquine therapy and secondary prophylaxis against Pneumocystis carinii pneumonia in patients with AIDS. *South Med J* 1990; **83:** 403–4.

Rosacea. Topical clindamycin[1] has improved the inflammatory episodes of rosacea (p.1076), although other features of the skin disorder may not respond.

1. Wilkin JK, DeWitt S. Treatment of rosacea: topical clindamycin versus oral tetracycline. *Int J Dermatol* 1993; **32:** 65–7.

Toxoplasmosis. Primaquine with clindamycin has been used for the treatment of toxoplasmosis (p.576) instead of the more usual treatment with pyrimethamine plus sulphadiazine, in patients unable to tolerate sulphonamides. A suggested dose has been clindamycin 600 mg by mouth every 6 hours for at least 3 weeks, then maintenance therapy with at least 1200 mg daily;[1] patients also received pyrimethamine. Luft *et al.*[2] gave oral clindamycin 600 mg four times daily together with pyrimethamine 75 mg daily for 6 weeks to patients with AIDS and toxoplasmic encephalitis. Acute therapy with pyrimethamine and clindamycin, 600 mg four times a day by mouth[3] or 1200 mg every 6 hours intravenously,[4] was as effective as pyrimethamine and sulphadiazine, but maintenance therapy with pyrimethamine and clindamycin 300 mg four times daily by mouth was less effective than pyrimethamine and sulphadiazine at preventing relapses in a population followed for 3 years or more.[3] Clindamycin with fluorouracil produced beneficial responses in a study involving 16 patients.[5]

In contrast, another study comparing clindamycin alone [in lower doses—300 mg twice daily by mouth] with pyrimethamine alone for prophylaxis of toxoplasmic encephalitis reported an unacceptably high incidence of adverse effects with clindamycin which forced premature termination of the clindamycin arm—see under Precautions, above.

1. Remington JS, Vildé JL. Clindamycin for toxoplasma encephalitis in AIDS. *Lancet* 1991; **338:** 1142–3.
2. Luft BJ, *et al.* Toxoplasmic encephalitis in patients with the acquired immunodeficiency syndrome. *N Engl J Med* 1993; **329:** 995–1000.
3. Katlama C, *et al.* Pyrimethamine-clindamycin vs pyrimethamine-sulphadiazine as acute and long-term therapy for toxoplasmic encephalitis in patients with AIDS. *Clin Infect Dis* 1996; **22:** 268–75.
4. Dannemann B, *et al.* Treatment of toxoplasmic encephalitis in patients with AIDS: a randomized trial comparing pyrimethamine plus clindamycin to pyrimethamine plus sulfadiazine. *Ann Intern Med* 1992; **116:** 33–43.
5. Dhiver C, *et al.* 5-Fluoro-uracil-clindamycin for treatment of cerebral toxoplasmosis. *AIDS* 1993; **7:** 143–4.

Preparations

BP 1998: Clindamycin Capsules; Clindamycin Injection;
USP 23: Clindamycin for Injection; Clindamycin Hydrochloride Capsules; Clindamycin Injection; Clindamycin Palmitate Hydrochloride for Oral Solution; Clindamycin Phosphate Gel; Clindamycin Phosphate Topical Solution; Clindamycin Phosphate Topical Suspension; Clindamycin Phosphate Vaginal Cream.

Proprietary Preparations (details are given in Part 3)
Aust.: Cleocin; Dalacin; Lanacine; ***Austral.:*** Cleocin; Clindatech; Dalacin C; Dalacin V; ***Belg.:*** Dalacin C; Dalacin T; Dalacin Vaginal; ***Canad.:*** Dalacin C; Dalacin T; Dalacin Vaginal; ***Fr.:*** Dalacine; Dalacine T; ***Ger.:*** Aclinda; Basocin; Clin-Sanorania; Clinda; Clinda-saar; Clindahexal; Clindastad; Sobelin; Turimycin; ***Irl.:*** Dalacin; Dalacin C; Dalacin T; ***Ital.:*** Cleocin; Dalacin C; Dalacin T; ***Neth.:*** Dalacin C; Dalacin T; ***Norw.:*** Dalacin; ***S.Afr.:*** Dalacin C; Dalacin T; Dalacin VC; ***Spain:*** Clinwas; Dalacin; ***Swed.:*** Dalacin; ***Switz.:*** Dalacin C; Dalacin T; Dalacin V; ***UK:*** Dalacin; Dalacin C; Dalacin T; ***USA:*** C/T/S; Cleocin; Cleocin T; Clinda-Derm.

Clioquinol (4770-t)

Clioquinol (BAN, rINN).

Chinoform; Chloroiodoquine; Cliochinolum; Iodochlorhydroxyquin; Iodochlorhydroxyquinoline; Quiniodochlor. 5-Chloro-7-iodoquinolin-8-ol.

C_9H_5ClINO = 305.5.

CAS — 130-26-7.

Pharmacopoeias. In *Aust., Br., It., Swiss,* and *US.*

A yellowish-white to brownish-yellow, voluminous powder with a slight characteristic odour. It darkens on exposure to light.

Practically **insoluble** in water; soluble 1 in 3500 of alcohol, 1 in 120 of chloroform, and 1 in 4500 of ether; freely soluble in dimethylformamide and in pyridine; soluble in hot ethyl acetate and in hot glacial acetic acid. **Store** in airtight containers. Protect from light.

Adverse Effects and Precautions

Clioquinol may rarely cause iodism in sensitive patients. Local application of clioquinol in ointments or creams may occasionally cause severe irritation or hypersensitivity and there may be cross-sensitivity with other halogenated hydroxyquinolines.

Clioquinol stains clothing and linen yellow on contact and may stain the skin and discolour fair hair.

Clioquinol given by mouth has been associated with severe neurotoxicity. In Japan, the epidemic development of subacute myelo-opticoneuropathy (SMON) in the 1960s was associated with the ingestion of normal or high doses of clioquinol for prolonged periods and the sale of clioquinol and related hydroxyquinolines was subsequently banned in Japan. Symptoms of subacute myelo-opticoneuropathy are principally those of peripheral neuropathy, including optic atrophy, and myelopathy. Abdominal pain and diarrhoea often precede neurological symptoms such as paraesthesias in the legs progressing to paraplegia in some patients and loss of visual acuity sometimes leading to blindness. A characteristic green pigment, a chelate of clioquinol with iron, is often seen on the tongue and in the urine and faeces. Cerebral disturbances, including confusion and retrograde amnesia, have also been reported. Although many patients improved when clioquinol was withdrawn, others had residual disablement.

It was suggested that the Japanese epidemic might be due to genetic susceptibility, but a few similar cases of subacute myelo-opticoneuropathy have been reported from several other countries in association with clioquinol or related hydroxyquinoline derivatives, such as broxyquinoline or di-iodohydroxyquinoline. Oral preparations of clioquinol have now been banned in most countries.

Absorption of clioquinol through the skin has been noted following topical application.[1,2] Significant toxicity has been found in *dogs* treated with 5 g of a 3% clioquinol topical preparation for 28 days.[3] The Committee on Drugs of the American Academy of Pediatrics[4] considered that there was a potential risk of toxicity to infants and children from clioquinol and di-iodohydroxyquinoline applied topically. Since alternative effective preparations are available for dermatitis the Committee recommended that products containing either of these compounds should not be used.

1. Fischer T, Hartvig P. Skin absorption of 8-hydroxyquinolines. *Lancet* 1977; **i:** 603.
2. Stohs SJ, *et al.* Percutaneous absorption of iodochlorhydroxyquin in humans. *J Invest Dermatol* 1984; **82:** 195–8.
3. Ezzedeen FW, *et al.* Percutaneous absorption and disposition of iodochlorhydroxyquin in dogs. *J Pharm Sci* 1984; **73:** 1369–72.
4. Kauffman RE, *et al.* Clioquinol (iodochlorhydroxyquin, Vioform) and iodoquinol (diiodohydroxyquin): blindness and neuropathy. *Pediatrics* 1990; **86:** 797–8.

Abnormal coloration. Green discoloration of the tongue, urine, and faeces and yellow discoloration of the nails have been recognised with clioquinol.[1] Topical application of a clioquinol-containing corticosteroid preparation was associated with intense red discoloration of white hair in 2 patients with generalised dermatitis.

1. Bandmann H-J, Speer U. Red hair after application of chinoform. *Contact Dermatitis* 1984; **10:** 113.

Hypersensitivity. Classification of clioquinol as a contact allergen which can commonly cause sensitisation, especially when applied to eczematous skin; chlorquinaldol can also cause sensitisation, but less frequently.[1] It is important to include clioquinol and chlorquinaldol in routine patch testing since the clinical reaction may be relatively mild and sensitivity easily missed, particularly in the presence of a corticosteroid which suppresses or attenuates the reaction.

1. Anonymous. Skin sensitisers in topical corticosteroids. *Drug Ther Bull* 1986; **24:** 57–9.

Uses and Administration

Clioquinol is a halogenated hydroxyquinoline with antibacterial and antifungal activity and is used in creams and ointments, usually containing 3%, in the treatment of skin infections. It is applied together with a corticosteroid in inflammatory skin conditions complicated by bacterial or fungal infections. It is also used in ear drops for otitis externa. The treatment of bacterial and of fungal skin infections is described on p.142 and p.371 respectively.

For a discussion of the risks from topical application of clioquinol, see Adverse Effects and Precautions, above.

Clioquinol was formerly given by mouth in the treatment of intestinal amoebiasis. It was also formerly used for the prophylaxis and treatment of traveller's diarrhoea and similar infections but was of doubtful value. Oral preparations have now been withdrawn because of neurotoxicity (see Adverse Effects and Precautions, above).

Preparations

BP 1998: Betamethasone and Clioquinol Cream; Betamethasone and Clioquinol Ointment; Clioquinol Cream; Hydrocortisone and Clioquinol Cream; Hydrocortisone and Clioquinol Ointment;
USP 23: Clioquinol and Hydrocortisone Cream; Clioquinol and

Hydrocortisone Ointment; Clioquinol Cream; Clioquinol Ointment; Compound Clioquinol Topical Powder.

Proprietary Preparations (details are given in Part 3)
Austral.: Silic C†; Vioform†; ***Canad.:*** Vioform; ***Ger.:*** Linolasept; ***Switz.:*** Vioform; ***USA:*** Vioform.

Multi-ingredient: ***Aust.:*** Betnovate-C; Locacorten Vioform; ***Austral.:*** First Aid Antiseptic Powder†; Hydroform; Locacorten Vioform; Quinaband; Vioform-Hydrocortisone†; ***Belg.:*** Betnelan-VC; Locacortene Vioforme; ***Canad.:*** Aristoform†; Locacorten Vioform; Phenoris; Propaderm-C†; Vioform-Hydrocortisone; ***Fr.:*** Diprosept; Locacortene Vioforme†; ***Ger.:*** Locacorten Vioform; Millicorten-Vioform; Sermaform†; ***Irl.:*** Betnovate-C; Oralcer; Synalar C; Vioform-Hydrocortisone; ***Ital.:*** Dermadex Chinolinico†; Diproform; Locorten; Locorten Vioformio; Recto Menaderm†; Reticus Antimicotico†; Viobeta; Viocidina; ***Neth.:*** Betnelan Clioquinol†; Celestoform; Locacorten Vioform; ***Norw.:*** Betnovat med Chinoform; Locacorten Vioform; Synalar med Chinoform; ***S.Afr.:*** Betnovate-C; Locacorten Vioform; Manoderm†; Propaderm-C†; Quadriderm; Synalar C; ***Spain:*** Antiblef Eczem; Cuatroderm; Locortene Vioformo; Menaderm Clio; Menaderm Otologico; Recto Menaderm; Synobel; Triaformo†; ***Swed.:*** Betnovat med Chinoform; Celeston valerat med chinoform; Locacorten Vioform; Synalar med Chinoform†; ***Switz.:*** Betnovate-C; Locacorten Vioform†; Quadriderm; ***UK:*** Betnovate-C; Haelan-C†; Locorten Vioform; Oralcer; Quinaband; Synalar C; Vioform-Hydrocortisone; ***USA:*** 1 + 1-F; Ala-Quin; Albaform HC; Corque; Hysone; Iodo-Cortifair†; Pedi-Cort V; UAD Cream or Lotion†; Vioform-Hydrocortisone†.

Clofazimine (6553-m)

Clofazimine *(BAN, USAN, rINN)*.

B-663; G-30320; NSC-141046. 3-(4-Chloroanilino)-10-(4-chlorophenyl)-2,10-dihydro-2-phenazin-2-ylideneisopropylamine.

$C_{27}H_{22}Cl_2N_4$ = 473.4.

CAS — 2030-63-9.

Pharmacopoeias. In Br., Fr., Int. and US.

A fine reddish-brown, odourless or almost odourless powder or dark red crystals. Practically **insoluble** in water; slightly or sparingly soluble in alcohol; soluble in chloroform; sparingly soluble in acetone and in ethyl acetate; very slightly soluble in ether. **Store** in airtight containers. Protect from light.

Adverse Effects

Adverse effects to clofazimine are dose-related, the most common being red to brown discoloration of the skin especially on areas exposed to sunlight; leprotic lesions may become mauve to black. These changes are more noticeable in light-skinned people and may limit its acceptance. The conjunctiva and cornea may also show some signs of red to brown pigmentation. The generalised discoloration may take months to years to disappear after stopping therapy with clofazimine. Discoloration of hair, tears, sweat, sputum, breast milk, urine, and faeces may occur.

Gastro-intestinal effects are uncommon for doses of clofazimine less than 100 mg daily and usually are not severe. Symptoms of nausea, vomiting, and abdominal pain experienced shortly after the start of treatment may be due to direct irritation of the gastro-intestinal tract and such symptoms usually disappear on dose reduction. Administration of doses of 300 mg daily or more for several months sometimes produces abdominal pain, diarrhoea, weight loss, gastro-intestinal bleeding, and in severe cases the small bowel may become oedematous and symptoms of bowel obstruction may develop. This may be due to deposition of crystals of clofazimine in the wall of the small bowel and in the mesenteric lymph nodes. Crystal deposition may also occur in other organs including the liver and spleen and cause adverse effects. Symptoms usually regress on withdrawal of treatment.

Clofazimine may produce a dryness of the skin and ichthyosis as well as decreased sweat production and rashes. Pruritus and photosensitivity reactions have also been reported.

Eye irritation and decreased tear production may occur.

Headache, drowsiness, dizziness, and taste disorders have been reported rarely.

The incidence of adverse effects experienced with clofazimine was reviewed in 65 patients who were receiving or had received clofazimine in doses of either 700 mg per week or less as antimycobacterial therapy, or more than 700 mg per week as anti-inflammatory therapy.[1] Length of treatment ranged from 1 to 83 months. Adverse effects on the skin included discoloration in 20% of patients, pigmentation in 64.6%, dry skin in 35.4%, and pruritus in 5%. Ocular adverse effects experienced were conjunctival pigmentation in 49.2% of patients, subjective dimness of vision in 12.3%, and dry eyes, burning and other ocular irritation in 24.6%. Gastro-intestinal adverse effects included abdominal pain in 33.8% of patients, nausea in 9.2%, diarrhoea in 9.2%, and weight loss, vomiting, or loss of appetite in 13.8%. The different dose regimens for antimycobacterial therapy or anti-inflammatory effect had similar incidences of adverse effects. Skin pigmentation in 8 patients who had discontinued treatment with clofazimine disappeared on average 8.5 months after stopping therapy, the maximum time required being one year. Adverse effects of clofazimine were considered to be well tolerated.

In another report covering 540 patients receiving clofazimine 100 mg on alternate days or 300 mg daily, the most common adverse effect was skin pigmentation which occurred in 77.8% of the patients. Ichthyotic changes were reported in 66.7% and pruritus in 20.2%. Gastro-intestinal symptoms occurred in 20 patients (about 4%); other effects such as discoloration of sweat, urine, and tears were minor.[2]

1. Moore VJ. A review of side-effects experienced by patients taking clofazimine. *Lepr Rev* 1983; **54:** 327–35.
2. Kumar B, *et al.* More about clofazimine—3 years experience and review of the literature. *Indian J Lepr* 1987; **59:** 63–74.

Effects on the eyes. Accumulation of clofazimine crystals in the eye can lead to pigmentation of the cornea and conjunctiva. Degeneration of the retinal pigment epithelium has also been attributed to clofazimine therapy in one patient.[1] Slight repigmentation was observed following withdrawal of clofazimine.

1. Forster DJ, *et al.* Bull's eye retinopathy and clofazimine. *Ann Intern Med* 1992; **116:** 876–7.

Effects on the heart. A report of ventricular tachycardia, probably torsade de pointes, associated with clofazimine in one patient.[1]

1. Choudhri SH, *et al.* Clofazimine induced cardiotoxicity—a case report. *Lepr Rev* 1995; **66:** 63–8.

Splenic infarction. A case report.

1. McDougall AC, *et al.* Splenic infarction and tissue accumulation of crystals associated with the use of clofazimine (Lamprene; B663) in the treatment of pyoderma gangrenosum. *Br J Dermatol* 1980; **102:** 227–30.

Precautions

Clofazimine should be used with caution in patients with gastro-intestinal symptoms such as abdominal pain and diarrhoea. If gastro-intestinal symptoms develop during treatment with clofazimine, the dose should be reduced and, if necessary, the interval between doses increased, or the drug should be discontinued. It has been recommended that daily doses of more than 100 mg of clofazimine should not be administered for more than 3 months because of dose-related adverse effects on the gastro-intestinal tract; patients receiving doses greater than 100 mg daily should be under medical supervision.

The manufacturers recommend caution in patients with impaired liver or renal function.

Patients should be warned that clofazimine may cause a reddish-brown discoloration of skin, conjunctiva, tears, sputum, sweat, urine, and faeces.

As clofazimine crosses the placental barrier and is distributed into breast milk, neonates of women receiving clofazimine may have skin discoloration at birth or from breast feeding.

Pregnancy. Experience with clofazimine in pregnancy is limited. Farb and co-workers[1] reported 2 successful pregnancies in women who received clofazimine throughout pregnancy but noted that a literature review revealed 3 neonatal deaths in 13 pregnancies, although the deaths could not be directly attributed to clofazimine. Duncan and Oakey[2] have reported reduced urinary-oestrogen concentrations in pregnant leprosy patients receiving clofazimine and suggested that additional studies should be done. Although it has been suggested that administration of clofazimine should be avoided as far as possible in the first trimester of pregnancy,[3] treatment should not be interrupted in women who become pregnant, since leprosy is exacerbated during pregnancy.[4]

1. Farb H, *et al.* Clofazimine in pregnancy complicated by leprosy. *Obstet Gynecol* 1982; **59:** 122–3.
2. Duncan ME, Oakey RE. Reduced estrogen excretion due to clofazimine? *Int J Lepr* 1983; **51:** 112–13.
3. WHO. *A guide to leprosy control*. 2nd ed. Geneva: WHO, 1988.
4. WHO. *WHO model prescribing information: drugs used in mycobacterial diseases*. Geneva: WHO, 1991.

Interactions

The anti-inflammatory action of clofazimine in Type 2 lepra reactions has been reported to be reduced by dapsone although the antimycobacterial effect was not affected. For a report of the effect of clofazimine on rifampicin absorption, see p.244.

Antimicrobial Action

Clofazimine is weakly bactericidal against *Mycobacterium leprae*. The minimum inhibitory concentration for *Mycobacterium leprae* in mouse tissue has been estimated to lie between 0.1 and 1 μg per gram; uneven tissue distribution precludes a more accurate estimate. Tissue antimicrobial activity in humans cannot be demonstrated until after about 50 days of therapy.

Clofazimine is active *in vitro* against various other species of *Mycobacterium*.

Resistance has been reported rarely.

The MIC of clofazimine against most strains of *Mycobacterium avium* complex is reported to be 1.6 to 2 μg per mL. Although this is a concentration achievable in the serum clinical results have been disappointing. The disparity between *in vitro* and clinical results has led to the study of clofazimine's bactericidal action. Yajko and co-workers[1] determined a MBC of clofazimine against *M. avium* complex isolated from AIDS patients of 32 μg per mL versus an MIC of 0.5 to 2 μg per mL. Their experiments demonstrated that while clofazimine was inhibitory *in vitro*, it was not effective in killing the organism and little or no killing would occur at concentrations of clofazimine achievable in the serum.

Additional work by Lindholm-Levy and Heifets[2] demonstrated that the MIC for clofazimine against *M. avium* complex isolated from AIDS patients was pH-dependent. The average MICs at pH 6.8, 6.0, and 5.0 were 0.19 μg per mL, 3.0 μg per mL, and 4.0 μg per mL respectively; all MICs were lower than clofazimine concentrations achievable in macrophages. The MBC ranged from 64 to 256 times higher than the MIC.

Since *M. avium* complex concentrates and multiplies within macrophages, an effective therapeutic drug may need to concentrate in macrophages as does clofazimine, but whether clofazimine reaches a sufficient concentration within the macrophage for bactericidal activity has not been determined. A drug would also need to be effective in the acidic environment within the macrophage.

1. Yajko DM, *et al.* Therapeutic implications of inhibition versus killing of Mycobacterium avium complex by antimicrobial agents. *Antimicrob Agents Chemother* 1987; **31:** 117–20.
2. Lindholm-Levy PJ, Heifets LB. Clofazimine and other riminocompounds: minimal inhibitory and minimal bactericidal concentrations at different pHs for Mycobacterium avium complex. *Tubercle* 1988; **69:** 179–86.

Pharmacokinetics

Clofazimine is absorbed from the gastro-intestinal tract in amounts varying from 45 to 70%. Absorption is greatest when clofazimine is given in microcrystalline formulations and when it is taken immediately after food. The time to steady-state plasma concentrations has not been determined but exceeds 30 days.

Average plasma concentrations in leprosy patients receiving 100 or 300 mg daily are reported as 0.7 μg per mL and 1.0 μg per mL, respectively.

Because of its lipophilic nature, clofazimine is mainly distributed to fatty tissue and reticuloendothelial cells, including macrophages. Clofazimine is distributed to most organs and tissues and into breast milk; it crosses the placenta but not the blood-brain barrier.

The tissue half-life following a single dose has been reported to be about 10 days; that following multiple oral doses has been variously estimated to be between 25 and 90 days. Clofazimine accumulates in the body and is largely excreted unchanged in the faeces, both as unabsorbed drug and via biliary excretion. About 1% of the dose is excreted in 24 hours in the urine as unchanged clofazimine and metabolites. A small amount of clofazimine is also excreted through sebaceous and sweat glands.

References to the pharmacokinetics of clofazimine.

1. Holdiness MR. Clinical pharmacokinetics of clofazimine: a review. *Clin Pharmacokinet* 1989; **16:** 74–85.

Uses and Administration

Clofazimine is an antimycobacterial and is one of the main drugs used in regimens for the treatment of multibacillary leprosy (p.128), although because of its adverse effect on skin colour it may be replaced by, for example, ofloxacin or minocycline in light-skinned patients. It has anti-inflammatory properties and has been given in Type 2 lepra reactions and in a variety of skin disorders. It may also be used as a component of regimens for the treatment of opportunistic mycobacterial infections (p.133) due to *Mycobacterium avium* complex.

Clofazimine is administered orally immediately after a meal for optimum absorption.

For multibacillary leprosy, the most common regimen is that recommended by WHO in which rifampicin 600 mg and clofazimine 300 mg are both given once a month under supervision together with clofazimine 50 mg daily [or 100 mg every other day depending on what preparations are available] and dapsone 100 mg daily, both in self-administered doses; this treatment continues for 2 years. In children aged 10 to 14 years a suggested dose for clofazimine is 200 mg once a month and 50 mg on alternate days.

Clofazimine 50 mg daily is given in combination with ofloxacin and minocycline in patients with rifampicin-resistant leprosy. Clofazimine is not usually given in paucibacillary leprosy. However, it may be used in association with rifampicin instead of dapsone when the latter has caused severe toxicity.

Clofazimine has been used in the treatment of Type 2 lepra reactions, although the effect may not be evident for 4 to 6 weeks. A dose of up to 300 mg daily has been suggested but it should not be given for longer than 3 months. Corticosteroids may be given in conjunction with clofazimine, and standard antileprosy treatment should be continued. Clofazimine is not used in Type 1 lepra reactions.

In the treatment of opportunistic mycobacterial infections doses of 100 to 200 mg daily have been given and have been increased up to 300 mg daily in patients with AIDS and disseminated *M. avium* complex infection.

Preparations

BP 1998: Clofazimine Capsules;
USP 23: Clofazimine Capsules.

Proprietary Preparations (details are given in Part 3)
Austral.: Lamprene; ***Irl.:*** Lamprene; ***Neth.:*** Lampren; ***S.Afr.:*** Lamprene; ***Spain:*** Lampren; ***Switz.:*** Lamprene; ***UK:*** Lamprene; ***USA:*** Lamprene.

Multi-ingredient: ***S.Afr.:*** MB-Combi†.

Clofoctol (12586-t)

Clofoctol *(rINN)*.

2-(2,4-Dichlorobenzyl)-4-(1,1,3,3-tetramethylbutyl)phenol.

$C_{21}H_{26}Cl_2O = 365.3$.

CAS — 37693-01-9.

Clofoctol is an antimicrobial compound with bacteriostatic or bactericidal activity against Gram-positive organisms such as staphylococci and streptococci. It is given in doses of 20 to 40 mg per kg daily by the rectal route in the treatment of respiratory-tract infections.

Preparations

Proprietary Preparations (details are given in Part 3)
Fr.: Octofene; ***Ital.:*** Gramplus; Octofene.

Clometocillin Potassium (57-p)

Clometocillin Potassium *(rINNM)*.

3,4-Dichloro-α-methoxybenzylpenicillin Potassium; Penicillin 356 (clometocillin). Potassium (6*R*)-6-[2-(3,4-dichlorophenyl)-2-methoxyacetamido]penicillanate.

$C_{17}H_{17}Cl_2KN_2O_5S = 471.4$.

CAS — 1926-49-4 (clometocillin); 15433-28-0 (clometocillin potassium).

Clometocillin is a penicillin that has been given by mouth as the potassium salt in the treatment of susceptible bacterial infections.

Preparations

Proprietary Preparations (details are given in Part 3)
Belg.: Rixapen.

Cloxacillin (14777-t)

Cloxacillin *(BAN, rINN)*.

(6*R*)-6-[3-(2-Chlorophenyl)-5-methylisoxazole-4-carboxamido]penicillanic acid.

$C_{19}H_{18}ClN_3O_5S = 435.9$.

CAS — 61-72-3.

Cloxacillin Benzathine (12594-t)

Cloxacillin Benzathine *(BANM)*.

The *N,N'*-dibenzylethylenediamine salt of cloxacillin.

$C_{16}H_{20}N_2,(C_{19}H_{18}ClN_3O_5S)_2 = 1112.1$.

CAS — 23736-58-5; 32222-55-2.

Pharmacopoeias. In *US* for veterinary use only. Also in *BP(Vet)*.

A white or almost white powder. Slightly **soluble** in water, alcohol, and isopropyl alcohol; soluble in chloroform; freely soluble in methyl alcohol; sparingly soluble in acetone. The pH of a 1% suspension is 3.0 to 6.5. **Store** at a temperature not exceeding 25° in airtight containers.

Cloxacillin Sodium (60-m)

Cloxacillin Sodium *(BANM, USAN, rINNM)*.

BRL-1621; Cloxacilina Sódica; Cloxacillinum Natricum; P-25.

$C_{19}H_{17}ClN_3NaO_5S,H_2O = 475.9$.

CAS — 642-78-4 (anhydrous cloxacillin sodium); 7081-44-9 (cloxacillin sodium monohydrate).

Pharmacopoeias. In *Eur.* (see p.viii), *Int., Jpn, Pol.,* and *US. Chin.* includes anhydrous cloxacillin sodium.

A white or almost white, odourless, hygroscopic, crystalline powder. 1.09 g of monograph substance is approximately equivalent to 1 g of anhydrous cloxacillin. Each g of monograph substance represents about 2.1 mmol of sodium.

Freely **soluble** in water and in methyl alcohol; soluble in alcohol; slightly soluble in chloroform. A 10% solution in water has a pH of 5 to 7 and a 1% solution in water has a pH of 4.5 to 7.5.

Store at a temperature not exceeding 25° in airtight containers.

Cloxacillin sodium has been reported to be **incompatible** with aminoglycosides and a number of other antimicrobials.

Adverse Effects and Precautions

As for Flucloxacillin, p.209.

Effects on the kidneys. References.

1. García-Ortiz R, *et al.* Cloxacillin-induced acute tubulo interstitial nephritis. *Ann Pharmacother* 1992; **26:** 1241–2.

Effects on the liver. References.

1. Enat R, *et al.* Cholestatic jaundice caused by cloxacillin: macrophage inhibition factor test in preventing rechallenge with hepatotoxic drugs. *Br Med J* 1980; **280:** 982–3.
2. Konikoff F, *et al.* Cloxacillin-induced cholestatic jaundice. *Am J Gastroenterol* 1986; **81:** 1082–3.

Interactions

As for Benzylpenicillin, p.160.

Antimicrobial Action

As for Flucloxacillin, p.209.

Pharmacokinetics

Cloxacillin is incompletely absorbed from the gastro-intestinal tract after oral administration, and absorption is further reduced by the presence of food in the stomach. After an oral dose of 500 mg, a peak plasma concentration of 7 to 14 μg per mL is attained in fasting subjects in 1 to 2 hours. Absorption is more complete when given by intramuscular injection and peak plasma concentrations of about 15 μg per mL have been observed 30 minutes after a dose of 500 mg. Doubling the dose can double the plasma concentration. About 94% of cloxacillin in the circulation is bound to plasma proteins. Cloxacillin has been reported to have a plasma half-life of 0.5 to 1 hour. The half-life is prolonged in neonates.

Cloxacillin crosses the placenta and distributed into in breast milk. There is little diffusion into the CSF except when the meninges are inflamed. Therapeutic concentrations can be achieved in pleural and synovial fluids and in bone.

Cloxacillin is metabolised to a limited extent, and the unchanged drug and metabolites are excreted in the urine by glomerular filtration and renal tubular secretion. About 35% of an oral dose is excreted in the urine and up to 10% in the bile. Cloxacillin is not removed by haemodialysis.

Plasma concentrations are enhanced if probenecid is given concomitantly. Reduced concentrations in patients with cystic fibrosis have been attributed to enhanced nonrenal clearance of cloxacillin.

References.

1. Spino M, *et al.* Cloxacillin absorption and disposition in cystic fibrosis. *J Pediatr* 1984; **105:** 829–35.
2. Mattie H, *et al.* Diffusion of cloxacillin into synovial tissue. *Br J Clin Pharmacol* 1992; **34:** 275–7.
3. Schievink HI, *et al.* The passage of cloxacillin into cerebrospinal fluid in the absence of meningitis. *Br J Clin Pharmacol* 1993; **36:** 57–60.

Uses and Administration

Cloxacillin is an isoxazolyl penicillin used similarly to flucloxacillin (p.209) in the treatment of infections due to staphylococci resistant to benzylpenicillin.

It is administered by mouth or by injection as the sodium salt. By mouth it should be given at least 30 minutes before meals as the presence of food in the stomach reduces absorption. All doses are expressed in terms of the equivalent amount of cloxacillin.

Usual doses are 500 mg four times daily by mouth, or 250 mg by intramuscular injection every 4 to 6 hours or 500 mg may be given by slow intravenous injection over 3 to 4 minutes every 4 to 6 hours or by intravenous infusion. All systemic doses may be doubled in severe infections.

Cloxacillin sodium has also been administered by intra-articular, or intrapleural injection, and by inhalation.

Children up to 2 years of age may be given one-quarter the adult dose and those aged 2 to 10 years, one-half the adult dose.

Cloxacillin may be administered in combination with other antibacterials, including ampicillin, to produce a wider spectrum of activity. Cloxacillin benzathine is used in veterinary medicine.

Preparations

BP 1998: Cloxacillin Capsules; Cloxacillin Injection; Cloxacillin Oral Solution;
USP 23: Cloxacillin Sodium Capsules; Cloxacillin Sodium for Oral Solution.

Proprietary Preparations (details are given in Part 3)
Austral.: Alclox†; Orbenin†; ***Belg.:*** Orbenin; Penstapho N; ***Canad.:*** Apo-Cloxi; Novo-Cloxin; Nu-Cloxi; Orbenin†; Tegopen; ***Fr.:*** Orbenine; ***Irl.:*** Orbenin; ***Neth.:*** Orbenin; ***Norw.:*** Ekvacillin; ***S.Afr.:*** Clocillin; Cloxin; Orbenin; ***Spain:*** Anaclosil; Orbenin; ***Swed.:*** Ekvacillin; ***Switz.:*** Rivoclox†; ***UK:*** Orbenin†; ***USA:*** Cloxapen; Tegopen†.

Multi-ingredient: ***Irl.:*** Ampiclox; ***Ital.:*** Amplium; ***S.Afr.:*** Ampiclox; Apen; Cloxam; Megamox; ***Switz.:*** Pencloxin†; ***UK:*** Ampiclox†.

Colistin Sulphate (61-b)

Colistin Sulphate *(BANM, pINNM)*.

Colistin Sulfate; Colistini Sulfas; Polymyxin E Sulphate.

CAS — 1066-17-7 (colistin); 1264-72-8 (colistin sulphate).

Pharmacopoeias. In *Chin., Eur.* (see p.viii), *Pol.,* and *US.*

A mixture of the sulphates of polypeptides produced by certain strains of *Bacillus polymyxa* var. *colistinus* or obtained by any other means. A white to slightly yellow, odourless, hygroscopic powder. The Ph. Eur. specifies not less than 19 000 units per mg calculated on the dried substance; USP specifies not less than 500 μg of colistin per mg.

Freely **soluble** in water; slightly soluble in alcohol and in methyl alcohol; practically insoluble in acetone and in ether. A 1% solution in water has a pH of 4.0 to 7.0. The base is precipitated from aqueous solution above pH 7.5. **Store** in airtight containers. Protect from light.

Colistin Sulphomethate Sodium (62-v)

Colistin Sulphomethate Sodium *(BANM)*.

Colistimethate Sodium *(USAN, rINN)*; Colistimetato de Sódio; Colistimethatum Natrium; Colistineméthanesulfonate Sodique; Pentasodium Colistinmethanesulfonate; Sodium Colistimethate; Sodium Colistinmethanesulphonate; W-1929.

CAS — 30387-39-4 (colistin sulphomethate); 8068-28-8 (colistin sulphomethate sodium).

Pharmacopoeias. In *Eur.* (see p.viii), *Jpn, Pol.*, and *US*.

An antimicrobial substance prepared from colistin by the action of formaldehyde and sodium bisulphite, whereby amino groups are sulphomethylated. A white to slightly yellow, odourless, hygroscopic powder. The Ph. Eur. specifies not less than 11 500 units per mg calculated on the dried substance; USP specifies not less than 390 μg of colistin per mg. Very or freely **soluble** in water; slightly soluble in alcohol; soluble in methyl alcohol; practically insoluble in acetone and ether. A 1% solution in water has a pH of 6.2 to 8.5. **Store** in airtight containers. Protect from light.

Incompatibilities. Lack of compatibility has been reported with various drugs including other antibacterials.

Units

The first International Standard Preparation (1968) for colistin contains 20 500 units per mg of colistin sulphate and the first International Reference Preparation (1966) for colistin sulphomethate contains 12 700 units per mg of colistin sulphomethate.

Adverse Effects, Treatment, and Precautions

As for Polymyxin B Sulphate, p.239.

Colistin sulphate is poorly absorbed from the gastro-intestinal tract and adverse effects do not normally follow its administration in the usual oral doses. Bronchospasm may occur during inhalation. Overgrowth of non-susceptible organisms, particularly *Proteus* spp., may occur after prolonged administration. Pain and local irritation are reported to be less troublesome following intramuscular injection of colistin sulphomethate sodium than with polymyxin B.

Cystic fibrosis. Colistin sulphate was reported to be associated with a lower rate of severe nephrotoxicity among 19 patients with cystic fibrosis than has been previously reported in other patient populations.[1]

1. Bosso JA, *et al.* Toxicity of colistin in cystic fibrosis patients. *DICP Ann Pharmacother* 1991; **25:** 1168–70.

Porphyria. Colistin has been associated with clinical exacerbations of porphyria and is considered unsafe in porphyric patients.[1]

1. Moore MR, McColl KEL. *Porphyria: drug lists.* Glasgow: Porphyria Research Unit, University of Glasgow, 1991.

Interactions

As for Polymyxin B Sulphate, p.239.

Antimicrobial Action

The antimicrobial spectrum and mode of action of colistin is similar to that of polymyxin B (p.239) but the sulphate is slightly, and the sulphomethate significantly, less active. MICs for most sensitive species range from about 0.01 to 4 μg per mL; susceptible strains of *Pseudomonas aeruginosa* generally respond to concentrations below 8 μg per mL.

Pharmacokinetics

Colistin sulphate and colistin sulphomethate sodium are poorly absorbed from the gastro-intestinal tract. They are not absorbed through intact skin. Peak plasma activity usually occurs 2 to 3 hours after an intramuscular injection of colistin sulphomethate sodium. Some of the sulphomethate sodium may be hydrolysed to colistin *in vivo*. Colistin is reversibly bound to body tissues, but binding does not occur with the sulphomethate.

Colistin sulphomethate is mainly excreted by glomerular filtration as changed and unchanged drug and up to 80% of a parenteral dose may be recovered in the urine within 24 hours. Excretion is more rapid in children than in adults; it is diminished in patients with impaired kidney function.

Colistin diffuses across the placenta but diffusion into the CSF is negligible except occasionally in infants.

Neonates. The biological half-life of colistin sulphomethate sodium was variously reported as 9 hours in newborn infants falling to 2.6 hours 3 or 4 days later and 2.3 to 2.6 hours (according to age) in premature infants.[1]

1. Ritschel WA. Biological half-lives of drugs. *Drug Intell Clin Pharm* 1970; **4:** 332–47.

Renal impairment. Colistin sulphomethate was administered intramuscularly in a dose of 75 mg to 10 healthy persons and 8 patients with renal impairment. The biological half-life was 4.8 hours in normal persons and 18 hours in patients with renal impairment. A substantial change in drug distribution occurred as indicated by the smaller volume of distribution in the patients with renal impairment.[1]

1. Gibaldi M, Perrier D. Drug distribution and renal impairment. *J Clin Pharmacol* 1972; **12:** 201–4.

Uses and Administration

Colistin is a polymyxin antibiotic that has been used in the treatment of severe Gram-negative infections, especially those due to *Pseudomonas aeruginosa*, although other drugs are usually preferred. It has been used by mouth as the sulphate for the treatment of gastro-intestinal infections and in combination with other drugs for the selective decontamination of the gastro-intestinal tract in patients at high risk of endogenous infections (see under Intensive Care, p.128). The sulphomethate sodium salt has been used by inhalation in the management of respiratory infections, especially in patients with cystic fibrosis (p.119).

In the UK the usual dose of colistin sulphate by mouth is 1.5 to 3 million units three times daily; children weighing up to 15 kg body-weight may be given 250 000 to 500 000 units three times daily, and those weighing 15 to 30 kg may be given 0.75 to 1.5 million units three times daily. In the USA, doses are expressed in terms of the equivalent amount of colistin in mg. A suggested dose for adults and children is 5 to 15 mg per kg body-weight daily in 3 divided doses.

Colistin has been given parenterally, as the sulphomethate sodium salt, by intramuscular injection or slow intravenous injection or infusion. In the UK usual doses have been 6 million units daily in divided doses. In the USA, the usual dose is 2.5 to 5 mg per kg daily in divided doses. Doses must be reduced in renal failure.

The UK manufacturers recommend 6 million units daily in divided doses by inhalation in respiratory infection but lower doses have been recommended by some; patients over 40 kg may be given 1 million units every 12 hours, those weighing less than 40 kg may be given 500 000 units every 12 hours.

Colistin sulphomethate sodium has also been given by subconjunctival injection and as a bladder instillation. Both the sulphate and the sulphomethate sodium salt have been applied topically, often with other antibacterials, in the management of ear, eye, and skin infections.

Preparations

BP 1998: Colistimethate Injection; Colistin Tablets;
USP 23: Colistimethate for Injection; Colistin and Neomycin Sulfates and Hydrocortisone Acetate Otic Suspension; Colistin Sulfate for Oral Suspension.

Proprietary Preparations (details are given in Part 3)
Austral.: Coly-Mycin M; ***Belg.:*** Colimycine; ***Canad.:*** Coly-Mycin M; ***Fr.:*** Colimycine; ***Ger.:*** Bakto-Diaront†; Diaront mono; ***Irl.:*** Colomycin; ***Ital.:*** Colimicina; ***Neth.:*** Belcomycine; Colimycine; ***Norw.:*** Colimycin; ***Spain:*** Colimicina; ***UK:*** Colomycin; ***USA:*** Coly-Mycin M.

Multi-ingredient: ***Aust.:*** AKZ; ***Austral.:*** Coly-Mycin†; ***Canad.:*** Coly-Mycin Otic†; ***Fr.:*** Bacicoline; Colicort; ***Ger.:*** Ecolicin; ***Ital.:*** Colbiocin; Colimicina†; Eubetal Antibiotico; Iducol; Otobiotic†; ***Neth.:*** Bacicoline-B; ***Switz.:*** AKZ; Bacicoline†; ***USA:*** Coly-Mycin S Otic; Cortisporin-TC.

Co-tetroxazine (12612-v)

Co-tetroxazine *(BAN)*.

CAS — 73173-12-3.

A mixture of tetroxoprim and sulphadiazine in the proportion of 2:5.

Co-tetroxazine has properties similar to those of co-trimoxazole (below) and is used similarly, mainly in the treatment of infections of the respiratory and urinary tracts. It is given by mouth in an initial dose of 700 mg (tetroxoprim 200 mg or its equivalent as the embonate and sulphadiazine 500 mg), followed by 350 mg twice daily.

Preparations

Proprietary Preparations (details are given in Part 3)
Ger.: Sterinor; ***Ital.:*** Oxosint; Sterinor; Tibirox†.

Co-trifamole (4902-z)

Co-trifamole *(BAN)*.

CN-3123.

A mixture of 5 parts of sulphamoxole and 1 part of trimethoprim.

Co-trifamole has properties similar to those of co-trimoxazole (below) and has been used similarly by mouth in an initial dose of 960 mg (trimethoprim 160 mg and sulphamoxole 800 mg) followed by 480 mg every 12 hours.

Preparations

Proprietary Preparations (details are given in Part 3)
Fr.: Supristol†; ***S.Afr.:*** Supristol†; ***Spain:*** Supristol†.

Co-trimazine (4903-c)

Co-trimazine *(BAN)*.

CAS — 39474-58-3.

A mixture of 5 parts of sulphadiazine and 1 part of trimethoprim.

Co-trimazine has properties similar to those of co-trimoxazole (below) and is used similarly. It is given by mouth in a usual dose of 480 mg (trimethoprim 80 mg and sulphadiazine 400 mg) twice daily.

Preparations are available in some countries which contain trimethoprim and sulphadiazine in proportions different to co-trimazine.

Preparations

Proprietary Preparations (details are given in Part 3)
Fr.: Antrima.

Multi-ingredient: ***Ital.:*** Kombinax.

Co-trimoxazole (4904-k)

Co-trimoxazole *(BAN)*.

CAS — 8064-90-2.

A mixture of 5 parts of sulphamethoxazole and 1 part of trimethoprim.

Diluted infusion solutions of co-trimoxazole have a limited stability and eventually form a precipitate: this happens more rapidly at higher concentrations. The manufacturers recommend a dilution of 480 mg in 130 mL, which is usually stable for up to 6 hours, but more concentrated solutions should be used within shorter periods of time, and a dilution of 480 mg in 80 mL should be used within 2 hours. The usual diluent is 5% glucose, although other solutions, including 0.9% sodium chloride, have been stated to be compatible for adequate periods.

Co-trimoxazole is reported to be incompatible with verapamil hydrochloride.

Adverse Effects and Treatment

The adverse effects of co-trimoxazole are those of its components (see Sulphamethoxazole, p.254, and Trimethoprim, p.265). Gastro-intestinal disturbances (mainly nausea and vomiting) and skin reactions are the most common adverse effects. There have been occasional deaths, especially in elderly patients, mainly due to blood dyscrasias or severe skin reactions.

A high incidence of adverse effects has been reported in AIDS patients; desensitisation may sometimes be considered (see under Immunocompromised Patients, in Precautions, below).

There has been concern over the safety of co-trimoxazole. In 1985, reporting on 85 deaths associated with the use of co-trimoxazole[1] and predominantly due to blood dyscrasias (50 reports) and skin reactions (14 reports), the Committee on

Safety of Medicines (CSM) in the UK found that fatalities showed a marked increase with age: below 40 years, there were 0.25 reported deaths per million prescriptions, but for patients over 65 years of age the number of reported deaths per million prescriptions was more than 15-fold greater. However, at that time the CSM felt that it would be unwise to assume that trimethoprim was substantially less liable than co-trimoxazole to cause fatal adverse reactions.[1] It was suggested by Lacey and colleagues[2] that most of the deaths associated with the use of co-trimoxazole were typical of sulphonamide toxicity and that the indications for the use of co-trimoxazole should be reduced; this included the suggestion that it should be contra-indicated in the elderly. The CSM stated that their main message was that the risks of treatment of co-trimoxazole were more apparent in the elderly, but that there was no significant difference between the numbers of reports received for serious adverse reactions to trimethoprim and co-trimoxazole when corrected for prescription volumes.[3] In practice, despite further occasional reports of fatalities in elderly patients,[4] there did not appear to have been a marked reduction in the prescribing of this drug in the UK.[5] A similar warning of increased risk from co-trimoxazole in elderly patients was issued by the Adverse Drug Reactions Advisory Committee in Australia.[6]

More recently, a large population-based follow-up study in the UK[7] indicated that the risks of serious liver, blood, skin, and kidney disorders with either co-trimoxazole, trimethoprim, or cephalexin were small and were similar to those with many other antibacterials. Although in 1995 the CSM did restrict the use of co-trimoxazole on the grounds that its place in therapy had changed[8] (see under Uses and Administration, below), they also noted that co-trimoxazole continued to show a similar pattern of serious suspected adverse reactions to that reported 10 years earlier and that adverse drug reactions with trimethoprim were similar; blood dyscrasias and generalised skin disorders were the most serious reactions in each case and remained predominantly in elderly patients.

1. Committee on Safety of Medicines. Deaths associated with co-trimoxazole, ampicillin and trimethoprim. *Current Problems 15* 1985.
2. Lacey RW, *et al.* Co-trimoxazole toxicity. *Br Med J* 1985; **291:** 481.
3. Goldberg A. Co-trimoxazole toxicity. *Br Med J* 1985; **291**: 673.
4. Whittington RM. Toxic epidermal necrolysis and co-trimoxazole. *Lancet* 1989; **ii**: 574.
5. Carmichael AJ, Tan CY. Fatal toxic epidermal necrolysis associated with co-trimoxazole. *Lancet* 1989; **ii**: 808–9.
6. Adverse Drug Reactions Advisory Committee. Trimethoprim-sulphamethoxazole warning on elderly. *Aust Adverse Drug React Bull* February 1990.
7. Jick H, Derby LE. Is co-trimoxazole safe? *Lancet* 1995; **345:** 1118–19.
8. Committee on Safety of Medicines. Revised indications for co-trimoxazole (Septrin, Bactrim, various generic preparations). *Current Problems* 1995; **21:** 6.

Precautions

As for Sulphamethoxazole, p.255 and Trimethoprim, p.265.

Co-trimoxazole should not be given to patients with a history of hypersensitivity to it or to the sulphonamides or trimethoprim. It is contra-indicated in patients with severe hepatic failure and should be used with caution in patients with lesser degrees of hepatic impairment. Like its components, co-trimoxazole should be used with caution in impaired renal function, and dosage adjustment may be necessary; it should not be used in severe renal impairment without monitoring of plasma drug concentrations. An adequate fluid intake should be maintained to reduce the risk of crystalluria, but alkalinisation of the urine, although it increases urinary excretion of the sulphamethoxazole component, decreases urinary trimethoprim excretion. Regular blood counts and urinalyses and renal function tests should be carried out in patients receiving prolonged treatment with co-trimoxazole. Elderly patients may be more susceptible to adverse effects (see above). Folate supplementation may be necessary in patients predisposed to folate deficiency, such as elderly patients and when high doses of co-trimoxazole are given for a prolonged period.

Glucose 6-phosphate dehydrogenase deficiency. Some have expressed the opinion that co-trimoxazole should be avoided by people with glucose 6-phosphate dehydrogenase deficiency.[1]

1. WHO. Glucose-6-phosphate dehydrogenase deficiency. *Bull WHO* 1989; **67**: 601–11.

Immunocompromised patients. An extraordinarily high frequency of adverse reactions to co-trimoxazole has been reported in patients with AIDS being treated for *Pneumocystis carinii* pneumonia. Masur[1] commented that, when therapeutic doses of co-trimoxazole are used, hypersensitivity rashes and leucopenia each develop in 30% of patients compared with less than 5% for each complication in patients without AIDS but other studies have reported an even higher incidence of toxicity, and the overall incidence of adverse effects, including fever, malaise, and hepatitis, may be 80% or more.[2-4] Adverse reactions also appear to be unusually frequent when prophylactic doses are used.[4]

The occurrence of high serum concentrations of trimethoprim and sulphamethoxazole in patients has been proposed as a contributing factor to the high incidence of adverse effects,[5,6] and Sattler and colleagues[5] reported that adverse effects, and in particular myelosuppression, were kept to tolerable levels in a group of patients in whom the dose of co-trimoxazole was adjusted to maintain serum trimethoprim concentrations at 5 to 8 μg per mL. However, McLean and others[7] demonstrated no difference in the frequency of side-effects when the sulphamethoxazole dose was modified. A lower frequency of cutaneous reactions has been reported among African, Haitian, and American black AIDS patients compared with white AIDS patients suggesting a genetic susceptibility for such reactions.[8]

Some workers have used diphenhydramine alone or with adrenaline to manage hypersensitivity reactions associated with co-trimoxazole therapy thus allowing continuation of treatment,[9,10] and other workers have tried desensitisation to co-trimoxazole in patients with AIDS.[11-15] For mention of desensitisation to sulphonamides in patients with AIDS, see under Sulphamethoxazole, p.255. Van der Ven and others[16] have suggested that it is the reactive hydroxylamine metabolites of sulphamethoxazole which produce the adverse effects in HIV-infected individuals and that acetylcysteine, which would address the glutathione deficiency in these patients and thus perhaps enable increased scavenging of such metabolites, might be of benefit.

An increased incidence of myelosuppression, although not, apparently, of other adverse effects, has been reported in patients with leukaemia receiving maintenance chemotherapy.[17,18]

1. Masur H. Treatment of infections and immune defects. In: Fauci AS, moderator. Acquired immunodeficiency syndrome: epidemiologic, clinical, immunologic, and therapeutic considerations. *Ann Intern Med* 1984; **100**: 92–106.
2. Gordin FM, *et al.* Adverse reactions to trimethoprim-sulfamethoxazole in patients with the acquired immunodeficiency syndrome. *Ann Intern Med* 1984; **100**: 495–9.
3. Jaffe HS, *et al.* Complications of co-trimoxazole in treatment of AIDS-associated Pneumocystis carinii pneumonia in homosexual men. *Lancet* 1983; **ii**: 1109–11.
4. Mitsuyasu R, *et al.* Cutaneous reaction to trimethoprim-sulfamethoxazole in patients with AIDS and Kaposi's sarcoma. *N Engl J Med* 1983; **308**: 1535.
5. Sattler FR, *et al.* Trimethoprim-sulfamethoxazole compared with pentamidine for treatment of Pneumocystis carinii pneumonia in the acquired immunodeficiency syndrome. *Ann Intern Med* 1988; **109**: 280–7.
6. Stevens RC, *et al.* Pharmacokinetics and adverse effects of 20-mg/kg/day trimethoprim and 100-mg/kg/day sulfamethoxazole in healthy adult subjects. *Antimicrob Agents Chemother* 1991; **35**: 1884–90.
7. McLean I, *et al.* Modified trimethoprim-sulphamethoxazole doses in Pneumocystis carinii pneumonia. *Lancet* 1987; **ii**: 857–8.
8. Colebunders R, *et al.* Cutaneous reactions to trimethoprim-sulfamethoxazole in African patients with the acquired immunodeficiency syndrome. *Ann Intern Med* 1987; **107**: 599–600.
9. Gibbons RB, Lindauer JA. Successful treatment of Pneumocystis carinii pneumonia with trimethoprim-sulfamethoxazole in hypersensitive AIDS patients. *JAMA* 1985; **253**: 1259–60.
10. Toma E, Fournier S. Adverse reactions to co-trimoxazole in HIV infection. *Lancet* 1991; **338:** 954.
11. Kreuz W, *et al.* "Treating through" hypersensitivity to co-trimoxazole in children with HIV infection. *Lancet* 1990; **336**: 508–9.
12. Carr A, *et al.* Efficacy and safety of rechallenge with low-dose trimethoprim-sulphamethoxazole in previously hypersensitive HIV-infected patients. *AIDS* 1993; **7**: 65–71.
13. Absar N, *et al.* Desensitization to trimethoprim/sulfamethoxazole in HIV-infected patients. *J Allergy Clin Immunol* 1994; **93:** 1001–5.
14. Cortese LM, *et al.* Trimethoprim/sulfamethoxazole desensitization. *Ann Pharmacother* 1996; **30:** 184–6.
15. Caumes E, *et al.* Efficacy and safety of desensitization with sulfamethoxazole and trimethoprim in 48 previously hypersensitive patients infected with human immunodeficiency virus. *Arch Dermatol* 1997; **133:** 465–9.
16. van der Ven AJAM, *et al.* Adverse reactions to co-trimoxazole in HIV infection. *Lancet* 1991; **338**: 431–3.
17. Woods WG, *et al.* Myelosuppression associated with co-trimoxazole as a prophylactic antibiotic in the maintenance phase of childhood acute lymphocytic leukemia. *J Pediatr* 1984; **105**: 639–44.
18. Drysdale HC, Jones LF. Co-trimoxazole prophylaxis in leukaemia. *Lancet* 1982; **i**: 448.

Interference with diagnostic tests. Cohen and others[1,2] have reported that co-trimoxazole causes a small reduction in serum thyroxine and tri-iodothyronine concentrations, probably due to the sulphonamide component,[2] and suggest that although co-trimoxazole cannot be concluded to be a cause of hypothyroidism (as all concentrations remained within the normal range), tests of thyroid function should be interpreted with care in patients on such treatment.

1. Cohen HN, *et al.* Effects on human thyroid function of sulphonamide and trimethoprim combination drugs. *Br Med J* 1980; **281**: 646–7.
2. Cohen HN, *et al.* Trimethoprim and thyroid function. *Lancet* 1981; **i**: 676–7.

Porphyria. See under Sulphamethoxazole, p.255, and Trimethoprim, p.265.

Interactions

Any of the drug interactions reported with sulphamethoxazole (p.255), or trimethoprim (p.265), may occur with co-trimoxazole.

Antimicrobial Action

The actions and spectrum of activity of co-trimoxazole are essentially those of its components, sulphamethoxazole (p.255) and trimethoprim (p.265).

Because they act at different points of the folate metabolic pathway a potent synergy exists between its components *in vitro* with an increase of up to about 10-fold in antibacterial activity, and a frequently bactericidal action where the components individually are generally bacteriostatic. The optimum effect against most organisms is seen at a ratio of 1 part trimethoprim to 20 of sulphamethoxazole: although co-trimoxazole is formulated as a 1 to 5 ratio, differences in the pharmacokinetics of the two drugs mean that the ratio of the peak concentrations is approximately 1:20. However, it is not clear that the optimum ratio is achieved at all sites, and given that both drugs are present in therapeutic concentrations the contribution of synergy to the effects of co-trimoxazole *in vivo* is uncertain.

Resistance to co-trimoxazole develops more slowly *in vitro* than to either component alone. Resistance has increased, and although initially slow, a more rapid increase was seen in many countries during the 1980s, occurring in both Gram-positive and Gram-negative organisms. Resistance has occurred notably among Enterobacteriaceae. Resistant strains of *Haemophilus influenzae*, streptococci, and *Vibrio cholerae* have been reported rarely. Although resistant organisms are usually resistant to both components of the mixture, strains resistant to either the sulphonamide or trimethoprim and with a reduced sensitivity to co-trimoxazole have been reported.

Pharmacokinetics

See sulphamethoxazole (p.256) and trimethoprim (p.266). When co-trimoxazole is administered by mouth, plasma concentrations of trimethoprim and sulphamethoxazole are generally around the optimal ratio of 1:20, although they may vary from 1:2 to 1:30 or more. The ratio of the two drugs is usually much lower in the tissues (often around 1:2 to 1:5) since trimethoprim, the more lipophilic drug, penetrates many tissues better than sulphamethoxazole and has a much larger volume of distribution. In urine the ratio may vary from 1:1 to 1:5 depending on the pH.

Uses and Administration

Co-trimoxazole is a mixture of the sulphonamide, sulphamethoxazole, and trimethoprim, and has been used in a wide variety of infections due to susceptible organisms, particularly those of the urinary, respiratory, and gastro-intestinal tracts, although the indications for its use were restricted recently in the UK (see below). Its main use now is in *Pneumocystis carinii* pneumonia, toxoplasmosis, and nocardiosis.

Its other uses have included the treatment of: acne; biliary-tract infections; brucellosis (generally in combination with other drugs); cat scratch disease; chancroid; *Burkholderia (Pseudomonas) cepacia* infections in cystic fibrosis; some forms of AIDS-associated diarrhoea such as the protozoal infection isosporiasis; gonorrhoea; granuloma inguinale; the prophylaxis of infections in immunocompromised patients and selective decontamination for patients in intensive care; listeriosis; melioidosis; mycetoma; otitis media; pertussis; typhoid and paratyphoid fever; and Whipple's disease. For details of the bacterial infections listed above and their treatment, see under Choice of Antibacterial, p.116.

Co-trimoxazole is usually given by mouth in a dose of 960 mg (trimethoprim 160 mg and sulphamethoxazole 800 mg) twice daily; in severe infections 2.88 g daily in 2 divided doses may be given. Lower doses are given for long-term treatment and in patients with renal impairment; half the usual dosage has been suggested in patients with a creatinine clearance between 30 and 15 mL per minute, but co-trimoxazole is generally not recommended when the creatinine clearance is less than 15 mL per minute unless facilities for haemodialysis are available.

Suggested doses of co-trimoxazole to be given twice daily to children are: from 6 weeks to 5 months of age, 120 mg; 6 months to 5 years, 240 mg; 6 to 12 years, 480 mg. Co-trimoxazole should not be given to infants below 6 weeks of age because of the risk of kernicterus from the sulphonamide component (see Pregnancy and Breast Feeding, under Precautions of Sulphamethoxazole, p.255).

Higher doses of co-trimoxazole of up to 120 mg per kg body-weight daily given in two to four divided doses for 14 to 21 days are used in the treatment of *Pneumocystis carinii* pneumonia; serum concentrations should be monitored and consideration of folate supplementation has been suggested (but see Pneumocystis carinii Pneumonia, below). For prophylaxis in patients with AIDS, the standard dose of co-trimoxazole (960 mg twice daily) may be given, but has been associated with a high incidence of adverse effects (see under Precautions, above). Alternatively the following dose regimens may be used: 960 mg daily (7 days each week); 960 mg daily on alternate days (3 days each week); or 960 mg twice daily on alternate days (3 days each week).

For serious infections, if oral administration is not possible, co-trimoxazole may be given initially by intravenous infusion diluted immediately before use in a suitable diluent. The contents of each ampoule containing 480 mg of co-trimoxazole in 5 mL are added to 125 mL of diluent and infused over 60 to 90 minutes, unless fluid restriction is required, in which case the manufacturers permit the use of only 75 mL of diluent. Dosage is similar to that by mouth.

The current place of co-trimoxazole in therapy was reviewed by the UK Committee on Safety of Medicines (CSM) in 1995 (see also under Adverse Effects and Treatment, above).[1] As a result they recommended that its use should be limited to: *Pneumocystis carinii* pneumonia, toxoplasmosis, and nocardiosis; urinary-tract infections and acute exacerbations of chronic bronchitis, but only when there is bacteriological evidence of sensitivity to co-trimoxazole and good reason to prefer it to a single antibiotic; and acute otitis media in children, but again only when there is good reason to prefer the combination.

1. Committee on Safety of Medicines. Revised indications for co-trimoxazole (Septrin, Bactrim, various generic preparations). *Current Problems* 1995; **21:** 6.

Blastocystis infection. For a mention of the use of co-trimoxazole in the treatment of *Blastocystis hominis* infection, see p.574.

Cyclosporiasis. Patients with *Cyclospora* infection (p.574) have responded to treatment with co-trimoxazole.[1,2]

1. Pape JW, *et al.* Cyclospora infection in adults infected with HIV: clinical manifestations, treatment and prophylaxis. *Ann Intern Med* 1994; **121:** 654–7.
2. Hoge CW, *et al.* Placebo-controlled trial of co-trimoxazole for cyclospora infections among travellers and foreign residents in Nepal. *Lancet* 1995; **345:** 691–3. Correction. *ibid.*: 1060.

Granulomatous diseases. Although co-trimoxazole appears to be effective in reducing the incidence of bacterial infection in patients with chronic granulomatous disease,[1-4] a disorder of leucocyte function associated with recurrent life-threatening infection and granuloma formation, its use in systemic vasculitis is much more controversial. There have been a number of reports of benefit from co-trimoxazole in patients with Wegener's granulomatosis (p.1031),[5-7] but even where benefit has been reported relapse appears to be common,[7] and Hoffman and others,[8] reporting the experience of the USA National Institutes of Health in 158 patients are sceptical of its value: only 1 of 9 patients given 960 mg twice daily by mouth had any prolonged improvement.

More recently evidence has emerged that addition of co-trimoxazole to maintenance regimens in patients already in remission reduces the incidence of relapse.[9]

1. Gallin JI, *et al.* Recent advances in chronic granulomatous disease. *Ann Intern Med* 1983; **99:** 657–74.
2. Mouy R, *et al.* Incidence, severity, and prevention of infections in chronic granulomatous disease. *J Pediatr* 1989; **114:** 555–60.
3. Margolis DM, *et al.* Trimethoprim-sulfamethoxazole prophylaxis in the management of chronic granulomatous disease. *J Infect Dis* 1990; **162:** 723–6.
4. Gallin JI, Malech HL. Update on chronic granulomatous diseases of childhood: immunotherapy and potential for gene therapy. *JAMA* 1990; **263:** 1533–7.
5. DeRemee RA, *et al.* Wegener's granulomatosis: observations on treatment with antimicrobial agents. *Mayo Clin Proc* 1985; **60:** 27–32.
6. Bowden FJ, Griffiths H. Co-trimoxazole in the treatment of Wegener's granulomatosis. *Med J Aust* 1989; **151:** 303–4.
7. Valeriano-Marcet J, Spiera H. Treatment of Wegener's granulomatosis with sulfamethoxazole-trimethoprim. *Arch Intern Med* 1991; **151:** 1649–52.
8. Hoffman GS, *et al.* Wegener granulomatosis: an analysis of 158 patients. *Ann Intern Med* 1992; **116:** 488–98.
9. Stegeman CA, *et al.* Trimethoprim-sulfamethoxazole (co-trimoxazole) for the prevention of relapses of Wegener's granulomatosis. *N Engl J Med* 1996; **335:** 16–20.

Isosporiasis. In isosporiasis (p.575) WHO recommends co-trimoxazole 960 mg four times daily for 10 days by mouth for treatment;[1] such a regimen followed by 960 mg twice daily for 3 weeks has been reported to be initially effective in patients with AIDS suffering from isosporiasis, with resolution of diarrhoea within 2 days of beginning treatment, but was associated with a high rate of recurrence.[2] A shorter initial regimen followed by indefinite prophylaxis may be preferable in persons with AIDS.

1. WHO. *WHO model prescribing information: drugs used in parasitic diseases.* Geneva: WHO, 1995.
2. DeHovitz JA, *et al.* Clinical manifestations and therapy of Isospora belli infection in patients with the acquired immunodeficiency syndrome. *N Engl J Med* 1986; **315:** 87–90.

Nocardiosis. Co-trimoxazole is used in the treatment of nocardiosis (p.133). There is no consensus on the optimum dosage; doses of 2.88 to 3.84 g daily in divided doses for up to 3 months have been used.

Pneumocystis carinii pneumonia. Co-trimoxazole is used for both the treatment and prophylaxis of *Pneumocystis carinii* pneumonia (p.370). Various studies[1-4] have shown intermittent dosing (such as 960 mg three times a week on alternate days) is effective for the prophylaxis of pneumonia and is better tolerated than daily dosing; the addition of folinic acid had no effect on tolerability and may be associated with a higher rate of therapeutic failure (see p.1343). A single daily dose of 480 mg may also be effective and better tolerated.[5]

1. Wormser GP, *et al.* Low-dose intermittent trimethoprim-sulfamethoxazole for prevention of Pneumocystis carinii pneumonia in patients with human immunodeficiency virus infection. *Arch Intern Med* 1991; **151:** 688–92.
2. Stein DS, *et al.* Use of low-dose trimethoprim-sulfamethoxazole thrice weekly for primary and secondary prophylaxis of Pneumocystis carinii pneumonia in human immunodeficiency virus-infected patients. *Antimicrob Agents Chemother* 1991; **35:** 1705–9.
3. Ruskin J, LaRiviere M. Low-dose co-trimoxazole for prevention of Pneumocystis carinii pneumonia in human immunodeficiency virus disease. *Lancet* 1991; **337:** 468–71.
4. Bozzette SA, *et al.* The tolerance for zidovudine plus thrice weekly or daily trimethoprim-sulfamethoxazole with and without leucovorin for primary prophylaxis in advanced HIV disease. *Am J Med* 1995; **98:** 177–82.
5. Centers for Disease Control. 1997 USPHS/IDSA guidelines for the prevention of opportunistic infections in persons infected with human immunodeficiency virus. *MMWR* 1997; **46** (RR-12): 1–48.

Toxoplasmosis. There is some evidence that administration of co-trimoxazole for prophylaxis of *Pneumocystis carinii* pneumonia produces an additional benefit in acting prophylactically against toxoplasmic encephalitis in persons with AIDS,[1-4] but the evidence (as for other drugs) has been largely anecdotal or from small retrospective studies.[4] In the retrospective study by Carr *et al.*,[3] prophylaxis with co-trimoxazole 960 mg twice daily every Monday and Thursday appeared to be effective. More recently 960 mg twice daily on 3 days per week (Monday, Wednesday, and Friday) was considered effective prophylaxis against toxoplasmosis and *Pneumocystis carinii* pneumonia in patients with HIV infection.[5]

For a discussion of toxoplasmosis and its treatment, see p.576.

1. Centers for Disease Control. 1997 USPHS/IDSA guidelines for the prevention of opportunistic infections in persons infected with human immunodeficiency virus. *MMWR* 1997; **46** (RR-12): 1–48.
2. Zangerle R, Allerberger F. Effect of prophylaxis against pneumocystis carinii on toxoplasma encephalitis. *Lancet* 1991; **337:** 1232.
3. Carr A, *et al.* Low-dose trimethoprim-sulfamethoxazole prophylaxis for toxoplasmic encephalitis in patients with AIDS. *Ann Intern Med* 1992; **117:** 106–11.
4. Beaman MH, *et al.* Prophylaxis for toxoplasmosis in AIDS. *Ann Intern Med* 1992: **117:** 163–4.
5. Podzamczer D, *et al.* Intermittent trimethoprim-sulfamethoxazole compared with dapsone-pyrimethamine for the simultaneous primary prophylaxis of pneumocystis pneumonia and toxoplasmosis in patients infected with HIV. *Ann Intern Med* 1995; **122:** 755–61.

Preparations

BP 1998: Co-trimoxazole Intravenous Infusion; Co-trimoxazole Oral Suspension; Co-trimoxazole Tablets; Dispersible Co-trimoxazole Tablets; Paediatric Co-trimoxazole Oral Suspension; Paediatric Co-trimoxazole Tablets;
USP 23: Sulfamethoxazole and Trimethoprim Injection; Sulfamethoxazole and Trimethoprim Oral Suspension; Sulfamethoxazole and Trimethoprim Tablets.

Proprietary Preparations (details are given in Part 3)
Aust.: Bactrim; Cotribene; Eusaprim; Oecotrim; Supracombin; Trimetho comp; ***Austral.:*** Bactrim; Resprim; Septrin; ***Belg.:*** Bactrim; Eusaprim; ***Canad.:*** Apo-Sulfatrim; Bactrim; Novo-Trimel; Nu-Cotrimox; Roubac; Septra; ***Fr.:*** Bactekod†; Bactrim; Cotrimazol; Eusaprim; ***Ger.:*** Bactoreduct; Bactrim; Berlocid; Cotrim-Tablinen; Cotim; Cotrim; Cotrim Holsten; Cotrim-basan†; Cotrim-Diolan; Cotrim-Hefa; Cotrim-Puren; Cotrim-Riker†; Cotrimhexal; Cotrimox-Wolff; Cotrimstada; Drylin; Duobiocin†; duratrimet†; Eusaprim; Jenamoxazol; Kepinol; Linaris; Microtrim; Nymix-amid N†; Omsat†; Sigaprim; Sulfacet†; Sulfotrimin†; Supracombin; TMS; Trigonyl†; ***Irl.:*** Antrimox; Bactrim; Cotrimel; Duobact; Septrin; Tricomox; ***Ital.:*** Abacin; Bacterial; Bactrim; Chemitrim; Eusaprim; Gantaprim†; Gantrim; Isotrim; Medixin; Oxaprim†; Strepto-Plus; Sulmen†; Suprin†; Trim†; ***Jpn:*** Baktar†; ***Neth.:*** Bactrimel; Eusaprim; Sulfotrim†; Trimoxol; ***Norw.:*** Bactrim; Eusaprim†; ***S.Afr.:*** Acuco; Arcanaprim; Bactrim; Bencole; Briscotrim†; Cocydal; Cotrivan†; Cozole; Doctrim; Duotrim†; Durobac; Dynazole; Fabubac; Mezenol†; Microbac†; Norisep†; Partrim†; Purbac; Septran; Spectrim; Thoxaprim†; Tri-Co; Trimethox; Trimoks; Trimzol; Troxazole; Ultrasept†; Ultrazole; Xerazole; Xeroprim; ***Spain:*** Abactrim; Azosulfin†; Bactifor; Bridotrim; Brongenit; Eduprim; Gobens Trim; Momentol; Salvatrim; Septrin; Toose; ***Swed.:*** Bactrim; Eusaprim; Triferm-Sulfa†; Trimetoprim-Sulfa†; ***Switz.:*** Bactrim; Cotrim; Escoprim; Eusaprim; Groprim; Helveprim; Imexim; Nopil; Pharmaprim†; Sigaprim; Supracombin; TMS†; ***UK:*** Bactrim†; Chemotrim; Comixco; Comox†; Fectrim; Laratrim; Septrin; ***USA:*** Bactrim; Cotrim; Septra; SMZ-TMP; Sulfamethoprim; Sulfatrim DS; Uroplus.

Multi-ingredient: ***Ital.:*** Pulmotrim†; ***Spain:*** Abactrim Balsamico†; Bactopumon; Balsoprim; Bronco Aseptilex Fuerte; Bronco Bactifor; Bronco Sergo; Broncorema; Broncovir NF; Bronquicisteina; Bronquidiazina CR; Bronquimar; Bronquimucil; Bronquium; Eduprim Mucolitico; Libetusin†; Lotusix; Mucorama TS; Neumopectolina; Pulmo Menal; Pulmosterin Duo; Tosdetan; Traquivan; Tresium.

Cycloserine (64-q)

Cycloserine *(BAN, rINN)*.

Cicloserina; D-Cycloserin; Cycloserinum. (+)-(*R*)-4-Aminoisoxazolidin-3-one.

$C_3H_6N_2O_2$ = 102.1.

CAS — 68-41-7.

Pharmacopoeias. In *It.*, *Jpn*, and *US*.

An antimicrobial substance produced by the growth of certain strains of *Streptomyces orchidaceus* or *S. garyphalus*, or obtained by synthesis.

A white or pale yellow, hygroscopic, crystalline powder, odourless or with a slight odour. Its activity diminishes on absorbing water. Freely **soluble** in water. A 10% solution in water has a pH of 5.5 to 6.5. **Store** in airtight containers.

Adverse Effects and Treatment

The most frequent adverse effects with cycloserine involve the CNS and include anxiety, confusion, disorientation, depression, psychoses possibly with suicidal tendencies, aggression, irritability, and paranoia. Vertigo, headache, drowsiness, speech difficulties, tremor, paresis, hyperreflexia, peripheral neuropathies, coma, and convulsions may also occur. Neurological reactions are dose related and may be reduced by keeping plasma concentrations below 30 μg per mL. It has been reported that up to 30% of patients have experienced side-effects. These reactions usually subside when cycloserine is discontinued or the dosage is reduced. Pyridoxine has been used in an attempt to treat or prevent neurological reactions but its value is unproven.

Hypersensitivity reactions including skin reactions and photosensitivity occur rarely. Serum aminotransferase values may be raised, especially in patients with a history of liver disease. Folate and vitamin B_{12} deficiency, megaloblastic anaemia, and sideroblastic anaemia have been reported occasionally when cycloserine has been administered with other antituberculous drugs. Heart failure has occurred in patients receiving doses of 1 g or more daily.

Precautions

Cycloserine is contra-indicated in patients with epilepsy, depression, psychosis, severe anxiety, severe renal insufficiency, or in those who abuse alcohol. Cycloserine should be discontinued or the dose reduced if allergic dermatitis or symptoms of CNS toxicity develop.

Cycloserine has a low therapeutic index, and dosage should be adjusted according to plasma concentrations which should be monitored at least weekly in patients with renal impairment, those taking doses greater than 500 mg daily, and in patients showing signs of neurological toxicity. Plasma concentrations should be maintained below 30 μg per mL. Patients with renal impairment require lower doses.

Porphyria. Cycloserine has been associated with clinical exacerbations of porphyria and is considered unsafe in porphyric patients.[1]

1. Moore MR, McColl KEL. *Porphyria: drug lists.* Glasgow: Porphyria Research Unit, University of Glasgow, 1991.

Interactions

Patients receiving cycloserine with alcohol are at increased risk of convulsions. Neurotoxic effects may be potentiated by concurrent administration of cycloserine and ethionamide, and increased CNS toxicity, such as dizziness and drowsiness, may occur in patients receiving cycloserine and isoniazid. For a mention of increased blood-alcohol concentrations in patients receiving cycloserine, see p.1100.

Antimicrobial Action

Cycloserine interferes with bacterial cell wall synthesis by competing with D-alanine for incorporation into the cell wall. It has variable activity against Gram-positive and Gram-negative bacteria including *Escherichia coli* and *Staphylococcus aureus*.

Cycloserine is active against *Mycobacterium tuberculosis* and some other mycobacteria. Minimum inhibitory concentrations *in vitro* for *M. tuberculosis* range from 5 to 20 μg per mL. Resistance develops if cycloserine is used alone.

Pharmacokinetics

Cycloserine is readily and almost completely absorbed from the gastro-intestinal tract. Peak plasma concentrations of 10 μg per mL have been obtained 3 to 4 hours after a dose of 250 mg rising to 20 to 30 μg per mL on repeating the dose every 12 hours. The plasma half-life is about 10 hours and is prolonged in patients with renal impairment.

Cycloserine is widely distributed in body tissues and fluids including the CSF, the placenta, and breast milk.

Cycloserine is excreted largely unchanged by glomerular filtration. About 50% of a single 250-mg dose is excreted unchanged in the urine within 12 hours and about 70% is excreted within 72 hours. As negligible amounts of cycloserine appear in the faeces it is assumed that the remainder of a dose is metabolised to unidentified metabolites. It is removed by haemodialysis.

Pregnancy and breast feeding. Cycloserine has been shown to pass to the fetus, amniotic fluid,[1] and into breast milk.[2] Concentrations in breast milk after 250 mg four times daily have been reported to range from 6 to 19 μg per mL.[2]

1. Holdiness MR. Transplacental pharmacokinetics of the antituberculosis drugs. *Clin Pharmacokinet* 1987; **13:** 125–9.
2. Snider DE, Powell KE. Should women taking antituberculosis drugs breast-feed? *Arch Intern Med* 1984; **144:** 5 89–90.

Uses and Administration

Cycloserine is a second-line antimycobacterial that may be used in the treatment of tuberculosis (p.146) as part of a multi-drug regimen when resistance to or toxicity from primary drugs has developed. It has been used in urinary-tract infections although less toxic drugs are preferred.

The usual dose in tuberculosis is 0.5 to 1 g daily by mouth in divided doses. The maximum daily dose is 1 g. Some recommend an initial dose of 250 mg twice daily for 2 weeks. Experience in children is limited; an initial paediatric dose of 10 mg per kg body-weight daily has been suggested. Dosage in patients with renal impairment should be reduced and doses for all patients should be adjusted by monitoring plasma concentrations (see Precautions, above).

L-Cycloserine (levcycloserine) has been investigated for the treatment of Gaucher disease (p.1544).

Preparations

USP 23: Cycloserine Capsules.

Proprietary Preparations (details are given in Part 3)
Austral.: Closina; ***Canad.:*** Seromycin; ***UK:*** Cycloserine; ***USA:*** Seromycin.

Danofloxacin Mesylate (10962-e)

Danofloxacin Mesylate *(BANM, USAN)*.

Danofloxacin Mesilate *(rINNM)*; CP-76136 (danofloxacin); CP-76136-27 (danofloxacin mesylate).

$C_{19}H_{20}FN_3O_3,CH_4O_3S$ = 453.5.

CAS — 112398-08-0 (danofloxacin); 119478-55-6 (danofloxacin mesylate).

Danofloxacin is a fluoroquinolone antibacterial used as the mesylate in veterinary medicine.

Dapsone (6554-b)

Dapsone *(BAN, USAN, rINN)*.

DADPS; Dapsonum; DDS; Diaminodiphenylsulfone; Diaphenylsulfone; Disulone; NSC-6091; Sulphonyldianiline. Bis(4-aminophenyl) sulphone.

$C_{12}H_{12}N_2O_2S$ = 248.3.

CAS — 80-08-0.

Pharmacopoeias. In *Chin., Eur.* (see p.viii), *Int.*, and *US.*

A white or slightly yellowish-white odourless crystalline powder. Ph. Eur. **solubilities** are: very slightly soluble in water; sparingly soluble in alcohol; freely soluble in acetone. USP solubilities are: very slightly soluble in water, freely soluble in alcohol and soluble in acetone. Both pharmacopoeias state soluble in dilute mineral acids. **Protect** from light.

Adverse Effects

Varying degrees of dose-related haemolysis and methaemoglobinaemia are the most frequently reported adverse effects of dapsone and occur in most subjects given more than 200 mg daily; doses of up to 100 mg daily do not cause significant haemolysis but subjects deficient in glucose-6-phosphate dehydrogenase are affected by doses above about 50 mg daily.

Although agranulocytosis has been reported rarely with dapsone when used alone, reports have been more common when dapsone has been used with other drugs in the prophylaxis of malaria.

Rash and pruritus may develop. Serious cutaneous hypersensitivity reactions occur rarely and include maculopapular rash, exfoliative dermatitis, toxic epidermal necrolysis, and Stevens-Johnson syndrome. Fixed drug eruptions have occurred.

A 'dapsone syndrome' may occur and resembles mononucleosis in its presentation (see below).

Peripheral neuropathy with motor loss has been reported in patients on dapsone for dermatological conditions. Peripheral neuropathy may occur as part of leprosy reaction states and is not an indication to discontinue dapsone.

Other adverse effects occur infrequently and include nausea, vomiting, anorexia, headache, hepatitis, and psychosis.

Carcinogenicity. A survey of 1678 leprosy patients admitted for treatment to the National Hansen's Disease Center in Carville between 1939 and 1977 indicated that, although dapsone has been implicated as a carcinogen in *animals*, the use of dapsone did not appear to affect significantly the risk of any cancer in these patients.[1]

1. Brinton LA, *et al.* Cancer mortality among patients with Hansen's disease. *J Natl Cancer Inst* 1984; **72:** 109–14.

Effects on the blood. Haemolysis is the most frequent serious adverse effect of dapsone and may occur at doses of 200 mg or higher daily.[1] Red blood cells may contain Heinz bodies and there is a reduction in their life span. Well-known risk factors include glucose-6-phosphate deficiency, methaemoglobin reductase deficiency, and haemoglobin M trait; haemoglobin E trait may also increase susceptibility to haemolytic reactions.[2] Haemolytic anaemia has been reported in a neonate following ingestion of dapsone in breast milk.[3]

Methaemoglobinaemia, though common, is rarely symptomatic.[1]

Agranulocytosis has occurred rarely following dapsone use in leprosy and skin disease. More cases have been observed when used for malaria prophylaxis[4] (see also under Pyrimethamine, p.437) and dermatitis herpetiformis.[5] The reaction is usually self-limiting once the drug is withdrawn, but fatalities have occurred.[5,6]

Aplastic anaemia has been reported.[7,8] Of 11 fatalities attributed to dapsone reported to the British and Swedish adverse reaction registers[9] between 1968 and 1988, 7 were due to white blood cell dyscrasias; none were attributed to red cell dyscrasias although such reactions formed almost half of all serious reactions reported for dapsone.

Thrombocytosis was reported in a patient with AIDS receiving dapsone prophylactically.[10]

See also **Hypoalbuminaemia**, below.

1. Jopling WH. Side-effects of antileprosy drugs in common use. *Lepr Rev* 1983; **54:** 261–70.
2. Lachant NA, Tanaka KR. Case report: dapsone-associated Heinz body hemolytic anemia in a Cambodian woman with hemoglobin E trait. *Am J Med Sci* 1987; **294:** 364–8.
3. Sanders SW, *et al.* Hemolytic anemia induced by dapsone transmitted through breast milk. *Ann Intern Med* 1982; **96:** 465–6.
4. Firkin FC, Mariani AF. Agranulocytosis due to dapsone. *Med J Aust* 1977; **2:** 247–51.
5. Cockburn EM, *et al.* Dapsone-induced agranulocytosis: spontaneous reporting data. *Br J Dermatol* 1993; **128:** 702–3.
6. Barss P. Fatal dapsone agranulocytosis in a Melanesian. *Lepr Rev* 1986; **57:** 63–6.
7. Foucauld J, *et al.* Dapsone and aplastic anemia. *Ann Intern Med* 1985; **102:** 139.
8. Meyerson MA, Cohen PR. Dapsone-induced aplastic anaemia in a woman with bullous systemic lupus erythematosus. *Mayo Clin Proc* 1994; **69:** 1159–62.
9. Björkman A, Phillips-Howard PA. Adverse reactions to sulfa drugs: implications for malaria chemotherapy. *Bull WHO* 1991; **69:** 297–304.
10. Wynn RF, *et al.* Case report of dapsone-related thrombocytosis in an AIDS patient. *Am J Med* 1995; **98:** 602.

Effects on the eyes. Eye damage associated with acute or subacute dapsone poisoning.[1,2]

1. Daneshmend TK. The neurotoxicity of dapsone. *Adverse Drug React Acute Poisoning Rev* 1984; **3:** 43–58.
2. Alexander TA, *et al.* Presumed DDS ocular toxicity. *Indian J Ophthalmol* 1989; **37:** 150–1.

Effects on the lungs. Pulmonary eosinophilia occurred on 2 occasions in a women receiving dapsone for urticaria.[1] On each occasion symptoms resolved when dapsone was stopped.

1. Jaffuel D, *et al.* Eosinophilic pneumonia induced by dapsone. *Br Med J* 1998; **317:** 181.

Effects on mental state. Psychosis has been reported in leprosy patients on dapsone but the role of dapsone in this effect is poorly defined.[1] Manic depressive reactions have been reported in 2 patients with skin disorders. These reactions appear to be idiosyncratic reactions to dapsone.[2,3]

1. Daneshmend T. Idiosyncratic dapsone induced manic depression. *Br Med J* 1989; **299:** 324.
2. Carmichael AJ, Paul CJ. Idiosyncratic dapsone induced manic depression. *Br Med J* 1989; **298:** 1524. Correction. *ibid.*; **299:** 56.
3. Gawkrodger D. Manic depression induced by dapsone in patient with dermatitis herpetiformis. *Br Med J* 1989; **299:** 860.

Effects on the nervous system. Clinical details of 13 patients who experienced dapsone-induced neuropathy. Patients received a mean dose of 115 g (range 6 to 380 g) over 19 months for various dermatological conditions.[1] All patients had motor weakness and some experienced sensory impairment. Most recovered within several months of discontinuing dapsone.

1. Daneshmend TK. The neurotoxicity of dapsone. *Adverse Drug React Acute Poisoning Rev* 1984; **3:** 43–58.

Effects on taste. A persistent sweet taste and tingling of the face and lips was described in a patient receiving dapsone for ocular cicatricial pemphigoid.[1] The symptoms resolved when dapsone was stopped.

1. Stafanous SN, Morgan SJ. A previously unrecognised side effect of dapsone. *Br J Ophthalmol* 1997; **81:** 1113–14.

Hyperpigmentation. Hyperpigmented macules were reported in 32 of approximately 800 children who received dapsone with pyrimethamine for 3 months or more for malaria prophylaxis.[1] The reaction was attributed to the dapsone component.

1. David KP, *et al.* Hyperpigmented dermal macules in children following the administration of Maloprim for malaria chemoprophylaxis. *Trans R Soc Trop Med Hyg* 1997; **91:** 204–8.

Hypersensitivity reactions. DAPSONE SYNDROME. This syndrome is a rare hypersensitivity reaction although it has been suggested[1] that the incidence has increased since the introduction of multidrug therapy for leprosy. It occurs in the first 6 weeks of therapy and symptoms include rash, which is always present, fever, jaundice, and eosinophilia. The syndrome has occurred in leprosy patients,[2-4] in patients with skin disorders,[5,6] and in a patient on weekly dapsone (in association with pyrimethamine) for malaria prophylaxis.[7] Fatalities have occurred.[3,8] Desensitisation has been successfully carried out in several patients with AIDS who exhibited hypersensitivity to dapsone.[9]

1. Richardus JH, Smith TC. Increased incidence in leprosy of hypersensitivity reactions to dapsone after introduction of multidrug therapy. *Lepr Rev* 1989; **60:** 267–73.
2. Joseph MS. Hypersensitivity reaction to dapsone. *Lepr Rev* 1985; **56:** 315–20.
3. Jamrozik K. Dapsone syndrome occurring in two brothers. *Lepr Rev* 1986; **57:** 57–62.
4. Hortaleza AR, *et al.* Dapsone syndrome in a Filipino man. *Lepr Rev* 1995; **66:** 307–13.
5. Tomecki KJ, Catalano CJ. Dapsone hypersensitivity: the sulfone syndrome revisited. *Arch Dermatol* 1981; **117:** 38–9.
6. Kromann NP, *et al.* The dapsone syndrome. *Arch Dermatol* 1982; **118:** 531–2.
7. Grayson ML, *et al.* Severe dapsone syndrome due to weekly Maloprim. *Lancet* 1988; **i:** 531.
8. Frey HM, *et al.* Fatal reaction to dapsone during treatment of leprosy. *Ann Intern Med* 1981; **94:** 777–9.
9. Metroka CE, *et al.* Desensitization to dapsone in HIV-positive patients. *JAMA* 1992; **267:** 512.

Hypoalbuminaemia. Severe and often life-threatening hypoalbuminaemia has been reported rarely in patients taking dapsone for extended periods for dermatitis herpetiformis.[1-3] Hypoalbuminaemia usually resolves rapidly once dapsone is withdrawn.

1. Kingham JGC, *et al.* Dapsone and severe hypoalbuminaemia. *Lancet* 1979; **ii:** 662–4 and 1018.
2. Foster PN, Swan CHJ. Dapsone and fatal hypoalbuminaemia. *Lancet* 1981; **ii:** 806–7.
3. Sinclair SA, *et al.* Life threatening hypoalbuminaemia associated with dapsone therapy. *Br J Dermatol* 1996; **135** (suppl 47): 45.

Photosensitivity. Photosensitivity has been reported in 6 patients taking dapsone.[1]

1. Dhanapaul S. DDS-induced photosensitivity with reference to six case reports. *Lepr Rev* 1989; **60:** 147–50.

Treatment of Adverse Effects

In severe overdosage the stomach should be emptied by lavage. Administration of activated charcoal by mouth has been shown to enhance the elimination of dapsone and its monoacetyl metabolite. Methaemoglobinaemia has been treated with slow intravenous injections of methylene blue 1 to 2 mg per kg body-weight repeated after one hour if necessary. Methylene blue should not be administered to patients with glucose-6-phosphate dehydrogenase deficiency since it will not be effective. Haemolysis has been treated by infusion of concentrated human red blood cells to replace the damaged cells. Supportive therapy includes administration of oxygen and fluids.

References to the treatment of dapsone overdose.[1-3]

1. Dawson AH, Whyte IM. Management of dapsone poisoning complicated by methaemoglobinaemia. *Med Toxicol Adverse Drug Exp* 1989; **4:** 387–92.
2. Endre ZH, *et al.* Successful treatment of acute dapsone intoxication using charcoal hemoperfusion. *Aust N Z J Med* 1983; **13:** 509–12.
3. Hoetelmans RMW, *et al.* Combined dapsone and clofazimine intoxication. *Hum Exp Toxicol* 1996; **15:** 625–8.

Prevention of haemotoxicity. Administration of cimetidine with dapsone may reduce the incidence or severity of dapsone-induced methaemoglobinaemia and haemolysis, probably by reducing *N*-hydroxylation.[1,2] Other strategies, such as the use of the antoxidant alpha tocopherol, were considered less successful.[3]

1. Coleman MD, *et al.* The use of cimetidine as a selective inhibitor of dapsone N-hydroxylation in man. *Br J Clin Pharmacol* 1990; **30:** 761–7.
2. Rhodes LE, *et al.* Cimetidine improves the therapeutic/toxic ratio of dapsone in patients on chronic dapsone therapy. *Br J Dermatol* 1995; **132:** 257–62.
3. Coleman MD, Coleman NA. Drug-induced methaemoglobinaemia: treatment issues. *Drug Safety* 1996; **14:** 394–405.

Precautions

Dapsone should not be used in patients with severe anaemia. It is recommended that regular blood counts be performed during treatment. Patients deficient in glucose-6-phosphate dehydrogenase, or methaemoglobin reductase, or with haemoglobin M are more susceptible to the haemolytic effects of dapsone.

It is now generally considered that the benefits of dapsone in the treatment of leprosy outweigh any potential risk to the pregnant patient. Some leprologists recommend folic acid 5 mg daily for leprosy patients receiving dapsone during pregnancy. Dapsone is distributed into breast milk and there has been a report of haemolytic anaemia in a breast fed infant (see Effects on the Blood, under Adverse Effects, above). While some feel that dapsone should not be used in mothers who are breast feeding, in general treatment for leprosy is continued in such patients.

Porphyria. Dapsone has been associated with clinical exacerbations of porphyria and is considered unsafe in porphyric patients.[1]

1. Moore MR, McColl KEL. *Porphyria: drug lists.* Glasgow: Porphyria Research Unit, University of Glasgow, 1991.

Interactions

Serum concentrations of dapsone are increased, with a consequent increased risk of adverse effects, during concurrent administration of probenecid, probably as a result of reduced renal excretion of dapsone. Increased dapsone concentrations have also been reported in patients receiving trimethoprim, and patients receiving this combination may be at increased risk of dapsone toxicity. Rifampicin reduces serum concentrations of dapsone to a level that may compromise efficacy in infections other than leprosy. Rifampicin concentrations are generally unaffected. Dapsone may antagonise the anti-inflammatory properties of clofazimine (p.194).

Pyrimethamine. Although some manufacturers warn that dapsone-induced haematotoxicity could be potentiated by folic acid antagonists such as pyrimethamine, the tolerability of dapsone plus pyrimethamine was similar to dapsone alone when each treatment was given on a once-weekly basis to patients with HIV.[1] Dapsone concentrations were not significantly higher in patients receiving dapsone plus pyrimethamine than in those receiving dapsone alone.

1. Falloon J, *et al.* Pharmacokinetics and safety of weekly dapsone and dapsone plus pyrimethamine for prevention of pneumocystis pneumonia. *Antimicrob Agents Chemother* 1994; **38:** 1580–7.

Trimethoprim. In a study of AIDS patients with *Pneumocystis carinii* pneumonia, the mean peak serum concentrations of dapsone were 1.5 μg per mL following 100 mg daily for 7 days and 2.1 μg per mL following dapsone in combination with trimethoprim 20 mg per kg body-weight daily; concentrations of trimethoprim were also increased.[1] Elevated dapsone concentrations may contribute to the toxicity and the efficacy of this combination.

1. Lee BL, *et al.* Dapsone, trimethoprim, and sulfamethoxazole plasma levels during treatment of pneumocystis pneumonia in patients with the acquired immuno deficiency syndrome (AIDS). *Ann Intern Med* 1989; **110:** 606–11.

Antimicrobial Action

Dapsone is a sulphone active against a wide range of bacteria but it is mainly employed for its action against *Mycobacterium leprae*. Its mechanism of action is probably similar to that of the sulphonamides which involves inhibition of folic acid synthesis in susceptible organisms. It is usually considered to be bacteriostatic against *M. leprae* although it may also possess weak bactericidal activity. It is also active against *Plasmodium* and *Pneumocystis carinii*. As with the sulphonamides antibacterial activity is inhibited by *p*-aminobenzoic acid.

Using the mouse foot-pad technique the minimum inhibitory concentration for *M. leprae* has been reported to be less than 10 ng per mL.

Secondary (acquired) dapsone resistance of *Mycobacterium leprae* is mainly associated with dapsone being used on its own. Primary dapsone resistance has also been reported with increasing frequency in areas with secondary resistance. Resistance of *M. leprae* to dapsone should be suspected whenever a patient relapses clinically and bacteriologically.

Combinations of dapsone with the folate antagonists sulphadimidine,[1] cycloguanil,[1] or pyrimethamine[2] showed synergistic activity against *Mycobacterium avium* complex *in vitro*.

1. Gonzalez AH, *et al.* In-vitro activity of dapsone and two potentiators against Mycobacterium avium complex. *J Antimicrob Chemother* 1989; **24:** 19–22.
2. Shah LM, *et al.* Enhanced in vitro activity of pyrimethamine in combination with dapsone against Mycobacterium avium complex. *Antimicrob Agents Chemother* 1996; **40:** 2426–7.

MULTIDRUG RESISTANCE. Strains of *Mycobacterium leprae* with multiple resistance to rifampicin, ofloxacin, and dapsone have been isolated from patients who have previously received dapsone monotherapy followed by treatment with rifampicin in combination with ofloxacin.[1]

1. Cambau E, *et al.* Multidrug-resistance to dapsone, rifampicin, and ofloxacin in Mycobacterium leprae. *Lancet* 1997; **349:** 103–4.

Pharmacokinetics

Dapsone is almost completely absorbed from the gastro-intestinal tract with peak plasma concentrations occurring from 2 to 8 hours after a dose. Steady-state concentrations are not attained until after at least 8 days of daily administration; doses of 100 mg daily provide trough concentrations of 0.5 μg per mL which are well in excess of the MIC for *M. leprae*. About 50 to 80% of dapsone in the circulation is bound to plasma proteins and nearly 100% of its monoacetylated metabolite is bound.

Dapsone undergoes enterohepatic recycling. It is widely distributed; it is present in saliva and breast milk and crosses the placenta. The half-life ranges from 10 to 50 hours.

Dapsone is acetylated to monoacetyldapsone, the major metabolite, and other mono and diacetyl derivatives. Acetylation exhibits genetic polymorphism. Hydroxylation is the other major metabolic pathway resulting in hydroxylamine dapsone which may be responsible for dapsone-associated methaemoglobinaemia and haemolysis.

Dapsone is mainly excreted in the urine, only 20% of a dose as unchanged drug.

References.

1. Zuidema J, *et al.* Clinical pharmacokinetics of dapsone. *Clin Pharmacokinet* 1986; **11:** 299–315.
2. Pieters FAJM, Zuidema J. The pharmacokinetics of dapsone after oral administration to healthy volunteers. *Br J Clin Pharmacol* 1986; **22:** 491–4.
3. May DG, *et al.* The disposition of dapsone in cirrhosis. *Clin Pharmacol Ther* 1992; **51:** 689–700.
4. Mirochnick M, *et al.* Pharmacokinetics of dapsone in children. *J Pediatr* 1993; **122:** 806–9.
5. Opravil M, *et al.* Levels of dapsone and pyrimethamine in serum during once-weekly dosing for prophylaxis of Pneumocystis carinii pneumonia and toxoplasmic encephalitis. *Antimicrob Agents Chemother* 1994; **38:** 1197–9.
6. Gatti G, *et al.* Pharmacokinetics of dapsone in human immunodeficiency virus-infected children. *Antimicrob Agents Chemother* 1995; **39:** 1101–6.
7. Gatti G, *et al.* Population pharmacokinetics of dapsone administered biweekly to human immunodeficiency virus-infected patients. *Antimicrob Agents Chemother* 1996; **40:** 2743–8.
8. Gatti G, *et al.* Penetration of dapsone into cerebrospinal fluid of patients with AIDS. *J Antimicrob Chemother* 1997; **40:** 113–15.

Uses and Administration

Dapsone is used as part of multi-drug regimens in the treatment of all forms of leprosy (p.128). It has also been used in the prophylaxis of leprosy and in the management of household contacts of leprosy patients. Dapsone is used as an alternative to cotrimoxazole for the treatment and prophylaxis of *Pneumocystis carinii* pneumonia (p.370), and in combination with pyrimethamine for the prophylaxis of malaria (see under Pyrimethamine, p.438). It is also used in dermatitis herpetiformis and other dermatoses (below), and has been tried for the prophylaxis of toxoplasmosis (p.576) and for the treatment of cutaneous leishmaniasis (p.575) and actinomycetoma (p.132).

Dapsone is usually given by mouth. There are some reports of it being given by intramuscular injection but such injections can be painful and cause abscess formation.

The most common regimens for leprosy are those recommended by WHO. For multibacillary leprosy rifampicin 600 mg and clofazimine 300 mg are both given once a month under supervision together with dapsone 100 mg and clofazimine 50 mg both daily in self-administered doses for 2 years. Doses of all 3 drugs are reduced in children and in those aged 10 to 14 years daily doses of dapsone 50 mg, or 1 to 2 mg per kg if their body-weight is low, are given. Adults weighing less than 35 kg also receive reduced doses of rifampicin and dapsone and in such patients the dapsone dose is 50 mg or 1 to 2 mg per kg daily.

The WHO regimen for paucibacillary leprosy consists of rifampicin 600 mg under supervision once a month and dapsone 100 mg self-administered daily; both are given for 6 months. Doses are reduced in children and low-weight patients as for multibacillary leprosy.

For the prophylaxis of *Pneumocystis carinii* pneumonia, dapsone may be given alone or in combination with pyrimethamine in a suggested dose of 100 mg daily. For treatment, the same dose of dapsone is given with trimethoprim.

The adult dose of dapsone for malaria prophylaxis is 100 mg weekly with pyrimethamine 12.5 mg weekly.

The dose required for the treatment of dermatitis herpetiformis has to be titrated for individual patients but it is usual to start with 50 mg daily by mouth gradually increased to 300 mg daily or more if required. This dose should be reduced to a minimum as soon as possible. Maintenance dosage can often be reduced in patients receiving a gluten-free diet.

Kaposi's sarcoma. For a report of the control of non-epidemic (not HIV-related) Kaposi's sarcoma by the use of dapsone, see p.496.

Connective tissue disorders. Dapsone has been used in a number of inflammatory disorders. Relapsing polychondritis (p.1027) has responded to dapsone, as has Behçet's syndrome (p.1018) and systemic lupus erythematosus (p.1029). Vasculitic syndromes such as hypersensitivity vasculitis (p.1022) have also responded to dapsone.

Skin disorders. Dapsone is used in a variety of skin disorders. The mechanism of action is unknown but unrelated to its antimicrobial activity. These uses include the suppression of skin lesions in dermatitis herpetiformis (p.1073) and symptomatic treatment of erythema multiforme in patients who fail to respond to aciclovir (p.1074). Reports, generally involving small numbers of patients, suggest that dapsone may also be beneficial for cicatricial pemphigoid, bullous pemphigoid (p.1075), pyoderma gangrenosum (p.1076), and urticaria (p.1076).

Spider bites. As discussed on p.1534, necrotic araneism resulting from the bite of spiders of the genus *Loxosceles* is usually treated conservatively with surgical repair of any persistent defect. A prospective clinical study of 31 patients with brown recluse spider bites indicated[1] that treatment with dapsone 100 mg daily for 14 days followed by delayed surgical intervention if necessary reduced the incidence of wound complications and residual scarring compared with treatment by immediate surgical excision. A dose of 100 mg twice daily has also been given for 14 days.[2]

1. Rees RS, *et al.* Brown recluse spider bites: a comparison of early surgical excision versus dapsone and delayed surgical excision. *Ann Surg* 1985; **202:** 659–63.
2. King LE, Rees RS. Dapsone treatment of a brown recluse bite. *JAMA* 1983; **250:** 648.

Preparations

BP 1998: Dapsone Tablets;
USP 23: Dapsone Tablets.

Proprietary Preparations (details are given in Part 3)
Canad.: Avlosulfon; ***Spain:*** Sulfona.

Multi-ingredient: ***Aust.:*** Isoprodian; ***Austral.:*** Maloprim; ***Belg.:*** Maloprim†; ***Fr.:*** Disulone; ***Ger.:*** Isoprodian; ***Irl.:*** Maloprim; ***S.Afr.:*** Isoprodian†; Maloprim; MB-Combi†; ***UK:*** Maloprim.

Daptomycin (3854-z)

Daptomycin *(BAN, USAN, rINN).*

Ly-146032. *N*-Decanoyl-L-tryptophyl-L-asparaginyl-L-aspartyl-L-threonylglycyl-L-ornithyl-L-aspartyl-D-alanyl-L-aspartylglycyl-D-seryl-*threo*-3-methyl-L-glutamyl-3-anthraniloyl-L-alanine 1.13-3.4-lactone.

$C_{72}H_{101}N_{17}O_{26}$ = 1620.7.

CAS — 103060-53-3.

Daptomycin is a lipopeptide antibacterial that is reported to have a spectrum of antibacterial activity similar to that of vancomycin (p.268) and greater potency against many bacterial strains *in vitro*. Its action *in vitro* is potentiated by the presence of calcium ions, and it is reported to show antimicrobial synergy with the aminoglycosides against enterococci and *Staphylococcus aureus*. It has been investigated in patients with Gram-positive infections at doses of 2 mg per kg body-weight daily by intravenous infusion. Results in *animals* given higher doses suggest that it has nephrotoxic potential.

References.

1. Pryka RD, *et al.* Clinical pharmacokinetics of daptomycin. *DICP Ann Pharmacother* 1990; **24:** 255–6.
2. Kreft B, *et al.* Experimental studies on nephrotoxicity and pharmacokinetics of LY 146032 (daptomycin) in rats. *J Antimicrob Chemother* 1990; **25:** 635–43.
3. Lamp KC, *et al.* In vitro pharmacodynamic effects of concentration, pH, and growth phase on serum bactericidal activities of daptomycin and vancomycin. *Antimicrob Agents Chemother* 1992; **36:** 2709–14.
4. Woodworth JR, *et al.* Single-dose pharmacokinetics and antibacterial activity of daptomycin, a new lipopeptide antibiotic, in healthy volunteers. *Antimicrob Agents Chemother* 1992; **36:** 318–25.
5. Lamp KC, Rybak MJ. Teicoplanin and daptomycin bactericidal activities in the presence of albumin or serum under controlled conditions of pH and ionized calcium. *Antimicrob Agents Chemother* 1993; **37:** 605–9.
6. Woodworth JR, *et al.* Tobramycin and daptomycin disposition when co-administered to healthy volunteers. *J Antimicrob Chemother* 1994; **33:** 655–9.

Demeclocycline (65-p)

Demeclocycline *(BAN, rINN).*

Demethylchlortetracycline. (4*S*,4a*S*,5a*S*,6*S*,12a*S*)-7-Chloro-4-dimethylamino-1,4,4a,5,5a,6,11,12a-octahydro-3,6,10,12,12a-pentahydroxy-1,11-dioxonaphthacene-2-carboxamide; 7-Chloro-6-demethyltetracycline.

$C_{21}H_{21}ClN_2O_8$ = 464.9.

CAS — 127-33-3 (demeclocycline); 13215-10-6 (demeclocycline sesquihydrate).

Pharmacopoeias. In *US.*

A yellow odourless crystalline powder. Sparingly **soluble** in water; soluble 1 in 200 of alcohol and 1 in 40 of methyl alcohol; soluble in 3N hydrochloric acid and in alkaline solutions. A 1% solution in water has a pH of 4 to 5.5. **Store** in airtight containers. Protect from light.

Demeclocycline Hydrochloride (66-s)

Demeclocycline Hydrochloride *(BANM, rINNM).*

Demeclocyclini Hydrochloridum.

$C_{21}H_{21}ClN_2O_8,HCl$ = 501.3.

CAS — 64-73-3.

Pharmacopoeias. In *Eur.* (see p.viii) and *US.*

An antimicrobial substance produced by the growth of certain strains of *Streptomyces aureofaciens* or by any other means.

A yellow, odourless, crystalline powder. **Soluble** 1 in 60 of water and 1 in 50 of methyl alcohol; slightly soluble in alcohol; very slightly soluble or practically insoluble in acetone; practically insoluble in chloroform and in ether; sparingly soluble in solutions of alkali hydroxides and carbonates. A 1% solution in water has a pH of 2 to 3. **Store** in airtight containers. Protect from light.

Adverse Effects and Precautions

As for Tetracycline Hydrochloride, p.259.

Phototoxic reactions occur more frequently with demeclocycline than with other tetracyclines and patients should avoid exposure to direct sunlight.

Reversible nephrogenic diabetes insipidus with polyuria, polydipsia, and weakness may occur in patients treated with demeclocycline. Plasma creatinine should be monitored in patients receiving demeclocycline for long periods for inappropriate secretion of antidiuretic hormone since tetracycline-induced renal impairment may not otherwise be apparent in the absence of oliguria. For a comment that the usefulness of demeclocycline for this indication may be limited by nephrotoxicity in patients with cardiac or hepatic disease, see under Uses, below.

Interactions

As for Tetracycline Hydrochloride, p.260.

Antimicrobial Action

As for Tetracycline Hydrochloride, p.260. Demeclocycline is stated to be somewhat more active against certain strains of some organisms including *Neisseria gonorrhoeae* and *Haemophilus influenzae*, as well as to being the most active of the tetracyclines *in vitro* against *Brucella* spp.

Pharmacokinetics

As for Tetracycline Hydrochloride, p.260.

Peak plasma concentrations of about 1.5 to 1.7 μg per mL have been reported 3 to 4 hours after a single oral dose of 300 mg of demeclocycline but higher plasma concentrations may be achieved with repeated dosage. Its biological half-life is about 12 hours. The renal clearance of demeclocycline is about half that of tetracycline.

Uses and Administration

Demeclocycline is a tetracycline derivative with uses similar to those of tetracycline (p.261). It is excreted more slowly and effective blood concentrations are maintained for a longer period.

It is given by mouth as the hydrochloride in a usual adult dosage of 600 mg daily in 2 or 4 divided doses preferably one hour before or 2 hours after meals; 900 mg daily in divided doses may be given for atypical pneumonia. Older children have been given 6 to 12 mg per kg body-weight daily in divided doses, but the effect of tetracyclines on teeth and bones should be considered.

Demeclocycline may be given to adults in the treatment of chronic hyponatraemia associated with the inappropriate secretion of antidiuretic hormone, when water restriction has proved ineffective. Initially demeclocycline hydrochloride 0.9 to 1.2 g is given daily in divided doses, reduced to maintenance doses of 0.6 to 0.9 g daily.

Like other tetracyclines, demeclocycline should be avoided in patients with renal impairment and doses reduced if it has to be given. Patients with liver disease should not receive more than 1 g daily.

The calcium and magnesium salts of demeclocycline are also used.

Syndrome of inappropriate ADH secretion (SIADH). Demeclocycline may be given in the treatment of the syndrome of inappropriate ADH (antidiuretic hormone) secretion (SIADH) (p.1241) to antagonise the effect of ADH on the renal tubules; lithium has been given as an alternative. Both lithium and demeclocycline act by interfering with the cellular action of ADH to produce nephrogenic diabetes insipidus. Since Forrest and colleagues[1] reported that demeclocycline was superior to lithium, demeclocycline became the preferred treatment for chronic SIADH if water restriction was unsuccessful,[2] although fluid restriction is probably still the treatment of choice. However, since nephrotoxicity has been reported in patients with cardiac or hepatic disease, its usefulness in the treatment of hyponatraemic states might be limited; this view was supported by studies in patients with heart failure[3] and cirrhosis.[4]

1. Forrest JN, *et al.* Superiority of demeclocycline over lithium in the treatment of chronic syndrome of inappropriate secretion of antidiuretic hormone. *N Engl J Med* 1978; **298:** 173–7.
2. Schrier RW. Treatment of hyponatremia. *N Engl J Med* 1985; **312:** 1121–2.
3. Zegers de Beyl D, *et al.* Demeclocycline treatment of water retention in congestive heart failure. *Br Med J* 1978; **1:** 760.
4. Miller PD, *et al.* Plasma demeclocycline levels and nephrotoxicity: correlation in hyponatremic cirrhotic patients. *JAMA* 1980; **243:** 2513–15.

Preparations

BP 1998: Demeclocycline Capsules;
USP 23: Demeclocycline Hydrochloride and Nystatin Capsules; Demeclocycline Hydrochloride and Nystatin Tablets; Demeclocycline Hydrochloride Capsules; Demeclocycline Hydrochloride Tablets; Demeclocycline Oral Suspension.

Proprietary Preparations (details are given in Part 3)
Aust.: Ledermycin; ***Austral.:*** Ledermycin; ***Belg.:*** Ledermycin; ***Canad.:*** Declomycin; ***Irl.:*** Ledermycin; ***Ital.:*** Bioterciclin†; Clortetrin†; Detravis†; Diuciclin†; Fidocin†; Ledermicina; ***Neth.:*** Ledermycin; ***S.Afr.:*** Ledermycin†; ***Spain:*** Provimicina†; ***UK:*** Ledermycin; ***USA:*** Declomycin.

Multi-ingredient: ***Aust.:*** Ledermix; ***Irl.:*** Deteclo; Ledermix; ***Ital.:*** Bioterciclin†; Deciclina†; Demebronc†; Rubrociclina; Varibiotic†; ***S.Afr.:*** Ledermix; Tritet; ***Spain:*** Varibiotic; ***Switz.:*** Ledermix; ***UK:*** Deteclo; Ledermix.

Dibekacin Sulphate (67-w)

Dibekacin Sulphate *(BANM, rINNM).*

3′,4′-Dideoxykanamycin B. 6-*O*-(3-Amino-3-deoxy-α-D-glucopyranosyl)-2-deoxy-4-*O*-(2,6-diamino-2,3,4,6-tetradeoxy-α-D-*erythro*-hexopyranosyl)-streptamine sulphate.

$C_{18}H_{37}N_5O_8,xH_2SO_4$ = 451.5 (dibekacin).

CAS — 34493-98-6 (dibekacin); 58580-55-5 (dibekacin sulphate).

Pharmacopoeias. In *Jpn.*

Dibekacin is an aminoglycoside derived from kanamycin with actions and uses similar to those of gentamicin (p.212). It has been given as the sulphate, intramuscularly or intravenously in doses of 1 to 3 mg of dibekacin per kg body-weight daily in divided doses; doses in the upper half of this range are mostly recommended in Europe while those in the lower half have been preferred in the Far East. Dosage should be adjusted based on serum-dibekacin concentration monitoring. It is also used topically for eye infections.

Preparations

Proprietary Preparations (details are given in Part 3)
Belg.: Dikacine; ***Fr.:*** Debekacyl; Icacine†; ***Ital.:*** Kappabi†; ***Jpn:*** Panimycin; ***Spain:*** Klobamicina†.

Dicloxacillin (14178-t)

Dicloxacillin *(BAN, USAN, rINN).*

BRL-1702; R-13423. (6*R*)-6-[3-(2,6-Dichlorophenyl)-5-methylisoxazole-4-carboxamido]penicillanic acid.

$C_{19}H_{17}Cl_2N_3O_5S$ = 470.3.

CAS — 3116-76-5.

Dicloxacillin Sodium (68-e)

Dicloxacillin Sodium *(BANM, USAN, rINNM)*.

Dicloxacilina Sódica; Dicloxacillinum Natricum; P-1011. Sodium dicloxacillin monohydrate.

$C_{19}H_{16}Cl_2N_3NaO_5S,H_2O = 510.3$.

CAS — 343-55-5 (dicloxacillin sodium, anhydrous); 13412-64-1 (dicloxacillin sodium, monohydrate).

Pharmacopoeias. In *Eur.* (see p.viii), *Int.*, *Jpn*, and *US*.

A white or almost white hygroscopic crystalline powder. 1.09 g of monograph substance is approximately equivalent to 1 g of anhydrous dicloxacillin. Each g of monograph substance represents approximately 2 mmol of sodium. Freely **soluble** in water; soluble in alcohol and in methyl alcohol. A 10% solution in water has a pH of 5.0 to 7.0 and a 1% solution in water has a pH of 4.5 to 7.5. **Store** at a temperature not exceeding 25° in airtight containers.

Adverse Effects and Precautions

As for Flucloxacillin, p.209.

Effects on the liver. References.

1. Kleinman MS, Presberg JE. Cholestatic hepatitis after dicloxacillin-sodium therapy. *J Clin Gastroenterol* 1986; **8:** 77–8.

Interactions

As for Benzylpenicillin, p.160.

Antimicrobial Action

As for Flucloxacillin, p.209.

Pharmacokinetics

Dicloxacillin, like flucloxacillin, is about twice as well absorbed from the gastro-intestinal tract as cloxacillin but absorption is also reduced by the presence of food in the stomach. After an oral dose of 500 mg, peak plasma concentrations of 10 to 18 µg per mL in about 1 hour have been reported in fasting subjects. Doubling the dose can double the plasma concentration. About 97% of dicloxacillin in the circulation is bound to plasma proteins. Dicloxacillin has been reported to have a plasma half-life of 0.5 to 1 hour. The half-life is prolonged in neonates.

The distribution of dicloxacillin in body tissues and fluids is similar to that of cloxacillin (p.195).

Dicloxacillin is metabolised to a limited extent and the unchanged drug and metabolites are excreted in the urine by glomerular filtration and renal tubular secretion. About 60% of a dose given by mouth is excreted in the urine. Only small amounts are excreted in the bile. Dicloxacillin is not removed by haemodialysis.

Plasma concentrations are enhanced if probenecid is given concomitantly. Reduced concentrations have been reported in patients with cystic fibrosis.

Uses and Administration

Dicloxacillin is an isoxazolyl penicillin used similarly to flucloxacillin (p.209) in the treatment of infections due to staphylococci resistant to benzylpenicillin.

It is administered by mouth, as the sodium salt, at least 1 hour before or 2 hours after meals since the presence of food in the stomach reduces absorption. Doses are expressed in terms of the equivalent amount of dicloxacillin. The usual dose is 125 to 250 mg of dicloxacillin every 6 hours. Children may be given 12.5 to 25 mg per kg body-weight daily in divided doses. Doses may be increased in severe infections. Dicloxacillin sodium has also been given parenterally.

Preparations

USP 23: Dicloxacillin Sodium Capsules; Dicloxacillin Sodium for Oral Suspension.

Proprietary Preparations (details are given in Part 3)
Austral.: Diclocil; Distaph; ***Belg.:*** Diclocil†; ***Fr.:*** Diclocil†; ***Ger.:*** Dichlor-Stapenor; ***Ital.:*** Diclo; Diclocillin†; Dicloxan†; Diflor†; Novapen†; ***Neth.:*** Diclocil†; ***Norw.:*** Diclocil; ***Swed.:*** Diclocil; ***USA:*** Dycill; Dynapen; Pathocil.

Multi-ingredient: ***Aust.:*** Totocillin†; ***Ger.:*** Totocillin†; ***Ital.:*** Ampiplus; Diamplicil; Dicil†; Duplamox†; Duplexcillina; Duplexil; Velamox D†.

Difloxacin (19232-m)

Difloxacin *(rINN)*.

A-56619 (difloxacin hydrochloride); Abbott-56619 (difloxacin hydrochloride). 6-Fluoro-1-(p-fluorophenyl)-1,4-dihydro-7-(4-methyl-1-piperazinyl)-4-oxo-3-quinolinecarboxylic acid.

$C_{21}H_{19}F_2N_3O_3 = 399.4$.

CAS — 98106-17-3 (difloxacin); 91296-86-5 (difloxacin hydrochloride).

NOTE. Difloxacin Hydrochloride is *USAN*.

Difloxacin is a fluoroquinolone antibacterial used, as the hydrochloride, in veterinary medicine. It was formerly used in humans but was associated with an unacceptably high incidence of adverse CNS effects.

Dihydrostreptomycin Sulphate (71-g)

Dihydrostreptomycin Sulphate *(BANM, rINNM)*.

Dihydrostreptomycini Sulfas. *O*-2-Deoxy-2-methylamino-α-L-glucopyranosyl-(1→2)-*O*-5-deoxy-3-*C*-hydroxymethyl-α-L-lyxofuranosyl-(1→4)-N^1,N^3-diamidino-D-streptamine sulphate.

$(C_{21}H_{41}N_7O_{12})_2,3H_2SO_4 = 1461.4$.

CAS — 128-46-1 (dihydrostreptomycin); 5490-27-7 (dihydrostreptomycin sulphate).

Pharmacopoeias. In *Eur.* (see p.viii). Also in *US* for veterinary use only.

A white or almost white powder; it may be hygroscopic. 1.25 g of monograph substance is approximately equivalent to 1 g of dihydrostreptomycin.

Freely **soluble** in water; practically insoluble in alcohol, acetone, chloroform, and methyl alcohol. A 25% solution in water has a pH of 5 to 7. **Store** at a temperature not exceeding 30° in airtight containers. Protect from light.

Dihydrostreptomycin is an aminoglycoside antibacterial with actions similar to those of streptomycin (p.249). Since it is more likely than streptomycin to cause partial or complete loss of hearing it is not used parenterally in humans, although it is used as the sulphate in veterinary medicine. As it is not absorbed following oral administration it has been given by this route for gastro-intestinal infections.

Preparations

Proprietary Preparations (details are given in Part 3)

Multi-ingredient: ***Fr.:*** Entercine†; ***Ger.:*** Penimycin†; ***Ital.:*** Diarstop†; ***Spain:*** Cilinafosal DHD Estrep; Citrocil; Cunticina Adultos†; Cunticina Infantil†; Enterowas†; Estreptoenterol; Estreptosirup†; Kolotanino†; Salitanol Estreptomicina; Sorbitoxin†; Sulfintestin Neomicina.

Dirithromycin (18782-h)

Dirithromycin *(BAN, USAN, rINN)*.

ASE-136BS; Dirithromycinum; LY-237216. (1*R*,2*R*,3*R*,6*R*,7*S*,8*S*,9*R*,10*R*,12*R*,13*S*,15*R*,17*S*)-7-(2,6-Dideoxy-3-*C*,3-*O*-dimethyl-α-L-*ribo*-hexopyranosyloxy)-3-ethyl-2,10-dihydroxy-15-(2-methoxyethoxymethyl)-2,6,8,10,12,17-hexamethyl-9-(3,4,6-trideoxy-3-dimethylamino-β-L-*xylo*-hexopyranosyloxy)-4,16-dioxa-14-azabicyclo[11.3.1]heptadecan-5-one; (9*S*)-9-Deoxo-11-deoxy-9,11-{imino[(1*R*)-2-(2-methoxyethoxy)-ethylidene]oxy} erythromycin.

$C_{42}H_{78}N_2O_{14} = 835.1$.

CAS — 62013-04-1.

Pharmacopoeias. In *Eur.* (see p.viii).

A white or almost white powder. It exhibits polymorphism. Very slightly **soluble** in water; very soluble in methyl alcohol and in dichloromethane.

Adverse Effects and Precautions

As for Erythromycin, p.204. Dirithromycin should be used with caution in patients with moderate to severe hepatic impairment since its metabolite erythromycylamine is primarily eliminated in the bile.

Interactions

For a discussion of drug interactions with macrolide antibacterials, see Erythromycin, p.205.

Antimicrobial Action

As for Erythromycin, p.205. Dirithromycin is reported to have little activity against some strains of *Haemophilus influenzae*.

References.

1. Counter FT, *et al.* Synthesis and antimicrobial evaluation of dirithromycin (AS-E 136; LY237216), a new macrolide antibiotic derived from erythromycin. *Antimicrob Agents Chemother* 1991; **335:** 1116–26.
2. Segreti J, Kapell KS. In vitro activity of dirithromycin against Chlamydia trachomatis. *Antimicrob Agents Chemother* 1994; **38:** 2213–14.
3. Kirst HA, *et al.* Antimicrobial characterization and interrelationships of dirithromycin and epidirithromycin. *Antimicrob Agents Chemother* 1995; **39:** 1436–41.

Pharmacokinetics

Dirithromycin is readily absorbed following oral administration and undergoes rapid non-enzymatic hydrolysis to erythromycylamine. Absorption is enhanced by food. Bioavailability is about 10%. Daily administration of dirithromycin 500 mg produces peak plasma concentrations of erythromycylamine of about 0.4 µg per mL.

Erythromycylamine is widely distributed and tissue concentrations exceed those in plasma. Protein binding is 15 to 30%. Erythromycylamine is mainly excreted unchanged in the bile with only about 2% in the urine. The mean plasma half-life is about 8 hours and the mean urinary terminal elimination half-life is about 44 hours.

References.

1. Sides GD, *et al.* Pharmacokinetics of dirithromycin. *J Antimicrob Chemother* 1993; **31** (suppl C): 65–75.
2. LaBreque D, *et al.* Pharmacokinetics of dirithromycin in patients with impaired hepatic function. *J Antimicrob Chemother* 1993; **32:** 741–50.

Uses and Administration

Dirithromycin is a prodrug of the macrolide antibiotic erythromycylamine, which has similar properties to those of erythromycin (p.204) and is used in pulmonary, skin, and soft tissue infections caused by susceptible organisms.

Dirithromycin is given by mouth in a usual dose of 500 mg once daily.

General references.

1. Various. Dirithromycin: a new once-daily macrolide. *J Antimicrob Chemother* 1993; **31** (suppl C): 1–185.
2. Brogden RN, Peters DH. Dirithromycin: a review of its antimicrobial activity, pharmacokinetic properties and therapeutic efficacy. *Drugs* 1994; **48:** 599–616.

Preparations

Proprietary Preparations (details are given in Part 3)
Aust.: Dimac; ***Belg.:*** Unibac; ***Fr.:*** Dynabac; ***Ital.:*** Dinabac; ***Spain:*** Balodin; Noriclan; Nortron; ***USA:*** Dynabac.

Doxycycline (72-q)

Doxycycline *(BAN, USAN, rINN)*.

Doxycycline Monohydrate; Doxycyclinum; GS-3065. (4*S*,4a*R*,5*S*,5a*R*,6*S*,12a*S*)-4-Dimethylamino-1,4,4a,5,5a,6,11,12a-octahydro-3,5,10,12,12a-pentahydroxy-6-methyl-1,11-dioxonaphthacene-2-carboxamide monohydrate; 6-Deoxy-5β-hydroxytetracycline monohydrate.

$C_{22}H_{24}N_2O_8,H_2O = 462.4$.

CAS — 564-25-0 (anhydrous doxycycline); 17086-28-1 (doxycycline monohydrate).

Pharmacopoeias. In *Eur.* (see p.viii) and *US*.

A yellow crystalline powder. Very slightly **soluble** in water; sparingly or very slightly soluble in alcohol; practically insoluble in chloroform and in ether; freely soluble in dilute acids and alkali hydroxides and carbonates. A 1% aqueous suspension has a pH of 5.0 to 6.5. **Store** in airtight containers. Protect from light.

Doxycycline Calcium (73-p)

Doxycycline Calcium *(BANM, rINNM)*.

A complex prepared from doxycycline hydrochloride and calcium chloride.

Doxycycline Fosfatex (18633-l)

Doxycycline Fosfatex *(BAN, USAN)*.

AB-08; DMSC. 6-Deoxy-5β-hydroxytetracycline—metaphosphoric acid—sodium metaphosphate in the ratio 3:3:1.

$(C_{22}H_{24}N_2O_8)_3(HPO_3)_3NaPO_3 = 1675.2$.

CAS — 83038-87-3.

Doxycycline Hydrochloride (74-s)

Doxycycline Hydrochloride *(BANM)*.

Doxycycline Hyclate *(rINNM)*; Dossiciclina Iclato; Doxycyclini Hyclas. Doxycycline hydrochloride hemiethanolate hemihydrate.

$C_{22}H_{24}N_2O_8,HCl,\frac{1}{2}C_2H_5OH,\frac{1}{2}H_2O = 512.9$.

CAS — 10592-13-9 ($C_{22}H_{24}N_2O_8,HCl$); 24390-14-5 ($C_{22}H_{24}N_2O_8,HCl,\frac{1}{2}C_2H_5OH,\frac{1}{2}H_2O$).

Pharmacopoeias. In *Chin.*, *Eur.* (see p.viii), *Int.*, *Jpn*, *Pol.*, and *US*.

A yellow hygroscopic crystalline powder. Doxycycline hydrochloride 115 mg is approximately equivalent to 100 mg of doxycycline. Ph. Eur. **solubilities** are: freely soluble in water and in methyl alcohol; sparingly soluble in alcohol; practically insoluble in ether; dissolves in solutions of alkali hydroxides and carbonates. USP solubilities are: soluble in water; slightly soluble in alcohol; practically insoluble in chloroform and in ether; soluble in solutions of alkali hydroxides and carbonates. A 1% solution in water has a pH of 2 to 3. **Store** in airtight containers. Protect from light.

Incompatibilities. Preparations of doxycycline hydrochloride have an acid pH and incompatibility may reasonably be expected with alkaline preparations or with drugs unstable at low pH. Reduced antimicrobial activity has been reported *in vitro* when doxycycline hydrochloride was mixed with riboflavine.

Adverse Effects and Precautions

As for Tetracycline Hydrochloride, p.259.

Gastro-intestinal disturbances are reported to be less frequent than with tetracycline and doxycycline may also cause less tooth discoloration.

Oesophageal ulceration may be a particular problem if capsules or tablets are taken with insufficient fluid or in a recumbent posture: doxycycline should be taken with at least half a glass of water, in an upright position, and one hour or more before retiring to bed. There is some evidence from studies in *animals* that preparations of the base, which have a higher pH, cause less oesophageal damage than those of the more acid hydrochloride. Dispersible tablets or liquid formulations should be used in elderly patients, who may be at greater risk of oesophageal injury.

Unlike many tetracyclines, doxycycline does not appear to accumulate in patients with impaired renal function, and aggravation of renal impairment may be less likely.

Anosmia. Anosmia or dysosmia (absent or impaired sense of smell) have occasionally been reported in patients receiving doxycycline, although the association has not been definitely established.[1]

1. Bleasel AF, *et al.* Anosmia after doxycycline use. *Med J Aust* 1990; **152:** 440.

Porphyria. For the suggestion that doxycycline might be porphyrinogenic, see under Tetracycline Hydrochloride, p.260.

Interactions

As for Tetracycline Hydrochloride, p.260.

Doxycycline has a lower affinity for binding with calcium than many tetracyclines. In consequence its absorption is less likely to be affected by milk or food, although it is still affected by antacids and iron preparations.

The metabolism of doxycycline may be accelerated by drugs that induce hepatic enzymes such as alcohol (chronic use); antiepileptics including carbamazepine, phenobarbitone, and phenytoin; and rifampicin. It has been suggested that doxycycline could increase cyclosporin concentrations, but evidence for this seems to be scant.

Antimicrobial Action

As for Tetracycline Hydrochloride, p.260. Doxycycline is more active than tetracycline against many bacterial species including the enterococci and various anaerobes. Cross-resistance is common although some tetracycline-resistant *Staphylococcus aureus* respond to doxycycline. Doxycycline is also reported to be more active against protozoa, particularly *Plasmodium* spp.

Pharmacokinetics

For the general pharmacokinetics of the tetracyclines, see Tetracycline Hydrochloride, p.260.

Doxycycline hydrochloride is readily and almost completely absorbed from the gastro-intestinal tract and absorption is not significantly affected by the presence of food in the stomach or duodenum. Mean peak plasma concentrations of 2.6 μg per mL have been reported 2 hours after a 200-mg dose by mouth, falling to 1.45 μg per mL at 24 hours. After intravenous infusion of the same dose peak plasma concentrations are briefly somewhat higher, but become very similar to those after oral administration following equilibration into the tissues.

From 80 to 95% of doxycycline in the circulation is reported to be bound to plasma proteins. Its biological half-life varies from about 12 to 24 hours. Doxycycline is more lipid-soluble than tetracycline. It is widely distributed in body tissues and fluids.

In patients with normal renal function about 40% of a dose is slowly excreted in the urine although more is excreted by this route if urine is made alkaline. However, the majority of a dose of doxycycline is excreted in the faeces following chelation in the intestines. Although doxycycline has been reported to undergo some inactivation in the liver, some sources consider this doubtful; however, the kinetics of doxycycline have been reportedly altered in patients receiving drugs which induce hepatic metabolism.

Doxycycline is stated not to accumulate significantly in patients with renal impairment although excretion in the urine is reduced; increased amounts of doxycycline are excreted in the faeces in these patients. Nevertheless there have been reports of some accumulation in renal failure. Removal of doxycycline by haemodialysis is insignificant.

Review.

1. Saivin S, Houin G. Clinical pharmacokinetics of doxycycline and minocycline. *Clin Pharmacokinet* 1988; **15:** 355–66.

Distribution. Concentrations of doxycycline in CSF of patients with neurological manifestations of Lyme disease receiving doxycycline 200 mg daily by mouth ranged from 0.4 to 2.5 μg per mL at 4 hours after a dose.[1] This represented 3 to 36% of the serum concentration at that time and was reported to be adequate for the treatment of the infection.

1. Karlsson M, *et al.* Concentrations of doxycycline and penicillin G in sera and cerebrospinal fluid of patients treated for neuroborreliosis. *Antimicrob Agents Chemother* 1996; **40:** 1104–7.

Uses and Administration

Doxycycline is a tetracycline derivative with uses similar to those of tetracycline (p.261). It may sometimes be preferred to other tetracyclines in the treatment of sensitive infections because of its fairly reliable absorption and its long half-life which permits less frequent (often once daily) dosage. It also has the advantage that it can be given (with care) to patients with renal insufficiency. However, relatively high doses may need to be given for urinary-tract infections because of its low renal excretion.

Doxycycline is normally administered by mouth as doxycycline or its various derivatives. Doses are expressed in terms of doxycycline. The usual dose is 200 mg of doxycycline on the first day (as a single dose or 100 mg repeated after 12 hours), followed by 100 mg daily. Older children weighing 45 kg or less may be given 4 mg per kg body-weight initially and thereafter 2 mg per kg daily but the effect of tetracyclines on teeth and bones should be considered. In severe infections the initial dosage is maintained throughout the course of treatment. In patients with sensitive gonococcal infections doxycycline has occasionally been given in a single dose of 300 mg, alone or followed by a second similar dose one hour later. For syphilis, doxycycline 200 or 300 mg is given daily for at least 15 or 10 days, respectively. In the treatment of acne a dose of 50 mg daily may be adequate. For relapsing fever and louse-borne typhus, doxycycline 100 or 200 mg may be given as a single dose. For prophylaxis of scrub typhus, 200 mg may be taken as a single dose.

Doxycycline capsules and tablets should be given with plenty of fluid, with the patient in an upright position, and well before retiring for the night. It may be given with food or milk if gastric irritation occurs. Dispersible tablets or liquid formulations are advisable in elderly patients.

In patients in whom oral therapy is not feasible doxycycline may be given, as the hydrochloride, by slow intravenous infusion of a solution containing 0.1 to 1 mg per mL, in doses equivalent to those by mouth. Infusions should be given over 1 to 4 hours.

Solutions of doxycycline are also used for treating malignant effusions (p.484).

Malaria. Doxycycline is used in some areas for the treatment of chloroquine-resistant falciparum malaria (p.422) in a dose of 200 mg daily for at least 7 days in combination with quinine. Doxycycline 100 mg daily has been used for prophylaxis in areas of high risk where other drugs are likely to be ineffective, but it is not suitable for extended prophylactic use.

Preparations

BP 1998: Doxycycline Capsules;
USP 23: Doxycycline Calcium Oral Suspension; Doxycycline Capsules; Doxycycline for Injection; Doxycycline for Oral Suspension; Doxycycline Hyclate Capsules; Doxycycline Hyclate Delayed-release Capsules; Doxycycline Hyclate Tablets.

Proprietary Preparations (details are given in Part 3)
Aust.: Biocyclin; Dotur; Doxybene; Doxyderm; Doxydyn; Doxylan; Gewacyclin†; Mundicycline; Sigadoxin; Supracyclin; Vibramycin; Vibravenos; ***Austral.:*** Doryx; Doxsig; Doxy; Doxylin; Vibra-Tabs; Vibramycin; Vizam; ***Belg.:*** Dagramycine; Doxyfim; Doxylets; Doxymycine†; Doxytab†; Logamicyl†; Roxyne†; Unidox; Vibracare; Vibramycine; Vibratab; ***Canad.:*** Apo-Doxy; Doryx; Doxycin; Doxytec; Novo-Doxylin; Vibra-Tabs; Vibramycin; ***Fr.:*** Doxy; Doxygram; Doxylets; Granudoxy; Monocline; Spanor; Tolexine; Vibramycine N; Vibraveineuse; ***Ger.:*** Azudoxat; Azudoxat-T†; Bactidox; Clinofug D; Doxakne; Doxy; Doxy Komb; Doxy M; Doxy Pohl†; Doxy S+K; Doxy-basan†; Doxy-Diolan; Doxy-HP; Doxy-N-Tablinen; Doxy-P; Doxy-Puren; Doxy-Tablinen; Doxy-Wolff; Doxybiocin†; Doxyderma; Doxyhexal; Doxymono; Doxyremed†; Doxytem; duradoxal; Ichthraletten Doxy†; Jenacyclin; Mespafin; Neodox; Nymix-cyclin N†; Remicyclin D†; Sigacyclat†; Sigadoxin; Supracyclin; Vibramycin; Vibravenos; ***Irl.:*** Vibramycin; ***Ital.:*** Abadox†; Bassado; Doxicento†; Doxifin†; Doxilen†; Doxina; Doxivis†; Esadoxi†; Farmodoxi†; Germiciclin†; Ghimadox†; Gram-Val; Iclados†; Minidox†; Miraclin; Monodoxin; Philcociclina†; Radox†; Samecin†; Semelciclina†; Stamicina†; Unacil; Ximicina†; ***Neth.:*** Dagracycline; Doxy-Dagra; Doxymycin†; Dumoxin†; Neo-Dagracycline; Unidox; Vibra-S; Vibramycin; ***Norw.:*** Doxylin; Dumoxin; Vibramycin; ***S.Afr.:*** Acne-Cy-Clean†; Bok-C-Lin†; Cyclidox; Doryx; Doxyclin†; Doxycyl; Doxylets†; Doxymycin†; Dumoxin; Viacin; Vibramycin; ***Spain:*** Clisemina; Docostyl; Dosil; Doxi Crisol; Doxi Sergo; Doxiclat; Doxinate; Doxiten; Doxiten Bio; Novelciclina; Retens; Solupen; Tetrasan; Vibracina; Vibravenosa; ***Swed.:*** Doryx; Doxyferm; Idocyklin†; Vibramycin; ***Switz.:*** Diocimex; Doxy-basan; Doxycline; Doxylag†; Doxysol; Helvedoclyn; Rudocycline; Servidoxyne†; Sigadoxin; Supracycline; Vibramycine; Vibraveineuse; Zadorine; ***UK:*** Cyclodox; Demix; Doxylar; Nordox†; Ramysis; Vibramycin; Vibramycin D; ***USA:*** Bio-Tab; Doryx; Doxy; Doxy-Tabs†; Doxychel; Monodox; Vibra-Tabs; Vibramycin.

Multi-ingredient: ***Aust.:*** Mucotectan; Vibrabron; ***Ger.:*** Ambrodoxy; Ambroxol AL comp; Ambroxol comp; Amdox-Puren; Azudoxat comp; Codidoxal†; Doxam; Doximucol; Doxy Comp; Doxy Lindoxyl; Doxy Plus; Doxy-duramucal; Doxy-Wolff Mucolyt; Doxysolvat; Eftapan Doxy†; Jenabroxol comp; Mibrox comp†; Mucotectan; Sagittamuc; Sigamuc; Terelit; Vibratussal†; ***Ital.:*** Ribociclina; ***Spain:*** Dosil Enzimatico; Doxiten Enzimatico; Duo Gobens; Pulmotropic; Solupen Enzimatico; Sorciclina.

Enoxacin (16623-k)

Enoxacin *(BAN, USAN, rINN)*.

AT-2266; CI-919; PD-107779. 1-Ethyl-6-fluoro-1,4-dihydro-4-oxo-7-(1-piperazinyl)-1,8-naphthyridine-3-carboxylic acid.

$C_{15}H_{17}FN_4O_3$ = 320.3.

CAS — 74011-58-8.

Pharmacopoeias. In *Jpn.*

Adverse Effects and Precautions

As for Ciprofloxacin, p.186.

Interactions

As for Ciprofloxacin, p.187.

Of the fluoroquinolones, enoxacin has been reported to cause the strongest interaction with theophylline (p.768) and with caffeine (p.750).

Antimicrobial Action

As for Ciprofloxacin, p.187, although enoxacin is less potent *in vitro*.

Pharmacokinetics

Peak plasma concentrations of 2 to 3 μg per mL are achieved 1 to 2 hours after a 400-mg dose of enoxacin by mouth. A plasma half-life of about 4 to 6 hours has been reported. In renal impairment the half-life of enoxacin may be prolonged and the oxometabolite may accumulate. Plasma protein binding has ranged from 18 to 57%. Enoxacin appears to be widely distributed in the body and concentrations higher than those in plasma have been reported in tissues such as lung, kidney, and prostate. High concentrations are achieved in bile, but the extent of biliary excretion is not completely clear.

Enoxacin is eliminated from the body mainly by urinary excretion, but also by metabolism. The major metabolite, 3-oxo-enoxacin, has some antibacterial activity. Urinary excretion of enoxacin is by both tubular secretion and glomerular filtration and may be reduced by probenecid. High concentrations are achieved in the urine since about 60% of an oral dose of enoxacin appears unchanged in the urine within 24 hours; about 10% is recovered as 3-oxo-enoxacin.

Uses and Administration

Enoxacin is a fluoroquinolone antibacterial with properties similar to those of ciprofloxacin (p.185) but it is generally less potent *in vitro*. It is used mainly in the treatment of urinary-tract infections (p.149) and gonorrhoea (p.126).

For urinary-tract infections enoxacin is given by mouth in doses of 200 to 400 mg twice daily. A single 400-mg dose may be given for uncomplicated gonorrhoea.

Half the usual dose is recommended in renal impairment when the creatinine clearance is 30 mL or less per minute.

References.

1. Henwood JM, Monk JP. Enoxacin: a review of its antibacterial activity, pharmacokinetic properties and therapeutic use. *Drugs* 1988; **36:** 32–66.
2. Jaber LA, *et al.* Enoxacin: a new fluoroquinolone. *Clin Pharm* 1989; **8:** 97–107.
3. Patel SS, Spencer CM. Enoxacin: a reappraisal of its clinical efficacy in the treatment of genitourinary tract infections. *Drugs* 1996; **51:** 137–60.

Preparations

Proprietary Preparations (details are given in Part 3)
Aust.: Gyramid; ***Austral.:*** Enoxin; ***Fr.:*** Enoxor; ***Ger.:*** Enoxor; Gyramid†; ***Ital.:*** Bactidan; Enoxen; ***Jpn:*** Flumark; ***S.Afr.:*** Bactidron; ***Spain:*** Almitil; ***UK:*** Comprecin†; ***USA:*** Penetrex.

Enrofloxacin (2489-h)

Enrofloxacin *(BAN, USAN, rINN).*

BAY-Vp-2674. 1-Cyclopropyl-7-(4-ethylpiperazin-1-yl)-6-fluoro-1,4-dihydro-4-oxoquinoline-3-carboxylic acid.

$C_{19}H_{22}FN_3O_3$ = 359.4.

CAS — 93106-60-6.

Enrofloxacin is a fluoroquinolone antibacterial that is used in veterinary practice.

Erythromycin (77-l)

Erythromycin *(BAN, rINN).*

Eritromicina; Erythromycinum. Erythromycin A is (2*R*,3*S*,4*S*,5*R*,6*R*,8*R*,10*R*,11*R*,12*S*,13*R*)-5-(3-amino-3,4,6-trideoxy-*N*,*N*-dimethyl-β-D-*xylo*-hexopyranosyloxy)-3-(2,6-dideoxy-3-*C*,3-*O*-dimethyl-α-L-*ribo*-hexopyranosyloxy)-13-ethyl-6,11,12-trihydroxy-2,4,6,8,10,12-hexamethyl-9-oxotridecan-13-olide.

$C_{37}H_{67}NO_{13}$ = 733.9.

CAS — 114-07-8.

Pharmacopoeias. In *Chin., Eur.* (see p.viii), *Int., Jpn, Pol.,* and *US.*

Erythromycin is produced by the growth of a strain of *Streptomyces erythreus* and is a mixture of macrolide antibiotics consisting largely of erythromycin A.

It occurs as white or slightly yellow, odourless or almost odourless, slightly hygroscopic crystals or powder. Slightly **soluble** in water but less soluble at higher temperatures; soluble to freely soluble in alcohol; soluble in chloroform, in ether, and in methyl alcohol. It dissolves in dilute hydrochloric acid. A 0.067% solution in water has a pH of 8.0 to 10.5. **Store** in airtight containers at a temperature not exceeding 30°. Protect from light.

Erythromycin Acistrate (2798-z)

Erythromycin Acistrate *(USAN, rINN).*

Acetylerythromycin Stearate. Erythromycin 2′-acetate stearate.

$C_{39}H_{69}NO_{14},C_{18}H_{36}O_2$ = 1060.4.

CAS — 96128-89-1.

Erythromycin Estolate (78-y)

Erythromycin Estolate *(BAN, USAN, rINNM).*

Erythromycin Propionate Lauryl Sulfate; Erythromycin Propionate Lauryl Sulphate; Erythromycini Estolas; Propionylerythromycin Lauryl Sulphate. Erythromycin 2′-propionate dodecyl sulphate.

$C_{40}H_{71}NO_{14},C_{12}H_{26}O_4S$ = 1056.4.

CAS — 3521-62-8.

Pharmacopoeias. In *Chin., Eur.* (see p.viii), *Pol.,* and *US.*

A white, odourless or almost odourless, crystalline powder. The Ph. Eur. specifies not less than 610 units per mg and the USP specifies a potency equivalent to not less than 600 μg of erythromycin per mg, both calculated on the anhydrous basis. 1.44 g of monograph substance is approximately equivalent to 1 g of erythromycin.

Practically **insoluble** in water; soluble to freely soluble in alcohol; soluble 1 in 10 of chloroform and 1 in 15 of acetone; practically insoluble in dilute hydrochloric acid. A saturated solution in water has a pH of 4.5 to 7.0. **Store** in airtight containers at a temperature not exceeding 30°. Protect from light.

Erythromycin Ethyl Succinate (80-q)

Erythromycin Ethyl Succinate *(BANM).*

Erythromycin Ethylsuccinate; Erythromycini Ethylsuccinas. Erythromycin 2′-(ethylsuccinate).

$C_{43}H_{75}NO_{16}$ = 862.1.

CAS — 41342-53-4.

NOTE. Compounded preparations of erythromycin ethyl succinate (erythromycin ethylsuccinate) and acetyl sulphafurazole (sulfisoxazole acetyl) in USP 23 may be represented by the name Co-erynsulfisox.

Pharmacopoeias. In *Chin., Eur.* (see p.viii), *Int., Jpn, Pol.,* and *US.*

A white or slightly yellow, odourless or almost odourless, hygroscopic crystalline powder. The Ph. Eur. specifies not less than 780 units per mg and the USP specifies a potency equivalent to not less than 765 μg of erythromycin per mg, both calculated on the anhydrous basis. 1.17 g of monograph substance is approximately equivalent to 1 g of erythromycin.

Practically **insoluble** or very slightly soluble in water; freely soluble in alcohol, dehydrated alcohol, acetone, chloroform, macrogol 400, and methyl alcohol. A 1% suspension in water has a pH of 6.0 to 8.5. **Store** in airtight containers at a temperature not exceeding 30°. Protect from light.

Erythromycin Gluceptate (81-p)

Erythromycin Gluceptate *(BANM, rINNM).*

Erythromycin glucoheptonate.

$C_{37}H_{67}NO_{13},C_7H_{14}O_8$ = 960.1.

CAS — 304-63-2; 23067-13-2.

Pharmacopoeias. In *US.*

A white, odourless or almost odourless, slightly hygroscopic powder. It has a potency equivalent to not less than 600 μg of erythromycin per mg calculated on the anhydrous basis. 1.3 g of monograph substance is approximately equivalent to 1 g of erythromycin.

Freely **soluble** in water, alcohol, and methyl alcohol; slightly soluble in acetone and chloroform; practically insoluble in ether. A 2.5% solution in water has a pH of 6 to 8.

Erythromycin Lactobionate (82-s)

Erythromycin Lactobionate *(BANM, rINNM).*

Erythromycini Lactobionas. Erythromycin mono(4-*O*-β-D-galactopyranosyl-D-gluconate).

$C_{37}H_{67}NO_{13},C_{12}H_{22}O_{12}$ = 1092.2.

CAS — 3847-29-8.

Pharmacopoeias. In *Chin., Eur.* (see p.viii), *Pol.,* and *US.*

White or slightly yellow hygroscopic powder. The USP specifies a potency equivalent to not less than 525 μg of erythromycin per mg, calculated on the anhydrous basis. 1.5 g of monograph substance is approximately equivalent to 1 g of erythromycin.

Soluble in water; freely soluble in dehydrated alcohol and in methyl alcohol; very slightly soluble in acetone and in dichloromethane; practically insoluble in ether. A 2 to 5% solution in water has a pH of 6.5 to 7.5. **Store** in an airtight container at a temperature not exceeding 25°.

Erythromycin Propionate (83-w)

Erythromycin Propionate *(BANM, USAN, rINNM).*

Erythromycin Propanoate; Propionylerythromycin. Erythromycin 2′-propionate.

$C_{40}H_{71}NO_{14}$ = 790.0.

CAS — 134-36-1.

Pharmacopoeias. In *Fr.*

1.08 g of monograph substance is approximately equivalent to 1 g of erythromycin.

Erythromycin Stearate (84-e)

Erythromycin Stearate *(BANM, rINNM).*

Erythromycini Stearas. Erythromycin octadecanoate.

$C_{37}H_{67}NO_{13},C_{18}H_{36}O_2$ = 1018.4.

CAS — 643-22-1.

Pharmacopoeias. In *Eur.* (see p.viii), *Int., Jpn, Pol.,* and *US.*

The stearate of erythromycin with some uncombined stearic acid.

White or slightly yellow crystals or powder, odourless or with a slight earthy odour. The Ph. Eur. specifies not less than 600 units per mg and the USP specifies a potency equivalent to not less than 550 μg of erythromycin per mg, both calculated on the anhydrous basis. 1.39 g of monograph substance is approximately equivalent to 1 g of erythromycin.

Practically **insoluble** in water; soluble in alcohol, dehydrated alcohol, acetone, chloroform, ether, and methyl alcohol. Solutions in acetone, dehydrated alcohol, chloroform, and methyl alcohol may be opalescent. A 1% aqueous suspension has a pH of 6 to 11. **Store** in airtight containers at a temperature below 30°. Protect from light.

Incompatibilities. The stability of erythromycin derivatives is dependent upon pH, with particularly rapid degradation occurring at a pH greater than 10 or less than 5.5. Incompatibility might reasonably be expected, therefore, when erythromycin preparations are mixed with drugs or preparations that have a highly acidic or alkaline pH. In practice, reports of incompatibility are not always consistent, and other factors such as the temperature and concentration of solutions, and the diluents used, may play a role.

Adverse Effects

Erythromycin and its salts and esters are generally well-tolerated and serious adverse effects are rare. Probably because of the stimulant activity of erythromycin on the gut gastro-intestinal disturbances such as abdominal discomfort and cramp, nausea, vomiting, and diarrhoea are fairly common after both oral and parenteral administration. Gastro-intestinal effects are dose-related and appear to be more common in young than in older subjects. Supra-infection with resistant organisms may occur and pseudomembranous colitis has been reported.

Hypersensitivity reactions appear to be uncommon, having been reported in about 0.5% of patients and include pruritus, urticaria and skin rash as well as occasional cases of anaphylaxis. Hypersensitivity or irritation may occur following topical application of erythromycin.

A hypersensitivity reaction may also be responsible for the hepatotoxicity sometimes reported in patients receiving erythromycin or its derivatives. Symptoms indicative of cholestasis, including upper abdominal pain (sometimes very severe), nausea and vomiting, abnormal liver function values, raised serum bilirubin and usually jaundice, may be accompanied by rash, fever, and eosinophilia. Symptoms usually occur initially in patients who have been receiving the drug for more than 10 days, although they may develop more quickly in patients given the drug in a previous course of treatment. Erythromycin may interfere with tests for serum aspartate aminotransferase (SGOT), which might make diagnosis of hepatotoxicity more difficult.

The majority of reports of liver dysfunction have been in patients receiving the estolate, and it has been suggested that the propionyl ester linkage is particularly associated with hepatotoxicity, but symptoms have been reported in patients receiving the base and most of the other derivatives, both by mouth and parenterally. Hepatic dysfunction seems to be rare in children. The effects of erythromycin on the liver are generally reversible on discontinuing treatment.

A generally reversible sensorineural deafness, sometimes with tinnitus, has been reported in patients receiving erythromycin and appears to be related to serum concentration, with an increased likelihood of such effects in patients given doses of 4 g or more daily of base or its equivalent, in those given intravenous therapy, and in those with renal or hepatic impairment.

Other adverse effects that have been reported in patients receiving erythromycin include agranulocytosis, arrhythmias, central neurotoxicity including psychotic reactions and nightmares, a myasthenia-like syndrome, and pancreatitis. Parenteral formulations of erythromycin are irritant and intravenous administration may produce thrombophlebitis, particularly at high doses. Intramuscular injection is generally avoided as it may produce severe pain.

General reviews.

1. Periti P, *et al.* Adverse effects of macrolide antibacterials. *Drug Safety* 1993; **9:** 346–64.

Effects on body temperature. A report of 2 cases of hypothermia associated with oral erythromycin in children.[1] Symptoms resolved on withdrawal of the medication. The children were cousins, perhaps indicating a genetic predisposition to the effect.

1. Hassel B. Hypothermia from erythromycin. *Ann Intern Med* 1991; **115:** 69–70.

Effects on the gastro-intestinal tract. Comparison in patients with upper respiratory-tract infections has suggested that erythromycin ethylsuccinate was associated with less abdominal pain than an equivalent dosage of erythromycin base;

the ethylsuccinate and acistrate did not differ in their gastro-intestinal tolerability.[1] Another study has indicated that there was no significant difference in gastro-intestinal symptoms between plain and enteric-coated formulations of erythromycin base.[2] Severe nausea and vomiting following rapid intravenous infusion of erythromycin lactobionate ceased in 2 patients converted to erythromycin base or ethylsuccinate by mouth, but the adverse effects with the lactobionate may have been due to the rate of administration, since in 2 further patients symptoms resolved when the lactobionate was given more slowly as a more dilute solution.[3]

For reference to the stimulant effects of erythromycin on the gastro-intestinal tract, see Decreased Gastro-intestinal Motility under Uses and Administration, below.

1. Saloranta P, *et al.* Erythromycin ethylsuccinate, base and acistrate in the treatment of upper respiratory tract infection: two comparative studies of tolerability. *J Antimicrob Chemother* 1989; **24:** 455–62.
2. Ellsworth AJ, *et al.* Prospective comparison of patient tolerance to enteric-coated vs non-enteric-coated erythromycin. *J Fam Pract* 1990; **31:** 265–70.
3. Seifert CF, *et al.* Intravenous erythromycin lactobionate-induced severe nausea and vomiting. *DICP Ann Pharmacother* 1989; **23:** 40–4.

Effects on the heart. References to prolongation of the QT interval and associated arrhythmias in patients receiving erythromycin intravenously.

1. McComb JM, *et al.* Recurrent ventricular tachycardia associated with QT prolongation after mitral valve replacement and its association with intravenous administration of erythromycin. *Am J Cardiol* 1984; **54:** 922–3.
2. Schoenenberger RA, *et al.* Association of intravenous erythromycin and potentially fatal ventricular tachycardia with Q-T prolongation (torsades de pointes). *Br Med J* 1990; **330:** 1375–6.
3. Nattel S, *et al.* Erythromycin-induced long QT syndrome: concordance with quinidine and underlying cellular electrophysiologic mechanism. *Am J Med* 1990; **89:** 235–8.
4. Gitler B, *et al.* Torsades de pointes induced by erythromycin. *Chest* 1994; **105:** 368–72.
5. Gouyon JB, *et al.* Cardiac toxicity of intravenous erythromycin lactobionate in preterm infants. *Pediatr Infect Dis J* 1994; **13:** 840–1.

Effects on the skin. A report of Stevens-Johnson syndrome possibly caused by erythromycin.[1]

1. Lestico MR, Smith AD. Stevens-Johnson syndrome following erythromycin administration. *Am J Health-Syst Pharm* 1995; **52:** 1805–7.

Overdosage. Acute pancreatitis was reported in a 12-year-old girl after ingestion of about 5 g of erythromycin base.[1]

1. Berger TM, *et al.* Acute pancreatitis in a 12-year-old girl after an erythromycin overdose. *Pediatrics* 1992; **90:** 624–6.

Precautions

Erythromycin and its derivatives should be avoided in those known to be hypersensitive to it, or in those who have previously developed liver disorders while receiving it. All forms of erythromycin should be used with care in patients with existing liver disease or hepatic impairment, and the estolate is best avoided in such patients. Repeated courses of the estolate or administration for longer than 10 days increase the risk of hepatotoxicity. It has been suggested that erythromycin should be used with care in patients with a history of arrhythmias or a prolonged QT interval.

Erythromycin may interfere with some diagnostic tests including measurements of urinary catecholamines and 17-hydroxycorticosteroids. The estolate has been associated with falsely-elevated serum aspartate aminotransferase (SGOT) values when measured colorimetrically, although genuine elevations of this enzyme, due to hepatotoxicity, also occur.

Erythromycin is irritant; solutions for parenteral administration should be suitably diluted and administered by intravenous infusion over up to 60 minutes to reduce the incidence of thrombophlebitis.

Porphyria. Erythromycin has been associated with acute attacks of porphyria and is considered unsafe in patients with acute porphyria.[1]

1. Moore MR, McColl KEL. *Porphyria: drug lists.* Glasgow: Porphyria Research Unit, University of Glasgow, 1991.

Pregnancy. Of 298 pregnant women who took erythromycin estolate, clindamycin, or placebo for 3 weeks or longer, about 14, 4, and 3% respectively had abnormally high serum aspartate aminotransferase (SGOT) values.[1] Erythromycin estolate should probably not be given to pregnant women.

1. McCormack WM, *et al.* Hepatotoxicity of erythromycin estolate during pregnancy. *Antimicrob Agents Chemother* 1977; **12:** 630–5.

Interactions

Erythromycin and other macrolides have the potential to interact with a large number of drugs through their action on hepatic cytochrome P450 isoenzymes, particularly CYP1A2 and CYP3A4. Macrolides inhibit drug metabolism by microsomal cytochromes by competitive inhibition and by the formation of inactive complexes. Such interactions can result in severe adverse effects, including ventricular arrhythmias with the non-sedative antihistamines astemizole and terfenadine and with the prokinetic drug cisapride. Enzyme inhibition is reported to be particularly pronounced with macrolides such as erythromycin and triacetyloleandomycin. Clarithromycin is less likely to inhibit the hepatic metabolism of other drugs, although those undergoing first-pass metabolism may still be affected. Other macrolides such as azithromycin and dirithromycin are reported to have little or no effect on hepatic cytochromes, and consequently may produce fewer interactions.

Other mechanisms by which macrolides cause interactions include suppression of the gastro-intestinal flora responsible for the intraluminal metabolism of digoxin and possibly oral contraceptives, and the stimulant effect of macrolides on gastro-intestinal motility which is believed to be responsible for the interaction between spiramycin and levodopa.

Cimetidine is one of the few drugs reported to affect erythromycin (see below).

The effect on antimicrobial action when erythromycin is given with other antimicrobials is discussed under Antimicrobial Action, below.

For reference to the effects of erythromycin and other macrolides on other drugs, see p.13 (alfentanil), p.1133 (bromocriptine), p.341 (carbamazepine), p.393 (colchicine), p.521 (cyclosporin), p.851 (digoxin), p.446 (dihydroergotamine), p.859 (disopyramide), p.446 (ergotamine), p.1275 (lovastatin), p.663 (midazolam and triazolam), p.354 (phenytoin), p.940 (quinidine), p.242 (rifabutin), p.563 (tacrolimus), p.418 (terfenadine), p.768 (theophylline), p.363 (valproate), p.966 (warfarin), and p.699 (zopiclone).

In the case of astemizole, cisapride, and terfenadine the Committee on Safety of Medicines (CSM) in the UK has warned that there is a risk of inducing ventricular arrhythmias if erythromycin, or possibly other macrolides, are given concomitantly.[1,2]

1. Committee on Safety of Medicines. Ventricular arrhythmias due to terfenadine and astemizole. *Current Problems 35* 1992.
2. Committee on Safety of Medicines/Medicines Control Agency. Cisapride (Prepulsid, Alimax): interactions with antifungals and antibiotics can lead to ventricular arrhythmias. *Current Problems* 1996; **22:** 1.

Cimetidine. The concomitant administration of cimetidine may increase plasma concentrations of erythromycin and was associated with deafness in one patient.[1]

1. Mogford N, *et al.* Erythromycin deafness and cimetidine treatment. *Br Med J* 1994; **309:** 1620.

Mechanism. In *rats* and humans, triacetyloleandomycin, and erythromycin and some of its derivatives, induce microsomal enzymes; the nitrosoalkane metabolites so formed produce stable inactive complexes with the iron of cytochrome P450. Eventually the oxidative metabolism of other drugs may be decreased. These effects are marked after administration of triacetyloleandomycin, moderate after erythromycin, small after oleandomycin, and absent or negligible after josamycin, midecamycin, or spiramycin.[1,2]

1. Pessayre D, *et al.* Drug interactions and hepatitis produced by some macrolide antibiotics. *J Antimicrob Chemother* 1985; **16** (suppl A): 181–94.
2. Periti P, *et al.* Pharmacokinetic drug interactions of macrolides. *Clin Pharmacokinet* 1992; **23:** 106–31.

Antimicrobial Action

Erythromycin is a macrolide antibiotic with a broad and essentially bacteriostatic action against many Gram-positive and to a lesser extent some Gram-negative bacteria, as well as other organisms including mycoplasmas, spirochaetes, chlamydias, and rickettsias.

Mechanism of action. Erythromycin and other macrolides bind reversibly to the 50S subunit of the ribosome, resulting in blockage of the transpeptidation or translocation reactions, inhibition of protein synthesis, and hence inhibition of cell growth. Its action is predominantly bacteriostatic, but high concentrations are slowly bactericidal against the more sensitive strains. Because of the ready penetration of macrolides into white blood cells and macrophages there has been some interest in their potential synergy with host defence mechanisms *in vivo*. Its actions are increased at moderately alkaline pH (up to about 8.5), particularly in Gram-negative species, probably because of the improved cellular penetration of the nonionised form of the drug.

Spectrum of activity. Erythromycin has a broad spectrum of activity. The following pathogenic organisms are usually sensitive to erythromycin (but see also Resistance, below).

Gram-positive cocci, particularly streptococci such as *Streptococcus pneumoniae* and *Str. pyogenes.* Most strains of *Staphylococcus aureus* remain susceptible, although resistance can emerge rapidly, and some enterococcal strains are also susceptible.

Many other Gram-positive organisms respond to erythromycin, including *Bacillus anthracis*, *Corynebacterium diphtheriae*, *Erysipelothrix rhusiopathiae*, and *Listeria monocytogenes*. Anaerobic *Clostridium* spp. are also usually susceptible, as is *Propionibacterium acnes*. *Nocardia* spp. vary in their susceptibility.

Gram-negative cocci including *Neisseria meningitidis* and *N. gonorrhoeae*, and *Moraxella (Branhamella) catarrhalis* are usually sensitive.

Other Gram-negative organisms vary in their susceptibility, but *Bordetella* spp., some *Brucella* strains, *Flavobacterium*, and *Legionella* spp. are usually susceptible. *Haemophilus ducreyi* is reportedly susceptible, but *H. influenzae* is somewhat less so. The Enterobacteriaceae are not susceptible in general, although some strains may respond at alkaline pH. *Helicobacter pylori* and most strains of *Campylobacter jejuni* are sensitive (about 10% of the latter are reported to be resistant).

Among the Gram-negative anaerobes more than half of all strains of *Bacteroides fragilis* and many *Fusobacterium* strains are resistant.

Other organisms usually sensitive to erythromycin include *Actinomyces*, *Chlamydia*, rickettsias, spirochaetes such as *Treponema pallidum* and *Borrelia burgdorferi*, some mycoplasmas (notably *Mycoplasma pneumoniae*) and some of the opportunistic mycobacteria: *Mycobacterium scrofulaceum* and *M. kansasii* are usually susceptible but *M. intracellulare* is often resistant and *M. fortuitum* usually so.

Fungi, yeasts, and viruses are resistant to erythromycin.

Minimum inhibitory concentrations (MICs) of erythromycin may be as little as 0.001 μg per mL for the most sensitive strains of *Str. pneumoniae* and *Mycoplasma pneumoniae* but MICs for these and other organisms most sensitive to erythromycin (such as *Str. pyogenes*, *Listeria*, the more sensitive strains of *Neisseria gonorrhoeae* and *Corynebacterium diphtheriae*, *Moraxella catarrhalis*, and *Bordetella pertussis*) range from about 0.01 to 0.25 μg per mL. Organisms with MICs up to about 0.5 μg per mL are considered sensitive, and those with MICs between about 0.5 and 2 μg per mL of moderate sensitivity.

Activity with other antimicrobials. As with other bacteriostatic antimicrobials, the possibility of an antagonistic effect if erythromycin is given with a bactericide exists, and some antagonism has been shown *in vitro* between erythromycin and various penicillins and cephalosporins or gentamicin. However, in practice the results of such concurrent use are complex, and depend on the organism; in some cases synergy has been seen. Because of the adjacency of their binding sites on the ribosome erythromycin may competitively inhibit the effects of chloramphenicol or lincosamides such as clindamycin. A synergistic effect has been seen when erythromycin was combined with a sulphonamide, notably against *Haemophilus influenzae*. Erythromycin has also been reported to enhance the antiplasmodial actions of chloroquine.

Resistance. Several mechanisms of acquired resistance to erythromycin have been reported of which the most common is a plasmid-mediated ability to methylate ribosomal RNA, resulting in decreased binding of the antimicrobial drug. This can result in cross-resistance between erythromycin, other macrolides, lincosamides, and streptogramin B because they share a common binding site on the ribosome and this pattern of resistance is referred to as the MLS_B phenotype. It is seen in staphylococci, and to a somewhat lesser extent in streptococci, as well as in a variety of other species including *Bacteroides fragilis*, *Clostridium perfringens*, *Corynebacterium diphtheriae*, *Listeria*, and *Legionella* spp.

Decreased binding of antimicrobial agent to the ribosome may also occur as a result of a chromosomal mutation, resulting in an alteration of the ribosomal proteins in the 50S subunit, which conveys one-step high-level erythromycin resistance. This form of resistance has been demonstrated in *Escherichia coli* and some strains of *Str. pyogenes*, and probably occurs in *Staphylococcus aureus*.

Other forms of erythromycin resistance may be due to the elaboration of a plasmid-determined erythromycin esterase which can inactivate the drug, or to decreased drug penetration. The latter may be partly responsible for the intrinsic resistance of Gram-negative bacteria like the Enterobacteriaceae, but has also been shown to be acquired as a plasmid-mediated determinant in some organisms; production of a protein which increases drug efflux from the cell is thought to explain the MS form of resistance in which organisms are resistant to 14-carbon ring macrolides and streptogramins but retain sensitivity to 16-carbon ring macrolides and lincosamides.

The incidence of resistance varies greatly with the area and the organism concerned, and although the emergence of resistance is rarely a problem in the short-term treatment of infection it is quite common in conditions requiring prolonged treatment, such as endocarditis due to *Staph. aureus*. The incidence of resistance in *Staph. aureus* has been reported to be about 30 to 40% among hospital isolates and 5 to 10% in general practice. The incidence of resistance in streptococci is generally lower but shows geographical variation and may be increasing in some countries including the UK. In addition, localised outbreaks of resistant strains may occur and produce a much higher incidence of resistance.

References to erythromycin resistance.

1. Eady EA, *et al.* Multiple mechanisms of erythromycin resistance. *J Antimicrob Chemother* 1990; **26:** 461–5.
2. Seppälä H, *et al.* Resistance to erythromycin in group A streptococci. *N Engl J Med* 1992; **326:** 292–7.
3. Lonks JR, Medeiros AA. High rate of erythromycin and clarithromycin resistance among Streptococcus pneumoniae isolates from blood cultures from Providence, RI. *Antimicrob Agents Chemother* 1993; **37:** 1742–5.
4. Soriano F, Fernández-Roblas R. High rates of erythromycin-resistance Streptococcus pneumoniae among penicillin-resistant strains. *J Antimicrob Chemother* 1993; **31:** 440.
5. Sutcliffe J, *et al.* Streptococcus pneumoniae and Streptococcus pyogenes resistant to macrolides but sensitive to clindamycin: a common resistance pattern mediated by an efflux system. *Antimicrob Agents Chemother* 1996; **40:** 1817–24.
6. Eady EA, *et al.* Antibiotic resistant propionibacteria in acne: need for policies to modify antibiotic usage. *Br Med J* 1993; **306:** 555–6.
7. Barry AL, *et al.* Macrolide resistance among Streptococcus pneumoniae and Streptococcus pyogenes isolated from out-patients in the USA. *J Antimicrob Chemother* 1997; **40:** 139–40.

Pharmacokinetics

Erythromycin base is unstable in gastric acid, and absorption is therefore variable and unreliable. In consequence, the base is usually administered in film- or enteric-coated preparations, or one of the more acid-stable salts or esters is employed. Food may reduce the absorption of the base or the stearate, although this depends to some extent on the formulation, but the esters are generally more reliably and quickly absorbed and their absorption is little affected by food, obviating any need to take them before food.

Peak plasma concentrations generally occur between 1 and 4 hours after administration, and have been reported to range between about 0.3 and 0.5 μg per mL after 250 mg of erythromycin base, and from 0.3 to 1.9 μg per mL after 500 mg. Similar concentrations have been seen after equivalent doses of the stearate. Somewhat higher peak concentrations may be achieved on repeated administration four times daily. Higher total concentrations are achieved after oral administration of the acistrate, estolate, or ethyl succinate, but only about 20 to 35% of acistrate or estolate, or 55% of ethyl succinate is present as the active base, the rest being present as the ester (in the case of the estolate, as the propionate). Peak concentrations of about 0.5 μg per mL of erythromycin base have been reported following 250 mg of the acistrate or estolate, or 500 mg of the ethyl succinate. A peak of 3 to 4 μg per mL can be achieved after intravenous administration of 200 mg of gluceptate or lactobionate.

Erythromycin is widely distributed throughout body tissues and fluids, although it does not cross the blood-brain barrier well and concentrations in CSF are low. Relatively high concentrations are found in the liver and spleen, and some is taken up into polymorphonuclear lymphocytes and macrophages. Around 70 to 75% of the base is protein bound, but after administration as the estolate the propionate ester is stated to be about 95% protein bound. Erythromycin crosses the placenta: fetal plasma concentrations are variously stated to be 5 to 20% of those in the mother. It is distributed into breast milk.

Erythromycin is excreted in high concentrations in the bile and 2 to 5% of an oral dose is excreted in the urine. As much as 12 to 15% of an intravenous dose may be excreted by the urinary route. Some erythromycin is demethylated in the liver but its metabolic fate has not been completely determined. The half-life of erythromycin is usually reported to be roughly in the range 1.5 to 2.5 hours, although this may be somewhat longer in patients with renal impairment.

Uses and Administration

Erythromycin is a macrolide antibiotic with a wide spectrum of activity, that has been used in the treatment of a wide variety of infections caused by susceptible organisms (see Antimicrobial Action, above).

Its uses have included bronchitis, severe campylobacter enteritis, chancroid, diphtheria, legionnaire's disease and other *Legionella* infections, neonatal conjunctivitis, pertussis, pneumonia (mycoplasmal and other atypical pneumonias as well as streptococcal), sinusitis, and trench fever, and, combined with neomycin, for the prophylaxis of surgical infection in patients undergoing bowel surgery.

Erythromycin is used as an alternative to penicillin in penicillin-allergic patients with various conditions including anthrax, actinomycosis, the prophylaxis of endocarditis (although no longer recommended for this in the UK), leptospirosis, listeriosis, otitis media (usually with a sulphonamide such as sulphafurazole), pharyngitis, the prevention of perinatal streptococcal infections, rheumatic fever, and infections in splenectomised patients, and staphylococcal and streptococcal skin infections. It has also been used in the treatment of penicillin-allergic patients with syphilis, but there are doubts about its efficacy. In penicillin-allergic patients in the early stages of Lyme disease erythromycin may be employed as an alternative to a tetracycline. It is also used as an alternative to the tetracyclines in patients with chlamydial infections (such as epididymitis, lymphogranuloma venereum, nongonococcal urethritis, chlamydial pneumonia, pelvic inflammatory disease, psittacosis, and trachoma), and in Q fever.

For details of all these infections and their treatment, see under Choice of Antibacterial, p.116.

Both oral and topical erythromycin may be employed in acne (see Skin Disorders, below).

Administration and dosage. Erythromycin may be given as the base or its salts or esters; doses are expressed in terms of the base. The usual oral dose is the equivalent of erythromycin 1 to 2 g daily in 2 to 4 divided doses; for severe infections this may be increased to up to 4 g daily in divided doses. A maximum of 1.5 g daily has been suggested for patients with severe renal impairment. For children the dose is usually about 30 to 50 mg per kg body-weight daily although it may be doubled in severe infections; a recommended dose for children aged 2 to 8 years is 1 g daily in divided doses, and for infants and children up to 2 years of age, 500 mg daily in divided doses.

In the patient who is unable to take erythromycin by mouth and in severely ill patients in whom it is necessary to attain an immediate high blood concentration, erythromycin may be given intravenously in the form of one of its more soluble salts such as the gluceptate or the lactobionate, in doses equivalent to those by mouth.

To reduce the risk of venous irritation it should be administered only by continuous or intermittent intravenous infusion of a solution containing not more than 0.5% of erythromycin. Intermittent infusions should be given every 6 hours over 20 to 60 minutes.

For the preparation of solutions of erythromycin gluceptate or lactobionate for infusion, a primary solution containing not more than 5% of erythromycin should be prepared with water. Sodium chloride or other inorganic salt solution should not be used in preparing the primary solution. It should be further diluted before intravenous administration with 0.9% sodium chloride or other suitable intravenous fluid. Acidic solutions, such as glucose, should only be used if buffered with sodium bicarbonate.

Other routes. Erythromycin was formerly given by intramuscular injection, but such injections are painful and are no longer generally recommended. Erythromycin is used as a 0.5 to 1% ophthalmic ointment for the treatment and prophylaxis of infections of the eye, particularly of neonatal conjunctivitis. It may also be applied topically as a 2 or 4% solution for the treatment of acne vulgaris.

Propionyl erythromycin mercaptosuccinate is also used. Erythromycin salnacedin, a prodrug of erythromycin, acetylcysteine, and salicylic acid, is under investigation for the treatment acne. Erythromycin thiocyanate and erythromycin phosphate are used in veterinary medicine.

Administration. A discussion of the significance of different formulations and salts used for oral preparations of erythromycin concluded that there was no clear evidence that any was superior in terms of clinical effect.[1]

1. Anonymous. Giving erythromycin by mouth. *Drug Ther Bull* 1995; **33:** 77–9.

Decreased gastro-intestinal motility. Erythromycin stimulates gut motility, apparently by acting as a motilin receptor agonist although it has been suggested that it may have other actions as well.[1] It has been tried, with some success, for its prokinetic action in a small number of patients with decreased gastro-intestinal motility (p.1168) including those with gastroparesis,[2-5] reflux ileus,[6] acute colonic pseudo-obstruction (Ogilvie's syndrome),[6,7] delayed gastric emptying following pancreatic-duodenal surgery,[8] and neonatal postoperative intestinal dysmotility.[9] However, side-effects associated with the long-term use of erythromycin necessary in, for example, diabetic gastroparesis, may be problematic.[10]

1. Catnach SM, Fairclough PD. Erythromycin and the gut. *Gut* 1992; **33:** 397–401.
2. Janssens J, *et al.* Improvement of gastric emptying in diabetic gastroparesis by erythromycin: preliminary studies. *N Engl J Med* 1990; **322:** 1028–31.

3. Dull JS, *et al.* Successful treatment of gastroparesis with erythromycin in a patient with progressive systemic sclerosis. *Am J Med* 1990; **89:** 528–30.
4. Wadhwa NK, *et al.* Intraperitoneal erythromycin for gastroparesis. *Ann Intern Med* 1991; **114:** 912.
5. Richards RD, *et al.* The treatment of idiopathic and diabetic gastroparesis with acute intravenous and chronic oral erythromycin. *Am J Gastroenterol* 1993; **88:** 203–7.
6. Armstrong DN, *et al.* Erythromycin for reflux ileus in Ogilvie's syndrome. *Lancet* 1991; **337:** 378.
7. Bonacini M, *et al.* Erythromycin as therapy for acute colonic pseudo-obstruction (Ogilvie's syndrome). *J Clin Gastroenterol* 1991; **13:** 475–6.
8. Yeo CJ, *et al.* Erythromycin accelerates gastric emptying after pancreaticoduodenectomy: a prospective, randomized, placebo-controlled trial. *Ann Surg* 1993; **218:** 229–38.
9. Simkiss DE, *et al.* Erythromycin in neonatal postoperative intestinal dysmotility. *Arch Dis Child* 1994; **71:** F128–9.
10. Tanis AA, *et al.* Side-effects of oral erythromycin for treatment of diabetic gastroparesis. *Lancet* 1993; **342:** 1431.

Skin disorders. ACNE. Erythromycin may be used topically or orally in the treatment of acne (p.1072). Oral erythromycin may be used as an alternative to a tetracycline in moderate acne. Topical erythromycin may be used as first-line treatment for mild acne and as adjunctive treatment in more severe acne. Erythromycin is also available as a complex with zinc (as the acetate) that has been reported to be more effective than topical erythromycin alone[1] or oral minocycline.[2] However, development of antibiotic resistance by the skin flora may be a problem. Combination therapy with benzoyl peroxide and erythromycin has been reported to be helpful in preventing the selection of antibiotic-resistant mutants[3,4] and to be more effective than topical clindamycin alone.[5] It has also been recommended that courses of topical antibiotics be restricted to 10 to 12 weeks, repeated if necessary after a few weeks, and that concomitant treatment with different oral and topical antibiotics or antibiotic rotation be avoided.[6]

1. Habbema L, *et al.* A 4% erythromycin and zinc combination (Zineryt®) versus 2% erythromycin (Eryderm®) in acne vulgaris: a randomized, double-blind comparative study. *Br J Dermatol* 1989; **121:** 497–502.
2. Stainforth J, *et al.* A single-blind comparison of topical erythromycin/zinc lotion and oral minocycline in the treatment of acne vulgaris. *J Dermatol Treat* 1993; **4:** 119–22.
3. Eady EA, *et al.* Effects of benzoyl peroxide and erythromycin alone and in combination against antibiotic-sensitive and -resistant skin bacteria from acne patients. *Br J Dermatol* 1994; **131:** 331–6.
4. Eady EA, *et al.* The effects of acne treatment with a combination of benzoyl peroxide and erythromycin on skin carriage of erythromycin-resistant propionibacteria. *Br J Dermatol* 1996; **134:** 107–13.
5. Packman AM, *et al.* Treatment of acne vulgaris: combination of 3% erythromycin and 5% benzoyl peroxide in a gel compared to clindamycin phosphate lotion. *Int J Dermatol* 1996; **35:** 209–11.
6. Eady EA, *et al.* Antibiotic resistant propionibacteria in acne: need for policies to modify antibiotic usage. *Br Med J* 1993; **306:** 555–6.

Preparations

BP 1998: Erythromycin Estolate Capsules; Erythromycin Ethyl Succinate Oral Suspension; Erythromycin Ethyl Succinate Tablets; Erythromycin Lactobionate Intravenous Infusion; Erythromycin Stearate Tablets; Erythromycin Tablets;
USP 23: Erythromycin and Benzoyl Peroxide Topical Gel; Erythromycin Delayed-release Capsules; Erythromycin Delayed-release Tablets; Erythromycin Estolate and Sulfisoxazole Acetyl Oral Suspension; Erythromycin Estolate Capsules; Erythromycin Estolate for Oral Suspension; Erythromycin Estolate Oral Suspension; Erythromycin Estolate Tablets; Erythromycin Ethylsuccinate and Sulfisoxazole Acetyl for Oral Suspension; Erythromycin Ethylsuccinate for Oral Suspension; Erythromycin Ethylsuccinate Injection; Erythromycin Ethylsuccinate Oral Suspension; Erythromycin Ethylsuccinate Tablets; Erythromycin Lactobionate for Injection; Erythromycin Ointment; Erythromycin Ophthalmic Ointment; Erythromycin Pledgets; Erythromycin Stearate Tablets; Erythromycin Tablets; Erythromycin Topical Gel; Erythromycin Topical Solution; Sterile Erythromycin Ethylsuccinate; Sterile Erythromycin Gluceptate; Sterile Erythromycin Lactobionate.

Proprietary Preparations (details are given in Part 3)
Aust.: Akne; Aknemycin; Emuvin; Ery-Maxin; Eryaknen; Erybesan; Erycinum; Erysolvan; Erythrocin; Ilosone; Meromycin; Monomycin; Stiemycine; ***Austral.:*** E-Mycin; EES; Emu-V; Eryacne; Eryc; Erythrocin; Ilosone; ***Belg.:*** Acneryne; Aknemycin; Eryderm; Erythrocine; Erythroforte; Ilosone†; Inderm; Macromycine†; ***Canad.:*** Diomycin; E-Mycin; EES; Erybid; Eryc; Eryped†; Erysol; Erythrocin; Erythromid†; Ilosone; Ilotycin; Novo-Rythro; PCE; Staticin; T-Stat; ***Fr.:*** Abboticine; Biolid†; Egery; Ery; Erycocci; Eryfluid; Erythrophar†; Erythrocine; Erythrogel; Erythrogram; Logecine; Propiocine; Stimycine; ***Ger.:*** Akne Cordes; Aknederm Ery; Aknefug-EL; aknemago; Aknemycin; Aknin; Bisolvonat Mono; Clinofug Gel; duraerythromycin; durapaediat; Ery-Diolan; Ery-Reu; Eryaknen; Erybeta; Erycinum; Erydermec; Eryhexal; Erysec; Erythro; erythro-basan†; Erythro-Hefa; Erythrocin; Erythrocin Neo; Erythrogenat; Erytop; Eupragin; Inderm; Infectomycin; Lederpaediat; Medismon; Monomycin; Paediathrocin; Pharyngocin†; Praecimycin†; Sanasepton; Semibiocin†; Sigapedil†; Skid E; Stiemycine; Togiren†; Udima Ery; ***Irl.:*** Erycen†; Erymax; Erythrocin; Erythromid; Erythroped; Ilosone; Primacine; Stiemycin; Tiprocin; ***Ital.:*** Eritrobios†; Eritrocina; Eritrocist; Erytrociclin; Ilosone; Lauromicina; Marocid†; Proterytrin†; Rossomicina†; Roxochemil†; Stellamicina; Zalig; ***Neth.:*** Aknemycin; Eryacne; Eryc; Eryderm; Erythrocine; Inderm; Stiemycin; ***Norw.:*** Abboticin; Ery-Max; ***S.Afr.:*** Acu-Erylate S; Arcanamycin; Betamycin; E-Mycin; Emu-K†; Emu-V; Eromel; Eromel-S; Erycette; Eryderm; Erymax; Erymin S†; Erymycin; Erystat; Erythrocin; Erythromid; Erythroped; Estomycin; Ethimycin†; Ilosone; Ilotycin; Infectocin†; Macrolate†; Purmycin; Rubimycin†; Ryped; Spectrasone; Stiemycin; Succilate; Succin; Xeramel; ***Spain:*** Bio Exazol; Bronsema; Deripil; Doranol†; Eridosis; Eriprodin†; Eritrogobens; Eritroveinte; Ery-Max; Euskin; Iloticina Anti Acne†; Iloticina†; Lagarmicin; Lederpax; Liferitin†; Loderm; Neo Iloticina; Pantodrin; Pantomicina; Taleilcina†; Tolerabiotico†; ***Swed.:*** Abboticin; Ery-Max; ***Switz.:*** Aknemycin; Aknilox; Cimetrin; Erios; Eritrolag†; Ery; Eryaknen; Eryderm; Erymax†; Erythrocine; Erytran; Helvemycin; Ilosone†; Ilotycin; Inderm; Monomycine; Pharmatrocin†; Propiocine†; Servitrocin; Staticine; ***UK:*** Arpimycin; Eryacne; Erycen; Erymax; Erymin; Erythrocin; Erythromid; Erythroped; Ilosone; Retcin; Rommix; Ronmix; Stiemycin; Tiloryth; ***USA:*** Ak-Mycin; Aknemycin; ATS; Del-Mycin; E-Base; E-Mycin; E/Gel; EES; Emgel; Eramycin; Ery-sol†; Ery-Tab; Eryc; Erycette; Eryderm; Erygel; Erymax; Eryped; Erythra-Derm; Erythrocin; ETS†; Ilosone; Ilotycin; PCE; Robimycin Robitabs; Romycin†; Staticin; T-Stat; Theramycin Z; Wyamycin†.

Multi-ingredient: ***Aust.:*** Aknemycin compositum; AKZ; ***Belg.:*** Benzamycin; Zineryt; ***Canad.:*** Pediazole; Sans-Acne; Stievamycin; ***Fr.:*** Antibio-Aberel; Pediazole; ***Ger.:*** Aknemycin; Bisolvonat; Clinesfar; Ecolicin; Synergomycin; Zineryt; ***Irl.:*** Benzamycin; Zineryt; ***Ital.:*** Lauromicina; Mucolysin Antibiotico†; Rubrociclina; Zineryt; ***Neth.:*** Zineryt; ***S.Afr.:*** Benzamycine; Pediazole; ***Spain:*** Albiron†; Bio Exazol Balsamico†; Broncoliticì†; Bronsema Balsamico; Erifoscin; Tododermil Compuesto; Tosdiazina; ***Switz.:*** Aknemycin; AKZ; Pediazole; Stiemycine; ***UK:*** Benzamycin; Isotrexin; Zineryt; ***USA:*** Benzamycin; Eryzole; ESP†; Pediazole.

Ethambutol Hydrochloride (7556-j)

Ethambutol Hydrochloride (*BANM, USAN, rINNM*).

CL-40881; Ethambutoli Hydrochloridum. (*S,S*)-*N,N'*-Ethylenebis(2-aminobutan-1-ol) dihydrochloride.

$C_{10}H_{24}N_2O_2$,2HCl = 277.2.

CAS — 74-55-5 (ethambutol); 1070-11-7 (ethambutol hydrochloride).

Pharmacopoeias. In *Chin., Eur.* (see p.viii), *Int., Jpn, Pol.,* and *US.*

A white, odourless or almost odourless crystalline powder. Freely **soluble** in water; soluble in alcohol and in methyl alcohol; slightly soluble in chloroform; slightly or very slightly soluble in ether. A 2% solution in water has a pH of 3.7 to 4.0. **Store** in airtight containers.

Adverse Effects and Treatment

The most important adverse effect of ethambutol is retrobulbar neuritis with a reduction in visual acuity, constriction of visual field, central or peripheral scotoma, and green-red colour blindness. One or both eyes may be affected. The degree of visual impairment appears to depend on the dose and duration of therapy; toxicity is observed most frequently at daily doses of 25 mg per kg body-weight and after 2 months of therapy. Recovery of vision usually takes place over a period of a few weeks or months but in rare cases it may take up to one year or more or the effect may be permanent. Retinal haemorrhage has occurred rarely.

Renal clearance of urate may be reduced and acute gout has been precipitated rarely.

Hypersensitivity reactions including skin rashes, pruritus, leucopenia, fever, and joint pains appear to be rare with ethambutol. Other adverse effects which have been reported include confusion, disorientation, hallucinations, headache, dizziness, malaise, jaundice or transient liver dysfunction, peripheral neuritis, thrombocytopenia, and gastrointestinal disturbances such as nausea, vomiting, anorexia, and abdominal pain.

Teratogenicity has been observed in *animals.*

Blood concentrations of ethambutol following overdosage may be reduced by haemodialysis or peritoneal dialysis.

Effects on the blood. Neutropenia has been reported in a patient on ethambutol, isoniazid, and rifampicin.[1] Each drug induced neutropenia individually on rechallenge. Thrombocytopenia attributable to ethambutol has been reported in 2 patients.[2,3]

1. Jenkins PF, *et al.* Neutropenia with each standard antituberculosis drug in the same patients. *Br Med J* 1980; **280:** 1069–70.
2. Rabinovitz M, *et al.* Ethambutol-induced thrombocytopenia. *Chest* 1982; **81:** 765–6.
3. Prasad R, Mukerji PK. Ethambutol-induced thrombocytopaenia. *Tubercle* 1989; **70:** 211–12.

Effects on the eyes. In a discussion of ethambutol's ocular toxicity Citron and Thomas[1] reported that ophthalmic effects were found in 10 of 2184 patients receiving ethambutol in doses of 25 mg or less per kg body-weight daily, although few of the 10 patients complained of symptoms. In 9 of the 10 patients, ocular changes occurred after the second month of treatment. In the 928 patients who only received 2 months of ethambutol therapy, ocular toxicity was not reported. While short-term use of ethambutol is usually safe, deterioration of vision leading to long-term blindness has been reported after only a few doses of ethambutol;[2] it was suspected that this was an idiosyncratic reaction. Rapid onset reversible ocular toxicity has also occurred.[3] Visual defects occurring with ethambutol generally resolve when the drug is discontinued; for long-term visual loss hydroxocobalamin or cyanocobalamin[2,4,5] have been used with varying success.

1. Citron KM, Thomas GO. Ocular toxicity from ethambutol. *Thorax* 1986; **41:** 737–9.
2. Karnik AM, *et al.* A case of ocular toxicity to ethambutol—an idiosyncratic reaction? *Postgrad Med J* 1985; **61:** 811–13.
3. Schild HS, Fox BC. Rapid-onset reversible ocular toxicity from ethambutol therapy. *Am J Med* 1991; **90:** 404–6.
4. Harada T, *et al.* Ocular toxicity with ethambutol. *Jpn J Clin Ophthalmol* 1979; **33:** 1345–55.
5. Guerra R, Casu L. Hydroxycobalamin for ethambutol-induced optic neuropathy. *Lancet* 1981; **ii:** 1176.

Effects on the kidneys. Interstitial nephritis has been reported in 5 patients on ethambutol and isoniazid.[1,2] Three patients were also receiving additional antimycobacterials.

1. Collier J, *et al.* Two cases of ethambutol nephrotoxicity. *Br Med J* 1976; **2:** 1105–6.
2. Stone WJ, *et al.* Acute diffuse interstitial nephritis related to chemotherapy of tuberculosis. *Antimicrob Agents Chemother* 1976; **10:** 164–72.

Effects on the liver. Although transient abnormalities in liver function commonly occur during the early stages of antituberculosis treatment, drugs other than ethambutol are generally considered responsible. Ethambutol has generated fewer reports of hepatotoxicity to the Committee on Safety of Medicines in the UK than rifampicin, isoniazid, or pyrazinamide,[1] and the use of regimens containing ethambutol has been recommended for patients unable to tolerate standard regimens due to hepatotoxicity.[1-3]

1. Ormerod LP, *et al.* Hepatotoxicity of antituberculosis drugs. *Thorax* 1996; **51:** 111–13.
2. Ormerod LP. Chemotherapy and management of tuberculosis in the United Kingdom: recommendations of the Joint Tuberculosis Committee of the British Thoracic Society. *Thorax* 1990; **45:** 403–8.
3. WHO. *TB/HIV: a clinical manual.* Geneva: WHO, 1996.

Effects on the skin. Details of one patient in whom toxic epidermal necrolysis was associated with the use of ethambutol.[1] The manufacturer notes that isolated cases of photosensitive lichenoid eruptions, Stevens-Johnson syndrome, and bullous dermatitis have also occurred.

1. Pegram PS, *et al.* Ethambutol-induced toxic epidermal necrolysis. *Arch Intern Med* 1981; **141:** 1677–8.

Hyperuricaemia. In a controlled study of 71 patients receiving ethambutol 20 mg per kg body-weight daily by mouth with other antimycobacterials, serum-uric acid concentrations increased in 66, mainly in the first 2 weeks of treatment.[1] One patient experienced arthralgia and another acute gouty arthritis. Serum-uric acid concentrations did not change in 60 control patients receiving other antimycobacterials.

1. Khanna BK, Gupta VP. Ethambutol-induced hyperuricaemia. *Tubercle* 1984; **65:** 195–9.

Precautions

Ethambutol is generally contra-indicated in patients with optic neuritis. It should be given in reduced dosage to patients with impaired kidney function and dosage adjustments may need to be made according to serum concentrations of ethambutol. It should be used with great care in patients with visual defects, the elderly, and in children in whom evaluation of changes in visual acuity may be difficult; it should generally not be used in children under 6 years of age and some consider that it should not be used in children under 13 years of age nor in patients with visual defects. Ocular examination is recommended before treatment with ethambutol and some consider that regular examinations are necessary during treatment especially in children. Patients should be advised to report visual disturbances immediately and to discontinue ethambutol pending visual evaluation.

Ethambutol may precipitate attacks of gout.

Although ethambutol crosses the placenta and may be teratogenic in *animals,* problems in humans have not been documented. It is generally considered that the benefits of ethambutol in the treatment of tuberculosis outweigh any potential risks in pregnancy.

Antimicrobial Action

Ethambutol is bacteriostatic against *Mycobacterium tuberculosis* with an MIC of 0.5 to 8 μg per mL; it is bactericidal at higher concentrations. It possesses little sterilising activity. Resistant strains of *M. tuberculosis* are readily produced if ethambutol is used alone.

Mycobacterium avium complex. Strains of *Mycobacterium avium* complex have been reported to be resistant *in vitro* to ethambutol[1] but appear to be susceptible to a combination of ethambutol and rifampicin[2] or ethambutol and ciprofloxacin.[3]

Studies have suggested that ethambutol increases the effectiveness of other antibacterial drugs by increasing cell-wall permeability.[4] Other investigators have proposed inhibition of synthesis of the outermost layer of the cell envelope by ethambutol as a mechanism for the increased drug susceptibility of *M. avium* complex.[5]

1. Kiehn TE, *et al.* Infections caused by Mycobacterium avium complex in immunocompromised patients: diagnosis by blood culture and fecal examination, antimicrobial susceptibility tests, and morphological and seroagglutination characteristics. *J Clin Microbiol* 1985; **21:** 168–73.
2. Zimmer BL, *et al.* In vitro synergistic activity of ethambutol, isoniazid, kanamycin, rifampin, and streptomycin against Mycobacterium avium-intracellulare complex. *Antimicrob Agents Chemother* 1982; **22:** 148–50.
3. Hoffner SE, *et al.* In-vitro synergistic activity between ethambutol and fluorinated quinolones against Mycobacterium avium complex. *J Antimicrob Chemother* 1989; **24:** 317–24.
4. Hoffner SE, *et al.* Microcalorimetric studies of the initial interaction between antimycobacterial drugs and Mycobacterium avium. *J Antimicrob Chemother* 1990; **25:** 353–9.
5. Rastogi N, *et al.* Enhancement of drug susceptibility of Mycobacterium avium by inhibitors of cell envelope synthesis. *Antimicrob Agents Chemother* 1990; **34:** 759–64.

Pharmacokinetics

About 80% of an oral dose of ethambutol is absorbed from the gastro-intestinal tract, and the remainder appears in the faeces unchanged. Absorption is not significantly impaired by food. After a single dose of 25 mg per kg body-weight, peak plasma concentrations of up to 5 μg per mL appear within 4 hours, and are less than 1 μg per mL by 24 hours.

Ethambutol is distributed to most tissues, including the lungs, kidneys, and erythrocytes. It diffuses into the CSF when the meninges are inflamed. It has been reported to cross the placenta and is distributed into breast milk. The elimination half-life following oral administration is about 3 to 4 hours.

Ethambutol is partially metabolised in the liver to the aldehyde and dicarboxylic acid derivatives which are inactive and then excreted in the urine. Most of a dose appears in the urine within 24 hours as unchanged drug and 8 to 15% as the inactive metabolites.

Distribution. In a study of the absorption of ethambutol[1] given in a dose of 25 mg per kg body-weight to 13 healthy subjects and to 21 patients with tuberculous meningitis, mean serum concentrations measured at 3 hours were 4.1 μg per mL (range 2.6 to 6.6) and 4.9 μg per mL (range 3.4 to 8) respectively. A CSF concentration of 0.07 μg per mL was measured at 3 hours in 2 of 5 healthy subjects, no ethambutol being detected in the other 3. The mean CSF concentration at 3 hours was 0.48 μg per mL (0.05 to 1.6) in 4 of 5 patients, no ethambutol being detected in the fifth.

1. Pilheu JA, *et al.* Concentrations of ethambutol in the cerebrospinal fluid after oral administration. *Tubercle* 1971; **52:** 117–22.

Oral administration. In patients with HIV infections receiving standard multi-drug therapy for tuberculosis, serum concentrations of ethambutol were low or very low compared with those expected.[1]

1. Peloquin CA, *et al.* Low antituberculosis drug concentrations in patients with AIDS. *Ann Pharmacother* 1996; **30:** 919–25.

Pregnancy and breast feeding. Ethambutol crosses the placenta and is present in fetal tissue in amounts of at least 74.5% of the maternal serum concentration.[1] Use of ethambutol during pregnancy has not been associated with fetal abnormalities.[2]

Ethambutol diffuses into breast milk to produce concentrations similar to those in plasma.[3]

1. Holdiness MR. Transplacental pharmacokinetics of the antituberculosis drugs. *Clin Pharmacokinet* 1987; **13:** 125–9.
2. Snider DE, *et al.* Treatment of tuberculosis during pregnancy. *Am Rev Respir Dis* 1980; **122:** 65–79.
3. Snider DE, Powell KE. Should women taking antituberculosis drugs breast-feed? *Arch Intern Med* 1984; **144:** 589–90.

Uses and Administration

Ethambutol is used with other antituberculous drugs in the primary treatment of pulmonary and extrapulmonary tuberculosis (p.146) to suppress emergence of resistance to the other drugs used in the regimens. It has also been used as a component of regimens for the treatment of opportunistic mycobacterial infections (p.133).

In the treatment of tuberculosis, ethambutol is given, as the hydrochloride, usually with isoniazid, rifampicin, and pyrazinamide in the initial 8-week phase and sometimes in combinations with isoniazid and rifampicin in the continuation phase. It is given by mouth in a single daily dose of 15 mg per kg body-weight daily or 30 mg per kg three times weekly or 45 mg per kg twice weekly. Ethambutol has also been used occasionally with other drugs for prophylaxis if the likelihood of resistance to isoniazid is high, when daily doses of 15 mg per kg have been employed, for 6 months or more. If it is used in patients with renal impairment (see Precautions, above), then doses should be adjusted according to serum concentrations.

Preparations

BP 1998: Ethambutol Tablets;
USP 23: Ethambutol Hydrochloride Tablets.

Proprietary Preparations (details are given in Part 3)
Aust.: Etibi; Myambutol; ***Austral.:*** Myambutol; ***Belg.:*** Myambutol; ***Canad.:*** Etibi; Myambutol; ***Fr.:*** Dexambutol; Myambutol; ***Ger.:*** EMB; Myambutol; ***Irl.:*** Myambutol; ***Ital.:*** Etapiam; Etibi; Miambutol; ***Neth.:*** Myambutol; ***S.Afr.:*** Myambutol; Mycrol†; ***Spain:*** Cidanbutol†; Inagen†; Myambutol; ***Swed.:*** Myambutol; ***Switz.:*** Myambutol; Servambutol†; ***UK:*** Myambutol†; ***USA:*** Myambutol.

Multi-ingredient: ***Aust.:*** Myambutol-INH; ***Fr.:*** Dexambutol-INH; ***Ger.:*** EMB-INH; Myambutol-INH; ***Ital.:*** Etanicozid B6; Etibi-INH; Miazide; Miazide B6; ***S.Afr.:*** Mynah; Myrin; Tuberol; ***Spain:*** Isoetam; ***Switz.:*** Myambutol-INH; ***UK:*** Mynah†.

Ethionamide (7557-z)

Ethionamide *(BAN, USAN, rINN).*

Ethionamidum; Etionamide; 1314-TH. 2-Ethylpyridine-4-carbothioamide.

$C_8H_{10}N_2S$ = 166.2.

CAS — 536-33-4.

Pharmacopoeias. In *Eur.* (see p.viii), *Int., Jpn, Pol.,* and *US.*

Yellow crystals or a yellow crystalline powder with a slight sulphide-like odour. The Ph. Eur. specifies practically **insoluble** in water while the USP states slightly soluble. Sparingly soluble in alcohol and propylene glycol; slightly soluble in chloroform, and in ether; soluble in methyl alcohol. **Store** in airtight containers.

Adverse Effects and Treatment

Many patients cannot tolerate therapeutic doses of ethionamide and have to discontinue treatment. The most common adverse effects are dose-related gastro-intestinal disturbances, including anorexia, excessive salivation, a metallic taste, nausea, vomiting, abdominal pain, and diarrhoea.

Mental disturbances including depression, anxiety, and psychosis have been provoked. Dizziness, drowsiness, headache, postural hypotension, and asthenia may also occur occasionally. Peripheral and optic neuropathy and a pellagra-like syndrome have occurred. Pyridoxine or nicotinamide have been suggested for the treatment or prevention of neurotoxic effects. Although jaundice is rare hepatitis may occur. The incidence of hepatotoxicity is increased when ethionamide is given in association with rifampicin.

Other side-effects reported include hypersensitivity reactions, alopecia, dermatitis (including photodermatitis), endocrine disturbances, hypoglycaemia, and hypothyroidism with or without goitre.

Teratogenic effects have been reported in *animals.*

Effects on the liver. Use of ethionamide or prothionamide with rifampicin for the treatment of multibacillary leprosy has been associated with a high incidence of hepatotoxicity. A hepatitis incidence of 4.5 to 5% has been reported for patients on ethionamide or prothionamide, rifampicin, and either dapsone or clofazimine.[1,2] In these studies, diagnosis of hepatitis was based on clinical assessment. When laboratory monitoring was used, an incidence of 13% was reported with a regimen of ethionamide or prothionamide with rifampicin and dapsone.[3] A regimen of prothionamide, dapsone, rifampicin, and clofazimine has been associated with a 22% incidence based on laboratory monitoring.[4] Administration of ethionamide in association with pyrazinamide has also resulted in a high incidence of abnormal liver function tests.[5]

In the above studies rifampicin was administered daily during part or all of the regimens. The incidence of hepatotoxicity when ethionamide or prothionamide is administered in association with once-monthly rifampicin may be lower; hepatotoxicity was not reported in patients receiving monthly rifampicin and daily prothionamide, isoniazid, and dapsone.[6]

1. Pattyn SR, *et al.* Hepatotoxicity of the combination of rifampin-ethionamide in the treatment of multibacillary leprosy. *Int J Lepr* 1984; **52:** 1–6.
2. Pattyn SR, *et al.* Combined regimens of one year duration in the treatment of multibacillary leprosy—II: combined regimens with rifampicin administered during 6 months. *Lepr Rev* 1989; **60:** 118–23.
3. Cartel J-L, *et al.* Hepatitis in leprosy patients treated by a daily combination of dapsone, rifampin, and a thioamide. *Int J Lepr* 1983; **51:** 461–5.
4. Ji B, *et al.* Hepatotoxicity of combined therapy with rifampicin and daily prothionamide for leprosy. *Lepr Rev* 1984; **55:** 283–9.
5. Schless JM, *et al.* The use of ethionamide in combined drug regimens in the re-treatment of isoniazid-resistant pulmonary tuberculosis. *Am Rev Respir Dis* 1965; **91:** 728–37.
6. Ellard GA, *et al.* Long-term prothionamide compliance: a study carried out in India using a combined formulation containing prothionamide, dapsone and isoniazid. *Lepr Rev* 1988; **59:** 163–75.

Precautions

Ethionamide should not be given to patients with severe liver disease. Liver function tests should be carried out before and during treatment with ethionamide.

Caution is necessary in administering ethionamide to patients with depression or other psychiatric illness. Difficulty may be experienced in the management of diabetes mellitus. Ethionamide is best avoided during pregnancy.

Interactions

The side-effects of other antimycobacterials may be increased when ethionamide is administered concomitantly (see above, and under Cycloserine, p.199).

Antimicrobial Action

Ethionamide is active only against mycobacteria including *Mycobacterium tuberculosis, M. kansasii, M. leprae,* and some strains of *M. avium* complex. Most susceptible organisms are inhibited by 10 μg or less per mL. It is considered to be bactericidal against *M. leprae* and an MIC of 0.05 μg per mL has been reported.

Resistance develops rapidly if used alone and there is complete cross-resistance between ethionamide and prothionamide. Despite the structural similarity cross-resistance does not occur with isoniazid but may occur with thiacetazone.

Pharmacokinetics

Ethionamide is readily absorbed from the gastro-intestinal tract, and peak plasma concentrations of about 2 μg per mL occur 2 hours after an oral dose of 250 mg. It is widely distributed throughout body tissues and fluids. It crosses the placenta and penetrates the uninflamed meninges, appearing in the CSF in concentrations equivalent to those in serum. The half-life is reported to be 2 to 3 hours. Ethionamide is extensively metabolised, probably in the liver, to the active sulphoxide and other inactive metabolites and less than 1% of a dose appears in the urine as unchanged drug.

Following single oral doses of ethionamide 15 or 20 mg per kg body-weight in children with tuberculous meningitis, the peak spinal fluid concentration was reached in 1½ to 2½ hours.[1] A wide range of concentrations was reported but doses of 20 mg per kg were more likely to produce spinal fluid concentrations above 2.5 μg per mL, the concentration considered by the authors to be essential for therapeutic success.

1. Donald PR, Seifart HI. Cerebrospinal fluid concentrations of ethionamide in children with tuberculous meningitis. *J Pediatr* 1989; **115:** 483–6.

Uses and Administration

Ethionamide is a thioamide derivative considered to be interchangeable with prothionamide. It has been used in combination with other antituberculous drugs for the treatment of tuberculosis (p.146), when resistance to or toxicity from primary drugs has developed. It has also been used, as a substitute for clofazimine, in regimens for the treatment of leprosy (p.128) but less toxic alternatives are now preferred.

In the treatment of resistant tuberculosis adults may be given 250 mg every 8 to 12 hours (maximum 1 g daily) while for children 4 to 5 mg per kg body-weight every 8 hours has been suggested (maximum 750 mg daily). It may be given in divided doses with meals to minimise gastro-intestinal adverse effects, or as a single daily dose after the evening meal or at bedtime. Similar doses were used for the treatment of leprosy.

Ethionamide has also been administered as rectal suppositories; the hydrochloride has been given intravenously.

Preparations

USP 23: Ethionamide Tablets.

Proprietary Preparations (details are given in Part 3)
S.Afr.: Ethatyl; ***USA:*** Trecator.

Faropenem Sodium (17297-b)

Faropenem Sodium *(rINNM)*.

Fropenem Sodium. Sodium (+)-(5*R*,6*S*)-6-[(1*R*)-1-hydroxyethyl]-7-oxo-3-[(2*R*)-tetrahydro-2-furyl]-4-thia-1-azabicyclo[3.2.0]hept-2-ene-2-carboxylate.

$C_{12}H_{15}NaNO_5S$ = 308.3.

CAS — 106560-14-9 (faropenem); 122547-49-3 (faropenem sodium).

Faropenem is a penem antibacterial that is given by mouth as the sodium salt for the treatment of susceptible infections.

References.

1. Woodcock JM, *et al.* The in-vitro activity of faropenem, a novel oral penem. *J Antimicrob Chemother* 1997; **39:** 35–43.

Fleroxacin (2953-w)

Fleroxacin *(BAN, USAN, rINN)*.

AM-833; Ro-23-6240; Ro-23-6240/000. 6,8-Difluoro-1-(2-fluoroethyl)-1,4-dihydro-7-(4-methyl-1-piperazinyl)-4-oxo-3-quinolinecarboxylic acid.

$C_{17}H_{18}F_3N_3O_3$ = 369.3.

CAS — 79660-72-3.

Fleroxacin is a fluoroquinolone antibacterial with actions and uses similar to those of ciprofloxacin (p.185), but is reported to have greater systemic bioavailability and a longer half-life. It is given by mouth or by intravenous infusion for the treatment of susceptible infections in usual doses of 200 or 400 mg once daily.

The incidence of adverse effects associated with fleroxacin has been relatively high.

General references.

1. Leigh D, *et al.* eds. Fleroxacin, a long acting fluoroquinolone with broad spectrum activity. *J Antimicrob Chemother* 1988; **22** (suppl D): 1–234.
2. Balfour JA, *et al.* Fleroxacin: a review of its pharmacology and therapeutic efficacy in various infections. *Drugs* 1995; **49:** 794–850.

Toxicity.

1. Bowie WR, *et al.* Adverse reactions in a dose-ranging study with a new long-acting fluoroquinolone, fleroxacin. *Antimicrob Agents Chemother* 1989; **33:** 1778–82.

Preparations

Proprietary Preparations (details are given in Part 3)
Aust.: Quinodis; ***Belg.:*** Quinodis; ***Ger.:*** Quinodis; ***Jpn:*** Megalocin; ***Switz.:*** Quinodis.

Flomoxef (1792-n)

Flomoxef *(rINN)*.

6315-S. 7*R*-7-[2-(Difluoromethylthio)acetamido]-3-[1-(2-hydroxyethyl)-1*H*-tetrazol-5-ylthiomethyl]-7-methoxy-1-oxa-3-cephem-4-carboxylic acid.

$C_{15}H_{18}F_2N_6O_7S_2$ = 496.5.

CAS — 99665-00-6.

Flomoxef is an oxacephalosporin or oxacephem antibiotic with properties similar to latamoxef (p.221). It is given by intravenous injection as the sodium salt.

Preparations

Proprietary Preparations (details are given in Part 3)
Jpn: Flumarin.

Florfenicol (824-p)

Florfenicol *(BAN, USAN, rINN)*.

Sch-25298. 2,2-Dichloro-*N*-[(αS,βR)-α-(fluoromethyl)-β-hydroxy-4-methanesulfonylphenethyl]acetamide.

$C_{12}H_{14}Cl_2FNO_4S$ = 358.2.

CAS — 76639-94-6.

Florfenicol, a fluorinated analogue of chloramphenicol, is an antibacterial used in veterinary medicine.

Flucloxacillin (12125-y)

Flucloxacillin *(BAN, rINN)*.

BRL-2039; Floxacillin *(USAN)*. (6*R*)-6-[3-(2-Chloro-6-fluorophenyl)-5-methylisoxazole-4-carboxamido]penicillanic acid.

$C_{19}H_{17}ClFN_3O_5S$ = 453.9.

CAS — 5250-39-5.

NOTE. Compounded preparations of equal parts by weight of flucloxacillin and ampicillin have the British Approved Name Co-fluampicil.

Flucloxacillin Magnesium (3868-r)

Flucloxacillin Magnesium *(BANM, rINNM)*.

$(C_{19}H_{16}ClFN_3O_5S)_2Mg,8H_2O$ = 1074.2.

CAS — 58486-36-5.

Pharmacopoeias. In Br.

A white or almost white powder. 2.4 g of monograph substance is approximately equivalent to 1 g of anhydrous flucloxacillin. Each g of monograph substance represents about 0.9 mmol of magnesium.

Slightly **soluble** in water and in chloroform; freely soluble in methyl alcohol. A 0.5% solution in water has a pH of 4.5 to 6.5. **Store** at a temperature not exceeding 25°. Protect from moisture.

Flucloxacillin Sodium (85-l)

Flucloxacillin Sodium *(BANM, rINNM)*.

Flucloxacilina Sódica; Flucloxacillinum Natricum.

$C_{19}H_{16}ClFN_3NaO_5S,H_2O$ = 493.9.

CAS — 1847-24-1.

Pharmacopoeias. In Eur. (see p.viii).

A white or almost white crystalline hygroscopic powder. 1.09 g of monograph substance is approximately equivalent to 1 g of anhydrous flucloxacillin. Each g of monograph substance represents about 2 mmol of sodium.

Freely **soluble** in water and in methyl alcohol; soluble in alcohol. A 10% solution in water has a pH of 5 to 7. **Store** at a temperature not exceeding 25° in airtight containers.

As with other penicillins, flucloxacillin sodium is **incompatible** with aminoglycosides.

Adverse Effects and Precautions

As for Benzylpenicillin p.159.

Hepatitis and cholestatic jaundice have been reported occasionally with flucloxacillin and may be delayed in onset; older patients and those receiving flucloxacillin for more than two weeks are at greater risk. Agranulocytosis and neutropenia have been associated rarely with isoxazolyl penicillins such as flucloxacillin. Phlebitis has followed intravenous infusion.

Effects on the liver. References.

1. Bengtsson F, *et al.* Flucloxacillin-induced cholestatic liver damage. *Scand J Infect Dis* 1985; **17:** 125–8.
2. Turner IB, *et al.* Prolonged hepatic cholestasis after flucloxacillin therapy. *Med J Aust* 1989; **151:** 701–5.
3. Fairley CK, *et al.* Flucloxacillin jaundice. *Lancet* 1992; **339:** 679.
4. Committee on Safety of Medicines. Flucloxacillin-induced cholestatic jaundice. *Current Problems 35* 1992.
5. Fairley CK, *et al.* Risk factors for development of flucloxacillin associated jaundice. *Br Med J* 1993; **306:** 233–5. Correction. *ibid.*; **307:** 1179.

Interactions

As for Benzylpenicillin, p.160.

Antimicrobial Action

Flucloxacillin is bactericidal with a mode of action similar to that of benzylpenicillin, but is resistant to staphylococcal penicillinase. It is active therefore against penicillinase-producing and non-penicillinase-producing staphylococci, with minimum inhibitory concentrations in the range of 0.25 to 0.5 µg per mL. Its activity against streptococci such as *Streptococcus pneumoniae* and *Str. pyogenes* is less than that of benzylpenicillin but sufficient to be useful when these organisms are present with penicillin-resistant staphylococci. Flucloxacillin is virtually ineffective against *Enterococcus faecalis*.

Resistance. The resistance of staphylococci to flucloxacillin and other penicillinase-resistant penicillins is described under methicillin (p.225).

Pharmacokinetics

Flucloxacillin like dicloxacillin, is about twice as well absorbed from the gastro-intestinal tract as cloxacillin, but absorption is also reduced by the presence of food in the stomach. After an oral dose of 250 mg to 1 g, in fasting subjects, peak plasma concentrations in about 1 hour are usually in the range of 5 to 15 µg per mL. Plasma concentrations following the intramuscular injection of flucloxacillin sodium are similar, but peak concentrations are achieved in about 30 minutes. Doubling the dose can double the plasma concentration. About 95% of flucloxacillin in the circulation is bound to plasma proteins. Flucloxacillin has been reported to have a plasma half-life of approximately 1 hour. The half-life is prolonged in neonates.

The distribution of flucloxacillin into body tissues and fluids is similar to that of cloxacillin (p.195).

Flucloxacillin is metabolised to a limited extent and the unchanged drug and metabolites are excreted in the urine by glomerular filtration and renal tubular secretion. About 50% of a dose by mouth and up to 90% of an intramuscular dose is excreted in the urine within 6 hours. Only small amounts are excreted in the bile. Flucloxacillin is not removed by haemodialysis.

Plasma concentrations are enhanced if probenecid is given concomitantly.

References.

1. Anderson P, *et al.* Pharmacokinetics and distribution of flucloxacillin in pacemaker patients. *Eur J Clin Pharmacol* 1985; **27:** 713–19.
2. Herngren L, *et al.* Pharmacokinetics of free and total flucloxacillin in newborn infants. *Eur J Clin Pharmacol* 1987; **32:** 403–9.

Uses and Administration

Flucloxacillin is an isoxazolyl penicillin used primarily for the treatment of infections due to staphylococci resistant to benzylpenicillin. These include bone and joint infections, endocarditis, peritonitis (associated with continuous ambulatory peritoneal dialysis), pneumonia, skin infections (including soft-tissue infections), and toxic shock syndrome. For discussions of these infections and their treatment, see under Choice of Antibacterial, p.116.

Administration and dosage. Flucloxacillin is administered by mouth as the sodium or magnesium salt. It should be taken at least 30 minutes before meals as the presence of food in the stomach reduces absorption. It is administered parenterally as the sodium salt. All doses are expressed as flucloxacillin. In severe renal impairment a reduction in dosage may be necessary.

The usual dose by mouth or by intramuscular injection is 250 mg four times daily. It is administered intravenously in a dose of 250 mg to 1 g four times daily by slow injection over 3 to 4 minutes or by intravenous infusion. All systemic doses may be doubled in severe infections; doses of up to 8 g daily have been suggested for endocarditis or osteomyelitis.

Flucloxacillin has been administered by other routes in conjunction with systemic therapy. It has been administered in a dose of 250 to 500 mg daily by intra-articular injection, dissolved if necessary in a 0.5% solution of lignocaine hydrochloride, and by intrapleural injection in a dose of 250 mg daily. Using powder for injection, 125 to 250 mg has been dissolved in 3 mL of sterile water and inhaled by nebuliser 4 times daily.

Children up to 2 years of age may be given one-quarter the adult dose and those aged 2 to 10 years, one-half the adult dose.

Flucloxacillin may be administered in combination with other antibacterials, including ampicillin (known as co-fluampicil), to produce a wider spectrum of activity. If flucloxacillin is used concurrently with an aminoglycoside the two drugs should not be mixed.

Preparations

BP 1998: Co-fluampicil Capsules; Co-fluampicil Oral Suspension; Flucloxacillin Capsules; Flucloxacillin Injection; Flucloxacillin Oral Solution; Flucloxacillin Oral Suspension.

Proprietary Preparations (details are given in Part 3)
Aust.: Floxapen; ***Austral.:*** Flopen; Floxapen; Flucil; Staphylex; ***Belg.:*** Floxapen; Staphycid; ***Canad.:*** Fluclox†; ***Ger.:*** Staphylex; ***Irl.:*** Floxapen; Flucillin; Fluclon; Geriflox; Ladropen; Stafoxil; ***Ital.:*** Betabiotic; ***Neth.:*** Floxapen; Stafoxil; ***S.Afr.:*** Floxapen; Flucillin; ***Swed.:*** Heracillin; Isoxapen†; ***Switz.:*** Floxapen; Flucloxin; ***UK:*** Floxapen; Fluclomix; Galfloxin; Ladropen†; Stafoxil; Staphlipen†.

Multi-ingredient: ***Aust.:*** Fluxapril; ***Ger.:*** Flanamox; Fluxapril; ***Ital.:*** Flanamox†; Infectrin; ***S.Afr.:*** Flumox; Macropen; Megapen; Suprapen; ***UK:*** Flu-Amp; Magnapen; Zoxin.

Flumequine (12757-f)

Flumequine *(BAN, USAN, rINN)*.

R-802. 9-Fluoro-6,7-dihydro-5-methyl-1-oxo-1*H*,5*H*-pyrido[3,2,1-*ij*]quinoline-2-carboxylic acid.

$C_{14}H_{12}FNO_3$ = 261.2.

CAS — 42835-25-6.

Flumequine is a 4-quinolone antibacterial with actions and uses similar to those of nalidixic acid (p.228). It may be more active *in vitro* against some Enterobacteriaceae. In the treatment of urinary-tract infections doses of 400 mg are given three times daily by mouth.

Preparations

Proprietary Preparations (details are given in Part 3)
Belg.: Apurone; ***Fr.:*** Apurone; ***Ital.:*** Flumural.

Flurithromycin (3075-e)

Flurithromycin *(rINN)*.

CI-932; P-0501A. (8*S*)-8-Fluoroerythromycin.

$C_{37}H_{66}FNO_{13}$ = 751.9.

CAS — 82664-20-8.

Flurithromycin is a fluorinated macrolide antibiotic derived from erythromycin (p.204). It is given by mouth as the ethyl succinate in the treatment of susceptible infections.

References.

1. Saverino D, *et al.* Antibacterial profile of flurithromycin, a new macrolide. *J Antimicrob Chemother* 1992; **30:** 261–72.

Preparations

Proprietary Preparations (details are given in Part 3)
Ital.: Flurizic; Ritro.

Formosulphathiazole (4905-a)

Formaldehyde-sulphathiazole; Formosulfathiazole; Methylenesulfathiazole.

CAS — 13968-86-0.

A condensation product of sulphathiazole with formaldehyde.

Formosulphathiazole is a sulphonamide with properties similar to those of sulphamethoxazole (p.254). It is poorly absorbed and is given for its antibacterial action in the gastro-intestinal tract, often in combination with other antibacterials.

Preparations

Proprietary Preparations (details are given in Part 3)

Multi-ingredient: ***Ger.:*** Diaront NN†; ***Spain:*** Estreptosirup†; Sorbitoxin†; Sulfintestin Neom; Sulfintestin Neomicina.

Fosfomycin (179-a)

Fosfomycin *(BAN, USAN, rINN)*.

MK-955; Phosphomycin; Phosphonomycin. (1*R*,2*S*)-1,2-Epoxypropylphosphonic acid.

$C_3H_7O_4P$ = 138.1.

CAS — 23155-02-4 (fosfomycin); 26016-98-8 (fosfomycin calcium); 26016-99-9 (fosfomycin disodium); 78964-85-9 (fosfomycin trometamol).

Pharmacopoeias. Eur. (see p.viii) and *Jpn* include Fosfomycin Calcium and Fosfomycin Sodium.

An antibiotic isolated from *Streptomyces fradiae* and other *Streptomyces* spp. or produced synthetically.

Adverse Effects and Precautions

Gastro-intestinal disturbances including nausea and diarrhoea, transient increases in serum concentrations of aminotransferases, headache, visual disturbances, and skin rashes have been reported following the use of fosfomycin. Eosinophilia and, rarely, aplastic anaemia, have also occurred.

Antimicrobial Action

Fosfomycin is a bactericidal antibacterial. Following active uptake into the cell it is reported to interfere with the first step in the synthesis of bacterial cell walls. It is active *in vitro* against a range of Gram-positive and Gram-negative bacteria including *Staphylococcus aureus*, some streptococci, most Enterobacteriaceae, *Haemophilus influenzae*, *Neisseria* spp., and some strains of *Pseudomonas aeruginosa* although some are resistant. *Bacteroides* spp. are not sensitive. MICs are very variable and depend on the type of test media used as well as inoculum size: glucose 6-phosphate potentiates its activity *in vitro* but MICs determined in the presence of glucose 6-phosphate correlate better with activity *in vivo*. MICs for the most sensitive strains have been reported to range from about 1 to 4 µg per mL, but organisms with MICs up to about 16 µg per mL have been considered sensitive and those with MICs between about 16 and 64 µg per mL of moderate sensitivity. Bacterial resistance to fosfomycin has been reported and can be chromosomal or, in some organisms, transferred by plasmids encoding multiple resistance (for example in *Serratia marcescens*). However, there appears to be little cross resistance with other antibacterials.

Fosfomycin has been reported to demonstrate antimicrobial synergy with a wide range of antibacterials against organisms such as enterococci, methicillin-resistant *Staph. aureus*, and the enterobacteria. Such synergistic effects have been reported particularly with the beta lactams, but also with aminoglycosides, macrolides, tetracyclines, chloramphenicol, rifamycin, and lincomycin. Antimicrobial antagonism with a beta lactam has also been reported.

There is some suggestion that co-administration of fosfomycin with an aminoglycoside may also reduce the nephrotoxicity of the latter *in vivo*.

References.

1. Barry AL, Brown SD. Antibacterial spectrum of fosfomycin trometamol. *J Antimicrob Chemother* 1995; **35:** 228–30.

Pharmacokinetics

Fosfomycin or fosfomycin calcium are poorly absorbed from the gastro-intestinal tract. Peak plasma concentrations about 4 hours after a 1-g dose of fosfomycin are around 7 µg per mL, and bioavailability has been calculated at about 30 to 40%. Similar bioavailability has been reported for the trometamol salt, and plasma concentrations of about 22 to 32 µg per mL have been reported 2 hours after a dose of 50 mg per kg body-weight (about 3 g fosfomycin). Fosfomycin disodium is administered by the intramuscular or intravenous routes: intravenous infusion of a 3-g dose results in peak serum concentrations of around 220 µg per mL. The plasma half-life is about 2 hours. Fosfomycin does not appear to be bound to plasma proteins. It diffuses across the placenta and is widely distributed in body fluids including the CSF; small amounts have been found in breast milk and bile. The majority of a parenteral dose is excreted unchanged in the urine, by glomerular filtration, within 24 hours.

Following oral administration of fosfomycin trometamol, urinary concentrations of 3 mg per mL have been reported within 2 to 4 hours of a 3-g dose; therapeutic concentrations are maintained for about 36 hours following a single oral dose.

References.

1. Bergan T, *et al.* Pharmacokinetic profile of fosfomycin trometamol. *Chemotherapy* 1993; **39:** 297–301.

Uses and Administration

Fosfomycin is a phosphonic acid antibacterial administered by mouth as the trometamol salt in the treatment of acute uncomplicated infections of the urinary tract. It is given to adults as a single dose equivalent to 3 g of fosfomycin; children over 5 years may be given 2 g. For a discussion of urinary-tract infections and their treatment, see p.149.

Fosfomycin trometamol has also been used for the prophylaxis of infection in transurethral surgical procedures; the equivalent of 3 g of fosfomycin has been given by mouth 3 hours before and repeated 24 hours after the procedure. For a discussion of surgical infections and their prophylaxis and treatment, see p.144.

Fosfomycin has also been given by mouth as the calcium salt and intramuscularly or intravenously as the disodium salt in the treatment of a variety of bacterial infections due to susceptible organisms. Doses are calculated in terms of the base. The usual adult dose by mouth is 1 g of fosfomycin every 6 to 8 hours. Higher doses have been given parenterally, with up to 20 g daily of fosfomycin being given intravenously in severe infection.

Fosfomycin has been administered as an ingredient of combination preparations also containing a beta lactam.

References.

1. Reeves DS. Fosfomycin trometamol. *J Antimicrob Chemother* 1994; **34:** 853–8.
2. Patel SS, *et al.* Fosfomycin tromethamine: a review of its antibacterial activity, pharmacokinetic properties and therapeutic efficacy as a single-dose oral treatment for acute uncomplicated lower urinary tract infections. *Drugs* 1997; **53:** 637–56.

Preparations

Proprietary Preparations (details are given in Part 3)

Aust.: Monuril; ***Belg.:*** Fosfocin†; Monuril; ***Fr.:*** Fosfocine; Monuril; Uridoz; ***Ger.:*** Fosfocin; Monuril; ***Irl.:*** Monuril; ***Ital.:*** Afos; Biocin; Biofos†; Endociclina†; Faremicin; Fonofos; Fosfobiotic†; Fosfocin; Fosfogram†; Fosforal; Foximin†; Francital; Gram-Micina†; Ipamicina; Lancetina†; Lofoxin; Monuril; Neofocin†; Palmofen†; Priomicina†; Ultramicina; Vastocin†; ***Jpn:*** Fosmicin-S; Fosmicin†; ***Neth.:*** Monuril; ***S.Afr.:*** Urizone; ***Spain:*** Fosfocina; Monofoscin; Monurol; Solufos; ***Swed.:*** Fosfocin†; ***Switz.:*** Fosfocin; Monuril; ***UK:*** Monuril†; ***USA:*** Monurol.

Multi-ingredient: ***Ital.:*** Focet†; Fosfolexin†; Kufaprim†; Moxacin†; Moxiprim†; ***Spain:*** Erifoscin.

Framycetin Sulphate (86-y)

Framycetin Sulphate *(BANM, rINNM)*.

Framycetini Sulfas; Neomycin B Sulphate. 2-Deoxy-4-*O*-(2,6-diamino-2,6-dideoxy-α-D-glucopyranosyl)-5-*O*-[3-*O*-(2,6-diamino-2,6-dideoxy-β-L-idopyranosyl)-β-D-ribofuranosyl]streptamine sulphate.

$C_{23}H_{46}N_6O_{13},xH_2SO_4$.

CAS — 119-04-0 (framycetin); 4146-30-9 (framycetin sulphate).

Pharmacopoeias. In *Eur.* (see p.viii).

Framycetin is an antimicrobial substance produced by certain strains of *Streptomyces fradiae* or *Streptomyces decaris* or by any other means. It contains not more than 3% of neomycin C (p.229) and loses not more than 8% of its weight on drying. A white or yellowish-white, hygroscopic powder containing not less than 630 units of neomycin B per mg after drying. Freely **soluble** in water; very slightly soluble in alcohol; practically insoluble in acetone and in ether. A 1% solution in water has a pH of 6 to 7. **Store** in airtight containers. Protect from light.

Framycetin is an aminoglycoside antibiotic which forms the major component of neomycin (p.229) and has similar actions and uses. It is used as the sulphate and is administered topically in the treatment of infections of the skin, eye, and ear. It is often used in combination with other antibacterials and corticosteroids in topical preparations.

Framycetin sulphate is poorly absorbed and has been given by mouth for the treatment of gastro-intestinal infections and pre-operatively for bowel preparation. It has sometimes been given prophylactically as part of regimens for the selective decontamination of the digestive tract in patients in intensive care.

Preparations

Proprietary Preparations (details are given in Part 3)
Aust.: Sofra-Tull; ***Austral.:*** Sofra-Tulle; Soframycin; ***Belg.:*** Soframycine; ***Canad.:*** Sofra-Tulle; Soframycin; ***Fr.:*** Framitulle†; Framybiotal; Isofra; Rhinalene a la framycetine; Soframycine; ***Ger.:*** Leukase N; Sofra-Tull; Tuttomycin†; ***Irl.:*** Sofra-Tulle; Soframycin; ***Ital.:*** Sofra-Tulle†; ***Neth.:*** Sofra-Tulle; Soframycin; ***Norw.:*** Sofra-Tulle; ***S.Afr.:*** Sofra-Tulle; Soframycin; ***Swed.:*** Sofra-Tulle; ***Switz.:*** Frakitacine; Sofra-Tulle; Soframycin; ***UK:*** Sofra-Tulle; Soframycin.

Multi-ingredient: ***Aust.:*** Leukase; Leukase-Kegel; ***Austral.:*** Otodex; Sofradex; Soframycin; ***Belg.:*** Dexa-Sol Soframycine†; Sofraline; Sofrasolone; ***Canad.:*** Proctosedyl; Sofracort; Soframycin; ***Fr.:*** Anti-Rhinyl†; Corticetine; Cortifra†; Dermocalm; Dexapolyfra†; Dulcimyxine†; Frakidex; Frazoline; Neoparyl Framycetine; Polyfra; Rhinotrophyl; Rhinyl; Soframycine Hydrocortisone; Soframycine Naphazoline; Topifram; ***Ger.:*** Dexabiotan in der Ophtiole†; Leukase N; Leukase†; Soframycin†; ***Irl.:*** Proctosedyl; Sofradex; Soframycin; ***Ital.:*** Sinrinal†; Topicort Composto†; ***Neth.:*** Proctosedyl; Sofradex; ***Norw.:*** Proctosedyl; Sofradex; ***S.Afr.:*** Proctosedyl; Sofradex; Soframycin†; ***Spain:*** Abrasone; Aldo Otico; Aldoderma; Cusispray†; Nesfare Antibiotico; Otomidrin; ***Swed.:*** Proctosedyl; Sofradex; ***Switz.:*** Corticetine; Dexalocal-F; Frakidex; Proctosedyl†; Pulpomixine; Sofradex; ***UK:*** Sofradex; Soframycin.

Furaltadone Hydrochloride (14192-k)

Furaltadone Hydrochloride *(BANM, rINNM)*.

(±)-5-Morpholinomethyl-3-(5-nitrofurfurylideneamino)oxazolidin-2-one hydrochloride.

$C_{13}H_{16}N_4O_6,HCl$ = 360.8.

CAS — 139-91-3 (furaltadone); 59302-14-6 (±-furaltadone).

Pharmacopoeias. Fr. includes Furaltadone for veterinary use.

Furaltadone was formerly administered by mouth as an antibacterial but was later withdrawn owing to its toxic effects. Furaltadone hydrochloride is still used topically in preparations for external ear disorders.

Furaltadone has been used in veterinary medicine.

Preparations

Proprietary Preparations (details are given in Part 3)

Multi-ingredient: ***Spain:*** Panotile.

Fusafungine (87-j)

Fusafungine *(BAN, rINN)*.

CAS — 1393-87-9.

A depsipeptide antibiotic produced by *Fusarium lateritium* strain 437.

Fusafungine is active against some Gram-positive and Gram-negative organisms and *Candida albicans*. It has also been stated to possess anti-inflammatory activity.

It is used in the form of an aerosol spray in the treatment of infections of the upper respiratory tract in usual doses of 500 µg by inhalation every 4 hours. It has also been given intranasally.

Preparations

Proprietary Preparations (details are given in Part 3)
Aust.: Locabiosol; ***Belg.:*** Locabiotal; ***Fr.:*** Locabiotal; ***Ger.:*** Locabiosol; ***Irl.:*** Locabiotal; ***Ital.:*** Locabiotal; ***S.Afr.:*** Locabiotal; ***Spain:*** Fusaloyos; ***Switz.:*** Locabiotal; ***UK:*** Locabiotal.

Fusidic Acid (88-z)

Fusidic Acid *(BAN, USAN, rINN).*

Acidum Fusidicum; SQ-16603. *ent*-16α-Acetoxy-3β-dihydroxy-4β,8β,14α-trimethyl-18-nor-5β,10α-cholesta-(17*Z*)-17(20),24-dien-21-oic acid hemihydrate.

$C_{31}H_{48}O_6,\frac{1}{2}H_2O$ = 525.7.

CAS — 6990-06-3 (anhydrous fusidic acid).

Pharmacopoeias. In *Eur.* (see p.viii).

An antimicrobial substance produced by the growth of certain strains of *Fusidium coccineum.*

A white or almost white crystalline powder. Practically **insoluble** in water; freely soluble in alcohol. **Store** at a temperature of 2° to 8°. Protect from light.

Sodium Fusidate (154-s)

Sodium Fusidate *(BANM, rINNM).*

Fusidate Sodium *(USAN)*; Natrii Fusidas; SQ-16360.

$C_{31}H_{47}NaO_6$ = 538.7.

CAS — 751-94-0.

Pharmacopoeias. In *Eur.* (see p.viii).

A white or almost white, slightly hygroscopic, crystalline powder. 1 g of monograph substance is approximately equivalent to 0.98 g of fusidic acid.

Freely **soluble** in water and in alcohol. A 1.25% solution in water has a pH of 7.5 to 9.0. **Store** in airtight containers at a temperature of 2° to 8°. Protect from light.

Incompatibility. The UK manufacturers state that the reconstituted sodium fusidate injection is incompatible with infusion solutions containing glucose 20% or more, and that precipitation may occur in solutions with a pH of less than 7.4.

Adverse Effects and Precautions

Apart from mild gastro-intestinal upsets fusidic acid or sodium fusidate appear to be well tolerated when given by mouth. Treatment with fusidates, by mouth or especially by the intravenous route, has been associated with jaundice and changes in liver function; normal liver function is usually restored when treatment is discontinued. Therefore, fusidates should be given with caution to patients with impaired liver function, and periodic monitoring of hepatic function is recommended in these patients and in those receiving high or prolonged oral doses.

Venospasm, thrombophlebitis, and haemolysis have occurred in patients given fusidates intravenously. To reduce this it is recommended that solutions be buffered and that the solution should be given as a slow infusion into a large vein where there is a good blood-flow. Hypocalcaemia has occurred after intravenous administration of doses above those recommended, and has been attributed to the phosphate-citrate buffer in the preparation. Intramuscular or subcutaneous administration may lead to tissue necrosis and is contra-indicated.

Hypersensitivity reactions in the form of rashes and irritation may occur after the topical administration of fusidates; rash is rare after systemic administration. Fusidic acid or its derivatives should be avoided in patients known to be hypersensitive to fusidates.

Fusidic acid competes with bilirubin for binding to albumin *in vitro* and caution has been advised if it is given to premature, jaundiced, acidotic or seriously-ill neonates because of the possible risk of kernicterus.

Effects on the blood. There have been occasional reports of granulocytopenia[1-3] and one case of thrombocytopenia[3] following the use of systemic doses of fusidic acid.

1. Revell P, *et al.* Granulocytopenia due to fusidic acid. *Lancet* 1988; **ii:** 454–5.
2. Evans DIK. Granulocytopenia due to fusidic acid. *Lancet* 1988; **ii:** 851.
3. Leibowitz G, *et al.* Leukopenia and thrombocytopenia due to fusidic acid. *Postgrad Med J* 1991; **67:** 591–2.

Antimicrobial Action

Fusidic acid is a steroidal antibiotic with a bacteriostatic or bactericidal activity mainly against Gram-positive bacteria.

Mechanism of action. Fusidic acid inhibits bacterial protein synthesis, although, in contrast to drugs such as the macrolides or tetracyclines it does not bind to the bacterial ribosome, but inhibits a factor necessary for translocation of peptide subunits and elongation of the peptide chain. It is capable of inhibiting protein synthesis in mammalian cells but exerts a selective action against susceptible infecting organisms because of poor penetration into the host cell.

Spectrum of activity. Fusidic acid is very active against staphylococci, notably *Staph. aureus* and *Staph. epidermidis* (including methicillin-resistant strains). *Nocardia asteroides* and many clostridial strains are also highly susceptible. The streptococci and enterococci are less susceptible.

Most Gram-negative bacteria are intrinsically resistant but fusidic acid is active against *Neisseria* spp. and *Bacteroides fragilis.* It has some activity against strains of *Mycobacterium tuberculosis* and *M. leprae.*

Fungi are resistant, but fusidic acid has some activity against a range of protozoa including *Giardia lamblia* and *Plasmodium falciparum.* High concentrations of fusidate are reported to inhibit viral growth *in vitro*, including that of HIV, although it is unclear whether this represents a surfactant effect, a general cytotoxic effect, or a genuine antiviral action.

Minimum inhibitory concentrations (MICs) for susceptible *Staph. aureus* isolates are reported to range from about 0.03 to 0.1 μg per mL; up to 16 μg per mL may be required to inhibit streptococci. The activity is reduced in the presence of protein. Fusidic acid is bactericidal for many strains at concentrations close to the MIC, but in most methicillin-resistant *Staph. aureus* the ratio of the bactericidal to the inhibitory concentration is much greater.

Activity with other antimicrobials. No synergy has been demonstrated *in vitro* in most studies between fusidic acid and rifampicin or vancomycin, and antagonism of the effects of ciprofloxacin has been reported. Interactions with the penicillins are complex, with either antagonism of the effect of one or both drugs, or no interaction. However, the combination of an antistaphylococcal penicillin with fusidic acid may prevent the emergence of fusidic acid-resistant staphylococcal mutants, and such combinations may be clinically effective.

Resistance. Resistant strains of staphylococci are readily selected *in vitro*, and occasionally during therapy, but the number of clinical isolates that are initially resistant remains relatively low at about 1 to 2% overall, despite widespread topical use. Resistance may be chromosomally mediated, representing altered protein synthesis, or plasmid-mediated, which appears to be due to reduced penetration of active drug into the cell.

Pharmacokinetics

Sodium fusidate is well absorbed from the gastro-intestinal tract, and a single 500-mg dose is reported to produce mean plasma concentrations of about 30 μg per mL 2 to 4 hours after administration, although there is considerable interindividual variation. Oral suspensions of fusidic acid are less well absorbed, and a 500-mg dose of such a suspension is reported to produce peak plasma concentrations of about 23 μg per mL. Absorption may be delayed by food, but may be more rapid in children than adults. Some accumulation occurs with repeated administration and plasma concentrations of 100 μg per mL or more have been reported following 500 mg of sodium fusidate three times daily for 4 days.

Fusidate is widely distributed into tissues and body fluids, including bone, pus, and synovial fluid; it penetrates cerebral abscesses but does not enter CSF in appreciable amounts. It has been found in the fetal circulation and in breast milk. About 95% or more of fusidate in the circulation is bound to plasma protein.

Fusidate has a plasma half-life that has been variously reported as 5 to 6 and 10 to 15 hours. It is excreted in the bile, almost entirely as metabolites some of which have weak antimicrobial activity. About 2% appears unchanged in the faeces. Little is excreted in the urine or removed by haemodialysis.

References.

1. Reeves DS. The pharmacokinetics of fusidic acid. *J Antimicrob Chemother* 1987; **20:** 467–76.
2. Peter J-D, *et al.* Pharmacokinetics of intravenous fusidic acid in patients with cholestasis. *Antimicrob Agents Chemother* 1993; **37:** 501–6.
3. Brown NM, *et al.* The pharmacokinetics and protein-binding of fusidic acid in patients with severe renal failure requiring either haemodialysis or continuous ambulatory peritoneal dialysis. *J Antimicrob Chemother* 1997; **39:** 803–9.

Uses and Administration

Fusidic acid and its salts are antibiotics used mainly in the treatment of staphylococcal infections, often in conjunction with other drugs. They have been used in the treatment of abscess, including brain abscess, in bone and joint infections, in staphylococcal infections in patients with cystic fibrosis, in the treatment of staphylococcal endocarditis, and topically in eye infections and infections of the skin. For details of these infections and their treatment see under Choice of Antibacterial, p.116.

Administration and dosage. The fusidates are given by mouth or topically as fusidic acid or sodium fusidate, or intravenously as sodium fusidate. The diethanolamine salt has also been used intravenously. Sodium fusidate is administered as tablets in a usual dose of 500 mg by mouth every 8 hours, although this dose may be doubled in severe infection. Because of differences in absorption (see Pharmacokinetics, above) 250 mg of fusidic acid is therapeutically equivalent to only 175 mg of the sodium salt, so doses of fusidic acid suspension appear relatively higher. Suggested doses are: up to 1 year, 50 mg per kg body-weight daily in 3 divided doses; 1 to 5 years, 250 mg three times daily; 5 to 12 years, 500 mg three times daily; over 12 years, 750 mg three times daily.

In severe infections sodium fusidate 500 mg is given three times daily by slow intravenous infusion. Each 500-mg dose is usually administered as a buffered solution (pH 7.4 to 7.6) diluted to 500 mL with sodium chloride or other suitable intravenous solution. For children and adults weighing less than 50 kg a dose of 6 to 7 mg per kg body-weight three times daily is recommended.

Sodium fusidate as an ointment (2%) or medicated dressing, or fusidic acid as a cream or gel (2%), are used in the local treatment of skin infections. A sterile gel of fusidic acid (2%) has been used for the treatment of abscesses and 1% eye drops of fusidic acid may be used in eye infections. Topical use may lead to problems of resistance.

Preparations

BP 1998: Fusidic Acid Oral Suspension; Sodium Fusidate Ointment.

Proprietary Preparations (details are given in Part 3)
Aust.: Fucidin; Fucithalmic; ***Austral.:*** Fucidin; ***Belg.:*** Fucidin; Fucithalmic; ***Canad.:*** Fucidin; ***Fr.:*** Fucidine; Fucithalmic; ***Ger.:*** Fucidine; Fucithalmic; ***Irl.:*** Fucidin; Fucithalmic; ***Ital.:*** Fucidin†; Fucithalmic; Stafusid Antibiotico†; ***Neth.:*** Fucidin; Fucithalmic; ***Norw.:*** Fucidin; Fucithalmic; ***S.Afr.:*** Fucidin; Fucithalmic; ***Spain:*** Fucidine; Fucithalmic; ***Swed.:*** Fucidin; Fucithalmic; ***Switz.:*** Fucidine; Fucithalmic; ***UK:*** Fucidin; Fucithalmic.

Multi-ingredient: ***Belg.:*** Fucicort; ***Ger.:*** Fucicort; Fucidine H†; Fucidine plus; ***Irl.:*** Fucibet; Fucidin H; ***Ital.:*** Tibicorten F†; ***S.Afr.:*** Fucidin H; ***Spain:*** Fucibet; ***Swed.:*** Fucidin-Hydrocortison; ***Switz.:*** Fucicort; ***UK:*** Fucibet; Fucidin H.

Gentamicin Sulphate (89-c)

Gentamicin Sulphate (BANM, pINNM).

Gentamicin Sulfate (USAN); Gentamicini Sulfas; NSC-82261; Sch-9724.

CAS — 1403-66-3 (gentamicin); 1405-41-0 (gentamicin sulphate).

NOTE. GNT is a code approved by the BP for use on single unit doses of eye drops containing gentamicin sulphate where the individual container may be too small to bear all the appropriate labelling information.

Pharmacopoeias. In *Chin., Eur.* (see p.viii), *Int., Jpn, Pol.,* and *US.*

The sulphates of a mixture of antimicrobial substances produced by *Micromonospora purpurea*. Gentamicin sulphate is a complex mixture of the sulphates of gentamicin C_1, gentamicin C_{1A}, and gentamicin C_2. Some commercial samples may contain significant quantities of the minor components gentamicin C_{2A} and gentamicin C_{2B}. It contains when dried not less than 590 units of gentamicin per mg.

A white to buff powder. Freely **soluble** in water; practically insoluble in alcohol, acetone, chloroform, and ether. A 4% solution in water has a pH of 3.5 to 5.5. The powder has been sterilised by irradiation. **Store** in airtight containers.

Incompatibilities. The aminoglycosides are inactivated *in vitro* by various penicillins and cephalosporins via an interaction with the beta-lactam ring, the extent of inactivation depending on temperature, concentration, and duration of contact. The different aminoglycosides vary in their stability, with amikacin apparently the most resistant and tobramycin the most susceptible to inactivation; gentamicin and netilmicin are of intermediate stability. The beta lactams also vary in their ability to produce inactivation, with ampicillin, benzylpenicillin, and antipseudomonal penicillins such as carbenicillin and ticarcillin producing marked inactivation. Inactivation has also been reported with clavulanic acid.

Gentamicin is also incompatible with frusemide, heparin, sodium bicarbonate (the acid pH of gentamicin solutions may liberate carbon dioxide), and some solutions for parenteral nutrition. Interactions with preparations having an alkaline pH, or drugs unstable at acid pH, might reasonably be expected.

Given their potential for incompatibility, gentamicin and other aminoglycosides should not generally be mixed with other drugs in syringes or infusion solutions nor given through the same intravenous line. When aminoglycosides are given with a beta lactam administration should generally be at separate sites.

References to the incompatibility of aminoglycosides with beta lactams.

1. Tindula RJ, *et al.* Aminoglycoside inactivation by penicillins and cephalosporins and its impact on drug-level monitoring. *Drug Intell Clin Pharm* 1983; **17:** 906–8.
2. Henderson JL, *et al.* In vitro inactivation of gentamicin, tobramycin, and netilmicin by carbenicillin, azlocillin, or mezlocillin. *Am J Hosp Pharm* 1981; **38:** 1167–70.
3. Wright DN, *et al.* In vitro inactivation of aminoglycosides by apalcillin. *Antimicrob Agents Chemother* 1986; **29:** 353–4.
4. Navarro AS, *et al.* In-vitro interaction between dibekacin and penicillins. *J Antimicrob Chemother* 1986; **17:** 83–9.
5. Courcol RJ, Martin GR. Comparative aminoglycoside inactivation by potassium clavulanate. *J Antimicrob Chemother* 1986; **17:** 682–4.

Stability. There was an average 16% potency loss of gentamicin sulphate from solutions containing 10 and 40 mg per mL when stored at 4° or 25° in plastic disposable syringes for 30 days, and a brown precipitate formed in several. Storage in glass disposable syringes for 30 days produced an average 7% potency loss, which was considered acceptable, but storage for longer resulted in precipitate formation in some cases and was not recommended.[1]

1. Weiner B, *et al.* Stability of gentamicin sulfate injection following unit dose repackaging. *Am J Hosp Pharm* 1976; **33:** 1254–9.

Adverse Effects

The aminoglycosides can produce irreversible, cumulative ototoxicity affecting both the cochlea (manifest as hearing loss, initially of higher tones, and which, because speech recognition relies greatly on lower frequencies, may not be at first apparent) and the vestibular system (manifest as dizziness or vertigo). The incidence and relative toxicity with different aminoglycosides is a matter of some dispute, but netilmicin is probably less cochleotoxic than gentamicin or tobramycin, and amikacin more so, and netilmicin also exhibits less vestibular toxicity than gentamicin, tobramycin, or amikacin while streptomycin produces a high incidence of vestibular damage. Vestibular damage is more common than hearing loss in patients receiving gentamicin.

Reversible nephrotoxicity may occur and acute renal failure has been reported, often in association with the concurrent administration of other nephrotoxic drugs. Renal impairment is usually mild, although acute tubular necrosis and interstitial nephritis have occurred. Decreased glomerular filtration rate is usually seen only after several days, and may even occur after therapy has been discontinued. Electrolyte disturbances (notably hypomagnesaemia, but also hypocalcaemia and hypokalaemia) have occurred. The nephrotoxicity of gentamicin is reported to be largely due to the gentamicin C_2 component.

Although particularly associated with high plasma concentrations, many risk factors have been suggested for ototoxicity and nephrotoxicity in patients receiving aminoglycosides—see Precautions below.

Aminoglycosides possess a neuromuscular blocking action and respiratory depression and muscular paralysis have been reported, notably after absorption from serous surfaces. Neomycin has the most potent action and several deaths have been associated with its use.

Hypersensitivity reactions have occurred, especially after local use, and cross-sensitivity between aminoglycosides may occur. Very rarely, anaphylactic reactions to gentamicin have occurred. Some hypersensitivity reactions have been attributed to the presence of sulphites in parenteral formulations, and endotoxic shock has also been reported.

Infrequent effects reported for gentamicin include blood dyscrasias, purpura, nausea and vomiting, stomatitis, and signs of liver dysfunction such as increased serum aminotransferase values, and increased serum-bilirubin concentrations. Neurotoxicity has occurred, with both peripheral neuropathies and central symptoms being reported including encephalopathy, confusion, lethargy, hallucinations, convulsions, and mental depression. There have been isolated reports of meningeal irritation, arachnoiditis, polyradiculitis, and ventriculitis following the intrathecal, intracisternal, or intraventricular administration of aminoglycosides. Subconjunctival injection of gentamicin may lead to pain, hyperaemia, and conjunctival oedema, while severe retinal ischaemia has followed intra-ocular injection.

Effects on the ears. Reviews and references to aminoglycoside-induced ototoxicity.

1. Cone LA. A survey of prospective, controlled clinical trials of gentamicin, tobramycin, amikacin, and netilmicin. *Clin Ther* 1982; **5:** 155–62.
2. Kahlmeter G, Dahlager JI. Aminoglycoside toxicity—a review of clinical studies published between 1975 and 1982. *J Antimicrob Chemother* 1984; **13** (suppl A): 9–22.
3. Brummett RE, Fox KE. Aminoglycoside-induced hearing loss in humans. *Antimicrob Agents Chemother* 1989; **33:** 797–800.
4. Mattie H, *et al.* Determinants of efficacy and toxicity of aminoglycosides. *J Antimicrob Chemother* 1989; **24:** 281–93.

Effects on the kidney. Some references and reviews on aminoglycoside-induced nephrotoxicity.

1. Cone LA. A survey of prospective, controlled clinical trials of gentamicin, tobramycin, amikacin, and netilmicin. *Clin Ther* 1982; **5:** 155–62.
2. Lietman PS, Smith CR. Aminoglycoside nephrotoxicity in humans. *Rev Infect Dis* 1983; **5** (suppl 2): S284–93.
3. Kahlmeter G, Dahlager JI. Aminoglycoside toxicity—a review of clinical studies published between 1975 and 1982. *J Antimicrob Chemother* 1984; **13** (suppl A): 9–22.
4. Kohlapp SJ, *et al.* Nephrotoxicity of the constituents of the gentamicin complex. *J Infect Dis* 1984; **149:** 605–14.
5. Mattie H, *et al.* Determinants of efficacy and toxicity of aminoglycosides. *J Antimicrob Chemother* 1989; **24:** 281–93.
6. Appel GB. Aminoglycoside nephrotoxicity. *Am J Med* 1990; **88** (suppl 3C): 16S–20S.
7. Bertino JS, *et al.* Incidence of and significant risk factors for aminoglycoside-associated nephrotoxicity in patients dosed by using individualized pharmacokinetic monitoring. *J Infect Dis* 1993; **167:** 173–9.

Treatment of Adverse Effects

Aminoglycosides may be removed by haemodialysis or to a much lesser extent by peritoneal dialysis. Calcium salts given intravenously have been used to counter neuromuscular blockade; the effectiveness of neostigmine has been variable.

For the suggestion that calcium-channel blockers may reduce aminoglycoside-related nephrotoxicity, see Kidney Disorders, under Uses of Verapamil, p.963.

Precautions

Gentamicin is contra-indicated in patients with a known history of allergy to it, and probably in those allergic to other aminoglycosides. Great care is required in patients with myasthenia gravis, parkinsonism, and other conditions characterised by muscular weakness.

Because the risk of ototoxicity and nephrotoxicity is increased at high plasma concentrations, it is generally desirable to determine dosage requirements of the aminoglycosides by individual monitoring. In patients receiving gentamicin, dosage should be adjusted to avoid peak plasma concentrations above 10 to 12 μg per mL, or trough concentrations (immediately before next dose) exceeding 2 μg per mL. Monitoring is particularly important in patients receiving high doses or prolonged courses, in infants and the elderly, and in patients with impaired renal function, who generally require reduced doses. Some authorities consider that monitoring is also important in obese patients and those with cystic fibrosis. See Pharmacokinetics below for other patient groups in whom pharmacokinetics may be altered. Impaired hepatic function or auditory function, bacteraemia, fever, and perhaps exposure to loud noises have also been reported to increase the risk of ototoxicity, while volume depletion or hypotension, liver disease, or female sex have been reported as additional risk factors for nephrotoxicity. Regular assessment of auditory and renal function is particularly necessary in patients with additional risk factors.

Topical application of gentamicin is contra-indicated in patients with known or suspected perforation of the ear drum.

Use of aminoglycosides during pregnancy may damage the 8th cranial nerve of the fetus.

Interference with assay procedures. The implications of drug interference with assays for aminoglycosides have been reviewed by Yosselson-Superstine.[1] A number of other antimicrobials and antineoplastics may alter the results of microbiological assays but this might be overcome by selection of an appropriate assay organism. Microbiological assays for aminoglycosides in samples also containing imipenem could be accomplished by using cysteine hydrochloride to inactivate imipenem since it is stable to most beta-lactamases and resistant strains are extremely rare.[2] Because aminoglycosides may be inactivated by penicillins and cephalosporins it has been recommended that aminoglycoside sampling times should be chosen to coincide with a trough plasma concentration for the beta lactam. Samples should be frozen if there is to be a delay before they are assayed[3] or a penicillinase added. However, one group of workers have reported loss of gentamicin activity after storage at −60° before assay.[4] Furthermore, there have been reports that concentrations of aminoglycosides in patients also receiving beta lactams have been overestimated using a homogeneous enzyme immunoassay, probably because of an inability to differentiate between active drug and inactivated products.[5,6] The radionuclide gallium-67 interferes with radio-enzymatic assays and it has been suggested that an agar diffusion method should be used in patients who have received a gallium scan.[7,8] Heparin has been shown to produce underestimation of aminoglycoside concentrations when using microbiological, enzymatic, or immunoassays.[9-11] It has been recommended that either serum should be used or that blood samples should not be collected in heparinised tubes or from indwelling catheter lines. Some consider that concentrations of heparin reached in the blood of patients receiving heparin are too low to affect gentamicin.[12] Falsely low concentrations have also been reported in microbiological assays in the presence of zinc salts.[13] Heat treatment of whole blood to inactivate human immunodeficiency virus leads to an increase in the concentration of gentamicin subsequently found on assay.[14]

1. Yosselson-Superstine S. Drug interferences with plasma assays in therapeutic drug monitoring. *Clin Pharmacokinet* 1984; **9:** 67–87.
2. McLeod KM, *et al.* Gentamicin assay in the presence of imipenem. *J Antimicrob Chemother* 1986; **17:** 828–9.
3. Tindula RJ, *et al.* Aminoglycoside inactivation by penicillins and cephalosporins and its impact on drug-level monitoring. *Drug Intell Clin Pharm* 1983; **17:** 906–8.

4. Carlson LG, *et al.* Potential liabilities of gentamicin homogeneous enzyme immunoassay. *Antimicrob Agents Chemother* 1982; **21:** 192–4.
5. Ebert SC, Clementi WA. In vitro inactivation of gentamicin by carbenicillin, compared by Emit and microbiological assays. *Drug Intell Clin Pharm* 1983; **17:** 451.
6. Dalmady-Israel C, *et al.* Ticarcillin and assay of tobramycin. *Ann Intern Med* 1984; **100:** 460.
7. Bhattacharya I, *et al.* Effects of radiopharmaceuticals on radioenzymatic assays of aminoglycoside antibiotics: interference by gallium-67 and its elimination. *Antimicrob Agents Chemother* 1978; **14:** 448–53.
8. Shannon K, *et al.* Interference with gentamicin assays by gallium-67. *J Antimicrob Chemother* 1980; **6:** 285–300.
9. Nilsson L. Factors affecting gentamicin assay. *Antimicrob Agents Chemother* 1980; **17:** 918–21. Correction. *ibid.*; **18:** 839.
10. Nilsson L, *et al.* Inhibition of aminoglycoside activity by heparin. *Antimicrob Agents Chemother* 1981: **20:** 155–8.
11. O'Connell MB, *et al.* Heparin interference with tobramycin, netilmicin, and gentamicin concentrations determined by Emit. *Drug Intell Clin Pharm* 1984; **18:** 503–4.
12. Regamey C, *et al.* Inhibitory effect of heparin on gentamicin concentrations in blood. *Antimicrob Agents Chemother* 1972; **1:** 329–32.
13. George RH, Healing DE. The effect of zinc on aminoglycoside assay. *J Antimicrob Chemother* 1978; **4:** 186.
14. Eley A, *et al.* Effect of heat on gentamicin assays. *Lancet* 1987; **ii:** 335–6.

Interactions

Concurrent use of other nephrotoxic drugs, including other aminoglycosides, vancomycin, some of the cephalosporins, cyclosporin, and cisplatin, or potentially ototoxic drugs such as ethacrynic acid and perhaps frusemide, may increase the risk of aminoglycoside toxicity. It has been suggested that concurrent use of an antiemetic such as dimenhydrinate may mask the early symptoms of vestibular ototoxicity. Care is also required if other drugs with a neuromuscular blocking action are given concomitantly (p.1306). The neuromuscular blocking properties of aminoglycoside may be sufficient to provoke severe respiratory depression in patients receiving general anaesthetics or opioids.

There is a theoretical possibility that the antibacterial effects of aminoglycosides could be reduced by use with a bacteriostatic antibacterial, but such combinations have been used successfully in practice.

Since aminoglycosides have been shown to be incompatible with some beta lactams *in vitro* (see Incompatibility, above) these antibacterials should be administered separately if both are required; antagonism *in vivo* has been reported only in a few patients with severe renal impairment, in whom aminoglycoside activity was diminished. Aminoglycosides exhibit synergistic activity with a number of beta lactams *in vivo* (below).

For a report of severe hypocalcaemia in a patient receiving aminoglycosides and bisphosphonates, see p.735.

Antimicrobial Action

Gentamicin is an aminoglycoside antibiotic and has a bactericidal action against many Gram-negative aerobes and against some strains of staphylococci.

Mechanism of action. Aminoglycosides are taken up into sensitive bacterial cells by an active transport process which is inhibited in anaerobic, acidic, or hyperosmolar environments. Within the cell they bind to the 30S, and to some extent to the 50S subunits of the bacterial ribosome, inhibiting protein synthesis and generating errors in the transcription of the genetic code. The manner in which cell death is brought about is imperfectly understood, and other mechanisms may contribute, including effects on membrane permeability.

Spectrum of activity. The following pathogenic organisms are usually sensitive to gentamicin (but see also Resistance, below).

Many strains of Gram-negative bacteria including species of *Brucella, Calymmatobacterium, Campylobacter, Citrobacter, Escherichia, Enterobacter, Klebsiella, Proteus, Providencia, Pseudomonas, Serratia, Vibrio*, and *Yersinia*. Some activity has been reported against isolates of *Neisseria* although aminoglycosides are rarely used clinically in neisserial infections.

Among the Gram-positive organisms many strains of *Staphylococcus aureus* are highly sensitive to gentamicin. *Listeria monocytogenes* and some strains of *Staph. epidermidis* may also be sensitive to gentamicin, but enterococci and streptococci are insensitive to gentamicin.

Some actinomycetes and mycoplasmas have been reported to be sensitive to gentamicin but mycobacteria are insensitive at clinically achievable concentrations; anaerobic organisms, yeasts, and fungi are resistant.

Minimum inhibitory concentrations (MICs) of gentamicin for the most sensitive organisms (some staphylococci, enterobacteria, sensitive *Pseudomonas aeruginosa* strains) are 0.03 to 2 μg per mL; the aminoglycosides are usually bactericidal at concentrations not far above the MIC. Organisms with MICs up to about 8 μg per mL are generally considered sensitive to gentamicin. Bacterial regrowth does not resume immediately the concentration of gentamicin falls below the MIC, and this prolonged postantibiotic effect is the basis for once-daily dosing (see below).

Activity with other antimicrobials. Gentamicin exhibits synergy with beta lactams, probably because the effects of the latter on bacterial cell walls enhance aminoglycoside penetration. Enhanced activity has been demonstrated with a penicillin (such as ampicillin or benzylpenicillin) and gentamicin against the enterococci, and gentamicin has been combined with an antipseudomonal penicillin such as ticarcillin for enhanced activity against *Pseudomonas* spp., and with vancomycin for enhanced activity against staphylococci and streptococci.

Resistance to the aminoglycosides may be acquired by three main mechanisms. The first is by mutation of ribosomal target sites leading to reduced affinity for binding; this type of resistance is generally only relevant for streptomycin and, even then, it appears to be rare in Gram-negative bacteria. Secondly, penetration of aminoglycosides into bacterial cells is by an oxygen-dependent active transport process and resistance may occur because of elimination or reduction of this uptake; when it occurs this generally results in cross resistance to all aminoglycosides. Thirdly, and by far the most important cause of resistance to the aminoglycosides, is inactivation by enzymatic modification. Three main classes of enzyme conferring resistance have been found, operating by phosphorylation, acetylation, or addition of a nucleotide group, usually adenyl. Enzyme production is usually plasmid-determined and resistance can therefore be transferred between bacteria, even of different species. Resistance to other antibacterials may be transferred at the same time. In *Staph. aureus* such transfer of resistance is reportedly facilitated when these drugs are used topically. Each type of enzyme produces characteristic patterns of resistance, but their overlapping and variable affinities for their substrates result in a wide range of permutations of cross resistance to the different aminoglycosides.

The different enzymes vary in their distribution and prevalence in different locations, and at different time, presumably with variations in antibacterial usage, but relationships to the use of specific aminoglycosides are difficult to establish. These variations in drug sensitivity require local testing to determine resistance and establish susceptibility of bacteria to the aminoglycoside being used.

Because of such local variations, estimates of the incidence of resistance are of limited value. In general, the occurrence of resistant pathogens seems to be greater in Southern than in Northern Europe, and perhaps greater in the USA than in Europe. There has been particular concern over the increasing incidence of high-level gentamicin resistance among enterococci (in up to 50% of isolates from some centres) since they already possess inherent or acquired resistance to many drugs, including vancomycin in some cases; a similar problem exists with gentamicin resistance in methicillin-resistant strains of *Staph. aureus*. Such multiply-resistant strains pose a major therapeutic problem in those centres where they occur, since the usual synergistic combinations with other antibacterials are ineffective. However, results from some centres indicate that rational use of a wider range of aminoglycosides (including amikacin which is not affected by most of the aminoglycoside degrading enzymes) has resulted in a modest decline in overall aminoglycoside resistance.

Pharmacokinetics

Gentamicin and other aminoglycosides are poorly absorbed from the gastro-intestinal tract but are rapidly absorbed after intramuscular injection. Average peak plasma concentrations of about 4 μg per mL have been attained in patients with normal renal function 30 to 60 minutes after intramuscular administration of a dose equivalent to 1 mg of gentamicin per kg body-weight, which is similar to concentrations achieved after intravenous infusion. There may be considerable individual variation. Several doses are required before plasma equilibrium concentrations occur and this may represent the saturation of binding sites in body tissues such as the kidney. Binding of gentamicin to plasma proteins is usually low.

Following parenteral administration gentamicin and other aminoglycosides diffuse mainly into extracellular fluids. However, there is little diffusion into the CSF and even when the meninges are inflamed effective concentrations may not be achieved; diffusion into the eye is also poor. Aminoglycosides diffuse readily into the perilymph of the inner ear. They cross the placenta but only small amounts have been reported in breast milk.

Systemic absorption of gentamicin and other aminoglycosides has been reported after topical use on denuded skin and burns and following instillation into, and irrigation of, wounds, body-cavities, and joints, but not the urinary bladder.

The plasma elimination half-life for gentamicin has been reported to be 2 to 3 hours though it may be considerably longer in neonates and patients with renal impairment. Gentamicin and other aminoglycosides do not appear to be metabolised and are excreted virtually unchanged in the urine by glomerular filtration. At steady-state at least 70% of a dose may be recovered in the urine in 24 hours and urine concentrations in excess of 100 μg per mL may be achieved. However, gentamicin and the other aminoglycosides appear to accumulate in body tissues to some extent, mainly in the kidney, although the relative degree to which this occurs may vary with different aminoglycosides. Release from these sites is slow and small amounts of aminoglycosides may be detected in the urine for up to 20 days or more after administration ceases. Small amounts of gentamicin appear in the bile.

The pharmacokinetics of the aminoglycosides are affected by many factors, which may become significant because of the relatively small difference between therapeutic and toxic concentrations, reinforcing the need for monitoring. Absorption from intramuscular sites may be reduced in critically-ill patients, especially in conditions that reduce perfusion such as shock. Plasma concentrations may also be reduced in patients with conditions which expand extracellular fluid volume or increase renal clearance including ascites, cirrhosis, heart failure, malnutrition, spinal cord injury, burns, cystic fibrosis, and possibly leukaemia. Clearance is also reportedly increased in intravenous drug abusers, and in patients who are febrile. In contrast, renal impairment or reduced renal clearance for any reason (for example in neonates with immature renal function, or in the elderly in whom glomerular function tends to decline with age) can result in markedly increased plasma concentrations and/or prolonged half-lives (although in neonates initial plasma concentrations may actually be reduced, due to a larger volume of distribution). Plasma concentrations may also be higher than expected for a given dose in obese patients (in whom extracellular volume is lower, relative to weight), and in patients with anaemia.

Renal clearance, and hence plasma concentrations, of aminoglycosides may vary according to a circadian cycle, and it has been suggested that this should be taken into account when determining and comparing plasma aminoglycoside concentrations.

Uses and Administration

Gentamicin is an aminoglycoside antibiotic used, usually in combination, to treat severe systemic infections due to sensitive Gram-negative and other organisms (see Antimicrobial Action above). They include biliary-tract infections (acute cholecystitis or cholangitis), brucellosis, cat scratch disease, cystic fibrosis, endocarditis (in the treatment and prophylaxis of endocarditis due to streptococci, enterococci, or staphylococci), endometritis, gastroenteritis, granuloma inguinale, listeriosis, meningitis, otitis externa, otitis media, pelvic inflammatory disease, peritonitis, plague, pneumonia, septicaemia, skin infections such as in burns or ulcers (given systemically for pseudomonal and other Gram-negative infections), and urinary-tract infections (acute pyelonephritis), as well as in the prophylaxis of surgical infection and the treatment of immunocompromised patients and those in intensive care. For details of these infections and their treatment, see under Choice of Antibacterial, p.116.

Gentamicin is often used concomitantly with other antibacterials to extend its spectrum of efficacy or increase its effectiveness, e.g. with a penicillin for enterococcal and streptococcal infections, or an antipseudomonal beta lactam for pseudomonal infections, or with metronidazole or clindamycin for mixed aerobic-anaerobic infections.

Administration and dosage. Gentamicin is used as the sulphate but doses are expressed in terms of gentamicin base. In the management of many of the infections above it is commonly given intramuscularly every 8 hours to provide a total daily dose of 3 to 5 mg of gentamicin per kg body-weight. Slightly lower doses have been suggested in the prophylaxis and treatment of streptococcal endocarditis: in the UK a dose of 60 to 80 mg of gentamicin, given twice daily in association with penicillin or vancomycin has been suggested for treatment, and 120 mg before induction of anaesthesia, with a penicillin or vancomycin or teicoplanin, in prophylaxis for high-risk patients. For urinary-tract infections, if renal function is not impaired, 160 mg once daily may be used.

Gentamicin sulphate may also be given intravenously in similar doses to those used intramuscularly, but there is some disagreement as to the appropriate method. In the USA, intravenous infusion over 30 minutes to 2 hours is favoured, but sources in the UK differ, with some manufacturers recommending infusion over no more than 20 minutes, in a limited fluid volume, while others suggest that it should not be given by infusion, recommending bolus injection over 2 to 3 minutes, and yet others recommend administration in a similar way to the USA. Both methods present problems: intravenous infusion has been associated with both subtherapeutic and excessive trough concentrations of gentamicin, while bolus injection may increase the risk of neuromuscular blockade.

The course of treatment should generally be limited to 7 to 10 days. As gentamicin is poorly distributed into fatty tissue some authorities suggest that dosage calculations should be based on an estimate of lean body-weight.

Doses in infants and children are usually somewhat higher than those in adults but exact dosage recommendations vary. One suggested dose is 3 mg of gentamicin per kg every 12 hours in premature infants and those up to 2 weeks of age, with older neonates and children receiving 2 mg per kg every 8 hours. Alternatively, 2.5 mg per kg every 12 hours in the first week of life (increased to every 18 hours in those of less than 35 weeks gestation); 2.5 mg per kg every 8 hours in infants and neonates; and 2.0 to 2.5 mg per kg every 8 hours in children has been suggested.

Dose adjustment and monitoring. It is recommended that dosage should be adjusted in all patients according to plasma-gentamicin concentrations, and this is particularly important where factors such as age, renal impairment, or high dose may predispose to toxicity, or where there is a risk of subtherapeutic concentrations (see Pharmacokinetics, above, for factors that may affect plasma concentrations). Although there has been some dispute about the relationship between plasma concentrations and toxicity it is generally recommended that trough plasma concentrations (measured just before the next dose) should be less than 2 μg per mL, and peak concentrations should reach at least 4 μg per mL but not exceed 10 to 12 μg per mL. In the UK peak concentrations are generally measured one hour after intramuscular and intravenous administration, but the latter has varied between centres and countries and may lead to difficulties in comparing figures.

Various methods, none universally accepted, have been proposed for calculating aminoglycoside dosage requirements. Predictive nomograms, although possibly valuable in determining an initial dose, for example in renal impairment, are considered to be unsuitable for further dose determination, and methods based on the use of individualised pharmacokinetic parameters are recommended. Good results have been reported with the method of Sawchuk and Zaske, or with methods using Bayesian statistics which may be somewhat simpler to implement (for references see below).

Once-daily dosage. Some sources consider, in contrast to what has been the accepted view, that there may be advantages to administering the total daily requirement as a single dose (see below). However, it is not yet clear whether once-daily dosage is as effective as conventional dosage regimens in all cases, particularly in children, or in patients with endocarditis, renal impairment, or who are immunocompromised. With once-daily dosage, traditional methods of monitoring peak and trough plasma concentrations may not be applicable and advice on dosage and plasma concentrations should be sought.

Other routes. Gentamicin has sometimes been given by mouth for enteric infections and to suppress intestinal flora and has occasionally been given by inhalation in cystic fibrosis. In meningitis it has been administered intrathecally or intraventricularly usually in doses of 1 to 5 mg daily in conjunction with intramuscular therapy. Doses of 20 to 40 mg have been given by subconjunctival injection.

A bone cement impregnated with gentamicin is used in orthopaedic surgery. Acrylic beads containing gentamicin and threaded on to surgical wire are implanted in the management of bone infections.

Gentamicin is also used topically for skin infections in concentrations of 0.1 to 0.3%, but as topical use may lead to the emergence of resistance it is considered inadvisable. Similar concentrations are used in preparations for topical application to the eyes and ears.

A liposomal formulation of gentamicin is under investigation.

Administration and dosage. CONCENTRATION MONITORING. References to the problems of drug concentration monitoring of the aminoglycosides, and the difficulty in correlating concentrations with toxicity.

1. Scott DK, *et al.* Aminoglycoside trough levels: a source of error. *Lancet* 1982; **ii:** 441–2.
2. Wenk M, *et al.* Serum level monitoring of antibacterial drugs: a review. *Clin Pharmacokinet* 1984; **9:** 475–92.
3. Rodvold KA, *et al.* Aminoglycoside pharmacokinetic monitoring: an integral part of patient care? *Clin Pharm* 1988; **7:** 608–13.
4. Banks BEC. Monitoring of aminoglycosides. *J Antimicrob Chemother* 1990; **26:** 145–8.
5. McCormack JP, *et al.* A critical reevaluation of the therapeutic range of aminoglycosides. *Clin Infect Dis* 1992; **14:** 320–39.
6. Aronson JK, Reynolds DJM. Aminoglycoside antibiotics. *Br Med J* 1992; **305;** 1421–4.

DOSAGE CALCULATION. References to methods of dosage calculation for aminoglycosides including nomograms[1-6] and pharmacokinetic methods,[7-16] such as those of Sawchuk and Zaske,[7,8] and Bayesian analysis.[9-11,17,18]

1. Hull JH, Sarubbi FA. Gentamicin serum concentrations: pharmacokinetic predictions. *Ann Intern Med* 1976; **85:** 183–9.
2. Sarubbi FA, Hull JH. Amikacin serum concentrations: prediction of levels and dosage guidelines. *Ann Intern Med* 1978; **89:** 612–18.
3. Chan RA, *et al.* Gentamicin therapy in renal failure: a nomogram for dosage. *Ann Intern Med* 1972; **76:** 773–8.
4. Lesar TS, *et al.* Gentamicin dosing errors with four commonly used nomograms. *JAMA* 1982; **248:** 1190–3.
5. Platt DR, *et al.* Comparison of four methods of predicting serum gentamicin concentrations in adult patients with impaired renal function. *Clin Pharm* 1982; **1:** 361–5.
6. Watling SM, Kisor DF. Population pharmacokinetics: development of a medical intensive care unit-specific gentamicin dosing nomogram. *Ann Pharmacother* 1993; **27:** 151–4.
7. Sawchuk RJ, Zaske DE. Pharmacokinetics of dosing regimens which utilize multiple intravenous infusions: gentamicin in burn patients. *J Pharmacokinet Biopharm* 1976; **4:** 183–95.
8. Sawchuk RJ, *et al.* Kinetic model for gentamicin dosing with the use of individual patient parameters. *Clin Pharmacol Ther* 1977; **21:** 362–9.
9. Burton ME, *et al.* A Bayesian feedback method of aminoglycoside dosing. *Clin Pharmacol Ther* 1985; **37:** 349–57.
10. Koup JR, *et al.* Multiple-dose non-linear regression analysis program: aminoglycoside dose prediction. *Clin Pharmacokinet* 1983; **8:** 456–62.
11. Chrystyn H. Validation of the use of Bayesian analysis in the optimization of gentamicin therapy from the commencement of dosing. *Drug Intell Clin Pharm* 1988; **22:** 49–53.
12. Lackner TE, *et al.* A nonexponential, nonlogarithmic pharmacokinetic dosing method for gentamicin. *Clin Pharm* 1991; **10:** 706–10.
13. Burton ME, *et al.* Accuracy of Bayesian and Sawchuk-Zaske dosing methods for gentamicin. *Clin Pharm* 1986; **5:** 143–9.
14. Rodvold KA, *et al.* Aminoglycoside pharmacokinetics monitoring: an integral part of patient care? *Clin Pharm* 1988; **7:** 608–13.
15. Erdman SM, *et al.* An updated comparison of drug dosing methods part III: aminoglycoside antibiotics. *Clin Pharmacokinet* 1991; **20:** 374–88.
16. Watling SM, Dasta JF. Aminoglycoside dosing considerations in intensive care unit patients. *Ann Pharmacother* 1993; **27:** 351–7.
17. Radomski KM, *et al.* General versus subpopulation values in Bayesian prediction of aminoglycoside pharmacokinetics in hematology-oncology patients. *Am J Health-Syst Pharm* 1997; **54:** 541–4.
18. Duffull SB, *et al.* Comparison of two Bayesian approaches to dose-individualization for once-daily aminoglycoside regimens. *Br J Clin Pharmacol* 1997; **43:** 125–35.

IN NEONATES AND INFANTS. References.

1. Gennrich JL, Nitake M. Devising an aminoglycoside dosage regimen for neonates seven to ninety days chronological age. *Neonatal Pharmacol Q* 1992; **1:** 45–50.
2. Sidhu JS, *et al.* Assessment of bioelectrical impedance for individualising gentamicin therapy in neonates. *Eur J Clin Pharmacol* 1993; **44:** 253–8.
3. Weber W, *et al.* Population kinetics of gentamicin in neonates. *Eur J Clin Pharmacol* 1993; **44** (suppl 1): S23–S25.
4. Isemann BT, *et al.* Optimal gentamicin therapy in preterm neonates includes loading doses and early monitoring. *Ther Drug Monit* 1996; **18:** 549–55.
5. Logsdon BA, Phelps SJ. Routine monitoring of gentamicin serum concentrations in pediatric patients with normal renal function is unnecessary. *Ann Pharmacother* 1997; **31:** 1514–18.3

IN PATIENTS WITH NON-IDEAL BODY-WEIGHT. References.

1. Traynor AM, *et al.* Aminoglycoside dosing weight correction factors for patients of various body sizes. *Antimicrob Agents Chemother* 1995; **39:** 545–8.

IN RENAL IMPAIRMENT. Although a number of nomograms, schedules, and rules have been devised for the calculation of aminoglycoside dosage in renal impairment, where possible dosage modification should be based on the monitoring of individual pharmacokinetic parameters. Standard dosage calculation methods should not be used for patients undergoing dialysis as they may require supplementary post-dialysis doses.

ONCE-DAILY DOSAGE. The concept of administering aminoglycosides once daily rather than in divided doses is attractive on the grounds of convenience and economy. The rationale cited by proponents of single daily doses for preferring high intermittent plasma concentrations includes the prolonged postantibiotic effect of aminoglycosides (persistent antibacterial activity after plasma concentrations have fallen below the MIC), potentially higher antibacterial concentrations at the site of infection, and theoretical reductions in the incidence of adaptive resistance, with no apparent increase in nephrotoxicity. There have been numerous clinical and *animal* studies but clinical studies have generally included small numbers of patients with uncomplicated infections and have excluded patients with altered pharmacokinetic profiles. Despite the deficiencies of these studies, several meta-analyses have been published which have concluded that once-daily administration appears to be at least as effective as, and no more toxic than, multiple daily dosing in such patient populations.[1-7] Some have questioned the validity of these conclusions[8] while others take a more optimistic view.[9] Several methods for calculating doses and monitoring treatment have been proposed[10-12] but consensus is still needed on appropriate treatment regimens and suitable target serum concentrations.[10,13,14] There is currently insufficient information for paediatric or geriatric patients, pregnant or breast-feeding women, or patients with burns, cystic fibrosis, or impaired renal or hepatic function,[10,13,14] although some patient populations are being assessed.[15] Once daily dosage may be inappropriate for the treatment of enterococcal endocarditis.[10]

1. Barza M, *et al.* Single or multiple daily doses of aminoglycosides: a meta-analysis. *Br Med J* 1996; **312:** 338–45.
2. Hatala R, *et al.* Once-daily aminoglycoside dosing in immunocompetent adults: a meta-analysis. *Ann Intern Med* 1996; **124:** 717–25.
3. Ferriols-Lisart R, Alos-Almiñana M. Effectiveness and safety of once-daily aminoglycosides: a meta-analysis. *Am J Health-Syst Pharm* 1996; **53:** 1141–50.
4. Munckhof WJ, *et al.* A meta-analysis of studies on the safety and efficacy of aminoglycosides given either once daily or as divided doses. *J Antimicrob Chemother* 1996; **37:** 645–63.
5. Bailey TC, *et al.* A meta-analysis of extended-interval dosing versus multiple daily dosing of aminoglycosides. *Clin Infect Dis* 1997; **24:** 786–95.
6. Ali MZ, Goetz MB. A meta-analysis of the relative efficacy and toxicity of single daily dosing versus multiple daily dosing of aminoglycosides. *Clin Infect Dis* 1997; **24:** 796–809.
7. Hatala R, *et al.* Single daily dosing of aminoglycosides in immunocompromised adults: a systematic review. *Clin Infect Dis* 1997; **24:** 810–15.
8. Bertino JS, *et al.* Single daily dosing of aminoglycosides—a concept whose time has not yet come. *Clin Infect Dis* 1997; **24:** 820–3.
9. Gilbert DN. Meta-analyses are no longer required for determining the efficacy of single daily dosing of aminoglycosides. *Clin Infect Dis* 1997; **24:** 816–19.
10. Freeman CD, *et al.* Once-daily dosing of aminoglycosides: review and recommendations for clinical practice. *J Antimicrob Chemother* 1997; **39:** 677–86.
11. Begg EJ, *et al.* A suggested approach to once-daily aminoglycoside dosing. *Br J Clin Pharmacol* 1995; **39:** 605–9.
12. Prins JM, *et al.* Validation and nephrotoxicity of a simplified once-daily aminoglycoside dosing schedule and guidelines for monitoring therapy. *Antimicrob Agents Chemother* 1996; **40:** 2494–9.
13. Rodvold KA, *et al.* Single daily doses of aminoglycosides. *Lancet* 1997; **350:** 1412.
14. Anonymous. Aminoglycosides once daily? *Drug Ther Bull* 1997; **35:** 36–7.
15. Finnell DL, *et al.* Validation of the Hartford nomogram in trauma surgery patients. *Ann Pharmacother* 1998; **32:** 417–21.

Ménière's disease. Gentamicin and streptomycin have been used for medical ablation in advanced Ménière's disease (p.400). Although gentamicin given systemically is considered to be more ototoxic than streptomycin evidence from *animal* studies suggests that intratympanic administration may be less ototoxic. This and a higher incidence of side-effects with streptomycin has meant that intratympanic gentamicin is now preferred. Intratympanic gentamicin has been reported to control vertigo symptoms in 91% of patients, though 19% experienced a worsening of their hearing loss immediately after treatment.[1] Other workers using similar methods have also had successful outcomes.[2,3] Although the ideal regimen for intratympanic gentamicin has yet to be defined, its use is considered promising in the treatment of Ménière's disease.

1. Beck C. Intratympanic application of gentamicin for treatment of Menière's disease. *Keio J Med* 1986; **35:** 36–41.
2. Nedzelski JM, *et al.* Chemical labyrinthectomy: local application of gentamicin for the treatment of unilateral Meniere's disease. *Am J Otol* 1992; **13:** 18–22.
3. Pyykkö I, *et al.* Intratympanic gentamicin in bilateral Meniere's disease. *Otolaryngol Head Neck Surg* 1994; **110:** 162–7.

Preparations

BP 1998: Gentamicin Cream; Gentamicin Eye Drops; Gentamicin Injection; Gentamicin Ointment;
USP 23: Gentamicin and Prednisolone Acetate Ophthalmic Ointment; Gentamicin and Prednisolone Acetate Ophthalmic Suspension; Gentamicin Injection; Gentamicin Sulfate Cream; Gentamicin Sulfate Ointment; Gentamicin Sulfate Ophthalmic Ointment; Gentamicin Sulfate Ophthalmic Solution.

Proprietary Preparations (details are given in Part 3)
Aust.: Gentax; Refobacin; Sulmycin; ***Austral.:*** Cidomycin†; Garamycin; Genoptic; ***Belg.:*** Alcomicin†; Genoptic†; Gentamytrex; Geomycine; ***Canad.:*** Alcomicin; Cidomycin; Diogent; Garamycin; Garatec; Gentacidin; Ocugram; RO-Gentycin†; ***Fr.:*** Gentabilles; Gentalline; Martigenta†; Ophtagram; ***Ger.:*** Dispagent; duragentamt†; duragentamicin; Gencin; Gent-Ophtal; Genta; Gentamix†; Gentamytrex; Ophtagram; Refobacin; Sulmycin; ***Irl.:*** Cidomycin; Genticin; ***Ital.:*** Gentalyn; Gentamen; Gentibioptal; Genticol; Gentomil; Megental Pediatrico†; Ribomicin; Septopal†; ***Neth.:*** Garacol; Garamycin; Gentamytrex; Gentogram†; ***Norw.:*** Garamycin; Gensumycin; ***S.Afr.:*** Cidomycin; Fermentmycin; Garamycin; Gencin; Genoptic; Sabax Gentamix; ***Spain:*** Biogent†; Coliriocilina Gentam; Genoptic†; Genta Gobens; Gentallorens†; Gentalodina; Gentamedical; Gentamin†; Gentamival; Gentamorgens†; Genticina; Gentisum†; Gentralay; Gevramycin; Gevramycina Topica; Hosbogen†; Lantogent; Rexgenta; Supragenta†; ***Swed.:*** Garamycin; Gensumycin; ***Switz.:*** Garamycin; Ophtagram; Servigenta; Yedoc; ***UK:*** Cidomycin; Garamycin; Genticin; ***USA:*** G-Myticin; Garamycin; Genoptic; Gentacidin; Gentafair†; Gentak; Gentasol; Gentrasul†; Jenamicin†.

Multi-ingredient: ***Aust.:*** Decoderm compositum; Decoderm trivalent; Diprogenta; Refobacin-Palacos R; Septopal; Terra-Cortril mit Gentamicin; ***Austral.:*** Celestone VG; Palacos E with Garamycin; Palacos R with Garamycin; Septopal; ***Belg.:*** Decoderm Comp; Duracoll; Garasone; Septopal; ***Canad.:*** Diprogen; Garasone; Valisone-G; ***Fr.:*** Gentasone; Palacos avec Gentamicine; Palacos R Gentamicine; ***Ger.:*** Betagentam; Corti-Refobacin†; Decoderm Comp; Decoderm trivalent†; Dexa-Gentamicin; Dexamytrex; Diprogenta; durabetagent†; Inflanegent; Refobacin-Palacos R; Septopal; Sulmycin mit Celestan-V; ***Irl.:*** Genticin HC†; Gentisone HC; Palacos R with Gentamicin; Septopal; ***Ital.:*** Citrizan Antibiotico; Diprogenta; Formomicin; Genalfa; Genatrop; Gentacort; Gentalyn Beta; Vasosterone Oto; Voltamicin; ***Neth.:*** Celestoderm met Garamycin†; Dexamytrex; Palacos R met gentamicine; Septopal; ***Norw.:*** Palacos cum gentamicin; Septopal; ***S.Afr.:*** Celestoderm-V with Garamycin; Diprogenta; Garasone†; Palacos R with Garamycin; Pred G; Quadriderm; Septopal; ***Spain:*** Celestoderm Gentamicina; Cuatroderm; Diprogenta; Flutenal Gentamicina; Interderm; Novoter Gentamicina; ***Swed.:*** Celeston valerat med gentamicin; Corticoderm comp†; Palacos cum gentamicin; Septopal; ***Switz.:*** Decoderm compositum†; Decoderm trivalent†; Diprogenta; Infectoflam; Ophtasone; Palacos avec Garamycin; Pred G; Quadriderm; Septopal; Triderm; Voltamicin; ***UK:*** Genticin HC†; Gentisone HC; Palacos LV with Gentamicin; Palacos R with Gentamicin; Septopal; Vipsogal; ***USA:*** Pred G.

Gramicidin (90-s)

Gramicidin *(BAN, rINN).*

Gramicidin D; Gramicidin (Dubos); Gramicidinum.

CAS — 1405-97-6 (gramicidin); 113-73-5 (gramicidin S).

NOTE. The name gramicidin was formerly applied to tyrothricin.

Pharmacopoeias. In *Eur.* (see p.viii) and *US.*

A mixture consisting mainly of three pairs of linear polypeptides produced by the growth of *Bacillus brevis* Dubos; it may be obtained from tyrothricin (p.267), of which it is one of the principal components. The Ph. Eur. specifies a potency of not less than 900 units per mg calculated on the dried substance.

It occurs as a white or almost white, odourless, crystalline, slightly hygroscopic powder. Practically **insoluble** in water; sparingly soluble to soluble in alcohol; practically insoluble in cyclohexane. **Store** in airtight containers.

Gramicidin has properties similar to those of tyrothricin (p.267) and is too toxic to be administered systemically. It has been used for the local treatment of susceptible infections usually in combination with other antibacterials such as neomycin and polymyxin B, and frequently with a corticosteroid as well.

Gramicidin sulphate has also been used. Gramicidin S or 'Soviet gramicidin' ($C_{60}H_{92}N_{12}O_{10}$ = 1141.4) has been used.

Preparations

USP 23: Neomycin and Polymyxin B Sulfates and Gramicidin Cream; Neomycin and Polymyxin B Sulfates and Gramicidin Ophthalmic Solution; Neomycin and Polymyxin B Sulfates, Gramicidin, and Hydrocortisone Acetate Cream; Neomycin Sulfate and Gramicidin Ointment; Nystatin, Neomycin Sulfate, Gramicidin, and Triamcinolone Acetonide Cream; Nystatin, Neomycin Sulfate, Gramicidin, and Triamcinolone Acetonide Ointment.

Proprietary Preparations (details are given in Part 3)
Fr.: Argicilline; Pharmacilline.

Multi-ingredient: ***Aust.:*** Mycostatin V; Topsym polyvalent; Volon A antibiotikahaltig; ***Austral.:*** Aristocomb; Graneodin†; Kenacomb; Neosporin; Otocomb Otic; Otodex; Sofradex; Soframycin; ***Belg.:*** Dexa-Sol Soframycine†; Fungispect†; Graneodine; Mycolog; ***Canad.:*** Diosporin; Kenacomb; Lidecomb†; Lidosporin; Neosporin; Optimyxin; Optimyxin Plus; Polycidin; Polysporin; Polysporin Burn Formula; Polysporin Triple Antibiotic; Sofracort; Soframycin; Triacomb; Viaderm-KC; ***Fr.:*** Topifram; ***Ger.:*** Heliomycort†; Kombi-Stulln; Polyspectran; Soframycin†; Ultexiv; ***Irl.:*** Graneodin; Kenacomb; Neosporin; Sofradex; Soframycin; ***Ital.:*** Assocort; Combiderm†; Eta Biocortilen VC; Neogram; Sprayrin†; Vasosterone Antibiotico; ***Neth.:*** Mycolog; Neosporin†; Polyspectran G†; Sofradex; ***Norw.:*** Polysporin†; Sofradex; ***S.Afr.:*** Kenacomb; Sofradex; Soframycin†; ***Spain:*** Deltasiton; Flodermol; Fludronef; Intradermo Cort Ant Fung; Midacina; Oftalmo†; Oftalmowell; Poxider; Spectrocin; Tivitis; Trigon Topico; ***Swed.:*** Bafucin; Kenacombin†; Kenacort-T med Graneodin†; Sofradex; ***Switz.:*** Angidine; Mycolog; Neosporin; Sofradex; Topsym polyvalent; Tyrothricine + Gramicidine; ***UK:*** Adcortyl with Graneodin; Graneodin; Neosporin; Sofradex; Soframycin; Tri-Adcortyl; ***USA:*** Ak-Spore; Alba-3; Neosporin; Ocutricin.

Grepafloxacin Hydrochloride

(17086-c)

Grepafloxacin Hydrochloride *(BANM, USAN, rINNM).*

OPC-17116. (±)-1-Cyclopropyl-6-fluoro-1,4-dihydro-5-methyl-7-(3-methyl-1-piperazinyl)-4-oxo-3-quinolinecarboxylic acid monohydrochloride.

$C_{19}H_{22}FN_3O_3$,HCl = 395.9.

CAS — 119914-60-2 (grepafloxacin); 161967-81-3 (grepafloxacin hydrochloride).

Adverse Effects and Precautions

As for Ciprofloxacin, p.186.

Interactions

As for Ciprofloxacin, p.187.

Antimicrobial Action

As for Ciprofloxacin, p.187, although grepafloxacin is reported to have greater activity against Gram-positive bacteria, including *Streptococcus pneumoniae.*

Pharmacokinetics

Grepafloxacin is rapidly absorbed from the gastro-intestinal tract following oral administration with a reported bioavailability of about 70%. Peak plasma concentrations are achieved within 2 hours of a dose. Grepafloxacin is widely distributed into body tissues and is reported to be 50% bound to plasma proteins. It is extensively metabolised, primarily in the liver, and several metabolites have been identified, some possessing weak antibacterial activity. The elimination half-life of grepafloxacin ranges from 10 to 16 hours. It is excreted mainly in bile but also in the urine.

Uses and Administration

Grepafloxacin is a fluoroquinolone antibacterial with actions and uses similar to those of ciprofloxacin (p.188). It is used as the hydrochloride in the treatment of community-acquired pneumonia and acute bacterial exacerbations of chronic bronchitis; it is also used in chlamydial urethritis and cervicitis, and in gonorrhoea. Doses are expressed in terms of grepafloxacin base. For bronchitis the usual adult dose is 400 mg once daily by mouth and for pneumonia 600 mg once daily; in both conditions treatment may be given for up to 10 days. For chlamydial urethritis and cervicitis, 400 mg once daily is given for 7 days. In acute uncomplicated gonorrhoea a single dose of 400 mg is used.

General references.

1. Wagstaff AJ, Balfour JA. Grepafloxacin. *Drugs* 1997; **53:** 817–24.

Preparations

Proprietary Preparations (details are given in Part 3)
UK: Raxar; ***USA:*** Raxar.

Halquinol (4785-m)

Halquinol *(BAN).*

Chlorhydroxyquinoline; Chlorquinol; Halquinols *(USAN)*; SQ-16401. A mixture of the chlorinated products of quinolin-8-ol containing 57 to 74% of 5,7-dichloroquinolin-8-ol (chloroxine), 23 to 40% of 5-chloroquinolin-8-ol (cloxyquin), and not more than 4% of 7-chloroquinolin-8-ol.

CAS — 8067-69-4 (halquinol); 773-76-2 (5,7-dichloroquinolin-8-ol).

Halquinol is a halogenated hydroxyquinoline with properties similar to those of clioquinol (p.193). It is used topically in infected skin conditions and one of its constituents, 5,7-dichloroquinolin-8-ol (chloroxine), is also applied as a 2% cream in the treatment of dandruff and seborrhoeic dermatitis of the scalp.

Preparations

Proprietary Preparations (details are given in Part 3)
UK: Valpeda; ***USA:*** Capitrol.

Multi-ingredient: ***Aust.:*** Decoderm trivalent; ***Ger.:*** Decoderm trivalent†; Diaront NN†; Dignoquine†; Hylakombun N†; ***Ital.:*** Beben Clorossina; ***Norw.:*** Kenacutan; ***Spain:*** Decoderm Trivalente; Deltasiton; *Swed.:* Kenacutan; *Switz.:* Decoderm trivalent†; *UK:* Antiseptic Foot Balm; Tardrox†.

Hetacillin (183-j)

Hetacillin *(BAN, USAN, pINN).*

BL-P-804; BRL-804; Hetacillinum; Isopropylidene-aminobenzylpenicillin; Phenazacillin. (6*R*)-6-(2,2-Dimethyl-5-oxo-4-phenylimidazolidin-1-yl)penicillanic acid.

$C_{19}H_{23}N_3O_4S$ = 389.5.

CAS — 3511-16-8.

Pharmacopoeias. In *Fr.*

Hetacillin Potassium (92-e)

Hetacillin Potassium *(BANM, USAN, pINNM).*

Hetacillinum Kalicum; Isopropylideneaminobenzylpenicillin Potassium.

$C_{19}H_{22}KN_3O_4S$ = 427.6.

CAS — 5321-32-4.

Pharmacopoeias. In *US.*

A white to light buff crystalline powder. 1.1 g of monograph substance is approximately equivalent to 1 g of hetacillin and 900 mg of ampicillin. Each g of monograph substance represents about 2.3 mmol of potassium. Freely **soluble** in water; soluble in alcohol. A 1% solution in water has a pH of 7 to 9. **Store** in airtight containers.

Hetacillin has properties similar to those of ampicillin (p.153), to which it is rapidly converted after administration by mouth or by injection. It has been given as the acid or potassium salt by mouth or as the potassium salt by injection in the treatment of susceptible infections.

Preparations

Proprietary Preparations (details are given in Part 3)
Spain: Etaciland†.

Hexamine (5657-m)

Methenamine *(rINN)*; Aminoform; E239; Esametilentetrammina; Esammina; Formine; Hexamethylenamine; Metenammina; Urotropine. Hexamethylenetetramine; 1,3,5,7-Tetraazatricyclo[3.3.1.1^{3,7}]decane.

$C_6H_{12}N_4$ = 140.2.

CAS — 100-97-0.

Pharmacopoeias. In *Aust., Belg., Chin., Ger., Neth., Pol., Swiss,* and *US.*

Almost odourless, colourless, lustrous crystals or white crystalline powder.

Soluble 1 in 1.5 of water, 1 in 12.5 of alcohol, 1 in 10 of chloroform, and 1 in 320 of ether. Solutions in water are alkaline to litmus.

Hexamine Hippurate (5660-r)

Hexamine Hippurate *(BAN).*

Methenamine Hippurate *(USAN, rINNM).* Hexamethylenetetramine hippurate.

$C_6H_{12}N_4,C_9H_9NO_3$ = 319.4.

CAS — 5714-73-8.

Pharmacopoeias. In *US.*

Hexamine Mandelate (5661-f)

Methenamine Mandelate *(rINNM)*; Hexamine Amygdalate; Mandelato de Metenamina. Hexamethylenetetramine mandelate.

$C_6H_{12}N_4,C_8H_8O_3$ = 292.3.

CAS — 587-23-5.

Pharmacopoeias. In *US.*

A white crystalline almost odourless powder.

Very **soluble** in water; soluble 1 in 10 of alcohol, 1 in 20 of chloroform, and 1 in 350 of ether. Solutions in water have a pH of about 4.

Adverse Effects and Precautions

Hexamine and its salts are generally well tolerated but may cause gastro-intestinal disturbances such as nausea, vomiting, and diarrhoea. Skin rashes, and occasionally other hypersensitivity reactions, may occur.

Comparatively large amounts of the active moiety formaldehyde may be formed during prolonged administration or when large doses are used, and may give rise to irritation and inflammation of the urinary tract especially the bladder, painful and frequent micturition, haematuria, and proteinuria. The effect of the formaldehyde may be diluted by administering alkalinising drugs such as sodium bicarbonate or large quantities of water but it is then less effective.

Hexamine and its salts are contra-indicated in patients with hepatic insufficiency because of the liberation of ammonia in the gastro-intestinal tract. Although hexamine itself is not contra-indicated in renal insufficiency, the salts should be avoided, at any rate in severe insufficiency, because of the risk of mandelate or hippurate crystalluria. They should also be avoided in patients with severe dehydration, metabolic acidosis, or gout.

Interference with laboratory estimations for catecholamines, 17-hydroxycorticosteroids, and oestrogens in the urine has been reported.

Interactions

The concomitant use of agents that alkalinise the urine, including some antacids, potassium citrate, and diuretics such as acetazolamide or the thiazides should be avoided because the activation of hexamine to formaldehyde may be inhibited.

The concomitant administration of hexamine and sulphonamides may increase the risk of crystalluria since hexamine requires low urinary pH for its effect, at which sulphonamides and their metabolites are poorly soluble; hexamine may also form poorly soluble compounds with some sulphonamides.

Antimicrobial Action

Hexamine owes its antibacterial properties to formaldehyde, a non-specific bactericide, which is slowly liberated by hydrolysis at acid pH. Most Gram-positive and Gram-negative organisms and fungi are susceptible, usually at MICs of around 20 μg per mL. Hippuric and mandelic acids have some antibacterial activity *in vitro* but their contribution to the antibacterial action of the salts *in vivo*, beyond assisting the maintenance of low urinary pH, is uncertain. Urea-splitting organisms such as *Proteus* and some *Pseudomonas* spp. tend to increase urinary pH and inhibit the release of formaldehyde thereby decreasing the effectiveness of hexamine. The concomitant use of acetohydroxamic acid, a potent inhibitor of bacterial urease, has been suggested for urinary infections due to these organisms. True resistance to formaldehyde does not appear to be a problem in clinical use.

Pharmacokinetics

Hexamine is readily absorbed from the gastro-intestinal tract and widely distributed in the body. Under acid conditions hexamine is slowly hydrolysed to formaldehyde and ammonia: about 10 to 30% of the administered dose may be converted in the stomach unless it is given as an enteric coated preparation. Almost no hydrolysis of hexamine takes place at physiological pH, and it is therefore virtually inactive in the body. The half-life is reported to be approximately 4 hours. Hexamine is rapidly and almost completely eliminated in the urine, and provided this is suitably acid (preferably below pH 5.5) bactericidal concentrations of formaldehyde are achieved; because of the time taken for hydrolysis, however, these are not achieved until the urine reaches the bladder, with peak concentrations up to 2 hours after administration. Absorption, and hence excretion, may be somewhat delayed in patients given enteric-coated formulations.

Small amounts of hexamine may be distributed into breast milk.

The mandelate and hippurate moieties are also rapidly absorbed and are excreted in urine by tubular secretion as well as glomerular filtration.

Uses and Administration

Hexamine is used, usually as the hippurate or mandelate, in the prophylaxis and treatment of chronic or recurrent, uncomplicated, lower urinary-tract infections and asymptomatic bacteriuria. It has been considered suitable for long-term use because acquired resistance does not appear to develop.

Hexamine and its salts should not be used in upper urinary-tract infections because it is eliminated too rapidly to exert an effect, nor in acute urinary infections. It is only active in acid urine (pH below 5.5), when formaldehyde is released, and although hippuric or mandelic acid helps to acidify the urine, administration of ammonium chloride or ascorbic acid may be tried. If urea-splitting bacteria such as *Proteus* or some *Pseudomonas* spp. are present they may produce so much ammonia that the urine cannot be acidified (see also Antimicrobial Action, above).

The usual dose of hexamine or hexamine mandelate is 1 g by mouth four times daily; a dose of about 15 mg per kg bodyweight four times daily has been suggested in children up to 6 years of age and 0.5 g four times daily in those aged 6 to 12 years. Hexamine hippurate is given in a usual dose of 1 g twice daily, or 0.5 to 1 g twice daily in children 6 to 12 years of age. Topically, hexamine has been used in deodorant preparations, since in the presence of acid sweat it liberates formaldehyde. Hexamine calcium thiocyanate has been used in combination with other ingredients in preparations for upper respiratory-tract disorders.

Preparations

USP 23: Methenamine and Monobasic Sodium Phosphate Tablets; Methenamine Elixir; Methenamine Hippurate Tablets; Methenamine Mandelate Delayed-release Tablets; Methenamine Mandelate for Oral Solution; Methenamine Mandelate Oral Suspension; Methenamine Mandelate Tablets; Methenamine Tablets.

Proprietary Preparations (details are given in Part 3)
Aust.: Antihydral†; Hiprex; *Austral.:* Hiprex; Mandelamine†; *Belg.:* Hiprex; *Canad.:* Dehydral; Hiprex; Mandelamine; Urasal; *Ger.:* Aci-steril†; Antihydral; Hiprex†; Mandelamine; Urotractan; *Irl.:* Hiprex; *Neth.:* Reflux; Urocedulamin†; *Norw.:* Hiprex; *S.Afr.:* Hippramine; *Swed.:* Hippuran†; Hiprex; *Switz.:* Antihydral; Mandelamine; *UK:* Hiprex; *USA:* Hiprex; Mandelamine†; Urex.

Multi-ingredient: *Aust.:* Antihydral M†; *Belg.:* Carbobel; Mictasol; *Fr.:* Aerophagyl†; Aromalgyl; Intesticarbine†; Mictasol; Saprol†; Uraseptine Rogier†; Uromil; *Ger.:* Antihydral M; Mucidan†; *Ital.:* Cinarbile†; Mictasol†; *S.Afr.:* Azo-Mandelamine†; *Swed.:* Mucidan†; *Switz.:* Antihydral M; *USA:* Atrosept; Cystex; Dolsed; Prosed/DS; Thiacide†; Trac Tabs 2X; UAA; Uridon Modified; Urimar-T; Urised; Urisedamine; Uro-Phosphate; Urogesic Blue; Uroqid-Acid.

Imipenem (16849-l)

Imipenem *(BAN, USAN, rINN).*

N-Formimidoyl Thienamycin; Imipemide; MK-787; MK-0787. (5*R*,6*S*)-6-[(*R*)-1-Hydroxyethyl]-3-(2-iminomethylaminoethylthio)-7-oxo-1-azabicyclo[3.2.0]hept-2-ene-2-carboxylic acid monohydrate.

$C_{12}H_{17}N_3O_4S,H_2O$ = 317.4.

CAS — 64221-86-9 (anhydrous imipenem); 74431-23-5 (imipenem monohydrate).

Pharmacopoeias. In *Eur.* (see p.viii) and *US.*

The *N*-formimidoyl derivative of thienamycin, an antibiotic produced by *Streptomyces cattleya*.

A white, almost white, or light yellow to tan-coloured crystalline powder. Sparingly **soluble** in water; slightly soluble in methyl alcohol. A 0.5% solution in water has a pH of 4.5 to 7.0. Imipenem is unstable at alkaline or acidic pH and the commercially available injection of imipenem with cilastatin sodium for intravenous use, is buffered to provide, when reconstituted, a solution with pH 6.5 to 7.5. The manufacturers advise against mixing with other antibacterials. **Store** in airtight containers at a temperature of 2° to 8°.

References.

1. Bigley FP, *et al.* Compatibility of imipenem-cilastatin sodium with commonly used intravenous solutions. *Am J Hosp Pharm* 1986; **43:** 2803–9.
2. Smith GB, *et al.* Stability and kinetics of degradation of imipenem in aqueous solution. *J Pharm Sci* 1990; **79:** 732–40.

Adverse Effects

Imipenem is only given in association with the enzyme inhibitor cilastatin and thus clinical experience relates to the combination.

Adverse effects with imipenem-cilastatin are similar in general to those with other beta-lactams (see benzylpenicillin, p.159, and cephalothin, p.179). They include hypersensitivity reactions such as skin rashes, urticaria, eosinophilia, fever, and rarely, anaphylaxis; gastro-intestinal effects such as nausea, vomiting, diarrhoea, and altered taste; and superinfection with non-susceptible organisms such as *Enterococcus faecium*, strains of *Pseudomonas aeruginosa* with acquired resistance, and *Candida*. Pseudomembranous colitis may develop. Toxic epidermal necrolysis has been reported rarely. Increases in liver enzymes and abnormalities in haematological parameters, including a positive Coombs' test, have been noted.

Local reactions such as pain or thrombophlebitis may occur following injection.

Seizures or convulsions have been reported with imipenem-cilastatin, particularly in patients with a history of CNS lesions and/or poor renal function, but sometimes in those without predisposing factors for seizures given recommended doses.

Cilastatin has protected against the nephrotoxicity seen with high doses of imipenem given experimentally to *animals*.

Effects on the nervous system. References.

1. Eng RH, *et al.* Seizure propensity with imipenem. *Arch Intern Med* 1989; **149:** 1881–3.
2. Brown RB, *et al.* Seizure propensity with imipenem. *Arch Intern Med* 1990; **150:** 1551.
3. Job ML, Dretler RH. Seizure activity with imipenem therapy: incidence and risk factors. *DICP Ann Pharmacother* 1990; **24:** 467–9.
4. Leo RJ, Ballow CH. Seizure activity associated with imipenem use: clinical case reports and review of the literature. *DICP Ann Pharmacother* 1991; **25:** 351–4.
5. Duque A, *et al.* Vertigo caused by intravenous imipenem/cilastatin. *DICP Ann Pharmacother* 1991; **25:** 1009.
6. Lucena M, *et al.* Imipenem/cilastatin-associated hiccups. *Ann Pharmacother* 1992; **26:** 1459.
7. Norrby SR. Neurotoxicity of carbapenem antibacterials. *Drug Safety* 1996; **15:** 87–90.

Superinfection. References.

1. Gray JW, *et al.* Enterococcal superinfection in paediatric oncology patients treated with imipenem. *Lancet* 1992; **339:** 1487–8.

Precautions

Imipenem-cilastatin should not be given to patients known to be hypersensitive to it, and should be administered with caution to patients known to be hypersensitive to penicillins, cephalosporins, or other beta-lactams because of the possibility of cross-sensitivity.

It should be given with caution to patients with renal impairment, and the dose reduced appropriately. Particular care is necessary in patients with CNS disorders such as epilepsy.

Interactions

Seizures have been reported in patients receiving ganciclovir concomitantly with imipenem-cilastatin.

Antimicrobial Action

Imipenem is bactericidal and acts similarly to the penicillins by inhibiting synthesis of the bacterial cell wall. It has a very broad spectrum of activity *in vitro*, including activity against Gram-positive and Gram-negative aerobic and anaerobic organisms, and is stable to hydrolysis by beta-lactamases produced by most bacterial species. Cilastatin, the enzyme inhibitor given in association with imipenem, appears to have no antibacterial activity.

Most Gram-positive cocci are sensitive to imipenem (MIC_{90} ranging from 0.01 to 0.1 μg per mL) including most streptococci, and both penicillinase- and non-penicillinase-producing staphylococci, although its activity against methicillin-resistant *Staphylococcus aureus* is variable. Imipenem has good to moderate activity against *Enterococcus faecalis*, but most *E. faecium* are resistant. *Nocardia*, *Rhodococcus*, and *Listeria* spp. are also sensitive.

Among Gram-negative bacteria, imipenem is active against many of the Enterobacteriaceae (MIC_{90} ranging from 0.1 to 8 μg per mL) including *Citrobacter* and *Enterobacter* spp., *Escherichia coli, Klebsiella, Proteus, Providencia, Salmonella, Serratia, Shigella,* and *Yersinia* spp. Its activity against *Pseudomonas aeruginosa* is similar to that of ceftazidime and the MIC_{90} has ranged from 2 to 8 μg per mL. Imipenem is also active against *Acinetobacter* spp. and *Campylobacter jejuni*, and also against *Haemophilus influenzae* and *Neisseria* spp., including beta-lactamase-producing strains.

Many anaerobic bacteria, including *Bacteroides* spp., are sensitive to imipenem, but *Clostridium difficile* is only moderately susceptible.

It is not active against *Chlamydia trachomatis, Mycoplasma* spp., fungi, or viruses.

There have been reports of antagonism between imipenem and other beta-lactams *in vitro*. Imipenem and aminoglycosides often act synergistically.

Imipenem is a potent inducer of beta-lactamases of some Gram-negative bacteria, but generally remains stable to them. Acquired resistance has been reported in *Ps. aeruginosa* during treatment with imipenem.

Resistance. References.

1. King A, *et al.* Resistance to imipenem in Pseudomonas aeruginosa. *J Antimicrob Chemother* 1995; **36:** 1037–41.
2. Ballestero S, *et al.* Carbapenem resistance in Pseudomonas aeruginosa from cystic fibrosis patients. *J Antimicrob Chemother* 1996; **38:** 39–45.
3. Rasmussen BA, Bush K. Carbapenem-hydrolyzing β-lactamases. *Antimicrob Agents Chemother* 1997; **41:** 223–32.
4. Livermore DM. Acquired carbapenemases. *J Antimicrob Chemother* 1997; **39:** 673–6.
5. MacKenzie FM, *et al.* Emergence of a carbapenem-resistant Klebsiella pneumoniae. *Lancet* 1997; **350:** 783.
6. Pikis A, *et al.* Decreased susceptibility to imipenem among penicillin-resistant Streptococcus pneumoniae. *J Antimicrob Chemother* 1997; **40:** 105–8.
7. Mainardi J-L, *et al.* Carbapenem resistance in a clinical isolate of Citrobacter freundii. *Antimicrob Agents Chemother* 1997; **41:** 2352–4.

Pharmacokinetics

Imipenem is not appreciably absorbed from the gastro-intestinal tract and is administered parenterally.

It is excreted primarily in the urine by glomerular filtration and tubular secretion and undergoes partial metabolism in the kidneys by dehydropeptidase I, an enzyme in the brush border of the renal tubules, to inactive, nephrotoxic metabolites, with only 5 to 45% of a dose excreted in the urine as unchanged active drug. Imipenem is administered in conjunction with cilastatin sodium (p.185), a dehydropeptidase inhibitor, resulting in increased urinary-imipenem concentrations. Cilastatin does not affect serum concentrations of imipenem.

The pharmacokinetics of imipenem and cilastatin are similar and both have plasma half-lives of approximately one hour; half-lives may be prolonged in neonates and in patients with renal impairment, especially those of cilastatin. Following intramuscular administration of imipenem with cilastatin peak plasma concentrations of 10 to 12 μg per mL are achieved at about 2 hours and prolonged absorption results in plasma concentrations of above 2 μg per mL for 6 to 8 hours. The bioavailability of imipenem following intramuscular injection is about 75%. Up to 20% of imipenem and 40% of cilastatin in the circulation is bound to plasma proteins. Imipenem is widely distributed in body tissues and fluids and crosses the placenta. Information on penetration into the CSF is limited, but concentrations appear to be relatively low.

When given with cilastatin about 70% of an intravenous dose of imipenem is recovered unchanged in the urine within 10 hours. A total of 50% of an intramuscular dose is recovered in the urine and concentrations above 10 μg per mL are maintained for 12 hours following a dose of 500 or 750 mg. Cilastatin is also excreted mainly in the urine, the majority as unchanged drug and about 12% as *N*-acetyl cilastatin. Both imipenem and cilastatin are removed by haemodialysis.

About 1% of imipenem is excreted via the bile in the faeces.

Reviews.

1. Drusano GL. An overview of the pharmacology of imipenem/cilastatin. *J Antimicrob Chemother* 1986; **18** (suppl E): 79–92.
2. Watson ID, *et al.* Clinical pharmacokinetics of enzyme inhibitors in antimicrobial chemotherapy. *Clin Pharmacokinet* 1988; **15:** 133–64.

Pharmacokinetics in the elderly.

1. Finch RG, *et al.* Pharmacokinetic studies of imipenem/cilastatin in elderly patients. *J Antimicrob Chemother* 1986; **18** (suppl E): 103–7.

Pharmacokinetics in liver disease.

1. Rolando N, *et al.* The penetration of imipenem/cilastatin into ascitic fluid in patients with chronic liver disease. *J Antimicrob Chemother* 1994; **33:** 163–7.

Pharmacokinetics in pregnancy and the neonate.

1. Reed MD, *et al.* Clinical pharmacology of imipenem and cilastatin in premature infants during the first week of life. *Antimicrob Agents Chemother* 1990; **34:** 1172–7.
2. Heikkilä A, *et al.* Pharmacokinetics and transplacental passage of imipenem during pregnancy. *Antimicrob Agents Chemother* 1992; **36:** 2652–5.

Pharmacokinetics in renal impairment.

1. Verbist L, *et al.* Pharmacokinetics and tolerance after repeated doses of imipenem/cilastatin in patients with severe renal failure. *J Antimicrob Chemother* 1986; **18** (suppl E): 115–20.
2. Alarabi AA, *et al.* Pharmacokinetics of intravenous imipenem/cilastatin during intermittent haemofiltration. *J Antimicrob Chemother* 1990; **26:** 91–8.
3. Pietroski NA, *et al.* Steady-state pharmacokinetics of intramuscular imipenem-cilastatin in elderly patients with various degrees of renal function. *Antimicrob Agents Chemother* 1991; **35:** 972–5.
4. Konishi K, *et al.* Removal of imipenem and cilastatin by hemodialysis in patients with end-stage renal failure. *Antimicrob Agents Chemother* 1991; **35:** 1616–20.
5. Chan CY, *et al.* Pharmacokinetics of parenteral imipenem/cilastatin in patients on continuous ambulatory peritoneal dialysis. *J Antimicrob Chemother* 1991; **27:** 225–32.

Uses and Administration

Imipenem is a carbapenem beta-lactam antibiotic, differing from the penicillins in that the 5-membered ring is unsaturated and contains a carbon rather than a sulphur atom. Since imipenem is metabolised in the kidney by the enzyme dehydropeptidase I it is administered only in association with cilastatin (p.185), an inhibitor of the enzyme; this enhances urinary concentrations of active drug and was found to protect against the nephrotoxicity of high doses of imipenem in *animals*.

Imipenem is used for the treatment of infections caused by susceptible organisms (see Antimicrobial Action, above). They include infections in immunocompromised patients (with neutropenia), intra-abdominal infections, bone and joint infections, skin and soft-tissue infections, urinary-tract infections, biliary-tract infections, hospital-acquired pneumonia, and septicaemia. It may also be used for the treatment of gonorrhoea and for surgical infection (prophylaxis). For details of these infections and their treatment, see under Choice of Antibacterial, p.116. It is not indicated for meningitis.

Administration and dosage. Commercial preparations contain imipenem and cilastatin, as the sodium salt, in a ratio of 1 to 1. Doses of the combination are expressed in terms of the amount of anhydrous imipenem. Imipenem is administered by intravenous infusion or deep intramuscular injection. When administered intravenously, doses of 250 or 500 mg are infused over 20 to 30 minutes, and doses of 750 mg or 1 g over 40 to 60 minutes. The usual intravenous dose in adults is 1 to 2 g daily in divided doses every 6 or 8 hours, depending on the severity of the infection. A maximum daily dose of 4 g or 50 mg per kg body-weight is advised.

Children of 3 months or more and weighing less than 40 kg may be given 15 mg per kg every 6 hours by intravenous infusion; the total daily dose should not exceed 2 g.

For surgical infection prophylaxis in adults, imipenem 1 g may be given intravenously on induction of anaesthesia, followed by a further 1 g three hours later, with additional doses of 500 mg at 8 and 16 hours if necessary.

Imipenem may be administered intramuscularly in adults with mild to moderate infections in doses of 500 or 750 mg every 12 hours. A single 500-mg intramuscular dose may be given in uncomplicated gonorrhoea.

Doses should be reduced in patients with renal impairment. The manufacturers have recommended the following maximum *intravenous* doses in patients with a creatinine clearance of 70 mL per minute or less: mild impairment (creatinine clearance 31 to 70 mL per minute), 500 mg every 6 to 8 hours; moderate impairment (creatinine clearance 21 to 30 mL per minute), 500 mg every 8 to 12 hours; and severe impairment (creatinine clearance 6 to 20 mL per minute), 250 mg (or 3.5 mg per kg, which ever is the lower) or occasionally 500 mg every 12 hours. Patients with a creatinine clearance of 5 mL per minute or less should only be given imipenem if haemodialysis is started within 48 hours. Imipenem and cilastatin are cleared from the body by haemodialysis and doses should be given after a dialysis session and then every 12 hours. Information is lacking on the safety or effectiveness of the intramuscular route in patients with renal impairment.

General reviews.

1. Buckley MM, *et al.* Imipenem/cilastatin: a reappraisal of its antibacterial activity, pharmacokinetic properties and therapeutic efficacy. *Drugs* 1992; **44:** 408–44. Correction. *ibid.*; 1012.
2. Balfour JA, *et al.* Imipenem/cilastatin: an update of its antibacterial activity, pharmacokinetics and therapeutic efficacy in the treatment of serious infections. *Drugs* 1996; **51:** 99–136.

Preparations

USP 23: Imipenem and Cilastatin for Injectable Suspension; Imipenem and Cilastatin for Injection.

Proprietary Preparations (details are given in Part 3)

Multi-ingredient: ***Aust.:*** Zienam; ***Austral.:*** Primaxin; ***Belg.:*** Tienam; ***Canad.:*** Primaxin; ***Fr.:*** Tienam; ***Ger.:*** Zienam; ***Ital.:*** Imipem; Tenacid; Tienam; ***Neth.:*** Tienam; ***Norw.:*** Tienam; ***S.Afr.:*** Tienam; ***Spain:*** Tienam; ***Swed.:*** Tienam; ***Switz.:*** Tienam; ***UK:*** Primaxin; ***USA:*** Primaxin.

Isepamicin (2173-v)

Isepamicin *(BAN, USAN, rINN)*.

HAPA-B; HAPA-gentamicin B; Sch-21420. 4-*O*-(6-Amino-6-deoxy-α-D-glucopyranosyl)-1-*N*-(3-amino-L-lactoyl)-2-deoxy-6-*O*-(3-deoxy-4-*C*-methyl-3-methylamino-β-L-arabinopyranosyl)streptamine; 1*N*-(*S*-3-Amino-2-hydroxypropionyl)-gentamicin B.

$C_{22}H_{43}N_5O_{12}$ = 569.6.

CAS — 58152-03-7.

Isepamicin is a semisynthetic aminoglycoside with actions and uses similar to those of gentamicin (p.212). It is reported not to be degraded by many of the enzymes responsible for aminoglycoside resistance. It is given by intramuscular injection or intravenous infusion as the sulphate in a dose of 15 mg per kg body-weight daily in 2 divided doses. Dosage should be adjusted based on serum-isepamicin concentration monitoring.

References.

1. Kuranari M, *et al.* Effect of hemodialysis on serum concentration of isepamicin in a patient with endstage renal failure. *Ann Pharmacother* 1993; **27:** 1284–5.
2. Lin C-C, *et al.* Pharmacokinetics of intravenously administered isepamicin in men. *Antimicrob Agents Chemother* 1995; **39:** 2774–8.
3. Tod M, *et al.* Population pharmacokinetic study of isepamicin with intensive care unit patients. *Antimicrob Agents Chemother* 1996; **40:** 983–7.
4. Radwanski E, *et al.* Pharmacokinetics of isepamicin following a single administration by intravenous infusion or intramuscular injections. *Antimicrob Agents Chemother* 1997; **41:** 1794–6.
5. Nomeir AA, *et al.* Single-dose pharmacokinetics of isepamicin in young and geriatric volunteers. *J Clin Pharmacol* 1997; **37:** 1021–30.

Preparations

Proprietary Preparations (details are given in Part 3)

Fr.: Isepalline; ***Ital.:*** Isepacin; Vizax.

Isoniazid (7559-k)

Isoniazid *(BAN, pINN)*.

INAH; INH; Isoniazidum; Isonicotinic Acid Hydrazide; Isonicotinylhydrazide; Isonicotinylhydrazine; Tubazid. Isonicotinohydrazide.

$C_6H_7N_3O$ = 137.1.

CAS — 54-85-3.

NOTE. The name Isopyrin, which has been applied to isoniazid, has also been applied to isopropylaminophenazone.

Pharmacopoeias. In *Chin., Eur.* (see p.viii), *Int., Jpn, Pol.,* and *US.*

Colourless, odourless crystals, or white crystalline powder. **Soluble** 1 in 8 of water, 1 in 50 of alcohol; slightly soluble in chloroform; very slightly soluble in ether. A 5% solution in water has a pH of 6.0 to 8.0. Solutions are **sterilised** by autoclaving.

Incompatible with sugars. **Store** in airtight containers. Protect from light.

Adverse Effects

Isoniazid is generally well tolerated at currently recommended doses. However, patients who are slow acetylators of isoniazid appear to have a higher incidence of some adverse effects. Also patients whose nutrition is poor are at risk of peripheral neuritis which is one of the commonest adverse effects of isoniazid. Other neurological adverse effects include psychotic reactions and convulsions. Pyridoxine may be given to prevent or treat these adverse effects. Optic neuritis has also been reported.

Transient increases in liver enzymes occur in 10 to 20% of patients during the first few months and usually return to normal despite continued treatment. Elevated liver enzymes associated with clinical signs of hepatitis such as nausea and vomiting, or fatigue may indicate hepatic damage; in these circumstances, isoniazid should be stopped pending evaluation and if damage is confirmed should only be reintroduced cautiously once hepatic function has recovered. The incidence of liver damage is highest in patients over 35 years of age. The influence of acetylator status is uncertain. Fatalities have occurred following liver necrosis.

Haematological effects reported following use of isoniazid include various anaemias, agranulocytosis, thrombocytopenia, and eosinophilia.

Hypersensitivity reactions occur infrequently and include skin eruptions (including erythema multiforme), fever, and vasculitis.

Other adverse effects include nausea, vomiting, pellagra, hyperglycaemia, lupus-like syndrome, urinary retention, and gynaecomastia.

Symptoms of overdosage include slurred speech, metabolic acidosis, hyperglycaemia, convulsions, and coma; fatalities can occur.

Carcinogenicity. Concern about the carcinogenicity of isoniazid arose in the 1970s when Miller[1,2] and others[3] reported an increased risk of bladder cancer in patients treated with isoniazid. However, no evidence to support a carcinogenic effect of isoniazid was found in more than 25 000 patients followed up for 9 to 14 years in studies organised by the USA Public Health Service[4] and in 3842 patients followed up for 16 to 24 years in the UK.[5]

1. Miller CT. Isoniazid and cancer risks. *JAMA* 1974; **230:** 1254.
2. Miller CT, *et al.* Relative importance of risk factors in bladder carcinogenesis. *J Chron Dis* 1978; **31:** 51–6.
3. Kerr WK, Chipman ML. The incidence of cancer of bladder and other sites after INH therapy. *Am J Epidemiol* 1976; **104:** 335–6.
4. Glassroth JL, *et al.* An assessment of the possible association of isoniazid with human cancer deaths. *Am Rev Respir Dis* 1977; **116:** 1065–74.
5. Stott H, *et al.* An assessment of the carcinogenicity of isoniazid in patients with pulmonary tuberculosis. *Tubercle* 1976; **57:** 1–15.

Effects on the blood. In addition to the effects mentioned above, rare reports of adverse effects of isoniazid on the blood include bleeding associated with acquired inhibition of fibrin stabilisation[1] or of factor XIII[2] and red cell aplasia.[3-5]

For a reference to neutropenia, see Effects on the Blood under Ethambutol Hydrochloride, p.207.

1. Otis PT, *et al.* An acquired inhibitor of fibrin stabilization associated with isoniazid therapy: clinical and biochemical observations. *Blood* 1974; **44:** 771–81.
2. Krumdieck R, *et al.* Hemorrhagic disorder due to an isoniazid-associated acquired factor XIII inhibitor in a patient with Waldenström's macroglobulinemia. *Am J Med* 1991; **90:** 639–45.
3. Claiborne RA, Dutt AK. Isoniazid-induced pure red cell aplasia. *Am Rev Respir Dis* 1985; **131:** 947–9.
4. Lewis CR, Manoharan A. Pure red cell hypoplasia secondary to isoniazid. *Postgrad Med J* 1987; **63:** 309–10.
5. Veale KS, *et al.* Pure red cell aplasia and hepatitis in a child receiving isoniazid therapy. *J Pediatr* 1992; **120:** 146–8.

Effects on the CNS. References.

1. Blumberg EA, Gil RA. Cerebellar syndrome caused by isoniazid. *DICP Ann Pharmacother* 1990; **24:** 829–31.
2. Pallone KA, *et al.* Isoniazid-associated psychosis: case report and review of the literature. *Ann Pharmacother* 1993; **27:** 167–70.
3. Cheung WC, *et al.* Isoniazid induced encephalopathy in dialysis patients. *Tubercle Lung Dis* 1993; **74:** 136–9.
4. Shah BR, *et al.* Acute isoniazid neurotoxicity in an urban hospital. *Pediatrics* 1995; **95:** 700–4.

Effects on the liver. In a review of hepatotoxicity of antituberculous regimens containing isoniazid, Girling[1] stressed that hepatitis occurring during chemotherapy may be due to the disease itself, alcoholism, cirrhosis, or other infections. When treatment is implicated, it may not be possible to identify which drug or drugs are responsible.

A multicentre study[2] considered the incidence of hepatotoxicity from a short-term regimen of daily isoniazid, rifampicin, and pyrazinamide for 8 weeks in the initial phase followed by daily isoniazid and rifampicin for 16 weeks in the continuing phase. Analysis from 617 patients showed an incidence of hepatotoxic reactions of 1.6%; the incidence of elevated aspartate aminotransferase was 23.2%. In the same study, 445 patients on a nine-month regimen of daily isoniazid and rifampicin had a 1.2% incidence of hepatotoxicity and 27.1% incidence of elevated liver enzymes. Dutt *et al.*[3] had reported a similar incidence of hepatitis of 1.4% among 350 patients on a 9-month regimen of rifampicin and isoniazid. A retrospective analysis[4] of 430 children on isoniazid and rifampicin revealed hepatotoxic reactions in 3.3%, the highest incidence being in children with severe disease.

While increasing age,[5-8] high isoniazid doses, and pre-existing hepatic disease appear to increase the risk of isoniazid-induced hepatotoxicity, the influence of other factors is less certain. Speculation that fast acetylators of isoniazid could be at increased risk of hepatotoxicity due to production of a hepatotoxic hydrazine metabolite have not been supported;[9] in fact, slow acetylators have generally been found to have a higher risk than fast.[7,10] This could reflect a reduced rate of subsequent metabolism to non-toxic compounds. In addition, concentrations of hydrazine in the blood have not been found to correlate with acetylator status.[11,12]

The Joint Tuberculosis Committee of the British Thoracic Society is anxious that fears over the safety of treatment regimens do not compromise adequate therapy of the disease itself. In an update to their guidelines,[13] they make recommendations for initial measurement of liver function in all patients and regular monitoring in patients with known chronic liver disease. Tests should be repeated if symptoms of liver dysfunction occur, and details are given concerning the response to deteriorating liver function depending on the clinical situation, and include guidelines for prompt reintroduction of appropriate antituberculosis therapy once normal liver function is restored.

1. Girling DJ. The hepatic toxicity of antituberculosis regimens containing isoniazid, rifampicin and pyrazinamide. *Tubercle* 1978; **59:** 13–32.
2. Combs DL, *et al.* USPHS tuberculosis short-course chemotherapy trial 21: effectiveness, toxicity, and acceptability: the report of final results. *Ann Intern Med* 1990; **112:** 397–406.
3. Dutt AK, *et al.* Short-course chemotherapy for extrapulmonary tuberculosis: nine years' experience. *Ann Intern Med* 1986; **104:** 7–12.
4. O'Brien RJ, *et al.* Hepatotoxicity from isoniazid and rifampin among children treated for tuberculosis. *Pediatrics* 1983; **72:** 491–9.
5. Black M, *et al.* Isoniazid-associated hepatitis in 114 patients. *Gastroenterology* 1975; **69:** 289–302.
6. Stead WW, *et al.* Benefit-risk considerations in preventive treatment for tuberculosis in elderly persons. *Ann Intern Med* 1987; **107:** 843–5.
7. Dickinson DS, *et al.* Risk factors for isoniazid (INH)-induced liver dysfunction. *J Clin Gastroenterol* 1981; **3:** 271–9.
8. Døssing M, *et al.* Liver injury during antituberculosis treatment: an 11-year study. *Tubercle Lung Dis* 1996; **77:** 335–40.
9. Gurumurthy P, *et al.* Lack of relationship between hepatic toxicity and acetylator phenotype in three thousand South Indian patients during treatment with isoniazid for tuberculosis. *Am Rev Respir Dis* 1984; **129:** 58–61.
10. Pande JN, *et al.* Risk factors for hepatotoxicity from antituberculosis drugs: a case-control study. *Thorax* 1996; **51:** 132–6.
11. Gent WL, *et al.* Factors in hydrazine formation from isoniazid by paediatric and adult tuberculosis patients. *Eur J Clin Pharmacol* 1992; **43:** 131–6.
12. Donald PR, *et al.* Hydrazine production in children receiving isoniazid for the treatment of tuberculous meningitis. *Ann Pharmacother* 1994; **28:** 1340–3.
13. Ormerod LP, *et al.* Hepatotoxicity of antituberculosis drugs. *Thorax* 1996; **51:** 111–13.

Effects on the pancreas. Pancreatitis was associated with isoniazid therapy in 2 patients.[1,2] Chronic pancreatic insufficiency was reported in 1 patient following administration of isoniazid, rifampicin, ethambutol, and pyrazinamide.[3]

1. Chan KL, *et al.* Recurrent acute pancreatitis induced by isoniazid. *Tubercle Lung Dis* 1994; **75:** 383–5.
2. Rabassa AA, *et al.* Isoniazid-induced acute pancreatitis. *Ann Intern Med* 1994; **121:** 433–4.
3. Liu BA, *et al.* Pancreatic insufficiency due to antituberculosis therapy. *Ann Pharmacother* 1997; **31:** 724–6.

Effects on the skin and hair. Isoniazid causes cutaneous drug reactions in less than 1% of patients.[1,2] These reactions include urticaria, purpura, acneform syndrome,[3] a lupus erythematosus-like syndrome (see below),[4] and exfoliative dermatitis.[5] Pellagra is also associated with isoniazid.[6] Isoniazid was considered the most likely cause of alopecia in 5 patients receiving antituberculosis regimens which also included rifampicin, ethambutol, and pyrazinamide.[7]

1. Arndt KA, Jick H. Rates of cutaneous reactions to drugs: a report from the Boston Collaborative Drug Surveillance Program. *JAMA* 1976; **235:** 918–23.
2. Bigby M, *et al.* Drug-induced cutaneous reactions: a report from the Boston Collaborative Drug Surveillance Program on 15 438 consecutive inpatients, 1975 to 1982. *JAMA* 1986; **256:** 3358–63.
3. Thorne N. Skin reactions to systemic drug therapy. *Practitioner* 1973; **211:** 606–13.
4. Smith AG. Drug-induced photosensitivity. *Adverse Drug React Bull* 1989; **136:** 508–11.
5. Rosin MA, King LE. Isoniazid-induced exfoliative dermatitis. *South Med J* 1982; **75:** 81.
6. Ishii N, Nishihara Y. Pellagra encephalopathy among tuberculous patients: its relation to isoniazid therapy. *J Neurol Neurosurg Psychiatry* 1985; **48:** 628–34.
7. FitzGerald JM, *et al.* Alopecia side-effect of antituberculosis drugs. *Lancet* 1996; **347:** 472–3.

Lupus. Antinuclear antibodies have been reported to occur in up to 22% of patients receiving isoniazid; however, patients are usually asymptomatic and overt lupoid syndrome is rare.[1] The incidence of antibody induction has been reported to be higher in slow acetylators than in fast acetylators[2] but the difference was not statistically significant and acetylator phenotype is not considered an important determinant of the risk of isoniazid-induced lupus.[1,3] Sim and co-workers[4] have demonstrated that the syndrome appeared to be due to isoniazid itself rather than its metabolite acetylisoniazid.

1. Hughes GRV. Recent developments in drug-associated systemic lupus erythematosus. *Adverse Drug React Bull* 1987; **123:** 460–3.
2. Alarcon-Segovia D, *et al.* Isoniazid acetylation rate and development of antinuclear antibodies upon isoniazid treatment. *Arthritis Rheum* 1971; **14:** 748–52.
3. Clark DWJ. Genetically determined variability in acetylation and oxidation: therapeutic implications. *Drugs* 1985; **29:** 342–75.
4. Sim E, *et al.* Drugs that induce systemic lupus erythematosus inhibit complement component C4. *Lancet* 1984; **ii:** 422–4.

Treatment of Adverse Effects

Pyridoxine hydrochloride 10 mg daily has been recommended in the UK for prophylaxis of peripheral neuritis although some authorities have suggested using up to 50 mg daily. A dose of 100 to 200 mg daily has been suggested for treatment if peripheral neuritis develops.

Nicotinamide has been given, usually in association with pyridoxine, in patients who develop pellagra.

Treatment of overdosage is symptomatic and supportive and consists of gastric lavage, control of convulsions, and correction of metabolic acidosis. Large doses of pyridoxine may be needed intravenously. Isoniazid is removed by haemodialysis.

Pyridoxine deficiency associated with isoniazid in doses of 5 mg per kg body-weight daily is uncommon. Patients at risk of developing pyridoxine deficiency include those with diabetes, uraemia, alcoholism, HIV infection, and malnutrition.[1,2] Supplementation with pyridoxine should be considered for this at-risk group as well as for pregnant women and patients with seizure disorders.[1] It is common practice to give a dose of 10 mg daily, although a dose of 6 mg daily might be sufficient.[3]

1. American Thoracic Society and the Centers for Disease Control. Treatment of tuberculosis and tuberculosis infection in adults and children. *Am J Respir Crit Care Med* 1994; **149:** 1359–74.
2. Joint Tuberculosis Committee of the British Thoracic Society. Chemotherapy and management of tuberculosis in the United Kingdom: recommendations 1998. *Thorax* 1998; **53:** 536–48.
3. Snider DE. Pyridoxine supplementation during isoniazid therapy. *Tubercle* 1980; **61:** 191–6.

Overdosage. Isoniazid doses of 6 g or more are associated with severe toxicity and doses above 15 g may be fatal without appropriate treatment. Symptoms may not occur until 2 hours after ingestion. Treatment includes early removal of the drug from the stomach, supportive treatment, and intravenous administration of pyridoxine in a dose at least equal to the amount of isoniazid ingested. Diazepam may be given intravenously to assist seizure control and sodium bicarbonate for metabolic acidosis. Dialysis has been used but may not be necessary.[1] Forced diuresis has also been tried.[2] Sievers and Herrier[3] recommend an initial dose of pyridoxine hydrochloride 5 g (even if the amount of isoniazid ingested is unknown) given intravenously over 3 to 5 minutes. This dose is repeated at 5 to 20 minute intervals until the dose greatly exceeds that of ingested isoniazid, seizures cease, or consciousness is regained. Other methods of pyridoxine administration have been proposed. Wason *et al.*[4] suggest administration of the total amount of pyridoxine as a single intravenous infusion in glucose 5% over 30 to 60 minutes. A maximum dose of pyridoxine has not been set; doses in the range of 70 to 357 mg per kg body-weight over 1 hour[4] and 52 g intravenously[3] have been used in isoniazid overdosage without pyridoxine toxicity.

1. Cameron WF. Isoniazid overdose. *Can Med Assoc J* 1978; **118:** 1413–15.
2. Brown CV. Acute isoniazid poisoning. *Am Rev Respir Dis* 1972; **105:** 206–16.
3. Sievers ML, Herrier RN. Treatment of acute isoniazid toxicity. *Am J Hosp Pharm* 1975; **32:** 202–6.
4. Wason S, *et al.* Single high-dose pyridoxine treatment for isoniazid overdose. *JAMA* 1981; **246:** 1102–4.

Precautions

Isoniazid should be administered with caution to patients with convulsive disorders, a history of psychosis, or hepatic or renal dysfunction. Patients who are at risk of neuropathy or pyridoxine deficiency, including those who are diabetic, alcoholic, malnourished, uraemic, or pregnant, should receive pyridoxine usually in a dose of 10 mg daily. If symptoms of hepatitis such as malaise, fatigue, anorexia, and nausea develop isoniazid should be discontinued pending evaluation.

Liver function should be checked before treatment with isoniazid and special care should be taken in alcoholic patients or those with pre-existing liver disease. Regular monitoring of liver function is recommended in patients with pre-existing liver disease, and isoniazid treatment should be suspended if serum aminotransferase concentrations are elevated to 5 times the normal upper limit or the bilirubin concentration rises. Careful monitoring should be considered for black and Hispanic women, in whom there may be an increased risk of fatal hepatitis.

Periodic eye examinations during isoniazid treatment have also been suggested.

Porphyria. Isoniazid was considered to be unsafe in patients with acute porphyria although there was conflicting experimental evidence of porphyrinogenicity.[1]

1. Moore MR, McColl KEL. *Porphyria: drug lists.* Glasgow: Porphyria Research Unit, University of Glasgow, 1991.

Pregnancy and the neonate. Snider *et al.*[1] in a review of antituberculous treatment in pregnant patients reported that over 95% of 1480 pregnancies in which isoniazid had been given resulted in a normal term infant. Slightly more than 1% of the infants/fetuses were abnormal and many of these abnormalities were CNS related. Isoniazid is therefore recognised as being suitable for use in regimens for the **treatment** of tuberculosis in **pregnant** patients.[2,3] Pyridoxine supplementation is recommended[2] (see Treatment of Adverse Effects, above). Preventive therapy with isoniazid is generally delayed until after delivery unless other risk factors are present.[2]

Isoniazid crosses the placenta and average fetal concentrations of 61.5 and 72.8% of maternal serum or plasma concentration have been reported.[4] The half-life of isoniazid may be prolonged in neonates.[4]

Isoniazid is distributed into breast milk. Peak concentrations of 6 μg per mL of milk following isoniazid doses of 5 mg per kg body-weight and 16.6 μg per mL of milk following a 300-mg dose have been reported.[5] Adverse effects on infants during **breast feeding** have not been reported,[6] although such infants should be monitored for toxic reactions.[5]

Isoniazid is also suitable for use in the **neonate**.[2]

1. Snider DE, *et al.* Treatment of tuberculosis during pregnancy. *Am Rev Respir Dis* 1980; **122:** 65–79.
2. American Thoracic Society and the Centers for Disease Control. Treatment of tuberculosis and tuberculosis infection in adults and children. *Am J Respir Crit Care Med* 1994; **149:** 1359–74.
3. Joint Tuberculosis Committee of the British Thoracic Society. Chemotherapy and management of tuberculosis in the United Kingdom: recommendations 1998. *Thorax* 1998; **53:** 536–48.
4. Holdiness MR. Transplacental pharmacokinetics of the antituberculosis drugs. *Clin Pharmacokinet* 1987; **13:** 125–9.
5. Snider D, Powell KE. Should women taking antituberculosis drugs breast-feed? *Arch Intern Med* 1984; **144:** 589–90.
6. Committee on Drugs. Transfer of drugs and other chemicals into human milk. *Pediatrics* 1989; **84:** 924–36.

Interactions

The risk of hepatotoxicity may be increased in patients receiving isoniazid in combination with rifampicin or other potentially hepatotoxic drugs.

Isoniazid can inhibit the hepatic metabolism of a number of drugs, in some cases leading to increased toxicity. These include the antiepileptics carbamazepine (p.341), ethosuximide (p.345), and phenytoin (p.354), the benzodiazepines diazepam and triazolam (p.663), chlorzoxazone (p.1313), and theophylline (p.768). The metabolism of enflurane (p.1222) may be increased in patients receiving isoniazid, resulting in potentially nephrotoxic levels of fluoride. Isoniazid has been associated with increased toxicity of cycloserine (p.199) and warfarin (p.966).

For interactions affecting isoniazid, see below.

Alcohol. The metabolism of isoniazid may be increased in chronic alcoholics: this may lead to reduced isoniazid effectiveness.[1] These patients may also be at increased risk of developing isoniazid-induced peripheral neuropathies and hepatic damage (see Precautions, above).

1. Anonymous. Interaction of drugs with alcohol. *Med Lett Drugs Ther* 1981; **23:** 33–4.

Antacids. Oral absorption of isoniazid is reduced by aluminium-containing antacids; isoniazid should be given one hour before the antacid.[1]

1. Hurwitz A, Schluzman DL. Effects of antacids on gastrointestinal absorption of isoniazid in rat and man.

Corticosteroids. Administration of prednisolone 20 mg to 13 slow acetylators and 13 fast acetylators receiving isoniazid 10 mg per kg body-weight reduced plasma concentrations of isoniazid by 25 and 40% respectively.[1] Renal clearance of isoniazid was also enhanced in both acetylator phenotypes and the rate of acetylation increased in slow acetylators only.[1] The clinical significance of this effect is not established.

1. Sarma GR, *et al.* Effect of prednisolone and rifampin on isoniazid metabolism in slow and rapid inactivators of isoniazid. *Antimicrob Agents Chemother* 1980; **18:** 661–6.

Food. Palpitations, headache, conjunctival irritation, severe flushing, tachycardia, tachypnoea, and sweating have been reported in patients taking isoniazid following ingestion of cheese, red wine,[1] and some fish.[2,3] Accumulation of tyramine[1] or histamine[2] has been proposed as the cause of these food-related reactions, and they could be mistaken for anaphylaxis.[3]

1. Toutoungi M, *et al.* Cheese, wine, and isoniazid. *Lancet* 1985; **ii:** 671.
2. Kottegoda SR. Cheese, wine and isoniazid. *Lancet* 1985; **ii:** 1074.
3. O'Sullivan TL. Drug-food interaction with isoniazid resembling anaphylaxis. *Ann Pharmacother* 1997; **31:** 928.

Ketoconazole. Serum concentrations of isoniazid were below the limits of detection in a patient also receiving rifampicin and ketoconazole.[1]

1. Abadie-Kemmerly S, *et al.* Failure of ketoconazole treatment of Blastomyces dermatitidis due to interaction of isoniazid and rifampin. *Ann Intern Med* 1988; **109:** 844–5. Correction. *ibid.* 1989; **111:** 96.

Zalcitabine. The clearance of isoniazid was approximately doubled when zalcitabine was given to 12 HIV-positive patients.[1] In addition, care is needed since zalcitabine also causes peripheral neuropathy.

1. Lee BL, *et al.* The effect of zalcitabine on the pharmacokinetics of isoniazid in HIV-infected patients. *Intersci Conf Antimicrob Agents Chemother* 1994; **34:** 3(A4).

Antimicrobial Action

Isoniazid is highly active against *Mycobacterium tuberculosis* which it inhibits *in vitro* at concentrations of 0.02 to 0.2 μg per mL. Isoniazid may have activity against some strains of other mycobacteria including *M. kansasii*.

Although it is rapidly bactericidal against actively dividing *M. tuberculosis* it is considered to be only bacteriostatic against semi-dormant organisms and has less sterilising activity than rifampicin or pyrazinamide.

Resistance to isoniazid develops rapidly if it is used alone in the treatment of clinical infection, and may be due in some strains to loss of the gene for catalase production. Resistance is delayed or prevented by combination with other antimycobacterials and it appears to be highly effective in preventing emergence of resistance to other antituberculous drugs. Resistance does not appear to be a problem when isoniazid is used alone in prophylaxis, probably because the bacillary load is low.

Mycobacterium avium complex. Synergistic activity of isoniazid plus streptomycin and, to a lesser degree, isoniazid plus clofazimine against *Mycobacterium avium* complex (MAC) has been demonstrated *in vitro* and *in vivo*.[1]

1. Reddy MV, *et al.* In vitro and in vivo synergistic effect of isoniazid with streptomycin and clofazimine against Mycobacterium avium complex (MAC). *Tubercle Lung Dis* 1994; **75:** 208–12.

Pharmacokinetics

Isoniazid is readily absorbed from the gastro-intestinal tract and following intramuscular injection. Peak concentrations of about 3 to 8 μg per mL appear in blood 1 to 2 hours after a fasting dose of 300 mg by mouth. The rate and extent of absorption of isoniazid is reduced by food. Isoniazid is not considered to be bound appreciably to plasma proteins and diffuses into all body tissues and fluids, including the CSF. It appears in fetal blood if given during pregnancy and in breast milk (see above).

The plasma half-life for isoniazid ranges from about 1 to 6 hours, those who are fast acetylators having shorter half-lives. The primary metabolic route is the acetylation of isoniazid to acetylisoniazid by *N*-acetyltransferase found in the liver and small intestine. Acetylisoniazid is then hydrolysed to isonicotinic acid and monoacetylhydrazine; isonicotinic acid is conjugated with glycine to isonicotinyl glycine (isonicotinuric acid) and monoacetylhydrazine is further acetylated to diacetylhydrazine. Some unmetabolised isoniazid is conjugated to hydrazones. The metabolites of isoniazid have no tuberculostatic activity and, apart from possibly monoacetylhydrazine, they are also less toxic. The rate of acetylation of isoniazid and monoacetylhydrazine is genetically determined and there is a bimodal distribution of persons who acetylate them either slowly or rapidly. Various ethnic groups, especially Eskimos, Japanese, and Chinese, are predominantly rapid acetylators whereas in populations of Caucasians, Negroes, and Indians (Madras), proportions of slow and rapid acetylators are similar. When isoniazid is administered daily or 2 or 3 times weekly, clinical effectiveness is not influenced by acetylator status.

In patients with normal renal function, over 75% of a dose appears in the urine in 24 hours, mainly as metabolites. Small amounts of drug are also excreted in the faeces. Isoniazid is removed by dialysis.

Distribution. Therapeutic concentrations of isoniazid have been detected in cerebrospinal fluid[1,2] and synovial fluid[3] several hours after oral administration. Diffusion into saliva is good and it has been suggested that salivary concentrations could be used in place of serum concentrations in pharmacokinetic studies.[4]

1. Forgan-Smith R, *et al.* Pyrazinamide and other drugs in tuberculous meningitis. *Lancet* 1973; **ii:** 374.
2. Miceli JN, *et al.* Isoniazid (INH) kinetics in children. *Fedn Proc* 1983; **42:** 1140.
3. Mouries D, *et al.* Passage articulaire de l'isoniazide et de l'éthambutol: deux observations de synovite tuberculeuse du genou. *Nouv Presse Med* 1975; **4:** 2734.
4. Gurumurthy P, *et al.* Salivary levels of isoniazid and rifampicin in tuberculous patients. *Tubercle* 1990; **71:** 29–33.

Oral administration. Malabsorption of isoniazid may occur in patients with HIV infection. However, it is not clear whether this is related to the infection itself or associated diarrhoea. In a report of treatment failure during observed antituberculosis therapy in 2 patients with HIV infection serum concentrations of isoniazid in 1 patient were low or undetectable for up to 12 hours after a dose.[1] However, serum concentrations of isoniazid in 26 HIV-positive patients undergoing intermittent antituberculosis treatment were generally regarded as adequate in a single sample taken 2 hours after a dose.[2] A pharmacokinetic study in volunteers without tuberculosis indicated that the presence of diarrhoea had a greater influence on absorption than either the presence or severity of HIV infection.[3]

1. Patel KB, *et al.* Drug malabsorption and resistant tuberculosis in HIV-infected patients. *N Engl J Med* 1995; **332:** 336–7.
2. Peloquin CA, *et al.* Low antituberculosis drug concentrations in patients with AIDS. *Ann Pharmacother* 1996; **30:** 919–25.
3. Sahai J, *et al.* Reduced plasma concentrations of antituberculosis drugs in patients with HIV infection. *Ann Intern Med* 1997; **127:** 289–93.

Uses and Administration

Isoniazid is a hydrazide derivative that is the mainstay of the primary treatment of pulmonary and extrapulmonary tuberculosis (p.146). It is administered with other antituberculous drugs such as rifampicin and pyrazinamide. Isoniazid is also used in high risk subjects for the prophylaxis of tuberculosis. It was formerly given in regimens for the treatment of opportunistic mycobacterial infections (p.133) attributable to the *Mycobacterium avium* complex.

Isoniazid is given in the initial and continuation phases of short-course tuberculosis regimens. The usual adult dose is 300 mg daily by mouth on an empty stomach. Children's doses vary between 5 mg per kg body-weight daily (WHO and UK) and 10 to 20 mg per kg daily (USA), all with a maximum of 300 mg daily. For intermittent therapy, WHO recommend 10 mg per kg three times a week or 15 mg per kg twice a week, while the recommended dose in the UK is 15 mg per kg three times a week. In the USA 15 mg per kg two or three times a week is recommended for adults and 20 to 40 mg per kg two or three times a week for children (maximum 900 mg). Doses may need to be reduced in patients with hepatic impairment or moderate to severe renal impairment.

Similar doses to those used orally may be given by intramuscular injection when isoniazid cannot be taken by mouth; it may also be given by intravenous injection. Isoniazid has also been given intrathecally and intrapleurally.

In tuberculosis prophylaxis, daily doses of 300 mg are given for at least 6 months and sometimes for up to 1 year. Alternatively it may be given with rifampicin for 3 months. Doses of 5 to 10 mg per kg isoniazid daily to a maximum of 300 mg daily have been suggested for prophylaxis in children in the UK.

Isoniazid aminosalicylate (pasiniazid) and isoniazid sodium glucuronate have also been used in the treatment of tuberculosis.

Preparations

BP 1998: Isoniazid Injection; Isoniazid Tablets;
USP 23: Isoniazid Injection; Isoniazid Syrup; Isoniazid Tablets; Rifampin and Isoniazid Capsules.

Proprietary Preparations (details are given in Part 3)
Belg.: Nicotibine; Rimifon†; ***Canad.:*** Isotamine; ***Fr.:*** Rimifon; ***Ger.:*** Dipasic†; Glurонazid†; Isozid; Isozid-compositum; Tb-Phlogin cum B_6†; tebesium; tebesium-s; ***Ital.:*** Cin†; Nicazide†; Nicizina; Nicozid; ***Spain:*** Cemidon; Cemidon B6; Dipasic†; Duplicalcio 150; Pyreazid; Rimifon; ***Swed.:*** Tibinide; ***Switz.:*** Rimifon; ***UK:*** Rimifon; ***USA:*** Laniazid; Nydrazid.

Multi-ingredient: ***Aust.:*** Isoprodian; Myambutol-INH; Rifater; Rifoldin INH; Rimactan + INH; ***Canad.:*** Rifater; ***Fr.:*** Dexambutol-INH; Rifater; Rifinah; ***Ger.:*** EMB-INH; Iso-Eremfat; Isoprodian; Myambutol-INH; Rifa/INH†; Rifater; Rifinah; ***Irl.:*** Rifater; Rifinah; Rimactazid; ***Ital.:*** Emozide B6†; Etanicozid B6; Etibi-INH; Miazide; Miazide B6; Rifanicozid; Rifater; Rifinah; ***Neth.:*** Rifinah; ***S.Afr.:*** Isoprodian†; Mynah; Myrin; Pyrifin; Rifater; Rifinah; Tuberol; ***Spain:*** Amiopia; Duplicalcio; Duplicalcio B12; Duplicalcio Hidraz; Isoetam; Poli Biocatines†; Rifater; Rifazida†; Rifinah; Rimactazid; Victogon; ***Switz.:*** Myambutol-INH; Rifater; Rifinah; Rifoldine-INH†; Rimactazide; Rimactazide + Z; ***UK:*** Mynah†; Rifater; Rifinah; Rimactazid; ***USA:*** Rifamate; Rifater; Rimactane/INH Dual Pack†.

Josamycin (94-y)

Josamycin (*USAN, rINN*).

EN-141; Leucomycin A_3. A stereoisomer of 7-(formylmethyl)-4,10-dihydroxy-5-methoxy-9,16-dimethyl-2-oxo-oxacyclohexadeca-11,13-dien-6-yl 3,6-dideoxy-4-*O*-(2,6-dideoxy-3-*C*-methyl-α-L-*ribo*-hexopyranosyl)-3-(dimethylamino)-β-D-glucopyranoside 4′-acetate 4″-isovalerate.

$C_{42}H_{69}NO_{15}$ = 828.0.

CAS — 16846-24-5; 56689-45-3.

Pharmacopoeias. In *Fr.* and *Jpn.*

Josamycin Propionate (18281-b)

Josamycin Propionate (*rINNM*).

YS-20P. Josamycin 10-propionate.

$C_{45}H_{73}NO_{16}$ = 884.1.

CAS — 56111-35-4.

Pharmacopoeias. In *Fr.* and *Jpn.*

Josamycin is derived from *Streptomyces narvonensis* var. *josamyceticus.* 1.07 mg of josamycin propionate is approximately equivalent to 1 mg of josamycin base.

Adverse Effects and Precautions

As for Erythromycin, p.204. Josamycin is reported to produce less gastro-intestinal disturbance than comparable doses of erythromycin.

A case of josamycin-induced pedal oedema has been reported.[1]

1. Bosch X, *et al.* Josamycin-induced pedal oedema. *Br Med J* 1993; **307:** 26.

Interactions

For a discussion of drug interactions with macrolide antibacterials, see Erythromycin, p.205.

Antimicrobial Action

As for Erythromycin, p.205. Some reports suggest that josamycin may be more active against some strains of anaerobic species such as *Bacteroides fragilis.*

Uses and Administration

Josamycin is a macrolide antibiotic with actions and uses similar to those of erythromycin (p.206). It is given by mouth as the base or the propionate but doses are calculated in terms of the base. Usual doses are 1 to 2 g daily of josamycin (or its equivalent), in 2 or more divided doses.

Preparations

Proprietary Preparations (details are given in Part 3)
Aust.: Josalid; ***Fr.:*** Josacine; ***Ger.:*** Wilprafen; ***Ital.:*** Iosalide; Josaxin; ***Jpn:*** Josamy; ***Spain:*** Josamina; Josaxin; ***Switz.:*** Josacine.

Kanamycin Acid Sulphate (95-j)

Kanamycin Acid Sulphate (*BANM*).

Kanamycini Sulfas Acidus.

Pharmacopoeias. In *Eur.* (see p.viii).

A form of kanamycin sulphate prepared by adding sulphuric acid to a solution of kanamycin sulphate and drying by a suitable method. A white or almost white, hygroscopic powder containing not less than 670 units per mg and 23 to 26% of sulphate, calculated on the dried material. 1.34 g of monograph substance is approximately equivalent to 1 g of kanamycin. **Soluble** 1 in 1 of water; practically insoluble in alcohol, acetone, and ether. A 1% solution in water has a pH of 5.5 to 7.5.

Kanamycin Sulphate (96-z)

Kanamycin Sulphate (*BANM, rINNM*).

Kanamycin A Sulphate; Kanamycin Monosulphate; Kanamycini Monosulfas. 6-*O*-(3-Amino-3-deoxy-α-D-glucopyranosyl)-4-*O*-(6-amino-6-deoxy-α-D-glucopyranosyl)-2-deoxystreptamine sulphate monohydrate.

$C_{18}H_{36}N_4O_{11},H_2SO_4,H_2O$ = 600.6.

CAS — 59-01-8 (kanamycin); 25389-94-0 (kanamycin sulphate, anhydrous).

Pharmacopoeias. In *Chin., Eur.* (see p.viii), *Jpn, Pol.,* and *US.*

The sulphate of an antimicrobial substance produced by the growth of *Streptomyces kanamyceticus.*

A white or almost white, odourless or almost odourless, crystalline powder. The Ph. Eur. specifies not less than 750 units per mg and 15.0 to 17.0% of sulphate, calculated on the dried material; USP specifies not less than 750 μg per mg. 1.2 g of monograph substance is approximately equivalent to 1 g of kanamycin.

Soluble 1 in 8 of water; practically insoluble in alcohol, acetone, ether, and ethyl acetate. A 1% solution in water has a pH of 6.5 to 8.5. **Store** in airtight containers.

Incompatibilities. For discussion of the incompatibility of aminoglycosides such as kanamycin with beta lactams, see under Gentamicin Sulphate, p.212. Kanamycin is also reported to be incompatible with various other drugs including some other antimicrobials as well as with some electrolytes.

Adverse Effects, Treatment, and Precautions

As for Gentamicin Sulphate, p.212.

Peak plasma concentrations of kanamycin greater than 30 μg per mL, and trough concentrations greater than 10 μg per mL should be avoided. Auditory (cochlear) toxicity is more frequent than vestibular toxicity.

Local pain and inflammation, as well as bruising and haematoma have been reported at the site of intramuscular injections.

Gastro-intestinal disturbances and a malabsorption syndrome, similar to that seen with oral neomycin (p.229), have occurred following administration of kanamycin by mouth. Oral kanamycin (local therapy) should be avoided in patients with gastro-intestinal ulceration.

Antimicrobial Action

As for Gentamicin Sulphate, p.213. It is active against a similar range of organisms although it is not active against *Pseudomonas* spp. Some strains of *Mycobacterium tuberculosis* are sensitive. MICs of kanamycin for the most sensitive organisms range from about 0.5 to 4 μg per mL but organisms with MICs less than about 8 μg per mL are considered sensitive.

Resistance has been reported in strains of many of the organisms normally sensitive to kanamycin, and at one time was widespread, but a decline in the use of kanamycin has meant that resistance has become somewhat less prevalent. Cross-resistance occurs between kanamycin and neomycin, framycetin and paromomycin, and partial cross-resistance has been reported between kanamycin and streptomycin.

References.

1. Ho YII, *et al.* In-vitro activities of aminoglycoside-aminocyclitols against mycobacteria. *J Antimicrob Chemother* 1997; **40:** 27–32.

Pharmacokinetics

As for Gentamicin Sulphate, p.213.

Less than 1% of an oral dose is absorbed, although this may be significantly increased if the gastro-intestinal mucosa is inflamed or ulcerated.

After intramuscular injection peak plasma concentrations of kanamycin of about 20 and 30 μg per mL are attained in about 1 hour following doses of 0.5 and 1 g respectively. A plasma half-life of about 3 hours has been reported. Absorption after intraperitoneal instillation is similar to that from intramuscular administration.

Kanamycin is rapidly excreted by glomerular filtration and most of a parenteral dose appears in the urine within 24 hours. It has been detected in cord blood and in breast milk.

Uses and Administration

Kanamycin is an aminoglycoside antibacterial with actions similar to those of gentamicin (p.214). It has been used in the treatment of susceptible Gram-negative and staphylococcal infections, including gonorrhoea (p.126) and neonatal gonococcal eye infections (p.132), although its use has declined in many centres because of the development of resistance. As with gentamicin it may be used with penicillins and with cephalosporins; the injections should be given at separate sites. Kanamycin has also been used as a second-line drug in tuberculosis (p.146), but other, safer drugs are usually preferred.

The sulphate or acid sulphate salts are often used: in the USA preparations containing the bisulphate ($C_{18}H_{36}N_4O_{11},2H_2SO_4$), but referred to as the sulphate, are available. Doses are expressed in terms of kanamycin base. It is usually administered by intramuscular injection and in acute infections adults may be given 15 mg per kg body-weight daily, to a maximum of 1.5 g daily, given in 2 to 4 divided doses. The same doses may be given by slow intravenous infusion of a 0.25 to 0.5% solution over 30 to 60 minutes; in the UK the manufacturers suggest that up to 30 mg per kg daily may be given by this route in overwhelming infection. Similar doses are used in children. Treatment should preferably not continue for longer than 7 to 10 days or exceed a cumulative dose of 10 g kanamycin. A single intramuscular dose of 2 g has been used in the treatment of penicillin-resistant gonorrhoea. A dose of 3 to 4 g weekly has been suggested by the UK manufacturers for patients with chronic bacterial infections, up to a cumulative dose not to exceed 50 g, but prolonged administration increases the risk of nephrotoxicity and is not generally recommended.

In the treatment and prophylaxis of neonatal gonococcal infections in infants born to mothers with gonorrhoea the equivalent of kanamycin 25 mg per kg, up to a maximum of 75 mg, may be given as a single intramuscular dose.

Peak plasma concentrations of greater than 30 μg per mL and trough concentrations greater than 10 μg per mL should be avoided. It is recommended that dosage should be adjusted in all patients according to plasma-kanamycin concentrations, and this is particularly important where factors such as age, renal impairment, or dose may predispose to toxicity, or where there is a risk of subtherapeutic concentrations. For discussion of the methods of calculating aminoglycoside dosage requirements, see p.214.

Kanamycin has been used by mouth similarly to neomycin (p.230), for the suppression of intestinal flora. For pre-operative use, the equivalent of 1 g of kanamycin may be given every hour for 4 hours, then 1 g every 6 hours for 36 to 72 hours. In the management of hepatic encephalopathy 8 to 12 g daily in divided doses may be given.

Kanamycin has also been administered in doses equivalent to 250 mg as a nebulised inhalation, 2 to 4 times daily. Solutions of kanamycin 0.25% have been used for the irrigation of body cavities.

Kanamycin tannate has also been used.

Preparations

BP 1998: Kanamycin Injection;
USP 23: Kanamycin Injection; Kanamycin Sulfate Capsules.

Proprietary Preparations (details are given in Part 3)
Belg.: Kanamytrex†; ***Fr.:*** Kamycine; ***Ger.:*** Kan-Ophtal; Kana-Stulln; Kanamytrex; ***Irl.:*** Kannasyn; ***Ital.:*** Keimicina; Tannamicina†; ***Spain:*** Kanacolirio; Kanescin; Kantrex; ***UK:*** Kannasyn; ***USA:*** Kantrex.

Multi-ingredient: ***Fr.:*** Sterimycine; ***Ital.:*** Dermaflogil; Desagamma K†; Fluomicetina; Fluorocortisol K†; Kanaderm†; Kanatrombina†; Kanazone; Roseomix†; ***S.Afr.:*** Kantrexil; ***Spain:*** Kanafosal; Kanafosal Predni; Kanapomada; Lysokana; Naso Pekamin; Tasumicina†.

Kitasamycin (97-c)

Kitasamycin *(BAN, USAN, rINN).*
Leucomycin.
CAS — 1392-21-8.
Pharmacopoeias. In *Jpn* which also includes Acetylkitasamycin.

An antimicrobial substance produced by *Streptomyces kitasatoensis*, consisting mainly of kitasamycins A_4 and A_5.

Kitasamycin is a macrolide antibiotic with actions and uses similar to those of erythromycin (p.204). It has been administered by mouth as kitasamycin base or intravenously as the tartrate. Acetylkitasamycin has also been administered by mouth.

Latamoxef Disodium (186-k)

Latamoxef Disodium *(BANM, rINNM).*
LY-127935; Moxalactam Disodium *(USAN)*; 6059-S. (7*R*)-7-[2-Carboxy-2-(4-hydroxyphenyl)acetamido]-7-methoxy-3-(1-methyl-1*H*-tetrazol-5-ylthiomethyl)-1-oxa-3-cephem-4-carboxylic acid, disodium salt.
$C_{20}H_{18}N_6Na_2O_9S$ = 564.4.
CAS — 64952-97-2 (latamoxef); 64953-12-4 (latamoxef disodium).
Pharmacopoeias. In *Jpn.*

1.08 g of monograph substance is approximately equivalent to 1 g of latamoxef. Each g of monograph substance represents about 3.5 mmol of sodium.

Latamoxef is an oxacephalosporin antibiotic differing from the cephalosporins in that the sulphur atom of the 7-aminocephalosporanic acid nucleus is replaced by oxygen. Like cephamandole, it has a methylthiotetrazole side-chain and may cause hypoprothrombinaemia. Serious bleeding episodes have been reported with latamoxef and, in addition to hypoprothrombinaemia, inhibition of platelet function and more rarely immune-mediated thrombocytopenia may be responsible for interference with haemostasis. As with the methylthiotetrazole-containing cephalosporins, a disulfiram-like reaction with alcohol may occur.

Latamoxef has antimicrobial activity similar to that of the third-generation cephalosporin cefotaxime (p.168), although it is generally less active against Gram-positive bacteria and more active against *Bacteroides fragilis.*

It has been given intramuscularly or intravenously as the disodium salt in the treatment of susceptible infections. Doses have been expressed in terms of the equivalent amount of latamoxef and have usually ranged from 0.5 to 4 g daily in two divided doses. Higher doses have been associated with an increased risk of bleeding. Prophylaxis with vitamin K has been recommended during treatment with latamoxef and bleeding time monitored in patients on higher doses. Reduced dosage has been employed in patients with impaired renal function.

Preparations

USP 23: Moxalactam Disodium for Injection.

Proprietary Preparations (details are given in Part 3)
Fr.: Moxalactam†; ***Ger.:*** Festamoxin†; Moxalactam†; ***Ital.:*** Baxal†; Betalactam†; Latoxacef†; Mactam; Moxacef†; Moxatres†; Oxacef†; Polimoxal†; Priolatt†; Sectam; ***Jpn:*** Shiomarin.

Lenampicillin Hydrochloride (16873-l)

Lenampicillin Hydrochloride *(rINNM).*
KBT-1585. 2,3-Dihydroxy-2-butenyl(2*S*,5*R*,6*R*)-6-[(*R*)-2-amino-2-phenylacetamido]-3,3-dimethyl-7-oxo-4-thia-1-azabicyclo[3.2.0]heptane-2-carboxylate, cyclic carbonate, hydrochloride.
$C_{21}H_{23}N_3O_7S,HCl$ = 497.9.
CAS — 86273-18-9 (lenampicillin); 80734-02-7 (lenampicillin hydrochloride).

Lenampicillin is an ester of ampicillin (p.153) to which it is hydrolysed *in vivo*. It is administered by mouth, as the hydrochloride, in the treatment of susceptible infections.

Preparations

Proprietary Preparations (details are given in Part 3)
Jpn: Takacillin†; Varacillin†.

Levofloxacin (15283-v)

Levofloxacin *(BAN, USAN, rINN).*
DR-3355; HR-355; RWJ-25213; S-(−)-Ofloxacin. (−)-(S)-9-Fluoro-2,3-dihydro-3-methyl-10-(4-methyl-1-piperazinyl)-7-oxo-7*H*-pyrido[1,2,3-*de*]-1,4-benzoxazine-6-carboxylic acid.
$C_{18}H_{20}FN_3O_4$ = 361.4.
CAS — 100986-85-4 (levofloxacin); 138199-71-0 (levofloxacin hemihydrate).

Adverse Effects and Precautions

As for Ciprofloxacin, p.186.

Interactions

As for Ciprofloxacin, p.187.

References.

1. Liao S, *et al.* Absence of an effect of levofloxacin on warfarin pharmacokinetics and anticoagulation in male volunteers. *J Clin Pharmacol* 1996; **36:** 1072–7.
2. Gisclon LG, *et al.* Absence of a pharmacokinetic interaction between intravenous theophylline and orally administered levofloxacin. *J Clin Pharmacol* 1997; **37:** 744–50.
3. Doose DR, *et al.* Levofloxacin does not alter cyclosporine disposition. *J Clin Pharmacol* 1998; **38:** 90–3.

Antimicrobial Action

As for Ciprofloxacin, p.187.

Levofloxacin is generally considered to be about twice as active as its isomer, ofloxacin (p.233). It has a broad spectrum of activity which includes Gram-positive bacteria.

References.

1. George J, Morrissey I. The bactericidal activity of levofloxacin compared with ofloxacin, D-ofloxacin, ciprofloxacin, sparfloxacin and cefotaxime against Streptococcus pneumoniae. *J Antimicrob Chemother* 1997; **39:** 719–23.
2. Licata L, *et al.* Comparison of the postantibiotic and postantibiotic sub-MIC effects of levofloxacin and ciprofloxacin on Staphylococcus aureus and Streptococcus pneumoniae. *Antimicrob Agents Chemother* 1997; **41:** 950–5.
3. Entenza JM, *et al.* Levofloxacin versus ciprofloxacin, flucloxacillin, or vancomycin for treatment of experimental endocarditis due to methicillin-susceptible or -resistant Staphylococcus aureus. *Antimicrob Agents Chemother* 1997; **41:** 1662–7.
4. Spangler SK, *et al.* Postantibiotic effect and postantibiotic sub-MIC effect of levofloxacin compared to those of ofloxacin, ciprofloxacin, erythromycin, azithromycin, and clarithromycin against 20 pneumococci. *Antimicrob Agents Chemother* 1998; **42:** 1253–5.

Pharmacokinetics

Levofloxacin is rapidly and almost completely absorbed following oral administration with peak plasma concentrations achieved within an hour of a dose. It is distributed into body tissues including the bronchial mucosa and lungs, but penetration into CSF is relatively poor. Levofloxacin is approximately 30 to 40% bound to plasma proteins. It is only metabolised to a small degree to inactive metabolites. The elimination half-life of levofloxacin is 6 to 8 hours, although this may be prolonged in patients with renal impairment. Levofloxacin is excreted largely unchanged, primarily in the urine.

References.

1. Fish DN, Chow AT. The clinical pharmacokinetics of levofloxacin. *Clin Pharmacokinet* 1997; **32:** 101–19.
2. Chien S-C, *et al.* Pharmacokinetic profile of levofloxacin following once-daily 500-milligram oral or intravenous doses. *Antimicrob Agents Chemother* 1997; **41:** 2256–60.
3. Preston SL, *et al.* Pharmacodynamics of levofloxacin: a new paradigm for early clinical trials. *JAMA* 1998; **279:** 125–9.
4. Chien S-C, *et al.* Double-blind evaluation of the safety and pharmacokinetics of multiple oral once-daily 750-milligram and 1-gram doses of levofloxacin in healthy volunteers. *Antimicrob Agents Chemother* 1998; **42:** 885–8.

Uses and Administration

Levofloxacin is the *S*-(−)-isomer of the fluoroquinolone antibacterial ofloxacin (p.233). It is given by mouth or intravenously for the treatment of susceptible infections in a usual dose of 250 or 500 mg once or twice daily. Doses should be reduced in patients with renal impairment.

Reviews.

1. Davis R, Bryson HM. Levofloxacin: a review of its antibacterial activity, pharmacokinetics and therapeutic efficacy. *Drugs* 1994; **4:** 677–700.
2. Martin SJ, *et al.* Levofloxacin and sparfloxacin: new quinolone antibiotics. *Ann Pharmacother* 1998; **32:** 320–36.
3. Langtry HD, Lamb HM. Levofloxacin: its use in infections of the respiratory tract, skin, soft tissues and urinary tract. *Drugs* 1998; **56:** 487–515.

Preparations

Proprietary Preparations (details are given in Part 3)
Jpn: Cravit; ***UK:*** Tavanic; ***USA:*** Levaquin.

Lincomycin Hydrochloride (98-k)

Lincomycin Hydrochloride (*BANM, rINNM*).

Lincomycini Hydrochloridum; NSC-70731; U-10149 (lincomycin). Methyl 6-amino-6,8-dideoxy-*N*-[(2*S*,4*R*)-1-methyl-4-propylprolyl]-1-thio-α-D-*erythro*-D-*galacto*-octopyranoside hydrochloride monohydrate.

$C_{18}H_{34}N_2O_6S,HCl,H_2O$ = 461.0.

CAS — 154-21-2 (lincomycin); 859-18-7 (lincomycin hydrochloride, anhydrous); 7179-49-9 (lincomycin hydrochloride, monohydrate).

NOTE. Lincomycin is *USAN*.

Pharmacopoeias. In *Chin., Eur.* (see p.viii), *Jpn, Pol.*, and *US*.

An antimicrobial substance produced by the growth of *Streptomyces lincolnensis* var. *lincolnensis* or by any other means. A white or almost white crystalline powder, odourless or with a slight odour. It contains not more than 5% of lincomycin B. 1.13 g of monograph substance is approximately equivalent to 1 g of lincomycin. Very or freely **soluble** in water; slightly soluble in alcohol; soluble in dimethylformamide; very slightly soluble in acetone; practically insoluble in ether. A 10% solution of lincomycin hydrochloride in water has a pH of 3.0 to 5.5. **Store** at a temperature not exceeding 30° in airtight containers.

Incompatibilities. Solutions of lincomycin hydrochloride have an acid pH and incompatibility may be expected with alkaline preparations, or with drugs unstable at low pH.

Adverse Effects, Treatment, and Precautions

As for Clindamycin, p.191.

Hypotension, ECG changes, and on rare occasions cardiac arrest, have followed rapid intravenous injections. Other adverse reactions reported rarely with lincomycin include aplastic anaemia, pancytopenia, and tinnitus.

Interactions

As for Clindamycin, p.191.

Absorption of lincomycin is reduced by adsorbent antidiarrhoeals and cyclamate sweeteners.

Antimicrobial Action

As for Clindamycin (p.191) but it is less potent. The minimum inhibitory concentrations of lincomycin have been reported to range from 0.05 to 2 μg per mL for the most sensitive organisms. There is complete cross-resistance between clindamycin and lincomycin.

Pharmacokinetics

About 20 to 30% of a dose of lincomycin given by mouth is absorbed from the gastro-intestinal tract and following a 500-mg dose, peak plasma concentrations of 2 to 7 μg per mL are reached within 2 to 4 hours. Food markedly reduces the rate and extent of absorption. The intramuscular injection of 600 mg produces peak plasma concentrations of 8 to 18 μg per mL usually within 30 minutes.

The biological half-life of lincomycin is about 5 hours. Lincomycin is widely distributed in the tissues including bone and body fluids but diffusion into the CSF is poor, although it may be slightly better when the meninges are inflamed. It diffuses across the placenta and is distributed into breast milk. Lincomycin is partially inactivated in the liver; unchanged drug and metabolites are excreted in the urine, bile, and faeces. Lincomycin is not effectively removed from the blood by dialysis.

Uses and Administration

Lincomycin is a lincosamide antibiotic with actions and uses similar to those of its chlorinated derivative, clindamycin (p.192). Clindamycin is usually preferred to lincomycin because of its greater activity and better absorption. However, the usefulness of both drugs is limited by their potential to cause pseudomembranous colitis.

Lincomycin hydrochloride is administered by mouth in doses equivalent to 500 mg of lincomycin 3 or 4 times daily taken at least 1 hour before food; by intramuscular injection, 600 mg once or twice daily; by slow intravenous infusion over not less than one hour, 600 mg to 1 g two or three times daily in at least 100 mL of diluent. Higher doses have been given in very severe infections, up to a total daily dose of about 8 g. Children over the age of 1 month may be given 20 to 60 mg per kg bodyweight daily in divided doses by mouth or 10 to 20 mg per kg daily in divided doses by intramuscular injection or intravenous infusion. Doses may need to be reduced in patients with severe renal impairment: a reduction to 25 to 30% of the usual dose has been recommended.

Lincomycin hydrochloride may be administered into the eye by subconjunctival injection in a dose equivalent to 75 mg of lincomycin.

Preparations

BP 1998: Lincomycin Capsules; Lincomycin Injection;
USP 23: Lincomycin Hydrochloride Capsules; Lincomycin Hydrochloride Syrup; Lincomycin Injection.

Proprietary Preparations (details are given in Part 3)
Austral.: Lincocin; ***Belg.:*** Lincocin; ***Canad.:*** Lincocin; ***Fr.:*** Lincocine; ***Ger.:*** Albiotic; ***Irl.:*** Lincocin†; ***Ital.:*** Cillimicina†; Lincocin; ***Neth.:*** Lincocin; ***Norw.:*** Lincocin†; ***S.Afr.:*** Lincocin; ***Spain:*** Cillimicina; Lincocin; ***Swed.:*** Lincocin; ***Switz.:*** Lincocin; ***USA:*** Lincocin; Lincorex.

Lomefloxacin Hydrochloride (5472-k)

Lomefloxacin Hydrochloride (*BANM, USAN, rINNM*).

NY-198; SC-47111; SC-47111A (lomefloxacin); SC-47111B (lomefloxacin mesylate). (*RS*)-1-Ethyl-6,8-difluoro-1,4-dihydro-7-(3-methylpiperazin-1-yl)-4-oxoquinoline-3-carboxylic acid hydrochloride.

$C_{17}H_{19}F_2N_3O_3,HCl$ = 387.8.

CAS — 98079-51-7 (lomefloxacin); 98079-52-8 (lomefloxacin hydrochloride); 114394-67-1 (lomefloxacin mesylate).

Adverse Effects and Precautions

As for Ciprofloxacin, p.186.

Concern has been expressed over the relatively high incidence of phototoxicity reactions in patients receiving lomefloxacin. Patients should be advised to avoid exposure to sunlight during, and for a few days after, lomefloxacin therapy, and to discontinue the drug immediately if phototoxicity occurs.

Interactions

As for Ciprofloxacin, p.187. Lomefloxacin does not appear to interact significantly with theophylline or caffeine.

Antimicrobial Action

As for Ciprofloxacin, p.187. Most streptococci, including *Streptococcus pneumoniae*, are relatively resistant to lomefloxacin. Cross-resistance between lomefloxacin and other quinolones has been reported.

References.

1. Van der Auwera P, *et al.* In-vitro activity of lomefloxacin in comparison with pefloxacin and ofloxacin. *J Antimicrob Chemother* 1989; **23:** 209–19.
2. Chambers ST, *et al.* Antimicrobial effects of lomefloxacin in vitro. *J Antimicrob Chemother* 1991; **27:** 481–9.
3. Leigh DA, *et al.* Antibacterial activity of lomefloxacin. *J Antimicrob Chemother* 1991; **27:** 589–98.
4. Banerjee DK, *et al.* In-vitro activity of lomefloxacin against pathogenic and environmental mycobacteria. *J Antimicrob Chemother* 1992; **30:** 236–8.

Pharmacokinetics

Lomefloxacin is rapidly and almost completely absorbed following oral administration, peak plasma concentrations of about 3 μg per mL being attained about 1 to 1.5 hours after a 400-mg dose. Lomefloxacin is approximately 10% bound to plasma proteins. It is widely distributed into body tissues including the lungs and prostate.

The elimination half-life of lomefloxacin is about 7 to 8 hours, and is prolonged in patients with renal impairment. Lomefloxacin is excreted in the urine, mainly as unchanged drug but also in small amounts as the glucuronide and other metabolites. Small amounts are also eliminated unchanged in the faeces.

References.

1. Leroy A, *et al.* Lomefloxacin pharmacokinetics in subjects with normal and impaired renal function. *Antimicrob Agents Chemother* 1990; **34:** 17–20.
2. Gros I, Carbon C. Pharmacokinetics of lomefloxacin in healthy volunteers: comparison of 400 milligrams once daily and 200 milligrams twice daily given orally for 5 days. *Antimicrob Agents Chemother* 1990; **34:** 150–2.
3. Blum RA, *et al.* Pharmacokinetics of lomefloxacin in renally compromised patients. *Antimicrob Agents Chemother* 1990; **34:** 2364–8.
4. Cowling P, *et al.* The pharmacokinetics of lomefloxacin in elderly patients with urinary tract infection following daily dosing with 400 mg. *J Antimicrob Chemother* 1991; **28:** 101–7.
5. Kovarik JM, *et al.* Steady-state pharmacokinetics and sputum penetration of lomefloxacin in patients with chronic obstructive pulmonary disease and acute respiratory tract infections. *Antimicrob Agents Chemother* 1992; **36:** 2458–61.
6. Freeman CD, *et al.* Lomefloxacin clinical pharmacokinetics. *Clin Pharmacokinet* 1993; **25:** 6–19.

Uses and Administration

Lomefloxacin is a fluoroquinolone antibacterial with actions and uses similar to those of ciprofloxacin (p.188).

It is given by mouth, as the hydrochloride, for the treatment of susceptible infections, including bronchitis due to *Haemophilus influenzae* or *Moraxella catarrhalis* and urinary-tract infections. The usual dose is the equivalent of 400 mg of lomefloxacin base once daily. Evening administration may minimise the risk of phototoxicity reactions.

Dosage should be reduced in patients with moderate to severe renal impairment.

General references.

1. Wadworth AN, Goa KL. Lomefloxacin: a review of its antibacterial activity, pharmacokinetic properties and therapeutic use. *Drugs* 1991; **42:** 1018–60.
2. Neu HC, ed. Lomefloxacin: development of a once-a-day quinolone. *Am J Med* 1992; **92** (suppl 4A): 1S–137S.
3. Symonds WT, Nix DE. Lomefloxacin and temafloxacin: two new fluoroquinolone antimicrobials. *Clin Pharm* 1992; **11:** 753–66.

Preparations

Proprietary Preparations (details are given in Part 3)
Aust.: Uniquin; ***Fr.:*** Logiflox; ***Ital.:*** Chimono; Maxaquin; Uniquin; ***Jpn:*** Bareon; Lomeflon; ***S.Afr.:*** Maxaquin; Uniquin; ***Switz.:*** Maxaquin; Okacin; ***USA:*** Maxaquin.

Loracarbef (5477-f)

Loracarbef (*BAN, USAN, rINN*).

LY-163892. (6*R*,7*S*)-3-Chloro-8-oxo-7-D-phenylglycylamino-1-azabicyclo[4.2.0]oct-2-ene-2-carboxylic acid monohydrate.

$C_{16}H_{16}ClN_3O_4,H_2O$ = 367.8.

CAS — 76470-66-1 (anhydrous loracarbef); 121961-22-6 (loracarbef monohydrate).

Pharmacopoeias. In *US*.

Approximately 105 mg of loracarbef monohydrate is equivalent to 100 mg of anhydrous loracarbef. A 10% suspension in water has a pH of 3.0 to 5.5. **Store** in airtight containers.

Adverse Effects and Precautions

Adverse effects of loracarbef are generally similar to those of other beta-lactams (see Benzylpenicillin, p.159, and Cephalothin, p.179). They include gastro-intestinal disturbances particularly diarrhoea and hypersensitivity reactions such as skin rashes. Increases in liver enzymes and abnormalities in haematological parameters have been reported.

Loracarbef should not be given to patients known to be hypersensitive to it or to other beta-lactams because of the possibility of cross-sensitivity. It should be given with caution in patients with impaired renal function; a dosage reduction may be required.

Effects on the kidneys. References.

1. Thieme RE, *et al.* Acute interstitial nephritis associated with loracarbef therapy. *J Pediatr* 1995; **127:** 997–1000.

Interactions

Probenecid decreases the renal excretion of loracarbef thereby increasing its plasma concentrations.

Antimicrobial Action

Loracarbef is bactericidal with antibacterial activity similar to that of cefaclor (p.163).

References.

1. Knapp CC, Washington JA. In vitro activities of LY-163892, cefaclor, and cefuroxime. *Antimicrob Agents Chemother* 1988; **32:** 131–3.
2. Cao C, *et al.* In-vitro activity and β-lactamase stability of LY-163892. *J Antimicrob Chemother* 1988; **22:** 155–65.
3. Jones RN, Barry AL. Antimicrobial activity of LY-163892, an orally administered 1-carbacephem. *J Antimicrob Chemother* 1988; **22:** 315–20.
4. Howard AJ, Dunkin KT. Comparative in-vitro activity of a new oral carbacephem, LY-163892. *J Antimicrob Chemother* 1988; **22:** 445–56.
5. Shelton S, Nelson JD. In vitro susceptibilities of common pediatric pathogens to LY-163892. *Antimicrob Agents Chemother* 1988; **32:** 268–70.
6. Doern GV, *et al.* In vitro activity of loracarbef (LY-163892), a new oral carbacephem antimicrobial agent, against respiratory isolates of Haemophilus influenzae and Moraxella catarrhalis. *Antimicrob Agents Chemother* 1991; **35:** 1504–7.
7. Arguedas AG, *et al.* In-vitro activity of cefprozil (BMY-28100) and loracarbef (LY-163892) against pathogens obtained from middle ear fluid. *J Antimicrob Chemother* 1991; **27:** 311–18.

Pharmacokinetics

Loracarbef is well absorbed from the gastro-intestinal tract with a bioavailability of 90%. Peak plasma concentrations following 200- and 400-mg doses as capsules are about 8 and 14 μg per mL respectively at 1.2 hours. Peak concentrations are achieved more rapidly following administration as oral suspension and the paediatric dose of 15 mg per kg body-weight produces a concentration of approximately 19 μg per mL at 0.8 hours. Absorption is delayed by the presence of food. A plasma half-life of about 1 hour has been reported which may be prolonged in renal impairment. About 25% is bound to plasma proteins.

Loracarbef is excreted largely unchanged in the urine, and therapeutic concentrations are maintained in the urine for up to 12 hours. Probenecid delays excretion. Loracarbef is removed by haemodialysis.

References.

1. Nelson JD, *et al.* Pharmacokinetics of LY-163892 in infants and children. *Antimicrob Agents Chemother* 1988; **32:** 1738–9.
2. Kusmiesz H, *et al.* Loracarbef concentrations in middle ear fluid. *Antimicrob Agents Chemother* 1990; **34:** 2030–1.
3. Therasse DG, *et al.* Effects of renal dysfunction on the pharmacokinetics of loracarbef. *Clin Pharmacol Ther* 1993; **54:** 311–16.
4. Lees AS, *et al.* The pharmacokinetics, tissue penetration and in-vitro activity of loracarbef, a β-lactam antibiotic of the carbacephem class. *J Antimicrob Chemother* 1993; **32:** 853–9.
5. Hill SL, *et al.* Sputum and serum pharmacokinetics of loracarbef (LY163892) in patients with chronic bronchial sepsis. *J Antimicrob Chemother* 1994; **33:** 129–36.
6. Sitar DS, *et al.* Pharmacokinetic disposition of loracarbef in healthy young men and women at steady state. *J Clin Pharmacol* 1994; **34:** 924–9.

Uses and Administration

Loracarbef is an oral carbacephem antibiotic. The carbacephems are closely related to the cephalosporins, but replacement of the S atom in the 7-aminocephalosporanic acid nucleus by a methylene group is said to enhance stability. It is used similarly to cefaclor in the treatment of susceptible infections of the respiratory and urinary tracts and of skin and soft tissue. For details of these infections and their treatment, see under Choice of Antibacterial, p.116.

Loracarbef is given as the monohydrate. Doses are expressed in terms of the equivalent amount of anhydrous loracarbef. The usual adult dose is 200 to 400 mg every 12 hours. In uncomplicated urinary-tract infections a dose of 200 mg daily may be adequate. A suggested dose for children is 7.5 mg per kg body-weight every 12 hours for uncomplicated infections or 15 mg per kg every 12 hours for acute otitis media. Loracarbef should be given an hour before food or on an empty stomach. Doses should be reduced in patients with renal function impairment.

General references.

1. Moellering RC, Jacobs NF. Advances in outpatient antimicrobial therapy: loracarbef. *Am J Med* 1992; **92** (suppl 6A): 1S–103S.
2. Brogden RN, McTavish D. Loracarbef: a review of its antimicrobial activity, pharmacokinetic properties and therapeutic efficacy. *Drugs* 1993; **45:** 716–36.

Preparations

USP 23: Loracarbef Capsules; Loracarbef for Oral Suspension.

Proprietary Preparations (details are given in Part 3)
Aust.: Lorabid; Lorax; ***Ger.:*** Lorafem; ***Ital.:*** Carbem; ***Neth.:*** Lorax; ***S.Afr.:*** Lorabid; ***Swed.:*** Lorabid; ***USA:*** Lorabid.

Lymecycline (100-a)

Lymecycline *(BAN, rINN).*

Limeciclina; Tetracyclinemethylene lysine.

$C_{29}H_{38}N_4O_{10}$ = 602.6.

CAS — 992-21-2.

Pharmacopoeias. In *Br.*

A water-soluble combination of tetracycline, lysine, and formaldehyde. A yellow very hygroscopic powder. Lymecycline 407 mg is approximately equivalent to 300 mg of tetracycline and to 325 mg of tetracycline hydrochloride. Very **soluble** in water; slightly soluble in alcohol; practically insoluble in acetone, chloroform, and ether. It contains not more than 5% by weight of water. A 1% solution in water has a pH of 7.8 to 8.1. **Store** at a temperature not exceeding 25°. Protect from light.

Lymecycline is a tetracycline derivative with general properties similar to those of tetracycline (p.259).

Doses are expressed in terms of the equivalent amount of tetracycline base. The usual adult dose is the equivalent of 300 mg of tetracycline administered twice daily by mouth; in severe infections doses of up to the equivalent of 1.2 g may be given over 24 hours. In the treatment of acne, the equivalent of 300 mg of tetracycline may be given daily.

Preparations

BP 1998: Lymecycline Capsules.

Proprietary Preparations (details are given in Part 3)
Aust.: Tetralysal; ***Belg.:*** Tetralysal; ***Fr.:*** Tetralysal; ***Ital.:*** Tralisin†; ***Norw.:*** Tetralysal; ***S.Afr.:*** Tetralysal; ***Swed.:*** Tetralysal; ***UK:*** Tetralysal.

Multi-ingredient: ***Spain:*** Tetralfa†.

Mafenide Acetate (4908-r)

Mafenide Acetate *(BANM, rINNM).*

NSC-34632 (mafenide). α-Aminotoluene-*p*-sulphonamide acetate.

$C_7H_{10}N_2O_2S,C_2H_4O_2$ = 246.3.

CAS — 138-39-6 (mafenide); 13009-99-9 (mafenide acetate).

NOTE. Mafenide is *USAN.*

Pharmacopoeias. In *Chin.* and *US.* .

A white to pale yellow crystalline powder. 11.2 g of monograph substance is approximately equivalent to 8.5 g of mafenide. Freely **soluble** in water. A 10% solution in water has a pH of 6.4 to 6.8. **Store** in airtight containers. Protect from light.

Adverse Effects, Treatment, and Precautions

Mafenide is absorbed to some extent following topical application and may produce systemic effects similar to those of other sulphonamides (see Sulphamethoxazole, p.254).

Mafenide acetate cream may cause pain or a burning sensation on application to the burnt area, with occasional bleeding or excoriation. The separation of the eschar may be delayed and fungal invasion of the wound has been reported. By its action in inhibiting carbonic anhydrase mafenide may cause metabolic acidosis and hyperventilation; acid-base balance should therefore be monitored, particularly in patients with extensive burns, or with pulmonary or renal impairment, and treatment should be temporarily suspended and continuous fluid therapy given if persistent acidosis occurs.

Pharmacokinetics

Mafenide is absorbed from wounds into the circulation and is metabolised to *p*-carboxybenzenesulphonamide which is excreted in the urine. The metabolite has no antibacterial action but retains the ability to inhibit carbonic anhydrase.

Uses and Administration

Mafenide is a sulphonamide that is not inactivated by *p*-aminobenzoic acid or by pus and serum. The acetate is used as a cream, containing the equivalent of mafenide 8.5%, in conjunction with debridement, for the prevention and treatment of infection, including *Pseudomonas aeruginosa,* in second- and third-degree burns (p.1073). Mafenide hydrochloride and mafenide propionate have also been used.

Preparations

USP 23: Mafenide Acetate Cream.

Proprietary Preparations (details are given in Part 3)
USA: Sulfamylon.

Multi-ingredient: ***Ger.:*** Combiamid; ***Spain:*** Pental Forte; Pentalmicina.

Magainins (5484-r)

The magainins are a group of antimicrobial peptides derived from amphibians. A number of semisynthetic derivatives including MSI-78, MSI-93, and MSI-94 are under development as topical anti-infectives.

References.

1. Chopra I. The magainins: antimicrobial peptides with potential for topical application. *J Antimicrob Chemother* 1993; **32:** 351–3.
2. Levison ME, *et al.* The bactericidal activity of magainins against Pseudomonas aeruginosa and Enterococcus faecium. *J Antimicrob Chemother* 1993; **32:** 577–85.
3. Fuchs PC, *et al.* In vitro antimicrobial activity of MSI-78, a magainin analog. *Antimicrob Agents Chemother* 1998; **42:** 1213–16.

Mandelic Acid (5662-d)

Amygdalic Acid; Phenylglycolic Acid; Racemic Mandelic Acid. 2-Hydroxy-2-phenylacetic acid.

$C_8H_8O_3$ = 152.1.

CAS — 90-64-2; 17199-29-0 ((+)-mandelic acid); 611-72-3 ((±)-mandelic acid); 611-71-2 ((−)-mandelic acid).

Pharmacopoeias. In *Neth.* and *US.*

White to yellowish-white, almost odourless, crystals or crystalline powder. Gradually turns yellow and decomposes on prolonged exposure to light. Freely **soluble** in water; very soluble in alcohol; freely soluble in ether and in isopropyl alcohol; soluble in chloroform. **Protect** from light.

Mandelic acid has bacteriostatic properties and has been given by mouth in the treatment of urinary-tract infections, usually as the ammonium or calcium salt. It is excreted unchanged in the urine and has been effective against uncomplicated infections due to Gram-negative and a few Gram-positive species, provided that the pH is maintained below 5.5. Mandelic acid is also used as a 1% flushing solution for the maintenance of indwelling urinary catheters.

Gastro-intestinal disturbances, dizziness and tinnitus, and dysuria or haematuria have been reported occasionally following ingestion of mandelic acid or its salts. It is contra-indicated in patients with impaired renal function.

Mandelic acid is a component of hexamine mandelate (p.216).

Preparations

Proprietary Preparations (details are given in Part 3)
Multi-ingredient: ***Fr.:*** Intesticarbine†; ***Ger.:*** Urodil N†.

Marbofloxacin (15416-h)

Marbofloxacin *(BAN, rINN).*

9-Fluoro-2,3-dihydro-3-methyl-10-(4-methyl-1-piperazinyl)-7-oxo-7*H*-pyrido[3,2,1-*ij*][4,1,2]benzoxadiazine-6-carboxylic acid.

$C_{17}H_{19}FN_4O_4$ = 362.4.

CAS — 115550-35-1.

Marbofloxacin is a fluoroquinolone antibacterial used in veterinary medicine.

Mecillinam (102-x)

Mecillinam *(BAN, rINN).*

Amdinocillin *(USAN)*; FL-1060; Ro-10-9070. (6*R*)-6-(Perhydroazepin-1-ylmethyleneamino)penicillanic acid.

$C_{15}H_{23}N_3O_3S$ = 325.4.

CAS — 32887-01-7.

Pharmacopoeias. In *US.*

Freely **soluble** in water and in methyl alcohol. A 10% solution in water has a pH of 4.0 to 6.2. **Store** in airtight containers.

Adverse Effects and Precautions

As for Benzylpenicillin, p.159.

Interactions

As for Benzylpenicillin, p.160.

Antimicrobial Action

Mecillinam is a derivative of amidinopenicillanic acid. Unlike benzylpenicillin and related antibiotics, it is active against many Gram-negative bacteria, in particular Enterobacteriaceae including *Escherichia coli, Enterobacter, Klebsiella, Salmonella,* and *Shigella* spp.; indole-positive *Proteus* and *Serratia marcescens* are generally resistant. It is less active against *Neisseria* spp. and *Haemophilus influenzae. Pseudomonas aeruginosa* and *Bacteroides* spp. are considered to be resistant. It is much less active against Gram-positive bacteria; enterococci including *Enterococcus faecalis* are resistant.

Mecillinam interferes with the synthesis of the bacterial cell wall by binding with a different penicillin-binding protein from benzylpenicillin. This difference in mode of action may explain the synergism against many Gram-negative organisms that has been reported *in vitro* between mecillinam and various penicillins or cephalosporins.

Mecillinam is inactivated by beta-lactamases, but is more stable than ampicillin.

Pharmacokinetics

Mecillinam is poorly absorbed from the gastro-intestinal tract. Peak plasma concentrations of about 6 and 12 μg per mL have been achieved half an hour after intramuscular doses of 200 and 400 mg, respectively. The usual plasma half-life of about 1 hour has been reported to be prolonged to 3 or 4 hours in severe renal failure. Between 5 and 10% of mecillinam is bound to plasma proteins. Mecillinam is widely distributed into body tissues and fluids; little passes into the CSF unless the meninges are inflamed. It crosses the placenta into the fetal circulation; little appears to be distributed into breast milk.

Mecillinam is metabolised to only a limited extent. From 50 to 70% of a parenteral dose may be excreted in the urine within 6 hours by glomerular filtration and tubular secretion. Renal tubular secretion can be reduced by the concomitant use of probenecid. Some mecillinam is excreted in bile where high concentrations are achieved.

Mecillinam is removed by haemodialysis.

References.

1. Heikkilä A, *et al.* The pharmacokinetics of mecillinam and pivmecillinam in pregnant and non-pregnant women. *Br J Clin Pharmacol* 1992; **33:** 629–33.

Uses and Administration

Mecillinam is a semisynthetic penicillin with a substituted amidino group at the 6-position of the penicillanic acid nucleus. It is given by slow intravenous injection, by intravenous infusion, or intramuscularly in the treatment of susceptible Gram-negative infections (see under Antimicrobial Action, above).

For urinary-tract infections a typical dose of 5 to 10 mg per kg body-weight has been given every 6 to 8 hours. A total dose of up to 60 mg per kg daily has been suggested for very severe infections.

Mecillinam has been administered in combination with other beta-lactams, particularly ampicillin (p.153), to extend the spectrum of antimicrobial activity to Gram-positive organisms and because of reported synergism against Gram-negative bacteria *in vitro*.

The pivaloyloxymethyl ester of mecillinam, pivmecillinam, is used orally (see p.239).

References.

1. Neu HC. Amdinocillin: a novel penicillin: antibacterial activity, pharmacology and clinical use. *Pharmacotherapy* 1985; **5:** 1–10.

Preparations

USP 23: Amdinocillin for Injection.

Proprietary Preparations (details are given in Part 3)
Norw.: Selexid; ***Swed.:*** Selexid; ***UK:*** Selexidin†.

Meclocycline Sulfosalicylate (103-r)

Meclocycline Sulfosalicylate *(USAN)*.

GS-2989 (meclocycline); Meclocycline Sulphosalicylate; NSC-78502 (meclocycline). (4S,4aR,5S,5aR,6S,12aS)-7-Chloro-4-dimethylamino-1,4,4a,5,5a,6,11,12a-octahydro-3,5,10,12,12a-pentahydroxy-6-methylene-1,11-dioxonaphthacene-2-carboxamide 5-sulphosalicylate; 7-Chloro-6-demethyl-6-deoxy-5β-hydroxy-6-methylenetetracycline 5-sulphosalicylate.

$C_{22}H_{21}ClN_2O_8,C_7H_6O_6S$ = 695.0.

CAS — 2013-58-3 (meclocycline); 73816-42-9 (meclocycline sulfosalicylate).

NOTE. Meclocycline is *BAN*, *USAN*, and *rINN*.

Pharmacopoeias. In US.

A 1% solution in water has a pH of 2.5 to 3.5. **Store** in airtight containers. Protect from light.

Meclocycline is a tetracycline antibiotic derived from oxytetracycline (p.235). It is applied topically as the sulfosalicylate for the treatment of acne vulgaris and superficial skin infections. Potency is expressed in terms of meclocycline. Preparations containing the equivalent of 1 or 2% are available. Meclocycline sulfosalicylate has also been given as a pessary in the treatment of vulvovaginal infections.

Preparations

USP 23: Meclocycline Sulfosalicylate Cream.

Proprietary Preparations (details are given in Part 3)
Ger.: Meclosorb; ***Ital.:*** Meclocil Ovuli†; Mecloderm; Mecloderm Antiacne; Mecloderm Ovuli; Mecloderm Polvere Aspersoria; Meclutin Semplice; Novacnyl; Traumatociclina; ***Spain:*** Quoderm; ***USA:*** Meclan.

Multi-ingredient: ***Ital.:*** Anti-Acne; Meclocil Desa†; Meclocil†; Mecloderm F; Meclutin.

Meropenem (5491-x)

Meropenem *(BAN, USAN, rINN)*.

ICI-194660; SM-7338. (4R,5S,6S)-3-[(3S,5S)-5-Dimethylcarbamoylpyrrolidin-3-ylthio]-6-[(R)-1-hydroxyethyl]-4-methyl-7-oxo-1-azabicyclo[3.2.0]hept-2-ene-2-carboxylic acid trihydrate.

$C_{17}H_{25}N_3O_5S,3H_2O$ = 437.5.

CAS — 96036-03-2 (meropenem); 119478-56-7 (meropenem trihydrate).

Adverse Effects and Precautions

As for Imipenem, p.216.

Meropenem is more stable to renal dehydropeptidase I than imipenem and administration with cilastatin, which inhibits this enzyme, is not required. Meropenem may have less potential to induce seizures than imipenem (see also below).

Effects on the nervous system. *Animal* studies have indicated that meropenem induces fewer seizures than imipenem-cilastatin and clinical data from the manufacturer have substantiated this.[1] Comparison of data from 3125 patients with a variety of infections (sometimes including meningitis) treated with meropenem with that from 2886 patients who received other antibacterials, principally cephalosporin-based regimens or imipenem-cilastatin, showed that meropenem was not associated with any greater risk of seizures than the other antibacterials and was likely to have less neurotoxic potential than imipenem-cilastatin making it a suitable drug to use in the treatment of meningitis.

1. Norrby SR, *et al.* Safety profile of meropenem: international clinical experience based on the first 3125 patients treated with meropenem. *J Antimicrob Chemother* 1995; **36** (suppl A): 207–23.

Interactions

Probenecid inhibits the renal excretion of meropenem thereby increasing its plasma concentrations and prolonging its elimination half-life.

Antimicrobial Action

As for Imipenem, p.217.

Meropenem is slightly more active than imipenem against Enterobacteriaceae and slightly less active against Gram-positive organisms.

Pharmacokinetics

Following intravenous injection of meropenem 0.5 and 1.0 g over 5 minutes, peak plasma concentrations of about 50 and 112 μg per mL respectively are attained. The same doses infused over 30 minutes produce peak plasma concentrations of 23 and 49 μg per mL, respectively.

Meropenem has a plasma elimination half-life of about one hour; this may be prolonged in patients with renal impairment and is also slightly prolonged in children. Meropenem is widely distributed into body tissues and fluids including the CSF and bile. It is more stable to renal dehydropeptidase I than imipenem and is mainly excreted in the urine by tubular secretion and glomerular filtration. About 70% of a dose is recovered unchanged in the urine over a 12-hour period and urinary concentrations above 10 μg per mL are maintained for up to 5 hours after a 500-mg dose. Meropenem has one inactive metabolite which is excreted in the urine.

Meropenem is removed by haemodialysis.

References.

1. Hextall A, *et al.* Intraperitoneal penetration of meropenem. *J Antimicrob Chemother* 1991; **28:** 314–16.
2. Leroy A, *et al.* Pharmacokinetics of meropenem (ICI 194,660) and its metabolite (ICI 213,689) in healthy subjects and in patients with renal impairment. *Antimicrob Agents Chemother* 1992; **36:** 2794–8.
3. Chimata M, *et al.* Pharmacokinetics of meropenem in patients with various degrees of renal function, including patients with end-stage renal disease. *Antimicrob Agents Chemother* 1993; **37:** 229–33.
4. Bergogne-Bérézin E, *et al.* Concentration of meropenem in serum and in bronchial secretions in patients undergoing fibreoptic bronchoscopy. *Eur J Clin Pharmacol* 1994; **46:** 87–8. Correction. *ibid.*; 282.
5. Dagan R, *et al.* Penetration of meropenem into the cerebrospinal fluid of patients with inflamed meninges. *J Antimicrob Chemother* 1994; **34:** 175–9.
6. Mouton JW, Van den Anker JN. Meropenem clinical pharmacokinetics. *Clin Pharmacokinet* 1995; **28:** 275–86.
7. Blumer JL, *et al.* Sequential, single-dose pharmacokinetic evaluation of meropenem in hospitalized infants and children. *Antimicrob Agents Chemother* 1995; **39:** 1721–5.
8. Novelli A, *et al.* Clinical pharmacokinetics of meropenem after the first and tenth intramuscular administration. *J Antimicrob Chemother* 1996; **37:** 775–81.

Uses and Administration

Meropenem is a carbapenem beta-lactam antibiotic with actions and uses similar to those of imipenem (p.217). It is more stable to renal dehydropeptidase I than imipenem and need not be given in association with an enzyme inhibitor such as cilastatin. It is used in the treatment of susceptible infections including intra-abdominal infections, meningitis, respiratory-tract infections (including in cystic fibrosis patients), septicaemia, skin infections, urinary-tract infections, and infections in immunocompromised patients. For details of these infections and their treatment, see under Choice of Antibacterial, p.116.

Meropenem is administered intravenously as the trihydrate, but doses are expressed in terms of the amount of anhydrous meropenem. It is given by slow injection over 3 to 5 minutes or by infusion over 15 to 30 minutes in a usual adult dose of 0.5 to 1 g every 8 hours, increased to 2 g every 8 hours for meningitis; doses of up to 2 g every 8 hours have also been used in cystic fibrosis. Doses should be reduced in patients with renal impairment (creatinine clearance of less than 51 mL per minute).

Children over 3 months of age and weighing less than 50 kg may be given 10 to 20 mg per kg body-weight every 8 hours, increased to 40 mg per kg every 8 hours for meningitis. Doses of 25 to 40 mg per kg every 8 hours have been used in children with cystic fibrosis.

Reviews.

1. Pryka RD, Haig GM. Meropenem: a new carbapenem antimicrobial. *Ann Pharmacother* 1994; **28:** 1045–54.
2. Wiseman LR, *et al.* Meropenem: a review of its antibacterial activity, pharmacokinetic properties and clinical efficacy. *Drugs* 1995; **50:** 73–101.
3. Finch RG, *et al.* eds. Meropenem: focus on clinical performance. *J Antimicrob Chemother* 1995; **36** (suppl A): 1–223.

Preparations

Proprietary Preparations (details are given in Part 3)
Aust.: Optinem; ***Austral.:*** Merrem; ***Belg.:*** Meronem; ***Canad.:*** Merrem; ***Ger.:*** Meronem; ***Irl.:*** Meronem; ***Ital.:*** Merrem; ***Jpn:*** Meropen; ***Neth.:*** Meronem; ***S.Afr.:*** Meronem; ***Spain:*** Meronem; ***Swed.:*** Meronem; ***Switz.:*** Meronem; ***UK:*** Meronem; ***USA:*** Merrem.

Metampicillin (185-c)

Metampicillin *(rINN)*.

(6R)-6-(D-2-Methyleneamino-2-phenylacetamido)penicillanic acid.

$C_{17}H_{19}N_3O_4S$ = 361.4.

CAS — 6489-97-0.

Metampicillin Sodium (104-f)

Metampicillin Sodium *(rINNM)*.

$C_{17}H_{18}N_3NaO_4S$ = 383.4.

CAS — 6489-61-8.

Metampicillin has actions and uses similar to those of ampicillin (p.153).

After oral administration it is almost completely hydrolysed to ampicillin. When given parenterally however, a proportion of the administered dose exists in the circulation as unchanged metampicillin which has some antibacterial activity of its own.

Metampicillin has been given by mouth or by intramuscular or intravenous injection in usual doses of 1 to 2 g daily in 2 to 4 divided doses as metampicillin or the sodium salt.

Preparations

Proprietary Preparations (details are given in Part 3)
Fr.: Suvipen; ***Spain:*** Amilprats†; Dompil; Janopen†; Meta Framan; Metaclarben†; Metakes; Metalcor†; Metamas†; Neo Togram†; Pirobiotic†; Serfabiotic; Tampilen†.

Multi-ingredient: ***Spain:*** Dompil Balsamico†; Maxilase Antibiotica†; Pulmosterin Meta.

Methacycline Hydrochloride (105-d)

Methacycline Hydrochloride *(BANM)*.

Metacycline Hydrochloride *(pINNM)*; GS-2876 (methacycline); Metacyclini Chloridum; Méthylènecycline Chlorhydrate; 6-Methyleneoxytetracycline Hydrochloride. (4S,4aR,5S,5aR,6S,12aS)-4-Dimethylamino-1,4,4a,5,5a,6,11,12a-octahydro-3,5,10,12,12a-pentahydroxy-6-methylene-1,11-dioxonaphthacene-2-carboxamide hydrochloride; 6-Demethyl-6-deoxy-5β-hydroxy-6-methylenetetracycline hydrochloride.

$C_{22}H_{22}N_2O_8,HCl$ = 478.9.

CAS — 914-00-1 (methacycline); 3963-95-9 (methacycline hydrochloride).

NOTE. Methacycline is *USAN*.

Pharmacopoeias. In *Pol.* and *US.*

A yellow crystalline powder. Methacycline 92 mg is approximately equivalent to 100 mg of methacycline hydrochloride. **Soluble** 1 in 100 of water, 1 in 300 of alcohol, and 1 in 390 of acetone; very slightly soluble in chloroform and ether; soluble in dilute solutions of sodium hydroxide. A 1% solution in water has a pH of 2 to 3. **Store** in airtight containers. Protect from light.

Adverse Effects and Precautions

As for Tetracycline Hydrochloride, p.259. Pigment deposition in the eyes as well as the skin has been reported.

Interactions

As for Tetracycline Hydrochloride, p.260.

Antimicrobial Action

As for Tetracycline Hydrochloride, p.260.

Pharmacokinetics

As for Tetracycline Hydrochloride, p.260.

Around 60% of a dose by mouth is absorbed. About 80 to 90% of methacycline in the circulation is bound to plasma proteins. Plasma concentrations of up to 2.6 μg per mL have been reported 4 hours after a 300-mg dose of methacycline. Its biological half-life is about 14 to 15 hours. About 60% of a dose is slowly excreted unchanged in the urine.

Uses and Administration

Methacycline is a tetracycline derivative with uses similar to those of tetracycline (p.261). Like demeclocycline it is excreted more slowly than tetracycline and effective blood concentrations are maintained for longer periods.

Methacycline hydrochloride is administered by mouth in a usual dose of 600 mg daily in 2 or 4 divided doses, preferably one hour before or 2 hours after meals. Children over 8 years of age have been given 150 mg twice daily, but the effect of tetracyclines on teeth and bones should be considered.

Preparations

USP 23: Methacycline Hydrochloride Capsules; Methacycline Hydrochloride Oral Suspension.

Proprietary Preparations (details are given in Part 3)
Aust.: Optimycin; ***Austral.:*** Rondomycin; ***Belg.:*** Rondomycine†; ***Fr.:*** Lysocline; Physiomycine; ***Ital.:*** Benciclina†; Esarondil; Franciclina†; Francomicina†; Medomycin†; Metadomus†; Metamicina†; Paveciclina†; Quickmicina†; Rotilen; Stafilon; Treis-Ciclina†; Wassermicina†; ***Swed.:*** Rondomycin†.

Multi-ingredient: ***Aust.:*** Optimycin S; ***Switz.:*** Lysocline†.

Methaniazide (7562-l)

Methaniazide *(rINN)*.

Isoniazid Mesylate; Isoniazid Methanesulfonate. 2-Isonicotinoylhydrazinomethanesulphonic acid.

$C_7H_9N_3O_4S$ = 231.2.

CAS — 13447-95-5 (methaniazide); 6059-26-3 (calcium methaniazide); 3804-89-5 (sodium methaniazide).

Methaniazide is a derivative of isoniazid (p.218). It has been administered as the sodium or calcium salt in the treatment of tuberculosis.

Preparations

Proprietary Preparations (details are given in Part 3)
Aust.: Neo-Tizide; ***Ital.:*** Neo-Tizide†.

Methicillin Sodium (106-n)

Methicillin Sodium *(BANM, USAN)*.

Meticillin Sodium *(pINNM)*; BRL-1241; Dimethoxyphenecillin Sodium; Dimethoxyphenyl Penicillin Sodium; Meticillinum Natricum; SQ-16123; X-1497. Sodium (6R)-6-(2,6-dimethoxybenzamido)penicillanate monohydrate.

$C_{17}H_{19}N_2NaO_6S,H_2O$ = 420.4.

CAS — 61-32-5 (methicillin); 132-92-3 (anhydrous methicillin sodium); 7246-14-2 (methicillin sodium monohydrate).

Pharmacopoeias. In *It.* and *US.*

A fine white crystalline powder, odourless or with a slight odour. 1.11 g of monograph substance is approximately equivalent to 1 g of anhydrous methicillin. Each g of monograph substance represents about 2.4 mmol of sodium.

Freely **soluble** in water and methyl alcohol; slightly soluble in amyl alcohol, chloroform, and propyl alcohol; practically insoluble in ether and acetone. A 1% solution in water has a pH of 5.0 to 7.5. **Store** in airtight containers.

Methicillin sodium has been reported to be **incompatible** with aminoglycosides and a number of other antimicrobials. It has also been reported to be incompatible with acidic and alkaline drugs.

Adverse Effects and Precautions

As for Benzylpenicillin, p.159.

Methicillin is the penicillin most commonly associated with acute interstitial nephritis.

Effects on the kidneys. References.

1. Sanjad SA, *et al.* Nephropathy, an underestimated complication of methicillin therapy. *J Pediatr* 1974; **84:** 873–7.
2. Galpin JE, *et al.* Acute interstitial nephritis due to methicillin. *Am J Med* 1978; **65:** 756–65.

Interactions

As for Benzylpenicillin, p.160.

Antimicrobial Action

Methicillin has a mode of action similar to that of benzylpenicillin (p.160) but it is resistant to staphylococcal penicillinase. There is evidence that methicillin is more stable to staphylococcal penicillinase than the other penicillinase-resistant penicillins.

Methicillin is active against both penicillinase-producing and non-penicillinase-producing staphylococci, and also against *Streptococcus pyogenes* (group A beta-haemolytic streptococci), *Str. pneumoniae*, and some viridans streptococci. It is virtually ineffective against *Enterococcus faecalis*.

The minimum inhibitory concentration against susceptible penicillinase-producing and non-penicillinase-producing staphylococci, is usually within the range of 1 to 4 μg per mL. Its activity against penicillin-sensitive staphylococci and streptococci is less than that of benzylpenicillin.

Resistance of staphylococci to methicillin is due to the expression of an altered penicillin-binding protein and is not dependent on penicillinase production. There is cross-resistance with other penicillins, including the penicillinase-resistant penicillins cloxacillin, dicloxacillin, flucloxacillin, nafcillin, and oxacillin, and with the cephalosporins. Methicillin-resistant staphylococci are also frequently resistant to other antibacterials including aminoglycosides, chloramphenicol, ciprofloxacin, clindamycin, erythromycin, and tetracycline. The incidence of such resistance has varied considerably. However, both endemic (restricted to one hospital) and epidemic (affecting more than one hospital) strains of methicillin-resistant *Staphylococcus aureus* (MRSA) are now recognised and infections are a problem in many hospitals. There have been fewer studies on coagulase-negative staphylococci, but patterns of methicillin resistance in *Staph. epidermidis* are similar to those for MRSA and the frequency of resistance may be higher.

For further details on methicillin-resistant staphylococci and the management of infections, see under Staphylococcal Infections, p.144.

References to methicillin-resistant staphylococci.

1. Hackbarth CJ, Chambers HF. Methicillin-resistant staphylococci: genetics and mechanisms of resistance. *Antimicrob Agents Chemother* 1989; **33:** 991–4.
2. Maple PAC, *et al.* World-wide antibiotic resistance in methicillin-resistant Staphylococcus aureus. *Lancet* 1989; **i:** 537–40.
3. Mouton RP, *et al.* Correlations between consumption of antibiotics and methicillin resistance in coagulase negative staphylococci. *J Antimicrob Chemother* 1990; **26:** 573–83.
4. Marples RR, Reith S. Methicillin-resistant Staphylococcus aureus in England and Wales. *Commun Dis Rep* 1992; **2:** R25–R29.
5. de Lencastre H, *et al.* Molecular aspects of methicillin resistance in Staphylococcus aureus. *J Antimicrob Chemother* 1994; **33:** 7–24.

Pharmacokinetics

Methicillin is inactivated by gastric acid and must be given by injection. Peak plasma concentrations are attained within 0.5 to 1 hour of an intramuscular injection; concentrations of up to 18 μg per mL have been achieved after a dose of 1 g. A half-life of 0.5 to 1 hour has been reported, although this may be increased to 3 to 6 hours in renal impairment. About 40% of the methicillin in the circulation is bound to plasma proteins. It is widely distributed in body fluids and in tissues, but there is little diffusion into the CSF unless the meninges are inflamed. Methicillin also crosses the placenta and appears in breast milk. Relatively high concentrations are achieved in bile compared with plasma, although only small amounts are excreted in bile. The majority is rapidly excreted by tubular secretion and glomerular filtration; up to 80% of an injected dose has been detected unchanged in the urine.

Plasma concentrations are enhanced if probenecid is given concomitantly. They may be reduced in patients with cystic fibrosis.

Uses and Administration

Methicillin is a penicillinase-resistant penicillin and has been used similarly to flucloxacillin (p.209) in the treatment of staphylococcal infections resistant to benzylpenicillin.

It is not active by mouth and is given by injection as the sodium salt. In severe renal impairment a reduction in dosage may be necessary.

The usual dosage of methicillin sodium is 1 g every 4 to 6 hours intramuscularly, or intravenously by slow injection over 3 to 4 minutes or by intravenous infusion. In severe infections up to 12 g daily may be given intravenously in divided doses.

Children up to 2 years of age may be given one-quarter the adult dose and those aged 2 to 10 years, one-half the adult dose.

Preparations

USP 23: Methicillin for Injection.

Proprietary Preparations (details are given in Part 3)
Ital.: Staficyn; ***UK:*** Celbenin†; ***USA:*** Staphcillin†.

Mezlocillin Sodium (107-h)

Mezlocillin Sodium *(BANM, rINNM)*.

BAY-f-1353. Sodium (6R)-6-[D-2-(3-mesyl-2-oxoimidazolidine-1-carboxamido)-2-phenylacetamido]penicillanate monohydrate.

$C_{21}H_{24}N_5NaO_8S_2,H_2O$ = 579.6.

CAS — 51481-65-3 (mezlocillin); 42057-22-7 (anhydrous mezlocillin sodium); 59798-30-0 (anhydrous mezlocillin sodium).

NOTE. Mezlocillin is *USAN*.

Pharmacopoeias. In *US.*

A white to pale yellow crystalline powder. 1.07 g of monograph substance is approximately equivalent to 1 g of anhydrous mezlocillin. Each g of monograph substance represents about 1.7 mmol of sodium. Freely **soluble** in water. A 10% solution in water has a pH of 4.5 to 8.0. **Store** in airtight containers.

Incompatibility has been reported with aminoglycosides, ciprofloxacin, metronidazole, and tetracyclines.

Adverse Effects and Precautions

As for Carbenicillin Sodium, p.162.

As mezlocillin sodium has a lower sodium content than carbenicillin sodium, hypernatraemia and hypokalaemia are less likely to occur. Prolongation of bleeding time has been less frequent and less severe than with carbenicillin.

Interactions

As for Benzylpenicillin, p.160.

For the effect of mezlocillin on the clearance of cefotaxime, see p.168.

See also above for incompatibilities.

Antimicrobial Action

Mezlocillin has a similar antimicrobial action to piperacillin (p.237). Its activity against *Pseudomonas aeruginosa* is less than that of azlocillin or piperacillin.

Pharmacokinetics

Mezlocillin is not absorbed from the gastro-intestinal tract to any significant extent. It is well absorbed after intramuscular administration, peak plasma concentrations of 15 to 25 µg per mL having been observed 45 to 90 minutes after a single dose of 1 g. It is reported to have nonlinear dose-dependent pharmacokinetics. Between 16 and 42% of mezlocillin in the circulation is bound to plasma proteins. Mezlocillin is reported to have a plasma half-life of about one hour, but longer in neonates; in patients with renal impairment half-lives of up to about 6 hours have been reported.

Mezlocillin is widely distributed in body tissues and fluids. It crosses the placenta into the fetal circulation and small amounts are distributed into breast milk. There is little diffusion into CSF except when the meninges are inflamed.

Mezlocillin is reported to be metabolised to a limited extent. About 55% of a dose is excreted unchanged in the urine by glomerular filtration and tubular secretion within 6 hours of administration, hence achieving high urinary concentrations. High concentrations are also found in the bile; up to 30% of a dose has been reported to be excreted by this route.

Plasma concentrations are enhanced if probenecid is administered concomitantly.

Mezlocillin is removed by haemodialysis, and to some extent by peritoneal dialysis.

Uses and Administration

Mezlocillin is a ureidopenicillin with uses similar to those of piperacillin (p.238). It is commonly administered in association with an aminoglycoside; however they should be administered separately as they have been shown to be incompatible.

Administration and dosage. Mezlocillin is given by injection as the sodium salt. Doses are expressed in terms of the equivalent amount of mezlocillin. Dosage may need to be reduced in severe renal impairment. It may be administered by slow intravenous injection over 3 to 5 minutes, by intravenous infusion over 30 minutes, or by deep intramuscular injection. Single intramuscular doses should not exceed 2 g.

For the treatment of serious infections 200 to 300 mg per kg body-weight daily in divided doses may be administered intravenously; usual doses are 4 g every 6 hours or 3 g every 4 hours. For life-threatening infections up to 350 mg per kg daily may be given, but the total daily dose should not normally exceed 24 g. For uncomplicated urinary-tract infections a dose of 1.5 to 2 g may be given intramuscularly or intravenously every 6 hours.

Uncomplicated gonorrhoea may be treated by a single intramuscular or intravenous dose of mezlocillin 1 to 2 g. Probenecid 1 g by mouth may be given at the same time or up to half-an-hour before the injection.

For the prophylaxis of infection during surgery an intravenous pre-operative dose of mezlocillin 4 g, followed by 2 postoperative doses at 6-hourly intervals may be given.

Preparations

USP 23: Mezlocillin for Injection.

Proprietary Preparations (details are given in Part 3)
Aust.: Baypen; ***Fr.:*** Baypen; ***Ger.:*** Baypen; Melocin; ***Ital.:*** Baypen; ***Spain:*** Baypen; ***USA:*** Mezlin.

Multi-ingredient: ***Aust.:*** Optocillin; ***Ger.:*** Optocillin.

Micronomicin Sulphate (736-p)

Micronomicin Sulphate *(pINNM).*

Gentamicin C_{2B} Sulphate; KW-1062 (micronomicin); 6'*N*-Methylgentamicin C_{1A} Sulphate; Sagamicin Sulphate. *O*-2-Amino-2,3,4,6-tetradeoxy-6-(methylamino)-α-D-*erythro*-hexopyranosyl-(1→4)-*O*-[3-deoxy-4-*C*-methyl-3-(methylamino)-β-L-arabinopyranosyl-(1→6)]-2-deoxy-D-streptamine hemipentasulphate.

$(C_{20}H_{41}N_5O_7)_2,5H_2SO_4$ = 1417.5.

CAS — 52093-21-7 (micronomicin).

Pharmacopoeias. In *Jpn.*

Micronomicin is an aminoglycoside with general properties similar to those of gentamicin (p.212). It may be given as the sulphate by intramuscular injection or by intravenous infusion over 0.5 to 1 hour in doses of 120 to 240 mg daily in 2 or 3 divided doses. Dosage should be adjusted based on serum micronomicin concentration monitoring. It is also used topically for infections of the eye.

Preparations

Proprietary Preparations (details are given in Part 3)
Ital.: Sagamicina; ***Jpn:*** Sagamicin; ***Mon.:*** Microphta.

Midecamycin (108-m)

Midecamycin *(rINN).*

Midecamycin A_1; Mydecamycin. 7-(Formylmethyl)-4,10-dihydroxy-5-methoxy-9,16,-dimethyl-2-oxo-oxacyclohexadeca-11,13-dien-6-yl 3,6-dideoxy-4-*O*-(2,6-dideoxy-3-*C*-methyl-α-L-*ribo*-hexopyranosyl)-3-(dimethylamino)-β-D-glucopyranoside 4′,4″-dipropionate.

$C_{41}H_{67}NO_{15}$ = 814.0.

CAS — 35457-80-8 (midecamycin); 55881-07-7 (midecamycin acetate).

Pharmacopoeias. In *Jpn* which also includes Midecamycin Acetate.

Midecamycin is a macrolide antibiotic produced by the growth of *Streptomyces mycarofaciens* and with actions and uses similar to those of erythromycin (p.204) but somewhat less active. It has been given by mouth as midecamycin or midecamycin acetate.

Preparations

Proprietary Preparations (details are given in Part 3)
Fr.: Mosil; ***Ital.:*** Macroral; Midecin; Miocamen; Miokacin; ***Jpn:*** Medemycin; ***Spain:*** Momicine; Myoxam; Normicina.

Minocycline Hydrochloride (109-b)

Minocycline Hydrochloride *(BANM, rINNM).*

Minocyclini Hydrochloridim. (4*S*,4a*R*,5a*R*,6*S*,12a*S*)-4,7-Bis(dimethylamino)-1,4,4a,5,5a,6,11,12a-octahydro-3,10,12,12a-tetrahydroxy-6-methyl-1,11-dioxonaphthacene-2-carboxamide hydrochloride; 6-Demethyl-6-deoxy-7-dimethylaminotetracycline hydrochloride.

$C_{23}H_{27}N_3O_7$,HCl = 493.9.

CAS — 10118-90-8 (minocycline); 13614-98-7 (minocycline hydrochloride).

NOTE. Minocycline is *USAN.*

Pharmacopoeias. In *Eur.* (see p.viii), *Jpn,* and *US.*

A yellow hygroscopic crystalline powder. Minocycline hydrochloride 108 mg is approximately equivalent to 100 mg of minocycline. Sparingly **soluble** or soluble in water; slightly soluble in alcohol; practically insoluble in chloroform and in ether; dissolves in solutions of alkali hydroxides and carbonates. A 1% solution in water has a pH of 3.5 to 4.5. **Store** in airtight containers. Protect from light.

Incompatibilities. Preparations of minocycline hydrochloride have an acid pH and incompatibility may reasonably be expected with alkaline preparations or with drugs unstable at low pH.

Adverse Effects and Precautions

As for Tetracycline Hydrochloride, p.259.

Vestibular side-effects including dizziness or vertigo may occur with minocycline, particularly in women. Patients should be advised not to drive or operate machinery if affected.

Severe adverse effects including erythema nodosum, hepatitis, and systemic lupus erythematosus have been reported, often in patients taking the drug long-term for acne. Hypersensitivity reactions may include arthralgia, myalgia, pulmonary infiltration, and anaphylaxis. Other adverse effects include alopecia, myocarditis, and vasculitis.

Minocycline has also been associated with pigmentation of the skin and other tissues. Three patterns of skin pigmentation have been described: blue-black macules occurring in areas of inflammation and scarring and possibly due to an iron chelate of minocycline within macrophages; blue-grey macules or hyperpigmentation affecting normal skin and which may be due to a break-down product of minocycline; or a greyish-brown discoloration occurring particularly in sun-exposed areas of skin ('muddy skin syndrome'), apparently due to melanin deposition. Skin pigmentation appears to resolve slowly on discontinuing the drug although recovery may be incomplete.

Unlike many tetracyclines, minocycline does not appear to accumulate in patients with impaired renal function, and aggravation of renal impairment may be less likely.

There have been several reports of severe complications in patients receiving minocycline for acne including serum-sickness-like disease,[1,2] lupus erythematosus,[3] and hepatitis.[3,4] The number of cases reported probably reflects the widespread use of this drug and the true incidence of such adverse effects is difficult to assess.[5] A study of 700 patients receiving minocycline for acne revealed adverse effects in 13.6%, mostly benign.[6] Gastro-intestinal disturbances and vestibular disturbances were the most common, each occurring in about 2% of patients, and pigmentation in up to 4% of patients. Another problem is that of assessing the incidence of severe adverse effects relative to other antibacterials commonly used in acne such as tetracycline and erythromycin. Nevertheless, minocycline should probably be regarded as a second-line oral antibacterial for the treatment of acne until further evidence is available.[3,5]

1. Knowles SR, *et al.* Serious adverse reactions induced by minocycline: report of 13 patients and review of the literature. *Arch Dermatol* 1996; **132:** 934–9.
2. Harel L, *et al.* Serum-sickness-like reaction associated with minocycline therapy in adolescents. *Ann Pharmacother* 1996; **30:** 481–3.
3. Gough A, *et al.* Minocycline induced autoimmune hepatitis and systemic lupus erythematosus-like syndrome. *Br Med J* 1996; **312:** 169–72.
4. Australian Adverse Drug Reactions Advisory Committee. Minocycline and the liver, the CNS, the skin. *Aust Adverse Drug React Bull* 1996; **15:** 14.
5. Seukeran DC, *et al.* Benefit-risk assessment of acne therapies. *Lancet* 1997; **349:** 1251–2.
6. Goulden V, *et al.* Safety of long-term high-dose minocycline in the treatment of acne. *Br J Dermatol* 1996; **134:** 693–5.

Effects on the lungs. References to minocycline-induced pneumonitis.

1. Guillon J-M, *et al.* Minocycline-induced cell-mediated hypersensitivity pneumonitis. *Ann Intern Med* 1992; **117:** 476–81.
2. Bridges AJ. Minocycline-induced pneumonia. *Ann Intern Med* 1993; **118:** 749–50.
3. Sigmann P. Minocycline-induced pneumonia. *Ann Intern Med* 1993; **118:** 750.
4. Sitbon O, *et al.* Minocycline pneumonitis and eosinophilia: a report on 8 patients. *Arch Intern Med* 1994; **154:** 1633–40.
5. Dykhuizen RS, *et al.* Minocycline and pulmonary eosinophilia. *Br Med J* 1995; **310:** 1520–1.

Effects on the nervous system. Some references to the vestibular adverse effects of minocycline.

1. Williams DN, *et al.* Minocycline: possible vestibular side-effects. *Lancet* 1974; **ii:** 744–6.
2. Nicol CS, Oriel JD. Minocycline: possible vestibular side-effects. *Lancet* 1974; **ii:** 1260.
3. Yeadon A. Chemoprophylaxis of meningococcal infection. *Lancet* 1975; **i:** 109.
4. Fanning WL, *et al.* Side effects of minocycline: a double-blind study. *Antimicrob Agents Chemother* 1977; **11:** 712–17.
5. Gump DW, *et al.* Side effects of minocycline: different dosage regimens. *Antimicrob Agents Chemother* 1977; **12:** 642–6.
6. Greco TP, *et al.* Minocycline toxicity: experience with an altered dosage regimen. *Curr Ther Res* 1979; **25:** 193–201.

Hyperpigmentation. References to skin and tissue pigmentation in patients receiving minocycline.

1. Attwood HD, Dennett X. A black thyroid and minocycline treatment. *Br Med J* 1976; **2:** 1109–10.
2. Fenske NA, *et al.* Minocycline-induced pigmentation at sites of cutaneous inflammation. *JAMA* 1980; **244:** 1103–6.
3. Ridgway HA, *et al.* Hyperpigmentation associated with oral minocycline. *Br J Dermatol* 1982; **107:** 95–102.
4. Zijdenbos AM, Balmus KJ. Pigmentation secondary to minocycline therapy. *Br J Dermatol* 1984; **110:** 117–18.
5. Basler RSW. Minocycline-related hyperpigmentation. *Arch Dermatol* 1985; **121:** 606–8.
6. Noble JG, *et al.* The black thyroid: an unusual finding during neck exploration. *Postgrad Med J* 1989; **65:** 34–5.
7. Dwyer CM, *et al.* Skin pigmentation due to minocycline treatment of facial dermatoses. *Br J Dermatol* 1993; **129:** 158–62.
8. Okada N, *et al.* Characterization of pigmented granules in minocycline-induced cutaneous pigmentation: observations using fluorescence microscopy and high-performance liquid chromatography. *Br J Dermatol* 1993; **129:** 403–7.

Interactions

As for Tetracycline Hydrochloride, p.260.

Minocycline has a lower affinity for binding with calcium than tetracycline. In a consequence its absorption is less affected by milk and food, although it is still affected by iron salts and antacids.

Antimicrobial Action

Minocycline has a spectrum of activity and mode of action similar to that of tetracycline (p.260) but it is more active against many species including *Staphylococcus aureus*, streptococci, *Neisseria meningitidis*, various enterobacteria, *Acinetobacter*, *Bacteroides*, *Haemophilus*, *Nocardia*, and some mycobacteria, including *M. leprae*.

Partial cross-resistance exists between minocycline and other tetracyclines but some strains resistant to other drugs of the group remain sensitive to minocycline, perhaps because of better cell-wall penetration.

Pharmacokinetics

For the general pharmacokinetics of the tetracyclines, see Tetracycline Hydrochloride, p.260.

Minocycline is readily absorbed from the gastro-intestinal tract and is not significantly affected by the presence of food or moderate amounts of milk. Oral doses of 200 mg followed by 100 mg every 12 hours are reported to produce plasma concentrations within the range of 2 to 4 μg per mL. It is more lipid-soluble than doxycycline and the other tetracyclines and is widely distributed in body tissues and fluids with high concentrations being achieved in the hepatobiliary tract, lungs, sinuses and tonsils, as well as in tears, saliva, and sputum. Penetration into the CSF is relatively poor, although a higher ratio of CSF to blood concentrations has been reported with minocycline than with doxycycline. It crosses the placenta and is distributed into breast milk. About 75% of minocycline in the circulation is bound to plasma proteins. It has a low renal clearance: only about 5 to 10% of a dose is excreted in the urine and up to about 34% is excreted in the faeces. However, in contrast to most tetracyclines it appears to undergo some metabolism in the liver, mainly to 9-hydroxyminocycline. Sources differ as to whether the normal plasma half-life of 11 to 26 hours is prolonged, with a consequent risk of accumulation, in patients with renal impairment, but hepatic impairment does not appear to lead to accumulation. Little minocycline is removed by dialysis.

Review.

1. Saivin S, Houin G. Clinical pharmacokinetics of doxycycline and minocycline. *Clin Pharmacokinet* 1988; **15:** 355–66.

Uses and Administration

Minocycline is a tetracycline derivative with uses similar to those of tetracycline (p.261). It is also a component of multidrug regimens for the treatment of leprosy (p.128) and has been used in the prophylaxis of meningococcal infection (see under Meningitis, p.130) to eliminate the carrier state, but the high incidence of vestibular disturbances means that it is not the drug of choice for the latter. Despite some conflicting pharmacokinetic data, patients with impaired renal function do not usually require adjustment of minocycline dosage, although this may be considered if renal impairment is severe.

Minocycline is normally given by mouth as the hydrochloride. Doses are expressed in terms of minocycline base. The usual dose is 200 mg of minocycline daily in divided doses, usually every 12 hours. An initial loading dose of 200 mg may be given. A dose of 50 mg twice daily or 100 mg once daily by mouth is used for the treatment of acne. For leprosy, minocycline 100 mg daily is recommended (by WHO) as a substitute for clofazimine in the standard multidrug regimen for multibacillary disease. In asymptomatic meningococcal carriers 100 mg may be given twice daily for 5 days, usually followed by a course of rifampicin.

Older children have been given 4 mg per kg bodyweight initially followed by 2 mg per kg every 12 hours but the effect of tetracyclines on teeth and bones should be considered.

In patients in whom oral therapy is not feasible minocycline may be given as the hydrochloride, by slow intravenous infusion in doses equivalent to those by mouth. In some countries it has also been given by intramuscular injection.

Minocycline is applied as a 2% gel for periodontal infections.

Musculoskeletal and joint disorders. For reference to the use of minocycline in the treatment of rheumatoid arthritis, see under Tetracycline Hydrochloride, p.261.

Preparations

BP 1998: Minocycline Tablets;
USP 23: Minocycline for Injection; Minocycline Hydrochloride Capsules; Minocycline Hydrochloride Oral Suspension; Minocycline Hydrochloride Tablets.

Proprietary Preparations (details are given in Part 3)
Aust.: Klinoc; Minocin; Oracyclin; ***Austral.:*** Akamin; Minomycin; ***Belg.:*** Klinotab†; Mino-50; Minocin; Minotab; ***Canad.:*** Minocin; ***Fr.:*** Logryx†; Mestacine; Minolis; Mynocine; ***Ger.:*** Akne-Puren; Aknereduct; Aknin-Mino; Aknosan; durakne; Icht-Oral; Klinomycin; Lederderm; Minakne; Mino-Wolff; Minoclir; Minogalen; Minoplus; Skid; Udima; ***Irl.:*** Dentomycin; Minocin; Minox; ***Ital.:*** Minocin; ***Neth.:*** Aknemin; Minocin; Minotab; ***S.Afr.:*** Cyclimycin; Mino T; Minomycin; Minotabs; Romin; Triomin; ***Spain:*** Minocin; ***Switz.:*** Aknin-N; Aknoral; Dentomycine; Minocin; ***UK:*** Aknemin; Blemix; Cyclomin; Dentomycin; Minocin; Minogal; ***USA:*** Dynacin; Minocin; Vectrin.

Morinamide (7563-y)

Morinamide *(pINN)*.

Morphazinamide. *N*-Morpholinomethylpyrazine-2-carboxamide.

$C_{10}H_{14}N_4O_2$ = 222.2.
CAS — 952-54-5.

Morinamide has been used in the treatment of tuberculosis. It has been given by mouth as the hydrochloride.

Preparations

Proprietary Preparations (details are given in Part 3)
Ital.: Piazofolina.

Mupirocin (16906-v)

Mupirocin *(BAN, USAN, rINN)*.

BRL-4910A; Pseudomonic Acid. 9-[(2*E*)-4-[(2*S*,3*R*,4*R*,5*S*)-5-[(2*S*,3*S*,4*S*,5*S*)-2,3-Epoxy-5-hydroxy-4-methylhexyl]tetrahydro-3,4-dihydroxypyran-2-yl]-3-methylbut-2-enoyloxy]nonanoic acid.

$C_{26}H_{44}O_9$ = 500.6.
CAS — 12650-69-0.

Pharmacopoeias. In *US.*

An antibiotic produced by *Pseudomonas fluorescens*.

A white to off-white crystalline solid. Very slightly **soluble** in water; freely soluble in dehydrated alcohol, in acetone, in chloroform, and in methyl alcohol; slightly soluble in ether. A saturated solution in water has a pH of 3.5 to 4.5 **Store** in airtight containers.

Adverse Effects and Precautions

Mupirocin is usually well tolerated but local reactions such as burning, stinging, and itching may occur after the application of mupirocin to the skin.

Some mupirocin products are formulated in a macrogol base: such formulations are not suitable for application to mucous membranes and should be used with caution in patients with extensive burns or wounds because of the possibility of macrogol toxicity. Care is also required in patients with renal impairment.

Antimicrobial Action

Mupirocin is an antibiotic which inhibits bacterial protein synthesis by binding to isoleucyl transfer RNA synthetase. It is primarily bacteriostatic at low concentrations, although it is usually bactericidal in the high concentrations achieved on the skin. At these concentrations it may have some activity against organisms reported to be relatively resistant to mupirocin *in vitro*.

It is mainly active against Gram-positive aerobes. Most strains of staphylococci (including methicillin-resistant and multiply-resistant *Staph. aureus*) and streptococci are susceptible *in vitro*, although the enterococci are relatively resistant. Mupirocin is also active against *Listeria monocytogenes* and *Erysipelothrix rhusiopathiae*. The Gram-negative organisms are generally insensitive, but *Haemophilus influenzae*, *Neisseria* spp. and a few others are sensitive. Anaerobic organisms, both Gram-positive and Gram-negative, are generally resistant, and activity against fungi is low.

MICs for the most sensitive strains of staphylococci range between about 0.01 to 0.25 μg per mL and those for sensitive streptococcal strains from around 0.06 to 0.5 μg per mL; *Listeria* is inhibited by 8 μg per mL. Mupirocin is more active *in vitro* at acid pH than in alkaline conditions.

Naturally resistant strains of *Staph. aureus* occur rarely but resistance, including high-level plasmid-mediated transferable resistance, has emerged, particularly during long-term treatment. With as many as 8% of staphylococcal strains from some centres proving resistant there has been some concern that inappropriate prescribing of mupirocin has led to steadily increasing resistance.

Activity against fungi. Activity of mupirocin 2% against *Candida albicans in vitro* was comparable to that of other commonly used topical antifungals. Although MICs were considerably in excess of those reported for susceptible bacteria, clinical responses in 10 patients suggested that adequate concentrations of mupirocin were achieved following topical application.[1]

1. Rode H, *et al.* Efficacy of mupirocin in cutaneous candidiasis. *Lancet* 1991; **338:** 578.

Activity with other drugs. Polymyxin B nonapeptide, a potent disruptor of the outer membrane of the Enterobacteriaceae, produced marked antimicrobial synergy with mupirocin against *Salmonella typhimurium in vitro*, presumably by increasing penetration of mupirocin to the organism.[1]

1. Vaara M. The outer membrane as the penetration barrier against mupirocin in Gram-negative enteric bacteria. *J Antimicrob Chemother* 1992; **29:** 221–2.

Resistance. Reports and discussions of mupirocin resistance.

1. Rahman M, *et al.* Transmissible mupirocin resistance in Staphylococcus aureus. *Epidemiol Infect* 1989; **102:** 261–70.
2. Cookson BD. Mupirocin resistance in staphylococci. *J Antimicrob Chemother* 1990; **25:** 497–503.
3. Wise R, Johnson J. Mupirocin resistance. *Lancet* 1991; **338:** 578.
4. Cookson B, *et al.* Mupirocin-resistant Staphylococcus aureus. *Lancet* 1992; **339:** 625.
5. Gilbart J, *et al.* High-level mupirocin resistance in Staphylococcus aureus: evidence for two distinct isoleucyl-tRNA synthetases. *Antimicrob Agents Chemother* 1993; **37:** 32–8.
6. Janssen DA, *et al.* Detection and characterization of mupirocin resistance in staphylococcus aureus. *Antimicrob Agents Chemother* 1993; **37:** 2003–6.
7. Cookson BD. The emergence of mupirocin resistance: a challenge to infection control and antibiotic prescribing practice. *J Antimicrob Chemother* 1998; **41:** 11–18.

Pharmacokinetics

Only very small amounts of topically applied mupirocin are absorbed into the systemic circulation where it is rapidly metabolised to monic acid.

Uses and Administration

Mupirocin is an antibiotic which is applied topically as a 2% ointment in a macrogol basis in the treatment of various bacterial skin infections. It should be applied up to three times a day for up to 10 days. This ointment is not suitable for application to mucous membranes, and mupirocin 2%, as the calcium salt, in a paraffin basis is used for eradication of the nasal carriage of *Staphylococcus aureus*, particularly epidemic methicillin-resistant strains.

For further details of skin infections and staphylococcal infections and their treatment, see under Choice of Antibacterial, p.142.

Preparations

USP 23: Mupirocin Ointment.

Proprietary Preparations (details are given in Part 3)
Aust.: Bactroban; ***Austral.:*** Bactroban; ***Belg.:*** Bactroban; ***Canad.:*** Bactroban; ***Fr.:*** Bactroban; ***Ger.:*** Eismycin†; Turixin; ***Irl.:*** Bactroban; ***Ital.:*** Bactroban; ***Neth.:*** Bactroban; ***S.Afr.:*** Bactroban; ***Spain:*** Bactroban; Celefer†; Plasimine; ***Swed.:*** Bactroban; ***Switz.:*** Bactroban; ***UK:*** Bactroban; ***USA:*** Bactroban.

Nadifloxacin (15296-w)

Nadifloxacin *(BAN, rINN).*

Jinofloxacin; OPC-7251. (±)-9-Fluoro-6,7-dihydro-8-(4-hydroxypiperidino)-5-methyl-1-oxo-1*H*,5*H*-benzo[*ij*]quinolizine-2-carboxylic acid.

$C_{19}H_{21}FN_2O_4$ = 360.4.

CAS — 124858-35-1.

Nadifloxacin is a fluoroquinolone antibacterial. It is applied topically in the treatment of acne.

Preparations

Proprietary Preparations (details are given in Part 3)
Jpn: Acuatim.

Nafcillin Sodium (110-x)

Nafcillin Sodium *(BANM, USAN, rINNM).*

Nafcillinum Natricum; Wy-3277. Sodium (6*R*)-6-(2-ethoxy-1-naphthamido)penicillanate monohydrate.

$C_{21}H_{21}N_2NaO_5S,H_2O$ = 454.5.

CAS — 147-52-4 (nafcillin); 985-16-0 (nafcillin sodium, anhydrous); 7177-50-6 (nafcillin sodium, monohydrate).

Pharmacopoeias. In *US.*

A white to yellowish-white powder with not more than a slight characteristic odour. 1.1 g of monograph substance is approximately equivalent to 1 g of anhydrous nafcillin. Each g of monograph substance represents 2.2 mmol of sodium.

Freely **soluble** in water and chloroform; soluble in alcohol. A 3% solution in water has a pH of 5 to 7. **Store** in airtight containers.

Nafcillin sodium has been reported to be **incompatible** with aminoglycosides and a number of other antibacterials. It has also been reported to be incompatible with acidic and alkaline drugs.

Adverse Effects and Precautions

As for Benzylpenicillin, p.159.

Thrombophlebitis may occur when nafcillin is given by intravenous injection, and tissue damage has been reported on extravasation.

Effects on the kidneys. References.

1. Lestico MR, *et al.* Hepatic and renal dysfunction following nafcillin administration. *Ann Pharmacother* 1992; **26:** 985–90.
2. Guharoy SR, *et al.* Suspected nafcillin-induced interstitial nephritis. *Ann Pharmacother* 1993; **27:** 170–3.

Effects on the liver. References.

1. Lestico MR, *et al.* Hepatic and renal dysfunction following nafcillin administration. *Ann Pharmacother* 1992; **26:** 985–90.

Interactions

As for Benzylpenicillin, p.160.

For the effect of nafcillin on *cyclosporin,* see p.521, and on *warfarin,* see p.966.

Antimicrobial Action

As for Flucloxacillin, p.209.

Pharmacokinetics

Nafcillin is incompletely and irregularly absorbed from the gastro-intestinal tract, especially when administered after a meal. After intramuscular injection it is absorbed more reliably, an injection of 0.5 to 1 g producing peak plasma concentrations of 5 to 8 μg per mL within about 0.5 to 2 hours. Up to 90% of nafcillin in the circulation is bound to plasma proteins. Nafcillin has been reported to have a plasma half-life of about 0.5 to 1 hour. The half-life is prolonged in neonates.

Nafcillin crosses the placenta into the fetal circulation and is distributed into breast milk. There is little diffusion into the CSF except when the meninges are inflamed. Therapeutic concentrations can be achieved in pleural and synovial fluids and in bone.

Nafcillin differs from most other penicillins in that it is largely inactivated by hepatic metabolism. It is excreted via the bile though some reabsorption takes place in the small intestine. Only about 10% of a dose given by mouth before food and about 30% of a dose given intramuscularly is excreted in the urine.

Plasma concentrations are enhanced if probenecid is given concomitantly.

Uses and Administration

Nafcillin is a penicillinase-resistant penicillin used similarly to flucloxacillin (p.209) in the treatment of infections due to staphylococci resistant to benzylpenicillin.

It is administered by mouth or by injection as the sodium salt. Doses are expressed in terms of the equivalent amount of nafcillin. By intramuscular injection the usual dose is 500 mg of nafcillin every 4 to 6 hours. Children may be given 25 mg per kg body-weight twice daily, and neonates 10 mg per kg twice daily. Nafcillin sodium may also be given intravenously by slow injection over 5 to 10 minutes or by slow infusion; adult doses are 0.5 to 1.5 g of nafcillin every 4 hours, although it is usually recommended that it be used for not more than 24 to 48 hours because of the risk of thrombophlebitis.

The dose by mouth for adults is 0.25 to 1 g of nafcillin every 4 to 6 hours; for children it is 6.25 to 12.5 mg per kg four times daily; and for neonates it is 10 mg per kg three or four times daily. It should preferably be given at least one hour before or 2 hours after meals.

Preparations

USP 23: Nafcillin for Injection; Nafcillin Injection; Nafcillin Sodium Capsules; Nafcillin Sodium for Oral Solution; Nafcillin Sodium Tablets.

Proprietary Preparations (details are given in Part 3)
Canad.: Unipen†; ***USA:*** Nafcil; Nallpen; Unipen.

Nalidixic Acid (5663-n)

Nalidixic Acid *(BAN, USAN, rINN).*

Acidum Nalidixicum; Nalidixinic Acid; NSC-82174; Win-18320. 1-Ethyl-1,4-dihydro-7-methyl-4-oxo-1,8-naphthyridine-3-carboxylic acid.

$C_{12}H_{12}N_2O_3$ = 232.2.

CAS — 389-08-2.

Pharmacopoeias. In *Chin., Eur.* (see p.viii), *Jpn, Pol.,* and *US.*

White to very pale yellow odourless crystalline powder.

Practically **insoluble** or very slightly soluble in water; soluble 1 in 910 of alcohol and 1 in 29 of chloroform; slightly soluble in acetone, in methyl alcohol, and in toluene; very slightly soluble in ether; soluble in dichloromethane and in solutions of fixed alkali hydroxides and carbonates.

Store in airtight containers. Protect from light.

Adverse Effects

The most frequent adverse reactions to nalidixic acid involve the gastro-intestinal tract, skin, and central nervous system. Gastro-intestinal effects have been reported in about 8% of patients and include nausea, vomiting, diarrhoea, and abdominal pain.

Neurological side-effects include visual disturbances, headache, dizziness or vertigo, drowsiness, and sometimes confusion, depression, excitement, and hallucinations. Toxic psychoses or convulsions have occurred, especially after large doses; convulsions are most likely in patients with predisposing factors such as cerebrovascular insufficiency, parkinsonism, or epilepsy. There have been reports of intracranial hypertension especially in infants and young children and also of metabolic acidosis. Peripheral neuropathies, muscular weakness, and myalgia are occasional side-effects.

Adverse effects on the skin include photosensitivity reactions with erythema and bullous eruptions, allergic rashes, urticaria, and pruritus. Eosinophilia, fever, angioedema, and, rarely, anaphylactoid reactions have occurred. Arthralgia has been reported (degenerative changes in weight-bearing joints of young *animals* are documented). Tendon damage has occasionally been associated with related compounds, the fluoroquinolones (see under Ciprofloxacin: Effects on the Musculoskeletal System, p.186).

Cholestatic jaundice, thrombocytopenia, and leucopenia have occurred rarely, as has haemolytic anaemia in patients who may or may not be deficient in glucose-6-phosphate dehydrogenase. There have been isolated reports of fatal autoimmune haemolytic anaemia in elderly patients.

Precautions

Nalidixic acid should be avoided in patients subject to convulsions. It should be given with care to patients with impaired renal or hepatic function or with glucose-6-phosphate dehydrogenase deficiency. Blood counts and renal and hepatic function should be monitored if treatment continues for more than 2 weeks.

It should be avoided in babies less than 3 months old. Since nalidixic acid and related antimicrobials have been shown to cause degenerative changes in weight-bearing joints of young *animals*, it has been suggested that these compounds should not be used in children, adolescents, pregnant women, or during lactation. Treatment should be discontinued if symptoms of arthralgia occur.

Exposure to strong sunlight or sunlamps should be avoided during treatment with nalidixic acid.

Nalidixic acid may cause false-positive reactions in urine tests for glucose using copper reduction methods.

Porphyria. Nalidixic acid has been associated with clinical exacerbations of porphyria and is considered unsafe in porphyric patients.[1]

1. Moore MR, McColl KEL. *Porphyria: drug lists.* Glasgow: Porphyria Research Unit, University of Glasgow, 1991.

Interactions

The excretion of nalidixic acid is reduced and plasma concentrations increased by the concomitant administration of probenecid. Nitrofurantoin and nalidixic acid are antagonistic *in vitro* and should not be used together. Serious gastro-intestinal toxicity has been associated with the concomitant use of nalidixic acid and melphalan (p.545). There is a possible risk of increased nephrotoxicity when nalidixic acid is administered with cyclosporin.

Nalidixic acid is reported to enhance the effect of oral anticoagulants such as warfarin (p.966); this may be due in part to displacement of anticoagulant from its plasma binding sites. The dose of anticoagulant may need to be reduced.

For the effect of some quinolone antibacterials on xanthines, see under Caffeine, p.750, and Theophylline, p.768.

Convulsions may be precipitated by the administration of some quinolones with NSAIDs (p.187), although this has not been reported with nalidixic acid.

Antimicrobial Action

Nalidixic acid is considered to act by interfering with the replication of bacterial DNA, probably by inhibiting DNA gyrase (topoisomerase) activity. It is active against Gram-negative bacteria including *Escherichia coli, Klebsiella* spp., *Proteus* spp., *Enterobacter* spp., *Salmonella* spp., and *Shigella* spp., and is usually bactericidal. Most susceptible organisms are inhibited by 16 μg or less per mL. *Pseudomonas aeruginosa*, Gram-positive bacteria, and anaerobes are not generally susceptible.

Bacterial resistance may develop rapidly, sometimes within a few days of commencing treatment, but it does not appear to be transferable or R-plasmid mediated (see also below). Cross-resistance occurs with oxolinic acid and cinoxacin.

The antibacterial activity of nalidixic acid is not significantly affected by differences in urinary pH. Antagonism between nitrofurantoin and nalidixic acid has been demonstrated *in vitro*.

Bacterial plasmid-mediated resistance to quinolones had not been seen by the late 1980s.[1] A report of such resistance to nalidixic acid in *Shigella dysenteriae* responsible for an epidemic of shigellosis in Bangladesh in 1987,[2] was questioned at the time.[3] On reinspection of the data, chromosomal mutation rather than plasmid-mediated resistance was confirmed as the mechanism responsible so far for resistance to quinolones.[1]

1. Courvalin P. Plasmid-mediated 4-quinolone resistance: a real or apparent absence? *Antimicrob Agents Chemother* 1990; **34:** 681–4.
2. Munshi MH, *et al.* Plasmid-mediated resistance to nalidixic acid in Shigella dysenteriae type 1. *Lancet* 1987; **ii:** 419–21.
3. Crumplin GC. Plasmid-mediated resistance to nalidixic acid and new 4-quinolones? *Lancet* 1987; **ii:** 854–5.

Pharmacokinetics

Nalidixic acid is rapidly and almost completely absorbed from the gastro-intestinal tract and peak plasma concentrations of 20 to 50 μg per mL have been reported 2 hours after the administration of 1 g by mouth. Plasma half-lives of about 1 to 2.5 hours have been reported (but see below).

Nalidixic acid is partially metabolised to hydroxynalidixic acid, which has antibacterial activity similar to that of nalidixic acid and accounts for about 30% of active drug in the blood. About 93% of nalidixic acid and 63% of hydroxynalidixic acid are bound to plasma proteins. Both nalidixic acid and hydroxynalidixic acid are rapidly metabolised to inactive glucuronide and dicarboxylic acid derivatives; the major inactive metabolite carboxynalidixic acid is usually only detected in urine.

Nalidixic acid and its metabolites are excreted rapidly in the urine, nearly all of a dose being eliminated within 24 hours. About 80 to 90% of the drug excreted in the urine is as inactive metabolites but urinary concentrations of unchanged drug and active metabolite ranging from 25 to 250 μg per mL are achieved after a single 1-g dose. Hydroxynalidixic acid accounts for about 80 to 85% of activity in the urine. Urinary excretion is reduced by probenecid.

Traces of nalidixic acid appear in breast milk and appear to cross the placenta. About 4% of a dose is excreted in the faeces.

Although a plasma half-life of 1 to 2.5 hours is generally cited for nalidixic acid, values of 6 to 7 hours have been reported for active drug (nalidixic acid and hydroxynalidixic acid) after using more specific and sensitive assay techniques and longer sampling periods than previously.[1]

The elimination rate of nalidixic acid appears to be not markedly altered by renal insufficiency, but the elimination of hydroxynalidixic acid is significantly reduced. 7-Carboxynalidixic acid has appeared in the plasma of patients with renal insufficiency.[2] Plasma concentrations of active drug were higher and the half-life prolonged in elderly subjects.[3]

1. Ferry N, *et al.* Nalidixic acid kinetics after single and repeated oral doses. *Clin Pharmacol Ther* 1981; **29:** 695–8.
2. Cuisinaud G, *et al.* Nalidixic acid kinetics in renal insufficiency. *Br J Clin Pharmacol* 1982; **14:** 489–93.
3. Barbeau G, Belanger P-M. Pharmacokinetics of nalidixic acid in old and young volunteers. *J Clin Pharmacol* 1982; **22:** 490–6.

Uses and Administration

Nalidixic acid is a 4-quinolone antibacterial used in the treatment of uncomplicated lower urinary-tract infections due to Gram-negative bacteria other than *Pseudomonas* spp. (p.149). It has also been used to treat shigellosis (bacillary dysentery) (p.125).

The usual adult dose is 4 g daily by mouth in 4 divided doses for at least 7 days in acute infections. Since bacterial resistance may develop rapidly it has been suggested that if treatment with nalidixic acid has not resulted in a negative urine culture within 48 hours another antimicrobial should be used. If therapy continues for longer than 2 weeks the dose should usually be halved. Children have been given 50 to 55 mg per kg body-weight daily in 4 divided doses reduced to 30 to 33 mg per kg daily for prolonged treatment (but see Precautions, above).

Although the antibacterial activity of nalidixic acid does not appear to be influenced by urinary pH, the concomitant administration of sodium bicarbonate or sodium citrate does increase the concentration of active drug in the urine. A suggested adult dose of nalidixic acid, in conjunction with sodium citrate, is 660 mg three times daily for 3 days.

Preparations

BP 1998: Nalidixic Acid Oral Suspension; Nalidixic Acid Tablets; ***USP 23:*** Nalidixic Acid Oral Suspension; Nalidixic Acid Tablets.

Proprietary Preparations (details are given in Part 3)
Austral.: Negram; ***Canad.:*** NegGram; ***Fr.:*** Negram; ***Ger.:*** Nogram†; ***Irl.:*** Negram; ***Ital.:*** Betaxina; Faril†; Nalicidin†; Nalidixin; Naligram; Nalissina; NegGram; Uralgin; Uri-Flor; Urogram; Uropan†; ***Neth.:*** Negram†; ***Norw.:*** Negram; ***S.Afr.:*** Puromylon; Winlomylon; ***Spain:*** Wintomylon†; ***Swed.:*** Negram†; ***Switz.:*** Negram†; ***UK:*** Negram; Uriben; ***USA:*** NegGram.

Multi-ingredient: ***Irl.:*** Mictral; ***UK:*** Mictral.

Neomycin (111-r)

Neomycin *(BAN, rINN).*

CAS — 1404-04-2 (neomycin); 3947-65-7 (neomycin A); 119-04-0 (neomycin B); 66-86-4 (neomycin C).

A mixture of 2 isomers, neomycin B ($C_{23}H_{46}N_6O_{13}$ = 614.6) and neomycin C ($C_{23}H_{46}N_6O_{13}$ = 614.6) with neomycin A (neamine, $C_{12}H_{26}N_4O_6$ = 322.4); neomycins B and C are glycoside esters of neamine and neobiosamines B and C. Framycetin (p.210) consists of neomycin B.

The BP states that when Neomycin is prescribed or demanded, Neomycin Sulphate must be dispensed or supplied.

Neomycin Sulphate (112-f)

Neomycin Sulphate *(BANM, rINNM).*

Fradiomycin Sulfate; Neomycini Sulfas.

CAS — 1405-10-3.

NOTE. NEO is a code approved by the BP for use on single unit doses of eye drops containing neomycin sulphate where the individual container may be too small to bear all the appropriate labelling information.

Pharmacopoeias. In *Chin., Eur.* (see p.viii), *Int., Jpn, Pol.,* and *US.*

Neomycin sulphate is a mixture of the sulphates of the antimicrobial substances produced by the growth of certain selected strains of *Streptomyces fradiae*. The Ph. Eur. specifies not less than 680 units per mg.

Neomycin sulphate occurs as a white or yellowish-white, odourless or almost odourless, hygroscopic powder. Very or freely **soluble** in water; very slightly soluble in alcohol; practically insoluble in acetone, chloroform, and ether. A 1% solution in water has a pH of 5.0 to 7.5. **Store** in airtight containers. Protect from light.

Neomycin Undecenoate (113-d)

Neomycin Undecenoate *(BANM).*

Neomycin Undecylenate *(USAN, rINNM).* The 10-undecenoate salt of neomycin.

CAS — 1406-04-8.

Adverse Effects and Treatment

As for Gentamicin Sulphate, p.212.

Neomycin has particularly potent nephrotoxic and ototoxic properties which have led to the general abandonment of parenteral administration. However, sufficient may be absorbed by other routes, e.g. following oral administration, instillation into cavities or open wounds or topical administration to damaged skin, to produce irreversible partial or total deafness. The effect is dose-related and is enhanced by renal impairment. Nephrotoxic effects may also occur.

When given by mouth neomycin in large doses causes nausea, vomiting, and diarrhoea. Prolonged oral therapy may cause a malabsorption syndrome with steatorrhoea and diarrhoea which can be very severe. Supra-infection may occur, especially with prolonged oral treatment.

Neomycin has a neuromuscular blocking action similar to but stronger than that of other aminoglycosides and respiratory depression and arrest has followed the intraperitoneal instillation of neomycin. Fatalities have occurred.

Hypersensitivity reactions, such as rashes, pruritus, and sometimes drug fever or even anaphylaxis, occur frequently during local treatment with neomycin and may be masked by the combined use of a corticosteroid. Cross-sensitivity with other aminoglycoside antibiotics may occur.

Precautions

As for Gentamicin Sulphate, p.212. Parenteral administration of neomycin, or its use for irrigation of wounds or serous cavities such as the peritoneum, is no longer recommended.

Neomycin is contra-indicated for intestinal disinfection when an obstruction is present and in patients with a known history of allergy to aminoglycosides. It should be used with great care in patients with kidney or liver disease or neuromuscular disorders and in those with impaired hearing. The topical use of neomycin in patients with extensive skin damage or perforated tympanic membranes may result in deafness. Neomycin sulphate should not be applied topically or for urological purposes in doses greater than 1 g daily; it should not be used urologically for longer than 10 days.

Prolonged local use should be avoided as it may lead to skin sensitisation and possible cross-sensitivity to other aminoglycosides.

Neomycin was thought to be responsible for a hypersensitivity reaction in a child given measles mumps and rubella vaccine containing neomycin 25 μg.[1] However there is also a report of successful vaccination with measles mumps and rubella vaccine in a neomycin-sensitive child.[2] Although the vaccine may contain small amounts of neomycin or kanamycin, and sensitivity to either is considered a contra-indication to its use, it is only rarely necessary to withold it once appropriate expert advice has been taken. There is little logic to intradermal testing since test solutions contain 4 to 40 times as much neomycin as the vaccine.[2]

1. Kwittken PL, *et al.* MMR vaccine and neomycin allergy. *Am J Dis Child* 1993; **147:** 128–9.
2. Elliman D, Dhanraj B. Safe MMR vaccination despite neomycin allergy. *Lancet* 1991; **337:** 365.

Interactions

As for Gentamicin Sulphate, p.213. Absorption following oral or local administration may be sufficient to produce interactions with other drugs administered systemically.

Neomycin, taken by mouth, has been reported to impair the absorption of other drugs including phenoxymethylpenicillin, digoxin, methotrexate, and some vitamins; the efficacy of oral contraceptives might be reduced. The effects of acarbose (p.317) may be enhanced by oral neomycin.

Antimicrobial Action

Neomycin has a mode of action and spectrum of activity similar to that of gentamicin (p.213) but it lacks activity against *Pseudomonas aeruginosa.* It is reported to be active against *Mycobacterium tuberculosis.*

Because of its extensive topical use resistance has been reported to be relatively widespread, notably among staphylococci, and some *Salmonella, Shigella,* and *Escherichia coli* strains. Cross-resistance with kanamycin, framycetin, and paromomycin occurs.

Pharmacokinetics

Neomycin is poorly absorbed from the alimentary tract, about 97% of an orally administered dose being excreted unchanged in the faeces. Doses of 3 g by mouth produce peak plasma concentrations of up to 4 μg per mL and absorption is similar after administration by enema. Absorption may be increased in conditions which damage or inflame the mucosa. Absorption has also been reported to occur from the peritoneum, respiratory tract, bladder, wounds, and inflamed skin.

Once neomycin is absorbed it is rapidly excreted by the kidneys in active form. It has been reported to have a half-life of 2 to 3 hours.

Uses and Administration

Neomycin is an aminoglycoside antibiotic used topically in the treatment of infections of the skin, ear, and eye due to susceptible staphylococci and other organisms. Most preparations contain the sulphate, but neomycin undecenoate or hydrochloride are also used. Neomycin is often used in combination with another antibacterial such as bacitracin, colistin, gramicidin, or polymyxin B. Such combinations have been used topically in the eye before ophthalmic surgery for infection prophylaxis (p.144) and, in conjunction with propamidine isethionate, in the treatment of acanthamoeba keratitis (p.573). A cream containing neomycin sulphate and chlorhexidine hydrochloride has been used for application to the nostrils in the treatment of staphylococcal nasal carriers (p.144) but, as with other topical antibacterial preparations, development of resistance may be a problem. Neomycin is often combined with topical corticosteroid preparations, but such combinations should only be used under supervision because of the risk that signs of resistant infection may be suppressed. Care must also be taken where there is skin trauma because of the risk of increased absorption and toxicity. For details of bacterial skin infections and their treatment, see p.142.

Because neomycin sulphate is poorly absorbed from the gastro-intestinal tract, it has been given by mouth for bowel preparation before abdominal surgery, often in combination with erythromycin (p.144). Neomycin sulphate is also used in combination with other antibacterials and antifungals in the selective decontamination of the digestive tract (SDD) in patients in intensive care (p.128).

Neomycin is rarely used in the treatment of existing gastro-intestinal infections. Although it may be useful in the treatment of diarrhoea due to infection with enteropathogenic *Escherichia coli* (EPEC) (p.124) the use of neomycin in children with other forms of acute diarrhoea is not recommended.

Neomycin sulphate may be given by mouth to patients with incipient hepatic encephalopathy (p.1170) to reduce the flora of the gastro-intestinal tract.

Neomycin has lipid regulating properties and has occasionally been given by mouth in the treatment of hyperlipidaemias (see below). It has also been used for the irrigation of wounds and body cavities but such use is no longer recommended because of the risk of toxicity.

Administration and dosage. For pre-operative use, 1 g of neomycin sulphate has been given hourly for 4 hours and then every 4 hours for a day or more before surgery, up to a maximum of 3 days; suggested doses in children, given every 4 hours, are 1 g in those aged over 12 years and 250 to 500 mg in those aged 6 to 12 years.

As an adjunct in the management of hepatic encephalopathy, 4 to 12 g may be given daily in divided doses, usually for 5 to 7 days; children may be given 50 to 100 mg per kg body-weight daily in divided doses. Prolonged administration may cause malabsorption.

Topical preparations typically contain the equivalent of 0.35% neomycin base.

Hyperlipidaemias. Neomycin has been given in doses of up to 2 g daily by mouth in the treatment of hypercholesterolaemia (p.1265). It is thought to reduce intestinal absorption of cholesterol through its action on microbial flora, resulting in greater catabolism of low-density lipoproteins in the body.[1] However, more effective and safer drugs are preferred

1. Illingworth DR. Lipid-lowering drugs: an overview of indications and optimum use. *Drugs* 1987, **33:** 259–79.

Preparations

BP 1998: Hydrocortisone Acetate and Neomycin Ear Drops; Hydrocortisone Acetate and Neomycin Eye Drops; Hydrocortisone Acetate and Neomycin Eye Ointment; Hydrocortisone and Neomycin Cream; Neomycin Eye Drops; Neomycin Eye Ointment; Neomycin Oral Solution; Neomycin Tablets;
USP 23: Colistin and Neomycin Sulfates and Hydrocortisone Acetate Otic Suspension; Neomycin and Polymyxin B Sulfates and Bacitracin Ointment; Neomycin and Polymyxin B Sulfates and Bacitracin Ophthalmic Ointment; Neomycin and Polymyxin B Sulfates and Bacitracin Zinc Ointment; Neomycin and Polymyxin B Sulfates and Bacitracin Zinc Ophthalmic Ointment; Neomycin and Polymyxin B Sulfates and Dexamethasone Ophthalmic Ointment; Neomycin and Polymyxin B Sulfates and Dexamethasone Ophthalmic Suspension; Neomycin and Polymyxin B Sulfates and Gramicidin Cream; Neomycin and Polymyxin B Sulfates and Gramicidin Ophthalmic Solution; Neomycin and Polymyxin B Sulfates and Hydrocortisone Acetate Cream; Neomycin and Polymyxin B Sulfates and Hydrocortisone Acetate Ophthalmic Suspension; Neomycin and Polymyxin B Sulfates and Hydrocortisone Ophthalmic Suspension; Neomycin and Polymyxin B Sulfates and Hydrocortisone Otic Solution; Neomycin and Polymyxin B Sulfates and Hydrocortisone Otic Suspension; Neomycin and Polymyxin B Sulfates and Lidocaine Cream; Neomycin and Polymyxin B Sulfates and Prednisolone Acetate Ophthalmic Suspension; Neomycin and Polymyxin B Sulfates Cream; Neomycin and Polymyxin B Sulfates Ophthalmic Ointment; Neomycin and Polymyxin B Sulfates Ophthalmic Solution; Neomycin and Polymyxin B Sulfates Solution for Irrigation; Neomycin and Polymyxin B Sulfates, Bacitracin Zinc, and Hydrocortisone Acetate Ophthalmic Ointment; Neomycin and Polymyxin B Sulfates, Bacitracin Zinc, and Hydrocortisone Ointment; Neomycin and Polymyxin B Sulfates, Bacitracin Zinc, and Hydrocortisone Ophthalmic Ointment; Neomycin and Polymyxin B Sulfates, Bacitracin Zinc, and Lidocaine Ointment; Neomycin and Polymyxin B Sulfates, Bacitracin, and Hydrocortisone Acetate Ointment; Neomycin and Polymyxin B Sulfates, Bacitracin, and Hydrocortisone Acetate Ophthalmic Ointment; Neomycin and Polymyxin B Sulfates, Bacitracin, and Lidocaine Ointment; Neomycin and Polymyxin B Sulfates, Gramicidin, and Hydrocortisone Acetate Cream; Neomycin for Injection; Neomycin Sulfate and Bacitracin Ointment; Neomycin Sulfate and Bacitracin Zinc Ointment; Neomycin Sulfate and Dexamethasone Sodium Phosphate Cream; Neomycin Sulfate and Dexamethasone Sodium Phosphate Ophthalmic Ointment; Neomycin Sulfate and Dexamethasone Sodium Phosphate Ophthalmic Solution; Neomycin Sulfate and Fluocinolone Acetonide Cream; Neomycin Sulfate and Fluorometholone Ointment; Neomycin Sulfate and Flurandrenolide Cream; Neomycin Sulfate and Flurandrenolide Lotion; Neomycin Sulfate and Flurandrenolide Ointment; Neomycin Sulfate and Gramicidin Ointment; Neomycin Sulfate and Hydrocortisone Acetate Cream; Neomycin Sulfate and Hydrocortisone Acetate Lotion; Neomycin Sulfate and Hydrocortisone Acetate Ointment; Neomycin Sulfate and Hydrocortisone Acetate Ophthalmic Ointment; Neomycin Sulfate and Hydrocortisone Acetate Ophthalmic Suspension; Neomycin Sulfate and Hydrocortisone Cream; Neomycin Sulfate and Hydrocortisone Ointment; Neomycin Sulfate and Hydrocortisone Otic Suspension; Neomycin Sulfate and Methylprednisolone Acetate Cream; Neomycin Sulfate and Prednisolone Acetate Ointment; Neomycin Sulfate and Prednisolone Acetate Ophthalmic Ointment; Neomycin Sulfate and Prednisolone Acetate Ophthalmic Suspension; Neomycin Sulfate and Prednisolone Sodium Phosphate Ophthalmic Ointment; Neomycin Sulfate and Triamcinolone Acetonide Cream; Neomycin Sulfate and Triamcinolone Acetonide Ophthalmic Ointment; Neomycin Sulfate Cream; Neomycin Sulfate Ointment; Neomycin Sulfate Ophthalmic Ointment; Neomycin Sulfate Oral Solution; Neomycin Sulfate Tablets; Neomycin Sulfate, Sulfacetamide Sodium, and Prednisolone Acetate Ophthalmic Ointment; Nystatin, Neomycin Sulfate, Gramicidin, and Triamcinolone Acetonide Cream; Nystatin, Neomycin Sulfate, Gramicidin, and Triamcinolone Acetonide Ointment.

Proprietary Preparations (details are given in Part 3)

Aust.: Bykomycin; ***Austral.:*** Neosulf; Siguent Neomycin; ***Belg.:*** Fradyl†; ***Canad.:*** Mycifradin; Myciguent; ***Ger.:*** Bykomycin; Cysto-Myacyne N; Glycomycin†; Myacyne; Nebacetin N; Uro-Nebacetin N; Vagicillin; ***Irl.:*** Mycifradin; Myciguent†; ***Ital.:*** Endomixin†; ***Jpn:*** Francetin†; ***S.Afr.:*** Mycifradin; ***Switz.:*** Uro-Beniktol N; ***UK:*** Mycifradin; Nivemycin; ***USA:*** Mycifradin; Myciguent; Neo-fradin; Neo-Tabs.

Multi-ingredient: ***Aust.:*** Baneocin; Betnesol-N; Betnovate-N; Cicatrex; Conjunctin-S†; Conjunctin†; Decadron mit Neomycin†; Dexa-Rhinospray; Dolothricin; Dorithricin; Ecomytrin; Ecomytrin-Hydrocortison; Hydoftal; Hydrocortimycin; Locacorten mit Neomycin; Mycostatin V; Nebacetin; Neo-Delphicort; Neocones; Otosporin; Polybactrin; Riker Antibiotic-Spray; Synalar N; Topsym polyvalent; Tropoderm; Tyrothricin comp; Ulcurilen; Volon A antibiotikahaltig; ***Austral.:*** Aristocomb; Cicatrin; Coly-Mycin†; Graneodin†; Kenacomb; Mycitracin†; Nemdyn; Neo-Medrol; Neosporin; Otocomb Otic; Spersin; ***Belg.:*** Betnelan-VN; Conjunctin†; De Icin; Decadron avec Neomycine; Dexa-Rhinospray; Flogocid; Fungispec†; Graneodine; Ledercort†; Maxitrol; Mycolog; Nebacetine†; Neo-Synalar†; Neobacitracine; Neodexon; Otosporin; Panotile; Pimafucort; Plastenan Neomycine†; Polydexa; Polygynax; Predmycin; Pulvo Neomycine; Rhinovalon Neomycine; Rikosol†; Spitalen; Statrol; Synalar Bi-Ophtalmic†; Synalar Bi-Otic; ***Canad.:*** Betnovate-N†; Cicatrin; Coly-Mycin Otic†; Cortisporin; Dioptrol; Diospor HC; Diosporin; FML Neo Liquifilm†; Halcicomb†; Kaomycin†; Kenacomb; Lidecomb†; Maxitrol; Metimyd†; Neo-Cortef; Neo-Medrol Acne; Neo-Medrol Veriderm; NeoDecadron; Neosporin; Neotopic; Optimyxin Plus; Proctosone; Synalar Bi-Otic†; Triacomb; Viaderm-KC; ***Fr.:*** Antibio-Synalar; Antibiotulle Lumiere; Atebemyxine; Bacteomycine; Betneval-Neomycine; Cebemyxine; Chibro-Cadron; Cidermex; Corticotulle Lumiere; Cortneo†; Dexagrane; Diprosone Neomycine; Dulcicortine†; Halog Neomycine; Locacortene†; Madecassol Neomycine Hydrocortisone; Martisol†; Maxidrol; Myco-Ultralan; Mycolog; Optidex†; Panotile; Penticort Neomycine; Pimafucort†; Pivalone Neomycine; Plastenan Neomycine; Polydexa; Polydexa a la Phenylephrine; Polygynax; Polygynax Virgo; Pulvo 47 Neomycine; Synalar Neomycine; Tergynan; Topsyne Neomycine; Trofoseptine†; ***Ger.:*** Antibiotulle Lumiere; Batrax; Betnesol-VN†; Bivacyn; Bykomycin F†; Chibro-Cadron; Cicatrex; Corticotulle Lumiere; Cortidexason comp; Dexa Polyspectran N; Dispadex comp; Dontisolon M Mundheilpaste†; Dontisolon M Zylinderampullen†; Efflumycin; Eustoporin†; Farco-Uromycin; Ficortril Lotio m. Neomycin†; Halog Tri; Heliomycort†; Isopto Max; Jellin polyvalent; Jellin-Neomycin; Jellisoft-Neomycin; Kaopectate N†; Kombi-Stulln; Korticoid c. Neomycin-ratiopharm†; Linola-H-compositum N; Lokalison-antimikrobiell Creme N; Medicreme†; Medicrucin-blau†; Medicrucin-gelb N†; Medicrucin-rose†; Myacyne; Mycinopred†; Nebacetin; Neo-Medrate Akne-Lotio†; Neobac; Neotracin; Otosporin; Pimafucort; Polybactrin†; Polyfen†; Polygynax; Polyspectran; Polyspectran OS†; Predni aquos. in der Ophtiole†; Prednitracin; Pulvo Neomycin; Sermaka N†; Tampovagan C-N N†; Topoderm N; Topsym polyvalent; Tyzine compositum†; Ulcurilen N; Ultexiv; Uromycin†; Vibrocil cN†; Volon A antibiotikahaltig N; ***Irl.:*** Audicort; Betnesol-N; Betnovate-N; Biotrin†; Cicatrin; Dexa-Rhinaspray; FML Neo†; Graneodin; Kenacomb; Maxitrol; Naseptin; Neo-Cortef; Neo-Medrone; Neosporin; Otomize; Otosporin; Polybactrin; Polybactrin Soluble†; Synalar N; Vibrocil†; Vista-Methasone N; ***Ital.:*** Abiostil; Anauran; Anfocort; Antibioptal; Antibioticoedermin B†; Assocort; Bimixin; Bio-Delta Cortilen; Cicatrene; Combiderm†; Demicina†; Dermadex Neomicina†; Dermocur†; Desalfa; Desamix-Neomicina; Doricum; Drenison con Neomicina†; Ecoval con Neomicina; Enterocantril†; Enterostop; Eta Biocortilen; Eta Biocortilen VC; Etamicina†; Halciderm Combi; Idracemi; Idrocet; Idroneomicil; Idustatin; Kataval; Localyn; Localyn-Neomicina; Locorten; Locorten Neomicina†; Menaderm; Mixotone; Mycocur†; Nasomixin; Nefluan; Neo-Audiocort; Neo-Cortofen; Neo-Cortofen "Antrax"†; Neo-Medrol Lozione Antiacne†; Neo-Medrol Veriderm; Neocortigamma†; Neocortovol†; Neodes†; Neogram; Oftalmosporin†; Oftisone†; Orobicin; Otobiotic†; Otomicetina; Otosporin; Pimafucort†; Prednigamma†; Rinojet SF; Solprene; Sprayrin†; Streptosil con Neomicina-Fher; Topsyn Neomicina†; Trofodermin; Uretral†; Vasosterone Antibiotico; Vasosterone Collirio; ***Neth.:*** Betnelan Neomycine†; Celestoderm met Neomycine; Decadron met neomycine; Maxitrol†; Mycolog; Nebacetin†; Neosporin†; Otosporin; Panotile; Pimafucort; Polyspectran B†; Polyspectran G†; Predmycin-P Liquifilm†; Synalar Bi-Otic; ***Norw.:*** Ecomytrin-Hydrocortison†; Maxitrol; Polysporin†; ***S.Afr.:*** Betnesol-N; Betnovate-N†; Cicatrin; Covomycin; Covomycin-D; FML Neo; Kaomycin†; Kaoneo†; Kenacomb; Maxitrol; Naseptin; Nasomixin; Nebacetin†; Neo-Medrol; Neoderm; Neopan; Neopec†; Neosporin; Otoseptil†; Otosporin; Synalar N; Trialone; Vibrocil; ***Spain:*** Alantomicina; Alantomicina Complex; Anasilpiel; Antihemorr; Antihemorroidal; Bacisporin; Banedif; Betamatil con Neomicina; Bexicortil; Bio Hubber; Bio Hubber Fuerte; Blastoestimulina; Cilinafosal Hidrocort; Cilinafosal Neomicina; Cilinavagin Neomicina; Coliriocilina Espectro; Coliriocilina Prednisona; Creanolona; Decadran Neomicina; Decoderm Trivalente; Deltacina; Deltasiton; Derbitan Antibiotico; Dermisone Hidroc Neomic†; Dermisone Tri Antibiotic; Dermo Hubber; Dermomycose Talco; Drenison Neomicina; Ecomitrin†; Enterowas†; Estreptosirup†; Flodermol; Fludronef; Fluo Vasoc; FML Neo; Gingilone; Gingilone Comp†; Gramicidin†; Grietalgen Hidrocort; Heridasone†; Hidroc Neomic; Idasal Antibiotico†; Indertal†; Infalina†; Intradermo Cort Ant Fung; Iruxol Neo; Leuco Hubber; Linitul Antibiotico; Liquipom Dexa Antib; Maxitrol; Menaderm; Midacina; Mirantal; Nasokey†; Nasotic Oto; Neo Analsona; Neo Bacitrin; Neo Bacitrin Hidrocortis; Neo Hubber; Neo Moderin; Neo Synalar; Neocones; Neodemusin†; Neodexa; Neodexaplast†; Oftalmo; Oftalmowell; Ophtacortine†; Oto Difusor; Oto Neomicin Calm; Oto Vitna†; Otogen Hydrocortisona†; Otogen Prednisolona†; Otonina; Otosporin; Oxidermiol Enzima; Panotile; Pentalmicina; Phonal; Plaskine Neomicina; Plastenan Neomicina†; Polirino†; Poly Pred; Pomada Antibiotica; Positon; Poxider; Prednis Neomic; Pulverodil†; Puodermina Hidrocor†; Rino Dexa; Rino Vitna†; Rinobanedif; Rinoblanco Dexa Antibio; Rinocusi Descong†; Rinovel; Saleton†; Salvacolina NN†; Sorbitoxin†; Spectrocin; Statrol; Sulfintestin Neom; Sulfintestin Neomicina; Synalar Nasal; Synalar Neomicina; Synalar Otico; Tisuderma; Tivitis; Tricin†; Trigon Topico; Tulgrasum Antibiotico; Tyroneomicin; Vasocon Ant; Vinciseptil Otico; Wasserdermina†; Xilorroidal†; ***Swed.:*** Betnovat med neomycin; Celeston valerat comp.; Decadron cum neomycin; Ecomytrin-Hydrocortison†; Ecomytrin†; Isopto Biotic; Kenacombin†; Kenacort-T med Graneodin†; Nebacetin†; ***Switz.:*** Bacimycine; Baneopol; Batramycine; Betnovate-N; Cicatrex; Cloptison-N; Cortifluid N; Cortimycine; Decadron a la neomycine†; Dermovate-NN; Dexa-Rhinospray†; Dontisolon M†; Ecomytrin-Hydrocortison†; Flogocid NN; FML Neo; Halciderm comp†; Kaomycine†; Locacorten c. Neomycin†; Maxitrol; Mycinopred; Mycolog; Nebacetin†; Neo-Hydro; Neo-Medrol†; Neocones; Neosporin; Neosporin-B†; Neotracin; Otosporin; Otospray; Panotile; Pivalone compositum; Polybactrin Solubile†; Polybactrin†; Polydexa; Prednitracin; Riccomycine; Septomixine; Spersapolymyxin; Statrol†; Synalar N; Topsym polyvalent; Tyrocombine; Urethra-Steril†; Vistajunctin†; ***UK:*** Adcortyl with Graneodin; Audicort; Betnesol-N; Betnovate-N; Cicatrin; Cloburate-N†; Dermovate-NN; Dexa-Rhinaspray†; FML Neo Liquifilm; Graneodin; Gregoderm; Maxitrol; Naseptin; Neo-Cortef; Neo-Medrone†; Neosporin; Otomize; Otosporin; Polybactrin†; Predsol-N; Synalar N; Tri-Adcortyl; Tri-Cicatrin†; Tribiotic†; Uniroid; Vibrocil†; Vista-Methasone N; ***USA:*** Ak-Neo-Dex; Ak-Spore; Ak-Spore HC; Ak-Trol; Alba-3; AntibiOtic; Bacticort; Bactine First Aid Antibiotic Plus Anesthetic; Campho-Phenique Antibiotic Plus Pain Reliever Ointment; Clomycin; Coly-Mycin S Otic; Coracin; Cortatrigen; Cortisporin; Cortisporin-TC; Dexacidin; Dexasporin; Drotic†; Ear-Eze; Infectrol†; Lanabiotic; LazerSporin-C; Maxitrol; Medi-Quik†; Mycitracin; Mycitracin Plus; Neo-Cortef†; Neo-Dexair; Neo-Dexameth; Neo-Synalar†; Neocin; NeoDecadron; Neomixin; Neosporin; Neosporin GU; Neosporin Plus; Neotal; Neotricin HC; Neotricin†; Octicair; Ocutricin; Otic-Care; Oticin HC; OtiTricin; Otocort; Otomycin-HPN; Otosporin; Pediotic; Poly-Dex; Poly-Pred; Septa; Spectrocin Plus; Storz-N-D; Storz-N-P-D; Topisporin†; Tribiotic Plus; Triple Antibiotic; UAD-Otic.

Netilmicin Sulphate (114-n)

Netilmicin Sulphate (*BANM, rINNM*).

N^1-Ethylsissomicin; Netilmicin Sulfate (*USAN*); Netilmicini Sulfas; Sch-20569. 4-*O*-[(2*R*,3*R*)-*cis*-3-Amino-6-aminomethyl-3,4-dihydro-2*H*-pyran-2-yl]-2-deoxy-6-*O*-(3-deoxy-4-*C*-methyl-3-methylamino-β-L-arabinopyranosyl)-1-*N*-ethyl-streptamine sulphate.

$(C_{21}H_{41}N_5O_7)_2,5H_2SO_4$ = 1441.6.

CAS — 56391-56-1 (netilmicin); 56391-57-2 (netilmicin sulphate).

Pharmacopoeias. In *Eur.* (see p.viii), *Jpn, Pol.*, and *US*.

A semisynthetic derivative of sissomicin. 1.5 g of monograph substance is approximately equivalent to 1 g of netilmicin.

A white to pale yellowish-white very hygroscopic powder. Very or freely **soluble** in water; practically insoluble in alcohol, in dehydrated alcohol, in acetone, and in ether. A 4% solution in water has a pH between 3.5 and 5.5. **Store** in airtight containers. Protect from light.

Incompatibilities. For discussion of the incompatibility of aminoglycosides, including netilmicin, with beta lactams, see under Gentamicin Sulphate, p.212. Netilmicin is also reported to be incompatible with frusemide, heparin, and vitamin B complex.

Adverse Effects, Treatment, and Precautions

As for Gentamicin Sulphate, p.212. Some studies suggest that netilmicin is less nephrotoxic and ototoxic than gentamicin or tobramycin, although others have not found any significant differences in their toxic effects.

Peak plasma concentrations of netilmicin greater than 16 µg per mL, and trough concentrations greater than 4 µg per mL should be avoided and some sources suggest that peaks below 12 µg per mL and troughs below 2 µg per mL are preferable.

Effects on the cardiovascular system. Severe hypotension was associated with administration of netilmicin in a patient undergoing artificial ventilation.[1] Hypotensive episodes were of short duration and coincided with netilmicin injection. They almost disappeared when sedation was stopped.

1. Rygnestad T. Severe hypotension associated with netilmicin treatment. *Br Med J* 1997; **315:** 31.

Interactions

As for Gentamicin Sulphate, p.213.

Antimicrobial Action

As for Gentamicin Sulphate, p.213. It is active against a similar range of organisms although it is also reported to have some activity against *Nocardia*. It may be somewhat less effective against *Pseudomonas aeruginosa*. MICs of netilmicin for the most sensitive organisms range from about 0.25 to 2 µg per mL, but organisms with MICs less than about 8 µg per mL are considered sensitive. It is not degraded by all of the enzymes responsible for aminoglycoside resistance, and may be active against some strains resistant to gentamicin or tobramycin, but this is less marked than with amikacin: for example, gentamicin-resistant *Proteus, Providencia, Pseudomonas*, and *Serratia* are usually also netilmicin-resistant. Between about 5 and 20% of Gram-negative isolates are reported to be resistant to netilmicin.

Pharmacokinetics

As for Gentamicin Sulphate, p.213.

Following intramuscular injection of netilmicin, peak plasma concentrations are achieved within half to 1 hour, and concentrations of about 7 µg per mL have been reported following doses of 2 mg per kg body-weight; similar concentrations are obtained after intravenous infusion of the same dose over 1 hour. Peak concentrations following rapid intravenous injection may transiently be 2 or 3 times higher than those following infusion. Administration of standard, once-daily doses may produce transient peak concentrations of 20 to 30 µg per mL. In multiple dosing studies, administration of netilmicin in usual doses every 12 hours produced steady-state concentrations on the second day which were less than 20% higher than those seen after the first dose.

The half-life of netilmicin is usually 2.0 to 2.5 hours. About 80% of a dose is excreted in the urine within 24 hours.

Uses and Administration

Netilmicin is a semisynthetic aminoglycoside antibiotic with actions and uses similar to those of gentamicin (p.214). It may be used as an alternative to amikacin (p.150) in the treatment of infections caused by susceptible bacteria that are resistant to gentamicin and tobramycin. As with gentamicin, netilmicin may be used with penicillins and with cephalosporins; the injections should be given separately.

Netilmicin is given as the sulphate but doses are expressed in terms of the equivalent amount of base. It is usually given intramuscularly in doses equivalent to netilmicin 4 to 6 mg per kg body-weight daily as a single dose; alternatively, it may be given in equally divided doses every 8 or 12 hours; for the control of life-threatening infections, up to 7.5 mg per kg may be given daily in divided doses every 8 hours for short periods. In the management of urinary-tract infections regimens consisting of either a single daily dose of 150 mg or of 3 to 4 mg per kg daily in divided doses every 12 hours have been suggested. A single dose of 300 mg has been suggested for gonorrhoea (p.126) although it is not recommended in current treatment guidelines.

The same doses may be given by slow intravenous injection over 3 to 5 minutes or infused intravenously over half to 2 hours in 50 to 200 mL of infusion fluid; proportionately less fluid should be given to children.

Treatment with netilmicin is usually given for 7 to 14 days. Prolonged peak plasma concentrations greater than 16 µg per mL and trough plasma concentrations greater than 4 µg per mL should be avoided. Some sources suggest peaks below 12 µg per mL and troughs below 2 µg per mL for divided daily dose regimens.

Dosage recommendations in infants and children vary somewhat. One suggested regimen is the equivalent of 7.5 to 9.0 mg of netilmicin per kg daily in infants and neonates older than 1 week, and 6.0 to 7.5 mg per kg daily in older children, both given in divided doses every 8 hours. Premature infants, and neonates less than 1 week old, would be given 6 mg per kg daily in divided doses of 3 mg per kg every 12 hours. An alternative regimen is 4 to 6.5 mg per kg daily in neonates less than 6 weeks of age, in divided doses every 12 hours, and 5.5 to 8.0 mg per kg daily in divided doses every 8 or 12 hours in older infants and children.

It is recommended that dosage should be adjusted in all patients according to plasma-netilmicin concentrations, and this is particularly important where factors such as age, renal impairment or dose may predispose to toxicity, or where there is a risk of subtherapeutic concentrations. For discussion of the methods of calculating aminoglycoside dosage requirements, see p.214.

Preparations

USP 23: Netilmicin Sulfate Injection.

Proprietary Preparations (details are given in Part 3)
Aust.: Certomycin; ***Austral.:*** Netromycin; ***Belg.:*** Netromycine; ***Canad.:*** Netromycin; ***Fr.:*** Netromicine; ***Ger.:*** Certomycin; ***Irl.:*** Netillin; ***Ital.:*** Nettacin; Zetamicin; ***Neth.:*** Netromycine; ***Norw.:*** Netilyn; ***S.Afr.:*** Netromycin; ***Spain:*** Dalinar; Netrocin; Vivicil†; ***Swed.:*** Netilyn; ***Switz.:*** Netromycine; ***UK:*** Netillin; ***USA:*** Netromycin.

Nifuroxazide (13014-j)

Nifuroxazide (*rINN*).

2′-(5-Nitrofurfurylidene)-4-hydroxybenzohydrazide.

$C_{12}H_9N_3O_5$ = 275.2.

CAS — 965-52-6.

Pharmacopoeias. In *Fr.*

Nifuroxazide is an antibacterial that has been given by mouth in a dose of 800 mg daily in the treatment of colitis and diarrhoea. It is poorly absorbed from the gastro-intestinal tract.

Preparations

Proprietary Preparations (details are given in Part 3)
Belg.: Bacifurane; Ercefuryl; ***Fr.:*** Ambatrol; Antinal; Bacifurane†; Ercefuryl; Lumifurex; Nifur; Panfurex; ***Ital.:*** Diarret; Ercefuryl; ***Spain:*** Ercefuril†; ***Switz.:*** Antinal†.

Nifurtoinol (13016-c)

Nifurtoinol (*rINN*).

Hydroxymethylnitrofurantoin. 3-Hydroxymethyl-1-(5-nitrofurfurylideneamino)hydantoin.

$C_9H_8N_4O_6$ = 268.2.

CAS — 1088-92-2.

Nifurtoinol is a nitrofuran antibacterial with properties similar to those of nitrofurantoin (p.231) and is used in the treatment of urinary-tract infections. It is given by mouth in doses of up to 300 mg daily in divided doses.

Preparations

Proprietary Preparations (details are given in Part 3)
Belg.: Urfadyn PL; ***Fr.:*** Urfadyn†; ***Ital.:*** Urfadyn†; ***Neth.:*** Uridurine†; ***Switz.:*** Urfadyne.

Multi-ingredient: ***Ital.:*** Fultrexin†.

Nifurzide (19569-v)

Nifurzide (*rINN*).

5-Nitro-2-thiophenecarboxylic acid [3-(5-nitro-2-furyl)allylidene]hydrazide.

$C_{12}H_8N_4O_6S$ = 336.3.

CAS — 39978-42-2.

Nifurzide is an antibacterial that has been given by mouth in a dose of 450 mg daily in the treatment of diarrhoea. It is poorly absorbed from the gastro-intestinal tract.

Preparations

Proprietary Preparations (details are given in Part 3)
Fr.: Ricridene.

Nisin (13021-y)

234.

CAS — 1414-45-5.

Nisin is a polypeptide antibiotic produced by *Streptococcus lactis* which is used as a preservative for foods.

It is under investigation for treating various infections including those caused by *Helicobacter pylori* and *Clostridium difficile*.

A study of the mode of action of nisin suggesting that its primary target is the cytoplasmic membrane and that membrane disruption accounts for its bactericidal action.[1]

1. Ruhr E, Sahl H-G. Mode of action of the peptide antibiotic nisin and influence on the membrane potential of whole cells and on cytoplasmic and artificial membrane vesicles. *Antimicrob Agents Chemother* 1985; **27:** 841–5.

Nitrofurantoin (5651-x)

Nitrofurantoin (*BAN, rINN*).

Furadoninum; Nitrofurantoinum. 1-(5-Nitrofurfurylideneamino)hydantoin; 1-(5-Nitrofurfurylideneamino)imidazolidine-2,4-dione.

$C_8H_6N_4O_5$ = 238.2.

CAS — 67-20-9 (anhydrous nitrofurantoin); 17140-81-7 (nitrofurantoin monohydrate).

Pharmacopoeias. In *Chin.* and *Eur.* (see p.viii).
Int. and *US* specify anhydrous or monohydrate.

Yellow odourless or almost odourless crystals or fine crystalline powder. It is discoloured by alkalis and by exposure to light and decomposes on contact with metals other than stainless steel or aluminium.

Very slightly **soluble** in water and in alcohol; soluble in dimethylformamide. **Store** at a temperature not exceeding 25° in airtight containers. Protect from light.

Nitrofurantoin Sodium (5652-r)

Nitrofurantoin Sodium *(BANM, rINNM)*.

$C_8H_5N_4NaO_5$ = 260.1.

CAS — 54-87-5.

Adverse Effects

The estimated incidence of adverse effects with nitrofurantoin has varied enormously, but may be around 10% overall; an incidence of serious reactions of about 0.001% for pulmonary, and 0.0007% for neurological reactions has been suggested. The most common adverse effects encountered with nitrofurantoin involve the gastro-intestinal tract. They are dose-related and generally include nausea, vomiting, and anorexia; abdominal pain and diarrhoea occur less frequently. It has been reported that adverse effects on the gastro-intestinal tract are less common when nitrofurantoin is administered in a macrocrystalline form or with food.

Neurological adverse effects include headache, drowsiness, vertigo, dizziness, nystagmus, and intracranial hypertension. Severe and sometimes irreversible peripheral polyneuropathy has developed, particularly in patients with impaired renal function and in those given prolonged therapy.

Hypersensitivity reactions such as skin rashes, urticaria, pruritus, fever, and angioedema may occur. Anaphylaxis, erythema multiforme, Stevens-Johnson syndrome, exfoliative dermatitis, pancreatitis, a lupus-like syndrome, myalgia, and arthralgia have also been reported. Patients with a history of asthma may experience acute asthmatic attacks.

Acute pulmonary sensitivity reactions characterised by sudden onset of fever, chills, eosinophilia, cough, chest pain, dyspnoea, pulmonary infiltration or consolidation, and pleural effusion may occur within hours to a few days of beginning therapy, but they usually resolve on discontinuation.

Subacute or chronic pulmonary symptoms including interstitial pneumonitis and pulmonary fibrosis may develop more insidiously in patients on long-term therapy and the latter are not always reversible, particularly if therapy is continued after onset of symptoms.

Hepatotoxicity including cholestatic jaundice and hepatitis may develop rarely, particularly in women, and probably represents a hypersensitivity reaction. Other adverse effects include megaloblastic anaemia, leucopenia, granulocytopenia or agranulocytosis, thrombocytopenia, aplastic anaemia, and haemolytic anaemia in persons with a genetic deficiency of glucose-6-phosphate dehydrogenase. Transient alopecia has been reported.

There is limited evidence from *animal* studies that nitrofurantoin may be carcinogenic, although this has not been demonstrated conclusively in humans.

References.

1. Koch-Weser J, *et al.* Adverse reactions to sulfisoxazole, sulfamethoxazole, and nitrofurantoin: manifestations and specific reaction rates during 2118 courses of therapy. *Arch Intern Med* 1971; **128:** 399–404.
2. Holmberg L, *et al.* Adverse reactions to nitrofurantoin: analysis of 921 reports. *Am J Med* 1980; **69:** 733–8.
3. Penn RG, Griffin JP. Adverse reactions to nitrofurantoin in the United Kingdom, Sweden, and Holland. *Br Med J* 1982; **284:** 1440–2.
4. D'Arcy PF. Nitrofurantoin. *Drug Intell Clin Pharm* 1985; **19:** 540–7.

Precautions

Nitrofurantoin should not be given to patients with impaired renal function since antibacterial concentrations in the urine may not be attained and toxic concentrations in the plasma can occur. Nitrofurantoin is also contra-indicated in patients known to be hypersensitive to nitrofurans, in those with a deficiency of glucose-6-phosphate dehydrogenase, and in infants less than three months old. It has been suggested that nitrofurantoin should not be used in pregnant patients at term because of the possibility of producing haemolytic anaemia in the neonate, and that it should be avoided or used with caution in nursing mothers of infants with a deficiency of glucose-6-phosphate dehydrogenase since traces are found in breast milk.

Nitrofurantoin should be used with care in the elderly, who may be at increased risk of toxicity, particularly acute pulmonary reactions. All patients undergoing prolonged therapy should be monitored for changes in pulmonary function, and the drug withdrawn at the first signs of pulmonary damage. Care is required in patients with pre-existing pulmonary, hepatic, neurological or allergic disorders, and in those with conditions (such as anaemia, diabetes mellitus, electrolyte imbalance, debility, or vitamin B deficiency) which may predispose to peripheral neuropathy. Nitrofurantoin should be withdrawn if signs of peripheral neuropathy develop.

Nitrofurantoin may cause false positive reactions in urine tests for glucose using copper reduction methods.

Nitrofurantoin may cause a brownish discoloration of the urine.

Porphyria. Nitrofurantoin was considered to be unsafe in patients with acute porphyria although there is conflicting experimental evidence on porphyrinogenicity.[1]

1. Moore MR, McColl KEL. *Porphyria: drug lists.* Glasgow: Porphyria Research Unit, University of Glasgow, 1991.

Interactions

Nitrofurantoin and the quinolone antibacterials are antagonistic *in vitro* and their concomitant use is not recommended. The antibacterial activity of nitrofurantoin may be decreased in the presence of carbonic anhydrase inhibitors and other drugs that alkalinise the urine.

Probenecid or sulphinpyrazone may reduce the excretion of nitrofurantoin and should not be given concomitantly. Magnesium trisilicate may reduce the absorption of nitrofurantoin but it is not clear whether this applies to other antacids.

For reference to the effect of nitrofurantoin on phenytoin, see p.354. For mention of a possible decrease in contraceptive efficacy when nitrofurantoin was given concomitantly with oral contraceptives, see under Hormonal Contraceptives, p.1433.

Antimicrobial Action

Nitrofurantoin is bactericidal *in vitro* to most Gram-positive and Gram-negative urinary-tract pathogens. The mode of action is uncertain but appears to depend on the formation of reactive intermediates by reduction; this process occurs more efficiently in bacterial than in mammalian cells.

It is effective against the enterococci *in vitro*, as well as various other Gram-positive species including staphylococci, streptococci, and corynebacteria, although this is of little clinical significance. Most strains of *Escherichia coli* are particularly sensitive to nitrofurantoin but *Enterobacter* and *Klebsiella* spp. are less susceptible and some may be resistant. *Pseudomonas aeruginosa* is resistant as are most strains of *Proteus* spp.

Organisms with MICs below 32 μg per mL are usually considered susceptible, as such concentrations are readily achievable in urine, while strains with MICs above about 128 μg per mL are considered resistant. Nitrofurantoin is generally bactericidal at concentrations not much above the MIC. It is most active in acid urine, and if the pH exceeds 8 most of the antibacterial activity is lost. Resistance rarely develops during nitrofurantoin treatment but may occur during prolonged treatment. Plasmid-encoded resistance has been reported in *E. coli*. Resistance may be due to the loss of nitrofuran reductases which generate the active intermediates.

Pharmacokinetics

Nitrofurantoin is readily absorbed from the gastro-intestinal tract. The absorption rate is dependent on crystal size. The macrocrystalline form has slower dissolution and absorption rates, produces lower serum concentrations than the microcrystalline form, and takes longer to achieve peak concentrations in the urine. The presence of food in the gastro-intestinal tract may increase the bioavailability of nitrofurantoin and prolong the duration of therapeutic urinary concentrations. Preparations of nitrofurantoin from different sources may not be bioequivalent, and care may be necessary if changing from one brand to another.

Following absorption, concentrations in blood and body tissues are low because of rapid elimination, and antibacterial concentrations are not achieved. Nitrofurantoin crosses the placenta and the blood-brain barrier and traces have been detected in breast milk. There is some disagreement about the degree of protein binding, and although figures of up to about 60% are quoted by some sources, others suggest that the figure should be as much as 90 to 95%. The plasma half-life is reported to range from 0.3 to 1 hour.

Nitrofurantoin is metabolised in the liver and most body tissues while about 30 to 40% of a dose is excreted rapidly in the urine as unchanged nitrofurantoin. Some tubular reabsorption may occur in acid urine. Average doses give a concentration of 50 to 200 μg per mL in the urine in patients with normal renal function.

Uses and Administration

Nitrofurantoin is a nitrofuran derivative which is used in the treatment of uncomplicated lower urinary-tract infections (p.149), including for prophylaxis or long-term suppressive therapy in recurrent infection.

It is given by mouth usually in a dose of 50 to 100 mg four times daily, with food or milk. In uncomplicated infection 100 mg twice daily may be adequate. Treatment is usually continued for 7 days. A usual long-term prophylactic dose is 50 to 100 mg at bedtime.

Infants over 3 months of age and older children may be given 3 mg per kg body-weight daily in 4 divided doses by mouth. For long-term prophylactic therapy 1 mg per kg once daily may be adequate.

Preparations

BP 1998: Nitrofurantoin Oral Suspension; Nitrofurantoin Tablets; ***USP 23:*** Nitrofurantoin Capsules; Nitrofurantoin Oral Suspension; Nitrofurantoin Tablets.

Proprietary Preparations (details are given in Part 3)
Aust.: Furadantin; Urolong; ***Austral.:*** Furadantin; Macrodantin; ***Belg.:*** Furadantine; ***Canad.:*** Macrobid; Macrodantin; Novo-Furan; ***Fr.:*** Furadantine; Furadoine; Microdoine; ***Ger.:*** Cystit; Furadantin; ituran†; Nierofu†; Nifurantin; Nifuretten; Phenurin†; Uro-Selz†; Uro-Tablinen; Urodil†; Urolong†; ***Irl.:*** Furadantin; Macrobid; Macrodantin; ***Ital.:*** Cistofuran; Furadantin; Furedan; Furil; Macrodantin; Neo-Furadantin; Nitrofurin G.W.†; Urolisa†; ***Neth.:*** Furabid; Furadantine MC; ***Norw.:*** Furadantin; ***S.Afr.:*** Furadantin; Macrodantin; Urantin; ***Spain:*** Chemiofurin; Furantoina; Furobactina; ***Swed.:*** Furadantin; ***Switz.:*** Furadantine; Trocurine†; Urodin; Urolong†; Uvamine retard; ***UK:*** Furadantin; Macrobid; Macrodantin; Urantoin; ***USA:*** Furadantin; Macrobid; Macrodantin.

Multi-ingredient: ***Aust.:*** Spasmo-Urolong; Urospasmon sine phenazopyridino; ***Ger.:*** Nifurantin B 6; Nitrofurantoin comp.†; Spasmo Nierofu†; Spasmo-Uroclear†; Spasmo-Urolong†; Sulfa-Uro-Tablinen†; Sulfa-Urolong†; Uroclear†; Urospasmon; Urospasmon sine; ***Spain:*** Furantoina Sedante†; Urogobens Antiespasmo; ***Switz.:*** Spasmo-Urolong†; Trocurine†; Urospasmon†.

Nitrofurazone (1626-w)

Nitrofurazone *(BAN)*.

Nitrofural *(pINN)*; Furacilinum; Nitrofuralum. 5-Nitro-2-furaldehyde semicarbazone.

$C_6H_6N_4O_4$ = 198.1.

CAS — 59-87-0.

Pharmacopoeias. In *Eur.* (see p.viii), *Pol.*, and *US.*

A lemon to brownish-yellow odourless, crystalline powder. It slowly darkens on exposure to light and discolours on contact with alkalis.

Soluble 1 in 4200 of water, 1 in 590 of alcohol, and 1 in 350 of propylene glycol; soluble in dimethylformamide; practically insoluble in chloroform and ether. The filtrate from a 1%

suspension in water has a pH of 5.0 to 7.5. **Store** at a temperature not exceeding 40° in airtight containers. Protect from light.

Autoclaving gauze dressings impregnated with nitrofurazone, as recommended by the US manufacturer of the preparation, resulted in a greater than 10% loss of the drug.[1] Since the spectroscopic assay used may not distinguish between nitrofurazone and some of its degradation products, it is possible that the degree of degradation was greater than this.

1. Phillips C, Fisher E. Effect of autoclaving on stability of nitrofurazone soluble dressing. *Am J Health-Syst Pharm* 1996; **53:** 1169–71.

Adverse Effects

Sensitisation and generalised allergic skin reactions may be produced by the topical application of nitrofurazone.

Nitrofurazone is a toxic drug when given by mouth and serious adverse effects include severe peripheral neuropathy; haemolysis may occur in patients with a deficiency of glucose-6-phosphate dehydrogenase. Nitrofurazone in high oral doses is carcinogenic in *rats*.

Precautions

Topical preparations of nitrofurazone are contra-indicated in patients with known hypersensitivity. Those preparations containing macrogols should be used with caution in patients with renal dysfunction since macrogols can be absorbed and their accumulation in such patients may result in symptoms of progressive renal impairment.

Because of the risk of haemolysis nitrofurazone by mouth should be used with caution in patients with glucose-6-phosphate dehydrogenase deficiency.

Antimicrobial Action

Nitrofurazone is a nitrofuran derivative with a broad spectrum of antibacterial activity, but with little activity against *Pseudomonas* spp. It also has antitrypanosomal activity.

Uses and Administration

Nitrofurazone is a nitrofuran derivative which is used as a local application for wounds, burns, ulcers, and skin infections, and for the preparation of surfaces before skin grafting. It is usually applied in a concentration of 0.2% in a water-soluble or water-miscible basis. A solution of nitrofurazone was formerly used for bladder irrigation.

Preparations

USP 23: Nitrofurazone Cream; Nitrofurazone Ointment; Nitrofurazone Topical Solution.

Proprietary Preparations (details are given in Part 3)
Belg.: Furacine; ***Ger.:*** Furacin-Sol; Nifucin; ***Ital.:*** Furacin; ***Neth.:*** Furacine†; ***S.Afr.:*** Furacin; Furasept; Furex; Germex†; ***Spain:*** Furacin; ***USA:*** Furacin.

Multi-ingredient: ***Ger.:*** Furacin-Otalgicum†; Nifucin; ***Ital.:*** Furanvit; Furotricina; ***Spain:*** Dertrase.

Nitroxoline (5664-h)

Nitroxoline *(BAN, pINN)*.

5-Nitroquinolin-8-ol.

$C_9H_6N_2O_3$ = 190.2.

CAS — 4008-48-4.

Nitroxoline is a drug with antibacterial and antifungal properties used in the treatment of urinary-tract infections in usual doses of 600 mg daily by mouth in divided doses before food. It has also been given in combination with sulphamethizole.

Preparations

Proprietary Preparations (details are given in Part 3)
Fr.: Nibiol; ***Ger.:*** Nicene forte†; ***Ital.:*** Uro-Coli†; ***Spain:*** Nibiol†.

Multi-ingredient: ***Ger.:*** Nicene N†; ***S.Afr.:*** Nicene.

Norfloxacin (12349-g)

Norfloxacin *(BAN, USAN, rINN)*.

AM-715; MK-366; Norfloxacinum. 1-Ethyl-6-fluoro-1,4-dihydro-4-oxo-7-(piperazin-1-yl)quinoline-3-carboxylic acid.

$C_{16}H_{18}FN_3O_3$ = 319.3.

CAS — 70458-96-7.

Pharmacopoeias. In *Chin., Eur.* (see p.viii), *Pol.,* and *US.*

A white to pale yellow hygroscopic, crystalline powder. Slightly **soluble** or very slightly soluble in water; slightly soluble in alcohol and in acetone; freely soluble in acetic acid; sparingly soluble in chloroform; very slightly soluble in methyl alcohol and in ethyl acetate; practically insoluble in ether. **Store** in airtight containers. Protect from light.

Adverse Effects and Precautions

As for Ciprofloxacin, p.186.

Effects on the kidneys. References.

1. Hestin D, *et al.* Norfloxacin-induced nephrotic syndrome. *Lancet* 1995; **345:** 732–3.

Interactions

As for Ciprofloxacin, p.187.

Antimicrobial Action

As for Ciprofloxacin, p.187, although norfloxacin is less potent *in vitro*. Norfloxacin is not active against *Chlamydia* spp., mycoplasmas, or mycobacteria.

Pharmacokinetics

About 30 to 40% of an oral dose of norfloxacin is absorbed. Peak plasma concentrations of about 1.5 µg of norfloxacin per mL have been achieved 1 to 2 hours after the administration of a 400-mg dose by mouth; the presence of food can delay absorption. The plasma half-life is about 4 hours and may be prolonged in renal impairment; a value of 6.5 hours or more has been reported when creatinine clearance is below 30 mL per minute. Norfloxacin has been reported to be 14% bound to plasma proteins. It is probably widely distributed, but information is limited. Norfloxacin penetrates well into tissues of the genito-urinary tract. It crosses the placenta. Relatively high concentrations are achieved in bile.

About 30% of a dose is excreted unchanged in the urine within 24 hours producing high urinary concentrations; norfloxacin is least soluble at a urinary pH of 7.5. Urinary excretion is by tubular secretion and glomerular filtration and is reduced by probenecid although plasma concentrations of norfloxacin are not generally affected. Some metabolism occurs, possibly in the liver, and several metabolites have been identified in urine, some with antibacterial activity. About 30% of an oral dose is recovered from the faeces.

References.

1. Norrby SR. Pharmacokinetics of norfloxacin: clinical implications. *Eur J Chemother Antibiot* 1983; **3:** 19–25.
2. Swanson BN, *et al.* Norfloxacin disposition after sequentially increasing oral doses. *Antimicrob Agents Chemother* 1983; **23:** 284–8.
3. Fillastre JP, *et al.* Pharmacokinetics of norfloxacin in renal failure. *J Antimicrob Chemother* 1984; **14:** 439.
4. Arrigo G, *et al.* Pharmacokinetics of norfloxacin in chronic renal failure. *Int J Clin Pharmacol Ther Toxicol* 1985; **23:** 491–6.
5. MacGowan AP, *et al.* The pharmacokinetics of norfloxacin in the aged. *J Antimicrob Chemother* 1988; **22:** 721–7.
6. Kelly JG, *et al.* Chronic dose urinary and serum pharmacokinetics of norfloxacin in the elderly. *Br J Clin Pharmacol* 1988; **26:** 787–90.

Uses and Administration

Norfloxacin is a fluoroquinolone antibacterial with properties similar to those of ciprofloxacin, but it is generally less potent *in vitro*.

Norfloxacin is used mainly in the treatment of urinary-tract infections (p.149). It is also used for the treatment of gonorrhoea (p.126).

Norfloxacin is administered by mouth. In urinary-tract infections the usual dose is 400 mg twice daily for 3 to 10 days. Treatment may need to be continued for up to 12 weeks in chronic relapsing urinary-tract infections; it may be possible to reduce the dose to 400 mg once daily if there is an adequate response within the first 4 weeks.

Doses may need to be reduced in renal impairment; 400 mg once daily has been suggested when the creatinine clearance is 30 mL or less per minute.

A single oral dose of 800 mg is given in the treatment of uncomplicated gonorrhoea.

Eye drops containing 0.3% of norfloxacin are used to treat eye infections topically.

Reviews.

1. Holmes B, *et al.* Norfloxacin: a review of its antibacterial activity, pharmacokinetic properties and therapeutic use. *Drugs* 1985; **30:** 482–513.
2. Wolfson JS, Hooper DC. Norfloxacin: a new targeted fluoroquinolone antimicrobial agent. *Ann Intern Med* 1988; **108:** 238–51.

Preparations

USP 23: Norfloxacin Tablets.

Proprietary Preparations (details are given in Part 3)
Aust.: Urobacid; Zoroxin; ***Austral.:*** Noroxin; ***Belg.:*** Chibroxol; Zoroxin; ***Canad.:*** Noroxin; ***Fr.:*** Chibroxine; Noroxine; ***Ger.:*** Barazan; Chibroxin; ***Ital.:*** Flossac; Fulgram; Noroxin; Sebercim; Utinor; ***Jpn:*** Baccidal; ***Neth.:*** Chibroxol; Noroxin; ***S.Afr.:*** Noroxin; ***Spain:*** Amicrobin; Baccidal; Chibroxin; Esclebin; Espeden; Nalion; Noroxin; Senro; Uroctal; Vicnas; ***Swed.:*** Lexinor; ***Switz.:*** Chibroxol; Noroxin; ***UK:*** Noroxin†; Utinor; ***USA:*** Chibroxin; Noroxin.

Novobiocin (115-h)

Novobiocin *(BAN, rINN)*.

Crystallinic Acid; PA-93; Streptonivicin; U-6591. 4-Hydroxy-3-[4-hydroxy-3-(3-methylbut-2-enyl)benzamido]-8-methylcoumarin-7-yl 3-*O*-carbamoyl-5,5-di-*C*-methyl-α-L-lyxofuranoside.

$C_{31}H_{36}N_2O_{11}$ = 612.6.

CAS — 303-81-1.

An antimicrobial substance produced by the growth of *Streptomyces niveus* and *S. spheroides* or related organisms.

Novobiocin Calcium (116-m)

Novobiocin Calcium *(BANM, rINNM)*.

Calcium Novobiocin; Novobiocinum Calcium.

$(C_{31}H_{35}N_2O_{11})_2Ca$ = 1263.3.

CAS — 4309-70-0.

Novobiocin Sodium (117-b)

Novobiocin Sodium *(BANM, rINNM)*.

Novobiocinum Natricum; Sodium Novobiocin.

$C_{31}H_{35}N_2NaO_{11}$ = 634.6.

CAS — 1476-53-5.

Pharmacopoeias. In *Fr., Int.,* and *US.*

White or yellowish-white, odourless, hygroscopic crystalline powder. It contains not less than the equivalent of 850 µg per mg of novobiocin, calculated on the dried substance. 1.04 g of monograph substance is approximately equivalent to 1 g of novobiocin. Each g of monograph substance represents about 1.6 mmol of sodium. Freely **soluble** in water, alcohol, methyl alcohol, glycerol, and propylene glycol; slightly soluble in butyl acetate; practically insoluble in acetone, chloroform, or ether. A 2.5% solution in water has a pH of 6.5 to 8.5. **Store** in airtight containers.

Novobiocin is an antimicrobial which is structurally related to coumarin. It is active against Gram-positive bacteria such as *Staphylococcus aureus* (including methicillin-resistant strains) and other staphylococci; the enterococci are usually resistant. Some Gram-negative organisms including *Haemophilus influenzae* and *Neisseria* spp. are also susceptible, as are some strains of *Proteus*, but most of the Enterobacteriaceae are resistant. Its action is primarily bacteriostatic, although it may be bactericidal against more sensitive species at high concentrations. It is an inhibitor of DNA gyrase and is effective in eliminating plasmids, but resistance to novobiocin develops readily *in vitro* and during therapy.

Although novobiocin has been used alone or with other drugs such as rifampicin or tetracycline in the treatment of infections due to staphylococci and other susceptible organisms, it has been largely superseded by other drugs because of the problems of resistance and toxicity.

Novobiocin is a potent sensitiser and hypersensitivity reactions are relatively common; they include rashes, fever, and pruritus, and more serious reactions such as Stevens-Johnson syndrome and pneumonitis. Jaundice and liver damage have occurred, although apparent jaundice may be due to a yellow metabolite of the drug rather than hyperbilirubinaemia. Other adverse effects include eosinophilia, leucopenia, thrombocytopenia, and haemolytic anaemia; gastro-intestinal disturbances are common.

Porphyria. Novobiocin has been associated with clinical exacerbations of porphyria and is considered unsafe in porphyric patients.[1]

1. Moore MR, McColl KEL. *Porphyria: drug lists.* Glasgow: Porphyria Research Unit, University of Glasgow, 1991.

Preparations

USP 23: Novobiocin Sodium Capsules.

Proprietary Preparations (details are given in Part 3)
USA: Albamycin.

Multi-ingredient: ***Spain:*** Tetra Tripsin.

Ofloxacin (16935-w)

Ofloxacin *(BAN, USAN, rINN)*.

DL-8280; HOE-280. (±)-9-Fluoro-2,3-dihydro-3-methyl-10-(4-methyl-1-piperazinyl)-7-oxo-7*H*-pyrido[1,2,3-*de*]-1,4-benzoxazine-6-carboxylic acid.

$C_{18}H_{20}FN_3O_4$ = 361.4.

CAS — 82419-36-1; 83380-47-6.

Pharmacopoeias. In *US.*

Protect from light.

Adverse Effects and Precautions

As for Ciprofloxacin, p.186.

Interactions

As for Ciprofloxacin, p.187.

Antimicrobial Action

As for Ciprofloxacin, p.187.

Ofloxacin is more active than ciprofloxacin against *Chlamydia trachomatis*. It is also active against *Mycobacterium leprae* as well as *M. tuberculosis* and some other *Mycobacterium* spp. Synergistic activity against *M. leprae* has been reported between ofloxacin and rifabutin.

The optically active *S*-(–)-isomer levofloxacin (p.221) has twice the activity of the racemate ofloxacin.

Resistance has been reported in some strains of *Neisseria gonorrhoeae*.

References.

1. Dhople AM, *et al.* In vitro synergistic activity between ofloxacin and ansamycins against Mycobacterium leprae. *Arzneimittelforschung* 1993; **43:** 384–6.
2. Kam K-M, *et al.* Ofloxacin susceptibilities of 5667 Neisseria gonorrhoea strains isolated in Hong Kong. *Antimicrob Agents Chemother* 1993; **37:** 2007–8.
3. Kam KM, *et al.* Quinolone-resistant Neisseria gonorrhoeae in Hong Kong. *Sex Transm Dis* 1996; **23:** 103–8.
4. Cambau E, *et al.* Multidrug-resistance to dapsone, rifampicin, and ofloxacin in Mycobacterium leprae. *Lancet* 1997; **349:** 103–4.

Pharmacokinetics

Ofloxacin is rapidly and well absorbed from the gastro-intestinal tract. Oral bioavailability is almost 100% and a peak plasma concentration of 3 to 4 μg per mL is achieved 1 to 2 hours after a dose of 400 mg by mouth. Absorption may be delayed by the presence of food, but the extent of absorption is not substantially affected. The plasma half-life ranges from 5 to 8 hours; in renal impairment values of 15 to 60 hours have been reported.

About 25% is bound to plasma proteins. Ofloxacin is widely distributed in body fluids, including the CSF, and tissue penetration is good. It crosses the placenta and is distributed into breast milk. Relatively high concentrations are achieved in bile.

There is limited metabolism to desmethyl and *N*-oxide metabolites; desmethyl ofloxacin has moderate antibacterial activity. However, ofloxacin is eliminated mainly by the kidneys. Excretion is by tubular secretion and glomerular filtration and 75 to 80% of a dose is excreted unchanged in the urine over 24 to 48 hours, resulting in high urinary concentrations. Less than 5% is excreted in the urine as metabolites. From 4 to 8% of a dose may be excreted in the faeces.

Only small amounts of ofloxacin are removed by haemodialysis.

References.

1. Lamp KC, *et al.* Ofloxacin clinical pharmacokinetics. *Clin Pharmacokinet* 1992; **22:** 32–46.
2. Flor SC, *et al.* Bioequivalence of oral and intravenous ofloxacin after multiple-dose administration to healthy male volunteers. *Antimicrob Agents Chemother* 1993; **37:** 1468–72.
3. Nau R, *et al.* Kinetics of ofloxacin and its metabolites in cerebrospinal fluid after a single intravenous infusion of 400 milligrams of ofloxacin. *Antimicrob Agents Chemother* 1994; **38:** 1849–53.
4. Tang-Liu DD-S, *et al.* Comparative tear concentrations over time of ofloxacin and tobramycin in human eyes. *Clin Pharmacol Ther* 1994; **55:** 284–92.
5. Bethell DB, *et al.* Pharmacokinetics of oral and intravenous ofloxacin in children with multidrug-resistant typhoid fever. *Antimicrob Agents Chemother* 1996; **40:** 2167–72.
6. Dermaz B, *et al.* Aqueous humor penetration of topically applied ciprofloxacin, ofloxacin and tobramycin. *Arzneimittelforschung* 1997; **47:** 413–15.
7. McMullin CM, *et al.* The pharmacokinetics of once-daily oral 400 mg ofloxacin in patients with peritonitis complicating continuous ambulatory peritoneal dialysis. *J Antimicrob Chemother* 1997; **39:** 829–31.

Uses and Administration

Ofloxacin is a fluoroquinolone antibacterial used similarly to ciprofloxacin (p.188). It is also used in chlamydial infections such as nongonococcal urethritis (p.149) and in the treatment of mycobacterial infections such as leprosy (p.128).

Ofloxacin is given by mouth as the base or intravenously as the hydrochloride. All doses are expressed in terms of the base.

The adult oral or intravenous dose ranges from 200 mg daily to 400 mg twice daily depending on the severity and the nature of the infection. Oral doses up to 400 mg may be given as a single dose, preferably in the morning. For intravenous use a 0.2% solution is infused over 30 minutes or a 0.4% solution over 60 minutes. A single 400-mg dose may be given by mouth for uncomplicated gonorrhoea. A dose of 400 mg daily by mouth has been recommended (by WHO) as part of an alternative multidrug therapy regimen for leprosy.

Lower doses may be necessary in patients with impaired renal function. Following a normal initial dose, subsequent doses are halved to 100 to 200 mg daily or the usual dose is given every 24 hours in patients with a creatinine clearance of 20 to 50 mL per minute and reduced to 100 mg every 24 hours when the creatinine clearance is less than 20 mL per minute. Patients on dialysis may be given 100 mg every 24 hours.

Ofloxacin is also employed as 0.3% eye drops.

Reviews.

1. Todd PA, Faulds D. Ofloxacin: a reappraisal of its antimicrobial activity, pharmacology and therapeutic use. *Drugs* 1991; **42:** 825–76.

Preparations

Proprietary Preparations (details are given in Part 3)
Aust.: Floxal; Tarivid; ***Austral.:*** Ocuflox; Oflocet; ***Belg.:*** Tarivid; Trafloxal; ***Canad.:*** Floxin; Ocuflox; ***Fr.:*** Exocine; Oflocet; ***Ger.:*** Floxal; Tarivid; Uro-Tarivid; ***Irl.:*** Exocin; Tarivid; ***Ital.:*** Exocin; Flobacin; Oflocin; ***Jpn:*** Tarivid; ***Neth.:*** Tarivid; Trafloxal; ***Norw.:*** Tarivid; ***S.Afr.:*** Exocin; Tarivid; ***Spain:*** Oflovir; Surnox; Tarivid; ***Swed.:*** Tarivid; ***Switz.:*** Floxal; Tarivid; ***UK:*** Exocin; Tarivid; ***USA:*** Floxin; Ocuflox.

Oleandomycin Phosphate (118-v)

Oleandomycin Phosphate *(BANM, rINNM)*.

PA-105 (oleandomycin).

(2*R*,3*S*,4*R*,5*S*,6*S*,8*R*,10*R*,11*S*,12*R*,13*R*)-3-(2,6-Dideoxy-3-*O*-methyl-α-L-*arabino*-hexopyranosyloxy)-8,8-epoxymethano-11-hydroxy-2,4,6,10,12,13-hexamethyl-9-oxo-5-(3,4,6-trideoxy-3-dimethylamino-β-D-*xylo*-hexopyranosyloxy)tridecan-13-olide phosphate.

$C_{35}H_{61}NO_{12},H_3PO_4$ = 785.9.

CAS — 3922-90-5 (oleandomycin); 7060-74-4 (oleandomycin phosphate).

Oleandomycin is a macrolide antibiotic produced by the growth of certain strains of *Streptomyces antibioticus* with actions and uses similar to those of erythromycin (p.204). It has antimicrobial activity weaker than that of erythromycin. It has been given by mouth or intravenously as the phosphate.

The triacetyl ester, triacetyloleandomycin (p.265), has also been used.

Ormetoprim (6350-z)

Ormetoprim *(USAN, rINN)*.

NSC-95072; Ro-5-9754. 5-(4,5-Dimethoxy-2-methylphenyl)methyl-2,4-pyrimidinediamine.

$C_{14}H_{18}N_4O_2$ = 274.3.

CAS — 6981-18-6.

Ormetoprim is a diaminopyrimidine antibacterial used in veterinary medicine in combination with sulphadimethoxine.

Oxacillin Sodium (119-g)

Oxacillin Sodium *(BANM, USAN, rINNM)*.

(5-Methyl-3-phenyl-4-isoxazolyl)penicillin Sodium; Oxacillinum Natricum; Oxacillinum Natrium; P-12; SQ-16423. Sodium (6*R*)-6-(5-methyl-3-phenylisoxazole-4-carboxamido)-penicillanate monohydrate.

$C_{19}H_{18}N_3NaO_5S,H_2O$ = 441.4.

CAS — 66-79-5 (oxacillin); 1173-88-2 (oxacillin sodium, anhydrous); 7240-38-2 (oxacillin sodium, monohydrate).

Pharmacopoeias. In Chin. and US.

A fine white crystalline powder, odourless or with a slight odour. 1.1 g of monograph substance is approximately equivalent to 1 g of anhydrous oxacillin. Each g of monograph substance represents about 2.3 mmol of sodium.

Freely **soluble** in water, in methyl alcohol, and in dimethyl sulphoxide; slightly soluble in dehydrated alcohol and in chloroform; practically insoluble in ether and in ethyl acetate. A 3% solution in water has a pH of 4.5 to 7.5. **Store** at a temperature between 15° and 30° in airtight containers.

Oxacillin sodium has been reported to be **incompatible** with aminoglycosides and tetracyclines.

Adverse Effects and Precautions

As for Flucloxacillin, p.209.

Effects on the liver. References.

1. Onorato IM, Axelrod JL. Hepatitis from intravenous high-dose oxacillin therapy: findings in an adult inpatient population. *Ann Intern Med* 1978; **89:** 497–500.
2. Saliba B, Herbert PN. Oxacillin hepatotoxicity in HIV-infected patients. *Ann Intern Med* 1994; **120:** 1048.

Interactions

As for Benzylpenicillin, p.160.

Antimicrobial Action

As for Flucloxacillin, p.209.

The isolation of pneumococci resistant to oxacillin but sensitive to benzylpenicillin has been reported.[1,2] The resistance was due to acquisition of a low-affinity penicillin-binding protein and conferred cross-resistance to methicillin and cloxacillin, and, to a lesser degree, to cefotaxime.

1. Johnson AP, *et al.* Oxacillin-resistant pneumococci sensitive to penicillin. *Lancet* 1993; **341:** 1222.
2. Dowson CG, *et al.* Genetics of oxacillin resistance in clinical isolates of Streptococcus pneumoniae that are oxacillin resistant and penicillin susceptible. *Antimicrob Agents Chemother* 1994; **38:** 49–53.

Pharmacokinetics

Oxacillin is incompletely absorbed from the gastro-intestinal tract. Absorption is reduced by the presence of food in the stomach and is less than with cloxacillin. Peak plasma concentrations of 3 to 6 μg per mL have been achieved 1 hour after a dose of 500 mg given by mouth to fasting subjects. Following the intramuscular injection of 500 mg peak plasma concentrations of up to 15 μg per mL have been achieved after 30 minutes. Doubling the dose can double the plasma concentration. About 93% of the oxacillin in the circulation is bound to plasma proteins. Oxacillin has been reported to have a plasma half-life of 0.5 to 1 hour. The half-life is prolonged in neonates.

The distribution of oxacillin into body tissues and fluids is similar to that of cloxacillin (p.195).

Oxacillin undergoes some metabolism, and the unchanged drug and metabolites are excreted in the urine by glomerular filtration and renal tubular secretion.

About 20 to 30% of an oral dose and more than 40% of an intramuscular dose is rapidly excreted in the urine. Oxacillin is also excreted in the bile.

Plasma concentrations are enhanced if probenecid is given.

Uses and Administration

Oxacillin is an isoxazolyl penicillin used similarly to flucloxacillin (p.209) in the treatment of infections due to staphylococci resistant to benzylpenicillin.

Oxacillin is administered by mouth as the sodium salt, preferably at least 1 hour before or 2 hours after meals, or by injection. Doses are expressed in terms of the equivalent amount of oxacillin. Usual oral doses are 500 mg to 1 g of oxacillin every 4 to 6 hours. Similar doses may be given by intramuscular injection, by slow intravenous injection over about 10 minutes, or by intravenous infusion.

Children weighing less than 40 kg may be given 50 to 100 mg per kg body-weight daily in divided doses by mouth or parenterally.

Doses may be increased in severe infections.

Preparations

USP 23: Oxacillin for Injection; Oxacillin Injection; Oxacillin Sodium Capsules; Oxacillin Sodium for Oral Solution.

Proprietary Preparations (details are given in Part 3)
Aust.: Stapenor; ***Belg.:*** Penstapho; ***Fr.:*** Bristopen; ***Ger.:*** Stapenor; ***Ital.:*** Penstapho; ***USA:*** Bactocill; Prostaphlin†.

Multi-ingredient: ***Aust.:*** Optocillin; Totocillin†; ***Ger.:*** Optocillin; Totocillin†.

Oxolinic Acid (5665-m)

Oxolinic Acid *(BAN, USAN, rINN).*

Acidum Oxolinicum; NSC-110364; W-4565. 5-Ethyl-5,8-dihydro-8-oxo-1,3-dioxolo[4,5-g]quinoline-7-carboxylic acid.

$C_{13}H_{11}NO_5$ = 261.2.

CAS — 14698-29-4.

Pharmacopoeias. In *Eur.* (see p.viii).

An almost white or pale yellow crystalline powder. Practically **insoluble** in water and in alcohol; very slightly soluble in dichloromethane; dissolves in dilute solutions of alkali hydroxides. **Protect** from light.

Oxolinic acid is a 4-quinolone antibacterial with properties similar to those of nalidixic acid (p.228), although adverse effects on the CNS may be more frequent. It is given in the treatment of urinary-tract infections in a usual dose of 750 mg by mouth every 12 hours, preferably after food.

Preparations

Proprietary Preparations (details are given in Part 3)
Belg.: Uritrate; ***Fr.:*** Urotrate; ***Ital.:*** Ossian†; Pelvis†; Tilvis†; Tiurasin†; Uritrate†; ***Spain:*** Oribiox; Oxoinex.

Oxytetracycline (121-d)

Oxytetracycline *(BAN, rINN).*

Glomycin; Hydroxytetracycline; Oxytetracyclinum; Riomitsin; Terrafungine. 4S,4aR,5S,5aR,6S,12aS-4-Dimethylamino-1,4,4a,5,5a,6,11,12a-octahydro-3,5,6,10,12,12a-hexahydroxy-6-methylene-1,11-dioxonaphthacene-2-carboxamide; 5β-Hydroxytetracycline.

$C_{22}H_{24}N_2O_9$ = 460.4.

CAS — 79-57-2 (anhydrous oxytetracycline); 6153-64-6 (oxytetracycline dihydrate).

Pharmacopoeias. In *Eur.* (see p.viii), which specifies a variable amount of water; *Pol.* and *US* allow the anhydrous substance or the dihydrate ($C_{22}H_{24}N_2O_9,2H_2O$ = 496.5); *Int.* includes the dihydrate.

An antimicrobial substance produced by the growth of certain strains of *Streptomyces rimosus*, or by any other means. It contains a variable quantity of water. It occurs as an odourless yellow to tan-coloured crystalline powder. Stable in air but darkens on exposure to strong sunlight. Oxytetracycline dihydrate 1.08 g is approximately equivalent to 1 g of oxytetracycline.

Soluble 1 in 4150 of water, 1 in 66 of dehydrated alcohol, and 1 in 6250 of ether; sparingly soluble in alcohol; freely soluble in dilute acids and alkalis. A 1% suspension in water has a pH of 4.5 to 7.5. It deteriorates in solutions having a pH of less than 2 and is rapidly destroyed by alkali hydroxide solutions. **Store** in airtight containers. Protect from light.

Oxytetracycline Calcium (120-f)

Oxytetracycline Calcium *(BANM, rINNM).*

$C_{44}H_{46}CaN_4O_{18}$ = 958.9.

CAS — 15251-48-6 (xCa).

Pharmacopoeias. In *Br.* and *US.*

A pale yellow to greenish-fawn or light brown crystalline powder. Oxytetracycline calcium 1.04 g is approximately equivalent to 1 g of oxytetracycline.

Practically **insoluble** in water; soluble 1 in more than 1000 of alcohol, chloroform, and ether; soluble in dilute acids and in dilute solutions of sodium hydroxide; dissolves slowly in dilute ammonia solution. A 2.5% suspension in water has a pH of about 6.0 to 8.0. **Store** at a temperature not exceeding 15° in airtight containers. Protect from light.

Oxytetracycline Hydrochloride (122-n)

Oxytetracycline Hydrochloride *(BANM, rINNM).*

Oxytetracyclini Hydrochloridum.

$C_{22}H_{24}N_2O_9,HCl$ = 496.9.

CAS — 2058-46-0.

Pharmacopoeias. In *Chin., Eur.* (see p.viii), *Int., Jpn, Pol.,* and *US.*

A yellow, odourless, hygroscopic, crystalline powder. Oxytetracycline hydrochloride 1.08 g is approximately equivalent to 1 g of oxytetracycline. It decomposes above 180°. It darkens on exposure to sunlight or to moist air above 90°, but there is little loss of potency.

Freely **soluble** in water; sparingly soluble in alcohol and in methyl alcohol; less soluble in dehydrated alcohol; practically insoluble in chloroform and in ether. A 1% solution in water has a pH of 2.0 to 3.0.

Solutions in water become turbid on standing owing to hydrolysis and precipitation of oxytetracycline base. Oxytetracycline hydrochloride deteriorates in solutions having a pH of less than 2 and is rapidly destroyed by alkali hydroxide solutions. **Store** in airtight containers. Protect from light.

Incompatibilities. Oxytetracycline injections have an acid pH and incompatibility may reasonably be expected with alkaline preparations, or with drugs unstable at low pH. Tetracyclines can chelate metal cations to produce insoluble complexes, and incompatibility has been reported with solutions containing metallic salts.

Reports of incompatibility are not always consistent, and other factors, such as the strength and composition of the vehicles used, may play a role.

Adverse Effects and Precautions

As for Tetracycline Hydrochloride, p.259.

Oxytetracycline may produce less tooth discoloration than some other tetracyclines but gastro-intestinal symptoms tend to be more severe.

Porphyria. For the suggestion that oxytetracycline might be porphyrinogenic, see under Tetracycline Hydrochloride, p.260.

Interactions

As for Tetracycline Hydrochloride, p.260.

Antimicrobial Action

As for Tetracycline Hydrochloride, p.260. It is somewhat less active against many organisms.

Pharmacokinetics

As for Tetracycline Hydrochloride, p.260. A dose of 500 mg every 6 hours by mouth is reported to produce steady-state plasma concentrations of 3 to 4 μg per mL.

Uses and Administration

Oxytetracycline is a tetracycline derivative with actions and uses similar to those of tetracycline (p.261).

Oxytetracycline dihydrate or hydrochloride are usually used in tablets and capsules, and for injections, and the calcium salt in aqueous oral suspensions; all three are also used in topical preparations. Doses have been expressed as anhydrous oxytetracycline, the dihydrate, or the hydrochloride but in practice this appears to make little difference.

Oxytetracycline is usually given in doses of 250 to 500 mg four times daily by mouth, usually one hour before food or 2 hours after food. Older children have been given 25 to 50 mg per kg body-weight daily by mouth, in 4 divided doses, but the effect of tetracyclines on teeth and bones should be considered.

Oxytetracycline is sometimes given intramuscularly, in doses of 250 to 300 mg daily, but this route may be painful and produces lower blood concentrations than oral administration in the recommended doses. It has also been given by intravenous infusion, in usual doses of 250 to 500 mg every 12 hours, although up to 2 g daily in divided doses may be given.

Oxytetracycline and its salts have been applied topically, often in combination with other agents, as a variety of eye and ear drops, ointments, creams, and sprays.

Preparations

BP 1998: Oxytetracycline Capsules; Oxytetracycline Tablets;
USP 23: Oxytetracycline and Nystatin Capsules; Oxytetracycline and Nystatin for Oral Suspension; Oxytetracycline and Phenazopyridine Hydrochlorides and Sulfamethizole Capsules; Oxytetracycline Calcium Oral Suspension; Oxytetracycline for Injection; Oxytetracycline Hydrochloride and Hydrocortisone Acetate Ophthalmic Suspension; Oxytetracycline Hydrochloride and Hydrocortisone Ointment; Oxytetracycline Hydrochloride and Polymyxin B Sulfate Ointment; Oxytetracycline Hydrochloride and Polymyxin B Sulfate Ophthalmic Ointment; Oxytetracycline Hydrochloride and Polymyxin B Sulfate Topical Powder; Oxytetracycline Hydrochloride and Polymyxin B Sulfate Vaginal Tablets; Oxytetracycline Hydrochloride Capsules; Oxytetracycline Injection; Oxytetracycline Tablets.

Proprietary Preparations (details are given in Part 3)
Aust.: Tetra-Tablinen; ***Belg.:*** Terramycine†; ***Fr.:*** Innolyre†; Posicycline; Terramycine Solu-Retard; Terramycine†; ***Ger.:*** Aknin†; BTH-S (Broncho-Tetra-Holz)†; duratetracyclin†; Macocyn†; Tetra-Tablinen; Tetracycletten N†; ***Irl.:*** Berkmycen; Clinimycin; Imperacin†; ***Norw.:*** Oxy-Dumocyclin†; Oxytetral; ***S.Afr.:*** Acu-Oxytet; Be-Oxytet; Betacycline†; Cotet†; Dynoxytet; O-4 Cycline; O-Tet; Oxy; Oxymycin†; Oxypan; Rocap; Roxy; Spectratet; Terramycin†; Tetracem; Tetramel; ***Spain:*** Terramicina; ***Swed.:*** Oxy-Dumocyclin†; Oxytetral; ***Switz.:*** Aknin†; Terramycine†; ***UK:*** Berkmycen; Imperacin†; Oxymycin; Oxytetramix; Terramycin; ***USA:*** Terramycin; Uri-Tet†.

Multi-ingredient: ***Aust.:*** Bisolvomycin; Terra-Cortril; Terra-Cortril mit Gentamicin; Terra-Cortril mit Polymyxin B-Sulfat; Terramycin mit Polymyxin-B-Sulfat; Tetra-Gelomyrtol; ***Belg.:*** Eoline; Terra-Cortril; Terramycine; ***Fr.:*** Auricularum; Primyxine; Ster-Dex; Tetranase; ***Ger.:*** Bisolvomycin; BTH-N Broncho-Tetra-Holz†; Corti Biciron N; Incut†; Oxy Biciron; Terracortril; Terramycin; Tetra-Gelomyrtol; ***Irl.:*** Terra-Cortril; Terra-Cortril Nystatin; ***Ital.:*** Bisolvomicin†; Chemyterral†; Cosmiciclina; Geomix†; Proteroxyna†; Terramicina con Polimixina B Pomata Dermica†; ***Neth.:*** Terra-Cortril Gel Steraject met polymyxine-B; Terra-Cortril met polymyxine-B; Terra-Cortril†; Terramycin met polymyxine-B; ***Norw.:*** Corticyklin†; Terra-Cortril; Terra-Cortril Polymyxin B; Terramycin Polymyxin B; ***S.Afr.:*** Bisolvomycin; Cotet; Terra-Cortril; Terramycin; Vernacycline-V†; ***Spain:*** Bisolvon Ciclina†; Bronquinflamatoria†; Coliriocilina Espectro; Pulmonilo Synergium; Terra-Cortril; Terramicina; ***Swed.:*** Terracortril; Terracortril med polymyxin B; Terramycin Polymyxin B; ***Switz.:*** Terracortril; Terramycine; ***UK:*** Terra-Cortril; Terra-Cortril Nystatin; Terra-Cortril†; Trimovate; ***USA:*** Terra-Cortril; Terramycin with Polymyxin B†; Urobiotic-250†.

Panipenem (15342-d)

Panipenem *(rINN).*

(+)-(5R,6S)-3-[[(S)-1-Acetimidoyl-3-pyrrolidinyl]thio}-6-[(R)-1-hydroxyethyl]-7-oxo-1-azabicyclo[3.2.0]hept-2-ene-2-carboxylic acid.

$C_{15}H_{21}N_3O_4S$ = 339.4.

CAS — 87726-17-8.

Panipenem is a carbapenem beta-lactam antibiotic similar to imipenem (p.216). It is given by injection in combination with betamipron (p.161) to reduce adverse renal effects.

Preparations

Proprietary Preparations (details are given in Part 3)
Multi-ingredient: ***Jpn:*** Carbenin.

Paromomycin Sulphate (123-h)

Paromomycin Sulphate *(BANM, rINNM).*

Aminosidin Sulphate; Aminosidine Sulphate; Catenulin Sulphate; Crestomycin Sulphate; Estomycin Sulphate; Hydroxymycin Sulphate; Monomycin A Sulphate; Neomycin E Sulphate; Paucimycin Sulphate. O-2,6-Diamino-2,6-dideoxy-β-L-idopyranosyl-(1→3)-O-β-D-ribofuranosyl-(1→5)-O-[2-amino-2-deoxy-α-D-glucopyranosyl-(1→4)]-2-deoxystreptamine sulphate.

$C_{23}H_{45}N_5O_{14},xH_2SO_4$ = 615.6 (paromomycin).

CAS — 7542-37-2; 59-04-1 (both paromomycin); 1263-89-4 (paromomycin sulphate).

Pharmacopoeias. In *Chin., Int., It.,* and *US.*

A mixture of the sulphates of the antimicrobial substances produced by the growth of certain strains of *Streptomyces rimosus* var. *paromomycinus.*

A creamy-white to light yellow, odourless or almost odourless, hygroscopic powder. It loses not more than 5% of its weight on drying. Very **soluble** in water; practically insoluble in alcohol, chloroform, and ether. A 3% solution in water has a pH of 5.0 to 7.5. **Store** in airtight containers.

Adverse Effects, Treatment, and Precautions

As for Neomycin Sulphate, p.229.

Effects on the pancreas. Pancreatitis was associated with paromomycin administration during treatment of cryptosporidiosis in a patient with HIV infection.[1]

1. Tan WW, *et al.* Paromomycin-associated pancreatitis in HIV-related cryptosporidiosis. *Ann Pharmacother* 1995; **29:** 22–4.

Interactions

As for Neomycin Sulphate, p.229.

Antimicrobial Action

Paromomycin has an antibacterial spectrum similar to that of neomycin (p.229) but is also active against some protozoa, including *Leishmania* spp., *Entamoeba histolytica*, and *Cryptosporidium* spp., and has anthelmintic properties against tapeworms.

There is cross-resistance between paromomycin and kanamycin, framycetin, neomycin, and streptomycin.

Antimycobacterial activity. References.

1. Kanyok TP, *et al.* Activity of aminosidine (paromomycin) for Mycobacterium tuberculosis and Mycobacterium avium. *J Antimicrob Chemother* 1994; **33:** 323–7.
2. Piersimoni C, *et al.* Bacteriostatic and bactericidal activities of paromomycin against Mycobacterium avium complex isolates. *J Antimicrob Chemother* 1994; **34:** 421–4.
3. Kanyok TP, *et al.* In vivo activity of paromomycin against susceptible and multidrug-resistant Mycobacterium tuberculosis and M. avium complex strains. *Antimicrob Agents Chemother* 1994; **38:** 170–3.

Pharmacokinetics

Paromomycin is poorly absorbed from the gastro-intestinal tract and most of the dose is eliminated unchanged in the faeces.

Uses and Administration

Paromomycin is an aminoglycoside antibiotic that has been administered by mouth as the sulphate in the treatment of intestinal protozoal infections, including amoebiasis, cryptosporidiosis, and giardiasis. It has also been tried parenterally for visceral, and topically for cutaneous, leishmaniasis. For details of these infections and their treatment, see under Choice of Antiprotozoal, p.573. It has also been used in the treatment of tapeworm infection but it is not the treatment of choice (see Taeniasis, p.96), and, similarly to neomycin (p.230), has been used in the suppression of intestinal flora both pre-operatively and in the management of hepatic encephalopathy.

In intestinal amoebiasis a recommended dose for both adults and children is the equivalent of 25 to 35 mg of paromomycin per kg body-weight daily in 3 divided doses with meals for 5 to 10 days. Similar doses have been tried in cryptosporidiosis.

In taeniasis and other tapeworm infections, a dose of 1 g every 15 minutes to a total of 4 g has been given, except for infection due to *Hymenolepis nana*, in which 45 mg per kg has been given daily as a single dose for 5 to 7 days.

A suggested dose for hepatic encephalopathy is 4 g daily given in divided doses at regular intervals for 5 to 6 days.

Preparations

USP 23: Paromomycin Sulfate Capsules; Paromomycin Sulfate Syrup.

Proprietary Preparations (details are given in Part 3)
Aust.: Humatin; ***Belg.:*** Gabbroral; ***Canad.:*** Humatin; ***Fr.:*** Humagel†; ***Ger.:*** Humatin; ***Ital.:*** Gabbroral; Humatin; Sinosid†; ***Spain:*** Gabbroral†; Humagel†; Humatin; ***Switz.:*** Humatin; ***USA:*** Humatin.

Pefloxacin Mesylate (10363-e)

Pefloxacin Mesylate *(BANM, USAN).*

Pefloxacin Mesilate *(rINNM)*; EU-5306 (pefloxacin); 1589-RB (pefloxacin); 41982-RP. 1-Ethyl-6-fluoro-1,4-dihydro-7-(4-methyl-1-piperazinyl)-4-oxo-3-quinolinecarboxylic acid methanesulphonate dihydrate.

$C_{17}H_{20}FN_3O_3,CH_4O_3S,2H_2O$ = 465.5.

CAS — 70458-92-3 (pefloxacin); 70458-95-6 (pefloxacin mesylate).

Pharmacopoeias. In *Pol.*

Pefloxacin is a fluoroquinolone antibacterial with actions and uses similar to those of ciprofloxacin (p.185). It also has bactericidal activity against *Mycobacterium leprae* and has been tried in the treatment of leprosy (p.128).

Pefloxacin has a longer plasma half-life than ciprofloxacin (about 8 to 13 hours) and is also extensively metabolised, the principal metabolite being *N*-desmethyl pefloxacin which is otherwise known as norfloxacin (p.233).

Pefloxacin is given by mouth or by intravenous infusion as the mesylate in the treatment of susceptible infections. Doses are expressed in terms of the equivalent amount of pefloxacin and are usually 400 mg twice daily by mouth or by intravenous infusion.

Fluoroquinolones have caused adverse effects on the musculoskeletal system (see under Ciprofloxacin, p.186) and in the case of pefloxacin this has led to certain restrictions in some countries.

General references.

1. Gonzalez JP, Henwood JM. Pefloxacin: a review of its antibacterial activity, pharmacokinetic properties and therapeutic use. *Drugs* 1989; **37:** 628–68.
2. Bint AJ, *et al.* eds. Pefloxacin in clinical practice. *J Antimicrob Chemother* 1990; **26**(suppl B): 1–229.

Adverse effects.

1. Chevalier X, *et al.* A case of destructive polyarthropathy in a 17-year-old youth following pefloxacin treatment. *Drug Safety* 1992; **7:** 310–14.
2. Al-Hedaithy MA, Noreddin AM. Hypersensitivity anaphylactoid reaction to pefloxacin in a patient with AIDS. *Ann Pharmacother* 1996; **30:** 612–14.

Pharmacokinetics.

1. Bressolle F, *et al.* Pefloxacin clinical pharmacokinetics. *Clin Pharmacokinet* 1994; **27:** 418–46.

Preparations

Proprietary Preparations (details are given in Part 3)
Aust.: Peflacine†; ***Belg.:*** Peflacine; ***Fr.:*** Peflacine; ***Ger.:*** Peflacin; ***Ital.:*** Peflacin; Peflox; ***Neth.:*** Peflacin†; ***Spain:*** Azuben; Peflacine.

Phenethicillin Potassium (129-p)

Phenethicillin Potassium *(BANM).*

Pheneticillin Potassium *(rINNM)*; Penicillin B; Pheneticillinum Kalicum; Potassium α-Phenoxyethylpenicillin. A mixture of the D(+)- and L(−)-isomers of potassium (6*R*)-6-(2-phenoxypropionamido)penicillanate.

$C_{17}H_{19}KN_2O_5S$ = 402.5.

CAS — 147-55-7 (phenethicillin); 132-93-4 (phenethicillin potassium).

Phenethicillin is a phenoxypenicillin with actions and uses similar to those of phenoxymethylpenicillin (below). It has been given by mouth, as the potassium salt, for the treatment of susceptible mild to moderate infections. Phenethicillin sodium has also been used.

Preparations

Proprietary Preparations (details are given in Part 3)
Austral.: Pensig†; ***Ital.:*** Penicilloral†; ***Neth.:*** Broxil; ***Spain:*** Bendralan†.

Phenoxymethylpenicillin (130-n)

Phenoxymethylpenicillin *(BAN, rINN).*

Fenoximetilpenicilina; Penicillin, Phenoxymethyl; Penicillin V *(USAN)*; Phénomycilline; Phenoxymethyl Penicillin; Phenoxymethylpenicillinum. (6*R*)-6-(2-Phenoxyacetamido)penicillanic acid.

$C_{16}H_{18}N_2O_5S$ = 350.4.

CAS — 87-08-1.

Pharmacopoeias. In *Eur.* (see p.viii), *Int.*, *Pol.*, and *US.*

Phenoxymethylpenicillin is an antimicrobial acid produced by the growth of certain strains of *Penicillium notatum* or related organisms on a culture medium containing an appropriate precursor, or obtained by any other means.

It is a white crystalline slightly hygroscopic powder. Very slightly **soluble** in water; freely soluble in acetone; freely soluble or soluble in alcohol; practically insoluble in fixed oils and liquid paraffin. Suspensions in water have a pH of 2.4 to 4.0. **Store** in airtight containers.

Phenoxymethylpenicillin Calcium (131-h)

Phenoxymethylpenicillin Calcium *(BANM, rINNM).*

Penicillin V Calcium; Phenoxymethylpenicillinum Calcicum.

$(C_{16}H_{17}N_2O_5S)_2Ca,2H_2O$ = 774.9.

CAS — 147-48-8 (anhydrous phenoxymethylpenicillin calcium); 73368-74-8 (phenoxymethylpenicillin calcium dihydrate).

Pharmacopoeias. In *Int.*

A white crystalline powder. 2.2 g of monograph substance is approximately equivalent to 1 g of phenoxymethylpenicillin. Each g of monograph substance represents about 1.3 mmol of calcium.

Phenoxymethylpenicillin Potassium (132-m)

Phenoxymethylpenicillin Potassium *(BANM, rINNM).*

Fenoximetilpenicilina Potássica; Penicillin V Potassium *(USAN)*; Phenoxymethylpenicillinum Kalicum.

$C_{16}H_{17}KN_2O_5S$ = 388.5.

CAS — 132-98-9.

Pharmacopoeias. In *Eur.* (see p.viii), *Int.*, *Jpn*, *Pol.*, and *US.*

A white crystalline powder. 1.1 g of monograph substance is approximately equivalent to 1 g of phenoxymethylpenicillin. Each g of monograph substance represents about 2.6 mmol of potassium.

Freely **soluble** in water; the USP states that it is soluble 1 in 150 of alcohol but the Ph. Eur. claims that it is practically insoluble in alcohol; practically insoluble in acetone, in ether, in fixed oils, and in liquid paraffin. A 0.5% solution in water has a pH of 5.5 to 7.5 and a 3% solution in water has a pH of 4.0 to 7.5. **Store** in airtight containers.

Units

The first International Standard Preparation (1957) of phenoxymethylpenicillin contained 1695 units per mg but was discontinued in 1968. Despite this, doses of phenoxymethylpenicillin are still expressed in units in some countries.

Phenoxymethylpenicillin 250 mg is approximately equivalent to 400 000 units.

Adverse Effects and Precautions

As for Benzylpenicillin, p.159.

Phenoxymethylpenicillin is usually well tolerated but may occasionally cause transient nausea and diarrhoea.

Interactions

As for Benzylpenicillin, p.160.

Guar gum may reduce the absorption of phenoxymethylpenicillin. Reduced absorption was also reported when phenoxymethylpenicillin was given following a course of *neomycin* by mouth.[1] *Beta blockers* might have potentiated anaphylactic reactions in 2 patients on nadolol and propranolol, respectively, who died following a dose of phenoxymethylpenicillin.[2]

1. Cheng SH, White A. Effect of orally administered neomycin on the absorption of penicillin V. *N Engl J Med* 1962; **267:** 1296–7.
2. Berkelman RL, *et al.* Beta-adrenergic antagonists and fatal anaphylactic reactions to oral penicillin. *Ann Intern Med* 1986; **104:** 134.

Antimicrobial Action

Phenoxymethylpenicillin has a range of antimicrobial activity similar to that of benzylpenicillin (p.160) and a similar mode of action. It may be less active against some susceptible organisms particularly Gram-negative bacteria.

The mechanisms and patterns of resistance to phenoxymethylpenicillin are similar to those of benzylpenicillin.

Pharmacokinetics

Phenoxymethylpenicillin is more resistant to inactivation by gastric acid and is more completely absorbed than benzylpenicillin from the gastro-intestinal tract following administration by mouth. Absorption is usually rapid, although variable, with about 60% of an oral dose being absorbed. The calcium and potassium salts are better absorbed than the free acid. Peak plasma concentrations of 3 to 5 µg per mL have been observed 30 to 60 minutes after a dose of 500 mg. The effect of food on absorption appears to be slight. The plasma half-life of phenoxymethylpenicillin is about 30 to 60 minutes and may be increased to about 4 hours in severe renal impairment. About 80% is reported to be protein bound. The distribution and elimination of phenoxymethylpenicillin is similar to that of benzylpenicillin (p.161). It is metabolised in the liver to a greater extent than benzylpenicillin; several metabolites have been identified including penicilloic acid. The unchanged drug and metabolites are excreted rapidly in the urine. Only small amounts are excreted in the bile.

References.

1. Roos K, Brorson J-E. Concentration of phenoxymethylpenicillin in tonsillar tissue. *Eur J Clin Pharmacol* 1990; **39:** 417–18.
2. Sjöberg I, *et al.* Accumulation of penicillin in vaginal fluid. *Obstet Gynecol* 1990; **75:** 18–21.
3. Heikkilä AM, *et al.* The need for adjustment of dosage regimen of penicillin V during pregnancy. *Obstet Gynecol* 1993; **81:** 919–21.

Uses and Administration

Phenoxymethylpenicillin is used similarly to benzylpenicillin (p.161) in the treatment or prophylaxis of infections caused by susceptible organisms, especially streptococci. It is used only for the treatment of mild to moderate infections, and not for chronic, severe, or deep-seated infections since absorption can be unpredictable. Patients treated initially with parenteral benzylpenicillin may continue treatment with phenoxymethylpenicillin by mouth once a satisfactory clinical response has been obtained. Specific indications for phenoxymethylpenicillin include anthrax (mild uncomplicated infections), Lyme disease (early stage in pregnant women or young children), pharyngitis or tonsillitis, rheumatic fever (primary and secondary prophylaxis), streptococcal skin infections, and spleen disorders (pneumococcal infection prophylaxis). For details of these infections and their treatment, see under Choice of Antibacterial, p.116.

Administration and dosage. Phenoxymethylpenicillin is administered by mouth, usually as the potassium or calcium salt, preferably at least 30 minutes before or 2 hours after food. Benzathine phenoxymethylpenicillin (p.159) and hydrabamine phenoxymethylpenicillin have also been used.

Doses are expressed in terms of the equivalent amount of phenoxymethylpenicillin.

Usual adult doses have been 250 to 500 mg every 6 hours, but authorities in the UK now recommend 500 to 750 mg every 6 hours. Children may be given the following doses every 6 hours: up to 1 year, 62.5 mg; 1 to 5 years, 125 mg; and 6 to 12 years, 250 mg. Dosage may need to be modified in severe renal impairment.

To prevent recurrences of rheumatic fever WHO and other authorities recommend 250 mg twice daily.

Preparations

BP 1998: Phenoxymethylpenicillin Oral Solution; Phenoxymethylpenicillin Tablets;
USP 23: Penicillin V for Oral Suspension; Penicillin V Potassium for Oral Solution; Penicillin V Potassium Tablets; Penicillin V Tablets.

Proprietary Preparations (details are given in Part 3)
Aust.: Cliacil; Mack Pen; Megacillin; Ospen; Penbene; Star-Pen; ***Austral.:*** Abbocillin-VK; Cilicaine VK; Cilopen VK; LPV; PVK; ***Belg.:*** Peni-Oral†; ***Canad.:*** Apo-Pen-VK; Ledercillin VK; Nadopen-V; Novo-Pen-VK; Nu-Pen-VK; Pen-Vee; PVFK; V-Cillin K; ***Fr.:*** Oracilline; Ospen; ***Ger.:*** Antibiocin†; Arcasin; Dignopenicillin†; durapenicillin; Infectocillin; Isocillin; Ispenoral; Jenacillin V; Megacillin oral; Ospen†; P-Mega-Tablinen; Pen-BASF; pen-V-basan†; Penbeta; Penhexal; Penicillat; V-Tablopen; ***Irl.:*** Calvepen; V-Cil-K†; ***Ital.:*** Fenospen; ***Neth.:*** Acipen; Acipen-V; ***Norw.:*** Apocillin; Calcipen; Femepen; Rocilin; Weifapenin; ***S.Afr.:*** Betacillin†; Betapen; Copen†; Darocillin; Deltacillin†; Dynapen; Len V.K.; Novo V-K; Oracillin VK†; Orapen†; V-Cil-K; Veekay†; ***Spain:*** Penilevel; ***Swed.:*** Abbopen†; Calciopen; Fenoxypen†; Kavepenin; Penferm†; Roscopenin†; Tikacillin; Vepenicillin†; ***Switz.:*** Arcasin; Brunocilline; Cliacil†; Fenoxypen; Megacilline; Monocilline; Ospen; Penadur VK Mega†; Penisol; Phenocillin; Rivopen-V; Stabicilline; ***UK:*** Apsin VK; Distaquaine V-K; Rimapen; Stabillin V-K†; ***USA:*** Beepen-VK; Betapen-VK†; Ledercillin VK†; Pen-V†; Pen-Vee K; Robicillin VK†; V-Cillin K†; Veetids.

Multi-ingredient: ***Spain:*** Penilevel Retard.

Phthalylsulphathiazole (4912-k)

Phthalylsulphathiazole *(BAN)*.

Phthalylsulfathiazole *(rINN)*; Ftalilsulfatiazol; Phthalazolum; Phthalylsulfathiazolum; Sulfaphtalylthiazol. 4′-(1,3-Thiazol-2-ylsulphamoyl)phthalanilic acid.

$C_{17}H_{13}N_3O_5S_2$ = 403.4.

CAS — 85-73-4.

Pharmacopoeias. In *Eur.* (see p.viii).

White or yellowish-white crystalline powder.

Practically **insoluble** in water and in ether; slightly soluble in alcohol and in acetone; freely soluble in dimethylformamide. **Protect** from light.

Phthalylsulphathiazole is a sulphonamide with properties similar to those of sulphamethoxazole (p.254). It is poorly absorbed, about 95% remaining in the intestine and only about 5% being slowly hydrolysed to sulphathiazole and absorbed.

It is given for its antibacterial action in the gastro-intestinal tract, in combination with other antibacterials, for the treatment of infections and for bowel decontamination before surgery.

Preparations

Proprietary Preparations (details are given in Part 3)
Austral.: Phthazol†; ***Ital.:*** Colicitina†.

Multi-ingredient: ***Aust.:*** Hylakombun; ***Ger.:*** Diaront NN†; ***S.Afr.:*** Diastat†; ***Spain:*** Biocortison†; Cunticina Adultos†; Cunticina Infantil†; Derbitan Antibiotico; Enterowas†; Estreptoenterol; Kolotanino†; Sulfathalidin Estrepto†.

Pipemidic Acid (5666-b)

Pipemidic Acid *(rINN)*.

Piperamic Acid; 1489-RB. 8-Ethyl-5,8-dihydro-5-oxo-2-(piperazin-1-yl)pyrido[2,3-*d*]pyrimidine-6-carboxylic acid.

$C_{14}H_{17}N_5O_3$ = 303.3.

CAS — 51940-44-4.

Pharmacopoeias. In *Chin.* and *Jpn* (both as the trihydrate).

Pipemidic acid is a 4-quinolone antibacterial with properties similar to those of nalidixic acid (p.228), but is more active *in vitro* against some bacteria, including *Pseudomonas aeruginosa*.

Doses of 400 mg (as the trihydrate) by mouth twice daily are used in the treatment of urinary-tract infections.

For the effect of pipemidic acid on the clearance of xanthines, see under Caffeine, p.750, and Theophylline, p.768.

Preparations

Proprietary Preparations (details are given in Part 3)
Aust.: Deblaston; ***Belg.:*** Pipram; ***Fr.:*** Pipram; ***Ger.:*** Deblaston; ***Ital.:*** Acipem; Biopim; Cistomid; Diperpen; Faremid; Filtrax; Impresial†; Pipeacid; Pipedac; Pipedase†; Pipefort; Pipemid; Pipram; Pipurin; Pro-Uro; Solupemid†; Tractur; Urodene; Uropimid; Urosan; Urosetic; Urosten†; Urotractin; Uroval; ***Jpn:*** Dolcol; ***Neth.:*** Pipram; ***S.Afr.:*** Deblaston; Septidron; ***Spain:*** Galusan; Nuril; Urisan; Uropipedil; ***Switz.:*** Deblaston.

Piperacillin (14850-l)

Piperacillin *(BAN, rINN)*.

Piperacillinum. (6*R*)-6-[*R*-2-(4-Ethyl-2,3-dioxopiperazine-1-carboxamido)-2-phenylacetamido]penicillanic acid monohydrate; 3-Dimethyl-7-oxo-4-thia-1-azabicyclo[3.2.0]heptane-2-carboxylic acid monohydrate.

$C_{23}H_{27}N_5O_7S,H_2O$ = 535.6.

CAS — 61477-96-1 (anhydrous piperacillin); 66258-76-2 (piperacillin monohydrate).

Pharmacopoeias. In *Chin., Eur.* (see p.viii), and *US.*

A white or off-white crystalline powder. Very slightly **soluble** or slightly soluble in water; freely or very soluble in methyl alcohol; sparingly soluble in isopropyl alcohol; slightly soluble in ethyl acetate.

Piperacillin Sodium (133-b)

Piperacillin Sodium *(BANM, USAN, rINNM)*.

CL-227193; Piperacillinum Natricum; T-1220.

$C_{23}H_{26}N_5NaO_7S$ = 539.5.

CAS — 59703-84-3.

Pharmacopoeias. In *Eur.* (see p.viii), *Jpn, Pol.,* and *US.*

A white or almost white hygroscopic powder. 1.04 g of monograph substance is approximately equivalent to 1 g of piperacillin. Each g of monograph substance represents 1.85 mmol of sodium. A 40% solution in water has a pH of 5.5 to 7.5. Freely **soluble** in water, in alcohol, and in methyl alcohol; practically insoluble in ethyl acetate. **Store** in airtight containers.

Incompatibility has been reported with aminoglycosides and sodium bicarbonate.

Adverse Effects and Precautions

As for Carbenicillin Sodium, p.162.

As piperacillin sodium has a lower sodium content than carbenicillin sodium, hypernatraemia and hypokalaemia are less likely to occur. Prolongation of bleeding time has been less frequent and less severe than with carbenicillin.

Hypersensitivity. In the mid 1980s there were reports of a relatively high incidence of adverse reactions to piperacillin, especially fever, in patients with cystic fibrosis.[1-3] However, the manufacturers[4] considered such patients to be particularly prone to allergy and cited reactions with other semisynthetic penicillins including carbenicillin and azlocillin.

Similar apparent hypersensitivity reactions have been reported in patients taking high doses of piperacillin and other ureidopenicillins, over long periods for other indications,[5] and with other penicillins in patients with cystic fibrosis,[6] although piperacillin does appear to be most frequently implicated.[6]

1. Stead RJ, *et al.* Adverse reactions to piperacillin in cystic fibrosis. *Lancet* 1984; **i:** 857–8.
2. Strandvik B. Adverse reactions to piperacillin in patients with cystic fibrosis. *Lancet* 1984; **i:** 1362.
3. Stead RJ, *et al.* Adverse reactions to piperacillin in adults with cystic fibrosis. *Thorax* 1985; **40:** 184–6.
4. Brock PG, Roach M. Adverse reactions to piperacillin in cystic fibrosis. *Lancet* 1984; **i:** 1070–1.
5. Lang R, *et al.* Adverse reactions to prolonged treatment with high doses of carbenicillin and ureidopenicillins. *Rev Infect Dis* 1991; **13:** 68–72.
6. Pleasants RA, *et al.* Allergic reactions to parenteral beta-lactam antibiotics in patients with cystic fibrosis. *Chest* 1994; **106:** 1124–8.

Interactions

As for Benzylpenicillin, p.160.

Neuromuscular blockers. Piperacillin and other ureidopenicillins are reported to prolong the action of competitive muscle relaxants such as vecuronium (p.1306).

Antimicrobial Action

Piperacillin has a similar antimicrobial action to carbenicillin (p.162) and ticarcillin (p.263) but is active against a wider range of Gram-negative organisms including *Klebsiella pneumoniae*. It is also generally more active *in vitro*, especially against *Pseudomonas aeruginosa* and the Enterobacteriaceae, against Gram-positive *Enterococcus faecalis* and possibly against *Bacteroides fragilis*. There is, however, an inoculum effect, i.e. minimum inhibitory concentrations of piperacillin increase with the size of the inoculum.

Combinations of piperacillin and aminoglycosides have been shown to be synergistic *in vitro* against *Ps. aeruginosa* and Enterobacteriaceae. The effect of combining piperacillin with other beta lactams has been less predictable. The activity of piperacillin against some organisms, resistant because of the production of beta-lactamases, may be restored by tazobactam, a beta-lactamase inhibitor. Such organisms include beta-lactamase-producing strains of staphylococci, *Escherichia coli*, *Haemophilus influenzae*, and *Bacteroides* spp.; the activity of piperacillin against *Ps. aeruginosa* is not enhanced by tazobactam.

Resistance has developed in *Ps. aeruginosa* during treatment with piperacillin, especially when used alone. There may be some cross-resistance with other antipseudomonal penicillins.

References.

1. Fass RJ, Prior RB. Comparative in vitro activities of piperacillin-tazobactam and ticarcillin-clavulanate. *Antimicrob Agents Chemother* 1989; **33:** 1268–74.
2. Kuck NA, *et al.* Comparative in vitro and in vivo activities of piperacillin combined with the β-lactamase inhibitors tazobactam, clavulanic acid, and sulbactam. *Antimicrob Agents Chemother* 1989; **33:** 1964–9.
3. Higashitani F, *et al.* Inhibition of β-lactamases by tazobactam and in-vitro antibacterial activity of tazobactam combined with piperacillin. *J Antimicrob Chemother* 1990; **25:** 567–74.
4. Mehtar S, *et al.* The in-vitro activity of piperacillin/tazobactam, ciprofloxacin, ceftazidime and imipenem against multiple resistant Gram-negative bacteria. *J Antimicrob Chemother* 1990; **25:** 915–19.
5. Kempers J, MacLaren DM. Piperacillin/tazobactam and ticarcillin/clavulanic acid against resistant Enterobacteriaceae. *J Antimicrob Chemother* 1990; **26:** 598–9.
6. Kadima TA, Weiner JH. Mechanism of suppression of piperacillin resistance in enterobacteria by tazobactam. *Antimicrob Agents Chemother* 1997; **41:** 2177–83.

Pharmacokinetics

Piperacillin is not absorbed from the gastro-intestinal tract. It is well absorbed after intramuscular administration, peak plasma concentrations of 30 to 40 μg per mL being observed 30 to 50 minutes after a dose of 2 g. The pharmacokinetics of piperacillin are reported to be nonlinear and dose-dependent. The plasma half-life is about one hour, but is prolonged in neonates. In patients with severe renal insufficiency there may be a threefold increase in half-life; in those with end-stage renal failure half-lives of 4 to 6 hours have been reported and in those with both renal and hepatic impairment much longer half-lives may result. About 20% of piperacillin in the circulation is bound to plasma proteins.

Piperacillin is widely distributed in body tissues and fluids. It crosses the placenta into the fetal circulation and small amounts are distributed into breast milk. There is little diffusion into the CSF except when the meninges are inflamed.

About 60 to 80% of a dose is excreted unchanged in the urine by glomerular filtration and tubular secretion within 24 hours, achieving high concentrations.

High concentrations are also found in the bile and about 20% of a dose may be excreted by this route.

Plasma concentrations are enhanced if probenecid is administered concomitantly.

Piperacillin is removed by haemodialysis.

Piperacillin with tazobactam. The pharmacokinetics of piperacillin do not appear to be altered by the coadministration of tazobactam, but piperacillin reduces the renal clearance of tazobactam.

References.

1. Heikkilä A, Erkkola R. Pharmacokinetics of piperacillin during pregnancy. *J Antimicrob Chemother* 1991; **28:** 419–23.
2. Wise R, *et al.* Pharmacokinetics and tissue penetration of tazobactam administered alone and with piperacillin. *Antimicrob Agents Chemother* 1991; **35:** 1081–4.
3. Johnson CA, *et al.* Single-dose pharmacokinetics of piperacillin and tazobactam in patients with renal disease. *Clin Pharmacol Ther* 1992; **51:** 32–41.
4. Dupon M, *et al.* Plasma levels of piperacillin and vancomycin used as prophylaxis in liver transplant patients. *Eur J Clin Pharmacol* 1993; **45:** 529–34.
5. Sörgel F, Kinzig M. The chemistry, pharmacokinetics and tissue distribution of piperacillin/tazobactam. *J Antimicrob Chemother* 1993; **31** (suppl A): 39–60.
6. Reed MD, *et al.* Single-dose pharmacokinetics of piperacillin and tazobactam in infants and children. *Antimicrob Agents Chemother* 1994; **38:** 2817–26.
7. Bourget P, *et al.* Clinical pharmacokinetics of piperacillin-tazobactam combination in patients with major burns and signs of infection. *Antimicrob Agents Chemother* 1996; **40:** 139–45.
8. Occhipinti DJ, *et al.* Pharmacokinetics and pharmacodynamics of two multiple-dose piperacillin-tazobactam regimens. *Antimicrob Agents Chemother* 1997; **41:** 2511–17.

Uses and Administration

Piperacillin is a ureidopenicillin that is used similarly to ticarcillin (p.263) for the treatment of infections caused by *Pseudomonas aeruginosa*, and also infections due to other susceptible bacteria (see Antimicrobial Action, above). It has been used particularly in immunocompromised patients (neutropenic patients) and for biliary-tract infections (cholangitis). Other indications have included uncomplicated gonorrhoea due to penicillin-sensitive gonococci, surgical infection prophylaxis, and urinary-tract infections. For details of these infections and their treatment, see under Choice of Antibacterial, p.116.

For the treatment of serious infections piperacillin is commonly given with an aminoglycoside, but they should be administered separately because of possible incompatibility.

Administration and dosage. Piperacillin is given by injection as the sodium salt. Doses are expressed in terms of the equivalent amount of piperacillin. Doses should generally be reduced in moderate to severe renal impairment.

Piperacillin may be administered by slow intravenous injection over 3 to 5 minutes, by intravenous infusion over 20 to 40 minutes, or by deep intramuscular injection. Single doses of more than 2 g for adults or 0.5 g for children should not be given by the intramuscular route.

For the treatment of serious or complicated infections, piperacillin 200 to 300 mg per kg body-weight daily in divided doses may be given intravenously; the usual dose is 4 g every 6 or 8 hours. In life-threatening infections, particularly those caused by *Pseudomonas* or *Klebsiella* spp., it should be given in a dose of not less than 16 g daily. The usual maximum daily dose is 24 g, although this has been exceeded.

For mild or uncomplicated infections, 100 to 150 mg per kg daily may be given; usual doses are 2 g of piperacillin every 6 or 8 hours, or 4 g every 12 hours, by intravenous administration, or 2 g every 8 or 12 hours by intramuscular injection.

Uncomplicated gonorrhoea may be treated by a single intramuscular dose of 2 g. Probenecid 1 g by mouth may be given half an hour before the injection.

For the prophylaxis of infection during surgery, 2 g of piperacillin just before the procedure, or when the umbilical cord is clamped in caesarean section, followed by at least 2 doses of 2 g at intervals of 4 or 6 hours may be given.

The intravenous route is preferred for infants and children. Those aged over 1 month to 12 years may be given 100 to 300 mg per kg body-weight daily in 3 or 4 divided doses. Neonates less than 7 days old or weighing less than 2 kg may be given 150 mg per kg daily in 3 divided doses. Those more than 7 days old and weighing more than 2 kg may be given 300 mg per kg daily in 3 or 4 divided doses.

Piperacillin with tazobactam. Piperacillin has also been administered in association with tazobactam (p.257), a beta-lactamase inhibitor, to widen its antibacterial spectrum to organisms usually resistant because of the production of beta-lactamases. It is given intravenously in a ratio of piperacillin (as the sodium salt) 8 parts to 1 part of tazobactam (as the sodium salt). Doses of the combination, calculated on piperacillin content, are similar to those of piperacillin alone.

References.

1. Greenwood D, Finch RG, eds. Piperacillin/tazobactam: a new β-lactam/β-lactamase inhibitor combination. *J Antimicrob Chemother* 1993; **31** (suppl A): 1–124.
2. Bryson HM, Brogden RN. Piperacillin/tazobactam: a review of its antibacterial activity, pharmacokinetic properties and therapeutic potential. *Drugs* 1994; **47:** 506–35.
3. Schoonover LL, *et al.* Piperacillin/tazobactam: a new beta-lactam/beta-lactamase inhibitor combination. *Ann Pharmacother* 1995; **29:** 501–14.

Preparations

USP 23: Piperacillin for Injection.

Proprietary Preparations (details are given in Part 3)
Aust.: Pipril; ***Austral.:*** Pipril; ***Belg.:*** Pipcil; ***Canad.:*** Pipracil; ***Fr.:*** Piperilline; ***Ger.:*** Pipril; ***Irl.:*** Pipril; ***Ital.:*** Avocin; Eril; Peracil; Picillin; Piperital; Pipracin; ***Neth.:*** Pipcil; ***S.Afr.:*** Pipril; ***Spain:*** Piperzam; Pipril; ***Swed.:*** Ivacin; ***Switz.:*** Pipril; ***UK:*** Pipril; ***USA:*** Pipracil.

Multi-ingredient: ***Aust.:*** Fluxapril; Tazonam; ***Austral.:*** Tazocin; ***Belg.:*** Tazocin; ***Canad.:*** Tazocin; ***Fr.:*** Tazocilline; ***Ger.:*** Fluxapril; Tazobac; ***Irl.:*** Tazocin; ***Ital.:*** Tazobac; Tazocin; ***Neth.:*** Tazocin; ***S.Afr.:*** Tazocin; ***Spain:*** Tazocel; ***Swed.:*** Tazocin; ***Switz.:*** Tazobac; ***UK:*** Tazocin; ***USA:*** Zosyn.

Piromidic Acid (5667-v)

Piromidic Acid *(rINN)*.

PD-93. 8-Ethyl-5,8-dihydro-5-oxo-2-(pyrrolidin-1-yl)pyrido[2,3-*d*]pyrimidine-6-carboxylic acid.

$C_{14}H_{16}N_4O_3$ = 288.3.

CAS — 19562-30-2.

Piromidic acid is a 4-quinolone antibacterial with actions and uses similar to those of nalidixic acid (p.228). It is used in the treatment of susceptible infections in doses of up to 3 g daily by mouth in divided doses.

Preparations

Proprietary Preparations (details are given in Part 3)
Ital.: Enterol†; Enteromix; Pirodal†; Uropir†.

Pivampicillin (188-t)

Pivampicillin *(BAN, rINN)*.

MK-191. Pivaloyloxymethyl (6*R*)-6-(α-D-phenylglycylamino)penicillanate.

$C_{22}H_{29}N_3O_6S$ = 463.5.

CAS — 33817-20-8.

Pharmacopoeias. In *Eur.* (see p.viii).

A white or almost white crystalline powder. 1.3 g of monograph substance is approximately equivalent to 1 g of ampicillin. Practically **insoluble** in water; soluble in dehydrated alcohol; freely soluble in methyl alcohol. It dissolves in dilute acids. **Store** in airtight containers.

Pivampicillin Hydrochloride (135-g)

Pivampicillin Hydrochloride *(BANM, USAN, rINNM)*.

$C_{22}H_{29}N_3O_6S,HCl$ = 500.0.

CAS — 26309-95-5.

1.43 g of monograph substance is approximately equivalent to 1 g of ampicillin.

Adverse Effects and Precautions

As for Ampicillin, p.153. Pivampicillin is reported to cause a lower incidence of diarrhoea than ampicillin, although upper gastro-intestinal discomfort may be more frequent. These effects appear to be more common when pivampicillin is taken on an empty stomach.

Pivaloyloxymethyl esters such as pivampicillin have been associated with the induction of carnitine deficiency (see below).

Carnitine deficiency has been reported following the administration of pivampicillin and pivmecillinam.[1] It is thought that the pivalic acid liberated on hydrolysis of these pivaloyloxymethyl esters *in vivo* is excreted as pivaloyl-carnitine with a consequent depletion in plasma and muscle concentrations of carnitine.[2] In one patient, low plasma-carnitine concentrations persisted after discontinuing pivampicillin, despite 6 weeks of replacement therapy with carnitine 1g daily by mouth. She had originally presented with skeletal myopathy after receiving pivampicillin for 3 months. A more intensive carnitine replacement regimen might be necessary in such patients.[3]

1. Holme E, *et al.* Carnitine deficiency induced by pivampicillin and pivmecillinam therapy. *Lancet* 1989; **ii:** 469–73.
2. Anonymous. Carnitine deficiency. *Lancet* 1990; **335:** 631–3.
3. Rose SJ, *et al.* Carnitine deficiency associated with long-term pivampicillin treatment: the effect of a replacement therapy regime. *Postgrad Med J* 1992; **68:** 932–4.

Porphyria. Pivampicillin has been associated with acute attacks of porphyria and is considered unsafe in patients with acute porphyria.[1]

1. Moore MR, McColl KEL. *Porphyria: drug lists.* Glasgow: Porphyria Research Unit, University of Glasgow, 1991.

Interactions

As for Benzylpenicillin, p.160.

There is a theoretical possibility that carnitine deficiency may be increased in patients receiving pivampicillin and valproate.

Antimicrobial Action

Pivampicillin has the antimicrobial activity of ampicillin to which it is hydrolysed *in vivo* (p.153).

Pharmacokinetics

Pivampicillin is acid-stable and is readily absorbed from the gastro-intestinal tract. On absorption it is rapidly and almost completely hydrolysed to ampicillin, pivalic acid, and formaldehyde. Plasma-ampicillin concentrations 1 hour after administration are 2 to 3 times those attained after an equivalent dose of ampicillin. The absorption of pivampicillin is generally not significantly affected by food. About 70% of a dose is excreted in the urine as ampicillin within 6 hours.

Uses and Administration

Pivampicillin is the pivaloyloxymethyl ester of ampicillin (p.154) and has similar uses. It may be given by mouth in doses of 0.5 g twice daily with food. Suggested doses in children are: under 1 year of age, 40 to 60 mg per kg body-weight daily; 1 to 5 years, 350 to 525 mg daily; 6 to 10 years, 525 to 700 mg daily all in 2 or 3 divided doses. Doses may be doubled in severe infections. In gonorrhoea a single dose of 1.5 to 2 g has been given, often in association with probenecid 1 g, in areas where gonococci remain sensitive.

Pivampicillin hydrochloride is used in some countries.

Pivampicillin has also been administered in association with pivmecillinam hydrochloride (p.238).

Preparations

Proprietary Preparations (details are given in Part 3)
Aust.: Pondocillin; ***Canad.:*** Pondocillin; ***Fr.:*** Proampi; ***Irl.:*** Pondocillin; ***Norw.:*** Pondocillin; ***S.Afr.:*** Pondocillin; ***Spain:*** Inacilin†; Lervipan; Pivamiser; ***Swed.:*** Pondocillin; ***UK:*** Pondocillin†.

Multi-ingredient: ***Aust.:*** Miraxid†; ***Ger.:*** Miraxid†; ***Swed.:*** Miraxid†; ***Switz.:*** Miraxid†; ***UK:*** Miraxid†; Pondocillin Plus†.

Pivcephalexin Hydrochloride (13138-m)

Cephalexin Pivoxil Hydrochloride; Pivcefalexin Hydrochloride; ST-21. Pivaloyloxymethyl (7*R*)-3-methyl-7-(α-D-phenylglycylamino)-3-cephem-4-carboxylate hydrochloride.

$C_{22}H_{27}N_3O_6S,HCl$ = 498.0.

CAS — 27726-31-4.

Pivcephalexin is the pivaloyloxymethyl ester of cephalexin (p.178). It is administered by mouth as the hydrochloride.

For reference to carnitine deficiency occurring after the administration of some pivaloyloxymethyl esters, see under Adverse Effects and Precautions of Pivampicillin, above.

Preparations

Proprietary Preparations (details are given in Part 3)
Ital.: Bencef†; Cefalen†; Pivacef†.

Pivmecillinam (136-q)

Pivmecillinam *(BAN, rINN)*.

Amdinocillin Pivoxil *(USAN)*; FL-1039; Pivamdinocillin; Ro-10-9071. Pivaloyloxymethyl (6*R*)-6-(perhydroazepin-1-ylmethyleneamino)penicillanate.

$C_{21}H_{33}N_3O_5S$ = 439.6.

CAS — 32886-97-8.

Pivmecillinam Hydrochloride (137-p)

Pivmecillinam Hydrochloride *(BANM, rINNM)*.

Pivmecillinami Hydrochloridum.

$C_{21}H_{33}N_3O_5S,HCl = 476.0$.

CAS — 32887-03-9.

Pharmacopoeias. In *Eur.* (see p.viii) and *Jpn.*

A white or almost white crystalline powder. Freely **soluble** in water, in dehydrated alcohol, and in methyl alcohol; slightly soluble in acetone. A 10% solution has a pH of 2.8 to 3.8. **Store** at a temperature of 2° to 8°. Protect from light. Pivmecillinam 1.35 g and pivmecillinam hydrochloride 1.46 g are each approximately equivalent to 1 g of mecillinam.

Adverse Effects and Precautions

As for Benzylpenicillin, p.159.

Pivaloyloxymethyl esters such as pivmecillinam have been associated with the induction of carnitine deficiency (see Pivampicillin, p.238).

Administration. Oesophageal injury has been associated rarely with pivmecillinam tablets.[1,2] Patients are advised to take them during a meal, while sitting or standing, and washed down with at least half a glass of water.[3]

1. Committee on Safety of Medicines. Pivmecillinam and oesophageal injury. *Current Problems 19* 1987.
2. Mortimer Ö, Wilholm B-B. Oesophageal injury associated with pivmecillinam tablets. *Eur J Clin Pharmacol* 1989; **37:** 605–7.
3. Anonymous. CSM warning on pivmecillinam. *Pharm J* 1987; **238:** 443.

Interactions

As for Benzylpenicillin, p.160.

Antimicrobial Action

Pivmecillinam has the antimicrobial activity of mecillinam (p.223) to which it is hydrolysed *in vivo*.

Pharmacokinetics

Pivmecillinam is well absorbed from the gastro-intestinal tract and is rapidly hydrolysed to the active drug mecillinam (p.224), pivalic acid, and formaldehyde. The presence of food in the stomach does not appear to have a significant effect on absorption. Peak plasma concentrations of mecillinam of up to 5 µg per mL have been achieved 1 to 2 hours after a 400-mg dose of pivmecillinam.

About 45% of a dose may be excreted in the urine as mecillinam, mainly within the first 6 hours.

References.

1. Heikkilä A, *et al.* The pharmacokinetics of mecillinam and pivmecillinam in pregnant and non-pregnant women. *Br J Clin Pharmacol* 1992; **33**; 629–33.

Uses and Administration

Pivmecillinam is the pivaloyloxymethyl ester of mecillinam (p.224), to which it is hydrolysed on oral administration. It has been used principally in the treatment of urinary-tract infections (p.149).

Doses of pivmecillinam are expressed in a confusing manner since no differentiation is made between the hydrochloride, used in tablets, and the base, used in suspensions for oral use.

In urinary-tract infections the usual dose has been 200 to 400 mg taken two or three times daily.

Pivmecillinam should preferably be taken with food (see also under Adverse Effects and Precautions, above).

Pivmecillinam has been administered in combination with other beta lactams, particularly pivampicillin (p.238), to extend the spectrum of antimicrobial activity to Gram-positive organisms and because of reported synergism against Gram-negative bacteria *in vitro*.

For parenteral administration, mecillinam is used.

Preparations

Proprietary Preparations (details are given in Part 3)
Aust.: Selexid; ***Belg.:*** Selexid†; ***Canad.:*** Selexid; ***Fr.:*** Selexid; ***Irl.:*** Selexid†; ***Norw.:*** Selexid; ***Spain:*** Selecid†; ***Swed.:*** Selexid; ***Switz.:*** Selexid†; ***UK:*** Selexid†.

Multi-ingredient: ***Aust.:*** Miraxid†; ***Ger.:*** Miraxid†; ***Swed.:*** Miraxid†; ***Switz.:*** Miraxid†; ***UK:*** Miraxid†; Pondocillin Plus†.

Polymyxin B Sulphate (139-w)

Polymyxin B Sulphate *(BANM, rINNM)*.

Polymyxin B Sulfate; Polymyxini B Sulfas.

CAS — 1404-26-8 (polymyxin B); 1405-20-5 (polymyxin B sulphate).

Pharmacopoeias. In *Eur.* (see p.viii), *Jpn, Pol.*, and *US.*

A mixture of the sulphates of polypeptides produced by the growth of certain strains of *Bacillus polymyxa* or obtained by other means. A white or buff-coloured, hygroscopic powder, odourless or with a slight odour. The Ph. Eur. specifies that it contains not less than 6500 units per mg and the USP specifies not less than 6000 units of polymyxin B per mg both calculated on the dried substance.

Soluble or freely soluble in water; slightly soluble in alcohol. A 2% solution in water has a pH of 5 to 7 and a 0.5% solution has a pH of 5.0 to 7.5. **Store** in airtight containers. Protect from light.

Incompatibilities. Lack of compatibility has been reported with many other drugs including antimicrobials. Polymyxin B sulphate is rapidly inactivated by strong acids and alkalis.

Units

The second International Standard Preparation (1969) of polymyxin B sulphate contains 8403 units per mg.

NOTE. The available forms of polymyxin B sulphate are generally less pure than the International Standard Preparation and doses are sometimes stated in terms of pure polymyxin base; 100 mg of pure polymyxin B is considered to be equivalent to 1 million units (1 mega unit).

Adverse Effects, Treatment, and Precautions

When given parenterally the major adverse effects of the polymyxins are dose-related neurotoxicity and nephrotoxicity. Hypersensitivity reactions are rare, although rashes and fever have been reported, and polymyxins cause histamine release which may lead to bronchoconstriction and other anaphylactoid symptoms.

Neurotoxic reactions include both peripheral effects such as circumoral and 'stocking-glove' pattern paraesthesias, visual disturbances, and dizziness, ataxia, confusion, drowsiness, and other central effects. The polymyxins are potent neuromuscular blockers, and respiratory paralysis and apnoea may result, especially in patients with impaired renal function or pre-existing disorders of neuromuscular transmission such as myasthenia gravis, in whom particular care is needed. Neostigmine or calcium salts are of little value in reversing neuromuscular blockade and artificial ventilation may be required if it develops.

Nephrotoxicity may occur in up to 20% of patients following parenteral use and may be marked by nitrogen retention, haematuria, proteinuria, and tubular necrosis. Electrolyte disturbances frequently occur. Patients with pre-existing renal impairment are at particular risk and require dosage reduction. Renal function should be monitored. Signs of increasing nitrogen retention are an indication for dosage reduction in all patients and the drugs should be withdrawn if oliguria occurs. Although polymyxin B is stated to be more nephrotoxic than colistin on a weight-for-weight basis their effects on the kidney seem to be similar at therapeutically equivalent doses.

Polymyxin B is irritant and pain following intramuscular injection may be severe. Meningeal irritation may follow the intrathecal administration of polymyxin B.

Polymyxins should be avoided in patients with a history of hypersensitivity to any of the group. Serum concentrations of polymyxins should be monitored in patients receiving parenteral therapy.

Ear drops containing polymyxins should not be used in patients with perforated ear drums, and topical application to large areas of broken skin should be avoided, because of the risk of systemic absorption.

Interactions

Polymyxins may enhance the action of neuromuscular blockers (p.1306). Additive nephrotoxicity may occur if polymyxins are given with other potentially nephrotoxic drugs including aminoglycosides and cephalothin.

Antimicrobial Action

Polymyxin B and the other polymyxin antibiotics act primarily by binding to membrane phospholipids and disrupting the bacterial cytoplasmic membrane. Polymyxin B has a bactericidal action on most Gram-negative bacilli except *Proteus* spp. It is particularly effective against *Pseudomonas aeruginosa.* Of the other Gram-negative organisms, *Acinetobacter* spp., *Escherichia coli, Enterobacter* and *Klebsiella* spp., *Haemophilus influenzae, Bordetella pertussis, Salmonella,* and *Shigella* spp. are sensitive. Classical *Vibrio cholerae* is sensitive but the El Tor and O139 biotypes are resistant. *Serratia marcescens, Providencia* spp., and *Bacteroides fragilis* are usually resistant. It is not active against *Neisseria* spp., obligate anaerobes, and Gram-positive bacteria. Some fungi such as *Coccidioides immitis* are susceptible but most are resistant.

Polymyxins have been reported to demonstrate antimicrobial synergy with a variety of other drugs, including chloramphenicol, tetracyclines, and the sulphonamides and trimethoprim.

MICs for the most sensitive species generally range from about 0.01 to 4 µg per mL. The action of polymyxin B is reduced by divalent cations such as calcium and magnesium, and so activity *in vivo* is less marked than *in vitro*.

Acquired resistance to polymyxin B is uncommon, although adaptive resistance may develop in enterobacteria exposed to sublethal concentrations. There is complete cross-resistance between polymyxin B and colistin.

Pharmacokinetics

Polymyxin B sulphate is not absorbed from the gastro-intestinal tract, except in the newborn. It is not absorbed through the intact skin.

Peak plasma concentrations after intramuscular administration are usually obtained within 2 hours, but are variable and it is partially inactivated by serum. It is widely distributed and extensively bound to cell membranes in the tissues. Accumulation may occur after repeated doses. Polymyxin B is reported to have a half-life of about 6 hours. There is no diffusion into the CSF.

Polymyxin B sulphate is excreted mainly by the kidneys, up to 60% being recovered in the urine, but there is a time lag of 12 to 24 hours before polymyxin B is recovered in the urine.

Uses and Administration

Polymyxin B sulphate is used topically, often in combination with other drugs, in the treatment of skin, ear, and eye infections due to susceptible organisms. Eye drops of polymyxin B with neomycin and gramicidin have been used for the prophylaxis of infection in patients undergoing ocular surgery (p.144) and, in combination with propamidine isethionate, for the treatment of acanthamoeba keratitis (p.573). Polymyxin B has been given orally for oropharyngeal decontamination or the suppression of intestinal flora in patients at high risk of endogenous infections (see under Intensive Care, p.128). Polymyxin B has also been used parenterally for the treatment of infections due to susceptible Gram-negative bacteria, especially *Pseudomonas aeruginosa,* but other drugs are generally preferred.

For topical application polymyxin B is usually available as a 0.1% solution or ointment. Parenteral doses have ranged from 15 000 to 25 000 units (about 1.5 to 2.5 mg) per kg body-weight daily, preferably by intravenous infusion, although the intramuscular route has been used despite the severe pain which may be associated with it. Higher doses have been given to neonates, but dosage must be reduced in patients with impaired renal function.

Polymyxin B has also been given intrathecally in meningeal infection, and by subconjunctival injection for eye infections.

Preparations

BP 1998: Polymyxin and Bacitracin Eye Ointment;
USP 23: Bacitracin and Polymyxin B Sulfate Topical Aerosol; Bacitracin Zinc and Polymyxin B Sulfate Ointment; Bacitracin Zinc and Polymyxin B Sulfate Ophthalmic Ointment; Chloramphenicol and Polymyxin B Sulfate Ophthalmic Ointment; Chloramphenicol, Polymyxin B Sulfate, and Hydrocortisone Acetate

Ophthalmic Ointment; Neomycin and Polymyxin B Sulfates and Bacitracin Ointment; Neomycin and Polymyxin B Sulfates and Bacitracin Ophthalmic Ointment; Neomycin and Polymyxin B Sulfates and Bacitracin Zinc Ointment; Neomycin and Polymyxin B Sulfates and Bacitracin Zinc Ophthalmic Ointment; Neomycin and Polymyxin B Sulfates and Dexamethasone Ophthalmic Ointment; Neomycin and Polymyxin B Sulfates and Dexamethasone Ophthalmic Suspension; Neomycin and Polymyxin B Sulfates and Gramicidin Cream; Neomycin and Polymyxin B Sulfates and Gramicidin Ophthalmic Solution; Neomycin and Polymyxin B Sulfates and Hydrocortisone Acetate Cream; Neomycin and Polymyxin B Sulfates and Hydrocortisone Acetate Ophthalmic Suspension; Neomycin and Polymyxin B Sulfates and Hydrocortisone Ophthalmic Suspension; Neomycin and Polymyxin B Sulfates and Hydrocortisone Otic Solution; Neomycin and Polymyxin B Sulfates and Hydrocortisone Otic Suspension; Neomycin and Polymyxin B Sulfates and Lidocaine Cream; Neomycin and Polymyxin B Sulfates and Prednisolone Acetate Ophthalmic Suspension; Neomycin and Polymyxin B Sulfates Cream; Neomycin and Polymyxin B Sulfates Ophthalmic Ointment; Neomycin and Polymyxin B Sulfates Ophthalmic Solution; Neomycin and Polymyxin B Sulfates Solution for Irrigation; Neomycin and Polymyxin B Sulfates, Bacitracin Zinc, and Hydrocortisone Acetate Ophthalmic Ointment; Neomycin and Polymyxin B Sulfates, Bacitracin Zinc, and Hydrocortisone Ointment; Neomycin and Polymyxin B Sulfates, Bacitracin Zinc, and Hydrocortisone Ophthalmic Ointment; Neomycin and Polymyxin B Sulfates, Bacitracin Zinc, and Lidocaine Ointment; Neomycin and Polymyxin B Sulfates, Bacitracin, and Hydrocortisone Acetate Ointment; Neomycin and Polymyxin B Sulfates, Bacitracin, and Hydrocortisone Acetate Ophthalmic Ointment; Neomycin and Polymyxin B Sulfates, Bacitracin, and Lidocaine Ointment; Neomycin and Polymyxin B Sulfates, Gramicidin, and Hydrocortisone Acetate Cream; Oxytetracycline Hydrochloride and Polymyxin B Sulfate Ointment; Oxytetracycline Hydrochloride and Polymyxin B Sulfate Ophthalmic Ointment; Oxytetracycline Hydrochloride and Polymyxin B Sulfate Topical Powder; Oxytetracycline Hydrochloride and Polymyxin B Sulfate Vaginal Tablets; Polymyxin B for Injection; Polymyxin B Sulfate and Bacitracin Zinc Topical Aerosol; Polymyxin B Sulfate and Bacitracin Zinc Topical Powder; Polymyxin B Sulfate and Hydrocortisone Otic Solution.

Proprietary Preparations (details are given in Part 3)

Canad.: Aerosporin; ***Irl.:*** Aerosporin†; ***UK:*** Aerosporin†; ***USA:*** Aerosporin†.

Multi-ingredient: ***Aust.:*** Conjunctin-S†; Conjunctin†; Neocones; Otosporin; Polybactrin; Polytrim; Riker Antibiotic-Spray; Terra-Cortril mit Polymyxin B-Sulfat; Terramycin mit Polymyxin-B-Sulfat; ***Austral.:*** Chloromyxin†; Mycitracin†; Neosporin; Spersin; ***Belg.:*** Conjunctin†; De Icin; Maxitrol; Ophtalmotrim; Otosporin; Panotile; Polydexa; Polygynax; Polytrim; Predmycin; Rikosol†; Statrol; Synalar Bi-Ophtalmic†; Synalar Bi-Otic; Terra-Cortril; Terramycine; ***Canad.:*** Antibiotic Ointment; Antibiotique Onguent; Bacimyxin; Bioderm; Cortisporin; Dioptrol; Diospor HC; Diosporin; Lanabiotic; Lidomyxin; Lidosporin; Maxitrol; Neo Bace; Neosporin; Neotopic; Ophthocort; Optimyxin; Optimyxin Plus; Ozonol Antibiotic Plus; Polycidin; Polyderm; Polysporin; Polysporin Burn Formula; Polysporin Triple Antibiotic; Polytopic; Polytracin; Polytrim; Synalar Bi-Otic†; Webber Antibiotic Cold Sore Ointment; ***Fr.:*** Antibio-Synalar; Antibiotulle Lumiere; Atebemyxine; Auricularum; Cebemyxine; Corticotulle Lumiere; Dexapolyfra†; Dulcimyxine†; Maxidrol; Optidex†; Panotile; Polydexa; Polydexa a la Phenylephrine; Polyfra; Polygynax; Polygynax Virgo; Primyxine; Sterimycine; ***Ger.:*** Antibiotulle Lumiere; Corticotulle Lumiere; Dexa Polyspectran N; Dexabiotan in der Ophtiole†; Eustoporin†; Isopto Max; Kombi-Stulln; Mycinopred†; Otosporin; Panotile N; Polybactrin†; Polygynax; Polyspectran; Polyspectran HC; Polyspectran OS†; Terracortril; Terramycin; ***Irl.:*** Maxitrol; Neosporin; Otosporin; Polybactrin; Polybactrin Soluble†; Polyfax; ***Ital.:*** Anauran; Aurizone†; Dermobios; Dermobios Oto†; Mixotone; Oftalmosporin†; Otosporin; Polytrim†; Rinojet SF; Roseomix†; Terramicina con Polimixina B Pomata Dermica†; ***Neth.:*** Maxitrol†; Neosporin†; Otosporin; Panotile; Polyspectran B†; Polyspectran G†; Polytrim; Predmycin-P Liquifilm†; Synalar Bi-Otic; Terra-Cortril Gel Steraject met polymyxine-B; Terra-Cortril met polymyxine-B; Terramycin met polymyxine-B; ***Norw.:*** Maxitrol; Polysporin†; Terra-Cortril Polymyxin B; Terramycin Polymyxin B; ***S.Afr.:*** Maxitrol; Neosporin; Otosporin; Polysporin; Polytrim; Terra-Cortril; Terramycin; ***Spain:*** Bacisporin; Blastoestimulina; Creanolona; Dermisone Tri Antibiotic; Idasal Antibiotico†; Linitul Antibiotico; Liquipom Dexa Antib; Maxitrol; Nasotic Oto; Neocones; Oftalmo†; Oftalmotrim; Oftalmotrim Dexa; Oftalmowell; Otix; Otocusi Enzimatico†; Otosporin; Panotile; Phonal; Poliantib; Poly Pred; Pomada Antibiotica; Statrol; Synalar Nasal; Synalar Otico; Terra-Cortril; Terramicina; Tivitis; Tulgrasum Antibiotico; Vinciseptil Otico; ***Swed.:*** Isopto Biotic; Terracortril med polymyxin B; Terramycin Polymyxin B; ***Switz.:*** Baneopol; Maxitrol; Mycinopred; Neocones; Neosporin; Neosporin-B†; Otosporin; Panotile; Polybactrin Solubile†; Polybactrin†; Polydexa; Pulpomixine; Septomixine; Spersapolymyxin; Statrol†; Terracortril; Terramycine; Vistajunctin†; ***UK:*** Gregoderm; Maxitrol; Neosporin; Otosporin; Polybactrin†; Polyfax; Polytrim; Terra-Cortril†; Tribiotic†; Uniroid; ***USA:*** Ak-Poly-Bac; Ak-Spore; Ak-Spore HC; Ak-Trol; Alba-3; AntibiOtic; Aquaphor Antibiotic; Bacticort; Bactine First Aid Antibiotic Plus Anesthetic; Betadine First Aid Antibiotics + Moisturizer; Betadine Plus First Aid Antibiotics & Pain Reliever; Campho-Phenique Antibiotic Plus Pain Reliever Ointment; Clomycin; Coracin; Cortatrigen; Cortisporin; Dexacidin; Dexasporin; Drotic†; Ear-Eze; Infectrol†; Lanabiotic; LazerSporin-C; Maxitrol; Medi-Quik†; Mycitracin; Mycitracin Plus; Neocin; Neomixin; Neosporin; Neosporin GU; Neosporin Plus; Neotal; Neotricin HC; Neotricin†; Octicair; Ocutricin; Ophthocort†; Otic-Care; Oticin HC; OtiTricin; Otobiotic; Otocort; Otomycin-HPN; Otosporin; Pediotic; Poly-Dex; Poly-Pred; Polycin-B; Polysporin; Polytrim; Pyocidin-Otic†; Septa; Spectrocin Plus; Storz-N-P-D; Terramycin with Polymyxin B†; Topisporin†; Tribiotic Plus; Triple Antibiotic; UAD-Otic.

Pristinamycin (140-m)

Pristinamycin *(BAN, rINN).*

RP-7293.

CAS — 11006-76-1.

Pristinamycin is a streptogramin antibiotic produced by the growth of *Streptomyces pristina spiralis*, with actions and uses similar to those of virginiamycin (p.269). It is administered by mouth in the treatment of susceptible infections (particularly staphylococcal infections) in a dose of 2 to 4 g daily in divided doses. Children have been given 50 to 100 mg per kg body-weight daily.

Pristinamycin is a naturally occurring mixture of two synergistic components, pristinamycin I which is a macrolide, and pristinamycin II which is a depsipeptide.[1] It has been available for many years as an oral anti-staphylococcal drug, and also acts against streptococci. It is effective against strains showing resistance to erythromycin; resistance to pristinamycin is currently rare, although resistance in staphylococci has been reported.[2,3] It is effective against methicillin-resistant *Staphylococcus aureus* (MRSA) but its usefulness in severe infection is limited by its poor solubility, which prevents development of an intravenous formulation. Mixtures of water-soluble derivatives of pristinamycins I and II, including RP-59500 (p.247), are under investigation.

1. Hamilton-Miller JMT. From foreign pharmacopoeias: 'new' antibiotics from old? *J Antimicrob Chemother* 1991; **27:** 702–5.
2. Loncle V, *et al.* Analysis of pristinamycin-resistant Staphylococcus epidermidis isolates responsible for an outbreak in a Parisian hospital. *Antimicrob Agents Chemother* 1993; **37:** 2159–65.
3. Allignet J, *et al.* Distribution of genes encoding resistance to streptogramin A and related compounds among staphylococci resistant to these antibiotics. *Antimicrob Agents Chemother* 1996; **40:** 2523–8.

Preparations

Proprietary Preparations (details are given in Part 3)
Belg.: Pyostacine; ***Fr.:*** Pyostacine.

Procaine Penicillin (141-b)

Procaine Penicillin *(BAN).*

Benzylpenicillin Novocaine; Benzylpenicillinum Procainum; Penicillin G Procaine; Procaine Benzylpenicillin; Procaine Penicillin G; Procaini Benzylpenicillinum. 2-(4-Aminobenzoyloxy)ethyldiethylammonium (6*R*)-6-(2-phenylacetamido)penicillanate monohydrate.

$C_{13}H_{20}N_2O_2,C_{16}H_{18}N_2O_4S,H_2O = 588.7.$

CAS — 54-35-3 (anhydrous procaine penicillin); 6130-64-9 (procaine penicillin monohydrate).

Pharmacopoeias. In *Chin., Eur.* (see p.viii), *Int., Pol.,* and *US.*

A white, crystalline powder. Procaine penicillin 600 mg is approximately equivalent to 360 mg of benzylpenicillin (600 000 units).

Slightly **soluble** in water; sparingly soluble in alcohol. A 0.33% solution in water has a pH of 5.0 to 7.5. **Store** in airtight containers.

Adverse Effects and Precautions

As for Benzylpenicillin, p.159.

Procaine penicillin should not be given to patients known to be hypersensitive to either component.

Severe, usually transient, reactions with symptoms of severe anxiety and agitation, psychotic reactions, including visual and auditory hallucinations, seizures, tachycardia and hypertension, cyanosis, and a sensation of impending death have occasionally been reported with procaine penicillin and may be due to accidental intravascular injection. Since similar reactions have also occurred with other depot penicillin preparations that do not contain procaine, its presence is unlikely to be the major cause of such reactions, but may be a contributory factor, especially after injection of high doses. They have been termed non-allergic, pseudoallergic, pseudoanaphylactic, or Hoigné's syndrome and the term embolic-toxic reaction has also been proposed.

Procaine penicillin should not be injected intravascularly since ischaemic reactions may occur.

Interactions

As for Benzylpenicillin, p.160.

Pharmacokinetics

When procaine penicillin is given by intramuscular injection, it forms a depot from which it is slowly released and hydrolysed to benzylpenicillin. Peak plasma concentrations are produced in 1 to 4 hours, and effective concentrations of benzylpenicillin are usually maintained for 12 to 24 hours. However, plasma concentrations are lower than those following an equivalent dose of benzylpenicillin potassium or sodium.

Distribution into the CSF is reported to be poor.

Uses and Administration

Procaine penicillin has the same antimicrobial action as benzylpenicillin (p.160) to which it is hydrolysed gradually following deep intramuscular injection. This results in a prolonged effect, but because of the relatively low blood concentrations produced, its use should be restricted to infections caused by micro-organisms that are highly sensitive to penicillin. Procaine penicillin should not be used as the sole treatment for severe acute infections, and when bacteraemia is present.

It is used mainly in the treatment of syphilis; other indications have included anthrax, pneumonia (in children in developing countries), and Whipple's disease. For details of these infections and their treatment, see under Choice of Antibacterial, p.116.

Administration and dosage. Procaine penicillin is administered by deep intramuscular injection in usual doses of 0.6 to 1.2 g daily.

Patients with syphilis are given procaine penicillin 1.2 g daily for 10 to 15 days; infants up to 2 years of age with congenital syphilis may be given 50 mg per kg body-weight daily. Treatment may be continued for 3 weeks in patients with late syphilis.

Procaine penicillin is also administered in combined preparations with other penicillins, including benzylpenicillin, benzathine penicillin, and benethamine penicillin.

Preparations

BP 1998: Fortified Procaine Benzylpenicillin Injection; Procaine Benzylpenicillin Injection;
USP 23: Penicillin G Benzathine and Penicillin G Procaine Injectable Suspension; Penicillin G Procaine for Injectable Suspension; Penicillin G Procaine Injectable Suspension; Penicillin G Procaine with Aluminum Stearate Injectable Oil Suspension; Sterile Penicillin G Procaine.

Proprietary Preparations (details are given in Part 3)

Austral.: Cilicaine Syringe; ***Canad.:*** Ayercillin; Wycillin†; ***Ger.:*** Jenacillin O; ***S.Afr.:*** Novocillin; Procillin; Quick-Cillin†; ***Spain:*** Aqucilina; Farmaproina; Fradicilina; Provipen Procaina†; ***USA:*** Crysticillin; Pfizerpen-AS†; Wycillin.

Multi-ingredient: ***Aust.:*** Fortepen; Retarpen compositum; ***Austral.:*** Bicillin All Purpose†; ***Belg.:*** Combicilline†; ***Canad.:*** Bicillin A-P; ***Fr.:*** Bipenicilline†; ***Ger.:*** Bipensaar; Depotpen†; Hydracillin; Jenacillin A; Retacillin; ***Ital.:*** Tri-Wycillina; ***Neth.:*** Bicilline; Penidural D/F; ***S.Afr.:*** Penilente Forte; Ultracillin; ***Spain:*** Aqucilina D A; Benzetacil Compuesta; Broncosolvente EP†; Cepacilina; Cilina 400†; Davurmicin†; Neocepacilina; Penibiot Retard†; Peniroger Procain†; Provipen†; ***Switz.:*** Penadur 6-3-3†; ***UK:*** Bicillin; ***USA:*** Bicillin C-R.

Propicillin Potassium (142-v)

Propicillin Potassium *(BANM, pINNM).*

Potassium α-Phenoxypropylpenicillin; Propicillinum Kalicum. A mixture of the D(+)- and L(−)-isomers of potassium (6*R*)-6-(2-phenoxybutyramido)penicillanate.

$C_{18}H_{21}KN_2O_5S = 416.5.$

CAS — 551-27-9 (propicillin); 1245-44-9 (propicillin potassium).

Propicillin is a phenoxypenicillin with actions and uses similar to those of phenoxymethylpenicillin (p.236). It is given by mouth, as the potassium salt, for the treatment of susceptible mild to moderate infections.

Preparations

Proprietary Preparations (details are given in Part 3)
Ger.: Baycillin; Oricillin†.

Prothionamide (7567-k)

Prothionamide *(BAN)*.

Protionamide *(rINN)*; RP-9778; TH-1321. 2-Propylpyridine-4-carbothioamide.

$C_9H_{12}N_2S$ = 180.3.

CAS — 14222-60-7.

Pharmacopoeias. In *Chin., Int.,* and *Jpn.*

Adverse Effects, Precautions, and Antimicrobial Action

As for Ethionamide, p.208; it may be better tolerated than ethionamide.

Pharmacokinetics

Prothionamide is readily absorbed from the gastro-intestinal tract and produces peak plasma concentrations about 2 hours after a dose by mouth. It is widely distributed throughout body tissues and fluids, including the CSF. Prothionamide is metabolised to the active sulphoxide and other inactive metabolites and less than 1% of a dose appears in the urine as unchanged drug.

Uses and Administration

Prothionamide is a thioamide derivative considered to be interchangeable with ethionamide (p.208). Complete cross-resistance occurs between the two drugs. Prothionamide has been administered by mouth in doses similar to those used for ethionamide. It has also been administered as rectal suppositories; prothionamide hydrochloride has been given intravenously. Like ethionamide, it has generally been replaced by less toxic antimycobacterials.

Preparations

Proprietary Preparations (details are given in Part 3)
Austral.: Trevintix†; ***Ger.:*** ektebin; Peteha.

Multi-ingredient: ***Aust.:*** Isoprodian; ***Ger.:*** Isoprodian; Peteha; ***S.Afr.:*** Isoprodian†.

Prulifloxacin (15200-s)

Prulifloxacin *(rINN)*.

NM-441. (±)-7-{4-[(*Z*)-2,3-Dihydroxy-2-butenyl]-1-piperazinyl}-6-fluoro-1-methyl-4-oxo-1*H*,4*H*-[1,3]thiazeto[3,2-*a*]quinoline-3-carboxylic acid cyclic carbonate.

$C_{21}H_{20}FN_3O_6S$ = 461.5.

CAS — 123447-62-1.

Prulifloxacin is a fluoroquinolone antibacterial.

Pyrazinamide (7568-a)

Pyrazinamide *(BAN, rINN)*.

Pyrazinamidum; Pyrazinoic Acid Amide. Pyrazine-2-carboxamide.

$C_5H_5N_3O$ = 123.1.

CAS — 98-96-4.

Pharmacopoeias. In *Chin., Eur.* (see p.viii), *Int., Jpn, Pol.,* and *US.*

A white or almost white, odourless or almost odourless, crystalline powder. **Soluble** 1 in 67 of water, 1 in 175 of dehydrated alcohol, 1 in 135 of chloroform, 1 in 1000 of ether, and 1 in 72 of methyl alcohol; slightly soluble in alcohol and in dichloromethane.

Adverse Effects and Treatment

Hepatotoxicity is the most serious side-effect of pyrazinamide therapy and its frequency appears to be related to dose. However, in currently recommended doses, when given in association with isoniazid and rifampicin, the incidence of hepatitis has been reported to be less than 3%. Patients may experience a transient increase in liver enzyme values; more seriously hepatomegaly, splenomegaly, and jaundice may develop and on rare occasions death has occurred.

Hyperuricaemia commonly occurs and may lead to attacks of gout.

Other side-effects are anorexia, nausea, vomiting, arthralgia, malaise, fever, sideroblastic anaemia, and dysuria. Photosensitivity and skin rashes have been reported on rare occasions.

Effects on blood pressure. Acute hypertension was associated with pyrazinamide administration in a previously normotensive woman.[1]

1. Goldberg J, *et al.* Acute hypertension as an adverse effect of pyrazinamide *JAMA* 1997; **277:** 1356.

Effects on the liver. The risk of hepatitis with antituberculous regimens containing pyrazinamide may be lower than suggested by early studies, in which large doses were used, often for long periods. The incidence of hepatitis in studies of short-course regimens containing pyrazinamide has ranged from 0.2% in Africa, to 0.6% in Hong Kong, to 2.8% in Singapore.[1] These and later studies[2-4] have shown that hepatotoxicity is not increased when pyrazinamide is added to the initial phase of short-term chemotherapy containing rifampicin and isoniazid. Nevertheless, a report[5] of four cases of fulminant hepatic failure in patients given triple therapy with the potentially hepatotoxic drugs rifampicin, isoniazid, and pyrazinamide (one patient also received ethambutol) highlighted the importance of strict liver function monitoring and this was reinforced by others. However, the Joint Tuberculosis Committee of the British Thoracic Society is anxious that fears over the safety of treatment regimens do not compromise adequate therapy of the disease itself. In an update to their guidelines,[6] they recommend initial measurement of liver function in all patients and regular monitoring in patients with known chronic liver disease. Tests should be repeated if symptoms of liver dysfunction occur, and details are given concerning the response to deteriorating liver function and include guidelines for prompt re-introduction of appropriate antituberculosis therapy once normal liver function is restored.

1. Girling DJ. The role of pyrazinamide in primary chemotherapy for pulmonary tuberculosis. *Tubercle* 1984; **65:** 1–4.
2. Parthasarathy R, *et al.* Hepatic toxicity in South Indian patients during treatment of tuberculosis with short-course regimens containing isoniazid, rifampicin and pyrazinamide. *Tubercle* 1986; **67:** 99–108.
3. Combs DL, *et al.* USPHS tuberculosis short-course chemotherapy trial 21: effectiveness, toxicity, and acceptability: the report of final results. *Ann Intern Med* 1990; **112:** 397–406.
4. LeBourgeois M, *et al.* Good tolerance of pyrazinamide in children with pulmonary tuberculosis. *Arch Dis Child* 1989; **64:** 177–8.
5. Mitchell I, *et al.* Anti-tuberculous therapy and acute liver failure. *Lancet* 1995; **345:** 555–6.
6. Ormerod LP, *et al.* Hepatotoxicity of antituberculosis drugs. *Thorax* 1996; **51:** 111–13.

Effects on the nervous system. Convulsions which developed in a 2-year-old child receiving antituberculous therapy appeared to be due to pyrazinamide.[1] Pyrazinamide had been administered in a dose of 250 mg daily.

1. Herlevsen P, *et al.* Convulsions after treatment with pyrazinamide. *Tubercle* 1987; **68:** 145–6.

Hyperuricaemia. Hyperuricaemia during therapy with pyrazinamide may be due to inhibition of uric acid excretion by pyrazinoic acid, the main metabolite of pyrazinamide.[1]

In a large multicentre study,[2] the incidence of elevated serum concentrations of uric acid for patients on rifampicin, isoniazid, and pyrazinamide was 52.2% at 8 weeks while the incidence for patients on rifampicin and isoniazid was 5.4%. Arthralgia was reported in 6 of 617 patients on rifampicin, isoniazid, and pyrazinamide, but in none of the 445 patients on rifampicin and isoniazid.

Slight increases in plasma concentrations of uric acid occurred in 9 of 43 children after one month's treatment with rifampicin, isoniazid, ethambutol, and pyrazinamide. Arthralgias and gout did not occur. Uric acid concentrations were normal on completion of treatment with pyrazinamide.[3] Some studies have suggested a relationship between elevated serum uric acid levels and arthralgia,[4] but this has not been confirmed.[5]

1. Ellard GA, Haslam RM. Observations on the reduction of the renal elimination of urate in man caused by the administration of pyrazinamide. *Tubercle* 1976; **57:** 97–103.
2. Combs DL, *et al.* USPHS tuberculosis short-course chemotherapy trial 21: effectiveness, toxicity, and acceptability: the report of final results. *Ann Intern Med* 1990; **112:** 397–406.
3. Le Bourgeois M, *et al.* Good tolerance of pyrazinamide in children with pulmonary tuberculosis. *Arch Dis Child* 1989; **64:** 177–8.
4. Hong Kong Tuberculosis Treatment Services/British MRC. Adverse reactions to short-course regimens containing streptomycin, isoniazid, pyrazinamide and rifampicin in Hong Kong. *Tubercle* 1976; **57:** 81–95.
5. Jenner PJ, *et al.* Serum uric acid concentrations and arthralgia among patients treated with pyrazinamide-containing regimens in Hong Kong and Singapore. *Tubercle* 1981; **62:** 175–9.

Pellagra. Pellagra, probably due to pyrazinamide developed in a 26-year-old woman receiving antituberculous therapy.[1] Symptoms regressed, without stopping therapy, on administration of nicotinamide.

1. Jørgensen J. Pellagra probably due to pyrazinamide: development during combined chemotherapy of tuberculosis. *Int J Dermatol* 1983; **22:** 44–5.

Precautions

Pyrazinamide is contra-indicated by the manufacturers in patients with liver damage, although some consider that it can be used with care when the liver damage is not severe. Liver function should be assessed before and regularly during treatment. The British Thoracic Society recommends that, in patients with chronic liver disease, pyrazinamide treatment should be suspended if serum aminotransferase concentrations are elevated to 5 times the normal upper limit or the bilirubin concentration rises. Although the manufacturer recommends that pyrazinamide should not be restarted in patients with evidence of hepatocellular damage, the UK guidelines allow cautious re-introduction of antimycobacterial drugs, including pyrazinamide, once liver function has returned to normal.

Caution should be observed in patients with impaired renal function or a history of gout. Increased difficulty has been reported in controlling diabetes mellitus when diabetics are given pyrazinamide.

Porphyria. Pyrazinamide has been associated with acute attacks of porphyria and is considered unsafe in patients with acute porphyria.[1]

1. Moore MR, McColl KEL. *Porphyria: drug lists.* Glasgow: Porphyria Research Unit, University of Glasgow, 1991.

Pregnancy. Although the American Thoracic Society[1,2] considers that there is insufficient teratogenicity data to recommend the routine use of pyrazinamide during pregnancy, others, including the IUAT[3] and the British Thoracic Society,[4] do not contra-indicate pyrazinamide in pregnant patients.

For details on distribution into breast milk, see Pharmacokinetics, below.

1. American Thoracic Society. Treatment of tuberculosis and tuberculosis infection in adults and children. *Am Rev Respir Dis* 1986; **134:** 355–63.
2. American Thoracic Society and the Centers for Disease Control. Treatment of tuberculosis and tuberculosis infection in adults and children. *Am J Respir Crit Care Med* 1994; **149:** 1359–74.
3. Anonymous. Antituberculosis regimens of chemotherapy: recommendations from the Committee on Treatment of the International Union Against Tuberculosis and Lung Disease. *Bull Int Union Tuberc Lung Dis* 1988; **63:** 60–4.
4. Joint Tuberculosis Committee of the British Thoracic Society. Chemotherapy and management of tuberculosis in the United Kingdom: recommendations 1998. *Thorax* 1998; **53:** 536–48.

Interactions

Probenecid. A study of the complex interactions occurring when pyrazinamide and probenecid are given to patients with gout.[1] Urinary excretion of urate depends on the relative size and timing of doses of the two drugs. Probenecid is known to block the excretion of pyrazinamide.

1. Yü TF, *et al.* The effect of the interaction of pyrazinamide and probenecid on urinary uric acid excretion in man. *Am J Med* 1977; **63:** 723–8.

Zidovudine. Low or undetectable concentrations of pyrazinamide occurred in 4 patients also taking zidovudine.[1] In the same study, 6 of 7 patients with HIV infections taking pyrazinamide without zidovudine had normal serum pyrazinamide concentrations.

1. Peloquin CA, *et al.* Low antituberculosis drug concentrations in patients with AIDS. *Ann Pharmacother* 1996; **30:** 919–25.

Antimicrobial Action

Pyrazinamide has a bactericidal effect on *Mycobacterium tuberculosis* but appears to have no activity against other mycobacteria or micro-organisms *in vitro*. The MIC for *M. tuberculosis* is less than 20 μg per mL at pH 5.6; it is almost completely inactive at a neutral pH. Pyrazinamide is effective against persisting tubercle bacilli within the acidic intracellular environment of the macrophages. The initial inflammatory response to chemotherapy increases the number of organisms in the acidic environment. As inflammation subsides and pH increases, the sterilising activity of pyrazinamide decreases. This pH-dependent activity explains the clinical effectiveness of pyrazinamide as part of the initial 8-week phase in short-course treatment regimens.

Resistance to pyrazinamide rapidly develops when it is used alone.

Although the antimicrobial activity of pyrazinamide has been recognised since the 1950s, the mode of action has not been determined. Methodologic advances and the increased clinical importance of pyrazinamide have led to renewed investigations. One proposal is that pyrazinoic acid is the active moiety. Pyrazinamidase produced by the tubercle bacilli is known to convert pyrazinamide to pyrazinoic acid. Salfinger and colleagues[1] using a radiometric method for susceptibility testing (BACTEC) and an *in-vitro* system of cultured human blood macrophages have further proposed that the pyrazinoic acid formed within the macrophage would be trapped, thereby lowering intracellular pH to levels toxic to tubercle bacilli.

1. Salfinger M, *et al.* Pyrazinamide and pyrazinoic acid activity against tubercle bacilli in cultured human macrophages and in the BACTEC system. *J Infect Dis* 1990; **162:** 201–7.

Activity with other antimicrobials. Pyrazinamide exhibited synergistic activity against *Mycobacterium tuberculosis* with clarithromycin.[1]

1. Mor N, Esfandiari A. Synergistic activities of clarithromycin and pyrazinamide against Mycobacterium tuberculosis in human macrophages. *Antimicrob Agents Chemother* 1997; **41:** 2035–6.

Pharmacokinetics

Pyrazinamide is readily absorbed from the gastro-intestinal tract. Peak serum concentrations occur about 2 hours after a dose by mouth and have been reported to be about 35 μg per mL after 1.5 g, and 66 μg per mL after 3 g. Pyrazinamide is widely distributed in body fluids and tissues and diffuses into the CSF. The half-life has been reported to be about 9 to 10 hours. It is metabolised primarily in the liver by hydrolysis to the major active metabolite pyrazinoic acid which is subsequently hydroxylated to the major excretory product 5-hydroxypyrazinoic acid. It is excreted through the kidney mainly by glomerular filtration. About 70% of a dose appears in the urine within 24 hours mainly as metabolites and 4 to 14% as unchanged drug. Pyrazinamide is removed by dialysis. Pyrazinamide is distributed into breast milk.

Lacroix and his colleagues[1] reported a short distribution phase and an elimination phase of 9.6 hours in healthy subjects following a single oral dose of pyrazinamide 27 mg per kg body-weight; the half-life for the major metabolite pyrazinoic acid was 11.8 hours.

In the major metabolic pathway, pyrazinamide was deaminated to pyrazinoic acid which was hydroxylated to hydroxypyrazinoic acid; in the minor pathway, pyrazinamide was hydroxylated to hydroxypyrazinamide which was then deaminated to hydroxypyrazinoic acid. The limiting step was deamination; oxidation by xanthine oxidase occurred very quickly.

A similar study was carried out in 10 patients with cirrhosis of the liver.[2] Following a dose of 19.3 mg per kg, the elimination phase was 15.07 hours for pyrazinamide and 24 hours for pyrazinoic acid.

1. Lacroix C, *et al.* Pharmacokinetics of pyrazinamide and its metabolites in healthy subjects. *Eur J Clin Pharmacol* 1989; **36:** 395–400.
2. Lacroix C, *et al.* Pharmacokinetics of pyrazinamide and its metabolites in patients with hepatic cirrhotic insufficiency. *Arzneimittelforschung* 1990; **40:** 76–9.

Bioavailability. The oral bioavailability of rifampicin and isoniazid, but not of pyrazinamide, was decreased by food in many patients.[1]

1. Zent C, Smith P. Study of the effect of concomitant food on the bioavailability of rifampicin, isoniazid and pyrazinamide. *Tubercle Lung Dis* 1995; **76:** 109–13.

Breast feeding. The peak concentration of pyrazinamide in breast milk of a 29-year-old woman was 1.5 μg per mL 3 hours after administration of a 1-g dose of pyrazinamide.[1] The peak plasma concentration was 42 μg per mL after 2 hours.

1. Holdiness MR. Antituberculosis drugs and breast-feeding. *Arch Intern Med* 1984; **144:** 1888.

Distribution. Pyrazinamide was given to 28 patients with suspected tuberculous meningitis in doses of 34 to 41 mg per kg body-weight. The mean concentration of pyrazinamide in the CSF 2 hours after administration was 38.6 μg per mL and represented about 75% of that in serum; concentrations at 5 and 8 hours were 44.5 and 31.0 μg per mL respectively and were about 10% higher than those in serum.[1] The use of corticosteroids appeared to have no influence on penetration of pyrazinamide into the CSF of patients with tuberculous meningitis.[2]

1. Ellard GA, *et al.* Penetration of pyrazinamide into the cerebrospinal fluid in tuberculous meningitis. *Br Med J* 1987; **294:** 284–5.
2. Woo J, *et al.* Cerebrospinal fluid and serum levels of pyrazinamide and rifampicin in patients with tuberculous meningitis. *Curr Ther Res* 1987; **42:** 235–42.

Uses and Administration

Pyrazinamide is used as part of multi-drug regimens for the treatment of tuberculosis (p.146), primarily in the initial 8-week phase of short-course treatment. Pyrazinamide is usually given daily or 2 or 3 times a week. In the UK recommended doses by mouth for adults and children are up to 35 mg per kg body-weight daily (maximum daily dose is 3 g) or 50 mg per kg three times a week, or up to 75 mg per kg twice a week. To standardise administration, the usual dose for patients under 50 kg is 1.5 g daily, 2.0 g three times a week, or 3.0 g twice a week. For patients 50 kg or greater, the usual dose is 2.0 g daily, 2.5 g three times a week, or 3.5 g twice a week. The recommended doses in the USA are 15 to 30 mg per kg daily (maximum 2 g) or 50 to 70 mg per kg 3 times a week (maximum 3 g each day) or twice a week (maximum 4 g each day). WHO recommends 25 mg per kg daily or 35 mg per kg three times a week or 50 mg per kg twice a week.

Administration in hepatic impairment. See under Precautions, above.

Administration in renal impairment. The manufacturer in the UK suggests that dosage reductions may be necessary in patients with impaired renal function.

In a study of 6 patients on haemodialysis[1] the average amount of pyrazinamide and its metabolites removed during a dialysis session was 926 mg after an oral dose of 1700 mg. It was recommended that the usual pyrazinamide dose be given to patients on dialysis as the risk of accumulation was negligible, and that the dose on dialysis days be given after the procedure.

1. Lacroix C, *et al.* Haemodialysis of pyrazinamide in uraemic patients. *Eur J Clin Pharmacol* 1989; **37:** 309–11.

Preparations

BP 1998: Pyrazinamide Tablets;
USP 23: Pyrazinamide Tablets.

Proprietary Preparations (details are given in Part 3)
Aust.: Pyrafat; ***Austral.:*** Zinamide; ***Belg.:*** Tebrazid; ***Canad.:*** Tebrazid; ***Fr.:*** Pirilene; ***Ger.:*** pezetamid†; Pyrafat; ***Irl.:*** Zinamide; ***Ital.:*** Piraldina; ***S.Afr.:*** Isopas†; Pyrazide; Rozide; ***UK:*** Zinamide.

Multi-ingredient: ***Aust.:*** Rifater; ***Canad.:*** Rifater; ***Fr.:*** Rifater; ***Ger.:*** Rifater; ***Irl.:*** Rifater; ***Ital.:*** Rifater; ***S.Afr.:*** Pyrifin; Rifater; ***Spain:*** Rifater; ***Switz.:*** Rifater; Rimactazide + Z; ***UK:*** Rifater; ***USA:*** Rifater.

Ramoplanin (3759-c)

Ramoplanin *(USAN, rINN)*.
A-16686; MDL-62198.
CAS — 76168-82-6.

Ramoplanin is a glycopeptide antibiotic with a spectrum of activity *in vitro* similar to that of vancomycin (p.268) but considerably more potent. It is also active against *Bacteroides* spp. It is under investigation as an antibacterial, notably in the topical treatment of acne and skin infections, and to reduce nasal carriage of staphylococci.

Ribostamycin Sulphate (144-q)

Ribostamycin Sulphate *(BANM, rINNM)*.
SF-733 (ribostamycin). 2-Deoxy-4-*O*-(2,6-diamino-2,6-dideoxy-α-D-glucopyranosyl)-5-*O*-(β-D-ribofuranosyl)-streptamine sulphate.
$C_{17}H_{34}N_4O_{10},xH_2SO_4$ = 454.5 (ribostamycin).
CAS — 25546-65-0 (ribostamycin); 53797-35-6 (ribostamycin sulphate).
Pharmacopoeias. In *Jpn.*

An aminoglycoside antibiotic derived from *Streptomyces ribosidificus* or prepared synthetically.

Ribostamycin is an aminoglycoside with actions and uses similar to those of gentamicin (p.212). It has been given as the sulphate by intramuscular injection in a suggested dose of 1 g daily, in divided doses, and by mouth in usual doses of 1.5 to 3 g daily.

Preparations

Proprietary Preparations (details are given in Part 3)
Ital.: Ribomed†; Ribostamin†; Ribostat; ***Jpn:*** Vistamycin.

Rifabutin (16512-w)

Rifabutin *(BAN, USAN, rINN)*.
Ansamicin; Ansamycin; LM-427; Rifabutine.
(9*S*,12*E*,14*S*,15*R*,16*S*,17*R*,18*R*,19*R*,20*S*,21*S*,22*E*,24*Z*)-6,16,18,20-Tetrahydroxy-1′-isobutyl-14-methoxy-7,9,15,17,19,21,25-heptamethylspiro[9,4-(epoxypentadeca[1,11,13]trienimino)-2*H*-furo-[2′,3′:7,8]naphth[1,2-*d*]imidazole-2,4′-piperidine]-5,10,26-(3*H*,9*H*)-trione-16-acetate.
$C_{46}H_{62}N_4O_{11}$ = 847.0.
CAS — 72559-06-9.
Pharmacopoeias. In *US.*

An amorphous red-violet powder. Very slightly **soluble** in water; sparingly soluble in alcohol; soluble in chloroform and methyl alcohol. **Protect** from light and from excessive heat.

Adverse Effects and Precautions

As for Rifampicin, p.243. It produces a syndrome of polyarthralgia-arthritis at doses greater than 1 g daily. Uveitis has been reported, especially in patients also receiving clarithromycin or fluconazole.

A polyarthralgia-arthritis syndrome has been reported in 9 of 10 patients receiving a daily dose of rifabutin greater than 1 g.[1] The syndrome did not occur in patients receiving less than 1 g daily and disappeared on drug withdrawal. Two patients with polyarthralgia-arthritis symptoms developed uveitis (see also below under Effects on the Eyes) and aphthous stomatitis at doses of approximately 1.8 g per day.

An orange-tan skin pigmentation has been reported to occur in most patients receiving rifabutin.[1] Urine may be discoloured.[2] An influenza-like syndrome has been reported in 2 of 12 patients given 300 mg daily for Crohn's disease,[3] in 1 of 16 HIV-infected patients on continuous rifabutin,[1] and in 8 of 15 HIV-infected patients receiving increasing doses of rifabutin.[2]

Other reported adverse effects include hepatitis,[1] leucopenia[2] (including neutropenia[4]), epigastric pain,[3] rash,[3] erythema,[2] and ageusia.[5]

Rash, fever, and vomiting occurred in 1 of 2 children receiving 6.5 mg per kg body-weight per day.[6]

1. Siegal FP, *et al.* Dose-limiting toxicity of rifabutin in AIDS-related complex: syndrome of arthralgia/arthritis. *AIDS* 1990; **4:** 433–41.
2. Torseth J, *et al.* Evaluation of the antiviral effect of rifabutin in AIDS-related complex. *J Infect Dis* 1989; **159:** 1115–18.
3. Basilisco G, *et al.* Controlled trial of rifabutin in Crohn's disease. *Curr Ther Res* 1989; **46:** 245–50.
4. Apseloff G, *et al.* Severe neutropenia caused by recommended prophylactic doses of rifabutin. *Lancet* 1996; **348:** 685.
5. Morris JT, Kelly JW. Rifabutin-induced ageusia. *Ann Intern Med* 1993; **119:** 171–2.
6. Levin RH, Bolinger AM. Treatment of nontuberculous mycobacterial infections in pediatric patients. *Clin Pharm* 1988; **7:** 545–51.

Effects on the eyes. Uveitis may occur a few weeks or months after starting rifabutin, and generally necessitates withdrawal of the drug and treatment with topical or systemic corticosteroids and cycloplegics.[1] The Committee on Safety of Medicines (CSM) in the UK was aware of 48 reports of uveitis in patients taking rifabutin.[2] Most patients were also receiving clarithromycin for treatment of AIDS-related *Mycobacterium avium* complex (MAC) infection and some were also receiving fluconazole (see Interactions, below). A dosage reduction to 300 mg rifabutin daily is now recommended in patients also receiving macrolides or triazole antifungals[2,3] and is reported to produce a satisfactory response in MAC infections.[4]

1. Tseng AL, Walmsley SL. Rifabutin-associated uveitis. *Ann Pharmacother* 1995; **29:** 1149–55.
2. Committee on Safety of Medicines. Rifabutin (Mycobutin)–uveitis. *Current Problems 20* 1994.
3. Committee on Safety of Medicines. Revised indications and drug interactions of rifabutin. *Current Problems* 1997; **23:** 14.
4. Shafran SD, *et al.* A comparison of two regimens for the treatment of Mycobacterium avium complex bacteremia in AIDS; rifabutin, ethambutol, and clarithromycin versus rifampin, ethambutol, clofazimine, and ciprofloxacin. *N Engl J Med* 1996; **335:** 377–83.

Interactions

As for Rifampicin, p.244. Rifabutin is reported to be a less potent inducer of microsomal enzymes than rifampicin, but similar interactions should nevertheless be anticipated.

Plasma concentrations of rifabutin are increased by concurrent administration of clarithromycin (and possibly other macrolides) and fluconazole resulting in increased rifabutin toxicity, in particular uveitis and neutropenia (see also above).

Antiretroviral drugs. Rifabutin interacts with HIV-protease inhibitors, decreasing their plasma concentrations but increasing its own, with a possible risk of uveitis. Most clinical experience appears to have been gained with rifabutin in combination with indinavir. The manufacturer of indinavir suggests that the dose of rifabutin should be reduced to half the usual dose, and that of indinavir increased to 1000 to 1200 mg every 8 hours in patients taking the two drugs together. Rifabutin should not be given with ritonavir. A similar interaction may occur with delavirdine.

Although rifabutin is reported to reduce the plasma concentrations of zidovudine, the manufacturer suggests that the reduction may not be clinically relevant.

Antimicrobial Action

Rifabutin possesses a spectrum of antibacterial activity similar to that of rifampicin (p.245). However, most investigations have concentrated on its action against mycobacteria. Cross-resistance is common with rifampicin.

Antimycobacterial action. Rifabutin possesses activity against most species of mycobacteria. Dickinson and Mitchison[1] have reported that the MIC of rifabutin against rifampicin-sensitive *Mycobacterium tuberculosis* strains is 8 times lower than that of rifampicin. At a concentration of 0.6 μg per mL, 69% of *Mycobacterium avium* complex strains were sensitive to rifabutin while 35% were sensitive to this concentration of rifampicin.

Another study has reported the MIC for rifabutin against clinical isolates of *M. avium* complex as 1.53 μg per mL for an agar dilution method and 1.25 μg per mL for a radiometric broth method.[2]

Rifabutin has been reported to be active in *animal* assays against *Mycobacterium leprae*,[3] including a rifampicin-resistant strain.[4] Synergistic activity against *M. leprae* has been reported[5] *in vitro* for rifabutin with clinafloxacin and rifabutin with sparfloxacin.

1. Dickinson JM, Mitchison DA. In vitro activity of new rifamycins against rifampicin-resistant M. tuberculosis and MAIS-complex mycobacteria. *Tubercle* 1987; **68:** 177–82.
2. Heifets LB, *et al.* Determination of ansamycin MICs for Mycobacterium avium complex in liquid medium by radiometric and conventional methods. *Antimicrob Agents Chemother* 1985; **28:** 570–5.
3. Hastings RC, Jacobson RR. Activity of ansamycin against Mycobacterium leprae in mice. *Lancet* 1983; **ii:** 1079–80. Correction. *ibid.*: 1210.
4. Hastings RC, *et al.* Ansamycin activity against rifampicin-resistant Mycobacterium leprae. *Lancet* 1984; **i:** 1130.
5. Dhople AM, Ibanez MA. In-vitro activity of three new fluoroquinolones and synergy with ansamycins against Mycobacterium leprae. *J Antimicrob Chemother* 1993; **32:** 445–51.

Resistance. Rifampicin-resistant strains of *Mycobacterium tuberculosis* have been identified in 2 patients receiving rifabutin alone as prophylaxis against *M. avium* complex.[1,2] It is therefore important to exclude *M. tuberculosis* infection before beginning rifabutin prophylaxis.

Rifampicin-resistant *M. kansasii* has also been reported in a patient receiving rifabutin.[3]

1. Weltman AC, *et al.* Rifampicin-resistant Mycobacterium tuberculosis. *Lancet* 1995; **345:** 1513.
2. Bishai WR, *et al.* Brief report: rifampin-resistant tuberculosis in a patient receiving rifabutin prophylaxis. *N Engl J Med* 1996; **334:** 1573–6.
3. Meynard JL, *et al.* Rifampin-resistant Mycobacterium kansasii infection in a patient with AIDS who was receiving rifabutin. *Clin Infect Dis* 1997; **24:** 1262–3.

Pharmacokinetics

Rifabutin is poorly absorbed from the gastro-intestinal tract, but is widely distributed. Approximately 70% is bound to plasma proteins. Both hepatic and renal clearance occurs. A terminal half-life of 36 hours has been reported.

The pharmacokinetics of rifabutin were studied in HIV-infected patients with normal renal and hepatic function.[1] A two-compartment open pharmacokinetic model was proposed. Rifabutin was rapidly but incompletely absorbed from the gastro-intestinal tract and bioavailability was poor; being 20% on day one of the study and 12% on day 28. Mean peak plasma concentrations occurred 2 to 3 hours following oral doses and were about 350, 500, and 900 ng per mL following doses of 300, 600, and 900 mg respectively. The peak and trough concentrations following 600 mg twice daily were about 900 and 200 ng per mL respectively. Rifabutin was approximately 70% bound to plasma proteins. The area under the curve showed a decrease on repeated dosage which might be explained by the induction of drug-metabolising liver enzymes. A large volume of distribution of 8 to 9 L per kg, indicative of extensive tissue distribution, and a mean terminal half-life of 32 to 38 hours were reported.

This study[1] also showed that the peak plasma concentration of the major metabolite, 25-deacetylrifabutin, was 10% of the parent compound. Only 4% of unchanged rifabutin was excreted in the urine following oral administration and between 6 to 14% following intravenous administration. Total urinary excretion of rifabutin and metabolite 72 hours after intravenous administration was 44%; total faecal excretion was between 30 and 49%.

Peak and trough concentrations at steady state were reported as 900 and 200 ng per mL respectively in one patient with tuberculosis given rifabutin 450 mg daily.[2] While these figures are the same as those previously reported with 600 mg twice daily,[1] that earlier study[1] showed that there is considerable interpatient variability.

CSF concentrations in 5 patients with AIDS on rifabutin 450 mg daily ranged from 36 to 70% of serum concentrations.[3]

1. Skinner MH, *et al.* Pharmacokinetics of rifabutin. *Antimicrob Agents Chemother* 1989; **33:** 1237–41.
2. Gillespie SH, *et al.* The serum rifabutin concentrations in a patient successfully treated for multi-resistant mycobacterium tuberculosis infection. *J Antimicrob Chemother* 1990; **25:** 490–1. Correction. *ibid.* 1991; **27:** 877.
3. Siegal FP, *et al.* Dose-limiting toxicity of rifabutin in AIDS-related complex: syndrome of arthralgia/arthritis. *AIDS* 1990; **4:** 433–41.

Uses and Administration

Rifabutin is a rifamycin antibiotic used for the *prophylaxis* of *Mycobacterium avium* complex (MAC) infection in immunocompromised patients and for the *treatment* of opportunistic mycobacterial infections (including those due to MAC) (p.133) and tuberculosis (p.146). When used for treatment, rifabutin, like rifampicin should be given in combination with other antibacterials to prevent the emergence of resistant organisms.

Rifabutin is given by mouth as a single daily dose. The recommended dose for the prophylaxis of *M. avium* complex infection is 300 mg daily. For the treatment of opportunistic mycobacterial infections the dose is 450 to 600 mg daily and for pulmonary tuberculosis the dose is 150 to 450 mg daily, in each case as part of a multi-drug regimen. Doses should be reduced to 300 mg daily in patients also receiving macrolides or azole antifungals (see under Adverse Effects, Effects on the Eyes, above).

Reviews.

1. Brogden RN, Fitton A. Rifabutin: a review of its antimicrobial activity, pharmacokinetic properties and therapeutic efficacy. *Drugs* 1994; **47:** 983–1009.

Cryptosporidiosis. Rifabutin may have a potential prophylactic effect against cryptosporidiosis (p.574).

Inflammatory bowel disease. Rifabutin, in combination with azithromycin or clarithromycin, has been studied in the treatment of Crohn's disease (see Inflammatory Bowel Disease, p.1171). The rationale for this use is based on the putative involvement of *Mycobacterium paratuberculosis* as a causative factor for the disease.

Preparations

USP 23: Rifabutin Capsules.

Proprietary Preparations (details are given in Part 3)
Aust.: Mycobutin; ***Austral.:*** Mycobutin; ***Canad.:*** Mycobutin; ***Fr.:*** Ansatipine; ***Ger.:*** Mycobutin; ***Ital.:*** Mycobutin; ***Neth.:*** Mycobutin; ***S.Afr.:*** Mycobutin; ***Spain:*** Ansatipin; ***Swed.:*** Ansatipin; ***Switz.:*** Mycobutine; ***UK:*** Mycobutin; ***USA:*** Mycobutin.

Rifampicin (7569-t)

Rifampicin *(BAN, rINN)*.

Ba-41166/E; L-5103; NSC-113926; Rifaldazine; Rifampicinum; Rifampin *(USAN)*; Rifamycin AMP. 3-(4-Methylpiperazin-1-yliminomethyl)rifamycin SV; (12*Z*,14*E*,24*E*)-(2*S*,16*S*,17*S*,18*R*,19*R*,20*R*,21*S*,22*R*,23*S*)-1,2-Dihydro-5,6,9,17,19-pentahydroxy-23-methoxy-2,4,12,16,18,20,22-heptamethyl-8-(4-methylpiperazin-1-yliminomethyl)-1,11-dioxo-2,7-(epoxypentadeca[1,11,13]trienimino)naphtho[2,1-*b*]furan-21-yl acetate.

$C_{43}H_{58}N_4O_{12}$ = 822.9.

CAS — 13292-46-1.

Pharmacopoeias. In *Chin., Eur.* (see p.viii), *Int., Jpn, Pol.,* and *US.*

A practically odourless reddish brown or brownish red crystalline powder. Slightly or very slightly **soluble** in water; slightly soluble in acetone, alcohol, and ether; freely soluble in chloroform; soluble in ethyl acetate and methyl alcohol. A 1% suspension in water has a pH of 4.5 to 6.5. **Store** at a temperature not exceeding 25° in airtight containers in an atmosphere of nitrogen. Protect from light.

Stability. The method employed when preparing an oral liquid from commercial rifampicin capsules influenced the dispersion of the powder and consequently the measured concentration of rifampicin in the final product.

1. Nahata MC, *et al.* Effect of preparation method and storage on rifampin concentration in suspensions. *Ann Pharmacother* 1994; **28:** 182–5.

Adverse Effects

Rifampicin is usually well tolerated. Adverse effects are more common during intermittent therapy or after restarting interrupted treatment.

Some patients may experience a cutaneous syndrome which presents 2 to 3 hours after a daily or intermittent dose as facial flushing, itching, rash, or rarely eye irritation. A 12-hour 'flu' syndrome of fever, chills, bone pain, shortness of breath, and malaise has been associated with intermittent administration. It usually occurs after 3 to 6 months of intermittent treatment and has a higher incidence with doses of 20 mg or more per kg body-weight given once weekly than with currently recommended regimens. Anaphylaxis or shock has occurred rarely.

Gastro-intestinal adverse effects include nausea, vomiting, anorexia, diarrhoea, and epigastric distress. Administration on an empty stomach is recommended for maximal absorption, but this has to be balanced against administration after a meal to minimise gastro-intestinal intolerance. Pseudomembranous colitis has been reported. Rifampicin produces transient abnormalities in liver function. Hepatitis occurs rarely. Fatalities due to hepatotoxicity have been reported occasionally (see below).

Rifampicin can cause thrombocytopenia and purpura, usually when administered as an intermittent regimen, and if this occurs further administration of rifampicin is contra-indicated. Other haematological adverse effects include eosinophilia, leucopenia, and haemolytic anaemia.

Alterations in kidney function and renal failure have occurred, particularly during intermittent therapy. Menstrual disturbances have been reported.

Nervous system adverse effects include headache, drowsiness, ataxia, dizziness, numbness, and muscular weakness.

Thrombophlebitis has occurred following prolonged intravenous infusion.

Rifampicin causes a harmless orange-red discoloration of the urine and other body fluids.

Effects on the blood. Thrombocytopenia may occur in patients taking rifampicin, most commonly as intermittent therapy, and probably has an immunological basis. The platelet count may fall within 3 hours of a dose and return to normal within 36 hours, if additional doses are not given.[1] There may also be a risk of thrombocytopenia when re-introducing rifampicin to patients who have interrupted their treatment.[2] Thrombocytopenia has also been reported in a patient taking rifampicin for the first time for meningococcal prophylaxis.[3] Fatalities have occurred when rifampicin was not withdrawn once thrombocytopenic purpura had developed or when treatment with rifampicin was resumed in patients who had experienced purpura.[1] However, there is a report of the successful re-introduction of rifampicin in a patient who developed thrombocytopenia without rifampicin-dependent antibodies.[4]

Bleeding from the oral cavity not associated with thrombocytopenia was reported in one patient taking rifampicin.[5] Leucopenia[6,7] and haemolysis or haemolytic anaemia[8] or red cell aplasia[9] have occurred. Disseminated intravascular coagulation has been reported in one patient receiving intermittent rifampicin therapy.[10] The incidence of deep vein thrombosis increased in one group of hospitalised tuberculosis patients when rifampicin was introduced as standard therapy,[11] but data from others have not supported a causal relationship.[12]

1. Girling DJ. Adverse effects of antituberculosis drugs. *Drugs* 1982; **23:** 56–74.
2. Burnette PK, *et al.* Rifampin-associated thrombocytopenia secondary to poor compliance. *Drug Intell Clin Pharm* 1989; **23:** 382–4.
3. Hall AP, *et al.* New hazard of meningococcal chemoprophylaxis. *J Antimicrob Chemother* 1993; **31:** 451.
4. Bhasin DK, *et al.* Can rifampicin be restarted in patients with rifampicin-induced thrombocytopenia? *Tubercle* 1991; **72:** 306–7.
5. Sule RR. An unusual reaction to rifampicin in a once monthly dose. *Lepr Rev* 1996; **67:** 227–33.
6. Van Assendelft AHW. Leucopenia in rifampicin chemotherapy. *J Antimicrob Chemother* 1985; **16:** 407–8.
7. Vijayakumaran P, *et al.* Leucocytopenia after rifampicin and ofloxacin therapy in leprosy. *Lepr Rev* 1997; **68:** 10–15.
8. Lakshminarayan S, *et al.* Massive haemolysis caused by rifampicin. *Br Med J* 1973; **2:** 282–3.
9. Mariette X, *et al.* Rifampicin-induced pure red cell aplasia. *Am J Med* 1989; **87:** 459–60.
10. Souza CS, *et al.* Disseminated intravascular coagulopathy as an adverse reaction to intermittent rifampin schedule in the treatment of leprosy. *Int J Lepr* 1997; **65:** 366–71.
11. White NW. Venous thrombosis and rifampicin. *Lancet* 1989; **ii:** 434–5.
12. Cowie RL, *et al.* Deep-vein thrombosis and pulmonary tuberculosis. *Lancet* 1989; **ii:** 1397.

Effects on the gastro-intestinal tract. In addition to symptoms of gastro-intestinal intolerance, gastro-intestinal bleeding and erosive gastritis,[1] ulcerative colitis,[2] and eosinophilic colitis[3] have been reported in patients receiving rifampicin.

1. Zargar SA, *et al.* Rifampicin-induced upper gastrointestinal bleeding. *Postgrad Med J* 1990; **66:** 310–11.
2. Tajima A, *et al.* Rifampicin-associated ulcerative colitis. *Ann Intern Med* 1992; **116:** 778–9.
3. Lange P, *et al.* Eosinophilic colitis due to rifampicin. *Lancet* 1994; **344:** 1296–7.

Effects on the immune system. Symptoms including malaise, arthralgia, arthritis, and oedema of the extremities occurring in 4 patients taking rifampicin and 3 taking rifabutin were considered to be due to drug-induced lupus syndrome.[1] All had positive anti-nuclear antibody titres.

1. Berning SE, Iseman MD. Rifamycin-induced lupus syndrome. *Lancet* 1997; **349:** 1521–2.

Effects on the liver. Transient abnormalities in liver function are common during the early stages of antituberculous treatment with rifampicin and other drugs, but sometimes there is more serious hepatotoxicity that may require a change of treatment especially in patients with pre-existing liver disease.

The use of rifampicin daily with ethionamide or prothionamide for the treatment of multibacillary leprosy has long been associated with a high incidence of hepatotoxicity (see p.208) and ethionamide and prothionamide are no longer recommended for the treatment of leprosy because of their severe hepatotoxicity. However, hepatic reactions have also been reported with rifampicin, isoniazid, and pyrazinamide, the drugs most commonly used to treat tuberculosis, and have occasionally proved fatal. A report[1] of four cases of fulminant hepatic failure in patients given triple therapy with the potentially hepatotoxic drugs rifampicin, isoniazid, and pyrazinamide (one patient also received ethambutol) highlighted the importance of strict liver function monitoring and this was reinforced by others.

The Joint Tuberculosis Committee of the British Thoracic Society is nevertheless anxious that fears over the safety of treatment regimens do not compromise adequate therapy of the disease itself. In an update to their guidelines,[2] they make recommendations for initial measurement of liver function in all patients and regular monitoring in patients with pre-existing liver disease. Tests should be repeated if symptoms of liver dysfunction occur, and details are given concerning the response to deteriorating liver function and include guidelines for prompt re-introduction of appropriate antituberculosis therapy once normal liver function is restored.

1. Mitchell I, *et al.* Anti-tuberculous therapy and acute liver failure. *Lancet* 1995; **345:** 555–6.
2. Ormerod LP, *et al.* Hepatotoxicity of antituberculosis drugs. *Thorax* 1996; **51:** 111–13.

Effects on the lungs. Pulmonary fibrosis in an elderly man was attributed to rifampicin.[1]

1. Umeki S. Rifampicin and pulmonary fibrosis. *Arch Intern Med* 1988; **148:** 1663, 7.

Effects on the pancreas. Chronic pancreatic insufficiency was reported in 1 patient following administration of rifampicin, isoniazid, ethambutol, and pyrazinamide.[1]

1. Liu BA, *et al.* Pancreatic insufficiency due to antituberculosis therapy. *Ann Pharmacother* 1997; **31:** 724–6.

Effects on the skin. Skin reactions to rifampicin are usually mild, irrespective of it being given daily or intermittently.[1] However, there have been a few isolated reports of severe reactions.[2-4] Contact dermatitis has been observed.[5]

1. Girling DJ. Adverse reactions to rifampicin in antituberculosis regimens. *J Antimicrob Chemother* 1977; **3:** 115–32.
2. Okano M, *et al.* Toxic epidermal necrolysis due to rifampicin. *J Am Acad Dermatol* 1987; **17:** 303–4.
3. Goldin HM, *et al.* Rifampin and exfoliative dermatitis. *Ann Intern Med* 1987; **107:** 789.
4. Mimouni A, *et al.* Fixed drug eruption following rifampin treatment. *DICP Ann Pharmacother* 1990; **24:** 947–8.
5. Anker N, Da Gunha Bang F. Long-term intravenous rifampicin treatment: advantages and disadvantages. *Eur J Respir Dis* 1981; **62:** 84–6.

Hypersensitivity. References.

1. Girling DJ. Adverse reactions to rifampicin in antituberculosis regimens. *J Antimicrob Chemother* 1977; **3:** 115–32.
2. Wurtz RM, *et al.* Anaphylactoid drug reactions to ciprofloxacin and rifampicin in HIV-infected patients. *Lancet* 1989; **i:** 955–6.
3. Harland RW, *et al.* Anaphylaxis from rifampin. *Am J Med* 1992; **92:** 581–2.
4. Criudde F, Leynadier F. The diagnosis of allergy to rifampicin confirmed by skin test. *Am J Med* 1994; **97:** 403–4.

Overdosage. Cases of skin pigmentation induced by rifampicin overdose have been reviewed.[1] Reddish-orange discoloration of the skin appeared within a few hours of drug administration; urine, mucous membranes, and sclera were also discoloured. Periorbital or facial oedema, pruritus, and gastro-intestinal intolerance occurred in most patients. Treatment was supportive and clinical symptoms resolved in most patients over 3 to 4 days, although fatalities occurred with doses over 14 g.

1. Holdiness MR. A review of the redman syndrome and rifampicin overdosage. *Med Toxicol Adverse Drug Exp* 1989; **4:** 444–51.

Precautions

Liver function should be checked before and during treatment with rifampicin and special care should be taken in alcoholic patients or those with pre-existing liver disease who require regular checks during therapy. Some manufacturers contra-indicate its use in patients with jaundice. A self-limiting hyperbilirubinaemia may occur in the first 2 or 3 weeks of treatment. Alkaline phosphatase values may be raised moderately due to rifampicin's enzyme inducing capacity. When other liver function tests are within normal limits, hyperbilirubinaemia in the first few weeks or moderately elevated alkaline phosphatase are not indications to withdraw rifampicin. However, dose adjustment is necessary when there is other evidence of hepatic function impairment and treatment should be suspended when there is evidence of more serious liver toxicity.

Blood counts should be monitored during prolonged treatment and in patients with hepatic disorders. Should thrombocytopenia or purpura occur then rifampicin should be withdrawn permanently. Some manufacturers also recommend such withdrawal in patients who develop haemolytic anaemia or renal failure.

Administration of rifampicin following interruption of treatment has been associated with increased risk of serious adverse effects.

Patients should be advised that rifampicin may colour faeces, saliva, sputum, sweat, tears, urine, and other body-fluids orange-red. Soft contact lenses worn by patients receiving rifampicin may become permanently stained.

Rifampicin should not be given by the intramuscular or subcutaneous route. When given by intravenous infusion care should be taken to avoid extravasation.

Adrenocortical insufficiency. Acute adrenal crisis has been precipitated by rifampicin in patients with adrenal insufficiency[1] and induction of microsomal enzymes may be enough to compromise even patients with mildly impaired cortisol production. Critical hypotension has also developed in non-Addisonian patients within a week to 10 days of starting rifampicin therapy. However, it has not been necessary to suspend the use of rifampicin if patients are treated with corticosteroids.[2] The effectiveness of corticosteroid therapy can be reduced by rifampicin (see under Interactions, below).

1. Elansary EH, Earis JE. Rifampicin and adrenal crisis. *Br Med J* 1983; **286:** 1861–2.
2. Boss G. Rifampicin and adrenal crisis. *Br Med J* 1983; **287:** 62.

Porphyria. Porphyria cutanea tarda[1] and porphyria variegata[2] have been precipitated by rifampicin. Moore and McColl[3] consider rifampicin to be unsafe for use in patients with acute porphyria.

1. Millar JW. Rifampicin-induced porphyria cutanea tarda. *Br J Dis Chest* 1980; **74:** 405–8.
2. Igual J-P, *et al.* Poussée aiguë de Porphyrie variegata: rôle de la rifampicine? *Nouv Presse Med* 1982; **11:** 2846.
3. Moore MR, McColl KEL. *Porphyria: drug lists.* Glasgow: Porphyria Research Unit, University of Glasgow, 1991.

Pregnancy and breast feeding. Authorities such as the International Union Against Tuberculosis[1] and the WHO Expert Committee on Leprosy[2] recommend **treatment** of **pregnant** patients with the same rifampicin-containing multidrug regimens as would be used in nonpregnant patients. Of the standard drugs recommended for leprosy or tuberculosis, only streptomycin has proven teratogenicity.[3] While administration of rifampicin to pregnant patients is generally considered to be safe, the drug does cross into the fetus[4] and malformations and bleeding tendencies have been reported.[3] From a literature review of tuberculosis regimens, Snider and co-workers[3] reported 386 normal term infants and 29 elective terminations out of 446 pregnancies in patients who took rifampicin in association with other antimycobacterial drugs. A variety of malformations were reported; there were 14 abnormal infants or fetuses, 2 premature births, 9 still-births and 7 spontaneous abortions. Snider *et al.* did not consider that rifampicin increased the overall risk of congenital malformations.

Bleeding disorders in 2 mothers shortly after delivery, and scalp haemorrhage, anaemia, and shock in one of the infants have been reported.[5] The authors recommended blood coagulation monitoring and prophylactic administration of vitamin K to mothers and neonates when the mother has received rifampicin during pregnancy.

Rifampicin is present in small amounts in breast milk; 1 to 3 μg per mL has been reported.[6] The American Academy of Pediatrics considers that mothers taking rifampicin may **breast feed**.[7]

1. Committee on Treatment of the International Union against Tuberculosis and Lung Disease. Antituberculosis regimens of chemotherapy. *Bull Int Union Tuberc Lung Dis* 1988; **63:** 60–4.
2. WHO. WHO expert committee on leprosy: sixth report. *WHO Tech Rep Ser 768* 1988.
3. Snider DE, *et al.* Treatment of tuberculosis during pregnancy. *Am Rev Respir Dis* 1980; **122:** 65–79.
4. Holdiness MR. Transplacental pharmacokinetics of the antituberculosis drugs. *Clin Pharmacokinet* 1987; **13:** 125–9.
5. Chouraqui JP, *et al.* Hémorragie par avitaminose K chez la femme enceinte et le nouveau-né: rôle éventuel de la rifampicine: a propos de 2 observations. *Therapie* 1982; **37:** 447–50.
6. Vorherr H. Drug excretion in breast milk. *Postgrad Med* 1974; **56:** 97–104.
7. American Academy of Pediatrics, Committee on Drugs. The transfer of drugs and other chemicals into human milk. *Pediatrics* 1989; **84:** 924–36.

Interactions

Rifampicin accelerates the metabolism of some drugs by inducing microsomal liver enzymes and possibly by interfering with hepatic uptake. A number of drugs have been reported to be affected but the clinical significance of some of these interactions remains to be determined. Although most drugs involved may require an increase in dosage to maintain effectiveness women taking oral contraceptives should change to another form of contraception (see p.1433). Other drugs reported to be affected include atovaquone, azathioprine, chloramphenicol, cimetidine, clofibrate, corticosteroids, coumarin anticoagulants, cyclosporin, dapsone, diazepam and other benzodiazepines, doxycycline, fluconazole, haloperidol, hexobarbitone, HIV-protease inhibitors, itraconazole, ketoconazole, methadone, oral hypoglycaemics, phenytoin, quinine, sulphasalazine, thyroid, theophylline, zidovudine, and several cardiovascular drugs including beta blockers, digitoxin, digoxin, and antiarrhythmics such as disopyramide, lorcainide, mexiletine, propafenone, quinidine, tocainide, and verapamil and other calcium-channel blockers.

Some interactions affecting the activity of rifampicin are discussed below.

Reviews.

1. Venkatesan K. Pharmacokinetic drug interactions with rifampicin. *Clin Pharmacokinet* 1992; **22:** 47–65.
2. Borcherding SM, *et al.* Update on rifampin drug interactions II. *Arch Intern Med* 1992; **152:** 711–16.
3. Grange JM, *et al.* Clinically significant drug interactions with antituberculosis agents. *Drug Safety* 1994; **11:** 242–51.

Antacids. The bioavailability of rifampicin measured by a urinary excretion method was significantly reduced when administered simultaneously with magnesium trisilicate, aluminium hydroxide, or sodium bicarbonate.[1]

1. Khalil SAH, *et al.* Effect of antacids on oral absorption of rifampicin. *Int J Pharmaceutics* 1984; **20:** 99–106.

Antiretroviral drugs. Rifamycins can induce the metabolism of zidovudine, delavirdine, and HIV-protease inhibitors including indinavir, ritonavir, and saquinavir resulting in potentially subtherapeutic plasma concentrations. In addition HIV-protease inhibitors inhibit the metabolism of rifamycins resulting in elevated plasma-rifamycin concentrations and an increased incidence of adverse effects.[1] In general, rifampicin and HIV-protease inhibitors should not be used concurrently. See also p.242 for comment on the interaction of HIV-protease inhibitors with rifabutin.

1. Anonymous. Clinical update: impact of HIV protease inhibitors on the treatment of HIV-infected tuberculosis patients with rifampin. *MMWR* 1996; **45:** 921–5.

Clofazimine. Concomitant administration of clofazimine to leprosy patients receiving rifampicin with or without dapsone may decrease the rate of absorption of rifampicin and increase the time to peak plasma level.[1] In patients receiving clofazimine, rifampicin, and dapsone, the rifampicin area under the curve was reduced.[1] However, a multiple dose study showed that pharmacokinetics of rifampicin were similar after 7 days treatment with rifampicin and dapsone or rifampicin, dapsone, and clofazimine.[2]

1. Mehta J, *et al.* Effect of clofazimine and dapsone on rifampicin (Lositril) pharmacokinetics in multibacillary and paucibacillary leprosy cases. *Lepr Rev* 1986; **57** (suppl 3): 67–76.
2. Venkatesan K, *et al.* The effect of clofazimine on the pharmacokinetics of rifampicin and dapsone in leprosy. *J Antimicrob Chemother* 1986; **18:** 715–18.

Isoniazid. It has been shown that there is little significant pharmacokinetic interaction between rifampicin and isoniazid.[1] Although lower blood concentrations of rifampicin have been reported with concomitant isoniazid administration, the effect is not considered clinically significant.[2]

Since both drugs are hepatotoxic, concurrent administration could be associated with an increased incidence of hepatic damage, although the benefits of using this combination are considered to outweigh any potential risks.

1. Acocella G, *et al.* Kinetics of rifampicin and isoniazid administered alone and in combination to normal subjects and patients with liver disease. *Gut* 1972; **13:** 47–53.

2. Mouton RP, *et al.* Blood levels of rifampicin, desacetylrifampicin and isoniazid during combined therapy. *J Antimicrob Chemother* 1979; **5:** 447–54.

Ketoconazole. Concomitant administration of rifampicin, ketoconazole, and isoniazid have produced low serum concentrations of each drug resulting in failure of antifungal treatment.[1] Rifampicin serum concentrations are reduced when rifampicin is given concurrently with ketoconazole;[2] separation of the doses by 30 minutes[3] to 12 hours[2] may result in similar rifampicin concentrations to those attained when rifampicin is given alone, although serum concentrations of ketoconazole remain depressed regardless of the time of administration.

1. Abadie-Kemmerly S, *et al.* Failure of ketoconazole treatment of Blastomyces dermatitidis due to interaction of isoniazid and rifampin. *Ann Intern Med* 1988; **109:** 844–5. Correction. *ibid.* 1989; **111:** 96.
2. Engelhard D, *et al.* Interaction of ketoconazole with rifampin and isoniazid. *N Engl J Med* 1984; **311:** 1681–3.
3. Doble N, *et al.* Pharmacokinetic study of the interaction between rifampicin and ketoconazole. *J Antimicrob Chemother* 1988; **21:** 633–5.

Probenecid. Although one study[1] showed that concomitant administration of probenecid could increase serum-rifampicin concentrations, another[2] subsequently found that the effect was uncommon and inconsistent and concluded that probenecid had no place as an adjunct to routine rifampicin therapy.

1. Kenwright S, Levi AJ. Impairment of hepatic uptake of rifamycin antibiotics by probenecid and its therapeutic implications. *Lancet* 1973; **ii:** 1401–5.
2. Fallon RJ, *et al.* Probenecid and rifampicin serum levels. *Lancet* 1975; **ii:** 792–4.

Antimicrobial Action

Rifampicin is bactericidal against a wide range of micro-organisms and interferes with their synthesis of nucleic acids by inhibiting DNA-dependent RNA polymerase. It has the ability to kill intracellular organisms. It is active against mycobacteria, including *Mycobacterium tuberculosis* and *M. leprae* and, having high sterilising activity against these organisms, it possesses the ability to eliminate semi-dormant or persisting organisms. Rifampicin is active against Gram-positive bacteria, especially staphylococci, but less active against Gram-negative organisms. The most sensitive Gram-negative bacteria include *Neisseria meningitidis*, *N. gonorrhoeae*, *Haemophilus influenzae*, and *Legionella* spp. Rifampicin also has activity against *Chlamydia trachomatis* and some anaerobic bacteria. At high concentrations it is active against some viruses. Rifampicin has no effect on fungi but has been reported to enhance the antifungal activity of amphotericin.

Minimum inhibitory concentrations tend to vary with the medium used; MICs for the most sensitive organisms (chlamydia, staphylococci) tend to range from about 0.01 to 0.02 μg per mL, while the MIC for most susceptible mycobacteria ranges from 0.1 to 2 μg per mL. The concomitant use of other antimicrobials may enhance or antagonise the bactericidal activity of rifampicin.

Strains of *Mycobacterium tuberculosis*, *M. leprae* and other usually susceptible bacteria have demonstrated resistance, both initially and during treatment. Thus in tuberculosis and leprosy regimens, rifampicin is used in combination with other drugs to delay or prevent the development of rifampicin resistance. There does not appear to be cross-resistance apart from that between rifampicin and other rifamycins. However, there have been isolated reports of the emergence of multidrug-resistant strains of *M. leprae* (see below).

MULTIDRUG RESISTANCE. Strains of *Mycobacterium leprae* with multiple resistance to rifampicin, ofloxacin, and dapsone have been isolated from patients who have previously received dapsone monotherapy followed by treatment with rifampicin in combination with ofloxacin.[1,2]

1. Cambau E, *et al.* Multidrug-resistance to dapsone, rifampicin, and ofloxacin in Mycobacterium leprae. *Lancet* 1997; **349:** 103–4.
2. Ji B, *et al.* High relapse rate among lepromatous leprosy patients treated with rifampicin plus ofloxacin daily for 4 weeks. *Antimicrob Agents Chemother* 1997; **41:** 1953–6.

Pharmacokinetics

Rifampicin is readily absorbed from the gastro-intestinal tract and peak plasma concentrations of about 7 to 10 μg per mL have been reported 2 to 4 hours after a dose of 600 mg but there may be considerable interindividual variation. Food may reduce and delay absorption. Rifampicin is approximately 80% bound to plasma proteins. It is widely distributed in body tissues and fluids and diffusion into the CSF is increased when the meninges are inflamed. Rifampicin crosses the placenta and is distributed into breast milk (see Pregnancy and Breast Feeding, under Precautions, above). Half-lives for rifampicin have been reported to range initially from 2 to 5 hours, the longest elimination times occurring after the largest doses. However, as rifampicin induces its own metabolism, elimination time may decrease by up to 40% during the first 2 weeks resulting in half-lives of about 1 to 3 hours. The half-life is prolonged in patients with liver disease.

Rifampicin is rapidly metabolised in the liver mainly to active desacetylrifampicin; rifampicin and desacetylrifampicin are excreted in the bile. Rifampicin, but not its main metabolite, is then reabsorbed. About 60% of a dose eventually appears in the faeces. The amount excreted in the urine increases with increasing doses and up to 30% of a dose of 900 mg may be excreted in the urine, about half of it within 24 hours. The metabolite formylrifampicin is also excreted in the urine. In patients with impaired renal function the half-life of rifampicin is not prolonged at doses of 600 mg or less.

Distribution. Rifampicin is widely distributed in most body tissues and fluids following oral or intravenous administration.[1] Rifampicin is also able to penetrate into polymorphonuclear leucocytes to kill intracellular pathogens.[2] Rifampicin does not appear to diffuse well through the uninflamed meninges[3] but therapeutic concentrations have been attained in the CSF following daily doses of 600 and 900 mg when the meninges are inflamed;[4] concentrations in the CSF are about 10 to 20% of simultaneous serum concentrations, and approximately represent the fraction unbound to plasma proteins. Administration of corticosteroids does not appear to influence the penetration of rifampicin into the CSF of patients with tuberculous meningitis.[5]

1. Holdiness MR. Clinical pharmacokinetics of the antituberculosis drugs. *Clin Pharmacokinet* 1984; **9:** 511–44.
2. Prokesch RC, Hand WL. Antibiotic entry into human polymorphonuclear leukocytes. *Antimicrob Agents Chemother* 1982; **21:** 373–80.
3. Sippel JE, *et al.* Rifampin concentrations in cerebrospinal fluid of patients with tuberculous meningitis. *Am Rev Respir Dis* 1974; **109:** 579–80.
4. D'Oliveira JJG. Cerebrospinal fluid concentrations of rifampin in meningeal tuberculosis. *Am Rev Respir Dis* 1972; **106:** 432–7
5. Woo J, *et al.* Cerebrospinal fluid and serum levels of pyrazinamide and rifampicin in patients with tuberculous meningitis. *Curr Ther Res* 1987; **42:** 235–42.

Intravenous administration. Mean peak plasma concentrations of 10 μg per mL following administration of 600 mg of rifampicin by intravenous infusion over 3 hours have been reported. Peak plasma concentrations declined with repeated administration but to a less marked extent than occurs with oral administration.[1] Mean peak plasma concentrations of 27 μg per mL have been reported in children following doses of 11.5 mg per kg body-weight infused over 30 minutes. Mean concentrations of 1.9 μg per mL were reported 8 hours following the dose.[2]

1. Acocella G, *et al.* Serum and urine concentrations of rifampicin administered by intravenous infusion in man. *Arzneimittelforschung* 1977; **27:** 1221–6.
2. Koup JR, *et al.* Pharmacokinetics of rifampin in children I. Multiple dose intravenous infusion. *Ther Drug Monit* 1986; **8:** 11–16.

Oral administration. Gastro-intestinal absorption of rifampicin is considered good. However, analysis of serum-rifampicin concentrations in children indicated that only 50 ± 22% of a freshly prepared suspension was absorbed following oral administration.[1] Also varying oral bioavailability from capsule formulations has been reported and could result in ineffective therapy[2] or higher than needed serum concentrations.[3]

The oral bioavailability of rifampicin and isoniazid, but not of pyrazinamide, was decreased by food in many patients.[4]

Subtherapeutic plasma rifampicin concentrations have been reported in patients with HIV infection, possibly related to impaired absorption.[5-7]

1. Koup JR, *et al.* Pharmacokinetics of rifampin in children II. Oral bioavailability. *Ther Drug Monit* 1986; **8:** 17–22.
2. Holdiness MR. Clinical pharmacokinetics of the antituberculosis drugs. *Clin Pharmacokinet* 1984; **9:** 511–44.
3. Ganiswarna SG, *et al.* Bioavailability of rifampicin caplets (600 mg and 450 mg) in healthy Indonesian subjects. *Int J Clin Pharmacol Ther Toxicol* 1986; **24:** 60–4.
4. Zent C, Smith P. Study of the effect of concomitant food on the bioavailability of rifampicin, isoniazid and pyrazinamide. *Tubercle Lung Dis* 1995; **76:** 109–13.
5. Patel KB, *et al.* Drug malabsorption and resistant tuberculosis in HIV-infected patients. *N Engl J Med* 1995; **332:** 336–7.
6. Peloquin CA, *et al.* Low antituberculosis drug concentrations in patients with AIDS. *Ann Pharmacother* 1996; **30:** 919–25.
7. Sahai J, *et al.* Reduced plasma concentrations of antituberculosis drugs in patients with HIV infection. *Ann Intern Med* 1997; **127:** 289–93.

Uses and Administration

Rifampicin belongs to the rifamycin group of antimycobacterials (p.113) and is used in the treatment of various infections due to mycobacteria and other susceptible organisms (see Antimicrobial Action, above). It is usually given combined with other antibacterials to prevent the emergence of resistant organisms.

Rifampicin is used, notably in combination with isoniazid and pyrazinamide, as a component of multidrug regimens for the treatment of tuberculosis, and with dapsone and clofazimine in the treatment of leprosy. It is a component of various regimens for the treatment of opportunistic mycobacterial infections.

Other uses include brucellosis, chancroid, chlamydial infections, the treatment of staphylococcal endocarditis, penicillin-resistant pneumococcal meningitis, prophylaxis of epiglottitis due to *Haemophilus influenzae*, Legionnaires' disease, the prophylaxis of meningococcal and *H. influenzae* meningitis, mycetoma, the eradication of pharyngeal streptococcal carriage in pharyngitis, Q fever, and in various staphylococcal infections for treatment or prophylactically to reduce staphylococcal carriage. For discussions of all these infections and their treatment, see under Choice of Antibacterial, p.116.

The usual adult dose of rifampicin is 600 mg daily by mouth, preferably on an empty stomach, or by intravenous infusion as the base or the sodium salt; higher doses are sometimes employed (see below).

Rifampicin is used in the initial and continuation phases of short-course **tuberculosis** regimens (p.146) in combination with other antimycobacterials. Rifampicin is administered orally on an empty stomach in single daily doses of 10 mg per kg body-weight (maximum 600 mg) to children and adults or may be given intermittently two or three times weekly in doses of 10 or 15 mg per kg (maximum 900 mg) to children and adults. Alternatively doses may be expressed as follows: with daily administration, adults weighing less than 50 kg receive 450 mg and those over 50 kg receive 600 mg; with intermittent administration, adults receive 600 to 900 mg 2 or 3 times weekly. The maximum recommended dose is considered to be 900 mg because a greater incidence of adverse effects is associated with doses above 900 mg.

In **leprosy** regimens (p.128), rifampicin is usually given with dapsone for paucibacillary leprosy, and with dapsone and clofazimine for multibacillary leprosy. Rifampicin is given once monthly in a usual adult dose of 600 mg by mouth; it may also be given daily in the same dose. Guidelines for monthly doses in low-body-weight adults and in children are rifampicin 450 mg for adults weighing less than 35 kg and children 10 to 14 years old. Low body-weight children may be given 12 to 15 mg per kg monthly. Single-dose treatment with rifampicin, ofloxacin, and minocycline may be an alternative in patients with single-lesion paucibacillary leprosy.

For **prophylaxis** against meningococcal meningitis and the treatment of meningococcal carriers, rifampicin is usually given in a dose of 600 mg twice daily by mouth for 2 days; recommended doses to be given to children twice daily for 2 days are 10 mg per kg for children between 1 and 12 years of age and 5 mg per kg for children under 12 months. For prophylaxis against meningitis due to *Haemophilus influenzae* a dose of 20 mg per kg is given once daily by mouth for 4 days with a maximum daily dose of 600 mg. This dose is suitable for adults and children over 3 months of age; recommendations regarding use in infants vary and are discussed in detail below (p.246).

In the treatment of **brucellosis**, **Legionnaires' disease**, and serious **staphylococcal infections** a dose of 600 to 1200 mg daily in divided doses has been recommended in combination with other drugs.

Administration in hepatic and renal impairment. See under Precautions, above.

Meningitis prophylaxis. HAEMOPHILUS INFLUENZAE MENINGITIS PROPHYLAXIS. Meningeal infection with *Haemophilus influenzae* type b (Hib) in children is associated with substantial morbidity, but the incidence has decreased since the introduction of immunisation with *H. influenzae* type b vaccine. Although a world-wide problem, the disease and its prophylaxis has been studied mainly in the USA, where it has been shown that children under 4 years of age form the highest risk group for primary infection while children under 2 years of age form the highest risk group for secondary infection.[1] The goal of prophylaxis in close contacts is to eliminate carriage of the organism to prevent spread to young children. Risk of infection to young children with recent household contact to the primary case of infection with *Haemophilus influenzae* type b is increased 600- to 800-fold,[1,2] but only increased 20-fold[3] from day-care or school contact. The risk may be higher when more than 1 index patient is identified.

Rifampicin in doses of 20 mg per kg per day once daily for 4 days (maximum dose 600 mg) has been shown to eradicate Hib nasopharyngeal carriage in at least 95% of contacts of the primary case.[4] There is some evidence from a study involving 68 families of patients with Hib infection that rifampicin 20 mg per kg daily for 2 days may be as effective as a 4-day course in eradicating Hib pharyngeal colonisation.[5] Rifampicin prophylaxis appears to be successful in preventing infection in household contacts, but benefit in school settings where there has been a single index case has not been established.[3]

Various recommendations have been made for rifampicin prophylaxis. Administration of rifampicin to all persons, regardless of vaccine status, with close, recent (within 2 weeks) contact to the primary case and who are likely to be exposed to susceptible children has been endorsed by the American Academy of Pediatrics;[6] similar recommendations have been made in the UK.[2] Rifampicin should also be given to the primary case since treatment of the infection does not eradicate nasopharyngeal carriage.[2,6] Rifampicin prophylaxis following exposure through day-care or school contact may be given and has been endorsed by the American Centers for Disease Control.[7]

In the UK prophylaxis is recommended for all room contacts when 2 or more cases of *H. influenzae* disease have occurred in a playgroup or nursery within 120 days.[2]

Rifampicin prophylaxis is not recommended for pregnant women,[2,6] and in the UK prophylaxis is not recommended in breast-feeding mothers.[2] Recommendations for prophylaxis in infants differ between the USA and the UK. Infants under 3 months of age are excluded from UK recommendations[2] while in the USA all neonates are considered eligible for prophylaxis.[6]

1. Casto DT, Edwards DL. Preventing Haemophilus influenzae type b disease. *Clin Pharm* 1985; **4:** 637–48.
2. Cartwright KAV, *et al.* Chemoprophylaxis for Haemophilus influenzae type b: rifampicin should be given to close contacts. *Br Med J* 1991; **302:** 546–7.
3. ASHP Commission on Therapeutics. ASHP therapeutic guidelines on nonsurgical antimicrobial prophylaxis. *Clin Pharm* 1990; **9:** 423–45.
4. Band JD, *et al.* Prevention of Hemophilus influenzae type b disease. *JAMA* 1984; **251:** 2381–6.
5. Green M, *et al.* Duration of rifampin chemoprophylaxis for contacts of patients infected with Haemophilus influenzae type B. *Antimicrob Agents Chemother* 1992; **36:** 545–7.
6. American Academy of Pediatrics. Revision of recommendation for use of rifampin prophylaxis of contacts of patients with Haemophilus influenzae infection. *Pediatrics* 1984; **74:** 301–2.
7. Broome CV, *et al.* Use of chemoprophylaxis to prevent the spread of Hemophilus influenzae b in day-care facilities. *N Engl J Med* 1987; **36:** 1226–8.

MENINGOCOCCAL MENINGITIS PROPHYLAXIS. *Neisseria meningitidis* is an important cause of bacterial meningitis; all age groups are at risk during epidemics but children are usually at highest risk during endemic outbreaks. Vaccines are available for meningococci groups A and C but not for group B, therefore antimicrobial prophylaxis remains important in preventing the spread of the disease. The aim of prophylaxis is to eliminate nasopharyngeal carriage of the organism. Sulphadiazine and minocycline are no longer used because of resistance and adverse effects. The current antibacterial of choice is rifampicin; rates of 70 to 90% have been reported for eradication of nasal carriage.[1] Rifampicin is given for 2 days in doses of 600 mg twice daily (1200 mg per day) for adults, 10 mg per kg body-weight twice daily for children aged 1 to 12 years, and 5 mg per kg twice daily for children under 12 months.[1,2] Alternative drugs are ceftriaxone and ciprofloxacin. Once a meningococcal infection occurs, the risk of infection in household contacts increases 500- to 1200-fold.[2] Antibacterial prophylaxis should be given as soon as possible to household contacts and persons exposed to the patient's oral secretions (ideally within 24 hours of diagnosis of the index case). It is also recommended for child care or nursery school contacts in the USA,[1] but is not usually advised for this group in the UK following a single case.[2] The index patient should also receive rifampicin or other prophylaxis since treatment with penicillin does not necessarily eradicate nasopharyngeal carriage.

Treatment of meningococcal meningitis is discussed on p.130.

1. Committee on Infectious Diseases of the American Academy of Pediatrics, Infectious Diseases and Immunization Committee of the Canadian Pediatric Society. Meningococcal disease prevention and control strategies for practice-based physicians. *Pediatrics* 1996; **97:** 404–11.
2. PHLS Meningococcal Infections Working Group and Public Health Medicine Environmental Group. Control of meningococcal disease: guidance for consultants in communicable disease control. *Commun Dis Rep* 1995; **5** (review 13): R189–R195.

Preparations

BP 1998: Rifampicin Capsules; Rifampicin Oral Suspension;
USP 23: Rifampin and Isoniazid Capsules; Rifampin Capsules; Rifampin for Injection; Rifampin Oral Suspension.

Proprietary Preparations (details are given in Part 3)
Aust.: Eremfat; Rifoldin; Rimactan; ***Austral.:*** Rifadin; Rimycin; ***Belg.:*** Rifadine; Rimactan; ***Canad.:*** Rifadin; Rimactane; Rofact; ***Fr.:*** Rifadine; Rimactan; ***Ger.:*** Eremfat; Rifa; Rimactan; ***Irl.:*** Rifadin; Rimactane; ***Ital.:*** Rifadin; Rifapiam; Rimactan†; ***Neth.:*** Rifadin; Rimactan; ***Norw.:*** Rifadin; Rimactan; ***S.Afr.:*** Rifadin; Rifcin; Rimactane; ***Spain:*** Diabacil†; Dinoldin†; Rifagen; Rifaldin; Rifocina; Rimactan; ***Swed.:*** Rifadin; Rimactan; ***Switz.:*** Rifoldine; Rimactan; ***UK:*** Rifadin; Rimactane; ***USA:*** Rifadin; Rimactane.

Multi-ingredient: ***Aust.:*** Rifater; Rifoldin INH; Rimactan + INH; ***Canad.:*** Rifater; ***Fr.:*** Rifater; Rifinah; ***Ger.:*** Iso-Eremfat; Rifa/INH†; Rifater; Rifinah; ***Irl.:*** Rifater; Rifinah; Rimactazid; ***Ital.:*** Rifanicozid; Rifater; Rifinah; ***Neth.:*** Rifinah; ***S.Afr.:*** MB-Combi†; Myrin; Pyrifin; Rifater; Rifinah; ***Spain:*** Rifater; Rifazida†; Rifinah; Rimactazid; ***Switz.:*** Rifater; Rifinah; Rifoldine-INH†; Rimactazide; Rimactazide + Z; ***UK:*** Rifater; Rifinah; Rimactazid; ***USA:*** Rifamate; Rifater; Rimactane/INH Dual Pack†.

Rifamycin Sodium (146-s)

Rifamycin Sodium *(BANM, rINNM)*.

M-14 (rifamycin); Rifamicina; Rifamycin SV Sodium; Rifamycinum Natricum. Sodium (12*Z*,14*E*,24*E*)-(2*S*,16*S*,17*S*,18*R*,19*R*,20*R*,21*S*,22*R*,23*S*)-21-acetoxy-1,2-dihydro-6,9,17,19-tetrahydroxy-23-methoxy-2,4,12,16,18,20,22-heptamethyl-1,11-dioxo-2,7-(epoxypentadeca-1,11,13-trienimino)-naphtho[2,1-*b*]furan-5-olate.

$C_{37}H_{46}NNaO_{12}$ = 719.8.

CAS — 6998-60-3 (rifamycin); 14897-39-3; 15105-92-7 (both rifamycin sodium).

Pharmacopoeias. In *Eur.* (see p.viii) and *Pol.*

The monosodium salt of rifamycin SV, a substance obtained by chemical transformation of rifamycin B which is produced during growth of certain strains of *Amycolatopsis mediterranei* (*Nocardia mediterranei*; *Streptomyces mediterranei*). Rifamycin SV may also be obtained directly from certain mutants of *Amycolatopsis mediterranei*. Rifamycin sodium contains not less than 900 units per mg calculated on the anhydrous substance. A red, fine or slightly granular powder. **Soluble** in water; freely soluble in dehydrated alcohol; practically insoluble in ether. A 5% solution has a pH of 6.5 to 8.0. **Store** in airtight containers at a temperature of 2° to 8°. Protect from light.

Adverse Effects and Precautions

Some gastro-intestinal side-effects have occurred following injections of rifamycin. High doses may produce alterations in liver function. Hypersensitivity reactions including rashes, pruritus, and occasional anaphylaxis have occurred rarely, but prolonged administration increases the risk of sensitisation. A reddish coloration of the urine has been reported. It should be used with care in patients with hepatic dysfunction.

Antimicrobial Action

Rifamycin has similar antimicrobial actions to those of rifampicin (p.245).

Pharmacokinetics

Rifamycin is not effectively absorbed from the gastro-intestinal tract. Plasma concentrations of 2 μg per mL have been achieved 2 hours after a dose of 250 mg by intramuscular injection. The plasma half-life is reported to be about 1 hour. It is excreted mainly in the bile and only small amounts appear in the urine.

Uses and Administration

Rifamycin is a rifamycin antibacterial that has been used in the treatment of infections caused by susceptible organisms such as staphylococci. It has been given as the sulphate by intramuscular injection and by slow intravenous infusion and is also administered by local instillation and topical application.

Preparations

Proprietary Preparations (details are given in Part 3)
Aust.: Rifocin; ***Belg.:*** Rifocine; ***Fr.:*** Otofa; Rifocine; ***Ger.:*** Chibro-Rifamycin†; ***Ital.:*** Rifocin; ***Switz.:*** Otofa; Rifocine†.

Rifapentine (16978-r)

Rifapentine *(BAN, USAN, rINN)*.

DL-473; DL-473-IT; L-11473; MDL-473. 3-[*N*-(4-Cyclopentyl-1-piperazinyl)formimidoyl]rifamycin.

$C_{47}H_{64}N_4O_{12}$ = 877.0.

CAS — 61379-65-5.

Rifapentine is a rifamycin antibacterial (see Rifampicin, p.243) that is used, in combination with other antimycobacterials, for the treatment of tuberculosis. It is under investigation for the prophylaxis of *Mycobacterium avium* complex infections in patients with AIDS.

Rifapentine is given by mouth in a dose of 600 mg twice a week during the initial phase, then once weekly during the continuation phase of treatment.

Preparations

Proprietary Preparations (details are given in Part 3)
USA: Priftin.

Rifaximin (503-j)

Rifaximin *(USAN, rINN)*.

L-105; Rifaxidin; Rifaximine. (2*S*,16*Z*,18*E*,20*S*,21*S*,22*R*,23*R*,24*R*,25*S*,26*S*,27*S*,28*E*)-5,6,21,23,25-Pentahydroxy-27-methoxy-2,4,11,16,20,22,24,26-octamethyl-2,7-(epoxypentadeca[1,11,13]trienimino)benzofuro[4,5-e]pyrido[1,2-*a*]benzimidazole-1,15(2*H*)-dione 25-acetate.

$C_{43}H_{51}N_3O_{11}$ = 785.9.

CAS — 80621-81-4.

NOTE. The code L-105 has also been applied to a cephalosporin under investigation.

Rifaximin is a rifamycin antibacterial with antimicrobial actions similar to those of rifampicin (p.245), but which is poorly absorbed from the gastro-intestinal tract. It has been given by mouth in the treatment of gastro-intestinal infections, for surgical infection prophylaxis, and in hepatic encephalopathy. Suggested doses have ranged from 10 to 15 mg per kg body-weight daily in adults. It has also been used topically as a 5% ointment.

References.

1. Gillis JC, Brogden RN. Rifaximin: a review of its antibacterial activity, pharmacokinetic properties and therapeutic potential in conditions mediated by gastrointestinal bacteria. *Drugs* 1995; **49:** 467–84.

Preparations

Proprietary Preparations (details are given in Part 3)
Ital.: Dermodis; Normix; Redactiv; Rifacol.

Rokitamycin (2827-b)

Rokitamycin *(rINN)*.

M-19-Q; 3″-Propionyl-leucomycin A_5; Rikamycin; TMS-19Q. [(4*R*,5*S*,6*S*,7*R*,9*R*,10*R*,11*E*,13*E*,16*R*)-7-(Formylmethyl)-4,10-dihydroxy-5-methoxy-9,16-dimethyl-2-oxooxacyclohexadeca-11,13-dien-6-yl]-3,6-dideoxy-4-*O*-(2,6-dideoxy-3-*C*-methyl-α-L-*ribo*-hexopyranosyl)-3-(dimethylamino)-β-D-glucopyranoside 4″-butyrate 3″-propionate.

$C_{42}H_{69}NO_{15}$ = 828.0.

CAS — 74014-51-0.

Rokitamycin is a macrolide antibiotic with actions and uses similar to those of erythromycin (p.204). It has been given by mouth in doses of 400 mg twice daily.

Preparations

Proprietary Preparations (details are given in Part 3)
Ital.: Paidocin; Rokital.

Rolitetracycline (149-l)

Rolitetracycline *(BAN, USAN, rINN).*

PMT; Pyrrolidinomethyltetracycline; SQ-15659. N^2-(Pyrrolidin-1-ylmethyl)tetracycline.

$C_{27}H_{33}N_3O_8$ = 527.6.

CAS — 751-97-3.

Pharmacopoeias. In *It.*

Rolitetracycline Nitrate (150-v)

Rolitetracycline Nitrate *(BANM, USAN, rINNM).*

Pyrrolidinomethyltetracycline Nitrate Sesquihydrate.

$C_{27}H_{33}N_3O_8,HNO_3,1\frac{1}{2}H_2O$ = 617.6.

CAS — 20685-78-3; 7681-32-5 (both anhydrous rolitetracycline nitrate); 26657-13-6 (rolitetracycline nitrate sesquihydrate).

1.17 mg of rolitetracycline nitrate is approximately equivalent to 1 mg of rolitetracycline.

Stability. Rolitetracycline is unstable in the presence of water: aqueous solutions of the base or the nitrate are hydrolysed in solution to tetracycline,[1,2] more than 50% being so converted in 3 hours at 25° according to one report,[1] while 15% of a reconstituted injection of the base has been reported to be lost in 21 to 25 hours when stored at 5°.[2]

1. Hughes DW, *et al.* Stability of rolitetracycline in aqueous solution. *J Pharm Pharmacol* 1974; **26:** 79–80.
2. Wilson WL, *et al.* Chemical stability of reconstituted rolitetracycline formulations. *Can J Pharm Sci* 1976; **11:** 126–8.

Adverse Effects and Precautions

As for Tetracycline Hydrochloride, p.259.

Shivering and more rarely rigor due to a Herxheimer-like reaction may be associated with the first few injections of rolitetracycline in infections due to organisms highly sensitive to tetracyclines. Injections may be followed by a peculiar taste sensation, often similar to ether. Rapid intravenous injection may cause transient giddiness, hot flushes, reddening of the face and, occasionally, peripheral circulatory failure.

Symptoms of myasthenia gravis have been exacerbated by the intravenous administration of rolitetracycline although it has been suggested that this may be due to magnesium ions in the formulation.

Interactions

As for Tetracycline Hydrochloride, p.260.

Antimicrobial Action

As for Tetracycline Hydrochloride, p.260.

Pharmacokinetics

As for Tetracycline Hydrochloride, p.260.

Rolitetracycline is not absorbed from the gastro-intestinal tract. When administered by injection about 50% of rolitetracycline in the circulation is bound to plasma proteins. Peak plasma concentrations of about 4 to 6 µg per mL have been reported about 0.5 to 1 hour after a dose of 350 mg given intramuscularly while after intravenous administration they may be as high as 20 µg per mL. The half-life has been reported to range from about 5 to 8 hours. About 50% of a dose is excreted in the urine.

Uses and Administration

Rolitetracycline is a tetracycline derivative with uses similar to those of tetracycline (p.261). It is given by slow intravenous injection. It has also been given by deep intramuscular injection. Treatment with an oral tetracycline should be substituted as soon as possible. It is also included in some topical eye preparations.

Adults may be given 275 mg once daily by slow intravenous injection over 2 to 3 minutes; in severe infections the dose may be given up to 3 times daily. Extravasation into subcutaneous tissues should be avoided.

Older children have been given 10 mg per kg body-weight daily but the effect of tetracyclines on teeth and bones should be considered.

Rolitetracycline citrate has also been used.

Preparations

Proprietary Preparations (details are given in Part 3)
Aust.: Reverin; ***Austral.:*** Reverin†; ***Belg.:*** Reverin†; ***Canad.:*** Reverin; ***Ger.:*** Reverin†; ***Irl.:*** Reverin†; ***Ital.:*** Reverin†; ***S.Afr.:*** Reverin†.

Multi-ingredient: ***Ital.:*** Colbiocin; Eubetal Antibiotico; Iducol; Vitecaf.

Roxithromycin (680-p)

Roxithromycin *(USAN, rINN).*

Roxithromycinum; RU-965; RU-28965. Erythromycin 9-{*O*-[(2-methoxyethoxy)methyl]oxime}.

$C_{41}H_{76}N_2O_{15}$ = 837.0.

CAS — 80214-83-1.

Pharmacopoeias. In *Eur.* (see p.viii).

A white crystalline powder. It exhibits polymorphism. Very slightly **soluble** in water; freely soluble in alcohol, in acetone, and in dichloromethane; slightly soluble in dilute hydrochloric acid. **Store** in airtight containers.

Adverse Effects and Precautions

As for Erythromycin, p.204. Gastro-intestinal disturbances are the most frequent adverse effect, but are less frequent than with erythromycin. Increases in liver enzyme values and hepatitis have been reported. Rashes and other hypersensitivity reactions, headache, dizziness, weakness, and changes in blood cell counts have also occurred.

Effects on the pancreas. Acute pancreatitis, with duodenal inflammation, pain, pancreatic enlargement and raised serum-amylase developed within 24 hours of substitution of roxithromycin for erythromycin ethyl succinate in a patient being treated for respiratory-tract infection.[1] Symptoms resolved rapidly once roxithromycin was withdrawn.

1. Souweine B, *et al.* Acute pancreatitis associated with roxithromycin therapy. *DICP Ann Pharmacother* 1991; **25:** 1137.

Eosinophilia. For a report of an eosinophilic syndrome in a patient following treatment with azithromycin or roxithromycin, see Azithromycin, p.155.

Interactions

For a discussion of drug interactions with macrolide antibacterials, see Erythromycin, p.205.

Antimicrobial Action

As for Erythromycin, p.205. It is reported to be as active or slightly less active than erythromycin.

Pharmacokinetics

Following oral administration roxithromycin is absorbed, with a bioavailability of about 50%. Peak plasma concentrations of about 6 to 8 µg per mL occur around 2 hours after a single dose of 150 mg. The mean peak plasma concentration at steady state after a dose of 150 mg twice daily is 9.3 µg per mL. Absorption is reduced when taken after, but not before, a meal. It is widely distributed in tissues and body fluids. It is reported to be about 96% bound to plasma protein (mainly α_1-acid glycoprotein) at trough concentrations, but binding is saturable, and only about 86% is bound at usual peak concentrations. Small amounts of roxithromycin are metabolised in the liver, and the majority of a dose is excreted in the faeces as unchanged drug and metabolites; about 7 to 12% is excreted in urine, and up to 15% via the lungs. The elimination half-life is reported to range between about 8 and 13 hours, but may be more prolonged in patients with impaired hepatic or renal function and in children.

References.

1. Puri SK, Lassman HB. Roxithromycin: a pharmacokinetic review of a macrolide. *J Antimicrob Chemother* 1987; **20** (suppl B): 89–100.
2. Periti P, *et al.* Clinical pharmacokinetic properties of the macrolide antibiotics: effects of age and various pathophysiological states (part II). *Clin Pharmacokinet* 1989; **16:** 261–82.

Uses and Administration

Roxithromycin is a macrolide antibiotic with actions and uses similar to those of erythromycin (p.206). It is given by mouth in a dose of 150 mg twice daily or sometimes 300 mg once daily, before meals, in the treatment of susceptible infections.

References to roxithromycin.

1. Phillips I, *et al.*, eds. Roxithromycin: a new macrolide. *J Antimicrob Chemother* 1987; **20** (suppl B): 1–187.
2. Young RA, *et al.* Roxithromycin: a review of its antibacterial activity, pharmacokinetic properties and clinical efficacy. *Drugs* 1989; **37:** 8–41. Correction. *ibid.*, (No. 3, contents page).
3. Bahal N, Nahata MC. The new macrolide antibiotics: azithromycin, clarithromycin, dirithromycin, and roxithromycin. *Ann Pharmacother* 1992; **26:** 46–55.
4. Williams JD, Sefton AM. Comparison of macrolide antibiotics. *J Antimicrob Chemother* 1993; **31** (suppl C): 11–26.
5. Markham A, Faulds D. Roxithromycin: an update of its antimicrobial activity, pharmacokinetic properties and therapeutic use. *Drugs* 1994; **48:** 297–326.
6. Young LS, Lode H, eds. Roxithromycin: first of a new generation of macrolides: update and perspectives. *Infection* 1995; **23** (suppl 1): S1–S52.
7. Lovering AM, *et al.*, eds. Roxithromycin—additional therapeutic potential. *J Antimicrob Chemother* 1998; **41** (suppl B): 1–97.

Preparations

Proprietary Preparations (details are given in Part 3)

Aust.: Rulide; ***Austral.:*** Biaxin†; Biaxsig; Rulide; ***Belg.:*** Claramid; Rulid; ***Fr.:*** Claramid; Rulid; ***Ger.:*** Rulid; ***Ital.:*** Assoral; Overal; Rossitrol; Rulid; ***Neth.:*** Rulide; ***S.Afr.:*** Rulide; ***Spain:*** Macrosil; Rotesan; Rotramin; Rulide; ***Swed.:*** Cirumycin†; Surlid; ***Switz.:*** Rulid.

RP-59500 (12225-k)

Quinupristin/dalfopristin.

CAS — 126602-89-9; 176861-85-1.

Dalfopristin (15265-m)

Dalfopristin *(BAN, USAN, rINN).*

RP-54476. (3*R*,4*R*,5*E*,10*E*,12*E*,14*S*,26*R*,26a*S*)-26-{[2-(Diethylamino)ethyl]sulfonyl}-8,9,14,15,24,25,26,26a-octahydro-14-hydroxy-3-isopropyl-4,12-dimethyl-3*H*-21,18-nitrilo-1*H*,22*H*-pyrrolo[2.1-c][1,8,4,19]dioxadiazacyclotetracosine-1,7,16,22(4*H*,17*H*)-tetrone; (26*R*,27*S*)-26-{[2-(Diethylamino)-ethyl]sulfonyl}-26,27-dihydrovirginiamycin M_1.

$C_{34}H_{50}N_4O_9S$ = 690.9.

CAS — 112362-50-2.

Quinupristin (15345-m)

Quinupristin *(BAN, USAN, rINN).*

RP-57.699; RP-57669. *N*-{(6*R*,9*S*,10*R*,13*S*,15a*S*,18*R*,22*S*,24a*S*)-22-[*p*-(Dimethylamino)benzyl]-6-ethyldocosahydro-10,23-dimethyl-5,8,12,15,17,21,24-heptaoxo-13-phenyl-18-{[(3*S*)-3-quinuclidinylthio]methyl}-12*H*-pyrido[2,1-*f*]pyrrolo[2,1-*l*][1,4,7,10,13,16]-oxapentaazacyclononadecin-9-yl}-3-hydroxy-picolinamide; 4-[4-(Dimethylamino)-*N*-methyl-L-phenylalamine]-5-(*cis*-5-{[(*S*)-1-azabicyclo[2.2.2]oct-3-ylthio]methyl}-4-oxo-L-2-piperidinecarboxylic acid)-virginiamycin S_1.

$C_{53}H_{67}N_9O_{10}S$ = 1022.2.

CAS — 120138-50-3.

RP-59500 is a streptogramin antibacterial with activity against a wide range of Gram-positive bacteria including vancomycin-resistant enterococci and methicillin-resistant *Staphylococcus aureus*. It is a synergistic mixture of two pristinamycin derivatives, dalfopristin and quinupristin, in the ratio of 70 to 30 and, being water soluble, can be given parenterally.

References.

1. Finch RG. Antibacterial activity of quinupristin/dalfopristin: rationale for clinical use. *Drugs* 1996; **51** (suppl 1): 31–7.
2. Bryson HM, Spencer CM. Quinupristin-dalfopristin. *Drugs* 1996; **52:** 406–15.
3. Bayston R, *et al.*, eds. Quinupristin/dalfopristin—update on the first injectable streptogramin. *J Antimicrob Chemother* 1997; **39** (suppl A): 1–151.

Rufloxacin (3763-l)

Rufloxacin *(BAN, rINN).*

MF-934. 9-Fluoro-2,3-dihydro-10-[4-methylpiperazin-1-yl]-7-oxo-7*H*-pyrido[1,2,3-*de*]-1,4-benzothiazine-6-carboxylic acid.

$C_{17}H_{18}FN_3O_3S$ = 363.4.

CAS — 101363-10-4.

Rufloxacin is a fluoroquinolone antibacterial with properties similar to those of ciprofloxacin (p.185). It is given by mouth as the hydrochloride in the treatment of susceptible infections in an initial dose of 400 mg followed by 200 mg daily. A plasma half-life of 30 hours or more has been reported.

Preparations

Proprietary Preparations (details are given in Part 3)
Ital.: Qari; Tebraxin.

Silver Sulphadiazine (4913-a)

Silver Sulfadiazine *(USAN)*; Sulfadiazine Silver; Sulphadiazine Silver.

$C_{10}H_9AgN_4O_2S$ = 357.1.

CAS — 22199-08-2.

Pharmacopoeias. In *Chin.*, *Jpn*, and *US*.

A white or creamy-white, odourless or almost odourless crystalline powder. It becomes yellow on exposure to light. Slightly **soluble** in acetone; practically insoluble in alcohol, in chloroform, or in ether; freely soluble in 30% ammonia solution. It decomposes in moderately strong mineral acids. **Protect** from light.

Adverse Effects, Treatment, and Precautions

Silver sulphadiazine may be absorbed following topical application and produce systemic effects similar to those of other sulphonamides (see Sulphamethoxazole, p.254).

Local pain or irritation are uncommon; the separation of the eschar may be delayed and fungal invasion of the wound may occur.

Transient leucopenia does not usually require withdrawal of silver sulphadiazine, but blood counts should be monitored to ensure they return to normal within a few days. Systemic absorption of silver, resulting in argyria, can occur when silver sulphadiazine is applied to large area wounds or over prolonged periods.

Argyria. A report of argyria, with discoloration of the skin and sensorimotor neuropathy, caused by excessive application of silver sulphadiazine 1% cream to extensive leg ulcers.[1]

1. Payne CMER, *et al.* Argyria from excessive use of topical silver sulphadiazine. *Lancet* 1992; **340:** 126.

Interactions

As for Sulphamethoxazole, p.255.

Silver sulphadiazine is not antagonised by *p*-aminobenzoic acid or related compounds. The silver content of silver sulphadiazine may inactivate enzymatic debriding agents.

Antimicrobial Action

Silver sulphadiazine has broad antimicrobial activity against Gram-positive and Gram-negative bacteria including *Pseudomonas aeruginosa*, and some yeasts and fungi. Silver sulphadiazine has a bactericidal action; in contrast to sulphadiazine, the silver salt acts primarily on the cell membrane and cell wall and its action is not antagonised by *p*-aminobenzoic acid. Resistance to silver sulphadiazine has been reported and may develop during therapy.

Pharmacokinetics

Silver sulphadiazine slowly releases sulphadiazine when in contact with wound exudates. Up to about 10% of the sulphadiazine may be absorbed; concentrations in blood of 10 to 20 μg per mL have been reported although higher concentrations may be achieved when extensive areas of the body are treated. Some silver may also be absorbed.

Uses and Administration

Silver sulphadiazine is a sulphonamide that is used, in conjunction with debridement, as a 1% cream for the prevention and treatment of infection in severe burns (p.1073).

Silver sulphadiazine has also been used in other skin conditions, such as leg ulcers (p.1076), where infection may prevent healing and for the prophylaxis of infection in skin grafting.

Preparations

USP 23: Silver Sulfadiazine Cream.

Proprietary Preparations (details are given in Part 3)
Aust.: Flammazine; ***Belg.:*** Flammazine; ***Canad.:*** Dermazin; Flamazine; SSD; ***Fr.:*** Flammazine; Sicazine; ***Ger.:*** Brandiazin; Flammazine; ***Irl.:*** Flamazine; ***Ital.:*** Sofargen; Ustionil†; ***Neth.:*** Flammazine; ***Norw.:*** Flamazine; ***S.Afr.:*** Argent-Eze; Bactrazine; Flamazine; ***Spain:*** Flammazine; Plusdermona†; Silvederma; ***Switz.:*** Flammazine; Silvadene; Silvertone; ***UK:*** Flamazine; ***USA:*** Silvadene; SSD; Thermazene.

Multi-ingredient: ***Austral.:*** Silvazine; ***Belg.:*** Flammacerium; ***Canad.:*** Flamazine C; ***Fr.:*** Flammacerium; ***Ital.:*** Connettivina Plus; ***Neth.:*** Flammacerium; ***Spain:*** Unitul Complex; ***Switz.:*** Ialugen Plus.

Sissomicin Sulphate (152-q)

Sissomicin Sulphate *(BANM).*

Sisomicin Sulphate *(rINNM)*; Antibiotic 6640 (sissomicin); Rickamicin Sulphate; Sch-13475 (sissomicin); Sisomicin Sulfate *(USAN)*. 4-*O*-[(2*R*,3*R*)-*cis*-3-Amino-6-aminomethyl-3,4-dihydro-2*H*-pyran-2-yl]-2-deoxy-6-*O*-(3-deoxy-4-*C*-methyl-3-methylamino-β-L-arabinopyranosyl)streptamine sulphate; 2-Deoxy-6-*O*-(3-deoxy-4-*C*-methyl-3-methylamino-β-L-arabinopyranosyl)-4-*O*-(2,6-diamino-2,3,4,6-tetradeoxy-D-*glycero*-hex-4-enopyranosyl)streptamine sulphate.

$(C_{19}H_{37}N_5O_7)_2,5H_2SO_4$ = 1385.5.

CAS — 32385-11-8 (sissomicin); 53179-09-2 (sissomicin sulphate).

Pharmacopoeias. In *Jpn* and *US.*

Sissomicin is an antibiotic produced by *Micromonospora inyoensis* and closely related to gentamicin C_{1A}.

It loses not more than 15% of its weight on drying. 1.5 g of monograph substance is approximately equivalent to 1 g of sissomicin. A 4% solution has a pH of 3.5 to 5.5. **Store** in airtight containers.

Sissomicin is an aminoglycoside with general properties similar to those of gentamicin (p.212). It is given as the sulphate and the usual dose for adults is the equivalent of 3 mg of sissomicin per kg body-weight daily given intramuscularly in 2 or 3 divided doses. Sissomicin may be given by intravenous infusion if necessary. Peak plasma concentrations greater than 12 μg per mL and trough concentrations above 2 μg per mL should be avoided.

It is recommended that dosage should be adjusted in all patients according to plasma-sissomicin concentrations, and this is particularly important where factors such as age, renal impairment, or dose may predispose to toxicity, or where there is a risk of subtherapeutic concentrations. Dosage may be adjusted using schedules developed for gentamicin. For discussion of the methods of calculating aminoglycoside dosage requirements, see p.214.

Preparations

USP 23: Sisomicin Sulfate Injection.

Proprietary Preparations (details are given in Part 3)
Fr.: Sisolline†; ***Ital.:*** Mensiso; Sisobiotic†; Sisomin†; ***Spain:*** Sisomina.

Sparfloxacin (9355-r)

Sparfloxacin *(BAN, USAN, rINN).*

AT-4140; CI-978. 5-Amino-1-cyclopropyl-7-(*cis*-3,5-dimethylpiperazin-1-yl)-6,8-difluoro-1,4-dihydro-4-oxoquinoline-3-carboxylic acid.

$C_{19}H_{22}F_2N_4O_3$ = 392.4.

CAS — 110871-86-8.

Adverse Effects and Precautions

As for Ciprofloxacin, p.186.

Concern over phototoxicity associated with sparfloxacin has led to restriction of its use in some countries; patients should be advised to avoid exposure to sunlight during, and for a few days after, sparfloxacin therapy, and to discontinue the drug immediately if phototoxicity occurs.

Sparfloxacin may prolong the QT interval and various cardiac arrhythmias have been reported.

Interactions

As for Ciprofloxacin, p.187.

As sparfloxacin may prolong the QT interval it should not be administered concomitantly with other drugs known to have this effect (such as the antihistamines astemizole and terfenadine, cisapride, erythromycin, pentamidine, phenothiazines, or tricyclic antidepressants).

Sparfloxacin does not appear to interact with theophylline or caffeine, nor with warfarin or cimetidine. Probenecid does not alter the pharmacokinetics of sparfloxacin.

Antimicrobial Action

As for Ciprofloxacin, p.187.

Sparfloxacin is reported to be more active *in vitro* than ciprofloxacin against mycobacteria and against Gram-positive bacteria, including *Streptococcus pneumoniae* and other streptococci and staphylococci.

References.

1. Richard MP, *et al.* Sensitivity to sparfloxacin and other antibiotics, of Streptococcus pneumoniae, Haemophilus influenzae and Moraxella catarrhalis strains isolated from adult patients with community-acquired lower respiratory tract infections: a European multicentre study. *J Antimicrob Chemother* 1998; **41:** 207–14.

Pharmacokinetics

Sparfloxacin is well absorbed from the gastro-intestinal tract following oral administration with a reported bioavailability of about 90%. Peak plasma concentrations are achieved 3 to 6 hours after a dose. Sparfloxacin is widely distributed into body tissues and fluids, including respiratory tissues, but is only about 45% bound to plasma proteins. It is metabolised in the liver by glucuronidation and has an elimination half-life of about 20 hours. It is excreted in equal amounts in the faeces and urine as unchanged drug and as the glucuronide metabolite.

References.

1. Shimada J, *et al.* Clinical pharmacokinetics of sparfloxacin. *Clin Pharmacokinet* 1993; **25:** 358–69.
2. Fillastre JP, *et al.* Pharmacokinetics of sparfloxacin in patients with renal impairment. *Antimicrob Agents Chemother* 1994; **38:** 733–7.
3. Trautmann M, *et al.* Pharmacokinetics of sparfloxacin and serum bactericidal activity against pneumococci. *Antimicrob Agents Chemother* 1996; **40:** 776–9.

Uses and Administration

Sparfloxacin is a fluoroquinolone antibacterial with actions similar to those of ciprofloxacin (p.188). It is used for the treatment of community-acquired pneumonia and acute bacterial exacerbations of chronic bronchitis including those caused by pneumococci. The usual dose by mouth is 400 mg initially followed by 200 mg daily.

Doses should be reduced in patients with renal impairment. A suggested maintenance dose is 200 mg on alternate days.

General references.

1. Finch RG, *et al.*, eds. Sparfloxacin: focus on clinical performance. *J Antimicrob Chemother* 1996; **37** (suppl A): 1–167.
2. Goa KL, *et al.* Sparfloxacin: a review of its antibacterial activity, pharmacokinetic properties, clinical efficacy and tolerability in lower respiratory tract infections. *Drugs* 1997; **53:** 700–25.
3. Martin SJ, *et al.* Levofloxacin and sparfloxacin: new quinolone antibiotics. *Ann Pharmacother* 1998; **32:** 320–36.

Preparations

Proprietary Preparations (details are given in Part 3)

Fr.: Zagam; ***Jpn:*** Spara; ***S.Afr.:*** Zagam; ***Switz.:*** Zagam; ***USA:*** Zagam.

Spectinomycin (155-w)

Spectinomycin *(BAN, rINN).*

Actinospectacin. Perhydro-4a,7,9-trihydroxy-2-methyl-6,8-bis(methylamino)pyrano[2,3-*b*][1,4]benzodioxin-4-one.

$C_{14}H_{24}N_2O_7$ = 332.3.

CAS — 1695-77-8.

An antimicrobial substance produced by the growth of *Streptomyces spectabilis* or by any other means.

Spectinomycin Hydrochloride (157-l)

Spectinomycin Hydrochloride *(BANM, USAN, rINNM).*

M-141; Spectinomycini Hydrochloridum; U-18409AE. Spectinomycin dihydrochloride pentahydrate.

$C_{14}H_{24}N_2O_7,2HCl,5H_2O$ = 495.3.

CAS — 21736-83-4 (anhydrous spectinomycin hydrochloride); 22189-32-8 (spectinomycin hydrochloride pentahydrate).

Pharmacopoeias. In *Eur.* (see p.viii), *Int.*, and *US.*

A white or almost white to pale buff slightly hygroscopic crystalline powder. 1.5 g of monograph substance is approximately equivalent to 1 g of spectinomycin. Freely **soluble** in water; very slightly soluble or practically insoluble in alcohol; practically insoluble in chloroform and in ether. A solution in water (1 to 10%) has a pH of 3.8 to 5.6. **Store** at a temperature not exceeding 30° in airtight containers.

Adverse Effects and Precautions

Nausea, headache, dizziness, fever and chills, insomnia, and urticaria have occasionally occurred with single doses of spectinomycin. Anaphylaxis has occurred rarely. Mild to moderate pain has been reported following intramuscular injections. Alterations in kidney and liver function and a decrease in haemoglobin and haematocrit have occasionally been observed with repeated doses. Although a reduction in urine output has occasionally been seen after single and multiple dose administration, spectinomycin has not been observed to produce functional changes indicative of nephrotoxicity.

Spectinomycin is ineffective in the treatment of syphilis and patients being treated for gonorrhoea should be observed for evidence of syphilis.

Interactions

Lithium. For the effect of spectinomycin on lithium, see p.293.

Antimicrobial Action

Spectinomycin is an aminocyclitol antibiotic that acts by binding to the 30S subunit of the bacterial ribosome and inhibiting protein synthesis. Its activity is generally modest, particularly against Gram-positive organisms. Anaerobic organisms are mostly resistant. Various Gram-negative organisms are sensitive, including many enterobacteria and also *Haemophilus ducreyi*, and it is particularly effective against *Neisseria gonorrhoeae*. Although generally bacteriostatic, spectinomycin is bactericidal against susceptible gonococci at concentrations not much above the MIC. Most strains of *N. gonorrhoeae* are inhibited by concentrations in the range 2 to 20 μg per mL.

Resistance may develop by chromosomal mutation or may be plasmid-mediated in some organisms; resistant gonococci have been reported clinically, notably in the Far East, but in most parts of the world resistant neisserial strains have been uncommon to date.

Pharmacokinetics

Spectinomycin is poorly absorbed by mouth but is rapidly absorbed following the intramuscular injection of the hydrochloride. A 2-g dose produces peak plasma concentrations of about 100 μg per mL at 1 hour while a 4-g dose produces peak concentrations of about 160 μg per mL at 2 hours. Therapeutic plasma concentrations are maintained for up to 8 hours. Distribution into saliva is poor (which limits its value in pharyngeal gonorrhoea). It is poorly bound to plasma proteins. Spectinomycin is excreted in an active form in the urine and up to 100% of a dose has been recovered within 48 hours. A half-life of about 1 to 3 hours has been reported. The half-life is prolonged in patients with impaired renal function. Spectinomycin is partially removed by dialysis.

Uses and Administration

Spectinomycin is used as an alternative to cephalosporins or fluoroquinolones in the treatment of gonorrhoea (p.126) although poor distribution into saliva limits its usefulness in pharyngeal infections. It has also been used in the treatment of chancroid (p.118).

Spectinomycin is administered as the hydrochloride but doses are calculated in terms of the base. In the treatment of gonorrhoea it is given by deep intramuscular injection as a single dose equivalent to 2 g of spectinomycin, although a dose of 4 g may sometimes be required divided between two injection sites. Multiple-dose courses have been used for the treatment of disseminated infections.

Spectinomycin is not effective against syphilis or chlamydial infections and additional therapy for these infections may be given concomitantly.

Doses equivalent to spectinomycin 40 mg per kg body-weight have been administered to children.

Preparations

BP 1998: Spectinomycin Injection;
USP 23: Spectinomycin for Injectable Suspension.

Proprietary Preparations (details are given in Part 3)

Aust.: Trobicin; ***Austral.:*** Trobicin; ***Belg.:*** Trobicin; ***Canad.:*** Trobicin; ***Fr.:*** Trobicine; ***Ger.:*** Stanilo; ***Irl.:*** Trobicin; ***Ital.:*** Trobicin; ***Norw.:*** Trobicin†; ***S.Afr.:*** Trobicin; ***Spain:*** Kempi; ***Swed.:*** Trobicin; ***Switz.:*** Trobicin; ***UK:*** Trobicin; ***USA:*** Trobicin.

Spiramycin (158-y)

Spiramycin *(BAN, USAN, rINN)*.

Espiramicina; IL-5902; NSC-55926; NSC-64393 (hydrochloride); RP-5337; Spiramycinum. A mixture comprised principally of (4*R*,5*S*,6*S*,7*R*,9*R*,10*R*,16*R*)-(11*E*,13*E*)-6-[(*O*-2,6-dideoxy-3-*C*-methyl-α-L-*ribo*-hexopyranosyl)-(1→4)-(3,6-dideoxy-3-dimethylamino-β-D-glucopyranosyl)oxy]-7-formylmethyl-4-hydroxy-5-methoxy-9,16-dimethyl-10-[(2,3,4,6-tetradeoxy-4-dimethylamino-D-*erythro*-hexopyranosyl)oxy]oxacyclohexadeca-11,13-dien-2-one (Spiramycin I).

$C_{43}H_{74}N_2O_{14}$ = 843.1.

CAS — 8025-81-8.

Pharmacopoeias. In *Eur.* (see p.viii). *Jpn* includes Acetylspiramycin.

A macrolide antibiotic produced by the growth of certain strains of *Streptomyces ambofaciens* or obtained by any other means.

A white or slightly yellowish slightly hygroscopic powder. It contains not less than 3900 units per mg, calculated with reference to the dried substance. Slightly **soluble** in water; freely soluble in alcohol, acetone, and methyl alcohol; sparingly soluble in ether. A 0.5% solution in methyl alcohol and water has a pH of 8.5 to 10.5. **Store** in airtight containers.

Units

3200 units of spiramycin are contained in 1 mg of the first International Reference Preparation (1962).

Adverse Effects and Precautions

As for Erythromycin, p.204. The most frequent adverse effects are gastro-intestinal disturbances; skin hypersensitivity reactions have also occurred. Transient paraesthesia has been reported during parenteral administration.

Interactions

For a discussion of drug interactions with macrolide antibacterials, see Erythromycin, p.205.

Antimicrobial Action

As for Erythromycin, p.205, although it is somewhat less active *in vitro* against many species. It is active against *Toxoplasma gondii*.

Pharmacokinetics

Spiramycin is incompletely absorbed from the gastro-intestinal tract and is widely distributed in the tissues. A dose of 2 g produces peak blood concentrations of about 3 μg per mL after 3 hours; concentrations fall with a half-life of about 8 hours. High tissue concentrations are achieved and persist long after the plasma concentration has fallen to low levels but it does not diffuse into the CSF to an appreciable extent.

Spiramycin is metabolised in the liver to active metabolites; substantial amounts are excreted in the bile and about 10% in the urine. It is distributed into breast milk.

Uses and Administration

Spiramycin is a macrolide antibiotic that has been used similarly to erythromycin (p.206) in the treatment of susceptible bacterial infections. It has also been used in the protozoal infections cryptosporidiosis (p.574) and toxoplasmosis (p.576).

Spiramycin is given by mouth as the base or rectally or intravenously as the adipate; doses are calculated in terms of the base. The usual adult dose is 2 to 3 g by mouth daily, in 2 divided doses. Doses of 4 to 5 g have been given daily in divided doses for severe infections. A dose equivalent to about 500 mg of spiramycin may be given by slow intravenous infusion every 8 hours; in severe infection 1 g may be given every 8 hours. Children may be given 50 to 100 mg per kg body-weight daily in divided doses by mouth.

Acetylspiramycin is also used.

Preparations

Proprietary Preparations (details are given in Part 3)

Aust.: Rovamycin; ***Belg.:*** Rovamycine; ***Canad.:*** Rovamycine; ***Fr.:*** Rovamycine; ***Ger.:*** Rovamycine; Selectomycin; ***Ital.:*** Bykomycetin†; Rovamicina; ***Neth.:*** Rovamycine; ***Norw.:*** Rovamycin; ***Spain:*** Dicorvin; Rovamycine; ***Swed.:*** Rovamycin†; ***Switz.:*** Rovamycine.

Multi-ingredient: ***Fr.:*** Rodogyl; ***Spain:*** Rhodogil.

Stearylsulfamide (14888-m)

Stearylsulfamide *(rINN)*.

N-Sulphanilylstearamide.

$C_{24}H_{42}N_2O_3S$ = 438.7.

CAS — 498-78-2.

Stearylsulfamide is a sulphonamide used topically in the treatment of skin disorders.

Preparations

Proprietary Preparations (details are given in Part 3)

Multi-ingredient: ***Spain:*** Crema Neutra†.

Streptomycin (160-q)

Streptomycin *(BAN, rINN)*.

Estreptomicina. *O*-2-Deoxy-2-methylamino-α-L-glucopyranosyl-(1→2)-*O*-5-deoxy-3-*C*-formyl-α-L-lyxofuranosyl-(1→4)-N^3,N^3-diamidino-D-streptamine.

$C_{21}H_{39}N_7O_{12}$ = 581.6.

CAS — 57-92-1.

An antimicrobial organic base produced by the growth of certain strains of *Streptomyces griseus*, or by any other means.

Streptomycin Hydrochloride (162-s)

Streptomycin Hydrochloride *(BANM, rINNM)*.

$C_{21}H_{39}N_7O_{12}$,3HCl = 691.0.

CAS — 6160-32-3.

1.19 g of monograph substance is approximately equivalent to 1 g of streptomycin.

Streptomycin Sulphate (163-w)

Streptomycin Sulphate *(BANM, rINNM)*.

Streptomycin Sesquisulphate; Streptomycini Sulfas; Sulfato de Estreptomicina.

$(C_{21}H_{39}N_7O_{12})_2$,$3H_2SO_4$ = 1457.4.

CAS — 3810-74-0.

Pharmacopoeias. In *Chin., Eur.* (see p.viii), *Int., Jpn, Pol.,* and *US.*

A white or almost white, odourless or almost odourless, hygroscopic powder. The Ph. Eur. specifies not less than 720 units per mg calculated on the dried substance; the USP specifies not less than 650 μg and not more than 850 μg of streptomycin per mg. 1.25 g of monograph substance is approximately equivalent to 1 g of streptomycin.

Ph. Eur. **solubilities** are: very soluble in water; practically insoluble in dehydrated alcohol, and in ether. USP solubilities are: freely soluble in water; very slightly soluble in alcohol; practically insoluble in chloroform. A 25% solution in water has a pH of 4.5 to 7.0. **Incompatible** with acids and alkalis. **Store** in airtight containers and protect from moisture.

CAUTION. *Streptomycin may cause severe dermatitis in sensitised persons, and pharmacists, nurses, and others who handle the drug frequently should wear masks and rubber gloves.*

Adverse Effects, Treatment, and Precautions

As for Gentamicin Sulphate, p.212. Like gentamicin the ototoxic effects of streptomycin are manifested mainly on vestibular rather than auditory function. Ototoxicity has been observed in infants whose mothers had been given streptomycin during pregnancy. However, streptomycin is reported to be somewhat less nephrotoxic than the other aminoglycosides.

Paraesthesia in and around the mouth is not uncommon after intramuscular injection of streptomycin, and other neurological symptoms, including peripheral neuropathies, optic neuritis, and scotoma have occasionally occurred. Intrathecal administration has resulted in symptoms of meningeal inflammation including radiculitis, arachnoiditis, nerve root pain, and paraplegia, and some authorities recommend that such administration be avoided.

Hypersensitivity skin reactions are reported in about 5% of patients, and eosinophilia may occur. There have been reports of severe exfoliative dermatitis and anaphylaxis. Sensitisation is common among those who handle streptomycin occupationally. Topical and inhalational use of streptomycin should be avoided. If necessary, hypersensitivity can usually be overcome by desensitisation. Aplastic anaemia and agranulocytosis have been reported rarely.

Although sources differ, it is usually suggested that peak plasma concentrations greater than about 40 μg per mL, and trough concentrations greater than 3 to 5 μg per mL should be avoided; in the UK it has been suggested that trough concentrations in excess of 1 μg per mL should be avoided in elderly tubercular patients. A total cumulative dose in excess of 100 g may be associated with a higher incidence of adverse effects.

Interactions

As for Gentamicin Sulphate, p.213.

Antimicrobial Action

Streptomycin has a mode of action and antimicrobial spectrum similar to that of gentamicin (p.213), although most strains of *Pseudomonas aeruginosa* are resistant. It is effective against *Yersinia pestis, Francisella tularensis*, and *Brucella* spp. Streptomycin has particular activity against *Mycobacterium tuberculosis*.

The MIC of streptomycin for most susceptible organisms is in the range of 1 to 8 μg per mL. Resistance has commonly been reported in many of the species normally sensitive to streptomycin, and may develop in strains which are initially sensitive within a few days or weeks of beginning therapy. The widespread emergence of resistance has largely put paid to its use in infections due to the common Gram-negative aerobes. Primary resistance in *M. tuberculosis* is relatively uncommon in the UK and USA but may be seen in a third or more of cases in the Far East.

Both low-level and high-level resistance have been reported; the latter is thought to be due to mutation of the ribosomal binding site of the antibiotic and cannot be overcome by the synergistic use of another drug such as a beta lactam, whereas strains with moderate resistance due to decreased uptake or permeability of streptomycin may respond to combined use.

Organisms resistant to framycetin, kanamycin, neomycin, and paromomycin usually show cross-resistance to streptomycin, although streptomycin-resistant strains sometimes respond to one of these drugs.

References.

1. Honoré N, Cole ST. Streptomycin resistance in mycobacteria. *Antimicrob Agents Chemother* 1994; **38:** 238–42.
2. Cooksey RC, *et al.* Characterization of streptomycin resistance mechanisms among Mycobacterium tuberculosis isolates from patients in New York City. *Antimicrob Agents Chemother* 1996; **40:** 1186–8.
3. Ho YII, *et al.* In-vitro activities of aminoglycoside-aminocyclitols against mycobacteria. *J Antimicrob Chemother* 1997; **40:** 27–32.

Pharmacokinetics

As for Gentamicin Sulphate, p.213. After intramuscular injection of streptomycin, maximum concentration in the blood is reached in 0.5 to 2 hours but the time taken and the concentration attained, which may be as high as about 50 μg per mL after a dose of 1 g, vary considerably. The half-life of streptomycin is about 2½ hours. About one-third of streptomycin in the circulation is bound to plasma proteins. It is rapidly excreted by glomerular filtration and the concentration of streptomycin in the urine is often very high with about 30 to 90% of a dose usually being excreted within 24 hours.

Uses and Administration

Streptomycin is an aminoglycoside antibacterial mainly used in conjunction with other antimycobacterials, in the treatment of tuberculosis, when drug resistance is thought likely. It may be classified as a first-line or primary antituberculous drug. Streptomycin has been used as an alternative to gentamicin in combination with a penicillin in the treatment of bacterial endocarditis. Streptomycin is effective in the treatment of plague, tularaemia, and, in conjunction with a tetracycline, in brucellosis. It has also been used, in combination with other drugs, in various other infections including mycetoma and Whipple's disease. For details of these infections and their treatment, see under Choice of Antibacterial, p.116.

Streptomycin is mostly used as the sulphate but doses are expressed in terms of the base. It is given by intramuscular injection as a solution in water or sodium chloride 0.9%; solutions more concentrated than 500 mg per mL should not be used.

In the treatment of tuberculosis streptomycin is given during the initial phase of short-course regimens in usual doses of 15 mg per kg body-weight daily, up to a maximum of 1 g daily. A reduction in the maximum dose to 500 to 750 mg in adults aged over 40 years, and in those weighing less than 50 kg has been suggested. Streptomycin may also be given as part of an intermittent regimen 2 or 3 times weekly. It has been given by the intrathecal route, together with intramuscular administration, for tuberculous meningitis but this is no longer recommended.

Children with tuberculosis may also be given streptomycin 15 to 20 mg per kg daily (to a maximum of 1 g daily).

In the treatment of non-tuberculous infections streptomycin has been given in usual doses of 1 to 2 g daily, and occasionally up to 4 g daily in divided doses, depending on the susceptibility and severity of infection; children may be given up to 40 mg per kg daily (maximum 1 g daily), usually in divided doses.

The course of treatment (other than in tuberculosis) should usually be limited to 7 to 14 days, and peak plasma concentrations greater than 40 μg per mL and trough concentrations greater than 3 to 5 μg per mL should be avoided. In all patients dosage should preferably be adjusted according to plasma-streptomycin concentrations, and particularly where factors such as age, renal impairment, or high dose may predispose to toxicity. For discussion of the methods used to calculate aminoglycoside dosage requirements, see under Gentamicin Sulphate, p.214.

Streptomycin has also been used as the pantothenate and as a complex with calcium chloride.

Administration and dosage. A report of the successful use of streptomycin 7 to 15 mg per kg body-weight as an intravenous infusion over half to one hour in 4 patients with tuberculosis. Despite the view that streptomycin should be given intramuscularly because of the greater risk of toxicity with the intravenous route, this study was considered to indicate that intravenous administration was feasible in selected patients unable to tolerate the intramuscular route.[1]

1. Driver AG, Worden JP. Intravenous streptomycin. *DICP Ann Pharmacother* 1990; **24:** 826–8.

Ménière's disease. Streptomycin and gentamicin have been used for medical ablation in advanced Ménière's disease (p.400). Systemic treatment has generally been limited by the development of chronic ataxia and oscillopsia (oscillating vision). However, streptomycin sulphate 1 g twice daily by intramuscular injection on 5 days a week for 2 weeks, repeated as necessary to a total dose of up to 60 g, has produced improvements in vestibular symptoms without hearing loss in patients with bilateral Ménière's disease.[1,2] Local (intratympanic) injections have also been tried,[3] but gentamicin is considered to be less toxic and is now generally preferred.

1. Graham MD, *et al.* Titration streptomycin therapy for bilateral Meniere's disease: a preliminary report. *Otolaryngol Head Neck Surg* 1984; **92:** 440–7.
2. Shea JJ, *et al.* Long-term results of low dose intramuscular streptomycin for Ménière's disease. *Am J Otol* 1994; **15:** 540–4.
3. Beck C, Schmidt CL. 10 Years of experience with intratympanally applied streptomycin (gentamycin) in the therapy of Morbus Menière. *Arch Otorhinolaryngol* 1978; **221:** 149–52.

Preparations

BP 1998: Streptomycin Injection;
USP 23: Streptomycin for Injection; Streptomycin Injection.

Proprietary Preparations (details are given in Part 3)
Ger.: Strepto-Fatol; ***Ital.:*** Streptocol; ***S.Afr.:*** Novostrep; Solustrep; ***Spain:*** Cidan Est†.

Multi-ingredient: ***Ital.:*** Streptan†; ***S.Afr.:*** Diastat†; ***Spain:*** Bio Hubber; Bio Hubber Fuerte; Derbitan Antibiotico; Estrepto P H†; Neodualestrepto†; Sulfathalidin Estrepto†.

Succinylsulphathiazole (4914-t)

Succinylsulphathiazole *(BAN).*

Succinylsulfathiazole *(rINN)*; Succinilsolfatiazolo; Succinylsulfathiazolum. 4'-(1,3-Thiazol-2-ylsulphamoyl)succinanilic acid monohydrate.

$C_{13}H_{13}N_3O_5S_2,H_2O$ = 373.4.

CAS — 116-43-8 (anhydrous succinylsulphathiazole).

Pharmacopoeias. In *Eur.* (see p.viii).

White or yellowish-white crystalline powder.

Very slightly **soluble** in water; slightly soluble in acetone and in alcohol; practically insoluble in ether; dissolves in aqueous solutions of alkali hydroxides and carbonates. **Protect** from light.

Succinylsulphathiazole is a sulphonamide with properties similar to those of sulphamethoxazole (p.254). It is poorly absorbed, and has been given for its antibacterial activity in the gastro-intestinal tract.

Sulbactam (13275-l)

Sulbactam *(BAN, rINN).*

CP-45899. Penicillanic acid 1,1-dioxide; (2*S*,5*R*)-3,3-Dimethyl-7-oxo-4-thia-1-azabicyclo[3.2.0]heptane-2-carboxylic acid 4,4-dioxide.

$C_8H_{11}NO_5S$ = 233.2.

CAS — 68373-14-8.

Sulbactam Sodium (11563-b)

Sulbactam Sodium *(BANM, USAN, rINNM).*

CP-45899-2.

$C_8H_{10}NNaO_5S$ = 255.2.

CAS — 69388-84-7.

Pharmacopoeias. In *US.*

A white to off-white crystalline powder. 1.09 g of sulbactam sodium is approximately equivalent to 1 g of sulbactam. Freely **soluble** in water and in dilute acid; sparingly soluble in acetone, in chloroform, and in ethyl acetate. **Store** in airtight containers.

Sulbactam is a penicillanic acid sulphone with beta-lactamase inhibitory properties. It generally has only weak antibacterial activity, except against Neisseriaceae, but it is an irreversible inhibitor of many plasmid-mediated and some chromosomal beta-lactamases and has a similar spectrum of beta-lactamase inhibition to clavulanic acid (p.190), although it is regarded as less potent. Sulbactam can therefore enhance the activity of penicillins and cephalosporins against many resistant strains of bacteria.

It is given in association with ampicillin (p.153) in the treatment of various infections where beta-lactamase production is suspected. Sulbactam is poorly absorbed from the gastro-intestinal tract and is given by injection as the sodium salt. The pharmacokinetics of parenteral sulbactam and ampicillin are similar. For oral administration the mutual prodrug sultamicillin (p.257) is available in some countries. Sulbactam has also been given with cefoperazone.

General references.

1. Campoli-Richards DM, Brogden RN. Sulbactam/ampicillin: a review of its antibacterial activity, pharmacokinetic properties, and therapeutic use. *Drugs* 1987; **33:** 577–609.
2. Payne DJ, *et al.* Comparative activities of clavulanic acid, sulbactam, and tazobactam against clinically important β-lactamases. *Antimicrob Agents Chemother* 1994; **38:** 767–72.
3. Nicolas-Chanoine MH. Inhibitor-resistant β-lactamases. *J Antimicrob Chemother* 1997; **40:** 1–3.

Pharmacokinetics references.

1. Foulds G, *et al.* Pharmacokinetics of sulbactam in humans. *Antimicrob Agents Chemother* 1983; **23:** 692–9.
2. Watson ID, *et al.* Clinical pharmacokinetics of enzyme inhibitors in antimicrobial chemotherapy. *Clin Pharmacokinet* 1988; **15:** 133–64.
3. Alexov M, *et al.* Efficacy of ampicillin-sulbactam is not dependent upon maintenance of a critical ratio between components: sulbactam pharmacokinetics in pharmacodynamic interactions. *Antimicrob Agents Chemother* 1996; **40:** 2468–77.

Preparations

USP 23: Ampicillin and Sulbactam for Injection; Sterile Sulbactam Sodium.

Proprietary Preparations (details are given in Part 3)
Aust.: Combactam; ***Fr.:*** Betamaze; ***Ger.:*** Combactam.

Multi-ingredient: ***Aust.:*** Sulperazon†; Unasyn; ***Fr.:*** Unacim; ***Ger.:*** Unacid; ***Ital.:*** Bethacil; Loricin; Unasyn; ***Spain:*** Bacimex†; Galotam; Unasyn; ***UK:*** Dicapen†; ***USA:*** Unasyn.

Sulbenicillin Sodium (164-e)

Sulbenicillin Sodium *(rINNM).*

α-Sulfobenzylpenicillin Sodium; Sulfocillin Sodium. The disodium salt of (6*R*)-6-(2-phenyl-2-sulphoacetamido)penicillanic acid.

$C_{16}H_{16}N_2Na_2O_7S_2$ = 458.4.

CAS — 34779-28-7; 41744-40-5 (both sulbenicillin).

Pharmacopoeias. In *Chin.* and *Jpn.*

Sulbenicillin sodium has actions and uses similar to those of carbenicillin sodium (p.162). It is given by intramuscular or intravenous injection usually in doses equivalent to sulbenicillin 2 to 4 g daily in divided doses. Higher doses may be necessary for severe infections.

Preparations

Proprietary Preparations (details are given in Part 3)
Ital.: Kedacillina; ***Jpn:*** Lilacillin.

Sulfabenzamide (4915-x)

Sulfabenzamide *(BAN, USAN, rINN)*.

N-Sulphanilylbenzamide.

$C_{13}H_{12}N_2O_3S$ = 276.3.

CAS — 127-71-9.

Pharmacopoeias. In US.

A fine, white, practically odourless powder. Practically **insoluble** in water and in ether; soluble in acetone, alcohol, and sodium hydroxide 4% solution. **Protect** from light.

Sulfabenzamide is a sulphonamide with properties similar to those of sulphamethoxazole (p.254). It is reported to exert an optimal bacteriostatic action at pH 4.6. It is used with sulphacetamide and sulphathiazole in pessaries or a vaginal cream for the treatment of bacterial vaginosis, although its value has been questioned by some authorities. The vaginal cream is also used for the prevention of bacterial infection following cervical and vaginal surgery.

Preparations

USP 23: Triple Sulfa Vaginal Cream; Triple Sulfa Vaginal Tablets.

Proprietary Preparations (details are given in Part 3)

Multi-ingredient: ***Austral.:*** Sultrin; ***Belg.:*** Sultrin; ***Canad.:*** Sultrin; ***Ger.:*** Neosultrin†; ***Irl.:*** Sultrin; ***S.Afr.:*** Sultrin; ***Switz.:*** Sultrin†; ***UK:*** Sultrin; ***USA:*** Alba Gyn; Dayto Sulf; Gyne-Sulf; Sultrin; Triple Sulfa; Trysul; VVS.

Sulfacytine (4916-r)

Sulfacytine *(BAN, USAN)*.

Sulfacitine *(pINN)*; CI-636. 1-Ethyl-*N*-sulphanilylcytosine; *N*[1]-(1-Ethyl-1,2-dihydro-2-oxopyrimidin-4-yl)sulphanilamide.

$C_{12}H_{14}N_4O_3S$ = 294.3.

CAS — 17784-12-2.

Sulfacytine is a short-acting sulphonamide with properties similar to those of sulphamethoxazole (p.254). It has been used in the treatment of urinary-tract infections.

Preparations

Proprietary Preparations (details are given in Part 3)

USA: Renoquid.

Sulfadicramide (13277-j)

Sulfadicramide *(rINN)*.

N′-(3,3-Dimethylacroyl)sulphanilamide.

$C_{11}H_{14}N_2O_3S$ = 254.3.

CAS — 115-68-4.

Sulfadicramide is a sulphonamide with properties similar to those of sulphamethoxazole (p.254). It is applied as a 15% ointment for superficial infections of the eye.

Preparations

Proprietary Preparations (details are given in Part 3)

Ger.: Irgamid†; ***Neth.:*** Irgamid; ***Switz.:*** Irgamid.

Sulfadoxine (4917-f)

Sulfadoxine *(BAN, USAN, rINN)*.

Ro-4-4393; Sulfadoxinum; Sulformethoxine; Sulforthomidine; Sulphormethoxine; Sulphorthodimethoxine. *N*[1]-(5,6-Dimethoxypyrimidin-4-yl)sulphanilamide.

$C_{12}H_{14}N_4O_4S$ = 310.3.

CAS — 2447-57-6.

Pharmacopoeias. In *Eur.* (see p.viii), *Int.*, and *US*.

A white or yellowish-white crystalline powder. Very slightly **soluble** in water; slightly soluble in alcohol and in methyl alcohol; practically insoluble in ether. It dissolves in solutions of alkali hydroxides and in dilute mineral acids. **Protect** from light.

Adverse Effects, Treatment, and Precautions

As for Sulphamethoxazole, p.254. For reference to the adverse effects of a combination of sulfadoxine and pyrimethamine, see Pyrimethamine, p.437.

If side-effects occur, sulfadoxine has the disadvantage that several days are required for elimination from the body.

Interactions

As for Sulphamethoxazole, p.255.

Antimicrobial Action

As for Sulphamethoxazole, p.255. Synergy exists between sulfadoxine and pyrimethamine, which act against folate metabolism at different points of the metabolic cycle.

Resistance to the combination of sulfadoxine and pyrimethamine in plasmodia, first noted in Thailand in the late 1970s, has become widespread in many malarious areas of the world. For further details of resistance to antimalarial drugs, see p.422.

Pharmacokinetics

Sulfadoxine is readily absorbed from the gastro-intestinal tract. High concentrations in the blood are reached in about 4 hours; the half-life in the blood is about 4 to 9 days. About 90 to 95% is reported to be bound to plasma proteins.

Sulfadoxine is widely distributed to body tissues and fluids; it passes into the fetal circulation and has been detected in low concentrations in breast milk. Sulfadoxine is excreted very slowly in urine, primarily unchanged.

Uses and Administration

Sulfadoxine is a long-acting sulphonamide that has been used in the treatment of various infections but is now rarely used alone.

It is given as a fixed-dose combination of 20 parts sulfadoxine with 1 part pyrimethamine (Fansidar) in the treatment of falciparum malaria resistant to other therapies (p.422), usually following a course of quinine. Although formerly used in the prophylaxis of malaria, the risk of toxicity from the combination is now generally considered to outweigh its value.

In the treatment of malaria, the usual dose by mouth is 1.5 g of sulfadoxine with 75 mg of pyrimethamine as a single dose; this should not be repeated for at least 7 days. Suggested oral doses for children are: 5 to 10 kg body-weight, 250 mg sulfadoxine with 12.5 mg pyrimethamine; 11 to 20 kg, 500 mg sulfadoxine with 25 mg pyrimethamine; 21 to 30 kg, 750 mg sulfadoxine with 37.5 mg pyrimethamine; 31 to 45 kg, 1 g sulfadoxine with 50 mg pyrimethamine.

The combination of sulfadoxine with pyrimethamine may also be administered intramuscularly.

Sulfadoxine with pyrimethamine has also been tried in the treatment of actinomycetomas (see Mycetoma p.132), and for prophylaxis of *Pneumocystis carinii* pneumonia in immunocompromised patients (see p.370 for the more usual prophylactic regimens).

A mixture of 5 parts of sulfadoxine with 1 part trimethoprim is used in veterinary medicine.

Administration. The combination of sulfadoxine and pyrimethamine has been administered by the intramuscular route,[1-5] but its role in the treatment of falciparum malaria is not clear.

1. Harinasuta T, *et al.* Parenteral Fansidar® in falciparum malaria. *Trans R Soc Trop Med Hyg* 1988; **82:** 694.
2. Salako LA, *et al.* Parenteral sulfadoxine-pyrimethamine (Fansidar): an effective and safe but under-used method of anti-malarial treatment. *Trans R Soc Trop Med Hyg* 1990; **84:** 641–3.
3. Simão F, *et al.* Comparison of intramuscular sulfadoxine-pyrimethamine and intramuscular quinine for the treatment of falciparum malaria in children. *Trans R Soc Trop Med Hyg* 1991; **85:** 341–4.
4. Winstanley PA, *et al.* The disposition of oral and intramuscular pyrimethamine/sulphadoxine in Kenyan children with high parasitaemia but clinically non-severe falciparum malaria. *Br J Clin Pharmacol* 1992; **33:** 143–8.
5. Newton CRJC, *et al.* A single dose of intramuscular sulfadoxine-pyrimethamine as an adjunct to quinine in the treatment of severe malaria: pharmacokinetics and efficacy. *Trans R Soc Trop Med Hyg* 1993; **87:** 207–10.

Preparations

USP 23: Sulfadoxine and Pyrimethamine Tablets.

Proprietary Preparations (details are given in Part 3)

Ital.: Fanasil.

Multi-ingredient: ***Aust.:*** Fansidar; ***Austral.:*** Fansidar; ***Belg.:*** Fansidar; ***Canad.:*** Fansidar; ***Fr.:*** Fansidar; ***Ger.:*** Fansidar†; ***Irl.:*** Fansidar; ***Neth.:*** Fansidar†; ***Norw.:*** Fansidar†; ***S.Afr.:*** Fansidar; ***Swed.:*** Fansidar; ***Switz.:*** Fansidar; Fansimef; ***UK:*** Fansidar; ***USA:*** Fansidar.

Sulfamerazine (4918-d)

Sulfamerazine *(BAN, rINN)*.

RP-2632; Solfamerazina; Sulfamerazinum; Sulfamethyldiazine; Sulfamethylpyrimidine; Sulphamerazine. *N*[1]-(4-Methylpyrimidin-2-yl)sulphanilamide.

$C_{11}H_{12}N_4O_2S$ = 264.3.

CAS — 127-79-7.

Pharmacopoeias. In *Eur.* (see p.viii), *Pol.*, and *US*.

A white or faintly pinkish- or yellowish-white, odourless or almost odourless, crystalline powder or crystals; it slowly darkens on exposure to light.

Soluble 1 in 6250 of water at 20° and 1 in 3300 of water at 37°; sparingly soluble in acetone; slightly soluble in alcohol; very slightly soluble in chloroform, in dichloromethane, and in ether; dissolves in dilute mineral acids and in solutions of alkali hydroxides. **Protect** from light.

Sulfamerazine Sodium (4919-n)

Sulfamerazine Sodium *(BANM, rINN)*.

Soluble Sulphamerazine; Sulfamerazinum Natricum; Sulphamerazine Sodium.

$C_{11}H_{11}N_4NaO_2S$ = 286.3.

CAS — 127-58-2.

Pharmacopoeias. In *Aust.* .

1.08 g of monograph substance is approximately equivalent to 1 g of sulfamerazine.

Sulfamerazine is a short-acting sulphonamide with properties similar to those of sulphamethoxazole (p.254). It is usually administered in conjunction with other sulphonamides.

Preparations

USP 23: Sulfamerazine Tablets; Trisulfapyrimidines Oral Suspension; Trisulfapyrimidines Tablets.

Proprietary Preparations (details are given in Part 3)

Multi-ingredient: ***Canad.:*** Trisulfaminic; ***Ger.:*** Berlocombin; ***S.Afr.:*** Tersulpha†; Trisulpha†; ***USA:*** Neotrizine†; Triple Sulfa No 2†.

Sulfamethylthiazole (14272-k)

Methylsulfathiazole. 4-Amino-*N*-(4-methyl-2-thiazolyl)benzenesulfonamide.

$C_{10}H_{11}N_3O_2S_2$ = 269.3.

CAS — 515-59-3.

Sulfamethylthiazole is a sulphonamide with properties similar to those of sulphamethoxazole (p.254). It is applied topically in combination with tetracycline in the treatment of eye infections.

Preparations

Proprietary Preparations (details are given in Part 3)

Multi-ingredient: ***Ital.:*** Pensulvit.

Sulfametopyrazine (4920-k)

Sulfametopyrazine *(BAN)*.

Sulfalene *(USAN, pINN)*; AS-18908; NSC-110433; Solfametopirazina; Solfametossipirazina; Sulfamethoxypyrazine; Sulfapirazinmetossina; Sulfapyrazin Methoxyne; Sulphalene. *N*[1]-(3-Methoxypyrazin-2-yl)sulphanilamide.

$C_{11}H_{12}N_4O_3S$ = 280.3.

CAS — 152-47-6.

Pharmacopoeias. In *It.*

Adverse Effects, Treatment, and Precautions

As for Sulphamethoxazole, p.254.

If side-effects occur, sulfametopyrazine has the disadvantage that several days are required for its elimination from the body.

Interactions

As for Sulphamethoxazole, p.255.

Antimicrobial Action

As for Sulphamethoxazole, p.255.

Pharmacokinetics

Sulfametopyrazine is readily absorbed from the gastro-intestinal tract; 60 to 80% is bound to plasma proteins. Only about 5% of a dose is metabolised to the acetyl derivative. It is slowly excreted in the urine. The biological half-life has been reported to be about 60 to 65 hours.

Uses and Administration

Sulfametopyrazine is a long-acting sulphonamide that has been used in the treatment of respiratory- and urinary-tract infections due to sensitive organisms. It is usually given by mouth in a single dose of 2 g once a week.

Sulfametopyrazine is given in the ratio 4 parts of sulfametopyrazine to 5 parts of trimethoprim as a combination with uses similar to co-trimoxazole (p.197). It is also given with pyrimethamine (p.438) in the treatment of falciparum malaria.

Preparations

Proprietary Preparations (details are given in Part 3)
Belg.: Kelfizina; Longum; ***Ger.:*** Longum; ***Irl.:*** Kelfizine W; ***Ital.:*** Kelfizina; ***Spain:*** Longum†; ***UK:*** Kelfizine W.

Multi-ingredient: ***Ital.:*** Kelfiprim; Metakelfin; Trimed†.

Sulfametrole (4921-a)

Sulfametrole *(BAN, rINN).*

N^1-(4-Methoxy-1,2,5-thiadiazol-3-yl)sulphanilamide.

$C_9H_{10}N_4O_3S_2$ = 286.3.

CAS — 32909-92-5.

Sulfametrole is a sulphonamide with properties similar to those of sulphamethoxazole (p.254). It is given in the ratio of 5 parts of sulfametrole to 1 part of trimethoprim as a combination with uses similar to co-trimoxazole (p.197). Usual doses are 960 mg (800 mg of sulfametrole and 160 mg of trimethoprim) twice daily by mouth. It has also been given by intravenous infusion.

Preparations

Proprietary Preparations (details are given in Part 3)

Multi-ingredient: ***Aust.:*** Lidaprim; ***Ger.:*** Lidaprim†; ***Ital.:*** Lidaprim; ***Switz.:*** Maderan.

Sulfaquinoxaline (4924-r)

Sulfaquinoxaline *(BAN, rINN).*

Sulfabenzpyrazine; Sulphaquinoxalina; Sulphaquinoxaline. N^1-(Quinoxalin-2-yl)sulphanilamide.

$C_{14}H_{12}N_4O_2S$ = 300.3.

CAS — 59-40-5 (sulfaquinoxaline); 967-80-6 (sulfaquinoxaline sodium).

Pharmacopoeias. In *Fr.* Also in *BP(Vet)* and in *US* for veterinary use only.

Fr. also includes Sulfaquinoxaline Sodium, $C_{14}H_{11}N_4NaO_2S$ = 322.3.

A yellow, odourless or almost odourless, powder. Practically **insoluble** in water; very slightly soluble in alcohol; practically insoluble in ether. It dissolves in aqueous solutions of alkalis. **Protect** from light.

Sulfaquinoxaline is a sulphonamide antibacterial used in veterinary medicine.

Sulfasuccinamide (13570-t)

Sulfasuccinamide *(rINN).*

4′-Sulphamoylsuccinanilic acid.

$C_{10}H_{12}N_2O_5S$ = 272.3.

CAS — 3563-14-2.

Sulfasuccinamide is a sulphonamide with properties similar to those of sulphamethoxazole (p.254). It is applied topically as the base or the sodium salt in the treatment of local infections of the ear, nose, and throat.

Preparations

Proprietary Preparations (details are given in Part 3)

Multi-ingredient: ***Fr.:*** Otoralgyl sulfamide; RhinATP; ***Switz.:*** Otoralgyl.

Sulfatroxazole (8641-t)

Sulfatroxazole *(BAN, rINN).*

N^1-(4,5-Dimethyl-1,2-oxazol-3-yl)- sulfanilamide.

$C_{11}H_{13}N_3O_3S$ = 267.3.

CAS — 23256-23-7.

Sulfatroxazole is a sulphonamide antibacterial used in combination with trimethoprim in veterinary medicine.

Sulfenazone (3943-c)

Sulfamazone. α-{*p*-[(6-Methoxy-3-pyridazinyl)sulfamoyl]anilino}-2,3-dimethyl-5-oxo-1-phenyl-3-pyrazoline-4-methanesulphonic acid.

$C_{22}H_{24}N_6O_7S_2$ = 548.6.

CAS — 65761-24-2 (sulfenazone); 13061-27-3 (sulfenazone sodium).

Sulfenazone is an antibacterial with antipyretic activity that is given as the sodium salt, by mouth or rectally, in infections of the upper respiratory tract.

Preparations

Proprietary Preparations (details are given in Part 3)
Ital.: Marespin.

Sulphacetamide (4927-n)

Sulphacetamide *(BAN).*

Sulfacetamide *(rINN)*; Acetosulfaminum. *N*-Sulphaniloylacetamide.

$C_8H_{10}N_2O_3S$ = 214.2.

CAS — 144-80-9.

Pharmacopoeias. In *Aust., Int., Neth.,* and *US.*

A white, odourless, crystalline powder.

Slightly **soluble** in water and in ether; soluble in alcohol; very slightly soluble in chloroform; freely soluble in dilute mineral acids and in solutions of alkali hydroxides. Solutions in water are acid to litmus and sensitive to light; they are unstable when acidic or strongly alkaline. **Protect** from light.

Sulphacetamide Sodium (4928-h)

Sulphacetamide Sodium *(BANM).*

Sulfacetamide Sodium *(rINNM)*; Soluble Sulphacetamide; Sulfacetamidum Natricum; Sulfacylum; Sulphacetamidum Sodium.

$C_8H_9N_2NaO_3S,H_2O$ = 254.2.

CAS — 127-56-0 (anhydrous sulphacetamide sodium); 6209-17-2 (sulphacetamide sodium monohydrate).

NOTE. SULF is a code approved by the BP for use on single unit doses of eye drops containing sulphacetamide sodium where the individual container may be too small to bear all the appropriate labelling information.

Pharmacopoeias. In *Chin., Eur.* (see p.viii), *Int., Pol.,* and *US.*

White or yellowish-white, odourless crystalline powder. 1.19 g of monograph substance is approximately equivalent to 1 g of sulphacetamide. **Soluble** 1 in 2.5 of water; sparingly soluble in alcohol; slightly soluble in dehydrated alcohol; practically insoluble in chloroform and in ether. A 5% solution in water has a pH of 8.0 to 9.5. **Store** in airtight containers. Protect from light.

When solutions are heated, hydrolysis occurs forming sulphanilamide which may be deposited as crystals, especially from concentrated solutions and under cold storage conditions.

Adverse Effects, Treatment, and Precautions

As for Sulphamethoxazole, p.254.

Local application of sulphacetamide sodium to the eye may cause burning or stinging but this is rarely severe enough to necessitate discontinuance of treatment.

Antimicrobial Action

As for Sulphamethoxazole, p.255.

Pharmacokinetics

When sulphacetamide sodium is applied to the eye it penetrates into ocular tissues and fluids; sulphonamide may be absorbed into the blood when the conjunctiva is inflamed.

Uses and Administration

Sulphacetamide is a sulphonamide which is used with sulfabenzamide and sulphathiazole in preparations for vaginal use, and is applied, as the sodium salt, in infections or injuries of the eyes although it is rarely of much value. Eye drops containing sulphacetamide sodium 10% to 30% and eye ointments containing up to 10% have been used. The sodium salt is also applied topically in the treatment of skin infections.

Preparations

BP 1998: Sulfacetamide Eye Drops; Sulfacetamide Eye Ointment;

USP 23: Neomycin Sulfate, Sulfacetamide Sodium, and Prednisolone Acetate Ophthalmic Ointment; Sulfacetamide Sodium and Prednisolone Acetate Ophthalmic Ointment; Sulfacetamide Sodium and Prednisolone Acetate Ophthalmic Suspension; Sulfacetamide Sodium Ophthalmic Ointment; Sulfacetamide Sodium Ophthalmic Solution; Triple Sulfa Vaginal Cream; Triple Sulfa Vaginal Tablets.

Proprietary Preparations (details are given in Part 3)
Aust.: Beocid Puroptal; Blephasulf†; Cetazin; ***Austral.:*** Acetopt; Bleph-10; Optamide; ***Belg.:*** Anginamide; Antebor; Isopto Cetamide; Sulfa 10; Ultra; ***Canad.:*** Bleph-10 Liquifilm; Cetamide; Diosulf; Ophtho-Sulf; Sodium Sulamyd; Sulfex; ***Fr.:*** Antebor; Vitaseptine; ***Ger.:*** Albucid; Sulfableph N Liquifilm†; ***Irl.:*** Bleph-10†; ***Ital.:*** Prontamid; ***S.Afr.:*** Albucid†; Bleph-10; Covosulf; Opticet†; Spersamide; ***Spain:*** Sulfacet; Sulfacetam; ***Switz.:*** Antebor†; Spersacet; ***UK:*** Albucid†; ***USA:*** Ak-Sulf; Bleph-10; Cetamide; Isopto Cetamide; Klaron; Ocusulf-10; Sebizon; Sodium Sulamyd; Storz-Sulf; Sulf-10; Sulfac.

Multi-ingredient: ***Aust.:*** Blephamide; ***Austral.:*** Blephamide; Sultrin; ***Belg.:*** Cetapred†; Isopto Cetapred; Neo-Golaseptine†; Sultrin; ***Canad.:*** Blephamide; Celestone S†; Dioptimyd; Metimyd; Sulfacet-R; Sultrin; Vasocidin; Vasosulf; ***Fr.:*** Antebor B_6; ***Ger.:*** Blefcon; Blephamide; Blephamide N Liquifilm; Combiamid; Dexabiotan in der Ophtiole†; Neosultrin†; ***Irl.:*** Blephamide†; Corticid†; Sultrin; ***Ital.:*** Antisettico Astringente Sedativo; Aureomix; Brumeton Colloidale S; Chemyterral†; Cosmiciclina; Visublefarite; ***S.Afr.:*** Blephamide; Covancaine; Covosan; Spersacet C; Sultrin; ***Spain:*** Amidrin Bio†; Betamida; Celestone S; Liquipom Dexamida; Oto Neomicin Calm; Pomada Llorens Sulfaclor†; Visublefarite; ***Swed.:*** Blefcon; Metimyd; ***Switz.:*** Antebor B_6†; Blephamide; Cetapred†; Isopto Cetapred†; Spersacet C; Sultrin†; ***UK:*** Sultrin; ***USA:*** Ak-Cide; Alba Gyn; Blephamide; Cetapred; Dayto Sulf; FML-S; Gyne-Sulf; Isopto Cetapred; Metimyd; Novacet; Optimyd; Sulfacet-R; Sulphrin†; Sulster; Sultrin; Triple Sulfa; Trysul; Vasocidin; Vasosulf; VVS.

Sulphachlorpyridazine (4929-m)

Sulphachlorpyridazine *(BAN).*

N^1-(6-Chloropyridazin-3-yl)sulphanilamide.

$C_{10}H_9ClN_4O_2S$ = 284.7.

CAS — 80-32-0.

Pharmacopoeias. In *US* for veterinary use only.

Sulphachlorpyridazine is a sulphonamide antibacterial used in veterinary medicine, sometimes in combination with trimethoprim.

Sulphadiazine (4930-t)

Sulphadiazine *(BAN).*

Sulfadiazine *(rINN)*; Solfadiazina; Solfapirimidina; Sulfadiazinum. N^1-(Pyrimidin-2-yl)sulphanilamide.

$C_{10}H_{10}N_4O_2S$ = 250.3.

CAS — 68-35-9.

NOTE. Sulphadiazine may be given with tetroxoprim or trimethoprim; such combinations have been given approved names Co-tetroxazine (p.196) and Co-trimazine (p.196) respectively.

Pharmacopoeias. In *Chin., Eur.* (see p.viii), and *US.*

White, yellowish-white, or pinkish-white, odourless or almost odourless, crystals or crystalline powder, slowly darkening on exposure to light.

Soluble 1 in 13 000 of water; slightly to sparingly soluble in acetone; very slightly to sparingly soluble in alcohol; it dissolves in dilute mineral acids and in solutions of alkali hydroxides. **Protect** from light.

Sulphadiazine Sodium (4931-x)

Sulphadiazine Sodium *(BANM).*

Sulfadiazine Sodium *(rINN)*; Sodium Sulfadiazine; Soluble Sulphadiazine; Sulfadiazinum Natricum.

$C_{10}H_9N_4NaO_2S$ = 272.3.

CAS — 547-32-0.

Pharmacopoeias. In *Aust., Chin.,* and *US.*

A white powder. 1.09 g of monograph substance is approximately equivalent to 1 g of sulphadiazine.

Soluble 1 in 2 of water; slightly soluble in alcohol. On prolonged exposure to humid air it absorbs carbon dioxide with the liberation of sulphadiazine and becomes incompletely soluble in water. **Store** in airtight containers. Protect from light.

Incompatibilities. Solutions of sulphadiazine sodium are alkaline, and incompatibility may reasonably be expected with acidic drugs or with preparations unstable at high pH.

Adverse Effects, Treatment, and Precautions

As for Sulphamethoxazole, p.254.

Because of the low solubilities of sulphadiazine and its acetyl derivative in urine, crystalluria is more likely after administration of sulphadiazine than after sulphamethoxazole.

Sulphadiazine sodium solution is strongly alkaline; it should therefore be administered intravenously in a strength not exceeding 5% to reduce the risk of thrombosis of the vein; extravasation may cause sloughing and necrosis. For the same reason, intramuscular injections are painful and sulphadiazine sodium should not be given by intrathecal or subcutaneous injection.

Carnitine deficiency. A case of hyperammonaemia and carnitine deficiency in an immunosuppressed patient receiving sulphadiazine and pyrimethamine for the treatment of toxoplasmosis.[1]

1. Sekas G, Harbhajan SP. Hyperammonemia and carnitine deficiency in a patient receiving sulfadiazine and pyrimethamine. *Am J Med* 1993; **95:** 112–13.

Effects on the eyes. Numerous white stone-like concretions of sulphadiazine occurred in the conjunctiva of a woman who had used sulphadiazine eye drops for about one year.[1]

1. Boettner EA, *et al.* Conjunctival concretions of sulfadiazine. *Arch Ophthalmol* 1974; **92:** 446–8

Effects on the kidneys. Reports of crystalluria and renal failure associated with the use of sulphadiazine in patients with AIDS,[1-4] including the suggestion that such patients may be particularly prone to sulphadiazine-induced renal toxicity.[3]

1. Goadsby PJ, *et al.* Acquired immunodeficiency syndrome (AIDS) and sulfadiazine-associated acute renal failure. *Ann Intern Med* 1987; **107:** 784–5.

2. Ventura MG, *et al.* Sulfadiazine revisited. *J Infect Dis* 1989; **160:** 556–7.
3. Simon DI, *et al.* Sulfadiazine crystalluria revisited: the treatment of Toxoplasma encephalitis in patients with acquired immunodeficiency syndrome. *Arch Intern Med* 1990; **150:** 2379–84.
4. Díaz F, *et al.* Sulfadiazine-induced multiple urolithiasis and acute renal failure in a patient with AIDS and Toxoplasma encephalitis. *Ann Pharmacother* 1996; **30:** 41–2.

Effects on the salivary glands. Enlargement of the salivary glands (sialadenitis) has been reported in a patient who received a preparation containing sulphadiazine; complete recovery followed within 3 days of discontinuing therapy. Oral rechallenge confirmed that sulphadiazine was the causative agent.

1. Añíbarro B, Fontela JL. Sulfadiazine-induced sialadenitis. *Ann Pharmacother* 1997; **31:** 59–60.

Interactions

As for Sulphamethoxazole, p.255.

Antimicrobial Action

As for Sulphamethoxazole, p.255.

Pharmacokinetics

Sulphadiazine is readily absorbed from the gastro-intestinal tract, peak blood concentrations being reached 3 to 6 hours after a single dose; 20 to 55% has been reported to be bound to plasma proteins. It penetrates into the CSF to produce therapeutic concentrations, which may be more than half of those in the blood, within 4 hours of administration by mouth. Up to 40% of sulphadiazine in the blood is present as the acetyl derivative. The half-life of sulphadiazine is about 10 hours; it is prolonged in renal impairment.

About 50% of a single dose of sulphadiazine given by mouth is excreted in the urine in 24 hours; 15 to 40% is excreted as the acetyl derivative.

The urinary excretion of sulphadiazine and the acetyl derivative is dependent on pH. About 30% is excreted unchanged in both fast and slow acetylators when the urine is acidic whereas about 75% is excreted unchanged by slow acetylators when the urine is alkaline. The half-life of sulphadiazine ranges from 7 to 12 hours and that of its metabolite from 8 to 12 hours.[1]

1. Vree TB, *et al.* Determination of the acetylator phenotype and pharmacokinetics of some sulphonamides in man. *Clin Pharmacokinet* 1980; **5:** 274–94.

Uses and Administration

Sulphadiazine is a short-acting sulphonamide that has been used similarly to sulphamethoxazole (p.256) in the treatment of infections due to susceptible organisms. It has been used in the treatment of nocardiosis and lymphogranuloma venereum, and has been given for the prophylaxis of rheumatic fever in penicillin-allergic patients. For details of these infections and their treatment, see Choice of Antibacterial, p.116. Sulphadiazine is also given with pyrimethamine for the treatment of toxoplasmosis (p.576) and has been tried in disseminated *Acanthamoeba* infection (p.573).

In the treatment of susceptible infections sulphadiazine may be given by mouth in usual doses of 2 to 4 g followed by up to 6 g daily in divided doses, although up to 8 g daily has been suggested for toxoplasmosis; a suggested dose in children is 75 mg per kg body-weight initially then 150 mg per kg daily in divided doses to a maximum of 6 g daily. A concentration in the blood of 100 to 150 μg per mL is desirable. Sulphadiazine is used in infants less than 2 months of age for congenital toxoplasmosis. For the prophylaxis of rheumatic fever, patients weighing less than about 30 kg are given 500 mg once daily, while those over 30 kg may receive 1 g once daily.

Sulphadiazine is also given intravenously as the sodium salt. The usual dose is the equivalent of sulphadiazine 2 to 3 g initially, followed by 1 g four times daily for 2 days; subsequent treatment is given by mouth. Children and infants over 2 months of age may be given the equivalent of 50 mg per kg initially, followed by 25 mg per kg four times daily.

Intravenous doses of sulphadiazine sodium are given by infusion or by slow intravenous injection of a solution containing up to 5%. It may be diluted with sodium chloride 0.9%. Sulphadiazine sodium has been given by deep intramuscular injection but great care must be exercised to prevent damage to subcutaneous tissues and the intravenous route is preferred.

The use of sulphadiazine with trimethoprim is described under co-trimazine (p.196). Sulphadiazine has also been given in association with other sulphonamides, particularly sulfamerazine and sulphadimidine, to reduce the problems of low solubility in urine.

Preparations

BP 1998: Sulfadiazine Injection;
USP 23: Sulfadiazine Sodium Injection; Sulfadiazine Tablets; Trisulfapyrimidines Oral Suspension; Trisulfapyrimidines Tablets.

Proprietary Preparations (details are given in Part 3)
Fr.: Adiazine.

Multi-ingredient: ***Aust.:*** Bisolvonamid; Ophcillin N; Rhinon; Triglobe; Urospasmon sine phenazopyridino; ***Belg.:*** Trimatrim†; ***Canad.:*** Coptin; Ovoquinol†; Trisulfaminic; ***Fr.:*** Antrima; ***Ger.:*** Bisolvonamid†; Diben-amid†; Nitrofurantoin comp.†; Spasmo-Urolcear†; Sterinor; Sulfa-Uro-Tablinen†; Sulfa-Urolong†; sulfopecticept†; Triglobe; Uroclear†; Urospasmon; Urospasmon sine; ***Ital.:*** Chemiovis†; Geomix†; Kombinax; Oxosint; Sterinor; Sulfadrina†; Tibirox†; ***Norw.:*** Trisulfamid; ***S.Afr.:*** Tersulpha†; Trisulpha†; ***Spain:*** Bio Hubber; Bio Hubber Fuerte; Bronco Aseptilex; Broncomicin Bals; Triglobe; ***Swed.:*** Trimin sulfa; ***Switz.:*** Urospasmon†; ***USA:*** Neotrizine†; Triple Sulfa No 2†.

Sulphadimethoxine (4932-r)

Sulphadimethoxine *(BAN).*

Sulfadimethoxine *(rINN)*; Solfadimetossina; Solfadimetossipirimidina. N^1-(2,6-Dimethoxypyrimidin-4-yl)sulphanilamide.

$C_{12}H_{14}N_4O_4S$ = 310.3.

CAS — 122-11-2.

Pharmacopoeias. In *Fr.* and *It.*

Sulphadimethoxine is a long-acting sulphonamide with properties similar to those of sulphamethoxazole (p.254). It is readily absorbed from the gastro-intestinal tract, and about 98 to 99% is bound to plasma proteins. Half-lives of about 30 to 40 hours have been reported. It has been given by mouth.

Preparations

Proprietary Preparations (details are given in Part 3)
Ital.: Chemiosalfa†; Deltin†; Risulpir†; Ritarsulfa†; Sulfadren†; Sulfastop†; ***S.Afr.:*** Sulfathox†.

Sulphadimidine (4933-f)

Sulphadimidine *(BAN).*

Sulfadimidine *(rINN)*; Solfametazina; Sulfadimerazine; Sulfadimezinum; Sulfadimidinum; Sulfamethazine; Sulphadimethylpyrimidine; Sulphamethazine. N^1-(4,6-Dimethylpyrimidin-2-yl)sulphanilamide.

$C_{12}H_{14}N_4O_2S$ = 278.3.

CAS — 57-68-1.

NOTE. Sulfadimethylpyrimidine has been used as a synonym for sulphasomidine (p.257). Care should be taken to avoid confusion between the two compounds, which are isomeric.

Pharmacopoeias. In *Chin., Eur.* (see p.viii), *Int.,* and *US.*

White or yellowish-white, almost odourless, crystals or powder. It may darken on exposure to light.

Very slightly **soluble** in water; soluble in acetone; slightly soluble in alcohol; very slightly soluble in ether; it dissolves in dilute mineral acids and in aqueous solutions of alkali hydroxides. **Protect** from light.

Sulphadimidine Sodium (4934-d)

Sulphadimidine Sodium *(BANM).*

Soluble Sulphadimidine; Sulfadimidine Sodium; Sulfamethazine Sodium.

$C_{12}H_{13}N_4NaO_2S$ = 300.3.

CAS — 1981-58-4.

Pharmacopoeias. In *Aust., Br.,* and *Int.*

White or creamy-white, odourless or almost odourless, hygroscopic crystals or powder. 1.08 g of monograph substance is approximately equivalent to 1 g of sulphadimidine.

Freely **soluble** in water; sparingly soluble in alcohol. A 10% solution has a pH of 10 to 11. **Protect** from light.

Sulphadimidine is a short-acting sulphonamide with properties similar to those of sulphamethoxazole (p.254).

It is well absorbed from the gastro-intestinal tract and about 80 to 90% has been stated to be bound to plasma protein. Reported half-lives have ranged from 1.5 to 4 hours in fast and 5.5 to 8.8 hours in slow acetylators. Because of the relatively high solubility of the drug and its acetyl metabolite crystalluria may be less likely than with sulphamethoxazole.

In the treatment of susceptible infections sulphadimidine is given by mouth in an initial dose of 2 g, followed by 0.5 to 1.0 g every 6 to 8 hours. It has also been given parenterally as the sodium salt.

Sulphadimidine has also been used with trimethoprim similarly to co-trimoxazole (p.197) and in association with other sulphonamides, particularly sulfamerazine and sulphadiazine.

Because its pharmacokinetics differ in fast and slow acetylators, sulphadimidine has been used to determine acetylator status.

Preparations

BP 1998: Paediatric Sulfadimidine Oral Suspension; Sulfadimidine Injection; Sulfadimidine Tablets;
USP 23: Trisulfapyrimidines Oral Suspension; Trisulfapyrimidines Tablets.

Proprietary Preparations (details are given in Part 3)
Irl.: Sulphamezathine†.

Multi-ingredient: ***Canad.:*** Trisulfaminic; ***Norw.:*** Trisulfamid; ***S.Afr.:*** Tersulpha†; ***USA:*** Neotrizine†; Triple Sulfa No 2†.

Sulphafurazole (4936-h)

Sulphafurazole *(BAN).*

Sulfafurazole *(pINN)*; Sulfafurazolum; Sulfisoxazole; Sulphafuraz. N^1-(3,4-Dimethylisoxazol-5-yl)sulphanilamide.

$C_{11}H_{13}N_3O_3S$ = 267.3.

CAS — 127-69-5.

Pharmacopoeias. In *Eur.* (see p.viii), *Jpn, Pol.,* and *US.*

A white or yellowish-white, odourless crystalline powder or crystals.

Soluble 1 in 7700 of water, 1 in 10 of boiling alcohol; sparingly soluble in alcohol; slightly soluble in dichloromethane and in ether; it dissolves in solutions of alkali hydroxides and in dilute mineral acids. **Store** in airtight containers. Protect from light.

Acetyl Sulphafurazole (4937-m)

Sulfisoxazole Acetyl. N^1-Acetyl Sulphafurazole; *N*-(3,4-Dimethylisoxazol-5-yl)-*N*-sulphanilylacetamide.

$C_{13}H_{15}N_3O_4S$ = 309.3.

CAS — 80-74-0.

NOTE. Acetyl sulphafurazole is to be distinguished from the N^4-acetyl derivative formed from sulphafurazole by conjugation in the body.

Compounded preparations of erythromycin ethyl succinate (erythromycin ethylsuccinate) and acetyl sulphafurazole (sulfisoxazole acetyl) in USP 23 may be represented by the name Co-erynsulfisox.

Pharmacopoeias. In *US.*

A white to slightly yellow crystalline powder. 1.16 g of monograph substance is approximately equivalent to 1 g of sulphafurazole.

Practically **insoluble** in water; soluble 1 in about 180 of alcohol, 1 in 35 of chloroform, 1 in about 200 of methyl alcohol, and 1 in about 1100 of ether. **Store** in airtight containers. Protect from light.

Sulphafurazole Diethanolamine (4938-b)

Sulfafurazole Diolamine *(pINNM)*; NU-445; Sulfisoxazole Diolamine *(USAN)*; Sulphafurazole Diolamine. The 2,2′-iminobisethanol salt of sulphafurazole.

$C_{11}H_{13}N_3O_3S,C_4H_{11}NO_2$ = 372.4.

CAS — 4299-60-9.

Pharmacopoeias. In *US.*

An odourless, white to off-white, fine, crystalline powder. 1.39 g of monograph substance is approximately equivalent to 1 g of sulphafurazole.

Soluble 1 in 2 of water, 1 in 16 of alcohol, 1 in 1000 of chloroform, 1 in 4 of methyl alcohol, and 1 in 250 of isopropyl alcohol; practically insoluble in ether. **Store** in airtight containers. Protect from light.

Adverse Effects, Treatment, and Precautions

As for Sulphamethoxazole, p.254.

Sulphafurazole and its acetyl derivative are relatively soluble in urine and the risk of crystalluria is generally slight, but nevertheless adequate fluid intake is recommended.

Interactions

As for Sulphamethoxazole, p.255.

Sulphafurazole has been reported to increase the anaesthetic effect of thiopentone sodium.

Eye preparations of sulphafurazole diethanolamine should not be applied concomitantly with preparations of silver salts.

Antimicrobial Action

As for Sulphamethoxazole, p.255.

Pharmacokinetics

Sulphafurazole is readily absorbed from the gastro-intestinal tract with peak plasma concentrations occurring 1 to 4 hours after a dose by mouth. Acetyl sulphafurazole (the N^1-acetyl derivative) is broken down to sulphafurazole in the gastro-intestinal tract before absorption, resulting in delayed and somewhat lower peak concentrations. Following absorption about 85 to 90% is bound to plasma proteins. Sulphafurazole readily diffuses into extracellular fluid, but very little diffuses into cells. Concentrations in the CSF are about one-third of those in the blood. It crosses the placenta into the fetal circulation and is distributed into breast milk. About 30% of sulphafurazole in the blood and in the urine is in the form of the N^4-acetyl derivative.

It is excreted rapidly, up to 95% of a single dose being eliminated in 24 hours. The half-life is reported to range from about 5 to 8 hours. Both sulphafurazole and its N^4-acetyl derivative are more soluble than many other sulphonamides in urine.

Uses and Administration

Sulphafurazole is a short-acting sulphonamide that is used similarly to sulphamethoxazole (p.256), notably in the treatment of chlamydial infections such as lymphogranuloma venereum, chlamydial pneumonia, urethritis, and trachoma. It is used, usually with erythromycin, in the treatment of otitis media. For details of these infections and their treatment see Choice of Antibacterial, p.116.

It is usually administered by mouth. In the treatment of susceptible infections sulphafurazole is given in an initial dose of 2 to 4 g followed by 4 to 8 g daily in divided doses every 4 to 6 hours. For children, the dose is 75 mg per kg body-weight initially, followed by 150 mg per kg daily in divided doses to a maximum of 6 g daily. Dosage modification may be necessary in patients with renal impairment. Acetyl sulphafurazole is tasteless and is used in liquid oral preparations of the drug; doses are expressed in terms of sulphafurazole.

Sulphafurazole diethanolamine has been used, as an ophthalmic ointment or solution containing the equivalent of 4% of sulphafurazole, in the topical treatment of susceptible eye infections.

Sulphafurazole diethanolamine has also been given parenterally.

Preparations

USP 23: Erythromycin Estolate and Sulfisoxazole Acetyl Oral Suspension; Erythromycin Ethylsuccinate and Sulfisoxazole Acetyl for Oral Suspension; Sulfisoxazole Acetyl Oral Suspension; Sulfisoxazole Diolamine Injection; Sulfisoxazole Diolamine Ophthalmic Ointment; Sulfisoxazole Diolamine Ophthalmic Solution; Sulfisoxazole Tablets.

Proprietary Preparations (details are given in Part 3)
Canad.: Novo-Soxazole; ***USA:*** Gantrisin†; SS-Tab.

Multi-ingredient: ***Canad.:*** Azo Gantrisin†; Pediazole; ***Fr.:*** Pediazole; ***Ital.:*** Fultrexin†; ***S.Afr.:*** Pediazole; ***Switz.:*** Pediazole; ***USA:*** Azo Gantrisin†; Eryzole; ESP†; Pediazole.

Sulphaguanidine (4939-v)

Sulphaguanidine *(BAN)*.

Sulfaguanidine *(rINN)*; Solfaguanidina; Sulfaguanidinum; Sulfamidinum; Sulginum. 1-Sulphanilylguanidine; N'-Amidinosulphanilamide monohydrate.

$C_7H_{10}N_4O_2S,H_2O$ = 232.3.

CAS — 57-67-0 (anhydrous sulphaguanidine); 6190-55-2 (sulphaguanidine monohydrate).

Pharmacopoeias. In *Aust., Fr., Ger., It., Pol.,* and *Swiss.*

Sulphaguanidine is a sulphonamide with properties similar to those of sulphamethoxazole (p.254). It is absorbed to a limited extent from the gastro-intestinal tract and may therefore be more likely to cause systemic effects than less well-absorbed drugs such as phthalylsulphathiazole and succinylsulphathiazole. It is used, usually in combination with other drugs, in the treatment of gastro-intestinal infections, and has also been applied locally to the skin and throat.

Preparations

Proprietary Preparations (details are given in Part 3)
Fr.: Ganidan†.

Multi-ingredient: ***Aust.:*** Carboguan†; ***Fr.:*** Entercine†; Litoxol; ***Ger.:*** Jacosulfon†; ***Spain:*** Angileptol; Kolotanino†.

Sulphamethizole (4941-f)

Sulphamethizole *(BAN)*.

Sulfamethizole *(rINN)*; Sulfamethizolum. N^1-(5-Methyl-1,3,4-thiadiazol-2-yl)sulphanilamide.

$C_9H_{10}N_4O_2S_2$ = 270.3.

CAS — 144-82-1.

Pharmacopoeias. In *Eur.* (see p.viii), *Jpn,* and *US.*

Almost odourless, white or yellowish-white crystalline powder or crystals.

Soluble 1 in 2000 of water, 1 in 38 of alcohol, 1 in 13 of acetone, and 1 in 1900 of chloroform and of ether; it dissolves in solutions of alkali hydroxides and in dilute mineral acids. **Protect** from light.

Adverse Effects, Treatment, and Precautions

As for Sulphamethoxazole, p.254.

Sulphamethizole and its acetyl derivative are relatively soluble in urine, and the risk of crystalluria is quite low, but an adequate fluid intake should generally be maintained.

Interactions

As for Sulphamethoxazole, p.255.

Antimicrobial Action

As for Sulphamethoxazole, p.255.

Pharmacokinetics

Sulphamethizole is readily absorbed from the gastro-intestinal tract; about 90% has been reported to be bound to plasma proteins. Its half-life has been reported to range from about 1.5 to 3 hours. It is only slightly acetylated in the body and is rapidly excreted, about 60% of a dose being eliminated in the urine in 5 hours and around 90% within 10 hours. Sulphamethizole and its acetyl derivative are readily soluble in urine over a wide pH range. Only low concentrations are achieved in blood and tissues because of its rapid excretion.

Uses and Administration

Sulphamethizole is a short-acting sulphonamide that is given by mouth in the treatment of infections of the urinary tract, sometimes in combination with other antibacterials; it is unsuitable for the treatment of systemic infection since only relatively low concentrations of drug are achieved in the blood and tissues.

It is given in adult doses of 1.5 to 4 g daily in 3 to 4 divided doses. A suggested dose for children is 30 to 45 mg per kg body-weight daily in 4 divided doses.

Sulphamethizole monoethanolamine has also been used.

Preparations

USP 23: Oxytetracycline and Phenazopyridine Hydrochlorides and Sulfamethizole Capsules; Sulfamethizole Oral Suspension; Sulfamethizole Tablets.

Proprietary Preparations (details are given in Part 3)
Aust.: Lucosil; Urolucosil; ***Austral.:*** Urolucosil†; ***Belg.:*** Lucosil†; Urolucosil†; ***Fr.:*** Rufol; ***Ital.:*** Rufol†; ***Norw.:*** Lucosil†; ***Spain:*** Tiosulfan†; ***Switz.:*** Urolucosil†; ***USA:*** Thiosulfil Forte.

Multi-ingredient: ***Ger.:*** Harnosal; Nicene N†; ***S.Afr.:*** Nicene; ***Spain:*** Dorsect†; Micturol Sedante; ***USA:*** Urobiotic-250†.

Sulphamethoxazole (4942-d)

Sulphamethoxazole *(BAN)*.

Sulfamethoxazole *(USAN, rINN)*; Ro-4-2130; Sulfamethoxazolum; Sulfisomezole. N^1-(5-Methylisoxazol-3-yl)sulphanilamide.

$C_{10}H_{11}N_3O_3S$ = 253.3.

CAS — 723-46-6.

NOTE. Sulphamethoxazole may be given with trimethoprim and a preparation of such a combination has been given the approved name Co-trimoxazole, p.196.

Pharmacopoeias. In *Chin., Eur.* (see p.viii), *Int., Jpn, Pol.,* and *US.*

A white or off-white, almost odourless, crystalline powder.

Soluble 1 in 3400 of water; soluble 1 in 50 of alcohol; freely soluble in acetone; slowly and usually incompletely soluble 1 in 2 of carbon disulphide; soluble 1 in 1000 of chloroform and of ether; it dissolves in dilute solutions of sodium hydroxide. **Protect** from light.

Adverse Effects and Treatment

Nausea, vomiting, anorexia, and diarrhoea are relatively common following the administration of sulphamethoxazole and other sulphonamides.

Hypersensitivity reactions to sulphonamides have proved a problem. Fever is relatively common, and reactions involving the skin may include rashes, pruritus, photosensitivity reactions, exfoliative dermatitis, and erythema nodosum. Severe, potentially fatal, skin reactions including toxic epidermal necrolysis and the Stevens-Johnson syndrome, have occurred in patients treated with sulphonamides. Dermatitis may also occur from contact of sulphonamides with the skin. Systemic lupus erythematosus, particularly exacerbation of pre-existing disease, has also been reported.

Nephrotoxic reactions including interstitial nephritis and tubular necrosis, which may result in renal failure, have been attributed to hypersensitivity to sulphamethoxazole. Lumbar pain, haematuria, oliguria, and anuria may also occur due to crystallisation in the urine of sulphamethoxazole or its less soluble acetylated metabolite. The risk of crystalluria can be reduced by the administration of fluids to maintain a high urine output. If necessary, alkalinisation of the urine by administration of sodium bicarbonate may increase solubility and aid the elimination of sulphonamides.

Blood disorders have occasionally occurred during treatment with the sulphonamides including sulphamethoxazole, and include agranulocytosis, aplastic anaemia, thrombocytopenia, leucopenia, hypoprothrombinaemia, and eosinophilia. Many of these effects on the blood may result from hypersensitivity reactions. Sulphonamides may rarely cause cyanosis due to methaemoglobinaemia. Acute haemolytic anaemia is a rare complication which may be associated with glucose-6-phosphate dehydrogenase deficiency.

Other adverse effects which may be manifestations of a generalised hypersensitivity reaction to sulphonamides include a syndrome resembling serum sickness, liver necrosis, hepatomegaly and jaundice, myocarditis, pulmonary eosinophilia and fibrosing alveolitis, and vasculitis including polyarteritis nodosa. Anaphylaxis has been reported only very rarely.

Other adverse reactions that have been reported after the administration of sulphamethoxazole or other sulphonamides include hypoglycaemia, hypothyroidism, neurological reactions including aseptic meningitis, ataxia, benign intracranial hypertension, convulsions, dizziness, drowsiness, fatigue, headache, insomnia, mental depression, peripheral or optic neuropathies, psychoses, tinnitus, vertigo, and pancreatitis.

Sulphonamides may displace serum-bound bilirubin, resulting in jaundice and kernicterus in premature neonates.

As with other antimicrobials, sulphamethoxazole may cause alterations of the bacterial flora in the gastro-intestinal tract. There is, therefore, the possibility, although it appears to be small, that pseudomembranous colitis may occur.

Slow acetylators of sulphamethoxazole may be at greater risk of adverse reactions than fast acetylators.

Precautions

In patients receiving sulphamethoxazole, adequate fluid intake is necessary to reduce the risk of crystalluria; the daily urine output should be 1200 to 1500 mL or more. The administration of compounds which render the urine acid may increase the risk of crystalluria; the risk may be reduced with alkaline urine.

Treatment with sulphonamides should be discontinued immediately a rash appears because of the danger of severe allergic reactions such as the Stevens-Johnson syndrome.

Sulphamethoxazole should be given with care to patients with renal or hepatic impairment and is contra-indicated in patients with severe renal or hepatic failure or with blood disorders. Dosage reduction may be necessary in renal impairment. Complete blood counts and urinalyses with microscopic examination should be carried out particularly during prolonged therapy. Sulphamethoxazole should not be given to patients with a history of hypersensitivity to sulphonamides as cross-sensitivity may occur between drugs of this group. Care is generally advisable in patients with a history of allergy or asthma. Caution is also needed in the elderly, who may be more likely to have other risk factors for reactions. Sulphamethoxazole should not be given to patients with acute porphyria as it may cause exacerbations of the disease and some authorities consider it contra-indicated in lupus erythematosus for similar reasons. Patients with glucose 6-phosphate dehydrogenase deficiency may be at risk of haemolytic reactions.

Sulphamethoxazole and other sulphonamides are not usually given to infants within 1 to 2 months of birth because of the risk of producing kernicterus; for the same reason, they are generally contra-indicated in women prior to delivery or in nursing mothers.

Patients with AIDS may be particularly prone to adverse reactions, especially when sulphamethoxazole is given in combination with trimethoprim as co-trimoxazole.

Sulphonamides have been reported to interfere with some diagnostic tests including those for urea, creatinine, and urinary glucose and urobilinogen.

Immunocompromised patients. Sulphamethoxazole is mainly conjugated in the liver to the N^4-acetyl derivative, but is also oxidised, to a limited extent, to the hydroxylamine,[1-5] and this metabolite has been implicated in the development of adverse reactions to sulphonamides. The metabolite appears to be produced through cytochrome P450 oxidative metabolism and it has been suggested that slow acetylators of sulphamethoxazole exhibit increased oxidation compared with other metabolic routes.[1] AIDS patients also exhibit increased oxidation since they may be depleted of substrated such as acetylcoenzyme A or glutathione necessary for acetylation or detoxification, and this may explain their susceptibility to sulphamethoxazole toxicity.[2,3]

There have been attempts to inhibit the formation of the hydroxylamine metabolite by competitive inhibition of cytochrome P450 enzymes, notably with fluconazole and ketoconazole.[4,5] Encouraging results have been obtained with fluconazole in healthy volunteers, but the potential for clinical benefit in AIDS patients requires further study.[5]

However, one successful method of overcoming adverse effects in AIDS patients has been desensitisation. Desensitisation by administration of initial doses of 4 mg of sulphamethoxazole or 5 mg of sulphadiazine every 6 hours, doubled at 24-hour intervals until the desired dose was reached, was uneventful in 9 of 13 patients with AIDS requiring sulphonamide treatment for opportunistic infections.[6] The remaining 4 had cutaneous reactions with fever, but in 2 of these reactions were successfully managed with an antihistamine. Although there is a risk of anaphylaxis, patients with AIDS can be successfully treated with sulphonamides if desensitisation is employed.

See also under Immunocompromised Patients in Precautions of Co-trimoxazole, p.197.

1. Cribb AE, Spielberg SP. Sulfamethoxazole is metabolized to the hydroxylamine in humans. *Clin Pharmacol Ther* 1992; **51:** 522–6.
2. Lee BL, *et al.* The hydroxylamine of sulfamethoxazole and adverse reactions in patients with acquired immunodeficiency syndrome. *Clin Pharmacol Ther* 1994; **56:** 184–9.
3. van der Ven AJA, *et al.* Urinary recovery and kinetics of sulphamethoxazole and its metabolites in HIV-seropositive patients and healthy volunteers after a single oral dose of sulphamethoxazole. *Br J Clin Pharmacol* 1995; **39:** 621–5.
4. Mitra AK, *et al.* Inhibition of sulfamethoxazole hydroxylamine formation by fluconazole in human liver microsomes and healthy volunteers. *Clin Pharmacol Ther* 1996; **59:** 332–40.
5. Gill HJ, *et al.* The effect of fluconazole and ketoconazole on the metabolism of sulphamethoxazole. *Br J Clin Pharmacol* 1996; **42:** 347–53.
6. Torgovnick J, Arsura E. Desensitization to sulfonamides in patients with HIV infection. *Am J Med* 1990; **88:** 548–9.

Porphyria. Sulphonamides have been associated with clinical exacerbations of porphyria and are considered unsafe in porphyric patients.[1]

1. Moore MR, McColl KEL. *Porphyria: drug lists.* Glasgow: Porphyria Research Unit, University of Glasgow, 1991.

Pregnancy and breast feeding. Some sulphonamides have been shown to cause fetal abnormalities including cleft palate in *animals*, but fears of teratogenic effects in humans do not appear to be substantiated. Sulphonamides are probably safe in the first trimester of pregnancy although throughout pregnancy they should be used only in the absence of a suitable alternative drug.[1] Sulphonamides may displace serum-bound bilirubin and they should be avoided close to delivery because of the risk of kernicterus in the neonate. The risk of drug-induced bilirubin displacement has been reviewed by Walker.[2] The initial evidence suggesting a kernicterus-promoting effect of drugs in neonates was reported for sulphafurazole and this drug now serves as a standard displacing agent against which other drugs are evaluated. Although all sulphonamides are highly protein bound, each has a different capacity to displace bilirubin. Sulphadiazine and sulphanilamide have been found to be the least displacing of the sulphonamides and the effects of sulphadiazine on bilirubin may not be clinically significant; an increased incidence of hyperbilirubinaemia and kernicterus has not been demonstrated following its use for prophylaxis of rheumatic fever during pregnancy. Sulphasalazine should theoretically cause significant bilirubin displacement, but studies suggest that the drug may be given to pregnant and lactating patients with Crohn's disease. Metabolites of sulphonamides have also been evaluated for kernicterus-promoting effects; glucuronide metabolites are expected to compete for binding sites less effectively than the parent compound, whereas acetylated metabolites of some sulphonamides appear to be more potent bilirubin displacers.

1. Wise R. Prescribing in pregnancy: antibiotics. *Br Med J* 1987; **294:** 42–4.
2. Walker PC. Neonatal bilirubin toxicity: a review of kernicterus and the implications of drug-induced bilirubin displacement. *Clin Pharmacokinet* 1987; **13:** 26–50.

Interactions

The action of sulphonamides may be antagonised by *p*-aminobenzoic acid and compounds derived from it, particularly potassium aminobenzoate and the procaine group of local anaesthetics.

Sulphamethoxazole and other sulphonamides may potentiate the effects of some drugs, such as oral anticoagulants (p.966), methotrexate (p.549), and phenytoin (p.354); this may be due to displacement of the drug from plasma protein binding sites or to inhibition of metabolism. However, the clinical significance of these interactions appears to depend on the particular sulphonamide involved. The possibility of interactions with other highly protein-bound drugs such as NSAIDs should be considered.

High doses of sulphonamides have been reported to have a hypoglycaemic effect; the antidiabetic effect of the sulphonylurea compounds may be enhanced by the concomitant administration of sulphonamides (p.332). Sulphonamides given intravenously, but not orally, have been associated with a decrease in plasma-cyclosporin concentrations when used concomitantly (p.521). Isolated reports have described possible failures of hormonal contraceptives resulting in pregnancy in patients given sulphonamides (p.1433).

Antimicrobial Action

Sulphamethoxazole and other sulphonamides have a similar structure to *p*-aminobenzoic acid and interfere with the synthesis of nucleic acids in sensitive micro-organisms by blocking the conversion of *p*-aminobenzoic acid to the co-enzyme dihydrofolic acid, a reduced form of folic acid; in man, dihydrofolic acid is obtained from dietary folic acid so sulphonamides do not affect human cells. Their action is primarily bacteriostatic, although they may be bactericidal where concentrations of thymine are low in the surrounding medium. The sulphonamides have a broad spectrum of action, but the development of widespread resistance (see below) has greatly reduced their usefulness, and susceptibility often varies widely even among nominally sensitive pathogens. The following strains may demonstrate sensitivity.

Gram-positive cocci, particularly the Group A streptococci and some strains of *Streptococcus pneumoniae*, and to a lesser extent staphylococci. Enterococci and many of the clostridia are more or less resistant although strains of *Clostridium perfringens* are moderately susceptible. Among other Gram-positive organisms that have been reported to be sensitive are *Bacillus anthracis* and many strains of Nocardia, especially *N. asteroides*.

The Gram-negative cocci *Neisseria meningitidis* and *N. gonorrhoeae* were formerly extremely susceptible to sulphonamides but most strains are now resistant. Susceptibility is often seen in *Haemophilus influenzae* and *H. ducreyi* but varies widely among the Enterobacteriaceae: strains of *Escherichia coli*, *Klebsiella*, *Proteus*, *Salmonella*, and *Serratia* are sometimes sensitive but few strains of *Shigella* are now susceptible. *Vibrio cholerae* may be sensitive.

Other organisms that have been reported to be sensitive include *Actinomyces* spp., *Brucella*, *Calymmatobacterium granulomatis*, *Legionella*, and *Yersinia pestis*. Chlamydia are sensitive, but not mycoplasmas, rickettsias, or spirochaetes, nor in general the mycobacteria. *Pseudomonas aeruginosa* is resistant although sulphonamides may be effective against *Burkholderia* (*Pseudomonas*) *pseudomallei*.

Sulphonamides have some activity against the protozoa *Plasmodium falciparum* and *Toxoplasma gondii*. They are also active against *Pneumocystis carinii*, but are ineffective against most fungi.

Sulphamethoxazole and other sulphonamides demonstrate synergy with the dihydrofolate reductase inhibitors pyrimethamine and trimethoprim which inhibit a later stage in folic acid synthesis. For reports of the antimicrobial activity of sulphamethoxazole with trimethoprim, see Co-trimoxazole, p.197.

The *in vitro* antimicrobial activity of sulphamethoxazole is very dependent on both the culture medium and size of inoculum used.

Resistance. Acquired resistance to sulphonamides is common and widespread among formerly susceptible organisms, particularly *Neisseria* spp., *Shigella* and some other enterobacteria, staphylococci and streptococci.

There appear to be several mechanisms of resistance including alteration of dihydropteroate synthetase, the enzyme inhibited by sulphonamides, to a less sensitive form, or an alteration in folate biosynthesis to an alternative pathway; increased production of *p*-aminobenzoic acid; or decreased uptake or enhanced metabolism of sulphonamides.

Resistance may result from chromosomal alteration, or may be plasmid mediated and transferable, as in many resistant strains of enterobacteria. High-level resistance is usually permanent and irreversible.

There is complete cross-resistance between the different sulphonamides.

Pharmacokinetics

Sulphamethoxazole is readily absorbed from the gastro-intestinal tract and peak plasma concentrations are reached after about 2 hours. Doses of 1 g twice daily should produce blood concentrations of unconjugated sulphamethoxazole in excess of 50 μg per mL. About 65% is bound to plasma proteins and the plasma half-life is about 6 to 12 hours; it is prolonged in patients with severe renal impairment.

Sulphamethoxazole, like most sulphonamides, diffuses freely throughout the body tissues and may be detected in the urine, saliva, sweat, and bile, in the cerebrospinal, peritoneal, ocular, and synovial fluids, and in pleural and other effusions. It crosses the placenta into the fetal circulation, and low concentrations have been detected in breast milk.

Sulphamethoxazole undergoes conjugation mainly in the liver, chiefly to the inactive N^4-acetyl derivative; this metabolite represents about 15% of the total amount of sulphamethoxazole in the blood. Metabolism is increased in patients with renal impairment and decreased in those with hepatic impairment. Elimination in the urine is dependent on pH. About 80 to 100% of a dose is excreted in the urine, of which about 60% is in the form of the acetyl derivative, with the remainder as unchanged drug and glucuronide.

Sulphamethoxazole is also oxidised to the hydroxylamine, a metabolite that has been implicated in adverse reactions to sulphonamides (see also Immunocompromised Patients, under Precautions, above).

Uses and Administration

The use of sulphamethoxazole and other sulphonamides has been limited by the increasing incidence of resistant organisms. Their main use has been in the treatment of acute, uncomplicated urinary-tract infections, particularly those caused by *Escherichia coli*. They have also been used in nocardiosis, and in some other bacterial infections such as otitis media, chlamydial infections, and prophylaxis of meningococcal meningitis but have largely been replaced by other drugs: even where pathogens retain some sensitivity to sulphonamides a combination such as co-trimoxazole (sulphamethoxazole with trimethoprim) has often been preferred. The usual treatment of these infections is discussed under Choice of Antibacterial, p.116. Sulphonamides are also used, often in combination with pyrimethamine or trimethoprim, in the treatment of protozoal infections, particularly malaria (p.422) and toxoplasmosis (p.576); they are also used similarly in *Pneumocystis carinii* pneumonia (p.370).

Sulphamethoxazole is an intermediate-acting sulphonamide given by mouth in a usual dose of 2 g initially, followed by 1 g twice daily. In severe infections 1 g three times daily may be given.

A suggested dose for children is 50 to 60 mg per kg body-weight initially, followed by 25 to 30 mg per kg twice daily. A total daily dose of 75 mg per kg should not be exceeded.

Reduction of dosage may be required in patients with renal impairment.

For the uses and dosage of sulphamethoxazole with trimethoprim, see Co-trimoxazole, p.197.

Sulphamethoxazole lysine has also been used.

Administration. The USA manufacturers of sulphamethoxazole have recommended that blood concentrations be measured in patients receiving sulphonamides for serious infections. The following concentrations of free sulphonamide in the blood were considered to be therapeutically effective: for most infections, 50 to 150 μg per mL, and for serious infections, 120 to 150 μg per mL. Concentrations of 200 μg per mL should not be exceeded since the incidence of adverse reactions may be increased.

Preparations

BP 1998: Co-trimoxazole Intravenous Infusion; Co-trimoxazole Oral Suspension; Co-trimoxazole Tablets; Dispersible Co-trimoxazole Tablets; Paediatric Co-trimoxazole Oral Suspension; Paediatric Co-trimoxazole Tablets;
USP 23: Sulfamethoxazole and Trimethoprim Injection; Sulfamethoxazole and Trimethoprim Oral Suspension; Sulfamethoxazole and Trimethoprim Tablets; Sulfamethoxazole Oral Suspension; Sulfamethoxazole Tablets.

Proprietary Preparations (details are given in Part 3)
USA: Gantanol; Urobak.

Multi-ingredient: ***Aust.:*** Bactrim; Cotribene; Eusaprim; Oecotrim; Supracombin; Trimetho comp; ***Austral.:*** Bactrim; Resprim; Septrin; ***Belg.:*** Bactrim; Eusaprim; ***Canad.:*** Apo-Sulfatrim; Bactrim; Novo-Trimel; Nu-Cotrimox; Roubac; Septra; ***Fr.:*** Bactekod†; Bactrim; Cotrimazol; Eusaprim; ***Ger.:*** Bactoreduct; Bactrim; Berlocid; Co-trim-Tablinen; Cotim; Cotrim; Cotrim Holsten; Cotrim-basan†; Cotrim-Diolan; Cotrim-Hefa; Cotrim-Puren; Cotrim-Riker†; Cotrimhexal; Cotrimox-Wolff; Cotrimstada; Drylin; Duobiocin†; duratrimet†; Eusaprim; Jenamoxazol; Kepinol; Linaris; Microtrim; Nymix-amid N†; Omsat†; Sigaprim; Sulfacet†; Sulfotrimin†; Supracombin; TMS; Trigonyl†; ***Irl.:*** Antrimox; Bactrim; Cotrimel; Duobact; Septrin; Tricomox; ***Ital.:*** Abacin; Bacterial; Bactrim; Chemitrim; Eusaprim; Gantaprim†; Gantrim; Isotrim; Medixin; Oxaprim†; Pulmotrim†; Strepto-Plus; Sulmen†; Suprin†; Trim†; ***Jpn:*** Baktar†; ***Neth.:*** Bactrimel; Eusaprim; Sulfotrim†; Trimoxol; ***Norw.:*** Bactrim; Eusaprim†; ***S.Afr.:*** Acuco; Arcanaprim; Bactrim; Bencole; Briscotrim†; Cocydal; Cotrivan†; Cozole; Doctrim; Duotrim†; Durobac; Dynazole; Fabubac; Mezenol†; Microbac†; Norisept†; Partrim†; Purbac; Septran; Spectrim; Thoxaprim†; Tri-Co; Trimethox; Trimoks; Trimzol; Troxazole; Ultrasept†; Ultrazole; Xerazole; Xeroprim; ***Spain:*** Abactrim; Abactrim Balsamico†; Azosulfin†; Bactifor; Bactopumon; Balsoprim; Bridotrim; Bronco Aseptilex Fuerte; Bronco Bactifor; Bronco Sergo; Broncorema; Broncovir NF; Brongenit; Bronquicisteina; Bronquidiazina CR; Bronquimar; Bronquimucil; Bronquium; Eduprim; Eduprim Mucolitico; Gobens Trim; Libetusin†; Lotusix; Momentol; Mucorama TS; Neumopectolina; Pulmo Menal; Pulmosterin Duo; Salvatrim; Septrin; Soltrim; Toose; Tosdetan; Traquivan; Tresium; ***Swed.:*** Bactrim; Eusaprim; Triferm-Sulfa†; Trimetoprim-Sulfa†; ***Switz.:*** Bactrim; Cotrim; Escoprim; Eusaprim; Groprim; Helveprim; Imexim; Nopil; Pharmaprim†; Sigaprim; Supracombin; TMS†; ***UK:*** Bactrim†; Chemotrim; Comixco; Comox†; Fectrim; Laratrim; Septrin; ***USA:*** Azo Gantanol†; Bactrim; Cotrim; Septra; SMZ-TMP; Sulfamethoprim; Sulfatrim DS; Uroplus.

Sulphamethoxypyridazine (4944-h)

Sulphamethoxypyridazine *(BAN)*.

Sulfamethoxypyridazine *(rINN)*; Solfametossipiridazina; Sulfamethoxypyridazinum. N^1-(6-Methoxypyridazin-3-yl)sulphanilamide.

$C_{11}H_{12}N_4O_3S$ = 280.3.
CAS — 80-35-3.

Pharmacopoeias. In *Eur.* (see p.viii) and *Int.*

A white or slightly yellowish crystalline powder which colours slowly on exposure to light.

Practically **insoluble** in water; slightly soluble in alcohol; sparingly soluble in acetone; very slightly soluble in dichloromethane; dissolves in dilute mineral acids and solutions of alkali hydroxides. **Protect** from light.

Acetyl Sulphamethoxypyridazine (4945-m)

Sulfamethoxypyridazine Acetyl. *N*-(6-Methoxypyridazin-3-yl)-*N*-sulphanilylacetamide.

$C_{13}H_{14}N_4O_4S$ = 322.3.
CAS — 3568-43-2.

NOTE. Acetyl sulphamethoxypyridazine is to be distinguished from the N^4-acetyl derivative formed from sulphamethoxypyridazine by conjugation in the body.

1.15 g of monograph substance is approximately equivalent to 1 g of sulphamethoxypyridazine.

Sulphamethoxypyridazine is a long-acting sulphonamide with properties similar to those of sulphamethoxazole (p.254). It is rapidly absorbed from the gastro-intestinal tract and excreted slowly in urine, partly as the N^4-acetyl metabolite; it remains detectable for up to 7 days after a dose. It is used with trimethoprim similarly to co-trimoxazole.

Acetyl sulphamethoxypyridazine, which is hydrolysed in the gastro-intestinal tract forming sulphamethoxypyridazine, and sulphamethoxypyridazine sodium have also been used.

Skin disorders. Sulphamethoxypyridazine in doses of 0.25 to 1.5 g daily by mouth provided satisfactory control of dermatitis herpetiformis (p.1073) in 33 of 37 patients and was an effective alternative to dapsone. Five patients were withdrawn due to adverse effects. The sulphonamide also produced benefit in 3 patients with linear IgA disease and 10 of 15 with cicatricial pemphigoid (p.1075), although one patient in the latter group developed alveolitis.[1]

1. McFadden JP, *et al.* Sulphamethoxypyridazine for dermatitis herpetiformis, linear IgA disease and cicatricial pemphigoid. *Br J Dermatol* 1989; **121:** 759–62.

Preparations

Proprietary Preparations (details are given in Part 3)
Ital.: Sulfalex†.

Multi-ingredient: ***Ital.:*** Velaten.

Sulphamoxole (4946-b)

Sulphamoxole *(BAN)*.

Sulfamoxole *(USAN, rINN)*; Sulphadimethyloxazole. N^1-(4,5-Dimethyloxazol-2-yl)sulphanilamide.

$C_{11}H_{13}N_3O_3S$ = 267.3.
CAS — 729-99-7.

NOTE. Sulphamoxole may be given with trimethoprim and a preparation of such a combination has been given the approved name Co-trifamole, p.196.

Pharmacopoeias. In *Fr.*

Sulphamoxole is a sulphonamide with properties similar to those of sulphamethoxazole (p.254). It has been used in combination with trimethoprim as co-trifamole (p.196).

Preparations

Proprietary Preparations (details are given in Part 3)

Multi-ingredient: ***Fr.:*** Supristol†; ***S.Afr.:*** Supristol†; ***Spain:*** Supristol†.

Sulphanilamide (4947-v)

Sulfanilamide *(rINN)*; Solfammide; Streptocidum; Sulfaminum; Sulfanilamidum. 4-Aminobenzenesulphonamide; *p*-Sulphamidoaniline.

$C_6H_8N_2O_2S$ = 172.2.
CAS — 63-74-1.

Pharmacopoeias. In *Aust.*, *Belg.*, and *Fr.* Also in *BP(Vet)*.

A white, or almost white, odourless or almost odourless crystalline powder.

Slightly **soluble** in water and in alcohol; practically insoluble in chloroform and in ether; dissolves in solutions of alkali hydroxides. **Protect** from light.

Sulphanilamide is a short-acting sulphonamide with properties similar to those of sulphamethoxazole (p.254). Its antibacterial activity is less than that of sulphamethoxazole. It has been used topically, including as pessaries or as a vaginal cream, for the treatment of susceptible infections, often in combination with other drugs. The sodium, sodium mesylate, and camsylate salts have also been used.

Preparations

Proprietary Preparations (details are given in Part 3)
Belg.: Astreptine; Paraseptine†; ***Canad.:*** AVC; ***Fr.:*** Exoseptoplix; ***Ger.:*** Defonamid†; ***Spain:*** Azol; Pomada Sulfamida Orravan†; ***USA:*** AVC.

Multi-ingredient: ***Belg.:*** Angichrome†; Mucorhinyl; Polyseptol; Pyal; Rhinamide†; Sulfa-Sedemol†; Sulfaryl; ***Canad.:*** AVC/Dienestrol†; ***Fr.:*** Rhinamide; ***Ger.:*** Acetonal Vaginale†; Gynaedron†; Jacosulfon†; Oestro-Gynaedron†; Pyodron†; ***Ital.:*** Chemiovis†; Otocaina†; ***S.Afr.:*** Achromide; Daromide†; Ung Vernleigh; ***Spain:*** Amidrin; Azol†; Buco Regis; Cilinafosal; Cilinafosal DHD Estrep; Cilinafosal Hidrocort; Cilinavagin Neomicina; Dorsec†; Faderma†; Frikton†; Gargaril Sulfamida†; Kanafosal; Kanafosal Predni; Mentol Sedans Sulfamidad†; Nasopomada; Odontocromil c Sulfamida; Oto Difusor; Otonasal; Pental Forte; Pentalmicina; Polvos Wilfe; Pomada Heridas; Pomada Wilfe; Quimpe Amida; Rinosular†; Vitavox Pastillas; ***Switz.:*** Oestro-Gynaedron†; Ovuthricinol†; ***USA:*** Alasulf; Benegyn†; Deltavac; DIT1-2.

Sulphapyridine (4949-q)

Sulphapyridine *(BAN)*.

Sulfapyridine *(rINN)*. N^1-(2-Pyridyl)sulphanilamide.

$C_{11}H_{11}N_3O_2S$ = 249.3.
CAS — 144-83-2.

Pharmacopoeias. In *Fr.* and *US.* Also in *BP(Vet)*.

A white or yellowish-white, odourless or almost odourless, crystalline powder or granules. It slowly darkens on exposure to light.

Soluble 1 in 3500 of water, 1 in 440 of alcohol, 1 in 65 of acetone; dissolves in dilute mineral acids and aqueous solutions of alkali hydroxides. **Protect** from light.

Sulphapyridine is a short- or intermediate-acting sulphonamide, with properties similar to those of sulphamethoxazole (p.254). It is slowly and incompletely absorbed from the gastro-intestinal tract and excreted in urine; sulphapyridine and its acetyl metabolite are poorly soluble in urine and the risk of crystalluria is relatively high. Adverse effects are common, and gastro-intestinal disturbances may preclude continued therapy. Because of its toxicity, sulphapyridine is now little used except occasionally for dermatitis herpetiformis and related skin disorders where alternative treatment cannot be used; doses of up to 1 g four times daily by mouth are given initially, reduced to the minimum effective maintenance dose once improvement occurs.

For reference to another, and possibly less toxic, sulphonamide in the treatment of dermatitis herpetiformis and similar dermatoses, see Sulphamethoxypyridazine, p.256.

As with sulphamethoxypyridazine, benefit has also been seen with sulphapyridine in cicatricial pemphigoid.[1]

1. Elder MJ, *et al.* Sulphapyridine—a new agent for the treatment of ocular cicatricial pemphigoid. *Br J Ophthalmol* 1996; **80:** 549–52.

Preparations

USP 23: Sulfapyridine Tablets.

Proprietary Preparations (details are given in Part 3)
Canad.: Dagenan.

Multi-ingredient: *Fr.:* Pommade Lelong; *Ger.:* Jacosulfon†.

Sulphasomidine (4952-h)

Sulphasomidine *(BAN).*

Sulfisomidine *(rINN)*; Sulfa-isodimérazine; Sulfaisodimidine; Sulfasomidine; Sulfisomidinum. N^1-(2,6-Dimethylpyrimidin-4-yl)sulphanilamide.

$C_{12}H_{14}N_4O_2S$ = 278.3.

CAS — 515-64-0.

NOTE. Sulfadimethylpyrimidine has been used as a synonym for sulphasomidine, and sulphadimethylpyrimidine is sometimes used as a synonym for sulphadimidine (p.253). Care should be taken to avoid confusion between the two compounds, which are isomeric.

Pharmacopoeias. In *Eur.* (see p.viii).

White or yellowish-white powder or crystals. Very slightly **soluble** in water; slightly soluble in alcohol and in acetone; dissolves in dilute aqueous solutions of alkali hydroxides and in dilute mineral acids. **Protect** from light.

Sulphasomidine is a short-acting sulphonamide with properties similar to those of sulphamethoxazole (p.254). It has been applied topically for skin or vaginal infections and administered by mouth. The sodium salt has also been used.

Preparations

Proprietary Preparations (details are given in Part 3)
Aust.: Aristamid†; *Ger.:* Aristamid†.

Multi-ingredient: *S.Afr.:* Gynedron†; Moni-Gynedron†; Oestro-Gynedron†; Poly-Gynedron†; Tricho-Gynedron†.

Sulphathiazole (4953-m)

Sulphathiazole *(BAN).*

Sulfathiazole *(rINN)*; M & B 760; Norsulfazole; RP-2090; Solfatiazolo; Sulfanilamidothiazolum; Sulfathiazolum; Sulfonazolum. N^1-(1,3-Thiazol-2-yl)sulphanilamide.

$C_9H_9N_3O_2S_2$ = 255.3.

CAS — 72-14-0.

Pharmacopoeias. In *Eur.* (see p.viii) and *US.*

A white or yellowish-white, almost odourless, crystalline powder.

Practically **insoluble** or very slightly soluble in water; slightly soluble in alcohol; soluble in acetone; practically insoluble in dichloromethane and in ether; dissolves in dilute mineral acids and solutions of alkali hydroxides. **Protect** from light.

Sulphathiazole Sodium (4954-b)

Sulphathiazole Sodium *(BANM).*

Sulfathiazole Sodium *(rINNM)*; Soluble Sulphathiazole; Sulfathiazolum Natricum.

$C_9H_8N_3NaO_2S_2,5H_2O$ = 367.4.

CAS — 144-74-1 (anhydrous sulphathiazole sodium); 6791-71-5 (sulphathiazole sodium pentahydrate).

Pharmacopoeias. In *Aust.* ($1\frac{1}{2}H_2O$). Also in *BP(Vet)* ($1\frac{1}{2}H_2O$ or $5H_2O$).

A white or yellowish-white, odourless or almost odourless, crystalline powder or granules. 1.44 g of monograph substance is approximately equivalent to 1 g of sulphathiazole.

Freely **soluble** in water; soluble in alcohol. A solution in water containing the equivalent of 1% of the anhydrous substance has a pH of 9 to 10. **Protect** from light.

Sulphathiazole is a short-acting sulphonamide with properties similar to those of sulphamethoxazole (p.254). It is now rarely used systemically due to its toxicity.

Sulphathiazole is used with other sulphonamides, usually sulfabenzamide and sulphacetamide, in preparations for the topical treatment of vaginal infections and is also applied in combination with other drugs in the treatment of skin infections.

Sulphathiazole sodium has been applied topically with other drugs in the treatment of eye infections.

Preparations

USP 23: Triple Sulfa Vaginal Cream; Triple Sulfa Vaginal Tablets.

Proprietary Preparations (details are given in Part 3)

Multi-ingredient: *Austral.:* Sultrin; *Belg.:* Pyal; Sultrin; *Canad.:* Sultrin; *Ger.:* Neosultrin†; Peniazol†; Tampovagan C-N N†; *Irl.:* Sultrin; *Ital.:* Chemiovis†; Propiazol†; Streptosil con Neomicina-Fher; *S.Afr.:* Sultrin; Trisulpha†; *Spain:* Bucodrin; Cremsol; Polvos Wilfe; Pomada Wilfe; Rinotiazol Fenilefri†; Sabanotropico; Salitanol Estreptomicina; Sulfatiazol Dr. Andreu†; *Switz.:* Sultrin†; Tyrocombine†; Urethra-Steril†; *UK:* Sultrin; *USA:* Alba Gyn; Dayto Sulf; Gyne-Sulf; Sultrin; Triple Sulfa; Trysul; VVS.

Sulphaurea (4956-g)

Sulphaurea *(BAN).*

Sulfacarbamide *(rINN)*; Sulfanilcarbamide; Sulphacarbamide; Sulphanilylurea; Urosulphanum. Sulphanilylurea monohydrate.

$C_7H_9N_3O_3S,H_2O$ = 233.2.

CAS — 547-44-4 (anhydrous sulphaurea); 6101-35-5 (sulphaurea monohydrate).

Pharmacopoeias. In *Pol.*

Sulphaurea is a sulphonamide with properties similar to those of sulphamethoxazole (p.254). It was formerly used in the treatment of urinary-tract infections, sometimes in conjunction with phenazopyridine.

Preparations

Proprietary Preparations (details are given in Part 3)

Multi-ingredient: *Norw.:* Trisulfamid.

Sultamicillin (17000-k)

Sultamicillin *(BAN, USAN, rINN).*

CP-49952. Penicillanoyloxymethyl (6*R*)-6-(D-2-phenylglycylamino)penicillanate *S′,S′*-dioxide.

$C_{25}H_{30}N_4O_9S_2$ = 594.7.

CAS — 76497-13-7.

Sultamicillin is a prodrug of ampicillin (p.153) and the beta-lactamase inhibitor sulbactam (p.250); it consists of the two compounds linked chemically as a double ester. During absorption from the gastro-intestinal tract it is hydrolysed, releasing equimolar quantities of ampicillin and sulbactam.

Sultamicillin is given by mouth as tablets containing sultamicillin tosylate or as oral suspension containing sultamicillin. It is used in the treatment of infections where beta-lactamase-producing organisms might occur, including uncomplicated gonorrhoea, otitis media, respiratory-tract and urinary-tract infections. The usual dose is 375 to 750 mg of sultamicillin (equivalent to 147 to 294 mg of sulbactam and 220 to 440 mg of ampicillin) twice daily. A single dose of sultamicillin 2.25 g together with probenecid 1 g may be used for uncomplicated gonorrhoea.

When parenteral therapy is necessary a combined preparation of ampicillin with sulbactam is given.

References.

1. Friedel HA, *et al.* Sultamicillin: a review of its antibacterial activity, pharmacokinetic properties and therapeutic use. *Drugs* 1989; **37:** 491–522.

Preparations

Proprietary Preparations (details are given in Part 3)
Aust.: Dynapen†; Unasyn; *Fr.:* Unacim; *Ger.:* Unacid PD; *Ital.:* Bethacil; Unasyn; *Spain:* Bacimex; Unasyn; *Switz.:* Unacide†; *UK:* Unasyn†.

Taurolidine (17001-a)

Taurolidine *(BAN, rINN).*

4,4′-Methylenebis(perhydro-1,2,4-thiadiazine 1,1-dioxide).

$C_7H_{16}N_4O_4S_2$ = 284.4.

CAS — 19388-87-5.

Taurolidine is a broad-spectrum antimicrobial that is hydrolysed in aqueous solution to its monomeric form taurultam and other metabolites, with the release of what was originally thought to be formaldehyde but are now thought to be activated methylene glycol or methylol groups, from which it is believed to derive its activity. Its antibacterial activity *in vitro* is modest but is reported to be enhanced in the presence of serum or urine: it is active against a variety of pathogens including *Staphylococcus aureus*, *Escherichia coli*, and *Pseudomonas aeruginosa*. Taurolidine is also reported to inactivate bacterial endotoxin.

It is applied topically for intraperitoneal irrigation; solutions containing 0.5 and 2% are available. Taurolidine has been given experimentally as an intravenous infusion in the treatment of severe sepsis or endotoxic shock and in pancreatitis.

Preparations

Proprietary Preparations (details are given in Part 3)
Aust.: Taurolin; *Ger.:* Taurolin; *Neth.:* Taurolin†; *Switz.:* Taurolin.

Tazobactam Sodium (10443-e)

Tazobactam Sodium *(BANM, USAN, rINNM).*

CL-307579; CL-298741 (tazobactam); YTR-830; YTR-830H (tazobactam). Sodium (2*S*,3*S*,5*R*)-3-methyl-7-oxo-3-(1*H*-1,2,3-triazol-1-ylmethyl)-4-thia-1-azabicyclo[3.2.0]-heptane-2-carboxylate 4,4-dioxide.

$C_{10}H_{11}N_4NaO_5S$ = 322.3.

CAS — 89786-04-9 (tazobactam); 89785-84-2 (tazobactam sodium).

Tazobactam is a penicillanic acid sulphone derivative with beta-lactamase inhibitory properties similar to those of sulbactam (p.250) although it is regarded as more potent. It has the potential to enhance the activity of beta-lactam antibacterials against beta-lactamase-producing bacteria.

The combination of piperacillin sodium (p.237) with tazobactam sodium is given intravenously for the treatment of bacterial infections. The pharmacokinetics of tazobactam and piperacillin are similar.

References.

1. Bush K, *et al.* Kinetic interactions of tazobactam with β-lactamases from all major structural classes. *Antimicrob Agents Chemother* 1993; **37:** 851–8.
2. Payne DJ, *et al.* Comparative activities of clavulanic acid, sulbactam, and tazobactam against clinically important β-lactamases. *Antimicrob Agents Chemother* 1994; **38:** 767–72.

Preparations

Proprietary Preparations (details are given in Part 3)

Multi-ingredient: *Aust.:* Tazonam; *Austral.:* Tazocin; *Belg.:* Tazocin; *Canad.:* Tazocin; *Fr.:* Tazocilline; *Ger.:* Tazobac; *Irl.:* Tazocin; *Ital.:* Tazobac; Tazocin; *Neth.:* Tazocin; *S.Afr.:* Tazocin; *Spain:* Tazocel; *Swed.:* Tazocin; *Switz.:* Tazobac; *UK:* Tazocin; *USA:* Zosyn.

Teicoplanin (18689-v)

Teicoplanin *(BAN, USAN, rINN).*

A-8327; DL-507-IT; L-12507; MDL-507; Teichomycin A_2.

CAS — 61036-62-2 (teichomycin); 61036-64-4 (teichomycin A_2).

A glycopeptide antibiotic obtained from cultures of *Actinoplanes teichomyceticus* or the same substance obtained by any other means.

Adverse Effects and Precautions

Fever and chills, skin rash and pruritus, and occasional bronchospasm and anaphylaxis have been reported in patients receiving teicoplanin, but, in comparison with vancomycin (p.267), it appears to be better tolerated when given by rapid intravenous injection and, although erythema and flushing of the upper body have occurred, the 'red-man syndrome' has been reported less often. In addition, unlike vancomycin, teicoplanin does not appear to cause tissue necrosis and can be administered by intramuscular injection. Other hypersensitivity reactions have included rigors, angioedema and, rarely, severe skin reactions including exfoliative dermatitis, erythema multiforme, Stevens-Johnson syndrome, and toxic epidermal necrolysis.

Other reported reactions include gastro-intestinal disturbances, dizziness, headache, thrombocytopenia (especially at high doses), leucopenia, neutropenia, eosinophilia, disturbances in liver enzyme values, and pain, erythema, and thrombophlebitis or abscess at the site of administration. Rare cases of agranulocytosis have occurred. Impairment of renal function, and ototoxicity, have been reported but both appear to be less frequent than with vancomycin.

Renal and auditory function should be monitored during prolonged therapy in patients with pre-existing renal insufficiency, and in those receiving other ototoxic or nephrotoxic drugs concurrently, although opinions conflict on whether increased risk of nephrotoxicity has been demonstrated from combined therapy with drugs such as the aminoglycosides. In general, periodic blood counts and liver and renal function tests are advised during treatment.

No relationship has yet been established between plasma concentration and toxicity, and plasma-concentration monitoring is not generally considered necessary. Dosage adjustment is required in renal impairment.

Hypersensitivity. Although there have been occasional reports of cross-sensitivity to teicoplanin in patients hypersensitive to vancomycin,[1,2] the majority of reports suggest that cross-sensitivity is very rare and teicoplanin can usually be used in patients intolerant of vancomycin.[3-5]

1. McElrath MJ, *et al.* Allergic cross-reactivity of teicoplanin and vancomycin. *Lancet* 1986; **i:** 47.
2. Grek V, *et al.* Allergic cross-reaction of teicoplanin and vancomycin. *J Antimicrob Chemother* 1991; **28:** 476–7.
3. Smith SR, *et al.* Teicoplanin administration in patients experiencing reactions to vancomycin. *J Antimicrob Chemother* 1989; **23:** 810–12.
4. Schlemmer B, *et al.* Teicoplanin for patients allergic to vancomycin. *N Engl J Med* 1988; **318:** 1127–8.
5. Wood G, Whitby M. Teicoplanin in patients who are allergic to vancomycin. *Med J Aust* 1989; **150:** 668.

Red-man syndrome. Although teicoplanin is believed[1,2] to be less likely than vancomycin to induce the red-man syndrome, symptoms consistent with the syndrome have nevertheless been reported following intravenous administration.[3]

1. Sahai J, *et al.* Comparison of vancomycin- and teicoplanin-induced histamine release and "red man syndrome". *Antimicrob Agents Chemother* 1990; **34:** 765–9.
2. Rybak MJ, *et al.* Absence of "red man syndrome" in patients being treated with vancomycin or high-dose teicoplanin. *Antimicrob Agents Chemother* 1992; **36:** 1204–7.
3. Dubettier S, *et al.* Red man syndrome with teicoplanin. *Rev Infect Dis* 1991; **13:** 770.

Antimicrobial Action

As for Vancomycin Hydrochloride, p.268. It may be more active *in vitro* against enterococci and some anaerobic organisms, including strains of *Clostridium,* but some coagulase-negative staphylococci are less sensitive to teicoplanin than to vancomycin. MICs for the most sensitive organisms such as sensitive strains of *Staphylococcus aureus* or *Streptococcus pneumoniae* range from about 0.03 to 0.25 μg per mL, but organisms with MICs below 8 μg per mL are generally considered sensitive, and those with MICs between about 8 and 16 μg per mL of intermediate sensitivity. There have been difficulties in the determination of the MIC for coagulase-negative staphylococci.

Acquired resistance to teicoplanin has developed in staphylococci during treatment with teicoplanin. Cross-resistance with vancomycin has occurred in staphylococci and enterococci.

Pharmacokinetics

Teicoplanin is poorly absorbed from the gastro-intestinal tract. Following intravenous administration of a 400-mg dose peak plasma concentrations one hour later are reported to be in the range 20 to 50 μg per mL. It is well absorbed following intramuscular injection with a bioavailability of about 90%; following administration of 3 mg per kg body-weight intramuscularly, peak plasma concentrations of 7 μg per mL have been reported after 2 hours.

The pharmacokinetics of teicoplanin are triphasic, with a biphasic distribution and a prolonged elimination. Penetration into the CSF is poor. It is taken up into white blood cells, and about 90 to 95% of teicoplanin in plasma is protein bound. It is excreted almost entirely by glomerular filtration in the urine, as unchanged drug. The terminal half-life is prolonged, but reported half-lives have ranged from about 30 to over 160 hours, depending on the sampling time; an effective clinical half-life of about 60 hours has been suggested for use in calculating dosage regimens. Half-life is prolonged in patients with reduced or impaired renal function. Teicoplanin is not removed by haemodialysis.

Teicoplanin is a mixture of several components, the pharmacokinetics of which have been shown to vary slightly, depending on their lipophilicity.

References.

1. Rowland M. Clinical pharmacokinetics of teicoplanin. *Clin Pharmacokinet* 1990; **18:** 184–209.
2. Bernareggi A, *et al.* Pharmacokinetics of individual components of teicoplanin in man. *J Pharmacokinet Biopharm* 1990; **18:** 525–43.
3. Lam YWF, *et al.* The pharmacokinetics of teicoplanin in varying degrees of renal function. *Clin Pharmacol Ther* 1990; **47:** 655–61.
4. Steer JA, *et al.* Pharmacokinetics of a single dose of teicoplanin in burn patients. *J Antimicrob Chemother* 1996; **37:** 545–53.
5. Reed MD, *et al.* The pharmacokinetics of teicoplanin in infants and children. *J Antimicrob Chemother* 1997; **39:** 789–96.

Uses and Administration

Teicoplanin is a glycopeptide antibiotic that may be used as an alternative to vancomycin (p.269) in the treatment of serious Gram-positive infections where other drugs cannot be used, including in the treatment and prophylaxis of infective endocarditis, in peritonitis associated with continuous ambulatory peritoneal dialysis, and in suspected infection in neutropenic or otherwise immunocompromised patients. Teicoplanin, administered orally, has been suggested as a possible alternative to vancomycin or metronidazole in antibiotic-associated colitis. For details of these infections and their treatment, see under Choice of Antibacterial, p.116.

Teicoplanin is given intravenously, as a bolus dose or by infusion over 30 minutes, or else by intramuscular injection. The usual dose is 400 mg (or 6 mg per kg body-weight) intravenously initially, followed by 200 mg (or 3 mg per kg) intravenously or intramuscularly on each subsequent day of treatment. In more severe infections, 400 mg may be given intravenously every 12 hours for the first 3 doses, followed by maintenance doses of 400 mg daily. Higher doses of up to 12 mg per kg daily have been given occasionally.

For the prophylaxis of endocarditis in high-risk penicillin-allergic patients undergoing dental or other procedures, teicoplanin may be given in a single dose of 400 mg by intravenous injection together with gentamicin, before the procedure. A similar dose of teicoplanin is given for prophylaxis in orthopaedic surgery at induction of anaesthesia.

In children, loading doses of 10 mg per kg every 12 hours for 3 doses may be followed by 6 to 10 mg per kg daily, depending on the severity of infection. In neonates, a loading dose of 16 mg per kg on the first day may be followed by maintenance doses of 8 mg per kg daily given by intravenous infusion.

Dosage should be adjusted in patients with impaired renal function. A suggested regimen is the administration of usual doses for the first 3 days of therapy, followed by half the normal daily dose in patients with mild renal insufficiency (creatinine clearance between 40 and 60 mL per minute) or one-third of the normal dose in those with more marked insufficiency (creatinine clearance below 40 mL per minute). Alternatively, dosage may be adjusted by giving the usual daily dose only every 2 or 3 days.

Reviews.

1. Brogden RN, Peters DH. Teicoplanin: a reappraisal of its antimicrobial activity, pharmacokinetic properties and therapeutic efficacy. *Drugs* 1994; **47:** 823–54.
2. Murphy S, Pinney RJ. Teicoplanin or vancomycin in the treatment of Gram-positive infections? *J Clin Pharm Ther* 1995; **20:** 5–11.
3. de Lalla F, Tramarin A. A risk-benefit assessment of teicoplanin in the treatment of infections. *Drug Safety* 1995; **13:** 317–28.
4. Periti P, *et al.* Antimicrobial prophylaxis in orthopaedic surgery: the role of teicoplanin. *J Antimicrob Chemother* 1998; **41:** 329–40.

Preparations

Proprietary Preparations (details are given in Part 3)
Aust.: Targocid; ***Austral.:*** Targocid; ***Belg.:*** Targocid; ***Fr.:*** Targocid; ***Ger.:*** Targocid; ***Irl.:*** Targocid; ***Ital.:*** Targosid; Teicomid; ***Neth.:*** Targocid; ***Norw.:*** Targocid; ***S.Afr.:*** Targocid; ***Spain:*** Targocid; ***Swed.:*** Targocid; ***Switz.:*** Targocid; ***UK:*** Targocid.

Temafloxacin (5794-l)

Temafloxacin *(BAN, rINN).*

A-62254; Abbott-62254. (*RS*)-1-(2,4-Difluorophenyl)-6-fluoro-1,4-dihydro-7-(3-methylpiperazin-1-yl)-4-oxoquinoline-3-carboxylic acid.

$C_{21}H_{18}F_3N_3O_3$ = 417.4.
CAS — 108319-06-8 (temafloxacin); 105784-61-0 (temafloxacin hydrochloride).

NOTE. Temafloxacin Hydrochloride is *USAN.*

Temafloxacin is a fluoroquinolone antibacterial with properties similar to those of ciprofloxacin (p.185). It was formerly given by mouth in the treatment of susceptible infections but was withdrawn worldwide in 1992 following reports of serious adverse events, mainly in the USA. These adverse effects included symptoms of severe hypoglycaemia, hepatic dysfunction, haemolytic anaemia, renal dysfunction sometimes requiring dialysis, anaphylaxis, and death.

Preparations

Proprietary Preparations (details are given in Part 3)
Swed.: Temac†.

Temocillin Sodium (17002-t)

Temocillin Sodium *(BANM, rINNM).*

BRL-17421; Temocillin Disodium. The disodium salt of (6*S*)-6-[2-carboxy-2-(3-thienyl)acetamido]-6-methoxypenicillanic acid.

$C_{16}H_{16}N_2Na_2O_7S_2$ = 458.4.

CAS — 66148-78-5 (temocillin); 61545-06-0 (temocillin disodium).

NOTE. Temocillin is *USAN.*

Incompatibility has been reported with aminoglycosides.

Adverse Effects and Precautions

As for Benzylpenicillin, p.159.

Interactions

As for Benzylpenicillin, p.160.

Antimicrobial Action

Temocillin is bactericidal and highly resistant to a wide range of beta-lactamases produced by Gram-negative bacteria, including those inactivating third-generation cephalosporins. It is active *in vitro* against the majority of Gram-negative aerobic bacteria, including many of the Enterobacteriaceae, *Haemophilus influenzae, Moraxella (Branhamella) catarrhalis,* and *Neisseria gonorrhoeae.* It exhibits no significant activity against *Pseudomonas aeruginosa,* although some strains of *Burkholderia (Pseudomonas) cepacia* may be susceptible. It is not active against Gram-negative anaerobes such as *Bacteroides fragilis* or against Gram-positive organisms.

MICs for susceptible Enterobacteriaceae are generally in the range of 1 to 16 μg per mL. Unlike some other beta-lactams, temocillin does not appear to induce the production of beta lactamases.

Pharmacokinetics

Temocillin is not absorbed from the gastro-intestinal tract. Its pharmacokinetics appear to be nonlinear. After intramuscular and intravenous administration, high and prolonged plasma concentrations are obtained. It has a plasma half-life of about 4.5 hours, which is longer than for most penicillins; half-lives of 18 hours or more have been reported in severe renal failure. About 85% of temocillin in the circulation is bound to plasma proteins. Temocillin is widely distributed in the body, but like other penicillins penetration in the CSF is poor. Small amounts have been detected in breast milk.

A small proportion of temocillin is metabolised, but about 70 to 80% of a dose is excreted unchanged in the urine within 24 hours, mainly by glomerular filtration. Some is excreted in the bile.

Temocillin is removed by haemodialysis.

Uses and Administration

Temocillin is a semisynthetic penicillin used for the treatment of infections caused by beta-lactamase-producing strains of Gram-negative aerobic bacteria (see Antimicrobial Action, above).

It is given by injection as the sodium salt. Doses are expressed in terms of the equivalent amount of temocillin. Administration is by slow intravenous injection over 3 to 4 minutes, by intravenous infusion over 30 to 40 minutes, or by intramuscular injection. The usual dose is 1 to 2 g every 12 hours. For uncomplicated urinary-tract infections 1 g daily may be given.

In patients with impaired renal function the interval between doses may need to be increased.

References.

1. Lode H, *et al.* eds. First international workshop on temocillin. *Drugs* 1985; **29** (suppl 5): 1–243.
2. Teham S, Whittaker J. Temocillin (Temopen®): a review of UK clinical trial results. *Clin Trials J* 1989; **28:** 1–8.
3. Spencer RC. Temocillin. *J Antimicrob Chemother* 1990; **26:** 735–7.
4. Anonymous. Temocillin injection for gram-negative infections only. *Drug Ther Bull* 1991; **29:** 55–6.

Preparations

Proprietary Preparations (details are given in Part 3)
Belg.: Negaban; ***Ger.:*** Temopen†; ***UK:*** Temopen†.

Terizidone (13309-g)

Terizidone *(rINN)*.

B-2360. 4,4'-[*p*-Phenylenebis(methyleneamino)]bis(isoxazolidin-3-one).

$C_{14}H_{14}N_4O_4$ = 302.3.

CAS — 25683-71-0.

Terizidone has been used in the treatment of infections of the urinary tract and of pulmonary and extrapulmonary tuberculosis.

Preparations

Proprietary Preparations (details are given in Part 3)
Aust.: Terivalidin; ***Ger.:*** Terizidon†; ***Ital.:*** Urovalidin†; ***S.Afr.:*** Terivalidin†.

Tetracycline (168-z)

Tetracycline *(BAN, rINN)*.

Tetraciclina; Tetracyclinum. A variably hydrated form of (4S,4aS,5aS,6S,12aS)-4-Dimethylamino-1,4,4a,5,5a,6,11,12a-octahydro-3,6,10,12,12a-pentahydroxy-6-methyl-1,11-dioxonaphthacene-2-carboxamide.

$C_{22}H_{24}N_2O_8$ = 444.4.

CAS — 60-54-8 (anhydrous tetracycline); 6416-04-2 (tetracycline trihydrate).

Pharmacopoeias. In *Eur.* (see p.viii), *Jpn*, and *US*.

A yellow, odourless, crystalline powder. It darkens in strong sunlight in a moist atmosphere. Tetracycline (anhydrous) 1 g is approximately equivalent to 1.08 g of tetracycline hydrochloride.

Soluble 1 in 2500 of water and 1 in 50 of alcohol; soluble in methyl alcohol; sparingly soluble in acetone; practically insoluble in chloroform and in ether; freely soluble in dilute acids and in alkali hydroxide solutions. It loses not more than 13% of its weight on drying. A 1% suspension in water has a pH of 3.0 to 7.0. The potency of tetracycline is reduced in solutions having a pH below 2 and it is rapidly destroyed in solutions of alkali hydroxides. **Store** in airtight containers. Protect from light.

Tetracycline Phosphate Complex (170-s)

Tetracycline Phosphate Complex *(BAN)*.

CAS — 1336-20-5.

Pharmacopoeias. In *US*.

Jpn includes Tetracycline Metaphosphate ($C_{22}H_{24}N_2O_8$,HPO_3,⅙$NaPO_3$ = 544.8).

A complex of sodium metaphosphate and tetracycline. A yellow crystalline powder with a faint characteristic odour A 1% aqueous suspension has a pH of 2 to 4. **Soluble** 1 in 31 of water, 1 in 130 of alcohol; slightly soluble in methyl alcohol; very slightly soluble in acetone. **Store** in airtight containers. Protect from light.

Tetracycline Hydrochloride (169-c)

Tetracycline Hydrochloride *(BANM, rINNM)*.

Tetracyclini Hydrochloridum.

$C_{22}H_{24}N_2O_8$,HCl = 480.9.

CAS — 64-75-5.

Pharmacopoeias. In *Chin., Eur.* (see p.viii), *Int., Jpn, Pol.,* and *US*.
US also includes Epitetracycline Hydrochloride.

A yellow, odourless, hygroscopic, crystalline, powder. Tetracycline hydrochloride darkens in moist air when exposed to strong sunlight.

Soluble 1 in 10 of water and 1 in 100 of alcohol; practically insoluble in acetone, in chloroform, and in ether; soluble in aqueous solutions of alkali hydroxides and carbonates, although it is rapidly destroyed by alkali hydroxide solutions. A 1% solution in water has a pH of 1.8 to 2.8. The potency of tetracycline hydrochloride is reduced in solutions having a pH below 2. Solutions in water become turbid on standing owing to hydrolysis and precipitation of tetracycline.

Store in airtight containers. Protect from light.

Incompatibilities. Tetracycline injections have an acid pH and incompatibility may reasonably be expected with alkaline preparations, or with drugs unstable at low pH. Tetracyclines can chelate metal cations to produce insoluble complexes, and incompatibility has been reported with solutions containing metallic salts. Reports of incompatibility are not always consistent, and other factors, such as the strength and composition of the vehicles used, may play a role.

Stability. Tetracycline undergoes reversible epimerisation in solution to the less active 4-epitetracycline;[1,2] the degree of epimerisation is dependent on pH, and is greatest at a pH of about 3, with conversion of some 55% to the epimer at equilibrium.[1] The rate at which epimerisation occurs is affected by a variety of factors including temperature and the presence of phosphate or citrate ions.[1] Intravenous solutions of tetracycline hydrochloride with a pH between 3 and 5 have been reported to be stable for 6 hours, but to lose approximately 8 to 12% of their potency in 24 hours at room temperature.[3] Although epimerisation has been observed to be the dominant degradation reaction at pH 2.5 to 5, outside this pH range other reactions become important, with the pH-dependent formation of anhydrotetracycline at very low pH, and oxidation to isotetracycline at alkaline pH.[4]

In contrast to the case in solution, suspensions of tetracycline hydrochloride are stable for at least 3 months[2] at pHs between 4 and 7, because epimerisation, which continues until an equilibrium is achieved between tetracycline and its epimer, depends only on the portion in solution, and the solubility of tetracycline at these pHs is low.

The stability of solid dosage forms and powder at various temperatures and humidities has also been studied; tetracycline hydrochloride was fairly stable when stored at 37° and 66% humidity for 2 months, with about a 10% loss of potency, but the phosphate was rather less stable, with potency losses of 25 to 40% and the formation of potentially toxic degradation products.[5] Comparison with other tetracyclines indicated that tetracycline was less stable than demeclocycline and more stable than rolitetracycline.[5] However, although this study, and an accelerated stability study carried out by the WHO[6] indicate that there is a risk of deterioration of solid dose tetracycline, in practice a study of its stability during shipment to the tropics found that deterioration was not a problem.[7]

1. Remmers EG, *et al.* Some observations on the kinetics of the C4 epimerization of tetracycline. *J Pharm Sci* 1963; **52:** 752–6.
2. Grobben-Verpoorten A, *et al.* Determination of the stability of tetracycline suspensions by high performance liquid chromatography. *Pharm Weekbl (Sci)* 1985; **7:** 104–8.
3. Parker EA. Solution additive chemical incompatibility study. *Am J Hosp Pharm* 1967; **24:** 434–9.
4. Vej-Hansen B, Bundgaard H. Kinetic study of factors affecting the stability of tetracycline in aqueous solution. *Arch Pharm Chemi (Sci)* 1978; **6:** 201–14.
5. Walton VC, *et al.* Anhydrotetracycline and 4-epianhydrotetracycline in market tetracyclines and aged tetracycline products. *J Pharm Sci* 1970; **59:** 1160–4.
6. WHO. WHO expert committee on specifications for pharmaceutical preparations: thirty-first report. *WHO Tech Rep Ser 790* 1990.
7. Hogerzeil HV, *et al.* Stability of essential drugs during shipment to the tropics. *Br Med J* 1992; **304:** 210–14.

Adverse Effects

The side-effects of tetracycline are common to all tetracyclines. Gastro-intestinal effects including nausea, vomiting, and diarrhoea are common especially with high doses and most are attributed to irritation of the mucosa. Other effects that have been reported include dry mouth, glossitis and discoloration of the tongue, stomatitis, and dysphagia. Oesophageal ulceration has also been reported, particularly after ingestion of capsules or tablets with insufficient water at bedtime.

Oral candidiasis, vulvovaginitis, and pruritus ani occur mainly due to overgrowth with *Candida albicans* and there may be overgrowth of resistant coliform organisms, such as *Pseudomonas* spp. and *Proteus* spp., causing diarrhoea. More seriously, enterocolitis due to superinfection with resistant staphylococci and pseudomembranous colitis due to *Clostridium difficile* have occasionally been reported. It has been suggested that disturbances in the intestinal flora are more common with tetracycline than better absorbed analogues such as doxycycline.

Usual therapeutic doses given to patients with renal disease increase the severity of uraemia with increased excretion of nitrogen and losses of sodium, accompanied by acidosis and hyperphosphataemia. These effects are related to the dose and the severity of renal impairment and are probably due to the anti-anabolic effects of the tetracycline.

Severe and sometimes fatal hepatotoxicity associated with fatty changes in the liver and pancreatitis has been reported in pregnant women given tetracycline intravenously for pyelonephritis, and in patients with renal impairment or those given high doses.

Tetracyclines are deposited in deciduous and permanent teeth during their formation, causing discoloration and enamel hypoplasia. They are also deposited in calcifying areas in bone and the nails and interfere with bone growth when given in therapeutic doses to young infants or pregnant women. An increase in intracranial pressure with headache, visual disturbances, and papilloedema has been reported in patients given tetracyclines; the use of tetracyclines in infants has been associated with a bulging fontanelle. If raised intracranial pressure occurs tetracycline treatment should be stopped.

Hypersensitivity to the tetracyclines is much less common than to the beta-lactams, but hypersensitivity reactions, including rashes, fixed drug eruptions, exfoliative dermatitis, toxic epidermal necrolysis, drug fever, pericarditis, angioedema, urticaria, and asthma have been reported; anaphylaxis has occurred very rarely. Photosensitivity, which has been reported with most tetracyclines but particularly with demeclocycline and other long-acting analogues, appears to be phototoxic rather than photoallergic in nature. Paraesthesia may be an early sign of impending phototoxicity. Nail discoloration and onycholysis may occur. Abnormal pigmentation of the skin and eye has occurred rarely: permanent discoloration of the cornea has been reported in infants born to mothers given tetracycline in high doses during pregnancy. Myopia in patients taking tetracyclines may be due to transient hydration of the lens. Local pain and irritation can occur when tetracyclines are given parenterally and thrombophlebitis may follow intravenous injections. A Jarisch-Herxheimer-like reaction occurs commonly in patients with relapsing fever treated with tetracycline.

Although rare, haemolytic anaemia, eosinophilia, neutropenia, and thrombocytopenia have been reported. Tetracyclines may produce hypoprothrombinaemia. They have also been associated with reductions in serum-vitamin B concentrations, including a case of folate deficiency and concomitant megaloblastic anaemia.

The use of out-of-date or deteriorated tetracyclines has been associated with the development of a reversible Fanconi-type syndrome characterised by polyuria and polydipsia with nausea, glycosuria, aminoaciduria, hypophosphataemia, hypokalaemia, and hyperuricaemia with acidosis and proteinuria; these effects have been attributed to the presence of degradation products, in particular anhydroepitetracycline.

Other adverse effects that have occasionally been reported in patients receiving tetracyclines include increased muscle weakness in patients with myasthenia gravis and provocation of lupus erythematosus.

Precautions

The tetracyclines are contra-indicated in patients hypersensitive to any of this group of antibacterials, since cross-sensitivity may occur. They should be avoided in patients with systemic lupus erythematosus. In general the tetracyclines, with the exception of doxycycline and perhaps minocycline, are considered to be contra-indicated in renal impairment, particularly if severe: if they must be given, doses should be reduced.

Tetracyclines should not be used during pregnancy because of the risk of hepatotoxicity in the mother as well as the effects on the developing fetus. They should also be avoided during breast feeding and in children up to the age of 8, or some authorities say 12, years. Use in pregnancy, potentially during breast feeding, or in childhood, may result in impaired bone growth and permanent discoloration of the child's teeth.

Care should be taken if tetracyclines are given to patients with impaired liver function and high doses should be avoided. Patients who may be exposed to direct sunlight should be warned of the risk of photosensitivity. Care is advisable in patients with myasthenia gravis, who may be at risk of neuromuscular blockade. Serum-monitoring of tetracyclines may be helpful in patients with risk factors receiving parenteral therapy: it has been suggested that serum concentrations of tetracycline should not exceed 15 μg per mL.

Tetracycline may interfere with some diagnostic tests including determination of urinary catecholamines or glucose.

Porphyria. Tetracyclines were considered to be probably safe in patients with acute porphyria, although there was conflicting experimental evidence of porphyrinogenicity, with results from *animals* or *in-vitro* systems suggesting that doxycycline or oxytetracycline might be porphyrinogenic.[1]

1. Moore MR, McColl KEL. *Porphyria: drug lists*. Glasgow: Porphyria Research Unit, University of Glasgow, 1991.

Interactions

The absorption of the tetracyclines is reduced by divalent and trivalent cations such as aluminium, bismuth, calcium, iron, magnesium, and zinc, and therefore concomitant administration of tetracyclines with antacids, iron preparations, some foods such as milk and dairy products, or other preparations containing such cations, whether as active ingredients or excipients, may result in subtherapeutic serum concentrations of the antibacterial. Sodium bicarbonate, colestipol, and kaolin-pectin are also reported to reduce tetracycline absorption, but potential reductions due to cimetidine or sucralfate are probably of little clinical significance.

The nephrotoxic effects of tetracyclines may be exacerbated by diuretics, methoxyflurane, or other potentially nephrotoxic drugs. Potentially hepatotoxic drugs should be used with caution in patients receiving tetracyclines. An increased incidence of benign intracranial hypertension has been reported when retinoids and tetracyclines are given together. Tetracyclines have been reported to produce increased concentrations of lithium, digoxin, and theophylline (although these interactions are not strongly established); the effects of oral anticoagulants may also be increased. There have been occasional reports of tetracyclines increasing the toxic effects of ergot alkaloids and methotrexate. Tetracyclines may decrease plasma-atovaquone concentrations. Ocular inflammation has occurred following the use of ocular preparations preserved with thiomersal in some patients receiving tetracyclines. Tetracyclines may decrease the effectiveness of oral contraceptives.

Because of possible antagonism of the action of the penicillins by predominantly bacteriostatic tetracyclines it has been recommended that the two types of drug should not be given concomitantly, especially when a rapid bactericidal action is necessary.

Antimicrobial Action

The group of tetracycline antibiotics is mainly bacteriostatic, with a broad spectrum of antimicrobial activity including chlamydias, mycoplasmas, rickettsias, and spirochaetes, and also many aerobic and anaerobic Gram-positive and Gram-negative pathogenic bacteria, and some protozoa.

Mechanism of action. Tetracyclines are taken up into sensitive bacterial cells by an active transport process. Once within the cell they bind reversibly to the 30S subunit of the ribosome, preventing the binding of aminoacyl transfer RNA and inhibiting protein synthesis and hence cell growth. Although tetracyclines also inhibit protein synthesis in mammalian cells they are not actively taken up, permitting selective effects on the infecting organism.

Spectrum of activity. The following pathogenic organisms are usually sensitive to tetracyclines.

Gram-positive cocci including some strains of *Staphylococcus aureus* and coagulase-negative staphylococci, and streptococci including *Str. pneumoniae, Str. pyogenes* (group A), some *Str. agalactiae* (group B), and some viridans streptococci. Enterococci are essentially resistant.

Other sensitive Gram-positive bacteria include strains of *Actinomyces israelii, Bacillus anthracis, Erysipelothrix rhusiopathiae, Listeria monocytogenes*, and among the anaerobes some *Clostridium* spp. *Nocardia* spp. are generally much less susceptible although some are sensitive to minocycline. *Propionibacterium acnes* is susceptible although the action of the tetracyclines in acne is complex and benefit may be seen even at subinhibitory concentrations.

Gram-negative cocci including *Neisseria meningitidis* (meningococci) and *N. gonorrhoeae* (gonococci), *Acinetobacter* spp., and *Moraxella (Branhamella) catarrhalis*.

Other sensitive Gram-negative aerobes include *Bordetella pertussis, Brucella* spp., *Calymmatobacterium granulomatis, Campylobacter* spp., *Eikenella corrodens, Francisella tularensis, Haemophilus influenzae* and some strains of *Haemophilus ducreyi, Legionella, Pasteurella multocida, Streptobacillus moniliformis*, and various members of the Vibrionaceae including *Aeromonas hydrophila, Plesiomonas shigelloides, Vibrio cholerae* and *Vibrio parahaemolyticus*. Although many of the Enterobacteriaceae, including *Salmonella, Shigella*, and *Yersinia* spp., are susceptible, resistant strains are common; *Proteus* and *Providencia* spp. are not susceptible. *Pseudomonas aeruginosa* is not susceptible either, although some other species formerly classified as *Pseudomonas* respond, including *Burkholderia mallei, B. pseudomallei*, and *Stenotrophomonas (Xanthomonas) maltophilia*.

Among the Gram-negative anaerobes *Bacteroides fragilis* may sometimes be susceptible, although wild strains are often resistant, and *Fusobacterium* may also be sensitive.

Other organisms usually sensitive to tetracyclines include *Helicobacter pylori, Chlamydia* spp., *Rickettsia* and *Coxiella* spp., many spirochaetes including *Borrelia burgdorferi, Leptospira*, and *Treponema pallidum*, atypical mycobacteria such as *Mycobacterium marinum*, and mycoplasmas including *Mycoplasma pneumoniae* and *Ureaplasma urealyticum*. In addition the tetracyclines are active against some protozoa including *Plasmodium falciparum* and *Entamoeba histolytica*.

Fungi, yeasts, and viruses are generally resistant.

Minimum inhibitory concentrations (MICs) of tetracycline for the most sensitive organisms (*Streptococci, Neisseria*, sensitive *Shigella* and *Salmonella* spp., *Bacteroides fragilis*) range from about 0.25 to 2 μg per mL, but organisms with MICs up to about 4 μg per mL are considered sensitive. MICs for the other tetracyclines are generally similar, although minocycline, and to a lesser extent doxycycline, are somewhat more active *in vitro* against many susceptible organisms than the other tetracyclines.

Resistance. Resistance to the tetracyclines is usually plasmid-mediated and transferable. It is often inducible and appears to be associated with the ability to prevent accumulation of the antibiotic within the bacterial cell both by decreasing active transport of the drug into the cell and by increasing tetracycline efflux.

Unsurprisingly, given the widespread use of the tetracyclines (including as components of animal feeds, although this is now banned in some countries) resistant strains of the majority of sensitive species have now been reported. Resistance has increased particularly among Enterobacteriaceae such as *Escherichia coli, Enterobacter, Salmonella*, and *Shigella* spp., especially in hospital isolates, and multiple resistance is common. Staphylococci are commonly resistant, although doxycycline or minocycline are occasionally effective against tetracycline-resistant strains. Resistance is now also common among the streptococci, with reported resistance rates of 15 to 62% among group A, and even more among group B streptococci; resistance among pneumococci is reported to range from 3 to 23%, with multiple drug resistance becoming common. Emergence of high-level tetracycline-resistant strains of *Neisseria gonorrhoeae* is common in some areas. Frequent resistance is also seen in clostridia, and in *Bacteroides fragilis* (among more than 60% of isolates in some countries), while increasing resistance amongst *Haemophilus ducreyi* has limited the value of tetracyclines in chancroid.

As the genetic determinants of tetracycline resistant organisms have been elucidated it has become clear that the same or very similar genes are responsible for resistance in a number of different genera.[1] More than a dozen distinguishable resistance determinants have been described but most of these can be grouped into 3 major families, each of which presumably evolved from an ancestral determinant, possibly originally derived from tetracycline-producing *Streptomyces* spp. The families represented by classes A to E, and K and L, respectively both code for an active efflux system which keeps intracellular tetracycline concentrations below inhibitory values; the former family are common among Gram-negative genera, while the latter have only been found in Gram-positive organisms to date. A third family of determinants, represented by classes M and O, specifies resistance by a cytoplasmic factor which protects the ribosome. Other tetracycline resistance determinants have yet to have their mechanism identified. As more and more determinants are identified it is clear that they have evolved over millennia to serve some function in the bacterial cell; identification of that role might suggest steps to control their persistence and spread.

1. Levy SB. Evolution and spread of tetracycline resistance determinants. *J Antimicrob Chemother* 1989; **24:** 1–3.

Pharmacokinetics

Most tetracyclines are incompletely absorbed from the gastro-intestinal tract, about 60 to 80% of a dose of tetracycline usually being available. The degree of absorption is diminished by the presence of divalent and trivalent metal ions, with which tetracyclines form stable insoluble complexes, and to a variable degree by milk or food. However, the more lipophilic analogues doxycycline and minocycline are almost completely absorbed (more than 90%), and they are little affected by food. Formulation with phosphate may enhance the absorption of tetracycline.

Administration of tetracycline 500 mg by mouth every 6 hours generally produces steady-state concentrations of 4 to 5 μg per mL, whereas with doxycycline a dose of 200 mg is sufficient to produce peak concentrations of about 3 μg per mL. Peak plasma concentrations occur about 1 to 3 hours after ingestion. Higher concentrations can be achieved after intravenous administration; concentrations may be higher in women than in men.

In the circulation, tetracyclines are bound to plasma proteins in varying degrees, but reported values differ considerably ranging from about 20 to 40% for oxytetracycline, 20 to 65% for tetracycline, about 45% for chlortetracycline, 35 to 90% for demeclocycline, 75% for minocycline, and about 80 to 95% for methacycline and doxycycline.

The tetracyclines are widely distributed throughout the body tissues and fluids. Concentrations in CSF are relatively low, but may be raised if the meninges are inflamed. Small amounts appear in saliva, and the fluids of the eye and lung; higher concentrations are achieved with more lipid-soluble analogues such as minocycline and doxycycline. Tetracyclines appear in breast milk where concentrations may be 60% or more of those in the plasma. They diffuse across the placenta and appear in the fetal circulation in concentrations of about 25 to 75% of those in the maternal blood. Tetracyclines are retained at sites of new bone formation and recent calcification and in developing teeth.

The tetracyclines have been classified in terms of their duration of action in the body, although the divisions appear to overlap somewhat. Of the 'short-acting' derivatives, chlortetracycline has a reported half-life of about 6 hours, oxytetracycline 9 hours, and tetracycline 8 hours, although reported values for the latter two range from about 6 to 12 hours. The 'intermediate-acting' tetracyclines, demeclocycline and methacycline have reported half-lives of about 12 and 14 hours respectively, although various sources cite values of 7 to 17 hours, and the 'long-acting' minocycline and doxycycline have half-lives of about 16 to 18 hours, with reported values anywhere between 11 to 26 and 12 to 24 hours respectively.

The tetracyclines are excreted in the urine and in the faeces. Renal clearance is by glomerular filtration. Up to 60% of an intravenous dose of tetracycline and up to 55% of a dose by mouth is eliminated unchanged in the urine; concentrations in the urine of up to 300 μg per mL of tetracycline may be reached 2 hours after a usual dose is taken and be maintained for up to 12 hours. For most tetracyclines between about 40 to 70% of a dose is excreted in the urine, but for chlortetracycline, doxycycline, and minocycline, rather less is eliminated by this route since chlortetracycline and minocycline undergo metabolism, and doxycycline is excreted extensively via the digestive tract. Urinary excretion is increased if urine is alkalinised.

The tetracyclines are excreted in the bile where concentrations 5 to 25 times those in plasma can occur. Since there is some enterohepatic reabsorption complete elimination is slow. Considerable quantities occur in the faeces after administration by mouth and lesser amounts after administration by injection.

Uses and Administration

The tetracyclines are bacteriostatic antibiotics with a wide spectrum of activity and have been used in the treatment of a large number of infections caused by susceptible organisms (see Antimicrobial Action, above). With the emergence of bacterial resistance and the development of other antibacterials their use has become more restricted, but they remain the usual drugs of choice in rickettsial infections, including ehrlichiosis, typhus, spotted fevers, trench fever, and Q fever; chlamydial infections, including psittacosis, lymphogranuloma venereum, trachoma, non-gonococcal urethritis, chlamydial conjunctivitis, and pharyngitis, sinusitis, or pneumonia due to *Chlamydia pneumoniae*; and mycoplasmal infections, especially pneumonia caused by *Mycoplasma pneumoniae*. They are widely used as part of regimens for pelvic inflammatory disease. A tetracycline is often used in the treatment of cholera, in conjunction with fluid and electrolyte replacement, and is usually the treatment of choice in relapsing fever and in the early stages of Lyme disease. They are also used in the oral treatment of acne (below) and rosacea. Tetracyclines may be of benefit in the treatment of melioidosis. They may be used for mouth infections, especially in destructive forms of periodontal disease. Tetracyclines are used, often in association with streptomycin or rifampicin, in the treatment of brucellosis, and may be given with streptomycin in plague, and as an alternative to streptomycin in the treatment of tularaemia. Tetracyclines are used as an alternative to other drugs in the treatment of actinomycosis, infected animal bites, anthrax, bronchitis, gastro-enteritis (due to *Campylobacter* or *Yersinia enterocolitica*), granuloma inguinale, leptospirosis, and syphilis. Opinions differ as to their value in listeriosis. There are now relatively few areas where tetracycline-resistant gonococci are uncommon, which limits the value of tetracyclines in gonorrhoea, but they are often given with antigonorrhoeal therapy to treat concomitant chlamydial infections, and they retain some value in the prophylaxis and treatment of neonatal gonococcal conjunctivitis by topical application. For details of these infections and their treatment, see under Choice of Antibacterial, p.116.

Tetracycline has antiprotozoal actions and may be given in conjunction with quinine in the management of falciparum malaria resistant to chloroquine (below). Tetracyclines are the usual treatment for balantidiasis (p.574) and they have been used in amoebiasis in association with an amoebicide in the treatment of severe amoebic dysentery and in *Dientamoeba fragilis* infections (p.573).

Tetracycline has been used in the management of malabsorption syndromes such as tropical sprue.

Tetracycline is instilled as a sclerosant solution for pleurodesis and in the management of malignant effusions (p.484).

Administration and dosage. In the treatment of systemic infections the tetracyclines are usually administered by mouth. In severe acute infections they may be given by slow intravenous infusion or, rarely, by intramuscular injection; parenteral therapy should be substituted by oral administration as soon as practicable. Doses of tetracycline base and tetracycline hydrochloride are expressed in terms of tetracycline hydrochloride.

The usual adult dosage of tetracycline hydrochloride is 250 or 500 mg every 6 hours by mouth, preferably one hour before or 2 hours after meals. Higher doses, up to 4 g daily have occasionally been given in resistant infection, but increase the risk of adverse effects. Modified release formulations are available in some countries. In severe infections, tetracycline hydrochloride may be administered by slow intravenous infusion every 12 hours as a solution containing not more than 0.5%. The usual dose is 1 g daily but up to 2 g daily has been given to patients with normal renal function. If the intramuscular route is to be used, tetracycline hydrochloride has been given in a dosage of 200 to 300 mg daily in divided doses. As intramuscular injections are painful, procaine hydrochloride is usually included in the solution.

In children, the effects on teeth should be considered and tetracyclines only used when absolutely essential. Tetracycline hydrochloride has been given to older children in doses of 25 to 50 mg per kg bodyweight daily by mouth in divided doses and in doses of up to 10 mg per kg daily by intravenous infusion. If the intramuscular route is used, the dose should not exceed 250 mg daily.

Care is required if tetracyclines are given to the elderly. They should be avoided if possible in renal impairment (with the exception of doxycycline) and doses reduced if they must be used.

Other routes. Although topical application carries the risk of sensitisation and may contribute to the development of resistance tetracycline hydrochloride has been applied as a 3% ointment; a 0.2% solution has been used in acne but systemic treatment appears to produce better results. A 1% eye ointment or eye drops are used in the treatment of ocular infections due to sensitive organisms. For the treatment of pleural effusions, 500 mg of tetracycline hydrochloride may be dissolved in 30 to 50 mL of sodium chloride 0.9% and instilled into the pleural space. For periodontal disease, fibres that release tetracycline are available in some countries; they are inserted into the periodontal pocket.

Review.

1. Chopra I, *et al.* Tetracyclines, molecular and clinical aspects. *J Antimicrob Chemother* 1992; **29:** 245–77.

Administration. Tetracycline may cause oesophagitis or oesophageal ulceration and tablets or capsules should therefore be given with at least 100 mL of water while the patient is in an upright sitting position.[1]

1. Vong SK, Parekh RK. Swallowing tablets and capsules. *Pharm J* 1987; **238:** 5.

Malaria. In areas where chloroquine-resistant *Plasmodium falciparum* may also be resistant to quinine, tetracycline has been used in combination with quinine to treat malaria.[1,2] Tetracyclines are active against both blood and tissue forms of the parasite, and high cure rates have been obtained with such combinations, although WHO has suggested they be reserved for when quinine resistance has been reported and for patients in whom pyrimethamine-sulfadoxine is contra-indicated. The action of tetracycline is relatively slow and it should never be used alone to treat malaria. For a detailed discussion of the treatment and prophylaxis of malaria, see p.422.

The dose of tetracycline hydrochloride given by mouth with quinine on days 1 to 3 has varied; doses of 1 to 2 g daily have been given for 7 days or 1 g daily for 7 to 10 days. The total daily dose should be divided and that usually recommended is 250 mg four times daily although 500 mg twice daily may be more practical in the field. If the patient is too ill for oral medication quinine should be given parenterally until the oral therapy can be begun; tetracycline should not be administered parenterally. Although tetracycline therapy is normally contra-indicated in pregnant women and children below 8 years, it may have to be given if the risk of withholding the drug is judged to outweigh the risk to developing teeth and bones.

Tetracycline is not considered suitable for extended prophylactic use, although doxycycline 100 mg daily has been used for short-term prophylaxis in areas of high risk where other drugs are likely to be ineffective.

1. WHO. Practical chemotherapy of malaria: report of a WHO scientific group. *WHO Tech Rep Ser 805* 1990.
2. WHO. *WHO model prescribing information: drugs used in parasitic diseases.* 2nd ed. Geneva: WHO, 1995.

Mouth ulceration. Ulceration of the oral mucosa (aphthous ulcer or aphthous stomatitis) (p.1172) may be idiopathic and self-limiting, but it may also be caused by mechanical trauma, nutritional deficiencies, drug reactions, or underlying disease.

In recurrent aphthous stomatitis tetracyclines, used as mouthwashes, reportedly reduce ulcer pain and duration,[1] but their potential for adverse effects if swallowed must be borne in mind, and their acidity may damage tooth enamel if poorly formulated. Topical application of a tetracycline has been considered the treatment of choice for oral ulceration associated with Behçet's syndrome (p.1018).

1. Henricsson V, Axéll T. Treatment of recurrent aphthous ulcers with Aureomycin mouth rinse or Zendium dentifrice. *Acta Odontol Scand* 1985; **43:** 47–52.

Peptic ulcer disease. Tetracycline may be used as part of triple therapy to eradicate *Helicobacter pylori* in patients with peptic ulcer disease (p.1174). The usual dose of tetracycline in these regimens is 500 mg four times daily for 2 weeks.

Rheumatic disorders. Tetracyclines, usually minocycline, are among the wide range of drugs tried in rheumatoid arthritis (p.2). A 48-week study[1] indicated that minocycline hydrochloride 100 mg twice daily was of benefit in patients with mild to moderate rheumatoid arthritis. Its mechanism of action, whether antibacterial or anti-inflammatory, remained to be determined.[2] There has been speculation over the role of infection as a cause of rheumatoid arthritis.[3]

The role of antibacterials is also uncertain in reactive arthritis (p.117), although long-term treatment with a tetracycline in addition to an NSAID has been reported to shorten the duration of reactive arthritis resulting from *Chlamydia trachomatis* infection.[4]

1. Tilley BC, *et al.* Minocycline in rheumatoid arthritis: a 48-week, double-blind, placebo-controlled trial. *Ann Intern Med* 1995; **122:** 81–9.
2. Paulus HE. Minocycline treatment of rheumatoid arthritis. *Ann Intern Med* 1995; **122:** 147–8.
3. McKendry RJR. Is rheumatoid arthritis caused by an infection? *Lancet* 1995; **345:** 1319–20.
4. Lauhio A. Reactive arthritis: consider combination treatment. *Br Med J* 1994; **308:** 1302–3.

Skin disorders. ACNE. Tetracyclines may be used topically or orally in the treatment of acne (p.1072). In acne, antibacterials appear to act by suppressing the growth of *Propionibacterium acnes*, but also by suppressing inflammation. Topical tetracycline is used for mild acne and as an adjunct to systemic treatment in more severe forms. Tetracyclines, given orally, are the drugs of choice for moderate acne and may be considered, in high doses, for severe acne. A suggested dosage regimen for oral treatment of moderate acne is tetracycline 500 mg twice daily for 3 months, reduced to 250 mg twice daily for a further 3 months or changed to another antibacterial if there has been no improvement. Maximum improvement is said to occur after 4 to 6 months, but treatment may need to continue for 2 or more years.

Oxytetracycline and minocycline have also been widely used. Minocycline has been reported to have superior antibacterial activity against *P. acnes* and a reduced incidence of resistance,[1] and has also been more effective than erythromycin against oxytetracycline-resistant acne.[2] However, it can cause skin pigmentation and may be associated rarely with immunologically mediated reactions[3] and some dermatologists do not favour its use. The usual dose of minocycline is 100 mg daily in one or two divided doses; some patients may need up to 200 mg daily.[4] Another alternative is doxycycline 50 mg daily.

1. Eady EA, *et al.* Superior antibacterial action and reduced incidence of bacterial resistance in minocycline compared to tetracycline-treated acne patients. *Br J Dermatol* 1990; **122:** 233–44.
2. Knaggs HE, *et al.* The role of oral minocycline and erythromycin in tetracycline therapy-resistant acne—a retrospective study and a review. *J Dermatol Treat* 1993; **4:** 53–6.
3. Ferner RE, Moss C. Minocycline for acne. *Br Med J* 1996; **312:** 138.

4. Goulden V, *et al.* Safety of long-term high-dose minocycline in the treatment of acne. *Br J Dermatol* 1996; **134:** 693–5.

PEMPHIGUS AND PEMPHIGOID. Corticosteroids are generally given to control the blistering in pemphigus and pemphigoid (p.1075), although there have been reports[1-3] suggesting that a tetracycline (often minocycline) may be of value in controlling the lesions associated with various types of pemphigus and pemphigoid.

1. Sawai T, *et al.* Pemphigus vegetans with oesophageal involvement: successful treatment with minocycline and nicotinamide. *Br J Dermatol* 1995; **132:** 668–70.
2. Poskitt L, Wojnarowska F. Minimizing cicatricial pemphigoid orodynia with minocycline. *Br J Dermatol* 1995; **132:** 784–9.
3. Kolbach DN, *et al.* Bullous pemphigoid successfully controlled by tetracycline and nicotinamide. *Br J Dermatol* 1995; **133:** 88–90.

ROSACEA. Tetracycline is the oral antibacterial of choice for the treatment of rosacea (p.1076). Long-term treatment is usually necessary. Tetracycline and doxycycline have also been shown to improve ocular manifestations of rosacea.[1]

1. Frucht-Pery J, *et al.* Efficacy of doxycycline and tetracycline in ocular rosacea. *Am J Ophthalmol* 1993; **116:** 88–92.

Preparations

BP 1998: Tetracycline Capsules; Tetracycline Intravenous Infusion; Tetracycline Tablets;
USP 23: Sterile Tetracycline Phosphate Complex; Tetracycline Hydrochloride and Nystatin Capsules; Tetracycline Hydrochloride Capsules; Tetracycline Hydrochloride for Injection; Tetracycline Hydrochloride for Topical Solution; Tetracycline Hydrochloride Ointment; Tetracycline Hydrochloride Ophthalmic Ointment; Tetracycline Hydrochloride Ophthalmic Suspension; Tetracycline Hydrochloride Tablets; Tetracycline Oral Suspension; Tetracycline Phosphate Complex Capsules; Tetracycline Phosphate Complex for Injection.

Proprietary Preparations (details are given in Part 3)
Aust.: Achromycin; Actisite; Hostacyclin; Latycin; Steclin; Tetrarco; ***Austral.:*** Achromycin; Achromycin V; Latycin; Mysteclin; Panmycin P†; Steclin-V†; Tetramykoin†; Tetrex; ***Belg.:*** Hostacycline; ***Canad.:*** Achromycin; Achromycin V; Apo-Tetra; Novo-Tetra; Nu-Tetra; Tetracyn; ***Fr.:*** Florocycline; Hexacycline†; Tetramig†; ***Ger.:*** Achromycin; Akne-Pyodron Kur†; Akne-Pyodron oral†; Dispatetrin; Hostacyclin; Imex; Quimocyclin N†; Sagittacin N; Steclin†; Supramycin; Tefilin; Tetrabakat†; Tetrablet†; Tetracitro S†; Tetralution; ***Irl.:*** Achromycin; Hostacycline; Tetrachel†; ***Ital.:*** Acromicina; Ambramicina; Calociclina; Ibicyn†; Spaciclina; Tetra-Proter†; Tetrabioptal; Tetrafosammina; ***Neth.:*** Tetrarco†; ***S.Afr.:*** Achromycin; Arcanacycline; Gammatet; Hostacycline†; Rotet; Tetrex; ***Spain:*** Actisite; Ambramicina; Bristaciclina; Kinciclina; Quimpe Antibiotico; Tetra Hubber; Tetralen†; Tetrarco Simple†; ***Swed.:*** Achromycin; Actisite; ***Switz.:*** Achromycine; Actisite; Servitet†; Tetraseptine; Triphacycline; ***UK:*** Achromycin; Economycin; Sustamycin†; Tetrabid-Organon†; Tetrachel; ***USA:*** Achromycin V†; Achromycin†; Actisite; Nor-Tet; Panmycin; Robitet Robicaps†; Sumycin; Teline†; Tetracap; Tetralan†; Tetram†.

Multi-ingredient: ***Aust.:*** Eftapan Tetra; Fluorex Plus; Mysteclin; ***Austral.:*** Helidac; Mysteclin-V; Tetrex-F†; ***Belg.:*** Topicycline†; ***Canad.:*** Achrocidin†; ***Fr.:*** Abiosan†; Amphocycline; Aphlomycine†; Colicort; ***Ger.:*** Achromycin†; Duotal†; Eftapan Tetra†; Makatussin Tetra†; Mysteclin; Polcortolon TC; Polycid N†; Tetra-Ozothin†; Traumanase-cyclin†; ***Irl.:*** Chymocyclar†; Deteclo; Mysteclin-F†; Topicycline; ***Ital.:*** Alfaflor; Chimotetra†; Colbiocin; Cortilen TC†; Dermobios; Dermobios Oto†; Desonix†; Eubetal Antibiotico; Flumetol Antibiotico; Iducol; Mictasone; Pensulvit; Talsutin†; Vitecaf; ***Neth.:*** Amphocycline†; ***S.Afr.:*** Mysteclin-V†; Riostatin; Tetrex-F; Tritet; Vagmycin; ***Spain:*** Bristaciclina Dental; Broncofenil Forte†; Bronquinflamatoria; Chymocyclar†; Finegosan†; Gine Heyden; Mucorex Ciclin; Nasopomada; Otocusi Enzimatico†; Sanicel; Tantum Ciclina; Terranilo; Tetra Tripsin; ***Switz.:*** Amphocycline†; Cervicaletten†; Chymocycline†; ***UK:*** Deteclo; Mysteclin†; Topicycline; ***USA:*** Helidac; Topicycline.

Tetroxoprim (13315-b)

Tetroxoprim *(BAN, USAN, rINN)*.

5-[3,5-Dimethoxy-4-(2-methoxyethoxy)benzyl]pyrimidine-2,4-diyldiamine.

$C_{16}H_{22}N_4O_4$ = 334.4.

CAS — 53808-87-0.

NOTE. Tetroxoprim may be given with sulphadiazine and a preparation of such a combination has been given the approved name Co-tetroxazine, p.196.

Tetroxoprim is a dihydrofolate reductase inhibitor similar to, but less active than, trimethoprim (p.265). It is used, in conjunction with sulphadiazine, as co-tetroxazine (p.196).

Tetroxoprim embonate has also been used.

Preparations

Proprietary Preparations (details are given in Part 3)

Multi-ingredient: ***Ger.:*** Sterinor; ***Ital.:*** Oxosint; Sterinor; Tibirox†.

Thenoic Acid (13319-p)

Tenoic Acid; 2-Thiophenic Acid. Thiophene-2-carboxylic acid.

$C_5H_4O_2S$ = 128.2.

CAS — 527-72-0.

Thenoic acid has been administered by mouth, rectally, or as nasal drops as the sodium salt, and by mouth as the lithium salt, in the treatment of respiratory-tract infections. The ethanolamine salt has been used as a mucolytic.

Preparations

Proprietary Preparations (details are given in Part 3)
Fr.: Soufrane; Thiopheol†; ***Spain:*** Trophires.

Multi-ingredient: ***Fr.:*** Glossithiase; Rhinotrophyl; Trophires; Trophires Compose; ***Spain:*** Broncofenil Forte†; Trophires; Trophires Rectal Lact†.

Thiacetazone (7572-j)

Thiacetazone *(BAN)*.

Thioacetazone *(rINN)*; Amithiozone; TBI/698; Tebezonum. 4-Acetamidobenzaldehyde thiosemicarbazone.

$C_{10}H_{12}N_4OS$ = 236.3.

CAS — 104-06-3.

Pharmacopoeias. In *Int.*

Adverse Effects

Gastro-intestinal disorders, hypersensitivity reactions including skin rashes, conjunctivitis, and vertigo are the side-effects most frequently reported with thiacetazone although the incidence appears to vary from country to country. Toxic epidermal necrolysis, exfoliative dermatitis, which has sometimes been fatal, and the Stevens-Johnson syndrome have been reported. Thiacetazone may cause bone-marrow depression with leucopenia, agranulocytosis, and thrombocytopenia. Acute haemolytic anaemia may occur and a large percentage of patients will have some minor degree of anaemia. Hepatotoxicity with jaundice may also develop. Cerebral oedema has been reported.

In a 10-year series of 1212 patients with tuberculosis who were treated with a regimen of streptomycin, isoniazid, and thiacetazone, 171 (14%) had adverse reactions associated with thiacetazone. The most common side-effects were giddiness (10%), occurring mainly in association with streptomycin, and skin rashes (3%) including exfoliation and the Stevens-Johnson syndrome.[1]

1. Pearson CA. Thiacetazone toxicity in the treatment of tuberculosis patients in Nigeria. *J Trop Med Hyg* 1978; **81:** 238–42.

Effects on the nervous system. Acute peripheral neuropathy which occurred in a 50-year-old man on 2 separate occasions within 15 minutes of administration of thiacetazone may have been due to an allergic reaction.[1]

1. Gupta PK, *et al.* Acute severe peripheral neuropathy due to thiacetazone. *Indian J Tuberc* 1984; **31:** 126–7.

Effects on the skin. A high incidence of severe and sometimes fatal cutaneous hypersensitivity reactions to thiacetazone has been reported in patients with HIV infection being treated for tuberculosis.[1,2] WHO advised that thiacetazone should be avoided in such patients.[3] Unfortunately, thiacetazone has been one of the mainstays of tuberculosis treatment in the developing world because of its relatively low cost.[4] Some have supported a change to rifampicin-based regimens in, for example, parts of Africa with a high incidence of HIV infection.[5] Others have found a lower frequency of fatalities from adverse cutaneous reactions to thiacetazone than reported previously and have suggested that improved management might allow retention of thiacetazone in tuberculosis programmes.[6] This was rejected by other workers who considered that better and more cost-effective regimens were available than those containing thiacetazone.[7] A pragmatic approach may be to adopt a strategy depending upon the prevailing incidence of HIV infection in the population.[8] Thus, where the incidence of HIV infection is high, ethambutol should be substituted for thiacetazone; where the incidence is moderate, routine HIV testing could be used to identify patients at risk; and where the incidence is low, education of patients on the risks of skin reaction would be adequate.

1. Nunn P, *et al.* Cutaneous hypersensitivity reactions due to thiacetazone in HIV-1 seropositive patients treated for tuberculosis. *Lancet* 1991; **337:** 627–30.
2. Chintu C, *et al.* Cutaneous hypersensitivity reactions due to thiacetazone in the treatment of tuberculosis in Zambian children infected with HIV-I. *Arch Dis Child* 1993; **68:** 665–8.
3. Raviglione MC, *et al.* HIV-associated tuberculosis in developing countries: clinical features, diagnosis, and treatment. *Bull WHO* 1992; **70:** 515–26.
4. Nunn P, *et al.* Thiacetazone—avoid like poison or use with care? *Trans R Soc Trop Med Hyg* 1993; **87:** 578–82.
5. Okwera A, *et al.* Randomised trial of thiacetazone and rifampicin-containing regimens for pulmonary tuberculosis in HIV-infected Ugandans. *Lancet* 1994; **344:** 1323–8.
6. Ipuge YAI, *et al.* Adverse cutaneous reactions to thiacetazone for tuberculosis treatment in Tanzania. *Lancet* 1995; **346:** 657–60.
7. Elliott AM, *et al.* Treatment of tuberculosis in developing countries. *Lancet* 1995; **346:** 1098–9.
8. van Gorkom J, Kibuga DR. Cost-effectiveness and total costs of three alternative strategies for the prevention and management of severe skin reactions attributable to thiacetazone in the treatment of human immunodeficiency virus positive patients with tuberculosis in Kenya. *Tubercle Lung Dis* 1996; **77:** 30–6.

Hypertrichosis. Hypertrichosis occurred in 2 children and was associated with the use of thiacetazone.[1]

1. Nair LV, Sugathan P. Thiacetazone induced hypertrichosis. *Indian J Dermatol Venereol* 1982; **48:** 161–3.

Precautions

The efficacy and toxicity of a regimen of treatment which includes thiacetazone should be determined in a community before it is used widely since there appear to be geographical differences.

Thiacetazone should not be given to patients with liver impairment. It has also been suggested that because thiacetazone has a low therapeutic index and is excreted mainly in the urine, it should not be given to patients with renal impairment. It should probably be avoided in HIV-positive patients because they are at increased risk of severe adverse effects (see Effects on the Skin, above).

Interactions

Thiacetazone may enhance the ototoxicity of streptomycin.

Antimicrobial Action

Thiacetazone is bacteriostatic. It is effective against most strains of *Mycobacterium tuberculosis*, although sensitivity varies in different parts of the world. The MIC for sensitive strains is 1 μg per mL.

Thiacetazone is also bacteriostatic against *Mycobacterium leprae*. Resistance to thiacetazone develops when used alone. Cross-resistance can develop between thiacetazone and ethionamide, or prothionamide.

Pharmacokinetics

Thiacetazone is absorbed from the gastro-intestinal tract and peak plasma concentrations of 1 to 2 μg per mL have been obtained about 4 to 5 hours after a 150-mg dose. About 20% of a dose is excreted unchanged in the urine. A half-life of about 12 hours has been reported.

Uses and Administration

Thiacetazone has been used in association with other antimycobacterials in the initial and continuation treatment phases of tuberculosis (p.146). Thiacetazone-containing regimens are less effective than the short-course regimens recommended by WHO and are used in long-term regimens combined with isoniazid in some developing countries to reduce drug costs. However, thiacetazone is not generally recommended for use in HIV-positive patients because of the risk of severe adverse reactions (but see Effects on the Skin, above).

Thiacetazone has been used in the treatment of leprosy (p.128), but WHO now considers that such use is no longer justified.

In the treatment of tuberculosis thiacetazone has been given orally in doses of 150 mg daily or 2.5 mg per kg body-weight daily. Thiacetazone may be used with isoniazid usually in the continuation phase of some longer treatment regimens to prevent emergence of isoniazid resistance. Thiacetazone has also been used in the initial phase in association with streptomycin and isoniazid. Daily administration is recommended as the drug is less effective when given intermittently.

Thiamphenicol (171-w)

Thiamphenicol *(BAN, USAN, rINN)*.

CB-8053; Dextrosulphenidol; Thiamfenicol; Thiamphenicolum; Thiophenicol; Tiamfenicolo; Win-5063-2; Win-5063 (racephenicol). (αR,βR)-2,2-Dichloro-N-(β-hydroxy-α-hydroxymethyl-4-methylsulphonylphenethyl)acetamide.

$C_{12}H_{15}Cl_2NO_5S$ = 356.2.

CAS — 15318-45-3 (thiamphenicol); 847-25-6 (racephenicol).

NOTE. Racephenicol, the racemic form of thiamphenicol, is *USAN*.

Pharmacopoeias. In *Eur.* (see p.viii).

A fine white to yellowish-white odourless crystalline powder or crystals. Slightly **soluble** in water, ether, and ethyl acetate; soluble in methyl alcohol; sparingly soluble in dehydrated alcohol and acetone; freely soluble in dimethylformamide and acetonitrile; very soluble in dimethylacetamide. **Protect** from light and moisture.

Thiamphenicol Glycinate Hydrochloride (172-e)

Thiamphenicol Aminoacetate Hydrochloride; Tiamfenicolo Glicinato Cloridrato.

$C_{14}H_{18}Cl_2N_2O_6S,HCl$ = 449.7.

CAS — 2393-92-2 (thiamphenicol glycinate); 2611-61-2 (thiamphenicol glycinate hydrochloride).

Pharmacopoeias. In *It.*

1.26 g of monograph substance is approximately equivalent to 1 g of thiamphenicol.

Adverse Effects and Precautions

As for Chloramphenicol, p.182.

Thiamphenicol is probably more liable to cause dose-dependent reversible depression of the bone marrow than chloramphenicol but it is not usually associated with aplastic anaemia. Thiamphenicol also appears to be less likely to cause the 'grey syndrome' in neonates.

Doses of thiamphenicol should be reduced in patients with renal impairment. It is probably not necessary to reduce doses in patients with impaired liver function.

Interactions

As for Chloramphenicol, p.183.

Although thiamphenicol is not metabolised in the liver and might not be expected to be affected by drugs which induce hepatic enzymes, it is reported to inhibit hepatic microsomal enzymes and may affect the metabolism of other drugs.

Antimicrobial Action

Thiamphenicol has a broad spectrum of activity resembling that of chloramphenicol (p.183). Although in general it is less active than chloramphenicol it is reported to be equally effective, and more actively bactericidal, against *Haemophilus* and *Neisseria* spp. MICs for the most sensitive strains range from about 0.1 to 2 µg per mL.

Cross-resistance has been reported between thiamphenicol and chloramphenicol. However, some strains resistant to chloramphenicol may be susceptible to thiamphenicol.

Pharmacokinetics

Thiamphenicol is absorbed from the gastro-intestinal tract following oral administration and peak serum concentrations of 3 to 6 µg per mL have been achieved about 2 hours after a 500-mg dose.

Thiamphenicol has been reported to diffuse into the CSF, across the placenta, into breast milk, and to penetrate well into the lungs. About 10% is bound to plasma proteins. The half-life of thiamphenicol is around 2 to 3 hours but unlike chloramphenicol the half-life is increased in patients with renal impairment. It is excreted in the urine, about 70% of a dose being excreted in 24 hours as unchanged drug. It undergoes little or no conjugation with glucuronic acid in the liver. A small amount is excreted in the bile and the faeces.

Uses and Administration

Thiamphenicol has been used similarly to chloramphenicol (p.184) in the treatment of susceptible infections, including sexually transmitted diseases. The usual adult dose is 1.5 g daily by mouth in divided doses; up to 3 g daily has been given initially in severe infections. A daily dose of 30 to 100 mg per kg body-weight has been suggested in children. Equivalent doses may be administered by intramuscular or intravenous injection as the more water-soluble glycinate.

Thiamphenicol has also been used as thiamphenicol glycine acetylcysteinate, thiamphenicol sodium glycinate isophthalolate, and thiamphenicol palmitate.

Preparations

Proprietary Preparations (details are given in Part 3)
Belg.: Fluimucil Antibiotic; Urfamycine; ***Fr.:*** Fluimucil Antibiotic; Thiophenicol; ***Ger.:*** Urfamycine†; ***Ital.:*** Flogotisol; Fluimucil Antibiotico; Glitisol; ***Spain:*** Fluimucil Antibiotico; Urfamycin; ***Switz.:*** Fluimucil Antibiotic†; Urfamycine.

Multi-ingredient: ***Ital.:*** Fultrexin†.

Thiocarlide (7573-z)

Thiocarlide *(BAN)*.

Tiocarlide *(rINN)*. 4,4'-Bis(isopentyloxy)thiocarbanilide.

$C_{23}H_{32}N_2O_2S$ = 400.6.

CAS — 910-86-1.

Thiocarlide has been used for the treatment of pulmonary tuberculosis.

Preparations

Proprietary Preparations (details are given in Part 3)
Spain: Isoxyl†.

Thiostrepton (8708-f)

$C_{72}H_{85}N_{19}O_{18}S_5$ = 1664.9.

CAS — 1393-48-2.

Pharmacopoeias. In *US* for veterinary use only.

A white to off-white crystalline powder. Practically **insoluble** in water, in the lower alcohols, in nonpolar organic solvents, and in dilute aqueous acids and alkalis; soluble in glacial acetic acid, in chloroform, in dimethylformamide, in dimethyl sulphoxide, in dioxan, and in pyridine. **Store** in airtight containers.

Thiostrepton is an antibacterial produced by strains of *Streptomyces azureus*. It is included in topical antibacterial preparations for veterinary use.

Tiamulin Fumarate (13337-w)

Tiamulin Fumarate *(BANM, USAN, rINNM)*.

81723-hfu; SQ-14055 (tiamulin); SQ-22947 (tiamulin fumarate). 11-Hydroxy-6,7,10,12-tetramethyl-1-oxo-10-vinylperhydro-3a,7-pentanoinden-8-yl (2-diethylaminoethylthio)acetate hydrogen fumarate.

$C_{28}H_{47}NO_4S,C_4H_4O_4$ = 609.8.

CAS — 55297-95-5 (tiamulin); 555297-96-6 (tiamulin fumarate).

Tiamulin fumarate is an antibacterial used in veterinary medicine.

Ticarcillin Sodium (173-l)

Ticarcillin Sodium *(BANM, pINNM)*.

BRL-2288; Ticarcillin Disodium *(USAN)*; Ticarcillinum Natricum. The disodium salt of (6*R*)-6-[2-carboxy-2-(3-thienyl)acetamido]penicillanic acid.

$C_{15}H_{14}N_2Na_2O_6S_2$ = 428.4.

CAS — 34787-01-4 (ticarcillin); 3973-04-4 (ticarcillin); 4697-14-7 (ticarcillin disodium); 29457-07-6 (ticarcillin disodium); 74682-62-5 (ticarcillin monosodium).

Pharmacopoeias. In *Eur.* (see p.viii), *Jpn*, and *US*.
US includes Ticarcillin Monosodium.

A white to pale yellow hygroscopic powder. 1.1 g of monograph substance is approximately equivalent to 1 g of ticarcillin. Each g of monograph substance represents about 4.7 mmol of sodium.

Freely **soluble** in water; soluble in methyl alcohol; practically insoluble in ether. A solution in water containing about 1% has a pH of 6 to 8. A 5% solution in water has a pH of 5.5 to 7.5. **Store** in airtight containers at 2° to 8°.

Incompatibility has been reported with aminoglycosides.

References.

1. Swenson E, *et al.* Compatibility of ticarcillin disodium clavulanate potassium with commonly used intravenous solutions. *Curr Ther Res* 1990; **48:** 385–94.

Adverse Effects and Precautions

As for Carbenicillin Sodium, p.162.

Cholestatic jaundice and hepatitis have been reported with the combination ticarcillin with clavulanic acid; the clavulanic acid component has been implicated.

Effects on the liver. Cholestatic jaundice and hepatitis have been associated with combined preparations of a penicillin and clavulanic acid (see Amoxycillin, p.152) and 2 cases had been reported to the UK Committee on Safety of Medicines in association with ticarcillin and clavulanic acid.[1] It appeared that the clavulanic acid was probably responsible.

1. Committee on Safety of Medicines/Medicines Control Agency. Cholestatic jaundice with co-amoxiclav. *Current Problems* 1993; **19:** 2.

Interactions

As for Benzylpenicillin, p.160.

Antimicrobial Action

Ticarcillin is bactericidal and has a mode of action and range of activity similar to that of carbenicillin (p.162) but is reported to be 2 to 4 times more active against *Pseudomonas aeruginosa*.

Combinations of ticarcillin and aminoglycosides have been shown to be synergistic *in vitro* against *Ps. aeruginosa* and Enterobacteriaceae.

The activity of ticarcillin against organisms usually resistant because of the production of certain beta-lactamases is enhanced by clavulanic acid, a beta-lactamase inhibitor. Such organisms have included staphylococci, many Enterobacteriaceae, *Haemophilus influenzae*, and *Bacteroides* spp.; the activity of ticarcillin against *Ps. aeruginosa* is not enhanced by clavulanic acid. Resistance to ticarcillin with clavulanic acid has been reported.

There is cross-resistance between carbenicillin and ticarcillin.

References.

1. Pulverer G, *et al.* In-vitro activity of ticarcillin with and without clavulanic acid against clinical isolates of Gram-positive and Gram-negative bacteria. *J Antimicrob Chemother* 1986; **17** (suppl C): 1–5.
2. Masterton RG, *et al.* Timentin resistance. *Lancet* 1987; **ii:** 975–6.
3. Fass RJ, Prior RB. Comparative in vitro activities of piperacillin-tazobactam and ticarcillin-clavulanate. *Antimicrob Agents Chemother* 1989; **33:** 1268–74.
4. Kempers J, MacLaren DM. Piperacillin/tazobactam and ticarcillin/clavulanic acid against resistant Enterobacteriaceae. *J Antimicrob Chemother* 1990; **26:** 598–9.

Pharmacokinetics

Ticarcillin is not absorbed from the gastro-intestinal tract. After intramuscular injection of 1 g peak plasma concentrations in the range of 20 to 30 µg per mL are achieved after 0.5 to 1 hour. About 50% of ticarcillin in the circulation is bound to plasma proteins. A plasma half-life of 70 minutes has been reported. A shorter half-life in patients with cystic fibrosis (about 50 minutes in one study) has been attributed to increased renal and non-renal elimination. The half-life is prolonged in neonates and also in patients with renal impairment especially if hepatic function is also impaired. A half-life of about 15 hours has been reported in severe renal impairment.

Distribution of ticarcillin in the body is similar to that of carbenicillin. Relatively high concentrations have been reported in bile, but ticarcillin is excreted principally by glomerular filtration and tubular secretion. Concentrations of 2 to 4 mg per mL are achieved in the urine after the intramuscular injection of 1 or 2 g. Ticarcillin is metabolised to a limited extent. Up to 90% of a dose is excreted unchanged in the urine mostly within 6 hours after administration. The concomitant administration of probenecid produces higher plasma-ticarcillin concentrations.

Ticarcillin is removed by haemodialysis and, to some extent, by peritoneal dialysis.

Ticarcillin with clavulanic acid. The pharmacokinetics of ticarcillin and clavulanic acid (p.190) are broadly similar and neither appears to affect the other to any great extent.

References.

1. Staniforth DH, *et al.* Pharmacokinetics of parenteral ticarcillin formulated with clavulanic acid: Timentin. *Int J Clin Pharmacol Ther Toxicol* 1986; **24:** 123–9.
2. Brogard JM, *et al.* Biliary elimination of ticarcillin plus clavulanic acid (Claventin®): experimental and clinical study. *Int J Clin Pharmacol Ther Toxicol* 1989; **27:** 135–44.
3. de Groot R, *et al.* Pharmacokinetics of ticarcillin in patients with cystic fibrosis: a controlled prospective study. *Clin Pharmacol Ther* 1990; **47:** 73–8.
4. Wang J-P, *et al.* Disposition of drugs in cystic fibrosis IV: mechanisms for enhanced renal clearance of ticarcillin. *Clin Pharmacol Ther* 1993; **54:** 293–302.
5. Burstein AH, *et al.* Ticarcillin-clavulanic acid pharmacokinetics in preterm neonates with presumed sepsis. *Antimicrob Agents Chemother* 1994; **38:** 2024–8.

Uses and Administration

Ticarcillin is a carboxypenicillin used in the treatment of severe Gram-negative infections, especially those due to *Pseudomonas aeruginosa*. Pseudomonal infections where ticarcillin is used include those in cystic fibrosis (respiratory-tract infections), immunocompromised patients (neutropenia), peritonitis, and septicaemia. Other infections that may be due to *Ps. aeruginosa* include bone and joint infections, meningitis, otitis media (chronic), skin infections (burns, ecthyma gangrenosum, ulceration), and urinary-tract infections. For details of these infections and their treatment, see under Choice of Antibacterial, p.116.

Administration and dosage. Ticarcillin is given by injection as the sodium salt. Doses are expressed in terms of the equivalent amount of ticarcillin. They may need to be reduced in renal impairment.

Ticarcillin is given to adults and children in a dose of 200 to 300 mg per kg body-weight daily by intravenous infusion in divided doses every 4 or 6 hours.

In adults the concomitant administration of probenecid 1 g three times daily by mouth may achieve higher and more prolonged plasma concentrations of ticarcillin but caution is advised in patients with impaired renal function.

In the treatment of complicated urinary-tract infections adults and children may be given a dose of ticarcillin 150 to 200 mg per kg daily by intravenous infusion in divided doses every 4 or 6 hours. In uncomplicated urinary-tract infections the usual adult dose is ticarcillin 1 g every 6 hours intramuscularly or by slow intravenous injection. Children with uncomplicated urinary-tract infections may be given 50 to 100 mg per kg body-weight daily in divided doses. Not more than 2 g of ticarcillin should be injected intramuscularly into one site.

In patients with cystic fibrosis ticarcillin has been administered by nebuliser in the management of respiratory-tract infections.

Ticarcillin is often used with an aminoglycoside but the injections must be administered separately because of possible incompatibility.

Ticarcillin with clavulanic acid. Ticarcillin may be administered in a combination preparation with clavulanic acid (p.190), a beta-lactamase inhibitor, to widen its antibacterial spectrum to organisms usually resistant because of the production of beta-lactamases. This combination is administered by intravenous infusion in a ratio of 15 or 30 parts of ticarcillin (as the sodium salt) to 1 part of clavulanic acid (as the potassium salt). Doses are according to the content of ticarcillin, similar to those specified above.

Preparations

USP 23: Ticarcillin and Clavulanic Acid for Injection; Ticarcillin and Clavulanic Acid Injection; Ticarcillin for Injection.

Proprietary Preparations (details are given in Part 3)
Austral.: Tarcil; Ticillin†; ***Belg.:*** Triacilline; ***Canad.:*** Ticar; ***Fr.:*** Ticarpen; ***Neth.:*** Ticarpen; ***Spain:*** Ticarpen; ***UK:*** Ticar†; ***USA:*** Ticar.

Multi-ingredient: ***Aust.:*** Timenten; ***Austral.:*** Timentin; ***Belg.:*** Timentin; ***Canad.:*** Timentin; ***Fr.:*** Claventin; ***Ger.:*** Betabactyl; ***Irl.:*** Timentin; ***Ital.:*** Clavucar; Timentin; ***Neth.:*** Timentin; ***Switz.:*** Timenten; ***UK:*** Timentin; ***USA:*** Timentin.

Tilmicosin (3769-a)

Tilmicosin *(BAN, USAN, rINN).*

EL-870; LY-177370. 4^A-*O*-De(2,6-dideoxy-3-*C*-methyl-α-L-*ribo*-hexopyranosyl)-20-deoxo-20-(*cis*-3,5-dimethyl-piperidino)tylosin.

$C_{46}H_{80}N_2O_{13}$ = 869.1.

CAS — 108050-54-0.

NOTE. Tilmicosin Phosphate is *USAN.*

Pharmacopoeias. In US.

Tilmicosin is a macrolide antibacterial used in veterinary medicine.

Tobramycin (18310-c)

Tobramycin *(BAN, USAN, rINN).*

47663; Nebramycin Factor 6; Tobramycinum. 6-*O*-(3-Amino-3-deoxy-α-D-glucopyranosyl)-2-deoxy-4-*O*-(2,6-diamino-2,3,6-trideoxy-α-D-*ribo*-hexopyranosyl)streptamine.

$C_{18}H_{37}N_5O_9$ = 467.5.

CAS — 32986-56-4.

Pharmacopoeias. In Eur. (see p.viii), *Jpn,* Pol., and US.

An antibiotic substance produced by the growth of *Streptomyces tenebrarius* or by any other means.

A white or almost white hygroscopic powder. Freely **soluble** in water; very slightly soluble in alcohol; practically insoluble in chloroform and in ether. Contains not more than 8.0% w/w of water. A 10% solution in water has a pH of 9.0 to 11.0. **Store** at a temperature not exceeding 25° in airtight containers.

Tobramycin Sulphate (174-y)

Tobramycin Sulphate *(BANM, rINNM).*

$(C_{18}H_{37}N_5O_9)_2,5H_2SO_4$ = 1425.4.

CAS — 49842-07-1 ($C_{18}H_{37}N_5O_9,xH_2SO_4$); 79645-27-5 (($C_{18}H_{37}N_{5}O_{9})_2,5H_2SO_4$).

Pharmacopoeias. In Pol. and US.

1.5 g of monograph substance is approximately equivalent to 1 g of tobramycin. A 4% solution in water has a pH of 6.0 to 8.0. **Store** in airtight containers.

Incompatibilities. For discussion of the incompatibility of aminoglycosides, including tobramycin, with beta lactams, see under Gentamicin Sulphate, p.212. Tobramycin is also reported to be incompatible with various other drugs and, as injections have an acid pH, incompatibility with alkaline preparations or with drugs unstable at acid pH may reasonably be expected.

Adverse Effects, Treatment, and Precautions

As for Gentamicin Sulphate, p.212. Some studies suggest that tobramycin is slightly less nephrotoxic than gentamicin but others have not found any significant difference in their effects on the kidney.

Peak plasma-tobramycin concentrations greater than 12 μg per mL (some suggest 10 μg per mL) and trough concentrations greater than 2 μg per mL should be avoided.

Interactions

As for Gentamicin Sulphate, p.213.

Antimicrobial Action

As for Gentamicin Sulphate, p.213. Tobramycin is reported to be somewhat more effective *in vitro* than gentamicin against *Pseudomonas aeruginosa* and less effective against *Serratia,* staphylococci, and enterococci; however these differences do not necessarily translate into differences in clinical effectiveness. MICs are generally similar to those of gentamicin.

Cross-resistance between tobramycin and gentamicin is generally seen, but about 10% of strains resistant to gentamicin are susceptible to tobramycin.

References to activity against *Pseudomonas aeruginosa.*[1,2]

1. Barclay ML, *et al.* Adaptive resistance to tobramycin in Pseudomonas aeruginosa lung infection in cystic fibrosis. *J Antimicrob Chemother* 1996; **37:** 1155–64.
2. den Hollander JG, *et al.* Synergism between tobramycin and ceftazidime against a resistant Pseudomonas aeruginosa strain, tested in an in vitro pharmacokinetic model. *Antimicrob Agents Chemother* 1997; **41:** 95–100.

Pharmacokinetics

As for Gentamicin Sulphate, p.213.

Following intramuscular administration of tobramycin peak plasma concentrations are achieved within 30 to 90 minutes and concentrations of about 4 μg per mL have been reported following doses of 1 mg per kg body-weight. Administration of usual doses by slow intravenous injection may result in plasma concentrations which briefly exceed 12 μg per mL. A plasma half-life of 2 to 3 hours has been reported.

Inhalation. References.

1. Touw DJ, *et al.* Pharmacokinetics of aerosolized tobramycin in adult patients with cystic fibrosis. *Antimicrob Agents Chemother* 1997; **41:** 184–7.

Uses and Administration

Tobramycin is an aminoglycoside antibiotic with actions and uses similar to those of gentamicin (p.214). It is used, usually as the sulphate, particularly in the treatment of pseudomonal infections.

As with gentamicin, tobramycin may be used with penicillins or cephalosporins; the injections should be administered separately.

Doses of tobramycin sulphate are expressed in terms of tobramycin base, and are similar to those of gentamicin, with the usual adult dose ranging from 3 to 5 mg of tobramycin per kg daily in 3 or 4 divided doses. For mild to moderate urinary-tract infections a dose of 2 to 3 mg per kg once daily may be effective. In patients with cystic fibrosis, doses of 8 to 10 mg per kg daily in divided doses may be necessary to achieve therapeutic plasma concentrations.

A suggested dose for children is 6 to 7.5 mg per kg daily in 3 or 4 divided doses. Premature and full-term neonates may be given 2 mg per kg every 12 hours. See under Gentamicin Sulphate (p.214) for reference to once-daily dosage of aminoglycosides.

Tobramycin sulphate is given by intramuscular injection, or by intravenous infusion over 20 to 60 minutes in 50 to 100 mL of sodium chloride 0.9% or glucose 5% injection; proportionately less fluid should be given to children. It has also been given slowly by direct intravenous injection.

Treatment should generally be limited to 7 to 10 days, and peak plasma concentrations greater than 12 μg per mL (some suggest 10 μg per mL) or trough concentrations greater than 2 μg per mL should be avoided. In all patients, dosage should be adjusted according to plasma-tobramycin concentrations and particularly where factors such as age, renal impairment, or high dose may predispose to toxicity (see Gentamicin Sulphate, p.214).

Tobramycin may be administered into the eye as a 0.3% ointment or drops in the treatment of eye infections, and has been given by inhalation in patients with cystic fibrosis.

Administration and dosage. BY INHALATION. Tobramycin has been administered by inhalation to patients with cystic fibrosis (p.119) and *Pseudomonas aeruginosa* infection. A nebulised solution containing 600 mg of tobramycin in 30 mL of saline 0.45% was given three times daily for 4 to 8 weeks.[1] The short-term administration of such high doses by ultrasonic nebuliser appeared to be safe and effective. Tobramycin has also been given in combination with other inhaled antibacterials such as colistin or ticarcillin.

1. Ramsey BW, *et al.* Efficacy of aerosolized tobramycin in patients with cystic fibrosis. *N Engl J Med* 1993; **328:** 1740–6.

Preparations

BP 1998: Tobramycin Injection;
USP 23: Tobramycin and Dexamethasone Ophthalmic Ointment; Tobramycin and Dexamethasone Ophthalmic Suspension; Tobramycin and Fluorometholone Acetate Ophthalmic Suspension; Tobramycin for Injection; Tobramycin Injection; Tobramycin Ophthalmic Ointment; Tobramycin Ophthalmic Solution.

Proprietary Preparations (details are given in Part 3)
Aust.: Brulamycin; Tobrasix; Tobrex; ***Austral.:*** Nebcin; Tobrex; ***Belg.:*** Obracin; Tobrex; ***Canad.:*** Nebcin; Tobrex; ***Fr.:*** Nebcine; Tobrex; ***Ger.:*** Brulamycin; Gernebcin; Tobra-cell; Tobramaxin; ***Irl.:*** Nebcin; Tobralex; ***Ital.:*** Nebicina; Tobral; Tobrex; ***Neth.:*** Obracin; Tobrex†; ***Norw.:*** Nebcina; ***S.Afr.:*** Mytobrin; Nebcin; Tobrex; ***Spain:*** Tobra Gobens; Tobra Laf†; Tobradistin; Tobrex; ***Swed.:*** Nebcina; ***Switz.:*** Obracin; Tobrex; ***UK:*** Nebcin; Tobralex†; ***USA:*** AkTob; Defy; Nebcin; Tobi; Tobrasol; Tobrex.

Multi-ingredient: ***Belg.:*** Tobradex; ***Canad.:*** Tobradex; ***Ital.:*** Tobradex; ***Neth.:*** Tobradex†; ***S.Afr.:*** Tobradex; ***Switz.:*** Tobradex; ***USA:*** Tobradex.

Tosufloxacin (10456-c)

Tosufloxacin *(USAN, rINN).*

Abbott-61827. (±)-7-(3-Amino-1-pyrrolidinyl)-1-(2,4-difluorophenyl)-6-fluoro-1,4-dihydro-4-oxo-1,8-naphthyridine-3-carboxylic acid.

$C_{19}H_{15}F_3N_4O_3$ = 404.3.

CAS — 108138-46-1 (anhydrous tosufloxacin); 107097-79-0 (tosufloxacin monohydrate).

Tosufloxacin is a fluoroquinolone antibacterial with properties similar to those of ciprofloxacin (p.185). It has been given by mouth as the tosylate in the treatment of susceptible infections.

Triacetyloleandomycin (175-j)

Triacetyloleandomycin *(BAN).*

Troleandomycin *(USAN, rINN)*; NSC-108166. The triacetyl ester of oleandomycin.

$C_{41}H_{67}NO_{15}$ = 814.0.

CAS — 2751-09-9.

Pharmacopoeias. In *Fr.* and US.

A white, odourless, crystalline powder. It contains the equivalent of not less than 750 μg of oleandomycin per mg. 1.18 g of monograph substance is approximately equivalent to 1 g of oleandomycin. Freely **soluble** in alcohol; soluble in chloroform; slightly soluble in ether and in water. A 10% solution in alcohol (50%) has a pH of 7.0 to 8.5. **Store** in airtight containers.

Adverse Effects and Precautions

As for Erythromycin, p.204. After administration of triacetyloleandomycin for 2 weeks or more, or in repeated courses, hepatotoxicity with transient disturbances of liver function and jaundice, as described for erythromycin, have occurred and liver function should be monitored in patients who receive the drug for more than 14 days or in repeated courses. It should be used with care in patients with hepatic impairment and avoided in those who have previously developed liver toxicity on receiving it.

Interactions

For a discussion of drug interactions with macrolide antibacterials, see Erythromycin, p.205.

For the effect of triacetyloleandomycin on serum concentrations of *carbamazepine*, see p.341 and for its effect on *triazolam*, see under Diazepam, p.663. The concomitant administration of triacetyloleandomycin and *cisapride* can increase plasma concentrations of cisapride which may result in serious ventricular arrhythmias. Triacetyloleandomycin has a more potent effect on hepatic cytochrome P450 than erythromycin (p.205), and interactions reported between drugs such as *astemizole*, the *ergot alkaloids*, *terfenadine*, or *theophylline* and other macrolides are at least as likely if they are taken with triacetyloleandomycin.

For the effects of triacetyloleandomycin on *methylprednisolone*, see Administration in Asthma under Uses, below.

Antimicrobial Action

Triacetyloleandomycin is hydrolysed *in vivo* to oleandomycin (p.234) which has a range of activity similar to but, in general, less effective than that of erythromycin (p.205). It has a similar pattern of resistance to erythromycin.

Pharmacokinetics

Triacetyloleandomycin is more rapidly and completely absorbed from the gastro-intestinal tract than is oleandomycin, to which it is hydrolysed *in vivo*. Peak plasma-oleandomycin concentrations of about 2 μg per mL are attained 2 hours after a single dose of 500 mg, and detectable amounts are present in plasma after 12 hours. It is excreted in the faeces via the bile; about 20% of the dose can be recovered in active form from the urine.

Uses and Administration

Triacetyloleandomycin is a macrolide antibiotic with actions similar to those of erythromycin (p.206). It has been given by mouth in the treatment of susceptible infections although more effective antibacterials are generally preferred. The usual adult dose is the equivalent of 1 to 2 g daily of oleandomycin in divided doses by mouth. Children have been given the equivalent of about 25 to 45 mg per kg body-weight daily.

Administration in asthma. Triacetyloleandomycin inhibits the elimination of methylprednisolone[1] and has been given to children with corticosteroid-dependent asthma, being treated with methylprednisolone by mouth to permit a reduction in corticosteroid dosage.[2-4] It is unclear whether triacetyloleandomycin has actions in asthma beyond its effect on methylprednisolone metabolism; there is some evidence that it may reduce airway hyperresponsiveness,[3] and there is a report of a patient in whom the corticosteroid component of her regimen was tapered to zero, and who was successfully maintained on triacetyloleandomycin alone.[5]

The role of corticosteroids in the treatment of asthma is discussed on p.745.

1. Szefler SJ, *et al.* Dose- and time-related effect of troleandomycin on methylprednisolone elimination. *Clin Pharmacol Ther* 1982; **32:** 166–71.
2. Eitches RW, *et al.* Methylprednisolone and troleandomycin in treatment of steroid-dependent asthmatic children. *Am J Dis Child* 1985; **139:** 264–8.
3. Ball BD, *et al.* Effect of low-dose troleandomycin on glucocorticoid pharmacokinetics and airway hyperresponsiveness in severely asthmatic children. *Ann Allergy* 1990; **65:** 37–45.
4. Kamada AK, *et al.* Efficacy and safety of low-dose troleandomycin therapy in children with severe, steroid-requiring asthma. *J Allergy Clin Immunol* 1993; **91:** 873–82.
5. Rosenberg SM, *et al.* Use of TAO without methylprednisolone in the treatment of severe asthma. *Chest* 1991; **100:** 849–50.

Preparations

USP 23: Troleandomycin Capsules.

Proprietary Preparations (details are given in Part 3)
Belg.: TAO†; ***Ital.:*** Treis-Micina†; Triocetin; Viamicina†; ***USA:*** TAO.

Trimethoprim (1401-c)

Trimethoprim *(BAN, USAN, rINN)*.

BW-56-72; NSC-106568; Trimethoprimum; Trimethoxyprim. 5-(3,4,5-Trimethoxybenzyl)pyrimidine-2,4-diamine.

$C_{14}H_{18}N_4O_3$ = 290.3.

CAS — 738-70-5.

NOTE. Trimethoprim may be given with various sulphonamides and some preparations of such combinations have been given approved names: see Co-trifamole, p.196; Co-trimazine, p.196; and Co-trimoxazole, p.196.

Pharmacopoeias. In *Chin., Eur.* (see p.viii), *Int., Pol.,* and *US.*

White or yellowish-white, odourless crystals or crystalline powder. It exhibits polymorphism. Very slightly **soluble** in water; slightly soluble in alcohol and in acetone; sparingly soluble in chloroform and in methyl alcohol; soluble in benzyl alcohol; practically insoluble in ether and in carbon tetrachloride. **Store** in airtight containers. Protect from light.

Incompatibility. The UK manufacturers state that trimethoprim injections (containing the lactate) should not be mixed with solutions of other antibacterials including sulphonamides because of incompatibility. Although a former such preparation stated that it should not be diluted in chloride-containing infusion solutions, because of the risk of precipitating trimethoprim hydrochloride, others are stated to be compatible with sodium chloride 0.9% and some other chloride-containing solutions including Ringer's solution. Injections are considered compatible with glucose 5% and with sodium lactate.

Adverse Effects and Treatment

Trimethoprim is reasonably well tolerated in general, and the most frequent adverse effects at usual doses are pruritus and skin rash (in about 3 to 7% of patients) and mild gastro-intestinal disturbances including nausea, vomiting, and sore mouth.

Rarely, more severe effects have been reported. Sulphonamide-like skin reactions including exfoliative dermatitis, erythema multiforme, Stevens-Johnson syndrome, and toxic epidermal necrolysis have occurred. Disturbances of liver enzyme values and cholestatic jaundice have been associated with trimethoprim. Rises in serum creatinine and blood-urea nitrogen have been reported although it is unclear whether this represents genuine renal dysfunction or inhibition of tubular secretion of creatinine. Fever is not uncommon but occasionally hypersensitivity reactions may be severe and manifest as anaphylaxis. Cases of aseptic meningitis have also been reported.

Trimethoprim may cause a depression of haemopoiesis due to interference of the drug in the metabolism of folic acid, particularly when given over a prolonged period or in high doses. This may manifest as megaloblastic anaemia, or as thrombocytopenia and leucopenia; methaemoglobinaemia has also been seen. Calcium folinate 5 to 15 mg daily by mouth may be given to counter this effect. Trimethoprim is teratogenic in *animals*.

For reports of adverse effects of trimethoprim when used with sulphamethoxazole, see Co-trimoxazole, p.196.

Hyperkalaemia. Trimethoprim has been reported to induce hyperkalaemia,[1] particularly in HIV-infected patients being treated for *Pneumocystis carinii* pneumonia[2,3] or in the elderly.[4-7] The hyperkalaemia may be due to amiloride-like potassium-sparing properties of trimethoprim,[8] and may be potentiated by ACE inhibitors.[7]

1. Smith GW, Cohen SB. Hyperkalaemia and non-oliguric renal failure associated with trimethoprim. *Br Med J* 1994; **308:** 454.
2. Choi MJ, *et al.* Brief report: trimethoprim-induced hyperkalemia in a patient with AIDS. *N Engl J Med* 1993; **328:** 703–6.
3. Greenberg S, *et al.* Trimethoprim-sulfamethoxazole induces reversible hyperkalemia. *Ann Intern Med* 1993; **119:** 291–5.
4. Modest GA, *et al.* Hyperkalemia in elderly patients receiving standard doses of trimethoprim-sulfamethoxazole. *Ann Intern Med* 1994; **120:** 437.
5. Pennypacker LC, *et al.* Hyperkalemia in elderly patients receiving standard doses of trimethoprim-sulfamethoxazole. *Ann Intern Med* 1994; **120:** 437.
6. Canaday DH, Johnson JR. Hyperkalemia in elderly patients receiving standard doses of trimethoprim-sulfamethoxazole. *Ann Intern Med* 1994; **120:** 437–8.
7. Thomas RJ. Severe hyperkalemia with trimethoprim-quinapril. *Ann Pharmacother* 1996; **30:** 413–14.
8. Velázquez H, *et al.* Renal mechanism of trimethoprim-induced hyperkalemia. *Ann Intern Med* 1993; **119:** 296–301.

Precautions

Trimethoprim should not be given to patients with a history of hypersensitivity to the drug, and it should be discontinued if a skin rash appears. Care is necessary in administering trimethoprim to patients with impaired renal function to avoid accumulation and toxicity: it should not be given in severe renal impairment unless blood concentrations can be monitored. It should be used with caution in patients with severe hepatic damage as changes may occur in the absorption and metabolism of trimethoprim.

It is suggested that regular haematological examination should be made during prolonged courses of treatment; trimethoprim should not usually be given to patients with serious haematological disorders and particularly not in megaloblastic anaemia secondary to folate depletion. Caution should be taken in patients with actual or possible folate deficiency and administration of folinic acid should be considered. Trimethoprim should be avoided during pregnancy. Trimethoprim appears in breast milk and care is required when it is used in nursing mothers. Elderly patients may be more susceptible to adverse effects and a lower dosage may be advisable.

Trimethoprim may interfere with some diagnostic tests including serum-methotrexate assay where dihydrofolate reductase is used, and the Jaffé reaction for creatinine.

For reports dealing with precautions for trimethoprim given with sulphamethoxazole, see Co-trimoxazole, p.197.

Fragile X syndrome. A warning that trimethoprim and other folate antagonists should be avoided in children with the fragile X chromosome which is associated with mental retardation and is folate sensitive.[1] Trimethoprim should also be avoided in pregnant women who are at risk of having a child with fragile X chromosome, until more is known about the expression of this chromosome.

1. Hecht F, Glover TW. Antibiotics containing trimethoprim and the fragile X chromosome. *N Engl J Med* 1983; **308:** 285–6.

Porphyria. Trimethoprim has been associated with clinical exacerbations of porphyria and is considered unsafe in porphyric patients.[1]

1. Moore MR, McColl KEL. *Porphyria: drug lists.* Glasgow: Porphyria Research Unit, University of Glasgow, 1991.

Interactions

Trimethoprim may increase serum concentrations and potentiate the effect of a number of drugs, including phenytoin, digoxin, and procainamide. The effect may be due to competitive inhibition of renal excretion, decreased metabolism, or both. It has been suggested that trimethoprim may potentiate the effects of warfarin. Trimethoprim has been reported to reduce the renal excretion and increase blood concentrations of zidovudine and lamivudine. Trimethoprim and dapsone increase each other's serum concentrations when given concomitantly, whereas rifampicin may decrease trimethoprim concentrations.

An increased risk of nephrotoxicity has been reported with the use of trimethoprim or co-trimoxazole and cyclosporin. Intravenous administration of trimethoprim and sulphonamides may reduce cyclosporin concentrations in blood. In patients given trimethoprim who were also receiving diuretics hyponatraemia has been reported (an increased risk of thrombocytopenia has been seen in elderly patients given co-trimoxazole with diuretics, although it is unclear which component is responsible).

Administration of trimethoprim with other depressants of bone marrow function may increase the likelihood of myelosuppression and there may be a particular risk of megaloblastic anaemia if it is given with other folate inhibitors such as pyrimethamine or methotrexate.

Antimicrobial Action

Trimethoprim is a dihydrofolate reductase inhibitor. It inhibits the conversion of bacterial dihydrofolic acid to tetrahydrofolic acid which is necessary for the synthesis of certain amino acids, purines, thymidine, and ultimately DNA synthesis. It acts in the same metabolic pathway as the sulphonamides. It exerts its selective action because of a far greater affinity for the bacterial than the mammalian enzyme. Trimethoprim may be bacteriostatic or bactericidal depending on growth conditions; pus, for example, may inhibit the action of trimethoprim because of the presence of thymine and thymidine.

Spectrum of activity. Trimethoprim is active against a wide range of Gram-negative and Gram-positive aerobes, as well as some protozoa. The following species are usually susceptible (but see also Resistance, below).

Many Gram-positive cocci, including *Staphylococcus aureus*, streptococci including *Streptococcus pyogenes*, *Str. pneumoniae*, and the viridans streptococci, and to a variable extent enterococci, although their sensitivity is reduced in the presence of folate.

Other sensitive Gram-positive organisms include strains of *Listeria*, *Corynebacterium diphtheriae*, and the Gram-positive bacilli.

Among the Gram-negative organisms most of the Enterobacteriaceae are susceptible, or moderately so, including *Citrobacter*, *Enterobacter*, *Escherichia coli*, *Hafnia*, *Klebsiella*, *Proteus mirabilis*, *Providencia*, *Salmonella*, some *Serratia*, *Shigella*, and *Yersinia*. *Legionella* and *Vibrio* are also sensitive, and so are *Haemophilus influenzae* and *H. ducreyi*.

Anaerobic species are usually resistant, and so, to varying degrees are *Brucella* spp., *Neisseria*, and *Nocardia*. *Mycobacterium tuberculosis* is resistant although *M. marinum* may not be. *Pseudomonas aeruginosa* is resistant, and so are the chlamydias, mycoplasmas, and rickettsias, as well as the spirochaetes.

Trimethoprim has some activity against *Pneumocystis carinii* and against some protozoa such as *Naegleria*, *Plasmodium*, and *Toxoplasma*.

Minimum inhibitory concentrations (MICs) vary considerably with the medium; in particular the media should contain minimal amounts of thymine or thymidine. MICs for the most sensitive strains range from about 0.01 to 0.5 μg per mL; in the treatment of urinary tract infectious organisms with MICs up to about 8 μg per mL are considered sensitive and those with MICs between 8 and 16 μg per mL of moderate sensitivity, but since concentrations in blood are lower than those in urine such MICs would not indicate sensitivity in systemic infections.

Activity with other antimicrobials. Because their modes of action are complementary, affecting different stages in folate metabolism, a potent synergistic effect exists between trimethoprim and sulphonamides against many organisms *in vitro*. The effect is most marked when the two drugs are present in the ratio of their MICs: i.e. an organism susceptible to 1 μg per mL of trimethoprim and 20 μg per mL of sulphonamide will be maximally inhibited by a 1:20 mixture.

Fixed-dose combinations of trimethoprim with various sulphonamides are available, of which co-trimoxazole (trimethoprim with sulphamethoxazole in a 1:5 mixture) is the most widely used. For further details on the antimicrobial action of co-trimoxazole, see p.197.

Synergy has also been reported with rifampicin, and with the polymyxins.

Resistance. Resistance to trimethoprim may be due to several mechanisms. Clinical resistance is often due to plasmid-mediated dihydrofolate reductases that are resistant to trimethoprim: such genes may become incorporated into the chromosome via transposons. Resistance may also be due to overproduction of dihydrofolate reductase, changes in cell permeability, or bacterial mutants which are intrinsically resistant to trimethoprim because they depend on exogenous thymine and thymidine for growth. Despite fears of a rapid increase in resistance if trimethoprim was used alone there is little evidence that this has been any worse than in areas where it has been used in combination with sulphonamides. Nonetheless, trimethoprim resistance has been reported in many species, and very high frequencies of resistance have been seen in some developing countries, particularly among the Enterobacteriaceae.

References.

1. Huovinen P, *et al.* Trimethoprim and sulfonamide resistance. *Antimicrob Agents Chemother* 1995; **39:** 279–89.

Pharmacokinetics

Trimethoprim is rapidly and almost completely absorbed from the gastro-intestinal tract and peak concentrations in the circulation occur about 1 to 4 hours after an oral dose; peak plasma concentrations of about 1 μg per mL have been reported after a single dose of 100 mg. About 45% is bound to plasma proteins. Trimethoprim is widely distributed to various tissues and fluids including kidneys, liver, lung and bronchial secretions, saliva, aqueous humour, prostatic tissue and fluid, and vaginal secretions; concentrations in many of these tissues are reported to be higher than serum concentrations but concentrations in the CSF are about one-quarter to one-half of those in the blood. Trimethoprim readily crosses the placenta and it appears in breast milk. The half-life is about 8 to 11 hours in adults and somewhat less in children, but is prolonged in severe renal impairment and in neonates, whose renal function is immature.

Trimethoprim is excreted primarily by the kidneys through glomerular filtration and tubular secretion. About 10 to 20% of trimethoprim is metabolised in the liver and small amounts are excreted in the faeces via the bile, but most is excreted in urine, predominantly as unchanged drug. About 40 to 60% of a dose is excreted in urine within 24 hours. Trimethoprim is removed from the blood by haemodialysis to some extent.

Uses and Administration

Trimethoprim is a diaminopyrimidine antibacterial that is used for the treatment of infections due to sensitive organisms, including gastro-enteritis, respiratory-tract infections, and in particular the treatment and prophylaxis of urinary-tract infections. For details of these infections and their treatment, see Choice of Antibacterial, p.116.

Trimethoprim is also used in conjunction with sulphonamides. The most common combination is co-trimoxazole (trimethoprim with sulphamethoxazole) (p.196). Other combinations are co-trimazine (with sulphadiazine) and co-trifamole (with sulphamoxole); trimethoprim is also used with sulfamerazine, sulfametopyrazine, sulfametrole, and sulphamethoxypyridazine, and, in veterinary practice, with sulfadoxine, sulfaquinoxaline, sulfatroxazole, or sulphachlorpyridazine.

The combination of trimethoprim with sulphamethoxazole (co-trimoxazole) or with dapsone is used in the management of *Pneumocystis carinii* pneumonia (p.370).

The usual dose of trimethoprim in acute infection is 100 or 200 mg twice daily by mouth; doses of 200 or 300 mg daily as a single dose are also used. For the dosage of trimethoprim when given with sulphamethoxazole, see under Co-trimoxazole, p.197. Up to 20 mg per kg body-weight daily may be given in combination with dapsone for the treatment of *Pneumocystis carinii* pneumonia.

Children may be given 6 to 8 mg per kg daily of trimethoprim in 2 divided doses: suggested regimens for children are, 6 to 12 years, 100 mg twice daily; 6 months to 5 years, 50 mg twice daily; 6 weeks to 5 months, 25 mg twice daily.

For long-term prophylaxis the usual dose is 100 mg at night for adults; children aged 6 to 12 years may be given 50 mg at night and those aged 6 months to 5 years, 25 mg at night.

Trimethoprim is also administered intravenously by injection or infusion as the lactate although doses are in terms of the base. The usual dose is 200 mg every 12 hours in adults; children may be given 8 mg per kg daily in 2 or 3 divided doses. Initial doses may be higher or given more frequently in severely ill patients.

Care should be taken in patients with moderate to severe renal impairment and doses generally should be reduced; plasma concentrations should be monitored in patients with severe renal impairment.

Combinations of trimethoprim and polymyxin B have been used topically in the treatment and prophylaxis of eye infections. Trimethoprim sulphate is also used.

Administration. SINGLE-DOSE THERAPY. Although there are obvious advantages to a single-dose regimen, Nolan and others[1] found that treatment with trimethoprim in a single dose of 75 to 450 mg, depending on age, in 50 children with confirmed urinary-tract infection, although it apparently eliminated infection, was associated with about a 1 in 4 risk of recurrence within 10 days, often asymptomatic. The problems with a single-dose regimen were confirmed by Österberg and colleagues[2] in a study involving 344 evaluated cases of cystitis in 306 women. Only 122 of 173 cases treated with trimethoprim 320 mg as a single dose were evaluated as cured after 5 weeks, compared with 149 of 171 given 160 mg twice daily for 1 week (71 versus 87%). Again, these results suggest that about one patient in 4 would have to be re-treated.

1. Nolan T, *et al.* Single dose trimethoprim for urinary tract infection. *Arch Dis Child* 1989; **64:** 581–6.
2. Österberg E, *et al.* Efficacy of single-dose versus seven-day trimethoprim treatment of cystitis in women: a randomized double-blind study. *J Infect Dis* 1990; **161:** 942–7.

Preparations

BP 1998: Co-trimoxazole Intravenous Infusion; Co-trimoxazole Oral Suspension; Co-trimoxazole Tablets; Dispersible Co-trimoxazole Tablets; Paediatric Co-trimoxazole Oral Suspension; Paediatric Co-trimoxazole Tablets; Trimethoprim Tablets;
USP 23: Sulfamethoxazole and Trimethoprim Injection; Sulfamethoxazole and Trimethoprim Oral Suspension; Sulfamethoxazole and Trimethoprim Tablets; Trimethoprim Tablets.

Proprietary Preparations (details are given in Part 3)
Aust.: Alprimol†; Monoprim; Motrim; Solotrim; Triprim; Wellcoprim; ***Austral.:*** Alprim; Triprim; ***Belg.:*** Wellcoprim; ***Canad.:*** Proloprim; ***Fr.:*** Wellcoprim; ***Ger.:*** Infectotrimet; TMP-ratiopharm; Trimanyl†; Trimono; Uretrim; ***Irl.:*** Ipral; Monotrim; ***Ital.:*** Abaprim; ***Neth.:*** Monotrim†; Wellcoprim; ***Norw.:*** Wellcoprim†; ***S.Afr.:*** Monotrim†; Proloprim†; Triprim; ***Spain:*** Syraprim†; Tediprima; ***Swed.:*** Idotrim; Wellcoprim†; ***Switz.:*** Monotrim; Primosept; ***UK:*** Ipral†; Monotrim; Tiempe; Trimogal; Trimopan; Triprimix; ***USA:*** Proloprim; Trimpex.

Multi-ingredient: ***Aust.:*** Bactrim; Cotribene; Eusaprim; Lidaprim; Oecotrim; Polytrim; Supracombin; Triglobe; Trimetho comp; ***Austral.:*** Bactrim; Resprim; Septrin; ***Belg.:*** Bactrim; Eusaprim; Ophtalmotrim; Polytrim; Trimatrim†; ***Canad.:*** Apo-Sulfatrim; Bactrim; Coptin; Novo-Trimel; Nu-Cotrimox; Polytrim; Roubac; Septra; ***Fr.:*** Antrima; Bactekod†; Bactrim; Cotrimazol; Eusaprim; Supristol†; ***Ger.:*** Bactoreduct; Bactrim; Berlocid; Berlocombin; Co-trim-Tablinen; Cotim; Cotrim; Cotrim Holsten; Cotrim-basan†; Cotrim-Diolan; Cotrim-Hefa; Cotrim-Puren; Cotrim-Riker†; Cotrimhexal; Cotrimox-Wolff; Cotrimstada; Drylin; Duobiocin†; duratrimet†; Eusaprim; Jenamoxazol; Kepinol; Lidaprim†; Linaris; Microtrim; Nymix-amid N†; Omsat†; Sigaprim; Sulfacet†; Sulfotrimin†; Supracombin; TMS; Triglobe; Trigonyl†; ***Irl.:*** Antrimox; Bactrim; Cotrimel; Duobact; Septrin; Tricomox; ***Ital.:*** Abacin; Bacterial; Bactrim; Chemitrim; Eusaprim; Gantaprim†; Gantrim; Isotrim; Kelfiprim; Kombinax; Lidaprim; Medixin; Oxaprim†; Polytrim†; Pulmotrim†; Strepto-Plus; Sulmen†; Suprin†; Trim†; Trimed†; Velaten; ***Jpn:*** Baktar†; ***Neth.:*** Bactrimel; Eusaprim; Polytrim; Sulfotrim†; Trimoxol; ***Norw.:*** Bactrim; Eusaprim†; ***S.Afr.:*** Acuco; Arcanaprim; Bactrim; Bencole; Briscotrim†; Cocydal; Cotrivan†; Cozole; Doctrim; Duotrim†; Durobac; Dynazole; Fabubac; Mezenol†; Microbac†; Norisep†; Partrim†; Polytrim; Purbac; Septran; Spectrim; Supristol†; Thoxaprim†; Tri-Co; Trimethox; Trimoks; Trimzol; Troxazole; Ultrasept†; Ultrazole; Xerazole; Xeroprim; ***Spain:*** Abactrim; Abactrim Balsamico†; Azosulfin†; Bactifor; Bactopumon; Balsoprim; Bridotrim; Bronco Aseptilex Fuerte; Bronco Bactifor; Bronco Sergo; Broncorema; Broncovir NF; Brongenit; Bronquicisteina; Bronquidiazina CR; Bronquimar; Bronquimucil; Bronquium; Eduprim; Eduprim Mucolitico; Gobens Trim; Libetusin†; Lotusix; Momentol; Mucorama TS; Neumopectolina; Oftalmotrim; Oftalmotrim Dexa; Otix; Pulmo Menal; Pulmosterin Duo; Salvatrim; Septrin; Soltrim; Supristol†; Toose; Tosdetan; Traquivan; Tresium; Triglobe; ***Swed.:*** Bactrim; Eusaprim; Triferm-Sulfa†; Trimetoprim-Sulfa†; Trimin sulfa; ***Switz.:*** Bactrim; Cotrim; Escoprim; Eusaprim; Groprim; Helveprim; Imexim; Maderan; Nopil; Pharmaprim†; Sigaprim; Supracombin; TMS†; ***UK:*** Bactrim†; Chemotrim; Comixco; Comox†; Fectrim; Laratrim; Polytrim; Septrin; ***USA:*** Bactrim; Cotrim; Polytrim; Septra; SMZ-TMP; Sulfamethoprim; Sulfatrim DS; Uroplus.

Trospectomycin Sulphate (1363-m)

Trospectomycin Sulphate *(BANM, rINNM)*.

Trospectomycin Sulfate *(USAN)*; U-63366 (trospectomycin); U-63366F. (2*R*,4a*R*,5a*R*,6*S*,7*S*,8*R*,9*S*,9a*R*,10a*S*)-2-Butyl-4a,7,9-trihydroxy-6,8-bis(methylamino)perhydropyrano[2,3-*b*][1,4]benzodioxin-4-one sulphate pentahydrate.

$C_{17}H_{30}N_2O_7,H_2SO_4,5H_2O$ = 562.6.

CAS — 88669-04-9 (trospectomycin); 88851-61-0 (trospectomycin sulphate).

Trospectomycin is a water-soluble derivative of spectinomycin (p.248) but is more active against Gram-positive organisms, *Haemophilus influenzae*, and *Chlamydia trachomatis* as well as *Neisseria*. It has been investigated in various infections and given as the sulphate in a dose equivalent to 1 g of the base intramuscularly. Reported adverse effects include perioral paraesthesia, pain at the injection site, nausea, and dizziness.

References.

1. Novak E, *et al.* Human safety and pharmacokinetics of a single intramuscular dose of a novel spectinomycin analog, trospectomycin (U-63366F). *Antimicrob Agents Chemother* 1990; **34:** 2342–7.
2. Nichols DJ, *et al.* Pharmacokinetics of trospectomycin sulphate in healthy subjects after single intravenous and intramuscular doses. *Br J Clin Pharmacol* 1991; **32:** 255–7.
3. Keefer MC, *et al.* Single-dose trospectomycin for chlamydial urethritis in men. *Antimicrob Agents Chemother* 1991; **35:** 986–7.
4. Beam TR, *et al.* In-vitro activity of trospectromycin [sic] against Gram-positive cocci. *J Antimicrob Chemother* 1995; **36:** 874–8.

Trovafloxacin Mesylate (17529-b)

Trovafloxacin Mesylate *(USAN)*.

Trovafloxacin Mesilate *(rINNM)*; CP-99219-27; CP-99219 (trovafloxacin). 7-[(1*R*,5*S*,6*S*)-6-Amino-3-azabicyclo[3.1.0]hex-3-yl]-1-(2,4-difluorophenyl)-6-fluoro-1,4-dihydro-4-oxo-1,8-naphthyridine-3-carboxylic acid monomethanesulphonate.

$C_{20}H_{15}F_3N_4O_3,CH_4O_3S = 512.5.$

CAS — 147059-72-1 (trovafloxacin); 147059-75-4 (trovafloxacin mesylate).

Adverse Effects and Precautions

As for Ciprofloxacin, p.186.

Dizziness is the most common adverse effect reported with trovafloxacin.

Antimicrobial Action

As for Ciprofloxacin, p.187.

Uses and Administration

Trovafloxacin is a fluoroquinolone antibacterial with actions and uses similar to those of ciprofloxacin (p.188). It is given as the mesylate by mouth for the treatment of susceptible infections. The prodrug alatrofloxacin (p.150) is used as the mesylate for intravenous infusion. Doses of both trovafloxacin mesylate and alatrofloxacin mesylate are expressed in terms of trovafloxacin base. Usual daily doses are the equivalent of 100 to 200 mg of trovafloxacin by mouth and 200 to 300 mg intravenously.

General references.

1. Haria M, Lamb HM. Trovafloxacin. *Drugs* 1997; **54:** 435–45.

Preparations

Proprietary Preparations (details are given in Part 3)
USA: Trovan.

Tylosin (13388-r)

Tylosin *(BAN, rINN)*.

$C_{46}H_{77}NO_{17} = 916.1.$

CAS — 1401-69-0.

Pharmacopoeias. In *Eur.* (see p.viii) and *US* for veterinary use.

A mixture of antimicrobial macrolides, produced by the growth of certain strains of *Streptomyces fradiae* or by any other means. It consists largely of tylosin A, but tylosin B (desmycosin), tylosin C (macrocin), and tylosin D (relomycin) may also be present.

An almost white to buff-coloured powder. Slightly **soluble** in water; soluble in alcohol, in amyl acetate, and in chloroform; freely soluble in dehydrated alcohol, in dichloromethane, and in methyl alcohol; dissolves in dilute mineral acids. A 2.5% suspension in water has a pH of 8.5 to 10.5. It loses not more than 5% of its weight on drying. **Protect** from light, moisture, and excessive heat.

Tylosin Tartrate (13389-f)

Tylosin Tartrate *(BANM, rINNM)*.

$(C_{46}H_{77}NO_{17})_2,C_4H_6O_6 = 1982.3.$

CAS — 1405-54-5.

Pharmacopoeias. In *Eur.* (see p.viii) for veterinary use.

An almost white or slightly yellow hygroscopic powder. 1.1 g of monograph substance is approximately equivalent to 1 g of tylosin. Freely **soluble** in water; slightly soluble in dehydrated alcohol; freely soluble in dichloromethane; dissolves in dilute mineral acids. A 2.5% solution in water has a pH of 5.0 to 7.2. **Store** in airtight containers. Protect from light.

Tylosin is a macrolide antibiotic with actions similar to those of erythromycin (p.204). Tylosin and its phosphate and tartrate salts are used in veterinary medicine in the prophylaxis and treatment of various infections caused by susceptible organisms.

Tylosin and tylosin phosphate are added to animal feeding stuffs as growth promoters for pigs.

Tyrothricin (176-z)

Tyrothricin *(BAN, rINN)*.

Tirotricina.

CAS — 1404-88-2.

Pharmacopoeias. In *Fr., Swiss,* and *US.*

An antimicrobial substance produced by the growth of *Bacillus brevis* Dubos. It is a mixture consisting chiefly of gramicidin and tyrocidine, the latter being usually present as the hydrochloride. Both components are mixtures of polypeptides.

Store in airtight containers.

Adverse Effects and Precautions

Tyrothricin is too toxic to be administered systemically; effects that have been reported include liver and kidney damage as well as Stevens-Johnson syndrome. It damages the sensory epithelium of the nose and instances of prolonged loss of smell have occurred after its use as a nasal spray or instillation. Tyrothricin should not be instilled into the nasal cavities or into closed body cavities.

Uses and Administration

Tyrothricin is unsuitable for systemic treatment. It is active *in vitro* against many Gram-positive bacteria and has been used either alone or in conjunction with other antibacterials in the local treatment of infections mainly of the skin and mouth.

Preparations

Proprietary Preparations (details are given in Part 3)
Belg.: Hydrotricine†; ***Fr.:*** Codetricine; ***Ger.:*** Tyrosur; ***Ital.:*** Faringotricina; Ginotricina†; Hydrotricine; Rinotricina; Solutricina†.

Multi-ingredient: ***Aust.:*** Dolothricin; Dorithricin; Lemocin; Neocones; Recessan; Sanoral; Tongill; Tyrosolvin; Tyrothricin comp; ***Belg.:*** Glottyl†; Lemocin; n-Tricidine†; Tricidine; Tyro-Drops; ***Canad.:*** Emercreme No 4; Soropon; Webber Antibiotic Cold Sore Ointment; ***Fr.:*** A 313; Bronpax; Codetricine vitamine C; Collunovar; Maxi-Tyro†; Pharyngine a la Vitamine C†; Solutricine Tetracaine; Solutricine Vitamine C; TOM†; Tyrcine; Tyrothricine Lafran; Veybirol-Tyrothyricine; ***Ger.:*** Anginomycin; Dori; Dorithricin; Ekzemex†; Enzym-Tyrosolvetten†; Inspirol Halsschmerztabletten; Lemocin; Mandro-Angin†; Myacyne; Nordathricin N; Pellit Wund- und Heilsalbe; Peniazol†; Penimycin†; Polycid N†; Sirit†; Stas Halstabletten†; Trachisan; Tyrosirinal†; Tyrosur; ***Irl.:*** Tyrozets; ***Ital.:*** Antibioticoedermin B†; Bio-Arscolloid; Colimicina†; Deltavagin; Furotricina; Golamixin; Kinogen; Rinocidina; ***S.Afr.:*** Otoseptil†; Tyrogel†; ***Spain:*** Anginovag; Bucometasona; Cavum Pediatrico†; Cicatral; Cohortan; Cohortan Antibiotico; Diformiltricina; Forunculone†; Gradin Del D Andreu; Gramicidin†; Hemodren Compuesto; Infalina†; Miozets; Neocones; Otogen Hydrocortisona†; Otogen Prednisolona†; Otosedol Biotico; Oxidermiol Antihist; Pastillas Koki Ment Tivo; Piorlis; Piorreol†; Pulverodil†; Roberfarin; Sedofarin; Super Koki†; Timpanalgesic†; Venoflavan†; Viberol Tirotricina; Wasserdermina†; ***Switz.:*** GEM†; Larocal†; Lemocin; Mebucaine; Neocones; Otothricinol; Ovuthricinol†; Rhinothricinol; Sangerol; Septomixine; Solutricine; Trachisan; Tyliculine†; Tyrocombine; Tyroqualine; Tyrosolvin†; Tyrothricin; Tyrothricine + Gramicidine; ***UK:*** Tyrocane†; Tyrozets; Ulcaid†.

Vancomycin Hydrochloride (177-c)

Vancomycin Hydrochloride *(BANM, rINNM)*.

Vancomycini Hydrochloridum. (S_a)-(3*S*,6*R*,7*R*,22*R*,23*S*,26*S*,36*R*,38a*R*)-44-{[2-*O*-(3-Amino-2,3,6-trideoxy-3-*C*-methyl-α-L-*lyxo*-hexopyranosyl)-β-D-glucopyranosyl]oxy}-3-(carbamoylmethyl)-10,19-dichloro-2,3,4,5,6,7,23,24,25,26,36,37,38,38a-tetradecahydro-7,22,28,30,32-pentahydroxy-6-[(2*R*)-4-methyl-2-(methylamino)valeramido]-2,5,24,38,39-pentaoxo-22*H*-8,11:18,21-dietheno-23,36-(iminomethano)-13,16:31,35-dimetheno-1*H*,16*H*-[1,6,9]oxadiazacyclohexadecino[4,5-*m*][10,2,16]-benzoxadiazacyclotetracosine-26-carboxylic acid, monohydrochloride.

$C_{66}H_{75}Cl_2N_9O_{24},HCl = 1485.7.$

CAS — 1404-90-6 (vancomycin); 1404-93-9 (vancomycin hydrochloride).

Pharmacopoeias. In *Eur.* (see p.viii), *Jpn, Pol.* and *US.*
US also includes vancomycin base.

A glycopeptide antimicrobial substance or mixture of glycopeptides produced by the growth of certain strains of *Amycolatopsis orientalis* (*Nocardia orientalis, Streptomyces orientalis*), or by any other means. A white, almost white, or tan to brown, hygroscopic, odourless powder. 1.03 g of monograph substance is approximately equivalent to 1 g of vancomycin. Freely **soluble** in water; slightly soluble in alcohol; practically insoluble in ether and in chloroform. A 5% solution in water has a pH of 2.5 to 4.5.

Store in airtight containers. Protect from light. Solutions are most stable at pH 3 to 5; the manufacturers recommend that they should be stored in a refrigerator.

Incompatibilities. Solutions of vancomycin hydrochloride have an acid pH and incompatibility may reasonably be expected with alkaline preparations, or with drugs unstable at low pH. Reports of incompatibility are not always consistent, and other factors such as the strength of solution, and composition of the vehicles used, may play a part.

Stability. Although the manufacturers recommend storage at 2° to 8°, solutions of vancomycin hydrochloride in various diluents (sodium chloride 0.9%, glucose 5%, and peritoneal dialysis solution) have been found to be stable for at least 14 days at room temperature.[1-3]

1. Das Gupta V, *et al.* Stability of vancomycin hydrochloride in 5% dextrose and 0.9% sodium chloride injections. *Am J Hosp Pharm* 1986; **43:** 1729–31.
2. Walker SE, Birkhans B. Stability of intravenous vancomycin. *Can J Hosp Pharm* 1988; **41:** 233–8.
3. Mauhinuey WM, *et al.* Stability of vancomycin hydrochloride in peritoneal dialysis solution. *Am J Hosp Pharm* 1992; **49:** 137–9.

Adverse Effects

The intravenous administration of vancomycin may be associated with the so-called 'red-neck' or 'red-man' syndrome, characterised by erythema, flushing, or rash over the face and upper torso, and sometimes by hypotension and shock-like symptoms. The effect appears to be due in part to the release of histamine and is usually related to rapid infusion.

Hypersensitivity reactions may occur in about 5% of patients and include rashes, fever, chills, and rarely, anaphylactoid reactions, exfoliative dermatitis, Stevens-Johnson syndrome, toxic epidermal necrolysis, and vasculitis. Many reactions have become less frequent with the availability of more highly purified preparations. Reversible neutropenia, eosinophilia and rarely thrombocytopenia and agranulocytosis have been reported; neutropenia is stated to be more common in patients who have received a total dose of 25 g or more. Nephrotoxicity may occur, particularly at high doses or in patients with predisposing factors, but has declined in frequency with greater awareness of the problem and appropriate monitoring of plasma concentrations and renal function.

Ototoxicity is also associated with vancomycin administration, and is more likely in patients with high plasma concentrations. It may progress after drug withdrawal, and may be irreversible. Hearing loss may be preceded by tinnitus, which must be regarded as a sign to discontinue treatment.

Vancomycin is irritant; intravenous administration may be associated with thrombophlebitis, although this can be minimised by the slow infusion of dilute solutions, and by using different infusion sites. Extravasation may cause tissue necrosis.

Because of its poor absorption, relatively few adverse effects have been reported after the oral administration of vancomycin, although mild gastro-intestinal disturbances have occurred.

Effects on the ears. Reviews of ototoxicity associated with vancomycin therapy:[1,2] the actual number of cases is quite small, and close examination suggests that in most cases where hearing loss occurred patients had also received an aminoglycoside. The degree, and the reversibility, of ototoxicity associated with vancomycin alone is uncertain.

1. Bailie GR, Neal D. Vancomycin ototoxicity and nephrotoxicity: a review. *Med Toxicol* 1988; **3:** 376–86.
2. Brummett RE, Fox KE. Vancomycin- and erythromycin-induced hearing loss in humans. *Antimicrob Agents Chemother* 1989; **33:** 791–6.

Effects on the gastro-intestinal tract. A 25-year-old woman developed *Clostridium difficile* colitis following a course of vancomycin and metronidazole, both by mouth, for pelvic inflammatory disease.[1] The condition resolved after treatment with vancomycin given alone.

1. Bingley PJ, Harding GM. Clostridium difficile colitis following treatment with metronidazole and vancomycin. *Postgrad Med J* 1987; **63:** 993–4.

Effects on the heart. A report[1] of cardiac arrest associated with inadvertent and rapid intravenous administration of vancomycin 150 mg to a neonate.

1. Boussemart T, *et al.* Cardiac arrest associated with vancomycin in a neonate. *Arch Dis Child* 1995; **73:** F123.

Effects on the kidneys. Nephrotoxicity was seen in 14 of 101 patients assigned to vancomycin 1 g before and after vascular surgery for infection prophylaxis, compared with 2 of 99 assigned to saline placebo in one study,[1] suggesting that even short regimens of vancomycin can affect renal function. In a study involving 224 patients, nephrotoxicity was seen in 8 of 168 given vancomycin alone, 14 of 63 given vancomycin with an aminoglycoside, and 11 of 103 given an aminoglycoside without vancomycin.[2] This latter study found that concomitant aminoglycoside therapy, trough serum concentrations of vancomycin greater than 10 μg per mL, and prolonged vancomycin therapy (for more than 21 days) were associated with an increased risk of nephrotoxicity. In both studies nephrotoxicity was defined in terms of increased serum-creatinine.

1. Gudmundsson GH, Jensen LJ. Vancomycin and nephrotoxicity. *Lancet* 1989; **i:** 625.
2. Rybak MJ, *et al.* Nephrotoxicity of vancomycin, alone and with an aminoglycoside. *J Antimicrob Chemother* 1990; **25:** 679–87.

Effects on the nervous system. Reports of encephalopathy[1] (associated with high CSF concentrations after oral administration) and peripheral neuropathy[2] associated with vancomycin.

1. Thompson CM, *et al.* Absorption of oral vancomycin—possible associated toxicity. *Int J Pediatr Nephrol* 1983; **4:** 1–4.
2. Leibowitz G, *et al.* Mononeuritis multiplex associated with prolonged vancomycin treatment. *Br Med J* 1990; **300:** 1344.

Effects on the skin. Skin reactions associated with vancomycin have commonly been rash, erythema, or pruritus but there have also been reports of linear IgA dermatosis,[1] Stevens-Johnson-like reaction,[2] bullous eruption,[3] and exfoliative dermatitis.[3] In one analysis, risk factors for adverse cutaneous reactions were suggested to be age under 40 years and duration of therapy greater than 7 days.[3]

1. Piketty C, *et al.* Linear IgA dermatosis related to vancomycin. *Br J Dermatol* 1994; **130:** 130–1.
2. Laurencin CT, *et al.* Stevens-Johnson-like reaction with vancomycin treatment. *Ann Pharmacother* 1992; **26:** 1520–1.
3. Korman TM, *et al.* Risk factors for adverse cutaneous reactions associated with intravenous vancomycin. *J Antimicrob Chemother* 1997; **39:** 371–81.

Local reactions. Garrelts and colleagues[1] have reported that despite the view that thrombophlebitis is less frequent with more highly purified preparations of vancomycin it may still be common: in 6 patients receiving vancomycin as solutions containing 4 or 5 mg per mL a total of 35 sites were used and phlebitis developed at 32. The intraperitoneal infusion of vancomycin has been associated with chemical peritonitis, and it has been suggested that it might be associated with less highly purified brands of the drug,[2] but others have failed to confirm such reports.[3]

1. Garrelts JC, *et al.* Phlebitis associated with vancomycin therapy. *Clin Pharm* 1988; **7:** 720–1.
2. Smith TA, *et al.* Chemical peritonitis associated with intraperitoneal vancomycin. *DICP Ann Pharmacother* 1991; **25:** 602–3.
3. Abel SR. Lack of chemical peritonitis after intraperitoneal use of two brands of vancomycin hydrochloride. *Clin Pharm* 1989; **8:** 91–2.

Red-man syndrome. References to the 'red-man syndrome',[1-13] including the suggestion that pretreatment with an antihistamine can provide significant protection against it.[8,10] Similar reactions do not appear to be a problem with teicoplanin and substitution of teicoplanin for vancomycin may be a viable alternative in patients at risk.[12-14] Skin tests are reported[15] to be of little value in predicting the severity of 'red-man syndrome'.

1. Southorn PA, *et al.* Adverse effects of vancomycin administered in the perioperative period. *Mayo Clin Proc* 1986; **61:** 721–4.
2. Pau AK, Khakoo R. "Red-neck" syndrome with slow infusion of vancomycin. *N Engl J Med* 1985; **313:** 756–7.
3. Davis RL, *et al.* The "red man's syndrome" and slow infusion of vancomycin. *Ann Intern Med* 1986; **104:** 285–6.
4. Best CJ, *et al.* Perioperative complications following the use of vancomycin in children: a report of two cases. *Br J Anaesth* 1989; **62:** 576–7.
5. Healy DP, *et al.* Vancomycin-induced histamine release and "red man syndrome": comparison of 1- and 2-hour infusions. *Antimicrob Agents Chemother* 1990; **34:** 550–4.
6. Levy M, *et al.* Vancomycin-induced red man syndrome. *Pediatrics* 1990; **86:** 572–80.
7. Bailie GR, *et al.* Red-neck syndrome associated with intraperitoneal vancomycin. *Clin Pharm* 1990; **9:** 671–2.
8. Wallace MR, *et al.* Red man syndrome: incidence, etiology, and prophylaxis. *J Infect Dis* 1991; **164:** 1180–5.
9. Rybak MJ, *et al.* Absence of "red man syndrome" in patients being treated with vancomycin or high-dose teicoplanin. *Antimicrob Agents Chemother* 1992; **36:** 1204–7.
10. Sahai J, *et al.* Influence of antihistamine pretreatment on vancomycin-induced red-man syndrome. *J Infect Dis* 1989; **160:** 876–81.
11. Anonymous. Red men should go: vancomycin and histamine release. *Lancet* 1990; **335:** 1006–7.
12. Sahai J, *et al.* Comparison of vancomycin- and teicoplanin-induced histamine release and "red man syndrome". *Antimicrob Agents Chemother* 1990; **34:** 765–9.
13. Polk RE. Anaphylactoid reactions to glycopeptide antibiotics. *J Antimicrob Chemother* 1991; **27** (suppl B): 17–29.
14. Smith SR. Vancomycin and histamine release. *Lancet* 1990; **335:** 1341.
15. Polk RE, *et al.* Vancomycin skin tests and prediction of "red man syndrome" in healthy volunteers. *Antimicrob Agents Chemother* 1993; **37:** 2139–43.

AFTER ORAL ADMINISTRATION. Reports of rash[1] and 'red-man syndrome'[2,3] following oral administration of vancomycin.

1. McCullough JM, *et al.* Oral vancomycin-induced rash: case report and review of the literature. *DICP Ann Pharmacother* 1991; **25:** 1326–8.
2. Killian AD, *et al.* Red man syndrome after oral vancomycin. *Ann Intern Med* 1991; **115:** 410–11.
3. Bergeron L, Boucher FD. Possible red-man syndrome associated with systemic absorption of oral vancomycin in a child with normal renal function. *Ann Pharmacother* 1994; **28:** 581–4.

Precautions

Vancomycin should not be given to patients who have experienced a hypersensitivity reaction to it. It should not be given intramuscularly, and care should be taken when it is given intravenously to avoid extravasation, because of the risk of tissue necrosis. The adverse effects of infusion may be minimised by dilution of each 500 mg of vancomycin in at least 100 mL of fluid, and by infusion of doses over not less than 60 minutes.

Because the risk of ototoxicity and nephrotoxicity is thought to be increased at high plasma concentrations it may be desirable to adjust dosage requirements according to plasma-vancomycin concentrations. It has been suggested that dosage should be adjusted to avoid peak plasma concentrations above 30 to 40 μg per mL and trough concentrations exceeding 10 μg per mL, although uncertainty about the optimum methods and sampling times for monitoring, as well as some uncertainty about the degree of risk, means that there is less general agreement than for the aminoglycosides. It is agreed, however, that vancomycin should be generally avoided in patients with a history of deafness and that particular care is necessary in patients with renal impairment, in neonates (especially if premature), and in the elderly, all of whom may be at increased risk of toxicity. Renal function and blood counts should be monitored regularly in all patients, and monitoring of auditory function is advisable, especially in patients with the risk factors mentioned. Vancomycin should be discontinued in patients who develop tinnitus.

Since vancomycin is poorly absorbed, toxicity is much less of a problem following oral administration than with the intravenous route but care is required in patients with inflammatory gastro-intestinal disorders, including antibiotic-associated colitis, in whom absorption may be enhanced.

Interactions

Other ototoxic or nephrotoxic drugs, such as the aminoglycosides and loop diuretics, markedly increase the risk of toxicity and should be given concomitantly with vancomycin only with great caution.

Some of the adverse effects of vancomycin may be enhanced by the concurrent use of general anaesthetics; it has been suggested that, where patients require both, vancomycin infusions should be completed before the induction of anaesthesia.

Vancomycin may increase neuromuscular blockade produced by drugs such as suxamethonium or vecuronium.

Antimicrobial Action

Vancomycin is a glycopeptide antibiotic with a primarily bactericidal action against a variety of Gram-positive bacteria.

Mechanism of action. It exerts its action by inhibiting the formation of the peptidoglycan polymers of the bacterial cell wall. Unlike penicillins which act primarily to prevent the cross-linking of peptidoglycans which gives the cell wall its strength, vancomycin prevents the transfer and addition of the muramylpentapeptide building blocks that make up the peptidoglycan molecule itself. Vancomycin may also exert some effects by damaging the cytoplasmic membrane of the protoplast, and by inhibiting bacterial RNA synthesis.

Spectrum of activity. Staphylococci, notably *Staph. aureus* and *Staph. epidermidis* (including methicillin-resistant strains), *Streptococcus pneumoniae, Str. pyogenes*, and some strains of Group B streptococci are reported to be susceptible to vancomycin. The viridans streptococci, and enterococci such as *Enterococcus faecalis*, are often 'tolerant', i.e. inhibition, but no bactericidal effect, can be achieved at usual plasma concentrations (but see Activity with other Antimicrobials and Resistance, below).

Clostridium difficile is usually highly susceptible but other clostridia vary somewhat in their susceptibility; *Actinomyces* spp., *Bacillus anthracis*, *Corynebacterium* spp., some lactobacilli, and *Listeria* are usually susceptible. Virtually all Gram-negative organisms, as well as mycobacteria and fungi, are intrinsically resistant.

Minimum inhibitory concentrations (MICs) of vancomycin for the most susceptible organisms range from about 0.1 to 2 μg per mL; for most organisms it is bactericidal at concentrations not far above the MIC. Organisms with MICs up to about 4 μg per mL are generally considered sensitive to vancomycin, and those with MICs between about 4 and 16 μg per mL of intermediate sensitivity.

Activity with other antimicrobials. Vancomycin exhibits synergy with the aminoglycosides against enterococci; such combinations are usually bactericidal, even against vancomycin-tolerant strains. The synergistic effect is reported to be greater with gentamicin than with streptomycin. Combinations with an aminoglycoside are also reported to demonstrate synergy against *Staph. aureus*; however, variable results, including antimicrobial antagonism, or lack of synergy, have been reported against strains of *Staph. aureus* when vancomycin was combined with rifampicin. Synergy has been reported with the third-generation cephalosporins against *Staph. aureus* and enterococci.

Resistance to vancomycin in normally susceptible organisms has until recently remained relatively uncommon, although high-level intrinsic resistance has been seen in some species of *Lactobacillus*, *Leuconostoc*, and *Erysipelothrix*. However, there are an increasing number of reports of high-level acquired resistance amongst enterococci, apparently plasmid-mediated and transferable to other Gram-positive organisms, notably *Staph. aureus*, which are causing considerable concern. Organisms exhibiting high-level vancomycin resistance demonstrate cross-resistance to teicoplanin. Low-level resistance has also been reported in enterococci, but these organisms remain sensitive to teicoplanin, and this form of resistance does not appear to be transferable. Low-level vancomycin resistance has also been seen rarely among some staphylococcal strains: in contrast to the enterococci, these are often cross-resistant to teicoplanin. The mechanism of acquired resistance is uncertain, although it appears to be associated with the development of novel cell-membrane proteins.

Reference[1] to increasing resistance to vancomycin amongst enterococci, including its possible transferral to *Staphylococcus aureus*, and guidelines to prevent its spread.[2,3]

1. Murray BE. Vancomycin-resistant enterococci. *Am J Med* 1997; **102:** 284–93.
2. Edmond MB, *et al.* Vancomycin-resistant Staphylococcus aureus: perspectives on measures needed for control. *Ann Intern Med* 1996; **124:** 329–34.
3. Hospital Infection Control Practices Advisory Committee (HICPAC). Recommendations for preventing the spread of vancomycin resistance. *Infect Control Hosp Epidemiol* 1995; **16:** 105–13.

Pharmacokinetics

Vancomycin is only poorly absorbed from the gastro-intestinal tract although absorption may be somewhat greater when the gastro-intestinal tract is inflamed. Intramuscular administration is associated with pain and tissue necrosis; systemic doses are therefore given intravenously. Infusion of a 1-g dose intravenously over 60 minutes has reportedly been associated with plasma concentrations of up to about 60 μg per mL immediately after completion of the infusion, and about 25 μg per mL 2 hours later, falling to under 10 μg per mL after 11 hours. However, there may be considerable interindividual variation in the pharmacokinetics of vancomycin: a range of half-lives between 3 and 13 hours has been reported, with an average of about 6 hours, in patients with normal renal function. Half-life may be prolonged in patients with renal impairment, to 7 days or more in anephric patients. About 55% is bound to plasma proteins though large variations have been reported.

Vancomycin diffuses into extracellular fluid, including pleural, pericardial, ascitic, and synovial fluid. Small amounts are found in bile. However, there is little diffusion into the CSF and even when the meninges are inflamed effective concentrations may not be achieved. Vancomycin crosses the peritoneal cavity; about 60% of an intraperitoneal dose is reported to be absorbed in 6 hours. It is reported to cross the placenta. It is also distributed into breast milk.

Little or no metabolism of vancomycin is thought to take place. It is excreted unchanged by the kidneys, mostly by glomerular filtration. Some 80 to 90% of the dose is excreted in urine within 24 hours. There appears to be a small amount of non-renal clearance, although the mechanism for this has not been determined.

As for the aminoglycosides, the pharmacokinetics of vancomycin may be altered by conditions which affect renal clearance: clearance of vancomycin has been reported to be enhanced in burn patients, whereas in those with renal impairment, or reduced renal function (such as neonates or the elderly) clearance is reduced, and plasma-concentrations and half-lives increased. Dosage adjustment is often necessary in patients with reduced or impaired renal function; ideally, this should be based on plasma-concentration monitoring. Although clearance is also altered in hepatic impairment, it has been suggested that dosage adjustment is not necessary in the absence of other factors.

Plasma concentrations of vancomycin are reported to be little affected by conventional haemodialysis, although the use of high-flux membranes may significantly reduce vancomycin concentrations. Peritoneal dialysis, although it may decrease concentrations, is also held not to do so by significant amounts, but haemoperfusion or haemofiltration effectively removes vancomycin from the blood.

Uses and Administration

Vancomycin is a glycopeptide antibiotic that is used in the treatment of serious staphylococcal or other Gram-positive infections where other drugs such as the penicillins cannot be used because of resistance or patient intolerance. It is used particularly in the treatment of methicillin-resistant staphylococcal infections (p.144), in conditions such as brain abscess, staphylococcal meningitis, peritonitis associated with continuous ambulatory peritoneal dialysis, and septicaemia. It is used alone, or in combination with another drug such as an aminoglycoside, in the treatment and prophylaxis of endocarditis, for the prophylaxis of surgical infection, and in intensive care and the management of immunocompromised patients. It is also used (by mouth) in the treatment of antibiotic-associated colitis (see under Gastro-enteritis, p.123). For details of all these infections and their treatment, see under Choice of Antibacterial, p.116.

Vancomycin may be used concomitantly with other antibacterials to extend the spectrum of efficacy or increase effectiveness, notably with gentamicin or other aminoglycosides, or with rifampicin (but see Antimicrobial Action, above).

Administration and dosage. Vancomycin is given as the hydrochloride but doses are expressed in terms of the base. It is administered intravenously, preferably by intermittent infusion, although continuous infusion has been used. For intermittent infusion, a concentrated solution containing the equivalent of 500 mg of vancomycin in 10 mL of water is prepared and then added to glucose 5% or sodium chloride 0.9% to produce a diluted solution containing not more than 5 mg per mL; this diluted solution is then infused over at least 60 minutes for a 500-mg dose or 100 minutes for a 1-g dose. Final concentrations of up to 10 mg per mL may be used for patients requiring fluid restriction, although there is an increased risk of adverse events. For continuous intravenous infusion, the equivalent of 1 to 2 g is added to a sufficiently large volume of glucose or sodium chloride to permit the daily dose to be given over a period of 24 hours.

The usual adult dose is the equivalent of 500 mg of vancomycin every 6 hours or 1 g every 12 hours. Response is generally seen within 48 to 72 hours in sensitive infections. In patients with staphylococcal endocarditis treatment for at least 3 weeks has been recommended.

For the prophylaxis of endocarditis in high-risk penicillin-allergic patients undergoing dental or other procedures, vancomycin may be given before the procedure in a single dose of 1 g by intravenous infusion over at least 100 minutes followed by intravenous gentamicin.

Doses in infants and children. Children may be given 10 mg per kg body-weight every 6 hours. Neonates may be given an initial dose of 15 mg per kg followed by 10 mg per kg every 12 hours in the first week of life, and every 8 hours up to the age of one month.

For the prophylaxis of endocarditis in children a single dose of 20 mg per kg has been suggested.

Dose adjustment and monitoring. It has been recommended that dosage should be adjusted if necessary according to plasma-vancomycin concentrations, and this is particularly important where factors such as age or renal impairment may predispose to toxicity, or where there is a risk of subtherapeutic concentrations. There has been some dispute about the relationship between plasma concentrations and toxicity, and this, complicated by differences in the sampling time after the end of infusion and by differences in the regimens administered and assay method used, has meant that suggested peak and trough concentrations have varied considerably. However in order to avoid toxic concentrations immediately after the end of infusion the consensus appears to be that concentrations of not more than 30 to 40 μg per mL should be aimed for 1 to 2 hours after completion of infusion. It is usually recommended that trough concentrations (measured just before the next dose) should be below 10 μg per mL, but a number of centres seem to accept trough concentrations below 15 μg per mL, and this may permit improved therapeutic activity against less-sensitive staphylococci.

Various methods, including predictive nomograms based on creatinine clearance and pharmacokinetic methods such as those using Bayesian statistics have been suggested for calculating vancomycin dosage requirements in patients with reduced renal function (see also below). One suggested approach has been a loading dose of 15 mg per kg followed by a daily dose in mg equivalent to about 15 times the glomerular filtration rate in mL per minute; or in anuric patients a dose of 1 g every 7 to 10 days. However, individualised dosage based on plasma concentrations is generally to be preferred.

Other routes. Vancomycin hydrochloride is administered by mouth in the treatment of staphylococcal enterocolitis and antibiotic-associated colitis including pseudomembranous colitis associated with the overgrowth of *Clostridium difficile*. It is given in a dose of 0.5 to 2.0 g daily in 3 or 4 divided doses for 7 to 10 days; the lowest dose of 0.5 g daily is often considered adequate. A dose for children is 40 mg per kg body-weight daily in 3 or 4 divided doses; some authorities suggest that half this dose is adequate.

In meningitis or other CNS infections vancomycin has sometimes been given by the intrathecal or intraventricular route in order to ensure adequate CSF concentrations of antibiotic. Vancomycin has also been applied topically to the eye or given by subconjunctival or intravitreal injection; it has also been given by inhalation.

Administration. References to methods of determining vancomycin dosage and the necessity for monitoring plasma concentrations.

1. Nielsen HE, *et al.* Renal excretion of vancomycin in kidney disease. *Acta Med Scand* 1975; **197:** 261–4.
2. Moellering RC, *et al.* Vancomycin therapy in patients with impaired renal function: a nomogram for dosage. *Ann Intern Med* 1981; **94:** 343–6.
3. Rotschafer JC, *et al.* Pharmacokinetics of vancomycin; observations in 28 patients and dosage recommendations. *Antimicrob Agents Chemother* 1982; **22:** 391–4.
4. Matzke GR, *et al.* Pharmacokinetics of vancomycin in patients with various degrees of renal function. *Antimicrob Agents Chemother* 1984; **25:** 433–7.
5. Matzke GR, *et al.* Evaluation of the vancomycin-clearance: creatinine-clearance relationship for predicting vancomycin dosage. *Clin Pharm* 1985; **4:** 311–15.
6. Rybak MJ, Boike SC. Monitoring vancomycin therapy. *Drug Intell Clin Pharm* 1986; **20:** 757–61.
7. Healy DP, *et al.* Comparison of steady-state pharmacokinetics of two dosage regimens of vancomycin in normal volunteers. *Antimicrob Agents Chemother* 1987; **31:** 393–7.
8. Rodvold KA, *et al.* Evaluation of a two-compartment Bayesian forecasting program for predicting vancomycin concentrations. *Ther Drug Monit* 1989; **11:** 269–75.
9. Pryka RD, *et al.* Individualizing vancomycin dosage regimens: one- vs two-compartment Bayesian models. *Ther Drug Monit* 1989; **11:** 450–4.
10. Pryka RD, *et al.* An updated comparison of drug dosing methods part IV: vancomycin. *Clin Pharmacokinet* 1991; **20:** 463–76.
11. Gabriel MH, *et al.* Prospective evaluation of a vancomycin dosage guideline for neonates. *Clin Pharm* 1991; **10:** 129–32.
12. Ackerman BH, Vanmier AM. Necessity of a loading dose when using vancomycin in critically ill patients. *J Antimicrob Chemother* 1992; **29:** 460–1.
13. Freeman CD, *et al.* Vancomycin therapeutic drug monitoring: is it necessary? *Ann Pharmacother* 1993; **27:** 594–8.
14. Saunders NJ. Why monitor peak vancomycin concentrations? *Lancet* 1994; **344:** 1748–50. [Subsequent correspondence. *ibid.* 1995; **345:** 645–7.]
15. Leader WG, *et al.* Pharmacokinetic optimisation of vancomycin therapy. *Clin Pharmacokinet* 1995; **28:** 327–42.
16. Marra F, *et al.* Vancomycin serum concentration monitoring: the middle ground is best. *Clin Drug Invest* 1996; **12:** 105–18.
17. Shackley F, *et al.* Trough-only monitoring of serum vancomycin concentrations in neonates. *J Antimicrob Chemother* 1998; **41:** 141–2.

Preparations

BP 1998: Vancomycin Injection;
USP 23: Sterile Vancomycin Hydrochloride; Vancomycin Hydrochloride Capsules; Vancomycin Hydrochloride for Injection; Vancomycin Hydrochloride for Oral Solution; Vancomycin Injection.

Proprietary Preparations (details are given in Part 3)
Austral.: Vancocin; Vancoled; ***Belg.:*** Vancocin; ***Canad.:*** Vancocin; ***Fr.:*** Vancocine; ***Ger.:*** VANCO; ***Irl.:*** Vancocin; ***Ital.:*** Vancocina; ***Neth.:*** Vancocin; ***Norw.:*** Vancocin; ***S.Afr.:*** Vancocin; ***Spain:*** Diatracin; ***Swed.:*** Vancocin; Vancoled†; Vancoscand; ***Switz.:*** Vancocin; ***UK:*** Vancocin; ***USA:*** Lyphocin; Vancocin; Vancoled; Vancor†.

Virginiamycin (178-k)

Virginiamycin *(BAN, USAN, rINN).*

Antibiotic 899; SKF-7988; Virgimycin.

CAS — 11006-76-1; 21411-53-0 (virginiamycin M_1*); 23152-29-6 (virginiamycin* S_1*).*

A mixture consisting principally of 2 antimicrobial substances, virginiamycin M_1, and virginiamycin S_1, produced by the growth of *Streptomyces virginiae.*

Adverse Effects

Virginiamycin may cause gastro-intestinal disturbances including diarrhoea and vomiting. A few instances of hypersensitivity have been observed.

Antimicrobial Action

Virginiamycin has a spectrum of antimicrobial activity similar to that of erythromycin (p.205). It is active against staphylococci and some streptococci; *Neisseria gonorrhoeae* and *Haemophilus influenzae* are reported to be sensitive.

Cross-resistance is often observed between streptogramins, macrolides, and lincosamides.

References to the action of streptogramins (synergistins, synergimycins) such as virginiamycin, and the synergistic interaction of their macrolide and depsipeptide components.

1. Le Goffic F. Structure activity relationships in lincosamide and streptogramin antibiotics. *J Antimicrob Chemother* 1985; **16** (suppl A): 13–21.

2. Duval J. Evolution and epidemiology of MLS resistance. *J Antimicrob Chemother* 1985; **16** (suppl A): 137–49.
3. Di Giambattista M, *et al.* The molecular basis of the inhibitory activities of type A and type B synergimycins and related antibiotics on ribosomes. *J Antimicrob Chemother* 1989; **24:** 485–507.

Resistance. References.

1. Welton LA, *et al.* Antimicrobial resistance in enterococci isolated from turkey flocks fed virginiamycin. *Antimicrob Agents Chemother* 1998; **42:** 705–8.

Pharmacokinetics

Virginiamycin is incompletely absorbed following a dose by mouth. Concentrations of about 1 μg per mL are found in the blood around one hour after ingestion of a dose of 500 mg. It is widely distributed in tissues and body fluids but does not cross the blood-brain barrier. It is metabolised in the liver and excreted in the bile; about 13% of a dose is excreted in the urine. The half-life is reported to be about 5 hours.

Uses and Administration

Virginiamycin is a streptogramin antibiotic used for the treatment of infections due to sensitive organisms, particularly Gram-positive cocci. The usual dose by mouth is 2 to 3 g daily in divided doses increased to 4 g daily if necessary in severe infections. Children have been given 50 to 100 mg per kg body-weight daily. It has been applied locally in a dusting-powder or 0.5% ointment.

Virginiamycin is used in animal feeding stuffs as a production enhancer.

Preparations

Proprietary Preparations (details are given in Part 3)
Fr.: Staphylomycine†.

Multi-ingredient: *Belg.:* Spitalen.

Xibornol (14022-f)

Xibornol *(BAN, rINN)*.

CP3H; IHP; IBX. 6-(Isoborn-2-yl)-3,4-xylenol; 6-[(1*R*,2*S*,4*S*)-Born-2-yl]-3,4-xylenol.

$C_{18}H_{26}O$ = 258.4.

CAS — 38237-68-2; 13741-18-9.

Xibornol is an antimicrobial that is reported to have a bacteriostatic action on Gram-positive organisms such as staphylococci and streptococci, as well as activity against *Haemophilus influenzae*. It is given by mouth in doses of 1 to 1.5 g daily; it has also been given rectally.

Preparations

Proprietary Preparations (details are given in Part 3)
Fr.: Nanbacine; *Ital.:* Bracen†.

Multi-ingredient: *Spain:* Xibornol Prodes.

Antidepressants

This chapter describes drugs used principally in the treatment of affective disorders. Affective disorders are disorders of mood that may manifest as *depression* or *mania* or, in some cases, as *mixed affective states* in which depressive and manic episodes may coexist or alternate.

The core features of depressive disorders are low mood, anhedonia (the loss of interest in former pleasures or activities), pessimism, and lethargy. They were formerly classified either as *endogenous*, in which the symptoms were independent of external factors and considered to be a consequence of factors within the patient, or *reactive*, in which depressive symptoms were a result of external stressors (i.e. exogenous). It is now recognised that depressive disorders are composed of both endogenous and reactive factors. Similarly, the classification of *neurotic depression* is no longer considered useful because it encompasses several different syndromes. Depressive episodes are classified according to severity as mild, moderate, severe, or severe with psychosis. *Recurrent brief depression* is defined as depressive episodes of a few days duration that recur regularly. Depression is often accompanied by characteristic *somatic* symptoms, including anorexia, weight loss, insomnia, early morning waking, and psychomotor retardation. Symptoms associated with *atypical depression* include overeating and oversleeping.

The main symptoms of *mania* are overactivity, mood changes ranging from elation to irritability, expansive ideas, and inflated self-importance. Manic episodes are classified according to severity in a similar manner to depressive disorders: namely, mild, moderate, severe, or severe with psychosis. *Hypomania* is differentiated from mania in terms of a reduction in intensity of symptoms and social incapacity.

Alternating episodes of mania and depression are termed *manic depression* (or more precisely *bipolar disorder*). Since it is very rare for repeated episodes of mania to occur without alternating episodes of depression, it is accepted practice to include mania without depression within the bipolar category. The term *unipolar disorder* (*unipolar depression*) is reserved for depressive disorders without mania.

Persistent but mild disturbances of mood exist in which the symptoms are not severe enough to meet the criteria for classification as a major depressive or hypomanic disorder, but may nevertheless cause considerable suffering to the patient. *Dysthymia* is the term used to describe a chronic depressive state whereas *cyclothymia* has some similarity to bipolar disorder, the instability characterised by long periods of milder elation and milder depression.

The term *seasonal affective disorder* has been applied to depressive disorders repeatedly occurring seasonally, but not related to seasonal stressful life events; the depressive symptoms usually occur during the autumn and winter months. There have also been reports of patients developing seasonal bipolar disorder with hypomania or mania occurring in the summer months.

Anxiety is often associated with depressive disorders at all levels of severity and it may be difficult to distinguish between the two conditions, especially in the milder forms. *Mixed anxiety and depressive disorder* defines a state in which anxiety and depressive symptoms coexist but neither component is severe enough to merit classification as an anxiety disorder or a depressive disorder.

Classification of antidepressants. Antidepressants are classified into different groups either structurally or depending on which central neurotransmitters they act upon. The older tricyclic and related cyclic antidepressants and the monoamine oxidase inhibitors (MAOIs) have now been joined by the selective serotonin reuptake inhibitors (SSRIs), the reversible inhibitors of monoamine oxidase type A (RIMAs) (e.g. moclobemide), and more recently by the serotonin and noradrenaline reuptake inhibitors (SNRIs) (e.g. venlafaxine). Other antidepressants that do not fit exactly into these groups include bupropion, mirtazapine, nefazodone, reboxetine, trazodone, and viloxazine.

Lithium salts provide a source of lithium ions that compete with sodium ions at various sites in the body and thus have an action and side-effects distinct and separate from those of other antidepressants.

Depression

Clinical depression (unipolar depression) is a disturbance of mood that is distinguishable from the usual mood fluctuations of everyday life. A depressed mood is usually the major symptom, which may be accompanied by a variety of other mental or somatic symptoms representing several depressive syndromes.

The aetiology of depression is unknown but it may represent an interaction between psychological and biochemical mechanisms rather than any single factor. The symptoms appear to be mediated through alterations in levels of some central neurotransmitters, although it is not certain that this represents a cause of the disorder. However, it is at this level that the antidepressant drugs currently in clinical use exert their action.

There are several approaches to the treatment of depression depending on the severity of the condition and the risks to the patient, and these have been summarised in consensus statements in the UK[1,2] and the USA.[3] Although the most common form of treatment is with an antidepressant drug, other forms of treatment may also be of value in some situations. Psychosocial or psychotherapeutic management may be effective alone in mild depressive disorders or may be used in conjunction with antidepressants[1,3] or following electroconvulsive therapy (ECT). ECT is used in severe depression or when the patient has not responded to drug therapy; it has been given in repeated courses without evidence of brain damage.[4] ECT is of particular value when a rapid improvement in symptoms is essential (e.g. patients at high risk of suicide), and for patients with depressive psychosis or psychomotor retardation.[3,4] Light therapy appears to be effective in patients with seasonal affective disorder.[5] Exposure to bright artificial light may take place at any time of the day,[3] and the therapy should continue until the natural seasonal remission of the disorder; antidepressant drugs may also be used.[3]

CHOICE OF ANTIDEPRESSANT. Tricyclic antidepressants have long been preferred over MAOIs for the treatment of depressive episodes[6] because of the problem of drug interactions and the need for strict dietary precautions required for the latter group. Unfortunately, the traditional tricyclics such as amitriptyline are associated with adverse effects that can limit their use or cause patient distress, and because of their cardiotoxicity they are associated with a high risk of fatality in patients taking overdoses with suicidal intent. The emergence of new antidepressants over the last few years has improved the treatment options for patients.[6,7] Several drugs related to the tricyclic group such as lofepramine and mianserin are less cardiotoxic than the earlier tricyclics.[2] Subsequently, selective serotonin reuptake inhibitors (SSRIs) such as fluoxetine were developed and provided further important improvements in adverse effect profile and safety. More recently serotonin and noradrenaline reuptake inhibitors (SNRIs) such as venlafaxine have been developed, as well as reversible inhibitors of monoamine oxidase type A (RIMAs) such as moclobemide. Antidepressants such as nefazodone, mirtazapine, and reboxetine, which have slightly different biochemical profiles from the major groups, have also been recently introduced.

While such improvements are welcome, they have not been accompanied by any marked improvement in antidepressant activity. This has led to much debate about the choice of antidepressant therapy, most of that debate focussing on the choice between a tricyclic or an SSRI. There are arguments supporting the first-choice use of SSRIs because of fewer unpleasant side-effects,[8] although they do cause a different range of adverse effects which may be a problem in some patients; the same arguments can also be applied to the SNRIs, RIMAs, and other new antidepressants. Nevertheless, the tricyclics remain the preferred first choice of many practitioners because of wide experience with their use and familiarity with their pharmacological actions.[1,2,9] Tricyclics with *sedative properties* may be more suitable for agitated and anxious patients, whereas those with *less sedative properties* may be preferred for withdrawn and apathetic patients. Tricyclics have *antimuscarinic* and *cardiotoxic* side-effects to varying degrees, and these properties will preclude their use in some patients, for whom the SSRIs may be a safer choice. However, the SSRIs themselves have characteristic side-effects; *gastro-intestinal symptoms* such as nausea and vomiting may be a problem, and *sleep disturbances* and *anxiety* may be exacerbated at the start of treatment. Moreover, those in current clinical use *interact to varying degrees* with cytochrome P450 isoenzymes, which carries a potential for interaction with a wide range of compounds.[6]

MAOIs are rarely used as first-choice antidepressants, but are particularly effective in atypical depression.[2,3] RIMAs offer a safer alternative to the MAOIs and fewer dietary restrictions are necessary.[10]

The sedative properties of some of the antidepressants may adversely affect the performance of potentially hazardous tasks such as *driving and the operation of machinery*. It would therefore be prudent to select one of the less sedative antidepressants where appropriate, although caution is warranted in this respect with all psychotropic drugs, especially at the start of treatment.

An area of particular concern with regard to initial choice of antidepressant drug is the most appropriate drug for patients considered to be a high suicide risk.[11] Varying relative risks of *toxicity in overdosage* for different groups of antidepressant have been assessed:[12-14] older tricyclics and maprotiline[15] appear to be more toxic in overdosage than mianserin[16] and the SSRIs;[14] MAOIs have an intermediate risk.[17] Within the tricyclic group, desipramine[12,13] has been reported to be associated more frequently with fatal overdosage whereas lofepramine[18] may be one of the safer tricyclics. Although such analyses cannot determine to what extent the data reflect prescribing patterns and patient selection as opposed to drug toxicity[12,13,18] it is widely accepted that the older tricyclics are toxic in overdosage, and that safer options are the SSRIs[19,20] and the newer tricyclic and related cyclic antidepressants.[20] In practice, it is often difficult to identify patients at high risk for suicide, and it has therefore been suggested that a routine strategy should be to initiate antidepressant therapy in all patients with drugs that have low toxicity in overdose.[11,20] However, whichever antidepressant is chosen, all patients should be closely monitored during early therapy until improvement in depression has been observed and limited quantities of antidepressants should be prescribed at any one time.

Several options exist for those who show no response to an adequate trial of the first-choice antidepressant. A drug with a different biochemical profile may be substituted;[3] alternatively, some patients may respond preferentially to another drug within the same group.[21,22] MAOIs can be tried in patients who are refractory to or intolerant of treatment with other antidepressants. Lithium may be used for the prophylaxis of recurrent unipolar depression as an alternative to standard antidepressants, although it is more commonly used in the management of bipolar disorder (see Manic Depression below); its role in unipolar depression is more usually to augment the effect of standard antidepressants in drug-resistant patients. Other drugs that have been used in augmentation strategies for resistant depression include thyroid hormones (liothyronine) and central stimulants[3] such as methylphenidate. Pindolol has also been studied as an augmentation agent in combination with several SSRIs and other serotonergic antidepressants. Because of an association with the eosinophilia-myalgia syndrome, the use of tryptophan is severely restricted; in the UK, it is reserved for use as an adjunct only, in patients with severe and disabling depression refractory to other treatment (see p.310).

Antidepressant effects may also be augmented by coadministration of a second antidepressant with a different mechanism of action.[3] Although combination therapy with differing classes of antidepressants has been used successfully in the treatment of drug-resistant depression, it may result in enhanced adverse reactions or interactions and is therefore considered unsuitable or controversial by some authorities; it should only ever be employed under expert supervision. For further details of the interactions between different antidepressants when coadministered, see under Interactions of Phenelzine, p.305.

Other drugs used in the treatment of depression include flupenthixol, the antidepressant dose of which is lower than that used for the treatment of psychoses. Ademetionine, the active derivative of methionine, has been tried in depressive disorders, and extracts of the plant hypericum (St John's wort) (*Hypericum perforatum*) are widely used in Germany for depression.[23,24]

MANAGEMENT OF ANTIDEPRESSANT THERAPY. Although the adverse effects of antidepressant drugs appear soon after treatment is initiated, there is a delay of about two weeks before any therapeutic benefit is observed, and at least six weeks before maximum improvement in depressive symptoms occurs.[6] Claims of a fast onset of action have been made for several antidepressants, but in a review[25] of data relating to onset of action with currently available antidepressants, none has been shown conclusively to work faster than any other. The delay in onset of antidepressant effect may relate to a combination of pharmacokinetic and neurochemical factors.

In order to minimise adverse effects, antidepressant therapy is usually initiated with a low dose, which is then increased gradually over 1 to 2 weeks until an adequate response is observed.[1] However, this approach must be balanced against the need to obtain a full therapeutic effect as soon as possible. Gradual introduction of treatment is of particular importance in the elderly who may be more susceptible to adverse effects. Patients should not be considered resistant to the chosen drug until they have been maintained at an adequate dose for 6 to 8 weeks.[3] Treatment failure is often due to subtherapeutic doses being used,[2] particularly with the older tricyclics whose adverse effects limit maximum tolerable doses in many patients.[26] Therapeutic drug monitoring is not usually considered necessary or even useful for routine antidepressant therapy, although there are instances when it may be of value such as when a patient's compliance is uncertain.[3]

If response to the drug is good, the patient should continue with the same drug for at least 4 to 6 months;[1-3] symptoms are likely to recur if treatment is discontinued prematurely.[27] It is often recommended that doses should be reduced for maintenance treatment but this view has been challenged and the recommendation made that the dose closest to that which achieved clinical response should be used unless adverse effects are intolerable.[1-3] Continuation of antidepressant therapy beyond this phase[28] is a matter of clinical judgement. Prophylactic maintenance therapy should be considered for recurrent depressive disorders,[1-3,27,29] and may be necessary for several years in some cases. Again, full therapeutic doses are recommended for prophylaxis rather than reduced doses.[29]

When changing a patient from one type of antidepressant to another due regard should be given to allowing the appropriate drug-free interval between the 2 drugs. An MAOI (including a RIMA) should not be started until at least one week after stopping a tricyclic antidepressant, an SSRI, or any related antidepressant; in the case of the SSRIs paroxetine and sertraline the drug-free interval is extended to two weeks, and for fluoxetine, to five weeks because of their longer half-lives. Conversely, two weeks should elapse between discontinuing MAOI therapy and starting patients on a tricyclic antidepressant, an SSRI, or any related antidepressant. A drug-free interval is not necessary following discontinuation of a RIMA. Sudden discontinuation of antidepressant therapy after regular administration for 8 weeks or more may precipitate withdrawal symptoms,[30,31] which can be minimised by a gradual reduction in dosage; most authorities recommend reducing the dose over a period of about 4 weeks.

DEPRESSION IN CHILDREN. Depressive disorders may arise in childhood and adolescence, the prevalence increasing with age.[32] Treatment generally commences with psychosocial and psychotherapeutic methods, followed by antidepressant therapy if no improvement is seen after 4 to 6 weeks.[32,33] SSRIs[32-34] and lofepramine[32] are considered the optimum first choices in children and adolescents because they are less toxic in overdose. The older tricyclics are reserved for refractory cases in adolescents and may be augmented with lithium;[33] ECT may be used in severe depression.[32] Some authorities recommend avoiding desipramine because of reports of death due to cardiac toxicity in 4 children.[34]

DEPRESSION IN THE ELDERLY. Depression in the elderly may be particularly severe and the suicide risk higher compared with younger adults.[35,36] Altered metabolism and urinary excretion in elderly patients may increase the risks of adverse effects with tricyclic antidepressants; the cardiotoxicity of this particular group of drugs may also be a problem.[37] In this respect, the SSRIs offer many significant advantages for the management of elderly depressed patients.[38,39] Lower initial doses of antidepressant drugs are often recommended in the elderly to minimise adverse effects but individual differences in metabolism and excretion may mean that some patients are undertreated.[36] The elderly tend to respond more slowly to antidepressants than younger patients and therefore concomitant psychosocial or psychotherapeutic management may be warranted. ECT is a safe and effective treatment in the elderly,[37] although temporary memory impairment after treatment in some patients may limit its use to those at high risk for suicide or who are refractory to or intolerant of antidepressant drugs. Depression late in life may require long-term antidepressant treatment beyond the recovery phase, even after first episodes of depression and should be a continuation of the treatment that was successful in the initial acute phase.[39]

DEPRESSION IN PREGNANCY. Treatment of women with depressive disorders during and after pregnancy raises concerns about the risk of teratogenicity, fetal growth retardation, or perinatal problems; the ratio of risk to benefit must therefore be considered very carefully before antidepressant drugs are administered.[40,41] Maternal mood disorders in the immediate postpartum period are related to hormonal changes, particularly falling progesterone levels; the symptoms are mild and resolve spontaneously after several days, therefore no treatment is required.[42,43] Of greater concern are major depressive episodes that occur beyond this initial phase, which are clinically identical to depressive disorders in general and call for the same principles of management.[43] These depressive episodes have been found to be related to the presence of immediate postpartum mood disorders, although no hormonal basis to this association has been identified.[44] Nevertheless, there is interest in the use of oestrogen as a treatment.[45]

As with administration of any medication to nursing mothers, the risks to the infant from drugs distributed into breast milk must be considered. The American Academy of Pediatrics[46,47] considers that all antidepressants are drugs whose effect on nursing infants could be of concern.

DEPRESSION WITH ANXIETY. Symptoms of anxiety and depression often coexist, and although it may be difficult to distinguish which is the predominant disorder, especially in milder forms, patients usually require an antidepressant. Anxiolytics and antipsychotics can be useful adjuncts in agitated depression, but a sedative antidepressant might be preferable. Combination preparations of antidepressants with antipsychotics or anxiolytics should not be used because the dosage of the individual components should be adjusted separately. Also, anxiolytics should only be prescribed on a short-term basis whereas antidepressants are given for several months.

DEPRESSION IN CHRONIC FATIGUE SYNDROME. Although no randomised double-blind studies assessing the efficacy of antidepressants in chronic fatigue syndrome have been published it has been suggested that antidepressant therapy should be tried in depressed patients.[48] Controlled trials of antidepressants in non-depressed patients with chronic fatigue syndrome are particularly needed.[48]

1. Paykel ES, Priest RG. Recognition and management of depression in general practice: consensus statement. *Br Med J* 1992; **305:** 1198–1202.
2. Montgomery SA, *et al.* Guidelines for treating depressive illness with antidepressants: a statement from the British Association for Psychopharmacology. *J Psychopharmacol* 1993; **7:** 19–23.
3. American Psychiatric Association. Practice guidelines for major depressive disorder in adults. *Am J Psychiatry* 1993; **150** (suppl): 1–26.
4. Scott AIF. Contemporary practice of electroconvulsive therapy. *Br J Hosp Med* 1994; **51:** 334–8.
5. Partonen T, Lönnqvist J. Seasonal affective disorder. *Lancet* 1998; **352:** 1369–74.
6. Richelson E. Pharmacology of antidepressants—characteristics of the ideal drug. *Mayo Clin Proc* 1994; **69:** 1069–81.
7. Möller H-J, Volz H-P. Drug treatment of depression in the 1990s: an overview of achievements and future possibilities. *Drugs* 1996; **52:** 625–38.
8. Harrison G. New or old antidepressants: new is better. *Br Med J* 1994; **309:** 1280–1.
9. Owens D. New or old antidepressants: benefits of new drugs are exaggerated. *Br Med J* 1994; **309:** 1281–2.
10. Lecrubier Y. Risk-benefit assessment of newer versus older monoamine oxidase (MAO) inhibitors. *Drug Safety* 1994; **10:** 292–300.
11. Henry JA. Epidemiology and relative toxicity of antidepressant drugs in overdose. *Drug Safety* 1997; **16:** 374–90.
12. Beaumont G. The toxicity of antidepressants. *Br J Psychiatry* 1989; **154:** 454–8.
13. Kapur S, *et al.* Antidepressant medications and the relative risk of suicide attempt and suicide. *JAMA* 1992; **268:** 3441–5.
14. de Jonghe F, Swinkels JA. The safety of antidepressants. *Drugs* 1992; **43** (suppl 2): 40–7.
15. Knudsen KAI, Heath A. Effects of self poisoning with maprotiline. *Br Med J* 1984; **288:** 601–3.
16. Inman WHW. Blood disorders and suicide in patients taking mianserin or amitriptyline. *Lancet* 1988; **ii:** 90–2.
17. Cassidy S, Henry J. Fatal toxicity of antidepressant drugs in overdose. *Br Med J* 1987; **295:** 1021–4.
18. Malmvik J, *et al.* Antidepressants in suicide: differences in fatality and drug utilisation. *Eur J Clin Pharmacol* 1994; **46:** 291–4.
19. Henry JA, *et al.* Relative mortality from overdose of antidepressants. *Br Med J* 1995; **310:** 221–4. Correction. *ibid.;* 911.
20. Freemantle N, *et al.* Prescribing selective serotonin reuptake inhibitors as strategy for prevention of suicide. *Br Med J* 1994; **309:** 249–53.
21. Brown WA, Harrison W. Are patients who are intolerant to one serotonin selective reuptake inhibitor intolerant to another? *J Clin Psychiatry* 1995; **56:** 30–4.
22. Joffe RT, *et al.* Response to an open trial of a second SSRI in major depression. *J Clin Psychiatry* 1996; **57:** 114–15.
23. Linde K, *et al.* St John's wort for depression—an overview and meta-analysis of randomised clinical trials. *Br Med J* 1996; **313:** 253–8.
24. de Smet PAGM, Nolen WA. St John's wort as an antidepressant. *Br Med J* 1996; **313:** 241–2.
25. Soares JC, Gershon S. Prospects for the development of new treatments with a rapid onset of action in affective disorders. *Drugs* 1996; **52:** 477–82.
26. Kendrick T. Prescribing antidepressants in general practice. *Br Med J* 1996; **313:** 829–30.
27. Angst J. A regular review of the long term follow up of depression. *Br Med J* 1997; **315:** 1143–6.
28. Edwards JG. Long term pharmacotherapy of depression. *Br Med J* 1998; **316:** 1180–1.
29. Montgomery SA. Prophylactic treatment of depression. *Br J Hosp Med* 1994; **52:** 5–7.
30. Dilsaver SC. Withdrawal phenomena associated with antidepressant and antipsychotic agents. *Drug Safety* 1994; **10:** 103–114.
31. Haddad P, *et al.* Antidepressant discontinuation reactions. *Br Med J* 1998; **316:** 1105–6.
32. Mirza KAH, Michael A. Major depression in children and adolescents. *Br J Hosp Med* 1996; **55:** 57–61.
33. Harrington R. Depressive disorder in adolescence. *Arch Dis Child* 1995; **72:** 193–5.
34. Carrey NJ, *et al.* Pharmacological treatment of psychiatric disorders in children and adolescents: focus on guidelines for the primary care practitioner. *Drugs* 1996; **51:** 750–9.
35. Wattis J. What an old age psychiatrist does. *Br Med J* 1996; **313:** 101–4.
36. Waern M, *et al.* High rate of antidepressant treatment in elderly people who commit suicide. *Br Med J* 1996; **313:** 1118.
37. Mendels J. Clinical management of the depressed geriatric patient: current therapeutic options. *Am J Med* 1993; **94** (suppl 5A): 13S–18S.
38. Preskorn SH. Recent pharmacologic advances in antidepressant therapy for the elderly. *Am J Med* 1993; **94** (suppl 5A): 2S–12S.
39. Lebowitz BD, *et al.* Diagnosis and treatment of depression in late life: consensus statement update. *JAMA* 1997; **278:** 1186–90.
40. Robert E. Treating depression in pregnancy. *N Engl J Med* 1996; **335:** 1056–8.
41. Schou M. Treating recurrent affective disorders during and after pregnancy: what can be taken safely? *Drug Safety* 1998; **18:** 143–52.
42. Harris B, *et al.* Maternity blues and major endocrine changes: Cardiff puerperal mood and hormone study II. *Br Med J* 1994; **308:** 949–53.
43. Murray D. Oestrogen and postnatal depression. *Lancet* 1996; **347:** 918–19.
44. Cooper PJ, Murray L. Postnatal depression. *Br Med J* 1998; **316:** 1884–6.
45. Gregoire AJP, *et al.* Transdermal oestrogen for treatment of severe postnatal depression. *Lancet* 1996; **347:** 930–3.
46. American Academy of Pediatrics Committee on Drugs. The transfer of drugs and other chemicals into human milk. *Pediatrics* 1994; **93:** 137–50.

47. Berlin CM. American Academy of Pediatrics Committee on Drugs. Drugs and breast milk. *Pediatrics* 1995; **95:** 957–8.
48. The Royal Colleges of Physicians, Psychiatrists and General Practitioners. *Chronic Fatigue Syndrome*. London, 1997.

Manic depression

Bipolar disorder (manic depression) is a mixed affective disorder in which the patient experiences alternating episodes of hypomania or mania and depression. Although isolated episodes of mania may occur, they are more usually part of bipolar disorder; for the purposes of classification, mania without depression is therefore included in the bipolar category. Bipolar disorder is usually treated with mood-stabilising drugs, the most important of which is lithium. Electroconvulsive therapy (ECT) is also effective and is used for example in patients for whom lithium treatment is unsuitable or in patients refractory to lithium or other drugs.

Drug therapy of the manic phase is directed at controlling the acute attack, maintaining that response, and preventing further attacks. Lithium is effective in acute mania but it may take a few days before an antimanic effect is seen. Treatment in acutely agitated manic patients is therefore usually initiated with an antipsychotic to produce a rapid tranquillising effect; typical drugs include the phenothiazine chlorpromazine and the butyrophenones droperidol and haloperidol. The antipsychotic may be used in conjunction with lithium, and then gradually withdrawn once lithium becomes effective, but due consideration should be given to the risks from interactions between antipsychotics and lithium (see under Interactions of Lithium, p.294). Alternatively, initiation of lithium therapy may be postponed until the acute attack has been stabilised with the antipsychotic. Benzodiazepines have also been used until lithium has achieved its full effect; they should not be used for long periods owing to the risk of dependence.

Once the acute phase has been brought under control drug treatment should continue until it is safe to expect that the patient will not suffer a relapse; this might entail maintaining treatment for several months. High doses of lithium are usually required to control the acute phase, but as the margin between the therapeutic and the toxic concentration of lithium is narrow, the dose should be reduced to maintenance levels as soon as practicable. Regular monitoring of serum concentrations of lithium is essential during the initial and maintenance phases of therapy to minimise the risks of lithium toxicity (see under Pharmacokinetics of Lithium, p.294).

Depression follows the manic phase in bipolar disorder, and patients receiving an antipsychotic may also require antidepressant treatment, as may those on lithium even though it possesses antidepressant activity. Treatment of the depressive phase of bipolar disorder is essentially similar to that of unipolar depression (see above), but extra caution is warranted because some antidepressant drugs may precipitate hypomania or mania. Antidepressants have also been implicated in the induction of rapid cycling, in which there are four or more affective episodes in a year. Some authorities recommend that, if the use of an antidepressant drug is necessary, it should be given in the lowest effective dose and for the shortest time possible, or should not be given long term without the cover of a mood-stabilising drug.

Patients with recurrent episodes of bipolar disorder may require prophylactic therapy with lithium. Sometimes prophylaxis may be instituted following treatment of a first episode where there is an expectation of repeated attacks. Lithium prophylaxis usually entails extending the maintenance treatment and continuing to monitor serum concentrations as before; it may need to be continued for a prolonged period. Some authorities have also given antipsychotics, either alone or with lithium, for prophylaxis.

When lithium therapy is to be discontinued, withdrawal should be gradual over a period of weeks to allay any concerns about relapse.

Should the above treatments fail in an acute attack of mania or in the prophylaxis of bipolar disorder, then antiepileptics offer another approach. Those that have been used include carbamazepine and valproate. Carbamazepine is used in the prophylaxis of bipolar disorder and appears to be particularly effective in rapid cycling. Valproate is used in the treatment of the acute manic phase; safety and efficacy for long-term use in excess of three weeks remains to be established.

References.

1. Aronson JK, Reynolds DJM. Lithium. *Br Med J* 1992; **305:** 1273–6.
2. Goodwin GM. Drug treatment in mania. *Prescribers' J* 1994; **34:** 19–26.
3. Price LH, Heninger GR. Lithium in the treatment of mood disorders. *N Engl J Med* 1994; **331:** 591–8.
4. American Psychiatric Association. Practice guideline for the treatment of patients with bipolar disorder. *Am J Psychiatry* 1994; **151** (suppl): 1–36.
5. Silverstone T, Romans S. Long term treatment of bipolar disorder. *Drugs* 1996; **51:** 367–82.
6. Anonymous. Drugs for psychiatric disorders. *Med Lett Drugs Ther* 1997; **39:** 33–40.
7. Swann AC, *et al.* Depression during mania: treatment response to lithium or divalproex. *Arch Gen Psychiatry* 1997; **54:** 37–42.
8. Daly I. Mania. *Lancet* 1997; **349:** 1157–60.

Mania

Although isolated episodes of mania may occur, mania is usually followed by depression when it is considered to be part of bipolar disorder (manic depression). It is accepted practice to include mania without depression within the bipolar category. The treatment of acute attacks of mania and their prophylaxis are therefore described under Manic Depression, above.

Amesergide (14579-y)

Amesergide *(USAN, rINN)*.

LY-237733. *N*-Cyclohexyl-1-isopropyl-6-methylergoline-8β-carboxamide.

$C_{25}H_{35}N_3O$ = 393.6.

CAS — 121588-75-8.

Amesergide is a selective serotonin antagonist under investigation for the treatment of depression.

Amesergide was found to be a potent inhibitor of the debrisoquine/sparteine hydroxylase CYP2D6.[1] Pharmacokinetic interactions are therefore to be expected between amesergide and substrates of CYP2D6, which include most tricyclic antidepressants and many antipsychotics of the phenothiazine and butyrophenone types.

1. Baumann P, *et al.* Influence of amesergide treatment on the dextromethorphan test. *Br J Clin Pharmacol* 1994; **38:** 151–2.

Amineptine Hydrochloride (12358-q)

Amineptine Hydrochloride *(rINNM)*.

S-1694. 7-[(10,11-Dihydro-5*H*-dibenzo[*a*,*d*]cyclohepten-5-yl)amino]heptanoic acid hydrochloride.

$C_{22}H_{27}NO_2$,HCl = 373.9.

CAS — 57574-09-1 (amineptine); 30272-08-3 (amineptine hydrochloride).

Amineptine hydrochloride is a tricyclic antidepressant (see Amitriptyline, below). Amineptine hydrochloride has been given by mouth in the treatment of depression in doses of 100 to 200 mg daily.

Hepatic adverse effects seem to be more common than with most other tricyclic antidepressants (see Effects on the Liver, p.274). Also amineptine has been subject to abuse and withdrawal has been both prolonged and difficult.

In 5 patients very severe acne-type lesions were associated with the chronic self-increased administration of high doses of amineptine (200 to 1000 mg daily).[1] The presence of an unusual lactam form of metabolites was detected in all patients and in 2 these metabolites were still present, along with the lesions, 3 months after therapy had been withdrawn.

1. Vexiau P, *et al.* Severe acne-like lesions caused by amineptine overdose. *Lancet* 1988; **i:** 585.

Preparations

Proprietary Preparations (details are given in Part 3)
Fr.: Survector; ***Ital.:*** Maneon; Survector; ***Spain:*** Survector.

Amitriptyline (12293-g)

Amitriptyline *(BAN, rINN)*.

3-(10,11-Dihydro-5*H*-dibenzo[*a*,*d*]cyclohepten-5-ylidene)propyldimethylamine; 10,11-Dihydro-*N*,*N*-dimethyl-5*H*-dibenzo[*a*,*d*]cycloheptene-$\Delta^{5,\gamma}$-propylamine.

$C_{20}H_{23}N$ = 277.4.

CAS — 50-48-6.

Amitriptyline Embonate (2501-v)

Amitriptyline Embonate *(BANM, rINNM)*.

$(C_{20}H_{23}N)_2,C_{23}H_{16}O_6$ = 943.2.

CAS — 17086-03-2.

Pharmacopoeias. In *Br.*

A pale yellow to brownish-yellow, odourless or almost odourless powder. Amitriptyline embonate 1.5 g is approximately equivalent to 1 g of amitriptyline hydrochloride and 0.88 g of amitriptyline. Practically **insoluble** in water; slightly soluble in alcohol; freely soluble in chloroform. **Protect** from light.

Amitriptyline Hydrochloride (2502-g)

Amitriptyline Hydrochloride *(BANM, rINNM)*.

Amitriptylini Hydrochloridum.

$C_{20}H_{23}N$,HCl = 313.9.

CAS — 549-18-8.

Pharmacopoeias. In *Chin., Eur.* (see p.viii), *Int., Jpn, Pol.,* and *US.*

Odourless or almost odourless, colourless crystals or white or almost white powder.

Freely **soluble** in water, in alcohol, in chloroform, in dichloromethane, and in methyl alcohol; practically insoluble in ether. A 1% solution in water has a pH of 5.0 to 6.0. **Protect** from light.

Stability. Decomposition occurred when solutions of amitriptyline hydrochloride in water or phosphate buffers were autoclaved at 115° to 116° for 30 minutes in the presence of excess oxygen.[1] The decomposition of amitriptyline as the hydrochloride in buffered aqueous solution was accelerated by metal ions particularly from amber glass ampoules.[2] Disodium edetate 0.1% significantly reduced the decomposition rate of these amitriptyline solutions but propyl gallate and hydroquinone were less effective. Sodium metabisulphite produced an initial lowering of amitriptyline concentration and subsequently an acceleration of decomposition.

Solutions of amitriptyline hydrochloride in water are stable for at least 8 weeks at room temperature if protected from light either by storage in a cupboard or in amber containers.[3] Decomposition to ketone and, to a lesser extent, other unidentified products was found to occur on exposure to light.

1. Enever RP, *et al.* Decomposition of amitriptyline hydrochloride in aqueous solution: identification of decomposition products. *J Pharm Sci* 1975; **64:** 1497–9.
2. Enever RP, *et al.* Factors influencing decomposition rate of amitriptyline hydrochloride in aqueous solution. *J Pharm Sci* 1977; **66:** 1087–9.
3. Buckles J, Walters V. The stability of amitriptyline hydrochloride in aqueous solution. *J Clin Pharm* 1976; **1:** 107–12.

Adverse Effects

Many side-effects of amitriptyline and similar tricyclic antidepressants are caused by their antimuscarinic actions. The antimuscarinic side-effects are relatively common and occur before an antidepressant effect is obtained. Tolerance is often achieved if treatment is continued and side-effects may be less troublesome if treatment is initiated with small doses and then increased gradually, although this may delay the clinical response. Antimuscarinic effects include dry mouth, constipation occasionally leading to paralytic ileus, urinary retention, blurred vision and disturbances in accommodation, increased intra-ocular pressure, and hyperthermia.

Drowsiness may also be a common side-effect. Conversely, a few tricyclic antidepressants possess little or no sedative potential and nervousness and insomnia may occur.

Other neurological adverse effects include headache, peripheral neuropathy, tremor, ataxia, epileptiform seizures, tinnitus, and occasional extrapyramidal symptoms including speech difficulties; confusion or delirium may occur, particularly in the elderly. Gastro-intestinal complaints include sour or metallic taste, stomatitis, and gastric irritation with nausea and vomiting.

Various effects on the cardiovascular system have been reported and are discussed in more detail under Effects on the Cardiovascular System, below. Orthostatic hypotension and tachycardia may occur in patients without a history of cardiovascular disease, and may be particularly troublesome in the elderly.

Hypersensitivity reactions, such as urticaria and angioedema, and photosensitisation have been reported and, rarely, cholestatic jaundice and blood disorders, including eosinophilia, bone-marrow depression, thrombocytopenia, leucopenia, and agranulocytosis.

Endocrine effects include testicular enlargement, gynaecomastia and breast enlargement, and galactorrhoea. Sexual dysfunction may also occur. Changes in blood sugar concentrations may also occur, and, very occasionally, hyponatraemia associated with inappropriate secretion of antidiuretic hormone.

Other side-effects that have been reported are increased appetite with weight gain (or occasionally anorexia with weight loss). Sweating may be a problem.

Symptoms of **overdosage** may include excitement and restlessness with marked antimuscarinic effects, including dryness of the mouth, dilated pupils, tachycardia, urinary retention, and intestinal stasis. Severe symptoms include unconsciousness, convulsions and myoclonus, hyperreflexia, hypotension, acidosis, and respiratory and cardiac depression, with life-threatening cardiac arrhythmias that may recur some days after apparent recovery.

Tricyclics and other antidepressants with high affinity for muscarinic receptors are more likely to cause antimuscarinic side-effects than those with low affinity.[1] Studies *in vitro* showed antidepressant affinities for human muscarinic acetylcholine receptors to be, in descending order: amitriptyline, protriptyline, clomipramine, trimipramine, doxepin, imipramine, nortriptyline, desipramine, amoxapine, maprotiline, trazodone. The effect of affinities for other receptor sites was less certain, although those antidepressants with high affinity for histamine H_1 receptors might be expected to be more sedating. Affinities for *murine* histamine H_1 receptors in descending order were: doxepin, trimipramine, amitriptyline, maprotiline, amoxapine, nortriptyline, imipramine, clomipramine, protriptyline, trazodone, desipramine.

1. Richelson E. Antimuscarinic and other receptor-blocking properties of antidepressants. *Mayo Clin Proc* 1983; **58:** 40–6.

Effects on the blood. Following a case report of agranulocytosis linked with imipramine, review of the literature suggested that agranulocytosis associated with tricyclic antidepressant use was a rare idiosyncratic condition, resulting from a direct toxic effect rather than an allergic mechanism, and particularly affected the elderly from 4 to 8 weeks after beginning treatment.[1]

Neutropenia reported[2] in a patient after separate exposure to two tricyclic antidepressants, namely imipramine and nortriptyline, indicated that there may be cross-intolerance between the tricyclic antidepressants and if neutropenia developed with one member of the group the use of others on future occasions should be avoided.

Between 1963 and 1993 the UK Committee on Safety of Medicines had received 912 reports of drug-induced agranulocytosis of which 38 were due to tricyclic antidepressants (12 fatal) and 1499 cases of neutropenia of which 46 were due to tricyclics (0 fatal).[3]

In a report[4] on a patient who developed aplastic anaemia associated with concomitant therapy with remoxipride and dothiepin it was noted that up to May 1993 the UK Committee on Safety of Medicines had received 11 reports of aplastic anaemia secondary to dothiepin treatment.

1. Albertini RS, Penders TM. Agranulocytosis associated with tricyclics. *J Clin Psychiatry* 1978; **39:** 483–5.
2. Draper BM, Manoharan A. Neutropenia with cross-intolerance between two tricyclic antidepressant agents. *Med J Aust* 1987; **146:** 452–3.
3. Committee on Safety of Medicines/Medicines Control Agency. Drug-induced neutropenia and agranulocytosis. *Current Problems* 1993; **19:** 10–11.
4. Philpott NJ, *et al.* Aplastic anaemia and remoxipride. *Lancet* 1993; **342:** 1244–5.

Effects on the cardiovascular system. The cardiotoxic potential of tricyclic antidepressants after overdosage is widely acknowledged; symptoms include arrhythmias, conduction defects, and hypotension. This factor was, in part, responsible for the development of antidepressants with different chemical structures and pharmacological properties that are less cardiotoxic. It also led to some concern over whether tricyclic antidepressants had adverse effects on the heart or cardiovascular system when used in usual therapeutic doses.

Since the introduction of the tricyclic antidepressants, several reports, often anecdotal, have been published of adverse cardiovascular effects and have included malignant hypertension with amitriptyline,[1] and cardiomyopathy in a patient who had received amitriptyline and imipramine.[2] Sudden cardiac death in patients with pre-existing cardiac disease has been linked with amitriptyline[3-5] or imipramine,[4] although the Boston Collaborative Drug Surveillance Program failed to substantiate these findings.[6]

Re-evaluations and reviews of this topic[7,8] concluded that the only significant or serious cardiovascular side-effects, seen in patients with no previous history of cardiovascular disease given therapeutic doses of tricyclic antidepressants, are orthostatic hypotension and tachycardia, and that these effects may be particularly troublesome in elderly patients. However, there have been reports of sudden death in 4 children given desipramine when plasma concentrations were not above therapeutic values;[9,10] it was known that one of the children had no cardiac abnormality.

In patients with overt heart disease it was considered[7] that the only ones likely to be at increased risk were those with intraventricular conduction abnormalities; in patients with a history of myocardial infarction or angina, but free of conduction defects, the use of tricyclics appeared to be primarily limited by the degree to and frequency with which they developed orthostatic hypotension. In a re-evaluation of the risks/benefits of tricyclics in patients with ischaemic heart disease no consensus was reached.[11] In practice the authors used selective serotonin reuptake inhibitors (SSRIs) or bupropion as first-choice therapy in patients with ischaemic heart disease who were mildly or moderately depressed; tricyclics were reserved for patients not responding and were also used as first-choice therapy for patients with more severe depression despite cardiac risks.

1. Dunn FG. Malignant hypertension associated with use of amitriptyline hydrochloride. *South Med J* 1982; **75:** 1124–5.
2. Howland JS, *et al.* Cardiomyopathy associated with tricyclic antidepressants. *South Med J* 1983; **76:** 1455–6.
3. Coull DC, *et al.* Amitriptyline and cardiac disease. *Lancet* 1970; **ii:** 590–1.
4. Moir DC, *et al.* Cardiotoxicity of amitriptyline. *Lancet* 1972; **ii:** 561–4.
5. Moir DC, *et al.* Medicines evaluation and monitoring group: a follow-up study of cardiac patients receiving amitriptyline. *Eur J Clin Pharmacol* 1973; **6:** 98–101.
6. Boston Collaborative Drug Surveillance Program. Adverse reactions to the tricyclic-antidepressant drugs: report from Boston Collaborative Drug Surveillance Program. *Lancet* 1972; **i:** 529–31.
7. Glassman AH. Cardiovascular effects of tricyclic antidepressants. *Annu Rev Med* 1984; **35:** 503–11.
8. Mortensen SA. Cyclic antidepressants and cardiotoxicity. *Practitioner* 1984; **228:** 1180–3.
9. Anonymous. Sudden death in children treated with a tricyclic antidepressant. *Med Lett Drugs Ther* 1990; **32:** 53.
10. Riddle MA, *et al.* Another sudden death in a child treated with desipramine. *J Am Acad Child Adolesc Psychiatry* 1993; **32:** 792–7.
11. Glassman AH, *et al.* The safety of tricyclic antidepressants in cardiac patients: risk-benefit reconsidered. *JAMA* 1993; **269:** 2673–5.

EFFECTS ON THE PERIPHERAL CIRCULATION. Painful vasospastic episodes, characterised by cold and blue hands and feet, have been reported in one woman each time she received imipramine 150 mg daily but only with amitriptyline when the dose was increased to 200 mg daily.[1] This led the authors to suggest that the ability of tricyclic antidepressants to induce vasospasm was not limited to imipramine and that the effect may be partly dose-dependent. Additionally, acrocyanosis of the hands and feet has occurred in a child receiving imipramine for nocturnal enuresis.[2]

1. Appelbaum PS, Kapoor W. Imipramine-induced vasospasm: a case report. *Am J Psychiatry* 1983; **140:** 913–15.
2. Anderson RP, Morris BAP. Acrocyanosis due to imipramine. *Arch Dis Child* 1988; **63:** 204–5.

Effects on the endocrine system. The *syndrome of inappropriate antidiuretic hormone secretion with hyponatraemia* has been reported in patients receiving tricyclics and other antidepressants. The Committee on Safety of Medicines in the UK, commenting on reports it had received of hyponatraemia associated with the antidepressants (fluoxetine, paroxetine, lofepramine, clomipramine, and imipramine), considered that it was likely to occur with any antidepressant and usually involved elderly patients.[1] Case reports of hyponatraemia in 24 patients treated with tricyclics and 20 patients treated with other antidepressants have been summarised.[2]

In a review covering the effects of drugs on *prolactin secretion*[3] it was stated that antidepressants could affect prolactin secretion by disturbing the balance of catecholaminergic inhibition and serotonergic stimulation of prolactin release, although any change is less than with antipsychotic therapy. Clomipramine and nortriptyline had been reported to stimulate prolactin release whereas amitriptyline, desipramine, and imipramine had been reported to be without effect. Such stimulation may account for symptoms of galactorrhoea or amenorrhoea reported with some tricyclics.

1. Committee on Safety of Medicines/Medicines Control Agency. Antidepressant-induced hyponatraemia. *Current Problems* 1994; **20:** 5–6.
2. Spigset O, Hedenmalm K. Hyponatraemia and the syndrome of inappropriate antidiuretic hormone secretion (SIADH) induced by psychotropic drugs. *Drug Safety* 1995; **12:** 209–25.
3. Hell K, Wernze H. Drug-induced changes in prolactin secretion: clinical implications. *Med Toxicol* 1988; **3:** 463–98.

Effects on the gastro-intestinal tract. By 1978 the Committee on Safety of Medicines in the UK had been notified of cases of ileus, probably resulting from the antimuscarinic effects of tricyclic antidepressants.[1] Various tricyclics were taken by different patients, there being no suggestion that any one was especially liable to cause ileus. Fortunately the complication appeared to be rare.

1. Committee on Safety of Medicines. *Current Problems 3* 1978.

Effects on the kidneys and urine. Haematuria has been observed in a patient receiving amitriptyline and carbamazepine;[1] amitriptyline was implicated as carbamazepine had been taken alone for an extensive period without producing this symptom.

Mention has also been made of amitriptyline producing a blue-green colour in urine,[2] although it was considered to be a rare phenomenon.

1. Gillman MA, Sandyk R. Hematuria following tricyclic therapy. *Am J Psychiatry* 1984; **141:** 463–4.
2. Beeley L. *Br Med J* 1986; **293:** 750.

Effects on the liver. Of 91 cases of hepatitis due to antidepressant therapy (including tricyclic antidepressants), 63 occurred in patients receiving amineptine, sometimes with other psychotropic agents; in approximately 50% of these amineptine cases, benzodiazepines had also been taken and it was postulated that the benzodiazepines may have increased the oxidation of amineptine to a toxic metabolite.[1] Most patients presented with abdominal pain and mixed liver damage with predominant cholestasis. One died after myocardial infarction, but all the others recovered. The mean amineptine dosage was 200 mg daily. In comparison, only 10 of the 91 cases were attributed to other tricyclic antidepressants, being amitriptyline (4), clomipramine (3), demexiptiline (2), and dibenzepin (1). Cross hepatotoxicity has also been reported in one patient between amineptine and clomipramine.[2]

Hepatotoxicity has also been noted with lofepramine. The UK Committee on Safety of Medicines had by the end of 1987 received 57 reports of abnormal liver function tests associated with lofepramine.[3] They included hepatic failure (1), jaundice (9), and hepatitis (5). All reactions occurred within the first 8 weeks of treatment and all were reversible on discontinuation of the drug.

1. Lefebure B, *et al.* Hépatites aux antidépresseurs. *Therapie* 1984; **39:** 509–16.
2. Larrey D, *et al.* Cross hepatotoxicity between tricyclic antidepressants. *Gut* 1986; **27:** 726–7.
3. Committee on Safety of Medicines. Lofepramine (Gamanil) and abnormal blood tests of liver function. *Current Problems 23* 1988.

Effects on the mouth. The inhibition of salivation caused by tricyclic antidepressants (in this case clomipramine) has been implicated in dental caries formation.[1]

1. deVries MW, Peeters F. Dental caries with longterm use of antidepressants. *Lancet* 1995; **346:** 1640.

Effects on the nervous system. In addition to drowsiness, especially with those with antihistaminic activity, a variety of effects on the nervous system have been attributed to tricyclic antidepressants, including peripheral neuropathy, tremor, ataxia, confusion, and delirium. Of particular concern is a reduction in the seizure threshold (see Epileptogenic Effect, below). Extrapyramidal effects and neuroleptic malignant syndrome (see below) may also occasionally occur.

Effects on sexual function. Loss of libido and impotence are common symptoms of depression, often making the role of drugs in producing sexual dysfunction difficult to assess.[1]

Sedation due to tricyclic antidepressants may lead to loss of libido and many of the tricyclics have been reported to cause impotence.[1,2] Amitriptyline, clomipramine, desipramine, doxepin, nortriptyline, and trimipramine have been stated to delay or inhibit ejaculation, and amoxapine, imipramine, and protriptyline, also to cause painful ejaculation. However, some tricyclics have been used for their effect on ejaculation to treat patients for premature ejaculation (see Clomipramine, p.282).

In women, anorgasmia or delayed orgasm has been reported with amitriptyline, amoxapine, clomipramine, and imipramine,[1-3] although spontaneous orgasm associated with yawning has been reported with clomipramine.[4]

1. Beeley L. Drug-induced sexual dysfunction and infertility. *Adverse Drug React Acute Poisoning Rev* 1984; **3:** 23–42.
2. Anonymous. Drugs that cause sexual dysfunction. *Med Lett Drugs Ther* 1987; **29:** 65–70.
3. Shen WW, Sata LS. Inhibited female orgasm resulting from psychotropic drugs: a clinical review. *J Reprod Med* 1983; **28:** 497–9.
4. McLean JD, *et al.* Unusual side effects of clomipramine associated with yawning. *Can J Psychiatry* 1983; **28:** 569–70.

Effects on the skin. Hypersensitivity reactions to tricyclic antidepressants are said to be uncommon.[1] Urticaria and angioedema have occurred, the urticaria occasionally clearing without drug withdrawal. Pruritus is also uncommon, but may be associated with transient erythema. Photosensitivity reactions are far less common than with phenothiazines, but have been reported. Rarely exfoliative dermatitis has developed, and purpura, pigmentation, and lichen planus have been noted in isolated reports. Hypersensitivity reactions to antidepressants usually occur between 14 and 60 days after the start of treatment.[2]

With regard to photosensitivity reactions protriptyline has been the tricyclic most frequently implicated.[3,4]

Toxic epidermal necrolysis has been reported in a patient 2 weeks after commencing therapy with amoxapine.[5]

Amitriptyline and fluoxetine have been implicated in the development of atypical cutaneous lymphoid hyperplasia in 8 patients, 7 of whom either had an underlying immunosuppressant systemic disease or were receiving concomitant therapy with immunomodulatory drugs.[6] The lesions improved or resolved on discontinuation of the antidepressant, although in some patients other factors may have contributed to lesional resolution.

1. Almeyda J. Drug reactions XIII: cutaneous reactions to imipramine and chlordiazepoxide. *Br J Dermatol* 1971; **84:** 298–9.
2. Quitkin F. Cross-tolerance of tricyclic antidepressant drugs. *JAMA* 1979; **241:** 1625.
3. Smith AG. Drug-induced photosensitivity. *Adverse Drug React Bull* 1989; **136** (June): 508–11.
4. Harth Y, Rapoport M. Photosensitivity associated with antipsychotics, antidepressants and anxiolytics. *Drug Safety* 1996; **14:** 252–9.
5. Camisa C, Grines C. Amoxapine: a cause of toxic epidermal necrolysis? *Arch Dermatol* 1983; **119:** 709–10.
6. Crowson AN, Magro CM. Antidepressant therapy: a possible cause of atypical cutaneous lymphoid hyperplasia. *Arch Dermatol* 1995; **131:** 925–9.

Epileptogenic effect. In a detailed review[1] of drug-induced seizures the following points were made regarding tricyclic antidepressants. Seizures have been reported after normal therapeutic doses of tricyclic antidepressants as well as after overdosage, although the mechanism by which the seizures are induced is unclear. Seizures usually appear within a few days of starting the drug or changing to a higher dose but in patients with no previous history of epilepsy or no predisposing medical condition the frequency seems to be very low with an incidence of approximately 1 in 1000. Jick *et al.*[2] reported an incidence of 0.4 per 1000 based on 16 cases out of an estimated group of 42 000 patients receiving tricyclics and who had no predisposing factors. However, in another review[3] Rosenstein *et al.* considered that a reasonable estimate of the incidence was 3 to 6 per 1000. Thus there are variations in the reported incidence of seizures in patients without predisposing factors. However, it is widely agreed that they should be used very cautiously in patients with epilepsy or those with a low convulsive threshold.

In a retrospective analysis of 1313 cases[4] of overdosage involving cyclic antidepressants, seizures occurred more commonly with the tricyclics amoxapine (24.5%) and desipramine (17.9%), and the tetracyclic maprotiline (12.2%). In another analysis of 302 consecutive cases of tricyclic overdosage Buckley *et al.*[5] found a higher rate of seizures with dothiepin in overdosage (13%) than other tricyclics.

1. Zaccara G, *et al.* Clinical features, pathogenesis and management of drug-induced seizures. *Drug Safety* 1990; **5:** 109–51.
2. Jick SS, *et al.* Antidepressants and convulsions. *J Clin Psychopharmacol* 1992; **12:** 241–5.
3. Rosenstein DL, *et al.* Seizures associated with antidepressants: a review. *J Clin Psychiatry* 1993; **54:** 289–99.
4. Wedin GP, *et al.* Relative toxicity of cyclic antidepressants. *Ann Emerg Med* 1986; **15:** 797–804.
5. Buckley NA, *et al.* Greater toxicity in overdose of dothiepin than of other tricyclic antidepressants. *Lancet* 1994: **343:** 159–62.

Extrapyramidal effects. Various extrapyramidal effects such as orofacial and choreoathetoid movements, and dyskinesias have been attributed to treatment with tricyclic antidepressants. Mention has been made of the sensitivity to imipramine of some patients with panic disorder, developing symptoms of insomnia, jitteriness, and irritability.[1] These symptoms have also been observed in patients with panic disorder treated with low doses of desipramine although the symptoms usually subsided when the dose of the tricyclic was gradually increased. It has been suggested[2] that these symptoms may be related to akathisia and are more likely to occur with those tricyclics that have a more potent effect on inhibition of noradrenaline reuptake.

Dysarthria has been reported[3] and was said to be not uncommon in those taking higher doses of tricyclic antidepressants, but unusual at lower doses.[4]

Reviews of adverse effects of drugs on the nervous system have also listed acute torsion dystonias and tremors[5] as being caused or exacerbated by tricyclic antidepressants.

1. Yeragani VK, *et al.* Tricyclic induced jitteriness—a form of akathisia? *Br Med J* 1986; **292:** 1529.
2. Cole JO, Bodkin JA. Antidepressant drug side effects. *J Clin Psychiatry* 1990; **51** (suppl): 21–6.
3. Quader SE. Dysarthria: an unusual side effect of tricyclic antidepressants. *Br Med J* 1977; **2:** 97.
4. Saunders M. Dysarthria with tricyclic antidepressants. *Br Med J* 1977; **2:** 317.
5. Lane RJM, Routledge PA. Drug-induced neurological disorders. *Drugs* 1983; **26:** 124–47.

Hypersensitivity. See under Effects on the Skin, above.

Neuroleptic malignant syndrome. Of 16 cases of neuroleptic malignant syndrome reported to the UK Committee on Safety of Medicines by July 1986, 3 cases occurred in patients receiving a tricyclic antidepressant; a combination of amitriptyline and perphenazine had been taken by one patient and dothiepin or clomipramine alone by two other patients. The clomipramine case was fatal.[1] Amoxapine has also been involved.[2] Another report associating the syndrome with the combined use of clomipramine and triazolam has been published[3] where it was postulated that the inhibition or antagonism of dopaminergic systems may be involved.

1. Committee on Safety of Medicines. Neuroleptic malignant syndrome—an underdiagnosed condition? *Current Problems 18* 1986.
2. Madakasira S. Amoxapine-induced neuroleptic malignant syndrome. *DICP Ann Pharmacother* 1989; **23:** 50–1.
3. Domingo P, *et al.* Benign type of malignant syndrome. *Lancet* 1989; **i:** 50.

Overdosage. Tricyclic antidepressants have been associated with a higher risk of fatality following suicide attempts by drug overdose than have non-tricyclics.[1] Some consider desipramine to be associated more frequently than other tricyclic antidepressants with fatal overdosage.[2]

1. Anonymous. Antidepressant drugs and the risk of suicide. *WHO Drug Inf* 1993; **7:** 18–20.
2. Amitai Y, Frischer H. The toxicity and dose of desipramine hydrochloride. *JAMA* 1994; **272:** 1719–20.

Treatment of Adverse Effects

The basis of the management of tricyclic antidepressant poisoning is intensive supportive care and symptomatic therapy.

Since tricyclic antidepressants slow gastro-intestinal transit time, absorption may be delayed in overdosage. Following ingestion of an overdose of a tricyclic antidepressant the stomach may be emptied by emesis or lavage. The use of activated charcoal by mouth as an adjunct to gastric lavage has been suggested. Supportive therapy alone may then suffice for patients who are not severely poisoned. In particular the patient should be monitored for cardiac arrhythmias. One authority has advised that although cardiac arrhythmias are of concern some will respond to correction of hypoxia and acidosis and that the use of antiarrhythmic drugs is best avoided.

Convulsions can be managed by giving diazepam intravenously. Diazepam by mouth is usually adequate to sedate delirious patients, although large doses may be needed.

Physostigmine salicylate has been reported to be beneficial in some forms of cardiotoxicity, and in convulsions and coma but its routine use cannot be recommended because of the serious adverse effects it may cause (see Antimuscarinic Poisoning in Uses of Physostigmine, p.1396). Peritoneal dialysis, haemodialysis, and measures to increase urine production are not of value in tricyclic antidepressant poisoning, and charcoal haemoperfusion is of doubtful benefit.

Precautions

The antimuscarinic effects of tricyclic antidepressants warrant their cautious use in patients with urinary retention, prostatic hyperplasia, or chronic constipation; caution has also been advised in untreated angle-closure glaucoma and in phaeochromocytoma.

The epileptogenic potential of tricyclic antidepressants leads to caution in administering them to patients with a history of epilepsy and their potential cardiotoxicity to caution in cardiovascular disease and avoidance in heart block, cardiac arrhythmias, or in the immediate recovery period after myocardial infarction.

Blood-sugar concentrations may be altered in diabetic patients.

Because tricyclic antidepressants are metabolised and inactivated in the liver they should be used with caution in patients with impaired liver function; they should be avoided in severe liver disease. Caution has also been recommended in patients with hyperthyroidism as administration of tricyclics may precipitate cardiac arrhythmias.

Patients should be closely monitored during early antidepressant therapy until improvement in depression is observed because suicide is an inherent risk in depressed patients. For further details, see under Depression, p.271.

If tricyclic antidepressants are used for the depressive component of bipolar disorder (manic depression) mania may be precipitated; similarly, psychotic symptoms may be aggravated if tricyclics are used for a depressive component of schizophrenia.

Drowsiness is often experienced particularly at the start of therapy and patients, if affected, should not drive or operate machinery.

Regular dental check-ups are recommended for patients on long-term therapy with tricyclic antidepressants, particularly those with marked antimuscarinic actions.

Elderly patients can be particularly sensitive to the side-effects of tricyclic antidepressants and a reduced dose, especially initially, should be employed.

Tricyclic antidepressants are not recommended for depression in children. If they are used for nocturnal enuresis they should be limited to short courses with a full physical examination before subsequent courses.

Tricyclic antidepressants should be withdrawn gradually to reduce the risk of withdrawal symptoms (see below).

It has been recommended that, where possible, tricyclic antidepressants should be stopped some days before elective surgery; they should be used with caution in patients requiring concurrent electroconvulsive therapy (see also under Anaesthesia, below).

Anaesthesia. Patients receiving tricyclic antidepressants are at an increased risk of developing hypotension or cardiac arrhythmias during anaesthesia. Tricyclics may also dangerously potentiate the cardiovascular effects of vasopressor drugs such as sympathomimetics that may be required during anaesthesia. Although some manufacturers recommend stopping tricyclics several days before elective surgery where possible, this is considered by some authorities to be unnecessary as long as the anaesthetist is informed if they are not stopped.

Commenting on the anaesthetic considerations relevant to electroconvulsive therapy (ECT),[1] it was considered that concurrent therapy with tricyclic antidepressants should not be a contra-indication to anaesthesia for ECT. A major consideration, though, was said to be the interaction of tricyclics with barbiturates resulting in increased sleep time and duration of anaesthesia. This meant that lower doses of barbiturate anaesthetics should be employed.

1. Gaines GY, Rees DI. Electroconvulsive therapy and anesthetic considerations. *Anesth Analg* 1986; **65:** 1345–56.

Breast feeding. In general, only small amounts of tricyclic antidepressants are distributed into breast milk. Nevertheless, most manufacturers advise that tricyclics should be avoided by the mother during breast feeding.

Case reports indicate that amitriptyline and its metabolite, nortriptyline,[1,2] desipramine and its metabolite, 2-hydroxydesipramine,[3] dothiepin and its primary metabolites (nordothiepin, dothiepin-*S*-oxide, and nordothiepin-*S*-oxide),[4] doxepin and its metabolite, *N*-desmethyldoxepin,[5,6] imipramine and its metabolite, desipramine,[7] and maprotiline[8] are all present in breast milk in concentrations similar to those in maternal blood; amoxapine and its metabolite, 8-hydroxyamoxapine,[9] have also been detected in breast milk but in concentrations lower than in maternal blood. In the above cases all but one of the infants were breast fed without experiencing side-effects and tricyclics were undetectable in the infant's blood or present only in minute amounts. In the affected infant[6] adverse effects included sedation and shallow respiration. The infant's mother had received doxepin and, although doxepin was almost undetectable in the infant's serum, the desmethyl metabolite appeared to have accumulated. There were no data for the effects of amoxapine on breast-fed infants because the case reported[9] involved samples of milk taken from a woman experiencing galactorrhoea as an adverse effect of tricyclic administration. No adverse effects were seen during a 27-month follow-up of 14 breast-fed infants whose mothers had received imipramine 100 to 225 mg daily for 4 to 24 weeks.[10]

The American Academy of Pediatrics[11,12] considers that all antidepressants, including tricyclics, are drugs whose effect on nursing infants is unknown but may be of concern.

1. Bader TF, Newman K. Amitriptyline in human breast milk and the nursing infant's serum. *Am J Psychiatry* 1980; **137:** 855–6.
2. Brixen-Rasmussen L, *et al.* Amitriptyline and nortriptyline excretion in human breast milk. *Psychopharmacology (Berl)* 1982; **76:** 94–5.

3. Stancer HC, Reed KL. Desipramine and 2-hydroxydesipramine in human breast milk and the nursing infant's serum. *Am J Psychiatry* 1986; **143:** 1597–1600.
4. Ilett KF, *et al.* The excretion of dothiepin and its primary metabolites in breast milk. *Br J Clin Pharmacol* 1993; **33:** 635–9.
5. Kemp J, *et al.* Excretion of doxepin and N-desmethyldoxepin in human milk. *Br J Clin Pharmacol* 1985; **20:** 497–9.
6. Matheson I, *et al.* Respiratory depression caused by N-desmethyldoxepin in breast milk. *Lancet* 1985; **ii:** 1124.
7. Sovner R, Orsulak PJ. Excretion of imipramine and desipramine in human breast milk. *Am J Psychiatry* 1979; **136:** 451–2.
8. Lloyd AH. Practical considerations in the use of maprotiline (Ludiomil) in general practice. *J Int Med Res* 1977; **5** (suppl 4): 122–38.
9. Gelenberg AJ. Amoxapine, a new antidepressant, appears in human milk. *J Nerv Ment Dis* 1979; **167:** 635–6.
10. Misri S, Sivertz K. Tricyclic drugs in pregnancy and lactation: a preliminary report. *Int J Psychiatry Med* 1991; **21:** 157–71.
11. American Academy of Pediatrics Committee on Drugs. The transfer of drugs and other chemicals into human milk. *Pediatrics* 1994; **93:** 137–50.
12. Berlin CM. American Academy of Pediatrics Committee on Drugs. Drugs and breast milk. *Pediatrics* 1995; **95:** 957–8.

Cardiovascular disease. For comments on the potential cardiotoxicity of tricyclic antidepressants and precautions to be observed in patients with pre-existing cardiovascular disorders, see under Effects on the Cardiovascular System in Adverse Effects, above.

Contact lenses. Based on reports involving amitriptyline[1] and maprotiline[2] it has been considered that the antimuscarinic action of tricyclic antidepressants may decrease tear flow enough to cause corneal drying and staining of contact lenses.[3]

1. Litovitz GL. Amitriptyline and contact lenses. *J Clin Psychiatry* 1984; **45:** 188.
2. Troiano G. Amitriptyline and contact lenses. *J Clin Psychiatry* 1985; **46:** 199.
3. Anonymous. Drugs interfering with contact lenses. *Aust J Hosp Pharm* 1987; **17:** 55–6.

Diabetes mellitus. The fact that tricyclic antidepressants may cause alterations in blood-glucose concentrations has led to the recommendation that these drugs be used with caution in diabetic patients. Additionally, amitriptyline has been reported[1] to cause hypoglycaemic unawareness; one patient did not experience her usual adrenergic symptoms that preceded or accompanied a hypoglycaemic episode.

1. Sherman KE, Bornemann M. Amitriptyline and asymptomatic hypoglycemia. *Ann Intern Med* 1988; **109:** 683–4.

Driving. While affective disorders probably adversely affect driving skill,[1,2] treatment with antidepressant drugs may also be hazardous,[1] although patients may be safer drivers with medication than without.[2] Impairment of performance is largely related to sedative and antimuscarinic effects both of which are more pronounced at the start of treatment; sedative tricyclics, such as amitriptyline and doxepin, are likely to cause greater psychomotor impairment than less sedative tricyclics such as imipramine and nortriptyline.[1] However, a recent epidemiological study[4] was unable to confirm any increased risk of road-traffic accidents in those drivers receiving tricyclic antidepressants or selective serotonin reuptake inhibitors (SSRIs). In healthy subjects fluoxetine (an SSRI) and dothiepin appeared to have a similar but apparently small potential for impairing psychomotor and driving performance.[3]

It has been mentioned[2] that the UK Medical Commission on Accident Prevention has recommended that patients on long-term psychotropic medication are unsuitable to be drivers of heavy goods or public service vehicles.

1. Ashton H. Drugs and driving. *Adverse Drug React Bull* 1983; **98:** 360–3.
2. Cremona A. Mad drivers: psychiatric illness and driving performance. *Br J Hosp Med* 1986; **35:** 193–5.
3. Ramaekers JG, *et al.* A comparative study of acute and subchronic effects of dothiepin, fluoxetine and placebo on psychomotor and actual driving performance. *Br J Clin Pharmacol* 1995; **39:** 397–404.
4. Barbone F, *et al.* Association of road-traffic accidents with benzodiazepine use. *Lancet* 1998; **352:** 1331–6.

Electroconvulsive therapy. For comments concerning the precautions to be observed in patients receiving electroconvulsive therapy, see under Anaesthesia, above.

Epilepsy. For comments on the epileptogenic effect of tricyclic antidepressants and precautions to be observed in patients with a history of epilepsy or other risk factors for development of seizures, see under Epileptogenic Effect in Adverse Effects, above.

Gastro-oesophageal reflux disease. Mention has been made[1] that the antimuscarinic action of tricyclic antidepressants may cause relaxation of the lower oesophageal sphincter and could aggravate nocturnal symptoms of gastro-oesophageal reflux if given in the late evening.

1. Atkinson M. Use and misuse of drugs in the treatment of gastro-oesophageal reflux. *Prescribers' J* 1982; **22:** 129–36.

Glaucoma. It has been considered by the manufacturers that tricyclic antidepressants, because of their antimuscarinic actions, should be used with caution in patients with angle-closure glaucoma or raised intra-ocular pressure. There have been few reports of glaucoma associated with tricyclics, but recently acute angle-closure glaucoma was reported in 4 patients with narrow angles while taking imipramine in usual doses,[1] and similarly in another patient taking clomipramine.[2] In the latter case, the presenting sign was amaurosis fugax, caused by the combination of an abnormally large drop in blood pressure on standing and raised intra-ocular pressure.

1. Ritch R, *et al.* Oral imipramine and acute angle closure glaucoma. *Arch Ophthalmol* 1994; **112:** 67–8.
2. Schlingemann RO, *et al.* Amaurosis fugax on standing and angle-closure glaucoma with clomipramine. *Lancet* 1996; **347:** 465.

Phaeochromocytoma. Administration of imipramine[1,2] or desipramine[3] has caused adverse effects such as seizures and cardiovascular abnormalities (tachycardia and hypertension or hypotension) which have led to the recognition of a previously undiagnosed phaeochromocytoma. It has been suggested[3] that imipramine and its metabolite, desipramine, may be particularly effective in unmasking phaeochromocytoma and that this may be a reflection of their relative potency among the tricyclic antidepressants in inhibiting the noradrenaline reuptake mechanism.

1. Kaufmann JS. Pheochromocytoma and tricyclic antidepressants. *JAMA* 1974; **229:** 1282.
2. Mok J, Swann I. Diagnosis of phaeochromocytoma after ingestion of imipramine. *Arch Dis Child* 1978; **53:** 676–7.
3. Achong MR, Keane PM. Pheochromocytoma unmasked by desipramine therapy. *Ann Intern Med* 1981; **94:** 358–9.

Porphyria. Amitriptyline was considered to be unsafe in patients with acute porphyria, although there is conflicting experimental evidence of porphyrinogenicity.[1]

1. Moore MR, McColl KEL. *Porphyria: drug lists.* Glasgow: Porphyria Research Unit, University of Glasgow, 1991.

Pregnancy. Although there have been isolated reports[1] attributing *congenital malformations* to the use of tricyclic antidepressants during pregnancy, large-scale studies and case-control data[2,3] have failed to substantiate any such association. Indeed, one report[4] on experience in 8 pregnant women being treated with a tricyclic antidepressant suggested that the antidepressant dose might need to be increased during the second half of pregnancy to achieve a response.

Fetal tachyarrhythmia detected at 37 weeks of gestation was attributed to maternal ingestion of dothiepin during pregnancy. Following discontinuation of therapy by the mother no abnormalities in fetal heart rate were found and an uneventful labour followed with a healthy infant being delivered. However, the authors expressed concern that fetal tachycardias may result in *in-utero* cardiac failure and considered that tricyclic antidepressants should be used during pregnancy only if there were compelling reasons.[5]

Withdrawal syndromes manifesting as hypothermia and jitteriness[6] or convulsions[7,8] have been reported in neonates whose mothers took clomipramine during pregnancy. Management has been with phenobarbitone or clomipramine. The manufacturers advise that if it is justifiable to do so, clomipramine should be withdrawn at least 7 weeks before the calculated date of confinement.

1. Barson AJ. Malformed infant. *Br Med J* 1972; **2:** 45.
2. Greenberg G, *et al.* Maternal drug histories and congenital abnormalities. *Br Med J* 1977; **2:** 853–6.
3. Winship KA, *et al.* Maternal drug histories and central nervous system anomalies. *Arch Dis Child* 1984; **59:** 1052–60.
4. Wisner KL, *et al.* Tricyclic dose requirements across pregnancy. *Am J Psychiatry* 1993; **150:** 1541–2.
5. Prentice A, Brown R. Fetal tachyarrhythmia and maternal antidepressant treatment. *Br Med J* 1989; **298:** 190.
6. Musa AB, Smith CS. Neonatal effects of maternal clomipramine therapy. *Arch Dis Child* 1979; **54:** 405.
7. Cowe L, *et al.* Neonatal convulsions caused by withdrawal from maternal clomipramine. *Br Med J* 1982; **284:** 1837–8.
8. Bromiker R, Kaplan M. Apparent intrauterine fetal withdrawal from clomipramine hydrochloride. *JAMA* 1994; **272:** 1722–3.

Surgery. For comments regarding the precautions to be observed in patients undergoing surgery, see under Anaesthesia, above.

Withdrawal. Sudden discontinuation of antidepressant therapy after regular administration for 8 weeks or more may precipitate withdrawal symptoms. The symptoms associated with withdrawal of tricyclic antidepressants appear to form four distinct syndromes:[1] a range of gastro-intestinal disturbances and generalised somatic symptoms such as malaise, chills, headache, and increased perspiration, which may also be accompanied by anxiety and agitation; sleep disturbances characterised by insomnia followed by excessive and vivid dreams; parkinsonism or akathisia; and hypomania or mania. Tricyclic withdrawal has also resulted in cardiac arrhythmias in some patients. Withdrawal symptoms seem to be more common and more severe in children.[2]

Many of the symptoms associated with discontinuation of tricyclic therapy may be produced by cholinergic rebound[1] and can be minimised by a gradual reduction in antidepressant dosage. Some authorities recommend reducing the dose over a period of 4 weeks. If withdrawal symptoms do occur, they may be managed by reinstitution of the tricyclic in a dose sufficient to eliminate them, followed by gradual discontinuation thereafter.[1,2] On the occasions that it may be necessary to stop a tricyclic abruptly, the withdrawal symptoms may be treated with a centrally active antimuscarinic such as atropine or benztropine,[1] or alternatively, an antimuscarinic that does not cross the blood-brain barrier, such as propantheline, if the only withdrawal symptoms are gastro-intestinal in nature.[1] Awareness of the possibility of withdrawal syndromes helps to avoid misinterpreting new symptoms after withdrawal as evidence of relapse.

Tricyclic antidepressants have been included in some classifications as drugs of dependence because of their potential to produce withdrawal syndromes, but this concept has been challenged by Lichtigfeld and Gillman[3] after reviewing several substance abuse studies and finding no evidence of abuse or dependence of the barbiturate type developing with the tricyclics.

Withdrawal symptoms have been reported in neonates born to mothers who took tricyclic antidepressants during pregnancy (see under Pregnancy, above).

1. Dilsaver SC. Withdrawal phenomena associated with antidepressant and antipsychotic agents. *Drug Safety* 1994; **10:** 103–14.
2. Anonymous. Problems when withdrawing antidepressives. *Drug Ther Bull* 1986; **24:** 29–30.
3. Lichtigfeld FJ, Gillman MA. The possible abuse of and dependence on major tranquillisers and tricyclic antidepressants. *S Afr Med J* 1994; **84:** 5–6.

Interactions

Interactions involving tricyclic antidepressants often result from additive side-effects shared by each drug or from altered metabolism of one drug by the other.

Side-effects may be enhanced by the concurrent administration of antimuscarinic drugs or CNS depressants, including alcohol. Barbiturates and other enzyme inducers such as rifampicin and some antiepileptics can increase the metabolism of tricyclic antidepressants and may result in lowered plasma concentrations and reduced antidepressant response. Cimetidine, methylphenidate, antipsychotics, and calcium-channel blockers may reduce the metabolism of the tricyclics leading to the possibility of increased plasma concentrations and accompanying toxicity.

Patients taking thyroid preparations may show an accelerated response to tricyclic antidepressants and occasionally liothyronine has been employed to produce this effect in patients with refractory depression. However, concomitant administration of tricyclics with thyroid hormone therapy may precipitate cardiac arrhythmias.

The antihypertensive effects of bethanidine, debrisoquine, guanethidine, and possibly clonidine may be reduced by tricyclic antidepressants. The pressor effects of sympathomimetics, especially those of the direct-acting drugs adrenaline and noradrenaline, can be enhanced by tricyclic antidepressants; however, there is no clinical evidence of dangerous interactions between adrenaline-containing local anaesthetics and tricyclic antidepressants. Great care should however be taken to avoid inadvertent intravenous administration of the local anaesthetic preparation.

Halofantrine and antiarrhythmics which prolong the QT interval may increase the likelihood of ventricular arrhythmias. The risk of arrhythmias may also be increased when astemizole, terfenadine, cisapride, or sotalol are taken with tricyclic antidepressants.

Although different antidepressants have been used together under expert supervision in refractory cases of depression, severe adverse reactions including the serotonin syndrome (see p.303) may occur. For this reason an appropriate drug-free interval should elapse between discontinuing some types of antidepressant and starting another. Tricyclic antidepressants should not generally be given to patients receiving MAOIs or for at least two weeks after their discontinuation. No treatment-free period is necessary after stopping a reversible inhibitor of monoamine oxidase type A (RIMA) and starting a tricyclic. At least one week should elapse between withdrawing a tricyclic antidepressant and starting any drug liable to provoke a serious reaction (e.g. phenelzine).

Further details concerning some of the above interactions, and others, are given below.

Alcohol. For reference to the effect of alcohol on amitriptyline, see under CNS depressants, below.

Analgesics. Doubling of plasma-doxepin concentrations with associated lethargy has been reported in one patient following the addition of *dextropropoxyphene* to the tricyclic therapy.[1] This was consistent with previous studies indicating that dextropropoxyphene can impair the hepatic metabolism of other drugs.

For general reference to the effect of tricyclic antidepressants, notably amitriptyline and clomipramine, on opioid analgesics, see under Morphine, p.57.

1. Abernethy DR, *et al.* Impairment of hepatic drug oxidation by propoxyphene. *Ann Intern Med* 1982; **97:** 223–4.

Antiarrhythmics. Antiarrhythmics that prolong the QT interval may increase the likelihood of ventricular arrhythmias when given concomitantly with tricyclic antidepressants. There has been a report[1] of a patient receiving desipramine who had raised serum-desipramine concentrations and signs of toxicity after starting treatment with digoxin and *propafenone* for paroxysmal atrial fibrillation. It was considered that propafenone probably reduced the metabolism and clearance of desipramine.

1. Katz MR. Raised serum levels of desipramine with the antiarrhythmic propafenone. *J Clin Psychiatry* 1991; **52:** 432–3.

Anticoagulants. For the effect of tricyclic antidepressants on anticoagulants, see under Warfarin, p.967.

Antidepressants. Combination therapy with differing classes of antidepressants has been used successfully in the treatment of drug-resistant depression. It should be emphasised, however, that such combination may result in enhanced adverse reactions or interactions, and should be employed only under expert supervision. This practice is considered unsuitable or controversial by some authorities. For further details of the interactions between different antidepressants when coadministered, see under Interactions of Phenelzine, p.305. For details of the serotonin syndrome that can arise when two serotonergic drugs with different mechanisms of action are administered, see under Adverse Effects of Phenelzine, p.303.

Antidiabetics. For the effect of tricyclic antidepressants on sulphonylurea antidiabetics, see p.332.

Antiepileptics. Antidepressants may antagonise the activity of antiepileptics by lowering the convulsive threshold.

Reviewing drug interactions with *phenytoin*, Nation and colleagues[1] have observed that although there have been a number of reports of interactions between antiepileptics and tricyclic or related antidepressants, most involved enzyme-inducing antiepileptics other than phenytoin or phenytoin in combination with other drugs. In the only report they could identify where phenytoin was the sole antiepileptic used, 2 patients required high doses of desipramine to achieve an antidepressant effect and to maintain plasma-desipramine concentrations in the range usually associated with therapeutic efficacy.

Concomitant administration of nortriptyline and *carbamazepine* in one patient led to a decrease in serum-nortriptyline concentration; an increase in nortriptyline dose was required.[2]

Valproate has been reported to increase plasma concentrations of amitriptyline and its metabolite nortriptyline.[3]

The effects of tricyclic antidepressants on antiepileptics are reported under phenytoin, p.355.

1. Nation RL, *et al.* Pharmacokinetic drug interactions with phenytoin (part II). *Clin Pharmacokinet* 1990; **18:** 131–50.
2. Brøsen K, Kragh-Sørensen P. Concomitant intake of nortriptyline and carbamazepine. *Ther Drug Monit* 1993; **15:** 258–60.
3. Wong SL, *et al.* Effects of divalproex sodium on amitriptyline and nortriptyline pharmacokinetics. *Clin Pharmacol Ther* 1996; **60:** 48–53.

Antifungals. Increased serum concentrations of nortriptyline were observed in a patient also being given *fluconazole*.[1] Raised serum concentrations of nortriptyline and associated symptoms of intoxication occurred in a patient during concomitant treatment with *terbinafine*;[2] the interaction was confirmed on rechallenge.

1. Gannon RH. Fluconazole-nortriptyline drug interaction. *Ann Pharmacother* 1992; **26:** 1456.
2. van der Kuy P-HM, *et al.* Nortriptyline intoxication induced by terbinafine. *Br Med J* 1998; **316:** 441.

Antihypertensives. In general, the hypotensive effect of antihypertensives is enhanced by tricyclic antidepressants, but there is antagonism of the effect of *adrenergic neurone blockers* and of *clonidine*.

For reference to a suggestion that butriptyline may be less likely to inhibit the antihypertensive effect of adrenergic neurone blockers than other tricyclics, see under Sympathomimetics, below.

Antimalarials. *Halofantrine* prolongs the QT interval and increases the risk of ventricular arrhythmias if administered with tricyclic antidepressants.

Antineoplastics. For the effect of tricyclic antidepressants on *altretamine*, see p.502.

Antiprotozoals. *Furazolidone*, an antiprotozoal with monoamine oxidase inhibiting activity, resulted in a toxic psychosis when given with amitriptyline to one patient.[1]

1. Aderhold RM, Muniz CE. Acute psychosis with amitriptyline and furazolidone. *JAMA* 1970; **213:** 2080.

Antipsychotics. For a discussion of interactions between antipsychotics and tricyclic antidepressants, see Chlorpromazine (p.652).

Antivirals. HIV-protease inhibitors may increase the plasma concentrations of tricyclic antidepressants whose metabolism is mediated through common cytochrome P450 isoenzymes. Ritonavir has produced moderate increases for the area under the curve for desipramine and the manufacturer has predicted a similar increase for other tricyclics such as amitriptyline, clomipramine, imipramine, maprotiline, nortriptyline, and trimipramine. Monitoring of drug concentrations and/or adverse effects is recommended when these tricyclics are used with ritonavir.

Anxiolytics. For a suggestion that benzodiazepines may increase the oxidation of amineptine to a toxic metabolite, see under Effects on the Liver in Adverse Effects, above.

Barbiturates. For details of the interaction of tricyclics with barbiturate anaesthetics, see under Anaesthesia in Precautions, above.

Beta blockers. *Labetalol* increased the bioavailability of imipramine in healthy subjects and inhibited its metabolism.[1] The risk of ventricular arrhythmias may be increased when tricyclic antidepressants are taken with *sotalol*.

1. Hermann DJ, *et al.* Comparison of verapamil, diltiazem, and labetalol on the bioavailability and metabolism of imipramine. *J Clin Pharmacol* 1992; **32:** 176–83.

Calcium-channel blockers. *Diltiazem* and *verapamil* each increased the bioavailability of imipramine in healthy subjects.[1] Diltiazem increased the bioavailability of nortriptyline in one patient,[2] probably by reducing the first-pass metabolism of nortriptyline.

1. Hermann DJ, *et al.* Comparison of verapamil, diltiazem, and labetalol on the bioavailability and metabolism of imipramine. *J Clin Pharmacol* 1992; **32:** 176–83.
2. Krähenbühl S, *et al.* Pharmacokinetic interaction between diltiazem and nortriptyline. *Eur J Clin Pharmacol* 1996; **49:** 417–19.

CNS depressants. Drugs with depressant actions on the CNS may be expected to enhance the drowsiness and related effects produced by the sedating-type of tricyclic antidepressants. Such an interaction may occur between *alcohol* and tricyclic antidepressants and one study has shown that alcohol decreases the hepatic first-pass extraction of amitriptyline resulting in increased free plasma-amitriptyline concentrations, especially during the period of drug absorption.[1]

The problems that may be encountered with *barbiturate anaesthetics* are discussed under Anaesthesia in Precautions, above.

1. Dorian P, *et al.* Amitriptyline and ethanol: pharmacokinetic and pharmacodynamic interaction. *Eur J Clin Pharmacol* 1983; **25:** 325–31.

Disulfiram. Acute organic brain syndrome has been reported in 2 patients receiving disulfiram following the addition of amitriptyline to their treatment.[1] It was suspected that the syndrome was potentiated by the combined action of the two drugs and the synergistic elevation in dopamine concentration.

For a report of the enhancement of the disulfiram-alcohol reaction by amitriptyline, see p.1573.

1. Maany I, *et al.* Possible toxic interaction between disulfiram and amitriptyline. *Arch Gen Psychiatry* 1982; **39:** 743–4.

Dopaminergics. *Selegiline* (p.1144) is an irreversible selective inhibitor of monoamine oxidase type B used in Parkinson's disease. Serious adverse effects have been reported[1] when selegiline and tricyclic antidepressants have been used concomitantly, in some instances resembling the potentially fatal serotonin syndromes reported when tricyclics are administered together with non-selective MAOIs (see under Phenelzine, p.303).

Some authorities advise that tricyclic antidepressants should not generally be given to patients receiving selegiline, or for at least two weeks after it has been discontinued. Similarly, at least one week should elapse between withdrawing a tricyclic antidepressant and starting selegiline.

For reference to the effect of tricyclic antidepressants on *levodopa*, see p.1139.

1. Anonymous. Selegiline and antidepressants: risk of serious interactions. *WHO Drug Inf* 1995; **9:** 160–1.

Fenfluramine. Increases in steady-state plasma-amitriptyline concentrations have occurred in 3 patients given fenfluramine[1] and the manufacturers of fenfluramine have advised that it should not be used concurrently with antidepressants.

1. Gunne L-M, *et al.* Effect of fenfluramine on steady-state plasma levels of amitriptyline. *Postgrad Med J* 1975; **51** (suppl 1): 117.

Food. There has been a report of 3 patients in whom a high-fibre diet reduced or abolished the effectiveness of their tricyclic antidepressant therapy;[1] the tricyclics involved were doxepin in two patients and desipramine in one.

1. Stewart DE. High-fiber diet and serum tricyclic antidepressant levels. *J Clin Psychopharmacol* 1992; **12:** 438–40.

General anaesthetics. For the effect of amitriptyline on *enflurane*, see p.1222.

Histamine H_2-receptor antagonists. *Cimetidine* is a known inhibitor of hepatic metabolism of drugs and symptoms of tricyclic toxicity have been reported in patients receiving cimetidine concurrently with desipramine[1] and imipramine;[1] there has been a report of psychosis developing in a patient given imipramine in addition to cimetidine treatment.[2] Elevated tricyclic concentrations during combined therapy or reductions in tricyclic concentrations after withdrawal of cimetidine have been reported for imipramine[3] and nortriptyline.[4] Studies in healthy subjects have also indicated increased bioavailability and/or impaired hepatic metabolism of doxepin[5,6] and imipramine[7] during cimetidine therapy. This evidence points to the fact that adjustment of tricyclic antidepressant dosage may be required if cimetidine therapy is initiated or discontinued. *Ranitidine* has been reported not to alter the pharmacokinetics of amitriptyline,[8] doxepin,[6] or imipramine.[7]

1. Miller DD, Macklin M. Cimetidine-imipramine interaction: a case report. *Am J Psychiatry* 1983; **140:** 351–2.
2. Miller ME, *et al.* Psychosis in association with combined cimetidine and imipramine treatment. *Psychosomatics* 1987; **28:** 217–19.
3. Shapiro PA. Cimetidine-imipramine interaction: case report and comments. *Am J Psychiatry* 1984; **141:** 152.
4. Miller DD, *et al.* Cimetidine's effect on steady-state serum nortriptyline concentrations. *Drug Intell Clin Pharm* 1983; **17:** 904–5.
5. Abernethy DR, Todd EL. Doxepin-cimetidine interaction: increased doxepin bioavailability during cimetidine treatment. *J Clin Psychopharmacol* 1986; **6:** 8–12.
6. Sutherland DL, *et al.* The influence of cimetidine versus ranitidine on doxepin pharmacokinetics. *Eur J Clin Pharmacol* 1987; **32:** 159–64.
7. Wells BG, *et al.* The effect of ranitidine and cimetidine on imipramine disposition. *Eur J Clin Pharmacol* 1986; **31:** 285–90.
8. Curry SH, *et al.* Lack of interaction of ranitidine with amitriptyline. *Eur J Clin Pharmacol* 1987; **32:** 317–20.

Muscle relaxants. There has been an isolated report[1] of a patient taking *baclofen* for spasticity who experienced leg weakness and was unable to stand after starting treatment with nortriptyline. Symptoms improved on discontinuation of nortriptyline but recurred when imipramine was given.

1. Silverglat MJ. Baclofen and tricyclic antidepressants: possible interaction. *JAMA* 1981; **246:** 1659.

Sex hormones. There have been anecdotal reports of interactions between tricyclic antidepressants and oestrogens[1-3] resulting in either lack of antidepressant response or tricyclic toxicity; the significance of these interactions is not, however, established.

1. Prange AJ, *et al.* Estrogen may well affect response to antidepressant. *JAMA* 1972; **219:** 143–4.
2. Khurana RC. Estrogen-imipramine interaction. *JAMA* 1972; **222:** 702–3.
3. Somani SM, Khurana RC. Mechanism of estrogen-imipramine interaction. *JAMA* 1973; **223:** 560.

Smoking. Tobacco smoke has been reported to reduce the plasma levels of tricyclic antidepressants.[1-3] The clinical significance is not, however, fully established as the plasma concentration of unbound drug may not be affected.[3] The mechanism is probably by stimulation of hepatic drug metabolism by components present in cigarette smoke.

1. Perel JM, *et al.* Pharmacodynamics of imipramine in depressed patients. *Psychopharmacol Bull* 1975; **11:** 16–18.
2. John VA, *et al.* Effects of age, cigarette smoking and the oral contraceptive on the pharmacokinetics of clomipramine and its desmethyl metabolite during chronic dosing. *J Int Med Res* 1980; **8** (suppl 3): 88–95.
3. Perry PJ, *et al.* Effects of smoking on nortriptyline plasma concentrations in depressed patients. *Ther Drug Monit* 1986; **8:** 279–84.

Sympathomimetics. The pressor effects of sympathomimetics can be enhanced by tricyclic antidepressants.

Results of a study[1] in which butriptyline was shown not to inhibit the pressor effect of tyramine, suggested that interactions of butriptyline with direct-acting sympathomimetic amines such as noradrenaline and phenylephrine, and with adrenergic neurone blocking antihypertensive drugs such as guanethidine and bethanidine, may be less likely to occur than with tricyclic antidepressants such as desipramine.

For precautions to be observed in patients on tricyclic therapy who may require sympathomimetics during anaesthesia, see under Anaesthesia in Precautions, above.

1. Ghose K, *et al.* Some clinical pharmacological studies with butriptyline, an antidepressive drug. *Br J Clin Pharmacol* 1977; **4:** 91–3.

Pharmacokinetics

Amitriptyline is readily absorbed from the gastro-intestinal tract, peak plasma concentrations occurring within a few hours of oral administration.

Amitriptyline undergoes extensive first-pass metabolism and is demethylated in the liver to its primary active metabolite, nortriptyline. Other paths of metabolism of amitriptyline include hydroxylation (possibly to active metabolites) and *N*-oxidation; nortriptyline follows similar paths. Amitriptyline is excreted in the urine, mainly in the form of its metabolites, either free or in conjugated form.

Amitriptyline and nortriptyline are widely distributed throughout the body and are extensively bound to plasma and tissue protein. Amitriptyline has been estimated to have an elimination half-life ranging from about 9 to 36 hours, which may be considerably extended in overdosage. Plasma concentrations of amitriptyline and nortriptyline vary very widely between individuals and no simple correlation with therapeutic response has been established.

Amitriptyline and nortriptyline cross the placenta and are distributed into breast milk (see Breast Feeding under Precautions, above).

References.

1. Schulz P, *et al.* Discrepancies between pharmacokinetic studies of amitriptyline. *Clin Pharmacokinet* 1985; **10:** 257–68.
2. Task Force on the Use of Laboratory Tests in Psychiatry. Tricyclic antidepressants—blood level measurements and clinical outcome: an APA Task Force Report. *Am J Psychiatry* 1985; **142:** 155–62.
3. Caccia S, Garattini S. Formation of active metabolites of psychotropic drugs: an updated review of their significance. *Clin Pharmacokinet* 1990; **18:** 434–59.
4. Brøsen K, Gram LF. Clinical significance of the sparteine/debrisoquine oxidation polymorphism. *Eur J Clin Pharmacol* 1989; **36:** 537–47.
5. Llerena A, *et al.* Debrisoquin and mephenytoin hydroxylation phenotypes and CYP2D6 genotype in patients treated with neuroleptic and antidepressant agents. *Clin Pharmacol Ther* 1993; **54:** 606–11.
6. Wood AJJ, Zhou HH. Ethnic differences in drug disposition and responsiveness. *Clin Pharmacokinet* 1991; **20:** 350–73.

Uses and Administration

Tricyclic antidepressants such as amitriptyline were developed from phenothiazine compounds related to chlorpromazine and, as the name suggests, possess a 3-ring molecular structure. They inhibit the neuronal reuptake of noradrenaline in the CNS; some, in addition, inhibit the reuptake of serotonin (5-HT). Prevention of the reuptake of these monoamine neurotransmitters potentiates their action in the brain, which appears to be associated with antidepressant activity, although the precise mode of action of the tricyclics in depression remains to be elucidated. Tricyclic antidepressants also possess affinity for muscarinic and histamine H_1 receptors to varying degrees, see under Adverse Effects, above. Amitriptyline is one of the more sedating tricyclics.

Antidepressants with one, two, or four rings have also been developed, and these share only some of the properties of the tricyclics. While the sedative action and other adverse effects of amitriptyline and other tricyclics are soon apparent, it may be 2 to 4 weeks before the antidepressant effect is seen. After a response has been obtained, maintenance therapy should be continued for at least 4 to 6 months to avoid relapse on discontinuation of therapy.

Amitriptyline, a dibenzocycloheptadiene, is usually given by mouth as the hydrochloride; the hydrochloride may also be administered by intramuscular or intravenous injection.

In the treatment of depression, amitriptyline hydrochloride is given by mouth initially in a daily dose of 75 mg in divided doses (or as a single dose at night). Thereafter, the dose may be gradually increased, if necessary, to 150 mg daily, the additional doses being given in the late afternoon or evening. Therapy may also be initiated with a single dose of 50 to 100 mg at bedtime, increased by 25 or 50 mg as necessary to a total of 150 mg daily. In the USA, doses of up to 200 mg daily and, occasionally, up to 300 mg daily have been used in severely depressed patients in hospital.

Adolescent and elderly patients often have reduced tolerance to tricyclic antidepressants and initial doses of amitriptyline hydrochloride 30 to 75 mg daily may be adequate, given either as divided doses or as a single dose, preferably at bedtime. Half the usual maintenance dose will often be sufficient.

Amitriptyline may also be given by mouth in liquid form as the hydrochloride or the embonate with doses expressed in terms of the base. Amitriptyline oxide (amitriptylinoxide) is also given by mouth.

In the initial stages of treatment, if administration by mouth is impracticable or inadvisable, 10 to 20 mg of the hydrochloride may be given by intravenous or intramuscular injection four times daily, but oral administration should be substituted as soon as possible; in some countries only the intramuscular route is used for parenteral administration in doses of 20 to 30 mg of the hydrochloride four times daily.

Amitriptyline is also used for the treatment of nocturnal enuresis in children in whom organic pathology has been excluded. However, drug therapy for nocturnal enuresis should be reserved for when other methods have failed and should preferably only be given to cover periods away from home; tricyclic antidepressants are not recommended in children under 6 years of age (some authorities recommend that they should not be given until 7 years of age). Doses of amitriptyline that have been suggested are 10 to 20 mg at bedtime for children aged 6 to 10 years, and 25 to 50 mg at bedtime for children over 11 years of age. Depending on the dosage form used these doses may be for the hydrochloride or for the base when given as the embonate. Treatment, including the period of gradual withdrawal, should not continue for longer than 3 months. A full physical examination is recommended before a further course.

Tricyclic antidepressants including amitriptyline may be helpful in some disorders characterised by anxiety.

Amitriptyline should be withdrawn gradually to reduce the risk of withdrawal symptoms.

Alcohol dependence. See under Desipramine, p.282.

Anorexia nervosa. Counselling and psychotherapy form the major part of treatment of anorexia nervosa and there is little or no role for specific drug therapy. Antidepressants may be indicated when there is co-existing depression but malnourished anorexic patients may be more susceptible to adverse effects and less responsive than other patients with depression. Tricyclic antidepressants may add to the risk of cardiac arrhythmias and severe hypotension in these patients; clomipramine can sometimes cause severe nausea or intractable constipation.

Anxiety disorders. See under Clomipramine, p.282.

Bulimia nervosa. A combination of counselling, support, psychotherapy, and antidepressants is the usual treatment for bulimia nervosa. Antidepressants can help to reduce the frequency of overeating and some other symptoms of bulimia but relapse tends to occur on discontinuation. A wide range of antidepressants has been tried, but the tricyclic desipramine and the SSRI fluoxetine have been the most commonly used and are considered to be well tolerated.

Ciguatera poisoning. Amitriptyline has relieved some of the neurological symptoms associated with ciguatera poisoning (see Mannitol, p.901).

Cocaine dependence. See under Desipramine, p.282.

Depression. As discussed on p.271, there is very little difference in efficacy between the different groups of antidepressant drugs, and choice is often made on the basis of adverse effect profile. Tricyclic antidepressants have traditionally been the first choice for the treatment of depression, and often still are because of wide experience with their use and familiarity with their pharmacological actions. The more sedating tricyclics such as amitriptyline, clomipramine, dothiepin, doxepin, and trimipramine may be of value in depression with associated agitation or anxiety. The less sedating tricyclics such as desipramine, imipramine, lofepramine, nortriptyline, and protriptyline may be of value for withdrawn or apathetic depressed patients.

Combination therapy with differing classes of antidepressants, including the tricyclics, has been used in the treatment of refractory or drug-resistant depression. However, such therapy may result in enhanced adverse reactions or interactions and is considered unsuitable or controversial by some workers. For further details, see Antidepressants under Interactions of Phenelzine, p.305.

Headache. Tricyclic antidepressants can be effective in the management of some types of headache and although they are especially useful when the headache is accompanied by depression their beneficial effects appear to be independent of their antidepressant action. They are used for the prophylaxis of migraine (p.443) when drugs such as propranolol or pizotifen have proved ineffective or unsuitable and may be useful when additional treatment to simple analgesics is required for tension-type headache, being particularly effective in chronic forms of the condition (see p.444). Amitriptyline is the tricyclic usually used but others have been tried. A suggested dosage for amitriptyline in the prophylaxis of migraine is 10 mg at night increased to a maintenance dose of 50 to 75 mg at night; the need for continuing prophylaxis should be reviewed at intervals of about 6 months.

References.

1. Mathew NT. Prophylaxis of migraine and mixed headache: a randomized controlled study. *Headache* 1981; **21:** 105–9.
2. Pfaffenrath V, *et al.* Combination headache: practical experience with a combination of a β-blocker and an antidepressive. *Cephalalgia* 1986; **6** (suppl 5): 25–32.
3. Wörz R, Scherhag R. Treatment of chronic tension headache with doxepin or amitriptyline—results of a double-blind study. *Headache Q* 1990; **1:** 216–23.
4. Ziegler DK, *et al.* Propranolol and amitriptyline in prophylaxis of migraine: pharmacokinetic and therapeutic effects. *Arch Neurol* 1993; **50:** 825–30.
5. Pfaffenrath V, *et al.* Efficacy and tolerability of amitriptylinoxide in the treatment of chronic tension-type headache: a multicentre controlled study. *Cephalalgia* 1994; **14:** 149–55.

Hiccup. A protocol for the management of intractable hiccups may be found under Chlorpromazine, p.655. Amitriptyline is one of a wide range of drugs for which there are anecdotal reports[1] of success in the treatment of intractable hiccup.

1. Stalnikowicz R, *et al.* Amitriptyline for intractable hiccups. *N Engl J Med* 1986; **315:** 64–5.

Hyperactivity. When drug therapy is required for attention deficit hyperactivity disorder (p.1476), initial treatment is usually with central stimulants. Tricyclic antidepressants such as imipramine or desipramine are also used but, because of lower efficacy and associated adverse effects, are reserved as second-choice drugs for patients who fail to respond to or who are intolerant of stimulants. They may also be of use for selected patients with certain co-existing disorders.

Interstitial cystitis. Tricyclic antidepressants such as amitriptyline or imipramine have been found to be of benefit in the treatment of interstitial cystitis (p.1377) given at night in conjunction with hexamine hippurate during the day.[1]

1. Cardozo L. Postmenopausal cystitis. *Br Med J* 1996; **313:** 129.

Irritable bowel syndrome. The management of irritable bowel syndrome is discussed on p.1172 where reference is made to the response that may be achieved by some patients to a tricyclic antidepressant, particularly where bowel frequency is the presenting symptom, since the antimuscarinic properties of the tricyclics slow intestinal transit.

Micturition disorders. Tricyclic antidepressants are among the drugs used as an alternative or adjunct to nonpharmacological methods for the treatment of **nocturnal enuresis** in children (p.453) in whom organic pathology has been excluded. However, because of their potentially fatal toxicity in overdosage, there has been concern over the safety of using tricyclics in households with children. Most experience in nocturnal enuresis has been with imipramine, but other tricyclics such as amitriptyline, nortriptyline, and clomipramine have also been used. Their mechanism of action in nocturnal enuresis is unclear. It may be the result of a combination of their antimuscarinic and antispasmodic actions as well as their effect on sleep patterns and possible stimulation of antidiuretic hormone secretion. Imipramine appears to be most effective in older children, but many patients develop tolerance and increasingly higher doses are required.

Tricyclic antidepressants are also sometimes used in the management of **urinary incontinence** (p.454).

Narcoleptic syndrome. Tricyclic antidepressants are the primary treatment for cataplexy and sleep paralysis associated with narcolepsy (p.1476). Clomipramine and imipramine appear to be the most widely used for these symptoms. The onset of action is quicker than when used for depression and doses required appear to be lower. Doses should be titrated to provide maximal protection for the time of day when symptoms usually occur and evening doses should be avoided to minimise nocturnal arousal. Protriptyline has also been reported to be effective[1] and because of its stimulant properties may also be beneficial for sleepiness in patients who remain symptomatic or who cannot tolerate central nervous system stimulants, the primary form of therapy for this symptom.

1. Schmidt HS, *et al.* Protriptyline: an effective agent in the treatment of the narcolepsy-cataplexy syndrome and hypersomnia. *Am J Psychiatry* 1977; **134:** 183–5.

Pain. Tricyclic antidepressants, usually amitriptyline, are useful in alleviating some types of pain when given in subantidepressant doses. This is discussed with other methods of pain relief on p.4. Chronic neurogenic pain as seen in cancer (p.8), central post-stroke pain (p.8), diabetic neuropathy (p.9), phantom limb pain (p.10), and postherpetic neuralgia (p.10) responds to therapy with tricyclics. Tricyclics are also often of benefit in the treatment of idiopathic orofacial pain (p.10), and may be of value for patients with refractory reflex sympathetic dystrophy (p.11). Pain and sleep quality may be improved by tricyclics in patients with fibromyalgia, a condition that responds poorly to analgesics and anti-inflammatory drugs. Patients with migraine or chronic tension-type headache may also benefit from tricyclics (see Headache, above). There is little evidence for an analgesic effect of tricyclics in acute pain.

Some specific references to the use of amitriptyline for pain.

1. Watson CP, *et al.* Amitriptyline versus placebo in postherpetic neuralgia. *Neurology* 1982; **32:** 671–3.
2. Watson CPN. Therapeutic window for amitriptyline analgesia. *Can Med Assoc J* 1984; **130:** 105.
3. Carette S, *et al.* Evaluation of amitriptyline in primary fibrositis: a double-blind, placebo-controlled study. *Arthritis Rheum* 1986; **29:** 655–9.
4. Goldenberg DL, *et al.* A randomized, controlled trial of amitriptyline and naproxen in the treatment of patients with fibromyalgia. *Arthritis Rheum* 1986; **29:** 1371–7.
5. Max MB, *et al.* Amitriptyline relieves diabetic neuropathy pain in patients with normal or depressed mood. *Neurology* 1987; **37:** 589–96.
6. Max MB, *et al.* Amitriptyline, but not lorazepam, relieves postherpetic neuralgia. *Neurology* 1988; **38:** 1427–32.
7. Max MB, *et al.* Effects of desipramine, amitriptyline, and fluoxetine on pain in diabetic neuropathy. *N Engl J Med* 1992; **326:** 1250–6.
8. Onghena P, Van Houdenhove, B. Antidepressant-induced analgesia in chronic non-malignant pain: a meta-analysis of 39 placebo-controlled studies. *Pain* 1992; **49:** 205–19.
9. Watson CPN, *et al.* Amitriptyline versus maprotiline in postherpetic neuralgia: a randomized double-blind, crossover trial. *Pain* 1992; **48:** 29–36.
10. McQuay HJ, *et al.* Dose-response for analgesic effect of amitriptyline in chronic pain. *Anaesthesia* 1993; **48:** 281–5.
11. Eija K, *et al.* Amitriptyline effectively relieves neuropathic pain following treatment of breast cancer. *Pain* 1995; **64:** 293–302.
12. McQuay HJ, *et al.* A systematic review of antidepressants in neuropathic pain. *Pain* 1996; **68:** 217–27.
13. Godfrey RG. A guide to the understanding and use of tricyclic antidepressants in the overall management of fibromyalgia and other chronic pain syndromes. *Arch Intern Med* 1996; **156:** 1047–52.
14. McQuay HJ, Moore RA. Antidepressants and chronic pain. *Br Med J* 1997; **314:** 763–4.

Pathological crying or laughing. Pathological crying or laughing can result from lesions in certain areas of the brain. Attempts at treatment have mostly been with antidepressants and favourable results have been reported in double-blind studies with amitriptyline[1] and nortriptyline.[2]

1. Schiffer RB, *et al.* Treatment of pathologic laughing and weeping with amitriptyline. *N Engl J Med* 1985; **312:** 1480–2.
2. Robinson RG, *et al.* Pathological laughing and crying following stroke: validation of a measurement scale and a double-blind treatment study. *Am J Psychiatry* 1993; **150:** 286–93.

Premenstrual syndrome. See under Clomipramine, p.282.

Schizophrenia. Antidepressants such as the tricyclics are considered worth trying as an adjunct in the treatment of patients with schizophrenia (p.637) who develop depression during the recovery phase after an acute episode of psychosis. There is, however, no clear evidence that they are effective during acute psychotic episodes or for depression during periods of remission in patients with chronic schizophrenia.[1]

1. Anonymous. The drug treatment of patients with schizophrenia. *Drug Ther Bull* 1995; **33:** 81–6.

Sexual dysfunction. Impotence or ejaculatory problems have been reported as adverse effects of tricyclic antidepressants (see Effects on Sexual Function in Adverse Effects, above). Such properties have been studied as a potential form of treatment for men with premature ejaculation (see Clomipramine, p.282).

Skin disorders. See under Doxepin, p.283.

Smoking cessation. Tricyclic antidepressants are among the drugs that have been tried with varying degrees of success as alternatives to nicotine replacement therapy to alleviate the withdrawal syndrome associated with smoking cessation (p.1608).

Stuttering. See under Clomipramine, p.282.

Preparations

BP 1998: Amitriptyline Oral Suspension; Amitriptyline Tablets;
USP 23: Amitriptyline Hydrochloride Injection; Amitriptyline Hydrochloride Tablets; Chlordiazepoxide and Amitriptyline Hydrochloride Tablets; Perphenazine and Amitriptyline Hydrochloride Tablets.

Proprietary Preparations (details are given in Part 3)
Aust.: Saroten; Tryptizol; ***Austral.:*** Amitrol; Endep; Tryptanol; Tryptine; ***Belg.:*** Redomex; Tryptizol; ***Canad.:*** Elavil; Levate; Novo-Triptyn; ***Fr.:*** Elavil; Laroxyl; ***Ger.:*** Amineurin; Equilibrin; Euplit†; Laroxyl†; Novoprotect; Saroten; Sylvemid†; Syneudon; ***Irl.:*** Amyline†; Domical; Laroxyl†; Lentizol; Tryptizol; ***Ital.:*** Adepril; Amilit-IFI; Laroxyl; Neurarmonil†; Triptizol; ***Neth.:*** Sarotex; Tryptizol; ***Norw.:*** Sarotex; Tryptizol; ***S.Afr.:*** Endep; Noriline†; Saroten; Trepiline; Tryptanol; ***Spain:*** Tryptizol; ***Swed.:*** Saroten; Tryptizol; ***Switz.:*** Saroten; Tryptizol; ***UK:*** Domical; Elavil; Lentizol; Tryptizol; ***USA:*** Elavil; Endep†; Enovil†.

Multi-ingredient: ***Aust.:*** Limbitrol; Pantrop; ***Austral.:*** Mutabon D; ***Belg.:*** Limbitrol; ***Canad.:*** Elavil Plus; Etrafon; PMS-Levazine; Triavil; ***Ger.:*** Limbatril; Longopax†; Pantrop†; Parks-Plus†; ***Irl.:*** Limbitrol†; Triptafen; ***Ital.:*** Diapatol; Limbitryl; Mutabon; Sedans; ***Neth.:*** Limbitrol†; Mutabon A/D/F†; ***S.Afr.:*** Etrafon; Limbitrol; ***Spain:*** Deprelio; Mutabase; Nobritol; ***Switz.:*** Limbitrol; ***UK:*** Limbitrol†; Triptafen; ***USA:*** Etrafon; Limbitrol; Triavil.

Amoxapine (2503-q)

Amoxapine *(BAN, USAN, rINN).*

CL-67772. 2-Chloro-11-(piperazin-1-yl)dibenz[*b,f*][1,4]oxazepine.

$C_{17}H_{16}ClN_3O = 313.8.$

CAS — 14028-44-5.

Pharmacopoeias. In *Jpn* and *US.*

A white to yellowish white crystalline powder. Practically **insoluble** in water; freely soluble in chloroform; sparingly soluble in methyl alcohol and in toluene; slightly soluble in acetone; soluble in tetrahydrofuran. **Store** in airtight containers.

Adverse Effects, Treatment, and Precautions

As for tricyclic antidepressants in general (see Amitriptyline, p.273).

Amoxapine has also been associated with tardive dyskinesias and the neuroleptic malignant syndrome has been reported.

Antidopaminergic effects. Amoxapine is a derivative of the antipsychotic loxapine (p.677) and possesses some neuroleptic activity. It also demonstrates dopamine-receptor blocking properties as do its hydroxylated metabolites. A variety of adverse effects that are symptoms of such blockade have been reported and reviewed[1,2] and include akinesia, akathisia, withdrawal dyskinesia, reversible tardive dyskinesia, persistent dyskinesia, elevated serum concentration of prolactin, and galactorrhoea. Chorea[3] and oculogyric crisis[4] have also been reported.

1. Tao GK, *et al.* Amoxapine-induced tardive dyskinesia. *Drug Intell Clin Pharm* 1985; **19:** 548–9.
2. Devarajan S. Safety of amoxapine. *Lancet* 1989; **ii:** 1455.
3. Patterson JF. Amoxapine-induced chorea. *South Med J* 1983; **76:** 1077.
4. Hunt-Fugate AK, *et al.* Adverse reactions due to dopamine blockade by amoxapine. *Pharmacotherapy* 1984; **4:** 35–9.

Antimuscarinic effects. While amoxapine has been reported to produce in depressed patients adverse effects associated with antimuscarinic activity (such as constipation, blurred vision, and dry mouth), Bourne *et al.*[1] considered that such reports did not reflect *in-vitro* findings that amoxapine had considerably less affinity for muscarinic binding sites than amitriptyline and this was supported by their results in healthy subjects. The adverse effects described as antimuscarinic could possibly be explained by amoxapine affecting noradrenergic mechanisms.

1. Bourne M, *et al.* A comparison of the effects of single doses of amoxapine and amitriptyline on autonomic functions in healthy volunteers. *Eur J Clin Pharmacol* 1993; **44:** 57–62.

Effects on the endocrine system. Reversible nonketotic hyperglycaemia developed in a 49-year-old woman with no history of diabetes mellitus within 5 days of therapy with amoxapine 50 mg three times daily by mouth.[1] The patient had previously experienced nonketotic hyperglycaemic coma after loxapine 150 mg daily. 7-Hydroxyamoxapine, a metabolite common to both amoxapine and loxapine, was implicated.

1. Tollefson G, Lesar T. Nonketotic hyperglycemia associated with loxapine and amoxapine: case report. *J Clin Psychiatry* 1983; **44:** 347–8.

Overdosage. In overdosage, amoxapine is reported to cause acute renal failure with rhabdomyolysis,[1,2] coma, and seizures.[3-5] Although there has been some debate as to whether the incidence of seizures and death is higher with overdosage of amoxapine than other tricyclic antidepressants some[6] consider that evidence does seem to favour increased neurological consequences.

It has been reported that amoxapine is not cardiotoxic in overdosage[3] but again more recent evidence would suggest that there is cardiotoxic potential.[6,7]

1. Pumariega AJ, *et al.* Acute renal failure secondary to amoxapine overdose. *JAMA* 1982; **248:** 3141–2.
2. Jennings AE, *et al.* Amoxapine-associated acute renal failure. *Arch Intern Med* 1983; **143:** 1525–7.
3. Kulig K, *et al.* Amoxapine overdose: coma and seizures without cardiotoxic effects. *JAMA* 1982; **248:** 1092–4.
4. Litovitz TL, Troutman WG. Amoxapine overdose: seizures and fatalities. *JAMA* 1983; **250:** 1069–71.
5. Jefferson JW. Convulsions associated with amoxapine. *JAMA* 1984; **251:** 603–4.
6. Leonard BE. Safety of amoxapine. *Lancet* 1989; **ii:** 808.
7. Sørensen MR. Acute myocardial failure following amoxapine intoxication. *J Clin Psychopharmacol* 1988; **8:** 75.

Interactions

For interactions associated with tricyclic antidepressants, see Amitriptyline, p.276.

Pharmacokinetics

Amoxapine is readily absorbed from the gastro-intestinal tract. It bears a close chemical relationship to loxapine (p.677) and is similarly metabolised by hydroxylation. It is excreted in the urine, mainly as its metabolites in conjugated form as glucuronides.

Amoxapine has been reported to have a plasma half-life of 8 hours and its major metabolite, 8-hydroxyamoxapine, has been reported to have a biological half-life of 30 hours; another metabolite, 7-hydroxyamoxapine, has a half-life of 6.5 hours. Both metabolites are pharmacologically active. Amoxapine is extensively bound to plasma proteins.

Amoxapine and its metabolite 8-hydroxyamoxapine are distributed into breast milk (see Breast Feeding under Precautions for Amitriptyline, p.275).

Uses and Administration

Amoxapine, the *N*-desmethyl derivative of loxapine (p.677), is a dibenzoxazepine tricyclic antidepressant with actions and uses similar to those of amitriptyline (p.278). Amoxapine is one of the less sedating tricyclics and its antimuscarinic effects are mild; it also inhibits the reuptake of dopamine.

In the treatment of depression (p.271) amoxapine is given in oral doses of 50 mg two or three times daily initially, gradually increased up to 100 mg three times daily as necessary. Higher doses of up to 600 mg daily may be required in severely depressed patients in hospital. A suggested dose for the elderly is 25 mg two or three times daily initially, increased after 5 to 7 days to up to 150 mg daily as necessary; some patients may require further increases to a maximum of 300 mg daily.

Once-daily dosage regimens, usually given at night, are suitable for amoxapine up to 300 mg daily; divided-dosage regimens are recommended for doses above 300 mg daily.

It has been claimed that, in the treatment of depression, amoxapine has a more rapid onset of action than amitriptyline or imipramine with a clinical effect possibly appearing 4 to 7 days after the initiation of therapy, although this fact has sometimes been disputed.

Amoxapine should be withdrawn gradually to reduce the risk of withdrawal symptoms.

References.

1. Jue SG, *et al.* Amoxapine: a review of its pharmacology and efficacy in depressed states. *Drugs* 1982; **24:** 1–23.

Preparations

USP 23: Amoxapine Tablets.

Proprietary Preparations (details are given in Part 3)
Canad.: Asendin; ***Fr.:*** Defanyl; ***Irl.:*** Asendis; ***Spain:*** Demolox; ***UK:*** Asendis; ***USA:*** Asendin.

Befloxatone (15879-w)

Befloxatone *(rINN).*

(*R*)-5-(Methoxymethyl)-3-{*p*-[(*R*)-4,4,4-trifluoro-3-hydroxybutoxy]phenyl}-2-oxazolidinone.

$C_{15}H_{18}F_3NO_5 = 349.3.$

CAS — 134564-82-2.

Befloxatone, an oxazolidinone derivative, is a reversible inhibitor of monoamine oxidase type A (RIMA) (see Moclobemide, p.298) under investigation for the treatment of depression.

References.

1. Durrieu G, *et al.* Oral tyramine pressor effect after chronic treatment with befloxatone in healthy volunteers. *Br J Clin Pharmacol* 1995; **39:** 574P.
2. Patat A, *et al.* Pharmacodynamics and pharmacokinetics of two dose regimens of befloxatone, a new reversible and selective monoamine oxidase inhibitor, at steady state in healthy volunteers. *J Clin Pharmacol* 1996; **36:** 216–29.
3. Warot D, *et al.* Effects of befloxatone, a reversible selective monoamine oxidase-A inhibitor, on psychomotor function and memory in healthy subjects. *J Clin Pharmacol* 1996; **36:** 942–50.

Benactyzine Hydrochloride (7005-g)

Benactyzine Hydrochloride *(BANM, rINNM).*

2-Diethylaminoethyl benzilate hydrochloride.

$C_{20}H_{25}NO_3,HCl = 363.9.$

CAS — 302-40-9 (benactyzine); 57-37-4 (benactyzine hydrochloride).

Benactyzine has antidepressant and antimuscarinic activity. It has been used as the hydrochloride in the management of depression and associated anxiety. Methylbenactyzium bromide (p.465), the methobromide of benactyzine, has been used for its antimuscarinic activity in the treatment of gastro-intestinal spasm and nocturnal enuresis.

Preparations

Proprietary Preparations (details are given in Part 3)

Multi-ingredient: ***Ital.:*** Sirenitas†; ***USA:*** Deprol†.

Brofaromine (2840-n)

Brofaromine *(rINN).*

CGP-11305A (brofaromine hydrochloride). 4-(7-Bromo-5-methoxy-2-benzofuranyl)piperidine.

$C_{14}H_{16}BrNO_2 = 310.2.$

CAS — 63638-91-5.

Brofaromine is a reversible inhibitor of monoamine oxidase type A (RIMA) (see Moclobemide, p.298). It has been studied as an antidepressant but its development appears to have been stopped.

References.

1. Waldmeier PC, *et al.* Urinary excretion of O-methylated catecholamines, tyramine and phenyl-ethylamine by volunteers treated with tranylcypromine and CGP 11305 A. *Eur J Clin Pharmacol* 1983; **25:** 361–8.
2. Steiger A, *et al.* Results of an open clinical trial of brofaromine (CGP 11305 A), a competitive, selective, and short-acting inhibitor of MAO-A in major endogenous depression. *Pharmacopsychiatry* 1987; **20:** 262–9.
3. Fischer EK, *et al.* Selektive MAO-hemmung vs monoamin-wiederaufnahmehemmung: klinische studie mit brofaromin und imipramin. *Munch Med Wschr* 1990; **132** (suppl 1): S21–S24.
4. van Vliet IM, *et al.* MAO inhibitors in panic disorder: clinical effects of treatment with brofaromine: a double blind placebo controlled study. *Psychopharmacology (Berl)* 1993; **112:** 483–9.
5. Zeeh J, *et al.* Influence of age, frailty and liver function on the pharmacokinetics of brofaromine. *Eur J Clin Pharmacol* 1996; **49:** 387–91.

Bupropion Hydrochloride (12469-j)

Bupropion Hydrochloride *(BANM, USAN).*

Amfebutamone Hydrochloride *(rINNM)*; BW-323. (±)-2-(*tert*-Butylamino)-3′-chloropropiophenone hydrochloride.

$C_{13}H_{18}ClNO,HCl = 276.2.$

CAS — 34911-55-2 (bupropion); 31677-93-7 (bupropion hydrochloride).

Adverse Effects and Treatment

Agitation, anxiety, and insomnia often occur during the initial stages of bupropion therapy. Other side-effects reported with bupropion include dry mouth, headache or migraine, weight loss, nausea and vomiting, constipation, and tremor; skin rashes, anaphylactoid reactions (characterised by pruritus, angioedema, urticaria, and dyspnoea), and psychotic episodes have also been reported.

Seizures, which appear to be partially dose-related, may occur with bupropion and have been particularly notable in patients with anorexia nervosa or bulimia nervosa; the risk is also increased in patients with a history of seizure disorders or other predisposing factor.

Symptoms of overdosage include hallucinations, nausea and vomiting, tachycardia, loss of consciousness, and death (following massive overdose); seizures have occurred in approximately one-third of all bupropion overdose cases. Gastric lavage or administration of activated charcoal within the first 12 hours of ingestion may decrease absorption. Treatment is supportive. Benzodiazepines may be tried for seizures. Diuresis, dialysis, and haemoperfusion are unlikely to be of benefit.

Hypersensitivity. Eosinophilia has been reported[1] in a patient 12 days after bupropion was added to her existing treatment regimen of glibenclamide and tolmetin. The eosinophil count returned to normal after all medication was stopped. Bupropion appeared to be the causative drug.

1. Malesker MA, *et al.* Eosinophilia associated with bupropion. *Ann Pharmacother* 1995; **29:** 867–8.

Precautions

Bupropion is contra-indicated in patients with epilepsy and should be used with extreme caution in patients with a history of seizure disorders or other predisposing factors because of its propensity to induce seizures. It is also contra-indicated in patients with a current or prior history of anorexia nervosa or bulimia nervosa as a higher incidence of seizures has been noted in such patients treated with bupropion.

Bupropion should be used with caution in patients with bipolar disorder (manic depression) or psychoses because of the risk of precipitating mania. It should also be used cautiously in patients with a recent history of myocardial infarction or unstable heart disease, and in hepatic or renal impairment.

Patients should be closely monitored during early therapy until improvement in depression is observed because suicide is an inherent risk in depressed patients. For further details, see under Depression, p.271.

As with other CNS-active drugs, the ability to perform tasks requiring motor or cognitive skills or judgement may be impaired by bupropion, and patients, if affected, should not drive or operate machinery.

Bupropion is distributed into breast milk and therefore has the potential for serious adverse effects in the infant.

Interactions

Bupropion should not be given concurrently with or within 14 days of stopping an MAOI.

The use of alcohol with bupropion should be minimised or avoided completely because it may alter the seizure threshold. Similarly, other drugs that lower the seizure threshold, such as other antidepressants, antipsychotics, theophylline, or systemic corticosteroids, should be used with extreme caution together with bupropion.

Use of nicotine transdermal patches concurrently with bupropion has been associated with hypertension, and patients using this combination should therefore have their blood pressure monitored.

Caution has been advised in patients receiving levodopa because of reports of a higher incidence of adverse effects in patients receiving these two drugs concurrently.

Animal studies have indicated that bupropion may induce drug-metabolising enzymes and interactions with other drugs are therefore a possibility. It is itself metabolised by hepatic enzyme systems and drugs known to affect such systems (e.g. carbamazepine, cimetidine, phenobarbitone, and phenytoin) may interact with bupropion.

Antiepileptics. Undetectable plasma-bupropion concentrations developed in 2 patients who were also receiving carbamazepine; plasma concentrations of hydroxybupropion, an active metabolite of bupropion, were high.[1]

1. Popli AP, *et al.* Bupropion and anticonvulsant drug interactions. *Ann Clin Psychiatry* 1995; **7:** 99–101.

Pharmacokinetics

Bupropion is well absorbed from the gastro-intestinal tract but may undergo extensive first-pass metabolism. Several metabolites of bupropion are pharmacologically active and have longer half-lives than the parent compound. Hydroxybupropion is comparable in potency to bupropion; threohydrobupropion and erythrohydrobupropion are produced by hydroxylation and/or reduction and are about one-tenth to one-half the potency of the parent compound. Bupropion is 84% bound to plasma proteins. The terminal plasma half-life of bupropion is about 14 hours. The metabolites of bupropion are excreted primarily in the urine; less than 1% of the parent drug is excreted unchanged. Bupropion crosses the placenta and is distributed into breast milk.

References.

1. Sweet RA, *et al.* Pharmacokinetics of single- and multiple-dose bupropion in elderly patients with depression. *J Clin Pharmacol* 1995; **35:** 876–84.

Distribution into breast milk. There has been a report of accumulation of bupropion in human breast milk in concentrations higher than those in maternal plasma.[1] However, neither bupropion nor its metabolites were detected in the plasma of the infant breast-fed twice daily by the affected mother and no adverse effects were noted in the infant (but see Precautions, above).

1. Briggs GC, *et al.* Excretion of bupropion in breast milk. *Ann Pharmacother* 1993; **27:** 431–3.

Smoking. No clinically significant differences were observed for the pharmacokinetics of bupropion or its metabolites between cigarette smokers and non-smokers.[1]

1. Hsyu P-H, *et al.* Pharmacokinetics of bupropion and its metabolites in cigarette smokers versus nonsmokers. *J Clin Pharmacol* 1997; **37:** 737–43.

Uses and Administration

Bupropion is a chlorpropiophenone antidepressant chemically unrelated to other classes of antidepressants but similar in structure to the central stimulant diethylpropion (p.1479). It is a weak blocker of neuronal reuptake of serotonin and noradrenaline compared with tricyclic antidepressants; it also inhibits the neuronal reuptake of dopamine. The antidepressant effect may not be evident until after 4 weeks of therapy. Bupropion is also used as an aid to smoking cessation.

Bupropion is given by mouth as the hydrochloride. To minimise agitation, anxiety, and insomnia often experienced at the start of therapy, and to reduce the risk of seizures doses should be increased gradually; the total daily dose should be administered in equally divided doses and the maximum recommended single and total daily doses should not be exceeded. Insomnia at the start of therapy may be minimised by avoiding bedtime doses. Patients with renal or hepatic impairment should be given reduced doses and monitored for toxic effects.

In the treatment of depression bupropion hydrochloride is given in initial doses of 100 mg twice daily increased, if necessary, after at least 3 days to 100 mg three times daily. In severe cases, if no improvement has been observed after several weeks of therapy, the dose may be increased further to a maximum of 150 mg three times daily. Bupropion hydrochloride is also available as a modified-release preparation given in an initial dose of 150 mg once a day in the morning increased, if necessary, after at least 3 days to 150 mg twice daily; in severe cases, the dose of the modified-release preparation may be increased further after several weeks to 200 mg twice daily.

Bupropion hydrochloride is given as a modified-release preparation as an aid to smoking cessation in an initial dose of 150 mg once a day, increased after at least 3 days to 150 mg twice a day.

Depression. The management of depression is discussed on p.271. References to the use of bupropion in patients with depression are given below.

1. Anonymous. Bupropion for depression. *Med Lett Drugs Ther* 1989; **31:** 97–8.
2. Weisler RH, *et al.* Comparison of bupropion and trazodone for the treatment of major depression. *J Clin Psychopharmacol* 1994; **14:** 170–9.
3. Kavoussi RJ, *et al.* Double-blind comparison of bupropion sustained release and sertraline in depressed outpatients. *J Clin Psychiatry* 1997; **58:** 532–7.

Smoking cessation. The management of smoking cessation is discussed on p.1608. References to the use of bupropion in smoking cessation are given below.

1. Anonymous. Bupropion (Zyban) for smoking cessation. *Med Lett Drugs Ther* 1997; **39:** 77–8.
2. Benowitz NL. Treating tobacco addiction—nicotine or no nicotine? *N Engl J Med* 1997; **337:** 1230–1.
3. Hurt RD, *et al.* A comparison of sustained-release bupropion and placebo for smoking cessation. *N Engl J Med* 1997; **337:** 1195–1202.

Preparations

Proprietary Preparations (details are given in Part 3)

USA: Wellbutrin; Zyban.

Butriptyline Hydrochloride (2505-s)

Butriptyline Hydrochloride *(BANM, USAN, rINNM).*

AY-62014. (±)-3-(10,11-Dihydro-5*H*-dibenzo[*a,d*]cyclohepten-5-yl)-2-methylpropyldimethylamine hydrochloride.

$C_{21}H_{27}N,HCl = 329.9.$

CAS — 35941-65-2 (butriptyline); 5585-73-9 (butriptyline hydrochloride).

Butriptyline hydrochloride 28.1 mg is approximately equivalent to 25 mg of butriptyline.

Adverse Effects, Treatment, and Precautions

As for tricyclic antidepressants in general (see Amitriptyline, p.273).

Interactions

For interactions associated with tricyclic antidepressants, see Amitriptyline, p.276.

Uses and Administration

Butriptyline hydrochloride is a tricyclic antidepressant with actions and uses similar to those of amitriptyline (p.278). It is one of the less sedating tricyclics.

In the treatment of depression (p.271) it is given by mouth as the hydrochloride in doses equivalent to butriptyline 25 mg three times daily initially, gradually increased to a maximum of 150 mg daily as necessary.

Butriptyline should be withdrawn gradually to reduce the risk of withdrawal symptoms.

Preparations

Proprietary Preparations (details are given in Part 3)

Aust.: Evasidol; ***Belg.:*** Evadyne†; ***Irl.:*** Evadyne†; ***Ital.:*** Evadene; ***UK:*** Evadyne†.

Citalopram Hydrobromide (12575-c)

Citalopram Hydrobromide (*BANM, rINNM*).

Lu-10-171; Nitalapram Hydrobromide. 1-(3-Dimethylaminopropyl)-1-(4-fluorophenyl)-1,3-dihydroisobenzofuran-5-carbonitrile hydrobromide.

$C_{20}H_{21}FN_2O,HBr = 405.3$.

CAS — 59729-33-8 (citalopram); 59729-32-7 (citalopram hydrobromide).

Citalopram hydrochloride 22.25 mg and citalopram hydrobromide 24.99 mg are equivalent to 20 mg of citalopram.

Adverse Effects, Treatment, and Precautions

As for selective serotonin reuptake inhibitors (SSRIs) in general (see Fluoxetine, p.284).

Interactions

For interactions associated with selective serotonin reuptake inhibitors, see Fluoxetine, p.286.

Pharmacokinetics

Citalopram is readily absorbed from the gastro-intestinal tract and maximum plasma concentrations are reached 2 to 4 hours after oral administration. Citalopram is widely distributed throughout the body; protein binding is low. Citalopram is metabolised by demethylation, deamination, and oxidation to inactive metabolites. The elimination half-life of citalopram is reported to be about 33 hours. It is excreted in the urine and faeces. Citalopram is distributed into breast milk in very low concentrations.

Uses and Administration

Citalopram, a phthalane derivative, is a selective serotonin reuptake inhibitor (SSRI) with actions and uses similar to those of fluoxetine (p.287). Citalopram is given by mouth as citalopram hydrobromide, usually as a single dose. Doses are expressed in terms of citalopram.

In the treatment of depression, the dose of citalopram is 20 to 60 mg daily by mouth. Doses at the lower end of the therapeutic range should be employed in elderly patients and those with hepatic impairment. Citalopram has also been given as the hydrochloride by intravenous infusion in similar doses when the oral route is impracticable.

In the treatment of panic disorder with or without agoraphobia, the initial dose of citalopram is 10 mg daily by mouth increasing to 20 mg daily after one week. The dose may be increased thereafter as required up to a maximum of 60 mg daily.

Citalopram should be withdrawn gradually to reduce the risk of withdrawal symptoms.

Reviews.

1. Milne RJ, Goa KL. Citalopram: a review of its pharmacodynamic and pharmacokinetic properties, and therapeutic potential in depressive illness. *Drugs* 1991; **41:** 450–77.

Alcohol dependence. Studies[1,2] suggested that citalopram might reduce alcohol intake and the desire to drink in the short-term in patients with alcohol dependence (p.1099) but it appeared to be no more effective than placebo after 12 weeks of treatment.[2]

1. Naranjo CA, *et al.* Citalopram decreases desirability, liking, and consumption of alcohol in alcohol-dependent drinkers. *Clin Pharmacol Ther* 1992; **51:** 729–39.
2. Naranjo CA, *et al.* Effects of citalopram and a brief psychosocial intervention on alcohol intake, dependence and problems. *Addiction* 1995; **90:** 87–99.

Anxiety disorders. Citalopram has been given in a variety of anxiety disorders (p.635) including panic disorders, obsessive-compulsive disorder, and social phobia.

References.

1. Wade AG, *et al.* The effect of citalopram in panic disorder. *Br J Psychiatry* 1997; **170:** 549–53.
2. Koponen H, *et al.* Citalopram in the treatment of obsessive-compulsive disorder: an open pilot study. *Acta Psychiatr Scand* 1997; **96:** 343–6.
3. Bouwer C, Skin DJ. Use of the selective serotonin reuptake inhibitor citalopram in the treatment of generalized social phobia. *J Affective Disord* 1998; **49:** 79–82.

Depression. As discussed on p.271, there is very little difference in efficacy between the different groups of antidepressant drugs. Selective serotonin reuptake inhibitors (SSRIs) such as citalopram are increasingly being recognised as first-choice treatment because they offer advantages over the older tricyclics in terms of fewer unpleasant side-effects and safety in overdosage.

References.

1. Shaw DM, *et al.* A comparison of the antidepressant action of citalopram and amitriptyline. *Br J Psychiatry* 1986; **149:** 515–17.
2. Andersen G, *et al.* Effective treatment of poststroke depression with the selective serotonin reuptake inhibitor citalopram. *Stroke* 1994; **25:** 1099–1104.
3. Montgomery SA, *et al.* The optimal dosing regimen for citalopram—a meta-analysis of nine placebo-controlled studies. *Int Clin Psychopharmacol* 1994; **9** (suppl 1): 35–40.
4. Rosenberg C, *et al.* Citalopram and imipramine in the treatment of depressive patients in general practice: a Nordic Multicentre Clinical Study. *Int Clin Psychopharmacol* 1994; **9** (suppl 1): 41–8.
5. Patris M, *et al.* Citalopram versus fluoxetine: a double-blind, controlled, multicentre, phase III trial in patients with unipolar major depression treated in general practice. *Int Clin Psychopharmacol* 1996; **11:** 129–36.
6. Anonymous. Three new antidepressants. *Drug Ther Bull* 1996; **34:** 65–8.

Pathological crying or laughing. Inappropriate or uncontrolled crying or laughing can occur in patients with lesions in certain areas of the brain. Attempts at treatment have mostly been with antidepressant drugs, including selective serotonin reuptake inhibitors (SSRIs). Favourable results have been reported in a double-blind placebo-controlled study[1] with citalopram.

1. Andersen G, *et al.* Citalopram for post-stroke pathological crying. *Lancet* 1993; **342:** 837–9.

Schizophrenia. The treatment of schizophrenia consists mainly of a combination of social therapy and antipsychotic drugs (see p.637). In a preliminary placebo-controlled study[1] in 15 patients with chronic schizophrenia who exhibited signs of impulsive aggression, citalopram given in addition to existing antipsychotic therapy significantly reduced the frequency of aggressive incidents but not the average severity of the incidents.

1. Vartiainen H, *et al.* Citalopram, a selective serotonin reuptake inhibitor, in the treatment of aggression in schizophrenia. *Acta Psychiatr Scand* 1995; **91:** 348–51.

Preparations

Proprietary Preparations (details are given in Part 3)
Aust.: Seralgan; Seropram; ***Austral.:*** Cipramil; ***Belg.:*** Cipramil; ***Fr.:*** Seropram; ***Ger.:*** Cipramil; ***Irl.:*** Cipramil; ***Ital.:*** Elopram; Seropram; ***Neth.:*** Cipramil; ***Norw.:*** Cipramil; ***S.Afr.:*** Cipramil; ***Spain:*** Prisdal; Seropram; ***Swed.:*** Cipramil; ***Switz.:*** Seropram; ***UK:*** Cipramil; ***USA:*** Celexa.

Clomipramine Hydrochloride

(2507-e)

Clomipramine Hydrochloride (*BANM, USAN, rINNM*).

Chlorimipramine Hydrochloride; Clomipramini Hydrochloridum; G-34586; Monochlorimipramine Hydrochloride. 3-(3-Chloro-10,11-dihydro-5*H*-dibenz[*b,f*]azepin-5-yl)propyldimethylamine hydrochloride.

$C_{19}H_{23}ClN_2,HCl = 351.3$.

CAS — 303-49-1 (clomipramine); 17321-77-6 (clomipramine hydrochloride).

Pharmacopoeias. In *Eur.* (see p.viii) and *Jpn.*

A slightly hygroscopic white or slightly yellow crystalline powder. Freely **soluble** in water and in dichloromethane; soluble in alcohol; practically insoluble in ether. A 10% solution in water has a pH of 3.5 to 5.0. **Protect** from light.

Adverse Effects, Treatment, and Precautions

As for tricyclic antidepressants in general (see Amitriptyline, p.273).

Porphyria. Clomipramine was considered to be unsafe in patients with acute porphyria.[1]

1. Moore MR, McColl KEL. *Porphyria: drug lists.* Glasgow: Porphyria Research Unit, University of Glasgow, 1991.

Interactions

For interactions associated with tricyclic antidepressants, see Amitriptyline, p.276.

In relation to interactions with other antidepressants, it should be noted that the combination of clomipramine and tranylcypromine is particularly hazardous, and that the serotonin syndrome (p.303) has occurred in patients receiving clomipramine and moclobemide (see under Interactions of Antidepressants in Phenelzine, p.305).

Pharmacokinetics

Clomipramine is readily absorbed from the gastro-intestinal tract, and extensively demethylated during first-pass metabolism in the liver to its primary active metabolite, desmethylclomipramine.

Clomipramine and desmethylclomipramine are widely distributed throughout the body and are extensively bound to plasma and tissue protein. Clomipramine has been estimated to have a plasma elimination half-life of about 21 hours, which may be considerably extended in overdosage; that of desmethylclomipramine is longer.

Paths of metabolism of both clomipramine and desmethylclomipramine include hydroxylation and *N*-oxidation. Clomipramine is excreted in the urine, mainly in the form of its metabolites, either free or in conjugated form. Clomipramine crosses the placenta and is distributed into breast milk.

References.

1. Gex-Fabry M, *et al.* Clomipramine metabolism: model-based analysis of variability factors from drug monitoring data. *Clin Pharmacokinet* 1990; **19:** 241–55.
2. Balant-Gorgia AE, *et al.* Clinical pharmacokinetics of clomipramine. *Clin Pharmacokinet* 1991; **20:** 447–62.
3. Nielsen KK, *et al.* Single-dose kinetics of clomipramine: relationship to the sparteine and S-mephenytoin oxidation polymorphisms. *Clin Pharmacol Ther* 1994; **55:** 518–27.

Uses and Administration

Clomipramine is a dibenzazepine tricyclic antidepressant with actions and uses similar to those of amitriptyline (p.278). It has antimuscarinic properties and is also a potent serotonin reuptake inhibitor. Clomipramine is one of the more sedating tricyclics.

In the treatment of depression, clomipramine is given by mouth as the hydrochloride in doses of 10 mg daily initially, increasing gradually to 30 to 150 mg daily if required; up to 250 mg daily may be given in severe cases. A suggested initial dose for the elderly is 10 mg daily increasing gradually to 30 to 50 mg daily if required. Clomipramine may be given in divided doses throughout the day, but since it has a prolonged half-life, once-daily dosage regimens are also suitable, usually given at night.

In the treatment of obsessive-compulsive disorders and phobias, clomipramine hydrochloride may be given by mouth in an initial dose of 25 mg daily (or 10 mg daily for elderly patients) increased gradually over two weeks to 100 to 150 mg daily. In the USA, maximum doses of 250 mg daily have been used.

In the adjunctive treatment of cataplexy associated with narcolepsy, clomipramine hydrochloride is given by mouth in an initial dose of 10 mg daily and gradually increased until a satisfactory response occurs, usually within the range of 10 to 75 mg daily.

In the initial stages of treatment of depression or obsessional or phobic states only, if administration by mouth is impracticable or inadvisable clomipramine may be given by the intramuscular or intravenous routes. The daily dose of clomipramine hydrochloride by intramuscular injection is 25 to 50 mg, increasing by 25 mg a day up to a maximum of 100 to 150 mg daily; oral administration should be substituted as soon as possible. Clomipramine hydrochloride may also be given by intravenous infusion in initial doses of 25 to 50 mg diluted in 250 to 500 mL of sodium chloride 0.9% or glucose 5% and infused over 1.5 to 3 hours to assess tolerance; the dose may then be increased by 25 mg daily until an optimum therapeutic dose is achieved; this is usually about 100 mg daily, although more may be required. As the initial dose is gradually increased the volume of infusion fluid may be decreased to a minimum of 125 mL, and the duration of infusion decreased to a minimum of 45 minutes. When a satisfactory response to intravenous infusion has been obtained (usually after 7 to 10 days) oral therapy should be substituted, initially giving double the maximum intravenous dose by mouth and subsequently adjusting to a satisfactory maintenance dose if necessary. Patients must be carefully supervised during intravenous infusion of clomipramine hydrochloride and the blood pressure carefully monitored owing to the risk of hypotension.

Clomipramine should be withdrawn gradually to reduce the risk of withdrawal symptoms.

Anxiety disorders. Tricyclic antidepressants that are serotonin reuptake inhibitors such as clomipramine and imipramine have been given in the management of anxiety disorders (p.635) including obsessive-compulsive disorder, phobias, panic disorders, and trichotillomania.

References.

1. Insel TR, *et al.* Obsessive-compulsive disorder: a double-blind trial of clomipramine and clorgyline. *Arch Gen Psychiatry* 1983; **40:** 605–12.
2. Marks IM, *et al.* Clomipramine, self-exposure and therapist-aided exposure for obsessive-compulsive rituals. *Br J Psychiatry* 1988; **152:** 522–34.
3. Jenike MA, *et al.* Obsessive-compulsive disorder: a double-blind, placebo-controlled trial of clomipramine in 27 patients. *Am J Psychiatry* 1989; **146:** 1328–30.
4. Flament MF, *et al.* Clomipramine treatment of childhood obsessive-compulsive disorder: a double-blind controlled study. *Arch Gen Psychiatry* 1985; **42:** 977–83.
5. Leonard H, *et al.* Treatment of childhood obsessive compulsive disorder with clomipramine and desmethylimipramine: a double-blind crossover comparison. *Psychopharmacol Bull* 1988; **24:** 93–5.
6. McTavish D, Benfield P. Clomipramine: an overview of its pharmacological properties and a review of its therapeutic use in obsessive compulsive disorder and panic disorder. *Drugs* 1990; **39:** 136–53.
7. Kelly MW, Myers CW. Clomipramine: a tricyclic antidepressant effective in obsessive compulsive disorder. *DICP Ann Pharmacother* 1990; **24:** 739–44.
8. Swedo SE, *et al.* A double-blind comparison of clomipramine and desipramine in the treatment of trichotillomania (hair pulling). *N Engl J Med* 1989; **321:** 497–501.

Autism. There is an anecdotal report that clomipramine alleviated adventitious movements when tried in 5 boys with autistic disorder.[1]

1. Brasic JR, *et al.* Clomipramine ameliorates adventitious movements and compulsions in prepubertal boys with autistic disorder and severe mental retardation. *Neurology* 1994; **44:** 1309–12.

Depression. As discussed on p.271, there is very little difference in efficacy between the different groups of antidepressant drugs, and choice is often made on the basis of adverse effect profile. Tricyclic antidepressants such as clomipramine have traditionally been the first choice for the treatment of depression, and often still are because of wide experience with their use and familiarity with their pharmacological actions. Clomipramine is one of the more sedating tricyclics and consequently may be of value in depression with associated agitation or anxiety.

For specific mention of the use of clomipramine in combination with MAOIs, see Antidepressants under Interactions of Phenelzine, p.305.

Narcoleptic syndrome. Tricyclic antidepressants are the primary treatment for cataplexy and sleep paralysis associated with narcolepsy (p.1476). Clomipramine and imipramine appear to be the most widely used for these symptoms. The onset of action is quicker than when used for depression and doses required appear to be lower. Doses should be titrated to provide maximal protection for the time of day when symptoms usually occur and evening doses should be avoided to minimise nocturnal arousal.

Premenstrual syndrome. Clomipramine has been shown in a placebo-controlled trial[1] to be effective in reducing premenstrual irritability and depressed mood when administered during the luteal phase. Doses of clomipramine ranged from 25 to 75 mg daily. It was postulated that the efficacy of clomipramine in relieving premenstrual symptoms is related to its serotonin reuptake inhibitor activity. For the overall management of premenstrual syndrome, see p.1456.

1. Sundblad C, *et al.* Clomipramine administered during the luteal phase reduces the symptoms of premenstrual syndrome: a placebo-controlled trial. *Neuropsychopharmacology* 1993; **9:** 133–45.

Sexual dysfunction. Clomipramine has been used for its inhibitory effect on ejaculation to treat men for premature ejaculation.[1]

1. Hawton K. Erectile dysfunction and premature ejaculation. *Br J Hosp Med* 1988; **40:** 428–36.

Stuttering. Clomipramine was of modest success in a controlled study[1] of 17 patients with developmental stuttering (p.674). It was suggested that its efficacy may be related to its serotonin reuptake inhibitor activity.

1. Gordon CT, *et al.* A double-blind comparison of clomipramine and desipramine in the treatment of developmental stuttering. *J Clin Psychiatry* 1995; **56:** 238–42.

Preparations

BP 1998: Clomipramine Capsules.

Proprietary Preparations (details are given in Part 3)
Aust.: Anafranil; ***Austral.:*** Anafranil; Placil; ***Belg.:*** Anafranil; ***Canad.:*** Anafranil; Novo-Clopamine; ***Fr.:*** Anafranil; ***Ger.:*** Anafranil; Hydiphen; ***Irl.:*** Anafranil; ***Ital.:*** Anafranil; ***Neth.:*** Anafranil; ***Norw.:*** Anafranil; ***S.Afr.:*** Anafranil; ***Spain:*** Anafranil; ***Swed.:*** Anafranil; ***Switz.:*** Anafranil; ***UK:*** Anafranil; Tranquax; ***USA:*** Anafranil.

Clorgyline Hydrochloride (2508-l)

Clorgyline Hydrochloride *(BANM)*.

Clorgiline Hydrochloride *(rINNM)*; M & B-9302. 3-(2,4-Dichlorophenoxy)propyl(methyl)prop-2-ynylamine hydrochloride.

$C_{13}H_{15}Cl_2NO,HCl = 308.6$.

CAS — 17780-72-2 (clorgyline); 17780-75-5 (clorgyline hydrochloride).

Clorgyline hydrochloride, a propylamine derivative, is an irreversible inhibitor of monoamine oxidase type A (see Phenelzine, p.302) that has been tried in the treatment of depression. Although research and development as an antidepressant appears to have been abandoned clorgyline is sometimes used as a pharmacological tool.

Demexiptiline Hydrochloride (3933-j)

Demexiptiline Hydrochloride *(rINNM)*.

LM-2909. *O*-[2-(Methylamino)ethyl]oxime-5*H*-dibenzo[*a,d*]cyclohepten-5-one hydrochloride.

$C_{18}H_{18}N_2O,HCl = 314.8$.

CAS — 24701-51-7 (demexiptiline).

Demexiptiline hydrochloride is a tricyclic antidepressant (see Amitriptyline, p.273).

Preparations

Proprietary Preparations (details are given in Part 3)
Fr.: Tinoran†.

Desipramine Hydrochloride (2509-y)

Desipramine Hydrochloride *(BANM, USAN, rINNM)*.

Desipramini Hydrochloridum; Desmethylimipramine Hydrochloride; DMI; EX-4355; G-35020; JB-8181; NSC-114901; RMI-9384A. 3-(10,11-Dihydro-5*H*-dibenz[*b,f*]azepin-5-yl)propyl(methyl)amine hydrochloride.

$C_{18}H_{22}N_2,HCl = 302.8$.

CAS — 50-47-5 (desipramine); 58-28-6 (desipramine hydrochloride).

Pharmacopoeias. In Eur. (see p.viii) and US.

A white or almost white, crystalline powder. **Soluble** 1 in 12 of water, 1 in 14 of alcohol, and 1 in 3.5 of chloroform; practically insoluble in ether; freely soluble in methyl alcohol. **Store** in airtight containers. Protect from light.

Adverse Effects, Treatment, and Precautions

As for tricyclic antidepressants in general (see Amitriptyline, p.273).

Interactions

For interactions associated with tricyclic antidepressants, see Amitriptyline, p.276.

Pharmacokinetics

Desipramine is the principal active metabolite of imipramine (p.289).

Uses and Administration

Desipramine, the principal active metabolite of imipramine (p.289), is a dibenzazepine tricyclic antidepressant with actions and uses similar to those of amitriptyline (p.278). It is one of the less sedating tricyclics and its antimuscarinic effects are mild.

In the treatment of depression, desipramine is given as the hydrochloride by mouth in daily doses of 100 to 200 mg; higher doses of up to 300 mg daily may be required in severely depressed patients in hospital. Lower doses should be used in adolescents and the elderly and are usually 25 to 100 mg daily; higher doses of up to 150 mg daily may be required for severe depression. Initial doses should be at a lower level and gradually increased according to tolerance and clinical response. Therapy may initially be given as a single daily dose or in divided doses; maintenance therapy may be given as a single daily dose usually at night.

Desipramine should be withdrawn gradually to reduce the risk of withdrawal symptoms.

Alcohol dependence. Desipramine has been tried with some success to treat depression secondary to alcohol dependence in recently abstinent patients.[1] It was suggested that treatment of secondary depression may reduce the risk for drinking relapse in depressed patients. However, use of desipramine to prevent drinking relapse could not be extended to patients who are not depressed.

For a discussion of the management of alcohol withdrawal and abstinence, see p.1099.

1. Mason BJ, *et al.* A double-blind, placebo-controlled trial of desipramine for primary alcohol dependence stratified on the presence or absence of major depression. *JAMA* 1996; **275:** 761–7.

Cocaine dependence. The overall management of cocaine withdrawal symptoms is discussed on p.1291. Since dopamine depletion may be the cause of the depression often associated with cocaine craving and with relapse, drugs such as desipramine that interact with dopaminergic systems have been tried in managing cocaine withdrawal symptoms. However, studies[1-4] have provided conflicting results on the use of desipramine for the management of persons who abuse cocaine, and the idea of giving desipramine to cocaine-dependent persons has been both criticised[5] and defended.[6]

1. Giannini AJ, *et al.* Treatment of depression in chronic cocaine and phencyclidine abuse with desipramine. *J Clin Pharmacol* 1986; **26:** 211–14.
2. Weiss RD. Relapse to cocaine abuse after initiating desipramine treatment. *JAMA* 1988; **260:** 2545–6.
3. Gawin FH, *et al.* Desipramine facilitation of initial cocaine abstinence. *Arch Gen Psychiatry* 1989; **46:** 117–21.
4. Fischman MW, *et al.* Effects of desipramine maintenance on cocaine self-administration by humans. *J Pharmacol Exp Ther* 1990; **253:** 760–70.
5. Clark RJ. The treatment of chemical dependence. *JAMA* 1989; **261:** 3239.
6. Weiss RD. The treatment of chemical dependence. *JAMA* 1989; **261:** 3239.

Depression. As discussed on p.271, there is very little difference in efficacy between the different groups of antidepressant drugs, and choice is often made on the basis of adverse effect profile. Tricyclic antidepressants such as desipramine have traditionally been the first choice for the treatment of depression, and often still are because of wide experience with their use and familiarity with their pharmacological actions. Desipramine is one of the less sedating tricyclics and consequently may be of value for withdrawn or apathetic depressed patients.

Hyperactivity. When drugs are required for children with attention deficit hyperactivity disorder, initial treatment is usually with central stimulants (see p.1476). Tricyclic antidepressants such as imipramine or desipramine[1-3] are also used but, because of lower efficacy and associated adverse effects, are reserved for patients who fail to respond to, or who are intolerant of, stimulants. They may also be of use for selected patients with certain co-existing disorders.

1. Rapport MD, *et al.* Methylphenidate and desipramine in hospitalized children: I. separate and combined effects on cognitive function. *J Am Acad Child Adolesc Psychiatry* 1993; **32:** 333–42.
2. Pataki CS, *et al.* Side effects of methylphenidate and desipramine alone and in combination in children. *J Am Acad Child Adolesc Psychiatry* 1993; **32:** 1065–72.
3. Singer HS, *et al.* The treatment of attention-deficit hyperactivity disorder in Tourette's syndrome: a double-blind placebo-controlled study with clonidine and desipramine. *Pediatrics* 1995; **95:** 74–81.

Pain. Antidepressants, usually amitriptyline or another tricyclic, are useful in alleviating some types of pain (p.4) when given in subantidepressant doses.

References.

1. Kishore-Kumar R, *et al.* Desipramine relieves postherpetic neuralgia. *Clin Pharmacol Ther* 1990; **47:** 305–12.
2. Max MB, *et al.* Effects of desipramine, amitriptyline, and fluoxetine on pain in diabetic neuropathy. *N Engl J Med* 1992; **326:** 1250–6.
3. Coquoz D, *et al.* Central analgesic effects of desipramine, fluvoxamine, and moclobemide after single oral dosing: a study in healthy volunteers. *Clin Pharmacol Ther* 1993; **54:** 339–44.
4. Gordon NC, *et al.* Temporal factors in the enhancement of morphine analgesia by desipramine. *Pain* 1993; **53:** 273–6.

Preparations

BP 1998: Desipramine Tablets;
USP 23: Desipramine Hydrochloride Capsules; Desipramine Hydrochloride Tablets.

Proprietary Preparations (details are given in Part 3)
Aust.: Pertofran; ***Austral.:*** Pertofran; ***Belg.:*** Pertofran; ***Canad.:*** Norpramin; Pertofrane; ***Fr.:*** Pertofran; ***Ger.:*** Pertofran; Petylyl; ***Irl.:*** Pertofran†; ***Ital.:*** Nortimil; ***Neth.:*** Pertofran; ***Norw.:*** Sertofren†; ***S.Afr.:*** Pertofran†; ***Switz.:*** Pertofran†; ***UK:*** Pertofran†; ***USA:*** Norpramin; Pertofrane†.

Dibenzepin Hydrochloride (2510-g)

Dibenzepin Hydrochloride *(BANM, USAN, rINNM)*.

HF-1927. 10-(2-Dimethylaminoethyl)-5,10-dihydro-5-methyl-dibenzo[*b,e*][1,4]diazepin-11-one hydrochloride.

$C_{18}H_{21}N_3O,HCl = 331.8$.

CAS — 4498-32-2 (dibenzepin); 315-80-0 (dibenzepin hydrochloride).

Dibenzepin hydrochloride is a tricyclic antidepressant (see Amitriptyline, p.273).

In the treatment of depression dibenzepin hydrochloride is given by mouth in doses of 240 to 480 mg daily; higher doses of up to 720 mg daily may be required in some patients with severe depression.

Dibenzepin hydrochloride has also been given in doses of up to 360 mg daily by intravenous infusion.

Dibenzepin should be withdrawn gradually to reduce the risk of withdrawal symptoms.

References.

1. Wirtheim E, Bloch Y. Dibenzepin overdose causing pulmonary edema. *Ann Pharmacother* 1996; **30:** 789–90.

Preparations

Proprietary Preparations (details are given in Part 3)
Aust.: Noveril; ***Belg.:*** Noveril†; ***Ger.:*** Noveril; ***Ital.:*** Noveril†; ***Neth.:*** Noveril†; ***S.Afr.:*** Noveril†; ***Switz.:*** Noveril.

Dothiepin Hydrochloride (2512-p)

Dothiepin Hydrochloride *(BANM, USAN)*.

Dosulepin Hydrochloride *(rINNM)*; Dosulepini Hydrochloridum. 3-(Dibenzo[*b,e*]thiepin-11-ylidene)propyldimethylamine hydrochloride.

$C_{19}H_{21}NS,HCl = 331.9.$

CAS — 113-53-1 (dothiepin); 897-15-4 (dothiepin hydrochloride).

Pharmacopoeias. In *Eur.* (see p.viii).

A white to faintly yellow crystalline powder. It consists chiefly of the *E*-isomer. Freely **soluble** in water, in alcohol, and in dichloromethane. **Protect** from light.

Adverse Effects, Treatment, and Precautions

As for tricyclic antidepressants in general (see Amitriptyline, p.273).

Interactions

For interactions associated with tricyclic antidepressants, see Amitriptyline, p.276.

Pharmacokinetics

Dothiepin hydrochloride is readily absorbed from the gastro-intestinal tract, and extensively demethylated by first-pass metabolism in the liver to its primary active metabolite, desmethyldothiepin (also termed northiaden). Paths of metabolism also include *S*-oxidation.

Dothiepin is excreted in the urine, mainly in the form of its metabolites; small amounts are also excreted in the faeces. Elimination half-lives of about 14 to 24 and 23 to 46 hours have been reported for dothiepin and its metabolites respectively.

Dothiepin is distributed into breast milk (see Breast Feeding under Precautions in Amitriptyline, p.275).

References.

1. Maguire KP, *et al.* Clinical pharmacokinetics of dothiepin: single-dose kinetics in patients and prediction of steady-state concentrations. *Clin Pharmacokinet* 1983; **8:** 179–85.
2. Yu DK, *et al.* Pharmacokinetics of dothiepin in humans: a single dose dose-proportionality study. *J Pharm Sci* 1986; **75:** 582–5.
3. Ilett KF, *et al.* The excretion of dothiepin and its primary metabolites in breast milk. *Br J Clin Pharmacol* 1993; **33:** 635–9.

Uses and Administration

Dothiepin hydrochloride is a tricyclic antidepressant with actions and uses similar to those of amitriptyline (p.278). It is one of the more sedating tricyclics.

In the treatment of depression, dothiepin hydrochloride is given by mouth in doses of 25 mg three times daily initially, gradually increased to 50 mg three times daily if necessary; alternatively a single dose at night may be given. Higher doses of up to 225 mg daily have been given in severely depressed patients. The recommended initial dose for the elderly is 50 to 75 mg daily. Half the normal maintenance dose may be adequate.

Dothiepin should be withdrawn gradually to reduce the risk of withdrawal symptoms.

Depression. As discussed on p.271, there is very little difference in efficacy between the different groups of antidepressant drugs, and choice is often made on the basis of adverse effect profile. Tricyclic antidepressants such as dothiepin were formerly the first choice for the treatment of depression, and often still are because of wide experience with their use and familiarity with their pharmacological actions. Dothiepin is one of the more sedating tricyclics and consequently may be of value in depression with associated agitation or anxiety.

References.

1. Goldstein BJ, Claghorn JL. An overview of seventeen years experience with dothiepin in the treatment of depression in Europe. *J Clin Psychiatry* 1980; **41:** 64–70.
2. Lancaster SG, Gonzalez JP. Dothiepin: a review of its pharmacodynamic and pharmacokinetic properties, and therapeutic efficacy in depressive illness. *Drugs* 1989; **38:** 123–47.
3. Donovan S, *et al.* Dothiepin versus amitriptyline for depression: an analysis of comparative studies. *Drug Invest* 1991; **3:** 178–82.

Pain. Antidepressants, usually amitriptyline or another tricyclic, are useful in alleviating some types of pain (p.4) when given in subantidepressant doses.

References.

1. Feinmann C, *et al.* Psychogenic facial pain: presentation and treatment. *Br Med J* 1984; **288:** 436–8.
2. Caruso I, *et al.* Double-blind study of dothiepin versus placebo in the treatment of primary fibromyalgia syndrome. *J Int Med Res* 1987; **15:** 154–9.

Preparations

BP 1998: Dosulepin Capsules; Dosulepin Tablets.

Proprietary Preparations (details are given in Part 3)
Aust.: Xerenal; ***Austral.:*** Dothep; Prothiaden; ***Belg.:*** Prothiaden; ***Fr.:*** Prothiaden; ***Ger.:*** Idom; ***Irl.:*** Prothiaden; ***Ital.:*** Protiaden; ***Neth.:*** Prothiaden; ***S.Afr.:*** Jardin; Prothiaden; Thaden; ***Spain:*** Prothiaden; ***Switz.:*** Protiaden; ***UK:*** Prepadine; Prothiaden.

Multi-ingredient: ***Aust.:*** Harmomed.

Doxepin Hydrochloride (2513-s)

Doxepin Hydrochloride *(BANM, USAN, rINNM)*.

Doxepini Hydrochloridum; NSC-108160; P-3693A. 3-(Dibenz[*b,e*]oxepin-11-ylidene)propyldimethylamine hydrochloride.

$C_{19}H_{21}NO,HCl = 315.8.$

CAS — 1668-19-5 (doxepin); 1229-29-4 (doxepin hydrochloride); 4698-39-9 (doxepin hydrochloride, E-isomer); 25127-31-5 (doxepin hydrochloride, Z-isomer).

Pharmacopoeias. In *Eur.* (see p.viii), *Pol.*, and *US.*

A white or almost white crystalline powder with a slight amine-like odour. It consists of a mixture of *Z*- and *E*-isomers. Doxepin hydrochloride 113 mg is approximately equivalent to 100 mg of doxepin. Freely **soluble** in water, in alcohol, and in dichloromethane. **Protect** from light.

Adverse Effects, Treatment, and Precautions

As for tricyclic antidepressants in general (see Amitriptyline, p.273). Drowsiness and other systemic effects can also occur following topical application.

Interactions

For interactions associated with tricyclic antidepressants, see Amtriptyline, p.276.

Pharmacokinetics

Doxepin is readily absorbed from the gastro-intestinal tract, and extensively demethylated by first-pass metabolism in the liver, to its primary active metabolite, desmethyldoxepin. Doxepin is also absorbed through the skin following topical application.

Paths of metabolism of both doxepin and desmethyldoxepin include hydroxylation and *N*-oxidation. Doxepin is excreted in the urine, mainly in the form of its metabolites, either free or in conjugated form.

Doxepin and desmethyldoxepin are widely distributed throughout the body and are extensively bound to plasma and tissue protein. Doxepin has been estimated to have a plasma half-life ranging from 8 to 24 hours, which may be considerably extended in overdosage; that of desmethyldoxepin is longer.

Doxepin crosses the blood-brain barrier and the placenta. It is distributed into breast milk (see Breast Feeding under Precautions in Amitriptyline, p.275).

References.

1. Faulkner RD, *et al.* Multiple-dose doxepin kinetics in depressed patients. *Clin Pharmacol Ther* 1983; **34:** 509–15.
2. Joyce PR, Sharman JR. Doxepin plasma concentrations in clinical practice: could there be a pharmacokinetic explanation for low concentrations? *Clin Pharmacokinet* 1985; **10:** 365–70.

Uses and Administration

Doxepin is a dibenzoxepine tricyclic antidepressant with actions and uses similar to those of amitriptyline (p.278). It has moderate antimuscarinic and marked sedative properties and has serotonin re-uptake inhibitor activity.

In the treatment of depression doxepin is given by mouth as the hydrochloride in doses equivalent to doxepin 75 mg daily initially, gradually adjusted according to individual response. Doses of up to 300 mg daily may be required in severely depressed patients; mildly affected patients may respond to as little as 25 to 50 mg daily. Daily doses up to 100 mg may be given in divided doses or as a single dose at bedtime. If the total daily dose exceeds 100 mg, it should be given in divided doses, although the largest portion up to a maximum of 100 mg may be given at bedtime. In the USA, the maximum single dose is 150 mg. A suggested starting dose in the elderly is 10 to 50 mg daily. A satisfactory response may be obtained in many elderly patients at a daily dose of 30 to 50 mg.

Doxepin hydrochloride has also been given by intramuscular or intravenous injection.

Doxepin should be withdrawn gradually to reduce the risk of withdrawal symptoms.

Doxepin has histamine H_1- and H_2-receptor antagonist activity and is used topically in a cream containing 5% of the hydrochloride for the short-term (up to 8 days) relief of moderately severe pruritus associated with various types of dermatitis (see below).

Depression. As discussed on p.271, there is very little difference in efficacy between the different groups of antidepressant drugs, and choice is often made on the basis of adverse effect profile. Tricyclic antidepressants such as doxepin were formerly the first choice for the treatment of depression, and often still are because of wide experience with their use and familiarity with their pharmacological actions. Doxepin is one of the more sedating tricyclics and consequently may be of value in depression with associated agitation or anxiety.

Headache. Tricyclic antidepressants can be effective in the management of some types of headache and although they are especially useful when the headache is accompanied by depression their beneficial effects are independent of their antidepressant action.

References.

1. Wörz R, Scherhag R. Treatment of chronic tension headache with doxepin or amitriptyline—results of a double-blind study. *Headache Q* 1990; **1:** 216–23.

Skin disorders. Tricyclic antidepressants have a wide range of pharmacological activity and some members of the group have notable antihistaminic actions. Doxepin in particular has very potent antihistaminic activity. It has been shown to be an effective oral alternative to conventional H_1-antagonist antihistamines in the treatment of chronic urticaria,[1-3] and to be an effective oral treatment for idiopathic cold urticaria.[4,5] In the case of cold urticaria it was suggested that the action of doxepin was due to inhibition of platelet-activating factor-like lipid release.[5]

For an overview of the possible treatments for the various urticarias, including mention of the use of doxepin, see p.1076.

Doxepin has also been used topically for the relief of pruritus associated with various types of allergic and inflammatory skin disorders[6,7] but some authorities remain to be convinced of its efficacy.[8] Topical application of doxepin can also produce drowsiness and other systemic effects. The management of pruritus is briefly discussed on p.1075 but more details on the use of standard antihistamines in this condition can be found on p.400.

1. Greene SL, *et al.* Double-blind crossover study comparing doxepin with diphenhydramine for the treatment of chronic urticaria. *J Am Acad Dermatol* 1985; **12:** 669–75.
2. Harto A, *et al.* Doxepin in the treatment of chronic urticaria. *Dermatologica* 1985; **170:** 90–3.
3. Goldsobel AB, *et al.* Efficacy of doxepin in the treatment of chronic idiopathic urticaria. *J Allergy Clin Immunol* 1986; **78:** 867–73.
4. Neittaanmäki H, *et al.* Comparison of cinnarizine, cyproheptadine, doxepin, and hydroxyzine in treatment of idiopathic cold urticaria: usefulness of doxepin. *J Am Acad Dermatol* 1984; **11:** 483–9.
5. Grandel KE, *et al.* Association of platelet-activating factor with primary acquired cold urticaria. *N Engl J Med* 1985; **313:** 405–9.
6. Drake LA, *et al.* Relief of pruritus in patients with atopic dermatitis after treatment with topical doxepin cream. *J Am Acad Dermatol* 1994; **31:** 613–16.
7. Smith PF, Corelli RL. Doxepin in the management of pruritus associated with allergic cutaneous reactions. *Ann Pharmacother* 1997; **31:** 633–5.
8. Anonymous. Doxepin cream for pruritus. *Med Lett Drugs Ther* 1994; **36:** 99–100.

Preparations

BP 1998: Doxepin Capsules;
USP 23: Doxepin Hydrochloride Capsules; Doxepin Hydrochloride Oral Solution.

Proprietary Preparations (details are given in Part 3)
Aust.: Sinequan; ***Austral.:*** Deptran; Sinequan; ***Belg.:*** Quitaxon; Sinequan; ***Canad.:*** Sinequan; Triadapin; Zonalon; ***Fr.:*** Quitaxon; Sinequan; ***Ger.:*** Aponal; Desidox; Doneurin; Mareen; Sinquan; ***Irl.:*** Sinequan; ***Neth.:*** Sinequan; ***Norw.:*** Sinequan; ***Spain:*** Sinequan; ***Switz.:*** Sinquane; ***UK:*** Sinequan; Xepin; ***USA:*** Adapin†; Sinequan; Zonalon.

Duloxetine Hydrochloride (17135-s)

Duloxetine Hydrochloride *(USAN, rINNM).*

LY-248686 (duloxetine). (+)-(S)-N-Methyl-γ-(1-naphthyloxy)-2-thiophenepropylamine hydrochloride.

$C_{18}H_{19}NOS,HCl = 333.9.$

CAS — 116539-59-4 (duloxetine); 136434-34-9 (duloxetine hydrochloride).

Duloxetine hydrochloride is a serotonin and noradrenaline re-uptake inhibitor (SNRI) under investigation for the treatment of depression. It is also being studied in the management of urinary incontinence.

References.

1. Mulcahy JJ, *et al.* Efficacy and safety of duloxetine in stress incontinence patients. *Neurourol Urodyn* 1996; **15:** 395–6.
2. Berk M, *et al.* An open-label study of duloxetine hydrochloride, a mixed serotonin and noradrenaline reuptake inhibitor, in patients with DSM-111-R major depressive disorder. *Int Clin Psychopharmacol* 1997; **12:** 137–40.

Etoperidone Hydrochloride (12721-w)

Etoperidone Hydrochloride *(USAN, rINNM).*

Clopradone Hydrochloride; McN-A-2673-11; ST-1191 (etoperidone). 2-{3-[4-(3-Chlorophenyl)piperazin-1-yl]propyl}-4,5-diethyl-2,4-dihydro-3H-1,2,4-triazol-3-one hydrochloride.

$C_{19}H_{28}ClN_5O,HCl = 414.4.$

CAS — 52942-31-1 (etoperidone); 57775-22-1 (etoperidone hydrochloride).

Etoperidone hydrochloride is a triazolopyridine antidepressant related structurally to trazodone (p.308). It is used in the treatment of depression in doses of up to 150 mg daily by mouth.

References.

1. Aprile F, *et al.* Etoperidone, maprotiline and trazodone for the therapy of severe depressive conditions requiring hospital admission: a standard controlled study. *Acta Ther* 1983; **9:** 353–66.

Preparations

Proprietary Preparations (details are given in Part 3)
Spain: Centren†; Depraser.

Femoxetine (16802-x)

Femoxetine *(rINN).*

FG-4963 (hydrochloride). (+)-*trans*-3-[(p-Methoxyphenoxy)methyl]-1-methyl-4-phenylpiperidine.

$C_{20}H_{25}NO_2 = 311.4.$

CAS — 59859-58-4.

Femoxetine is a selective serotonin reuptake inhibitor (see Fluoxetine, below) with antidepressant properties.

References.

1. Dahl L-E, *et al.* Antidepressant effect of femoxetine and desipramine and relationship to the concentration of amine metabolites in cerebrospinal fluid. *Acta Psychiatr Scand* 1982; **66:** 9–17.
2. Skrumsager BK, Jeppesen K. Femoxetine and amitriptyline in general practice: a randomized double-blind group comparison. *Pharmacopsychiatry* 1986; **19:** 368–77.
3. Schrader H, *et al.* The treatment of accessory symptoms in narcolepsy: a double-blind cross-over study of a selective serotonin re-uptake inhibitor (femoxetine) versus placebo. *Acta Neurol Scand* 1986; **74:** 297–303.
4. Warrington SJ, *et al.* Cardiovascular (ECG and systolic time intervals) and anticholinergic effects of repeated doses of femoxetine—a comparison with amitriptyline and placebo in healthy men. *Br J Clin Pharmacol* 1989; **27:** 343–51.

Fluoxetine Hydrochloride (12763-x)

Fluoxetine Hydrochloride *(BANM, USAN, rINNM).*

Fluoxetini Hydrochloridum; LY-110140. (±)-N-Methyl-3-phenyl-3-(α,α,α-trifluoro-p-tolyloxy)propylamine hydrochloride.

$C_{17}H_{18}F_3NO,HCl = 345.8.$

CAS — 54910-89-3 (fluoxetine); 59333-67-4 (fluoxetine hydrochloride).

Pharmacopoeias. In *Eur.* (see p.viii) and *US.*

A white or almost white crystalline powder. Fluoxetine hydrochloride 22.4 mg is approximately equivalent to 20 mg of fluoxetine.

Sparingly **soluble** in water and in dichloromethane; freely soluble in alcohol and in methyl alcohol; practically insoluble in ether. A 1% solution in water has a pH of 4.5 to 6.5. **Store** in airtight containers.

References to the pharmaceutical properties of fluoxetine hydrochloride.

1. Peterson JA, *et al.* Stability of fluoxetine hydrochloride in fluoxetine solution diluted with common pharmaceutical diluents. *Am J Hosp Pharm* 1994; **51:** 1342–5.

Adverse Effects

Selective serotonin reuptake inhibitors (SSRIs) such as fluoxetine are less sedative than tricyclic antidepressants and have few antimuscarinic or cardiotoxic effects. Adverse effects reported with fluoxetine include dry mouth and gastro-intestinal disturbances such as nausea, vomiting, dyspepsia, constipation, and diarrhoea. Anorexia and weight loss may also occur. Neurological side-effects have included either anxiety, restlessness, nervousness, and insomnia, or drowsiness and fatigue; headache, tremor, dizziness, convulsions, extrapyramidal effects, and sexual dysfunction have also occurred. The concern that some SSRIs may be associated with increased suicidal ideation is discussed under Effects on Mental State, below.

Excessive sweating and pruritus or skin rashes such as urticaria have also been reported. In some patients who have developed rashes while taking fluoxetine, systemic events involving the lungs, kidneys, or liver, and possibly related to vasculitis, have developed; it has therefore been advised that fluoxetine therapy should be discontinued in any patient who develops a skin rash.

Hyponatraemia, possibly due to inappropriate secretion of antidiuretic hormone, has been associated with the use of antidepressants, particularly in the elderly.

Abnormal liver function tests have been reported.

In overdosage nausea, vomiting, and excitation of the CNS are considered to be prominent features; death has been reported.

In a report[1] from the Committee on Safety of Medicines (CSM) in June 1992 comparing reports received for fluoxetine with those for fluvoxamine the number of adverse reports so far received for fluvoxamine was 1236 (from about 280 000 prescriptions) and for fluoxetine was 2422 (from about 480 000 prescriptions). The overall adverse reactions profiles were similar for both antidepressants apart from dermatological reactions being more likely with fluoxetine and gastro-intestinal reactions with fluvoxamine. Reports of attempted suicide increased after the adverse publicity in 1990 and the number of reports per million prescriptions were similar for the 2 drugs (25 for fluoxetine and 20 for fluvoxamine); such figures were not disconcerting given that features of depression including attempted suicide can worsen after the introduction of any antidepressant.

1. Committee on Safety of Medicines. Safety of fluoxetine (Prozac): comparison with fluvoxamine (Faverin). *Current Problems 34* 1992.

Effects on the blood. Abnormalities in platelet aggregation were associated with fluoxetine given to a severely underweight patient.[1] Platelet activity returned to normal when fluoxetine was discontinued. Fluoxetine was suspected of being the cause of bruising in a patient whose blood clotting parameters were within normal limits.[2] The suggested mechanism was inhibition of uptake of serotonin into platelets, thereby disrupting platelet aggregation. The authors suggested that caution should be exercised when treating patients with thrombocytopenia or platelet dysfunction with fluoxetine.

1. Alderman CP, *et al.* Abnormal platelet aggregation associated with fluoxetine therapy. *Ann Pharmacother* 1992; **26:** 1517–19.
2. Pai VB, Kelly MW. Bruising associated with the use of fluoxetine. *Ann Pharmacother* 1996; **30:** 786–8.

Effects on the cardiovascular system. The selective serotonin reuptake inhibitors (SSRIs) are not associated with the same degree of cardiotoxicity as the tricyclic antidepressants (see p.274), although orthostatic hypotension has been reported in some patients. The manufacturers of fluvoxamine state that a decrease in heart rate with ECG changes has been noted. However, a study[1] on long-term fluvoxamine treatment in 311 patients followed for one year revealed no significant effect on ECG findings compared with patients treated with placebo.

Concern over the use of sertraline in patients with coronary heart disease was raised following a report[2] of a 53-year-old man with a history of coronary heart disease who experienced attacks of sudden precordial chest pain after starting treatment with sertraline. The pain responded to glyceryl trinitrate. The manufacturers[3] pointed out that there had been no ECG changes confirming an ischaemic origin of the disorder in this patient and that in studies sertraline had had no demonstrable clinical effects on intraventricular conduction or ECG intervals. Furthermore, no significant changes in cardiovascular indices had been recorded in patients who had taken overdoses of up to 6 g of sertraline. It was suggested that this might have been an effect on the gastro-intestinal tract possibly at the oesophageal level.

1. Hochberg HM, *et al.* Electrocardiographic findings during extended clinical trials of fluvoxamine in depression: one years experience. *Pharmacopsychiatry* 1995; **28:** 253–6.
2. Iruela LM. Sudden chest pain with sertraline. *Lancet* 1994; **343:** 1106.
3. Berti CA, Doogan DP. Sudden chest pain with sertraline. *Lancet* 1994; **343:** 1510–11.

Effects on the endocrine system. The syndrome of inappropriate antidiuretic hormone secretion (SIADH) with hyponatraemia has been reported in patients receiving antidepressants. The Committee on Safety of Medicines (CSM) in the UK, commenting on reports it had received of hyponatraemia associated with antidepressants (fluoxetine, paroxetine, lofepramine, clomipramine, and imipramine), considered that it was likely to occur with any antidepressant, and usually involved elderly patients.[1] Case reports of hyponatraemia in 16 patients treated with selective serotonin reuptake inhibitors (SSRIs) have been summarised.[2] A further review[3] of reports on 15 patients with hyponatraemia with SIADH induced by fluoxetine (12 cases), fluvoxamine (2), and paroxetine (1) showed that the risk was greatest during the early treatment phase. This is borne out by four single-case reports[4-7] of hyponatraemia with SIADH in elderly patients receiving sertraline.

1. Committee on Safety of Medicines/Medicines Control Agency. Antidepressant-induced hyponatraemia. *Current Problems* 1994; **20:** 5–6.
2. Spigset O, Hedenmalm K. Hyponatraemia and the syndrome of inappropriate antidiuretic hormone secretion (SIADH) induced by psychotropic drugs. *Drug Safety* 1995; **12:** 209–25.
3. Canadian Medical Association. Hyponatraemia and selective serotonin reuptake inhibitors. *Can Med Assoc J* 1996; **154:** 63.
4. Bluff DD. SIADH in a patient receiving sertraline. *Ann Intern Med* 1995; **123:** 811.
5. Adverse Drug Reactions Advisory Committee. Selective serotonin reuptake inhibitors and SIADH. *Med J Aust* 1996; **164:** 562.
6. Kessler J, Samuels SC. Sertraline and hyponatremia. *N Engl J Med* 1996; **335:** 524.
7. Robinson D, *et al.* SIADH—compulsive drinking or SSRI influence? *Ann Pharmacother* 1996; **30:** 885.

Effects on the eyes. Symptoms of glaucoma developed in a patient receiving fluoxetine; the symptoms subsided within 2 days of drug withdrawal.[1] Similar symptoms have been reported[4] with paroxetine. Intra-ocular pressure following fluoxetine administration was recorded in 20 patients in a placebo-controlled crossover double-blind study.[2] Significant increases were demonstrated in all patients 2 hours after receiving fluoxetine by mouth; some patients still had raised intra-ocular pressure after 8 hours.

There has been a report[3] of anisocoria (uneven pupillary dilatation) in one patient taking paroxetine and in another taking sertraline. It was noted that the UK Committee on Safety on Medicines had received 21 reports of mydriasis associated with paroxetine but it appeared that noticeably asymmetrical mydriasis as seen in these 2 patients had not previously been reported.

1. Ahmad S. Fluoxetine and glaucoma. *DICP Ann Pharmacother* 1991; **25:** 436.
2. Costagliola C, *et al.* Fluoxetine oral administration increases intraocular pressure. *Br J Ophthalmol* 1996; **80:** 678.
3. Barrett J. Anisocoria associated with selective serotonin reuptake inhibitors. *Br Med J* 1994; **309:** 1620.
4. Eke T, Carr S. Acute glaucoma, chronic glaucoma, and serotoninergic drugs. *Br J Ophthalmol* 1998; **82:** 976–7.

Effects on the hair. Ogilvie reported that he had seen 2 patients who experienced hair loss associated with the use of fluoxetine.[1] He had found 4 other published cases and had also ascertained that up to the end of 1991 the US manufacturers had received 498 reports of fluoxetine-associated alopecia.

1. Ogilvie AD. Hair loss during fluoxetine treatment. *Lancet* 1993; **342:** 1423.

Effects on mental state. There has been concern that fluoxetine increases *suicidal ideation* and there have been suggestions that there may be a link with akathisia[1] or dosage.[2] However meta-analyses[3,4] (criticism of statistical power not withstanding[5]) have not confirmed an increased risk and this appears to be supported by the results of prescription event monitoring,[6] and is the view of various regulatory authorities. However some reviewers consider that under certain conditions all antidepressants and antipsychotics can induce suicidal ideation in some individuals and comment that there does appear to be enough anecdotal evidence to indicate that fluoxetine may induce suicidal ideation on rare occasions.[7,8] It has been suggested that as suicidal ideation has been associated with induction of akathisia, agitation, or panic by fluoxetine, propranolol might be added to therapy to control these effects.[7,8] There has also been concern that fluvoxamine like fluoxetine may increase suicidal ideation and a suggestion that it might be dose-related.[9]

For a discussion of the choice of antidepressant with respect to safety in overdosage, see under Depression, p.271.

For further effects on mental function, see also under Withdrawal and under Mania in Precautions, below.

There have also been suggested links between the use of fluoxetine and *irritability, hostility, and aggression*.[10] However, one review[8] noted that an unpublished analysis by Heiligenstein *et al.* indicated that patients taking fluoxetine for a variety of disorders were not more likely to be aggressive than those taking placebo. Prescription event monitoring has also found no evidence to suggest that fluoxetine increases the frequency of aggression.[6]

Initiation of antidepressant therapy with paroxetine or sertraline has been associated with either worsening or a new onset of *flashback syndrome* in 2 patients with a history of lysergide abuse.[11]

1. Rothschild AJ, Locke CA. Reexposure to fluoxetine after serious suicide attempts by three patients: the role of akathisia. *J Clin Psychiatry* 1991; **52:** 491–3.
2. Fichtner CG, *et al.* Does fluoxetine have a therapeutic window? *Lancet* 1991; **338:** 520–1.
3. Beasley CM, *et al.* Fluoxetine and suicide: a meta-analysis of controlled trials of treatment for depression. *Br Med J* 1991; **303:** 685–92. Correction. *ibid.*: 968.
4. Goldstein DJ, *et al.* Analyses of suicidality in double-blind, placebo-controlled trials of pharmacotherapy for weight reduction. *J Clin Psychiatry* 1993; **54:** 309–16.
5. Li Wan Po A. Fluoxetine and suicide: meta-analysis and Monte-Carlo simulations. *Pharmacoepidemiol Drug Safety* 1993; **2:** 79–84.
6. Nakielny J. Fluoxetine and suicide. *Lancet* 1994; **343:** 1359.
7. Healy D. The fluoxetine and suicide controversy: a review of the evidence. *CNS Drugs* 1994; **1:** 223–31.
8. Power AC, Cowen PJ. Fluoxetine and suicidal behaviour; some clinical and theoretical aspects of a controversy. *Br J Psychiatry* 1992; **161:** 735–41.
9. Pitchot W, *et al.* Therapeutic window for 5-HT reuptake inhibitors. *Lancet* 1992; **339:** 689.
10. Anonymous. Fluoxetine, suicide and aggression. *Drug Ther Bull* 1992; **30:** 5–6.
11. Markel H, *et al.* LSD flashback syndrome exacerbated by selective serotonin reuptake inhibitor antidepressants in adolescents. *J Pediatr* 1994; **125:** 817–19.

Effects on sexual function. It has been considered that sexual dysfunction occurs in up to 1.9% of patients taking fluoxetine, with impotence or ejaculatory problems occurring in less than 1% of patients.[1] These figures were based on information supplied by the US manufacturer for the data sheet but have been disputed.[2,3] More recent studies and anecdotal reports quote rates of 7.8 to 75% for sexual dysfunction with fluoxetine but it appears that only small numbers of men were studied.[4] The reported frequency of sexual dysfunction is usually higher in men taking selective serotonin reuptake inhibitors (SSRIs) than in women; complaints include a decrease in or loss of libido, delayed ejaculation, erectile difficulty, or anorgasmia.[5] However, loss of libido, delayed orgasm, or anorgasmia have also been reported in women.[5,6]

Suggested[5] strategies for managing SSRI-induced sexual dysfunction include reducing the dosage of the SSRI or altering the timing of its administration or changing to another antidepressant. Various drugs have also been tried but evidence of efficacy is mainly anecdotal. Cyproheptadine is the drug most commonly reported to have been used but the SSRI may become less effective (see under Interactions, below) and patients should be monitored for worsening symptoms of depression.

The effects of the SSRIs on sexual function have been studied as a potential form of treatment for men with premature ejaculation, (see Sexual Dysfunction in Uses, below).

1. Hollander JB. Fluoxetine and sexual dysfunction. *JAMA* 1994; **272:** 242.
2. Balon R. Fluoxetine and sexual dysfunction. *JAMA* 1995; **273:** 1489.
3. Hopkins HS, Gelenberg AJ. Fluoxetine and sexual dysfunction. *JAMA* 1995; **273:** 1489–90.
4. Hollander JB. Fluoxetine and sexual dysfunction. *JAMA* 1995; **273:** 1490.
5. Frye CB, Berger JE. Treatment of sexual dysfunction induced by selective serotonin-reuptake inhibitors. *Am J Health-Syst Pharm* 1998; **55:** 1167–9.
6. Feiger A, *et al.* Nefazodone versus sertraline in outpatients with major depression: focus on efficacy, tolerability, and effects on sexual function and satisfaction. *J Clin Psychiatry* 1996; **57** (suppl 2): 53–62.

Effects on the skin. *Toxic epidermal necrolysis* developed in a 16-year-old girl 8 days after beginning fluvoxamine therapy.[1] Other drugs, which included metoclopramide, clorazepate, and clomipramine were discounted as possible causes.

Amitriptyline and fluoxetine have been implicated in the development of *atypical cutaneous lymphoid hyperplasia* in 8 patients, 7 of whom either had an underlying immunosuppressant systemic disease or were receiving concomitant therapy with immunomodulatory agents.[2] The lesions improved or resolved on discontinuation of the antidepressant, although in some patients other factors may have contributed to lesional resolution.

1. Wolkenstein P, *et al.* Toxic epidermal necrolysis after fluvoxamine. *Lancet* 1993; **342:** 304–5.
2. Crowson AN, Magro CM. Antidepressant therapy: a possible cause of atypical cutaneous lymphoid hyperplasia. *Arch Dermatol* 1995; **131:** 925–9.

Epileptogenic effect. Generalised seizures have been reported in two patients with no previous history of seizures following initiation of fluoxetine therapy.[1,2] Although convulsions have been noted in patients receiving fluvoxamine (see p.288), a small clinical study involving 35 depressed epileptic patients[3] found no change in the number of seizures or in their nature when fluvoxamine was given in doses of up to 200 mg daily.

For reference to the use of fluoxetine as adjunctive treatment for complex partial seizures, see Epilepsy under Uses and Administration, below.

1. Weber JJ. Seizure activity associated with fluoxetine therapy. *Clin Pharm* 1989; **8:** 296–8.
2. Ware MR, Stewart RB. Seizures associated with fluoxetine therapy. *DICP Ann Pharmacother* 1989; **23:** 428.
3. Harmant J, *et al.* Fluvoxamine: an antidepressant with low (or no) epileptogenic effect. *Lancet* 1990; **336:** 386.

Extrapyramidal effects. Extrapyramidal effects can occur with fluoxetine. For example, Eisenhauer and Jermain provide details of a boy who developed tics while receiving the drug.[1] Akathisia has also been associated with fluoxetine.[2,3] The UK Committee on Safety of Medicines had received 39 reports of extrapyramidal reactions with paroxetine including 15 of dystonia of the face and mouth.[4] It was observed that although extrapyramidal effects may occur with other selective serotonin reuptake inhibitors (SSRIs), orofacial dystonias appeared to be more common with paroxetine. However, evidence from monitoring prescriptions within the UK has shown that the overall incidence of extrapyramidal effects is the same for paroxetine as for other SSRIs.[5] Orofacial dystonias (teeth clenching) or dyskinesias (teeth grinding) with resultant severe damage to teeth and gums in the majority of cases have been reported[6] in 6 patients receiving fluoxetine, fluvoxamine, paroxetine, or sertraline. The authors conclude that these adverse effects were not specific for any particular SSRI.

1. Eisenhauer G, Jermain DM. Fluoxetine and tics in an adolescent. *Ann Pharmacother* 1993; **27:** 725–6.
2. Lipinski JF, *et al.* Fluoxetine-induced akathisia: clinical and theoretical implications. *J Clin Psychiatry* 1989; **50:** 339–42.
3. Rothschild AJ, Locke CA. Reexposure to fluoxetine after serious suicide attempts by three patients: the role of akathisia. *J Clin Psychiatry* 1991; **52:** 491–3.
4. Committee on Safety of Medicines/Medicines Control Agency. Dystonia and withdrawal symptoms with paroxetine (Seroxat). *Current Problems* 1993; **19:** 1.
5. Choo V. Paroxetine and extrapyramidal reactions. *Lancet* 1993; **341:** 624.
6. Fitzgerald K, Healy D. Dystonias and dyskinesias of the jaw associated with the use of SSRIs. *Hum Psychopharmacol Clin Exp* 1995; **10:** 215–19.

Neuroleptic malignant syndrome. The manufacturers of fluoxetine report that neuroleptic malignant syndrome-like events have occurred.

Overdosage. Selective serotonin reuptake inhibitors (SSRIs) are generally regarded as being less toxic in overdosage than tricyclic antidepressants or MAOIs. Of 41 cases of self-poisoning with fluvoxamine, only one patient died and even here fluvoxamine was not implicated.[1] Prolonged cerebral depression occurred in a patient following fluvoxamine overdose,[1] but this may have been due to an interaction with temazepam which the patient also took in overdose. One hour after taking 40 sertraline 50-mg tablets in a suicide attempt a 42-year-old woman was flushed, angry, emotionally labile, and easily distracted but not psychotic.[2] Apart from watery bowel movements recovery was mainly uneventful following treatment with gastric lavage, oral activated charcoal with sorbitol, and intravenous hydration.

Fatal overdose has been reported with citalopram in 6 patients,[3] although the suggested cause of death as cardiac dysfunction rather than seizures was disputed.[4]

For a discussion of choice of antidepressant with respect to safety in overdosage, see under Depression, p.271.

1. Banerjee AK. Recovery from prolonged cerebral depression after fluvoxamine overdose. *Br Med J* 1988; **296:** 1774.
2. Brown DF, Kerr HD. Sertraline overdose. *Ann Pharmacother* 1994; **28:** 1307.
3. Öström M, *et al.* Fatal overdose with citalopram. *Lancet* 1996; **348:** 339–40.
4. Brion F, *et al.* Fatal overdose with citalopram? *Lancet* 1996; **348:** 1380.

Treatment of Adverse Effects

Treatment of overdosage with a selective serotonin reuptake inhibitor (SSRI) involves emesis induction or gastric lavage followed by symptomatic and supportive therapy. The use of activated charcoal by mouth as an adjunct to gastric lavage has been suggested. Dialysis, haemoperfusion, exchange transfusion, and measures to increase urine production are considered unlikely to be of benefit.

Precautions

Fluoxetine and other selective serotonin reuptake inhibitors (SSRIs) that undergo hepatic metabolism and renal excretion should be used with caution and in reduced doses in patients with impaired hepatic or renal function and some authorities recommend that they should not be used in severe hepatic or renal failure. Because of their epileptogenic effect SSRIs should be used with caution in patients with epilepsy or a history of such disorders (and should be avoided if the epilepsy is poorly controlled). Fluoxetine may alter glycaemic control and therefore caution is also warranted in diabetic subjects. Fluoxetine should be discontinued in patients who develop a rash since systemic effects, possibly related to vasculitis, have occurred in such patients.

Patients should be closely monitored during early therapy until improvement in depression is observed because suicide is an inherent risk in depressed patients. For further details, see under Depression, p.271. For a discussion of the concern that SSRIs, particularly fluoxetine, may increase suicidal ideation, see Effects on Mental State in Adverse Effects, above.

If SSRIs are given for the depressive component of bipolar disorder, mania may be precipitated.

SSRIs may impair performance of skilled tasks and, if affected, patients should not drive or operate machinery.

Some authorities recommend reduced or less frequent dosage of SSRIs for elderly patients.

Significant amounts of fluoxetine are distributed into breast milk and the manufacturers have reported that adverse effects have been observed in a breast-fed infant; consequently fluoxetine is not recommended for nursing mothers. Similarly, the manufacturers of some other SSRIs have recommended that they should be avoided during breast feeding (fluvoxamine and paroxetine) or used with caution (citalopram).

SSRIs should be withdrawn gradually to reduce the risk of withdrawal symptoms.

Abuse. There have been occasional reports of individuals abusing fluoxetine.[1,2]

1. Tinsley JA, *et al.* Fluoxetine abuse. *Mayo Clin Proc* 1994; **69:** 166–8.
2. Pagliaro LA, Pagliaro AM. Fluoxetine abuse by an intravenous drug user. *Am J Psychiatry* 1993; **150:** 1898.

Blood disorders. For a reference recommending cautious use of fluoxetine in patients with thrombocytopenia or platelet dysfunction, see Effects on the Blood in Adverse Effects, above.

Breast feeding. Symptoms of colic were reported[1] in a 6-week-old infant whose mother was taking fluoxetine 20 mg daily. The concentrations of fluoxetine and its active metabolite norfluoxetine were 69 ng per mL and 90 ng per mL respectively in breast milk, and 340 ng per mL and 208 ng per mL respectively in the infant's plasma. The infant's symptoms resolved when he was formula fed. In a study[2] of 10 women taking fluoxetine while breast feeding 11 infants, breast milk concentrations of fluoxetine ranged from 17.4 to 293 ng per mL and of norfluoxetine from 23.4 to 379.1 ng per mL. No adverse effects were noted in the infants.

The excretion of fluvoxamine into breast milk was studied[3] in a woman who had been receiving fluvoxamine maleate 100 mg twice daily for 2 weeks. The concentration of fluvoxamine base 4.75 hours after a dose was 310 ng per mL in maternal plasma and 90 ng per mL in breast milk. It was estimated that an infant would ingest only 0.5% of the daily maternal intake. It was considered that these data supported the notion that administration of fluvoxamine to nursing mothers posed little risk to the infant.

Plasma concentrations of sertraline were undetectable in a breast-fed infant despite the presence of significant concentrations in the mother's breast milk, ranging from 8.8 to 43 ng per mL over a 24-hour period.[4] However, the authors pointed out that metabolite levels were not measured and that sertraline may have been present in the infant at a concentration below the level of sensitivity of the assay. Two further studies[5,6] detected desmethylsertraline in breast milk, which was also detected in the plasma of some of the infants in one of the studies[5] but not in any of the infants in the other study.[6]

Citalopram appears in breast milk in very low concentrations. Paroxetine is also distributed into breast milk.

1. Lester BM, *et al.* Possible association between fluoxetine hydrochloride and colic in an infant. *J Am Acad Child Adolesc Psychiatry* 1993; **32:** 1253–5.
2. Taddio A, *et al.* Excretion of fluoxetine and its metabolite, norfluoxetine, in human breast milk. *J Clin Pharmacol* 1996; **36:** 42–7.
3. Wright S, *et al.* Excretion of fluvoxamine in breast milk. *Br J Clin Pharmacol* 1991; **31:** 209.
4. Altshuler LL, *et al.* Breastfeeding and sertraline: a 24-hour analysis. *J Clin Psychiatry* 1995; **56:** 243–5.

5. Stowe ZN, *et al.* Sertraline and desmethylsertraline in human breast milk and nursing infants. *Am J Psychiatry* 1997; **154:** 1255–60.
6. Kristensen JH, *et al.* Distribution and excretion of sertraline and N-desmethylsertraline in human milk. *Br J Clin Pharmacol* 1998; **45:** 453–7.

Driving. While affective disorders probably adversely affect driving skill,[1,2] treatment with antidepressant drugs may also be hazardous,[1] although patients may be safer drivers with medication than without.[2] Impairment of performance is largely related to sedative and antimuscarinic effects, both of which are more pronounced with older antidepressants such as the tricyclic antidepressants than with the selective serotonin reuptake inhibitors (SSRIs), although a comparative study[3] of fluoxetine (an SSRI) and dothiepin (a tricyclic) in healthy subjects demonstrated a similar but apparently small potential for impairing psychomotor and driving performance. However, a recent epidemiological study[4] was unable to confirm any increased risk of road-traffic accidents in those drivers receiving tricyclic antidepressants or selective serotonin reuptake inhibitors (SSRIs).

It has been mentioned[2] that the UK Medical Commission on Accident Prevention has recommended that patients on long-term psychotropic medication are unsuitable to be drivers of heavy goods or public service vehicles.

1. Ashton H. Drugs and driving. *Adverse Drug React Bull* 1983; **98:** 360–3.
2. Cremona A. Mad drivers: psychiatric illness and driving performance. *Br J Hosp Med* 1986; **35:** 193–5.
3. Ramaekers JG, *et al.* A comparative study of acute and subchronic effects of dothiepin, fluoxetine and placebo on psychomotor and actual driving performance. *Br J Clin Pharmacol* 1995; **39:** 397–404.
4. Barbone F, *et al.* Association of road-traffic accidents with benzodiazepine use. *Lancet* 1998; **352:** 1331–6.

Mania. Hypomania or mania have been reported with some of the selective serotonin reuptake inhibitors (SSRIs).

Fluvoxamine has been associated with manic behaviour in 8 patients who were being treated for major depression;[1] three also had concurrent obsessive-compulsive disorder. Daily doses of fluvoxamine ranged from 75 to 300 mg and duration of therapy to development of manic behaviour from 2 to 6 weeks. The authors were unable to determine whether fluvoxamine had induced mania or unmasked latent bipolar disorder in these patients. However, they recommended that fluvoxamine-treated patients should be monitored for manic behaviour.

1. Dorevitch A, *et al.* Fluvoxamine-associated manic behavior: a case series. *Ann Pharmacother* 1993; **27:** 1455–7.

Pregnancy. An early prospective study[1] comparing 128 pregnant women exposed to a mean daily dose of about 26 mg of fluoxetine during their first trimester with control groups receiving tricyclic antidepressants or non-teratogens found the incidence of neonatal malformations to be similar in all groups and did not exceed that in the general population. However, there was a tendency for a higher incidence of miscarriages in the groups receiving fluoxetine or tricyclics. A more recent prospective study[2] comparing 228 pregnant women taking fluoxetine with a control group taking non-teratogens confirmed that there was no significant increased incidence in major fetal abnormalities in the fluoxetine group, but it did not reveal an increased risk of miscarriage. There was an increase in the incidence of minor fetal abnormalities in infants exposed to fluoxetine during the first trimester. Also, infants exposed to fluoxetine during the third trimester experienced more perinatal complications such as prematurity, low full-term birth-weight and length, and poor neonatal adaptation compared with infants exposed only during the first and second trimesters. However, the design of this study was criticised[3] because of several methodological problems such as unmatched controls and a higher maternal age in the fluoxetine group, which may partly explain the excess of poor perinatal outcomes. The manufacturer evaluated the outcome of 796 pregnancies in which the mother received fluoxetine during the first trimester and considered that it was unlikely that fluoxetine increased the risk of spontaneous abortion or fetal malformation.[7] The effects of fluoxetine on fetal neurodevelopment were studied[4] in 55 pregnant women by later assessing global IQ of the children; no differences were seen in those exposed to fluoxetine *in utero* compared with those exposed to tricyclic antidepressants or non-teratogens.

CNS toxicity and an increased heart rate were reported in a neonate whose mother had received 20 mg of fluoxetine daily throughout most of her pregnancy.[5] The neonate's symptoms resolved 96 hours after delivery.

A prospective controlled study[6] on pregnancy outcome in women exposed to fluvoxamine, paroxetine, or sertraline found that, when used in recommended doses, there appeared to be no increase in the risk of major congenital malformations, miscarriages, or still-births when compared with women exposed to non-teratogens.

1. Pastuszak A, *et al.* Pregnancy outcome following first-trimester exposure to fluoxetine (Prozac). *JAMA* 1993; **269:** 2246–8.
2. Chambers CD, *et al.* Birth outcomes in pregnant women taking fluoxetine. *N Engl J Med* 1996; **335:** 1010–15.
3. Robert E. Treating depression in pregnancy. *N Engl J Med* 1996; **335:** 1056–8.
4. Nulman I, *et al.* Neurodevelopment of children exposed in utero to antidepressant drugs. *N Engl J Med* 1997; **336:** 258–62.
5. Spencer MJ. Fluoxetine hydrochloride (Prozac) toxicity in a neonate. *Pediatrics* 1993; **92:** 721–2.
6. Kulin NA, *et al.* Pregnancy outcome following maternal use of the new selective serotonin reuptake inhibitors: a prospective controlled multicenter study. *JAMA* 1998; **279:** 609–10.
7. Goldstein DJ, *et al.* Effects of first-trimester fluoxetine exposure on the newborn. *Obstet Gynecol* 1997; **89:** 713–18.

Withdrawal. Withdrawal symptoms have been reported for SSRIs,[1-5] although the number of cases is greatest for paroxetine. The UK Committee on Safety of Medicines (CSM) has advised that normally paroxetine should not be discontinued abruptly.[1] Up to July 1994 the CSM had received 430 reports of symptoms occurring on withdrawal of paroxetine, including dizziness, sweating, nausea, insomnia, tremor, and confusion. The reactions, which had been reported more often with paroxetine than with other SSRIs, tended to start 1 to 4 days after stopping paroxetine and resolved in some patients on reinstating treatment. A retrospective analysis[5] has also found that withdrawal symptoms occur significantly more frequently in patients treated with the shorter half-life SSRIs, such as paroxetine, than in those receiving an SSRI with a longer half-life metabolite, such as fluoxetine. There has also been a report[2] of 2 patients without a history of major psychiatric disorder who developed severe behavioural symptoms when paroxetine was withdrawn. Discontinuation was abrupt in one patient and gradual, over a 12-day period, in the other. Symptoms were predominantly hypomanic over the first few days, followed by a period of escalated ego-dystonic aggression, behavioural dyscontrol, and suicidal intention.

Some authorities recommend that any antidepressant, including an SSRI, that has been administered regularly for 8 weeks or more should be discontinued gradually over a period of about 4 weeks.

1. Price JS, *et al.* A comparison of the post-marketing safety of four selective serotonin re-uptake inhibitors including the investigation of symptoms occurring on withdrawal. *Br J Clin Pharmacol* 1996; **42:** 757–63.
2. Bloch M, *et al.* Severe psychiatric symptoms associated with paroxetine withdrawal. *Lancet* 1995; **346:** 57.
3. Szabadi E. Fluvoxamine withdrawal syndrome. *Br J Psychiatry* 1992; **160:** 283–4.
4. Adverse Drug Reactions Advisory Committee (ADRAC). SSRI's and withdrawal syndrome. *Aust Adverse Drug React Bull* 1996; **15:** 3.
5. Coupland NJ, *et al.* Serotonin reuptake inhibitor withdrawal. *J Clin Psychopharmacol* 1996; **16:** 356–62.

Interactions

Selective serotonin reuptake inhibitors (SSRIs) interact with a range of other drugs mainly as a result of their inhibitory activity on hepatic cytochrome P450 isoenzymes. Individual SSRIs do not all exhibit the same degree of inhibition nor do they react with the same isoenzymes. The range of drugs inhibited by specific SSRIs varies according to which isoenzyme is affected.

The effects of alcohol may possibly be enhanced by SSRIs.

Although different antidepressants have been used together under expert supervision in refractory cases of depression, severe adverse reactions including the *serotonin syndrome* (see p.303) may occur. Sequential prescribing of different types of antidepressant may also produce adverse reactions, and an appropriate drug-free interval should elapse between discontinuing one type of antidepressant and starting another. SSRIs should not generally be given to patients receiving MAOIs or for at least two weeks after their discontinuation. No treatment-free period is necessary after stopping a reversible inhibitor of monoamine oxidase type A (RIMA) and starting an SSRI. At least one week should elapse between withdrawing an SSRI and starting any drug liable to provoke a serious reaction (e.g. phenelzine); in the case of the SSRIs paroxetine and sertraline the drug-free interval is extended to two weeks, and for fluoxetine five weeks, because of their longer half-lives.

Further details concerning some of these interactions, and others, are given below.

References.

1. Mitchell PB. Drug interactions of clinical significance with selective serotonin reuptake inhibitors. *Drug Safety* 1997; **17:** 390–406.
2. Sproule BA, *et al.* Selective serotonin reuptake inhibitors and CNS drug interactions: a critical review of the evidence. *Clin Pharmacokinet* 1997; **33:** 454–71.

Antibacterials. Rapid development of delirium was reported[1] in a patient when *clarithromycin* was added to his existing regimen of fluoxetine and nitrazepam. It was suggested that his delirium was a result of increased plasma-fluoxetine concentrations produced by the inhibition of cytochrome P450 enzymes by clarithromycin.

1. Pollak PT, *et al.* Delirium probably induced by clarithromycin in a patient receiving fluoxetine. *Ann Pharmacother* 1995; **29:** 486–8.

Anticoagulants. Selective serotonin reuptake inhibitors (SSRIs) may increase the anticoagulant activity of warfarin (see p.967).

Antidepressants. Combination therapy with differing classes of antidepressants has been used successfully in the treatment of drug-resistant depression. It should be emphasised, however, that such combinations may result in enhanced adverse reactions or interactions, and should be employed only under expert supervision. This practice is considered unsuitable or controversial by some authorities. For further details of the interactions between different antidepressants when coadministered, see under Interactions of Phenelzine, p.305. For details of the serotonin syndrome that can arise when two serotonergic drugs with different mechanisms of action are administered, see under Adverse Effects of Phenelzine, p.303.

Antiepileptics. Antidepressants may antagonise the activity of antiepileptics by lowering the convulsive threshold.

There has been a report of the serotonin syndrome (see p.303) developing in a patient 14 days after fluoxetine had been added to *carbamazepine* therapy.[1]

Phenobarbitone has been reported to reduce serum concentrations of paroxetine.[2] Steady-state serum concentrations of paroxetine were found to be lower in patients taking *phenytoin* than in those taking carbamazepine or *valproate*.[3]

Some selective serotonin reuptake inhibitors (SSRIs) have been reported to increase plasma concentrations of carbamazepine (see p.341) and phenytoin (see p.355).

1. Dursun SM, *et al.* Toxic serotonin syndrome after fluoxetine plus carbamazepine. *Lancet* 1993; **342:** 442–3.
2. Greb WH, *et al.* The effect of liver enzyme inhibition by cimetidine and enzyme induction by phenobarbitone on the pharmacokinetics of paroxetine. *Acta Psychiatr Scand* 1989; **80** (suppl 350): 95–8.
3. Andersen BB, *et al.* No influence of the antidepressant paroxetine on carbamazepine, valproate and phenytoin. *Epilepsy Res* 1991; **10:** 201–4.

Antihistamines. *Cyproheptadine* given to male and female patients as treatment for sexual dysfunction induced by fluoxetine or paroxetine produced re-emergence of previously controlled depressive symptoms[1,2] or bulimia nervosa.[3] Fluvoxamine could theoretically increase plasma concentrations of *astemizole* or *terfenadine* by inhibition of their hepatic cytochrome P450 metabolism. As this increases the risk of ventricular arrhythmias, the manufacturers of fluvoxamine advise against use of such a combination (see also under Astemizole, p.402 and Terfenadine, p.418). Cardiac abnormalities have been reported with concomitant administration of fluoxetine and terfenadine (see p.418).

1. Feder R. Reversal of antidepressant activity of fluoxetine by cyproheptadine in three patients. *J Clin Psychiatry* 1991; **52:** 163–4.
2. Christensen RC. Adverse interaction of paroxetine and cyproheptadine. *J Clin Psychiatry* 1995; **56:** 433–4.
3. Goldbloom DS, Kennedy SH. Adverse interaction of fluoxetine and cyproheptadine in two patients with bulimia nervosa. *J Clin Psychiatry* 1991; **52:** 261–2.

Antimigraine drugs. There is a risk of CNS toxicity with selective serotonin reuptake inhibitors (SSRIs) and sumatriptan (see p.451).

Antimuscarinics. For the effect of selective serotonin reuptake inhibitors (SSRIs) on benztropine, see p.458.

Antipsychotics. For reports of adverse effects in patients given concomitant treatment with selective serotonin reuptake inhibitors (SSRIs) and antipsychotics, see under Chlorpromazine, p.652.

Antivirals. Plasma concentrations of fluoxetine are possibly increased by HIV-protease inhibitors.

For the effect of fluoxetine on delavirdine, see p.607.

Anxiolytics. Fluoxetine and fluvoxamine increase plasma concentrations of some benzodiazepines (see under Diazepam, p.664).

Beta blockers. For the effect of fluoxetine and fluvoxamine on beta blockers, see p.830.

Cough suppressants. For the effect of fluoxetine and paroxetine on dextromethorphan, see p.1058.

Cyclosporin. For the effect of fluoxetine on cyclosporin, see p.521.

Dopaminergics. *Selegiline* is an irreversible selective inhibitor of monoamine oxidase type B. Serious adverse effects have been reported when selegiline and selective serotonin reuptake inhibitors (SSRIs) have been used concomitantly (see p.1144). In some instances, these reactions resemble the potentially fatal serotonin syndromes reported when SSRIs are administered together with non-selective MAOIs (see p.303).

Some authorities advise that SSRIs should not generally be given to patients receiving selegiline, or for at least two weeks after it has been discontinued. Similarly, at least one week should elapse between withdrawing an SSRI and starting selegiline; this interval should be increased to two weeks for paroxetine and sertraline, and to five weeks for fluoxetine because of their longer half-lives.

Hypnotics. A patient receiving paroxetine developed delirium following addition of *zolpidem* to her treatment.[1] Transient visual hallucinations have also been reported in at least one other patient but no causal relationship was established for this interaction.

1. Katz SE. Possible paroxetine-zolpidem interaction. *Am J Psychiatry* 1995; **152:** 1689.

Opioid analgesics. A possible case of serotonin syndrome (p.303) has been reported with coadministration of *tramadol* and sertraline.[1] For reference to selective serotonin reuptake inhibitors (SSRIs) enhancing the effects and toxicity of *methadone*, see p.54.

1. Mason BJ, Blackburn KH. Possible serotonin syndrome associated with tramadol and sertraline coadministration. *Ann Pharmacother* 1997; **31:** 175–7.

Parasympathomimetics. For the effect of fluvoxamine on *tacrine*, see p.1399.

Smoking. Serum concentrations of fluvoxamine were lower in smokers than non-smokers in a single-dose study.[1] It was proposed that the polycyclic hydrocarbons present in cigarette smoke stimulated hepatic metabolism of fluvoxamine by cytochrome P450 enzymes.

1. Spigset O, *et al.* Effect of cigarette smoking on fluvoxamine pharmacokinetics in humans. *Clin Pharmacol Ther* 1995; **58:** 399–403.

Theophylline. For the effect of fluvoxamine on theophylline, see p.768.

Pharmacokinetics

Fluoxetine is readily absorbed from the gastro-intestinal tract with peak plasma concentrations appearing about 6 to 8 hours after administration. The systemic bioavailability does not appear to be affected by food. It is extensively metabolised, by demethylation, in the liver to its primary active metabolite norfluoxetine. Excretion is mainly via the urine.

Fluoxetine used clinically is a racemic mixture consisting of *R* and *S* enantiomers in equal amounts. Both enantiomers are active according to *animal* studies, but *S*-fluoxetine is eliminated more slowly. Metabolism leads to *R* and *S* enantiomers of norfluoxetine with the *S* enantiomer being considered as active as the parent drug; the *R* enantiomer is considered to be much less active. This metabolism is subject to genetic polymorphism. While the small proportion of the population known as slow metabolisers do show a different spectrum of parent drug and metabolite, the overall activity does not appear to be altered.

Fluoxetine is widely distributed throughout the body and is extensively bound to plasma proteins.

Fluoxetine has a relatively long elimination half-life of about 1 to 3 days; that of its metabolite, norfluoxetine, is even longer, being about 4 to 16 days. These long half-lives have clinical implications. Steady-state plasma concentrations will only be attained after several weeks. Additionally, after discontinuation fluoxetine and its metabolites may persist for a considerable time and this has led to precautions concerning the subsequent administration of other serotonergic antidepressants (see Interactions, above).

Fluoxetine and norfluoxetine are distributed into breast milk (see Breast Feeding under Precautions, above).

References.

1. van Harten J. Clinical pharmacokinetics of selective serotonin reuptake inhibitors. *Clin Pharmacokinet* 1993; **24:** 203–20.
2. Altamura AC, *et al.* Clinical pharmacokinetics of fluoxetine. *Clin Pharmacokinet* 1994; **26:** 201–14.
3. Baumann P. Pharmacokinetic-pharmacodynamic relationship of the selective serotonin reuptake inhibitors. *Clin Pharmacokinet* 1996; **31:** 444–69.
4. Greenblatt DJ, *et al.* Inhibition of human cytochrome P450-3A isoforms by fluoxetine and norfluoxetine: in vitro and in vivo studies. *J Clin Pharmacol* 1996; **36:** 792–8.
5. Hamelin BA, *et al.* The disposition of fluoxetine but not sertraline is altered in poor metabolizers of debrisoquin. *Clin Pharmacol Ther* 1996; **60:** 512–21.
6. Preskorn SH. Clinically relevant pharmacology of selective serotonin reuptake inhibitors: an overview with emphasis on pharmacokinetics and effects on oxidative drug metabolism. *Clin Pharmacokinet* 1997; **32** (suppl 1): 1–21.

Uses and Administration

Selective serotonin reuptake inhibitors (SSRIs) such as fluoxetine preferentially inhibit the reuptake of serotonin compared with noradrenaline, and have limited direct action at other neurotransmitter sites, including muscarinic receptors. They therefore cause fewer antimuscarinic or sedative side-effects than the tricyclic antidepressants and are less cardiotoxic. Specific SSRIs differ in selectivity and potency for the reuptake of serotonin and the two parameters are not interdependent. Thus, citalopram is the most selective of the currently available serotonin reuptake inhibitors, whereas paroxetine is the most potent.

Prevention of the reuptake of monoamine transmitters such as serotonin potentiates their action in the brain, which appears to be associated with antidepressant activity, although the precise mode of action of SSRIs in depression remains to be elucidated.

SSRIs provide an alternative to the tricyclics for the treatment of depression. As with the tricyclics, it may be several weeks before an antidepressant effect is seen. After a response has been obtained, maintenance therapy should be continued for 4 to 6 months after the depression has resolved to avoid relapse on discontinuation of therapy.

Some SSRIs are also used as part of the management of obsessive-compulsive disorder and panic disorders with or without agoraphobia, and as part of the management of bulimia nervosa.

Fluoxetine, a phenylpropylamine derivative, is given by mouth as the hydrochloride; doses are expressed in terms of fluoxetine.

In the treatment of depression the usual dose of fluoxetine is 20 mg daily and some authorities recommend giving this dose in the morning. In the USA, it is recommended that if no clinical response is seen after several weeks, the daily dose may be gradually increased, up to a maximum of 80 mg daily. Doses above 20 mg a day may be administered in 2 divided doses, say in the morning and at noon.

Fluoxetine is used in doses of 60 mg daily in the management of bulimia nervosa.

In the management of obsessive-compulsive disorder the initial dose of fluoxetine is 20 mg daily increased after several weeks if there is no response to up to 60 mg daily. Up to 80 mg daily has been used in the USA where twice daily regimens are also employed.

Because fluoxetine is subject to hepatic metabolism, lower doses, such as alternate-day dosing, have been recommended in patients with significant hepatic impairment; some authorities recommend that SSRIs should be avoided if hepatic impairment is severe. Similar recommendations, because of renal excretion, have been made for patients with mild to moderate renal impairment; it should not, however, be used at all in patients with severe renal impairment. Some authorities recommend a lower or less frequent dosage in elderly patients.

It should be noted that the prolonged half-lives of fluoxetine and norfluoxetine will result in the need for several weeks of therapy to be employed before steady-state concentrations are attained; similarly after dosage adjustments a time lag will occur before steady-state concentrations are again achieved.

Fluoxetine should be withdrawn gradually to reduce the risk of withdrawal symptoms.

References.

1. Gram LF. Fluoxetine. *N Engl J Med* 1994; **331:** 1354–61.
2. Finley PR. Selective serotonin reuptake inhibitors: pharmacologic profiles and potential therapeutic distinctions. *Ann Pharmacother* 1994; **28:** 1359–69.
3. Hyttel J. Pharmacological characterization of selective serotonin reuptake inhibitors (SSRIs). *Int Clin Psychopharmacol* 1994; **9** (suppl 1): 19–26.

Alcohol dependence. Short-term studies[1,2] suggested that fluoxetine might initially have a small effect in reducing alcohol intake in patients with alcohol dependence (p.1099) but it appeared to be no more effective than placebo in reducing relapse when given for 12 weeks or longer.[3]

1. Naranjo CA, *et al.* Fluoxetine differentially alters alcohol intake and other consummatory behaviors in problem drinkers. *Clin Pharmacol Ther* 1990; **47:** 490–8.
2. Gorelick DA, Paredes A. Effect of fluoxetine on alcohol consumption in male alcoholics. *Alcohol Clin Exp Res* 1992; **16:** 261–5.
3. Kranzler HR, *et al.* Placebo-controlled trial of fluoxetine as an adjunct to relapse prevention in alcoholics. *Am J Psychiatry* 1995; **152:** 391–7.

Anorexia nervosa. Counselling and psychotherapy form the major part of treatment of anorexia nervosa and there is little or no role for specific drug therapy. Antidepressants may be indicated when there is co-existing depression but malnourished anorexic patients may be more susceptible to adverse effects and less responsive than other patients with depression. Fluoxetine has been tried with some success, although the efficacy and safety of selective serotonin reuptake inhibitors (SSRIs) (in this case citalopram) has been questioned.[1]

1. Bergh C, *et al.* Selective serotonin reuptake inhibitors in anorexia. *Lancet* 1996; **348:** 1459–60.

Anxiety disorders. Selective serotonin reuptake inhibitors (SSRIs) have been given in a variety of anxiety disorders (p.635) but their role in these disorders is most well established in the treatment of *obsessive-compulsive disorder.* Efficacy in obsessive-compulsive disorder appears to have been best demonstrated for fluvoxamine and fluoxetine but other SSRIs may also be effective and patients unresponsive to one SSRI may respond to another. SSRIs may also be of use in the treatment of *panic disorders*. Encouraging results have been obtained with various SSRIs in the treatment of *social phobia*. Fluoxetine has also been tried in the treatment of *post-traumatic stress disorder* and *trichotillomania*.

References.

1. Schneier FR, *et al.* Fluoxetine in panic disorder. *J Clin Psychopharmacol* 1990; **10:** 119–21.
2. Montgomery SA, *et al.* A double-blind, placebo-controlled study of fluoxetine in patients with DSM-III-R obsessive-compulsive disorder. *Eur Neuropsychopharmacol* 1993; **3:** 143–52.
3. Wood A, *et al.* Pharmacotherapy of obsessive compulsive disorder—experience with fluoxetine. *Int Clin Psychopharmacol* 1993; **8:** 301–6.
4. Van Ameringen M, *et al.* Fluoxetine efficacy in social phobia. *J Clin Psychiatry* 1993; **54:** 27–32.
5. Tollefson GD, *et al.* A multicenter investigation of fixed-dose fluoxetine in the treatment of obsessive-compulsive disorder. *Arch Gen Psychiatry* 1994; **51:** 559–67.
6. Yanchick JK, *et al.* Efficacy of fluoxetine in trichotillomania. *Ann Pharmacother* 1994; **28:** 1245–6.
7. van der Kolk BA, *et al.* Fluoxetine in posttraumatic stress disorder. *J Clin Psychiatry* 1994; **55:** 517–22.

Bulimia nervosa. A combination of counselling, support, psychotherapy, and antidepressants is the usual treatment for bulimia nervosa. Fluoxetine and the tricyclic desipramine have been suggested as the antidepressants of choice because they have been used extensively and are considered to be well tolerated. In a study[1] involving 398 patients, fluoxetine at a dose of 60 mg daily reduced the number of bulimic episodes more effectively than placebo. Antidepressants in general do not appear to alter the patient's disturbed self-image, although a study[2] by Goldbloom and Olmsted suggested that disturbed attitudes might improve during short-term therapy with fluoxetine.

1. Goldstein DJ, *et al.* Long-term fluoxetine treatment of bulimia nervosa. *Br J Psychiatry* 1995; **166:** 660–6.
2. Goldbloom DS, Olmsted MP. Pharmacotherapy of bulimia nervosa with fluoxetine: assessment of clinically significant attitudinal change. *Am J Psychiatry* 1993; **150:** 770–4.

Depression. As discussed on p.271, there is very little difference in efficacy between the different groups of antidepressant drugs, and choice is often made on the basis of adverse effect profile. Selective serotonin reuptake inhibitors (SSRIs) such as fluoxetine are increasingly being recognised as first-choice treatment because they offer advantages over the older tricyclics in terms of fewer unpleasant side-effects and safety in overdosage.

Combination therapy with differing classes of antidepressants, including the SSRIs, has been used in the treatment of drug-resistant depression. However, such therapy may result in enhanced adverse reactions or interactions and is considered unsuitable or controversial by some workers. For further details, see Antidepressants under Interactions of Phenelzine, p.305.

References to the use of SSRIs in general and to the use of fluoxetine are given below.

1. Song F, *et al.* Selective serotonin reuptake inhibitors: meta-analysis of efficacy and acceptability. *Br Med J* 1993; **306:** 683–7.
2. Edwards JG. Selective serotonin reuptake inhibitors in the treatment of depression. *Prescribers' J* 1994; **34:** 197–204.

3. Montgomery SA, *et al.* Selective serotonin reuptake inhibitors: meta-analysis of discontinuation rates. *Int Clin Psychopharmacol* 1994; **9:** 47–53.
4. Roose SP, *et al.* Comparative efficacy of selective serotonin reuptake inhibitors and tricyclics in the treatment of melancholia. *Am J Psychiatry* 1994; **151:** 1735–9.
5. Fava M, *et al.* Lithium and tricyclic augmentation of fluoxetine treatment for resistant major depression: a double blind, controlled study. *Am J Psychiatry* 1994; **151:** 1372–4.
6. Fava M, *et al.* Relapse in patients on long-term fluoxetine treatment: response to increased fluoxetine dose. *J Clin Psychiatry* 1995; **56:** 52–5.
7. Anderson IM, Tomenson BM. Treatment discontinuation with selective serotonin reuptake inhibitors compared with tricyclic antidepressants: a meta-analysis. *Br Med J* 1995; **310:** 1433–8.
8. Goodnick PJ, *et al.* Treatment of depression in patients with diabetes mellitus. *J Clin Psychiatry* 1995; **56:** 128–36.
9. Lam RW, *et al.* Multicenter, placebo-controlled study of fluoxetine in seasonal affective disorder. *Am J Psychiatry* 1995; **152:** 1765–70.
10. Brown WA, Harrison W. Are patients who are intolerant to one serotonin selective reuptake inhibitor intolerant to another? *J Clin Psychiatry* 1995; **56:** 30–4.
11. Joffe RT, *et al.* Response to an open trial of a second SSRI in major depression. *J Clin Psychiatry* 1996; **57:** 114–15.
12. Nobler MS, *et al.* Fluoxetine treatment of dysthymia in the elderly. *J Clin Psychiatry* 1996; **57:** 254–6.
13. Burke WJ, *et al.* Fluoxetine and norfluoxetine serum concentrations and clinical response in weekly versus daily dosing. *Psychopharmacol Bull* 1996; **32:** 27–32.
14. Mourilhe P, Stokes PE. Risks and benefits of selective serotonin reuptake inhibitors in the treatment of depression. *Drug Safety* 1998; **18:** 57–82.

Disturbed behaviour. Selective serotonin reuptake inhibitors (SSRIs) appear to have been of some benefit in controlling symptoms such as impulsiveness and aggression[1-3] when tried in various disorders for the management of disturbed behaviour (see p.636). There have been several case reports of fluoxetine being used with some success in the control of fantasies associated with various paraphilias.[4]

1. Coccaro EF, *et al.* Fluoxetine treatment of impulsive aggression in DSM-III-R personality disorder patients. *J Clin Psychopharmacol* 1990; **10:** 373–5.
2. Cornelius JR, *et al.* Fluoxetine trial in borderline personality disorder. *Psychopharmacol Bull* 1990; **26:** 151–4.
3. Vartiainen H, *et al.* Citalopram, a selective serotonin reuptake inhibitor, in the treatment of aggression in schizophrenia. *Acta Psychiatr Scand* 1995; **91:** 348–51.
4. Richer M, Crismon ML. Pharmacotherapy of sexual offenders. *Ann Pharmacother* 1993; **27:** 316–19.

Epilepsy. Preliminary data from an open-label study[1] of 17 patients with epilepsy suggest that fluoxetine, which was given as an adjunct to their normal drug regimen, may have an antiepileptic effect in complex partial seizures with or without secondary generalisation. However, there have been case reports of seizures associated with the use of fluoxetine (see Epileptogenic Effect in Adverse Effects, above). As with other antidepressants, it is recommended that selective serotonin reuptake inhibitors (SSRIs) should be used with caution in patients with epilepsy or a history of such disorders and should be avoided if epilepsy is poorly controlled.

1. Favale E, *et al.* Anticonvulsant effect of fluoxetine in humans. *Neurology* 1995; **45:** 1926–7.

Headache. Initial studies suggest that the selective serotonin reuptake inhibitors (SSRIs) fluoxetine and fluvoxamine may be of some benefit for chronic daily headache[1-3] but results in the prophylaxis of migraine have been conflicting.[3-5] Sertraline has been tried in the management of various types of headache[1,6] but efficacy has been variable and its use may be limited by frequent adverse effects.

Discussions of the overall management of migraine and tension-type headache can be found on p.443 and p.444.

1. Sosin D. Clinical efficacy of fluoxetine vs sertraline in a headache clinic population. *Headache* 1993; **33:** 284.
2. Manna V, *et al.* Chronic tension-type headache, mood depression and serotonin: therapeutic effects of fluvoxamine and mianserine. *Headache* 1994; **34:** 44–9.
3. Saper JR, *et al.* Double-blind trial of fluoxetine: chronic daily headache and migraine. *Headache* 1994; **34:** 497–502.
4. Adly C, *et al.* Fluoxetine prophylaxis of migraine. *Headache* 1992; **32:** 101–4.
5. Bánk J. A comparative study of amitriptyline and fluvoxamine in migraine prophylaxis. *Headache* 1994; **34:** 476–8.
6. Solomon GD, Pearson E. Sertraline in the management of headache. *Clin Pharmacol Ther* 1994; **55:** 130.

Hyperactivity. When drug therapy is indicated for attention deficit hyperactivity disorder (p.1476) initial treatment is usually with central stimulants. Fluoxetine has produced beneficial effects in small numbers of patients with comorbid disorders such as depression or obsessive-compulsive disorder when used as an adjunct to central stimulants.[1,2]

1. Gammon GD, Brown TE. Fluoxetine and methylphenidate in combination for treatment of attention deficit disorder and comorbid depressive disorder. *J Child Adolesc Psychopharmacol* 1993; **3:** 1–10.
2. Bussing R, Levin GM. Methamphetamine and fluoxetine treatment of a child with attention-deficit hyperactivity disorder and obsessive-compulsive disorder. *J Child Adolesc Psychopharmacol* 1993; **3:** 53–8.

Hypochondriasis. Fluoxetine in an initial dose of 20 mg daily gradually increased up to 80 mg daily produced some beneficial results in 10 of 14 patients with hypochondriasis who completed 12 weeks of treatment.[1] The general management of hypochondriasis is discussed on p.636.

1. Fallon BA, *et al.* Fluoxetine for hypochondriacal patients without major depression. *J Clin Psychopharmacol* 1993; **13:** 438–41.

Hypotension. Selective serotonin reuptake inhibitors (SSRIs) have been suggested for patients with neurally mediated hypotension refractory to standard treatment (see p.790).

Obesity. Fluoxetine has been tried with some success as part of the management of obesity (p.1476). Fluoxetine's mechanism of action in obesity is unknown. Serotonin is believed to be involved in the regulation of satiety[1] but fluoxetine has also been shown to increase resting energy expenditure and raise basal body temperature.[2] A common dose for fluoxetine in the management of obesity has been 60 mg daily; it appears that fluoxetine has a dose-related effect on weight loss.[3] Reviews[1,4] agree that fluoxetine can aid weight reduction in the short term but after 16 to 20 weeks some patients have started to regain weight and its long-term efficacy remains to be established. Troublesome adverse effects can occur.[1] Some patients treated with fluoxetine for depression have experienced an increase of appetite and some have gained weight. There has been a report[5] of a patient who lost weight during treatment with fluoxetine for depression despite an increased appetite and food intake.

1. Anonymous. Fluoxetine (Prozac) and other drugs for treatment of obesity. *Med Lett Drugs Ther* 1994; **36:** 107–8.
2. Bross R, Hoffer LJ. Fluoxetine increases resting energy expenditure and basal body temperature in humans. *Am J Clin Nutr* 1995; **61:** 1020–5.
3. Levine LR, *et al.* Use of fluoxetine, a selective serotonin-uptake inhibitor, in the treatment of obesity: a dose-response study. *Int J Obes* 1989; **13:** 635–45.
4. Bray GA. Use and abuse of appetite-suppressant drugs in the treatment of obesity. *Ann Intern Med* 1993; **119:** 707–13.
5. Fichtner CG, Braun BG. Hyperphagia and weight loss during fluoxetine treatment. *Ann Pharmacother* 1994; **28:** 1350–2.

Orthostatic hypotension. There has been a report[1] that fluoxetine 20 mg daily for 6 to 8 weeks produced beneficial effects in 4 of 5 patients with chronic symptomatic orthostatic hypotension refractory to other treatment. The treatment of orthostatic hypotension is discussed on p.1040.

1. Grubb BP, *et al.* Fluoxetine hydrochloride for the treatment of severe refractory orthostatic hypotension. *Am J Med* 1994; **97:** 366–8.

Pain. Fluoxetine has been reported to be of benefit as an alternative to tricyclic antidepressants in fibromyalgia, alone[1] or with cyclobenzaprine[2] or amitriptyline.[3]

See also Headache, above.

1. Geller SA. Treatment of fibrositis with fluoxetine hydrochloride (Prozac). *Am J Med* 1989; **87:** 594–5.
2. Cantini F, *et al.* Fluoxetina associata a ciclobenzaprina nel trattamento della fibromialgia. *Minerva Med* 1994; **85:** 97–100.
3. Goldenberg D, *et al.* A randomized, double-blind crossover trial of fluoxetine and amitriptyline in the treatment of fibromyalgia. *Arthritis Rheum* 1996; **39:** 1852–9.

Parkinsonism. It has been suggested that fluoxetine might be of use in the management of selected patients with Parkinson's disease who have levodopa-induced dyskinesias unresponsive to other measures.[1] However, although fluoxetine has been reported to have produced beneficial results in such patients[2] there has also been a report of increased disability in patients with Parkinson's disease given fluoxetine.[3] Extrapyramidal effects have also been reported in other patients taking fluoxetine (see under Adverse Effects, above). The overall management of parkinsonism is discussed on p.1128.

1. Giron LT, Koller WC. Methods of managing levodopa-induced dyskinesias. *Drug Safety* 1996; **14:** 365–74.
2. Durif F, *et al.* Levodopa-induced dyskinesias are improved by fluoxetine. *Neurology* 1995; **45:** 1855–8.
3. Steur ENHJ. Increase of Parkinson disability after fluoxetine medication. *Neurology* 1993; **43:** 211–3.

Pathological crying or laughing. Inappropriate or uncontrolled crying or laughing can occur in patients with lesions in certain areas of the brain. Attempts at treatment have mostly been with antidepressant drugs, including selective serotonin reuptake inhibitors (SSRIs). Beneficial effects have been claimed for fluoxetine in an uncontrolled study[1] and an anecdotal report.[2]

1. Seliger GM, *et al.* Fluoxetine improves emotional incontinence. *Brain Inj* 1992; **6:** 267–70.
2. Hanger HC. Emotionalism after stroke. *Lancet* 1993; **342:** 1235–6.

Peripheral vascular disease. There have been anecdotal reports of fluoxetine in a daily dose of 20 to 60 mg producing favourable therapeutic responses in patients with Raynaud's syndrome.[1,2] The usual management of peripheral vascular disease such as Raynaud's syndrome is discussed on p.794.

1. Bolte MA, Avery D. Case of fluoxetine-induced remission of Raynaud's phenomenon—a case report. *Angiology* 1993; **44:** 161–3.
2. Jaffe IA. Serotonin reuptake inhibitors in Raynaud's phenomenon. *Lancet* 1995; **345:** 1378.

Premenstrual syndrome. Fluoxetine has been shown in double-blind studies[1-4] to be effective in controlling both the psychological and somatic symptoms of women with premenstrual syndrome (p.1456) and has also been reported[5] to be more effective than tricyclic antidepressants. Long-term efficacy appears to be maintained.[6] A dose of 20 mg daily appears to be as effective as 60 mg daily but produces fewer adverse effects.[4]

1. Stone AB, *et al.* Fluoxetine in the treatment of late luteal phase dysphoric disorder. *J Clin Psychiatry* 1991; **52:** 290–3.
2. Menkes DB, *et al.* Fluoxetine treatment of severe premenstrual syndrome. *Br Med J* 1992; **305:** 346–7.
3. Wood SH, *et al.* Treatment of premenstrual syndrome with fluoxetine: a double-blind, placebo-controlled, crossover study. *Obstet Gynecol* 1992; **80:** 339–44.
4. Steiner M, *et al.* Fluoxetine in the treatment of premenstrual dysphoria. *N Engl J Med* 1995; **332:** 1539–34.
5. Mortola JF. A risk-benefit appraisal of drugs used in the management of premenstrual syndrome. *Drug Safety* 1994; **10:** 160–9.
6. Pearlstein TB, Stone AB. Long-term fluoxetine treatment of late luteal phase dysphoric disorder. *J Clin Psychiatry* 1994; **55:** 332–5.

Sexual dysfunction. Impotence or ejaculatory problems have been reported as adverse effects of selective serotonin reuptake inhibitors (SSRIs) (see Effects on Sexual Function in Adverse Effects, above). Such properties of the SSRIs have been studied as a potential form of treatment for men with premature ejaculation (see Paroxetine, p.302 and Sertraline, p.308).

Preparations

Proprietary Preparations (details are given in Part 3)
Aust.: Fluctine; Mutan; ***Austral.:*** Erocap; Lovan; Prozac; Zactin; ***Belg.:*** Prozac; ***Canad.:*** Prozac; ***Fr.:*** Prozac; ***Ger.:*** Fluctin; ***Irl.:*** Prozac; ***Ital.:*** Fluoxeren; Prozac; ***Neth.:*** Prozac; ***Norw.:*** Fontex; ***S.Afr.:*** Lorien; Prozac; Prozyn; Sanzur; ***Spain:*** Adofen; Docutrix†; Prozac; Reneuron; ***Swed.:*** Fontex; ***Switz.:*** Fluctine; ***UK:*** Prozac; ***USA:*** Prozac.

Fluvoxamine Maleate (12768-h)

Fluvoxamine Maleate *(BANM, USAN, rINNM).*

DU-23000. *(E)*-5-Methoxy-4′-trifluoromethylvalerophenone *O*-2-aminoethyloxime maleate.

$C_{15}H_{21}F_3N_2O_2,C_4H_4O_4$ = 434.4.

CAS — 54739-18-3 (fluvoxamine); 61718-82-9 (fluvoxamine maleate).

Pharmacopoeias. In Br.

A white to almost white crystalline powder. Sparingly **soluble** in water; freely soluble in alcohol and in methyl alcohol.

Adverse Effects, Treatment, and Precautions

As for selective serotonin reuptake inhibitors (SSRIs) in general (see Fluoxetine, p.284).

Bradycardia with ECG changes has been noted with fluvoxamine (see also Effects on the Cardiovascular System in Adverse Effects of Fluoxetine, p.284).

It is recommended that fluvoxamine should be withdrawn in patients who have an increase in serum concentrations of liver enzymes.

Fluvoxamine should be given in reduced dosage to patients with hepatic or renal impairment. Some also recommend similar reductions in the elderly.

Reviews.

1. Wagner W, *et al.* Fluvoxamine: a review of its safety profile in world-wide studies. *Int Clin Psychopharmacol* 1994; **9:** 223–7.

In the UK the Committee on Safety of Medicines (CSM) has reported[1] that between 25 September 1986 and 23 March 1988 it had received 961 reports of adverse reactions associated with the use of fluvoxamine and that these included 5 deaths. The most frequently reported reactions were nausea (183) and vomiting (101). Other reactions included dizziness, somnolence, agitation, headache, tremor, and, during the first few days, worsening of anxiety. There were 13 reports of convulsions. Reports of appetite stimulation and antimuscarinic reactions were unusual. The effects sometimes resolved with time or dose reduction.

For a comparison of the adverse reaction profile of fluoxetine with that of fluvoxamine, see under Adverse Effects of Fluoxetine, p.284.

1. Committee on Safety of Medicines. Fluvoxamine (Faverin): adverse reaction profile. *Current Problems 22* 1988.

Interactions

For interactions associated with selective serotonin reuptake inhibitors (SSRIs), see Fluoxetine, p.286.

Fluvoxamine can greatly increase plasma concentrations of theophylline (see p.768), and it is recommended that concomitant use should be avoided or, if this is not possible, the dose of theophylline should be halved and monitoring of plasma-theophylline concentrations instituted.

References.

1. Wagner W, Vause EW. Fluvoxamine: a review of global drug-drug interaction data. *Clin Pharmacokinet* 1995; **29** (suppl 1): 26–32.

Pharmacokinetics

Fluvoxamine is readily absorbed from the gastro-intestinal tract with peak plasma concentrations appearing 2 to 8 hours after administration. Systemic bioavailability does not appear to be affected by food. It is extensively metabolised, by oxidative demethylation and deamination, in the liver to inactive metabolites. Excretion is mainly in the urine. Fluvoxamine is widely distributed throughout the body and protein binding is reported to be about 80%; it has a plasma-elimination half-life of about 15 hours. Fluvoxamine is distributed into breast milk (see Breast Feeding under Precautions in Fluoxetine, p.285).

References.

1. De Bree H, *et al.* Fluvoxamine maleate: disposition in man. *Eur J Drug Metab Pharmacokinet* 1983; **8:** 175–9.
2. Overmars H, *et al.* Fluvoxamine maleate: metabolism in man. *Eur J Drug Metab Pharmacokinet* 1983; **8:** 269–80.
3. van Harten J, *et al.* Pharmacokinetics of fluvoxamine maleate in patients with liver cirrhosis after single-dose oral administration. *Clin Pharmacokinet* 1993; **24:** 177–82.
4. Perucca E, *et al.* Clinical pharmacokinetics of fluvoxamine. *Clin Pharmacokinet* 1994; **27:** 175–90.
5. van Harten J. Overview of the pharmacokinetics of fluvoxamine. *Clin Pharmacokinet* 1995; **29** (suppl 1): 1–9.
6. Xu Z-H, *et al.* In vivo inhibition of CYP2C19 but not CYP2D6 by fluvoxamine. *Br J Clin Pharmacol* 1996; **42:** 518–21.
7. Spigset O, *et al.* Non-linear fluvoxamine disposition. *Br J Clin Pharmacol* 1998; **45:** 257–63.

Uses and Administration

Fluvoxamine, an aralkylketone derivative, is a selective serotonin reuptake inhibitor (SSRI) with actions and uses similar to those of fluoxetine (p.287).

In the treatment of depression fluvoxamine is given by mouth as the maleate in doses of 100 to 200 mg daily; in some patients the dose may need to be gradually increased to a maximum of 300 mg daily. It is recommended that daily dosages exceeding 100 mg should be given in divided doses.

Fluvoxamine is also used in a similar dosage in the management of obsessive-compulsive disorder. It is recommended that if no improvement of symptoms is observed within 10 weeks, treatment with fluvoxamine should be re-assessed.

Reduced doses should be employed in patients with hepatic or renal impairment. In the USA, dose reductions are similarly recommended for elderly patients.

Fluvoxamine should be withdrawn gradually to reduce the risk of withdrawal symptoms.

Reviews.

1. Grimsley SR, Jann MW. Paroxetine, sertraline, and fluvoxamine: new selective serotonin reuptake inhibitors. *Clin Pharm* 1992; **11:** 930–57.
2. Mendlewicz J. Efficacy of fluvoxamine in severe depression. *Drugs* 1992; **43** (suppl 2): 32–9.
3. Wilde ME, *et al.* Fluvoxamine: an updated review of its pharmacology, and therapeutic use in depressive illness. *Drugs* 1993; **46:** 895–924.
4. Palmer KJ, Benfield P. Fluvoxamine: an overview of its pharmacological properties and review of its therapeutic potential in non-depressive disorders. *CNS Drugs* 1994; **1:** 57–87.

Anxiety disorders. Fluvoxamine has been given in a variety of anxiety disorders (p.635) including obsessive-compulsive disorder, panic disorders, and social phobia.

References.

1. Jenike MA, *et al.* A controlled trial of fluvoxamine in obsessive-compulsive disorder: implications for a serotonergic theory. *Am J Psychiatry* 1990; **147:** 1209–15.
2. Mallya GK, *et al.* Short- and long-term treatment of obsessive-compulsive disorder with fluvoxamine. *Ann Clin Psychiatry* 1992; **4:** 77–80.
3. Black DW, *et al.* A comparison of fluvoxamine, cognitive therapy, and placebo in the treatment of panic disorder. *Arch Gen Psychiatry* 1993; **50:** 44–50.
4. Hoehn-Saric R, *et al.* Effect of fluvoxamine on panic disorder. *J Clin Psychopharmacol* 1993; **13:** 321–6.
5. van Vliet IM, *et al.* Psychopharmacological treatment of social phobia: a double blind placebo controlled study with fluvoxamine. *Psychopharmacology (Berl)* 1994; **115:** 128–34.
6. Freeman CPL, *et al.* Fluvoxamine versus clomipramine in the treatment of obsessive compulsive disorder: a multicenter, randomized, double-blind, parallel group comparison. *J Clin Psychiatry* 1994; **55:** 301–5.
7. Greist JH, *et al.* Efficacy of fluvoxamine in obsessive-compulsive disorder: results of a multicentre, double blind, placebo-controlled trial. *Eur J Clin Res* 1995; **7:** 195–204.

Depression. As discussed on p.271, there is very little difference in efficacy between the different groups of antidepressant drugs. Selective serotonin reuptake inhibitors (SSRIs) such as fluvoxamine are increasingly being recognised as first-choice treatment because they offer advantages over the older tricyclics in terms of fewer unpleasant side-effects and safety in overdosage.

References.

1. Harris B, *et al.* Fluvoxamine versus amitriptyline in depressed hospital out-patients: a multicentre double-blind comparative trial. *Br J Clin Res* 1991; **2:** 89–99.
2. Ottevanger EA. The efficacy of fluvoxamine in patients with severe depression. *Br J Clin Res* 1991; **2:** 125–32.
3. Rahman MK, *et al.* A double-blind, randomised comparison of fluvoxamine with dothiepin in the treatment of depression in elderly patients. *Br J Clin Pract* 1991; **45:** 255–8.
4. Bougerol T, *et al.* Efficacy and tolerability of moclobemide compared with fluvoxamine in depressive disorder (DSM-III): a French/Swiss double-blind trial. *Psychopharmacology (Berl)* 1992; **106** (suppl): S102–S108.
5. Franchini L, *et al.* A 24-month follow-up study of unipolar subjects: a comparison between lithium and fluvoxamine. *J Affective Disord* 1994; **32:** 225–31.
6. Ansseau M, *et al.* Controlled comparison of paroxetine and fluvoxamine in major depression. *Hum Psychopharmacol Clin Exp* 1994; **9:** 329–36.
7. Franchini L, *et al.* Fluvoxamine and lithium in long-term treatment of unipolar subjects with high recurrence rate. *J Affective Disord* 1996; **38:** 67–9.

Headache. For reference to the use of selective serotonin reuptake inhibitors (SSRIs), including fluvoxamine, in the management of various types of headache, see under Fluoxetine, p.288.

Preparations

BP 1998: Fluvoxamine Tablets.

Proprietary Preparations (details are given in Part 3)

Aust.: Floxyfral; ***Austral.:*** Luvox; ***Belg.:*** Floxyfral; ***Canad.:*** Luvox; ***Fr.:*** Floxyfral; ***Ger.:*** Fevarin; ***Irl.:*** Faverin; ***Ital.:*** Dumirox; Fevarin; Maveral; ***Neth.:*** Fevarin; ***Norw.:*** Fevarin; ***S.Afr.:*** Luvox; ***Spain:*** Dumirox; ***Swed.:*** Fevarin; ***Switz.:*** Floxyfral; ***UK:*** Faverin; ***USA:*** Luvox.

Imipramine (2514-w)

Imipramine (*BAN, rINN*).

3-(10,11-Dihydro-5*H*-dibenz[*b,f*]azepin-5-yl)propyldimethylamine.

$C_{19}H_{24}N_2$ = 280.4.

CAS — 50-49-7.

Imipramine 0.88 g is approximately equivalent to 1 g of imipramine hydrochloride.

Imipramine Embonate (2515-e)

Imipramine Embonate (*BANM, rINNM*).

Imipramine Pamoate.

$(C_{19}H_{24}N_2)_2, C_{23}H_{16}O_6$ = 949.2.

CAS — 10075-24-8.

Imipramine embonate 1.5 g is approximately equivalent to 1 g of imipramine hydrochloride.

Imipramine Hydrochloride (2516-l)

Imipramine Hydrochloride (*BANM, rINNM*).

Imipram. Hydrochlor.; Imipramini Chloridum; Imipramini Hydrochloridum; Imizine.

$C_{19}H_{24}N_2$,HCl = 316.9.

CAS — 113-52-0.

Pharmacopoeias. In *Chin., Eur.* (see p.viii), *Int., Jpn, Pol.,* and *US.*

A white or slightly yellow, odourless or almost odourless, crystalline powder. Freely **soluble** in water and in alcohol; soluble in acetone; practically insoluble in ether. A 10% solution in water has a pH of 3.6 to 5.0. **Store** in airtight containers. Protect from light.

Adverse Effects, Treatment, and Precautions

As for tricyclic antidepressants in general (see Amitriptyline, p.273).

Porphyria. Imipramine has been associated with acute attacks of porphyria and is considered unsafe in patients with acute porphyria.[1]

1. Moore MR, McColl KEL. *Porphyria: drug lists.* Glasgow: Porphyria Research Unit, University of Glasgow, 1991.

Interactions

For interactions associated with tricyclic antidepressants, see Amitriptyline, p.276.

Pharmacokinetics

Imipramine is readily absorbed from the gastro-intestinal tract, and extensively demethylated by first-pass metabolism in the liver, to its primary active metabolite, desipramine.

Paths of metabolism of both imipramine and desipramine include hydroxylation and *N*-oxidation. Imipramine is excreted in the urine, mainly in the form of its metabolites, either free or in conjugated form; small amounts are excreted in the faeces via the bile.

Imipramine and desipramine are widely distributed throughout the body and are extensively bound to plasma and tissue protein. Imipramine has been estimated to have an elimination half-life ranging from 9 to 28 hours, which may be considerably extended in overdosage. Plasma concentrations of imipramine and desipramine vary very widely between individuals but some correlation with therapeutic response has been established.

Imipramine and desipramine cross the blood-brain barrier and placenta and are distributed into breast milk (see Breast Feeding under Precautions in Amitriptyline, p.275).

A detailed and extensive review of the clinical pharmacokinetics of imipramine and desipramine.[1]

Imipramine and desipramine are rapidly and completely absorbed when taken orally. Absorption occurs in the small intestine rather than from the stomach and food has no effect on absorption, peak drug concentration, or time to peak drug concentration for imipramine.

Both drugs are subject to extensive first-pass metabolism in the liver and probably also undergo enterohepatic recycling. Imipramine is mainly eliminated by demethylation to the active metabolite, desipramine and to a lesser extent by aromatic hydroxylation. Desipramine is metabolised by aromatic hydroxylation to 2-hydroxydesipramine. Other minor pathways of metabolism also occur.

The discovery of genetic polymorphism, namely the extensive and poor metaboliser phenotypes of sparteine and debrisoquine, has done much to explain the interindividual differences observed in the metabolism of imipramine and desipramine as first-pass metabolism is reduced in poor metabolisers.

Both imipramine and desipramine are highly bound to plasma proteins the ranges being 60 to 96% and 73 to 92% respectively.

Half-lives have usually been estimated from single-dose pharmacokinetic studies and values of about 12 hours and 22 hours have been reported in healthy young adults given imipramine and desipramine respectively. The sampling times have been different in the various studies and shorter elimination half-lives were reported initially compared with more recent work which indicates an elimination half-life nearly double that of previous estimates. Mean half-lives in alcoholic patients, the elderly, and children given imipramine have been reported to be 10.9, 28.6, and 14.5 hours respectively and in alcoholic patients and elderly subjects given desipramine to be 15.1 and 20.9 hours respectively.

Plasma concentration data after multiple doses comes mainly from studies in depressed patients and with a few exceptions support a fairly linear relationship between dose and steady-state concentration of imipramine. There is some evidence, however, that nonlinear rises in plasma concentration may occur with desipramine in doses above 150 mg daily and this effect may be clinically relevant with higher doses of either imipramine or desipramine in some patients, although the position is still not entirely clear.

The assumption of linear kinetics has also been used to predict steady-state concentrations and thus the dose ultimately required after giving a single test dose. Several investigators have successfully done so for both imipramine and desipramine but the possibility of nonlinear kinetics has been used as an argument against such procedures.

1. Sallee FR, Pollock BG. Clinical pharmacokinetics of imipramine and desipramine. *Clin Pharmacokinet* 1990; **18:** 346–64.

Uses and Administration

Imipramine is a dibenzazepine tricyclic antidepressant with actions and uses similar to those of amitriptyline (p.278). Imipramine is one of the less sedating tricyclics and has moderate antimuscarinic activity. Imipramine is usually given by mouth as the hydrochloride.

In the treatment of depression, the usual daily dose of imipramine hydrochloride is up to 75 mg in divided doses initially, gradually increased to 150 to 200 mg daily as necessary; higher doses of up to 300 mg daily may be required in severely depressed patients in hospital. A suggested initial dose for the elderly in the UK is 10 mg at night, gradually increasing to 30 to 50 mg daily. In the USA, daily doses of 25 to 50 mg are recommended for initial therapy in the elderly and adolescents increasing to a maximum of 100 mg daily as required. Since imipramine has a prolonged half-life, once-daily dosage regimens up to 150 mg are also suitable, usually given at night.

In the initial stages of treatment, if administration by mouth is impracticable or inadvisable, up to 100 mg of imipramine hydrochloride may be given daily in divided doses by intramuscular injection, but oral administration should be substituted as soon as possible.

Imipramine is also used for the treatment of nocturnal enuresis in children in whom organic pathology has been excluded. However, drug therapy for nocturnal enuresis should be reserved for those in whom other methods have failed and should preferably only be given to cover periods away from home; tricyclic antidepressants are not recommended in children under 6 years of age (some authorities recommend that they should not be given until 7 years of age). Suggested doses of imipramine hydrochloride are 25 mg for children aged 6 to 7 years (20 to 25 kg body-weight), 25 to 50 mg for children aged 8 to 11 years (25 to 35 kg body-weight), and 50 to 75 mg for children aged over 11 years (35 to 54 kg body-weight). The dose should be taken just before bedtime and treatment, including the gradual period of withdrawal, should not continue for longer than 3 months. A full physical examination is recommended before a further course.

Imipramine may also be given by mouth in liquid form as the embonate with doses expressed in terms of the hydrochloride. Imipramine oxide hydrochloride (imipraminoxide hydrochloride) is also used as an antidepressant and for nocturnal enuresis.

Imipramine should be withdrawn gradually to reduce the risk of withdrawal symptoms.

Alcohol dependence. Imipramine was shown to be an effective treatment for primary depression in actively drinking alcoholic patients, and may improve drinking behaviour in those whose depression responded to treatment.[1]

For a discussion of the management of alcohol withdrawal and abstinence, see p.1099.

1. McGrath PJ, *et al.* Imipramine treatment of alcoholics with primary depression: a placebo-controlled clinical trial. *Arch Gen Psychiatry* 1996; **53:** 232–40.

Anxiety disorders. See under Clomipramine, p.282.

Some references to the use of imipramine in anxiety disorders are given below.

1. Cross-National Collaborative Panic Study, Second Phase Investigators. Drug treatment of panic disorder: comparative efficacy of alprazolam, imipramine, and placebo. *Br J Psychiatry* 1992; **160:** 191–202.
2. Lepola UM, *et al.* Three-year follow-up of patients with panic disorder after short-term treatment with alprazolam and imipramine. *Int Clin Psychopharmacol* 1993; **8:** 115–18.
3. Rickels K, *et al.* Antidepressants for the treatment of generalised anxiety disorder: a placebo-controlled comparison of imipramine, trazodone, and diazepam. *Arch Gen Psychiatry* 1993; **50:** 884–95.
4. Clark DM, *et al.* A comparison of cognitive therapy, applied relaxation and imipramine in the treatment of panic disorder. *Br J Psychiatry* 1994; **164:** 759–69.

Depression. As discussed on p.271, there is very little difference in efficacy between the different groups of antidepressant drugs, and choice is often made on the basis of adverse effect profile. Tricyclic antidepressants such as imipramine have traditionally been the first choice for the treatment of depression, and often still are because of wide experience with their use and familiarity with their pharmacological actions. Imipramine is one of the less sedating tricyclics and consequently may be of value for withdrawn or apathetic depressed patients.

Hyperactivity. See under Desipramine, p.282.

Micturition disorders. For the use of tricyclic antidepressants, including imipramine, in the treatment of nocturnal enuresis, see under Amitriptyline, p.278.

Pain. Antidepressants, usually amitriptyline or another tricyclic, are useful in alleviating some types of pain (p.4) when given in subantidepressant doses.

In one study[1] imipramine was found to reduce the symptoms of patients who had chest pain despite a normal coronary angiogram.

Further references[2-5] to the use of imipramine as an analgesic are given below.

1. Cannon RO, *et al.* Imipramine in patients with chest pain despite normal coronary angiograms. *N Engl J Med* 1994; **330:** 1411–17.
2. Kvinesdal B, *et al.* Imipramine treatment of painful diabetic neuropathy. *JAMA* 1984; **251:** 1727–30.
3. Walsh TD. Controlled study of imipramine and morphine in chronic pain due to advanced cancer. *Proc Am Soc Clin Oncol* 1986; **5:** 237.
4. Hummel T, *et al.* A comparison of the antinociceptive effects of imipramine, tramadol and anpirtoline. *Br J Clin Pharmacol* 1994; **37:** 325–33.
5. Godfrey RG. A guide to the understanding and use of tricyclic antidepressants in the overall management of fibromyalgia and other chronic pain syndromes. *Arch Intern Med* 1996; **156:** 1047–52.

Preparations

BP 1998: Imipramine Tablets;
USP 23: Imipramine Hydrochloride Injection; Imipramine Hydrochloride Tablets.

Proprietary Preparations (details are given in Part 3)
Aust.: Tofranil; ***Austral.:*** Imiprin†; Melipramine; Tofranil; ***Belg.:*** Tofranil; ***Canad.:*** Impril; Novo-Pramine; Tofranil; ***Fr.:*** Tofranil; ***Ger.:*** Pryleugan; Tofranil; ***Irl.:*** Tofranil; ***Ital.:*** Surplix†; Tofranil; ***Neth.:*** Tofranil; ***Norw.:*** Tofranil; ***S.Afr.:*** Ethipramine†; Medipramine†; Mipralin†; Tofranil; ***Spain:*** Imiprex†; Tofranil; ***Swed.:*** Tofranil; ***Switz.:*** Tofranil; ***UK:*** Tofranil; ***USA:*** Imp-Tab; Janimine; Tofranil; Tofranil-PM.

Multi-ingredient: ***Spain:*** Paidenur†.

Iprindole Hydrochloride (2518-j)

Iprindole Hydrochloride (*BANM, rINNM*).
Pramindole Hydrochloride; Wy-3263 (iprindole). 5-(3-Dimethylaminopropyl)-6,7,8,9,10,11-hexahydrocyclooct[*b*]indole hydrochloride.
$C_{19}H_{28}N_2,HCl = 320.9$.
CAS — 5560-72-5 (iprindole); 20432-64-8 (iprindole hydrochloride).

NOTE. Iprindole is *USAN*.

Iprindole hydrochloride has actions and uses similar to those of amitriptyline (p.273), but it only has weak antimuscarinic and sedative effects. It has been used as an alternative to tricyclic antidepressants for the treatment of depression.

Preparations

Proprietary Preparations (details are given in Part 3)
Irl.: Prondol†; ***UK:*** Prondol†.

Iproniazid Phosphate (2520-p)

Iproniazid Phosphate (*BANM, rINNM*).
2′-Isopropylisonicotinohydrazide phosphate.
$C_9H_{13}N_3O,H_3PO_4 = 277.2$.
CAS — 54-92-2 (iproniazid); 305-33-9 (iproniazid phosphate).

Iproniazid phosphate 155 mg is approximately equivalent to 100 mg of iproniazid.

Adverse Effects, Treatment, and Precautions

As for MAOIs in general (see Phenelzine, p.302).

Effects on the liver. Of 91 cases of hepatitis due to antidepressant therapy, cytolytic reactions occurred in 11 treated with iproniazid.[1] Five patients died, 3 of them after involuntary rechallenge. High levels of antimitochondrial antibody were found in 5 patients.

1. Lefebure B, *et al.* Hépatites aux antidépresseurs. *Therapie* 1984; **39:** 509–16.

Porphyria. Iproniazid has been associated with clinical exacerbations of porphyria and is considered unsafe in porphyric patients.[1]

1. Moore MR, McColl KEL. *Porphyria: drug lists.* Glasgow: Porphyria Research Unit, University of Glasgow, 1991.

Interactions

For interactions associated with MAOIs, see Phenelzine, p.304.

Uses and Administration

Iproniazid, a hydrazine derivative, is an irreversible inhibitor of both monoamine oxidase types A and B with actions and uses similar to those of phenelzine (p.306).

Iproniazid is used in the treatment of depression, but as discussed on p.271 the risks associated with irreversible non-selective MAOIs usually mean that other antidepressants are preferred. It is given by mouth as the phosphate in doses equivalent to iproniazid 50 to 150 mg daily. Once a response has been obtained the dosage may be gradually reduced for maintenance therapy; some patients may respond to 25 to 50 mg daily or every other day.

Iproniazid should be withdrawn gradually to reduce the risk of withdrawal symptoms.

Iproniazid is the isopropyl derivative of isoniazid (see p.218) and was developed for use in tuberculosis, but owing to its toxicity is no longer used for this purpose.

Preparations

Proprietary Preparations (details are given in Part 3)
Fr.: Marsilid.

Isocarboxazid (2521-s)

Isocarboxazid (*BAN, rINN*).
Ro-5083l. 2′-Benzyl-5-methylisoxazole-3-carbohydrazide.
$C_{12}H_{13}N_3O_2 = 231.3$.
CAS — 59-63-2.

Pharmacopoeias. In *US.*

A white or practically white, crystalline powder with a slight characteristic odour. **Soluble** 1 in 2000 of water, 1 in 83 of alcohol, 1 in 2 of chloroform, and 1 in 58 of ether.

Adverse Effects, Treatment, and Precautions

As for MAOIs in general (see Phenelzine, p.302).

Interactions

For interactions associated with MAOIs, see Phenelzine, p.304.

Pharmacokinetics

Isocarboxazid is readily absorbed from the gastro-intestinal tract reaching peak plasma concentrations 3 to 5 hours after ingestion. It is metabolised by the liver, and is excreted in the urine mainly in the form of metabolites.

Uses and Administration

Isocarboxazid, a hydrazine derivative, is an irreversible inhibitor of both monoamine oxidase types A and B with actions and uses similar to those of phenelzine (p.306).

Isocarboxazid is used in the treatment of depression but as discussed on p.271 the risks associated with irreversible non-selective MAOIs usually mean that other antidepressants are preferred. It is given by mouth in an initial dose of 30 mg daily in single or divided doses. If no improvement occurs after 4 weeks, doses of up to 60 mg daily can be tried for up to 4 to 6 weeks. Once a response has been obtained the dosage may be gradually reduced to a maintenance of 10 to 20 mg daily, although doses of up to 40 mg daily may be needed in some patients. Half the normal maintenance dose may be adequate in the elderly.

Isocarboxazid should be withdrawn gradually to reduce the risk of withdrawal symptoms.

Preparations

USP 23: Isocarboxazid Tablets.

Proprietary Preparations (details are given in Part 3)
Irl.: Marplan†; ***Ital.:*** Marplan†; ***UK:*** Marplan; ***USA:*** Marplan.

Lithium Carbonate (5057-h)

Lithium Carbonate (*USAN*).
CP-15467-61; Lithii Carbonas; Lithium Carb.; NSC-16895.
$Li_2CO_3 = 73.89$.
CAS — 554-13-2.

NOTE. Commercially available lithium materials have atomic weights ranging from 6.94 to 6.99. The molecular weight of lithium carbonate of 73.89 given above has been calculated using the lowest atomic weight; using the highest figure would give a molecular weight of 73.99. This difference does not affect the figure of 27 mmol of lithium being provided by 1 g of lithium carbonate. Nor should it affect the outcome of assays of serum-lithium concentrations given the limits of error of the assay methods. However, while it is doubtful that there would be any discernible effect on serum concentrations resulting from this atomic weight variance in a patient changing to a different lithium preparation, the different pharmacokinetic characteristics still have to be considered.

Pharmacopoeias. In *Chin., Eur.* (see p.viii), *Int., Jpn, Pol.,* and *US.*

A white odourless granular powder. Each g represents 27 mmol of lithium.

Ph. Eur. **solubilities** are: slightly soluble in water; practically insoluble in alcohol. USP solubilities are: sparingly soluble in water, very slightly soluble in alcohol; dissolves, with effervescence, in dilute mineral acids. A saturated solution is alkaline to litmus.

Lithium Citrate (7058-t)

Lithii Citras.
$C_6H_5Li_3O_7,4H_2O = 282.0$.
CAS — 919-16-4 (anhydrous lithium citrate); 6080-58-6 (lithium citrate tetrahydrate).

NOTE. Commercially available lithium materials have atomic weights ranging from 6.94 to 6.99. The molecular weight of lithium citrate of 282.0 given above has been calculated using the lowest atomic weight; using the highest figure would give a molecular weight of 282.1. This difference does not affect the figure of 10.6 mmol of lithium being provided by 1 g of lithium citrate. Nor should it affect the outcome of assays of serum-lithium concentrations given the limits of error of the assay methods. However, while it is doubtful that there would be any discernible effect on serum concentrations resulting from this atomic weight variance in a patient changing to a different lithium preparation, the different pharmacokinetic characteristics still have to be considered.

Pharmacopoeias. In *Eur.* (see p.viii) and *US.*
US also includes lithium hydroxide.

A white or almost white odourless fine deliquescent crystalline powder or granules. Each g represents 10.6 mmol of lithium. Freely **soluble** in water; slightly soluble in alcohol. A 5% solution in water has a pH of 7.0 to 10.0. **Store** in airtight containers.

Adverse Effects

Many of the side-effects of lithium are dose-related and the margin between the therapeutic and toxic dose is narrow.

Initial adverse effects of lithium therapy include nausea, diarrhoea, vertigo, muscle weakness, and a dazed feeling; these effects often abate with continued therapy. Fine hand tremors, polyuria, and polydipsia may, however, persist. Other adverse effects that may occur at therapeutic serum-lithium concentrations include weight gain and oedema (which should not be treated with diuretics). Hypercalcaemia, hypermagnesaemia, and hyperparathyroidism have been reported. Skin disorders such as acne, psoriasis, and rashes may be exacerbated by lithium therapy. Leucocytosis is a relatively common adverse effect. Long-term adverse effects include hypothyroidism and/or goitre, rarely hyperthyroidism, and mild cognitive and memory impairment. Histological and functional changes in the kidney have been noted following long-term use of therapeutic concentrations of lithium (but see under Effects on the Kidneys, below).

Toxic effects may be expected at serum-lithium concentrations of about 1.5 mmol per litre, although they can appear at lower concentrations. They call for immediate withdrawal of treatment and should always be considered very seriously.

Signs of lithium toxicity include increasing diarrhoea, vomiting, anorexia, muscle weakness, lethargy, giddiness with ataxia, lack of coordination, tinnitus, blurred vision, coarse tremor of the extremities and lower jaw, muscle hyperirritability, choreoathetoid movements, dysarthria, and drowsiness. Symptoms of severe overdosage at serum-lithium concentrations above 2 mmol per litre include hyperreflexia and hyperextension of limbs, syncope, toxic psychosis, seizures, polyuria, renal failure, electrolyte imbalance, dehydration, circulatory failure, coma, and occasionally death. The hazards of lithium in pregnant patients are discussed under Pregnancy in Precautions, below.

Effects on the blood. There has been a recent report of a patient developing thrombocytopenia after restarting lithium therapy following a gap of some weeks.[1] Withdrawing the lithium led to an improvement in platelet count, but the count fell when lithium therapy was tried again. Leucocytosis is a recognised effect of lithium which this patient also experienced. Concerns about leukaemia induction have not been verified.

In discussing this instance of thrombocytopenia, Collins[1] cites early reports of aplastic and megaloblastic anaemia and a case of fatal haemolytic anaemia reported to the UK Committee on Safety of Medicines.

1. Collins S. Thrombocytopenia associated with lithium carbonate. *Br Med J* 1992; **305:** 159.

Effects on the cardiovascular system. Reports of adverse effects on the heart associated with lithium have included bradycardia due to sinus node dysfunction,[1] which has persisted after stopping lithium,[2] premature ventricular contractions,[3] atrioventricular block,[4] and T-wave depression.[5] For the adverse cardiac effects associated with lithium intoxication, see under Overdosage, below.

For mention of myocarditis associated with lithium therapy, see under Effects on the Musculoskeletal System, below.

1. Montalescot G, *et al.* Serious sinus node dysfunction caused by therapeutic doses of lithium. *Int J Cardiol* 1984; **5:** 94–6.
2. Palileo EV, *et al.* Persistent sinus node dysfunction secondary to lithium therapy. *Am Heart J* 1983; **106:** 1443–4.
3. Tangedahl TN, Gau GT. Myocardial irritability associated with lithium carbonate therapy. *N Engl J Med* 1972; **287:** 867–9.
4. Martin CA, Piascik MT. First degree A-V block in patients on lithium carbonate. *Can J Psychiatry* 1985; **30:** 114–16.
5. Demers RG, Heninger GR. Electrocardiographic T-wave changes during lithium carbonate treatment. *JAMA* 1971; **218:**381–6.

Effects on the endocrine system. Myers and West have reviewed the effects of lithium on the endocrine system.[1] Although the published prevalence figures have varied widely there is a small, but definite, risk that patients taking lithium in therapeutic doses will develop clinical *goitre*, *hypothyroidism*, or, rarely, both; the risk appears to be greatest during the first 2 years of lithium therapy.[2] Auto-immune atrophic thyroiditis is now thought to be one important pre-disposing factor.[1] Early goitre and lithium-induced hypothyroidism are both reversible if lithium is discontinued; if continued treatment with lithium is desirable the patient should be treated with thyroxine. There have been rare reports of *hyperthyroidism* in lithium-treated patients and the association may only be one of coincidence, although it is important to realise that hyperthyroidism can precipitate mania and can also be mistaken for an attack of mania.

Increases in serum concentrations of calcium and parathyroid hormone have been described in patients receiving lithium therapy. Myers and West[1] considered the increases to be slight. However some patients have experienced parathyroid hyperplasia.[3,4]

Cases of *diabetes mellitus* developing in patients treated with lithium have been reported but Myers and West[1] did not view this as being attributable to lithium, an opinion also expressed by Pandit *et al.*[5] who carried out another review of the literature.

1. Myers DH, West TET. Hormone systems. In: Johnson FN, ed. *Depression & mania: modern lithium therapy.* Oxford: IRL Press, 1987: 220–6.
2. Vincent A, *et al.* Lithium-associated hypothyroidism: a practical review. *Lithium* 1994; **5:** 73–4.
3. Nordenström J, *et al.* Hyperparathyroidism associated with treatment of manic-depressive disorders by lithium. *Eur J Surg* 1992; **158:** 207–11.
4. Taylor JW, Bell AJ. Lithium-induced parathyroid dysfunction: a case report and review of the literature. *Ann Pharmacother* 1993; **27:** 1040–3.
5. Pandit MK, *et al.* Drug-induced disorders of glucose tolerance. *Ann Intern Med* 1993; **118:** 529–39.

Effects on the eyes. The adverse effects of lithium on the eyes have been reviewed by Fraunfelder *et al.*[1] Decrease in accommodation has been reported in up to 10% of patients taking lithium but mainly younger patients are affected. Blurred vision may also occur, most commonly early in therapy, but this may improve with time. Lithium can affect extraocular muscles and produce diplopia. A reduction in dosage or discontinuation of therapy may be required. Lithium reduces lachrymal secretions and is excreted in tears in increased concentrations. In rare cases this may result in ocular irritation but this usually causes few problems when artificial tears are used. Photophobia, which occurs rarely with lithium therapy, may also be associated with the excretion of lithium in tears. Lithium can reduce dark adaptation due to a direct neural effect but whether this can progress further to cause irreversible macular or retinal degeneration is not proven. There are some rare but poorly documented reports of deposits in the cornea or conjunctiva. Fraunfelder *et al.* considered that on the evidence available it was unlikely that lithium increased the risk of developing senile cataracts.

Lithium can cause various forms of nystagmus, many of which are reversible on reducing the dose or withdrawal of the drug. However, downbeat nystagmus is a serious adverse effect and is often irreversible. Irreversible oscillopsia can occur rarely secondary to nystagmus. Oculogyric crisis has been associated with lithium therapy and may be exacerbated by concomitant treatment with haloperidol.

Some ocular effects may occur secondary to the effects of lithium on other systems. Exophthalmos and other thyroid-related eye disorders may occur rarely as a secondary effect of lithium on the thyroid. Lithium can also cause pseudotumour cerebri with papilloedema (benign intracranial hypertension). Most cases have occurred a few years after starting therapy but there has been one report of this condition after only 7 months of treatment. Ptosis has been reported, mainly associated with unmasking of myasthenia gravis.

1. Fraunfelder FT, *et al.* The effects of lithium on the human visual system. *J Toxicol Cutan Ocul Toxicol* 1992; **11:** 97–169.

Effects on the kidneys. Lithium is primarily excreted by renal mechanisms. Polyuria, with associated polydipsia, is the most common symptom that results from the effects of lithium on the kidney and Walker and Kincaid-Smith have mentioned[1] that the incidence in studies has ranged from 4 to 50%. The symptoms are associated with a decreased urinary concentrating ability and are believed to be due to a lithium-induced nephrogenic diabetes insipidus-like syndrome. The polyuria was originally assumed to be a reversible effect, but as a result of several studies showing persisting nephrogenic diabetes insipidus this was questioned and suggestions made that lithium may cause irreversible kidney damage. Patients were identified with renal histological changes that included tubular atrophy, focal interstitial nephropathy and focal fibrosis, and impairment of glomerular filtration rate. However, Walker and Kincaid-Smith have remarked that in many of these patients such effects were found either after suffering acute lithium toxicity or severe polyuria and that many of the non-specific histological lesions have also been identified in psychiatric patients who have never received lithium.[1] They concluded that patients on long-term maintenance lithium therapy do appear to be susceptible to the development of progressive impairment of urinary concentrating ability but that it was most noticeable in patients with a history of acute lithium toxicity. The risk of renal damage and impaired glomerular filtration rate was thought to be extremely small in patients on stable maintenance lithium therapy without prior episodes of acute lithium intoxication.

These conclusions were broadly similar to those published later by George who considered that, although it was necessarily an oversimplified view, many, and perhaps all, of the renal side-effects of lithium are induced by excessive dosage.[2] Schou[3,4] has also defended lithium with respect to its renal toxicity and stated that long-term therapy, if properly controlled, does not lead to chronic or irreversible renal damage.

1. Walker RG, Kincaid-Smith P. Kidneys and the fluid regulatory system. In: Johnson FN, ed. *Depression & mania: modern lithium therapy.* Oxford: IRL Press, 1987: 206–13.
2. George CRP. Renal aspects of lithium toxicity. *Med J Aust* 1989; **150:** 291–2.
3. Schou M. Serum lithium monitoring of prophylactic treatment: critical review and updated recommendations. *Clin Pharmacokinet* 1988; **15:** 283–6.
4. Schou M. Lithium treatment of manic-depressive illness: past, present, and perspectives. *JAMA* 1988; **259:** 1834–6.

Effects on the musculoskeletal system. Baandrup and colleagues have stated that knowledge about the effects of lithium on muscle is fragmentary.[1] The effects on skeletal muscle are represented mainly by varying degrees of weakness and tremor (for further details see under Effects on the Nervous and Neuromuscular Systems, below). Aggravation of myasthenia gravis has been reported. Acute or subacute painful proximal myopathy causing myalgia, cramps, myokymia, or weakness has also been described. Lithium has also been listed as causing toxic myocarditis but Baandrup *et al.* could only trace three cases possibly associated with lithium.

1. Baandrup U, *et al.* Muscle. In: Johnson FN, ed. *Depression & mania: modern lithium therapy.* Oxford: IRL Press, 1987: 236–8.

Effects on the nervous and neuromuscular systems. Neurotoxicity has long been recognised as a potential adverse effect of lithium. Sansone and Ziegler have listed the effects of lithium on the nervous system as either being minor (which can be minimised by reduction of lithium dose during maintenance therapy) or severe (which warrant immediate and complete withdrawal of the drug).[1] They considered the minor effects to include decreased concentration and comprehension, impaired short-term memory, restlessness and anxiety, depression, fine rapid tremors, and easy fatigue. Serious or severe effects included declining cognition and mental status, gait disturbances, movement disorders such as choreoathetosis, myoclonus, and parkinsonism, seizures, cerebellar signs, pseudotumour cerebri (although this was rare), neuroleptic malignant syndrome, myopathy, axonal neuropathy, a myasthenic syndrome, and exacerbation of underlying neuromuscular disease.

Commenting on lithium-induced tremor Johns and Harris[2] have emphasised that there are 2 types. The first is a coarse tremor occurring with impending and actual lithium toxicity and appears to have both cerebellar and parkinsonian components. It is often associated with incoordination, facial spasms, twitching of muscles and limbs, hyperactive reflexes, and more general systemic signs of toxicity. With this type of tremor it was mandatory to stop or decrease the dose of lithium. The second type, which is more common, is a fine tremor, usually occurring within normal therapeutic concentrations, either transiently within a few days of starting treatment or later as a long-standing side-effect. With this type of fine tremor there was evidence to show that a slight decrease in dose may be beneficial.

In addition to the effects mentioned above impairment of taste perception (mainly involving butter and celery)[3] and speech disturbances with few other signs of toxicity[4-6] have been reported.

Further details of the effects of lithium on the nervous system are under Effects on the Eyes, above, under Effects on the Musculoskeletal System, above, and under Epileptogenic Effect, below.

1. Sansone ME, Ziegler DK. Brain and nervous system. In: Johnson FN, ed. *Depression & mania: modern lithium therapy.* Oxford: IRL Press, 1987: 240–5.
2. Johns S, Harris B. Tremor. *Br Med J* 1984; **288:** 1309.

3. Himmelhoch JM, Hanin I. Side effects of lithium carbonate. *Br Med J* 1974; **4:** 233.
4. Solomon K, Vickers R. Dysarthria resulting from lithium carbonate: a case report. *JAMA* 1975; **231:** 280.
5. Worrall EP, Gillham RA. Lithium-induced constructional dyspraxia. *Br Med J* 1983; **286:** 189.
6. McGovern GP. Lithium induced constructional dyspraxia. *Br Med J* 1983; **286:** 646.

Effects on respiration. Lithium is not generally recognised as a respiratory depressant but an episode of reversible respiratory failure about 3 weeks after the start of lithium therapy has been described in a patient with stable chronic airways obstruction.[1] Recovery of consciousness and resolution of hypercapnia occurred within 24 to 36 hours of lithium discontinuation.

1. Weiner M, *et al.* Effect of lithium on the responses to added respiratory resistances. *N Engl J Med* 1983; **308:** 319–22.

Effects on sexual function and fertility. Lithium does not seem to interfere with sexual function in the majority of patients, but there have been isolated reports of impotence associated with loss of libido attributed to lithium therapy.[1]

Studies *in vitro* have demonstrated that in concentrations comparable with those reported to be achieved in semen lithium can inhibit sperm motility,[2] but concentrations found in cervico-vaginal mucus were considered unlikely to affect motility.[3]

1. Beeley L. Drug-induced sexual dysfunction and infertility. *Adverse Drug React Acute Poisoning Rev* 1984; **3:** 23–42.
2. Raoof NT, *et al.* Lithium inhibits human sperm motility in vitro. *Br J Clin Pharmacol* 1989; **28:** 715–17.
3. Salas IG, *et al.* Lithium carbonate concentration in cervico-vaginal mucus and serum after repeated oral dose administration. *Br J Clin Pharmacol* 1989; **28:** 751P.

Effects on the skin and hair. Cutaneous side-effects associated with lithium therapy have been reported by many investigators and these have been reviewed by Lambert and Dalac.[1] Approximately 1% of patients present with some kind of skin disorder though they are not necessarily serious or severe. Although the onset varies from 2 or 3 weeks to 7 or more years, a large number of reactions start to appear once optimal serum-lithium concentrations have been attained. Effects reported include psoriasis which may be severe and require lithium withdrawal. Seborrhoeic dermatitis and follicular keratosis are also encountered and can improve spontaneously or after discontinuation of lithium. Acneform eruptions are found in areas not usually affected by acne vulgaris; in general the face is less affected or not affected at all.

Hair loss, not always severe, is more frequent than cutaneous effects. About 6% of patients may be affected and all kinds of alopecias have been found. The onset occurs several weeks or months after the start of lithium therapy. The hair usually regrows despite continuing therapy but in some cases regrowth only occurs after withdrawal of lithium. Fraunfelder *et al.*,[2] in their review of the effects on the ocular system, stated that loss of eyebrows and eyelashes had been associated with lithium therapy but was a rare event. They advised that patients affected should have their thyroid function assessed as hair loss due to lithium-induced hypothyroidism could be corrected by medication.

For references to the association of lithium with lupus, see under Lupus, below.

1. Lambert D, Dalac S. Skin, hair and nails. In: Johnson FN, ed. *Depression & mania: modern lithium therapy.* Oxford: IRL Press, 1987: 232–4.
2. Fraunfelder FT, *et al.* The effects of lithium on the human visual system. *J Toxicol Cutan Ocul Toxicol* 1992; **11:** 97–169.

Epileptogenic effect. Seizures occurring during lithium therapy are usually indicative of toxicity or impending toxicity. There have, however, been a few isolated case reports describing seizures in patients with serum-lithium concentrations within the normally accepted therapeutic range.[1,2]

1. Demers R, *et al.* Convulsion during lithium therapy. *Lancet* 1970; **ii:** 315–16.
2. Massey EW, Folger WN. Seizures activated by therapeutic levels of lithium carbonate. *South Med J* 1984; **77:** 1173–5.

Lupus. Studies have demonstrated that antinuclear antibodies were more common in patients taking lithium carbonate than in controls.[1,2] The absence of anti-DNA antibodies indicated that they did not have true systemic lupus erythematosus but it was considered that patients ingesting lithium might be at risk. Dermatologic manifestations of lupus together with antinuclear antibodies have been reported in one patient during lithium therapy.[3]

1. Johnstone EC, Whaley K. Antinuclear antibodies in psychiatric illness: their relationship to diagnosis and drug treatment. *Br Med J* 1975; **2:** 724–5.
2. Presley AP, *et al.* Antinuclear antibodies in patients on lithium carbonate. *Br Med J* 1976; **2:** 280–1.
3. Shukla VR, Borison RL. Lithium and lupuslike syndrome. *JAMA* 1982; **248:** 921–2.

Overdosage. In a short discussion of lithium toxicity Proudfoot[1] has mentioned that nausea, vomiting, and diarrhoea are common early features and are followed by coarse tremor, increased muscle tone, cogwheel rigidity, fasciculation, and myoclonus. Coma and convulsions could occur in the most serious cases and cardiac effects (first-degree heart block and QRS and QT prolongation) have been described rarely. A patient may appear to be aware with open eyes but have an expressionless face and be unable to move or speak (coma vigil). Acute renal failure and nephrogenic diabetes insipidus may develop.

Amdisen[2] considered that the great majority of lithium intoxications reported had occurred in patients with an intercurrent reduction of renal function or in patients who had been treated with dosages of lithium that were, in fact, too high. The patient usually experiences a period of days to a few weeks with slight 'nervous' symptoms that have been termed the 'prodromal' symptoms, although they are signs of a manifest slight intoxication. At an unpredictable point renal function starts to deteriorate and within hours or at the most within a few days, the patient will become severely intoxicated with the symptomatology of an acute intoxication. By this point lithium should have been discontinued and efficient detoxification measures instituted if the patient is to make a complete recovery.

Lithium therapy should be controlled by measuring serum concentrations to ensure that values for lithium do not rise to levels associated with toxicity. However, some patients may have concentrations considered to be toxic without showing any symptoms; unfortunately other patients may develop signs of toxicity at serum concentrations deemed to be safe.[3]

In acute overdosage[2] vomiting often occurred within an hour of ingestion due to the high concentration of lithium in the stomach, but significant amounts of lithium could still reach the systemic circulation. The typical clinical symptoms often appeared after a latency period and gastro-intestinal symptoms could re-appear at a later time. The symptoms of overdosage were reported to be mainly related to the alimentary and nervous systems and included abdominal pain, anorexia, nausea, and vomiting, occasionally mild diarrhoea, giddiness, tremor, ataxia, slurring speech, myoclonus, twitching, asthenia, and depression; renal symptoms had also been noted by some investigators. Again efficient detoxification procedures should be instituted as rapidly as possible.

A series of 28 patients with lithium self-poisoning and therapeutic intoxication has been described by Dyson and co-workers and many of the features and symptoms mentioned in the above 2 reviews were noted in these patients.[4] Other workers[5] have also reported cases of lithium toxicity which illustrate the differences between acute and chronic toxicity encountered clinically.

Other symptoms that have been noted in case reports of lithium intoxication in individual patients include photophobia,[6] acute polyarthritis involving several large joints,[7] severe hypertension,[8] deep venous thrombophlebitis,[9] reduction of central temperature,[10] and severe leucopenia.[11]

1. Proudfoot AT. Acute poisoning with antidepressants and lithium. *Prescribers' J* 1986; **26:** 97–106.
2. Amdisen A. Clinical features and management of lithium poisoning. *Med Toxicol* 1988; **3:** 18–32.
3. Stern R. Lithium in the treatment of mood disorders. *N Engl J Med* 1995; **332:** 127–8.
4. Dyson EH, *et al.* Self-poisoning and therapeutic intoxication with lithium. *Hum Toxicol* 1987; **6:** 325–9.
5. Ananth J, *et al.* Acute and chronic lithium toxicity: case reports and a review. *Lithium* 1992; **3:** 139–45.
6. Caplan RP, Fry AH. Photophobia in lithium intoxication. *Br Med J* 1982; **285:** 1314–15.
7. Black DW, Waziri R. Arthritis associated with lithium toxicity: case report. *J Clin Psychiatry* 1984; **45:** 135–6.
8. Michaeli J, *et al.* Severe hypertension and lithium intoxication. *JAMA* 1984; **251:** 1680.
9. Lyles MR. Deep venous thrombophlebitis associated with lithium toxicity. *J Natl Med Assoc* 1984; **76:** 633–4.
10. Follézou J-Y, Bleibel J-M. Reduction of temperature and lithium poisoning. *N Engl J Med* 1985; **313:** 1609.
11. Green ST, Dunn FG. Severe leucopenia in fatal lithium poisoning. *Br Med J* 1985; **290:** 517.

Treatment of Adverse Effects

In the case of recent acute overdosage the stomach should be emptied by either induction of emesis or by lavage.

Further measures involve procedures aimed at enhancing the renal clearance of lithium or its active removal. Measures to increase urine production may be useful in patients with mild to moderate toxicity and normal or not severely impaired renal function, otherwise treatment is with haemodialysis. Peritoneal dialysis is less effective and only appropriate if haemodialysis facilities are not available. Haemofiltration has been tried to good effect.

Maintenance of fluid and electrolyte balance is particularly important, due to the risk of hypernatraemia. Supportive treatment also includes maintenance of renal function and control of seizures. Once the serum and dialysis fluid are free of lithium, it has been recommended that serum-lithium concentrations should be monitored for at least another week so that allowance can be made for delayed diffusion from body tissues.

As a result of the narrow margin between therapeutic and toxic serum concentrations lithium poisoning may also develop during the course of therapeutic lithium administration. In some instances temporary withdrawal of lithium therapy and administration of generous amounts of sodium and fluid may be all that is required while adverse effects abate. In any serious or severe case of intoxication active measures such as dialysis and supportive measures outlined above may need to be instituted.

References.

1. Gomolin IH. Coping with excessive doses. In: Johnson FN, ed. *Depression & mania: modern lithium therapy.* Oxford: IRL Press, 1987: 154–7.
2. Amdisen A. Clinical features and management of lithium poisoning. *Med Toxicol* 1988; **3:** 18–32.
3. Okusa MD, *et al.* Clinical manifestations and management of acute lithium intoxication. *Am J Med* 1994; **97:** 383–9.
4. Swartz CM, Jones P. Hyperlithemia correction and persistent delirium. *J Clin Pharmacol* 1994; **34:** 865–70.
5. Wells BG. Amiloride in lithium-induced polyuria. *Ann Pharmacother* 1994; **28:** 888–9.
6. Tyrer SP. Lithium intoxication: appropriate treatment. *CNS Drugs* 1996; **6:** 426–39.

Precautions

The margin between the therapeutic and the toxic concentration of lithium is narrow, therefore the decision to give lithium usually requires specialist advice and serum concentrations should be monitored regularly under controlled conditions.

Lithium should be avoided in patients with cardiac disease or renal impairment, and cardiac and renal function should be monitored regularly. It should also be avoided in Addison's disease or other conditions with a sodium imbalance and in severely debilitated or dehydrated patients.

Patients receiving lithium should be examined periodically for abnormal thyroid function, since goitre and hypothyroidism may develop. Lithium should be used with caution in patients with myasthenia gravis because exacerbation of this disorder has been reported (see Effects on the Musculoskeletal System in Adverse Effects, above).

Lithium should be used with particular care in the elderly since this group may be particularly susceptible to toxicity due to decreasing renal function.

Impaired driving performance or machine operation skills may occur in patients receiving lithium (see Driving, below).

Patients receiving lithium therapy should be taught to recognise the symptoms of early toxicity (see under Adverse Effects, above) and, should these occur, to discontinue therapy and request medical aid at once. Among other factors, lithium requirements may change during fever, infection, and when mood swings occur. Patients should also be instructed to maintain an adequate intake of fluid; they should be warned not to compensate for an omitted dose by subsequently taking a double dose. Additionally, patients should not be switched between different formulations or preparations of lithium without therapeutic monitoring as bioavailability may be different.

A temporary dose reduction or discontinuation of lithium therapy may be necessary in vomiting, diarrhoea, excessive sweating, or any other condition that causes excessive sodium loss, thereby increasing serum-lithium concentrations. Conversely, increased sodium levels are likely to reduce serum-lithium concentrations. Patients taking lithium should therefore maintain an adequate fluid intake and should avoid increasing or decreasing sodium intake through dietary changes or ingestion of sodium-containing medicaments. Significant changes in caffeine intake may affect serum-lithium concentrations (see Xanthines under Interactions, below).

Lithium therapy should, where possible, be withdrawn slowly over a period of weeks to allay any concerns about relapse (see below).

If lithium is used during pregnancy then dose adjustments will be required to compensate for the altered renal handling. The risks of using lithium in pregnant patients are described under Pregnancy, below.

Lithium should be withdrawn 2 days before major surgery to safeguard the patient from accumulation (see under Anaesthesia, below).

Anaesthesia. Schou and Hippus have provided guidelines for the management of patients on lithium who are to undergo major surgery.[1] Lithium should be discontinued 2 to 3 days before major surgery, but need not be discontinued for minor surgery. There is no clinical evidence of interaction between lithium and anaesthetics, although lithium may prolong the action of neuromuscular blockers. Lithium may accumulate due to reduced renal clearance associated with anaesthesia; lithium treatment should be resumed as soon as possible after surgery, when kidney function and fluid-electrolyte balance have become normal. Patients are often not allowed fluids or foods by mouth the night before surgery but patients with lithium-induced polyuria should be given fluids parenterally during the night before the operation, if they vomit copiously, or if they are unconscious for several hours.

1. Schou M, Hippus H. Guidelines for patients receiving lithium treatment who require major surgery. *Br J Anaesth* 1987; **59:** 809–10.

Breast feeding. Lithium is distributed into breast milk and most manufacturers in the UK suggest that mothers receiving lithium should bottle feed their babies. After reviewing the few rare cases of adverse effects associated with lithium in breast-fed infants Ananth[1] also concluded that it would be best to avoid breast feeding during lithium therapy. However Schou[2] questioned whether the advantages of such a course would be outweighed by the losses when breast feeding is avoided. Ananth did however recommend that if a mother did want to breast feed this should be done at times to avoid peak blood concentrations of lithium. It was also recommended that the infant should be carefully monitored. Medication should be withheld or breast feeding stopped if the infant developed an infection or dehydration as they would be more susceptible to the adverse effects of lithium.

1. Ananth J. Lithium during pregnancy and lactation. *Lithium* 1993; **4:** 231–7.
2. Schou M. Lithium treatment during pregnancy, delivery, and lactation: an update. *J Clin Psychiatry* 1990; **51:** 410–13.

Cystic fibrosis. Reduced renal excretion of lithium was demonstrated in eight patients with cystic fibrosis compared with healthy subjects.[1] The authors recommend caution when prescribing standard doses of lithium to patients with cystic fibrosis until more definitive data are available.

1. Brager NPD, *et al.* Reduced renal fractional excretion of lithium in cystic fibrosis. *Br J Clin Pharmacol* 1996; **41:** 157–9.

Driving. While affective disorders probably adversely affect driving skill,[1,2] treatment with antidepressant drugs, including lithium, may also be hazardous,[1] although patients may be safer drivers with medication than without.[2] Lithium has been reported[1] to adversely affect the choice reaction time (a test to assess the time taken to respond correctly to some signals but not others) to a level considered dangerous for driving.

It has been mentioned[2] that the UK Medical Commission on Accident Prevention has recommended that patients on long-term psychotropic medication are unsuitable to be drivers of heavy goods or public service vehicles.

1. Ashton H. Drugs and driving. *Adverse Drug React Bull* 1983; **98:** 360–3.
2. Cremona A. Mad drivers: psychiatric illness and driving performance. *Br J Hosp Med* 1986; **35:** 193–5.

Pregnancy. Case reports of mothers taking lithium during pregnancy pointed to an increased risk of congenital abnormalities with the heart being mainly affected.[1] Support for this increased risk came from a study by Källén and Tandberg[2] who investigated the records of 59 children born to women who had taken lithium during pregnancy. However, in a more recent study Jacobson *et al.*[3] prospectively followed 138 pregnant women being treated with lithium and did not identify any difference in pregnancy outcome between them and a control group. Jacobson *et al.* thus considered that lithium was not a major teratogen and felt that women with major affective disorders could continue lithium treatment during pregnancy provided that adequate fetal screening tests were carried out. In a subsequent review Cohen *et al.*[4] interpreted the evidence more cautiously. They considered that the teratogenic risk was lower than previously thought, but that it would still be wise for women who wished to become pregnant to discontinue lithium if at all possible, at least during the period of embryogenesis.

Schou[1] commented that although there was a study which suggested that lithium treatment during pregnancy may increase the risk of fetal macrosomia, premature delivery, and perinatal mortality, it had not been published in full.

The renal clearance of lithium by the mother is not constant during pregnancy; in the second half of the pregnancy clearance rises gradually by 30 to 50% but falls abruptly and significantly after delivery to pre-pregnancy values.[1,5] The increased doses of lithium that may be given during pregnancy to compensate for this increased clearance may result in lithium toxicity.[5] It is generally considered[1,6] advisable to discontinue lithium during the last few days of pregnancy to reduce the risk of maternal lithium toxicity due to accumulation of lithium but it should be started again a few days later after delivery at reduced dosage because of the increased postpartum risk of manic and depressive relapse.[1] *Polyhydramnios* (an excess of amniotic fluid) in the last trimester of pregnancy has been reported and has been attributed to fetal lithium toxicity (polyuria and diabetes insipidus).[7,8]

Reducing the dosage during the last few days of pregnancy also helps to reduce lithium concentrations in the neonate and avoid associated adverse effects.[1,6] Amongst adverse effects that have been reported in neonates exposed *in utero* to lithium Ananth[6] listed cyanosis, lethargy, flaccidity, hypotonia, poor gag and sucking reflexes, feeding problems, bradycardia, tachycardia, goitre, hypothyroidism, nephrogenic diabetes, and jaundice; withdrawal symptoms had also been observed.

1. Schou M. Lithium treatment during pregnancy, delivery, and lactation: an update. *J Clin Psychiatry* 1990; **51:** 410–13.
2. Källén B, Tandberg A. Lithium and pregnancy: a cohort study on manic-depressive women. *Acta Psychiatr Scand* 1983; **68:** 134–9.
3. Jacobson SJ, *et al.* Prospective multicentre study of pregnancy outcome after lithium exposure during first trimester. *Lancet* 1992; **339:** 530–3.
4. Cohen LS, *et al.* A reevaluation of risk of in utero exposure to lithium. *JAMA* 1994; **271:** 146–50.
5. Lemoine J-M. Pregnancy, delivery and lactation. In: Johnson FN, ed. *Depression & mania: modern lithium therapy.* Oxford: IRL Press, 1987: 139–46.
6. Ananth J. Lithium during pregnancy and lactation. *Lithium* 1993; **4:** 231–7.
7. Krause S, *et al.* Polyhydramnios with maternal lithium treatment. *Obstet Gynecol* 1990; **75:** 504–6.
8. Ang MS, *et al.* Maternal lithium therapy and polyhydramnios. *Obstet Gynecol* 1990; **76:** 517–19.

Surgery. For comments regarding the precautions to be observed in patients undergoing Surgery, see under Anaesthesia, above.

Withdrawal. Goodnick[1] has discussed the problems associated with stopping lithium treatment. A withdrawal syndrome consisting of symptoms such as anxiety, tremor, fatigue, nausea, sweating, headache, sleep disturbances, diarrhoea, or blurred vision, usually develops within days of sudden cessation of treatment with lithium. These may simply be a recurrence of symptoms of mood change. Uncontrolled studies of withdrawal symptoms have raised the possibility of a lithium-withdrawal state but controlled studies have been convincingly negative. It is, however, wise to reduce lithium dosage gradually rather than stop high-dosage treatment abruptly.

A frequent worry associated with the termination of lithium therapy is that of relapse. Most evidence has supported the view that any relapses occurring in the first weeks after lithium withdrawal are simply part of a pattern of recurrence of bipolar disorder in general and are not indicative of a higher rate of recurrence. Mander and Loudon,[2] however, have found the proportion of patients relapsing on sudden withdrawal of lithium therapy to be 50%, a figure they consider to be too high to be accounted for by the natural history of the disease process. They and others[3] advise that this risk should be considered when prescribing lithium for bipolar disorder. Faedda *et al.*[4] found that, in patients who previously had been stable on lithium for at least 18 months, the risk of early recurrence of bipolar disorder was higher when therapy was withdrawn rapidly in less than 2 weeks than when it was withdrawn gradually over 2 to 4 weeks.

1. Goodnick PJ. Terminating treatment. In: Johnson FN, ed. *Depression & mania: modern lithium therapy.* Oxford: IRL Press, 1987: 115–17.
2. Mander AJ, Loudon JB. Rapid recurrence of mania following abrupt discontinuation of lithium. *Lancet* 1988; **ii:** 15–17.
3. Goodwin GM. Recurrence of mania after lithium withdrawal. *Br J Psychiatry* 1994; **164:** 149–52.
4. Faedda GL, *et al.* Outcome after rapid vs gradual discontinuation of lithium treatment in bipolar disorders. *Arch Gen Psychiatry* 1993; **50:** 448–55.

Interactions

Concurrent administration of diuretics with lithium exerts a paradoxical antidiuretic effect, and diuretics are normally contra-indicated in patients receiving lithium therapy. Further interactions reported with lithium are discussed below.

Reviews of drug interactions with lithium.

1. Amdisen A. Lithium and drug interactions. *Drugs* 1982; **24:** 133–9.
2. Beeley L. Drug interactions with lithium. *Prescribers' J* 1986; **26:** 160–2.
3. Harvey NS, Merriman S. Review of clinically important drug interactions with lithium. *Drug Safety* 1994; **10:** 455–63.
4. Finley PR, *et al.* Clinical relevance of drug interactions with lithium. *Clin Pharmacokinet* 1995; **29:** 172–91.

ACE inhibitors. Concurrent administration of lithium with ACE inhibitors has been reported[1-5] to increase serum-lithium concentrations, although in a study[6] of enalapril and lithium in healthy volunteers, the lithium levels remained unchanged. ACE inhibitors such as *captopril*,[1] *enalapril*,[2-4] and *lisinopril*[4,5] have been implicated. The mechanism is unclear but it has been suggested[7] that suppression of the renin-angiotensin-aldosterone system by ACE inhibitors may be responsible. Lithium excretion by the kidney is dependent on both glomerular filtration and sodium concentration in the proximal tubule, both of which are reduced by ACE inhibitors. It has also been suggested[4] that inhibition of angiotensin II production may lead to reduced fluid intake through lack of activation of the thirst stimulus and this would enhance the tendency to volume depletion caused by natriuresis. Patients considered[7] to be at risk from this reaction would include those whose renal function is largely dependent on the effect of angiotensin II, those with congestive heart failure, and patients with volume depletion.

1. Pulik M, Lida H. Interaction lithium-inhibiteurs de l'enzyme de conversion. *Presse Med* 1988; **17:** 755.
2. Douste-Blazy P, *et al.* Angiotensin converting enzyme inhibitors and lithium treatment. *Lancet* 1986; **i:** 1448.
3. Navis GJ, *et al.* Volume homeostasis, angiotensin converting enzyme inhibition, and lithium therapy. *Am J Med* 1989; **86:** 621.
4. Correa FJ, Eiser AR. Angiotensin-converting enzyme inhibitors and lithium toxicity. *Am J Med* 1992; **93:** 108–9.
5. Baldwin CM, Safferman AZ. A case of lisinopril-induced lithium toxicity. *DICP Ann Pharmacother* 1990; **24:** 946–7.
6. DasGupta K, *et al.* The effect of enalapril on serum lithium levels in healthy men. *J Clin Psychiatry* 1992; **53:** 398–400.
7. Mignat C, Unger T. Ace inhibitors: drug interactions of clinical significance. *Drug Safety* 1995; **12:** 334–47.

Analgesics. See NSAIDs, below.

Antidepressants. Lithium has been used to augment the effect of other antidepressants in refractory depression. However, there have been reports of adverse reactions with some of these combinations. For further details, see Antidepressants under Interactions of Phenelzine, p.305.

Antiepileptics. Severe CNS toxicity despite 'normal' serum-lithium concentrations has been described in a patient also taking *phenytoin* together with *phenobarbitone*.[1] Symptoms indicative of lithium toxicity have also been reported in one patient receiving *phenytoin* concomitantly,[2] again where concentrations were not abnormal.

For reports of neurotoxicity in patients receiving *carbamazepine* and lithium, see p.341.

1. Speirs J, Hirsch SR. Severe lithium toxicity with "normal" serum concentrations. *Br Med J* 1978; **1:** 815–16.
2. MacCallum WAG. Interaction of lithium and phenytoin. *Br Med J* 1980; **280:** 610–11.

Antimicrobials. Lithium toxicity has been reported on isolated occasions in patients receiving *metronidazole*,[1] *spectinomycin*,[2] and *tetracycline*.[3]

However, it has been noted that lithium and tetracycline have been used concomitantly without serious problems in many patients and that additionally tetracycline has been used to treat the acneform skin eruptions induced by lithium.[4] These same authors investigating healthy subjects found that lithium concentrations were decreased, rather than increased, following the addition of tetracycline but considered this was probably of no clinical significance.

1. Teicher MH, *et al.* Possible nephrotoxic interaction of lithium and metronidazole. *JAMA* 1987; **257:** 3365–6.
2. Anonymous. Possible adverse drug-drug interaction report: lithium intoxication in a spectinomycin-treated patient. *Int Drug Ther Newslett* 1978; **13:** 15.
3. McGennis AJ. Lithium carbonate and tetracycline interaction. *Br Med J* 1978; **1:** 1183.
4. Fankhauser MP, *et al.* Evaluation of lithium-tetracycline interaction. *Clin Pharm* 1988; **7:** 314–17.

Antimigraine drugs. The UK manufacturers of *sumatriptan* recommend that lithium and sumatriptan should not be used together; there may be a risk of increased CNS toxicity (but see also, p.451).

Antineoplastics. Transient decreases in serum-lithium concentration occurred in a patient after administration of *cisplatin*.[1] The relative contributions of cisplatin itself, or the fluid loading procedure involving intravenous fluids and mannitol, or their combined effects were unclear. The interaction, however, had no apparent clinical significance in this patient although a risk of undertreatment with lithium may occur in other patients.

1. Pietruszka LJ, *et al.* Evaluation of cisplatin-lithium interaction. *Drug Intell Clin Pharm* 1985; **19:** 31–2.

Antipsychotics and anxiolytics. In the control of acute mania lithium is often too slow in onset to be used alone and therefore additional therapy with an antipsychotic may be necessary. It should be noted, however, that such combinations should be used with care as interactions and adverse reactions have occurred.

The renal excretion of lithium is increased during concurrent *chlorpromazine* treatment,[1] which means that subsequent withdrawal of chlorpromazine can result in an abrupt rise in serum-lithium concentrations.[2] The serum concentration of chlorpromazine can also be reduced by the concurrent administration of lithium,[3] and chlorpromazine toxicity may be precipitated by the abrupt withdrawal of lithium in patients previously stabilised on the two drugs together. Ventricular fibrillation has been described following withdrawal of lithium in a patient concurrently taking chlorpromazine;[4] it was suggested that the chlorpromazine dose should be reduced if lithium is to be discontinued.

There have been isolated reports of neurotoxicity or brain damage, characterised by delirium, seizures, encephalopathy, or an increased incidence of extrapyramidal symptoms in patients receiving lithium concomitantly with *flupenthixol decanoate*,[5] *fluphenazine decanoate*,[6] or high-dose *haloperidol*,[7-9] although two earlier retrospective studies of patients taking lithium with antipsychotics had failed to detect such adverse reactions.[10,11] However, neurological reactions have continued to be reported in patients receiving lithium concomitantly with *thioridazine*,[12,13] *sulpiride*,[14] *clozapine*,[15] and *risperidone*.[16] Although a causal relationship between these events and concomitant administration of lithium and antipsychotic has not been fully established, patients should be monitored for signs of neurotoxicity if receiving such combinations.

Ross and Coffey in a discussion of the interactions between lithium and antipsychotics[17] have made the following comments. The neurotoxicity induced by lithium and antipsychotics is a rare entity, about 40 cases being reported in the literature. There is controversy as to whether the combination produces any greater risk than either drug alone and there is controversy over whether the neurotoxicity is a distinct diagnostic entity or simply represents atypical cases of lithium toxicity or the neuroleptic malignant syndrome. They mentioned suggestions that have been made that the interaction between lithium and haloperidol represents a form of neuroleptic malignant syndrome while that between lithium and the phenothiazines, especially thioridazine, represents a form of lithium toxicity. They concluded that the risk from combination therapy was very small but that the clinician should, nevertheless, be aware of it.

Although lithium has been reported to interact with *diazepam* with the result of hypothermic episodes,[18] Ross and Coffey[17] considered that this was more likely to be an idiosyncratic response rather than a true drug interaction; they stated that in general it is considered quite safe to use lithium and benzodiazepines in combination.

1. Sletten I, *et al.* The effect of chlorpromazine on lithium excretion in psychiatric subjects. *Curr Ther Res* 1966; **8:** 441–6.
2. Pakes GE. Lithium toxicity with phenothiazine withdrawal. *Lancet* 1979; **ii:** 701.
3. Rivera-Calimlim L, *et al.* Effect of lithium on plasma chlorpromazine levels. *Clin Pharmacol Ther* 1978; **23:** 451–5.
4. Stevenson RN, *et al.* Ventricular fibrillation due to lithium withdrawal—an interaction with chlorpromazine? *Postgrad Med J* 1989; **65:** 936–8.
5. West A. Adverse effects of lithium treatment. *Br Med J* 1977; **2:** 642.
6. Singh SV. Lithium carbonate/fluphenazine decanoate producing irreversible brain damage. *Lancet* 1982; **ii:** 278.
7. Cohen WJ, Cohen NH. Lithium carbonate, haloperidol, and irreversible brain damage. *JAMA* 1974; **230:** 1283–7.
8. Loudon JB, Waring H. Toxic reactions to lithium and haloperidol. *Lancet* 1976; **ii:** 1088.
9. Thomas C, *et al.* Lithium/haloperidol combinations and brain damage. *Lancet* 1982; **i:** 626.
10. Baastrup PC, *et al.* Adverse reactions in treatment with lithium carbonate and haloperidol. *JAMA* 1976; **236:** 2645–6.
11. Prakash R. Lithium-haloperidol combination and brain damage. *Lancet* 1982; **i:** 1468–9.
12. Standish-Barry HMAS, Shelly MA. Toxic neurological reaction to lithium/thioridazine. *Lancet* 1983; **i:** 771.
13. Cantor CH. Encephalopathy with lithium and thioridazine in combination. *Med J Aust* 1986; **144:** 164–5.
14. Dinan TG, O'Keane V. Acute extrapyramidal reactions following lithium and sulpiride co-administration: two case reports. *Hum Psychopharmacol Clin Exp* 1991; **6:** 67–9.
15. Blake LM, *et al.* Reversible neurologic symptoms with clozapine and lithium. *J Clin Psychopharmacol* 1992; **12:** 297–9.
16. Swanson CL, *et al.* Effects of concomitant risperidone and lithium treatment. *Am J Psychiatry* 1995; **152:** 1096.
17. Ross DR, Coffey CE. Neuroleptics and anti-anxiety agents. In: Johnson FN, ed. *Depression & mania: modern lithium therapy.* Oxford: IRL Press, 1987: 167–71.
18. Naylor GJ, McHarg A. Profound hypothermia on combined lithium carbonate and diazepam treatment. *Br Med J* 1977; **2:** 22.

Benzodiazepines. See Antipsychotics and Anxiolytics, above.

Calcium-channel blockers. Neurotoxicity has been reported in one patient receiving lithium following the addition of *verapamil*.[1] Serum-lithium concentrations were still inside the accepted therapeutic range and it was considered that the similar actions of lithium and verapamil on neurosecretory processes may have been responsible. Verapamil has also been reported to decrease serum-lithium concentrations.[2] Neurotoxicity has also been reported in a patient receiving lithium and *diltiazem*[3] as well as other drugs. Psychosis, possibly induced by the use of diltiazem and lithium together, has been reported in another patient.[4]

1. Price WA, Giannini AJ. Neurotoxicity caused by lithium-verapamil synergism. *J Clin Pharmacol* 1986; **26:** 717–19.
2. Weinrauch LA, *et al.* Decreased serum lithium during verapamil therapy. *Am Heart J* 1984; **108:** 1378–80.
3. Valdiserri EV. A possible interaction between lithium and diltiazem: case report. *J Clin Psychiatry* 1985; **46:** 540–1.
4. Binder EF, *et al.* Diltiazem-induced psychosis and a possible diltiazem-lithium interaction. *Arch Intern Med* 1991; **151:** 373–4.

Central stimulants. There is a report of a woman who had been stabilised on lithium treatment for 15 months developing lithium toxicity within a few days of being given *mazindol*.[1]

1. Hendy MS, *et al.* Mazindol-induced lithium toxicity. *Br Med J* 1980; **280:** 684–5.

Diuretics. *Thiazide diuretics* produce sodium depletion by inhibiting distal tubular sodium reabsorption. The consequent increase in proximal tubular reabsorption frequently results in an increase in serum lithium concentrations.[1] Patients who are stabilised on lithium therapy and begin taking thiazide diuretics are at significant risk of developing lithium toxicity. Toxic lithium concentrations may be seen within 3 to 5 days of diuretic initiation. *Loop diuretics* (*frusemide, bumetanide,* and *ethacrynic acid*) seem less likely to cause lithium retention, although caution is warranted, especially with patients in whom dietary sodium is restricted.[1] *Amiloride*, and probably other potassium-sparing diuretics, have no effect on lithium excretion, but *acetazolamide* increases lithium excretion. However, the diuretic action of acetazolamide is short-lived and the interaction may therefore be transient.[1]

It has therefore been suggested that if diuretic therapy is necessary in patients stabilised on lithium a reduction of 25 to 50% of the lithium dose should be initiated,[1,2] lithium concentrations measured twice weekly until re-stabilisation occurs, and that perhaps loop diuretics such as bumetanide or frusemide would be preferable.

The topic of lithium-diuretic interaction and precautions to be observed has also been discussed by Grau.[3]

1. Beeley L. Drug interactions with lithium. *Prescribers' J* 1986; **26:** 160–3.
2. Ramsay LE. Interactions that matter: diuretics and antihypertensive drugs. *Prescribers' J* 1984; **24:** 60–5.
3. Grau E. Diuretics. In: Johnson FN, ed. *Depression & mania: modern lithium therapy.* Oxford: IRL Press, 1987: 180–3.

Gastro-intestinal drugs. Administration of *sodium bicarbonate* with lithium has led to reduced blood-lithium concentrations and has been attributed to increased renal excretion of the lithium cation in response to the extra load of bicarbonate anion to be excreted.[1] *Antacids* containing combinations of *aluminium and magnesium hydroxides* and *simethicone* had no effect on the dissolution and solubility of lithium carbonate *in vitro*[2] nor on its bioavailability *in vivo*.[3]

There has been one case report describing a possible interaction between lithium and *ispaghula* where the ispaghula may have inhibited intestinal absorption of lithium resulting in low serum concentrations.[4]

There is an increased risk of extrapyramidal effects and the possibility of neurotoxicity when drugs such as *metoclopramide* are given to patients receiving lithium.

1. McSwiggan C. A significant drug interaction. *Aust J Pharm* 1978; **59:** 6.
2. Schiessler DM, *et al.* Effect of antacids on lithium carbonate dissolution and solubility in vitro. *Am J Hosp Pharm* 1983; **40:** 825–8.
3. Goode DL, *et al.* Effect of antacid on the bioavailability of lithium carbonate. *Clin Pharm* 1984; **3:** 284–7.
4. Perlman BB. Interaction between lithium salts and ispaghula husk. *Lancet* 1990; **335:** 416.

Methyldopa. Lithium toxicity induced by concurrent administration of methyldopa has been described on a number of occasions.[1-3] Symptoms of toxicity may occur even though serum-lithium concentrations remain within the therapeutic range.

1. Byrd GJ. Methyldopa and lithium carbonate: suspected interaction. *JAMA* 1975; **233:** 320.
2. O'Regan JB. Adverse interaction of lithium carbonate and methyldopa. *Can Med Assoc J* 1976; **115:** 385–6.
3. Osanloo E, Deglin JH. Interaction of lithium and methyldopa. *Ann Intern Med* 1980; **92:** 433–4.

Muscle relaxants. For reports of prolongation of neuromuscular blockade by lithium see under Atracurium, p.1307. For further comments relating to surgery and anaesthesia, see under Anaesthesia in Precautions, above.

For reports of hypothermic episodes occurring during the concomitant administration of lithium and *diazepam* see under Antipsychotics and Anxiolytics, above.

Severe aggravation of hyperkinetic symptoms occurred in 2 patients with Huntington's chorea when *baclofen* was added to their treatment with lithium and haloperidol.[1]

1. Andén N-E, *et al.* Baclofen and lithium in Huntington's chorea. *Lancet* 1973; **ii:** 93.

NSAIDs. Decreased clearance and increased serum concentrations of lithium, resulting in toxicity on some occasions, have been reported after the concomitant administration of lithium with *diclofenac*,[1] *ibuprofen*,[2,3] *indomethacin*,[4,5] *naproxen*,[8] and *piroxicam*;[9,10] secondary sources have also implicated *ketoprofen* and *phenylbutazone*.[11] However, serum-lithium concentration is not increased by the concomitant administration of *sulindac*.[8,12,13] Although serum-lithium concentrations were increased in one patient receiving *aspirin*[14] this has not been substantiated by others and an interaction is considered unlikely;[5,15] it has also been pointed out that control of sodium balance is necessary in such studies[15] and in the report purporting to demonstrate an interaction the diet had not been controlled. In a discussion Furnell[11] has stated that for mild occasional aches, pains, and fever paracetamol is the preferred analgesic in patients receiving lithium, although occasional doses of aspirin are acceptable. Sulindac appeared to be the safest NSAID for long-term use. Diclofenac, ibuprofen, indomethacin, ketoprofen, naproxen, phenylbutazone, and piroxicam should be avoided where possible but if it was necessary to use one of these drugs the maintenance dose of lithium should be reduced. He also considered that perhaps other NSAIDs, for which no information was available at that time, should be regarded as having the potential to cause a rise in serum-lithium concentrations. Subsequent to Furnell's discussion, decreased renal clearance and increased serum concentrations of lithium, sometimes resulting in toxicity, have been found when lithium was taken with *ketorolac*[6,7] or *tiaprofenic acid*.[16]

1. Reimann IW, Frölich JC. Effects of diclofenac on lithium kinetics. *Clin Pharmacol Ther* 1981; **30:** 348–52.
2. Kristoff CA, *et al.* Effect of ibuprofen on lithium plasma and red blood cell concentrations. *Clin Pharm* 1986; **5:** 51–5.
3. Ragheb M. Ibuprofen can increase serum lithium level in lithium-treated patients. *J Clin Psychiatry* 1987; **48:** 161–3.
4. Frölich JC, *et al.* Indomethacin increases plasma lithium. *Br Med J* 1979; **1:** 1115–16.
5. Reimann IW, *et al.* Indomethacin but not aspirin increases plasma lithium ion levels. *Arch Gen Psychiatry* 1983; **40:** 283–6.
6. Langlois R, Paquette D. Increased serum lithium levels due to ketorolac therapy. *Can Med Assoc J* 1994; **150:** 1455–6.
7. Iyer V. Ketorolac (Toradol®) induced lithium toxicity. *Headache* 1994; **34:** 442–4.
8. Ragheb M, Powell AL. Lithium interaction with sulindac and naproxen. *J Clin Psychopharmacol* 1986; **6:** 150–4.
9. Kerry RJ, *et al.* Possible toxic interaction between lithium and piroxicam. *Lancet* 1983; **i:** 418–19.
10. Walbridge DG, Bazire SR. An interaction between lithium carbonate and piroxicam presenting as lithium toxicity. *Br J Psychiatry* 1985; **147:** 206–7.
11. Furnell MM. Non-steroidal anti-inflammatory drugs. In: Johnson FN, ed. *Depression & mania: modern lithium therapy.* Oxford: IRL Press, 1987: 183–6.
12. Furnell MM, Davies J. The effect of sulindac on lithium therapy. *Drug Intell Clin Pharm* 1985; **19:** 374–6.
13. Ragheb MA, Powell AL. Failure of sulindac to increase serum lithium levels. *J Clin Psychiatry* 1986; **47:** 33–4.
14. Bendz H, Feinberg M. Aspirin increases serum lithium ion levels. *Arch Gen Psychiatry* 1984; **41:** 310–11.
15. Reimann I. Aspirin increases serum lithium ion levels. *Arch Gen Psychiatry* 1984; **41:** 311.
16. Alderman CP, Lindsay KSW. Increased serum lithium concentration secondary to treatment with tiaprofenic acid and fosinopril. *Ann Pharmacother* 1996; **30:** 1411–3.

Parasympathomimetics. For the effect of lithium on parasympathomimetics, see p.1394.

Xanthines. It has been reported[1] that *theophylline* enhances the renal clearance of lithium, thus tending to reduce serum-lithium concentrations. Lithium blood concentrations increased by 24% when *caffeine* was eliminated from the diet of 11 patients taking lithium.[2] No toxicity was observed but these patients had been maintained on low base-line lithium concentrations; toxicity might occur in patients maintained at higher concentrations.

1. Cook BL, *et al.* Theophylline-lithium interaction. *J Clin Psychiatry* 1985; **46:** 278–9.
2. Mester R, *et al.* Caffeine withdrawal increases lithium blood levels. *Biol Psychiatry* 1995; **37:** 348–50.

Pharmacokinetics

Lithium is readily and completely absorbed from the gastro-intestinal tract when taken as one of its salts. Absorption can be affected by the formulation of preparation taken. Peak serum concentrations are obtained between 0.5 and 3 hours after ingestion from conventional tablets or capsules; following modified-release formulations peak concentrations are delayed and may occur between 3 and 12 hours after administration. Lithium is distributed throughout the body and distribution is complete within about 6 to 10 hours; higher concentrations occur in the bones, the thyroid gland, and portions of the brain, than in the serum.

Lithium is excreted unchanged, predominantly in the urine; only a small amount can be detected in the faeces, saliva, and sweat. It is not bound to plasma proteins. It crosses the placenta and is distributed into breast milk. The elimination half-life in patients with normal renal function is about 20 to 24 hours, but increases with decreasing renal function; half-lives of up to 36 hours have been reported for elderly patients and 40 to 50 hours for patients with renal impairment. Steady-state concentrations may not, therefore, be attained until 4 to 7 days after the initiation of treatment.

Following administration of lithium salts there is wide intersubject variation between both the serum concentrations obtained following a given dose, and between those required for therapeutic effect. Concentrations also vary considerably according to factors such as the dosage regimen (whether given in single or divided daily doses), renal function, the dietary regimen of the patient, the patient's state of health, the time at which the blood sample is taken, and concomitant medication, such as sodium salts or diuretics, as well as by formulation and bioavailability. Moreover, there is only a narrow margin between the therapeutic and the toxic serum concentration of lithium. Therefore, not only is individual titration of lithium dosage essential to ensure constant appropriate concentrations for the patient, but the conditions under which the blood samples are taken for monitoring must be carefully controlled. In practice, the lithium ion concentration is measured in the serum from a blood sample drawn 12 hours after the last dose of lithium in a patient who has been taking their daily lithium requirement at the scheduled hours for 4 to 7 days. Under these conditions the distribution of the last dose of lithium is complete and steady-state concentrations will have been attained. The usual maintenance therapeutic serum concentrations of lithium are 0.4 to 1.0 mmol per litre; toxic effects may be expected at concentrations exceeding 1.5 mmol per litre. For further details regarding monitoring of serum concentrations of lithium, see under Uses and Administration, below. Estimation of lithium concentrations in other body fluids such as saliva has been investigated as a less invasive method of monitoring. However, results have been equivocal and these methods have not replaced serum monitoring in general practice.

References.

1. Johnson FN, ed. *Depression & mania: modern lithium therapy.* Oxford: IRL Press, 1987.
2. Ward ME, *et al.* Clinical pharmacokinetics of lithium. *J Clin Pharmacol* 1994; **34:** 280–5.
3. Reiss RA, *et al.* Lithium pharmacokinetics in the obese. *Clin Pharmacol Ther* 1994; **55:** 392–8.

Administration. References concerning the pharmacokinetic methods of predicting lithium dosage requirements.

1. Williams PJ, *et al.* Bayesian forecasting of serum lithium concentrations: comparison with traditional methods. *Clin Pharmacokinet* 1989; **17:** 45–52.
2. Browne JL, *et al.* A comparison of pharmacokinetic versus empirical lithium dosing techniques. *Ther Drug Monit* 1989; **11:** 149–54.
3. Marken PA, *et al.* Preliminary comparison of predictive and empiric lithium dosing: impact on patient outcome. *Ann Pharmacother* 1994; **28:** 1148–52.

Cystic fibrosis. For a reference to reduced renal excretion of lithium in patients with cystic fibrosis, see Cystic Fibrosis in Precautions, above.

Distribution into breast milk. For references to the distribution of lithium into breast milk, see Breast Feeding in Precautions, above.

Pregnancy. For references to changes in renal clearance of lithium during pregnancy, see under Pregnancy in Precaution, above.

Uses and Administration

Lithium, as one of its salts, provides a source of lithium ions, which compete with sodium ions at various sites in the body. It thus has an action and side-effects distinct and separate from those of other antidepressants. Its mode of action is not understood, but it is effective in the treatment and prophylaxis of mania, and prophylaxis of manic depression (bipolar disorder) and recurrent unipolar depression. Since the margin between therapeutic and toxic serum concentrations is narrow the decision to give lithium is usually based on specialist advice; lithium should not be prescribed unless facilities for monitoring serum concentrations are available.

Lithium has a narrow therapeutic/toxic ratio. As toxic effects are associated with concentrations above 1.5 mmol per litre, and may occur with concentrations as low as 1.0 mmol per litre in susceptible patients such as the elderly, it is recommended that doses are adjusted to provide a serum-lithium concentration of 0.4 to 1.0 mmol per litre (at the lower end of the range for maintenance therapy and elderly patients). Treatment with lithium thus needs to be monitored through measurement of serum concentrations. It should be emphasised that serum concentrations should be adjusted for each individual patient to those that give a clinical response without evidence of toxicity. Patients must be taught to recognise the symptoms of early lithium intoxication in order to omit further doses of lithium and seek medical care should it be impending.

The dose of lithium given depends on the preparation chosen since different preparations of lithium salts vary widely in bioavailability. Recommended doses for some UK preparations are as follows:

- *Camcolit* tablets (Norgine, UK) containing lithium carbonate; for treatment, initially 1.5 to 2 g daily (elderly, 0.5 to 1 g daily); for prophylaxis, initially 0.5 to 1.2 g daily (elderly, 0.5 to 1 g daily). Film-coated tablets in divided doses; modified-release tablets in single or divided doses
- *Li-Liquid* oral solution (Rosemont, UK) containing lithium citrate; for treatment and prophylaxis, initially 1.018 to 3.054 g daily in two divided doses (elderly or patients less than 50 kg body-weight, 0.509 g twice daily)
- *Liskonum* tablets (SmithKline Beecham, UK) containing lithium carbonate; for treatment, initially 450 to 675 mg twice daily (elderly, 225 mg twice daily); for prophylaxis, initially 450 mg twice daily (elderly, 225 mg twice daily)
- *Litarex* tablets (Dumex, UK) containing lithium citrate; for treatment and prophylaxis, initially 564 mg twice daily
- *Priadel* tablets (Delandale, UK) containing lithium carbonate; for treatment and prophylaxis, initially 0.4 to 1.2 g daily as a single dose or in two divided doses (elderly or patients less than 50 kg body-weight, 0.4 g daily)
- *Priadel* syrup (Delandale, UK) containing lithium citrate; for treatment and prophylaxis, initially 1.04 to 3.12 g daily in two divided doses (elderly or patients less than 50 kg body-weight, 0.52 g twice daily).

Lithium is not recommended for use in children.

The initial dose given is adjusted after 4 to 7 days according to the results of serum-lithium estimations obtained under controlled conditions (samples being taken 12 hours after the preceding dose). Serum-lithium concentrations are then checked once a week to ensure that they remain within the therapeutic range for 4 weeks. The frequency of estimations can then be reduced to about once every 3 months. Should the patient's circumstances change such that the lithium pharmacokinetics or requirements might be affected, close control of serum concentrations should be reinstated until the concentrations stabilise once more. Such circumstances could involve a change of lithium preparation, an intercurrent illness (including a urinary-tract infection), a manic or depressive phase, a change in dietary regimen or body temperature, pregnancy, and concomitant administration of medication (in particular, sodium-containing preparations and diuretics). For further details see under Precautions, above. On long-term use lithium has been associated with thyroid disorders and mild cognitive and memory impairment. Therefore, long-term treatment should only be undertaken if it is definitely indicated. Patients need to be carefully reassessed after a period of 3 to 5 years and lithium continued only if the benefit persists.

Lithium is also used for the management of aggressive of self-mutilating behaviour.

The doses are similar to those used in the prophylaxis of recurrent affective disorders described above.

Lithium therapy should, where possible, be withdrawn slowly over a period of weeks to allay any concerns about relapse. For further details, see Withdrawal under Precautions, above.

Other lithium salts have been used in the treatment of psychiatric disorders and these include the acetate, bromide, gluconate, glutamate, and sulphate.

Lithium carbonate is used in homoeopathic medicines.

Reference to the use of lithium in non-psychiatric conditions.

1. Schou M. Use in non-psychiatric conditions. In: Johnson FN, ed. *Depression & mania: modern lithium therapy.* Oxford: IRL Press, 1987: 46–50.

Administration. A double-blind study in unipolar and bipolar patients on prophylactic lithium supported the trend towards using lithium in lower dosage.[1] It indicated that a plasma concentration as low as 0.45 mmol per litre was as effective as what had been the traditionally accepted concentration of 0.8 mmol per litre and above.

1. Abou-Saleh MT, Coppen A. The efficacy of low-dose lithium: clinical, psychological and biological correlates. *J Psychiatr Res* 1989; **23:** 157–62.

Depression. Lithium may be used in the treatment and prophylaxis of recurrent unipolar depression, usually when standard antidepressants have failed (p.271). Lithium is also used to augment the efficacy of other antidepressants in refractory cases.

References.

1. Franchini L, *et al.* Fluvoxamine and lithium in long-term treatment of unipolar subjects with high recurrence rate. *J Affective Disord* 1996; **38:** 67–9.

Headache. Lithium is one of a number of drugs tried in cluster headache (see p.443) to prevent headache attacks during cluster periods when ergotamine is ineffective or has otherwise had to be withdrawn. In a double-blind study[1] lithium and verapamil were found to be of similar efficacy for cluster headache prophylaxis although verapamil appeared to produce fewer adverse effects.

1. Bussone G, *et al.* Double blind comparison of lithium and verapamil in cluster headache prophylaxis. *Headache* 1990; **30:** 411–17.

Manic depression. The management of manic depression (bipolar disorder) is discussed on p.273 where the role of lithium is covered. Briefly, lithium's main role is in prophylaxis. It is sometimes used in the control of the acute manic stage, but, because of its slow onset of action, usually in conjunction with an antipsychotic drug.

References.

1. Johnson FN, ed. *Depression & mania: modern lithium therapy.* Oxford: IRL Press, 1987.
2. Aronson JK, Reynolds DJM. Lithium. *Br Med J* 1992; **305:** 1273–6.
3. Birch NJ, *et al.* Lithium prophylaxis: proposed guidelines for good clinical practice. *Lithium* 1993; **4:** 225–30.
4. Peet M, Pratt JP. Lithium: current status in psychiatric disorders. *Drugs* 1993; **46:** 7–17.
5. Price LH, Heninger GR. Lithium in the treatment of mood disorders. *N Engl J Med* 1994; **331:** 591–8.
6. Jensen HV, *et al.* Lithium prophylaxis of manic-depressive disorder: daily lithium dosing schedule versus every second day. *Acta Psychiatr Scand* 1995; **92:** 69–74.
7. Moncrieff J. Lithium revisited: a re-examination of the placebo-controlled trials of lithium prophylaxis in manic-depressive disorder. *Br J Psychiatry* 1995; **167:** 569–74.
8. Jensen HV, *et al.* Twelve-hour brain lithium concentration in lithium maintenance treatment of manic-depressive disorder: daily versus alternate-day dosing schedule. *Psychopharmacology (Berl)* 1996; **124:** 275–8.
9. Maj M, *et al.* Late non-responders to lithium prophylaxis in bipolar patients: prevalence and predictors. *J Affective Disord* 1996; **39:** 39–42.

Schizophrenia. The addition of lithium to antipsychotic treatment may be worthwhile in patients with schizophrenia (p.637) or schizoaffective disorders who fail to respond to an antipsychotic alone, but the danger of an interaction between the drugs should be borne in mind (see under Interactions, above). Although affective symptoms need not be present for patients with schizophrenia to respond to adjunctive lithium their presence does appear to predict a greater likelihood of response.[1]

1. Christison GW, *et al.* When symptoms persist: choosing among alternative somatic treatments for schizophrenia. *Schizophr Bull* 1991; **17:** 217–45.

Preparations

BP 1998: Lithium Carbonate Tablets; Slow Lithium Carbonate Tablets;
USP 23: Lithium Carbonate Capsules; Lithium Carbonate Extended-release Tablets; Lithium Carbonate Tablets; Lithium Citrate Syrup.

Proprietary Preparations (details are given in Part 3)
Aust.: Neurolepsin; Quilonorm; ***Austral.:*** Lithicarb; Priadel†; ***Belg.:*** Camcolit†; Maniprex; Neurolithium†; Priadel; ***Canad.:*** Carbolith; Duralith; Lithane; Lithizine; ***Fr.:*** Neurolithium; Tera-

lithe; *Ger.:* Hypnorex; leukominerase; Li 450; Quilonum; *Irl.:* Camcolit; Priadel; *Ital.:* Carbolithium; Demalit†; Manialit†; *Neth.:* Litarex†; Priadel; *Norw.:* Litarex; Lithionit; *S.Afr.:* Camcolit; Lentolith; Priadel†; Quilonum; *Spain:* Plenur; *Swed.:* Litarex†; Lithionit; *Switz.:* Hypnorex†; Litarex; Lithiofor; Neurolithium; Priadel; Quilonorm; *UK:* Camcolit; Li-Liquid; Liskonum; Litarex; Lithonate; Phasal†; Priadel; *USA:* Cibalith-S†; Eskalith; Lithobid; Lithonate; Lithotabs.

Multi-ingredient: *Aust.:* Togal; *Austral.:* Caprilate; *Fr.:* Lithines Magnesies†; Sommieres Au Pentavit B†; *Ger.:* NeyDop "N" (Revitorgan-Dilutionen "N" Nr. 97); Togal; *Spain:* Arthrisel†; Citinoides; Lithines†; Litinoides†; Otogen†.

Lofepramine Hydrochloride (2522-w)

Lofepramine Hydrochloride *(BANM, USAN, rINNM).*

Leo-640; Lopramine Hydrochloride; WHR-2908A. 5-{3-[*N*-(Chlorophenacyl)-*N*-methylamino]propyl}-10,11-5*H*-dihydrodibenz[*b,f*]azepine hydrochloride.

$C_{26}H_{27}ClN_2O,HCl = 455.4$.

CAS — 23047-25-8 (lofepramine); 26786-32-3 (lofepramine hydrochloride).

Adverse Effects, Treatment, and Precautions

As for tricyclic antidepressants in general (see Amitriptyline, p.273). Lofepramine should be avoided in patients with severe hepatic or renal impairment.

Effects on the liver. See under Amitriptyline, p.274.

Overdosage. Lofepramine is a newer tricyclic antidepressant that may be less toxic in overdosage than earlier tricyclics.[1]

1. Reid F, Henry JA. Lofepramine overdosage. *Pharmacopsychiatry* 1990; **23:** 23–27.

Porphyria. Lofepramine has been associated with clinical exacerbations of porphyria and is considered unsafe in porphyric patients.[1]

1. Moore MR, McColl KEL. *Porphyria: drug lists.* Glasgow: Porphyria Research Unit, University of Glasgow, 1991.

Interactions

For interactions associated with tricyclic antidepressants, see Amitriptyline, p.276.

Pharmacokinetics

Lofepramine is readily absorbed from the gastro-intestinal tract, and extensively demethylated by first-pass metabolism in the liver to its primary metabolite, desipramine (p.282). Since lofepramine slows gastro-intestinal transit time absorption can, however, be delayed, particularly in overdosage. Paths of metabolism also include *N*-oxidation and hydroxylation. Lofepramine is mainly excreted in the urine, chiefly in the form of its metabolites. It is highly bound to plasma proteins. Lofepramine is distributed into breast milk.

Uses and Administration

Lofepramine is a dibenzazepine tricyclic antidepressant with actions and uses similar to those of amitriptyline (p.278). One of its metabolites is desipramine (p.282). Lofepramine is one of the less sedating tricyclics.

In the treatment of depression lofepramine is given by mouth as the hydrochloride in divided doses equivalent to lofepramine 140 to 210 mg daily.

Lofepramine should be withdrawn gradually to reduce the risk of withdrawal symptoms.

References.

1. Lancaster SG, Gonzalez JP. Lofepramine: a review of its pharmacodynamic and pharmacokinetic properties, and therapeutic efficacy in depressive illness. *Drugs* 1989; **37:** 123–40.

Administration in the elderly. The UK manufacturer has suggested that some elderly patients may respond to lower than usual doses of lofepramine, but in a study[1] involving 46 elderly patients with various grades of depression lofepramine 70 mg once daily was no more effective than placebo at the end of 28 days of treatment.

1. Tan RSH, *et al.* The effect of low dose lofepramine in depressed elderly patients in general medical wards. *Br J Clin Pharmacol* 1994; **37:** 321–4.

Depression. As discussed on p.271, there is very little difference in efficacy between the different groups of antidepressant drugs, and choice is often made on the basis of adverse effect profile. Tricyclic antidepressants such as amitriptyline or imipramine have traditionally been the first choice for the treatment of depression, and often still are because of wide experience with their use and familiarity with their pharmacological actions. Lofepramine is one of the less sedating tricyclics and consequently may be of value for withdrawn or apathetic depressed patients.

Preparations

Proprietary Preparations (details are given in Part 3)

Aust.: Tymelyt; *Belg.:* Tymelyt; *Ger.:* Gamonil; *Irl.:* Gamanil; *Ital.:* Timelit†; *S.Afr.:* Emdalen; *Spain:* Deftan; *Swed.:* Tymelyt; *Switz.:* Gamonil; *UK:* Gamanil; Lomont.

Maprotiline Hydrochloride (2524-l)

Maprotiline Hydrochloride *(BANM, rINNM).*

Ba-34276; Maprotilini Hydrochloridum. 3-(9,10-Dihydro-9,10-ethanoanthracen-9-yl)propyl(methyl)amine hydrochloride.

$C_{20}H_{23}N,HCl = 313.9$.

CAS — 10262-69-8 (maprotiline); 10347-81-6 (maprotiline hydrochloride).

NOTE. Maprotiline is *USAN.*

Pharmacopoeias. In *Eur.* (see p.viii) and *US.*

A fine white to off-white practically odourless crystalline powder. It exhibits polymorphism. Slightly **soluble** in water; soluble in alcohol; freely soluble in methyl alcohol and in chloroform; sparingly soluble in dichloromethane; very slightly soluble in acetone. **Store** in airtight containers.

Adverse Effects, Treatment, and Precautions

As for tricyclic antidepressants in general (see Amitriptyline, p.273).

Skin rashes seem more common with maprotiline than with tricyclic antidepressants. Seizures have occurred in patients with no prior history of such disorders as well as in those with a history of epilepsy and the risk is increased if high doses of maprotiline are employed. It should not be used in patients with epilepsy or a lowered seizure threshold.

Maprotiline should be withdrawn gradually to reduce the risk of withdrawal symptoms.

By March 1985 the UK Committee on Safety of Medicines[1] had received reports of the following adverse reactions associated with maprotiline from a cumulative total of 2.5 million prescriptions: convulsions (124), hepatic reactions (4), and haematological reactions (8). There had also been 454 reports of skin rashes.

1. Committee on Safety of Medicines. Dangers of newer antidepressants. *Current Problems 15* 1985.

Effects on the skin. In addition to many recorded instances of skin rashes with maprotiline (see above) cutaneous vasculitis, which resolved on discontinuation of therapy, has also been observed.[1]

1. Oakley AMM, Hodge L. Cutaneous vasculitis from maprotiline. *Aust N Z J Med* 1985; **15:** 256–7.

Epileptogenic effect. In a retrospective review of 186 psychiatric patients with no history of prior seizures, 5 of 32 patients receiving maprotiline developed generalised tonic-clonic seizures, compared with 1 of 45 receiving a tricyclic antidepressant.[1] There were no seizures in the remaining patients who received other medications, or no drug treatment. Two of the 5 patients experiencing seizures with maprotiline were receiving doses of 75 to 150 mg daily, 2 were receiving daily doses of 200 to 300 mg, and one patient experienced partial complex seizures with a daily dose of 150 mg and generalised tonic-clonic seizures after increasing the daily dose to 300 mg.

1. Jabbari B, *et al.* Incidence of seizures with tricyclic and tetracyclic antidepressants. *Arch Neurol* 1985; **42:** 480–1.

Overdosage. Apart from seizures being more common with maprotiline, features of overdosage are similar to those experienced with tricyclic antidepressant poisonings (see under Adverse Effects of Amitriptyline, p.273).

For a discussion of choice of antidepressant with respect to safety in overdosage, see under Depression, p.271.

References.

1. Crome P, Newman B. Poisoning with maprotiline and mianserin. *Br Med J* 1977; **2:** 260.
2. Curtis RA, *et al.* Fatal maprotiline intoxication. *Drug Intell Clin Pharm* 1984; **18:** 716–20.
3. Knudsen K, Heath A. Effects of self poisoning with maprotiline. *Br Med J* 1984; **288:** 601–3.
4. Crome P, Ali C. Clinical features and management of self-poisoning with newer antidepressants. *Med Toxicol* 1986; **1:** 411–20.

Interactions

Interactions associated with maprotiline are similar to those associated with tricyclic antidepressants (see Amitriptyline, p.276).

Pharmacokinetics

Maprotiline is slowly but completely absorbed from the gastro-intestinal tract.

Maprotiline is extensively demethylated in the liver to its principal active metabolite, desmethylmaprotiline; paths of metabolism of both maprotiline and desmethylmaprotiline include *N*-oxidation, aliphatic and aromatic hydroxylation, and the formation of aromatic methoxy derivatives. In addition to desmethylmaprotiline, maprotiline-*N*-oxide is also reported to be pharmacologically active. The average elimination half-life of maprotiline is reported to be about 51 hours and that of its active metabolite even longer (range 60 to 90 hours). Maprotiline is excreted in the urine, mainly in the form of its metabolites, either in free or in conjugated form; appreciable amounts are also excreted in the faeces.

Maprotiline is widely distributed throughout the body and is extensively bound to plasma protein. Maprotiline is distributed into breast milk (see Breast Feeding under Precautions of Amitriptyline, p.275).

References.

1. Maguire KP, *et al.* An evaluation of maprotiline: intravenous kinetics and comparison of two oral doses. *Eur J Clin Pharmacol* 1980; **18:** 249–54.
2. Alkalay D, *et al.* Bioavailability and kinetics of maprotiline. *Clin Pharmacol Ther* 1980; **27:** 697–703.
3. Firkusny L, Gleiter H. Maprotiline metabolism appears to co-segregate with the genetically-determined CYP2D6 polymorphic hydroxylation of debrisoquine. *Br J Clin Pharmacol* 1994; **37:** 383–8.

Uses and Administration

Maprotiline is a tetracyclic antidepressant with actions and uses similar to those of tricyclic antidepressants (see Amitriptyline, p.278). It has moderate sedative and antimuscarinic properties. Like the tricyclics, maprotiline is an inhibitor of the reuptake of noradrenaline; it also has weak affinity for central adrenergic (α_1) receptors

In the treatment of depression (p.271) maprotiline is given by mouth as the hydrochloride in doses of 25 to 75 mg daily in three divided doses, gradually increased to 150 mg daily if necessary; up to 225 mg daily may be required in severely depressed patients in hospital. The dosage should be adjusted after 1 or 2 weeks according to response. Because of the prolonged half-life of maprotiline the total daily dose may also be given as a single dose, usually at night. A suggested initial dose for elderly patients is 10 mg three times daily or 30 mg at night gradually increased according to response over a period of 1 to 2 weeks to 25 mg three times daily or 75 mg at night.

Maprotiline has been given by injection as the mesylate and in oral drops as the resinate.

Maprotiline should be withdrawn gradually to reduce the risk of withdrawal symptoms.

Preparations

USP 23: Maprotiline Hydrochloride Tablets.

Proprietary Preparations (details are given in Part 3)

Aust.: Ludiomil; *Belg.:* Ludiomil; *Canad.:* Ludiomil; *Fr.:* Ludiomil; *Ger.:* Aneural; Delgian†; Depressase†; Deprilept; Kanopan†; Ludiomil; Mapro-GRY; Mapro-Tablinen†; Maprolu; Mirpan; Psymion; *Irl.:* Ludiomil†; *Ital.:* Ludiomil; Maprolit†; *Neth.:* Ludiomil; *S.Afr.:* Ludiomil; *Spain:* Ludiomil; *Swed.:* Ludiomil; *Switz.:* Ludiomil; *UK:* Ludiomil; *USA:* Ludiomil.

Medifoxamine (12920-k)

Medifoxamine *(rINN).*

NN-Dimethyl-2,2-diphenoxyethylamine.

$C_{16}H_{19}NO_2 = 257.3$.

CAS — 32359-34-5.

Medifoxamine is an antidepressant which is given by mouth in usual doses of 50 mg three times daily.

References.

1. Saleh S, *et al.* The serum protein binding of medifoxamine. *Br J Clin Pharmacol* 1989; **27:** 708P.
2. Saleh S, *et al.* Absolute bioavailability and pharmacokinetics of medifoxamine in healthy humans. *Br J Clin Pharmacol* 1990; **30:** 621–4.
3. Saleh S, Turner P. Ocular hypotensive effects of medifoxamine. *Br J Clin Pharmacol* 1992; **34:** 269–71.
4. Gainsborough N, *et al.* The pharmacokinetics and pharmacodynamics of medifoxamine after oral administration in healthy elderly volunteers. *Eur J Clin Pharmacol* 1994; **46:** 163–6.

Preparations

Proprietary Preparations (details are given in Part 3)

Fr.: Cledial.

Melitracen Hydrochloride (2526-j)

Melitracen Hydrochloride *(USAN, rINNM).*

N7001; U-24973A. 3-(9,10-Dihydro-10,10-dimethyl-9-anthrylidene)propyldimethylamine hydrochloride.

$C_{21}H_{25}N,HCl = 327.9$.

CAS — 5118-29-6 (melitracen); 10563-70-9 (melitracen hydrochloride).

Melitracen hydrochloride 28.1 mg is approximately equivalent to 25 mg of melitracen.

Melitracen hydrochloride is a tricyclic antidepressant (see Amitriptyline, p.273).

In the treatment of depression initial doses equivalent to melitracen 25 mg two to three times daily are given by mouth and gradually increased to a total of 225 mg daily if necessary. Elderly patients should generally be given reduced doses equivalent to melitracen 10 mg three times daily initially.

Melitracen should be withdrawn gradually to reduce the risk of withdrawal symptoms.

Preparations

Proprietary Preparations (details are given in Part 3)
Aust.: Dixeran; *Belg.:* Dixeran; *Ger.:* Trausabun†; *Ital.:* Melixeran†; *Switz.:* Dixeran.

Multi-ingredient: *Aust.:* Deanxit; *Belg.:* Deanxit; *Ital.:* Deanxit; *Spain:* Deanxit; *Switz.:* Deanxit.

Metapramine Fumarate (3936-k)

Metapramine Fumarate *(rINNM)*.

10,11-Dihydro-5-methyl-10-(methylamino)-5*H*-dibenz[*b,f*]azepine fumarate.

$C_{16}H_{18}N_2,C_4H_4O_4$ = 354.4.

CAS — 21730-16-5 (metapramine); 93841-84-0 (metapramine fumarate).

Metapramine fumarate is a tricyclic antidepressant (see Amitriptyline, p.273).

Mianserin Hydrochloride (2527-z)

Mianserin Hydrochloride *(BANM, USAN, rINNM)*.

Mianserini Hydrochloridum; Org-GB-94. 1,2,3,4,10,14b-Hexahydro-2-methyldibenzo[*c,f*]pyrazino[1,2-*a*]azepine hydrochloride.

$C_{18}H_{20}N_2,HCl$ = 300.8.

CAS — 24219-97-4 (mianserin); 21535-47-7 (mianserin hydrochloride).

Pharmacopoeias. In *Eur.* (see p.viii).

White or almost white crystals or crystalline powder. Sparingly **soluble** in water; slightly soluble in alcohol; soluble in dichloromethane. A 1% solution in water has a pH of 4.0 to 5.5. **Protect** from light.

Adverse Effects

The most common adverse effect associated with mianserin is drowsiness. Mianserin also causes bone-marrow depression usually presenting as leucopenia, granulocytopenia, or agranulocytosis; aplastic anaemia has been reported. These adverse haematological reactions generally occur during the first few weeks of therapy and especially in the elderly.

Other side-effects reported include convulsions, disturbances of liver function and jaundice, breast disorders (gynaecomastia, nipple tenderness, and non-puerperal lactation), dizziness, orthostatic hypotension, oedema, polyarthropathy, skin rash, sweating, and tremor.

Hyponatraemia, possibly due to inappropriate secretion of antidiuretic hormone, has been associated with the use of antidepressants, particularly in the elderly.

Antimuscarinic and cardiac side-effects are fewer and milder than with tricyclic antidepressants; mianserin may be associated with a lower risk of cardiotoxicity in overdosage.

Effects on the blood. Between 1976 and the end of 1988 the Committee on Safety of Medicines in the UK had received 239 reports of adverse haematological reactions associated with mianserin.[1] They included 68 reports of agranulocytosis and 84 reports of granulocytopenia or leucopenia where mianserin was considered to be the probable or possible cause; there had been 17 fatalities. Allowing for the pattern of prescribing there was a greater number of reports of white blood cell disorders in patients over 65 years of age but there was no sex difference. The data also indicated that the adverse reactions were most likely to develop during the first three months of therapy. By the end of 1992 the number of reports of mianserin-induced agranulocytosis received by the CSM had risen to 79 and the number of reports of mianserin-induced neutropenia was 105.[2]

A case of fatal aplastic anaemia associated with mianserin has also been reported.[3]

Proposed mechanisms of mianserin haematotoxicity have included a direct toxicity[4] and an immunologically-mediated mechanism.[5] Mianserin is administered as a racemic preparation and there is also evidence from *in vitro* studies that the metabolites of mianserin exhibit cytotoxicity. A significant correlation between the desmethyl metabolite and cytotoxicity was found and the formation of metabolites was greater with the *R*(−)-enantiomer than with the *S*(+)-enantiomer.[6]

1. Committee on Safety of Medicines. Mianserin and white blood cell disorders in the elderly. *Current Problems 25* 1989.
2. Committee on Safety of Medicines/Medicines Control Agency. Drug-induced neutropenia and agranulocytosis. *Current Problems* 1993; **19:** 10–11.
3. Durrant S, Read D. Fatal aplastic anaemia associated with mianserin. *Br Med J* 1982; **285:** 437.
4. O'Donnell JL, *et al.* Possible mechanism for mianserin induced neutropenia associated with saturable elimination kinetics. *Br Med J* 1985; **291:** 1375–6.
5. Stricker BHC, *et al.* Thrombocytopenia and leucopenia with mianserin-dependent antibodies. *Br J Clin Pharmacol* 1985; **19:** 102–4.
6. Riley RJ, *et al.* A stereochemical investigation of the cytotoxicity of mianserin metabolites in vitro. *Br J Clin Pharmacol* 1989; **27:** 823–30.

Effects on the cardiovascular system. Although mianserin is considered to be less cardiotoxic than the tricyclic antidepressants adverse effects have been noted in individual patients. Two elderly patients developed signs of disturbed cardiac function (cardiac failure, atrial and ventricular fibrillation, bradycardia, and frequent ventricular ectopic beats) which resolved after the drug was discontinued.[1] One of the patients also developed hypokalaemia which was possibly caused by mianserin. It was suggested that persons most likely to experience problems were the elderly with a past history of cardiovascular disorders. Further reports of mianserin-induced cardiac effects include recurrent ventricular fibrillation in a 61-year-old man after an overdose of mianserin[2] and bradycardia in a 50-year-old woman following a therapeutic dose.[3]

1. Whiteford H, *et al.* Disturbed cardiac function possibly associated with mianserin therapy. *Med J Aust* 1984; **140:** 166–7.
2. Haefeli WE, *et al.* Recurrent ventricular fibrillation in mianserin intoxication. *Br Med J* 1991; **302:** 415–16.
3. Carcone B, *et al.* Symptomatic bradycardia caused by mianserin at therapeutic doses. *Hum Exp Toxicol* 1991; **10:** 383–4.

Effects on the liver. By March 1985 the Committee on Safety of Medicines in the UK had received 57 reports of hepatic reactions associated with mianserin from a cumulative total of 5 million prescriptions. Reactions had included jaundice and other abnormalities of liver function, but no fatalities had been reported.[1]

Case reports have also been published concerning jaundice;[2-5] the liver function returned to normal after discontinuation of mianserin or dose reduction.

1. Committee on Safety of Medicines. Dangers of newer antidepressants. *Current Problems 15* 1985.
2. Adverse Drug Reactions Advisory Committee. Mianserin: a possible cause of neutropenia and agranulocytosis. *Med J Aust* 1980; **2:** 673–4.
3. Goldstraw PW, *et al.* Mianserin and jaundice. *N Z Med J* 1983; **96:** 985.
4. Zarski J-P, *et al.* Toxicité hépatique des nouveaux anti-dépresseurs: a propos d'une observation. *Gastroenterol Clin Biol* 1983; **7:** 220–1.
5. Otani K, *et al.* Hepatic injury caused by mianserin. *Br Med J* 1989; **299:** 519.

Effects on the musculoskeletal system. Hughes and Coote in describing one patient who developed an acute polyarthritis affecting the hands and feet 6 days after commencing therapy with mianserin[1] also mentioned that the UK Committee on Safety of Medicines had received 19 reports of arthritis and arthralgia associated with mianserin.

1. Hughes A, Coote J. Arthropathy associated with treatment with mianserin. *Br Med J* 1986; **292:** 1050.

Effects on the skin. Reports of adverse dermatological reactions in individual patients related to mianserin therapy have included toxic epidermal necrolysis[1] and erythema multiforme.[2,3]

1. Randell P. Tolvon and toxic epidermal necrolysis. *Med J Aust* 1979; **2:** 653.
2. Quraishy E. Erythema multiforme during treatment with mianserin—a case report. *Br J Dermatol* 1981; **104:** 481.
3. Cox NH. Erythema multiforme due to mianserin—a case against generic prescribing. *Br J Clin Pract* 1985; **39:** 293–4.

Effects on the tongue. Glossitis associated with mianserin therapy has been reported in 2 patients.[1] Additionally, glossitis accompanied by severe facial oedema has been noted in another patient.[2] In all cases symptoms resolved after withdrawal of mianserin.

1. de la Fuente JR, Berlanga C. Glossitis associated with mianserin. *Lancet* 1984; **i:** 233.
2. Leibovitch G, *et al.* Severe facial oedema and glossitis associated with mianserin. *Lancet* 1989; **ii:** 871–2.

Epileptogenic effect. By March 1985 the UK Committee on Safety of Medicines had received 64 reports of convulsions associated with mianserin from a total of 5 million prescriptions.[1]

In a previous review[2] concerning 40 of these cases it was considered that a causal connection could be established only in a minority. It was suggested that mianserin is no more epileptogenic than tricyclic antidepressants, an opinion that was also shared by other reviewers.[3]

1. Committee on Safety of Medicines. Dangers of newer antidepressants. *Current Problems 15* 1985.
2. Edwards JG, Glen-Bott M. Mianserin and convulsive seizures. *Br J Clin Pharmacol* 1983; **15:** 299S–311S.
3. Richens A, *et al.* Antidepressant drugs, convulsions and epilepsy. *Br J Clin Pharmacol* 1983; **15:** 295S–298S.

Overdosage. Experience with 100 consecutive cases of intoxication with mianserin[1] revealed that when it was the only drug ingested symptoms were mild and neither deep coma nor convulsions occurred. More serious symptoms were seen in patients who had taken multiple drug overdoses and there were 2 fatalities. The results suggested that following an acute overdose mianserin is less toxic than the tricyclic antidepressants. This conclusion was also supported by a large follow-up study[2] comparing the outcome of suicide attempts among patients who had taken mianserin in overdose with those who had taken amitriptyline.

1. Chand S, *et al.* One hundred cases of acute intoxication with mianserin hydrochloride. *Pharmakopsychiatrie* 1981; **14:** 15–17.
2. Inman WHW. Blood disorders and suicide in patients taking mianserin or amitriptyline. *Lancet* 1988; **ii:** 90–2.

Precautions

Mianserin is contra-indicated in patients with severe liver disease and in patients with mania. Patients with bipolar disorder may switch from a depressive to a manic phase during treatment with mianserin.

Although mianserin does not have the cardiotoxicity of the tricyclic antidepressants, it should be used with caution in patients with cardiovascular disorders, such as heart block, or after recent myocardial infarction. It should be used with caution in patients with diabetes mellitus, epilepsy, and hepatic or renal insufficiency. Patients with suicidal tendencies should be carefully supervised during early treatment. Patients with angle-closure glaucoma or prostatic hyperplasia should be monitored even though antimuscarinic effects are rare.

A full blood count is recommended every 4 weeks during the first 3 months of treatment, because of the risk of bone-marrow depression. Similarly, if a patient receiving mianserin develops fever, sore throat, stomatitis, or other signs of infection, treatment should be stopped and a full blood count obtained. The elderly are considered to be at special risk of blood disorders from mianserin. For further details see Effects on the Blood under Adverse Effects, above.

Drowsiness is often experienced at the start of mianserin therapy and patients if affected should not drive or operate machinery. For further details of the effects of antidepressant therapy on driving see under Amitriptyline, p.276.

The manufacturers warn that if surgery is required the anaesthetist should be informed that the patient has received mianserin (see also Anaesthesia under Amitriptyline, p.275).

The manufacturers recommend that mianserin should not be given during breast feeding, but some authorities consider the amount distributed into breast milk too small to be harmful.

Mianserin should be withdrawn gradually to reduce the risk of withdrawal symptoms.

Interactions

It is recommended that mianserin should not be given to patients receiving MAOIs or for at least 14 days after their discontinuation. At least one week should elapse between withdrawing mianserin and starting any drug liable to provoke a serious reaction (e.g. phenelzine). Unlike the tricyclics, mianserin does not diminish the effects of the antihypertensives guanethidine, hydralazine, propranolol, clonidine, or bethanidine. However, it is still recommended that blood pressure be monitored when mianserin is prescribed with antihypertensive therapy. Plasma-phenytoin concentrations should be monitored carefully in patients treated concurrently with mianserin; phenytoin has been reported to reduce concentrations of mianserin. There may be potentiation of effects when mianserin is given concomitantly with CNS depressants such as alcohol, anxiolytics, or antipsychotics.

Antiepileptics. Reduced plasma concentrations and half-lives of mianserin and desmethylmianserin were observed in 6 patients also receiving antiepileptic therapy consisting of phenytoin with either carbamazepine or phenobarbitone.[1]

Mianserin may antagonise the action of antiepileptics by lowering the convulsive threshold.

1. Nawishy S, *et al.* Kinetic interaction of mianserin in epileptic patients on anticonvulsant drugs. *Br J Clin Pharmacol* 1982; **13:** 612P–13P.

Pharmacokinetics

Mianserin is readily absorbed from the gastro-intestinal tract, but its bioavailability is reduced to about 70% by extensive first-pass metabolism in the liver.

Paths of metabolism of mianserin include aromatic hydroxylation, *N*-oxidation, and *N*-demethylation. Desmethylmianserin and 8-hydroxymianserin are pharmacologically active.

Mianserin is excreted in the urine, almost entirely as its metabolites, either free or in conjugated form; some is also found in the faeces.

Mianserin is widely distributed throughout the body and is extensively bound to plasma proteins. It has been found to have a biphasic plasma half-life with the duration of the terminal phase ranging from about 6 to 40 hours. Mianserin crosses the blood-brain barrier and the placenta. It is distributed into breast milk.

References.

1. Hrdina PD, *et al.* Mianserin kinetics in depressed patients. *Clin Pharmacol Ther* 1983; **33:** 757–62.
2. Pinder RM, Van Delft AML. The potential therapeutic role of enantiomers and metabolites of mianserin. *Br J Clin Pharmacol* 1983; **15:** 269S–276S.
3. Begg EJ, *et al.* Variability in the elimination of mianserin in elderly patients. *Br J Clin Pharmacol* 1989; **27:** 445–51.
4. Buist A, *et al.* Mianserin in breast milk. *Br J Clin Pharmacol* 1993; **36:** 133–4.
5. Dahl M-L, *et al.* Stereoselective disposition of mianserin is related to debrisoquin hydroxylation polymorphism. *Clin Pharmacol Ther* 1994; **56:** 176–83.

Uses and Administration

Mianserin is a tetracyclic antidepressant. It does not appear to have significant antimuscarinic properties, but has a marked sedative action. Unlike the tricyclic antidepressants, mianserin does not prevent the peripheral reuptake of noradrenaline; it blocks presynaptic adrenergic (α_2) receptors and increases the turnover of brain noradrenaline. Mianserin is also an antagonist of serotonin receptors in some parts of the brain.

In the treatment of depression (p.271) mianserin is given by mouth as the hydrochloride in initial doses of 30 to 40 mg daily increased gradually thereafter as necessary. The effective daily dosage is usually between 30 and 90 mg. The daily dosage may be divided throughout the day or given as a single dose at night. Divided daily dosages of up to 200 mg have been given. The recommended initial daily dose in the elderly is not more than 30 mg, which may be slowly increased if necessary.

Mianserin should be withdrawn gradually to reduce the risk of withdrawal symptoms.

General references.

1. Marshall RJ. The pharmacology of mianserin—an update. *Br J Clin Pharmacol* 1983; **15:** 263S-268S.

Preparations

BP 1998: Mianserin Tablets.

Proprietary Preparations (details are given in Part 3)
Aust.: Tolvon; ***Austral.:*** Lerivon; Lumin; Tolvon; ***Belg.:*** Lerivon; ***Fr.:*** Athymil; ***Ger.:*** Hopacem; Mianeurin; Prisma; Tolvin; ***Irl.:*** Tolvon; ***Ital.:*** Lantanon; ***Neth.:*** Tolvon; ***Norw.:*** Tolvon; ***S.Afr.:*** Lantanon; ***Spain:*** Lantanon; ***Swed.:*** Tolvon; ***Switz.:*** Lantanon†; Tolvon; ***UK:*** Bolvidon†; Norval†.

Milnacipran (19513-l)

Milnacipran *(BAN, rINN).*

F-2207; Midalcipran. (±)-*cis*-2-(Aminomethyl)-*N*,*N*-diethyl-1-phenylcyclopropanecarboxamide.

$C_{15}H_{22}N_2O = 246.3$.

CAS — 92623-85-3 (milnacipran); 101152-94-7 (milnacipran hydrochloride).

Milnacipran is a serotonin and noradrenaline reuptake inhibitor (SNRI) used for the treatment of depression (p.271). It is given by mouth as the hydrochloride in doses of 100 mg daily.

References.

1. Serre C, *et al.* An early clinical trial of midalcipran, 1-phenyl-1-diethyl aminocarbonyl 2-aminomethyl cyclopropane (2) hydrochloride, a potential fourth generation antidepressant. *Curr Ther Res* 1986; **39:** 156–64.
2. Ansseau M, *et al.* Controlled comparison of two doses of milnacipran (F2207) and amitriptyline in major depressive inpatients. *Psychopharmacology (Berl)* 1989; **98:** 163–8.
3. Palmier C, *et al.* Monoamine uptake inhibition by plasma from healthy volunteers after single oral doses of the antidepressant milnacipran. *Eur J Clin Pharmacol* 1989; **37:** 235–8.
4. Ansseau M, *et al.* Controlled comparison of milnacipran and fluoxetine in major depression. *Psychopharmacology (Berl)* 1994; **114:** 131–7.
5. Leinonen E, *et al.* Long-term efficacy and safety of milnacipran compared to clomipramine in patients with major depression. *Acta Psychiatr Scand* 1997; **96:** 497–504.
6. Tignol J, *et al.* Double-blind study of the efficacy and safety of milnacipran and imipramine in elderly patients with major depressive episode. *Acta Psychiatr Scand* 1998; **97:** 157–65.
7. Spencer CM, Wilde MI. Milnacipran: a review of its use in depression. *Drugs* 1998; **56:** 405–27.

Minaprine Hydrochloride (12963-v)

Minaprine Hydrochloride *(BANM, USAN, rINNM).*

AGR-1240 (minaprine); 30038CB (minaprine dihydrochloride); CB-30038 (minaprine dihydrochloride). *N*-(4-Methyl-6-phenylpyridazin-3-yl)-2-morpholinoethylamine dihydrochloride.

$C_{17}H_{22}N_4O,2HCl = 371.3$.

CAS — 25905-77-5 (minaprine); 25953-17-7 (minaprine dihydrochloride).

Minaprine hydrochloride is an antidepressant with stimulant properties that has been given by mouth for various psychiatric disorders.

References.

1. Mikus P, *et al.* A controlled study of minaprine and nomifensine in outpatients with masked depression. *Clin Trials J* 1985; **22:** 477–87.
2. Passeri M, *et al.* Minaprine for senile dementia. *Lancet* 1985; **i:** 824.
3. Bohacek N, *et al.* A double-blind comparison of minaprine and imipramine in the treatment of depressed patients. *J Clin Psychopharmacol* 1986; **6:** 320–1.
4. Amsterdam JD, *et al.* Double-blind, placebo-controlled, fixed dose trial of minaprine in patients with major depression. *Pharmacopsychiatry* 1989; **22:** 137–43.
5. Wheatley D. Minaprine: an anticholinergic-free antidepressant? Results of a controlled trial of mianserin. *Br J Psychiatry* 1989; **155:** 106–7.
6. Parnetti L, *et al.* Multicentre controlled randomised double-blind placebo study of minaprine in elderly patients suffering from prolonged depressive reaction. *Drug Invest* 1993; **6:** 181–8.

Preparations

Proprietary Preparations (details are given in Part 3)
Fr.: Cantor†; ***Ital.:*** Cantor†; ***Spain:*** Isopulsan†.

Mirtazapine (11022-r)

Mirtazapine *(BAN, USAN, rINN).*

Org-3770. (*RS*)-1,2,3,4,10,14b-Hexahydro-2-methylpyrazino-[2,1-*a*]pyrido[2,3-*c*][2]benzazepine.

$C_{17}H_{19}N_3 = 265.4$.

CAS — 61337-67-5.

Adverse Effects

Side-effects commonly reported with mirtazapine are an increase in appetite and weight; drowsiness or sedation generally occur during the first few weeks of treatment. Increases in liver enzyme levels have been reported less commonly, and oedema rarely. Other rarely reported side-effects include postural hypotension, mania, exanthema, convulsions, tremor, myoclonus, and reversible agranulocytosis, leucopenia, and granulocytopenia.

Hyponatraemia, possibly due to inappropriate secretion of antidiuretic hormone, has been associated with the use of antidepressants, particularly in the elderly.

Precautions

Mirtazapine should be used with caution in patients with epilepsy, hepatic or renal impairment, and cardiac disorders such as conduction disturbances, angina pectoris, and recent myocardial infarction, and also in patients with hypotension, diabetes mellitus, and in those with a history of manic depression (bipolar disorder). Treatment should be stopped if jaundice develops. Although mirtazapine has only weak antimuscarinic activity, caution should nevertheless be exercised in patients with micturition disturbances, angle-closure glaucoma, and raised intra-ocular pressure.

Patients should be advised to report any of the following symptoms during treatment: fever, sore throat, stomatitis, or other signs of infection; treatment should be stopped and a blood count performed.

Drowsiness is often experienced at the start of therapy and patients, if affected, should not drive or operate machinery.

Patients should be closely monitored during early therapy until improvement in depression is observed because suicide is an inherent risk in depressed patients. For further details, see under Depression, p.271.

Mirtazapine should be withdrawn gradually to reduce the risk of withdrawal symptoms.

Interactions

Mirtazapine should not be used concomitantly with or within two weeks of discontinuing an MAOI; at least one week should elapse between discontinuation of mirtazapine and starting any drug liable to provoke a serious reaction (e.g. phenelzine). Administration of mirtazapine concurrently with alcohol, anxiolytics, or hypnotics may potentiate sedative effects.

Pharmacokinetics

Mirtazapine is well absorbed from the gastro-intestinal tract with peak plasma levels occurring after about 2 hours. Plasma protein binding is about 85%. Mirtazapine is extensively metabolised in the liver and the major biotransformation pathways are demethylation and oxidation followed by glucuronide conjugation; cytochrome P450 isoenzymes involved are CYP2D6, CYP1A2, and CYP3A4. The *N*-desmethyl metabolite is pharmacologically active. Elimination is via urine (75%) and faeces (15%). The mean plasma elimination half-life is 20 to 40 hours. Data from *animal* studies indicate that mirtazapine crosses the placenta and is distributed into breast milk.

Uses and Administration

Mirtazapine, a piperazinoazepine, is an analogue of mianserin (p.297); it is a noradrenergic and specific serotonergic antidepressant. It enhances the release of noradrenaline and, indirectly, serotonin through blockade of central presynaptic adrenergic (α_2) receptors. The effects of released serotonin are mediated via 5-HT_1 receptors as mirtazapine blocks both 5-HT_2 and 5-HT_3 receptors. Mirtazapine is given as a racemic mixture: the S(+)-enantiomer blocks α_2 and 5-HT_2 receptors whereas the R(−)-enantiomer blocks 5-HT_3 receptors. Mirtazapine is also a potent antagonist at histamine (H_1) receptors which gives it sedative properties; it has very little antimuscarinic activity.

In the treatment of depression (p.271), mirtazapine is given by mouth in an initial daily dose of 15 mg, which may be increased gradually according to clinical response. Changes in dose should be made at intervals of at least 1 to 2 weeks because of the long half-life. The usual effective dose lies within the range of 15 to 45 mg. Daily doses may be given as a single dose, preferably at bedtime, or in 2 equally divided doses.

Mirtazapine should be withdrawn gradually to reduce the risk of withdrawal symptoms.

References.

1. Sitsen JMA, Moors J. Mirtazapine, a novel antidepressant, in the treatment of anxiety symptoms: results from a placebo-controlled trial. *Drug Invest* 1994; **8:** 339–44.
2. van Moffaert M, *et al.* Mirtazapine is more effective than trazodone: a double-blind controlled study in hospitalized patients with major depression. *Int Clin Psychopharmacol* 1995; **10:** 3–9.
3. Marttila M, *et al.* A double-blind study comparing the efficacy and tolerability of mirtazapine and doxepin in patients with major depression. *Eur Neuropsychopharmacol* 1995; **5:** 441–6.
4. Bremner JD. A double-blind comparison of Org 3770, amitriptyline, and placebo in major depression. *J Clin Psychiatry* 1995; **56:** 519–25.
5. Richou H, *et al.* A multicentre, double-blind, clomipramine-controlled efficacy and safety study of Org 3770. *Hum Psychopharmacol Clin Exp* 1995; **10:** 263–71.
6. Anonymous. Mirtazapine—a new antidepressant. *Med Lett Drugs Ther* 1996; **38:** 113–14.
7. Kasper S, *et al.* A risk-benefit assessment of mirtazapine in the treatment of depression. *Drug Safety* 1997; **17:** 251–64.
8. Puzantian T. Mirtazapine, an antidepressant. *Am J Health-Syst Pharm* 1998; **55:** 44–9.

Preparations

Proprietary Preparations (details are given in Part 3)
Aust.: Remeron; ***Ger.:*** Remergil; ***Irl.:*** Zispin; ***Ital.:*** Remeron; ***Neth.:*** Remeron; ***Swed.:*** Remeron; ***UK:*** Zispin; ***USA:*** Remeron.

Moclobemide (19529-x)

Moclobemide *(BAN, USAN, rINN).*

Ro-11-1163; Ro-11-1163/000. 4-Chloro-*N*-(2-morpholinoethyl)benzamide.

$C_{13}H_{17}ClN_2O_2 = 268.7$.

CAS — 71320-77-9.

Adverse Effects

Adverse effects reported to occur with moclobemide include sleep disturbances, dizziness, agitation, restlessness, irritability, and headache. Gastro-intestinal disturbances include dry mouth, diarrhoea, constipation, and nausea and vomiting. Paraesthesia, visual disturbances, and oedema have also been reported, and skin reactions include rash, pruritus, urticaria, and flushing. Confusional states that disappear rapidly on discontinuation of the drug have been observed. Raised liver enzymes have been reported.

Hyponatraemia, possibly due to inappropriate secretion of antidiuretic hormone, has been associated with the use of antidepressants, particularly in the elderly.

Effects on the cardiovascular system. Hypertension has been reported[1,2] rarely in patients taking moclobemide. In some of these cases, the patients were taking other drugs concomitantly although moclobemide was suspected to be the cause. Blood pressure usually returned to normal after discontinuation of moclobemide.

1. Coulter DM, Pillans PI. Hypertension with moclobemide. *Lancet* 1995; **346:** 1032.
2. Boyd IW. Hypertension with moclobemide. *Lancet* 1995; **346:** 1498.

Overdosage. Symptoms that have been reported with overdosage of moclobemide include agitation, aggression, and behavioural disturbances.

References.

1. Hetzel W. Safety of moclobemide taken in overdose for attempted suicide. *Psychopharmacology (Berl)* 1992; **106:** S127–S129.
2. Hackett LP, *et al.* Disposition and clinical effects of moclobemide and three of its metabolites following overdose. *Drug Invest* 1993; **5:** 281–4.
3. Myrenfors PG, *et al.* Moclobemide overdose. *J Intern Med* 1993; **233:** 113–15.

Precautions

Moclobemide is contra-indicated in patients with acute confusional states and in those with phaeochromocytoma. It should be avoided in excited or agitated patients and in those with severe hepatic impairment. Manic episodes may be provoked in patients with bipolar disorders. Care is also required in patients with thyrotoxicosis as moclobemide may theoretically precipitate a hypertensive reaction.

Patients should be closely monitored during early antidepressant therapy until improvement in depression is observed because suicide is an inherent risk in depressed patients. For further details, see under Depression, p.271.

Although impairment of mental alertness is generally not expected with moclobemide, caution should be exercised with respect to driving or operating machinery until individual reactions have been assessed.

Antidepressants, particularly MAOIs, should be withdrawn gradually to reduce the risk of withdrawal symptoms.

Although the amounts of moclobemide distributed into breast milk are reported to be small (see under Pharmacokinetics, below), the manufacturers advise caution and consideration of the benefits of moclobemide therapy to the mother against possible risks to the infant.

Interactions

The dietary restrictions that need to be followed with non-selective inhibitors of monoamine oxidase types A and B (see under Interactions of Phenelzine, p.304) are less stringent with selective reversible inhibitors of monoamine oxidase type A such as moclobemide. However, the manufacturers of moclobemide recommend that since some patients may be especially sensitive to tyramine, consumption of large amounts of tyramine-rich food should be avoided.

Medicines containing *sympathomimetics, dextromethorphan*, or *anorectics* should not be taken with moclobemide. Moclobemide should not be given with *other antidepressants* although a treatment-free period is unnecessary following its cessation. For further details, see Antidepressants under Interactions of Phenelzine, p.305. Therapy with moclobemide should not be started until at least a week following cessation of a tricyclic or related antidepressant or a selective serotonin reuptake inhibitor or related antidepressant (2 weeks in the case of paroxetine and sertraline; at least 5 weeks in the case of fluoxetine) or for at least a week after stopping treatment with MAOIs. CNS excitation or depression may occur if moclobemide is taken concomitantly with *opioid analgesics*, and there is also a risk of CNS toxicity if taken with *serotonin (5-HT_1) agonists*. Moclobemide may enhance the effects of *ibuprofen* and possibly *other NSAIDs*. There has also been a warning that a hypertensive crisis may occur if moclobemide and *levodopa* are used together. The metabolism of moclobemide is inhibited by *cimetidine*, leading to increased plasma concentrations.

Antimigraine drugs. For the effects of moclobemide on serotonin (5-HT_1) agonists, see under Sumatriptan, p.451.

Cimetidine. Administration of cimetidine 1 g daily for 2 weeks increased the mean maximum plasma concentration of moclobemide in 8 healthy subjects from 575 ng per mL to 787 ng per mL; several other parameters associated with moclobemide absorption and disposition were also affected.[1] It was suggested that a reduction in the dosage of moclobemide might be required.

1. Schoerlin M-P, *et al.* Cimetidine alters the disposition kinetics of the monoamine oxidase-A inhibitor moclobemide. *Clin Pharmacol Ther* 1991; **49:** 32–8.

Dopaminergics. Caution is required when *selegiline* and moclobemide are given together. Dietary restrictions (see under Phenelzine, p.304) are recommended by one manufacturer, whereas another advises that this combination should be avoided.

For the effects of moclobemide on *levodopa*, see p.1139, and on selegiline, see p.1144.

Opioid analgesics. Symptoms suggestive of a mild serotonin syndrome (p.303) developed in a 73-year-old woman taking moclobemide, nortriptyline, and lithium after she was given *pethidine* intravenously.[1]

1. Gillman PK. Possible serotonin syndrome with moclobemide and pethidine. *Med J Aust* 1995; **162:** 554.

Sympathomimetics. Symptoms resembling phaeochromocytoma occurred in an elderly woman who was receiving treatment with the reversible MAOI toloxatone;[1] the woman had also been receiving a preparation containing *phenylephrine* without ill-effect but the symptoms occurred after addition of *terbutaline* therapy. It was noted that such an interaction is more typical of older, irreversible, less selective MAOIs.

1. Lefebvre H, *et al.* Life-threatening pseudo-phaeochromocytoma after toloxatone, terbutaline, and phenylephrine. *Lancet* 1993; **341:** 555–6.

Pharmacokinetics

Moclobemide is readily absorbed from the gastrointestinal tract, peak plasma concentrations occurring within 1 to 2 hours of ingestion. Absorption is virtually complete but first-pass metabolism reduces bioavailability of the drug. Moclobemide is widely distributed throughout the body and undergoes extensive metabolism, mainly oxidation, in the liver. Metabolites of moclobemide and a small amount of unchanged drug are excreted in the urine. Moclobemide has a plasma elimination half-life of 1 to 2 hours. Moclobemide is distributed into breast milk.

References.

1. Mayersohn M, Guentert TW. Clinical pharmacokinetics of the monoamide oxidase-A inhibitor moclobemide. *Clin Pharmacokinet* 1995; **29:** 292–332.
2. Gram LF, *et al.* Moclobemide: a substrate of CYP2C19 and an inhibitor of CYP2C19, CYP2D6, and CYP1A2: a panel study. *Clin Pharmacol Ther* 1995; **57:** 670–7.

Distribution into breast milk. In a study[1] of the distribution of moclobemide into the breast milk of 6 lactating mothers given a single 300-mg dose of moclobemide, a mean of 0.057% of the dose appeared in breast milk as moclobemide and 0.031% as its major metabolite Ro-12-8095 within 24 hours of administration. It was considered that this small amount of moclobemide was unlikely to be hazardous to suckling infants.

1. Pons G, *et al.* Moclobemide excretion in human breast milk. *Br J Clin Pharmacol* 1990; **29:** 27–31.

Uses and Administration

Moclobemide, a benzamide derivative, is a reversible inhibitor of monoamine oxidase type A (RIMA) (see under Phenelzine, p.306) used for the treatment of depression and of social phobia.

In the treatment of depression the usual initial daily dose of moclobemide is 300 mg by mouth in divided doses. This may be increased to up to 600 mg daily according to response. In some patients, a maintenance dose of 150 mg daily may be sufficient.

In the treatment of social phobia, the initial daily dose of moclobemide is 300 mg increased after 3 days to 600 mg given in 2 divided doses. Treatment should be continued for 8 to 12 weeks to assess efficacy; patients should be periodically re-evaluated thereafter to determine the need for further treatment.

Moclobemide should be taken after food.

Doses in patients with severe hepatic impairment may need to be reduced by half to one-third.

Antidepressants, particularly MAOIs, should be withdrawn gradually to reduce the risk of withdrawal symptoms.

Reviews.

1. Fulton B, Benfield P. Moclobemide: an update of its pharmacological properties and therapeutic use. *Drugs* 1996; **52:** 450–74.

Anxiety disorders. The use of MAOIs in general in the management of anxiety disorders is discussed under Phenelzine on p.306. For a discussion of the overall treatment of anxiety disorders, see p.635.

Some references to the use of moclobemide in anxiety disorders are given below.

1. Versiani M, *et al.* Pharmacotherapy of social phobia: a controlled study with moclobemide and phenelzine. *Br J Psychiatry* 1992; **161:** 353–60.

Depression. As discussed on p.271 there is very little difference in efficacy between the different groups of antidepressant drugs, and choice is often made on the basis of adverse effects. The traditional MAOIs such as phenelzine are rarely used as first-choice antidepressants because of the dangers of dietary and drug interactions. Reversible inhibitors of monoamine oxidase type A (RIMAs) such as moclobemide offer a safer alternative to the irreversible non-selective MAOIs and fewer dietary restrictions are necessary.

References.

1. Fitton A, *et al.* Moclobemide: a review of its pharmacological properties and therapeutic use in depressive illness. *Drugs* 1992; **43:** 561–96.
2. Bougerol T, *et al.* Efficacy and tolerability of moclobemide compared with fluvoxamine in depressive disorder (DSM III): a French/Swiss double-blind trial. *Psychopharmacology (Berl)* 1992; **106** (suppl): S102–S108.
3. Angst J, Stabl M. Efficacy of moclobemide in different patient groups: a meta-analysis of studies. *Psychopharmacology (Berl)* 1992; **106** (suppl): S109–S113.
4. Angst J, *et al.* Efficacy of moclobemide in different patient groups: results of new subscales of the Hamilton Depression Rating Scale. *Clin Neuropharmacol* 1993; **16** (suppl 2): S55–S62.
5. Angst J, *et al.* Antidepressant therapy with moclobemide in primary care practice. *Hum Psychopharmacol Clin Exp* 1993; **8:** 319–25.
6. Freeman H. Moclobemide. *Lancet* 1993; **342:** 1528–32.
7. Lonnqvist J, *et al.* Moclobemide and fluoxetine in atypical depression: a double-blind trial. *J Affective Disord* 1994; **32:** 169–77.
8. Anonymous. Moclobemide for depression. *Drug Ther Bull* 1994; **32:** 6–8.
9. Norman TR, Burrows GD. A risk-benefit assessment of moclobemide in the treatment of depressive disorders. *Drug Safety* 1995; **12:** 46–54.
10. Roth M, *et al.* Moclobemide in elderly patients with cognitive decline and depression: an international double-blind, placebo-controlled trial. *Br J Psychiatry* 1996; **168:** 149–57.

Smoking cessation. Nicotine replacement therapy is one of the main methods of pharmacotherapy used to alleviate the withdrawal syndrome associated with smoking cessation (see p.1608). In a preliminary double-blind, placebo-controlled parallel-group study in 88 smokers, moclobemide facilitated smoking cessation in highly dependent smokers.[1]

1. Berlin I, *et al.* A reversible monoamine oxidase A inhibitor (moclobemide) facilitates smoking cessation and abstinence in heavy, dependent smokers. *Clin Pharmacol Ther* 1995; **58:** 444–52.

Preparations

Proprietary Preparations (details are given in Part 3)
Aust.: Aurorix; ***Austral.:*** Arima; Aurorix; ***Belg.:*** Aurorix; ***Canad.:*** Manerix; ***Fr.:*** Moclamine; ***Ger.:*** Aurorix; ***Irl.:*** Manerix; ***Ital.:*** Aurorix; ***Neth.:*** Aurorix; ***Norw.:*** Aurorix; ***S.Afr.:*** Aurorix; ***Spain:*** Manerix; ***Swed.:*** Aurorix; ***Switz.:*** Aurorix; ***UK:*** Manerix.

Nefazodone Hydrochloride (6275-x)

Nefazodone Hydrochloride *(BANM, USAN, rINNM)*.

BMY-13754; MJ-13754-1.

CAS — 83366-66-9 (nefazodone); 82752-99-6 (nefazodone hydrochloride).

Adverse Effects and Treatment

The most common adverse effects seen with nefazodone are weakness, dry mouth, nausea, constipation, somnolence, dizziness, and lightheadedness. Other effects which have occurred less frequently include chills, fever, orthostatic hypotension, vasodilatation, arthralgia, paraesthesia, confusion, memory impairment, abnormal dreams, ataxia, and amblyopia and other visual disturbances. Syncope has occurred rarely.

Hyponatraemia possibly due to inappropriate secretion of antidiuretic hormone has been associated with the use of antidepressants, particularly in the elderly.

In overdosage, the symptoms that have been reported most frequently include hypotension, nausea, vomiting, and drowsiness. Treatment of overdosage involves gastric lavage followed by symptomatic and supportive therapy.

Precautions

Nefazodone should be used with caution in patients with epilepsy, a history of hypomania or mania, severe renal impairment, or hepatic impairment and those with a recent history of myocardial infarction or unstable heart disease. It should also be used with caution in cardiovascular or cerebrovascular disease that could be exacerbated by hypotension, and in any condition such as dehydration or hypovolaemia that may predispose patients to hypotension.

Priapism has been associated with trazodone (see p.309), to which nefazodone is structurally related, and the manufacturer recommends that any patient developing inappropriate or prolonged penile erections should discontinue nefazodone immediately.

Patients should be closely monitored during early antidepressant therapy until improvement in depression is observed because suicide is an inherent risk in depressed patients. For further details, see under Depression, p.271. Nefazodone may impair performance of skilled tasks and, if affected, patients should not drive or operate machinery.

Antidepressants should be withdrawn gradually to reduce the risk of withdrawal symptoms.

Interactions

Nefazodone should not be given to patients receiving MAOIs or for at least 14 days after their discontinuation; it has also been recommended that any drug liable to provoke a serious reaction (e.g. phenelzine) should not be given within one week after discontinuation of nefazodone therapy. For further details on the coadministration of antidepressants, see Antidepressants under Interactions of Phenelzine, p.305.

Orthostatic hypotension can be a problem with nefazodone, and therefore a reduction in dose of antihypertensive drugs administered concomitantly may be required.

Nefazodone is an inhibitor of the cytochrome P450 isoenzyme responsible for the metabolism of the triazolobenzodiazepines, alprazolam and triazolam, and consequently produces clinically important increases in their plasma concentrations. The potential also exists for increased plasma concentrations of astemizole, cisapride, and terfenadine (which are metabolised by the same isoenzyme), and therefore there is a risk of inducing ventricular arrhythmias.

Plasma concentrations of digoxin are increased by the concomitant administration of nefazodone and it is recommended that, because of digoxin's narrow therapeutic index, plasma concentrations of digoxin should be monitored if coadministration with nefazodone is necessary. The potential for interaction between nefazodone and general anaesthetics exists and the manufacturer recommends that nefazodone should be stopped before elective surgery for as long as clinically feasible.

Pharmacokinetics

Nefazodone is readily absorbed from the gastro-intestinal tract and peak plasma concentrations have been obtained 1 to 3 hours after oral administration. Absorption is delayed and reduced by food but this is not considered to be clinically significant. Nefazodone undergoes extensive first-pass metabolism and is more than 99% bound to plasma proteins; it is widely distributed. It is extensively metabolised by N-dealkylation and hydroxylation in the liver to several metabolites, two of which are known to be pharmacologically active, hydroxynefazodone and *m*-chlorophenylpiperazine. Excretion is via the urine (approximately 55%) and the faeces (20 to 30%), predominately as metabolites in both cases. The plasma elimination half-life is 2 to 4 hours. Pharmacokinetic parameters are reported to be non-linear with increasing doses.

Reviews.

1. Greene DS, Barbhaiya RH. Clinical pharmacokinetics of nefazodone. *Clin Pharmacokinet* 1997; **33:** 260–75.

Uses and Administration

Nefazodone is a phenylpiperazine antidepressant structurally related to trazodone (see p.308). It blocks the reuptake of serotonin at presynaptic neurones and is an antagonist at postsynaptic 5-HT_2 receptors. Unlike trazodone, nefazodone inhibits the reuptake of noradrenaline. It blocks α_1-adrenoceptors but has no apparent effect on dopamine receptors. Nefazodone does not appear to have very significant antimuscarinic properties compared with tricyclic antidepressants.

Nefazodone is given by mouth as the hydrochloride for the treatment of depression in a usual initial dose of 50 to 100 mg twice daily, increased after 5 to 7 days to 200 mg twice daily. The dose may be increased gradually, if necessary, to a maximum of 300 mg twice daily. Elderly patients, especially females, may have higher plasma concentrations than other patients and a maximal therapeutic effect is usually achieved at doses of 100 to 200 mg twice daily. Initial doses should be restricted to 50 mg twice daily. Doses should be restricted to the lower end of the range in patients with hepatic or severe renal impairment.

Antidepressants should be withdrawn gradually to reduce the risk of withdrawal symptoms.

Reviews.

1. Ellingrod VL, Perry PJ. Nefazodone: a new antidepressant. *Am J Health-Syst Pharm* 1995; **52:** 2799–2812.

Anxiety disorders. Data from a preliminary study[1] involving 14 patients have suggested that nefazodone might be of benefit in panic disorder and panic disorder associated with depression or generalized anxiety. The overall management of panic disorder and other anxiety disorders is discussed on p.635.

1. DeMartinis NA, *et al.* An open-label trial of nefazodone in high comorbidity panic disorder. *J Clin Psychiatry* 1996; **57:** 245–8.

Depression. As discussed on p.271, there is very little difference in efficacy between the different groups of antidepressant drugs, and choice is often made on the basis of adverse effect profile. Nefazodone has a different biochemical profile from both the tricyclics and the SSRIs.

References.

1. Feiger A, *et al.* Nefazodone versus sertraline, in outpatients with major depression: focus an efficacy, tolerability, and effects on sexual function and satisfaction. *J Clin Psychiatry* 1996; **57** (suppl 2): 53–62.
2. Rickels K, *et al.* Nefazodone and imipramine in major depression: a placebo-controlled trial. *Br J Psychiatry* 1994; **164:** 802–5.
3. Fontaine R, *et al.* A double-blind comparison of nefazodone, imipramine, and placebo in major depression. *J Clin Psychiatry* 1994; **55:** 234–41.
4. Ansseau M, *et al.* Controlled comparison of nefazodone and amitriptyline in major depressive inpatients. *Psychopharmacology (Berl)* 1994; **115:** 254–60.
5. Anonymous. Nefazodone for depression. *Med Lett Drugs Ther* 1995; **37:** 33–4.
6. Baldwin DS, *et al.* A multicenter double-blind comparison of nefazodone and paroxetine in the treatment of outpatients with moderate-to-severe depression. *J Clin Psychiatry* 1996; **57** (suppl 2): 46–52.
7. Anonymous. Three new antidepressants. *Drug Ther Bull* 1996; **34:** 65–8.
8. Cyr M, Brown CS. Nefazodone: its place among antidepressants. *Ann Pharmacother* 1996; **30:** 1006–12.
9. Davis R, *et al.* Nefazodone: a review of its pharmacology and clinical efficacy in the management of major depression. *Drugs* 1997; **53:** 608–36.

Premenstrual syndrome. Nefazodone in doses ranging from 100 to 600 mg daily throughout the menstrual cycle has produced beneficial effects in an open study[1] involving 54 women with premenstrual syndrome (p.1456).

1. Freeman EW, *et al.* Nefazodone in the treatment of premenstrual syndrome: a preliminary study. *J Clin Psychopharmacol* 1994; **14:** 180–6.

Preparations

Proprietary Preparations (details are given in Part 3)
Austral.: Serzone; ***Canad.:*** Serzone; ***Irl.:*** Dutonin; ***Ital.:*** Reseril; ***Neth.:*** Dutonin; ***Norw.:*** Nefadar; ***S.Afr.:*** Serzone; ***Swed.:*** Nefadar; ***UK:*** Dutonin; ***USA:*** Serzone.

Nialamide (2528-c)

Nialamide *(BAN, rINN).*

N'-(2-Benzylcarbamoylethyl)isonicotinohydrazide.

$C_{16}H_{18}N_4O_2$ = 298.3.

CAS — 51-12-7.

Nialamide, a hydrazine derivative, is an irreversible inhibitor of monoamine oxidase types A and B (see Phenelzine, p.302). Nialamide is used in the treatment of depression, but as discussed on p.271, the risks associated with irreversible, non-selective MAOIs usually mean that other antidepressants are preferred. It is given in usual initial doses of 150 to 200 mg daily by mouth. The dose is adjusted according to response; usual maintenance doses are 75 to 150 mg daily. In severe depression doses of up to 300 mg daily may be given.

Nialamide should be withdrawn gradually to reduce the risk of withdrawal symptoms.

Preparations

Proprietary Preparations (details are given in Part 3)
Belg.: Niamid; ***Fr.:*** Niamide†.

Nomifensine Maleate (2529-k)

Nomifensine Maleate *(BANM, USAN, rINNM).*

36-984; Hoe-984. 1,2,3,4-Tetrahydro-2-methyl-4-phenylisoquinolin-8-ylamine maleate.

$C_{16}H_{18}N_2,C_4H_4O_4$ = 354.4.

CAS — 24526-64-5 (nomifensine); 32795-47-4 (nomifensine maleate).

Nomifensine maleate is a tetrahydroisoquinoline compound formerly used in the treatment of depression. Nomifensine maleate was withdrawn worldwide in January 1986 due to the risk of acute haemolytic anaemia with intravascular haemolysis. In some cases, renal failure also developed.

References.

1. Anonymous. Hoechst withdraws Merital: 'risks no longer outweighed by benefits'. *Pharm J* 1986; **236:** 113.
2. Committee on Safety of Medicines. CSM update: withdrawal of nomifensine. *Br Med J* 1986; **293:** 41.

Nortriptyline Hydrochloride

(2530-w)

Nortriptyline Hydrochloride *(BANM, USAN, rINNM).*

38489; Nortriptylini Hydrochloridum. 3-(10,11-Dihydro-5*H*-dibenzo[*a,d*]cyclohepten-5-ylidene)propyl(methyl)amine hydrochloride.

$C_{19}H_{21}N,HCl$ = 299.8.

CAS — 72-69-5 (nortriptyline); 894-71-3 (nortriptyline hydrochloride).

Pharmacopoeias. In *Eur.* (see p.viii), *Jpn,* and *US.*

A white or off-white powder with a slight characteristic odour. Nortriptyline hydrochloride 22.8 mg is approximately equivalent to 20 mg of nortriptyline.

Soluble 1 in 90 of water, 1 in 30 of alcohol, 1 in 20 of chloroform, and 1 in 10 of methyl alcohol; soluble in dichloromethane; practically insoluble in ether and in most other organic solvents. A 1% solution in water has a pH of about 5. **Store** in airtight containers. Protect from light.

Adverse Effects, Treatment, and Precautions

As for tricyclic antidepressants in general (see Amitriptyline, p.273).

Effects on ventilation. Severe hyperventilation developed in a 61-year-old man with end-stage renal disease after receiving nortriptyline 125 mg daily;[1] mechanical ventilation was necessary to correct severe respiratory alkalosis.

1. Sunderrajan S, *et al.* Nortriptyline-induced severe hyperventilation. *Arch Intern Med* 1985; **145:** 746–7.

Porphyria. Nortriptyline was considered to be unsafe in patients with acute porphyria, although there is conflicting experimental evidence of porphyrinogenicity.[1]

1. Moore MR, McColl KEL. *Porphyria: drug lists.* Glasgow: Porphyria Research Unit, University of Glasgow, 1991.

Interactions

For interactions associated with tricyclic antidepressants, see Amitriptyline, p.276.

Pharmacokinetics

Nortriptyline is the principal active metabolite of amitriptyline (p.277). Nortriptyline has been reported to have a longer plasma half-life than amitriptyline. Nortriptyline is subject to extensive first-pass metabolism in the liver to 10-hydroxynortriptyline, which is active.

Metabolism. There is evidence that individuals with a slow debrisoquine hydroxylation phenotype may be at greater risk of confusional states when taking nortriptyline.[1] This was thought to be because the polymorphic hydroxylation of debrisoquine and nortriptyline are mediated by similar enzymatic mechanisms, with slow oxidizers having higher plasma nortriptyline concentrations.[2,3] Jerling and Alván[4] observed during therapeutic drug monitoring that there was a nonlinear (dose-dependent) relationship between dose and plasma-nortriptyline concentrations in subjects who were considered to be extensive metabolisers of debrisoquine; nonlinearity did not appear to occur in poor metabolisers. There was no significant correlation between hydroxylation phenotype and amitriptyline concentrations, suggesting that demethylation and hydroxylation of tricyclic antidepressants are mediated by different cytochrome P-450 isoenzymes.[5]

The pharmacokinetics and pharmacological actions of 10-hydroxynortriptyline, the major active metabolite of nortriptyline, have been reviewed.[3]

1. Park BK, Kitteringham NR. Adverse reactions and drug metabolism. *Adverse Drug React Bull* 1987; **122:** 456–9.
2. Nordin C, *et al.* Plasma concentrations of nortriptyline and its 10-hydroxy metabolite in depressed patients—relationship to the debrisoquine hydroxylation metabolic ratio. *Br J Clin Pharmacol* 1985; **19:** 832–5.
3. Nordin C, Bertilsson L. Active hydroxymetabolites of antidepressants: emphasis on E-10-hydroxy-nortriptyline. *Clin Pharmacokinet* 1995; **28:** 26–40.
4. Jerling M, Alván G. Nonlinear kinetics of nortriptyline in relation to nortriptyline clearance as observed during therapeutic drug monitoring. *Eur J Clin Pharmacol* 1994; **46:** 67–70.
5. Bertilsson L, *et al.* Metabolism of various drugs in subjects with different debrisoquine and sparteine oxidation phenotypes. *Br J Clin Pharmacol* 1982; **14:** 602P.

Plasma concentrations. Nortriptyline appears to have a specific therapeutic window between 50 and 150 ng per mL within which favourable antidepressant responses occur. Above and below this specific plasma concentration range, there is a poor clinical response. Plasma concentration measurements were unequivocally useful in problem patients who did not respond to usual oral doses or in high-risk patients who, because of age or medical illness, would best be treated with the lowest possible effective dose of the drug.[1]

It has been suggested[2] that within this window of total nortriptyline concentrations there is a probability of an antidepressant response of 68% or more with free concentrations of 7 to 10 ng per mL.

For reference to dose-dependent kinetics of nortriptyline observed in individuals with a fast debrisoquine hydroxylation phenotype, see under Metabolism, above.

1. Task Force on the Use of Laboratory Tests in Psychiatry. Tricyclic antidepressants—blood level measurements and clinical outcome: an APA task force report. *Am J Psychiatry* 1985; **142:** 155–62.
2. Perry PJ, *et al.* The relationship of free nortriptyline levels to antidepressant response. *Drug Intell Clin Pharm* 1984; **18:** 510.

Uses and Administration

Nortriptyline is a dibenzocycloheptadiene tricyclic antidepressant with actions and uses similar to those of amitriptyline (p.278). It is the principal active metabolite of amitriptyline. Nortriptyline is one of the less sedating tricyclics and its antimuscarinic effects are mild.

In the treatment of depression nortriptyline is given by mouth as the hydrochloride starting with a low dose and gradually increasing to the equivalent of nortriptyline 75 to 100 mg daily in divided doses. Up to a maximum of 150 mg daily may be required in patients with severe depression. The manufacturers recommend that plasma concentrations of nortriptyline should be monitored when doses above 100 mg daily are given. Adolescents and the elderly may be given 30 to 50 mg daily in divided doses. Since nortriptyline has a prolonged half-life, once-daily dosage regimens are also suitable, usually given at night.

Nortriptyline is also used for the treatment of nocturnal enuresis in children in whom organic pathology has been excluded. However, drug therapy for nocturnal enuresis should be reserved for those in whom other methods have failed and should preferably only be given to cover periods away from home; tricyclic antidepressants are not recommended in children under 6 years of age (some authorities recommend that they should not be given until 7 years of age). Suggested doses are 10 mg for children aged 6 to 7 years, 10 to 20 mg for children aged 8 to 11 years, and 25 to 35 mg for children aged over 11 years. The dose should be given 30 minutes before bedtime and treatment should not continue for longer than 3 months, which should include a period of gradual withdrawal. A full physical examination is recommended before a further course.

Nortriptyline should be withdrawn gradually to reduce the risk of withdrawal symptoms.

Depression. As discussed on p.271, there is very little difference in efficacy between the different groups of antidepressant drugs, and choice is often made on the basis of adverse effect profile. Tricyclic antidepressants such as nortriptyline have traditionally been the first choice for the treatment of depression, and often still are because of wide experience with their use and familiarity with their pharmacological actions. Nortriptyline is one of the less sedating tricyclics and consequently may be of value for withdrawn or apathetic depressed patients.

Micturition disorders. See under Amitriptyline, p.278.

Pathological crying or laughing. See under Amitriptyline, p.279.

Preparations

BP 1998: Nortriptyline Capsules; Nortriptyline Tablets;
USP 23: Nortriptyline Hydrochloride Capsules; Nortriptyline Hydrochloride Oral Solution.

Proprietary Preparations (details are given in Part 3)
Aust.: Nortrilen; ***Austral.:*** Allegron; Nortab†; ***Belg.:*** Nortrilen; ***Canad.:*** Aventyl; ***Ger.:*** Nortrilen; ***Irl.:*** Aventyl; ***Ital.:*** Noritren; Vividyl; ***Neth.:*** Nortrilen; ***Norw.:*** Noritren; ***S.Afr.:*** Aventyl; ***Spain:*** Martimil; Paxtibi; ***Swed.:*** Noritren†; Sensaval; ***Switz.:*** Nortrilen; ***UK:*** Allegron; Aventyl†; ***USA:*** Aventyl; Pamelor.

Multi-ingredient: ***Fr.:*** Motival; ***Ger.:*** Benpon†; ***Irl.:*** Motipress; Motival; ***Ital.:*** Dominans; ***S.Afr.:*** Motival; ***Spain:*** Norfenazin; Tropargal; ***UK:*** Motipress; Motival.

Opipramol Hydrochloride (2532-l)

Opipramol Hydrochloride *(BANM, USAN, rINNM)*.

G-33040. 2-[4-(3-5*H*-Dibenz[*b,f*]azepin-5-ylpropyl)piperazin-1-yl]ethanol dihydrochloride.

$C_{23}H_{29}N_3O,2HCl = 436.4$.

CAS — 315-72-0 (opipramol); 909-39-7 (opipramol dihydrochloride).

Pharmacopoeias. In *Pol.*

Opipramol is a tricyclic antidepressant (see Amitriptyline, p.273). Opipramol hydrochloride is given by mouth in doses of 50 to 300 mg daily in the treatment of depression.

Opipramol should be withdrawn gradually to reduce the risk of withdrawal symptoms.

Preparations

Proprietary Preparations (details are given in Part 3)
Aust.: Insidon; ***Belg.:*** Insidon; ***Fr.:*** Insidon; ***Ger.:*** Insidon; ***Irl.:*** Insidon; ***Ital.:*** Insidon; ***Neth.:*** Insidon; ***Norw.:*** Insidon†; ***Swed.:*** Ensidon†; ***Switz.:*** Insidon.

Oxaflozane Hydrochloride (2295-z)

Oxaflozane Hydrochloride *(rINNM)*.

1766-Cerm (oxaflozane); CERM-1766 (oxaflozane). 4-Isopropyl-2-(α,α,α-trifluoro-*m*-tolyl)morpholine hydrochloride.

$C_{14}H_{18}F_3NO,HCl = 309.8$.

CAS — 26629-87-8 (oxaflozane); 26629-86-7 (oxaflozane hydrochloride).

Oxaflozane hydrochloride is an antidepressant given by mouth in doses of 15 to 30 mg daily; a suggested initial dose for elderly patients is 7.5 mg daily.

Preparations

Proprietary Preparations (details are given in Part 3)
Fr.: Conflictan.

Oxaprotiline Hydrochloride (13054-f)

Oxaprotiline Hydrochloride *(USAN, rINNM)*.

C-49802B-Ba. (±)-α-[(Methylamino)methyl]-9,10-ethanoanthracene-9(10*H*)-ethanol hydrochloride.

$C_{20}H_{23}NO,HCl = 329.9$.

CAS — 56433-44-4 (oxaprotiline); 39022-39-4 (oxaprotiline hydrochloride).

Oxaprotiline hydrochloride, a hydroxylated derivative of maprotiline hydrochloride (p.296), is a tetracyclic antidepressant.

References.

1. Roffman M, *et al.* A double-blind comparative study of oxaprotiline with amitriptyline and placebo in moderate depression. *Curr Ther Res* 1982; **32:** 247–56.
2. Giedke H, *et al.* Amitriptyline and oxaprotiline in the treatment of hospitalized depressive patients: clinical aspects, psychophysiology, and drug plasma levels. *Eur Arch Psychiatry Neurol Sci* 1986; **235:** 329–38.
3. Emrich HM, *et al.* Serotonin reuptake inhibition vs. norepinephrine reuptake inhibition: a double-blind differential-therapeutic study with fluvoxamine and oxaprotiline in endogenous and neurotic depressives. *Pharmacopsychiatry* 1987; **20:** 60–3.
4. Schmauss M, *et al.* Oxaprotiline versus maprotiline in inpatients with endogenous depression: a double-blind, controlled study. *Curr Ther Res* 1987; **41:** 342–50.

Oxitriptan (12836-r)

Oxitriptan *(rINN)*.

5-HTP; L-5-Hydroxytryptophan; Ro-0783/B. L-2-Amino-3-(5-hydroxy-1*H*-indol-3-yl)propionic acid.

$C_{11}H_{12}N_2O_3 = 220.2$.

CAS — 4350-09-8 (oxitriptan); 56-69-9 (DL-5-hydroxytryptophan).

Oxitriptan is the L form of 5-hydroxytryptophan, a precursor of serotonin. Like tryptophan (p.310) it is used in the treatment of depression; it is given in doses of up to 600 mg daily by mouth.

Oxitriptan is also used in myoclonic disorders especially posthypoxic myoclonus (p.338). It has also been employed in various neurological conditions including migraine, pain syndromes, and sleep disorders, and as an adjunct in epilepsy and parkinsonism.

DL-Oxitriptan has also been used as an antidepressant.

Preparations

Proprietary Preparations (details are given in Part 3)
Fr.: Levotonine; ***Ger.:*** Levothym; ***Ital.:*** Oxyfan; Serotonyl†; Serovit†; Trimag†; Tript-OH; Triptene†; ***Spain:*** Cincofarm; Telesol; ***Switz.:*** Tript-OH; Triptum†.

Paroxetine Hydrochloride (18670-k)

Paroxetine Hydrochloride *(BANM, rINNM)*.

BRL-29060 (paroxetine); BRL-29060A (paroxetine hydrochloride); FG-7051 (paroxetine). (−)-*trans*-5-(4-*p*-Fluorophenyl-3-piperidylmethoxy)-1,3-benzodioxole hydrochloride.

$C_{19}H_{20}FNO_3,HCl = 365.8$.

CAS — 61869-08-7 (paroxetine); 78246-49-8 (paroxetine hydrochloride).

NOTE. Paroxetine is *USAN*.

Paroxetine hydrochloride 22.2 mg is approximately equivalent to 20 mg of paroxetine.

Adverse Effects, Treatment, and Precautions

As for selective serotonin reuptake inhibitors (SSRIs) in general (see Fluoxetine, p.284).

Extrapyramidal reactions (including orofacial dystonias) and withdrawal symptoms associated with paroxetine have been reported to the Committee on Safety of Medicines in the UK more commonly than with other SSRIs. For further details, see Extrapyramidal Effects under Adverse Effects of Fluoxetine, p.285 and Withdrawal under Precautions, p.286.

There is a potential for worsening of panic symptoms during the initial treatment of panic disorder with paroxetine.

Interactions

For interactions associated with selective serotonin reuptake inhibitors (SSRIs), see Fluoxetine, p.286.

Pharmacokinetics

Paroxetine is readily absorbed from the gastro-intestinal tract with peak plasma concentrations occurring within about 5 hours of ingestion. It undergoes extensive first-pass metabolism in the liver. The main metabolic pathway is oxidation followed by methylation and formation of glucuronide and sulphate conjugates. Paroxetine is widely distributed throughout body tissues and is about 95% bound to plasma proteins. The elimination half-life of paroxetine is reported to be about 21 hours. Excretion is via the urine (approximately 64%) and the faeces (approximately 36%), mainly as metabolites in both cases. Paroxetine is distributed into breast milk.

References.

1. Dalhoff K, *et al.* Pharmacokinetics of paroxetine in patients with cirrhosis. *Eur J Clin Pharmacol* 1991; **41:** 351–4.

Uses and Administration

Paroxetine, a phenylpiperidine derivative, is a selective serotonin reuptake inhibitor (SSRI) with actions and uses similar to those of fluoxetine (p.287). Paroxetine is given by mouth as paroxetine hydrochloride, usually in the morning as a single dose with food. Doses are expressed in terms of paroxetine.

In the treatment of depression, the usual dose of paroxetine is 20 mg daily, increased gradually, if necessary, by increments of 10 mg to a maximum of 50 mg daily.

In the treatment of obsessive-compulsive disorder, the initial dose is 20 mg daily increased weekly in 10-mg increments to a usual maintenance dose of 40 mg daily; some patients may require up to 60 mg daily.

In the treatment of panic disorder with or without agoraphobia, the initial dose is 10 mg daily increased weekly in 10-mg increments according to clinical response; the usual recommended maintenance dose is 40 mg daily, although some patients may benefit from 60 mg daily. The initial dose for the treatment of social phobia is 20 mg daily increased after 2 weeks if necessary by increments of 10 mg at weekly intervals to a maximum of 50 mg daily.

A suggested maximum daily dose in elderly or debilitated patients is 40 mg. A recommended dose in the UK for patients with severe renal or severe hepatic impairment is 20 mg daily; incremental dosage if required should be restricted to the lower end of the range.

Paroxetine should be withdrawn gradually to reduce the risk of withdrawal symptoms. For further details, see Withdrawal under Precautions of Fluoxetine, p.286.

Reviews.

1. Dechant KL, Clissold SP. Paroxetine: a review of its pharmacodynamic and pharmacokinetic properties and therapeutic potential in depressive illness. *Drugs* 1991; **41:** 225–53.
2. Grimsley SR, Jann MW. Paroxetine, sertraline, and fluvoxamine: new selective serotonin reuptake inhibitors. *Clin Pharm* 1992; **11:** 930–57.
3. Anonymous. Paroxetine for treatment of depression. *Med Lett Drugs Ther* 1993; **35:** 24–5.
4. Caley CF, Weber SS. Paroxetine: a selective serotonin reuptake inhibiting antidepressant. *Ann Pharmacother* 1993; **27:** 1212–22.
5. Gunasekara NS, *et al.* Paroxetine: an update of its pharmacology and therapeutic use in depression and a review of its use in other disorders. *Drugs* 1998; **55:** 85–120.

Anxiety disorders. Paroxetine has been given in a variety of anxiety disorders (p.635) including obsessive-compulsive disorder, panic disorder, and social phobia. It has also been tried for adult night terrors.

References.

1. Oehrberg S, *et al.* Paroxetine in the treatment of panic disorder: a randomised, double-blind, placebo-controlled study. *Br J Psychiatry* 1995; **167:** 374–9.
2. Stein MB, *et al.* Paroxetine in the treatment of generalized social phobia: open-label treatment and double-blind placebo-controlled discontinuation. *J Clin Psychopharmacol* 1996; **16:** 218–22.
3. Zohar J, *et al.* Paroxetine versus clomipramine in the treatment of obsessive-compulsive disorder. *Br J Psychiatry* 1996; **169:** 468–74.
4. Lecrubier Y, *et al.* Long-term evaluation of paroxetine, clomipramine and placebo in panic disorder. *Acta Psychiatr Scand* 1997; **95:** 153–60.

5. Wilson SJ, *et al.* Adult night terrors and paroxetine. *Lancet* 1997; **350:** 185.
6. Stein MB, *et al.* Paroxetine treatment of generalized social phobia (social anxiety disorder). *JAMA* 1998; **280:** 708–13.

Depression. As discussed on p.271, there is very little difference in efficacy between the different groups of antidepressant drugs, and choice is often made on the basis of adverse effect profile. Selective serotonin reuptake inhibitors (SSRIs) such as paroxetine are increasingly being recognised as first-choice treatment because they offer advantages over the older tricyclics in terms of fewer unpleasant side-effects and safety in overdosage.

References.

1. De Wilde J, *et al.* A double-blind, comparative, multicentre study comparing paroxetine with fluoxetine in depressed patients. *Acta Psychiatr Scand* 1993; **87:** 141–5.
2. Arminen S-L, *et al.* A 12-week double-blind multi-centre study of paroxetine and imipramine in hospitalized depressed patients. *Acta Psychiatr Scand* 1994; **89:** 382–9.
3. Ansseau M, *et al.* Controlled comparison of paroxetine and fluvoxamine in major depression. *Hum Psychopharmacol Clin Exp* 1994; **9:** 329–36.
4. Montgomery SA, *et al.* Reduction of suicidal thoughts with paroxetine in comparison with reference antidepressants and placebo. *Eur Neuropsychopharmacol* 1995; **5:** 5–13.
5. Geretsegger C, *et al.* Multicenter double blind study of paroxetine and amitriptyline in elderly depressed inpatients. *Psychopharmacology (Berl)* 1995; **119:** 277–81.
6. Leyman S, *et al.* Paroxetine: post-marketing experience on 4024 depressed patients in Belgium. *Eur J Clin Res* 1995; **7:** 287–96.
7. Rodríguez-Ramos P, *et al.* Effects of paroxetine in depressed adolescents. *Eur J Clin Res* 1996; **8:** 49–61.
8. Schnyder U, Koller-Leiser A. A double-blind, multicentre study of paroxetine and maprotiline in major depression. *Can J Psychiatry* 1996; **41:** 239–44.
9. Moon C, Vince M. Treatment of major depression in general practice: a double-blind comparison of paroxetine and lofepramine. *Br J Clin Pract* 1996; **50:** 240–4.

Premenstrual syndrome. Paroxetine in doses ranging from 10 to 30 mg daily throughout the menstrual cycle has produced beneficial effects in controlling both the psychological and somatic symptoms of women with premenstrual syndrome;[1] it was more effective than the tetracyclic antidepressant maprotiline, a noradrenaline reuptake inhibitor.

For a discussion of the overall management of premenstrual syndrome, see p.1456.

1. Eriksson E, *et al.* The serotonin reuptake inhibitor paroxetin is superior to the noradrenaline reuptake inhibitor maprotiline in the treatment of premenstrual syndrome. *Neuropsychopharmacology* 1995; **12:** 167–76.

Sexual dysfunction. Impotence or ejaculatory problems have been reported as adverse effects of selective serotonin reuptake inhibitors (SSRIs) (see Effects on Sexual Function in Adverse Effects of Fluoxetine, p.285). Such properties of the SSRIs have been studied as a potential form of treatment for men with premature ejaculation. Paroxetine was found to be effective in delaying premature ejaculation in a study involving 17 patients with primary (lifelong) or a history of at least 2 years' premature ejaculation.[1]

1. Waldinger MD, *et al.* Paroxetine treatment of premature ejaculation: a double-blind, randomized, placebo-controlled study. *Am J Psychiatry* 1994; **151:** 1377–9.

Preparations

Proprietary Preparations (details are given in Part 3)
Aust.: Seroxat; ***Austral.:*** Aropax; ***Belg.:*** Aropax; Seroxat; ***Canad.:*** Paxil; ***Fr.:*** Deroxat; ***Ger.:*** Seroxat; Tagonis; ***Irl.:*** Seroxat; ***Ital.:*** Sereupin; Seroxat; ***Neth.:*** Seroxat; ***Norw.:*** Seroxat; ***S.Afr.:*** Aropax; ***Spain:*** Aropax†; Frosinor; Motivan; Seroxat; ***Swed.:*** Seroxat; ***Switz.:*** Deroxat; ***UK:*** Seroxat; ***USA:*** Paxil.

Phenelzine Sulphate (2533-y)

Phenelzine Sulphate (*BANM, pINNM*).

Phenelzine Sulfate. Phenethylhydrazine hydrogen sulphate.

$C_8H_{12}N_2,H_2SO_4 = 234.3.$

CAS — 51-71-8 (phenelzine); 156-51-4 (phenelzine sulphate).

Pharmacopoeias. In *Br.* and *US.*

A white to yellowish-white powder or pearly platelets with a pungent odour. Phenelzine sulphate 25.8 mg is approximately equivalent to 15 mg of phenelzine.

Freely **soluble** in water; practically insoluble in alcohol, in chloroform, and in ether. A 1% solution in water has a pH of between 1.4 and 1.9. **Store** in airtight containers. Protect from heat and light.

Adverse Effects

Adverse effects commonly associated with phenelzine and other MAOIs include orthostatic hypotension and attacks of dizziness. Other common side-effects include headache, dryness of the mouth, constipation and other gastro-intestinal disturbances (including nausea and vomiting), and oedema. Drowsiness, weakness, and fatigue are reported frequently although CNS stimulation may occur and symptoms include agitation, nervousness, euphoria, restlessness, insomnia, and convulsions. Psychotic episodes, with manic reactions, or toxic delirium, may be induced in susceptible persons.

Sweating and muscle tremors, twitching, or hyperreflexia may occur, which in overdosage may present as extreme hyperpyrexia and neuromuscular irritability. Other reported reactions include blurred vision, urinary retention or difficulty in micturition, skin rashes, leucopenia, sexual disturbances, and weight gain with inappropriate appetite. Jaundice has been reported with hydrazine MAOIs and, on rare occasions, fatal progressive hepatocellular necrosis. Peripheral neuropathies associated with the hydrazine derivatives may be caused by pyridoxine deficiency. Hyponatraemia, possibly due to inappropriate secretion of antidiuretic hormone, has been associated with the use of antidepressants, particularly in the elderly.

Symptoms of overdosage may be mild initially and progress over the ensuing 24 to 48 hours. Following mild overdosage and symptomatic and supportive therapy recovery may occur in 3 to 4 days, but following massive overdosage symptoms may persist for up to 2 weeks. Symptoms of CNS depression including drowsiness have been observed with overdosage, but CNS stimulation is more common and is manifested by irritability, hyperactivity, agitation, hallucinations, or convulsions. Respiratory depression and coma may ultimately occur. Cardiovascular effects include hypertension, sometimes with severe headache, although hypotension is more frequently observed; cardiac arrhythmias and peripheral collapse can also develop. Profuse sweating, hyperpyrexia, and neuromuscular excitation with hyperreflexia are also prominent features of overdosage.

MAOIs have been the most commonly implicated drugs in the serotonin syndrome (see below). A severe hypertensive crisis, sometimes fatal, may occur if an MAOI is given simultaneously with some other drugs or certain foods (see Interactions, below). These reactions are characterised by severe headache and a rapid and sometimes prolonged rise in blood pressure followed by intracranial haemorrhage or acute cardiac failure.

For the adverse effects of reversible inhibitors of monoamine oxidase type A (RIMAs), see Moclobemide, p.298.

A suspicion that the reported side-effects of MAOIs were both exaggerated and overemphasised prompted a comparative study in patients receiving phenelzine or imipramine.[1] The report noted that the dosages of phenelzine used were at the upper end of the usual therapeutic range (mean 77 mg daily) while those of imipramine were in the middle of the usual therapeutic range (mean 139 mg daily). A very similar profile of side-effects in the two groups was observed. With the exception of significantly increased incidence of drowsiness in the phenelzine-treated group, the 2 groups did not differ in the frequency of autonomic, CNS, cardiovascular, or psychological side-effects. However, a significantly greater number of phenelzine-treated patients had to discontinue their treatment because of the severity of the side-effects. Overall, it was considered that phenelzine was reasonably well-tolerated when compared with imipramine.

Rabkin and colleagues have also studied the side-effect profile of phenelzine and made comparisons with tranylcypromine and imipramine.[2,3] A retrospective review involving 198 patients led them to believe that although phenelzine was more likely than the other two drugs to induce side-effects, drug discontinuation because of side-effects was less likely to occur. This was probably because phenelzine showed clear-cut clinical efficacy resulting in prescribers being reluctant to discontinue therapy.

1. Evans DL, *et al.* Early and late side effects of phenelzine. *J Clin Psychopharmacol* 1982; **2:** 208–10.
2. Rabkin J, *et al.* Adverse reactions to monoamine oxidase inhibitors. Part I: a comparative study. *J Clin Psychopharmacol* 1984; **4:** 270–8.
3. Rabkin JG, *et al.* Adverse reactions to monoamine oxidase inhibitors. Part II: treatment correlates and clinical management. *J Clin Psychopharmacol* 1985; **5:** 2–9.

Effects on the cardiovascular system. MAOIs are generally considered to be relatively free of adverse cardiovascular effects. The hypertensive reaction that may follow interactions of MAOIs with foods or other drugs is well known (see Interactions, below) but it should not be forgotten that orthostatic hypotension may be encountered as a side-effect when these drugs are used on their own.

In one study[1] involving 14 patients it was found that phenelzine produced both a significant decrease in lying systolic blood pressure and significant orthostatic hypotension; in 2 patients these effects on blood pressure necessitated modification of treatment regimens. Differences between the effects of phenelzine and those reported for the tricyclic antidepressants were noted. Tricyclics were not known to affect lying systolic blood pressure and although both tricyclics and phenelzine could cause orthostatic hypotension, that occurring with the tricyclics typically reaches a maximum within the first week of treatment whereas with phenelzine the maximum effect was noted after 4 weeks. Additionally, the study provided some indication that the blood pressure effects of phenelzine may attenuate with time, a phenomenon that is not known to occur with the tricyclics.

1. Kronig MH, *et al.* Blood pressure effects of phenelzine. *J Clin Psychopharmacol* 1983; **3:** 307–10.

Effects on the endocrine system. Drug-induced *hyperprolactinaemia* may result from the administration of MAOIs[1] and this has led to galactorrhoea in women.[2] Occasionally, MAOIs may cause *dilutional hyponatraemia* due to a reduction in the renal excretion of free water mediated by both enhanced vasopressin release and increased antidiuretic action on the renal tubule.[3] The Committee on Safety of Medicines in the UK, commenting on reports[4] it had received of hyponatraemia with antidepressants (fluoxetine, paroxetine, lofepramine, clomipramine, and imipramine), considered that it was likely to occur with any antidepressant and usually involved elderly patients.

1. Slater SL, *et al.* Elevation of plasma-prolactin by monoamine-oxidase inhibitors. *Lancet* 1977; **ii:** 275–6.
2. Segal M, Heys RF. Inappropriate lactation. *Br Med J* 1969; **4:** 236.
3. Baylis PH. Drug-induced endocrine disorders. *Adverse Drug React Bull* 1986; No 116: 432–5.
4. Committee on Safety of Medicines/Medicines Control Agency. Antidepressant-induced hyponatraemia. *Current Problems* 1994; **20:** 5–6.

Effects on the liver. Published case reports of hepatotoxic reactions to MAOIs have included jaundice in 4 patients[1] and hepatic failure progressing to encephalopathy in 2 patients;[2] this latter reaction was attributed to a hypersensitivity reaction.

Of 91 cases of hepatitis associated with antidepressants reported to French pharmacovigilance centres during the years 1977 to 1983 an MAOI (iproniazid) was implicated in 11. These 11 cases were associated with cytolytic reactions and 5 patients died.[3]

Two cases of fulminant hepatic failure have been reported[4] following administration of phenelzine for 4 months; all other causes of acute liver damage were ruled out. Both patients recovered after emergency liver transplantation.

1. Holdsworth CD, *et al.* Hepatitis caused by the newer amine-oxidase-inhibiting drugs. *Lancet* 1961; **ii:** 621–3.
2. Wilkinson SP, *et al.* Frequency and type of renal and electrolyte disorders in fulminant hepatic failure. *Br Med J* 1974; **1:** 186–9.
3. Lefebure B, *et al.* Hépatites aux antidépresseurs. *Therapie* 1984; **39:** 509–16.
4. Gómez-Gil E, *et al.* Phenelzine-induced fulminant hepatic failure. *Ann Intern Med* 1996; **124:** 692–3.

Effects on the nervous system. MAOIs produce a variety of effects on the nervous system. Drowsiness is frequently reported but symptoms of CNS stimulation, including agitation, nervousness, and euphoria may also occur; psychotic episodes may be induced in susceptible individuals. Further adverse neurological reactions are described under Epileptogenic Effect and Extrapyramidal Effects, below.

Peripheral neuropathies, sometimes associated with a documented pyridoxine deficiency, have been reported in patients receiving phenelzine.[1,2] In most of the patients the neuropathies developed 6 weeks to 4 months after the initiation of phenelzine,[2] although in one case symptoms did not occur for 11 years.[1] The symptoms also generally disappeared when pyridoxine was given together with continued phenelzine therapy.[2] The possibility that the dietary restrictions imposed on persons taking phenelzine might have contributed to a low pyridoxine intake was considered unlikely. The most probable mechanism for the induced pyridoxine deficiency was combination of the hydrazine moiety with the pyridoxal form of the vitamin to form an inactive compound.

A considerable number of drugs can inhibit transmission at the myoneural junction under experimental conditions and it has been said that phenelzine may cause postoperative respiratory depression, a common syndrome generally manifesting as a delay in re-establishing spontaneous respiration and perhaps due to a combined action of phenelzine with muscle relaxants.[3] For further details, see Anaesthesia under Precautions, below.

1. Heller CA, Friedman PA. Pyridoxine deficiency and peripheral neuropathy associated with long-term phenelzine therapy. *Am J Med* 1983; **75:** 887–8.
2. Stewart JW, *et al.* Phenelzine-induced pyridoxine deficiency. *J Clin Psychopharmacol* 1984; **4:** 225–6.
3. Lane RJM, Routledge PA. Drug-induced neurological disorders. *Drugs* 1983; **26:** 124–47.

Effects on sexual function. MAOIs such as phenelzine and tranylcypromine have been implicated in producing both impotence and failure of ejaculation.[1,2] Priapism has been reported with phenelzine.[3] There have also been several reports of anorgasmia in women attributed to MAOIs and in a review of these cases it was said that the effect seemed to be dose-related.[4] It should be remembered that loss of libido and impotence are common symptoms of depression, often making the role of drugs in producing sexual dysfunction difficult to assess.

1. Simpson GM, *et al.* Effects of anti-depressants on genito-urinary function. *Dis Nerv Syst* 1965; **26:** 787–9.
2. Wyatt RJ, *et al.* Treatment of intractable narcolepsy with a monoamine oxidase inhibitor. *N Engl J Med* 1971; **285:** 987–91.
3. Yeragani VK, Gershon S. Priapism related to phenelzine therapy. *N Engl J Med* 1987; **317:** 117–18.
4. Shen WW, Sata LS. Inhibited female orgasm resulting from psychotropic drugs: a clinical review. *J Reprod Med* 1983; **28:** 497–9.

Epileptogenic effect. Convulsions represent one of the less common, but nevertheless serious, adverse effects of MAOIs; they may be a feature of overdosage.

A typical grand-mal seizure with tonic-clonic convulsions has been reported in one patient with no history of epilepsy or predisposing factors shortly after the start of phenelzine therapy.[1] The point was made that phenelzine-induced seizures had rarely been observed.

1. Bhugra DK, Kaye N. Phenelzine induced grand mal seizure. *Br J Clin Pract* 1986; **40:** 173–4.

Extrapyramidal effects. A parkinsonian syndrome has been described in one patient who received phenelzine and the mechanisms by which phenelzine could have induced these effects were discussed.[1] The symptoms developed about 5 weeks after the start of therapy and gradually resolved over 10 days following the withdrawal of phenelzine.

1. Gillman MA, Sandyk R. Parkinsonism induced by a monoamine oxidase inhibitor. *Postgrad Med J* 1986; **62:** 235–6.

Lupus. A reversible lupus-like reaction has been reported in one patient who had been taking phenelzine sulphate for 8 months.[1]

1. Swartz C. Lupus-like reaction to phenelzine. *JAMA* 1978; **239:** 2693.

Overdosage. MAOIs in overdose rarely produce severe hypertension; the blood pressure may be high or low, or may alternate between the two. More commonly the patient gradually develops widespread muscle spasms, trismus, and opisthotonus with widely dilated pupils and a hot and sweating skin. By approximately 16 to 24 hours after ingestion body temperature may increase to a point where hyperthermia can be fatal, unless neuromuscular blocking drugs are given; temperatures of 42.1 to 43.8° have been recorded immediately before death. Disseminated intravascular coagulation, rhabdomyolysis, and acute tubular necrosis can also occur. It is recommended that the temperature of a patient who has taken an overdose of an MAOI should be closely monitored, and if the rectal temperature increases to more than 39°, the trachea should be intubated and the patient's lungs ventilated using pancuronium bromide as a neuromuscular blocking drug; this produces a dramatic decrease in temperature.[1]

1. Henry JA. Specific problems of drug intoxication. *Br J Anaesth* 1986; **58:** 223–33.

Serotonin syndrome. The serotonin syndrome most commonly results from an additive adverse effect between two or more drugs that enhance serotonergic activity at central receptors, usually by different mechanisms; the pathogenesis and management have been reviewed.[1-5] MAOIs have been the most commonly implicated drugs in this syndrome, and cases have been reported when MAOIs have been combined with other antidepressants such as the tricyclics, selective serotonin reuptake inhibitors (SSRIs), serotonin and noradrenaline reuptake inhibitors (SNRIs), trazodone, lithium, and tryptophan. MAOIs combined with the opioids dextromethorphan and pethidine have also produced the serotonin syndrome. The interaction can occur with both irreversible and reversible MAOIs, and with those selective for monoamine oxidase type A such as moclobemide as well as with non-selective MAOIs.[6] The selective inhibitor of monoamine oxidase type B, selegiline, may also pose problems at high doses as selectivity starts to diminish. As usage of the newer SSRIs increases, so too has the number of case reports of adverse reactions when these drugs have been combined with other serotonergic drugs.

Other drugs that may potentially cause serotonin syndrome in certain circumstances include buspirone, carbamazepine, and methylenedioxyamphetamine.[2] Rarely, a single serotonergic drug has produced the serotonin syndrome.[3]

Serotonergic potentiation may also occur if one serotonergic drug is administered following another without allowing a sufficient drug-free interval after discontinuation of the first. This is a particular problem when the first drug is an irreversible MAOI or a drug with a long half-life such as the SSRI fluoxetine.

The serotonin syndrome is characterised by the development of at least three of the following clinical features after a recent change in a treatment regimen involving serotonergic drugs: agitation, ataxia, diaphoresis, diarrhoea, fever, hyperreflexia, myoclonus, shivering, and changes in mental status. The onset of the syndrome may occur within minutes of the change, or several weeks later.[3] The occurrence and severity of the syndrome do not appear to be dose-related,[3] and it is distinct from the hypertensive crises produced by the interaction between MAOIs and tyramine (see below), and from the neuroleptic malignant syndrome (see p.651).[4]

The serotonin syndrome is relatively uncommon and in the majority of cases the symptoms are mild. However, severe complications including disseminated intravascular coagulation, severe hyperthermia, respiratory failure, and seizures have been reported; there have also been fatalities, hence the need for great caution when giving serotonergic drugs together. The use of combination therapy with serotonergic antidepressant drugs for the treatment of refractory or drug-resistant depression is discussed below.

Most cases of serotonin syndrome resolve within 24 hours following withdrawal of the offending drugs and administration of supportive therapy.[1-5] Paracetamol and external cooling may be used to reduce fever; development of hyperthermia requires aggressive cooling measures. Benzodiazepines may be of value to control myoclonus and seizures. Serotonin antagonists have been tried as specific drug therapy for the serotonin syndrome. The non-specific antagonists cyproheptadine and methysergide have been tried with some success.[3,4] Other drugs that have been tried but with inconsistent results include propranolol, chlorpromazine, and dantrolene.[3,4]

1. Sternbach H. The serotonin syndrome. *Am J Psychiatry* 1991; **148:** 705–13.
2. Nierenberg DW, Semprebon M. The central nervous system serotonin syndrome. *Clin Pharmacol Ther* 1993; **53:** 84–8.
3. Sporer KA. The serotonin syndrome: implicated drugs, pathophysiology and management. *Drug Safety* 1995; **13:** 94–104.
4. Corkeron MA. Serotonin syndrome—a potentially fatal complication of antidepressant therapy. *Med J Aust* 1995; **163:** 481–2.
5. Brown TM, *et al.* Pathophysiology and management of the serotonin syndrome. *Ann Pharmacother* 1996; **30:** 527–33.
6. Livingston MG. Interactions with selective MAOIs. *Lancet* 1995; **345:** 533–4.

Treatment of Adverse Effects

In cases of overdosage with MAOIs the stomach may be emptied by lavage or emesis. Management then largely involves intensive symptomatic and supportive therapy with particular attention being given to CNS effects, hyperpyrexia which may develop into malignant hyperthermia, and cardiovascular effects. It should not be forgotten that delayed effects, even in patients who are initially asymptomatic, may develop some time after the overdose and therefore prolonged monitoring is warranted. Other drugs taken with an overdose of MAOIs may complicate the features and result in the need for an even longer period of monitoring. Special care should be observed with any drug therapy used in the management of MAOI overdosage in view of the many known interactions which occur with this class of drugs.

Excitation of the CNS may necessitate the use of diazepam. Neuromuscular irritability may call for the use of a neuromuscular blocker such as pancuronium or intubation with assisted ventilation. Hyperpyrexia, which may be a particular problem, may respond to simple antipyretics such as paracetamol and external cooling, but if these measures fail the use of pancuronium has often been advocated; dantrolene has also been suggested. For further details of the treatment of drug-induced hyperthermia, see Fever and Hyperthermia, p.1.

Hypotension, which is a fairly common feature, should be managed by intravenous fluid therapy and volume expansion; vasopressors should be avoided. Conversely, a hypertensive crisis may occasionally occur following an overdose with MAOIs and can be managed with phentolamine given by slow intravenous injection.

Overdosage. Accompanying a case report of MAOI overdosage Linden and co-workers have discussed the pathophysiology of poisoning and the management of such patients.[1]

Good supportive care including correction of abnormalities of neuromuscular activity, temperature, blood pressure, and cardiac rhythm was considered to be the primary treatment. It was stressed that monitoring of asymptomatic patients should be prolonged to rule out the delayed and severe toxicity that is known to have occurred.

CNS excitation and neuromuscular irritability were best managed by diazepam or amylobarbitone if a barbiturate was chosen, phenytoin if seizures developed, and pancuronium if ventilation was impaired by neuromuscular hyperactivity.

It was considered that paracetamol and external cooling may be an effective measure for mild to moderate hyperpyrexia although in severe cases muscle paralysis with pancuronium may become necessary. If any of these measures failed dantrolene or bromocriptine were suggested as drugs that might be employed. Contrary to many other sources these authors did not advocate the use of phenothiazines, such as chlorpromazine, for neuromuscular hyperactivity and hyperpyrexia as the adverse effects of coma, hypotension, and cardiac arrest had been reported following their use.

Quite detailed discussion concerned the choice of drugs for the treatment of various cardiovascular effects. Phentolamine and nitroprusside were preferred for hypertension with beta blockers being a possibility. For hypotension unresponsive to volume expansion it was considered that vasopressors could be used with caution although the risk of precipitating a hypertensive crisis should be borne in mind; a direct-acting drug such as noradrenaline was thought preferable to an indirect-acting vasopressor. However, the usual advice is to avoid the use of vasopressors. Cardiac arrhythmias were said to be difficult to treat and suggestions were given for drugs that may be used in differing types of arrhythmias.

Little evidence was said to be available documenting the efficacy of diuresis or dialysis in reducing toxicity.

For a further comment regarding hyperthermia and the use of pancuronium, see Overdosage under Adverse Effects, above.

1. Linden CH, *et al.* Monoamine oxidase inhibitor overdose. *Ann Emerg Med* 1984; **13:** 1137–44.

Precautions

Phenelzine and other MAOIs should not be given to patients with liver disease or, because of their effects on blood pressure, to patients with cerebrovascular disease or phaeochromocytoma. They should be avoided or only used with great caution in patients with blood disorders or cardiovascular disease. MAOIs should similarly be avoided or used with great caution in elderly or agitated patients who may be particularly susceptible to their adverse effects. They should be given with caution to epileptic patients since they may influence the incidence of seizures and may therefore affect antiepileptic requirements; caution has also been advised in diabetic patients because of conflicting evidence as to whether glucose metabolism is altered or requirements of hypoglycaemics changed. MAOIs should be used with caution, if at all, in patients with hyperthyroidism because of increased sensitivity to pressor amines.

Patients should be closely monitored during early antidepressant therapy until improvement in depression is observed because suicide is an inherent risk in depressed patients. For further details, see under Depression, p.271.

MAOIs are not usually considered a suitable form of therapy for the depressive component of bipolar disorder (manic depression) as mania may be precipitated; similarly psychotic symptoms may be aggravated if they are used for a depressive component of schizophrenia.

MAOIs have a prolonged action so patients should not take any of the foods or drugs known to cause reactions (see below)for at least 14 days after stopping treatment. A similar drug-free period has been advised before any patient undergoes surgery since it may involve the use of drugs that can interact with MAOIs, although not all agree that this is necessary; caution has been advised in patients requiring MAOIs concurrently with electroconvulsive therapy; for further details see under Anaesthesia, below. Patients should carry cards giving details of their MAOI therapy; they and their relatives should be fully conversant with the implications of food and drug interactions and the precautions to be taken.

Patients liable to take charge of vehicles or other machinery should be warned that MAOIs may modify behaviour and state of alertness. Patients affected by drowsiness should not drive or operate machinery.

MAOIs should be withdrawn gradually to reduce the risk of withdrawal symptoms (see below).

For the precautions to be observed with reversible inhibitors of monoamine oxidase A (RIMAs), see Moclobemide, p.298.

Anaesthesia. The considerations given to patients receiving tricyclic antidepressants before receiving anaesthesia for electroconvulsive shock therapy (ECT) or surgery (see Amitriptyline, p.275) are also generally applicable to patients being treated with MAOIs; the manufacturer of phenelzine also warns that cardiovascular depression following ECT has been reported. The interactions of other drugs with MAOIs may be more numerous or more severe than those with tricyclics and the interaction with pethidine should not be forgotten.

Reviewing the potential problems of anaesthesia in patients receiving MAOIs Stack and colleagues have made the following points and comments.[1]

It is often not fully appreciated that the interaction between MAOIs and *opioid analgesics* has two distinct forms: an excitatory form, which may be due to central serotonergic overactivity, characterised by sudden agitation, unmanageable behaviour, headache, hypertension or hypotension, rigidity, hyperpyrexia, convulsions, and coma; and a depressive form consisting of respiratory depression, hypotension, and coma as a result of the inhibition of hepatic microsomal enzymes by the MAOI leading to accumulation of free opioid analgesic. *Pethidine* is the only commonly used opioid analgesic to have elicited the excitatory response which has frequently been severe and often fatal. For this reason, pethidine should never be administered to patients receiving MAOIs. *Morphine* does not block neuronal serotonin uptake but its narcotic effects may be potentiated in the presence of MAOIs and a single case report of the depressive type of reaction has been described. Thus, morphine is the opioid analgesic of choice but must be given in reduced dosage and the dosage carefully titrated against clinical response. *Phenoperidine* is probably best avoided as its metabolites are norpethidine and, to a lesser extent, pethidine. *Papaveretum* would appear to have no advantage over morphine and although interactions of MAOIs with *pentazocine* have occurred in animals, it is not clear if this occurs in man. *Methadone* has been used in a patient without mishap and there is also anecdotal evidence to support the safety of *fentanyl*. A case report[2] described the successful use of *alfentanil* (together with propofol and atracurium) mentioning that this was the first report of such use in patients receiving MAOIs. A further case report[3] described a patient who underwent successful anaesthesia with *sufentanil* (together with thiopentone, lignocaine, and vecuronium) while continuing to take an MAOI (tranylcypromine) as well as a tricyclic antidepressant (imipramine) and lorazepam.

With regard to induction agents,[1] the use of *ketamine* in patients receiving MAOIs should be avoided on theoretical grounds, although no interactions have been reported. Potentiation of *barbiturates* may be expected.

With neuromuscular blocking drugs, phenelzine has been shown to decrease plasma cholinesterase concentration and there have been case reports of a prolonged effect with *suxamethonium*; additionally this prolongation of the effect of suxamethonium may lead to apnoea and modification of the fit during electroconvulsive therapy. There appeared to be a theoretical hazard with *pancuronium bromide* since it releases stored adrenaline, but *alcuronium*, *atracurium*, or *vecuronium* would all appear to be suitable alternatives.

Enflurane, *halothane*, *isoflurane*, and *nitrous oxide* are all safe in the presence of MAOIs, although there is a theoretical possibility of an increased risk of hepatic damage with halothane.

Indirect-acting sympathomimetics pose a serious and possibly lethal hypertensive interaction but *direct-acting sympathomimetics*, such as *adrenaline*, *isoprenaline*, and *noradrenaline*, are reliable vasopressors in the presence of MAOIs although great care should be taken with their use because of enhanced receptor sensitivity.

In conclusion, these reviewers[1] considered that the advice that MAOIs should be stopped about 2 weeks before anaesthesia was unreasonable, as there was a wide range of safe and suitable anaesthetics available, but that the dangers of sympathetic overactivity must always be remembered. This view, that it is safe to continue MAOIs throughout the period of anaesthesia and surgery, has also been advocated by Hirshman and Lindeman[4,5] although others have registered disapproval.[6]

The anaesthetist should be informed of all drugs that the patient is or has been taking; this is particularly important when emergency surgery is required in a patient receiving MAOI therapy.

1. Stack CG, *et al.* Monoamine oxidase inhibitors and anaesthesia: a review. *Br J Anaesth* 1988; **60:** 222–7.
2. Powell H. Use of alfentanil in a patient receiving monoamine oxidase inhibitor therapy. *Br J Anaesth* 1990; **64:** 528.
3. O'Hara JF, *et al.* Sufentanil-isoflurane-nitrous oxide anesthesia for a patient treated with monoamine oxidase inhibitor and tricyclic antidepressant. *J Clin Anesth* 1995; **7:** 148–50.
4. Hirshman CA, Lindeman K. MAO inhibitors: must they be discontinued before anesthesia? *JAMA* 1988; **260:** 3507–8.
5. Hirshman CA, Lindeman KS. Anesthesia and monoamine oxidase inhibitors. *JAMA* 1989; **261:** 3407–8.
6. Gevirtz C. Anesthesia and monoamine oxidase inhibitors. *JAMA* 1989; **261:** 3407.

Driving. While affective disorders probably adversely affect driving skill,[1,2] treatment with antidepressant drugs may also be hazardous,[1] although patients may be safer drivers with medication than without.[2] Impairment of performance is largely related to sedative properties and some MAOIs can adversely affect psychomotor performance.[1,2]

It has been mentioned[2] that the UK Medical Commission on Accident Prevention has recommended that patients on long-term psychotropic medication are unsuitable to be drivers of heavy goods or public service vehicles.

1. Ashton H. Drugs and driving. *Adverse Drug React Bull* 1983; **98:** 360–3.
2. Cremona A. Mad drivers: psychiatric illness and driving performance. *Br J Hosp Med* 1986; **35:** 193–5.

Electroconvulsive therapy. For comments concerning the precautions to be observed in patients receiving electroconvulsive therapy, see under Anaesthesia, above.

Porphyria. Phenelzine was considered to be unsafe in patients with acute porphyria because it has been shown to be porphyrinogenic in *animals*.[1]

1. Moore MR, McColl KEL. *Porphyria: drug lists*. Glasgow: Porphyria Research Unit, University of Glasgow, 1991.

Surgery. For comments regarding the precautions to be observed in patients undergoing surgery, see under Anaesthesia, above.

Withdrawal. Sudden discontinuation of antidepressant therapy after regular administration for 8 weeks or more may precipitate withdrawal symptoms. The symptoms associated with withdrawal of MAOIs[1,2] include gastro-intestinal disturbances and generalised somatic symptoms such as nausea and vomiting, anorexia, chills, headache, and giddiness; sleep disturbances characterised by insomnia, severe nightmares, and somnolence; and a range of CNS symptoms including panic, anxiety, restlessness, agitation, cognitive impairment, mood swings, depression and suicidal ideation, hypomania, delusions, and hallucinations.

The pathophysiology of the MAOI withdrawal syndrome has not been fully elucidated, although it has been hypothesised that some of the symptoms represent adrenergic hyperactivity[1] produced by the release of excessive amounts of dopamine and noradrenaline as a consequence of abrupt discontinuation of MAOI therapy.[2] This withdrawal syndrome may be very severe; some of the symptoms may be ameliorated by reinstitution of the MAOI in low doses, but the best management is considered to be prevention by gradually discontinuing the drug.[2] Some authorities recommend reducing the dose over a period of 4 weeks.

With the exception of tranylcypromine, the withdrawal syndrome of MAOIs is not a consequence of drug dependence.[1] Tranylcypromine has been reported to produce dependence and tolerance in patients receiving high doses irrespective of whether or not they had a previous history of substance abuse. Tranylcypromine is similar in structure to amphetamine which may be responsible for its addictive properties.[1]

1. Anonymous. Problems when withdrawing antidepressives. *Drug Ther Bull* 1986; **24:** 29–30.
2. Dilsaver SC. Withdrawal phenomena associated with antidepressant and antipsychotic agents. *Drug Safety* 1994; **10:** 103–14.

Interactions of MAOIs with Foods

A major disadvantage of MAOIs such as phenelzine is that by inhibiting monoamine oxidase they cause an accumulation of amine neurotransmitters. This means that the pressor effects of *tyramine* (contained in a number of common foods and also metabolised by monoamine oxidase) can be dangerously enhanced. Reactions to foods rich in pressor amines such as tyramine can therefore occur in patients being treated with MAOIs producing hypertensive crises. Cheese, especially aged or matured cheeses, meat or yeast extracts, pickled herrings, smoked foods, and broad bean pods have caused such reactions. Patients should be warned not to eat any of these foods while being treated with an MAOI and for at least 14 days after its discontinuation. Some foods will only cause a reaction if large amounts are eaten, and foods may vary in tyramine content depending upon methods of manufacture and storage. Any protein-containing food such as meat, fish, or game subject to hydrolysis, fermentation, pickling, smoking, or spoilage could contain tyramine derived from tyrosine as a result of these processes or of deterioration. Patients taking MAOIs should therefore be advised to eat protein-containing foods only if fresh.

Alcoholic beverages, including wines, beers, and drinks that are de-alcoholised or are low in alcohol, contain variable amounts of tyramine and are best avoided.

The above dietary restrictions that need to be observed with MAOIs may be less stringent for reversible inhibitors of monoamine oxidase type A (RIMAs) such as moclobemide (see p.299), although the manufacturers recommend that since some patients may be especially sensitive to tyramine, consumption of large amounts of tyramine-rich food should be avoided.

MAOIs can, when taken in conjunction with certain foodstuffs, cause a hypertensive reaction which is sometimes fatal. This effect is accepted and well documented and has led to the publication of many lists of prohibited foods and drinks. Some workers have expressed the opinion that the dangers of the interaction may have been slightly overemphasised or exaggerated and that the published lists may have been overinclusive;[1-3] this may have led to reduced compliance in a number of patients.

Reviewing and discussing the MAOI interaction with tyramine Brown and colleagues[1] made the following observations and recommendations. The hyperadrenergic state resulting from this interaction consisted of three syndromes although significant overlap between them existed: paroxysmal headache of great severity; cardiovascular symptoms with paroxysmal hypertension; and intracerebral haemorrhage and death. The most common offending agent reported had been tranylcypromine at doses of 20 to 50 mg daily although a few reports had involved phenelzine.

Their critical review of the literature led them to suggest that only 4 foodstuffs clearly warranted total prohibition: aged cheese, pickled herring or fish, concentrated yeast extracts, and broad bean pods.

The ingestion of cheese was said to have been associated with 80% of all case reports and with virtually all fatalities. It was agreed that aged cheese should not be permitted, although cottage and cream cheese required no restriction. There was less agreement concerning dairy products such as yoghurt and sour cream and it was suggested that limited amounts were permissible.

Pickled herring or smoked fish were to be avoided because of several well-documented cases of hypertensive crisis as well as detection of high levels of tyramine. Any meat may become dangerous unless consumed while fresh as tyramine is formed from bacterial protein degradation.

Concentrated yeast extracts have a significant tyramine content and yeast vitamin supplements may also constitute a hazard; baker's yeast was considered to be safe.

Broad bean pods contain dopamine although the beans were stated to have little pressor activity and carried no prohibition.

Other foods which had been reported to have caused a hypertensive reaction but for which these authors considered that there was insufficient evidence to warrant dietary restriction were chocolate and caffeine-containing beverages, soy sauce, fresh fish, wild game, and fruits although caution was necessary with avocados and bananas.

Other reviews and lists of foods[2,4] give broadly similar recommendations.

The consumption of alcoholic beverages, and in particular Chianti wine, has frequently been advised against. However, sources have differed with respect to whether particular types of drink (white wine, red wine, spirits, or beer) are safe or not. Hannah, *et al.*[5] demonstrated no significant differences in mean free tyramine concentration between white wine, red wine, Chianti, and beer although within each category of wine there could be up to a fiftyfold variation even if from the same grape stock. Mention has also been made[6,7] that alcohol-free or low-alcohol beers are likely to contain similar amounts of tyramine as alcoholic beers. The consumption of alcoholic drinks with MAOIs still appears to be controversial with some advocating total abstinence while others permit a modest intake.

1. Brown C, *et al.* The monoamine oxidase inhibitor-tyramine interaction. *J Clin Pharmacol* 1989; **29:** 529–32.
2. Lippman SB, Nash K. Monoamine oxidase inhibitor update: potential adverse food and drug interactions. *Drug Safety* 1990; **5:** 195–204.
3. Folks DG. Monoamine oxidase inhibitors: reappraisal of dietary considerations. *J Clin Psychopharmacol* 1983; **3:** 249–52.

4. Anonymous. Foods interacting with MAO inhibitors. *Med Lett Drugs Ther* 1989; **31:** 11–12.
5. Hannah P, *et al.* Tyramine in wine and beer. *Lancet* 1988; **i:** 879.
6. Sandler M. Monoamine oxidase inhibitors and low alcohol or alcohol free drinks. *Br Med J* 1990; **300:** 1527.
7. Beswick DT, Rogers ML. Monoamine oxidase inhibitors and low alcohol or alcohol free drinks. *Br Med J* 1990; **301:** 179–80.

Interactions of MAOIs with other Drugs

MAOIs inhibit the metabolism of some *amine drugs* (notably indirect-acting sympathomimetics), which can lead to dangerous enhancement of their pressor effects. MAOIs also inhibit the metabolism of other drug-metabolising enzymes and are therefore responsible for a large number of *other drug interactions*. Moreover, they have an additive effect with serotonergic drugs which has led to the recognition of the *serotonin syndrome* (see above), an interactive adverse effect shared with some other antidepressants. As in the case of foods, the danger of an interaction persists for at least 14 days after treatment with an MAOI has been discontinued.

Severe hypertensive reactions due to enhancement of pressor activity have followed the administration of sympathomimetics such as *amphetamines, dopamine, ephedrine, levodopa, phenylephrine, phenylpropanolamine*, and *pseudoephedrine*. Reactions may also follow the use of anorectics and stimulants with sympathomimetic activity such as *fenfluramine, methylphenidate, pemoline*, and *phentermine*. There have been case reports of fatalities in patients who took cough preparations containing *dextromethorphan*. There is no clinical evidence of dangerous interactions between *adrenaline-containing local anaesthetics* and MAOIs. Great care should however be taken to avoid inadvertent intravenous administration of the local anaesthetic preparation. Significant rises in blood pressure have been reported following the use of *buspirone* with MAOIs.

Inhibition of drug-metabolising enzymes by MAOIs may enhance the effects of *barbiturates and possibly other hypnotics, hypoglycaemics*, and possibly *antimuscarinics*. *Alcohol* metabolism may be altered and its effects enhanced; see also under Interactions of MAOIs with Foods, above. *Antihypertensives including guanethidine, reserpine*, and *methyldopa* should be given with caution; hypotensive and hypertensive reactions have been suggested; the hypotensive effects of *beta blockers* and *thiazide diuretics* may be enhanced.

The administration of *pethidine and other opioid analgesics* to patients taking an MAOI has also been associated with very severe and sometimes fatal reactions. When it is considered essential to use an opioid analgesic a test dose of morphine should be given. It has been suggested that the test dose should be one-tenth to one-fifth of the normal dose and if this produces no untoward reaction, the dose of morphine can be gradually and carefully increased over a period of 2 to 3 hours. The use of opioid analgesics and other drugs employed during general anaesthesia in patients continuing to take MAOIs is discussed in Anaesthesia under Precautions, above.

Clozapine may enhance the CNS effects of MAOIs.

Although different antidepressants have been used together under expert supervision in refractory cases of depression, severe adverse reactions may occur. MAOIs should not generally be given to patients receiving *tricyclic antidepressants, selective serotonin reuptake inhibitors (SSRIs), serotonin and noradrenaline reuptake inhibitors (SNRIs)*, or *nefazodone* or *trazodone*. An appropriate drug-free interval should elapse between discontinuing one type of antidepressant and starting another. An MAOI should not be started until at least one week after stopping a tricyclic antidepressant, an SSRI, an SNRI, nefazodone, trazodone, or any related antidepressant; in the case of the SSRIs paroxetine and sertraline, the drug-free interval is extended to two weeks, and for fluoxetine, five weeks because of their longer half-lives. Conversely, two weeks should elapse between discontinuing MAOI therapy and starting patients on a tricyclic antidepressant, an SSRI, an SNRI, or any related antidepressant. For further warnings on the coadministration of antidepressants, see below. Interactions can also occur between MAOIs themselves.

For details of the less severe interactions associated with reversible inhibitors of monoamine oxidase A, see Interactions of Moclobemide, p.299.

References.

1. Bazire S. Interactions with monoamine oxidase inhibitors. *Pharm J* 1986; **236:** 418–9.
2. Gascoigne EW, Griffiths J. Hismanal and monoamine oxidase inhibitors. *Pharm J* 1986; **236:** 545–6.
3. Woods KL. Interactions that matter: monoamine oxidase inhibitors. *Prescribers' J* 1989; **29:** 75–9.
4. Lippman SB, Nash K. Monoamine oxidase inhibitor update: potential adverse food and drug interactions. *Drug Safety* 1990; **5:** 195–204.
5. Blackwell B. Monoamine oxidase inhibitor interactions with other drugs. *J Clin Psychopharmacol* 1991; **11:** 55–9.
6. Livingston MC, Livingston HM. Monoamine oxidase inhibitors: an update on drug interactions. *Drug Safety* 1996; **14:** 219–27.

Anticoagulants. For the effects of MAOIs on warfarin, see p.967.

Antidepressants. Combination therapy with differing classes of antidepressants has been used successfully in the treatment of drug-resistant depression. It should be emphasised, however, that such combination therapy may result in interactions or enhanced adverse reactions such as the serotonin syndrome (see above), and is therefore considered unsuitable or controversial by some authorities. Because combination therapy poses increased risks it should be employed only under expert supervision. Despite these drawbacks certain combinations of drugs have been found to be beneficial, although others are considered unsuitable; it should be noted that absence of information documenting unsuitability or hazard does not necessarily imply that the two drugs may be used safely together but may merely reflect an untried combination.

MAOIs have been used fairly frequently under expert supervision with tricyclics in refractory depression and it has been stated[1] that the risk of serious problems in combining tricyclic antidepressant and MAOI antidepressant therapy is almost exclusively limited to sequential prescribing, in particular the addition of a tricyclic to established treatment with an MAOI. The recommended procedure was said to be to allow a drug-free interval of at least one week and then to start both drugs together at a low dosage. The dosage of both drugs is then gradually increased to around half that normally prescribed for the drugs when given on their own. The dietary restrictions for MAOIs alone apply equally to the combined antidepressant regimen. Amitriptyline and trimipramine were considered to be the tricyclics least likely to produce side-effects in combination with MAOIs, while phenelzine and isocarboxazid were the safest MAOIs.

Two tricyclic antidepressants that have been considered particularly unsuitable for combination therapy with MAOIs are clomipramine, a tricyclic with serotonin reuptake inhibiting activity, and imipramine. Reports of interactions have occurred with both these drugs.[2,3] The combination of clomipramine with tranylcypromine is particularly dangerous. Symptoms suggestive of the serotonin syndrome occurred in an elderly patient due to an interaction between clomipramine and moclobemide, a reversible inhibitor of monoamine oxidase type A (RIMA).[4] Two fatalities due to serotonin syndrome have been reported following overdosage with clomipramine and moclobemide.[5] A 39-year-old woman developed the serotonin syndrome while taking imipramine with moclobemide, although it was suggested that an excessive dose of the tricyclic may have been ingested accidentally.[6]

In the UK the Committee on Safety of Medicines (CSM) has warned[7] that enhanced serotonergic effects may result from combination therapy of selective serotonin reuptake inhibitors (SSRIs), such as fluoxetine and fluvoxamine, with other antidepressants, including MAOIs. Although such an enhancement may be beneficial in some instances it can produce a life-threatening serotonin syndrome. Such reactions had later been reported in patients taking sertraline with MAOIs.[8-10] Three fatalities due to serotonin syndrome have been reported following overdosage with citalopram and moclobemide.[5] Bakish *et al.*[11] have reported good efficacy and tolerability with combinations of moclobemide and SSRIs. However, Hawley *et al.*[12] reported a high rate of adverse events with these combinations, although as significant improvement in depressive symptoms was observed in some patients, they suggest that the combination of moclobemide with SSRIs deserves consideration as an option for the treatment of refractory depression.

Combination therapy with a tricyclic antidepressant and an SSRI has sometimes been used to treat resistant depression. Fluvoxamine[13] and fluoxetine[14] have been reported to increase plasma concentrations of the tricyclic, although to varying degrees. Fluoxetine has been reported to produce three- to fourfold increases in plasma concentrations of desipramine and imipramine whereas fluvoxamine has a minimal effect on desipramine plasma levels, but produces a three- to fourfold increase in concentrations of imipramine.[15] Plasma-desipramine concentrations are elevated threefold by paroxetine but increases of only 30% are produced by sertraline.[15] Additionally, norfluoxetine, the active metabolite of fluoxetine, has a long half-life and is responsible for the continuing interaction with tricyclics for several days or weeks after fluoxetine has been withdrawn. Citalopram was reported to have no effect on plasma-tricyclic concentrations in one patient although antidepressant effects were augmented.[16]

Lithium and tryptophan have been used to augment the effect of other antidepressants in refractory depression. Phenelzine has been used successfully in combination with lithium and tryptophan[17] in patients with treatment-resistant chronic depression although such a regimen has probably been used less since the reports of the eosinophilia-myalgia syndrome associated with tryptophan (see p.310). There have, however, been several case reports of reactions similar to the serotonin syndrome in patients receiving MAOIs together with tryptophan.[18,19] Although lithium is often added to tricyclic antidepressant therapy in patients with refractory depression, epileptic seizures have been reported in one patient receiving amitriptyline when lithium was added.[20] Serotonin syndrome has been reported[28] in a patient given clomipramine and lithium. Severe neurotoxicity has been reported[21,22] in some patients receiving lithium and tricyclic or tetracyclic antidepressants together; adverse effects included tremor, memory impairment, disorganised thinking, and auditory hallucinations. One manufacturer of lithium preparations also reports symptoms of nephrogenic diabetes in patients receiving these combinations. By 1989 the CSM had received 19 reports of adverse reactions in patients treated with fluvoxamine and lithium; 5 reports concerned convulsions and 1 hyperthermia.[7] The risk of CNS toxicity is increased when lithium is administered together with fluoxetine, fluvoxamine, paroxetine, and sertraline. There has been a report[23] of one fatality when fluoxetine was replaced by tranylcypromine and tryptophan with no wash-out period; the patient was also receiving other drugs concurrently.

The combination of the serotonin and noradrenaline reuptake inhibitor (SNRI) venlafaxine with MAOIs is contraindicated by the manufacturers because of the risk of life-threatening adverse reactions. Serious adverse reactions have been reported when venlafaxine was combined with isocarboxazid,[24] phenelzine,[25] or tranylcypromine.[26]

Trazodone is chemically unrelated to other antidepressants but does have serotonergic actions. Serotonin syndrome has been reported when trazodone was combined with the SSRI paroxetine.[27]

1. Katona CLE, Barnes TRE. Pharmacological strategies in depression. *Br J Hosp Med* 1985; **34:** 168–71.
2. Beaumont G. Drug interactions with clomipramine (Anafranil). *J Int Med Res* 1973; **1:** 480–4.
3. Graham PM, *et al.* Combination monoamine oxidase inhibitor/tricyclic antidepressant interaction. *Lancet* 1982; **ii:** 440.
4. Spigset O, *et al.* Serotonin syndrome caused by a moclobemide-clomipramine interaction. *Br Med J* 1993; **306:** 248.
5. Neuvonen PJ, *et al.* Five fatal cases of serotonin syndrome after moclobemide-citalopram or moclobemide-clomipramine overdoses. *Lancet* 1993; **342:** 1419.
6. Brodribb TR, *et al.* Efficacy and adverse effects of moclobemide. *Lancet* 1994; **343:** 475.
7. Committee on Safety of Medicines. Fluvoxamine and fluoxetine-interaction with monoamine oxidase inhibitors, lithium and tryptophan. *Current Problems 26* 1989. Correction. *ibid. 27* 1989 [hypothermia should have read hyperthermia].
8. Brannan SK, *et al.* Sertraline and isocarboxazid cause a serotonin syndrome. *J Clin Psychopharmacol* 1994; **14:** 144–5.
9. Graber MA, *et al.* Sertraline-phenelzine drug interaction: a serotonin syndrome reaction. *Ann Pharmacother* 1994; **28:** 732–5.
10. Corkeron MA. Serotonin syndrome — a potentially fatal complication of antidepressant therapy. *Med J Aust* 1995; **163:** 481–2.
11. Bakish D, *et al.* Moclobemide and specific serotonin re-uptake inhibitor combination treatment of resistant anxiety and depressive disorders. *Hum Psychopharmacol Clin Exp* 1995; **10:** 105–9.
12. Hawley CJ, *et al.* Combining SSRIs and moclobemide. *Pharm J* 1996; **257:** 506.
13. Bertschy G, *et al.* Fluvoxamine-tricyclic antidepressant interaction: an accidental finding. *Eur J Clin Pharmacol* 1991; **40:** 119–20.
14. Westermeyer J. Fluoxetine-induced tricyclic toxicity: extent and duration. *J Clin Pharmacol* 1991; **31:** 388–92.
15. Ereshefsky L, *et al.* Antidepressant drug interactions and the cytochrome P450 system: the role of cytochrome P450 2D6. *Clin Pharmacokinet* 1995; **29** (suppl 1): 10–19.
16. Baettig D, *et al.* Tricyclic antidepressant plasma levels after augmentation with citalopram: a case study. *Eur J Clin Pharmacol* 1993; **44:** 403–5.

17. Barker WA, *et al.* The Newcastle chronic depression study: results of a treatment regime. *Int Clin Psychopharmacol* 1987; **2;** 261–72.
18. Pare CMB. Potentiation of monoamine oxidase inhibitors by tryptophan. *Lancet* 1963; **ii:** 527–8.
19. Price WA, *et al.* Serotonin syndrome: a case report. *J Clin Pharmacol* 1986; **26:** 77–8.
20. Solomon JG. Seizures during lithium-amitriptyline therapy. *Postgrad Med* 1979; **66:** 145–8.
21. Austin LS, *et al.* Toxicity resulting from lithium augmentation of antidepressant treatment in elderly patients. *J Clin Psychiatry* 1990; **51:** 344–5.
22. Lafferman J, *et al.* Lithium augmentation for treatment-resistant depression in the elderly. *J Geriatr Psychiatry Neurol* 1988; **1:** 49–52.
23. Kline SS, *et al.* Serotonin syndrome versus neuroleptic malignant syndrome as a cause of death. *Clin Pharm* 1989; **8:** 510–14.
24. Klysner R, *et al.* Toxic interaction of venlafaxine and isocarboxazid. *Lancet* 1995; **346:** 1298–9.
25. Heister MA, *et al.* Serotonin syndrome induced by administration of venlafaxine and phenelzine. *Ann Pharmacother* 1996; **30:** 84.
26. Hodgman MJ. Serotonin syndrome due to venlafaxine and maintenance tranylcypromine therapy. *Hum Exp Toxicol* 1997; **16:** 14–17.
27. Reeves RR, *et al.* Serotonin syndrome produced by paroxetine and low-dose trazodone. *Psychosomatics* 1995; **36:** 159.
28. Kojima H, *et al.* Serotonin syndrome during clomipramine and lithium treatment. *Am J Psychiatry* 1993; **150:** 1897.

Antiepileptics. Antidepressants may antagonise the activity of antiepileptics by lowering the convulsive threshold.

Antimigraine drugs. For the effect of MAOIs on serotonin ($5-HT_1$) agonists, see under Sumatriptan, p.451.

Antineoplastics. For the effect of MAOIs on altretamine, see p.502.

Dopaminergics. For the effect of MAOIs on amantadine, see p.1130, and on levodopa, see p.1139.

General anaesthetics. The problems that may be encountered with MAOIs and general anaesthetics are discussed under Anaesthesia in Precautions, above.

Insulin. For the effect of MAOIs on Insulin, see p.326.

Muscle relaxants. For the effects of MAOIs on suxamethonium, see p.1321. Problems that may be encountered with MAOIs and muscle relaxants used during anaesthesia are discussed under Precautions, above.

Opioid analgesics. The problems that may be encountered with MAOIs and opioid analgesics used during anaesthesia are discussed under Precautions, above.

Respiratory stimulants. For the effect of MAOIs on doxapram, see p.1480.

Pharmacokinetics

Phenelzine is readily absorbed from the gastro-intestinal tract reaching peak plasma concentrations 2 to 4 hours after ingestion. It is metabolised in the liver and is excreted in the urine almost entirely in the form of metabolites.

Uses and Administration

Monoamine oxidase inhibitors (MAOIs) inhibit the action of monoamine oxidase, the enzyme responsible for the metabolism of several biogenic amines. Monoamine oxidase exists in two forms: type A and type B. Monoamine oxidase type A preferentially de-aminates, by oxidation, adrenaline, noradrenaline, and serotonin whereas monoamine oxidase type B preferentially metabolises benzylamine and phenylethylamine; dopamine and tyramine are de-aminated by both forms of the enzyme. The traditional MAOIs such as phenelzine, iproniazid, isocarboxazid, nialamide, and tranylcypromine are inhibitors of both types; apart from tranylcypromine, all are hydrazine derivatives and bind irreversibly. Selective inhibitors include selegiline (p.1144), an irreversible inhibitor of monoamine oxidase type B used in the treatment of Parkinson's disease. Clorgyline is an irreversible selective type A inhibitor. Reversible inhibitors of monoamine oxidase type A (RIMAs) include brofaromine, moclobemide, and toloxatone. Antidepressant activity appears to reside predominantly with inhibition of monoamine oxidase type A although the mode of action of these drugs in depression is not fully understood. Advantages claimed for selective inhibitors are fewer or less severe side-effects than those experienced with non-selective inhibitors. As tyramine is de-aminated by both monoamine oxidase types A and B, inhibiting only one of the enzymes allows for continued, albeit reduced, de-amination. Thus the dietary precautions that need to be observed with non-selective inhibitors of both monoamine oxidase types A and B are less stringent with the selective inhibitors.

Phenelzine and other antidepressant MAOIs are used in the treatment of atypical depression, particularly where phobic features or associated anxiety are present, or in patients who have not responded to other antidepressants. However, the risks associated with irreversible non-selective MAOIs usually mean that other antidepressants are preferred. Up to a month may elapse before an antidepressant response is obtained with MAOIs. After a response has been obtained maintenance therapy may need to be continued for at least 4 to 6 months to avoid relapse on discontinuation of therapy. MAOI therapy is not generally indicated for children. Care should be taken in elderly patients because of an increased susceptibility to adverse effects. Moreover, therapy with the non-selective inhibitors is particularly unsuitable for patients considered unable to adhere to the strict dietary requirements necessary for its safe usage.

Phenelzine is given by mouth as the sulphate in doses equivalent to phenelzine 15 mg three times daily; if no response has been obtained after 2 weeks the dosage may be increased to 15 mg four times daily; severely depressed patients in hospital may be given up to 30 mg three times daily. Once a response has been obtained the dosage may be gradually reduced for maintenance therapy; some patients may continue to respond to 15 mg on alternate days.

Phenelzine should be withdrawn gradually to reduce the risk of withdrawal symptoms.

Anxiety disorders. Although tricyclic antidepressants and selective serotonin reuptake inhibitors are often the drugs of choice for the treatment of *panic disorder*, MAOIs also appear to be effective in blocking attacks. MAOIs also appear to be effective in *social phobias* and can improve anticipatory anxiety and functional disability. The major treatment for *post-traumatic stress disorder* is psychotherapy but MAOIs or tricyclic antidepressants can help to reduce traumatic recollections and nightmares and to repress flashbacks. For a discussion of anxiety disorders, including mention of the limited use of MAOIs, see p.635.

References.

1. Buigues J, Vallejo J. Therapeutic response to phenelzine in patients with panic disorder and agoraphobia with panic attacks. *J Clin Psychiatry* 1987; **48:** 55–9.
2. Frank JB, *et al.* A randomized clinical trial of phenelzine and imipramine for posttraumatic stress disorder. *Am J Psychiatry* 1988; **145:** 1289–91.

Depression. As discussed on p.271 there is very little difference in efficacy between the different groups of antidepressant drugs, and choice is often made on the basis of adverse effects. MAOIs are rarely used as first-choice antidepressants because of the dangers of dietary and drug interactions. Even in depressed patients with atypical, hypochondriacal, hysterical, or phobic features, for which MAOIs are particularly effective, it is often recommended that another antidepressant type should be tried first. Reversible inhibitors of monoamine oxidase type A (RIMAs) offer an alternative to the MAOIs and less strict dietary restrictions are necessary. They may be an effective first choice in a wide range of depressive disorders, although their relative efficacy in atypical depression remains to be established.

Combination therapy with differing classes of antidepressants, including the MAOIs, has been used in the treatment of drug-resistant depression. However, such therapy may result in enhanced adverse reactions or interactions and is considered unsuitable or controversial by some workers. For further details, see Antidepressants under Interactions, above.

Hyperactivity. When drug therapy is required for attention deficit hyperactivity disorder (p.1476), initial treatment is usually with central stimulants. MAOIs have been used successfully but problems with dietary restriction and potential drug interactions have limited their use.

Migraine. A number of drugs have been used for the prophylaxis of migraine (p.443), although propranolol or pizotifen are generally preferred. Antidepressants such as the tricyclics can be useful alternatives when these drugs are ineffective or unsuitable. MAOIs are best reserved for severe cases refractory to other prophylactic treatment.

Orthostatic hypotension. MAOIs together with a sympathomimetic to induce a pressor reaction for the management of orthostatic hypotension is considered to be controversial (see p.1040).

Preparations

BP 1998: Phenelzine Tablets;
USP 23: Phenelzine Sulfate Tablets.

Proprietary Preparations (details are given in Part 3)
Austral.: Nardil; ***Belg.:*** Nardelzine; ***Canad.:*** Nardil; ***Irl.:*** Nardil; ***Spain:*** Nardelzine†; ***UK:*** Nardil; ***USA:*** Nardil.

Pirlindole (14854-c)

Pirlindole *(rINN)*.

2,3,3a,4,5,6-Hexahydro-8-methyl-1*H*-pyrazino[3,2,1-*jk*]carbazole.

$C_{15}H_{18}N_2$ = 226.3.

CAS — 60762-57-4.

Pirlindole has been given in doses of up to a maximum of 400 mg daily by mouth in the treatment of depression.

Preparations

Proprietary Preparations (details are given in Part 3)
Spain: Lifril.

Pivagabine (15915-r)

Pivagabine *(rINN)*.

4-Pivalamidobutyric acid.

$C_9H_{17}NO_3$ = 187.2.

CAS — 69542-93-4.

Pivagabine has been used as an antidepressant in doses of 900 mg twice daily.

Preparations

Proprietary Preparations (details are given in Part 3)
Ital.: Tonerg; Zenit†.

Protriptyline Hydrochloride (2534-j)

Protriptyline Hydrochloride *(BANM, USAN, rINNM)*.

MK-240. 3-(5*H*-Dibenzo[*a,d*]cyclohept-5-enyl)propyl(methyl)amine hydrochloride.

$C_{19}H_{21}N,HCl$ = 299.8.

CAS — 438-60-8 (protriptyline); 1225-55-4 (protriptyline hydrochloride).

Pharmacopoeias. In *Br.* and *US.*

A white to yellowish white, odourless or almost odourless powder. **Soluble** 1 in 2 of water, 1 in 3.5 of alcohol, and 1 in 2.5 of chloroform; practically insoluble in ether. A 1% solution in water has a pH of 5.0 to 6.5.

Adverse Effects, Treatment, and Precautions

As for tricyclic antidepressants in general (see Amitriptyline, p.273).

Since protriptyline may have some stimulant properties anxiety and agitation may occur more frequently; cardiovascular effects such as tachycardia and hypotension may also be more frequent than with other tricyclics. Photosensitivity rashes have been noted more commonly with protriptyline than with other tricyclic antidepressants and patients taking it should avoid direct sunlight.

Interactions

For interactions associated with tricyclic antidepressants, see Amitriptyline, p.276.

Pharmacokinetics

Protriptyline is well but slowly absorbed after oral administration, peak plasma concentrations being achieved after several hours.

Paths of metabolism of protriptyline include *N*-oxidation and hydroxylation. Protriptyline is excreted in the urine, mainly in the form of its metabolites, either free or in conjugated form.

Protriptyline is widely distributed throughout the body and extensively bound to plasma and tissue protein. Protriptyline has been estimated to have a very prolonged elimination half-life ranging from 55 to 198 hours, which may be further prolonged in overdosage.

Uses and Administration

Protriptyline is a dibenzocycloheptatriene tricyclic antidepressant with actions and uses similar to those of amitriptyline (p.278). It has considerably less sedative properties than other tricyclics and may have a stimulant effect, thus making it particularly suitable for apathetic and withdrawn patients; its antimuscarinic properties are moderate.

In the treatment of depression, protriptyline is given by mouth as the hydrochloride in doses of 5 to 10 mg three or four times daily. It has been suggested that, because of its potential stimulant activity, any dosage increases should be added to the morning dose first and if insomnia occurs the last dose should be given no later than mid-afternoon. Higher doses of up to 60 mg daily may be required in severely depressed patients. A suggested initial dose for adolescents and the elderly is 5 mg three times daily; close monitoring of the cardiovascular system has been suggested if the dose exceeds a total of 20 mg daily in elderly subjects.

Protriptyline should be withdrawn gradually to reduce the risk of withdrawal symptoms.

Depression. As discussed on p.271, there is very little difference in efficacy between the different groups of antidepressant drugs, and choice is often made on the basis of adverse effect profile. Tricyclic antidepressants such as protriptyline have traditionally been the first choice for the treatment of depression, and often still are because of wide experience with their use and familiarity with their pharmacological actions. Protriptyline is one of the less sedating tricyclics and consequently may be of value for withdrawn or apathetic depressed patients.

Preparations

BP 1998: Protriptyline Tablets;
USP 23: Protriptyline Hydrochloride Tablets.

Proprietary Preparations (details are given in Part 3)
Canad.: Triptil; ***Irl.:*** Concordin; ***Swed.:*** Concordin; ***UK:*** Concordin; ***USA:*** Vivactil.

Quinupramine (13204-x)

Quinupramine *(rINN)*.

LM-208. 10,11-Dihydro-5-(quinuclidin-3-yl)-5*H*-dibenz[*b,f*]azepine.

$C_{21}H_{24}N_2$ = 304.4.

CAS — 31721-17-2.

Quinupramine is a tricyclic antidepressant (see Amitriptyline, p.273). It is given by mouth or by intravenous infusion in doses of 5 to 15 mg daily in the treatment of depression.

Quinupramine should be withdrawn gradually to reduce the risk of withdrawal symptoms.

Preparations

Proprietary Preparations (details are given in Part 3)
Aust.: Kevopril; ***Fr.:*** Kinupril.

Reboxetine (2881-w)

Reboxetine *(BAN, rINN)*.

FCE-20124. (±)-(2*R**)-2-[(α*R**)-α-(*o*-Ethoxyphenoxy)benzyl]morpholine; (±)-(2*RS*)-2-[(α*RS*)-α-(2-Ethoxyphenoxy)benzyl]morpholine.

$C_{19}H_{23}NO_3$ = 313.4.

CAS — 71620-89-8; 98769-81-4 (both reboxetine); 98769-82-5 (reboxetine mesylate).

Adverse Effects

Side-effects reported with reboxetine include insomnia, increased sweating, dizziness, postural hypotension, paraesthesia, impotence, and dysuria. Vertigo, dry mouth, constipation, tachycardia, and urinary retention (mainly in men) have also been reported. Reduced plasma-potassium concentrations have been observed in elderly patients following prolonged administration.

Hyponatraemia, possibly as a result of inappropriate secretion of antidiuretic hormone, has been associated with the use of antidepressants, particularly in the elderly.

Precautions

Reboxetine should be used with caution in patients with renal or hepatic impairment. It should also be used under close supervision in patients with bipolar disorder, urinary retention, benign prostatic hyperplasia, glaucoma, or a history of epilepsy or cardiac disorders.

Patients should be closely monitored during early therapy until improvement in depression is observed because suicide is an inherent risk in depressed patients. For further details, see under Depression, p.271.

Ability to perform tasks requiring motor or cognitive skills or judgement may be impaired by reboxetine and patients, if affected, should not drive or operate machinery.

Interactions

Reboxetine should not be taken together with, or within two weeks of discontinuing an MAOI; at least one week should elapse after discontinuing reboxetine therapy before starting any drug liable to provoke a serious reaction (e.g. phenelzine). Increases in blood pressure may occur when reboxetine and ergotamine are administered together. Caution should be exercised when reboxetine is given with other drugs that lower blood pressure because postural hypotension has occurred with reboxetine. Clinical data on interactions with reboxetine are limited but the manufacturer advises that concomitant administration with the following drugs should be avoided: antiarrhythmics, antipsychotics, cyclosporin, tricyclic antidepressants, fluvoxamine, azole antifungals, and macrolide antibacterials. The possibility of hypokalaemia if reboxetine is given with potassium-depleting diuretics should also be considered.

Pharmacokinetics

Reboxetine is well absorbed from the gastro-intestinal tract with peak plasma levels occurring after about 2 hours. Plasma protein binding is about 97% (92% in elderly subjects). Reboxetine is metabolised by dealkylation, hydroxylation, and oxidation followed by glucuronide or sulphate conjugation. Elimination is mainly via urine (78%) with 10% excreted as unchanged drug. The plasma elimination half-life is 13 hours. Data from *animal* studies indicate that reboxetine crosses the placenta and is distributed into breast milk.

References.

1. Dostert P, *et al.* Review of the pharmacokinetics and metabolism of reboxetine, a selective noradrenaline reuptake inhibitor. *Eur Neuropsychopharmacol* 1997; **7** (suppl 1): S23–S35.

Uses and Administration

Reboxetine is a selective and potent inhibitor of the reuptake of noradrenaline; it also has a weak effect on serotonin reuptake. Reboxetine has no significant affinity for muscarinic receptors. It is given by mouth as the mesylate for the treatment of depression with doses expressed as reboxetine. The daily dose of reboxetine is 8 mg in two divided doses, which may be increased after 3 to 4 weeks, if necessary, to 10 mg daily; the maximum daily dose should not exceed 12 mg. Lower doses of 4 mg daily in 2 divided doses are recommended in hepatic or renal impairment; doses may be increased thereafter according to tolerance. Reboxetine is not recommended for use in elderly patients.

References.

1. Berzewski H, *et al.* Efficacy and tolerability of reboxetine compared with imipramine in a double-blind study in patients suffering from major depressive episodes. *Eur Neuropsychopharmacol* 1997; **7** (suppl 1): S37–S47.
2. Anonymous. Reboxetine—another new antidepressant. *Drug Ther Bull* 1998; **36:** 86–8.

Preparations

Proprietary Preparations (details are given in Part 3)
Swed.: Edronax; ***UK:*** Edronax.

Rubidium Chloride (723-m)

RbCl = 120.9.

Rubidium chloride has been used in the treatment of depression.

Rubidium chloride (^{82}Rb) is used for cardiac imaging (see p.1424).

References.

1. Linter CM. Neuropsychiatric aspects of trace elements. *Br J Hosp Med* 1985; **34:** 361–5.
2. Placidi G, *et al.* Exploration of the clinical profile of rubidium chloride in depression: a systematic open trial. *J Clin Psychopharmacol* 1988; **8:** 184–8.

Preparations

Proprietary Preparations (details are given in Part 3)
Ital.: Rubinorm†.

Sertraline Hydrochloride (18681-x)

Sertraline Hydrochloride *(BANM, USAN, rINNM)*.

CP-51974-01; Cp-51974-1. (1*S*,4*S*)-4-(3,4-Dichlorophenyl)-1,2,3,4-tetrahydro-1-naphthyl(methyl)amine hydrochloride.

$C_{17}H_{17}Cl_2N,HCl$ = 342.7.

CAS — 79617-96-2 (sertraline); 79559-97-0 (sertraline hydrochloride).

Sertraline hydrochloride 56 mg is approximately equivalent to 50 mg of sertraline.

Adverse Effects, Treatment, and Precautions

As for selective serotonin reuptake inhibitors (SSRIs) in general (see Fluoxetine, p.284).

Interactions

For interactions associated with selective serotonin reuptake inhibitors (SSRIs), see Fluoxetine, p.286.

Pharmacokinetics

Sertraline is slowly absorbed from the gastro-intestinal tract with peak plasma concentrations occurring about 4.5 to 8.5 hours after ingestion. It undergoes extensive first-pass metabolism in the liver. The main pathway is demethylation to *N*-desmethylsertraline; further metabolism and glucuronide conjugation occurs. Sertraline is widely distributed throughout body tissues and is highly (about 98%) bound to plasma proteins. The plasma elimination half-life of sertraline is reported to be 24 to 26 hours. Sertraline is excreted in approximately equal amounts in the urine and faeces, mainly as metabolites. Sertraline is distributed into breast milk (see Breast Feeding under Precautions in Fluoxetine, p.285).

References.

1. Démolis J-L, *et al.* Influence of liver cirrhosis on sertraline pharmacokinetics. *Br J Clin Pharmacol* 1996; **42:** 394–7.
2. Preskorn SH, ed. Sertraline: a pharmacokinetic profile. *Clin Pharmacokinet* 1997; **32** (suppl 1): 1–55.

Uses and Administration

Sertraline, a naphthaleneamine derivative, is a selective serotonin reuptake inhibitor (SSRI) with actions and uses similar to those of fluoxetine (p.287). Sertraline is given by mouth as sertraline hydrochloride as a single dose in the morning or evening. Doses are expressed in terms of sertraline.

In the treatment of depression, the usual initial dose of sertraline is 50 mg daily increased, if necessary, in increments of 50 mg at intervals of at least a week to a maximum of 200 mg daily. Doses of 150 mg daily or more should not be given for longer than 8 weeks.

In the treatment of obsessive-compulsive disorder the usual initial dose of sertraline is 50 mg daily. In the treatment of panic disorder with or without agoraphobia, the usual initial dose is 25 mg daily increased after one week to 50 mg daily. Doses may be increased, if necessary, in increments of 50 mg at intervals of at least a week to a maximum of 200 mg daily.

Once the optimal therapeutic response is obtained dosage should be reduced to the lowest effective level for maintenance.

Lower or less frequent doses are recommended in patients with significant hepatic impairment, although some manufacturers recommend that sertraline should not be used at all. Caution is advised in patients with renal impairment.

Sertraline should be withdrawn gradually to reduce the risk of withdrawal symptoms.

Reviews.

1. Murdoch D, McTavish D. Sertraline: a review of its pharmacodynamic and pharmacokinetic properties, and therapeutic potential in depression and obsessive-compulsive disorder. *Drugs* 1992; **44:** 604–24.
2. Grimsley SR, Jann MW. Paroxetine, sertraline, and fluvoxamine: new selective serotonin reuptake inhibitors. *Clin Pharm* 1992; **11:** 930–57.

Anxiety disorders. Sertraline has been given in a variety of anxiety disorders (p.635) including obsessive-compulsive disorder, panic disorder, social phobia, and post-traumatic stress disorder.

References.

1. Jenike MA, *et al.* Sertraline in obsessive-compulsive disorder: a double-blind comparison with placebo. *Am J Psychiatry* 1990; **147:** 923–8.
2. Chouinard G, *et al.* Results of a double-blind placebo controlled trial of a new serotonin uptake inhibitor, sertraline, in the treatment of obsessive-compulsive disorder. *Psychopharmacol Bull* 1990; **26:** 279–84.

3. Greist J, *et al.* Double-blind parallel comparison of three dosages of sertraline and placebo in outpatients with obsessive-compulsive disorder. *Arch Gen Psychiatry* 1995; **52:** 289–95.
4. Katzelnick DJ, *et al.* Sertraline for social phobia: a double-blind, placebo-controlled crossover study. *Am J Psychiatry* 1995; **152:** 1368–71.
5. Brady KT, *et al.* Sertraline treatment of comorbid posttraumatic stress disorder and alcohol dependence. *J Clin Psychiatry* 1995; **56:** 502–5.

Depression. As discussed on p.271, there is very little difference in efficacy between the different groups of antidepressant drugs, and choice is often made on the basis of adverse effect profile. Selective serotonin reuptake inhibitors (SSRIs) such as sertraline are increasingly being recognised as first-choice treatment because they offer advantages over the older tricyclics in terms of fewer unpleasant side-effects and safety in overdosage.

References.

1. Haider A, *et al.* Clinical effect of converting antidepressant therapy from fluoxetine to sertraline. *Am J Health-Syst Pharm* 1995; **52:** 1317–19.
2. Bennie EH, *et al.* A double-blind multicenter trial comparing sertraline and fluoxetine in outpatients with major depression. *J Clin Psychiatry* 1995; **56:** 229–37.
3. Stowe ZN, *et al.* Sertraline in the treatment of women with postpartum major depression. *Depression* 1995; **3:** 49–55.

Headache. For reference to the use of selective serotonin reuptake inhibitors (SSRIs), including sertraline, in the management of various types of headache, see under Fluoxetine, p.288.

Premenstrual syndrome. Sertraline in doses ranging from 50 to 150 mg daily throughout the menstrual cycle has produced beneficial effects in controlling both the psychological and somatic symptoms of women with premenstrual syndrome.[1-3] Administration of sertraline in a dose of 50 mg daily solely during the luteal phase was also of benefit.[4]

For a discussion of the overall management of premenstrual syndrome, see p.1456.

1. Freeman EW, *et al.* Sertraline versus desipramine in the treatment of premenstrual syndrome: an open-label trial. *J Clin Psychiatry* 1996; **57:** 7–11.
2. Yonkers KA, *et al.* Sertraline in the treatment of premenstrual dysphoric disorder. *Psychopharmacol Bull* 1996; **32:** 41–6.
3. Yonkers KA, *et al.* Symptomatic improvement of premenstrual dysphoric disorder with sertraline treatment: a randomized controlled trial. *JAMA* 1997; **278:** 983–8.
4. Young SA, *et al.* Treatment of premenstrual dysphoric disorder with sertraline during the luteal phase: a randomized, double-blind, placebo-controlled crossover trial. *J Clin Psychiatry* 1998; **59:** 76–80.

Sexual dysfunction. Impotence or ejaculatory problems have been reported as adverse effects of selective serotonin reuptake inhibitors (SSRIs) (see Effects on Sexual Function in Adverse Effects of Fluoxetine, p.285). Such properties of the SSRIs have been studied as a potential form of treatment for men with premature ejaculation. Significant improvements were noted in a placebo-controlled trial[1] involving 52 men with self-reported premature ejaculation.

1. Mendels J, *et al.* Sertraline treatment for premature ejaculation. *J Clin Psychopharmacol* 1995; **15:** 341–6.

Preparations

Proprietary Preparations (details are given in Part 3)
Aust.: Gladem; Tresleen; Zoloft; ***Austral.:*** Zoloft; ***Belg.:*** Serlain; ***Canad.:*** Zoloft; ***Fr.:*** Zoloft; ***Irl.:*** Lustral; ***Ital.:*** Serad; Tatig; Zoloft; ***Neth.:*** Zoloft; ***Norw.:*** Zoloft; ***S.Afr.:*** Zoloft; ***Spain:*** Aremis; Besitran; ***Swed.:*** Zoloft; ***Switz.:*** Gladem; Zoloft; ***UK:*** Lustral; ***USA:*** Zoloft.

Setiptiline (2987-x)

Setiptiline *(rINN)*.

2,3,4,9-Tetrahydro-2-methyl-1*H*-dibenzo[3,4:6,7]cyclohepta[1,2-*c*]pyridine.

$C_{19}H_{19}N$ = 261.4.

CAS — 57262-94-9.

Setiptiline is an antidepressant used as the maleate in the treatment of depression.

Preparations

Proprietary Preparations (details are given in Part 3)
Jpn: Tecipul†.

Teniloxazine (2991-c)

Teniloxazine *(rINN)*.

(±)-2-{[(α-2-Thienyl-*o*-tolyl)oxy]methyl}morpholine.

$C_{16}H_{19}NO_2S$ = 289.4.

CAS — 62473-79-4.

Teniloxazine has antidepressant properties and is also being studied for use in the management of dementia.

References.

1. Ogura C, *et al.* Clinical pharmacology of a new antidepressant, Y-8894 in healthy young and elderly volunteers. *Br J Clin Pharmacol* 1987; **23:** 537–43.
2. Orlando R, *et al.* The pharmacokinetics of teniloxazine in healthy subjects and patients with hepatic cirrhosis. *Br J Clin Pharmacol* 1995; **39:** 445–8.
3. Aguglia E, *et al.* Comparison of teniloxazine and piracetam in Alzheimer-type or vascular dementia. *Curr Ther Res* 1995; **56:** 250–7.

Tianeptine Sodium (17007-n)

Tianeptine Sodium *(rINNM)*.

The sodium salt of 7-[(3-chloro-6,11-dihydro-6-methyldibenzo[*c,f*][1,2]thiazepin-11-yl)amino]heptanoic acid *S,S*-dioxide.

$C_{21}H_{25}ClN_2NaO_4S$ = 459.9.

CAS — 66981-73-5 (tianeptine).

Tianeptine sodium is an antidepressant reported to act by increasing (rather than inhibiting) the presynaptic reuptake of serotonin. It is given by mouth in doses of 12.5 mg three times daily in the treatment of depression. Doses should be reduced to a total of 25 mg daily in elderly patients and those with renal impairment, but it has been stated that no dose modification is necessary in patients with chronic alcoholism or cirrhosis.

Isolated cases of hepatitis have been reported during treatment with tianeptine.

References.

1. Royer RJ, *et al.* Tianeptine and its main metabolite: pharmacokinetics in chronic alcoholism and cirrhosis. *Clin Pharmacokinet* 1989; **16:** 186–91.
2. Carlhant D, *et al.* Pharmacokinetics and bioavailability of tianeptine in the elderly. *Drug Invest* 1990; **2:** 167–72.
3. Demotes-Mainard F, *et al.* Pharmacokinetics of the antidepressant tianeptine at steady state in the elderly. *J Clin Pharmacol* 1991; **31:** 174–8.
4. Wilde MI, Benfield P. Tianeptine: a review of its pharmacodynamic and pharmacokinetic properties, and therapeutic efficacy in depression and coexisting anxiety and depression. *Drugs* 1995; **49:** 411–39.

Preparations

Proprietary Preparations (details are given in Part 3)
Fr.: Stablon.

Toloxatone (3229-y)

Toloxatone *(rINN)*.

5-(Hydroxymethyl)-3-*m*-tolyl-2-oxazolidinone.

$C_{11}H_{13}NO_3$ = 207.2.

CAS — 29218-27-7.

Toloxatone is a reversible inhibitor of monoamine oxidase type A (RIMA) (see Moclobemide, p.298). It is used as an antidepressant in doses of 200 mg three times daily by mouth.

References.

1. Benedetti MS, *et al.* Pharmacokinetics of toloxatone in man following intravenous and oral administrations. *Arzneimittelforschung* 1982; **32:** 276–80.

Preparations

Proprietary Preparations (details are given in Part 3)
Fr.: Humoryl; ***Ital.:*** Umoril.

Tranylcypromine Sulphate (2537-k)

Tranylcypromine Sulphate *(BANM, rINNM)*.

SKF-385; Transamine Sulphate; Tranylcypromine Sulfate. (±)-*trans*-2-Phenylcyclopropylamine sulphate.

$(C_9H_{11}N)_2,H_2SO_4$ = 364.5.

CAS — 155-09-9 (tranylcypromine); 13492-01-8 (tranylcypromine sulphate).

Pharmacopoeias. In Br.

A white or almost white crystalline powder; odourless or with a faint odour of cinnamaldehyde. Tranylcypromine sulphate 13.7 mg is approximately equivalent to 10 mg of tranylcypromine. **Soluble** in water; very slightly soluble in alcohol and in ether; practically insoluble in chloroform.

Adverse Effects, Treatment, and Precautions

As for MAOIs in general (see Phenelzine, p.302).

Tranylcypromine has a stimulant action and insomnia is a common side-effect if it is taken in the evening.

Hypertensive reactions are more likely to occur with tranylcypromine than with other MAOIs, but severe liver damage occurs less frequently. Tranylcypromine should not be used in patients with hyperthyroidism.

Dependence. Dependence on tranylcypromine with tolerance has been reported in patients receiving high doses with or without a history of previous substance abuse. For further details, see Withdrawal under Precautions in Phenelzine, p.304.

Effects on the cardiovascular system. Although orthostatic hypotension is the more common effect of MAOIs on blood pressure, hypertension can occur. A hypertensive crisis has been described in two patients after only one dose of tranylcypromine.[1,2] In the first case it was thought possible that an autointeraction may have occurred between tranylcypromine and amphetamine to which it is partly metabolised. In the second case the provocation of hypertension led to the finding of a previously-undiagnosed phaeochromocytoma and it was suggested this may have been a possibility in previous reports of hypertension induced by MAOIs.

1. Gunn J, *et al.* Hypertensive crisis and broad complex bradycardia after a single dose of monoamine oxidase inhibitor. *Br Med J* 1989; **298:** 964.
2. Cook RF, Katritsis D. Hypertensive crisis precipitated by a monoamine oxidase inhibitor in a patient with phaeochromocytoma. *Br Med J* 1990; **300:** 614.

Porphyria. Tranylcypromine was considered to be unsafe in patients with acute porphyria because it has been shown to be porphyrinogenic in *animals*.[1]

1. Moore MR, McColl KEL. *Porphyria: drug lists.* Glasgow: Porphyria Research Unit, University of Glasgow, 1991.

Interactions

For interactions associated with MAOIs, see Phenelzine, p.304.

The concomitant administration of clomipramine with tranylcypromine is particularly hazardous.

Pharmacokinetics

Tranylcypromine is readily absorbed from the gastro-intestinal tract, peak plasma concentrations occurring about 1 to 3 hours after ingestion. It is excreted in the urine mainly in the form of metabolites. Tranylcypromine has a reported plasma elimination half-life of about 2.5 hours.

In 9 depressed patients, tranylcypromine absorption was rapid after oral dosing.[1] Absorption was biphasic in 7. Elimination was also rapid, with an elimination half-life of 1.54 to 3.15 hours. From 2 to 7 hours after dosing, standing systolic and diastolic blood pressures were lowered, and standing pulse was raised. The onset of the effect on standing systolic blood pressure correlated with the time of peak plasma tranylcypromine concentration. Maximum orthostatic drop of blood pressure and rise in pulse rate occurred 2 hours after dosing. Mean plasma tranylcypromine concentrations correlated with mean orthostatic drop of systolic blood pressure and rise of pulse rate. Patients experiencing clinically significant hypotensive reactions to tranylcypromine may benefit from changes in their dose regimen aimed at minimising peak concentrations.

1. Mallinger AG, *et al.* Pharmacokinetics of tranylcypromine in patients who are depressed: relationship to cardiovascular effects. *Clin Pharmacol Ther* 1986; **40:** 444–50.

Uses and Administration

Tranylcypromine, a cyclopropylamine derivative, is an MAOI with actions and uses similar to those of phenelzine (p.306). It produces a less prolonged inhibition of the enzymes than phenelzine.

Tranylcypromine is used in the treatment of depression, but as discussed on p.271 the risks associated with traditional non-selective MAOIs such as tranylcypromine usually mean that other antidepressants are preferred. It is given by mouth as the sulphate in doses equivalent to tranylcypromine 10 mg in the morning and 10 mg in the afternoon; if the response is inadequate after a week, 10 mg may be given additionally at midday; a dosage of 30 mg daily should only be exceeded with caution, although some authorities have allowed a maximum dose of 60 mg daily. Once a satisfactory response has been obtained the dosage may be gradually reduced for maintenance; some patients may continue to respond to 10 mg daily.

Tranylcypromine should be withdrawn gradually to reduce the risk of withdrawal symptoms.

Preparations

BP 1998: Tranylcypromine Tablets.

Proprietary Preparations (details are given in Part 3)
Austral.: Parnate; ***Canad.:*** Parnate; ***Ger.:*** Jatrosom N; Parnate; ***Irl.:*** Parnate; ***S.Afr.:*** Parnate; ***Spain:*** Parnate; ***UK:*** Parnate; ***USA:*** Parnate.

Multi-ingredient: ***Aust.:*** Jatrosom†; ***Austral.:*** Parstelin†; ***Irl.:*** Parstelin; ***Ital.:*** Parmodalin; ***UK:*** Parstelin.

Trazodone Hydrochloride (2541-y)

Trazodone Hydrochloride *(BANM, USAN, rINNM)*.

AF-1161. 2-[3-(4-*m*-Chlorophenylpiperazin-1-yl)propyl]-1,2,4-triazolo[4,3-*a*]pyridin-3(2*H*)-one hydrochloride.

$C_{19}H_{22}ClN_5O,HCl$ = 408.3.

CAS — 19794-93-5 (trazodone); 25332-39-2 (trazodone hydrochloride).

Pharmacopoeias. In Br. and US.

A white to off-white crystalline powder. Sparingly **soluble** to soluble in water; sparingly soluble in alcohol and in chloroform; practically insoluble in ether. A 1% solution in water has a pH of 3.9 to 4.5. **Store** in airtight containers. Protect from light.

Adverse Effects and Treatment

Trazodone has sedative properties and drowsiness may initially occur but usually disappears on continuing treatment. Other side-effects occasionally reported include dizziness, headache, nausea and vomiting, weakness, weight loss, tremor, dry mouth, bradycardia or tachycardia, orthostatic hypotension, oedema, constipation, diarrhoea, blurred vision, restlessness, confusional states, insomnia, and skin rash. Although some of these effects are typical of antimuscarinic activity it is reported that trazodone has little antimuscarinic activity compared with tricyclic antidepressants. *Animal* studies have also indicated that trazodone is less cardiotoxic than the tricyclics. Priapism has been reported on a number of occasions.

Agranulocytosis, thrombocytopenia, and anaemia have been reported rarely. Adverse effects on hepatic function, including jaundice and hepatocellular damage, which may sometimes be severe, have also been reported rarely.

Hyponatraemia possibly due to inappropriate secretion of antidiuretic hormone has been associated with the use of antidepressants, particularly in the elderly.

Symptoms of overdosage include drowsiness, dizziness, vomiting, priapism, respiratory arrest, seizures, and ECG changes. Treatment of overdosage involves gastric lavage followed by the administration of activated charcoal and symptomatic and supportive therapy.

Effects on the cardiovascular system. Although trazodone is considered to cause fewer adverse cardiovascular reactions than the tricyclic antidepressants, side-effects have, nevertheless, been reported in individual patients. In therapeutic doses it has been associated with heart block in a patient with pre-existing cardiovascular disease,[1] as well as in a patient with no ECG abnormalities.[2] Similarly, ventricular arrhythmias have been associated with therapeutic doses of trazodone both in patients with a history of cardiac problems,[3,4] and with no history of cardiac abnormalities.[5] Atrial fibrillation has been reported in one patient with ischaemic heart disease.[6]

1. Rausch JL, *et al.* Complete heart block following a single dose of trazodone. *Am J Psychiatry* 1984; **141:** 1472–3.
2. Lippmann S, *et al.* Trazodone cardiotoxicity. *Am J Psychiatry* 1983; **140:** 1383.
3. Janowsky D, *et al.* Ventricular arrhythmias possibly aggravated by trazodone. *Am J Psychiatry* 1983; **140:** 796–7.
4. Vlay SC, Friedling S. Trazodone exacerbation of VT. *Am Heart J* 1983; **106:** 604.
5. Johnson BA. Trazodone toxicity. *Br J Hosp Med* 1985; **33:** 298.
6. White WB, Wong SHY. Rapid atrial fibrillation associated with trazodone hydrochloride. *Arch Gen Psychiatry* 1985; **42:** 424.

Effects on the eyes. One patient receiving clomipramine and trazodone by mouth noted excessive blinking whenever the dose of trazodone exceeded or equalled that of clomipramine.[1] When trazodone, but not clomipramine, was withdrawn, blinking became normal within 3 weeks.

1. Cooper MA, Dening TR. Excessive blinking associated with combined antidepressants. *Br Med J* 1986; **293:** 1243.

Effects on the liver. A mixed hepatocellular-cholestatic liver enzyme pattern has been reported in one patient after about 3 weeks of treatment with trazodone in doses of up to 500 mg daily.[1] The enzyme abnormalities returned to normal 4 weeks after trazodone was discontinued but it was suggested that liver enzyme values should be monitored during the first 4 weeks of therapy. Another similar case apparently presenting as obstructive jaundice and hepatocellular inflammation, in which the patient had only been receiving 50 mg daily for 2 weeks, has also been described.[2] In this case it was believed that the patient suffered an idiosyncratic drug reaction to trazodone. Further reports of trazodone-induced liver injury include an elderly patient who developed chronic active hepatitis after receiving trazodone 150 mg daily for approximately 8 months.[3] A case of fatal hepatic necrosis reported in another elderly patient was considered to be due to treatment with trazodone and neuroleptics.[4] The authors of the report noted that up to August 1991 the UK Committee on Safety of Medicines had received 14 reports of adverse effects on the liver associated with trazodone including one episode of fatal hepatic necrosis.

1. Chu AG, *et al.* Trazodone and liver toxicity. *Ann Intern Med* 1983; **99:** 128–9.
2. Sheikh KH, Nies AS. Trazodone and intrahepatic cholestasis. *Ann Intern Med* 1983; **99:** 572.
3. Beck PL, *et al.* Chronic active hepatitis associated with trazodone therapy. *Ann Intern Med* 1993; **118:** 791–2.
4. Hull M, *et al.* Fatal hepatic necrosis associated with trazodone and neuroleptic drugs. *Br Med J* 1994; **309:** 378.

Effects on mental state. There have been reports of mania,[1,2] and paranoid psychosis with hallucinations[3] associated with the use of trazodone in depressed patients; delirium[4] in patients with bulimia nervosa; and possible psychosis or hypomania[5] in a patient receiving trazodone-tryptophan treatment of aggression.

1. Warren M, Bick PA. Two case reports of trazodone-induced mania. *Am J Psychiatry* 1984; **141:** 1103–4.
2. Arana GW, Kaplan GB. Trazodone-induced mania following desipramine-induced mania in major depressive disorders. *Am J Psychiatry* 1985; **142:** 386.
3. Kraft TB. Psychosis following trazodone administration. *Am J Psychiatry* 1983; **140:** 1383–4.
4. Damlouji NF, Ferguson JM. Trazodone-induced delirium in bulimic patients. *Am J Psychiatry* 1984; **141:** 434–5.
5. Patterson BD, Srisopark MM. Severe anorexia and possible psychosis or hypomania after trazodone-tryptophan treatment of aggression. *Lancet* 1989; **i:** 1017.

Effects on sexual function. Trazodone is notable for the number of reports of priapism that have been associated with its use.[1,2] In most cases, priapism occurred during treatment with standard doses after 1 to 3 weeks of therapy. Several patients required surgery and recovery was not always complete.[1] In a review[3] of priapism induced by psychotropic drugs, it was proposed that drug-induced priapism was related to blockade of alpha-adrenoceptors in the absence of sufficient antimuscarinic activity, criteria which the pharmacological profile of trazodone fulfills.

Trazodone has been tried in the treatment of impotence (see Sexual Dysfunction in Uses, below).

Inhibition of ejaculation has also been reported in one man[4] and an increase in libido in 3 women.[5]

1. Committee on Safety of Medicines. Priapism and trazodone (Molipaxin). *Current Problems 13* 1984.
2. Anonymous. Priapism with trazodone (Desyrel). *Med Lett Drugs Ther* 1984; **26:** 35.
3. Patel AG, *et al.* Priapism associated with psychotropic drugs. *Br J Hosp Med* 1996; **55:** 315–19.
4. Jones SD. Ejaculatory inhibition with trazodone. *J Clin Psychopharmacol* 1984; **4:** 279–81.
5. Gartrell N. Increased libido in women receiving trazodone. *Am J Psychiatry* 1986; **143:** 781–2.

Effects on the skin. Reports of adverse dermatological reactions in individual patients have included leucocytoclastic vasculitis,[1] erythema multiforme,[2] and exacerbation of psoriasis.[3]

1. Mann SC, *et al.* Leukocytoclastic vasculitis secondary to trazodone treatment. *J Am Acad Dermatol* 1984; **10:** 699–70.
2. Ford HE, Jenike MA. Erythema multiforme associated with trazodone therapy: case report. *J Clin Psychiatry* 1985; **46:** 294–5.
3. Barth JH, Baker H. Generalized pustular psoriasis precipitated by trazodone in the treatment of depression. *Br J Dermatol* 1986; **115:** 629–30.

Epileptogenic effect. Tonic-clonic seizures related to trazodone therapy have been reported in 2 patients[1,2] with no previous history of seizure disorders.

1. Bowdan ND. Seizure possibly caused by trazodone hydrochloride. *Am J Psychiatry* 1983; **140:** 642.
2. Lefkowitz D, *et al.* Seizures and trazodone therapy. *Arch Gen Psychiatry* 1985; **42:** 523.

Overdosage. Reviews of published and unpublished reports have indicated that the incidence of serious toxicity from trazodone overdose alone was low compared with tricyclic antidepressant overdose.[1-4]

In one review covering 149 overdose cases,[1] only 10 deaths had been reported and in only one case was trazodone the sole agent reported to be ingested; in this case autopsy revealed an acute myocardial infarction after the patient was stable. The remaining 9 patients also had histories of ingestion of unknown quantities of alcohol, benzodiazepines, or other sedative-hypnotics that may have contributed to their demise. In the surviving 139 patients, 2 cases of respiratory arrest, one case of priapism, one occurrence of seizure, 2 cases of right bundle-branch block, one case of atrioventricular block, and one T-wave inversion were reported. The remaining patients had minor CNS-depressant effects.

In the second review[2] no fatalities occurred in 39 of 88 cases of overdosage where trazodone alone was ingested. However 9 deaths occurred in the remaining 49 cases where trazodone was ingested with other drugs or alcohol.

For a discussion of choice of antidepressant with respect to safety in overdosage, see under Depression, p.271.

1. Hassan E, Miller DD. Toxicity and elimination of trazodone after overdose. *Clin Pharm* 1985; **4:** 97–100.
2. Gamble DE, Peterson LG. Trazodone overdose: four years of experience from voluntary reports. *J Clin Psychiatry* 1986; **47:** 544–6.
3. Crome P, Ali C. Clinical features and management of self-poisoning with newer antidepressants. *Med Toxicol* 1986; **1:** 411–20.
4. Gallant DM. Antidepressant overdose: symptoms and treatment. *Psychopathology* 1987; **20** (suppl 1): 75–81.

Precautions

Trazodone should be used with caution in patients with cardiovascular disorders, such as ischaemic heart disease and its use is not recommended in the immediate recovery phase after myocardial infarction. Similarly, it should be used with caution in patients with epilepsy and severe hepatic or renal insufficiency. Trazodone should be discontinued immediately if patients develop signs of hepatic dysfunction. Patients developing inappropriate or prolonged penile erections should discontinue trazodone immediately.

Patients should be closely monitored during early antidepressant therapy until improvement in depression is observed because suicide is an inherent risk in depressed patients. For further details, see under Depression, p.271.

Drowsiness is often experienced at the start of trazodone antidepressant therapy and patients, if affected, should not drive or operate machinery.

As with other antidepressants, trazodone therapy should be withdrawn gradually.

Breast feeding. In a study of 6 lactating women each given a single 50-mg dose of trazodone, it was concluded that exposure of babies to trazodone via breast milk is very small.[1] However, trazodone has been reported to form an active metabolite and it was not known to what extent this metabolite distributed into breast milk.

1. Verbeeck RK, *et al.* Excretion of trazodone in breast milk. *Br J Clin Pharmacol* 1986; **22:** 367–70.

Interactions

Trazodone should not be given to patients receiving MAOIs or for at least 14 days after their discontinuation. It has also been recommended that any drug liable to provoke a serious reaction (e.g. phenelzine) should not be given within one week after the discontinuation of trazodone therapy. For further details, see Antidepressants under Interactions of Phenelzine, p.305.

It is considered unlikely that trazodone will alter the effects of antihypertensives such as guanethidine; some interaction may, however, occur with clonidine. The dose of antihypertensives may need to be reduced if administered concomitantly with trazodone.

The sedative effects of trazodone may be enhanced by concurrent administration with alcohol or other CNS depressants. The potential for interaction between trazodone and general anaesthetics exists and the manufacturer recommends that trazodone should be stopped before elective surgery for as long as clinically feasible.

Trazodone can antagonise the effect of antiepileptic drugs. Trazodone may increase plasma concentrations of digoxin or phenytoin and the manufacturer recommends monitoring concentrations if used concurrently with trazodone.

Anticoagulants. For the effect of trazodone on *warfarin*, see p.967.

Antiepileptics. For the effect of trazodone on *phenytoin*, see p.355.

Pharmacokinetics

Trazodone is readily absorbed from the gastro-intestinal tract although absorption is affected by food. When trazodone is taken shortly after a meal there may be an increase in the amount absorbed, a decrease in the maximum concentration, and a lengthening in the time to maximum concentration compared with the fasting state; peak plasma concentrations occur about one hour after administration when taken on an empty stomach and after about 2 hours when taken with food. Protein binding is reported to be about 89 to 95%.

Trazodone is extensively metabolised in the liver and paths of metabolism include *N*-oxidation and hydroxylation. The metabolite *m*-chlorophenylpiperazine is active in *animals*. Trazodone is excreted predominantly in the urine almost entirely in the form of its metabolites, either in free or in conjugated form: some is excreted in the faeces via biliary elimination. The elimination of trazodone from the plasma is biphasic, with a terminal elimination half-life of 5 to 9 hours.

Small amounts of trazodone are distributed into breast milk (see under Breast Feeding in Precautions, above).

References.

1. Bayer AJ, *et al.* Pharmacokinetic and pharmacodynamic characteristics of trazodone in the elderly. *Br J Clin Pharmacol* 1983; **16:** 371–6.

Uses and Administration

Trazodone is a triazolopyridine antidepressant chemically unrelated to other classes of antidepressants. It blocks the reuptake of serotonin at presynaptic neurones and also has an action at 5-HT_1 receptors. Unlike the tricyclic antidepressants, trazodone does not inhibit the peripheral reuptake of noradrenaline, although it may indirectly facilitate neuronal release. Trazodone blocks central α_1-adrenoceptors and appears to have no effect on the central reuptake of dopamine. It does not appear to have very significant antimuscarinic properties, but has a marked sedative action.

Trazodone is given by mouth as the hydrochloride for the treatment of depression in doses of 150 mg daily initially; total daily dosage may be increased by 50 mg every 3 to 4 days to up to 300 to 400 mg daily if necessary. The daily dosage may be divided throughout the day after food or be given as a single dose at night. Divided daily dosages of up to 600 mg may be given in severe depression in hospitalised patients. A suggested initial dose in elderly and other susceptible patients is 100 mg daily, and total daily doses above 300 mg are unlikely to be needed in these patients.

As with other antidepressants, trazodone should be withdrawn gradually.

Anxiety disorders. Trazodone, like the tricyclic antidepressants, has been shown to produce beneficial effects in patients with generalised anxiety.[1] Although more studies are required to determine the role of antidepressants in the treatment of anxiety some consider them preferable to the use of benzodiazepines especially when medium- or long-term therapy is necessary or when depression is also present. For a discussion of the treatment of anxiety disorders, see p.635.

1. Rickels K, *et al.* Antidepressants for the treatment of generalized anxiety disorder: a placebo-controlled comparison of imipramine, trazodone, and diazepam. *Arch Gen Psychiatry* 1993; **50:** 884–95.

Depression. As discussed on p.271, there is very little difference in efficacy between the different groups of antidepressant drugs, and choice is often made on the basis of adverse effect profile. Trazodone has a different biochemical profile from both the tricyclics and the SSRIs.

References.

1. Weisler RH, *et al.* Comparison of bupropion and trazodone for the treatment of major depression. *J Clin Psychopharmacol* 1994; **14:** 170–9.

Disturbed behaviour. Trazodone has produced beneficial results[1-3] when tried in various disorders for the control of symptoms such as agitation, aggression, and disruptive behaviour (see under Disturbed Behaviour, p.636). Although adverse effects such as sedation and orthostatic hypotension can occur with trazodone and may be particularly problematical in the elderly, some[4] consider that, in the management of dementia, trazodone might be worth trying in nonpsychotic patients with disturbed behaviour, especially those with mild symptoms or those intolerant or unresponsive to antipsychotics.

1. Pasion RC, Kirby SG. Trazodone for screaming. *Lancet* 1993; **341:** 970.
2. Lebert F, *et al.* Behavioral effects of trazodone in Alzheimer's disease. *J Clin Psychiatry* 1994; **55:** 536–8.
3. Sultzer DL, *et al.* A double-blind comparison of trazodone and haloperidol for treatment of agitation in patients with dementia. *Am J Geriatr Psychiatry* 1997; **5:** 60–9.
4. American Psychiatric Association. Practice guideline for the treatment of patients with Alzheimer's disease and other dementias of late life. *Am J Psychiatry* 1997; **154** (suppl): 1–39.

Sexual dysfunction. Priapism can occur as an adverse effect of trazodone (see Effects on Sexual Function in Adverse Effects, above) and this has led to trials of oral trazodone for the treatment of erectile dysfunction (p.1614). Positive responses have been reported, either in conjunction with yohimbine[1] or alone.[2]

1. Montorsi F, *et al.* Effect of yohimbine-trazodone on psychogenic impotence: a randomized, double-blind, placebo-controlled study. *Urology* 1994; **44:** 732–6.
2. Lance R, *et al.* Oral trazodone as empirical therapy for erectile dysfunction: a retrospective review. *Urology* 1995; **46:** 117–20.

Substance dependence. The antidepressant and anxiolytic properties of trazodone have been reported to have been useful when tried in patients experiencing withdrawal syndromes from cocaine (p.1291)[1] or benzodiazepines (p.661).[2]

1. Small GW, Purcell JJ. Trazodone and cocaine abuse. *Arch Gen Psychiatry* 1985; **42:** 524.
2. Ansseau M, De Roeck J. Trazodone in benzodiazepine dependence. *J Clin Psychiatry* 1993; **54:** 189–91.

Preparations

USP 23: Trazodone Hydrochloride Tablets.

Proprietary Preparations (details are given in Part 3)
Aust.: Trittico; ***Belg.:*** Trazolan; ***Canad.:*** Desyrel; ***Fr.:*** Pragmarel†; ***Ger.:*** Thombran; ***Irl.:*** Molipaxin; ***Ital.:*** Trittico; ***Neth.:*** Trazolan; ***S.Afr.:*** Molipaxin; ***Spain:*** Deprax; ***Switz.:*** Trittico; ***UK:*** Molipaxin; ***USA:*** Desyrel; Trialodine†.

Trimipramine (2538-a)

Trimipramine *(BAN, USAN, rINN)*.

IL-6001; 7162-RP; Trimeprimine. Dimethyl{3-(10,11-dihydro-5*H*-dibenz[*b,f*]azepin-5-yl-2-methyl)propyl}amine.

$C_{20}H_{26}N_2$ = 294.4.

CAS — 739-71-9.

Trimipramine Maleate (2539-t)

Trimipramine Maleate *(BANM, USAN, rINNM)*.

Trimipramine Hydrogen Maleate; Trimipramini Maleas.

$C_{20}H_{26}N_2,C_4H_4O_4$ = 410.5.

CAS — 521-78-8.

Pharmacopoeias. In *Eur.* (see p.viii).

A white or almost white crystalline powder. Trimipramine maleate 34.9 mg is approximately equivalent to 25 mg of trimipramine. Slightly **soluble** in water and in alcohol; practically insoluble in ether. **Protect** from light.

Adverse Effects, Treatment, and Precautions

As for tricyclic antidepressants in general (see Amitriptyline, p.273).

Interactions

For interactions associated with tricyclic antidepressants, see Amitriptyline, p.276.

Pharmacokinetics

Trimipramine is readily absorbed after oral administration, peak plasma concentrations being obtained in 2 hours. It is metabolised in the liver to its major metabolite desmethyltrimipramine, which is active. Trimipramine is excreted in the urine mainly in the form of its metabolites. It is extensively bound to plasma proteins. The half-life is reported to be about 9 to 11 hours.

References.

1. Abernethy DR, *et al.* Trimipramine kinetics and absolute bioavailability: use of gas-liquid chromatography with nitrogen-phosphorus detection. *Clin Pharmacol Ther* 1984; **35:** 348–53.
2. Maurer H. Metabolism of trimipramine in man. *Arzneimittelforschung* 1989; **39:** 101–3.
3. Musa MN. Nonlinear kinetics of trimipramine in depressed patients. *J Clin Pharmacol* 1989; **29:** 746–7.

Uses and Administration

Trimipramine is a dibenzazepine tricyclic antidepressant with actions and uses similar to those of amitriptyline (p.278). It has marked antimuscarinic and sedative properties.

In the treatment of depression (p.271), trimipramine is given by mouth as the maleate in doses equivalent to 50 to 75 mg of trimipramine daily initially, gradually increased as necessary to 150 to 300 mg daily. A suggested initial dose for the elderly in the UK is 30 to 75 mg daily, gradually increased as necessary; half the normal maintenance dose may be sufficient. In the USA, the elderly and adolescents may be given 50 mg daily initially followed by gradual increments as necessary up to a maximum of 100 mg daily. Trimipramine may be given in divided doses during the day, but since it has a prolonged half-life, once-daily dosage regimens are also suitable, usually given at night.

Trimipramine has also been given orally as the hydrochloride and intramuscularly as the mesylate.

Trimipramine should be withdrawn gradually to reduce the risk of withdrawal symptoms.

Preparations

BP 1998: Trimipramine Tablets.

Proprietary Preparations (details are given in Part 3)
Aust.: Stangyl; ***Austral.:*** Surmontil; ***Belg.:*** Surmontil; ***Canad.:*** Apo-Trimip; Novo-Tripramine; Rhotrimine; Surmontil; ***Fr.:*** Surmontil; ***Ger.:*** Herphonal; Stangyl; ***Irl.:*** Surmontil; ***Ital.:*** Surmontil; ***Neth.:*** Surmontil; ***Norw.:*** Surmontil; ***S.Afr.:*** Surmontil; Tydamine; ***Spain:*** Surmontil; ***Swed.:*** Surmontil; ***Switz.:*** Surmontil; ***UK:*** Surmontil; ***USA:*** Surmontil.

Tryptophan (664-p)

Tryptophan *(USAN, rINN)*.

L-Tryptophan; Tryptophanum; W. L-2-Amino-3-(indol-3-yl)propionic acid.

$C_{11}H_{12}N_2O_2$ = 204.2.

CAS — 73-22-3.

Pharmacopoeias. In *Eur.* (see p.viii), *Jpn*, and *US*.

Fr. also includes DL-Tryptophan.

White to almost white or slightly yellowish-white crystals or crystalline or amorphous powder. Sparingly **soluble** in water; slightly soluble in alcohol or soluble in hot alcohol; practically insoluble in ether; soluble in dilute hydrochloric acid; dissolves in dilute solutions of alkali hydroxides and mineral acids. A 1% solution in water has a pH of 5.5 to 7.0. **Protect** from light.

Adverse Effects

Tryptophan-containing products have been associated with the eosinophilia-myalgia syndrome; for further details, see below.

Other side-effects that have been reported include nausea, headache, lightheadedness, and drowsiness.

An increased incidence of bladder tumours has been reported in *mice* given L-tryptophan orally as well as in cholesterol pellets embedded in the bladder lumen.

Eosinophilia-myalgia syndrome. In late 1989 the first notification linking the eosinophilia-myalgia syndrome with the use of tryptophan-containing products was made in the USA.[1] There followed a number of similar published case reports from the USA, Europe, and Japan. Reviews of tryptophan-associated eosinophilia-myalgia syndrome have noted that by early 1990 over 1500 cases were known in the USA.[2,3]

In early 1990 the Centers for Disease Control in the USA summarised the features and known reports concerning the syndrome.[4] As the name implies the characteristic features are an intense eosinophilia together with disabling fatigue and muscle pain, although multisystem organ involvement and inflammatory disorders affecting the joints, skin, connective tissue, lungs, heart, and liver have also been recorded. Symptoms have generally developed over several weeks and the syndrome has occurred in patients who had been receiving tryptophan for many years previously with no untoward effect. In most patients slow and gradual improvement in the degree of eosinophilia and other clinical manifestations has followed the withdrawal of tryptophan, but in some patients the disease has progressed despite withdrawal and there have been fatalities.[5-7] The inflammatory condition has necessitated the use of corticosteroids in some patients.

The eosinophilia-myalgia syndrome has been reported in patients taking both tryptophan-containing prescription products for depression and non-prescription dietary supplements for a number of disorders including insomnia, the premenstrual syndrome, and stress; it does not appear to have occurred in patients receiving amino-acid preparations containing tryptophan as part of total parenteral nutrition regimens. The recognition of this syndrome led to the withdrawal of tryptophan-containing products or severe restrictions being imposed upon their use in many countries during 1990.

Various theories were proposed as to the reason for the association of tryptophan with this syndrome. Confusion existed because the reports implicated a very wide range of products from different manufacturers. More recent evidence, however, appears to have confirmed that contaminated tryptophan has originated from a single manufacturer in Japan.[8-10] Bulk tryptophan is imported from Japan for manufacture into finished pharmaceutical dosage forms and it was noted in one of these reports[9] that a single product was often found to contain two or more lots of powdered tryptophan that were blended together during the production of tablets or capsules. Many trace contaminants have been found in batches of tryptophan associated with the syndrome.[11] One contaminant has been identified as 1,1′-ethylidenebis(tryptophan).[12] Its inclusion in bulk tryptophan powder appeared to coincide with alterations in the manufacturing conditions that involved a change in the strain of *Bacillus amyloliquefaciens* used in the fermentation process and a reduction in the amount of charcoal used for purification.[9] Other investigations indicated the presence of bacitracin-like peptides in batches of the contaminated tryptophan.[13] However, further work[14] has provided only weak support for an association between the syndrome and any one particular contaminant and the causative agent remains to be confirmed. Nonetheless, since the syndrome only appeared to be associated with tryptophan from one manufacturer, tryptophan preparations were reintroduced in the UK in 1994 for restricted use under carefully monitored conditions.[15]

1. Anonymous. Eosinophilia-myalgia syndrome—New Mexico. *MMWR* 1989; **38:** 765–7.
2. Troy JL. Eosinophilia-myalgia syndrome. *Mayo Clin Proc* 1991; **66:** 535–8.
3. Milburn DS, Myers CW. Tryptophan toxicity: a pharmacoepidemiologic review of eosinophilia-myalgia syndrome. *DICP Ann Pharmacother* 1991; **25:** 1259–62.
4. Kilbourne EM, *et al.* Interim guidance on the eosinophilia-myalgia syndrome. *Ann Intern Med* 1990; **112:** 85–6.
5. Anonymous. Eosinophilia-myalgia syndrome associated with ingestion of L-tryptophan—United States, through August 24, 1990. *JAMA* 1990; **264:** 1655.
6. Kaufman LD, *et al.* Clinical follow-up and immunogenetic studies of 32 patients with eosinophilia-myalgia syndrome. *Lancet* 1991; **337:** 1071–4.
7. Hertzman PA, *et al.* The eosinophilia-myalgia syndrome: status of 205 patients and results of treatment 2 years after onset. *Ann Intern Med* 1995; **122:** 851–5.
8. Slutsker L, *et al.* Eosinophilia-myalgia syndrome associated with exposure to tryptophan from a single manufacturer. *JAMA* 1990; **264:** 213–17.
9. Belongia EA, *et al.* An investigation of the cause of the eosinophilia-myalgia syndrome associated with tryptophan use. *N Engl J Med* 1990; **323:** 357–65.
10. Varga J, *et al.* The cause and pathogenesis of the eosinophilia-myalgia syndrome. *Ann Intern Med* 1992; **116:** 140–7.
11. Hill RH, *et al.* Contaminants in L-tryptophan associated with eosinophilia myalgia syndrome. *Arch Environ Contam Toxicol* 1993; **25:** 134–42.
12. Mayeno AN, *et al.* Characterization of "peak E", a novel amino acid associated with eosinophilia-myalgia syndrome. *Science* 1990; **250:** 1707–8.
13. Barnhart ER, *et al.* Bacitracin-associated peptides and contaminated L-tryptophan. *Lancet* 1990; **336:** 742.
14. Philen RM, *et al.* Tryptophan contaminants associated with eosinophilia-myalgia syndrome. *Am J Epidemiol* 1993; **138:** 154–9.
15. Committee on Safety of Medicines/Medicines Control Agency. L-Tryptophan (Optimax): limited availability for resistant depression. *Current Problems* 1994; **20:** 2.

Precautions

Tryptophan has been associated with eosinophilia-myalgia syndrome and it is therefore recommended that patients receiving tryptophan should be closely monitored with particular care being paid to eosinophil counts, haematological changes, and muscle symptomatology.

Patients taking tryptophan may experience drowsiness and if affected they should not drive or operate machinery. For further details of the effects of antidepressant therapy on driving see under Amitriptyline, p.276.

Abnormal metabolism of tryptophan may occur in patients with pyridoxine deficiency and tryptophan is thus sometimes given with pyridoxine supplements.

Interactions

Although tryptophan has been given as additional therapy to patients receiving MAOIs in the belief that clinical efficacy may be improved, it should be noted that the adverse effects of either drug may also be potentiated. For further details, see Antidepressants under Interactions of Phenelzine, p.305.

Use of tryptophan with drugs that inhibit the reuptake of serotonin may exacerbate the adverse effects of the latter and precipitate the serotonin syndrome (p.303).

There have been occasional reports of sexual disinhibition in patients taking tryptophan in conjunction with phenothiazines or benzodiazepines.

For a report of tryptophan reducing blood concentrations of levodopa, see Nutritional Agents under Interactions for Levodopa, p.1139.

Pharmacokinetics

Tryptophan is readily absorbed from the gastro-intestinal tract. Tryptophan is extensively bound to plasma albumin. It is metabolised in the liver by tryptophan pyrrolase. Metabolites include hydroxytryptophan, which is then converted to serotonin, and kynurenine derivatives. Some tryptophan is converted to nicotinic acid and nicotinamide. Pyridoxine and ascorbic acid are cofactors in the decarboxylation and hydroxylation respectively of tryptophan; pyridoxine apparently prevents the accumulation of the kynurenine metabolites.

References.

1. Green AR, *et al.* The pharmacokinetics of L-tryptophan following its intravenous and oral administration. *Br J Clin Pharmacol* 1985; **20:** 317–21.

Uses and Administration

Tryptophan is an amino acid which is an essential constituent of the diet. Tryptophan and DL-tryptophan have been used as dietary supplements.

Tryptophan is a precursor of serotonin. Because CNS depletion of serotonin is considered to be involved in depression, tryptophan has been used in its treatment. Although it has been given alone, evidence of effectiveness is scant and tryptophan has generally been used as adjunctive therapy in depression. Pyridoxine and ascorbic acid are involved in the metabolism of tryptophan to serotonin (see Pharmacokinetics, above) and have sometimes been given concomitantly.

In many countries preparations containing tryptophan have either been withdrawn from the market or their availability severely restricted or limited because of its association with the eosinophilia-myalgia syndrome. In the UK tryptophan is restricted to use by hospital specialists only as an adjunct to other antidepressant medication for patients with severe and disabling depressive illness of more than 2 years' continuous duration who have failed to respond to an adequate trial of standard antidepressant drug treatment.

In the treatment of depression the usual dose of tryptophan is 1 g given three times daily, but some patients may require up to 6 g daily in divided doses. Lower doses may be required in the elderly especially those with renal or hepatic impairment.

Depression. Tryptophan has only weak antidepressant properties itself but it has been used in combination with other antidepressants in the belief that it would potentiate their effects. Although beneficial effects have been reported in some patients given tryptophan with tricyclic antidepressants or MAOIs, alone or with lithium, evidence of efficacy is mainly limited to case reports and small controlled studies.[1,2]

Since the publication of reports linking the use of tryptophan with the eosinophilic-myalgia syndrome (see under Adverse Effects, above) preparations containing tryptophan for depression have either been withdrawn from the market or their availability severely restricted and limited in many countries. In the UK tryptophan is restricted to use by hospital specialists only as an adjunct to other antidepressant medication for patients with severe and disabling depressive illness of more than 2 years' continuous duration who have failed to respond to an adequate trial of standard antidepressant drug treatment.[3]

For a discussion of the treatment of depression, see p.271.

1. Barker WA, *et al.* The Newcastle chronic depression study: results of a treatment regime. *Int Clin Psychopharmacol* 1987; **2:** 261–72.
2. Smith S. Tryptophan in the treatment of resistant depression—a review. *Pharm J* 1998; **261:** 819–21.
3. Committee on Safety of Medicines/Medicines Control Agency. L-Tryptophan (Optimax): limited availability for resistant depression. *Current Problems* 1994; **20:** 2.

Dietary supplementation. The use of tryptophan as a dietary supplement has been reviewed.[1] However, because of its association with the eosinophilia-myalgia syndrome (see under Adverse Effects, above), the addition of tryptophan to food intended for human consumption is prohibited in some countries.

1. Li Wan Po A, Maguire T. Tryptophan: useful dietary supplement or a health hazard? *Pharm J* 1990; **244:** 484–5.

Insomnia. Tryptophan, sometimes in the form of dietary supplements, has enjoyed some popularity for the treatment of insomnia (p.638). However, the point has been made that in comparison with other hypnotics such as the benzodiazepines, the effects of tryptophan have been more difficult to substantiate and enthusiasm for tryptophan has waned considerably amongst sleep researchers.[1] It should also be noted that since the publication of reports linking the use of tryptophan with the eosinophilia-myalgia syndrome (see under Adverse Effects, above) preparations indicated for insomnia have been withdrawn from the market in many countries.

1. Lahmeyer HW. Tryptophan for insomnia. *JAMA* 1989; **262:** 2748.

Preparations

Proprietary Preparations (details are given in Part 3)
Canad.: Tryptan; ***Ger.:*** Ardeytropin; Kalma; Sedanoct†; ***UK:*** Optimax.

Multi-ingredient: ***Austral.:*** Trypto-Sleep†; ***Fr.:*** Vita-Dermacide; ***Irl.:*** Optimax; ***Spain:*** Calcioretard; ***USA:*** PDP Liquid Protein.

Venlafaxine Hydrochloride (10487-d)

Venlafaxine Hydrochloride *(BANM, USAN, rINNM)*.

Wy-45030. *(RS)*-1-(2-Dimethylamino-1-*p*-methoxyphenylethyl)cyclohexanol hydrochloride.

$C_{17}H_{27}NO_2,HCl = 313.9.$

CAS — 93413-69-5 (venlafaxine); 99300-78-4 (venlafaxine hydrochloride).

Venlafaxine hydrochloride 28.3 mg is approximately equivalent to 25 mg of venlafaxine.

Adverse Effects and Treatment

Adverse effects that have been reported most frequently with venlafaxine include nausea, headache, insomnia, somnolence, dry mouth, dizziness, constipation, asthenia, sweating, and nervousness. Orthostatic hypotension has been seen occasionally. Other adverse effects have included anorexia, dyspepsia, abdominal pain, anxiety, sexual dysfunction, visual disturbances, vasodilatation, vomiting, tremor, paraesthesia, chills, palpitations, weight gain, agitation, and skin rashes. Convulsions have also been reported. Reversible increases in liver enzymes and alterations in serum-cholesterol concentrations have also been seen. Dose-related increases in blood pressure have been observed in some patients. Activation of mania or hypomania has occasionally been reported.

Hyponatraemia possibly due to inappropriate secretion of antidiuretic hormone has been associated with the use of antidepressants, particularly in the elderly.

In overdosage, the symptoms that have reported include lethargy, somnolence, ECG changes, cardiac arrhythmias, and seizures. Treatment of overdosage includes emesis induction or gastric lavage followed by symptomatic and supportive therapy. The use of activated charcoal by mouth as an adjunct to gastric lavage has been suggested. Dialysis, haemoperfusion, exchange perfusion, and measures to increase urine production are considered unlikely to be of benefit.

Precautions

Venlafaxine should be used with caution in patients with hepatic or renal impairment and those with a history of myocardial infarction or unstable heart disease. Blood pressure monitoring may be advisable in patients taking more than 200 mg of venlafaxine daily. Venlafaxine should also be used with caution in patients with a history of epilepsy and should be discontinued in any patient developing a seizure. It should also be used cautiously in patients with a history of hypomania or mania. Venlafaxine should be discontinued in patients who develop a rash.

Patients should be closely monitored during early antidepressant therapy until improvement in depression is observed because suicide is an inherent risk in depressed patients. For further details, see under Depression, p.271.

As with other antidepressants, venlafaxine may impair performance of skilled tasks and if affected, patients should not drive or operate machinery.

Symptoms reported on abrupt discontinuation or dose reduction of venlafaxine therapy include fatigue, headache, nausea or vomiting, dizziness, dry mouth, diarrhoea, insomnia, nervousness, confusion, paraesthesia, sweating, and vertigo. It is therefore recommended that venlafaxine should be withdrawn gradually over at least one week after more than one week's therapy and the patient monitored to minimise the risk of withdrawal reactions.

Breast feeding. In one study[1] both venlafaxine and its metabolite *O*-desmethylvenlafaxine were detected in breast milk in significant quantities and there were measurable concentrations of desmethylvenlafaxine in the infants' plasma.

1. Ilett KF, *et al.* Distribution and excretion of venlafaxine and O-desmethylvenlafaxine in human milk. *Br J Clin Pharmacol* 1998; **45:** 459–62

Interactions

Venlafaxine should not be used concomitantly with MAOIs. At least 14 days should elapse between discontinuation of an MAOI and starting treatment with venlafaxine and at least 7 days should elapse between stopping venlafaxine and starting any drug liable to provoke a serious reaction (e.g. phenelzine). For further details, see Antidepressants under Interactions of Phenelzine, p.305.

Cimetidine inhibits the hepatic metabolism of venlafaxine but not its active metabolite *O*-desmethylvenlafaxine, which is present in the plasma in much greater concentrations. The manufacturer, therefore, recommends that clinical monitoring may only be necessary when cimetidine and venlafaxine are administered concomitantly to elderly patients and to those with hepatic impairment or pre-existing hypertension.

Pharmacokinetics

Venlafaxine is readily absorbed from the gastro-intestinal tract. Following oral administration it undergoes extensive first-pass metabolism in the liver mainly to the active metabolite *O*-desmethylvenlafaxine. Peak plasma concentrations of venlafaxine and *O*-desmethylvenlafaxine appear about 2 and 4 hours after administration, respectively. Protein binding of venlafaxine and *O*-desmethylvenlafaxine is low. The mean elimination half-life of venlafaxine and *O*-desmethylvenlafaxine is about 5 and 11 hours, respectively. Venlafaxine is excreted predominately in the urine, mainly in the form of its metabolites, either free or in conjugated form; about 2% is excreted in the faeces.

References.

1. Troy SM, *et al.* The pharmacokinetics of venlafaxine when given in a twice-daily regimen. *J Clin Pharmacol* 1995; **35:** 404–9.
2. Troy SM, *et al.* Pharmacokinetics and effect of food on the bioavailability of orally administered venlafaxine. *J Clin Pharmacol* 1997; **37:** 954–61.
3. Ball SE, *et al.* Venlafaxine: in vitro inhibition of CYP2D6 dependent imipramine and desipramine metabolism; comparative studies with selected SSRIs, and effects on human hepatic CYP3A4, CYP2C9 and CYP1A2. *Br J Clin Pharmacol* 1997; **43:** 619–26.

Distribution into breast milk. For reference to the distribution of venlafaxine and its metabolite into breast milk, see Breast Feeding under Precautions, above.

Renal impairment. The mean terminal disposition half-life of venlafaxine was prolonged from a mean of 3.8 hours in 18 healthy subjects to 5.8 hours in 12 patients with mild to moderate renal impairment (creatinine clearance 10 to 70 mL per minute) and 10.6 in patients requiring haemodialysis;[1] corresponding values for *O*-desmethylvenlafaxine, the active major metabolite of venlafaxine, were 11.8, 16.8, and 28.5 hours respectively. Because of the large intersubject variability the change in disposition for venlafaxine and its active metabolite was evident only in patients with a creatinine clearance of less than 30 mL per minute; drug clearance in these patients was reduced by about 55% and half-life more than doubled. It was calculated that for these patients half the usually daily dose could be given once daily.

1. Troy SM, *et al.* The effect of renal disease on the disposition of venlafaxine. *Clin Pharmacol Ther* 1994; **56:** 14–21.

Uses and Administration

Venlafaxine, a phenylethylamine derivative, is a serotonin and noradrenaline reuptake inhibitor (SNRI); it also weakly inhibits dopamine reuptake. It is reported to have little affinity for muscarinic, histaminergic, or α_1-adrenergic receptors *in vitro*.

Venlafaxine is used in the treatment of depression. It is given by mouth as the hydrochloride; doses are expressed in terms of venlafaxine. The initial daily dose is 75 mg in two or three divided doses with food, which may be increased, if necessary, after several weeks to 150 mg daily. Severely depressed or hospitalised patients may require an initial daily dose of 150 mg increased, if necessary, by up to 75 mg every 2 to 4 days to a maximum daily dose of 375 mg; the dosage should then be gradually reduced. Modified-release preparations are available for once daily dosing. Patients with renal or hepatic impairment may require a reduced dose. It has been suggested that for patients with moderate renal or hepatic impairment, the dose should be reduced by half and given once daily.

Venlafaxine should be withdrawn gradually to reduce the risk of withdrawal symptoms.

Reviews.

1. Montgomery SA. Venlafaxine: a new dimension in antidepressant pharmacotherapy. *J Clin Psychiatry* 1993; **54:** 119–26.
2. Anonymous. Venlafaxine—a new antidepressant. *Med Lett Drugs Ther* 1994; **36:** 49–50.
3. Ellingrod VL, Perry PJ. Venlafaxine: a heterocyclic antidepressant. *Am J Hosp Pharm* 1994; **51:** 3033–46.
4. Holliday SM, Benfield P. Venlafaxine: a review of its pharmacology and therapeutic potential in depression. *Drugs* 1995; **49:** 280–94.
5. Morton WA, *et al.* Venlafaxine: a structurally unique and novel antidepressant. *Ann Pharmacother* 1995; **29:** 387–95.

Anxiety disorders. Anecdotal reports and small studies have suggested that venlafaxine might be of use in the treatment of obsessive-compulsive disorder[1,2] and in panic disorder.[3,4] The overall management of anxiety disorders is discussed on p.635.

1. Ananth J, *et al.* Venlafaxine for treatment of obsessive-compulsive disorder. *Am J Psychiatry* 1995; **152:** 1832.
2. Rauch SL, *et al.* Open treatment of obsessive-compulsive disorder with venlafaxine: a series of ten cases. *J Clin Psychopharmacol* 1996; **16:** 81–4.
3. Geracioti TD. Venlafaxine treatment of panic disorder: a case series. *J Clin Psychiatry* 1995; **56:** 408–10.
4. Pollack MH, *et al.* Venlafaxine for panic disorder: results from a double-blind, placebo-controlled study. *Psychopharmacol Bull* 1996; **32:** 667–70.

Depression. As discussed on p.271, there is very little difference in efficacy between the different groups of antidepressant drugs, and choice is often made on the basis of adverse effect profile. Selective serotonin reuptake inhibitors (SSRIs) are increasingly being recognised as first-choice treatment because they offer advantages over the older tricyclics in terms of fewer unpleasant side-effects and safety in overdosage. Similar properties also favour the use of serotonin and noradrenaline reuptake inhibitors such as venlafaxine.

References.

1. Schweizer E, *et al.* Placebo-controlled trial of venlafaxine for the treatment of major depression. *J Clin Psychopharmacol* 1991; **11:** 233–6.
2. Mendels J, *et al.* Efficacy and safety of b i d doses of venlafaxine in a dose-response study. *Psychopharmacol Bull* 1993; **29:** 169–74.
3. Schweizer E, *et al.* Comparison of venlafaxine and imipramine in the acute treatment of major depression in outpatients. *J Clin Psychiatry* 1994; **55:** 104–8.
4. Cunningham LA, *et al.* A comparison of venlafaxine, trazodone, and placebo in major depression. *J Clin Psychopharmacol* 1994; **14:** 99–106.
5. Shrivastava RK, *et al.* Long-term safety and clinical acceptability of venlafaxine and imipramine in outpatients with major depression. *J Clin Psychopharmacol* 1994; **14:** 322–9.
6. Derivan A, *et al.* Venlafaxine: measuring the onset of antidepressant action. *Psychopharmacol Bull* 1995; **31:** 439–47.
7. Anonymous. Three new antidepressants. *Drug Ther Bull.* 1996; **34:** 65–8.

Hyperactivity. When drugs are indicated for attention deficit hyperactivity disorder (p.1476) initial treatment is usually with central stimulants. Antidepressants may be used for patients who fail to respond to, or who are intolerant of, central stimulants and venlafaxine has been reported[1,2] to be effective in a small number of adult patients.

1. Hedges D, *et al.* An open trial of venlafaxine in adult patients with attention deficit hyperactivity disorder. *Psychopharmacol Bull* 1995; **31:** 779–83.
2. Adler LA, *et al.* Open-label trial of venlafaxine in adults with attention deficit disorder. *Psychopharmacol Bull* 1995; **31:** 785–8.

Preparations

Proprietary Preparations (details are given in Part 3)
Aust.: Efexor; Trewilor; ***Austral.:*** Efexor; ***Canad.:*** Effexor; ***Ger.:*** Trevilor; ***Ital.:*** Efexor; ***Neth.:*** Efexor; ***S.Afr.:*** Efexor; ***Spain:*** Dobupal; Vandral; ***Swed.:*** Efexor; ***Switz.:*** Efexor; ***UK:*** Efexor; ***USA:*** Effexor.

Viloxazine Hydrochloride (2540-l)

Viloxazine Hydrochloride *(BANM, USAN, rINNM).*

ICI-58834. 2-(2-Ethoxyphenoxymethyl)morpholine hydrochloride.

$C_{13}H_{19}NO_3,HCl = 273.8.$

CAS — 46817-91-8 (viloxazine); 35604-67-2 (viloxazine hydrochloride).

Viloxazine hydrochloride 57.7 mg is approximately equivalent to 50 mg of viloxazine.

Adverse Effects

Nausea is commonly associated with viloxazine therapy, and vomiting and headache may also occur. Viloxazine has been associated with fewer antimuscarinic side-effects such as dry mouth, disturbance of accommodation, tachycardia, constipation, and difficulty with micturition than the tricyclic antidepressants. Exacerbation of anxiety, agitation, drowsiness, confusion, ataxia, dizziness, insomnia, tremor, paraesthesia, sweating, musculo-skeletal pain, mild hypertension, skin rashes, convulsions, and jaundice with elevated transaminases have also been reported less frequently.

It has also been stated that cardiac arrhythmias and severe hypotension are less likely to occur with viloxazine than with tricyclic antidepressants in high doses or in overdosage.

Epileptogenic effect. In a review[1] of 6 cases of convulsive seizures during treatment with viloxazine notified to the UK Committee on Safety of Medicines, and 2 other cases from Japan, critical study of the patients' histories suggested a possible causal connection in only 2. It was concluded that even if viloxazine did possess convulsive properties like other antidepressants, it was probably less epileptogenic than conventional tricyclics and was not contra-indicated in epileptics.

1. Edwards JG, Glen-Bott M. Does viloxazine have epileptogenic properties? *J Neurol Neurosurg Psychiatry* 1984; **47:** 960–4.

Precautions

Although viloxazine appears to be less cardiotoxic than the tricyclic antidepressants, it should be used with caution in patients with cardiovascular disease and should be avoided in the immediate recovery phase after myocardial infarction. Viloxazine is contra-indicated in patients with mania, severely impaired liver function, or a history of peptic ulcer. Caution is necessary in patients with epilepsy. Patients with suicidal tendencies should be carefully supervised during treatment. For further details, see under Depression, p.271.

Viloxazine is not recommended in patients who are breast feeding.

Withdrawal of viloxazine may occasionally be associated with malaise, headache, and vomiting.

Impaired alertness may be experienced with viloxazine antidepressant therapy and patients, if affected, should not drive or operate machinery. For further details of the effects of antidepressant therapy on driving see under Amitriptyline, p.276.

If surgery is required the anaesthetist should be informed that the patient has received viloxazine (see also Anaesthesia under Amitriptyline, p.275).

Migraine. Mention has been made that viloxazine may occasionally precipitate attacks in migrainous patients and in these circumstances should be discontinued.[1]

1. Nightingale S. Management of migraine. *Prescribers' J* 1985; **25:** 129–34.

Porphyria. Viloxazine hydrochloride was considered to be unsafe in patients with acute porphyria because it has been shown to be porphyrinogenic in *animals.*[1]

1. Moore MR, McColl KEL. *Porphyria: drug lists.* Glasgow: Porphyria Research Unit, University of Glasgow, 1991.

Interactions

Viloxazine should not be given to patients receiving MAOIs or for at least 14 days after their discontinuation. It has also been recommended that any drug liable to provoke a serious reaction (e.g. phenelzine) should not be given within one week after discontinuation of viloxazine therapy. Viloxazine may diminish the effects of antihypertensives, such as guanethidine, debrisoquine, and bethanidine; some interaction may also occur with clonidine and, in general, blood pressure should be monitored when viloxazine is prescribed with antihypertensive therapy. Interactions may occur with drugs that undergo hepatic metabolism increasing their plasma concentrations. The dosage of drugs such as phenytoin, carbamazepine, and theophylline may therefore need to be reduced, but it should also be noted that viloxazine has caused convulsions. Since viloxazine appears to have some influence on brain dopamine metabolism viloxazine should be given with caution to patients receiving levodopa. The CNS depressant action of alcohol may be enhanced by concurrent administration of viloxazine.

Pharmacokinetics

Viloxazine is readily absorbed from the gastro-intestinal tract and extensively metabolised. The principal paths of metabolism of viloxazine include hydroxylation and conjugation. Viloxazine is excreted in the urine, mainly in the form of its metabolites, either free or in conjugated form.

Unlike the tricyclic antidepressants, viloxazine has a short plasma half-life of about 2 to 5 hours.

Viloxazine is distributed into breast milk.

Uses and Administration

Viloxazine is a bicyclic antidepressant. It does not have marked antimuscarinic or sedative properties. Like the tricyclic antidepressants (see Amitriptyline, p.273), viloxazine is an inhibitor of the reuptake of noradrenaline; it may also enhance the release of serotonin from neuronal stores.

Viloxazine is given for the treatment of depression (p.271) by mouth as the hydrochloride in doses equivalent to viloxazine 300 mg daily, preferably taken as 200 mg in the morning and 100 mg at lunchtime; the last dose of the day should not be given later than 6 p.m. A total daily dose of 400 mg should not be exceeded. A suggested initial dose for the elderly is 100 mg daily cautiously increased if necessary. Half the normal maintenance dose may be adequate.

Viloxazine should be withdrawn gradually to reduce the risk of withdrawal symptoms.

Preparations

Proprietary Preparations (details are given in Part 3)
Aust.: Vivarint; ***Belg.:*** Vivalan; ***Fr.:*** Vivalan; ***Ger.:*** Vivalan; ***Ital.:*** Vicilan; ***Spain:*** Vivarint; ***UK:*** Vivalan.

Viqualine (1456-p)

Viqualine *(rINN).*

6-Methoxy-4-{3-[(3*R*,4*R*)-3-vinyl-4-piperidyl]propyl}quinoline.

$C_{20}H_{26}N_2O = 310.4.$

CAS — 72714-74-0.

Viqualine is reported to be a serotonin reuptake inhibitor with some serotonin-releasing effects. It is being studied as an antidepressant and has been tried as an adjunct to aid abstinence in alcohol-dependent patients.

References.

1. Kenny M, *et al.* The effect of PK5078, a new serotonin uptake inhibitor, on serotonin levels and uptake in human platelets, following administration to healthy volunteers. *Eur J Clin Pharmacol* 1983; **25:** 23–8.
2. Naranjo CA, *et al.* Differential effects of viqualine on alcohol intake and other consummatory behaviors. *Clin Pharmacol Ther* 1989; **46:** 301–9.

Zimeldine Hydrochloride (14028-v)

Zimeldine Hydrochloride *(BANM, USAN, rINNM).*

H-102/09 (zimeldine); Zimelidine Hydrochloride. (*Z*)-4-Bromo-γ-(3-pyridyl)cinnamyldimethylamine dihydrochloride monohydrate.

$C_{16}H_{17}BrN_2,2HCl,H_2O = 408.2.$

CAS — 56775-88-3 (zimeldine); 60525-15-7 (anhydrous zimeldine dihydrochloride); 61129-30-4 (zimeldine dihydrochloride monohydrate).

Zimeldine hydrochloride is a serotonin reuptake inhibitor that was formerly used in the treatment of depression. It was withdrawn worldwide in September 1983 because of the risk of Guillain-Barré syndrome associated with its use.

References.

1. Anonymous. Astra's zimeldine withdrawn because of neurological side effects. *Pharm J* 1983; **231:** 360.
2. Committee on Safety of Medicines. Zimeldine (Zelmid). *Current Problems 11* 1983.

Antidiabetics

This chapter describes diabetes mellitus and its management with antidiabetics. The oral drugs included in this chapter are classified in Table 1; insulin, which is given parenterally, is discussed on p.322 and classified in Table 2.

Diabetes mellitus

Diabetes mellitus is a group of disorders of carbohydrate metabolism in which the action of insulin is diminished or absent through altered secretion, decreased insulin activity, or a combination of both factors. It is characterised by hyperglycaemia. As the disease progresses tissue or vascular damage ensues leading to severe diabetic complications such as retinopathy, nephropathy, neuropathy, cardiovascular disease, and foot ulceration.

Diabetes mellitus may be categorised into several types but the two major types are type 1 (insulin-dependent diabetes mellitus; IDDM) and type 2 (non-insulin-dependent diabetes mellitus; NIDDM). The term juvenile-onset diabetes has sometimes been used for type 1 and maturity-onset diabetes for type 2. Another type of diabetes mellitus, malnutrition-related diabetes, is briefly discussed under Effects of Cassava, in Starch, p.1356.

Type 1 diabetes mellitus is present in patients who have little or no endogenous insulin secretory capacity and who therefore require exogenous insulin therapy for survival. This form of the disease has an auto-immune basis in most cases, and usually develops before adulthood. The associated hypoinsulinaemia and hyperglucagonaemia put such patients at risk of ketosis and ketoacidosis.

In **type 2 diabetes mellitus** the disease typically develops in later life. Insulin secretion may appear normal or even excessive (and type 2 patients are thus less prone to ketosis) but it is insufficient to compensate for insulin resistance. Obesity is present in the majority of type 2 patients; non-obese patients tend to have low insulin secretory capacity (although not as low as in type 1 diabetes) rather than appreciable insulin resistance.

Diagnosis of diabetes mellitus. Diagnosis is based upon blood-glucose concentrations exceeding set values under specified conditions. Criteria issued by WHO[1] in the 1980s advised that diabetes mellitus is likely if the glucose concentration in a random sample of venous whole blood exceeds 10.0 mmol per litre or 11.1 mmol per litre in capillary whole blood or in venous plasma. If there are accompanying symptoms the presence of marked hyperglycaemia is considered diagnostic of diabetes. In the absence of symptoms or if the elevation of blood-glucose concentration is less marked (more often the case with type 2 than with type 1 diabetes), the diagnosis needs to be confirmed either by repeated sampling or by an **oral glucose tolerance test** (OGTT). This test consists of an overnight fast followed by measurement of the fasting blood-glucose concentration, then the administration of a 75-g oral glucose load (in children 1.75 g per kg body-weight up to a maximum of 75 g), and further measurement of the blood-glucose concentration two hours later. WHO diagnostic values for measurements in venous whole blood are greater than or equal to 6.7 mmol per litre for the fasting state and 10.0 mmol per litre after the glucose load. The corresponding values for capillary whole blood are 6.7 and 11.1 mmol per litre, and for venous plasma 7.8 and 11.1 mmol per litre.[1,3] There has been some confusion at an international level as to whether the glucose load should be 75 g of the anhydrous form or the monohydrate. Sources at WHO have therefore suggested that the form should be standardised as 75 g of anhydrous glucose (anhydrous dextrose), which would be equivalent to 82.5 g of the monohydrate (glucose BP; dextrose monohydrate).

Table 1. Classification of oral antidiabetics.

Aldose Reductase Inhibitors	*Sulphonylureas*
Epalrestat	Acetohexamide
Sorbinil	Carbutamide
Tolrestat	Chlorpropamide
Alpha Glucosidase Inhibitors	Glibenclamide
Acarbose	Glibornuride
Emiglitate	Gliclazide
Miglitol	Glimepiride
Voglibose	Glipizide
Biguanides	Gliquidone
Buformin	Glisentide
Metformin	Glisolamide
Phenformin	Glisoxepide
Miscellaneous	Glyclopyramide
Glybuzole	Glycyclamide
Glymidine	Tolazamide
Guar Gum	Tolbutamide
Midaglizole	
Pioglitazone	
Repaglinide	
Troglitazone	

Modified diagnostic criteria have been proposed by the American Diabetes Association:[2] as an alternative to the WHO diagnostic values from an OGTT they recommend either a randomly sampled plasma-glucose concentration of 11.1 mmol or more per litre, or, for preference, a fasting plasma-glucose concentration of 7.0 mmol or more per litre as diagnostic of diabetes provided the diagnosis is confirmed by any of the 3 methods on a subsequent day. Patients with fasting plasma-glucose concentrations between 6.1 mmol per litre (the upper limit of normal) and 7.0 mmol per litre are considered to have impaired fasting glucose, the equivalent of impaired glucose tolerance. A subsequent provisional report[61] from WHO has suggested adoption of similar criteria. However, there has been some concern about the lack of agreement between these newer criteria and the previous ones, which may result in alterations in prevalence of diabetes.[62,63]

Other diagnostic methods, such as measurement of glycosylated haemoglobin have been investigated.[4] There is also some interest in using antibodies to insulin, to islet cells, or to the enzyme glutamic acid decarboxylase, as predictive tests for those patients likely to develop diabetes mellitus.[5]

Once the presence of diabetes has been confirmed the distinction between type 1 and type 2 is made on clinical grounds. Type 1 diabetes is characterised particularly by a rapid onset of symptoms and there is often associated ketosis; patients tend to be young. Type 2 diabetes usually occurs in older patients, has less abrupt onset of symptoms, and is commonly associated with obesity; ketosis is typically absent.

Management of diabetes mellitus.

DIETARY MODIFICATION. Dietary control is important in both type 1 and type 2 diabetes, and in the latter, possibly in association with increased exercise (see below), may sometimes correct the condition, at least temporarily. Eliminating sugar from the diet is not the only aim. Correction of obesity is desirable in all patients and in those with type 2 diabetes it will remove one of the factors associated with insulin resistance. Anorectic drugs are not effective in promoting weight loss in these patients.[6] A high fibre intake may also lower blood-sugar concentrations and additional fibre is sometimes taken in the form of guar gum (see p.321). The influence of diet on diabetes is such that all diabetic patients need to be aware of the composition of foods and to be able to make adjustments to their diet, especially to counteract treatment-induced hypoglycaemia. Controversy continues, however, as to the optimum composition of the diet in diabetics, and in particular as to what the relative contribution of calories from fat and from carbohydrate should be.

EXERCISE. All diabetic patients should be encouraged to exercise, according to their age and physical capability.[1] Exercise improves metabolism and enhances the action of insulin on the tissues. It is also a useful component of any weight reduction programme although diet is more effective in promoting weight loss and metabolic control.[6]

ORAL HYPOGLYCAEMICS. If patients with type 2 diabetes have not achieved suitable control after about 3 months of dietary modification and increased physical activity, then oral hypoglycaemics may be tried. The two major classes are the *sulphonylureas* and the *biguanides*. Sulphonylureas act mainly by increasing endogenous insulin secretion, while biguanides act chiefly by decreasing hepatic gluconeogenesis and increasing peripheral utilisation of glucose. Both types function only in the presence of some endogenous insulin production. Other drugs that can reduce blood-sugar concentrations when taken by mouth include the alpha-glucosidase inhibitors, such as acarbose and miglitol, and guar gum.

Oral treatment of type 2 diabetes is usually begun with a sulphonylurea.[7] Chlorpropamide and glibenclamide have long half-lives and hence an increased tendency to cause hypoglycaemia, although a recent large study[8] reported that hypoglycaemic episodes were less frequent with chlorpropamide than glibenclamide. They are best avoided in the elderly; a sulphonylurea with a short half-life, such as gliclazide, gliquidone, or tolbutamide, should be used instead.

There is evidence that the use of low-dose sulphonylurea therapy in patients with diagnosed type 2 diabetes but near-normoglycaemia due to early remission (the so-called honeymoon period) can delay the onset of hyperglycaemia.[9]

Sulphonylureas can cause weight gain and obese patients may be treated with the biguanide metformin rather than with a sulphonylurea. Results from the UK Prospective Diabetes Study (UKPDS) have suggested substantial benefits from the use of metformin to provide intensive blood-glucose control in overweight diabetic patients.[64] Metformin is as effective as the sulphonylureas in terms of blood-glucose control and is less likely to cause hypoglycaemia,[64] but has a rare tendency to cause lactic acidosis in patients with renal impairment,[10] in whom it should not be used.

Drug treatment may also involve an alpha-glucosidase inhibitor such as *acarbose* which acts by delaying the absorption of glucose from a carbohydrate load.[11] Combination of acarbose with a sulphonylurea and diet has also been shown to be more effective than diet and sulphonylurea therapy alone.[12] *Guar gum* may also be used as an adjunct to any of the oral hypoglycaemics to enhance the improvement in blood-sugar control.

Should treatment with one of the oral hypoglycaemics fail then a different type or in some instances combinations of different types may produce improvement. Alarming evidence[64] of an increased risk of death in UKPDS patients given intensive therapy with metformin in combination with a sulphonylurea was not borne out by further analysis, although some concern remains. Patients with type 2 diabetes who cannot be controlled adequately by oral therapy and diet need insulin either in addition to or in place of oral therapy. About 30% of those on sulphonylureas will be transferred to insulin treatment within 4 years, a change which now tends to be made earlier owing to increasingly strict criteria for glycaemic control (tight control of blood glucose has now been shown to decrease the risk of complications, see Diabetic Complications, below). There is evidence that therapy with insulin and a sulphonylurea is more effective than therapy with insulin alone in type 2 patients.[13] As insulin therapy is associated with more hypoglycaemic episodes and a greater tendency to weight gain it remains reasonable to begin with oral therapy in type 2 diabetes before proceeding to insulin.[14]

Insulin is also added to oral treatment to provide cover during periods of severe stress, as in severe infection, trauma, or major surgery. Type 2 patients who become pregnant should be switched from oral therapy to insulin (see Pregnancy, below).

INSULIN THERAPY. While insulin may not be a necessary part of the treatment of type 2 diabetes, it is essential in the treatment of patients with type 1, since they have little or no endogenous insulin secretory capacity.

The aim of insulin therapy is to achieve the best possible control of blood-glucose concentrations without the risk of the hypoglycaemia that can occur if too fine a degree of control is attempted. Tight control of blood-glucose concentrations can reduce the long-term complications of diabetes such as retinopathy, nephropathy, and neuropathy (see Diabetic Complications, below) but in some patients (such as the elderly, or those who lack motivation) it may be better merely to alleviate symptoms rather than attempt tight control. Exercise and dietary discipline are necessary to maintain normal sensitivity to insulin.

Insulin may be of beef or pork origin, or it may be human insulin produced by gene technology or by modification of porcine insulin. Human and porcine insulin are less immunogenic than bovine insulin and where possible most newly diagnosed type 1 patients are now given human insulin. Modified insulin analogues such as insulin lispro are now available.

Insulin is available in a range of preparations offering a short, intermediate, or long action on subcutaneous injection. Insulin dosage schedules make use of the varying durations of action, for example by incorporating a short-acting and intermediate-acting insulin into a daily schedule. Most patients with type 1 diabetes require two or three injections of insulin daily, or with intensive regimens even more. A once-daily regimen can be used if the patient is simply to be kept asymptomatic; this may also be successful in patients with type 2 diabetes not satisfactorily controlled by oral hypoglycaemics.

The various types of insulin may also be given intramuscularly but the subcutaneous route is usually preferred. Soluble insulin can also be given intravenously. Details of insulin administration and dosage schedules are given on p.327.

IMMUNOSUPPRESSION. Many patients with type 1 diabetes experience a temporary improvement in pancreatic beta-cell function soon after initial treatment with insulin. This produces a period of remission known as the honeymoon period during which a small dose of insulin is sufficient to maintain good control. Attempts to prolong the honeymoon period have included tight control immediately following diagnosis and also, given the probable auto-immune nature of the condition, administration of an immunosuppressant.[15-19]

PANCREATIC TRANSPLANTATION. Transplantation of the whole pancreas in patients with type 1 diabetes poorly controlled by insulin therapy has usually been carried out in association with kidney transplantation.[20,21] However, this is currently unlikely to be practicable for many patients, and transplantation of pancreatic islet cells has been investigated as an alternative.[21-25] Results in *animals* have suggested that a reasonable degree of glycaemic control may be achievable long term without immunosuppression, using a vascularised 'artificial pancreas' containing allogeneic or even xenogeneic islet cells.[26] However, few patients to date have remained independent of insulin within a year of islet-cell transplantation.[25]

OTHER DRUG TREATMENTS. Various other drugs have been tried for diabetes mellitus, particularly when conventional therapy has proved unsuccessful. *Troglitazone*, one of the thiazolidinediones, which appear to increase insulin sensitivity, has been the subject of much interest for type 2 diabetes and insulin resistance,[27,28] but hepatotoxicity has limited its value. Addition of the α-glucosidase inhibitor *miglitol* to diet and sulphonylurea therapy has been reported to improve glycaemic control in poorly controlled type 2 patients.[29] Addition of the amylin analogue *pramlintide* to insulin therapy has improved glycaemic control in patients with type 1 diabetes.[30] Other approaches under investigation include inhibition of fatty acid oxidation or the use of β_3-adrenoceptor agonists (selective agonists of β-receptors thought to be associated with lipolysis and thermogenesis) to stimulate energy expenditure.[27]

Mecasermin (insulin-like growth factor I; IGF-1) has been shown to improve metabolic control in patients with type 1 diabetes and insulin resistance (and in some type 2 patients).[31,32] *Glucagon-like peptide 1* (GLP-1; insulinotropin) improves glycaemic control in type 2 patients.[33] Improvements in insulin sensitivity have also been seen in insulin-resistant type 2 patients treated with a haemodialysate of calf blood,[34] while in other studies improved insulin sensitivity was seen following treatment with the *vanadium* salt, vanadyl sulphate,[35] or *chromium* supplementation.[36]

PROPHYLAXIS. Because overt diabetes is the culmination of a prolonged process some effort has gone into preventing its development, either by interventions aimed at modifying risk factors in populations or groups, or by targeting individuals thought to be at high risk.[3] Strategies under consideration for the prevention of type 1 diabetes include avoidance of cows' milk proteins (thought to be a possible environmental trigger) during infancy; administration of free radical scavengers such as nicotinamide;[37] administration of prophylactic insulin[38,39] (or possibly of oral hypoglycaemics) to allow 'beta cell rest'; encouraging the development of antigen tolerance, for example by the oral administration of antigens such as insulin, glutamic acid decarboxylase, or heat shock protein[39-41] (a similar approach using subcutaneous antigen has apparently extended the honeymoon period in *animal* studies[42]); or by immunosuppression (see above) or immunomodulation with agents such as BCG vaccine,[43] although some have found the latter ineffective.[44] Preventive strategies for insulin resistance and type 2 diabetes have tended to focus on weight loss and dietary modification.[3] However, prophylactic drug therapy may be possible: a study with troglitazone in nondiabetic obese subjects demonstrated reduced insulin resistance, and improved glucose tolerance in those in whom it was impaired.[45,46]

Monitoring of therapy. Monitoring of therapy is an integral part of the management of the diabetic patient. Detection of urinary glucose has generally been superseded by the monitoring of blood glucose (see Glucose Tests, p.1585). For adequate diabetic control, the aim is to reduce fasting blood-glucose concentrations to within the range 3.3 to 5.6 mmol per litre of venous whole blood, and postprandial concentrations to below 10 mmol per litre.[1] Many patients monitor their blood-glucose concentrations regularly at home and this is essential for intensified insulin regimens when tight control is required. The value of self-monitoring of blood-glucose concentrations in type 2 patients is more debatable,[47] although moves to more intensive therapy may make this desirable. Detection of urinary ketones is useful in diabetics prone to ketosis; this is usually performed in clinics. Diabetic clinics also often measure the degree of haemoglobin glycosylation (HbA_1 or HbA_{1c}) as an indicator of mean blood-glucose control. More recently the advanced glycation end-product (AGE) of haemoglobin has been found to be a useful indicator of long-term blood glucose control.[48] Techniques for continuous monitoring of blood glucose are under investigation.[49,50]

Pregnancy. Adverse pregnancy outcomes, including spontaneous abortion and congenital malformation, are more common in diabetic than in nondiabetic women. Improved management of the pregnant diabetic patient, particularly early in pregnancy, lessens the incidence of such events,[51,52] but an increased risk still exists.[53] Diabetic women are advised to plan their pregnancies so that glycaemic control can be improved before conception. Some may need to avoid pregnancy (most commonly because of renal disease),[54] but management has improved sufficiently for this to be rare.[52]

Insulin is the preferred treatment in pregnancy,[55] even in women with type 2 diabetes; patients taking oral hypoglycaemics should therefore be switched to insulin. Insulin regimens are similar to those nonpregnant patients, the dose being adjusted according to regular blood-glucose measurements. Insulin requirements may decrease during the first trimester but they increase during the latter two, reaching about twice prepregnancy requirements at term; they then fall once labour has begun and fall again after delivery.[55]

Pregnant diabetic patients are at risk of nocturnal hypoglycaemia owing to continued fetal glucose consumption while the mother is in a relatively fasting state. They are also prone to diabetic ketoacidosis which must be treated with great urgency because of the high risk of fetal loss.

Gestational diabetes, that is diabetes which develops during pregnancy, may simply be impaired glucose tolerance associated with pregnancy.[56] It is not clear whether treatment of gestational glucose intolerance significantly decreases perinatal mortality or birthweight.[57] There is, therefore, disagreement about the benefits of universal screening for gestational glucose intolerance.[2,56-58,65] Many women with gestational diabetes may be managed by diet alone or, if necessary, also with insulin. Some workers, however, have advocated prophylactic administration of insulin to women who could be managed by diet alone, in view of the metabolic effects of insulin.[59]

Surgery. Insulin-dependent diabetics who require surgery should be managed with a continuous intravenous insulin infusion. Insulin is given as normal the night before operation, and switched to either a variable-rate infusion via a syringe pump, together with a 5% glucose drip (with potassium chloride, provided the patient is not hyperkalaemic), or to a combined insulin-glucose infusion, on the day of operation. (Many anaesthetists prefer insulin and a sodium chloride infusion if blood glucose is already high.[60]) Subsequent conversion back to subcutaneous insulin should be undertaken before breakfast, giving the first subcutaneous dose 30 minutes before stopping continuous infusion. Non-insulin-dependent patients should have any oral treatment omitted on the day of operation, and may be given insulin by a similar regimen if control is poor or deteriorates as can happen with major surgery.

1. WHO. Diabetes mellitus: report of a WHO study group. *WHO Tech Rep Ser 727* 1985.
2. American Diabetes Association. Report of the Expert Committee on the Diagnosis and classification of Diabetes Mellitus. *Diabetes Care* 1997; **20:** 1183–97.
3. WHO. Prevention of diabetes mellitus: report of a WHO study group. *WHO Tech Rep Ser 844* 1994.
4. McCance DR, *et al.* Comparison of tests for glycated haemoglobin and fasting and two hour plasma glucose concentrations as diagnostic methods for diabetes. *Br Med J* 1994; **308:** 1323–8.
5. Palmer JP. What is the best way to predict IDDM? *Lancet* 1994; **343:** 1377–8.
6. Brown SA, *et al.* Promoting weight loss in type II diabetes. *Diabetes Care* 1996; **19:** 613–24.
7. Melander A, *et al.* Sulfonylureas: why, which and how? *Diabetes Care* 1990; **13** (suppl 3): 18–25.
8. United Kingdom Prospective Diabetes Study Group. United Kingdom prospective diabetes study (UKPDS) 13: relative efficacy of randomly allocated diet, sulphonylurea, insulin, or metformin in patients with newly diagnosed non-insulin dependent diabetes followed for three years. *Br Med J* 1995; **310:** 83–8.
9. Banerji MA, *et al.* Prolongation of near-normoglycemic remission in black NIDDM subjects with chronic low-dose sulfonylurea treatment. *Diabetes* 1995; **44:** 466–70.
10. Khan IH, *et al.* Severe lactic acidosis in patient receiving continuous ambulatory peritoneal dialysis. *Br Med J* 1993; **307:** 1056–7.
11. Buse J, *et al.* The PROTECT study: final results of a large multicenter postmarketing study in patients with type 2 diabetes. *Clin Ther* 1998; **20:** 257–69.
12. Coniff RF, *et al.* Multicenter, placebo-controlled trial comparing acarbose (BAY g 5421) with placebo, tolbutamide, and tolbutamide-plus-acarbose in non-insulin-dependent diabetes mellitus. *Am J Med* 1995; **98:** 443–51.
13. Johnson JL, *et al.* Efficacy of insulin and sulfonylurea combination therapy in type II diabetes: a meta-analysis of the randomized placebo-controlled trials. *Arch Intern Med* 1996; **156:** 259–64.
14. United Kingdom Prospective Diabetes Study Group. United Kingdom Prospective Diabetes Study 24: a 6-year, randomized, controlled trial comparing sulfonylurea, insulin, and metformin therapy in patients with newly diagnosed type 2 diabetes that could not be controlled with diet therapy. *Ann Intern Med* 1998; **128:** 165–75.
15. Pozzilli P, Maclaren NK. Immunotherapy at clinical diagnosis of insulin-dependent diabetes: an approach still worth considering. *Trends Endocrinol Metab* 1993; **4:** 101–5.
16. Bougneres PF, *et al.* Factors associated with early remission of type I diabetes in children treated with cyclosporine. *N Engl J Med* 1988; **318:** 663–70.
17. The Canadian-European Randomized Control Trial Group. Cyclosporin-induced remission of IDDM after early intervention: association of 1 yr of cyclosporin treatment with enhanced insulin secretion. *Diabetes* 1988; **37:** 1574–82.
18. Harrison LC, *et al.* Increase in remission rate in newly diagnosed type I diabetic subjects treated with azathioprine. *Diabetes* 1985; **34:** 1306–8.
19. Yilmaz MT, *et al.* Immunoprotection in spontaneous remission of type 1 diabetes: long-term follow-up results. *Diabetes Res Clin Pract* 1993; **19:** 151–62.
20. Remuzzi G, *et al.* Pancreas and kidney/pancreas transplants: experimental medicine or real improvement? *Lancet* 1994; **343:** 27–31.
21. Robertson RP. Pancreatic and islet transplantation for diabetes—cures or curiosities? *N Engl J Med* 1992; **327:** 1861–8.
22. Pyzdrowski KL, *et al.* Preserved insulin secretion and insulin dependence in recipients of islet autografts. *N Engl J Med* 1992; **327:** 220–6.
23. Gores PF, *et al.* Insulin independence in type I diabetes after transplantation of unpurified islets from single donor with 15-deoxyspergualin. *Lancet* 1993; **341:** 19–21.
24. Soon-Shiong P, *et al.* Insulin independence in a type 1 diabetic patient after encapsulated islet transplantation. *Lancet* 1994; **343:** 950–1.
25. Weir GC, Bonner-Weir S. Scientific and political impediments to successful islet transplantation. *Diabetes* 1997; **46:** 1247–56.
26. Maki T, *et al.* Novel delivery of pancreatic islet cells to treat insulin-dependent diabetes mellitus. *Clin Pharmacokinet* 1995; **28:** 471–82.
27. Petrie JR, Donnelly R. New pharmacological approaches to insulin and lipid metabolism. *Drugs* 1994; **47:** 701–10.
28. Suter SL, *et al.* Metabolic effects of new oral hypoglycemic agent CS-045 in NIDDM subjects. *Diabetes Care* 1992; **15:** 193–203.
29. Johnston PS, *et al.* Effects of the carbohydrase inhibitor miglitol in sulfonylurea-treated NIDDM patients. *Diabetes Care* 1994; **17:** 20–29.
30. Thompson RG, *et al.* Effects of pramlintide, an analog of human amylin, on plasma glucose profiles in patients with IDDM: results of a multicenter trial. *Diabetes* 1997; **46:** 632–6.
31. Moses AC, *et al.* Insulin-like growth factor I (rhIGF-I) as a therapeutic agent for hyperinsulinemic insulin-resistant diabetes mellitus. *Diabetes Res Clin Pract* 1995; **28** (suppl): S185–S194.

32. Acerini CL, *et al.* Randomised placebo-controlled trial of human recombinant insulin-like growth factor I plus intensive insulin therapy in adolescents with insulin-dependent diabetes mellitus. *Lancet* 1997; **350:** 1199–1204.
33. Todd JF, *et al.* Glucagon-like peptide-1 (GLP-1): a trial of treatment in non-insulin-dependent diabetes mellitus. *Eur J Clin Invest* 1997; **27:** 533–6.
34. Jacob S, *et al.* Improvement of glucose metabolism in patients with type II diabetes after treatment with a hemodialysate. *Arzneimittelforschung* 1996; **46:** 269–72.
35. Cohen N, *et al.* Oral vanadyl sulfate improves hepatic and peripheral insulin sensitivity in patients with non-insulin-dependent diabetes mellitus. *J Clin Invest* 1995; **95:** 2501–9.
36. Anderson RA, *et al.* Elevated intakes of supplemental chromium improve glucose and insulin variables in individuals with type 2 diabetes. *Diabetes* 1997; **46:** 1786–91.
37. Pozzilli P, *et al.* Meta-analysis of nicotinamide treatment in patients with recent onset insulin dependent diabetes. *Diabetes Care* 1996; **19:** 1357–63.
38. Keller RJ, *et al.* Insulin prophylaxis in individuals at high risk of type 1 diabetes. *Lancet* 1993; **341:** 927–8.
39. Alberti KGMM. Preventing insulin dependent diabetes mellitus. *Br Med J* 1993; **307:** 1435–6.
40. Williams G. IDDM: long honeymoon, sweet ending. *Lancet* 1994; **343:** 684–5.
41. Jones DB, Armstrong NW. Peptide therapy for diabetes. *Lancet* 1994; **343:** 1168–9.
42. Elias D, Cohen IR. Peptide therapy for diabetes in NOD mice. *Lancet* 1994; **343:** 704–6.
43. Shehadeh N, *et al.* Effect of adjuvant therapy on development of diabetes in mouse and man. *Lancet* 1994; **343:** 706–7.
44. Pozzilli P, *et al.* BCG vaccine in insulin-dependent diabetes mellitus. *Lancet* 1997; **349:** 1520–1.
45. Nolan JJ, *et al.* Improvement in glucose tolerance and insulin resistance in obese subjects treated with troglitazone. *N Engl J Med* 1994; **331:** 1188–93.
46. Keen H. Insulin resistance and the prevention of diabetes mellitus. *N Engl J Med* 1994; **331:** 1226–7.
47. Tattersall R. Self monitoring of blood glucose concentrations by non-insulin dependent diabetic patients. *Br Med J* 1992; **305:** 1171–2.
48. Wolffenbuttel BHR, *et al.* Long-term assessment of glucose control by haemoglobin-AGE measurement. *Lancet* 1996; **347:** 513–15.
49. Pickup JC. Sampling and sensing blood glucose. *Lancet* 1993; **342:** 1068.
50. Bolinder J, *et al.* Long-term continuous glucose monitoring with microdialysis in ambulatory insulin-dependent diabetic patients. *Lancet* 1993; **342:** 1080–5.
51. Steel JM, *et al.* Can prepregnancy care of diabetic women reduce the risk of abnormal babies? *Br Med J* 1990; **301:** 1070–4.
52. Steel JM, Johnstone FD. Guidelines for the management of insulin-dependent diabetes mellitus in pregnancy. *Drugs* 1996; **52:** 60–70.
53. Casson IF, *et al.* Outcomes of pregnancy in insulin dependent diabetic women: results of a five year population cohort study. *Br Med J* 1997; **315:** 275–8.
54. Pearson JF. Pregnancy and complicated diabetes. *Br J Hosp Med* 1993; **49:** 739–42.
55. Crombach G, *et al.* Insulin use in pregnancy: clinical pharmacokinetic considerations. *Clin Pharmacokinet* 1993; **24:** 89–100.
56. Jarrett RJ. Gestational diabetes: a non-entity? *Br Med J* 1993; **306:** 37–8.
57. Ales KL, Santini DL. Should all pregnant women be screened for gestational glucose intolerance? *Lancet* 1989; **i:** 1187–91.
58. Mazze RS, Krogh CL. Gestational diabetes mellitus: now is the time for detection and treatment. *Mayo Clin Proc* 1992; **67:** 995–1002.
59. Thompson DJ, *et al.* Prophylactic insulin in the management of gestational diabetes. *Obstet Gynecol* 1990; **75:** 960–4.
60. Eldridge AJ, Sear JW. Peri-operative management of diabetic patients: any changes for the better since 1985? *Anaesthesia* 1996; **51:** 45–51.
61. Alberti KGMM, Zimmet PZ. Definition, diagnosis, and classification of diabetes mellitus and its complications. Part I: diagnosis and classification of diabetes mellitus. Provisional report of a WHO consultation. *Diabetic Med* 1998; **15:** 539–53.
62. DECODE Study Group. Will new diagnostic criteria for diabetes mellitus change phenotype of patients with diabetes? Reanalysis of European epidemiological data. *Br Med J* 1998; **317:** 371–5.
63. Wahl PW, *et al.* Diabetes in older adults: comparison of 1997 American Diabetes Association classification of diabetes mellitus with 1985 WHO classification. *Lancet* 1998; **352:** 1012–15.
64. UK Prospective Diabetes Study Group. Effect of intensive blood-glucose control with metformin on complications in overweight patients with type 2 diabetes (UKPDS 34). *Lancet* 1998; **352:** 854–65.
65. Hoffman L, *et al.* Gestational diabetes mellitus—management guidelines [of] the Australasian Diabetes in Pregnancy Society. *Med J Aust* 1998; **169:** 93–7.

Diabetic complications

Much of the increased mortality and morbidity seen in diabetic patients is the result of various complications which develop with increasing duration of disease, particularly when glycaemic control is poor. Such complications may originate from increased glycation of proteins and other biological macromolecules in the hyperglycaemic environment, or from increased accumulation of sorbitol and other polyols via the aldose reductase pathway, but other factors play an important role in determining susceptibility. At the macrovascular level, diabetics are prone to hypertension and ischaemic heart disease, and heart disease is a major cause of death. Microvascular tissue damage is an important factor in the development of diabetic nephropathy and retinopathy; it may also contribute to the other major complication, diabetic neuropathy. Collagen abnormalities are also seen. Diabetics with poor glycaemic control also have an increased liability to severe bacterial or fungal infection. Sometimes several factors may interact; thus neuropathy, infection, and impaired blood flow due to macro- or microvascular disease may all play a role in the development of diabetic foot disease, a complication which can ultimately lead to amputation.

Prevention of diabetic complications. Much attention has been focussed on whether strict or tight glycaemic control can modify the development or progression of diabetic complications. In general, the longer-term studies have provided more encouraging results than initial results indicated, and meta-analysis of such studies[1] has suggested that intensive regimens may prevent microvascular complications.

The Diabetes Control and Complications Trial (DCCT)[2] confirmed this view in type 1 diabetes. It compared in selected patients the effects of conventional insulin therapy with those of continuous subcutaneous insulin infusion or multiple-injection regimens, on the development and progression of complications. The intensive treatment was aimed at keeping preprandial blood-glucose concentrations between 3.9 and 6.7 mmol per litre, postprandial concentrations at less than 10 mmol per litre, a weekly 3 a.m. measurement at greater than 3.6 mmol per litre, and the monthly glycosylated haemoglobin measurement at less than 6.05%. Intensive insulin therapy reduced the development and progression of retinopathy; it also reduced the occurrence of microalbuminuria, albuminuria, and clinical neuropathy. The major disadvantage of intensive insulin therapy was a threefold greater risk of hypoglycaemia; weight gain was also significantly greater.

While it is accepted that some patients will benefit from intensive insulin regimens, this approach requires caution in patients at risk of hypoglycaemia. Also such intensive treatment may not always be necessary, for example in patients known to maintain good control by conventional dosage schedules, or where improvement can be obtained by setting achievable targets and improving patient education.[3] However, intensive therapy can help sustain endogenous insulin secretion in type 1 diabetes, which is associated with improved metabolic control;[4] this would support initiation of intensive insulin therapy at an early stage.

The reports of the UK Prospective Diabetes Study (UKPDS) have provided similar evidence in patients with type 2 diabetes. This study has examined the benefits of intensive therapy, using a variety of drugs together with diet and exercise. Intensive therapy, which aimed at producing fasting plasma-glucose concentrations of below 6 mmol per litre, substantially decreased the risk of microvascular complications (particularly retinopathy). There was no difference in benefit between intensive therapy with sulphonylureas and with insulin.[5] Metformin also produced benefit in the overweight patients who received it.[6] The UKPDS did not provide unequivocal evidence of a reduction in macrovascular disease with improved glycaemic control, although there was some suggestion of a reduction in risk of myocardial infarction (in line with a small earlier Japanese study[9]). However, it did show that vigorous control of blood pressure, using captopril or atenolol as the first-line drugs, reduced the risk of both macrovascular and microvascular complications,[7,8] suggesting that this should have a high priority in the treatment of type 2 diabetes.

Diabetic eye disease. Diabetic patients are prone to potentially blinding eye disease, usually in the form of cataract or diabetic retinopathy. Cataract generally requires surgical extraction, particular care being taken to avoid infection. Diabetic retinopathy may take a 'background', non-proliferative form, or become a more serious proliferative retinopathy associated with neovascularisation, vitreous haemorrhage and retinal detachment.

Although strict glycaemic control has been shown to reduce the risk of developing retinopathy,[2,5] once proliferative retinopathy has developed, glycaemic control is not adequate to prevent worsening.[11] Moreover, transient early worsening may occur in patients transferred to more intensive regimens.[12]

Aldose reductase inhibitors such as epalrestat and sorbinil have also been investigated for the prevention of retinopathy, but despite some benefits results have generally been unimpressive.[13,14] The benefits of antiplatelet agents are also unclear; aspirin, dipyridamole, and ticlopidine appear to reduce the development of microaneurysms in diabetic patients,[15,16] but aspirin has not been shown to prevent the development of retinopathy.[17]

Once proliferative retinopathy has developed photocoagulation using an argon laser or a xenon arc is effective in limiting progression, while vitrectomy may be helpful for vitreous haemorrhage and retinal detachment. Interferon alfa-2a has been reported to slow the progression of proliferative diabetic retinopathy in 3 patients,[18] although all 3 experienced haemorrhage within 6 weeks of stopping the drug. Epoetin has also proved of benefit in a few patients,[19] and it has been suggested that oxpentifylline should be investigated.[20] Results from a large European study (EUCLID) demonstrated a reduction in the progression of retinopathy in patients with type 1 diabetes treated with an ACE inhibitor, lisinopril.[21] Improvement in retinal hard exudates has been seen in patients given the low-molecular-weight heparinoid danaparoid sodium.[22]

Diabetic heart disease. Most damage to the cardiac tissue in diabetic patients is due to accelerated ischaemic heart disease. Hypertension and hyperlipidaemias, both of which are prevalent in diabetes mellitus, contribute to this process. Symptoms of angina pectoris may be less marked or absent in diabetic patients. Management of ischaemic heart disease is, however, similar in diabetic and non-diabetic patients (see Angina, p.780), except that if a beta blocker is given it should be a selective one. Diabetic patients are more likely than non-diabetics to die after myocardial infarction, but it has been shown that treatment with an insulin-glucose infusion after myocardial infarction, followed by subcutaneous insulin for at least 3 months, improves long-term survival in patients with both type 1 and type 2 diabetes.[23] Despite concerns about the use of aspirin in diabetics there is strong evidence for its prophylactic value and indeed some suggestion that higher than usual doses (300 mg rather than 75 to 100 mg daily) may be required in diabetics.[24]

Diabetics may also develop a form of cardiomyopathy in the absence of ischaemic heart disease. Again, the condition is managed similarly to cardiomyopathy in non-diabetic patients (see p.785).

Cardiac autonomic neuropathy has been reported to be improved by thioctic acid (see Diabetic Neuropathy, below).

Diabetic nephropathy. Nephropathic changes associated with microvascular disease develop in up to 30% of patients with type 1 diabetes and up to 40% of those with type 2 disease; diabetic nephropathy, of which the first clinical sign is albuminuria, is one of the major causes of end-stage renal disease.

Results from the Diabetes Control and Complications Trial (DCCT) indicate that strict glycaemic control reduces the incidence of microalbuminuria in type 1 diabetes,[2] and a small study has suggested that extrapolation of this to patients with type 2 diabetes is justified.[9] However, while good control may prevent development of the initial lesion, it is not clear whether it can prevent progression in patients who are already microalbuminuric Some studies, including the DCCT, have suggested that this is the case;[2,9] others have failed to confirm it.[25]

Another approach is dietary protein restriction, which appears from a number of small studies to have a beneficial effect on disease progression.[26,27]

The most important approach to slowing the progression of diabetic nephropathy is aggressive antihypertensive control.[7,28,29] Although meta-analysis[30] has suggested that ACE inhibitors have an antiproteinuric effect over and above their antihypertensive properties, results from the UKPDS showed no difference between the effects of an ACE inhibitor and a beta blocker in reducing microalbuminuria in type 2 patients.[8] Beneficial effects have also been reported when ACE inhibitors are given to patients with microalbuminuria but without hypertension,[30,33-36] and it has been recommended that such patients receive ACE inhibitors, initially in small doses, to slow the progression of renal disease.[28] Some consider that small decreases in blood pressure associated with such therapy may be responsible for the benefit.[8] It is unclear whether ACE inhibition would be appropriate in normotensive diabetics without evidence of renal disease, in an attempt to prevent it ever developing.

The aldose reductase inhibitors have been investigated for their effects on nephropathy, but results have been, at best, ambiguous; a study in microalbuminuric patients given tolrestat did show a decrease in urinary albumin excretion but this was concomitant with a decrease in the (initially raised) glomerular filtration rate.[37] Pimagedine, which inhibits the formation of glycosylated end products, is also under investigation.

Diabetic neuropathy. A variety of peripheral neuropathies are common complications of diabetes mellitus. The intensity and extent of neurological abnormalities are proportional to the degree and duration of hyperglycaemia. Neuropathic symptoms include symmetrical sensory loss, particularly in the feet and lower limbs; the various features of autonomic neuropathy including gastroparesis, postural hypotension, impotence, and gustatory sweating; pain and cranial nerve palsy associated with mononeuropathies; and acute, painful, sensory neuropathy.

Results from the DCCT indicated that strict glycaemic control could substantially reduce the occurrence of clinical neuropathy in patients with type 1 diabetes,[2] and again there is reason to believe that this will also prove true of patients with type 2.[9]

Although some studies have suggested that the aldose reductase inhibitors such as epalrestat[38] and tolrestat[39] can reduce the severity of diabetic neuropathy, larger scale analysis has apparently failed to demonstrate any benefit. Interesting preliminary results have suggested that the ACE inhibitor lisinopril may also have benefits in diabetic neuropathy.[40]

Other management of diabetic neuropathy is essentially symptomatic. The pain, which can be severe, may be managed with tricyclic antidepressants, antiarrhythmics, antiepileptics, and topical capsaicin, as discussed on p.9.

Diabetic gastroparesis may respond to prokinetic drugs such as metoclopramide, cisapride, or domperidone;[41] an alternative is to try erythromycin.[42] Diarrhoea may respond to tetracycline (see below), while postural hypotension should be managed conventionally (see p.1040) although care may be required in the use of elastic stockings in patients with impaired blood flow to the feet. Results from a study using the antioxidant thioctic acid have suggested some improvement in cardiac autonomic neuropathy.[43]

Diarrhoea. Diabetic patients may develop intermittent bouts of watery diarrhoea, increasing in frequency as the condition worsens; autonomic neuropathy and abnormalities of digestion and bowel flora may play a role.[44] Beneficial results have been reported from the use of clonidine,[45,46] and of octreotide,[47,48] but a conventional antidiarrhoeal drug (usually codeine or diphenoxylate) or a broad spectrum antibiotic (especially tetracycline) may also be effective. The mechanism of action of tetracycline in diabetic diarrhoea is uncertain, but it has been suggested that one or two doses of tetracycline should be the first line of treatment.[49]

Foot disease. Various types of diabetic tissue damage, including circulatory impairment, neuropathy, collagen changes, and increased susceptibility to infection, may contribute to the foot lesions to which diabetics are prone. Ulceration and tissue necrosis at pressure-points may be followed by infection, gangrene, and sepsis. Management involves drainage and debridement of dead and infected tissue, and the use of antibiotics if necessary: broad spectrum cover should be given intravenously if there is systemic infection, and adapted once the results of bacteriological culture are available.[50] Local antiseptic therapy may be helpful, especially for infections with *Pseudomonas* or *Proteus* spp. Strict control of blood glucose is important and insulin should be given as required. Effective pain relief, together with bed rest, may be required, and surgical reconstruction to improve blood supply may be helpful in some cases. Ultimately, some patients require amputation of all or part of the foot. Preventive care, with regular visits to a chiropodist, is therefore particularly important.

Hyperlipidaemias. Insulin plays an important role in lipid metabolism and deficient insulin action results in impaired degradation of chylomicra and VLDL (very low-density lipoprotein) particles, increased availability of non-esterified fatty acids to the liver (where they act as a source of VLDL and ketone bodies), and decreased production of HDL (high-density lipoprotein) cholesterol. As a result, diabetics are prone to hypertriglyceridaemia and have a blood-lipid profile associated with an increased risk of atherosclerosis, and hence of macrovascular complications. Good glycaemic control is the most important means of controlling hyperlipidaemias, but dietary advice, and if necessary the use of lipid regulating drugs (see p.1265) may also be appropriate.[31]

Hypertension. Hypertension is twice as common in the diabetic as in the non-diabetic population, and is associated with both macrovascular complications and microvascular disease (especially diabetic nephropathy). Management of hypertension in diabetics follows the same principles as in the general population, but it should be treated aggressively with a view to retarding development of complications,[7,32,51,52] and the threshold for drug treatment is lower than in non-diabetic patients (see Hypertension, p.788). An ACE inhibitor or a beta blocker have been shown to be effective.[7,8] Addition of diuretic therapy, a calcium-channel blocker, or an alpha blocker may need to be considered in some cases;[7] the latter should however be avoided in patients with autonomic neuropathy where there is a risk of exacerbating postural hypotension.[10]

1. Wang PH, *et al.* Meta-analysis of effects of intensive blood-glucose control on late complications of type I diabetes. *Lancet* 1993; **341:** 1306–9.
2. The Diabetes Control and Complications Trial Research Group. The effect of intensive treatment of diabetes on the development and progression of long-term complications in insulin-dependent diabetes mellitus. *N Engl J Med* 1993; **329:** 977–86.
3. Short R. Implementing the lessons of DCCT. *Diabetic Med* 1994; **11:** 220–8.
4. The Diabetes Control and Complications Trial Research Group. Effect of intensive therapy on residual β-cell function in patients with type 1 diabetes in the Diabetes Control and Complications Trial: a randomized, controlled trial. *Ann Intern Med* 1998; **128:** 517–23.
5. UK Prospective Diabetes Study Group. Intensive blood-glucose control with sulphonylureas or insulin compared with conventional treatment and risk of complications in patients with type 2 diabetes (UKPDS 33). *Lancet* 1998; **352:** 837–53.
6. UK Prospective Diabetes Study (UKPDS) Group. Effect of intensive blood-glucose control with metformin on complications in overweight patients with type 2 diabetes (UKPDS 34). *Lancet* 1998; **352:** 854–65.
7. UK Prospective Diabetes Study Group. Tight blood pressure control and risk of macrovascular and microvascular complications in type 2 diabetes: UKPDS 38. *Br Med J* 1998; **317:** 703–13.
8. UK Prospective Diabetes Study Group. Efficacy of atenolol and captopril in reducing risk of macrovascular and microvascular complications in type 2 diabetes: UKPDS 39. *Br Med J* 1998; **317:** 713–20.
9. Ohkubo Y, *et al.* Intensive insulin therapy prevents the progression of diabetic microvascular complications in Japanese patients with non-insulin-dependent diabetes mellitus: a randomized prospective 6-year study. *Diabetes Res Clin Pract* 1995; **28:** 103–17.
10. Fatourechi V, *et al.* A practical guideline for management of hypertension in patients with diabetes. *Mayo Clin Proc* 1996; **71:** 53–8.
11. Esmatjes E, *et al.* Long-term evolution of diabetic retinopathy and renal function after pancreas transplantation. *Transplant Proc* 1992; **24:** 12–13.
12. Henricsson M, *et al.* The effect of glycaemic control and the introduction of insulin therapy on retinopathy in non-insulin-dependent diabetes mellitus. *Diabetic Med* 1997; **14:** 123–31.
13. Hotta N, *et al.* Epalrestat can truly prevent diabetic retinopathy in clinical double-blind study. *Diabetes* 1990; **39** (suppl 1): 61A.
14. Sorbinil Retinopathy Trial Research Group. A randomized trial of sorbinil, an aldose reductase inhibitor, in diabetic retinopathy. *Arch Ophthalmol* 1990; **108:** 1234–44.
15. The DAMAD Study Group. Effect of aspirin alone and aspirin plus dipyridamole in early diabetic retinopathy: a multicenter randomized controlled clinical trial. *Diabetes* 1989; **38:** 491–8.
16. The TIMAD Study Group. Ticlopidine treatment reduces the progression of nonproliferative diabetic retinopathy. *Arch Ophthalmol* 1990; **108:** 1577–83.
17. Early Treatment Diabetic Retinopathy Study Research Group. Effects of aspirin treatment on diabetic retinopathy: ETDRS report number 8. *Ophthalmology* 1991; **98** (suppl): 757–65.
18. Skowsky WR, *et al.* A pilot study of chronic recombinant interferon-alfa 2a for diabetic proliferative retinopathy: metabolic effects and ophthalmologic effects. *J Diabetes Complications* 1996; **10:** 94–9.
19. Friedman EA, *et al.* Erythropoietin in diabetic macular edema and renal insufficiency. *Am J Kidney Dis* 1995; **26:** 202–8.
20. Sebag J, *et al.* Effects of pentoxifylline on choroidal blood flow in nonproliferative diabetic retinopathy. *Angiology* 1994; **45:** 429–33.
21. Chaturvedi N, *et al.* Effect of lisinopril on progression of retinopathy in normotensive people with type 1 diabetes. *Lancet* 1998; **351:** 28–31.
22. van der Pijl JW, *et al.* Effect of danaparoid sodium on hard exudates in diabetic retinopathy. *Lancet* 1997; **350:** 1743–5.
23. Malmberg K, *et al.* Prospective randomised study of intensive insulin treatment on long term survival after acute myocardial infarction in patients with diabetes mellitus. *Br Med J* 1997; **314:** 1512–15.
24. Yudkin JS. Which diabetic patients should be taking aspirin? *Br Med J* 1995; **311:** 641–2.
25. Microalbuminuria Collaborative Study Group, United Kingdom. Intensive therapy and progression to clinical albuminuria in patients with insulin dependent diabetes mellitus and microalbuminuria. *Br Med J* 1995; **311:** 973–7.
26. Sugimoto T, *et al.* Effect of dietary protein restriction on proteinuria in non-insulin-dependent diabetic patients with nephropathy. *J Nutr Sci Vitaminol* 1991; **37** (suppl): S87–S92.
27. Zeller K, *et al.* Effect of restricting dietary protein on the progression of renal failure in patients with insulin-dependent diabetes mellitus. *N Engl J Med* 1991; **324:** 78–84.
28. Mogensen CE, *et al.* Prevention of diabetic renal disease with special reference to microalbuminuria. *Lancet* 1995; **346:** 1080–4.
29. Savage MW, *et al.* Therapeutic options in diabetic renal disease and hypertension. *Br J Hosp Med* 1995; **54:** 429–34.
30. Kasiske BL, *et al.* Effect of antihypertensive therapy on the kidney in patients with diabetes: a meta-regression analysis. *Ann Intern Med* 1993; **118:** 129–38.
31. American Diabetes Association. Management of dyslipidemia in adults with diabetes. *Diabetes Care* 1998; **21:** 179–82.
32. Haffner SM, *et al.* Mortality from coronary heart disease in subjects with type 2 diabetes and in nondiabetic subjects with and without prior myocardial infarction. *N Engl J Med* 1998; **339:** 229–34.
33. Laffel LMB, *et al.* The beneficial effect of angiotensin-converting enzyme inhibition with captopril on diabetic nephropathy in normotensive IDDM patients with microalbuminuria. *Am J Med* 1995; **99:** 497–504.
34. Ravid M, *et al.* Long-term stabilizing effect of angiotensin-converting enzyme inhibition on plasma creatinine and on proteinuria in normotensive type II diabetic patients. *Ann Intern Med* 1993; **118:** 577–81.
35. Mathiesen ER, *et al.* Efficacy of captopril in postponing nephropathy in normotensive insulin dependent diabetic patients with microalbuminuria: 8 years follow-up. *Diabetologia* 1995; **38:** 1746.
36. The EUCLID Study Group. Randomised placebo-controlled trial of lisinopril in normotensive patients with insulin-dependent diabetes and normoalbuminuria or microalbuminuria. *Lancet* 1997; **349:** 1787–92.
37. Passariello N, *et al.* Effect of aldose reductase inhibitor (tolrestat) on urinary albumin excretion rate and glomerular filtration rate in IDDM subjects with nephropathy. *Diabetes Care* 1993; **16:** 789–95.
38. Uchida K, *et al.* Effect of 24 weeks of treatment with epalrestat, an aldose reductase inhibitor, on peripheral neuropathy in patients with non-insulin-dependent diabetes mellitus. *Clin Ther* 1995; **17:** 460–6.
39. Boulton AJM, *et al.* A multicentre trial of the aldose-reductase inhibitor, tolrestat, in patients with symptomatic diabetic neuropathy. *Diabetologia* 1990; **33:** 431–7.
40. Reja A, *et al.* Is ACE inhibition with lisinopril helpful in diabetic neuropathy? *Diabetic Med* 1995; **12:** 307–9.
41. Drenth JPH, Engels LGJB. Diabetic gastroparesis: a critical reappraisal of new treatment strategies. *Drugs* 1992; **44:** 537–53.
42. Richards RD, *et al.* The treatment of idiopathic and diabetic gastroparesis with acute intravenous and chronic oral erythromycin. *Am J Gastroenterol* 1993; **88:** 203–7.
43. Ziegler D, *et al.* Effect of treatment with the antioxidant α-lipoic acid on cardiac autonomic neuropathy in non-insulin-dependent diabetic patients: a 4-month randomized controlled trial (DEKAN study). *Clin Auton Res* 1995; **5:** 323.
44. Ogbonnaya KI, Arem R. Diabetic diarrhea: pathophysiology, diagnosis, and management. *Arch Intern Med* 1990; **150:** 262–7.
45. Fedorak RN, *et al.* Treatment of diabetic diarrhea with clonidine. *Ann Intern Med* 1985; **102:** 197–9.
46. Sacerdote A. Topical clonidine for diabetic diarrhea. *Ann Intern Med* 1986; **105:** 139.
47. Michaels PE, Cameron RB. Octreotide is cost-effective therapy in diabetic diarrhea. *Arch Intern Med* 1991; **151:** 2469.
48. Mourad FH, *et al.* Effective treatment of diabetic diarrhoea with somatostatin analogue, octreotide. *Gut* 1992; **33:** 1578–80.
49. Clark CM, Lee DA. Prevention and treatment of the complications of diabetes mellitus. *N Engl J Med* 1995; **332:** 1210–17.
50. West NJ. Systemic antimicrobial treatment of foot infections in diabetic patients. *Am J Health-Syst Pharm* 1995; **52:** 1199–1207.
51. Barnett AH. Diabetes and hypertension. *Br Med Bull* 1994; **50:** 397–407.
52. Gilbert RE, *et al.* Diabetes and hypertension: Australian Diabetes Society position statement. *Med J Aust* 1995; **163:** 372–5.

Diabetic emergencies

Hypoglycaemia. The most frequent complication of insulin therapy is hypoglycaemia and patients taking insulin need to be educated about its cause, symptoms, and treatment. Most patients can recognise the early warning signs of hypoglycaemia and by taking sugar immediately can prevent more serious symptoms developing. Comatose patients need to be given intravenous glucose or, if this is not practicable, subcutaneous, intramuscular, or intravenous glucagon (although glucose is still required if there is no response within 10 minutes). Hypoglycaemia can also develop in patients taking oral hypoglycaemics, notably the sulphonylureas.

Some patients report loss of the warning signs of hypoglycaemia after transferring from animal to human insulin and these patients, if appropriate, may need to be transferred back to porcine insulin. However, a study suggests that the most significant factor in loss of hypoglycaemic warning signs may be exposure to hypoglycaemia itself, and that avoidance of hypoglycaemic episodes restores awareness.[1] This effect, which appears to be due to an adaptive conservation of glucose uptake in the brain,[2] is liable to be a particular problem in patients receiving intensive therapy. There is some evidence that caffeine may be useful in restoring awareness of hypoglycaemia.[3]

For further details on the treatment of insulin-induced hypoglycaemia, see p.323.

Diabetic ketoacidosis is caused by an absolute or relative lack of insulin and commonly occurs after failure to adjust insulin dosage in the presence of factors which increase insulin requirements (see p.325). Failure of an insulin pump may be a cause.[4] Also pregnant diabetic women are more prone to development of diabetic ketoacidosis.

Diabetic ketoacidosis is characterised by hyperglycaemia, hyperketonaemia, and acidaemia, with subsequent dehydration and electrolyte abnormalities. Onset may be rapid, or insidious over many days. Initial presenting symptoms such as thirst, polyuria, fatigue, and weight loss are those of any newly presenting insulin-dependent diabetic; they then progress to nausea, vomiting, abdominal pain, and impaired consciousness or coma, and, if untreated, death.[4-7]

Diabetic ketoacidosis is a medical emergency and should be treated immediately with fluid replacement and insulin.[4-9] Fluid requirements depend on the needs of the individual; over vigorous fluid replacement without severe dehydration carries the risk of precipitating cerebral oedema.[7-9]

Soluble insulin should also be administered immediately. Large doses were formerly used because of the presence of insulin resistance in diabetic ketoacidosis, probably related to the effects of acidaemia.[4] Lower-dose regimens have since been shown to provide adequate insulin concentrations and are now used routinely.[4,6] Ideally insulin should be given by the intravenous route,[4,6] although it may be given by the intramuscular route provided the circulatory state of the patient is satisfactory.[5,7]

Lack of response to insulin is generally a result of inadequate hydration but may occasionally be caused by genuine insulin resistance.[4,6] In this case the intravenous route is essential and the insulin dose doubled on a one- to two-hourly basis until an adequate response is obtained.[4] A case report has suggested that mecasermin may be useful if there is insulin resistance.[10]

When the blood-glucose concentration has fallen to less than 10 mmol per litre the dose of insulin may be reduced by about half and glucose is administered intravenously,[4] usually in a strength of 5% with saline[5,6] although some have advocated a glucose strength of 10%.[4] The administration of glucose enables insulin to be continued in order to clear ketone bodies without inducing hypoglycaemia; this is essential if a recurrence of ketoacidosis is to be avoided.[6] Once glucose concentrations have been controlled and acidosis has completely cleared, subcutaneous injections of insulin can be begun,[6,7] but intravenous insulin should be continued at a reduced rate for an hour during the change-over.[5]

Total body stores of potassium are depleted in patients with diabetic ketoacidosis. Insulin deficiency appears to be the main initiating factor for hyperkalaemia in diabetic ketoacidosis.[11] Although patients may present with raised, normal, or decreased serum-potassium concentrations, the concentrations will start to fall with the correction of acidosis. Potassium is added to the infusion fluid after initial fluid expansion and once insulin therapy is commenced.[5] In hyperkalaemic patients, potassium is administered once serum concentrations have fallen to within normal limits.[5-7]

Intravenous bicarbonate is now generally reserved for patients with severe acidaemia; a common practice is to give it to those with a pH of less than 7.0 with the aim of raising the pH to 7.1.[4-7]

Phosphate concentrations are affected in a similar manner to potassium concentrations in the ketoacidotic state, but there is less agreement on the need for routine phosphate administration. Phosphate concentrations should be monitored and phosphate administered if clinically significant hypophosphataemia occurs.[7]

Hyperosmolar hyperglycaemic nonketotic coma (HONK). This occurs mainly in elderly patients with type 2 diabetes and though much less common than diabetic ketoacidosis it carries a higher mortality. Patients may present in coma with severe hyperglycaemia but without ketosis; dehydration and renal impairment are common.[4] Treatment is similar to that of diabetic ketoacidosis (see above), although potassium requirements are lower and large amounts of fluid and less insulin may be required; some suggest the use of hypotonic fluid if necessary.[12] There is an increased likelihood of thrombotic events, so prophylactic anticoagulation should be considered.

1. Cranston I, *et al.* Restoration of hypoglycaemia awareness in patients with long-duration insulin-dependent diabetes. *Lancet* 1994; **344:** 283–7.
2. Boyle PJ, *et al.* Brain glucose uptake and unawareness of hypoglycemia in patients with insulin-dependent diabetes mellitus. *N Engl J Med* 1995; **333:** 1726–31.
3. Debrah K, *et al.* Effect of caffeine on recognition of and physiological responses to hypoglycaemia in insulin-dependent diabetes. *Lancet* 1996; **347:** 19–24.
4. Alberti KGMM. Diabetic emergencies. *Br Med Bull* 1989; **45:** 242–63.
5. Richardson JE, Donaldson MDC. Diabetic emergencies. *Prescribers' J* 1989; **29:** 174–83.
6. Sanson TH, Levine SN. Management of diabetic ketoacidosis. *Drugs* 1989; **38:** 289–300.
7. Lebovitz HE. Diabetic ketoacidosis. *Lancet* 1995; **345:** 767–72.
8. Adrogué HJ, *et al.* Salutary effects of modest fluid replacement in the treatment of adults with diabetic ketoacidosis: use in patients without extreme volume deficit. *JAMA* 1989; **262:** 2108–13.
9. Johnston C. Fluid replacement in diabetic ketoacidosis. *Br Med J* 1992; **305:** 522.
10. Usala A-L, *et al.* Brief report: treatment of insulin-resistant diabetic ketoacidosis with insulin-like growth factor I in an adolescent with insulin-dependent diabetes. *N Engl J Med* 1992; **327:** 853–7.
11. Anonymous. Hyperkalaemia in diabetic ketoacidosis. *Lancet* 1986; **ii:** 845–6.
12. Wright AD. Diabetic emergencies in adults. *Prescribers' J* 1989; **29:** 147–54.

Acarbose (12304-c)

Acarbose *(BAN, USAN, rINN).*

Bay-g-5421. *O*-{4-Amino-4,6-dideoxy-*N*-[(1*S*,4*R*,5*S*,6*S*)-4,5,6-trihydroxy-3-hydroxymethylcyclohex-2-enyl]-α-D-glucopyranosyl}-(1→4)-*O*-α-D-glucopyranosyl-(1→4)-D-glucopyranose.

$C_{25}H_{43}NO_{18}$ = 645.6.

CAS — 56180-94-0.

Adverse Effects

Acarbose may cause gastro-intestinal disturbances, including flatulence due to bacterial action on nonabsorbed carbohydrate in the colon. Abdominal distension, diarrhoea, and pain may occur. A decreased dosage of acarbose together with improved dietary habits may reduce these adverse effects. Hepatotoxicity may occur and may necessitate a reduction in dosage or withdrawal of the drug. Skin reactions have occurred rarely.

The manufacturers reported that the incidence of adverse effects in a postmarketing surveillance study of acarbose was lower than that seen in previous clinical trials;[1] this was held to represent better tailoring of individual doses to patient tolerability.

1. Spengler M, Cagatay M. The use of acarbose in the primary-care setting: evaluation of efficacy and tolerability of acarbose by postmarketing surveillance study. *Clin Invest Med* 1995; **18:** 325–31.

Effects on the liver. Reports of hepatocellular liver damage, with jaundice and elevated serum aminotransferases, in patients receiving acarbose.[1-3] Symptoms resolved on discontinuation of the drug.

1. Andrade RJ, *et al.* Hepatic injury caused by acarbose. *Ann Intern Med* 1996; **124:** 931.
2. Carrascosa M, *et al.* Acarbose-induced acute severe hepatotoxicity. *Lancet* 1997; **349:** 698–9.
3. Fujimoto Y, *et al.* Acarbose-induced hepatic injury. *Lancet* 1998; **351:** 340.

Precautions

Acarbose is contra-indicated in inflammatory bowel disease, particularly where there is associated ulceration, and in gastro-intestinal obstruction or patients predisposed to it. It should be avoided in conditions which may deteriorate as a result of increased gas formation, such as hernia.

Acarbose is also contra-indicated in patients with hepatic impairment and liver enzyme values should be monitored at high doses.

Acarbose is not appropriate for pregnant patients or for those who are breast feeding.

If hypoglycaemia should develop in a patient receiving acarbose it needs to be treated with glucose, since the action of acarbose inhibits the hydrolysis of disaccharides.

Interactions

Acarbose may enhance the effects of other hypoglycaemics, including insulin, and may necessitate a reduction in their dosage. Concomitant administration of gastro-intestinal adsorbents and digestive enzyme preparations may diminish the effects of acarbose and should be avoided. Neomycin and cholestyramine may enhance the effects of acarbose and a reduction in its dosage may be required.

Pharmacokinetics

Following oral administration of acarbose, the majority of active unchanged drug remains in the lumen of the gastro-intestinal tract to exert its pharmacological activity and is metabolised by intestinal enzymes and by the microbial flora. Ultimately about 35% of a dose is absorbed in the form of metabolites. Acarbose is excreted in the urine and faeces.

Uses and Administration

Acarbose is an inhibitor of alpha glucosidases, especially sucrase. Through this action it retards the digestion and absorption of carbohydrates in the small intestine and hence reduces the increase in blood-glucose concentrations after a carbohydrate load. It is given by mouth in the treatment of type 2 diabetes mellitus (p.313); usual initial doses are 25 or 50 mg daily at first and then increased to three times daily immediately before food. Doses up to 100 to 200 mg three times daily may be given if necessary. Some benefit has also been demonstrated when acarbose is used to supplement insulin therapy in type 1 diabetes mellitus.

Acarbose has also been studied for the treatment of reactive hypoglycaemia, the dumping syndrome, and certain types of hyperlipoproteinaemia.

References.

1. Clissold SP, Edwards C. Acarbose: a preliminary review of its pharmacodynamic and pharmacokinetic properties, and therapeutic potential. *Drugs* 1988; **35:** 214–43.
2. Hotta N, *et al.* Long-term effect of acarbose on glycaemic control in non-insulin-dependent diabetes mellitus: a placebo-controlled double-blind study. *Diabetic Med* 1993; **10:** 134–8.
3. Balfour JA, McTavish D. Acarbose: an update of its pharmacology and therapeutic use in diabetes mellitus. *Drugs* 1993; **46:** 1025–54.
4. Anonymous. Acarbose for non-insulin-dependent diabetes mellitus. *Drug Ther Bull* 1994; **32:** 51–3.
5. Chiasson J-L, *et al.* The efficacy of acarbose in the treatment of patients with non-insulin-dependent diabetes mellitus: a multicenter controlled clinical trial. *Ann Intern Med* 1994; **121:** 928–35.
6. Coniff RF, *et al.* Multicenter, placebo-controlled trial comparing acarbose (BAY g 5421) with placebo, tolbutamide, and tolbutamide-plus-acarbose in non-insulin-dependent diabetes mellitus. *Am J Med* 1995; **98:** 443–51.
7. Spengler M, Cagatay M. The use of acarbose in the primary-care setting: evaluation of efficacy and tolerability of acarbose by postmarketing surveillance study. *Clin Invest Med* 1995; **18:** 325–31.
8. Salvatore T, Giugliano D. Pharmacokinetic-pharmacodynamic relationships of acarbose. *Clin Pharmacokinet* 1996; **30:** 94–106.
9. Anonymous. Acarbose for diabetes mellitus. *Med Lett Drugs Ther* 1996; **38:** 9–10.
10. Hoffman J, Spengler M. Efficacy of 24-week monotherapy with acarbose, metformin, or placebo in dietary-treated NIDDM patients: the Essen-II study. *Am J Med* 1997; **103:** 483–90.
11. Hollander P, *et al.* Acarbose in the treatment of type I diabetes. *Diabetes Care* 1997; **20:** 248–53.
12. Buse J, *et al.* The PROTECT study: final results of a large multicenter postmarketing study in patients with type 2 diabetes. *Clin Ther* 1998; **20:** 257–69.

Preparations

Proprietary Preparations (details are given in Part 3)

Aust.: Glucobay; ***Austral.:*** Glucobay; ***Belg.:*** Glucobay; ***Canad.:*** Prandase; ***Fr.:*** Glucor; ***Ger.:*** Glucobay; ***Irl.:*** Glucobay; ***Ital.:*** Glicobase; Glucobay; ***Neth.:*** Glucobay; ***Norw.:*** Glucobay; ***S.Afr.:*** Glucobay; ***Spain:*** Glucobay; Glumida; ***Swed.:*** Glucobay; ***Switz.:*** Glucobay; ***UK:*** Glucobay.

Acetohexamide (7213-j)

Acetohexamide *(BAN, USAN, rINN)*.

Compound 33006. 1-(4-Acetylbenzenesulphonyl)-3-cyclohexylurea.

$C_{15}H_{20}N_2O_4S$ = 324.4.

CAS — 968-81-0.

Pharmacopoeias. In *Jpn*, and *US*.

A white, odourless or almost odourless, crystalline powder. Practically **insoluble** in water and in ether; soluble 1 in 230 of alcohol and 1 in 210 of chloroform; soluble in pyridine and dilute solutions of alkali hydroxides.

Acetohexamide is a sulphonylurea hypoglycaemic (p.331). Its duration of action is 12 hours or more. It is given by mouth in the treatment of type 2 diabetes mellitus (p.313) in a usual initial dose of 250 mg daily before breakfast. This may then be increased by increments of 250 to 500 mg daily at intervals of 5 to 7 days to a maintenance dose of up to 1.5 g daily; increasing the dose above 1.5 g does not usually lead to further benefit. Doses in excess of 1 g daily may be taken in 2 divided doses, before the morning and evening meals.

Preparations

USP 23: Acetohexamide Tablets.

Proprietary Preparations (details are given in Part 3)
Canad.: Dimelor; ***Ital.:*** Dimelor†; ***S.Afr.:*** Dimelor; ***USA:*** Dymelor.

Biguanide Antidiabetics (17495-w)

NOTE. Biguanide antidiabetics in this chapter are: Buformin (p.319); Metformin Hydrochloride (p.330); Phenformin Hydrochloride (p.330).

Adverse Effects

Gastro-intestinal adverse effects including anorexia, nausea, and diarrhoea may occur with biguanides; patients may experience a metallic taste and there may be weight loss. Absorption of various substances including vitamin B_{12} may be impaired.

Hypoglycaemia is rare with a biguanide given alone, although it may occur if other contributing factors or drugs are present.

Lactic acidosis, sometimes fatal, has occurred with biguanides, primarily with phenformin. When it has occurred with metformin it is generally accepted that the lactic acidosis was usually in patients whose condition contra-indicated the use of metformin, particularly those with renal impairment.

Phenformin has been implicated in the controversial reports of excessive cardiovascular mortality associated with oral hypoglycaemic therapy (see under Sulphonylureas, Effects on the Cardiovascular System, p.331).

A review of the adverse effects of biguanide therapy.[1]

1. Paterson KR, *et al.* Undesired effects of biguanide therapy. *Adverse Drug React Acute Poisoning Rev* 1984; **3:** 173–82.

Effects on the blood. See Malabsorption, under Effects on the Gastro-intestinal Tract, below.

Effects on the gastro-intestinal tract. DIARRHOEA. A retrospective survey of diarrhoea in diabetic patients.[1] Thirty of 265 diabetic patients reported diarrhoea or alternating diarrhoea and constipation, comprising: 11 of 54 taking metformin; 9 of 45 taking metformin with a sulphonylurea; 3 of 53 taking a sulphonylurea only; 5 of 78 on insulin therapy; 2 of 35 on diet alone. Among 150 nondiabetic controls 12 reported diarrhoea.

1. Dandona P, *et al.* Diarrhea and metformin in a diabetic clinic. *Diabetes Care* 1983; **6:** 472–4.

MALABSORPTION. Megaloblastic anaemia due to vitamin B_{12} malabsorption in a 58-year-old woman was associated with long-term treatment with metformin.[1]

In a survey of diabetic patients receiving biguanide therapy,[2] malabsorption of vitamin B_{12} was observed in 14 of 46 diabetics taking metformin or phenformin; metformin was more commonly to blame. Withdrawal of the drug resulted in normal absorption in only 7 of the 14.

1. Callaghan TS, *et al.* Megaloblastic anaemia due to vitamin B_{12} malabsorption associated with long-term metformin treatment. *Br Med J* 1980; **280:** 1214–15.
2. Adams JF, *et al.* Malabsorption of vitamin B_{12} and intrinsic factor secretion during biguanide therapy. *Diabetologia* 1983; **24:** 16–18.

Effects on the liver. A report of severe cholestatic hepatitis attributed to metformin.[1]

1. Babich MM, *et al.* Metformin-induced acute hepatitis. *Am J Med* 1998; **104:** 490–2.

Hypersensitivity. Vasculitis and pneumonitis in a 59-year-old woman was associated with administration of metformin.[1] Symptoms improved on withdrawal of metformin, but reappeared on its reintroduction.

1. Klapholz L, *et al.* Leucocytoclastic vasculitis and pneumonitis induced by metformin. *Br Med J* 1986; **293:** 483.

Hypoglycaemia. The UK manufacturers of metformin state that hypoglycaemia does not occur with metformin alone, even in overdosage, although it may occur if given concomitantly with alcohol or other hypoglycaemics. Interim results from the UK Prospective Diabetes Study,[1] however, indicate that metformin therapy was associated with fewer hypoglycaemic episodes than sulphonylurea or insulin treatment, but more than with diet alone. One or more hypoglycaemic episodes were reported in 6% of the patients receiving the biguanide in this study, although only 1 patient had a severe episode.

1. United Kingdom Prospective Diabetes Study Group. United Kingdom prospective diabetes study (UKPDS) 13: relative efficacy of randomly allocated diet, sulphonylurea, insulin, or metformin in patients with newly diagnosed non-insulin dependent diabetes followed for 3 years. *Br Med J* 1995; **310:** 83–8.

Lactic acidosis. References to lactic acidosis associated with administration of biguanide hypoglycaemics.[1-12] Most recent reports implicate metformin, the most widely used biguanide, although cases of phenformin-associated lactic acidosis still occur.[10,11] From 1995, when metformin was introduced in the USA, until June 1996, the FDA had received reports of metformin-associated lactic acidosis in 66 patients,[12] the diagnosis being confirmed in 47. This represented a rate of about 5 cases per 100 000. Almost all patients with confirmed lactic acidosis had 1 or more risk factors such as cardiac or chronic hypoxic pulmonary disease, or renal insufficiency.

1. Anonymous. Biguanides and lactic acidosis in diabetics. *Br Med J* 1977; **2:** 1436.
2. Misbin RI. Phenformin-associated lactic acidosis: pathogenesis and treatment. *Ann Intern Med* 1977; **87:** 591–5.
3. Bergman U, *et al.* Epidemiology of adverse drug reactions to phenformin and metformin. *Br Med J* 1978; **2:** 464–6.
4. Korhonen T, *et al.* Biguanide-induced lactic acidosis in Finland. *Eur J Clin Pharmacol* 1979; **15:** 407–10.
5. McGuiness ME, Talbert RL. Phenformin-induced lactic acidosis: a forgotten adverse drug reaction. *Ann Pharmacother* 1993; **27:** 1183–7.
6. Monson JP. Metformin and lactic acidosis. *Prescribers' J* 1993; **33:** 170–3.
7. Wilholm B-E, Myrhed M. Metformin-associated lactic acidosis in Sweden 1977–1991. *Eur J Clin Pharmacol* 1993; **44:** 589–91.
8. Khan IH, *et al.* Severe lactic acidosis in patient receiving continuous ambulatory peritoneal dialysis. *Br Med J* 1993; **307:** 1056–7.
9. Pearlman BL, *et al.* Metformin-associated lactic acidosis. *Am J Med* 1996; **101:** 109–10.
10. Rosand J, *et al.* Fatal phenformin-associated lactic acidosis. *Ann Intern Med* 1997; **127:** 170.
11. Enia G, *et al.* Lactic acidosis induced by phenformin is still a public health problem in Italy. *Br Med J* 1997; **315:** 1466–7.
12. Misbin RI, *et al.* Lactic acidosis in patients with diabetes treated with metformin. *N Engl J Med* 1998; **338:** 265–6.

Pancreatitis. References to acute pancreatitis associated with phenformin.

1. Wilde H. Pancreatitis and phenformin. *Ann Intern Med* 1972; **77:** 324.
2. Chase HS, Mogan GR. Phenformin-associated pancreatitis. *Ann Intern Med* 1977; **87:** 314–15.

Treatment of Adverse Effects

Acute poisoning with biguanides may lead to the development of lactic acidosis and calls for intensive supportive therapy. For a discussion of the treatment of acidoses, see p.1147. Glucose or glucagon may be required for hypoglycaemia, the general management of which is outlined in Insulin, p.323.

Precautions

Biguanides are inappropriate for patients with diabetic coma and ketoacidosis, or for those with severe infection, stress, trauma, or other severe conditions where the biguanide is unlikely to control the hyperglycaemia; insulin should be administered in such situations. Biguanides should not be given to patients with impairment of renal or hepatic function. Renal impairment may predispose patients to lactic acidosis and renal function should be monitored throughout therapy. Biguanides should also not be given to patients with heart failure, recent myocardial infarction, dehydration, alcoholism, or any other condition likely to predispose to lactic acidosis.

Insulin is preferred for the treatment of pregnant patients.

Owing to the possibility of decreased vitamin B_{12} absorption, annual monitoring of vitamin B_{12} concentrations is advisable during long-term treatment.

Driving. Patients with diabetes mellitus are required to declare their condition to the UK vehicle licensing centre who then assess their fitness to drive. The law treats hypoglycaemic episodes as being under the influence of a drug and patients using insulin are generally not permitted to drive vocationally. Driving is not permitted when hypoglycaemic awareness has been lost. Drivers should normally check their blood glucose concentration before setting out, and, on long journeys, at intervals of about 2 hours. If hypoglycaemia occurs, the driver should stop until recovery is complete.

Vocational drivers needing oral hypoglycaemic drugs have a difficult problem especially if they are on rotating shifts, if the amount of physical exercise varies greatly, or if they change jobs frequently.[1] If they are to be allowed to drive they should be taking a biguanide or a short-acting sulphonylurea.

1. Raffle PAB. Drugs and driving. *Prescribers' J* 1981; **21:** 197–204.

Interactions

Use of a biguanide concomitantly with other drugs that lower blood sugar concentrations increases the risk of hypoglycaemia, while drugs that increase blood glucose may reduce the effect of biguanide therapy.

In general fewer drug interactions have been reported with biguanides than with sulphonylureas. Alcohol may increase the risk of lactic acidosis as well as of hypoglycaemia. Care should be taken if biguanides are given concomitantly with drugs that may impair renal function.

Anticoagulants. For the effect of metformin on phenprocoumon, see p.967.

Cimetidine. Cimetidine administration resulted in increased plasma-metformin concentrations in 7 healthy subjects.[1] The renal clearance of metformin was reduced; competition for proximal tubular secretion was considered responsible. A reduction in metformin dosage may be required in patients taking metformin and cimetidine concomitantly in order to reduce the risk of lactic acidosis.

1. Somogyi A, *et al.* Reduction of metformin renal tubular secretion by cimetidine in man. *Br J Clin Pharmacol* 1987; **23:** 545–51.

Ketotifen. A report of a decrease in platelet counts among 10 diabetic patients receiving biguanides when they were also given ketotifen.[1] The fall, which was marked in 3, returned to normal a few days after the end of ketotifen therapy. However, the investigators did not consider the effect clinically significant.

1. Doleček R. Ketotifen in the treatment of diabetics with various allergic conditions. *Pharmatherapeutica* 1981; **2:** 568–74.

Sulphonylureas. For reference to an apparent increase in mortality with an intensive regimen of metformin plus a sulphonylurea, see p.333.

Uses and Administration

The biguanide antidiabetics are a class of hypoglycaemic drugs given by mouth in the treatment of type 2 diabetes mellitus (p.313). They are used to supplement treatment by diet modification when such modification has not proved effective on its own. Although sulphonylureas (p.331) are usually preferred, a biguanide is often added or given instead to patients who are not responding to a sulphonylurea. Since biguanides are not associated with weight gain they may be useful in obese patients who gain weight on sulphonylureas despite adequate dietary modification.

The mode of action of biguanides is not clear. They do not stimulate insulin release but require that some insulin be present in order to exert their hypoglycaemic effect. Possible mechanisms of action include delay in the absorption of glucose from the gastro-intestinal tract, an increase in insulin sensitivity and glucose uptake into cells, and inhibition of hepatic gluconeogenesis. Biguanides do not usually lower blood-glucose concentrations in non-diabetic subjects.

Hyperlipidaemias. The effect of biguanides on lipid metabolism is unclear although some studies have demonstrated a lowering of blood concentrations of very low-density-lipoprotein cholesterol and total cholesterol.[1] Such effects may be beneficial in the long-term treatment of type 2 diabetes mellitus with concomitant lipid disorders.[2,3] For a discussion of the treatment of hyperlipidaemias, see p.1265.

1. Schäfer G. Biguanides: a review of history, pharmacodynamics and therapy. *Diabete Metab* 1983; **9:** 148–63.
2. Rains SGH, *et al.* The reduction of low density lipoprotein cholesterol by metformin is maintained with long-term therapy. *J R Soc Med* 1989; **82:** 93–4.
3. Lalor BC, *et al.* Placebo-controlled trial of the effects of guar gum and metformin on fasting blood glucose and serum lipids in obese, type 2 diabetic patients. *Diabetic Med* 1990; **7:** 242–5.

Buformin (14764-j)

Buformin *(USAN, pINN).*

DBV; W-37. 1-Butylbiguanide.

$C_6H_{15}N_5$ = 157.2.

CAS — 692-13-7 (buformin); 1190-53-0 (buformin hydrochloride).

Buformin is a biguanide hypoglycaemic (p.318). It is given by mouth in the treatment of type 2 diabetes mellitus (p.313) in doses of up to 300 mg daily. The hydrochloride has also been used.

Preparations

Proprietary Preparations (details are given in Part 3)
Spain: Silubin Retard; ***Switz.:*** Silubin.

Carbutamide (7215-c)

Carbutamide *(BAN, rINN).*

BZ-55; Ca-1022; Glybutamide; U-6987. 1-Butyl-3-sulphanilylurea.

$C_{11}H_{17}N_3O_3S$ = 271.3.

CAS — 339-43-5.

Pharmacopoeias. In *It.*

Carbutamide is a sulphonylurea hypoglycaemic (p.331). It is given by mouth in the treatment of type 2 diabetes mellitus (p.313) in single daily doses of 0.5 to 1 g, but is more toxic than chlorpropamide.

Preparations

Proprietary Preparations (details are given in Part 3)
Aust.: Invenol; ***Fr.:*** Glucidoral; ***Ger.:*** Nadisan†.

Chlorpropamide (7216-k)

Chlorpropamide *(BAN, rINN).*

Chlorpropamidum. 1-(4-Chlorobenzenesulphonyl)-3-propylurea.

$C_{10}H_{13}ClN_2O_3S$ = 276.7.

CAS — 94-20-2.

Pharmacopoeias. In *Chin., Eur.* (see p.viii), *Jpn, Pol.,* and *US.*

A white, odourless or almost odourless, crystalline powder. It exhibits polymorphism. Practically **insoluble** in water; soluble in alcohol; freely soluble in acetone and in dichloromethane; sparingly soluble in chloroform; dissolves in aqueous solutions of alkali hydroxides. **Protect** from light.

Adverse Effects and Treatment

As for sulphonylureas in general, p.331.

Chlorpropamide may be more likely than other sulphonylureas to induce a syndrome of inappropriate secretion of antidiuretic hormone (SIADH) characterised by water retention, hyponatraemia, and CNS effects. Patients receiving chlorpropamide may develop facial flushing after drinking alcohol.

Precautions

As for sulphonylureas in general, p.332.

Chlorpropamide should be avoided in the elderly and in renal or hepatic impairment because its long half-life increases the risk of hypoglycaemia. Some manufacturers recommend that chlorpropamide should not be used in patients with severe impairment of thyroid function. The antidiuretic effect of chlorpropamide may cause problems in patients with conditions associated with fluid retention.

Porphyria. Chlorpropamide has been associated with acute attacks of porphyria and is considered unsafe in patients with acute porphyria.[1]

1. Moore MR, McColl KEL. *Porphyria: drug lists.* Glasgow: Porphyria Research Unit, University of Glasgow, 1991.

Interactions

As for sulphonylureas in general, p.332.

Chlorpropamide may produce profound facial flushing in association with alcohol ingestion.

Pharmacokinetics

Chlorpropamide is readily absorbed from the gastro-intestinal tract and is extensively bound to plasma proteins. The half-life is about 35 hours. About 80% of a dose is metabolised in the liver; metabolites and unchanged drug are excreted in the urine. Chlorpropamide crosses the placenta and has been detected in breast milk.

Uses and Administration

Chlorpropamide is a sulphonylurea hypoglycaemic (p.331). It has a duration of action of at least 24 hours, and is given by mouth in the treatment of type 2 diabetes mellitus (p.313) in an initial daily dose of 250 mg as a single dose with breakfast. It is usual to adjust this dose after 5 to 7 days to achieve an optimum maintenance dose which is usually in the range 100 to 500 mg daily; increasing the dose above 500 mg is unlikely to produce further benefit. Although a reduced dose range has been proposed for the elderly, use of chlorpropamide is inadvisable in this group.

Chlorpropamide, though not the other sulphonylureas, is also sometimes used in cranial diabetes insipidus (p.1237). It has been reported to act by sensitising the renal tubules to antidiuretic hormone. The dose has to be carefully adjusted to minimise the risk of hypoglycaemia. An initial dose of 100 mg daily, adjusted if necessary to a maximum of 350 mg daily has been recommended, although doses of up to 500 mg daily have been used.

Patients with type 2 diabetes whose blood glucose is adequately controlled at first by sulphonylureas often eventually experience treatment failure and loss of diabetic control. Results from the UK Prospective Diabetes Study[1] have suggested that the 6-year failure rate was higher in patients treated with glibenclamide (48%) than in those given chlorpropamide (40%). This difference was equivalent to delaying the requirement for additional therapy for a year in chlorpropamide-treated patients.

1. Matthews DR, *et al.* UKPDS 26: sulphonylurea failure in non-insulin-dependent diabetic patients over six years. *Diabetic Med* 1998; **15:** 297–303.

Preparations

BP 1998: Chlorpropamide Tablets;
USP 23: Chlorpropamide Tablets.

Proprietary Preparations (details are given in Part 3)
Austral.: Diabinese; ***Belg.:*** Diabinese; ***Canad.:*** Diabinese; Novo-Propamide; ***Fr.:*** Diabinese†; ***Irl.:*** Diabinese; ***Ital.:*** Diabemide; Diabexan; Diabinese†; Gliconorm†; Normoglic†; ***Norw.:*** Diabinese; ***S.Afr.:*** Diabinese; Diabitex†; Hypomide; ***Spain:*** Diabinese; ***Swed.:*** Diabines; ***Switz.:*** Diabinese; ***UK:*** Diabinese†; Glymese; ***USA:*** Diabinese.

Multi-ingredient: ***Ital.:*** Bidiabe; Bidiamet†; Pleiamide; ***Switz.:*** Diabiformine.

Emiglitate (18830-k)

Emiglitate *(BAN, rINN).*

Bay-o-1248. Ethyl 4-(2-[(2*R*,3*R*,4*R*,5*S*)-3,4,5-trihydroxy-2-(hydroxymethyl)piperidino]ethoxy)benzoate.

$C_{17}H_{25}NO_7$ = 355.4.

CAS — 80879-63-6.

Emiglitate is an alpha-glucosidase inhibitor similar in action to acarbose (p.317). It is given by mouth and has been investigated for the management of diabetes mellitus.

References.

1. Lembcke B, *et al.* Inhibition of sucrose- and starch-induced glycaemic and hormonal responses by the α-glucosidase inhibitor emiglitate (BAY o 1248) in healthy volunteers. *Eur J Clin Pharmacol* 1991; **41:** 561–7.

Epalrestat (2905-h)

Epalrestat *(rINN).*

ONO-2235. 5-[(*Z,E*)-β-Methylcinnamylidene]-4-oxo-2-thioxo-3-thiazolidineacetic acid.

$C_{15}H_{13}NO_3S_2$ = 319.4.

CAS — 82159-09-9.

Epalrestat is an aldose reductase inhibitor similar in action to tolrestat (p.333). It is given by mouth for the treatment of diabetic complications including neuropathy (p.315).

References.

1. Goto Y, *et al.* A placebo-controlled double-blind study of epalrestat (ONO-2235) in patients with diabetic neuropathy. *Diabetic Med* 1993; **10** (suppl 2): 39S–43S.
2. Ucluda K, *et al.* Effect of 24 weeks of treatment with epalrestat, an aldose reductase inhibitor, on peripheral neuropathy in patients with non-insulin-dependent diabetes mellitus. *Clin Ther* 1995; **17:** 460–6.

Preparations

Proprietary Preparations (details are given in Part 3)
Jpn: Kinedak.

Glibenclamide (7217-a)

Glibenclamide *(BAN, rINN).*

Glibenclamidum; Glybenclamide; Glybenzcyclamide; Glyburide *(USAN)*; HB-419; U-26452. 1-{4-[2-(5-Chloro-2-methoxybenzamido)ethyl]benzenesulphonyl}-3-cyclohexylurea.

$C_{23}H_{28}ClN_3O_5S$ = 494.0.

CAS — 10238-21-8.

NOTE. The name glibornuride has frequently but erroneously been applied to glibenclamide.

Pharmacopoeias. In *Chin., Eur.* (see p.viii), *Int., Jpn, Pol.,* and *US.*

A white or almost white, crystalline powder. Practically **insoluble** in water and in ether; slightly soluble in alcohol and in methyl alcohol; sparingly soluble in dichloromethane; dissolves in dilute solutions of alkali hydroxides. **Store** in airtight containers.

Adverse Effects, Treatment, and Precautions

As for sulphonylureas in general, p.331.

For a suggestion that the failure rate in type 2 diabetics treated with glibenclamide may be higher than that for those treated with chlorpropamide, see p.319.

Effects on the blood. References.

1. Nataas OB, Nesthus I. Immune haemolytic anaemia induced by glibenclamide in selective IgA deficiency. *Br Med J* 1987; **295:** 366–7.

Hypoglycaemia. Severe hypoglycaemia may occur in any patient treated with any sulphonylurea (see p.332); this potentially life-threatening complication requires prolonged and energetic treatment.[1] Glibenclamide has a relatively prolonged duration of action and appears to cause severe hypoglycaemia more often than shorter-acting sulphonylureas such as tolbutamide.

Asplund and colleagues reviewed 57 instances of hypoglycaemia associated with glibenclamide.[2] The median age of patients affected was 70 years; only one was less than 60 years old. Median daily dosage was 10 mg. Coma or disturbed consciousness was observed in 46 patients. Ten of these remained comatose despite alleviation of their hypoglycaemia and died up to 20 days after presentation. In discussing their review, the authors reported that, including the present series of 57 cases, there had been published reports on 101 severe hypoglycaemias with glibenclamide, 14 with a fatal outcome.

There has been a more recent report[3] of hypoglycaemic coma associated with the inhalation of glibenclamide by a worker at a pharmaceutical plant.

1. Ferner RE, Neil HAW. Sulphonylureas and hypoglycaemia. *Br Med J* 1988; **296:** 949–50.
2. Asplund K, *et al.* Glibenclamide-associated hypoglycaemia: a report on 57 cases. *Diabetologia* 1983; **24:** 412–17.
3. Albert F, *et al.* Hypoglycaemia by inhalation. *Lancet* 1993; **342:** 47–8.

Interactions

As for sulphonylureas in general, p.332.

Pharmacokinetics

Glibenclamide is readily absorbed from the gastro-intestinal tract, peak plasma concentrations usually occurring within 2 to 4 hours, and is extensively bound to plasma proteins. Absorption may be slower in hyperglycaemic patients and may differ according to the particle size of the preparation used. It is metabolised, almost completely, in the liver, the principal metabolite being only very weakly active. Approximately 50% of a dose is excreted in the urine and 50% via the bile into the faeces.

References.

1. Coppack SW, *et al.* Pharmacokinetic and pharmacodynamic studies of glibenclamide in non-insulin dependent diabetes mellitus. *Br J Clin Pharmacol* 1990; **29:** 673–84.
2. Jaber LA, *et al.* The pharmacokinetics and pharmacodynamics of 12 weeks of glyburide therapy in obese diabetics. *Eur J Clin Pharmacol* 1993; **45:** 459–63.
3. Hoffman A, *et al.* The effect of hyperglycaemia on the absorption of glibenclamide in patients with non-insulin-dependent diabetes mellitus. *Eur J Clin Pharmacol* 1994; **47:** 53–5.
4. Rydberg T, *et al.* Concentration-effect relations of glibenclamide and its active metabolites in man: modelling of pharmacokinetics and pharmacodynamics. *Br J Clin Pharmacol* 1997; **43:** 373–81.

Uses and Administration

Glibenclamide is a sulphonylurea hypoglycaemic (p.331). It is given by mouth in the treatment of type 2 diabetes mellitus (p.313) and has a duration of action of up to 24 hours.

The usual initial dose of conventional formulations in type 2 diabetes mellitus is 2.5 to 5 mg daily with breakfast, adjusted every 7 days by increments of 2.5 mg daily up to 15 mg daily. Although increasing the dose above 15 mg is unlikely to produce further benefit, doses of up to 20 mg daily have been given. Doses greater than 10 mg daily may be given in 2 divided doses. Because of the relatively long duration of action of glibenclamide, it is best avoided in the elderly.

In some countries micronised preparations of glibenclamide are available, in which the drug is formulated with a smaller particle size, and which have enhanced bioavailability. The usual initial dose of one such preparation (Glynase) is 1.5 to 3 mg daily, adjusted every 7 days by increments of 1.5 mg, up to a usual maximum of 12 mg daily. Doses greater than 6 mg daily may be given in 2 divided doses.

Action. Proceedings of a symposium on the mechanism of action of glibenclamide.[1]

1. Gavin JR, ed. Glyburide: new insights into its effects on the beta cell and beyond. *Am J Med* 1990; **89** (suppl 2A): 1–53S.

EFFECTS ON THE HEART. A reduced incidence of ventricular fibrillation has been reported in diabetics treated with glibenclamide who develop myocardial infarction, compared with those receiving other treatments or with nondiabetic patients with myocardial infarction.[1] However, it should be borne in mind that some evidence has also suggested that sulphonylureas may impair the adaptive responses of the heart to ischaemia—see p.331.

1. Lomuscio A, *et al.* Effects of glibenclamide on ventricular fibrillation in non-insulin-dependent diabetes with acute myocardial infarction. *Coron Artery Dis* 1994; **5:** 767–71.

Preparations

BP 1998: Glibenclamide Tablets;
USP 23: Glyburide Tablets.

Proprietary Preparations (details are given in Part 3)
Aust.: Dia-Eptal; Euglucon; Gewaglucon; Gilemal; Glucobene; Neogluconin; Normoglucon; Semi-Euglucon; ***Austral.:*** Daonil; Euglucon; Glimel; Semi-Daonil; ***Belg.:*** Bevoren; Daonil; Euglucon; ***Canad.:*** DiaBeta; Euglucon; Gen-Glybe; ***Fr.:*** Daonil; Euglucan; Hemi-Daonil; Miglucan; ***Ger.:*** Azuglucon; Bastiverit; dia-basan†; Dia-BASF; duraglucon N; Euglucon N; Gliben; Gliben-Puren N; Glibenhexal; Glimidstada; Gluco-Tablinen; Gluconorm; Glucoremed; Glukoreduct; Glukovital; glycolande N; Maninil; Orabetic†; Praeciglucon; Semi-Euglucon N; Semi-Gliben-Puren N; ***Irl.:*** Daonil; Euglucon†; Melbetese; Semi-Daonil; ***Ital.:*** Daonil; Euglucon; Gliben; Gliboral; ***Jpn:*** Euglucon; ***Neth.:*** Daonil; Euglucon; Hemi-Daonil; Semi-Euglucon; ***Norw.:*** Daonil; Euglucon; ***S.Afr.:*** Abbenclamide†; Clinibent†; Daonil; Euglucon; Glyben; Glycomin; Melix†; Semi-Daonil†; ***Spain:*** Daonil; Euglucon; Glucolon; Norglicem; ***Swed.:*** Daonil; Euglucon; ***Switz.:*** Daonil; Euglucon; gli-basan; Glibesifar; Gluco-Tablinen†; Melix†; Semi-Daonil; Semi-Euglucon; ***UK:*** Calabren; Daonil; Diabetamide; Euglucon; Libanil†; Malix; Semi-Daonil; ***USA:*** DiaBeta; Glynase; Micronase.

Multi-ingredient: ***Ital.:*** Bi-Euglucon; Bi-Euglucon M; Gliben F; Glibomet; Gliformin; Glucomide; Suguan; Suguan M.

Glibornuride (7218-t)

Glibornuride *(BAN, USAN, rINN).*

Ro-6-4563. 1-[(2S,3R)-2-Hydroxyborn-3-yl]-3-tosylurea; 1-[(2S,3R)-2-Hydroxyborn-3-yl]-3-*p*-tolylsulphonylurea.

$C_{18}H_{26}N_2O_4S = 366.5.$

CAS — 26944-48-9.

NOTE. The name glibornuride has frequently but erroneously been applied to glibenclamide.

Glibornuride is a sulphonylurea hypoglycaemic (p.331). It is given by mouth in the treatment of type 2 diabetes mellitus (p.313) in doses of 12.5 to 75 mg daily; up to 100 mg daily has occasionally been given. Daily doses of 50 mg or more are given in 2 divided doses.

Preparations

Proprietary Preparations (details are given in Part 3)
Aust.: Glutril; Glutril; ***Fr.:*** Glutril; ***Ger.:*** Gluborid; Glutril†; ***Ital.:*** Glutril†; ***Switz.:*** Gluborid; Glutril.

Gliclazide (7220-y)

Gliclazide *(BAN, rINN).*

Glyclazide; SE-1702. 1-(3-Azabicyclo[3.3.0]oct-3-yl)-3-tosylurea; 1-(3-Azabicyclo[3.3.0]oct-3-yl)-3-*p*-tolylsulphonylurea.

$C_{15}H_{21}N_3O_3S = 323.4.$

CAS — 21187-98-4.

Pharmacopoeias. In Br. and Fr.

A white or almost white powder. Practically **insoluble** in water; slightly soluble in alcohol; sparingly soluble in acetone; freely soluble in dichloromethane.

Adverse Effects, Treatment, and Precautions

As for sulphonylureas in general, p.331.

It has been suggested that gliclazide may be suitable for use in patients with renal impairment, but careful monitoring of blood-sugar concentration is essential. The UK manufacturers recommend that it should not be used in patients with severe renal impairment.

Interactions

As for sulphonylureas in general, p.332.

Pharmacokinetics

Gliclazide is readily absorbed from the gastro-intestinal tract. It is extensively bound to plasma proteins. The half-life is about 10 to 12 hours. Gliclazide is extensively metabolised in the liver to metabolites without significant hypoglycaemic activity. Metabolites and a small amount of unchanged drug are excreted in the urine.

References.

1. Kobayashi K, *et al.* Pharmacokinetics of gliclazide in healthy and diabetic subjects. *J Pharm Sci* 1984; **73:** 1684–7.
2. Palmer KJ, Brogden RN. Gliclazide: an update of its pharmacological properties and therapeutic efficacy in non-insulin-dependent diabetes mellitus. *Drugs* 1993; **46:** 92–125.

Uses and Administration

Gliclazide is a sulphonylurea hypoglycaemic (p.331). It is given by mouth in the treatment of type 2 diabetes mellitus (p.313) and has a duration of action of 12 hours or more. Because its effects are less prolonged than those of chlorpropamide or glibenclamide it may be more suitable for elderly patients, who are prone to hypoglycaemia with longer-acting sulphonylureas. The usual initial dose is 40 to 80 mg daily, gradually increased, if necessary, up to 320 mg daily. Doses of more than 160 mg daily are given in 2 divided doses.

References.

1. Holmes B, *et al.* Gliclazide: a preliminary review of its pharmacodynamic properties and therapeutic efficacy in diabetes mellitus. *Drugs* 1984; **27:** 301–27.
2. Palmer KJ, Brogden RN. Gliclazide: an update of its pharmacological properties and therapeutic efficacy in non-insulin-dependent diabetes mellitus. *Drugs* 1993; **46:** 92–125.
3. Harrower ADN, Wong C. Comparison of secondary failure rate between three second generation sulphonylureas. *Diabetes Res* 1990; **13:** 19–21.
4. Mailhot J. Efficacy and safety of gliclazide in the treatment of non-insulin-dependent diabetes mellitus: a Canadian multicenter study. *Clin Ther* 1993; **15:** 1060–8.

Preparations

BP 1998: Gliclazide Tablets.

Proprietary Preparations (details are given in Part 3)
Aust.: Diamicron; ***Austral.:*** Diamicron; ***Belg.:*** Diamicron; ***Canad.:*** Diamicron; ***Fr.:*** Diamicron; ***Ger.:*** Diamicron; ***Irl.:*** Diamicron; ***Ital.:*** Diabrezide; Diamicron; ***Neth.:*** Diamicron; ***S.Afr.:*** Diamicron; Ziclin; ***Spain:*** Diamicron; ***Switz.:*** Diamicron; ***UK:*** Diaglyk; Diamicron.

Glimepiride (2804-x)

Glimepiride *(BAN, USAN, rINN).*

HOE-490. 1-({*p*-[2-(3-Ethyl-4-methyl-2-oxo-3-pyrroline-1-carboxamido)ethyl]phenyl}sulfonyl)-3-(*trans*-4-methylcyclohexyl)urea.

$C_{24}H_{34}N_4O_5S = 490.6.$

CAS — 93479-97-1.

Glimepiride is a sulphonylurea hypoglycaemic (p.331). It is given by mouth for the treatment of type 2 diabetes mellitus (p.313). Doses of 1 to 2 mg daily by mouth initially may be increased if necessary to 4 mg daily for maintenance. The maximum recommended dose is 6 mg in the UK and 8 mg in the USA.

References.

1. Ratheiser K, *et al.* Dose relationship of stimulated insulin production following intravenous application of glimepiride in healthy man. *Arzneimittelforschung* 1993; **43:** 856–8.
2. Rosenkranz B, *et al.* Kinetics and efficacy of glimepiride in diabetic patients with kidney disease. *Clin Pharmacol Ther* 1994; **55:** 207.
3. Tsumura K-I. Clinical evaluation of glimepiride (HOE490) in NIDDM, including a double blind comparative study versus gliclazide. *Diabetes Res Clin Pract* 1995; **28** (suppl): S147–S149.
4. Sonnenberg GE, *et al.* Short-term comparison of once- versus twice-daily administration of glimepiride in patients with non-insulin-dependent diabetes mellitus. *Ann Pharmacother* 1997; **31:** 671–6.
5. Langtry HD, Balfour JA. Glimepiride: a review of its use in the management of type 2 diabetes mellitus. *Drugs* 1998; **55:** 563–84.

Preparations

Proprietary Preparations (details are given in Part 3)
Ger.: Amaryl; ***Irl.:*** Amaryl; ***Neth.:*** Amaryl; ***S.Afr.:*** Amaryl; ***Swed.:*** Amaryl; ***Switz.:*** Amaryl; ***UK:*** Amaryl; ***USA:*** Amaryl.

Glipizide (7222-z)

Glipizide *(BAN, USAN, pINN).*

CP-28720; Glipizidum; Glydiazinamide; K-4024. 1-Cyclohexyl-3-{4-[2-(5-methylpyrazine-2-carboxamido)ethyl]benzenesulphonyl}urea.

$C_{21}H_{27}N_5O_4S = 445.5.$

CAS — 29094-61-9.

Pharmacopoeias. In Eur. (see p.viii) and US.

A white or almost white crystalline powder. Practically **insoluble** in water and in alcohol; sparingly soluble in acetone; soluble in dichloromethane. It dissolves in dilute solutions of alkali hydroxides. **Store** in airtight containers. Protect from light.

Adverse Effects, Treatment, and Precautions

As for sulphonylureas in general, p.331.

Interactions

As for sulphonylureas in general, p.332.

Antacids. Magnesium hydroxide and sodium bicarbonate have been reported to increase the rate of absorption, although not the total amount absorbed, of a dose of glipizide in healthy subjects.[1,2] No such effect was seen with aluminium hydroxide.[2]

1. Kivisto KT, Neuvonen PJ. Enhancement of absorption and effect of glipizide by magnesium hydroxide. *Clin Pharmacol Ther* 1991; **49:** 39–43.
2. Kivisto KT, Neuvonen PJ. Differential effects of sodium bicarbonate and aluminium hydroxide on the absorption and activity of glipizide. *Eur J Clin Pharmacol* 1991; **40:** 383–6.

Pharmacokinetics

Glipizide is readily absorbed from the gastro-intestinal tract with peak plasma concentrations occurring 1 to 3 hours after a single dose. It is extensively bound to plasma proteins and has a half-life of approximately 2 to 4 hours. It is metabolised mainly in the liver and excreted chiefly in the urine, largely as inactive metabolites.

A study in 12 healthy subjects indicating that hyperglycaemia impairs the absorption of single doses of glipizide.[1] This is probably a result of an effect on gastric emptying and gastric motility.

1. Groop LC, *et al.* Hyperglycaemia and absorption of sulphonylurea drugs. *Lancet* 1989; **ii:** 129–30.

Uses and Administration

Glipizide is a sulphonylurea hypoglycaemic (p.331). It is given by mouth in the treatment of type 2 diabetes mellitus (p.313) and has a duration of action of up to 24 hours. The usual initial dose is 2.5 to 5 mg daily given as a single dose 15 to 30 minutes before breakfast. Dosage may be adjusted at intervals of several days by amounts of 2.5 to 5 mg daily, to a maximum of 40 mg daily. Doses larger than 15 mg daily are given in two divided doses before meals. Modified-release formulations of glipizide are available in some countries; one such preparation (Glucotrol XL) is given in doses of 5 to 10 mg daily as a single dose with breakfast.

Administration. Although glipizide may be given in doses up to a recommended maximum of 40 mg, evidence for the benefits of high doses is scanty. A small study in patients with type 2 diabetes mellitus found that not only did increases in glipizide doses to more than 10 mg daily produce little or no benefit, but that the higher doses were associated with reduced rises in plasma-insulin concentrations and a lesser reduction in plasma-glucose concentrations.[1] There is, however, some evidence that glycaemic control and insulin sensitivity can be improved by the use of a modified-release rather than a conventional formulation of glipizide.[2]

1. Stenman S, *et al.* What is the benefit of increasing the sulfonylurea dose? *Ann Intern Med* 1993; **118:** 169–72.
2. Berelowitz M, *et al.* Comparative efficacy of once-daily controlled-release formulation of glipizide and immediate-release glipizide in patients with NIDDM. *Diabetes Care* 1994; **17:** 1460–4.

Preparations

BP 1998: Glipizide Tablets;
USP 23: Glipizide Tablets.

Proprietary Preparations (details are given in Part 3)
Aust.: Glibenese; Minidiab; ***Austral.:*** Melizide; Minidiab; ***Belg.:*** Glibinese; Minidiab; ***Fr.:*** Glibenese; Minidiab; Ozidia; ***Ger.:*** Glibenese; ***Irl.:*** Glibenese; ***Ital.:*** Minidiab; ***Neth.:*** Glibenese; ***Norw.:*** Apamid; Mindiab; ***S.Afr.:*** Minidiab; ***Spain:*** Glibenese; Minodiab; ***Swed.:*** Apamid; Glibenese†; Mindiab; ***Switz.:*** Glibenese; ***UK:*** Glibenese; Minodiab; ***USA:*** Glucotrol.

Gliquidone (7223-c)

Gliquidone *(BAN, rINN).*

ARDF-26. 1-Cyclohexyl-3-{4-[2-(3,4-dihydro-7-methoxy-4,4-dimethyl-1,3-dioxo-2(1*H*)-isoquinolyl)ethyl]benzenesulphonyl}urea.

$C_{27}H_{33}N_3O_6S$ = 527.6.

CAS — 33342-05-1.

Pharmacopoeias. In Br.

A white or almost white powder. Practically **insoluble** in water; slightly soluble in alcohol and in methyl alcohol; soluble in acetone; freely soluble in dimethylformamide.

Adverse Effects, Treatment, and Precautions

As for sulphonylureas in general, p.331.

Since renal excretion plays little part in the elimination of gliquidone, it has been suggested that it may be suitable in patients with renal impairment, but careful monitoring of blood-sugar concentration is essential. The UK manufacturers recommend that it should not be used in patients with severe renal impairment.

Interactions

As for sulphonylureas in general, p.332.

Pharmacokinetics

Gliquidone is readily absorbed from the gastro-intestinal tract. It is extensively bound to plasma proteins and has a half-life of approximately 1.5 hours. It is extensively metabolised in the liver, the metabolites having no significant hypoglycaemic effect, and is eliminated chiefly in the faeces via the bile; only about 5% of a dose is excreted in the urine.

Uses and Administration

Gliquidone is a sulphonylurea hypoglycaemic (p.331). It is given by mouth in the treatment of type 2 diabetes mellitus (p.313) in a usual initial dosage of 15 mg daily given as a single dose up to 30 minutes before breakfast. Dosage may be adjusted by increments of 15 mg to a usual dose of 45 to 60 mg daily in 2 or 3 unequally divided doses, the largest dose being taken in the morning with breakfast. Single doses above 60 mg and daily doses above 180 mg are not recommended.

Preparations

BP 1998: Gliquidone Tablets.

Proprietary Preparations (details are given in Part 3)
Aust.: Glurenorm; ***Belg.:*** Glurenorm; ***Ger.:*** Glurenorm; ***Ital.:*** Glurenor; ***Spain:*** Glurenor; ***UK:*** Glurenorm.

Glisentide (12786-b)

Glisentide *(rINN).*

Glipentide. 1-Cyclopentyl-3-[*p*-(2-*o*-anisamidoethyl)benzenesulphonyl]urea.

$C_{22}H_{27}N_3O_5S$ = 445.5.

CAS — 32797-92-5.

Glisentide is a sulphonylurea hypoglycaemic (p.331). It is given by mouth in the treatment of type 2 diabetes mellitus (p.313) in doses of 2.5 to 20 mg daily.

Preparations

Proprietary Preparations (details are given in Part 3)
Spain: Staticum.

Glisolamide (12787-v)

Glisolamide *(rINN).*

1-Cyclohexyl-3-{*p*-[2-(5-methylisoxazole-3-carboxamido)ethyl]benzenesulphonyl}urea.

$C_{20}H_{26}N_4O_5S$ = 434.5.

CAS — 24477-37-0.

Glisolamide is a sulphonylurea hypoglycaemic (p.331). It is given by mouth in the treatment of type 2 diabetes mellitus (p.313) in doses of 5 to 20 mg daily.

Preparations

Proprietary Preparations (details are given in Part 3)
Ital.: Diabenor.

Glisoxepide (7224-k)

Glisoxepide *(BAN, rINN).*

Bay-b-4231; FBB-4231; Glisoxepid; RP-22410. 1-(Perhydroazepin-1-yl)-3-{4-[2-(5-methylisoxazole-3-carboxamido)ethyl]benzenesulphonyl}urea.

$C_{20}H_{27}N_5O_5S$ = 449.5.

CAS — 25046-79-1.

Glisoxepide is a sulphonylurea hypoglycaemic (p.331). It is given by mouth in the treatment of type 2 diabetes mellitus (p.313) in a usual initial dose of 2 to 4 mg daily at breakfast, increased if necessary to up to 16 mg daily in divided doses.

Preparations

Proprietary Preparations (details are given in Part 3)
Aust.: Pro-Diaban; ***Ger.:*** Pro-Diaban; ***Ital.:*** Glucoben†.

Glybuzole (7225-a)

Glybuzole *(rINN).*

AN-1324; Désaglybuzole; RP-7891. *N*-(5-*tert*-Butyl-1,3,4-thiadiazol-2-yl)benzenesulphonamide.

$C_{12}H_{15}N_3O_2S_2$ = 297.4.

CAS — 1492-02-0.

Glybuzole is an oral hypoglycaemic with a structure distinct from that of the sulphonylureas, biguanides, or sulphonamidopyrimidines.

Glyclopyramide (7226-t)

Glyclopyramide *(rINN).*

1-(4-Chlorobenzenesulphonyl)-3-(pyrrolidin-1-yl)urea.

$C_{11}H_{14}ClN_3O_3S$ = 303.8.

CAS — 631-27-6.

Glyclopyramide is a sulphonylurea hypoglycaemic (p.331). It is given by mouth in the treatment of type 2 diabetes mellitus.

Glycyclamide (7227-x)

Glycyclamide *(rINN).*

Gliciclamide; K-38; K-386; Tolcyclamide. 1-Cyclohexyl-3-tosylurea; 1-Cyclohexyl-3-*p*-tolylsulphonylurea.

$C_{14}H_{20}N_2O_3S$ = 296.4.

CAS — 664-95-9.

Glycyclamide is a sulphonylurea hypoglycaemic (p.331). It is given by mouth in the treatment of type 2 diabetes mellitus.

Preparations

Proprietary Preparations (details are given in Part 3)
Ital.: Diaborale.
Multi-ingredient: ***Ital.:*** Diabomet†.

Glymidine (7228-r)

Glymidine *(BAN).*

Glymidine Sodium *(USAN, rINN)*; Glycodiazine; SH-717. The sodium salt of *N*-[5-(2-methoxyethoxy)pyrimidin-2-yl]benzenesulphonamide.

$C_{13}H_{14}N_3NaO_4S$ = 331.3.

CAS — 3459-20-9 (sodium salt); 339-44-6 (base).

Glymidine is a sulphonamidopyrimidine hypoglycaemic; its actions and uses are similar to those of the sulphonylureas (p.331) and it has been given by mouth in the treatment of type 2 diabetes mellitus.

Preparations

Proprietary Preparations (details are given in Part 3)
Ger.: Redul†.

Guar Gum (5427-l)

E412; Guar Flour; Guar Galactomannan; Jaguar Gum.

CAS — 9000-30-0.

Pharmacopoeias. In Eur. (see p.viii). Also in USNF.

A gum obtained from the ground endosperms of the seeds of *Cyamopsis tetragonolobus* (=*C. psoraloides*) (Leguminosae).

Guar Galactomannan (Ph. Eur.) is described as a yellowish-white powder. It is **soluble** in cold and hot water; practically insoluble in organic solvents. Its main components are polysaccharides composed of D-galactose and D-mannose at molecular ratios of 1:1.4 to 1:2. The molecules consist of a linear main chain of β-(1→4)-glycosidically linked mannopyranoses and single α-(1→6)-glycosidically linked galactopyranoses.

Guar Gum (USNF 18) is a similar substance but slightly differently described. It is characterised as consisting chiefly of a high-molecular-weight hydrocolloidal polysaccharide, a galactomannan, composed of galactan and mannan units combined through glycosidic linkages. It is a white to yellowish-white almost odourless powder, dispersible in hot or cold water to form a colloidal solution.

Adverse Effects and Precautions

Guar gum can cause gastro-intestinal disturbance with flatulence, diarrhoea, or nausea, particularly at the start of treatment.

Because guar gum swells on contact with liquid it should always be washed down carefully with water and should not be taken immediately before going to bed. It should not be used in patients with oesophageal disease or intestinal obstruction.

Interactions

Guar gum may retard the absorption of other drugs given concomitantly; where this is likely to pose a problem the other drug should be taken at least an hour before administration of guar gum.

Uses and Administration

Guar gum is used in diabetes mellitus (p.313) as an adjunct to treatment with diet, insulin, or oral hypoglycaemics since it is considered to reduce both postprandial and fasting blood-glucose concentrations. It is given with or immediately before meals in doses of 5 g usually three times daily. Adverse gastro-intestinal effects may be decreased by initial administration of 5 g once daily. Each dose of guar gum granules should be taken stirred in about 200 mL of a cold drink. Alternatively it can be sprinkled over or mixed with food which must be taken accompanied by about 200 mL of fluid. Guar gum has also been incorporated into various foods.

Guar gum is also used to slow gastric emptying in some patients with the dumping syndrome (p.1169). It is being investigated in the treatment of hyperlipidaemias.

Guar gum is also used as a thickening and suspending agent, and as a tablet binder.

Guar gum is an example of a soluble fibre; wheat bran is an insoluble fibre.[1] On contact with water it forms a highly viscous gel, the viscosity of which varies with such factors as its plant source or the form in which it is administered.[2]

Fibres such as guar gum reduce postprandial and fasting blood-glucose concentrations as well as plasma-insulin concentrations in healthy subjects and diabetic patients.[1,3,4] Bran has little effect on glucose and insulin concentrations.[5] Possible mechanisms for these effects of guar gum include a delay in gastric emptying,[1,3-5] decreased small-bowel motility,[1,4] decreased glucose absorption resulting from increased viscosity of the contents of the gastro-intestinal tract,[1,3] or inhibition of gastro-intestinal hormones.[3]

Guar gum also lowers serum total cholesterol and low-density-lipoprotein (LDL) cholesterol concentrations; high-density-lipoprotein (HDL) cholesterol and triglyceride concentrations appear to be unaffected.[4] The most likely mechanism is binding of bile acids, reducing their enterohepatic circulation in a similar way to bile-acid sequestrants.[3,4]

Reductions in fasting and postprandial blood-glucose concentrations and in glycosylated haemoglobin have been demonstrated in both type 1 and type 2 **diabetics,** but they have generally been small.[3] Many studies have examined the effect of a high-fibre diet on diabetic control but have often used unspecified mixtures of soluble and insoluble fibres. Interpretation of these studies is further complicated by variations in the diet (such as carbohydrate and fat content),[1] the effect of the diet on body weight,[5] and the method of food preparation.[1] Most studies have shown some improvement, albeit modest, in glycaemic control and lipid values[1] but there have been a few studies showing either no change or deterioration in blood-glucose concentrations.[5,6] While it might be possible to prepare a palatable preparation of guar gum, gastro-intestinal effects can be a problem,[1,3] but can generally be ameliorated by gradual introduction.[1] Advantages of natural dietary fibres may reside in the simultaneous reduction in ingestion of saturated fats or quickly digested carbohydrate.[1] For further discussion of high-fibre diets see Bran, p.1181.

When used alone in patients with **hypercholesterolaemia** guar gum has generally produced a modest reduction in plasma-cholesterol and LDL-cholesterol concentrations although some studies have been unable to demonstrate an effect. A few studies have suggested that the cholesterol-lowering effect is attenuated after 8 to 12 weeks of treatment but a long-term study observed a 17% decrease in total serum cholesterol that was maintained for 24 months.[7] Preliminary studies have shown further reductions in cholesterol and LDL-cholesterol concentrations on addition of guar gum to therapy with other lipid regulating drugs. The usual treatment of hyperlipidaemias is discussed on p.1265.

There have been suggestions that guar gum reduces appetite by promoting a feeling of fullness, but studies have not demonstrated a consistent reduction in body weight.[4] Products containing guar gum have, however, been promoted as **slimming aids**. Their use cannot be advocated because of the risk of tablets swelling before reaching the stomach and causing oesophageal obstruction.

1. Hockaday TDR. Fibre in the management of diabetes 1: natural fibre useful as part of total dietary prescription. *Br Med J* 1990; **300:** 1334–6.
2. Ellis PR, *et al.* Guar gum: the importance of reporting data on its physico-chemical properties. *Diabetic Med* 1986; **3:** 490–1.
3. Anonymous. Guar gum: of help to diabetics? *Drug Ther Bull* 1987; **25:** 65–7.
4. Todd PA, *et al.* Guar gum: a review of its pharmacological properties, and use as a dietary adjunct in hypercholesterolaemia. *Drugs* 1990; **39:** 917–28.
5. Tattersall R, Mansell P. Fibre in the management of diabetes 2: benefits of fibre itself are uncertain. *Br Med J* 1990; **300:** 1336–7.
6. Mann J. Diabetic dietary prescriptions. *Br Med J* 1989; **298:** 1535–6.
7. Salenius J-P, *et al.* Long term effects of guar gum on lipid metabolism after carotid endarterectomy. *Br Med J* 1995; **310:** 95–6.

Preparations

Proprietary Preparations (details are given in Part 3)
Austral.: Guarina†; ***Belg.:*** Fibraguar†; ***Ger.:*** Glucotard; Guar Verlan; Guarem†; Lejguar; ***Irl.:*** Guarem; ***Ital.:*** Guargel†; Leiguar†; ***Spain:*** Biotropic; Fibraguar; ***Switz.:*** Glucotard†; Guarem†; Leiguar; Lubo†; ***UK:*** Guarem; Guarina†.

Multi-ingredient: ***Austral.:*** Diet Fibre Complex 1500†; ***Belg.:*** Mucipulgite; ***Fr.:*** Moxydar; Mucipulgite; Mulkine; ***Ital.:*** Cruscasohn; ***Switz.:*** Demosvelte N; Mucipulgite.

Insulin (7202-e)

Insulinum.

CAS — 9004-10-8 (insulin; neutral insulin); 11070-73-8 (bovine insulin); 12584-58-6 (porcine insulin); 11061-68-0 (human insulin); 8063-29-4 (biphasic insulin); 9004-21-1 (globin zinc insulin); 68859-20-1 (insulin argine); 8049-62-5 (insulin zinc suspensions); 53027-39-7 (isophane insulin); 9004-17-5 (protamine zinc insulin); 9004-12-0 (dalanated insulin); 51798-72-2 (bovine insulin defalan); 11091-62-6 (porcine insulin defalan); 133107-64-9 (insulin lispro).

Pharmacopoeias. Most pharmacopoeias define a variety of insulin preparations. See also below.

Definitions and Terminology

Insulin is a hormone produced by the beta cells of the islets of Langerhans of the pancreas and consists of 2 chains of amino acids, the A and B chains, connected by 2 disulphide bridges. Insulin produced by different species conforms to the same basic structure but has different sequences of amino acids in the chains. **Porcine insulin** ($C_{256}H_{381}N_{65}O_{76}S_6$ = 5777.6) differs from **human insulin** ($C_{257}H_{383}N_{65}O_{77}S_6$ = 5807.7) in only one amino acid in the B chain whereas **bovine insulin** ($C_{254}H_{377}N_{65}O_{75}S_6$ = 5733.6) differs from human insulin not only in this same amino acid in the B chain but also in 2 amino acids in the A chain.

The precursor of insulin in the pancreas is proinsulin which is a single polypeptide chain incorporating both the A and B chains of insulin connected by a peptide termed the C-peptide (or connecting-peptide). Although the insulins of various species may be similar in composition the proinsulins are not, in that the sequence and number of amino acids in the C-peptide may vary considerably.

Insulin (Ph. Eur., USP 23) is of either bovine or porcine origin; the USP also allows mixed bovine and porcine origin. **Human Insulin** (Ph. Eur.) is produced either by the enzymatic modification and suitable purification of porcine insulin or by recombinant DNA technology in micro-organisms. **Insulin Human** (USP 23) is produced similarly.

Early commercial insulins were obtained by extraction from bovine or porcine or mixed bovine and porcine pancreases and were purified by recrystallisation only. Insulins obtained by such methods were often termed '**conventional insulins**' to distinguish them from insulins which have undergone further purification processes. An extract which has been recrystallised only once can be separated into 3 components or fractions termed the 'a', 'b', and 'c' components. The 'a' component consists of high molecular weight substances and is only usually found in very impure preparations since repeated recrystallisation will remove most of it. The 'b' component consists largely of proinsulin and insulin dimers, and the 'c' component consists of insulin, insulin esters, arginine insulin, and desamidoinsulin. Other pancreatic peptides such as glucagon, pancreatic polypeptide, somatostatin, and vasoactive intestinal peptide are also usually found in products which have not undergone further purification. Gel filtration will substantially reduce the content of proinsulin but will not significantly reduce the content of insulin derivatives or pancreatic peptides; products purified by gel filtration are often termed '**single-peak insulins**'. Addition of ion-exchange chromatography to the purification methods will further reduce the proinsulin content and also reduce the contamination by insulin derivatives and pancreatic peptides. In the UK '**highly purified insulins**' and '**monocomponent insulins**' are terms sometimes applied to insulins which have undergone both gel filtration and ion-exchange chromatography. In the USA the Food and Drugs Administration (FDA) has designated the term '**purified insulins**' for preparations similarly prepared and containing less than 10 ppm of proinsulin.

Much of the insulin now produced has an amino-acid sequence identical to that of human insulin. **Human insulin (emp)** is produced by the enzymatic modification of insulin obtained from the porcine pancreas; it is also sometimes called **semisynthetic human insulin**. The term **human insulin (crb)** is used for insulin produced by the chemical combination of A and B chains which have been obtained from bacteria genetically modified by recombinant DNA technology. **Human insulin (prb)** is produced from proinsulin obtained from bacteria genetically modified by recombinant DNA technology. **Human insulin (pyr)** is insulin produced from a precursor obtained from a yeast genetically modified by recombinant DNA technology. Human insulin obtained by recombinant DNA technology is sometimes termed **biosynthetic human insulin**.

Insulin or human insulin is supplied in a variety of forms in solution or suspension for injection (see Table 2). Crystalline insulin may be prepared for therapeutic use merely by making a solution, either of acidic or neutral pH. **Soluble insulin** or '**neutral insulin**' is a short-acting preparation that can be given intravenously if necessary to cover emergencies. Soluble formulations are sometimes referred to as '**regular insulin**' or '**unmodified insulin**'; these names reflect the fact that the preparation has not been formulated in order to prolong the duration of action of the insulin.

In order to prolong the duration of action of insulin, preparations may be formulated as suspensions in 2 general ways. The first involves complexing insulin with a protein from which it is slowly released; examples are **protamine zinc insulin**, which contains an excess of protamine, and **isophane insulin**, which contains equimolecular amounts of insulin and protamine. The second method of prolonging the action of insulin is to modify the particle size and the various **insulin zinc suspensions** are in this category.

Biphasic insulins are mixtures providing for both immediate and prolonged action.

Chemical modification of the insulin molecule has resulted in insulins such as **dalanated insulin** (prepared by the removal of the C-terminal alanine from the B chain of insulin), **insulin defalan** (prepared by the removal of the terminal phenylalanine), and **sulphated insulin**, but these insulins have not been widely used. **Insulin argine** and **insulin lispro** have been developed recently; insulin lispro, in which the B28 and B29 amino acid residues of human insulin are replaced with lysine and proline, is now available as a rapidly acting alternative to soluble insulin. Recombinant DNA technology has enabled production of other insulin analogues with altered pharmacokinetic profiles; some of these are being evaluated clinically (see Insulin Analogues and Proinsulin under Uses, below).

Stability and Storage

Insulin in powder form should be stored in airtight containers and protected from light. Storage at a low temperature is also recommended. The Ph. Eur. advises storage at a temperature not exceeding −20° while the USP requires storage at −10° to −25°. It is stressed that this temperature is for the powder and not for the preparations; preparations should not be subjected to storage conditions that lead to freezing.

Both the Ph. Eur. and the USP recommend that insulin preparations be stored in a refrigerator at 2° to 8°, protected from light, and not be allowed to freeze. It is recognised that patients may not follow such stringent storage guidelines and most manufacturers of commercial insulin preparations consider that storage by the patient at a temperature of up to 25° would be acceptable for up to one month. Patients should still be advised not to expose their vials or cartridges to excessive heat or sunlight.

It is advisable to shake suspensions gently before a dose is withdrawn.

Adsorption. The adsorption of insulin onto glass and plastics used in administration sets has been decreased by the addition of albumin or polygeline to insulin solutions. Some workers consider this to be unnecessary since in practice insulin adsorption is not a major problem.[1,2] Running approximately 10 mL of the insulin solution through the intravenous tubing before beginning the infusion has been suggested by some.[2]

1. Alberti KGMM. Diabetic emergencies. *Br Med Bull* 1989; **45:** 242–63.
2. Sanson TH, Levine SN. Management of diabetic ketoacidosis. *Drugs* 1989; **38:** 289–300.

Aggregation. For discussion of the problems of insulin aggregation, see Intensive Administration Regimens under Uses, below.

Units

One unit of *bovine insulin* is contained in 0.03891 mg of the first International Standard (1986). One unit of *porcine insulin* is contained in 0.03846 mg of the first International Standard (1986). One unit of *human insulin* is contained in 0.03846 mg of the first International Standard (1986).

Adverse Effects

The most frequent complication of insulin therapy is hypoglycaemia, the speed of onset and duration of which may vary according to the type of preparation used and the route of administration. It is usually associated with an excessive dosage of insulin, the omission of a meal by the patient, or increased physical activity. Patients, especially the elderly or those with tightly controlled diabetes or diabetes of long standing, may not experience the typical early warning symptoms of a hypoglycaemic attack. There have been reports of hypoglycaemia, sometimes with decreased warning symptoms, in patients changing from animal (especially bovine) to human insulin (see under Hypoglycaemia, below). Symptoms of hypoglycaemia resulting from increased sympathetic activity include hunger, pallor, sweating, palpitations, anxiety, and tremulousness. Other symptoms include headache, visual disturbances such as blurred or double vision, slurred speech, paraesthesia of the mouth and fingers, alterations in behaviour, and impaired mental or intellectual ability. If untreated, hypoglycaemia may lead to convulsions and coma which should not be confused with hyperglycaemic coma.

Insulin, administered subcutaneously, may cause either lipoatrophy or lipohypertrophy. Lipoatrophy appears to occur less frequently with purified insulins than with conventional insulins; if it has occurred, it may be reversed by the injection of a purer animal insulin or human insulin into and around the atrophied site. Lipohypertrophy is usually associated with repeated injections at the same site and may usually be overcome by rotating the site of injection, although it should be remembered that absorption of insulin may vary from different anatomical areas. Prolonged insulin therapy may result in weight gain.

Insulin may occasionally cause local or systemic hypersensitivity reactions. Local reactions, characterised by erythema and pruritus at the injection site, usually disappear with continued treatment. Generalised hypersensitivity may produce urticaria, angioedema, and very rarely anaphylactic reactions; if continued therapy with insulin is essential hyposensitisation procedures may need to be performed. Again, hypersensitivity reactions are observed less frequently with purified than with conventional insulins and porcine insulin is less immunogenic than bovine insulin. Although hypersensitivity reactions have been reported in patients transferred from animal to human insulins, there are only isolated reports of such reactions in patients treated exclusively with human insulin.

Many patients treated with insulin, either animal or human insulin, develop antibodies but the significance of such antibody formation with regard to the clinical management of the patient is not entirely clear.

Of patients who received intensive insulin therapy for type 1 diabetes as part of the Diabetes Control and Complications Trial, those who experienced the greatest weight gain also had increased blood concentrations of triglycerides and low-density-lipoprotein cholesterol, and lowered high-density-lipoprotein cholesterol.[1] These lipid changes, together with higher blood pressure, increased waist-to-hip ratio, and greater insulin requirements, were held to be similar to the symptoms of insulin resistance and to indicate a possible increased risk of macrovascular disease. Results from the UK Prospective Diabetes Study indicated that type 2 diabetic patients treated with insulin had greater weight gain than those managed with other therapies,[2] but demonstrated no evidence of harmful cardiovascular effects.

For discussion of some of the specific problems associated with continuous infusion of insulin, see Intensive Administration Regimens under Uses, below.

1. Purnell JQ, *et al.* Effect of excessive weight gain with intensive therapy of type 1 diabetes on lipid levels and blood pressure: results from the DCCT. *JAMA* 1998; **280:** 140–6.
2. UK Prospective Diabetics Study (UKPDS) Group. Intensive blood-glucose control with sulphonylureas or insulin compared with conventional treatment and risk of complications in patients with type 2 diabetes (UKPDS 33). *Lancet* 1998; **352:** 837–53.

Antibody formation. A review of human insulin including a discussion on the clinical importance of insulin antibodies.[1] Both pork and human insulin are definitely less immunogenic than beef insulin producing fewer circulating insulin antibodies, but several studies have indicated no detectable change in antibody concentrations on switching from pork to human insulin or *vice versa*. Antibodies cause lipoatrophy and are responsible for the substantial insulin resistance seen in some patients, but with purified pork insulin in common use, both events became rare. Interest has been revived in the possible contribution of antibodies in modifying metabolic control. In the short term and under hospital conditions, they are known to prolong the intravenous half-life of injected insulin and to delay the appearance in the circulation of a subcutaneously administered bolus dose. Patients with moderate concentrations of antibodies are also reported to show delay in recovery from induced hypoglycaemia, but on the other hand to lose control less quickly after insulin withdrawal and thus may be relatively protected from ketoacidosis.

1. Pickup J. Human insulin. *Br Med J* 1986; **292:** 155–7.

Effects on the liver. For a report of hepatomegaly occurring after insulin overdosage, see under Abuse, in Precautions, below.

Effects on the skin. Delayed pressure urticaria, in the form of large wheals occurring 4 to 6 hours after prolonged pressure, and lasting for up to 24 hours, was seen in a patient with type 1 diabetes within 6 months of changing from animal to human insulin.[1] The condition improved following a switch back to insulin of animal origin, and became aggravated again following a second attempt to switch to human insulin.

1. Payne CMER, *et al.* True delayed pressure urticaria induced by human Monotard insulin. *Br J Dermatol* 1996; **134:** 184.

Hypersensitivity. Hypersensitivity reactions to insulin preparations may be caused not only by the insulin itself, but also by other components of the formulation such as zinc[1] or protamine.[2]

See also under Antibody Formation, above and under Precautions, below.

1. Feinglos MN, Jegasothy BV. "Insulin" allergy due to zinc. *Lancet* 1979; **i:** 122–4.
2. Sánchez MB, *et al.* Protamine as a cause of generalised allergic reactions to NPH insulin. *Lancet* 1982; **i:** 1243.

HYPOSENSITISATION. Following failure of standard hyposensitisation measures in a patient with cutaneous hypersensitivity to insulin, hyposensitisation was attempted by giving insulin by mouth.[1] Aspirin 1.3 g three times daily by mouth was also given to antagonise vascular mediators of the reaction. After one week subsequent hyposensitisation using insulin by injection was successful. When the patient stopped taking aspirin after 6 months the original hypersensitivity reactions recurred; aspirin was then given permanently in a dose of 1.3 g twice daily.

1. Holdaway IM, Wilson JD. Cutaneous insulin allergy responsive to oral desensitisation and aspirin. *Br Med J* 1984; **289:** 1565–6.

Hypoglycaemia. Hypoglycaemia is the major adverse effect of insulin treatment with severe hypoglycaemic episodes in up to a third of all insulin-treated patients at some point in their lives. Moves towards more intensive insulin therapy, in order to reduce the development of diabetic complications, increase the risk of hypoglycaemic episodes.[1] This may be connected with the fact that patients maintaining strict glycaemic control are prone to 'hypoglycaemia unawareness' in which the normal adrenergic counter-response to hypoglycaemia (characterised by symptoms such as pallor, sweating, and tremor) is reduced or lost,[2] so that hypoglycaemia can develop without warning. Such a loss of awareness of impending hypoglycaemia also seems to develop in diabetics as disease duration increases.[3] One of the primary factors in reducing awareness of hypoglycaemia is that repeated hypoglycaemic episodes seem to trigger an adaptive conservation of glucose concentrations in the brain, resulting in higher central than peripheral blood glucose values;[4] avoidance of hypoglycaemia helps restore awareness.

When recombinant human insulin became generally available in the late 1980s a number of patients complained of a loss of awareness of impending hypoglycaemia following transfer to human insulin,[5,6] and there were reports of severe or even fatal hypoglycaemia occurring in patients who had been well stabilised on animal insulins.[5-7]

This was, and remains, a somewhat controversial area. Despite some small studies suggesting a problem,[8-11] others failed to find evidence of a difference between animal and human insulins.[12-14] However, most commentators appear to consider that patients should continue to have access to animal insulins if desired, and that those well maintained on an animal insulin should not be transferred to human insulin without appropriate clinical grounds,[3,7,15-17] and then only with careful monitoring.

There has also been concern about possible long-term sequelae of hypoglycaemic episodes on the CNS. However, a recent report on patients participating in the Diabetes Control and Complications Trial (DCCT) suggested that the increased risk of hypoglycaemia seen with intensive therapy was not associated with neuropsychological impairment.[18]

For the treatment of insulin-induced hypoglycaemia, see below.

1. The Diabetes Control and Complications Trial Research Group. The effect of intensive treatment of diabetes on the development and progression of long-term complications in insulin-dependent diabetes mellitus. *N Engl J Med* 1993; **329:** 977–86.
2. Widom B, Simonson DC. Glycemic control and neuropsychologic function during hypoglycemia in patients with insulin-dependent diabetes mellitus. *Ann Intern Med* 1990; **112:** 904–12.
3. Everett J, Kerr D. Changing from porcine to human insulin. *Drugs* 1994; **47:** 286–96.
4. Cranston I, *et al.* Restoration of hypoglycaemia awareness in patients with long-duration insulin-dependent diabetes. *Lancet* 1994; **344:** 283–7.
5. Teuscher A, Berger WG. Hypoglycaemia unawareness in diabetics transferred from beef/porcine insulin to human insulin. *Lancet* 1987; **ii:** 382–5.
6. Pickup J. Human insulin: problems with hypoglycaemia in a few patients. *Br Med J* 1989; **299:** 991–3.
7. Gale EAM. Hypoglycaemia and human insulin. *Lancet* 1989; **ii:** 1264–6.
8. Berger W, *et al.* Warning symptoms of hypoglycaemia during treatment with human and porcine insulin in diabetes mellitus. *Lancet* 1989; **i:** 1041–4.
9. Heine RJ, *et al.* Responses to human and porcine insulin in healthy subjects. *Lancet* 1989; **ii:** 946–9.
10. Egger M, *et al.* Risk of severe hypoglycaemia in insulin treated diabetic patients transferred to human insulin: a case control study. *Br Med J* 1991; **303:** 617–21.
11. Egger M, *et al.* Influence of human insulin on symptoms and awareness of hypoglycaemia: a randomised double blind crossover trial. *Br Med J* 1991; **303:** 622–6.
12. Colagiuri S, *et al.* Double-blind crossover comparison of human and porcine insulins in patients reporting lack of hypoglycaemia awareness. *Lancet* 1992; **339:** 1432–5.
13. Patrick AW, *et al.* Human insulin and awareness of acute hypoglycaemic symptoms in insulin-dependent diabetes. *Lancet* 1991; **338:** 528–32.
14. Maran A, *et al.* Double blind clinical and laboratory study of hypoglycaemia with human and porcine insulin in diabetic patients reporting hypoglycaemia unawareness after transferring to human insulin. *Br Med J* 1993; **306:** 167–71.
15. Gerich JE. Unawareness of hypoglycaemia and human insulin. *Br Med J* 1992; **305:** 324–5.
16. Williams G, Patrick AW. Human insulin and hypoglycaemia: burning issue or hot air? *Br Med J* 1992; **305:** 355–7.
17. Teuscher A, Kiln MR. Patient-empowerment and free insulin market. *Lancet* 1994; **344:** 1299–1300.
18. The Diabetes Control and Complications Trial Research Group. Effects of intensive diabetes therapy on neuropsychological function in adults in the Diabetes Control and Complications Trial. *Ann Intern Med* 1996; **124:** 379–88.

Oedema. Severe, acute oedema is a rare adverse effect of insulin treatment, occurring most often at the initiation of therapy.[1-3] It should be distinguished from chronic and subacute forms of oedema which may be complications of the diabetic disease process.[2,3] Possible mechanisms of acute oedema are sodium retention resulting from a direct action of insulin on the renal tubule or an effect of insulin on vascular permeability.[1,3] The oedema usually responds to a decrease in insulin dosage.

1. Bleach NR, *et al.* Insulin oedema. *Br Med J* 1979; **2:** 177–8.
2. Lawrence JR, Dunnigan MG. Diabetic (insulin) oedema. *Br Med J* 1979; **2:** 445.
3. Evans DJ, *et al.* Insulin oedema. *Postgrad Med J* 1986; **62:** 665–8.

Treatment of Insulin-induced Hypoglycaemia

In the conscious and cooperative patient hypoglycaemia is treated by the oral administration of a readily absorbable form of carbohydrate, such as sugar lumps or a glucose-based drink and all diabetics should always carry a suitable sugar source by way of precaution.

If hypoglycaemic coma occurs, up to 50 mL of a 50% solution of glucose should be given intravenously. Glucose 10 or 20% may be used but larger volumes are required. Occasionally this may need to be repeated and an intravenous infusion of glucose initiated. If after about one hour, blood-glucose concentrations are normal and the patient has failed to regain consciousness, the possibility of cerebral oedema should be considered. In situations where the intravenous administration of glucose is impractical or not feasible, glucagon 0.5 to 1 mg by subcutaneous, intramuscular, or intravenous injection may arouse the patient sufficiently to allow oral glucose to be given. If the patient fails to respond to glucagon within about 10 to 15 minutes, then glucose has to be given intravenously despite any impracticalities.

Following a return to consciousness, carbohydrates by mouth may need to be given until the action of insulin has ceased which, for preparations with a relatively long duration of action such as isophane insulin, some insulin zinc suspensions, and protamine zinc insulin, may be several hours.

Carbohydrate. A comparative study[1] of 7 different preparations of oral carbohydrate for the treatment of hypoglycaemia in the conscious patient found no significant difference in effectiveness between glucose or sucrose in solution or tablet form; a hydrolysed polysaccharide solution containing glucose, maltose, and various more complex saccharides (Glucidex 19) was also roughly comparable. However, a glucose gel and orange juice were each less effective in treating hypoglycaemia.

1. Slama G, *et al.* The search for an optimized treatment of hypoglycemia: carbohydrates in tablets, solution, or gel for the correction of insulin reactions. *Arch Intern Med* 1990: **150:** 589–93.

Table 2. BP and USP insulin preparations.

Type	BP/USP Title	Synonyms	Description	pH	Common classification	Approximate action profile after subcutaneous administration: Onset	Time to peak	Duration
Soluble insulins (also known as regular or unmodified insulin)	Insulin Injection (BP 1998)	Neutral Insulin Neutral Insulin Injection Soluble Insulin	Solution of Insulin (BP 1998) or Human Insulin (BP 1998)	6.9 to 7.8	Short-acting	30 minutes to 1 hour	2 to 5 hours	6 to 8 hours
	Insulin Injection (USP 23)		Solution of Insulin (USP 23)	2.5 to 3.5 (acidified) 7.0 to 7.8 (neutral)				
	Insulin Human Injection (USP 23)		Solution of Insulin Human (USP 23)	7.0 to 7.8				
Biphasic insulins	Biphasic Insulin Injection (BP 1998)	Biphasic Insulin	Suspension of crystals containing bovine Insulin (BP 1998) in a solution of porcine Insulin (BP 1998)	6.6 to 7.2	Intermediate-acting	Within 2 hours	4 to 12 hours	Up to 24 hours
	Biphasic Isophane Insulin Injection (BP 1998)	Biphasic Isophane Insulin	Buffered suspension of porcine Insulin (BP 1998) or Human Insulin (BP 1998) complexed with protamine sulphate or other suitable protamine, in a solution of porcine Insulin (BP 1998) or Human Insulin (BP 1998) respectively. Contains the equivalent of 300 to 600μg of protamine sulphate per 100 units of insulin in the complex	6.9 to 7.8				
Insulin suspensions	Isophane Insulin Injection (BP 1998)	Isophane Insulin Isophane Insulin (NPH) Isophane Protamine Insulin Injection	Suspension of Insulin (BP 1998) or Human Insulin (BP 1998) complexed with protamine sulphate or another suitable protamine. Contains 300 to 600μg of protamine sulphate per 100 units of insulin	6.9 to 7.8				
	Isophane Insulin Suspension (USP 23)		Buffered aqueous suspension of zinc-insulin crystals and protamine sulphate, combined in a manner such that the solid phase of the suspension consists of crystals composed of insulin, protamine, and zinc	7.0 to 7.8				
	Isophane Insulin Human Suspension (USP 23)		Buffered aqueous suspension of zinc-insulin human crystals and protamine sulphate, combined in such a manner that the solid phase of the suspension consists of crystals composed of insulin human, protamine, and zinc	7.0 to 7.5				
	Insulin Zinc Suspension (Amorphous) (BP 1998)	Amorph. I.Z.S. Insulin Semilente Insulin Zinc Injectable Suspension (Amorphous)	Suspension of Insulin (BP 1998) complexed with a suitable zinc salt; the insulin is in a form insoluble in water	6.9 to 7.8				
	Prompt Insulin Zinc Suspension (USP 23)		Buffered aqueous suspension of Insulin (USP 23) modified by the addition of zinc chloride in a manner such that the solid phase is amorphous	7.0 to 7.8				

Table 2. BP and USP insulin preparations.

Type	BP/USP Title	Synonyms	Description	pH	Common classification	Approximate action profile after subcutaneous administration: Onset	Time to peak	Duration
Insulin suspensions *cont*	Insulin Zinc Suspension (BP 1998)	Insulin Lente I.Z.S. I.Z.S. (Mixed) Insulin Zinc Suspension (Mixed) Insulin Zinc Injectable Suspension	Suspension of Insulin (BP 1998) or a mixture of bovine and porcine insulin or Human Insulin (BP 1998) with a suitable zinc salt; the insulin is in a form insoluble in water. It may be produced by mixing Insulin Zinc Suspension (Amorphous) (BP 1998) and Insulin Zinc Suspension (Crystalline) (BP 1998) in a ratio of 3 to 7	6.9 to 7.8				
	Insulin Zinc Suspension (USP 23)	Insulin Zinc	Buffered aqueous suspension of Insulin (USP 23) modified by the addition of zinc chloride in a manner such that the solid phase of the suspension consists of a mixture of approximately 3 parts of amorphous insulin to 7 parts of crystalline insulin	7.0 to 7.8	Intermediate or long-acting	2 to 3 hours	6 to 15 hours	Up to 30 hours
	Insulin Human Zinc Suspension (USP 23)		Buffered aqueous suspension of Insulin Human (USP 23) modified by the addition of a suitable zinc salt in a manner such that the solid phase of the suspension consists of a mixture of approximately 3 parts of amorphous insulin to 7 parts of crystalline insulin	7.0 to 7.8				
	Insulin Zinc Suspension (Crystalline) (BP 1998)	Cryst. I.Z.S. Insulin Ultralente Insulin Zinc Injectable Suspension (Crystalline)	Suspension of Insulin (BP 1998) or Human Insulin (BP 1998) complexed with a suitable zinc salt; the insulin is in the form of crystals insoluble in water	6.9 to 7.8				
	Extended Insulin Zinc Suspension (USP 23)		Buffered aqueous suspension of Insulin (USP 23) modified by the addition of zinc chloride in a manner such that the solid phase is predominantly crystalline	7.0 to 7.8	Long-acting	4 hours	10 to 20 hours	Up to 36 hours
	Extended Insulin Human Zinc Suspension (USP 23)		Buffered aqueous suspension of Insulin Human (USP 23) modified by the addition of a suitable zinc salt in a manner such that the solid phase of the suspension is predominantly crystalline	7.0 to 7.8				

Glucagon. A discussion of the relative merits of parenteral glucose and glucagon in unconscious hypoglycaemic patients[1] suggested that glucagon should be encouraged as first-line treatment, although in practice (see above) parenteral glucose is usually preferred. The effect of glucagon relies upon the patient having adequate liver glycogen stores, which may not always be the case.

1. Gibbins RL. Treating hypoglycaemia in general practice. *Br Med J* 1993; **306:** 600–1.

Surgical excision. Reports[1,2] of the treatment of insulin overdosage by excision of tissue at the site of injection.

1. Campbell IW, Ratcliffe JG. Suicidal insulin overdose managed by excision of insulin injection site. *Br Med J* 1982; **285:** 408–9.
2. Levine DF, Bulstrode C. Managing suicidal insulin overdose. *Br Med J* 1982; **285:** 974–5.

Precautions

Dosage requirements of insulin may be altered by many factors. Increased doses are usually necessary during infection, emotional stress, accidental or surgical trauma, puberty, and the latter two trimesters of pregnancy, and decreased doses are usually necessary in patients with impaired renal or liver function or during the first trimester of pregnancy. Following initiation and stabilisation of therapy in newly diagnosed diabetic patients, a temporary decrease in requirements may also occur (the so-called honeymoon period).

Because of the possibility of differing responses to insulins from different species, care is recommended to avoid the inadvertent change from insulin of one species to another. Reduction in insulin dosage may be required on transfer from animal (especially bovine insulin) to human insulin. Hypoglycaemic problems associated with a change to human insulin are discussed under Adverse Effects, above. Care is also necessary during excessive exercise; hypoglycaemia caused by metabolic effects and increased insulin absorption is the usual response, but hyperglycaemia may sometimes occur.

The use of insulin necessitates monitoring of therapy, such as the testing of blood or urine for glucose concentrations and the urine for ketones, by the patient.

Drugs which have an effect on blood-glucose concentrations may alter glycaemic control with consequent need for a change in insulin dose (see under Interactions, below).

CAUTION. *Biphasic insulin, insulin zinc suspensions, isophane insulin, and protamine zinc insulin should never be given intravenously and they are not suitable for the emergency treatment of diabetic ketoacidosis.*

Abuse. Transient recurrent hepatomegaly associated with hypoglycaemia was associated with the surreptitious administration of additional insulin injections in an insulin-dependent diabetic. Increased storage of glycogen in the liver resulting from insulin excess was considered responsible for the hepatomegaly.[1]

Decreased plasma C-peptide concentrations or the presence of anti-insulin antibodies may be used to confirm insulin abuse as a cause of hypoglycaemia in patients who have never been treated with insulin medically.[2] Insulin has been abused by bodybuilders and other sportspersons;[3,4] severe brain damage after prolonged neuroglycopenia has resulted.[3]

1. Asherov J, *et al.* Hepatomegaly due to self-induced hyperinsulinism. *Arch Dis Child* 1979; **54:** 148–9.
2. Grunberger G, *et al.* Factitious hypoglycemia due to surreptitious administration of insulin: diagnosis, treatment, and long-term follow-up. *Ann Intern Med* 1988; **108:** 252–7.
3. Elkin SL, *et al.* Bodybuilders find it easy to obtain insulin to help them in training. *Br Med J* 1997; **314:** 1280.
4. Honour JW. Misuse of natural hormones in sport. *Lancet* 1997; **349:** 1786.

Accelerated absorption. Factors such as a hot bath, sauna, or use of a sunbed have been reported to accelerate the absorption of subcutaneous injection, presumably by an increase in skin blood flow.[1-4] There may, therefore, be a risk of hypoglycaemia.[4]

1. Koivisto VA. Sauna-induced acceleration in insulin absorption from subcutaneous injection site. *Br Med J* 1980; **280:** 1411–13.
2. Cüppers HJ, *et al.* Sauna-induced acceleration in insulin absorption? *Br Med J* 1980; **281:** 307.

3. Koivisto VA. Sauna-induced acceleration in insulin absorption. *Br Med J* 1980; **281:** 621–2.
4. Husband DJ, Gill GV. "Sunbed seizures": a hypoglycaemic hazard for insulin-dependent diabetics. *Lancet* 1984; **ii:** 1477.

Adrenocortical insufficiency. A report of 2 cases of recurrent severe hypoglycaemia in type 1 diabetics which persisted despite a reduction in insulin doses and proved to be due to Addison's disease.[1] Insulin requirements rose again in both patients following replacement therapy with fludrocortisone and hydrocortisone.

1. Armstrong L, Bell PM. Addison's disease presenting as reduced insulin requirement in insulin dependent diabetes. *Br Med J* 1996; **312:** 1601–2.

Driving. Patients in the UK with diabetes mellitus are required to declare their condition to the vehicle licensing centre who then assess their fitness to drive. The law treats hypoglycaemic episodes as being under the influence of a drug and patients taking insulin are generally not permitted to drive vocationally.[1] Driving is not permitted when hypoglycaemic awareness has been lost. Drivers should normally check their blood-glucose concentration before setting out, and, on long journeys, at intervals of about 2 hours. If hypoglycaemia occurs, the driver should stop until recovery is complete.

Regulations in other countries differ widely.[2]

1. Stevens AB, *et al.* Motor vehicle driving among diabetics taking insulin and non-diabetics. *Br Med J* 1989; **299:** 591–5.
2. DiaMond Project Group on Social Issues. Global regulations on diabetics treated with insulin and their operation of commercial motor vehicles. *Br Med J* 1993; **307:** 250–3.

Exercise. A discussion of the metabolic effects of exercise and the precautions to be taken by the exercising type 1 diabetic.[1]

1. Greenhalgh PM. Competitive sport and the insulin-dependent diabetic patient. *Postgrad Med J* 1990; **66:** 803–6.

Hypersensitivity to protamine. A retrospective survey has indicated that patients receiving isophane insulin, which contains protamine, have an increased risk of severe reactions simulating anaphylaxis when protamine is used to reverse systemic heparinisation after cardiac catheterisation.[1] A mechanism involving IgE and IgG antibodies to protamine has been proposed.[2]

See also Hypersensitivity under Adverse Effects, above.

1. Stewart WJ, *et al.* Increased risk of severe protamine reactions in NPH insulin-dependent diabetics undergoing cardiac catheterization. *Circulation* 1984; **70:** 788–92.
2. Weiss ME, *et al.* Association of protamine IgE and IgG antibodies with life-threatening reactions to intravenous protamine. *N Engl J Med* 1989; **320:** 886–92.

Infections. Decreased requirements of insulin, added to the dialysate, occurred in 6 diabetic patients undergoing continuous ambulatory peritoneal dialysis for chronic renal failure during episodes of severe bacterial peritonitis.[1] This was contrary to the increased insulin requirements exhibited by most diabetic patients during severe infections and probably resulted from increased absorption of insulin due to mesothelial damage.

1. Henderson IS, *et al.* Decreased intraperitoneal insulin requirements during peritonitis on continuous ambulatory peritoneal dialysis. *Br Med J* 1985; **290:** 1474.

Menstruation. Discussion on the control of diabetes during the menstrual cycle and the possible need to adjust insulin dosage regularly around the time of menstruation.[1]

1. Magos A, Studd J. Effects of the menstrual cycle on medical disorders. *Br J Hosp Med* 1985; **33:** 68–77.

Morning hyperglycaemia. Morning hyperglycaemia may be the result of mere waning of subcutaneously injected insulin. It may also be rebound hyperglycaemia (posthypoglycaemic hyperglycaemia or the Somogyi phenomenon) occurring after an episode of nocturnal hypoglycaemia. Morning hyperglycaemia has also been observed without antecedent hypoglycaemia even during constant intravenous infusion of insulin, when the waning of previously injected insulin would not be a factor and this is commonly referred to as the dawn phenomenon. Clinically, it is important to distinguish between the dawn phenomenon, simple waning of previously injected insulin, and rebound hyperglycaemia as a cause of early-morning hyperglycaemia because their treatment differs. Management of the dawn phenomenon and insulin waning generally consists of adjusting the evening dose of insulin to provide additional coverage between 4 a.m. and 7 a.m. Management of rebound hyperglycaemia consists of reducing insulin doses or providing additional late-evening carbohydrate, or both, to avoid nocturnal hypoglycaemia. Mistaking rebound hyperglycaemia for the dawn phenomenon or mere waning of injected insulin could result in more serious nocturnal hypoglycaemia, if evening doses of insulin were increased.[1]

1. Cryer PE, Gerich JE. Glucose counterregulation, hypoglycemia, and intensive insulin therapy in diabetes mellitus. *N Engl J Med* 1985; **313:** 232–41.

Pregnancy. For discussion of the precautions necessary in the management of diabetes mellitus during pregnancy, see p.313.

There has been a report of 2 cases of fetal malformation in the offspring of well-controlled diabetic women who received *insulin lispro*.[1] However, the incidence of fetal malformation is increased in infants of women with diabetes. Although the use of insulin lispro is not recommended during pregnancy the manufacturers were aware of 19 live births among women treated with insulin lispro, 1 of which exhibited a congenital abnormality.[2]

1. Diamond T, Kormas N. Possible adverse fetal effect of insulin lispro. *N Engl J Med* 1997; **337:** 1009.
2. Anderson JH, *et al.* Possible adverse fetal effect of insulin lispro. *N Engl J Med* 1997; **337:** 1010.

Renal impairment. See under Infections, above.

Smoking. Smoking has been reported to decrease the absorption of insulin and may contribute to metabolic instability in diabetic patients.[1] Dosage adjustment may be necessary.

Smoking is of course highly undesirable in diabetic patients, who already have an increased risk of cardiovascular disease.

1. Miller LG. Recent developments in the study of the effects of cigarette smoking on clinical pharmacokinetics and clinical pharmacodynamics. *Clin Pharmacokinet* 1989; **17:** 90–108.

Surgery. For a discussion of the management of diabetes mellitus during surgery, see p.313.

Transmission of prion disease. Studies of cattle with proven bovine spongiform encephalopathy (BSE) have not detected infectivity in the pancreas, from which bovine insulin is derived.[1]

1. Wickham EA. Potential transmission of BSE via medicinal products. *Br Med J* 1996; **312:** 988–9.

Travelling. Advice for the diabetic patient when travelling, including adjustment of insulin dosage when crossing time zones.[1,2] Since insulin solution or suspension must not be frozen, it should not be carried in the luggage hold of an aircraft.

1. Barry M, Bia F. Advice for the traveling diabetic. *JAMA* 1989; **261:** 1799.
2. Sane T, *et al.* Adjustment of insulin doses of diabetic patients during long distance flights. *Br Med J* 1990; **301:** 421–2.

Interactions

Many drugs have an effect on blood-glucose concentrations and may alter insulin requirements. Drugs with hypoglycaemic activity or which may decrease insulin requirements include ACE inhibitors, alcohol, anabolic steroids, aspirin, beta blockers (which may also mask the warning signs of hypoglycaemia), disopyramide, fenfluramine, guanethidine, some monoamine oxidase inhibitors, mebendazole, octreotide, some tetracyclines, and the tricyclic antidepressant amitriptyline.

On the other hand, increased requirements of insulin may possibly be seen with chlordiazepoxide, chlorpromazine, some calcium-channel blockers such as diltiazem or nifedipine, corticosteroids, diazoxide, lithium, thiazide diuretics, and thyroid hormones.

Both increased and decreased requirements may occur with cyclophosphamide, isoniazid, and oral contraceptives.

ACE inhibitors. Although ACE inhibitors are favoured for use in diabetic patients with hypertension or evidence of incipient nephropathy or both, they may increase insulin sensitivity and thus decrease insulin requirements when given concomitantly.[1,2] The need for oral hypoglycaemics may also be decreased.

1. Ferriere M, *et al.* Captopril and insulin sensitivity. *Ann Intern Med* 1985; **102:** 134–5.
2. McMurray J, Fraser DM. Captopril, enalapril, and blood glucose. *Lancet* 1986; **i:** 1035.

Alcohol. Severe hypoglycaemic episodes have been reported in type 1 diabetics following heavy drinking episodes.[1,2] Alcohol inhibits gluconeogenesis, and its effects are therefore likely to be greatest if taken without food; however, it seems to be generally agreed that diabetics need not abstain from a moderate alcohol intake with meals.

1. Arky RA, *et al.* Irreversible hypoglycemia. *JAMA* 1968; **206:** 575–8.
2. Potter J, *et al.* Insulin induced hypoglycaemia in an accident and emergency department: the tip of an iceberg. *Br Med J* 1982; **285:** 1180–2.

Aspirin. Aspirin produces a modest decrease in blood-glucose concentrations but a significant interaction at conventional analgesic doses appears to be unlikely. One study in children with type 1 diabetes found an average 15% decrease in blood glucose values following treatment with aspirin 1.2 to 2.4 g daily for 3 days, but there were no significant changes in insulin requirements.[1] However, high doses of aspirin can reduce or even replace the insulin dose required.[2] Other salicylates might be expected to have similar properties.

1. Kaye R, *et al.* Antipyretics in patients with juvenile diabetes mellitus. *Am J Dis Child* 1966; **112:** 52–5.
2. Reid J, Lightbody TD. The insulin equivalence of salicylate. *Br Med J* 1959; **1:** 897.

Beta blockers. There are a few reports of severe hypoglycaemia in patients, including insulin-treated diabetics, who were given propranolol or pindolol;[1-3] there is also a report of an interaction with timolol given as eye drops.[4] Some evidence exists of an interaction with metoprolol,[5] but little evidence for some of the more selective beta blockers. Because of the effects of beta blockers on the sympathetic nervous system the usual premonitory signs of hypoglycaemia may not occur, allowing a severe episode to develop before the patient is aware and able to counter it.

1. Kotler MN, *et al.* Hypoglycaemia precipitated by propranolol. *Lancet* 1966; **ii:** 1389–90.
2. McMurtry RJ. Propranolol, hypoglycemia, and hypertensive crisis. *Ann Intern Med* 1974; **80:** 669–70.
3. Samii K, *et al.* Severe hypoglycaemia due to beta-blocking drugs in haemodialysis patients. *Lancet* 1976; **i:** 545–6.
4. Angelo-Nielsen K. Timolol topically and diabetes mellitus. *JAMA* 1980; **244:** 2263.
5. Newman RJ. Comparison of propranolol, metoprolol, and acebutolol on insulin-induced hypoglycaemia. *Br Med J* 1976; **2:** 447–9.

Calcium-channel blockers. Diabetes worsened in an insulin-treated diabetic when given diltiazem.[1] The resultant intractable hyperglycaemia improved when the drug was withdrawn, and recurred, although at a more manageable level, when diltiazem was restarted at a lower dose. There are also reports of a diabetogenic effect of nifedipine.[2,3] However, reports of significant disturbances of metabolic control appear to be uncommon.

1. Pershadsingh HA, *et al.* Association of diltiazem therapy with increased insulin resistance in a patient with type I diabetes mellitus. *JAMA* 1987; **257:** 930–1.
2. Bhatnagar SK, *et al.* Diabetogenic effects of nifedipine. *Br Med J* 1984; **289:** 19.
3. Heyman SN, *et al.* Diabetogenic effect of nifedipine. *DICP Ann Pharmacother* 1989; **23:** 236–7.

Interferons. A report of markedly increased insulin requirements developing in a previously well controlled diabetic following treatment with interferon alfa 2a.[1] Insulin requirements rapidly fell once interferon therapy was discontinued.

1. Campbell S, *et al.* Rapidly reversible increase in insulin requirement with interferon. *Br Med J* 1996; **313:** 92.

Oral contraceptives. Both increases and decreases (mainly the former) in insulin requirements have been reported in insulin-dependent diabetics given various oral contraceptives.[1] However, it appears that in most cases the effects of a hormonal contraceptive on diabetic control are modest or insignificant: one study suggests that progestogen-only and combined oral contraceptives in general have little effect.[2]

1. Zeller WJ, *et al.* Verträglichkeit von hormonalen Ovulationskemmern bei Diabetikerinnen. *Arzneimittelforschung* 1974; **24:** 351–7.
2. Rådberg T, *et al.* Oral contraception in diabetic women: diabetes control, serum and high density lipoprotein lipids during low-dose progestogen, combined oestrogen/progestogen and non-hormonal contraception. *Acta Endocrinol (Copenh)* 1981; **98:** 246–51.

Pharmacokinetics

Insulin has no hypoglycaemic effect when administered by mouth since it is inactivated in the gastro-intestinal tract.

It is fairly rapidly absorbed from subcutaneous tissue following injection and although the half-life of unmodified insulin in blood is very short (being only a matter of minutes), the duration of action of most preparations is considerably longer due to their formulation (for further details see Uses and Administration, below). The rate of absorption from different anatomical sites may be different depending on local blood flow, with absorption from the abdomen being faster than that from the arm, and that from the arm faster than from buttock or thigh. Absorption may also be increased by exercise. The absorption of insulin after intramuscular administration is more rapid than that following subcutaneous administration. Human insulin may be absorbed slightly faster from subcutaneous tissue than porcine or bovine insulin.

Insulin is rapidly metabolised, mainly in the liver but also in the kidneys and muscle tissue. In the kidneys it is reabsorbed in the proximal tubule and either returned to venous blood or metabolised, with only a small amount excreted unchanged in the urine.

For discussion of factors which may affect the absorption of insulin, see under Precautions, Accelerated Absorption, above, and Uses, Administration Routes, below.

Resistance to Insulin

The term insulin resistance has traditionally been used to describe a state in which diabetic patients exhibit considerably increased insulin requirements. It is now used in a much wider sense, and is for instance also applied to patients in whom a subnormal biological response to insulin can be demonstrated, although many of these patients do not apparently present difficulties in their clinical management. Insulin resistance is found particularly in obese patients; resistance to endogenous insulin is thought to be linked to the development of type 2 diabetes in such patients. Insulin resistance is frequently associated with lipid disorders, hypertension, and ischaemic heart disease. In women, it may also be linked to polycystic ovary syndrome.

Insulin resistance of the type manifested by greatly increased insulin requirements may be due to a variety of factors, including antibody formation and inadequate absorption of insulin from subcutaneous sites.

References.

1. Moller DE, Flier JS. Insulin resistance—mechanisms, syndromes, and implications. *N Engl J Med* 1991; **325:** 938–48.
2. Eckel RH. Insulin resistance: an adaptation for weight maintenance. *Lancet* 1992; **340:** 1452–3.
3. Clausen JO, *et al.* Insulin resistance: interactions between obesity and a common variant of insulin receptor substrate-1. *Lancet* 1995; **346:** 397–402.
4. Davidson MB. Clinical implications of insulin resistance syndromes. *Am J Med* 1995; **99:** 420–6.
5. Krentz AJ. Insulin resistance. *Br Med J* 1996; **313:** 1385–9. Correction. *ibid.* 1997; **314:** 134.

Uses and Administration

Insulin is a hormone that plays a key role in regulating carbohydrate, protein, and fat metabolism. The main stimulus for its secretion is glucose, although many other factors including amino acids, catecholamines, cortisol, glucagon, and growth hormone and its hypothalamic release-inhibiting hormone (somatostatin), are involved in its regulation. The secretion of insulin is not constant and peaks occur in response to the intake of food.

The major effects of insulin on carbohydrate homoeostasis follow its binding to specific cell-surface receptors on insulin-sensitive tissues, notably the liver, muscles, and adipose tissue. It inhibits hepatic glucose production and enhances peripheral glucose disposal thereby reducing blood-glucose concentration. It also inhibits lipolysis thereby preventing the formation of ketone bodies.

Therapy with insulin is essential for the long-term survival of all patients with type 1 diabetes mellitus. It may also be necessary in some patients with type 2 disease. The management of diabetes mellitus and the role of insulin in type 1 and type 2 disease is discussed on p.313. Insulin is generally the treatment chosen for all types of diabetes mellitus during pregnancy.

Choice of insulin. The different types of insulin and their formulations are described under Definitions, above. In some countries including the UK the commercially available preparations have been standardised to a single strength containing 100 units per mL; a strength of 40 units per mL is still available in some other countries, and in others concentrated injections (500 units per mL) are available to enable high doses to be given subcutaneously in a small volume. All formulations can be given by subcutaneous injection, most by intramuscular injection, but only soluble insulins can be given by the intravenous route. The long-term management of diabetic patients usually involves the subcutaneous route. Syringes and needles for subcutaneous injection are preferably disposable. Pen-injector devices which hold the insulin in cartridge form and meter the required dose are becoming increasingly popular. Soluble insulin is often given by the intraperitoneal route to patients on continuous ambulatory peritoneal dialysis.

The various formulations of insulin are classified, according to their duration of action after subcutaneous injection, as short-, intermediate-, or long-acting. The exact duration of action for any particular preparation, however, is variable and may depend upon factors such as interindividual variation, the patient's antibody status, whether the insulin is of human or animal origin, the dose, and the site of injection. *Short-acting* insulins are the soluble insulins, which have an onset after about 30 minutes to 1 hour, a peak activity at about 2 to 5 hours, and a duration of about 6 to 8 hours. *Intermediate-acting* insulins include biphasic insulins, isophane insulins, and amorphous insulin zinc suspensions. In general these have an onset within about 2 hours, peak activity after about 4 to 12 hours, and a duration of up to 24 hours. Commercially available mixtures of soluble insulins and isophane insulins have activities which would normally place them within the intermediate-acting category. Mixed insulin zinc suspensions may be classified as either *intermediate- or long-acting* as the duration of action may be up to 30 hours; the onset of action is generally 2 to 3 hours and the time to peak activity 6 to 15 hours. *Long-acting* insulins include crystalline insulin zinc suspensions and protamine zinc insulins. These generally have an onset after about 4 hours, a peak activity at about 10 to 20 hours, and a duration of up to 36 hours. Following intramuscular injection, the onset of action of all insulins is generally more rapid and the duration of action shorter.

The type of formulation, its dose, and the frequency of administration are chosen to suit the needs of the individual patient. Whatever the formulation, human insulin is generally used for all newly diagnosed diabetics.

Control. The dosage of insulin must be determined for each patient and although a precise dose range cannot be given a total dose in excess of about 80 units daily would be unusual and may indicate the presence of a form of insulin resistance. The dose should be adjusted as necessary according to the results of regular monitoring of blood concentrations (or occasionally urine concentrations) of glucose by the patient.

The WHO has recommended that the glucose concentration of venous whole blood under fasting conditions should be kept within the range of 3.3 to 5.6 mmol per litre (60 to 100 mg per 100 mL) and after meals should not be allowed to exceed 10 mmol per litre (180 mg per 100 mL); blood-glucose concentrations should not be allowed to fall below 3 mmol per litre (55 mg per 100 mL). In practice it seems to be generally acceptable for patients to aim for blood-glucose concentrations between 4 and 10 mmol per litre, with the understanding that occasional variations outside this range may occur. It should be remembered that the glucose concentrations in venous plasma, venous whole blood, and capillary whole blood may be slightly different. Control may also be determined by monitoring of glycosylated haemoglobin concentrations; ideally the aim is an HbA_{1c} level of less than 7% or an HbA_1 of less than 8.8%, compared with normal ranges of 4 to 6% and 5 to 7.5% respectively. Insulin requirements may be altered by various factors (see Precautions, above). The aim of any regimen should be to achieve the best possible control of blood glucose by attempting to mimic as closely as possible the pattern of optimum endogenous insulin secretion. Many regimens involve the use of a short-acting soluble insulin together with an intermediate-acting insulin, such as isophane insulin or mixed insulin zinc suspension. Such a combination is often given twice daily with about two-thirds of the total daily requirement given before breakfast and the remaining third before the evening meal. It may sometimes be necessary, though, to give 3 or 4 injections daily to achieve good control and this typically involves the administration of a soluble insulin before meals together with an intermediate- or long-acting insulin given usually in the evening. A once-daily injection of an intermediate- or long-acting insulin is now generally considered to be acceptable only for those patients with type 2 diabetes mellitus who still retain some endogenous insulin secretion but nevertheless require insulin therapy, or for those patients with type 1 disease unable to cope satisfactorily with more intensive regimens. If a more intensive regimen is desired, continuous subcutaneous infusion may be employed using soluble insulin in an infusion pump. This delivers a constant basal infusion of insulin supplying about half of the total daily requirements, the remainder being provided by patient-activated bolus doses before each meal. The technique has a limited place in the management of diabetes; patients using it need to be well-motivated, reliable, and able to monitor their own blood glucose, and must have access to expert advice at all times. Formulations in which the insulin is in suspension are not suitable for administration by continuous subcutaneous infusion.

Ketoacidosis. Insulin is also an essential part of the emergency management of diabetic ketoacidosis, see below. Only short-acting soluble insulins should be used. Treatment includes adequate fluid replacement, usually by infusing sodium chloride 0.9% initially, and the administration of potassium salts to prevent or correct hypokalaemia. If possible, insulin should be given by continuous intravenous infusion and typical initial infusion rates range between 5 and 10 units per hour; if facilities for intravenous infusion are not available intramuscular injection may be employed, typically with a loading dose of 10 to 20 units, followed by injection of 5 units every hour. Since insulin normally corrects hyperglycaemia before ketosis it is usually necessary to continue administration of insulin once normoglycaemia has been achieved but to change the rehydration fluid to glucose-saline so that the additional glucose prevents the development of hypoglycaemia.

General reviews of insulin and its use.[1-7] It has been suggested that the plethora of insulin preparations available might sensibly be reduced,[7] although others dispute this.[8]

1. Brogden RN, Heel RC. Human insulin: a review of its biological activity, pharmacokinetics and therapeutic use. *Drugs* 1987; **34:** 350–71.
2. Fisher BM. Choosing an insulin. *Prescribers' J* 1988; **28:** 138–43 and 169 (correction).
3. Anonymous. Human insulins: an update. *Drug Ther Bull* 1989; **27:** 21–4.
4. Home PD, *et al.* Insulin treatment: a decade of change. *Br Med Bull* 1989; **45:** 92–110.
5. Zinman B. The physiologic replacement of insulin: an elusive goal. *N Engl J Med* 1989; **321:** 363–70.
6. MacPherson JN, Feely J. Insulin. *Br Med J* 1990; **300:** 731–6.
7. Anonymous. Insulin preparations—time to rationalise. *Drug Ther Bull* 1996; **34:** 11–14.
8. von Kriegstein E, *et al.* Need for many types of insulin. *Lancet* 1996; **347:** 1045.

Administration. ADMINISTRATION ROUTES. The long-term management of diabetic patients usually involves injection by the **subcutaneous** route. The advice to diabetics has been to inject their insulin using a full-depth perpendicular injection.[1] In many non-obese patients, however, such a technique may result in inadvertent intramuscular injection.[1,2] Since insulin is absorbed more rapidly after intramuscular than subcutaneous administration, such a change between routes may lead to greater day to day variability in blood-glucose control. In particular, overnight control may be inadequate if intermediate-acting preparations such as isophane insulin are used.[1] Some workers therefore consider that extended-action insulins should be injected at an angle into a raised skin fold. Although injection of soluble insulin into muscle may produce a more physiological action profile, until more data are available a technique that ensures subcutaneous administration may be prudent with soluble insulins as well.[1]

The anatomic *site* of subcutaneous insulin injection is usually rotated in an attempt to decrease local adverse effects (see Adverse Effects, above). However, the rate of absorption varies between sites and such a practice may also contribute to day-to-day variability in blood-glucose concentrations.[3] For example, large variations in blood-glucose concentrations have been reported following subcutaneous injection into the thigh.[4] Some workers have suggested rotation of injection sites within an anatomic region, or possibly use of the same anatomic region for injections given at a specific time of day.[3] *Jet injectors* deliver insulin at high pressure across the skin into the subcutaneous tissue without use of a needle.[5-7] The greater dispersion obtained gives more rapid absorption of short- and intermediate-acting insulins and consequently reduces the total duration of action.[5,7] Delayed pain and bleeding may be a problem.[5,7] Despite having been available for some years, there is little information about their benefits and risks[8] and they are not widely used.[7] However, results in a small study in women with gestational diabetes have suggested that jet injection may be associated with less variation in postprandial blood-glucose concentration and a lower incidence of insulin antibodies.[9]

Insulin preparations may also be administered by **intramuscular** injection. Absorption is more rapid than from a subcutaneous injection. However, exercise may produce considerable variations in insulin absorption after intramuscular administration.[1] Soluble insulins may be given **intravenously**; this route is used in diabetic ketoacidosis, and also in surgery and labour.[10] Intermittent pulsed intravenous insulin therapy added to a conventional subcutaneous regimen has been reported to improve symptoms of postural hypotension[11] and hypertension.[12]

The subcutaneous and intravenous routes, and, rarely, the intramuscular route have all been used for the continuous administration of insulin (see Intensive Administration Regimens, below).

Formulations of insulin for **intranasal** administration are under investigation.[6,13-15] Absorption enhancers such as deoxycholate or laureth 9 have been used to facilitate uptake of insulin from the nasal mucosa. Studies in type 2[16] and type 1[17,18] diabetes have investigated the use of intranasal insulin given less than 30 minutes before a meal; in type 1 patients this was as an adjunct to base-line subcutaneous insulin. Two studies considered intranasal insulin to be promising.[16,17] However, one study found higher plasma-glucose concentrations 120 to 150 minutes after intranasal than after preprandial subcutaneous insulin.[18] Although local reactions such as nasal irritation[16-18] and chronic rhinitis[18] have occurred, these problems may be decreased by the development of less irritant absorption enhancers.

Endogenous insulin is delivered into the portal venous system, and then passes immediately to the liver where a large fraction of the insulin is extracted. The above routes of administration all deliver insulin into the peripheral circulation, with the risk of peripheral hyperinsulinaemia which has been considered a risk factor for atherosclerotic complications.[19] Administration of insulin via the **intraperitoneal** or **oral** routes may overcome this problem to some extent. Peritoneal insulin is used routinely in diabetics undergoing chronic ambulatory peritoneal dialysis, but has also been used for continuous administration (see Intensive Administration Regimens, below). Various formulations of insulin for oral delivery are also under investigation.[6] Some success in controlling blood-glucose concentrations has been achieved in a limited number of diabetics using a microemulsion of insulin in a lipid phase of similar composition to chylomicra.[20] **Rectal** administration of insulin has also been tried,[6,21] as has an aerosol for oral **inhalation**.[22]

1. Thow J, Home P. Insulin injection technique: depth of injection is important. *Br Med J* 1990; **301:** 3–4.
2. Frid A, Linden B. Where do lean diabetics inject their insulin? A study using computed tomography. *Br Med J* 1986; **292:** 1638.
3. Bantle JP, *et al.* Rotation of the anatomic regions used for insulin injections and day-to-day variability of plasma glucose in type 1 diabetic subject. *JAMA* 1990; **263:** 1802–6.
4. Henriksen JE, *et al.* Impact of injection sites for soluble insulin on glycaemic control in type 1 (insulin-dependent) diabetic patients treated with a multiple insulin injection regimen. *Diabetologia* 1993; **36:** 752–8.
5. Anonymous. Jet injection of insulin. *Lancet* 1985; **i:** 1140.
6. Chien YW, Banga AK. Potential developments in systemic delivery of insulin. *Drug Dev Ind Pharm* 1989; **15:** 1601–34.
7. MacPherson JN, Feely J. Insulin. *Br Med J* 1990; **300:** 731–6.
8. Pickup J. The pursuit of perfect control in diabetes: better insulin better delivered. *Br Med J* 1988; **297:** 929–31.
9. Jovanovic-Peterson L, *et al.* Jet-injected insulin is associated with decreased antibody production and postprandial glucose variability when compared with needle-injected insulin in gestational diabetic women. *Diabetes Care* 1993; **16:** 1479–84.
10. Home PD, *et al.* Insulin treatment: a decade of change. *Br Med Bull* 1989; **45:** 92–110.
11. Aoki TT, *et al.* Chronic intermittent intravenous insulin therapy corrects orthostatic hypotension of diabetes. *Am J Med* 1995; **99:** 683–4.
12. Aoki TT, *et al.* Effect of chronic intermittent intravenous insulin therapy on antihypertensive medication requirements in IDDM subjects with hypertension and nephropathy. *Diabetes Care* 1995; **18:** 1260–5.
13. Pontiroli AE, *et al.* Intranasal drug delivery: potential advantages and limitations from a clinical pharmacokinetic perspective. *Clin Pharmacokinet* 1989; **17:** 299–307.
14. Illum L, Davis SS. Intranasal insulin: clinical pharmacokinetics. *Clin Pharmacokinet* 1992; **23:** 30–41.
15. Coates PA, *et al.* Intranasal insulin: the effects of three dose regimens on postprandial glycaemic profiles in type II diabetic subjects. *Diabetic Med* 1995; **12:** 235–9.
16. El-Etr M, *et al.* Preprandial intranasal insulin as adjuvant therapy in type II diabetics. *Lancet* 1987; **ii:** 1085–6.
17. Salzman R, *et al.* Intranasal aerosolized insulin: mixed-meal studies and long-term use in type I diabetes. *N Engl J Med* 1985; **312:** 1078–84.
18. Lassmann-Vague V, *et al.* Preprandial intranasal insulin. *Lancet* 1988; **i:** 367–8.
19. Zinman B. The physiologic replacement of insulin: an elusive goal. *N Engl J Med* 1989; **321:** 363–70.
20. Cho YW, Flynn M. Oral delivery of insulin. *Lancet* 1989; **ii:** 1518–19.
21. Nishihata T, *et al.* Effectiveness of insulin suppositories in diabetic patients. *J Pharm Pharmacol* 1989; **41:** 799–801.
22. Laube BL, *et al.* Preliminary study of the efficacy of insulin aerosol delivered by oral inhalation in diabetic patients. *JAMA* 1993; **269:** 2106–9.

INSULIN ANALOGUES AND PROINSULIN. Recombinant-DNA technology has enabled the production of insulin analogues with altered pharmacokinetic profiles.[1,2] Most of the insulin in pharmaceutical preparations is in the form of hexamers, which requires time to dissociate before absorption from a subcutaneous site. Substitution of amino-acid residues at the monomer-monomer interface has produced monomeric insulin analogues that retain the biological activity of insulin.[3] Good results have been reported with an analogue, **insulin lispro**,[4] in which the B28 and B29 residues are replaced with lysine and proline. In comparative studies of insulin lispro versus soluble insulin given before meals to patients also receiving a long-acting insulin, insulin lispro was reported to result in good glycaemic control,[5,6] and could be given immediately before meals (5 to 15 minutes) rather than 20 to 40 minutes before as with soluble insulin. There is a suggestion that it may result in fewer hypoglycaemic episodes in such regimens,[6] but it is not, in fact, clear that this is so, although postprandial glycaemic control is improved. There is also a report of benefit in a patient with severe insulin resistance.[7] Insulin lispro is commercially available and has been widely reviewed.[8-12]

Protein engineering has also been used to produce a range of soluble insulins with absorption half-lives greater than 24 hours and hence a prolonged action.[1,2] Development has however, been less impressive than with the rapid-acting analogues.[1]

Immunogenicity and possible unwanted metabolic effects of insulin analogues must be studied in addition to metabolic efficacy before they can be introduced into clinical use.[1,2]

Proinsulin (the natural precursor of insulin) appears to be more active than insulin in suppressing the hepatic production rather than the peripheral uptake of glucose.[2,13] It has therefore been studied particularly in patients with type 2 diabetes mellitus. However, development by some manufacturers has been suspended because of a higher rate of adverse cardiac effects in patients treated with proinsulin than in controls.[2]

Mecasermin (insulin-like growth factor; see p.1260) has been observed to reverse hyperglycaemia and ketoacidosis in patients with insulin resistance.[14,15]

1. Barnett AH, Owens DR. Insulin analogues. *Lancet* 1997; **349:** 47–51. Correction. *ibid.*; 656.
2. Zinman B. The physiologic replacement of insulin: an elusive goal. *N Engl J Med* 1989; **321:** 363–70.
3. Brange J, *et al.* Monomeric insulins obtained by protein engineering and their medical implications. *Nature* 1988; **333:** 679–82.
4. Desmet M, *et al.* [Lys (B28), Pro (B29)] human insulin (Lys-Pro): patients treated with LysPro vs human regular insulin—quality of life assessment. *Diabetes* 1994; **43** (suppl 1): 167A.
5. Howey DC, *et al.* [Lys(B28), Pro(B29)]-human insulin: effect of injection time on postprandial glycemia. *Clin Pharmacol Ther* 1995; **58:** 459–69.
6. Garg SK, *et al.* Pre-meal insulin analogue insulin lispro vs Humulin R insulin treatment in young subjects with type 1 diabetes. *Diabetic Med* 1996; **13:** 47–52.
7. Henrichs HR, *et al.* Severe insulin resistance treated with insulin lispro. *Lancet* 1996; **348:** 1248.
8. Anonymous. Lispro, a rapid-onset insulin. *Med Lett Drugs Ther* 1996; **38:** 97–8.
9. Campbell RK, *et al.* Insulin lispro: its role in the treatment of diabetes mellitus. *Ann Pharmacother* 1996; **30:** 1263–71.
10. Holleman F, Hoekstra JBL. Insulin lispro. *N Engl J Med* 1997; **337:** 176–83.
11. Anonymous. Humalog—a new insulin analogue. *Drug Ther Bull* 1997; **35:** 57–8.
12. Wilde MI, McTavish D. Insulin Lispro: a review of its pharmacological properties and therapeutic use in the management of diabetes mellitus. *Drugs* 1997; **54:** 597–614.
13. Goran EA. Human proinsulin—a new therapeutic agent? *Pharm J* 1986; **236:** 667.
14. Usala A-L, *et al.* Brief report: treatment of insulin-resistant diabetic ketoacidosis with insulin-like growth factor I in an adolescent with insulin-dependent diabetes. *N Engl J Med* 1992; **327:** 853–7.
15. Moses AC, *et al.* Insulin-like growth factor I (rhIGF-I) as a therapeutic agent for hyperinsulinemic insulin-resistant diabetes mellitus. *Diabetes Res Clin Pract* 1995; **28** (suppl): S185–S194.

INTENSIVE ADMINISTRATION REGIMENS. Intensive regimens for insulin administration aim to mimic more closely the physiological insulin pattern in which a basal insulin concentration is supplemented by a preprandial boost of insulin.[1-5] Such intensive regimens are used to provide tight control in an attempt to avoid long-term complications (see p.315).

In multiple-injection regimens, the basal insulin is provided by an injection of intermediate- or long-acting insulin given usually at night. Soluble insulin is administered before each main meal, perhaps with a pen-injector device.[6] Systems for continuous administration may be designed on an open-loop or closed-loop delivery system. Open-loop systems comprise an infusion pump with the infusion rate programmed or controlled manually according to manual blood-glucose monitoring. Closed-loop systems (the 'artificial pancreas') consist of an insulin pump, a glucose sensor, and a computer for analysis of blood-glucose data. Systems for continuous administration have most commonly used the subcutaneous route, but intraperitoneal, intravenous, or intramuscular infusion have also been used.

The most extensively investigated open-loop system is continuous subcutaneous insulin infusion using an external pump. A battery-powered pump infuses soluble insulin via a subcutaneous catheter which is resited every 1 to 3 days. A background infusion is given at a predetermined rate, and preprandial bolus doses given using an override switch or manual drive.[7] Complications include erythema, abscess, or cellulitis at the injection site and, rarely, systemic infection, hypersensitivity reactions to components of the administration set, pump malfunction, adsorption of insulin or preservative on to the administration set, or catheter obstruction.[7] If the pump fails, the onset of ketoacidosis may be more rapid and more likely to be associated with dangerous hyperkalaemia than with conventional administration regimens because there is no depot of insulin.[5] Although improved glycaemic control in intensive regimens may be associated with decreased hypoglycaemic awareness and more hypoglycaemic episodes, one study has reported fewer severe hypoglycaemic episodes in patients switched from multiple daily injections to continuous subcutaneous infusion of insulin.[8]

Further development of open-loop delivery systems has been in the design of implantable insulin pumps. The first pumps delivered insulin at a constant basal rate, but variable-rate models, such as the programmable implantable medication system (PIMS) are now available.[2,9] One of the major problems with implantable pumps has been the tendency for insulin to aggregate on prolonged exposure to body heat, movement, and contact with hydrophobic surfaces.[2] Insulin aggregates may occlude pumps and tubing,[2,9] and studies have suggested that their prolonged infusion may induce amyloidosis.[9] Insulin aggregation has been decreased by the development of insulin preparations containing calcium, glycerol, bicarbonate, or, most successfully, poloxamer.[2,9] Insulin pumps are implanted subcutaneously, usually in the abdomen, but the catheter is usually placed peritoneally or intravenously.[2,9] Glycaemic control has been good;[10,11] a French multicentre study involving 224 patients found that glycosylated haemoglobin fell on average from 7.4 to 6.8% six months after implantation.[12] Specific problems with hypoglycaemia or ketoacidosis do not appear to have been identified,[9-11] and indeed there is some evidence that the postprandial insulin profile is better and hypoglycaemia less frequent, in patients using implantable pumps for intraperitoneal or intravenous delivery compared with those receiving continuous subcutaneous infusion from an external pump.[13] Complications include mechanical failure of the system, infection (particularly of the implantation site) and skin necrosis over the implant. Peritoneal catheters may become obstructed by omental tissue.[9-11]

Closed-loop continuous infusion systems are generally confined to research and experimental work. External pumps are used since no glucose sensor suitable for implantation has yet been developed.[9] (However, results in *animals* have suggested that an alternative to such systems may be a vascularised artificial pancreas containing islet cells.[14])

Intensified insulin regimens have the advantage of improving the patient's lifestyle and allowing flexibility in timing of meals. However, careful dietary control must still be maintained and regular monitoring of blood-glucose concentrations is an important component of such regimens. Therefore patients must be well-motivated, reliable, and able to monitor their own blood glucose, and must have access to expert 24-hour help.[4-7] Although there are reports of success with intensive administration regimens in brittle (labile) diabetics,[15] these patients are generally unlikely to benefit from such regimens.[5]

1. Fisher BM. Choosing an insulin. *Prescribers' J* 1988; **28:** 138–43 and 169 (correction).
2. Pickup J. The pursuit of perfect control in diabetes: better insulin better delivered. *Br Med J* 1988; **297:** 929–31.
3. Home PD, *et al.* Insulin treatment: a decade of change. *Br Med Bull* 1989; **45:** 92–110.
4. Zinman B. The physiologic replacement of insulin: an elusive goal. *N Engl J Med* 1989; **321:** 363–70.
5. MacPherson JN, Feely J. Insulin. *Br Med J* 1990; **300:** 731–6.
6. Anonymous. Insulin pen: mightier than syringe? *Lancet* 1989; **i:** 307–8.
7. Anonymous. Continuous subcutaneous insulin infusion. *JAMA* 1989; **262:** 1239–43.
8. Bode BW, *et al.* Reduction in severe hypoglycemia with long-term continuous subcutaneous insulin infusion in type I diabetes. *Diabetes Care* 1996; **19:** 324–7.
9. Anonymous. Continuous peritoneal insulin infusion and implantable insulin infusion pumps for diabetic control. *JAMA* 1989; **262:** 3195–8.
10. Point Study Group. One-year trial of a remote-controlled implantable insulin infusion system in type I diabetic patients. *Lancet* 1988; **ii:** 866–9.

11. Saudek CD, *et al.* A preliminary trial of the programmable implantable medication system for insulin delivery. *N Engl J Med* 1989; **321:** 574–9.
12. Broussolle C, *et al.* French multicentre experience of implantable insulin pumps. *Lancet* 1994; **343:** 514–15.
13. Nathan DM, *et al.* Postprandial insulin profiles with implantable pump therapy may explain decreased frequency of severe hypoglycemia, compared with intensive subcutaneous regimens, in insulin-dependent diabetes mellitus patients. *Am J Med* 1996; **100:** 412–17.
14. Maki T, *et al.* Novel delivery of pancreatic islet cells to treat insulin-dependent diabetes mellitus. *Clin Pharmacokinet* 1995; **28:** 471–82.
15. Wood DF, *et al.* Management of "brittle" diabetes with a preprogrammable implanted pump delivering intraperitoneal insulin. *Br Med J* 1990; **301:** 1143–4.

MIXING OF INSULINS. There are studies indicating that the rapid effect of soluble insulin may be lost if mixed in the syringe immediately prior to injection with insulins containing high concentrations of free zinc.[1,2] Insulin manufacturers recommend immediate injection of mixtures prepared in the syringe; if delay is unavoidable a consistent routine is advised. The shorter-acting insulin should be drawn into the syringe first to prevent contamination of the vial by the longer-acting preparation. Insulins from different manufacturers should not be mixed since formulation differences, such as the buffer or preservative used, may render them incompatible.[3]

1. Mühlhauser I, *et al.* Miscibility of human and bovine ultralente insulin with soluble insulin. *Br Med J* 1984; **289:** 1656–7.
2. Heine RJ, *et al.* Mixing short and intermediate acting insulins in the syringe: effect on postprandial blood glucose concentrations in type I diabetics. *Br Med J* 1985; **290:** 204–5.
3. Fisher BM. Choosing an insulin. *Prescribers' J* 1988; **28:** 138–43 and 169 (correction).

Diabetes mellitus. Insulin is the mainstay of the treatment of type 1 diabetes mellitus. For a discussion of the treatment of diabetes mellitus, including the contexts in which insulin is used, see p.313. The possible role of tight glycaemic control with insulin to prevent the development of microvascular and macrovascular complications in patients with type 1 diabetes is discussed on p.315, while further discussion of specific regimens and approaches to insulin therapy is given under Administration, above.

DIABETIC EMERGENCIES. As discussed on p.316, diabetic ketoacidosis is a medical emergency and should be treated immediately with fluid replacement and insulin.[1-4] Potassium, and possibly phosphate, replacement may also be required, but bicarbonate should not be given unless acidaemia is very severe.

Soluble insulin is the form used in diabetic ketoacidosis, ideally by the intravenous route. Large doses were formerly used because of the presence of insulin resistance in diabetic ketoacidosis, probably related to the effects of acidaemia.[1] Lower-dose regimens have since been shown to provide adequate insulin concentrations and are now used routinely.[1,3] Adults are sometimes given an initial bolus injection of soluble insulin 5 to 20 units.[3,5] Soluble insulin, diluted to a concentration of 1 unit per mL,[1,2] is then administered continuously via an infusion pump at a rate of 5 to 10 units per hour.[3] Children have been given insulin intravenously as a bolus of 0.1 unit per kg body-weight followed by an infusion of 0.1 unit per kg per hour.[2]

Insulin may be given by the intramuscular route provided the circulatory state of the patient is satisfactory.[2,4] Adults may be given a bolus injection of 20 units followed by 5 units per hour.[1,4] Children may be given 0.25 unit per kg as a bolus followed by 0.1 unit per kg per hour.[1,2]

Lack of response to insulin is generally a result of inadequate hydration but may occasionally be caused by genuine insulin resistance.[1,3] In this case the intravenous route is essential[1] and the insulin dose needs to be doubled on a one- to two-hourly basis until an adequate response has been obtained.[1] A case report has suggested that mecasermin may be useful if there is insulin resistance.[6]

When the blood-glucose concentration has fallen to less than 10 mmol per litre the dose of insulin may be reduced by about half and glucose administered intravenously.[1] (A recent study reported benefit, however, from continuing insulin infusion at a rate of 5 units per hour until resolution of hyperketonaemia.[7]) Glucose is usually given in a strength of 5% with saline[2,3] although some have advocated a glucose strength of 10%.[1] The administration of glucose enables insulin to be continued in order to clear ketone bodies, without inducing hypoglycaemia; this is essential if a recurrence of ketoacidosis is to be avoided.[3] Once glucose concentrations have been controlled and acidosis has completely cleared, subcutaneous injections of insulin can be started,[3] but intravenous infusion should be continued at a reduced rate for an hour during the change-over.[2]

Hyperosmolar hyperglycaemic nonketotic coma (HONK) is much less common in type 1 diabetics than diabetic ketoacidosis.[1,2] It occurs mainly in elderly patients with type 2 diabetes and has a much higher mortality than diabetic ketoacidosis.[1] Patients may present in coma or be very drowsy with severe hyperglycaemia but without significant ketosis; dehydration and renal impairment are also major features and hypernatraemia is more common.[1] Treatment is similar to diabetic ketoacidosis; bicarbonate is not required[1] and potassium requirements are lower.[5] Less insulin but more fluid is usually required and some have advocated the use of hypotonic fluids.[5]

1. Alberti KGMM. Diabetic emergencies. *Br Med Bull* 1989; **45:** 242–63.
2. Richardson JE, Donaldson MDC. Diabetic emergencies. *Prescribers' J* 1989; **29:** 174–83.
3. Sanson TH, Levine SN. Management of diabetic ketoacidosis. *Drugs* 1989; **38:** 289–300.
4. Lebovitz HE. Diabetic ketoacidosis. *Lancet* 1995; **345:** 767–72.
5. Wright AD. Diabetic emergencies in adults. *Prescribers' J* 1989; **29:** 147–54.
6. Usala A-L, *et al.* Brief report: treatment of insulin-resistant diabetic ketoacidosis with insulin-like growth factor I in an adolescent with insulin-dependent diabetes. *N Engl J Med* 1992; **327:** 853–7.
7. Wiggam MI, *et al.* Treatment of diabetic ketoacidosis using normalization of blood 3-hydroxybutyrate concentration as the end point of emergency management. *Diabetes Care* 1997; **20:** 1347–52.

TYPE 2 DIABETES MELLITUS. Traditionally the use of insulin in patients with type 2 diabetes has tended to be reserved for those who cannot be controlled by diet and oral hypoglycaemics alone.[1,2] Given the possible association between circulating insulin and atherosclerotic cardiovascular symptoms[3] there has been some concern about the administration of exogenous insulin to insulin-resistant patients who are already hyperinsulinaemic. Furthermore, patients switched to insulin tend to gain weight[2] which is undesirable in a frequently obese patient group.

Although it is still the consensus that insulin should be reserved for those poorly controlled on diet and oral hypoglycaemic drugs,[4] insulin is nonetheless being used more frequently in type 2 patients. This is largely because of a trend toward more intensive regimens designed to produce tighter glycaemic control, on the hypothesis that, as in patients with type 1 disease, this will reduce the development and progression of diabetic complications. Results from the UK Prospective Diabetes Study,[5-7] show that insulin is an effective option in type 2 diabetes, and confirm the value of intensive therapy in retarding microvascular complications.[7]

In order to minimise the dose of insulin required, and any risks it may entail, it has been suggested that insulin therapy in type 2 diabetes should be combined with other measures including oral hypoglycaemic drugs.[8] There has long been debate about the value of combined therapy, but a recent meta-analysis indicated that glycaemic control was better, and insulin requirements lower, in type 2 diabetics who received insulin with a sulphonylurea.[9]

For further discussion of the management of type 2 diabetes mellitus see under Diabetes Mellitus, p.313.

1. Tattersall RB, Scott AR. When to use insulin in the maturity onset diabetic. *Postgrad Med J* 1987; **63:** 859–64.
2. Taylor R. Insulin for the non-insulin dependent? *Br Med J* 1988; **296:** 1015–16.
3. Stern MP. Do non-insulin-dependent diabetes mellitus and cardiovascular disease share common antecedents? *Ann Intern Med* 1996; **124** (suppl): 110–16.
4. Henry RR, Genuth S. Forum one: current recommendations about intensification of metabolic control in non-insulin-dependent diabetes mellitus. *Ann Intern Med* 1996; **124** (suppl): 175–7.
5. United Kingdom Prospective Diabetes Study Group. United Kingdom prospective diabetes study (UKPDS) 13: relative efficacy of randomly allocated diet, sulphonylurea, insulin, or metformin in patients with newly diagnosed non-insulin-dependent diabetes followed for three years. *Br Med J* 1995; **310:** 83–8.
6. Turner R, *et al.* United Kingdom Prospective Diabetes Study 17: a 9-year update of a randomized, controlled trial on the effect of improved metabolic control on complications in non-insulin-dependent diabetes mellitus. *Ann Intern Med* 1996; **124** (suppl): 136–45.
7. UK Prospective Diabetes Study Group. Intensive blood-glucose control with sulphonylureas or insulin compared with conventional treatment and risk of complications in patients with type 2 diabetes (UKPDS 33). *Lancet* 1998; **352:** 837–53.
8. Henry RR. Glucose control and insulin resistance in non-insulin-dependent diabetes mellitus. *Ann Intern Med* 1996; **124** (suppl): 97–103.
9. Johnson JL, *et al.* Efficacy of insulin and sulfonylurea combination therapy in type II diabetes: a meta-analysis of the randomized placebo-controlled trials. *Arch Intern Med* 1996; **156:** 259–64.

Diagnosis and testing. PITUITARY FUNCTION. Insulin-induced hypoglycaemia has been used to provide a stressful stimulus in order to assess hypothalamic-pituitary function. The insulin stress or insulin tolerance test has been used as a standard test for assessment of growth hormone or corticotrophin deficiency. However, it is unpleasant, expensive, and not without risk, and is contra-indicated in patients with angina, heart failure, cerebrovascular disease, or epilepsy; some workers recommend its use only when results of alternative tests are equivocal,[1,2] and it should only be performed in specialist units under strict surveillance.[3]

1. Clayton RN. Diagnosis of adrenal insufficiency. *Br Med J* 1989; **298:** 271–2.
2. Stewart PM, *et al.* A rational approach for assessing the hypothalamic-pituitary-adrenal axis. *Lancet* 1994; **343:** 1208–10.
3. Hindmarsh PC, Swift PGF. An assessment of growth hormone provocation tests. *Arch Dis Child* 1995; **72:** 362–8.

Hyperkalaemia. Insulin promotes the intracellular uptake of potassium. It is therefore used in the management of moderate to severe hyperkalaemia, when it is given with glucose (see p.1149).

Liver disorders. References[1,2] to the use of insulin and glucagon in the treatment of liver disorders based on their reported hepatotrophic effect. However, a small randomised study[3] found no benefit from insulin and glucagon infusions in fulminant hepatic failure.

1. Baker AL, *et al.* A randomized clinical trial of insulin and glucagon infusion for treatment of alcoholic hepatitis: progress report in 50 patients. *Gastroenterology* 1981; **80:** 1410–14.
2. Jaspan JB, *et al.* Insulin and glucagon infusion in the treatment of liver failure. *Arch Intern Med* 1984; **144:** 2075–8.
3. Harrison PM, *et al.* Failure of insulin and glucagon infusion to stimulate liver regeneration in fulminant hepatic failure. *J Hepatol* 1990; **10:** 332–6.

Myocardial infarction. Recent discussions on the effects of insulin with glucose and potassium in the ischaemic heart including its effect in reducing blood free fatty acids have emphasised its potential benefits in left ventricular failure and cardiogenic shock.[1,2] Glucose-insulin-potassium solutions have been investigated in only small numbers of patients with acute myocardial infarction although a meta-analysis of randomised controlled studies performed before the widespread use of thrombolytics found a reduction in mortality in recipients of these solutions and suggests that further investigation of its value in acute myocardial infarction may be warranted.[3] Insulin-glucose infusion followed by multiple daily subcutaneous insulin injections has been reported to reduce mortality in diabetics who suffered a myocardial infarction.[4,5]

For the conventional management of myocardial infarction see p.791.

1. Opie LH. Glucose and the metabolism of ischaemic myocardium. *Lancet* 1995; **345:** 1520–1.
2. Taegtmeyer H, *et al.* Metabolic support for the postischaemic heart. *Lancet* 1995; **345:** 1552–5.
3. Fath-Ordoubadi F, Beatt KJ. Glucose-insulin-potassium therapy for treatment of acute myocardial infarction: an overview of randomized placebo-controlled trials. *Circulation* 1997; **96:** 1152–6.
4. Malmberg K, *et al.* Randomized trial of insulin-glucose infusion followed by subcutaneous insulin treatment in diabetic patients with acute myocardial infarction (DIGAMI Study): effects on mortality at 1 year. *J Am Coll Cardiol* 1995; **26:** 57–65.
5. Malmberg K, *et al.* Prospective randomised study of intensive insulin treatment on long term survival after acute myocardial infarction in patients with diabetes mellitus. *Br Med J* 1997; **314:** 1512–15.

Neonatal hyperglycaemia. Hyperglycaemia is common in very immature neonates, although hypoglycaemia is more common in neonates born to diabetic mothers. Neonatal hyperglycaemia has been treated by glucose restriction until glucose tolerance improves. However, the use of an insulin infusion can allow normal glucose administration to continue.[1] It was suggested that insulin was best administered intravenously in a separate, easily titratable solution because of the frequent fluctuations of requirement in these infants. An alternative approach, namely subcutaneous injection of a long-acting insulin, has been reported to result in less fluctuation of blood-glucose concentrations,[2] and hence easier management.

1. Binder ND, *et al.* Insulin infusion with parenteral nutrition in extremely low birth weight infants with hyperglycemia. *J Pediatr* 1989; **114:** 273–80.
2. Mitamura R, *et al.* Ultralente insulin treatment of transient neonatal diabetes mellitus. *J Pediatr* 1996; **128:** 268–70.

Organ and tissue transplantation. Brief discussion of the possibility that administration of hormones, including insulin, to 'brain-dead' patients could improve the function of donated organs.[1]

1. Darby JM, *et al.* Approach to management of the heartbeating 'brain-dead' organ donor. *JAMA* 1989; **261:** 2222–8.

Preparations

Ph. Eur.: Biphasic Insulin Injection; Biphasic Isophane Insulin Injection; Insulin Injection *(Neutral Insulin; Neutral Insulin Injection; Soluble Insulin)*; Insulin Zinc Suspension *(Insulin Lente; I.Z.S)*; Insulin Zinc Suspension (Amorphous) *(Amorph. I.Z.S.; Insulin Semilente)*; Insulin Zinc Suspension (Crystalline) *(Cryst. I.Z.S.; Insulin Ultralente)*; Isophane Insulin Injection;

USP 23: Extended Insulin Human Zinc Suspension; Extended Insulin Zinc Suspension; Insulin Human Injection; Insulin Human Zinc Suspension; Insulin Injection; Insulin Zinc Suspension; Isophane Insulin Human Suspension; Isophane Insulin Suspension; Prompt Insulin Zinc Suspension.

Proprietary Preparations (details are given in Part 3)

Aust.: Actrapid HM; Depot-Insulin; Humalog; Huminsulin Basal; Huminsulin Long; Huminsulin Normal; Huminsulin Profil I; Huminsulin Ultralong; Insulatard HM; Insulatard†; Insuman Basal; Insuman Infusat; Insuman komb Typ 15; Insuman Rapid; Komb-Insulin; Lente MC; Mixtard 30/70†; Mixtard HM 10/90; Monotard HM; Rapitard MC†; Ultratard HM; Velosulin HM; Velosulin†; ***Austral.:*** Actraphane HM†; Actraphane MC†; Actrapid; Actrapid MC†; Humalog; Humulin 20/80; Humulin L; Humulin NPH; Humulin R; Humulin UL; Hypurin Isophane; Hypurin Neutral; Initard Human†; Insulin 2; Isotard MC; Lente MC; Mixtard 20/80; Monotard HM; Protamine Zinc Insulin MC†; Protaphane HM; Rapitard MC†; Semilente MC†; Ultralente MC; Ultratard HM; ***Belg.:*** Actrapid HM; Humuline 20/80; Humuline Long; Humuline NPH; Humuline Regular; Humuline Ultralong; Initard Humanum†; Insulatard HM; Insulatard-X Humanum†; Lente MC; Mixtard HM; Mixtard-X Humanum†; Monotard HM; Ultralente MC; Ultratard HM; Velosuline Humanum; *Canad.:* Humulin 10/90; Humulin L; Humulin N; Humulin R; Humulin U; Iletin II Pork Lente; Iletin II Pork NPH; Iletin II Pork Regular; Iletin Lente; Iletin NPH; Iletin Regular; Iletin Semilente†; Iletin Ultralente†; Initard 50/50†; Insulatard NPH Human†; Insulatard NPH†; Insulin-Toronto (Regular)†; Lente Insulin†; Mixtard 15/85†; Mixtard 30/70†; Novolin; Novolin Lente; Novolin NPH; Novolin Toronto; Novolin Ultralente; PZI Iletin†; Semilente Insulin†; Ultralente Insulin†; Velosulin (Regular)†; Velosulin Human†; *Fr.:* Actrapid HM; Endopancrine 100; Endopancrine 40; Endopancrine Protamine; Endopancrine Zinc Protamine; Humalog; Insulatard HM†; Insulatard Nordisk†; Insuline NPH†; Insuline Semi Tardum; Insuline Tardum MX; Insuline Ultra Tardum; Insuman Intermediaire 100%; Insuman Intermediaire 25/75; Insuman Rapide; Lente MC; Lillypen Profil; Lillypen Protamine Isophane; Lillypen Rapide; Mixtard HM; Mixtard Novolet; Mixtard†; Monotard HM; Orgasuline 30/70; Orgasuline N.P.H.; Orgasuline Rapide; Rapitard MC; Semilente MC; Ultralente MC; Ultratard HM; Umuline Profil 10; Umuline Protamine Isophane (NPH); Umuline Rapide; Umuline Zinc; Umuline Zinc Compose; Velosuline Humaine†; Velosuline†; *Ger.:* Actraphane HM; Actrapid HM; Basal-H-Insulin; Berlinsulin H 10/90; Berlinsulin H Basal; Berlinsulin H Normal; Depot-H-Insulin; Depot-H15-Insulin; Depot-Insulin; Depot-Insulin Horm†; Depot-Insulin S; H-Insulin; H-Tronin; Humalog; Huminsulin; Huminsulin Basal; Huminsulin Long; Huminsulin Normal; Huminsulin Profil I; Huminsulin Ultralong; Insulatard; Insulatard Human; Komb-H-Insulin; Komb-Insulin; Komb-Insulin S; L-Insulin; Lente†; Mixtard; Mixtard Human; Monotard HM; Protaphan HM; Rapitard; Semilente; Ultralente; Ultratard HM; Velasulin; Velasulin Human; *Irl.:* Actrapid; Humalog; Human Actraphane†; Human Initard 50/50†; Human Protaphane†; Human Velosulin†; Humulin I; Humulin Lente; Humulin M2; Humulin S; Humulin Zn; Insulatard; Insuman 25/75; Insuman Basal; Insuman Rapid; Mixtard 10; Monotard; Neulente†; Neuphane†; Ultratard; Velosulin†; *Ital.:* Actraphane HM; Actrapid HM; Bio-Insulin 10/90; Bio-Insulin I; Bio-Insulin L; Bio-Insulin R; Bio-Insulin U; Humulin 10/90; Humulin I; Humulin L; Humulin R; Humulin U; Lenta MC†; Monotard HM; Protaphane HM; Rapitard MC†; Ultratard HM; *Neth.:* Actrapid; Humaject 10/90; Humaject NPH; Humaject Regular; Humalog; Humuline 10/90; Humuline NPH; Humuline Regular; Humuline Zink†; Insulatard; Isuhuman Basal; Isuhuman Comb 15; Isuhuman Infusat; Isuhuman Rapid; Mixtard 10/90; Monotard; Ultratard; Velosulin; *Norw.:* Actrapid; Humalog; Humulin Mix; Humulin NPH; Humulin Regular; Insulatard; Insulin Basal; Insulin Infusat; Insulin Komb 25/75; Insulin Rapid; Mixtard 10/90; Monotard; Ultratard; Velosulin; *S.Afr.:* Actraphane HM; Actrapid HM; Humalog; Humulin 20/80; Humulin L; Humulin N; Humulin R; Humulin U; Mixtard 10/90; Monotard HM; Protaphane HM; Ultratard HM; *Spain:* Actrapid; Combitard Humana 15/85†; Humaplus 10/90; Humaplus NPH; Humaplus Regular; Humulina; Humulina Lenta; Humulina NPH; Humulina Regular; Humulina Ultralenta; Insulatard; Insulatard Humana†; Insulatard Novolet; Lente MC; Meztardia Humana 50/50†; Mixtard 10; Mixtard 30/70; Monotard; Ultratard; Velosulin Humana†; *Swed.:* Actrapid; Humalog; Humulin Mix 10/90; Humulin NPH; Humulin Regular; Humutard; Insulatard; Isuhuman Basal; Isuhuman Comb 25/75; Isuhuman Infusat; Isuhuman Rapid; Mixtard 10/90; Monotard; Ultratard; Velosulin; *Switz.:* Actraphane HM†; Actrapid HM; Actrapid MC; Humalog; Huminsulin Basal (NPH); Huminsulin Long; Huminsulin Normal; Huminsulin Profil I; Huminsulin Ultralong; Initard Humaine†; Initard†; Insulatard HM; Insulatard MC; Lente MC; Mixtard 30 MC; Mixtard HM; Monotard HM; Rapitard MC; Semilente MC; Ultralente MC; Ultratard HM; Velosulin HM; Velosulin MC; *UK:* Humaject I; Humaject M1; Humaject S; Humalog; Human Actraphane†; Human Actrapid; Human Initard 50/50†; Human Insulatard; Human Mixtard 10; Human Monotard; Human Ultratard; Human Velosulin; Humulin I; Humulin Lente; Humulin M1; Humulin S; Humulin Zn; Hypurin Biphasic 30/70; Hypurin Isophane; Hypurin Lente; Hypurin Neutral; Hypurin Protamine Zinc; Initard 50/50†; Insulatard; Lentard MC; PenMix 10/90†; Pork Mixtard 30; Pur-in Isophane†; Pur-in Mix 15/85†; Pur-in Neutral†; Rapitard MC†; Semitard MC†; Velosulin; *USA:* Humalog; Humulin 70/30; Humulin BR†; Humulin L; Humulin N; Humulin R†; Humulin U Ultralente; Insulatard NPH Human†; Insulatard NPH†; Lente; Lente Iletin I; Lente Iletin II; Lente L; Mixtard Human 70/30†; Mixtard†; Novolin 70/30; Novolin L; Novolin N; Novolin R; NPH Iletin I; NPH Iletin II; Regular Iletin I; Regular Iletin II; Semilente Iletin I†; Semilente†; Ultralente; Ultralente Iletin I†; Ultralente U†; Velosulin Human BR; Velosulin†.

Metformin Hydrochloride (7231-c)

Metformin Hydrochloride *(BANM, USAN, rINNM)*.

LA-6023; La-6023 (metformin); Metformini Hydrochloridum.

1,1-Dimethylbiguanide hydrochloride.

$C_4H_{11}N_5,HCl = 165.6.$

CAS — 657-24-9 (metformin); 1115-70-4 (metformin hydrochloride).

Pharmacopoeias. In Eur. (see p.viii) and Pol.

A white crystalline powder. Freely **soluble** in water; slightly soluble in alcohol; practically insoluble in acetone, and in dichloromethane.

Adverse Effects, Treatment, and Precautions

As for biguanides in general, p.318.

Interactions

As for biguanides in general, p.318.

Pharmacokinetics

Metformin hydrochloride is slowly and incompletely absorbed from the gastro-intestinal tract; the absolute bioavailability of a single 500- mg dose is reported to be about 50 to 60%, although this is reduced somewhat if taken with food. Following absorption plasma protein binding is negligible, and it is excreted unchanged in the urine. The plasma elimination half-life is reported to range from about 2 to 6 hours after oral administration.

References.

1. Scheen AJ. Clinical pharmacokinetics of metformin. *Clin Pharmacokinet* 1996; **30:** 359–71.
2. Sambol NC, *et al.* Pharmacokinetics and pharmacodynamics of metformin in healthy subjects and patients with noninsulin-dependent diabetes mellitus. *J Clin Pharmacol* 1996; **36:** 1012–21.

Uses and Administration

Metformin hydrochloride is a biguanide hypoglycaemic (p.318). It is given by mouth in the treatment of type 2 diabetes mellitus (p.313). Initial dosage is 500 mg two or three times daily or 850 mg once or twice daily with or after meals, gradually increased if necessary to 2 to 3 g daily; doses above 2 g daily are associated with an increased incidence of gastro-intestinal adverse effects.

Metformin is also used as the chlorophenoxyacetate and as the embonate.

General references.

1. Dunn CJ, Peters DH. Metformin: a review of its pharmacological properties and therapeutic use in non-insulin-dependent diabetes mellitus. *Drugs* 1995; **49:** 721–49.
2. Anonymous. Metformin for non-insulin-dependent diabetes mellitus. *Med Lett Drugs Ther* 1995; **37:** 41–2.
3. Bailey CJ, Turner RC. Metformin. *N Engl J Med* 1996; **334:** 574–9.
4. Melchior WR, Jaber LA. Metformin: an antihyperglycemic agent for treatment of type II diabetes. *Ann Pharmacother* 1996; **30:** 158–64.
5. Davidson MB, Peters AL. An overview of metformin in the treatment of type 2 diabetes mellitus. *Am J Med* 1997; **102:** 99–110.
6. Klepser TB, Kelly MW. Metformin hydrochloride: an antihyperglycemic agent. *Am J Health-Syst Pharm* 1997; **54:** 893–903. Correction. *ibid.*; 1335.

Action. A review of the action of metformin[1] suggested that the major action of metformin lay in increasing glucose transport across the cell membrane in skeletal muscle. There is also some evidence *in vitro* that it can inhibit the formation of advanced glycosylation end-products.[2]

1. Klip A, Leiter LA. Cellular mechanism of action of metformin. *Diabetes Care* 1990; **13:** 696–704.
2. Tanaka Y, *et al.* Inhibitory effect of metformin on formation of advanced glycation end products. *Curr Ther Res* 1997; **58:** 693–7.

Polycystic ovary syndrome. It has been suggested that hyperinsulinism may play a pathogenetic role in stimulating the abnormal androgen production from the ovary seen in women with polycystic ovary syndrome (PCO, p.1240). Two small studies have reported an improvement in androgen concentrations concomitant with a decrease in serum insulin following metformin treatment in women with the syndrome.[1,2] However, another study was unable to demonstrate a reduction in either insulin or circulating androgen concentrations when metformin was given.[3] Combination of metformin with clomiphene appears to improve ovulatory response, compared with clomiphene alone, in women with PCO; metformin also increased the rate of spontaneous ovulation.[4]

1. Velazquez EM, *et al.* Metformin therapy in polycystic ovary syndrome reduces hyperinsulinemia, insulin resistance, hyperandrogenemia, and systolic blood pressure, while facilitating normal menses and pregnancy. *Metabolism* 1994; **43:** 647–54.
2. Nestler JE, Jakubowicz DJ. Decreases in ovarian cytochrome P450c17α activity and serum free testosterone after reduction of insulin secretion in polycystic ovary syndrome. *N Engl J Med* 1996; **335:** 617–23.
3. Ehrmann DA, *et al.* Effects of metformin on insulin secretion, insulin action, and ovarian steroidogenesis in women with polycystic ovary syndrome. *J Clin Endocrinol Metab* 1997; **82:** 524–30.
4. Nestler JE, *et al.* Effects of metformin on spontaneous and clomiphene-induced ovulation in the polycystic ovary syndrome. *N Engl J Med* 1998; **338:** 1876–80.

Preparations

BP 1998: Metformin Tablets.

Proprietary Preparations (details are given in Part 3)
Aust.: Diabetex; Glucophage; Orabet; *Austral.:* Diabex; Diaformin; Glucophage; *Belg.:* Glucophage; *Canad.:* Glucophage; *Fr.:* Glucinan; Glucophage; Stagid; *Ger.:* Diabetase; Glucophage S; Mediabet; Meglucon; Mescorit; Siofor; *Irl.:* Glucophage; *Ital.:* Devian†; Diaberit†; Diabetosan†; Glucophage; Metforal; Metiguanide; *Neth.:* Glucophage; *Norw.:* Glucophage; *S.Afr.:* Dextin; Glucophage; *Spain:* Glucophage; *Swed.:* Glucophage; *Switz.:* Glucophage; *UK:* Glucamet; Glucophage; Orabet; *USA:* Glucophage.

Multi-ingredient: *Ital.:* Bi-Euglucon M; Bidiamet†; Diabomet†; Glibomet; Glucomide; Glucosulfa; Pleiamide; Suguan M; *Switz.:* Diabiformine.

Midaglizole (3694-z)

Midaglizole *(rINN)*.

DG-5128. (±)-2-[α-(2-Imidazolin-2-ylmethyl)benzyl]pyridine.

$C_{16}H_{17}N_3 = 251.3.$

CAS — 66529-17-7.

Midaglizole is under investigation as a hypoglycaemic. A proposed mode of action is stimulation of insulin secretion by antagonism of alpha$_2$-adrenoceptors. Midaglizole has also been investigated as a bronchodilator in asthma.

References.

1. Kawazu S, *et al.* Initial phase II clinical studies on midaglizole (DG-5128). *Diabetes* 1987; **36:** 221–6.
2. Yoshie Y, *et al.* The inhibitory effect of a selective α$_2$-adrenergic receptor antagonist on moderate- to severe-type asthma. *J Allergy Clin Immunol* 1989; **84:** 747–52.

Pharmacokinetics. A series of studies on the pharmacokinetics of midaglizole.[1] Peak plasma concentrations were achieved about one hour after single oral doses. Metabolites with hypoglycaemic activity were detected, but amounts appeared negligible. The elimination half-life in plasma was 2.5 to 2.9 hours and protein binding ranged from 54 to 69%. Midaglizole was excreted predominantly in the urine, but with a significant amount excreted in the faeces. No significant accumulation of midaglizole was detected after multiple dosing.

1. Nomura H, *et al.* Pharmacokinetics of midaglizole, a new hypoglycaemic agent in healthy subjects. *Biopharm Drug Dispos* 1990; **11:** 701–13.

Miglitol (18829-n)

Miglitol *(BAN, USAN, pINN)*.

Bay-m-1099. (2R,3R,4R,5S)-1-(2-Hydroxyethyl)-2-(hydroxymethyl)piperidine-3,4,5-triol.

$C_8H_{17}NO_5 = 207.2.$

CAS — 72432-03-2.

Miglitol is an alpha-glucosidase inhibitor similar in action to acarbose (p.317). It is given by mouth in the management of type 2 diabetes mellitus (p.313), alone or in combination with a sulphonylurea. Usual initial doses are 25 mg three times daily with meals, increased if necessary to a maximum of 100 mg three times daily.

References.

1. Katsilambros N, *et al.* A double-blind study on the efficacy and tolerance of a new α-glucosidase inhibitor in type-2 diabetics. *Arzneimittelforschung* 1986; **36:** 1136–8.
2. Kennedy FP, Gerich JE. A new alpha-glucosidase inhibitor (Bay-m-1099) reduces insulin requirements with meals in insulin dependent diabetes mellitus. *Clin Pharmacol Ther* 1987; **42:** 455–8.
3. Heinz G, *et al.* Reduction of postprandial blood glucose by the α-glucosidase inhibitor miglitol (BAY m 1099) in type II diabetes. *Eur J Clin Pharmacol* 1989; **37:** 33–6.
4. Dimitriadis G, *et al.* Effects of α-glucosidase inhibition on meal glucose tolerance and timing of insulin administration in patients with type I diabetes mellitus. *Diabetes Care* 1991; **14:** 393–8.
5. Lembcke B, *et al.* Inhibition of glycemic and hormonal responses after repetitive sucrose and starch loads by different doses of the α-glucosidase inhibitor miglitol (BAY m 1099) in man. *Pharmacology* 1991; **43:** 318–28.
6. Johnston PS, *et al.* Effects of the carbohydrase inhibitor miglitol in sulfonylurea-treated NIDDM patients. *Diabetes Care* 1994; **17:** 20–9.
7. Escobar-Jiménez F, *et al.* Efficacy and tolerability of miglitol in the treatment of patients with non-insulin-dependent diabetes mellitus. *Curr Ther Res* 1995; **56:** 258–68.

Preparations

Proprietary Preparations (details are given in Part 3)
USA: Glyset.

Phenformin Hydrochloride (7232-k)

Phenformin Hydrochloride *(BANM, pINNM)*.

Fenformina Cloridrato. 1-Phenethylbiguanide hydrochloride.

$C_{10}H_{15}N_5,HCl = 241.7.$

CAS — 114-86-3 (phenformin); 834-28-6 (phenformin hydrochloride).

Pharmacopoeias. In Chin.

Phenformin hydrochloride is a biguanide hypoglycaemic (p.318). Although it is generally considered to be associated with an unacceptably high incidence of lactic acidosis, often fatal, it is still available in some countries for the treatment by mouth of type 2 diabetes mellitus.

Phenformin was implicated in the controversial reports of excess cardiovascular mortality associated with oral hypoglycaemic therapy (see under Sulphonylureas, Effects on the Cardiovascular System, p.331).

Preparations

Proprietary Preparations (details are given in Part 3)

Multi-ingredient: ***Ital.:*** Bi-Euglucon; Bidiabe; Gliben F; Gliformin; Suguan; ***Spain:*** Diabis Activado†.

Pimagedine (17309-z)

Pimagedine *(rINN)*.

GER-11 (pimagedine hydrochloride). Aminoguanidine.

CH_6N_4 = 74.09.

CAS — 79-17-4.

NOTE. Pimagedine Hydrochloride is *USAN*.

Pimagedine reportedly inhibits the formation of glycosylated proteins (advanced glycosylation end-products) and has other actions including inhibition of aldose reductase. It is under investigation for the prevention of diabetic complications (p.315).

References.

1. Corbett JA, *et al.* Aminoguanidine, a novel inhibitor of nitric oxide formation, prevents diabetic vascular dysfunction. *Diabetes* 1992; **41:** 552–6.
2. Wolffenbuttel BHR, Huijberts MSP. Aminoguanidine, a potential drug for the treatment of diabetic complications. *Neth J Med* 1993; **42:** 205–8.

Pioglitazone Hydrochloride (10380-l)

Pioglitazone Hydrochloride *(USAN, rINNM)*.

AD-4833 (pioglitazone); U-72107A (hydrochloride); U-72107E (pioglitazone). (±)-5-{*p*-[2-(5-Ethyl-2-pyridyl)ethoxy]benzyl}-2,4-thiazolidinedione hydrochloride.

$C_{19}H_{20}N_2O_3S,HCl$ = 392.9.

CAS — 111025-46-8 (pioglitazone); 112529-15-4 (pioglitazone hydrochloride).

Pioglitazone is a thiazolidinedione oral hypoglycaemic similar to troglitazone (p.334). It has been tried in the management of type 2 diabetes mellitus (p.313).

Pramlintide (15583-k)

Pramlintide *(rINN)*.

AC-137; Pramlintida.

CAS — 151126-32-8.

Pramlintide is an analogue of amylin, a pancreatic peptide thought to play a role in the regulation of glucose homoeostasis. Pramlintide is under investigation in the management of diabetes mellitus (p.313).

References.

1. Thompson RG, *et al.* The human amylin analogue (AC137) reduces glucose following Sustacol (Rm) in patients with type II diabetes. *Diabetes* 1995; **44** (suppl 1): 127A.
2. Kolterman OG, *et al.* Reduction of postprandial hyperglycemia in subjects with IDDM by intravenous infusion of AC137, a human amylin analogue. *Diabetes Care* 1995; **18:** 1179–82.
3. Thompson RG, *et al.* Pramlintide: a human amylin analogue reduced postprandial plasma glucose, insulin, and C-peptide concentrations in patients with type 2 diabetes. *Diabetic Med* 1997; **14:** 547–55.
4. Thompson RG, *et al.* Effects of pramlintide, an analog of human amylin, on plasma glucose profiles in patients with IDDM: results of a multicenter trial. *Diabetes* 1997; **46:** 632–6.

Repaglinide (15410-t)

Repaglinide *(BAN, rINN)*.

AG-EE-6232W; AG-EE-623-ZW. (+)-2-Ethoxy-α-{[(*S*)-α-isobutyl-*o*-piperidinobenzyl]carbamoyl}-*p*-toluic acid; (*S*)-2-Ethoxy-4-{[1-(*o*-piperidinophenyl)-3-methylbutyl]carbamoylmethyl}benzoic acid.

$C_{27}H_{36}N_2O_4$ = 452.6.

CAS — 135062-02-1.

Repaglinide is a hypoglycaemic used for the treatment of type 2 diabetes mellitus (p.313). It has a chemical structure different from that of the sulphonylureas, but appears to have a similar mode of action.

Repaglinide is given by mouth up to 30 minutes before meals, in usual initial doses of 0.5 to 2 mg; initial doses of 1 mg or more are usually given to patients who have had previous hypoglycaemic treatment. The dose may be adjusted, at intervals of 1 to 2 weeks, up to a maximum of 4 mg before meals; a total of 16 mg daily should not be exceeded. Repaglinide is also given in combination with metformin in type 2 diabetes not adequately controlled by metformin alone.

Adverse effects appear to be similar to those of the sulphonylureas (p.331).

References.

1. Wolfenbuttel BHR, *et al.* Effects of a new oral hypoglycaemic agent, repaglinide, on metabolic control in sulphonylurea-treated patients with NIDDM. *Eur J Clin Pharmacol* 1993; **45:** 113–16.
2. Anonymous. Repaglinide for type 2 diabetes mellitus. *Med Lett Drugs Ther* 1998; **40:** 55–6.

Preparations

Proprietary Preparations (details are given in Part 3)

UK: Novonorm; ***USA:*** Prandin.

Rosiglitazone (10913-h)

Rosiglitazone *(rINN)*.

(±)-5-{*p*-[2-(Methyl-2-pyridylamino)ethoxy]benzyl}-2,4-thiazolidinedione.

$C_{18}H_{19}N_3O_3S$ = 357.4.

Rosiglitazone is a thiazolidinedione oral hypoglycaemic under investigation for the treatment of type 2 diabetes mellitus.

Sorbinil (16992-t)

Sorbinil *(BAN, USAN, rINN)*.

CP-45634. (*S*)-6-Fluorospiro(chroman-4,4′-imidazolidine)-2′,5′-dione.

$C_{11}H_9FN_2O_3$ = 236.2.

CAS — 68367-52-2.

Sorbinil is an aldose reductase inhibitor similar in action to tolrestat (p.333). It was tried mainly in the treatment of diabetic neuropathy, with conflicting results, and development appears to have been discontinued.

Severe skin reactions have been reported.

References.

1. Masson EA, Boulton AJM. Aldose reductase inhibitors in the treatment of diabetic neuropathy: a review of the rationale and clinical experience. *Drugs* 1990; **39:** 190–202.
2. Zenon GJ, *et al.* Potential use of aldose reductase inhibitors to prevent diabetic complications. *Clin Pharm* 1990; **9:** 446–57.
3. Dyck PJ, *et al.* Nerve glucose, fructose, sorbitol, myo-inositol, and fiber degeneration and regeneration in diabetic neuropathy. *N Engl J Med* 1988; **319:** 542–8.
4. Sima AAF, *et al.* Regeneration and repair of myelinated fibers in aural-nerve biopsy specimens from patients with diabetic neuropathy treated with sorbinil. *N Engl J Med* 1988; **319:** 548–55.
5. Asbury AK. Understanding diabetic neuropathy. *N Engl J Med* 1988; **319:** 577–8.

Sulphonylurea Antidiabetics

(17475-g)

NOTE. Sulphonylurea antidiabetics in this chapter are: Acetohexamide (p.318); Carbutamide (p.319); Chlorpropamide (p.319); Glibenclamide (p.319); Glibornuride (p.320); Gliclazide (p.320); Glimepiride (p.320); Glipizide (p.320); Gliquidone (p.321); Glisentide (p.321); Glisolamide (p.321); Glisoxepide (p.321); Glyclopyramide (p.321); Glycyclamide (p.321); Tolazamide (p.333); Tolbutamide (p.333).

Adverse Effects

Gastro-intestinal disturbances such as nausea, vomiting, heartburn, anorexia, diarrhoea, and a metallic taste may occur with sulphonylureas and are usually mild and dose-dependent; increased appetite and weight gain may occur. Skin rashes and pruritus may occur and photosensitivity has been reported. Rashes are usually hypersensitivity reactions and may progress to more serious disorders (see below). Facial flushing may develop in patients receiving sulphonylureas, particularly chlorpropamide, when alcohol is imbibed (see under Interactions, below).

Hypoglycaemia may occur 4 or more hours after food; this is usually an indication of overdosage and is relatively uncommon. Hypoglycaemia is more likely with long-acting sulphonylureas such as chlorpropamide, which has been associated with severe, prolonged, and sometimes fatal hypoglycaemia.

Other severe effects may be manifestations of a hypersensitivity reaction. They include cholestatic jaundice, leucopenia, thrombocytopenia, aplastic anaemia, agranulocytosis, haemolytic anaemia, erythema multiforme or the Stevens-Johnson syndrome, exfoliative dermatitis, and erythema nodosum.

The sulphonylureas, particularly chlorpropamide, occasionally induce a syndrome of inappropriate secretion of antidiuretic hormone (SIADH) characterised by water retention, hyponatraemia, and CNS effects. However, some sulphonylureas, such as glibenclamide, glipizide, and tolazamide are also stated to have mild diuretic actions.

Work on tolbutamide has suggested that the sulphonylureas might be associated with an increase in cardiovascular mortality; this has been the subject of considerable debate (see Effects on the Cardiovascular System, below).

A review of the adverse effects and precautions of sulphonylurea drugs.[1]

1. Paice BJ, *et al.* Undesired effects of the sulphonylurea drugs. *Adverse Drug React Acute Poisoning Rev* 1985; **4:** 23–36.

Effects on the cardiovascular system. A multicentre study carried out under the University Group Diabetes Program (UGDP) reported an increased incidence in mortality from cardiovascular complications in diabetic patients given tolbutamide as compared with those treated with diet alone or insulin;[1] a similar increase was also noted in patients given phenformin.[2] The reports from the UGDP aroused prolonged controversy which was not entirely settled by detailed reassessment of relevant studies.[3] Eventually in 1984 the FDA made it a requirement that sulphonylurea oral hypoglycaemics be labelled with a specific warning about the possibility of increased cardiovascular mortality associated with the use of these drugs.[4] Subsequently the cardiovascular effects of the sulphonylureas were reviewed by Huupponen.[5] More recently it has been hypothesised that the action of the sulphonylureas in preventing the opening of ATP-sensitive potassium channels in the myocardium may abolish adaptive changes (ischaemic preconditioning) that protect the heart against ischaemic insult.[6] However, results from the UK Prospective Diabetes Study did not demonstrate any adverse cardiovascular effects associated with sulphonylurea therapy.[7]

1. University Group Diabetes Program. Effects of hypoglycemic agents on vascular complications in patients with adult-onset diabetes III: clinical implications of UGDP results. *JAMA* 1971; **218:** 1400–10.
2. University Group Diabetes Program. Effects of hypoglycemic agents on vascular complications in patients with adult-onset diabetes IV: a preliminary report on phenformin results. *JAMA* 1971; **217:** 777–84.
3. Report of the Committee for the Assessment of Biometric Aspects of Controlled Trials of Hypoglycemic Agents. *JAMA* 1975; **231:** 583–600.
4. FDA. Class labeling for oral hypoglycemics. *FDA Drug Bull* 1984; **14:** 16–17.
5. Huupponen R. Adverse cardiovascular effects of sulphonylurea drugs: clinical significance. *Med Toxicol* 1987; **2:** 190–209.
6. Yellon DM, *et al.* Angina reassessed: pain or protector? *Lancet* 1996; **347:** 1159–62.
7. UK Prospective Diabetes Study (UKPDS) Group. Intensive blood-glucose control with sulphonylureas or insulin compared with conventional treatment and risk of complications in patients with type 2 diabetes (UKPDS 33). *Lancet* 1998; **352:** 837–53.

Effects on the eyes. When a diabetic patient who had experienced bilateral visual loss for several months and who had been taking chlorpropamide for one year stopped treatment, visual acuity improved and colour vision rapidly returned.[1] A 5-day challenge with chlorpropamide resulted in a mild decrease in acuity followed by return to base-line values when treatment was again stopped. Drug-induced optic neuropathy was considered to have occurred. There is also a report of a patient with type 2 diabetes mellitus who developed myopia two days after starting treatment with glibenclamide 10 mg daily.[2] Visual difficulties resolved a few days after stopping glibenclamide.

1. Wymore J, Carter JE. Chlorpropamide-induced optic neuropathy. *Arch Intern Med* 1982; **142:** 381.
2. Teller J, *et al.* Accommodation insufficiency induced by glybenclamide. *Ann Ophthalmol* 1989; **21:** 275–6.

Effects on the kidneys. A report in one patient of the nephrotic syndrome in association with chlorpropamide therapy.[1] Serological testing and renal biopsy demonstrated that the glomerular lesions were of an immune-complex nature. Both the nephrotic syndrome and the glomerulonephritis resolved after treatment was stopped. The patient also developed a skin eruption, hepatitis, and eosinophilia.

1. Appel GB, *et al.* Nephrotic syndrome and immune complex glomerulonephritis associated with chlorpropamide therapy. *Am J Med* 1983; **74:** 337–42.

Effects on the liver. A review of the patients admitted with drug-induced acute liver disease to a hospital in Jamaica over the years 1973 to 1988.[1] Chlorpropamide was implicated in 8 of the 53 cases. Hepatocanalicular cholestasis occurred in 5 and diffuse necrosis in 3 of these 8. One patient with massive hepatic necrosis died. Intrahepatic cholestasis,[2] and an acute hepatitis-like syndrome[3] have been described in patients receiving glibenclamide.

1. Lee MG, *et al.* Drug-induced acute liver disease. *Postgrad Med J* 1989; **65:** 367–70.

2. Wongpaitoon V, *et al.* Intrahepatic cholestasis and cutaneous bullae associated with glibenclamide therapy. *Postgrad Med J* 1981; **57:** 244–6.
3. Goodman RC, *et al.* Glyburide-induced hepatitis. *Ann Intern Med* 1987; **106:** 837–9.

Effects on the thyroid. See under Precautions, below.

Hypoglycaemia. Severe hypoglycaemia may occur in any patient treated with any sulphonylurea; this potentially life-threatening complication requires prolonged and energetic treatment.[1] Sulphonylureas with a prolonged duration of action such as chlorpropamide and glibenclamide appear to cause severe hypoglycaemia more often than shorter-acting drugs such as tolbutamide. Experience with newer drugs is limited.

A review of 1418 cases of drug-induced hypoglycaemia reported since 1940 has shown that sulphonylureas (especially chlorpropamide and glibenclamide), either alone or with a second hypoglycaemic or potentiating agent, account for 63% of all cases.[2] Another analysis,[3] of 185 children reported to 10 regional poison centres in the USA after ingesting sulphonylureas found that hypoglycaemia developed only in 56. A lack of hypoglycaemia during the first 8 hours after ingestion was predictive of a benign outcome, and it was recommended that suspected cases be observed for 8 hours with frequent blood glucose monitoring. Children who developed signs of hypoglycaemia, or in whom blood glucose fell below 3.3 mmol per litre could be given intravenous glucose if necessary.

See also under Abuse, below.

1. Ferner RE, Neil HAW. Sulphonylureas and hypoglycaemia. *Br Med J* 1988; **296:** 949–50.
2. Seltzer HS. Drug-induced hypoglycaemia. *Endocrinol Metab Clin North Am* 1989; **18:** 163–83.
3. Spiller HA, *et al.* Prospective multicenter study of sulfonylurea ingestion in children. *J Pediatr* 1997; **131:** 141–6.

Treatment of Adverse Effects

In acute poisoning the stomach should be emptied. Hypoglycaemia should be treated with urgency; the general management of hypoglycaemia is described under insulin (see p.323). The patient should be observed over several days in case hypoglycaemia recurs.

Studies *in vitro*[1] and in healthy subjects[2,3] have suggested that activated charcoal may be of benefit in acute poisoning with sulphonylureas.

1. Kannisto H, Neuvonen PJ. Adsorption of sulfonylureas onto activated charcoal in vitro. *J Pharm Sci* 1984; **73:** 253–6.
2. Neuvonen PH, Kärkkäinen S. Effects of charcoal, sodium bicarbonate, and ammonium chloride on chlorpropamide kinetics. *Clin Pharmacol Ther* 1983; **33:** 386–93.
3. Neuvonen PJ, *et al.* Effect of activated charcoal on absorption of tolbutamide and valproate in man. *Eur J Clin Pharmacol* 1983; **24:** 243–6.

Precautions

Sulphonylureas should not be used in type 1 diabetes mellitus. Use in type 2 diabetes mellitus is contra-indicated in patients with ketoacidosis and in those with severe infection, stress, trauma, or other severe conditions where the sulphonylurea is unlikely to control the hyperglycaemia; insulin should be administered in such situations.

Insulin is also preferred for the treatment of pregnant patients. Some sulphonylureas are excreted in breast milk and the class of drugs should be avoided during breast feeding.

Sulphonylureas with a long half-life such as chlorpropamide or glibenclamide are associated with an increased risk of hypoglycaemia. They should therefore be avoided in patients with impairment of renal or hepatic function, and a similar precaution would tend to apply in other groups with an increased susceptibility to this effect, such as the elderly, debilitated or malnourished patients, and those with adrenal or pituitary insufficiency. As with all diabetics changes in diet or prolonged exercise may also provoke hypoglycaemia. Where a sulphonylurea needs to be used in patients at increased risk of hypoglycaemia, a short-acting drug such as tolbutamide, gliquidone, or gliclazide may be preferred; these three sulphonylureas, being principally inactivated in the liver, are perhaps particularly suitable in renal impairment, although careful monitoring of blood-sugar concentration is essential.

Abuse. A report of severe hypoglycaemia, at first thought to be due to insulinoma but later found to be due to nesidioblastosis [proliferation of the islet cells], in a woman covertly taking chlorpropamide.[1]

1. Rayman G, *et al.* Hyperinsulinaemic hypoglycaemia due to chlorpropamide-induced nesidioblastosis. *J Clin Pathol* 1984; **37:** 651–4.

Administration. It has been suggested that continuously high plasma concentrations of sulphonylureas may lead to the development of tolerance, and that therefore the maximum recommended doses should be reduced.[1]

1. Melander A, *et al.* Is there a concentration-effect relationship for sulphonylureas? *Clin Pharmacokinet* 1998; **34:** 181–8.

Driving. Patients with diabetes mellitus are required to declare their condition to the UK vehicle licensing centre who then assess their fitness to drive. The law treats hypoglycaemic episodes as being under the influence of a drug and patients using insulin are generally not permitted to drive vocationally. Driving is not permitted when hypoglycaemic awareness has been lost. Drivers should normally check their blood glucose concentration before setting out, and, on long journeys, at intervals of about 2 hours. If hypoglycaemia occurs, the driver should stop until recovery is complete.

Vocational drivers needing oral hypoglycaemic drugs have a difficult problem especially if they are on rotating shifts, if the amount of physical exercise varies greatly, or if they change jobs frequently.[1] If they are to be allowed to drive they should be taking a biguanide or a short-acting sulphonylurea.

1. Raffle PAB. Drugs and driving. *Prescribers' J* 1981; **21:** 197–204.

Thyroid disorders. There are conflicting reports concerning the effects of sulphonylureas on thyroid function, with some studies suggesting an increased incidence of thyroid dysfunction in patients treated with tolbutamide or chlorpropamide,[1] while other suggest no antithyroid action.[2,3] Some manufacturers consequently recommend that chlorpropamide be avoided in patients with severe impairment of thyroid function. Changes in thyroid function may conversely affect glycaemic control—for mention of the possible effects of thyroid hormones on sulphonylurea requirements see under Interactions, below.

1. Hunton RB, *et al.* Hypothyroidism in diabetics treated with sulphonylurea. *Lancet* 1965; **ii:** 449–51.
2. Burke G, *et al.* Effect of long-term sulfonylurea therapy on thyroid function in man. *Metabolism* 1967; **16:** 651–7.
3. Feely J, *et al.* Antithyroid effect of chlorpropamide? *Hum Toxicol* 1983; **2:** 149–53.

Interactions

Numerous interactions have been reported with the sulphonylureas, largely representing either pharmacokinetic interactions (due to the displacement of the antidiabetic from plasma proteins or alteration in its metabolism or excretion) or pharmacological interactions with drugs having an independent effect on blood sugar. In the former class most reports concern older sulphonylureas such as chlorpropamide and tolbutamide, although the possibility of such reactions with newer should be borne in mind.

A diminished hypoglycaemic effect, possibly requiring an increased dose of sulphonylurea, has been seen or might be expected on theoretical grounds with adrenaline, aminoglutethimide, chlorpromazine, corticosteroids, diazoxide, oral contraceptives, rifamycins, and thiazide diuretics.

An increased hypoglycaemic effect has occurred or might be expected with ACE inhibitors, alcohol, allopurinol, some analgesics (notably azapropazone, phenylbutazone, and the salicylates), azole antifungals (fluconazole, ketoconazole, and miconazole), chloramphenicol, cimetidine, clofibrate and related compounds, coumarin anticoagulants, halofenate, heparin, MAOIs, octreotide (although this may also produce hyperglycaemia), ranitidine, sulphinpyrazone, sulphonamides (including co-trimoxazole), tetracyclines, tricyclic antidepressants, and thyroid hormones.

Beta blockers have been reported both to increase hypoglycaemia and to mask the typical sympathetic warning signs. There are sporadic and conflicting reports of a possible interaction with calcium-channel blockers, but overall any effect seems to be of little clinical significance.

In addition to producing hypoglycaemia alcohol can interact with chlorpropamide to produce an unpleasant flushing reaction. Such an effect is rare with other sulphonylureas and alcohol.

General references.

1. O'Byrne S, Feely J. Effects of drugs on glucose tolerance in non-insulin-dependent diabetics (part I). *Drugs* 1990; **40:** 6–18.
2. O'Byrne S, Feely J. Effects of drugs on glucose tolerance in non-insulin-dependent diabetics (part II). *Drugs* 1990; **40:** 203–19.
3. Girardin E, *et al.* Hypoglycémies induites par les sulfamides hypoglycémiants. *Ann Med Interne (Paris)* 1992; **143:** 11–17.

ACE inhibitors. There are sporadic reports of marked hypoglycaemia developing in patients taking a sulphonylurea who are given an ACE inhibitor (mainly captopril or enalapril).[1-4] However, studies in diabetic patients have failed to find much evidence of a problem,[5-7] suggesting that the incidence of such a reaction is low.

1. Rett K, *et al.* Hypoglycemia in hypertensive diabetic patients treated with sulfonylureas, biguanides, and captopril. *N Engl J Med* 1988; **319:** 1609.
2. Arauz-Pacheco C, *et al.* Hypoglycemia induced by angiotensin-converting enzyme inhibitors in patients with non-insulin-dependent diabetes receiving sulfonylurea therapy. *Am J Med* 1990; **89:** 811–13.
3. McMurray J, Fraser DM. Captopril, enalapril, and blood glucose. *Lancet* 1986; **i:** 1035.
4. Girardin E, *et al.* Hypoglycémies induites par les sulfamides hypoglycémiants. *Ann Med Interne (Paris)* 1992; **143:** 11–17.
5. Ferriere M, *et al.* Captopril and insulin sensitivity. *Ann Intern Med* 1985; **102:** 134–5.
6. Passa P, *et al.* Enalapril, captopril, and blood glucose. *Lancet* 1986; **i:** 1447.
7. Winocour P, *et al.* Captopril and blood glucose. *Lancet* 1986; **ii:** 461.

Alcohol. Sulphonylurea-induced alcohol intolerance is seen mainly but not exclusively with chlorpropamide; this is similar to the disulfiram-alcohol interaction, although it is not clear whether the mechanism is the same. Since the main symptom of the reaction (facial flushing) appears to occur more commonly in diabetic than non-diabetic subjects, it has been proposed that this symptom could be used as a diagnostic test for a certain subset of patients with type 2 diabetes mellitus.[1,2] However, some have not considered the test to be sufficiently specific[3-6] and despite a great deal having been published on the chlorpropamide-alcohol flushing test (CPAF), its value remains poorly defined. Alcohol, as well as provoking a flushing reaction with chlorpropamide, has been reported both to increase and to decrease the half-life of tolbutamide depending on whether the alcohol administration was acute or chronic.[7] Alcohol may also have a variable effect of its own on blood-glucose concentrations; there is a general tendency to increased hypoglycaemia when alcohol and sulphonylureas are taken concurrently.[6]

1. Leslie RDG, Pyke DA. Chlorpropamide-alcohol flushing: a dominantly inherited trait associated with diabetes. *Br Med J* 1978; **2:** 1519–21.
2. Pyke DA, Leslie RDG. Chlorpropamide-alcohol flushing: a definition of its relation to non-insulin-dependent diabetes. *Br Med J* 1978; **2:** 1521–2.
3. de Silva NE, *et al.* Low incidence of chlorpropamide-alcohol flushing in diet-treated, non-insulin-dependent diabetes. *Lancet* 1981; **i:** 128–31.
4. Fui SNT, *et al.* Epidemiological study of prevalence of chlorpropamide alcohol flushing in insulin dependent diabetes, non-insulin dependent diabetics, and non-diabetics. *Br Med J* 1983; **287:** 1509–12.
5. Fui SNT, *et al.* Test for chlorpropamide-alcohol flush becomes positive after prolonged chlorpropamide treatment in insulin-dependent and non-insulin-dependent diabetics. *N Engl J Med* 1983; **309:** 93–6.
6. Lao B, *et al.* Alcohol tolerance in patients with non-insulin-dependent (type 2) diabetes treated with sulphonylurea derivatives. *Arzneimittelforschung* 1994; **44:** 727–34.
7. Sellers EM, Holloway MR. Drug kinetics and alcohol ingestion. *Clin Pharmacokinet* 1978; **3:** 440–52.

Analgesics. Phenylbutazone[1,2] and related drugs such as azapropazone[3] have been associated with acute hypoglycaemic episodes when given to patients receiving sulphonylureas (in most reports, tolbutamide). Other analgesics may enhance the hypoglycaemic effect of sulphonylureas, including indobufen,[4] fenclofenac,[5] and the salicylates.[6,7]

1. Tannenbaum H, *et al.* Phenylbutazone-tolbutamide drug interaction. *N Engl J Med* 1974; **290:** 344.
2. Dent LA, Jue SG. Tolbutamide-phenylbutazone interaction. *Drug Intell Clin Pharm* 1976; **10:** 711.
3. Andreasen PB, *et al.* Hypoglycaemia induced by azapropazone-tolbutamide interaction. *Br J Clin Pharmacol* 1981; **12:** 581–3.
4. Elvander-Ståhl E, *et al.* Indobufen interacts with the sulphonylurea, glipizide, but not with the β-adrenergic receptor antagonists, propranolol and atenolol. *Br J Clin Pharmacol* 1984; **18:** 773–8.
5. Allen PA, Taylor RT. Fenclofenac and thyroid function tests. *Br Med J* 1980; **281:** 1642.
6. Richardson T, *et al.* Enhancement by sodium salicylate of the blood glucose lowering effect of chlorpropamide—drug interaction or summation of similar effects? *Br J Clin Pharmacol* 1986; **22:** 43–8.
7. Kubacka RT, *et al.* Effects of aspirin and ibuprofen on the pharmacokinetics and pharmacodynamics of glyburide in healthy subjects. *Ann Pharmacother* 1996; **30:** 20–6.

Antibacterials. Chloramphenicol markedly inhibits the metabolism of tolbutamide and increases its half-life,[1] which can result in hypoglycaemia. Sulphonamides,[2] including co-trimoxazole,[3,4] may also enhance the hypoglycaemic effects of the sulphonylureas, while rifampicin (and probably other rifamycins) can enhance the metabolism and decrease the effect of tolbutamide and chlorpropamide,[5,6] and dosage of the hypoglycaemic drug may need to be increased.

1. Christensen LK, Skovsted L. Inhibition of drug metabolism by chloramphenicol. *Lancet* 1969; **ii:** 1397–9.
2. Soeldner JS, Steinke J. Hypoglycemia in tolbutamide-treated diabetes: report of two cases with measurement of serum insulin. *JAMA* 1965; **193:** 148–9.
3. Wing LMH, Miners JO. Cotrimoxazole as an inhibitor of oxidative drug metabolism: effects of trimethoprim and sulphamethoxazole separately and combined on tolbutamide disposition. *Br J Clin Pharmacol* 1985; **20:** 482–5.
4. Johnson JF, Dobmeier ME. Symptomatic hypoglycemia secondary to a glipizide-trimethoprim/sulfamethoxazole drug interaction. *DICP Ann Pharmacother* 1990; **24:** 250–1.
5. Syvälahti EKG, *et al.* Rifampicin and drug metabolism. *Lancet* 1974; **ii:** 232–3.
6. Self TH, Morris T. Interaction of rifampin and chlorpropamide. *Chest* 1980; **77:** 800–1.

Anticoagulants. Dicoumarol increases serum concentrations and therefore the hypoglycaemic effects of tolbutamide, and possibly chlorpropamide. In addition, sulphonylureas may affect anticoagulant function (p.967).

Antiepileptics. For references to phenytoin toxicity when tolbutamide or tolazamide were given concurrently, see under Phenytoin p.355.

Antifungals. Increased plasma concentrations of tolbutamide have been reported when fluconazole was given concomitantly,[1] but there was no evidence of hypoglycaemia, and no hypoglycaemic symptoms were seen in 29 women receiving gliclazide or glibenclamide who were given fluconazole or clotrimazole for vulvovaginitis.[2] However, there are reports of hypoglycaemia in a patient who took fluconazole with glipizide,[3] and similar interactions have been reported for ketoconazole (with tolbutamide, in healthy subjects),[4] and miconazole (with tolbutamide, in a diabetic),[5] suggesting that such combinations should be regarded with caution.

1. Lazar JD, Wilner DK. Drug interactions with fluconazole. *Rev Infect Dis* 1990; **12** (suppl 3): S327–S333.
2. Rowe BR, *et al.* Safety of fluconazole in women taking oral hypoglycaemic agents. *Lancet* 1992; **339:** 255–6.
3. Fournier JP, *et al.* Coma hypoglycémique chez une patiente traitée par glipizide et fluconazole: une possible interaction? *Therapie* 1992; **47:** 446–7.
4. Krishnaiah YSR, *et al.* Interaction between tolbutamide and ketoconazole in healthy subjects. *Br J Clin Pharmacol* 1994; **37:** 205–7.
5. Meurice JC, *et al.* Interaction miconazole et sulfamides hypoglycémiants. *Presse Med* 1983; **12:** 1670.

Metformin. Results apparently suggesting increased mortality in patients who received intensive drug therapy with metformin in combination with a sulphonylurea were reported by the UK Prospective Diabetes Study.[1] This was considered to be artefactual, since it was not confirmed by epidemiological analysis, but some concern remains and further study is needed.

1. UK Prospective Diabetes Study Group. Effect of intensive blood-glucose control with metformin on complications in overweight patients with type 2 diabetes (UKPDS 34). *Lancet* 1998; **352:** 854–65.

Thyroid hormones. It has been suggested that initiation of thyroid replacement therapy may increase the requirement for insulin or oral hypoglycaemic drugs in diabetic patients,[1] which would not seem unreasonable given the stimulant effects of thyroid hormones on metabolic function. Patients stabilised on long-term thyroid replacement therapy are, however, unlikely to be at risk. For a discussion of the mooted effects of sulphonylureas on thyroid function, see Precautions, above.

1. Refetoff S. Thyroid hormone therapy. *Med Clin North Am* 1975; **59:** 1147–62.

Pharmacokinetics

Reviews.

1. Marchetti P, Navalesi R. Pharmacokinetic-pharmacodynamic relationships of oral hypoglycaemic agents: an update. *Clin Pharmacokinet* 1989; **16:** 100–28.

Uses and Administration

The sulphonylurea antidiabetics are a class of hypoglycaemic drugs given by mouth in the treatment of type 2 diabetes mellitus (p.313). They are used to supplement treatment by diet modification when such modification has not proved effective on its own.

Sulphonylureas appear to have several modes of action, apparently mediated by inhibition of ATP-sensitive potassium channels. Initially, secretion of insulin by functioning islet beta cells is increased. However, insulin secretion subsequently falls again but the hypoglycaemic effect persists and may be due to inhibition of hepatic glucose production and increased sensitivity to any available insulin; this may explain the observed clinical improvement in glycaemic control. The duration of action of sulphonylureas is variable; drugs such as gliclazide and tolbutamide are relatively short-acting (approximately 12 and 10 hours respectively) while chlorpropamide has a prolonged action (over 24 hours).

In patients who do not respond to a sulphonylurea, addition of metformin and/or acarbose or a trial of metformin or acarbose alone may be worthwhile before considering transfer to insulin therapy.

Tolazamide (7233-a)

Tolazamide *(BAN, USAN, rINN).*

NSC-70762; U-17835. 1-(Perhydroazepin-1-yl)-3-tosylurea; 1-(Perhydroazepin-1-yl)-3-*p*-tolylsulphonylurea.

$C_{14}H_{21}N_3O_3S$ = 311.4.

CAS — 1156-19-0.

Pharmacopoeias. In *Br., Jpn,* and *US.*

A white or almost white crystalline powder, odourless or with a slight odour. Very slightly **soluble** in water; slightly soluble in alcohol; soluble in acetone; freely soluble in chloroform.

Adverse Effects, Treatment, and Precautions

As for sulphonylureas in general, p.331.

Interactions

As for sulphonylureas in general, p.332.

Pharmacokinetics

Tolazamide is slowly absorbed from the gastro-intestinal tract, peak plasma concentrations occurring 4 to 8 hours after a dose by mouth, and is extensively bound to plasma proteins. It has a half-life of about 7 hours. It is metabolised in the liver to metabolites with some hypoglycaemic activity. About 85% of an oral dose is excreted in the urine, chiefly as metabolites.

Uses and Administration

Tolazamide is a sulphonylurea hypoglycaemic (p.331). It is given by mouth in the treatment of type 2 diabetes mellitus (p.313) and has a duration of action of at least 10 hours and sometimes up to 20 hours. The usual initial dose in type 2 diabetes mellitus is 100 to 250 mg daily by mouth given as a single dose with breakfast and increased if necessary at weekly intervals by 100 to 250 mg usually to a maximum of 1 g daily; no further benefit is likely to be gained with higher doses. Doses of 500 mg or more daily may be given in divided doses.

Preparations

BP 1998: Tolazamide Tablets;
USP 23: Tolazamide Tablets.

Proprietary Preparations (details are given in Part 3)
Belg.: Tolinase†; ***Ger.:*** Norglycin†; ***Irl.:*** Tolanase; ***Ital.:*** Diabewas†; ***Neth.:*** Tolinase†; ***Swed.:*** Tolinase; ***UK:*** Tolanase; ***USA:*** Tolinase.

Tolbutamide (7234-t)

Tolbutamide *(BAN, rINN).*

Butamidum; Tolbutamidum; Tolglybutamide. 1-Butyl-3-tosylurea; 1-Butyl-3-*p*-tolylsulphonylurea.

$C_{12}H_{18}N_2O_3S$ = 270.3.

CAS — 64-77-7 (tolbutamide); 473-41-6 (tolbutamide sodium).

Pharmacopoeias. In *Chin., Eur.* (see p.viii), *Int., Jpn, Pol.,* and *US.*

A white or almost white, almost odourless, crystalline powder. Practically **insoluble** in water; soluble in alcohol, in acetone, and in chloroform; slightly soluble in ether. It dissolves in dilute solutions of alkali hydroxides.

Tolbutamide sodium 1.08 g is approximately equivalent to 1 g of tolbutamide.

Adverse Effects, Treatment, and Precautions

As for sulphonylureas in general, p.331. Tolbutamide was implicated in the controversial reports of excess cardiovascular mortality associated with oral hypoglycaemic therapy (see under Sulphonylureas, Effects on the Cardiovascular System, p.331).

Thrombophlebitis has occurred following the intravenous injection of tolbutamide sodium; too rapid injection may cause a transient sensation of heat in the vein.

It has been suggested that tolbutamide may be suitable for use in patients with renal impairment, but careful monitoring of blood-sugar concentration is essential. The UK manufacturers recommend that it should not be used in patients with severe renal impairment.

Interactions

As for sulphonylureas in general, p.332.

Pharmacokinetics

Tolbutamide is readily absorbed from the gastro-intestinal tract and is extensively bound to plasma proteins; the half-life is generally within the range of 4 to 7 hours but may be considerably longer. Tolbutamide is metabolised in the liver and is excreted in the urine chiefly as metabolites with little hypoglycaemic activity. Tolbutamide has been detected in breast milk.

Uses and Administration

Tolbutamide is a sulphonylurea hypoglycaemic (p.331). It is given by mouth in the treatment of type 2 diabetes mellitus (p.313) and has a duration of action of about 10 hours.

The usual initial dose by mouth in type 2 diabetes mellitus may range from 1 to 2 g daily, given either as a single dose with breakfast or, more usually, in divided doses. Maintenance doses usually range from 0.25 to 2 g daily. Although it is unlikely that response will be improved by increasing the dose further, daily doses of 3 g have been given.

Tolbutamide sodium ($C_{12}H_{17}N_2NaO_3S$ = 292.3) has sometimes been used in the diagnosis of insulinoma as well as other pancreatic disorders including diabetes mellitus. The equivalent of 1 g of tolbutamide is given by intravenous injection as a 5% solution usually over 2 to 3 minutes.

Diagnosis and testing. References.

1. McMahon MM, *et al.* Diagnostic interpretation of the intravenous tolbutamide test for insulinoma. *Mayo Clin Proc* 1989; **64:** 1481–8.
2. Marks V. Diagnosis and differential diagnosis of hypoglycemia. *Mayo Clin Proc* 1989; **64:** 1558–61.

Preparations

BP 1998: Tolbutamide Tablets;
USP 23: Tolbutamide for Injection; Tolbutamide Tablets.

Proprietary Preparations (details are given in Part 3)
Aust.: Rastinon; ***Austral.:*** Rastinon; ***Belg.:*** Rastinon; ***Canad.:*** Mobenol†; Novo-Butamide; Orinase; ***Fr.:*** Dolipol; ***Ger.:*** Artosin; Guabeta N†; Orabet; Rastinon; ***Irl.:*** Rastinon; ***Ital.:*** Aglycid†; Diabeton Metilato†; Rastinon; ***Neth.:*** Artosin; Rastinon; ***S.Afr.:*** Rastinon; ***Spain:*** Rastinon; ***Swed.:*** Rastinon†; ***Switz.:*** Rastinon; ***UK:*** Glyconon; Rastinon†; ***USA:*** Orinase; Orinase Diagnostic; Tol-Tab.

Multi-ingredient: ***Ital.:*** Glucosulfa.

Tolrestat (17014-d)

Tolrestat *(BAN, USAN, rINN).*

AY-27773. *N*-[6-Methoxy-5-trifluoromethyl-1-naphthyl(thiocarbonyl)]-*N*-methylglycine.

$C_{16}H_{14}F_3NO_3S$ = 357.3.

CAS — 82964-04-3.

Tolrestat inhibits the enzyme aldose reductase which catalyses the conversion of glucose to sorbitol. It has been suggested that accumulation of sorbitol in certain cells, occurring only in conditions of hyperglycaemia and resulting in a hyperosmotic effect, may be involved in the pathogenesis of some diabetic complications. Aldose reductase inhibitors have no influence on blood-glucose concentrations.

Tolrestat was investigated in the management of diabetic complications, but was subsequently withdrawn by the manufacturers following reports of poor efficacy and adverse effects on the liver.

Preparations

Proprietary Preparations (details are given in Part 3)
Irl.: Alredase†; ***Ital.:*** Alredase†; Lorestat†.

Troglitazone (17121-m)

Troglitazone *(BAN, USAN, rINN)*.

CI-991; CS-045; GR-92132X. (±)-*all-rac*-5-{*p*-[(6-Hydroxy-2,5,7,8-tetramethyl-2-chromanyl)methoxy]benzyl}-2,4-thiazolidinedione.

$C_{24}H_{27}NO_5S$ = 441.5.

CAS — 97322-87-7.

Adverse Effects and Precautions

Troglitazone has been associated with severe hepatic reactions, sometimes fatal, which has led to its withdrawal in the UK. Regular monitoring of liver function during therapy, and withdrawal of the drug in any patient who develops jaundice or signs of liver dysfunction, is required. It should not be given to patients with pre-existing moderate or severe elevations of liver enzyme values, or active liver disease. Increased plasma volume has been reported in healthy subjects given troglitazone: it should be used with caution in patients with heart failure. Other adverse effects reported in patients receiving troglitazone include dizziness, headache, fatigue, musculoskeletal pain, and nausea and vomiting. There is no evidence of hypoglycaemia associated with the use of troglitazone alone.

Effects on the liver. The Committee on Safety of Medicines in the UK was aware of over 130 cases of hepatic reactions to troglitazone worldwide as of December 1997,[1] although only 1 had been in the UK. There had been 6 deaths. The average time to the onset of the reaction was 3 months, but the frequency of these reactions, and the existence of risk factors predisposing to them, were unclear. The manufacturers had voluntarily withdrawn the drug in the UK.

1. Committee on Safety of Medicines/Medicines Control Agency. Troglitazone (Romozin) withdrawn. *Current Problems* 1997; **23:** 13.

Interactions

Troglitazone may enhance the hypoglycaemic effects of sulphonylureas; dosage adjustment may be necessary. There is a possibility that troglitazone may enhance the metabolism of drugs metabolised by cytochrome CYP3A4, including some oral contraceptives and terfenadine.

Cholestyramine. Cholestyramine markedly impaired the absorption of troglitazone when the 2 drugs were given concomitantly.[1]

1. Young MA, *et al.* Concomitant administration of cholestyramine influences the absorption of troglitazone. *Br J Clin Pharmacol* 1998; **45:** 37–40.

Pharmacokinetics

Troglitazone is rapidly absorbed following oral administration, with peak plasma concentrations 1 to 3 hours after a dose. Bioavailability is about 53%; absorption is markedly increased in the presence of food. In the body, troglitazone is more than 99% bound to plasma albumin. It is extensively metabolised in the liver and excreted largely in faeces as metabolites; small amounts of metabolites are excreted in urine. Plasma elimination half-life ranges from 10 to 39 hours.

Uses and Administration

Troglitazone is a thiazolidinedione oral hypoglycaemic which is thought to act by increasing receptor sensitivity to insulin. It is given by mouth for the treatment of type 2 diabetes mellitus (p.313) in usual doses of 200 to 400 mg daily with food, although as mentioned above it has been withdrawn in the UK owing to hepatotoxicity. In the USA, doses of up to 600 mg daily may be given, but if response is still inadequate after 1 month at this dose, the drug should be withdrawn.

References.

1. Suter SL, *et al.* Metabolic effects of new oral hypoglycemic agent CS-045 in NIDDM subjects. *Diabetes Care* 1992; **15:** 193–203.
2. Onuma T, *et al.* The effect of a new oral hypoglycemic drug, CS-045, on glucose tolerance and serum lipids in nonobese Japanese patients with non-insulin-dependent diabetes mellitus: a pilot study. *Curr Ther Res* 1994; **55:** 416–21.
3. Nolan JJ, *et al.* Improvement in glucose tolerance and insulin resistance in obese subjects treated with troglitazone. *N Engl J Med* 1994; **331:** 1188–93.
4. Iwamoto Y, *et al.* Effects of troglitazone: a new hypoglycemic agent in patients with NIDDM poorly controlled by diet therapy. *Diabetes Care* 1996; **19:** 151–6.
5. Anonymous. Troglitazone for non-insulin-dependent diabetes mellitus. *Med Lett Drugs Ther* 1997; **39:** 49–51.
6. Spencer CM, Markham A. Troglitazone. *Drugs* 1997; **54:** 89–101.
7. Maggs DG, *et al.* Metabolic effects of troglitazone monotherapy in type 2 diabetes mellitus: a randomized, double-blind, placebo-controlled trial. *Ann Intern Med* 1998; **128:** 176–85.
8. Schwartz S, *et al.* Effect of troglitazone in insulin-treated patients with type II diabetes mellitus. *N Engl J Med* 1998; **338:** 861–6.
9. Inzucchi SE, *et al.* Efficacy and metabolic effects of metformin and troglitazone in type II diabetes mellitus. *N Engl J Med* 1998; **338:** 867–72.

Preparations

Proprietary Preparations (details are given in Part 3)
Jpn: Noscal; ***UK:*** Romozin†; ***USA:*** Rezulin.

Voglibose (15399-k)

Voglibose *(rINN)*.

AO-128. 3,4-Dideoxy-4-{[2-hydroxy-1-(hydroxymethyl)ethyl]amino}-2-*C*-(hydroxymethyl)-*D*-epi-inositol.

$C_{10}H_{21}NO_7$ = 267.3.

CAS — 83480-29-9.

Voglibose is an inhibitor of alpha-glucosidase with general properties similar to those of acarbose (p.317). It is used in the treatment of diabetes mellitus (p.313) in doses of 200 to 300 μg by mouth three times daily before meals.

Preparations

Proprietary Preparations (details are given in Part 3)
Jpn: Basen.

Antiepileptics

This chapter describes antiepileptic drugs and their use in the management of epilepsy, status epilepticus, and other convulsive disorders. The main antiepileptics are

- Acetylureas: Phenacemide
- Barbiturates: Phenobarbitone, primidone
- Benzodiazepines: Clonazepam
- GABA analogues: Gabapentin, vigabatrin
- Hydantoins: Phenytoin
- Iminostilbenes: Carbamazepine
- Succinimides: Ethosuximide
- Miscellaneous: Felbamate, lamotrigine, topiramate, valproate.

Epilepsy

Definitions and classification. An epileptic seizure has been defined as a paroxysmal discharge of cerebral neurones accompanied by clinical phenomena apparent to the patient or to an observer. The phenomena may be of a motor, sensory, or autonomic nature and there may also be impairment or complete loss of consciousness. Motor disturbances may include convulsions, which are involuntary, violent, and spasmodic or prolonged contraction of skeletal muscles. The word 'fit' is often used colloquially to describe an epileptic seizure. Epilepsy is defined as a condition characterised by a recurrence of such seizures. A patient should not be described as having epilepsy until a second non-febrile seizure occurs.

Effective management of a patient with epilepsy requires a detailed and accurate classification of seizure types. The following is a broad account of the classification of seizures based on the views of the Commission on Classification and Terminology of the International League Against Epilepsy in 1981[1] and 1989.[2]

- **Partial seizures** (focal seizures or localisation-related seizures) are epileptic seizures in which the neuronal discharges remain localised in one area of the brain. The phenomena associated with such a seizure depend on the site of origin of the discharge. If there is no loss of consciousness, the seizure is known as a *simple partial seizure* and includes Jacksonian epilepsy, which may be associated with motor or sensory disturbances. If there is impaired consciousness the seizure is referred to as a *complex partial seizure*. Partial seizures were formerly referred to as psychomotor epilepsy or temporal lobe epilepsy, but the terms are not synonymous and should be avoided. Partial seizures may become *secondarily generalised seizures* if the neuronal discharge spreads to involve the entire brain.
- **Generalised seizures** are characterised by neuronal discharges involving both cerebral hemispheres simultaneously from the outset. Subclassifications are based on the presence or absence of different types of convulsions. *Absences* (petit mal) are generalised seizures occurring in children characterised by a sudden loss of consciousness lasting for a few seconds. There is usually accompanying motor activity which may vary in degree from eyelid blinking to more extensive clonic body movements. *Atypical absence seizures* are those with a slower onset and longer duration. *Myoclonic seizures* are epileptic seizures in which the motor manifestation is myoclonus (see below). *Clonic seizures* are characterised by loss of consciousness, autonomic symptoms, and rhythmic clonic contractions of all muscles. *Tonic seizures* are also associated with loss of consciousness and autonomic symptoms accompanied by tonic contractions of the limbs. *Tonic-clonic seizures* (grand mal) are characterised by disordered contraction of muscles. During the tonic phase, all the muscles go into spasm followed up to a minute later by rhythmic clonic contractions. Finally, the patient enters a deep stupor followed by a period of confusion as consciousness is regained. *Atonic seizures* are characterised by loss of postural tone; the head sags or the patient falls down.

Within the categories of partial and generalised epilepsies, seizures have also been classified as idiopathic (formerly referred to as primary) in which no cause can be identified; symptomatic in which the seizures are associated with diagnosable underlying disorders; or cryptogenic in which the epilepsies are known or suspected to be symptomatic but the cause is not clear.

- A third category of **unclassified seizures** covers undetermined epilepsies and epileptic syndromes. Localisation-related syndromes include Rolandic and occipital epilepsies (both idiopathic), while generalised idiopathic syndromes include childhood absence epilepsies, and the cryptogenic or symptomatic generalised syndromes include infantile spasms (as for example in West's syndrome), Lennox-Gastaut syndrome, and epilepsy with myoclonic absences.
- **Special syndromes** include conditions such as febrile convulsions (see below) in which seizures are related to specific situations.

It has been suggested that classification based on seizure type is the most useful in choice of antiepileptic drug whereas the syndrome classification has more benefits in deciding an overall therapeutic strategy and assessing long-term prognosis.

Status epilepticus is generally recognised as a seizure lasting more than 30 minutes or several distinct episodes without restoration of consciousness in between (see below).

Other convulsive disorders, including alcohol withdrawal syndrome, eclampsia and pre-eclampsia, myoclonus, neonatal seizures, and porphyria, are discussed below.

Starting antiepileptic therapy. A single seizure does not constitute epilepsy and therefore does not necessarily warrant immediate treatment with antiepileptics. The consequences of starting antiepileptic therapy too early are that the patient may be unnecessarily exposed to the adverse effects of the drugs used. There are also the social implications of an erroneous epilepsy diagnosis to take into account, such as the loss of a patient's driving licence. However, the implications of delaying treatment must also be considered. The decision to start antiepileptic therapy should be based on whether the risks of further seizures outweigh the risks of treatment. Although there has long been concern that seizures may damage the brain and intellectual capabilities, or even cause death, there are insufficient data to support these claims. Status epilepticus rather than individual seizures or seizure frequency may be responsible for brain injury or death, although the risks of a newly diagnosed epileptic patient developing status epilepticus are unknown. The most compelling reasons for treatment are risk of personal injury or causing injury to others during a seizure, and consideration of the psychosocial consequences of untreated epilepsy such as low self-esteem, anxiety, and domestic and employment difficulties.

Prognosis of epilepsy is another factor frequently considered when implementing antiepileptic therapy. There has been a long-held belief that seizures beget seizures, and that untreated epilepsy would have a poor prognosis. Nevertheless, there is still uncertainty, especially in childhood, over whether or not antiepileptics can alter the natural progression of epilepsy. Thus, whether antiepileptic therapy should be started early to improve prognosis or delayed or avoided altogether remains contentious.[3,4] A study[5] involving 397 patients found that patients treated immediately after a first tonic-clonic seizure had a lower 2-year risk of recurrence than patients who were only started on treatment after a recurrence. In contrast, a decelerating disease process with successively longer intervals between seizures was shown[6] in untreated children with newly diagnosed tonic-clonic seizures followed up for 2 years. Results from another study[7] suggested that seizure control or the prospects for and success of eventual withdrawal of therapy is little influenced by the number of pretreatment seizures up to 10 seizures; above this number there was a reduced chance of completely controlling seizures. Shinnar *et al.*[8] commented that many of the differences in reported risks in seizure recurrence can be attributed to differences in methodology as well as different important risk factors in the populations studied; also, few studies have followed up patients for more than 2 to 4 years. In their prospective study of children identified at the time of a first unprovoked seizure, the risk of recurrence after 8 years of follow-up was found to be less than 50%. Sadzot[9] pointed out that epidemiological studies conducted in untreated patients in developing countries do not support the assumption that repeated seizures exacerbate epilepsy. However, some forms of epilepsy are clearly intractable and experimental evidence would suggest that certain seizure types can have a detrimental effect on prognosis.[10] Epilepsy is a heterogeneous disorder and further prospective studies on larger homogeneous groups are needed, as well as identification of the factors that contribute to the development of chronic and intractable seizures, in order to make firm conclusions.[9]

Some neurologists do not treat a first seizure but prefer to wait for evidence of recurrence unless clinical features such as more than one seizure type or a neurological deficit predispose to poor seizure control. However, it should be borne in mind that the first attack of many non-convulsive seizures may go undetected. Furthermore, as single partial seizures appear to occur less frequently than single generalised tonic-clonic seizures, many neurologists assume that the first detected attack of a non-convulsive seizure is in fact one of multiple seizures and institute treatment.

Choice of antiepileptic. Once a decision to treat has been made, the choice of antiepileptic is determined primarily by its effectiveness against the type of seizures experienced and its potential adverse effects.[11-17] Monotherapy is preferable to a multiple-drug regimen and treatment is therefore initiated with a single drug, increasing the dose gradually until seizures are brought under control or adverse effects become unacceptable. If treatment with the first drug fails, it is preferable to try alternative single first-line antiepileptics before giving combinations of drugs. The dose of the first drug should be gradually decreased as the dose of the second is increased. If combinations are necessary in intractable cases, regimens should avoid the inclusion, where possible, of sedating drugs such as the barbiturates or benzodiazepines. Many antiepileptics interact with each other through complex mechanisms and dosage adjustments may be necessary to maintain plasma concentrations within the therapeutic range; plasma monitoring is often advisable with combination therapy.

Simple and complex **partial seizures** with or without **secondary generalisation** may be treated with *carbamazepine*, *phenytoin* or *valproate*; the response rate is somewhat lower than for tonic-clonic seizures associated with primary generalised epilepsy (see below). *Phenobarbitone* or *primidone* are used less often; sedation can be a problem. *Acetazolamide, clobazam,* or *clonazepam*, or one of the newer antiepileptics such as *gabapentin, lamotrigine*, or *vigabatrin*, may be tried in refractory cases. Lamotrigine has been shown to be of equal efficacy to carbamazepine as monotherapy for partial seizures with or without secondary generalisation. Adjunctive therapy with *tiagabine* or *topiramate* is another option for refractory partial seizures, and in some countries *oxcarbazepine* is becoming more widely accepted as an effective and safe alternative to carbamazepine.[18] Calcium-channel blockers such as flunarizine, nifedipine, and nimodipine have been studied with equivocal results in patients with refractory epilepsy, particularly those with partial seizures.

The drugs used most often to treat **generalised** tonic-clonic seizures are *carbamazepine, phenytoin,* or *valproate*. For tonic-clonic seizures as part of the syndrome of primary generalised epilepsy, valproate is the drug of choice. *Phenobarbitone* and *primidone* may also be used, but sedation might be a problem. In refractory cases, *lamotrigine* and *vigabatrin* may be tried.

The drugs of choice for **absence seizures** are *ethosuximide* or *valproate*, both of which appear to be equally effective.[19] Since absence seizures occur primarily in children the precautions concerning valproate hepatotoxicity apply, and some prefer ethosuximide despite its potentially serious adverse effects (see p.344). However, where absence seizures are associated with tonic-clonic seizures valproate is the drug of choice since it is effective in both conditions; valproate is also preferred for atypical absence seizures.

Valproate is normally the drug of choice for **myoclonic seizures**, including those associated with juvenile myoclonic epilepsy.[20] *Clonazepam* is also used alone or in combination with valproate[21] but its sedative side-effects and the development of tolerance limit its use.[22] *Ethosuximide* and *methsuximide* have also been used as has *progabide*.

In **catamenial epilepsy** (epilepsy associated with menstruation) seizures can be predicted and intermittent therapy with *clobazam* may be useful.

Of the **unclassified seizures Lennox-Gastaut syndrome** begins in early childhood and is particularly difficult to treat because multiple seizure types co-exist; seizures rarely remit entirely. *Valproate* is most frequently used because of its broad spectrum of activity and *lamotrigine* is also effective. *Phenytoin, phenobarbitone,* and *carbamazepine* may be useful for tonic or tonic-clonic seizures, but they may exacerbate absence or myoclonic seizures. *Benzodiazepines* have also been used although development of tolerance is a problem. *Felbamate, progabide, topiramate,* and *vigabatrin* have also been shown to be effective.

Infantile spasms (as for example in **West's syndrome**) are generally unresponsive to conventional antiepileptics.[23,24] *Corticotrophin* and *corticosteroids* have been commonly used but they are associated with frequent and severe adverse effects, and there is controversy over whether they have a better effect on long-term outcome than antiepileptics. *Vigabatrin* is effective either as adjunctive or monotherapy, and many consider that it should replace corticotrophin or corticosteroids as the treatment of choice.[15,17,25] Other drugs that have been used include *nitrazepam* and *valproate*. *Felbamate* and *lamotrigine* have also been shown to be effective for infantile spasms.[26]

Choice of antiepileptics in children. The use of antiepileptics in general in children has been reviewed.[26-28] Again, appropriate treatment depends on seizure type, but there is a lack or evidence to support many therapeutic choices,[25,28] in part because of the difficulties in undertaking trials in this population. In addition, children may be particularly susceptible to some adverse effects, including effects on behaviour, cognition, and development; behavioural problems have been associated particularly with phenobarbitone.[29] Where control is not achieved with one antiepileptic others should be tried,[28,30] although the chances of remission are reduced somewhat.[30] Dietary modification (the ketogenic diet) may also be tried.

Withdrawal of antiepileptic therapy. The possibility of drug withdrawal arises in patients who achieve prolonged seizure-free periods on antiepileptic therapy. Concern over the potential adverse effects of antiepileptic therapy clearly makes withdrawal attractive; however, it should be borne in mind that the practical and social consequences of seizure recurrence may be considerable (for example, loss of driving licence and restricted employment prospects).

Several studies have addressed the prognosis for relapse following antiepileptic withdrawal in children in remission. Long-term follow-up in children whose therapy was withdrawn after seizures had been controlled for several years found that about 25 to 30% had seizure recurrence, in most cases within 2 years of withdrawal.[31,32] Another group reported a higher relapse rate when therapy was withdrawn after 1 year (46%) compared with 3 years (29%);[33] analysis by seizure type suggested that this was due particularly to a difference in outcome in children with complex partial seizures.[34] There is evidence from another prospective study that the remission rate may be as high as 80% among the general population of epileptic children (containing fewer refractory cases than those seen in epilepsy centres).[35]

There has been some uncertainty as to whether these results can be extrapolated to adults.[36] Berg and Shinnar did a meta-analysis[37] that included 25 studies and 5354 patients (children and adults). The overall rate of relapse in seizure-free patients following discontinuation of antiepileptic therapy was 25% at 1 year and 29% at 2 years. There was a higher risk for relapse in adolescent- and adult-onset epilepsy compared with childhood-onset epilepsy.

Although these findings indicate that it is often possible to withdraw therapy successfully, it is more difficult to offer an individual prognosis. Some consider that most adult patients whose livelihood or lifestyle depends on their being seizure-free would be ill advised to contemplate drug withdrawal.[38] Epilepsy of long duration before remission is achieved,[31,39] refractory epilepsy[39] or combined seizure types,[31] cerebral pathology[40] or mental or neurological deficit[41] may all be factors that increase the risk of relapse, and, as previously mentioned, there is a greater likelihood of relapse in adolescent- and adult-onset epilepsy. Seizure type also seems to be important in most studies, with partial seizures associated with a higher risk of relapse,[39] particularly if secondarily generalised;[39] the risk may also be increased in patients with a history of tonic-clonic seizures but the findings of studies are conflicting.[38] Withdrawal of treatment in juvenile myoclonic epilepsy is generally considered inappropriate as up to 90% of patients who are in remission will relapse if treatment is withdrawn.[42,43] Abnormal EEG before withdrawal is also reported in many studies, including the previously quoted meta-analysis,[37] to be prognostic of a poor outcome but this is not universally accepted.[40] Andersson *et al.*[33] found that in children who demonstrated abnormal EEG activity the overall risk of relapse on discontinuation of therapy was only slightly higher than in patients with no such activity, although certain abnormal activities were associated with higher relapse rates than others.

Treatment with more than one antiepileptic is a risk factor for poor prognosis.[38,44] One study has suggested that the type of drug withdrawn is significant, with a poorer prognosis for patients on valproate.[39] Interestingly, however, another study in patients receiving *combination* antiepileptic therapy, as opposed to monotherapy, indicated that a significant increase in seizures was more likely when the carbamazepine component was withdrawn.[45] It should be remembered that withdrawal of enzyme-inducing antiepileptics can result in changes in serum concentrations of other concomitantly administered antiepileptics.[46]

Limited data suggest that the longer the duration of remission before withdrawal, the lower the risk of relapse.[44] In practice seizure control for 2 to 3 years before withdrawal is attempted appears to be considered mandatory,[40,47] although some suggest that this may not be necessary with all seizure types.[34]

Several strategies for predicting the likely outcome after withdrawal of antiepileptic therapy in individuals have been published.[43,48,49] Recognising that epilepsy is a heterogeneous disorder, scoring systems to allow for various risk factors have been devised.[43,48]

When a decision to withdraw is made, it is agreed that drug withdrawal should be gradual to reduce the risk of provoking withdrawal seizures. Drugs should be withdrawn one at a time[50] but there is no agreement on the optimum rate of withdrawal for individual drugs. Shorvon[50] suggested that withdrawal of carbamazepine, barbiturates, or benzodiazepines should be carried out slowly whereas it may be possible to discontinue phenytoin or valproate quickly (over a few days in hospital) if necessary. Exacerbation of seizures may be brought under control by re-establishing the drug being withdrawn. Although it has been suggested that withdrawal over a long period may reduce the relapse rate, one study in children indicated no significant difference in seizure recurrence rate when various antiepileptics including barbiturates were withdrawn over 6 weeks or 9 months.[51]

1. Commission on Classification and Terminology of the International League against Epilepsy. Proposal for revised clinical and electroencephalographic classification of epileptic seizures. *Epilepsia* 1981; **22:** 489–501.
2. Commission on Classification and Terminology of the International League against Epilepsy. Proposal for revised classification of epilepsies and epileptic syndromes. *Epilepsia* 1989; **30:** 389–99.
3. Reynolds EH. Do anticonvulsants alter the natural course of epilepsy?: treatment should be started as early as possible. *Br Med J* 1995; **310:** 176–7.
4. Chadwick D. Do anticonvulsants alter the natural course of epilepsy?: case for early treatment is not established. *Br Med J* 1995; **310:** 177–8.
5. First Seizure Trial Group. Randomized clinical trial on the efficacy of antiepileptic drugs in reducing the risk of relapse after a first unprovoked tonic-clonic seizure. *Neurology* 1993; **43:** 478–83.
6. van Donselaar CA, *et al.* Clinical course of untreated tonic-clonic seizures in childhood: prospective, hospital based study. *Br Med J* 1997; **314:** 401–4.
7. Camfield C, *et al.* Does the number of seizures before treatment influence ease of control or remission of childhood epilepsy?: not if the number is 10 or less. *Neurology* 1996; **46:** 41–4.
8. Shinnar S, *et al.* The risk of seizure recurrence after a first unprovoked afebrile seizure in childhood: an extended follow-up. *Pediatrics* 1996; **98:** 216–25.
9. Sadzot B. Epilepsy: a progressive disease? *Br Med J* 1997; **314:** 391–2.
10. O'Donoghue M, Sander JWAS. Does early anti-epileptic drug treatment alter the prognosis for remission of the epilepsies? *J R Soc Med* 1996; **89:** 245–8.
11. Anonymous. Drugs for epilepsy. *Med Lett Drugs Ther* 1995; **37:** 37–40.
12. Sabers A, Gram L. Drug treatment of epilepsy in the 1990s: achievements and new developments. *Drugs* 1996; **52:** 483–93.
13. Brodie MJ, Dichter MA. Antiepileptic drugs. *N Engl J Med* 1996; **334:** 168–75.
14. Britton JW, So EL. Selection of antiepileptic drugs: a practical approach. *Mayo Clin Proc* 1996; **71:** 778–86.
15. Wallace SJ, *et al.* Epilepsy—a guide to medical treatment 1: antiepileptic drugs. *Hosp Med* 1998; **59:** 379–87.
16. Dichter MA, Brodie MJ. New antiepileptic drugs. *N Engl J Med* 1996; **334:** 1583–90.
17. Stephen LJ, Brodie MJ. New drug treatments for epilepsy. *Prescribers' J* 1998; **38:** 98–106.
18. Perucca E. The new generation of antiepileptic drugs: advantages and disadvantages. *Br J Clin Pharmacol* 1996; **42:** 531–43.
19. Mikati MA, Browne TR. Comparative efficacy of antiepileptic drugs. *Clin Neuropharmacol* 1988; **11:** 130–40.
20. Timmings PL, Richens A. Juvenile myoclonic epilepsy. *Br Med J* 1992; **305:** 4–5.
21. Anonymous. Diagnosing juvenile myoclonic epilepsy. *Lancet* 1992; **340:** 759–60.
22. Ashton H. Guidelines for the rational use of benzodiazepines: when and what to use. *Drugs* 1994; **48:** 25–40.
23. Appleton RE. Infantile spasms. *Arch Dis Child* 1993; **69:** 614–18.
24. Haines ST, Casto DT. Treatment of infantile spasms. *Ann Pharmacother* 1994; **28:** 779–91.
25. Appleton RE. The new antiepileptic drugs. *Arch Dis Child* 1996; **75:** 256–62. Correction. *ibid.* 1997; **76:** 81.
26. Morton LD, Pellock JM. Diagnosis and treatment of epilepsy in children and adolescents. *Drugs* 1996; **51:** 399–414.
27. Zupanc ML. Update on epilepsy in pediatric patients. *Mayo Clin Proc* 1996; **71:** 899–916.
28. Neville BGR. Epilepsy in childhood. *Br Med J* 1997; **315:** 924–30.
29. de Silva M, *et al.* Randomised comparative monotherapy trial of phenobarbitone, phenytoin, carbamazepine, or sodium valproate for newly diagnosed childhood epilepsy. *Lancet* 1996; **347:** 709–13.
30. Camfield PR, *et al.* If a first antiepileptic drug fails to control a child's epilepsy, what are the chances of success with the next drug? *J Pediatr* 1997; **131:** 821–4.
31. Thurston JH, *et al.* Prognosis in childhood epilepsy. *N Engl J Med* 1982; **306:** 831–6.
32. Shinnar S, *et al.* Discontinuing antiepileptic medication in children with epilepsy after two years without seizures. *N Engl J Med* 1985; **313:** 976–80.
33. Andersson T, *et al.* A comparison between one and three years of treatment in uncomplicated childhood epilepsy: a prospective study: II: the EEG as predictor of outcome after withdrawal of treatment. *Epilepsia* 1997; **38:** 225–32.
34. Braathen G, *et al.* Comparison between one and three years of treatment in uncomplicated childhood epilepsy: a prospective study: I: outcome in different seizure types. *Epilepsia* 1996; **37:** 822–32.
35. Bouma PAD, *et al.* Discontinuation of antiepileptic therapy: a prospective study in children. *J Neurol Neurosurg Psychiatry* 1987; **50:** 1579–83.
36. Pedley TA. Discontinuing antiepileptic drugs. *N Engl J Med* 1988; **318:** 982–4.
37. Berg AT, Shinnar S. Relapse following discontinuation of antiepileptic drugs: a meta-analysis. *Neurology* 1994; **44:** 601–8.
38. Anonymous. Antiepileptic drug withdrawal—hawks or doves? *Lancet* 1991; **337:** 1193–4.
39. Callaghan N, *et al.* Withdrawal of anticonvulsant drugs in patients free of seizures for two years: a prospective study. *N Engl J Med* 1988; **318:** 942–6.
40. Chadwick D. Drug withdrawal and epilepsy: when and how? *Drugs* 1988; **35:** 579–83.
41. Emerson R, *et al.* Stopping medication in children with epilepsy: predicators of outcome. *N Engl J Med* 1981; **304:** 1125–9.
42. Anonymous. Diagnosing juvenile myoclonic epilepsy. *Lancet* 1992; **340:** 759–60.
43. Medical Research Council Antiepileptic Drug Withdrawal Study Group. Prognostic index for recurrence of seizures after remission of epilepsy. *Br Med J* 1993; **306:** 1374–8.
44. Medical Research Council Antiepileptic Drug Withdrawal Study Group. Randomised study of antiepileptic drug withdrawal in patients in remission. *Lancet* 1991; **337:** 1175–80.
45. Duncan JS, *et al.* Discontinuation of phenytoin, carbamazepine, and valproate in patients with active epilepsy. *Epilepsia* 1990; **31:** 324–33.
46. Duncan JS, *et al.* Effects of discontinuation of phenytoin, carbamazepine, and valproate on concomitant antiepileptic medication. *Epilepsia* 1991; **32:** 101–15.
47. Anonymous. Withdrawing antiepileptic drugs. *Drug Ther Bull* 1989; **27:** 29–30.
48. Camfield C, *et al.* Outcome of childhood epilepsy: a population-based study with a simple predictive scoring system for those treated with medication. *J Pediatr* 1993; **122:** 861–8.
49. Shinnar S, *et al.* Discontinuing antiepileptic drugs in children with epilepsy: a prospective study. *Ann Neurol* 1994; **35:** 534–45.

50. Shorvon SD. Medical assessment and treatment of chronic epilepsy. *Br Med J* 1991; **302:** 363–6.
51. Tennison MB, *et al.* Discontinuing antiepileptic drugs in children with epilepsy: a comparison of a six-week and a nine-month taper period. *N Engl J Med* 1994; **330:** 1407–10.

Cognition. There has long been concern that antiepileptic therapy might affect mental function. Children are particularly vulnerable to cognitive impairment, which can develop insidiously and therefore be overlooked. However, cognitive impairment and learning problems in children may also be caused by underlying cerebral pathology responsible for the epilepsy or the seizures themselves. The relationship between cognitive impairment, antiepileptic drugs, and epilepsy is complex and poorly understood; psychosocial and environmental factors may also contribute. Many studies, including comparative studies, have assessed the effects of antiepileptics on cognitive function, but the results have often been variable. A major difficulty has been to distinguish subtle effects of drug therapy on mental function, if they exist, from those of sedation or the effect of the disease itself.

Although subtle effects on cognition have been most commonly reported with barbiturate antiepileptics such as phenobarbitone, they may also occur with other antiepileptics, and in adults as well as children. Benzodiazepines, phenobarbitone, and primidone are most frequently linked to sedative effects and behavioural problems whereas phenytoin, carbamazepine, and valproate are less problematic. Studies of effects on cognition have been conducted in healthy adults in an effort to separate any confounding factors of epilepsy and seizures, and standard antiepileptics have been shown to impair cognition in people with and without epilepsy. Results from recent studies in both groups have demonstrated that at therapeutic serum concentrations phenobarbitone, phenytoin, carbamazepine, oxcarbazepine, and valproate have similar adverse effects on cognitive function.[1] Most of the newer antiepileptics appear to be better tolerated, although zonisamide and topiramate produce some cognitive impairment. There is also limited evidence that gabapentin, lamotrigine, and vigabatrin may enhance cognitive function. However, further data are required for the newer antiepileptics before a definitive assessment can be made.[2]

There is wide interindividual variation in the effects that antiepileptics have on cognitive function; in some patients the effects may become apparent at low serum levels, whereas other tolerate high serum levels without apparent untoward effect.[2] Variable results from studies mean that it is difficult to make comparisons. It is, however, generally agreed that phenobarbitone is less desirable for use in children than other antiepileptics.

Most studies on the adverse effects of antiepileptics on cognitive function have had methodological flaws and have involved small numbers of patients; recommendations for future research have been made.[3] Future studies should assess antiepileptic use in different epileptic patient populations.[2]

In view of the potential effect of antiepileptics on cognition, the Committee on Drugs of the American Academy of Pediatrics[4] has made a number of recommendations, that include the following

- the relative influence of each antiepileptic on cognitive and behavioural function should be considered along with all other potential adverse effects;
- the child's behaviour and academic progress should be monitored through routine questioning of parents and teachers as well as by the physician's own observations of cognitive function, mood, and behaviour;
- should behavioural or cognitive changes occur in relation to starting antiepileptic therapy, the need for medication and/or possible alteration of medication must be reassessed.

1. Kälviäinen R, *et al.* Cognitive adverse effects of antiepileptic drugs: incidence, mechanisms and therapeutic implications. *CNS Drugs* 1996; **5:** 358–68.
2. Devinsky O. Cognitive and behavioral effects of antiepileptic drugs. *Epilepsia* 1995; **36** (suppl 2): S46–S65.
3. Aldenkamp AP, Vermeulen J. Phenytoin and carbamazepine: differential effects on cognitive function. *Seizure* 1995; **4:** 95–104.
4. Committee on Drugs of the American Academy of Pediatrics. Behavioral and cognitive effects of anticonvulsant therapy. *Pediatrics* 1995; **96:** 538–40.

Driving. Driving by patients with epilepsy is generally regulated[1,2] and restricted to those whose seizures are adequately controlled. Also, antiepileptic drugs may produce CNS-related adverse effects, including dizziness and drowsiness, that could impair a patient's ability to drive a vehicle or operate machinery, particularly during the initial stages of therapy.

1. Krumholz A, *et al.* Driving and epilepsy: a review and reappraisal. *JAMA* 1991; **265:** 622–6.
2. Shorvon S. Epilepsy and driving: British regulations have recently been eased. *Br Med J* 1995; **310:** 885–6.

Pregnancy. The management of epilepsy during pregnancy may present problems for both the mother and the fetus.[1-4]

The incidence of spontaneous abortion and still-births increases in women with epilepsy although the reason is unknown. A single generalised seizure does not usually pose clinical problems for the fetus, but both mother and fetus are at risk of serious trauma from maternal falls and intra-uterine deaths have been reported. Status epilepticus is associated with significant mortality in mother and fetus. The frequency of seizures increases during pregnancy in some women; this may be related to hormonal or other factors such as lack of sleep, but one of the main reasons is likely to be decreased plasma-antiepileptic concentrations due to a change in drug disposition as pregnancy progresses.

Although more than 90% of pregnant women receiving antiepileptic therapy will deliver normal infants, unequivocal teratogenic risks have been identified for all the major antiepileptics.[5] The risk appears to increase when 2 or more drugs are given together. Untreated epilepsy itself has been associated with an increase in fetal abnormalities,[6] although to a lesser degree than with antiepileptics. This does not appear to be associated with maternal seizures during pregnancy and, since some of these effects were also described before the use of antiepileptics became widespread, there may be a relationship with a genetic component of epilepsy.[5,6] A variety of syndromes, including craniofacial and digital abnormalities and, less commonly, cleft lip and palate, have been described with *carbamazepine, phenobarbitone, phenytoin, primidone, troxidone*, and *valproate*; congenital heart disease, microcephaly, and developmental delay may also occur with some antiepileptics. Specific syndromes have previously been ascribed to individual antiepileptics such as the 'fetal hydantoin syndrome' with phenytoin, but now it is recognised that there is some degree of overlap between the effects seen with different drugs, and the broader term 'fetal antiepileptic drug syndrome' is therefore considered to be more appropriate by some.[5,6] In some cases, the milder dysmorphic features become less apparent as the child grows older. There is still insufficient data to determine which of the older antiepileptics is more teratogenic.[5] Neural tube defects are associated with valproate and carbamazepine and the risk of spina bifida has been calculated to be about 1%,[7-9] which is about 20 times the rate in the general population. Additional problems that may occur with some antiepileptic therapies include neonatal sedation and drug dependence with phenobarbitone (see p.350) and benzodiazepines if given close to term. Neonatal bleeding is associated with the enzyme-inducing antiepileptics carbamazepine, phenobarbitone, and phenytoin, and has also been reported with valproate and other antiepileptics. Little is known of the effects of the newer antiepileptics on the fetus, although the manufacturers have reported congenital anomalies in the offspring of some mothers using *vigabatrin* during pregnancy and teratogenicity with *topiramate* and *vigabatrin* in *animals*. There appears to be little evidence of teratogenic potential for *felbamate, gabapentin*, or *lamotrigine* in *animal* studies to date, although there is a theoretical risk with lamotrigine because, like valproate, it is a folate antagonist.

Patients with epilepsy who wish to become pregnant require specialist advice. Withdrawal of antiepileptic therapy may be an option if the patient has been seizure-free for at least 2 years (for further details of drug withdrawal, see above); resumption of therapy may be considered after the end of the first trimester. If antiepileptics are to be continued throughout pregnancy, monotherapy is preferred using the lowest possible effective dose, although doses may have to be increased in response to changes in drug disposition during pregnancy, with the necessary readjustments being made after delivery. Since there is a risk of fetal malformations with all the established antiepileptics, and a lack of data for the newer ones, it is generally considered that as long as there is good seizure control there is little to be gained from changing a pregnant patient's antiepileptic treatment. If a patient becomes pregnant while taking carbamazepine, phenytoin, or valproate she should be counselled regarding the risk of neural tube and other defects and should be offered antenatal screening. Adequate supplementation of folic acid is advised before pregnancy and during the first trimester to counteract the risk of neural tube defects; it has been suggested that women receiving antiepileptics should be given folic acid in similar doses to those used in women who have previously given birth to an infant with neural tube defects (for further details, see Neural Tube Defects under Folic Acid, p.1341). Although folic acid can reduce serum-phenytoin concentrations this does not appear to be a problem in practice (see p.357).

To counteract the risk of neonatal bleeding associated with carbamazepine, phenobarbitone, and phenytoin, prophylactic vitamin K_1 is recommended for the mother from 36 weeks' gestation, and then for the neonate after delivery (for further details, see under Haemorrhagic Disease of the Newborn, p.1372).

Status epilepticus occurring during pregnancy should be treated in the same way as for the general population (see below). First seizures occurring during the second half of pregnancy may be part of eclampsia (see below) and should be differentiated from epilepsy.

Antiepileptics are generally distributed into breast milk (although this information is not always known for the newer ones), but for most of the older established drugs, the concentrations are lower than in maternal plasma, and **breast feeding** is considered to be safe for these antiepileptics when given in usual doses, with the possible exception of the barbiturates and ethosuximide.[1-3] Problems of neonatal sedation may occur with the benzodiazepines and barbiturates (including primidone) and breast feeding should be avoided when possible.[1] Ethosuximide is distributed in significant amounts into breast milk and breast feeding should be avoided; hyperexcitability and poor suckling have been reported in the infant. There is little data for the new antiepileptics regarding breast feeding, and therefore the manufacturers recommend that breast feeding should be avoided.

1. Brodie MJ. Management of epilepsy during pregnancy and lactation. *Lancet* 1990; **336:** 426–7.
2. Delgado-Escueta AV, Janz D. Consensus guidelines: preconception counseling, management, and care of the pregnant woman with epilepsy. *Neurology* 1992; **42** (suppl 5): 149–160.
3. Anonymous. Epilepsy and pregnancy. *Drug Ther Bull* 1994; **32:** 49–51.
4. Cleland PG. Management of pre-existing disorders in pregnancy: epilepsy. *Prescribers' J* 1996; **36:** 102–109.
5. Finnell RH, *et al.* Teratogenicity of antiepileptic drugs. In: Levy RH, *et al.* eds. *Antiepileptic drugs*. 4th ed. New York: Raven Press, 1995; 209–30.
6. Gaily E, *et al.* Minor anomalies in offspring of epileptic mothers. *J Pediatr* 1988; **112:** 520–9.
7. Lindhout D, Schmidt D. In-utero exposure to valproate and neural tube defects. *Lancet* 1986; **i:** 1392–3.
8. Oakeshott P, Hunt GM. Valproate and spina bifida. *Br Med J* 1989; **298:** 1300–1.
9. Rosa FW. Spina bifida in infants of women treated with carbamazepine during pregnancy. *N Engl J Med* 1991; **324:** 674–7.

Status epilepticus

Status epilepticus has been arbitrarily defined as a prolonged seizure, or a period of repeated seizures without restoration of normal consciousness in between, lasting for more than 30 minutes,[1] although it has been suggested that in practice prolonged or repeated seizure activity lasting more than 5 to 10 minutes can be regarded as status epilepticus and requires treatment.[2,3] Any type of seizure can lead to status epilepticus but generalised tonic-clonic status epilepticus is the most common and most dangerous type.[2,3] The longer seizures continue, the more difficult they are to control and the higher the morbidity and mortality; permanent neuronal damage can occur after 30 minutes of seizure activity.

Initial treatment consists of supporting respiration, including the provision of oxygen, and maintaining blood pressure. The aim is then to terminate the seizures as quickly as possible. Antiepileptic treatment differs slightly between centres and countries,[1-9] but in most cases treatment is started with *diazepam* to abort the attack followed by phenytoin (or alternatively phenobarbitone, chlormethiazole, or paraldehyde) to prevent recurrence. Diazepam is given by intravenous injection or rectally. (Rectal diazepam has also been used in the home setting to treat acute repetitive seizures, which may evolve into status epilepticus). Some prefer *lorazepam* to diazepam as the initial benzodiazepine because it combines rapid onset with prolonged duration of antiepileptic action. Other benzodiazepines used have included *clonazepam* and *midazolam*.

Once control of seizures is obtained *phenytoin sodium* may be given intravenously with monitoring of blood pressure and ECG. *Fosphenytoin sodium* is a prodrug of phenytoin sodium and has the advantage that it may be administered at a faster rate of intravenous infusion. Phenytoin has been considered to be more appropriate than a benzodiazepine for the management of status epilepticus or recurrent seizures in patients with head injuries or other acute neurological lesions. Phenytoin carries a lower risk of respiratory failure or loss of consciousness, and results in a longer-lasting control of seizures.[10] Alternatively, intravenous *phenobarbitone sodium* may be given if the patient has not recently received oral phenobarbitone or primidone; careful observation of respiration is mandatory as a large dose of diazepam may have been given previously.[1] Some workers have suggested that using phenobarbitone for the initial treatment of convulsive status epilepticus might be at least as effective, safe, and practical as using diazepam with phenytoin.[11] Other alternatives include *chlormethiazole edisylate* by intravenous infusion or *paraldehyde* rectally or by deep intramuscular injection. Another option is to give *lignocaine* intravenously.

If the above measures do not control seizures, anaesthesia should be instituted with a short-acting barbiturate such as *thiopentone*, and the patient ventilated;[1,4] *pentobarbitone* is used similarly.[2,3,6] Other anaesthetics have been tried in the treatment of intractable convulsive status epilepticus including *etomidate, isoflurane, midazolam,* and *propofol*.[3,4,6]

If cerebral neoplasm or arteritis is suspected high-dose *dexamethasone* therapy is started, provided meningitis or cerebral abscess is absent.[1] Alcoholics are given intravenous *thiamine*.[1,4]

Valproate administered intravenously in a small study was found to be effective in controlling status epilepticus of various types including that associated with generalised tonic-clonic and myoclonic seizures.[12]

The treatment of partial status epilepticus is similar to that of generalised tonic-clonic status epilepticus.[3] However, epilepsia partialis continua may be refractory to standard antiepileptics; it may respond to treatment with high doses of *corticosteroids*.[1]

Intravenous benzodiazepines are usually used for the initial treatment of absence status epilepticus[3] followed by oral administration of valproate or *ethosuximide*. Valproate is considered to be the drug of choice for the prevention of recurrence of absence status epilepticus.[13]

1. Brodie MJ. Status epilepticus in adults. *Lancet* 1990; **336:** 551–2.
2. Working Group on Status Epilepticus. Treatment of convulsive status epilepticus: recommendations of the Epilepsy Foundation of America's Working Group on Status Epilepticus. *JAMA* 1993; **270:** 854–9.
3. Bauer J, Elger CE. Management of status epilepticus in adults. *CNS Drugs* 1994; **i:** 26–44.
4. Anonymous. Stopping status epilepticus. *Drug Ther Bull* 1996; **34:** 73–5.
5. Rylance GW. Treatment of epilepsy and febrile convulsions in children. *Lancet* 1990; **336:** 488–91.
6. Cascino GD. Generalized convulsive status epilepticus. *Mayo Clin Proc* 1996; **71:** 787–92.
7. Shorvon S. Tonic clonic status epilepticus. *J Neurol Neurosurg Psychiatry* 1993; **56:** 125–34.
8. Tasker RC. Emergency treatment of acute seizures and status epilepticus. *Arch Dis Child* 1998; **79:** 78–83.
9. Lowenstein DH, Alldredge BK. Status epilepticus. *N Engl J Med* 1998; **338:** 970–6.
10. Eldridge PR, Punt JAG. Risks associated with giving benzodiazepines to patients with acute neurological injuries. *Br Med J* 1990; **300:** 1189–90.
11. Shaner DM, *et al.* Treatment of status epilepticus: a prospective comparison of diazepam and phenytoin versus phenobarbital and optional phenytoin. *Neurology* 1988; **38:** 202–7.
12. Giroud M, *et al.* Use of injectable valproic acid in status epilepticus: a pilot study. *Drug Invest* 1993; **5:** 154–9.
13. Berkovic SF, *et al.* Valproate prevents the recurrence of absence status. *Neurology* 1989; **39:** 1294–7.

Other convulsive disorders

Disorders that feature convulsions or epileptic seizures but are not considered to be forms of epilepsy are described below.

Alcohol withdrawal syndrome. For a discussion of the management of seizures associated with alcohol withdrawal syndrome, see p.1099.

Eclampsia and pre-eclampsia. Pre-eclampsia is a hypertensive disorder occurring in pregnancy that entails increased blood pressure together with proteinuria, and sometimes abnormal coagulation and liver function, and oedema; it may progress to eclampsia, which is a convulsive phase. The treatment of pre-eclampsia and eclampsia is primarily aimed at reducing hypertension (see Hypertension in Pregnancy, under Hypertension, p.788) and treating or preventing resultant seizures. Whether the treatment of the hypertension alone is sufficient to prevent the progression of pre-eclampsia to eclampsia is a matter of debate.[1] The management of seizures associated with eclampsia has been discussed.[2,3] It is difficult to identify those patients who will experience eclamptic seizures. Some give *antiepileptics* prophylactically to all women with advanced pre-eclampsia, but this is considered greatly to increase the risk of major adverse effects; others reserve antiepileptics for those who have had a first seizure. *'Lytic cocktails'* consisting of chlorpromazine, pethidine, and/or promethazine have been used in some countries in the management of pre-eclampsia and imminent eclampsia but they result in heavy sedation and the use of phenothiazines is generally not recommended late in pregnancy.

Eclampsia in the UK has been treated with *diazepam, chlormethiazole,* or *phenytoin*. However, for many years *magnesium sulphate* has been the preferred treatment of eclampsia in the USA and studies[4-6] have shown it to be more effective and to cause fewer adverse effects. A meta-analysis[7] of 9 randomised trials involving 2390 patients with pre-eclampsia and 1743 patients with eclampsia concluded that magnesium sulphate was more effective than phenytoin or no therapy in prevention of seizures in pre-eclamptic patients, but less effective than diazepam. In eclamptic patients, magnesium sulphate was superior to phenytoin, diazepam, or a lytic cocktail in terms of seizure recurrence. Thus, many in the UK now consider magnesium sulphate to be the preferred drug for the treatment of eclampsia,[8-11] but further studies may be necessary to establish its role for the prevention of eclampsia in pre-eclamptic patients.[8,11] Some commentators have suggested,[12] in the light of evidence of possible neonatal toxicity, that magnesium sulphate should be restricted to use in eclampsia or more severe pre-eclampsia.

1. Ramsay MM, *et al.* Are anticonvulsants necessary to prevent eclampsia. *Lancet* 1994; **343:** 540–1.
2. Redman CWG, Roberts JM. Management of pre-eclampsia. *Lancet* 1993; **341:** 1451–4.
3. Mushambi MC, *et al.* Recent developments in the pathophysiology and management of pre-eclampsia. *Br J Anaesth* 1996; **76:** 133–48.
4. Dommisse J. Phenytoin sodium and magnesium sulphate in the management of eclampsia. *Br J Obstet Gynaecol* 1990; **97:** 104–9.
5. The Eclampsia Trial Collaborative Group. Which anticonvulsant for women with eclampsia?: evidence from the Collaborative Eclampsia Trial. *Lancet* 1995; **345:** 1455–63. Correction. *ibid.*; **346:** 258.
6. Lucas MJ, *et al.* A comparison of magnesium sulfate with phenytoin for the prevention of eclampsia. *N Engl J Med* 1995; **333:** 201–5.
7. Chien PFW, *et al.* Magnesium sulphate in the treatment of eclampsia and pre-eclampsia: an overview of the evidence from randomised trials. *Br J Obstet Gynaecol* 1996; **103:** 1085–91.
8. Anthony J, *et al.* Role of magnesium sulfate in seizure prevention in patients with eclampsia and pre-eclampsia. *Drug Safety* 1996; **15:** 188–99.
9. Robson SC. Magnesium sulphate: the time of reckoning. *Br J Obstet Gynaecol* 1996; **103:** 99–102.
10. Duley L. Magnesium sulphate regimens for women with eclampsia: messages from the Collaborative Eclampsia Trial. *Br J Obstet Gynaecol* 1996; **103**: 103–5.
11. Gülmezoglu AM, Duley L. Use of anticonvulsants in eclampsia and pre-eclampsia: survey of obstetricians in the United Kingdom and Republic of Ireland. *Br Med J* 1998; **316:** 975–6.
12. Bennett P, Edwards D. Use of magnesium sulphate in obstetrics. *Lancet* 1997; **350:** 1491.

Febrile convulsions. Febrile convulsions have been defined[1] as epileptic seizures occurring between the ages of 6 months to 5 years and associated with a fever arising from an infectious illness outside the CNS. They usually occur during the rising phase of fever early in the course of the infection and are not considered to be a form of epilepsy.[2]

Febrile convulsions are considered to be benign if limited to a single tonic or tonic-clonic seizure lasting less than 15 minutes without any focal characteristics; the majority of patients are less than 3 years of age.[2] About one-third of children who have a benign febrile convulsion will experience a recurrence.[1,2] The risk of developing epilepsy is low, but nevertheless it is 2 to 3 times greater than the risk in the population as a whole.[2] Unless they are recurrent, benign febrile convulsions need only simple treatment to lower body temperature[1,2] such as that described under Fever and Hyperthermia, p.1.

Prolonged febrile convulsions lasting longer than 15 minutes and associated with some focal characteristics are not considered to be benign and further increases the risk of developing epilepsy.[2] When they are prolonged or recurrent they are treated with intravenous or rectal *diazepam* to prevent possible brain damage resulting from continued seizure activity, although any such affect appears to be rare.[3]

The prophylactic administration of *antiepileptics* to children thought to be at risk of recurrence of febrile convulsions remains controversial. Many consider that even if recurrences can be prevented there is no evidence that the risk of developing epilepsy is reduced.[1,2,4] A working group of the Royal College of Physicians and the British Paediatric Association considered that pooled analyses of studies of the prophylactic use of *phenobarbitone* or *sodium valproate* showed that long-term prophylaxis was rarely indicated, apart from occasional use for a child who has frequent recurrences.[1] A study which demonstrated lack of benefit and adverse effects on cognitive function with long-term prophylactic treatment with phenobarbitone[5] supported the view of the working group, and a later meta-analysis also considered that prophylaxis could not be recommended.[6] Although some workers have demonstrated that intermittent prophylaxis with phenobarbitone or diazepam[7] given at the onset of and during fever could prevent recurrence of febrile convulsions, the working group did not recommend their routine use in this way.[1] Other workers have found that administration of paracetamol as an antipyretic and the use of diazepam for intermittent prophylaxis failed to prevent recurrences of febrile convulsions.[8]

1. Joint Working Group of the Research Unit of the Royal College of Physicians and the British Paediatric Association. Guidelines for the management of convulsions with fever. *Br Med J* 1991; **303:** 634–6.
2. Smith MC. Febrile seizures: recognition and management. *Drugs* 1994; **47:** 933–44.
3. Verity CM. Do seizures damage the brain? The epidemiological evidence. *Arch Dis Child* 1998; **78:** 78–84.
4. Knudsen FU, *et al.* Long term outcome of prophylaxis for febrile convulsions. *Arch Dis Child* 1996; **74:** 13–18.
5. Farwell JR, *et al.* Phenobarbital for febrile seizures—effects on intelligence and on seizure recurrence. *N Engl J Med* 1990; **322:** 364–9.
6. Rantala H, *et al.* A meta-analytic review of the preventative treatment of recurrences of febrile seizures. *J Pediatr* 1997; **131:** 922–5.
7. Rosman NP, *et al.* A controlled trial of diazepam administered during febrile illnesses to prevent recurrence of febrile seizures. *N Engl J Med* 1993; **329:** 79–84.
8. Uhari M, *et al.* Effect of acetaminophen and of low intermittent doses of diazepam on prevention of recurrences of febrile seizures. *J Pediatr* 1995; **126:** 991–5.

Myoclonus. Myoclonus consists of brief, involuntary, jerky movements of sudden onset which may be focal, segmental, or generalised, and are caused by muscular contractions (positive myoclonus) or inhibitions (negative myoclonus). The term 'myoclonus' is nonspecific and classification as physiological (in normal subjects), essential (no known cause), epileptic (seizures dominate), or symptomatic (encephalopathy dominates; many causes including storage diseases, neurodegenerative syndromes, toxic and drug-induced syndromes, and hypoxia) is important in order to decide on treatment.[1]

Myoclonus may also be subdivided into cortical, reticular, or spinal forms. Cortical myoclonus is considered to be a subset of epilepsy and responds best to antiepileptics, usually *valproate* and/or *clonazepam*; *piracetam* is also used, usually as adjunctive therapy. In epileptic myoclonus, epileptic seizures (myoclonic seizures in which the motor manifestation is myoclonus) dominate. Their treatment is discussed under Epilepsy, above. Reticular myoclonus is usually caused by anoxia or acute encephalopathy and is treated with *clonazepam* or *serotonin*. Posthypoxic myoclonus occurring after hypoxic coma may respond to *oxitriptan* or *serotonin* combined with *carbidopa*; antiepileptics may help. Essential myoclonus may benefit from clonazepam.

1. Caviness JN. Myoclonus. *Mayo Clin Proc.* 1996; **71:** 679–88.

Neonatal seizures. Neonatal seizures differ from epilepsy and the definitions in the international classification of epilepsy and epileptic syndromes (see above) do not apply. They are frequently subtle and difficult to recognise. Causes include asphyxia, glucose or electrolyte imbalance, infection, CNS or cerebrovascular lesions, inborn errors of metabolism, and drug withdrawal or intoxication.

Neonatal seizures represent a neurological emergency in the newborn and rapid diagnosis and treatment is essential. Infusion of glucose or electrolytes may be of benefit. Current practice involves administration of antiepileptic drugs to control seizures, although there is no consensus on their use. *Phenobarbitone* and *phenytoin* are the most widely used. Some consider phenobarbitone to be the mainstay of treatment for all types of seizures in neonates, although response rates are variable. If seizures persist, phenytoin may be added to therapy. Other drugs that have been tried include *carbamazepine, benzodiazepines*, and *primidone*. Pyridoxine dependent seizures can be abolished by regular administration of large doses of the vitamin.

References.

1. Zupanc ML. Update on epilepsy in pediatric patients. *Mayo Clin Proc* 1996; **71:** 899–916.
2. Morton LD, Pellock JM. Diagnosis and treatment of epilepsy in children and adolescents. *Drugs* 1996; **51:** 399–414.
3. Singh B, *et al.* Treatment of neonatal seizures with carbamazepine. *J Child Neurol* 1996; **11:** 378–82.
4. Evans D, Levene M. Neonatal seizures. *Arch Dis Child Fetal Neonatal Ed* 1998; **78:** F70–F75.

Porphyria. Convulsions may occur at the peak of an acute attack of porphyria (p.983) but usually disappear as the attack resolves and therapy should be aimed at the underlying disease.[1] However, some patients continue to experience convulsions while in remission and their management poses a major therapeutic problem as all the first-line antiepileptics have been associated with acute attacks.[2] Barbiturates (*phenobarbitone, primidone*), hydantoins (*phenytoin, ethotoin*), and *carbamazepine* are considered unsafe,[1] as are *sulthiame* and *progabide*. There is limited evidence that the *benzodiazepines, sodium valproate*, and probably *valpromide* are porphyrinogenic but status epilepticus has been treated successfully with intravenous *diazepam*. Seizure prophylaxis may be undertaken as a calculated risk using sodium valproate or *clonazepam* if considered essential. *Magnesium sulphate* is safe. *Chlormethiazole* is also probably safe. *Gabapentin* and *vigabatrin* have each been tried in a few patients without ill-effect, although there has been a report of a bullous skin eruption in one patient given vigabatrin.[3] Other antiepileptics such as the succinimides (*ethosuximide, methsuximide, phensuximide*) and oxazolidinediones (*paramethadione, troxidone*) are considered to be unsafe.[1]

1. Moore MR, McColl KEL. *Porphyria: drug lists*. Glasgow: Porphyria Research Unit, University of Glasgow, 1991.
2. Gorchein A. Drug treatment in acute porphyria. *Br J Clin Pharmacol* 1997; **44:** 427–34.
3. Hommel L, *et al.* Acute bullous skin eruption after treatment with vigabatrine. *Dermatology* 1995; **191:** 181.

4-Amino-3-hydroxybutyric Acid (12360-n)

Buxamin; Gabob.

$C_4H_9NO_3$ = 119.1.

CAS — 352-21-6.

Aminohydroxybutyric acid has been claimed to be of value in a variety of neurological disorders including as an adjunct in the treatment of epilepsy. It should be distinguished from its isomer 3-amino-4-hydroxybutyric acid (Gobab) which is reported to possess anti-inflammatory and antifungal activity.

Preparations

Proprietary Preparations (details are given in Part 3)
Ital.: Gamibetal; ***Spain:*** Bogil.

Multi-ingredient: ***Ital.:*** Gamibetal Complex; Gamibetal Plus; Parvisedil; ***Spain:*** Cefabol; Disfil; Dorken; Gaboril Complex†; Gamalate B6; Paidenur†; Pertranquil; Plenumil†; Redutona.

Barbexaclone (12418-m)

Barbexaclone *(rINN).*

Compound of (−)-N,α-Dimethylcyclohexaneethylamine with 5-ethyl-5-phenylbarbituric acid.

$C_{12}H_{12}N_2O_3,C_{10}H_{21}N$ = 387.5.

CAS — 4388-82-3.

Barbexaclone is a compound of levopropylhexedrine (p.1485) with phenobarbitone (p.350). It is used in the treatment of various types of epilepsy (p.335). Usual adult doses are 200 to 400 mg daily given by mouth in divided doses.

Preparations

Proprietary Preparations (details are given in Part 3)
Aust.: Maliasin; ***Ger.:*** Maliasin; ***Ital.:*** Maliasin; ***Switz.:*** Maliasin.

Beclamide (6604-r)

Beclamide *(BAN, pINN).*

Benzchlorpropamide; Chlorethylphenamide. *N*-Benzyl-3-chloropropionamide.

$C_{10}H_{12}ClNO$ = 197.7.

CAS — 501-68-8.

Adverse Effects

Side-effects include dizziness, gastro-intestinal disturbances, loss of weight, skin rashes, transitory leucopenia, and renal disturbances.

Uses and Administration

Beclamide has been used as an antiepileptic for the control of tonic-clonic and simple partial seizures (p.335). It has also been used for the management of behaviour disorders (p.636).

Beclamide is given by mouth in a dosage of 1.5 to 3 g daily in divided doses. Suggested doses for children are: less than 5 years of age, 0.75 to 1 g daily; 5 to 10 years of age, 1.5 g daily.

Preparations

Proprietary Preparations (details are given in Part 3)
Ger.: Neuracen†; ***Spain:*** Posedrine.

Carbamazepine (6605-f)

Carbamazepine *(BAN, USAN, rINN).*

Carbamazepinum; G-32883. 5*H*-Dibenz[*b,f*]azepine-5-carboxamide.

$C_{15}H_{12}N_2O$ = 236.3.

CAS — 298-46-4.

Pharmacopoeias. In *Chin., Eur.* (see p.viii), *Int., Jpn, Pol.,* and *US.*

A white or almost white crystalline powder. It exhibits polymorphism.

Practically **insoluble** in water and in ether; soluble or sparingly soluble in alcohol and in acetone; freely soluble in dichloromethane. **Store** in airtight containers.

Incompatibility. Carbamazepine suspension should be mixed with an equal volume of diluent before nasogastric administration as undiluted suspension is adsorbed onto polyvinyl chloride nasogastric tubes.[1]

The FDA have received a report of a patient who passed an orange rubbery mass in his faeces the day after taking a carbamazepine suspension (Tegretol) followed immediately by chlorpromazine solution (Thorazine). Subsequent testing showed that mixing the same carbamazepine suspension with a thioridazine hydrochloride solution (Mellaril) also resulted in the precipitation of a rubbery orange mass.

1. Clark-Schmidt AL, *et al.* Loss of carbamazepine suspension through nasogastric feeding tubes. *Am J Hosp Pharm* 1990; **47:** 2034–7.

Stability. FDA studies indicate that carbamazepine tablets could lose up to one-third of their effectiveness if stored in humid conditions.[1] This appears to be due to formation of a dihydrate form which leads to hardening of the tablet resulting in poor dissolution and absorption.[2,3] As the dihydrate has also been detected after storage under ambient conditions some suggest that storage with silica gel sachets may be necessary to avoid physical deterioration of carbamazepine tablets.[2]

1. Anonymous. Moisture hardens carbamazepine tablets, FDA finds. *Am J Hosp Pharm* 1990; **47:** 958.
2. Lowes MMJ. More information on hardening of carbamazepine tablets. *Am J Hosp Pharm* 1991; **48:** 2130–1.
3. Wang JT, *et al.* Effects of humidity and temperature on in vitro dissolution of carbamazepine tablets. *J Pharm Sci* 1993; **82:** 1002–5.

Adverse Effects

Fairly common side-effects of carbamazepine, particularly in the initial stages of therapy, include dizziness, drowsiness, and ataxia. These effects may be minimised by starting therapy with a low dose. Drowsiness and disturbances of cerebellar and oculo-motor function (with ataxia, nystagmus, and diplopia) are also symptoms of excessive plasma concentrations of carbamazepine, and may disappear with continued treatment at reduced dosage.

Gastro-intestinal symptoms are reported to be less common, and include dry mouth, abdominal pain, nausea and vomiting, anorexia, and diarrhoea or constipation.

Generalised erythematous rashes may be severe and may necessitate withdrawal of treatment. Photosensitivity reactions, urticaria, exfoliative dermatitis, toxic epidermal necrolysis, erythema multiforme and the Stevens-Johnson syndrome, and systemic lupus erythematosus have also been reported.

Occasional reports of blood disorders include agranulocytosis, aplastic anaemia, eosinophilia, persistent leucopenia, leucocytosis, thrombocytopenia, and purpura. Lymphadenopathy, splenomegaly, pneumonitis, abnormalities of liver and kidney function, and cholestatic jaundice have occurred. Some or all of these symptoms as well as fever and rashes may represent a generalised hypersensitivity reaction to carbamazepine.

Other adverse effects reported include paraesthesia, headache, arrhythmias and heart block, heart failure, hyponatraemia and oedema, impotence, male infertility, gynaecomastia, galactorrhoea, and dystonias and dyskinesias with asterixis. Rectal administration has resulted in local irritation.

Overdosage may be manifested by many of the adverse effects listed above, especially those on the nervous system, and may result in stupor, coma, convulsions, respiratory depression, and death.

In rare cases, carbamazepine has been reported to exacerbate seizures in patients suffering from mixed-type epilepsy—see Precautions, below.

Congenital malformations have been reported in infants born to women who received carbamazepine during pregnancy.

Effects on the blood. Occasional reports of fatal haematological reactions associated with carbamazepine led the manufacturers to recommend extensive blood monitoring during therapy. However, because of the rarity of blood disorders due to carbamazepine these recommendations were questioned and the manufacturers subsequently modified their guidelines.

Case reports and studies of carbamazepine's haematological effects have been reviewed.[1] The incidence of haematological reactions to carbamazepine has been estimated to range between 1:10 800 and 1:38 000 per year while one group reported the rate of bone marrow suppression to be between 1:10 000 and 1:50 000 cases. The incidence of aplastic anaemia has been calculated to be 1:200 000 per year. Another investigator indicated that 2.2 deaths per million exposures were associated with aplastic anaemia and agranulocytosis. However, of 27 reports of aplastic anaemia (16 fatal) associated with carbamazepine many were found to have had coincidental disease or were receiving multiple-drug therapy. Benign or clinically insignificant leucopenia has occurred, usually during the first 3 months of treatment, in about 12% of children and 7% of adults but in most patients this resolved despite continuation of therapy. Mild transient thrombocytopenia has occurred in about 2% of patients; transient eosinophilia has also occurred.

The reviewers[1] suggested that all patients should have blood and platelet counts before treatment. Patients with low white cell and neutrophil counts are at risk of developing leucopenia and should be monitored every 2 weeks for the first 1 to 3 months. If counts fall further the dose should be reduced or treatment discontinued if necessary. Aplastic anaemia, agranulocytosis, and thrombocytopenia have a rapid onset and are best monitored by instructing the patient to report warning symptoms (see Precautions, below).

For a discussion of the effects of antiepileptics, including carbamazepine, on serum folate, see under Phenytoin, p.353.

1. Sobotka JL, *et al.* A review of carbamazepine's hematologic reactions and monitoring recommendations. *DICP Ann Pharmacother* 1990; **24:** 1214–19.

Effects on bone. For the effects of antiepileptics including carbamazepine on bone and on calcium and vitamin D metabolism, see under Phenytoin, p.353.

Effects on the endocrine system. There have been a number of reports of *hyponatraemia* or *water intoxication* in patients receiving carbamazepine.[1-6] One review[7] states that although hyponatraemia occurs in 10 to 15% of patients taking carbamazepine, it is seldom symptomatic or severe enough to cause fluid retention. However, care should be taken to distinguish the confusion, dizziness, nausea and headache of water intoxication from side-effects due to the central and gastro-intestinal effects of the drug.[2] The mechanism is uncertain; although some studies suggest an increase in secretion of antidiuretic hormone in subjects given carbamazepine,[3,4,6] others indicate the reverse,[5,8] and the fact that the hyponatraemic effects of carbamazepine can be partly reversed by demeclocycline[5] is cited as evidence for an effect on the kidney, either directly upon the distal tubule or by increasing sensitivity to the effects of antidiuretic hormone.

Carbamazepine may reduce serum concentrations of *thyroid* hormones through enzyme induction—see under Interactions of Thyroxine, p.1498.

For mention of the effects of antiepileptics on *sexual function* in male epileptic patients, see under Phenytoin, p.353.

1. Henry DA, *et al.* Hyponatraemia during carbamazepine treatment. *Br Med J* 1977; **1:** 83–4.
2. Stephens WP, *et al.* Water intoxication due to carbamazepine. *Br Med J* 1977; **1:** 754–5.
3. Ashton MG, *et al.* Water intoxication associated with carbamazepine treatment. *Br Med J* 1977; **1:** 1134–5.
4. Smith NJ, *et al.* Raised plasma arginine vasopressin concentration in carbamazepine-induced water intoxication. *Br Med J* 1977; **2:** 804.
5. Ballardie FW, Mucklow JC. Partial reversal of carbamazepine-induced water intolerance by demeclocycline. *Br J Clin Pharmacol* 1984; **17:** 763–5.
6. Sørensen PS, Hammer M. Effects of long-term carbamazepine treatment on water metabolism and plasma vasopressin concentration. *Eur J Clin Pharmacol* 1984; **26:** 719–22.
7. Mucklow J. Selected side-effects 2: carbamazepine and hyponatraemia. *Prescribers' J* 1991; **31:** 61–4.
8. Stephens WP, *et al.* Plasma arginine vasopressin concentrations and antidiuretic action of carbamazepine. *Br Med J* 1978; **1:** 1445–7.

Effects on the eyes. On rare occasions lenticular opacities have been associated with carbamazepine.[1] Retinotoxicity associated with long-term carbamazepine use has been reported[2] in 2 patients. Following discontinuation of the drug visual function and retinal morphological changes improved.

1. Anonymous. Adverse ocular effects of systemic drugs. *Med Lett Drugs Ther* 1976; **18:** 63–4.
2. Nielsen NV, Syversen K. Possible retinotoxic effect of carbamazepine. *Acta Ophthalmol (Copenh)* 1986; **64:** 287–90.

Effects on the heart. A review[1] of reports of cardiac effects associated with carbamazepine revealed that patients could be divided into 2 distinct groups based on their symptoms. One group consisted mainly of young patients with non life-threatening sinus tachycardia following carbamazepine overdosage while the other group was composed of older female patients with potentially life-threatening bradycardia or atrioventricular block associated with therapeutic or modestly raised blood concentrations of carbamazepine. However, there has been a report of fatal syncope, probably due to ventricular asystole, in a 20-year-old patient.[2] Carbamazepine should be avoided in patients who develop, or who are likely to develop, conduction abnormalities.[1]

Elevation of ventricular and atrial stimulation thresholds was reported in a 59-year-old man with a permanent dual-chamber pacemaker, 5 days after starting carbamazepine for mania.[3]

For a report of carbamazepine producing fatal eosinophilic myocarditis, see under Hypersensitivity, below.

1. Kasarkis EJ, *et al.* Carbamazepine-induced cardiac dysfunction: characterization of two distinct clinical syndromes. *Arch Intern Med* 1992; **152:** 186–91.
2. Stone S, Lange LS. Syncope and sudden unexpected death attributed to carbamazepine in a 20-year-old epileptic. *J Neurol Neurosurg Psychiatry* 1987; **49:** 1460–1.
3. Ambrosi P, *et al.* Carbamazepine and pacing threshold. *Lancet* 1993; **342:** 365.

Effects on the liver. Although adverse effects of carbamazepine on the liver are very rare, and often comprise only abnormal results from liver function tests,[1] they may occasionally be serious and deaths have occurred from liver failure[2] or hepatic necrosis.[3]

1. Hadžić N, *et al.* Acute liver failure induced by carbamazepine. *Arch Dis Child* 1990; **65:** 315–17.
2. Zucker P, *et al.* Fatal carbamazepine hepatitis. *J Pediatr* 1977; **91:** 667–8.
3. Smith DW, *et al.* Fatal hepatic necrosis associated with multiple anticonvulsant therapy. *Aust N Z J Med* 1988; **18:** 575–81.

Effects on mental function. Carbamazepine therapy has been associated in a few patients with the development of acute psychotic and paranoid symptoms[1-3] and with phobias[2] and mood disturbances, including mania[4] and melancholia.[5] One case of acute paranoid psychosis was associated with the addition of carbamazepine to long-term sodium valproate therapy in a patient subsequently diagnosed as having a schizotypal personality.[3] The problems of antiepileptic therapy adversely affecting cognition are discussed on p.337.

1. Berger H. An unusual manifestation of Tegretol® (carbamazepine) toxicity. *Ann Intern Med* 1971; **74:** 449–50.
2. Mathew G. Psychiatric symptoms associated with carbamazepine. *Br Med J* 1988; **296:** 1071.
3. McKee RJW, *et al.* Acute psychosis with carbamazepine and sodium valproate. *Lancet* 1989; **i:** 167.
4. Reiss AL, O'Donnell DJ. Carbamazepine-induced mania in two children: case report. *J Clin Psychiatry* 1984; **45:** 272–4.
5. Gardner DL, Cowdry RW. Development of melancholia during carbamazepine treatment in borderline personality disorder. *J Clin Psychopharmacol* 1986; **6:** 236–9.

Effects on the nervous system. ASEPTIC MENINGITIS. Aseptic meningitis has developed in a patient with Sjögren's syndrome given carbamazepine. It abated when the drug was withdrawn and symptoms recurred on rechallenge.[1] Aseptic meningitis has also been associated with carbamazepine in a patient without Sjögren's syndrome.[2]

1. Hilton E, Stroh EM. Aseptic meningitis associated with administration of carbamazepine. *J Infect Dis* 1989; **159:** 363–4.
2. Simon LT, *et al.* Carbamazepine-induced aseptic meningitis. *Ann Intern Med* 1990; **112:** 627–8.

EXTRAPYRAMIDAL EFFECTS. References to extrapyramidal effects associated with carbamazepine.

1. Crosley CJ, Swender PT. Dystonia associated with carbamazepine administration: experience in brain-damaged children. *Pediatrics* 1979; **63:** 612–15.
2. Jacome D. Carbamazepine-induced dystonia. *JAMA* 1979; **241:** 2263.
3. Joyce RP, Gunderson CH. Carbamazepine-induced orofacial dyskinesia. *Neurology* 1980; **30:** 1333–4.
4. Neglia JP, *et al.* Tics and vocalizations in children treated with carbamazepine. *Pediatrics* 1984; **73:** 841–4.

Effects on the skin. A report[1] of erythema multiforme following substitution of a generic for a proprietary brand of carbamazepine. Skin lesions resolved when the patient stopped taking the generic formulation and did not recur when the proprietary brand was restarted. A 6-year-old boy developed Stevens-Johnson syndrome 5 weeks after carbamazepine was added to valproic acid, which he had been taking as sole antiepileptic therapy for several weeks.[2] Carbamazepine was discontinued and the patient eventually made a full recovery; administration of valproic acid was continued because it was not thought to be the causative agent (but see under Valproate, p.362).

For a reference to successful desensitisation in patients who developed skin rashes on exposure to carbamazepine, see Hypersensitivity Reactions under Treatment of Adverse Effects, below.

1. Busch RL. Generic carbamazepine and erythema multiforme: generic-drug nonequivalency. *N Engl J Med* 1989; **321:** 692–3.
2. Keating A, Blahunka P. Carbamazepine-induced Stevens-Johnson syndrome in a child. *Ann Pharmacother* 1995; **29:** 538–9.

Hypersensitivity. A syndrome comprising lymphadenopathy, fever, and rash and less commonly hepatosplenomegaly and eosinophilia has been associated with carbamazepine.[1] Although a literature search was only able to find 20 published cases to 1986, 22 cases had been reported to the Australian Adverse Drug Reactions Advisory Committee between 1975 and 1990. A positive rechallenge in 2 patients tested suggests that the syndrome is due to a hypersensitivity reaction. Most reactions occurred within 30 days of the start of administration.

Carbamazepine antibodies were detected in an 8-year-old child who developed symptoms of serum sickness including fever, skin rash, oedema, and lymphadenopathy during treatment with carbamazepine.[2] Hypersensitivity to carbamazepine with multisystem effects clinically resembling a mononucleosis syndrome was reported in a 15-year-old boy 2 weeks after starting monotherapy with carbamazepine.[3] All symptoms resolved after discontinuation of carbamazepine and treatment with prednisone.

A hypersensitivity reaction producing fatal eosinophilic myocarditis has been reported in a 13-year-old patient; initial symptoms mimicked scarlet fever.[4]

For references to successful desensitisation in patients sensitive to carbamazepine, see Hypersensitivity Reactions under Treatment of Adverse Effects, below.

1. Anonymous. Anticonvulsants and lymphadenopathy. *WHO Drug Inf* 1991; **5:** 11.
2. Hosoda N, *et al.* Anticarbamazepine antibody induced by carbamazepine in a patient with severe serum sickness. *Arch Dis Child* 1991; **66:** 722–3.
3. Merino N, *et al.* Multisystem hypersensitivity reaction to carbamazepine. *Ann Pharmacother* 1994; **28:** 402–3.
4. Salzman MB, *et al.* Carbamazepine and fatal eosinophilic myocarditis. *N Engl J Med* 1997; **336:** 878–9.

Systemic lupus erythematosus. A review[1] of 80 cases of systemic lupus erythematosus-like syndromes associated with carbamazepine that had been reported to the manufacturer suggested that the frequency of reports (less than 0.001%) was below that for idiopathic lupus. The symptoms due to carbamazepine usually resolved on discontinuation of treatment whereas persistence would have implied a diagnosis of idiopathic disease.

1. Jain KK. Systemic lupus erythematosus (SLE)-like syndromes associated with carbamazepine therapy. *Drug Safety* 1991; **6:** 350–60.

Treatment of Adverse Effects

In the treatment of carbamazepine overdosage the stomach should be emptied by lavage; repeated doses of activated charcoal may be given with the aim not only of preventing absorption but also of aiding elimination. Supportive and symptomatic therapy alone may then suffice; haemoperfusion has been suggested for the management of the more severely poisoned patient (but see below).

Hypersensitivity reactions. Successful desensitisation to carbamazepine was reported[1] in a 12-year-old boy who was sensitive to carbamazepine, sodium valproate, and phenytoin. Starting with a low dose of carbamazepine 0.1 mg daily the dose was doubled, generally every 2 days, up to 100 mg daily. The dose was then gradually increased over 4 weeks to a maintenance dose of 200 mg twice daily. The same technique was used to desensitise 7 patients all of whom developed dramatic skin rashes when first exposed to carbamazepine.[2] Carbamazepine treatment in full doses was achieved without problem in about 6 weeks.

1. Smith H, Newton R. Adverse reactions to carbamazepine managed by desensitisation. *Lancet* 1985; **i:** 753.
2. Eames P. Adverse reactions to carbamazepine managed by desensitisation. *Lancet* 1989; **i:** 509–10.

Overdosage. Carbamazepine poisoning and its management has been reviewed.[1,2] Gastric lavage may be particularly useful in carbamazepine overdosage as the antimuscarinic effects delay gastric emptying. In patients who are comatose or who have lost the gag reflex gastric lavage may be performed via a large-bore orogastric tube following endotracheal intubation. In alert patients at low risk of loss of consciousness emesis may be induced with ipecacuanha [although UK authorities consider this to be of very limited value]. Supportive measures such as management of airways, ventilation and monitoring of cardiovascular function and electrolyte balance are most important. Administration of activated charcoal, via a nasogastric tube is effective and should be continued until the patient is free of symptoms.[1] Although charcoal haemoperfusion is also of value, repeated oral doses of activated charcoal seem to be as effective and less invasive.

A report[3] of the use of plasmapheresis in the treatment of an acute overdose of carbamazepine concluded that plasmapheresis removed a very small percentage of the total body load of carbamazepine and could not be recommended.

Death due to carbamazepine overdosage does occasionally occur and the cause reported in two cases was aspiration of gastric contents;[2] the authors considered this to be a major danger of carbamazepine overdosage.

1. Durelli L, *et al.* Carbamazepine toxicity and poisoning: incidence, clinical features and management. *Med Toxicol Adverse Drug Exp* 1989; **4:** 95–107.
2. Denning DW, *et al.* Death due to carbamazepine self-poisoning: remedies reviewed. *Hum Toxicol* 1985; **4:** 255–60.
3. Kale PB, *et al.* Evaluation of plasmapheresis in the treatment of an acute overdose of carbamazepine. *Ann Pharmacother* 1993; **27:** 866–70.

Precautions

Carbamazepine should be avoided in patients with atrioventricular conduction abnormalities. It should not be given to patients with a history of bone marrow depression. Carbamazepine should be given with caution to patients with a history of blood disorders or of cardiac, hepatic, or renal disease. Patients or their carers should be told how to recognise signs of blood, liver, and skin toxicity and they should be advised to seek immediate medical attention if symptoms such as fever, sore throat, rash, mouth ulcers, bruising, or bleeding develop. Carbamazepine should be withdrawn, if necessary under cover of a suitable alternative antiepileptic, if leucopenia which is severe, progressive, or associated with clinical symptoms develops. Care is required in identifying patients with mixed seizure disorders that include generalised absence or atypical absence seizures, who may be at risk of an increase in generalised seizures if given carbamazepine. It may also exacerbate absence and myoclonic seizures.

Care is required when withdrawing carbamazepine therapy—see also under Uses and Administration, below.

Since carbamazepine has mild antimuscarinic properties caution should be observed in patients with glaucoma or raised intra-ocular pressure; scattered punctate lens opacities occur rarely with carbamazepine and it has been suggested that patients should be examined periodically for eye changes.

Abuse. Overdosage requiring hospital admission has been reported following abuse of carbamazepine.[1]

1. Crawford PJ, Fisher BM. Recreational overdosage of carbamazepine in Paisley drug abusers. *Scott Med J* 1997; **42:** 44–5.

Breast feeding. For comment on antiepileptic therapy and breast feeding, see under Pregnancy on p.337.

Driving. For comment on antiepileptic drugs and driving, see p.337.

Porphyria. Carbamazepine has been associated with acute attacks of porphyria and is considered unsafe in patients with acute porphyria.[1]

1. Moore MR, McColl KEL. *Porphyria: drug lists*. Glasgow: Porphyria Research Unit, University of Glasgow, 1991.

Pregnancy. For comments on the management of epilepsy during pregnancy, see p.337.

There is an increased risk of neural tube defects in infants exposed *in utero* to antiepileptics including carbamazepine and a variety of syndromes such as craniofacial and digital abnormalities and, less commonly, cleft lip and palate have been described. Exposure to carbamazepine has been calculated to carry a 1% risk of spina bifida.[1] A 'carbamazepine syndrome' characterised by facial dysmorphic features and mild mental retardation has been described.[2] There is also a risk of neonatal bleeding.

1. Rosa FW. Spina bifida in infants of women treated with carbamazepine during pregnancy. *N Engl J Med* 1991; **324:** 674–7.
2. Ornoy A, Cohen E. Outcome of children born to epileptic mothers treated with carbamazepine during pregnancy. *Arch Dis Child* 1996; **75:** 517–20.

Interactions

There are complex interactions between antiepileptics and toxicity may be enhanced without a corresponding increase in antiepileptic activity. Such interactions are very variable and unpredictable and plasma monitoring is often advisable with combination therapy.

The metabolism of carbamazepine is reported to be less susceptible to inhibition by other drugs than that of phenytoin but a few drugs are reported to inhibit its metabolism, resulting in raised plasma concentrations and associated toxicity.

Carbamazepine is a hepatic enzyme inducer and induces its own metabolism as well as that of a number of other drugs, including some antibacterials (notably, doxycycline), anticoagulants, and sex hormones (notably, oral contraceptives). Carbamazepine and phenytoin may also mutually enhance one another's metabolism. The metabolism of carbamazepine is similarly enhanced by enzyme inducers such as phenobarbitone.

General references.

1. Spina E, *et al.* Clinically significant pharmacokinetic drug interactions with carbamazepine: an update. *Clin Pharmacokinet* 1996; **31:** 198–214.

Alcohol. Alcohol may exacerbate the CNS side-effects of carbamazepine.

Analgesics. *Dextropropoxyphene* has been reported to cause substantial elevation of serum-carbamazepine concentrations[1] and carbamazepine toxicity[1,2] when the two drugs are given together, probably due to inhibition of carbamazepine metabolism.[1]

1. Dam M, Christiansen J. Interaction of propoxyphene with carbamazepine. *Lancet* 1977; **ii:** 509.
2. Yu YL, *et al.* Interaction between carbamazepine and dextropropoxyphene. *Postgrad Med J* 1986; **62:** 231–3.

Anthelmintics. For the effect of carbamazepine on *mebendazole* and *praziquantel*, see p.104 and p.108, respectively.

Antibacterials. The antimycobacterial *isoniazid*[1,2] and macrolides such as *triacetyloleandomycin*[3,4] and *erythromycin*[4-7] have been reported to cause substantial elevations of serum concentrations of carbamazepine and symptoms of carbamazepine toxicity[1-4,6,7] when given to patients concomitantly with the antiepileptic. *Clarithromycin* has also been reported to increase serum concentrations of carbamazepine.[8]

Carbamazepine may enhance the metabolism of *doxycycline*.[9]

1. Valsalan VC, Cooper GL. Carbamazepine intoxication caused by interaction with isoniazid. *Br Med J* 1982; **285:** 261–2.
2. Wright JM, *et al.* Isoniazid-induced carbamazepine toxicity and vice versa. *N Engl J Med* 1982; **307:** 1325–7.
3. Dravet C, *et al.* Interaction between carbamazepine and triacetyloleandomycin. *Lancet* 1977; **i:** 810–11.
4. Mesdjian E, *et al.* Carbamazepine intoxication due to triacetyloleandomycin administration in epileptic patients. *Epilepsia* 1980; **21:** 489–96.
5. Wong YY, *et al.* Effect of erythromycin on carbamazepine kinetics. *Clin Pharmacol Ther* 1983; **33:** 460–4.
6. Hedrick R, *et al.* Carbamazepine-erythromycin interaction leading to carbamazepine toxicity in four epileptic children. *Ther Drug Monit* 1983; **5:** 405–7.
7. Mitsch RA. Carbamazepine toxicity precipitated by intravenous erythromycin. *Drug Intell Clin Pharm* 1989; **23:** 878–9.
8. Albani F, *et al.* Clarithromycin-carbamazepine interaction: a case report. *Epilepsia* 1993; **34:** 161–2.
9. Neuvonen PJ, *et al.* Effect of antiepileptic drugs on the elimination of various tetracycline derivatives. *Eur J Clin Pharmacol* 1975; **9:** 147–54.

Anticoagulants. For the effect of carbamazepine on warfarin, see p.967.

Antidepressants. As with all antiepileptics, antidepressants may antagonise the antiepileptic activity of carbamazepine by lowering the convulsive threshold.

Antidepressants such as *fluoxetine*,[1] *fluvoxamine*,[2] and *viloxazine*[3] increase plasma concentrations of carbamazepine and may induce carbamazepine toxicity. A toxic serotonin syndrome has been reported in a patient who received *fluoxetine* and carbamazepine concomitantly.[4] Severe neurotoxicity reported during concomitant therapy with *lithium* and carbamazepine[5,6] may be due to a synergistic effect as reports indicate that either drug was tolerated when not administered with the other and measured plasma concentrations did not indicate overdosage.[6]

Because of the structural similarity to tricyclic antidepressants the manufacturers have suggested that carbamazepine should not be given to patients taking an *MAOI* or within 14 days of stopping such treatment.

For the effect of carbamazepine on antidepressants, see Mianserin (p.297) and Amitriptyline (p.277).

1. Pearson HJ. Interaction of fluoxetine with carbamazepine. *J Clin Psychiatry* 1990; **51:** 126.
2. Fritze J, *et al.* Interaction between carbamazepine and fluvoxamine. *Acta Psychiatr Scand* 1991; **84:** 583–4.
3. Scarpello JHB, Cottrell N. Overuse of monitoring of blood concentrations of antiepileptic drugs. *Br Med J* 1987; **294:** 1355.
4. Dursun SM, *et al.* Toxic serotonin syndrome after fluoxetine plus carbamazepine. *Lancet* 1993; **342:** 442–3.
5. Andrus PF. Lithium and carbamazepine. *J Clin Psychiatry* 1984; **45:** 525.
6. Chaudhry RP, Waters BGH. Lithium and carbamazepine interaction: possible neurotoxicity. *J Clin Psychiatry* 1983; **44:** 30–1.

Antiepileptics. Interactions of varying degrees of clinical significance have been reported between carbamazepine and other antiepileptics.

Serum concentrations of carbamazepine are reported to be reduced by *phenobarbitone*, but without loss of seizure control;[1,2] this reduction is probably due to induction of carbamazepine metabolism.

The interaction with *phenytoin* is somewhat more complex and the consequences vary. There is evidence of a lowering of serum-carbamazepine concentrations, presumably due to induction of metabolism by phenytoin;[1-3] in return carbamazepine has been reported both to lower and increase serum phenytoin—see p.355. Again, these reports do not indicate a loss of seizure control or toxicity resulting from the interaction, although the possibility presumably exists. Gradually withdrawing phenytoin from 2 patients who had been receiving carbamazepine and phenytoin as combination antiepileptic therapy resulted in a dramatic increase in plasma-carbamazepine concentrations;[4] one patient exhibited neurotoxic symptoms. The authors recommended that plasma-carbamazepine monitoring should be carried out whenever phenytoin administration is discontinued in patients receiving these two drugs together.

Valproic acid produces an increase in serum concentrations of the active epoxide metabolite of carbamazepine. This is usually attributed to inhibition of its hydrolysis by epoxide hydrolase,[5] although an additional proposed mechanism[6] is inhibition of the glucuronidation of carbamazepine-10,11-trans-diol, the compound that the epoxide is converted to under normal circumstances. Adverse effects may be a problem if unusually high epoxide concentrations arise but, in general, this interaction is of limited clinical significance. However, *valpromide*, the amide derivative of valproic acid is a much more powerful inhibitor of epoxide hydrolase than valproic acid,[7-9] and therefore produces greater increases in epoxide plasma concentrations with clinical signs of toxicity.[8] Switching from sodium valproate to valpromide has resulted in toxicity in patients also receiving carbamazepine.[8] Neither valproic acid nor valpromide have any significant effect on plasma concentrations of the parent drug, carbamazepine. *Valnoctamide,* an isomer of valpromide, appears to be at least as potent as valpromide in inhibiting the elimination of the epoxide metabolite of carbamazepine.[10] Valnoctamide is used as an anxiolytic preparation, although it does appear to possess some antiepileptic activity. For a report of acute psychosis associated with the combination of carbamazepine and sodium valproate, see Effects on Mental Function under Adverse Effects, above. For the effects of carbamazepine on valproic acid, see p.363.

For the effects of carbamazepine on *ethosuximide*, see p.345.

Of the newer antiepileptics *stiripentol*[11] has been reported to inhibit carbamazepine metabolism, while *felbamate* causes a significant fall in plasma-carbamazepine concentrations which may require an increase in the dose of carbamazepine.[12] However, another study[13] has shown a significant increase in plasma-concentrations of the active epoxide metabolite, which may counteract the effect of the decrease in plasma concentrations of the parent compound. Neurotoxicity has been observed following use of carbamazepine with *lamotrigine*.[14] The suggestion that this was due to raised concentrations of carbamazepine epoxide was not confirmed in a controlled study in which the 2 drugs were used together safely and effectively.[15] *Progabide* has been reported to increase plasma concentrations of the epoxide metabolite, probably due to inhibition of microsomal epoxide hydrolase.[16] For the effects of carbamazepine on *topiramate*, see p.360.

For interactions with benzodiazepines, see below.

1. Cereghino JJ, *et al.* The efficacy of carbamazepine combinations in epilepsy. *Clin Pharmacol Ther* 1975; **18:** 733–41.
2. Rane A, *et al.* Kinetics of carbamazepine and its 10,11-epoxide metabolite in children. *Clin Pharmacol Ther* 1976; **19:** 276–83.
3. Christiansen J, Dam M. Influence of phenobarbital and diphenylhydantoin on plasma carbamazepine levels in patients with epilepsy. *Acta Neurol Scand* 1973; **49:** 543–6.
4. Chapron DJ, *et al.* Unmasking the significant enzyme-inducing effects of phenytoin on serum carbamazepine concentrations during phenytoin withdrawal. *Ann Pharmacother* 1993; **27:** 708–11.
5. Kerr BM, Levy RH. Carbamazepine epoxide. In: Levy RH, *et al.* eds. *Antiepileptic drugs*. 4th ed. New York: Raven Press, 1995: 529–41.
6. Bernus I, *et al.* The mechanism of the carbamazepine-valproate interaction in humans. *Br J Clin Pharmacol* 1997; **44:** 21–7.
7. Levy RH, *et al.* Inhibition of carbamazepine epoxide elimination by valpromide and valproic acid. *Epilepsia* 1986; **27:** 592.
8. Meijer JWA, *et al.* Possible hazard of valpromide-carbamazepine combination therapy in epilepsy. *Lancet* 1984; **i:** 802.
9. Pisani F, *et al.* Effect of valpromide on the pharmacokinetics of carbamazepine-10,11-epoxide. *Br J Clin Pharmacol* 1988; **25:** 611–13.
10. Pisani F, *et al.* Impairment of carbamazepine-10,11-epoxide elimination by valnoctamide, a valpromide isomer, in healthy subjects. *Br J Clin Pharmacol* 1992; **34:** 85–7.
11. Levy RH, *et al.* Stiripentol level-dose relationship and interaction with carbamazepine in epileptic patients. *Epilepsia* 1985; **26:** 544–5.
12. Albani F, *et al.* Effect of felbamate on plasma levels of carbamazepine and its metabolites. *Epilepsia* 1991; **32:** 130–2.
13. Wagner ML, *et al.* Effect of felbamate on carbamazepine and its major metabolites. *Clin Pharmacol Ther* 1993; **53:** 536–43.
14. Warner T, *et al.* Lamotrigine-induced carbamazepine toxicity: an interaction with carbamazepine-10,11-epoxide. *Epilepsy Res* 1992; **11:** 147–50.
15. Stolarek I, *et al.* Vigabatrin and lamotrigine in refractory epilepsy. *J Neurol Neurosurg Psychiatry* 1994; **57:** 921–4.
16. Kroetz DL, *et al.* In vivo and in vitro correlation of microsomal epoxide hydrolase inhibition by progabide. *Clin Pharmacol Ther* 1993; **54:** 485–97.

Antifungals. Malaise, myoclonus, and trembling are reported[1] to have developed in a patient receiving carbamazepine following the addition of *miconazole* to therapy. For the effect of carbamazepine on *itraconazole*, see p.382.

1. Loupi E, *et al.* Interactions médicamenteuses et miconazole. *Therapie* 1982; **37:** 437–41.

Antihistamines. *Terfenadine* and carbamazepine are both highly protein bound and therefore may compete for protein binding sites. An 18-year-old woman receiving carbamazepine as an antiepileptic experienced symptoms of neurotoxicity shortly after starting treatment with terfenadine for rhinitis.[1] The concentration of free carbamazepine in the plasma was higher than normal and returned to normal on discontinuation of terfenadine.

1. Hirschfeld S, Jarosinski P. Drug interaction of terfenadine and carbamazepine. *Ann Intern Med* 1993; **118:** 907–8.

Antimalarials. *Chloroquine* and *mefloquine* may antagonise the antiepileptic activity of carbamazepine by lowering the convulsive threshold.

Antiprotozoals. A patient receiving carbamazepine for bipolar disorder developed dizziness, diplopia, and nausea four days after the addition of *metronidazole* for diverticulitis.[1]

1. Patterson BD. Possible interaction between metronidazole and carbamazepine. *Ann Pharmacother* 1994; **28:** 1303–4.

Antipsychotics. As with all antiepileptics, antipsychotics may antagonise the antiepileptic activity of carbamazepine by lowering the convulsive threshold. Increased plasma concentrations of carbamazepine epoxide have been reported to occur during concomitant therapy with carbamazepine and *loxapine*, possibly due to induction of carbamazepine metabolism or inhibition of metabolism of the epoxide.[1] Raised serum concentrations of carbamazepine have also been reported in patients receiving *haloperidol*.[2] For the effect of carbamazepine on haloperidol, see under Chlorpromazine, p.653.

1. Collins DM, *et al.* Potential interaction between carbamazepine and loxapine: case report and retrospective review. *Ann Pharmacother* 1993; **27:** 1180–3.
2. Iwahashi K, *et al.* The drug-drug interaction effects of haloperidol on plasma carbamazepine levels. *Clin Neuropharmacol* 1995; **18:** 233–6.

Antivirals. *Ritonavir* inhibits several microsomal liver enzymes and therefore may potentially interact with antiepileptics such as carbamazepine. The manufacturer of ritonavir advises that such combinations may require patient monitoring or should be avoided.

Anxiolytics. For a discussion of the potential interaction between carbamazepine and the anxiolytic *valnoctamide*, an isomer of the antiepileptic valpromide, see under Antiepileptics, above.

See also under Benzodiazepines, below.

Benzodiazepines. The metabolism of benzodiazepines may be enhanced in patients who have received long-term therapy with carbamazepine due to induction of hepatic drug-metabolising enzymes; the benzodiazepine plasma concentrations are reduced, its half-life is shorter, and clearance is increased.[1,2] Some benzodiazepines may also affect carbamazepine. One group of workers reported that after addition of *clobazam* to carbamazepine therapy a dose reduction for the latter was required due to increased blood concentrations.[3] In a later study[4] it appeared that clobazam could produce a moderate increase in the metabolism of carbamazepine. The plasma ratio of metabolites of carbamazepine, including carbamazepine-10,11-epoxide, to parent compound was increased in patients taking clobazam and carbamazepine.

1. Dhillon S, Richens A. Pharmacokinetics of diazepam in epileptic patients and normal volunteers following intravenous administration. *Br J Clin Pharmacol* 1981; **12:** 841–4.
2. Lai AA, *et al.* Time-course of interaction between carbamazepine and clonazepam in normal man. *Clin Pharmacol Ther* 1978; **24:** 316–23.
3. Franceschi M, *et al.* Clobazam in drug-resistant and alcoholic withdrawal seizures. *Clin Trials J* 1983; **20:** 119–25.
4. Muñoz JJ, *et al.* The effect of clobazam on steady state plasma concentrations of carbamazepine and its metabolites. *Br J Clin Pharmacol* 1990; **29:** 763–5.

Calcium-channel blockers. Six patients with steady-state carbamazepine concentrations experienced symptoms of neurotoxicity consistent with carbamazepine intoxication within 36 to 96 hours of the administration of the first dose of *verapamil.*[1] In 5 patients, in whom plasma concentrations were measured, there was a mean increase of 46% in total carbamazepine and 33% in free carbamazepine; no effect on the plasma protein binding of carbamazepine was observed. The results suggested that verapamil inhibits the metabolism of carbamazepine to an extent likely to have important clinical repercussions. There has also been a report[2] of a patient in whom *diltiazem*, but not *nifedipine*, precipitated carbamazepine neurotoxicity.

For the effect of carbamazepine on dihydropyridine calcium-channel blockers, see under Nifedipine, p.918.

1. Macphee GJA, *et al.* Verapamil potentiates carbamazepine neurotoxicity: a clinically important inhibitory interaction. *Lancet* 1986; **i:** 700–703.
2. Brodie MJ, Macphee GJA. Carbamazepine neurotoxicity precipitated by diltiazem. *Br Med J* 1986; **292:** 1170–1.

Corticosteroids. For the effect of carbamazepine on corticosteroids, see p.1014.

Cyclosporin. For the effect of carbamazepine on cyclosporin, see p.521.

Danazol. Co-administration of *danazol* with carbamazepine has been reported to increase the half-life and decrease clearance of carbamazepine,[1] resulting in increases in plasma-carbamazepine concentrations of up to 100%[1,2] and resultant toxicity in a number of patients.[2]

1. Krämer G, *et al.* Carbamazepine-danazol drug interaction: its mechanism examined by a stable isotope technique. *Ther Drug Monit* 1986; **8:** 387–92.
2. Zielinski JJ, *et al.* Clinically significant danazol-carbamazepine interaction. *Ther Drug Monit* 1987; **9:** 24–7.

Dermatological drugs. In one patient stabilised on carbamazepine therapy addition of *isotretinoin* appeared to reduce plasma concentrations of carbamazepine and its active epoxide metabolite.[1] However, no adverse events were noted during a 6-week period of treatment with isotretinoin.

1. Marsden JR. Effect of isotretinoin on carbamazepine pharmacokinetics. *Br J Dermatol* 1988; **119:** 403–4.

Diuretics. There has been a report of symptomatic hyponatraemia associated with concomitant use of carbamazepine and a diuretic (*hydrochlorothiazide* or *frusemide*).[1] Carbamazepine serum concentrations are increased by concomitant administration of *acetazolamide*.[2]

1. Yassa R, *et al.* Carbamazepine, diuretics, and hyponatremia: a possible interaction. *J Clin Psychiatry* 1987; **48:** 281–3.
2. McBride MC. Serum carbamazepine levels are increased by acetazolamide. *Ann Neurol* 1984; **16:** 393.

Gastro-intestinal drugs. *Cimetidine* is reported to produce a transient increase in plasma-carbamazepine concentrations, followed by a return to pre-cimetidine values within about a week;[1] some increase in side-effects was seen. *Ranitidine* does not appear to affect plasma-carbamazepine concentrations.[2] Neurotoxicity has been observed in a patient receiving carbamazepine and *metoclopramide*.[3]

1. Dalton MJ, *et al.* Cimetidine and carbamazepine: a complex drug interaction. *Epilepsia* 1986; **27:** 553–8.
2. Dalton MJ, *et al.* Ranitidine does not alter single-dose carbamazepine pharmacokinetics in healthy adults. *Drug Intell Clin Pharm* 1985; **19:** 941–4.
3. Sandyk R. Carbamazepine and metoclopramide interaction: possible neurotoxicity. *Br Med J* 1984; **288:** 830.

Grapefruit juice. The bioavailability and plasma concentrations of carbamazepine have been reported[1] to be increased by grapefruit juice.

1. Garg SK, *et al.* Effect of grapefruit juice on carbamazepine bioavailability in patients with epilepsy. *Clin Pharmacol Ther* 1998; **64:** 286–8.

Neuromuscular blockers. For the effect of carbamazepine on *suxamethonium*, see p.1321 and on *competitive neuromuscular blockers*, see under Atracurium, p.1306.

Sex hormones. For the effect of carbamazepine on sex hormones, particularly in oral contraceptives, see p.1433.

Theophylline. A decrease in serum-carbamazepine concentrations of about 50% was reported[1] in an epileptic patient given theophylline. The patient experienced seizures and the proposed mechanism was that theophylline had increased the metabolism of carbamazepine.

For the effect of carbamazepine on theophylline, see p.769.

1. Mitchell EA, *et al.* Interaction between carbamazepine and theophylline. *N Z Med J* 1986; **99:** 69–70.

Thyroxine. For the effect of carbamazepine on thyroxine, see p.1498.

Vitamins. The plasma concentration of carbamazepine was increased in 2 patients given *nicotinamide*.[1] For the effect of antiepileptics, including carbamazepine, on *vitamin D* concentrations, see Effects on Bone under the Adverse Effects of Phenytoin, p.353.

1. Bourgeois BFD, *et al.* Interactions between primidone, carbamazepine, and nicotinamide. *Neurology* 1982; **32:** 1122–6.

Pharmacokinetics

Carbamazepine is slowly and irregularly absorbed from the gastro-intestinal tract. It is extensively metabolised in the liver and one of its primary metabolites, carbamazepine-10,11-epoxide is also active. Carbamazepine is excreted in the urine almost entirely in the form of its metabolites; some is also excreted in faeces. Elimination of carbamazepine is reported to be more rapid in children and accumulation of the active metabolite may often be higher than in adults.

Carbamazepine is widely distributed throughout the body and is extensively bound (about 75%) to plasma proteins. It induces its own metabolism so that the plasma half-life may be considerably reduced after repeated administration. Estimation of the mean plasma half-life of carbamazepine on repeated administration is about 10 to 20 hours; it appears to be considerably shorter in children than in adults. Moreover, the metabolism of carbamazepine is readily induced by drugs which induce hepatic microsomal enzymes (see under Interactions, above).

Monitoring of plasma concentrations may be performed as an aid in assessing control and the therapeutic range of total plasma-carbamazepine is usually quoted as being about 4 to 12 µg per mL (16 to 50 µmol per litre), although this is subject to considerable variation. It has been suggested by some, but not all investigators, that measurement of free carbamazepine concentrations in plasma may prove more reliable, and measurement of concentrations in saliva or tears, which contain only free carbamazepine, has also been performed.

Carbamazepine crosses the placental barrier and is distributed into breast milk.

The pharmacokinetics of carbamazepine are affected by the concomitant administration of other antiepileptics (see under Interactions, above).

References.

1. Schmidt D, Haenel F. Therapeutic plasma levels of phenytoin, phenobarbital, and carbamazepine: individual variation in relation to seizure frequency and type. *Neurology* 1984; **34:** 1252–5.
2. Bertilsson L, Tomson T. Clinical pharmacokinetics and pharmacological effects of carbamazepine and carbamazepine-10,11-epoxide: an update. *Clin Pharmacokinet* 1986; **11:** 177–98.
3. Gilman JT. Carbamazepine dosing for pediatric seizure disorders: the highs and lows. *DICP Ann Pharmacother* 1991; **25:** 1109–12.
4. Kodama Y, *et al.* In vivo binding characteristics of carbamazepine and carbamazepine-10,11-epoxide to serum proteins in paediatric patients with epilepsy. *Eur J Clin Pharmacol* 1993; **44:** 291–3.
5. Bernus I, *et al.* Early stage autoinduction of carbamazepine metabolism in humans. *Eur J Clin Pharmacol* 1994; **47:** 355–60.
6. Caraco Y, *et al.* Carbamazepine pharmacokinetics in obese and lean subjects. *Ann Pharmacother* 1995; **29:** 843–7.
7. Mahmood I, Chamberlin N. A limited sampling method for the estimation of AUC and C_{max} of carbamazepine and carbamazepine epoxide following a single and multiple dose of a sustained-release product. *Br J Clin Pharmacol* 1998; **45:** 241–6.
8. Cohen H, *et al.* Feasibility and pharmacokinetics of carbamazepine oral loading doses. *Am J Health-Syst Pharm* 1998; **55:** 1134–40.

Uses and Administration

Carbamazepine is a dibenzazepine derivative with antiepileptic and psychotropic properties. It is used to control secondarily generalised tonic-clonic seizures and partial seizures. Carbamazepine is also used in the treatment of trigeminal neuralgia and has been tried with variable success in glossopharyngeal neuralgia and other severe pain syndromes associated with neurological disorders such as tabes dorsalis and multiple sclerosis. Another use of carbamazepine is in the prophylaxis of manic depression (bipolar disorder) unresponsive to lithium.

In the treatment of **epilepsy**, the dose of carbamazepine should be adjusted to the needs of the individual patient to achieve adequate control of seizures; this usually requires total plasma-carbamazepine concentrations of about 4 to 12 µg per mL (16 to 50 µmol per litre). A low initial dose of carbamazepine is recommended to minimise side-effects. The suggested initial oral dose is 100 to 200 mg once or twice daily gradually increased by increments of 100 to 200 mg every 2 weeks to a usual maintenance dose of 0.8 to 1.2 g daily in divided doses; up to 2 g daily may occasionally be necessary. The usual oral dosage in children based on body-weight is 10 to 20 mg per kg daily in divided doses. Alternatively the dose may be expressed in terms of the age of the child and suggested daily doses are: up to 1 year of age, 100 to 200 mg; 1 to 5 years, 200 to 400 mg; 5 to 10 years, 400 to 600 mg; 10 to 15 years, 0.6 to 1 g.

Oral daily doses are divided and carbamazepine is usually given 2 to 4 times daily. A twice-daily regimen may be associated with improved compliance but may produce widely fluctuating plasma-carbamazepine concentrations leading to intermittent side-effects. However, twice-daily administration may be suitable for patients receiving carbamazepine as monotherapy, and without peak-related side-effects. Also modified-release formulations can minimise fluctuations in plasma concentration and may allow effective twice-daily administration. Different preparations vary in bioavailability and it may be prudent to avoid changing the formulation.

The time and manner of taking carbamazepine should be standardised for the patient since variations might affect absorption with consequent fluctuations in the plasma concentrations.

Carbamazepine may be given by the rectal route in doses up to a maximum of 250 mg every 6 hours to patients for whom oral treatment is temporarily not possible. The dosage should be increased by about 25% when changing from an oral formulation to suppositories, and it is recommended that the rectal route should not be used for longer than 7 days.

As with other antiepileptics, withdrawal of carbamazepine therapy or transition to or from another type of antiepileptic therapy should be made gradually to avoid precipitating an increase in the frequency of seizures. For a discussion on whether or not to withdraw antiepileptic therapy in seizure-free patients, see p.335.

In the treatment of **trigeminal neuralgia** the initial dose of carbamazepine is 100 mg once or twice daily by mouth increased gradually as necessary; the usual maintenance dose is 400 to 800 mg daily in 2 to 4 divided doses but up to 1.6 g daily may be required. When pain relief has been obtained attempts should be made to reduce and ultimately discontinue the therapy, until another attack occurs.

For the prophylaxis of **manic depression**, carbamazepine is given in an initial oral dose of 400 mg daily in divided doses, increased gradually as necessary up to a maximum of 1.6 g daily; the usual maintenance dose range is 400 to 600 mg daily.

Administration. A modified-release formulation of carbamazepine produced a substantial reduction in intra-dose fluctuations in carbamazepine concentrations[1] and tolerability and seizure control in patients with epilepsy may be improved.[2,3] However, bioavailability appeared to be slightly less than conventional preparations and dosage adjustments may be required when changing between formulations.[1] A modified-release formulation should be considered in patients receiving high doses who suffer intermittent adverse effects such as diplopia, nausea, dizziness and tiredness, and may offer the opportunity to convert a three or four times daily regimen to twice- or even, in some patients, once-daily administration.[2,4]

1. McKee PJW, *et al.* Monotherapy with conventional and controlled-release carbamazepine: a double-blind, double-dummy comparison in epileptic patients. *Br J Clin Pharmacol* 1991; **32:** 99–104.
2. Anonymous. Carbamazepine update. *Lancet* 1989; **ii:** 595–7.
3. Ryan SW, *et al.* Slow release carbamazepine in treatment of poorly controlled seizures. *Arch Dis Child* 1990; **65:** 930–5.
4. McKee PJW, *et al.* Double dummy comparison between once and twice daily dosing with modified-release carbamazepine in epileptic patients. *Br J Clin Pharmacol* 1993; **36:** 257–61.

Diabetes insipidus. Cranial diabetes insipidus is usually treated by replacement therapy with antidiuretic hormone (ADH) in the form of desmopressin (see p.1237). Carbamazepine is one of a variety of other drugs that have been tried to promote ADH secretion, although some consider that it is usually ineffective and has unwanted effects.[1,2] Doses of 200 to 400 mg daily by mouth have been given. See also Effects on the Endocrine System under Adverse Effects, above.

1. Seckl J, Dunger D. Postoperative diabetes insipidus. *Br Med J* 1989; **298:** 2–3.
2. Singer I, *et al.* The management of diabetes insipidus in adults. *Arch Intern Med* 1997; **157:** 1293–1301.

Epilepsy. Carbamazepine is one of the drugs of choice for partial seizures with or without secondary generalisation and for tonic-clonic seizures secondary to a focal discharge (see p.335). It should not be used for tonic-clonic seizures that are part of the syndrome of primary generalised epilepsy and may exacerbate absence and myoclonic seizures.

References.

1. Mattson RH, *et al.* Comparison of carbamazepine, phenobarbital, phenytoin, and primidone in partial and secondarily generalised tonic-clonic seizures. *N Engl J Med* 1985; **313:** 145–51.
2. Mattson RH, *et al.* A comparison of valproate with carbamazepine for the treatment of complex partial seizures and secondarily generalized tonic-clonic seizures in adults. *N Engl J Med* 1992; **327:** 765–71.
3. Richens A, *et al.* A multicentre comparative trial of sodium valproate and carbamazepine in adult onset epilepsy. *J Neurol Neurosurg Psychiatry* 1994; **57:** 682–7.
4. Heller AJ, *et al.* Phenobarbitone, phenytoin, carbamazepine, or sodium valproate for newly diagnosed adult epilepsy: a randomised comparative monotherapy trial. *J Neurol Neurosurg Psychiatry* 1995; **58:** 44–50.
5. Verity CM, *et al.* A multicentre comparative trial of sodium valproate and carbamazepine in paediatric epilepsy. *Dev Med Child Neurol* 1995; **37:** 97–108.
6. de Silva M, *et al.* Randomised comparative monotherapy trial of phenobarbitone, phenytoin, carbamazepine, or sodium valproate for newly diagnosed childhood epilepsy. *Lancet* 1996; **347:** 709–13.

Hiccup. A protocol for the management of intractable hiccups may be found under Chlorpromazine, p.655. Carbamazepine may be of value for the treatment of neurogenic hiccups such as those that occur in multiple sclerosis.[1] Carbamazepine has also been reported to have been of benefit in 3 patients with diaphragmatic flutter,[2] a rare disorder associated with involuntary contractions of the diaphragm.

1. McFarling DA, Susac JO. Hoquet diabolique: intractable hiccups as a manifestation of multiple sclerosis. *Neurology* 1979; **29:** 797–801.
2. Vantrappen G, *et al.* High-frequency diaphragmatic flutter: symptoms and treatment by carbamazepine. *Lancet* 1992; **339:** 265–7.

Hyperactivity. When drugs are indicated for attention deficit hyperactivity disorder (p.1476) initial treatment is usually with central stimulants but meta-analysis of a small number of trials has provided preliminary evidence that carbamazepine may be an effective alternative.[1]

1. Silva RR, *et al.* Carbamazepine use in children and adolescents with features of attention-deficit hyperactivity disorder: a meta-analysis. *J Am Acad Child Adolesc Psychiatry* 1996; **35:** 352–8.

Manic depression. Carbamazepine is an alternative to lithium in patients with bipolar disorder (p.273) and seems to be particularly effective in those who have rapid-cycling manic-depressive illness with 4 or more affective episodes a year. Although clearly effective in the majority of patients in the short-term,[1,2] at least one study showed a much lower response rate in the long-term[2] and claims that carbamazepine is as effective as lithium in this condition have been criticised.[3] In another study lithium appeared to be more effective than carbamazepine in the acute phase of mania but there was no significant difference in the follow-up phase;[4] men tended to respond better to carbamazepine than women. Mania appears to respond better than depression.[1]

Carbamazepine has been tried in combination with lithium,[1,5] particularly in patients unresponsive to one drug alone. This combination may produce a more rapid response than lithium alone[6] but is associated with a potential risk of serious neurotoxicity—see Antidepressants under Interactions, above.

1. Ballenger JC. The clinical use of carbamazepine in affective disorders. *J Clin Psychiatry* 1988; **49** (suppl): 13–19.
2. Frankenburg FR, *et al.* Long-term response to carbamazepine: a retrospective study. *J Clin Psychopharmacol* 1988; **8:** 130–2.
3. Murphy DJ, *et al.* Carbamazepine in bipolar affective disorder. *Lancet* 1989; **ii:** 1151–2.
4. Lusznat RM, *et al.* Carbamazepine vs lithium in the treatment and prophylaxis of mania. *Br J Psychiatry* 1988; **153:** 198–204.
5. Kramlinger KG, Post RM. Adding lithium carbonate to carbamazepine: antimanic efficacy in treatment-resistant mania. *Acta Psychiatr Scand* 1989; **79:** 378–85.
6. Di Costanzo E, Schifano F. Lithium alone or in combination with carbamazepine for the treatment of rapid-cycling bipolar affective disorder. *Acta Psychiatr Scand* 1991; **83:** 456–9.

Movement disorders. Carbamazepine is one of many drugs that have been tried in the symptomatic treatment of *chorea* (p.636); these have been anecdotal reports of benefit in both non-hereditary[1] and hereditary choreas.[2] Carbamazepine is also among the drugs that have been tried in the treatment of *dystonias* that have not responded to levodopa or antimuscarinics (p.1141). Although some patients may benefit from carbamazepine, it is not generally recommended because of a relatively low success rate and the possibility of adverse effects.[3]

Carbamazepine has also been used in resistant cases of *tardive dyskinesia* (see under Extrapyramidal Disorders, p.650).

1. Roig M, *et al.* Carbamazepine: an alternative drug for the treatment of nonhereditary chorea. *Pediatrics* 1988; **82:** 492–5.
2. Roulet E, Deonna T. Successful treatment of hereditary dominant chorea with carbamazepine. *Pediatrics* 1989; **83:** 1077.
3. Anonymous. Dystonia: underdiagnosed and undertreated? *Drug Ther Bull* 1988; **26:** 33–6.

Neonatal seizures. Carbamazepine has been tried in the management of neonatal seizures (p.338).

Pain. As well as being used to ease the pain of trigeminal neuralgia (see below) carbamazepine may be of use in other neurogenic pain including that associated with diabetic neuropathy. Chronic burning pain in the feet of a former prisoner of war, a result of neuropathic beriberi, was virtually abolished by treatment with carbamazepine 200 mg three times daily.[1]

1. Skelton WP. Neuropathic beriberi and carbamazepine. *Ann Intern Med* 1988; **109:** 598–9.

Psychiatric disorders. Carbamazepine has psychotropic properties and has been tried in the management of several psychiatric disorders, particularly in patients with *manic depression (bipolar disorder)* (see above). Carbamazepine has also been used with mixed results in various disorders for the control of symptoms such as agitation, aggression, and rage[1-4] (see under Disturbed Behaviour, p.636). It may produce modest benefit when used as an adjunct to antipsychotics in the management of refractory schizophrenia (p.637) but any improvement appears to be related to its mood stabilising effect.[5] However, carbamazepine also has the potential to reduce serum concentrations of antipsychotics, resulting in clinical deterioration (see under Interactions for Chlorpromazine, p.653). Carbamazepine has also been tried in *post-traumatic stress disorder*[6] (see p.635).

1. Mattes JA. Comparative effectiveness of carbamazepine and propranolol for rage outbursts. *J Neuropsychiatr Clin Neurosci* 1990; **2:** 159–64.
2. Gleason RP, Schneider LS. Carbamazepine treatment of agitation in Alzheimer's outpatients refractory to neuroleptics. *J Clin Psychiatry* 1990; **51:** 115–18.
3. Tariot PN, *et al.* Carbamazepine treatment of agitation in nursing home patients with dementia: a preliminary study. *J Am Geriatr Soc* 1994; **42:** 1160–6.
4. Cueva JE, *et al.* Carbamazepine in aggressive children with conduct disorder: a double-blind and placebo-controlled study. *J Am Acad Child Adolesc Psychiatry* 1996; **35:** 480–90.
5. Okuma T. Use of antiepileptic drugs in schizophrenia: a review of efficacy and tolerability. *CNS Drugs* 1994; **1:** 269–84.
6. Wolf ME, *et al.* Posttraumatic stress disorder in Vietnam veterans: clinical and EEG findings; possible therapeutic effects of carbamazepine. *Biol Psychiatry* 1988; **23:** 642–4.

Restless legs syndrome. The aetiology of restless legs syndrome (p.639) is obscure and treatment has been largely empirical. In a double-blind study involving 174 patients carbamazepine appeared to be more effective than placebo.[1]

1. Telstad W, *et al.* Treatment of the restless legs syndrome with carbamazepine: a double blind study. *Br Med J* 1984; **288:** 444–6.

Tinnitus. Treatment of tinnitus (p.1297) is difficult, and many drugs have been tried. Although carbamazepine has been reported to be effective in some patients, it is rarely used because of its adverse effects.

Trigeminal neuralgia. Carbamazepine is the drug of choice in the treatment of trigeminal neuralgia (p.12). Satisfactory pain relief may be achieved in 70% or more of patients, although increasingly larger doses may be required and side-effects can be troublesome.

Withdrawal syndromes. Carbamazepine has been tried in the prophylaxis and treatment of various withdrawal syndromes including that associated with cocaine[1] (p.1291). It has been reported[2,3] to be of benefit in some patients during benzodiazepine withdrawal but such adjunct therapy is not usually indicated (see p.661). Carbamazepine has been shown[4,5] to be effective in the treatment of symptoms of the alcohol withdrawal syndrome (p.1099) but as there are limited data on its efficacy in preventing associated delirium tremens and seizures it is usually recommended that it should only be used as an adjunct to benzodiazepine therapy. Carbamazepine is also being studied[6] as an aid in the treatment of alcohol dependence.

1. Halikas JA, *et al.* Cocaine reduction in unmotivated crack users using carbamazepine versus placebo in a short-term, double-blind crossover design. *Clin Pharmacol Ther* 1991; **50:** 81–95.
2. Schweizer E, *et al.* Carbamazepine treatment in patients discontinuing long-term benzodiazepine therapy: effects on withdrawal severity and outcome. *Arch Gen Psychiatry* 1991; **48:** 448–52.
3. Klein E, *et al.* Alprazolam withdrawal in patients with panic disorder and generalized anxiety disorder: vulnerability and effect of carbamazepine. *Am J Psychiatry* 1994; **151:** 1760–6.
4. Malcolm R, *et al.* Double-blind controlled trial comparing carbamazepine to oxazepam treatment of alcohol withdrawal. *Am J Psychiatry* 1989; **146:** 617–21.
5. Stuppaeck CH, *et al.* Carbamazepine versus oxazepam in the treatment of alcohol withdrawal: a double-blind study. *Alcohol Alcohol* 1992; **27:** 153–8.
6. Mueller TI, *et al.* A double-blind, placebo-controlled pilot study of carbamazepine for the treatment of alcohol dependence. *Alcohol Clin Exp Res* 1997; **21:** 86–92.

Preparations

BP 1998: Carbamazepine Tablets;
USP 23: Carbamazepine Oral Suspension; Carbamazepine Tablets.

Proprietary Preparations (details are given in Part 3)
Aust.: Neurotop; Sirtal; Tegretol; ***Austral.:*** Tegretol; Teril; ***Belg.:*** Tegretol; ***Canad.:*** Novo-Carbamaz; Tegretol; ***Fr.:*** Tegretol; ***Ger.:*** Carba; Carbagamma; Carbium; Finlepsin; Fokalepsin; Sirtal; Tegretal; Timonil; ***Irl.:*** Gericarb; Tegretol; Temporol; ***Ital.:*** Tegretol; ***Neth.:*** Tegretol; ***Norw.:*** Tegretol; Trimonil; ***S.Afr.:*** Carpaz; Degranol; Prozine; Tegretol; Temporol†; ***Spain:*** Tegretol; ***Swed.:*** Hermolepsin; Tegretol; Trimonil; ***Switz.:*** Tegretol; Timonil; ***UK:*** Epimaz; Tegretol; Teril; Timonil; ***USA:*** Atretol; Epitol; Tegretol.

Clonazepam (6606-d)

Clonazepam *(BAN, USAN, rINN).*

Clonazepamum; Ro-5-4023. 5-(2-Chlorophenyl)-1,3-dihydro-7-nitro-1,4-benzodiazepin-2-one.

$C_{15}H_{10}ClN_3O_3$ = 315.7.

CAS — 1622-61-3.

Pharmacopoeias. In *Eur.* (see p.viii), *Jpn, Pol.,* and *US.*

A light yellow crystalline powder with a faint odour. Practically **insoluble** in water; slightly soluble in alcohol and in methyl alcohol; sparingly soluble in acetone and in chloroform; very slightly to slightly soluble in ether. **Store** in airtight containers. Protect from light.

Dependence and Withdrawal

As for Diazepam, p.661.

Withdrawal. A study[1] of the withdrawal of clonazepam therapy in 40 epileptic children found that 19 exhibited withdrawal symptoms of increased seizure frequency, either alone or with other symptoms but that this effect was transient. Withdrawal seizures and status may become an obstacle to the removal of useless or even deleterious therapy with clonazepam because the transient nature of these effects is not always recognised. Clonazepam should not be prescribed for more than 3 to 6 months and should be discontinued if clear and lasting therapeutic benefit cannot be demonstrated.

See also under Uses and Administration, below.

1. Specht U, *et al.* Discontinuation of clonazepam after long-term treatment. *Epilepsia* 1989; **30:** 458–63.

Adverse Effects, Treatment, and Precautions

As for the benzodiazepines, p.661.

The principal adverse effect of clonazepam is drowsiness, which occurs in about 50% of all patients on starting therapy. Salivary or bronchial hypersecretion may cause respiratory problems in children.

Care is required when withdrawing clonazepam therapy—see above.

Breast feeding. Benzodiazepines, such as clonazepam, given to the mother may cause neonatal sedation and breast feeding should be avoided. For comments on antiepileptic therapy and breast feeding, see under Pregnancy on p.337.

Driving. For a comment on antiepileptic drugs and driving, see p.337.

Effects on the endocrine system. Precocious development of secondary sexual characteristics occurred in a 15-month-old girl 2 months after starting treatment with clonazepam 500 μg twice daily for convulsions.[1] Symptoms regressed upon withdrawal of clonazepam.

1. Choonara IA, *et al.* Clonazepam and sexual precocity. *N Engl J Med* 1985; **312:** 185.

Effects of sexual function. Sexual dysfunction was reported briefly[1] in male patients receiving clonazepam for the treatment of post-traumatic stress disorder; symptoms resolved when therapy was changed to diazepam.

1. Fossey MD, Hamner MB. Clonazepam induced sexual dysfunction in male veterans with PTSD. *Biol Psychiatry* 1994; **35:** 656.

Extrapyramidal disorders. For reference to extrapyramidal disorders associated with the administration of benzodiazepines including clonazepam, see under Effects on the Nervous System in Diazepam, p.662. However, clonazepam is also used in the treatment of some extrapyramidal disorders as discussed under Uses and Administration, below.

Porphyria. For comments on the use of benzodiazepines in porphyria, see p.339.

Pregnancy. For comments on the management of epilepsy during pregnancy, see p.337.

Tolerance. For evidence suggesting that the benzodiazepine antagonist flumazenil may reverse tolerance to the anticonvulsant effects of benzodiazepines, see under Benzodiazepine Tolerance in the Uses and Administration of Flumazenil, p.981.

Interactions

Concomitant administration of hepatic enzyme inducers, such as carbamazepine, phenobarbitone, or phenytoin, may accelerate the metabolism of clonazepam. Concomitant intake of alcohol may affect the patient's response to clonazepam. Clonazepam may be expected to have the sedative interactions associated with benzodiazepines in general (see under Interactions of Diazepam, p.663).

Antiarrhythmics. For reference to an interaction between clonazepam and amiodarone, see under Diazepam, p.663.

Antiepileptics. For reference to possible interactions between clonazepam and other antiepileptics, see under Diazepam, p.664 and Benzodiazepines under Interactions of Phenytoin, p.356.

Pharmacokinetics

Clonazepam is well absorbed following oral administration and peak plasma concentrations have been reported to occur within 4 hours. It is extensively metabolised in the liver, its principal metabolite being 7-aminoclonazepam, which probably has little antiepileptic activity; minor metabolites are the 7-acetamido- and 3-hydroxy- derivatives. It is excreted in the urine almost entirely as its metabolites in free or conjugated form. It is about 86% bound to plasma protein and estimations of its plasma half-life range from about 20 to 40 hours, and occasionally more.

A therapeutic range of plasma concentrations has not been established.

Clonazepam crosses the placental barrier.

Bioavailability. It has been suggested, on the basis of anecdotal evidence,[1] that there may be differences in bioavailability, and hence in clinical effect, between formulations of clonazepam.

1. Rapaport MH. Clinical differences between the generic and nongeneric forms of clonazepam. *J Clin Psychopharmacol* 1997; **17:** 424.

Uses and Administration

Clonazepam is a benzodiazepine derivative similar to diazepam (p.666), with marked antiepileptic properties.

It may be used in the treatment of all types of epilepsy and seizures (p.335) but its usefulness is sometimes limited by the development of tolerance and by sedation, and other antiepileptics are often preferred. It may also be used in myoclonus (p.338) and associated abnormal movements. Clonazepam is also employed for the treatment of panic disorder.

Treatment is initiated with small doses that are progressively increased to an optimum dose according to the response of the patient. In the UK the initial adult dose is 1 mg (500 μg in the elderly) by mouth at night for 4 nights gradually increased over 2 to 4 weeks to a usual maintenance dose of 4 to 8 mg daily in 3 or 4 divided doses; in the USA it is recommended that the total dose should not exceed 20 mg daily. In the UK initial daily doses in children are 250 μg for children up to 5 years of age and 500 μg for children 5 to 12 years of age; usual daily maintenance doses, given in 3 or 4 divided doses, are: infants, 0.5 to 1 mg; children 1 to 5 years, 1 to 3 mg; children 5 to 12 years, 3 to 6 mg. In the USA it is recommended that the total dose should not exceed 200 μg per kg body-weight daily in children. There is little value in routinely monitoring plasma-clonazepam concentrations.

Clonazepam is also used as an alternative to other benzodiazepines in the emergency management of status epilepticus (p.337). The usual dose is 1 mg given by intravenous injection over about 30 seconds or by intravenous infusion, repeated if necessary; the dose in infants and children is 500 μg.

As with other antiepileptics, withdrawal of clonazepam therapy or transition to or from another type of antiepileptic therapy should be made gradually to avoid precipitating an increase in the frequency of seizures. For a discussion on whether or not to withdraw antiepileptic therapy in seizure-free patients, see p.335 and above.

In the treatment of panic disorder, clonazepam is given in an initial dose of 250 μg twice daily by mouth. This may be increased after 3 days to a total of 1 mg daily; a few patients may benefit from further increases, up to a maximum of 4 mg daily. In order to minimise drowsiness, dosage may be taken as a single dose at bedtime. Withdrawal should again be gradual.

Administration. Serum concentrations of clonazepam following administration via the buccal, intranasal, or intravenous routes were measured in a crossover study[1] in 7 healthy males. The results demonstrated that intranasal clonazepam may offer an alternative to buccal administration in patients with serial seizures but the initial concentrations were too low to recommend its use as an alternative to intravenous clonazepam in the management of status epilepticus. The nasal formulation used in this study contained dimethyl-β-cyclodextrin as a solubiliser and absorption enhancer.

1. Schols-Hendriks MWG, *et al.* Absorption of clonazepam after intranasal and buccal administration. *Br J Clin Pharmacol* 1995; **39:** 449–51.

Extrapyramidal disorders. Clonazepam may be of benefit in some extrapyramidal disorders. It has been tried in the management of patients with *tic disorders* such as *Tourette's syndrome* (p.636) but evidence of efficacy from controlled studies is limited.[1] Some use clonazepam in preference to haloperidol[2] since it does not carry the risk of tardive dyskinesia associated with such antipsychotics. There is also limited evidence of benefit in antipsychotic-induced *akathisia*[3,4] and *tardive dyskinesia*[5] (see under Extrapyramidal Disorders, p.650), and of improvement in *dysarthria* in a study in patients with parkinsonism.[6]

1. Goetz CG. Clonidine and clonazepam in Tourette syndrome. *Adv Neurol* 1992; **58:** 245–51.
2. Truong DD, *et al.* Clonazepam, haloperidol, and clonidine in tic disorders. *South Med J* 1988; **81:** 1103–5.
3. Kutcher S, *et al.* Successful clonazepam treatment of neuroleptic-induced akathisia in older adolescents and young adults: a double-blind, placebo-controlled study. *J Clin Psychopharmacol* 1989; **9:** 403–6.
4. Pujalte D, *et al.* A double-blind comparison of clonazepam and placebo in the treatment of neuroleptic-induced akathisia. *Clin Neuropharmacol* 1994; **17:** 236–42.
5. Thaker GK, *et al.* Clonazepam treatment of tardive dyskinesia: a practical GABAmimetic strategy. *Am J Psychiatry* 1990: **147:** 445–51.
6. Biary N, *et al.* A double-blind trial of clonazepam in the treatment of parkinsonian dysarthria. *Neurology* 1988; **38:** 255–8.

Hiccup. A protocol for the management of intractable hiccups may be found under Chlorpromazine, p.655. Clonazepam might also be of value, especially in neurogenic hiccups.

Parasomnias. Treatment of parasomnias (p.639) including sleep behaviour disorder, restless legs syndrome, and periodic movements in sleep is largely empirical, but benzodiazepines such as clonazepam are often employed.[1] Small double-blind studies have provided some evidence for benefit with clonazepam therapy.[2,3]

1. Schenck CH, Mahowald MW. Long-term, nightly benzodiazepine treatment of injurious parasomnias and other disorders of disrupted nocturnal sleep in 170 adults. *Am J Med* 1996; **100:** 333–7.
2. Montagna P, *et al.* Clonazepam and vibration in restless legs syndrome. *Acta Neurol Scand* 1984; **69:** 428–30.
3. Peled R, Lavie P. Double-blind evaluation of clonazepam on periodic leg movements in sleep. *J Neurol Neurosurg Psychiatry* 1987; **50:** 1679–81.

Phantom limb pain. The management of phantom limb pain (p.10) can be difficult, and antidepressants and antiepileptics are used for the neurogenic components of the pain. Rapid and marked pain relief was achieved in 2 patients with lancinating phantom limb pain following treatment with clonazepam with or without amitriptyline.[1]

1. Bartusch SL, *et al.* Clonazepam for the treatment of lancinating phantom limb pain. *Clin J Pain* 1996; **12:** 59–62.

Psychiatric disorders. Clonazepam has been tried in a variety of psychiatric disorders. A beneficial response has been reported in patients with *panic disorders*[1] (see under Anxiety Disorders, p.635), perhaps suggesting a similar action to alprazolam (p.641).

1. Tesar GE, *et al.* Double-blind, placebo-controlled comparison of clonazepam and alprazolam for panic disorder. *J Clin Psychiatry* 1991; **52:** 69–76.

Stiff-man syndrome. Clonazepam has been used as an alternative to diazepam in the management of stiff-man syndrome (p.667) and is reported[1] to be effective for familial startle disease, a rare congenital form of stiff-man syndrome.

1. Ryan SG, *et al.* Startle disease, or hyperekplexia: response to clonazepam and assignment of the gene (STHE) to chromosome 5q by linkage analysis. *Ann Neurol* 1992; **31:** 663–8.

Trigeminal neuralgia. Although carbamazepine is the drug of choice in the treatment of trigeminal neuralgia (p.12), clonazepam may be used in carbamazepine-intolerant patients.

Preparations

BP 1998: Clonazepam Injection;
USP 23: Clonazepam Tablets.

Proprietary Preparations (details are given in Part 3)
Aust.: Rivotril; ***Austral.:*** Paxam; Rivotril; ***Belg.:*** Rivotril; ***Canad.:*** Rivotril; ***Fr.:*** Rivotril; ***Ger.:*** Antelepsin; Rivotril; ***Irl.:*** Rivotril; ***Ital.:*** Rivotril; ***Neth.:*** Rivotril; ***Norw.:*** Rivotril; ***S.Afr.:*** Rivotril; ***Spain:*** Rivotril; ***Swed.:*** Iktorivil; ***Switz.:*** Rivotril; ***UK:*** Rivotril; ***USA:*** Klonopin.

Ethadione (9445-d)

3-Ethyl-5,5-dimethyl-2,4-oxazolidinedione.
$C_7H_{11}NO_3$ = 157.2.
CAS — 520-77-4.

Ethadione is an oxazolidinedione antiepileptic with actions and uses similar to those of troxidone (p.361); like troxidone it appears to owe its action to metabolism to dimethadione. It has been used to treat epilepsy (p.335) in patients with absence seizures resistant to other therapy. Usual initial doses are 500 mg daily by mouth, increased gradually to up to 2 g daily if necessary.

Preparations

Proprietary Preparations (details are given in Part 3)
Aust.: Petidion; ***Switz.:*** Petidion.

Ethosuximide (6611-x)

Ethosuximide *(BAN, USAN, rINN).*

CI-366; CN-10395; NSC-64013; PM-671. 2-Ethyl-2-methylsuccinimide.

$C_7H_{11}NO_2$ = 141.2.
CAS — 77-67-8.

Pharmacopoeias. In *Chin., Eur.* (see p.viii), *Int., Jpn,* and *US.*

A white or off-white powder or waxy solid with a characteristic odour. Freely **soluble** in water and in chloroform; very soluble in alcohol, in dichloromethane, and in ether; very slightly soluble in petroleum spirit. **Store** in airtight containers. Protect from light.

Adverse Effects

Gastro-intestinal side-effects including nausea, vomiting, anorexia, gastric upset, and abdominal pain occur fairly frequently with ethosuximide. Other side-effects which may occur include headache, fatigue, lethargy, drowsiness, dizziness, ataxia, hiccup, and euphoria.

More rarely dyskinesias, personality changes, depression, psychosis, skin rashes, erythema multiforme or Stevens-Johnson syndrome, systemic lupus erythematosus, photophobia, gum hypertrophy, tongue swelling, myopia, and vaginal bleeding have been reported. There are a few reports of blood disorders including eosinophilia, leucopenia, agranulocytosis, thrombocytopenia, pancytopenia, and aplastic anaemia; fatalities have occurred.

Abnormal renal and liver function values have been recorded.

Precautions

Ethosuximide should be used with caution in patients with impaired hepatic or renal function. The manufacturers recommend regular hepatic and renal function tests (and some suggest blood counts) during treatment with ethosuximide, although some authorities question the practical value of such monitoring. Patients or their carers should be told how to recognise signs of blood toxicity and they should be advised to seek immediate medical attention if symptoms such as fever, sore throat, mouth ulcers, bruising, or bleeding develop.

Care is required when withdrawing ethosuximide therapy—see also under Uses and Administration, below.

Breast feeding. Ethosuximide is distributed in significant amounts into breast milk and breast feeding should be avoided; hyperexcitability and poor suckling have been reported in the infant. For comment on antiepileptic therapy and breast feeding, see under Pregnancy on p.337.

Driving. For a comment on antiepileptic drugs and driving, see p.337.

Porphyria. Ethosuximide has been associated with clinical exacerbations of porphyria and is considered unsafe in porphyric patients.[1]

1. Moore MR, McColl KEL. *Porphyria: drug lists.* Glasgow: Porphyria Research Unit, University of Glasgow, 1991.

Pregnancy. For comments on the management of epilepsy during pregnancy, see p.337.

Interactions

There are complex interactions between antiepileptics and toxicity may be enhanced without a corresponding increase in antiepileptic activity. Such interactions are very variable and unpredictable and plasma monitoring is often advisable with combination therapy.

Isoniazid raises the plasma concentration and increases the risk of toxicity of ethosuximide. Psychotic behaviour has been reported[1] in a patient stabilised on ethosuximide and sodium valproate, following the introduction of *isoniazid*. Serum-ethosuximide concentrations rose substantially until both ethosuximide and isoniazid were discontinued.

Since ethosuximide has a limited spectrum of antiepileptic action, patients with mixed seizure syndromes may require concomitant administration of other antiepileptics. *Carbamazepine, phenobarbitone*, and *phenytoin* have all been shown[2] to increase the clearance of ethosuximide and thus reduce plasma concentrations. This interaction is likely to be clinically relevant and higher ethosuximide dosages may be necessary to achieve therapeutic drug levels. Although ethosuximide has been used in combination with *valproic acid* quite frequently there is little evidence of an interaction. However, in one study 4 of 5 patients receiving a combination regimen including ethosuximide experienced a marked increase in serum ethosuximide concentrations when valproic acid was added,[3] and there is evidence for a decrease in ethosuximide clearance and consequent prolongation in its half-life when the two drugs are given together, although the effect seems to vary between individuals, with some unaffected.[4]

It has been suggested that *antidepressants* and *antipsychotics* may antagonise the antiepileptic activity of ethosuximide by lowering the convulsive threshold.

For the effects of ethosuximide on *oral contraceptives*, see p.1433.

1. van Wieringen A, Vrijlandt CM. Ethosuximide intoxication caused by interaction with isoniazid. *Neurology* 1983; **33:** 1227–8.
2. Giaccone M, *et al.* Effect of enzyme inducing anticonvulsants on ethosuximide pharmacokinetics in epileptic patients. *Br J Clin Pharmacol* 1996; **41:** 575–9.
3. Mattson RH, Cramer JA. Valproic acid and ethosuximide interaction. *Ann Neurol* 1980; **7:** 583–4.
4. Pisani F, *et al.* Valproic acid-ethosuximide interaction: a pharmacokinetic study. *Epilepsia* 1984; **25:** 229–33.

Pharmacokinetics

Ethosuximide is readily absorbed from the gastrointestinal tract and extensively hydroxylated in the liver to its principal metabolite which is reported to be inactive. It is excreted in the urine mainly in the form of its metabolites either free or in conjugated form but about 20% is also excreted as unchanged ethosuximide.

Ethosuximide is widely distributed throughout the body, but is not significantly bound to plasma proteins. A half-life of about 60 hours has been reported for adults with a shorter half-life of about 30 hours in children.

Monitoring of plasma concentrations has been suggested as an aid in assessing control and the therapeutic range of ethosuximide is usually quoted as being 40 to 100 μg per mL (about 300 to 700 μmol per litre); measurement of concentrations in saliva and tears has also been performed.

Ethosuximide crosses the placental barrier, and is distributed into breast milk.

The pharmacokinetics of ethosuximide are affected by the concomitant administration of other antiepileptics (see under Interactions, above).

Uses and Administration

Ethosuximide is a succinimide antiepileptic used in the treatment of absence seizures. It may also be used for myoclonic seizures. Ethosuximide is ineffective against tonic-clonic seizures and may unmask them if given alone in mixed seizure types.

A plasma-ethosuximide concentration of 40 to 100 μg per mL (about 300 to 700 μmol per litre) appears to be generally necessary. The initial dose for patients of 6 years and over is 500 mg daily by mouth. The dosage is then adjusted by increments, usually of 250 mg every 4 to 7 days, according to the response of the patient. For children up to 6 years of age the initial dose is 250 mg daily increased gradually in small increments every few days to a usual dose of 20 mg per kg body-weight; one manufacturer recommends that the dose should not exceed 1 g. Sometimes doses of up to 2 g may be necessary in adults and older children; strict supervision is necessary when the dose exceeds 1.5 g.

As with other antiepileptics, withdrawal of ethosuximide therapy or transition to or from another type of antiepileptic therapy should be made gradually to avoid precipitating an increase in the frequency of seizures. For a discussion on whether or not to withdraw antiepileptic therapy in seizure-free patients, see p.335.

Epilepsy. Ethosuximide is a drug of choice in the treatment of absence seizures; it may also be used for myoclonic, atonic, and tonic seizures but is ineffective in other forms of epilepsy (p.335). Ethosuximide may be administered with other antiepileptics in the treatment of mixed-seizure syndromes that include absences. It has been suggested that ethosuximide may provoke tonic-clonic seizures, but there is not a great deal of evidence for this. One early report indicated that 22 of 85 patients receiving a regimen of ethosuximide, methsuximide, and troxidone for absence seizures developed tonic-clonic seizures[1] and another of similar vintage reported exacerbation of mixed-seizure types in 7 patients receiving ethosuximide.[2] However, it is known that up to half of all patients with absence seizures experience generalised tonic-clonic seizures at some point[3] and it would presumably be difficult to distinguish such attacks from any putative effect of ethosuximide. Furthermore, ethosuximide is not effective against tonic-clonic seizures, and in patients with mixed-seizure types it might be expected to unmask the non-absence components of the disease.

Ethosuximide has also been tried in the management of absence status epilepticus (p.337).

1. Friedel B, Lempp R. Grand-mal-provokation beider behandlung kindlicher petit-mal mit oxazolidinen oder succinimiden und ihre therapeutischen konsequenzen. *Z Kinderheilk* 1962; **87:** 42–51.
2. de Haas AML, Kuilman M. Ethosuximide (α-ethyl-α-methylsuccinimide) and grand mal. *Epilepsia* 1964; **5:** 90–6.
3. Sherwin AL. Ethosuximide: clinical use. In: Levy RH, *et al.*, eds. *Antiepileptic drugs* 4th ed. New York: Raven Press, 1995: 667–73.

Preparations

BP 1998: Ethosuximide Capsules; Ethosuximide Oral Solution; *USP 23:* Ethosuximide Capsules.

Proprietary Preparations (details are given in Part 3)
Aust.: Petinimid; Simatin; Suxinutin; ***Austral.:*** Zarontin; ***Belg.:*** Zarontin; ***Canad.:*** Zarontin; ***Fr.:*** Zarontin; ***Ger.:*** Petnidan; Pyknolepsinum; Suxilep; Suxinutin; ***Irl.:*** Zarontin; ***Ital.:*** Zarontin; ***Neth.:*** Zarontin; ***Norw.:*** Zarondan; ***S.Afr.:*** Zarontin; ***Spain:*** Simatin†; Zarontin; ***Swed.:*** Suxinutin; ***Switz.:*** Petinimid; Suxinutin; ***UK:*** Emeside; Zarontin; ***USA:*** Zarontin.

Multi-ingredient: ***Aust.:*** Acrisuxin; ***Ger.:*** Acrisuxin†; ***Switz.:*** Acrisuxin.

Ethotoin (6612-r)

Ethotoin *(BAN, rINN)*.
3-Ethyl-5-phenylhydantoin.
$C_{11}H_{12}N_2O_2$ = 204.2.
CAS — 86-35-1.
Pharmacopoeias. In US.

A white crystalline powder. Practically **insoluble** in water; freely soluble in dehydrated alcohol and in chloroform; soluble in ether. **Store** in airtight containers.

Ethotoin is a hydantoin antiepileptic with actions similar to those of phenytoin (p.352), but it is reported to be both less toxic and less effective; it is not one of the main drugs used to treat epilepsy (p.335).

Ethotoin is given by mouth in an initial dosage of up to 1 g daily, increased gradually at intervals of several days to 2 to 3 g daily, given in 4 to 6 divided doses after meals. A suggested maintenance dose for children is 0.5 to 1 g daily.

A study[1] of the pharmacokinetics of ethotoin given at more convenient intervals of every 8 hours.

1. Browne TR, Szabo GK. A pharmacokinetic rationale for three times daily administration of ethotoin (Peganone). *J Clin Pharmacol* 1989; **29:** 270–1.

Porphyria. Ethotoin has been associated with clinical exacerbations of porphyria and is considered unsafe in porphyric patients.[1]

1. Moore MR, McColl KEL. *Porphyria: drug lists.* Glasgow: Porphyria Research Unit, University of Glasgow, 1991.

Preparations

USP 23: Ethotoin Tablets.

Proprietary Preparations (details are given in Part 3)
Norw.: Peganone†; ***USA:*** Peganone.

Felbamate (2858-e)

Felbamate *(USAN, rINN)*.
AD-03055; W-554. 2-Phenyl-1,3-propanediol dicarbamate.
$C_{11}H_{14}N_2O_4$ = 238.2.
CAS — 25451-15-4.

Adverse Effects

The most frequently reported adverse effects with felbamate are anorexia, weight loss, nausea and vomiting, rash, insomnia, headache, dizziness, somnolence, and diplopia. Aplastic anaemia or acute liver failure, sometimes fatal, have occurred rarely.

Precautions

Felbamate is contra-indicated in patients with a history of blood disorders or hepatic impairment. It should be used only in the treatment of severe epilepsy refractory to other antiepileptics because of the risk of fatal aplastic anaemia or acute liver failure. Complete blood counts should be carried out before the patient starts treatment and regularly during treatment. Aplastic anaemia can occur after felbamate has been discontinued so patients should continue to be monitored for some time. Liver function tests are also recommended before commencing and regularly during treatment. Patients should be advised of the symptoms of aplastic anaemia and be told to report immediately should any such symptoms develop. Felbamate should be discontinued if there is any evidence of bone marrow depression or liver abnormalities. Felbamate may cause photosensitivity reactions and patients should be advised to take protective measures against exposure to UV radiation.

Care is required when withdrawing felbamate therapy—see also under Uses and Administration, below.

Elderly. Following single doses of felbamate, plasma concentrations and half-lives were greater and mean clearance lower in elderly than in young subjects, whereas pharmacokinetic parameters following multiple dosing schedules were similar.[1] Thus, the elderly may require lower initial doses of felbamate and slower dose titration.

1. Richens A, *et al.* Single and multiple dose pharmacokinetics of felbamate in the elderly. *Br J Clin Pharmacol* 1997; **44:** 129–34.

Pregnancy. For comments on the management of epilepsy during pregnancy, see p.337.

Renal impairment. A single-dose pharmacokinetic study[1] indicated that in patients with renal impairment the initial dose of felbamate may need to be lower and increases made more cautiously than in patients with normal renal function.

1. Glue P, *et al.* Single-dose pharmacokinetics of felbamate in patients with renal dysfunction. *Br J Clin Pharmacol* 1997; **44:** 91–3.

Interactions

The metabolism of felbamate is enhanced by enzyme inducers such as phenytoin and carbamazepine. Felbamate inhibits or enhances the metabolism of several other antiepileptics and care is required when it is added to therapy.

For some references to the effect of felbamate on other antiepileptics, see under Carbamazepine, p.341, Phenobarbitone, p.351, Phenytoin, p.355, and Valproate p.363.

For the effect of felbamate on warfarin, see p.967.

Pharmacokinetics

Felbamate is well absorbed from the gastro-intestinal tract and peak plasma concentrations have been reported 1 to 6 hours after oral administration. Protein binding is reported to be low (about 22 to 36%). It is partly metabolised in the liver by hydroxylation and conjugation to inactive metabolites. Felbamate is excreted in the urine as metabolites and unchanged drug (40 to 50%); less than 4% appears in the faeces. The elimination half-life is reported to be between 14 and 23 hours.

The pharmacokinetics of felbamate are reported to be linear at the doses used clinically. Therapeutic plasma concentrations have been reported to be between 30 and 80 μg per mL.

See under Precautions (above) for mention of pharmacokinetic studies of felbamate in the elderly and in patients with renal impairment.

Uses and Administration

Felbamate is a carbamate structurally related to meprobamate (p.678). It is used in the treatment of epilepsy.

Felbamate is given to adults as monotherapy or adjunctive therapy for refractory partial seizures with or without secondary generalisation. It is used in children as adjunctive therapy in controlling the seizures associated with the Lennox-Gastaut syndrome. Because of its toxicity felbamate should only be used in severe cases unresponsive to other drugs.

The initial adult dose is 1.2 g daily by mouth in 3 or 4 divided doses. The dose should be increased gradually under close supervision up to a maximum of 3.6 g daily. The initial dose in children is 15 mg per kg body-weight daily in 3 or 4 divided doses gradually increased up to a maximum of 45 mg per kg daily.

As with other antiepileptics, withdrawal of felbamate therapy or transition to or from another type of antiepileptic therapy should be made gradually to avoid precipitating an increase in the frequency of seizures. For a discussion on whether or not to withdraw antiepileptic therapy in seizure-free patients, see p.335.

Epilepsy. Although felbamate was well tolerated in clinical trials, rare but serious adverse effects were noted during early postmarketing use.[1,2] Aplastic anaemia and serious hepatotoxic reactions, sometimes with fatal outcomes, developed in some patients. Patients taking felbamate should have frequent blood counts and monitoring of liver enzymes. Even if detected early, aplastic anaemia and hepatic impairment may not be reversible.[1] Usage in the USA is restricted to patients with refractory partial seizures with or without secondary generalisation. It is also used as adjunctive therapy for children with Lennox-Gastaut Syndrome.

The efficacy of felbamate as adjunctive therapy in refractory partial seizures in both adults[3] and children,[4] and in patients with the Lennox-Gastaut syndrome[5,6] has been demonstrated, although there appears to be an increased rate of drug clearance in younger children.[4] Felbamate also appears to be useful as adjunctive therapy in refractory absence seizures.[7]

The overall management of epilepsy is discussed on p.335.

1. Dichter MA, Brodie MJ. New antiepileptic drugs. *N Engl J Med* 1996; **334:** 1583–90.
2. Appleton RE. The new antiepileptic drugs. *Arch Dis Child* 1996; **75:** 256–62.
3. Bourgeois B, *et al.* Felbamate: a double-blind controlled trial in patients undergoing presurgical evaluation of partial seizures. *Neurology* 1993; **43:** 693–6.
4. Carmant L, *et al.* Efficacy of felbamate in therapy for partial epilepsy in children. *J Pediatr* 1994; **125:** 481–6.
5. The Felbamate Study Group in Lennox-Gastaut Syndrome. Efficacy of felbamate in childhood epileptic encephalopathy (Lennox-Gastaut Syndrome). *N Engl J Med* 1993; **328:** 29–33.
6. Dodson WE. Felbamate in the treatment of Lennox-Gastaut syndrome: results of a 12-month open-label study following a randomized clinical trial. *Epilepsia* 1993; **34** (suppl 7): S18–S24.
7. Devinsky O, *et al.* Felbamate for refractory absence seizures. *J Epilepsy* 1994; **7:** 189–94.

Preparations

Proprietary Preparations (details are given in Part 3)
Aust.: Taloxa; ***Fr.:*** Taloxa; ***Ger.:*** Taloxa; ***Ital.:*** Taloxa; ***Neth.:*** Taloxa; ***Norw.:*** Taloxoral; ***Spain:*** Taloxa; ***Swed.:*** Taloxa; ***USA:*** Felbatol.

Fosphenytoin Sodium (17705-b)

Fosphenytoin Sodium *(BANM, USAN, rINNM).*

ACC-9653; ACC-9653-010; CI-982 (fosphenytoin or fosphenytoin sodium); PD-135711-15B. 5,5-Diphenyl-3-[(phosphonooxy)methyl]-2,4-imidazolidinedione, disodium salt; 3-(Hydroxymethyl)-5,5-diphenylhydantoin, disodium phosphate (ester); 2,5-Dioxo-4,4-diphenylimidazolidin-1-ylmethyl phosphate disodium.

$C_{16}H_{13}N_2Na_2O_6P$ = 406.2.

CAS — 93390-81-9 (fosphenytoin); 92134-98-0 (fosphenytoin sodium).

Each mmol of fosphenytoin yields one mmol of phenytoin. Fosphenytoin sodium 75 mg is approximately equivalent to phenytoin sodium 50 mg.

Stability. References.

1. Fischer JH, *et al.* Stability of fosphenytoin sodium with intravenous solutions in glass bottles, polyvinyl chloride bags, and polypropylene syringes. *Ann Pharmacother* 1997; **31:** 553–9.

Adverse Effects and Precautions

As for Phenytoin, p.352.

Severe burning, itching, and paraesthesia, particularly in the groin area, have been reported following intravenous administration of fosphenytoin; reducing the rate of, or temporarily stopping, the infusion may relieve the discomfort.

Caution should be exercised when administering fosphenytoin to patients with severe renal impairment and others in whom phosphate restriction is necessary. The rate of metabolism of fosphenytoin to phenytoin may be increased following intravenous administration to patients with hepatic or renal disease, or in those with hypoalbuminaemia, and consequently there is an increased risk of adverse effects in such patients.

Interactions

As for Phenytoin, p.354.

Pharmacokinetics

Plasma concentrations of fosphenytoin are maximal at the end of intravenous infusion and about 30 minutes after intramuscular injection. Protein binding of fosphenytoin is high (95 to 99%) and is saturable; fosphenytoin displaces phenytoin from protein binding sites. Fosphenytoin is completely metabolised to phenytoin; other metabolites include phosphate and formaldehyde. Metabolites of phenytoin are excreted in the urine.

Uses and Administration

Fosphenytoin is a prodrug of phenytoin (p.352) used similarly as part of the emergency treatment of status epilepticus (p.337). It is also used for the prevention and treatment of seizures developing during neurosurgery and as a short-term parenteral substitute for oral phenytoin in the management of epilepsy (p.335).

Fosphenytoin is administered in the form of the sodium salt and doses of fosphenytoin sodium are expressed as phenytoin sodium equivalents; therefore no adjustment in dosage is necessary when substituting fosphenytoin for phenytoin or vice versa. The maximum rate of intravenous infusion of fosphenytoin sodium is 150 mg phenytoin sodium equivalents per minute and should not be exceeded.

In the treatment of tonic-clonic status epilepticus, the loading dose administered by intravenous infusion is 15 to 20 mg phenytoin sodium equivalents per kg body-weight. The intramuscular route is not appropriate for the management of status epilepticus because peak phenytoin concentrations will not be reached quickly enough. The loading dose for the treatment of seizures other than in status epilepticus is 10 to 20 mg phenytoin sodium equivalents per kg given intravenously or intramuscularly. Initial maintenance doses are 4 to 6 mg phenytoin sodium equivalents per kg daily. Continuous monitoring of the ECG and blood pressure is recommended during intravenous administration.

Fosphenytoin given intravenously or intramuscularly may be substituted for oral phenytoin at the same equivalent total daily dose for up to 5 days.

Withdrawal of antiepileptic therapy or transition to or from another type of antiepileptic therapy should be made gradually to avoid precipitating an increase in the frequency of seizures. For a discussion on whether or not to withdraw antiepileptic therapy in seizure-free patients, see p.335.

References.

1. Wilder BJ, *et al.* Safety and tolerance of multiple doses of intramuscular fosphenytoin substituted for oral phenytoin in epilepsy or neurosurgery. *Arch Neurol* 1996; **53:** 764–8.

Preparations

Proprietary Preparations (details are given in Part 3)
USA: Cerebyx.

Gabapentin (3797-f)

Gabapentin *(BAN, USAN, rINN).*

CI-945; GOE-3450. 1-(Aminomethyl)cyclohexaneacetic acid.

$C_9H_{17}NO_2$ = 171.2.

CAS — 60142-96-3.

Adverse Effects and Precautions

The most commonly reported adverse effects associated with gabapentin are somnolence, dizziness, ataxia, fatigue, nystagmus, headache, tremor, diplopia, amblyopia, rhinitis, and nausea and vomiting. Pharyngitis, dysarthria, weight gain, dyspepsia, amnesia, nervousness, coughing, and myalgia may occur less frequently. Rarely, pancreatitis, altered liver function tests, and Stevens-Johnson syndrome have been reported.

Gabapentin should be used with caution in patients with impaired renal function. False positive readings have been reported with some urinary protein tests in patients taking gabapentin.

Care is required when withdrawing gabapentin therapy—see also under Uses and Administration, below.

Carcinogenicity. It had been reported[1] that studies on gabapentin had been temporarily stopped in 1990 when pancreatic tumours were seen in *rodent* studies. However, the tumours were benign, occurred only with large doses, and were not thought to relate to humans.

1. Ramsay RE. Clinical efficacy and safety of gabapentin. *Neurology* 1994; **44** (suppl 5): S23–S30.

Driving. For a comment on antiepileptic drugs and driving, see p.337.

Effects on mental state. There have been isolated reports of depression, aggression, confusion, delusions, and hallucinations in patients receiving gabapentin.[1]

1. Anonymous. Gabapentin—a new antiepileptic drug. *Drug Ther Bull* 1994; **32:** 29–30.

Pregnancy. For comments on the management of epilepsy during pregnancy, see p.337.

Renal impairment. The manufacturer recommends that the dosage of gabapentin should be adjusted in patients with reduced renal function or those undergoing haemodialysis.

Suggested maintenance doses are: 400 mg three times daily for patients with a creatinine clearance of 60 to 90 mL per minute; 300 mg twice daily for a clearance of 30 to 60 mL per minute; 300 mg once daily for a clearance of 15 to 30 mL per minute; and 300 mg on alternate days for a clearance of less than 15 mL per minute. Patients undergoing haemodialysis can be given a loading dose of 300 to 400 mg followed by maintenance doses of 200 to 300 mg following each 4 hours of haemodialysis.

Interactions

The absorption of gabapentin from the gastro-intestinal tract is reduced by antacids and concomitant administration is therefore not recommended. Cimetidine has been reported to reduce the renal clearance of gabapentin but the manufacturers do not consider this to be of clinical importance. For reference to a possible interaction with other antiepileptics, see under Phenytoin, p.355.

Pharmacokinetics

Gabapentin is absorbed from the gastro-intestinal tract by means of a saturable mechanism. Following multiple dosing peak plasma concentrations are usually achieved within 2 hours of administration and steady state achieved within 1 to 2 days. Gabapentin is not appreciably metabolised and most of a dose is excreted unchanged in the urine with the remainder appearing in the faeces. Gabapentin is widely distributed throughout the body but binding to plasma proteins is minimal. The elimination half-life has been reported to be about 5 to 7 hours.

References.

1. Blum RA, *et al.* Pharmacokinetics of gabapentin in subjects with various degrees of renal function. *Clin Pharmacol Ther* 1994; **56:** 154–9.
2. Elwes RDC, Binnie CD. Clinical pharmacokinetics of newer antiepileptic drugs: lamotrigine, vigabatrin, gabapentin and oxcarbazepine. *Clin Pharmacokinet* 1996; **30:** 403–15.

Uses and Administration

Gabapentin is an antiepileptic effective in the treatment of partial seizures with or without secondary generalisation and is used as adjunctive therapy in patients unresponsive to or intolerant of standard antiepileptic drugs. It is not generally considered effective for absence seizures. Although gabapentin is an analogue of gamma-aminobutyric acid (GABA), it is neither a GABA agonist nor antagonist and its mechanism of action is unknown.

The initial adult dose of gabapentin is 300 mg by mouth on the first day of treatment, 300 mg twice daily on the second day, and 300 mg three times daily on the third day; thereafter the dose may be increased until effective antiepileptic control is achieved. The usual maximum dose is 2.4 g daily in divided doses, but the usual range is 0.9 to 1.8 g daily. Higher doses of up to 3.6 g daily administered for a short period have been reported to be well tolerated. The total daily dose should be taken in three equally divided doses and the maximum dosage interval should not exceed 12 hours. Dosage adjustment is necessary in the presence of impaired renal function (see above).

As with other antiepileptics, withdrawal of gabapentin therapy or transition to or from another type of antiepileptic therapy should be made gradually to avoid precipitating an increase in the frequency of seizures. The manufacturers recommend reducing the dose gradually over at least 7 days. For a discussion on whether or not to withdraw antiepileptic therapy in seizure-free patients, see p.335.

Epilepsy. Gabapentin is used in epilepsy (p.335) as adjunctive therapy for partial seizures with or without secondary generalisation in patients refractory to standard antiepileptics.[1-5] In double-blind placebo-controlled studies[6-9] in such patients seizure frequency was reduced when gabapentin was added to treatment. Long-term efficacy has been encouraging.[10-12] It appears to have similar efficacy to other adjunctive antiepileptics.[3] However, gabapentin may cause fewer adverse effects and its lack of potential for interactions with other antiepileptics is considered to make it particularly suitable for adjunctive treatment. Dosage is adjusted against clinical response rather than by monitoring blood concentrations. Experience of its use as monotherapy in partial epilepsy[13,14] is limited and its efficacy as adjunctive treatment in generalised seizures also remains to be determined.

Although experience with gabapentin in children is also limited it has been found to be effective as adjunctive therapy in an open-label trial[15] involving 32 children aged between 2 and 16 years with refractory partial seizures with or without secondary generalisation when given in doses of up to 50 mg per kg body-weight daily. Gabapentin was well tolerated by most of the children; the major adverse effects were behavioural, although these were associated with the occurrence of base-line mental retardation and attention deficit.

1. Goa KL, Sorkin EM. Gabapentin: a review of its pharmacological properties and clinical potential in epilepsy. *Drugs* 1993; **46:** 409–27.
2. Chadwick D. Gabapentin. *Lancet* 1994; **343:** 89–91.
3. Anonymous. Gabapentin—a new antiepileptic drug. *Drug Ther Bull* 1994; **32:** 29–30.
4. Ramsay RE. Clinical efficacy and safety of gabapentin. *Neurology* 1994; **44** (suppl 5): S23–S30.
5. Andrews CO, Fischer JH. Gabapentin: a new agent for the management of epilepsy. *Ann Pharmacother* 1994; **28:** 1188–96.
6. UK Gabapentin Study Group. Gabapentin in partial epilepsy. *Lancet* 1990; **335:** 1114–17.
7. Sivenius J, *et al.* Double-blind study of gabapentin in the treatment of partial seizures. *Epilepsia* 1991; **32:** 539–42.
8. US Gabapentin Study Group. Gabapentin as add-on therapy in refractory partial epilepsy: a double-blind, placebo-controlled, parallel-group study. *Neurology* 1993; **43:** 2292–8.
9. Anhut H, *et al.* International Gabapentin Study Group. Gabapentin (Neurontin) as add-on therapy in patients with partial seizures: a double-blind, placebo-controlled study. *Epilepsia* 1994; **35:** 795–801.
10. US Gabapentin Study Group. The long-term safety and efficacy of gabapentin (Neurontin®) as add-on therapy in drug-resistant partial epilepsy. *Epilepsy Res* 1994; **18:** 67–73.
11. Sivenius J, *et al.* Long-term study with gabapentin in patients with drug-resistant epileptic seizures. *Arch Neurol* 1994; **51:** 1047–50.
12. Anhut H, *et al.* Long-term safety and efficacy of gabapentin (Neurontin) as add-on therapy in patients with refractory partial seizures. *J Epilepsy* 1995; **8:** 44–50.
13. Ojemann LM, *et al.* Long-term treatment with gabapentin for partial epilepsy. *Epilepsy Res* 1992; **13:** 159–65.
14. Beydoun A, *et al.* Gabapentin monotherapy II: a 26-week, double-blind, dose-controlled multicenter study of conversion from polytherapy in outpatients with refractory complex partial or secondarily generalized seizures. *Neurology* 1997; **49:** 746–52.
15. Khurana DS, *et al.* Efficacy of gabapentin therapy in children with refractory partial seizures. *J Pediatr* 1996; **128:** 829–33.

Motor neurone disease. For mention of interest in the use of gabapentin in patients with motor neurone disease, see p.1625.

Pain. Neurogenic pain is often insensitive to opioid analgesics, and various drugs, including antiepileptics, have been tried (see p.4). Carbamazepine appears to be the antiepileptic most frequently used. There have been anecdotal reports of the successful use of gabapentin in the treatment of patients with intractable neurogenic pain,[1] including central pain[2] (see p.8) and postherpetic neuralgia[3] (see p.10).

1. Rosner H, *et al.* Gabapentin adjunctive therapy in neuropathic pain states. *Clin J Pain* 1996; **12:** 56–8.
2. Schachter SC, Sauter MK. Treatment of central pain with gabapentin: case reports. *J Epilepsy* 1996; **9:** 223–5.
3. Segal AZ, Rodorf G. Gabapentin as a novel treatment for postherpetic neuralgia. *Neurology* 1996; **46:** 1175–6.

Parkinsonism. While some overall ratings of Parkinson's disease (p.1128) appeared to be improved by gabapentin in a double-blind study involving 19 patients with advanced parkinsonism, improvements in individual signs and symptoms were not significant.[1] It was also reported that 5 of 6 other patients with progressive supranuclear palsy had experienced worsening of their disease when given gabapentin.

1. Olson WL, *et al.* Gabapentin for parkinsonism: a double-blind, placebo-controlled, crossover trial. *Am J Med* 1997; **102:** 60–6.

Preparations

Proprietary Preparations (details are given in Part 3)
Aust.: Neurontin; ***Austral.:*** Neurontin; ***Canad.:*** Neurontin; ***Fr.:*** Neurontin; ***Ger.:*** Neurontin; ***Irl.:*** Neurontin; ***Ital.:*** Aclonium; ***Norw.:*** Neurontin; ***S.Afr.:*** Neurontin; ***Spain:*** Neurontin; ***Swed.:*** Neurontin; ***Switz.:*** Neurontin; ***UK:*** Neurontin; ***USA:*** Neurontin.

Lamotrigine (18658-r)

Lamotrigine *(BAN, USAN, rINN)*.

BW-430C. 6-(2,3-Dichlorophenyl)-1,2,4-triazine-3,5-diyldiamine.

$C_9H_7Cl_2N_5$ = 256.1.

CAS — 84057-84-1.

Adverse Effects

Skin rashes may occur during therapy with lamotrigine; severe skin reactions including Stevens-Johnson syndrome and toxic epidermal necrolysis have been reported, especially in children, and usually occur within 8 weeks of starting lamotrigine. Symptoms such as fever, malaise, influenza-like symptoms, drowsiness, lymphadenopathy, facial oedema and, rarely, hepatic dysfunction, leucopenia, and thrombocytopenia have also been reported in conjunction with rashes as part of a hypersensitivity syndrome. Other adverse effects include angioedema and photosensitivity; diplopia, blurred vision, and conjunctivitis; and dizziness, drowsiness, insomnia, headache, ataxia, tiredness, nausea and vomiting, irritability and aggression, tremor, agitation, and confusion.

The manufacturers report that there have been rare instances of death following a rapidly progressive illness with status epilepticus, multi-organ dysfunction, and disseminated intravascular coagulation in patients receiving therapy with multiple antiepileptics including lamotrigine, although the role of lamotrigine remains to be established. It has been suggested[1] that multi-organ failure and disseminated intravascular coagulation, with associated rhabdomyolysis, are complications of severe convulsive seizures rather than of lamotrigine therapy. However, Schaub *et al.*[2] reported a patient with no history of generalised seizures who developed a syndrome of disseminated intravascular coagulation, rhabdomyolysis, renal failure, maculopapular rash, and ataxia 14 days after lamotrigine was added to her antiepileptic regimen.

1. Yuen AWC, Bihari DJ. Multiorgan failure and disseminated intravascular coagulation in severe convulsive seizures. *Lancet* 1992; **340:** 618.
2. Schaub JEM, *et al.* Multisystem adverse reaction to lamotrigine. *Lancet* 1994; **344:** 481.

Effects on the blood. Septic shock secondary to leucopenia occurred in a patient when lamotrigine was added to therapy with sodium valproate.[1]

1. Nicholson RJ, *et al.* Leucopenia associated with lamotrigine. *Br Med J* 1995; **310:** 504.

Effects on the liver. Fatal fulminant hepatic failure has been reported[1] in one patient following addition of lamotrigine to an antiepileptic regimen comprising sodium valproate and carbamazepine.

1. Makin AJ, *et al.* Fulminant hepatic failure induced by lamotrigine. *Br Med J* 1995; **311:** 292.

Effects on the skin. Rashes account for withdrawal from therapy in about 2% of those given lamotrigine,[1,2] and serious skin reactions including Stevens-Johnson syndrome and toxic epidermal necrolysis occur in about 1 in 1000 adult patients.[3,4] The main risk factors appear to be concomitant use with valproate, and exceeding the recommended initial dose of lamotrigine or the recommended rate of dose escalation. The risk appears to be greater in children[1,4,5] and has been estimated to be between 1 in 50 and 1 in 300. These skin reactions usually occur within 8 weeks of starting therapy with lamotrigine, but onset as early as the first day and as late as 2 years has been noted.[6]

1. Mackay FJ, *et al.* Safety of long-term lamotrigine in epilepsy. *Epilepsia* 1997; **38:** 881–6.
2. Messenheimer J, *et al.* Safety review of adult clinical trial experience with lamotrigine. *Drug Safety* 1998; **18:** 281–96.
3. Committee on Safety of Medicines/Medicines Control Agency. Lamotrigine (Lamictal) and serious skin reactions. *Current Problems* 1996; **22:** 12.
4. Committee on Safety of Medicines/Medicines Control Agency. Lamotrigine (Lamictal): increased risk of serious skin reactions in children. *Current Problems* 1997; **23:** 8.
5. Mitchell P. Paediatric lamotrigine use hit by rash reports. *Lancet* 1997; **349:** 1080.
6. Adverse Drug Reactions Advisory Committee (ADRAC). Lamotrigine and severe skin reactions. *Aust Adverse Drug React Bull* 1997; **16:** 3.

Overdosage. No serious toxicity was observed in a patient who deliberately took an overdose of 1.35 g of lamotrigine and was subsequently treated with gastric lavage and activated charcoal.[1] Symptoms at presentation one hour after ingestion had included nystagmus and muscle hypertonicity. ECG monitoring had revealed widening of the QRS interval.

1. Buckley NA, *et al.* Self-poisoning with lamotrigine. *Lancet* 1993; **342:** 1552–3.

Precautions

Lamotrigine is contra-indicated in patients with hepatic impairment until more information is available. Caution is advised when there is renal impairment. Patients receiving lamotrigine should be closely monitored and changes in hepatic, renal, and clotting functions looked for. They should be warned to see their doctor immediately if rashes or influenza-like symptoms associated with hypersensitivity develop. Withdrawal of lamotrigine should be considered if rash, fever, influenza-like symptoms, drowsiness, or worsening of seizure control occurs. Care is required when withdrawing lamotrigine therapy—see also under Uses and Administration, below. Abrupt withdrawal should be avoided unless serious skin reactions have occurred. To minimise the risk of developing serious skin reactions, dosage recommendations should not be exceeded. Children's body-weight should be monitored and the dose reviewed if necessary.

Driving. For a comment on antiepileptic drugs and driving, see p.337.

Intellectual impairment. Aggressive behaviour has been reported in intellectually impaired patients given lamotrigine.[1] Of 19 such patients given lamotrigine, aggressive behaviour developed in 9; the drug was discontinued in 5, and stopped but reintroduced in a further 2, together with psychiatric management. One patient responded to a reduction in lamotrigine dosage.

1. Beran RG, Gibson RJ. Aggressive behaviour in intellectually challenged patients with epilepsy treated with lamotrigine. *Epilepsia* 1998; **39:** 280–2.

Pregnancy. For comments on the management of epilepsy during pregnancy, see p.337. There appears to be little evidence of teratogenic potential for lamotrigine in *animal* studies to date, although there is a theoretical risk with lamotrigine because it is a folate antagonist.

Renal impairment. Results from a pharmacokinetic study[1] indicated that impaired renal function was likely to have little effect on plasma concentrations of lamotrigine. The drug is mainly cleared by metabolism and although the glucuronide metabolite accumulates it is inactive. Nevertheless, there is limited clinical experience with lamotrigine in such patients and caution was recommended.

1. Wootton R, *et al.* Comparison of the pharmacokinetics of lamotrigine in patients with chronic renal failure and healthy volunteers. *Br J Clin Pharmacol* 1997; **43:** 23–7.

Interactions

There are complex interactions between antiepileptics and toxicity may be enhanced without a corresponding increase in antiepileptic activity. Such interactions are very variable and unpredictable and plasma monitoring is often advisable with combination therapy. The metabolism of lamotrigine is enhanced by the enzyme inducers carbamazepine, phenytoin, phenobarbitone, and primidone, and inhibited by valproate (see below).

Analgesics. Concomitant administration of *paracetamol* affects the metabolic disposition of lamotrigine but the clinical significance of this interaction remains to be determined.[1] Paracetamol reduced the area under the plasma concentration-time curve for lamotrigine, reduced lamotrigine's half-life, and increased the percentage of lamotrigine recovered in the urine.

1. Depot M, *et al.* Kinetic effects of multiple oral doses of acetaminophen on a single oral dose of lamotrigine. *Clin Pharmacol Ther* 1990; **48:** 346–55.

Antiepileptics. *Valproate* can inhibit the metabolism of lamotrigine resulting in increased concentrations of lamotrigine. This effect can be beneficial in the control of certain seizures, although careful monitoring is required as toxicity may occur. Disabling tremor occurred in 3 patients receiving such a combination which resolved when the dose of lamotrigine or valproate was reduced.[1]

Other reported symptoms of toxicity, that resolved on reduction of the lamotrigine dose, were sedation, ataxia, and fatigue.[2] Reversible encephalopathy has been reported[3] when sodium valproate was substituted for phenytoin in a patient also receiving lamotrigine, although her clinical condition had been satisfactory on this new regimen for several months. Symptoms improved when the doses of both valproate and lamotrigine were reduced. Pharmacokinetic studies[4,5] in healthy adults have attempted to elucidate the mechanism of the interaction between lamotrigine and valproate. The clearance of lamotrigine was found to be reduced, and the area under the curve and elimination half-life increased when valproate was administered concomitantly. Renal elimination was not affected and the investigators[4] suggested that there was hepatic competition for glucuronidation between valproate and lamotrigine. However, there was no substantial alteration in the linear kinetics of lamotrigine in the presence of therapeutic plasma concentrations of valproate.[5] Similar observations were made when lamotrigine was added to existing antiepileptic regimens in children,[6] although the clinical relevance of the influence of age on the pharmacokinetics remains to be determined. Both young age and concomitant administration of valproate are risk factors for lamotrigine-induced dermatological toxicity—see Effects on the Skin, above.

For details of dosage reductions required for lamotrigine when given together with valproate, see Uses and Administration, below.

Apart from valproate, other antiepileptics also affect plasma concentrations of lamotrigine when given concomitantly. May *et al.*[7] confirmed that, while valproate inhibited its elimination, *carbamazepine, phenytoin,* or *phenobarbitone* all markedly induced the elimination of lamotrigine. Others have confirmed a reduction in plasma-lamotrigine concentrations when given with phenytoin and other enzyme-inducing antiepileptics.[8]

For the effect of lamotrigine on the pharmacokinetics of carbamazepine, see p.341.

1. Reutens DC, *et al.* Disabling tremor after lamotrigine with sodium valproate. *Lancet* 1993; **342:** 185–6.
2. Pisani F, *et al.* Interaction of lamotrigine with sodium valproate. *Lancet* 1993; **341:** 1224.
3. Hennessy MJ, Wiles CM. Lamotrigine encephalopathy. *Lancet* 1996; **347:** 974–5.
4. Yuen AWC, *et al.* Sodium valproate acutely inhibits lamotrigine metabolism. *Br J Clin Pharmacol* 1992; **33:** 511–13.
5. Anderson GD, *et al.* Bidirectional interaction of valproate and lamotrigine in healthy subjects. *Clin Pharmacol Ther* 1996; **60:** 145–56.
6. Vauzelle-Kervroëdan F, *et al.* Influence of concurrent antiepileptic medication on the pharmacokinetics of lamotrigine as add-on therapy in epileptic children. *Br J Clin Pharmacol* 1996; **41:** 325–30.
7. May TW, *et al.* Serum concentrations of lamotrigine in epileptic patients: the influence of dose and comedication. *Ther Drug Monit* 1996; **18:** 523–31.
8. Battino D, *et al.* Lamotrigine plasma concentrations in children and adults: influence of age and associated therapy. *Ther Drug Monit* 1997; **19:** 620–7.

Pharmacokinetics

Lamotrigine is well absorbed from the gastro-intestinal tract and peak plasma concentrations have been reported 2.5 hours after oral administration. It is widely distributed in the body and is reported to be about 55% bound to plasma protein. It is extensively metabolised in the liver and excreted almost entirely in urine, principally as a glucuronide conjugate. It slightly induces its own metabolism and the half-life at steady state is reported to be about 24 hours.

The pharmacokinetics of lamotrigine are affected by the concomitant administration of other antiepileptics (see Interactions, above).

General references.

1. Rambeck B, Wolf P. Lamotrigine clinical pharmacokinetics. *Clin Pharmacokinet* 1993; **25:** 433–43.
2. Elwes RDC, Binnie CD. Clinical pharmacokinetics of newer antiepileptic drugs: lamotrigine, vigabatrin, gabapentin and oxcarbazepine. *Clin Pharmacokinet* 1996; **30:** 403–15.

In a study of newly diagnosed or poorly controlled epileptic patients[1] there appeared to be little relationship between plasma concentrations of lamotrigine and either its efficacy or the onset of adverse effects. Thus a 'target' range of concentrations for lamotrigine was considered to be inappropriate and routine therapeutic drug monitoring not to be useful.

1. Kilpatrick ES, *et al.* Concentration-effect and concentration-toxicity relations with lamotrigine: a prospective study. *Epilepsia* 1996; **37:** 534–8.

Renal impairment. See under Precautions, above.

Uses and Administration

Lamotrigine, a phenyltriazine compound, is an antiepileptic used as monotherapy and as an adjunct to treatment with other antiepileptics for partial seizures and primary and secondarily generalised tonic-clonic seizures. It is also used for seizures associated with the Lennox-Gastaut syndrome.

In the UK the initial **adult** dose for use as *monotherapy* is 25 mg once daily by mouth for 2 weeks followed by 50 mg once daily for 2 weeks; thereafter the dose is increased by a maximum of 50 to 100 mg every 1 to 2 weeks to usual maintenance doses of 100 to 200 mg daily, given as a single dose or in 2 divided doses. Some patients have required up to 500 mg daily.

The initial adult dose of lamotrigine for use as an *adjunct* to therapy with enzyme-inducing antiepileptics (but *not with valproate*) is 50 mg once daily for 2 weeks followed by 50 mg twice daily for 2 weeks; thereafter the daily dose is increased by a maximum of 100 mg every 1 to 2 weeks to usual maintenance doses of 200 to 400 mg daily given in 2 divided doses. Some patients have required up to 700 mg daily. In adults *taking valproate* the initial dose of lamotrigine is 25 mg every other day for 2 weeks followed by 25 mg once daily for 2 weeks; thereafter the daily dose is increased by a maximum of 25 to 50 mg every 1 to 2 weeks to usual maintenance doses of 100 to 200 mg daily given as a single dose or in 2 divided doses.

The doses above are permitted in the UK in **children** over 12 years of age; the use of lamotrigine as *monotherapy* is not recommended for children under 12 years of age. For children aged 2 to 12 years the initial dose of lamotrigine as an *adjunct* to therapy with enzyme-inducing antiepileptics (but *not with valproate*) is 2 mg per kg body-weight daily in 2 divided doses for 2 weeks followed by 5 mg per kg daily in 2 divided doses for 2 weeks; thereafter the dose is increased as necessary by a maximum of 2 to 3 mg per kg every 1 to 2 weeks; usual maintenance doses are 5 to 15 mg per kg daily in 2 divided doses. In children *taking valproate*, the initial dose of lamotrigine is 0.2 mg per kg once daily for 2 weeks followed by 0.5 mg per kg once daily for 2 weeks; thereafter the dose is increased by a maximum of 0.5 to 1 mg per kg every 1 to 2 weeks to usual maintenance doses of 1 to 5 mg per kg, which may be given once daily or in 2 divided doses. Children weighing 12.5 to 25 kg may be given 5 mg on alternate days for the first 2 weeks of therapy.

As with other antiepileptics, withdrawal of lamotrigine therapy or transition to or from another type of antiepileptic therapy should be made gradually to avoid precipitating an increase in the frequency of seizures. For a discussion on whether or not to withdraw antiepileptic therapy in seizure-free patients, see p.335. The manufacturers recommend that the withdrawal of lamotrigine should be tapered over at least 2 weeks.

Epilepsy. Lamotrigine is used in the treatment of epilepsy (p.335) where control is difficult to obtain. It has been used for both partial and secondarily generalised tonic-clonic seizures refractory to standard antiepileptic therapy.[1-6] About 30% of patients may experience a 50% reduction in seizure frequency and a relatively small percentage will become seizure-free.[4] Some patients may become sufficiently stabilised to allow withdrawal of concomitant antiepileptic therapy.[3] Lamotrigine has shown comparable efficacy to carbamazepine as monotherapy for partial seizures with or without secondary generalisation and primary generalised tonic-clonic seizures in newly diagnosed patients.[7] It also appears to be an effective adjunctive treatment in children with the Lennox-Gastaut syndrome.[8,9] There are anecdotal reports suggesting efficacy in patients with other types of seizures including atypical absence seizures, atonic seizures, primary generalised tonic-clonic seizures, myoclonic jerks, and status epilepticus; preliminary studies of lamotrigine given with valproate for absence seizures[10] and infantile spasms[11] showed promising results. Lamotrigine as adjunctive therapy has been found to be effective and well tolerated in paediatric patients with refractory epilepsy including those with developmental impairment;[12] it was particularly effective in absence and atypical seizures in this open-label study. However, despite all these encouraging views concerning the role of lamotrigine, the authors of a follow-up study[13] were less optimistic. They followed up 124 patients who had participated in an open-label trial of lamotrigine as adjunctive therapy for refractory epilepsy 6 to 8 years earlier and concluded that lamotrigine had only marginal benefit on the long-term prognosis of severe refractory epilepsy.

1. Richens A, Yuen AWC. Overview of the clinical efficacy of lamotrigine. *Epilepsia* 1991; **32** (suppl 2): S13–S16.
2. Brodie MJ. Lamotrigine. *Lancet* 1992; **339:** 1397–1400.
3. Goa KL, *et al.* Lamotrigine: a review of its pharmacological properties and clinical efficacy in epilepsy. *Drugs* 1993; **46:** 152–76.
4. Brodie MJ. Drugs in focus: 10. Lamotrigine. *Prescribers' J* 1993; **33:** 212–16.
5. Gilman JT. Lamotrigine: an antiepileptic agent for the treatment of partial seizures. *Ann Pharmacother* 1995; **29:** 144–51.
6. Anonymous. Lamotrigine for epilepsy. *Med Lett Drugs Ther* 1995; **37:** 21–3.
7. Brodie MJ, *et al.* UK Lamotrigine/Carbamazepine Monotherapy Trial Group. Double-blind comparison of lamotrigine and carbamazepine in newly diagnosed epilepsy. *Lancet* 1995; **345:** 476–9.
8. Donaldson JA, *et al.* Lamotrigine adjunctive therapy in childhood epileptic encephalopathy (the Lennox Gastaut Syndrome). *Epilepsia* 1997; **38:** 68–73.
9. Motte J, *et al.* Lamotrigine for generalized seizures associated with the Lennox-Gastaut syndrome. *N Engl J Med* 1997; **337:** 1807–12. Correction. *ibid.* 1998; **339:** 851–2.
10. Ferrie CD, *et al.* Lamotrigine as an add-on drug in typical absence seizures. *Acta Neurol Scand* 1995; **91:** 200–202.
11. Veggiotti P, *et al.* Lamotrigine in infantile spasms. *Lancet* 1994; **344:** 1375–6.

12. Besag FMC, *et al.* Lamotrigine for the treatment of epilepsy in childhood. *J Pediatr* 1995; **127:** 991–7.
13. Walker MC, *et al.* Long term use of lamotrigine and vigabatrin in severe refractory epilepsy: audit of outcome. *Br Med J* 1996; **313:** 1184–5.

Preparations

Proprietary Preparations (details are given in Part 3)
Aust.: Lamictal; ***Austral.:*** Lamictal; ***Belg.:*** Lamictal; ***Canad.:*** Lamictal; ***Fr.:*** Lamictal; ***Ger.:*** Lamictal; ***Irl.:*** Lamictal; ***Ital.:*** Lamictal; ***Neth.:*** Lamictal; ***Norw.:*** Lamictal; ***S.Afr.:*** Lamicitin; ***Spain:*** Labileno; Lamictal; ***Swed.:*** Lamictal; ***Switz.:*** Lamictal; ***UK:*** Lamictal; ***USA:*** Lamictal.

Methoin (6613-f)

Methoin *(BAN).*

Mephenytoin *(USAN, rINN)*; Mephenetoin; Methantoin; NSC-34652; Phenantoin. 5-Ethyl-3-methyl-5-phenylhydantoin.

$C_{12}H_{14}N_2O_2$ = 218.3.

CAS — 50-12-4.

Pharmacopoeias. In *Aust.* and *US.*

A white crystalline powder. **Soluble** 1 in 1400 of water, 1 in 15 of alcohol, 1 in 3 of chloroform, and 1 in 90 of ether; soluble in aqueous solutions of alkali hydroxides.

Methoin is a hydantoin antiepileptic with actions similar to those of phenytoin (p.352), but it is more toxic. Because of its potential toxicity it is not one of the main drugs used in the treatment of epilepsy (p.335) and is given only to patients unresponsive to other treatment. Some of the side-effects of methoin may be due to the metabolite, 5-ethyl-5-phenylhydantoin (also termed nirvanol). Like phenytoin the rate of metabolism of methoin is subject to genetic polymorphism.

Methoin is given in an initial daily dose by mouth of 50 to 100 mg for one week; thereafter the daily dose is increased by 50 to 100 mg at weekly intervals until the optimum dose is reached, which is usually between 200 and 600 mg daily for an adult and 100 and 400 mg daily for a child; daily maintenance doses are usually taken in 3 divided doses.

Preparations

USP 23: Mephenytoin Tablets.

Proprietary Preparations (details are given in Part 3)
Aust.: Epilan; ***Canad.:*** Mesantoin†; ***USA:*** Mesantoin.

Methsuximide (6614-d)

Methsuximide *(BAN).*

Mesuximide *(rINN)*; PM-396. *N*,2-Dimethyl-2-phenylsuccinimide.

$C_{12}H_{13}NO_2$ = 203.2.

CAS — 77-41-8.

Pharmacopoeias. In *US.*

A white to greyish-white crystalline powder; odourless or with a slight odour. M.p. 50° to 56°. **Soluble** 1 in 350 of water, 1 in 3 of alcohol, 1 in less than 1 of chloroform, and 1 in 2 of ether. **Store** in airtight containers.

Methsuximide is a succinimide antiepileptic with actions similar to those of ethosuximide (p.344), but with some activity in complex partial seizures. It is thought to owe its activity to its major metabolite *N*-desmethylmethsuximide. It is usually only given to patients unresponsive to other antiepileptic treatment.

The usual initial dosage is a single dose of 300 mg daily by mouth for the first week, and this is increased by 300 mg at weekly intervals to an optimum dosage, according to the patient's response. The suggested maximum daily dose is 1.2 g in divided doses.

Epilepsy. Methsuximide is used for absence seizures that are refractory to less toxic antiepileptics such as ethosuximide or valproate, which are the usual drugs to try (see p.335). Methsuximide has also been tried in complex partial seizures and myoclonic seizures.

References.

1. Tennison MB, *et al.* Methsuximide for intractable childhood seizures. *Pediatrics* 1991; **87:** 186–9.

Porphyria. Methsuximide has been associated with clinical exacerbations of porphyria and is considered unsafe in porphyric patients.[1]

1. Moore MR, McColl KEL. *Porphyria: drug lists.* Glasgow: Porphyria Research Unit, University of Glasgow, 1991.

Preparations

USP 23: Methsuximide Capsules.

Proprietary Preparations (details are given in Part 3)
Aust.: Petinutin; ***Austral.:*** Celontin†; ***Belg.:*** Celontin†; ***Canad.:*** Celontin; ***Ger.:*** Petinutin; ***Neth.:*** Celontin; ***S.Afr.:*** Celontin†; ***Switz.:*** Petinutin; ***USA:*** Celontin.

Methylphenobarbitone (4050-w)

Methylphenobarbitone *(BAN).*

Methylphenobarbital *(rINN)*; Enphenemalum; Mephobarbital; Methylphenobarbitalum; Phemitone. 5-Ethyl-1-methyl-5-phenylbarbituric acid.

$C_{13}H_{14}N_2O_3$ = 246.3.

CAS — 115-38-8.

Pharmacopoeias. In *Eur.* (see p.viii) and *US.*

Odourless colourless crystals or a white crystalline powder. Very slightly **soluble** or practically insoluble in water; very slightly soluble in alcohol, in dehydrated alcohol, and in ether; soluble 1 in 50 of chloroform; it forms water-soluble compounds with alkali hydroxides and carbonates and with aqueous ammonia. A saturated solution in water is acid to litmus.

Dependence and Withdrawal, Adverse Effects, Treatment, and Precautions

As for Phenobarbitone, p.350.

Interactions

As for Phenobarbitone, p.351.

Pharmacokinetics

Methylphenobarbitone is incompletely absorbed from the gastro-intestinal tract. It is demethylated to phenobarbitone in the liver.

Uses and Administration

Methylphenobarbitone is used similarly to phenobarbitone (p.351) in the treatment of epilepsy (p.335). It is given in usual doses of 200 to 400 mg daily by mouth; up to 600 mg daily may be given if required. It has also been used as a sedative.

Preparations

USP 23: Mephobarbital Tablets.

Proprietary Preparations (details are given in Part 3)
Austral.: Prominal; ***Spain:*** Prominal; ***UK:*** Prominal; ***USA:*** Mebaral.

Multi-ingredient: ***Belg.:*** Mathoine; ***Canad.:*** Ancatropine Gel†; ***Ital.:*** Dintoinale; Dintospina†; Metinal-Idantoina; Metinal-Idantoina L; ***Spain:*** Comital L.

Oxcarbazepine (19623-a)

Oxcarbazepine *(rINN).*

GP-47680. 10,11-Dihydro-10-oxo-5*H*-dibenz[*b,f*]azepine-5-carboxamide.

$C_{15}H_{12}N_2O_2$ = 252.3.

CAS — 28721-07-5.

Adverse Effects, Treatment, and Precautions

As for Carbamazepine, p.339.

Skin rashes occur less frequently with oxcarbazepine than with carbamazepine and a large proportion of patients with skin reactions to carbamazepine are able to tolerate oxcarbazepine. However, oxcarbazepine reduces plasma-sodium concentrations to a greater extent than carbamazepine.

Hyponatraemia. Hyponatraemia associated with oxcarbazepine therapy has been reported by a number of workers and it appears to be more pronounced at clinical doses of oxcarbazepine than with carbamazepine. Pendlebury *et al.*[1] reported hyponatraemia in 12 of 15 patients in whom oxcarbazepine was substituted for carbamazepine therapy. The fall in plasma-sodium concentrations appeared to be related to the dose of oxcarbazepine. Another group of workers[2] reported hyponatraemia in 23% of 350 patients whose serum-sodium concentrations were monitored. Most patients remain asymptomatic but some may experience drowsiness, increase in seizure frequency, and impaired consciousness.[3] It has been suggested that serum-sodium concentrations should be measured before the start of therapy but routine repeated determinations may be indicated only in elderly patients or if a high dosage is used.[4]

1. Pendlebury SC, *et al.* Hyponatraemia during oxcarbazepine therapy. *Hum Toxicol* 1989; **8:** 337–44.
2. Friis ML, *et al.* Therapeutic experiences with 947 epileptic outpatients in oxcarbazepine treatment. *Acta Neurol Scand* 1993; **87:** 224–7.
3. Steinhoff BJ, *et al.* Hyponatraemic coma under oxcarbazepine therapy. *Epilepsy Res* 1992; **11;** 67–70.
4. Kälviäinen R, *et al.* Place of newer antiepileptic drugs in the treatment of epilepsy. *Drugs* 1993; **46:** 1009–24.

Renal impairment. In a study[1] to assess the effect of renal impairment on the pharmacokinetics of oxcarbazepine and its metabolites, the following suggestions were made: no special dose adjustment appears necessary in patients with a creatinine clearance of greater than 30 mL per minute; the maximum target dose of oxcarbazepine given during the titration phase should be halved and the titration phase prolonged in patients with a clearance of 10 to 30 mL per minute; the glucuronides of oxcarbazepine and its monohydroxy metabolite are likely to accumulate during repeated administration in patients with a clearance of less than 10 mL per minute, but dosage adjustment in such patients could not be proposed from this study.

1. Rouan MC, *et al.* The effect of renal impairment on the pharmacokinetics of oxcarbazepine and its metabolites. *Eur J Clin Pharmacol* 1994; **47:** 161–7.

Interactions

Compared with carbamazepine (p.341) there appear to be fewer reports of drug interactions involving oxcarbazepine.

Antiepileptics. In a study[1] of epileptic patients receiving monotherapy the area under the concentration-time curve for *carbamazepine, phenytoin,* or *valproate* was unchanged when oxcarbazepine was added to treatment; only carbamazepine affected the pharmacokinetics of oxcarbazepine, producing a reduction in the area under the curve for the active metabolite hydroxycarbazepine. It was considered that there was unlikely to be any clinically relevant pharmacokinetic interaction if oxcarbazepine was used as adjunctive therapy with any of these antiepileptics, including carbamazepine.

1. McKee PJW, *et al.* A double-blind, placebo-controlled interaction study between oxcarbazepine and carbamazepine, sodium valproate and phenytoin in epileptic patients. *Br J Clin Pharmacol* 1994; **37:** 27–32.

Pharmacokinetics

Oxcarbazepine is well absorbed from the gastro-intestinal tract. It is widely distributed in the body and is reported to be about 40% bound to plasma protein. It is rapidly and extensively metabolised in the liver to the principal metabolite 10,11-dihydro-10-hydroxy-carbamazepine, which possesses antiepileptic activity. Oxcarbazepine is excreted in the urine mainly as metabolites; less than 1% is excreted as unchanged drug. The elimination half-life has been reported to be 1.0 to 2.5 hours for oxcarbazepine, and about 8 to 14 hours for the monohydroxy metabolite. Oxcarbazepine and its monohydroxy derivative cross the placental barrier and are distributed into breast milk.

References.

1. Dickinson RG, *et al.* First dose and steady-state pharmacokinetics of oxcarbazepine and its 10-hydroxy metabolite. *Eur J Clin Pharmacol* 1989; **37:** 69–74.
2. Patsalos PN, *et al.* Protein binding of oxcarbazepine and its primary active metabolite, 10-hydroxycarbazepine, in patients with trigeminal neuralgia. *Eur J Clin Pharmacol* 1990; **39:** 413–15.
3. Kumps A, Wurth C. Oxcarbazepine disposition: preliminary observations in patients. *Biopharm Drug Dispos* 1990; **11:** 365–70.
4. van Heiningen PNM, *et al.* The influence of age on the pharmacokinetics of the antiepileptic agent oxcarbazepine. *Clin Pharmacol Ther* 1991; **50:** 410–19.
5. Isojärvi JIT, *et al.* Serum sex hormone levels after replacing carbamazepine with oxcarbazepine. *Eur J Clin Pharmacol* 1995; **47:** 461–4.
6. Elwes RDC, Binnie CD. Clinical pharmacokinetics of newer antiepileptic drugs: lamotrigine, vigabatrin, gabapentin and oxcarbazepine. *Clin Pharmacokinet* 1996; **30:** 403–15.

Renal impairment. See above.

Uses and Administration

Oxcarbazepine is a derivative of carbamazepine (p.342) with similar actions. It is used as an antiepileptic in the treatment of partial and generalised tonic-clonic seizures. Oxcarbazepine appears to be an effective substitute for carbamazepine in patients experiencing untoward adverse effects or significant drug interactions. The initial dose in the treatment of epilepsy is 300 mg daily by mouth, which is gradually increased until the optimal clinical effect is observed. Maintenance doses are usually in the range of 600 to 1200 mg daily given in 2 or 3 divided doses. Doses should be reduced by about half in patients with moderate to severe renal impairment (see above).

As with other antiepileptics, withdrawal of oxcarbazepine therapy or transition to or from another type of antiepileptic therapy should be made gradually to avoid precipitating an increase in the frequency of seizures. For a discussion on whether or not to withdraw antiepileptic therapy in seizure-free patients, see p.335.

Epilepsy. Oxcarbazepine is used in the treatment of epilepsy (p.335) and may be a useful alternative in patients unable to tolerate carbamazepine.

The actions and uses of oxcarbazepine have been reviewed.[1-3] The efficacy of oxcarbazepine appears to be similar to that of carbamazepine and it may have a lower propensity to produce adverse effects on the CNS, and allergic reactions, although hyponatraemia is likely to be troublesome. Oxcarbazepine appears to induce hepatic enzymes to a lesser extent than carbamazepine[4,5] and may therefore produce fewer interactions. Oxcarbazepine has a different pharmacokinetic profile to that of carbamazepine and is reduced to a pharmacologically active 10-hydroxy metabolite.[1-3]

In a double-blind trial[6] involving newly diagnosed adult patients, oxcarbazepine was of similar efficacy and tolerability to valproate for partial or generalised tonic-clonic seizures.

1. Grant SM, Faulds D. Oxcarbazepine: a review of its pharmacology and therapeutic potential in epilepsy, trigeminal neuralgia and affective disorders. *Drugs* 1992; **43:** 873–88.
2. Kälviäinen R, *et al.* Place of newer antiepileptic drugs in the treatment of epilepsy. *Drugs* 1993; **46:** 1009–24.

3. Patsalos PN, Sander JWAS. Newer antiepileptic drugs: towards an improved risk-benefit ratio. *Drug Safety* 1994; **11:** 37–67.
4. Patsalos PN, *et al.* Dose dependent enzyme induction by oxcarbazepine? *Eur J Clin Pharmacol* 1990; **39:** 187–8.
5. Larkin JG, *et al.* Lack of enzyme induction with oxcarbazepine (600 mg daily) in healthy subjects. *Br J Clin Pharmacol* 1991; **31:** 65–71.
6. Christe W, *et al.* A double-blind controlled clinical trial: oxcarbazepine versus sodium valproate in adults with newly diagnosed epilepsy. *Epilepsy Res* 1997; **26:** 451–60.

Preparations

Proprietary Preparations (details are given in Part 3)
Aust.: Trileptal; ***Ital.:*** Trileptal; ***Neth.:*** Trileptal; ***S.Afr.:*** Trileptal; ***Switz.:*** Trileptal.

Paramethadione (6615-n)

Paramethadione *(BAN, rINN).*

5-Ethyl-3,5-dimethyl-1,3-oxazolidine-2,4-dione.

$C_7H_{11}NO_3$ = 157.2.

CAS — 115-67-3.

Paramethadione is an oxazolidinedione antiepileptic with actions similar to those of troxidone (p.361). Because of its potential toxicity it was given only to patients unresponsive to other antiepileptics.

Preparations

Proprietary Preparations (details are given in Part 3)
USA: Paradione†.

Phenacemide (6616-h)

Phenacemide *(BAN, rINN).*

Carbamidum Phenylaceticum. (Phenylacetyl)urea.

$C_9H_{10}N_2O_2$ = 178.2.

CAS — 63-98-9.

Pharmacopoeias. In *US.*

An odourless or practically odourless, white or practically white, fine crystalline powder. Very slightly **soluble** in water, in alcohol, in chloroform, and in ether; slightly soluble in acetone; soluble 1 in 500 of warm alcohol and 1 in 300 of methyl alcohol. **Store** in airtight containers.

Phenacemide is an acetylurea antiepileptic which is the straight-chain analogue of a hydantoin. It has been used in the treatment of epilepsy (p.335), especially in complex partial seizures; because of its potential toxicity it is not one of the main antiepileptics used and should be employed only in patients whose seizures are impossible to control with other recognised antiepileptics.

Severe adverse effects reported with phenacemide include psychoses and personality changes, blood disorders including aplastic anaemia, and liver and kidney damage; extreme caution is advised in giving phenacemide to patients with a history of such disorders.

Serum-creatinine concentrations should not be used as a measure of renal function in patients receiving phenacemide as it can increase creatinine concentrations in the absence of renal impairment.[1]

1. Cahen R, *et al.* Creatinine metabolism impairment by an anticonvulsant drug, phenacemide. *Ann Pharmacother* 1994; **28:** 49–51.

Preparations

USP 23: Phenacemide Tablets.

Proprietary Preparations (details are given in Part 3)
USA: Phenurone†.

Pheneturide (6617-m)

Pheneturide *(BAN, rINN).*

Ethylphenacemide; S-46. (2-Phenylbutyryl)urea.

$C_{11}H_{14}N_2O_2$ = 206.2.

CAS — 90-49-3.

Pheneturide is an acetylurea antiepileptic used in the treatment of epilepsy (p.335). Doses of 0.5 to 1.5 g daily have been given by mouth.

Preparations

Proprietary Preparations (details are given in Part 3)
Belg.: Laburide; ***Switz.:*** Benuride.

Multi-ingredient: ***Belg.:*** Trinuride†.

Phenobarbitone (4060-l)

Phenobarbitone *(BAN).*

Phenobarbital *(rINN)*; Fenobarbital; Phenemalum; Phenobarbitalum; Phenylethylbarbituric Acid; Phenylethylmalonylurea. 5-Ethyl-5-phenylbarbituric acid.

$C_{12}H_{12}N_2O_3$ = 232.2.

CAS — 50-06-6.

Pharmacopoeias. In *Chin., Eur.* (see p.viii), *Int., Jpn, Pol.,* and *US.*

Colourless crystals or a white odourless crystalline powder. It may exhibit polymorphism.

Soluble 1 in 1000 of water and 1 in 10 of alcohol; sparingly soluble in chloroform; soluble in ether; it forms water-soluble compounds with alkali hydroxides and carbonates and with ammonia. A saturated solution in water has a pH of about 5.

Phenobarbitone Sodium (4061-y)

Phenobarbitone Sodium *(BANM).*

Phenobarbital Sodium *(rINN)*; Fenobarbital Sódico; Phenemalnatrium; Phenobarbitalum Natricum; Sodium Phenylethylbarbiturate; Soluble Phenobarbitone. Sodium 5-ethyl-5-phenylbarbiturate.

$C_{12}H_{11}N_2NaO_3$ = 254.2.

CAS — 57-30-7.

Pharmacopoeias. In *Chin., Eur.* (see p.viii), *Int., Pol.,* and *US.*

A white odourless crystalline hygroscopic powder, granules, or flakes. It loses not more than 7% of its weight when dried. Very **soluble** in water (Ph. Eur. states that it is freely soluble in carbon dioxide-free water but a small amount may be insoluble); soluble in alcohol; practically insoluble in chloroform, in ether, and in dichloromethane. A 10% solution in water has a pH of 9.2 to 10.2.

Phenobarbitone sodium is **incompatible** with many other drugs and phenobarbitone may be precipitated from mixtures containing phenobarbitone sodium. This precipitation is dependent upon the concentration and the pH, and also on the presence of other solvents. Solutions of phenobarbitone sodium decompose on standing. **Store** in airtight containers.

Dependence and Withdrawal

As for the barbiturates (see Amylobarbitone, p.641).

Adverse Effects

The most frequent adverse effect following administration of phenobarbitone is sedation, but this often becomes less marked with continued administration. Like some of the other antiepileptics, phenobarbitone may produce subtle mood changes and impairment of cognition and memory that may not be apparent without testing. Depression may occur.

Prolonged administration may occasionally result in folate deficiency; rarely, megaloblastic anaemia has been reported. There is some evidence that phenobarbitone interferes with vitamin D metabolism.

At high doses nystagmus and ataxia may occur and the typical barbiturate-induced respiratory depression may become severe. Overdosage can prove fatal; toxic effects include coma, severe respiratory and cardiovascular depression, with hypotension and shock leading to renal failure. Hypothermia may occur, with associated pyrexia during recovery. Skin blisters (bullae) reportedly occur in about 6% of patients with barbiturate overdose.

Owing to their extreme alkalinity necrosis has followed subcutaneous injection or extravasation of sodium salts of barbiturates. Intravenous injections can be hazardous and cause hypotension, shock, laryngospasm, and apnoea.

Hypersensitivity reactions occur in a small proportion of patients; skin reactions are reported in 1 to 3% of patients receiving phenobarbitone, and are most commonly maculopapular, morbilliform, or scarlatiniform rashes. More severe reactions such as exfoliative dermatitis, Stevens-Johnson syndrome, and toxic epidermal necrolysis are extremely rare. Hepatitis and disturbances of liver function have been reported.

Paradoxical excitement, restlessness, and confusion may sometimes occur in the elderly, and irritability and hyperactivity may occur in children.

Neonatal drug dependence and symptoms resembling vitamin K deficiency have been reported in infants born to mothers who received phenobarbitone during pregnancy. Congenital malformations have been reported in children of women who received phenobarbitone during pregnancy but the causal role of the drug is a matter of some debate.

Effects on the blood. For the effects of antiepileptics, including phenobarbitone, on serum folate, see under Phenytoin, p.353.

Effects on bone. For the effects of antiepileptics including phenobarbitone on bone and on calcium and vitamin D metabolism, see under Phenytoin, p.353.

Effects on the endocrine system. For mention of the effects of antiepileptics on *sexual function* in male epileptic patients, see under Phenytoin, p.353.

Barbiturates may reduce serum concentrations of *thyroid* hormones through enzyme induction—see under Interactions of Thyroxine, p.1498.

Effects on the liver. For mention of the effects of phenobarbitone on the liver, see under Phenytoin, p.353.

Effects on mental function. For a review of the effects of antiepileptic therapy including phenobarbitone on *cognition*, see p.337.

DEPRESSION. Follow-up of 28 patients aged 6 to 16 who had received phenobarbitone or carbamazepine for epilepsy indicated that the rate of major depression was significantly higher in those receiving phenobarbitone.[1] Treatment with phenobarbitone should be avoided particularly in patients with a personal or family history of an affective disorder and patients who do receive it should be monitored for symptoms of depression.

1. Brent DA, *et al.* Phenobarbital treatment and major depressive disorder in children with epilepsy: a naturalistic follow-up. *Pediatrics* 1990; **85:** 1086–91.

Hypersensitivity. Knutsen *et al.*[1] have provided details of hypersensitivity reactions to phenobarbitone in 7 children, occurring usually 1 to 2 weeks after initiation of phenobarbitone therapy. The condition began with fever, sometimes extreme, and was followed by an intensely pruritic rash; adenopathy or conjunctivitis was also seen in 5 patients. Lymphocyte studies *in vitro* suggested a cell-mediated reaction to phenobarbitone. It was considered that cross-reactivity among the major antiepileptic agents presented a real risk and that if a patient demonstrated a hypersensitivity reaction a chemically dissimilar drug should be substituted.

1. Knutsen AP, *et al.* Immunologic aspects of phenobarbital hypersensitivity. *J Pediatr* 1984; **105:** 558–63.

Treatment of Adverse Effects

Following the recent ingestion of an overdose of a barbiturate the stomach may be emptied by lavage; repeated doses of activated charcoal may be given with the aim not only of preventing absorption but also of aiding elimination. The prime objectives of management are then intensive symptomatic and supportive therapy with particular attention being paid to the maintenance of cardiovascular, respiratory, and renal functions and to the maintenance of the electrolyte balance.

Several other methods aimed at the active removal of a barbiturate with a long elimination half-life such as phenobarbitone have been employed and include forced diuresis, haemodialysis, peritoneal dialysis, and charcoal haemoperfusion, but with the possible exception of charcoal haemoperfusion the hazards of such procedures are generally considered to outweigh any purported benefits.

Precautions

Phenobarbitone and other barbiturates should be used with care in children and elderly patients, in those in acute pain, and in those with mental depression. Also they should be given cautiously to patients with impaired hepatic, renal, or respiratory function and may be contra-indicated when the impairment is severe.

Care is required when withdrawing phenobarbitone therapy—see also under Uses and Administration, below.

Phenobarbitone and other barbiturates cause drowsiness and patients receiving them, if affected, should not take charge of vehicles or machinery where loss of attention could cause accidents.

Driving. For a comment on antiepileptic drugs and driving, see p.337.

Neonates. Care should be taken when giving phenobarbitone orally as the elixir to neonates as regular dosing could result in alcohol toxicity [the BP formulation contains 38% v/v alcohol].[1] Aqueous preparations are more readily made using the sodium salt than the acid.[2]

1. Colquhoun-Flannery W, Wheeler R. Treating neonatal jaundice with phenobarbitone: the inadvertent administration of significant doses of ethyl alcohol. *Arch Dis Child* 1992; **67:** 152.
2. Leach F. Treating neonatal jaundice with phenobarbitone: the inadvertent administration of significant doses of ethyl alcohol. *Arch Dis Child* 1992; **67:** 152.

Porphyria. Phenobarbitone has been associated with acute attacks of porphyria and is considered unsafe in patients with acute porphyria.[1]

1. Moore MR, McColl KEL. *Porphyria: drug lists*. Glasgow: Porphyria Research Unit, University of Glasgow, 1991.

Pregnancy and breast feeding. For comments on the management of epilepsy during pregnancy and comments on breast feeding, see p.337.

Congenital craniofacial and digital abnormalities and, less commonly, cleft lip and palate have been described with antiepileptics including phenobarbitone. *In utero* exposure to phenobarbitone might result in neonatal sedation and drug dependence and also in neonatal bleeding.

Phenobarbitone given to the mother may cause neonatal sedation and breast feeding should be avoided.

Interactions

There are complex interactions between antiepileptics and toxicity may be enhanced without a corresponding increase in antiepileptic activity. Such interactions are very variable and unpredictable and plasma monitoring is often advisable with combination therapy. Valproate and phenytoin have been reported to cause rises in phenobarbitone (and primidone) concentrations in plasma.

The effects of phenobarbitone and other barbiturates are enhanced by the concurrent administration of other CNS depressants including alcohol.

Phenobarbitone and other barbiturates may reduce the activity of many drugs by increasing the rate of metabolism through induction of drug-metabolising enzymes in liver microsomes.

Analgesics. Administration of *dextropropoxyphene* 65 mg three times daily to 4 epileptic patients stabilised on phenobarbitone therapy resulted in increases in serum-phenobarbitone concentration ranging from 8 to 29% but the increase was not considered of major importance in the light of the normally accepted therapeutic range for phenobarbitone.[1]

For the effect of phenobarbitone on *methadone* and *pethidine*, see p.54 and p.77, respectively.

1. Hansen BS, *et al.* Influence of dextropropoxyphene on steady state serum levels and protein binding of three anti-epileptic drugs in man. *Acta Neurol Scand* 1980; **61:** 357–67.

Antiarrhythmics. For the effect of phenobarbitone on *disopyramide* and on *lignocaine*, see p.859 and p.1294, respectively.

Antibacterials. Serum concentrations of phenytoin and phenobarbitone in a previously stabilised patient were increased when he took *chloramphenicol* concomitantly.[1] Subsequent monitoring revealed a similar effect when chloramphenicol was taken with phenobarbitone alone. In turn, phenobarbitone may affect serum concentrations of chloramphenicol (see p.183).

Barbiturates such as phenobarbitone and primidone may enhance the metabolism of *doxycycline*.[2]

1. Koup JR, *et al.* Interaction of chloramphenicol with phenytoin and phenobarbital. *Clin Pharmacol Ther* 1978; **24:** 571–5.
2. Neuvonen PJ, *et al.* Effect of antiepileptic drugs on the elimination of various tetracycline derivatives. *Eur J Clin Pharmacol* 1975; **9:** 147–54.

Anticoagulants. For the effect of barbiturates such as phenobarbitone and primidone on warfarin, see p.967.

Antidepressants. As with all antiepileptics, antidepressants may antagonise the antiepileptic activity of phenobarbitone by lowering the convulsive threshold.

For the effect of phenobarbitone on antidepressants, see Mianserin (p.297) and under Fluoxetine (p.286).

Inhibition of drug-metabolising enzymes by MAOIs may enhance the effects of barbiturates.

Antiepileptics. Interactions may occur if phenobarbitone is given with other antiepileptics, of which probably the most significant is the interaction with *valproate*. Valproate results in an increase in plasma-phenobarbitone concentration that has been reported to range from 17 to 48%,[1] and it may be necessary to reduce the dose of phenobarbitone in some patients.[1,2] The mechanism for the increase appears to be inhibition of the metabolism of phenobarbitone, resulting in reduced clearance;[2,3] valproate appears to inhibit both the direct *N*-glucosidation of phenobarbitone and the *O*-glucuronidation of *p*-hydroxyphenobarbitone.[4] However, it is worthy of note that phenobarbitone reciprocally increases the clearance of valproate, thus potentially requiring the valproate dose to be adjusted too.[5]

A similarly complex interaction exists between phenobarbitone and *phenytoin*. Phenytoin may cause a rise in plasma concentrations of phenobarbitone in some patients[6] since the two drugs compete for metabolism by the same enzyme system, but other evidence suggests that where this occurs it is rarely of significant magnitude.[7] Similarly, although phenobarbitone induces the metabolism of phenytoin it is also, as stated, a competitive inhibitor and in practice the two effects appear to balance out, with rarely any need for dose adjustment.[7-9] However, dosage adjustment of phenobarbitone may be crucial for some patients.[10] Measurement of serum concentrations of phenytoin and phenobarbitone in one patient[10] showed that, in her case, large increases in serum-phenobarbitone concentrations resulted from concomitant administration of phenytoin; the increases were concentration-dependent.

The GABA-agonist, *progabide* has also been reported to cause a significant increase in phenobarbitone concentrations when the two were given together to healthy subjects,[11] and the possibility exists that dosage adjustment might be necessary if progabide were added to phenobarbitone therapy.

Neurotoxicity, attributed to an increase in plasma concentrations of phenobarbitone, has been observed[12] in one patient receiving phenobarbitone and sodium valproate when *felbamate* was added to treatment. The dosage of phenobarbitone had already been reduced before treatment with felbamate was started. Data from a pharmacokinetic study[13] indicated that the interaction may result from the inhibition of phenobarbitone hydroxylation by felbamate.

Vigabatrin has been reported to lower plasma concentrations of phenobarbitone in some patients,[14] although dosage changes were not necessary in these patients.

For the effect of phenobarbitone on the metabolism of other antiepileptics, see under Carbamazepine, p.341, clonazepam, p.344, Ethosuximide, p.345, and Lamotrigine, p.348.

1. Richens A, Ahmad S. Controlled trial of sodium valproate in severe epilepsy. *Br Med J* 1975; **4:** 255–6.
2. Patel IH, *et al.* Phenobarbital-valproic acid interaction. *Clin Pharmacol Ther* 1980; **27:** 515–21.
3. Kapetanović IM, *et al.* Mechanism of valproate-phenobarbital interaction in epileptic patients. *Clin Pharmacol Ther* 1981; **29:** 480–6.
4. Bernus I, *et al.* Inhibition of phenobarbitone N-glucosidation by valproate. *Br J Clin Pharmacol* 1994; **38:** 411–16.
5. Perucca E, *et al.* Disposition of sodium valproate in epileptic patients. *Br J Clin Pharmacol* 1978; **5:** 495–9.
6. Morselli PL, *et al.* Interaction between phenobarbital and diphenylhydantoin in animals and in epileptic patients. *Ann N Y Acad Sci* 1971; **179:** 88–107.
7. Eadie MJ, *et al.* Factors influencing plasma phenobarbitone levels in epileptic patients. *Br J Clin Pharmacol* 1977; **4:** 541–7.
8. Cucinell SA, *et al.* Drug interactions in man: lowering effect of phenobarbital on plasma levels of bishydroxycoumarin (Dicumarol) and diphenylhydantoin (Dilantin). *Clin Pharmacol Ther* 1965; **6:** 420–9.
9. Booker HE, *et al.* Concurrent administration of phenobarbital and diphenylhydantoin: lack of an interference effect. *Neurology* 1971; **21:** 383–5.
10. Kuranari M, *et al.* Effect of phenytoin on phenobarbital pharmacokinetics in a patient with epilepsy. *Ann Pharmacother* 1995; **29:** 83–4.
11. Bianchetti G, *et al.* Pharmacokinetic interactions of progabide with other antiepileptic drugs. *Epilepsia* 1987; **28:** 68–73.
12. Gidal BE, Zupanc ML. Potential pharmacokinetic interaction between felbamate and phenobarbital. *Ann Pharmacother* 1994; **28:** 455–8.
13. Reidenberg P, *et al.* Effects of felbamate on the pharmacokinetics of phenobarbital. *Clin Pharmacol Ther* 1995; **58:** 279–87.
14. Browne TR, *et al.* A multicentre study of vigabatrin for drug-resistant epilepsy. *Br J Clin Pharmacol* 1989; **27** (suppl): 95S–100S.

Antifungals. For the effect of phenobarbitone on griseofulvin, see p.380, and on itraconazole, see p.382.

Antiprotozoals. For the effect of phenobarbitone on metronidazole, see p.586.

Antipsychotics. As with all antiepileptics, antipsychotics may antagonise the antiepileptic activity of phenobarbitone by lowering the convulsive threshold.

For the effect of phenobarbitone on antipsychotics, see under Chlorpromazine, p.653.

Beta blockers. For the effect of barbiturates on beta blockers, see under Anxiolytics and Antipsychotics, p.830.

Calcium-channel blockers. For the effect of phenobarbitone on dihydropyridine calcium-channel blockers, see under Nifedipine, p.918, and on verapamil, see p.962.

Corticosteroids. For the effect of phenobarbitone on corticosteroids, see p.1014.

Cyclosporin. For the effect of phenobarbitone on cyclosporin, see p.521.

Diuretics. Serum-phenobarbitone concentrations were raised in 8 of 10 epileptic patients taking phenobarbitone and additional antiepileptics when given *frusemide* 40 mg three times daily for 4 weeks.[1] This might have been the cause of drowsiness in 5 of 14 patients, 3 of whom had to discontinue frusemide.

1. Ahmad S, *et al.* Controlled trial of frusemide as an antiepileptic drug in focal epilepsy. *Br J Clin Pharmacol* 1976; **3:** 621–5.

Sex hormones. For the effect of phenobarbitone on sex hormones, particularly in oral contraceptives, see p.1433.

Theophylline. For the effect of phenobarbitone on theophylline, see p.769.

Thyroxine. For the effects of barbiturates on thyroxine, see p.1498.

Vaccines. *Influenza vaccination* can cause prolonged rises in serum-phenobarbitone concentrations in some patients.[1]

1. Jann MW, Fidone GS. Effect of influenza vaccine on serum anticonvulsant concentrations. *Clin Pharm* 1986; **5:** 817–20.

Vitamins. *Pyridoxine* reduced serum-phenobarbitone concentrations in 5 patients.[1] For the effect of antiepileptics, including phenobarbitone, on *vitamin D* concentrations, see Effects on Bone under the Adverse Effects of Phenytoin, p.353.

1. Hansson O, Sillanpaa M. Pyridoxine and serum concentration of phenytoin and phenobarbitone. *Lancet* 1976; **i:** 256.

Pharmacokinetics

Like other barbiturates phenobarbitone is readily absorbed from the gastro-intestinal tract, although it is relatively lipid-insoluble and may require an hour or longer to achieve effective concentrations.

Phenobarbitone is about 45% bound to plasma proteins and is only partly metabolised in the liver. About 25% of a dose is excreted in the urine unchanged at normal urinary pH. The plasma half-life is about 90 to 100 hours in adults but is greatly prolonged in neonates, and shorter (about 65 to 70 hours) in children. There is considerable interindividual variation in phenobarbitone kinetics.

Monitoring of plasma concentrations has been performed as an aid in assessing control and the therapeutic range of plasma-phenobarbitone is usually quoted as being 15 to 40 μg per mL (65 to 170 μmol per litre).

Phenobarbitone crosses the placental barrier and is distributed into breast milk.

The pharmacokinetics of phenobarbitone are affected by the concomitant administration of other antiepileptics (see under Interactions, above).

Uses and Administration

Phenobarbitone is a barbiturate that may be used as an antiepileptic to control partial and generalised tonic-clonic seizures.

The dose should be adjusted to the needs of the individual patient to achieve adequate control of seizures; this usually requires plasma concentrations of 15 to 40 μg per mL (65 to 170 μmol per litre). The usual dose by mouth is 60 to 180 mg daily, taken at night, and a suggested dose for children is up to 8 mg per kg body-weight daily.

Phenobarbitone sodium may be given parenterally as part of the emergency management of acute seizures or status epilepticus. Doubts have been expressed as to the efficacy of the intramuscular route owing to the delay in achieving adequate blood concentrations and the subcutaneous route may cause tissue necrosis. Intravenous injections should be given slowly and well diluted. Doses of 50 to 200 mg have been given by intramuscular or intravenous injection to adults, repeated after 6 hours if necessary up to a maximum of 600 mg daily. Injections for intravenous administration should be diluted 1 in 10 and given at a rate not exceeding 100 mg per minute until seizures stop or until a maximum of 15 mg per kg has been given.

As with other antiepileptics, withdrawal of phenobarbitone therapy or transition to or from another type of antiepileptic therapy should be made gradually to avoid precipitating an increase in the frequency of seizures. For a discussion on whether or not to withdraw antiepileptic therapy in seizure-free patients, see p.335.

Phenobarbitone has also been used as a hypnotic and sedative but drugs such as the benzodiazepines are preferred.

Phenobarbitone stimulates the enzymes in hepatic microsomes responsible for the metabolism of some drugs and normal body constituents including bilirubin, and for this reason it has been used to reduce hyperbilirubinaemia in neonatal jaundice.

Phenobarbitone magnesium and phenobarbitone diethylamine have also been used.

Cerebral malaria. Phenobarbitone is used to prevent convulsions in patients with cerebral malaria. In an early study[1] a single intramuscular injection of phenobarbitone sodium 3.5 mg per kg body-weight, or 200 mg in patients over 60 kg was effective. Since then a dose of 10 to 15 mg per kg has been suggested.[2] The optimal dose, particularly in children, awaits confirmation from a randomised controlled trial. For a discussion of the antimalarial treatment of malaria, see p.422.

1. White NJ, *et al.* Single dose phenobarbitone prevents convulsions in cerebral malaria. *Lancet* 1988; **ii:** 64–6.
2. Gilles HM. *Management of severe and complicated malaria.* Geneva: WHO, 1991.

Epilepsy. Phenobarbitone is used in the treatment of epilepsy (p.335) for partial seizures with or without secondary generalisation and for primary generalised tonic-clonic seizures. It may also be tried for atypical absence, atonic, and tonic seizures but is not effective in absence seizures. However, the usefulness of phenobarbitone is limited by problems of sedation in adults and paradoxical excitement in children. There is also concern about its effects on behaviour and cognition in children. Phenobarbitone is therefore usually reserved for use in cases unresponsive to other antiepileptics, although some have suggested that its low cost and broad efficacy make it a suitable first-line drug in developing countries.

References.

1. Mattson RH, *et al.* Comparison of carbamazepine, phenobarbital, phenytoin, and primidone in partial and secondarily generalised tonic-clonic seizures. *N Engl J Med* 1985; **313:** 145–51.
2. Heller AJ, *et al.* Phenobarbitone, phenytoin, carbamazepine, or sodium valproate for newly diagnosed adult epilepsy: a randomised comparative monotherapy trial. *J Neurol Neurosurg Psychiatry* 1995; **58:** 44–50.
3. de Silva M, *et al.* Randomised comparative monotherapy trial of phenobarbitone, phenytoin, carbamazepine, or sodium valproate for newly diagnosed childhood epilepsy. *Lancet* 1996; **347:** 709–13.
4. Pal DK, *et al.* Randomised controlled trial to assess acceptability of phenobarbital for childhood epilepsy in rural India. *Lancet* 1998; **351:** 19–23.

Febrile convulsions. Phenobarbitone has been used prophylactically in children thought to be at risk of recurrence of febrile convulsions (p.338), but routine use of antiepileptics is no longer recommended.

References.

1. Newton RW. Randomised controlled trials of phenobarbitone and valproate in febrile convulsions. *Arch Dis Child* 1988; **63:** 1189–91.
2. Farwell JR, *et al.* Phenobarbital for febrile seizures: effects on intelligence and on seizure recurrence. *N Engl J Med* 1990; **322:** 364–9. Correction. *ibid.* 1992; **326:** 144.

Neonatal intraventricular haemorrhage. Phenobarbitone is one of several drugs that have been tried to prevent the development of neonatal intraventricular haemorrhage (p.709). Studies of administration to neonates have shown inconsistent results. Initial studies[1-3] of antenatal administration to the mother were more promising, although a larger randomised study[4] in 610 women failed to show any effect of antenatal phenobarbitone on incidence or severity of intraventricular haemorrhage.

1. Kaempf JW, *et al.* Antenatal phenobarbital for the prevention of periventricular and intraventricular hemorrhage: a double-blind, randomized, placebo-controlled, multihospital trial. *J Pediatr* 1990; **117:** 933–8.
2. Barnes ER, Thompson DF. Antenatal phenobarbital to prevent or minimize intraventricular hemorrhage in the low-birth-weight neonate. *Ann Pharmacother* 1993; **27:** 49–52.
3. Thorp JA, *et al.* Antepartum vitamin K and phenobarbital for preventing intraventricular hemorrhage in the premature newborn: a randomized, double-blind, placebo-controlled trial. *Obstet Gynecol* 1994; **83:** 70–6.
4. Shankaran S, *et al.* The effect of antenatal phenobarbital therapy on neonatal intracranial hemorrhage in preterm infants. *N Engl J Med* 1997; **337:** 466–71.

Neonatal seizures. Some consider phenobarbitone to be the mainstay of treatment for all types of neonatal seizures (p.338). In a study[1] in 120 neonates with clinical seizure activity of varying aetiology, 48 were controlled by an initial intravenous loading dose of phenobarbitone 15 to 20 mg per kg body-weight over 10 to 15 minutes, and a further 37 were controlled by sequential bolus doses of phenobarbitone 5 to 10 mg per kg every 20 to 30 minutes up to a serum concentration of 40 μg per mL. Of the remaining 35 neonates only 7 responded when the serum-phenobarbitone concentration was increased to 100 μg per mL, 13 required addition of a second antiepileptic (phenytoin or lorazepam) and 4 were controlled by addition of a third drug. Phenobarbitone alone can effectively control seizures in the majority of neonates with recurrent seizure activity.

Phenobarbitone administered prophylactically as a single dose of about 40 mg per kg body-weight intravenously over one hour has also been shown to be effective in reducing the incidence of seizures in 15 infants with severe perinatal asphyxia compared with a control group who only received phenobarbitone if there was clinical evidence of seizures.[2] Subsequent follow-up over 3 years suggested that prophylactic phenobarbitone might also improve later neurological outcome.[2]

1. Gilman JT, *et al.* Rapid sequential phenobarbital treatment of neonatal seizures. *Pediatrics* 1989; **83:** 674–8.
2. Hall RT, *et al.* High-dose phenobarbital therapy in term newborn infants with severe perinatal asphyxia: a randomized, prospective study with three-year follow-up. *J Pediatr* 1998; **132:** 345–8.

Status epilepticus. Phenobarbitone given intravenously is an alternative to intravenous phenytoin in the management of status epilepticus (p.337) to prevent the recurrence of seizures once they have been brought under control with a benzodiazepine. Phenobarbitone should not be used in patients who have recently received oral phenobarbitone or primidone.

One study[1] suggested that phenobarbitone might be at least as effective, safe, and practical as diazepam with phenytoin for the initial treatment of convulsive status epilepticus.

1. Shaner DM, *et al.* Treatment of status epilepticus: a prospective comparison of diazepam and phenytoin versus phenobarbital and optional phenytoin. *Neurology* 1988; **38:** 202–7.

Preparations

BP 1998: Phenobarbital Elixir; Phenobarbital Injection; Phenobarbital Sodium Tablets; Phenobarbital Tablets;
USP 23: Ephedrine Sulfate and Phenobarbital Capsules; Phenobarbital Elixir; Phenobarbital Sodium for Injection; Phenobarbital Sodium Injection; Phenobarbital Tablets; Theophylline, Ephedrine Hydrochloride, and Phenobarbital Tablets.

Proprietary Preparations (details are given in Part 3)
Belg.: Ereclase†; Gardenal; ***Fr.:*** Aparoxal; Gardenal; ***Ger.:*** Lepinal; Lepinaletten; Luminal; Luminaletten; Nervolitan S†; Phenaemal; Phenaemaletten; Valocordin†; ***Ital.:*** Comizial; Gardenale; Luminale; Luminalette; Ritmosedina†; ***Norw.:*** Fenemal; ***S.Afr.:*** Gardenal; Lethyl; ***Spain:*** Gardenal; Gratusminal; Luminal; Luminaletas; ***Swed.:*** Fenemal; ***Switz.:*** Aphenylbarbit; Luminal; ***UK:*** Gardenal; ***USA:*** Luminal; Solfoton.

Multi-ingredient: ***Belg.:*** Asperal-B†; Dactil†; Dystonal; Epipropane; Migraine-Kranit†; Octonox; Perphyllone†; Spasmosedine; Trinuride†; Vethoine; ***Canad.:*** Bellergal; Dilantin with Phenobarbital; Donnatal; Phenaphen with Codeine; Tedral; ***Fr.:*** Aeine†; Alepsal; Anxoral; Asthmasedine†; Atrium; Canteine Bouteille†; Cardiocalm; Coquelusedal; Dinacode; Enuretine; Epanal†; Febrectol; Felisedine†; Garaspirine†; Kaneuron; Natisedine; Neurocalcium; Neuropax†; Nuidor†; Ortenal; Prenoxan au phenobarbital; Sedatonyl; Sedibaine; Spasmidenal; Spasmosedine; Sympaneurol; Sympathyl; Tedralan; Vericardine; ***Ger.:*** Adenopurin†; Adenovasin†; Antisacer comp.†; Baldronit forte N†; bella sanol†; Bellaravil-retard†; Bellaravil†; Bellergal†; Circovegetalin compositum†; Coritrat†; Coropar†; Digi-Pulsnorma†; Euklimant†; Govil†; Keldrin†; Myocardetten†; Nervo.opt†; Pulsnorma†; Rhythmochin II (cum sedativo)†; Secafobell†; Seda Nitro Mack†; Seda-Movicard†; Sediomed S†; Steno-Valocordin†; Ulcumel†; Vegomed†; ***Hung.:*** Triospan; ***Ital.:*** Bellergil; Brolumin†; Gamibetal Complex; Metinal-Idantoina L; Neurobiol; Sedital†; Sedonerva†; Sedotiren†; Teofilcolina Sedativa†; ***S.Afr.:*** Adco-Phenobarbitone Vitalet; Analgen-SA; Belladenal†; Bellatard; Bellavern†; Bellergal; Depain Plus; Donnatal; Framol†; Garoin; Menoflush + ¼; Millerspas; Pedriachol; Peterphyllin Co.†; Phenobarb Vitalet†; Propain Forte; Tedral†; Tropax†; ***Spain:*** Bellergal†; Comital L; Disfil; Distovagal; Epanutin Fenobarbitona†; Epilantin; Equidan†; Gaboril Complex†; Navarrofilina†; Oasil Relax†; Redutona; Sinergina S†; Solufilina Sedante; Tedral†; Winasma†; ***Switz.:*** Atrium; Bellergal; ***USA:*** Antispasmodic Elixir; Antrocol; Arco-Lase Plus; Barbidonna; Bel-Phen-Ergot S; Bellacane; Bellatal; Bellergal-S; Bronkolixir†; Bronkotabs†; Byclomine with Phenobarbital†; Chardonna-2; Donna-Sed; Donnamor; Donnapine†; Donnatal; Folergot-DF; Gustase Plus; Hyosophen; Kinesed†; Levsin with Phenobarbitone; Lufyllin-EPG; Malatal†; Mudrane; Mudrane GG; Phenerbel-S; Quadrinal; Relaxadon†; Spasmophen†; Spasquid†; Susano; Tedral†; Tedrigen; Theodrine.

Phensuximide (6618-b)

Phensuximide *(BAN, rINN).*

N-Methyl-2-phenylsuccinimide.

$C_{11}H_{11}NO_2 = 189.2.$

CAS — 86-34-0.

Pharmacopoeias. In *US.*

A white to off-white, odourless or almost odourless, crystalline powder. **Soluble** 1 in 210 of water, 1 in 11 of alcohol, 1 in less than 1 of chloroform, and 1 in 19 of ether. **Store** in airtight containers.

Phensuximide is a succinimide antiepileptic with actions similar to those of ethosuximide (p.344), but it is reported to be less effective; it is not one of the main drugs used (see p.335).

Phensuximide is given in the treatment of absence seizures in usual doses of 0.5 to 1 g two or three times daily by mouth.

Porphyria. Phensuximide has been associated with clinical exacerbations of porphyria and is considered unsafe in porphyric patients.[1]

1. Moore MR, McColl KEL. *Porphyria: drug lists.* Glasgow: Porphyria Research Unit, University of Glasgow, 1991.

Preparations

USP 23: Phensuximide Capsules.

Proprietary Preparations (details are given in Part 3)
Austral.: Milontin†; ***USA:*** Milontin.

Phenytoin (6601-a)

Phenytoin *(BAN, USAN, rINN).*

Diphenylhydantoin; Fenitoina; Phenantoinum; Phenytoinum. 5,5-Diphenylhydantoin; 5,5-Diphenylimidazolidine-2,4-dione.

$C_{15}H_{12}N_2O_2 = 252.3.$

CAS — 57-41-0.

Pharmacopoeias. In *Eur.* (see p.viii), *Int., Jpn, Pol.,* and *US.*

A white, or almost white, odourless, crystalline powder. Phenytoin 92 mg is approximately equivalent to 100 mg of phenytoin sodium (but see also under Uses and Administration, below). Practically **insoluble** in water; soluble in hot alcohol; slightly soluble to sparingly soluble in cold alcohol; slightly soluble in chloroform and in ether; very slightly soluble in dichloromethane; dissolves in dilute solutions of alkali hydroxides. **Store** in airtight containers.

Phenytoin Sodium (6602-t)

Phenytoin Sodium *(BANM, rINNM).*

Diphenin; Phenytoinum Natricum; Soluble Phenytoin.

$C_{15}H_{11}N_2NaO_2 = 274.2.$

CAS — 630-93-3.

Pharmacopoeias. In *Chin., Eur.* (see p.viii), *Int., Jpn, Pol.,* and *US.*

A white, odourless, slightly hygroscopic crystalline powder which on exposure to air gradually absorbs carbon dioxide with the liberation of phenytoin.

Soluble to freely soluble in water, the solution showing some turbidity due to partial hydrolysis and absorption of carbon dioxide; also soluble in alcohol; practically insoluble in chloroform, in dichloromethane, and in ether. **Store** in airtight containers.

Incompatibility. Phenytoin sodium only remains in solution when the pH is considerably alkaline (about 10 to 12) and there have been reports of loss of clarity or precipitation of phenytoin crystals when solutions of phenytoin sodium for injection have been mixed with a variety of drugs[1-6] or added to intravenous infusion fluids,[7-10] while binding has been reported following addition to enteral nutrition solutions.[11] A phenytoin precipitate has been reported to occlude implanted central venous access devices following the inadvertent admixture of phenytoin sodium with glucose 5% or glucose in sodium chloride (pH 4);[12,13] it may be successfully cleared by the local instillation of sodium bicarbonate 8.4% to increase the pH of the medium.

1. Misgen R. Compatibilities and incompatibilities of some intravenous solution admixtures. *Am J Hosp Pharm* 1965; **22:** 92–4.
2. Patel JA, Phillips GL. A guide to physical compatibility of intravenous drug admixtures. *Am J Hosp Pharm* 1966; **23:** 409–11.
3. Klamerus KJ, *et al.* Stability of nitroglycerin in intravenous admixtures. *Am J Hosp Pharm* 1984; **41:** 303–5.
4. Hasegawa GR, Eder JF. Visual compatibility of dobutamine hydrochloride with other injectable drugs. *Am J Hosp Pharm* 1984; **41:** 949–51.
5. Gayed AA, *et al.* Visual compatibility of diltiazem injection with various diluents and medications during simulated Y-site injection. *Am J Health-Syst Pharm* 1995; **52:** 516–20.
6. Trissel LA, *et al.* Compatibility of propofol injectable emulsion with selected drugs during simulated Y-site administration. *Am J Health-Syst Pharm* 1997; **54:** 1287–92.
7. Bauman JL, *et al.* Phenytoin crystallization in intravenous fluids. *Drug Intell Clin Pharm* 1977; **11:** 646–9.
8. Bauman JL, Siepler JK. Intravenous phenytoin (concluded). *N Engl J Med* 1977; **296:** 111.
9. Cloyd JC, *et al.* Concentration-time profile of phenytoin after admixture with small volumes of intravenous fluids. *Am J Hosp Pharm* 1978; **35:** 45–8.
10. Giacona N, *et al.* Crystallization of three phenytoin preparations in intravenous solutions. *Am J Hosp Pharm* 1982; **39:** 630–4.
11. Miller SW, Strom JG. Stability of phenytoin in three enteral nutrient formulas. *Am J Hosp Pharm* 1988; **45:** 2529–32.
12. Akinwande KI, Keehn DM. Dissolution of phenytoin precipitate with sodium bicarbonate in an occluded central various access device. *Ann Pharmacother* 1995; **29:** 707–9.
13. Tse CST, Abdullah R. Dissolving phenytoin precipitate in central venous access device. *Ann Intern Med* 1998; **128:** 1049.

Adverse Effects

Side-effects are fairly frequent in patients receiving phenytoin, but some remit with dose reduction or continued administration. Often reported are lack of appetite, headache, dizziness, transient nervousness, insomnia, and gastro-intestinal disturbances such as nausea, vomiting, and constipation. Tenderness and hyperplasia of the gums often occurs, particularly in younger patients, while acne, hirsutism, and coarsening of the facial features may be particularly undesirable in adolescents and women.

Phenytoin toxicity may be manifested as a syndrome of cerebellar, vestibular, and ocular effects, notably nystagmus, diplopia, and ataxia. Mental confusion, sometimes severe, may occur, and dyskinesias and exacerbations of seizure frequency have been noted. Hyperglycaemia has been associated with toxic concentrations.

Overdosage may result in hypotension, coma, and respiratory depression. Hypotension and CNS depression may also follow intravenous administration, if too rapid, as may cardiac arrhythmias and impaired cardiac conduction. Solutions for injection are very alkaline and may result in irritation at the injection site or phlebitis.

Prolonged therapy may produce subtle effects on mental function and cognition, especially in children. In addition there is some evidence that phenytoin interferes with vitamin D and folate metabolism. Rickets and osteomalacia have occurred in a few patients not exposed to adequate sunlight, although the causal role of phenytoin is debatable. A proportion of patients develop peripheral neuropathies, usually mild, and occasional cases of megaloblastic anaemia have been seen.

Mild hypersensitivity reactions are common, with skin rashes, often morbilliform, sometimes accompanied by fever. Bullous, exfoliative, or purpuric rashes may be symptoms of rare but severe reactions such as lupus erythematosus, erythema multiforme, Stevens-Johnson syndrome, or toxic epidermal necrolysis. Eosinophilia, lymphadenopathy, hepatitis, and blood disorders such as aplastic anaemia, leucopenia, thrombocytopenia, and agranulocytosis, have occurred rarely; some of these conditions may also represent hypersensitivity reactions.

Hypoprothrombinaemia of the newborn following administration of phenytoin during pregnancy has been reported. Congenital malformations have been seen in the offspring of mothers receiving phenytoin during pregnancy (see under Precautions, below).

Effects on the blood. AGRANULOCYTOSIS. Fatal agranulocytosis has been reported[1] in a patient 17 years after starting therapy with phenytoin and primidone. In the report it was stated that since 1963 the UK Committee on Safety of Medicines had received reports of 3 previous cases of fatal agranulocytosis associated with phenytoin and none associated with primidone. The most likely cause was considered to be a direct toxic effect of phenytoin although other possible mechanisms included the ability of both drugs to produce folate deficiency. For a discussion of the effect of antiepileptics on serum folate, see below.

1. Laurenson IF, *et al.* Delayed fatal agranulocytosis in an epileptic taking primidone and phenytoin. *Lancet* 1994, **344:** 332–3.

FOLIC ACID DEFICIENCY. Antiepileptic therapy has long been associated with folate deficiency and some studies have suggested that more than half of all patients on long-term therapy with drugs such as phenytoin, phenobarbitone, and primidone have subnormal serum-folate concentrations;[1,2] megaloblastic haemopoiesis is often present,[3] but clinical megaloblastic anaemia appears to be rare.

The relative importance of individual antiepileptics in causing folate deficiency and macrocytosis has been difficult to establish, because of the tendency to use combination regimens; with greater emphasis on single drug therapy there is evidence that monotherapy may produce less significant changes.[4,5] Despite suggestions that carbamazepine has relatively little effect on folic acid concentrations, Goggin *et al.* found its effects to be comparable with those of phenytoin;[5] in this study only valproate had little or no effect on red-cell folate concentrations.

The mechanism by which phenytoin and similar antiepileptics reduce serum folate is uncertain; there is good evidence for a reduction in absorption of glutamate both *in vitro*[6] and *in vivo*,[7] but the drugs associated with subnormal serum folate are all enzyme inducers and it has been suggested that enzyme induction and enhanced folate metabolism may also play a role.[2,5] Adverse blood changes also result from hypersensitivity (see below).

1. Horwitz SJ, *et al.* Relation of abnormal folate metabolism to neuropathy developing during anticonvulsant drug therapy. *Lancet* 1968; **i:** 563–5.
2. Maxwell JD, *et al.* Folate deficiency after anticonvulsant drugs: an effect of hepatic enzyme induction? *Br Med J* 1972; **1:** 297–9.
3. Wickramasinghe SN, *et al.* Megaloblastic erythropoiesis and macrocytosis in patients on anticonvulsants. *Br Med J* 1975; **4:** 136–7.
4. Dellaportas DI, *et al.* Chronic toxicity in epileptic patients receiving single-drug treatment. *Br Med J* 1982; **285:** 409–10.
5. Goggin T, *et al.* A comparative study of the relative effects of anticonvulsant drugs and dietary folate on the red cell folate status of patients with epilepsy. *Q J Med* 1987; **247:** 911–9.
6. Hoffbrand AV, Necheles TF. Mechanism of folate deficiency in patients receiving phenytoin. *Lancet* 1968; **ii:** 528–30.
7. Rosenberg IH, *et al.* Impairment of intestinal deconjugation of dietary folate. *Lancet* 1968; **ii:** 530–2.

Effects on bone. The effects of phenytoin and other antiepileptics on the skeletal system are a matter of some debate. There are numerous reports indicating effects on bone and on calcium and vitamin D metabolism. Gough *et al.*, in a study involving 226 outpatients with epilepsy,[1] found a reduction in serum-calcium concentration to hypocalcaemic values, significant reduction in 25-hydroxycholecalciferol concentrations, and elevated alkaline phosphatase associated with *carbamazepine, phenobarbitone,* or *phenytoin* therapy, although not with *valproate*. These effects were significantly greater in the group of patients receiving polytherapy, and there was limited evidence that these biochemical changes were exacerbated by reduced exposure to sunlight. Also measurements of bone mineral density in a study of 26 children revealed a reduction in density in those taking *valproate* but no reduction with *carbamazepine*.[2]

Nonetheless, despite these findings, reports of clinical osteomalacia are rare.[3] A study in 20 epileptic outpatients who had received antiepileptic therapy for a mean of 14½ years failed to show any clinical evidence of osteomalacia although there was some evidence of altered calcium metabolism.[4] Similarly osteomalacia was seen in only 1 of 19 elderly inpatients in another study,[5] a rate similar to that previously seen in elderly patients with acute illness not receiving antiepileptic therapy.

1. Gough H, *et al.* A comparative study of the relative influence of different anticonvulsant drugs, UV exposure and diet on vitamin D and calcium metabolism in out-patients with epilepsy. *Q J Med* 1986; **230:** 569–77.
2. Sleth RD, *et al.* Effect of carbamazepine and valproate on bone mineral density. *J Pediatr* 1995; **127:** 256–62.
3. Beghi E, *et al.* Adverse effects of anticonvulsant drugs: a critical review. *Adverse Drug React Acute Poisoning Rev* 1986; **2:** 63–86.
4. Fogelman I, *et al.* Do anticonvulsant drugs commonly induce osteomalacia? *Scott Med J* 1982; **27:** 136–42.
5. Harrington MG, Hodkinson HM. Anticonvulsant drugs and bone disease in the elderly. *J R Soc Med* 1987; **80:** 425–7.

Effects on the endocrine system and metabolism. Antiepileptics diminish *sexual potency* and *fertility* in young male epileptics.[1] Phenytoin is excreted in human semen in small quantities and this may possibly affect sperm morphology and motility. Reduced plasma concentrations of free testosterone have been detected in male epileptic patients receiving one or more of the following: carbamazepine, phenytoin, primidone, and sodium valproate.[2] *Gynaecomastia* has been reported[3] in 5 men receiving long-term antiepileptic treatment; one also complained of impotence but libido was stated to be normal in all 5. Phenytoin was a component of treatment in all patients and was the sole drug used in one.

Phenytoin may cause reversible *hyperglycaemia* at toxic doses but it does not appear to produce long-term effects on glucose tolerance when used in therapeutic doses.[4] Paradoxically, phenytoin has also been reported to improve insulin resistance in some patients.

Phenytoin may reduce serum concentrations of *thyroid* hormones through enzyme induction—see under Interactions of Thyroxine, p.1498.

1. Anonymous. [A brief summary]. *Br Med J* 1979; **2:** 1118.
2. Dana-Haeri J, *et al.* Reduction of free testosterone by antiepileptic drugs. *Br Med J* 1982; **284:** 85–6.
3. Monson JP, Scott DF. Gynaecomastia induced by phenytoin in men with epilepsy. *Br Med J* 1987; **294:** 612.
4. Hurel SJ, Taylor R. Drugs and glucose tolerance. *Adverse Drug React Bull* 1995; **174:** 659–62.

Effects on the liver. There have been occasional reports of liver damage, probably due to hypersensitivity, associated with phenobarbitone and phenytoin; however, Aiges *et al.* considered that such drugs need not be withdrawn if there were merely transient elevations in transaminase values.[1]

1. Aiges HW, *et al.* The effects of phenobarbital and diphenylhydantoin on liver function and morphology. *J Pediatr* 1980; **97:** 22–6.

Effects on the lungs. Pulmonary eosinophilia and acute respiratory failure requiring mechanical ventilation have been reported[1] in a patient receiving phenytoin; other pulmonary symptoms associated with phenytoin were reviewed.

1. Mahatma M, *et al.* Phenytoin-induced acute respiratory failure with pulmonary eosinophilia. *Am J Med* 1989; **87:** 93–4.

Effects on mental function. For a review of the effects of antiepileptic therapy including phenytoin on cognition, see p.337.

Effects on the skin. Skin reactions produced by phenytoin are discussed under Hypersensitivity, below. Rare, but severe reactions such as Stevens-Johnson syndrome and toxic epidermal necrolysis have also occurred.

For reference to cutaneous manifestations of zinc deficiency, possibly due to chelation with phenytoin, see under Valproate, p.362.

Gingival hyperplasia. Gingival hyperplasia, characterised by inflammation and a marked fibrotic response, may affect up to 50% of patients receiving phenytoin. It usually becomes apparent within the first few months of therapy and is observed more frequently in children; there is no increase in alveolar bone loss. The mechanism underlying its development is unknown, although the main metabolite of phenytoin, 5-(4-hydroxyphenyl)-5-phenylhydantoin, has been implicated.[1-3]

1. Ball DE, *et al.* Plasma and saliva concentrations of phenytoin and 5-(4-hydroxyphenyl)-5-phenylhydantoin (HPPH) in relation to gingival overgrowth in epileptic patients. *Br J Clin Pharmacol* 1995; **39:** 539P–588P.
2. Ieiri I, *et al.* Effect of 5-(p-hydroxyphenyl)-5-phenylhydantoin (p-HPPH) enantiomers, major metabolites of phenytoin, on the occurrence of chronic-gingival hyperplasia: in vivo and in vitro study. *Eur J Clin Pharmacol* 1995; **49:** 51–6.
3. Zhou LX, *et al.* Metabolism of phenytoin by the gingiva of normal humans: the possible role of reactive metabolites of phenytoin in the initiation of gingival hyperplasia. *Clin Pharmacol Ther* 1996; **60:** 191–8.

Hypersensitivity. In a prospective study[1] of 306 patients given phenytoin there was an overall incidence of 8.5% of morbilliform rash, but there was a marked seasonal incidence with most reactions occurring during the summer months. The results did not appear to be due to photosensitivity and might represent seasonal alterations in the immune system.

The acute hypersensitivity syndrome to phenytoin is well-recognised and is typically characterised by fever, skin eruptions, lymphadenopathy, and hepatitis;[2] other clinical manifestations which may occur include interstitial nephritis, anaemia, interstitial pulmonary infiltrates, thrombocytopenia, eosinophilia, myopathy, and diffuse intravascular coagulation. This distinctive syndrome occurs mainly in black male patients and should not be confused with more common mild general hypersensitivity reactions. Most cases resolve spontaneously following withdrawal of phenytoin and symptomatic management. The use of corticosteroids in the management of severe cases remains controversial in the absence of controlled double-blind studies of their effectiveness.

Phenytoin-induced pseudolymphoma mimicking cutaneous T-cell lymphoma occurred in a 25-year-old black male.[3] The cutaneous eruption and lymphadenopathy persisted after withdrawal of phenytoin for one year when the patient eventually became asymptomatic. However, it was considered that the risk of developing a true malignant lymphoma remained.

1. Leppik IE, *et al.* Seasonal incidence of phenytoin allergy unrelated to plasma levels. *Arch Neurol* 1985; **42:** 120–2.
2. Flowers FP, *et al.* Phenytoin hypersensitivity syndrome. *J Emerg Med* 1987; **5:** 103–8.
3. Harris DWS, *et al.* Phenytoin-induced pseudolymphoma: a report of a case and review of the literature. *Br J Dermatol* 1992; **127:** 403–6.

Peripheral neuropathies. Electrophysiological abnormalities following prolonged phenytoin treatment are common, but clinically significant peripheral neuropathy is rare.[1] The neuropathy usually involves sensory nerves and lesions are generally mild and asymptomatic.[2] Much of the reported clinical neuropathy has been associated with multiple drug therapy of epilepsy and with exposure to toxic concentrations of phenytoin.[1] Although an association with folate deficiency has been suggested, a study in 52 patients receiving long-term antiepileptic therapy failed to find any convincing evidence of a relationship between serum-folate concentration and peripheral neuropathy.[3]

1. Bruni J. Phenytoin toxicity. In: Levy RH, *et al.* eds. *Antiepileptic drugs*. 4th ed. New York: Raven Press, 1995: 345–50.
2. Argov Z, Mastaglia FL. Drug-induced peripheral neuropathies. *Br Med J* 1979; **1:** 663–6.
3. Horwitz SJ, *et al.* Relation of abnormal folate metabolism to neuropathy developing during anticonvulsant drug therapy. *Lancet* 1968; **i:** 563–5.

Treatment of Adverse Effects

Treatment of poisoning with phenytoin tends to be supportive. Gastric lavage may be tried in severe cases.

Multiple oral doses of activated charcoal may reduce the absorption of phenytoin[1,2] but the value of charcoal haemoperfusion in the management of phenytoin overdosage is debatable. A review of haemoperfusion included data from 2 patients who ingested phenytoin[3] but although it was suggested that haemoperfusion should contribute significantly to drug removal results are difficult to evaluate in these patients who had also ingested phenobarbitone. An evaluation in a patient who had also taken primidone[4] suggested that although initial clearance of phenytoin was promising the system rapidly became saturated and there was little overall benefit. Neither haemodialysis[5] nor peritoneal dialysis[6] is considered worthwhile.

1. Weidle PJ, *et al.* Multiple-dose activated charcoal as adjunct therapy after chronic phenytoin intoxication. *Clin Pharm* 1991; **10:** 711–14.
2. Dolgin JG, *et al.* Pharmacokinetic simulation of the effect of multiple-dose activated charcoal in phenytoin poisoning—report of two pediatric cases. *DICP Ann Pharmacother* 1991; **25:** 646–9.
3. Pond S, *et al.* Pharmacokinetics of haemoperfusion for drug overdose. *Clin Pharmacokinet* 1979; **4:** 329–54.
4. Baehler RW, *et al.* Charcoal hemoperfusion in the therapy for methsuximide and phenytoin overdose. *Arch Intern Med* 1980; **140:** 1466–8.
5. Rubinger D, *et al.* Inefficiency of haemodialysis in acute phenytoin intoxication. *Br J Clin Pharmacol* 1979; **7:** 405–7.
6. Czajka PA, *et al.* A pharmacokinetic evaluation of peritoneal dialysis for phenytoin intoxication. *J Clin Pharmacol* 1980; **20:** 565–9.

Precautions

Phenytoin is metabolised in the liver and should be given with care to patients with impaired liver function. Caution is also required in diabetic patients because of the potential effects of phenytoin on blood sugar.

Protein binding may be reduced in certain disease states such as uraemia, and in certain patient populations such as neonates and the elderly. However, this elevation of free phenytoin (pharmacologically active) is reported to be of little clinical significance, provided that hepatic function is not impaired, because the free phenytoin is extensively distributed, metabolised, and excreted so that the concentration of free drug in the plasma remains more or less unchanged. Thus, an alteration in protein binding would not necessarily require a change in dosage of phenytoin to be made although, when plasma concentrations are being monitored, relatively lower total plasma-phenytoin concentrations will be found to be effective since there is less bound (pharmacologically inactive) phenytoin available for measurement.

Intravenous phenytoin must be given slowly and extravasation must be avoided. Phenytoin should not be given intravenously to patients with sinus bradycardia, heart block, or Stokes-Adams syndrome, and should be used with caution in patients with hypotension, heart failure, and myocardial infarction; monitoring of blood pressure and the ECG is recommended during intravenous therapy.

Patients or their carers should be told how to recognise signs of blood or skin toxicity and they should be advised to seek immediate medical attention if symptoms such as fever, sore throat, rash, mouth ulcers, bruising, or bleeding develop. Phenytoin should be withdrawn, if necessary under cover of a suitable alternative antiepileptic, if leucopenia which is severe, progressive, or associated with clinical symptoms develops. It should also be discontinued if a skin rash develops; in the case of mild rashes phenytoin may be reintroduced cautiously, but should be discontinued immediately if the rash recurs.

Care is required when withdrawing phenytoin therapy—see also under Uses and Administration, below.

Phenytoin may interfere with some tests of thyroid function as it can reduce free and circulating concentrations of tetra-iodothyronine, mainly by enhanced conversion to tri-iodothyronine, and it may also produce lower than normal values for dexamethasone and metyrapone suppression tests.

Breast feeding. For comment on antiepileptic therapy and breast feeding, see under Pregnancy on p.337.

Driving. For comment on antiepileptic drugs and driving, see p.337.

Infections. A 52-year-old woman previously well-controlled on phenytoin 400 mg daily suffered phenytoin toxicity after a viral infection;[1] her plasma-phenytoin concentration had increased from 16 μg per mL to 51 μg per mL. Six weeks later she had recovered and was re-stabilised on phenytoin 400 mg daily.

1. Levine M, Jones MW. Toxic reaction to phenytoin following a viral infection. *Can Med Assoc J* 1983; **128:** 1270–1.

AIDS. Renal abnormalities or hypoalbuminaemia associated with AIDS may increase the risk of elevated free phenytoin concentrations and subsequent toxicity. Altered protein binding resulted in marked phenytoin toxicity, with lethargy and seizure-like activity, in an HIV-positive patient with profound hypoalbuminaemia and moderate renal insufficiency.[1] Therapeutic drug monitoring in 21 patients with AIDS indicated that although total serum concentrations of phenytoin were lower than in a reference population, the fraction of unbound drug was higher.[2] These changes might be attributed to hypoalbuminaemia and it was suggested that free rather than total phenytoin concentrations should be measured in HIV-infected patients with hypoalbuminaemia.

Phenytoin itself was associated with reversible hypogammaglobulinaemia in an HIV-positive patient who previously had borderline hypergammaglobulinaemia.[3]

1. Toler SM, *et al.* Severe phenytoin intoxication as a result of altered protein binding in AIDS. *DICP Ann Pharmacother* 1990; **24:** 698–700.
2. Burger DM, *et al.* Therapeutic drug monitoring of phenytoin in patients with the acquired immunodeficiency syndrome. *Ther Drug Monit* 1994; **16:** 616–20.
3. Britigan BE. Diphenylhydantoin-induced hypogammaglobulinemia in a patient infected with human immunodeficiency virus. *Am J Med* 1991; **90:** 524–7.

Porphyria. Phenytoin has been associated with acute attacks of porphyria and is considered unsafe in patients with acute porphyria.[1]

1. Moore MR, McColl KEL. *Porphyria: drug lists.* Glasgow: Porphyria Research Unit, University of Glasgow, 1991.

Pregnancy. For comments on the management of epilepsy during pregnancy, see p.337.

There is an increased risk of neural tube defects in infants exposed *in utero* to antiepileptics including phenytoin and a variety of syndromes such as craniofacial and digital abnormalities and, less commonly, cleft lip and palate have been described. Specific syndromes such as the 'fetal hydantoin syndrome' with phenytoin have been linked to individual antiepileptics. However, there is overlap between the effects seen with different antiepileptics and some consider the broader term 'fetal antiepileptic drug syndrome' to be more appropriate. There is also a risk of neonatal bleeding with phenytoin.

Interactions

There are complex interactions between antiepileptics and toxicity may be enhanced without a corresponding increase in antiepileptic activity. Such interactions are very variable and unpredictable and plasma monitoring is often advisable with combination therapy.

Since phenytoin is extensively bound to plasma proteins it can be displaced by drugs competing for protein-binding sites, thus liberating more free (pharmacologically active) phenytoin into the plasma. However, elevation of free phenytoin is reported to be of little clinical significance provided hepatic function is not impaired (see Precautions, above). A potentially more serious type of interaction may occur because phenytoin metabolism is saturable: toxic concentrations of phenytoin can develop in patients given drugs which inhibit phenytoin metabolism even to quite a minor degree. Phenytoin is a potent enzyme inducer, and induces the metabolism of a number of drugs, including some antibacterials, anticoagulants, corticosteroids, quinidine, and sex hormones (notably, oral contraceptives). The hypotensive properties of dopamine and the cardiac depressant properties of drugs such as lignocaine may be dangerously enhanced by intravenous administration of phenytoin.

General references.

1. Nation RL, *et al.* Pharmacokinetic drug interactions with phenytoin. *Clin Pharmacokinet* 1990; **18:** 37–60 and 131–150.

Anaesthetics. A 10-year-old girl with epilepsy who had been treated with phenytoin 100 mg three times daily for 5 years and who had lateral nystagmus developed symptoms of phenytoin intoxication following anaesthesia with *halothane*.[1] The plasma concentration of phenytoin 72 hours after anaesthesia was 41 μg per mL. It was suggested that temporary liver dysfunction was responsible for impaired metabolism of phenytoin.

1. Karlin JM, Kutt H. Acute diphenylhydantoin intoxication following halothane anesthesia. *J Pediatr* 1970; **76:** 941–4.

Analgesics. Various analgesics may interact with phenytoin. *Aspirin* is reported to displace phenytoin from plasma binding[1,2] but there is no evidence of any effect on metabolism and effects are unlikely to be clinically significant.[3,4] *Paracetamol* is reported to have no significant effect on serum-phenytoin concentrations.[4] Alterations of pharmacokinetic parameters have been reported with *bromfenac*, but it was thought unlikely that a change in phenytoin dose would be necessary.[5]

Other analgesic and anti-inflammatory drugs may have clinically significant effects. *Phenylbutazone* has been reported to cause an initial decrease in serum phenytoin, followed by an increase;[4] in addition to effects on protein binding it inhibits phenytoin metabolism[6] and severe phenytoin toxicity may result.[7] *Azapropazone* appears to be a competitive inhibitor of phenytoin metabolism and has also been implicated in interactions resulting in toxicity.[8,9] Substantial increases in serum phenytoin have been demonstrated in healthy subjects given *phenyramidol*,[10] indicating a potential for toxicity. There is a single report of toxicity in a patient receiving *ibuprofen* with phenytoin[11] but in a study in 9 healthy subjects, ibuprofen had no effect on the pharmacokinetics of phenytoin.[12]

The opioid analgesic *dextropropoxyphene* has also been reported to affect phenytoin metabolism, with the resultant development of toxic blood-phenytoin concentrations;[13] however, the patient in this case was taking relatively high doses of dextropropoxyphene (650 mg daily). For the effect of phenytoin on *methadone* and *pethidine*, see p.54 and p.77, respectively.

1. Fraser DG, *et al.* Displacement of phenytoin from plasma binding sites by salicylate. *Clin Pharmacol Ther* 1980; **27:** 165–9.
2. Paxton JW. Effects of aspirin on salivary and serum phenytoin kinetics in healthy subjects. *Clin Pharmacol Ther* 1980; **27:** 170–7.
3. Leonard RF, *et al.* Phenytoin-salicylate interaction. *Clin Pharmacol Ther* 1981; **29:** 56–60.
4. Neuvonen PJ, *et al.* Antipyretic analgesics in patients on antiepileptic drug therapy. *Eur J Clin Pharmacol* 1979; **15:** 263–8.
5. Gumbhir-Shah K, *et al.* Evaluation of pharmacokinetic interaction between bromfenac and phenytoin in healthy males. *J Clin Pharmacol* 1997; **37:** 160–8.
6. Andreasen PB, *et al.* Diphenylhydantoin half-life in man and its inhibition by phenylbutazone: the role of genetic factors. *Acta Med Scand* 1973; **193:** 561–4.
7. Kristensen MB. Drug interactions and clinical pharmacokinetics. *Clin Pharmacokinet* 1976; **1:** 351–72.
8. Roberts CJC, *et al.* Anticonvulsant intoxication precipitated by azapropazone. *Postgrad Med J* 1981; **57:** 191–2.
9. Geaney DP, *et al.* Interaction of azapropazone with phenytoin. *Br Med J* 1982; **284:** 1373.
10. Solomon HM, Schrogie JJ. The effect of phenyramidol on the metabolism of diphenylhydantoin. *Clin Pharmacol Ther* 1967; **8:** 554–6.
11. Sandyk R. Phenytoin toxicity induced by interaction with ibuprofen. *S Afr Med J* 1982; **62:** 592.
12. Townsend RJ, *et al.* The effects of ibuprofen on phenytoin pharmacokinetics. *Drug Intell Clin Pharm* 1985; **19:** 447–8.
13. Kutt H. Interactions between anticonvulsants and other commonly prescribed drugs. *Epilepsia* 1984; **25** (suppl 2): S118–S131.

Anthelmintics. For report of an interaction between phenytoin and *levamisole* with fluorouracil, see under Antineoplastics, below. For the effect of phenytoin on *mebendazole* and *praziquantel,* see p.104 and p.108, respectively.

Antiarrhythmics. There have been reports of phenytoin toxicity associated with substantial rises in serum-phenytoin concentrations following addition of *amiodarone* to the therapeutic regimen.[1,2] For the effect of phenytoin on amiodarone, see p.821.

For the effect of phenytoin on lignocaine, see p.1294.

1. Gore JM, *et al.* Interaction of amiodarone and diphenylhydantoin. *Am J Cardiol* 1984; **54:** 1145.
2. McGovern B, *et al.* Possible interaction between amiodarone and phenytoin. *Ann Intern Med* 1984; **101:** 650.

Antibacterials. Interactions, some clinically significant, may occur between phenytoin and various antibacterials. Concurrent administration of chloramphenicol with phenytoin has resulted in moderate[1] to marked[2] elevation of serum-phenytoin concentrations due to inhibition of phenytoin metabolism;[2] toxicity has resulted.[3,4] In turn, phenytoin may affect serum concentrations of chloramphenicol (see p.183).

Phenytoin may enhance the metabolism of *doxycycline*.[5]

There is limited evidence of an interaction with *erythromycin*[6] but this was subject to considerable interindividual variation and is of unknown clinical significance.

The interaction with *isoniazid* is well documented and potentially significant in slow acetylators of isoniazid. Some 10 to 20% of subjects receiving this combination may develop raised phenytoin concentrations and signs of toxicity;[7,8] in at least one case, death has resulted.[9] The effect is due to inhibition of hepatic microsomal enzymes by isoniazid; poor metabolisers of isoniazid may develop sufficient blood-isoniazid concentrations for this inhibition to become marked.

There have been conflicting reports of the effect of *ciprofloxacin* on serum concentrations of phenytoin. While some report no effect[10] others have reported reduced[11-13] or increased[14,15] concentrations of phenytoin in patients given ciprofloxacin. A fall in serum-phenytoin concentrations, and resultant loss of seizure control has been reported in a patient in whom *nitrofurantoin* was added to therapy.[16] The mechanism of this interaction is unknown although a combination of impaired absorption and increased metabolism of the phenytoin was suggested. Something similar was reported in a patient given *oxacillin* in whom plasma-phenytoin concentrations dropped markedly and status epilepticus developed.[17] This effect was thought to be due to impaired phenytoin absorption.

Rifampicin can also reduce plasma-phenytoin concentrations and markedly increase its clearance;[18,19] this is in marked contrast to the effects of isoniazid, and when given together it overrides the effects of isoniazid on phenytoin, even in slow acetylators.[19]

Various sulphonamides are reported to interact with phenytoin, reducing clearance and prolonging half-life: *sulphaphenazole* is reportedly the strongest inhibitor of phenytoin metabolism but *sulphamethizole* also inhibits phenytoin metabolism and the latter has been implicated in producing phenytoin toxicity.[20] *Co-trimoxazole* reportedly inhibits phenytoin metabolism to a modest degree; a case of phenytoin toxicity in a child given co-trimoxazole has been reported[21] but the role of the co-trimoxazole is uncertain since the patient was also receiving sulthiame.

See also under Antiprotozoals, below.

1. Koup JR, *et al.* Interaction of chloramphenicol with phenytoin and phenobarbital. *Clin Pharmacol Ther* 1978; **24:** 571–5.
2. Christensen LK, Skovsted L. Inhibition of drug metabolism by chloramphenicol. *Lancet* 1969; **ii:** 1397–9.
3. Ballek RE, *et al.* Inhibition of diphenylhydantoin metabolism by chloramphenicol. *Lancet* 1973; **i:** 150.
4. Rose JQ, *et al.* Intoxication caused by interaction of chloramphenicol and phenytoin. *JAMA* 1977; **237:** 2630–1.
5. Neuvonen PJ, *et al.* Effect of antiepileptic drugs on the elimination of various tetracycline derivatives. *Eur J Clin Pharmacol* 1975; **9:** 147–54.
6. Bachmann K, *et al.* Single dose phenytoin clearance during erythromycin treatment. *Res Commun Chem Pathol Pharmacol* 1984; **46:** 207–17.
7. Brennan RW, *et al.* Diphenylhydantoin intoxication attendant to slow inactivation of isoniazid. *Neurology* 1970; **20:** 687–93.
8. Kutt H, *et al.* Diphenylhydantoin intoxication: a complication of isoniazid therapy. *Am Rev Respir Dis* 1970; **101:** 377–84.
9. Johnson J, Freeman HL. Death due to isoniazid and phenytoin. *Br J Psychiatry* 1975; **129:** 511.
10. Slavich IL, *et al.* Grand mal epileptic seizures during ciprofloxacin therapy. *JAMA* 1989; **261:** 558–9.
11. Dillard ML, *et al.* Ciprofloxacin-phenytoin interaction. *Ann Pharmacother* 1992; **26:** 263.
12. Pollak PT, Slayter KL. Hazards of doubling phenytoin dose in the face of an unrecognized interaction with ciprofloxacin. *Ann Pharmacother* 1997; **31:** 61–4.
13. Brouwers PJ, *et al.* Ciprofloxacin-phenytoin interaction. *Ann Pharmacother* 1997; **31:** 498.
14. Schroeder D, *et al.* Effect of ciprofloxacin on serum phenytoin concentrations in epileptic patients. *Pharmacotherapy* 1991; **11:** 276.
15. Hull RL. Possible phenytoin-ciprofloxacin interaction. *Ann Pharmacother* 1993; **27:** 1283.
16. Heipertz R, Pilz H. Interaction of nitrofurantoin with diphenylhydantoin. *J Neurol* 1978; **218:** 297–301.
17. Fincham RW, *et al.* Use of phenytoin serum levels in a case of status epilepticus. *Neurology* 1976; **26:** 879–81.
18. Wagner JC, Slama TG. Rifampin-phenytoin drug interaction. *Drug Intell Clin Pharm* 1984; **18:** 497.
19. Kay L, *et al.* Influence of rifampicin and isoniazid on the kinetics of phenytoin. *Br J Clin Pharmacol* 1985; **20:** 323–6.
20. Siersbaek-Nielsen K, *et al.* Sulfamethizole-induced inhibition of diphenylhydantoin and tolbutamide metabolism in man. *Clin Pharmacol Ther* 1973; **14:** 148.
21. Gillman MA, Sandyk R. Phenytoin toxicity and co-trimoxazole. *Ann Intern Med* 1985; **102:** 559.

Anticoagulants. Serum-phenytoin concentrations have been reported to be markedly elevated by concurrent administration of *dicoumarol*[1,2] and elevated to a lesser extent by *phenprocoumon*;[2] however, although *warfarin* has been implicated in a report of phenytoin toxicity,[3] other evidence suggests that it has no effect on serum-phenytoin concentrations in most patients.[2]

For the effect of phenytoin on anticoagulants such as dicoumarol and warfarin, see p.967.

1. Hansen JM, *et al.* Dicoumarol-induced diphenylhydantoin intoxication. *Lancet* 1966; **ii:** 265–6.
2. Skovsted L, *et al.* The effect of different oral anticoagulants on diphenylhydantoin and tolbutamide metabolism. *Acta Med Scand* 1976; **199:** 513–5.
3. Rothermich NO. Diphenylhydantoin intoxication. *Lancet* 1966; **ii:** 640.

Antidepressants. As with all antiepileptics, antidepressants may antagonise the antiepileptic activity of phenytoin by lowering the convulsive threshold.

Plasma-phenytoin concentrations rose in 2 epileptic patients also receiving *imipramine* 75 mg daily for about 3 months for depression.[1] In one patient the concentration gradually increased over several weeks to more than twice the pretreatment figure and he showed mild signs of phenytoin intoxication which remitted after imipramine was stopped. Increased serum-phenytoin concentration and phenytoin toxicity has been described[2] in one patient, possibly precipitated by addition of *trazodone*. Elevated plasma-phenytoin concentrations, in some cases accompanied by signs and symptoms of phenytoin toxicity, have also been reported with *fluoxetine*[3] and with *viloxazine*.[4] The manufacturer of *mianserin* recommends that plasma concentrations of phenytoin should be monitored carefully during concomitant therapy.

For the effects of phenytoin on antidepressants, see under Amitriptyline (p.277), Fluoxetine (p.286), and Lithium (p.293).

1. Perucca E, Richens A. Interaction between phenytoin and imipramine. *Br J Clin Pharmacol* 1977; **4:** 485–6.
2. Dorn JM. A case of phenytoin toxicity possibly precipitated by trazodone. *J Clin Psychiatry* 1986; **47:** 89–90.
3. Nightingale SL. Fluoxetine labeling revised to identify phenytoin interaction and to recommend against use in nursing mothers. *JAMA* 1994; **271:** 1067.
4. Pisani F, *et al.* Elevation of plasma phenytoin by viloxazine in epileptic patients: a clinically significant interaction. *J Neurol Neurosurg Psychiatry* 1992; **55:** 126–7.

Antidiabetics. Transient rises in the amount of non-protein-bound phenytoin were observed in 17 patients when *tolbutamide* was given in addition to phenytoin, but none developed signs of intoxication.[1] Toxic symptoms were reported in another patient given phenytoin and tolbutamide concomitantly, although she had tolerated this combination on a previous occasion.[2]

Symptoms of phenytoin toxicity are known to have occurred[1] in one patient receiving *tolazamide* and phenytoin.

1. Wesseling H, Mols-Thürkow I. Interaction of diphenylhydantoin (DPH) and tolbutamide in man. *Eur J Clin Pharmacol* 1975; **8:** 75–8.
2. Beech E, *et al.* Phenytoin toxicity produced by tolbutamide. *Br Med J* 1988; **297:** 1613–14.

Antiepileptics. Interactions may occur when phenytoin is given concomitantly with other antiepileptics, but these are often variable in their effect and difficult to predict. *Phenobarbitone* both induces the metabolism of phenytoin and competes with it for metabolism by the same enzyme system; in practice there is rarely sufficient alteration for a change in phenytoin dosage to be necessary.[1-3] For the effect of phenytoin on phenobarbitone, see p.351.

Carbamazepine has been generally reported to lower serum-phenytoin concentrations,[4,5] although reports exist of elevated serum-phenytoin concentrations when the two were given concurrently.[6] It should be noted that phenytoin also reduces serum-carbamazepine values—see p.341. These studies have not indicated any loss of seizure control due to this interaction.

The interaction between phenytoin and *valproate* is complex. Valproate displaces phenytoin from serum binding sites and may inhibit its metabolism;[7] the former effect increases the concentration of free drug but reduces total serum phenytoin.[8,9] Most studies seem to suggest that the dose of phenytoin need only rarely be adjusted, but the possibility of loss of seizure control, or phenytoin toxicity, does exist.[7] Interestingly there is some evidence that the interactions may be affected by circadian variations in valproate concentrations.[10] Total plasma-phenytoin concentrations rose significantly in 9 of 11 patients, 2 of whom developed toxic symptoms, when the formulation of sodium valproate that they were receiving concurrently with phenytoin was changed from a standard tablet to a slow-release form.[11] The authors hypothesised that the reduced diurnal fluctuations in plasma-valproate concentrations due to the use of slow-release tablets reduced the displacement interaction between phenytoin and valproate, thereby increasing total plasma-phenytoin concentrations. Phenytoin may also cause a fall in serum concentrations of Valproate—see p.363.

For the effects of phenytoin on *ethosuximide*, see p.345.

For a discussion of the effect of *benzodiazepines* on plasma concentrations of phenytoin, see under Benzodiazepines, below.

Sulthiame causes substantial increases in plasma-phenytoin concentrations, in some cases resulting in phenytoin toxicity;[12] the dose of phenytoin may therefore require adjustment if these drugs are given together.

Interactions may also occur between phenytoin and some of the newer antiepileptics becoming available. *Progabide* may increase blood-phenytoin concentrations[13] and *stiripentol* appears to produce a dose-dependent reduction in phenytoin clearance.[14] *Felbamate* has also caused increases in serum-phenytoin concentrations, and in some cases toxicity requiring a reduction in phenytoin dose.[15,16] Phenytoin reduces plasma concentrations of *lamotrigine* as described on p.348.

Gradual or delayed reductions in plasma-phenytoin concentrations have been observed in several studies in patients given *vigabatrin*;[17] one review[17] states that concentrations have been reduced by 20 to 30%. The manufacturer of vigabatrin considers that this is unlikely to be of clinical significance although in one study the reduction was considered to compromise seizure control.[18]

Increased plasma concentrations of phenytoin with symptoms of toxicity have been reported in one patient receiving phenytoin, carbamazepine, and clobazam after *gabapentin* was added to treatment.[19]

Modest increases in plasma-phenytoin concentrations have been observed in some patients when *topiramate* was added to therapy, but it was considered that dosage adjustments were unlikely to be necessary.[20] For the effect of phenytoin on topiramate, see p.360.

1. Morselli PL, *et al.* Interaction between phenobarbital and diphenylhydantoin in animals and in epileptic patients. *Ann N Y Acad Sci* 1971; **179:** 88–107.
2. Cucinell SA, *et al.* Drug interactions in man: 1. lowering effect of phenobarbital on plasma levels of bishydroxycoumarin (Dicumarol) and diphenylhydantoin (Dilantin). *Clin Pharmacol Ther* 1965; **6:** 420–9.
3. Booker HE, *et al.* Concurrent administration of phenobarbital and diphenylhydantoin: lack of an interference effect. *Neurology* 1971; **21:** 383–5.
4. Hansen JM, *et al.* Carbamazepine-induced acceleration of diphenylhydantoin and warfarin metabolism in man. *Clin Pharmacol Ther* 1971; **12:** 539–43.
5. Windorfer A, Sauer W. Drug interactions during anticonvulsant therapy in childhood: diphenylhydantoin, primidone, phenobarbitone, clonazepam, nitrazepam, carbamazepin, and dipropylacetate. *Neuropadiatrie* 1977; **8:** 29–41.
6. Zielinski JJ, *et al.* Carbamazepine-phenytoin interaction: elevation of plasma phenytoin concentrations due to carbamazepine comedication. *Ther Drug Monit* 1985; **7:** 51–3.
7. Levy RH, Koch KM. Drug interactions with valproic acid. *Drugs* 1982; **24:** 543–56.
8. Monks A, Richens A. Effect of single doses of sodium valproate on serum phenytoin levels and protein binding in epileptic patients. *Clin Pharmacol Ther* 1980; **27:** 89–95.
9. Perucca E, *et al.* Interaction between phenytoin and valproic acid: plasma protein binding and metabolic effects. *Clin Pharmacol Ther* 1980; **28:** 779–89.
10. Riva R, *et al.* Time-dependent interaction between phenytoin and valproic acid. *Neurology* 1985; **35:** 510–15.
11. Suzuki Y, *et al.* Interaction between valproate formulation and phenytoin concentrations. *Eur J Clin Pharmacol* 1995; **48:** 61–3.
12. Hansen JM, *et al.* Sulthiame (Ospolot) as inhibitor of diphenylhydantoin metabolism. *Epilepsia* 1968; **9:** 17–22.
13. Bianchetti G, *et al.* Pharmacokinetic interactions of progabide with other antiepileptic drugs. *Epilepsia* 1987; **28:** 68–73.
14. Levy RH, *et al.* Stiripentol kinetics in epileptic patients: nonlinearity and interactions. *Epilepsia* 1984; **25:** 657.
15. Sheridan PH, *et al.* Open pilot study of felbamate (ADD03055) in partial seizures. *Epilepsia* 1986; **27:** 649.
16. Wilensky AJ, *et al.* Pharmacokinetics of W-554 (ADD 03055) in epileptic patients. *Epilepsia* 1985; **26:** 602–6.
17. Grant SM, Heel RC. Vigabatrin: a review of its pharmacodynamic and pharmacokinetic properties, and therapeutic potential in epilepsy and disorders of motor control. *Drugs* 1991; **41:** 889–926.
18. Browne TR, *et al.* Vigabatrin for refractory complex partial seizures: multicenter single-blind study with long-term follow-up. *Neurology* 1987; **37:** 184–9.
19. Tyndel F. Interaction of gabapentin with other antiepileptics. *Lancet* 1994; **343:** 1363–4.
20. Bourgeois BFD. Drug interaction profile of topiramate. *Epilepsia* 1996; **37** (suppl 2): S14–S17.

Antifungals. There have been several reports of interactions, sometimes resulting in phenytoin toxicity, between imidazole antifungals and phenytoin. The drug most frequently implicated is *miconazole*.[1-3] The related triazole antifungal *fluconazole* is also reported to interact with phenytoin,[4-6] possibly due to dose-related inhibition of cytochrome P450 by fluconazole.[4]

1. Bourgoin B, *et al.* Interaction pharmacocinétique possible phénytoïne-miconazole. *Therapie* 1981; **36:** 347–9.
2. Loupi E, *et al.* Interactions médicamenteuses et miconazole. *Therapie* 1982; **37:** 437–41.
3. Rolan PE, *et al.* Phenytoin intoxication during treatment with parenteral miconazole. *Br Med J* 1983; **287:** 1760.
4. Mitchell AS, Holland JT. Fluconazole and phenytoin: a predictable interaction. *Br Med J* 1989; **298:** 1315.
5. Howitt KM, Oziemski MA. Phenytoin toxicity induced by fluconazole. *Med J Aust* 1989; **151:** 603–4.
6. Cadle RM, *et al.* Fluconazole-induced symptomatic phenytoin toxicity. *Ann Pharmacother* 1994; **28:** 191–5.

Antigout drugs. The manufacturer of *sulphinpyrazone* states that it displaces phenytoin from its protein-binding sites, and also inhibits microsomal liver enzymes. The net result is an increase in plasma-phenytoin concentrations and a prolonged half-life, which is potentially hazardous.

A case has been described[1] in which reduced doses of phenytoin were necessary to avoid toxicity when *allopurinol* was added to the therapy of a child with the Lesch-Nyhan syndrome. Although the authors thought caution was advisable in using these two drugs together, they did emphasise that overgeneralisation may be dangerous since the child also received other antiepileptics and the contribution his disease may have played was unknown.

1. Yokochi K, *et al.* Phenytoin-allopurinol interaction: Michaelis-Menten kinetic parameters of phenytoin with and without allopurinol in a child with Lesch-Nyhan syndrome. *Ther Drug Monit* 1982; **4:** 353–7.

Antihistamines. A young woman developed drowsiness, ataxia, diplopia, tinnitus, and episodes of occipital headaches associated with vomiting after concomitant administration of phenytoin sodium and *chlorpheniramine*.[1] Chlorpheniramine might have delayed the hepatic metabolism of phenytoin thereby increasing the plasma concentrations.

1. Pugh RNH, *et al.* Interaction of phenytoin with chlorpheniramine. *Br J Clin Pharmacol* 1975; **2:** 173–4.

Antihypertensives. In 2 patients with hypoglycaemia associated with hyperinsulinism, therapeutic serum-phenytoin concentrations could not be achieved while they were also receiving *diazoxide*.[1] It was suggested that an increased rate of metabolism, and possibly a decreased binding, of phenytoin induced by diazoxide might have been responsible.

1. Roe TF, *et al.* Drug interaction: diazoxide and diphenylhydantoin. *J Pediatr* 1975; **87:** 480–4.

Antimalarials. Antimalarials may antagonise the antiepileptic activity of phenytoin by lowering the convulsive threshold.

Antineoplastics. There have been reports of decreased plasma-phenytoin concentrations associated with cancer chemotherapy,[1-4] resulting in some cases in loss of seizure control.[2-4] The effect appears to be due to impaired absorption of phenytoin arising from antineoplastic damage to the gastro-intestinal mucosa. In one patient a mean of 32% of an oral dose of phenytoin was absorbed following therapy with *cisplatin, vinblastine,* and *bleomycin*; this compared with a reported oral bioavailability of 80% or more.[3] Increased plasma-phenytoin concentrations were reported[5] in one patient when *tacrolimus* was added to existing therapy. Phenytoin was discontinued until levels were within the therapeutic range and then restarted at a lower dose, tacrolimus therapy continuing throughout; phenytoin levels remained stable thereafter.

The US manufacturer of levamisole reports that increased plasma-phenytoin concentrations have been observed in patients taking phenytoin concomitantly with *levamisole* administered as an adjuvant to *fluorouracil* therapy. For the effect of phenytoin on busulphan see under Effects on the Nervous System under Adverse Effects of Busulphan, p.509.

1. Fincham RW, Schottelius DD. Decreased phenytoin levels in antineoplastic therapy. *Ther Drug Monit* 1979; **1:** 277–83.
2. Bollini P, *et al.* Decreased phenytoin level during antineoplastic therapy: a case report. *Epilepsia* 1983; **24:** 75–8.
3. Sylvester RK, *et al.* Impaired phenytoin bioavailability secondary to cisplatinum, vinblastine, and bleomycin. *Ther Drug Monit* 1984; **6:** 302–5.
4. Grossman SA, *et al.* Decreased phenytoin levels in patients receiving chemotherapy. *Am J Med* 1989; **87:** 505–10.
5. Thompson PA, Mosley CA. Tacrolimus-phenytoin interaction. *Ann Pharmacother* 1996; **30:** 544.

Antiprotozoals. Conflicting results have been reported with *metronidazole*: while one study has suggested only minimal effects on phenytoin concentrations and metabolism,[1] another has indicated inhibition of the metabolism of phenytoin.[2] For the effect of phenytoin an metronidazole, see p.586.

1. Jensen JC, Gugler R. Interaction between metronidazole and drugs eliminated by oxidative metabolism. *Clin Pharmacol Ther* 1985; **37:** 407–10.
2. Blyden GT, *et al.* Metronidazole impairs clearance of phenytoin but not of alprazolam or lorazepam. *Clin Pharmacol Ther* 1986; **39:** 181.

Antipsychotics. As with all antiepileptics, antipsychotics may antagonise the antiepileptic activity of phenytoin by lowering the convulsive threshold. Two cases of phenytoin toxicity and elevated plasma-phenytoin concentrations associated with concurrent administration of the phenothiazine *thioridazine* have been reported;[1] but another study indicated that concurrent treatment with *thioridazine, chlorpromazine,* or *mesoridazine* reduced serum-phenytoin concentrations.[2]

The non-phenothiazine antipsychotic *loxapine* has also been implicated as producing a fall in serum-phenytoin concentration.[3] For the effect of phenytoin on clozapine, see p.659.

1. Vincent FM. Phenothiazine-induced phenytoin intoxication. *Ann Intern Med* 1980; **93:** 56–7.
2. Haidukewych D, Rodin EA. Effect of phenothiazines on serum antiepileptic drug concentrations in psychiatric patients with seizure disorder. *Ther Drug Monit* 1985; **7:** 401–4.
3. Ryan GM, Matthews PA. Phenytoin metabolism stimulated by loxapine. *Drug Intell Clin Pharm* 1977; **11:** 428–9.

Antivirals. *Zidovudine* may possibly reduce or increase plasma-concentrations of phenytoin.

Anxiolytics. See under Benzodiazepines, below.

Benzodiazepines. The metabolism of benzodiazepines may be enhanced in patients who have received long-term therapy with phenytoin due to induction of hepatic drug-metabolising enzymes. In comparison with healthy subjects, half-lives have been shorter and clearance increased.[1,2]

There are sporadic reports of interactions between phenytoin and benzodiazepines, but the evidence is conflicting. One group of workers[3] found some evidence of elevated plasma concentrations of phenytoin in patients given *diazepam* or *chlordiazepoxide* but, in contrast, another study suggested that these drugs produced a significant fall in serum-phenytoin concentrations.[4] There have been reports suggesting that phenytoin intoxication could result from the impaired metabolism associated with the combination[3,5] but in practice this seems to be very rare. There are similar conflicting reports for *clonazepam*.[6-8]

1. Dhillon S, Richens A. Pharmacokinetics of diazepam in epileptic patients and normal volunteers following intravenous administration. *Br J Clin Pharmacol* 1981; **12:** 841–4.
2. Scott AK, *et al.* Oxazepam pharmacokinetics in patients with epilepsy treated long-term with phenytoin alone or in combination with phenobarbitone. *Br J Clin Pharmacol* 1983; **16:** 441–4.
3. Vajda FJE, *et al.* Interaction between phenytoin and the benzodiazepines. *Br Med J* 1971; **1:** 346.
4. Houghton GW, Richens A. The effect of benzodiazepines and pheneturide on phenytoin metabolism in man. *Br J Clin Pharmacol* 1974; **1:** 344P–345P.
5. Kutt H, McDowell F. Management of epilepsy with diphenylhydantoin sodium: dosage regulation for problem patients. *JAMA* 1968; **203:** 969–72.
6. Eeg-Oloffson O. Experiences with Rivotril® in treatment of epilepsy—particularly minor motor epilepsy—in mentally retarded children. *Acta Neurol Scand* 1973; **49** (suppl 53): 29–31.
7. Johannessen SI, *et al.* Lack of effect of clonazepam on serum levels of diphenylhydantoin, phenobarbital and carbamazepine. *Acta Neurol Scand* 1977; **55:** 506–12.
8. Saavedra IN, *et al.* Phenytoin/clonazepam interaction. *Ther Drug Monit* 1985; **7:** 481–4.

Calcium-channel blockers. Raised serum-phenytoin concentration with phenytoin toxicity developed in a patient who had been taking *nifedipine* in addition to phenytoin for 3 weeks;[1] symptoms resolved completely after nifedipine withdrawal. The mechanism of interaction appeared to be complex. Similar effects have been reported with *diltiazem*.[2]

1. Ahmad S. Nifedipine-phenytoin interaction. *J Am Coll Cardiol* 1984; **3:** 1582.
2. Bahls FH, *et al.* Interactions between calcium channel blockers and the anticonvulsants carbamazepine and phenytoin. *Neurology* 1991; **41:** 740–2.

Cardiac glycosides. For the effect of phenytoin on cardiac glycosides, see under Digoxin, p.851.

Corticosteroids. Serum concentrations of phenytoin have been elevated[1] or reduced[2,3] following concurrent administration of *dexamethasone* and adjustment of phenytoin dosage may be required.[2,3] For the effect of phenytoin on corticosteroids, see p.1014.

1. Lawson LA, *et al.* Phenytoin-dexamethasone interaction: a previously unreported observation. *Surg Neurol* 1981; **16:** 23–4.
2. Wong DD, *et al.* Phenytoin-dexamethasone: a possible drug-drug interaction. *JAMA* 1985; **254:** 2062–3.
3. Recuenco I, *et al.* Effect of dexamethasone on the decrease of serum phenytoin concentrations. *Ann Pharmacother* 1995; **29:** 935.

Cyclosporin. For the effect of phenytoin on cyclosporin, see p.521.

Dermatological drugs. For the effect of phenytoin on methoxsalen, see p.1087.

Disulfiram. A well-documented interaction exists between phenytoin and *disulfiram*, which may result in clinical phenytoin toxicity.[1,2] The effect appears to be due to non-competitive inhibition of the metabolism of phenytoin by disulfiram,[2] which results in a substantial increase in phenytoin half-life and a decrease in its clearance.[3]

1. Dry J, Pradalier A. Intoxication par la phénytoïne au cours d'une association thérapeutique avec le disulfirame. *Therapie* 1973; **28:** 799–802.
2. Taylor JW, *et al.* Mathematical analysis of a phenytoin-disulfiram interaction. *Am J Hosp Pharm* 1981; **38:** 93–5.
3. Svendsen TL, *et al.* The influence of disulfiram on the half-life and metabolic clearance rate of diphenylhydantoin and tolbutamide in man. *Eur J Clin Pharmacol* 1976; **9:** 439–41.

Diuretics. Severe osteomalacia in 2 previously active young women taking *acetazolamide* in association with phenytoin or primidone and phenobarbitone has been reported.[1]

For the effect of antiepileptics such as phenytoin on frusemide, see p.872.

1. Mallette LE. Anticonvulsants, acetazolamide and osteomalacia. *N Engl J Med* 1975; **293:** 668.

Enteral and parenteral nutrition. Therapeutic plasma concentrations of phenytoin may be difficult to achieve in patients receiving enteral or total parenteral nutrition.[1,2] Incompatibility studies which indicate that phenytoin probably binds to components of the feed (see under Incompatibility, above) might explain this interaction when both are given together nasogastrically, but the same effect has also been reported when they were administered separately by the intravenous route.[2]

1. Summers VM, Grant R. Nasogastric feeding and phenytoin interaction. *Pharm J* 1989; **243:** 181.
2. Messahel FM, *et al.* Does total parenteral nutrition lower serum phenytoin levels? *Curr Ther Res* 1990; **47:** 1017–20.

Gastro-intestinal drugs. Evidence for an interaction between phenytoin and *antacids* is conflicting. Some studies have shown a decrease in the bioavailability of phenytoin given with various antacid mixtures[1,2] but others have failed to find any evidence of reduced absorption.[3] Furthermore even those studies which recorded decreased absorption varied in their results with regard to particular drugs, suggesting for example that calcium carbonate both does[1] and does not[2] reduce phenytoin bioavailability. The clinical significance of this data is uncertain but it has been suggested that if antacids and phenytoin are both required their doses should be spaced several hours apart.[4,5]

Another drug used in the therapy of peptic ulcer, *sucralfate*, is also reported to reduce phenytoin absorption.[6]

A well documented interaction exists between phenytoin and *cimetidine*, which produces a dose-dependent reduction in phenytoin clearance[7] and a significant elevation of serum-phenytoin concentration.[8] There are reports of phenytoin toxicity following cimetidine administration to epileptic patients[9,10] including a report of severe granulocytopenia associated with the combination.[11] Although some studies have found that neither *ranitidine*[12] nor *famotidine*[13] appear to affect the pharmacokinetics of phenytoin significantly, there have been isolated reports of raised plasma concentrations of phenytoin associated with concurrent use of ranitidine[14-16] or famotidine.[17]

Omeprazole 40 mg daily can decrease the plasma clearance of phenytoin[18] and increase the area under the serum-phenytoin concentration-time curve,[19] but one study[20] suggests that the dosage of 20 mg daily usually used for peptic ulcer is unlikely to produce a clinically significant effect on the steady-state plasma concentrations of phenytoin in patients with epilepsy.

1. Garnett WR, *et al.* Bioavailability of phenytoin administered with antacids. *Ther Drug Monit* 1979; **1:** 435–6.
2. Kulshrestha VK, *et al.* Interaction between phenytoin and antacids. *Br J Clin Pharmacol* 1978; **6:** 177–9.
3. O'Brien LS, *et al.* Failure of antacids to alter the pharmacokinetics of phenytoin. *Br J Clin Pharmacol* 1978; **6:** 176–7.
4. Cacek AT. Review of alterations in oral phenytoin bioavailability associated with formulation, antacids, and food. *Ther Drug Monit* 1986; **8:** 166–71.
5. D'Arcy PF, McElnay JC. Drug-antacid interactions: assessment of clinical importance. *Drug Intell Clin Pharm* 1987; **21:** 607–17.
6. Smart HL, *et al.* The effects of sucralfate upon phenytoin absorption in man. *Br J Clin Pharmacol* 1985; **20:** 238–40.
7. Bartle WR, *et al.* Dose-dependent effect of cimetidine on phenytoin kinetics. *Clin Pharmacol Ther* 1983; **33:** 649–55.
8. Iteogu MO, *et al.* Effect of cimetidine on single-dose phenytoin kinetics. *Clin Pharm* 1983; **2:** 302–4.
9. Phillips P, Hansky J. Phenytoin toxicity secondary to cimetidine administration. *Med J Aust* 1984; **141:** 602.
10. Hetzel DJ, *et al.* Cimetidine interaction with phenytoin. *Br Med J* 1981; **282:** 1512.
11. Sazie E, Jaffe JP. Severe granulocytopenia with cimetidine and phenytoin. *Ann Intern Med* 1980; **93:** 151–2.
12. Watts RW, *et al.* Lack of interaction between ranitidine and phenytoin. *Br J Clin Pharmacol* 1983; **15:** 499–500.
13. Sambol NC, *et al.* A comparison of the influence of famotidine and cimetidine on phenytoin elimination and hepatic blood flow. *Br J Clin Pharmacol* 1989; **27:** 83–7.
14. Bramhall D, Levine M. Possible interaction of ranitidine with phenytoin. *Drug Intell Clin Pharm* 1988; **22:** 979–80.
15. Tse CST, *et al.* Phenytoin concentration elevation subsequent to ranitidine administration. *Ann Pharmacother* 1993; **27:** 1448–51.
16. Tse CST, Iagmin P. Phenytoin and ranitidine interaction. *Ann Intern Med* 1994; **120:** 892–3.
17. Shinn AF. Unrecognized drug interactions with famotidine and nizatidine. *Arch Intern Med* 1991; **151:** 814.
18. Gugler R, Jensen JC. Omeprazole inhibits oxidative drug metabolism: studies with diazepam and phenytoin in vivo and 7-ethoxycoumarin in vitro. *Gastroenterology* 1985; **89:** 1235–41.
19. Prichard PJ, *et al.* Oral phenytoin pharmacokinetics during omeprazole therapy. *Br J Clin Pharmacol* 1987; **24:** 543–5.
20. Andersson T, *et al.* A study of the interaction between omeprazole and phenytoin in epileptic patients. *Ther Drug Monit* 1990; **12:** 329–33.

Muscle relaxants. An increase in serum concentrations of phenytoin has been reported[1] in a patient when *tizanidine* was added to therapy.

1. Ueno K, *et al.* Phenytoin-tizanidine interaction. *DICP Ann Pharmacother* 1991; **25:** 1273.

Neuromuscular blockers. For the effect of phenytoin on *suxamethonium*, see p.1321 and on *competitive neuromuscular blockers*, see under Atracurium, p.1306.

Sex hormones. For the effect of phenytoin on sex hormones, particularly in oral contraceptives, see p.1433.

Stimulants and anorectics. Although there has been a report of elevated phenytoin and primidone serum concentrations in a 5-year-old following addition of *methylphenidate* to therapy[1] there was no similar elevation in 2 other children receiving phenobarbitone and phenytoin in the same report, nor in 11 patients of varying ages given methylphenidate with antiepileptic therapy as part of a controlled study.[2] The likelihood of an interaction seems small in the majority of patients.

1. Garrettson LK, *et al.* Methylphenidate interaction with both anticonvulsants and ethyl biscoumacetate. *JAMA* 1969; **207:** 2053–6.
2. Kupferberg HJ, *et al.* Effect of methylphenidate on plasma anticonvulsant levels. *Clin Pharmacol Ther* 1972; **13:** 201–4.

Theophylline. Although most reports of an interaction between phenytoin and *theophylline* concern effects on theophylline concentrations, one study in 14 healthy subjects suggested that concurrent administration of the two could produce lowered serum-phenytoin concentrations, with a subsequent rise in concentration on discontinuing theophylline.[1] The mechanism was suggested to be enzyme induction by the xanthine resulting in increased phenytoin metabolism.

For the effect of phenytoin on theophylline, see p.769.

1. Taylor JW, *et al.* The interaction of phenytoin and theophylline. *Drug Intell Clin Pharm* 1980; **14:** 638.

Ticlopidine. Acute phenytoin toxicity has been reported in a well-stabilised patient following introduction of ticlopidine to prevent restenosis after placement of a coronary stent.[1] The patient also received metoprolol, aspirin, and for a short period lovastatin, but inhibition of the cytochrome P450 isoenzyme CYP2C19 by ticlopidine was considered the most likely cause of the patient's elevated serum phenytoin.

1. Donahue SR, *et al.* Ticlopidine inhibition of phenytoin metabolism mediated by potent inhibition of CYP2C19. *Clin Pharmacol Ther* 1997; **62:** 572–7.

Vaccines. Contradictory results have been reported for the effects of *influenza vaccine* on serum-phenytoin concentrations. Jann and Fidone[1] reported a significant elevation in total phenytoin concentration following vaccination, which was suggested to be due to interferon induction and concomitant inhibition of cytochrome P450. In contrast, other reports have suggested that any increase in serum-phenytoin concentration was temporary and not significant overall[2] or even that there was a slight fall in serum-phenytoin concentration.[3] One study reported a significant increase in total phenytoin concentration two days after vaccination, followed by a return to previous values but this was accompanied by evidence of a gradual and prolonged fall in free phenytoin concentrations.[4] The possibility of either phenytoin toxicity or loss of seizure control may exist in some epileptic patients given influenza vaccine during phenytoin therapy.[5]

1. Jann MW, Fidone GS. Effect of influenza vaccine on serum anticonvulsant concentrations. *Clin Pharm* 1986; **5:** 817–20.
2. Levine M, *et al.* Increased serum phenytoin concentration following influenza vaccination. *Clin Pharm* 1984; **3:** 505–9.
3. Sawchuk RJ, *et al.* Effect of influenza vaccination on plasma phenytoin concentrations. *Ther Drug Monit* 1979; **1:** 285–8.
4. Smith CD, *et al.* Effect of influenza vaccine on serum concentrations of total and free phenytoin. *Clin Pharm* 1988; **7:** 828–32.
5. Grabenstein JD. Drug interactions involving immunologic agents, part 1. vaccine-vaccine, vaccine-immunoglobulin, and vaccine-drug interactions. *DICP Ann Pharmacother* 1990; **24:** 67–80.

Vitamins. *Pyridoxine* given in large doses produced a reduction in serum-phenytoin concentrations in 7 patients,[1] perhaps reflecting increased activity by pyridoxal phosphate-dependent enzymes involved in phenytoin metabolism.

Correction of antiepileptic-associated folate deficiency with *folic acid* has been reported to result in a decrease in serum-phenytoin concentrations and an increase in seizure frequency.[2,3] The effect has been reported to be most marked in subjects with high initial serum-phenytoin concentrations[4] and is associated with an increased phenytoin metabolism.[5] However, in the majority of patients the effect is unlikely to assume clinical significance,[2,4] and there is some evidence that very low doses of folic acid may be used to maintain normal serum-folate values without an increase in seizure frequency.[3] Information regarding the dual and interdependent interaction between phenytoin and folic acid has been reviewed.[6] Although limited numbers of patients and healthy subjects were involved, evaluation of the data suggested that initiation of phenytoin and folic acid concomitantly prevents decreased folate levels and steady-state concentrations of phenytoin are reached sooner.

For the effect of antiepileptics, including phenytoin, on *vitamin D* concentrations, see Effects on Bone under Adverse Effects, above.

1. Hansson O, Sillanpaa M. Pyridoxine and serum concentration of phenytoin and phenobarbitone. *Lancet* 1976; **i:** 256.
2. Baylis EM, *et al.* Influence of folic acid on blood-phenytoin levels. *Lancet* 1971; **i:** 62–4.
3. Inoue F. Clinical implications of anticonvulsant-induced folate deficiency. *Clin Pharm* 1982; **1:** 372–3.
4. Furlanut M, *et al.* Effects of folic acid on phenytoin kinetics in healthy subjects. *Clin Pharmacol Ther* 1978; **24:** 294–7.
5. Berg MJ, *et al.* Phenytoin and folic acid interaction: a preliminary report. *Ther Drug Monit* 1983; **5:** 389–94.
6. Lewis DP, *et al.* Phenytoin-folic acid interaction. *Ann Pharmacother* 1995; **29:** 726–35.

Pharmacokinetics

Phenytoin is slowly but almost completely absorbed from the gastro-intestinal tract. It is largely insoluble at the acid pH of the stomach, most being absorbed from the upper intestine; the rate of absorption is variable and is reported to be affected by the presence of food. Absorption from the intramuscular site is even slower than that from the gastro-intestinal tract.

Phenytoin is extensively metabolised in the liver to inactive metabolites, chiefly 5-(4-hydroxyphenyl)-5-phenylhydantoin. The rate of metabolism appears to be subject to genetic polymorphism and may also be influenced by racial characteristics; it is reported to be increased during pregnancy and menstruation and to decrease with age. Phenytoin hydroxylation is saturable and is therefore readily inhibited by drugs that compete for its metabolic pathways; this is also the reason why small increments in dose may produce large rises in plasma concentration. Phenytoin undergoes enterohepatic recycling and is excreted in the urine, mainly as its hydroxylated metabolite, in either free or conjugated form.

Phenytoin is widely distributed throughout the body. It is extensively bound (about 90%) to plasma protein, although this may be reduced in certain disease states and in certain patient populations (see under Precautions, above). It has a very variable, dose-dependent half-life, but the mean plasma half-life appears to be about 22 hours at steady-state; because phenytoin inhibits its own metabolism it may sometimes be several weeks before a steady-state plasma-phenytoin concentration is attained.

Monitoring of plasma concentrations may be performed as an aid in assessing control, and the therapeutic range of total plasma-phenytoin concentrations is usually quoted as being 10 to 20 μg per mL (40 to 80 μmol per litre); some patients, however, are controlled at concentrations outside this range. It has been suggested that, because of differences in protein binding, measurement of free phenytoin concentrations in plasma may prove more reliable; measurement of concentrations in saliva, which contains only free phenytoin, has also been performed.

Phenytoin crosses the placental barrier and small amounts are distributed into breast milk.

The pharmacokinetics of phenytoin are affected by the concomitant administration of other antiepileptics (see Interactions, above).

Uses and Administration

Phenytoin is a hydantoin antiepileptic used to control partial and generalised tonic-clonic seizures. It is also used as part of the emergency treatment of status epilepticus and has been used for the prophylactic control of seizures developing during or after neurosurgery or following severe traumatic injury to the head. Phenytoin has also been used in the treatment of trigeminal neuralgia. It is a class Ib antiarrhythmic and has been used to treat cardiac arrhythmias.

Doses may be expressed in terms of phenytoin or phenytoin sodium; although phenytoin 92 mg is approximately equivalent to 100 mg of phenytoin sodium these molecular equivalents are not necessarily biologically equivalent. In the UK an oral suspension of phenytoin 90 mg in 15 mL may be considered approximately equivalent in therapeutic effect to capsules or tablets containing phenytoin sodium 100 mg. In the USA a suspension containing phenytoin 125 mg in 5 mL is available.

For **epilepsy** the dose of phenytoin should be adjusted to the needs of the individual patient to achieve adequate control of seizures, preferably with monitoring of plasma concentrations; in many patients control requires total plasma-phenytoin concentrations of 10 to 20 μg per mL (40 to 80 μmol per litre), but some are controlled at concentrations outside this range. A suggested initial dose by mouth of phenytoin or phenytoin sodium given as a single dose or in divided doses is 3 to 4 mg per kg body-weight daily or 150 to 300 mg daily progressively increased with care to 600 mg daily if necessary; the suggested minimum interval between increments has ranged from about 7 to 10 days. Particular care is needed at higher doses, where saturation of metabolism may mean that a small increment produces a large rise in plasma concentrations. A usual maintenance dose is 200 to 500 mg daily.

A suggested initial dose for children is 5 mg per kg body-weight daily in 2 or 3 divided doses up to a maximum of 300 mg daily; a suggested maintenance dose is 4 to 8 mg per kg daily in divided doses. Young children may require a higher dose per kg body-weight than adults due to more rapid metabolism.

The practice of starting phenytoin therapy with initial small doses means that more than a week may be required before therapeutic plasma concentrations are attained; it has been reported that it may even be several weeks before a steady-state concentration is established. Some workers therefore prefer to give an initial loading dose in order to reach the recommended plasma concentrations sooner. A suggested oral loading dose for adults is 0.6 to 1 g of phenytoin divided into 2 or 3 doses administered over 6 hours with the usual maintenance dosage being instituted 24 hours after the loading dose. Once the patient is stabilised the long half-life of phenytoin may permit the total daily dose to be given in two daily divisions, or perhaps as a single dose, usually at night.

Although clinical evidence is lacking, different brands of phenytoin, as well as different formulations from the same manufacturer, may vary in their bioavailability and patients may need to be restabilised in the event of a change.

In order to lessen gastric irritation, phenytoin should be taken with or after food. The time and manner of taking phenytoin should be standardised for the patient since variations might affect absorption with consequent fluctuations in the plasma concentrations.

As with other antiepileptics, withdrawal of phenytoin therapy or transition to or from another type of antiepileptic therapy should be made gradually to avoid precipitating an increase in the frequency of seizures. For a discussion on whether or not to withdraw antiepileptic therapy in seizure-free patients, see p.335.

In the treatment of tonic-clonic **status epilepticus** a benzodiazepine such as diazepam is usually given initially intravenously or rectally followed by the administration of phenytoin sodium intravenously. A suggested dose of phenytoin sodium has been 10 to 15 mg per kg body-weight given by slow intravenous injection or by intermittent infusion at a uniform rate of not more than 50 mg per minute. Thereafter maintenance doses of 100 mg by mouth or intravenously are given every 6 to 8 hours; the rate and dose should be reduced according to body-weight. The intravenous dose for neonates is 15 to 20 mg per kg body-weight at a rate not exceeding 1 to 3 mg per kg per minute. A suggested dose in children is 15 mg per kg given at a rate of 1 mg per kg per minute, not to exceed 50 mg per minute. Deaths have been caused by the over-rapid intravenous injection of phenytoin sodium and continuous monitoring of the ECG and blood pressure is recommended whenever phenytoin sodium is given intravenously.

Phenytoin sodium is absorbed slowly and erratically from the intramuscular site and therefore intramuscular injections are not appropriate for the emergency arrest of status epilepticus. They may, however, be used in certain situations to maintain or establish therapeutic plasma concentrations of phenytoin in patients who are unconscious or otherwise unable to take phenytoin by mouth. Owing to the slower absorption of phenytoin from intramuscular sites, patients stabilised on the oral route require an increase in the intramuscular dose of about 50%; it is recommended that, if possible, intramuscular injections of phenytoin sodium should not be continued for longer than one week. On transfer back to the oral route the patient should receive 50% of the original oral dose for the same period of time as intramuscular injections were given, to allow for continued absorption of the residual phenytoin in the intramuscular sites. In a patient who has not previously received phenytoin sodium, a suggested intramuscular dose is 100 to 200 mg.

Administration. IN CHILDREN AND NEONATES. A comparison of methods[1] for the prediction of required phenytoin dosage in paediatric patients indicated that all methods produced a sizeable number of predictions with an error of more than 10% and that close monitoring of serum concentrations and clinical status was recommended regardless of the method chosen to adjust dosage. Loughnan *et al.*[2] came to similar conclusions on the need to monitor plasma concentrations of phenytoin in the newborn and young infants.

1. Yuen GJ, *et al.* Phenytoin dosage predictions in paediatric patients. *Clin Pharmacokinet* 1989; **16:** 254–60.
2. Loughnan PM, *et al.* Pharmacokinetic observations of phenytoin disposition in the newborn and young infant. *Arch Dis Child* 1977; **52:** 302–9.

IN THE ELDERLY. Pharmacokinetic studies in elderly patients have shown reduced binding to plasma protein which was not itself an indication for dosage change,[1] but a study showing a decreased metabolism[2] did indicate that elderly patients may need lower doses of phenytoin than younger adults to maintain similar serum concentrations.

1. Patterson M, *et al.* Plasma protein binding of phenytoin in the aged: in vivo studies. *Br J Clin Pharmacol* 1982; **13:** 423–5.
2. Bauer LA, Blouin RA. Age and phenytoin kinetics in adult epileptics. *Clin Pharmacol Ther* 1982; **31:** 301–4.

IN HEPATIC IMPAIRMENT. For comments regarding the administration of phenytoin in hepatic impairment, see Precautions above.

Cardiac arrhythmias. Phenytoin has been given intravenously in the treatment of ventricular arrhythmias (p.782), especially those caused by overdosage with cardiac glycosides, but this use now appears to be obsolete.

A usual dose of phenytoin sodium was 3.5 to 5 mg per kg body-weight administered by slow intravenous injection at a uniform rate of not more than 50 mg per minute, repeated once if necessary.

Eclampsia and pre-eclampsia. Phenytoin has been used for eclampsia but now treatment with magnesium sulphate is preferred, see p.338.

Epidermolysis bullosa. There have been reports[1,2] of a favourable but variable clinical response to phenytoin in patients with recessive dystrophic epidermolysis bullosa (p.1074), a condition for which there is no truly effective treatment. However, a double-blind placebo-controlled study[3] concluded that phenytoin is not an effective treatment and offered no overall benefit when compared with placebo.

1. Bauer EA, *et al.* Phenytoin therapy of recessive dystrophic epidermolysis bullosa. *N Engl J Med* 1980; **303:** 776–81.
2. Cooper TW, Bauer EA. Therapeutic efficacy of phenytoin in recessive dystrophic epidermolysis. *Arch Dermatol* 1984; **120:** 490–5.
3. Caldwell-Brown D, *et al.* Lack of efficacy of phenytoin in recessive dystrophic epidermolysis bullosa. *N Engl J Med* 1992; **327:** 163–7.

Epilepsy. Phenytoin is one of the drugs of choice in the treatment of partial seizures with or without secondary generalisation and in primarily generalised tonic-clonic seizures (see p.335). It is also effective in other forms of epilepsy with the exception of absence and myoclonic seizures.

The non-linear pharmacokinetics of phenytoin make it difficult to use, particularly at higher doses, because small increases in doses may produce large rises in plasma concentrations. Phenytoin may be unsuitable for adolescents or for women because of potential coarsening of the facial features, acne, or hirsutism. Gingival hyperplasia and tenderness can also be a problem.

References.

1. Mattson RH, *et al.* Comparison of carbamazepine, phenobarbital, phenytoin, and primidone in partial and secondarily generalised tonic-clonic seizures. *N Engl J Med* 1985; **313:** 145–51.
2. Heller AJ, *et al.* Phenobarbitone, phenytoin, carbamazepine, or sodium valproate for newly diagnosed adult epilepsy: a randomised comparative monotherapy trial. *J Neurol Neurosurg Psychiatry* 1995; **58:** 44–50.
3. de Silva M, *et al.* Randomised comparative monotherapy trial of phenobarbitone, phenytoin, carbamazepine, or sodium valproate for newly diagnosed childhood epilepsy. *Lancet* 1996; **347:** 709–13.

Hiccup. Phenytoin may be of value for the treatment of intractable hiccups,[1] especially those of neurogenic origin. A protocol for the management of intractable hiccups may be found under Chlorpromazine, p.655.

1. Petroski D, Patel AN. Diphenylhydantoin for intractable hiccups. *Lancet* 1974; **i:** 739.

Neonatal seizures. Phenytoin is one of the antiepileptics that may be used in the management of neonatal seizures (p.338).

Post-traumatic seizures. In a double-blind study[1] in patients with serious head trauma, only 7 of 208 assigned to receive phenytoin experienced seizures within 1 week of commencing treatment, compared with 26 of 196 assigned to placebo. On follow-up for 2 years, however, the differences between the groups were not significant. Phenytoin, given in an initial loading dose of 20 mg per kg body-weight intravenously, and subsequently given in doses adequate to maintain a high therapeutic concentration, appeared to reduce the incidence of seizures in the first week after major head trauma but not thereafter. However, in another study involving 86 similar patients only 6% of those who had received phenytoin had developed post-traumatic epilepsy at the 2-year follow-up compared with 42% of the untreated patients.[2]

1. Temkin NR, *et al.* A randomized, double-blind study of phenytoin for the prevention of post-traumatic seizures. *N Engl J Med* 1990; **323:** 497–502.
2. Pechadre JC, *et al.* Prévention de l'épilepsie post-traumatique tardive par phénytoïne dans les traumatismes crâniens graves: suivi durant 2 ans. *Presse Med* 1991; **20:** 841–5.

Status epilepticus. Administration of a benzodiazepine is the most usual method used to abort an attack of status epilepticus (p.337). Once seizures have been brought under control, phenytoin may be given by intravenous infusion. Phenytoin has been considered more appropriate than a benzodiazepine for the management of status epilepticus in patients with head injuries or other acute neurological lesions.[1]

1. Eldridge PR, Punt JAG. Risks associated with giving benzodiazepines to patients with acute neurological injuries. *Br Med J* 1990; **300:** 1189–90.

Syndrome of inappropriate ADH secretion. Phenytoin has been used occasionally to inhibit pituitary antidiuretic hormone (ADH) secretion in patients with the syndrome of inappropriate ADH secretion (SIADH), the management of which is discussed on p.1241.

Tinnitus. Treatment of tinnitus (p.1297) is difficult and a wide variety of drugs has been tried including phenytoin which, though it has been reported to be effective in some patients is rarely used because of problems with adverse effects.

Trigeminal neuralgia. Phenytoin is used alone or added to treatment in trigeminal neuralgia (p.12) in patients unresponsive to or intolerant of carbamazepine.

Withdrawal syndromes. Phenytoin has little place in the management of seizures associated with the alcohol withdrawal syndrome (p.1099). Prophylaxis with phenytoin has been shown[1,2] to be ineffective for prevention of recurrent alcohol-related seizures and therapy drugs such as the benzodiazepines or chlormethiazole, which are effective both for the treatment and prophylaxis of such seizures, are preferred.

Results from a double-blind study[3] indicated that phenytoin was associated with a reduction in cocaine abuse compared with placebo. The abuse of cocaine is discussed on p.1290 and treatment of cocaine withdrawal on p.1291.

1. Chance JF. Emergency department treatment of alcohol withdrawal seizures with phenytoin. *Ann Emerg Med* 1991; **20:** 520–2.
2. Rathlev NK, *et al.* The lack of efficacy of phenytoin in the prevention of recurrent alcohol-related seizures. *Ann Emerg Med* 1994; **23:** 513–8.
3. Crosby RD, *et al.* Phenytoin in the treatment of cocaine abuse: a double-blind study. *Clin Pharmacol Ther* 1996; **59:** 458–68.

Wounds and ulcers. The use of phenytoin to promote wound healing (p.1076) was stimulated by the observation that phenytoin causes gingival hyperplasia. Topical application of phenytoin has produced encouraging results in the healing of various types of ulcers[1-4] and large abscess cavities.[5] It has been suggested that phenytoin may reduce bacterial colonisation by changing the pH or by a direct antibacterial effect.[2] The enhanced wound healing may also be due to increased fibroblast proliferation and increased collagen content.[2] Limited absorption from the wound site may occur[6,7] and patients may need to be monitored for signs of toxicity.

1. Muthukumarasamy MG, *et al.* Topical phenytoin in diabetic foot ulcers. *Diabetes Care* 1991; **14:** 909–11.
2. Pendse AK, *et al.* Topical phenytoin in wound healing. *Int J Dermatol* 1993; **32:** 214–17.
3. Anstead GM, *et al.* Phenytoin in wound healing. *Ann Pharmacother* 1996; **30:** 768–75.
4. Adjei O, *et al.* Phenytoin in the treatment of Buruli ulcer. *Trans R Soc Trop Med Hyg* 1998; **92:** 108–9.
5. Lodha SC, *et al.* Role of phenytoin in healing of large abscess cavities. *Br J Surg* 1991; **78:** 105–8.
6. Gore R, *et al.* Topical phenytoin. *Pharm J* 1991; **247:** 620.
7. Lewis WG, Rhodes RS. Systemic absorption of topical phenytoin sodium. *Ann Pharmacother* 1994; **28:** 961.

Preparations

BP 1998: Phenytoin Capsules; Phenytoin Injection; Phenytoin Oral Suspension; Phenytoin Tablets;
USP 23: Extended Phenytoin Sodium Capsules; Phenytoin Oral Suspension; Phenytoin Sodium Injection; Phenytoin Tablets; Prompt Phenytoin Sodium Capsules.

Proprietary Preparations (details are given in Part 3)
Aust.: Epanutin; Epilan-D; Phenhydan; ***Austral.:*** Dilantin; ***Belg.:*** Di-Hydan; Diphantoine; Epanutin; ***Canad.:*** Dilantin; ***Fr.:*** Di-Hydan; Pyoredol; ***Ger.:*** Epanutin; Phenhydan; Zentropil; ***Irl.:*** Epanutin; ***Ital.:*** Aurantin; Dintoina; ***Jpn:*** Aleviatin; ***Neth.:*** Epanutin; ***Norw.:*** Epinat; ***S.Afr.:*** Epanutin; ***Spain:*** Epanutin; Neosidantoina; Sinergina; ***Swed.:*** Epanutin; Fenantoin; Lehydan; ***Switz.:*** Antisacer†; Epanutin; Epilantine; Phenhydan; ***UK:*** Epanutin; Pentran; ***USA:*** Dilantin; Diphenylan†.

Multi-ingredient: ***Belg.:*** Mathoine; Trinuride†; Vethoine; ***Canad.:*** Dilantin with Phenobarbital; ***Ger.:*** Antisacer comp.†; ***Ital.:*** Dintoinale; Dintospina†; Gamibetal Complex; Metinal-Idantoina; Metinal-Idantoina L; Sedital†; ***S.Afr.:*** Garoin; ***Spain:*** Bonifen H†; Comital L; Disfil; Epanutin Fenobarbitona†; Epilantin; Equidan†; Gaboril Complex†; Redutona; Sinergina S†.

Primidone (6619-v)

Primidone (*BAN, rINN*).

Hexamidinum; Primaclone; Primidonum. 5-Ethyl-5-phenylperhydropyrimidine-4,6-dione.

$C_{12}H_{14}N_2O_2$ = 218.3.

CAS — 125-33-7.

Pharmacopoeias. In *Chin., Eur.* (see p.viii), *Jpn, Pol.,* and *US.*

A white or almost white odourless crystalline powder. **Soluble** 1 in 2000 of water and 1 in 200 of alcohol; very slightly soluble or practically insoluble in most organic solvents.

Adverse Effects, Treatment, and Precautions

As for Phenobarbitone, p.350. Adverse effects may be more frequent than with phenobarbitone. Most patients rapidly develop tolerance to the adverse CNS effects of primidone, including ataxia, drowsiness, headache, nausea and vomiting, nystagmus, and visual disturbances.

Care is required when withdrawing primidone therapy—see also under Uses and Administration, below.

It was noted that patients receiving primidone for essential tremor have a high incidence of acute adverse reactions following small initial doses.[1] This could be due to the absence of induced hepatic enzymes in these patients previously not exposed to antiepileptics.

1. Findley LJ, *et al.* Primidone in essential tremor of the hands and head: a double blind controlled clinical study. *J Neurol Neurosurg Psychiatry* 1985; **48:** 911–15.

Effects on the blood. For a report of delayed agranulocytosis in a patient treated with phenytoin and primidone, see p.353.

Effects on the endocrine system. For mention of the effects of antiepileptics on *sexual function* in male epileptic patients, see under Phenytoin, p.353.

Overdosage. Crystalluria has been reported[1] following acute overdosage of primidone and 7 other reported cases were also reviewed. Based on these few reports, crystalluria appears to be associated with serum-primidone concentrations in excess of 80 μg per mL. There is evidence from 2 reports of renal damage associated with crystal formation *in vivo*. Vigorous hydration, with or without forced alkaline diuresis, is recommended in patients at risk, in order to lessen the potential for renal toxicity and improve elimination.

1. Lehmann DF. Primidone crystalluria following overdose: a report of a case and an analysis of the literature. *Med Toxicol* 1987; **2:** 383–7.

Porphyria. Primidone has been associated with acute attacks of porphyria and is considered unsafe in patients with acute porphyria.[1]

1. Moore MR, McColl KEL. *Porphyria: drug lists.* Glasgow: Porphyria Research Unit, University of Glasgow, 1991.

Interactions

Primidone is metabolised in the body in part to phenobarbitone and interactions recorded for phenobarbitone (p.351) might potentially occur in patients receiving primidone. In addition, enzyme-inducing drugs enhance this metabolism and have the potential to produce elevated phenobarbitone concentrations.

Antiepileptics. Both *phenytoin*[1,2] and *carbamazepine*[3] have been reported to enhance the metabolism of primidone to phenobarbitone and when primidone was combined with phenytoin there have been instances of phenobarbitone toxicity.[2] *Vigabatrin* has been reported[4] to lower plasma concentrations of primidone in some patients, although it is unlikely that dosage changes would be necessary. *Valproate* may increase plasma concentrations of primidone and phenobarbitone, but patient response seems to be inconsistent.

1. Reynolds EH, *et al.* Interaction of phenytoin and primidone. *Br Med J* 1975; **2:** 594–5.
2. Fincham RW, Schottelius DD. Primidone: interactions with other drugs. In: Levy RH, *et al.*, (eds). *Antiepileptic drugs.* (4th ed.) New York: Raven Press, 1995: 467–75.
3. Baciewicz AM. Carbamazepine drug interactions. *Ther Drug Monit* 1986; **8:** 305–17.
4. Browne TR, *et al.* A multicentre study of vigabatrin for drug-resistant epilepsy. *Br J Clin Pharmacol* 1989; **27** (suppl): 95S–100S.

Pharmacokinetics

Primidone is readily absorbed from the gastro-intestinal tract and is reported to have a plasma half-life ranging from 10 to 15 hours, which is shorter than those of its principal metabolites phenylethylmalonamide and phenobarbitone, both of which are active. It is excreted in urine as unchanged drug (40%) and metabolites.

Primidone is widely distributed but is only partially bound to plasma protein; it has been suggested that it exhibits variable binding of up to about 20%. It crosses the placenta and is distributed into breast milk.

Uses and Administration

Primidone is an antiepileptic that is partially metabolised to phenobarbitone (p.351), but is also considered to have some antiepileptic activity in its own right. It may be given to control partial (especially complex partial) and generalised tonic-clonic seizures. Primidone is also used in the management of essential tremor.

In the treatment of epilepsy the dose of primidone should be adjusted according to the response of the patient; a limited correlation with plasma concentrations has suggested that concentrations of 5 to 12 μg per mL (23 to 55 μmol per litre) are usually necessary, but some sources suggest that monitoring of phenobarbitone concentrations may be adequate.

Suggested initial doses are 125 mg daily by mouth at bedtime increased, if necessary, by 125 mg every 3 days to a total of 500 mg daily given in 2 divided doses; if necessary, the daily dose may be increased further every 3 days by 250 mg in adults up to a maximum of 1.5 g daily given in divided doses; in children under 9 years of age the dose may be increased by increments of 125 mg. Usual maintenance doses in adults and children over 9 years of age are 0.75 to 1.5 g daily. Suggested maintenance doses for children are: up to 2 years, 250 to 500 mg daily; 2 to 5 years, 500 to 750 mg daily; 6 to 9 years, 0.75 to 1 g daily. Maintenance doses are usually given as 2 divided doses.

As with other antiepileptics, withdrawal of primidone therapy or transition to or from another type of antiepileptic therapy should be made gradually to avoid precipitating an increase in the frequency of seizures. For a discussion on whether or not to withdraw antiepileptic therapy in seizure-free patients, see p.335.

For essential tremor primidone is given in usual initial doses of 50 mg daily by mouth, increased gradually over 2 to 3 weeks if necessary, to a maximum of 750 mg daily.

Epilepsy. Primidone, like its metabolite phenobarbitone, is used in the treatment of epilepsy (p.335) for partial seizures with or without secondary generalisation and for primary generalised tonic-clonic seizures. However, because of problems of sedation, it is usually reserved for use in cases unresponsive to other antiepileptics.

Neonatal apnoea. Methylxanthines such as caffeine and theophylline are the main drugs used in the treatment of neonatal apnoea (p.773) in patients with no underlying seizure disorder; doxapram may be considered as an alternative in patients who do not respond to xanthines. Results from a preliminary study have suggested that adjunctive treatment with primidone[1] may be of value in neonates resistant to xanthine therapy alone.

1. Miller CA, *et al.* The use of primidone in neonates with theophylline-resistant apnea. *Am J Dis Child* 1993; **147:** 183–6.

Neonatal seizures. Primidone has been tried in the management of neonatal seizures (p.338).

Tremor. A beta blocker is often the first drug used in patients with essential tremor who require regular treatment (p.831) but primidone[1] may also be tried. A high incidence of acute adverse reactions has been reported following initial doses (see above). There has been concern that long-term use may produce tolerance to primidone's effects, although a small study has found a reduced response in only a few patients.[2]

1. Koller WC, Royse VL. Efficacy of primidone in essential tremor. *Neurology* 1986; **36:** 121–4.
2. Sasso E, *et al.* Primidone in the long-term treatment of essential tremor: a prospective study with computerized quantitative analysis. *Clin Neuropharmacol* 1990; **13:** 67–76.

Preparations

BP 1998: Primidone Oral Suspension; Primidone Tablets;
USP 23: Primidone Oral Suspension; Primidone Tablets.

Proprietary Preparations (details are given in Part 3)
Aust.: Cyral; Mysoline; ***Austral.:*** Mysoline; ***Belg.:*** Mysoline; ***Canad.:*** Mysoline; ***Fr.:*** Mysoline; ***Ger.:*** Liskantin; Mylepsinum; Resimatil; ***Irl.:*** Mysoline; ***Ital.:*** Mysoline; ***Neth.:*** Mysoline; ***Norw.:*** Mysoline; ***S.Afr.:*** Mysoline; ***Spain:*** Mysoline; ***Swed.:*** Mysoline; ***Switz.:*** Mysoline; ***UK:*** Mysoline; ***USA:*** Mysoline.

Progabide (16968-t)

Progabide *(BAN, USAN, rINN)*.

Halogabide; SL-76-002. 4-(4′-Chloro-5-fluoro-2-hydroxybenzhydrylideneamino)butyramide.

$C_{17}H_{16}ClFN_2O_2$ = 334.8.

CAS — 62666-20-0.

Adverse Effects and Precautions

Liver disorders, indicated by elevation of liver enzyme values, are reported to occur in about 9% of patients receiving progabide, usually in the first few months of treatment, and have progressed to jaundice, hepatitis, encephalopathy and death in some patients. Progabide is contra-indicated in patients with pre-existing liver disorders, and patients should undergo regular monitoring of liver function, particularly in the first 6 months of treatment.

Drowsiness, dizziness, fatigue, and gastro-intestinal disturbances, usually transient and dose-related, may occur, particularly at the beginning of treatment. Irritability and mood changes have been reported. Care is required when withdrawing progabide therapy—see also under Uses and Administration, below.

Progabide should be used with caution in patients with impaired renal function.

Driving. For a comment on antiepileptic drugs and driving, see p.337.

Porphyria. Progabide has been associated with acute attacks of porphyria and is considered unsafe in patients with acute porphyria.[1]

1. Moore MR, McColl KEL. *Porphyria: drug lists.* Glasgow: Porphyria Research Unit, University of Glasgow, 1991.

Interactions

There are complex interactions between antiepileptics and toxicity may be enhanced without a corresponding increase in antiepileptic activity. Such interactions are very variable and unpredictable and plasma monitoring is often advisable with combination therapy.

Antiepileptics. For the effects of progabide on other antiepileptics, see Carbamazepine, p.341; Phenobarbitone, p.351; and Phenytoin, p.355.

Pharmacokinetics

Progabide is reported to be well absorbed following oral administration; studies in *animals* suggest that it undergoes first-pass metabolism. The bioavailability of an oral dose is reported to be about 60%. It is extensively metabolised, in part by hydrolysis of the amide group to the corresponding carboxylic acid (PGA; SL-75-102) which is also active. Progabide is about 95% bound to plasma proteins. It is excreted in urine, chiefly as metabolites.

Uses and Administration

Progabide is an analogue of gamma-aminobutyric acid (GABA) and is believed to owe its antiepileptic properties to its action as an agonist at central GABA receptors. It is used in the treatment of partial and generalised tonic-clonic seizures resistant to other therapy. It has been employed for myoclonic seizures and in the Lennox-Gastaut and West's syndromes.

The dose is gradually increased to usual maintenance doses of 25 to 35 mg per kg body-weight daily given by mouth, divided into 3 doses. Higher maintenance doses of 35 to 45 mg per kg daily may be employed in children.

Doses should be reduced in patients with renal impairment.

As with other antiepileptics, withdrawal of progabide therapy or transition to or from another type of antiepileptic therapy should be made gradually to avoid precipitating an increase in the frequency of seizures. For a discussion on whether or not to withdraw antiepileptic therapy in seizure-free patients, see p.335.

Reviews.

1. Bergmann KJ. Progabide: a new GABA-mimetic agent in clinical use. *Clin Neuropharmacol* 1985; **8:** 13–26.

Epilepsy. Progabide is used in epilepsy (p.335) as monotherapy or adjuvant therapy for patients with refractory epilepsy. It is effective in the management of generalised tonic-clonic seizures, including secondarily generalised seizures, and also in simple and complex partial seizures. It is also effective in atonic and myoclonic seizures, but does not appear to be of benefit in absence seizures. It has been used in West's syndrome and Lennox-Gastaut syndrome.

Preparations

Proprietary Preparations (details are given in Part 3)
Fr.: Gabrene.

Stiripentol (3634-m)

Stiripentol *(USAN, rINN)*.

BCX-2600. 4,4-Dimethyl-1-[(3,4-methylenedioxy)phenyl]-1-penten-3-ol.

$C_{14}H_{18}O_3$ = 234.3.

CAS — 49763-96-4.

Adverse Effects and Precautions

Insomnia, occasional psychotic reactions, and gastro-intestinal disturbances have been reported in patients receiving stiripentol.

Interactions

Stiripentol is a potent inhibitor of hepatic microsomal drug metabolism, and interactions are possible when it is given with other drugs.

Stiripentol appears to inhibit several cytochrome P450 isoenzymes, including CYP1A2 and CYP3A4.[1] For interactions of stiripentol with other antiepileptics, see under Carbamazepine, p.341 and Phenytoin, p.355.

1. Tran A, *et al.* Influence of stiripentol on cytochrome P450-mediated metabolic pathways in humans: in vitro and in vivo comparison and calculation of in vivo inhibition constants. *Clin Pharmacol Ther* 1997; **62:** 490–504.

Pharmacokinetics

Stiripentol is incompletely absorbed following oral administration, and undergoes hepatic first-pass metabolism; as a result bioavailability of an oral dose is reported to be only about 20%. Its pharmacokinetics are non-linear, clearance decreasing with increasing dosage. Stiripentol is reported to be more than 99% protein bound. It is extensively metabolised and excreted in urine almost entirely as metabolites. Elimination is biphasic with a rapid initial and a prolonged terminal phase.

Uses and Administration

Stiripentol is an antiepileptic that has been investigated in various types of epilepsy. It has been given by mouth. It is thought to be less potent than some conventional antiepileptics, but may reduce their adverse effects when used together.

Reviews.

1. Bebin M, Bleck TP. New anticonvulsant drugs: focus on flunarizine, fosphenytoin, midazolam and stiripentol. *Drugs* 1994; **48:** 153–71.
2. Patsalos PN, Sander JWAS. Newer antiepileptic drugs: towards an improved risk-benefit ratio. *Drug Safety* 1994; **11:** 37–67.

Epilepsy. A 24-week study[1] in 10 children demonstrated that stiripentol might be effective as adjunctive therapy for the treatment of atypical absence seizures (p.335).

1. Farwell JR, *et al.* Stiripentol in atypical absence seizures in children: an open trial. *Epilepsia* 1993; **34:** 305–11.

Sulthiame (6621-f)

Sulthiame *(BAN, USAN)*.

Sultiame *(rINN)*; Riker-594. 4-(Tetrahydro-2*H*-1,2-thiazin-2-yl)benzenesulphonamide *S,S*-dioxide.

$C_{10}H_{14}N_2O_4S_2$ = 290.4.

CAS — 61-56-3.

Pharmacopoeias. In *Jpn.*

Sulthiame is a carbonic anhydrase inhibitor that has been used as an antiepileptic in most forms of epilepsy (p.335) except absence seizures. It has usually been given in conjunction with other antiepileptics and it is believed that much of its activity is due to the inhibition of metabolism of the other drugs.

Sulthiame is given by mouth in initial doses of 100 mg twice daily or 50 mg three times daily gradually increased according to response to 200 mg three times daily.

Interactions. For the effect of sulthiame on phenytoin, see under Phenytoin, p.355.

Porphyria. Sulthiame has been associated with clinical exacerbations of porphyria and is considered unsafe in porphyric patients.[1]

1. Moore MR, McColl KEL. *Porphyria: drug lists.* Glasgow: Porphyria Research Unit, University of Glasgow, 1991.

Preparations

Proprietary Preparations (details are given in Part 3)
Austral.: Ospolot; ***Ger.:*** Ospolot; ***Ital.:*** Ospolot†.

Tiagabine Hydrochloride (14669-z)

Tiagabine Hydrochloride *(USAN, rINNM).*
Abbott-70569.1; ABT-569; NNC-05-0328; NO-05-0328.
(−)-(*R*)-1-[4,4-Bis(3-methyl-2-thienyl)-3-butenyl]nipecotic acid hydrochloride.
$C_{20}H_{25}NO_2S_2,HCl = 412.0.$
CAS — 115103-54-3 (tiagabine); 145821-59-6 (tiagabine hydrochloride).

Tiagabine hydrochloride 55 mg is approximately equivalent to 50 mg of tiagabine.

Adverse Effects

The most common adverse effects include dizziness, nervousness, somnolence, and tremor. Other reported adverse effects include confusion, depression, difficulties in concentration, diarrhoea, nausea, ataxia, and nystagmus. Bruising, rashes, speech difficulties, and an influenza-like syndrome of chills, fever, myalgia, and headache have also been reported.

In a meta-analysis[1] of 5 double-blind trials involving approximately 1000 patients receiving tiagabine as adjunctive therapy for refractory partial seizures, discontinuation resulting from adverse effects was infrequent and occurred in 15% of patients receiving tiagabine compared with 5% receiving placebo. Adverse effects were usually associated with dose titration, and were generally mild to moderate in severity, and transient.

1. Leppike IE. Tiagabine: the safety landscape. *Epilepsia* 1995; **36** (suppl 6): S10–S13.

Precautions

Hepatic metabolism of tiagabine is reduced in patients with hepatic impairment, and dosage should therefore be reduced and/or the dosage intervals increased. It should not be used in patients with severely impaired hepatic functions.

Care is required when withdrawing tiagabine therapy—see Uses and Administration, below.

Driving. For comment on antiepileptic drugs and driving, see p.337.

Interactions

The hepatic metabolism of tiagabine is accelerated by concomitant administration of antiepileptics that induce enzymes of the cytochrome P450 system such as carbamazepine, phenobarbitone, phenytoin, or primidone. Plasma concentrations of tiagabine may be reduced by up to threefold by concomitant use.

Pharmacokinetics

Tiagabine is readily absorbed after oral administration. Food reduces the rate but not the extent of absorption. The absorption and elimination pharmacokinetics of tiagabine are linear within the therapeutic dosage range.

Tiagabine is widely distributed throughout the body and plasma protein binding is high (96%).

Tiagabine is extensively metabolised in the liver and excreted as metabolites in the faeces or, to a lesser extent, in the urine; only 2% of a dose is eliminated as unchanged drug. The plasma-elimination half-life is 7 to 9 hours, although this may be reduced to 2 to 3 hours by concomitant administration of liver enzyme-inducing drugs.

References.

1. Gustavson LE, Mengel HB. Pharmacokinetics of tiagabine, a γ-aminobutyric acid-uptake inhibitor, in healthy subjects after single and multiples doses. *Epilepsia* 1995; **36:** 605–11.
2. So EL, *et al.* Pharmacokinetics of tiagabine as add-on therapy in patients taking enzyme-inducing antiepilepsy drugs. *Epilepsy Res* 1995; **22:** 221–6.
3. Snel S, *et al.* The pharmacokinetics of tiagabine in healthy elderly volunteers and elderly patients with epilepsy. *J Clin Pharmacol* 1997; **37:** 1015–20.

Uses and Administration

Tiagabine hydrochloride is a nipecotic acid derivative used in the treatment of epilepsy (p.335) as adjunctive therapy for refractory partial seizures with or without secondary generalisation. It inhibits the uptake of GABA into neuronal and glial cells, and therefore increases the availability of GABA at receptor sites.

In the UK, the initial dose of tiagabine hydrochloride as adjunctive therapy in adults and children over 12 years of age is the equivalent of tiagabine 5 mg twice daily by mouth for 1 week, increased as necessary by weekly increments of 5 to 10 mg daily. The usual maintenance dose is 30 to 45 mg daily, in three divided doses, in patients receiving enzyme-inducing antiepileptics; in patients not taking enzyme-inducing drugs an initial maintenance dosage of 15 to 30 mg daily is suggested. Doses should be taken with food to avoid rapid rises in plasma concentrations, thereby reducing the incidence of adverse effects.

As with other antiepileptics, withdrawal of tiagabine therapy or transition to or from another type of antiepileptic therapy should be made gradually to avoid precipitating an increase in the frequency of seizures. For a discussion on whether or not to withdraw antiepileptic therapy in seizure-free patients, see p.335.

References.

1. Leach JP, Brodie MJ. Tiagabine. *Lancet* 1998; **351:** 203–7.
2. Adkins JC, Noble S. Tiagabine: a review of its pharmacodynamic and pharmacokinetic properties and therapeutic potential in the management of epilepsy. *Drugs* 1998; **55:** 437–60.

Preparations

Proprietary Preparations (details are given in Part 3)
Austral.: Gabitril; ***Irl.:*** Gabitril; ***UK:*** Gabitril; ***USA:*** Gabitril.

Topiramate (3130-h)

Topiramate *(BAN, USAN, rINN).*
McN-4853; RWJ-17021. 2,3:4,5-Di-*O*-isopropylidene-β-D-fructopyranose sulphamate.
$C_{12}H_{21}NO_8S = 339.4.$
CAS — 97240-79-4.

Adverse Effects

Adverse effects associated with topiramate therapy include ataxia, impaired concentration, confusion, dizziness, fatigue, paraesthesia, drowsiness, and difficulties with memory or cognition. Agitation, emotional lability (with behavioural disturbances), and depression may also occur. Other reported adverse effects include abdominal pain, anorexia, asthenia, diplopia, leucopenia, nausea, nystagmus, psychomotor retardation, speech disorder, altered taste, visual disturbances, and weight loss. The risk of nephrolithiasis is increased, especially in predisposed patients.

Precautions

Topiramate should be used with caution in patients with renal or hepatic impairment. There is a risk of renal calculi formation, especially in predisposed patients, and adequate hydration is recommended to reduce the risk.

Care is required when withdrawing topiramate therapy—see also under Uses and Administration, below.

Driving. For a comment on antiepileptic drugs and driving, see p.337.

Pregnancy. For comments on the management of epilepsy during pregnancy, see p.337.

Interactions

There are complex interactions between antiepileptics and toxicity may be enhanced without a corresponding increase in antiepileptic activity. Such interactions are very variable and unpredictable and plasma monitoring is often advisable with combination therapy.

Antiepileptics. In pharmacokinetic studies[1] *phenytoin* and *carbamazepine* decreased the plasma concentration of topiramate by about 50%.

For the effect of topiramate on phenytoin, see p.355.

1. Bourgeois BFD. Drug interaction profile of topiramate. *Epilepsia* 1996; **37:** (suppl 2): S14–S17.

Cardiac glycosides. For the effect of topiramate on *digoxin*, see p.851.

Sex hormones. For the effects of antiepileptics including topiramate on *oral contraceptives*, see p.1433.

Pharmacokinetics

Topiramate is readily absorbed following oral administration with peak plasma concentrations achieved about 2 hours after a dose. Bioavailability is not affected by the presence of food. The volume of distribution in women is approximately half that in men. Up to 50% of a dose may undergo metabolism in the liver. It is eliminated chiefly in urine, as unchanged drug and metabolites; mean plasma elimination half-life is about 21 hours. Steady state concentrations are achieved after about 4 to 8 days in patients with normal renal function. Clearance is decreased in patients with impaired renal or hepatic function, and steady state plasma concentrations may not be achieved for 10 to 15 days in the former. Children exhibit a higher clearance and shorter elimination half-life than adults.

References.

1. Perucca E, Bialer M. The clinical pharmacokinetics of the newer antiepileptic drugs: focus on topiramate, zonisamide, and tiagabine. *Clin Pharmacokinet* 1996; **31:** 29–46.

Uses and Administration

Topiramate, a sulphamate-substituted monosaccharide, is an antiepileptic used as adjunctive therapy for refractory partial seizures with or without secondary generalisation, seizures associated with the Lennox-Gastaut syndrome, and primary generalised tonic-clonic seizures.

The initial dose of topiramate is 50 mg once daily by mouth for one week increased thereafter by increments of 50 mg at weekly intervals until the effective dose is reached, which is usually within the range of 200 to 400 mg daily taken in 2 divided doses; some patients may require up to 800 mg daily. A lower initial dose, smaller increments, or longer intervals between increments may be necessary if patients cannot tolerate the above regimen.

The recommended dose in the UK for children aged 2 to 16 years is about 5 to 9 mg per kg body-weight daily given in 2 divided doses. Dosage is begun with 25 mg nightly for the first week and increased at intervals of 1 to 2 weeks by increments of 1 to 3 mg per kg daily.

Daily doses of more than 50 mg should be taken in 2 divided doses. Patients with moderate or severe renal impairment take longer to reach steady-state plasma concentrations than patients with normal renal function (see under Pharmacokinetics, above). It has been recommended that doses be halved in such patients.

As with other antiepileptics, withdrawal of topiramate therapy or transition to or from another type of antiepileptic therapy should be made gradually to avoid precipitating an increase in the frequency of seizures. For a discussion on whether or not to withdraw antiepileptic therapy in seizure-free patients, see p.335. The manufacturers have suggested decreasing the dose by 100 mg daily at weekly intervals.

Reviews.

1. Langtry HD, *et al.* Topiramate: a review of its pharmacodynamic and pharmacokinetic properties and clinical efficacy in the management of epilepsy. *Drugs* 1997; **54:** 752–73.
2. Privitera MD. Topiramate: a new antiepileptic drug. *Ann Pharmacother* 1997; **31:** 1164–73.
3. Markind JE. Topiramate: a new antiepileptic drug. *Am J Health-Syst Pharm* 1998; **55:** 554–62.
4. Sachdeo RC, *et al.* Topiramate: clinical profile in epilepsy. *Clin Pharmacokinet* 1998; **34:** 335–46.

Epilepsy. Topiramate is used in epilepsy (p.335) as adjunctive therapy for refractory partial seizures;[1,2] monotherapy with topiramate appeared to be safe and effective in one study.[3]

Topiramate is also used in patients with the Lennox-Gastaut syndrome and with primary generalised tonic-clonic seizures.

1. Ben-Menachem E, *et al.* Double-blind, placebo-controlled trial of topiramate as add-on therapy in patients with refractory partial seizures. *Epilepsia* 1996; **37:** 539–43.
2. Sharief M, *et al.* Double-blind, placebo-controlled study of topiramate in patients with refractory partial epilepsy. *Epilepsy Res* 1996; **25:** 217–24.
3. Sachdeo RC, *et al.* Topiramate monotherapy for partial onset seizures. *Epilepsia* 1997; **38:** 294–300.

Preparations

Proprietary Preparations (details are given in Part 3)
Austral.: Topamax; ***Irl.:*** Topamax; ***Norw.:*** Topimax; ***S.Afr.:*** Topamax; ***Swed.:*** Topimax; ***Switz.:*** Topamax; ***UK:*** Topamax; ***USA:*** Topamax.

Troxidone (6622-d)

Troxidone *(BAN)*.

Trimethadione *(rINN)*; Trimetadiona; Trimethadionum; Trimethinum. 3,5,5-Trimethyl-1,3-oxazolidine-2,4-dione.

$C_6H_9NO_3$ = 143.1.

CAS — 127-48-0.

Pharmacopoeias. In *Eur.* (see p.viii), *Int., Jpn,* and *US.*

Colourless or white granular crystals with a slightly camphoraceous odour. M.p. 45° to 47°. **Soluble** in water; freely to very soluble in alcohol, in chloroform, and in ether. **Store** in airtight containers. Protect from light.

Adverse Effects

Many adverse effects of troxidone are serious and call for prompt discontinuation of therapy. Common side-effects include drowsiness, which may subside on continuation of therapy, and photophobia and hemeralopia (blurring of vision in bright light), which is more frequent in adults.

Other side-effects include nausea and vomiting, abdominal pain, anorexia, weight loss, hiccups, malaise, insomnia, vertigo, headache, alopecia, paraesthesias, changes in blood pressure, and personality changes. Blood disorders include neutropenia (which does not call for withdrawal of therapy provided that it remains moderate), thrombocytopenia, pancytopenia, agranulocytosis, and aplastic anaemia. Lymphadenopathy, a lupus erythematosus syndrome, the nephrotic syndrome, and hepatitis may also occur. Skin rashes may lead to exfoliative dermatitis and erythema multiforme. A syndrome resembling myasthenia gravis has also been reported.

Symptoms of acute overdosage include drowsiness, nausea, dizziness, ataxia, visual disturbances, and coma.

Characteristic congenital malformations, termed the fetal troxidone syndrome, have been associated with the use of troxidone in pregnancy.

Precautions

Troxidone is contra-indicated in patients with severe hepatic or renal disease or with severe blood disorders. It should be used with caution in patients with disease of the retina or optic nerve and should be withdrawn if scotomata occur. Frequent examinations of blood, urine, and hepatic function should be carried out in patients receiving troxidone, and therapy should be withdrawn promptly at signs of renal or hepatic dysfunction, severe neutropenia or other blood disorders, or drug hypersensitivity. Troxidone should also be discontinued, at least temporarily, on the appearance of any skin disorder, however mild.

Care is required when withdrawing troxidone therapy—see also under Uses and Administration, below. Abrupt withdrawal should be avoided unless serious adverse effects have occurred, in which case substitution by an alternative antiepileptic may be necessary.

Administration of troxidone in pregnancy has been associated with a high incidence of congenital malformations.

Porphyria. Troxidone has been associated with clinical exacerbations of porphyria and is considered unsafe in porphyric patients.[1]

1. Moore MR, McColl KEL. *Porphyria: drug lists.* Glasgow: Porphyria Research Unit, University of Glasgow, 1991.

Pregnancy. For comments on the management of epilepsy during pregnancy, see p.337.

Pharmacokinetics

Troxidone is readily absorbed from the gastro-intestinal tract and extensively demethylated in the liver to its active metabolite, dimethadione, which is primarily responsible for the activity of troxidone on chronic administration.

Troxidone is very slowly excreted in the urine, over a period of several days, almost entirely in the form of dimethadione.

Troxidone is reported not to be significantly bound to plasma proteins.

Some correlation has been found between plasma concentrations of dimethadione exceeding 700 μg per mL and therapeutic response.

Uses and Administration

Troxidone is an oxazolidinedione antiepileptic that has been used in the treatment of absence seizures refractory to other antiepileptics. However, because of its potential toxicity, other antiepileptics are preferred (see under Epilepsy, p.335).

The initial dose of troxidone was 900 mg daily in divided doses, increased gradually according to the patient's response, to a recommended maximum dose of 2.4 g daily. Suggested doses of troxidone for children were 300 to 900 mg daily.

As with other antiepileptics, withdrawal of troxidone therapy or transition to or from another type of antiepileptic therapy should be made gradually to avoid precipitating an increase in the frequency of seizures. For a discussion on whether or not to withdraw antiepileptic therapy in seizure-free patients, see p.335.

Preparations

USP 23: Trimethadione Capsules; Trimethadione Oral Solution; Trimethadione Tablets.

Proprietary Preparations (details are given in Part 3)
Ger.: Tridione†; ***USA:*** Tridione.

Valproate (10447-z)

Valproate is a generic term applied to valproic acid, its salts and esters.

Valproic Acid (6623-n)

Valproic Acid *(BAN, USAN, rINN)*.

Abbott-44089; Acidum Valproicum. 2-Propylvaleric acid; 2-Propylpentanoic acid.

$C_8H_{16}O_2$ = 144.2.

CAS — 99-66-1.

Pharmacopoeias. In *Eur.* (see p.viii) and *US.*

A colourless to pale yellow, slightly viscous, clear liquid with a characteristic odour. Slightly to very slightly **soluble** in water; freely soluble in acetone, in alcohol, in chloroform, in ether, and in methyl alcohol; miscible with dichloromethane. Dissolves in dilute solutions of alkali hydroxides. **Store** in airtight glass containers.

Semisodium Valproate (16983-a)

Semisodium Valproate *(BAN)*.

Valproate Semisodium *(rINN)*; Abbott-50711; Divalproex Sodium *(USAN)*. 2-Propylvaleric acid—Sodium 2-propylvalerate (1:1); Sodium hydrogen bis(2-propylvalerate) oligomer.

$C_{16}H_{31}NaO_4$ = 310.4.

CAS — 76584-70-8.

Sodium Valproate (6608-h)

Sodium Valproate *(BANM, rINNM)*.

Abbott-44090; Natrii Valproas; Valproate Sodium *(USAN)*. Sodium 2-propylvalerate; Sodium 2-propylpentanoate.

$C_8H_{15}NaO_2$ = 166.2.

CAS — 1069-66-5.

Pharmacopoeias. In *Chin., Eur.* (see p.viii), *Int.,* and *Jpn.*

A white or almost white, crystalline, hygroscopic, powder. Very **soluble** in water and in alcohol; practically insoluble in ether. **Store** in airtight containers.

Valproate Pivoxil (2480-c)

Valproate Pivoxil *(rINN)*.

Hydroxymethyl 2-propylvalerate pivalate.

$C_{14}H_{26}O_4$ = 258.4.

CAS — 77372-61-3.

Valpromide (6624-h)

Valpromide *(rINN)*.

Dipropylacetamide. 2-Propylvaleramide.

$C_8H_{17}NO$ = 143.2.

CAS — 2430-27-5.

Adverse Effects

The most frequently reported adverse effects associated with valproate therapy are gastro-intestinal disturbances, particularly on initiation of therapy; use of enteric-coated formulations, administration with meals, and commencement of therapy with low doses may minimise symptoms.

Less common adverse effects include increased appetite and weight gain, oedema, headache, reversible prolongation of bleeding time, and thrombocytopenia. Leucopenia and bone marrow depression have been reported. Neurological adverse effects including ataxia, tremor, sedation, lethargy, confusion, and more rarely encephalopathy and coma, have occasionally been reported, although these are often associated with too high a starting dose, increasing doses too rapidly, or concomitant use of other antiepileptics. Reversible dementia associated with cerebral atrophy has been reported. Increased alertness may occur, which is generally considered beneficial, but occasionally aggression, hyperactivity, and behavioural disturbances have been reported in children. Hearing loss has been reported. There may occasionally be rashes, and, rarely, toxic epidermal necrolysis and Stevens-Johnson syndrome or erythema multiforme. Transient hair loss, sometimes with regrowth of curly hair, has occurred. Irregular periods, amenorrhoea, and gynaecomastia have been reported rarely.

Liver dysfunction including hepatic failure has occasionally been reported, usually in the first few months of treatment, and necessitates valproate withdrawal; there have been fatalities. Elevation of liver enzyme values is common but normally transient and dose-related. Hyperammonaemia has occurred, even in the absence of overt hepatic failure and is sometimes associated with neurological symptoms; hyperglycinaemia has also been reported. Pancreatitis has also been reported; plasma amylase should be measured if there is acute abdominal pain. In a few patients there have been reports of reversible defects in renal tubular function (Fanconi's syndrome).

Congenital malformations have been reported in infants born to women who had received antiepileptics including valproate during pregnancy.

Side-effects were present in 71 of 88 children receiving sodium valproate monotherapy[1] and, although average doses in these patients were significantly higher than in the 17 with no side-effects, no difference in the plasma concentrations was observed between the 2 groups. Behavioural alterations seen in 56 included irritability, longer and deeper sleep, superficial sleep, hyperactivity, being more alert, lassitude, drowsiness, being more sociable, calmness, being happier, absent mindedness, being sadder, aggressiveness, being more skillful, and docility; it was emphasised that stimulatory reactions were as frequent as depressant effects. Digestive disorders occurred in 43 children with anorexia, abdominal pain, and nausea and vomiting being the most frequent; diarrhoea, constipation, an increase in appetite, and a gain in weight also occurred. Neurological changes in the form of tremor, paraesthesia, or ataxia, occurring in only 4 patients, were less frequent than either behavioural or digestive reactions. Miscellaneous reactions including polydipsia, polyuria, diaphoresis, enuresis, hair loss, change in hair colour or texture, and rash were seen in 23 children. Of the 71 children experiencing reactions therapy continued unchanged in 56, was changed in 3 either by altering the pharmaceutical formulation (syrup, tablets, granules), by changing the frequency of dosing, or by reducing the dose in 6, and in the remaining 9 children valproate therapy was discontinued. With the exception of a temporary increase in plasma transaminase concentrations in 2 patients, hepatic or pancreatic dysfunction was not seen.

1. Herranz JL, *et al.* Side effects of sodium valproate in monotherapy controlled by plasma levels: a study in 88 pediatric patients. *Epilepsia* 1982; **23:** 203–14.

Effects on the blood. A number of reports have implicated valproate as a cause of occasional neutropenia,[1,2] leucopenia,[3] and thrombocytopenia.[2] A 1-year prospective study involving 45 patients found that absolute neutropenia developed in 12 and thrombocytopenia in 15, but that the disorders were transient and self-limiting.[2] However, neutropenia has occasionally been sufficiently severe to warrant withdrawal of valproate.[4] Red cell aplasia has also been associated with valproate therapy.[5,6] Kreuz *et al.*[7] in a study involving 30 children found that valproate might produce symptoms similar to those of von Willebrand's disease; 19 of the 30 had a history of minor haemorrhage during therapy, and 7 had abnormal bleeding times. They felt that factor VIII therapy may need to be given in patients receiving valproate who undergo surgery or in whom bleeding is severe.

For a discussion of the effects of antiepileptics, including valproate, on serum folate, see under Phenytoin, p.353.

1. Jaeken J, *et al.* Neutropenia during sodium valproate treatment. *Arch Dis Child* 1979; **54:** 986–7.
2. Barr RD, *et al.* Valproic acid and immune thrombocytopenia. *Arch Dis Child* 1982; **57:** 681–4.
3. Coulter DL, *et al.* Valproic acid therapy in childhood epilepsy. *JAMA* 1980; **244:** 785–8.
4. Symon DNK, Russell G. Sodium valproate and neutropenia. *Arch Dis Child* 1983; **58:** 235.

5. MacDougall LG. Pure red cell aplasia associated with sodium valproate therapy. *JAMA* 1982; **247:** 53–4.
6. Watts RG, *et al.* Valproic acid-induced cytopenias: evidence for a dose-related suppression of hematopoiesis. *J Pediatr* 1990; **117:** 495–9.
7. Kreuz W, *et al.* Induction of von Willebrand disease type I by valproic acid. *Lancet* 1990; **335:** 1350–1.

Effects on bone. For the effects of antiepileptics including valproate on bone and on calcium and vitamin D metabolism, see under Phenytoin, p.353.

Effects on the endocrine system. *Menstrual disturbances* occurred more frequently with valproate than other antiepileptics in a study of 238 women with epilepsy.[1] The disturbances were attributed to valproate-associated reproductive endocrine disorders, namely polycystic ovaries and elevated serum-testosterone concentrations.

For mention of the effects of antiepileptics on *sexual function* in male epileptic patients, see under Phenytoin, p.353.

1. Isojärvi JIT, *et al.* Polycystic ovaries and hyperandrogenism in women taking valproate for epilepsy. *N Engl J Med* 1993; **329:** 1383–8.

Effects on the liver. One review[1] of the hepatotoxicity of valproate included an analysis of 42 cases with fatal hepatitis, 3 cases with a Reye's-like syndrome, and 22 instances of hyperammonaemia. In 19 clinical trials the incidence of *abnormal serum aminotransferase* activity has ranged from 0 to 44% with an overall incidence of 11% in the 1197 patients monitored; in the non-fatal cases activity was usually between one and three times the upper limit of normal and was not usually, except in the most severe cases, accompanied by rises in serum bilirubin or alkaline phosphatase. In the 42 cases of *hepatitis* with a fatal outcome the age at presentation ranged from 2.5 months to 34 years with 69% aged 10 years or less. Below the age of 15 years the proportion of males was 62.5% but above this age it was 30%; the disproportionate vulnerability of young individuals, particularly boys, does not appear to be a reflection of prescribing habits in that age group. In more than two-thirds of these patients with a fatal outcome, prodromal symptoms comprised anorexia and vomiting, loss of epilepsy control, impaired consciousness, and ataxia; in about one-third there were signs of liver damage with fever, jaundice, ascites, peripheral oedema, and easy bruising. In all of the patients hepatic coma developed. In 36 patients on whom data were available the onset of hepatic illness in one-third occurred between 1 and 2 months and in only 2 patients did the onset occur after more than 5 months. Of these 42 patients with fatal hepatotoxicity 36 had received other drugs, mostly antiepileptics, concurrently. The 3 children with the *Reye's-like syndrome* all died within 3 weeks of the first occurrence of symptoms as a result of cerebral oedema (2) or aspiration pneumonia (1). In the 22 patients with symptomatic *hyperammonaemia*, characterised usually by impaired consciousness and ataxia, but without overt liver disease, withdrawal of valproate resulted in all becoming asymptomatic and biochemical abnormalities returned to normal. Hyperammonaemia has also been reported in asymptomatic patients. It was considered by the authors that measurement of serum aminotransferase would be of most value during the first three months of therapy and should be mandatory in the apparently predisposed patient with mental retardation, structural brain damage, or metabolic disorders and particular care should be given to those patients on multiple drug therapy. Testing at monthly intervals would then be reasonable and in those patients in whom an abnormality of aminotransferase developed the dose of valproate should be reduced; if values failed to normalise or continued to rise drug therapy should be withdrawn. It was felt likely though, that despite these precautions, a small number of severe reactions related to individual idiosyncrasy would not be prevented. Various hypotheses for the cause of valproate hepatotoxicity have been discussed in detail.[2]

Analysis of deaths in the USA attributed to valproate liver toxicity identified a decline in the incidence of fatalities as use in young children and use concurrently with other antiepileptics declined.[3]

1. Powell-Jackson PR, *et al.* Hepatotoxicity to sodium valproate: a review. *Gut* 1984; **25:** 673–81.
2. Eadie MJ, *et al.* Valproate-associated hepatotoxicity and its biochemical mechanisms. *Med Toxicol* 1988; **3:** 85–106.
3. Dreifuss FE, *et al.* Valproic acid hepatic fatalities: II US experience since 1984. *Neurology* 1989; **39:** 201–7.

Effects on mental function. For a review of the effects of antiepileptic therapy including sodium valproate on cognition, see p.337.

Effects on the nervous system. An *extrapyramidal* syndrome of tremor and rigidity, unresponsive to benztropine or benzhexol, developed in a 52-year-old man with schizophrenia given a therapeutic trial of sodium valproate 1 to 2 g daily.[1] Administration of sodium valproate to a man with dystonic movements of the neck and spine produced a severe subjective and objective deterioration in his symptoms which returned to their previous severity on withdrawal of the drug.[2]

A *stuporous state* associated with EEG abnormalities has been described[3] during valproate therapy for complex partial seizures and it was suggested that in certain forms of epilepsy valproate may exhibit a paradoxical epileptogenic effect. Other findings[4] have argued against an epileptic origin for valproate-induced stupor.

1. Lautin A, *et al.* Extrapyramidal syndrome with sodium valproate. *Br Med J* 1979; **2:** 1035–6.
2. Dick DJ, Saunders M. Extrapyramidal syndrome with sodium valproate. *Br Med J* 1980; **280:** 189.
3. Marescaux C, *et al.* Stuporous episodes during treatment with sodium valproate: report of seven cases. *Epilepsia* 1982; **23:** 297–305.
4. Aguglia U, *et al.* Negative myoclonus during valproate-related stupor: neurophysiological evidence of a cortical non-epileptic origin. *Electroencephalogr Clin Neurophysiol* 1995; **94:** 103–8.

Effects on the pancreas. Wyllie *et al.* reported 4 cases of pancreatitis associated with valproic acid therapy and reviewed 10 previously published cases.[1] None of the 14 patients suffered other symptoms of a toxic reaction to valproic acid. Pancreatitis was not a dose-related complication and had developed as early as one week and as late as 4.5 years following the introduction of therapy. Of the 14 patients, 2 died; 7 had been rechallenged with valproic acid and of these, 6 had recurrence of pancreatitis. It would seem, therefore, that the development of valproate-induced pancreatitis is a relative contra-indication to further therapy but that routine monitoring of serum-amylase concentrations in asymptomatic patients is not necessary. In February 1994 the Committee on Safety of Medicines in the UK commented[2] in a review of drug-induced pancreatitis that they had received 29 reports of pancreatitis, including 2 fatalities, associated with sodium valproate.

1. Wyllie E, *et al.* Pancreatitis associated with valproic acid therapy. *Am J Dis Child* 1984; **138:** 912–14.
2. Committee on Safety of Medicines/Medicines Control Agency. Drug-induced pancreatitis. *Current Problems* 1994; **20:** 2–3.

Effects on the skin and hair. Five of 250 patients developed curly hair during treatment with sodium valproate 1 g daily;[1] in 3 patients this effect followed temporary alopecia. Another report of hair curling in a patient who received sodium valproate in doses up to 3 g daily for 30 months commented that her hair started to revert to the former straight style 9 months after discontinuing the drug.[2]

Valproate-induced nicotinic-acid deficiency with an associated pellagra-like syndrome has been reported in a young boy;[3] the condition responded dramatically to the administration of nicotinamide.

Reduced serum-zinc concentrations and cutaneous manifestations of zinc deficiency were found in 2 patients receiving antiepileptic drugs.[4] It was postulated that deficiency occurred as a result of chelation by sodium valproate, and possibly phenytoin, in association with malabsorption and that, in one case, malabsorption was initiated by valproate.

Cutaneous vasculitis has been reported[5] in 2 patients taking sodium valproate. The reaction recurred on rechallenge.

Valproate might share the same order of risk as other antiepileptics for the development of Stevens-Johnson syndrome and toxic epidermal necrolysis,[6] although it had previously been regarded as safer in this respect.

1. Jeavons PM, *et al.* Valproate and curly hair. *Lancet* 1977; **i:** 359.
2. Gupta AK. 'Perming' effects associated with chronic valproate therapy. *Br J Clin Pract* 1988; **42:** 75–7.
3. Gillman MA, Sandyk R. Nicotinic acid deficiency induced by sodium valproate. *S Afr Med J* 1984; **65:** 986.
4. Lewis-Jones MS, *et al.* Cutaneous manifestations of zinc deficiency during treatment with anticonvulsants. *Br Med J* 1985; **290:** 603–4.
5. Kamper AM, *et al.* Cutaneous vasculitis induced by sodium valproate. *Lancet* 1991; **337:** 497–8.
6. Anonymous. Drugs as risk factors in severe cutaneous diseases. *WHO Drug Inf* 1996; **10:** 33–5.

Enuresis. Nocturnal enuresis associated with sodium valproate therapy has been reported[1] in 2 children. Remission of the enuresis was achieved either by reducing or redistributing the doses. Choonara[2] commented that several studies have recorded enuresis as a side-effect of valproate in children, the frequency being between 1 and 7%. The 2 most likely explanations are that it is secondary to a central effect on the thirst centre resulting in polydipsia or is a consequence of the increased depth of sleep associated with valproate.

1. Panayiotopoulos CP. Nocturnal enuresis associated with sodium valproate. *Lancet* 1985; **i:** 980–1.
2. Choonara IA. Sodium valproate and enuresis. *Lancet* 1985; **i:** 1276.

Treatment of Adverse Effects

Following overdosage the stomach may be emptied by lavage, although it has been suggested that this may be of limited value in view of the rapid absorption of valproic acid and its salts. Supportive therapy alone may then suffice.

Supportive measures provided sufficient treatment for a patient who had taken 25 g of sodium valproate.[1] Although a variety of active treatments including forced diuresis, naloxone, and haemodialysis or haemoperfusion have been advocated this case lends support to the view that questions the need for, and the efficacy of, such active measures.

1. Lakhani M, McMurdo MET. Survival after severe self poisoning with sodium valproate. *Postgrad Med J* 1986; **62:** 409–10.

Precautions

Valproate is contra-indicated in patients with pre-existing liver disease or a family history of severe hepatic dysfunction. Children under 3 years of age and those with congenital metabolic disorders, organic brain disease, or severe seizure disorders associated with mental retardation may be at particular risk of hepatotoxicity and the drug should be used with particular caution in these groups. Combination with other antiepileptics, which may also increase the risks of liver damage, should be avoided if possible. Liver function tests should be carried out, particularly in those most at risk, before and during the first 6 months of therapy.

Patients should be monitored for platelet function before major elective surgery; some sources suggest regular monitoring before and during therapy. Raised liver enzymes are not uncommon during treatment and are usually transient but patients should be reassessed clinically and liver function, including prothrombin time, monitored until they return to normal. An abnormally prolonged prothrombin time, particularly in association with other relevant abnormalities, requires discontinuation of treatment.

Patients or their carers should be told how to recognise signs of blood and liver toxicity and they should be advised to seek immediate medical attention if symptoms develop. It has also been recommended that pancreatic function should be monitored in the presence of acute abdominal pain. Valproate should be used with caution if systemic lupus erythematosus is suspected.

Care is required when withdrawing valproate therapy—see also under Uses and Administration, below.

It should be noted that the protein binding of valproate is saturable and thus shows concentration dependency with significant increases in free drug occurring at high total plasma concentrations.

Because valproate is partly excreted in the form of ketone bodies, it may cause false positives in urine tests for diabetes mellitus. Dosage adjustments may be necessary in severe renal impairment.

Breast feeding. Thrombocytopenic purpura and anaemia occurred in a breast-fed infant whose mother was being treated with valproate.[1] The baby recovered when breast feeding was stopped. For comment on antiepileptic therapy and breast feeding, see under Pregnancy on p.337.

1. Stahl MMS, *et al.* Thrombocytopenic purpura and anemia in a breast-fed infant whose mother was treated with valproic acid. *J Pediatr* 1997; **130:** 1001–3.

Driving. For a comment on antiepileptic drugs and driving, see p.337.

Porphyria. There is limited evidence that valproate is porphyrinogenic.[1] For comments on its use in porphyria, see p.339.

1. Moore MR, McColl KEL. *Porphyria: drug lists.* Glasgow: Porphyria Research Unit, University of Glasgow, 1991.

Pregnancy. For comments on the management of epilepsy during pregnancy see p.337.

There is an increased risk of neural tube defects in infants exposed *in utero* to antiepileptics including valproate and a variety of syndromes such as craniofacial and digital abnormalities and, less commonly, cleft lip and palate have been described. In an unselected series[1] of 17 infants whose epileptic mothers had received valproate during pregnancy, 9 had minor abnormalities and of these 5 had major abnormalities the most common (in 4) being a congenital heart defect. Neonatal bleeding, attributed to fibrinogen depletion and sometimes fatal, has been reported following exposure *in utero* to valproate.[2,3]

1. Thisted E, Ebbesen F. Malformations, withdrawal manifestations, and hypoglycaemia after exposure to valproate in utero. *Arch Dis Child* 1993; **69:** 288–91.
2. Majer RV, Green PJ. Neonatal afibrinogenaemia due to sodium valproate. *Lancet* 1987; **ii:** 740–1.
3. Bavoux F, *et al.* Neonatal fibrinogen depletion caused by sodium valproate. *Ann Pharmacother* 1994; **28:** 1307.

Interactions

There are complex interactions between antiepileptics and toxicity may be enhanced without a corresponding increase in antiepileptic activity. Such interactions are very variable and unpredictable and plasma monitoring is often advisable with combination therapy. Caution is recommended when administering valproate with other drugs liable to interfere with blood coagulation, such as aspirin or warfarin. Administration with other hepatotoxic drugs should be avoided.

General references.

1. Levy RH, Koch KM. Drug interactions with valproic acid. *Drugs* 1982; **24:** 543–56.

Analgesics. The valproic acid free fraction was reported to be increased, as was the half-life, when *aspirin* was given concomitantly in a study in 6 epileptic children;[1] this suggests that salicylates may inhibit the metabolism of valproate in addition to displacing it from protein binding sites. Furthermore, salicylates have been associated with an increased risk of Reye's syndrome (p.17) in children, and combination with another hepatotoxic drug such as valproate is clearly undesirable. In addition, both aspirin and valproate affect blood coagulation and platelet function.

Naproxen has also been reported to produce a slight displacement of protein-bound valproic acid but the effect is probably not sufficiently marked for it to have a clinical effect.[2]

1. Orr JM, *et al.* Interaction between valproic acid and aspirin in epileptic children: serum protein binding and metabolic effects. *Clin Pharmacol Ther* 1982; **31:** 642–9.
2. Grimaldi R, *et al.* In vivo plasma protein binding interaction between valproic acid and naproxen. *Eur J Drug Metab Pharmacokinet* 1984; **9:** 359–63.

Antibacterials. A patient receiving valproate therapy was reported[1] to have had raised valproate blood concentrations and symptoms consistent with valproate toxicity during concomitant therapy with *erythromycin*. There is a theoretical possibility that carnitine deficiency may be increased in patients receiving *pivampicillin* and valproate.

1. Redington K, *et al.* Erythromycin and valproate interaction. *Ann Intern Med* 1992; **116:** 877–8.

Antidepressants. As with all antiepileptics, antidepressants may antagonise the antiepileptic activity of valproate by lowering the convulsive threshold. For the effect of valproate on amitriptyline, see p.277.

Antiepileptics. The barbiturate antiepileptic *phenobarbitone* is reported to decrease serum-valproate concentrations when given concomitantly,[1] apparently by induction of valproate metabolism.[2] This effect is overshadowed, however, by the marked increase in serum-phenobarbitone concentrations caused by valproate inhibition of phenobarbitone metabolism—see p.351.

Carbamazepine and *phenytoin* are also enzyme-inducing drugs and, as might be expected, are reported to increase the metabolism and decrease the serum concentration of valproate.[3-5] The effect may be clinically significant.[6] The reciprocal effects of valproate on both drugs are complex, with conflicting effects on metabolism and protein binding, and the clinical outcome is difficult to predict. For more details see under Carbamazepine, p.341 and Phenytoin, p.355.

Raised serum concentrations of valproic acid have been reported in patients given *felbamate.*[7]

Valproate inhibits the metabolism of *lamotrigine* which may result in serious toxic reactions—see p.348. There is limited evidence that valproic acid may inhibit the metabolism of *ethosuximide* in some patients—see p.345.

For interactions with benzodiazepines, see under Diazepam, p.664.

1. Perucca E. Pharmacokinetic interactions with antiepileptic drugs. *Clin Pharmacokinet* 1982; **7:** 57–84.
2. Levy RH, Koch KM. Drug interactions with valproic acid. *Drugs* 1982; **24:** 543–56.
3. Panesar SK, *et al.* The effect of carbamazepine on valproic acid disposition in adult volunteers. *Br J Clin Pharmacol* 1989; **27:** 323–8.
4. Reunanen MI, *et al.* Low serum valproic acid concentrations in epileptic patients on combination therapy. *Curr Ther Res* 1980; **28:** 456–62.
5. Cramer JA, *et al.* Variable free and total valproic acid concentrations in sole- and multi-drug therapy. *Ther Drug Monit* 1986; **8:** 411–15.
6. Jann MW, *et al.* Increased valproate serum concentrations upon carbamazepine cessation. *Epilepsia* 1988; **29:** 578–81.
7. Wagner ML, *et al.* The effect of felbamate on valproic acid disposition. *Clin Pharmacol Ther* 1994; **56:** 494–502.

Antimalarials. Low serum concentrations of valproate have been reported[1] in patients taking *mefloquine.* Also, mefloquine and *chloroquine* may antagonise the antiepileptic activity of valproate by lowering the convulsive threshold.

1. Anonymous. Mefloquine for malaria. *Med Lett Drugs Ther* 1990; **32:** 13–14.

Antineoplastics. A marked reduction in serum-valproate concentration occurred in a 6-year-old child following a high-dose 24-hour infusion of *methotrexate.*[1]

1. Schrøder H, Østergaard JR. Interference of high-dose methotrexate in the metabolism of valproate? *Pediatr Hematol Oncol* 1994; **11:** 445–9.

Antipsychotics. As with all antiepileptics, antipsychotics may antagonise the antiepileptic activity of valproate by lowering the convulsive threshold. For the effect of valproate on *clozapine*, see p.659.

Antivirals. For the effect of valproate on *zidovudine,* see p.632.

Benzodiazepines. For interactions between valproate and benzodiazepines, see under Diazepam, p.664.

Cholestyramine. Cholestyramine may decrease the absorption of valproate.

Gastro-intestinal drugs. Administration with an *antacid* (aluminium and magnesium hydroxides) has been shown to increase significantly the bioavailability of a valproic acid preparation in healthy subjects;[1] other antacids in this study (calcium carbonate and an aluminium magnesium trisilicate mixture) had a lesser, insignificant effect.

Cimetidine significantly increased the half-life and decreased the clearance of sodium valproate in another study;[2] *ranitidine* had no effect on valproate pharmacokinetics.[2]

These interactions have not been reported to be of clinical significance, although the possibility must exist, particularly in patients on high-dose therapy.

1. May CA, *et al.* Effects of three antacids on the bioavailability of valproic acid. *Clin Pharm* 1982; **1:** 244–7.
2. Webster LK, *et al.* Effect of cimetidine and ranitidine on carbamazepine and sodium valproate pharmacokinetics. *Eur J Clin Pharmacol* 1984; **27:** 341–3.

Pharmacokinetics

Valproic acid and its salts are rapidly and completely absorbed from the gastro-intestinal tract; the rate, but not the extent, of absorption is delayed by administration with or after food.

Valproic acid is extensively metabolised in the liver, a large part by glucuronidation and the rest by a variety of complex pathways. It does not appear to enhance its own metabolism, but metabolism may be enhanced by other drugs which induce hepatic microsomal enzymes. It is excreted in the urine almost entirely in the form of its metabolites; small amounts are excreted in faeces and expired air.

Valproic acid is extensively bound to plasma protein. The extent of protein binding is concentration dependent and is stated to be about 90 to 95% at total concentrations of 50 μg per mL, falling to about 80 to 85% at 100 μg per mL. Reported half-lives for valproic acid have ranged from about 5 to 20 hours; the shorter half-lives have generally been recorded in epileptic patients receiving multiple drug therapy.

The 'target' range of total plasma-valproic acid is usually quoted as being 40 to 100 μg per mL (280 to 700 μmol per litre) but routine monitoring of plasma concentrations is not generally considered to be of use as an aid to assessing control.

Valproic acid crosses the placental barrier and small amounts are distributed into breast milk.

Valpromide is an amide derivative of valproic acid and its absorption is slower and its bioavailability somewhat less than that of valproic acid. Valpromide is rapidly and almost completely metabolised in the liver to valproic acid.

The pharmacokinetics of valproate are affected by the concomitant administration of other antiepileptics (see under Interactions, above).

References.

1. Zaccara G, *et al.* Clinical pharmacokinetics of valproic acid—1988. *Clin Pharmacokinet* 1988; **15:** 367–89.
2. Bialer M. Clinical pharmacology of valpromide. *Clin Pharmacokinet* 1991; **20:** 114–22.
3. Cloyd JC, *et al.* Valproic acid pharmacokinetics in children IV: effects of age and antiepileptic drugs on protein binding and intrinsic clearance. *Clin Pharmacol Ther* 1993; **53:** 22–9.
4. Yukawa E, *et al.* Population-based investigation of valproic acid relative clearance using nonlinear mixed effects modeling: influence of drug-drug interaction and patient characteristics. *J Clin Pharmacol* 1997; **37:** 1160–7.

Absorption. For a reference to the pharmacokinetics of rectal and oral administration of valproic acid, see under Uses and Administration, below.

Uses and Administration

Valproate, available as valproic acid, its salts and esters, is an antiepileptic used particularly in the treatment of primary generalised seizures, and notably absence and myoclonic seizures, and also for partial seizures. Its actions are complex and its mode of action in epilepsy is not fully understood. Valproate is also used to treat the acute manic phase of bipolar disorder (manic depression) and for the prophylaxis of migraine.

It can be given in a variety of forms including the sodium salts (semisodium valproate and sodium valproate), the amide derivative (valpromide), or as valproic acid. Magnesium valproate has also been tried as has calcium valproate. Valproate should preferably be taken with or after food.

In the treatment of **epilepsy** the dose should be adjusted to the needs of the individual patient to achieve adequate control of seizures. Plasma concentrations of valproate (see Pharmacokinetics, above) are not considered to be a useful index of efficacy and thus their routine monitoring is generally not helpful. A suggested initial oral dose of *sodium valproate* for *adults* is 600 mg daily in 2 divided doses, increased every 3 days by 200 mg daily to a usual range of 1 to 2 g daily (20 to 30 mg per kg body-weight daily); further increases up to a maximum of 2.5 g daily may be necessary if adequate control has not been achieved.

A suggested initial oral dose of sodium valproate for *children* weighing more than 20 kg is 400 mg daily (irrespective of weight) in 2 divided doses, gradually increased until control is achieved, with a usual range of 20 to 30 mg per kg daily; further increases to a maximum of 35 mg per kg daily may be necessary if adequate control has not been achieved. Children weighing less than 20 kg may be given 20 mg per kg daily, which may be increased to 40 mg per kg daily in severe cases, but only if it is possible to monitor the patient's plasma-valproate concentrations; it has been recommended that if the dose exceeds 40 mg per kg daily, the patient's clinical chemistry and haematological parameters should also be monitored.

When the oral route is not possible, sodium valproate may be given *intravenously* to initiate therapy or to continue therapy previously given orally. A suggested dose to *initiate* therapy in *adults* is up to 10 mg per kg body-weight by intravenous injection over 3 to 5 minutes followed by intravenous infusion, as necessary, up to a total of 2.5 g daily. The usual intravenous dose for *children* is in the range of 20 to 30 mg per kg daily. To *continue* therapy intravenously doses are the same as the patient's previous oral dose. In the USA, intravenous sodium valproate is given in doses similar to those used for semisodium valproate by mouth.

A suggested initial oral dose of *valproic acid* is 15 mg per kg daily increased at one-week intervals by 5 to 10 mg per kg daily. The maximum recommended dose of valproic acid in the UK is 30 mg per kg daily whereas in the USA it is 60 mg per kg daily. Valproic acid may be given in 2 to 4 divided doses. *Semisodium valproate* is given in similar doses to valproic acid.

The amide derivative of valproic acid, *valpromide*, is also used in some countries. Usual doses have ranged from 600 mg to 1.8 g by mouth daily, in divided doses.

As with other antiepileptics, withdrawal of valproate or transition to or from another type of antiepileptic therapy should be made gradually to avoid precipitating an increase in the frequency of seizures. For a discussion on whether or not to withdraw antiepileptic therapy in seizure-free patients, see p.335.

In the treatment of acute manic episodes of **manic depression**, semisodium valproate is given by mouth in an initial dose equivalent to valproic acid 750 mg daily in divided doses. Thereafter, the dose is increased as rapidly as possible to achieve the optimal response, up to a maximum of 60 mg per kg body-weight daily.

In the prophylaxis of **migraine** semisodium valproate is given by mouth in a dose equivalent to valproic acid 250 mg twice daily; up to 1 g daily may be necessary in some patients.

Administration. The pharmacokinetics of rectal and oral valproic acid have been compared;[1] rectal absorption does not show the slight circadian variation present when the drug is absorbed via the oral route and the rectal route appears to be an effective means of administration.

1. Yoshiyama Y, *et al.* Chronopharmacokinetic study of valproic acid in man: comparison of oral and rectal administration. *J Clin Pharmacol* 1989; **29:** 1048–52.

Cushing's syndrome. Sodium valproate has been used with metyrapone to reduce cortisol secretion in the management of Cushing's syndrome (p.1236).

Epilepsy. Valproate is one of the drugs of choice in primary generalised tonic-clonic seizures, absence seizures, and myoclonic seizures (see p.335). It is also the drug of choice in epileptic syndromes such as the Lennox-Gastaut syndrome because of its wide therapeutic spectrum, and it may be useful in infantile spasms. It is often used in partial seizures and controlled trials have suggested similar efficacy to the first-line drugs carbamazepine and phenytoin.

References.

1. Mattson RH, *et al.* A comparison of valproate with carbamazepine for the treatment of complex partial seizures and secondarily generalized tonic-clonic seizures in adults. *N Engl J Med* 1992; **327:** 765–71.
2. Davis R, *et al.* Valproic acid: a reappraisal of its pharmacological properties and clinical efficacy in epilepsy. *Drugs* 1994; **47:** 332–72.
3. Richens A, *et al.* A multicentre trial of sodium valproate and carbamazepine in adult onset epilepsy. *J Neurol Neurosurg Psychiatry* 1994; **57:** 682–7.
4. Heller AJ, *et al.* Phenobarbitone, phenytoin, carbamazepine, or sodium valproate for newly diagnosed adult epilepsy: a randomised comparative monotherapy trial. *J Neurol Neurosurg Psychiatry* 1995; **58:** 44–50.
5. Verity CM, *et al.* A multicentre comparative trial of sodium valproate and carbamazepine in paediatric epilepsy. *Dev Med Child Neurol* 1995; **37:** 97–108.
6. de Silva M, *et al.* Randomised comparative monotherapy trial of phenobarbitone, phenytoin, carbamazepine, or sodium valproate for newly diagnosed childhood epilepsy. *Lancet* 1996; **347:** 709–13.
7. Beydoun A, *et al.* and the Depakote Monotherapy for Partial Seizures Study Group. Safety and efficacy of divalproex sodium monotherapy in partial epilepsy: a double-blind, concentration-response design clinical trial. *Neurology* 1997; **48:** 182–8.

Extrapyramidal disorders. Valproate is one of several drugs with GABAergic action that has been tried with encouraging results in the management of tardive dyskinesia (see under Extrapyramidal Disorders on p.650).

Febrile convulsions. Sodium valproate has been used prophylactically in children thought to be at risk of recurrence of febrile convulsions (p.338), but routine use of antiepileptics is no longer recommended.

References.

1. Newton RW. Randomised controlled trials of phenobarbitone and valproate in febrile convulsions. *Arch Dis Child* 1988; **63:** 1189–91.

Headache. Propranolol is considered by many to be the prophylactic drug of choice for the prevention of *migraine* (p.443) and pizotifen to be the main alternative. However, many other drugs have been tried. Valproate has shown some success in several studies,[1-5] and may be an effective alternative in patients refractory to other drugs. It has also been tried in the prophylaxis of persistent chronic daily headache including *tension-type headache* (p.444) unresponsive to other drugs.[6]

1. Sørensen KV. Valproate: a new drug in migraine prophylaxis. *Acta Neurol Scand* 1988; **78:** 346–8.
2. Hering R, Kuritzky A. Sodium valproate in the prophylactic treatment of migraine: a double-blind study versus placebo. *Cephalalgia* 1992; **12:** 81–4.
3. Coria F, *et al.* Low-dose sodium valproate in the prophylaxis of migraine. *Clin Neuropharmacol* 1994; **17:** 569–73.
4. Mathew NT, *et al.* Migraine prophylaxis with divalproex. *Arch Neurol* 1995; **52:** 281–6.
5. Kaniecki RG. A comparison of divalproex with propranolol and placebo for the prophylaxis of migraine without aura. *Arch Neurol* 1997; **54:** 1141–5.
6. Mathew NT, Ali S. Valproate in the treatment of persistent chronic daily headache: an open label study. *Headache* 1991; **31:** 71–4.

Hiccup. Valproic acid may be of value in the treatment of intractable hiccups,[1] especially those of neurogenic origin. A protocol for the management of intractable hiccups may be found under Chlorpromazine, p.655.

1. Jacobson PL, *et al.* Treatment of intractable hiccups with valproic acid. *Neurology* 1981; **31:** 1458–60.

Manic depression. Valproate, usually as semisodium valproate, is used to treat the acute manic phase of bipolar disorder (p.273). It may have a useful role in patients who do not respond to lithium or cannot tolerate it, and in mixed manic states.

References.

1. Pope HG, *et al.* Valproate in the treatment of acute mania: a placebo-controlled study. *Arch Gen Psychiatry* 1991; **48:** 62–8.
2. Keck PE, *et al.* Valproate oral loading in the treatment of acute mania. *J Clin Psychiatry* 1993; **54:** 305–8.
3. Joffe RT. Valproate in bipolar disorder: the Canadian perspective. *Can J Psychiatry* 1993; **38** (suppl 2): S46–S50.
4. McElroy SL, Keck PE. Treatment guidelines for valproate in bipolar and schizoaffective disorders. *Can J Psychiatry* 1993; **38** (suppl 2): S62–S66.
5. Schaff MR, *et al.* Divalproex sodium in the treatment of refractory affective disorders. *J Clin Psychiatry* 1993; **54:** 380–4.
6. Nurnberg HG, *et al.* Response to anticonvulsant substitution among refractory bipolar manic patients. *J Clin Psychopharmacol* 1994; **14:** 207–9.
7. Anonymous. Valproate for bipolar disorder. *Med Lett Drugs Ther* 1994; **36:** 74–5.
8. Bowden CL, *et al.* Efficacy of divalproex vs lithium and placebo in the treatment of mania. *JAMA* 1994; **271:** 918–24. Correction. *ibid.*; 1830.
9. Stoll AL, *et al.* Neurologic factors predict a favorable valproate response in bipolar and schizoaffective disorders. *J Clin Psychopharmacol* 1994; **14:** 311–13.
10. Swann AC, *et al.* Depression during mania: treatment response to lithium or divalproex. *Arch Gen Psychiatry* 1997; **54:** 37–42.

Muscle spasm. The mainstay of management of *spasticity* is physiotherapy and an antispastic drug (see p.1303). Valproate has been tried for its GABAergic activity and case reports[1] of 4 patients with spastic conditions of various aetiologies indicated that the addition of valproate to the existing regimen of antispastic drugs might produce improvements in spasticity and pain; further studies are warranted.

Valproate has also been tried[2] in the management of *stiff-man syndrome* (p.667) unresponsive to diazepam.

1. Zachariah SB, *et al.* Positive response to oral divalproex sodium (Depakote) in patients with spasticity and pain. *Am J Med Sci* 1994; **308:** 38–40.
2. Spehlmann R, *et al.* Improvement of stiff-man syndrome with sodium valproate. *Neurology* 1981; **31:** 1162–3.

Myoclonus. Valproate is used alone or in combination with clonazepam for cortical myoclonus (see p.338).

Psychiatric disorders. Valproate has psychotropic properties and has been used in the management of manic depression (bipolar disorder) (see above). Valproate has also been tried in various disorders for the control of symptoms such as agitation, aggression, and rage;[1,2] (see under Disturbed Behaviour, p.636). It has also been tried in anxiety disorders (p.635) such as panic disorders,[3-5] and post-traumatic stress disorder.[6]

1. Geracioti TD. Valproic acid treatment of episodic explosiveness related to brain injury. *J Clin Psychiatry* 1994; **55:** 416–17.
2. Narayan M, *et al.* Treatment of dementia with behavioral disturbances using divalproex or a combination of divalproex and a neuroleptic. *J Clin Psychiatry* 1997; **58:** 351–4.
3. Primeau F, *et al.* Valproic acid and panic disorder. *Can J Psychiatry* 1990; **35:** 248–50.
4. Keck PE, *et al.* Valproate treatment of panic disorder and lactate-induced panic attacks. *Biol Psychiatry* 1993; **33:** 542–6.
5. Woodman CL, Noyes R. Panic disorder: treatment with valproate. *J Clin Psychiatry* 1994; **55:** 134–6.
6. Fesler FA. Valproate in combat-related posttraumatic stress disorder. *J Clin Psychiatry* 1991; **52:** 361–4.

Status epilepticus. Valproate is not usually given in the management of status epilepticus (p.337). However, it has been used in absence status epilepticus once the initial attack has been brought under control with intravenous benzodiazepines[1] and has been considered to be the drug of choice for the prevention of recurrence of absence status epilepticus.[2] In a small study it was effective in controlling status epilepticus associated with generalised tonic-clonic and myoclonic seizures.[3]

1. Bauer J, Elger CE. Management of status epilepticus in adults. *CNS Drugs* 1994; **1:** 26–44.
2. Berkovic SF, *et al.* Valproate prevents the recurrence of absence status. *Neurology* 1989; **39:** 1294–7.
3. Giroud M, *et al.* Use of injectable valproic acid in status epilepticus: a pilot study. *Drug Invest* 1993; **5:** 154–9.

Trigeminal neuralgia. Although carbamazepine is the drug of choice in the treatment of trigeminal neuralgia (p.12), sodium valproate is an alternative antiepileptic that may be used in carbamazepine-intolerant patients.

Preparations

BP 1998: Sodium Valproate Enteric-coated Tablets; Sodium Valproate Oral Solution; Sodium Valproate Tablets;
USP 23: Valproic Acid Capsules; Valproic Acid Syrup.

Proprietary Preparations (details are given in Part 3)
Aust.: Convulex; Depakine; Depakine Chrono; Ergenyl†; Leptilanil; ***Austral.:*** Epilim; Valpro; ***Belg.:*** Convulex; Depakine; ***Canad.:*** Depakene; Epival; ***Fr.:*** Depakine; Depakine Chrono; Depamide; ***Ger.:*** Convulex; Convulsofin; Ergenyl; Ergenyl Chrono; Leptilan; Mylproin; Orfiril; ***Irl.:*** Epilim; Epilim Chrono; ***Ital.:*** Depakin; Depamag; Depamide; Epicon†; ***Jpn:*** Depakene; Selenica; ***Neth.:*** Convulex; Depakine; Depakine Chrono; ***Norw.:*** Deprakine; Orfiril; ***S.Afr.:*** Convulex; Epilim; ***Spain:*** Depakine; Depamide; ***Swed.:*** Absenor; Ergenyl; Leptilen†; Orfiril; ***Switz.:*** Convulex; Depakine; Depakine Chrono; Orfiril; ***UK:*** Convulex; Epilim; Epilim Chrono; Orlept; ***USA:*** Depa†; Depacon; Depakene; Depakote; Deproic†.

Vigabatrin (17030-d)

Vigabatrin *(BAN, USAN, rINN).*

4-Amino-5-hexenoic Acid; MDL-71754; RMI-71754; γ-Vinyl Aminobutyric Acid; γ-Vinyl-GABA. 4-Aminohex-5-enoic acid.

$C_6H_{11}NO_2$ = 129.2.

CAS — 60643-86-9.

Pharmacopoeias. In Br.

A white to almost white powder. Very **soluble** in water.

Adverse Effects and Precautions

The most common adverse effects associated with vigabatrin therapy are drowsiness and fatigue, although in children excitation and agitation occur more frequently. Other CNS-related adverse effects include dizziness, nervousness, irritability, headache, nystagmus, ataxia, paraesthesia, tremor, and impaired concentration. Less commonly, confusion, memory disturbances, and visual disturbances such as diplopia have been reported. Some patients receiving vigabatrin have developed irreversible visual field defects, retinal disorders such as peripheral retinal atrophy, or very rarely optic neuritis or atrophy (see also below). Visual field function should be assessed before beginning treatment and during routine follow-up, and patients should be warned to report any new visual symptoms that develop during therapy. Psychiatric reactions such as agitation, aggression, depression, and paranoid reactions have occurred in patients with or without a psychiatric history; psychosis or mania have been reported rarely. Other reported adverse effects include weight gain, gastro-intestinal disturbances, oedema, alopecia, and skin rash. Haemoglobin and liver enzyme values may be decreased.

The manufacturers recommend that patients receiving vigabatrin should be observed carefully for any signs of adverse effects on neurological function. Caution is warranted in patients with a history of psychosis or behavioural problems.

Vigabatrin may exacerbate myoclonic or absence seizures.

Vigabatrin should be given with caution to the elderly and patients with renal impairment.

Care is required when withdrawing vigabatrin therapy—see also under Uses and Administration, below.

Driving. For a comment on antiepileptic drugs and driving, see p.337.

Effects on the eye. A report of 3 patients who developed bilateral severely constricted visual fields 2 to 3 years after vigabatrin was added to their antiepileptic regimens[1] prompted publication of similar anecdotal reports.[2-5] Peripheral retinal atrophy rather than optic nerve damage appeared to be the cause. Symptoms showed no improvement on discontinuation of the drug, although there was no further deterioration. The manufacturers replied[6] stating that it was a rare occurrence (less than 0.1%) and was being monitored in further clinical trials. The UK Committee on Safety of Medicines subsequently stated[7] (in March 1998) that it had received 41 reports of visual field defects since December 1989, which persisted in most cases despite discontinuation of treatment. The evidence suggested that the onset of symptoms varied from 1 month to several years after starting vigabatrin. The manufacturers advise visual field testing before treatment and during follow-up, although the CSM commented that no consensus existed on the best method of testing. Opinion amongst some paediatricians[8] is that the risk of developing visual field defects had to be weighed against the potential benefit of seizure control. In very young patients, in whom monitoring of vision was impossible, the benefits of vigabatrin in the treatment of infantile spasms are felt by some to outweigh this risk.[9] However, it is recommended[8] that children who have or who are at risk of developing a visual field defect should not be given vigabatrin; continued use in those who developed a visual defect would depend on the overall clinical situation.

1. Eke T, *et al.* Severe persistent visual field constriction associated with vigabatrin. *Br Med J* 1997; **314:** 180–1.
2. Wilson EA, Brodie MJ. Severe persistent visual field constriction associated with vigabatrin. *Br Med J* 1997; **314:** 1693.
3. Wong ICK, *et al.* Severe persistent visual field constriction associated with vigabatrin. *Br Med J* 1997; **314:** 1693–4.
4. Blackwell N, *et al.* Severe persistent visual field constriction associated with vigabatrin. *Br Med J* 1997; **314:** 1694.
5. Harding GFA. Severe persistent visual field constriction associated with vigabatrin. *Br Med J* 1997; **314:** 1694.
6. Backstrom JT, *et al.* Severe persistent visual field constriction associated with vigabatrin. *Br Med J* 1997; **314:** 1694–5.
7. Committee of Safety of Medicines/Medicines Control Agency. Vigabatrin (Sabril) and visual field defects. *Current Problems* 1998; **24:** 1.
8. Appleton RE. Guideline may help in prescribing vigabatrin. *Br Med J* 1998; **317:** 1322.
9. Harding GFA. Severe persistent visual field constriction associated with vigabatrin. *Br Med J* 1998; **316:** 232–3.

Effects on the liver. Vigabatrin has demonstrated *in-vivo* and *in-vitro* inhibition of plasma-alanine transaminase activity, which may mask signs of early underlying hepatic disease if only transaminase levels are evaluated.[1]

1. Richens A, *et al.* Evidence for both in vivo and in vitro interaction between vigabatrin and alanine transaminase. *Br J Clin Pharmacol* 1997; **43:** 163–8.

Effects on mental function. Behavioural disturbances ranging from irritability and confusion to psychotic reactions have been reported in patients receiving vigabatrin.[1-7] Psychiatric reactions were usually reversible when doses were reduced or gradually discontinued, but sometimes persisted after cessation of therapy. In 2 patients[8,9] psychosis developed following sudden withdrawal of vigabatrin; mental state improved when the drug was reinstated. Most patients who experienced psychotic reactions to vigabatrin are said to have had a previous history of behavioural disturbances or brain damage[6] and vigabatrin should be used with caution in such patients. However, a retrospective study[10] in the UK indicated that vigabatrin-induced behavioural disturbances could occur with a similar frequency in patients with no such history. Also, using low doses of vigabatrin to initiate therapy did not reduce the incidence of disturbances.

The problems of antiepileptic therapy adversely affecting cognition are discussed on p.337.

1. Sander JWAS, Hart YM. Vigabatrin and behaviour disturbances. *Lancet* 1990; **335:** 57.
2. Dam M. Vigabatrin and behaviour disturbances. *Lancet* 1990; **335:** 605.
3. Betts T, Thomas L. Vigabatrin and behaviour disturbances. *Lancet* 1990; **335:** 605–6.
4. Johnston SJ. Vigabatrin and behaviour disturbances. *Lancet* 1990; **335:** 606.
5. Robinson MK, *et al.* Vigabatrin and behaviour disturbances. *Lancet* 1990; **336:** 504.
6. Martínez AC, *et al.* Vigabatrin-associated reversible acute psychosis in a child. *Ann Pharmacother* 1995; **29:** 1115–17.
7. Naumann M, *et al.* Bipolar affective psychosis after vigabatrin. *Lancet* 1994; **343:** 606–7.
8. Ring HA, Reynolds EH. Vigabatrin and behaviour disturbance. *Lancet* 1990; **335:** 970.
9. Brodie MJ, McKee PJW. Vigabatrin and psychosis. *Lancet* 1990; **335:** 1279.
10. Wong ICK. Retrospective study of vigabatrin and psychiatric behavioural disturbances. *Epilepsy Res* 1995; **21:** 227–30.

Effects on the nervous system. Two patients developed disturbances of motor behaviour associated with the addition of vigabatrin to therapy for intractable seizures.[1]

Acute encephalopathy was reported[2] in two patients after starting vigabatrin in addition to carbamazepine; symptoms of stupor, dysphoria, and irritability were present in both and their EEG background activity was slowed. Clinical symptoms could not be related to intoxication with carbamazepine or its epoxide but it was not know whether an interaction between carbamazepine and vigabatrin had caused the acute encephalopathy. In a further report[3] vigabatrin was associated with the development of encephalopathy in 3 patients already receiving a variety of antiepileptic drugs other than carbamazepine; withdrawal of vigabatrin led to full recovery. The authors suggested that acute encephalopathy after vigabatrin may be related to a pre-existing cerebral abnormality.

1. Jongsma MJ, *et al.* Reversible motor disturbances induced by vigabatrin. *Lancet* 1991; **338:** 893.
2. Sälke-Kellermann A, Baier H. Acute encephalopathy with vigabatrin. *Lancet* 1993; **342:** 185.
3. Sharief MK, *et al.* Acute encephalopathy with vigabatrin. *Lancet* 1993; **342:** 619.

Interference with diagnostic tests. Vigabatrin can cause changes in the urinary excretion of amino acids which could be potentially misleading in patients undergoing investigation for metabolic disorders.[1,2]

1. Bonham JR, *et al.* Pyroglutamicaciduria from vigabatrin. *Lancet* 1989; **i:** 1452–3.
2. Shih VE, Tenanbaum A. Aminoaciduria due to vinyl-gaba administration. *N Engl J Med* 1990; **323:** 1353.

Porphyria. For comment on the use of vigabatrin in porphyria, see p.339.

Pregnancy. For comments on the management of epilepsy in pregnancy, see p.337.

Little is known of the effects of newer antiepileptics such as vigabatrin on the fetus, although congenital anomalies have been reported in the offspring of some mothers using vigabatrin during pregnancy.

Interactions

There are complex interactions between antiepileptics and toxicity may be enhanced without a corresponding increase in antiepileptic activity. Such interactions are very variable and unpredictable and plasma monitoring is often advisable with combination therapy.

Antiepileptics. For the effect of vigabatrin on plasma concentrations of other antiepileptics, see Phenobarbitone, p.351; Phenytoin, p.355; and Primidone, p.358.

Pharmacokinetics

Vigabatrin is well absorbed following oral administration of the racemate; the inactive *R*(-)-enantiomer is reported to be present at much higher plasma concentrations than the active *S*(+)-enantiomer, perhaps indicating a difference in bioavailability. Most of an oral dose is excreted in urine as unchanged drug. The elimination half-life is reported to be 5 to 7 hours. Vigabatrin is not significantly bound to plasma proteins.

There does not appear to be any correlation between plasma concentrations of vigabatrin and its efficacy or toxicity.

References.

1. Rey E, *et al.* Vigabatrin: clinical pharmacokinetics. *Clin Pharmacokinet* 1992; **23:** 267–78.
2. Hoke JF, *et al.* Pharmacokinetics of vigabatrin following single and multiple oral doses in normal volunteers. *J Clin Pharmacol* 1993; **33:** 458–62.
3. Elwes RDC, Binnie CD. Clinical pharmacokinetics of newer antiepileptic drugs: lamotrigine, vigabatrin, gabapentin and oxcarbazepine. *Clin Pharmacokinet* 1996; **30:** 403–15.
4. Vauzelle-Kervroëdan F, *et al.* Pharmacokinetics of the individual enantiomers of vigabatrin in neonates with uncontrolled seizures. *Br J Clin Pharmacol* 1996; **42:** 779–81.
5. Jacqz-Aigrain E, *et al.* Pharmacokinetics of the S(+) and R(−) enantiomers of vigabatrin during chronic dosing in a patient with renal failure. *Br J Clin Pharmacol* 1997; **44:** 183–5.

Uses and Administration

Vigabatrin is an analogue of gamma-aminobutyric acid (GABA) that acts as an irreversible inhibitor of GABA-transaminase, the enzyme responsible for the catabolism of GABA. It is used as an adjunctive antiepileptic in patients with epilepsy unresponsive to other therapy, but it may exacerbate myoclonic or absence seizures. It is also used as monotherapy for infantile spasms (as for example in West's syndrome).

The recommended initial dose of vigabatrin as adjunctive therapy in adults is 1 g daily by mouth, increased if necessary in increments of 0.5 g at weekly intervals to a maximum of 4 g daily. Higher doses should only be used in exceptional circumstances with close monitoring for adverse effects, and should not exceed 6 g daily. A recommended initial dose in children is 40 mg per kg body-weight daily increased to 80 to 100 mg per kg daily. Alternatively, doses for children may be expressed according to body-weight range as: 10 to 15 kg body-weight, 0.5 to 1 g daily; 15 to 30 kg, 1 to 1.5 g daily; 30 to 50 kg, 1.5 to 3 g daily; and 50 kg or more, adult dose. For infantile spasms the dose of vigabatrin as monotherapy is 60 to 100 mg per kg daily, depending on the severity of the spasms, adjusted according to response over 7 days. Up to 150 mg per kg daily has been used in some patients. Doses may be divided and given twice daily or taken as a single daily dose. Dosage reductions may be required in the elderly and in patients with renal impairment.

As with other antiepileptics, withdrawal of vigabatrin therapy or transition to or from another type of antiepileptic therapy should be made gradually to avoid precipitating an increase in the frequency of seizures. For a discussion on whether or not to withdraw antiepileptic therapy in seizure-free patients, see p.335. The manufacturers recommend gradually reducing the dose of vigabatrin over 2 to 4 weeks.

Epilepsy. Vigabatrin is used in the treatment of epilepsy (p.335) as adjunctive therapy for refractory seizures. Reviews[1-5] of vigabatrin have considered it to be most effective in the treatment of complex partial seizures with or without secondary generalisation; it may, however, exacerbate myoclonic or absence seizures. Efficacy as adjunctive therapy in refractory partial seizures was demonstrated by 2 multicentre studies[6,7] involving 228 patients (including 46 children) and a study[8] involving 52 patients being assessed for epilepsy surgery. However, in a follow-up study[9] of 120 patients who had participated in an open-label trial of vigabatrin as adjunctive therapy for refractory epilepsy 6 to 8 years earlier, it was considered that vigabatrin had had only marginal benefit on the long-term prognosis of severe refractory epilepsy, despite favourable results from the original trial.

Vigabatrin was compared with carbamazepine as monotherapy for patients with newly diagnosed epilepsy in an open-label randomised trial[10] involving 100 patients. Vigabatrin was discontinued more often than carbamazepine because of lack of efficacy and fewer of the successfully treated patients receiving vigabatrin achieved total freedom from seizures. However, discontinuation because of adverse effects occurred less often with vigabatrin than with carbamazepine and vigabatrin had a less deleterious effect on cognition.

Vigabatrin is also of value in infantile spasms (as for example in West's syndrome). In an assessment of vigabatrin as monotherapy in 192 infants with infantile spasms who were followed up for an average of 7.6 months,[11] there was complete cessation of spasms in 131 patients, a decrease in cluster frequency in 37, and no improvement in 24 (including deterioration in one infant). A crossover study comparing vigabatrin with corticotrophin in 42 infants found that both drugs produced some benefit.[12]

1. Anonymous. Vigabatrin—a new anti-convulsant. *Drug Ther Bull* 1990; **28:** 95–6.
2. Grant SM, Heel RC. Vigabatrin: a review of its pharmacodynamic and pharmacokinetic properties, and therapeutic potential in epilepsy and disorders of motor control. *Drugs* 1991; **41:** 889–926.
3. Brodie M. Drugs in focus I: vigabatrin. *Prescribers' J* 1992; **32:** 21–6.
4. Connelly JF. Vigabatrin. *Ann Pharmacother* 1993; **27:** 197–204.
5. Srinivasan J, Richens A. A risk-benefit assessment of vigabatrin in the treatment of neurological disorders *Drug Safety* 1994; **10:** 395–405.
6. Dalla Bernadina B, *et al.* Efficacy and tolerability of vigabatrin in children with refractory partial seizures: a single-blind dose-increasing study. *Epilepsia* 1995; **36:** 687–91.
7. French JA, *et al.* A double-blind, placebo-controlled study of vigabatrin three g/day in patients with uncontrolled complex partial seizures. *Neurology* 1996; **46:** 54–61.
8. Malmgren K, *et al.* Cost analysis of epilepsy surgery and of vigabatrin treatment in patients with refractory partial epilepsy. *Epilepsy Res* 1996; **25:** 199–207.
9. Walker MC, *et al.* Long term use of lamotrigine and vigabatrin in severe refractory epilepsy: audit of outcome. *Br Med J* 1996; **313:** 1184–5.
10. Kälviäinen R, *et al.* Vigabatrin vs carbamazepine monotherapy in patients with newly diagnosed epilepsy: a randomized, controlled study. *Arch Neurol* 1995; **52:** 989–96.
11. Aicardi J, *et al.* Sabril IS Investigator and Peer Review Groups. Vigabatrin as initial therapy for infantile spasms: a European retrospective survey. *Epilepsia* 1996; **37:** 638–42.
12. Vigevano F, Cilio MR. Vigabatrin versus ACTH as first-line treatment for infantile spasms: a randomized, prospective study. *Epilepsia* 1997; **38:** 1270–4.

Metabolic disorders. Vigabatrin, an irreversible inhibitor of GABA-transaminase, has been tried in GABA metabolic disorders not accompanied by epilepsy,[1-4] with ambivalent results. Data from 23 case reports of patients with succinic semialdehyde dehydrogenase deficiency indicated that vigabatrin was only clinically beneficial in about one-third of patients.[4]

1. Jaeken J, *et al.* Vigabatrin in GABA metabolism disorders. *Lancet* 1989; **i:** 1074.
2. Gibson KM, *et al.* Vigabatrin therapy in patient with succinic semialdehyde dehydrogenase deficiency. *Lancet* 1989; **ii:** 1105–6.
3. Stephenson JBP. Vigabatrin for startle-disease with altered cerebrospinal-fluid free gamma-aminobutyric acid. *Lancet* 1992; **340:** 430–1.
4. Gibson KM, *et al.* The clinical phenotype of succinic semialdehyde dehydrogenase deficiency (4-hydroxybutyric aciduria): case reports of 23 new patients. *Pediatrics* 1997; **99:** 567–74.

Stiff-man syndrome. There have been anecdotal reports[1,2] of improvement of stiff-man syndrome (p.667) with vigabatrin in patients unable to tolerate benzodiazepine therapy.

1. Vermeij FH, *et al.* Improvement of stiff-man syndrome with vigabatrin. *Lancet* 1996; **348:** 612.
2. Prevett MC, *et al.* Improvement of stiff-man syndrome with vigabatrin. *Neurology* 1997; **48:** 1133–4.

Preparations

BP 1998: Vigabatrin Oral Powder; Vigabatrin Tablets.

Proprietary Preparations (details are given in Part 3)
Aust.: Sabril; ***Austral.:*** Sabril; ***Belg.:*** Sabril; ***Canad.:*** Sabril; ***Fr.:*** Sabril; ***Ger.:*** Sabril; ***Irl.:*** Sabril; ***Ital.:*** Sabril; ***Neth.:*** Sabril; ***Norw.:*** Sabrilex; ***S.Afr.:*** Sabril; ***Spain:*** Sabrilex; ***Swed.:*** Sabrilex; ***Switz.:*** Sabril; ***UK:*** Sabril.

Zonisamide (1668-x)

Zonisamide (*BAN, USAN, rINN*).

AD-810; CI-912; PD-110843. 1-(1,2-Benzoxazol-3-yl)methanesulphonamide.

$C_8H_8N_2O_3S$ = 212.2.

CAS — 68291-97-4.

Zonisamide, a benzisoxazole derivative, is an antiepileptic used in patients with epilepsy unresponsive to other therapy, particularly for partial seizures. It is given by mouth in an initial dose of 100 to 200 mg daily, gradually increasing up to a maximum of 600 mg daily.

Epilepsy. Zonisamide is used in the treatment of refractory epilepsy (p.335). Most studies have been conducted in Japan and the available data do not support its use in patients outside Japan.[1,2] Clinical experience in Japan demonstrated its efficacy mainly in the treatment of partial seizures with or without secondary generalisation. Efficacy in primary generalised and mixed-seizure epilepsies appeared to be more variable, although it may be of value in refractory myoclonic seizures. Zonisamide might also be of use in the treatment of epileptic syndromes such as Lennox-Gastaut syndrome and West's syndrome, although only a small number of patients with the latter condition have been studied. The relatively few studies[3,4] conducted outside Japan appeared to confirm the efficacy of zonisamide as an adjunct in the treatment of partial epilepsies. However, patients treated with zonisamide in the USA and Europe may have had a higher incidence of renal calculi than those treated in Japan. In one US study, 4 of 113 patients (3.5%) receiving long-term treatment with zonisamide developed renal calculi,[2] but a familial relationship was found for 2. In pooled data from earlier studies, renal calculi had been reported in 13 of 700 patients (1.9%) treated in the USA and Europe compared with 2 of 1008 patients (0.2%) in Japan.[1] Clinical trials were temporarily suspended in the USA, but as the causal relationship between zonisamide and renal calculi was disputed, studies were resumed to clarify the issue. Pharmacokinetic differences between Japanese and non-Japanese patients could further complicate the use of zonisamide outside Japan and additional pharmacokinetic studies were awaited.

1. Peters DH, Sorkin EM. Zonisamide: a review of its pharmacodynamic and pharmacokinetic properties, and therapeutic potential in epilepsy. *Drugs* 1993; **45:** 760–87.
2. Patsalos PN, Sander JWAS. Newer antiepileptic drugs: towards an improved risk-benefit ratio. *Drug Safety* 1994; **11:** 37–67.
3. Leppik IE, *et al.* Efficacy and safety of zonisamide: results of a multicenter study. *Epilepsy Res* 1993; **14:** 165–73.
4. Schmidt D, *et al.* Zonisamide for add-on treatment of refractory partial epilepsy: a European double-blind trial. *Epilepsy Res* 1993; **15:** 67–73.

Preparations

Proprietary Preparations (details are given in Part 3)
Jpn: Excegran.

Antifungals

This chapter describes those drugs that are used mainly in the treatment and prophylaxis of fungal infections (mycoses). They include the allylamines (naftifine and terbinafine), several polyene antibiotics (including amphotericin and nystatin), other antifungal antibiotics (for example griseofulvin), azole derivatives, including imidazoles (such as ketoconazole) and triazoles (such as fluconazole and itraconazole), and a number of other compounds among them amorolfine, ciclopirox olamine, flucytosine, haloprogin, tolnaftate, and undecenoic acid and its salts.

Choice of Antifungal

Fungi may be classified as either yeasts or moulds according to their appearance and means of growth. Yeast-like fungi involved in infections include *Candida* spp., *Blastomyces dermatitidis, Coccidioides immitis, Histoplasma capsulatum, Sporothrix schenckii,* and the infective agents of chromoblastomycosis. Examples of pathogenic moulds include *Aspergillus* spp., the dermatophytes, and the Mucorales fungi.

Some fungi are true pathogens and can cause disease in any individual. Other fungi such as *Candida* species and *Pneumocystis carinii* (once thought to be a protozoan but now considered to be a fungus) are of low pathogenicity and require an alteration in the normal defence mechanisms for disease to occur; such disease is called opportunistic.

Fungal infections may be classified as **superficial**, affecting only the skin, hair, nails, or mucous membranes, or **systemic**, affecting the body as a whole; systemic infections tend to occur more frequently in immunocompromised individuals such as those with AIDS. Fungal infections may also be described as **local** when they are restricted to one body area, as **invasive** when there is spread into the tissues, or as **disseminated** when the infection has spread from the primary site to other organs throughout the body.

Ideally antifungal treatment should be chosen after the infecting organism has been identified but it is often necessary to start treatment before the pathogen can be cultured and identified especially in immunocompromised patients in whom infections are rapidly progressive.

The choice of treatment for the important fungal diseases is described below.

Aspergillosis

Aspergillosis is an infection caused by fungi of the genus *Aspergillus*, usually *A. fumigatus* although *A. flavus* and *A. niger* are also important species. Aspergillosis is usually acquired by inhalation and most commonly causes non-invasive disease of the respiratory tract. Other sites of infection include the eye following trauma or cataract surgery. Invasive disease of tissues adjacent to the site of infection, for example spread from the paranasal sinus to the orbit, and dissemination to distant organs may occur, predominantly in immunocompromised patients. In severely immunocompromised patients aspergillosis usually presents as severe acute pneumonia. Other organs affected may include the heart (particularly damaged or prosthetic valves), kidneys, bone, brain, liver, and skin.

In general the response of **invasive** aspergillosis to treatment is poor and early initiation of treatment is essential. Surgical excision may be necessary. High intravenous doses of amphotericin remain the antifungal treatment of choice.[1-3] However, the overall response rate to conventional amphotericin is reported to be only 30 to 35%,[3] although this may be improved by the use of liposomal amphotericin.[4-6] Combination therapy with amphotericin and flucytosine has also been suggested[7] and may be useful in cerebral, meningeal, or endocardial infections.[3] However, itraconazole by mouth[8] is emerging as the main alternative to amphotericin.

A number of approaches to reducing the incidence of aspergillosis in immunocompromised patients have been discussed, including chemoprophylaxis with either low-dose intravenous, intranasal, or nebulised amphotericin, or oral itraconazole[9,10] or a combination of these.[11]

Non-invasive forms of aspergillosis include allergic bronchopulmonary aspergillosis, a hypersensitivity reaction to *Aspergillus* usually occurring in asthmatic patients, and aspergilloma, a fungal mass or ball developing within the pulmonary cavity or paranasal sinus.

Allergic bronchopulmonary aspergillosis is usually treated with corticosteroids although oral itraconazole may be a useful adjunct. The treatment of **aspergilloma** depends on the severity of symptoms, and includes conservative management, antifungal therapy, or surgical resection. Oral itraconazole or intravenous amphotericin are once again the most effective drugs. Direct intracavitary instillation of antifungals has also been advocated for patients at particularly high risk of complications.[12] Inhaled amphotericin aerosol was reported to be poorly tolerated and of little value in preventing invasive pulmonary aspergillosis in granulocytopenic patients.[13]

Chronic locally invasive infections have been reported to respond to prolonged treatment with itraconazole;[14] in this small study, itraconazole produced clinical improvements but not mycological cure.

Aspergillosis of the **eye**, like other fungal eye infections, is difficult to treat; antifungals are generally not well absorbed following topical application and infections extending into the vitreous or anterior chamber require subconjunctival, intra-ocular, and/or systemic treatment. Systemic treatment is necessary for ocular manifestations of disseminated disease. When systemic therapy is required intravenous amphotericin is usually given; an oral azole compound may be given for less severe infections. For superficial eye infections a number of antifungals have been applied topically, including natamycin, amphotericin, azole compounds, and silver sulphadiazine when they have been given alone or as an adjunct to systemic therapy. Surgical excision of infected tissue may be necessary in severe infections.

1. Anonymous. Essential drugs: systemic mycoses. *WHO Drug Inf* 1991; **5:** 129–36.
2. Anonymous. Systemic antifungal drugs. *Med Lett Drugs Ther* 1997; **39:** 86–8.
3. Denning DW. Treatment of invasive aspergillosis. *J Infect* 1994; **28** (suppl 1): 25–33.
4. Ringdén O, *et al.* Efficacy of amphotericin B encapsulated in liposomes (AmBisome) in the treatment of invasive fungal infections in immunocompromised patients. *J Antimicrob Chemother* 1991; **28** (suppl B): 73–82.
5. Chopra R, *et al.* Liposomal amphotericin B (AmBisome) in the treatment of fungal infections in neutropenic patients. *J Antimicrob Chemother* 1991; **28** (suppl B): 93–104.
6. Mills W, *et al.* Liposomal amphotericin B in the treatment of fungal infections in neutropenic patients: a single-centre experience of 133 episodes in 116 patients. *Br J Haematol* 1994; **86:** 754–60.
7. Saral R. Candida and aspergillus infections in immunocompromised patients: an overview. *Rev Infect Dis* 1991; **13:** 487–92.
8. Denning DW, *et al.* NIAID mycoses study group multicenter trial of oral itraconazole therapy for invasive aspergillosis. *Am J Med* 1994; **97:** 135–44. Correction. *ibid.*; 497.
9. Beyer J, *et al.* Strategies in prevention of invasive pulmonary aspergillosis in immunosuppressed or neutropenic patients. *Antimicrob Agents Chemother* 1994; **38:** 911–17.
10. Cafferkey MT. Chemoprophylaxis of invasive pulmonary aspergillosis. *J Antimicrob Chemother* 1994; **33:** 917–24.
11. Todeschini G, *et al.* Oral itraconazole plus nasal amphotericin B for prophylaxis of invasive aspergillosis in patients with hematological malignancies. *Eur J Clin Microbiol Infect Dis* 1993; **12:** 614–18.
12. Kauffman CA. Quandary about treatment of aspergillomas persists. *Lancet* 1996; **347:** 1640.
13. Erjavec Z, *et al.* Tolerance and efficacy of amphotericin B inhalations for prevention of invasive pulmonary aspergillosis in haematological patients. *Eur J Clin Microbiol Infect Dis* 1997; **16:** 364–8.
14. Caras WE, Pluss JL. Chronic necrotizing pulmonary aspergillosis: pathologic outcome after itraconazole therapy. *Mayo Clin Proc* 1996; **71:** 25–30.

Blastomycosis

Blastomycosis (not to be confused with South American blastomycosis, see Paracoccidioidomycosis, below) is an infection caused by the fungus *Blastomyces dermatitidis.* Infection may be through the lungs and is usually followed by dissemination; the skin, skeleton, and genito-urinary system often becoming infected. Blastomycosis has been reported only rarely in patients with AIDS, but when it occurs it may be widely disseminated with CNS involvement and a high mortality.[1]

Intravenous amphotericin, once the mainstay of treatment is reserved for severe cases, CNS disease, cases unresponsive to other treatment, and infections in immunocompromised patients. Mild to moderate disease is treated with an oral azole, usually itraconazole,[2] fluconazole,[3] or ketoconazole. Patients with AIDS may require prolonged suppressive treatment, preferably with an oral azole, after a clinical response has been achieved.[1]

1. Pappas PG, *et al.* Blastomycosis in patients with the acquired immunodeficiency syndrome. *Ann Intern Med* 1992; **116:** 847–53.
2. Dismukes WE, *et al.* Itraconazole therapy for blastomycosis and histoplasmosis. *Am J Med* 1992; **93:** 489–97.
3. Pappas PG, *et al.* Treatment of blastomycosis with fluconazole: a pilot study. *Clin Infect Dis* 1995; **20:** 267–71.

Candidiasis

Candida spp. are commensal fungi commonly found in the gastro-intestinal tract, mouth, and vagina; they become pathogenic only when natural defence mechanisms fail. *C. albicans* is the species most commonly associated with infection, although infections with other species notably *C. (Torulopsis) glabrata, C. krusei, C. parapsilosis,* and *C. tropicalis* also occur. Predisposing factors for pathogenic *Candida* infection include antibacterial therapy, skin trauma, debility, diabetes mellitus, pregnancy, and immunodeficiency; candidiasis often occurs in patients with HIV infection.

Candidiasis (or candidosis), the general term for pathogenic infection with *Candida,* spp. can be superficial, deep local invasive, or disseminated.

Superficial candidiasis includes infection of the oropharynx, vagina, and skin. Oropharyngeal and vulvovaginal infections are commonly known as thrush. Superficial infections can usually be treated topically with an antifungal although the rare chronic mucocutaneous candidiasis syndrome normally requires systemic treatment. Antifungals used topically include amphotericin, nystatin, terbinafine, and the azole derivatives butoconazole, clotrimazole, econazole, isoconazole, miconazole, terconazole, and tioconazole. The choice of drug is determined by the availability of a suitable formulation for the site of infection as well as by toxicity and duration of treatment.

For **oropharyngeal** infections, agents such as chlorhexidine and povidone-iodine may be useful. Crystal violet has also been used,[1,2] but as well as being cosmetically less acceptable its use has become restricted due to fears over possible carcinogenicity.

Oesophageal infections are not normally accessible to topical therapy and should be treated with oral azoles.

Vulvovaginal candidiasis responds well to short courses of treatment (typically 3 to 14 days) with a topical antifungal as a cream or pessary,[3] although single-dose local treatment is not routinely recommended; longer courses may be necessary for recurrent infections. Single-dose or short-course oral therapy with fluconazole or itraconazole is also effective, but in general, oral treatment of such superficial infections is reserved for patients who do not respond to or are intolerant of topical therapy.

Topical therapy of superficial candidiasis in general may not be adequate in patients with intractable immunodepression, and oral azole therapy should also be considered in these patients.[4] Patients who either do not respond to or do not tolerate oral therapy, or those at risk of developing disseminated disease, may require intravenous amphotericin.[1,2,4]

Relapse after treatment of superficial candidiasis is common especially in patients with predisposing factors for infection. Recurrence may result from inadequate initial treatment. (In recurrent vulvovaginal candidiasis reinfection from other body sites or by sexual transmission from an untreated partner is not thought to be implicated.[5]) Patients with frequent recurrences usually require systemic treatment. Although long-term or intermittent administration of oral antifungals, usually fluconazole, has been recommended to reduce recurrences in immunocompromised patients,[4,6] there is growing concern over the increasing incidence of drug resistance.[7-9] Resistance may be a consequence of the selection of resistant strains of *C. albicans* or of intrinsically less sensitive species such as *C. krusei*.[9-12] In the USA, although primary prophylaxis against candidiasis is not recommended for patients with advanced HIV infection, it may be considered for patients with frequent or severe recurrent candidiasis.[13]

Preparations, such as yogurt, containing *Lactobacillus* spp. have been used in the treatment and prevention of vaginal candidiasis in an attempt to displace *Candida* from the vagina but evidence to support their use is limited. Other novel treatments have included the adjuvant use of granulocyte-macrophage colony-stimulating factors.[14,15]

Deep and disseminated candidiasis requires systemic antifungal treatment. Intravenous amphotericin, with or without flucytosine, has been regarded as the initial treatment of choice in most infections, although there has been some concern regarding the use of flucytosine in AIDS patients because of its bone-marrow toxicity. Treatment with an azole such as fluconazole and itraconazole may be an effective alternative. Fluconazole has been shown to be as effective as intravenous amphotericin.[16,17] Fluconazole is emerging as a first-line option for clinically stable patients with uncomplicated candidaemia, provided that they have not recently been treated with an azole.[18] However consensus has not been reached on how to treat patients in an unstable clinical condition or those with non-*albicans* candidal infections.[19] As with superficial infections, the emergence of resistant *Candida* is causing concern, especially in intensive care settings and in severely immunocompromised patients.[20] Prophylactic antifungal treatment is not recommended routinely[18,21] although some would consider it in critically ill patients or those receiving bone-marrow transplants at high risk of infection.[18] Empirical treatment before confirmation of disseminated candidiasis has been recommended for patients with heavy colonisation and a deteriorating condition.[18,21]

1. WHO. *Global programme on AIDS: guidelines for the clinical management of HIV infection in children.* Geneva: WHO, 1993.
2. Garber GE. Treatment of oral candida mucositis infections. *Drugs* 1994; **47:** 734–40.
3. Anonymous. Topical drugs for vaginal candidiasis. *Med Lett Drugs Ther* 1991; **33:** 81.
4. British Society for Antimicrobial Chemotherapy Working Party. Antifungal chemotherapy in patients with acquired immunodeficiency syndrome. *Lancet* 1992; **340:** 648–51.
5. Working Group of the British Society for Medical Mycology. Management of genital candidiasis. *Br Med J* 1995; **310:** 1241–4.
6. Working Party of the British Society for Antimicrobial Chemotherapy. Chemoprophylaxis for candidosis and aspergillosis in neutropenia and transplantation: a review and recommendations. *J Antimicrob Chemother* 1993; **32:** 5–21.
7. Powderly WG. Resistant candidiasis. *AIDS Res Hum Retroviruses* 1994; **10:** 925–9.
8. Sangeorzan JA, *et al.* Epidemiology of oral candidiasis in HIV-infected patients: colonization, infection, treatment, and emergence of fluconazole resistance. *Am J Med* 1994; **97:** 339–46.
9. Johnson EM, Warnock DW. Azole drug resistance in yeasts. *J Antimicrob Chemother* 1995; **36:** 751–5.
10. Millon L, *et al.* Émergence de Candida glabrata et Candida krusei chez des patients séropositifs pour le VIH atteints de candidose oropharyngée, traités de façon prolongée par le fluconazole. *J Mycol Med* 1994; **4:** 90–2.
11. Law D, *et al.* High prevalence of antifungal resistance in Candida spp from patients with AIDS. *J Antimicrob Chemother* 1994; **34:** 659–68.
12. Denning DW. Can we prevent azole resistance in fungi? *Lancet* 1995; **346:** 454–5.
13. Centers for Disease Control. USPHS/IDSA guidelines for the prevention of opportunistic infections in persons infected with human immunodeficiency virus: a summary. *Ann Intern Med* 1996; **124:** 348–68.
14. Shahar E, *et al.* White cell enhancement in the treatment of severe candidosis. *Lancet* 1995; **346:** 974–5.
15. Capetti A, *et al.* Employment of recombinant human granulocyte-macrophage colony stimulating factor in oesophageal candidiasis in AIDS patients. *AIDS* 1995; **9:** 1378–9.
16. Rex JH, *et al.* A randomized trial comparing fluconazole with amphotericin B for the treatment of candidemia in patients without neutropenia. *N Engl J Med* 1994; **331:** 1325–30.
17. Anaissie EJ, *et al.* Management of invasive candidal infections: results of a prospective, randomized, multicenter study of fluconazole versus amphotericin B and review of the literature. *Clin Infect Dis* 1996; **23:** 964–72.
18. Edwards JE, *et al.* International conference for the development of a consensus on the management and prevention of severe candidal infections. *Clin Infect Dis* 1997; **25:** 43–59.
19. Graybill JR. Editorial response: can we agree on the treatment of candidiasis? *Clin Infect Dis* 1997; **25:** 60–2.
20. Nguyen MH, *et al.* The changing face of candidemia: emergence of non-Candida albicans species and antifungal resistance. *Am J Med* 1996; **100:** 617–23.
21. British Society for Antimicrobial Chemotherapy Working Party. Management of deep Candida infection in surgical and intensive care unit patients. *Intensive Care Med* 1994; **20:** 522–8.

Chromoblastomycosis

Chromoblastomycosis (chromomycosis) is an infection caused by a number of opportunistic fungi, including *Fonsecaea compacta (Phialophora compacta), F. pedrosoi (P. pedrosoi), Phialophora verrucosa, Cladosporium carrionii,* and *Rhinocladiella aquaspersa*, following invasion of skin trauma sites. It occurs worldwide but is more common in tropical and subtropical climates. The disease is characterised by chronic cutaneous and subcutaneous lesions. In its early stages, when lesions are small, surgical excision or cryotherapy are the treatments of choice, although it has been suggested that there is some risk of spreading the lesion during surgery. In advanced cases drug treatment is necessary. There are reports of flucytosine,[1] itraconazole,[2-4] saperconazole,[5] terbinafine,[6] and thiabendazole[7] each having been used with some success. However, recurrence and drug resistance has been a problem with monotherapy. Local heat treatment aids healing and may be a useful adjunct to drug therapy.

1. Lopes CF, *et al.* Six years' experience in treatment of chromomycosis with 5-fluorocytosine. *Int J Dermatol* 1978; **17:** 414–18.
2. Borelli D. A clinical trial of itraconazole in the treatment of deep mycoses and leishmaniasis. *Rev Infect Dis* 1987; **9** (suppl 1): S57–S63.
3. Smith CH, *et al.* A case of chromoblastomycosis responding to treatment with itraconazole. *Br J Dermatol* 1993; **128:** 436–9.
4. Kullavanijaya P, Rojanavanich V. Successful treatment of chromoblastomycosis due to Fonsecaea pedrosoi by the combination of itraconazole and cryotherapy. *Int J Dermatol* 1995; **34:** 804–7.
5. Franco L, *et al.* Saperconazole in the treatment of systemic and subcutaneous mycoses. *Int J Dermatol* 1992; **31:** 725–9.
6. Esterre P, *et al.* Treatment of chromomycosis with terbinafine: preliminary results of an open pilot study. *Br J Dermatol* 1996; **134** (suppl 46): 33–6.
7. Ollé-Goig JE, Domingo J. A case of chromomycosis treated with thiabendazole. *Trans R Soc Trop Med Hyg* 1983; **77:** 773–4.

Coccidioidomycosis

Coccidioidomycosis is an infection caused by inhalation of the spores of *Coccidioides immitis*, a fungus found in the soil in arid and semi-desert areas mainly of North, Central, and South America. Patients may experience acute or chronic lung infections, meningitis, and disseminated disease. Common names for the infection include valley fever, desert fever, and desert rheumatism.

Acute pulmonary coccidioidomycosis is usually self-limiting and resolves spontaneously without specific chemotherapy; in 60% of cases the infection is asymptomatic or mild. In some patients the infection progresses to chronic pulmonary coccidioidomycosis with granulomatous lesions, fibrosis, and cavitation. A small proportion of patients develop acute progressive pneumonia which is commonly fatal if untreated, or disseminated disease usually involving the skin, bone, meninges, and joints. Severe pulmonary and disseminated infections are more likely in pregnant women, dark-skinned races, diabetics, and immunocompromised patients.

Antifungal therapy for severe or disseminated infections is with either intravenous amphotericin or an oral azole.[1] Ketoconazole,[2] itraconazole,[3] and fluconazole[4] have all been reported to be at least moderately effective in non-meningeal infections. Fluconazole is effective in meningeal infections[5] and is the most frequently recommended azole for this indication, although itraconazole has also produced beneficial responses;[6] intrathecal amphotericin may also be used, especially in aggressive infections.[7] The incidence of relapses following treatment is high, and lifelong therapy is now recommended following coccidioidal meningitis.[8] In patients with HIV infection, lifelong suppressive therapy with fluconazole, itraconazole, or amphotericin is recommended following treatment of either meningeal or non-meningeal coccidioidomycosis.[9,10]

1. Stevens DA. Coccidioidomycosis. *N Engl J Med* 1995; **332:** 1077–82.
2. Galgiani JN, *et al.* Ketoconazole therapy of progressive coccidioidomycosis: comparison of 400- and 800-mg doses and observations at higher doses. *Am J Med* 1988; **84:** 603–10.
3. Graybill JR, *et al.* Itraconazole treatment of coccidioidomycosis. *Am J Med* 1990; **89:** 282–90.
4. Catanzaro A, *et al.* Fluconazole in the treatment of chronic pulmonary and nonmeningeal disseminated coccidioidomycosis. *Am J Med* 1995; **98:** 249–56.
5. Galgiani JN, *et al.* Fluconazole therapy for coccidioidal meningitis. *Ann Intern Med* 1993; **119:** 28–35.
6. Tucker RM, *et al.* Itraconazole therapy for chronic coccidioidal meningitis. *Ann Intern Med* 1990; **112:** 108–12.
7. Anonymous. Systemic antifungal drugs. *Med Lett Drugs Ther* 1997; **39:** 86–8.
8. Dewsnup DH, *et al.* Is it ever safe to stop azole therapy for Coccidioides immitis meningitis? *Ann Intern Med* 1996; **124:** 305–10.
9. Anonymous. Drugs for AIDS and associated infections. *Med Lett Drugs Ther* 1995; **37:** 87–94.
10. Centers for Disease Control. 1997 USPHS/IDSA guidelines for the prevention of opportunistic infections in persons infected with human immunodeficiency virus. *MMWR* 1997; **46:** (RR-12): 1–45.

Cryptococcosis

Cryptococcosis is an infection caused by inhalation of the fungus *Cryptococcus neoformans*. It is rare in immunocompetent individuals, but is an important life-threatening disease in immunocompromised patients, especially those with AIDS, occurring principally as **cryptococcal meningitis**.

The choice of antifungal treatment depends on the immune status of the patient. In the immunocompetent, usual treatment is with amphotericin, with or without flucytosine;[1] itraconazole is a possible alternative.

In those, such as AIDS patients, with irreversible immunosuppression it is more difficult to achieve a cure, and the aim of treatment is long-term suppression. In these patients, initial therapy, usually with amphotericin alone or with flucytosine,[2] is generally followed by prolonged or lifelong therapy with fluconazole.[1-3] Itraconazole may be a suitable alternative for continuation therapy.[2-5] Fluconazole with flucytosine is an alternative when amphotericin with or without flucytosine cannot be given. An encouraging response was reported following initial treatment with fluconazole alone when compared with amphotericin,[6] although others found it to be inferior to amphotericin with flucytosine.[7] In another study, high dose intravenous therapy with fluconazole appeared to be effective.[8]

Fluconazole has been reported to be effective for primary prophylaxis in patients with HIV infection,[9] although in general prophylaxis against cryptococcosis is not recommended for such patients.[5] When prophylaxis is considered to be appropriate, fluconazole is preferred to amphotericin, and itraconazole is a possible alternative, but there are concerns about the emergence of resistant strains.[5,10]

Cryptococcal infection at other sites is reported to respond to fluconazole[11-13] although infection of the respiratory tract in immunocompetent patients often resolves without antifungal treatment.

1. Anonymous. Systemic antifungal drugs. *Med Lett Drugs Ther* 1997; **39:** 86–8.
2. British Society for Antimicrobial Chemotherapy Working Party. Antifungal chemotherapy in patients with acquired immunodeficiency syndrome. *Lancet* 1992; **340:** 648–51.
3. van der Horst CM, *et al.* Treatment of cryptococcal meningitis associated with the acquired immunodeficiency syndrome. *N Engl J Med* 1997; **337:** 15–21.

4. de Gans J, *et al.* Itraconazole as maintenance treatment for cryptococcal meningitis in the acquired immune deficiency syndrome. *Br Med J* 1988; **296:** 339.
5. Centers for Disease Control. 1997 USPHS/IDSA guidelines for the prevention of opportunistic infections in persons infected with human immunodeficiency virus. *MMWR* 1997; **46** (RR-12): 1–45.
6. Saag MS, *et al.* Comparison of amphotericin B with fluconazole in the treatment of acute AIDS-associated cryptococcal meningitis. *N Engl J Med* 1992; **326:** 83–9.
7. Larsen RA, *et al.* Fluconazole compared with amphotericin B plus flucytosine for cryptococcal meningitis in AIDS: a randomized trial. *Ann Intern Med* 1990; **113:** 183–7.
8. Menichetti F, *et al.* High-dose fluconazole therapy for cryptococcal meningitis in patients with AIDS. *Clin Infect Dis* 1996; **22:** 838–40.
9. Quagliarello VJ, *et al.* Primary prevention of cryptococcal meningitis by fluconazole in HIV-infected patients. *Lancet* 1995; **345:** 548–52.
10. Viard J-P, *et al.* Fulminant cryptococcal infections in HIV-infected patients on oral fluconazole. *Lancet* 1995; **346:** 118.
11. Bozzette SA, *et al.* Fluconazole treatment of persistent Cryptococcus neoformans prostatic infection in AIDS. *Ann Intern Med* 1991; **115:** 285–6.
12. Shuttleworth D, *et al.* Cutaneous cryptococcosis: treatment with oral fluconazole. *Br J Dermatol* 1989; **120:** 683–7.
13. Meyohas MC, *et al.* Treatment of non-meningeal cryptococcosis in patients with AIDS. *J Infect* 1996; **33:** 7–10.

Dermatophytoses

See under Skin Infections, below.

Endocarditis

Infective endocarditis caused by fungi such as *Aspergillus* or *Candida* is much less common than that caused by bacteria (see p.120). Fungal endocarditis is usually treated with intravenous amphotericin; surgical removal of an infected valve may be required.[1] Long-term survival was reported[2] in a patient with endocarditis due to *C. parapsilosis* who was not suitable for surgery. Treatment was initially with amphotericin, replaced by fluconazole after 27 days because of renal dysfunction. At the time of publication, the patient remained free of disease having received fluconazole for 26 months.

1. Ellis M. Fungal endocarditis. *J Infect* 1997; **35:** 99–103.
2. Czerwiec FS, *et al.* Long-term survival after fluconazole therapy of candidal prosthetic valve endocarditis. *Am J Med* 1993; **94:** 545–6.

Eye infections

Fungal infections of the eye are less common than infections with bacteria or viruses, but are usually severe and may lead to loss of vision. Diagnosis may be delayed due to a gradual onset of symptoms and empirical treatment with antibacterials. Infections may involve the cornea (keratitis), the interior of the eye (endophthalmitis), or the orbit and may occur following trauma (including surgery) or systemic disseminated infection. Patients with impaired host resistance such as diabetics or immunocompromised patients are particularly at risk. The most common fungi causing eye infections are *Aspergillus, Candida,* and *Fusarium*; others include *Blastomyces, Cryptococcus,* and *Sporothrix.* Infections of the orbit usually occur by spread from an infection of the paranasal sinus, commonly mucormycosis or aspergillosis.

Fungal infections of the eye are difficult to treat. Antifungals are generally not well absorbed following topical application and infections extending to the vitreous or anterior chamber require subconjunctival, intra-ocular, and/or systemic treatment. Systemic treatment is necessary for ocular manifestations of disseminated disease. When systemic therapy is required intravenous amphotericin is usually given; an oral azole compound may be given for less severe infections. Superficial infections may respond to topical treatment. Amphotericin or natamycin are most commonly used. An azole compound such as miconazole is sometimes used, or flucytosine in combination with another antifungal. Topical treatment may also be used as an adjunct to systemic therapy. Surgical excision of infected tissue may be necessary in severe infections.

Histoplasmosis

Histoplasmosis is a systemic infection caused by *Histoplasma capsulatum,* a fungus found in the soil in endemic areas, particularly at sites with heavy accumulations of bird or bat excrement. Infection is by inhalation of spores. Two types of histoplasmosis occur: classic histoplasmosis due to infection with *H. capsulatum* var. *capsulatum* and African histoplasmosis due to infection with *H. capsulatum* var. *duboisii.*

The major endemic area for *H. capsulatum* var. *capsulatum* is central USA. In endemic regions most of the population is infected and mild infections are generally asymptomatic. However, acute pulmonary infection can occur. Massive infection can be fatal. Chronic pulmonary histoplasmosis can result in lung fibrosis and cavitation. Histoplasmosis may also present as an acute or chronic disseminated infection involving widespread infiltration of the reticuloendothelial system and is primarily seen in immunodeficient or immunocompromised patients.

Histoplasma capsulatum var. *duboisii* is found in central Africa and causes a chronic disseminated form of histoplasmosis with focal lesions predominantly in skin and bone.

Antifungal therapy for classic or African histoplasmosis is necessary in patients with severe pulmonary infections, chronic fibrotic or cavitary disease, or disseminated infection. Infections which are not life-threatening may be treated with an oral azole in both immunocompetent and immunocompromised patients.[1] Ketoconazole has been largely replaced by itraconazole as the preferred antifungal.[2,3] Fluconazole is also reported to be moderately effective.[4,5] Patients with life-threatening infections or those not responding to oral treatment are given amphotericin intravenously. Patients with HIV infection should continue maintenance therapy with itraconazole daily or amphotericin weekly;[1,6] fluconazole, in doses of above 200 mg daily, has been tried as an alternative.[7] Primary prophylaxis with itraconazole may be considered for patients with advanced AIDS who live in an endemic area.[6]

1. Anonymous. Systemic antifungal drugs. *Med Lett Drugs Ther* 1997; **39:** 86–8.
2. Dismukes WE, *et al.* Itraconazole therapy for blastomycosis and histoplasmosis. *Am J Med* 1992; **93:** 489–97.
3. Wheat J, *et al.* Itraconazole treatment of disseminated histoplasmosis in patients with the acquired immunodeficiency syndrome. *Am J Med* 1995; **98:** 336–42.
4. McKinsey DS, *et al.* Fluconazole therapy for histoplasmosis. *Clin Infect Dis* 1996; **23:** 996–1001.
5. Wheat J, *et al.* Treatment of histoplasmosis with fluconazole in patients with acquired immunodeficiency syndrome. *Am J Med* 1997; **103:** 223–32.
6. Centers for Disease Control. 1997 USPHS/IDSA guidelines for the prevention of opportunistic infections in persons infected with human immunodeficiency virus. *MMWR* 1997; **46** (RR-12): 1–45.
7. Norris S, *et al.* Prevention of relapse of histoplasmosis with fluconazole in patients with the acquired immunodeficiency syndrome. *Am J Med* 1994; **96:** 504–8.

Infections in immunocompromised patients

Patients with a defective immune system are at special risk of infections, including those caused by fungi. Primary immune deficiency is rare, whereas secondary deficiency is more common; immunosuppressive therapy, cancer and its treatment, HIV infection, and splenectomy may all cause neutropenia and impaired humoral and cellular immunity in varying degrees. Fungi most commonly associated with infection in these patients include *Cryptococcus neoformans* and species of *Aspergillus* and *Candida. Pneumocystis carinii,* now considered to have characteristics of fungi, is an important cause of pneumonia in patients with AIDS. In areas in which they are endemic, coccidioidomycosis, histoplasmosis, and *Penicillium marneffei* infections are also more common in immunocompromised patients. A fungal cause of infection should be considered in immunocompromised patients with fever of unknown origin who have not responded to broad spectrum antibacterials. Fungal infection in patients with immune deficiency usually occurs as a widely disseminated disease and treatment should be commenced as early as possible. If the infection has not been identified, empirical treatment with intravenous amphotericin has been attempted but the effects on overall mortality remain uncertain.

Long-term suppression of fungal infection has been recommended for immunocompromised patients although this might allow development of resistance and the overgrowth of species not susceptible to the antifungals used. This is of particular concern with fluconazole, one of the drugs that has been most widely used for this purpose (see p.378). Antifungals are also used in selective digestive tract decontamination (see Intensive Care, p.128).

Treatment and prophylaxis of specific fungal infections in immunocompromised patients is discussed under the appropriate headings—see Aspergillosis, Candidiasis, Coccidioidomycosis, Cryptococcosis, and Histoplasmosis (above), and *Pneumocystis carinii* Pneumonia (below).

1. British Society for Antimicrobial Chemotherapy Working Party. Antifungal chemotherapy in patients with acquired immunodeficiency syndrome. *Lancet* 1992; **340:** 648–51.
2. Working Party of the British Society for Antimicrobial Chemotherapy. Chemoprophylaxis for candidosis and aspergillosis in neutropenia and transplantation: a review and recommendations. *J Antimicrob Chemother* 1993; **32:** 5–21.
3. American Thoracic Society. Fungal infection in HIV-infected persons. *Am J Respir Crit Care Med* 1995; **152:** 816–22.
4. Warnock DW. Fungal complications of transplantation: diagnosis, treatment and prevention. *J Antimicrob Chemother* 1995; **36** (suppl B): 73–90.
5. Meunier F. Targeting fungi: a challenge. *Am J Med* 1995; **99** (suppl 6A): 60S–67S.
6. Hood S, Denning DW. Treatment of fungal infections in AIDS. *J Antimicrob Chemother* 1996; **37**(suppl B): 71–85.
7. Gøtzsche PC, Johansen HK. Meta-analysis of prophylactic or empirical antifungal treatment versus placebo or no treatment in patients with cancer complicated by neutropenia. *Br Med J* 1997; **314:** 1238–44.
8. Centers for Disease Control. 1997 USPHS/IDSA guidelines for the prevention of opportunistic infections in persons infected with human immunodeficiency virus. *MMWR* 1997; **46** (RR–12): 1–45.
9. Working Party of the British Society for Antimicrobial Chemotherapy. Therapy of deep fungal infection in haematological malignancy. *J Antimicrob Chemother* 1997; **40:** 779–88.

Meningitis

Fungal diseases associated with meningitis include candidiasis, coccidioidomycosis, cryptococcosis, and histoplasmosis (see above). The treatment of each infection is discussed under the appropriate heading, but in general the initial drug of choice in fungal meningitis is intravenous amphotericin, sometimes with flucytosine.

Mucormycosis

Mucormycosis, a rare but serious infection caused by Mucorales fungi, is a type of zygomycosis, a term which is sometimes used synonymously. Mucormycosis usually occurs in poorly controlled diabetic patients or in immunocompromised patients. Patients receiving desferrioxamine may also be at increased risk of infection (see p.976). Infections of the mucosa of the respiratory tract or gastro-intestinal tract, or of abraded skin, usually with *Rhizopus* or *Rhizomucor* spp., can result in local invasion of deeper tissues including bone and the CNS with extensive tissue destruction. Disseminated disease may also occur.

Amphotericin intravenously can be effective in mucormycosis and is usually combined with aggressive surgical debridement of infected tissue. Invasive disease is difficult to treat and is usually fatal.

1. Boelaert JR. Mucormycosis (zygomycosis): is there news for the clinician? *J Infect* 1994; **28** (suppl 1): 1–6.

Mycetoma

Mycetoma is seen especially in the tropics and subtropics and involves subcutaneous tissue, bone, and skin. The term Madura foot is used for mycetoma affecting the foot. Organisms enter the tissues via local skin trauma. Mycetomas caused by fungi such as *Madurella mycetomatis, M. grisea,* or *Pseudallescheria boydii* are called eumycetomas. Those caused by the filamentous bacteria, actinomycetes, are called actinomycetomas and are discussed on p.132. Eumycetomas are often unresponsive to treatment. Some infections have responded to prolonged treatment with ketoconazole[1,2] and itraconazole has also been tried.[2]

1. Mahgoub ES, Gumaa SA. Ketoconazole in the treatment of eumycetoma due to Madurella mycetomii. *Trans R Soc Trop Med Hyg* 1984; **78:** 376–9.
2. Restrepo A. Treatment of tropical mycoses. *J Am Acad Dermatol* 1994; **31:** S91–S102.

Nail infections

See under Skin Infections, below.

Paracoccidioidomycosis

Paracoccidioidomycosis (South American blastomycosis) is caused by an infection with the fungus *Paracoccidioides brasiliensis.* The disease occurs predominantly in inhabitants or former inhabitants of regions of Central and South America and may remain dormant for long periods. Infection is thought to be by inhalation. While most primary infections are subclinical, some may be progressive and severe, particularly in immunocompromised patients. The lungs may be affected, the disease usually presenting as a chronic infection. Disseminated disease affects the skin, mucous membranes, gastro-intestinal tract, reticuloendothelial system, and adrenals, and may be either acute or chronic.

Treatment is usually with itraconazole, ketoconazole, or intravenous amphotericin for patients with severe infection.[1] Sulphonamides are now rarely used. Other azole derivatives may prove effective. Treatment may need to be continued for months or years to prevent relapse.

1. Anonymous. Systemic antifungal drugs. *Med Lett Drugs Ther* 1997; **39:** 86–8.

Peritonitis

Fungal peritonitis occasionally occurs in patients undergoing continuous ambulatory peritoneal dialysis or abdominal surgery, or in trauma. It is usually caused by yeasts such as *Candida*. Amphotericin has been the treatment of choice and is given intravenously rather than intraperitoneally since the latter route is painful.[1] Fluconazole may also be effective.[2,3] However, fungal peritonitis is a difficult infection to treat and it has a high morbidity and mortality.[1]

1. Working Party of the British Society for Antimicrobial Chemotherapy. Diagnosis and management of peritonitis in continuous ambulatory peritoneal dialysis. *Lancet* 1987; **i:** 845–9.
2. Levine J, *et al.* Fungal peritonitis complicating continuous ambulatory peritoneal dialysis: successful treatment with fluconazole, a new orally active antifungal agent. *Am J Med* 1989; **86:** 825–7.
3. Aguado JM, *et al.* Successful treatment of candida peritonitis with fluconazole. *J Antimicrob Chemother* 1994; **34:** 847.

Pityriasis versicolor

See under Skin Infections, below.

Pneumocystis carinii pneumonia

Pneumocystis carinii is an opportunistic unicellular pathogen which has been classified both with the protozoa and with the fungi, although more recent evidence suggests that it is probably a fungus. It appears to be acquired by the airborne route, but in persons with normally functioning immune systems clinical infection resolves spontaneously. However, in immunosuppressed patients it can produce interstitial pneumonia with progressive damage to the alveolar walls and accumulation of exudate in the air spaces; if untreated, the disease is almost always fatal. With the advent of AIDS (p.599), *Pneumocystis carinii* pneumonia (PCP) has become an increasing problem.

Treatment of acute disease is primarily with either co-trimoxazole or pentamidine.[1] Co-trimoxazole is the preferred drug,[2-4] given intravenously in severe infections and orally in mild infections. Intravenous pentamidine is generally reserved for patients who do not respond to or cannot tolerate co-trimoxazole. Combination therapy with co-trimoxazole and pentamidine is not more effective and is potentially more toxic than either drug alone.[5] Some centres prefer trimethoprim with dapsone for second line therapy[3] although the combination is only effective in patients with mild or moderately severe infections.[4] Dapsone should probably not be used alone for treatment of PCP,[3] but may be useful for prophylaxis (see below). Other alternatives include primaquine plus clindamycin,[6,7] and trimetrexate plus folinic acid.[8,9] Atovaquone may be used to treat mild to moderate infections.[4,10,11] Nebulised pentamidine is occasionally suggested for mild infections but is now generally reserved for prophylaxis (see below). Studies suggest that there is probably little difference in efficacy between these regimens, and ultimately the choice will be based on adverse effects and availability.[12] Initial studies of eflornithine have also produced beneficial responses.[13,14] Although it has been suggested that folinic acid could be administered with co-trimoxazole to reduce the risk of haematotoxicity,[3] increased therapeutic failure has been reported in patients receiving this combination.[15]

Prompt additional treatment with a corticosteroid is now of established value for patients with moderate or severe disease and is started at the same time as the antipneumocystis treatment is begun.[4,16,17] Adjuvant treatment with corticosteroids reduces morbidity and mortality[4] but exacerbation of cytomegalovirus infection has been reported.[18]

Prophylaxis is used in high-risk patients, especially among those with compromised immunity due to HIV infection. Primary prophylaxis is attempted in all HIV-infected adults with a CD4+ T lymphocyte count below 200 per μL or those with unexplained fever or candidiasis regardless of CD4+ T lymphocyte count.[19] In infants and young children, in whom the CD4+ T lymphocyte count is normally higher than in adults and in whom PCP commonly occurs at CD4+ T lymphocyte counts of greater than 200 per μL, separate guidelines proposed prophylaxis at age-specific CD4+ T lymphocyte count thresholds.[20] However, some children at risk of infection have not received appropriate prophylaxis.[21,22] USA guidelines now recommend that infants of HIV-positive mothers should receive prophylaxis beginning at 4 to 6 weeks of age and continued until they are shown to be seronegative, or for at least 1 year initially.[19]

Secondary prophylaxis is given to all patients with a history of PCP. Recommendations for prophylaxis in patients without HIV infection are not widely publicised, but is has been suggested that prophylaxis should be considered for patients who are immunosuppressed due to an underlying disorder or to immunosuppressant drug therapy.[23,24]

Co-trimoxazole by mouth is currently preferred for primary and secondary prophylaxis.[4,19] Pentamidine administered by an appropriate jet nebuliser or dapsone (alone or with pyrimethamine) are the usual alternatives in patients unable to tolerate co-trimoxazole.[4,19] A meta-analysis found that co-trimoxazole was the most effective drug of the three.[25] However, co-trimoxazole is not well tolerated and long-term studies suggest that, on an intention-to-treat basis, the efficacy of dapsone[26] or inhaled pentamidine[26,27] may be comparable, at least in patients with CD4+ T lymphocyte counts of more than 100 per μL. For secondary prophylaxis dapsone was found to be less effective than nebulised pentamidine in a study in patients with AIDS,[28] but the efficacy of regimens for secondary prophylaxis has not yet been fully evaluated. Regimens containing co-trimoxazole or dapsone also protect against toxoplasmosis, an increasingly common opportunistic infection in AIDS patients.[19,29,30]

Co-trimoxazole and dapsone are usually administered daily for prophylaxis of PCP,[19] but intermittent administration has been tried in an attempt to improve tolerance without compromising efficacy; co-trimoxazole given on three days a week[25,31] or dapsone plus pyrimethamine on two days a week[31] have produced promising results. A low dose of co-trimoxazole 480 mg daily is better tolerated than the usual dose of 960 mg daily and equally effective.[25] Response to inhaled pentamidine can be influenced by the choice of nebuliser;[32] commonly used nebulisers include the Fisoneb and Respirgard II. Patients receiving inhaled pentamidine may be prone to extrapulmonary *Pneumocystis* infection.[33,34] Other alternative prophylactic regimens include intermittent parenteral administration of pentamidine, pyrimethamine with sulfadoxine, clindamycin with primaquine, atovaquone, trimetrexate, and dapsone with trimethoprim.[4,19]

It has been suggested that the development of new drugs for PCP need to be accelerated, as there is some evidence that resistance to co-trimoxazole, mediated by mutations in the target dihydropteroate synthase enzyme, may be developing.[35]

1. Masur H. Prevention and treatment of pneumocystis pneumonia. *N Engl J Med* 1992; **327:** 1853–60. Correction. *ibid.* 1993; **328:** 1136.
2. Anonymous. Drugs for parasitic infections. *Med Lett Drugs Ther* 1998; **40:** 1–12.
3. Peters BS, *et al.* Adverse effects of drugs used in the management of opportunistic infections associated with HIV infection. *Drug Safety* 1994; **10:** 439–54.
4. Miller RF, *et al.* Pneumocystis carinii infection: current treatment and prevention. *J Antimicrob Chemother* 1996; **37** (suppl B): 33–53.
5. Glatt AE, Chirgwin K. Pneumocystis carinii pneumonia in human immunodeficiency virus-infected patients. *Arch Intern Med* 1990; **150:** 271–9.
6. Toma E, *et al.* Clindamycin/primaquine versus trimethoprim-sulfamethoxazole as primary therapy for Pneumocystis carinii pneumonia in AIDS: a randomized, double-blind pilot trial. *Clin Infect Dis* 1993; **17:** 178–84.
7. Black JR, *et al.* Clindamycin and primaquine therapy for mild-to-moderate episodes of Pneumocystis carinii pneumonia in patients with AIDS: AIDS Clinical Trials Group 044. *Clin Infect Dis* 1994; **18:** 905–13.
8. Amsden GW, *et al.* Trimetrexate for Pneumocystis carinii pneumonia in patients with AIDS. *Ann Pharmacother* 1992; **26:** 218–26.
9. Sattler FR, *et al.* Trimetrexate with leucovorin versus trimethoprim-sulfamethoxazole for moderate to severe episodes of Pneumocystis carinii pneumonia in patients with AIDS: a prospective, controlled multicenter investigation of the AIDS Clinical Trials Group Protocol 029/031. *J Infect Dis* 1994; **170:** 165–72.
10. Hughes W, *et al.* Comparison of atovaquone (566C80) with trimethoprim-sulfamethoxazole to treat Pneumocystis carinii pneumonia in patients with AIDS. *N Engl J Med* 1993; **328:** 1521–7.
11. Dohn MN, *et al.* Oral atovaquone compared with intravenous pentamidine for Pneumocystis carinii pneumonia in patients with AIDS. *Ann Intern Med* 1994; **121:** 174–80.
12. Safrin S, *et al.* Comparison of three regimens for treatment of mild to moderate Pneumocystis carinii pneumonia in patients with AIDS: a double-blind, randomized trial of oral trimethoprim-sulfamethoxazole, dapsone-trimethoprim, and clindamycin-primaquine. *Ann Intern Med* 1996; **124:** 792–802.
13. Smith D, *et al.* Pneumocystis carinii pneumonia treated with eflornithine in AIDS patients resistant to conventional therapy. *AIDS* 1990; **4:** 1019–21.
14. Smith DE, *et al.* Eflornithine versus cotrimoxazole in the treatment of Pneumocystis carinii pneumonia in AIDS patients. *AIDS* 1992; **6:** 1489–93.
15. Safrin S, *et al.* Adjunctive folinic acid with trimethoprim-sulfamethoxazole for Pneumocystis carinii pneumonia in AIDS patients is associated with an increased risk of therapeutic failure and death. *J Infect Dis* 1994; **170:** 912–17.
16. McGowan JE, *et al.* Report by the Working Group on Steroid Use, Antimicrobial Agents Committee, Infectious Diseases Society of America: Guidelines for the use of systemic glucocorticosteroids in the management of selected infections. *J Infect Dis* 1992; **165:** 1–13.
17. Bye MR, *et al.* Markedly reduced mortality associated with corticosteroid therapy of Pneumocystis carinii pneumonia in children with acquired immunodeficiency syndrome. *Arch Pediatr Adolesc Med* 1994; **148:** 638–41.
18. Nelson MR, *et al.* Treatment with corticosteroids—a risk factor for the development of clinical cytomegalovirus disease in AIDS. *AIDS* 1993; **7:** 375–8.
19. Centers for Disease Control. 1997 USPHS/IDSA guidelines for the prevention of opportunistic infections in persons infected with human immunodeficiency virus. *MMWR* 1997; **46** (RR-12): 1–45.
20. Centers for Disease Control. Guidelines for prophylaxis against Pneumocystis carinii pneumonia for children infected with human immunodeficiency virus. *JAMA* 1991; **265:** 1637–44.
21. Kovacs JA, Kovacs AAS. PCP prophylaxis in paediatric HIV infection: time for a change? *Lancet* 1994; **344:** 5–6.
22. Simonds RJ, *et al.* Prophylaxis against Pneumocystis carinii pneumonia among children with perinatally acquired human immunodeficiency virus infection in the United States. *N Engl J Med* 1995; **332:** 786–90.
23. Sepkowitz KA, *et al.* Pneumocystis carinii pneumonia without acquired immunodeficiency syndrome: more patients, same risk. *Arch Intern Med* 1995; **155:** 1125–8.
24. Yale SH, Limper AH. Pneumocystis carinii pneumonia in patients without acquired immunodeficiency syndrome: associated illnesses and prior corticosteroid therapy. *Mayo Clin Proc* 1996; **71:** 5–13.
25. Ioannidis JP, *et al.* A meta-analysis of the relative efficacy and toxicity of Pneumocystis carinii prophylactic regimens. *Arch Intern Med* 1996; **156:** 177–88.
26. Bozzette SA, *et al.* A randomised trial of three antipneumocystis agents in patients with advanced human immunodeficiency virus infection. *N Engl J Med* 1995; **332:** 693–9.
27. Rizzardi GP, *et al.* Risks and benefits of aerosolized pentamidine and cotrimoxazole in primary prophylaxis of Pneumocystis carinii pneumonia in HIV-1-infected patients: a two-year Italian multicentric randomized controlled trial. *J Infect* 1996; **32:** 123–31.
28. Salmon-Ceron D, *et al.* Lower survival in AIDS patients receiving dapsone compared with aerosolized pentamidine for secondary prophylaxis of Pneumocystis carinii pneumonia. *J Infect Dis* 1995; **172:** 656–64.
29. Girard P-M, *et al.* Dapsone–pyrimethamine compared with aerosolized pentamidine as primary prophylaxis against Pneumocystis carinii pneumonia and toxoplasmosis in HIV infection. *N Engl J Med* 1993; **328:** 1514–20.
30. Torres RA, *et al.* Randomized trial of dapsone and aerosolized pentamidine for the prophylaxis of Pneumocystis carinii pneumonia and toxoplasmosis encephalitis. *Am J Med* 1993; **95:** 573–83.
31. Podzamczer D, *et al.* Intermittent trimethoprim-sulfamethoxazole compared with dapsone-pyrimethamine for the simultaneous primary prophylaxis of pneumocystis pneumonia and toxoplasmosis in patients infected with HIV. *Ann Intern Med* 1995; **122:** 755–61.
32. Miller R, Steel S. Nebulized pentamidine as prophylaxis for Pneumocystis carinii pneumonia. *J Antimicrob Chemother* 1991; **27:** 153–7.
33. Witt K, *et al.* Dissemination of Pneumocystis carinii in patients with AIDS. *Scand J Infect Dis* 1991; **23:** 691–5.
34. Sha BE, *et al.* Pneumocystis carinii choroiditis in patients with AIDS: clinical features, response to therapy, and outcome. *J Acquir Immune Defic Syndr Hum Retrovirol* 1992; **5:** 1051–8.
35. Mei Q, *et al.* Failure of co-trimoxazole in Pneumocystis carinii infection and mutations in dihydropteroate synthase gene. *Lancet* 1998; **351:** 1631–2.

Protothecosis

Protothecosis is an infection with algae of the *Prototheca* spp., usually *P. wickerhamii.* Infection may follow minor trauma or surgery leading to a chronic skin lesion and occasionally dissemination. There are case reports of amphotericin with tetracycline[1] or of itraconazole[2] being used successfully in protothecosis.

1. Venezio FR, *et al.* Progressive cutaneous protothecosis. *Am J Clin Pathol* 1982; **77:** 485–93.
2. Tang WYM, *et al.* Cutaneous protothecosis: report of a case in Hong Kong. *Br J Dermatol* 1995; **133:** 479–82.

Respiratory-tract infections

A number of pathogenic fungi enter the body by inhalation and colonise the respiratory tract. Fungal infections of the respiratory tract include aspergillosis, blastomycosis, coccidioidomycosis, cryptococcosis, histoplasmosis, and paracoccidioidomycosis (see above). *Pneumocystis carinii,* now considered to have characteristics of fungi, is an important cause of pneumonia in HIV-infected patients (see above). Other fungi reported to produce respiratory-tract infections mainly in immunocompromised patients include *Fusarium* spp., *Penicillium marneffei, Pseudoallescheria boydii,* and Zygomycetes such as *Rhizopus arrhizus.* Acute pulmonary fungal infections in immunocompetent individuals are mostly self-limiting conditions that resolve without treatment. Severe, persistent, or progressive infections, or infections in immunocompromised patients, require treatment. Intravenous amphotericin is usually the drug of choice but mild to moderate infection can be treated with an oral azole such as fluconazole, itraconazole, or ketoconazole. Pulmonary granulomas may require surgical removal. Chronic suppressive treatment is recommended for patients with immunosuppression due to HIV infection.

Candida can cause respiratory-tract infections in immunocompromised patients; treatment is with intravenous amphotericin.

Skin infections

The most common fungal skin infections are the dermatophytoses, pityriasis versicolor, and candidiasis. The first two are described here; candidiasis is described on p.367. Other fungal skin infections are discussed under the appropriate headings: blastomycosis, chromoblastomycosis, mycetoma, mucormycosis, protothecosis (above), and sporotrichosis (below). Fungal infections that may involve the skin by dissemination include aspergillosis, coccidioidomycosis, cryptococcosis, histoplasmosis, and paracoccidioidomycosis (above). Less common fungi causing skin infections include *Penicillium marneffei.* Sometimes the infection may affect mucous membranes, nails, or subcutaneous tissue, and there can be spread to deeper tissue and dissemination especially in immunosuppressed patients. The term superficial fungal infections includes those involving the skin, nails, and mucous membranes. Antifungal treatment may be topical or systemic.[1,2]

Dermatophytoses (ringworm, tinea) are infections by dermatophytes, a group of fungi which includes soil-dwelling organisms and human and animal pathogens from 3 genera — *Epidermophyton, Microsporum,* and *Trichophyton.* Dermatophytoses are encouraged by hot and humid conditions and poor hygiene and occur throughout tropical and temperate regions of the world.

Dermatophytoses are classified according to the body site affected. They include

- tinea barbae (beard)
- tinea capitis (scalp)
- tinea corporis (body)
- tinea cruris (groin)
- tinea manuum (hand)
- tinea pedis (athlete's foot)
- tinea unguium (nail)

A chronic infection most commonly seen in the tropics is known as favus (tinea favosa) and a variant of tinea corporis known as tinea imbricata (tokelau) is caused by *T. concentricum* and is endemic in parts of the Far East and Central and South America. A severe form of dermatophytosis caused by animal pathogens with deep, suppurant, inflammatory lesions is known as kerion.

Deep infections may occur rarely in immunocompromised patients and may spread to involve lymph nodes, liver, and brain, and may be fatal.

Mild localised superficial dermatophytoses of hairless skin sites will often respond to *topical* therapy.[3,4] Non-specific agents that have a long history of topical use include benzoic acid, crystal violet, selenium sulphide, and salicylic acid. Many of these agents are effective, and while some older preparations such as compound benzoic acid ointment may be less cosmetically acceptable than modern products, they still have a role in the treatment of minor infections, particularly in the tropics.[5] However, the use of crystal violet is restricted due to fears over possible carcinogenicity (see p.1111).

There are a number of specific topical antifungals that are active against dermatophytes. The azoles used topically include clotrimazole, econazole, ketoconazole, and miconazole. Ciclopirox olamine[6] and the allylamine antifungals naftifine and terbinafine[7] appear to have similar activity. Chlorphenesin, tolnaftate, and undecenoic acid salts are all effective in uncomplicated dermatophytoses, but there are few comparative studies of their relative efficacy. Amorolfine has also been shown to be effective in skin infections, although its major application is in nail infections (see below).

Infections of some body sites respond poorly to topical therapy, as do extensive infections or those in heavily keratinised areas.[4] *Systemic* therapy may be appropriate in these cases as well as in disseminated disease. Griseofulvin, ketoconazole, and itraconazole are the drugs most widely used. Griseofulvin has proved to have few major toxic effects during long-term therapy and is useful for tinea capitis, extensive or disseminated infections, and nail infections in selected patients. However, since it has a narrow spectrum of activity largely confined to the dermatophytes, accurate diagnosis is essential particularly before embarking on a prolonged treatment course when no immediate response is anticipated. Ketoconazole has a broader spectrum of activity, but severe adverse effects can occur on prolonged administration and its place is likely to be taken by itraconazole which appears to produce a rapid response and thus requires shorter treatment periods.[4] Other azoles such as fluconazole may also be effective.[8] Terbinafine has been reported to be more effective than itraconazole in some forms of tinea[9,10] and also requires only short-duration therapy.[11,12] However, efficacy is reported to depend on the infecting organism.[13] Selenium sulphide shampoo may be a useful adjunct to oral therapy for tinea capitis to improve efficacy and limit the spread of infection.[14,15] A suitable topical antifungal is used in individuals suspected of carrying infection.[16]

Infections of the **nails (onychomycoses)** are notoriously difficult to treat.[17] Infections of the fingernails take up to 6 months to respond to oral griseofulvin and those of the toenails, a year or longer, but about 60% of nail infections fail to respond or relapse after the initial treatment course. The newer oral antifungals, terbinafine, itraconazole, and fluconazole, produce persistent fungicidal concentrations in the nail more rapidly than griseofulvin.[17,18] Terbinafine[19-22] and itraconazole[23] have been most widely studied. Both are reported to produce clinical and mycological cures in a high proportion of patients more quickly than griseofulvin — generally after 12 weeks' treatment or less. Long-term follow-up has demonstrated that the response to terbinafine is maintained.[24] Terbinafine has been reported to be more effective than itraconazole[25,26] but some have considered there to be no significant difference between them.[18] Although topical treatments are generally ineffective in nail infections amorolfine applied as a lacquer has produced encouraging results.[27] Another approach has been the dissolution of the nail plate with 40% urea paste, usually in combination with bifonazole.[28]

Pityriasis versicolor (tinea versicolor) is a superficial infection caused by the commensal yeast *Malassezia furfur (Pityrosporum orbiculare).* It is more common in tropical than in temperate latitudes and sun exposure may trigger the infection. Pityriasis versicolor will often respond to topical treatment with an azole antifungal or with selenium sulphide. Terbinafine administered topically (but not orally) is an alternative. Immunocompromised patients, including those receiving corticosteroids, may develop extensive infections. In addition, these fungi have caused septicaemia in patients receiving parenteral nutrition.[29] Severe infections require oral treatment with an azole.[30] Griseofulvin is not effective.

Other infections in which *Malassezia* yeasts are implicated include seborrhoeic dermatitis and pityrosporum folliculitis both of which may present in a more severe form in patients with AIDS. Topical or systemic azole antifungals are effective in these conditions and are the main drugs used (see p.1076). However, relapses are common.[31]

1. Gupta AK, *et al.* Antifungal agents: an overview, part II. *J Am Acad Dermatol* 1994; **30:** 911–33.
2. Piérard GE, *et al.* Treatment and prophylaxis of tinea infections. *Drugs* 1996; **52:** 209–24.
3. Smith EB. Topical antifungal drugs in the treatment of tinea pedis, tinea cruris, and tinea corporis. *J Am Acad Dermatol* 1993; **28:** S24–S28.
4. Degreef HJ, DeDoncker PRG. Current therapy of dermatophytosis. *J Am Acad Dermatol* 1994; **31:** S25–S30.
5. Gooskens V, *et al.* Treatment of superficial mycoses in the tropics: Whitfield's ointment versus clotrimazole. *Int J Dermatol* 1994; **33:** 738–42.
6. Bogaert H, *et al.* Multicentre double-blind clinical trials of ciclopirox olamine cream 1% in the treatment of tinea corporis and tinea cruris. *J Int Med Res* 1986; **14:** 210–16.
7. Evans EGV, *et al.* Comparison of terbinafine and clotrimazole in treating tinea pedis. *Br Med J* 1993; **307:** 645–7.
8. Faergemann J, *et al.* A multicentre (double-blind) comparative study to assess the safety and efficacy of fluconazole and griseofulvin in the treatment of tinea corporis and tinea cruris. *Br J Dermatol* 1997; **136:** 575–7.
9. Budimulja U, *et al.* A double-blind, randomized, stratified controlled study of the treatment of tinea imbricata with oral terbinafine or itraconazole. *Br J Dermatol* 1994; **130** (suppl 43): 29–31.
10. De Keyser P, *et al.* Two-week oral treatment of tinea pedis, comparing terbinafine (250 mg/day) with itraconazole (100 mg/day): a double-blind, multicentre study. *Br J Dermatol* 1994; **130** (suppl 43): 22–25.
11. Farag A, *et al.* One-week therapy with oral terbinafine in cases of tinea cruris/corporis. *Br J Dermatol* 1994; **131:** 684–6.
12. Hay RJ, *et al.* A comparison of 2 weeks of terbinafine 250 mg/day with 4 weeks of itraconazole 100 mg/day in plantar-type tinea pedis. *Br J Dermatol* 1995; **132:** 604–8.
13. Baudraz-Rosselet F, *et al.* Efficacy of terbinafine treatment of tinea capitis in children varies according to the dermatophyte species. *Br J Dermatol* 1996; **135:** 1011–12.
14. Allen HB, *et al.* Selenium sulfide: adjunctive therapy for tinea capitis. *Pediatrics* 1982; **69:** 81–3.
15. Givens TG, *et al.* Comparison of 1% and 2.5% selenium sulfide in the treatment of tinea capitis. *Arch Pediatr Adolesc Med* 1995; **149:** 808–11.
16. Anonymous. Management of scalp ringworm. *Drug Ther Bull* 1996; **34:** 5–6.
17. Denning DW, *et al.* Fungal nail disease: a guide to good practice (report of a working group of the British Society for Medical Mycology). *Br Med J* 1995; **311:** 1277–81.
18. Gupta AK, Scher RK. Oral antifungal agents for onychomycosis. *Lancet* 1998; **351:** 541–2.
19. Goodfield MJD, *et al.* Treatment of dermatophyte infection of the finger- and toe-nails with terbinafine (SF 86-327, Lamisil), an orally active fungicidal agent. *Br J Dermatol* 1989; **121:** 753–7.
20. Goodfield MJD, *et al.* Short term treatment of dermatophyte onychomycosis with terbinafine. *Br Med J* 1992; **304:** 1151–4.
21. Tausch I, *et al.* Evaluation of 6 weeks treatment of terbinafine in tinea unguium in a double-blind trial comparing 6 and 12 weeks therapy. *Br J Dermatol* 1997; **136:** 737–42.
22. Watson A, *et al.* Terbinafine in onychomycosis of the toenail: a novel treatment protocol. *J Am Acad Dermatol* 1995; **33:** 775–9.
23. Piepponen T, *et al.* Efficacy and safety of itraconazole in the long-term treatment of onychomycosis. *J Antimicrob Chemother* 1992; **29:** 195–205.
24. De Cuyper C. Long-term evaluation of terbinafine 250 and 500 mg daily in a 16-week oral treatment for toenail onychomycosis. *Br J Dermatol* 1996; **135:** 156–7.
25. De Backer M, *et al.* A 12-week treatment for dermatophyte toe onychomycosis: terbinafine 250 mg/day vs itraconazole 200 mg/day—a double-blind comparative trial. *Br J Dermatol* 1996; **134** (suppl 46): 16–17.
26. Bräutigam M, *et al.* Randomised double blind comparison of terbinafine and itraconazole for treatment of toenail tinea infection. *Br Med J* 1995; **311:** 919–22. Correction. *ibid.*; 1350.
27. Reinel D. Topical treatment of onychomycosis with amorolfine 5% nail lacquer: comparative efficacy and tolerability of once and twice weekly use. *Dermatology* 1992; **184** (suppl 1): 21–4.
28. Roberts DT, *et al.* Topical treatment of onychomycosis using bifonazole 1% urea/40% paste. *Ann N Y Acad Sci* 1988; **544:** 586–7.
29. Dankner WM, *et al.* Malassezia fungemia in neonates and adults: complication of hyperalimentation. *Rev Infect Dis* 1987; **9:** 743–53.
30. Goodless DR, *et al.* Ketoconazole in the treatment of pityriasis versicolor: international review of clinical trials. *DICP Ann Pharmacother* 1991; **25:** 395–8.
31. McGrath J, Murphy GM. The control of seborrhoeic dermatitis and dandruff by antipityrosporal drugs. *Drugs* 1991: **41:** 178–84.

Sporotrichosis

Sporotrichosis is a disease caused by *Sporothrix schenckii,* a fungus found in soil and vegetation, and seen in the Americas and Africa. It may be divided into cutaneous or extracutaneous infection. The cutaneous form is the more common. It probably follows entry of the organism through skin abrasions and usually presents as a single skin lesion, although infection may spread along lymphatic channels causing a series of skin lesions. Extracutaneous sporotrichosis usually presents as osteoarticular infection. Pulmonary infections are occasionally seen and, rarely, CNS and ocular infections.

Potassium iodide by mouth has traditionally been used for cutaneous infections although the mode of action is unclear since potassium iodide does not demonstrate antifungal activity *in vitro.* Itraconazole by mouth is also reported to be effective.[1-3] Oral treatment with terbinafine[4,5] or fluconazole[6] has been tried and may be effective.

Extracutaneous sporotrichosis is treated with amphotericin given intravenously or with itraconazole by mouth; fluconazole is an alternative.[1]

1. Anonymous. Systemic antifungal drugs. *Med Lett Drugs Ther* 1997; **39:** 86–8.
2. Sharkey-Mathis PK, *et al.* Treatment of sporotrichosis with itraconazole. *Am J Med* 1993; **95:** 279–85.
3. Restrepo A, *et al.* Itraconazole therapy in lymphangitic and cutaneous sporotrichosis. *Arch Dermatol* 1986; **122:** 413–17.
4. Hull PR, Vismer HP. Treatment of cutaneous sporotrichosis with terbinafine. *J Dermatol Treat* 1992; **3** (suppl 1): 35–8.
5. Kudoh K, *et al.* Successful treatment of cutaneous sporotrichosis with terbinafine. *J Dermatol Treat* 1996; **7:** 33–5.
6. Castro LGM, *et al.* Successful treatment of sporotrichosis with oral fluconazole: a report of three cases. *Br J Dermatol* 1993; **128:** 352–6.

Tinea

See under Skin Infections, above.

Amorolfine Hydrochloride (15828-f)

Amorolfine Hydrochloride *(BANM, rINNM)*.

Ro-14-4767-000 (amoralfine); Ro-14-4767/002 (amorolfine hydrochloride). (±)-*cis*-2,6-Dimethyl-4-[2-methyl-3-(*p*-*tert*-pentylphenyl)propyl]morpholine hydrochloride.

$C_{21}H_{35}NO,HCl = 354.0$.

CAS — 78613-35-1 (amorolfine); 78613-38-4 (amorolfine hydrochloride).

NOTE. Amorolfine is USAN.

Adverse Effects

Skin irritation, presenting as erythema, pruritus, or a burning sensation, and, rarely, more severe skin reactions have been reported following topical application of amorolfine.

Antimicrobial Action

Amorolfine is a morpholine derivative with antifungal activity. It appears to act be interfering with the synthesis of sterols essential for the functioning of fungal cell membranes.

Amorolfine is active *in vitro* against a wide variety of pathogenic and opportunistic fungi including dermatophytes, *Blastomyces dermatitidis*, *Candida* spp., *Histoplasma capsulatum*, and *Sporothrix schenckii*. It also has variable activity against *Aspergillus* spp. However, despite its *in vitro* activity, amorolfine is inactive when given systemically and this limits its use to topical application for superficial infections.

Uses and Administration

Amorolfine is a morpholine derivative applied topically as the hydrochloride in the treatment of fungal nail and skin infections (see p.371). After topical application, systemic absorption of amorolfine is negligible.

For the treatment of nail infections caused by dermatophytes, yeasts, and moulds a lacquer containing the equivalent of 5% amorolfine is painted onto the affected nail once or sometimes twice a week until the nail has regenerated. Treatment generally needs to be continued for 6 to 12 months.

For the treatment of skin infections, including various forms of tinea, a cream containing the equivalent of 0.25% amorolfine is applied once daily until clinical cure is achieved and then for a further 3 to 5 days.

References.

1. Anonymous. Amorolfine – putting a gloss on infected nails. *Drug Ther Bull* 1992; **30:** 19.
2. Haria M, Bryson HM. Amorolfine: a review of its pharmacological properties and therapeutic potential in the treatment of onychomycosis and other superficial fungal infections. *Drugs* 1995; **49:** 103–20.

Preparations

Proprietary Preparations (details are given in Part 3)

Aust.: Loceryl; ***Austral.:*** Loceryl; ***Belg.:*** Loceryl; ***Fr.:*** Loceryl; ***Ger.:*** Loceryl; ***Irl.:*** Loceryl; ***Norw.:*** Loceryl; ***S.Afr.:*** Loceryl; ***Spain:*** Locetar; Odenil Unas; ***Swed.:*** Loceryl; ***Switz.:*** Loceryl; ***UK:*** Loceryl.

Amphotericin (2562-a)

Amphotericin *(BAN)*.

Amphotericin B *(rINN)*; Anfotericina B.

$C_{47}H_{73}NO_{17} = 924.1$.

CAS — 1397-89-3.

Pharmacopoeias. In *Chin., Eur.* (see p.viii), *Int., Jpn, Pol.,* and *US.*

A mixture of antifungal polyenes produced by the growth of certain strains of *Streptomyces nodosus* or by any other means. It consists largely of amphotericin B. It occurs as a yellow to orange, odourless or almost odourless powder. The Ph. Eur. material contains not less than 750 units per mg with reference to the dried substance and not more than 10% of tetraenes, or not more than 5% if intended for use in parenteral dosage forms. The USP specifies not less than 750 µg of $C_{47}H_{73}NO_{17}$ per mg, and, for material intended for oral or topical use, not more than 15% of amphotericin A, both calculated on the dried substance.

Practically **insoluble** in water, alcohol, dehydrated alcohol, ether, and toluene; slightly soluble or soluble in dimethylformamide; slightly or very slightly soluble in methyl alcohol; soluble in dimethyl sulphoxide and propylene glycol.

Amphotericin is inactivated at low pH values.

Store at 2° to 8° in airtight containers. Protect from light.

Injections typical of conventional amphotericin formulations, are a complex of amphotericin and deoxycholate with suitable buffers which forms a colloidal dispersion when reconstituted. Other formulations of amphotericin for injection include a liposomal formulation, a colloidal dispersion of amphotericin and sodium cholesteryl sulphate, and a complex with phospholipids.

Preparation of solutions for injection. Lyophilised formulations for injection are prepared by reconstitution of amphotericin with sterile water for injection without preservatives, then dilution with glucose injection 5% with a pH above 4.2 to the desired final concentration. Mixture with sodium chloride injection 0.9% would precipitate the amphotericin.

Incompatibilities. Because of the wide range of incompatibilities reported with conventional amphotericin preparations it is generally advisable not to mix them with any other drug. Most incompatibilities are caused by precipitation of amphotericin due to a change in pH or by the disruption of the colloidal suspension. Precipitation can occur if amphotericin is added to sodium chloride 0.9% or to electrolyte solutions.

Although heparin is generally reported to be compatible with conventional amphotericin injection care should be taken if heparin flush solutions, which are diluted with sodium chloride solution, are used to maintain the patency of intravenous lines in patients receiving amphotericin. Flushing the intravenous line with 5% glucose solution has been suggested.

References.

1. Kintzel PE, Smith GH. Practical guidelines for preparing and administering amphotericin B. *Am J Hosp Pharm* 1992; **49:** 1156–64.

Compatibility with lipid emulsions. Mixtures of conventional amphotericin in commercial lipid emulsions have been reported to be unstable,[1-3] although others have reported satisfactory stability.[4-6] In one study[6] vigorous agitation of the mixtures enhanced their stability when compared to gentle mixing.

1. Ericsson O, *et al.* Amphotericin B is incompatible with lipid emulsions. *Ann Pharmacother* 1996; **30:** 298.
2. Ranchère JY, *et al.* Amphotericin B intralipid formulation: stability and particle size. *J Antimicrob Chemother* 1996; **37:** 1165–9.
3. Heide PE. Precipitation of amphotericin B from iv fat emulsion. *Am J Health-Syst Pharm* 1997; **54:** 1449.
4. Lopez RM, *et al.* Stability of amphotericin B in an extemporaneously prepared iv fat emulsion. *Am J Health-Syst Pharm* 1996; **53:** 2724–7.
5. Owens D, *et al.* Stability of amphotericin B 0.05 and 0.5 mg/mL in 20% fat emulsion. *Am J Health-Syst Pharm* 1997; **54:** 683–6.
6. Shadbhan Y, *et al.* The use of commercially available lipid emulsions for the preparation of amphotericin B-lipid admixtures. *J Antimicrob Chemother* 1997; **39:** 655–8.

Adverse Effects

Amphotericin for intravenous administration was originally only available in a conventional colloidal form; liposomal and other formulations have been developed to reduce toxicity. The following adverse effects apply to the **conventional** form. Common adverse effects which occur during or following intravenous infusion of amphotericin include headache, nausea, vomiting, chills, fever, malaise, muscle and joint pains, anorexia, diarrhoea, and gastro-intestinal cramp. Hypertension, hypotension, cardiac arrhythmias including ventricular fibrillation and cardiac arrest, skin rashes, anaphylactoid reactions, blurred vision, tinnitus, hearing loss, vertigo, gastro-intestinal bleeding, liver disorders, peripheral neuropathy, and convulsions have been reported occasionally.

Nephrotoxicity occurs in almost all patients receiving amphotericin intravenously. Both tubular and glomerular damage occur; there may be improvement on cessation of therapy, but there is a risk of permanent impairment of renal function, particularly in patients receiving large cumulative doses (over 5 g). Renal tubular acidosis without systemic acidosis may develop. Amphotericin administration is associated with increased urinary excretion of potassium and magnesium resulting in hypokalaemia and hypomagnesaemia respectively. Uric acid excretion is increased and nephrocalcinosis can occur. Limited data indicate that renal toxicity may be associated with sodium depletion; strategies to improve sodium load are discussed under Treatment of Adverse Effects, below.

A reversible, normocytic, normochromic anaemia develops in most patients receiving amphotericin, possibly due to a direct suppressive effect on erythropoietin production. There are rare reports of thrombocytopenia, leucopenia, agranulocytosis, eosinophilia, and coagulation defects.

Leucoencephalopathy has been reported rarely in patients also receiving total body irradiation.

Solutions of amphotericin irritate the venous endothelium and may cause pain and thrombophlebitis at the injection site. Extravasation may cause tissue damage.

After intrathecal injection amphotericin may also cause irritation of the meninges, neuropathy with pain, impaired vision, and retention of urine.

Topical application may produce local irritation, pruritus, and skin rash.

In general, adverse effects of **nonconventional** amphotericin have been similar to those of conventional amphotericin, but are less frequent and less severe. Brief reversible episodes of renal impairment have been observed but nonconventional formulations have been considered to be safe enough to use in patients with renal impairment who could not be given conventional amphotericin. Anaphylaxis has been reported rarely.

Effects on the eyes. Rapid loss of vision resulting in permanent bilateral blindness occurred in a patient with lupus erythematosus and cryptococcal meningitis after receiving a 1-mg test-dose of amphotericin.[1] Amphotericin was considered to be the causative agent as visual disturbances associated with cryptococcal meningitis are usually progressive in nature and acute blindness with normal funduscopic appearance has not previously been reported.

1. Li PKT, Lai KN. Amphotericin B induced ocular toxicity in cryptococcal meningitis. *Br J Ophthalmol* 1989; **73:** 397–8.

Effects on the heart. Ventricular arrhythmias in 2 patients, resulting in fatal sudden cardiac arrest in 1, were associated with both conventional and liposomal formulations of amphotericin at conventional doses and infusion rates,[1] but cardiac toxicity is more commonly associated with high doses or rapid infusion rates (see under Administration, below). Cardiac arrests in 5 infants and children, fatal in 4 cases, were associated with overdoses of conventional amphotericin of between 3.8 and 40.8 mg per kg body-weight.[2] An increased risk of arrhythmia and cardiac arrest has been reported in patients with evidence of antimony-induced myocardial damage who were switched to amphotericin treatment for visceral leishmaniasis.[3] A rest period of at least 10 days was advised before beginning amphotericin in such patients.

1. Aguado JM, *et al.* Ventricular arrhythmias with conventional and liposomal amphotericin. *Lancet* 1993; **342:** 1239.
2. Cleary JD, *et al.* Amphotericin B overdose in pediatric patients with associated cardiac arrest. *Ann Pharmacother* 1993; **27:** 715–19.
3. Thakur CP. Sodium antimony gluconate, amphotericin, and myocardial damage. *Lancet* 1998; **351:** 1928–9.

Effects on the kidneys. See Nephrotoxicity under Treatment of Adverse Effects, below.

Effects on the liver. Amphotericin has only rarely been associated with adverse effects on the liver. Carnecchia and Kurtzke[1] reported fatal liver failure in one patient after administration of a total dose of 4.82 g given intermittently over one year. The patient had been given a potentially incompatible intravenous admixture of amphotericin and diphenhydramine.

There have been a few reports of abnormal liver-function tests during amphotericin therapy;[2,3] in such cases amphotericin should be discontinued.

1. Carnecchia BM, Kurtzke JF. Fatal toxic reaction to amphotericin B in cryptococcal meningo-encephalitis. *Ann Intern Med* 1960; **53:** 1027–36.
2. Miller MA. Reversible hepatotoxicity related to amphotericin B. *Can Med Assoc J* 1984; **131:** 1245–7.
3. Abajo FJ, Carcas AJ. Amphotericin B hepatotoxicity. *Br Med J* 1986; **293:** 1243.

Effects on the lungs. Reports implicating concomitant administration of leucocytes[1] or other blood products[2] in the development of pulmonary reactions in patients receiving amphotericin have been refuted by the findings of other workers.[3,4] However, a report by Roncoroni *et al.*[5] indicates that amphotericin can produce pulmonary toxicity in the absence of blood products.

1. Wright DG, *et al.* Lethal pulmonary reactions associated with the combined use of amphotericin B and leukocyte transfusions. *N Engl J Med* 1981; **304:** 1185–9.
2. Haber RH, *et al.* Acute pulmonary decompensation due to amphotericin B in the absence of granulocyte transfusions. *N Engl J Med* 1986; **315:** 836.
3. Forman SJ, *et al.* Pulmonary reactions associated with amphotericin B and leukocyte transfusions. *N Engl J Med* 1981; **305:** 584–5.
4. Bow EJ, *et al.* Pulmonary complications in patients receiving granulocyte transfusions and amphotericin B. *Can Med Assoc J* 1984; **130:** 593–7.
5. Roncoroni AJ, *et al.* Bronchiolis obliterans possibly associated with amphotericin B. *J Infect Dis* 1990; **161:** 589.

Effects on potassium homoeostasis. In addition to the hypokalaemia known to be associated with amphotericin and due to increased urinary excretion of potassium, hyperkalaemia has been reported in a patient with severely impaired renal function who received a rapid infusion of amphotericin (see under Administration, below).

Hypersensitivity. Anaphylactoid reactions have occurred with conventional amphotericin. However, anaphylactic reactions have been associated with liposomal amphotericin,[1,2] including a report in 2 patients who subsequently tolerated conventional amphotericin.[1]

1. Laing RBS, *et al.* Anaphylactic reactions to liposomal amphotericin. *Lancet* 1994; **344:** 682.
2. Torre I, *et al.* Anaphylactic reaction to liposomal amphotericin B in children. *Ann Pharmacother* 1996; **30:** 1036–7.

Red man syndrome. Red man syndrome (see Vancomycin, p.267) occurred in one patient on 2 occasions following a test-dose of amphotericin 1 mg.[1]

1. Ellis ME, Tharpe W. Red man syndrome associated with amphotericin B. *Br Med J* 1990; **300:** 1468.

Treatment of Adverse Effects

To reduce febrile reactions antipyretics such as aspirin or paracetamol, and antihistamines such as diphenhydramine may be given before the intravenous infusion of conventional amphotericin. Hydrocortisone given intravenously before or during amphotericin infusion may reduce febrile reactions. However, corticosteroids should not be given indiscriminately to patients receiving amphotericin (see under Interactions, below) and dosage should be kept to a minimum. In the UK the advice is to give antipyretics or hydrocortisone prophylactically, but only to patients who have previously experienced acute adverse reactions and in whom continued treatment with intravenous amphotericin is essential. Pethidine has been given intravenously to treat amphotericin-induced shaking chills. Antiemetics may also be required. Amphotericin is not removed by haemodialysis. Hypokalaemia and hypomagnesaemia should be corrected, and adequate hydration and sodium supplements may reduce the severity of renal impairment. Liposomal, lipid complexed, or nonconventional colloidal amphotericin can be substituted for conventional amphotericin if the latter cannot be tolerated.

Heparin has been added to conventional amphotericin infusions to reduce the incidence of thrombophlebitis.

The value of prophylaxis against generalised reactions to amphotericin infusion was questioned after a retrospective study in 397 patients.[1] The most commonly used drugs were diphenhydramine, corticosteroids, paracetamol, and heparin. The authors concluded that patients who had experienced an adverse reaction following amphotericin administration should receive appropriate premedication before subsequent amphotericin infusions, but that empirical premedication was not justified.

1. Goodwin SD, *et al.* Pretreatment regimens for adverse events related to infusion of amphotericin B. *Clin Infect Dis* 1995; **20:** 755–61.

Anaemia. Amphotericin appears to produce a normochromic, normocytic anaemia by suppression of erythropoietin production.[1,2] Discontinuation of amphotericin reverses the suppression but if the anaemia is severe or treatment with amphotericin cannot be stopped, blood transfusions may be required. Recombinant erythropoietin may prove an alternative to blood transfusions in patients who need to continue treatment with amphotericin.

1. MacGregor RR, *et al.* Erythropoietin concentrations in amphotericin B-induced anemia. *Antimicrob Agents Chemother* 1978; **14:** 270–3.
2. Lin AC, *et al.* Amphotericin B blunts erythropoietin response to anemia. *J Infect Dis* 1990; **161:** 348–51.

Nephrotoxicity. There are limited reports indicating that correction of sodium depletion may reverse amphotericin-induced nephrotoxicity.[1] However, assessment of sodium status and correction of deficiency should precede amphotericin administration.[2,3] Use of mannitol as a protective agent is controversial and is not recommended.[2-4] Diuretics in general should be avoided.[5] Some have recommended supplementation with 150 mmol sodium for suitable patients.[3] However, routine prophylactic administration of sodium is not advised.[6] A randomised study in a small number of patients has suggested that prophylactic sodium supplementation could be beneficial, but that it enhances potassium loss.[7] Administration of amphotericin on alternate days is widely practised although it has never been proven to reduce nephrotoxicity.[2,3] A review of strategies for limiting the toxicity of amphotericin concluded that sodium balance should be monitored and sodium replacement implemented if necessary and that, where possible, salt restriction and drugs which potentiate sodium loss or nephrotoxicity should be avoided.[8]

More recently, liposomal, nonconventional colloidal, and lipid complexes and emulsion formulations have been reported to overcome most problems of chronic nephrotoxicity, even in patients with impaired renal function following previous treatment with conventional amphotericin (see under Uses and Administration, Administration, Alternative Formulations, below).

1. Heidemann HT, *et al.* Amphotericin B nephrotoxicity in humans decreased by salt repletion. *Am J Med* 1983; **75:** 476–81.
2. Warda J, Barriere SL. Amphotericin B nephrotoxicity. *Drug Intell Clin Pharm* 1985; **19:** 25–6.
3. Sabra R, Branch RA. Amphotericin B nephrotoxicity. *Drug Safety* 1990; **5:** 94–108.
4. Bullock WE, *et al.* Can mannitol reduce amphotericin B nephrotoxicity? Double-blind study and description of a new vascular lesion in kidneys. *Antimicrob Agents Chemother* 1976; **10:** 555–63.
5. Fisher MA, *et al.* Risk factors for amphotericin B-associated nephrotoxicity. *Am J Med* 1989; **87:** 547–52.
6. Gardner ML, *et al.* Sodium loading treatment for amphotericin B-induced nephrotoxicity. *DICP Ann Pharmacother* 1990; **24:** 940–6.
7. Llanos A, *et al.* Effect of salt supplementation on amphotericin B nephrotoxicity. *Kidney Int* 1991; **40:** 302–8.
8. Khoo SH, *et al.* Administering amphotericin B—a practical approach. *J Antimicrob Chemother* 1994; **33:** 203–13.

Precautions

Although anaphylaxis is rare following intravenous administration of amphotericin, it is advisable to administer a test dose and then to observe the patient carefully for about 30 minutes before starting treatment. Patients experiencing acute toxic reactions in whom treatment is essential may be given prophylactic antipyretics, antihistamines, or corticosteroids (see Treatment of Adverse Effects, above). To reduce the risk of vein irritation and infusion-related adverse effects, the rate of intravenous infusion of conventional amphotericin should be slow. For a discussion of the relation between infusion rate and adverse effects, see under Uses and Administration, Administration, Infusion Rate, below. Patients receiving any parenteral form of amphotericin should be monitored for changes in renal function, liver function, serum electrolytes, and haematological status. If the BUN or creatinine concentrations increase to clinically significant levels amphotericin therapy should be interrupted or the dose reduced until renal function is restored. Alternatively, a nonconventional amphotericin preparation may be substituted. Treatment should be discontinued if liver function tests are abnormal.

Care should be taken not to confuse the dosage regimens for individual preparations, and in particular those of conventional and non-conventional formulations.

Pregnancy. There are case reports of amphotericin having been used successfully to treat fungal infections in pregnant women without any adverse effects on the infant.[1,2]

1. Ismail MA, Lerner SA. Disseminated blastomycosis in a pregnant woman. *Am Rev Respir Dis* 1982; **126:** 350–3.
2. Peterson CM, *et al.* Coccidiodal meningitis and pregnancy: a case report. *Obstet Gynecol* 1989; **73:** 835–6.

Interactions

Most interactions have been observed during treatment with conventional amphotericin. Since nonconventional formulations appear to be less toxic, they may be anticipated to produce fewer serious interactions. Concomitant administration of nephrotoxic antibiotics, cyclosporin or other nephrotoxic immunosuppressants, or parenteral pentamidine may lead to an increased risk of nephrotoxicity. If possible amphotericin should not be given to patients receiving antineoplastics. Diuretics should generally be avoided in patients taking amphotericin. If a diuretic has to be given then volume and electrolyte depletion should be monitored carefully. The potassium-depleting effect of amphotericin may enhance the effects of neuromuscular blocking drugs and may increase the toxicity of digitalis glycosides; corticosteroids may enhance the depletion of potassium and their immunosuppressive effects may be detrimental in patients with severe fungal infections. Amphotericin may increase the toxicity of flucytosine, but the combination is used in severe infections for its synergistic activity. For information on synergistic and antagonistic effects with other antimicrobials, see under Antimicrobial Action, below. For an increased risk of cardiac arrhythmias and arrest when amphotericin was given to patients with myocardial damage induced by an antimony compound see Effects on the Heart, under Adverse Effects, above.

Antimicrobial Action

Amphotericin is a polyene antifungal antibiotic which appears to act mainly by interfering with the permeability of the cell membrane of sensitive fungi by binding to sterols, chiefly ergosterol. It is reported to be fungistatic at concentrations achieved clinically. It is active against *Absidia* spp., *Aspergillus* spp., *Basidiobolus* spp., *Blastomyces dermatitidis, Candida* spp., *Coccidioides immitis, Conidiobolus* spp., *Cryptococcus neoformans, Histoplasma capsulatum, Mucor* spp., *Paracoccidioides brasiliensis, Rhizopus* spp., *Rhodotorula* spp., and *Sporothrix schenckii*. Minimum inhibitory concentrations range from 0.03 to 1 μg per mL for many of these organisms. Other organisms that have been reported to be sensitive to amphotericin include the algal *Prototheca* spp. and *Leishmania* and *Naegleria* protozoa. It is inactive against bacteria, rickettsias, and viruses.

Some resistant strains of *Candida* have been isolated from immunocompromised patients receiving prolonged treatment with amphotericin.

Immunomodulating effects. *In vitro* and *animal* studies have shown amphotericin to have both immunostimulant and immunosuppressive properties.[1,2]

1. Bistoni F, *et al.* Immunoadjuvant activity of amphotericin B as displayed in mice infected with Candida albicans. *Antimicrob Agents Chemother* 1985; **27:** 625–31.
2. Abruzzo GK, *et al.* Influence of six antifungal agents on the chemiluminescence response of mouse spleen cells. *Antimicrob Agents Chemother* 1986; **29:** 602–7.

Microbiological interactions. Until recently, assessment of antifungal activity has depended largely upon empirical observations based on clinical experience. The development of a standard *in-vitro* method of susceptibility testing should improve the comparability of test results obtained from different laboratories, but the correlation of *in-vitro* results with clinical outcome has still to be determined, especially in relation to drug combinations.[1]

Azoles. Although there have been occasional reports of synergy between amphotericin and the azole antifungals,[2] greater emphasis has been placed on possible antagonism. Studies *in vitro* have supported theoretical concerns that the action of amphotericin (which depends on binding to ergosterol in the fungal cell membrane) would be antagonised by azoles (which inhibit ergosterol synthesis).[3,4] *Animal* studies appear to have confirmed antagonism between amphotericin and the imidazole ketoconazole, but not between amphotericin and the triazoles fluconazole or itraconazole.[1] Available clinical evidence seems to indicate that azoles given concurrently or as continuation therapy after induction therapy with amphotericin are effective in severe infections although reduced plasma concentrations of itraconazole have been reported in some patients while receiving amphotericin.[5] However, strains of *Candida albicans* resistant to both amphotericin and fluconazole have emerged in patients who have received repeated or prolonged courses of fluconazole.[6,7]

Flucytosine. Despite the results of an *in-vitro* study which demonstrated antagonism between amphotericin and flucytosine,[3] this combination is used clinically in severe systemic fungal infections and is generally considered to be synergistic.

Rifampicin. *In-vitro* studies have shown rifampicin to increase the antifungal activity of amphotericin against various *Aspergillus* spp.[8]

Tetracyclines. Minocycline may enhance amphotericin's activity against *Aspergillus* spp. *in vitro*.[9]

Zidovudine. Amphotericin may inhibit the metabolism of zidovudine, see p.631.

1. Sugar AM. Use of amphotericin B with azole antifungal drugs: what are we doing? *Antimicrob Agents Chemother* 1995; **39:** 1907–12.
2. Smith D, *et al.* Effect of ketoconazole and amphotericin B on encapsulated and non-encapsulated strains of Cryptococcus neoformans. *Antimicrob Agents Chemother* 1983; **24:** 851–5.
3. Martin E, *et al.* Antagonistic effects of fluconazole and 5-fluorocytosine on candidacidal action of amphotericin B in human serum. *Antimicrob Agents Chemother* 1994; **38:** 1331–8.
4. Sud IJ, Feingold DS. Effect of ketoconazole on the fungicidal action of amphotericin B in Candida albicans. *Antimicrob Agents Chemother* 1983; **23:** 185–7.
5. Pennick GJ, *et al.* Concomitant therapy with amphotericin B and itraconazole: does this combination affect the serum concentration of itraconazole? *Intersci Conf Antimicrob Agents Chemother* 1994; **34:** 39 (A34).
6. Kelly SL, *et al.* Resistance to fluconazole and amphotericin in Candida albicans from AIDS patients. *Lancet* 1996; **348:** 1523–4.
7. Nolte FS, *et al.* Isolation and characterization of fluconazole- and amphotericin B-resistant Candida albicans from blood of two patients with leukemia. *Antimicrob Agents Chemother* 1997; **44:** 196–9.
8. Hughes CE, *et al.* In vitro activities of amphotericin B in combination with four antifungal agents and rifampin against Aspergillus spp. *Antimicrob Agents Chemother* 1984; **25:** 560–2.
9. Hughes CE, *et al.* Enhancement of the in vitro activity of amphotericin B against Aspergillus spp. by tetracycline analogs. *Antimicrob Agents Chemother* 1984; **26:** 837–40.

Pharmacokinetics

There is little or no absorption of amphotericin from the gastro-intestinal tract. When administered intravenously in the conventional colloidal form and in the usual increasing dosage regimens, peak plasma concentrations of 0.5 to 4 μg per mL have been reported; the average plasma concentration with maintenance doses of 400 to 600 μg per kg body-weight daily tends to be 0.5 μg per mL. It is reported to be highly bound to plasma proteins and is widely distributed but passes into the CSF only in small quantities. The plasma half-life has been reported to be about 24 hours; with long-term administration the terminal half-life increases to 15 days.

Unchanged amphotericin is excreted in small amounts slowly in the urine. Traces have been reported to be present in the serum and urine several weeks after completion of treatment. Amphotericin is not removed by haemodialysis.

The pharmacokinetics of the nonconventional formulations differ considerably from the conventional formulation and from each other.

At the doses used clinically, liposomal amphotericin produces higher peak plasma concentrations (10 to 35 μg per mL after a dose of 3 mg per kg) than conventional amphotericin. A colloidal formulation with sodium cholesteryl sulphate produces lower maximum plasma concentrations of between 1 and 2.5 μg per mL after doses of 0.25 to 1.5 mg per kg. At a dose of 5 mg per kg per day, a phospholipid complex formulation is reported to produce mean maximum plasma concentrations of 1.7 μg per mL. *Animal* studies have shown that concentrations in the kidney following the nonconventional formulations are several times lower than those following the conventional formulation.

References.

1. Janknegt R, *et al.* Liposomal and lipid formulations of amphotericin B: clinical pharmacokinetics. *Clin Pharmacokinet* 1992; **23:** 279–91.

Children and neonates. Serum-amphotericin concentrations ranged from 0.78 to 10.02 μg per mL in 12 children (many with leukaemia) aged 4 months to 14 years following the intravenous infusion of conventional amphotericin 0.25 to 1.5 mg per kg body-weight daily. Serum concentrations did not correlate with dose. The elimination half-life was 18.1 ± 6.65 hours. There was an inverse relationship between age and total clearance, suggesting that children older than 9 years may require lower doses.[1]

The pharmacokinetics of amphotericin have also been studied in a group of 13 neonates with systemic fungal infections.[2] Conventional amphotericin was infused over 4 to 6 hours every 24 hours. Ten of the infants started treatment with 100 μg per kg increased over 4 to 6 days to 500 μg per kg. Three infants were started on a dose of 800 μg to 1 mg per kg reduced to 500 μg per kg daily. All infants were maintained on 500 μg per kg daily; total doses ranged from 17.3 to 28.6 mg per kg. Serum-amphotericin concentrations were measured after the first dose in 3 infants in the first group and 2 in the second; no serum-amphotericin could be detected in the 3 infants who had received 100 μg per kg. After 5 days' treatment peak serum-amphotericin concentrations ranged from 0.5 to 4.0 μg per mL and this was considered to be the range that could be achieved with the daily maintenance dose of 500 μg per kg. The elimination half-life was 14.8 hours. Drug elimination between doses was not detected in 4 of the infants; one was in oliguric renal failure and the other 3 had developed increases in serum-creatinine concentrations. CSF-amphotericin concentrations in 5 of the neonates ranged from 40 to 90% of simultaneous serum concentrations. These authors considered that an initial dose of 500 μg per kg was well tolerated and could produce therapeutic serum concentrations more quickly than a regimen which consisted of 100 μg per kg on day one increased over 4 to 6 days to 500 μg per kg daily.

1. Benson JM, Nahata MC. Pharmacokinetics of amphotericin B in children. *Antimicrob Agents Chemother* 1989; **33:** 1989–93.
2. Baley JE, *et al.* Pharmacokinetics, outcome of treatment, and toxic effects of amphotericin B and 5-fluorocytosine in neonates. *J Pediatr* 1990; **116:** 791–7.

Distribution. Amphotericin concentrations in various organs and tissues were determined in 13 cancer patients who had received conventional amphotericin before death.[1] Concentrations were determined by high-pressure liquid chromatography (HPLC) and bioassay. Mean recovery by HPLC reported as a percentage of total dose given was liver 27.5%, spleen 5.2%, lungs 3.2%, kidney 1.5%, heart 0.4%, brain 0.3% and pancreas 0.2%; each organ had a specific accumulation pattern. The mean total recovery was 38.8%. Reported median bile concentration was 7.3 μg per mL. The drug concentrations obtained by bioassay were much lower than those measured by HPLC. As the HPLC-determined concentrations of amphotericin were higher than the MICs for the pathogens in patients with candidiasis or aspergillosis, the poor clinical outcome in these patients suggested that amphotericin in the tissue lacked antifungal activity.

In another report amphotericin was not detected in the CSF of 4 AIDS patients with cryptococcal meningitis on intravenous maintenance conventional doses of 350 μg to 1.89 mg per kg body-weight given 1 to 7 times weekly.[2] The authors remarked that clinical success of amphotericin for this indication could not be explained by measurable CSF drug concentrations.

Concentrations of amphotericin have been measured in fetal-cord serum in one infant and were 37.5% of maternal serum concentration.[3]

1. Collette N, *et al.* Tissue concentrations and bioactivity of amphotericin B in cancer patients treated with amphotericin B-deoxycholate. *Antimicrob Agents Chemother* 1989; **33:** 362–8.
2. Dugoni BM, *et al.* Amphotericin B concentrations in cerebrospinal fluid of patients with AIDS and cryptococcal meningitis. *Clin Pharm* 1989; **8:** 220–1.
3. Ismail MA, Lerner SA. Disseminated blastomycosis in a pregnant woman. *Am Rev Respir Dis* 1982; **126:** 350–3.

Half-life. The terminal half-life for amphotericin was reported to be 15 days in 2 patients on completion of conventional amphotericin infusion therapy for disseminated histoplasmosis.[1] Another report provides a half-life of 21.5 hours (based on the exponential phase of disappearance from the blood) in a 65-year-old patient on a maintenance conventional dose of 500 μg per kg body-weight infused over one hour every other day.[2] Serum concentrations appeared to plateau at about 600 ng per mL 36 to 48 hours after each dose. This suggested that alternate-day administration might be effective.

1. Atkinson AJ, Bennett JE. Amphotericin B pharmacokinetics in humans. *Antimicrob Agents Chemother* 1978; **13:** 271–6.
2. Hoeprich PD. Elimination half-life of amphotericin B. *J Infect* 1990; **20:** 173–5.

Uses and Administration

Amphotericin is a polyene antifungal antibiotic. It is fungistatic at concentrations achieved clinically. Amphotericin is administered by intravenous infusion in the treatment of severe *systemic* fungal infections including aspergillosis, blastomycosis, candidiasis, coccidioidomycosis, cryptococcosis, histoplasmosis, mucormycosis, paracoccidioidomycosis, and sporotrichosis, and is the usual treatment of choice in fungal endocarditis, meningitis, peritonitis, or severe respiratory-tract infections. Many of these infections are most likely to occur in immunocompromised patients.

Amphotericin is also used for the *local* treatment of superficial candidiasis. It is taken by mouth for intestinal candidiasis, sometimes as part of regimens for selective decontamination of the digestive tract in patients at special risk of infection, such as those in intensive care (see p.128).

The role of amphotericin in the treatment of the above systemic and local infections is discussed under Choice of Antifungal, p.367.

Amphotericin also has antiprotozoal activity. It is used for primary amoebic meningoencephalitis caused by *Naegleria* spp. and for the treatment of visceral and mucocutaneous leishmaniasis.

Administration and dosage. Amphotericin is administered by *intravenous* infusion conventionally as a colloidal complex with sodium deoxycholate. There is also a liposomal form and other complexes of amphotericin available for administration by infusion when conventional amphotericin is contra-indicated because of toxicity, especially nephrotoxicity. Before starting therapy with any form of intravenous amphotericin a test dose should be given and the patient observed carefully for about 30 minutes.

Details of intravenous administration and dosage vary according to the formulation being used. Therapy has sometimes continued for several months depending on the infection. Doses are expressed in terms of amphotericin.

- *Conventional amphotericin* (e.g. Fungizone, UK). After an initial test dose (1 mg infused over 20 to 30 minutes) treatment usually starts with a daily dose of 250 μg per kg body-weight, increased gradually to a maximum of 1 mg per kg daily; in seriously ill patients up to 1.5 mg per kg daily or on alternate days may be necessary. If treatment is stopped for longer than 7 days, it should be resumed at a dose of 250 μg per kg daily and increased gradually. The daily dose is infused over 2 to 4 hours at a concentration of 100 μg per mL in glucose 5%. Slower infusion, over up to 6 hours, may be necessary to reduce the incidence of acute toxic effects.
- *Liposomal amphotericin* (e.g. AmBisome, UK). After an initial test dose (1 mg infused over 10 minutes), the usual dose is 1 mg per kg daily, increased gradually to 3 mg per kg if necessary. The daily dose is infused over 30 to 60 minutes at a concentration of 200 to 2000 μg per mL in glucose 5%.
- *Sodium cholesteryl sulphate-amphotericin complex* (e.g. Amphocil, UK). After an initial test dose (2 mg infused over 10 minutes) the usual dose is 1 mg per kg daily, increased gradually to 3 to 4 mg per kg daily if necessary; doses of up to 6 mg per kg daily have been given. The daily dose is infused at a rate of 1 to 2 mg per kg per hour at a concentration of 625 μg per mL in glucose 5%.
- *Phospholipid-amphotericin complex* (e.g. Abelcet, UK). After an initial test dose (1 mg infused over 15 minutes) the usual dose is 5 mg per kg daily. The daily dose is infused at a rate of 2.5 mg per kg per hour as a diluted suspension containing 1 mg per mL in glucose 5%.

Intrathecal injection of conventional amphotericin is used for patients with severe meningitis especially when intravenous therapy has been ineffective. Commencing with 25 μg, the dose is gradually increased to the maximum that can be tolerated without excessive discomfort. The usual dosage is 0.25 to 1 mg two to four times each week.

Amphotericin is also used *orally* as 10-mg lozenges or as a suspension containing 100 mg per mL for oral or perioral candidiasis. The suspension is given in a dose of 1 mL four times daily; it should be retained in the mouth for a minimum of 1 minute before swallowing. The lozenges are intended to be dissolved in the mouth and are given four times daily, increased to eight lozenges daily if necessary. Doses of 100 to 200 mg are given four times daily by mouth as tablets or suspension to suppress intestinal *Candida*.

Amphotericin has been given for candiduria by continuous bladder irrigation daily at a suggested concentration of 50 mg in 1000 mL of sterile water. Intermittent irrigation has also been tried.

Amphotericin has also been administered into the lung by nebulised solution, into the eye topically or by subconjunctival or intravitreal injection, by topical application to the skin, and into joint spaces by intra-articular injection.

Administration. ALTERNATIVE FORMULATIONS. A number of lipid formulations of amphotericin have been developed in an attempt to minimise renal toxicity and acute toxic reactions. Three lipid-based formulations of amphotericin available commercially in some countries are: liposomes (e.g. AmBisome, UK), a lipid complex with L-α-dimyristoylphosphatidylcholine and L-α-dimyristoylphosphatidylglycerol (e.g. Abelcet, UK), and a colloidal dispersion with sodium cholesteryl sulphate (e.g. Amphocil, UK).[1,2] The aim of reducing renal toxicity has largely been achieved, and in some cases patients unable to tolerate conventional amphotericin have subsequently been successfully treated with one of the lipid-based formulations. Experience with the liposomal formulation suggests that it also produces fewer acute toxic reactions.[1] Clinical studies with these formulations are generally encouraging,[1-5] but they differ in their pharmacokinetics and dosage and there are few formal comparisons of their efficacy.

Conventional amphotericin dispersed in lipid emulsions has been tried as a less expensive alternative to these commercial formulations.[6] However, such dispersions require vigorous mixing to incorporate the amphotericin into the lipid phase and several have been shown to be unstable (see above). While some clinical successes have been achieved, cases of nephrotoxicity have been observed.[7,8] There is currently insufficient evidence to recommend their use.[9]

1. Tollemar J, Ringdén O. Lipid formulations of amphotericin B: less toxicity but at what economic cost? *Drug Safety* 1995; **13:** 207–18.
2. Graybill JR. Lipid formulations for amphotericin B: does the emperor need new clothes? *Ann Intern Med* 1996; **124:** 921–3.
3. Hay RJ. Liposomal amphotericin B, AmBisome. *J Infect* 1994; **28** (suppl 1): 35–43.
4. Stevens DA. Overview of amphotericin B colloidal dispersion (Amphocil). *J Infect* 1994: **28** (suppl 1): 45–9.
5. de Marie S, *et al.* Clinical use of liposomal and lipid-complexed amphotericin B. *J Antimicrob Chemother* 1994; **33:** 907–16.
6. Cleary JD. Amphotericin B formulated in a lipid emulsion. *Ann Pharmacother* 1996; **30:** 409–12.
7. Gales MA, *et al.* Acute renal failure with amphotericin B in lipid emulsion. *Ann Pharmacother* 1996; **30:** 1036.
8. Joly V, *et al.* Amphotericin B in a lipid emulsion for the treatment of cryptococcal meningitis in AIDS patients. *J Antimicrob Chemother* 1996; **38:** 117–26.
9. Sievers TM, *et al.* Safety and efficacy of Intralipid emulsions of amphotericin B. *J Antimicrob Chemother* 1996; **38:** 333–47.

INFUSION RATE. Conventional amphotericin is usually given by intravenous infusion over 2 to 6 hours. A long infusion time is inconvenient for outpatients and often impractical in patients receiving other intravenous medications. This may be overcome by using one of the nonconventional formulations that can be infused over 30 to 120 minutes. Shorter infusion times have been tried with conventional amphotericin with varying results. In studies in small numbers patients without pre-existing renal impairment rapid infusion over 1 hour was generally no more toxic than infusion over 4 hours in two studies,[1,2] whereas others[3] found infusion over 45 minutes to be more toxic than a 4-hour infusion during the first 5 to 7 days of treatment. Cardiac toxicity reported in patients receiving rapid infusions includes atrial fibrillation in a patient with pre-existing cardiac disease,[2] ventricular fibrillation associated with hyperkalaemia in a patient with severely impaired renal function,[4] and bradycardia[5] and dilated cardiomyopathy[6] in patients without apparent risk factors. Bowler and colleagues[7] did not observe any ventricular dysrhythmias in patients with adequate renal function. In general, there is not sufficient evidence to justify reducing infusion times for conventional amphotericin to below 2 hours.

1. Oldfield EC, *et al.* Randomized, double-blind trial of 1- versus 4-hour amphotericin B infusion durations. *Antimicrob Agents Chemother* 1990; **34:** 1402–6.
2. Cruz JM, *et al.* Rapid intravenous infusion of amphotericin B: a pilot study. *Am J Med* 1992; **93:** 123–30.
3. Ellis ME, *et al.* Double-blind randomized study of the effect of infusion rates on toxicity of amphotericin B. *Antimicrob Agents Chemother* 1992; **36:** 172–9.
4. Craven PC, Gremillion DH. Risk factors of ventricular fibrillation during rapid amphotericin B infusion. *Antimicrob Agents Chemother* 1985; **27:** 868–71.
5. Soler JA, *et al.* Bradycardia after rapid intravenous infusion of amphotericin B. *Lancet* 1993; **341:** 372–3.
6. Arswa EL, *et al.* Amphotericin B-induced dilated cardiomyopathy. *Am J Med* 1994; **97:** 560–2.
7. Bowler WA, *et al.* Risk of ventricular dysrhythmias during 1-hour infusions of amphotericin B in patients with preserved renal function. *Antimicrob Agents Chemother* 1992; **36:** 2542–3.

Administration in neonates. Although the most appropriate dose of liposomal amphotericin for low-birth-weight preterm infants has yet to be established reports of a few cases suggest that it may be safe and effective even at relatively high doses. Lackner and colleagues[1] reported the use of doses of liposomal amphotericin of up to 5 mg per kg body-weight to be effective and well tolerated in 2 infants. No adverse effects on renal or hepatic function were observed. da Silva and colleagues[2] reported successful treatment of systemic candidiasis with lower doses of 1.25 mg per kg in 2 infants. Reversible abnormalities in hepatic enzymes occurred in one infant, but renal function was not impaired. Low doses of 0.5 or 1.0 mg per kg daily until blood cultures became negative and then on alternate days for up to 14 doses were well tolerated in a retrospective analysis of 36 mostly extremely low-birth-weight premature infants.[3] Candidaemia was fatal in 2 infants, and 4 others died of unrelated causes.

1. Lackner H, *et al.* Liposomal amphotericin-B (AmBisome) for treatment of disseminated fungal infections in two infants of very low birth weight. *Pediatrics* 1992; **89:** 1259–61.
2. da Silva LP, *et al.* Which is the most appropriate dosage of liposomal amphotericin-B (AmBisome) for the treatment of fungal infections in infants of very low birth weight? *Pediatrics* 1993; **91:** 1217–18.
3. Glick C, *et al.* Neonatal fungemia and amphotericin B. *South Med J* 1993; **86:** 1368–71.

Leishmaniasis. The treatment of visceral and mucocutaneous leishmaniasis including the use of amphotericin is described on p.575.

VISCERAL LEISHMANIASIS. Evidence of declining responsiveness to pentavalent antimonials has led to the evaluation of intravenous amphotericin as an alternative for first-line therapy. WHO has included liposomal amphotericin 3 mg per kg body-weight daily on each of five consecutive days and a sixth dose six days later among the regimens suggested for first-line therapy of Mediterranean visceral leishmaniasis in immunocompetent patients.[5] Amphotericin is also being evaluated in other parts of the world. In India, conventional amphotericin in modest doses (0.5 mg per kg on alternate days) produced good responses both in patients unresponsive to antimonials[1,2] and as first-line therapy.[3] Liposomal amphotericin 2 mg per kg daily on three, five, or seven days over a 10-day period all produced clinical cures and minimal toxicity[6] as did amphotericin lipid complex 1, 2, or 3 mg per kg daily for 5 days,[7] although relapses occurred in some patients taking the lower doses in this latter study. In Brazil, colloidal amphotericin with sodium cholesteryl sulphate in a dose of 2 mg per kg daily for 5 days produced cures in 10 patients although one subsequently relapsed.[8] Responses to liposomal amphotericin were reported to be slower in immunocompromised patients, and relapses occurred in 8 of 11 patients despite treatment with liposomal amphotericin 1.38 to 1.85 mg per kg daily for 21 days.[4] Increasing the dose to 4 mg per kg daily given on 10 days over a 38-day period did not improve the long-term outcome, although initial responses were good.[9]

MUCOCUTANEOUS LEISHMANIASIS. Amphotericin is used in mucocutaneous leishmaniasis unresponsive to antimonials. Successful treatment with liposomal amphotericin has been reported.[10]

1. Giri OP. Amphotericin B therapy in kala-azar. *J Indian Med Assoc* 1993; **91:** 91–3.
2. Mishra M, *et al.* Amphotericin versus pentamidine in antimony-unresponsive kala-azar. *Lancet* 1992; **340:** 1256–7.
3. Mishra M, *et al.* Amphotericin versus sodium stibogluconate in first-line treatment of Indian kala-azar. *Lancet* 1994; **344:** 1599–1600.
4. Davidson RN, *et al.* Liposomal amphotericin B (AmBisome) in Mediterranean visceral leishmaniasis: a multi-centre trial. *Q J Med* 1994; **87:** 75–81.
5. Gradoni L, *et al.* Treatment of Mediterranean visceral leishmaniasis. *Bull WHO* 1995; **73:** 191–7.
6. Thakur CP, *et al.* Comparison of three treatment regimens with liposomal amphotericin B (AmBisome) for visceral leishmaniasis in India: a randomized dose-finding study. *Trans R Soc Trop Med Hyg* 1996; **90:** 319–22.
7. Sundar S, *et al.* Short-course, low-dose amphotericin B lipid complex therapy for visceral leishmaniasis unresponsive to antimony. *Ann Intern Med* 1997; **127:** 133–7.
8. Dietze R, *et al.* Treatment of kala-azar in Brazil with Amphocil (amphotericin B cholesterol dispersion) for 5 days. *Trans R Soc Trop Med Hyg* 1995; **89:** 309–11.
9. Russo R, *et al.* Visceral leishmaniasis in HIV infected patients: treatment with high dose liposomal amphotericin B (AmBisome). *J Infect* 1996; **32:** 133–7.
10. Sampaio RNR, Marsden PD. Mucosal leishmaniasis unresponsive to glucantime therapy successfully treated with AmBisome. *Trans R Soc Trop Med Hyg* 1997; **91:** 77.

Primary amoebic meningoencephalitis. Although amphotericin is active *in vitro* against *Naegleria fowleri* and has been recommended for the treatment of primary amoebic meningoencephalitis (p.574) caused by this amoeba, there have been few reports of survival after its use. One patient who survived was treated with intravenous and intrathecal amphotericin.[1] Another survivor received both amphotericin and miconazole by the intravenous and intrathecal routes, and rifampicin and sulphafurazole by mouth.[2] In a third, aggressive therapy with intravenous and intrathecal amphotericin together with high-dose oral rifampicin was successful.[3]

1. Anderson K, Jamieson A. Primary amoebic meningoencephalitis. *Lancet* 1972; **i:** 902–3.
2. Seidel JS, *et al.* Successful treatment of primary amebic meningoencephalitis. *N Engl J Med* 1982; **306:** 346–8.
3. Brown RL. Successful treatment of primary amebic meningoencephalitis. *Arch Intern Med* 1991; **151:** 1201–2.

Preparations

BP 1998: Amphotericin Lozenges;
USP 23: Amphotericin B Cream; Amphotericin B for Injection; Amphotericin B Lotion; Amphotericin B Ointment.

Proprietary Preparations (details are given in Part 3)
Aust.: AmBisome; Ampho-Moronal; Amphocil; ***Austral.:*** Fungilin; Fungizone; ***Belg.:*** AmBisome; Fungizone; ***Canad.:*** Fungizone; ***Fr.:*** Fungizone; ***Ger.:*** Ampho-Moronal; ***Irl.:*** Abelcet; Amphocil; Fungizone; ***Ital.:*** AmBisome; Amphocil; Fungilin; Fungizone; ***Neth.:*** AmBisome; Amphocil; Fungizone; ***Norw.:*** Fungizone; ***S.Afr.:*** Fungizone; ***Spain:*** Abelcet; AmBisome; Funganiline; Fungizona; ***Swed.:*** Abelcet; AmBisome; Amphocil; Fungizone; ***Switz.:*** Ampho-Moronal; Fungizone; ***UK:*** Abelcet; AmBisome; Amphocil; Fungilin; Fungizone; ***USA:*** AmBisome; Fungizone.

Multi-ingredient: ***Aust.:*** Mysteclin; ***Belg.:*** Fungispec†; ***Fr.:*** Amphocycline; ***Ger.:*** Ampho-Moronal V; Ampho-Moronal V N†; Mysteclin; ***Irl.:*** Mysteclin-F†; ***Ital.:*** Anfocort; Talsutin†; ***Neth.:*** Amphocycline†; ***S.Afr.:*** Mysteclin-V†; Vagmycin; ***Spain:*** Gine Heyden; Sanicel; Trigon Topico; ***Switz.:*** Amphocycline†; Neo Amphocort†.

Bifonazole (12444-v)

Bifonazole *(BAN, USAN, rINN)*.

Bay-h-4502. 1-(α-Biphenyl-4-ylbenzyl)imidazole.

$C_{22}H_{18}N_2$ = 310.4.

CAS — 60628-96-8.

Pharmacopoeias. In *Jpn.*

Bifonazole is an imidazole antifungal with a broad spectrum of activity; sensitive fungi include dermatophytes, *Malassezia furfur*, and *Candida* spp. It also has antibacterial activity *in vitro* against some Gram-positive cocci.

Bifonazole is mainly used by topical application in the treatment of fungal skin and nail infections (p.371). It is applied topically once daily as a 1% cream, powder, solution, or gel. Treatment is usually continued for 2 to 4 weeks. More prolonged treatment is necessary for nail infections and bifonazole may be applied initially with a 40% urea paste to soften the nail.

Local reactions including burning and itching have been reported.

The need for caution when using an azole antifungal in pregnant or lactating patients is discussed under Fluconazole, p.378.

References.

1. Lackner TE, Clissold SP. Bifonazole: a review of its antimicrobial activity and therapeutic use in superficial mycoses. *Drugs* 1989; **38:** 204–25.

Preparations

Proprietary Preparations (details are given in Part 3)
Aust.: Fungiderm; Mycosporin; ***Austral.:*** Mycospor; ***Belg.:*** Mycospor; ***Fr.:*** Amycor; ***Ger.:*** Bifomyk; Mycospor; ***Ital.:*** Azolmen; Bifazol; ***Neth.:*** Mycospor; ***Norw.:*** Mycospor; ***S.Afr.:*** Mycospor; ***Spain:*** Bifokey; Dermokey†; Moldina; Monostop; Mycospor; ***Swed.:*** Mycosporan.

Multi-ingredient: ***Fr.:*** Amycor Onychoset; ***Ger.:*** Mycospor Nagelset; ***Norw.:*** Mycospor Carbamid; ***Spain:*** Mycospor Onicoset; ***Swed.:*** Mycosporan-Karbamid.

Bromochlorosalicylanilide (2212-t)

5-Bromo-4′-chlorosalicylanilide; 5-Bromo-*N*-(4-chlorophenyl)-2-hydroxybenzamide.

$C_{13}H_9BrClNO_2$ = 326.6.

Bromochlorosalicylanilide is a bromsalan antifungal applied topically. Photosensitivity may occur. See also Bromsalans, p.1104.

Preparations

Proprietary Preparations (details are given in Part 3)
Aust.: Multifungin.

Multi-ingredient: ***Aust.:*** Multifungin; ***Ger.:*** Multifungin†; ***Irl.:*** Multifungin H†; Multifungin†; ***S.Afr.:*** Multifungin†; ***Spain:*** Multifungin†.

Buclosamide (2564-x)

Buclosamide *(BAN, rINN)*.

N-Butyl-4-chlorosalicylamide; *N*-Butyl-4-chloro-2-hydroxybenzamide.

$C_{11}H_{14}ClNO_2$ = 227.7.

CAS — 575-74-6.

Buclosamide is an antifungal which has been applied topically in association with salicylic acid in the treatment of fungal skin infections. Photosensitivity has occurred.

Butenafine Hydrochloride (17893-n)

Butenafine Hydrochloride *(BANM, USAN, rINNM)*.

KP-363. *N*-(*p*-*tert*-Butylbenzyl)-*N*-methyl-1-naphthalenemethylamine hydrochloride; 4-*tert*-Butylbenzyl(methyl)(1-naphthalenemethyl)amine hydrochloride.

$C_{23}H_{27}N,HCl$ = 353.9.

CAS — 101828-21-1 (butenafine); 101827-46-7 (butenafine hydrochloride).

Butenafine is a benzylamine antifungal with actions similar to those of the allylamine antifungal terbinafine (p.387). The hydrochloride is used topically as a 1% cream for the treatment of superficial dermatophyte infections (p.371).

References.

1. Anonymous. Topical butenafine for tinea pedis. *Med Lett Drugs Ther* 1997; **39:** 63–4.

Preparations

Proprietary Preparations (details are given in Part 3)
Jpn: Mentax; ***USA:*** Mentax.

Butoconazole Nitrate (16554-x)

Butoconazole Nitrate *(BANM, USAN, rINNM)*.

RS-35887; RS-35887-00-10-3. 1-[4-(4-Chlorophenyl)-2-(2,6-dichlorophenylthio)butyl]imidazole mononitrate.

$C_{19}H_{17}Cl_3N_2S,HNO_3$ = 474.8.

CAS — 64872-76-0 (butoconazole); 64872-77-1 (butoconazole nitrate).

Pharmacopoeias. In *US.*

A white to off-white crystalline powder. Practically **insoluble** in water; sparingly soluble in methyl alcohol; very slightly soluble in ethyl acetate; slightly soluble in acetone, acetonitrile, dichloromethane, and in tetrahydrofuran. **Protect** from light.

Adverse Effects and Precautions

Local reactions including burning and irritation may occur when butoconazole is applied vaginally.

For information about the use of butoconazole during pregnancy and lactation, see under Pregnancy in Fluconazole, Precautions, p.378.

Effects on the blood. Severe reversible thrombocytopenia was associated with treatment with intravaginal butoconazole in one patient.[1] The patient had previously experienced a drop in white cell count following treatment with intravaginal clotrimazole, suggestive of an idiosyncratic reaction to imidazoles.

1. Maloley PA, *et al.* Severe reversible thrombocytopenia resulting from butoconazole cream. *DICP Ann Pharmacother* 1990; **24:** 143–4.

Antimicrobial Action

Butoconazole is an imidazole antifungal with antimicrobial activity similar to that of ketoconazole (p.383) including activity against *Candida* spp.

Pharmacokinetics

Approximately 5% of a dose of butoconazole is absorbed following vaginal administration. The plasma half-life is 21 to 24 hours.

Uses and Administration

Butoconazole nitrate is an imidazole antifungal used locally in the treatment of vulvovaginal candidiasis (p.367). It is administered intravaginally as a 100-mg pessary or as 5 g of a 2% cream for 3 to 6 consecutive nights.

Preparations

USP 23: Butoconazole Nitrate Cream.

Proprietary Preparations (details are given in Part 3)
Belg.: Gynomyk; ***Fr.:*** Gynomyk; ***Neth.:*** Gynomyk; ***Switz.:*** Femstat†; ***USA:*** Femstat.

Candicidin (2566-f)

Candicidin *(BAN, USAN, rINN)*.

NSC-94219.

CAS — 1403-17-4.

Pharmacopoeias. In *US.*

A mixture of antifungal heptaenes produced by *Streptomyces griseus*. It occurs as a yellow to brown powder. It contains not less than 1000 μg per mg, calculated on the dried substance. **Soluble** 1 in 75 of water, 1 in 260 of alcohol, 1 in 10 000 of chloroform, 1 in 33 000 of ether, and 1 in 50 of dimethyl sulphoxide; very slightly soluble in acetone and butyl alcohol. A 1% aqueous suspension has a pH of 8 to 10. **Store** at 2° to 8° in airtight containers.

Candicidin is a polyene antibiotic with antifungal actions. It has been used in the treatment of vaginal candidiasis.

Preparations

USP 23: Candicidin Ointment; Candicidin Vaginal Tablets.

Chlordantoin (2568-n)

Chlordantoin *(BAN, USAN)*.

Clodantoin *(rINN)*. 5-(1-Ethylpentyl)-3-(trichloromethylthio)hydantoin; 5-(1-Ethylpentyl)-3-(trichloromethylthio)imidazolidine-2,4-dione.

$C_{11}H_{17}Cl_3N_2O_2S$ = 347.7.

CAS — 5588-20-5.

Chlordantoin is an antifungal used locally for vulvovaginal infections.

Preparations

Proprietary Preparations (details are given in Part 3)
Multi-ingredient: ***Spain:*** Blastoestimulina.

Chlormidazole Hydrochloride (2569-h)

Chlormidazole Hydrochloride *(BANM, rINNM)*.

Clomidazole Hydrochloride. 1-(4-Chlorobenzyl)-2-methylbenzimidazole hydrochloride.

$C_{15}H_{13}ClN_2,HCl$ = 293.2.

CAS — 3689-76-7 (chlormidazole); 54118-67-1 (chlormidazole hydrochloride).

Chlormidazole hydrochloride is an imidazole antifungal used topically in the treatment of fungal infections of the skin.

The need for caution when using an azole antifungal in pregnant or lactating patients is discussed under Fluconazole, p.378.

Preparations

Proprietary Preparations (details are given in Part 3)
Multi-ingredient: ***Aust.:*** Myco-Synalar; ***Ger.:*** Myco-Jellin†; Polycid N†; ***Spain:*** Myco-Synalar; ***Switz.:*** Myco-Synalar.

Chlorphenesin (2570-a)

Chlorphenesin *(BAN, pINN)*.

3-(4-Chlorophenoxy)propane-1,2-diol.

$C_9H_{11}ClO_3$ = 202.6.

CAS — 104-29-0.

Chlorphenesin has antifungal and antibacterial properties. It is applied locally in mild uncomplicated dermatophyte and other cutaneous infections and in vaginal infections.

Chlorphenesin carbamate (p.1313) is used as a skeletal muscle relaxant.

Preparations

Proprietary Preparations (details are given in Part 3)
Aust.: Adermykon; ***Austral.:*** Mycil; Nappy Rash Powder; ***Canad.:*** Mycil; ***Ger.:*** Soorphenesin; ***S.Afr.:*** Mycil†.

Multi-ingredient: ***Aust.:*** Aleot; ***Austral.:*** ZSC; ***Canad.:*** Anivy; ***Ger.:*** Gynaedron†; Oestro-Gynaedron†; OestroTricho N†; Poly-Gynaedron†; ***Switz.:*** Antipririt†; Oestro-Gynaedron†; ***UK:*** Cutinea†.

Ciclopirox Olamine (2572-x)

Ciclopirox Olamine *(BANM, USAN, rINNM)*.

HOE-296. The 2-aminoethanol salt of 6-Cyclohexyl-1-hydroxy-4-methyl-2-pyridone.

$C_{12}H_{17}NO_2,C_2H_7NO$ = 268.4.

CAS — 29342-05-0 (ciclopirox); 41621-49-2 (ciclopirox olamine).

Pharmacopoeias. In *Eur.* (see p.viii) and *US.*

A white or pale yellow crystalline powder. It exhibits polymorphism. Slightly **soluble** in water; very soluble in alcohol and in dichloromethane; slightly soluble in ethyl acetate; practically insoluble in cyclohexane. A 1% aqueous solution has a pH of 8.0 to 9.0. **Protect** from light.

Adverse Effects

Irritation and pruritus have been reported after topical application of ciclopirox olamine.

Antimicrobial Action

Ciclopirox olamine has a wide spectrum of antifungal activity. It inhibits most *Candida, Epidermophyton, Microsporum,* and *Trichophyton* spp. and is also active against *Malassezia furfur*. It has some antibacterial activity.

Uses and Administration

Ciclopirox olamine is an antifungal which is applied topically twice daily as a 1% cream, solution, or powder in the treatment of cutaneous candidiasis (p.367), and other fungal skin infections, namely dermatophytosis and pityriasis versicolor (p.371). It has also been used in the treatment of vaginal candidiasis.

References.

1. Jue SG, *et al.* Ciclopirox olamine 1% cream: a preliminary review of its antimicrobial activity and therapeutic use. *Drugs* 1985; **29:** 330–41.

Preparations

USP 23: Ciclopirox Olamine Cream; Ciclopirox Olamine Topical Suspension.

Proprietary Preparations (details are given in Part 3)
Aust.: Batrafen; ***Canad.:*** Loprox; ***Fr.:*** Mycoster; ***Ger.:*** Batrafen; Nagel Batrafen; ***Irl.:*** Batrafen; ***Ital.:*** Batrafen; Biroxol; Brumixol; Dafnegin; Miclast; Micomicen; Micoxolamina; ***Neth.:*** Loprox; ***Spain:*** Batrafen; Ciclochem; Fungowas; Mikium†; Rimafungol; ***Switz.:*** Batrafen; ***USA:*** Loprox.

Cilofungin (5475-x)

Cilofungin *(USAN, rINN)*.

LY-121019. 1-[(4*R*,5*R*)-4,5-Dihydroxy-N^2-[*p*-(octyloxy)benzoyl]-L-ornithine]echinocandin B.

$C_{49}H_{71}N_7O_{17}$ = 1030.1.

CAS — 79404-91-4.

Cilofungin is a lipopeptide agent under investigation for the treatment of systemic fungal infections.

References.

1. Galgiani JN, *et al.* Activity of cilofungin against Coccidioides immitis: differential in vitro effects on mycelia and spherules correlated with in vivo studies. *J Infect Dis* 1990; **162:** 944–8.
2. Smith KR, *et al.* Comparison of cilofungin and amphotericin B for therapy of murine candidiasis. *Antimicrob Agents Chemother* 1990; **34:** 1619–21.
3. Denning DW, Stevens DA. Efficacy of cilofungin alone and in combination with amphotericin B in a murine model of disseminated aspergillosis. *Antimicrob Agents Chemother* 1991; **35:** 1329–33.
4. Khardori N, *et al.* Comparative efficacies of cilofungin (Ly 121019) and amphotericin B against disseminated Candida albicans infections in normal and granulocytopenic mice. *Antimicrob Agents Chemother* 1993; **37:** 729–36.

Clotrimazole (2573-r)

Clotrimazole *(BAN, USAN, rINN)*.

BAY-5097; Clotrimazolum; FB-5097. 1-(α-2-Chlorotrityl)imidazole.

$C_{22}H_{17}ClN_2$ = 344.8.

CAS — 23593-75-1.

NOTE. Compounded preparations of clotrimazole and betamethasone dipropionate in USP 23 may be represented by the name Co-climasone.

Pharmacopoeias. In *Chin., Eur.* (see p.viii), *Jpn, Pol.,* and *US.*

A white to pale yellow crystalline powder. Practically **insoluble** in water; soluble to freely soluble in alcohol; soluble in dichloromethane; slightly soluble in ether; freely soluble in acetone, in chloroform, and in methyl alcohol. **Store** in airtight containers. Protect from light.

Adverse Effects and Precautions

Gastro-intestinal disturbance, elevation of liver enzymes, dysuria, and mental depression have been reported after administration of clotrimazole by mouth. Local reactions including irritation and a burning sensation may occur in patients treated topically; contact allergic dermatitis has been reported.

For information about the use of clotrimazole during pregnancy and lactation, see under Pregnancy in Fluconazole, Precautions, p.378.

Antimicrobial Action

Clotrimazole is an imidazole antifungal with antimicrobial activity similar to that of ketoconazole (p.383). A high proportion of fungi sensitive to clotrimazole are inhibited by concentrations of 3 μg per mL. The protozoan *Trichomonas vaginalis* requires up to 100 μg per mL for inhibition.

Pharmacokinetics

When applied topically clotrimazole penetrates the epidermis but there is little if any systemic absorption. Absorption of 3 to 10% of a dose has been reported following vaginal administration. Clotrimazole is metabolised in the liver to inactive compounds and excreted in the faeces and urine.

Uses and Administration

Clotrimazole is an imidazole antifungal used topically in superficial candidiasis (p.367), and in the skin infections pityriasis versicolor and dermatophytosis (p.371). It may also be used occasionally in the treatment of the protozoal infection trichomoniasis when other drugs are contra-indicated (see p.577).

Clotrimazole is applied topically two or three times daily for 2 to 4 weeks as a 1% cream, lotion, or solution in the treatment of fungal skin infections; a 1% powder may be used in conjunction with the cream or solution and has been applied to prevent re-infection. The 1% solution is also used topically for fungal otitis externa. Clotrimazole is given as pessaries in dosage regimens of 100 mg for 6 days, 200 mg for 3 days, or a single dose of 500 mg in the treatment of vulvovaginal candidiasis; similar doses are given as a 1, 2, or 10% vaginal cream.

Lozenges of clotrimazole 10 mg are dissolved in the mouth for treatment or prophylaxis of oral candidiasis and may be administered five times daily for 14 days. Clotrimazole has also been administered by mouth but has now been largely superseded by other azole drugs.

Seborrhoeic dermatitis. Topical preparations containing an imidazole such as clotrimazole, ketoconazole, or miconazole usually together with hydrocortisone are used in the management of seborrhoeic dermatitis (see p.1076).

Sickle-cell disease. Oral clotrimazole has been investigated[1] in the treatment of sickle-cell disease (p.703).

1. Brugnara C, *et al.* Therapy with oral clotrimazole induces inhibition of the Gardos channel and reduction of erythrocyte dehydration in patients with sickle cell disease. *J Clin Invest* 1996; **97:** 1227–34.

Preparations

BP 1998: Clotrimazole Cream; Clotrimazole Pessaries;
USP 23: Clotrimazole and Betamethasone Dipropionate Cream; Clotrimazole Cream; Clotrimazole Lotion; Clotrimazole Lozenges; Clotrimazole Topical Solution; Clotrimazole Vaginal Tablets.

Proprietary Preparations (details are given in Part 3)
Aust.: Candibene; Canesten; Mycofug†; Myko Cordes; Pedikurol; ***Austral.:*** Canesten; Clonea; Gyne-Lotrimin; Hiderm; Lotremin†; Tinaderm Extra; ***Belg.:*** Canestene; Gyno-Canestene; ***Canad.:*** Canesten; Clotrimaderm; Myclo-Derm; Myclo-Gyne; Neo-Zol; ***Fr.:*** Trimysten†; ***Ger.:*** Antifungol; Antimyk†; Apocanda; Aru C; Azutrimazol; Benzoderm Myco; Canesten; Canifug; Clotri OPT; Clotrifug; Clotrigalen; Contrafungin†; cutistad; Dignotrimazol; durafungol; Fungizid; Gilt; Gyno-Canesten; Holfungin; Imazol; Jenamazol; KadeFungin; Logomed Hautpilz-Salbe; Lokalicid; Mono Baycuten†; Mycofug; Mycohaug C; Myko Cordes; Mykofungin; Mykohaug; Onymyken†; Ovis Neu; Pedisafe; Radikal; SD-Hermal; Stiemazol†; Uromykol; ***Irl.:*** Canesten; ***Ital.:*** Antimicotico; Canesten; Gyno-Canesten; ***Neth.:*** Canesten; ***Norw.:*** Canesten; Fungisten; ***S.Afr.:*** Canalba; Candaspor; Candizole; Canesten; Canex; Clomaderm; Closcript†; Covospor; Dynaspor; Gynezol; Medaspor; Micomisan; Mycoban; Normospor; Stiemazol†; Xeraspor; ***Spain:*** Canesten; Fungidermo; Ictan; Micomisan†; Micoter†; ***Swed.:*** Canesten; Clotriferm†; ***Switz.:*** Acnecolor; Canestene; Clocim; clot-basan†; cutistad; Eurosan; Fungotox; Gromazol; Imazol; ***UK:*** Athletes Foot Cream; Canesten; Canesten Combi; Fungederm; Masnoderm; Mycil Gold; ***USA:*** Femcare†; Fungoid; Gyne-Lotrimin; Lotrimin; Lotrimin AF; Mycelex; Mycelex-7 Combination Pack; Prescription Strength Desenex.

Multi-ingredient: ***Aust.:*** Myko Cordes; ***Austral.:*** Hydrozole; ***Belg.:*** Lotriderm; ***Canad.:*** Lotriderm; ***Ger.:*** Baycuten; Canesten HC; Fungidexan; Imazol; Imazol comp; Lotricomb; Myko Cordes Plus; ***Irl.:*** Canesten HC; Lotriderm; ***Ital.:*** Desamix Effe; Meclon; ***S.Afr.:*** Lotriderm; ***Spain:*** Beta Micoter; Clotrasone; ***Switz.:*** Imacort; Imazol; Triderm; ***UK:*** Canesten HC; Lotriderm; ***USA:*** Lotrisone.

Croconazole Hydrochloride (1983-p)

Croconazole Hydrochloride *(rINNM)*.

Cloconazole Hydrochloride; 710674-S (croconazole). 1-(1-{o-[(*m*-Chlorobenzyl)oxy]phenyl}vinyl)imidazole hydrochloride.

$C_{18}H_{15}ClN_2O,HCl = 347.2$.

CAS — 77175-51-0 (croconazole).

Pharmacopoeias. In *Jpn*.

Croconazole hydrochloride is an imidazole antifungal used topically in the treatment of superficial cutaneous candidiasis, dermatophytosis, and pityriasis versicolor.

The need for caution when using an azole antifungal in pregnant or lactating patients is discussed under Fluconazole, p.378.

Preparations

Proprietary Preparations (details are given in Part 3)
Aust.: Pilzcin; ***Ger.:*** Pilzcin; ***Jpn:*** Pilzcin.

Eberconazole (15271-n)

Eberconazole *(rINN)*.

WAS-2160. (±)-1-(2,4-Dichloro-10,11-dihydro-5*H*-dibenzo[*a*,*d*]cyclohepten-5-yl)imidazole.

$C_{18}H_{14}Cl_2N_2 = 329.2$.

CAS — 128326-82-9.

Eberconazole is an imidazole antifungal under investigation for the topical treatment of superficial fungal skin infections.

Econazole Nitrate (2579-b)

Econazole Nitrate *(BANM, USAN, rINNM)*.

C-C2470; Econazoli Nitras; R-14827; SQ-13050. (±)-1-[2,4-Dichloro-β-(4-chlorobenzyloxy)phenethyl]imidazole nitrate.

$C_{18}H_{15}Cl_3N_2O,HNO_3 = 444.7$.

CAS — 27220-47-9 (econazole); 24169-02-6 (econazole nitrate); 68797-31-9 ((±)-econazole nitrate).

Pharmacopoeias. In *Eur.* (see p.viii) and *US*.

A white or almost white, almost odourless, crystalline powder. Very slightly **soluble** in water; soluble in methyl alcohol; slightly soluble in alcohol; sparingly soluble in chloroform and dichloromethane; very slightly soluble to practically insoluble in ether. **Protect** from light.

Adverse Effects and Precautions

Local reactions including burning and irritation may occur when econazole nitrate is applied topically. Contact dermatitis has been reported rarely.

For information about the use of econazole during pregnancy and lactation, see under Pregnancy in Fluconazole, Precautions, p.378.

Porphyria. Econazole nitrate has been associated with clinical exacerbations of porphyria and is considered unsafe in porphyric patients.[1]

1. Moore MR, McColl KEL. *Porphyria: drug lists.* Glasgow: Porphyria Research Unit, University of Glasgow, 1991.

Antimicrobial Action

Econazole is an imidazole antifungal with antimicrobial activity similar to that of ketoconazole (p.383).

Pharmacokinetics

Absorption is not significant when econazole nitrate is applied to the skin or vagina.

Uses and Administration

Econazole is an imidazole antifungal used topically in the treatment of superficial candidiasis (see p.367) and in dermatophytosis and pityriasis versicolor (see Skin Infections, p.371).

Econazole nitrate is applied topically up to 3 times daily as a 1% cream, lotion, powder, or solution in the treatment of fungal skin infections. Treatment is continued for 2 to 4 weeks. It is also used in the treatment of vaginal candidiasis as pessaries of 150 mg once daily at bedtime for 3 consecutive nights; a single dose of 150 mg in a long-acting formulation has also been used. A 1% cream has been used for vulvovaginitis. It may also be applied to the male consort's genital area to prevent re-infection.

Econazole nitrate has also been administered as eye or ear drops.

Bacterial infections. Econazole nitrate 1% applied twice daily was effective in erosive interdigital bacterial infections when compared with placebo.[1]

1. Kates SG, *et al.* The antibacterial efficacy of econazole nitrate in interdigital toe web infections. *J Am Acad Dermatol* 1990; **22:** 583–6.

Preparations

BP 1998: Econazole Cream; Econazole Pessaries.

Proprietary Preparations (details are given in Part 3)
Aust.: Gyno-Pevaryl; Pevalip; Pevaryl; ***Austral.:*** Dermazole; Ecostatin; Pevaryl; ***Belg.:*** Gyno-Pevaryl; Pevaryl; ***Canad.:*** Ecostatin; ***Fr.:*** Dermazol; Furazanol; Gyno-Pevaryl; Pevaryl; ***Ger.:*** Epi-Pevaryl; Epi-Pevaryl Pv; Gyno-Pevaryl; ***Irl.:*** Ecostatin; Gyno-Pevaryl; Pevaryl; ***Ital.:*** Amicel; Biodermin†; Chemionazolo; Dermazol†; Eccelium; Eco Mi; Ecodergin†; Ecorex; Ifenec; Micogin; Micos; Micosten†; Pargin; Pevaryl; Polinazolo; Skilar†; ***Neth.:*** Pevaryl; ***Norw.:*** Pevaryl; ***S.Afr.:*** Gyno-Pevaryl; Pevaryl; ***Spain:*** Ecotam; Etramon; Gyno-Pevaryl; Micoespec; Micoseptil; Pevaryl; ***Swed.:*** Pevaryl; ***Switz.:*** Gyno-Pevaryl; Pevaryl; ***UK:*** Ecostatin; Gyno-Pevaryl; Pevaryl; ***USA:*** Spectazole.

Multi-ingredient: ***Aust.:*** Pevaryl; Pevisone; ***Belg.:*** Pevisone; ***Fr.:*** Pevisone; ***Ger.:*** Epi-Pevaryl Heilpaste; Epipevisone; ***Ital.:*** Pevisone; ***Norw.:*** Pevisone; ***S.Afr.:*** Pevisone; ***Swed.:*** Pevisone; ***Switz.:*** Pevisone; ***UK:*** Econacort; Pevaryl TC.

Enilconazole (12690-t)

Enilconazole *(BAN, USAN, rINN)*.

R-23979. (±)-1-(β-Allyloxy-2,4-dichlorophenethyl)imidazole.

$C_{14}H_{14}Cl_2N_2O = 297.2$.

CAS — 35554-44-0.

Enilconazole is an imidazole antifungal used in veterinary medicine as a 0.2% solution for the treatment of fungal skin infections in cattle, horses, and dogs.

Fenticlor (2580-x)

Fenticlor *(BAN, USAN, rINN)*.

D-25; HL-1050; NSC-4112; Ph-549; S-7. 2,2′-Thiobis(4-chlorophenol).

$C_{12}H_8Cl_2O_2S = 287.2$.

CAS — 97-24-5.

Fenticlor is an antifungal applied topically in the treatment of dermatophyte infections.

Photosensitivity reactions have been reported.

Preparations

Proprietary Preparations (details are given in Part 3)
Multi-ingredient: ***Spain:*** Dermisdin.

Fenticonazole Nitrate (16806-n)

Fenticonazole Nitrate *(BANM, USAN, rINNM)*.

Fenticonazoli Nitras; Rec-15/1476. (±)-1-[2,4-Dichloro-β-{[*p*-(phenylthio)benzyl]oxy}phenethyl]imidazole mononitrate.

$C_{24}H_{20}Cl_2N_2OS,HNO_3 = 518.4$.

CAS — 73151-29-8 (fenticonazole nitrate); 72479-26-6 (fenticonazole).

Pharmacopoeias. In *Eur.* (see p.viii).

A white or almost white, crystalline powder. Practically **insoluble** in water; sparingly soluble in dehydrated alcohol; freely soluble in methyl alcohol and in dimethylformamide. **Protect** from light.

Adverse Effects and Precautions

Burning and itching have been reported following the application of fenticonazole nitrate.

The need for caution when using an azole antifungal in pregnant or lactating patients is discussed under Fluconazole, p.378.

References.

1. Pigatto P, *et al.* Evaluation of skin irritation and contact sensitizing potential of fenticonazole. *Arzneimittelforschung* 1990; **40:** 329–31.

Antimicrobial Action

Fenticonazole is an imidazole antifungal active against a range of organisms including dermatophyte pathogens, *Malassezia furfur*, and *Candida albicans*.

References to antibacterial activity.

1. Jones BM, *et al.* Comparison of the in vitro activities of fenticonazole, other imidazoles, metronidazole, and tetracycline against organisms associated with bacterial vaginosis and skin infections. *Antimicrob Agents Chemother* 1989; **33:** 970–2.

Uses and Administration

Fenticonazole nitrate is an imidazole antifungal used topically in the treatment of vulvovaginal candidiasis (p.367). A 200-mg pessary is inserted into the vagina at bedtime for 3 nights or a 600-mg pessary is inserted once only at bedtime. Fenticonazole nitrate is also applied topically for the treatment of fungal skin infections.

Preparations

Proprietary Preparations (details are given in Part 3)
Aust.: Fenizolan; Lomexin; ***Fr.:*** Lomexin; ***Ger.:*** Fenizolan; Lomexin; ***Ital.:*** Falvin; Fentiderm; Fentigyn; Lomexin; ***Switz.:*** Mycodermil; ***UK:*** Lomexin.

Fluconazole (18642-y)

Fluconazole *(BAN, USAN, rINN)*.

UK-49858. 2-(2,4-Difluorophenyl)-1,3-bis(1*H*-1,2,4-triazol-1-yl)propan-2-ol.

$C_{13}H_{12}F_2N_6O$ = 306.3.

CAS — 86386-73-4.

Compatibility and stability studies with fluconazole.

1. Lor E, *et al.* Visual compatibility of fluconazole with commonly used injectable drugs during simulated Y-site administration. *Am J Hosp Pharm* 1991; **48:** 744–6.
2. Couch P, *et al.* Stability of fluconazole and amino acids in parenteral nutrient solutions. *Am J Hosp Pharm* 1992; **49:** 1459–62.
3. Hunt-Fugate AK, *et al.* Stability of fluconazole in injectable solutions. *Am J Hosp Pharm* 1993; **50:** 1186–7.
4. Ishisaka DY. Visual compatibility of fluconazole with drugs given by continuous infusion. *Am J Hosp Pharm* 1994; **51:** 2290 and 2292.

Adverse Effects

Adverse effects reported with fluconazole most commonly affect the gastro-intestinal tract and include abdominal pain, diarrhoea, flatulence, nausea, and vomiting. Other adverse effects include headache, dizziness, leucopenia, thrombocytopenia, and raised liver enzyme values. Serious hepatic toxicity has been reported in patients with severe underlying disease. Anaphylaxis and angioedema have been reported rarely.

Skin reactions are rare but exfoliative cutaneous reactions such as toxic epidermal necrolysis and Stevens-Johnson syndrome have occurred, more commonly in patients with AIDS.

Alopecia. Alopecia has occasionally been reported in patients receiving fluconazole, especially during prolonged treatment.[1,2]

1. Weinroth SE, Tuazon CU. Alopecia associated with fluconazole treatment. *Ann Intern Med* 1993; **119:** 637.
2. Pappas PG, *et al.* Alopecia associated with fluconazole therapy. *Ann Intern Med* 1995; **123:** 354–7.

Effect on electrolyte balance. Hypokalaemia was associated with fluconazole administration in 3 patients with acute myeloid leukaemia.[1]

1. Kidd D, *et al.* Hypokalaemia in patients with acute myeloid leukaemia after treatment with fluconazole. *Lancet* 1989; **i:** 1017.

Effects on the liver. Although severe hepatic reactions to fluconazole are rare they have been reported, especially in patients with severe underlying diseases or hepatic dysfunction.[1,2] Elevation of liver enzymes is commonly encountered and there have been reports of jaundice associated with fluconazole treatment.[3,4]

1. Wells C, Lever AML. Dose-dependent fluconazole hepatotoxicity proven on biopsy and rechallenge. *J Infect* 1992; **24:** 111–12.
2. Jacobson MA, *et al.* Fatal acute hepatic necrosis due to fluconazole. *Am J Med* 1994; **96:** 188–90.
3. Holmes J, Clements D. Jaundice in HIV positive haemophiliac. *Lancet* 1989; **i:** 1027.
4. Franklin IM, *et al.* Fluconazole-induced jaundice. *Lancet* 1990; **336:** 565.

Precautions

Fluconazole should be used with caution in patients with impaired renal or hepatic function.

Teratogenicity has occurred in *animals* given high doses of fluconazole and its use is not recommended in pregnancy. See below under Pregnancy. It should not be given to breast-feeding women.

Pregnancy. High (toxic) doses of fluconazole, itraconazole, and ketoconazole have been reported to be teratogenic in *rodents*. Although there is little information about the use of these drugs in human pregnancy there is a report of a woman who had received fluconazole 400 mg daily throughout pregnancy and who gave birth to an infant with severe craniofacial and limb abnormalities.[1] The abnormalities resembled those associated with the Antley-Bixler syndrome, a genetic disorder, but a teratogenic effect could not be excluded. However, prescription-event-monitoring studies of fluconazole did not reveal adverse effects on the fetus.[2,3] Nevertheless, the manufacturers recommend that fluconazole, itraconazole, and ketoconazole should be avoided during pregnancy. These drugs are also distributed into breast milk and should be avoided in lactating mothers.

Other azole antifungals including butoconazole, clotrimazole, econazole, miconazole, sulconazole, terconazole, and tioconazole are reported to be embryotoxic but not teratogenic in *rodents* given high doses. Their distribution into milk is often unknown. Many of these drugs are used topically or intravaginally and the systemic absorption from these routes of administration varies. While these drugs may not necessarily be contra-indicated in pregnancy and lactating mothers, consideration should be given to these potential risks when choosing antifungal therapy for such patients.

1. Lee BE, *et al.* Congenital malformations in an infant born to a woman treated with fluconazole. *Pediatr Infect Dis J* 1992; **11:** 1062–4.
2. Rubin PC, *et al.* Fluconazole and pregnancy: results of a prescription event-monitoring study. *Int J Gynecol Obstet* 1992; **37** (suppl): 25–7.
3. Inman W, *et al.* Safety of fluconazole in the treatment of vaginal candidiasis: a prescription-event monitoring study, with special reference to the outcome of pregnancy. *Eur J Clin Pharmacol* 1994; **46:** 115–18.

Renal impairment. For dose adjustments in renal impairment, see under Uses and Administration, below.

Interactions

Concomitant administration of rifampicin with fluconazole results in reduced plasma concentrations of fluconazole. Administration of hydrochlorothiazide and fluconazole has resulted in clinically insignificant increases in plasma-fluconazole concentrations.

Fluconazole may interfere with the metabolism of some drugs if given concomitantly, presumably through inhibition of cytochrome P450 (CYP3A4). This may account for the reported increases in plasma concentrations of phenytoin and sulphonylurea hypoglycaemics and reductions in the production of a toxic metabolite of sulphamethoxazole. Increases in plasma concentrations of cyclosporin, nortriptyline, rifabutin, tacrolimus, and zidovudine have also been reported.

Increases in terfenadine concentrations following high doses of fluconazole have been associated with ECG abnormalities. A similar effect may be anticipated with astemizole. Concurrent administration of fluconazole and cisapride could result in increased cisapride concentrations and associated toxicity. The concomitant use of fluconazole with astemizole, cisapride, or terfenadine should be avoided because of the risk of cardiac arrhythmias.

Fluconazole may also increase the effect of some oral anticoagulants and reduce the clearance of theophylline. The efficacy of oral contraceptives may be reduced.

Antimicrobial Action

Fluconazole is a triazole antifungal drug which in sensitive fungi inhibits cytochrome P-450 dependent enzymes resulting in impairment of ergosterol synthesis in fungal cell membranes. It is active against *Blastomyces dermatitidis*, *Candida* spp., *Coccidioides immitis*, *Cryptococcus neoformans*, *Epidermophyton* spp., *Histoplasma capsulatum*, *Microsporum* spp., and *Trichophyton* spp.

Resistance has developed in some *Candida* spp. following long-term prophylaxis with fluconazole, and cross-resistance with other azoles has been reported.

Microbiological interactions. A synergistic antifungal effect was seen *in vitro* with terbinafine and fluconazole against strains of *Candida albicans*.[1] For effects on the antifungal activity of fluconazole when given with amphotericin, see p.373.

1. Barchiesi F, *et al.* In vitro activities of terbinafine in combination with fluconazole and itraconazole against isolates of Candida albicans with reduced susceptibility to azoles. *Antimicrob Agents Chemother* 1997; **41:** 1812–14.

Resistance. The emergence of strains of *Candida* spp. resistant to fluconazole is increasingly important, particularly in immunocompromised patients receiving long-term prophylaxis with fluconazole.[1] In addition to resistance in *C. albicans*,[2,3] infections with *C. glabrata* and *C. krusei*, both of which are less sensitive to fluconazole than *C. albicans*, are becoming more common in these patients,[4,5] and secondary resistance of *C. glabrata* has been reported during fluconazole therapy.[6] Resistance to fluconazole is reported to occur more frequently than resistance to either ketoconazole or itraconazole and may be related to the widespread use of this drug.[3,5] Cross-resistance with other azoles[7] and with amphotericin[8,9] has been reported.

Fluconazole resistance has also been reported in *Cryptococcus neoformans*[10] and *Histoplasma capsulatum*.[11] Histoplasmosis developed during treatment with fluconazole in a patient with HIV infection.[12]

1. Rex JH, *et al.* Resistance of Candida species to fluconazole. *Antimicrob Agents Chemother* 1995; **39:** 1–8.
2. Sandven P, *et al.* Susceptibilities of Norwegian Candida albicans strains to fluconazole: emergence of resistance. *Antimicrob Agents Chemother* 1993; **37:** 2443–8.
3. Johnson EM, *et al.* Emergence of azole drug resistance in Candida species from HIV-infected patients receiving prolonged fluconazole therapy for oral candidosis. *J Antimicrob Chemother* 1995; **35:** 103–14.
4. Price MF, *et al.* Fluconazole susceptibilities of Candida species and distribution of species recovered from blood cultures over a 5-year period. *Antimicrob Agents Chemother* 1994; **38:** 1422–4.
5. Odds FC. Resistance of yeasts to azole-derivative antifungals. *J Antimicrob Chemother* 1993; **31:** 463–71.
6. Hitchcock CA, *et al.* Fluconazole resistance in Candida glabrata. *Antimicrob Agents Chemother* 1993; **37:** 1962–5.
7. Martinez-Suarez JV, Rodriguez-Tudela JL. Patterns of in vitro activity of itraconazole and imidazole antifungal agents against Candida albicans with decreased susceptibility to fluconazole from Spain. *Antimicrob Agents Chemother* 1995; **39:** 1512–16.
8. Kelly SL, *et al.* Resistance to fluconazole and amphotericin in Candida albicans from AIDS patients. *Lancet* 1996; **348:** 1523–4.
9. Nolte FS, *et al.* Isolation and characterization of fluconazole- and amphotericin B-resistant Candida albicans from blood of two patients with leukemia. *Antimicrob Agents Chemother* 1997; **41:** 196–9.
10. Venkateswarlu K, *et al.* Fluconazole tolerance in clinical isolates of Cryptococcus neoformans. *Antimicrob Agents Chemother* 1997; **41:** 748–51.
11. Wheat J, *et al.* Hypothesis on the mechanism of resistance to fluconazole in Histoplasma capsulatum. *Antimicrob Agents Chemother* 1997; **41:** 410–14.
12. Pottage JC, Sha BE. Development of histoplasmosis via human immunodeficiency virus infected patient receiving fluconazole. *J Infect Dis* 1991; **164:** 622–3.

Pharmacokinetics

Fluconazole is well absorbed following oral administration, bioavailability from the oral route being 90% or more of that from the intravenous route. Mean peak plasma concentrations of 6.72 μg per mL have been reported in healthy subjects following a 400-mg oral dose. Peak concentrations are reached within 1 to 2 hours of oral administration. Plasma concentrations are proportional to the dose over a range of 50 to 400 mg. Multiple dosing leads to increases in peak plasma concentrations; steady-state concentrations are reached in 6 to 10 days but may be attained on day 2 if a loading dose is given.

Fluconazole is widely distributed and the apparent volume of distribution is close to that of total body water. Concentrations in breast milk, joint fluid, saliva, sputum, vaginal fluids, and peritoneal fluid are similar to those achieved in plasma. Concentrations in the cerebrospinal fluid range from 50 to 90% of plasma concentrations, even in the absence of meningeal inflammation. Protein binding is only about 12%.

Eighty percent or more of fluconazole is excreted unchanged in the urine; about 11% is excreted as metabolites. The elimination half-life of fluconazole is about 30 hours and is increased in patients with impaired renal function. Fluconazole is removed by dialysis.

Reviews.

1. Debruyne D, Ryckelynek J-P. Clinical pharmacokinetics of fluconazole. *Clin Pharmacokinet* 1993; **24:** 10–27.
2. Debruyne D. Clinical pharmacokinetics of fluconazole in superficial and systemic mycoses. *Clin Pharmacokinet* 1997; **33:** 52–77.

Children and neonates. References.

1. Saxén H, *et al.* Pharmacokinetics of fluconazole in very low birth weight infants during the first two weeks of life. *Clin Pharmacol Ther* 1993; **54:** 269–77.
2. Nahata MC, Brady MT. Pharmacokinetics of fluconazole after oral administration in children with human immunodeficiency virus infection. *Eur J Clin Pharmacol* 1995; **48:** 291–3.

Distribution. Salivary concentrations of fluconazole following oral administration should be adequate for the treatment of oropharyngeal and oesophageal candidiasis[1,2] even in patients with AIDS who may have decreased salivation.[3] Treatment failures are more likely to be due to inadequate dosage or resistant organisms than to decreased salivary secretion.[3]

1. Force RW, Nahata MC. Salivary concentrations of ketoconazole and fluconazole: implications for drug efficacy in oropharyngeal and esophageal candidiasis. *Ann Pharmacother* 1995; **29:** 10–15.
2. Koks CHW, *et al.* Pharmacokinetics of fluconazole in saliva and plasma after administration of an oral suspension and capsules. *Antimicrob Agents Chemother* 1996; **40:** 1935–7.
3. Garcia-Hermoso D, *et al.* Fluconazole concentrations in saliva from AIDS patients with oropharyngeal candidosis refractory to treatment with fluconazole. *Antimicrob Agents Chemother* 1995; **39:** 656–60.

HIV-infected patients. Plasma clearance of fluconazole may be lower in patients with HIV infection than in immunocompetent patients, and the half-life may be prolonged.[1,2]

1. Tett S, *et al.* Pharmacokinetics and bioavailability of fluconazole in two groups of males with human immunodeficiency virus (HIV) infection compared with those in a group of males without HIV infection. *Antimicrob Agents Chemother* 1995; **39:** 1835–41.
2. McLachlan AJ, Tett SE. Pharmacokinetics of fluconazole in people with HIV infection: a population analysis. *Br J Clin Pharmacol* 1996; **41:** 291–8.

Uses and Administration

Fluconazole is a triazole antifungal administered by mouth or by intravenous infusion in similar doses. It is used for superficial mucosal (oropharyngeal, oesophageal, or vaginal) candidiasis and for fungal skin infections. It is also given for systemic infections including systemic candidiasis, coccidioidomycosis, and cryptococcosis, and has been tried in blastomycosis, chromoblastomycosis, histoplasmosis, and sporotrichosis. The place of fluconazole in the treatment of fungal infections is discussed under Choice of Antifungal, p.367.

For superficial mucosal candidiasis (other than genital candidiasis) the usual dose of fluconazole in the UK is 50 mg daily, although 100 mg daily may be given if necessary. Treatment usually continues for 7 to 14 days in oropharyngeal candidiasis (except in severely immunocompromised patients), for 14 days in atrophic oral candidiasis associated with dentures, and for 14 to 30 days in other mucosal candidal infections including oesophagitis. Higher doses are recommended in the USA where an initial dose of fluconazole 200 mg is followed by 100 mg daily and where the minimum treatment period is 14 days for oropharyngeal infection, or a minimum of 21 days and at least 14 days after resolution of symptoms for oesophageal infections; doses of up to 400 mg daily may be used for oesophageal candidiasis if necessary.

Fluconazole 150 mg by mouth as a single dose may be used for vaginal candidiasis or candidal balanitis.

Dermatophytosis, pityriasis versicolor, and *Candida* infections of the skin may be treated with fluconazole 50 mg daily for up to 6 weeks.

Systemic candidiasis, cryptococcal meningitis, and other cryptococcal infections may be treated with an initial dose of fluconazole 400 mg followed by 200 to 400 mg daily. Duration of therapy is based on clinical and mycological response, but is usually at least 6 to 8 weeks in cryptococcal meningitis. Fluconazole may also be used in daily doses of 100 to 200 mg to prevent relapse following a primary course of antifungal treatment for acute cryptococcal meningitis in patients with AIDS.

In immunocompromised patients at risk of fungal infections fluconazole may be given prophylactically in a dose of 50 to 400 mg daily.

Suggested doses for children over 4 weeks of age are 3 mg per kg daily for superficial infections (a loading dose of 6 mg per kg may be used on the first day if necessary), and 6 to 12 mg per kg daily for systemic infections. For prophylaxis in immunocompromised children, a dose of 3 to 12 mg per kg daily has been recommended. For infants under 2 weeks of age, these doses should be given once every 72 hours; for children aged between 2 and 4 weeks, the doses should be given every 48 hours. A maximum dose of 400 mg daily should not be exceeded in children, or 12 mg per kg at appropriate intervals in infants.

Patients with renal impairment may require dosage reduction. Normal loading or initial doses should be given on the first day of treatment and subsequent doses of fluconazole should be adjusted according to creatinine clearance. If the creatinine clearance is more than 50 mL per minute, the standard dose can be given. If the creatinine clearance is 11 to 50 mL per minute, half the standard dose can be given. Patients on regular haemodialysis should receive a standard dose of fluconazole after every dialysis session. No dosage adjustment is needed in patients with renal impairment given single-dose therapy.

Reviews of fluconazole.

1. Grant SM, Clissold SP. Fluconazole: a review of its pharmacodynamic and pharmacokinetic properties, and therapeutic potential in superficial and systemic mycoses. *Drugs* 1990; **39:** 877–916. Correction. *ibid.* **40:** 862.
2. Anonymous. Fluconazole. *Med Lett Drugs Ther* 1990; **32:** 50–2.
3. Kowalsky SF, Dixon DM. Fluconazole: a new antifungal agent. *Clin Pharm* 1991; **10:** 179–94.
4. Goa KL, Barradell LB. Fluconazole: an update of its pharmacodynamic and pharmacokinetic properties and therapeutic use in major superficial and systemic mycoses in immunocompromised patients. *Drugs* 1995; **50:** 658–90.

Administration. *High doses* of fluconazole of up to 1000 mg daily have been tried in the treatment of cryptococcal meningitis. In a study of 11 patients who received fluconazole 800 to 1000 mg daily intravenously for 3 weeks then orally until the CSF culture became negative, 6 patients had responded at 10 weeks and another 2 improved clinically.[1]

1. Menichetti F, *et al.* High-dose fluconazole therapy for cryptococcal meningitis in patients with AIDS. *Clin Infect Dis* 1996; **22:** 838–40.

Concern has been expressed about the increasingly widespread use of fluconazole[1] and, in particular, about the impact of continuous fluconazole therapy in immunodeficient patients on the development of resistance (see above). Nevertheless, fluconazole remains popular for primary and secondary prophylaxis. Some investigators have suggested the use of *intermittent doses*[2,3] although this could further increase the risk of infections with resistant organisms.

1. Mangino JE, *et al.* When to use fluconazole. *Lancet* 1995; **345:** 6–7.
2. Singh N, *et al.* Low-dose fluconazole as primary prophylaxis for cryptococcal infection in AIDS patients with CD4 cell counts of ≤ 100/mm³: demonstration of efficacy in a prospective, multicenter trial. *Clin Infect Dis* 1996; **23:** 1282–6.
3. Schuman P, *et al.* Weekly fluconazole for the prevention of mucosal candidiasis in women with HIV infection: a randomized, double-blind, placebo-controlled trial. *Ann Intern Med* 1997; **126:** 689–96.

Preparations

Proprietary Preparations (details are given in Part 3)
Aust.: Diflucan; Fungata; ***Austral.:*** Diflucan; ***Belg.:*** Diflucan; ***Canad.:*** Diflucan; ***Fr.:*** Triflucan; ***Ger.:*** Diflucan; Fungata; ***Irl.:*** Diflucan; ***Ital.:*** Biozolene; Diflucan; Elazor; ***Neth.:*** Diflucan; ***Norw.:*** Diflucan; ***S.Afr.:*** Diflucan; ***Spain:*** Diflucan; Lavisa; Loitin; Nesporac†; Solacap; ***Swed.:*** Diflucan; ***Switz.:*** Diflucan; ***UK:*** Diflucan; ***USA:*** Diflucan.

Flucytosine (2582-f)

Flucytosine (*BAN, USAN, rINN*).

5-FC; Flucytosinum; Ro-2-9915. 5-Fluorocytosine; 4-Amino-5-fluoropyrimidin-2(1*H*)-one.

$C_4H_4FN_3O$ = 129.1.

CAS — 2022-85-7.

Pharmacopoeias. In Eur. (see p.viii), *Int., Jpn,* and *US.*

A white to off-white crystalline powder, odourless or with a slight odour. Sparingly **soluble** in water; slightly soluble in alcohol and in dehydrated alcohol; practically insoluble in chloroform and ether. **Store** in airtight containers. Protect from light.

A solution of flucytosine for intravenous infusion should be stored between 18° and 25°. Precipitation may occur at lower temperatures and decomposition, with the formation of fluorouracil, at higher temperatures.

References.

1. Biondi L, Nairn JG. Stability studies of 5-fluorocytosine in aqueous solutions. *J Parenter Sci Technol* 1985; **39:** 200–4.
2. Biondi L, Nairn JG. Stability of 5-fluorouracil and flucytosine in parenteral solutions. *Can J Hosp Pharm* 1986; **39:** 60–6.
3. McPhail DC, *et al.* Stability and bioavailability of a flucytosine suspension. *Int J Pharm Pract* 1994; **2:** 235–9.
4. Wintermeyer SM, Nahata MC. Stability of flucytosine in an extemporaneously compounded oral liquid. *Am J Health-Syst Pharm* 1996; **53:** 407–9.

Adverse Effects

Side-effects of flucytosine include nausea, vomiting, diarrhoea, and skin rashes. Less frequently reported side-effects include confusion, hallucinations, convulsions, headache, sedation, and vertigo, and also allergic reactions, toxic epidermal necrolysis, and cardiotoxicity. Alterations in liver function tests are generally dose-related and reversible; hepatotoxicity may also occur. There have been a few reports of peripheral neuropathy.

Bone-marrow depression, especially leucopenia and thrombocytopenia, is associated with blood concentrations of flucytosine greater than 100 μg per mL, with concurrent amphotericin administration, and with renal function impairment. Fatal agranulocytosis and aplastic anaemia have been reported.

Effects on the blood. Bone marrow toxicity associated with flucytosine has been attributed to its conversion to fluorouracil, possibly by intestinal flora.[1]

1. Pirmohamed M, *et al.* The role of active metabolites in drug toxicity. *Drug Safety* 1994; **11:** 114–44.

Precautions

Flucytosine should be administered with great care to patients with renal impairment, or with blood disorders or bone marrow depression. Tests of renal and hepatic function and blood counts should be performed throughout therapy (at least weekly in patients with renal impairment or blood disorders). In patients with renal impairment, doses should be reduced and blood concentrations of flucytosine should be checked regularly. Monitoring is best done by measuring trough concentrations, thus blood samples should be taken just before an injection in patients undergoing a course of treatment with flucytosine. Care should be taken in patients receiving radiation therapy or other drugs which depress bone marrow.

Flucytosine is teratogenic in *rats* and this should be taken into account if pregnant women or those of childbearing age are to be treated. It should be avoided in breast-feeding women.

AIDS. High incidences of bone marrow toxicity have been reported in patients with AIDS during flucytosine therapy.[1] However, in a study in 381 patients, no additional haematotoxicity was reported in patients receiving amphotericin plus flucytosine compared with those receiving amphotericin alone.[2] The toxicity could be minimised by monitoring serum concentrations[3] and the British Society for Antimicrobial Chemotherapy has suggested that these should be maintained within 25 to 50 μg per mL in patients with AIDS.[4]

1. Chuck SL, Sande MA. Infections with Cryptococcus neoformans in the acquired immunodeficiency syndrome. *N Engl J Med* 1989; **321:** 794–9.
2. van der Horst CM, *et al.* Treatment of cryptococcal meningitis associated with the acquired immunodeficiency syndrome. *N Engl J Med* 1997; **337:** 15–21.
3. Viviani MA. Flucytosine—what is its future? *J Antimicrob Chemother* 1995; **35:** 241–4.
4. British Society for Antimicrobial Chemotherapy Working Party. Antifungal chemotherapy in patients with acquired immunodeficiency syndrome. *Lancet* 1992; **340:** 648–51.

Renal impairment. For dosage recommendations, see under Uses, below.

Interactions

Flucytosine is commonly given in combination with amphotericin. Amphotericin can cause a deterioration in renal function, which can result in raised flucytosine blood concentrations and increased toxicity. However, the two drugs are generally regarded as having synergistic antifungal activity. Cytarabine has been claimed to reduce blood concentrations of flucytosine and to antagonise its antifungal activity, although the evidence has been limited.

Antimicrobial Action

Flucytosine is a fluorinated pyrimidine antifungal which in susceptible fungi is converted to fluorouracil by cytosine deaminase. Fluorouracil is then incorporated in place of uracil into fungal RNA and disrupts protein synthesis. The activity of thymidilate synthetase is also inhibited and this effect interferes with fungal DNA synthesis.

Flucytosine is active against *Candida* spp., *Cryptococcus neoformans*, *Cladosporium* spp., and *Fonsecaea* spp. Some *Aspergillus* spp. have also been reported to be sensitive. There is synergy between flucytosine and amphotericin against *Candida* spp. and *Cryptococcus neoformans*.

There is a high incidence of primary resistance to flucytosine among isolates of *Candida* spp. and *Cryptococcus neoformans*. Resistance also develops during treatment with flucytosine and has been reported rarely from combination therapy with flucytosine and amphotericin.

Microbiological interactions. Although flucytosine is generally regarded as having synergistic activity with amphotericin, antagonism of the *in vitro* antifungal activity of *amphotericin* against *Candida* spp. by flucytosine has been reported.[1]

Enhanced antifungal activity against *Cryptococcus neoformans* has been reported using a combination of flucytosine and *fluconazole* in *animal* studies.[2,3]

1. Martin E, *et al.* Antagonistic effects of fluconazole and 5-fluorocytosine on candidacidal action of amphotericin B in human serum. *Antimicrob Agents Chemother* 1994; **38:** 1331–8.
2. Larsen RA, *et al.* Effect of fluconazole on fungicidal activity of flucytosine in murine cryptococcal meningitis. *Antimicrob Agents Chemother* 1996; **40:** 2178–82.
3. Nguyen MH, *et al.* Combination therapy with fluconazole and flucytosine in the murine model of cryptococcal meningitis. *Antimicrob Agents Chemother* 1997; **41:** 1120–3.

Pharmacokinetics

Flucytosine is absorbed rapidly and almost completely from the gastro-intestinal tract. After oral doses of 37.5 mg per kg body-weight every 6 hours, peak plasma concentrations of 70 to 80 µg per mL have been achieved within 2 hours; similar concentrations have been achieved but more rapidly, after an intravenous dose. The plasma-flucytosine concentration for optimum response is 25 to 50 µg per mL. Flucytosine is distributed widely through the body tissues and fluids and diffuses into the CSF; concentrations in the CSF have been reported to be 65 to 90% of those in serum. About 2 to 4% of flucytosine is protein bound.

About 90% of a dose is excreted unchanged by glomerular filtration; a small amount of flucytosine may be metabolised to fluorouracil. The small amount of an oral dose of flucytosine not absorbed from the gastro-intestinal tract is eliminated unchanged in the faeces. The elimination half-life is 2.5 to 6 hours in patients with normal renal function but increases with decreasing renal function. Flucytosine is removed by haemodialysis or peritoneal dialysis.

References.

1. Daneshmend TK, Warnock DW. Clinical pharmacokinetics of systemic antifungal agents. *Clin Pharmacokinet* 1983; **8:** 17–42.
2. Baley JE, *et al.* Pharmacokinetics, outcome of treatment, and toxic effects of amphotericin B and 5-fluorocytosine in neonates. *J Pediatr* 1990; **116:** 791–7.

Uses and Administration

Flucytosine is a fluorinated pyrimidine antifungal used in the treatment of systemic fungal infections. It is mainly used in combination with amphotericin in the treatment of severe systemic candidiasis and cryptococcal meningitis, or with fluconazole in cryptococcal meningitis. It has also been tried in other infections due to susceptible fungi including chromoblastomycosis. The various treatments for the above infections are discussed under Choice of Antifungal, p.367.

Flucytosine is given by *intravenous infusion* as a 1% solution over 20 to 40 minutes. A suggested dose is 200 mg per kg body-weight daily in 4 divided doses; a dose of 100 to 150 mg per kg daily may be sufficient in some patients. Dosage should be adjusted to produce plasma concentrations of 25 to 50 µg per mL. This is particularly important in patients with AIDS who are at increased risk of bone marrow toxicity. Parenteral treatment is rarely given for more than 7 days, except for cryptococcal meningitis when it is continued for at least 4 months.

Because flucytosine is mainly excreted by the kidneys, the dose must be adjusted in patients with renal impairment. One suggested regimen is to give 50 mg per kg every 12 hours to patients with a creatinine clearance of 20 to 40 mL per minute and every 24 hours to patients with a creatinine clearance of 10 to 20 mL per minute. Patients with a creatinine clearance of less than 10 mL per minute may be given a single dose of 50 mg per kg; further doses should be based on plasma concentrations which should not exceed 80 µg per mL.

Flucytosine is given by *mouth* in usual doses of 50 to 150 mg per kg daily in four divided doses. Again, blood concentrations should be monitored and dosage adjusted in patients with renal impairment to avoid accumulation of the drug.

Flucytosine has been used *topically*, but such use may increase problems of resistance.

Administration. Flucytosine has almost always been used in combination with another antifungal, usually amphotericin, since resistance can develop rapidly if it is used alone.[1] Combinations of flucytosine with azole antifungals such as fluconazole have produced encouraging responses in *animal*[2,3] and clinical studies.[4]

1. Viviani MA. Flucytosine—what is its future? *J Antimicrob Chemother* 1995; **35:** 241–4.
2. Larsen RA, *et al.* Effect of fluconazole on fungicidal activity of flucytosine in murine cryptococcal meningitis. *Antimicrob Agents Chemother* 1996; **40:** 2178–82.
3. Nguyen MH, *et al.* Combination therapy with fluconazole and flucytosine in the murine model of cryptococcal meningitis. *Antimicrob Agents Chemother* 1997; **41:** 1120–3.
4. Barbaro G, *et al.* Fluconazole vs itraconazole-flucytosine association in the treatment of esophageal candidiasis in AIDS patients: a double-blind, multicenter placebo-controlled study. *Chest* 1996; **110:** 1507–14.

Preparations

BP 1998: Flucytosine Tablets;
USP 23: Flucytosine Capsules.

Proprietary Preparations (details are given in Part 3)
Aust.: Ancotil; ***Austral.:*** Ancotil†; ***Canad.:*** Ancotil†; ***Fr.:*** Ancotil; ***Ger.:*** Ancotil†; ***Irl.:*** Alcobon; ***Ital.:*** Ancotil; ***Neth.:*** Ancotil; ***Norw.:*** Ancotil; ***S.Afr.:*** Alcobon†; ***Swed.:*** Ancotil; ***Switz.:*** Ancotil; ***UK:*** Alcobon; ***USA:*** Ancobon.

Flutrimazole (10991-c)

Flutrimazole *(BAN, rINN)*.

Flutrimazolum; UR-4056. 1-[*o*-Fluoro-α-(*p*-fluorophenyl)-α-phenylbenzyl]imidazole; (*RS*)-1-(2,4′-Difluorotrityl)imidazole.

$C_{22}H_{16}F_2N_2$ = 346.4.

CAS — 119006-77-8.

Flutrimazole is an imidazole antifungal used topically in the treatment of superficial fungal infections.

The need for caution when using an azole antifungal in pregnant or lactating patients is discussed under Fluconazole, p.378.

References.

1. Alomar A, *et al.* Flutrimazole 1% dermal cream in the treatment of dermatomycoses: a multicentre, double-blind, randomized, comparative clinical trial with bifonazole 1% cream: efficacy of flutrimazole 1% dermal cream in dermatomycoses. *Dermatology* 1995; **190:** 295–300.

Preparations

Proprietary Preparations (details are given in Part 3)
Spain: Flusporan; Funcenal; Micetal.

Genaconazole (10423-q)

Sch-39304; SM-8668. [*R*-(*R**,*R**)]-α-(2,4-Difluorophenyl)-α[1-(methylsulphonyl)ethyl]-1*H*-1,2,4-triazole-1-ethanol.

$C_{13}H_{15}F_2N_3O_3S$ = 331.3.

CAS — 121650-83-7.

Genaconazole is a triazole antifungal under investigation for systemic use.

Griseofulvin (2561-k)

Griseofulvin *(BAN, rINN)*.

Curling Factor; Griseofulvina; Griseofulvinum. (2*S*,4′*R*)-7-Chloro-2′,4,6-trimethoxy-4′-methylspiro[benzofuran-2(3*H*),3′-cyclohexene]-3,6′-dione.

$C_{17}H_{17}ClO_6$ = 352.8.

CAS — 126-07-8.

Pharmacopoeias. In *Chin., Eur.* (see p.viii), *Int., Jpn, Pol.,* and *US.*

An antifungal substance produced by the growth of certain strains of *Penicillium griseofulvum*, or by any other means. It is a white to creamy- or yellowish-white, odourless or almost odourless powder. The Ph. Eur. specifies that the particles of the powder are generally up to 5 µm in maximum dimension, though larger particles, which may occasionally exceed 30 µm, may be present; USP describes material with a predominance of particles of the order of 4 µm in diameter.

The Ph. Eur. specifies 97 to 102% of $C_{17}H_{17}ClO_6$, calculated on the dried substance; the USP specifies not less than 900 µg of $C_{17}H_{17}ClO_6$ per mg.

Ph. Eur. **solubilities** are: practically insoluble in water; slightly soluble in dehydrated alcohol and in methyl alcohol; freely soluble in dimethylformamide and in tetrachloroethane. USP solubilities are: very slightly soluble in water; sparingly soluble in alcohol; soluble in acetone, chloroform, and dimethylformamide. **Store** in airtight containers.

Adverse Effects

Side-effects are usually mild and transient and consist of headache, skin rashes, dryness of the mouth, an altered sensation of taste, and gastro-intestinal disturbances. Angioedema, erythema multiforme, toxic epidermal necrolysis, proteinuria, leucopenia and other blood dyscrasias, oral candidiasis, peripheral neuropathy, photosensitisation, and severe headache have been reported occasionally. Depression, confusion, dizziness, insomnia, and fatigue have also been reported. Griseofulvin may precipitate or aggravate systemic lupus erythematosus.

There have been a few reports of hepatotoxicity attributed to griseofulvin.

Effects on the skin. A report of fatal toxic epidermal necrolysis in a 19-year-old woman.[1] The reaction was attributed to griseofulvin which she had taken for 6 days; she had also received metronidazole for one day. Erythema multiforme occurred in 3 patients taking griseofulvin for 3 to 10 days.[2]

1. Mion G, *et al.* Fatal toxic epidermal necrolysis after griseofulvin. *Lancet* 1989; **ii:** 1331.
2. Rustin MHA, *et al.* Erythema multiforme due to griseofulvin. *Br J Dermatol* 1989; **120:** 455–8.

Precautions

Griseofulvin is contra-indicated in patients with porphyria, liver failure, or systemic lupus erythematosus.

Griseofulvin is embryotoxic and teratogenic in *rats*. It is contra-indicated in pregnancy. Women should not become pregnant during or within one month of stopping griseofulvin treatment. Since griseofulvin may reduce the effectiveness of oral contraceptives, additional contraceptive precautions should be taken during this time. The manufacturers also warn that men receiving griseofulvin should not father children within six months of treatment. The warning is based on data from *in-vitro* studies using mammalian cells which demonstrated aneuploidy.

Griseofulvin may impair the ability to drive or operate machinery, and has been reported to enhance the effects of alcohol.

Porphyria. Griseofulvin has been associated with acute attacks of porphyria and is considered unsafe in patients with acute porphyria.[1]

1. Moore MR, McColl KEL. *Porphyria: drug lists.* Glasgow: Porphyria Research Unit, University of Glasgow, 1991.

Interactions

Phenobarbitone has been reported to decrease the gastro-intestinal absorption of griseofulvin.

Griseofulvin may increase the rate of metabolism and diminish the effects of some drugs such as coumarin anticoagulants and oral contraceptives. Griseofulvin has also been reported to reduce plasma concentrations of salicylate in a patient taking aspirin (see p.18).

Griseofulvin may enhance the effects of alcohol.

Alcohol. In addition to reports of griseofulvin enhancing the effects of alcohol, a severe disulfiram-like reaction to alcohol has been reported in a patient taking griseofulvin.[1]

1. Fett DL, Vukov LF. An unusual case of severe griseofulvin-alcohol interaction. *Ann Emerg Med* 1994; **24:** 95–7.

Bromocriptine. For a report that griseofulvin can block the response to bromocriptine, see p.1134.

Antimicrobial Action

Griseofulvin is a fungistatic antibiotic which inhibits fungal cell division by disruption of the mitotic spindle structure. It may also interfere with DNA production. It is active against the common dermatophytes, including some species of *Epidermophyton, Microsporum*, or *Trichophyton*.

Pharmacokinetics

Absorption of griseofulvin from the gastro-intestinal tract is variable and incomplete, but is enhanced by reducing the particle size and by administration with a fatty meal.

Griseofulvin is about 84% bound to plasma proteins. It is deposited in keratin precursor cells and is concentrated in the stratum corneum of the skin and in the nails and hair, thus preventing fungal invasion of newly formed cells. Concentrations of 12 to 25 μg per g are maintained in skin during long-term administration, while concurrent plasma concentrations remain at about 1 to 2 μg per mL. Griseofulvin has an elimination half-life of 9 to 24 hours, and is metabolised by the liver mainly to 6-demethylgriseofulvin and its glucuronide conjugate which are excreted in the urine. A large amount of a dose of griseofulvin of reduced particle size appears unchanged in the faeces; less than 1% is excreted unchanged in the urine; some is excreted in the sweat.

Uses and Administration

Griseofulvin is an antifungal administered by mouth in the treatment of dermatophyte infections. It is generally given for such infections that involve the scalp, hair, nails, and skin and which do not respond to topical treatment (see p.371); infections of the soles of the feet, the palms of the hands, and the nails respond slowly.

The usual dose of griseofulvin is 0.5 to 1 g daily in single or divided doses; children may be given 10 mg per kg body-weight daily. These recommended doses are for preparations of griseofulvin of reduced particle size, sometimes known as microcrystalline or microsize griseofulvin, but the doses have been reduced by one third to one half when preparations, available in some countries, containing ultramicrocrystalline or ultramicrosize griseofulvin are used. Griseofulvin is probably best given with or after meals.

The duration of treatment depends on the thickness of the keratin layer: 2 to 6 weeks for infections of the hair and skin, up to 6 months for infections of the fingernails, and 12 months or more for infections of the toenails.

Administration. Although griseofulvin is usually given systemically, beneficial responses have been reported with some topical formulations[1,2] in fungal skin infections.

1. Macasaet EN, Pert P. Topical (1%) solution of griseofulvin in the treatment of tinea corporis. *Br J Dermatol* 1991; **124:** 110–11.
2. Aly R, *et al.* Topical griseofulvin in the treatment of dermatophytoses. *Clin Exp Dermatol* 1994; **19:** 43–6.

Non-infective skin disorders. Lichen planus is usually treated with corticosteroids, cyclosporin, or retinoids (see p.1075) but griseofulvin has been suggested as an alternative to topical corticosteroids in erosive disease.[1] However, some researchers have found it to be of no value.[2]

Dramatic responses of pigmented purpuric dermatoses to griseofulvin 500 to 750 mg daily have been reported in 5 patients.[3]

1. Lamey P-J, Lewis MAO. Oral medicine in practice: white patches. *Br Dent J* 1990; **168:** 147–52.
2. Bagan JV, *et al.* Treatment of lichen planus with griseofulvin. *Oral Surg Oral Med Oral Pathol* 1985; **60:** 608–10.
3. Tamaki K, *et al.* Successful treatment of pigmented purpuric dermatosis with griseofulvin. *Br J Dermatol* 1995; **132:** 159–60.

Preparations

BP 1998: Griseofulvin Tablets;
USP 23: Griseofulvin Capsules; Griseofulvin Oral Suspension; Griseofulvin Tablets; Ultramicrosize Griseofulvin Tablets.

Proprietary Preparations (details are given in Part 3)
Aust.: Biogrisin†; Fulcin†; Griseomed; Grisovin; ***Austral.:*** Fulcin; Griseostatin; Grisovin; ***Canad.:*** Fulvicin; Grisovin FP; ***Fr.:*** Fulcine; Grisefuline; ***Ger.:*** Fulcin S; Gricin; Griseo; Likuden M; Polygris†; ***Irl.:*** Fulcin; Grisederm†; ***Ital.:*** Delmofulvina†; Fulcin; Grisovina FP; ***Neth.:*** Fulcin†; ***Norw.:*** Fulcin; Fungivin†; Lamoryl; ***S.Afr.:*** Fulcin; Grisovin†; Microcidal; ***Spain:*** Fulcin; Fulvicina†; Greosin; Sulvina†; ***Swed.:*** Fulcin; Grisovin†; Lamoryl†; ***Switz.:*** Fulcin; Gris-PEG†; Grisol; Grisovin†; ***UK:*** Fulcin; Grisovin; ***USA:*** Fulvicin P/G; Fulvicin U/F; Grifulvin V; Gris-PEG; Grisactin; Grisactin Ultra.

Hachimycin (2583-d)

Hachimycin (*BAN, pINN*).
Trichomycin; Trichomycinum.
CAS — 1394-02-1.
Pharmacopoeias. In *Jpn.*

Hachimycin is a polyene antifungal antibiotic produced by *Streptomyces hachijoensis*. It is used locally and by mouth in the treatment of candidiasis, in the protozoal infection trichomoniasis, and in some fungal skin infections including those caused by *Trichophyton* spp.

Preparations

Proprietary Preparations (details are given in Part 3)
Spain: Tricomicin†.

Haloprogin (2585-h)

Haloprogin (*USAN, rINN*).
M-1028; NSC-100071. 3-Iodoprop-2-ynyl 2,4,5-trichlorophenyl ether.
$C_9H_4Cl_3IO = 361.4.$
CAS — 777-11-7.
Pharmacopoeias. In *US.*

Store in airtight containers and protect from light.

Adverse Effects

Local reactions may occur and include irritation, pruritus, and vesiculation.

Antimicrobial Action

Haloprogin is reported to inhibit *Epidermophyton, Microsporum, Trichophyton,* and *Candida* spp. and *Malassezia furfur.*

Uses and Administration

Haloprogin is an antifungal used in the treatment of dermatophytosis and pityriasis versicolor. It is applied topically as a 1% cream or solution twice daily for 2 to 4 weeks.

Preparations

USP 23: Haloprogin Cream; Haloprogin Topical Solution.

Proprietary Preparations (details are given in Part 3)
Ital.: Hycaden†; ***S.Afr.:*** Mycanden†; ***USA:*** Halotex.

Hydroxystilbamidine Isethionate (2588-v)

Hydroxystilbamidine Isethionate (*BANM*).
Hydroxystilbamidine Isetionate (*rINNM*). 2-Hydroxystilbene-4,4′-dicarboxamidine bis(2-hydroxyethanesulphonate).
$C_{16}H_{16}N_4O,2C_2H_6O_4S = 532.6.$
CAS — 495-99-8 (hydroxystilbamidine); 533-22-2 (hydroxystilbamidine isethionate).

Hydroxystilbamidine isethionate is an antifungal formerly used in the treatment of blastomycosis and in the protozoal infection leishmaniasis.

Isoconazole (11423-z)

Isoconazole (*BAN, USAN, rINN*).
Isoconazolum. 1-[2,4-Dichloro-β-(2,6-dichlorobenzyloxy)phenethyl]imidazole.
$C_{18}H_{14}Cl_4N_2O = 416.1.$
CAS — 27523-40-6.
Pharmacopoeias. In *Eur.* (see p.viii).

A white or almost white powder. Practically **insoluble** in water; freely soluble in alcohol; very soluble in methyl alcohol. **Protect** from light.

Isoconazole Nitrate (12868-g)

Isoconazole Nitrate (*BANM, rINNM*).
Isoconazoli Nitras; R-15454.
$C_{18}H_{14}Cl_4N_2O,HNO_3 = 479.1.$
CAS — 24168-96-5 (isoconazole mononitrate); 40036-10-0 (isoconazole nitrate).
Pharmacopoeias. In *Eur.* (see p.viii).

A white or almost white powder. Very slightly **soluble** in water; slightly soluble in alcohol; soluble in methyl alcohol. **Protect** from light.

Adverse Effects and Precautions

Local reactions including burning or itching may occur following the application of isoconazole. The need for caution when using an azole antifungal in pregnant or lactating patients is discussed under Fluconazole, p.378.

Antimicrobial Action

Isoconazole is an imidazole antifungal active against a wide spectrum of fungi including *Candida* spp., dermatophytes, and *Malassezia furfur.* It is also active against some Gram-positive bacteria.

Uses and Administration

Isoconazole nitrate is an imidazole antifungal used locally in the treatment of vaginal mycoses, particularly due to *Candida* spp. (p.367) and in fungal skin infections (p.371). For vaginal infections it is usually administered in a single dose of 600 mg or 300 mg daily for 3 days, in the form of pessaries. For skin infections a 2% cream or other topical formulation has been used.

Preparations

Proprietary Preparations (details are given in Part 3)
Aust.: Gyno-Travogen; Travogen; ***Austral.:*** Gyno-Travogen†; Travogen†; ***Belg.:*** Gyno-Travogen; Travogen; ***Fr.:*** Fazol; Fazol G; ***Ger.:*** Travogen; ***Irl.:*** Gyno-Travogen†; Travogen†; ***Ital.:*** Isogyn; Travogen; ***Neth.:*** Gyno-Travogen†; Travogen†; ***S.Afr.:*** Gyno-Travogen†; Travogen†; ***Switz.:*** Gyno-Travogen; Travogen; ***UK:*** Travogyn.

Multi-ingredient: ***Aust.:*** Travocort; ***Belg.:*** Travocort; ***Ger.:*** Bi-Vaspit; Travocort; ***Irl.:*** Travocort; ***Ital.:*** Travocort; ***S.Afr.:*** Travocort; ***Switz.:*** Travocort.

Itraconazole (18657-x)

Itraconazole (*BAN, USAN, rINN*).
Oriconazole; R-51211. (±)-2-sec-Butyl-4-[4-(4-{4-[(2R*,4S*)-2-(2,4-dichlorophenyl)-2-(1*H*-1,2,4-triazol-1-ylmethyl)-1,3-dioxolan-4-ylmethoxy]phenyl}-piperazin-1-yl)phenyl]-2,4-dihydro-1,2,4-triazol-3-one.
$C_{35}H_{38}Cl_2N_8O_4 = 705.6.$
CAS — 84625-61-6.
Pharmacopoeias. In *Eur.* (see p.viii).

A white or almost white powder. Practically **insoluble** in water; very slightly soluble in alcohol; freely soluble in dichloromethane; sparingly soluble in tetrahydrofuran. **Protect** from light.

An extemporaneously prepared oral liquid formulation of itraconazole was stable at 4° for 35 days,[1] but the bioavailability of this formulation was questioned.[2] A commercial oral liquid preparation is available in some countries.

1. Jacobson PA, *et al.* Stability of itraconazole in an extemporaneously compounded oral liquid. *Am J Health-Syst Pharm* 1995; **52:** 189–91.
2. Villarreal JD, Erush SC. Bioavailability of itraconazole from oral liquids in question. *Am J Health-Syst Pharm* 1995; **52:** 1707–8.

Adverse Effects

The most common adverse effects associated with itraconazole include dyspepsia, abdominal pain, nausea, constipation, diarrhoea (with the oral liquid), headache, and dizziness. Others include allergic reactions such as pruritus, rash, urticaria, and angioedema. Isolated cases of the Stevens-Johnson syndrome have been associated with itraconazole. An increase in liver enzyme values has occurred in some patients and cases of hepatitis and cholestatic jaundice have been observed, especially in those treated for more than one month. Alopecia, oedema, and hypokalaemia have also been associated with prolonged treatment. Endocrine effects, such as adrenal suppression and menstrual disorders, and peripheral neuropathy have been reported in a few patients usually when high doses were given.

Itraconazole 50 to 400 mg daily for a median of 5 months was considered to be well tolerated in 189 patients with systemic fungal infections.[1] Eighty-six patients had underlying disease including 49 with AIDS, 16 with diabetes, and 23 with malignancy. Nausea and vomiting occurred in 19 patients, hypertriglyceridaemia in 16 patients, hypokalaemia in 11 patients, and elevated liver enzyme values in 13 patients. The role of itraconazole in hypertriglyceridaemia could not be assessed because all the samples were not drawn in the fasting state and hypertriglyceridaemia is a complication of HIV infection. Gynaecomastia occurred in 2 patients, one receiving concurrent spironolactone. Rash occurred in 4 patients.

Of 49 patients receiving 100 to 400 mg itraconazole daily for up to 39 months, 23 patients did not experience adverse effects during treatment.[2] Six patients had nausea and vomiting. Five patients developed oedema and 2 patients developed hypertension; 3 of the patients who developed oedema and one who became hypertensive were diabetic. Three patients discontinued itraconazole; one due to vomiting, one to leucopenia, and one to nephrotic syndrome. The patient with nephrotic syndrome had pre-existing oedema and hypertension; the syndrome cleared when itraconazole was discontinued.

1. Tucker RM, *et al.* Adverse events associated with itraconazole in 189 patients on chronic therapy. *J Antimicrob Chemother* 1990; **26:** 561–6.
2. Graybill JR, *et al.* Itraconazole treatment of coccidioidomycosis. *Am J Med* 1990; **89:** 282–90.

Precautions

Itraconazole has caused abnormalities in fetal development in *rodents* and is therefore contra-indicated in pregnancy. Breast feeding while receiving itraconazole is not recommended. For further information, see under Pregnancy in Fluconazole, Precautions, p.378. Itraconazole should be avoided in patients with liver disease. Liver function should be monitored if treatment lasts more than one month or if there are symptoms suggestive of hepatitis. Treatment should be stopped if abnormal liver function is detected. Itraconazole plasma concentrations should be monitored in patients with hepatic cirrhosis and the dosage adjusted if necessary. Dose adjustments may also be required in some patients with renal insufficiency, for example those receiving continuous ambulatory peritoneal dialysis. Hypochlorhydria, which may be present in patients with AIDS, can reduce absorption of itraconazole. In this case absorption may be improved by administering itraconazole with an acidic drink, such as a cola beverage.

Interactions

Enzyme-inducing drugs such as rifampicin, carbamazepine, phenytoin, or phenobarbitone may decrease plasma concentrations of itraconazole. Concomitant administration of drugs that reduce stomach acidity, such as antimuscarinics, antacids, proton pump inhibitors, and histamine H_2-receptor antagonists, may reduce the absorption of itraconazole.

Itraconazole may interfere with drugs metabolised by hepatic microsomal enzymes, especially cytochrome P450 (CYP3A4), hence the warnings that plasma concentrations of astemizole, cisapride, cyclosporin, felodipine, statins such as lovastatin or simvastatin, midazolam, quinidine, terfenadine, triazolam, and warfarin may be increased. Concentrations of HIV-protease inhibitors such as indinavir or ritonavir may also be increased; itraconazole plasma concentrations may be increased in turn. The effects of digoxin and of vincristine may be increased by itraconazole but the efficacy of oral contraceptives might be reduced.

There is a risk of cardiac arrhythmias if itraconazole is used concomitantly with astemizole, cisapride, or terfenadine and such combinations should be avoided.

References.

1. Tucker RM, *et al.* Interaction of azoles with rifampin, phenytoin, and carbamazepine: in vitro and clinical observations. *Clin Infect Dis* 1992; **14:** 165–74.
2. Bonay M, *et al.* Possible interaction between phenobarbital, carbamazepine and itraconazole. *Drug Safety* 1993; **9:** 309–11.

Didanosine. Didanosine in a formulation containing buffering agents could reduce the absorption of itraconazole due to the resultant increase in gastric pH.[1]

1. Moreno F, *et al.* Itraconazole-didanosine excipient interaction. *JAMA* 1993; **269:** 1508.

Antimicrobial Action

Itraconazole is a triazole antifungal drug which in sensitive fungi inhibits cytochrome P-450 dependent enzymes resulting in impairment of ergosterol synthesis in fungal cell membranes. It has a slightly wider spectrum of activity than ketoconazole. It is active against *Aspergillus* spp., *Blastomyces dermatitidis*, *Candida* spp., *Coccidioides immitis*, *Cryptococcus neoformans*, *Epidermophyton* spp., *Histoplasma capsulatum*, *Malassezia furfur*, *Microsporum* spp., *Paracoccidioides brasiliensis*, *Sporothrix schenckii*, and *Trichophyton* spp. Itraconazole also has some antiprotozoal activity against *Leishmania* spp.

Acquired resistance to itraconazole is rare but ketoconazole-resistant strains of *Candida albicans* have been found to be cross resistant to itraconazole.

Microbiological interactions. A synergistic antifungal effect was seen *in vitro* with terbinafine and itraconazole against strains of *Candida albicans*.[1] For effects on the antifungal activity of azoles when given with amphotericin, see p.373.

1. Barchiesi F, *et al.* In vitro activities of terbinafine in combination with fluconazole and itraconazole against isolates of Candida albicans with reduced susceptibility to azoles. *Antimicrob Agents Chemother* 1997; **41:** 1812–14.

Resistance. For a discussion of increasing resistance of *Candida* spp. to azoles see Fluconazole, Antimicrobial Action, p.378. *Aspergillus fumigatus* resistant to itraconazole has also been identified.[1]

1. Denning DW, *et al.* Itraconazole resistance in Aspergillus fumigatus. *Antimicrob Agents Chemother* 1997; **41:** 1364–8.

Pharmacokinetics

Itraconazole is well absorbed when given by mouth after food. Mean peak plasma concentrations can be reached within 4 hours and for a 100-mg daily dose can range from 400 to 600 ng per mL at steady state which can be reached within 14 days. Bioavailability increases with doses of 100 to 400 mg in such a manner as to suggest that itraconazole undergoes saturable metabolism. Itraconazole is highly protein bound; only 0.2% circulates as free drug. Itraconazole is widely distributed but only small amounts diffuse into the CSF. Concentrations attained in the skin, sebum, pus, and female genital tissues are several times higher than simultaneous plasma concentrations. Therapeutic concentrations of itraconazole remain in the skin and mucous membranes for 1 to 4 weeks after the drug is discontinued.

Small amounts are distributed into breast milk.

Itraconazole is metabolised in the liver to inactive compounds which are excreted in the bile or urine; 3 to 18% is excreted in the faeces as unchanged drug. Small amounts are eliminated in the stratum corneum and hair. Itraconazole is not removed by dialysis.

The elimination half-life following a single 100-mg dose has been reported as 20 hours; the half-life increases to 30 hours with continued administration.

References.

1. Baelaert J, *et al.* Itraconazole pharmacokinetics in patients with renal dysfunction. *Antimicrob Agents Chemother* 1988; **32:** 1595–7.
2. Cauwenbergh G, *et al.* Pharmacokinetic profile of orally administered itraconazole in human skin. *J Am Acad Dermatol* 1988; **18:** 263–8.
3. Zimmermann T, *et al.* Influence of concomitant food intake on the oral absorption of two triazole antifungal agents, itraconazole and fluconazole. *Eur J Clin Pharmacol* 1994; **46:** 147–50.
4. Prentice AG, *et al.* Multiple dose pharmacokinetics of an oral solution of itraconazole in autologous bone marrow transplant recipients. *J Antimicrob Chemother* 1994; **34:** 247–52.
5. Coronel B, *et al.* Itraconazole concentrations during continuous haemodiafiltration. *J Antimicrob Chemother* 1994; **34:** 448–9.
6. Kintzel PE, *et al.* Low itraconazole serum concentrations following administration of itraconazole suspension to critically ill allogeneic bone marrow transplant recipients. *Ann Pharmacother* 1995; **29:** 140–3.
7. Prentice AG, *et al.* Multiple dose pharmacokinetics of an oral solution of itraconazole in patients receiving chemotherapy for acute myeloid leukaemia. *J Antimicrob Chemother* 1995; **36:** 657–63.
8. Patterson TF, *et al.* Systemic availability of itraconazole in lung transplantation. *Antimicrob Agents Chemother* 1996; **40:** 2217–20.

Uses and Administration

Itraconazole is a triazole antifungal given by mouth for the treatment of oropharyngeal and vulvovaginal candidiasis, for pityriasis versicolor, for dermatophytoses unresponsive to topical treatment, and for systemic infections including aspergillosis, blastomycosis, systemic candidiasis, chromoblastomycosis, coccidioidomycosis, cryptococcosis, histoplasmosis, paracoccidioidomycosis, and sporotrichosis. It is also given for the prophylaxis of fungal infections in immunocompromised patients. The place of itraconazole in the treatment of fungal infections is discussed under Choice of Antifungal, p.367.

The dose of itraconazole in oropharyngeal candidiasis is 100 mg (or 200 mg in patients with AIDS or neutropenia) daily by mouth for 15 days. Vulvovaginal candidiasis may be treated with itraconazole 200 mg by mouth twice daily for one day. Pityriasis versicolor may be treated with itraconazole 200 mg daily for 7 days. For dermatophytoses the dose is 100 mg daily for 15 days or 200 mg daily for 7 days in tinea corporis or tinea cruris, or 100 mg daily for 30 days in tinea pedis or tinea manuum. For nail infections the dose is 200 mg daily for 3 months or pulse therapy with 200 mg twice daily for 7 days repeated once (for fingernails) or twice (for toenails) after intervals of 21 days is suggested.

For systemic infections, itraconazole is given by mouth in usual doses of 100 to 200 mg once daily, increased to 200 mg twice daily for invasive or disseminated infections, including cryptococcal meningitis. In life-threatening infections a loading dose of 200 mg three times a day for 3 days has been suggested. A dose of 200 mg daily is recommended for primary or secondary prophylaxis in neutropenic patients or those with AIDS.

Reviews.

1. Haria M, *et al.* Itraconazole: a reappraisal of its pharmacological properties and therapeutic use in the management of superficial fungal infections. *Drugs* 1996; **51:** 585–620.

Administration. Doses of itraconazole 600 mg daily in two divided doses for periods of 3 to 16 months were used in 8 patients with systemic mycoses resistant to conventional therapy.[1] Two patients with AIDS and cryptococcal meningitis failed to respond and two who responded initially later relapsed or developed progressive disease when the dose was reduced. The main adverse effects were hypokalaemia, hypertension, and oedema possibly associated with adrenal suppression.

In a patient with cerebral aspergillosis, itraconazole 800 mg daily for 5 months then 400 mg daily for a further 4½ months produced complete resolution of cerebral lesions.[2]

1. Sharkey PK, *et al.* High-dose itraconazole in the treatment of severe mycoses. *Antimicrob Agents Chemother* 1991; **35:** 707–13.
2. Sánchez C, *et al.* Treatment of cerebral aspergillosis with itraconazole: do high doses improve the prognosis? *Clin Infect Dis* 1995; **21:** 1485–7.

INTERMITTENT ADMINISTRATION. Intermittent or pulse therapy comprising treatment with itraconazole for one week each month has been used successfully in nail infections.[1,2] A similar protocol using 5 mg per kg body-weight daily for one week in every 3 has been reported to be effective in the treatment of tinea capitis in children.[3]

1. De Doncker P, *et al.* Antifungal pulse therapy for onychomycosis: a pharmacokinetic and pharmacodynamic investigation of monthly cycles of 1-week pulse therapy with itraconazole. *Arch Dermatol* 1996; **132:** 34–41.
2. Tosti A, *et al.* Treatment of dermatophyte nail infections: an open randomized study comparing intermittent terbinafine therapy with continuous terbinafine treatment and intermittent itraconazole therapy. *J Am Acad Dermatol* 1996; **34:** 595–600.
3. Gupta AK, *et al.* Itraconazole pulse therapy is effective in the treatment of tinea capitis in children: an open multicentre study. *Br J Dermatol* 1997; **137:** 251–4.

Administration in neonates. Itraconazole was administered to two premature infants with disseminated candidiasis in a dose of 10 mg per kg body-weight daily in two divided doses for 3 or 4 weeks without adverse effects.[1] Treatment was successful in both infants.

1. Bhandari V, Narang A. Oral itraconazole therapy for disseminated candidiasis in low birth weight infants. *J Pediatr* 1992; **120:** 330.

Amoebic infections. Itraconazole has been suggested for *Acanthamoeba* keratitis, when it is given orally in combination with topical miconazole (see p.573).

Leishmaniasis. When systemic therapy is required for the treatment of cutaneous leishmaniasis, pentavalent antimonials are most commonly used (see p.575). The successful use of itraconazole has been reported in a few patients[1,2] but infections with *Leishmania aethiopica* may not respond.[3]

1. Albanese G, *et al.* Cutaneous leishmaniasis: treatment with itraconazole. *Arch Dermatol* 1989; **125:** 1540–2.
2. Pialoux G, *et al.* Cutaneous leishmaniasis in an AIDS patient: cure with itraconazole. *J Infect Dis* 1990; **162:** 1221–2.
3. Akuffo H, *et al.* The use of itraconazole in the treatment of leishmaniasis caused by Leishmania aethiopica. *Trans R Soc Trop Med Hyg* 1990; **84:** 532–4.

Preparations

Proprietary Preparations (details are given in Part 3)

Aust.: Sporanox; ***Austral.:*** Sporanox; ***Belg.:*** Sporanox; ***Canad.:*** Sporanox; ***Fr.:*** Sporanox; ***Ger.:*** Sempera; Siros; ***Irl.:*** Sporanox; ***Ital.:*** Sporanox; Triasporin; ***Neth.:*** Trisporal; ***Norw.:*** Sporanox; ***S.Afr.:*** Sporanox; ***Spain:*** Canadiol; Hongoseril; Sporanox; ***Swed.:*** Sporanox; ***Switz.:*** Sporanox; ***UK:*** Sporanox; ***USA:*** Sporanox.

Ketoconazole (2589-g)

Ketoconazole *(BAN, USAN, rINN)*.

Ketoconazolum; R-41400. (±)-*cis*-1-Acetyl-4-{4-[2-(2,4-dichlorophenyl)-2-imidazol-1-ylmethyl-1,3-dioxolan-4-yl-methoxy]phenyl}piperazine.

$C_{26}H_{28}Cl_2N_4O_4$ = 531.4.

CAS — 65277-42-1.

Pharmacopoeias. In *Eur.* (see p.viii) and *US.*

A white or almost white powder. Practically **insoluble** in water; sparingly soluble in alcohol; soluble in methyl alcohol; freely soluble in dichloromethane. **Protect** from light.

Adverse Effects

Gastro-intestinal disturbances are the most frequently reported adverse effect following the oral administration of ketoconazole. Nausea and vomiting have been reported in 3 to 10% of patients, and abdominal pain in about 1%. These adverse effects are dose-related and may be minimised by giving ketoconazole with food. Asymptomatic, transient elevations in serum concentrations of liver enzymes may occur in about 10% of patients. Hepatitis has been reported and the risk appears to increase if treatment with ketoconazole is continued for longer than 2 weeks; it is usually reversible on discontinuation of ketoconazole but fatalities have occurred. Ketoconazole interferes with steroid biosynthesis and reported adverse endocrine effects include gynaecomastia, oligospermia, and adrenal cortex suppression.

Other adverse effects include allergic reactions such as urticaria and angioedema, pruritus, rash, alopecia, headache, dizziness, and somnolence. Thrombocytopenia, paraesthesia, and photophobia have been reported rarely.

After topical administration of ketoconazole, irritation, dermatitis, or a burning sensation has occurred.

Effects on endocrine function. References.

1. DeFelice R, *et al.* Gynecomastia with ketoconazole. *Antimicrob Agents Chemother* 1981; **19:** 1073–4.
2. Pont A, *et al.* High-dose ketoconazole therapy and adrenal and testicular function in humans. *Arch Intern Med* 1984; **144:** 2150–3.
3. White MC, Kendall-Taylor P. Adrenal hypofunction in patients taking ketoconazole. *Lancet* 1985; **i:** 44–5.
4. Dandona P, *et al.* Non-suppression of cortisol secretion by long term treatment with ketoconazole in patients with acute leukaemia. *J Clin Pathol* 1985; **38:** 677–8.
5. Pillans PI, *et al.* Hyponatraemia and confusion in a patient taking ketoconazole. *Lancet* 1985; **i:** 821–2.
6. McCance DR, *et al.* Acute hypoadrenalism and hepatotoxicity after treatment with ketoconazole. *Lancet* 1987; **i:** 573.
7. Best TR, *et al.* Persistent adrenal insufficiency secondary to low-dose ketoconazole therapy. *Am J Med* 1987; **82:** 676–80.
8. Khosla S, *et al.* Adrenal crisis in the setting of high-dose ketoconazole therapy. *Arch Intern Med* 1989; **149:** 802–4.

Effects on the liver. Transient minor elevations of liver enzymes without clinical signs or symptoms of hepatic disease occur in about 10% of patients given ketoconazole and may occur at any stage of treatment. Although this reaction is not usually clinically important it may signal the onset of more serious hepatic injury and indicates the need for close monitoring of liver function. Symptomatic hepatic reactions are much rarer occurring in less than 0.1% of patients but are potentially fatal. There is usually a hepatocellular pattern of damage and sometimes cholestasis. Patients at increased risk of hepatic injury include those with a history of liver disease, those aged over 50, especially women, and those requiring prolonged treatment. It is important to monitor liver function during treatment as well as to limit the length of treatment. If liver enzyme values continue to rise or jaundice or hepatitis occur, ketoconazole should be withdrawn immediately since fatalities have occurred in patients who continued treatment after signs of hepatic injury developed.

References.

1. Janssen PA, Symoens JE. Hepatic reactions during ketoconazole treatment. *Am J Med* 1983; **74:** 80–5.
2. Lewis JH, *et al.* Hepatic injury associated with ketoconazole therapy. *Gastroenterology* 1984; **86:** 503–13.
3. Lake-Bakaar G, *et al.* Hepatic reactions associated with ketoconazole in the United Kingdom. *Br Med J* 1987; **294:** 419–21.

Precautions

Since ketoconazole has been reported to cause hepatotoxicity it should not be administered to patients with pre-existing liver disease. Patients receiving ketoconazole should be monitored for symptoms of hepatitis; also, liver function tests should be performed before commencement of treatment with ketoconazole lasting for more than 14 days and then at least monthly throughout treatment.

Ketoconazole has been shown to be teratogenic in *animal* studies and its use is generally not recommended during pregnancy. It should be avoided in breast-feeding women. For further information, see under Pregnancy in Fluconazole, Precautions, p.378.

AIDS. Hypochlorhydria, which may be present in patients with AIDS, can reduce the absorption of ketoconazole. As demonstrated in healthy subjects,[1] absorption may be improved by administering the ketoconazole with an acidic cola beverage.

1. Chin TWF, *et al.* Effects of an acidic beverage (Coca-Cola) on absorption of ketoconazole. *Antimicrob Agents Chemother* 1995; **39:** 1671–5.

Porphyria. Ketoconazole was considered to be unsafe in patients with acute porphyria because it has been shown to be porphyrinogenic in *animals* or *in vitro* systems.[1]

1. Moore MR, McColl KEL. *Porphyria: drug lists.* Glasgow: Porphyria Research Unit, University of Glasgow, 1991.

Interactions

Concomitant administration of drugs that reduce stomach acidity, such as antimuscarinics, antacids, histamine H_2-receptor antagonists, and proton pump inhibitors, may reduce the absorption of ketoconazole. Absorption of ketoconazole may also be reduced by sucralfate. Concomitant administration of ketoconazole with enzyme-inducing drugs such as rifampicin, isoniazid, or phenytoin may reduce plasma-ketoconazole concentrations. Concentrations of isoniazid and rifampicin may also be reduced by ketoconazole. Ketoconazole inhibits certain hepatic oxidase enzymes especially cytochrome P450 (CYP3A4) and may account for increases in plasma concentrations of some hepatically metabolised drugs such as alfentanil, the antihistamines astemizole and terfenadine, benzodiazepines, cisapride, corticosteroids, cyclosporin, delavirdine, HIV-protease inhibitors such as indinavir or ritonavir (which may increase plasma concentrations of ketoconazole in turn), oral anticoagulants, paclitaxel, sertindole, statins such as lovastatin or simvastatin, tacrolimus, tolbutamide, and zidovudine.

There is a risk of cardiac arrhythmias if ketoconazole is used concomitantly with astemizole, cisapride, or terfenadine and such combinations should be avoided.

A disulfiram-like reaction may occur in patients taking ketoconazole after drinking alcohol. The efficacy of oral contraceptives may be reduced.

Antimicrobial Action

Ketoconazole is an imidazole antifungal which interferes with ergosterol synthesis and therefore alters the permeability of the cell membrane of sensitive fungi. It is reported to be fungistatic at concentrations achieved clinically. Ketoconazole has a wide spectrum of antimicrobial activity including activity against *Blastomyces dermatitidis, Candida* spp., *Coccidioides immitis, Epidermophyton floccosum, Histoplasma capsulatum, Malassezia furfur, Microsporum canis, Paracoccidioides brasiliensis, Trichophyton mentagrophytes,* and *T. rubrum.* Some strains of *Aspergillus* spp., *Cryptococcus neoformans,* and *Sporothrix schenckii* are sensitive. MIC values for ketoconazole are dependent on the method used for their determination, and are not always predictive of *in vivo* activity. Ketoconazole has activity against some Gram-positive bacteria and some antiprotozoal activity against *Leishmania* spp. There are rare reports of *Candida albicans* acquiring resistance to ketoconazole.

Microbiological interactions. For the effect of imidazoles and amphotericin on each other's antimicrobial activity, see Amphotericin, p.373.

Resistance. For a discussion of increasing resistance of *Candida* spp. to azoles see Fluconazole, Antimicrobial Action, p.378.

Pharmacokinetics

The absorption of ketoconazole from the gastro-intestinal tract is variable and increases with decreasing stomach pH. It is recommended that ketoconazole is given with food to increase absorption and reduce gastro-intestinal disturbances, although reduced rate and extent of absorption have occurred when given after a meal. Mean peak plasma concentrations of about 3.5 μg per mL have been obtained 2 hours after administration of 200 mg by mouth. Systemic absorption following topical or vaginal application in healthy subjects is minimal. Ketoconazole is more than 90% bound to plasma proteins, mainly albumin. It is widely distributed and appears in breast milk. Penetration into the CSF is poor. The elimination of ketoconazole is reported to be biphasic, with an initial half-life of 2 hours and a terminal half-life of about 8 hours.

Ketoconazole is metabolised in the liver to inactive metabolites. It is excreted as metabolites and unchanged drug chiefly in the faeces; some is excreted in the urine.

References.

1. Daneshmend TK, Warnock DW. Clinical pharmacokinetics of ketoconazole. *Clin Pharmacokinet* 1988; **14:** 13–34.
2. Lelawongs P, *et al.* Effect of food and gastric acidity on absorption of orally administered ketoconazole. *Clin Pharm* 1988; **7:** 228–35.
3. Lake-Bakaar G, *et al.* Gastropathy and ketoconazole malabsorption in the acquired immunodeficiency syndrome (AIDS). *Ann Intern Med* 1988; **109:** 471–3.
4. Daneshmend TK. Diseases and drugs but not food decrease ketoconazole 'bioavailability'. *Br J Clin Pharmacol* 1990; **29:** 783–4.

Uses and Administration

Ketoconazole is an imidazole antifungal administered topically or by mouth. It is given by mouth in chronic mucocutaneous candidiasis, in fungal infections of the gastro-intestinal tract, in dermatophyte infections of the skin and fingernails not responding to topical treatment, and in systemic infections including blastomycosis, candidiasis, coccidioidomycosis, histoplasmosis, and paracoccidioidomycosis. It has been given for the prophylaxis of fungal infections in immunocompromised patients although fluconazole or itraconazole are usually preferred. It has been recommended that because of its erratic absorption and slow therapeutic response, ketoconazole should not be used for the treatment of life-threatening fungal infections including fungal meningitis or for severe infections in immunocompromised patients. Also because of the risk of hepatotoxicity with ketoconazole, its use in nonsystemic fungal infections tends to be restricted to serious infections resistant to other treatment.

The place of ketoconazole in the treatment of fungal infections is discussed under Choice of Antifungal, p.367.

The usual oral dose for treatment and prophylaxis of fungal infections is 200 mg once daily taken with food. This may be increased to 400 mg daily if an adequate response is not obtained; in some infections even higher doses have been used. Children may be given approximately 3 mg per kg body-weight daily, or 50 mg for those aged 1 to 4 years and 100 mg for children aged 5 to 12 years. Treatment should usually be continued for 14 days and for at least one week after symptoms have cleared and cultures have become negative. Some infections may require several months' treatment and administering ketoconazole for such prolonged periods may increase the risk of liver toxicity.

A dose of 400 mg once daily for 5 days is used for the treatment of chronic vaginal candidiasis.

Ketoconazole is applied topically as a 2% cream in the treatment of candidal or dermatophyte infections of the skin, or in the treatment of pityriasis versicolor. It is applied once or twice daily and continued for at least a few days after the disappearance of symptoms. A shampoo containing 2% ketoconazole is applied twice weekly for 2 to 4 weeks in the treatment of seborrhoeic dermatitis or once daily for up to 5 days in pityriasis versicolor.

Acanthamoeba infections. Although there is currently no established treatment for granulomatous amoebic encephalitis, ketoconazole may have some activity against the *Acanthamoeba* spp. responsible for this infection and has been applied topically to skin lesions. Ketoconazole has also been suggested for *Acanthamoeba* keratitis (p.573), when it has been given orally in combination with topical miconazole.

Acute respiratory distress syndrome. Ketoconazole is one of a number of agents which has been shown in preliminary studies to prevent or reduce the development of acute respiratory distress syndrome (ARDS) in patients with sepsis. For a discussion of the overall management of ARDS, see p.1017. In two small double-blind, controlled trials,[1,2] the development of ARDS and mortality rates were lower in high-risk patients who received ketoconazole than in those who received placebo. In an accompanying editorial,[3] Slotman commented that the achievement of adequate blood concentrations appeared to be essential. The mode of action could be associated with inhibition of leukotriene and thromboxane synthesis.[2,3]

1. Slotman GJ, *et al.* Ketoconazole prevents acute respiratory failure in critically ill surgical patients. *J Trauma* 1988; **28:** 648–54.
2. Yu M, Tomasa G. A double-blind, prospective, randomized trial of ketoconazole, a thromboxane synthetase inhibitor, in the prophylaxis of the adult respiratory distress syndrome. *Crit Care Med* 1993; **21:** 1635–42.
3. Slotman GJ. Ketoconazole: maybe it isn't the magic potion, but ... *Crit Care Med* 1993; **21:** 1642–4.

Endocrine disorders and malignant neoplasms. Ketoconazole has been reported to impair steroid hormone synthesis[1] and to blunt the response of cortisone to adrenocorticotrophic hormone (ACTH)[2] and has been tried in the management of a number of endocrine disorders.

In **Cushing's syndrome** (p.1236) there have been a few reports of patients responding to ketoconazole in doses of 600 to 1200 mg daily,[3,4] including regression of a metastatic adrenal carcinoma in 1 patient.[5] Definitive treatment is usually aimed at correcting the underlying pathology, and drug therapy often has an adjuvant or palliative role. Good results have been reported from the use of ketoconazole as an adjuvant to pituitary radiotherapy.[12]

Treatment of **hirsutism** is usually with an anti-androgen (see p.1441), but ketoconazole has been tried in small numbers of women at a dose of 400 mg daily with variable results.[6,7]

Ketoconazole was reported to produce a beneficial response in 3 boys with a form of **precocious puberty** (p.1241) that does not generally respond to gonadorelin analogues.[8]

The anti-androgenic effects of ketoconazole have also been found useful in the management of **prostatic cancer** (p.491) in selected patients.[9-11] However, the usual dose of ketoconazole of 1200 mg daily given in 3 doses is frequently poorly tolerated, and other drugs are generally preferred.

1. Pont A, *et al.* Ketoconazole blocks adrenal steroid synthesis. *Ann Intern Med* 1982; **97:** 370–2.
2. White MC, Kendall-Taylor P. Adrenal hypofunction in patients taking ketoconazole. *Lancet* 1985; **i:** 44–5.
3. Angeli A, Frairia R. Ketoconazole therapy in Cushing's disease. *Lancet* 1985; **i:** 821.
4. Shepherd FA, *et al.* Ketoconazole: use in the treatment of ectopic adrenocorticotropic hormone production and Cushing's syndrome in small-cell lung cancer. *Arch Intern Med* 1985; **145:** 863–4.
5. Contreras P, *et al.* Regression of metastatic adrenal carcinoma during palliative ketoconazole treatment. *Lancet* 1985; **ii:** 151–2.
6. Sonino N, *et al.* Low-dose ketoconazole treatment in hirsute women. *J Endocrinol Invest* 1990; **13:** 35–40.
7. Venturoli S, *et al.* Ketoconazole therapy for women with acne and/or hirsutism. *J Clin Endocrinol Metab* 1990; **71:** 335–9.
8. Holland FJ, *et al.* Ketoconazole in the management of precocious puberty not responsive to LHRH-analogue therapy. *N Engl J Med* 1985; **312:** 1023–8.
9. Williams G, *et al.* Objective responses to ketoconazole therapy in patients with relapsed progressive prostatic cancer. *Br J Urol* 1986; **58:** 45–51.
10. Lowe FC, Bamberger MH. Indications for use of ketoconazole in management of metastatic prostate cancer. *Urology* 1990; **36:** 541–5.
11. Mahler C, *et al.* Ketoconazole and liarozole in the treatment of advanced prostatic cancer. *Cancer* 1993; **71:** 1068–73.
12. Estrada J, *et al.* The long-term outcome of pituitary irradiation after unsuccessful transsphenoidal surgery in Cushing's disease. *N Engl J Med* 1997; **336:** 172–7.

Leishmaniasis. As discussed on p.575, ketoconazole has been tried as an alternative to conventional first- and second-line therapy for visceral leishmaniasis[1,2] although reports of treatment have not all been favourable.[3,8]

It has also been tried in cutaneous leishmaniasis. Weinrauch *et al.*[4] reported a cure rate of 70% in over 100 patients with *Leishmania major* infections treated with ketoconazole 200 to 400 mg daily by mouth for 4 to 6 weeks. Ketoconazole was not considered to be effective in infections due to *L. tropica*, *L. aethiopica*,[4] or *L. guyanensis*.[5] Ketoconazole 600 mg daily for 28 days has produced similar results to sodium stibogluconate intramuscularly for 20 days in patients with cutaneous leishmaniasis due to *L. panamensis*.[6] In a Guatemalan study,[7] ketoconazole was less effective than sodium stibogluconate when cutaneous leishmaniasis was due to *L. braziliensis*, but more effective when *L. mexicana* was the cause.

1. Wali JP, *et al.* Ketoconazole in treatment of visceral leishmaniasis. *Lancet* 1990; **330:** 810–11.
2. Wali JP, *et al.* Ketoconazole in the treatment of antimony- and pentamidine-resistant Kala-azar. *J Infect Dis* 1992; **166:** 215–16.
3. Sundar S, *et al.* Ketoconazole in visceral leishmaniasis. *Lancet* 1990; **336:** 1582–3.
4. Weinrauch L, *et al.* Ketoconazole in cutaneous leishmaniasis. *Br J Dermatol* 1987; **117:** 666–7.
5. Dedet J-P, *et al.* Failure to cure Leishmania braziliensis guyanensis cutaneous leishmaniasis with oral ketoconazole. *Trans R Soc Trop Med Hyg* 1986; **80:** 176.
6. Saenz RE, *et al.* Efficacy of ketoconazole against Leishmania braziliensis panamensis cutaneous leishmaniasis. *Am J Med* 1990; **89:** 147–55.
7. Navin TR, *et al.* Placebo-controlled clinical trial of sodium stibogluconate (Pentostam) versus ketoconazole for treating cutaneous leishmaniasis in Guatemala. *J Infect Dis* 1992; **165:** 528–34.
8. Rashid JR, *et al.* The efficacy and safety of ketoconazole in visceral leishmaniasis. *East Afr Med J* 1994; **71:** 392–5.

Seborrhoeic dermatitis. Ketoconazole 2% cream or shampoo is effective in seborrhoeic dermatitis[1,2] where it is usually used together with hydrocortisone (see p.1076).

1. Green CA, *et al.* Treatment of seborrhoeic dermatitis with ketoconazole II: response of seborrhoeic dermatitis of the face, scalp and trunk to topical ketoconazole. *Br J Dermatol* 1987; **116:** 217–21.
2. Katsambas A, *et al.* A double-blind trial of treatment of seborrhoeic dermatitis with 2% ketoconazole cream compared with 1% hydrocortisone cream. *Br J Dermatol* 1989; **121:** 353–7.

Preparations

USP 23: Ketoconazole Tablets.

Proprietary Preparations (details are given in Part 3)
Aust.: Beltop; Nizoral; ***Austral.:*** Nizoral; ***Belg.:*** Nizoral; ***Canad.:*** Nizoral; ***Fr.:*** Ketoderm; Nizoral; ***Ger.:*** Nizoral; Terzolin; ***Irl.:*** Nizoral; ***Ital.:*** Nizoral; Triatop; ***Neth.:*** Nizoral; ***Norw.:*** Fungoral; ***S.Afr.:*** Nizcreme; Nizoral; Nizovules; Nizshampoo; ***Spain:*** Fungarest; Fungo-Hubber; Ketoisdin; Micoticum; Panfungol; ***Swed.:*** Fungoral; ***Switz.:*** Nizoral; ***UK:*** Neutrogena Long Lasting Dandruff Control; Nizoral; ***USA:*** Nizoral.

Lanoconazole (15901-z)

Lanoconazole (*rINN*).

Latoconazole; NND-318; TJN-318. (±)-α-[(*E*)-4-(o-Chlorophenyl)-1,3-dithiolan-2-ylidene]imidazole-1-acetonitrile.

$C_{14}H_{10}ClN_3S_2$ = 319.8.

CAS — 101530-10-3.

Lanoconazole is an imidazole antifungal used topically in the treatment of fungal skin infections. The need for caution when using an azole antifungal in pregnant or lactating patients is discussed under Fluconazole, p.378.

Preparations

Proprietary Preparations (details are given in Part 3)
Jpn: Astat†.

Loflucarban (2576-n)

Loflucarban (*rINN*).

Clofluonide; Dichlorofluorothiocarbanilide. 3,5-Dichloro-4′-fluorothiocarbanilide.

$C_{13}H_9Cl_2FN_2S$ = 315.2.

CAS — 790-69-2.

Loflucarban is an antibacterial and antifungal used as a 1% powder in the treatment of dermatophytosis and pyoderma.

Preparations

Proprietary Preparations (details are given in Part 3)
Austral.: Fluonilid†.

Mepartricin (2590-f)

Mepartricin (*BAN, USAN, rINN*).

Methylpartricin; SN-654; SPA-S-160.

CAS — 11121-32-7.

A mixture of the methyl esters of 2 related polyene antibiotics obtained from a strain of *Streptomyces aureofaciens* or by any other means.

Mepartricin has antifungal and antiprotozoal activity and has been used in vaginal candidiasis and trichomoniasis as pessaries, as a vaginal cream, and as oral tablets. A cream and oral suspension are also available for the treatment of superficial and oral candidiasis. Mepartricin sodium lauryl sulphate is also used.

Mepartricin has been given by mouth in the treatment of benign prostatic hyperplasia (see p.1446 for the more usual treatment).

References.

1. De Bernardi M, *et al.* Pharmacologic treatment of benign prostatic hyperplasia. *Curr Ther Res* 1988; **43:** 1159–72.
2. Lotti T, *et al.* Observations on some hormone fractions in patients with benign prostatic hyperplasia treated with mepartricin. *Curr Ther Res* 1988; **44:** 402–9.
3. Tavanti A, *et al.* Changes in the plasma pattern of sex steroids in patients with liver cirrhosis treated with mepartricin. *J Int Med Res* 1989; **17:** 212–17.
4. Tosto A, *et al.* A double-blind study of the effects of mepartricin in the treatment of obstruction due to benign prostatic hyperplasia. *Curr Ther Res* 1995; **56:** 1270–75.

Preparations

Proprietary Preparations (details are given in Part 3)
Aust.: Iperplasin; ***Belg.:*** Gyno-Montril†; Montricin; Tricandil; ***Ital.:*** Ipertrofan; Montricin; Tricandil; ***Switz.:*** Candidal†; Tricandil†.

Miconazole (2591-d)

Miconazole (*BAN, rINN*).

Miconazolum; R-18134. 1-[2,4-Dichloro-β-(2,4-dichlorobenzyloxy)phenethyl]imidazole.

$C_{18}H_{14}Cl_4N_2O$ = 416.1.

CAS — 22916-47-8.

Pharmacopoeias. In Eur. (see p.viii), Jpn, and US.

White to pale cream powder. Very slightly **soluble** to practically insoluble in water; soluble 1 in 9.5 of alcohol, 1 in 2 of chloroform, 1 in 15 of ether, 1 in 4 of isopropyl alcohol, 1 in 5.3 of methyl alcohol, and 1 in 9 of propylene glycol; freely soluble in acetone and in dimethylformamide. **Protect** from light.

Incompatibility. Leaching of the potentially toxic plasticising agent diethylhexyl phthalate was reported when solutions containing miconazole were stored in PVC containers.[1]

1. Pearson SD, *et al.* Leaching of diethylhexyl phthalate from polyvinyl chloride containers by selected drugs and formulation components. *Am J Hosp Pharm* 1993; **50:** 1405–9.

Stability. Miconazole in castor oil or arachis oil is stable to dry heat sterilisation at 160° for 90 minutes.[1]

1. Lee RLH. Stability of miconazole on dry heating in vegetable oils. *Aust J Hosp Pharm* 1985; **15:** 233–4.

Miconazole Nitrate (2592-n)

Miconazole Nitrate (*BANM, USAN, rINNM*).

Miconazoli Nitras; R-14889.

$C_{18}H_{14}Cl_4N_2O,HNO_3$ = 479.1.

CAS — 22832-87-7.

Pharmacopoeias. In Eur. (see p.viii), Int., Jpn, and US.

A white or almost white, almost odourless, crystalline powder. **Soluble** 1 in 6250 of water, 1 in 312 of alcohol, 1 in 75 of methyl alcohol, 1 in 525 of chloroform, 1 in 119 of propylene glycol, 1 in 1408 of isopropyl alcohol; freely soluble in dimethyl sulphoxide; soluble in dimethylformamide; practically insoluble in ether. **Protect** from light.

Adverse Effects

After the intravenous infusion of miconazole, phlebitis, nausea, vomiting, diarrhoea, anorexia, pruritus, rash, febrile reactions, flushes, drowsiness, and hyponatraemia have been reported. Other effects include hyperlipidaemia, aggregation of erythrocytes, anaemia, and thrombocytosis. Transient tachycardia and other cardiac arrhythmias have followed the rapid intravenous injection of miconazole. Rare adverse effects include acute psychosis, arthralgia, and anaphylaxis. Many of these adverse effects have been associated with the injection vehicle which contains polyethoxylated castor oil (see p.1326).

After administration by mouth, nausea and vomiting have been reported, and also diarrhoea (usually on long-term treatment). There have been allergic reactions, rarely, and isolated reports of hepatitis.

Local irritation and sensitivity reactions may occur when miconazole nitrate is used topically; contact dermatitis has been reported.

Effects on the heart. Bradycardia, progressing to fatal ventricular fibrillation and cardiac arrest, occurred in a heart transplant patient during intravenous infusion of miconazole for an invasive fungal infection.[1]

1. Coley KC, Crain JL. Miconazole-induced fatal dysrhythmia. *Pharmacotherapy* 1997; **17:** 379–82.

Overdosage. A report[1] of a generalised tonic-clonic convulsion in an infant occurring 10 to 15 minutes after infusion of miconazole. A dose of 500 mg rather than the prescribed dose of 50 mg had inadvertently been administered.

1. Coulthard K, *et al.* Convulsions after miconazole overdose. *Med J Aust* 1987; **146:** 57–8.

Precautions

Miconazole should be avoided in patients with hepatic impairment. When administered intravenously the manufacturer recommends that daily doses of up to 2.4 g of miconazole should be diluted to a concentration of 1 mg per mL and infused at a rate of 100 mg per hour to minimise cardiorespiratory toxicity. Haematocrit, haemoglobin, and serum electrolytes and lipids should be monitored regularly.

The basis in miconazole nitrate pessaries and intravaginal cream may interact with latex products including contraceptive diaphragms and condoms.

Miconazole has been fetotoxic at high doses in *animals* and its use is generally not recommended during pregnancy. For further information, see under Pregnancy in Fluconazole, Precautions, p.378.

Porphyria. Miconazole was considered to be unsafe in patients with acute porphyria because it has been shown to be porphyrinogenic in *animals* or *in vitro* systems.[1]

1. Moore MR, McColl KEL. *Porphyria: drug lists.* Glasgow: Porphyria Research Unit, University of Glasgow, 1991.

Interactions

Miconazole may enhance the activity of oral anticoagulants, sulphonylurea hypoglycaemics, or phenytoin. Adverse effects have been reported when miconazole was given concomitantly with carbamazepine. Miconazole could be expected to have effects similar to those of ketoconazole (see p.383) on other drugs metabolised by cytochrome P450 (CYP3A4).

There is a risk of cardiac arrhythmias if miconazole is used concomitantly with astemizole, cisapride, or terfenadine and such combinations should be avoided.

Antimicrobial Action

Miconazole is an imidazole antifungal with similar antimicrobial activity to that of ketoconazole. It also has some activity against *Aspergillus* spp., *Cryptococcus neoformans, Pseudallescheria boydii,* and some Gram-positive bacteria including staphylococci and streptococci.

Microbiological interactions. A study *in vitro* indicating antimicrobial synergism of miconazole and benzoyl peroxide against *Staphylococcus* spp. and *Propionibacterium acnes*.[1]

For the effect on antifungal activity of giving azoles and amphotericin together, see p.373.

1. Vanden Bossche H, *et al*. Synergism of the antimicrobial agents miconazole and benzoyl peroxide. *Br J Dermatol* 1982; **107:** 343–8.

Pharmacokinetics

Miconazole is incompletely absorbed from the gastro-intestinal tract. Doses above 9 mg per kg body-weight by intravenous infusion usually produce peak plasma concentrations above 1 μg per mL. Penetration into the cerebrospinal fluid and sputum is poor but miconazole diffuses well into infected joints. Over 90% is reported to be bound to plasma proteins.

Miconazole is metabolised in the liver to inactive metabolites. From 10 to 20% of an oral or intravenous dose is excreted in the urine as metabolites. About 50% of an oral dose may be excreted mainly unchanged in the faeces. Following intravenous infusion, the elimination pharmacokinetics of miconazole have been described as triphasic, with an initial half-life of about 0.4 hours, an intermediate half-life of about 2.5 hours, and an elimination half-life of about 24 hours.

Very little miconazole is removed by haemodialysis.

There is little absorption through skin or mucous membranes when miconazole nitrate is applied topically.

Reviews.

1. Daneshmend TK, Warnock DW. Clinical pharmacokinetics of systemic antifungal drugs. *Clin Pharmacokinet* 1983; **8:** 17–42.

Uses and Administration

Miconazole is an imidazole antifungal used (sometimes as miconazole lactate or nitrate) in the treatment of superficial candidiasis (p.367), and of the skin infections dermatophytosis and pityriasis versicolor (p.371). It has also been given intravenously in the treatment of disseminated fungal infections, but other azoles are now more commonly used.

Miconazole may be given by mouth in a dose of 120 to 240 mg as oral gel four times daily after food for the treatment of oropharyngeal and intestinal candidiasis. Children aged over 6 years may be given 120 mg four times daily; aged 2 to 6 years, 120 mg twice daily; under 2 years, 60 mg twice daily. For the treatment of oral lesions the oral gel is applied directly. A sustained release lacquer is available for dentures.

Miconazole nitrate is applied once or twice daily as a 2% cream, lotion, or powder in the treatment of fungal infections of the skin including candidiasis, dermatophytosis, and pityriasis versicolor. In the treatment of vaginal candidiasis, 5 g of a 2% intravaginal cream is inserted into the vagina once daily for 10 to 14 days or twice daily for 7 days, or tampons coated with miconazole nitrate 100 mg are inserted daily for 5 days. Miconazole nitrate pessaries may be inserted in dosage regimens of 100 mg once or twice daily for 7 days, 200 or 400 mg daily for 3 days, or in a single dose of 1200 mg.

Intravenous doses of miconazole have ranged from 0.2 g daily to 1.2 g three times daily, depending on the sensitivity and severity of the infection. It should be diluted in sodium chloride 0.9% or glucose 5% and given by slow infusion; the manufacturer recommends that daily doses up to 2.4 g should be diluted to a concentration of 1 mg per mL and infused at a rate of 100 mg per hour, in order to reduce toxicity. Children over 1 year of age may be given 20 to 40 mg per kg body-weight daily but no more than 15 mg per kg of miconazole should be given at each infusion.

Acanthamoeba keratitis. Miconazole has been applied topically in *Acanthamoeba* keratitis (p.573) in combination with systemic treatment with either ketoconazole or itraconazole.

Skin disorders. Topical preparations containing an imidazole such as clotrimazole, ketoconazole, or miconazole usually together with hydrocortisone are used in the management of *seborrhoeic dermatitis* (p.1076). A cream containing miconazole nitrate 2% and benzoyl peroxide 5% has been used topically in the treatment of *acne* (p.1072).

Preparations

BP 1998: Miconazole Cream;
USP 23: Miconazole Injection; Miconazole Nitrate Cream; Miconazole Nitrate Topical Powder; Miconazole Nitrate Vaginal Suppositories.

Proprietary Preparations (details are given in Part 3)
Aust.: Acnidazil; Daktarin; Gyno-Daktarin; Mycoderm†; ***Austral.:*** Daktarin; Fungo; Gyno-Daktarin; Monistat; ***Belg.:*** Albistat; Daktar Duo†; Daktarin; Gyno-Daktarin; ***Canad.:*** Micatin; Monistat; ***Fr.:*** Britane; Daktarin; Gyno-Daktarin; ***Ger.:*** Castellani Neu; Daktar; Derma-Mykotral; Dumicoat; Epi-Monistat; Fungur M; Gyno-Daktar; Gyno-Monistat; Gyno-Mykotral; Infectosoor; Micotar; Mykotin mono; ***Irl.:*** Daktarin; Gyno-Daktarin; ***Ital.:*** Andergin; Daktarin; Fungiderm; Lampomicol†; Micoderm; Micomax; Miconal; Micotef; Miderm; Nizacol; Pivanozolo; Prilagin; ***Jpn:*** Florid-F†; ***Neth.:*** Daktarin; Dermacure; Gyno-Daktarin; ***Norw.:*** Daktar; Dumicoat; ***S.Afr.:*** Daktarin; Gyno-Daktarin; Gynospor; ***Spain:*** Daktarin; Funginazol†; Fungisdin; ***Swed.:*** Daktar; Dumicoat; ***Switz.:*** Daktar†; Daktarin; Dumicoat; Monistat; ***UK:*** Daktarin; Dumicoat; Femeron; Gyno-Daktarin; ***USA:*** Absorbine Antifungal Foot Powder; Anusol Antifungal Foot Powder; Breezee Mist Antifungal; Femizol-M; Fungoid; Lotrimin AF; M-Zole 7 Dual Pack; Maximum Strength Desenex Antifungal; Micatin; Monistat; Ony-Clear; Prescription Strength Desenex; ZeaSorb AF.

Multi-ingredient: ***Aust.:*** Daktacort; Mycocort†; ***Austral.:*** Daktozin; Fungo; ***Belg.:*** Acnidazil; Daktacort; Daktozin; ***Fr.:*** Daktacort; ***Ger.:*** Acnidazil; Daktar-Hydrocortison†; Decoderm tri; ***Irl.:*** Daktacort; ***Ital.:*** Acnidazil; Daktacort†; ***Neth.:*** Acnecure; Acnidazil; Daktacort; ***Norw.:*** Daktacort; ***S.Afr.:*** Acneclear; Acnidazil; Daktacort; Trialone; ***Spain:*** Bexicortil; Brentan; Dermisdin; Nutracel; ***Swed.:*** Cortimyk; Daktacort; ***Switz.:*** Acne Creme Plus; Acnidazil; Daktacort; Decoderm bivalent; ***UK:*** Acnidazil; Daktacort; ***USA:*** Fungoid HC.

Naftifine Hydrochloride (12995-y)

Naftifine Hydrochloride *(BANM, USAN, rINNM).*

AW-105-843; Naftifungin Hydrochloride; SN-105-843 (naftifine). (*E*)-*N*-Cinnamyl-*N*-methyl(1-naphthylmethyl)amine hydrochloride.

$C_{21}H_{21}N,HCl = 323.9.$

CAS — 65472-88-0 (naftifine); 65473-14-5 (naftifine hydrochloride).

Pharmacopoeias. In *US.*

Naftifine hydrochloride is an allylamine derivative (see Terbinafine Hydrochloride, p.387) which is reported to be fungicidal against dermatophytes, but only fungistatic against *Candida* spp.

Naftifine hydrochloride 1% is applied topically once or twice daily for fungal skin infections particularly dermatophytosis and pityriasis versicolor (p.371).

Local adverse reactions such as burning or stinging may occur.

Preparations

USP 23: Naftifine Hydrochloride Cream; Naftifine Hydrochloride Gel.

Proprietary Preparations (details are given in Part 3)
Aust.: Benecut; Exoderil; ***Canad.:*** Naftin; ***Ger.:*** Exoderil; ***Ital.:*** Suadian; ***Spain:*** Micosona; ***Switz.:*** Exoderil†; ***USA:*** Naftin.

Multi-ingredient: ***Aust.:*** Exoderil Zinkpaste; Naftifin Zinkpaste.

Natamycin (2593-h)

Natamycin *(BAN, USAN, pINN).*

Antibiotic A-5283; CL-12625; Pimaricin.

$C_{33}H_{47}NO_{13} = 665.7.$

CAS — 7681-93-8.

Pharmacopoeias. In *Pol.* and *US.*

A polyene antibiotic produced by the growth of *Streptomyces natalensis*. It is an off-white to cream-coloured powder. It may contain up to 3 moles of water.

Practically **insoluble** in water; slightly soluble in methyl alcohol; soluble in glacial acetic acid and dimethylformamide. A 1% aqueous suspension has a pH of 5.0 to 7.5. **Store** in airtight containers. Protect from light.

Adverse Effects and Precautions

Gastro-intestinal disturbances have occurred after the administration of natamycin by mouth. Local application of natamycin has sometimes produced irritation.

Porphyria. Natamycin has been associated with clinical exacerbations of porphyria and is considered unsafe in porphyric patients.[1]

1. Moore MR, McColl KEL. *Porphyria: drug lists.* Glasgow: Porphyria Research Unit, University of Glasgow, 1991.

Antimicrobial Action

Natamycin is a polyene antifungal active against *Candida* and *Fusarium* spp. In addition it is active against the protozoan *Trichomonas vaginalis*.

Pharmacokinetics

Natamycin is poorly absorbed from the gastro-intestinal tract. It is not absorbed through the skin or mucous membranes when applied topically. Following ocular administration, natamycin is present in therapeutic concentrations in corneal stroma but not in intra-ocular fluid; systemic absorption does not usually occur.

Uses and Administration

Natamycin is a polyene antifungal antibiotic used for the local treatment of candidiasis (p.367) and fungal keratitis (p.369). It has also been used in vaginal trichomoniasis (p.577).

A 5% ophthalmic suspension or a 1% ointment of natamycin is used in the treatment of blepharitis, conjunctivitis, or keratitis due to susceptible fungi, including *Fusarium solani*.

Natamycin is given by mouth for the treatment of intestinal candidiasis in a dose of up to 400 mg daily in divided doses, and as 10-mg lozenges or 2.5% drops for oral candidiasis.

Natamycin is used topically for fungal skin infections and for candidal and trichomonal infections of the vagina. Natamycin pessaries have been used.

Preparations

USP 23: Natamycin Ophthalmic Suspension.

Proprietary Preparations (details are given in Part 3)
Belg.: Pimafucin; ***Ger.:*** Deronga Heilpaste; Pima Biciron N; Pimafucin; ***Ital.:*** Natafucin; ***S.Afr.:*** Natacyn; ***UK:*** Pimafucin†; Tymasil†; ***USA:*** Natacyn.

Multi-ingredient: ***Belg.:*** Pimafucort; ***Fr.:*** Pimafucort†; ***Ger.:*** Incut†; Pima Biciron†; Pimafucort; Pimarektal†; ***Ital.:*** Pimafucort†; ***Neth.:*** Pimafucort.

Neticonazole Hydrochloride (4989-z)

Neticonazole Hydrochloride *(rINNM)*.

SS-717. (*E*)-1-{2-(Methylthio)-1-[o-(pentyloxy)phenyl]vinyl}imidazole hydrochloride.

$C_{17}H_{22}N_2OS,HCl = 338.9$.

CAS — 130726-68-0 (neticonazole); 130773-02-3 (neticonazole hydrochloride);.

Neticonazole hydrochloride is an imidazole antifungal used topically in the treatment of superficial fungal infections. The need for caution when using an azole antifungal in pregnant or lactating patients is discussed under Fluconazole, p.378.

Preparations

Proprietary Preparations (details are given in Part 3)
Jpn: Atolant; Methitoral; Newral.

Nifuroxime (2594-m)

Nifuroxime *(rINN)*.

5-Nitro-2-furaldehyde oxime.

$C_5H_4N_2O_4 = 156.1$.

CAS — 6236-05-1.

Nifuroxime is a nitrofuran antimicrobial and has been used with furazolidone to treat vaginal candidiasis and trichomoniasis.

Preparations

Proprietary Preparations (details are given in Part 3)
Multi-ingredient: ***Ital.:*** Ginecofuran; Tricofur†.

Nystatin (2596-v)

Nystatin *(BAN, USAN, rINN)*.

Fungicidin; Nistatina; Nystatinum.

CAS — 1400-61-9.

Pharmacopoeias. In *Eur.* (see p.viii), *Int., Pol.,* and *US* which specify not less than 4400 units per mg. Also in *Jpn* which does not specify potency.

An antifungal substance produced by the growth of certain strains of *Streptomyces noursei*. It contains mainly tetraenes, the principal component being nystatin A_1. It is a yellow to light brown hygroscopic powder with a characteristic odour suggestive of cereals, containing not less than 4400 units per mg of the dried substance. The USP states that nystatin intended for use in extemporaneous preparation of oral suspensions should contain not less than 5000 units per mg.

Very slightly **soluble** to practically insoluble in water; practically insoluble in alcohol, in chloroform, and in ether; freely soluble in dimethylformamide; slightly to sparingly soluble in methyl alcohol, in *n*-propyl alcohol, and in *n*-butyl alcohol. A 3% suspension in water has a pH of 6.0 to 8.0. **Store** in airtight containers at a temperature between 2 and 8° and protect from light.

Adverse Effects

Nausea, vomiting, and diarrhoea have occasionally been reported after the oral administration of nystatin. Oral irritation or sensitisation may occur. Rashes, including urticaria, and rarely the Stevens-Johnson syndrome have been reported. Irritation may occur rarely after the topical use of nystatin.

Effects on the skin. Generalised pustular eruptions were reported in 3 patients following oral administration of nystatin.[1] Subsequent sensitivity testing revealed delayed (type IV) hypersensitivity to nystatin.

1. Küchler A, *et al.* Acute generalized exanthematous pustulosis following oral nystatin therapy: a report of three cases. *Br J Dermatol* 1997; **137:** 808–11.

Antimicrobial Action

Nystatin is a polyene antifungal antibiotic which interferes with the permeability of the cell membrane of sensitive fungi by binding to sterols, chiefly ergosterol. Its main action is against *Candida* spp.

Pharmacokinetics

Nystatin is poorly absorbed from the gastro-intestinal tract. It is not absorbed through the skin or mucous membranes when applied topically.

Administration. In a study in 5 healthy subjects high salivary nystatin concentrations were maintained throughout a 2-hour period during which a controlled-release delivery system was retained in the mouth; concentrations exceeded those achieved with a nystatin pastille.[1] However, a further study[2] found that fungicidal nystatin concentrations were maintained in saliva 5 hours after nystatin pastilles had been used, whereas concentrations were undetectable 2 hours after using an oral suspension.

1. Encarnacion M, Chin I. Salivary nystatin concentrations after administration of an osmotic controlled release tablet and a pastille. *Eur J Clin Pharmacol* 1994; **46:** 533–5.
2. Millns B, Martin MV. Nystatin pastilles and suspension in the treatment of oral candidosis. *Br Dent J* 1996; **181:** 209–11.

Uses and Administration

Nystatin is a polyene antifungal antibiotic used for the prophylaxis and treatment of candidiasis of the skin and mucous membranes (see p.367). It has been administered with antibiotics in various regimens to suppress the overgrowth of gastro-intestinal flora and as part of selective decontamination regimens (see p.128).

For the treatment of intestinal or oesophageal candidiasis, nystatin is given in doses of 500 000 or 1 000 000 units by mouth 3 or 4 times a day. In infants and children a dosage of 100 000 units or more may be given 4 times daily.

For the treatment of lesions of the mouth, pastilles or a suspension may be given in a dosage of 100 000 units four times daily. Higher doses of, for example, 500 000 units four times daily, may be needed in immunocompromised patients. The formulation should be kept in contact with the affected area for as long as possible, and patients should avoid taking food or drink earlier than one hour after a dose. In the USA doses of 400 000 to 600 000 units four times daily of the suspension, or 200 000 to 400 000 units four or five times daily as lozenges, are used.

For prophylaxis of intestinal candidiasis in patients receiving broad-spectrum antibiotics, a total dose of 1 000 000 units daily may be given. A suggested prophylactic dose for infants born to mothers with vaginal candidiasis is 100 000 units daily.

For the treatment of vaginal infections nystatin is administered in a dosage of 100 000 to 200 000 units daily for 14 days as pessaries or vaginal cream. For cutaneous lesions, ointment, gel, cream, or dusting powder containing 100 000 units per g may be applied 2 to 4 times daily.

A liposomal formulation of nystatin for *parenteral* administration is under investigation.

Administration. LIPOSOMAL FORMULATIONS. References.

1. Wasan KM, *et al.* Physical characteristics and lipoprotein distribution of liposomal nystatin in human plasma. *Antimicrob Agents Chemother* 1997; **41:** 1871–5.

Preparations

BP 1998: Nystatin Ointment; Nystatin Oral Suspension; Nystatin Pessaries; Nystatin Tablets;
USP 23: Demeclocycline Hydrochloride and Nystatin Capsules; Demeclocycline Hydrochloride and Nystatin Tablets; Nystatin and Triamcinolone Acetonide Cream; Nystatin and Triamcinolone Acetonide Ointment; Nystatin Cream; Nystatin for Oral Suspension; Nystatin Lotion; Nystatin Lozenges; Nystatin Ointment; Nystatin Oral Suspension; Nystatin Tablets; Nystatin Topical Powder; Nystatin Vaginal Suppositories; Nystatin Vaginal Tablets; Nystatin, Neomycin Sulfate, Gramicidin, and Triamcinolone Acetonide Cream; Nystatin, Neomycin Sulfate, Gramicidin, and Triamcinolone Acetonide Ointment; Oxytetracycline and Nystatin Capsules; Oxytetracycline and Nystatin for Oral Suspension; Tetracycline Hydrochloride and Nystatin Capsules.

Proprietary Preparations (details are given in Part 3)
Aust.: Candio; Mycostatin; ***Austral.:*** Mycostatin; Nilstat; ***Belg.:*** Nilstat; ***Canad.:*** Candistatin; Mycostatin; Nadostine; Nilstat; Nyaderm; ***Fr.:*** Mycostatine; ***Ger.:*** Adiclair; Biofanal; Candida-Lokalicid†; Candio; Cordes Nystatin Soft; Fungireduct; Lederlind; Moronal; Mykoderm; MykoPosterine N; Mykundex; Mykundex Ovula†; Nystaderm; ***Irl.:*** Mycostatin; ***Ital.:*** Mycostatin; ***Norw.:*** Mycostatin; ***S.Afr.:*** Canstat; Mycostatin; Nystacid; ***Spain:*** Mycostatin; ***Swed.:*** Mycostatin; ***Switz.:*** Candio; Mycostatine; Rivostatin; ***UK:*** Infestat; Nyspes; Nystamont; Nystan; Nystatin-Dome; ***USA:*** Mycostatin; Nilstat; Nystex; Nystop.

Multi-ingredient: ***Aust.:*** Mycostatin V; Mycostatin-Zinkoxid; Topsym polyvalent; ***Austral.:*** Aristocomb; Kenacomb; Mysteclin-V; Otocomb Otic; Tetrex-F†; ***Belg.:*** Eoline; Flogocid; Mycolog; Polygynax; ***Canad.:*** Flagystatin; Halcicomb†; Kenacomb; Lidecomb†; Triacomb; Viaderm-KC; ***Fr.:*** Auricularum; Myco-Ultralan; Mycolog; Mycomnes; Polygynax; Polygynax Virgo; Tergynan; ***Ger.:*** Aureomycin N; Candio E comp N; Halog Tri; Heliomycort†; Jellin polyvalent; Lokalison-antimikrobiell Creme N; Moronal V; Moronal V N†; Moronal†; Multilind; Myco-Intradermi†; mykoproct sine; mykoproct†; Mykundex Heilsalbe; Nystaderm Comp; Nystalocal; Polygynax; Topsym polyvalent; Volonimat Plus N; ***Irl.:*** Flagyl Compak; Kenacomb; Nystaform; Nystaform-HC; Terra-Cortril Nystatin; Timodine; Tinaderm-M; ***Ital.:*** Assocort; Combiderm†; Desalfa; Fasigin N; Halciderm Combi; Macmiror Complex; Mycocur†; ***Neth.:*** Mycolog; ***S.Afr.:*** Duoderm†; Hiconcil-NS; Kenacomb; Pentrex-F†; Riostatin; Tetrex-F; ***Spain:*** Deltasiton; Interderm; Intradermo Cort Ant Fung; Milrosina Nistatina; Positon; Pulverodil†; Sudermin†; Tododermil Compuesto; ***Swed.:*** Kenacombin Novum; Kenacombin†; ***Switz.:*** Candio E†; Cervicaletten†; Dafnegil; Dermovate-NN; Flogocid NN; Halciderm comp†; Multilind; Mycolog; Nystacortone; Nystalocal; Topsym polyvalent; ***UK:*** Dermovate-NN; Flagyl Compak; Gregoderm; Mysteclin†; Nystadermal; Nystaform; Nystaform-HC; Nystaform†; Terra-Cortril Nystatin; Timodine; Tinaderm-M; Tri-Adcortyl; Tri-Cicatrin†; Trimovate; ***USA:*** Myco-Biotic II; Myco-Triacet II; Mycogen II; Mycolog-II; Myconel; Mytrex; NGT; Pedi-Dri; Tri-Statin II.

Omoconazole Nitrate (5542-z)

Omoconazole Nitrate *(USAN, rINNM)*.

10-80-07. (*Z*)-1-{2,4-Dichloro-β-[2-(*p*-chlorophenoxy)ethoxy]-α-methylstyryl}imidazole nitrate.

$C_{20}H_{17}Cl_3N_2O_2,HNO_3 = 486.7$.

CAS — 74512-12-2 (omoconazole); 83621-06-1 (omoconazole nitrate).

Omoconazole nitrate is an imidazole antifungal used locally for fungal skin infections (p.371) and for vaginal candidiasis (p.367). It is applied topically as a 1% cream, powder, or solution in the treatment of cutaneous candidiasis, dermatophytosis, and pityriasis versicolor. For vaginal candidiasis, omoconazole nitrate is given as pessaries in doses of 150 mg daily for 6 days, 300 mg daily for 3 days, or 900 mg as a single dose.

The need for caution when using an azole antifungal in pregnant or lactating patients is discussed under Fluconazole, p.378.

Preparations

Proprietary Preparations (details are given in Part 3)
Aust.: Azameno; ***Belg.:*** Fongarex; ***Fr.:*** Fongamil; Fongarex; ***Ger.:*** Fungisan; ***Ital.:*** Afongan; ***Spain:*** Afongan; Fongamil; ***Switz.:*** Azameno.

Oxiconazole Nitrate (16940-q)

Oxiconazole Nitrate *(BANM, USAN, rINNM)*.

Ro-13-8996; Ro-13-8996/001; Ro-13-8996/000 (oxiconazole); SGD-301-76; ST-813. 2′,4′-Dichloro-2-imidazol-1-ylacetophenone (*Z*)-*O*-(2,4-dichlorobenzyl)oxime mononitrate.

$C_{18}H_{13}Cl_4N_3O,HNO_3 = 492.1$.

CAS — 64211-46-7 (oxiconazole nitrate); 64211-45-6 (oxiconazole).

Oxiconazole nitrate is an imidazole antifungal applied topically as a cream, solution, or powder equivalent to oxiconazole 1% in the treatment of fungal infections of the skin (p.371). It is also given as a 600-mg pessary in the treatment of vaginal candidiasis (p.367).

Local reactions including burning and itching have been reported.

The need for caution when using an azole antifungal in pregnant or lactating patients is discussed under Fluconazole, p.378.

Reviews.

1. Jegasothy BV, Pakes GE. Oxiconazole nitrate: pharmacology, efficacy, and safety of a new imidazole antifungal agent. *Clin Ther* 1991; **13:** 126–41.

Preparations

Proprietary Preparations (details are given in Part 3)
Aust.: Gyno Oceral; Gyno-Liderman; Liderman; Oceral; ***Fr.:*** Fonx; ***Ger.:*** Myfungar; Oceral GB; ***Spain:*** Salongo; ***Switz.:*** Gyno-Myfungar; Myfungar; Oceral; ***USA:*** Oxistat.

Pentamycin (3000-z)

$C_{35}H_{58}O_{12} = 670.8$.

CAS — 6834-98-6.

Pentamycin is a polyene antifungal obtained from *Streptomyces pentaticus*. It is used in the treatment of vaginal candidiasis and for the protozoal infection trichomoniasis. One or two 3-mg vaginal pessaries are inserted for 5 to 10 consecutive days.

Preparations

Proprietary Preparations (details are given in Part 3)
Ital.: Cantricin†; Pentacin†; ***Switz.:*** Pentacine.

Propionic Acid (3001-c)

E280; E282 (calcium propionate); E283 (potassium propionate). Propanoic acid.

$C_2H_5.CO_2H = 74.08$.

CAS — 79-09-4.

Pharmacopoeias. In *Fr.* Also in *USNF.*

An oily liquid having a slight pungent, rancid odour. **Miscible** with water, alcohol, and various other organic solvents. **Store** in airtight containers.

Sodium Propionate (3005-x)

E281. Sodium propanoate.

$C_3H_5NaO_2 = 96.06$.

CAS — 137-40-6 (anhydrous sodium propionate); 6700-17-0 (sodium propionate hydrate).

Pharmacopoeias. In *Fr.* Also in *BP(Vet)* and *USNF.*

Colourless transparent crystals or white granular crystalline powder; odourless or with a slight characteristic odour. Deliquescent in moist air. **Soluble** 1 in 1 of water, 1 in 0.65 of boiling water, and 1 in 24 of alcohol; practically insoluble in chloroform and ether. **Store** in airtight containers.

Propionic acid and its salts are antifungals.

Sodium propionate has been used topically, usually in combination with other antimicrobial agents for the treatment of dermatophyte infections. Eye drops containing sodium propionate have also been used.

Propionic acid and its calcium, sodium, and potassium salts are used in the baking industry as inhibitors of moulds.

Preparations

Proprietary Preparations (details are given in Part 3)
Ital.: Propionat.

Multi-ingredient: ***Aust.:*** Dermowund; ***Austral.:*** Mycoderm; Oticane†; ***Canad.:*** Amino-Cerv; ***Fr.:*** Angispray; Anti-Rhinyl†; Dermacide; Rhinyl; ***Ger.:*** Onymyken S†; ***Ital.:*** Propiazol†; Undetin†; ***S.Afr.:*** Neopan; ***Spain:*** Undehache†; ***USA:*** Amino-Cerv; Prophyllin.

Protiofate (14254-z)

Protiofate *(rINN).*

Dipropyl 3,4-dihydroxy-2,5-thiophenedicarboxylate.

$C_{12}H_{16}O_6S = 288.3$.

CAS — 58416-00-5.

Protiofate is a thiophene derivative with antifungal and antiprotozoal activity. It has been used locally in the treatment of vaginal candidiasis and trichomoniasis.

Preparations

Proprietary Preparations (details are given in Part 3)
Ital.: Atrimycon†.

Pyrrolnitrin (3002-k)

Pyrrolnitrin *(USAN, rINN).*

52230; NSC-107654. 3-Chloro-4-(3-chloro-2-nitrophenyl)pyrrole.

$C_{10}H_6Cl_2N_2O_2 = 257.1$.

CAS — 1018-71-9.

Pyrrolnitrin is an antifungal antibiotic isolated from *Pseudomonas pyrrocinia* and applied topically in the treatment of superficial fungal infections.

Preparations

Proprietary Preparations (details are given in Part 3)
Ital.: Micutrin.

Multi-ingredient: ***Ital.:*** Micomplex†; Micutrin Beta.

Saperconazole (6498-l)

Saperconazole *(BAN, USAN, rINN).*

R-66905. 2-*sec*-Butyl-4-[4-(4-{4-[(2*RS*,4*SR*)-2-(2,4-difluorophenyl)-2-(1*H*-1,2,4-triazol-1-ylmethyl)-1,3-dioxolan-4-ylmethoxy]phenyl}piperazin-1-yl)phenyl]-2,4-dihydro-1,2,4-triazol-3-one.

$C_{35}H_{38}F_2N_8O_4 = 672.7$.

CAS — 110588-57-3.

Saperconazole is a triazole derivative under investigation for the treatment of systemic fungal infections.

The need for caution when using an azole antifungal in pregnant or lactating patients is discussed under Fluconazole, p.378.

References.

1. Odds FC. Antifungal activity of saperconazole (R66905) in vitro. *J Antimicrob Chemother* 1989; **24:** 533–7.
2. Franco L, *et al.* Saperconazole in the treatment of systemic and subcutaneous mycoses. *Int J Dermatol* 1992; **31:** 725–9.

Sertaconazole Nitrate (17275-r)

Sertaconazole Nitrate *(rINNM).*

Sertaconazoli Nitras. (±)-1-{2,4-Dichloro-β-[(7-chlorobenzo[*b*]thien-3-yl)methoxy]phenethyl}imidazole nitrate.

$C_{20}H_{15}Cl_3N_2OS,HNO_3 = 500.8$.

CAS — 99592-32-2 (sertaconazole); 99592-39-9 (sertaconazole nitrate).

Pharmacopoeias. In *Eur.* (see p.viii).

A white or almost white powder. Practically **insoluble** in water; sparingly soluble in alcohol and in dichloromethane; soluble in methyl alcohol. **Protect** from light.

Sertaconazole nitrate is an imidazole antifungal used topically in the treatment of superficial candidiasis, dermatophytosis, and pityriasis versicolor.

The need for caution when using an azole antifungal in pregnant or lactating patients is discussed under Fluconazole, p.378.

Preparations

Proprietary Preparations (details are given in Part 3)
Ger.: Zalain; ***Spain:*** Dermofix; Dermoseptic; Zalain.

Sulbentine (3006-r)

Sulbentine *(rINN).*

Dibenzthion; Sulbentinum. 3,5-Dibenzyltetrahydro-2*H*-1,3,5-thiadiazine-2-thione.

$C_{17}H_{18}N_2S_2 = 314.5$.

CAS — 350-12-9.

Sulbentine is an antifungal that was applied topically as a nail lacquer in the treatment of fungal nail infections.

Preparations

Proprietary Preparations (details are given in Part 3)
Ger.: Fungiplex†.

Sulconazole Nitrate (16999-m)

Sulconazole Nitrate *(BANM, USAN, rINNM).*

RS-44872; RS-44872-00-10-3. 1-[2,4-Dichloro-β-(4-chlorobenzyl)thiophenethyl]imidazole nitrate.

$C_{18}H_{15}Cl_3N_2S,HNO_3 = 460.8$.

CAS — 61318-90-9 (sulconazole); 61318-91-0 (sulconazole nitrate).

Pharmacopoeias. In *Fr.* and *US.*

White to almost white crystalline powder. **Soluble** 1 in 3333 of water, 1 in 100 of alcohol, 1 in 130 of acetone, 1 in 333 of chloroform, 1 in 286 of dichloromethane, 1 in 2000 of dioxan, 1 in 71 of methyl alcohol, 1 in 10 of pyridine, and 1 in 2000 of toluene. **Protect** from light.

Adverse Effects and Precautions

Local reactions including burning, itching, and erythema have been reported following sulconazole use.

For information about the use of sulconazole during pregnancy and lactation see under Pregnancy in Fluconazole, Precautions, p.378.

Antimicrobial Action

Sulconazole is an imidazole antifungal with activity against dermatophytes, *Candida* spp., and *Malassezia furfur.*

Uses and Administration

Sulconazole nitrate is an imidazole antifungal applied topically once or twice daily as a 1% cream or solution in the treatment of fungal skin infections including dermatophyte infections and pityriasis versicolor (p.371), and candidiasis (p.367).

Reviews.

1. Benfield P, Clissold SP. Sulconazole: a review of its antimicrobial activity and therapeutic use in superficial dermatomycoses. *Drugs* 1988; **35:** 143–53.

Preparations

Proprietary Preparations (details are given in Part 3)
Belg.: Myk-1; ***Fr.:*** Myk; ***Irl.:*** Exelderm; ***Ital.:*** Exelderm; ***Neth.:*** Myk-1; ***UK:*** Exelderm; ***USA:*** Exelderm.

Terbinafine Hydrochloride (14747-y)

Terbinafine Hydrochloride *(BANM, rINNM).*

SF-86-327 (terbinafine). (*E*)-6,6-Dimethylhept-2-en-4-ynl(methyl)-(1-naphthylmethyl)amine hydrochloride.

$C_{21}H_{26}ClN = 327.9$.

CAS — 91161-71-6 (terbinafine); 78628-80-5 (terbinafine hydrochloride).

NOTE. Terbinafine is *USAN.*

Adverse Effects

The most frequent adverse effects following oral administration of terbinafine hydrochloride are gastro-intestinal disturbances such as nausea, diarrhoea, anorexia, and mild abdominal pain; headache; and skin reactions including rash or urticaria sometimes with arthralgia or myalgia. Severe skin reactions including cutaneous lupus erythematosus, pustulosis, Stevens-Johnson syndrome and toxic epidermal necrolysis have occurred rarely. Loss or disturbance of taste, photosensitivity, and liver dysfunction with isolated reports of cholestasis, hepatitis, and jaundice, have occurred.

There may be local reactions after topical use of terbinafine.

Postmarketing surveillance of about 10 000 patients[1] suggested the following incidences of adverse effects to oral terbinafine: gastro-intestinal symptoms, 4.7%; dermatological effects, 3.3%; CNS symptoms (commonly headache), 1.8%; taste disturbances, 0.6%; and transient disturbances in liver function, 0.1%. Serious adverse effects possibly or probably related to terbinafine included angioedema, bronchospasm, erythema multiforme, extended stroke, and unilateral leg oedema.

1. O'Sullivan DP, *et al.* Postmarketing surveillance of oral terbinafine in the UK: report of a large cohort study. *Br J Clin Pharmacol* 1996; **42:** 559–65.

Effects on the blood. Neutropenia in one patient and pancytopenia in a second were associated with oral terbinafine and resolved once the drug was withdrawn.[1]

1. Kovacs MJ, *et al.* Neutropenia and pancytopenia associated with oral terbinafine. *J Am Acad Dermatol* 1994; **31:** 806.

Effects on the eyes. The US manufacturer has noted that changes in the lens and retina of the eye have sometimes been associated with oral terbinafine, although the significance of these changes was not known.

Precautions

Terbinafine should be used with caution in patients with impaired hepatic or renal function. It should not be given during breast feeding.

Psoriasis. It has been suggested that terbinafine may provoke or exacerbate psoriasis,[1] and that it should be avoided in patients with this disorder.

1. Wilson NJE, Evans S. Severe pustular psoriasis provoked by oral terbinafine. *Br J Dermatol* 1998; **139:** 168.

Interactions

Plasma concentrations of terbinafine may be increased by drugs that inhibit its metabolism by cytochrome P450, such as *cimetidine*, and decreased by drugs that induce cytochrome P450, such as *rifampicin*. For the effect of terbinafine on *nortriptyline*, see p.277.

Antimicrobial Action

Terbinafine is an allylamine derivative reported to have a broad spectrum of antifungal activity. It is considered to act through inhibition of fungal sterol synthesis. Terbinafine is fungicidal against dermatophytes and some yeasts but only fungistatic against *Candida albicans.*

References.

1. Petranyi G, *et al.* Antifungal activity of the allylamine derivative terbinafine in vitro. *Antimicrob Agents Chemother* 1987; **31:** 1365–8.
2. Schuster I, Ryder NS. Allylamines—mode and selectivity of action compared to azole antifungals and biological fate in mammalian organisms. *J Dermatol Treat* 1990; **1** (suppl 2): 7–9.
3. Clayton YM. Relevance of broad-spectrum and fungicidal activity of antifungals in the treatment of dermatomycoses. *Br J Dermatol* 1994; **130** (suppl 43): 7–8.
4. Leeming JP, *et al.* Susceptibility of Malassezia furfur subgroups to terbinafine. *Br J Dermatol* 1997; **137:** 764–7.

Microbiological interactions. Additive and synergistic activity was reported with terbinafine in combination with fluconazole or itraconazole against strains of *Candida albicans* that had reduced susceptibility to azoles *in vitro*.[1] Terbinafine was also reported to enhance the activity of azoles against the protozoan *Leishmania braziliensis*.[2]

1. Barchiesi F, *et al.* In vitro activities of terbinafine in combination with fluconazole and itraconazole against isolates of Candida albicans with reduced susceptibility to azoles. *Antimicrob Agents Chemother* 1997; **41:** 1812–14.
2. Rangel H, *et al.* Naturally azole-resistant Leishmania braziliensis promastigotes are rendered susceptible in the presence of terbinafine: comparative study with azole-susceptible Leishmania mexicana promastigotes. *Antimicrob Agents Chemother* 1996; **40:** 2785–91. Correction. *ibid.* 1997; **41:** 496.

Pharmacokinetics

Terbinafine hydrochloride is well absorbed from the gastro-intestinal tract. About 40% of a dose undergoes first-pass hepatic metabolism. Mean peak plasma concentrations of about 1 μg per mL are reported within 2 hours of a single oral dose of 250 mg. Steady state concentrations are about 25% higher than those seen after a single dose and are reached in 10 to 14 days. Terbinafine is extensively bound to plasma proteins. Terbinafine is distributed into the stratum corneum of the skin, the nail plate, and hair where it reaches concentrations considerably higher than those found in plasma. It appears in breast milk. Less than 5% of a topical dose of terbinafine hydrochloride is absorbed.

Terbinafine is metabolised in the liver to inactive metabolites which are excreted mainly in the urine. A plasma elimination half-life varying from 11 to 17 hours has been reported and a terminal elimination half-life of up to 400 hours in patients receiving prolonged therapy, probably representing elimination from skin and adipose tissue. Fungicidal concentrations in nails are maintained for several weeks after therapy is discontinued. The elimination rate may be altered in patients with liver disease or kidney disease.

References.

1. Kovarik JM, *et al.* Multiple-dose pharmacokinetics and distribution in tissue of terbinafine and metabolites. *Antimicrob Agents Chemother* 1995; **39:** 2738–41.

Uses and Administration

Terbinafine hydrochloride is an allylamine antifungal given by mouth in the treatment of dermatophyte infections of the skin and nails (p.371). It is also applied to the skin in dermatophytoses, in pityriasis versicolor (p.371), and in cutaneous candidiasis (p.367).

Terbinafine 250 mg as the hydrochloride is given once daily by mouth for 2 to 4 weeks for tinea cruris; treatment may be continued for 6 weeks for tinea pedis infections; a 4-week course is used in tinea corporis infections. A cream containing 1% terbinafine hydrochloride is applied once or twice daily for 1 to 2 weeks to treat tinea corporis and tinea cruris; a 1-week course is recommended for tinea pedis. A 2-week course of treatment is used in cutaneous candidiasis and pityriasis versicolor.

Dermatophyte infections of the nails are treated with terbinafine 250 mg by mouth, as the hydrochloride, once daily for 6 to 12 weeks although longer treatment may be necessary in toe-nail infections.

Reviews.

1. Balfour JA, Faulds D. Terbinafine: a review of its pharmacodynamic and pharmacokinetic properties, and therapeutic potential in superficial mycoses. *Drugs* 1992; **43:** 259–84.
2. Anonymous. Terbinafine for onychomycosis. *Med Lett Drugs Ther* 1996; **38:** 72–4.
3. Abdel-Rahman SM, Nahata MC. Oral terbinafine: a new antifungal agent. *Ann Pharmacother* 1997; **31:** 445–56.

Administration. INTERMITTENT OR SHORT-COURSE ADMINISTRATION. Intermittent or pulse therapy using terbinafine 1000 mg once every two weeks for 2 or 3 doses[1] or 500 mg daily for one week each month[2] has produced good responses in some patients with fungal nail infections. Similar responses have been reported using terbinafine in conventional doses for 2 weeks.[3] However, patients given a single 1000-mg dose did not respond.[1]

1. Shuster S, Munro CS. Single dose treatment of fungal nail disease. *Lancet* 1992; **339:** 1066.
2. Tosti A, *et al.* Treatment of dermatophyte nail infections: an open randomized study comparing intermittent terbinafine therapy with continuous terbinafine treatment and intermittent itraconazole therapy. *J Am Acad Dermatol* 1996; **34:** 595–600.
3. Wong C-K, Cho Y-L. Very short duration therapy with oral terbinafine for fingernail onychomycosis. *Br J Dermatol* 1995; **133:** 329–31.

Administration in children. Although terbinafine has not generally been recommended for use in children it has been tried in children over 2 years of age in doses of 125 mg daily by mouth for those weighing 20 to 40 kg and 62.5 mg daily for those weighing less than 20 kg.[1]

1. Jones TC. Overview of the use of terbinafine (Lamisil) in children. *Br J Dermatol* 1995; **132:** 683–9.

Administration in hepatic and renal impairment. The manufacturer recommends that patients with chronic stable liver dysfunction or with renal dysfunction (creatinine clearance of less than 50 mL per minute or serum-creatinine concentration of more than 300 μmol per litre) should receive half the usual dose of terbinafine.

Non-dermatophyte fungal infections. Beneficial responses to oral terbinafine have been reported in candidal nail infections,[1,2] aspergillosis,[3] chromoblastomycosis,[4] and sporotrichosis.[5,6]

1. Nolting S, *et al.* Terbinafine in onychomycosis with involvement by non-dermatophytic fungi. *Br J Dermatol* 1994; **130** (suppl 43): 16–21.
2. Segal R, *et al.* Treatment of Candida nail infection with terbinafine. *J Am Acad Dermatol* 1996; **35:** 958–61.
3. Schiraldi GF, *et al.* Refractory pulmonary aspergillosis: compassionate trial with terbinafine. *Br J Dermatol* 1996; **134** (suppl 46): 25–9.
4. Esterre P, *et al.* Treatment of chromomycosis with terbinafine: preliminary results of an open pilot study. *Br J Dermatol* 1996; **134** (suppl 46): 33–6.
5. Hull PR, Vismer HP. Treatment of cutaneous sporotrichosis with terbinafine. *J Dermatol Treat* 1992; **3** (suppl 1): 35–8.
6. Kudoh K, *et al.* Successful treatment of cutaneous sporotrichosis with terbinafine. *J Dermatol Treat* 1996; **7:** 33–5.

Preparations

Proprietary Preparations (details are given in Part 3)
Aust.: Daskil; Lamisil; ***Austral.:*** Lamisil; ***Belg.:*** Lamisil; ***Canad.:*** Lamisil; ***Fr.:*** Lamisil; ***Ger.:*** Lamisil; ***Irl.:*** Lamisil; ***Ital.:*** Daskil; Lamisil; ***Neth.:*** Lamisil; ***Norw.:*** Lamisil; ***S.Afr.:*** Lamisil; ***Spain:*** Lamisil; ***Swed.:*** Lamisil; ***Switz.:*** Lamisil; ***UK:*** Lamisil; ***USA:*** Lamisil.

Terconazole (13307-b)

Terconazole *(BAN, USAN, rINN)*.

R-42470; Terconazolum; Triaconazole. 1-{4-[[2-(2,4-Dichlorophenyl)-*r*-2-(1*H*-1,2,4-triazol-1-ylmethyl)-1,3-dioxolan-*c*-4-yl]methoxy]phenyl}-4-isopropylpiperazine.

$C_{26}H_{31}Cl_2N_5O_3$ = 532.5.

CAS — 67915-31-5.

Pharmacopoeias. In *Eur.* (see p.viii).

A white or almost white powder. Practically **insoluble** in water; sparingly soluble in alcohol; soluble in acetone; freely soluble in dichloromethane. **Protect** from light.

Adverse Effects

Local reactions including burning and itching have been reported with vaginal use of terconazole. Other adverse effects have included dysmenorrhoea and abdominal pain. A flu-like syndrome with headache, fever, chills, and hypotension has been reported in some patients and may be more prevalent with vaginal pessaries providing doses larger than 80 mg.

Flu syndrome. References.

1. Moebius UM. Influenza-like syndrome after terconazole. *Lancet* 1988; **ii:** 966–7.

Precautions

The pessary basis may interact with latex products including contraceptive diaphragms and condoms.

For information about the use of terconazole during pregnancy and lactation, see under Pregnancy in Fluconazole, Precautions, p.378.

Antimicrobial Action

Terconazole is a triazole derivative that binds to fungal cytochrome P450, thus disrupting ergosterol synthesis. Terconazole is active *in vitro* against *Candida* spp. and other fungi. It has some antibacterial activity *in vitro* but not against usual vaginal flora such as lactobacilli.

Pharmacokinetics

Following intravaginal administration, 5 to 16% of terconazole is absorbed. Systemically absorbed drug is metabolised by the liver and excreted in urine and faeces.

Uses and Administration

Terconazole is a triazole antifungal used in the local treatment of vulvovaginal candidiasis (p.367). Intravaginal dosage regimens are terconazole 40 mg (by 0.8% vaginal cream) or 80 mg (by pessary) at bedtime for 3 consecutive nights or 20 mg (by 0.4% cream) at bedtime for 7 consecutive nights.

Preparations

Proprietary Preparations (details are given in Part 3)
Belg.: Gyno-Terazol; ***Canad.:*** Terazol; ***Ital.:*** Terazol†; Terconal; ***Neth.:*** Gyno-Terazol; ***S.Afr.:*** Terazol; ***Swed.:*** Terazol; ***Switz.:*** Gyno-Terazol; ***USA:*** Terazol.

Tioconazole (13348-y)

Tioconazole *(BAN, USAN, rINN)*.

UK-20349. 1-[2,4-Dichloro-β-(2-chloro-3-thenyloxy)phenethyl]imidazole.

$C_{16}H_{13}Cl_3N_2OS$ = 387.7.

CAS — 65899-73-2.

Pharmacopoeias. In *US*.

Store in airtight containers.

Adverse Effects and Precautions

Local reactions to tioconazole including burning, itching, and erythema have been reported.

The ointment basis may interact with rubber or latex products such as condoms and contraceptive diaphragms.

For information about the use of tioconazole during pregnancy and lactation, see under Pregnancy in Fluconazole, Precautions, p.378.

Hypersensitivity. Tioconazole, an imidazole antifungal widely used in Finland, appeared to be an important cause of contact allergy in that country, since an incidence of more than 1% was reported in patients undergoing routine patch testing.[1] There may be cross-reactivity with other commonly used imidazole derivatives.

1. Heikkilä H, *et al.* A study of 72 patients with contact allergy to tioconazole. *Br J Dermatol* 1996; **134:** 678–80.

Antimicrobial Action

Tioconazole is an imidazole antifungal with a broad spectrum of activity including action against dermatophytes, *Malassezia furfur*, and *Candida albicans*. Tioconazole is active *in vitro* against some Gram-positive bacteria.

Uses and Administration

Tioconazole is an imidazole antifungal used in the treatment of superficial candidiasis (p.367), and dermatophytoses and pityriasis versicolor (p.371).

For vaginal candidiasis it is used as pessaries or vaginal cream or ointment in a dose of 100 mg on three consecutive days or as a single 300-mg dose.

It has been applied topically as a 1% cream, lotion, or powder in the treatment of superficial fungal infections. Tioconazole has also been used for nail infections as a 28% w/w topical solution, although systemic treatment is generally preferred.

Reviews.

1. Clissold SP, Heel RC. Tioconazole: a review of its antimicrobial activity and therapeutic use in superficial mycoses. *Drugs* 1986; **31:** 29–51.

Preparations

USP 23: Tioconazole Cream.

Proprietary Preparations (details are given in Part 3)
Aust.: Gyno-Trosyd; Trosyd; ***Canad.:*** Gynecure; Gyno-Trosyd†; Trosyd; ***Fr.:*** Gyno-Trosyd; Trosyd; ***Ger.:*** Fungibacid; Mykontral; ***Irl.:*** Trosyl; ***Ital.:*** Trosyd; Zoniden†; ***S.Afr.:*** Gyno-Trosyd; Trosyd; ***Spain:*** Trosid; ***Switz.:*** Gyno-Trosyd; Trosyd; ***UK:*** Trosyl; ***USA:*** Vagistat.

Multi-ingredient: ***Switz.:*** Trosyd†.

Tolciclate (3008-d)

Tolciclate *(USAN, rINN)*.

K-9147; KC-9147. *O*-(1,2,3,4-Tetrahydro-1,4-methano-6-naphthyl) *m*,*N*-dimethylthiocarbanilate.

$C_{20}H_{21}NOS$ = 323.5.

CAS — 50838-36-3.

Tolciclate is an antifungal with activity against *Epidermophyton*, *Microsporum*, and *Trichophyton* spp. It has been used topically as a 1% cream, lotion, or ointment, or as a 0.5% powder in the treatment of various dermatophyte infections and in pityriasis versicolor.

Preparations

Proprietary Preparations (details are given in Part 3)
Ger.: Fungifos; ***Ital.:*** Tolmicen; ***Switz.:*** Kilmicene†.

Tolnaftate (3009-n)

Tolnaftate *(BAN, USAN, rINN).*

Sch-10144; Tolnaftatum. *O*-2-Naphthyl *m,N*-dimethylthiocarbanilate.

$C_{19}H_{17}NOS$ = 307.4.

CAS — 2398-96-1.

Pharmacopoeias. In *Eur.* (see p.viii), *Jpn*, and *US*.

A white to creamy-white fine powder, odourless or with a slight odour. Practically **insoluble** in water; slightly or very slightly soluble in alcohol; freely soluble in acetone, in chloroform, and in dichloromethane; sparingly soluble in ether. **Store** in airtight containers. Protect from light.

Adverse Effects

Skin reactions occur rarely with tolnaftate and include irritation and contact dermatitis.

Antimicrobial Action

Tolnaftate inhibits the growth of the dermatophytes *Epidermophyton, Microsporum, Trichophyton* spp., and *Malassezia furfur*, but is not active against *Candida* spp. or bacteria.

Uses and Administration

Tolnaftate is an antifungal used topically as a 1% solution, powder, or cream in the treatment or prophylaxis of superficial dermatophyte infections and of pityriasis versicolor (see p.371). Tolnaftate is applied twice daily for 2 to 6 weeks. Repeat treatment may be required.

Like other topical antifungals, tolnaftate is not considered suitable for deep infections in nail beds or hair follicles but it may be used concomitantly with a systemic drug.

Preparations

USP 23: Tolnaftate Cream; Tolnaftate Gel; Tolnaftate Topical Aerosol Powder; Tolnaftate Topical Powder; Tolnaftate Topical Solution.

Proprietary Preparations (details are given in Part 3)

Aust.: Sorgoran; ***Austral.:*** Antifungal Foot Deodorant; Curatin; Pediderm†; Ringworm Ointment; Tinacare†; Tinacidin†; Tinaderm; Tineafax; ***Canad.:*** Absorbine Antifungal; Pitrex; Scholl Athlete's Foot Preparations; Tinactin; Tritin†; ZeaSorb AF; ***Fr.:*** Pedimycose†; Sporiline; ***Ger.:*** Chlorisept N†; Sorgoa; Tinatox; Tonoftal; ***Irl.:*** Mycil; Tinaderm; ***Ital.:*** Tinaderm; ***S.Afr.:*** Tinaderm; ***Spain:*** Devorfungi; Tinaderm; ***UK:*** Athlete's Foot; Mycil; Tinaderm; Tineafax†; ***USA:*** Absorbine Antifungal†; Aftate; Blis-To-Sol; Breezee Mist Antifungal; Desenex†; Dr Scholl's Athlete's Foot; Dr Scholl's Tritin Antifungal Powder; Genaspor; NP-27†; Quinsana Plus; Tinactin; Ting.

Multi-ingredient: ***Aust.:*** Focusan; ***Austral.:*** Curatin; ***Canad.:*** Absorbine Jr Antifungal; ***Irl.:*** Mycil; Tinaderm-M; ***Neth.:*** Focusan†; ***Norw.:*** Focusan†; ***S.Afr.:*** Duoderm†; Quadriderm; ***Spain:*** Cuatroderm; Wasserdermina†; ***Switz.:*** Focusan†; Quadriderm; Undex†; ***UK:*** Mycil; Tinaderm-M; ***USA:*** Absorbine Athletes Foot Care; Dermasept Antifungal; SteriNail.

Triacetin (3010-k)

Triacetin *(rINN).*

Glycerol Triacetate; Glycerolum Triacetas; Glyceryl Triacetate. 1,2,3-Propanetriol triacetate.

$C_9H_{14}O_6$ = 218.2.

CAS — 102-76-1.

Pharmacopoeias. In *Eur.* (see p.viii) and *US*.

A clear, colourless somewhat oily liquid with a slight fatty odour. **Soluble** in water; slightly soluble in carbon disulphide; miscible with alcohol, with chloroform, with dehydrated alcohol, with ether, and with toluene. **Store** in well-filled airtight containers.

Triacetin is reported to possess fungistatic properties based on the liberation of acetic acid. It has been applied topically in the treatment of superficial dermatophyte infections. It has also been used as a plasticiser in oral preparations.

Triacetin may destroy rayon fabric. It should not come into contact with metals.

Undecenoic Acid (3012-t)

Acidum Undecylenicum; 10-Hendecenoic Acid; Undecylenic Acid. Undec-10-enoic acid.

$C_{11}H_{20}O_2$ = 184.3.

CAS — 112-38-9.

Pharmacopoeias. In *Chin., Eur.* (see p.viii), and *US*.

A colourless or pale yellow clear liquid or a white to very pale yellow crystalline mass with a characteristic odour.

Practically **insoluble** in water; freely soluble in, or miscible with, alcohol and ether; freely soluble in fatty and essential oils; miscible with chloroform, and fixed and volatile oils. **Store** in airtight, non-metallic containers at a temperature of 8 to 15°. Protect from light.

Calcium Undecenoate (16172-g)

Calcium Undecylenate *(USAN).* Calcium di(undec-10-enoate).

$(C_{11}H_{19}O_2)_2Ca$ = 406.6.

Pharmacopoeias. In *US*.

A fine white powder with a characteristic odour. Practically **insoluble** in water, in cold alcohol, in acetone, in chloroform, and in ether; slightly soluble in hot alcohol.

Zinc Undecenoate (3014-r)

Undecilinato de Zinco; Zinc Undecylenate; Zinci Undecylenas. Zinc di(undec-10-enoate).

$(C_{11}H_{19}O_2)_2Zn$ = 431.9.

CAS — 557-08-4.

Pharmacopoeias. In *Chin., Eur.* (see p.viii), and *US*.

A fine white or almost white powder. Practically **insoluble** in water, alcohol, and ether. **Protect** from light.

Adverse Effects

Irritation may rarely occur after the topical application of undecenoic acid or its salts.

Antimicrobial Action

Undecenoic acid and its derivatives are active against some pathogenic fungi, including the dermatophytes *Epidermophyton, Trichophyton,* and *Microsporum* spp.

Uses and Administration

Undecenoic acid and its zinc salt are applied topically in the prophylaxis and treatment of superficial dermatophytoses, particularly tinea pedis (p.371). Typical concentrations are undecenoic acid 2 to 5% and zinc undecenoate 20%. They are used in creams, ointments, or powders, often in conjunction with each other. Calcium undecenoate is used as a 10 or 15% powder.

Methyl and propyl undecenoate, sodium sulphosuccinated undecenoic acid monoethanolamide, and undecenoic acid monoethanolamide are used similarly.

Preparations

USP 23: Compound Undecylenic Acid Ointment.

Proprietary Preparations (details are given in Part 3)

Aust.: Mayfung; Pelsano; Umadren; ***Canad.:*** Caldesene; Cruex; ***Fr.:*** Mycodecyl; ***Ger.:*** Benzoderm†; ***Irl.:*** Caldesene; ***Switz.:*** Lubex; Turexan Douche; ***USA:*** Blis-To-Sol; Caldesene; Cruex; Decylenes; Fungoid AF; Protectol.

Multi-ingredient: ***Aust.:*** Crino Cordes; Dequafungan; Mycopol; Mykozem; Pelsano; Salvyl; Tineafax; Umadren; ***Austral.:*** Acnederm; Egomycol; Mycoderm; Pedoz; Sebitar; Seborrol; ***Belg.:*** Pelsano; ***Canad.:*** Athletes Foot Antifungal; Cruex; Desenex; Ovoquinol†; ***Fr.:*** Mycodecyl; Paps; ***Ger.:*** Benzoderm†; Dermaethyl-H†; Dermaethyl†; Fungiderm N†; Gehwol Fungizid; Gehwol Fungizid Creme N; Gehwol Nagelpilz; Kytta-Nagelsalbe†; Mediphon†; Onymyken S†; Psorispray†; Skinman Soft; ***Irl.:*** Ceanel; Desenex; Genisol; Monphytol; Pedamed†; ***Ital.:*** Balta Intimo Soluzione; Genisol; Neo Zeta-Foot; Sideck Shampoo Antiforfora†; Sulfadeck†; Undecilendermina†; Undetin†; Zeta-Foot†; ***S.Afr.:*** AF; Ceanel; Mycota; Pedil; ***Spain:*** Acnosan; Infalina†; Pentoderm†; ***Switz.:*** Crimanex; Fungex; Pelsano; Pruri-med; Sebo Shampooing; Trosyd†; Turexan Creme; Turexan Emulsion; Undex†; ***UK:*** Ceanel; Genisol†; Healthy Feet; Monphytol; Mycota; Phytocil†; ***USA:*** Dermasept Antifungal; Desenex; Gordochom; Pedi-Pro; Phicon-F; SteriNail.

Voriconazole (18393-l)

Voriconazole *(BAN, rINN).*

UK-109496; Voriconazol. (2*R*,3*S*)-2-(2,4-Difluorophenyl)-3-(5-fluoropyrimidin-4-yl)-1-(1,2,4-triazol-1-yl)butan-2-ol.

$C_{16}H_{14}N_5F_3O$ = 349.3.

CAS — 137234-62-9.

Voriconazole is a triazole antifungal under investigation for systemic use.

References.

1. Radford SA, *et al.* In vitro studies of activity of voriconazole (UK-109,496), a new triazole antifungal agent, against emerging and less-common mold pathogens. *Antimicrob Agents Chemother* 1997; **41:** 841–3.
2. Ruhnke M, *et al.* In vitro activities of voriconazole (UK-109,496) against fluconazole-susceptible and -resistant Candida albicans isolates from oral cavities of patients with human immunodeficiency virus infection. *Antimicrob Agents Chemother* 1997; **41:** 575–7.
3. McGinnis MR, *et al.* In vitro evaluation of voriconazole against some clinically important fungi. *Antimicrob Agents Chemother* 1997; **41:** 1832–4.
4. Schwartz S, *et al.* Successful treatment of cerebral aspergillosis with a novel triazole (voriconazole) in a patient with acute leukaemia. *Br J Haematol* 1997; **97:** 663–5.

Antigout Drugs

This chapter deals with the treatment of gout and hyperuricaemia and the drugs used mainly for these disorders.

Gout and hyperuricaemia

Uric acid is the final product of the metabolism of endogenous and exogenous purine in man. An excess of uric acid, measured in the plasma as sodium urate, constitutes **hyperuricaemia**. This excess may be caused by an overproduction or underexcretion of urate. It may be primary (mainly idiopathic) or secondary when contributing factors include a range of diseases such as some enzyme deficiency states, cancer (and its treatment), renal impairment, and hypertension; other factors include obesity, alcohol, and some drugs, especially thiazide diuretics.

When plasma-urate concentrations exceed 0.42 mmol per litre (7 mg per 100 mL) there is a risk of crystals of monosodium urate monohydrate being formed and deposited in synovial fluid and various tissues. However, some subjects may have supersaturated plasma-urate concentrations without any crystal deposits, while others may suffer from deposits at concentrations of 0.42 mmol or less per litre. The presence of urate crystals in the synovial fluid leads to an inflammatory response in the affected joint, often the big toe. The ensuing pain, tenderness, and swelling constitute the symptoms of **acute inflammatory gouty arthritis**. An untreated acute attack usually subsides after several days. Unfortunately many patients suffer repeated acute attacks with a build up of crystal deposits at various sites including in and around the affected joint leading to **chronic gout**. The deposits, known as **tophi**, release urate crystals into the synovial fluid following various stimuli and so cause further acute attacks. The tophi in chronic gout can also lead to joint deterioration. Rarely, the kidney can be affected by urate deposits producing a gouty nephropathy and by uric acid calculi or stones (uric acid nephrolithiasis or urolithiasis).

Treatment

Plasma-urate concentrations may be reduced by control of obesity and modification of diet and alcohol intake. Drug treatment should be considered for hyperuricaemia only if there are recurrent attacks of gout or there is renal involvement, and such treatment (which is described under Chronic Gout, below) should not be started until after an acute attack has completely subsided.

Acute gout. An attack of acute inflammatory gouty arthritis is best treated as soon as possible with an NSAID. Aspirin or other salicylates are not suitable since they may increase plasma-urate concentrations. Treatment is started with high doses of an NSAID, the doses being reduced as the patient responds. Usually treatment can be withdrawn within a week. Colchicine has a role in treating patients in whom NSAIDs are contra-indicated. Patients who do not respond to NSAIDs or colchicine, or for whom these drugs are contraindicated, may be treated with a systemic corticosteroid. Intra-articular corticosteroids are effective in acute monoarticular gout. Drugs used for chronic gout (allopurinol or the uricosurics) should not be started during an acute attack since they can exacerbate and prolong it (see below). However, if an acute attack occurs during maintenance therapy with these drugs, they are usually continued and the acute attack treated in its own right.

Chronic gout. If the patient suffers frequent acute attacks or develops tophaceous gout, or has renal complications as a result of urate overproduction, then the hyperuricaemia will need to be treated, but not until 2 to 3 weeks after the patient has recovered from the latest acute attack. There are two approaches to this drug treatment (known as **interval treatment**) of hyperuricaemia: inhibiting the production of uric acid with allopurinol or enhancing the urinary excretion of uric acid with a uricosuric such as benzbromarone, probenecid, or sulphinpyrazone.

Allopurinol inhibits the enzyme xanthine oxidase and so blocks the metabolism of hypoxanthine to xanthine and of xanthine to uric acid leading to a reduction in the plasma-urate concentration. The intermediates hypoxanthine and xanthine can be cleared effectively by the kidney. The uricosurics inhibit renal tubular uric acid reabsorption. Therefore hyperuricaemia associated with underexcretion of uric acid can be treated with either allopurinol or a uricosuric and sometimes a combination of both treatments has been used. Hyperuricaemia due to overproduction of urate is treated with allopurinol; such patients excrete more than 700 or 800 mg of uric acid in their urine over 24 hours. Allopurinol should also be used for patients with renal urate deposits or with uric acid renal calculi.

As the plasma-urate concentration falls with either treatment there is mobilisation of urate crystals from established tophi which can trigger further acute attacks of gout. Patients are thus also given prophylaxis with an NSAID or colchicine from the start of interval treatment until at least a month after the plasma-urate has been reduced to an acceptable concentration; 3 or 4 months of prophylactic cover appears to be common. Once the hyperuricaemia is corrected, the patient continues to receive maintenance therapy indefinitely. If an acute attack occurs during maintenance therapy, this therapy should be continued and the acute attack treated in its own right.

Finally, surgery may have to be considered for patients severely affected by chronic tophaceous gout.

General references to gout and its management are given below.

1. Star VL, Hochberg MC. Prevention and management of gout. *Drugs* 1993; **45:** 212–22.
2. Snaith ML. Gout, hyperuricaemia, and crystal arthritis. *Br Med J* 1995; **310:** 521–4.
3. Emmerson BT. The management of gout. *N Engl J Med* 1996; **334:** 445–51.

Allopurinol (1004-m)

Allopurinol *(BAN, USAN, rINN)*.

Allopurinolum; BW-56-158; HPP; NSC-1390. 1*H*-Pyrazolo[3,4-*d*]pyrimidin-4-ol; 1,5-Dihydro-4*H*-pyrazolo[3,4-*d*]pyrimidin-4-one.

$C_5H_4N_4O$ = 136.1.

CAS — 315-30-0 (allopurinol); 17795-21-0 (allopurinol sodium).

Pharmacopoeias. In *Chin., Eur.* (see p.viii), *Int., Jpn, Pol.*, and *US.*

A white or off-white, almost odourless powder. It is a tautomeric mixture of 1*H*-pyrazolo[3,4-*d*]pyrimidin-4-ol and 1,5-dihydro-4*H*-pyrazolo[3,4-*d*]pyrimidin-4-one. Very slightly **soluble** in water and in alcohol; practically insoluble in chloroform and in ether; dissolves in dilute solutions of alkali hydroxides.

Incompatibility. Allopurinol sodium as a 3 mg per mL solution in 0.9% sodium chloride was visually incompatible with a number of drugs including amikacin sulphate, amphotericin, carmustine, cefotaxime sodium, chlorpromazine hydrochloride, cimetidine hydrochloride, clindamycin phosphate, cytarabine, dacarbazine, daunorubicin hydrochloride, diphenhydramine hydrochloride, doxorubicin hydrochloride, doxycycline hydrochloride, droperidol, floxuridine, gentamicin sulphate, haloperidol lactate, hydroxyzine hydrochloride, idarubicin hydrochloride, imipenem with cilastatin sodium, methylprednisolone sodium succinate, metoclopramide hydrochloride, minocycline hydrochloride, mustine hydrochloride, nalbuphine hydrochloride, netilmicin sulphate, ondansetron hydrochloride, pethidine hydrochloride, prochlorperazine edisylate, promethazine hydrochloride, sodium bicarbonate, streptozocin, tobramycin sulphate, and vinorelbine tartrate.[1]

1. Trissel LA, Martinez JF. Compatibility of allopurinol sodium with selected drugs during simulated Y-site administration. *Am J Hosp Pharm* 1994; **51:** 1792–9.

Adverse Effects

The most common side-effect of allopurinol is skin rash. Rashes are generally maculopapular or pruritic, but more serious hypersensitivity reactions may occur and include exfoliative rashes, the Stevens-Johnson syndrome, and toxic epidermal necrolysis. It is therefore recommended that allopurinol be withdrawn immediately if a rash occurs (see under Precautions below). Further symptoms of hypersensitivity include fever and chills, leucopenia or leucocytosis, eosinophilia, arthralgia, and vasculitis leading to renal and hepatic damage. These hypersensitivity reactions may be severe, even fatal, and patients with hepatic or renal impairment are at special risk.

Hepatotoxicity and signs of altered liver function may also be found in patients not exhibiting hypersensitivity.

Many other side-effects, usually of a less serious nature, have been noted and include paraesthesia, peripheral neuropathy, alopecia, hypertension, taste disturbances, nausea, vomiting, abdominal pain, diarrhoea, headache, drowsiness, and vertigo.

Patients with gout may experience an increase in acute attacks on beginning treatment with allopurinol, although attacks usually subside after several months.

A Boston Collaborative Drug Surveillance Program of 29 524 hospitalised patients revealed that, with the exception of skin reactions, of 1835 patients treated with allopurinol 33 (1.8%) experienced adverse effects. These effects were dose-related and the most frequent were haematological (11 patients, 0.6%), diarrhoea (5 patients, 0.3%), and drug fever (5 patients, 0.3%). Hepatotoxicity was reported in 3 patients (0.2%). Two patients developed possible hypersensitivity reactions to allopurinol.[1]

A further analysis involving 1748 outpatients indicated no instances of acute blood disorders, skin diseases, or hypersensitivity that warranted hospital treatment. Liver disease, although found, was considered to be unassociated with allopurinol. There were only 2 patients in whom renal disease could possibly have been caused by allopurinol.[2]

1. McInnes GT, *et al.* Acute adverse reactions attributed to allopurinol in hospitalised patients. *Ann Rheum Dis* 1981; **40:** 245–9.
2. Jick H, Perera DR. Reactions to allopurinol. *JAMA* 1984; **252:** 1411.

Effects on the blood. In addition to the haematological abnormalities of leucopenia, thrombocytopenia, haemolytic anaemia, and clotting abnormalities noted in the Boston Collaborative Drug Surveillance Program,[1] aplastic anaemia has also been reported, sometimes in patients with impaired renal function.[2]

1. McInnes GT, *et al.* Acute adverse reactions attributed to allopurinol in hospitalised patients. *Ann Rheum Dis* 1981; **40:** 245–9.
2. Anonymous. Allopurinol and aplastic anaemia. *WHO Drug Inf* 1989; **3:** 26.

Effects on the eyes. Although case reports have suggested an association between allopurinol use and the development of cataracts,[1] a detailed ophthalmological survey which involved 51 patients who had taken allopurinol failed to confirm this possible adverse effect.[2]

1. Fraunfelder FT, *et al.* Cataracts associated with allopurinol therapy. *Am J Ophthalmol* 1982; **94:** 137–40.
2. Clair WK, *et al.* Allopurinol use and the risk of cataract formation. *Br J Ophthalmol* 1989; **73:** 173–6.

Effects on the skin. Skin reactions are the most common side-effects of allopurinol.

An Australian report calculated that of 215 adverse effects noted over a 16-year period 188 (87.4%) were related to the skin or mucous membranes.[1] An analysis by the Boston Collaborative Drug Surveillance Program in the USA, of data on 15 438 patients hospitalised between 1975 and 1982 detected 6 allergic skin reactions attributed to allopurinol among 784 recipients of the drug.[2]

Serious skin reactions to allopurinol may occur as part of a generalised hypersensitivity reaction. A review of the literature between 1970 and the end of 1990 revealed 101 cases of allopurinol hypersensitivity syndrome, 94 of which involved the skin.[3] Skin reactions included erythema multiforme, Stevens-Johnson syndrome, toxic epidermal necrolysis, or a diffuse maculopapular or exfoliative dermatitis; 27 of the 101 patients died. The relative risk of toxic epidermal necrolysis or Stevens-Johnson syndrome occurring with allopurinol was high (calculated to be 5.5) in a case-control study including 13 patients with these cutaneous reactions who had received allopurinol.[4] This risk was not constant over time, being higher during the first 2 months of treatment. During these 2 months the estimated excess risk was 1.5 cases per million users per week.

1. Vinciullo C. Allopurinol hypersensitivity. *Med J Aust* 1984; **141:** 449–50.
2. Bigby M, *et al.* Drug-induced cutaneous reactions. *JAMA* 1986; **256:** 3358–63.
3. Arellano F, Sacristán JA. Allopurinol hypersensitivity syndrome: a review. *Ann Pharmacother* 1993; **27:** 337–43.
4. Roujeau J-C, *et al.* Medication use and the risk of Stevens-Johnson syndrome or toxic epidermal necrolysis. *N Engl J Med* 1995; **333:** 1600–1607.

Hypersensitivity. For mention of the allopurinol hypersensitivity syndrome, see Effects on the Skin, above.

Precautions

Allopurinol should not be used for the treatment of an acute attack of gout; additionally, allopurinol therapy should not be initiated for any purpose during an acute attack. However, allopurinol is continued when acute attacks occur in patients already receiving the drug, and the acute attack is treated separately.

Treatment should be stopped if any skin reactions or other signs of hypersensitivity develop. A cautious reintroduction at a low dose may be attempted when mild skin reactions have cleared; allopurinol should not be reintroduced in those patients who have experienced other forms of hypersensitivity reaction. Dosage should be reduced in renal impairment (see below). Allopurinol should also be administered with care to patients with hepatic impairment, and doses may need to be reduced. To reduce the risk of renal xanthine deposition an adequate fluid intake (2 to 3 litres daily) is required. In addition, a neutral or slightly alkaline urine may be desirable.

Allopurinol should be used with caution in nursing mothers as it has been reported to be distributed into breast milk.

Renal impairment. Excretion of allopurinol and its active metabolite oxypurinol is primarily via the kidneys and therefore the dosage should be reduced if renal function is impaired.

In the USA the manufacturer (Glaxo Wellcome) suggests a daily dose of 200 mg for patients with a creatinine clearance of 10 to 20 mL per minute and a maximum daily dose of 100 mg for a clearance of under 10 mL per minute with consideration being given to a longer dosing interval if the clearance falls below 3 mL per minute.

In the UK the manufacturer (Wellcome) recommends a maximum initial daily dosage of 100 mg for those with impaired renal function, increased only if the response is inadequate. Doses less than 100 mg daily or 100 mg at intervals longer than 1 day are recommended for those with severe renal insufficiency. Because of the imprecision of low creatinine clearance values, they suggest that, if facilities are available for monitoring, the allopurinol dose should be adjusted to maintain plasma-oxypurinol concentrations below 100 μmol per litre (15.2 μg per mL).

Interactions

Drugs that can increase uric acid concentrations may decrease the efficacy of allopurinol. Aspirin and the salicylates possess this activity and should be avoided in hyperuricaemia and gout. An increase in hypersensitivity reactions, and possibly also other adverse effects, has been reported in patients receiving allopurinol with thiazide diuretics, particularly in patients with impaired renal function.

The metabolism of azathioprine and mercaptopurine is inhibited by allopurinol and their doses should be reduced to one-quarter to one-third of the usual dose when either of them is given with allopurinol to avoid potentially life-threatening toxicity. There have also been reports of allopurinol enhancing the activity of, and possibly increasing the toxicity of, a number of other drugs including some antibacterials, some anticoagulants, some antineoplastics, captopril, cyclosporin, theophylline, and vidarabine.

ACE inhibitors. An apparent interaction between allopurinol and *captopril* has been reported in patients with chronic renal failure (CRF). In one patient fatal Stevens-Johnson syndrome developed and it was suggested that the reaction was secondary to the introduction of allopurinol potentiated by the presence of captopril.[1] In the second patient hypersensitivity, characterised by fever, arthralgia, and myalgia, occurred and in this case the cause was believed to be captopril, or one of its metabolites, potentiated by the addition of allopurinol.[2] The authors of both reports considered that the combination of allopurinol and captopril should be prescribed with care, especially in patients with CRF.

1. Pennell DJ, *et al.* Fatal Stevens-Johnson syndrome in a patient on captopril and allopurinol. *Lancet* 1984; **i:** 463.
2. Samanta A, Burden AC. Fever, myalgia, and arthralgia in a patient on captopril and allopurinol. *Lancet* 1984; **i:** 679.

Antacids. Allopurinol failed to reduce blood-uric-acid concentrations when administered at the same time as *aluminium hydroxide* in 3 patients on chronic haemodialysis. However, if allopurinol was given 3 hours before aluminium hydroxide the expected decrease in uric acid concentration did occur.[1]

1. Weissman I, Krivoy N. Interaction of aluminium hydroxide and allopurinol in patients on chronic hemodialysis. *Ann Intern Med* 1987; **107:** 787.

Antibacterials. Although an increased incidence of skin rashes has been noted when allopurinol has been used with *ampicillin* or *amoxycillin*, data currently available are insufficient to confirm whether this is due to allopurinol or not. For further details, see Ampicillin, p.153.

Anticoagulants. For the effect of allopurinol on *dicoumarol, phenprocoumon,* or *warfarin*, see Warfarin, p.967.

Antiepileptics. For a report of allopurinol possibly inhibiting the metabolism of *phenytoin*, see p.355.

Antigout drugs. Uricosuric drugs are likely to increase the renal elimination of oxypurinol (the major active metabolite of allopurinol). For example, concurrent administration of allopurinol and *benzbromarone* was found to lower plasma concentrations of oxypurinol by some 40%, although plasma concentrations of allopurinol itself were not affected.[1] The interaction was not clinically significant, since the combination was more effective than allopurinol alone in lowering serum concentrations of uric acid. The manufacturer recommends reassessing the dosage of allopurinol on an individual basis when a uricosuric drug is added.

Probenecid has been reported to decrease the clearance of orally administered allopurinol riboside.[2]

1. Müller FO, *et al.* The effect of benzbromarone on allopurinol/oxypurinol kinetics in patients with gout. *Eur J Clin Pharmacol* 1993; **44:** 69–72.
2. Were JBO, Shapiro TA. Effects of probenecid on the pharmacokinetics of allopurinol riboside. *Antimicrob Agents Chemother* 1993; **37:** 1193–6.

Antineoplastics and immunosuppressants. Allopurinol inhibits the metabolism of *azathioprine* and *mercaptopurine* and marked dosage reduction of these drugs is required if either is given concomitantly with allopurinol (p.506 and p.546, respectively). There are also reports of interactions between allopurinol and other antineoplastics. Mild chronic allopurinol-induced hepatotoxicity has been reported in one male patient to have been exacerbated by *tamoxifen*.[1] Hypersensitivity vasculitis resulting in the death of one patient receiving allopurinol and *pentostatin* has been described. Although it could not be ascertained whether this effect was due to one of the drugs alone or to an interaction it was believed that this combination should not be employed.[2]

For a report of an increased incidence of bone-marrow toxicity in patients given allopurinol with *cyclophosphamide*, see p.517. The effects of allopurinol on *cyclosporin* concentrations (a marked increase) are reported on p.521.

1. Shah KA, *et al.* Allopurinol hepatotoxicity potentiated by tamoxifen. *N Y State J Med* 1982; **82;** 1745–6.
2. Steinmetz JC, *et al.* Hypersensitivity vasculitis associated with 2-deoxycoformycin and allopurinol therapy. *Am J Med* 1989; **86:** 499.

Antivirals. For a report of vidarabine neurotoxicity in patients receiving allopurinol and *vidarabine*, see p.628.

Xanthines. For the effect of allopurinol on *theophylline* pharmacokinetics, see p.769.

Pharmacokinetics

Up to 90% of a dose of allopurinol is absorbed from the gastro-intestinal tract after oral administration; its plasma half-life is about 1 to 3 hours. Allopurinol's major metabolite is oxypurinol (alloxanthine) which is also an inhibitor of xanthine oxidase with a plasma half-life of about 15 or more hours in patients with normal renal function, although this is prolonged by renal impairment. Both allopurinol and oxypurinol are conjugated to form their respective ribonucleosides. Allopurinol and oxypurinol are not bound to plasma proteins.

Excretion is mainly through the kidney, but it is slow since oxypurinol undergoes tubular reabsorption. About 70% of a daily dose may be excreted in the urine as oxypurinol and up to 10% as allopurinol; prolonged administration may alter these proportions due to allopurinol inhibiting its own metabolism. The remainder of the dose is excreted in the faeces. Allopurinol and oxypurinol have also been detected in breast milk.

References.

1. Murrell GAC, Rapeport WG. Clinical pharmacokinetics of allopurinol. *Clin Pharmacokinet* 1986; **11:** 343–53.
2. McGaurn SP, *et al.* The pharmacokinetics of injectable allopurinol in newborns with the hypoplastic left heart syndrome. *Pediatrics* 1994; **94:** 820–3.

Uses and Administration

Allopurinol is used to treat hyperuricaemia (p.390) associated with chronic gout, acute uric acid nephropathy, recurrent uric acid stone formation, enzyme disorders, and cancer or cancer chemotherapy. It is not used for asymptomatic hyperuricaemia. Allopurinol is also used in the management of renal calculi caused by the deposition of calcium oxalate (in the presence of hyperuricosuria) and of 2,8-dihydroxyadenine (see below). It may have the potential to reduce oxidative injury by blocking the production of free radicals and is an ingredient of kidney preservation solutions. In addition allopurinol has antiprotozoal activity and has been used in leishmaniasis and American trypanosomiasis.

Allopurinol's use in **gout and hyperuricaemia** derives from its inhibitory action on the enzyme xanthine oxidase and the resultant reduction of the oxidation of hypoxanthine to xanthine and xanthine to uric acid. The urinary purine load, normally almost entirely uric acid, is thereby divided between hypoxanthine, xanthine, and uric acid, each with its independent solubility. This results in the reduction of urate and uric acid concentrations in plasma and urine, ideally to such an extent that deposits of monosodium urate monohydrate or uric acid are dissolved or prevented from forming. At low concentrations allopurinol acts as a competitive inhibitor of xanthine oxidase and at higher concentrations as a non-competitive inhibitor. However, most of its activity is due to the metabolite oxypurinol which is a non-competitive inhibitor of xanthine oxidase.

Allopurinol is used in patients with chronic gout to correct hyperuricaemia thereby reducing the likelihood of acute attacks and preventing the sequelae of chronic gout. It is not used to treat acute attacks of gout and may exacerbate and prolong them if given during attacks. Allopurinol should not be started until an acute attack has completely subsided. In the first few months of treatment with allopurinol there may be an increase in the frequency of acute attacks due to the release of urate from tophi; it is therefore recommended that treatment should be started with a low dose increased gradually and that an NSAID or colchicine should also be given during the first few months.

A suggested starting dose of allopurinol is 100 mg daily by mouth, gradually increased by 100 mg for example at weekly intervals until the concentration of urate in plasma is reduced to 0.36 mmol per litre (6 mg per 100 mL) or less. A daily dose range of 100 to 300 mg may be adequate for those with mild to moderate gout and up to 600 mg for those with moderately severe tophaceous gout. The maximum recommended daily dose is 800 mg in the USA and 900 mg in the UK. Up to 300 mg may be taken as a single daily dose; larger amounts should be taken in divided doses to reduce the risk of gastric irritation. Taking allopurinol after food will also minimise gastric irritation. Patients should maintain an adequate fluid intake to prevent renal xanthine deposition.

Doses of allopurinol should be reduced in patients with impaired renal function (see Precautions, above)

When used for the prevention of uric acid nephropathy associated with cancer therapy 600 to 800 mg may be given daily generally for 2 or 3 days and starting before the cancer treatment. A high fluid intake is essential. In hyperuricaemia secondary to cancer or cancer chemotherapy, maintenance doses of allopurinol are similar to those used in gout and are given according to the response.

The main use of allopurinol in children is for hyperuricaemia associated with cancer or cancer chemotherapy or with enzyme disorders. The suggested dose varies: in the UK a dose of 10 to 20 mg per kg body-weight daily or 100 to 400 mg daily is recommended for children under 15 years of age, while in the USA the dose is 150 mg daily for children under 6 years of age and 300 mg daily for those aged 6 to 10 years, adjusted if necessary after 48 hours.

Allopurinol has been given as the sodium salt by intravenous infusion in sodium chloride 0.9% or glucose 5% to patients (usually cancer patients) unable to take allopurinol by mouth. Doses have ranged from the equivalent of 300 to 700 mg of allopurinol every 24 hours.

Diagnosis and testing. Deficiency of the enzyme ornithine carbamoyltransferase can result in severe central nervous system dysfunction or even in death, and identification of women at risk of being carriers of this genetic enzyme deficiency has been described.[1] The enzyme deficiency causes carbamoyl phosphate to accumulate, which stimulates the synthesis of orotidine. The test relies on the administration of a single dose of allopurinol, which will, in carriers, greatly increase the urinary excretion of orotidine.

1. Hauser ER, *et al.* Allopurinol-induced orotidinuria. *N Engl J Med* 1990; **322:** 1641–5.

Duchenne muscular dystrophy. Controversy has surrounded the use of allopurinol in Duchenne muscular dystrophy (p.1025) since the initial favourable reports by Thomson and Smith.[1,2] Allopurinol was used in an attempt to increase the ATP levels in muscle which are depleted in this muscular dystrophy. Although others have reported similar results,[3] double-blind studies[4-6] failed to show any benefit from treatment. Despite these findings, some interest in the use of allopurinol for this disorder has continued.[7]

1. Thomson WHS, Smith I. X-linked recessive (Duchenne) muscular dystrophy (DMD) and purine metabolism: effects of oral allopurinol and adenylate. *Metabolism* 1978; **27:** 151–63.
2. Thomson WHS, Smith I. Allopurinol in Duchenne's muscular dystrophy. *N Engl J Med* 1978; **299:** 101.
3. Castro-Gago M, *et al.* Allopurinol in Duchenne muscular dystrophy. *Lancet* 1980; **i;** 1358–9.
4. Stern LM, *et al.* The progression of Duchenne muscular dystrophy: clinical trial of allopurinol therapy. *Neurology* 1981; **31:** 422–6.
5. Hunter JR, *et al.* Effects of allopurinol in Duchenne's muscular dystrophy. *Arch Neurol* 1983; **40:** 1294–9.
6. Bertorini TE, *et al.* Chronic allopurinol and adenine therapy in Duchenne muscular dystrophy: effects on muscle function, nucleotide degradation, and muscle ATP and ADP content. *Neurology* 1985; **35:** 61–5.
7. Castro-Gago M, *et al.* Long-term effects of xanthine-oxidase inhibitor (allopurinol) in Duchenne muscular dystrophy. *Int Pediatr* 1994; **9:** 15–20.

Epilepsy. Reduction in the frequency of seizures has been described in some patients with severe or intractable epilepsy (p.335) when allopurinol was added to their existing antiepileptic therapy.[1-3] Although the mode of action was not known it was noted that the patients were not hyperuricaemic and that allopurinol did not affect plasma concentrations of existing antiepileptics.[1]

1. DeMarco P, Zagnoni P. Allopurinol and severe epilepsy. *Neurology* 1986; **36:** 1538–9.
2. Tada H, *et al.* Clinical effects of allopurinol on intractable epilepsy. *Epilepsia* 1991; **32:** 279–83.
3. Zagnoni PG, *et al.* Allopurinol as an add-on therapy in refractory epilepsy—a double-blind placebo-controlled randomised study. *Epilepsia* 1994; **35:** 107–12.

Fluorouracil toxicity. Allopurinol has been used to reduce fluorouracil toxicity in patients receiving chemotherapy (see under Treatment of Adverse Effects in Fluorouracil, p.535).

Organ transplantation. Allopurinol 25 mg on alternate days has been added to the immunosuppressive treatment given to the patient after renal transplantation,[1] and is reported to reduce the frequency of acute rejection. One possible explanation for this effect is allopurinol's ability to suppress the production of free radicals (see Oxidative Injury, below). Organ and tissue transplantation, and the more usual drugs used in immunosuppressive regimens are discussed on p.498. It should be noted that allopurinol interacts with azathioprine and cyclosporin (see above).

1. Chocair P, *et al.* Low-dose allopurinol plus azathioprine/cyclosporin/prednisolone, a novel immunosuppressive regimen. *Lancet* 1993; **342:** 83–4.

Oxidative injury. Allopurinol through its inhibition of xanthine oxidase can block the development of superoxide free radicals during reperfusion after an ischaemic episode. Consequently, the ability of allopurinol to reduce oxidative injury has been investigated in a number of clinical situations.

In patients undergoing coronary artery bypass graft surgery, perioperative allopurinol administration reduced the number of ischaemic events and reduced the amount of dopamine required.[1,2] However, allopurinol failed to reduce the incidence of periventricular leucomalacia (thought to represent ischaemic infarction of the developing brain) in preterm infants compared with placebo in a large study.[3] Similarly, allopurinol did not reduce the incidence of infarct extension in patients with acute myocardial infarction.[4]

The possibility that allopurinol limits the production of free radicals has also led to allopurinol sodium being included as an ingredient of the University of Wisconsin (UW) solution, which is used for the preservation of organs for transplantation.[5]

1. Sisto T, *et al.* Pretreatment with antioxidants and allopurinol diminishes cardiac onset events in coronary artery bypass grafting. *Ann Thorac Surg* 1995; **59:** 1519–23.
2. Coghlan JG, *et al.* Allopurinol pretreatment improves postoperative recovery and reduces lipid peroxidation in patients undergoing coronary artery bypass grafting. *J Thorac Cardiovasc Surg* 1994; **107:** 248–56.
3. Russell GAB, Cooke RWI. Randomised controlled trial of allopurinol prophylaxis in very preterm infants. *Arch Dis Child* 1995; **73:** F27–F31.
4. Parmley LF, *et al.* allopurinol therapy of ischemic heart disease with infarct extension. *Can J Cardiol* 1992; **8:** 280–6.
5. Southard JH, Belzer FO. Organ preservation. *Annu Rev Med* 1995; **46:** 235–47.

Protozoal infections. Beneficial results have been reported in patients with *visceral leishmaniasis* (p.575) when allopurinol was added to their therapy;[1,2] these studies involved patients who either had a poor or no response to antimonial drugs or included untreated patients from areas where unresponsive cases were frequent. Positive results in leishmaniasis have also been described in patients with AIDS.[3,4] Variable responses in American *cutaneous leishmaniasis* have been reported.[5,8,9]

Some beneficial results have been noted in indeterminate and chronic Chagas' disease *(American trypanosomiasis, p.578)*.[6,10]

The selective antiparasitic action of allopurinol is believed to be due to its incorporation into the protozoal, but not the mammalian, purine salvage pathway. This leads to the formation of 4-aminopyrazolopyrimidine ribonucleotide triphosphate, a highly toxic analogue of adenosine triphosphate, that is incorporated into ribonucleic acid. This action of allopurinol is shared by allopurinol riboside, one of the minor metabolites in man but not by oxypurinol, the major human metabolite. Thus, some studies are now being conducted with allopurinol riboside, rather than allopurinol, in an attempt to enhance activity by avoiding host-mediated inactivation.[7]

1. Chunge CN, *et al.* Visceral leishmaniasis unresponsive to antimonial drugs: successful treatment using a combination of sodium stibogluconate plus allopurinol. *Trans R Soc Trop Med Hyg* 1985; **79:** 715–18.
2. di Martino L, *et al.* Low dosage combination of meglumine antimoniate plus allopurinol as first choice treatment of infantile visceral leishmaniasis in Italy. *Trans R Soc Trop Med Hyg* 1990; **84:** 534–5.
3. Dellamonica P, *et al.* Allopurinol for treatment of visceral leishmaniasis in patients with AIDS. *J Infect Dis* 1989; **160:** 904–5.
4. Smith D, *et al.* Visceral leishmaniasis (kala azar) in a patient with AIDS. *AIDS* 1989; **3:** 41–3.
5. Martinez S, Marr JJ. Allopurinol in the treatment of American cutaneous leishmaniasis. *N Engl J Med* 1992; **326:** 741–4.
6. Gallerano RH, *et al.* Therapeutic efficacy of allopurinol in patients with chronic Chagas' disease. *Am J Trop Med Hyg* 1990; **43:** 159–66.
7. Shapiro TA, *et al.* Pharmacokinetics and metabolism of allopurinol riboside. *Clin Pharmacol Ther* 1991; **49:** 506–14.
8. Velez I, *et al.* Inefficacy of allopurinol as monotherapy for Colombian cutaneous leishmaniasis: a randomized, controlled trial. *Ann Intern Med* 1997; **126:** 232–6.
9. Martinez S, *et al.* Treatment of cutaneous leishmaniasis with allopurinol and stibogluconate. *Clin Infect Dis* 1997; **24:** 165–9.
10. Sá G, *et al.* Treatment with allopurinol and itraconazole changes lytic activity in patients with chronic, low grade Trypanosoma cruzi infection. *Trans R Soc Trop Med Hyg* 1995; **89:** 438–9.

Renal calculi. Patients with recurrent calcium oxalate stones are usually treated with thiazide diuretics (p.888). Allopurinol has been suggested as an alternative, particularly where there is also hyperuricosuria; the recommended dose of allopurinol is 200 to 300 mg per day adjusted on the basis of subsequent 24-hour urinary urate excretion. However, there have been conflicting reports of the value of allopurinol in such patients.[1,2] Allopurinol is also advocated for the management of 2,8-dihydroxyadenine (2,8-DHA) renal stones associated with deficient activity of the enzyme adenine phosphoribosyltransferase.

1. Ettinger B, *et al.* Randomized trial of allopurinol in the prevention of calcium oxalate calculi. *N Engl J Med* 1986; **315:** 1386–9.
2. Tiselius H-G, *et al.* Clinical results of allopurinol treatment in the prevention of calcium oxalate stone formation. *J Urol (Baltimore)* 1986; **136:** 50–3.

Sarcoidosis. Although corticosteroids remain the mainstay of drug therapy for sarcoidosis, and other drugs are very much second line, there are reports of benefit in cutaneous disease from the use of allopurinol, as mentioned on p.1028.

Preparations

BP 1998: Allopurinol Tablets;
USP 23: Allopurinol Tablets.

Proprietary Preparations (details are given in Part 3)
Aust.: Apurin; Gewapurol; Gichtex; Purinol; Urosin; Zyloric; ***Austral.:*** Alloremed†; Allorin; Capurate; Progout; Zygout; Zyloprim; ***Belg.:*** Zyloric; ***Canad.:*** Novo-Purol; Purinol†; Zyloprim; ***Fr.:*** Xanturic†; Zyloric; ***Ger.:*** Allo; Allo-300-Tablinen; Allo-Efeka; Allo-Puren; Allobeta; Allohexal; Allop-Gry†; Allpargin; Apulonga†; Bleminol; Cellidrin; Dabroson†; dura AL; Embarin†; Epidropal†; Foligan; Jenapurinol; Milurit; Pureduct; Remid; Suspendol†; Uribenz; Uripurinol; Urosin; Urtias; Zyloric; ***Irl.:*** Caplenal; Purinol; Tipuric; Zyloric; ***Ital.:*** Allurit; Uricemil; Zyloric; ***Neth.:*** Apurin†; Zyloric; ***Norw.:*** Allopur; Arturic; Zyloric; ***S.Afr.:*** Abburic†; Be-Uric; Ethipurinol†; Lo-Uric; Lonol; Puricos; Pyrazol†; Redurate; Urinol†; Urozyl-SR; Zyloprim; ***Spain:*** Allural†; Zyloric; ***Swed.:*** Zyloric; ***Switz.:*** Allo-300-Tablinen†; allo-basan; Allopur; Cellidrine; Foligan; Lysuron; Mephanol; Sigapurol; Uredimin; Uriconorme; Zyloric; ***UK:*** Aloral; Caplenal; Cosuric; Hamarin†; Rimapurinol; Xanthomax; Zyloric; ***USA:*** Lopurin†; Zyloprim.

Multi-ingredient: ***Aust.:*** Allobenz; Duovitan; Gichtex plus; Uroplus; ***Belg.:*** Comburic; ***Fr.:*** Desatura; ***Ger.:*** Acifugan; allo.comp.-ratiopharm; Allomaron; Harpagin; Uricovac comp†; ***Ital.:*** Uricodue; Urifugan†; ***S.Afr.:*** Allomaron; ***Spain:*** Acifugan; Biuricowas†; Facilit; ***Switz.:*** Acifugan.

Benzbromarone (1005-b)

Benzbromarone *(BAN, USAN, rINN)*.

Benzbromaronum; L-2214; MJ-10061. 3,5-Dibromo-4-hydroxyphenyl 2-ethylbenzofuran-3-yl ketone.

$C_{17}H_{12}Br_2O_3$ = 424.1.

CAS — 3562-84-3.

Pharmacopoeias. In *Fr., Jpn,* and *Swiss.*

Adverse Effects

Benzbromarone may cause gastro-intestinal side-effects, especially diarrhoea. It may precipitate an acute attack of gout and cause uric acid renal calculi and renal colic.

Effects on the liver. A case of benzbromarone-induced liver damage has been reported.[1]

1. Van Der Klauw MM, *et al.* Hepatic injury caused by benzbromarone. *J Hepatol* 1994; **20:** 376–9.

Precautions

Benzbromarone should be avoided in patients with severe renal impairment, in those with uric acid renal calculi, and in those with urinary uric acid excretion rates of greater than 700 mg per 24 hours. Like other uricosurics, treatment with benzbromarone should not be started during an acute attack of gout. Similarly, an adequate fluid intake should be maintained to reduce the risk of uric acid renal calculi; additionally alkalinisation of the urine may be considered.

Interactions

Aspirin and other salicylates antagonise the effect of benzbromarone. Benzbromarone, in doses in excess of those normally used therapeutically, may increase the anticoagulant activity of coumarin oral anticoagulants.

Antigout drugs. For mention of the effects of benzbromarone on the clearance of oxypurinol, the major active metabolite of *allopurinol*, and the view that this was not clinically significant, see p.391.

Pharmacokinetics

Benzbromarone is only partially absorbed from the gastro-intestinal tract, reaching peak plasma concentrations about 6 hours after a dose by mouth. It is metabolised in the liver, and is excreted mainly in the faeces; a small amount appears in the urine.

References.

1. Maurer H, Wollenberg P. Urinary metabolites of benzbromarone in man. *Arzneimittelforschung* 1990; **40:** 460–2.
2. Walter-Sack I, *et al.* Variation of benzbromarone elimination in man—a population study. *Eur J Clin Pharmacol* 1990; **39:** 173–6.

Uses and Administration

Benzbromarone is a uricosuric drug which reduces plasma concentrations of uric acid by blocking renal tubular reabsorption. It has been suggested that benzbromarone may also increase the intestinal elimination of uric acid. It is used to treat hyperuricaemia including that associated with chronic gout (p.390).

Benzbromarone is not used to treat acute attacks of gout and may exacerbate and prolong them if given during an attack; treatment should not start therefore until an acute attack has subsided.

The usual dose is 50 to 300 mg daily by mouth. An NSAID or colchicine should be given initially to reduce the risk of precipitating acute gout. An adequate fluid intake should be maintained. Lower doses of benzbromarone (20 or 25 mg) are also used in the form of a combination product with allopurinol.

Preparations

Proprietary Preparations (details are given in Part 3)
Aust.: Uricovac; *Belg.:* Desuric; *Fr.:* Desuric; *Ger.:* Azubromaron†; Harolan†; Narcaricin; *Neth.:* Desuric; *S.Afr.:* Minuric; *Spain:* Urinorm; *Switz.:* Desuric; Obaron.

Multi-ingredient: *Aust.:* Allobenz; Duovitan; Gichtex plus; Uroplus; *Belg.:* Comburic; *Fr.:* Desatura; *Ger.:* Acifugan; allo.comp.-ratiopharm; Allomaron; Harpagin; Uricovac comp†; *Ital.:* Urifugan†; *S.Afr.:* Allomaron; *Spain:* Acifugan; Facilit; *Switz.:* Acifugan.

Benziodarone (9211-v)

Benziodarone *(BAN, rINN).*

L-2329. 2-Ethylbenzofuran-3-yl 4-hydroxy-3,5-di-iodophenyl ketone.

$C_{17}H_{12}I_2O_3$ = 518.1.

CAS — 68-90-6.

Benziodarone is a uricosuric drug structurally related to benzbromarone (see above) that is used to reduce hyperuricaemia in chronic gout. It was formerly used as a vasodilator.

Benziodarone has been associated with jaundice and thyroid disorders.

Preparations

Proprietary Preparations (details are given in Part 3)
Ital.: Plexocardio†; *Spain:* Dilafurane.

Multi-ingredient: *Ital.:* Uricodue; *Spain:* Biuricowas†.

Colchicine (1001-d)

Colchicinum. (S)-N-(5,6,7,9-Tetrahydro-1,2,3,10-tetramethoxy-9-oxobenzo[α]heptalen-7-yl)acetamide.

$C_{22}H_{25}NO_6$ = 399.4.

CAS — 64-86-8.

Pharmacopoeias. In *Chin., Eur.* (see p.viii), *Int., Jpn,* and *US. Chin.* also has a monograph for colchicine amide.

An alkaloid obtained from various *Colchicum* spp. It occurs as pale yellow to greenish-yellow, odourless or almost odourless amorphous scales or crystalline powder. It darkens on exposure to light.

Ph. Eur. states that it is very **soluble** (1 in less than 1) in water, rapidly recrystallising from concentrated solutions as the sesquihydrate, but the USP has soluble 1 in 25 of water. Freely soluble in alcohol; soluble 1 in 220 of ether; freely soluble in chloroform. **Store** in airtight containers. Protect from light.

Adverse Effects and Treatment

The most frequent adverse effects of oral colchicine are those involving the gastro-intestinal tract and may be associated with its antimitotic action. Diarrhoea, nausea, vomiting, and abdominal pain are often the first signs of toxicity and are usually an indication that colchicine therapy should be stopped or the dose reduced.

Bone marrow depression with agranulocytosis, thrombocytopenia, and aplastic anaemia have occurred on prolonged treatment as have peripheral neuropathy, myopathy, rashes, and alopecia.

Adverse effects after intravenous administration include cardiac arrhythmias and local reactions such as thrombophlebitis and neuritis. Extravasation may cause tissue necrosis.

Symptoms of acute **overdosage** with oral colchicine often do not appear for at least several hours. The first symptoms are most commonly nausea, vomiting, and diarrhoea. The diarrhoea may be severe and haemorrhagic. These symptoms, coupled with vascular damage, may lead to dehydration, hypotension, and shock. Multiple organ failure may occur and may be manifest as CNS toxicity, bone marrow depression, hepatocellular damage, muscle damage, respiratory distress, myocardial injury, and renal damage. Death may be due to respiratory depression, cardiovascular collapse, or bone marrow depression. In surviving patients, alopecia, rebound leucocytosis, and stomatitis may occur about 10 days after the acute overdose. The lethal dose varies: 7 mg of colchicine has caused death, yet recovery has occurred after much larger doses.

When treating colchicine overdosage or acute poisoning patients should be carefully monitored for some time to take account of the delayed onset of symptoms. In acute poisoning the stomach should be emptied by lavage and/or activated charcoal administered. Treatment is primarily symptomatic and supportive with attention being given to the control of respiration, maintenance of blood pressure and the circulation, and correction of fluid and electrolyte imbalance. Colchicine specific antibody (Fab) fragments have been used successfully in severe overdosage.

Effects on the neuromuscular system. Colchicine-induced myoneuropathy may be a common but unrecognised condition in patients with *reduced* renal function who receive usual doses of colchicine.[1] Although both skeletal muscles and peripheral nerves are affected, myopathy is most prominent and associated axonal neuropathy is mild. The condition usually presents with proximal muscle weakness and is always accompanied by elevations in serum creatine kinase concentrations. Withdrawal of colchicine leads to spontaneous remission of these symptoms within a few weeks but resolution of the polyneuropathy is slow. Examination of proximal muscles shows marked abnormal spontaneous activity and, because of the features of the condition, it is often initially misdiagnosed as probable polymyositis or uraemic myopathy.

A further report described a patient with *normal* renal function but chronic alcohol-induced liver disease who developed an unusual form of myoneuropathy after receiving only a short course of colchicine. This patient was also taking tolbutamide, the microsomal enzyme-inhibiting activity of which may have exacerbated the toxicity of colchicine.[2]

1. Kuncl RW, *et al.* Colchicine myopathy and neuropathy. *N Engl J Med* 1987; **316:** 1562–8.
2. Besana C, *et al.* Colchicine myoneuropathy. *Lancet* 1987; **ii:** 1271–2.

Overdosage. Some references to overdosage with colchicine.

1. Davies HO, *et al.* Massive overdose of colchicine. *Can Med Assoc J* 1988; **138:** 335–6.
2. Simons RJ, Kingma DW. Fatal colchicine toxicity. *Am J Med* 1989; **86:** 356–7.
3. Katz R, *et al.* Use of granulocyte colony-stimulating factor in the treatment of pancytopenia secondary to colchicine overdose. *Ann Pharmacother* 1992; **26:** 1087–8.
4. McIntyre IM, *et al.* Death following colchicine poisoning. *J Forensic Sci* 1994; **39:** 280–6.
5. Hood RL. Colchicine poisoning. *J Emerg Med* 1994; **12:** 171–7.
6. Baud FJ, *et al.* Brief report: treatment of severe colchicine overdose with colchicine-specific Fab fragments. *N Engl J Med* 1995; **332:** 642–5.

Precautions

Colchicine should be given with great care to old and debilitated patients who may be particularly susceptible to cumulative toxicity. It should also be used with caution in patients with cardiac, hepatic, renal, or gastro-intestinal disease. Care should also be exercised if treating pregnant patients since colchicine is known to be teratogenic in *animals* and there have also been some suggestions of a risk of fetal chromosome damage (trisomy 21) in humans.

Colchicine should not be administered by subcutaneous or intramuscular injection as it causes severe local irritation.

Interactions

Cyclosporin. Several workers have highlighted the need for caution if colchicine is used concomitantly with cyclosporin. Myopathies or rhabdomyolysis, especially in patients with renal impairment, may be a problem with this combination.[1,2] In addition, increased blood-cyclosporin concentrations and nephrotoxicity have developed in a renal transplant patient after the introduction of colchicine therapy.[3]

1. Rumpf KW, Henning HV. Is myopathy in renal transplant patients induced by cyclosporin or colchicine? *Lancet* 1990; **335:** 800–1.
2. Arellano F, Krupp P. Muscular disorders associated with cyclosporin. *Lancet* 1991; **337:** 915.
3. Menta R, *et al.* Reversible acute cyclosporin nephrotoxicity induced by colchicine administration. *Nephrol Dial Transplant* 1987; **2:** 380–1.

Erythromycin. Life-threatening colchicine toxicity has been described after 2 weeks of concomitant erythromycin administration in a patient with hepatic and renal impairment.[1]

1. Caraco Y, *et al.* Acute colchicine intoxication—possible role of erythromycin administration. *J Rheumatol* 1992; **19:** 494–6.

Pharmacokinetics

Peak plasma concentrations of colchicine are reached within 2 hours of oral administration. Colchicine is partially deacetylated in the liver and the unchanged drug and its metabolites are excreted in the bile and undergo intestinal reabsorption. Colchicine is found in high concentrations in leucocytes, kidneys, the liver, and spleen. Most of the drug is excreted in the faeces but 10 to 20% is excreted in the urine and this proportion rises in patients with liver disorders.

References.

1. Rochdi M, *et al.* Toxicokinetics of colchicine in humans: analysis of tissue, plasma and urine data in ten cases. *Hum Exp Toxicol* 1992; **11:** 510–16.
2. Chappey ON, *et al.* Colchicine disposition in human leukocytes after single and multiple oral administration. *Clin Pharmacol Ther* 1993; **54:** 360–7.
3. Rochdi M, *et al.* Pharmacokinetics and absolute bioavailability of colchicine after iv and oral administration in healthy human volunteers and elderly subjects. *Eur J Clin Pharmacol* 1994; **46:** 351–4.
4. Ferron GM, *et al.* Oral absorption characteristics and pharmacokinetics of colchicine in healthy volunteers after single and multiple doses. *J Clin Pharmacol* 1996; **36:** 874–83.

Uses and Administration

Colchicine is used for the relief of acute gout (p.390) and for the prophylaxis of acute attacks, particularly during the first few months of treatment with allopurinol or uricosurics. Colchicine produces a dramatic response in acute gout, probably by reducing the inflammatory reaction to urate crystals; this effect might be due to several actions including decreased leucocyte mobility. It is not an analgesic and has no effect on blood concentrations of uric acid, or on the excretion of uric acid. Colchicine also has an antimitotic action.

Colchicine has also been used in several other conditions including amyloidosis, Behçet's syndrome, familial Mediterranean fever, idiopathic thrombocytopenic purpura, pericarditis, primary biliary cirrhosis, and pyoderma gangrenosum.

If colchicine is used for acute attacks of **gout**, then treatment should be started as soon as possible and an effect may be expected within 12 hours. The recommended oral dose in the UK is 1 mg initially then 0.5 mg every 2 to 3 hours until pain relief is obtained or gastro-intestinal adverse effects occur; the total dose should not exceed 10 mg. At least 3 days should elapse before another course is given. In the USA the dose by mouth is 0.5 to 1.2 mg initially, then 0.5 or 0.6 mg every 1 to 2 hours or 1 or 1.2 mg every 2 hours until pain is relieved or gastro-intestinal adverse effects occur; the maximum total dose is 6 mg. Colchicine has sometimes been given intravenously in a dose of 1 or 2 mg over 2 to 5 minutes with additional doses of 0.5 or 1 mg every 6 to 24 hours as required to a total dose of not more than 4 mg in one course; once this amount of colchicine has been given further doses should not then be given by any route for at least 7 days.

When used for the short-term prophylaxis of gout doses by mouth are 0.5 or 0.6 mg one to three times daily.

Consideration should be given to using reduced dosages in patients with mild to moderate renal impairment.

Amyloidosis. Colchicine is well known to have a useful role in secondary amyloidosis in familial Mediterranean fever, where results have unexpectedly suggested the possibility of reversing nephropathic changes due to renal amyloid deposition (see below), and it may be beneficial in some other forms of amyloidosis,[1-6] especially when combined with other drugs. The mechanism of the anti-amyloid effect of colchicine is not clear. Amyloidosis and its management are discussed further on p.497.

1. Cohen AS, *et al.* Survival of patients with primary (AL) amyloidosis: colchicine-treated cases from 1976 to 1983 compared with cases seen in previous years (1961 to 1973). *Am J Med* 1987; **82:** 1182–90.
2. Benson MD. Treatment of AL amyloidosis with melphalan, prednisone, and colchicine. *Arthritis Rheum* 1986; **29:** 683–7.
3. Fritz DA, *et al.* Unusual longevity in primary systemic amyloidosis: a 19-year survivor. *Am J Med* 1989; **86:** 245–8.
4. Schattner A, *et al.* Primary amyloidosis with unusual bone involvement: reversibility with melphalan, prednisone, and colchicine. *Am J Med* 1989; **86:** 347–8.
5. Skinner M, *et al.* Treatment of 100 patients with primary amyloidosis: a randomised trial of melphalan, prednisone, and colchicine versus colchicine only. *Am J Med* 1996; **100:** 290–8.
6. Kyle RA, *et al.* A trial of three regimens for primary amyloidosis: colchicine alone, melphalan and prednisone, and melphalan, prednisone, and colchicine. *N Engl J Med* 1997; **336:** 1202–7.

Behçet's syndrome. Behçet's syndrome (p.1018) has been treated with numerous drugs. Where possible, topical treatment of local lesions should be attempted before embarking on systemic therapy. Corticosteroids are favoured for systemic treatment in many countries, but colchicine has also been widely employed and beneficial responses have been described for most of the symptoms including the ocular and cutaneous manifestations.[1-4] The mechanism of action in this condition is believed to be based on the effect on polymorphonuclear leucocytes and other cellular effects.[5] Colchicine has also been used in combination with corticosteroids for acute exacerbations, followed by colchicine maintenance;[6] colchicine with aspirin has also been recommended in acute disease,[7] and colchicine with benzathine penicillin has been tried.[8]

1. Mizushima Y, *et al.* Colchicine in Behçet's disease. *Lancet* 1977; **ii:** 1037.
2. Miyachi Y, *et al.* Colchicine in the treatment of the cutaneous manifestations of Behçet's disease. *Br J Dermatol* 1981; **104:** 67–9.
3. Benezra D, Cohen E. Treatment and visual prognosis in Behçet's disease. *Br J Ophthalmol* 1986; **70;** 589–92.
4. Masuda K, *et al.* Double-masked trial of cyclosporin versus colchicine and long term open study of cyclosporin in Behçet's disease. *Lancet* 1989; **i:** 1093–6.
5. Schattner A. Colchicine—expanding horizons. *Postgrad Med J* 1991; **67:** 223–6.
6. Rakover Y, *et al.* Behcet disease: long-term follow-up of three children and review of the literature. *Pediatrics* 1989; **83:** 986–92.
7. Wechsler B, Piette JC. Behçet's disease. *Br Med J* 1992; **304:** 1199–1200.
8. Çalgüneri M, *et al.* Effect of prophylactic benzathine penicillin on mucotaneous symptoms of Behçet's disease. *Dermatology* 1996; **192:** 125–8.

Familial Mediterranean fever. Familial Mediterranean fever is the most widely used term for an inherited disorder more accurately termed recurrent or paroxysmal polyserositis. It primarily affects Sephardic Jews or persons of Arab, Armenian, and Turkish ancestry, and is characterised by attacks of acute abdominal pain, fever, and signs of peritonitis, which resolve spontaneously, usually in 24 to 48 hours. Pleuritic chest pain, arthritis, skin rash, pericarditis, and headache may occur. The most dangerous complication, however, is type AA amyloidosis (see also p.497), which can lead to nephrotic syndrome, renal failure, and death.

Familial Mediterranean fever is treated with colchicine. Although a course of the drug may abort an acute attack if given early enough in its development, most patients receive prophylactic treatment, usually with a daily dose in adults of about 0.5 to 2 mg. Such treatment reduces the frequency of attacks and the development of amyloidosis;[1,2] some reversal of established renal problems may also be possible.[3,4] Preliminary evidence suggests interferon alfa may abort acute attacks.[5]

1. Zemer D, *et al.* Colchicine in the prevention and treatment of the amyloidosis of familial Mediterranean fever. *N Engl J Med* 1986; **314:** 1001–5.
2. Majeed HA, *et al.* Long-term colchicine prophylaxis in children with familial Mediterranean fever (recurrent hereditary polyserositis). *J Pediatr* 1990; **116:** 997–9.
3. Zemer D, *et al.* Reversal of the nephrotic syndrome by colchicine in amyloidosis of familial Mediterranean fever. *Ann Intern Med* 1992; **116:** 426.
4. Fak AS, *et al.* Colchicine and secondary amyloidosis. *Ann Intern Med* 1992; **117:** 795–6.
5. Tunca M, *et al.* The efficacy of interferon alpha on colchicine-resistant familial Mediterranean fever attacks: a pilot study. *Br J Rheumatol* 1997; **36:** 1005–8.

Idiopathic thrombocytopenic purpura. Case reports have described a few patients with idiopathic thrombocytopenic purpura (p.1023) who had partial or complete responses to colchicine.[1-3] A trial of colchicine has been suggested in adult patients with disease refractory to standard therapy who also do not respond to danazol or vinca alkaloids.[4]

1. Strother SV, *et al.* Colchicine therapy for refractory idiopathic thrombocytopenic purpura. *Arch Intern Med* 1984; **144:** 2198–2200.
2. Jim RTS. Therapeutic use of colchicine in thrombocytopenia. *Hawaii Med J* 1986; **45:** 221–6.
3. Baker RI, Manoharan A. Colchicine therapy for idiopathic thrombocytopenic purpura—an inexpensive alternative. *Aust N Z J Med* 1989; **19:** 412–13.
4. McMillian R. Therapy for adults with refractory chronic immune thrombocytopenic purpura. *Ann Intern Med* 1997; **126:** 307–14.

Interstitial lung disease. For reference to the use of colchicine as a potential alternative to corticosteroid therapy in patients with cryptogenic fibrosing alveolitis, see p.1024.

Pericarditis. Administration of colchicine produced an improvement in a few patients who required corticosteroid therapy to control recurrent episodes of pericarditis.[1,2] Corticosteroid therapy was withdrawn about 2 months after starting treatment with colchicine and the patients had been free of further attacks for up to 54 months. Colchicine was also used successfully in most of a series of 19 patients with recurrent pericarditis who had not yet received corticosteroids, suggesting that it might be tried before corticosteroids and after treatment with NSAIDs had failed.[3]

1. de la Serna AR, *et al.* Colchicine for recurrent pericarditis. *Lancet* 1987; **ii:** 1517.
2. Guindo J, *et al.* Recurrent pericarditis: relief with colchicine. *Circulation* 1990; **82:** 1117–20.
3. Millaire A, *et al.* Treatment of recurrent pericarditis with colchicine. *Eur Heart J* 1994; **15:** 120–4.

Primary biliary cirrhosis. Primary biliary cirrhosis (p.497) is a chronic progressive liver disease with no specific treatment, and in general drug therapy has been poor or largely ineffective. Reviewers have noted[1-3] that several trials have been conducted with colchicine, and, although biochemical parameters were improved, a beneficial effect on clinical symptoms or liver histology was not found, and only one study showed improved survival of the patients.[4] Some commentators consider that combination therapy with colchicine, methotrexate, and ursodeoxycholic acid may be more promising than single-agent therapy,[5] but others have noted that preliminary experience with such combinations has not been encouraging.[6]

1. Bateson MC. New directions in primary biliary cirrhosis. *Br Med J* 1990; **301:** 1290–1.
2. Stavinoha MW, Soloway RD. Current therapy of chronic liver disease. *Drugs* 1990; **39:** 814–40.
3. Neuberger J, *et al.* Primary biliary cirrhosis. *Gut* 1991; **32** (suppl): S73–S78.
4. Kaplan MM, *et al.* A prospective trial of colchicine for primary biliary cirrhosis. *N Engl J Med* 1986; **315:** 1448–54.
5. Goddard CJR, Warnes TW. Primary biliary cirrhosis: how should we evaluate new treatments? *Lancet* 1994; **343:** 1305–6.
6. Lim AG. Evaluation of new treatment for primary biliary cirrhosis. *Lancet* 1994; **344:** 61.

Pyoderma gangrenosum. Pyoderma gangrenosum (p.1076) associated with inflammatory bowel disease has been successfully treated with colchicine in 2 patients.[1,2] Colchicine was also of benefit in 3 patients with pyoderma associated with familial Mediterranean fever.[3]

1. Paolini O, *et al.* Treatment of pyoderma gangrenosum with colchicine. *Lancet* 1995; **345:** 1057–8.
2. Rampal P, *et al.* Colchicine in pyoderma gangrenosum. *Lancet* 1998; **351:** 1134–5.
3. Lugassy G, Ronnen M. Severe pyoderma associated with familial Mediterranean fever: favourable response to colchicine in three patients. *Am J Med Sci* 1992; **304:** 29–31.

Scleroderma. For mention of colchicine as a possible alternative to penicillamine in the management of scleroderma, see p.501.

Preparations

BP 1998: Colchicine Tablets;
USP 23: Colchicine Injection; Colchicine Tablets; Probenecid and Colchicine Tablets.

Proprietary Preparations (details are given in Part 3)
Austral.: Colgout.

Multi-ingredient: ***Fr.:*** Colchimax; Gripponyl†; ***Spain:*** Colchimax; ***USA:*** ColBenemid†; Proben-C†.

Colchicum (1003-h)

Colchique.

The dried ripe seeds or dried corm of the meadow saffron, *Colchicum autumnale.*

Colchicum contains colchicine (p.393) and has been used similarly for the relief of acute gout.

It is also included in several herbal and homoeopathic preparations.

Preparations

Proprietary Preparations (details are given in Part 3)
Fr.: Teinture de Cocheux†; ***Ger.:*** Colchysat.

Multi-ingredient: ***Fr.:*** Antigoutteux Rezall; ***Ger.:*** Colchicum-Strath†; Unguentum Lymphaticum.

Isobromindione (12866-b)

Isobromindione *(rINN).*

5-Bromo-2-phenyl-indan-1,3-dione.

$C_{15}H_9BrO_2$ = 301.1.

CAS — 1470-35-5.

Isobromindione is a uricosuric drug used by mouth in gout and hyperuricaemia. Bromindione used to be given as an anticoagulant.

Preparations

Proprietary Preparations (details are given in Part 3)
Ital.: Uridion.

Probenecid (1008-q)

Probenecid *(BAN, rINN).*

Probenecidum. 4-(Dipropylsulphamoyl)benzoic acid.

$C_{13}H_{19}NO_4S$ = 285.4.

CAS — 57-66-9.

Pharmacopoeias. In *Chin., Eur.* (see p.viii), *Int., Jpn,* and *US.*

A white or almost white, almost odourless, crystalline powder or small crystals. Practically **insoluble** in water; soluble in alcohol; sparingly soluble in dehydrated alcohol; soluble in acetone and in chloroform; slightly soluble or very slightly soluble in ether; practically insoluble in dilute acids; soluble dilute alkali.

Adverse Effects

Probenecid may cause nausea, vomiting, anorexia, headache, sore gums, flushing, dizziness, and urinary frequency. Hypersensitivity reactions, with fever, dermatitis, pruritus, urticaria, and, rarely, anaphylaxis have occurred and there have been reports of hepatic necrosis, the nephrotic syndrome, and aplastic anaemia. Haemolytic anaemia has also occurred, and may be associated with glucose-6-phosphate dehydrogenase deficiency.

When used in chronic gout, and particularly during the first few months of therapy, probenecid may precipitate acute attacks, and uric acid renal calculi with or without haematuria and renal colic may occur.

In massive overdosage probenecid causes stimulation of the central nervous system, with convulsions and death from respiratory failure. Severe overdosage should be managed by emesis or lavage and symptomatic treatment.

Precautions

Probenecid therapy should not be started during an acute attack of gout; however treatment is usually continued when acute attacks occur in patients already receiving the drug, and the acute attack is treated separately. Probenecid should not be given to patients with a history of uric acid renal calculi, blood disorders, or porphyria. It is not recommended for children under 2 years of age. Probenecid is also unsuitable for the control of hyperuricaemia secondary to cancer or cancer chemotherapy. It should be used with caution in patients with a history of peptic ulceration. Probenecid should not be used as an antibacterial adjunct in patients with known renal impairment, and it is ineffective in gout in patients with severe renal impairment.

To reduce the risk of uric acid renal calculi in patients with gout an adequate fluid intake (2 to 3 litres daily) is required, and, if necessary, especially during the first few months of treatment, sodium bicarbonate or potassium citrate may be given to render the urine alkaline.

A reducing substance has been found in the urine of some patients taking probenecid, and may give false positive results with some tests for glucose in the urine. Probenecid reduces the excretion of some iodinated contrast media and may interfere with laboratory tests by decreasing the excretion of aminohippuric acid, phenolsulphonphthalein, and sulphobromophthalein.

Abuse. It has been alleged that some athletes using banned anabolic steroids have also been taking probenecid in an attempt to inhibit the urinary excretion of steroid metabolites in order to avoid detection by urine screening tests.[1]

1. Anonymous. Does probenecid mask steroid use? *Pharm J* 1987; **239:** 299.

Interactions

The dose of probenecid may need to be increased if patients are also given drugs such as *diuretics* or *pyrazinamide* that increase the blood concentration of uric acid. Salicylates, including *aspirin*, and probenecid are mutually antagonistic and should not be given together.

Probenecid may also affect many of other drugs given concomitantly. By inhibiting renal tubular secretion, probenecid has the potential to increase the toxicity and/or to enhance the therapeutic efficacy of drugs excreted by that route. In some instances a reduction in dose is essential to counteract an increase in toxicity, as is the case with *methotrexate*. Some combinations, such as that with *ketorolac* should be avoided. Conversely, probenecid may be given with some *antibacterials* such as the penicillins and cephalosporins (other than cephaloridine) to increase their effects.

Altered excretion may also increase serum concentrations of other antibacterials (aminosalicylic acid, conjugated sulphonamides, dapsone, quinolones, rifampicin), some *antivirals* (aciclovir, possibly famciclovir and ganciclovir, zalcitabine, zidovudine), *captopril, lorazepam,* some *NSAIDs* (indomethacin, ketoprofen, meclofenamate, naproxen), *paracetamol,* and *sulphonylurea hypoglycaemic drugs*. The clinical significance of such interactions is not entirely clear although the possibility of the need for a reduction in dosage of these drugs should be borne in mind.

It has been reported that patients receiving probenecid require lower doses of *thiopentone* for induction of anaesthesia.

Reducing the urinary concentration of some drugs could diminish their activity in certain diseases as might happen with *nitrofurantoin* or some *quinolones* in urinary-tract infections and *penicillamine* in cystinuria.

Pharmacokinetics

Probenecid is completely absorbed from the gastro-intestinal tract with peak plasma concentrations achieved 2 to 4 hours after a dose. It is extensively bound to plasma proteins (85 to 95%). The plasma half-life is dose-dependent and ranges from less than 5 to more than 8 hours. Probenecid crosses the placenta. It is metabolised by the liver, and excreted in the urine mainly as metabolites. Excretion is increased in alkaline urine.

References.

1. Ho JC, *et al.* Probenecid disposition by parallel Michaelis-Menten and dose-dependent pseudo-first-order processes. *J Pharm Sci* 1986; **75:** 664–8.
2. Emanuelsson B-M, *et al.* Non-linear elimination and protein binding of probenecid. *Eur J Clin Pharmacol* 1987; **32:** 395–401.

Uses and Administration

Probenecid is a uricosuric drug used to treat hyperuricaemia (p.390) associated with chronic gout and diuretic therapy. It is also used as an adjunct to some antibacterial drugs to reduce their renal tubular excretion and has been given with the antiviral cidofovir (p.607) to reduce nephrotoxicity.

Probenecid's use in **chronic gout and hyperuricaemia** derives from its inhibition of the renal tubular reabsorption of uric acid so increasing the urinary excretion of uric acid. Probenecid is therefore of value in hyperuricaemia caused by decreased uric acid excretion rather than increased urate production, and so is not used for hyperuricaemia associated with cancer or cancer therapy. The increased excretion of uric acid leads to a lowering of plasma-urate concentrations which in turn leads to a reduction in urate deposits in the tissues, although this may take some time.

Probenecid has no analgesic or anti-inflammatory action and is of no value in acute gout. Treatment with probenecid should not be started until an acute attack has subsided as the attack may be prolonged and exacerbated. The risk of an attack occurring during the first few months of treatment with probenecid may be reduced by the concurrent administration of an NSAID or colchicine.

It is usual to start treatment for gout with doses of 250 mg twice daily by mouth increased after a week to 500 mg twice daily and later, if the therapeutic effects are inadequate, by 500-mg increments every 4 weeks, up to 2 g daily. Probenecid may not be effective in chronic renal impairment particularly when the glomerular filtration rate is less than 30 mL per minute. An adequate fluid intake is required to reduce the risk of uric acid renal calculi.

When the patient has been free from acute attacks for at least 6 months, and provided that the plasma-urate concentration is within acceptable limits, the daily dose may be gradually reduced, by 500 mg every 6 months, to the lowest effective maintenance dose which is then given indefinitely.

Probenecid may also be used as an **adjunct to antibacterial therapy** particularly when treating severe or resistant infections. It reduces the tubular excretion of penicillins and most cephalosporins and may increase their plasma concentrations up to fourfold; it does not affect cephaloridine. The usual dosage for reducing tubular excretion of penicillins and cephalosporins is 500 mg four times daily, or less in elderly patients with suspected renal impairment. When renal impairment is sufficient to retard the excretion of antibacterials, probenecid should not be given concurrently.

The dosage for children over 2 years of age and weighing less than 50 kg is 25 mg per kg body-weight (700 mg per m^2 body-surface) initially, followed by 10 mg per kg (300 mg per m^2) every 6 hours.

Single doses of probenecid 1 g are given together with an oral antibacterial, or 30 minutes before an injected antibacterial, in the single-dose treatment of gonorrhoea.

Preparations

BP 1998: Probenecid Tablets;
USP 23: Ampicillin and Probenecid Capsules; Ampicillin and Probenecid for Oral Suspension; Probenecid and Colchicine Tablets; Probenecid Tablets.

Proprietary Preparations (details are given in Part 3)
Austral.: Benemid; ***Canad.:*** Benemid; Benuryl; ***Fr.:*** Benemide†; ***Irl.:*** Benemid; ***Ital.:*** Solpurin†; Urocid†; ***Neth.:*** Benemid†; ***Norw.:*** Probecid; ***S.Afr.:*** Benemid; Proben†; ***Swed.:*** Probecid; ***Switz.:*** Benemid; ***UK:*** Benemid; ***USA:*** Benemid†; Probalan†.

Multi-ingredient: ***USA:*** ColBenemid†; Proben-C†.

Used as an adjunct in: ***Fr.:*** Prototapen†; ***Spain:*** Blenox; ***USA:*** Polycillin-PRB†; Principen with Probenecid†.

Sulphinpyrazone (1009-p)

Sulphinpyrazone *(BAN)*.

Sulfinpyrazone *(rINN)*; G-28315; Sulfinpyrazonum; Sulphoxyphenylpyrazolidine. 1,2-Diphenyl-4-(2-phenylsulphinylethyl)pyrazolidine-3,5-dione.

$C_{23}H_{20}N_2O_3S$ = 404.5.

CAS — 57-96-5.

Pharmacopoeias. In *Eur.* (see p.viii), *Jpn*, and *US*.

A white or off-white powder. Ph. Eur. **solubilities** are: very slightly soluble in water; sparingly soluble in alcohol; slightly soluble in ether; dissolves in dilute solutions of alkali hydroxides. USP solubilities are: practically insoluble in water and in petroleum spirit; soluble in alcohol and in acetone; and sparingly soluble in dilute solutions of alkalis. **Protect** from light.

Adverse Effects

The most frequent adverse effects of sulphinpyrazone involve the gastro-intestinal tract, and include nausea, vomiting, and abdominal pain. It may cause gastric bleeding and aggravate existing peptic ulcers. Skin rashes have been reported, and may be associated with a hypersensitivity reaction. Anaemia, agranulocytosis, leucopenia, and thrombocytopenia have been reported rarely as have raised liver enzyme values, jaundice, and hepatitis, impaired renal function, salt and water retention, and acute renal failure.

When used in chronic gout, particularly during the first few months of treatment, sulphinpyrazone may precipitate acute attacks and there is a risk of uric acid renal calculi developing.

Symptoms of overdosage include hypotension, acute renal failure, arrhythmias, respiratory disorders, convulsions, and coma, as well as gastro-intestinal effects. Treatment of overdose involves gastric lavage followed by symptomatic and supportive therapy.

Effects on the kidneys. Although renal failure has been reported occasionally in patients receiving sulphinpyrazone for gout[1] many of the cases have occurred in patients given the drug after a myocardial infarction.[2,3] Acute renal failure may also occur after overdose.[4]

1. Durham DS, Ibels LS. Sulphinpyrazone-induced acute renal failure. *Br Med J* 1981; **282:** 609.
2. Boelaert J, *et al.* Sulphinpyrazone-induced decrease in renal function: a review of reports with discussion of pathogenesis. *Acta Clin Belg* 1982; **37:** 368–75.
3. Lijnen P, *et al.* Decrease in renal function due to sulphinpyrazone treatment early after myocardial infarction. *Clin Nephrol* 1983; **19:** 143–6.
4. Florkowski CM, *et al.* Acute non-oliguric renal failure secondary to sulphinpyrazone overdose. *J Clin Pharm Ther* 1992; **17:** 71.

Precautions

Sulphinpyrazone should not be started during an acute attack of gout; however, treatment is usually continued when acute attacks occur in patients already receiving the drug, and the acute attack is treated separately. It should not be given to patients with uric acid renal calculi or an active peptic ulcer or a history of such disorders; use is also contra-indicated in patients with blood dyscrasias or blood coagulation disorders, porphyria, and in those with severe kidney or liver damage. Sulphinpyrazone should not be given to patients hypersensitive to it or to other pyrazole derivatives such as phenylbutazone; nor should it be given to patients in whom hypersensitivity reactions have been provoked by aspirin or by other drugs with prostaglandin-synthetase inhibiting activity. Sulphinpyrazone is not suitable for the control of hyperuricaemia associated with cancer or cancer chemotherapy. It should be given with care to patients whose renal function is impaired and to those with heart failure.

To reduce the risk of uric acid renal calculi an adequate fluid intake (2 to 3 litres daily) is required; alkalinising the urine with sodium bicarbonate or potassium citrate may also be considered. It is recommended that patients have periodic full blood counts to detect any haematological abnormalities.

Renal function tests involving aminohippuric acid or phenolsulphonphthalein may be invalidated.

Interactions

Doses of sulphinpyrazone may need to be increased if it is given with other drugs such as *diuretics* or *pyrazinamide* that increase uric acid concentrations. Sulphinpyrazone and salicylates including *aspirin* are mutually antagonistic and should not be used together. There may also be an increased risk of bleeding when sulphinpyrazone is used with other drugs such as aspirin that inhibit platelet function.

Sulphinpyrazone's renal tubular secretion is inhibited by probenecid although with little clinical effect. Since sulphinpyrazone, like probenecid, inhibits the tubular secretion of weak organic acids, interactions can be expected with penicillins although the effect is not considered to be clinically useful.

Sulphinpyrazone can inhibit the metabolism of some drugs leading to an increase in their activity. The most significant interaction of this type involves *warfarin, nicoumalone*, and possibly other coumarin anticoagulants (p.967). Patients receiving sulphinpyrazone and such an anticoagulant should have their prothrombin times monitored and the anticoagulant dosage reduced as appropriate. Similarly, sulphinpyrazone may potentiate the effects of *phenytoin* (see p.355), and possibly some *sulphonamides* and *sulphonylureas* (p.332).

The activity of *theophylline* may be diminished by sulphinpyrazone increasing its metabolism (p.769).

Pharmacokinetics

Sulphinpyrazone is readily absorbed from the gastro-intestinal tract. About 98% of the sulphinpyrazone in the circulation is bound to plasma proteins. It has been reported to have a plasma half-life of about 2 to 4 hours. Sulphinpyrazone is partly metabolised in the liver and some of the metabolites are active. On long-term therapy, sulphinpyrazone appears to induce its own metabolism. Unchanged drug and metabolites are mainly excreted in the urine.

References.

1. Bradbrook ID, *et al.* Pharmacokinetics of single doses of sulphinpyrazone and its major metabolites in plasma and urine. *Br J Clin Pharmacol* 1982; **13:** 177–85.
2. Schlicht F, *et al.* Pharmacokinetics of sulphinpyrazone and its major metabolites after a single dose and during chronic treatment. *Eur J Clin Pharmacol* 1985; **28:** 97–103.

Uses and Administration

Sulphinpyrazone is a uricosuric drug used to treat hyperuricaemia associated with chronic gout (p.390). It also has some antiplatelet activity.

Sulphinpyrazone's use in chronic gout derives from its inhibition of the renal tubular reabsorption of uric acid so increasing the urinary excretion of uric acid. It is therefore of value in hyperuricaemia caused by decreased uric acid excretion rather than increased urate production and so is not used for hyperuricaemia associated with cancer or cancer therapy. The increased excretion of uric acid leads to a lowering of plasma-urate concentrations which in turn leads to a reduction in urate deposits in the tissues, although this may take some time. Sulphinpyrazone has little analgesic or anti-inflammatory action and is of no value in acute gout. Treatment with sulphinpyrazone should not be started until an acute attack has subsided as the attack may be exacerbated and prolonged. At the beginning of treatment with sulphinpyrazone acute episodes of gout may be precipitated. An NSAID or colchicine may be given during the first few months of treatment to reduce the incidence of such attacks.

The initial dose of sulphinpyrazone is 100 to 200 mg once or twice daily, taken with meals or milk. This may be gradually increased over 1 to 3 weeks until a daily dosage of 600 mg is reached; up to 800 mg daily may be given if necessary. After the plasma-urate concentration has been controlled, the daily maintenance dose may be reduced to as low as 200 mg. An adequate fluid intake is required to prevent formation of uric acid renal calculi.

Antiplatelet therapy. Sulphinpyrazone inhibits platelet function, thereby inhibiting thrombosis. A meta-analysis of trials, conducted by the Antiplatelet Trialists' Collaboration, has shown that sulphinpyrazone reduces the risk of myocardial infarction, stroke, or vascular death in patients at high risk of occlusive vascular disease.[1] Similarly, sulphinpyrazone reduces the risk of occlusion in patients undergoing arterial reperfusion and revascularisation procedures.[2] However, aspirin is the most widely tested antiplatelet therapy, as discussed on p.797.

1. Antiplatelet Trialists' Collaboration. Collaborative overview of randomised trials of antiplatelet therapy—I: prevention of death, myocardial infarction, and stroke by prolonged antiplatelet therapy in various categories of patients. *Br Med J* 1994; **308:** 81–106.
2. Antiplatelet Trialists' Collaboration. Collaborative overview of randomised trials of antiplatelet therapy—II: maintenance of vascular graft or arterial patency by antiplatelet therapy. *Br Med J* 1994; **308:** 159–68.

Preparations

BP 1998: Sulfinpyrazone Tablets;
USP 23: Sulfinpyrazone Capsules; Sulfinpyrazone Tablets.

Proprietary Preparations (details are given in Part 3)
Aust.: Anturan; ***Austral.:*** Anturan; ***Canad.:*** Anturan; Novo-Pyrazone; ***Ger.:*** Anturano†; ***Irl.:*** Anturan†; ***Ital.:*** Enturen; ***S.Afr.:*** Anturan†; ***Spain:*** Falizal†; ***Switz.:*** Anturan; ***UK:*** Anturan; ***USA:*** Anturane.

Tisopurine (1010-n)

Tisopurine (*rINN*).
MPP. 1*H*-Pyrazolo[3,4-*d*]pyrimidine-4-thiol.
$C_5H_4N_4S$ = 152.2.
CAS — 5334-23-6.

Tisopurine, an analogue of allopurinol, is an inhibitor of uric acid synthesis. It is used in the treatment of disorders associated with hyperuricaemia (p.390), including gout, in doses of 100 to 400 mg daily.

Preparations

Proprietary Preparations (details are given in Part 3)
Aust.: Exuracid; ***Fr.:*** Thiopurinol†.

Urate Oxidase (14002-a)

CB-8129; Uricase.
CAS — 9002-12-4.

Urate oxidase oxidises uric acid to allantoin and is used in the treatment of disorders associated with severe hyperuricaemia. It is given by intramuscular or intravenous injection.

Hypersensitivity reactions, including anaphylactic reactions, have occurred after injections of urate oxidase[1] (utilising *Aspergillus flavus* as a source). In an attempt to reduce immunogenicity, urate oxidase (derived from *Arthrobacter protoformiae*) covalently attached to polyethylene glycol has been used;[2] in the patient who received this the product was effective and non-toxic.

1. Leaustic M, *et al.* Manifestation allergique a type de bronchospasme aprés injection intraveineuse d'urate oxydase chez une patiente traitée pour myélome. *Rev Rhum* 1983; **50:** 553–5.
2. Chua CC, *et al.* Use of polyethylene glycol-modified uricase (PEG-uricase) to treat hyperuricaemia in a patient with non-Hodgkin lymphoma. *Ann Intern Med* 1988; **109:** 114–17.

Preparations

Proprietary Preparations (details are given in Part 3)
Fr.: Uricozyme; ***Ital.:*** Uricozyme.

Antihistamines

The effects of histamine are considered to be mediated by 2 sets of receptors termed H_1 and H_2. Those effects which are mediated by the H_1 receptors include the contraction of smooth muscle and the dilatation and increased permeability of the capillaries. The effects of histamine on vascular smooth muscle are mediated by the H_2 as well as the H_1 receptors. Other effects that are mediated by the H_2 receptors include cardiac accelerating effects and, in particular, the stimulating action of histamine on the secretion of gastric acid. An H_3 receptor has also been identified in a number of systems including the CNS and peripheral nerves. It is thought that H_3 receptors are involved in the autoregulation of the release of histamine and other neurotransmitters from neurones.

The term 'antihistamines' is normally reserved for histamine H_1-receptor antagonists and this is the convention used in *Martindale*. Histamine H_2-receptor antagonists are described in the chapter on Gastro-intestinal Drugs (p.1167). Presently, no H_3-receptor antagonists have been developed for clinical use.

The older antihistamines are associated with troublesome sedative and antimuscarinic effects. To distinguish them from the newer antihistamines, which are essentially devoid of these effects, they are often termed 'sedating antihistamines' and this is the convention used in *Martindale*. The newer antihistamines are correspondingly termed 'non-sedating antihistamines'.

On the basis of their chemical structure most antihistamines can be classified into one of the following 6 groups:

- *Alkylamines:* drugs within this group possess significant sedative actions, although paradoxical stimulation can occur, especially in children. They are highly potent H_1-receptor antagonists. Brompheniramine and chlorpheniramine are typical alkylamines; acrivastine is a non-sedating alkylamine antihistamine.
- *Ethanolamines:* ethanolamine derivatives have pronounced sedative and antimuscarinic actions but a low incidence of gastro-intestinal effects. Examples include clemastine and diphenhydramine.
- *Ethylenediamines:* these antihistamines are selective H_1-receptor antagonists. They cause moderate sedation (despite having weak CNS effects), gastric disturbances, and skin sensitisation. Antazoline and pyrilamine are examples.
- *Phenothiazines:* phenothiazine antihistamines have significant sedative, and pronounced antiemetic and antimuscarinic effects. Photosensitivity reactions have occurred. Promethazine is a typical phenothiazine.
- *Piperazines:* this group of antihistamines possesses moderate sedative and significant antiemetic actions. Piperazine derivatives include cetirizine, cyclizine, and hydroxyzine. Cetirizine causes less sedation than other members of this group.
- *Piperidines:* piperidines cause moderate or low sedation and are highly selective for H_1 receptors. Examples include azatadine, cyproheptadine, and the non-sedating antihistamines astemizole, loratadine, and terfenadine.

Although characteristic pharmacological properties have been described for members of each group it should be noted that many of the effects of antihistamines vary as much with each patient as with each drug and that, in particular, some of the newer non-sedating antihistamines may share the chemical structure of a group in which the other members have sedative effects.

References.

1. Hill SJ, *et al.* International Union of Pharmacology. XIII. Classification of histamine receptors. *Pharmacol Rev* 1997; **49:** 253–78.

Hypersensitivity. Hypersensitivity may be defined as an exaggerated or inappropriate immune response causing tissue damage. Hypersensitivity reactions are generally classified into 4 types (types I to IV) although this may be considered an over simplification and more than one type can often be postulated for a patient's hypersensitivity. In each of the 4 types, prior sensitisation of the patient to the specific antigen is required. The term *'allergy'* by definition originally covered all types of hypersensitivity reactions as well as the induction of immunity in an individual. Nowadays, the term is more commonly applied to type I hypersensitivity reactions.

Type I, immediate hypersensitivity reactions occur after exposure to an antigen (the allergen) in a sensitised subject in whom the initial exposure to the antigen has caused the production of specific antibodies, mainly IgE, which are bound to the surface of mast cells and basophils. At this subsequent exposure, antigen binds to antibody resulting in degranulation of mast cells and basophils with release of mediators. These include preformed mediators such as histamine and chemotactic factors, and newly synthesised mediators such as leukotrienes, platelet-activating factor, and prostaglandins. Although type I reactions are usually described as being acute and short-lived, clinically there may often also be a late-phase and more prolonged reaction affecting the skin and bronchi. Examples of type I hypersensitivity reactions include allergic conjunctivitis (below), allergic rhinitis (below), urticaria and angioedema (below), and anaphylactic shock (below).

Type II, cell-surface hypersensitivity reactions are caused by the interaction of circulating antibodies, mainly IgG and IgM, with antigens that are on the surface of specific cells or tissues. This interaction results in activation of complement and of phagocytic and killer cells leading to cell damage or lysis. Type II reactions are responsible for blood transfusion reactions, some drug-induced blood disorders, and many auto-immune disorders.

Type III, immune complex hypersensitivity reactions are caused by the interaction of fixed or circulating antigens, with circulating antibodies, mainly IgG and IgM (either soluble or particulate) resulting in formation of immune complexes. The immune complexes trigger a variety of inflammatory processes including complement activation, mediator release from mast cells and basophils, and platelet aggregation. Examples of type III reactions include serum sickness, some auto-immune and neoplastic disorders, type 2 lepra reactions, and reactions, particularly in the lung, to some particulate antigens such as micro-organisms.

Type IV, cell-mediated or delayed hypersensitivity reactions, are caused by interaction of an antigen with sensitised T lymphocytes; lymphokines are released by T lymphocytes and inflammation ensues. Type IV reactions usually occur at least 24 hours after contact with the antigen. A type IV reaction is responsible for tuberculin reactions used for sensitivity testing, contact dermatitis, and some reactions to chronic infectious disease for example type 1 lepra reactions (p.128).

An **anaphylactoid** (pseudoallergic) reaction produces similar symptoms to those of anaphylaxis (see below), but is caused by direct release of histamine provoked by an unclear, non-immune mechanism. There is thus no requirement for prior exposure to the triggering factor, commonly a drug.

Adverse Effects of Antihistamines

The most common side-effect of the *sedating antihistamines* is CNS depression, with effects varying from slight drowsiness to deep sleep, and including lassitude, dizziness, and incoordination (although paradoxical stimulation may occasionally occur, especially in children). These sedative effects, when they occur, may diminish after a few days of treatment. A major advantage of the *non-sedating antihistamines* is that they cause little or no drowsiness.

Other side-effects that are more common with the *sedating antihistamines* include headache, psychomotor impairment, and antimuscarinic effects, such as dry mouth, thickened respiratory-tract secretions, blurred vision, urinary difficulty or retention, constipation, and increased gastric reflux. Another major advantage of the *non-sedating antihistamines* is that most have little or no antimuscarinic effect.

Occasional gastro-intestinal side-effects of antihistamines include nausea, vomiting, diarrhoea, or epigastric pain. Those with antiserotonin actions, such as cyproheptadine, may cause an increase in appetite with resultant weight gain, whereas anorexia has been reported with some other antihistamines.

Palpitations and arrhythmias have been reported occasionally with most antihistamines, but a major disadvantage of the *non-sedating antihistamines* astemizole and terfenadine is the rare occurrence of hazardous ventricular arrhythmias which has led to important restrictions on their use (see under Precautions, below).

Administration of antihistamines may sometimes cause rashes and hypersensitivity reactions (including bronchospasm, angioedema, and anaphylaxis) and cross-sensitivity to related drugs may occur. Photosensitivity can be a problem, particularly with the phenothiazine antihistamines.

Blood disorders, including agranulocytosis, leucopenia, haemolytic anaemia, and thrombocytopenia, although rare, have been reported. Jaundice has also been observed, particularly with the phenothiazine antihistamines.

Other adverse effects that have been reported with the antihistamines include convulsions, sweating, myalgia, paraesthesias, extrapyramidal effects, tremor, sleep disturbances, depression, tinnitus, hypotension, and hair loss.

Despite reports suggesting a possibility of human fetal abnormalities resulting from the use of some antihistamines, especially the piperazine derivatives, a causal relationship has largely been rejected; for details see under Precautions, below.

Some antihistamines have been abused for their mental effects.

Antihistamines available as preparations for application to the skin may occasionally cause skin sensitisation; systemic side-effects have been reported after topical application to large areas of the skin.

Overdosage with *sedating antihistamines* is associated with antimuscarinic, extrapyramidal, and CNS effects. In infants and children, CNS stimulation predominates over CNS depression, causing ataxia, excitement, tremors, psychoses, hallucinations, and convulsions; hyperpyrexia may also occur. Deepening coma and cardiorespiratory collapse may follow. In adults, CNS depression is more common with drowsiness, coma, and convulsions, progressing to respiratory failure and cardiovascular collapse. In the case of the *non-sedating antihistamines*, antimuscarinic effects are less marked, but hazardous ventricular arrhythmias may be a special problem even with doses not far in excess of those recommended for therapeutic use.

Reviews.

1. Simons FER. H_1-receptor antagonists: comparative tolerability and safety. *Drug Safety* 1994; **10:** 350–80.

Arrhythmias. Ventricular arrhythmias have been reported rarely with astemizole and terfenadine particularly in association with increased blood concentrations. For full details and specific warnings see under Astemizole, p.402, and Terfenadine, p.418.

The suspicion that such life-threatening arrhythmias may be a class effect of the non-sedating antihistamines has so far proven unfounded. Although recent data[1] from the WHO adverse drug reaction database showed that cardiac events had been reported with the 5 most widely prescribed non-sedating antihistamines (acrivastine, astemizole, cetirizine, loratadine, and terfenadine), other centres[2] have argued that definitive causality has only been proven for astemizole and terfenadine. In addition, a possible mechanism for drug-induced cardiac toxicity has only been demonstrated with astemizole and terfenadine;[3] both drugs have been shown to block cardiac potassium channels *in vitro*, a phenomenon that results in prolongation of the QT interval, which is a risk factor for developing ventricular arrhythmias. Studies[4] with loratadine and cetirizine have demonstrated that neither drug blocked potassium channels *in vitro*.

1. Lindquist M, Edwards IR. Risks of non-sedating antihistamines. *Lancet* 1997; **349:** 1322. Correction. *ibid.;* 1482.
2. Himmel MH, *et al.* Dangers of non-sedating antihistamines. *Lancet* 1997; **350:** 69.
3. Salata JJ, *et al.* Cardiac electrophysiological actions of the histamine H_1-receptor antagonists astemizole and terfenadine compared with chlorpheniramine and pyrilamine. *Circ Res* 1995; **76:** 110–19.
4. Woosley RL. Cardiac actions of antihistamines. *Ann Rev Pharmacol Toxicol* 1996; **36:** 233–52.

Reye's syndrome. For criticism of a suggested link in children between antihistamines and Reye's syndrome, see p.17.

Sedation. CNS depression is a common adverse effect of the sedating antihistamines and sedative effects can range from slight drowsiness to deep sleep. Daytime sedation can be a problem especially for those who have to drive or operate machinery. When sedative effects do occur they are most apparent at the start of treatment and often diminish after a few days despite continued administration. Sedation caused by alcohol or other CNS depressants is enhanced. Many studies have attempted to quantify and compare the sedative effects of the older antihistamines, but results vary widely and classifications are difficult to make. Theoretically, the onset, degree, and persistence of sedation depend on factors such as penetration of the blood-brain barrier and on the relative affinity for central and peripheral histamine H_1 receptors. In general, antihistamines of the ethanolamine and phenothiazine classes cause the most sedation.

In view of these problems, non-sedating antihistamines have been developed. These compounds have poor penetration into the CNS and/or higher affinity for peripheral rather than central histamine H_1 receptors. Studies with acrivastine,[1] astemizole,[2] loratadine,[3] and terfenadine[4] have generally indicated a lower incidence of sedation and related CNS effects than that observed with older antihistamines and comparable with that of placebo. In a study[5] to compare the effects of acrivastine, terfenadine, and diphenhydramine on driving performance, terfenadine had no significant effect on driving performance. Acrivastine's effects were dose-related, but with little effect at the normal therapeutic dose, whereas diphenhydramine profoundly impaired all the measures of driving performance. Studies with terfenadine[4] suggest that the incidence of sedation does not increase significantly with increased dose or duration of administration. Cetirizine appears to be more sedating than loratadine or terfenadine but less sedating than older antihistamines; the effect appears to be dose dependent.[6] Limited data with azelastine[7] indicate a similar incidence of drowsiness to that with terfenadine. An incidence of sedation comparable with that caused by terfenadine has also been observed for mequitazine when given in the recommended dosage of 5 mg twice daily.[4] Sedation has, however, occurred after doses of 10 mg twice daily.[8] Other newer antihistamines claimed to produce no troublesome sedation include ebastine, epinastine, fexofenadine, mizolastine, setastine, and temelastine.

A number of studies have indicated that the non-sedating antihistamines do not seem to enhance the effects of alcohol and other CNS depressants.

A few patients treated with non-sedating antihistamines have experienced drowsiness. Therefore it is prudent to exercise caution before driving or operating machinery; the effect of a drug on a particular patient can be ascertained after the first few doses.

1. Bojkowski CJ, *et al.* Acrivastine in allergic rhinitis: a review of clinical experience. *J Int Med Res* 1989; **17** (suppl 2): 54B–68B.
2. Anonymous. Astemizole—another non-sedating antihistamine. *Med Lett Drugs Ther* 1989; **31:** 43–4.
3. Clissold SP, *et al.* Loratadine: a preliminary review of its pharmacodynamic properties and therapeutic efficacy. *Drugs* 1989; **37:** 42–57.
4. McTavish D, *et al.* Terfenadine: an updated review of its pharmacological properties and therapeutic efficacy. *Drugs* 1990; **39:** 552–74.
5. Ramaekers JG, O'Hanlon JF. Acrivastine, terfenadine and diphenhydramine effects on driving performance as a function of dose and time after dosing. *Eur J Clin Pharmacol* 1994; **47:** 261–6.
6. Spencer CM, *et al.* Cetirizine: a reappraisal of its pharmacological properties and therapeutic use in selected allergic disorders. *Drugs* 1993; **46:** 1055–80.
7. McTavish D, Sorkin EM. Azelastine: a review of its pharmacodynamic and pharmacokinetic properties, and therapeutic potential. *Drugs* 1989; **38:** 778–800.
8. Brandon ML. Newer non-sedating antihistamines: will they replace older agents? *Drugs* 1985; **30:** 377–81.

Precautions for Antihistamines

Drowsiness is a major problem with the *sedating antihistamines* and those affected should not drive or operate machinery; alcohol should be avoided. In the case of *non-sedating antihistamines*, although drowsiness is rare, it can occur and it may affect the performance of skilled tasks.

Because of their antimuscarinic actions the *sedating antihistamines* should be used with care in conditions such as angle-closure glaucoma, urinary retention, prostatic hyperplasia, or pyloroduodenal obstruction; antimuscarinic side-effects are not a significant problem with the *non-sedating antihistamines*. Occasional reports of convulsions in patients taking antihistamines also calls for caution in patients with epilepsy.

Many antihistamines are excreted in the urine in the form of active metabolites so that dosage reduction may be necessary in renal impairment (see individual monographs for specific advice). Caution is also needed in hepatic impairment, notably in the case of phenothiazine antihistamines (for further details, see under Chlorpromazine on p.650) and, above all, in the case of the *non-sedating antihistamines*, astemizole and terfenadine, since hazardous ventricular arrhythmias may occur in the presence of excessive blood concentrations. Other important cautions that relate to astemizole and terfenadine include avoidance of concomitant administration of drugs liable to interfere with their hepatic metabolism (see under Interactions, below) and contra-indication in patients with cardiac disease, known or suspected prolongation of the QT interval, or hypokalaemia or other electrolyte imbalances. For full details see under Astemizole, p.402, and Terfenadine, p.418.

Antihistamines should not be given to neonates owing to their increased susceptibility to antimuscarinic effects. It has also been recommended that antihistamines, in particular phenothiazines (see Promethazine, p.416 and Trimeprazine, p.419), should be avoided in young children. Elderly patients are also more susceptible to many of the adverse effects of antihistamines and, in particular, their inappropriate use for postural giddiness should be avoided.

Topical preparations containing antihistamines should not be used on broken or eczematous skin.

A number of large studies have failed to demonstrate any strong associations between fetal abnormalities and antihistamines taken during pregnancy (see under Pregnancy, below).

Asthma. Antihistamines have been considered ineffective in the management of asthma despite demonstrated bronchodilator and histamine-blocking effects.[1] There has also been concern that antihistamines may cause airway obstruction and hence their use has often been contra-indicated in patients with asthma. Such obstruction appears to be a result of bronchoconstriction rather than mucus retention, since it can be reversed by bronchodilators. However, antihistamine-induced airway obstruction has rarely been noted clinically and many patients with asthma tolerate concurrent treatment with antihistamines without obvious adverse effects. Therefore the American Academy of Allergy and Immunology has recommended that antihistamines are not contra-indicated in patients with asthma, unless an adverse reaction has previously been demonstrated and the Food and Drug Administration (FDA) has since removed the warning against the use of over-the-counter antihistamines by people with asthma.[2]

1. Meltzer EO. To use or not to use antihistamines in patients with asthma. *Ann Allergy* 1990; **64:** 183–6.
2. Food and Drug Administration. Cold, cough, allergy, bronchodilator, and antiasthmatic drug products for over-the-counter human use: final monograph for OTC antihistamine drug products: final rule. *Fed Regist* 1992; **57:** 58369–70.

Pregnancy. Considerable anxiety has surrounded the issue of whether there is any risk to the fetus from antiemetic therapy during pregnancy. The most widely studied preparation was Debendox which contained doxylamine, dicyclomine, and pyridoxine, and was known as Bendectin in some countries. Dicyclomine was removed from the preparation in 1976 in the USA and subsequently in other countries, and the product was withdrawn from the market in 1983 because of threatened litigation.[1] By that time Debendox had been used for over 27 years and in over 33 million pregnancies worldwide.[1]

Evidence against Debendox initially came from anecdotal reports of malformations in infants whose mothers had taken the preparation during pregnancy.[2,3] Eskenazi and Bracken[4] found evidence of an association between prenatal exposure to the 3-component formulation of Bendectin and an increased risk of pyloric stenosis and possibly also defective heart valves in a study of 1369 malformed infants and 2968 healthy control cases. Other studies have suggested an increased incidence of oral clefts,[5] gastro-intestinal atresia,[6] and genital tract disorders,[7] but generally such increases have been small. No overall pattern of malformations appears to have emerged, and many large studies have failed to confirm an association between doxylamine use and congenital malformations.[8-13]

A prospective study of 11 481 pregnancies found no increased incidence of either severe congenital abnormalities or perinatal mortality rates in women who had been prescribed prochlorperazine, meclozine, cyclizine, or Bendectin during pregnancy, although there was some evidence of an excess number of congenital abnormalities in patients taking trimethobenzamide.[14]

The Collaborative Perinatal Project monitored the mothers of 50 282 children between 1958 and 1965.[15] Of these, 5401 were exposed to antihistamines and 1309 to phenothiazines during the first 4 months of pregnancy. There was no evidence to suggest that exposure to these drugs was related to malformations, although there were slight suggestions of associations between respiratory malformations and pheniramine, inguinal hernia and meclozine, inguinal hernia or genito-urinary malformations and diphenhydramine, and cardiovascular deformities and phenothiazines. Slone *et al.*[16] reporting on the same study, found no effects of phenothiazines on perinatal mortality, birth-weight, or IQ scores at the age of 4 years. The Collaborative Perinatal Project also noted a relationship between cardiovascular defects and inguinal hernia and dimenhydrinate exposure.[15]

Both the Committee on Safety of Medicines in the UK[17] and the Food and Drugs Administration in the USA[18] reviewed the available literature in 1981 and concluded that while the scientific evidence did not demonstrate an increase in birth defects with the Debendox combination, the risk of teratogenicity could not be completely excluded. There has been a study indicating that vomiting itself is not teratogenic.[19]

A number of other studies have been carried out on meclozine prompted by reports of fetal abnormalities in 10 patients associated with a preparation of meclozine and pyridoxine;[20] these studies have not supported the original reports.[21-23]

1. Merrell Pharmaceuticals. Production of Debendox to stop. *Lancet* 1983; **i:** 1395.
2. Paterson DC. Congenital deformities associated with Bendectin. *Can Med Assoc J* 1977; **116:** 1348.
3. Donnai D, Harris R. Unusual fetal malformations after antiemetics in early pregnancy. *Br Med J* 1978; **1:** 691–2.
4. Eskenazi B, Bracken MB. Bendectin (Debendox) as a risk factor for pyloric stenosis. *Am J Obstet Gynecol* 1982; **144:** 919–24.
5. Golding J, *et al.* Maternal anti-nauseants and clefts of lip and palate. *Hum Toxicol* 1983; **2:** 63–73.
6. Jick H, *et al.* First-trimester drug use and congenital disorders. *JAMA* 1981; **246:** 343–6.
7. Gibson GT, *et al.* Congenital anomalies in relation to the use of doxylamine/dicyclomine and other antenatal factors: an ongoing prospective study. *Med J Aust* 1981; **i:** 410–4.

8. Shapiro S, *et al.* Antenatal exposure to doxylamine succinate and dicyclomine hydrochloride (Bendectin) in relation to congenital malformations: perinatal mortality rate, birth weight, and intelligence quotient score. *Am J Obstet Gynecol* 1977; **128:** 480–5.
9. Harron DWG, *et al.* Debendox and congenital malformations in Northern Ireland. *Br Med J* 1980; **281:** 1379–81.
10. Fleming DM, *et al.* Debendox in early pregnancy and fetal malformation. *Br Med J* 1981; **283:** 99–101.
11. Mitchell AA, *et al.* Birth defects related to Bendectin use in pregnancy 1: Oral clefts and cardiac defects. *JAMA* 1981; **245:** 2311–14.
12. Mitchell AA, *et al.* Birth defects in relation to Bendectin use in pregnancy. *Am J Obstet Gynecol* 1983; **147:** 737–42.
13. Winship KA, *et al.* Maternal drug histories and central nervous system anomalies. *Arch Dis Child* 1984; **59:** 1052–9.
14. Milkovich L, van den Berg BJ. An evaluation of the teratogenicity of certain antinauseant drugs. *Am J Obstet Gynecol* 1976; **125:** 244–8.
15. Heinonen OP, *et al. Birth defects and drugs in pregnancy.* Massachusetts: Publishing Sciences Group, 1977.
16. Slone D, *et al.* Antenatal exposure to the phenothiazines in relation to congenital malformations, perinatal mortality rate, birth weight, and intelligence quotient score. *Am J Obstet Gynecol* 1977; **128:** 486–8.
17. Committee on Safety of Medicines. Data sheet change—Debendox. *Current Problems 6* 1981.
18. Food and Drugs Administration. Indications for Bendectin narrowed. *FDA Drug Bull* 1981; **11** (1).
19. Klebanoff MA, Mills JL. Is vomiting during pregnancy teratogenic? *Br Med J* 1986; **292:** 724–6.
20. Watson GI. Meclozine ("Ancoloxin") and foetal abnormalities: preliminary report by the epidemic observation unit of the College of General Practitioners. *Br Med J* 1962; **ii:** 1446.
21. Lenz W. How can the teratogenic action of a factor be established in man? *South Med J* 1971; **64** (suppl 1): 41–7.
22. Greenberg G, *et al.* Maternal drug histories and congenital abnormalities. *Br Med J* 1977; **2:** 853–6.
23. Shapiro S, *et al.* Meclizine in pregnancy in relation to congenital malformations. *Br Med J* 1978; **i:** 483.

Interactions of Antihistamines

Sedating antihistamines may enhance the sedative effects of CNS depressants including alcohol, barbiturates, hypnotics, opioid analgesics, anxiolytic sedatives, and antipsychotics. Sedative interactions apply to a lesser extent with the *non-sedating antihistamines*; they do not appear to potentiate the effects of alcohol, but it should be avoided in excess.

Sedating antihistamines have an additive antimuscarinic action with other antimuscarinic drugs, such as atropine and some antidepressants (both tricyclics and MAOIs).

Potentially hazardous ventricular arrhythmias have occurred when the *non-sedating antihistamines* astemizole and terfenadine have been given concomitantly with drugs liable to interfer with their hepatic metabolism, with other potentially arrhythmogenic drugs, and with those likely to cause electrolyte imbalance. For full details see under Astemizole, p.402, and Terfenadine, p.418.

It has been suggested that some *sedating antihistamines* could mask the warning signs of damage caused by ototoxic drugs such as aminoglycoside antibiotics.

Antihistamines may suppress the cutaneous histamine response to allergen extracts and should be stopped several days before skin testing.

Uses of Antihistamines

Histamine H_1-receptor antagonists (termed 'antihistamines' in *Martindale*) diminish or abolish the major actions of histamine in the body by competitive, reversible blockade of histamine H_1-receptor sites on tissues; they do not inactivate the histamine or prevent its synthesis or release. Histamine H_1 receptors are responsible for vasodilatation, increased capillary permeability, flare and itch reactions in the skin, and to some extent for contraction of smooth muscle in the bronchi and gastro-intestinal tract.

Many of the *sedating antihistamines* also possess antimuscarinic, adrenaline-antagonising, serotonin-antagonising, and local anaesthetic effects. Some also have calcium-channel blocking activity.

Antihistamines are used primarily for the alleviation of conditions (such as urticarial rashes and nasal allergy) that are characterised by type I hypersensitivity (see above), but by virtue of their associated pharmacological actions they are also used to alleviate the symptoms of a wide range of other conditions (such as pruritus and nausea and vomiting).

The antihistamines can improve or relieve the symptoms of seasonal allergic rhinitis ('hay fever') in a high percentage of patients. They alleviate rhinorrhoea and sneezing (and ocular symptoms such as conjunctivitis) but may be less effective for nasal congestion. The relief obtained is dependent on the severity and nature of the symptoms, being greater in the milder stages. The *non-sedating antihistamines* are preferred for daytime control, but a *sedating antihistamine* may be preferred at night. Antihistamines may also be of value in vasomotor rhinitis, despite the fact that this is not primarily an allergic condition.

Antihistamines are of value in preventing urticaria and are used to treat urticarial rashes and mild angioedema. They are also used as adjuncts to adrenaline in the emergency treatment of anaphylaxis and severe angioedema. The use of an antihistamine is not appropriate for the control of blood transfusion reactions caused by ABO incompatibility.

The *sedating antihistamines* are of value in the alleviation of pruritus both of allergic and of non-allergic origin; they have a major role in pruritus associated with atopic eczema. The *non-sedating antihistamines* do not alleviate pruritus of non-allergic origin owing to their poor penetration of the blood-brain barrier.

Sedating antihistamines have marked antiemetic activity and are used to control nausea and vomiting caused by a variety of vestibular disorders. In the case of motion sickness a sedating antihistamine, such as dimenhydrinate or promethazine, is used if severe drowsiness (or even sleep) is not considered undesirable, but generally a less sedative antihistamine, such as cyclizine or cinnarizine may be preferred. Sedating antihistamines are similarly used to control the vertigo and nausea associated with Ménière's disease and related conditions, with cinnarizine promoted as a specific treatment. Sedating antihistamines also have an important role in the alleviation of the nausea and vomiting of migraine, and buclizine is marketed in some countries in a combination preparation for this purpose; cyproheptadine, by virtue of its significant serotonin antagonist and its calcium-channel blocking activity, may be of value in the prophylaxis of migraine. Sedating antihistamines have a very limited role in the short-term management of vomiting of pregnancy but are no longer considered appropriate for nausea alone. *Sedating antihistamines* have also been widely used for premedication in anaesthetic practice and still have a major role in the prevention of postoperative nausea and vomiting.

Some of the antihistamines with very pronounced sedative effects, such as diphenhydramine and promethazine, have been marketed for occasional insomnia but their long duration of action can cause hangover effects. *Sedating antihistamines* are also widely marketed, often with a decongestant, in compound preparations for the symptomatic treatment of coughs and colds although there is little evidence of value. Some antihistamines are also available as preparations for topical application for the alleviation of insect bites, but there is little evidence of any real value and such use may be associated with sensitisation.

Anaesthesia

Phenothiazine antihistamines have been used for anaesthetic premedication and during surgical and obstetric procedures to relieve anxiety in apprehensive patients although benzodiazepines are now used more routinely. However, sedating antihistamines such as promethazine and cyclizine do have a role in the control of postoperative vomiting (below). Trimeprazine is still used for premedication in children, although when given alone, it may cause postoperative restlessness when pain is present. For a discussion of the wide range of drugs that may be used to achieve and maintain conditions suitable for surgery, see p.1220.

Anaphylaxis

Anaphylaxis is commonly a type I (immediate) hypersensitivity reaction (see above) to various allergens such as drugs, foods, and insect venoms. A clinically identical reaction can, however, be provoked by a type II (cell-surface) mechanism, as in blood transfusion reactions, by a type III (immune complex) mechanism, as in drug-induced serum sickness reactions, or by non-immune mechanisms (an anaphylactoid reaction). Symptoms of anaphylaxis and anaphylactoid reactions include erythema, pruritus, urticaria, and angioedema often of the eyes, lips, or tongue; respiratory obstruction may result from oedema of the larynx or epiglottis. Gastro-intestinal disturbances, bronchospasm, hypotension, and coma can occur in severe reactions.

Patients with severe anaphylactic or anaphylactoid reactions should be given immediate treatment with adrenaline. Addition of a parenteral antihistamine such as chlorpheniramine maleate or diphenhydramine hydrochloride and a corticosteroid such as hydrocortisone after the acute episode may decrease the duration and severity of symptoms and prevent relapse. This adjunctive role of parenteral antihistamine therapy is discussed further under Anaphylactic Shock, on p.816. The use of antihistamines in treating the symptoms of milder forms of anaphylaxis is discussed under individual symptoms such as Pruritus (below) and Urticaria and Angioedema (below).

Angioedema

See under Urticaria and Angioedema, below.

Asthma

Antihistamines, with the possible exception of ketotifen, appear to have no place in the treatment of asthma (p.745). A meta-analysis[1] of double-blind randomised placebo-controlled trials published since 1980 did not support the use of antihistamines in the treatment of asthma, although the quality of the studies was generally considered to be poor.

1. Van Ganse E, *et al.* Effects of antihistamines in adult asthma: a meta-analysis of clinical trials. *Eur Respir J* 1997; **10:** 2216–24.

Conjunctivitis

Allergic conjunctivitis is a type I hypersensitivity reaction (above). It is usually seasonal but perennial attacks due to allergens such as house dust mites can occur. Itching, tears, and burning are common symptoms and frequently rhinitis (below) will co-exist. Conjunctivitis can also be caused by pathogenic micro-organisms (p.122).

Avoidance of unnecessary exposure to aeroallergens is of prime importance in the management of allergic conjunctivitis.[1,2] Since a large number of inflammatory mediators are involved in its pathogenesis no single drug will be completely effective. Systemic sedating and non-sedating antihistamines are effective in reducing allergic symptoms and preventing attacks and the choice of drug depends on the degree of sedation required. Ophthalmic antihistamine preparations such as antazoline, levocabastine, and olopatadine may also be used for acute attacks. Ophthalmic corticosteroids may reduce inflammation, but use should be restricted to severe cases only and limited to 5 to 7 days' duration because of the risk of local adverse effects such as cataract or raised intra-ocular pressure. Mast-cell stabilisers including lodoxamide and sodium cromoglycate have been widely used for prophylaxis. Ketorolac eye drops are available for the treatment of allergic conjunctivitis. Combined preparations of astringents such as zinc sulphate and sympathomimetics such as naphazoline may also be used for symptomatic relief.

1. Ciprandi G, *et al.* Drug treatment of allergic conjunctivitis: a review of the evidence. *Drugs* 1992; **43:** 154–76.
2. Hingorani M, Lightman S. Therapeutic options in ocular allergic disease. *Drugs* 1995; **50:** 208–21.

Coughs and colds

Sedating antihistamines are frequently used in combination preparations for the treatment of coughs and colds (p.1052 and p.595 respectively). The mechanism of their antitussive action may involve reduction in cholinergic nerve transmission or may simply result from their sedative effects; reduction of nasal secretions may be of value in treating cough caused by postnasal drip. Antihistamines should not be used to treat productive coughs because reduction in bronchial secretions may cause formation of viscid mucus plugs. The sedative effects of antihistamines may prove troublesome for daytime use but may be a short-term advantage for night coughs.

Food allergy

The term food allergy (food hypersensitivity) should be reserved for instances in which an immune mechanism for the reaction is proven; food intolerance is used to describe a non-immune reaction. Food allergy may be the result of a type I (immediate), or possibly a type III (immune complex), reaction (see above). Management revolves around the identification of the provoking food allergen and its subsequent avoidance. Individualised diets are designed and patients are educated about possible hidden sources of the allergen. Drug therapy has a very limited role in the prevention of food allergy; oral sodium cromoglycate has been used but efficacy has not been unequivocally established.

Inadvertent exposure to an allergen resulting in anaphylactic shock (p.816) is managed symptomatically. Milder symptoms may be controlled by antihistamines and corticosteroids. Hyposensitisation plays no role in the routine management of food allergy (see p.1545).

References.

1. Hunter JO. Food allergy and intolerance. *Prescribers' J* 1997; **37:** 193–8.
2. Sampson HA. Food allergy. *JAMA* 1997; **278:** 1888–94.
3. Bindslev-Jensen C. Food allergy. *Br Med J* 1998; **316:** 1299–1302.

Hay fever

Hay fever is a seasonal form of allergic rhinitis in which symptoms of conjunctivitis are also present. Management is symptomatic and therapies used are discussed under Conjunctivitis, above and Rhinitis, below.

Insomnia

If a hypnotic has to be used for insomnia (p.638) then the choice usually falls on a benzodiazepine. However, some of the older sedating antihistamines including diphenhydramine and promethazine, have been promoted to the public for occasional insomnia, although their long duration of action may cause hangover effects. Promethazine was formerly popular for children but the use of hypnotics in this age group is not usually justified. Moreover a possible association between phenothiazines and sudden infant death syndrome (see under the Adverse Effects of Promethazine, p.416) contributed to the recommendation that such antihistamines should not be used in young children.

Ménière's disease

Ménière's disease is a disorder of the labyrinth (the inner ear) characterised by recurrent attacks of vertigo, hearing loss, and tinnitus. It usually presents in middle age and may equally affect men and women. The predominant pathological feature is an excess of endolymph fluid producing an increase in pressure in the membranous labyrinth (endolymphatic hydrops). It is progressive and attacks occur in clusters over a few weeks with periods of remission lasting weeks or months. Episodic vertigo is the most disabling symptom initially and is associated with nausea and vomiting, which improves as the disease progresses and hearing loss becomes more apparent. As the disease progresses the hearing loss becomes irreversible. Tinnitus (p.1297) worsens with each attack and becomes persistent and distressing.

The aims of treatment of Ménière's disease are to alleviate symptoms and preserve hearing if possible. It is therefore important to assess how far the disease has progressed, particularly in terms of hearing loss. In addition to conventional hearing tests, cochlear dysfunction may be assessed pharmacologically. Hypertonic glycerol has been administered orally to reduce the endolymphatic fluid volume by osmotic diuresis, any temporary improvement in hearing indicating reversible impairment. However, this test is associated with side-effects that some consider unacceptable. Urea has been used as an alternative to glycerol. Intravenous acetazolamide has been used diagnostically to increase endolymphatic pressure temporarily in order to produce transient hearing loss in patients in the reversible stages of the disease.

Acute attacks of vertigo in the early stages may be treated with the same drugs used for vertigo of any cause (see below).

Vasodilators have been advocated for maintenance treatment because ischaemia of the labyrinth has been postulated as a factor in the aetiology. Betahistine, a histamine analogue, is used. Restriction of dietary sodium and administration of diuretics, such as chlorthalidone, frusemide, and hydrochlorothiazide, has also been used traditionally to reduce the amount of fluid in the endolymphatic spaces.

As the disease progresses, medical ablation with aminoglycosides may be indicated. Systemic streptomycin has been used but the risk of ototoxicity and other serious adverse effects has limited its use. Intratympanic administration of gentamicin is now preferred although ototoxic effects have also been seen with this method albeit at a lower incidence than that with systemic streptomycin.

Surgical treatment remains an option for patients with Ménière's disease refractory to medical interventions.

References.

1. Saeed SR, *et al.* Ménière's disease. *Br J Hosp Med* 1994; **51:** 603–12.
2. Brookes GB. The pharmacological treatment of Ménière's disease. *Clin Otolaryngol* 1996; **21:** 3–11.
3. Claes J, Van de Heyning PH. Medical treatment of Ménière's disease: a review of literature. *Acta Otolaryngol (Stockh)* 1997; suppl 526: 37–42.
4. Saeed SR. Diagnosis and treatment of Ménière's disease. *Br Med J* 1998; **316:** 368–72.

Migraine

Antihistamines have a number of uses in the management of migraine (p.443). Those with antiemetic activity such as buclizine and cyclizine are used to alleviate the nausea and vomiting associated with migraine; they are common ingredients of compound analgesic preparations given for the initial treatment of migraine.

Those antihistamines with antiserotonin actions, including cyproheptadine and flunarizine have been used for the prophylaxis of migraine.

Nausea and vomiting

The older antihistamines such as cinnarizine, cyclizine, dimenhydrinate, meclozine, and promethazine are among the principal drugs used in the treatment of **motion sickness**. They are all of similar efficacy but may differ in onset and duration of action and in the extent of side-effects such as drowsiness and antimuscarinic effects. If a sedative effect is desired dimenhydrinate and promethazine are useful, otherwise a slightly less sedating antihistamine such as cinnarizine, cyclizine, or meclozine may be preferred. The aim is to prevent rather than treat the motion sickness since antiemetics are more effective if given prophylactically than after nausea and vomiting have developed. Antihistamines may be slightly less effective against motion sickness than the antimuscarinic hyoscine (p.462), but are often better tolerated. Non-sedating antihistamines such as astemizole and terfenadine, which penetrate poorly into the CNS, do not appear to be effective against motion sickness.

Diphenhydramine has been included in antiemetic regimens for the control of nausea and vomiting associated with **cancer chemotherapy** to reduce the extrapyramidal reactions associated with metoclopramide; it may also improve overall antiemetic control.

Cyclizine is given as a supplement to opioids for premedication and has been effective prophylactically as well as in established **postoperative nausea and vomiting**. Promethazine has also been used for the prevention and treatment of postoperative nausea and vomiting, but has marked sedative effects.

Nausea in the first trimester of **pregnancy** does not require drug therapy, but on rare occasions if vomiting is severe an antihistamine such as promethazine may be required pending specialist advice. See under Precautions for Antihistamines, above, for a discussion of the risks of antiemetic therapy during pregnancy.

The treatment of various types of nausea and vomiting is discussed in detail on p.1172.

Otitis media

Antihistamines and decongestants, alone or in combination, have been widely used in children for the treatment of symptoms of acute otitis media and associated respiratory symptoms, but the benefits of this practice have been questioned.[1-3] Acute otitis media and otitis media with effusion may resolve without treatment although, as discussed on p.134, antibacterials are often given.

1. Bain DJG. Can the clinical course of acute otitis media be modified by systemic decongestant or antihistamine treatment? *Br Med J* 1983; **287:** 654–6.
2. Cantekin EI, *et al.* Lack of efficacy of a decongestant-antihistamine combination for otitis media with effusion ("secretory" otitis media) in children. *N Engl J Med* 1983; **308:** 297–301.
3. Mandel EM, *et al.* Efficacy of amoxicillin with and without decongestant-antihistamine for otitis media with effusion in children: results of a double-blind, randomized trial. *N Engl J Med* 1987; **316:** 432–7.

Pruritus

The sedating antihistamines are commonly used to relieve pruritus (itching) (p.1075) including that associated with dermatoses such as atopic eczema (p.1073). They are useful to control nocturnal itching, particularly in children, but have also been used during the day.

The exact pathophysiology of itching remains unclear.[1-3] Although histamine release is associated with itching in atopic eczema different inflammatory mediators are involved in other dermatoses. The CNS is also thought to play a part in the perception of itch. Hence, the relative role of CNS sedation and peripheral histamine-receptor blockade in the mode of action of antihistamines in these conditions is a matter of debate, although sedation has generally been considered the more important. Studies with non-sedating antihistamines have been inconclusive; some[1] have indicated no benefit in the treatment of pruritus while one has shown a slight benefit from the addition of acrivastine or terfenadine to treatment with a topical corticosteroid and an emollient.[4] In addition, clemastine has been reported to provide no antipruritic benefit, yet it induced significant sedation. Thus the role of the antihistamines in the relief of itching associated with atopic eczema and other dermatoses remains to be defined.

1. Krause L, Shuster S. Mechanism of action of antipruritic drugs. *Br Med J* 1983; **287:** 1199–1200.
2. Advenier C, Queille-Roussel C. Rational use of antihistamines in allergic dermatological conditions. *Drugs* 1989; **38:** 634–44.
3. Greaves MW, Wall PD. Pathophysiology of itching. *Lancet* 1996; **348:** 938–40.
4. Doherty V, *et al.* Treatment of itching in atopic eczema with antihistamines with a low sedative profile. *Br Med J* 1989; **298:** 96.

Rhinitis

Rhinitis may be allergic or non-allergic in origin. Allergic rhinitis is a type I hypersensitivity reaction (see above); both early (sneezing, rhinorrhoea and nasal congestion) and late (nasal congestion) reactions may be provoked. It may be seasonal (as in hay fever) or perennial and, in some patients, will frequently co-exist with conjunctivitis (above). Non-allergic rhinitis may be divided into eosinophilic non-allergic rhinitis or non-eosinophilic non-allergic rhinitis. The term vasomotor rhinitis has been used to describe the latter although its use is best avoided since no vasomotor dysfunction has been clearly identified.

In the management of **allergic rhinitis**, avoidance of unnecessary exposure to aeroallergens is of prime importance. However in most sufferers this is not possible and some form of drug therapy will be necessary. A large number of inflammatory mediators are involved in the pathogenesis of rhinitis and no single drug is completely effective in the alleviation of symptoms. Nevertheless some antihistamines may be useful and any antimuscarinic effect may be of additional value in reducing secretions. They are also useful for controlling nasal itching, sneezing, and ocular symptoms, such as conjunctivitis but are less effective for relief of nasal congestion. Antihistamines are the drugs of choice for the treatment of mild and/or intermittent allergic rhinitis and they are also employed for the management of breakthrough symptoms in those sufferers using prophylactic intranasal corticosteroids or sodium cromoglycate (see below). Since the maximum effect of antihistamines occurs several hours after peak serum concentrations have been obtained, they should be given in anticipation of a reaction to achieve the maximum response. Studies of acrivastine, astemizole, cetirizine, loratadine, and terfenadine have generally indicated comparable efficacy to that of the older antihistamines.

Most antihistamines are unsuitable for topical use in the nose or eye since they are generally ineffective at the concentrations suitable for local therapy; also there is the potential for sensitisation. However, some antihistamines, such as antazoline salts, azelastine, and levocabastine have been used topically in the nose for control of symptoms. Some, but not all, studies have suggested that concomitant treatment with an H_2-receptor antagonist may be more effective than an H_1-receptor antagonist alone.

The actions of topical corticosteroids in allergic rhinitis include relief of inflammation, a decrease in capillary permeability and in mucus production, and vasoconstriction; they inhibit both the early and late response to allergen exposure. Corticosteroids are first-line treatment for the prophylaxis of moderate and/or persistent allergic rhinitis. In seasonal allergic rhinitis, they should be started at least 2 weeks before the pollen season and taken regularly throughout the season. Those applied intranasally include beclomethasone, budesonide, flunisolide, and fluticasone. At recommended dosage, local adverse effects are mild and transient and systemic effects not a risk; aqueous sprays may cause less local effects than pressurised aerosols. Treatment of allergic rhinitis with oral or parenteral corticosteroids has been reserved for short-term treatment in special circumstances only, although some have contested even this practice.

Mast-cell stabilisers such as ketotifen, nedocromil, and sodium cromoglycate are thought to act primarily by preventing release of inflammatory mediators from sensitised mast cells through stabilisation of mast-cell membranes. They are an alternative to corticosteroids in the prophylactic treatment of allergic rhinitis and are often preferred to the use of a corticosteroid as first-choice therapy in children. They may also be useful in controlling mild to moderate symptoms. Intranasal sympathomimetics such as phenylephrine, naphazoline, oxymetazoline, and xylometazoline may be useful for short-term treatment of allergic rhinitis to relieve severe nasal congestion which can be painful and may impede delivery of sodium cromoglycate or a corticosteroid to the mucosal surfaces. Oral sympathomimetic decongestants such as pseudoephedrine and phenylpropanolamine are less effective than topical sympathomimetics and adverse effects may be troublesome.

Hyposensitisation (see p.1545) is generally only indicated in severe allergic rhinitis when sensitivity testing demonstrates sensitivity to one allergen and when exposure to the allergen is unavoidable or symptomatic treatment has failed.

The management of **non-allergic rhinitis** is similar to that of allergic rhinitis despite different mechanisms being involved in its aetiology. Corticosteroids are often first-line therapy especially if nasal congestion is a dominant feature. The role of antihistamines is more limited; sedating antihistamines are useful in reducing nasal secretions because of their antimuscarinic actions; however, non-sedating antihistamines are relatively ineffective. In those patient where rhinorrhoea is a particular problem, intranasal administration of the antimuscarinic ipratropium is of value. Although intranasal decongestants have also been used they should generally be avoided because of the risk of rebound congestion. Oral decongestants are largely ineffective.

Other therapies tried include topical capsaicin, to induce local desensitisation, and nasal douching with a saline and sodium bicarbonate solution.

References

1. Horak F. Seasonal allergic rhinitis: newer treatment approaches. *Drugs* 1993; **45:** 518–27.
2. International Rhinitis Management Working Group. International consensus report on the diagnosis and management of rhinitis. *Allergy* 1994; **49** (suppl 19): 1–34.
3. Scadding GK. Chronic non-infectious, non-allergic rhinitis. *Prescribers' J* 1996; **36:** 93–101.
4. Parikh A, Scadding GK. Seasonal allergic rhinitis. *Br Med J* 1997; **314:** 1392–5.
5. Naclerio R, Soloman W. Rhinitis and inhalant allergens. *JAMA* 1997; **278:** 1842–8.
6. Durham S. Summer hay fever. *Br Med J* 1998; **316:** 843–5.
7. Mackay IS, Durham SR. Perennial rhinitis. *Br Med J* 1998; **316:** 917–20.

Urticaria and angioedema

The role of antihistamines and other drugs used in the treatment of urticaria and angioedema is discussed on p.1076.

Most patients with urticaria or angioedema derive some benefit from oral antihistamines,[1,2] especially in relief of pruritus. However, patients who are severely affected, particularly those with laryngeal oedema, should be treated as an allergic emergency and require treatment with adrenaline (see under Anaphylactic Shock, p.816). Also large doses of antihistamines are sometimes required and urticarias with a type I immunological origin and iatrogenic urticarias respond better than physical urticarias. If attacks of urticaria are frequent, antihistamines may be given prophylactically. Sedating antihistamines such as chlorpheniramine and diphenhydramine have been widely used in the treatment of urticaria. Hydroxyzine has been used particularly in dermographism and cholinergic urticaria. Cyproheptadine has generally been considered the drug of choice for cold urticaria, although appetite stimulation may be a problem.

However, non-sedating antihistamines[2-4] are probably the first line of treatment for urticaria now.

Some drugs with both H_1-antagonist and mast-cell stabilising actions, such as ketotifen, oxatomide, and azatadine have shown efficacy in the treatment of urticaria; the role of mast-cell stabilisation is unknown.[5]

Topical treatment is rarely effective except for cases of mild urticaria; topical antihistamines carry a risk of sensitisation.

1. Advenier C, Queille-Roussel C. Rational use of antihistamines in allergic dermatological conditions. *Drugs* 1989; **38:** 634–44.
2. Greaves MW, Sabroe RA. Allergy and the skin: urticaria. *Br Med J* 1998; **316:** 1147–50.
3. Mann KV, *et al.* Nonsedating histamine H_1-receptor antagonists. *Clin Pharm* 1989; **8:** 331–44.
4. Monroe EW. Chronic urticaria: review of nonsedating H_1 antihistamines in treatment. *J Am Acad Dermatol* 1988; **19:** 842–9.
5. Theoharides TC. Histamine$_2$ (H_2)-receptor antagonists in the treatment of urticaria. *Drugs* 1989; **37:** 345–55.

Vertigo

Vertigo is a symptom of vestibular disorders. It is characterised by a sensation of rotation of the surroundings or of movement of static objects. Dizziness is considered to be a wider term, although some use it as a synonym for vertigo.

A variety of disorders may affect the vestibular system and produce vertigo, including cerebrovascular disorders, epilepsy, head injury, malignant neoplasms, Ménière's disease (above), migraine, multiple sclerosis, and infections. Motion sickness can induce vertigo. Ototoxic drugs may also cause vestibular damage.

The management of vertigo has been reviewed.[1-4] Patients should undergo thorough investigations to identify any underlying cause. Simple measures to improve the integration of sensory input from visual, proprioceptive, and vestibular receptors may prove effective, especially in the elderly, in whom the inappropriate prescribing of drugs for postural instability needs to be avoided. Such measures include improving visual acuity, balance exercises, and the use of walking aids.

The mainstay of the pharmacological treatment of acute vertigo remains antihistamines, although their mechanism of action is unclear. They may have a direct action on the inner ear besides acting centrally. Antimuscarinic actions may contribute to their activity; antimuscarinics, especially hyoscine, have a long history of use in vertigo. Antihistamines used in the treatment of vertigo include buclizine, cyclizine, dimenhydrinate, diphenhydramine, meclozine, and promethazine. Cinnarizine and flunarizine are also used for vertigo although they are devoid of any significant antimuscarinic actions; their activity may be due to calcium-channel blockade. Phenothiazines such as prochlorperazine are also used to control any associated vomiting. Benzodiazepines including diazepam have been given in acute severe attacks. However their prolonged use in those with chronic symptoms is of questionable value.

Vasodilators may be of benefit in the treatment of vertigo of vascular aetiology. Parenteral or sublingual histamine was formerly widely used, and betahistine is still advocated. Nicotinyl alcohol has also been used.

1. Rascol O, *et al.* Antivertigo medications and drug-induced vertigo: a pharmacological review. *Drugs* 1995; **50:** 777–91.
2. Luxon LM. Vertigo: new approaches to diagnosis and management. *Br J Hosp Med* 1996; **56:** 519–20 and 537–41.
3. Luxon LM. Assessment and management of vertigo. *Prescribers' J* 1998; **38:** 87–97.
4. Baloh RW. Vertigo. *Lancet* 1998; **352:** 1841–6.

Acrivastine (16017-a)

Acrivastine *(BAN, USAN, rINN)*.

BW-825C. (*E*)-3-{6-[(*E*)-3-Pyrrolidin-1-yl-1-*p*-tolylprop-1-enyl]-2-pyridyl}acrylic acid.

$C_{22}H_{24}N_2O_2$ = 348.4.

CAS — 87848-99-5.

Adverse Effects and Precautions

As for the non-sedating antihistamines in general, p.397.

Interactions

As for the non-sedating antihistamines in general, p.399.

Pharmacokinetics

Acrivastine is well absorbed from the gastro-intestinal tract; peak plasma concentrations are achieved in about 1.5 hours. The plasma half-life of acrivastine is about 1.5 hours and the drug does not appear to cross the blood-brain barrier to a significant extent. Acrivastine along with an active metabolite is excreted principally in the urine.

Uses and Administration

Acrivastine is a non-sedating antihistamine structurally related to triprolidine. It does not have any significant sedative or antimuscarinic actions. It is used for the symptomatic relief of allergic conditions such as rhinitis (p.400) and various types of urticaria (p.401) when it is given by mouth in doses of 8 mg three times daily.

References.

1. Clinical experience with acrivastine— a new antihistamine. *J Int Med Res* 1989; **17** (suppl 2): 1B–68B (a series of papers on the use of acrivastine in skin disorders and rhinitis).
2. Brogden RN, McTavish D. Acrivastine: a review of its pharmacological properties and therapeutic efficacy in allergic rhinitis, urticaria and related disorders. *Drugs* 1991; **41:** 927–40.

Preparations

Proprietary Preparations (details are given in Part 3)
Aust.: Semprex; *Ital.:* Semprex; *Neth.:* Semprex; *S.Afr.:* Semprex; *Swed.:* Semprex; *UK:* Benadryl; Semprex.

Multi-ingredient: *Aust.:* Duact; *USA:* Semprex-D.

Antazoline Hydrochloride (6104-n)

Antazoline Hydrochloride *(BANM, rINNM)*.

Antazolini Hydrochloridum; Antazolinium Chloride; Imidamine Hydrochloride; Phenazolinum. *N*-Benzyl-*N*-(2-imidazolin-2-ylmethyl)aniline hydrochloride.

$C_{17}H_{19}N_3,HCl$ = 301.8.

CAS — 91-75-8 (antazoline); 2508-72-7 (antazoline hydrochloride).

Pharmacopoeias. In *Eur.* (see p.viii) and *Pol.*

A white or almost white crystalline powder. Sparingly **soluble** in water; soluble in alcohol; slightly soluble in dichloromethane.

Antazoline Mesylate (6105-h)

Antazoline Mesylate *(BANM)*.

Antazoline Mesilate *(rINNM)*; Antazoline Methanesulphonate; Imidamine Mesylate.

$C_{17}H_{19}N_3,CH_3SO_3H$ = 361.5.

CAS — 3131-32-6.

Antazoline Phosphate (6106-m)

Antazoline Phosphate *(BANM, rINNM)*.

Imidamine Phosphate.

$C_{17}H_{19}N_3,H_3PO_4$ = 363.3.

CAS — 154-68-7.

Pharmacopoeias. In *US.*

A white to off-white crystalline powder. **Soluble** in water; sparingly soluble in methyl alcohol; practically insoluble in ether. A 2% solution in water has a pH of 4 to 5. **Store** in airtight containers.

Antazoline Sulphate (10003-w)

Antazoline Sulphate *(BANM, rINNM).*

Antazoline Sulfate; Imidamine Sulphate.

$(C_{17}H_{19}N_3)_2H_2SO_4,2H_2O$ = 664.8.

CAS — 24359-81-7 (anhydrous antazoline sulphate).

NOTE. The above molecular formula is that provided in the *It. P.* Other sources give a molecular formula of $C_{17}H_{19}N_3,H_2SO_4$.

Pharmacopoeias. In *It.*

Adverse Effects and Precautions

As for the antihistamines in general, p.397.

Hypersensitivity. Reports of acute interstitial pneumonitis (with fever, rash, and dyspnoea)[1] and of immune thrombocytopenic purpura[2] were attributed to hypersensitivity reactions following the oral administration of antazoline.

1. Pahissa A, *et al.* Antazoline-induced allergic pneumonitis. *Br Med J* 1979; **2:** 1328.
2. Nielsen JL, *et al.* Immune thrombocytopenia due to antazoline (Antistina). *Allergy* 1981; **36:** 517–19.

Uses and Administration

Antazoline, an ethylenediamine derivative, is an antihistamine used topically for the treatment of allergic conjunctivitis (p.399). It is used as the hydrochloride, phosphate, or sulphate in eye drops, most commonly in a concentration of 0.5%; the mesylate has also been used. Antazoline salts are often used with a vasoconstrictor such as naphazoline hydrochloride or nitrate or xylometazoline hydrochloride.

Antazoline hydrochloride is used in a strength of up to 2% in a cream or ointment for the treatment of minor skin irritations, but as with other antihistamines there is a risk of sensitisation. The hydrochloride has also been given by mouth.

Preparations

Proprietary Preparations (details are given in Part 3)
Ger.: Visuphrine N in der Ophtiole†; ***UK:*** Insect Bite Ointment†; Wasp-Eze.

Multi-ingredient: ***Aust.:*** Histophtal; ***Austral.:*** Albalon-A Liquifilm; Allergy Eyes; Antistine-Privine; In A Wink Allergy; Optazine A†; ***Belg.:*** Zincfrin Antihistaminicum; ***Canad.:*** Albalon-A Liquifilm; Cooper AR; Ophtrivin-A; Vasocon-A; Zincfrin-A; ***Ger.:*** Allergopos N; Antistin-Privin; Digi-Pulsnorma†; duraforte†; Ophtalmin; Pulsnorma†; Solupen†; Spersallerg; ***Irl.:*** Otrivine-Antistin; RBC; ***Ital.:*** Antistin-Privina; Eubetal; Zincoimidazyl†; ***Norw.:*** Antistin-Privin†; Spersallerg; ***S.Afr.:*** Albalon-A; Antistin-Privin; Covosan; Gemini; Spersallerg; Zincfrin-A†; ***Spain:*** Alergoftal; Rinobanedif; ***Swed.:*** Antasten-Privin; ***Switz.:*** Antistin-Privin; Nospilin†; Spersallerg; Zincfrin-A†; ***UK:*** Modantis; Otrivine-Antistin; RBC; Vasocon-A†; ***USA:*** Antazoline-V; Vasocon-A.

Astemizole (12403-t)

Astemizole *(BAN, USAN, rINN).*

Astemizolum; R-43512. 1-(4-Fluorobenzyl)-2-{[1-(4-methoxyphenethyl)-4-piperidyl]amino}benzimidazole.

$C_{28}H_{31}FN_4O$ = 458.6.

CAS — 68844-77-9.

Pharmacopoeias. In *Eur.* (see p.viii) and *US.*

A white or almost white powder. Practically **insoluble** in water; soluble in alcohol; freely soluble in dichloromethane and in methyl alcohol. **Store** in airtight containers. Protect from light.

Adverse Effects and Precautions

As for the non-sedating antihistamines, p.397. Increased appetite and weight gain have been reported with astemizole.

Ventricular arrhythmias, including torsade de pointes, have occurred rarely with astemizole, particularly in association with raised blood concentrations (see Arrhythmias below). To reduce the risk of developing such arrhythmias the recommended dose should not be exceeded and astemizole should be avoided in patients with cardiac or significant hepatic disease, with known or suspected hypokalaemia or other electrolyte imbalance, or with known or suspected prolonged QT interval. The concomitant administration of drugs liable to interfere with the hepatic metabolism of astemizole, of other potentially arrhythmogenic drugs, and of drugs likely to cause electrolyte imbalance should be avoided (see under Interactions below). If syncope occurs astemizole should be withdrawn and the patient investigated for potential arrhythmias.

Arrhythmias. Although severe life-threatening cardiovascular effects including torsade de pointes and other ventricular arrhythmias were initially reported mainly after substantial overdoses of astemizole, such reactions have also occurred rarely with doses as low as 20 to 30 mg daily and even as low as 10 mg daily in those with possible predisposing factors. There is a report[1] of astemizole-induced torsade de pointes in a 15-year-old girl who claimed to have taken 10 mg daily for 10 weeks but pharmacokinetic data were more consistent with acute ingestion of higher doses. There have been several reports of cardiotoxicity following accidental overdosage with astemizole in children.[2-4]

A number of recommendations have been made to reduce the risk of developing serious arrhythmias, including those from the Committee on Safety of Medicines (CSM) in the UK[5,6] (see above for details). Astemizole should be discontinued immediately in patients who experience syncope, and appropriate clinical evaluation including ECG monitoring instituted because syncope has preceded or accompanied severe arrhythmias in some cases. Convulsions in patients taking astemizole may also be related to cardiovascular effects.[7]

Studies have suggested that astemizole induces ventricular arrhythmias by inhibiting cardiac potassium channels which results in prolongation of the QT interval, a risk factor for developing arrhythmias.[8]

1. Simons FER, *et al.* Astemizole-induced torsade de pointes. *Lancet* 1988; **ii:** 624.
2. Hoppu K, *et al.* Accidental astemizole overdose in young children. *Lancet* 1991; **338:** 538–40.
3. Tobin JR, *et al.* Astemizole-induced cardiac conduction disturbances in a child. *JAMA* 1991; **266:** 2737–40.
4. Wiley JF, *et al.* Cardiotoxic effects of astemizole overdose in children. *J Pediatr* 1992; **120:** 799–802.
5. Committee on Safety of Medicines. Ventricular arrhythmias due to terfenadine and astemizole. *Current Problems 35* 1992.
6. Committee on Safety of Medicines/Medicines Control Agency. Drug-induced prolongation of the QT interval. *Current Problems* 1996; **22:** 2.
7. Clark A, Love H. Astemizole-induced ventricular arrhythmias: an unexpected cause of convulsions. *Int J Cardiol* 1991; **33:** 165–7.
8. Rankin AC. Non-sedating antihistamines and cardiac arrhythmia. *Lancet* 1997; **350:** 1115–16.

Overdosage. Severe cardiac events have been associated with astemizole overdosage (see under Arrhythmias, above); management is mainly supportive. The absorption of astemizole from the gastro-intestinal tract can be prevented by administration of activated charcoal[1] but because astemizole is rapidly absorbed it would need to be given as soon as possible after poisoning. Haemodialysis does not appear to increase the clearance of astemizole.

1. Laine K, *et al.* The effect of activated charcoal on the absorption and elimination of astemizole. *Hum Exp Toxicol* 1994; **13:** 502–5.

Sedation. For discussion of the sedative effects of the older antihistamines, and the lack of such effects with the non-sedating antihistamines, including astemizole, see p.398.

Interactions

As for the non-sedating antihistamines in general, p.399.

Astemizole should not be given with drugs that inhibit its hepatic metabolism because of the increased risk of serious ventricular arrhythmias. These drugs include *itraconazole, ketoconazole*, and possibly other *imidazole and triazole antifungals*, and the macrolide antibacterials *clarithromycin, erythromycin*, and *triacetyloleandomycin*. Others, similarly to terfenadine (p.418), may include *serotonin reuptake inhibitors, HIV-protease inhibitors*, and *zileuton*. The metabolism of astemizole may also be inhibited by *grapefruit juice* and concomitant use should be avoided.

Concomitant administration with other potentially arrhythmogenic drugs such as *antiarrhythmics, tricyclic antidepressants*, the antimalarials *halofantrine* and *quinine, antipsychotics, cisapride*, and the beta blocker *sotalol* should be avoided, as should co-administration of *diuretics* that cause electrolyte imbalances such as hypokalaemia. The use of *terfenadine* and astemizole together is not recommended.

Pharmacokinetics

Absorption of astemizole from the gastro-intestinal tract is rapid and is reduced by food. First-pass metabolism is extensive, therefore plasma concentrations of unchanged drug are very low. The plasma concentration of astemizole plus metabolites takes about 4 to 8 weeks to reach steady state. The metabolism of astemizole is mediated through the cytochrome P450 enzyme system, mainly by the isoenzyme CYP3A4 and to a lesser extent by the isoenzymes CYP2D6 and CYP2A6. The elimination half-life of astemizole and its metabolites at steady state is about 19 days. Unchanged astemizole is highly bound to plasma proteins and does not appear to cross the blood-brain barrier to a significant extent. Desmethylastemizole, the major metabolite of astemizole, has histamine-H_1 blocking activity. The metabolites of astemizole are excreted slowly in the urine and faeces, and undergo enterohepatic recycling. Virtually none of an oral dose is excreted as unchanged drug.

Uses and Administration

Astemizole, a piperidine derivative, is a non-sedating antihistamine with a very long duration of action. It does not have significant sedative or antimuscarinic actions. Astemizole is used for the symptomatic relief of allergic conditions including rhinitis (p.400) and conjunctivitis (p.399), and skin disorders such as urticaria (p.401).

Astemizole is given by mouth in a dose of 10 mg once daily. Children aged 6 to 12 years may be given 5 mg daily. These doses must not be exceeded because of the risk of cardiac arrhythmias with higher doses. To ensure optimal absorption, astemizole should be given at least one hour before or two hours after a meal.

Reviews.

1. Richards DM, *et al.* Astemizole: a review of its pharmacodynamic properties and therapeutic efficacy. *Drugs* 1984; **28:** 38–61.
2. Krstenansky PM, Cluxton RJ. Astemizole: a long-acting, nonsedating antihistamine. *Drug Intell Clin Pharm* 1987; **21:** 947–53.

Preparations

USP 23: Astemizole Tablets.

Proprietary Preparations (details are given in Part 3)
Aust.: Hismanal; Pollonis; ***Austral.:*** Hismanal; ***Belg.:*** Hismanal; ***Canad.:*** Hismanal; ***Fr.:*** Hismanal; ***Ger.:*** Hismanal; ***Irl.:*** Hismanal; ***Ital.:*** Hismanal; Histamen; ***Neth.:*** Hismanal; ***S.Afr.:*** Hismanal; ***Spain:*** Alermizol; Esmacen; Hismanal; Histaminos; Hubermizol; Laridal; Paralergin; Retolen; Rifedot; Rimbol; Romadin; Simprox; Urdrim; ***Switz.:*** Hismacap†; Hismanal; ***UK:*** Hismanal; Pollon-eze; ***USA:*** Hismanal.

Multi-ingredient: ***Aust.:*** Hismadrin; ***Ital.:*** Histamen-D†; ***S.Afr.:*** Hismanal-D†.

Azatadine Maleate (6107-b)

Azatadine Maleate *(BANM, USAN, rINNM).*

Sch-10649. 6,11-Dihydro-11-(1-methyl-4-piperidylidene)-5*H*-benzo[5,6]cyclohepta[1,2-*b*]pyridine dimaleate.

$C_{20}H_{22}N_2,2C_4H_4O_4$ = 522.5.

CAS — 3964-81-6 (azatadine); 3978-86-7 (azatadine maleate).

Pharmacopoeias. In *US.*

A white to light cream-coloured, odourless powder. Freely **soluble** in water, in alcohol, in chloroform, and in methyl alcohol; practically insoluble in ether.

Adverse Effects and Precautions

As for the sedating antihistamines in general, p.397.

Extrapyramidal disorders. An acute dystonic reaction was reported in a patient who had taken azatadine maleate 20 to 30 mg by mouth over a 24-hour period.[1] The condition was reversed by intravenous injection of benztropine 2 mg.

1. Joske DJL. Dystonic reaction to azatadine. *Med J Aust* 1984; **141:** 449.

Interactions

As for the sedating antihistamines in general, p.399.

Pharmacokinetics

Azatadine maleate is readily absorbed from the gastro-intestinal tract and is partly metabolised. Peak plasma concentrations are achieved in about 4 hours. The elimination half-life has been reported to be 9 to 12 hours. Excretion of unchanged drug and metabolites is via the urine.

Uses and Administration

Azatadine maleate is a piperidine derivative closely related to cyproheptadine. It is a sedating antihistamine with a long duration of action; it also has antimuscarinic and antiserotonin properties.

Azatadine maleate is used for the symptomatic relief of allergic conditions including rhinitis (p.400) and urticaria (p.401);

it is also used for other pruritic skin disorders as well as reactions to insect bites and stings. It is given by mouth, usually in doses of 1 mg twice daily; if necessary 2 mg twice daily may be given. Children aged 6 to 12 years may be given 0.5 to 1 mg twice daily, and children aged 1 to 6 years, 0.25 mg twice daily.

Preparations

USP 23: Azatadine Maleate Tablets.

Proprietary Preparations (details are given in Part 3)
Austral.: Zadine; ***Belg.:*** Optimine; ***Canad.:*** Optimine; ***Ger.:*** Optimine†; ***Irl.:*** Optimine; ***Ital.:*** Idulian†; ***S.Afr.:*** Optimine; ***Spain:*** Lergocil; ***UK:*** Optimine; ***USA:*** Optimine.

Multi-ingredient: ***Canad.:*** Trinalin; ***Neth.:*** Congestan†; ***Spain:*** Atiramin; Idulanex; ***USA:*** Trinalin.

Azelastine Hydrochloride (15943-h)

Azelastine Hydrochloride *(BANM, USAN, rINNM).*

A-5610 (azelastine or azelastine hydrochloride); E-0659 (azelastine or azelastine hydrochloride); W-2979M (azelastine or azelastine hydrochloride). 4-(*p*-Chlorobenzyl)-2-(hexahydro-1-methyl-1*H*-azepin-4-yl)-1(2*H*)-phthalazinone monohydrochloride.

$C_{22}H_{24}ClN_3O,HCl$ = 418.4.

CAS — 58581-89-8 (azelastine); 79307-93-0 (azelastine hydrochloride).

Pharmacopoeias. In *Br.*

A white, crystalline powder. Slightly **soluble** in water; soluble in dehydrated alcohol; practically insoluble in ether, in *n*-hexane, and in toluene. **Store** in airtight containers. Protect from light.

Adverse Effects and Precautions

As for the antihistamines in general, p.397.

When administered intranasally irritation of the nasal mucosa and taste disturbances have been reported; somnolence, headache, and dry mouth have also been noted in some patients. Taste disturbance can occur after ophthalmic administration.

Pharmacokinetics

When administered intranasally, approximately 40% of the dose of azelastine reaches the systemic circulation. Elimination is via hepatic metabolism with excretion mainly in the faeces.

Azelastine is rapidly and almost completely absorbed after administration *by mouth*, peak plasma concentrations being achieved in 4 to 5 hours. Azelastine undergoes hepatic metabolism; the major metabolite, demethylazelastine, has antihistamine activity. The elimination half-life of azelastine is about 25 hours, increasing to 35.5 hours after multiple oral doses, possibly as a result of accumulation of the demethyl metabolite. Azelastine and its metabolites are excreted predominantly in the faeces and also in urine.

Uses and Administration

Azelastine hydrochloride is an antihistamine, which in addition to its histamine H_1-receptor-blocking activity, appears to inhibit the release of inflammatory mediators from mast cells. It is used topically in the symptomatic relief of allergic conditions including rhinitis (p.400) and conjunctivitis (p.399).

In rhinitis, the usual dose in the UK is 140 μg by nasal spray into each nostril twice daily. In conjunctivitis the usual dose is one drop of a 0.05% solution into each eye twice daily; this may be increased to four times daily in severe conditions.

Azelastine hydrochloride has also been given by mouth.

References.

1. McTavish D, Sorkin EM. Azelastine: a review of its pharmacodynamic and pharmacokinetic properties, and therapeutic potential. *Drugs* 1989; **38:** 778–800 (oral and nasal administration).
2. Busse WW, *et al.* Corticosteroid-sparing effect of azelastine in the management of bronchial asthma. *Am J Respir Crit Care Med* 1996; **153:** 122–7 (oral).
3. Wober W, *et al.* Efficacy and tolerability of azelastine nasal spray in the treatment of allergic rhinitis: large scale experience in community practice. *Curr Med Res Opin* 1997; **13:** 617–26 (nasal).
4. McNeely W, Wiseman LR. Intranasal azelastine: a review of its efficacy in the management of allergic rhinitis. *Drugs* 1998; **56:** 91–114.

Preparations

Proprietary Preparations (details are given in Part 3)
Aust.: Allergodil; Lasticom; ***Belg.:*** Allergodil; ***Fr.:*** Allergodil; ***Ger.:*** Allergodil; Rhinolast; ***Irl.:*** Rhinolast; ***Ital.:*** Allergodil; ***Jpn:*** Azeptin; ***Neth.:*** Allergodil; ***S.Afr.:*** Rhinolast; ***Spain:*** Afluon; Alferos; ***Switz.:*** Allergodil; ***UK:*** Optilast; Rhinolast; ***USA:*** Astelin.

Bamipine (6108-v)

Bamipine *(BAN, rINN).*

N-Benzyl-*N*-(1-methyl-4-piperidyl)aniline.

$C_{19}H_{24}N_2$ = 280.4.

CAS — 4945-47-5.

Bamipine is a sedating antihistamine with pronounced sedative effects.

Bamipine and its salts are used mainly for the symptomatic relief of allergic conditions such as urticaria (p.401) and in pruritic skin disorders. Bamipine hydrochloride is given by mouth in a dose of 50 to 100 mg three to four times daily. Bamipine, bamipine lactate, and bamipine salicylate have all been applied topically.

Preparations

Proprietary Preparations (details are given in Part 3)
Aust.: Soventol; ***Ger.:*** Soventol; ***Neth.:*** Soventol†.

Multi-ingredient: ***Aust.:*** Multifungin; ***Ger.:*** Multifungin†; Soventol C†; ***Irl.:*** Multifungin H†; Multifungin†; ***S.Afr.:*** Multifungin†; ***Spain:*** Multifungin†.

Bromodiphenhydramine Hydrochloride (6109-g)

Bromodiphenhydramine Hydrochloride *(BANM).*

Bromazine Hydrochloride *(rINNM).* 2-(4-Bromobenzhydryloxy)-*NN*-dimethylethylamine hydrochloride.

$C_{17}H_{20}BrNO,HCl$ = 370.7.

CAS — 118-23-0 (bromodiphenhydramine); 1808-12-4 (bromodiphenhydramine hydrochloride).

Pharmacopoeias. In *US.*

A white to pale buff-coloured, crystalline powder with a faint odour. **Soluble** 1 in less than 1 of water, 1 in 2 of alcohol and of chloroform, 1 in 31 of isopropyl alcohol, and 1 in 3500 of ether; practically insoluble in petroleum spirit. **Store** in airtight containers.

Bromodiphenhydramine hydrochloride, an ethanolamine derivative, is a sedating antihistamine with antimuscarinic and marked sedative actions.

It is used in combination preparations for the symptomatic treatment of coughs and the common cold (p.400) in a dose by mouth of 12.5 to 25 mg every 4 to 6 hours. The recommended maximum dose in such preparations is 150 mg daily. Children over 6 years of age may be given 6.25 to 12.5 mg every 6 hours.

Preparations

USP 23: Bromodiphenhydramine Hydrochloride Capsules; Bromodiphenhydramine Hydrochloride Elixir.

Proprietary Preparations (details are given in Part 3)

Multi-ingredient: ***Canad.:*** Ambenyl; ***USA:*** Ambenyl Cough Syrup; Amgenal Cough; Bromotuss with Codeine.

Brompheniramine Maleate (6110-f)

Brompheniramine Maleate *(BANM, rINNM).*

Brompheniramini Maleas; Parabromdylamine Maleate. (±)-3-(4-Bromophenyl)-*NN*-dimethyl-3-(2-pyridyl)propylamine hydrogen maleate.

$C_{16}H_{19}BrN_2,C_4H_4O_4$ = 435.3.

CAS — 86-22-6 (brompheniramine); 980-71-2 (brompheniramine maleate).

Pharmacopoeias. In *Eur.* (see p.viii) and *US.*

A white or almost white odourless crystalline powder. Ph. Eur. **solubilities** are: soluble in water; freely soluble in alcohol, in dichloromethane, and in methyl alcohol. USP solubilities are: soluble 1 in 5 of water, 1 in 15 of alcohol and of chloroform; slightly soluble in ether. A 1% solution in water has a pH of 4.0 to 5.0. **Store** in airtight containers. Protect from light.

Incompatibility has been reported with some diatrizoate, iodipamide, and iothalamate salts.

Dexbrompheniramine Maleate (6126-q)

Dexbrompheniramine Maleate *(BANM, rINNM).*

CAS — 2391-03-9.

Pharmacopoeias. In *US.*

A white odourless crystalline powder. **Soluble** 1 in 1.2 of water, 1 in 2.5 of alcohol, 1 in 2 of chloroform, and 1 in 3000 of ether. A 1% solution has a pH of about 5. **Store** in airtight containers. Protect from light.

Adverse Effects and Precautions

As for the sedating antihistamines in general, p.397.

Effects on the blood. A report[1] that agranulocytosis in a 34-year-old alcoholic man was possibly associated with brompheniramine therapy.

1. Hardin AS, Padilla F. Agranulocytosis during therapy with a brompheniramine-medication. *J Arkansas Med Soc* 1978; **75:** 206–8.

Extrapyramidal disorders. Facial dyskinesias have been reported[1,2] after administration of antihistamines including brompheniramine or dexbrompheniramine maleate.

1. Thach BT, *et al.* Oral facial dyskinesia associated with prolonged use of antihistaminic decongestants. *N Engl J Med* 1975; **293:** 486–7 (brompheniramine maleate, chlorpheniramine maleate, and phenindamine tartrate).
2. Barone DA, Raniolo J. Facial dyskinesia from overdose of an antihistamine. *N Engl J Med* 1980; **303:** 107 (dexbrompheniramine maleate).

Withdrawal. Withdrawal symptoms have been reported[1] following discontinuation of long-term therapy with brompheniramine maleate. The patient had been taking 48 mg almost every day for 20 years and developed tremor, nausea, depression, and apyrexial sweating within 48 hours of stopping treatment; symptoms resolved over the following weeks.

1. Kavanagh GM, *et al.* Withdrawal symptoms after discontinuation of long-acting brompheniramine maleate. *Br J Dermatol* 1994; **131:** 913–14.

Interactions

As for the sedating antihistamines in general, p.399.

Pharmacokinetics

After oral administration brompheniramine maleate appears to be well absorbed from the gastro-intestinal tract. Peak plasma concentrations are achieved within about 5 hours. An elimination half-life of about 25 hours has been reported. Brompheniramine maleate undergoes metabolism, unchanged drug and metabolites being excreted primarily in the urine.

References.

1. Simons FER, *et al.* The pharmacokinetics and antihistaminic effects of brompheniramine. *J Allergy Clin Immunol* 1982; **70:** 458–64.
2. Paton DM, Webster DR. Clinical pharmacokinetics of H_1-receptor antagonists (the antihistamines). *Clin Pharmacokinet* 1985; **10:** 477–97.

Uses and Administration

Brompheniramine maleate, an alkylamine derivative, is a sedating antihistamine with antimuscarinic and moderate sedative actions.

Dexbrompheniramine is the dextrorotatory isomer of brompheniramine, which is racemic, and has approximately twice the activity of brompheniramine by weight. Brompheniramine maleate and dexbrompheniramine maleate are used for the symptomatic relief of allergic conditions, mainly rhinitis (p.400) and conjunctivitis (p.399). They are common ingredients of compound preparations for the symptomatic treatment of coughs and the common cold (p.400).

Brompheniramine maleate is given by mouth usually in doses of 4 to 8 mg three or four times daily. Children up to 3 years of age have been given brompheniramine maleate 0.4 to 1 mg per kg bodyweight over 24 hours in four divided doses. Children aged 3 to 6 years may be given 1 to 2 mg three or four times daily and those aged 6 to 12 years 2 to 4 mg three or four times daily.

Brompheniramine maleate has also been given by subcutaneous, intramuscular, or slow intravenous injection; the dose is usually 5 to 20 mg every 6 to 12 hours as necessary and the total parenteral dose should not exceed 40 mg in 24 hours.

Dexbrompheniramine maleate is normally given as an ingredient of decongestant preparations containing pseudoephedrine. The dose of dexbrompheniramine maleate by mouth in these combinations is 2 mg up to four times daily. Children over 6 years may be given 1 mg up to four times a day.

Modified-release oral preparations of brompheniramine maleate or dexbrompheniramine maleate are available in some countries; dosage is specific to a particular formation.

Preparations

BP 1998: Brompheniramine Tablets;
USP 23: Brompheniramine Maleate and Pseudoephedrine Sulfate Syrup; Brompheniramine Maleate Elixir; Brompheniramine Maleate Injection; Brompheniramine Maleate Tablets; Dexbrompheniramine Maleate and Pseudoephedrine Sulfate Oral Solution.

Proprietary Preparations (details are given in Part 3)
Austral.: Dimetane†; ***Canad.:*** Dimetane; ***Fr.:*** Dimegan; ***Ger.:*** Dimegan; ***Irl.:*** Dimotane; ***Ital.:*** Antial†; Gammistin†; ***Swed.:*** Dimetane†; ***UK:*** Dimotane; ***USA:*** Bromarest†; Cophene-B†; Diamine TD†; Dimetane; Histaject†; Nasahist B†; ND Stat†; Oraminic II; Sinusol-B; Veltane.

Multi-ingredient: ***Aust.:*** Disophrol; ***Austral.:*** Dimetapp; Dimetapp DM; Dimetapp Elixir-Plus†; Dimetapp LA†; ***Belg.:*** Nasapert; Rinafort; ***Canad.:*** Centracol; Cold & Allergy Relief; Decongestant Antihistaminic Syrup; Dimetane Expectorant; Dimetane Expectorant-C; Dimetane Expectorant-DC; Dimetapp; Dimetapp Chewables; Dimetapp Clear; Dimetapp Cough & Cold Liqui-Gels; Dimetapp DM; Dimetapp Liqui-Gels; Dimetapp Oral Infant Drops; Dimetapp-C; Drixoral; Drixoral Day/Night; Drixtab; Pharmetapp; Tantapp; ***Fr.:*** Dimetane; Martigene; Rupton Chronules; ***Ger.:*** Ilvico N; Ilvico†; ***Irl.:*** Dimotane Co; Dimotane Expectorant; Dimotane Plus†; Dimotapp; Ilvico; ***Ital.:*** Exit†; ***Neth.:*** Nasapert†; ***Norw.:*** Lunerin†; ***S.Afr.:*** Dimetapp; Ilvico; ***Spain:*** Disofrol; Ilvico; ***Swed.:*** Disofrol; Lunerin; ***Switz.:*** Dimetapp; Disofrol; Rupton Chronules; ***UK:*** Dimotane Co; Dimotane Expectorant; Dimotane Plus; Dimotapp; ***USA:*** 12 Hour Antihistamine Nasal Decongestant; 12 Hour Cold; Alka-Seltzer Plus Night-Time Cold; Alka-Seltzer Plus Sinus Allergy; Allent; Allerhist†; Ami-Drix; Brofed; Bromadine-DM; Bromaline; Bromaline Plus; Bromanate; Bromarest DC†; Bromarest DX; Bromatane DX; Bromatapp; Bromfed; Bromfed-DM; Bromfed-PD; Bromfenex; Bromophen TD; Bromphen DX Cough; Bromphen†; Brompheniramine Cough; Brompheniramine DC Cough; Brotane DX†; Cheracol Sinus†; Dallergy-JR; Dexaphen-SA; Dimaphen; Dimetane Decongestant; Dimetane-DC; Dimetane-DX; Dimetapp; Dimetapp Cold & Allergy Chewable; Dimetapp Cold & Flu; Dimetapp DM; Disobrom; Disophrol; Dristan Allergy; Dristan Cold Maximum Strength Multi-symptom Formula; Drixomed; Drixoral; Drixoral Cold & Allergy; Drixoral Cold & Flu; Drixoral Plus; Endafed; ENT†; Histine DM; Iofed; Iohist DM; Liqui-Histine DM; Lodrane; Maximum Strength Dristan Cold; Myphetane DC; Myphetane DX; Myphetapp; Par-Drix†; Partapp TD; Poly-Histine CS CV; Poly-Histine DM; Respahist; Rondec Chewable; Siltapp; Tamine SR; Touro A & H; ULTRAbrom PD; Vicks DayQuil Allergy Relief.

Buclizine Hydrochloride (6111-d)

Buclizine Hydrochloride *(BANM, USAN, rINNM).*

NSC-25141; UCB-4445. *(RS)* 1-(4-*tert*-Butylbenzyl)-4-(4-chlorobenzhydryl)piperazine dihydrochloride.

$C_{28}H_{33}ClN_2,2HCl = 505.9.$

CAS — 82-95-1 (buclizine); 129-74-8 (buclizine hydrochloride).

Pharmacopoeias. In *Br.*

A white or slightly yellowish, crystalline powder. Practically **insoluble** in water; very slightly soluble in alcohol; sparingly soluble in chloroform and in propylene glycol.

Adverse Effects and Precautions

As for the sedating antihistamines in general, p.397.

Interactions

As for the sedating antihistamines in general, p.399.

Uses and Administration

Buclizine hydrochloride, a piperazine derivative, is a sedating antihistamine with antimuscarinic and moderate sedative actions. It is used mainly for its antiemetic action, particularly in the prevention of motion sickness (p.400) and in the treatment of migraine in combination with analgesics (p.443). In some countries it is given in the management of allergic conditions and in pruritic skin disorders (p.400). Buclizine has also been used in the treatment of vertigo (p.401) associated with disorders of the vestibular system, although its value in these conditions remains to be established.

To prevent motion sickness, buclizine hydrochloride is given at least 30 minutes before travelling in a dose of 50 mg by mouth, which may be repeated, if necessary, after 4 to 6 hours. The usual dose to alleviate nausea is 50 mg given up to three times daily.

In the treatment of migraine, buclizine hydrochloride is given in usual doses of 12.5 mg at the start of an attack or when one is known to be imminent.

In pruritic skin disorders the usual dose of buclizine hydrochloride is 25 to 50 mg daily.

Preparations

Proprietary Preparations (details are given in Part 3)
Belg.: Longifene; ***Fr.:*** Aphilan; ***S.Afr.:*** Longifene; ***Switz.:*** Longifene; ***USA:*** Bucladin-S Softab.

Multi-ingredient: ***Austral.:*** Migrex Pink†; ***Belg.:*** Agyrax; ***Ger.:*** Migralave N; ***Irl.:*** Migraleve; ***S.Afr.:*** Vomifene; ***Spain:*** Migraleve; ***Switz.:*** Hexafene; Migraleve; ***UK:*** Migraleve; Migralift.

Carbinoxamine Maleate (6113-h)

Carbinoxamine Maleate *(BANM, rINNM).*

2-[4-Chloro-α-(2-pyridyl)benzyloxy]-*NN*-dimethylethylamine hydrogen maleate.

$C_{16}H_{19}ClN_2O,C_4H_4O_4 = 406.9.$

CAS — 486-16-8 (carbinoxamine); 3505-38-2 (carbinoxamine maleate).

Pharmacopoeias. In *US.*

A white odourless crystalline powder. **Soluble** 1 in less than 1 of water, 1 in 1.5 of alcohol and of chloroform, and 1 in 8300 of ether. A 1% solution in water has a pH of 4.6 to 5.1. **Store** in airtight containers. Protect from light.

Adverse Effects and Precautions

As for the sedating antihistamines in general, p.397.

Interactions

As for the sedating antihistamines in general, p.399.

Uses and Administration

Carbinoxamine maleate, an ethanolamine derivative, is a sedating antihistamine with antimuscarinic, significant sedative, and serotonin antagonist effects. Carbinoxamine maleate is used for the relief of allergic conditions such as rhinitis (p.400), and is a common ingredient of compound preparations for symptomatic treatment of coughs and the common cold (p.400).

The dose of carbinoxamine maleate by mouth, used alone or in combination preparations, is usually in the range of 2 to 4 mg three to four times daily. Children may be given half the adult dose. Carbinoxamine polistirex has also been given by mouth.

Preparations

USP 23: Carbinoxamine Maleate Tablets.

Proprietary Preparations (details are given in Part 3)
Fr.: Allergefon; ***Ger.:*** Polistin Pad; Polistin T-Caps.

Multi-ingredient: ***Aust.:*** Capramin; Co-Tylenol; Rhinopront; ***Belg.:*** Rhinopront; ***Fr.:*** Humex; ***Ger.:*** Naldecol†; Rhinopront; Rhinotussal; Tylex†; ***Ital.:*** Rondec; Torfan; ***S.Afr.:*** Coryretard-C†; Coryretard-S†; Rhinotussal†; Rondec†; ***Spain:*** Rhinocap†; Rinoretard; Rondec; Toscal; Toscal Compuesto; ***Switz.:*** Co-Tylenol†; Rhinopront; Rhinotussal; ***UK:*** Davenol†; ***USA:*** Biohist-LA; Carbinoxamine Compound; Carbiset; Carbodec; Carbodec DM; Cardec DM Pediatric; Cardec-S; Pseudo-Car DM; Rondamine-DM; Rondec; Rondec-DM; Sildec-DM; Tussafed.

Cetirizine Hydrochloride (18617-l)

Cetirizine Hydrochloride *(BANM, USAN, rINNM).*

Cetirizini Dihydrochloridum; P-071; UCB-P071. The dihydrochloride of 2-[4-(4-chlorobenzhydryl)piperazin-1-yl]ethoxyacetic acid.

$C_{21}H_{25}ClN_2O_3,2HCl = 461.8.$

CAS — 83881-51-0 (cetirizine); 83881-52-1 (cetirizine hydrochloride).

Pharmacopoeias. In *Eur.* (see p.viii).

A white or almost white powder. Freely **soluble** in water; practically insoluble in acetone and in dichloromethane. A 5% solution in water has a pH of 1.2 to 1.8. **Protect** from light.

Adverse Effects and Precautions

As for the non-sedating antihistamines in general, p.397. Reduced dosage is recommended for patients with renal impairment.

Arrhythmias. The ECG effects of cetirizine were studied[1] in normal subjects and administration of doses of up to six times the usual recommended dose did not prolong the QT_c interval. Additionally, workers from the FDA[2] in the USA and representatives of the manufacturers[3] in Belgium have not found any association so far between cetirizine and the development of ventricular arrhythmias.

1. Sale ME, *et al.* The electrocardiographic effects of cetirizine in normal subjects. *Clin Pharmacol Ther* 1994; **56:** 295–301.
2. Himmel MH, *et al.* Dangers of non-sedating antihistamines. *Lancet* 1997; **350:** 69.
3. Coulie P, *et al.* Non-sedating antihistamines and cardiac arrhythmias. *Lancet* 1998; **351:** 451.

Sedation. For discussion of the sedative effects of antihistamines, including those of cetirizine, see p.398.

Interactions

As for the non-sedating antihistamines in general, p.399. However, some interactions are less likely with cetirizine than with non-sedating antihistamines such as astemizole and terfenadine, since cetirizine appears to have low hepatic metabolism and little arrhythmogenic potential (see Arrhythmias, above).

Anticoagulants. For a report of an interaction between cetirizine and *nicoumalone*, see under Interactions in Warfarin, p.967.

Pharmacokinetics

Cetirizine is rapidly absorbed from the gastro-intestinal tract after oral administration, peak plasma concentrations being attained in about one hour. Food delays the time to peak plasma concentrations but does not decrease the amount of drug absorbed. It is highly bound to plasma proteins and has an elimination half-life of about 10 hours. Cetirizine has been detected in breast milk. Cetirizine is excreted primarily in the urine mainly as unchanged drug. Cetirizine does not appear to cross the blood-brain barrier to a significant extent.

References.

1. Awni WM, *et al.* Effect of haemodialysis on the pharmacokinetics of cetirizine. *Eur J Clin Pharmacol* 1990; **38:** 67–9.
2. Desager JP, *et al.* A pharmacokinetic evaluation of the second-generation H_1-receptor antagonist cetirizine in very young children. *Clin Pharmacol Ther* 1993; **53:** 431–5.

Uses and Administration

Cetirizine hydrochloride, a piperazine derivative and metabolite of hydroxyzine (p.411), is described as a non-sedating antihistamine reported to be long-acting and with some mast-cell stabilising activity. It appears to have a low potential for drowsiness in usual doses and to be virtually free of antimuscarinic activity. It is used for the symptomatic relief of allergic conditions including rhinitis (p.400) and chronic urticaria (p.401).

In adults and children of 6 years and over, cetirizine hydrochloride is given by mouth in a dose of 10 mg once daily or 5 mg twice daily. In children aged 2 to 6 years old a dose of 5 mg once daily or 2.5 mg twice daily may be used for seasonal allergic rhinitis.

In patients with renal impairment it is recommended that the dosage is reduced to half the usual daily dose.

References.

1. Spencer CM, *et al.* Cetirizine: a reappraisal of its pharmacological properties and therapeutic use in selected allergic disorders. *Drugs* 1993; **46:** 1055–80.
2. Barnes CL, *et al.* Cetirizine: a new, nonsedating antihistamine. *Ann Pharmacother* 1993; **27:** 464–70.
3. Breneman D, *et al.* Cetirizine and astemizole therapy for chronic idiopathic urticaria: a double-blind placebo-controlled, comparative trial. *J Am Acad Dermatol* 1995; **33:** 192–8.
4. Breneman DL. Cetirizine versus hydroxyzine and placebo in chronic idiopathic urticaria. *Ann Pharmacother* 1996; **30:** 1075–9.
5. Anonymous. Cetirizine—a new antihistamine. *Med Lett Drugs Ther* 1996; **38:** 21–3.

Preparations

Proprietary Preparations (details are given in Part 3)
Aust.: Zyrtec; ***Austral.:*** Zyrtec; ***Belg.:*** Zyrtec; ***Canad.:*** Reactine; ***Fr.:*** Virlix; Zyrtec; ***Ger.:*** Zyrtec; ***Irl.:*** Zirtek; ***Ital.:*** Formistin; Virlix; Zirtec; ***Neth.:*** Zyrtec; ***Norw.:*** Zyrtec; ***S.Afr.:*** Zyrtec; ***Spain:*** Alerlisin; Virlix; Voltric; Zyrtec; ***Swed.:*** Zyrlex; ***Switz.:*** Zyrtec; ***UK:*** Zirtek.

Multi-ingredient: ***Belg.:*** Cirrus.

Chlorcyclizine Hydrochloride (6114-m)

Chlorcyclizine Hydrochloride *(BANM, rINNM).*

Chlorcyclizini Hydrochloridum; Chlorcyclizinium Chloride. 1-(4-Chlorobenzhydryl)-4-methylpiperazine hydrochloride.

$C_{18}H_{21}ClN_2,HCl = 337.3.$

CAS — 82-93-9 (chlorcyclizine); 1620-21-9 (chlorcyclizine hydrochloride).

Pharmacopoeias. In *Eur.* (see p.viii).

A white, crystalline powder. Freely **soluble** in water; soluble in alcohol; freely soluble in dichloromethane; practically insoluble in ether. A 1% solution in water has a pH of 5.0 to 6.0. **Protect** from light.

Chlorcyclizine hydrochloride, a piperazine derivative, is a sedating antihistamine. It is given by mouth in a dose of 50 mg three times daily for the symptomatic relief of hypersensitivity reactions; it is also used as an antiemetic. It has been used at a strength of 2% in topical preparations, although as with other antihistamines, there is a risk of sensitisation.

Chlorcyclizine dibunate (naftoclizine) has been administered as a cough suppressant similarly to sodium dibunate (p.1070).

Preparations

Proprietary Preparations (details are given in Part 3)
Ital.: Bechitus†; Bexedan†; ***Norw.:*** Trihistan; ***Swed.:*** Di-Paralene†.

Multi-ingredient: ***Belg.:*** Primatour†; ***Neth.:*** Primatour; ***Norw.:*** Anervan; ***Spain:*** Diminex Antitusigeno; Diminex Balsamico; ***Swed.:*** Anervan; Exolyt; ***USA:*** Mantadil†.

Chloropyrilene Citrate (6115-b)

Chloropyrilene Citrate *(BANM, rINNM).*

Chloromethapyrilene Citrate; Chlorothen Citrate; Chlorpyrilen Citrate. *N*-(5-Chloro-2-thenyl)-*N'N'*-dimethyl-*N*-(2-pyridyl)ethylenediamine dihydrogen citrate.

$C_{14}H_{18}ClN_3S,C_6H_8O_7$ = 488.0.

CAS — 148-65-2 (chloropyrilene); 148-64-1 (chloropyrilene citrate).

Chloropyrilene citrate, an ethylenediamine derivative, is a sedating antihistamine that has been used in the treatment of allergic conditions.

Preparations

Proprietary Preparations (details are given in Part 3)

Multi-ingredient: ***Canad.:*** Achrocidin†.

Chlorpheniramine Maleate (6116-v)

Chlorpheniramine Maleate *(BANM).*

Chlorphenamine Maleate *(rINNM)*; Chlorphenamini Maleas; Chlorprophenpyridamine Maleate. (±)-3-(4-Chlorophenyl)-*NN*-dimethyl-3-(2-pyridyl)propylamine hydrogen maleate.

$C_{16}H_{19}ClN_2,C_4H_4O_4$ = 390.9.

CAS — 132-22-9 (chlorpheniramine); 113-92-8 (chlorpheniramine maleate).

Pharmacopoeias. In *Chin., Eur.* (see p.viii), *Int., Jpn,* and *US.*

A white odourless crystalline powder. **Soluble** 1 in 4 of water and 1 in 10 of alcohol and of chloroform; slightly soluble in ether. **Store** in airtight containers. Protect from light.

Incompatibility has been reported with calcium chloride, kanamycin sulphate, noradrenaline acid tartrate, pentobarbitone sodium, and iodipamide meglumine.

Dexchlorpheniramine Maleate (6127-p)

Dexchlorpheniramine Maleate *(rINNM).*

Dexchlorpheniramini Maleas.

CAS — 25523-97-1 (dexchlorpheniramine); 2438-32-6 (dexchlorpheniramine maleate).

Pharmacopoeias. In *Eur.* (see p.viii), *Jpn,* and *US.*

A white odourless crystalline powder. **Soluble** 1 in 1.1 of water, 1 in 2 of alcohol, 1 in 1.7 of chloroform, and 1 in 2500 of ether; freely soluble in methyl alcohol and in dichloromethane. A 1% solution in water has a pH of 4.0 to 5.5. **Store** in airtight containers. Protect from light.

Adverse Effects and Precautions

As for the sedating antihistamines in general, p.397.

Injections may be irritant and cause transient hypotension or stimulation of the CNS.

Effects on the blood. There are several old and isolated reports of blood dyscrasias after administration of chlorpheniramine maleate; these include agranulocytosis,[1,2] thrombocytopenia,[3] pancytopenia,[4] and aplastic anaemia.[5] Haemolytic anaemia has occurred after administration of dexchlorpheniramine maleate.[6] The association with antihistamine administration has been questioned in some of these cases.[7]

1. Shenfield G, Spry CJF. Unusual cause of agranulocytosis. *Br Med J* 1968; **ii:** 52–3.
2. Hardin AS. Chlorpheniramine and agranulocytosis. *Ann Intern Med* 1988; **108:** 770.
3. Eisner EV, *et al.* Chlorpheniramine-dependent thrombocytopenia. *JAMA* 1975; **231:** 735–6.
4. Deringer PM, Maniatis A. Chlorpheniramine-induced bone-marrow suppression. *Lancet* 1976; **i:** 432.
5. Kanoh T, *et al.* Aplastic anaemia after prolonged treatment with chlorpheniramine. *Lancet* 1977; **i:** 546–7.
6. Duran-Suarez JR, *et al.* The I antigen as an immune complex receptor in a case of haemolytic anaemia induced by an antihistaminic agent. *Br J Haematol* 1981; **49:** 153–4.
7. Spry CJF. Chlorpheniramine-induced bone-marrow suppression. *Lancet* 1976; **i:** 545.

Effects on the senses. Chlorpheniramine has been reported to affect the senses of smell and taste.[1]

1. Schiffman SS. Taste and smell in disease. *N Engl J Med* 1983; **308:** 1275–9.

Extrapyramidal disorders. Facial dyskinesias have been reported[1,2] after administration of chlorpheniramine maleate by mouth.

1. Thach BT, *et al.* Oral facial dyskinesia associated with prolonged use of antihistaminic decongestants. *N Engl J Med* 1975; **293:** 486–7.
2. Davis WA. Dyskinesia associated with chronic antihistamine use. *N Engl J Med* 1976; **294:** 113.

Interactions

As for the sedating antihistamines in general, p.399.

Antiepileptics. For a report of the effect of chlorpheniramine on phenytoin, see p.355.

Pharmacokinetics

Chlorpheniramine maleate is absorbed relatively slowly from the gastro-intestinal tract, peak plasma concentrations occurring about 2.5 to 6 hours after administration by mouth. Bioavailability is low, values of 25 to 50% having been reported. Chlorpheniramine appears to undergo considerable first-pass metabolism. About 70% of chlorpheniramine in the circulation is bound to plasma proteins. There is wide interindividual variation in the pharmacokinetics of chlorpheniramine; values ranging from 2 to 43 hours have been reported for the half-life. Chlorpheniramine is widely distributed in the body, including passage into the CNS.

Chlorpheniramine maleate is extensively metabolised. Metabolites include desmethyl- and didesmethylchlorpheniramine. Unchanged drug and metabolites are excreted primarily in the urine; excretion is dependent on urinary pH and flow rate. Only trace amounts have been found in the faeces.

A duration of action of 4 to 6 hours has been reported; this is shorter than may be predicted from pharmacokinetic parameters.

More rapid and extensive absorption, faster clearance, and a shorter half-life have been reported in children.

References.

1. Rumore MM. Clinical pharmacokinetics of chlorpheniramine. *Drug Intell Clin Pharm* 1984; **18:** 701–7.
2. Paton DM, Webster DR. Clinical pharmacokinetics of H_1-receptor antagonists (the antihistamines). *Clin Pharmacokinet* 1985; **10:** 477–97.

Uses and Administration

Chlorpheniramine maleate, an alkylamine derivative, is a sedating antihistamine that causes a moderate degree of sedation; it also has antimuscarinic activity.

Dexchlorpheniramine is the dextrorotatory isomer of chlorpheniramine, which is racemic, and has approximately twice the activity of chlorpheniramine.

Chlorpheniramine maleate and dexchlorpheniramine maleate are used for the symptomatic relief of allergic conditions including urticaria and angioedema (p.401), rhinitis (p.400), and conjunctivitis (p.399), and in pruritic skin disorders (p.400). They are common ingredients of compound preparations for symptomatic treatment of coughs and the common cold (p.400). Chlorpheniramine may be administered intravenously as an adjunct in the emergency treatment of anaphylactic shock (p.399).

Chlorpheniramine maleate is given by mouth in doses of 4 mg every 4 to 6 hours up to a maximum of 24 mg daily. Doses recommended for children are: 1 to 2 years, 1 mg twice daily; 2 to 5 years, 1 mg every 4 to 6 hours (maximum 6 mg daily); 6 to 12 years, 2 mg every 4 to 6 hours (maximum 12 mg daily).

Chlorpheniramine maleate may be given by intramuscular, by subcutaneous, or by slow intravenous injection over a period of 1 minute. The usual dose is 10 to 20 mg and the total dose given by these routes in 24 hours should not normally exceed 40 mg. For children, doses of 87.5 μg per kg bodyweight subcutaneously four times daily have been suggested.

Dexchlorpheniramine maleate is given by mouth in doses of 2 mg every 4 to 6 hours up to a maximum of 12 mg daily. Children aged 2 to 5 years may be given 0.5 mg every 4 to 6 hours (maximum 3 mg daily), and those aged 6 to 12 years, 1 mg every 4 to 6 hours (maximum 6 mg daily).

Modified-release oral preparations of chlorpheniramine maleate or dexchlorpheniramine maleate are available in some countries; dosage is specific to a particular formulation.

Chlorpheniramine polistirex (a chlorpheniramine and sulphonated diethenylbenzene-ethenylbenzene copolymer complex) and chlorpheniramine tannate are given by mouth and used similarly to chlorpheniramine maleate.

Malaria. Chlorpheniramine may be tried in patients with malaria who experience chloroquine-induced pruritus (see p.427), but additionally it has been shown to have some promise as an adjunct in the treatment of chloroquine-resistant malaria itself. Early studies indicated that chlorpheniramine was only one of a number of drugs, that reversed chloroquine resistance *in vitro* in isolates of *Plasmodium falciparum*. Later clinical studies in children in Nigeria demonstrated enhanced efficacy when chlorpheniramine was given with chloroquine.[1-4] The overall management of malaria is discussed on p.422.

1. Sowunmi A, *et al.* Enhanced efficacy of chloroquine-chlorpheniramine combination in acute uncomplicated falciparum malaria in children. *Trans R Soc Trop Med Hyg* 1997; **91:** 63–7.
2. Sowunmi A, Oduola AMJ. Comparative efficacy of chloroquine/chlorpheniramine combination and mefloquine for the treatment of chloroquine-resistant Plasmodium falciparum malaria in Nigerian children. *Trans R Soc Trop Med Hyg* 1997; **91:** 689–93.
3. Sowunmi A, *et al.* Comparative efficacy of chloroquine plus chlorpheniramine and pyrimethamine/sulfadoxine in acute uncomplicated falciparum malaria in Nigerian children. *Trans R Soc Trop Med Hyg* 1998; **92:** 77–81.
4. Sowunmi A, *et al.* Comparative efficacy of chloroquine plus chlorpheniramine and halofantrine in acute uncomplicated falciparum malaria in Nigerian children. *Trans R Soc Trop Med Hyg* 1998; **92:** 441–5.

Otitis media. For studies questioning the use of chlorpheniramine maleate with decongestants in children with acute otitis media, see p.400.

Preparations

BP 1998: Chlorphenamine Injection; Chlorphenamine Oral Solution; Chlorphenamine Tablets;
USP 23: Chlorpheniramine Maleate and Pseudoephedrine Hydrochloride Oral Solution; Chlorpheniramine Maleate Extended-release Capsules; Chlorpheniramine Maleate Injection; Chlorpheniramine Maleate Syrup; Chlorpheniramine Maleate Tablets; Dexchlorpheniramine Maleate Syrup; Dexchlorpheniramine Maleate Tablets.

Proprietary Preparations (details are given in Part 3)
Aust.: Polaramin; Polaronil; ***Austral.:*** Allergex†; Piriton†; Polaramine; ***Belg.:*** Bronchalene; Polaramine; ***Canad.:*** Chlor-Tripolon; Histalon; Novo-Pheniram; Polaramine; ***Fr.:*** Polaramine; ***Ger.:*** Polaronil; ***Irl.:*** Anti-Hist; Piriton; ***Ital.:*** Clorten†; Lentostamin†; Polamin; Polaramin; Trimeton; ***Neth.:*** Polaramine; ***Norw.:*** Phenamin; Polaramin; ***S.Afr.:*** Allergex; Allerhist†; Chlorhist; Chlortrimeton; Histamed; Polaramine; ***Spain:*** Antihist; Polaramine; ***Swed.:*** Polaramin; ***Switz.:*** Polaramine; ***UK:*** Calimal; Piriton; Rimarin; ***USA:*** Aller-Chlor; Allergy; Chlo-Amine; Chlor; Chlor-Pro; Chlor-Trimeton; Chlorate†; Chlorspan; Chlortab†; Dexchlor†; Diabetic Tussin Allergy Relief; Efidac 24-Chlorpheniramine; Gen-Allerate; PediaCare Allergy Formula; Pfeiffer's Allergy; Phenetron†; Poladex†; Polaramine; Ricobid H; Telachlor†; Teldrin.

Multi-ingredient: numerous preparations are listed in Part 3.

Chlorphenoxamine Hydrochloride (353-c)

Chlorphenoxamine Hydrochloride *(BANM, rINNM).*

2-(4-Chloro-α-methylbenzhydryloxy)-*NN*-dimethylethylamine hydrochloride.

$C_{18}H_{22}ClNO,HCl$ = 340.3.

CAS — 77-38-3 (chlorphenoxamine); 562-09-4 (chlorphenoxamine hydrochloride).

Chlorphenoxamine, a congener of diphenhydramine (see p.409), has antimuscarinic and antihistaminic properties. It has been used in nausea, vomiting, and vertigo, and was formerly used in the symptomatic treatment of parkinsonism. Chlorphenoxamine has also been used in hypersensitivity reactions.

Preparations

Proprietary Preparations (details are given in Part 3)
Aust.: Systral; ***Fr.:*** Systral†; ***Ger.:*** Systral.

Multi-ingredient: ***Aust.:*** Calcilin compositum; Longtussin; Rodavan; Spirbon; Systral C; Systrason; ***Ger.:*** Rodavan; Systral C†; ***S.Afr.:*** Analgen-SA.

Cinnarizine (6118-q)

Cinnarizine *(BAN, USAN, rINN)*.

Cinnarizinum; 516-MD; R-516; R-1575. 1-Benzhydryl-4-cinnamylpiperazine; (*E*)-1-(Diphenylmethyl)-4-(3-phenylprop-2-enyl)piperazine.

$C_{26}H_{28}N_2$ = 368.5.

CAS — 298-57-7.

Pharmacopoeias. In *Eur.* (see p.viii), *Jpn*, and *Pol.*

A white or almost white powder. Practically **insoluble** in water; slightly soluble in alcohol and in methyl alcohol; soluble in acetone; freely soluble in dichloromethane. **Protect** from light.

Adverse Effects and Precautions

As for the sedating antihistamines in general, p.397.

There have been rare reports of extrapyramidal symptoms after cinnarizine, sometimes associated with depressive feelings.

High doses of cinnarizine should be used with caution in patients with hypotension because of the possibility of decreasing blood pressure further.

Extrapyramidal disorders. For reference to extrapyramidal disorders associated with the use of cinnarizine, see Flunarizine, p.411.

Hypersensitivity. A report[1] of immunologically-defined lichen planus pemphigoides in a 72-year-old woman taking cinnarizine. Lesions began to clear when treatment was stopped but challenge with cinnarizine provoked severe itching and reactivation of pigmented lesions.

1. Miyagawa S, *et al.* Lichen planus pemphigoides-like lesions induced by cinnarizine. *Br J Dermatol* 1985; **112:** 607–13.

Porphyria. Cinnarizine was considered to be unsafe in patients with acute porphyria because it has been shown to be porphyrinogenic in *animals* and *in-vitro* systems.[1]

1. Moore MR, McColl KEL. *Porphyria: drug lists.* Glasgow: Porphyria Research Unit, University of Glasgow, 1991.

Tinnitus. The Spanish System of Pharmacovigilance had received reports[1] of tinnitus associated with calcium-channel blockers; some of the reports, including the one relating to cinnarizine, were in patients also receiving other ototoxic drugs. WHO was said to have additional reports of tinnitus associated with calcium-channel blockers including cinnarizine.

1. Narváez M, *et al.* Tinnitus with calcium-channel blockers. *Lancet* 1994; **343:** 1229–30.

Weight gain. There has been a report[1] of weight gain in four patients who had taken cinnarizine for one to two years; in all cases the weight gain was associated with increased appetite.

1. Navarro-Badenes J, *et al.* Weight-gain associated with cinnarizine. *Ann Pharmacother* 1992; **26:** 928–30.

Interactions

As for the sedating antihistamines in general, p.399.

Pharmacokinetics

Cinnarizine is absorbed from the gastro-intestinal tract, peak plasma concentrations occurring 2 to 4 hours after oral administration. It undergoes metabolism and has a half-life of 3 to 6 hours. Cinnarizine is excreted in the faeces mainly as unchanged drug, and in the urine predominantly as metabolites.

Uses and Administration

Cinnarizine is a piperazine derivative with antihistamine, sedative, and calcium-channel blocking activity. It is used for the symptomatic treatment of nausea and vertigo caused by Ménière's disease and other vestibular disorders (p.401) and for the prevention and treatment of motion sickness (p.400). It is also used in the management of various peripheral and cerebral vascular disorders.

The usual dose for vertigo and vestibular disorders is 30 mg three times daily by mouth. For motion sickness a dose of 30 mg may be taken two hours before the start of the journey and 15 mg every 8 hours during the journey. Children aged 5 to 12 years may be given half the adult dose for both indications. In European countries other than the UK, a dose of 75 mg one or two times daily has been given for vertigo and vestibular disorders. Doses of 75 mg may also be given one to three times daily for cerebrovascular disorders and 2 or 3 times daily for peripheral vascular disorders.

References.

1. Shupak A, *et al.* Cinnarizine in the prophylaxis of seasickness: laboratory vestibular evaluation and sea study. *Clin Pharmacol Ther* 1994; **55:** 670–80.

Preparations

Proprietary Preparations (details are given in Part 3)
Aust.: Cinnabene; Pericephal; Stutgeron; ***Belg.:*** Stugeron; ***Ger.:*** Cerepar†; Cinnacet; Gigantén†; Stutgeron; ***Irl.:*** Stugeron; ***Ital.:*** Cinazyn; Senoger†; Stugeron; Toliman; ***Neth.:*** Cinnipirine; ***S.Afr.:*** Antimet; Purazine†; Stugeron; ***Spain:*** Pervasum; Stugeron; ***Swed.:*** Glanil†; ***Switz.:*** Cerepar; Cinnaforte†; Cinnageron; Ixertol†; Stugeron; ***UK:*** Cinaziere; Marzine RF†; Stugeron.

Multi-ingredient: ***Aust.:*** Cinnarplus; ***Belg.:*** Primatour†; Rinomar; Touristil; ***Fr.:*** Sureptil; ***Ger.:*** Arlevert; Stutgeron-Digoxin†; ***Ital.:*** Sureptil†; Vertigex†; ***Neth.:*** Primatour; ***Norw.:*** Rinomar; ***Spain:*** Clinadil; Clinadil Compositum; Diclamina; Ederal; Neorgine; Ornade; ***Swed.:*** Rinomar.

Clemastine Fumarate (6119-p)

Clemastine Fumarate *(BANM, USAN, rINNM)*.

Clemastini Fumaras; HS-592 (clemastine); Meclastine Fumarate; Mecloprodine Fumarate. (+)-(2*R*)-2-{2-[(*R*)-4-Chloro-α-methylbenzhydryloxy]ethyl}-1-methylpyrrolidine hydrogen fumarate.

$C_{21}H_{26}ClNO,C_4H_4O_4$ = 460.0.

CAS — 15686-51-8 (clemastine); 14976-57-9 (clemastine fumarate).

Pharmacopoeias. In *Eur.* (see p.viii), *Jpn, Pol.,* and *US.*

A white or almost white or colourless to faintly yellow, odourless, crystalline powder. Clemastine fumarate 1.34 mg is approximately equivalent to 1 mg of clemastine base.

Very slightly **soluble** in water; sparingly soluble in alcohol (70%); slightly soluble in alcohol (50%) and in methyl alcohol; very slightly soluble in chloroform. A 10% w/v suspension in water has a pH of 3.2 to 4.2. **Store** in airtight containers at a temperature not exceeding 25°. Protect from light.

Adverse Effects and Precautions

As for the sedating antihistamines in general, p.397.

Breast feeding. Drowsiness, irritability, and refusal to feed in a 10-week-old breast-fed baby occurred 12 hours after her mother started treatment with clemastine.[1] Clemastine was detected in the mother's breast milk. The baby recovered and was feeding normally on the day after the drug was stopped.

1. Kok THHG, *et al.* Drowsiness due to clemastine transmitted in breast milk. *Lancet* 1982; **i:** 914–15.

Porphyria. Clemastine has been associated with clinical exacerbations of porphyria and is considered unsafe in porphyric patients.[1]

1. Moore MR, McColl KEL. *Porphyria: drug lists.* Glasgow: Porphyria Research Unit, University of Glasgow, 1991.

Interactions

As for the sedating antihistamines in general, p.399.

Pharmacokinetics

Clemastine fumarate is rapidly and almost completely absorbed from the gastro-intestinal tract; peak plasma concentrations are achieved in 2 to 4 hours. Unchanged drug and metabolites are excreted principally in the urine. An elimination half-life of about 21 hours has been reported. Clemastine is distributed into breast milk.

References.

1. Schran HF, *et al.* The pharmacokinetics and bioavailability of clemastine and phenylpropanolamine in single-component and combination formulations. *J Clin Pharmacol* 1996; **36:** 911–22.

Uses and Administration

Clemastine fumarate, an ethanolamine derivative, is a sedating antihistamine with antimuscarinic and moderate sedative properties. It has been reported to have a duration of action of about 10 to 12 hours. It is used for the symptomatic relief of allergic conditions including urticaria and angioedema (p.401), rhinitis (p.400) and conjunctivitis (p.399), and in pruritic skin disorders (p.400).

Doses of clemastine fumarate are expressed in terms of the equivalent amount of clemastine base. The usual dose by mouth is 1 mg twice daily. Up to 6 mg daily has been given, particularly for urticaria and angioedema. Children aged 1 to 3 years may be given 0.25 to 0.5 mg twice daily; those aged 3 to 6 years, 0.5 mg twice daily; and those aged 6 to 12 years 0.5 to 1 mg twice daily.

Clemastine fumarate may be given by intramuscular or slow intravenous injection in a total daily dose equivalent to 2 to 4 mg of clemastine for acute allergic reactions; for prophylaxis 2 mg is given by intravenous injection. The dose for children is 25 μg per kg body-weight daily in two divided doses by intramuscular injection.

Clemastine fumarate has also been used topically, although there is a risk of sensitisation.

Preparations

BP 1998: Clemastine Oral Solution; Clemastine Tablets;
USP 23: Clemastine Fumarate Tablets.

Proprietary Preparations (details are given in Part 3)
Aust.: Tavegyl; ***Austral.:*** Tavegyl†; ***Canad.:*** Tavist; ***Ger.:*** Tavegil; ***Irl.:*** Tavegil; ***Ital.:*** Tavegil; ***Neth.:*** Tavegil; ***Norw.:*** Tavegyl; ***S.Afr.:*** Tavegyl; ***Spain:*** Tavegil; ***Swed.:*** Tavegyl; ***Switz.:*** Tavegyl; ***UK:*** Aller-eze; Tavegil; ***USA:*** Antihist-1; Contac 12 Hour Allergy; Tavist; Tavist-1.

Multi-ingredient: ***Canad.:*** Tavist-D; ***Ger.:*** Corto-Tavegil; ***S.Afr.:*** Rhinergal†; ***Spain:*** Dexa Tavegil; ***Switz.:*** Rhinergal†; ***UK:*** Aller-eze Plus; ***USA:*** Antihist-D; Tavist-D.

Clemizole Hydrochloride (6120-n)

Clemizole Hydrochloride *(BANM, rINNM)*.

AL-20. 1-(4-Chlorobenzyl)-2-(pyrrolidin-1-ylmethyl)benzimidazole hydrochloride.

$C_{19}H_{20}ClN_3,HCl$ = 362.3.

CAS — 442-52-4 (clemizole); 1163-36-6 (clemizole hydrochloride).

Clemizole hydrochloride is a sedating antihistamine. It has been used for the symptomatic relief of allergic conditions, in pruritic skin disorders, and in combination preparations for the treatment of symptoms of the common cold. Clemizole has also been applied topically as the hexachlorophane, the sodium sulphate, and the undecanoate derivatives in topical and rectal preparations combined with corticosteroids and local anaesthetics, although there is a risk of hypersensitivity from the topical use of antihistamines.

See p.191 for the use of clemizole penicillin.

Preparations

Proprietary Preparations (details are given in Part 3)
Ital.: Allerpant†; ***Spain:*** Alercur†.

Multi-ingredient: ***Aust.:*** Apracur; Scheriproct; Ultraproct; ***Austral.:*** Scheriproct; Ultraproct; ***Belg.:*** Scheriproct; Ultraproct; ***Irl.:*** Scheriproct; Ultralan†; Ultraproct; ***Norw.:*** Scheriproct; ***S.Afr.:*** Scheriproct; ***Spain:*** Ultraproct†.

Clocinizine Hydrochloride (12583-c)

Clocinizine Hydrochloride *(rINNM)*.

Chlorcinnazine Dihydrochloride. 1-(4-Chlorobenzhydryl)-4-cinnamylpiperazine dihydrochloride.

$C_{26}H_{27}ClN_2,2HCl$ = 475.9.

CAS — 298-55-5 (clocinizine).

Clocinizine hydrochloride, a piperazine derivative, is an antihistamine given by mouth in combination preparations for the symptomatic treatment of upper respiratory-tract disorders, often with a decongestant.

Preparations

Proprietary Preparations (details are given in Part 3)

Multi-ingredient: ***Belg.:*** Denoral; ***Fr.:*** Denoral; ***Ital.:*** Denoral; ***Spain:*** Senioral; Senioral Comp†.

Cyclizine (6121-h)

Cyclizine *(BAN, rINN)*.

1-Benzhydryl-4-methylpiperazine.

$C_{18}H_{22}N_2$ = 266.4.

CAS — 82-92-8.

Pharmacopoeias. In *Br.* and *US.*

A white or creamy-white, almost odourless, crystalline powder. M.p. 106° to 109°. **Soluble** 1 in 11 000 of water, 1 in 6 of alcohol and of ether, and 1 in 0.9 of chloroform; dissolves in most organic solvents and in dilute acids. A saturated solution in water has a pH of 7.6 to 8.6. **Store** in airtight containers. Protect from light.

Cyclizine Hydrochloride (6122-m)

Cyclizine Hydrochloride *(BANM, rINNM)*.

Cyclizini Hydrochloridum.

$C_{18}H_{22}N_2,HCl = 302.8.$

CAS — 303-25-3.

Pharmacopoeias. In *Eur.* (see p.viii) and *US*.

A white, odourless or almost odourless, crystalline powder, or small colourless crystals. **Soluble** 1 in 115 of water and of alcohol and 1 in 75 of chloroform; practically insoluble in ether. A 2% solution in alcohol 2 vol. and water 3 vol. has a pH of 4.5 to 5.5. **Store** in airtight containers. Protect from light.

Cyclizine Lactate (6123-b)

Cyclizine Lactate *(BANM, rINNM)*.

$C_{18}H_{22}N_2,C_3H_6O_3 = 356.5.$

CAS — 5897-19-8.

Pharmacopoeias. Br. and *US* include injections of cyclizine lactate.

Cyclizine lactate is reported to be **incompatible** with oxytetracycline hydrochloride, chlortetracycline hydrochloride, benzylpenicillin, and solutions with a pH of 6.8 or more.

Cyclizine Tartrate (10006-y)

Cyclizine Tartrate *(BANM, rINNM)*.

$C_{18}H_{22}N_2,C_4H_6O_6 = 416.5.$

Adverse Effects and Precautions

As for the sedating antihistamines in general, p.397. Cyclizine may aggravate severe heart failure. Hypotension may occur on injection.

Abuse. Cyclizine tablets have been abused either alone or in conjunction with opioids for their euphoric effects.[1-5] They have been taken by mouth or used to make injections. It has been suggested that cyclizine dependence may occur when it is used with opioids in the treatment of chronic pain.[6]

1. Gott PH. Cyclizine toxicity—intentional drug abuse of a proprietary antihistamine. *N Engl J Med* 1968; **279:** 596.
2. Kahn A, Harvey GJ. Increasing misuse of cyclizine. *Pharm J* 1985; **235:** 706.
3. Atkinson MK. Misuse of cyclizine. *Pharm J* 1985; **235:** 773.
4. Halpin D. Misuse of cyclizine. *Pharm J* 1985; **235:** 773.
5. Council of the Pharmaceutical Society of Great Britain. Sales of preparations containing cyclizine. *Pharm J* 1985; **235:** 797.
6. Hughes AM, Coote J. Cyclizine dependence. *Pharm J* 1986; **236:** 130.

Effects on the blood. A report[1] of agranulocytosis occurring in one patient after six weeks of treatment with cyclizine 50 mg three times daily. The blood count returned to normal once cyclizine was withdrawn.

1. Collier PM. Agranulocytosis associated with oral cyclizine. *Br Med J* 1986; **292:** 174.

Effects on the heart. In a study[1] of 11 patients with severe heart failure, cyclizine produced detrimental haemodynamic effects including increased systemic and pulmonary artery pressures and ventricular filling pressures, and negated the vasodilator effects of diamorphine. It was suggested that the use of cyclizine should be avoided in patients with acute myocardial infarction or severe heart failure.

1. Tan LB, *et al.* Detrimental haemodynamic effects of cyclizine in heart failure. *Lancet* 1988; **i:** 560–1.

Effects on the liver. An 8-year-old girl developed jaundice on 2 occasions after taking cyclizine hydrochloride 25 mg daily by mouth. 'Hypersensitivity hepatitis' was considered responsible.[1]

1. Kew MC, *et al.* "Hypersensitivity hepatitis" associated with administration of cyclizine. *Br Med J* 1973; **2:** 307.

Pregnancy. For discussion of the use of antihistamines in pregnancy, including studies involving cyclizine, see p.398.

Interactions

As for the sedating antihistamines in general, p.399. Cyclizine may counteract the haemodynamic benefits of opioids and this should be considered before using preparations that contain a combination of cyclizine and an opioid analgesic.

General anaesthetics. For a possible interaction between cyclizine premedication and *barbiturate anaesthetics* see under Thiopentone, p.1233.

Pharmacokinetics

Cyclizine is absorbed from the gastro-intestinal tract and has an onset of action within two hours. The duration of action is reported to be approximately 4 hours. Cyclizine is metabolised in the liver to the relatively inactive metabolite, norcyclizine. Both cyclizine and norcyclizine have plasma elimination half-lives of 20 hours. Less than 1% of the total oral dose is eliminated in the urine.

Uses and Administration

Cyclizine, a piperazine derivative, is a sedating antihistamine with antimuscarinic activity, although the sedative effects are not marked.

It is used as an antiemetic in the management of nausea and vomiting (p.400) including in motion sickness, irradiation sickness, postoperative nausea and vomiting, and drug-induced nausea and vomiting. It is included as an antiemetic in combination preparations for the treatment of migraine attacks (p.443). Cyclizine is also used for the symptomatic treatment of vertigo (p.401) caused by Ménière's disease and other vestibular disturbances.

In the management of nausea and vomiting, cyclizine hydrochloride is given by mouth in a usual dose of 50 mg up to three times daily, although up to 200 mg may be given in 24 hours if necessary. For the prevention of motion sickness, the first dose should be given about 30 minutes before travelling. Children aged 6 to 12 years may be given 25 mg up to three times daily.

Cyclizine is given intramuscularly or intravenously as the lactate. Doses of cyclizine lactate are similar to those of cyclizine hydrochloride given by mouth. For the prevention of postoperative nausea and vomiting the first dose of cyclizine lactate should be given about 20 minutes before the anticipated end of surgery.

Cyclizine tartrate is administered parenterally in combination with morphine tartrate in doses similar to those of cyclizine hydrochloride. Cyclizine is also administered as the hydrochloride by mouth in combination with dipipanone hydrochloride; the use of such fixed-combination opioid preparations is considered to be unsuitable for prolonged treatment as is required in palliative care. See also under Interactions, above.

Preparations

BP 1998: Cyclizine Injection; Cyclizine Tablets; Dipipanone and Cyclizine Tablets;
USP 23: Cyclizine Hydrochloride Tablets; Cyclizine Lactate Injection.

Proprietary Preparations (details are given in Part 3)
Aust.: Echnatol; Fortravel; Marzine; ***Canad.:*** Marzine; ***Fr.:*** Marzine†; ***Irl.:*** Valoid; ***Ital.:*** Marzine†; ***Neth.:*** Marzine†; ***Norw.:*** Marzine; ***S.Afr.:*** Aculoid; Covamet; Emitex; Medazine; Nauzine; Norizine†; Ryccard; Triazine†; Valoid; ***Swed.:*** Marzine; ***Switz.:*** Marzine; ***UK:*** Valoid; ***USA:*** Marezine.

Multi-ingredient: ***Aust.:*** Echnatol B_6; Migril; ***Austral.:*** Migral; ***Belg.:*** Migril†; ***Canad.:*** Megral; ***Fr.:*** Migwell; ***Ger.:*** Migrane-Kranit spezial N†; ***Irl.:*** Cyclimorph; Diconal; Migril; ***Neth.:*** Migril†; ***S.Afr.:*** Cyclimorph; Migril; Wellconal; ***Spain:*** Igril; ***Switz.:*** Migril; ***UK:*** Cyclimorph; Diconal; Femigraine†; Migril.

Cyproheptadine Hydrochloride

(6124-v)

Cyproheptadine Hydrochloride *(BANM, rINNM)*.

Cyproheptadini Hydrochloridum. 4-(5*H*-Dibenzo[*a,d*]cyclohepten-5-ylidene)-1-methylpiperidine hydrochloride sesquihydrate.

$C_{21}H_{21}N,HCl,1\frac{1}{2}H_2O = 350.9.$

CAS — 129-03-3 (cyproheptadine); 969-33-5 (anhydrous cyproheptadine hydrochloride); 41354-29-4 (cyproheptadine hydrochloride sesquihydrate).

Pharmacopoeias. In *Chin., Eur.* (see p.viii), *Jpn*, and *US*.

A white to slightly yellow, odourless or almost odourless, crystalline powder. Anhydrous cyproheptadine hydrochloride 10 mg is approximately equivalent to 11 mg of cyproheptadine hydrochloride sesquihydrate. **Soluble** 1 in 275 of water, 1 in 35 of alcohol, 1 in 26 of chloroform, and 1 in 1.5 of methyl alcohol; practically insoluble in ether. **Protect** from light.

Adverse Effects and Precautions

As for the sedating antihistamines in general, p.397. Increased appetite and weight gain may occur with cyproheptadine.

Abuse. A report[1] of dependence developing in a patient who had taken approximately 180 mg of cyproheptadine daily by mouth for 5 years.

1. Craven JL, Rodin GM. Cyproheptadine dependence associated with an atypical somatoform disorder. *Can J Psychiatry* 1987; **32:** 143–5.

Interference with diagnostic tests. Cyproheptadine reduced hypoglycaemia-induced growth hormone secretion by between 5 and 97% in 8 healthy subjects.[1] It was suggested that if patients receiving cyproheptadine were given a pituitary function test which used growth hormone response to insulin-induced hypoglycaemia, then cyproheptadine therapy should be stopped before the test.

1. Bivens CH, *et al.* Inhibition of hypoglycaemia-induced growth hormone secretion by the serotonin antagonists cyproheptadine and methysergide. *N Engl J Med* 1973; **289:** 236–9.

Interactions

As for the sedating antihistamines in general, p.399.

Antidepressants. For reports suggesting that cyproheptadine can reduce the effectiveness of *selective serotonin reuptake inhibitors*, see under Fluoxetine, p.286.

Pharmacokinetics

After absorption from the gastro-intestinal tract, cyproheptadine hydrochloride undergoes almost complete metabolism. Metabolites are excreted principally in the urine as conjugates, and also in the faeces.

Uses and Administration

Cyproheptadine, a piperidine derivative, is a sedating antihistamine with antimuscarinic, serotonin-antagonist, and calcium-channel blocking actions. It is used for the symptomatic relief of allergic conditions including urticaria and angioedema (p.401), rhinitis (p.400) and conjunctivitis (p.399), and in pruritic skin disorders (p.400). Other uses include the management of migraine (p.443).

For allergic conditions and pruritus the dose in adults, expressed as anhydrous cyproheptadine hydrochloride, is initially 4 mg three times a day by mouth, adjusted as necessary. The average dose requirement is 12 to 16 mg per day in three or four divided doses, but daily doses of up to 32 mg may occasionally be necessary. The dose for children aged 2 to 6 years is 2 mg two or three times a day increasing to a maximum of 12 mg per day and for children aged 7 to 14 years, 4 mg two or three times a day up to a maximum of 16 mg per day. Cyproheptadine is not recommended in debilitated elderly patients.

A dose of 4 mg is used for both prophylaxis and treatment of vascular headaches (including migraine) and may be repeated after 30 minutes; patients who respond usually obtain relief with 8 mg, and this dose should not be exceeded within a 4- to 6-hour period. A maintenance dose of 4 mg may be given every 4 to 6 hours.

Other cyproheptadine salts that have been given by mouth include the acetylaspartate, aspartate, cyclamate, orotate, acephyllinate (7-theophyllineacetate), and the pyridoxal phosphate salt (dihexazine).

Cyproheptadine was used to induce rapid and complete resolution of the serotonin syndrome (p.303) in a patient who had taken a single dose of sertraline 11 days after discontinuing treatment with isocarboxazid for depression.[1]

1. Lappin RI, Auchincloss EL. Treatment of the serotonin syndrome with cyproheptadine. *N Engl J Med* 1994; **331:** 1021–2.

Angina pectoris. Cyproheptadine was used successfully to treat 2 patients with Prinzmetal's angina[1] refractory to standard treatment with calcium-channel blockers and nitrates. Serotonin is an important endocrine mediator of coronary vasospasm and the beneficial effects of cyproheptadine were attributed to its activity as a serotonin antagonist. For a discussion of the usual management of Prinzmetal's angina, see under Angina Pectoris on p.780.

1. Schecter AD, *et al.* Refractory Prinzmetal angina treated with cyproheptadine. *Ann Intern Med* 1994; **121:** 113–14.

Appetite disorders. Cyproheptadine has been widely used as an appetite stimulant in a variety of conditions including anorexia nervosa and cachexia but in the long-term appears to have little value in producing weight gain and such use is no longer generally recommended. There has been concern that cyproheptadine was being promoted and used inappropriately as an appetite stimulant in some developing countries.[1]

1. Anonymous. Cyproheptadine: no longer promoted as an appetite stimulant. *WHO Drug Inf* 1994; **8:** 66.

Carcinoid syndrome. In patients with carcinoid syndrome, circulating tumour products, including serotonin, give rise to flushing, diarrhoea, and sometimes wheezing and progressive right heart failure.[1,2] The management of carcinoid tumours (p.477) is largely symptomatic. Cyproheptadine hydrochloride, a serotonin antagonist, has been helpful in relieving the diarrhoea;[1,2] doses of 4 to 8 mg have been given every 6 hours.[1] It has been used successfully with fenclonine, aprotinin, methylprednisolone, and antibacterials to prevent complications arising from release of tumour metabolites during hepatic embolisation, a procedure sometimes used to relieve the symptoms of carcinoid syndrome.[3] There have been a few reports of tumour regression, in addition to symptomatic control, after treatment of carcinoid tumours with cyproheptadine.[4,5]

1. Maton PN. The carcinoid syndrome. *JAMA* 1988; **260:** 1602–5.
2. Hodgson HJF. Controlling the carcinoid syndrome. *Br Med J* 1988; **297:** 1213–14.
3. Maton PN, *et al.* Role of hepatic arterial embolisation in the carcinoid syndrome. *Br Med J* 1983; **287:** 932–5. Correction to dosage. ibid.; 1664.
4. Harris AL, Smith IE. Regression of carcinoid tumour with cyproheptadine. *Br Med J* 1982; **285:** 475.
5. Leitner SP, *et al.* Partial remission of carcinoid tumor in response to cyproheptadine. *Ann Intern Med* 1989; **111:** 760–1.

Endocrine disorders. Cyproheptadine hydrochloride has been tried in a variety of disorders with a possible endocrine origin. Individual reports have suggested a beneficial response in some patients with Cushing's disease,[1,2] virilising congenital adrenal hyperplasia,[3] or galactorrhoea-amenorrhoea syndrome.[4] One study has suggested efficacy of cyproheptadine in a subgroup of depressed patients with abnormalities of cortisol secretion similar to those of Cushing's disease.[5] Reports of the beneficial effects of cyproheptadine in Cushing's syndrome (p.1236) have not been substantiated. The management of congenital adrenal hyperplasia (p.1020) is normally with corticosteroid therapy.

A favourable response to oral cyproheptadine and topical corticosteroids has been described in one patient with acanthosis nigricans associated with adenocarcinomas of the stomach and prostate.[6] The action of cyproheptadine in these disorders is unclear, although antagonism of serotonin has been postulated.

1. Marek J, *et al.* Cyproheptadine in Cushing's syndrome. *Lancet* 1977; **ii:** 653–4.
2. Griffith DN, Ross EJ. Pregnancy after cyproheptadine treatment for Cushing's disease. *N Engl J Med* 1981; **305:** 893–4.
3. Hsu T-H. Management of virilizing congenital adrenal hyperplasia with cyproheptadine. *Ann Intern Med* 1980; **92:** 628–30.
4. Wortsman J, *et al.* Cyproheptadine in the management of the galactorrhea-amenorrhea syndrome. *Ann Intern Med* 1979; **90:** 923–5.
5. Bansal S, Brown WA. Cyproheptadine in depression. *Lancet* 1983; **ii** 803.
6. Greenwood R, Tring FC. Treatment of malignant acanthosis nigricans with cyproheptadine. *Br J Dermatol* 1982; **106:** 697–8.

Sexual dysfunction. Cyproheptadine has been tried in the management of sexual dysfunction induced by selective serotonin reuptake inhibitors (SSRIs) (see Effects on Sexual Function under Fluoxetine, p.285) but may possibly reduce the effectiveness of the SSRI.

Preparations

BP 1998: Cyproheptadine Tablets;
USP 23: Cyproheptadine Hydrochloride Syrup; Cyproheptadine Hydrochloride Tablets.

Proprietary Preparations (details are given in Part 3)
Aust.: Periactin; ***Austral.:*** Periactin; ***Belg.:*** Periactin; ***Canad.:*** Periactin; ***Fr.:*** Periactine; ***Ger.:*** Nuran†; Periactinol†; Peritol; ***Irl.:*** Periactin; ***Ital.:*** Periactin; ***Neth.:*** Periactin; ***Norw.:*** Periactin†; ***S.Afr.:*** Periactin; ***Spain:*** Klarivitina; Periactin; Viternum; ***Swed.:*** Periactin; ***Switz.:*** Periactin; ***UK:*** Periactin; ***USA:*** Periactin.

Multi-ingredient: ***Ger.:*** Nuran BC forte†; Nurdelin†; ***Ital.:*** Carpantin; ***S.Afr.:*** Periactin B-C†; Periactin Vita†; ***Spain:*** Actilevol Orex; Anti Anorex Triple; Biomax†; Childrevit; Cobamas†; Covitasa B12; Desarrol; Enoton; Glotone; Medenorex; Pantobamin; Pranzo; Stolina; Tonico Juventus; Tres Orix Forte; Trimetabol; Troforex Pepsico; Vita Menal.

Deptropine Citrate (6125-g)

Deptropine Citrate *(BANM, rINNM)*.

Deptropini Citras; Dibenzheptropine Citrate. (1*R*,3*r*,5*S*)-3-(10,11-Dihydro-5*H*-dibenzo[*a*,*d*]cycloheptene-5-yloxy)tropane dihydrogen citrate.

$C_{23}H_{27}NO,C_6H_8O_7$ = 525.6.

CAS — 604-51-3 (deptropine); 2169-75-7 (deptropine citrate).

Pharmacopoeias. In *Eur.* (see p.viii).

A white or almost white, microcrystalline powder. Very slightly **soluble** in water and in alcohol; practically insoluble in dichloromethane and in ether. A 1% suspension in water has a pH of 3.7 to 4.5. **Protect** from light.

Deptropine citrate is a sedating antihistamine with a marked antimuscarinic action. It is mainly used in the treatment of respiratory-tract disorders.

Deptropine citrate is given by mouth in doses of 0.5 to 1 mg twice daily.

Preparations

Proprietary Preparations (details are given in Part 3)
Ital.: Brontin.

Dimenhydrinate (6128-s)

Dimenhydrinate *(BAN, rINN)*.

Chloranautine; Dimenhydrinatum; Diphenhydramine Teoclate; Diphenhydramine Theoclate. The diphenhydramine salt of 8-chlorotheophylline.

$C_{17}H_{21}NO,C_7H_7ClN_4O_2$ = 470.0.

CAS — 523-87-5.

Pharmacopoeias. In *Chin., Eur.* (see p.viii), *Jpn, Pol.,* and *US.*

A white odourless crystalline powder or colourless crystals. M.p. 102° to 107°. Slightly **soluble** in water; freely soluble in alcohol and in chloroform; sparingly soluble in ether.

Dimenhydrinate has been reported in early studies to be **incompatible** in solution with a wide range of compounds; those most likely to be encountered with dimenhydrinate include: aminophylline, glycopyrronium bromide, hydrocortisone sodium succinate, hydroxyzine hydrochloride, iodipamide, meglumine, some phenothiazines, and some soluble barbiturates.

Adverse Effects and Precautions

As for the sedating antihistamines in general, p.397.

Effects on the eyes. Dimenhydrinate 100 mg, given at 4-hourly intervals for 3 doses, was found to affect colour discrimination, night vision, reaction time, and stereopsis.[1]

1. Luria SM, *et al.* Effects of aspirin and dimenhydrinate (Dramamine) on visual processes. *Br J Clin Pharmacol* 1979; **7:** 585–93.

Porphyria. Dimenhydrinate has been associated with acute attacks of porphyria and is considered unsafe in patients with acute porphyria.[1]

1. Moore MR, McColl KEL. *Porphyria: drug lists.* Glasgow: Porphyria Research Unit, University of Glasgow, 1991.

Pregnancy. For discussion of the use of antihistamines in pregnancy, including a suggestion of a relationship between cardiovascular defects or inguinal hernia and dimenhydrinate exposure, see p.398.

Interactions

As for the sedating antihistamines in general, p.399.

Uses and Administration

Dimenhydrinate, an ethanolamine derivative, is a sedating antihistamine with antimuscarinic and significant sedative effects. It is used mainly as an antiemetic in the prevention and treatment of motion sickness (p.400). It is also used for the symptomatic treatment of nausea and vertigo caused by Ménière's disease and other vestibular disturbances (p.401).

The usual dose of dimenhydrinate by mouth is 50 to 100 mg, given either 2 to 3 times daily as in the UK, or every 4 to 6 hours to a maximum of 400 mg in 24 hours as in the USA. For the prevention of motion sickness, the first dose should be given at least 30 minutes before travelling. The doses for children are: 1 to 6 years, 12.5 to 25 mg two to three times daily; 7 to 12 years, 25 to 50 mg two to three times daily.

Dimenhydrinate may be given parenterally, a concentration of 5% being used for intramuscular injection and 0.5% for slow intravenous injection (usually over 2 minutes). Parenteral doses are similar to those given by mouth. Children have been given dimenhydrinate by intramuscular or slow intravenous injection in a dose of 1.25 mg per kg body-weight four times daily to a maximum of 300 mg daily.

Dimenhydrinate has also been administered by the rectal route.

Preparations

BP 1998: Dimenhydrinate Tablets;
USP 23: Dimenhydrinate Injection; Dimenhydrinate Syrup; Dimenhydrinate Tablets.

Proprietary Preparations (details are given in Part 3)
Aust.: Emedyl; Nausex; Travel-Gum; Vertirosan; ***Austral.:*** Andrumin; Dramamine; ***Belg.:*** Dramamine; Vagomine; ***Canad.:*** Childrens Motion Sickness Liquid; Gravol; Nauseatol; Nausex; Novo-Dimenate; Travamine; Travel Aid; Travel Tabs; Travelmate; Traveltabs; ***Fr.:*** Dramamine; Nausicalm; ***Ger.:*** Dimen; Epha-retard†; Logomed Reise-Tabletten; Mandros Reise; Monotrean; Novomina†; Reisegold; Reisetabletten-ratiopharm; Superpep; Vertigo-Vomex; Vomacur; Vomex A; ***Irl.:*** Dramamine; ***Ital.:*** Lomarin; Motozina; Travelgum; Valontan; Xamamina; ***Neth.:*** Dramamine; ***S.Afr.:*** Dramamine†; ***Spain:*** Biodramina; Cinfamar; Contramareo; Travel Well; Valontan†; ***Swed.:*** Amosyt; ***Switz.:*** Antemin; Demodenal; Dramamine; Reise Superpep-K; Trawell; ***UK:*** Dramamine; ***USA:*** Calm-X; Dimetabs; Dinate; DMH; Dramamine; Dramanate; Dramilin; Dramoject†; Dymenate; Hydrate; Marmine; Tega-Vert; Triptone; Vertab.

Multi-ingredient: ***Aust.:*** Neo-Emedyl; Synkapton; Vertirosan Vitamin B_6; ***Austral.:*** Travacalm; ***Belg.:*** Analergyl†; R Calm + B6; ***Canad.:*** Gravergol; ***Fr.:*** Mercalm; ***Ger.:*** Arlevert; Dimenhydrinat comp†; Dimenhydrinat retard†; Migraeflux N; Migraeflux orange N; Novomina infant†; Vomex A†; ***Ital.:*** Kine B6†; ***Spain:*** Acetuber; Biodramina Cafeina; Cinfamar Cafeina; Dramamine Cafeina†; Saldeva; Salvarina; Sin Mareo x 4; ***Switz.:*** Antemin compositum; Demodenal compositum; Dragees contre les maux de voyage no 537; Dramamine-compositum; Medramine retard; Medramine-B_6 Rectocaps; Migraeflux†; Rhinocap; Viaggio.

Dimethindene Maleate (6129-w)

Dimethindene Maleate *(BANM, USAN)*.

Dimetindene Maleate *(rINNM)*; Dimethpyrindene Maleate; Dimethylpyrindene Maleate; NSC-107677; Su-6518. *NN*-Dimethyl-2-{3-[1-(2-pyridyl)ethyl]-1*H*-inden-2-yl}ethylamine hydrogen maleate.

$C_{20}H_{24}N_2,C_4H_4O_4$ = 408.5.

CAS — 5636-83-9 (dimethindene); 3614-69-5 (dimethindene maleate).

Dimethindene maleate, an alkylamine derivative, is a sedating antihistamine; it is mildly sedative and is reported to have mast-cell stabilising properties. It is used for the symptomatic relief of allergic conditions including urticaria and angioedema (p.401), rhinitis (p.400), and in pruritic skin disorders (p.400). It is also used in compound preparations for the symptomatic treatment of coughs and the common cold (p.400).

Dimethindene maleate is given by mouth in a dose of 1 to 2 mg three times daily; modified-release preparations for once or twice daily administration are also available. It may also be given by the intravenous route. Dimethindene maleate is applied topically as a 0.1% gel, although as with any antihistamine there is a risk of sensitisation. It is used in a strength of 0.025% in compound nasal preparations.

Preparations

Proprietary Preparations (details are given in Part 3)
Aust.: Fenistil; ***Belg.:*** Fenistil; ***Ger.:*** Fenistil; ***Irl.:*** Fenostil†; ***Ital.:*** Fengel†; Fenistil; ***Neth.:*** Fenistil; ***Norw.:*** Fenistil; ***Spain:*** Fenistil; ***Swed.:*** Fenistil†; ***Switz.:*** Fenistil; ***UK:*** Fenostil†.

Multi-ingredient: ***Aust.:*** Trimedil; Vibrocil; ***Belg.:*** Trimedil†; Vibrocil; ***Ger.:*** Fenipectum†; Fenistil Plus†; Ralena†; Trimedil N†; Vibrocil; Vibrocil cN†; ***Irl.:*** Vibrocil†; ***Ital.:*** Vibrocil; ***S.Afr.:*** Vibrocil; Vibrocil-S; ***Switz.:*** Trimedil†; Vibrocil; ***UK:*** Vibrocil†.

Dimethothiazine Mesylate (6130-m)

Dimethothiazine Mesylate *(BANM)*.

Dimetotiazine Mesilate *(rINNM)*; Fonazine Mesylate *(USAN)*; IL-6302 (dimethothiazine); 8599-RP (dimethothiazine). 10-(2-Dimethylaminopropyl)-*NN*-dimethylphenothiazine-2-sulphonamide methanesulphonate.

$C_{19}H_{25}N_3O_2S_2,CH_3SO_3H$ = 487.7.

CAS — 7456-24-8 (dimethothiazine); 7455-39-2 (dimethothiazine mesylate).

Dimethothiazine mesylate, a phenothiazine derivative, is a sedating antihistamine. It has been used for the symptomatic relief of hypersensitivity reactions, in pruritic skin disorders, and in the management of various headaches including migraine.

Preparations

Proprietary Preparations (details are given in Part 3)
Canad.: Promaquid†; ***Ital.:*** Alius†; ***S.Afr.:*** Banistyl†; ***Spain:*** Migristene.

Diphenhydramine (10007-j)

Diphenhydramine *(BAN, rINN).*

Benzhydramine. 2-Benzhydryloxy-*NN*-dimethylethylamine.

$C_{17}H_{21}NO = 255.4.$

CAS — 58-73-1.

Pharmacopoeias. In *Jpn.*

Diphenhydramine Citrate (18347-g)

Diphenhydramine Citrate *(BANM, rINNM).*

Benzhydramine Citrate.

$C_{17}H_{21}NO,C_6H_8O_7 = 447.5.$

CAS — 88637-37-0.

Pharmacopoeias. In *US.*

Diphenhydramine citrate 15.3 mg is approximately equivalent to diphenhydramine hydrochloride 10 mg. **Store** in airtight containers. Protect from light.

Diphenhydramine Di(acefyllinate) (12669-f)

Benzhydramine Di(acefyllinate); Bietanautine; Diphenhydramine Di(acephyllinate). Diphenhydramine bis(theophyllin-7-ylacetate).

$C_{17}H_{21}NO,2C_9H_{10}N_4O_4 = 731.8.$

CAS — 6888-11-5.

NOTE. The name Etanautine has been applied both to diphenhydramine monoacefyllinate and to ethylbenzhydramine, an antimuscarinic formerly used in the symptomatic treatment of parkinsonism.

Diphenhydramine di(acefyllinate) 25.1 mg is approximately equivalent to diphenhydramine hydrochloride 10 mg.

Diphenhydramine Hydrochloride (6131-b)

Diphenhydramine Hydrochloride *(BANM, rINNM).*

Benzhydramine Hydrochloride; Dimedrolum; Diphenhydramini Hydrochloridum; Diphenhydraminium Chloride.

$C_{17}H_{21}NO,HCl = 291.8.$

CAS — 147-24-0.

Pharmacopoeias. In *Chin., Eur.* (see p.viii), *Jpn, Pol.,* and *US. Jpn* also includes Diphenhydramine Tannate.

A white or almost white, odourless, crystalline powder. It slowly darkens on exposure to light. Ph. Eur. **solubilities** are: very soluble in water; freely soluble in alcohol; practically insoluble in ether. USP solubilities are: soluble 1 in 1 of water, 1 in 2 of alcohol and of chloroform, and 1 in 50 of acetone; very slightly soluble in ether. A 5% solution in water has a pH of 4 to 6. **Store** in airtight containers. Protect from light.

Incompatibility has been reported with amphotericin, cefmetazole sodium, cephalothin sodium, hydrocortisone sodium succinate, some soluble barbiturates, some contrast media, and solutions of alkalis or strong acids.

Adverse Effects and Precautions

As for the sedating antihistamines in general, p.397.

Abuse. Reports of the abuse of diphenhydramine hydrochloride.

1. Anonymous. Is there any evidence that Benylin syrup is addictive? *Br Med J* 1979; **1:** 459.
2. Smith SG, Davis WM. Nonmedical use of butorphanol and diphenhydramine. *JAMA* 1984; **252:** 1010.
3. Feldman MD, Behar M. A case of massive diphenhydramine abuse and withdrawal from use of the drug. *JAMA* 1986; **255:** 3119–20.
4. de Nesnera AP. Diphenhydramine dependence: a need for awareness. *J Clin Psychiatry* 1996; **57:** 136–7.
5. Dinndorf PA, *et al.* Risk of abuse of diphenhydramine in children and adolescents with chronic illnesses. *J Pediatr* 1998; **133:** 293–5.

Extrapyramidal disorders. Reports[1-3] of dystonic extrapyramidal reactions to diphenhydramine.

1. Lavenstein BL, Cantor FK. Acute dystonia: an unusual reaction to diphenhydramine. *JAMA* 1976; **236:** 291.
2. Santora J, Rozek S. Diphenhydramine-induced dystonia. *Clin Pharm* 1989; **8:** 471.
3. Roila F, *et al.* Diphenhydramine and acute dystonia. *Ann Intern Med* 1989; **111:** 92–3.

Overdosage. In an evaluation of 136 cases, one fatal, of intoxication with diphenhydramine there was correlation between plasma concentration and frequency or extent of symptoms.[1] The most common symptom was impaired consciousness; additionally, psychosis, seizures, antimuscarinic symptoms such as mydriasis, tachycardia, and tachyarrhythmias, and respiratory failure were observed. Another report[2] describes rhabdomyolysis as an effect of oral diphenhydramine overdosage in one patient. The liberal application of a lotion containing diphenhydramine produced acute delirium with visual and auditory hallucinations in a 9-year-old boy[3] and similar effects were seen in 3 children with varicella-zoster infection following the topical application of diphenhydramine (2 of these children also received oral diphenhydramine).[4]

1. Köppel C, Tenczer J. Clinical symptomatology of diphenhydramine overdose: an evaluation of 136 cases in 1982 to 1985. *Clin Toxicol* 1987; **25:** 53–70.
2. Hampel G, *et al.* Myoglobinuric renal failure due to drug-induced rhabdomyolysis. *Hum Toxicol* 1983; **2:** 197–203.
3. Filloux F. Toxic encephalopathy caused by topically applied diphenhydramine. *J Pediatr* 1986; **108:** 1018–20.
4. Chan CYJ, Wallander KA. Diphenhydramine toxicity in three children with varicella-zoster infection. *DICP Ann Pharmacother* 1991; **25:** 130–2.

Porphyria. Diphenhydramine has been associated with clinical exacerbations of porphyria and is considered unsafe in porphyric patients.[1]

1. Moore MR, McColl KEL. *Porphyria: drug lists.* Glasgow: Porphyria Research Unit, University of Glasgow, 1991.

Pregnancy. For discussion of the use of antihistamines in pregnancy, including a suggestion of a relationship between inguinal hernia or genito-urinary malformations and diphenhydramine exposure, see p.398. See also under Interactions, below, for a report of perinatal death possibly associated with temazepam and diphenhydramine.

A pregnant woman who was receiving diphenhydramine hydrochloride 150 mg daily for a pruritic rash gave birth to an infant who developed diarrhoea and generalised tremulousness 5 days later.[1] The delay in appearance of withdrawal symptoms was considered to be due to absence of full activity of glucuronyl conjugating enzymes in the first few days of life.

1. Parkin DE. Probable Benadryl withdrawal manifestations in a new-born infant. *J Pediatr* 1974; **85:** 580.

Interactions

As for the sedating antihistamines in general, p.399.

Benzodiazepines. There has been a report[1] suggesting that a reduction in *temazepam* metabolism caused by diphenhydramine may have contributed to perinatal death after ingestion of these drugs by the mother.

1. Kargas GA, *et al.* Perinatal mortality due to interaction of diphenhydramine and temazepam. *N Engl J Med* 1985; **313:** 1417–18.

Pharmacokinetics

Diphenhydramine hydrochloride is well absorbed from the gastro-intestinal tract, though high first-pass metabolism appears to affect systemic availability. Peak plasma concentrations are achieved about 1 to 4 hours after administration by mouth. Diphenhydramine is widely distributed throughout the body including the CNS. It crosses the placenta and has been detected in breast milk. Diphenhydramine is highly bound to plasma proteins. Metabolism is extensive. Diphenhydramine is excreted mainly in the urine as metabolites; little is excreted as unchanged drug.

References.

1. Glazko AJ, *et al.* Metabolic disposition of diphenhydramine. *Clin Pharmacol Ther* 1974; **16:** 1066–76.
2. Paton DM, Webster DR. Clinical pharmacokinetics of H_1-receptor antagonists (the antihistamines). *Clin Pharmacokinet* 1985; **10:** 477–97 (includes studies indicating a correlation between plasma concentrations and both antihistaminic and sedative effects).
3. Simons KJ, *et al.* Diphenhydramine: pharmacokinetics and pharmacodynamics in elderly adults, young adults, and children. *J Clin Pharmacol* 1990; **30:** 665–71.
4. Scavone JM, *et al.* Pharmacokinetics and pharmacodynamics of diphenhydramine 25 mg in young and elderly volunteers. *J Clin Pharmacol* 1998; **38:** 603–9.

Uses and Administration

Diphenhydramine, an ethanolamine derivative, is a sedating antihistamine with antimuscarinic and pronounced sedative properties. It is used for the symptomatic relief of allergic conditions including urticaria and angioedema (p.401), rhinitis (p.400) and conjunctivitis (p.399), and in pruritic skin disorders (p.400). It is also used for its antiemetic properties in the treatment of nausea and vomiting (p.400), particularly in the prevention and treatment of motion sickness when it should be given at least 30 minutes before travelling, and in the treatment of vertigo of various causes (p.401). Diphenhydramine is used for its antimuscarinic properties in the control of parkinsonism (p.1128) and drug-induced extrapyramidal disorders (p.650) (although the possibility that diphenhydramine itself may cause extrapyramidal symptoms should be remembered). Diphenhydramine has pronounced central sedative properties and may be used as a hypnotic in the short-term management of insomnia (p.400). It is a common ingredient of compound preparations for symptomatic treatment of coughs and the common cold (p.400). Diphenhydramine may be administered parenterally as an adjunct in the emergency treatment of anaphylactic shock (p.399) and when oral therapy is not feasible.

For most indications, diphenhydramine hydrochloride is given by mouth in usual doses of 25 to 50 mg three to four times daily. The dose for children is 6.25 to 25 mg three to four times a day, or a total daily dose of 5 mg per kg body-weight may be given in divided doses. The maximum dose in adults and children is 300 mg daily. A dose of 20 to 50 mg may be used as a hypnotic in adults and children over 12 years old.

When oral therapy is not feasible, diphenhydramine hydrochloride may be administered by deep intramuscular injection or by intravenous injection using concentrations of 1% or 5%. Usual doses are 10 to 50 mg, though doses of 100 mg have been given. No more than 400 mg should be given in 24 hours. Diphenhydramine hydrochloride is applied topically, usually in preparations containing 1 to 2% although, as with other antihistamines, there is a risk of sensitisation.

Diphenhydramine citrate is administered by mouth in combination preparations for its hypnotic action; it is given in a dose of 76 mg at night. Diphenhydramine di(acefyllinate) is given by mouth as an antiemetic for the prevention and treatment of motion sickness and of nausea and vomiting; the usual dose is 90 to 135 mg. Other diphenhydramine salts that have been used include the polistirex, the salicylate, and the tannate administered by mouth, the methylbromide given rectally, and the methylsulphate applied topically.

Dimenhydrinate (p.408) is diphenhydramine theoclate and mefenidramium methylsulphate (p.413) is diphenhydramine methylsulphomethylate.

Preparations

BP 1998: Diphenhydramine Oral Solution;
USP 23: Acetaminophen and Diphenhydramine Citrate Tablets; Acetaminophen, Diphenhydramine Hydrochloride, and Pseudoephedrine Hydrochloride Tablets; Diphenhydramine and Pseudoephedrine Capsules; Diphenhydramine Hydrochloride Capsules; Diphenhydramine Hydrochloride Elixir; Diphenhydramine Hydrochloride Injection.

Proprietary Preparations (details are given in Part 3)

Aust.: Dermodrin; Dibondrin; Histaxin; Prurex; ***Austral.:*** Benadryl†; Nytol†; Unisom; ***Belg.:*** Benylin Antihistaminicum; Diphamine; Nuicalm; R Calm; ***Canad.:*** Aller-Aide; Allerdryl; Allergy Elixir; Allergy Tablets; Allernix; Benadryl; Calmex; Clear Caladryl Spray†; Dormex; Dormiphen; Insomnal; Nytol; Sleep Aid; Sleep-Eze D; Sominex; Unisom; Unisom-C; ***Fr.:*** Benylin†; Butix; Nautamine; ***Ger.:*** Benadryl N; Dolestan; Dormigoa N; Dormutil N; Emesan; Halbmond; Hevert-Dorm; Logomed Allergie-Gel†; Logomed Beruhigungs-Tabletten; Logomed Juckreiz; Lupovalin; Moradorm-A†; nervo OPT N; Nytol; Pellisal-Gel; Pellit Insektenstich; Pheramin N; S.8; Sediat; Sedopretten; Sedovegan Novo; Sekundal-D†; Vivinox Stark; ***Ital.:*** Allergan; Allergina†; Benadryl; ***Neth.:*** Benylin-Difenhydraminehydrochloride; ***S.Afr.:*** Betasleep; Dihydral†; ***Spain:*** Benadryl; Dormplus; ***Swed.:*** Benylan; Desentol; ***Switz.:*** Bedorma Nouvelle formulation; Benadryl†; Benocten; Benylin Paediatric; Comprimes somniferes "S"; Comprimes somniferes no 533 nouvelle formule; Dobacen; Neo-Synodorm; ***UK:*** Aller-eze; Histergan; Medinex; Nytol; Sleep Aid; Sleepia; ***USA:*** 40 Winks; Allerdryl†; AllerMax; Banophen; Belix†; Ben-Allergin†; Bena-D†; Benadryl; Benahist†; Benoject†; Bydramine Cough†; Compoz Night-time Sleep Aid; Dermamycin; Dihydrex; Diphen AF; Diphen Cough; Diphenhist; Dormarex 2†; Dormin; DPH†; Dytuss; Genahist; Hydramyn†; Hyrexin; Maximum Strength Sleepinal; Maximum Strength Unisom SleepGels; Miles Nervine; MouthKote P/R; Nidryl†; Nordryl; Nytol; Phendry; Scot-Tussin Allergy; Siladryl; Silphen; Sleep-eze 3; Sleepwell 2-nite; Snooze Fast; Sominex; Tusstat; Twilite; Uni-Bent Cough; Wehdryl†.

Multi-ingredient: numerous preparations are listed in Part 3.

Diphenylpyraline Hydrochloride (6132-v)

Diphenylpyraline Hydrochloride *(BANM, rINNM).*

4-Benzhydryloxy-1-methylpiperidine hydrochloride.

$C_{19}H_{23}NO,HCl = 317.9.$

CAS — 147-20-6 (diphenylpyraline); 132-18-3 (diphenylpyraline hydrochloride).

Pharmacopoeias. In *Br.*

A white or almost white, odourless or almost odourless powder. Freely **soluble** in water, in alcohol, and in chloroform; practically insoluble in ether.

Adverse Effects and Precautions

As for the sedating antihistamines in general, p.397.

Interactions

As for the sedating antihistamines in general, p.399.

Pharmacokinetics

References.

1. Graham G, Bolt AG. Half-life of diphenylpyraline in man. *J Pharmacokinet Biopharm* 1974; **2:** 191–5 (ranged from 24 to 40 hours).

Uses and Administration

Diphenylpyraline hydrochloride, a piperidine derivative, is a sedating antihistamine with antimuscarinic and significant sedative properties.

It is used for the symptomatic relief of allergic conditions including rhinitis (p.400), and in pruritic skin disorders (p.400). It is also used in compound preparations for the symptomatic treatment of coughs and the common cold (p.400).

Diphenylpyraline hydrochloride has been given by mouth in a dose of up to 20 mg daily in 3 or 4 divided doses. Diphenylpyraline and diphenylpyraline hydrochloride have been applied topically although as with any antihistamine there is a risk of sensitisation.

Diphenylpyraline theoclate is piprinhydrinate (p.416).

Preparations

Proprietary Preparations (details are given in Part 3)
Austral.: Histalert†; ***Ger.:*** Arbid N; Lyssipoll†; ***Irl.:*** Histryl†; ***UK:*** Histryl†; Lergoban†.

Multi-ingredient: ***Aust.:*** Arbid; Astronautal; Eucillin; Prurimix; Tropoderm; ***Austral.:*** Sinuzets Cold and Flu Capsules with Antihistamine†; ***Belg.:*** Rhinamide†; Tri-Cold; ***Canad.:*** Biohisdex DM; Biohisdine DM; Creo-Rectal; Emercreme No 4; Sinugex; Vito Bronches; ***Ger.:*** Arbid†; Doregrippin S†; Pectinfant N†; Perdiphen; Poikicin†; Proctospre; Rhinoinfant†; Ricolind†; Tempil N; Topoderm N; Vomistop†; ***Irl.:*** Eskornade†; ***S.Afr.:*** Actophlem; Eskornade; Solphyllex; Theophen Comp; ***Spain:*** Ornasec†; ***Switz.:*** Arbid; Proctospre; ***UK:*** Eskornade.

Doxylamine Succinate (6133-g)

Doxylamine Succinate *(BANM, rINNM)*.

Doxylaminium Succinate; Histadoxylamine Succinate. *NN*-Dimethyl-2-[α-methyl-α-(2-pyridyl)benzyloxy]ethylamine hydrogen succinate.

$C_{17}H_{22}N_2O,C_4H_6O_4$ = 388.5.

CAS — 469-21-6 (doxylamine); 562-10-7 (doxylamine succinate).

Pharmacopoeias. In US.

A white or creamy-white powder with a characteristic odour. **Soluble** 1 in 1 of water, 1 in 2 of alcohol and of chloroform, and 1 in 370 of ether. **Protect** from light.

Adverse Effects and Precautions

As for the sedating antihistamines in general, p.397. The controversy surrounding the use in pregnancy of combination products of doxylamine is discussed on p.398.

Overdosage. In an evaluation of 109 cases of intoxication with doxylamine,[1] no correlation was found between the amount ingested or plasma concentration and the frequency or extent of symptoms. The most common symptom was impaired consciousness. Additionally, psychotic behaviour, seizures, and antimuscarinic symptoms such as tachycardia and mydriasis were observed. Rhabdomyolysis occurred in one patient and was accompanied by transient impairment of renal function. These authors have further commented[2] that rhabdomyolysis had been noted in 7 of 442 cases of doxylamine overdosage, with an associated rise in plasma creatine kinase and myoglobinuria. They suggest that doxylamine has a direct toxic effect on striated muscle.

1. Köppel C, *et al.* Poisoning with over-the-counter doxylamine preparations: an evaluation of 109 cases. *Hum Toxicol* 1987; **6:** 355–9.
2. Köppel C, *et al.* Rhabdomyolysis in doxylamine overdose. *Lancet* 1987; **i:** 442–3.

Interactions

As for the sedating antihistamines in general, p.399.

Pharmacokinetics

Following oral administration of doxylamine succinate peak plasma concentrations occur after 2 to 3 hours. An elimination half-life of about 10 hours has been reported.

References.

1. Friedman H, *et al.* Clearance of the antihistamine doxylamine: reduced in elderly men but not in elderly women. *Clin Pharmacokinet* 1989; **16:** 312–16.

Uses and Administration

Doxylamine succinate, an ethanolamine derivative, is a sedating antihistamine with antimuscarinic and pronounced sedative effects.

Doxylamine succinate is given by mouth for the symptomatic relief of hypersensitivity reactions, in pruritic skin disorders (p.400), as a hypnotic in the short-term treatment of insomnia (p.400), and as an ingredient of compound preparations for symptomatic treatment of coughs and the common cold (p.400).

In general it is no longer used in the management of nausea and vomiting of early pregnancy (see p.398 for the controversy that has surrounded the use in pregnancy of combination products of doxylamine).

Doses of up to 25 mg of doxylamine succinate have been given every 4 to 6 hours to a maximum of 150 mg daily. The usual hypnotic dose is 25 mg at night.

Preparations

USP 23: Acetaminophen, Dextromethorphan Hydrobromide, Doxylamine Succinate, and Pseudoephedrine Hydrochloride Oral Solution; Doxylamine Succinate Syrup; Doxylamine Succinate Tablets.

Proprietary Preparations (details are given in Part 3)
Austral.: Dozile; Restaid†; Restavit; ***Belg.:*** Mereprine; ***Canad.:*** Unisom-2; ***Fr.:*** Donormyl; Mereprine; ***Ger.:*** Alsadorm†; Gittalun; Hoggar N; Mereprine; Munleit; Sedaplus; ***Ital.:*** Doxised†; ***S.Afr.:*** Restwell; Somnil; ***Spain:*** Donormyl; Dormacil†; Dormidina; Duebien; Unisom; ***Switz.:*** Mereprine; Sanalepsi N; ***USA:*** Doxysom†; Unisom Nighttime Sleep-Aid.

Multi-ingredient: ***Aust.:*** Wick Erkaltungs-Saft fur die Nacht; Wick Hustensaft; ***Austral.:*** Codral Tension Headache†; Dimetapp Cold, Cough & Flu; Fiorinal; Mersyndol; Ordov Migradol; Panadeine Plus; Panalgesic; ***Belg.:*** Pholco-Mereprine; Vicks Formule 44†; ***Canad.:*** Calmydone; Diclectin; Mercodol with Decapryn; Mersyndol with Codeine; Nighttime Cold & Flu; Nyquil; ***Ger.:*** Abiadin†; Ditenate†; Paedisup; Wick Medinait; ***Irl.:*** Syndol; ***Ital.:*** Vicks Medinait; ***S.Afr.:*** Abflex; Acurate; Adco-Dol; Asic; Betapyn; Cepacol; Dolerax; Forpyn; Lusadol†; Nethaprin Dospan; Nethaprin Expectorant; Paxidal; Pynstop; Sedapain; Sedinol; Syndette; Syndol; Tensopyn; Xerotens; ***Spain:*** Cariban; Medinait; Upsadex; Vicks Medinait†; ***Switz.:*** Pholprin†; Vicks Medinait; ***UK:*** Syndol; Vicks Medinite; ***USA:*** Alka-Seltzer Plus Night-Time Cold; All-Nite Cold Formula; Genite; Nite Time Cold Formula; NyQuil Hot Therapy; NyQuil Nighttime Cold/Flu; Nytcold Medicine; Pertussin All-Night PM†; Vicks NyQuil Liqui-Caps; Vicks NyQuil Multi-Symptom Cold Flu Relief.

Ebastine (2738-m)

Ebastine *(BAN, USAN, rINN)*.

LAS-W-090. 4′-*tert*-Butyl-4-[4-(diphenylmethoxy)piperidino]butyrophenone.

$C_{32}H_{39}NO_2$ = 469.7.

CAS — 90729-43-4.

Ebastine, a piperidine derivative, is a non-sedating antihistamine with a long duration of action. It does not have significant sedative or antimuscarinic actions.

Ebastine is given by mouth for the symptomatic relief of allergic conditions including rhinitis (p.400) and in pruritic skin disorders (p.400). The usual dose is 10 mg daily; children over 6 years of age may be given 5 mg daily.

References.

1. Wiseman LR, Faulds D. Ebastine: a review of its pharmacological properties and clinical efficacy in the treatment of allergic disorders. *Drugs* 1996; **51:** 260–77.

Preparations

Proprietary Preparations (details are given in Part 3)
Neth.: Kestine; ***Norw.:*** Kestine; ***Spain:*** Bromselon; Ebastel; ***Swed.:*** Kestine.

Multi-ingredient: ***Spain:*** Rino Ebastel; Tundrax.

Embramine Hydrochloride (6134-q)

Embramine Hydrochloride *(BANM, rINNM)*.

Embraminium Chloratum; Mebrophenhydramine Hydrochloride; Mebrophenhydraminium Chloratum. 2-(4-Bromo-α-methylbenzhydryloxy)-*NN*-dimethylethylamine hydrochloride.

$C_{18}H_{22}BrNO,HCl$ = 384.7.

CAS — 3565-72-8 (embramine); 13977-28-1 (embramine hydrochloride).

Embramine hydrochloride, an ethanolamine derivative, is a sedating antihistamine. Embramine hydrochloride and embramine theoclate have been administered by mouth for their antihistamine and antiemetic properties.

Emedastine Fumarate (6475-v)

Emedastine Fumarate *(BANM, rINNM)*.

AL-3432A; Emedastine Difumarate *(USAN)*. 1-(2-Ethoxyethyl)-2-(hexahydro-4-methyl-1*H*-1,4-diazepin-1-yl)benzimidazole fumarate (1:2).

$C_{17}H_{26}N_4O,2C_4H_4O_4$ = 534.6.

CAS — 87233-61-2 (emedastine); 87233-62-3 (emedastine fumarate).

Emedastine is an antihistamine with mast-cell stabilising properties. Emedastine 0.05%, as the fumarate, is used topically as eye drops for the symptomatic relief of allergic conjunctivitis (p.399).

Preparations

Proprietary Preparations (details are given in Part 3)
USA: Emadine.

Epinastine Hydrochloride (2906-m)

Epinastine Hydrochloride *(rINNM)*.

WAL-801-Cl. 3-Amino-9,13b-dihydro-1*H*-dibenz[*c,f*]imidazo[1,5-*a*]azepine hydrochloride.

$C_{16}H_{15}N_3,HCl$ = 285.8.

CAS — 80012-43-7 (epinastine).

Epinastine hydrochloride is an antihistamine reported to have no significant sedative activity. It has been given in the management of asthma, allergic rhinitis, and pruritic skin disorders in doses of up to 20 mg daily by mouth.

References.

1. Adamus WS, *et al.* Antihistamine activity and central effects of WAL 801 CL in man. *Eur J Clin Pharmacol* 1987; **33:** 381–5.
2. Adamus WS, *et al.* Pharmacodynamics of the new H_1-antagonist 3-amino-9,13b-dihydro-1H-dibenz[c,f]imidazo[1,5-a]azepine hydrochloride in volunteers. *Arzneimittelforschung* 1987; **37:** 569–72.

Preparations

Proprietary Preparations (details are given in Part 3)
Jpn: Alesion.

Fexofenadine Hydrochloride (3887-n)

Fexofenadine Hydrochloride *(BANM, USAN, rINNM)*.

MDL-16455A; Terfenadine Carboxylate Hydrochloride. (±)-*p*-{1-Hydroxy-4-[4-(hydroxydiphenylmethyl)-piperidino]butyl}-α-methylhydratropic acid hydrochloride.

$C_{32}H_{39}NO_4,HCl$ = 538.1.

CAS — 138452-21-8.

Adverse Effects and Precautions

As for the non-sedating antihistamines in general, p.397.

Interactions

As for the non-sedating antihistamines in general, p.399.

Plasma concentrations of fexofenadine have been increased after the concomitant administration of erythromycin or ketoconazole, but, unlike, terfenadine, the manufacturer has stated that this was not associated with adverse effects on the QT interval.

Antacids containing aluminium and magnesium hydroxide have reduced the absorption of fexofenadine.

Pharmacokinetics

Fexofenadine is rapidly absorbed after oral administration with peak plasma concentrations being reached in 2 to 3 hours. About 5% of the total dose is metabolised, mostly by the intestinal mucosa, with only 0.5 to 1.5% of the dose undergoing hepatic biotransformation. Elimination half-lives of about 14 hours have been reported although these may be prolonged in patients with renal impairment. Excretion is mainly in the faeces with only 10% being present in the urine. Fexofenadine does not appear to cross the blood-brain barrier.

Fexofenadine is a metabolite of terfenadine and as such has been detected in breast milk after the administration of terfenadine.

Uses and Administration

Fexofenadine, an active metabolite of terfenadine (p.418), is a non-sedating antihistamine. It does not possess significant sedative or antimuscarinic actions. Fexofenadine is used as the hydrochloride in the symptomatic relief of allergic conditions including rhinitis (p.400) and urticaria (p.401).

In the management of seasonal allergic rhinitis, fexofenadine hydrochloride is given by mouth in a dose of 120 mg daily either as a single dose or in two divided doses. Higher doses of 180 mg are recommended in urticaria.

It has been suggested that patients with renal impairment should receive an initial dose of 60 mg daily.

References.

1. Markham A, Wagstaff AJ. Fexofenadine. *Drugs* 1998; **55:** 269–74.

Preparations

Proprietary Preparations (details are given in Part 3)
Austral.: Telfast; ***Swed.:*** Telfast; ***UK:*** Telfast; ***USA:*** Allegra.
Multi-ingredient: ***USA:*** Allegra-D.

Flunarizine Hydrochloride (12759-n)

Flunarizine Hydrochloride *(BANM, USAN, rINNM).*

R-14950. *trans*-1-Cinnamyl-4-(4,4′-difluorobenzhydryl)piperazine dihydrochloride.

$C_{26}H_{26}F_2N_2,2HCl = 477.4.$

CAS — 52468-60-7 (flunarizine); 30484-77-6 (flunarizine hydrochloride).

Pharmacopoeias. In *Belg.*

Flunarizine dihydrochloride 11.8 mg is approximately equivalent to 10 mg of flunarizine.

Adverse Effects and Precautions

As for the sedating antihistamines in general, p.397. Adverse effects observed after administration of flunarizine also include weight gain, extrapyramidal symptoms (sometimes associated with depression), and, rarely, galactorrhoea.

Extrapyramidal disorders. Extrapyramidal motor signs (including parkinsonism, orofacial tardive dyskinesia, and akathisia) have been reported in 12 patients given flunarizine 10 to 40 mg daily for between 3 weeks and 15 months; 11 also had mental depression.[1] Partial or complete improvement of symptoms occurred after withdrawal of flunarizine. There have been other reports of similar effects,[2-4] but the association with flunarizine has not always been certain. Some workers have commented that flunarizine is often used in patients at increased risk of depression (migraine and geriatric patients) or extrapyramidal symptoms (geriatric patients)[2,5] or that flunarizine may unmask subclinical idiopathic Parkinson's disease.[5,6]

Extrapyramidal signs, including parkinsonism, have also been associated with the related drug, cinnarizine.[3,4] It has been suggested that such effects may be less likely to occur with cinnarizine than with flunarizine because of its shorter half-life and lower lipophilicity.[3]

1. Chouza C, *et al.* Parkinsonism, tardive dyskinesia, akathisia, and depression induced by flunarizine. *Lancet* 1986; **i:** 1303–4.
2. Meyboom RHB, *et al.* Parkinsonism, tardive dyskinesia, akathisia, and depression induced by flunarizine. *Lancet* 1986; **ii:** 292.
3. Laporte J-R, Capella D. Useless drugs are not placebos: lessons from flunarizine and cinnarizine. *Lancet* 1986; **ii:** 853–4.
4. Laporte J-R, Capella D. Useless drugs are not placebos. *Lancet* 1987; **i:** 1324.
5. Amery W. Side-effects of flunarizine. *Lancet* 1986; **i:** 1497.
6. Benvenuti F, *et al.* Side-effects of flunarizine. *Lancet* 1986; **ii:** 464.

Interactions

As for the sedating antihistamines in general, p.399.

Hepatic enzyme inducers such as carbamazepine, phenytoin, and valproate may interact with flunarizine by increasing its metabolism; an increase in dosage of flunarizine may be required.

Pharmacokinetics

Flunarizine hydrochloride is well absorbed from the gastro-intestinal tract, peak plasma concentrations occurring 2 to 4 hours after oral administration. Flunarizine hydrochloride is very lipophilic and is more than 90% bound to plasma proteins. It appears to undergo extensive metabolism; metabolites are excreted principally in the bile. Flunarizine hydrochloride has an elimination half-life of about 18 days.

Uses and Administration

Flunarizine is the difluorinated derivative of cinnarizine. It has antihistamine, sedative, and calcium-channel blocking activity. Flunarizine hydrochloride is used for migraine prophylaxis, for vertigo and vestibular disorders, and for peripheral and cerebral vascular disorders. It has also been tried as adjunctive antiepileptic therapy in patients refractory to standard regimens.

Flunarizine hydrochloride is given by mouth; doses are expressed in terms of the equivalent amount of flunarizine. The usual dose is 5 to 10 mg daily, usually given at night to minimise the effects of drowsiness.

Reviews.

1. Todd PA, Benfield P. Flunarizine: a reappraisal of its pharmacological properties and therapeutic use in neurological disorders. *Drugs* 1989; **38:** 481–99.

Epilepsy. Flunarizine has demonstrated antiepileptic activity in *animal* models, but the mechanism of action is unclear; calcium entry blockade or an effect on sodium channels has been postulated.[1] Most clinical studies have evaluated its use as adjunctive therapy in epileptic patients with partial seizures resistant to conventional treatment (see p.335). Doses of flunarizine of 15 to 20 mg daily by mouth appeared to provide the best response when given as part of multiple-drug antiepileptic regimens.[1] However, studies using fixed doses of flunarizine have been considered unsatisfactory because of flunarizine's variable clearance and long elimination half-life. Pledger *et al.*[2] overcame this by using a parallel group design and adjusting doses to achieve a constant plasma concentration of 60 ng per mL. They found flunarizine to have modest antiepileptic efficacy as adjunctive therapy for partial seizures. Even so, others[3] have concluded that the pharmacokinetic profile of flunarizine is too complex for its clinical use as an antiepileptic.

1. Todd PA, Benfield P. Flunarizine: a reappraisal of its pharmacological properties and therapeutic use in neurological disorders. *Drugs* 1989; **38:** 481–99.
2. Pledger GW, *et al.* Flunarizine for treatment of partial seizures: results of a concentration-controlled trial. *Neurology* 1994; **44:** 1830–6.
3. Hoppu K, *et al.* Flunarizine of limited value in children with intractable epilepsy. *Pediatr Neurol* 1995; **13:** 143–7.

Migraine. Flunarizine is used for the prophylaxis of migraine in some countries. As noted in reviews,[1,2] placebo-controlled studies have confirmed the efficacy of flunarizine in reducing the frequency of migraine attacks in both adult and paediatric patients. Also, comparative studies suggested it to be at least as effective as several other prophylactic antimigraine drugs including those generally preferred, pizotifen and propranolol (see p.443); subsequent studies appeared to confirm this opinion.[3,4] However, flunarizine is more likely to be reserved for use when first-line drugs have proved to be ineffective or unsuitable. Doses of flunarizine reported to be used for migraine prophylaxis are 10 mg daily for adults and 5 mg daily for children. Its mode of action in migraine is unclear; possible mechanisms are inhibition of vasospasm induced by mediators such as serotonin and prostaglandins, inhibition of cellular hypoxia, and improved blood viscosity and erythrocyte deformability. Calcium-channel blocking activity might have a role, but evidence for the efficacy of other calcium-channel blockers in migraine prophylaxis (see Nifedipine, p.921) is less convincing than for flunarizine.

Case reports have indicated benefit with flunarizine in the prophylaxis of the rare disorder of alternating hemiplegia in childhood.[5,6] While subsequent studies in 12 children did not produce conclusive findings, further investigation with flunarizine was considered to be warranted.[7]

The role of antihistamines in general in the management of migraine is discussed briefly on p.400.

1. Todd PA, Benfield P. Flunarizine: a reappraisal of its pharmacological properties and therapeutic use in neurological disorders. *Drugs* 1989; **38:** 481–99.
2. Andersson K-E, Vinge E. β-Adrenoceptor blockers and calcium antagonists in the prophylaxis and treatment of migraine. *Drugs* 1990; **3:** 355–73.
3. Gawel MJ, *et al.* Comparison of the efficacy and safety of flunarizine to propranolol in the prophylaxis of migraine. *Can J Neurol Sci* 1992; **19:** 340–5.
4. Soelberg Sørensen P, *et al.* Flunarizine versus metoprolol in migraine prophylaxis: a double-blind, randomized parallel group study of efficacy and tolerability. *Headache* 1991; **31:** 650–7.
5. Casaer P, Azou M. Flunarizine in alternating hemiplegia in childhood. *Lancet* 1984; **ii:** 579.
6. Curatolo P, Cusmai R. Drugs for alternating hemiplegic migraine. *Lancet* 1984; **ii:** 980.
7. Casaer P. Flunarizine in alternating hemiplegia in childhood. An international study in 12 children. *Neuropediatrics* 1987; **18:** 191–5.

Tourette's syndrome. Tourette's syndrome is a disorder characterised by motor and vocal tics and behavioural disturbances (see p.636). When symptoms are severe enough to cause discomfort or embarrassment treatment is usually with dopamine blockers such as haloperidol or pimozide but flunarizine is one of several drugs that have also been tried. A small unblinded study[1] involving 7 patients has suggested that flunarizine is more effective than placebo.

1. Micheli F, *et al.* Treatment of Tourette's syndrome with calcium antagonists. *Clin Neuropharmacol* 1990; **13:** 77–83.

Vertigo. Antihistamines are the mainstay of the treatment of vertigo (see p.401). However, their antimuscarinic side-effects may prove troublesome, particularly in the elderly, and they produce central sedation. Flunarizine is a calcium-channel blocker and an antihistamine that is devoid of antimuscarinic properties, although it may produce central sedation.

Preparations

Proprietary Preparations (details are given in Part 3)
Aust.: Amalium; Sibelium; ***Belg.:*** Sibelium; ***Canad.:*** Sibelium; ***Fr.:*** Sibelium; ***Ger.:*** Sibelium; ***Irl.:*** Sibelium; ***Ital.:*** Flugeral; Flunagen; Fluxarten; Gradient; Issium; Sibelium; Vasculene†; ***Neth.:*** Sibelium; ***S.Afr.:*** Sibelium; ***Spain:*** Flerudin; Flurpax; Sibelium; ***Switz.:*** Sibelium.

Halopyramine Hydrochloride (6135-p)

Halopyramine Hydrochloride *(BANM).*

Chloropyramine Hydrochloride *(rINNM). N*-(4-Chlorobenzyl)-*N′N′*-dimethyl-*N*-(2-pyridyl)ethylenediamine hydrochloride.

$C_{16}H_{20}ClN_3,HCl = 326.3.$

CAS — 59-32-5 (halopyramine); 6170-42-9 (halopyramine hydrochloride).

Halopyramine hydrochloride, an ethylenediamine derivative, is an antihistamines. It has been given by mouth and by injection.

Preparations

Proprietary Preparations (details are given in Part 3)
Hung.: Suprastin.

Histapyrrodine (11406-j)

Histapyrrodine *(rINN).*

N-Benzyl-*N*-phenyl-2-(pyrrolidin-1-yl)ethylamine.

$C_{19}H_{24}N_2 = 280.4.$

CAS — 493-80-1.

Histapyrrodine Hydrochloride (6136-s)

Histapyrrodine Hydrochloride *(rINNM).*

$C_{19}H_{24}N_2,HCl = 316.9.$

CAS — 6113-17-3.

Histapyrrodine, an ethylenediamine derivative, is a sedating antihistamine with antimuscarinic and moderate sedative properties. Histapyrrodine has been used for the symptomatic relief of hypersensitivity reactions and in pruritic skin disorders. It has been given by mouth as the hydrochloride and has been applied topically as the base or hydrochloride although, as with any antihistamine, there is a risk of sensitisation.

Preparations

Proprietary Preparations (details are given in Part 3)
Fr.: Domistan†.
Multi-ingredient: ***Fr.:*** Creme Domistan a la vitamine F†.

Homochlorcyclizine Hydrochloride (6137-w)

Homochlorcyclizine Hydrochloride *(BANM, rINNM).*

1-(4-Chlorobenzhydryl)perhydro-4-methyl-1,4-diazepine dihydrochloride.

$C_{19}H_{23}ClN_2,2HCl = 387.8.$

CAS — 848-53-3 (homochlorcyclizine); 1982-36-1 (homochlorcyclizine hydrochloride).

Pharmacopoeias. In *Jpn.*

Homochlorcyclizine hydrochloride, a piperazine derivative, is a sedating antihistamine with antimuscarinic and moderate sedative properties. It is used for the symptomatic relief of allergic conditions including urticaria (p.401) and rhinitis (p.400), and in pruritic skin disorders (p.400). It is given by mouth in doses of 10 to 20 mg three times daily.

Preparations

Proprietary Preparations (details are given in Part 3)
Jpn: Homoclomin.

Hydroxyzine Embonate (6138-e)

Hydroxyzine Embonate *(BANM, rINNM).*

Hydroxyzine Pamoate. 2-{2-[4-(4-Chlorobenzhydryl)piperazin-1-yl]ethoxy}ethanol 4,4′-methylenebis(3-hydroxy-2-naphthoate).

$C_{21}H_{27}ClN_2O_2,C_{23}H_{16}O_6 = 763.3.$

CAS — 68-88-2 (hydroxyzine); 10246-75-0 (hydroxyzine embonate).

Pharmacopoeias. In *Jpn* and *US.*

A light yellow almost odourless powder. Hydroxyzine embonate 170 mg is approximately equivalent to 100 mg of hydroxyzine hydrochloride. **Solubilities** are: practically insoluble in water and in methyl alcohol; very slightly soluble in chloroform and in ether; soluble 1 in 700 of alcohol, 1 in 10 of dimethylformamide, and 1 in 3.5 of 10M sodium hydroxide solution. **Store** in airtight containers.

Hydroxyzine Hydrochloride (6139-l)

Hydroxyzine Hydrochloride *(BANM, rINNM)*.

Hydroxyzini Hydrochloridum.

$C_{21}H_{27}ClN_2O_2,2HCl = 447.8$.

CAS — 2192-20-3.

Pharmacopoeias. In *Eur.* (see p.viii), *Jpn*, and *US*.

A white or almost white, hygroscopic, odourless crystalline powder. **Soluble** 1 in 1 of water, 1 in 4.5 of alcohol, and 1 in 13 of chloroform; slightly soluble in acetone; very slightly soluble to practically insoluble in ether. **Store** in airtight containers and protect from light.

Incompatibility has been reported with aminophylline, benzylpenicillin salts, chloramphenicol sodium succinate, dimenhydrinate, doxorubicin hydrochloride (in a liposomal formulation), thioridazine, and some soluble barbiturates.

A mixture of hydroxyzine hydrochloride, chlorpromazine hydrochloride, and pethidine hydrochloride stored in glass or plastic syringes was found[1] to be stable for 366 days at 4° and 25°.

1. Conklin CA, *et al.* Stability of an analgesic-sedative combination in glass and plastic single-dose syringes. *Am J Hosp Pharm* 1985; **42:** 339–42.

Adverse Effects and Precautions

As for the sedating antihistamines in general, p.397.

Intramuscular injection of hydroxyzine has been reported to cause marked local discomfort. Intravenous administration has been associated with haemolysis.

There has been a report[1] of accidental intra-arterial injection of hydroxyzine that led to necrosis of the extremity necessitating amputation of the digits of the affected limb.

1. Hardesty WH. Inadvertent intra-arterial injection. *JAMA* 1970; **213:** 872.

Effects on the heart. ECG abnormalities, particularly alterations in T-waves, were associated with anxiolytic doses of hydroxyzine hydrochloride, and, were similar to those produced by thioridazine and tricyclic antidepressants.[1]

1. Hollister LE. Hydroxyzine hydrochloride: possible adverse cardiac interactions. *Psychopharmacol Comm* 1975; **1:** 61–5.

Effects on sexual function. A 32-year-old man experience prolonged penile erections (priapism) after taking two separate doses of hydroxyzine for a skin rash.[1] The authors suggest that the effect may be due to a hydroxyzine metabolite which was found to be structurally similar to a metabolite of trazodone, a drug known to induce penile erections.

1. Thavundayil JX. *et al.* Prolonged penile erections induced by hydroxyzine: possible mechanism of action. *Neuropsychobiology* 1994; **30:** 4–6.

Effects on the skin. Four children given hydroxyzine hydrochloride for restlessness developed a fixed drug eruption of the penis.[1] All recovered on drug withdrawal and subsequently had positive rechallenges.

1. Cohen HA, *et al.* Fixed drug eruption of the penis due to hydroxyzine hydrochloride. *Ann Pharmacother* 1997; **31:** 327–9.

Liver disorders. A study[1] has suggested that hydroxyzine should only be administered once daily for the relief of pruritus in patients with primary biliary cirrhosis. The mean serum elimination half-lives of hydroxyzine and its metabolite cetirizine in 8 patients with primary biliary cirrhosis were 36.6 and 25.0 hours respectively.

1. Simons FER, *et al.* The pharmacokinetics and pharmacodynamics of hydroxyzine in patients with primary biliary cirrhosis. *J Clin Pharmacol* 1989; **29:** 809–15.

Porphyria. Hydroxyzine has been associated with clinical exacerbations of porphyria and is considered unsafe in porphyric patients.[1]

1. Moore MR, McColl KEL. *Porphyria: drug lists.* Glasgow: Porphyria Research Unit, University of Glasgow, 1991.

Interactions

As for the sedating antihistamines in general, p.399.

Pharmacokinetics

Hydroxyzine is rapidly absorbed from the gastro-intestinal tract and is metabolised. Metabolites include cetirizine (p.404) which has antihistamine activity. An elimination half-life of about 20 hours has been reported.

References.

1. Paton DM, Webster DR. Clinical pharmacokinetics of H_1-receptor antagonists (the antihistamines). *Clin Pharmacokinet* 1985; **10:** 477–97.

Liver disorders. For reference to a prolonged half-life of hydroxyzine in patients with primary biliary cirrhosis, see under Adverse Effects and Precautions, above.

Uses and Administration

Hydroxyzine, a piperazine derivative, is a sedating antihistamine with antimuscarinic and significant sedative properties; it is also an antiemetic. Its main use is as an anxiolytic (p.635). It is also used as an adjunct to pre- and postoperative medication (p.399) and in the management of pruritus (p.400) and urticaria (p.401) and has been used as an adjunct to opioid analgesia in the management of cancer pain (p.8).

Hydroxyzine may be given by mouth as the hydrochloride or the embonate; doses are expressed in terms of the equivalent amount of hydroxyzine hydrochloride.

The usual doses by mouth are: 50 to 100 mg four times a day for the short-term management of anxiety; for pruritus an initial dose of 25 mg given at night, increased if necessary to 25 mg three or four times daily; and 50 to 100 mg for pre- or postoperative sedation. For children over 6 years the initial dose is 15 to 25 mg daily increased if necessary to 50 to 100 mg daily in divided doses; for children 6 months to 6 years old the initial dose is 5 to 15 mg daily increased if necessary to 50 mg daily in divided doses. The pre- or postoperative sedative dose in children is 600 μg per kg body-weight.

Hydroxyzine hydrochloride may also be given by deep intramuscular injection. For prompt control of anxious or agitated adults 50 to 100 mg is injected intramuscularly initially, and the dose may be repeated every four to six hours as required. For other indications when oral administration is not practical, the intramuscular dose is 25 to 100 mg for adults and 1.1 mg per kg for children. Hydroxyzine should not be given by intravenous injection since haemolysis may result.

Preparations

USP 23: Hydroxyzine Hydrochloride Injection; Hydroxyzine Hydrochloride Syrup; Hydroxyzine Hydrochloride Tablets; Hydroxyzine Pamoate Capsules; Hydroxyzine Pamoate Oral Suspension.

Proprietary Preparations (details are given in Part 3)

Aust.: Atarax; ***Austral.:*** Atarax; ***Belg.:*** Atarax; ***Canad.:*** Atarax; Multipax; ***Fr.:*** Atarax; ***Ger.:*** AH 3 N; Atarax; Elroquil N; Masmoran†; ***Irl.:*** Atarax; ***Ital.:*** Atarax; Atazina†; ***Neth.:*** Atarax; Navicalm; ***Norw.:*** Atarax; ***S.Afr.:*** Aterax; ***Spain:*** Atarax; ***Swed.:*** Atarax; Vistaril†; ***Switz.:*** Atarax; ***UK:*** Atarax; Ucerax; ***USA:*** Anxanil†; Atarax; E-Vista†; Hyzine†; Neucalm 50†; Quiess†; Rezine; Vistacon†; Vistaject†; Vistaquel†; Vistaril; Vistazine.

Multi-ingredient: ***Aust.:*** Diligan; ***Belg.:*** Agyrax; Diligan†; Vesparax; ***Ger.:*** Diligan; ***Ital.:*** Vesparax†; ***Neth.:*** Vesparax; ***S.Afr.:*** Diligan†; Enarax†; Geratar; Vesparax; ***Spain:*** Calmoplex; Difilina Asmorax; Dolodens; Somatarax; ***Swed.:*** Histilos; Kombistrat†; ***Switz.:*** Hexafene; ***USA:*** Hydrophed; Marax; Theomax DF.

Isothipendyl Hydrochloride (6140-v)

Isothipendyl Hydrochloride *(BANM, rINNM)*.

NN-Dimethyl-1-(pyrido[3,2-*b*][1,4]benzothiazin-10-ylmethyl)ethylamine hydrochloride.

$C_{16}H_{19}N_3S,HCl = 321.9$.

CAS — 482-15-5 (isothipendyl); 1225-60-1 (isothipendyl hydrochloride).

Isothipendyl hydrochloride, an azaphenothiazine derivative, is an antihistamine that has been applied topically for hypersensitivity and pruritic skin disorders although as with any antihistamine there is a risk of sensitisation. It has also been administered by mouth and by the rectal route.

Preparations

Proprietary Preparations (details are given in Part 3)

Belg.: Andantol; ***Fr.:*** Apaisyl; Istamyl; ***Ital.:*** Andantol†; Calmogel; ***S.Afr.:*** Andantol†.

Multi-ingredient: ***Ger.:*** Transpulmin†; ***S.Afr.:*** Cothera Compound†.

Levocabastine Hydrochloride

(15953-b)

Levocabastine Hydrochloride *(BANM, USAN, rINNM)*.

R-50547. (−)-*trans*-1-[*cis*-4-Cyano-4-(*p*-fluorophenyl)cyclohexyl]-3-methyl-4-phenylisonipecotic acid hydrochloride.

$C_{26}H_{29}FN_2O_2,HCl = 457.0$.

CAS — 79516-68-0 (levocabastine); 79547-78-7 (levocabastine hydrochloride); 79449-98-2 (cabastine).

NOTE. The racemate of levocabastine, cabastine, is *rINN*.

Adverse Effects and Precautions

As for the antihistamines in general, p.397. The most common adverse effects reported with levocabastine eye drops are transient stinging and burning of the eyes, urticaria, dyspnoea, drowsiness, and headache. Following nasal administration headache, nasal irritation, somnolence, and fatigue have been noted. The use of levocabastine nasal spray is not recommended in those with significant renal impairment.

Pharmacokinetics

Levocabastine is absorbed following both nasal and ocular administration. Systemic availability has been estimated at 60 to 80% after nasal administration and 30 to 60% after ocular application. However absolute peak plasma concentrations are low. Plasma protein binding is about 55%. An elimination half-life of 35 to 40 hours has been reported for all routes of delivery. Elimination of levocabastine is primarily renal with 70% excreted as unchanged drug and 10% as an inactive acetylglucuronide metabolite; the remaining 20% is excreted unchanged in the faeces.

Trace amounts of levocabastine have been found in breast milk after ocular and nasal administration.

References.

1. Heykants J, *et al.* The pharmacokinetic properties of topical levocabastine: a review. *Clin Pharmacokinet* 1995; **29:** 221–30.

Uses and Administration

Levocabastine, a piperidine derivative, is a long-acting and potent antihistamine with a rapid onset of action. Levocabastine hydrochloride equivalent to 0.05% levocabastine is used topically as eye drops or as nasal spray in the treatment of allergic conjunctivitis (p.399) and rhinitis (p.400).

In the treatment of conjunctivitis, 1 drop of 0.05% eye drops is instilled into each eye twice daily and in rhinitis 2 sprays of a 0.05% nasal suspension are delivered to each nostril twice daily. The frequency of the dose in both conditions may be increased to 3 or 4 times daily if necessary, but treatment should not continue for longer than 4 weeks. In conjunctivitis it is recommended that treatment should be restricted to a total of 4 weeks in any one year.

References.

1. Dechant KL, Goa KL. Levocabastine: a review of its pharmacological properties and therapeutic potential as a topical antihistamine in allergic rhinitis and conjunctivitis. *Drugs* 1991; **41:** 202–24.
2. Noble S, McTavish D. Levocabastine: an update of its pharmacology, clinically efficacy and tolerability in the topical treatment of allergic rhinitis and conjunctivitis. *Drugs* 1995; **50:** 1032–49.

Preparations

Proprietary Preparations (details are given in Part 3)

Aust.: Livostin; ***Austral.:*** Livostin; ***Belg.:*** Livostin; ***Canad.:*** Livostin; ***Fr.:*** Levophta; ***Ger.:*** Levophta; Livocab; ***Ital.:*** Levostab; Livostin; ***Neth.:*** Livocab; ***Norw.:*** Livostin; ***S.Afr.:*** Livostin; ***Spain:*** Bilina; Livocab; ***Swed.:*** Livostin; ***Switz.:*** Livostin; ***UK:*** Livostin; ***USA:*** Livostin.

Loratadine (18661-c)

Loratadine *(BAN, USAN, rINN)*.

Sch-29851. Ethyl 4-(8-chloro-5,6-dihydro-11*H*-benzo[5,6]cyclohepta[1,2-*b*]pyridin-11-ylidene)piperidine-1-carboxylate.

$C_{22}H_{23}ClN_2O_2$ = 382.9.

CAS — 79794-75-5.

Adverse Effects and Precautions

As for the non-sedating antihistamines in general, p.397.

Effects on the liver. Two patients[1] developed severe necroinflammatory liver injury after receiving loratadine 10 mg daily for allergic rhinitis. Although both recovered after drug withdrawal, one patient required a liver transplantation and recovery was prolonged.

The manufacturers note that abnormal hepatic function including jaundice, hepatitis, and hepatic necrosis have been reported rarely.

1. Schiano TD, *et al.* Subfulminant liver failure and severe hepatotoxicity caused by loratadine use. *Ann Intern Med* 1996; **125:** 738–40.

Sedation. For discussion of the sedative effects of antihistamines, including loratadine, see p.398.

Interactions

As for the non-sedating antihistamines in general, p.399.

Loratadine is metabolised by cytochrome P450 isoenzymes CYP3A4 and CYP2D6. Therefore concomitant administration of other drugs that inhibit or are metabolised by these hepatic enzymes may result in changes in plasma concentrations of either drug and, possibly, adverse effects. Drugs known to inhibit one or other of these enzymes include cimetidine, erythromycin, ketoconazole, quinidine, fluconazole, and fluoxetine.

Data held on file by the manufacturer show that *erythromycin* can inhibit the metabolism of loratadine. However, even when given in large doses loratadine does not appear to cause the cardiac conduction disorders associated with the non-sedating antihistamines astemizole (see p.402) and terfenadine (see p.418).[1] Similarly, *clarithromycin* seemed to inhibit the metabolism of loratadine and its active metabolite descarboethoxyloratadine.[2]

Ketoconazole also appears to be able to inhibit the metabolism of loratadine and at therapeutic doses, is approximately 3 times more inhibitory than erythromycin.[3] However, the concentrations of ketoconazole required are reported to be much higher than those required to inhibit the metabolism of astemizole or terfenadine.

Cimetidine also appears to have an inhibitory effect on the metabolism of loratadine and all 4 drugs also attenuate the clearance of its active metabolite descarboethoxyloratadine although no clinically significant consequences were observed in these studies.[2,3]

1. Affrime MB, *et al.* Three month evaluation of electrocardiographic effects of loratadine in humans. *J Allergy Clin Immunol* 1993; **91:** 259.
2. Carr RA, *et al.* Steady-state pharmacokinetics and electrocardiographic pharmacodynamics of clarithromycin and loratadine after individual or concomitant administration. *Antimicrob Agents Chemother* 1998; **42:** 1176–80.
3. Brannan MD, *et al.* Effects of various cytochrome P450 inhibitors on the metabolism of loratadine. *Clin Pharmacol Ther* 1995; **57:** 193.

Pharmacokinetics

Loratadine is rapidly absorbed from the gastro-intestinal tract after oral administration, peak plasma concentrations being attained in about one hour. Bioavailability is increased and time to peak plasma concentrations is delayed when administered with food. Loratadine undergoes extensive metabolism. The major metabolite, descarboethoxyloratadine (desloratadine), has potent antihistamine activity. Reported mean elimination half-lives for loratadine and descarboethoxyloratadine are 8.4 and 28 hours respectively. Loratadine is about 98% bound to plasma proteins; descarboethoxyloratadine is less extensively bound. Loratadine and its metabolites have been detected in breast milk, but do not appear to cross the blood-brain barrier to a significant extent. Most of a dose is excreted equally in the urine and faeces, mainly in the form of metabolites.

Renal impairment. The disposition of loratadine does not appear to be significantly altered in patients with severe renal insufficiency and haemodialysis does not appear to be an effective means of removing loratadine or its metabolite descarboethoxyloratadine from the body.[1]

1. Matzke GR, *et al.* Pharmacokinetics of loratadine in patients with renal insufficiency. *J Clin Pharmacol* 1990; **30:** 364–71.

Uses and Administration

Loratadine, a piperidine derivative related to azatadine, is a long-acting, non-sedating antihistamine with no significant sedative or antimuscarinic activity. It is used for the symptomatic relief of allergic conditions including rhinitis (p.400) and chronic urticaria (p.401).

Loratadine is given by mouth in a dose of 10 mg once daily. The US manufacturer recommends that patients with hepatic failure or renal impairment should be given 10 mg on alternate days initially. Children aged 2 to 5 years may be given 5 mg once daily and those aged 6 to 12 years may be given 10 mg once daily.

References.

1. Barenholtz HA, McLeod DC. Loratadine: a nonsedating antihistamine with once-daily dosing. *DICP Ann Pharmacother* 1989; **23:** 445–50.
2. Simons FER. Loratadine, a non-sedating H_1-receptor antagonist (antihistamine). *Ann Allergy* 1989; **63:** 266–8.
3. Haria M, *et al.* Loratadine: a reappraisal of its pharmacological properties and therapeutic use in allergic disorders. *Drugs* 1994; **48:** 617–37.

Preparations

Proprietary Preparations (details are given in Part 3)
Aust.: Clarityn; ***Austral.:*** Claratyne; Lorastyne; ***Belg.:*** Claritine; Sanelor; ***Canad.:*** Claritin; ***Fr.:*** Clarityne; ***Ger.:*** Lisino; ***Irl.:*** Clarityn; ***Ital.:*** Clarityn; Fristamin; ***Neth.:*** Allerfre; Claritine; ***Norw.:*** Clarityn; Versal; ***S.Afr.:*** Clarityne; Polaratyne; ***Spain:*** Civeran; Clarityne; Optimin; Velodan; Viatine; ***Swed.:*** Clarityn; Versal; ***Switz.:*** Claritine; ***UK:*** Clarityn; ***USA:*** Claritin.

Multi-ingredient: ***Aust.:*** Clarinase; ***Austral.:*** Clarinase; ***Belg.:*** Clarinase; ***Canad.:*** Chlor-Tripolon ND; Claritin Extra; ***Fr.:*** Clarinase; ***S.Afr.:*** Clarityne D; Demazin NS; Polaratyne D; ***Spain:*** Clarinase; Logradin; Narine; ***USA:*** Claritin-D.

Mebhydrolin (12145-k)

Mebhydrolin *(BAN, rINN)*.

5-Benzyl-1,2,3,4-tetrahydro-2-methyl-γ-carboline.

$C_{19}H_{20}N_2$ = 276.4.

CAS — 524-81-2.

Mebhydrolin Napadisylate (6141-g)

Mebhydrolin Napadisylate *(BANM)*.

Mebhydrolin Napadisilate *(rINNM)*; Diazolinum; Mebhydrolin Naphthalenedisulphonate. Mebhydrolin naphthalene-1,5-disulphonate.

$(C_{19}H_{20}N_2)_2,C_{10}H_8O_6S_2$ = 841.1.

CAS — 6153-33-9.

Mebhydrolin napadisylate 152 mg is approximately equivalent to 100 mg of mebhydrolin.

Adverse Effects and Precautions

As for the sedating antihistamines in general, p.397. Granulocytopenia and agranulocytosis have been reported.

Interactions

As for the sedating antihistamines in general, p.399.

Pharmacokinetics

Mebhydrolin is absorbed slowly from the gastro-intestinal tract. It is extensively metabolised; only small amounts of unchanged drug are recovered in the urine. The manufacturers of mebhydrolin give a plasma half-life of about 4 hours.

Uses and Administration

Mebhydrolin, an ethylenediamine derivative, is a sedating antihistamine with antimuscarinic and sedative properties. It has been used for the symptomatic relief of allergic conditions including urticaria (p.401) and rhinitis (p.400), and in pruritic skin disorders (p.400).

Mebhydrolin is administered by mouth as the base or as the napadisylate salt. Doses are expressed in terms of the equivalent amount of mebhydrolin base and the usual dose has been 50 to 100 mg three times daily.

Preparations

Proprietary Preparations (details are given in Part 3)
Austral.: Fabahistin†; ***Ger.:*** Omeril; ***Irl.:*** Fabahistin†; ***Ital.:*** Incidal; ***Neth.:*** Incidal†; ***S.Afr.:*** Fabahistin†; ***UK:*** Fabahistin†.

Multi-ingredient: ***Ital.:*** Refagan†.

Meclozine Hydrochloride (6142-q)

Meclozine Hydrochloride *(BAN, pINNM)*.

Meclizine Hydrochloride; Meclizinium Chloride; Meclozini Hydrochloridum; Parachloramine Hydrochloride. 1-(4-Chlorobenzhydryl)-4-(3-methylbenzyl)piperazine dihydrochloride.

$C_{25}H_{27}ClN_2,2HCl$ = 463.9.

CAS — 569-65-3 (meclozine); 1104-22-9 (anhydrous meclozine hydrochloride); 31884-77-2 (meclozine hydrochloride, monohydrate).

Pharmacopoeias. In *Eur.* (see p.viii).
US specifies the monohydrate.

A white to yellow crystalline powder with a slight odour. **Solubilities** for the anhydrous salt are: slightly soluble in water; soluble in alcohol and in dichloromethane; practically insoluble in ether. Solubilities for the monohydrate salt are: practically insoluble in water and in ether; freely soluble in chloroform and in acid-alcohol-water mixtures; slightly soluble in dilute acids and in alcohol. **Store** in airtight containers.

Adverse Effects and Precautions

As for the sedating antihistamines in general, p.397. For reports of the use of antihistamines, including meclozine, in pregnancy, see p.398.

Interactions

As for the sedating antihistamines in general, p.399.

Uses and Administration

Meclozine hydrochloride, a piperazine derivative, is a sedating antihistamine with antimuscarinic and moderate sedative properties. It is mainly used for its antiemetic action which may last for up to 24 hours. Meclozine hydrochloride is used in the prevention and treatment of nausea and vomiting associated with a variety of conditions including motion sickness (p.400) and for the symptomatic treatment of vertigo (p.401) caused by Ménière's disease and other vestibular disorders. Meclozine hydrochloride has also been used for the symptomatic relief of hypersensitivity reactions and pruritic skin disorders (p.400).

The usual dose of meclozine hydrochloride for motion sickness is 25 to 50 mg by mouth taken about one hour before travelling and repeated every 24 hours if necessary; up to 100 mg daily in divided doses has been given for the treatment of vertigo and vestibular disorders. Both meclozine hydrochloride and meclozine base have been administered by the rectal route; doses are similar to those given by mouth.

Preparations

USP 23: Meclizine Hydrochloride Tablets.

Proprietary Preparations (details are given in Part 3)
Austral.: Ancolan†; ***Belg.:*** Postafene; ***Canad.:*** Bonamine; ***Fr.:*** Agyrax; ***Ger.:*** Bonamine; Calmonal†; Peremesin; Peremesin N; Postadoxin N; Postafen; ***Ital.:*** Neo-Istafene†; ***Neth.:*** Suprimal; ***Norw.:*** Postafen; ***Spain:*** Chiclida; Dramine; Navicalm; ***Swed.:*** Postafen; ***Switz.:*** Duremesan; Peremesine†; ***UK:*** Sea-legs; ***USA:*** Antivert; Antrizine; Bonine; Dizmiss; Dramamine II; Meni-D; Nico-Vert; Ru-Vert-M; Vergon; Vertin.

Multi-ingredient: ***Aust.:*** Contravert B_6; Diligan; ***Belg.:*** Diligan†; Postadoxine; ***Canad.:*** Antivert; ***Ger.:*** Diligan; Postadoxin†; ***Neth.:*** Emesafene; Neo-Cranimal†; ***Norw.:*** Peremesin; ***S.Afr.:*** Diligan†; Geratar; ***Swed.:*** Histilos; ***Switz.:*** Duremesan; Itinerol B_6; Peremesine†.

Mefenidramium Methylsulphate (2750-f)

Mefenidramium Metilsulfate *(rINN)*; Diphenhydramine Methylsulphomethylate; Mefenidramium Methylsulfate. [2-(Diphenylmethoxy)ethyl]trimethylammonium methyl sulphate.

$C_{19}H_{27}NO_5S$ = 381.5.

CAS — 4858-60-0.

Mefenidramium methylsulphate, an ethanolamine derivative, is a sedating antihistamine. It has antimuscarinic and significant sedative properties. Mefenidramium has been given for the symptomatic relief of hypersensitivity reactions and in pruritic skin disorders.

Preparations

Proprietary Preparations (details are given in Part 3)
Fr.: Allerga†.

Mepyramine Hydrochloride (13752-h)

Mepyramine Hydrochloride (*BANM, rINNM*).

Pyranisamine Hydrochloride; Pyrilamine Hydrochloride. *N-p*-Anisyl-*N'N'*-dimethyl-*N*-(2-pyridyl)ethylenediamine hydrochloride.

$C_{17}H_{23}N_3O,HCl = 321.8$.

CAS — 91-84-9 (mepyramine); 6036-95-9 (mepyramine hydrochloride).

Mepyramine Maleate (6144-s)

Mepyramine Maleate (*BANM, rINNM*).

Mepyramini Maleas; Pyranisamine Maleate; Pyrilamine Maleate. Mepyramine hydrogen maleate.

$C_{17}H_{23}N_3O,C_4H_4O_4 = 401.5$.

CAS — 59-33-6.

Pharmacopoeias. In *Eur.* (see p.viii) and *US*.

A white or slightly yellowish crystalline powder with a slight odour. M.p. 99° to 103°. **Solubilities** are: soluble 1 in 0.5 of water, 1 in 3 of alcohol, 1 in 15 of dehydrated alcohol, and 1 in 2 of chloroform; slightly to very slightly soluble in ether. A 2% solution in water has a pH of 4.9 to 5.2. **Store** in airtight containers. Protect from light.

Adverse Effects and Precautions

As for the sedating antihistamines in general, p.397.

Interactions

As for the sedating antihistamines in general, p.399.

Uses and Administration

Mepyramine, an ethylenediamine derivative, is a sedating antihistamine with antimuscarinic and sedative properties. Mepyramine maleate is used for the symptomatic relief of hypersensitivity reactions and in pruritic skin disorders (p.400). Mepyramine maleate is also a common ingredient of compound preparations for the symptomatic treatment of coughs and colds (p.400).

In the USA a usual dose of mepyramine maleate by mouth is 25 to 50 mg given three or four times daily; in some countries up to 1 g has been given daily in divided doses. Mepyramine maleate has also been used in eye drops. In some countries mepyramine maleate is available for parenteral use.

A cream containing 2% mepyramine maleate has been used locally for insect bites or stings, and for hypersensitivity and pruritic skin conditions, but as with any antihistamine there is a risk of sensitisation.

Mepyramine hydrochloride may be administered parenterally or by the rectal route. Mepyramine tannate and mepifylline (mepyramine acephyllinate) have been given by mouth.

Preparations

BP 1998: Mepyramine Tablets;
USP 23: Pyrilamine Maleate Tablets.

Proprietary Preparations (details are given in Part 3)
Austral.: Anthisan; Relaxa-Tabs; ***Irl.:*** Anthisan; ***Ital.:*** Antemesyl; ***S.Afr.:*** Anthisan; Histamed†; Mepyrimal; Pyramine†; Pyriped†; ***Spain:*** Fluidasa; ***UK:*** Anthisan.

Multi-ingredient: ***Aust.:*** Prefrin A; ***Austral.:*** Hycomine; Neo-Diophen; ***Belg.:*** Nortussine; Triaminic†; ***Canad.:*** Antitussive Decongestant Antihistamine Syrup; Bronchodex DM; Bronchosirum; Caldomine-DH; Centracol DM; Dristan Formula P†; Hycomine; IDM Solution; Jack and Jill Cough Syrup; Lemon Time; Midol Extra Strength†; Midol Multi-Symptom; Midol PMS Extra Strength; Pamprin; Pharmacol DM; Pharminicol DM; Prefrin A; Tantacol DM; Theo-Bronc; Trendar PMS; Triaminic; Triaminic Expectorant DH; Triaminicin; Trisulfaminic; Tussaminic C; Tussaminic DH; ***Fr.:*** Nortussine; Triaminic; ***Ger.:*** Praecimal†; ***Irl.:*** Prefrin A†; ***Ital.:*** Antemesyl; Balsamina Kroner; Cletanol C†; Cletanol†; Decongene†; Triaminic; Triaminicol†; Vasofen; ***S.Afr.:*** Antiflu; Ascold; Bronchiflu; Bronchilate†; Bronchistop; Cetamine; Cetrispect; Codef; Codomill; Colcaps; Coughcod; Degoran†; Docsed; Dykatuss Co; Efcod†; Expectco†; Expectotussin "C"; Flucol; Histodor; Kiddiekof; Medituss; Metaxol; Monotussin; Prefrin A†; Pyracod†; Triami†; Triaminic; ***Spain:*** Amplidermis; Bronquiasmol†; Diptol Antihist†; Pectobal Dextro; Triominic; ***Swed.:*** Prefrinal med mepyramin†; ***Switz.:*** Calpred; Demoderhin; Escogripp sans codeine; Escogripp†; Euceta Pic†; Histacyl Compositum; Histacylettes; No Grip; Stilex; Stix†; Triaminic†; ***UK:*** Anthisan Plus; Wasp-Eze; ***USA:*** 4-Way Fast Acting; A-Caine; Albatussin NN; Atrohist Pediatric; Calamycin; Codimal DH; Codimal DM; Codimal PH; Covangesic; Derma-Pax; Fiogesic†; HC Derma-Pax; Hemet†; Hemocaine†; Histalet Forte; Histosal; Hydrophene DH; Iohist D; Kisitan; Maximum Strength Midol Multi-Symptom Formula†; Maximum Strength Midol PMS†; Medacote; Midol Maximum Strength Multi-Symptom Menstrual; Midol PMS; Myci-Spray; ND-Gesic; Original Midol Multi-Symptom Formula†; Pamprin; Phanadex Cough; Poly-Histine; Poly-Histine D; Premsyn PMS; R-Tannamine; R-Tannate; Rectagene Medicated Rectal Balm; Rhinatate; Robitussin Night Relief; Rolatuss with Hydrocodone; Ru-Tuss with Hydrocodone; Rynatan; Soothaderm; Statuss Green; Tanoral; Tri-Tannate; Triaminic Expectorant DH; Triaminic Oral Infant; Tricodene Cough & Cold; Triotann; Tritan; Vanex Forte; Vetuss HC; Vitanumonyl.

Mequitazine (6145-w)

Mequitazine (*BAN, rINN*).

LM-209. 10-(Quinuclidin-3-ylmethyl)phenothiazine.

$C_{20}H_{22}N_2S = 322.5$.

CAS — 29216-28-2.

Adverse Effects and Precautions

As for the sedating antihistamines in general, p.397.

Sedation. For discussion of the sedative effects of antihistamines, see p.398. When mequitazine is given in the recommended dosage of 5 mg twice daily the incidence of sedation appears comparable with that of terfenadine. Sedation has, however, occurred after doses of 10 mg twice daily.

Interactions

As for the sedating antihistamines in general, p.399.

Pharmacokinetics

After absorption from the gastro-intestinal tract, mequitazine is metabolised. Unchanged drug and metabolites are excreted principally in the bile.

Uses and Administration

Mequitazine, a phenothiazine derivative, is a sedating antihistamine with antimuscarinic and mild sedative properties.

Mequitazine is used for the symptomatic relief of allergic conditions including urticaria (p.401), rhinitis (p.400) and conjunctivitis (p.399), and in pruritic skin disorders (p.400).

Mequitazine is given in usual doses of 5 mg twice daily by mouth.

Preparations

Proprietary Preparations (details are given in Part 3)
Aust.: Metaplexan; ***Belg.:*** Mircol; ***Fr.:*** Butix; Primalan; ***Ger.:*** Metaplexan; ***Irl.:*** Primalan; ***Ital.:*** Primalan; ***Neth.:*** Mircol†; ***Spain:*** Mircol; ***Switz.:*** Vigigan†; ***UK:*** Primalan.

Methapyrilene (20146-a)

Methapyrilene (*BAN*).

Thenylpyramine. *NN*-Dimethyl-*N'*-(2-pyridyl)-*N'*-(2-thenyl)ethylenediamine.

$C_{14}H_{19}N_3S = 261.4$.

CAS — 91-80-5 (methapyrilene); 33032-12-1 (methapyrilene fumarate); 135-23-9 (methapyrilene hydrochloride).

Methapyrilene, an ethylenediamine derivative, is an antihistamine that was withdrawn following reports of carcinogenicity in *rats*. It was used as the fumarate or the hydrochloride.

Methdilazine (6148-y)

Methdilazine (*BAN, rINN*).

10-(1-Methylpyrrolidin-3-ylmethyl)phenothiazine.

$C_{18}H_{20}N_2S = 296.4$.

CAS — 1982-37-2.

Pharmacopoeias. In *US*.

A light tan crystalline powder with a characteristic odour. Methdilazine 7.2 mg is equivalent to approximately 8 mg of methdilazine hydrochloride. Practically **insoluble** in water; soluble 1 in 2 of alcohol, 1 in 1 of chloroform, 1 in 8 of ether, and 1 in 40 of 0.1M hydrochloric acid; freely soluble in 3M hydrochloric acid and practically insoluble in 0.1M sodium hydroxide. **Store** in airtight containers. Protect from light.

Methdilazine Hydrochloride (6149-j)

Methdilazine Hydrochloride (*BANM, rINNM*).

$C_{18}H_{20}N_2S,HCl = 332.9$.

CAS — 1229-35-2.

Pharmacopoeias. In *US*.

A light tan crystalline powder with a slight characteristic odour. **Soluble** 1 in 2 of water and of alcohol, and 1 in 6 of chloroform; practically insoluble in ether; soluble 1 in 1 of 0.1M hydrochloric acid and 0.1M sodium hydroxide solution. A 1% solution in water has a pH of 4.8 to 6.0. **Store** in airtight containers. Protect from light.

Adverse Effects and Precautions

As for the sedating antihistamines in general, p.397.

Interactions

As for the sedating antihistamines in general, p.399.

Uses and Administration

Methdilazine, a phenothiazine derivative, is a sedating antihistamine with antimuscarinic and sedative activity. Methdilazine is also reported to have serotonin-antagonist properties.

Methdilazine hydrochloride is used for the symptomatic relief of hypersensitivity reactions and particularly for the control of pruritic skin disorders (p.400); it has also been given for migraine prophylaxis (p.443), but is usually reserved for use after other prophylactic drugs have proved to be ineffective or unsuitable. It is given by mouth in doses of 8 mg 2 to 4 times daily. Children over 3 years of age have been given half the adult dose. Methdilazine base has been used in similar doses.

Preparations

USP 23: Methdilazine Hydrochloride Syrup; Methdilazine Hydrochloride Tablets; Methdilazine Tablets.

Proprietary Preparations (details are given in Part 3)
Austral.: Dilosyn; ***USA:*** Tacaryl†.

Mizolastine (15293-q)

Mizolastine (*BAN, rINN*).

SL-85.0324-00. 2-{1-[1-(4-Fluorobenzyl)-1*H*-benzimidazol-2-yl]-4-piperidyl(methyl)amino}pyrimidin-4(1*H*)-one.

$C_{24}H_{25}FN_6O = 432.5$.

CAS — 108612-45-9.

Adverse Effects and Precautions

As for the non-sedating antihistamines in general, p.397. Mizolastine has only a weak potential to prolong the QT interval and has not been associated with arrhythmias. However, the manufacturers have warned against the use of mizolastine in patients with significant cardiac or hepatic disease, with known or suspected hypokalaemia or other electrolyte imbalance, or with known or suspected QT prolongation. The concomitant administration of drugs liable to interfere with the hepatic metabolism of mizolastine and of other potentially arrhythmogenic drugs should also be avoided (see under Interactions, below).

Interactions

As for the non-sedating antihistamines in general, p.399. Moderate increases in plasma concentrations of mizolastine have been reported following administration of *erythromycin* and *ketoconazole*; their concurrent use is contra-indicated by the manufacturer. They also advise against the concurrent use of drugs known to prolong the QT interval, such as class I and III antiarrhythmics, with mizolastine.

Other potent inhibitors or substrates for the hepatic metabolism of mizolastine include cimetidine, cyclosporin, and nifedipine; caution is advised with concurrent administration.

Pharmacokinetics

Mizolastine is rapidly absorbed from the gastro-intestinal tract with peak plasma concentrations being reached after about 1.5 hours. Plasma protein binding is about 98%. The mean elimination half-life is 13 hours. Mizolastine is mainly metabolised by glucuronidation although other metabolic pathways are involved, including metabolism by the cytochrome P450 isoenzyme CYP3A4, with the formation of inactive hydroxylated metabolites.

References.

1. Rosenzweig P, *et al.* Pharmacodynamics and pharmacokinetics of mizolastine (SL 85.0324), a new nonsedative H_1 antihistamine. *Ann Allergy* 1992; **69:** 135–9.

Uses and Administration

Mizolastine is a non-sedating antihistamine with a long duration of action. It does not have significant sedative or antimuscarinic actions; it is reported to have mast-cell stabilising properties. Mizolastine is used for the symptomatic relief of allergic conditions including rhinitis (p.400), conjunctivitis (p.399), and skin disorders such as urticaria (p.401). The dose, by mouth, is 10 mg daily.

References.

1. Leynadier F, *et al.* Efficacy and safety of mizolastine in seasonal allergic rhinitis. *Ann Allergy Asthma Immunol* 1996; **76:** 163–8.
2. Stern MA, *et al.* Can an antihistamine delay appearance of hay-fever symptoms when given prior to pollen season? *Allergy* 1997; **52:** 440–4.

Preparations

Proprietary Preparations (details are given in Part 3)
Neth.: Mizollen; ***UK:*** Mistamine; Mizollen.

Niaprazine (13006-j)

Niaprazine *(rINN)*.

1709-CERM. *N*-[3-(4-*p*-Fluorophenylpiperazin-1-yl)-1-methylpropyl]nicotinamide.

$C_{20}H_{25}FN_4O = 356.4$.
CAS — 27367-90-4.

Niaprazine, a piperazine derivative, is an antihistamine used in children for its sedative and hypnotic properties. The usual dose by mouth is 1 mg per kg body-weight at night.

Preparations

Proprietary Preparations (details are given in Part 3)
Fr.: Nopron; ***Ital.:*** Nopron.

Olopatadine Hydrochloride (15042-e)

Olopatadine Hydrochloride *(USAN, pINNM)*.

ALO-4943A; KW-4679. 11-[(*Z*)-3-(Dimethylamino)propylidene]-6,11-dihydrodibenz[*b,e*]oxepin-2-acetic acid hydrochloride.

$C_{21}H_{23}NO_3,HCl = 373.9$.
CAS — 113806-05-6 (olopatadine); 140462-76-6 (olopatadine hydrochloride).

Olopatadine hydrochloride is an antihistamine with mast-cell stabilising properties. It is used as eye drops containing the equivalent of 0.1% of olopatadine base in allergic conjunctivitis (p.399). Headache and stinging or burning of the eye have occurred after administration.

References.

1. Anonymous. Olopatadine for allergic conjunctivitis. *Med Lett Drugs Ther* 1997; **39:** 108–9.

Preparations

Proprietary Preparations (details are given in Part 3)
USA: Patanol.

Oxatomide (13056-n)

Oxatomide *(BAN, USAN, rINN)*.

R-35443. 1-[3-(4-Benzhydrylpiperazin-1-yl)propyl]benzimidazolin-2-one.

$C_{27}H_{30}N_4O = 426.6$.
CAS — 60607-34-3.

Adverse Effects and Precautions

As for the sedating antihistamines in general, see p.397. Increased appetite and weight gain have been reported, particularly at higher doses.

Oxatomide should be given with caution in patients with hepatic impairment.

Acute dystonic reactions and long-lasting impaired consciousness were associated with oxatomide therapy in 6 children.[1] Impaired consciousness varied from lethargy and somnolence to a clinical picture resembling encephalitis and persisted for 2 days or more in three patients. Plasma-oxatomide concentrations were measured in three patients and found to be high, although two of these had been given the recommended dose.

1. Casteels-Van Daele M, *et al.* Acute dystonic reactions and long-lasting impaired consciousness associated with oxatomide in children. *Lancet* 1986; **i:** 1204–5.

Interactions

As for the sedating antihistamines in general, p.399.

Pharmacokinetics

Peak plasma concentrations of oxatomide are achieved within 4 hours of administration by mouth. More than 90% of oxatomide in the circulation is bound to plasma proteins. Oxatomide is extensively metabolised; unchanged drug and metabolites are excreted in the urine and the faeces. Reported values for the terminal elimination half-life have generally been in the range of 20 to 30 hours.

References.

1. Paton DM, Webster DR. Clinical pharmacokinetics of H_1-receptor antagonists (the antihistamines). *Clin Pharmacokinet* 1985; **10:** 477–97.

Uses and Administration

Oxatomide, a piperazine derivative, is a sedating antihistamine that has also been reported to have mast-cell stabilising properties.

Oxatomide is used for the symptomatic relief of allergic conditions including urticaria (p.401), rhinitis (p.400), and conjunctivitis (p.399). Oxatomide is given by mouth as the anhydrous substance or as the monohydrate. The usual dose of anhydrous oxatomide is 30 mg twice daily although up to 60 mg twice daily may be necessary in some cases.

References.

1. Richards DM, *et al.* Oxatomide: a review of its pharmacodynamic properties and therapeutic efficacy. *Drugs* 1984; **27:** 210–31.

Preparations

Proprietary Preparations (details are given in Part 3)
Aust.: Tinset; ***Belg.:*** Tinset; ***Fr.:*** Tinset; ***Ger.:*** Tinset; ***Ital.:*** Tinset; ***Neth.:*** Tinset; ***S.Afr.:*** Tinset; ***Spain:*** Atoxan†; Cobiona; Oxatokey; Oxleti; Tanzal; ***Switz.:*** Tinset†; ***UK:*** Tinset†.

Oxomemazine (6151-p)

Oxomemazine *(rINN)*.

RP-6847; Trimeprazine *SS*-Dioxide. 10-(3-Dimethylamino-2-methylpropyl)phenothiazine 5,5-dioxide.

$C_{18}H_{22}N_2O_2S = 330.4$.
CAS — 3689-50-7.

Oxomemazine Hydrochloride (6152-s)

Oxomemazine Hydrochloride *(rINNM)*.

$C_{18}H_{22}N_2O_2S,HCl = 366.9$.
CAS — 4784-40-1.

Pharmacopoeias. In *Fr.*

Oxomemazine hydrochloride 11.1 mg is approximately equivalent to 10 mg of oxomemazine.

Oxomemazine, a phenothiazine derivative, is a sedating antihistamine used for the symptomatic relief of hypersensitivity reactions and in pruritic skin disorders (p.400). It is also an ingredient of compound preparations for the symptomatic treatment of coughs and the common cold (p.400).

It is given by mouth in doses equivalent to 10 to 40 mg of oxomemazine daily. Oxomemazine may also be administered by the rectal route. Oxomemazine hydrochloride has been used similarly by mouth.

Preparations

Proprietary Preparations (details are given in Part 3)
Belg.: Doxergan; ***Neth.:*** Doxergan†.

Multi-ingredient: ***Aust.:*** Aplexil; ***Belg.:*** Rectoplexil; Toplexil; ***Fr.:*** Rectoplexil; Toplexil; ***Ger.:*** Aplexil†; ***Neth.:*** Toplexil; ***Switz.:*** Toplexil.

Phenindamine Tartrate (6153-w)

Phenindamine Tartrate *(BANM, USAN, rINNM)*.

Phenindamine Acid Tartrate; Phenindamini Tartras; Phenindaminium Tartrate. 1,2,3,4-Tetrahydro-2-methyl-9-phenyl-2-azafluorene hydrogen tartrate; 2,3,4,9-Tetrahydro-2-methyl-9-phenyl-1*H*-indeno[2,1-*c*]pyridine hydrogen tartrate.

$C_{19}H_{19}N,C_4H_6O_6 = 411.4$.
CAS — 82-88-2 (phenindamine); 569-59-5 (phenindamine tartrate).

Pharmacopoeias. In *Br.*

A white or almost white, odourless or almost odourless, voluminous powder. Sparingly **soluble** in water; slightly soluble in alcohol; practically insoluble in chloroform and in ether. A 1% solution in water has a pH of 3.4 to 3.9. **Protect** from light.

Adverse Effects and Precautions

As for the sedating antihistamines in general, see p.397. Phenindamine tartrate may have a stimulant effect in certain individuals; to avoid the possibility of insomnia patients may be advised to take the last dose of the day several hours before retiring.

Interactions

As for the sedating antihistamines in general, p.399.

Uses and Administration

Phenindamine, a piperidine derivative, is a sedating antihistamine; however it may be mildly stimulating in certain individuals. It is used as the tartrate for the symptomatic relief of allergic conditions including urticaria (p.401) and rhinitis (p.400), and as an ingredient of compound preparations for coughs and the common cold (p.400).

Phenindamine tartrate is given in doses of 25 to 50 mg up to three times daily. Children over 6 years of age have been given up to 75 mg daily in divided doses.

Preparations

BP 1998: Phenindamine Tablets.

Proprietary Preparations (details are given in Part 3)
Irl.: Thephorin; ***UK:*** Thephorin; ***USA:*** Nolahist.

Multi-ingredient: ***USA:*** Nolamine; P-V-Tussin.

Pheniramine (14746-l)

Pheniramine *(BAN, rINN)*.

Prophenpyridamine. *NN*-Dimethyl-3-phenyl-3-(2-pyridyl)propylamine.

$C_{16}H_{20}N_2 = 240.3$.
CAS — 86-21-5.

Pheniramine Aminosalicylate (10013-l)

Pheniramine *p*-Aminosalicylate; Pheniramine 4-Aminosalicylate; Pheniramine Para-aminosalicylate. Pheniramine 4-amino-2-hydroxybenzoate.

$C_{16}H_{20}N_2,C_7H_7NO_3 = 393.5$.
CAS — 3269-83-8.

Pheniramine Maleate (6154-e)

Pheniramine Maleate *(BANM, USAN, rINNM)*.

Pheniramini Maleas; Pheniraminium Maleate; Prophenpyridamine Maleate. Pheniramine hydrogen maleate.

$C_{16}H_{20}N_2,C_4H_4O_4 = 356.4$.
CAS — 132-20-7.

Pharmacopoeias. In *Eur.* (see p.viii) and *US.*

A white crystalline powder; odourless or with a slight odour. M.p. 106° to 109°. Ph. Eur. **solubilities**: very soluble in water; freely soluble in alcohol, in dichloromethane, and in methyl alcohol. USP solubilities: soluble in water and in alcohol. A 1% solution in water has a pH of 4.5 to 5.5. **Protect** from light.

Adverse Effects and Precautions

As for the sedating antihistamines in general, p.397.

Abuse. References to the abuse of pheniramine by mouth.

1. Jones IH, *et al.* Pheniramine as an hallucinogen. *Med J Aust* 1973; **1:** 382–6.
2. Csillag ER, Landauer AA. Alleged hallucinogenic effect of a toxic overdose of an antihistamine preparation. *Med J Aust* 1973; **1:** 653–4.
3. Buckley NA, *et al.* Pheniramine—a much abused drug. *Med J Aust* 1994; **160:** 188–92.

Interactions

As for the sedating antihistamines in general, p.399.

Pharmacokinetics

The pharmacokinetics of pheniramine and its metabolites, *N*-desmethylpheniramine and *N*-didesmethylpheniramine, were investigated in 6 healthy subjects.[1] After oral administration of pheniramine aminosalicylate, peak-plasma pheniramine concentrations were reached in 1 to 2.5 hours. The terminal half-life ranged between 8 and 17 hours after intravenous administration (pheniramine maleate) and 16 and 19 hours after oral administration. The total recovery of pheniramine as unchanged drug and metabolites from the urine was 68 to 94% of the intravenous dose and 70 to 83% of the oral dose.

1. Witte PU, *et al.* Pharmacokinetics of pheniramine (Avil®) and metabolites in healthy subjects after oral and intravenous administration. *Int J Clin Pharmacol Ther Toxicol* 1985; **23:** 59–62.

Uses and Administration

Pheniramine, an alkylamine derivative, is a sedating antihistamine with antimuscarinic and moderate sedative properties.

It is used as the maleate or aminosalicylate for the symptomatic relief of allergic conditions including urticaria and angioedema (p.401), rhinitis (p.400), and conjunctivitis (p.399), and in pruritic skin disorders (p.400). It has also been used for its antiemetic properties in the prevention and control of motion sickness (p.400). Pheniramine maleate is used as an ingredient of compound preparations for the symptomatic treatment of coughs and the common cold (p.400). It is also used in combination with a decongestant in eye and nasal preparations.

Pheniramine maleate is given by mouth in a dose of 15 to 30 mg two or three times daily. In some countries pheniramine maleate has been administered parenterally.

Usual doses of the aminosalicylate are 25 to 50 mg two or three times daily by mouth.

The hydrochloride and the tannate have also been used.

Preparations

Proprietary Preparations (details are given in Part 3)

Aust.: Avil; ***Austral.:*** Aller-G†; Avil; Avilettes†; Fenamine; ***Belg.:*** Avil; ***Ger.:*** Avil; Aviletten†; ***Irl.:*** Daneral; ***Ital.:*** Inhiston; ***S.Afr.:*** Avil†; ***UK:*** Daneral†.

Multi-ingredient: ***Aust.:*** Neo Citran; Peremin; ***Austral.:*** Avil Decongestant; Avil†; Naphcon-A; ***Belg.:*** Naphcon-A†; Triaminic†; ***Canad.:*** Ak-Vernacon; Antitussive Decongestant Antihistamine Syrup; Bronchodex D; Bronchodex Pediatrique; Bronchosirum; Caldomine-DH; Calmylin Ace; Centracol DM; Centracol Pediatrique; Citron Chaud; Citron Chaud DM; Cold Decongestant; Contac Night-Time Hot Drink†; Diopticon A; Dirouget†; Dristan; Hot Lemon Relief; Naphcon-A; Neo Citran; Neo Citran A; Neo Citran DM; Neo Citran Nutrasweet; Opcon-A; Pharmacol DM; Pharminicol DM; Pulmorphan; Pulmorphan Pediatrique; Robitussin AC; Robitussin with Codeine; Tantacol DM; Triaminic; Triaminic Expectorant DH; Triaminicin; Trisulfaminic; Tussaminic C; Tussaminic DH; ***Fr.:*** Febrispir†; Fervex; Triaminic; ***Ger.:*** Cosavil†; Konjunktival Thilo; Rhinosovil; ***Irl.:*** Triominic; ***Ital.:*** Medramil; Senodin-AN; Tetramil; Triaminic; Triaminicflu; Triaminicol†; ***S.Afr.:*** Allertac; Calasthetic; Coff-Up; Degoran; Triami†; Triaminic; ***Spain:*** Triominic; ***Switz.:*** Nasello; Neo Citran; Neo-Urtisan; Triaminic†; ***UK:*** Triominic; ***USA:*** Ak-Con-A; Dristan Nasal Spray; Fiogesic†; Iohist D; Nafazair A; Naphazole-A; Naphazoline Plus; Naphcon-A; Naphoptic-A; Opcon-A; Poly-Histine; Poly-Histine D; Rolatuss with Hydrocodone; Ru-Tuss with Hydrocodone; S-T Forte; Scot-Tussin Original 5-Action; Statuss Green; Triaminic Expectorant DH; Triaminic Oral Infant; Tussirex; Vetuss HC.

Phenyltoloxamine Citrate (6155-l)

Phenyltoloxamine Citrate *(BANM, rINNM).*

C-5581H (phenyltoloxamine); Phenyltolyloxamine Citrate; PRN (phenyltoloxamine). 2-(2-Benzylphenoxy)-*NN*-dimethylethylamine dihydrogen citrate.

$C_{17}H_{21}NO,C_6H_8O_7$ = 447.5.

CAS — 92-12-6 (phenyltoloxamine); 1176-08-5 (phenyltoloxamine citrate).

Phenyltoloxamine citrate, an ethanolamine derivative, is a sedating antihistamine. It is usually given by mouth in combination preparations with a decongestant or analgesic. Phenyltoloxamine citrate has been used in nasal preparations. Phenyltoloxamine polistirex has also been administered by mouth.

Preparations

Proprietary Preparations (details are given in Part 3)

Multi-ingredient: ***Aust.:*** Codipront; Codipront cum Expectorans; ***Austral.:*** Sinutab with Codeine†; ***Belg.:*** Sinutab; ***Canad.:*** Omni-Tuss; Sinutab SA; Tussionex; ***Fr.:*** Biocidan; Netux; Rinurel; Rinutan; ***Ger.:*** Codipront; Codipront cum Expectorans†; ergo sanol spezial†; Naldecol†; ***Ital.:*** Codipront; ***S.Afr.:*** Adco-Sinal Co; Decon†; Pholtex; Sinustop with Codeine†; Sinustop†; Sinutab; Sinutab with Codeine; Suncodin†; ***Spain:*** Codipront; ***Switz.:*** Codipront; Codipront cum Expectorans; Ergosanol special; Ergosanol special a la cafeine; ***UK:*** Sinutab Nightime; ***USA:*** Aceta-Gesic; Biotab†; Comhist LA; Decongestabs; Decongestant; Decongestant SR; Flextra; Iohist D; Kutrase; Lobac; Magsal; Major-gesic; Medatussin Plus†; Menoplex; Mobigesic; Momentum; Myogesic; Naldec Pediatric†; Naldecon; Nalgest; Nalspan Pediatric; New Decongestant Pediatric; Norel Plus; Par Decon†; Percogesic; Phena-Chlor†; Phenylgesic; Poly-Histine; Poly-Histine D; Quadra Hist; Tri-Phen-Chlor TR; Uni-Decon.

Pimethixene (13118-f)

Pimethixene *(rINN).*

BP-400; Pimetixene. 9-(1-Methyl-4-piperidylidene)thioxanthene.

$C_{19}H_{19}NS$ = 293.4.

CAS — 314-03-4.

Pimethixene is reported to be a sedating antihistamine and an inhibitor of serotonin. It is given by mouth to children as a sedative and for the treatment of respiratory disorders.

Preparations

Proprietary Preparations (details are given in Part 3)

Fr.: Calmixene; ***Switz.:*** Sedosil.

Piprinhydrinate (6156-y)

Piprinhydrinate *(BAN, rINN).*

Diphenylpyraline Teoclate; Diphenylpyraline Theoclate. The diphenylpyraline salt of 8-chlorotheophylline; 4-Benzhydryloxy-1-methylpiperidine salt of 8-chlorotheophylline.

$C_{19}H_{23}NO,C_7H_7ClN_4O_2$ = 496.0.

CAS — 606-90-6.

Piprinhydrinate, a piperidine derivative, is an antihistamine given by mouth as an ingredient of compound preparations for the symptomatic relief of coughs and the common cold.

Preparations

Proprietary Preparations (details are given in Part 3)

Multi-ingredient: ***Aust.:*** Influvidon; ***Ger.:*** Kolton grippale N.

Promethazine (6101-r)

Promethazine *(BAN, rINN).*

Dimethyl (1-methyl-2-phenothiazin-10-ylethyl)amine.

$C_{17}H_{20}N_2S$ = 284.4.

CAS — 60-87-7.

Promethazine Hydrochloride (6102-f)

Promethazine Hydrochloride *(BANM, rINNM).*

Diprazinum; Proazamine Chloride; Promethazini Hydrochloridum; Promethazinium Chloride.

$C_{17}H_{20}N_2S,HCl$ = 320.9.

CAS — 58-33-3.

Pharmacopoeias. In *Chin., Eur.* (see p.viii), *Int., Jpn, Pol.,* and *US.*

A white or faintly yellow, practically odourless, crystalline powder. On prolonged exposure to air it is slowly oxidised, becoming blue in colour. **Solubilities** are: very to freely soluble in water; freely soluble in alcohol, in hot dehydrated alcohol, in chloroform, and in dichloromethane; practically insoluble in acetone, in ether, and in ethyl acetate. Both a 5% and a 10% solution in water have a pH of 4 to 5. **Store** in airtight containers. Protect from light.

Solutions of promethazine hydrochloride are **incompatible** with alkaline substances, which precipitate the insoluble promethazine base. Compounds reported to be incompatible with promethazine hydrochloride include aminophylline, barbiturates, benzylpenicillin salts, carbenicillin sodium, chloramphenicol sodium succinate, chlorothiazide sodium, cefmetazole sodium, cefoperazone sodium, cefotetan disodium, dimenhydrinate, doxorubicin hydrochloride (in a liposomal formulation), frusemide, heparin sodium, hydrocortisone sodium succinate, methicillin sodium, morphine sulphate, nalbuphine hydrochloride, and some contrast media and parenteral nutrient solutions.

Adsorption. References[1-4] to studies of the adsorption of promethazine hydrochloride onto various glass and plastic containers and infusion systems. Factors affecting the degree of adsorption included the particular material tested and the pH of the solution.

1. Kowaluk EA, *et al.* Interactions between drugs and polyvinyl chloride infusion bags. *Am J Hosp Pharm* 1981; **38:** 1308–14.
2. Kowaluk EA, *et al.* Interactions between drugs and intravenous delivery systems. *Am J Hosp Pharm* 1982; **39:** 460–7.
3. Rhodes RS, *et al.* Stability of meperidine hydrochloride, promethazine hydrochloride, and atropine sulfate in plastic syringes. *Am J Hosp Pharm* 1985; **42:** 112–5.
4. Martens HJ, *et al.* Sorption of various drugs in polyvinyl chloride, glass, and polyethylene-lined infusion containers. *Am J Hosp Pharm* 1990; **47:** 369–73.

Promethazine Theoclate (6103-d)

Promethazine Theoclate *(BAN).*

Promethazine Teoclate *(rINN).* The promethazine salt of 8-chlorotheophylline.

$C_{17}H_{20}N_2S,C_7H_7ClN_4O_2$ = 499.0.

CAS — 17693-51-5.

Pharmacopoeias. In *Br.*

A white or almost white odourless or almost odourless powder. Promethazine theoclate 1.5 mg is approximately equivalent to 1 mg of promethazine hydrochloride.

Very slightly **soluble** in water; sparingly soluble in alcohol; freely soluble in chloroform; practically insoluble in ether. **Protect** from light.

Adverse Effects

As for the sedating antihistamines in general, see p.397.

Cardiovascular side-effects are more commonly seen after injection, and bradycardia, tachycardia, transient minor increases in blood pressure, and occasional hypotension have all been reported with promethazine hydrochloride. Jaundice and blood dyscrasias have been reported, and extrapyramidal effects may occur at high doses.

Venous thrombosis has been reported at the site of intravenous injections, and arteriospasm and gangrene may follow inadvertent intra-arterial injection.

Overdosage. A toxic neurological syndrome which included CNS depression, acute excitomotor manifestations, ataxia and visual hallucinations, plus peripheral antimuscarinic effects developed in 2 children aged 44 months and 16 months after topical application of a 2% promethazine cream providing between 12.9 and 26 mg per kg body-weight.[1] The older child had also received hydroxyzine 10 mg by mouth 1 hour earlier.

1. Shawn DH, McGuigan MA. Poisoning from dermal absorption of promethazine. *Can Med Assoc J* 1984; **130:** 1460–1.

Sudden infant death syndrome. Although some early reports raised the possibility of an association between the use of phenothiazine antihistamines and the sudden infant death syndrome (SIDS) this has not been confirmed. Following an initial report that 4 of 7 infants with SIDS had been given trimeprazine before death and that a series of severe apnoeic crises had been observed in the twin of a SIDS victim given promethazine,[1] the same workers studied 52 SIDS victims, 36 near-miss infants, and 175 control subjects to investigate the role of nasopharyngitis and phenothiazines in this syndrome.[2] It was found that there was no difference in the incidence of nasopharyngitis between the 3 groups, but that the proportion of infants given phenothiazines was higher in both the SIDS group (23%) and the near-miss group (22%) than in the control group (2%). In a subsequent study,[3] they found that the incidence of central and obstructive sleep apnoeas was increased in 4 healthy infants given promethazine for 3 days, although the duration of the attacks was unaltered and generally short, with a range of 3 to 10 seconds. A report on behalf of the Commission of the European Communities,[4] stated that no link between sudden deaths in infants and drug administration had been confirmed by national drug monitoring centres. It was likely that the risk of apnoea was associated with all sedative drugs, especially in overdose.[4] Previously, phenothiazine-induced hyperthermia had been proposed as a contributory factor in SIDS.[5]

As recently as 1994 concern has been expressed[6] that promethazine was frequently prescribed for children under 2 years despite recommendations to the contrary. The current view in the UK and USA is that phenothiazine antihistamines such as promethazine and trimeprazine should not be given to children under 2 years of age, primarily because the safety of such use has not been established.

1. Kahn A, Blum D. Possible role of phenothiazines in sudden infant death. *Lancet* 1979; **ii:** 364–5.
2. Kahn A, Blum D. Phenothiazines and sudden infant death syndrome. *Pediatrics* 1982; **70:** 75–8.
3. Kahn A, *et al.* Phenothiazine-induced sleep apneas in normal infants. *Pediatrics* 1985; **75:** 844–7.
4. Cockfield. Phenergan, Theralene, Algotropyl—drugs responsible for the death of new-born babies. *Off J EC* 1986; **29:** C130/25–6.
5. Stanton AN. Sudden infant death syndrome and phenothiazines. *Pediatrics* 1983; **71:** 986–7.
6. Pollard AJ, Rylance G. Inappropriate prescribing of promethazine in infants. *Arch Dis Child* 1994; **70:** 357.

Precautions

As for the sedating antihistamines in general, p.398.

Intravenous injections of promethazine hydrochloride must be given slowly and extreme care must be taken to avoid extravasation or inadvertent intra-arterial injection, due to the risk of severe irritation. Promethazine should not be given by subcutaneous injection.

False negative and positive results have been reported with some pregnancy tests.

Anaesthesia. In 8 healthy subjects promethazine 25 mg intravenously decreased lower oesophageal sphincter pressure and increased the incidence of gastro-oesophageal reflux.[1] It might, therefore, increase the risk of regurgitation and aspiration of gastric contents during induction of and recovery from anaesthesia. The effect was attributed to the antimuscarinic properties of promethazine.

1. Brock-Utne JG, *et al.* The action of commonly used antiemetics on the lower oesophageal sphincter. *Br J Anaesth* 1978; **50:** 295–8.

Children. A possible association between phenothiazine sedatives and sudden infant death syndrome has been suggested, but has not been confirmed (see under Adverse Effects, above). The current view in the UK and USA is that promethazine should not be given to children under 2 years of age, primarily because the safety of such use has not been established.

Porphyria. Promethazine was considered to be unsafe in patients with acute porphyria although there is conflicting experimental evidence on porphyrinogenicity.[1]

1. Moore MR, McColl KEL. *Porphyria: drug lists.* Glasgow: Porphyria Research Unit, University of Glasgow, 1991.

Pregnancy. For discussion of the use of antihistamines in pregnancy, including studies involving phenothiazines, see p.398.

Renal impairment. Phenothiazine-induced toxic psychosis occurred in 5 patients with chronic renal failure; one had been given promethazine and 4 chlorpromazine.[1]

1. McAllister CJ, *et al.* Toxic psychosis induced by phenothiazine administration in patients with chronic renal failure. *Clin Nephrol* 1978; **10:** 191–5.

Interactions

As for the sedating antihistamines in general, p.399.

Pharmacokinetics

Promethazine is well absorbed after oral or intramuscular administration. Peak plasma concentrations have been observed 2 to 3 hours after administration by these routes, although there is low systemic bioavailability after oral administration, due to high first-pass metabolism in the liver. Promethazine is widely distributed; it enters the brain, crosses the placenta, and passes into breast milk. Values ranging from 76 to 93% have been reported for plasma-protein binding. Promethazine undergoes extensive metabolism, predominantly to promethazine sulphoxide, and also to *N*-desmethylpromethazine. It is excreted slowly via the urine and bile, chiefly as metabolites. Elimination half-lives of 5 to 14 hours have been reported.

References.

1. Taylor G, *et al.* Pharmacokinetics of promethazine and its sulphoxide metabolite after intravenous and oral administration to man. *Br J Clin Pharmacol* 1983; **15:** 287–93.
2. Paton DM, Webster DR. Clinical pharmacokinetics of H_1-receptor antagonists (the antihistamines). *Clin Pharmacokinet* 1985; **10:** 477–97.
3. Stavchansky S, *et al.* Bioequivalence and pharmacokinetic profile of promethazine hydrochloride suppositories in humans. *J Pharm Sci* 1987; **76:** 441–5.

Uses and Administration

Promethazine, a phenothiazine derivative, is a sedating antihistamine with antimuscarinic, significant sedative, and some serotonin-antagonist properties. It is usually given as the hydrochloride or theoclate. The antihistamine action has been reported to last for between 4 and 12 hours.

Promethazine hydrochloride is used for the symptomatic relief of allergic conditions including urticaria and angioedema (p.401), rhinitis (p.400) and conjunctivitis (p.399), and in pruritic skin disorders (p.400).

Promethazine hydrochloride and promethazine theoclate are used for their antiemetic action in the prevention and treatment of nausea and vomiting in conditions such as motion sickness, drug-induced vomiting, and postoperative vomiting (p.400). They are also used for the symptomatic treatment of nausea and vertigo caused by Ménière's disease and other vestibular disorders (p.401). Promethazine hydrochloride is also employed pre- and postoperatively in surgery and obstetrics for its sedative effects and for the relief of apprehension (p.399); it is often given in association with pethidine hydrochloride. Promethazine hydrochloride may be used for night-time sedation (p.400).

Promethazine hydrochloride is a common ingredient of compound preparations for the symptomatic treatment of coughs and the common cold (p.400).

For the treatment of allergic conditions promethazine hydrochloride is usually given by mouth in a dose of 25 mg at night increased to 25 mg twice daily if necessary; owing to its pronounced sedative effect it is preferably given at night but an alternative dose is 10 to 20 mg two or three times daily. Promethazine hydrochloride is given in doses of 20 to 50 mg at night for the short-term management of insomnia although its prolonged duration of action can lead to considerable drowsiness the following day. For the prevention of motion sickness promethazine hydrochloride can be given in a dose of 25 mg the night before travelling followed by a further 25 mg the following morning if necessary. Promethazine is also given as the theoclate for the prevention and treatment of nausea and vomiting. For the prevention of motion sickness the recommended dose of promethazine theoclate is 25 mg at night or 25 mg one to two hours before travelling. For nausea and vomiting arising from causes such as labyrinthitis a dose of 25 mg at night is usually adequate, but this may be increased to 25 mg two to three times daily if necessary to a maximum of 100 mg daily.

In children the following oral doses of promethazine hydrochloride have been recommended. For allergic conditions: 2 to 5 years, 5 to 15 mg daily in one or two divided doses; 5 to 10 years, 10 to 25 mg daily in one or two divided doses. For night sedation: 2 to 5 years, 15 to 20 mg; 5 to 10 years, 20 to 25 mg. For the prevention of motion sickness the following doses of promethazine hydrochloride may be given the night before the journey and repeated on the following morning if necessary: 2 to 5 years, 5 mg; 5 to 10 years, 10 mg. Promethazine theoclate may also be given to children aged 5 to 10 years for the prevention of motion sickness in a dose of 12.5 mg daily, starting either on the night before travelling for long journeys or one to two hours before short journeys.

Promethazine hydrochloride is also administered by the rectal route as suppositories. Doses are similar to those given by mouth.

Promethazine hydrochloride is given by deep intramuscular injection as a solution of 25 or 50 mg per mL. It may be given by slow intravenous injection or injected into the tubing of a freely running infusion in a concentration of not more than 25 mg per mL, although it is usually diluted to 2.5 mg per mL. The rate of infusion should not exceed 25 mg per minute. The usual parenteral dose for all indications apart from nausea and vomiting is 25 to 50 mg; a dose of 100 mg should not be exceeded. Doses of 12.5 to 25 mg, repeated at intervals of not less than 4 hours, may be given for the treatment of nausea and vomiting, although not more than 100 mg is usually given in 24 hours.

Children aged 5 to 10 years may be given 6.25 to 12.5 mg of promethazine hydrochloride by deep intramuscular injection.

Promethazine has been used topically to provide relief in hypersensitivity disorders of the skin and for burns but as with other antihistamines it may produce skin sensitisation.

Promethazine embonate and promethazine maleate have also been administered by mouth. Promethazine dioxide (Dioxopromethazine) has been used as the hydrochloride in eye and nose drops.

Eclampsia and pre-eclampsia. See under Sedation, below.

Sedation. Drug combinations known as lytic cocktails have been used in many countries for the management of pre-eclampsia and imminent eclampsia. The cocktail has usually consisted of a combination of chlorpromazine, pethidine, and/or promethazine.[1] However, phenothiazines are not generally recommended late in pregnancy. The more usual treatment of pre-eclampsia and eclampsia is primarily aimed at reducing hypertension (see Hypertension in Pregnancy, under Hypertension, p.788); the management of eclampsia, which is the convulsive phase, is discussed on p.338.

Lytic cocktails have also been used for sedation and analgesia in paediatric patients. However, there is a high rate of therapeutic failure as well as serious adverse effects with such combinations, and the American Academy of Pediatrics[2] has recommended that alternative sedatives and analgesics should be considered; guidelines have been drawn up should it be appropriate to use a lytic cocktail.

1. WHO. The hypertensive disorders of pregnancy: report of a WHO study group. *WHO Tech Rep Ser 758* 1987.
2. American Academy of Pediatrics Committee on Drugs. Reappraisal of Lytic cocktail/Demerol, Phenergan, and Thorazine (DPT) for the sedation of children. *Pediatrics* 1995; **95:** 598–602.

Preparations

BP 1998: Promethazine Hydrochloride Tablets; Promethazine Injection; Promethazine Oral Solution; Promethazine Teoclate Tablets;
USP 23: Promethazine Hydrochloride Injection; Promethazine Hydrochloride Suppositories; Promethazine Hydrochloride Syrup; Promethazine Hydrochloride Tablets.

Proprietary Preparations (details are given in Part 3)
Aust.: Phenergan†; ***Austral.:*** Avomine; Phenergan; Progant†; Prothazine†; ***Belg.:*** Phenergan; ***Canad.:*** Histantil; Phenergan; ***Fr.:*** Phenergan; ***Ger.:*** Atosil; Eusedon mono; Promkiddi†; Prothanon; Soporil†; ***Irl.:*** Avomine; Phenergan; ***Ital.:*** Allerfen; Crema Anitallergica Antipruriginosa†; Duplamin; Fargan; Farganesse; Fenazil; ***Neth.:*** Phenergan; ***Norw.:*** Phenergan; ***S.Afr.:*** Brunazine; Daralix; Lenazine; Phenergan; Prohist; Promahist†; Receptozine; ***Spain:*** Fenergan Topico; Frinova; Sayomol; ***Swed.:*** Lergigan; ***Switz.:*** Phenergan; ***UK:*** Avomine; Phenergan; Phenhalal; Q-Mazine; Sominex; ***USA:*** Anergan; K-Phen; Pentazine†; Phenameth†; Phenazine; Phenergan; Phenoject†; Pro; Promet 50†; Prometh†; Promethegan; Prorex†; Prothazine; V-Gan†.

Multi-ingredient: ***Austral.:*** Adalixin (New Formula)†; Adalixin C†; Painstop; Panadol Elixir with Promethazine†; Panquil; Phenergan†; Phensedyl; Prodalix Forte Cough Linctus-New Formula†; Prodalix Forte Cough Linctus†; Seda-Quell†; Tixylix; ***Belg.:*** Phenergan Expectorant; Quintex; Quintex Pediatrique; ***Canad.:*** Pamergan†; Phenergan Expectorant; Phenergan Expectorant with Codeine; Phenergan VC Expectorant; Phenergan VC Expectorant with Codeine; Promatussin DM; ***Fr.:*** Algotropyl; Fluisedal; Insomnyl†; Paxeladine Noctee; Quintopan Enfant; Rhinathiol Promethazine; Transmer†; Tussisedal; ***Ger.:*** Prothanon†; Prothazin; Pruriderm ultra†; Thesit P; ***Irl.:*** Night Nurse; Tixylix; ***Ital.:*** Difmetus Compositum; Nuleron; ***Neth.:*** Phenergan Expectorant†; ***S.Afr.:*** Acustop; Antituss; Ban Pain; Brunacod; Colcaps; Darosed; Dimiprol†; Dynapayne; End Pain†; Go-Pain; Goldgesic†; Histodor; Infacet†; Infapain Forte; Lenazine Forte; Lentogesic; Lesspain; Maxadol; Megapyn; Painagon; Pedigesic; Pedpain; Phenergan†; Phensedyl; Propain; Pynmed; Salterpyn; Sedlinct†; Stilpane†; Stopayne; Synaleve; Tenston; Tixylix; Vacudol; Xeramax; ***Spain:*** Actithiol Antihist; Antihemorroidal; Fenergan Expectorante; Hemotripsin†; Petigan Miro†; Sugarceton; ***Swed.:*** Lergigan comp; ***Switz.:*** Dobacen plus†; Linervidol; Lysedil; Lysedil compositum; Nardyl; Phenergan Expectorant; Rectoquintyl-Promethazine; Rhinathiol Promethazine; ***UK:*** Medised; Night Nurse; Pamergan P100; Phensedyl Plus; Phensedyl†; Ronpirin Cold Remedy; Tixylix Night-Time; ***USA:*** Mepergan; Para-Hist AT†; Pentazine VC with Codeine; Phenameth DM; Phenergan VC; Phenergan VC with Codeine; Phenergan with Codeine; Phenergan with Dextromethorphan; Phenergan-D†; Pherazine DM; Pherazine VC; Pherazine VC with Codeine; Pherazine with Codeine; Prometh VC Plain; Prometh with Dextromethorphan; Promethazine VC with Codeine; Promethist with Codeine.

Propiomazine Hydrochloride (6158-z)

Propiomazine Hydrochloride *(BANM, rINNM)*.

CB-1678 (propiomazine); Wy-1359 (propiomazine). 1-[10-(2-Dimethylaminopropyl)phenothiazin-2-yl]propan-1-one hydrochloride.

$C_{20}H_{24}N_2OS,HCl = 376.9$.

CAS — 362-29-8 (propiomazine); 1240-15-9 (propiomazine hydrochloride).

NOTE. Propiomazine is *USAN*.

Propiomazine Maleate (6159-c)

Propiomazine Maleate *(BANM, rINNM)*.

CB-1678; Propiomazine Hydrogen Maleate.

$C_{20}H_{24}N_2OS,C_4H_4O_4 = 456.6$.

CAS — 3568-23-8.

Propiomazine maleate 1.3 mg is approximately equivalent to 1 mg of propiomazine and 1.1 mg of propiomazine hydrochloride.

Adverse Effects and Precautions

As for the sedating antihistamines in general, see p.397. Local irritation may occur at the site of intravenous injection of propiomazine hydrochloride and there may be thrombophlebitis.

Interactions

As for the sedating antihistamines in general, p.399.

Uses and Administration

Propiomazine, a phenothiazine derivative, is a sedating antihistamine used for its sedative and antiemetic properties in insomnia (p.400) and nausea and vomiting (p.400).

It is given by mouth as the maleate as a hypnotic in doses equivalent to 25 to 50 mg of the base at night.

It is also given by intramuscular or slow intravenous injection in doses ranging from 10 to 40 mg of the hydrochloride for anaesthetic premedication and during surgical and obstetric procedures (p.399). Children weighing up to 27 kg have been given 0.55 to 1.1 mg per kg body-weight intramuscularly or intravenously. Alternatively, those aged 2 to 4 years have been given 10 mg; 4 to 6 years, 15 mg; 6 to 12 years, 25 mg.

Preparations

Proprietary Preparations (details are given in Part 3)
Swed.: Propavan; ***USA:*** Largon.

Setastine Hydrochloride (5686-p)

Setastine Hydrochloride *(rINNM)*.

EGYT-2062. 1-{2-[(*p*-Chloro-α-methyl-α-phenylbenzyl)oxy]ethyl}hexahydro-1*H*-azepine hydrochloride.

$C_{22}H_{28}ClNO,HCl = 394.4$.

CAS — 64294-95-7 (setastine).

Setastine hydrochloride, a derivative of clemastine, is an antihistamine claimed to have no sedative activity. It is given by mouth for the symptomatic relief of hypersensitivity disorders in doses of up to 6 mg daily.

Preparations

Proprietary Preparations (details are given in Part 3)
Hung.: Loderix.

Terfenadine (13308-v)

Terfenadine *(BAN, USAN, rINN).*

MDL-9918; RMI-9918; Terfenadinum. 1-(4-*tert*-Butylphenyl)-4-[4-(α-hydroxybenzhydryl)piperidino]butan-1-ol.

$C_{32}H_{41}NO_2$ = 471.7.

CAS — 50679-08-8.

Pharmacopoeias. In *Eur.* (see p.viii) and *US.*

A white to off-white crystalline powder; it is polymorphic. Ph. Eur. **solubilities** are: very slightly soluble in water and in dilute hydrochloric acid; soluble in methyl alcohol; freely soluble in dichloromethane. USP solubilities are: slightly soluble in water, in 0.1N hydrochloric acid, and in petroleum spirit; soluble in alcohol, in methyl alcohol, in octanol, and in toluene; freely soluble in chloroform. **Store** in airtight containers. Protect from light.

Adverse Effects and Precautions

As for the non-sedating antihistamines in general, p.397.

Ventricular arrhythmias, including torsade de pointes, have occurred rarely with terfenadine, particularly in association with raised blood concentrations (see Arrhythmias, below). To reduce the risk of developing such arrhythmias the recommended dose should not be exceeded and terfenadine should be avoided in patients with cardiac or significant hepatic disease, with known or suspected hypokalaemia or other electrolyte imbalance, or with known or suspected prolonged QT interval. The concomitant administration of drugs liable to interfere with the hepatic metabolism of terfenadine, of other potentially arrhythmogenic drugs, and of drugs likely to cause electrolyte imbalance should be avoided (see under Interactions, below). If palpitations, dizziness, syncope, or convulsions occur terfenadine should be withdrawn and the patient investigated for potential arrhythmias.

Alopecia. Hair loss was associated with terfenadine treatment in a 24-year-old patient.[1] Regrowth occurred when treatment was stopped.

1. Jones SK, Morley WN. Terfenadine causing hair loss. *Br Med J* 1985; **291:** 940.

Arrhythmias. Ventricular arrhythmias including torsade de pointes have occurred with terfenadine at doses greater than those recommended[1] and also normal doses in patients whose metabolism of terfenadine is impaired by drugs or by liver disease. Generalised convulsions and a quinine-like effect on the ECG has also been reported after a presumed overdose of terfenadine.[2] Consequently a number of recommendations have been made to reduce the risk of developing serious arrhythmias, including those from the Committee on Safety of Medicines (CSM) in the UK[3,4] (see above for details). Terfenadine should be discontinued immediately, and the patient evaluated for potential arrhythmias, in those who experience syncope after taking terfenadine.

Studies[5] have suggested that the ventricular arrhythmias are due to terfenadine itself rather than its active metabolite fexofenadine (p.410). Terfenadine has been shown to inhibit cardiac potassium channels which results in prolongation of the QT interval, a risk factor for developing arrhythmias, while the non-sedating antihistamines cetirizine, fexofenadine, and loratadine have had no demonstrable effect.[5,6]

1. MacConnell TJ, Stanners AJ. Torsades de pointes complicating treatment with terfenadine. *Br Med J* 1991; **302:** 1469.
2. Davies AJ, *et al.* Cardiotoxic effect with convulsions in terfenadine overdose. *Br Med J* 1989; **298:** 325.
3. Committee on Safety of Medicines. Ventricular arrhythmias due to terfenadine and astemizole. *Current Problems 35* 1992.
4. Committee on Safety of Medicines/Medicines Control Agency. Drug-induced prolongation of the QT interval. *Current Problems* 1996; **22:** 2.
5. Woolsey RL, *et al.* Mechanism of the cardiotoxic actions of terfenadine. *JAMA* 1993; **269:** 1532–6.
6. Rankin AC. Non-sedating antihistamines and cardiac arrhythmia. *Lancet* 1997; **350:** 1115–16.

Effects on the liver. Three episodes of acute hepatitis with jaundice occurred in a patient taking terfenadine intermittently over a period of 17 months.[1] Liver function tests returned to normal after interruption of drug administration. Two further cases[2] of cholestatic hepatitis associated with terfenadine administration have been reported. Again, liver function tests returned to normal after drug withdrawal. A study[3] by the Boston Collaborative Drug Surveillance Program of 210 683 patients who had received prescriptions for terfenadine concluded that the use of terfenadine was rarely associated with important idiopathic liver disease. The investigators found only 3 cases of acute liver disease where a causal connection to terfenadine could not be ruled out; all these patients had received a concomitant hepatotoxic drug and had made a full recovery.

1. Larrey D, *et al.* Terfenadine and hepatitis. *Ann Intern Med* 1985; **103:** 634.
2. Sahai A, Villeneuve JP. Terfenadine-induced cholestatic hepatitis. *Lancet* 1996; **348:** 552–3.
3. Myers MW, Jick H. Terfenadine and risk of acute liver disease. *Br J Clin Pharmacol* 1998; **46:** 251–3.

Effects on the nervous system. Non-sedating effects on the CNS have been reported after a single dose of terfenadine;[1] these have included anxiety, palpitations, and insomnia. The UK manufacturers commented that clinical studies suggest that the incidence of such effects is similar to that seen after placebo.[2]

Workers who had described a generalised tonic-clonic seizure in a patient taking terfenadine[3] later reported that the patient had subsequently had a second unprovoked seizure[4] and now considered that terfenadine may not have been the cause of his original seizure. Convulsions have been reported following overdosage with terfenadine (see under Arrhythmias, above).

The sedative effects of the older antihistamines and the lack of such effects with the non-sedating antihistamines including terfenadine are discussed under Sedation on p.398.

1. Napke E, Biron P. Nervous reactions after first dose of terfenadine in adults. *Lancet* 1989; **ii:** 615–16.
2. Masheter HC. Nervous reactions to terfenadine. *Lancet* 1989; **ii:** 1034.
3. Tidswell P, d'Assis-Fonseca A. Generalised seizure due to terfenadine. *Br Med J* 1993; **307:** 241.
4. Tidswell P, d'Assis-Fonseca A. Generalised seizure due to terfenadine. *Br Med J* 1993; **307:** 736.

Hypersensitivity. Terfenadine administration was associated with 108 reports of skin reactions, including rashes, urticaria, angioedema, photosensitivity reactions and peeling of the skin of the hands or feet.[1]

1. Stricker BHCh, *et al.* Skin reactions to terfenadine. *Br Med J* 1986; **293:** 536.

Porphyria. Terfenadine has been associated with clinical exacerbations of porphyria and is considered unsafe in porphyric patients.[1]

1. Moore MR, McColl KEL. *Porphyria: drug lists.* Glasgow: Porphyria Research Unit, University of Glasgow, 1991.

Interactions

As for the non-sedating antihistamines in general, p.399.

Terfenadine should not be given with drugs that inhibit its hepatic metabolism because of the increased risk of serious ventricular arrhythmias. These drugs include *itraconazole, ketoconazole*, and possibly other *imidazole* and *triazole antifungals*, the macrolide antibacterials *clarithromycin, erythromycin, josamycin*, and *triacetyloleandomycin*, the serotonin reuptake inhibitors *fluvoxamine, nefazodone,* and *sertraline*, the HIV-protease inhibitors *indinavir, nelfinavir, ritonavir,* and *saquinavir,* and *zileuton*. The metabolism of terfenadine may also be inhibited by grapefruit juice and concomitant use should be avoided.

Concomitant administration with other potentially arrhythmogenic drugs such as *antiarrhythmics, tricyclic antidepressants*, the antimalarials *halofantrine* and *quinine, antipsychotics, cisapride, probucol*, and the beta blocker *sotalol* should be avoided as should co-administration of *diuretics* that cause electrolyte imbalances especially hypokalaemia. The use of terfenadine and *astemizole* together is not recommended.

General references.

1. Kivistö KT, *et al.* Inhibition of terfenadine metabolism: pharmacokinetic and pharmacodynamic consequences. *Clin Pharmacokinet* 1994; **27:** 1–5.

Antibacterials. Pharmacokinetic studies have demonstrated that the macrolide antibiotics *erythromycin*[1] and *clarithromycin*[2] interfere with the metabolism of terfenadine leading to its accumulation. A high plasma-terfenadine concentration is associated with prolongation of the QT interval, and arrhythmias such as torsade de pointes have been reported in patients treated with therapeutic doses of terfenadine and erythromycin[3] or *triacetyloleandomycin*.[4]

1. Honig PK, *et al.* Changes in the pharmacokinetics and electrocardiographic pharmacodynamics of terfenadine with concomitant administration of erythromycin. *Clin Pharmacol Ther* 1992; **52:** 231–8.
2. Honig P, *et al.* Effect of erythromycin, clarithromycin and azithromycin on the pharmacokinetics of terfenadine. *Clin Pharmacol Ther* 1993; **53:** 161.
3. Biglin KE, *et al.* Drug-induced torsades de pointes: a possible interaction of terfenadine and erythromycin. *Ann Pharmacother* 1994; **28:** 282.
4. Fournier P, *et al.* Une nouvelle cause de torsades de pointes: association terfenadine et troleandomycine. *Ann Cardiol Angeiol (Paris)* 1993; **42:** 249–52.

Antidepressants. Cardiac abnormalities have been reported in 2 patients taking *fluoxetine* and terfenadine concomitantly.[1,2]

1. Swims MP. Potential terfenadine-fluoxetine interaction. *Ann Pharmacother* 1993; **27:** 1404–5.
2. Marchiando RJ, Cook MD. Probable terfenadine-fluoxetine-associated cardiac toxicity. *Ann Pharmacother* 1995; **29:** 937–8.

Antiepileptics. For reference to an interaction between terfenadine and *carbamazepine*, see p.341.

Antifungals. Pharmacokinetic studies have demonstrated that the imidazole antifungals *itraconazole*[1] and *ketoconazole*[2] interfere with the metabolism of terfenadine leading to its accumulation. A high plasma-terfenadine concentration is associated with prolongation of the QT interval, and arrhythmias such as torsade de pointes have been reported in patients treated with therapeutic doses of terfenadine and ketoconazole[3] or itraconazole.[1,4] While there has been a pharmacokinetic study[5] that suggested that the interaction between terfenadine and *fluconazole* might not be clinically significant, as the mechanism of the interaction appeared to involve the metabolite of terfenadine and did not lead to accumulation of the cardiotoxic parent compound, this may not always be the case. Studies in a small group of patients who exhibited abnormal patterns of terfenadine metabolism demonstrated increases in terfenadine concentrations associated with ECG abnormalities when terfenadine was administered with high doses of fluconazole.[6]

1. Pohjola-Sintonen S, *et al.* Itraconazole prevents terfenadine metabolism and increases risk of torsades de pointes ventricular tachycardia. *Eur J Clin Pharmacol* 1993; **45:** 191–3.
2. Honig PK, *et al.* Terfenadine-ketoconazole interaction: pharmacokinetic and electrocardiographic consequences. *JAMA* 1993; **269:** 1513–18.
3. Monahan BP, *et al.* Torsades de pointes occurring in association with terfenadine use. *JAMA* 1990; **264:** 2788–90.
4. Crane JK, *et al.* Syncope and cardiac arrhythmia due to an interaction between itraconazole and terfenadine. *Am J Med* 1993; **95:** 445–6.
5. Honig PK, *et al.* The effect of fluconazole on the steady-state pharmacokinetics and electrocardiographic pharmacodynamics of terfenadine in humans. *Clin Pharmacol Ther* 1993; **53:** 630–6.
6. Cantilena LR, *et al.* Fluconazole alters terfenadine pharmacokinetics and electrocardiographic pharmacodynamics. *Clin Pharmacol Ther* 1995; **57:** 185.

Calcium-channel blockers. For reference to an interaction between terfenadine and *nifedipine*, see p.918.

Grapefruit juice. A study[1] in healthy subjects given terfenadine and *grapefruit juice* concomitantly for 7 days demonstrated raised plasma-terfenadine concentrations and prolongation of the QT interval. These effects were less pronounced when terfenadine was administered 2 hours before grapefruit juice, but were nevertheless quantifiable in some subjects. In another study QT interval changes were not found in healthy subjects given single doses of terfenadine and grapefruit juice.[2] However the highly variable pharmacokinetics between individuals led the authors to conclude that prolongation of the QT interval was possible following single doses. The probable mechanism of the interaction is inhibition of the metabolism of terfenadine by the cytochrome P450 isoenzyme CYP3A4, although the component of grapefruit juice responsible is as yet unknown.

1. Benton RE, *et al.* Grapefruit juice alters terfenadine pharmacokinetics, resulting in prolongation of repolarization on the electrocardiogram. *Clin Pharmacol Ther* 1996; **59:** 383–8.
2. Rau SE, *et al.* Grapefruit juice-terfenadine single-dose interaction: magnitude, mechanism, and relevance. *Clin Pharmacol Ther* 1997; **61:** 401–9.

Pharmacokinetics

Terfenadine is rapidly absorbed from the gastro-intestinal tract; peak plasma concentrations are achieved within about 2 hours. It is a prodrug and undergoes extensive first-pass metabolism in the liver to its active metabolite the carboxylic acid derivative fexofenadine (p.410). The other main metabolite is an inactive piperidine-carbinol derivative. About 97% of terfenadine is bound to plasma proteins; fexofenadine is reported to be less extensively bound. Terfenadine does not appear to cross the blood-brain barrier to a significant extent; limited amounts of fexofenadine, but not the parent drug, have been detected in breast milk. An elimination half-life of 16 to 23 hours has been reported for terfenadine. The metabolites, and traces of unchanged drug, are excreted in the urine and the faeces.

References.

1. Eller MG, *et al.* Pharmacokinetics of terfenadine in healthy elderly subjects. *J Clin Pharmacol* 1992; **32:** 267–71.
2. Lucas BD, *et al.* Terfenadine pharmacokinetics in breast milk in lactating women. *Clin Pharmacol Ther* 1995; **57:** 398–402.

Uses and Administration

Terfenadine, a piperidine derivative, is a non-sedating antihistamine. It does not have significant sedative or antimuscarinic actions. It is used for the symptomatic relief of allergic conditions including rhinitis (p.400) and conjunctivitis (p.399) and skin disorders such as urticaria (p.401).

The maximum adult dose of terfenadine is 120 mg daily by mouth given either as 60 mg twice daily or 120 mg in the morning; a starting dose of 60 mg daily in a single dose or in two divided doses is recommended for rhinitis. Half the usual daily dose has been suggested for patients with impaired renal function. For children aged 3 to 12 years the recommended maximum dose is 1 mg per kg body-weight given twice daily; for rhinitis and conjunctivitis a starting dose of 1 mg per kg daily is recommended. Children who are over 12 years of age and weigh more than 50 kg may receive the usual adult dosage.

Reviews.

1. Sorkin EM, Heel RC. Terfenadine: a review of its pharmacodynamic properties and therapeutic efficacy. *Drugs* 1985; **29:** 34–56.
2. Mann KV, *et al.* Nonsedating histamine H_1-receptor antagonists. *Clin Pharm* 1989; **8:** 331–44.
3. McTavish D, *et al.* Terfenadine: an updated review of its pharmacological properties and therapeutic efficacy. *Drugs* 1990; **39:** 552–74.

Preparations

USP 23: Terfenadine Tablets.

Proprietary Preparations (details are given in Part 3)
Aust.: Terlane; Triludan; ***Austral.:*** Teldane; ***Belg.:*** Triludan; ***Canad.:*** Allergy Relief; Contac Allergy Formula; Seldane; ***Fr.:*** Teldane; ***Ger.:*** Balkis Spezial; Fomos; Heuschnupfen Systral†; Hisfedin; Histaterfen; Logomed Allergie-Tabletten; Logomed Juckreiz†; Teldane; Terfedura; Terfemundin; Terfen-Diolan†; Terfium; Vividrin mit Terfenadin; ***Irl.:*** Triludan; ***Ital.:*** Allerplus†; Teldane†; Triludan†; ***Neth.:*** Triludan; ***Norw.:*** Teldanex; ***S.Afr.:*** Fendin; Terfenor; Triludan; ***Spain:*** Aldira†; Alergist; Cyater; Rapidal; Ternadin; Triludan; ***Swed.:*** Teldanex; Terfex†; ***Switz.:*** Teldane; Triludan; ***UK:*** Aller-eze Clear†; Antihistamine Forte; Boots Hayfever Relief Antihistamine; Histafen; Seldane; Terfenor Antihistamine; Terfex; Triludan; ***USA:*** Seldane†.

Multi-ingredient: ***Aust.:*** Teldafed; ***Belg.:*** Teldafen; ***USA:*** Seldane-D†.

Thenyldiamine Hydrochloride (6165-j)

Thenyldiamine Hydrochloride *(BANM, rINNM).*

Thenyldiaminium Chloride. *NN*-Dimethyl-*N'*-(2-pyridyl)-*N'*-(3-thenyl)ethylenediamine hydrochloride.

$C_{14}H_{19}N_3S,HCl = 297.8.$

CAS — 91-79-2 (thenyldiamine); 958-93-0 (thenyldiamine hydrochloride).

Thenyldiamine hydrochloride, an ethylenediamine derivative, is an antihistamine. It is given by mouth as an ingredient of compound preparations for the symptomatic treatment of coughs and the common cold.

Preparations

Proprietary Preparations (details are given in Part 3)

Multi-ingredient: ***Ital.:*** NTR; ***Spain:*** Sinefricol.

Thiazinamium Methylsulphate (6166-z)

Thiazinamium Metilsulfate *(rINN)*; Methylpromethazinium Methylsulfuricum; WY-460E (thiazinamium chloride). Trimethyl[1-methyl-2-(phenothiazin-10-yl)ethyl]ammonium methyl sulphate.

$C_{19}H_{26}N_2O_4S_2 = 410.6.$

CAS — 2338-21-8 (thiazinamium); 4320-13-2 (thiazinamium chloride); 58-34-4 (thiazinamium methylsulphate).

NOTE. Thiazinamium Chloride is *USAN.*

Pharmacopoeias. In *Fr.*

Thiazinamium methylsulphate, a phenothiazine derivative, is an antihistamine that has been given in combination preparations for respiratory-tract disorders.

Thiethylperazine (17248-a)

Thiethylperazine *(BAN, USAN, rINN).*

2-Ethylthio-10-[3-(4-methylpiperazin-1-yl)-propyl]phenothiazine.

$C_{22}H_{29}N_3S_2 = 399.6.$

CAS — 1420-55-9.

Thiethylperazine Malate (7110-q)

Thiethylperazine Malate *(BANM, rINNM).*

$C_{22}H_{29}N_3S_2,2C_4H_6O_5 = 667.8.$

CAS — 52239-63-1.

Pharmacopoeias. In *US.*

Thiethylperazine malate 10.86 mg is approximately equivalent to 6.5 mg of thiethylperazine. A freshly prepared 1% solution in water has a pH of 2.8 to 3.8. **Store** in airtight containers. Protect from light.

Thiethylperazine Maleate (7111-p)

Thiethylperazine Maleate *(BANM, USAN, rINNM).*

GS-95; NSC-130044; Thiethylperazine Dimaleate.

$C_{22}H_{29}N_3S_2,2C_4H_4O_4 = 631.8.$

CAS — 1179-69-7.

Pharmacopoeias. In *Fr., Swiss,* and *US.*

A yellowish granular powder, odourless or with not more than a slight odour. Thiethylperazine maleate 10.28 mg is approximately equivalent to 6.5 mg of thiethylperazine.

Soluble 1 in 1700 of water and 1 in 530 of alcohol; slightly soluble in methyl alcohol; practically insoluble in chloroform and ether. A 0.1% solution in water has a pH of 2.8 to 3.8. **Store** in airtight containers. Protect from light.

Incompatibility. Incompatibility has been reported between injections of thiethylperazine maleate and nalbuphine hydrochloride.[1]

1. Jump WG, *et al.* Compatibility of nalbuphine hydrochloride with other preoperative medications. *Am J Hosp Pharm* 1982; **39:** 841–3.

Adverse Effects and Precautions

As for the sedating antihistamines in general, see p.397.

Interactions

As for the sedating antihistamines in general, p.399.

Uses and Administration

Thiethylperazine, a phenothiazine derivative with a piperazine side-chain, is a sedating antihistamine used as an antiemetic for the control of nausea and vomiting (p.400) associated with surgical procedures and cancer therapy. It has also been used for the management of vertigo (p.401) and motion sickness although there is some doubt over its efficacy for these indications.

Thiethylperazine is given in usual doses of 10 mg of the maleate up to three times daily by mouth; the maleate has also been given rectally. Where oral administration is impractical similar doses of the malate may be given by deep intramuscular injection.

Reduced doses of phenothiazines may be required in elderly patients. Thiethylperazine is not recommended for use in children.

Preparations

USP 23: Thiethylperazine Malate Injection; Thiethylperazine Maleate Suppositories; Thiethylperazine Maleate Tablets.

Proprietary Preparations (details are given in Part 3)
Aust.: Torecan; ***Austral.:*** Torecan†; ***Canad.:*** Torecan†; ***Ger.:*** Torecan; ***Irl.:*** Torecan†; ***Ital.:*** Torecan; ***Neth.:*** Torecan†; ***Norw.:*** Torecan†; ***Spain:*** Torecan; ***Swed.:*** Torecan; ***Switz.:*** Torecan; ***UK:*** Torecan†; ***USA:*** Norzine; Torecan.

Thonzylamine Hydrochloride (6167-c)

Thonzylamine Hydrochloride *(BANM, USAN, rINNM).*

N-*p*-Anisyl-*N'N'*-dimethyl-*N*-(pyrimidin-2-yl)ethylenediamine hydrochloride.

$C_{16}H_{22}N_4O,HCl = 322.8.$

CAS — 91-85-0 (thonzylamine); 63-56-9 (thonzylamine hydrochloride).

Thonzylamine hydrochloride, an ethylenediamine derivative, is an antihistamine given for the symptomatic relief of hypersensitivity disorders.

Preparations

Proprietary Preparations (details are given in Part 3)
Ital.: Tonamil.

Multi-ingredient: ***Ital.:*** Ascotodin; Collirio Alfa Antistaminico; Imidazyl Antistaminico; Narlisim; Pupilla Antistaminico; ***Spain:*** Angiofiline†; Normo Nar.

Tolpropamine Hydrochloride (6168-k)

Tolpropamine Hydrochloride *(BANM, rINNM).*

NN-Dimethyl-3-phenyl-3-*p*-tolylpropylamine hydrochloride.

$C_{18}H_{23}N,HCl = 289.8.$

CAS — 5632-44-0 (tolpropamine); 3339-11-5 (tolpropamine hydrochloride).

Tolpropamine hydrochloride, an alkylamine derivative, is an antihistamine. It used has been topically for the symptomatic relief of hypersensitivity and pruritic skin disorders, although as with any antihistamine there is a risk of skin sensitisation.

Preparations

Proprietary Preparations (details are given in Part 3)
Aust.: Pragman; ***Ger.:*** Pragman†; ***Ital.:*** Pragman†.

Trimeprazine Tartrate (6169-a)

Trimeprazine Tartrate *(BANM).*

Alimemazine Tartrate *(rINNM). NN*-Dimethyl-2-methyl-3-(phenothiazin-10-yl)propylamine tartrate.

$(C_{18}H_{22}N_2S)_2,C_4H_6O_6 = 747.0.$

CAS — 84-96-8 (trimeprazine); 4330-99-8 (trimeprazine tartrate).

Pharmacopoeias. In *Br., Fr., Jpn,* and *US.*

A white or slightly cream-coloured odourless or almost odourless crystalline powder. It darkens in colour on exposure to light. Trimeprazine tartrate 25 mg is approximately equivalent to 20 mg of trimeprazine.

BP **solubilities** are: freely soluble in water and in chloroform; sparingly soluble in alcohol; very slightly soluble in ether. USP solubilities are: soluble 1 in 2 of water, 1 in 20 of alcohol, 1 in 5 of chloroform, and 1 in 1800 of ether. A 2% solution in water has a pH of 5.0 to 6.5. **Store** in airtight containers. Protect from light.

Adverse Effects and Precautions

As for the sedating antihistamines in general, see p.397.

Children. There have been reports of adverse effects in children given trimeprazine tartrate by mouth. Fatal malignant hyperthermia[1] and severe cardiovascular depression[2] have occurred after its use for premedication, and severe respiratory and CNS depression[3] after use as a postoperative sedative. Doses in these 3 reports ranged from 2.4 to 4.4 mg per kg body-weight. A possible association between phenothiazine sedatives and sudden infant death syndrome has also been suggested, but has not been confirmed (see Promethazine Hydrochloride, p.416). The UK manufacturers no longer indicate trimeprazine tartrate for short-term sedation in children and recommend that it should not be used in infants less than 2 years of age. The maximum recommended dose for premedication for children aged 2 to 7 years is 2 mg per kg body-weight by mouth. There has recently been a warning[4] that the use of trimeprazine for deep sedation in diagnostic and therapeutic procedures in children is associated with prolonged drowsiness and that standards of monitoring, starvation, and postprocedural care should be similar to those with general anaesthesia.

1. Moyes DG. Malignant hyperpyrexia caused by trimeprazine. *Br J Anaesth* 1973; **45:** 1163–4.
2. Loan WB, Cuthbert D. Adverse cardiovascular response to oral trimeprazine in children. *Br Med J* 1985; **290:** 1548–9.
3. Mann NP. Trimeprazine and respiratory depression. *Arch Dis Child* 1981; **56:** 481–2.
4. Cray SH, Hinton W. Sedation for investigations: prolonged effect of chloral and trimeprazine. *Arch Dis Child* 1994; **71:** 179.

Pregnancy. For a discussion of the use of antihistamines in pregnancy, including studies involving phenothiazines, see p.398.

Interactions

As for the sedating antihistamines in general, p.399.

Uses and Administration

Trimeprazine, a phenothiazine derivative, is a sedating antihistamine with antiemetic activity and pronounced sedative effects. It also has some antimuscarinic actions. It is used mainly for its marked effect in the relief of pruritus (p.400) and, in the UK, for pre-operative medication in children. Trimeprazine may also be used in compound preparations for the symptomatic treatment of coughs (p.400).

Trimeprazine tartrate is administered by mouth; doses in the UK are given as the amount of trimeprazine tartrate; those in the USA are expressed in terms of the equivalent amount of trimeprazine. Even allowing for this, lower doses are used in the

USA. The dose of trimeprazine tartrate used in the UK for the relief of pruritus in adults is 10 mg two or three times daily; up to 100 mg daily has been given in refractory cases. Elderly patients are given 10 mg once or twice daily and children over 2 years of age 2.5 to 5 mg three or four times daily. In the USA the dose is the equivalent of trimeprazine 2.5 mg four times daily, or 5 mg twice daily as a modified-release preparation. Children in the USA between 2 and 3 years of age have been given 1.25 mg at night or three times daily; for older children this dose has been increased to 2.5 mg.

The usual recommended dose for premedication in children over 2 years is 2 mg per kg body-weight given by mouth about one to two hours before the operation.

Anaesthesia. Trimeprazine tartrate may be used for anaesthetic premedication (see p.399) in children when the oral route of administration is preferred to the more usual parenteral route of other phenothiazine antihistamines. Adverse effects have, however, been reported in children (see Administration in Children under Adverse Effects and Precautions, above). The UK manufacturers recommend that trimeprazine tartrate should not be used in infants less than 2 years of age.

Insomnia. Antihistamines such as trimeprazine tartrate have been used as alternatives to benzodiazepines for the treatment of insomnia (p.400), particularly for children. However, they are only indicated for short-term use, and antimuscarinic side-effects may prove troublesome.

Regimens involving a short course of trimeprazine tartrate in high dosage were tried in order to alter the sleep pattern of children with sleeping difficulties.[1,2] Adverse effects have, however, been reported in children (see Administration in Children under Adverse Effects and Precautions, above). The UK manufacturers no longer indicate trimeprazine tartrate for short-term sedation in children and recommend that it should not be used in infants less than 2 years of age.

1. Valman HB. ABC of 1 to 7 (revised): sleep problems. *Br Med J* 1987; **294:** 828–30.
2. Anonymous. What can be done for night waking in children? *Lancet* 1987; **ii:** 948–9.

Preparations

BP 1998: Alimemazine Tablets; Paediatric Alimemazine Oral Solution; Strong Paediatric Alimemazine Oral Solution;
USP 23: Trimeprazine Tartrate Syrup; Trimeprazine Tartrate Tablets.

Proprietary Preparations (details are given in Part 3)
Austral.: Vallergan; ***Belg.:*** Theralene; ***Canad.:*** Panectyl; ***Fr.:*** Theralene; ***Ger.:*** Repeltin; Theralene†; ***Irl.:*** Vallergan; ***Neth.:*** Nedeltran; ***Norw.:*** Vallergan; ***S.Afr.:*** Vallergan; ***Spain:*** Variargil; ***Swed.:*** Theralen; ***Switz.:*** Theralene†; ***UK:*** Vallergan; ***USA:*** Temaril†.

Multi-ingredient: ***Belg.:*** Theralene Pectoral; ***Fr.:*** Theralene Pectoral Nourrisson; Theralene Pectoral†; ***Spain:*** Efralen†.

Trimethobenzamide Hydrochloride (6170-e)

Trimethobenzamide Hydrochloride *(rINNM)*.

N-[4-(2-Dimethylaminoethoxy)benzyl]-3,4,5-trimethoxybenzamide hydrochloride.

$C_{21}H_{28}N_2O_5,HCl = 424.9.$

CAS — 138-56-7 (trimethobenzamide); 554-92-7 (trimethobenzamide hydrochloride).

Pharmacopoeias. In US.

A white crystalline powder with a slight phenolic odour. **Soluble** 1 in 2 of water, 1 in 59 of alcohol, 1 in 67 of chloroform, and 1 in 720 of ether.

Adverse Effects and Precautions

As for the sedating antihistamines in general, p.397.

Pain at the site of intramuscular injection and local irritation after rectal administration have been noted.

Pregnancy. For discussion of the use of antihistamines in pregnancy, including some evidence of an excess number of congenital abnormalities in infants born to mothers exposed to trimethobenzamide, see p.398.

Interactions

As for the sedating antihistamines in general, p.399.

Uses and Administration

Trimethobenzamide hydrochloride, an ethanolamine derivative, is a sedating antihistamine used as an antiemetic in the control of nausea and vomiting (p.400).

The usual dose is 250 mg by mouth or 200 mg by deep intramuscular injection or rectally three or four times daily. Children weighing more than 15 kg have been given 100 to 200 mg three or four times daily by the oral or rectal route.

Preparations

USP 23: Trimethobenzamide Hydrochloride Capsules; Trimethobenzamide Hydrochloride Injection.

Proprietary Preparations (details are given in Part 3)
Ital.: Anaus†; Ibikin†; ***USA:*** Arrestin; Stemetic†; T-Gen; Tebamide; Ticon; Tigan; Trimazide.

Multi-ingredient: ***USA:*** Emergent-Ez; Tigan; Triban.

Tripelennamine Citrate (6171-l)

Tripelennamine Citrate *(BANM, rINNM)*.

Tripelennaminium Citrate. N-Benzyl-N′N′-dimethyl-N-(2-pyridyl)ethylenediamine dihydrogen citrate.

$C_{16}H_{21}N_3,C_6H_8O_7 = 447.5.$

CAS — 91-81-6 (tripelennamine); 6138-56-3 (tripelennamine citrate).

Pharmacopoeias. In US.

A white crystalline powder. M.p. about 107°. Tripelennamine citrate 150 mg is approximately equivalent to 100 mg of tripelennamine hydrochloride. **Soluble** 1 in 1 of water; freely soluble in alcohol; very slightly soluble in ether; practically insoluble in chloroform. Solutions in water are acid to litmus. **Protect** from light.

Tripelennamine Hydrochloride (6172-y)

Tripelennamine Hydrochloride *(BANM, rINNM)*.

Tripelennaminium Chloride.

$C_{16}H_{21}N_3,HCl = 291.8.$

CAS — 154-69-8.

Pharmacopoeias. In US.

A white crystalline powder. M.p. 188 to 192°. It slowly darkens on exposure to light. **Soluble** 1 in 1 of water, 1 in 6 of alcohol and of chloroform, and 1 in 350 of acetone; practically insoluble in ether and in ethyl acetate. Solutions in water are practically neutral to litmus. **Protect** from light.

Adverse Effects and Precautions

As for the sedating antihistamines in general, p.397.

Abuse. A report[1] of the intravenous abuse of tripelennamine with pentazocine in the combination known as T's and blues.

1. Showalter CV. T's and blues: abuse of pentazocine and tripelennamine. *JAMA* 1980; **244:** 1224–5.

Overdosage. A severe toxic reaction, including agitation, hallucinations, and myoclonic jerks occurred in an 8-year-old child who was sprayed over the trunk and extremities with tripelennamine hydrochloride 2.1375 g in the treatment of severe poison ivy poisoning.[1] It was likely that inhalation of the fine mist of the aerosol spray contributed to the reaction but in this patient the initial reaction began 3 hours after exposure suggesting that percutaneous absorption through the multiple skin lesions probably contributed significantly. The original reaction was inadvertently prolonged by subsequent treatment with diphenhydramine hydrochloride and promethazine hydrochloride.

1. Schipior PG. An unusual case of antihistamine intoxication. *J Pediatr* 1967; **71:** 589–91.

Interactions

As for the sedating antihistamines in general, p.399.

Uses and Administration

Tripelennamine, an ethylenediamine derivative, is a sedating antihistamine with antimuscarinic and moderate sedative properties. It is used for the symptomatic relief of hypersensitivity reactions.

Tripelennamine hydrochloride is given by mouth in usual doses of 25 to 50 mg every 4 to 6 hours. Higher doses of up to 600 mg daily have been given. A recommended dose of the hydrochloride for children is 5 mg per kg body-weight daily in 4 to 6 divided doses; up to 300 mg daily has been given. Tripelennamine citrate has been used in equivalent doses in an elixir.

Tripelennamine hydrochloride has also been applied topically to the skin, although as with any antihistamine there is a risk of sensitisation.

Preparations

USP 23: Tripelennamine Citrate Elixir; Tripelennamine Hydrochloride Tablets.

Proprietary Preparations (details are given in Part 3)
Aust.: Azaron; ***Canad.:*** Pyribenzamine; Vaginex; ***Ger.:*** Azaron; ***Neth.:*** Azaron†; ***Spain:*** Azaron; ***USA:*** PBZ; Pelamine†; Vaginex.

Multi-ingredient: ***Ital.:*** Anticorizza; Lisabutina†; ***Spain:*** Oxidermiol Antihist; Polirino†; ***USA:*** Di-Delamine.

Triprolidine Hydrochloride (6173-j)

Triprolidine Hydrochloride *(BANM, rINNM)*.

(E)-2-[3-(Pyrrolidin-1-yl)-1-p-tolylprop-1-enyl]pyridine hydrochloride monohydrate.

$C_{19}H_{22}N_2,HCl,H_2O = 332.9.$

CAS — 486-12-4 (triprolidine); 550-70-9 (anhydrous triprolidine hydrochloride); 6138-79-0 (triprolidine hydrochloride, monohydrate).

Pharmacopoeias. In Br. and US.

A white crystalline powder, odourless or with a slight unpleasant odour. BP **solubilities** are: freely soluble in water and in alcohol; very soluble in chloroform; practically insoluble in ether. USP solubilities are: soluble 1 in 2.1 of water, 1 in 1.8 of alcohol, 1 in 1 of chloroform, and 1 in 2000 of ether. Solutions in water are alkaline to litmus. **Store** in airtight containers. Protect from light.

Adverse Effects and Precautions

As for the sedating antihistamines in general, p.397.

Interactions

As for the sedating antihistamines in general, p.399.

Pharmacokinetics

After absorption from the gastro-intestinal tract, triprolidine is metabolised; a carboxylated derivative accounts for about half the dose excreted in the urine. Reported half-lives vary from 3 to 5 hours or more.

General references.

1. Paton DM, Webster DR. Clinical pharmacokinetics of H_1-receptor antagonists (the antihistamines). *Clin Pharmacokinet* 1985; **10:** 477–97.
2. Miles MV, *et al.* Pharmacokinetics of oral and transdermal triprolidine. *J Clin Pharmacol* 1990; **30:** 572–5.

Distribution into breast milk. In a study[1] in 3 women of the excretion of triprolidine and pseudoephedrine, taken by mouth in a combined preparation, triprolidine was found to reach concentrations in breast milk similar to those found in plasma in one subject, and slightly lower than in plasma in the others. It was calculated that 0.06 to 0.2% of the ingested dose was excreted in breast milk over 24 hours. Concentrations of pseudoephedrine in breast milk exceeded those in plasma in all 3 women.

1. Findlay JWA, *et al.* Pseudoephedrine and triprolidine in plasma and breast milk of nursing mothers. *Br J Clin Pharmacol* 1984; **18:** 901–6.

Uses and Administration

Triprolidine hydrochloride, an alkylamine derivative, is a sedating antihistamine with antimuscarinic and mild sedative effects. It is used for the symptomatic relief of allergic conditions including urticaria (p.401) and rhinitis (p.400), and in pruritic skin disorders (p.400). It is often used in combination with pseudoephedrine hydrochloride for rhinitis and in other compound preparations for the symptomatic treatment of coughs and the common cold (p.400).

It is given by mouth, the usual dose for adults being 2.5 mg up to four times daily.

Triprolidine hydrochloride has also been applied topically to the skin, although as with any antihistamine there is a risk of sensitisation.

Otitis media. For studies questioning the use of triprolidine or pseudoephedrine in children with acute otitis media, see p.400.

Preparations

BP 1998: Triprolidine Tablets;
USP 23: Triprolidine and Pseudoephedrine Hydrochlorides Syrup; Triprolidine and Pseudoephedrine Hydrochlorides Tablets; Triprolidine Hydrochloride Syrup; Triprolidine Hydrochloride Tablets.

Proprietary Preparations (details are given in Part 3)
Aust.: Actidil; Pro-Actidil; ***Fr.:*** Actidilon†; ***Ger.:*** Pro-Actidil†; ***Irl.:*** Actidil†; Pro-Actidil†; ***Ital.:*** Actidil; ***S.Afr.:*** Pro-Actidil†; ***Spain:*** Pro-Actidil; ***Switz.:*** Pro-Actidil†; ***UK:*** Pro-Actidil†; ***USA:*** Myidyl†.

Multi-ingredient: ***Austral.:*** Actifed; Actifed CC Chesty; Actifed CC Dry; Actifed CC Junior; Codral Daytime/Nightime; Sudafed Plus; ***Belg.:*** Actifed; ***Canad.:*** Actifed; Actifed 12 Hour†; Actifed DM; Actifed Plus; CoActifed; Cotridin; Cotridin Expectorant; Triprofed; ***Fr.:*** Actidilon Hydrocortisone†; Actifed; Tussifed; ***Ger.:*** Actifed; Linctifed†; ***Irl.:*** Actifed; Actifed Compound; Actifed Expectorant; Linctifed†; ***Ital.:*** Actifed; Actifed Composto; Actigrip; ***S.Afr.:*** Actifed; Actifed Co; Actifed DM; Actigesic; Acuflu-P; Acugest; Acugest Co; Acutussive; Adco-Flupain; Adco-Muco Expect; Adco-Tussend; Arcana Cough Linctus†; Arcana Expectorant; Arcanafed; Coff-Rest; Emprazil-A; Endcol

Cough Linctus†; Endcol Decongestant†; Endcol Expectorant†; Fludactil; Fludactil Co; Fludactil Expectorant; Linctifed; Medifed; Neofed; Phendex; Rhinofed†; Trifen; ***Spain:*** Iniston; Iniston Antitusivo; Iniston Expectorante; ***UK:*** Actifed; Actifed Compound; Actifed Expectorant; Benylin Childrens Coughs & Colds; Sudafed Plus; ***USA:*** Actagen; Actagen-C Cough; Actifed; Actifed Plus; Actifed with Codeine†; Allercon; Allerfrim; Allerfrin with Codeine; Allergy Cold; Allerphed; Aprodine; Aprodine with Codeine; Bayer Select Night Time Cold; Cenafed Plus; Genac; Silafed; Sinu-Clear†; Triafed; Triafed with Codeine; Trifed; Trifed-C Cough; Triofed; Triposed.

Tritoqualine (13384-k)

Tritoqualine (*rINN*).

L-554. 7-Amino-4,5,6-triethoxy-3-(5,6,7,8-tetrahydro-4-methoxy-6-methyl-1,3-dioxolo[4,5-g]isoquinolin-5-yl)phthalide.

$C_{26}H_{32}N_2O_8$ = 500.5.

CAS — 14504-73-5.

Tritoqualine is stated to inhibit histidine decarboxylase which catalyses the conversion of histidine to histamine. It has the uses of antihistamines and is given by mouth for the symptomatic relief of hypersensitivity reactions and in pruritic skin disorders.

Preparations

Proprietary Preparations (details are given in Part 3)
Aust.: Hypostamin†; ***Fr.:*** Hypostamine; ***Ger.:*** Inhibostamin†; ***Ital.:*** Hypostamine†.

Antimalarials

This chapter describes the principal drugs used in the treatment and prophylaxis of malaria, one of the most serious protozoal infections in man. An estimated 40% of the world's population may be at risk of malaria; about 300 to 500 million develop clinical infection, which is often very severe, and over 1 million die each year. WHO produces guidelines for its strategic control and the management of malaria is under constant review. Measures required involve *protection* from mosquito bites, *prophylaxis* with antimalarial drugs, and *treatment* of any infection that develops. They also involve *vector control*; it is now recognised that for many countries vector eradication is an unrealistic aim.

Malaria and its aetiology

Malaria is caused by infection by any of four species of *Plasmodium. P. falciparum* causes falciparum (malignant tertian or subtertian) malaria which is the most serious form of malaria and can be rapidly fatal in non-immune individuals if not treated promptly. The other three species cause what are often termed 'benign' malarias; *P. vivax* causes vivax (benign tertian) malaria which is widespread but rarely fatal, although symptoms during the primary attack can be severe; *P. malariae* causes quartan malaria which is generally mild but can cause fatal nephrosis; and *P. ovale* causes ovale (ovale tertian) malaria which is the least common type of malaria, and produces clinical features similar to *P. vivax*.

The life cycle of *Plasmodium* is complex, comprising a sexual phase (sporogony) in the mosquito (vector) and an asexual phase (schizogony) in man (see Figure 1, below). Infection in man is usually caused by injection of *sporozoites* by the bite of an infected female anopheline mosquito. It may rarely be acquired in other ways such as through blood transfusion, congenitally via the placenta, through needlestick injuries, or after organ transplantation. Following an infected mosquito bite some of the sporozoites rapidly enter liver parenchymal cells where they undergo *exoerythrocytic* or *pre-erythrocytic schizogony*, forming *tissue schizonts* which mature and release thousands of *merozoites* into the blood on rupture of the cell. Some of these merozoites enter erythrocytes where they transform into *trophozoites*. These produce *blood schizonts* which, as they mature, rupture and release merozoites into the circulation which can infect other erythrocytes. This is termed the *erythrocytic cycle* and it is this periodic release of merozoites which is responsible for the characteristic periodicity of the fever in malaria. After several erythrocytic cycles, depending on the type of malaria, some erythrocytic forms develop into sexual *gametocytes*. It is ingestion of infected blood containing gametocytes by a biting female mosquito which allows the life cycle to be completed with the sexual phase in the mosquito. In *P. vivax* and *P. ovale* infections, some of the sporozoites entering the liver cells are thought to enter a latent tissue stage in the form of *hypnozoites* which are responsible for recurrence of malaria caused by these organisms. Recurrences resulting from the persistence of latent tissue forms are often referred to as *relapses* while renewed attacks caused by persistent residual erythrocytic forms are termed *recrudescences*. True relapses do not occur with falciparum or quartan malarias. Patients may sometimes be classified as *non-immune* if they have not previously or recently been exposed to *Plasmodium* infection and as *semi-immune* or *immune* if they have a history of prolonged exposure.

Clinical manifestations of malaria

The clinical symptoms of malaria are varied and non-specific but commonly include fever, fatigue, malaise, headache, myalgia, and sweating. Anaemia is a common complication due to haemolysis and in falciparum malaria serious complications such as acute renal failure, pulmonary oedema, and cerebral dysfunction can occur. Since none of the clinical features of malaria are diagnostic, a definitive diagnosis depends upon the demonstration of parasites in stained blood films. However, antimalarial drug treatment should not be withheld in the absence of positive blood films if there is clinical suspicion of malaria.

Antimalarial drugs

Antimalarial drugs can be classified by the stage of the parasitic life cycle they affect. Thus:

Blood schizontocides act on the erythrocytic stages of the parasite which are directly responsible for the clinical symptoms of the disease. They can produce a clinical cure or suppression of infection by susceptible strains of all four species of malaria parasite, but, since they have no effect on exoerythrocytic forms, do not produce a radical cure of relapsing forms of ovale or vivax malarias.

Tissue schizontocides act on the exoerythrocytic stages of the parasite and are used for causal prophylaxis to prevent invasion of the blood cells, or as anti-relapse drugs to produce radical cures of vivax and ovale malarias.

Gametocytocides destroy the sexual forms of the parasite to interrupt transmission of the infection to the mosquito vector.

Sporontocides have no direct effect on the gametocytes in the human host but prevent sporogony in the mosquito.

Antimalarial drugs can also be classified by the chemical group to which they belong, which in turn determines the stage of the life cycle they affect. The principal antimalarial drugs, classified according to *drug group* and *activity*, are listed in Table 1, p.423.

Other drugs with antimalarial activity being studied include the naphthyridine derivative, pyronaridine; the 4-piperazinoquinoline derivatives, piperaquine and hydroxypiperaquine; and a number of quinolone antibacterials. The 9-aminoacridines such as mepacrine are no longer used in the treatment of malaria.

The differing activities of antimalarial drugs allow the use of combinations of antimalarials to improve efficacy. Such combinations may have a simple additive effect or, more commonly, the drugs used may potentiate each other, for instance by acting at sequential steps in the parasite's folic acid pathway (e.g. pyrimethamine with sulfadoxine or dapsone). Alternatively, a combination may be complementary, when the drugs involved act against different stages in the life cycle of the parasite (e.g. the use of chloroquine with primaquine to produce radical cure of *P. vivax* or *P. ovale* infections). The rationale behind the use of such combinations may be to enhance efficacy, particularly when drug resistance is a problem (see below), or it may be an attempt to delay the development of resistance to one or more of the drugs concerned.

Resistance of *Plasmodium* to antimalarial drugs, in particular the spread of strains of *P. falciparum* resistant to chloroquine, is of great concern.

Chloroquine resistance in *P. falciparum* developed almost simultaneously in southern Asia and in South America at the end of the 1950s. Chloroquine resistance now affects most of Asia and the western Pacific islands with evidence of a westward spread. It is well established in South and Central America. Major and alarming changes in susceptibility have occurred in Africa, south of the Sahara and in islands off the eastern coast and there are now many reports of chloroquine resistance in West Africa.

Resistance in *P. falciparum* to proguanil and pyrimethamine first occurred in the early 1950s and is now apparent in many endemic areas. Cross resistance between proguanil and pyrimethamine may also occur.

Resistance in *P. falciparum* to the combination pyrimethamine-sulfadoxine (Fansidar) was first noted in the late 1970s in Thailand and has spread rapidly to other parts of the world including parts of South America and East Africa. Resistance to quinine, halofantrine, mefloquine, and artemisinin derivatives has also been noted. The emergence of multiple drug resistance in *P. falciparum* makes the selection of effective prophylaxis and treatment difficult.

Resistance in *P. vivax* to chloroquine and primaquine has also been reported in several parts of the world.[1]

A knowledge of the extent of resistance in terms of the geographical distribution and degree of resistance is important for the selection of appropriate control measures and for the development of policies for the rational use of antimalarial drugs. Effective drugs and drug combinations need to be selected according to local patterns of drug resistance. Indiscriminate and uncontrolled use of drugs should be prevented and adequate doses should be given to delay the selection of resistant strains. Malaria control strategies also need to involve other measures such as vector control and health education.

Treatment of malaria

Malaria is a serious and potentially fatal disease, particularly in the case of falciparum malaria (see below) and especially in non-immune individuals; prompt diagnosis and effective treatment are crucial.[2-4] Treatment is with a *blood schizontocide*, selected with due regard to the prevalence of specific patterns of drug resistance in the area of infection. In the case of vivax and ovale malarias (see below) subsequent treatment with a *tissue schizontocide* is needed where it is considered appropriate to prevent relapse.

Figure 1. Life cycle of the malaria parasite *Plasmodium*.

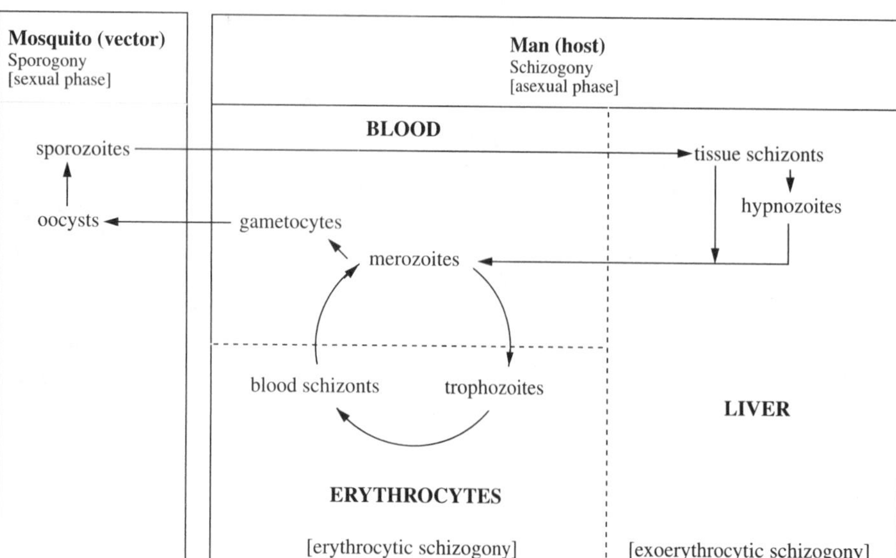

Table 1. Principal antimalarial drugs.

Antimalarial groups	Principal drugs	Activity
4-Methanolquinolines	Cinchona alkaloids Quinine Quinidine	Rapid-acting blood schizontocides. Some gametocytocidal activity.
	Mefloquine	Blood schizontocide.
4-Aminoquinolines	Chloroquine Hydroxychloroquine Amodiaquine	Rapid-acting blood schizontocides. Some gametocytocidal activity.
8-Aminoquinolines	Primaquine	Tissue schizontocide. Also gametocytocidal activity and some activity at other stages of the parasite's life-cycle.
Biguanides	Proguanil Chlorproguanil	Tissue schizontocides and slow-acting blood schizontocides. Some sporontocidal activity. Dihydrofolate reductase inhibitors.
Diaminopyrimidines	Pyrimethamine	Tissue schizontocide and slow-acting blood schizontocide. Some sporontocidal activity. Dihydrofolate reductase inhibitor. Usually used with antimalarials that inhibit different stages of folate synthesis (sulphonamides or sulphones) to form synergistic combinations.
Hydroxynaphthoquinones	Atovaquone	Blood schizontocide. Usually given in combination with proguanil.
9-Phenanthrenemethanols	Halofantrine	Blood schizontocide.
Sesquiterpene lactones	Artemisinin and its derivatives	Blood schizontocide.
Sulphonamides	Sulfadoxine Sulfametopyrazine	Blood schizontocides. Dihydropteroate and folate synthesis inhibitors. Usually given in combination with pyrimethamine.
Antibiotics	Tetracyclines Doxycycline Tetracycline Clindamycin	Blood schizontocides. Some tissue schizontocidal activity.
Sulphones	Dapsone	Blood schizontocide. Folate synthesis inhibitor. Usually given in combination with pyrimethamine.

Antimalarials are generally given by mouth, although in order to obtain a rapid response in patients with severe or complicated falciparum malaria (see below) it may be necessary to give parenteral therapy initially, the patient being transferred to oral therapy when feasible.[4]

Treatment of falciparum malaria. In most parts of the world *P. falciparum* is now resistant to chloroquine, therefore, apart from the rare circumstance of exposure in one of the few remaining areas of chloroquine sensitivity, chloroquine is **not** suitable for treatment. Instead, infections are treated with:

- quinine *and* (if quinine resistance is known or suspected) followed by *either* pyrimethamine-sulfadoxine (Fansidar) *or* (if Fansidar-resistant) by doxycycline *or* clindamycin

or alternatively with

- mefloquine

or

- atovaquone-proguanil (Malarone)

or

- halofantrine.

It is not necessary to give pyrimethamine-sulfadoxine (Fansidar), doxycycline, or clindamycin after the latter three treatments.

Resistance has already been reported in several countries to mefloquine or halofantrine; in addition cardiotoxicity is an important limitation on the use of halofantrine.

To combat the increasing problem of drug-resistant falciparum malaria, WHO has recommended that artemisinin and related compounds should be reserved solely for areas of multidrug-resistant malaria (and should not be used for prophylaxis); they are usually used in combination with mefloquine. A combination of artemether with benflumetol also shows promise. Pyronaridine is another drug that shows potential.

In the case of **severe or complicated falciparum malaria** including cerebral malaria parenteral treatment is required to produce adequate blood concentrations as quickly as possible.[2,4-6] Quinine is usually given intravenously, starting with a loading dose; quinidine has been used if quinine was not available. Patients of all ages need to be closely monitored while undergoing parenteral therapy and treatment is changed to an orally administered antimalarial as soon as the patient's condition permits. When there are only minimal health care facilities and parenteral therapy is not possible the nasogastric route may be used.[2,4] An artemisinin derivative may be considered in areas where quinine is known or found to be ineffective.[7] Intramuscular administration of the artemisinin derivative artemether has been reported to compare favourably with parenteral quinine in patients with severe disease (but see p.426). Supportive therapy in patients with severe or complicated malaria needs to be directed at reducing hyperpyrexia, controlling convulsions, maintaining fluid balance, and correcting hypoglycaemia.[2,4,5] Since iron might be involved in the pathogenesis of cerebral malaria, the iron chelator desferrioxamine has been tried in addition to standard antimalarial therapy, but any benefit is yet to be established. Anecdotal reports of the value of corticosteroids in cerebral malaria have not been substantiated by controlled studies and they have no place in the management of this condition. Other approaches such as the use of hyperimmune serum or monoclonal antibody to tumour necrosis factor have also been unsuccessful. White[8] emphasised the importance of achieving therapeutic concentrations of antimalarial drugs as early as possible.

Treatment of benign malarias. Benign malarias, which are usually caused by *P. vivax* and less commonly by *P. ovale* and *P. malariae*, can be debilitating but are usually less severe than falciparum malaria. Chloroquine is still the drug of choice (but chloroquine-resistant vivax infection has been reported from some areas—notably New Guinea and some adjacent islands). Chloroquine alone is adequate for *P. malariae* infections, but in the case of those caused by *P. vivax* or *P. ovale* a subsequent *radical cure* with a tissue schizontocide, usually primaquine, is needed to avoid the risk of relapse (caused by the presence of latent hypnozoites) months or years after the primary infection. Radical cure is inappropriate for patients living within an endemic area since re-infection is likely, therefore WHO recommends that it should be limited to patients resident in areas where transmission is *very low* or *absent* and to those treated *during an epidemic*; other patients should simply be treated with a further course of chloroquine in the event of relapse or re-infection. Mefloquine and halofantrine are also active in benign malarias but are not generally used.

Treatment of malaria during pregnancy. Malaria is especially dangerous during pregnancy and the seriousness of the disease usually outweighs any potential risk from treatment. Although fetal abnormalities have been associated with the use of high doses of chloroquine, extensive clinical experience suggests it is safe.[2,4] Quinine may be used for chloroquine-resistant malaria but care should be taken that patients do not become hypoglycaemic.[2,5] There may be difficulty if additional drugs are required as opinion varies over their suitability. Some consider that pyrimethamine combinations should be avoided,[2] especially during the first trimester (see under Pregnancy in Precautions of Pyrimethamine, p.437). The tetracyclines are contra-indicated on dental grounds and the safety of mefloquine, halofantrine, or atovaquone has not been fully assessed although mefloquine is now suggested for prophylactic use from the fourth month of pregnancy. For patients with vivax or ovale malaria during pregnancy radical cure with primaquine should be postponed until after delivery;[5,6] weekly chloroquine can be given during the remaining weeks of pregnancy.

Treatment of splenomegaly syndrome. A small number of individuals infected with *Plasmodium* develop chronic hyperreactive malarial splenomegaly syndrome, an aberrant immunological response formerly known as the tropical splenomegaly syndrome. Traditionally, patients have first received a full course of antimalarial chemotherapy appropriate to the causative species followed by lengthy and probably lifelong chemoprophylaxis.[9] However, a study in 312 patients suggested that pyrimethamine given with folinic acid for 30 days could produce a rapid reduction of splenomegaly which persisted for at least 3 months.[10]

Prophylaxis of malaria

Chemoprophylaxis of malaria may refer to absolute prevention of infection (*causal prophylaxis*) or to suppression of parasitaemia and its symptoms (*clinical prophylaxis*). Causal prophylaxis is provided by tissue schizontocides which destroy the exoerythrocytic forms of the parasite. Clinical prophylaxis is provided by blood schizontocides which, if continued until all exoerythrocytic forms of the parasite are destroyed, will ultimately produce a *suppressive cure*. In *P. falciparum* infections this would be achieved by about a month after the last infected bite, but relapses with *P. vivax* and *P. ovale* may still occur after standard clinical prophylactic regimens due to the presence of latent exoerythrocytic forms (hypnozoites).

The continuing increase in the prevalence of strains of *P. falciparum* resistant to chloroquine and other antimalarials along with growing evidence of toxicity of some regimens make recommendations for malaria prophylaxis increasingly difficult. Absolute protection cannot be guaranteed by any chemoprophylactic regimen currently in use and the importance and effectiveness of methods of avoiding bites from infected mosquitoes such as the use of *protective clothing, bed netting*, and *insect repellents* and *insecticides* must be stressed.[2,3] WHO recommends[3] the following measures to protect against mosquito bites:

- application of an insect repellent containing diethyltoluamide or dimethyl phthalate to exposed skin between dusk and dawn when mosquitoes commonly bite
- accommodation in buildings with screens over doors and windows
- use of mosquito nets at night, preferably impregnated with the pyrethroid insecticides permethrin or deltamethrin
- and use of anti-mosquito sprays or insecticide dispensers containing pyrethroids, or pyrethroid mosquito coils in bedrooms at night.

Recent studies in African children have demonstrated that pyrethroid-impregnated mosquito nets can reduce mortality substantially.[11-13] In addition to these measures, travellers should be advised, even if chemoprophylaxis has been taken regularly, to regard **any** fever *after the first week* and for *up to 1 year following possible exposure* as being caused by malaria and to seek medical advice **immediately**. Some authorities advise that travellers should also have antimalarial drugs ready for emergency self-treatment (*standby treatment*) when prompt medical attention is not available.

WHO considers that chemoprophylaxis should be reserved for those at high risk, notably *non-immune visitors*; widespread chemoprophylaxis in *immune or semi-immune* populations is no longer recommended except for women who are *pregnant*. Those such as the elderly, pregnant women, and adults who would need to take young children should consider very carefully whether it is absolutely necessary to travel to areas where falciparum malaria occurs; WHO specifically advises pregnant women not to travel on vacation to areas where transmission of *P. falciparum* occurs and also advises against taking babies and young children on holiday to malarious areas (particularly where there is transmission of *P. falciparum*).[2,3] Advice on chemoprophylaxis must be based on a knowledge of the occurrence and susceptibility of malaria strains in specific geographical areas. Local variations due to altitude, seasonal variations in temperature and rainfall, the degree of urbanisation, and many other factors further complicate the issue. WHO collates information provided by national health administrations and regularly publishes this information to assist in advising international travellers on the current situation; similar information is provided at national level by local institutes specialising in tropical diseases. However, the situation is so complex that advice differs. Recommendations issued by various authorities are usually for short-term stays and expert advice should be sought if long-term cover is required.

It is generally recommended that chemoprophylaxis should start about one week (or longer for mefloquine) before exposure to malaria, or if this is not possible at the earliest opportunity up to 1 or 2 days before exposure; this is partly to ensure that the patient is able to tolerate the drug. Chemoprophylaxis should continue throughout exposure and for at least 4 weeks after leaving the malarious area.

Prophylactic regimens. Depending upon the risk of infection and the availability and standard of local medical care WHO[2,3] has made various recommendations concerning chemoprophylaxis and/or standby treatment for non-immune travellers:

- in areas where *P. falciparum* is *absent* or still *sensitive to chloroquine*, travellers can either take chloroquine for prophylaxis or, if the infection risk is *very low*, not take prophylaxis at all
- in areas where *P. falciparum* is *resistant to chloroquine* but with a low risk of infection, chloroquine with proguanil is recommended as it may give some protection against *P. falciparum* and may alleviate the symptoms if an attack does occur; chloroquine given alone will only protect against *P. vivax* in these areas. Again if the infection risk is very low travellers may do without prophylaxis
- in areas of high risk or where there is multidrug resistance, mefloquine is recommended as first choice for prophylaxis, chloroquine with proguanil is recommended as second choice, with doxycycline as a further alternative in specified areas, depending on the patterns of drug resistance prevailing.

WHO also recommends that for the small number of travellers who would be unable to obtain prompt medical attention when malaria is suspected (within 24 hours of the onset of symptoms), it may be necessary to provide a course of treatment for self-administration (*standby treatment*). Clear instructions must be given and persons taking standby medication must seek medical advice as soon as possible. Also having completed the standby course they should resume any prophylaxis. The basis upon which the choice of prophylaxis is made (as detailed above) in turn broadly determines the appropriate choice of standby treatment. Thus:

- where *no prophylaxis* is deemed necessary, chloroquine is given for standby treatment in areas where there is chloroquine sensitivity, otherwise standby treatment is with pyrimethamine-sulfadoxine (Fansidar), or with mefloquine, or with quinine
- where prophylaxis is *with chloroquine* (either alone or with proguanil), standby treatment is with pyrimethamine-sulfadoxine (Fansidar), or with mefloquine, or with quinine
- where prophylaxis is *with mefloquine*, standby treatment is with pyrimethamine-sulfadoxine (Fansidar), or with quinine alone, or with quinine plus doxycycline or tetracycline
- where prophylaxis is *with doxycycline*, standby treatment is with mefloquine or with quinine plus tetracycline.

It should be noted that pyrimethamine-sulfadoxine (Fansidar) is appropriate *only for* areas such India and for Africa south of the Sahara. It should also be noted that halofantrine is no longer recommended for standby treatment.

In the USA recommendations for prophylaxis are provided by the Centers for Disease Control (CDC)[14-16] and other sources.[6] The recommendations for chloroquine-sensitive malaria are similar to those of WHO in that chloroquine alone is advised; hydroxychloroquine is suggested as an alternative. For all areas with chloroquine-resistant malaria, the use of mefloquine alone is recommended with alternatives being either doxycycline, or chloroquine (either with proguanil, or with pyrimethamine-sulfadoxine (Fansidar)) for standby treatment. Primaquine has also been advocated for prophylaxis. The use of primaquine has also been advocated during the last 2 weeks of prophylaxis to prevent relapses due to *P. vivax* or *P. ovale* in persons returning from prolonged exposure in areas where relapsing malaria is endemic.

UK experts[17] have also published guidelines for the prophylaxis of malaria and in most cases these are in broad agreement with those of WHO.

VACCINES. Malaria vaccines are under development and several are currently undergoing clinical evaluation (see p.1517).

Prophylaxis during pregnancy. The choice of drugs for prophylaxis during pregnancy is limited and whenever possible women who are pregnant or likely to become so should avoid travelling to malarious areas (see also above). In pregnant women who cannot avoid travelling to endemic areas, chloroquine may be given alone for prophylaxis in the few areas where *P. falciparum* is sensitive to chloroquine, or in combination with proguanil where resistance exists.[3] Mefloquine is normally avoided during the first trimester but may be given from the fourth month onwards; pyrimethamine-dapsone (Maloprim) is also contra-indicated in the first trimester. Folate supplements (folic acid 5 mg daily) need to be taken with proguanil and with pyrimethamine-dapsone (Maloprim).[17] In non-pregnant women of child-bearing potential, pregnancy needs to be avoided for 3 months after completing mefloquine prophylaxis. Doxycycline or primaquine is contra-indicated in pregnant women by most experts.

Pregnant women living in endemic areas commonly receive malaria chemoprophylaxis as a matter of policy since their susceptibility to the disease, especially among primigravidae, is believed to be increased. Routine prophylaxis has been shown to reduce anaemia and produce a trend towards higher birth-weights and lower perinatal mortality.[18-20] A study of chemoprophylaxis in 1049 pregnancies[21] suggested that multigravidae obtained less benefit than primigravidae and a follow-up study[22] found that the outcome of subsequent pregnancies was similar regardless of whether chemoprophylaxis or placebo had been given in the first pregnancy. This result suggested that it may be possible to restrict chemoprophylaxis to first pregnancies in endemic areas. A review of randomised studies[23] came to a similar conclusion.

Prophylaxis during breast feeding. Breast feeding by mothers taking mefloquine is usually contra-indicated although the amount ingested by the nursing infant may be too small to produce adverse effects. For other antimalarials it is generally accepted that the amount distributed into breast milk and consumed by nursing infants is too small to be harmful. However, these amounts are also too small to provide adequate protection and breast-fed infants still require chemoprophylaxis.

Prophylaxis in children. Chloroquine and proguanil may be given in scaled down doses to children of all ages but the choice of alternative drugs may be restricted especially in very young children and consideration should be given to whether their travel to malarious areas is absolutely necessary (see also above).

Prophylaxis in epilepsy. In subjects with a history of epilepsy the UK guidelines[17] advise that both chloroquine and mefloquine are unsuitable for prophylaxis. In areas without chloroquine resistance proguanil alone is recommended. In areas with a high risk of chloroquine resistance doxycycline may be considered, but its metabolism may be influenced by antiepileptics. Pyrimethamine-dapsone (Maloprim) may be an alternative; the UK guidelines mention folate supplementation (folic acid 5 mg daily) in those taking phenytoin or phenobarbitone.

Prophylaxis in HIV-infected travellers. HIV-infected travellers may take chloroquine routinely for antimalarial prophylaxis but its potential immunosuppressive effects should be recognised; proguanil, mefloquine, or doxycycline can also be used.[24,25] Although patients with AIDS may be at increased risk of adverse effects to sulphonamides a combination such as pyrimethamine-sulfadoxine (Fansidar) can be used for standby treatment if an alternative is not available.[24,25]

1. Whitby M. Drug resistant Plasmodium vivax malaria. *J Antimicrob Chemother* 1997; **40:** 749–52.
2. WHO. Practical chemotherapy of malaria: report of a WHO scientific group. *WHO Tech Rep Ser 805* 1990.
3. WHO. *International travel and health: vaccination requirements and health advice.* Geneva: WHO, 1998.
4. Gilles HM. *Management of severe and complicated malaria.* Geneva: WHO, 1991.
5. Molyneux M, Fox R. Diagnosis and treatment of malaria in Britain. *Br Med J* 1993; **306:** 1175–80.
6. Anonymous. Drugs for parasitic infections. *Med Lett Drugs Ther* 1998; **40:** 1–12.
7. Anonymous. Artemisinin and its derivatives: use as antimalarials. *WHO Drug Inf* 1993; **7:** 111–13.
8. White NJ. Not much progress in treatment of cerebral malaria. *Lancet* 1998; **352:** 594–5.
9. Cook GC. Prevention and treatment of malaria. *Lancet* 1988; **i:** 32–7.
10. Manenti F, *et al.* Treatment of hyperreactive malarial splenomegaly syndrome. *Lancet* 1994; **343:** 1441–2.
11. D'Alessandro U, *et al.* Mortality and morbidity from malaria in Gambian children after introduction of an impregnated bednet programme. *Lancet* 1995; **345:** 479–83.
12. Nevill CG, *et al.* Insecticide-treated bednets reduce mortality and severe morbidity from malaria among children on the Kenyan coast. *Trop Med Int Hlth* 1996; **1:** 139–46.
13. Binka FN, *et al.* Impact of permethrin impregnated bednets on child mortality in Kassena-Nankana district, Ghana: a randomized controlled trial. *Trop Med Int Hlth* 1996; **1:** 147–54.
14. Centers for Disease Control. Recommendations for the prevention of malaria among travelers. *MMWR* 1990; **39** (RR-3): 1–10.
15. Centers for Disease Control. Revised dosing regimen for malaria prophylaxis with mefloquine. *MMWR* 1990; **39:** 630.
16. Centers for Disease Control. Change of dosing regimen for malaria prophylaxis with mefloquine. *MMWR* 1991; **40:** 72–3.
17. Bradley DJ, *et al.* Guidelines for the prevention of malaria in travellers from the United Kingdom. *Commun Dis Rep Rev* 1997; **7:** R137–R152.
18. Greenwood AM, *et al.* The distribution of birth weights in Gambian women who received malaria chemoprophylaxis during their first pregnancy and in control women. *Trans R Soc Trop Med Hyg* 1994; **88:** 311–12.
19. Schultz LJ, *et al.* The efficacy of antimalarial regimens containing sulfadoxine-pyrimethamine and/or chloroquine in preventing peripheral and placental Plasmodium falciparum infection among pregnant women in Malawi. *Am J Trop Med Hyg* 1994; **51:** 515–22.
20. Nosten F, *et al.* Mefloquine prophylaxis prevents malaria during pregnancy: a double-blind, placebo-controlled study. *J Infect Dis* 1994; **169:** 595–603.
21. Greenwood BM, *et al.* The effects of malaria chemoprophylaxis given by traditional birth attendants on the course and outcome of pregnancy. *Trans R Soc Trop Med Hyg* 1989; **83:** 589–94.
22. Greenwood AM, *et al.* Can malaria chemoprophylaxis be restricted to first pregnancies? *Trans R Soc Trop Med Hyg* 1994; **88:** 681–2.
23. Garner P, Brabin B. A review of randomized controlled trials of routine antimalarial drug prophylaxis during pregnancy in endemic malarious areas. *Bull WHO* 1994; **72:** 89–99.
24. von Reyn CF, *et al.* International travel and HIV infection. *Bull WHO* 1990; **68:** 251–9.
25. Wilson ME, *et al.* Infections in HIV-infected travelers: risks and prevention. *Ann Intern Med* 1991; **114:** 582–92.

Amodiaquine (16289-t)

Amodiaquine *(BAN, rINN).*

4-(7-Chloro-4-quinolylamino)-2-(diethylaminomethyl)phenol.

$C_{20}H_{22}ClN_3O$ = 355.9.

CAS — 86-42-0.

Pharmacopoeias. In *Int.* and *US.*

Very pale yellow to light tan-yellow odourless powder. Practically **insoluble** in water; slightly soluble in alcohol; sparingly soluble in 0.1N hydrochloric acid. **Store** in airtight containers.

Amodiaquine Hydrochloride (1374-g)

Amodiaquine Hydrochloride *(BANM, rINNM).*

Amodiaquini Hydrochloridum. 4-(7-Chloro-4-quinolylamino)-2-(diethylaminomethyl)phenol dihydrochloride dihydrate.

$C_{20}H_{22}ClN_3O,2HCl,2H_2O$ = 464.8.

CAS — 69-44-3 (amodiaquine hydrochloride, anhydrous); 6398-98-7 (amodiaquine hydrochloride, dihydrate).

Pharmacopoeias. In *Fr., Int.,* and *US.*

A yellow, odourless, crystalline powder. Amodiaquine base 200 mg is approximately equivalent to 260 mg of amodiaquine hydrochloride. **Soluble** 1 in 25 of water and 1 in 78 of alcohol; very slightly soluble in chloroform and in ether. **Store** in airtight containers.

Sorption. For reference to loss of amodiaquine hydrochloride from solutions during membrane filtration, see Chloroquine, p.426.

Adverse Effects and Precautions

As for Chloroquine, p.426, but amodiaquine was associated with hepatitis and a much higher incidence of agranulocytosis when it was used for the prophylaxis of malaria.

Earlier isolated reports of amodiaquine causing severe neutropenia were usually when it had been used in anti-inflammatory doses for rheumatoid arthritis, but there was a cluster of cases in 1986 associated with its use in malaria prophylaxis.[1] In all, 23 cases of agranulocytosis, 7 of which were fatal, were reported in the UK, USA, and Switzerland during a 12-month period ending March 1986. Nearly all of these patients had used the drug at a dosage of 400 mg weekly and the periods of exposure ranged from 3 to 24 weeks.[1] Some of these patients also had evidence of liver damage[1] and there have been other reports of hepatotoxicity associated with the prophylactic use of amodiaquine.[2] Examination of data submitted to the UK Committee on Safety of Medicines[3] suggested that the frequency of adverse reactions to amodiaquine was about 1 in 1700 for serious reactions, 1 in 2200 for blood disorders, 1 in 15 650 for serious hepatic disorders, and 1 in 15 650 for fatal reactions. In contrast the frequency of agranulocytosis in users in France[4] has been estimated to be 1 in 25 000. Worldwide[4] the risk of severe reactions appears to be between 1 in 1000 and 1 in 5000. The manufacturers reportedly had 42 cases of serious adverse effects during amodiaquine prophylaxis, between 1985 and 1991; there were 28 cases of agranulocytosis (9 deaths) and 14 of hepatitis (3 deaths).[5] Whether there was significantly less risk when amodiaquine was given for treatment of malaria rather than prophylaxis was not certain.[6]

It has been suggested that an immunological reaction to amodiaquine quinone imine, which can be produced by autoxidation among other processes, may partially account for amodiaquine's greater tendency to induce agranulocytosis compared with chloroquine.[7,8]

The acute toxicity of amodiaquine appears to differ from that of chloroquine in that there have been no reports of cardiovascular symptoms following overdosage with amodiaquine[9] but intoxication with amodiaquine is also far less frequent than chloroquine poisoning. However, large doses of amodiaquine have been reported to produce syncope, spasticity, convulsions, and involuntary movements.[9]

1. Anonymous. Amodiaquine and agranulocytosis. *WHO Drug Inf* 1987; **1:** 5–6.
2. Larrey D, *et al.* Amodiaquine-induced hepatitis. *Ann Intern Med* 1986; **104:** 801–3.
3. Phillips-Howard PA, West LJ. Serious adverse drug reactions to pyrimethamine–sulphadoxine, pyrimethamine–dapsone and to amodiaquine in Britain. *J R Soc Med* 1990; **83:** 82–5.
4. Anonymous. Development of recommendations for the protection of short-stay travellers to malaria endemic areas: memorandum from two WHO meetings. *Bull WHO* 1988; **66:** 177–96.
5. Olliaro P, *et al.* Systematic review of amodiaquine treatment in uncomplicated malaria. *Lancet* 1996; **348:** 1196–1201.
6. White NJ. Can amodiaquine be resurrected? *Lancet* 1996; **348:** 1184–5.
7. Winstanley PA, *et al.* The toxicity of amodiaquine and its principal metabolites towards mononuclear leucocytes and granulocyte/monocyte colony forming units. *Br J Clin Pharmacol* 1990; **29:** 479–85.
8. Park BK, Kitteringham NR. Drug–protein conjugation and its immunological consequences. *Drug Metab Rev* 1990; **22:** 87–144.
9. Jaeger A, *et al.* Clinical features and management of poisoning due to antimalarial drugs. *Med Toxicol* 1987; **2:** 242–73.

Pharmacokinetics

Amodiaquine hydrochloride is readily absorbed from the gastro-intestinal tract. Amodiaquine is rapidly converted in the liver to the active metabolite desethylamodiaquine, only a negligible amount of amodiaquine being excreted unchanged in the urine. The plasma elimination half-life of desethylamodiaquine has varied from 1 to 10 days or more. Amodiaquine and desethylamodiaquine have been detected in the urine several months after administration.

References.

1. Winstanley P, *et al.* The disposition of amodiaquine in man after oral administration. *Br J Clin Pharmacol* 1987; **23:** 1–7.
2. White NJ, *et al.* Pharmacokinetics of intravenous amodiaquine. *Br J Clin Pharmacol* 1987; **23:** 127–35.
3. Winstanley PA, *et al.* The disposition of amodiaquine in Zambians and Nigerians with malaria. *Br J Clin Pharmacol* 1990; **29:** 695–701.
4. Krishna S, White NJ. Pharmacokinetics of quinine, chloroquine and amodiaquine: clinical implications. *Clin Pharmacokinet* 1996; **30:** 263–99.

Uses and Administration

Amodiaquine is a 4-aminoquinoline antimalarial with an action similar to that of chloroquine (p.429). It is as effective as chloroquine against chloroquine-sensitive strains of *Plasmodium falciparum* and is also effective against some chloroquine-resistant strains, although resistance to amodiaquine has developed and there may be partial cross-resistance between amodiaquine and chloroquine. Because of resistance and the risk of major toxicity amodiaquine is not recommended for the prophylaxis of malaria.

Amodiaquine is given by mouth as the hydrochloride, but doses are expressed in terms of amodiaquine base. For the treatment of falciparum malaria a total dose of 35 mg per kg body-weight has been given over 3 days.

References.

1. Olliaro P, *et al.* Systematic review of amodiaquine treatment in uncomplicated malaria. *Lancet* 1996; **348:** 1196–1201.

Preparations

USP 23: Amodiaquine Hydrochloride Tablets.

Proprietary Preparations (details are given in Part 3)
Fr.: Flavoquine.

Amopyroquine Hydrochloride (1375-q)

Amopyroquine Hydrochloride *(rINNM)*.

Amopyroquin Hydrochloride; CI-356; PAM-780; WR-4835. 4-(7-Chloro-4-quinolylamino)-2-(pyrrolidin-1-ylmethyl)phenol dihydrochloride.

$C_{20}H_{20}ClN_3O,2HCl = 426.8$.

CAS — 550-81-2 (amopyroquine); 10350-81-9 (amopyroquine dihydrochloride).

Amopyroquine is a 4-aminoquinoline antimalarial that is an analogue of amodiaquine (above). It has been administered as the hydrochloride by intramuscular injection or by mouth in the treatment of malaria.

References.

1. Verdier F, *et al.* Pharmacokinetics of intramuscular amopyroquin in healthy subjects and determination of a therapeutic regimen for Plasmodium falciparum malaria. *Antimicrob Agents Chemother* 1989; **33:** 316–21.
2. Gaudebout C, *et al.* Efficacy of intramuscular amopyroquin for treatment of Plasmodium falciparum malaria in the Gabon Republic. *Antimicrob Agents Chemother* 1993; **37:** 970–4.
3. Pussard E, *et al.* Pharmacokinetics and metabolism of amopyroquin after administration of two doses of 6 mg/kg im 24h apart to healthy volunteers. *J Antimicrob Chemother* 1994; **34:** 803–8.
4. Krishna S, White NJ. Pharmacokinetics of quinine, chloroquine and amodiaquine: clinical implications. *Clin Pharmacokinet* 1996; **30:** 263–99.

Artemisinin Derivatives (18783-m)

Arteether (9352-a)

Dihydroartemisinin Ethyl Ether; Dihydroqinghaosu Ethyl Ether; SM-227. (3*R*,5a*S*,6*R*,8a*S*,9*R*,10*S*,12*R*,12a*R*)-Decahydro-10-ethoxy-3,6,9-trimethyl-3,12-epoxy-12*H*-pyrano[4,3-*j*]-1,2-benzodioxepin.

$C_{17}H_{28}O_5 = 312.4$.

CAS — 75887-54-6.

Artemether (12024-p)

Artemether *(rINN)*.

Dihydroartemisinin Methyl Ether; Dihydroqinghaosu Methyl Ether; *o*-Methyldihydroartemisinin; SM-224. (3*R*,5a*S*,6*R*,8a*S*,9*R*,10*S*,12*R*,12a*R*)-Decahydro-10-methoxy-3,6,9-trimethyl-3,12-epoxy-12*H*-pyrano[4,3-*j*]-1,2-benzodioxepin.

$C_{16}H_{26}O_5 = 298.4$.

CAS — 71963-77-4.

Artemisinin (12023-q)

Artemisinin *(rINN)*.

Arteannuin; Artemisinine; Huanghuahaosu; Qinghaosu. (3*R*,5a*S*,6*R*,8a*S*,9*R*,12*S*,12a*R*)-Octahydro-3,6,9-trimethyl-3,12-epoxy-12*H*-pyrano[4,3-*j*]-1,2-benzodioxepin-10(3*H*)-one.

$C_{15}H_{22}O_5 = 282.3$.

CAS — 63968-64-9.

Sodium Artesunate (5761-m)

Sodium Artesunate *(rINNM)*.

Dihydroartemisinin Hemisuccinate Sodium; Dihydroqinghaosu Hemisuccinate Sodium; SM-804. (3*R*,5a*S*,6*R*,8a*S*,9*R*,10*S*,12*R*,12a*R*)-Decahydro-3,6,9-trimethyl-3,12-epoxy-12*H*-pyrano-[4,3-*j*]-1,2-benzodioxepin-10-ol hydrogen succinate sodium.

$C_{19}H_{27}O_8Na = 406.4$.

CAS — 88495-63-0 (artesunate).

Adverse Effects and Precautions

Treatment with artemisinin and its derivatives appears to be generally well tolerated, although there have been reports of mild gastro-intestinal disturbance, dizziness, tinnitus, neutropenia, elevated liver enzyme values, and ECG abnormalities including prolongation of the QT interval.

Evidence of severe neurotoxicity has been seen in *animals* given high doses.

Effects on the heart. Bradycardia was reported in 10 of 34 patients who received artemether orally for 4 days.[1]

1. Karbwang J, *et al.* Comparison of oral artemether and mefloquine in acute uncomplicated falciparum malaria. *Lancet* 1992; **340:** 1245–8.

Effects on the nervous system. Neurotoxicity has been reported in *animals* given arteether or artemether.[1] An *in vitro* study[2] has shown that dihydroartemisinin, the metabolite common to all artemisinin derivatives currently used, is neurotoxic. There has been a report[3] of acute cerebellar dysfunction manifesting as ataxia and slurred speech in a patient who took a 5-day course of artesunate by mouth.

1. Brewer TG, *et al.* Neurotoxicity in animals due to arteether and artemether. *Trans R Soc Trop Med Hyg* 1994; **88** (suppl 1): 33–6.
2. Wesche DL, *et al.* Neurotoxicity of artemisinin analogs in vitro. *Antimicrob Agents Chemother* 1994; **38:** 1813–19.
3. Miller LG, Panosian CB. Ataxia and slurred speech after artesunate treatment for falciparum malaria. *N Engl J Med* 1997; **336:** 1328.

Pregnancy. Artesunate or artemether was used to treat multidrug-resistant falciparum malaria in 83 pregnant women in Thailand; of 73 pregnancies resulting in live births none showed evidence of any congenital abnormality.[1] Sixteen of the women had received artesunate during the first trimester; of these, 12 had normal deliveries, 1 was lost to study, and 3 had spontaneous abortions. These preliminary findings were considered encouraging, and warranted further study of the safety of artemisinin derivatives in pregnancy.

1. McGready R, *et al.* Artemisinin derivatives in the treatment of falciparum malaria in pregnancy. *Trans R Soc Trop Med Hyg* 1998; **92:** 430–3.

Pharmacokinetics

Peak plasma concentrations have been achieved in about 3 hours following oral administration of artemether, in about 6 hours following intramuscular injection of artemether, and in about 11 hours following rectal administration of artemisinin. Artemisinin and its derivatives are all rapidly hydrolysed to the active metabolite dihydroartemisinin. Reported elimination half-lives have been about 45 minutes following intravenous administration of artesunate, about 4 hours following rectal artemisinin, and approximately 4 to 11 hours following intramuscular or oral artemether. There is very little published data on the pharmacokinetics of arteether, but its elimination half-life appears to be longer than that of artemether.

References.

1. Benakis A, *et al.* Pharmacokinetics of sodium artesunate after IM and IV administration. *Am J Trop Med Hyg* 1993; **49** (suppl): 293.
2. White NJ. Clinical pharmacokinetics and pharmacodynamics of artemisinin and derivatives. *Trans R Soc Trop Med Hyg* 1994; **88** (suppl 1): 41–3.
3. Bangchang KN, *et al.* Pharmacokinetics of artemether after oral administration to healthy Thai males and patients with acute, uncomplicated falciparum malaria. *Br J Clin Pharmacol* 1994; **37:** 249–53.
4. Hassan Alin M, *et al.* Multiple dose pharmacokinetics of oral artemisinin and comparison of its efficacy with that of oral artesunate in falciparum malaria patients. *Trans R Soc Trop Med Hyg* 1996; **90:** 61–5.
5. Teja-Isavadharm P, *et al.* Comparative bioavailability of oral, rectal, and intramuscular artemether in healthy subjects: use of simultaneous measurement by high performance liquid chromatography and bioassay. *Br J Clin Pharmacol* 1996; **42:** 599–604.
6. Dien TK, *et al.* Effect of food intake on pharmacokinetics of oral artemisinin in healthy Vietnamese subjects. *Antimicrob Agents Chemother* 1997; **41:** 1069–72.
7. Bethell DB, *et al.* Pharmacokinetics of oral artesunate in children with moderately severe Plasmodium falciparum malaria. *Trans R Soc Trop Med Hyg* 1997; **91:** 195–8.
8. Murphy SA, *et al.* The disposition of intramuscular artemether in children with cerebral malaria: a preliminary study. *Trans R Soc Trop Med Hyg* 1997; **91:** 331–4.
9. Batty KT, *et al.* A pharmacokinetic and pharmacodynamic study of intravenous vs oral artesunate in uncomplicated falciparum malaria. *Br J Clin Pharmacol* 1998; **45:** 123–9.
10. Karbwang J, *et al.* Pharmacokinetics of intramuscular artemether in patients with severe falciparum malaria with or without acute renal failure. *Br J Clin Pharmacol* 1998; **45:** 597–600.
11. Ashton M, *et al.* Artemisinin kinetics and dynamics during oral and rectal treatment of uncomplicated malaria. *Clin Pharmacol Ther* 1998; **63:** 482–92.

Uses and Administration

Artemisinin is a sesquiterpene lactone isolated from *Artemisia annua*, a herb that has traditionally been used in China for the treatment of malaria. It is a potent and rapidly acting blood schizontocide active against *Plasmodium vivax* and against both chloroquine-sensitive and chloroquine-resistant strains of *P. falciparum*.

Artemisinin and its derivatives artemether and sodium artesunate are used usually in combination with other antimalarials for the treatment of malaria resistant to conventional drugs.

The following doses are those suggested by the WHO for the treatment of malaria in areas of multidrug resistance. For oral administration in uncomplicated malaria, artemisinin or artesunate may be given as a 3-day course. The dose of artemisinin is 25 mg per kg body-weight on the first day with 12.5 mg per kg on the second and the third days. For artesunate, the initial dose is 5 mg per kg on the first day with 2.5 mg per kg on days two and three. In both cases a single dose of mefloquine 15 mg per kg (or occasionally 25 mg per kg if necessary) is given on the second day to effect radical cure. If the oral artemisinin compounds have to be used alone they should be given for a minimum of 5 days. For parenteral administration in severe malaria, artemether or artesunate are employed. The loading dose of artemether is 3.2 mg per kg intramuscularly followed by 1.6 mg per kg daily for a maximum of 7 days. The loading dose of artesunate is 2 mg per kg intramuscularly or intravenously followed after 4 hours and daily thereafter by a dose of 1 mg per kg again for a maximum of 7 days. For both drugs the patient should be transferred to oral therapy as soon as possible. Additionally a single oral dose of mefloquine should be given to effect radical cure.

Reviews.

1. de Vries PJ, Dien TK. Clinical pharmacology and therapeutic potential of artemisinin and its derivatives in the treatment of malaria. *Drugs* 1996; **52:** 818–36.

Administration of artemisinin derivatives. To overcome the poor solubility of *artemisinin* in water a number of dosage forms and routes of administration have been tried. Also, several more potent derivatives with more suitable pharmaceutical properties have been developed,[1-3] notably the methyl ether derivative, *artemether*, and the ethyl ether derivative, *arteether*, which are more lipid soluble; the sodium salt of the hemisuccinate ester, *sodium artesunate*, which is soluble in water but appears to have poor stability in aqueous solutions; and *sodium artelinate* which is both soluble and stable in water. Other derivatives which have been studied include *arteflene*. Several preparations of artemisinin derivatives are available either commercially or for studies organised by bodies such as WHO.[3] These include oral formulations of artemether, artesunate, artemisinin itself, and *dihydroartemisinin*; intramuscular formulations of arteether, artemether, and artesunate; intravenous formulations of *artelinic acid* and artesunate; and suppositories of artemisinin and artesunate.

1. Titulaer HAC, *et al.* Formulation and pharmacokinetics of artemisinin and its derivatives. *Int J Pharmaceutics* 1991; **69:** 83–92.
2. WHO. *WHO model prescribing information: drugs used in parasitic diseases.* 2nd ed. Geneva: WHO, 1995.
3. Olliaro PL, Trigg PI. Status of antimalarial drugs under development. *Bull WHO* 1995; **73:** 565–71.

Malaria. Artemisinin and its derivatives have been shown in many studies to be effective in the treatment of both acute uncomplicated and severe malaria, the overall management of which is discussed further on p.422. However, in an attempt to delay the development of resistance to these compounds WHO recommends[1-3] that their use be restricted to the treatment of malaria in areas of documented multidrug resistance, and that they should not be used at all for prophylaxis. Recrudescence rates are high when artemisinin compounds are given alone and they should therefore, when possible, be given with another antimalarial such as mefloquine in order to effect a radical cure.

In acute uncomplicated malaria the drugs are usually given by mouth. Those used have been artemisinin,[4] artemether[5-10] or artesunate[10-15] usually with mefloquine additionally. Artemether has also been used with benflumetol (see p.426). Arteether[16] has been given intramuscularly in acute malaria.

Parenteral therapy is generally necessary in severe malaria and good results in multidrug-resistant areas have been obtained with artemether,[17-19] arteether,[20] or artesunate[19,21] intramuscularly, usually followed by oral mefloquine. Artesunate has also been given intravenously.[19] Rectal administration of artesunate[22] or artemisinin,[19,21] followed by oral mefloquine, has been successful.

Alternatives to standard treatment of cerebral malaria with intravenous quinine have been sought, partly because of the problems associated with giving intravenous infusions in the field. Several studies have shown intramuscular artemether to be effective,[23-25] but the wisdom of such use when there is no multidrug resistance has been severely questioned[24,25] and is not endorsed by the WHO. Also, although artemether has compared favourably with quinine in the treatment of severe falciparum malaria,[17] in two larger studies[18,24] artemether, although an effective alternative to quinine, was associated with slightly longer coma-recovery times than quinine and did not reduce mortality significantly compared with quinine.

1. WHO. Practical chemotherapy of malaria: report of a WHO scientific group. *WHO Tech Rep Ser 805* 1990.
2. Anonymous. Artemisinin and its derivatives: use as antimalarials. *WHO Drug Inf* 1993; **7:** 111–13.
3. WHO. *WHO model prescribing information: drugs used in parasitic diseases.* 2nd ed. Geneva: WHO, 1995.
4. Hung LN, *et al.* Single dose artemisinin-mefloquine versus mefloquine alone for uncomplicated falciparum malaria. *Trans R Soc Trop Med Hyg* 1997; **91:** 191–4.
5. Karbwang J, *et al.* Comparison of oral artemether and mefloquine in acute uncomplicated falciparum malaria. *Lancet* 1992; **340:** 1245–8.
6. Bunnag D, *et al.* Artemether-mefloquine combination in multidrug resistant falciparum malaria. *Trans R Soc Trop Med Hyg* 1995; **89:** 213–15.
7. Karbwang J, *et al.* A comparative clinical trial of two different regimens of artemether plus mefloquine in multidrug resistant falciparum malaria. *Trans R Soc Trop Med Hyg* 1995; **89:** 296–8.
8. Karbwang J, *et al.* A comparative clinical trial of artemether and the sequential regimen of artemether-mefloquine in multidrug resistant falciparum malaria. *J Antimicrob Chemother* 1995; **36:** 1079–83.
9. Price RN, *et al.* Artesunate versus artemether in combination with mefloquine for the treatment of multidrug-resistant falciparum malaria. *Trans R Soc Trop Med Hyg* 1995; **89:** 523–7.
10. Bunnag D, *et al.* Artemether or artesunate followed by mefloquine as a possible treatment for multidrug resistant falciparum malaria. *Trans R Soc Trop Med Hyg* 1996; **90:** 415–17.
11. Looareesuwan S, *et al.* Randomized trial of mefloquine-doxycycline, and artesunate-doxycycline for treatment of acute uncomplicated falciparum malaria. *Am J Trop Med Hyg* 1994; **50:** 784–9.
12. Karbwang J, *et al.* Comparison of oral artesunate and quinine plus tetracycline in acute uncomplicated falciparum malaria. *Bull WHO* 1994; **72:** 233–8.
13. Luxemburger C, *et al.* Oral artesunate in the treatment of uncomplicated hyperparasitemic falciparum malaria. *Am J Trop Med Hyg* 1995; **53:** 522–5.
14. Looareesuwan S, *et al.* Comparative clinical trial of artesunate followed by mefloquine in the treatment of acute uncomplicated falciparum malaria: two- and three-day regimens. *Am J Trop Med Hyg* 1996; **54:** 210–13.
15. Price R, *et al.* Artesunate and mefloquine in the treatment of uncomplicated multidrug-resistant hyperparasitaemic falciparum malaria. *Trans R Soc Trop Med Hyg* 1998; **92:** 207–11.
16. Mishra SK, *et al.* Effectiveness of α,β-arteether in acute falciparum malaria. *Trans R Soc Trop Med Hyg* 1995; **89:** 299–301.
17. Karbwang J, *et al.* Comparison of artemether and quinine in the treatment of severe falciparum malaria in south-east Thailand. *Trans R Soc Trop Med Hyg* 1995; **89:** 668–71.
18. Hien TT, *et al.* A controlled trial of artemether or quinine in Vietnamese adults with severe falciparum malaria. *N Engl J Med* 1996; **335:** 76–83.
19. Vinh H, *et al.* Severe and complicated malaria treated with artemisinin, artesunate or artemether in Viet Nam. *Trans R Soc Trop Med Hyg* 1997; **91:** 465–7.
20. Mohanty S, *et al.* α,β-Arteether for the treatment of complicated falciparum malaria. *Trans R Soc Trop Med Hyg* 1997; **91:** 328–30.
21. Phuong CXT, *et al.* Comparison of artemisinin suppositories, intramuscular artesunate and intravenous quinine for the treatment of severe childhood malaria. *Trans R Soc Trop Med Hyg* 1997; **91:** 335–42.
22. Looareesuwan S, *et al.* Efficacy and tolerability of a sequential, artesunate suppository plus mefloquine, treatment of severe falciparum malaria. *Ann Trop Med Parasitol* 1995; **89:** 469–75.
23. Walker O, *et al.* An open randomized comparative study of intramuscular artemether and intravenous quinine in cerebral malaria in children. *Trans R Soc Trop Med Hyg* 1993; **87:** 564–6.
24. Boele van Hensbroek M, *et al.* A trial of artemether or quinine in children with cerebral malaria. *N Engl J Med* 1996; **335:** 69–75.
25. Murphy S, *et al.* An open randomized trial of artemether versus quinine in the treatment of cerebral malaria in African children. *Trans R Soc Trop Med Hyg* 1996; **90:** 298–301.

Preparations

Proprietary Preparations (details are given in Part 3)
Fr.: Paluther; ***Thai.:*** Artesunate.

Benflumetol (14735-s)

Benflumelol. 2,7-Dichloro-9-[(4-chlorophenyl)methylene]-α-[(dibutylamino)methyl]-9*H*-fluorene-4-methanol.

$C_{30}H_{32}Cl_3NO = 528.9.$

CAS — 82186-77-4.

Benflumetol is an antimalarial developed and used in China. It is given by mouth with artemether (p.425) for the treatment of falciparum malaria.

References to the use of benflumetol with artemether (CGP-56697) for the treatment of uncomplicated falciparum malaria.[1,2]

1. von Seidlein L, *et al.* Treatment of African children with uncomplicated falciparum malaria with a new antimalarial drug, CGP 56697. *J Infect Dis* 1997; **176:** 1113–16.
2. van Vugt M, *et al.* Randomized comparison of artemether-benflumetol and artesunate-mefloquine in treatment of multidrug-resistant falciparum malaria. *Antimicrob Agents Chemother* 1998; **42:** 135–9.

Chloroquine (1371-m)

Chloroquine *(BAN, rINN).*

Cloroquina. 4-(7-Chloro-4-quinolylamino)pentyldiethylamine; 7-Chloro-4-(4-diethylamino-1-methylbutylamino)quinoline.

$C_{18}H_{26}ClN_3 = 319.9.$

CAS — 54-05-7.

Pharmacopoeias. In US.

A white or slightly yellow odourless crystalline powder. Very slightly **soluble** in water; soluble in chloroform, ether, and dilute acids.

Chloroquine Hydrochloride (18496-t)

Chloroquine Hydrochloride *(BANM, rINNM).*

$C_{18}H_{26}ClN_3,2HCl = 392.8.$

CAS — 3545-67-3.

Pharmacopoeias. US includes the injection.

Chloroquine base 100 mg is approximately equivalent to 123 mg of chloroquine hydrochloride.

Chloroquine Phosphate (1372-b)

Chloroquine Phosphate *(BANM, rINNM).*

Chingaminum; Chlorochinium Phosphoricum; Chlorochinum Diphosphoricum; Chloroquini Diphosphas; Chloroquini Phosphas; Fosfato de Cloroquina; Quingamine; SN-7618.

$C_{18}H_{26}ClN_3,2H_3PO_4 = 515.9.$

CAS — 50-63-5.

Pharmacopoeias. In *Chin., Eur.* (see p.viii), *Int., Pol.,* and *US.*

A white or almost white, odourless, hygroscopic, crystalline powder which slowly discolours on exposure to light. It exists in two polymorphic forms, one melting at about 195° and the other at 215° to 218°. Chloroquine base 100 mg is approximately equivalent to 161 mg of chloroquine phosphate.

Freely **soluble** in water; very slightly soluble or practically insoluble in alcohol, in chloroform, and in ether; very slightly soluble in methyl alcohol. A 10% solution in water has a pH of 3.8 to 4.3. **Store** in airtight containers. Protect from light.

Chloroquine Sulphate (1373-v)

Chloroquine Sulphate *(BANM, rINNM).*

Chloroquini Sulfas; RP-3377; Sulfato de Cloroquina.

$C_{18}H_{26}ClN_3,H_2SO_4,H_2O = 436.0.$

CAS — 132-73-0 (anhydrous chloroquine sulphate).

Pharmacopoeias. In *Eur.* (see p.viii) and *Int.*

A white or almost white crystalline powder. Chloroquine base 100 mg is approximately equivalent to 136 mg of chloroquine sulphate. Freely **soluble** in water and in methyl alcohol; very slightly soluble in alcohol; practically insoluble in ether. An 8% solution in water has a pH of 4.0 to 5.0. **Store** in airtight containers. Protect from light.

Sorption. Various studies using low concentrations of chloroquine phosphate or chloroquine sulphate indicate that chloroquine exhibits pH-dependent binding to several materials used in medical equipment and membrane filters including soda glass and various plastics such as cellulose acetate, cellulose propionate, methacrylate butadiene styrene, polypropylene, polyvinyl chloride, ethylvinyl acetate, and polyethylene.[1-3] Although this effect may not be of relevance at doses used clinically[4] it is considered critical that laboratory workers undertaking assays and sensitivity testing should recognise that significant reductions in concentrations can occur when chloroquine is prepared or stored in equipment made from these materials.[2,3] As the effect of borosilicate glass or polystyrene appears to be minimal it has been suggested that they may be suitable for use in such procedures.[2,3]

Similar sorption has also been reported during membrane filtration of solutions of amodiaquine hydrochloride, mefloquine hydrochloride, or quinine sulphate.[1]

1. Baird JK, Lambros C. Effect of membrane filtration of antimalarial drug solutions on in vitro activity against Plasmodium falciparum. *Bull WHO* 1984; **62:** 439–44.
2. Yahya AM, *et al.* Binding of chloroquine to glass. *Int J Pharmaceutics* 1985; **25:** 217–23.
3. Yahya AM, *et al.* Investigation of chloroquine binding to plastic materials. *Int J Pharmaceutics* 1986; **34:** 137–43.
4. Martens HJ, *et al.* Sorption of various drugs in polyvinyl chloride, glass, and polyethylene-lined infusion containers. *Am J Hosp Pharm* 1990; **47:** 369–73.

Adverse Effects

Adverse effects experienced with dosage regimens of chloroquine used in the treatment and prophylaxis of malaria are generally less common and less severe than those associated with the larger doses used for prolonged periods in rheumatoid arthritis.

Frequent adverse effects of chloroquine include headache, various skin eruptions, pruritus, and gastro-intestinal disturbances such as nausea, vomiting, and diarrhoea. More rarely, mental changes including psychotic episodes, agitation, and personality changes may occur. Convulsions have been reported. Visual disturbances such as blurred vision and difficulties in focusing have occurred but these are more common with larger doses, when they may be associated with keratopathy or retinopathy, as discussed under Effects on the Eyes, below. Keratopathy usually occurs in the form of corneal opacities and is normally reversible when chloroquine is withdrawn. Retinopathy is the most serious adverse effect of chloroquine on the eyes and it can result in severe visual impairment. Changes may be irreversible and can even progress after chloroquine is discontinued. Those taking large doses of chloroquine for prolonged periods appear to be at greatest risk of developing retinopathy. Other uncommon adverse effects from prolonged use include loss of hair, bleaching of hair pigment, bluish-black pigmentation of the mucous membranes and skin, photosensitivity, tinnitus, reduced hearing, nerve deafness, neuromyopathy, and myopathy, including cardiomyopathy.

Blood disorders have been reported rarely. They include aplastic anaemia, reversible agranulocytosis, thrombocytopenia, and neutropenia.

Parenteral therapy with chloroquine can be hazardous and rapid intravenous administration or the use of large doses can result in cardiovascular toxicity and other symptoms of acute overdosage.

Acute overdosage with chloroquine is extremely dangerous and death can occur within a few hours. Initial effects include headache, gastro-intestinal disturbances, drowsiness, and dizziness. Hypokalaemia may occur within a few hours of ingestion of chloroquine. Visual disturbances may be dramatic with a sudden loss of vision. However, the main effect of overdosage with chloroquine is cardiovascular toxicity with hypotension and cardiac arrhythmias progressing to cardiovascular collapse, convulsions, cardiac and respiratory arrest, coma, and death.

Effects on the blood. Aplastic anaemia was associated with the use of chloroquine in 3 patients.[1] Two patients had received treatment over several months and one of these was later found to have acute myeloblastic leukaemia after receiving chloroquine treatment initially for discoid lupus erythematosus, and later for cerebral malaria. In the third patient aplastic anaemia developed 3 weeks after a short course of chloroquine for malaria.

1. Nagaratnam N, *et al.* Aplasia and leukaemia following chloroquine therapy. *Postgrad Med J* 1978; **54:** 108–12.

Effects on the eyes. The main adverse effects of chloroquine and hydroxychloroquine on the eye are keratopathy and retinopathy.

Keratopathy, characterised by corneal deposits, may occur within a few weeks of starting treatment. However, patients are often asymptomatic and fewer than 50% of affected patients complain of visual symptoms such as photophobia, haloes around lights, or blurred vision. Keratopathy is completely reversible on withdrawal of treatment and is not usually considered to be a contra-indication to continued treatment.[1]

Retinopathy is potentially more serious. The outcome following discontinuation of treatment is unpredictable and changes may be irreversible or may even progress.[2,3] Delayed-onset retinopathy has also been reported in patients many years after cessation of treatment.[4] The College of Ophthalmologists in the UK recommends eye examination before starting long-term treatment with chloroquine or hydroxychloroquine to establish a base-line, patients being told to stop treatment and seek expert advice if they note any disturbance of vision; when monitoring is considered necessary they have advocated Amsler testing by the patient once a month to detect premaculopathy which is often reversible. The reported incidence of retinopathy varies according to the methodology and criteria used.[1,5,6] From studies in patients on long-term antimalarial treatment, Bernstein[1] reported that an accumulation of 100 g of chloroquine [phosphate] (250 mg daily for 1 year) might cause retinopathy; the risk was significantly increased as the total dosage exceeded 300 g. Experience in rheumatology also indicates that the incidence of retinal toxicity is dose-related. While the total cumulative dose, the duration of treatment, and the age of the patient might all affect the incidence of retinal toxicity[7,8] the daily dose might be the most important factor.[9] It has been suggested that the risk of retinal damage is small with daily doses of up to 4.0 mg of chloroquine phosphate per kg body-weight (= chloroquine base approximately 2.5 mg per kg daily) or up to 6.5 mg of hydroxychloroquine sulphate per kg.[9] In obese patients, excessive dosage should be avoided by calculating dosage on the basis of lean body-weight. It appears that retinopathy is rarely, if ever, associated with the weekly dosages of chloroquine recommended for the prophylaxis of malaria.[10,11]

1. Bernstein HN. Ophthalmologic considerations and testing in patients receiving long-term antimalarial therapy. *Am J Med* 1983; **75** (suppl 1A): 25–34.
2. Ogawa S, *et al.* Progression of retinopathy long after cessation of chloroquine therapy. *Lancet* 1979; **i:** 1408.
3. Easterbrook M. Ocular effects and safety of antimalarial agents. *Am J Med* 1988; **85** (suppl 4A): 23–9.
4. Ehrenfeld M, *et al.* Delayed-onset chloroquine retinopathy. *Br J Ophthalmol* 1986; **70:** 281–3.
5. Finbloom DS, *et al.* Comparison of hydroxychloroquine and chloroquine use and the development of retinal toxicity. *J Rheumatol* 1985; **12:** 692–4.
6. Morsman CDG, *et al.* Screening for hydroxychloroquine retinal toxicity: is it necessary? *Eye* 1990; **4:** 572–6.
7. Elman A, *et al.* Chloroquine retinopathy in patients with rheumatoid arthritis. *Scand J Rheumatol* 1976; **5:** 161–6.
8. Marks JS, Power BJ. Is chloroquine obsolete in treatment of rheumatic disease? *Lancet* 1979; **i:** 371–3.
9. Mackenzie AH. Dose refinements in long-term therapy of rheumatoid arthritis with antimalarials. *Am J Med* 1983; **75** (suppl 1A): 40–5.
10. Breckenridge A. Risks and benefits of prophylactic antimalarial drugs. *Br Med J* 1989; **299:** 1057–8.
11. Lange WR, *et al.* No evidence for chloroquine-associated retinopathy among missionaries on long-term malaria chemoprophylaxis. *Am J Trop Med Hyg* 1994; **51:** 389–92.

Effects on glucose metabolism. While hypoglycaemia has occurred with quinine (see p.439), it was not generally thought to be associated with chloroquine; however, there has been a report of its occurrence in a patient with reactive hypoglycaemia.[1]

1. Abu-Shakra M, Lee P. Hypoglycemia: an unusual adverse reaction to chloroquine. *Clin Exp Rheumatol* 1994; **12:** 95.

Effects on the heart. Studies in patients with malaria[1] and in healthy subjects[2] indicate that the acute cardiovascular toxicity that may be associated with parenteral administration of chloroquine is related to transiently high plasma concentrations produced during the early part of the distribution phase; these findings appear to confirm that the rate of administration is a major determinant of this toxicity. Cardiac conduction abnormalities including heart block have also occurred in patients receiving long-term oral treatment with chloroquine[3] including use in lupus erythematosus[4] as well as after chloroquine overdosage or abuse.[5] Histological changes in endomyocardial biopsy specimens from 2 patients with cardiomyopathy associated with chloroquine or hydroxychloroquine therapy were found to be virtually identical to those seen in the skeletal muscle of patients with chloroquine-induced myopathy[6] (see also Effects on the Muscles, below).

1. White NJ, *et al.* Parenteral chloroquine for treating falciparum malaria. *J Infect Dis* 1987; **155:** 192–201.
2. Looareesuwan S, *et al.* Cardiovascular toxicity and distribution kinetics of intravenous chloroquine. *Br J Clin Pharmacol* 1986; **22:** 31–6.
3. Ogola ESN, *et al.* Chloroquine related complete heart block with blindness: case report. *East Afr Med J* 1992; **69:** 50–2.
4. Piette J-C, *et al.* Chloroquine cardiotoxicity. *N Engl J Med* 1987; **317:** 710–11.
5. Ihenacho HNC, Magulike E. Chloroquine abuse and heart block in Africans. *Aust N Z J Med* 1989; **19:** 17–21.
6. Ratliff NB, *et al.* Diagnosis of chloroquine cardiomyopathy by endomyocardial biopsy. *N Engl J Med* 1987; **316:** 191–3.

Effects on the muscles. Reviewing drug-induced myotoxicity Mastaglia made the following points concerning chloroquine.[1] The myopathy induced by chloroquine is characterised by progressive weakness and atrophy of proximal muscles and can develop insidiously after periods of therapy ranging from a few weeks to a few years. There are often mild sensory changes, depression of tendon reflexes, and abnormal nerve conduction studies suggestive of an associated peripheral neuropathy. The myopathy is reversible on withdrawal of treatment but recovery may take several months. Cardiomyopathy may also occur (see under Effects on the Heart, above). Similar effects have been reported with hydroxychloroquine.[2] In a retrospective review of 4405 patients with rheumatic disorders, 214 had received chloroquine or hydroxychloroquine and, of these, 3 developed myopathy.[3]

1. Mastaglia FL. Adverse effects of drugs on muscle. *Drugs* 1982; **24:** 304–21.
2. Estes ML, *et al.* Chloroquine neuromyotoxicity. *Am J Med* 1987; **82:** 447–55.
3. Avina-Zubieta JA, *et al.* Incidence of myopathy in patients treated with antimalarials: a report of three cases and a review of the literature. *Br J Rheumatol* 1995; **34:** 166–70.

Effects on the nervous system. Apart from neuropathies (see Effects on the Muscles, above) other adverse effects of chloroquine on the nervous system have included isolated reports of extrapyramidal symptoms and other involuntary movements[1,2] (in patients being treated for malaria), nystagmus[3] (in a patient on prolonged treatment for rheumatoid arthritis), and convulsions[4,5] and nonconvulsive status epilepticus[6] (in patients on malaria prophylaxis).

1. Umez-Eronini EM, Eronini EA. Chloroquine induced involuntary movements. *Br Med J* 1977; **1:** 945–6.
2. Singhi S, *et al.* Chloroquine-induced involuntary movements. *Br Med J* 1977; **2:** 520.
3. Marks JS. Motor polyneuropathy and nystagmus associated with chloroquine phosphate. *Postgrad Med J* 1979; **55:** 569.
4. Fish DR, Espir MLE. Convulsions associated with prophylactic antimalarial drugs: implications for people with epilepsy. *Br Med J* 1988; **297:** 526–7.
5. Fish DR, Espri MLE. Malaria prophylaxis and epilepsy. *Br Med J* 1988; **297:** 1267.
6. Mülhauser P, *et al.* Chloroquine and nonconvulsive status epilepticus. *Ann Intern Med* 1995; **123:** 76–7.

Effects on the skin. *Pruritus* is frequently reported in patients receiving chloroquine for the treatment of malaria and it may become so severe as to compromise treatment. The onset of itching occurs a few hours after administration but usually remits spontaneously within 72 hours. Although most workers consider that antihistamines are generally ineffective,[1,2] some patients may obtain some relief.[3] The incidence of pruritus is purported to be higher in black patients but this may only reflect the greater number of black patients surveyed. The aetiology of this reaction is unknown but the apparent higher incidence in black patients has prompted suggestions that it may have a genetic basis[4] or be related to the affinity of chloroquine for melanin.[2] Chloroquine's main metabolite monodesethylchloroquine has also been implicated.[5] One survey[1] in Nigeria found that of 1100 patients 74% had pruritus during antimalarial therapy; 61% of these reacted to chloroquine, 30% reacted to amodiaquine, 2.5% to Fansidar (pyrimethamine-sulfadoxine), and, 6.5% reacted to all three. In another study in Nigeria[4] the incidence of pruritus was reported to be 14% (8 of 56 patients) for chloroquine, 27% (14 of 52) for amodiaquine, and 13% (7 of 53) for halofantrine; none of 58 patients receiving quinine or 82 patients receiving mefloquine had pruritus.

There have been rare reports of more severe cutaneous reactions associated with chloroquine including *toxic epidermal necrolysis,*[6,7] *erythema multiforme,*[8] and *Stevens-Johnson syndrome*[9] although the causal role of chloroquine is not always clear as some of these patients also received other antimalarials, sometimes at an inappropriate dosage. In a more recent case of toxic epidermal necrolysis,[10] chloroquine given alone for malaria prophylaxis was the probable cause. For a discussion including the possible effect of chloroquine on the incidence of erythema multiforme in patients taking pyrimethamine with sulfadoxine, see under Pyrimethamine, p.437.

1. Ajayi AA, *et al.* Epidemiology of antimalarial-induced pruritus in Africans. *Eur J Clin Pharmacol* 1989; **37:** 539–40.
2. Osifo NG. Chloroquine-induced pruritus among patients with malaria. *Arch Dermatol* 1984; **120:** 80–2.
3. Okor RS. Responsiveness of chloroquine-induced pruritus to antihistamine therapy—clinical survey. *J Clin Pharm Ther* 1990; **15:** 147–50.
4. Sowunmi A, *et al.* Pruritus and antimalarial drugs in Africans. *Lancet* 1989; **ii:** 213.
5. Essien EE, *et al.* Chloroquine disposition in hypersensitive and non-hypersensitive subjects and its significance in chloroquine-induced pruritus. *Eur J Drug Metab Pharmacokinet* 1989; **14:** 71–7.
6. Kanwar AJ, Singh OP. Toxic epidermal necrolysis—drug induced. *Indian J Dermatol* 1976; **21:** 73–7.
7. Phillips-Howard PA, Warwick Buckler J. Idiosyncratic reaction resembling toxic epidermal necrolysis caused by chloroquine and Maloprim. *Br Med J* 1988; **296:** 1605.
8. Steffen R, Somaini B. Severe cutaneous adverse reactions to sulfadoxine-pyrimethamine in Switzerland. *Lancet* 1986; **i:** 610.
9. Bamber MG, *et al.* Fatal Stevens-Johnson syndrome associated with Fansidar and chloroquine. *J Infect* 1986; **13:** 31–3.
10. Boffa MJ, Chalmers RJG. Toxic epidermal necrolysis due to chloroquine phosphate. *Br J Dermatol* 1994; **131:** 444–5.

Overdosage. For adverse effects associated with chloroquine overdosage, see under Treatment of Adverse Effects, below.

Treatment of Adverse Effects

Acute overdosage with chloroquine can be rapidly lethal and intensive symptomatic supportive treatment should be commenced immediately. The first steps should be to maintain adequate respiration and to correct any cardiovascular disturbances. Early administration of adrenaline with diazepam (see below) may minimise the cardiotoxicity of chloroquine and control the arrhythmias. The stomach should be emptied by gastric lavage if ingestion has occurred recently; activated charcoal may be left in the stomach to limit any further absorption. Other methods to increase the elimination of chloroquine, such as dialysis, are probably of little use.

The clinical features and management of poisoning due to antimalarial drugs, including chloroquine, have been reviewed by Jaeger and colleagues.[1]

Chloroquine overdosage is the most severe and frequent cause of intoxications with antimalarial drugs and chloroquine is often used for suicide attempts. Severe toxic manifestations may occur within 1 to 3 hours and fatal outcomes usually occur within 2 to 3 hours of drug ingestion. The major clinical symptoms are of neurological, respiratory, and cardiovascular toxicity[1] though death is usually due to cardiac arrest related to the direct effect of chloroquine on the myocardium.[2] Chloroquine has a low safety margin: doses of 20 mg per kg body-weight are considered toxic and 30 mg per kg may be lethal. The mortality rate in published studies has ranged from 10 to 30% and is among the highest in clinical toxicology.[1] Gastric lavage should be carried out urgently, but preceded by correction of severe cardiovascular disturbances and institution of artificial ventilation because insertion of the stomach tube may induce sudden cardiac arrest or convulsions; induction of emesis is contra-indicated because of the risk of lung aspiration. Activated charcoal has been recommended to limit absorption of chloroquine that may be left in the gut.[3] There is no evidence to indicate that attempts to increase chloroquine elimination such as acidification of the urine, haemodialysis, peritoneal dialysis, or exchange transfusion, are effective in overdosage. Elimination in the urine is more dependent on haemodynamic status than on infusion of osmotic solutions or acidification. Any clearance achieved by haemoperfusion or haemodialysis is low in comparison with the normal total body clearance.[1]

It is not clear if correction of hypokalaemia is essential but administration of potassium should be avoided in the initial phases of intoxication when conduction disturbances still exist. The degree of hypokalaemia may be correlated with the severity of chloroquine intoxication and might be useful diagnostically.[4] However, chloroquine-induced hypokalaemia may be due to a transport-dependent mechanism rather than to true potassium depletion and overzealous correction could result in hyperkalaemia.[4]

Since there had been no effective treatment for severe chloroquine poisoning Riou *et al.*[2] tried treatment with early mechanical ventilation together with adrenaline and high doses of diazepam, both given intravenously, to counteract cardiotoxicity. Their results were encouraging. Diazepam had earlier been shown to decrease the cardiotoxicity of chloroquine in *animal* studies and there had been several clinical reports of beneficial responses. Riou *et al.* considered that routine administration of adrenaline before the onset of cardiac arrhythmia might be beneficial in the treatment of severe chloroquine poisoning.[2] The manufacturers of chloroquine have suggested giving adrenaline by intravenous infusion in a dose of 0.25 μg per kg body-weight per minute initially, with increments of 0.25 μg per kg per minute until adequate systolic blood pressure is restored, and diazepam by intravenous infusion in a dose of 2 mg per kg over 30 minutes as a loading dose, followed by 1 to 2 mg per kg per day for up to 2 to 4 days.

1. Jaeger A, *et al.* Clinical features and management of poisoning due to antimalarial drugs. *Med Toxicol* 1987; **2:** 242–73.
2. Riou B, *et al.* Treatment of severe chloroquine poisoning. *N Engl J Med* 1988; **318:** 1–6.
3. Neuvonen PJ, *et al.* Prevention of chloroquine absorption by activated charcoal. *Hum Exp Toxicol* 1992; **11:** 117–20.
4. Clemessy J-L, *et al.* Hypokalaemia related to acute chloroquine ingestion. *Lancet* 1995; **346:** 877–80.

Precautions

The eyes should be examined before starting long-term treatment with chloroquine or hydroxychloroquine and should be monitored subsequently; excessive doses of chloroquine and hydroxychloroquine are associated with retinal or visual field changes (for recommendations see Effects on the Eyes in Adverse Effects, above). There may be a temporary effect on visual accommodation.

Care is necessary in administering chloroquine to patients with impaired liver or renal function or to those with severe gastro-intestinal disorders, porphyria, a history of psoriasis, or a history of epilepsy (see below for advice not to use for malaria prophylaxis). Chloroquine should be used with caution in patients with myasthenia gravis as it may aggravate the condition. Patients with glucose-6-phosphate dehydrogenase deficiency should be observed for haemolytic anaemia during chloroquine treatment. Although there have been reports of fetal abnormalities associated with the use of chloroquine during pregnancy, the risks of malaria are considered to be greater and there appears to be no justification for withholding chloroquine for the treatment or prophylaxis of malaria.

It is important that when chloroquine is given intravenously it should be by slow infusion otherwise severe cardiotoxicity may develop.

Epilepsy. Since Fish and Espir[1,2] reported convulsions associated with the use of chloroquine for malaria prophylaxis in 4 previously healthy patients and in 2 patients with a history of seizures it has been suggested that prospective travellers who have a history of epilepsy should be warned of the risk. Although it was initially considered[3] that this should not restrict the use of chloroquine in epileptic patients, UK malaria experts have recommended that it should be avoided for malaria prophylaxis.[4]

1. Fish DR, Espir MLE. Convulsions associated with prophylactic antimalarial drugs: implications for people with epilepsy. *Br Med J* 1988; **297:** 526–7.
2. Fish DR, Espir MLE. Malaria prophylaxis and epilepsy. *Br Med J* 1988; **297:** 1267.
3. Hellgren U, Rombo L. Malaria prophylaxis and epilepsy. *Br Med J* 1988; **297:** 1267.
4. Bradley DJ, *et al.* Guidelines for the prevention of malaria in travellers from the United Kingdom. *Commun Dis Rep Rev* 1997; **7:** R137–R152.

Porphyria. The problem of prophylaxis and treatment of malaria in patients with porphyria has been discussed by Moore and McColl.[1] Although chloroquine is probably safe in porphyric patients some authorities consider its use to be contentious. Pyrimethamine is also probably safe in porphyric patients. Other drugs used for prophylaxis, such as dapsone and sulfadoxine and combinations containing them, are definitely contra-indicated in porphyric patients. Quinine is of proven safety in patients with porphyria and cell-culture tests have suggested that proguanil and mefloquine may also be safe.[1]

Chloroquine has been tried in the treatment of porphyria cutanea tarda but this is considered by some to be hazardous (see under Uses, below).

1. Moore MR, McColl KEL. *Porphyria: drug lists.* Glasgow: Porphyria Research Unit, University of Glasgow, 1991.

Pregnancy and breast feeding. There has been concern about the potential teratogenic effects of chloroquine because of a few case reports including defects in hearing and vision.[1] Two of 169 infants born to women who had received chloroquine 300 mg weekly throughout pregnancy had birth defects compared with 4 of 454 control infants whose mothers had not been exposed to antimalarials; the difference was not significant. The data suggested that chloroquine in the recommended prophylactic doses is not a strong teratogen and that its proved antimalarial benefits outweigh any possible risk of low-grade teratogenicity. Also it has been reported that chloroquine prophylaxis during pregnancy did not affect the birth-weight of neonates, compared with a control group.[2]

Chloroquine is distributed into breast milk, but not in an amount adequate to provide chemoprophylaxis against malaria for the infant (see under Pharmacokinetics, below).

1. Wolfe MS, Cordero JF. Safety of chloroquine in chemosuppression of malaria during pregnancy. *Br Med J* 1985; **290:** 1466–7.
2. Cot M, *et al.* Effect of chloroquine chemoprophylaxis during pregnancy on birth weight: results of a randomized trial. *Am J Trop Med Hyg* 1992; **46:** 21–7.

Psoriatic arthritis. It is recommended that chloroquine and hydroxychloroquine should not be used in the treatment of psoriatic arthritis as exacerbations of skin lesions can occur. Some patients may go on to develop generalised erythroderma with subsequent exfoliative dermatitis.[1] However, there has been controversy over the reported incidence of this adverse effect.[2,3]

1. Slagel GA, James WD. Plaquenil-induced erythroderma. *J Am Acad Dermatol* 1985; **12:** 857–62.
2. Luzar MJ. Hydroxychloroquine in psoriatic arthropathy: exacerbations of psoriatic skin lesions. *J Rheumatol* 1982; **9:** 462–4.
3. Sayers ME, Mazanec DJ. Use of antimalarial drugs for the treatment of psoriatic arthritis. *Am J Med* 1992; **93:** 474–5.

Renal impairment. Although the elimination of chloroquine is prolonged in renal impairment no dosage adjustment is required in the treatment of malaria. Similarly, dosage reduction is not required for chloroquine prophylaxis except in those with severe renal impairment. Doses tend to be reduced when it is given for longer periods to patients with impaired renal function.

Interactions

There is an increased risk of inducing ventricular arrhythmias if chloroquine is given together with halofantrine (see p.431) or other arrhythmogenic drugs such as amiodarone. There is an increased risk of convulsions when chloroquine is administered with mefloquine. The absorption of chloroquine can be reduced by concomitant administration of antacids and its metabolism may be inhibited by cimetidine.

For further details of interactions, see below.

Patients often wish to take chloroquine with food, antacids, or other gastro-intestinal drugs to alleviate gastro-intestinal irritation. However, *antacids* or *kaolin* can reduce the absorption of chloroquine and it is therefore recommended that they should be administered at least 4 hours apart.[1,2] Furthermore, cimetidine and chloroquine should be used with caution as *cimetidine* can significantly reduce the metabolism and elimination of chloroquine and increase its volume of distribution;[3] *ranitidine* might be more suitable if a histamine H_2-receptor antagonist is required as it appears to have little effect on the pharmacokinetics of chloroquine.[4] Administration with *food* may be beneficial as it appears to improve the absorption of chloroquine.[5,6]

Chloroquine should not be administered concurrently with *halofantrine* since the latter prolongs the QT interval and therefore there is an increased potential to induce arrhythmias (see p.431). Combination of chloroquine with *mefloquine* increases the risk of convulsions. Also concurrent administration of chloroquine and *proguanil* may increase the incidence of proguanil-associated mouth ulceration.[7] The activity of chloroquine may be affected when it is administered with other *antimalarials*. Mixtures of chloroquine with *quinine, mefloquine, amodiaquine, artemisinin,* or *pyrimethamine-sulfadoxine* were antagonistic *in vitro* against *Plasmodium falciparum*.[8] *Quinine* and chloroquine when used together may be antagonistic.[9]

Other *anti-infective drugs* that might interact with chloroquine include *metronidazole*; acute dystonic reactions occurred during concomitant therapy with metronidazole in a woman who had previously tolerated chloroquine alone.[10] Chloroquine may also reduce the gastro-intestinal absorption of *ampicillin* (see p.153) and possibly the bioavailability of *praziquantel* (see p.108).

Although concurrent antimalarial prophylaxis with chloroquine has been reported to reduce the antibody response to *human diploid rabies vaccine* (see p.1531), the immune response to other vaccines used in routine immunisation schedules (tetanus, diphtheria, measles, poliomyelitis, typhoid, and BCG) has not been found to be altered by chloroquine prophylaxis.[11,12]

Chloroquine may antagonise the antiepileptic activity of *carbamazepine* (see p.341) and *valproate* (see p.363).

Chloroquine has been reported to increase plasma concentrations of *cyclosporin* (see p.522) and to decrease concentrations of *thyroxine* (see p.1498).

Hydroxychloroquine has been reported to increase plasma concentrations of *digoxin* (see p.851).

1. McElnay JC, *et al.* In vitro experiments on chloroquine and pyrimethamine absorption in the presence of antacid constituents or kaolin. *J Trop Med Hyg* 1982; **85:** 153–8.
2. McElnay JC, *et al.* The effect of magnesium trisilicate and kaolin on the in vivo absorption of chloroquine. *J Trop Med Hyg* 1982; **85:** 159–63.
3. Ette EI, *et al.* Chloroquine elimination in humans: effect of low-dose cimetidine. *J Clin Pharmacol* 1987; **27:** 813–16.
4. Ette EI, *et al.* Effect of ranitidine on chloroquine disposition. *Drug Intell Clin Pharm* 1987; **21:** 732–4.
5. Tulpule A, Krishnaswamy K. Effect of food on bioavailability of chloroquine. *Eur J Clin Pharmacol* 1982; **23:** 271–3.
6. Lagrave M, *et al.* The influence of various types of breakfast on chloroquine levels. *Trans R Soc Trop Med Hyg* 1985; **79:** 559.
7. Drysdale SF, *et al.* Proguanil, chloroquine, and mouth ulcers. *Lancet* 1990; **335:** 164.
8. Stahel E, *et al.* Antagonism of chloroquine with other antimalarials. *Trans R Soc Trop Med Hyg* 1988; **82:** 221.
9. Hall AP. Quinine and chloroquine antagonism in falciparum malaria. *Trans R Soc Trop Med Hyg* 1973; **67:** 425.
10. Achumba JI, *et al.* Chloroquine-induced acute dystonic reactions in the presence of metronidazole. *Drug Intell Clin Pharm* 1988; **22:** 308–10.
11. Greenwood BM. Chloroquine prophylaxis and antibody response to immunisation. *Lancet* 1984; **ii:** 402–3.
12. Wolfe MS. Precautions with oral live typhoid (Ty 21a) vaccine. *Lancet* 1990; **336:** 631–2.

Pharmacokinetics

Chloroquine is rapidly and almost completely absorbed from the gastro-intestinal tract when given by mouth. Absorption is also rapid following intramuscular or subcutaneous administration. It is widely distributed into body tissues and has a large apparent volume of distribution. It accumulates in high concentrations in some tissues, such as the kidneys, liver, lungs, and spleen and is strongly bound in melanin-containing cells such as those in the eyes and the skin. It also crosses the placenta. Chloroquine is eliminated very slowly from the body and it may persist in tissues for months or even years after discontinuation of therapy.

Chloroquine is extensively metabolised in the liver, mainly to monodesethylchloroquine with smaller amounts of bisdesethylchloroquine (didesethylchloroquinine) and other metabolites being formed. Monodesethylchloroquine has been reported to have some activity against *Plasmodium falciparum*. Chloroquine and its metabolites are excreted in the urine, with about half of a dose appearing as unchanged drug and about 10% as the monodesethyl metabolite. Chloroquine and its monodesethyl metabolite are both distributed into breast milk.

Chloroquine is rapidly absorbed from the gastro-intestinal tract but peak plasma concentrations following oral administration can vary considerably.[1] A mean peak plasma concentration of 76 ng per mL has been obtained in healthy adults a mean of 3.6 hours after administration of the equivalent of 300 mg of chloroquine base by mouth as tablets.[2] In children with uncomplicated malaria given the equivalent of 10 mg per kg body-weight peak plasma concentrations of 250 ng per mL have been reached after 2 hours;[3] a mean peak of 134 ng per mL has been obtained after 5 hours in healthy children given a similar dose.[4] Nasogastric administration has also produced therapeutic concentrations in children with severe falciparum malaria.[5]

Oral bioavailability is increased if chloroquine is taken with food[6,7] and some beverages[8] and may also be affected by the state of health of the patient; mean values have ranged from about 70% in patients with malaria[9] to 78 or 89% in healthy adults.[2] Although oral bioavailability appears to be unaltered in moderately undernourished adults[10] it has been reported that it may be significantly reduced in children with kwashiorkor.[4]

Preliminary studies with chloroquine suppositories indicate that although rectal bioavailability is less than half of that of oral chloroquine, sustained therapeutic concentrations may be achieved.[11]

Absorption is also rapid following subcutaneous or intramuscular injection and mean peak plasma concentrations of chloroquine have been obtained within about 30 minutes.[5,9,12]

Chloroquine has a large apparent volume of distribution. A multicompartmental model appears to be necessary to describe the distribution kinetics of chloroquine.[2,13] Following intravenous administration there is a multi-exponential decline in plasma concentrations as chloroquine distributes out of a central compartment that has been estimated to be several orders of magnitude smaller than the total volume of distribution.[5,14] This slow distribution out of the central compartment produces transiently high cardiotoxic concentrations of chloroquine if the overall rate of parenteral delivery is not carefully controlled.

Reported mean values for protein binding have ranged from about 58 to 64%.[15,16] Chloroquine is also bound to platelets and granulocytes so that the plasma concentration is only 10 to 15% of that in whole blood.[17] If these cells are not removed by gentle centrifugation during analysis, erroneously high plasma concentrations will be reported. Furthermore, as chloroquine concentrations determined in serum are higher than those in plasma, probably due to release of chloroquine from platelets during coagulation, it is crucial to state whether analysis has been done on whole blood, serum, or properly separated plasma.

About 50% of a dose of chloroquine is metabolised in the liver mainly to the *N*-dealkylated metabolite monodesethylchloroquine; smaller amounts of bisdesethylchloroquine, 7-chloro-4-aminoquinoline, and *N*-oxidation products are formed. Some of these metabolites may contribute to the cardiotoxicity associated with chloroquine. In one study peak plasma concentrations of 7-chloro-4-aminoquinoline were found to be twice those of unchanged chloroquine despite the fact that only relatively small amounts are formed; this appears to be due to its fast rate of formation and long elimination half-life.[18]

A mean of 42 to 47% of a dose has been reported to be excreted in the urine as unchanged chloroquine and 7 to 12% as monodesethylchloroquine.[2] Various estimates of the terminal elimination half-life of chloroquine range from several days to up to 2 months but its slow release from tissues ensures that small amounts may still be detected after a year.[18,19]

The pharmacokinetics of chloroquine and their clinical implications have been reviewed.[20,21]

1. Hellgren U, *et al.* On the question of interindividual variations in chloroquine concentrations. *Eur J Clin Pharmacol* 1993; **45:** 383–5.
2. Gustafsson LL, *et al.* Disposition of chloroquine in man after single intravenous and oral doses. *Br J Clin Pharmacol* 1983; **15:** 471–9.
3. Adelusi SA, *et al.* Kinetics of the uptake and elimination of chloroquine in children with malaria. *Br J Clin Pharmacol* 1982; **14:** 483–7.
4. Walker O, *et al.* Single dose disposition of chloroquine in kwashiorkor and normal children—evidence for decreased absorption in kwashiorkor. *Br J Clin Pharmacol* 1987; **23:** 467–72.
5. White NJ, *et al.* Chloroquine treatment of severe malaria in children: pharmacokinetics, toxicity, and new dosage recommendations. *N Engl J Med* 1988; **319:** 1493–1500.
6. Tulpule A, Krishnaswamy K. Effect of food on bioavailability of chloroquine. *Eur J Clin Pharmacol* 1982; **23:** 271–3.
7. Lagrave M, *et al.* The influence of various types of breakfast on chloroquine levels. *Trans R Soc Trop Med Hyg* 1985; **79:** 559.
8. Mahmoud BM, *et al.* Significant reduction in chloroquine bioavailability following coadministration with the Sudanese beverages aradaib, karkadi and lemon. *J Antimicrob Chemother* 1994; **33:** 1005–9.
9. White NJ, *et al.* Parenteral chloroquine for treating falciparum malaria. *J Infect Dis* 1987; **155:** 192–201.
10. Tulpule A, Krishnaswamy K. Chloroquine kinetics in the undernourished. *Eur J Clin Pharmacol* 1983; **24:** 273–6.
11. WHO. Severe and complicated malaria. 2nd ed. *Trans R Soc Trop Med Hyg* 1990; **84** (suppl 2): 1–65.
12. Phillips RE, *et al.* Divided dose intramuscular regimen and single dose subcutaneous regimen for chloroquine: plasma concentrations and toxicity in patients with malaria. *Br Med J* 1986; **293:** 13–16.
13. Frisk-Holmberg M, *et al.* The single dose kinetics of chloroquine and its major metabolite desethylchloroquine in healthy subjects. *Eur J Clin Pharmacol* 1984; **26:** 521–30.
14. Looareesuwan S, *et al.* Cardiovascular toxicity and distribution kinetics of intravenous chloroquine. *Br J Clin Pharmacol* 1986; **22:** 31–6.
15. Walker O, *et al.* Characterization of chloroquine plasma protein binding in man. *Br J Clin Pharmacol* 1983; **15:** 375–7.
16. Ofori-Adjei D, *et al.* Protein binding of chloroquine enantiomers and desethylchloroquine. *Br J Clin Pharmacol* 1986; **22:** 356–8.
17. Gustafsson LL, *et al.* Pitfalls in the measurement of chloroquine concentrations. *Lancet* 1983; **i:** 126.
18. Ette EI, *et al.* Pharmacokinetics of chloroquine and some of its metabolites in healthy volunteers: a single dose study. *J Clin Pharmacol* 1989; **29:** 457–62.
19. Gustafsson LL, *et al.* Chloroquine excretion following malaria prophylaxis. *Br J Clin Pharmacol* 1987; **24:** 221–4.
20. Krishna S, White NJ. Pharmacokinetics of quinine, chloroquine and amodiaquine; clinical implications. *Clin Pharmacokinet* 1996; **30:** 263–99.
21. Ducharme J, Farinotti R. Clinical pharmacokinetics and metabolism of chloroquine: focus on recent advancements. *Clin Pharmacokinet* 1996; **31:** 257–74.

Distribution into breast milk. Studies[1,2] have suggested that it is safe for mothers to breast feed when they are receiving chloroquine for treatment of malaria. Although chloroquine and its monodesethyl metabolite are distributed into breast milk it has been estimated that the amount that would be consumed by an infant is well below the therapeutic range and separate chemoprophylaxis for the infant is required.

There appears to be no data on the excretion of hydroxychloroquine in milk after doses appropriate for the prevention or treatment of malaria but hydroxychloroquine has been detected in breast milk from 2 mothers receiving doses of 400 mg daily for systemic lupus erythematosus or rheumatoid arthritis.[3,4] One group of workers estimated that, calculated on a body-weight basis, a 9-month-old infant could receive about 2% of a maternal dose via breast feeding.[3]

1. Ogunbona FA, *et al.* Excretion of chloroquine and desethylchloroquine in human milk. *Br J Clin Pharmacol* 1987; **23:** 473–6.
2. Akintonwa A, *et al.* Placental and milk transfer of chloroquine in humans. *Ther Drug Monit* 1988; **10:** 147–9.
3. Nation RL, *et al.* Excretion of hydroxychloroquine in human milk. *Br J Clin Pharmacol* 1984; **17:** 368–9.
4. Østensen M, *et al.* Hydroxychloroquine in human breast milk. *Eur J Clin Pharmacol* 1985; **28:** 357.

Uses and Administration

Chloroquine is a 4-aminoquinoline antimalarial used in the treatment and prophylaxis of malaria. It has also been used in the treatment of hepatic amoebiasis, lupus erythematosus, light-sensitive skin eruptions, and rheumatoid arthritis.

Chloroquine is used for the prophylaxis and treatment of malaria due to susceptible strains of *Plasmodium falciparum, P. ovale, P. vivax*, and *P. malariae*, but widespread resistance in *P. falciparum* has greatly limited its value. It is a rapid-acting blood schizontocide with some gametocytocidal activity against *P. ovale, P. vivax, P. malariae*, and immature gametocytes of *P. falciparum*. Since it has no activity against exoerythrocytic forms, chloroquine does not produce a radical cure of vivax or ovale malarias. The mechanism of action of chloroquine against blood schizonts remains unclear but it may influence haemoglobin digestion by raising intravesicular pH in malaria parasite cells. It also interferes with synthesis of nucleoproteins by the parasite.

Chloroquine may be given as the phosphate, sulphate, or hydrochloride. Doses are normally expressed in terms of chloroquine base, and as a general guide chloroquine base 300 mg is approximately equivalent to chloroquine phosphate 500 mg or chloroquine sulphate 400 mg: chloroquine base 40 mg is approximately equivalent to chloroquine hydrochloride 50 mg.

For the *treatment of malaria* caused by *P. vivax, P. ovale, P. malariae*, and the few remaining strains of chloroquine-sensitive *P. falciparum* the usual total oral dose for adults and children is the equivalent of a total of about 25 mg of chloroquine base per kg body-weight given over 3 days. This total dose is given in a variety of ways. One way is to give 10 mg per kg followed after 6 to 8 hours by 5 mg per kg, then 5 mg per kg daily for the next 2 days; alternatively, 10 mg per kg may be given daily for the first 2 days and 5 mg per kg on the third day. Sometimes the adult doses are not expressed in terms of body-weight but as 600 mg followed after 6 to 8 hours by 300 mg, then 300 mg daily for the next 2 days. In severe and complicated malaria when the patient is unable to take oral medication and when chloroquine is to be used, then it can be given by injection. The intravenous route is preferred and a slow rate of infusion is essential, the required dose of 25 mg per kg being given in several infusions over 30 to 32 hours as described in further detail under Malaria, below. Should the patient recover sufficiently to be able to take chloroquine by mouth then the intravenous regimen should be halted and oral therapy commenced. It is important to bear in mind that in most parts of the world *P. falciparum* is now resistant to chloroquine which should *not* therefore be given for treatment.

For *prophylaxis of malaria* in areas where *P. falciparum* is absent or in one of the few remaining areas where it is still sensitive to chloroquine, a dose equivalent to 300 mg of chloroquine base is given once each week, beginning about one week before exposure and continuing throughout, and for at least 4 weeks after, exposure. For children, a weekly dose of 5 mg per kg has been recommended (but see also under Malaria, below). In areas of chloroquine-resistant malaria, but with a low risk of infection, chloroquine is administered with proguanil; where there is a high risk of infection alternative antimalarial regimens are recommended.

In the treatment of *hepatic amoebiasis* chloroquine is used with emetine or dehydroemetine. The usual dose is the equivalent of 600 mg of chloroquine base daily for 2 days then 300 mg daily for 2 or 3 weeks. A dose of 6 mg per kg daily up to a maximum of 300 mg daily has been suggested for children.

In *rheumatoid arthritis* response to treatment may not be apparent for up to 6 months, but if there is no improvement by then treatment should be discontinued. The usual dose is the equivalent of chloroquine base 150 mg daily (maximum 2.5 mg per kg daily) or up to 3 mg per kg daily in children. To avoid excessive dosage in obese patients, special care is needed to calculate the dosage on the basis of lean body-weight. For further details see under Effects on the Eyes, above.

In discoid and systemic *lupus erythematosus* chloroquine is used initially at a dose equivalent to 150 mg (maximum 2.5 mg per kg) of base daily, reducing gradually once symptoms have been controlled. Children are given a dose of up to 3 mg per kg daily.

In the management of *light-sensitive skin eruptions* adults are given the equivalent of 150 to 300 mg of chloroquine base daily during periods of intense light exposure; children are given up to 3 mg per kg.

Amoebiasis. For a discussion of the treatment of amoebiasis with mention of chloroquine for hepatic amoebiasis, see p.573.

Idiopathic pulmonary haemosiderosis. Chloroquine was reported to provide symptomatic improvement in two children with idiopathic pulmonary haemosiderosis,[1] a condition caused by extravascular destruction of blood in the lung. However, retinal changes necessitated withdrawal of chloroquine in one child.

1. Bush A, *et al.* Chloroquine in idiopathic pulmonary haemosiderosis. *Arch Dis Child* 1992; **67:** 625–7.

Inflammatory disorders. Chloroquine and hydroxychloroquine possess anti-inflammatory properties and they have been tried or used with some benefit in a range of inflammatory conditions which often have an immunological basis, although they rarely constitute first-line therapy in these disorders. Such conditions include rheumatoid arthritis (see under Hydroxychloroquine, p.432), ulcerative colitis,[1] infantile interstitial pneumonitis,[2,3] asthma,[4] giant cell arteritis,[5] and various skin disorders (see below). The mode of action in these conditions is unclear. Results of studies have been conflicting but it does appear that chloroquine and hydroxychloroquine might have some immunosuppressive effects.[6,7]

1. Mayer L, Sachar DB. Efficacy of chloroquine in the treatment of inflammatory bowel disease. *Gastroenterology* 1988; **94:** A293.

2. Springer C, *et al.* Chloroquine treatment in desquamative interstitial pneumonia. *Arch Dis Child* 1987; **62:** 76–7.
3. Kerem E, *et al.* Sequential pulmonary function measurements during treatment of infantile chronic interstitial pneumonitis. *J Pediatr* 1990; **116:** 61–7.
4. Charous BL. Open study of hydroxychloroquine in the treatment of severe symptomatic or corticosteroid-dependent asthma. *Ann Allergy* 1990; **65:** 53–8.
5. Le Guennec P, *et al.* Management of giant cell arteritis: value of synthetic antimalarial agents: a retrospective study of thirty six patients. *Rev Rhum* 1994; **61:** 423–8.
6. Bygbjerg IC, Flachs H. Effect of chloroquine on human lymphocyte proliferation. *Trans R Soc Trop Med Hyg* 1986; **80:** 231–5.
7. Prasad RN, *et al.* Immunopharmacology of chloroquine. *Trans R Soc Trop Med Hyg* 1987; **81:** 168–9.

Lupus erythematosus. Chloroquine can produce improvement in the skin and joint manifestations of discoid and systemic lupus erythematosus; its place in treatment is discussed on p.1029.

Malaria. The overall treatment and prophylaxis of malaria and the place of chloroquine in current recommendations are discussed on p.422.

TREATMENT. In the treatment of patients with chloroquine-sensitive falciparum malaria studies have found chloroquine to be at least as effective as quinine in both uncomplicated and severe infections.[1,2] However, few areas exist where *Plasmodium falciparum* remains sensitive to chloroquine. There are also reports of resistance to chloroquine in *P. vivax*.[3] There is limited evidence that chlorpheniramine might reverse chloroquine resistance in *P. falciparum* (see p.405).

Treatment with chloroquine is usually by mouth, adults and children being given the equivalent of 25 mg of chloroquine base per kg body-weight over 3 days. Any chloroquine lost through vomiting needs to be replaced by additional doses.[4] Encouraging results have also been obtained in a limited number of patients given the equivalent of 30 mg of chloroquine base per kg by mouth over 2 days in the form of a loading dose of 10 mg per kg followed by two doses of 5 mg per kg at intervals of 6 hours on the first day and two doses of 5 mg per kg at intervals of 12 hours on the second day.[5]

Parenteral therapy may be used if the infection is severe or oral administration is not possible. The parenteral regimen for adults and children recommended by WHO[6] consists of a loading dose equivalent to 10 mg of chloroquine base per kg body-weight given by constant rate intravenous infusion in sodium chloride injection over a period of at least 8 hours and followed by a further three 8-hour infusions each of 5 mg per kg during the next 24 hours. Alternatively the entire course may be given over 30 hours, each infusion of 5 mg per kg being given over 6 hours. There should be close monitoring for hypotension and other signs of cardiovascular toxicity.

The intramuscular or subcutaneous routes have been used if intravenous administration is not possible. Intramuscular or subcutaneous doses for adults and children are 3.5 mg per kg every 6 hours[4,6,7] or 2.5 mg per kg every 4 hours to a total dose equivalent to 25 mg of the base per kg body-weight.[4]

Whichever parenteral route is used, patients should be transferred to oral therapy as soon as possible and administration continued until a total dose equivalent to 25 mg of the base per kg body-weight has been given.

If injections cannot be given a chloroquine suspension or syrup appears to be well absorbed when given by nasogastric tube even in comatose patients. Rectal administration in young children has also produced promising responses.[8,9]

PROPHYLAXIS. The widespread prevalence of strains of *P. falciparum* resistant to chloroquine has considerably diminished the value of chloroquine for malaria chemoprophylaxis and has made recommendations increasingly complex (see p.422). If chloroquine is used for prophylaxis it is usually administered with proguanil. A dose equivalent to 300 mg of chloroquine base is given by mouth once each week, beginning about one week before exposure and continuing throughout, and for at least 4 weeks after, exposure. Some countries advise the use of 100 mg daily for 6 days a week. For children, a weekly dose of chloroquine base 5 mg per kg body-weight has been recommended, although UK malaria experts[10] have suggested the following prophylactic doses for children based on fractions of the adult dose of 300 mg weekly; from 0 to 5 weeks of age, one-eighth the adult dose; 6 to 52 weeks, one-quarter the adult dose; 1 to 5 years (10 to 19 kg body-weight), half the adult dose; 6 to 11 years (20 to 39 kg), three-quarters the adult dose; and 12 years of more (40 kg or more), the adult dose. They noted that body weight was a better guide to dosage than age for children over 6 months.

1. Watt G, *et al.* Chloroquine and quinine: a randomized, double-blind comparison of efficacy and side effects in the treatment of Plasmodium falciparum malaria in the Philippines. *Trans R Soc Trop Med Hyg* 1988; **82:** 205–8.
2. White NJ, *et al.* Open comparison of intramuscular chloroquine and quinine in children with severe chloroquine-sensitive falciparum malaria. *Lancet* 1989; **ii:** 1313–16.
3. Whitby M. Drug resistant Plasmodium vivax malaria. *J Antimicrob Chemother* 1997; **40:** 749–52.
4. WHO. *WHO model prescribing information: drugs used in parasitic diseases.* 2nd ed. Geneva: WHO, 1995.
5. Pussard E, *et al.* Efficacy of a loading dose of oral chloroquine in a 36-hour treatment schedule for uncomplicated Plasmodium falciparum malaria. *Antimicrob Agents Chemother* 1991; **35:** 406–9.
6. Gilles HM. *Management of severe and complicated malaria.* Geneva: WHO 1991.
7. WHO. Practical chemotherapy of malaria: report of a WHO scientific group. *WHO Tech Rep Ser 805* 1990.
8. Westman L, *et al.* Rectal administration of chloroquine for treatment of children with malaria. *Trans R Soc Trop Med Hyg* 1994; **88:** 446.
9. Antia-Obong OE, *et al.* Chloroquine phosphate suppositories in the treatment of childhood malaria in Calabar, Nigeria. *Curr Ther Res* 1995; **56:** 928–35.
10. Bradley DJ, *et al.* Guidelines for the prevention of malaria in travellers from the United Kingdom. *Commun Dis Rep Rev* 1997; **7:** R137–R152.

Porphyria cutanea tarda. Chloroquine and hydroxychloroquine have been used with some benefit in the treatment of porphyria cutanea tarda (p.983) and low doses (such as chloroquine phosphate 125 mg or hydroxychloroquine sulphate 200 mg given twice weekly) have been considered by some to be useful in patients unsuitable for phlebotomy.[1-3] However, the acute increase in urinary porphyrins and fall in hepatic porphyrin content produced by these drugs have been associated with a variable degree of hepatotoxicity[4] and others prefer to use desferrioxamine.[5]

1. Grossman ME, *et al.* Porphyria cutanea tarda. *Am J Med* 1979; **67:** 277–86.
2. Cainelli T, *et al.* Hydroxychloroquine versus phlebotomy in the treatment of porphyria cutanea tarda. *Br J Dermatol* 1983; **108:** 593–600.
3. Ashton RE, *et al.* Low-dose oral chloroquine in the treatment of porphyria cutanea tarda. *Br J Dermatol* 1984; **111:** 609–13.
4. Scholnick PL, *et al.* The molecular basis of the action of chloroquine in porphyria cutanea tarda. *J Invest Dermatol* 1973; **61:** 226–32.
5. Rocchi E. Treatment of porphyria cutanea tarda. *Br J Dermatol* 1987; **116:** 139–40.

Rheumatoid arthritis. For reference to the use of chloroquine in the treatment of rheumatoid arthritis, see under Hydroxychloroquine, p.432.

Sarcoidosis. Chloroquine and hydroxychloroquine have been tried in the management of sarcoidosis (p.1028) as alternatives or adjuncts to corticosteroid therapy. Some references to this use are given below.

1. DeSimone DP, *et al.* Granulomatous infiltration of the talus and abnormal vitamin D and calcium metabolism in a patient with sarcoidosis: successful treatment with hydroxychloroquine. *Am J Med* 1989; **87:** 694–6.
2. O'Leary TJ, *et al.* The effects of chloroquine on serum 1,25-dihydroxyvitamin D and calcium metabolism in sarcoidosis. *N Engl J Med* 1986; **315:** 727–30.
3. Adams JS, *et al.* Effective reduction in the serum 1,25-dihydroxyvitamin D and calcium concentration in sarcoidosis-associated hypercalcemia with short-course chloroquine therapy. *Ann Intern Med* 1989; **111:** 437–8.
4. Spiteri MA, *et al.* Lupus pernio: a clinico-radiological study of thirty-five cases. *Br J Dermatol* 1985; **112:** 315–22.
5. Jones E, Callen JP. Hydroxychloroquine is effective therapy for control of cutaneous sarcoidal granulomas. *J Am Acad Dermatol* 1990; **23:** 487–9.
6. Zic JA, *et al.* Treatment of cutaneous sarcoidosis with chloroquine: review of the literature. *Arch Dermatol* 1991; **127:** 1034–40.

Skin disorders. In addition to their use in lupus erythematosus hydroxychloroquine and chloroquine have been tried in a number of other skin disorders including polymorphic light eruptions,[1] lichen planus[2] (p.1075), cutaneous symptoms of dermatomyositis (p.1027), erythema nodosum,[3,4] and recurrent erythema multiforme (p.1074).

1. Murphy GM, *et al.* Hydroxychloroquine in polymorphic light eruption: a controlled trial with drug and visual sensitivity monitoring. *Br J Dermatol* 1987; **116:** 379–86.
2. Mostafa WZ. Lichen planus of the nail: treatment with antimalarials. *J Am Acad Dermatol* 1989; **20:** 289–90.
3. Alloway JA, Franks LK. Hydroxychloroquine in the treatment of chronic erythema nodosum. *Br J Dermatol* 1995; **132:** 661–2.
4. Jarrett P, Goodfield MJD. Hydroxychloroquine and chronic erythema nodosum. *Br J Dermatol* 1996; **134:** 373.

Preparations

BP 1998: Chloroquine Phosphate Tablets; Chloroquine Sulphate Injection; Chloroquine Sulphate Tablets;
USP 23: Chloroquine Hydrochloride Injection; Chloroquine Phosphate Tablets.

Proprietary Preparations (details are given in Part 3)
Aust.: Resochin; ***Austral.:*** Chlorquin; Nivaquine†; ***Belg.:*** Nivaquine; ***Canad.:*** Aralen; ***Fr.:*** Nivaquine; ***Ger.:*** Arthrabas; Resochin; Weimerquin; ***Irl.:*** Avloclor; Nivaquine; ***Ital.:*** Dichinalex†; ***Neth.:*** Nivaquine; ***S.Afr.:*** Anoclor; Daramal; Nivaquine; Plasmoquine; Promal†; ***Spain:*** Cidanchin†; Resochin; ***Switz.:*** Chlorochin; Nivaquine; Pharmaquine†; Resochine; ***UK:*** Avloclor; Malaviron; Nivaquine; ***USA:*** Aralen.

Multi-ingredient: ***Fr.:*** Savarine; ***S.Afr.:*** Daraclor†; ***USA:*** Aralen with Primaquine Phosphate†.

Chlorproguanil Hydrochloride (1376-p)

Chlorproguanil Hydrochloride *(BANM, rINNM).*

M-5943. 1-(3,4-Dichlorophenyl)-5-isopropylbiguanide hydrochloride.

$C_{11}H_{15}Cl_2N_5,HCl = 324.6.$

CAS — 537-21-3 (chlorproguanil); 15537-76-5 (chlorproguanil hydrochloride).

Chlorproguanil is a biguanide antimalarial with actions and uses similar to those of proguanil (p.435). It is sometimes given in combination with a sulphone such as dapsone.

References.

1. Keuter M, *et al.* Comparison of chloroquine, pyrimethamine and sulfadoxine, and chlorproguanil and dapsone as treatment for falciparum malaria in pregnant and non-pregnant women, Kakamega district, Kenya. *Br Med J* 1990; **301:** 466–70.
2. Rooth I, *et al.* Proguanil daily or chlorproguanil twice weekly are efficacious against falciparum malaria in a holoendemic area of Tanzania. *J Trop Med Hyg* 1991; **94:** 45–9.
3. Nevill CG, *et al.* Daily chlorproguanil is an effective alternative to daily proguanil in the prevention of Plasmodium falciparum malaria in Kenya. *Trans R Soc Trop Med Hyg* 1994; **88:** 319–20.
4. Winstanley P, *et al.* Chlorproguanil/dapsone for uncomplicated Plasmodium falciparum malaria in young children: pharmacokinetics and therapeutic range. *Trans R Soc Trop Med Hyg* 1997; **91:** 322–7.
5. Amukoye E, *et al.* Chlorproguanil-dapsone: effective treatment for uncomplicated falciparum malaria. *Antimicrob Agents Chemother* 1997; **41:** 2261–4.

Halofantrine Hydrochloride (16829-p)

Halofantrine Hydrochloride *(BANM, USAN, rINNM).*

WR-171669. (*RS*)-3-Dibutylamino-1-(1,3-dichloro-6-trifluoromethyl-9-phenanthryl)propan-1-ol hydrochloride; 1,3-Dichloro-α-[2-(dibutylamino)ethyl]-6-trifluoromethyl-9-phenanthrene-methanol hydrochloride.

$C_{26}H_{30}Cl_2F_3NO,HCl = 536.9.$

CAS — 69756-53-2 (halofantrine); 36167-63-2 (halofantrine hydrochloride); 66051-63-6 (±-halofantrine).

Adverse Effects and Precautions

Adverse effects associated with halofantrine include diarrhoea, abdominal pain, nausea, vomiting, pruritus, and skin rash. Transient elevation of serum transaminases, intravascular haemolysis, and hypersensitivity reactions have also been reported.

Halofantrine can adversely affect the heart and this is mainly seen as a prolongation of QT interval. Serious ventricular arrhythmias have been reported and fatalities have occurred. As a result it is contra-indicated in patients known to have a prolonged QT interval or those with cardiac disease or a family history of congenital QT prolongation, and also in those with unexplained syncopal attacks, thiamine deficiency, or electrolyte disturbances, or taking other arrhythmogenic drugs (see also under Effects on the Heart, below, and under Interactions, below).

Halofantrine is not recommended during pregnancy or in breast-feeding women. It should not be taken on a full stomach since this increases its bioavailability and thus the risk of toxicity; after taking halofantrine, fatty food should be avoided for 24 hours.

Effects on the blood. Halofantrine has been associated with acute intravascular haemolysis.[1,2]

1. Vachon F, *et al.* Halofantrine and acute intravascular haemolysis. *Lancet* 1992; **340:** 909–10.
2. Mojon M, *et al.* Intravascular haemolysis following halofantrine intake. *Trans R Soc Trop Med Hyg* 1994; **88:** 91.

Effects on the heart. Prolonged PR[1,2] and QT[1-5] intervals have been reported in patients given halofantrine and there are individual reports of fatal cardiac arrest[1,5] and of torsade de pointes.[4] In 1994, the UK Committee on Safety of Medicines (CSM)[6] noted that QT interval prolongation occurred at recommended doses of halofantrine in the majority of patients and that worldwide there had been 14 reports of cardiac arrhythmias associated with halofantrine; 8 patients were known to have died. To reduce the risk of arrhythmias they stressed that halofantrine should *not* be taken with meals, with other drugs that may induce arrhythmias (e.g. quinine, chloroquine, and mefloquine; tricyclic antidepressants; antipsychotics; certain antiarrhythmics; and the antihistamines terfenadine and astemizole), or with drugs causing electrolyte disturbances. Also, that it should *not* be administered to patients known to have prolongation of the QT interval or with any form of cardiac disease associated with QT intervals prolongation or ventricular arrhythmia (e.g. coronary heart disease, cardiomyopathy, or congenital heart disease). Monlun *et al.*[2] suggested ECG screening of all patients before starting treatment with halofantrine. Others[7] found pretreatment ECGs to be poorly predictive of QT lengthening during treatment. Children may experience serious cardiac effects at standard doses.[8]

1. Nosten F, *et al.* Cardiac effects of antimalarial treatment with halofantrine. *Lancet* 1993; **341:** 1054–6.
2. Monlun E, *et al.* Cardiac complications of halofantrine: a prospective study of 20 patients. *Trans R Soc Trop Med Hyg* 1995; **89:** 430–3.
3. Castot A, *et al.* Prolonged QT interval with halofantrine. *Lancet* 1993; **341:** 1541.
4. Monlun E, *et al.* Prolonged QT interval with halofantrine. *Lancet* 1993; **341:** 1541–2.
5. Anonymous. Halofantrine: revised data sheet. *WHO Drug Inf* 1993; **7:** 66–7.
6. Committee on Safety of Medicines/Medicines Control Agency. Cardiac arrhythmias with halofantrine (Halfan). *Current Problems* 1994; **20:** 6.
7. Matson PA, *et al.* Cardiac effects of standard-dose halofantrine therapy. *Am J Trop Med Hyg* 1996; **54:** 229–31.
8. Sowunmi A, *et al.* Cardiac effects of halofantrine in children suffering from acute uncomplicated falciparum malaria. *Trans R Soc Trop Med Hyg* 1998; **92:** 446–8.

Effects on the skin. For a comparison of the incidence of pruritus associated with halofantrine and other antimalarials, see Effects on the Skin under Adverse Effects of Chloroquine, p.427.

Interactions

Halofantrine prolongs the QT interval and should not be administered with other drugs that have the potential to induce cardiac arrhythmias, in particular the antimalarials mefloquine, chloroquine, and quinine, and also tricyclic antidepressants, phenothiazine antipsychotics, some antiarrhythmics (including amiodarone, disopyramide, flecainide, procainamide, quinidine, and the beta blocker sotalol), cisapride, and the antihistamines astemizole and terfenadine. Also, halofantrine should not be given with drugs that cause electrolyte disturbances (such as diuretics).

Pharmacokinetics

Halofantrine is slowly and erratically absorbed following administration by mouth, although it appears in the circulation within about one hour, peak concentrations occurring in 3 to 6 hours. Bioavailability of halofantrine is increased by administration with or after food, particularly food high in fat content, and it must therefore be taken on an empty stomach because of the risk of cardiac toxicity. The elimination half-life of halofantrine varies considerably between individuals, but is generally about 1 to 2 days. Halofantrine is metabolised in the liver, its major metabolite being desbutylhalofantrine which appears to be as active as the parent compound. Excretion of halofantrine is primarily via the faeces.

References.

1. Milton KA, *et al.* Pharmacokinetics of halofantrine in man: effects of food and dose size. *Br J Clin Pharmacol* 1989; **28:** 71–7.
2. Karbwang J, *et al.* Pharmacokinetics of halofantrine in healthy Thai volunteers. *Br J Clin Pharmacol* 1991; **32:** 639–40.
3. Veenendaal JR, *et al.* Pharmacokinetics of halofantrine and N-desbutylhalofantrine in patients with falciparum malaria following a multiple dose regimen of halofantrine. *Eur J Clin Pharmacol* 1991; **41:** 161–4.
4. Karbwang J, Na Bangchang K. Clinical pharmacokinetics of halofantrine. *Clin Pharmacokinet* 1994; **27:** 104–19.
5. Watkins WM, *et al.* Halofantrine pharmacokinetics in Kenyan children with non-severe and severe malaria. *Br J Clin Pharmacol* 1995; **39:** 283–7.
6. Ohrt C, *et al.* Pharmacokinetics of an extended-dose halofantrine regimen in patients with malaria and in healthy volunteers. *Clin Pharmacol Ther* 1995; **57:** 525–32.

Uses and Administration

Halofantrine is a 9-phenanthrenemethanol antimalarial used in the *treatment* of uncomplicated chloroquine-resistant falciparum and of chloroquine-resistant vivax malaria. Halofantrine is a blood schizontocide but has no activity against exoerythrocytic forms. Its value is limited by its unpredictable bioavailability and by cardiotoxicity. It should *not* be used where mefloquine has been used for prophylaxis (see under Malaria, below; and for cardiac hazard, see Effects on the Heart, above). Halofantrine should also *not* be used for malaria prophylaxis and is no longer recommended for standby treatment.

In the treatment of malaria, halofantrine hydrochloride is given by mouth as 3 doses of 500 mg at intervals of 6 hours, on an empty stomach. Dosage for children is based on 24 mg per kg body-weight divided into 3 doses. The following doses are recommended: 23 to 31 kg body-weight, 3 doses of 250 mg at intervals of 6 hours; 32 to 37 kg body-weight, 3 doses of 375 mg at intervals of 6 hours; over 37 kg body-weight, adult dose. A second course should be given after a week.

Reviews.

1. Bryson HM, Goa KL. Halofantrine: a review of its antimalarial activity, pharmacokinetic properties and therapeutic potential. *Drugs* 1992; **43:** 236–58.

Administration. A micronised oral formulation of halofantrine was developed in an attempt to improve bioavailability and allow a smaller administered dose,[1-5] although wide inter-individual variation in plasma concentrations was still seen.[1,5] A parenteral dosage form was also evaluated.[5]

1. Fadat G, *et al.* Efficacy of micronized halofantrine in semi-immune patients with acute uncomplicated falciparum malaria in Cameroon. *Antimicrob Agents Chemother* 1993; **37:** 1955–7.
2. Wildling E, *et al.* High dose chloroquine versus micronized halofantrine in chloroquine-resistant Plasmodium falciparum malaria. *J Antimicrob Chemother* 1994; **33:** 871–5.
3. Kremsner PG, *et al.* Comparison of micronized halofantrine with chloroquine-antibiotic combinations for treating Plasmodium falciparum malaria in adults from Gabon. *Am J Trop Med Hyg* 1994; **50:** 790–5.
4. Bouchaud O, *et al.* Clinical efficacy and pharmacokinetics of micronized halofantrine for the treatment of acute uncomplicated falciparum malaria in nonimmune patients. *Am J Trop Med Hyg* 1994; **51:** 204–13.
5. Krishna S, *et al.* Pharmacokinetics, efficacy and toxicity of parenteral halofantrine in uncomplicated malaria. *Br J Clin Pharmacol* 1993; **36:** 585–91.

Malaria. Halofantrine is one of the drugs that may be used for the treatment of falciparum malaria (p.422) where there is chloroquine resistance, but its value is limited by its unpredictable bioavailability and by cardiotoxicity. Halofantrine should not be used in patients in whom mefloquine treatment[1] or prophylaxis[2] has failed owing to cross-resistance between halofantrine and mefloquine (for cardiac hazard, see Effects on the Heart, above).

Halofantrine should not be used for malaria prophylaxis and is no longer recommended for standby treatment.

1. ter Kuile FO, *et al.* Halofantrine versus mefloquine in treatment of multidrug-resistant falciparum malaria. *Lancet* 1993; **341:** 1044–9.
2. Gay F, *et al.* Cross-resistance between mefloquine and halofantrine. *Lancet* 1990; **336:** 1262.

Preparations

Proprietary Preparations (details are given in Part 3)

Aust.: Halfan; ***Belg.:*** Halfan; ***Fr.:*** Halfan; ***Ger.:*** Halfan; ***Neth.:*** Halfan; ***S.Afr.:*** Halfan; ***Spain:*** Halfan; ***Switz.:*** Halfan; ***UK:*** Halfan; ***USA:*** Halfan.

Hydroxychloroquine Sulphate

(1380-b)

Hydroxychloroquine Sulphate *(BANM, rINNM).*

Hydroxychloroquine Sulfate; Oxichlorochin Sulphate; Sulfato de Hidroxicloroquina; Win-1258-2. 2-{*N*-[4-(7-Chloro-4-quinolylamino)pentyl]-*N*-ethylamino}ethanol sulphate.

$C_{18}H_{26}ClN_3O,H_2SO_4$ = 434.0.

CAS — 118-42-3 (hydroxychloroquine); 747-36-4 (hydroxychloroquine sulphate).

Pharmacopoeias. In *Br., Port.,* and *US.*

A white or almost white odourless or almost odourless crystalline powder. Hydroxychloroquine sulphate 100 mg is approximately equivalent to 77 mg of hydroxychloroquine base. Freely **soluble** in water; practically insoluble in alcohol, chloroform, and ether. A 1% solution in water has a pH of 3.5 to 5.5. **Protect** from light.

Adverse Effects, Treatment, and Precautions

As for Chloroquine, p.426.

Effects on the eyes. The main adverse effects of chloroquine and hydroxychloroquine on the eye are keratopathy and retinopathy. With respect to retinopathy, precautions should be observed in patients undergoing long-term treatment, as described under Chloroquine on p.427.

Interactions

As for Chloroquine, p.428.

Pharmacokinetics

The pharmacokinetics of hydroxychloroquine are similar to those of chloroquine (see p.428).

References.

1. Tett SE, *et al.* A dose-ranging study of the pharmacokinetics of hydroxychloroquine following intravenous administration to healthy volunteers. *Br J Clin Pharmacol* 1988; **26:** 303–13.
2. Tett SE, *et al.* Bioavailability of hydroxychloroquine tablets in healthy volunteers. *Br J Clin Pharmacol* 1989; **27:** 771–9.
3. Miller DR, *et al.* Steady-state pharmacokinetics of hydroxychloroquine in rheumatoid arthritis. *DICP Ann Pharmacother* 1991; **25:** 1302–5.
4. Ducharme J, *et al.* Enantioselective disposition of hydroxychloroquine after a single oral dose of the racemate to healthy subjects. *Br J Clin Pharmacol* 1995; **40:** 127–33.

Uses and Administration

Hydroxychloroquine sulphate is a 4-aminoquinoline antimalarial with actions similar to those of chloroquine (p.429), but is mainly used in the treatment of systemic and discoid lupus erythematosus and rheumatoid arthritis. It has also been used in the treatment of light-sensitive skin eruptions.

Hydroxychloroquine sulphate is given by mouth.

In *lupus erythematosus* and *rheumatoid arthritis* response to treatment may not be apparent for up to 6 months but if there is no improvement by then, treatment should be discontinued. In the UK treatment is usually started with 400 mg daily in divided doses with meals. In the USA recommended initial doses are 400 to 600 mg daily for rheumatoid arthritis and 400 mg once or twice daily for lupus erythematosus. Doses are reduced to the minimum effective dose for maintenance; this is usually 200 to 400 mg daily but should not exceed 6.5 mg per kg body-weight daily (or 400 mg daily whichever is the smaller). To avoid excessive dosage in obese patients, special care is needed to calculate the dosage on the basis of lean body-weight. For further details see under Effects on the Eyes in Chloroquine, p.427. In children the minimum effective dose should be used up to a maximum of 6.5 mg per kg body-weight daily (or 400 mg daily whichever is the smaller).

Hydroxychloroquine sulphate is also used in similar doses for the treatment of *light-sensitive skin eruptions*, but treatment should only be given during periods of maximum exposure to light.

Hydroxychloroquine sulphate may be used in *malaria* both for treatment and prophylaxis, when chloroquine is not available, with the same limitations as for chloroquine. In the USA the manufacturers recommend for *prophylaxis* of malaria a dose of 400 mg every 7 days; children may be given a weekly prophylactic dose of hydroxychloroquine sulphate 6.5 mg per kg body-weight (up to a maximum of 400 mg). In *treating* an acute malarial attack a dose of 800 mg has been used, followed after 6 to 8 hours by 400 mg and a further 400 mg on each of the 2 following days; in children an initial dose of hydroxychloroquine sulphate 13 mg per kg may be given, followed by 6.5 mg per kg 6 hours later and again on the second and third days.

HIV infection and AIDS. Preliminary evidence[1-3] for possible benefit with hydroxychloroquine in HIV infection. For the conventional management of HIV infection and AIDS, see p.599.

1. Sperber K, *et al.* Hydroxychloroquine treatment of patients with human immunodeficiency virus type 1. *Clin Ther* 1995; **17:** 622–36.
2. Ornstein MH, Sperber K. The antiinflammatory and antiviral effects of hydroxychloroquine in two patients with acquired immunodeficiency syndrome and active inflammatory arthritis. *Arthritis Rheum* 1996; **39:** 157–61.
3. Sperber K, *et al.* Comparison of hydroxychloroquine with zidovudine in asymptomatic patients infected with human immunodeficiency virus type 1. *Clin Ther* 1997; **19:** 913–23.

Inflammatory disorders. For the use of hydroxychloroquine and chloroquine in a range of inflammatory conditions, see under Chloroquine, p.429 and under Rheumatoid Arthritis, below.

Lipid regulation. Hydroxychloroquine has been reported to counter the adverse effects on lipid metabolism caused by corticosteroids in patients with rheumatoid arthritis[1] and systemic lupus erythematosus.[1,2] Hydroxychloroquine also showed antihyperlipidaemic properties in patients not receiving corticosteroids.[1]

1. Wallace DJ, *et al.* Cholesterol-lowering effect of hydroxychloroquine in patients with rheumatic disease: reversal of deleterious effects of steroids on lipids. *Am J Med* 1990; **89:** 322–6.
2. Hodis HN, *et al.* The lipid, lipoprotein, and apolipoprotein effects of hydroxychloroquine in patients with systemic lupus erythematosus. *J Rheumatol* 1993; **20:** 661–5.

Lupus erythematosus. One of hydroxychloroquine's main indications is lupus erythematosus (p.1029).

Malaria. The role of chloroquine and potentially therefore of hydroxychloroquine in the treatment and prophylaxis of malaria is discussed on p.422.

Porphyria cutanea tarda. For reference to the use of hydroxychloroquine in the treatment of porphyria cutanea tarda, see under the Uses and Administration of Chloroquine, p.430.

Rheumatoid arthritis. Hydroxychloroquine and chloroquine may be used as antirheumatic drugs in the management of *rheumatoid arthritis* (p.2) in an attempt to suppress the rate of cartilage erosion or alter the course of the disease. These antimalarials are considered to be less effective than the other disease modifying antirheumatic drugs (DMARDs) but they are better tolerated and so may be preferred in patients with milder forms of the disease.[1] For reference to precautions to reduce the incidence of retinopathy, see under Effects on the Eyes in Adverse Effects of Chloroquine, p.427.

Generally the minimum effective dose should be used for maintenance to minimise toxicity; for hydroxychloroquine sulphate this should not exceed 6.5 mg per kg lean body-weight daily. Daily doses of 200 or 400 mg are commonly used but one study indicates that there is little advantage in using the higher dose.[2] Although benefit has sometimes been obtained using antimalarials with other DMARDs such as gold[3] or penicillamine,[4] adverse effects are more common. Some workers have also tried hydroxychloroquine in combination with cyclophosphamide and azathioprine although the use of cyclophosphamide was discontinued after concern over a possible increased risk of malignancy.[5] Hydroxychloroquine has been reported to counter the adverse effects on lipid metabolism caused by corticosteroids being used to treat rheumatoid arthritis (see Lipid Regulation, above).

Experience with antimalarials to treat *juvenile rheumatoid arthritis* (p.2) is limited and the results have been variable.[6,7]

Chloroquine and hydroxychloroquine have also been reported to be of use in *palindromic rheumatism*.[8-10]

1. HERA Study Group. A randomized trial of hydroxychloroquine in early rheumatoid arthritis: the HERA study. *Am J Med* 1995; **98:** 156–68.
2. Pavelka K, *et al.* Hydroxychloroquine sulphate in the treatment of rheumatoid arthritis: a double blind comparison of two dose regimens. *Ann Rheum Dis* 1989; **48:** 542–6.
3. Scott DL, *et al.* Combination therapy with gold and hydroxychloroquine in rheumatoid arthritis: a prospective, randomized, placebo-controlled study. *Br J Rheumatol* 1989; **28:** 128–33.
4. Gibson T, *et al.* Combined D-penicillamine and chloroquine treatment of rheumatoid arthritis—a comparative study. *Br J Rheumatol* 1987; **26:** 279–84.
5. Csuka M, *et al.* Treatment of intractable rheumatoid arthritis with combined cyclophosphamide, azathioprine, and hydroxychloroquine: a follow-up study. *JAMA* 1986; **255:** 2315–19.
6. Brewer EJ, *et al.* Penicillamine and hydroxychloroquine in the treatment of severe juvenile rheumatoid arthritis. *N Engl J Med* 1986; **314:** 1269–76.
7. Grondin C, *et al.* Slow-acting antirheumatic drugs in chronic arthritis of childhood. *Semin Arthritis Rheum* 1988; **18:** 38–47.
8. Golding DN. D-Penicillamine in palindromic rheumatism. *Br Med J* 1976; **2:** 1382–3.
9. Richardson MR, Zalin AM. Treatment of palindromic rheumatism with chloroquine. *Br Med J* 1987; **294:** 741.
10. Hanonen P, *et al.* Treatment of palindromic rheumatism with chloroquine. *Br Med J* 1987; **294:** 1289.

Sarcoidosis. Chloroquine and hydroxychloroquine have been tried in the management of sarcoidosis (p.1028) as alternatives or adjuncts to corticosteroid therapy. For references to the use of hydroxychloroquine, see under Chloroquine, p.430.

Skin disorders. For reference to the use of hydroxychloroquine in a variety of skin disorders, see under Chloroquine, p.430.

Venous thrombo-embolism. Standard prophylaxis for surgical patients at high risk of venous thrombo-embolism is usually with an anticoagulant (see p.802). Hydroxychloroquine has been described by some as an antiplatelet agent[1] and although its mechanism of action is uncertain the incidence of fatal pulmonary embolism has been reduced in patients given hydroxychloroquine prophylactically after total hip replacement;[2] the usual daily divided dose was about 800 mg from the day before surgery until discharge; larger doses had been used.

1. Antiplatelet Trialists' Collaboration. Collaborative overview of randomised trials of antiplatelet therapy—III: reduction in venous thrombosis and pulmonary embolism by antiplatelet prophylaxis among surgical and medical patients. *Br Med J* 1994; **308:** 235–46.
2. Loudon JR. Hydroxychloroquine and postoperative thromboembolism after total hip replacement. *Am J Med* 1988; **85:** (suppl 4A): 57–61.

Preparations

BP 1998: Hydroxychloroquine Tablets;
USP 23: Hydroxychloroquine Sulfate Tablets.

Proprietary Preparations (details are given in Part 3)
Aust.: Plaquenil†; ***Austral.:*** Plaquenil; ***Belg.:*** Plaquenil; ***Canad.:*** Plaquenil; ***Fr.:*** Plaquenil; ***Ger.:*** Quensyl; ***Irl.:*** Plaquenil; ***Ital.:*** Plaquenil; ***Neth.:*** Plaquenil; ***Norw.:*** Ercoquin; Plaquenil; ***Swed.:*** Plaquenil; ***Switz.:*** Plaquenil; ***UK:*** Plaquenil; ***USA:*** Plaquenil.

Hydroxypiperaquine Phosphate (19318-s)

1,3-Bis[1-(7-chloro-4-quinolyl)-4-piperazinyl]-2-hydroxypropane phosphate.

$C_{29}H_{32}OCl_2N_6.4H_3PO_4$ = 943.5.

CAS — 74351-60-3.

Hydroxypiperaquine phosphate is a 4-piperazinoquinoline antimalarial which has been reported to be effective in the treatment of vivax malaria and chloroquine-sensitive and chloroquine-resistant falciparum malaria.

References.

1. Li Y, *et al.* Hydroxypiperaquine phosphate in treatment of falciparum malaria. *Chin Med J* 1981; **94:** 301–2.
2. Li Y, *et al.* Hydroxypiperaquine phosphate in treating chloroquine resistant falciparum malaria. *Chin Med J* 1981; **94:** 303–4.
3. Xu D, *et al.* Studies on the new antimalarial drug hydroxypiperaquine and its phosphate. *J Med Coll PLA* 1988; **3:** 5–12.
4. Chen L. Recent studies on antimalarial efficacy of piperaquine and hydroxypiperaquine. *Chin Med J* 1991; **104:** 161–3.

Mefloquine Hydrochloride (1381-v)

Mefloquine Hydrochloride *(BANM, USAN, rINNM).*

Mefloquini Hydrochloridum; Ro-21-5998 (mefloquine); Ro-21-5998/001 (mefloquine hydrochloride); WR-142490 (mefloquine). (*RS*)-[2,8-Bis(trifluoromethyl)-4-quinolyl]-(*SR*)-(2-piperidyl)methanol hydrochloride.

$C_{17}H_{16}F_6N_2O,HCl$ = 414.8.

CAS — 53230-10-7 (mefloquine); 51773-92-3 (mefloquine hydrochloride).

Pharmacopoeias. In Eur. (see p.viii).

A white or slightly yellow, crystalline powder. It shows polymorphism. Mefloquine base 250 mg is approximately equivalent to mefloquine hydrochloride 274 mg. Very slightly **soluble** in water; soluble in alcohol; freely soluble in methyl alcohol. **Protect** from light.

Sorption. For reference to loss of mefloquine hydrochloride from solutions during membrane filtration, see Chloroquine, p.426.

Stability. A report of the photolytic degradation of mefloquine hydrochloride in water.[1]

1. Tønnesen HH, Grislingaas A-L. Photochemical stability of biologically active compounds II: photochemical decomposition of mefloquine in water. *Int J Pharmaceutics* 1990; **60:** 157–62.

Adverse Effects

Since mefloquine has a long elimination half-life, adverse effects may occur or persist up to several weeks after the last dose.

The most frequent adverse effects of mefloquine are nausea, diarrhoea, vomiting, abdominal pain, anorexia, headache, dizziness, loss of balance, somnolence, and sleep disorders, notably insomnia and abnormal dreams.

Neurological or psychiatric disturbances have also been reported with mefloquine and include sensory and motor neuropathies, tremor, ataxia, visual disturbances, tinnitus, convulsions, anxiety, depression, confusion, hallucinations, panic attacks, emotional instability, aggression and agitation, and acute psychosis.

Other adverse effects include skin rashes, pruritus and urticaria, hair loss, muscle weakness, myalgia, liver function disturbances, and very rarely thrombocytopenia and leucopenia. There have been rare occurrences of erythema multiforme including the Stevens-Johnson syndrome. Cardiovascular effects have included hypotension, hypertension, tachycardia or palpitations, bradycardia, and other minor ECG changes. There have been isolated cases of atrioventricular block.

The frequencies of adverse effects in 134 soldiers who received mefloquine hydrochloride 250 mg weekly for malaria chemoprophylaxis were diarrhoea in 48%, nausea in 13%, vomiting in 2%, headache in 13%, and dizziness in 7%.[1] All of 7 healthy subjects who received a dose of mefloquine hydrochloride 15 mg per kg body-weight had symptoms which included vertigo, nausea, dizziness, and lightheadedness.[2] The manufacturers report that dizziness has occurred in 24% of patients with malaria treated with 750 mg of mefloquine, in 38% treated with 1000 mg, and in 96% treated with 1500 mg; splitting a dose into two doses given 8 hours apart can reduce the incidence of dizziness.[3] A prospective study involving 3673 patients found that anorexia, nausea, vomiting, dizziness, and sleep disorders were 1.1 to 1.4 times more frequent in patients receiving mefloquine 25 mg per kg for treatment of malaria than in those receiving 15 mg per kg, and that vomiting could be reduced by 40% if the higher dose was split and given as 15 mg per kg followed by a further 10 mg per kg after 16 to 24 hours.[4] The frequency of adverse effects is reported to be higher in subjects who become dehydrated.[5]

There has been concern that mefloquine's adverse effects, especially neuropsychiatric reactions, might limit its use for the prophylaxis of malaria, but as discussed under Effects on the Nervous System, below the incidence of adverse effects does not appear to be greater than with other prophylactic schedules.

1. Arthur JD, *et al.* Mefloquine prophylaxis. *Lancet* 1990; **335:** 972.
2. Patchen LC, *et al.* Neurologic reactions after a therapeutic dose of mefloquine. *N Engl J Med* 1989; **321:** 1415.
3. Stürchler D, *et al.* Neuropsychiatric side effects of mefloquine. *N Engl J Med* 1990; **322:** 1752–3.
4. ter Kuile FO, *et al.* Mefloquine treatment of acute falciparum malaria: a prospective study of non-serious adverse effects in 3673 patients. *Bull WHO* 1995; **73:** 631–42.
5. Perry IC. Malaria prophylaxis. *Br Med J* 1995; **310:** 1673.

Effects on the blood. A report of agranulocytosis in a patient with malaria 48 hours after treatment with a 1250-mg course of mefloquine. The patient had previously taken 250 mg of mefloquine weekly for 7 weeks without side-effects.[1]

1. Hennequin C, *et al.* Agranulocytosis during treatment with mefloquine. *Lancet* 1991; **337:** 984.

Effects on the nervous system. Neuropsychiatric reactions have been associated with the use of mefloquine although various figures have been reported for their frequency. In the UK the Committee on Safety of Medicines has quoted[1] figures of 1 in 10 000 to 1 in 20 000 for severe reactions to *prophylactic* doses and similarly the manufacturers report that 1 in 10 000 patients receiving mefloquine prophylaxis will experience serious problems. Others consider that the incidence of serious reactions is extremely low,[2] with a frequency of about 1 in 80 000. The manufacturers have also reported that most reactions in patients taking mefloquine for prophylaxis appear to occur after the first dose and have suggested that monitoring after the first dose could identify 40% of those at risk of neuropsychiatric effects.[3] Some authorities consider that over 75% of such reactions to mefloquine are apparent by the third dose.[4] This may allow for tolerability problems with mefloquine prophylaxis to be identified before travel. There has been much discussion on the comparative tolerability of antimalarials used for chemoprophylaxis. The incidence of adverse events, including neuropsychiatric events, was comparable for mefloquine and chloroquine in 2 uncontrolled questionnaire studies, one in tourists[5] and one in US Peace Corps volunteers.[6] However, in a more recent questionnaire in travellers,[7] although the incidence of reported adverse events was similar for mefloquine and chloroquine plus proguanil, neuropsychiatric adverse events were significantly more common in mefloquine recipients. In two randomised controlled trials,[8,9] both in military personnel, there was no difference between CNS symptoms in those receiving weekly mefloquine and those receiving chloroquine (with or without proguanil). In one of these studies,[9] a subgroup receiving a loading dose of mefloquine daily for 3 days initially had a higher incidence of CNS events. A review[10] of 10 controlled trials found no significant difference in the rates of withdrawal and overall incidence of adverse effects for mefloquine and alternative prophylactic regimens, but mefloquine was more likely than other drugs to cause insomnia and fatigue. Women may be at greater risk of adverse effects than men, and WHO has commented that adverse effects may limit the usefulness of mefloquine prophylaxis to highly motivated occupational subgroups or individuals at high risk of infection with chloroquine-resistant malaria.[16]

Neuropsychiatric reactions are more frequent following the higher doses of mefloquine used for *treatment* than those used for prophylaxis. Some workers have estimated that overall 1 in 8000 mefloquine users suffers from such reactions, with the incidence 60 times higher after treatment than after prophylaxis.[11] Other workers who have used mefloquine in nearly

14 000 treatments calculated that the overall frequency of serious neuropsychiatric reactions was 1 per 1754 treatments; serious neuropsychiatric reactions therefore appeared to be ten times more probable after treatment than with prophylactic use of mefloquine.[12]

A severe neurological syndrome associated with mefloquine treatment, with agitation, delirium, stupor, hyperpyrexia, mydriasis, and generalised rigors responded rapidly to treatment with physostigmine, suggesting a central anticholinergic aetiology.[13]

A discrete post-malaria neurological syndrome (including an acute confusional state or acute psychosis, convulsions, and tremor) has been observed following recovery from falciparum malaria and there appeared to be a strong association with mefloquine although it was not the only risk factor.[14] Nevertheless the risk was considered unacceptable by Mai *et al.*[14] who recommended that, where there was an effective alternative drug, mefloquine should not be used after initial treatment of severe malaria.

Emergence delirium during recovery from general anaesthesia after mefloquine prophylaxis has been reported in 3 cases.[15]

1. Committee on Safety of Medicines. Mefloquine (Lariam) and neuropsychiatric reactions. *Current Problems* 1996; **22:** 6.
2. Croft AMJ, World MJ. Neuropsychiatric reactions with mefloquine chemoprophylaxis. *Lancet* 1996; **347:** 326.
3. Stürchler D, *et al.* Neuropsychiatric side effects of mefloquine. *N Engl J Med* 1990; **322:** 1752–3.
4. Bradley DJ, *et al.* Guidelines for the prevention of malaria in travellers from the United Kingdom. *Commun Dis Rep Rev* 1997; **7:** R137–R152.
5. Steffen R, *et al.* Mefloquine compared with other malaria chemoprophylactic regimens in tourists visiting East Africa. *Lancet* 1993; **341:** 1299–1303.
6. Lobel HO, *et al.* Long-term malaria prophylaxis with weekly mefloquine. *Lancet* 1993; **341:** 848–51.
7. Barrett PJ, *et al.* Comparison of adverse events associated with use of mefloquine and combination of chloroquine and proguanil as antimalarial prophylaxis: postal and telephone survey of travellers. *Br Med J* 1996; **313:** 525–8. Correspondence. *ibid.*: 1552–4.
8. Croft AMJ, *et al.* Side effects of mefloquine prophylaxis for malaria: an independent randomized controlled trial. *Trans R Soc Trop Med Hyg* 1997; **91:** 199–203.
9. Boudreau E, *et al.* Tolerability of prophylactic Lariam regimens. *Trop Med Parasitol* 1993; **44:** 257–65.
10. Croft A, Garner P. Mefloquine to prevent malaria: a systematic review of trials. *Br Med J* 1997; **315:** 1412–16. Correspondence. *ibid.* 1998; **316:** 1980–1.
11. Weinke T, *et al.* Neuropsychiatric side effects after the use of mefloquine. *Am J Trop Med Hyg* 1991; **45:** 86–91.
12. Luxemburger C, *et al.* Mefloquine for multidrug-resistant malaria. *Lancet* 1991; **338:** 1268.
13. Speich R, Haller A. Central anticholinergic syndrome with the antimalarial drug mefloquine. *N Engl J Med* 1994; **331:** 57–8.
14. Mai NTH, *et al.* Post-malaria neurological syndrome. *Lancet* 1996; **348:** 917–21.
15. Gullahorn GM, *et al.* Anaesthesia emergence delirium after mefloquine prophylaxis. *Lancet* 1993; **341:** 632.
16. Anonymous. Mefloquine effectiveness impaired by high withdrawal rates. *WHO Drug Inf* 1998; **12:** 7–8.

Effects on the oesophagus. Oesophageal ulceration in one patient and discomfort in another 4 was attributed to swallowing mefloquine tablets with insufficient fluid.[1]

1. Phillips M. Antimalarial mefloquine. *Med J Aust* 1994; **161:** 227–8.

Effects on the skin. Single cases of Stevens-Johnson syndrome,[1] severe facial lesions,[2] exfoliative dermatitis,[3] toxic epidermal necrolysis,[4] and cutaneous vasculitis[5] have been associated with use of mefloquine for malaria prophylaxis.

For a comparison of the incidence of pruritus induced by various antimalarials, see under Chloroquine, p.427.

1. Van den Enden E, *et al.* Mefloquine-induced Stevens-Johnson syndrome. *Lancet* 1991; **337:** 683.
2. Shlim DR. Severe facial rash associated with mefloquine. *JAMA* 1991; **266:** 2560.
3. Martin GJ, *et al.* Exfoliative dermatitis during malarial prophylaxis with mefloquine. *Clin Infect Dis* 1993; **16:** 341–2.
4. McBride SR, *et al.* Fatal toxic epidermal necrolysis associated with mefloquine antimalarial prophylaxis. *Lancet* 1997; **349:** 101.
5. White AC, *et al.* Cutaneous vasculitis associated with mefloquine. *Ann Intern Med* 1995; **123:** 894.

Overdosage. Cardiac, hepatic, and neurological symptoms have been reported in a patient who inadvertently received 5.25 g of mefloquine over 6 days.[1] All symptoms disappeared rapidly when mefloquine was discontinued.

1. Bourgeade A, *et al.* Intoxication accidentelle à la méfloquine. *Presse Med* 1990; **19:** 1903.

Precautions

Tasks requiring fine coordination such as driving should not be undertaken during treatment with mefloquine or for at least 3 weeks afterwards; in the case of prophylactic use, care should be exercised while taking mefloquine and for at least 3 weeks after stopping it. The use of mefloquine for malaria prophylaxis is contra-indicated in patients with a history of psychiatric (including depression) or convulsive disorders and in those with severe hepatic impairment. Mefloquine is teratogenic in *animals* and its use during pregnancy is best avoided; however, in areas of chloroquine-resistant *Plasmodium falciparum* WHO and UK authorities suggest that mefloquine may be taken for malaria prophylaxis from the fourth month of pregnancy. It is recommended that women should also avoid becoming pregnant during and for 3 months after mefloquine use and that mothers should not breast feed while taking mefloquine. Mefloquine should be used with caution in patients with renal impairment and in those with cardiac conduction disorders.

Porphyria. For a discussion of the problems of prophylaxis and treatment of malaria in patients with porphyria and a comment that mefloquine may be safe for use in such patients, see under Precautions of Chloroquine, p.428.

Pregnancy. The manufacturers of mefloquine report that it is teratogenic in *rodents*. There is limited information on its effects in humans. One study in Thailand cited by WHO[1] found no difference between mefloquine and quinine in pregnancy outcome, but the numbers of treated patients who were in their first trimester were very small and its use should be kept to a minimum in that stage of pregnancy. Further spontaneous reports of exposure to mefloquine during the first trimester of pregnancy collected by the manufacturer revealed 24 fetal abnormalities and 17 spontaneous or missed abortions in 358 pregnancies, although a causal relationship was not established,[2] and a later study by the manufacturer involving 1627 reports of exposure during pregnancy appeared to show a similar incidence of congenital malformation to that in offspring of unexposed women.[6] In 53 army service women who inadvertently used mefloquine in pregnancy, and for whom pregnancy outcome was known, there were 17 elective abortions, 12 spontaneous abortions, one molar pregnancy, and 23 healthy live births, with no major congenital malformations.[3] The rate of spontaneous abortions was considered high.[3] A prospective cohort study involving 236 pregnant women who received an antimalarial in the first trimester did not demonstrate an increased risk of spontaneous abortion or anomaly in women who took mefloquine compared with other antimalarials, and the rate of spontaneous abortion was comparable with background rates.[7]

Confidence in the safety of mefloquine has increased, and mefloquine is now considered suitable for malaria prophylaxis in the second and third trimesters by both WHO[4] and authorities in the UK.[5] It should be avoided in the first trimester unless the risk of withholding mefloquine is considered greater, and pregnancy should be avoided during and for 3 months after prophylactic use.

1. WHO. Practical chemotherapy of malaria: report of a WHO scientific group. *WHO Tech Rep Ser 805* 1990.
2. Palmer KJ, *et al.* Mefloquine: a review of its antimalarial activity, pharmacokinetic properties and therapeutic efficacy. *Drugs* 1993; **45:** 430–75.
3. Smoak BL, *et al.* The effects of inadvertent exposure of mefloquine chemoprophylaxis on pregnancy outcomes and infants of US Army service women. *J Infect Dis* 1997; **176:** 831–3.
4. WHO. *International travel and health: vaccination requirements and health advice.* Geneva: WHO, 1998.
5. Bradley DJ, *et al.* Guidelines for the prevention of malaria in travellers from the United Kingdom. *Commun Dis Rep Rev* 1997; **7:** R137–R152.
6. Vanhauwere B, *et al.* Post-marketing surveillance of prophylactic mefloquine (Lariam®) use in pregnancy. *Am J Trop Med Hyg* 1998; **58:** 17–21.
7. Phillips-Howard PA, *et al.* Safety of mefloquine and other antimalarial agents in the first trimester of pregnancy. *J Travel Med* 1998; **5:** 121–6.

Interactions

Halofantrine should not be given with or after mefloquine because of the increased potential to induce hazardous cardiac arrhythmias, as discussed on p.430. There is an increased risk of convulsions when mefloquine is administered with chloroquine or quinine.

For further details of interactions, see below.

It is well established that the use of *halofantrine* with or after mefloquine is contra-indicated because of the risk of hazardous cardiac arrhythmias. Mefloquine and other related compounds such as *quinine*, *quinidine*, and *chloroquine* may be given concomitantly only under close medical supervision because of possible additive cardiac toxicity; there is also an increased risk of convulsions. It has been recommended[1] that extreme caution should be exercised in the use of mefloquine in patients also taking *beta blockers*, *calcium-channel blockers*, *digitalis*, or *antidepressants* until more was known about the risks of cardiotoxicity. More recently, WHO malaria prophylaxis guidelines[2] considered, in the light of information currently available, that although co-administration of mefloquine with *antiarrhythmic drugs*, *beta blockers*, *calcium-channel blockers*, *antihistamines*, *tricyclic antidepressants*, and *phenothiazines* might contribute to prolongation of QT intervals, it was not absolutely contra-indicated. Nevertheless an increased risk of ventricular arrhythmias has been reported when mefloquine is used concomitantly with *amiodarone* or *pimozide*.

Cardiopulmonary arrest has occurred after a single dose of mefloquine in a patient who was taking *propranolol*.[3]

A study in healthy subjects indicated that concurrent administration of *primaquine* could increase blood concentrations of mefloquine and might increase the incidence of adverse effects due to mefloquine,[4] but others reported no such interaction.[5] Studies in healthy subjects have also indicated that *ampicillin*,[6] *tetracycline*,[7] or *metoclopramide*[8] could increase blood concentrations of mefloquine.

There has been a case report[9] of a patient who experienced neuropsychiatric disturbances after consuming a large quantity of *alcohol* in conjunction with mefloquine; subsequent abstention from alcohol led to complete reversal of the reactions.

The manufacturers state that mefloquine-induced attenuation of immunisation produced by oral live *typhoid vaccines* cannot be excluded and therefore vaccination with such vaccines should be completed at least 3 days before taking mefloquine.

For the effect of mefloquine on *valproate*, see p.363. For its effect on *carbamazepine*, see p.341.

1. WHO. Practical chemotherapy of malaria: report of a WHO scientific group. *WHO Tech Rep Ser 805* 1990.
2. WHO. *International travel and health: vaccination requirements and health advice.* Geneva: WHO, 1998.
3. Anonymous. Mefloquine for malaria. *Med Lett Drugs Ther* 1990; **32:** 13–14.
4. MacLeod CM, *et al.* Interaction of primaquine with mefloquine in healthy males. *J Clin Pharmacol* 1990; **30:** 841.
5. Karbwang J, *et al.* Pharmacokinetics of mefloquine in the presence of primaquine. *Eur J Clin Pharmacol* 1992; **42:** 559–60.
6. Karbwang J, *et al.* Effect of ampicillin on mefloquine pharmacokinetics in Thai males. *Eur J Clin Pharmacol* 1991; **40:** 631–3.
7. Karbwang J, *et al.* Effect of tetracycline on mefloquine pharmacokinetics in Thai males. *Eur J Clin Pharmacol* 1992; **43:** 567–9.
8. Na Bangchang K, *et al.* The effect of metoclopramide on mefloquine pharmacokinetics. *Br J Clin Pharmacol* 1991; **32:** 640–1.
9. Wittes RC, Saginur R. Adverse reaction to mefloquine associated with ethanol ingestion. *Can Med Assoc J* 1995; **152:** 515–17.

Pharmacokinetics

The pharmacokinetics of mefloquine may be altered by malaria infection in a manner similar to those of quinine, the main effects being reductions in both its volume of distribution and its overall clearance.

Mefloquine is well absorbed from the gastro-intestinal tract but there is marked interindividual variation in the time required to achieve peak plasma concentrations. Mefloquine is about 98% bound to plasma proteins and high concentrations have been reported in red blood cells. It is widely distributed throughout the body. Mefloquine has a long elimination half-life; mean values of about 21 days have been reported for some patients, although like other pharmacokinetic data on mefloquine there is considerable variation in reported figures. Subtherapeutic concentrations of mefloquine may persist in the blood for several months. Mefloquine is metabolised in the liver. Little of a dose is excreted in the urine and animal studies suggest excretion of mefloquine and its metabolites is mainly in the bile and faeces.

Mefloquine is distributed into breast milk in small amounts.

Reviews of pharmacokinetic studies of mefloquine reveal considerable interindividual variation for several pharmacokinetic parameters and some evidence that there might be pharmacokinetic differences between ethnic groups.[1,2] Mefloquine is well absorbed by healthy subjects and by patients with uncomplicated malaria following oral administration.[3,4] In patients with complicated malaria adequate blood concentrations have been obtained using nasogastric administration but this route cannot be relied upon for seriously ill patients[5] as absorption may be incomplete.[1] Mefloquine has a large apparent volume of distribution but this is reduced in the presence of malaria.[6,7] In children who received mefloquine with sulfadoxine and pyrimethamine as tablets crushed and mixed with a glucose syrup, maximum blood-mefloquine concentrations were higher and reached in a shorter time compared with equivalent doses in adults.[8] In pregnant women with uncomplicated malaria blood concentrations were lower than in non-pregnant women and the apparent volume of distribution was larger.[9] Once-weekly prophylactic doses of mefloquine resulted in steady-state conditions at about 10 doses with no evidence of subsequent accumulation.[10] The manufacturer has stated that mefloquine is about 98% bound to plasma proteins. Mefloquine is metabolised in the liver[11] largely into 2,8-bis(trifluoromethyl)-4-quinoline carboxylic acid [Ro-21-5104][12] but this metabolite appears to be inactive against *Plasmodium falciparum*.[13] Only a small percentage of a dose is excreted in the urine[14] and studies in *animals* suggest excretion of mefloquine and its metabolites is primarily in the bile and faeces.[1] Mefloquine has an extremely long plasma elimination half-life; again there is considerable interindividual variation and mean values ranging from 13.9 to 27.5 days have been quoted, the smaller figure of the range referring to a formulation that did not provide as good absorption as the preparation now in use.[1]

Mefloquine is distributed into breast milk, but a single dose study in 2 women[15] indicated that the concentration of mefloquine in milk was only a small proportion of that seen in plasma.

1. Karbwang J, White NJ. Clinical pharmacokinetics of mefloquine. *Clin Pharmacokinet* 1990; **19:** 264–79.
2. Palmer KJ, *et al.* Mefloquine: a review of its antimalarial activity, pharmacokinetic properties and therapeutic efficacy. *Drugs* 1993; **45:** 430–75.
3. Karbwang J, *et al.* The pharmacokinetics of mefloquine when given alone or in combination with sulphadoxine and pyrimethamine in Thai male and female subjects. *Eur J Clin Pharmacol* 1987; **32:** 173–7.
4. Looareesuwan S, *et al.* Studies of mefloquine bioavailability and kinetics using a stable isotope technique: a comparison of Thai patients with falciparum malaria and healthy caucasian volunteers. *Br J Clin Pharmacol* 1987; **24:** 37–42.
5. Chanthavanich P, *et al.* Intragastric mefloquine is absorbed rapidly in patients with cerebral malaria. *Am J Trop Med Hyg* 1985; **34:** 1028–36.
6. Juma FD, Ogeto JO. Mefloquine disposition in normals and in patients with severe Plasmodium falciparum malaria. *Eur J Drug Metab Pharmacokinet* 1989; **14:** 15–17.
7. Karbwang J, *et al.* A comparison of the pharmacokinetics of mefloquine in healthy Thai volunteers and in Thai patients with falciparum malaria. *Eur J Clin Pharmacol* 1988; **35:** 677–80.
8. Singhasivanon V, *et al.* Pharmacokinetic study of mefloquine in Thai children aged 5-12 years suffering from uncomplicated falciparum malaria treated with MSP or MSP plus primaquine. *Eur J Drug Metab Pharmacokinet* 1994; **19:** 27–32.
9. Na Bangchang K, *et al.* Mefloquine pharmacokinetics in pregnant women with acute falciparum malaria. *Trans R Soc Trop Med Hyg* 1994; **88:** 321–3.
10. Pennie RA, *et al.* Steady state pharmacokinetics of mefloquine in long-term travellers. *Trans R Soc Trop Med Hyg* 1993; **87:** 459–62.
11. WHO. Severe and complicated malaria. 2nd ed. *Trans R Soc Trop Med Hyg* 1990; **84** (suppl 2): 1–65.
12. Panisko DM, Keystone JS. Treatment of malaria—1990. *Drugs* 1990; **39:** 160–89.
13. Håkanson A, *et al.* Comparison of the activity in vitro of mefloquine and two metabolites against Plasmodium falciparum. *Trans R Soc Trop Med Hyg* 1990; **84:** 503–4.
14. Schwartz DE, *et al.* Urinary excretion of mefloquine and some of its metabolites in African volunteers at steady state. *Chemotherapy* 1987; **33:** 305–8.
15. Edstein MD, *et al.* Excretion of mefloquine in human breast milk. *Chemotherapy* 1988; **34:** 165–9.

Uses and Administration

Mefloquine is a 4-methanolquinoline antimalarial related to quinine. It is a blood schizontocide effective against all forms of malaria including chloroquine- or multidrug-resistant strains of *Plasmodium falciparum*, although some strains are naturally resistant to mefloquine. It is used for the treatment of uncomplicated falciparum malaria and chloroquine-resistant vivax malaria, and also for malaria prophylaxis.

Mefloquine is administered by mouth as the hydrochloride but variation in the way doses for mefloquine are expressed could lead to confusion. In the UK and elsewhere doses are expressed in terms of the base and a dose of 250 mg base is approximately equivalent to 274 mg of mefloquine hydrochloride. In the USA doses are expressed in terms of the hydrochloride and a dose of 250 mg is therefore approximately equivalent to only 228 mg of mefloquine base. Doses in the USA could therefore be about 10% less than elsewhere.

Doses recommended in the UK are as follows. For the *treatment of malaria*, mefloquine base 20 to 25 mg per kg body-weight (up to a maximum of 1.5 g) as a single dose or preferably in 2 or 3 divided doses 6 to 8 hours apart. For the *prophylaxis of malaria*, a dose of mefloquine base 250 mg once weekly in adults and children over 45 kg. Children weighing 5 to 19 kg (age 3 months to 5 years) may be given one-quarter the adult dose; those weighing 20 to 30 kg (6 to 8 years), half the adult dose; and those weighing 31 to 45 kg (9 to 14 years), three-quarters the adult dose. Prophylaxis should be started 1 to 3 weeks before exposure and continued for 4 weeks after leaving the malarious area.

For other dosage recommendations, see under Malaria, below.

Malaria. The overall treatment and prophylaxis of malaria and the place of mefloquine in current recommendations are discussed on p.422.

TREATMENT. Clinical studies have shown mefloquine to be effective in the treatment of chloroquine- or multidrug-resistant falciparum malaria. It is also effective in benign malarias, but is not normally required since they usually respond to chloroquine.

Mefloquine is widely considered to be a suitable alternative to regimens using quinine for the treatment of chloroquine-resistant or multidrug-resistant strains of *Plasmodium falciparum*.[1-4] It may also be used in combination with an artemisinin derivative in regions of greatest multidrug resistance (see p.426). Other combinations are also being evaluated.[5,6]

As there is no parenteral formulation of mefloquine currently available it can only be used in patients who can take oral medication and is therefore unsuitable for sole treatment in severe infections. Mefloquine has produced adequate blood concentrations following nasogastric administration but this route cannot be relied upon in seriously ill patients.[7] If mefloquine is given to patients after parenteral administration of quinine, it is recommended that a period of 12 hours should be allowed after the last dose of quinine to avoid toxicity.[8]

In the UK the recommended dose for the treatment of malaria is the equivalent of 20 to 25 mg of mefloquine base per kg body-weight, as a single dose or preferably in two or three divided doses 6 to 8 hours apart, to a maximum of 1.5 g. The manufacturers recommend a lower dose of 15 mg per kg for the partially immune. In the USA the manufacturers recommend 1250 mg of mefloquine hydrochloride given as a single dose. WHO has recommended a dose of mefloquine base of 15 mg per kg (up to a maximum of 1000 mg).[2] However, in areas of multidrug-resistant malaria a dose of 25 mg per kg[9,10] has been shown to improve the response, and this dose is now recommended by WHO[11] for standby treatment in such areas (see below).

Mefloquine is one of the antimalarial drugs recommended by some experts to be carried as a *standby* for the emergency treatment of malaria. The adult dose recommended by WHO[11] for self-treatment is 15 mg per kg as a single dose, or 25 mg per kg (given as 15 mg per kg followed by 10 mg per kg 6 to 24 hours later) in areas of mefloquine resistance. In the USA mefloquine is not recommended for self-treatment.[12]

PROPHYLAXIS. It had been hoped that mefloquine could be reserved for the treatment of malaria, but increasing drug resistance to chemoprophylactic regimens has led to it being widely used for malaria prophylaxis. WHO recommends[11] that mefloquine should only be used in high-risk areas where chloroquine-resistant malaria is prevalent and authorities in the UK[13] and USA[14] endorse this. The equivalent of 250 mg of mefloquine base is given every week starting 1 to 3 weeks before departure and continuing throughout the period of exposure and for 4 weeks after leaving the malarious area. Starting mefloquine prophylaxis 2 to 3 weeks before exposure allows for detection of possible adverse effects before travelling (see Effects on the Nervous System, above, for concerns about neurotoxicity). It is now considered that mefloquine prophylaxis can be given for periods of up to one year[13] instead of the previous limit of 3 months.

Mefloquine is considered to be suitable for prophylaxis in women from the fourth month of pregnancy although it should be avoided during the first trimester and effective contraception should be used for three months after stopping the drug.[11]

Recommended dosages of mefloquine for prophylaxis in children have generally been based on 5 mg per kg body-weight as a single weekly dose in children over 15 kg body-weight[2,13] and above the age of 2 years.[13] However, the UK licensed doses are now for infants and children over 5 kg body-weight and above 3 months of age as follows: 5 to 19 kg (3 months to 5 years), one-quarter the adult dose; 20 to 30 kg (6 to 8 years), half the adult dose; 31 to 45 kg (9 to 14 years), three-quarters the adult dose. Similarly, WHO[11] recommends: 5 to 12 kg (3 to 23 months), one-quarter the adult dose; 13 to 16 kg (2 to 3 years), one-third the adult dose; 17 to 24 kg (4 to 7 years), half the adult dose; 25 to 35 kg (8 to 10 years), three-quarters the adult dose; 36 to 50 kg (11 to 13 years), the adult dose.

In the event of breakthrough malaria during malaria prophylaxis there may be a delay of up to several months before the onset of symptoms in contrast to that seen with other forms of prophylaxis.[15] Mefloquine should not be used for treatment if it has been used for prophylaxis.

1. WHO. Practical chemotherapy of malaria: report of a WHO scientific group. *WHO Tech Rep Ser 805* 1990.
2. WHO. *WHO model prescribing information: drugs used in parasitic diseases.* 2nd ed. Geneva: WHO, 1995.
3. Molyneux M, Fox R. Diagnosis and treatment of malaria in Britain. *Br Med J* 1993; **306:** 1175–80.
4. Anonymous. Drugs for parasitic infections. *Med Lett Drugs Ther* 1998; **40:** 1–12.
5. Looareesuwan S, *et al.* Randomized trial of mefloquine-doxycycline, and artesunate-doxycycline for treatment of acute uncomplicated falciparum malaria. *Am J Trop Med Hyg* 1994; **50:** 784–9.
6. Looareesuwan S, *et al.* Randomized trial of mefloquine-tetracycline and quinine-tetracycline for acute uncomplicated falciparum malaria. *Acta Trop (Basel)* 1994; **57:** 47–53.
7. Chanthavanich P, *et al.* Intragastric mefloquine is absorbed rapidly in patients with cerebral malaria. *Am J Trop Med Hyg* 1985; **34:** 1028–36.
8. Gilles HM. *Management of severe and complicated malaria.* Geneva: WHO, 1991.
9. ter Kuile FO, *et al.* High-dose mefloquine in the treatment of multidrug-resistant falciparum malaria. *J Infect Dis* 1992; **166:** 1393–1400.
10. Smithuis FM, *et al.* Comparison of two mefloquine regimens for treatment of Plasmodium falciparum malaria on the northeastern Thai-Cambodian border. *Antimicrob Agents Chemother* 1993; **37:** 1977–81.
11. WHO. *International travel and health: vaccination requirements and health advice.* Geneva: WHO, 1998.
12. Centers for Disease Control. Recommendations for the prevention of malaria among travelers. *MMWR* 1990; **39** (RR-3): 1–10.
13. Bradley DJ, *et al.* Guidelines for the prevention of malaria in travellers from the United Kingdom. *Commun Dis Rep Rev* 1997; **7:** R137–R152.
14. Centers for Disease Control. Change of dosing regimen for malaria prophylaxis with mefloquine. *MMWR* 1991; **40:** 72–3.
15. Day JH, Behrens RH. Delay in onset of malaria with mefloquine prophylaxis. *Lancet* 1995; **345:** 398.

Preparations

Proprietary Preparations (details are given in Part 3)
Aust.: Lariam; ***Austral.:*** Lariam; ***Belg.:*** Lariam; ***Canad.:*** Lariam; ***Fr.:*** Lariam; ***Ger.:*** Lariam; ***Irl.:*** Lariam; ***Ital.:*** Lariam; ***Neth.:*** Lariam; ***Norw.:*** Lariam; ***S.Afr.:*** Lariam; ***Swed.:*** Lariam; ***Switz.:*** Lariam; Mephaquine; ***UK:*** Lariam; ***USA:*** Lariam.

Multi-ingredient: ***Switz.:*** Fansimef.

Piperaquine Phosphate (19666-g)

Piperaquini Phosphas; 13228-RP. 1,3-Bis[1-(7-chloro-4-quinolyl)-4′-piperazinyl]propane.

$C_{29}H_{32}Cl_2N_6,4H_3PO_4,4H_2O$ = 999.6.

Pharmacopoeias. In *Chin.*

Piperaquine phosphate is a 4-piperazinoquinoline derivative which has been studied in the treatment and prophylaxis of falciparum malaria.

References.

1. Chen L, *et al.* Field observations on the antimalarial piperaquine. *Chin Med J* 1982; **95:** 281–6.
2. WHO. Advances in malaria chemotherapy: report of a WHO scientific group. *WHO Tech Rep Ser 711* 1984.
3. Lan C, *et al.* In vivo sensitivity of Plasmodium falciparum to piperaquine phosphate assayed in Linshui and Baisha counties, Hainan Province. *Chin J Parasitol Parasit Dis* 1989; **7:** 163–5.
4. Chen L. Recent studies on antimalarial efficacy of piperaquine and hydroxypiperaquine. *Chin Med J* 1991; **104:** 161–3.

Primaquine Phosphate (1387-e)

Primaquine Phosphate (*BANM, rINNM*).

Difosfato de Primaquina; Primachina Fosfato; Primachini Phosphas; Primaquine Diphosphate; Primaquini Diphosphas; Primaquinum Phosphoricum; SN-13,272. (*RS*)-8-(4-Amino-1-methylbutylamino)-6-methoxyquinoline diphosphate.

$C_{15}H_{21}N_3O,2H_3PO_4$ = 455.3.

CAS — 90-34-6 (primaquine); 63-45-6 (primaquine phosphate).

Pharmacopoeias. In *Chin., Eur.* (see p.viii), *Int.*, and *US.*

An orange-red, odourless, crystalline powder. Primaquine base 7.5 mg is approximately equivalent to 13.2 mg of primaquine phosphate. **Soluble** 1 in 15 of water; practically insoluble in alcohol, chloroform, and ether. Solutions are acid to litmus. **Protect** from light.

Adverse Effects

Adverse effects with therapeutic doses of primaquine are usually minimal but abdominal pain and gastric distress are more common if administered on an empty stomach. Larger doses may cause nausea and vomiting. Methaemoglobinaemia may occur occasionally. Haemolytic anaemia can occur in persons with a deficiency of glucose-6-phosphate dehydrogenase (G6PD) (see below). Other uncommon effects include mild anaemia and leucocytosis. Hypertension and cardiac arrhythmias have been reported on rare occasions. Primaquine may rarely produce leucopenia or agranulocytosis, usually following overdosage. Other effects associated with overdosage include gastro-intestinal symptoms, haemolytic anaemia, and methaemoglobinaemia with cyanosis.

A wide range of side-effects has been reported following the use of primaquine[1] but some, including pruritus and disturbances of visual accomodation, are considered to be inadequately documented or doubtfully attributed to the drug.

Acute intravascular haemolysis is the most serious toxic hazard of primaquine, especially in people with G6PD deficiency, other defects of the erythrocytic pentose phosphate pathway of glucose metabolism, or some types of haemoglobinopathy. In individuals with G6PD deficiency the severity of haemolysis is directly related to the degree of deficiency and to the quantity of primaquine administered. In patients with the African variant the standard course of primaquine generally produces a moderate and self-limiting anaemia, while in those with the Mediterranean and related Asian variants, haemolysis can result in progressive haemoglobinaemia and haemoglobinuria which can be fatal. Whenever possible, therapy with primaquine should be delayed until the acute stage of malaria has been brought under control by a blood schizontocide because of the risk of inducing haemolysis and compromising the gastro-intestinal tolerance of therapy.

1. Clyde DF. Clinical problems associated with the use of primaquine as a tissue schizontocidal and gametocytocidal drug. *Bull WHO* 1981; **59:** 391–5.

Precautions

Primaquine should be administered cautiously to acutely ill patients with any serious systemic disease characterised by a tendency to granulocytopenia such as rheumatoid arthritis or lupus erythematosus. It should also be used with care in patients with glucose-6-phosphate dehydrogenase deficiency. Primaquine should be withdrawn if signs of haemolysis or methaemoglobinaemia occur and the blood count should be monitored periodically.

Pregnancy. Radical cure of vivax or ovale malarias with primaquine should be delayed in pregnant women until after delivery.[1]

1. Panisko DM, Keystone JS. Treatment of malaria—1990. *Drugs* 1990; **39:** 160–89.

Interactions

Primaquine should not be administered concomitantly with drugs liable to induce haemolysis or bone marrow depression. Theoretically, mepacrine may increase the plasma concentrations of primaquine resulting in a higher risk of toxicity, and it has been recommended that these drugs should not be used concomitantly.

The pharmacokinetics of primaquine were not altered by the concurrent administration of mefloquine in healthy subjects,[1] although the effect of primaquine on mefloquine pharmacokinetics is uncertain (see under Mefloquine, p.433). In a study in patients with malaria, administration of quinine reduced the plasma concentrations of primaquine, although the clinical importance of the interaction was unclear.[1]

1. Edwards G, *et al.* Interactions among primaquine, malaria infection and other antimalarials in Thai subjects. *Br J Clin Pharmacol* 1993; **35:** 193–8.

Pharmacokinetics

Primaquine is readily absorbed from the gastro-intestinal tract. Peak plasma concentrations occur about 1 to 2 hours after a dose is taken and then rapidly diminish with a reported elimination half-life of 3 to 6 hours. It is widely distributed into body tissues.

Primaquine is rapidly metabolised in the liver, its major metabolite being carboxyprimaquine, and little unchanged drug is excreted in the urine. Carboxyprimaquine accumulates in the plasma on repeated administration.

References.

1. Fletcher KA, *et al.* Studies on the pharmacokinetics of primaquine. *Bull WHO* 1981; **59:** 407–12.
2. White NJ. Clinical pharmacokinetics of antimalarial drugs. *Clin Pharmacokinet* 1985; **10:** 187–215.
3. Mihaly GW, *et al.* Pharmacokinetics of primaquine in man, I: studies of the absolute bioavailability and effects of dose size. *Br J Clin Pharmacol* 1985; **19:** 745–50.
4. Ward SA, *et al.* Pharmacokinetics of primaquine in man, II: comparison of acute vs chronic dosage in Thai subjects. *Br J Clin Pharmacol* 1985; **19:** 751–5.
5. Bhatia SC, *et al.* Pharmacokinetics of primaquine in patients with P. vivax malaria. *Eur J Clin Pharmacol* 1986; **31:** 205–10.
6. Rønn A, Bygbjerg I. Unexpected high primaquine concentrations in acutely ill malaria patients. *Lancet* 1993; **341:** 305.

Uses and Administration

Primaquine is an 8-aminoquinoline antimalarial which is effective as a tissue schizontocide against intrahepatic forms of all types of malaria parasite and is used to produce radical cure of vivax and ovale malarias.

When used for radical cure of vivax and ovale malarias, a course of treatment with a blood schizontocide must be given first to kill any erythrocytic parasites. Primaquine phosphate is then administered by mouth, usually in a dose equivalent to 15 mg of the base daily for 14 days but higher doses or longer courses may be required to overcome resistance in some strains of *P. vivax* (see below); WHO has advised that a treatment period of 21 days should be employed to achieve radical cure in most of South-East Asia and Oceania. A suggested dose for children is 250 μg per kg body-weight daily for 14 days.

Regimens of 30 mg (children 500 to 750 μg per kg body-weight) once every 7 days for 8 weeks have been suggested to minimise haemolysis in patients with glucose-6-phosphate dehydrogenase deficiency (but see under Adverse Effects and Precautions, above).

Primaquine is also gametocytocidal and a single dose of 30 to 45 mg has been suggested to prevent transmission of falciparum malaria particularly in areas where there is potential for re-introduction of malaria.

Primaquine is also used in the treatment of *Pneumocystis carinii* pneumonia in AIDS patients in combination with clindamycin.

Malaria. The overall treatment and prophylaxis of malaria and the place of primaquine in current recommendations are described on p.422.

Despite the generally successful use of primaquine for radical cure of benign malarias,[1-3] there has been a report[4] of a patient weighing 84 kg who had relapse of vivax malaria after treatment including primaquine 15 mg given daily for 21 days; no further symptoms occurred after a second course of 15 mg given daily for 3 months. It was suggested that a daily dose of 15 mg might be inadequate for patients weighing more than 50 kg and that patients with vivax malaria who have relapsed after the standard course of primaquine and possibly those with vivax malaria acquired in South-East Asia or Melanesia should receive a total dose of 6 mg per kg body-weight in daily doses of 15 to 22.5 mg. A report from Thailand,[5] where primaquine-resistant strains of *Plasmodium vivax* are increasing, showed that a dose of primaquine 22.5 mg daily for 14 days was safe and more effective in preventing relapses than 15 mg daily in patients with an average body-weight of about 51 kg. There have been several other reports of primaquine-resistant *P. vivax*,[6-9] and the suggestion has been made that higher doses of primaquine (15 mg twice daily for 14 days, to give a total dose of 6 mg per kg assuming a body-weight of 70 kg) should be considered wherever the vivax malaria was acquired.[9]

Variable responses to primaquine in the Amazonian region were attributed to considerable variation in the content of primaquine both between and within batches of tablets; primaquine content ranged from 19 to 168% of the labelled content.[10]

In the USA, the CDC have suggested the use of primaquine during the last 2 weeks of prophylaxis to prevent relapses due to *P. vivax* or *P. ovale* in persons returning from prolonged exposure in areas where relapsing malaria is endemic.[11]

Primaquine has also been tried for prophylaxis of falciparum and vivax malaria; use for a year produced effective cover and was well tolerated by Javanese men without G6PD deficiency.[12] It was also effective for prophylaxis in Colombian military personnel; it was noted that primaquine prophylaxis could be stopped 1 week after departing the endemic area.[13]

1. WHO. Practical chemotherapy of malaria: report of a WHO scientific group. *WHO Tech Rep Ser 805* 1990.
2. WHO. *WHO model prescribing information: drugs used in parasitic diseases.* 2nd ed. Geneva: WHO, 1995.
3. Molyneux M, Fox R. Diagnosis and treatment of malaria in Britain. *Br Med J* 1993; **306:** 1175–80.
4. Luzzi GA, *et al.* Treatment of primaquine-resistant Plasmodium vivax malaria. *Lancet* 1992; **340:** 310.
5. Bunnag D, *et al.* High dose of primaquine in primaquine resistant vivax malaria. *Trans R Soc Trop Med Hyg* 1994; **88:** 218–19.
6. Collins WE, Jeffrey GM. Primaquine resistance in Plasmodium vivax. *Am J Trop Med Hyg* 1996; **55:** 243–9.
7. Signorini L, *et al.* Short report: primaquine-tolerant Plasmodium vivax in an Italian traveler from Guatemala. *Am J Trop Med Hyg* 1996; **55:** 472–3.
8. Smoak BL, *et al.* Plasmodium vivax infections in US Army troops: failure of primaquine to prevent relapse in studies from Somalia. *Am J Trop Med Hyg* 1997; **56:** 231–4.
9. Doherty JF, *et al.* Treatment of Plasmodium vivax malaria—time for a change? *Trans R Soc Trop Med Hyg* 1997; **91:** 76.
10. Petralanda I. Quality of antimalarial drugs and resistance to Plasmodium vivax in Amazonian region. *Lancet* 1995; **345:** 1433.
11. Centers for Disease Control. Recommendations for the prevention of malaria among travelers. *MMWR* 190; **39** (RR-3): 1–10.
12. Fryauff DJ, *et al.* Randomised placebo-controlled trial of primaquine for prophylaxis of falciparum and vivax malaria. *Lancet* 1995; **346:** 1190–3.
13. Soto J, *et al.* Primaquine prophylaxis against malaria in non-immune Colombian soldiers: efficacy and toxicity. *Ann Intern Med* 1998; **129:** 241–4.

Pneumocystis carinii pneumonia. Primaquine with clindamycin is used in the treatment of *Pneumocystis carinii* pneumonia as an alternative to co-trimoxazole or pentamidine (see p.370). Treatment has usually lasted 3 weeks with primaquine being given by mouth in daily doses equivalent to 30 mg of the base and clindamycin usually being given intravenously in doses of 600 mg four times daily or 300 to 450 mg four times daily by mouth.[1]

A randomised multicentre study[2] compared the use of a combination of primaquine (30 mg daily) and clindamycin (600 mg three times daily) with co-trimoxazole and with a combination of dapsone and trimethoprim in 181 AIDS patients who had confirmed mild to moderate *Pneumocystis carinii* pneumonia. Primaquine/clindamycin was as effective as the other two regimens, although the authors suggested that the combination might be best avoided in patients with severe myelosuppression.

Primaquine with clindamycin is not normally recommended for prophylaxis although there are reports of it being tried.[3]

1. Anonymous. Drugs for parasitic infections. *Med Lett Drugs Ther* 1998; **40:** 1–12.
2. Safrin S, *et al.* Comparison of three regimens for treatment of mild to moderate Pneumocystis carinii pneumonia in patients with AIDS: a double-blind, randomized trial of oral trimethoprim-sulfamethoxazole, dapsone-trimethoprim, and clindamycin-primaquine. *Ann Intern Med* 1996; **124:** 792–802.
3. Kay R, DuBois RE. Clindamycin/primaquine therapy and secondary prophylaxis against Pneumocystis carinii pneumonia in patients with AIDS. *South Med J* 1990; **83:** 403–4.

Preparations

USP 23: Primaquine Phosphate Tablets.

Proprietary Preparations (details are given in Part 3)

Multi-ingredient: *USA:* Aralen with Primaquine Phosphate†.

Proguanil Hydrochloride (1388-l)

Proguanil Hydrochloride (*BANM, rINNM*).

Bigumalum; Chloriguane Hydrochloride; Chloroguanide Hydrochloride; Proguanide Hydrochloride; Proguanili Hydrochloridum; RP-3359; SN-12,837. 1-(4-Chlorophenyl)-5-isopropylbiguanide hydrochloride.

$C_{11}H_{16}ClN_5,HCl = 290.2.$

CAS — 500-92-5 (proguanil); 637-32-1 (proguanil hydrochloride).

Pharmacopoeias. In *Br.* and *It.*

A white odourless or almost odourless crystalline powder. Slightly **soluble** in water, more soluble in hot water; sparingly soluble in alcohol; practically insoluble in chloroform and in ether. **Protect** from light.

Stability. Although the BP directs that proguanil hydrochloride should be protected from light, stability studies suggest that it is a very stable compound with only small amounts of its major decomposition product 4-chloroaniline being formed during thermal and photochemical stress.[1,2]

1. Owoyale JA, Elmarakby ZS. Effect of sunlight, ultraviolet irradiation and heat on proguanil. *Int J Pharmaceutics* 1989; **50:** 219–21.
2. Taylor RB, *et al.* A chemical stability study of proguanil hydrochloride. *Int J Pharmaceutics* 1990; **60:** 185–90.

Adverse Effects and Precautions

Apart from mild gastric intolerance, diarrhoea, and some reports of aphthous ulceration there appear to be few adverse effects associated with usual doses of proguanil hydrochloride. Haematological changes have been reported in patients with severe renal impairment. Overdosage may produce epigastric discomfort, vomiting, and renal irritation leading to haematuria.

Proguanil should be used with caution in patients with renal impairment; dosage should be reduced accordingly (see Uses and Administration, below).

Proguanil may be taken during pregnancy, but UK authorities recommend that folate supplements (folic acid 5 mg daily) should also be given.

Until 1985 proguanil was generally taken in a dose of 100 mg daily for malaria prophylaxis with few adverse effects. Although no serious adverse effects have been reported since the dose was increased to 200 mg daily, and it began to be used with chloroquine, there have been an increasing number of reports of reversible aphthous ulceration.[1] Chloroquine may exacerbate this effect.[2] There has also been a report of reversible alopecia in women and scaling of the skin in both men and women using proguanil.[3]

Megaloblastic anaemia and pancytopenia were associated with proguanil accumulation in 2 patients with renal failure receiving usual doses.[4]

1. Peto TEA. Toxicity of antimalarial drugs. *J R Soc Med* 1989; **82** (suppl 17): 30–4.
2. Drysdale SF, *et al.* Proguanil, chloroquine, and mouth ulcers. *Lancet* 1990; **335:** 164.
3. Hanson SN, *et al.* Hairloss and scaling with proguanil. *Lancet* 1989; **i:** 225.
4. Boots M, *et al.* Megaloblastic anemia and pancytopenia due to proguanil in patients with chronic renal failure. *Clin Nephrol* 1982; **18:** 106–8.

Porphyria. For a discussion of the problems of prophylaxis and treatment of malaria in patients with porphyria and a comment that proguanil may be safe for use in such patients, see under Precautions of Chloroquine, p.428.

Interactions

For a report of haematuria and high prothrombin ratio in a patient stabilised on warfarin who took proguanil for malaria prophylaxis, see p.967.

Pharmacokinetics

Proguanil is readily absorbed from the gastro-intestinal tract following administration by mouth, peak plasma concentrations occurring within about 4 hours. Proguanil is metabolised in the liver to the active metabolite cycloguanil. Peak plasma concentrations of cycloguanil occur approximately one hour after those of the parent drug. The elimination half-lives of both proguanil and cycloguanil are about 20 hours. Approximately 40 to 60% of proguanil is eliminated in the urine, of which 60% is unchanged and 30% cycloguanil. There is also some elimination via the faeces. Proguanil is distributed into breast milk in small amounts (which are not adequate to provide chemoprophylaxis for the infant).

Early studies found proguanil to be well absorbed from the gastro-intestinal tract with peak plasma concentrations occurring about 4 hours after administration.[1] In more recent studies, peak plasma concentrations of proguanil have been achieved within 2 to 4 hours.[2-4] Plasma protein binding for proguanil is stated to be 75%.[5] Proguanil behaves as an inactive prodrug. It is metabolised in the liver[3] to the active metabolite cycloguanil and to *p*-chlorophenylbiguanide which is inactive. Peak plasma concentrations of cycloguanil have been reported to occur about 5.3 hours after administration of proguanil.[4] Unlike proguanil and *p*-chlorophenylbiguanide, cycloguanil is not concentrated in erythrocytes and thus concentrations of cycloguanil in plasma and whole blood are similar.[4] The elimination half-lives for proguanil and cycloguanil are reported to be around 20 hours.[3,4] A review of early studies states that between 40 and 60% of a dose of proguanil was found to be excreted in the urine, 60% of this as the unchanged drug, 30% as cycloguanil, and 8% as *p*-chlorophenylbiguanide.[1] About 10% of a dose was excreted in the faeces.[1] However, these values can vary greatly and wide interindividual variations in the ability to metabolise proguanil to the active metabolite cycloguanil have been reported.[3,6,7] Malaria prophylaxis with proguanil might be less effective in poor metabolisers although this has not been proved conclusively[8] and, anyway, other factors such as lack of protection against mosquitoes and sensitivity of the malaria parasite might be more important.[9]

Plasma concentrations of cycloguanil may be reduced in the third trimester of pregnancy.[10]

1. White NJ. Clinical pharmacokinetics of antimalarial drugs. *Clin Pharmacokinet* 1985; **10:** 187–215.
2. Kelly JA, *et al.* The kinetics of proguanil during prophylaxis. *Trans R Soc Trop Med Hyg* 1986; **80:** 338.
3. Watkins WM, *et al.* Variability in the metabolism of proguanil to the active metabolite cycloguanil in healthy Kenyan adults. *Trans R Soc Trop Med Hyg* 1990; **84:** 492–5.
4. Wattanagoon Y, *et al.* Single dose pharmacokinetics of proguanil and its metabolites in healthy subjects. *Br J Clin Pharmacol* 1987; **24:** 775–80.
5. Jaeger A, *et al.* Clinical features and management of poisoning due to antimalarial drugs. *Med Toxicol* 1987; **2:** 242–73.
6. Ward SA, *et al.* Inter-subject variability in the metabolism of proguanil to the active metabolite cycloguanil in man. *Br J Clin Pharmacol* 1989; **27:** 781–7.
7. Helsby NA, *et al.* The multiple dose pharmacokinetics of proguanil. *Br J Clin Pharmacol* 1993; **35:** 653–6.
8. Mberu EK, *et al.* Japanese poor metabolizers of proguanil do not have an increased risk of malaria chemoprophylaxis breakthrough. *Trans R Soc Trop Med Hyg* 1995; **89:** 658–9.
9. Skjelbo E, *et al.* Chloroguanide metabolism in relation to the efficacy in malaria prophylaxis and the S-mephenytoin oxidation in Tanzanians. *Clin Pharmacol Ther* 1996; **59:** 304–11.
10. Wangboonskul J, *et al.* Single dose pharmacokinetics of proguanil and its metabolites in pregnancy. *Eur J Clin Pharmacol* 1993; **44:** 247–51.

Uses and Administration

Proguanil is a biguanide compound which has little antimalarial activity until metabolised in the body to the active antimalarial drug cycloguanil. Cycloguanil, like pyrimethamine, inhibits plasmodial dihydrofolate reductase and thus disrupts synthesis of nucleic acids in the parasite. Cycloguanil is active against pre-erythrocytic forms and is a slow blood schizontocide. It also has some sporontocidal activity, rendering the gametocytes non-infective to the mosquito vector.

The value of proguanil is limited by the rapid development of resistance.

Proguanil is used as the hydrochloride for the chemoprophylaxis of malaria, usually in association with chloroquine. Cycloguanil's schizontocidal activity on erythrocytic forms is too slow for cycloguanil or proguanil to be used alone for the treatment of malaria, but proguanil hydrochloride is given in combination with atovaquone (p.579) for the treatment of uncomplicated falciparum malaria.

For prophylaxis of malaria the usual adult daily dose of proguanil hydrochloride is 200 mg taken after food. It is generally recommended that chemoprophylaxis for travellers should start about one or two weeks before exposure to malaria, but if this is not possible it can be started 1 to 2 days prior to travel. Administration should continue throughout exposure and for at least 4 weeks after leaving a malarious area. For children's prophylactic doses, see under Administration in Children, below.

For the treatment of uncomplicated falciparum malaria, adult doses are proguanil hydrochloride 400 mg together with atovaquone 1000 mg, each by mouth as a single dose for 3 consecutive days. Children weighing 11 to 20 kg are given one-quarter the adult dose; those weighing 21 to 30 kg, half the adult dose; those weighing 31 to 40 kg, three-quarters the adult dose; and children over 40 kg, the adult dose.

Cycloguanil was formerly administered as an oily suspension of the embonate by intramuscular injection.

Administration in children. Dosage recommendations for proguanil (in association with chloroquine) for *malaria prophylaxis* in children have varied. A daily dose of proguanil hydrochloride 3 mg per kg body-weight has been recommended,[1,2] although UK malaria experts[1] have suggested the following prophylactic doses for children based on fractions of the adult dose of 200 mg daily: from 0 to 5 weeks of age, one-eighth the adult dose; 6 to 52 weeks, one-quarter the adult dose; 1 to 5 years (10 to 19 kg body-weight), half the adult dose; 6 to 11 years (20 to 39 kg), three-quarters the adult dose; and 12 years or more (40 kg or more), the adult dose. They noted that body-weight was a better guide to dosage than age for children over 6 months.

For doses of proguanil in combination with atovaquone for the *treatment* of malaria in children, see above.

1. Bradley DJ, *et al.* Guidelines for the prevention of malaria in travellers from the United Kingdom. *Commun Dis Rep Rev* 1997; **7:** R137–R152.
2. WHO. *International travel and health: vaccination requirements and health advice.* Geneva: WHO, 1998.

Administration in renal impairment. Proguanil is excreted by the kidneys and should be given in reduced dosage or avoided in patients with renal impairment. The following doses have been recommended based on creatinine clearance: creatinine clearance 20 to 59 mL per minute, 100 mg daily; 10 to 19 mL per minute, 50 mg every other day; less than 10 mL per minute, up to 50 mg once weekly.

Malaria. The overall treatment and prophylaxis of malaria and the place of proguanil in current recommendations are discussed on p.422.

TREATMENT. Proguanil alone is not suitable for the treatment of malaria. However, a combination of proguanil with atovaquone (Malarone) can be effective for the treatment of acute uncomplicated falciparum malaria,[1] including that produced by multidrug-resistant strains.[2] The combination has also been reported to be effective in benign malarias.[3]

PROPHYLAXIS. Proguanil has been used alone for the prophylaxis of malaria in very low risk areas of North Africa and the Middle East, but is more often given with chloroquine. However, the widespread prevalence of resistant strains of *Plasmodium falciparum* has considerably diminished the value of this regimen and has made recommendations for malaria prophylaxis increasingly complex. Studies using proguanil with a sulphonamide for chemoprophylaxis of malaria in Thailand produced encouraging results.[4,5] In a recent study, proguanil in combination with atovaquone (Malarone) appeared to be effective for prophylaxis in children living in an endemic area (Gabon).[6]

1. Radloff PD, *et al.* Atovaquone and proguanil for Plasmodium falciparum malaria. *Lancet* 1996; **347:** 1511–14.
2. Sabchareon A, *et al.* Efficacy and pharmacokinetics of atovaquone and proguanil in children with multidrug-resistant Plasmodium falciparum malaria. *Trans R Soc Trop Med Hyg* 1998; **92:** 201–6.
3. Radloff PD, *et al.* Atovaquone plus proguanil is an effective treatment for Plasmodium ovale and P. malariae malaria. *Trans R Soc Trop Med Hyg* 1996; **90:** 682.
4. Pang LW, *et al.* Malaria prophylaxis with proguanil and sulfisoxazole in children living in a malaria endemic area. *Bull WHO* 1989; **67:** 51–8.
5. Karwacki JJ, *et al.* Proguanil-sulphonamide for malaria prophylaxis. *Trans R Soc Trop Med Hyg* 1990; **84:** 55–7.
6. Lell B, *et al.* Randomised placebo-controlled study of atovaquone plus proguanil for malaria prophylaxis in children. *Lancet* 1998; **351:** 709–13.

Preparations

BP 1998: Proguanil Tablets.

Proprietary Preparations (details are given in Part 3)
Aust.: Paludrine; ***Austral.:*** Paludrine; ***Belg.:*** Paludrine; ***Canad.:*** Paludrine; ***Fr.:*** Paludrine; ***Ger.:*** Paludrine; ***Irl.:*** Paludrine; ***Ital.:*** Paludrine; ***Neth.:*** Paludrine; ***Norw.:*** Paludrine; ***S.Afr.:*** Paludrine; ***Swed.:*** Paludrine; ***Switz.:*** Paludrine; ***UK:*** Paludrine.

Multi-ingredient: ***Austral.:*** Malarone; ***Fr.:*** Savarine; ***Swed.:*** Malarone; ***UK:*** Malarone.

Pyrimethamine (1389-y)

Pyrimethamine *(BAN, rINN).*

BW-50-63; Pirimetamina; Pyrimethaminum; RP-4753. 5-(4-Chlorophenyl)-6-ethylpyrimidine-2,4-diyldiamine.

$C_{12}H_{13}ClN_4$ = 248.7.

CAS — 58-14-0.

Pharmacopoeias. In *Chin., Eur.* (see p.viii), *Int.*, and *US.*

A white or almost white, odourless, crystalline powder or colourless crystals. Practically **insoluble** in water; soluble 1 in 200 of alcohol and 1 in 125 of chloroform; slightly soluble in acetone; very slightly soluble in ether. **Store** in airtight containers. Protect from light.

Adverse Effects and Treatment

Administration of pyrimethamine for prolonged periods, as used to be the case when it was given alone for the prophylaxis of malaria, could cause depression of haematopoiesis due to interference with folic acid metabolism. Skin rashes and hypersensitivity reactions also occurred.

Larger doses, such as those employed in the treatment of toxoplasmosis, may cause gastro-intestinal symptoms such as atrophic glossitis, abdominal pain, and vomiting; haematological effects such as megaloblastic anaemia, leucopenia, thrombocytopenia, and pancytopenia are also more likely to occur. CNS effects including headache, dizziness, and insomnia have also been reported.

Pyrimethamine is used in combination with other antimalarials when patients may again experience the above adverse effects. Additionally pulmonary eosinophilia has been reported in patients receiving combinations that included pyrimethamine. Severe and sometimes fatal reactions have occurred when pyrimethamine has been used with *sulfadoxine* (Fansidar), including erythema multiforme and the Stevens-Johnson syndrome, and toxic epidermal necrolysis; there have also been isolated reports of hepatic toxicity. Agranulocytosis occurs more frequently when pyrimethamine is used with *dapsone* (Maloprim) and fatalities have been reported.

Acute overdosage with pyrimethamine can cause gastro-intestinal effects and CNS stimulation with vomiting, excitability, and convulsions. Tachycardia, respiratory depression, circulatory collapse, and death may follow. Treatment of overdosage is symptomatic.

Adverse effects with dapsone. Between 1972 and 1988 the Committee on Safety of Medicines in the UK received 76 reports of reactions that were attributed to the use of pyrimethamine with dapsone (Maloprim) of which 40 (53%) were considered to be serious including 6 deaths.[1] The incidence was estimated to be 1 in 9100 for serious reactions and 1 in 60 200 for fatalities. Serious blood disorders including agranulocytosis, granulocytopenia, or leucopenia occurred in 15 patients (estimated incidence of 1 in 20 000), five of whom died. The other death was in a patient with myocarditis. Three patients had cyanosis due to methaemoglobinaemia. Respiratory disorders such as pulmonary eosinophilia, influenza-like syndrome, and dyspnoea occurred in 6 patients. In 4 patients skin disorders were the principal effect and included epidermal necrolysis, angioedema, and bullous eruptions. Hepatic disorders were also reported in 4 patients. Three women using pyrimethamine-dapsone during pregnancy delivered malformed babies, one of them being stillborn. Other effects in 4 patients included convulsions, exacerbated epilepsy, pancreatitis, or a generalised allergic reaction.

In a review of 21 cases of agranulocytosis associated with pyrimethamine-dapsone Hutchinson *et al.*[2] concluded that although agranulocytosis can occur very rarely in patients taking pyrimethamine or dapsone alone, agranulocytosis due to the combination appears to be caused by an idiosyncratic reaction to dapsone exacerbated by the concurrent administration of pyrimethamine. Of the 18 individuals for whom dosage was certain, 12 had been taking one tablet of pyrimethamine-dapsone twice weekly. The recommended dose is one tablet taken once a week. Of the 9 patients who died, 6 had been taking one tablet twice weekly and one patient had taken one tablet once weekly; the dosage was uncertain in the remaining patients. The time of onset of symptoms had been 7 to 9 weeks after starting therapy in 16 of 19 of the patients.

According to Lee and Lau[3] pyrimethamine with dapsone may produce some degree of immunosuppression and render users more susceptible to common infections. They had found a higher incidence of non-specific upper respiratory-tract infections in military recruits receiving the combination than in those not receiving antimalarial prophylaxis.

Pulmonary eosinophilia has also occurred in patients taking pyrimethamine with dapsone, but, as there have also been similar reports of pulmonary toxicity in patients taking pyrimethamine with sulfadoxine (see below) or pyrimethamine with chloroquine, it has been suggested that pyrimethamine is probably the causative agent.[4]

1. Phillips-Howard PA, West LJ. Serious adverse drug reactions to pyrimethamine–sulphadoxine, pyrimethamine–dapsone and to amodiaquine in Britain. *J R Soc Med* 1990; **83:** 82–5.
2. Hutchinson DBA, *et al.* Agranulocytosis associated with Maloprim: review of cases. *Hum Toxicol* 1986; **5:** 221–7.
3. Lee PS, Lau EYL. Risk of acute non-specific upper respiratory tract infections in healthy men taking dapsone–pyrimethamine for prophylaxis against malaria. *Br Med J* 1988; **296:** 893–5.
4. Davidson AC, *et al.* Pulmonary toxicity of malaria prophylaxis. *Br Med J* 1988; **297:** 1240–1.

Adverse effects with sulphonamides. Severe and potentially fatal cutaneous reactions such as erythema multiforme and the Stevens-Johnson syndrome, and toxic epidermal necrolysis have been associated with the combined use of pyrimethamine with sulfadoxine (Fansidar) for malaria prophylaxis. The reported incidence of these reactions has varied with surveys in the UK,[1] USA,[2] and Sweden[3] yielding similar results and a survey from Switzerland[4] finding a much lower incidence. The overall rate of serious reactions to pyrimethamine-sulfadoxine in the UK has been estimated to be 1 in 2100. The estimates for severe cutaneous reactions were 1 in 4900 in the UK, 1 in 5000 to 1 in 8000 in the USA, 1 in 10 000 in Sweden, and 1 in 150 000 in Switzerland and the death rates were 1 in 11 100 in the UK, 1 in 11 000 to 1 in 25 000 in the USA, and 1 in 35 000 in Sweden; no fatalities were reported in Switzerland. Workers on the Swiss survey had suggested that the high incidence of cutaneous reactions reported in the USA might have been due to concurrent therapy with chloroquine but this has been disputed.[5] Phillips-Howard and West[1] suggested that the lower incidence reported in Switzerland may have been due to the different methods used to estimate the amount of drug usage. Whether this toxicity is due to the combined use of pyrimethamine and sulfadoxine is unclear as the estimated frequency of fatal reactions associated with the use of sulfadoxine alone in Mozambique was 1 in 50 000.[6]

There have been isolated reports of other severe or life-threatening reactions associated with the use of pyrimethamine-sulfadoxine when used alone or with chloroquine, including hepatotoxicity[7-9] (estimated incidence of 1 in 11 100 in the UK[1]), fatal multisystem toxicity,[10] drug fever and photodermatitis,[11] agranulocytosis,[11] and erythroderma resembling Sézary syndrome.[12] Severe pulmonary reactions have also occurred[3,13] but as similar reactions have also been reported when pyrimethamine has been used with other antimalarials including dapsone it has been suggested that pyrimethamine is the causative agent (see Adverse Effects with Dapsone, above). Hyperammonaemia and carnitine deficiency with deterioration in mental status has been reported in a patient receiving pyrimethamine and sulphadiazine for the treatment of toxoplasmosis.[14]

Severe megaloblastic anaemia in another patient receiving pyrimethamine and sulphadiazine for toxoplasmosis of the CNS[15] was treated by withdrawal of pyrimethamine and oral administration of folinic acid, together with a single platelet infusion.

For a comparison of the incidence of pruritus induced by various antimalarials including pyrimethamine with sulfadoxine, see Effects on the Skin under Chloroquine, p.427.

1. Phillips-Howard PA, West LJ. Serious adverse drug reactions to pyrimethamine–sulphadoxine, pyrimethamine–dapsone and to amodiaquine in Britain. *J R Soc Med* 1990; **83:** 82–5.
2. Miller KD, *et al.* Severe cutaneous reactions among American travelers using pyrimethamine–sulfadoxine (Fansidar®) for malaria prophylaxis. *Am J Trop Med Hyg* 1986; **35:** 451–8.
3. Hellgren U, *et al.* Adverse reactions to sulphadoxine–pyrimethamine in Swedish travellers: implications for prophylaxis. *Br Med J* 1987; **295:** 365–6.
4. Steffen R, Somaini B. Severe cutaneous adverse reactions to sulfadoxine–pyrimethamine in Switzerland. *Lancet* 1986; **i:** 610.
5. Rombo L, *et al.* Does chloroquine contribute to the risk of serious adverse reactions to Fansidar? *Lancet* 1985; **ii:** 1298–9.
6. Hernborg A. Stevens-Johnson syndrome after mass prophylaxis with sulfadoxine for cholera in Mozambique. *Lancet* 1985; **ii:** 1072–3.
7. Lazar HP, *et al.* Fansidar and hepatic granulomas. *Ann Intern Med* 1985; **102:** 722.
8. Wejstal R, *et al.* Liver damage associated with Fansidar. *Lancet* 1986; **i:** 854–5.
9. Zitelli BJ, *et al.* Fatal hepatic necrosis due to pyrimethamine–sulfadoxine (Fansidar). *Ann Intern Med* 1987; **106:** 393–5.
10. Selby CD, *et al.* Fatal multisystemic toxicity associated with prophylaxis with pyrimethamine and sulfadoxine (Fansidar). *Br Med J* 1985; **290:** 113–14.
11. Olsen VV, *et al.* Serious reactions during malaria prophylaxis with pyrimethamine–sulfadoxine. *Lancet* 1982; **ii:** 994.
12. Langtry JAA, *et al.* Erythroderma resembling Sézary syndrome after treatment with Fansidar and chloroquine. *Br Med J* 1986; **292:** 1107–8.
13. Svanbom M, *et al.* Unusual pulmonary reaction during short term prophylaxis with pyrimethamine–sulfadoxine (Fansidar). *Br Med J* 1984; **288:** 1876.
14. Sekas G, Harbhajan PS. Hyperammonemia and carnitine deficiency in a patient receiving sulfadiazine and pyrimethamine. *Am J Med* 1993; **95:** 112–13.
15. Chute JP, *et al.* Severe megaloblastic anemia complicating pyrimethamine therapy. *Ann Intern Med* 1995; **122:** 884–5.

Overdosage. Reports of overdosage with pyrimethamine in infants.

1. Akinyanju O, *et al.* Pyrimethamine poisoning. *Br Med J* 1973; **4:** 147–8.
2. Elmalem J, *et al.* Les accidents graves lors de la prescription de pyriméthamine chez les nourrissons traités pour une toxoplasmose. *Therapie* 1985; **40:** 357–9.

Precautions

Pyrimethamine may aggravate subclinical folic acid deficiency and it should not be given to patients with conditions associated with folate deficiency such as megaloblastic anaemia. Blood counts are required with prolonged treatment, and when large doses of pyrimethamine are used, as in the treatment of toxoplasmosis, blood counts should be checked twice weekly. Folinic acid, which does not interfere with the action of pyrimethamine against malaria or toxoplasmosis, has been given to prevent haematological toxicity due to pyrimethamine and its use is especially recommended if pyrimethamine is given during pregnancy (folic acid may be used as an alternative to folinic acid in malaria, but it interferes with the action of pyrimethamine against toxoplasmosis). Even if given with a folate supplement, some authorities consider it to be contra-indicated at least during the first trimester of pregnancy (see also under Pregnancy, below).

Pyrimethamine should be given with caution to patients with impaired renal or hepatic function. When patients with convulsive disorders need to receive large doses, as in the treatment of toxoplasmosis, it is recommended that small starting doses should be used.

When pyrimethamine is administered with sulphonamides or dapsone the general precautions applicable to those drugs should also be observed (see under Sulphamethoxazole, p.255 and under Dapsone, p.200) and treatment should be discontinued immediately if any skin reactions, sore throat, or shortness of breath occurs.

Breast feeding. Pyrimethamine is distributed into breast milk[1] but as no adverse effects have been reported in breast-fed infants, some authorities consider breast feeding to be compatible with the use of pyrimethamine for malaria prophylaxis.[2,3] However, administration of other folate antagonists to the infant should be avoided. The large doses of pyrimethamine used for treating toxoplasmosis may distribute into breast milk in sufficient quantities to interfere with folic acid metabolism in nursing infants.

1. Edstein MD, *et al.* Excretion of chloroquine, dapsone and pyrimethamine in human milk. *Br J Clin Pharmacol* 1986; **22:** 733–5.
2. American Academy of Pediatrics, Committee on Drugs. Transfer of drugs and other chemicals into human milk. *Pediatrics* 1989; **84:** 924–36.
3. Bennett PN, ed. *Drugs and human lactation.* Amsterdam: Elsevier, 1988.

Porphyria. For a discussion of the problems of prophylaxis and treatment of malaria in patients with porphyria and a comment that pyrimethamine is probably safe for use in such patients, see under Precautions of Chloroquine, p.428.

Pregnancy. There have been concerns over the use of pyrimethamine during pregnancy as it has been shown to be teratogenic in *animal* studies.[1] In one report severe congenital defects in a stillborn infant were attributed to the use of pyrimethamine in early pregnancy[2] but the association was considered to be questionable.[3] Other instances of congenital malformations with pyrimethamine and dapsone are given above under Adverse Effects with Dapsone. WHO generally considers the use of pyrimethamine combinations to be contra-indicated in malaria in pregnancy[4] but considers that they may be used after the first trimester in the treatment of toxoplasmosis.[5] UK experts[6] consider that pyrimethamine with dapsone (Maloprim) can be used cautiously for malaria prophylaxis after the first trimester if a visit to an area of transmission is unavoidable; a folate supplement (folic acid 5 mg daily) should be given.

1. Anonymous. Pyrimethamine combinations in pregnancy. *Lancet* 1983; **ii:** 1005–7. Correction. *ibid.*; 1378.
2. Harpey J-P, *et al.* Teratogenicity of pyrimethamine. *Lancet* 1983; **ii:** 399.
3. Smithells RW, Sheppard S. Teratogenicity of Debendox and pyrimethamine. *Lancet* 1983; **ii:** 623–4.
4. WHO. Practical chemotherapy of malaria: report of a WHO scientific group. *WHO Tech Rep Ser 805* 1990.
5. WHO. *WHO model prescribing information: drugs used in parasitic diseases.* 2nd ed. Geneva: WHO, 1995.
6. Bradley DJ, *et al.* Guidelines for the prevention of malaria in travellers from the United Kingdom. *Commun Dis Rep Rev* 1997; **7:** R137–R152.

Interactions

Administration of pyrimethamine with other folate antagonists such as co-trimoxazole, trimethoprim, methotrexate, or phenytoin may exacerbate bone marrow depression.

Signs of mild liver toxicity in 2 of 5 subjects who received *lorazepam* and pyrimethamine appeared to confirm earlier suspicions that concomitant administration of these drugs could cause hepatotoxicity. Both patients tolerated each drug when given separately.[1]

Studies *in vitro* and in *animals* suggest that *zidovudine* could reduce the effectiveness of pyrimethamine in the treatment of toxoplasmic encephalitis.[2] Furthermore, the dose of zidovudine may need to be altered if these drugs are used together as there has been a report that pyrimethamine with sulfadoxine (Fansidar) prolonged the serum half-life of zidovudine.[3]

1. Briggs M, Briggs M. Pyrimethamine toxicity. *Br Med J* 1974; **1:** 40.
2. Israelski DM, *et al.* Zidovudine antagonizes the action of pyrimethamine in experimental infection with Toxoplasma gondii. *Antimicrob Agents Chemother* 1989; **33:** 30–4.
3. Klein RS. Prophylaxis of opportunistic infections in individuals infected with HIV. *AIDS* 1989; **3** (suppl 1): S161–S173.

Pharmacokinetics

Pyrimethamine is almost completely absorbed from the gastro-intestinal tract and peak plasma concentrations of about 200 ng per mL are obtained 2 to 6 hours after oral administration of 25 mg by mouth. It is mainly concentrated in the kidneys, lungs, liver, and spleen and about 80 to 90% is bound to plasma proteins.

It is metabolised in the liver and slowly excreted via the kidney, the average half-life in plasma being about 4 days. Several metabolites have been detected in the urine. Pyrimethamine crosses the placenta. It is distributed into breast milk (see under Breast Feeding in Precautions, above).

References.

1. White NJ. Clinical pharmacokinetics of antimalarial drugs. *Clin Pharmacokinet* 1985; **10:** 187–215.

2. Cook IF, *et al.* Race-linked differences in serum concentrations of dapsone, monoacetyldapsone and pyrimethamine during malaria prophylaxis. *Trans R Soc Trop Med Hyg* 1986; **80:** 897–901.
3. Weiss LM, *et al.* Pyrimethamine concentrations in serum and cerebrospinal fluid during treatment of acute toxoplasma encephalitis in patients with AIDS. *J Infect Dis* 1988; **157:** 580–3.
4. Edstein MD, *et al.* Multiple-dose pharmacokinetics and in vitro antimalarial activity of dapsone plus pyrimethamine (Maloprim®) in man. *Br J Clin Pharmacol* 1990; **30:** 259–65.
5. Hellgren U, *et al.* Plasma concentrations of sulfadoxine-pyrimethamine, mefloquine and its main metabolite after regular malaria prophylaxis for two years. *Trans R Soc Trop Med Hyg* 1991; **85:** 356–7.
6. Winstanley PA, *et al.* The disposition of oral and intramuscular pyrimethamine/sulphadoxine in Kenyan children with high parasitaemia but clinically non-severe falciparum malaria. *Br J Clin Pharmacol* 1992; **33:** 143–8.
7. Newton CRJC, *et al.* A single dose of intramuscular sulfadoxine-pyrimethamine as an adjunct to quinine in the treatment of severe malaria: pharmacokinetics and efficacy. *Trans R Soc Trop Med Hyg* 1993; **87:** 207–10.
8. Jacobson JM, *et al.* Pyrimethamine pharmacokinetics in human immunodeficiency virus-positive patients seropositive for Toxoplasma gondii. *Antimicrob Agents Chemother* 1996; **40:** 1360–5.
9. Klinker H, *et al.* Plasma pyrimethamine concentrations during long-term treatment for cerebral toxoplasmosis in patients with AIDS. *Antimicrob Agents Chemother* 1996; **40:** 1623–7.
10. Trenque T, *et al.* Human maternofoetal distribution of pyrimethamine-sulphadoxine. *Br J Clin Pharmacol* 1998; **45:** 179–80.

Uses and Administration

Pyrimethamine is a diaminopyrimidine antimalarial used in the treatment and prophylaxis of malaria, in combination with a sulphonamide or dapsone. It is also used with a sulphonamide in the treatment of toxoplasmosis. Pyrimethamine with sulfadoxine has been tried in the treatment of actinomycetoma and for prophylaxis of *Pneumocystis carinii* pneumonia. Pyrimethamine alone or with sulfadoxine has also been tried in the treatment of isosporiasis.

Pyrimethamine exerts its antimalarial activity by inhibiting plasmodial dihydrofolate reductase thus indirectly blocking the synthesis of nucleic acids in the malaria parasite. It is active against pre-erythrocytic forms and is also a slow-acting blood schizontocide. It also has some sporontocidal activity; it does not prevent the formation of gametocytes but renders them non-infective to the mosquito vector. It is mainly effective against *Plasmodium falciparum* but has some activity against *P. vivax*.

The development of plasmodial resistance has rendered obsolete the use of pyrimethamine on its own in malaria. Combinations of pyrimethamine with long-acting sulphonamides, such as sulfadoxine or sulfametopyrazine, or with dapsone are now used, although resistance has also developed to them.

For *treatment of chloroquine-resistant or multidrug-resistant falciparum malaria*, pyrimethamine is usually given in combination with a long-acting sulphonamide, often following a course of quinine. Pyrimethamine in combination with sulfadoxine in a fixed dose ratio of 1 to 20 (Fansidar) is usually given by mouth. A single dose of pyrimethamine 75 mg with sulfadoxine 1.5 g is usually recommended. The dose should not be repeated for at least 7 days. The combination of pyrimethamine with sulfadoxine may also be administered intramuscularly. Suggested oral doses for children are: 5 to 10 kg body-weight 12.5 mg pyrimethamine and 250 mg sulfadoxine; 11 to 20 kg, 25 mg pyrimethamine and 500 mg sulfadoxine; 21 to 30 kg, 37.5 mg pyrimethamine and 750 mg sulfadoxine; 31 to 45 kg, 50 mg pyrimethamine and 1 g sulfadoxine. A combination of pyrimethamine with sulfametopyrazine is used similarly.

The combination of pyrimethamine with a sulphonamide, again usually sulfadoxine, may also be used in specified areas as *standby treatment* for malaria. For this purpose doses are similar to those given for standard treatment as described above.

For *prophylaxis of malaria*, a combined preparation of pyrimethamine and dapsone in a fixed ratio of 1 to 8 (Maloprim) is still occasionally used in areas of chloroquine or multidrug resistance although mefloquine is now generally preferred. The usual dose for adults is pyrimethamine 12.5 mg and dapsone 100 mg as a single weekly dose. Suggested doses for children are: 6 to 11 years (20 to 39 kg), half adult dose; 12 years or more (40 kg or more), adult dose. It is generally recommended that prophylaxis for travellers should start about one week before exposure to malaria and should continue throughout exposure and for at least 4 weeks after leaving a malarious area.

Pyrimethamine administered with a sulphonamide such as sulphadiazine is used in the *treatment of toxoplasmosis*. Alternatively, pyrimethamine may be given with clindamycin in AIDS patients with toxoplasmosis unable to tolerate a sulphonamide. For details of dosage regimens used, see below.

Isosporiasis. Isosporiasis (p.575) usually responds well to treatment with co-trimoxazole but there is a high incidence of recurrence in immunocompromised patients such as those with AIDS and some form of maintenance therapy is generally required. Pape *et al.*[1] found co-trimoxazole 960 mg given three times weekly or pyrimethamine 25 mg with sulfadoxine 500 mg given weekly to be equally effective maintenance regimens. Pyrimethamine given alone in daily doses of 50 to 75 mg with folate therapy may be of use in the treatment of patients sensitive to sulphonamides.[2]

1. Pape JW, *et al.* Treatment and prophylaxis of Isospora belli infection in patients with the acquired immunodeficiency syndrome. *N Engl J Med* 1989; **320:** 1044–7.
2. Weiss LM, *et al.* Isospora belli infection: treatment with pyrimethamine. *Ann Intern Med* 1988; **109:** 474–5.

Malaria. The overall treatment and prophylaxis of malaria and the place of pyrimethamine-sulfadoxine (Fansidar) and pyrimethamine-dapsone (Maloprim) in current recommendations are discussed on p.422.

TREATMENT. Resistance to combinations of pyrimethamine with sulfadoxine or sulfametopyrazine is now widespread, particularly in South-East Asia and South America and more recently in East and Central Africa, and it is generally considered that they should not be used alone in the treatment of falciparum malaria.[1-4] Pyrimethamine-sulfadoxine may be given in the treatment of falciparum malaria following a course of quinine, if quinine resistance is known or suspected. A formulation of pyrimethamine with sulfadoxine for intramuscular administration has been studied[5-8] but its role in the treatment of falciparum malaria is not clear.[1] WHO considers that a combination of mefloquine with pyrimethamine and sulfadoxine offers no therapeutic advantage over mefloquine alone and does not recommend this combination for treatment or for prophylaxis.[1]

PROPHYLAXIS. Owing to the development of resistance pyrimethamine is not effective on its own for prophylaxis.[9] Although resistance has developed to pyrimethamine with dapsone,[10] and the combination has been largely superseded by mefloquine, it remains useful for prophylaxis in some areas where other drugs are ineffective.[11] Chloroquine may be given in addition. The risk of toxicity with pyrimethamine in combination with a sulphonamide is considered too high for prophylactic use[1,11] but it may still be used in specified areas for standby treatment.[12]

1. WHO. Practical chemotherapy of malaria: report of a WHO scientific group. *WHO Tech Rep Ser 805* 1990.
2. Gilles HM. *Management of severe and complicated malaria.* Geneva: WHO, 1991.
3. WHO. *WHO model prescribing information: drugs used in parasitic diseases.* 2nd ed. Geneva: WHO, 1995.
4. Molyneux M, Fox R. Diagnosis and treatment of malaria in Britain. *Br Med J* 1993; **306:** 1175–80.
5. Harinasuta T, *et al.* Parenteral Fansidar® in falciparum malaria. *Trans R Soc Trop Med Hyg* 1988; **82:** 694.
6. Salako LA, *et al.* Parenteral sulphadoxine–pyrimethamine (Fansidar®): an effective and safe but under-used method of anti-malarial treatment. *Trans R Soc Trop Med Hyg* 1990; **84:** 641–3.
7. Simão F, *et al.* Comparison of intramuscular sulfadoxine-pyrimethamine and intramuscular quinine for the treatment of falciparum malaria in children. *Trans R Soc Trop Med Hyg* 1991; **85:** 341–4.
8. Newton CRJC, *et al.* A single dose of intramuscular sulfadoxine-pyrimethamine as an adjunct to quinine in the treatment of severe malaria: pharmacokinetics and efficacy. *Trans R Soc Trop Med Hyg* 1993; **87:** 207–10.
9. Nahlen BL, *et al.* Lack of efficacy of pyrimethamine prophylaxis in pregnant Nigerian women. *Lancet* 1989; **ii:** 830–4.
10. Cook IF. Inadequate prophylaxis of malaria with dapsone-pyrimethamine. *Med J Aust* 1985 **142:** 340–2.
11. Bradley DJ, *et al.* Guidelines for the prevention of malaria in travellers from the United Kingdom. *Commun Dis Rep Rev* 1997; **7:** R137–R152.
12. WHO. *International travel and health: vaccination requirements and health advice.* Geneva: WHO, 1998.

Mycetoma. For reference to the use of pyrimethamine as part of the treatment of actinomycetoma, see under Mycetoma, p.132.

Pneumocystis carinii pneumonia. For a mention of pyrimethamine in combination with dapsone or sulfadoxine for the prophylaxis of *Pneumocystis carinii* pneumonia, and a discussion of conventional prophylaxis and treatment, see p.370.

Toxoplasmosis. Pyrimethamine is given, usually in conjunction with sulphadiazine, in the treatment of toxoplasmosis (p.576). Folinic acid is also given to counteract the megaloblastic anaemia associated with these drugs. A suggested dosage regimen is pyrimethamine 50 to 200 mg daily with sulphadiazine 250 to 1000 mg every 6 hours for one or two days, then pyrimethamine 25 to 50 mg daily with sulphadiazine 125 to 500 mg every 6 hours for 2 to 4 weeks, or 4 to 6 weeks if the patient is immunocompromised. A suggested dose of pyrimethamine for children is 1 mg per kg body-weight daily for 1 to 3 days, then 0.5 mg per kg daily for 4 to 6 weeks, given with usual paediatric doses of sulphadiazine. Treatment may continue for 6 months to 1 year in infants with congenital toxoplasmosis.

Patients with AIDS may be given a loading dose of 100 to 200 mg pyrimethamine daily with sulphadiazine 500 to 1500 mg every 6 hours for one or two days, and then 50 to 100 mg pyrimethamine daily with the same dose of sulphadiazine for 3 to 6 weeks. Maintenance treatment for AIDS patients with pyrimethamine 25 to 50 mg daily and sulphadiazine 250 to 1000 mg every 6 hours may continue indefinitely. Pyrimethamine with clindamycin is an alternative in patients unable to tolerate a sulphonamide.

Other drugs tried in combination with pyrimethamine with promising results include azithromycin,[1] clarithromycin,[2] and doxycycline.[3,4]

Alternative regimens tried for long-term maintenance therapy in patients with AIDS include pyrimethamine plus sulphadiazine given twice weekly[5,6] or pyrimethamine alone in doses of 25 mg[7] or 50 mg[8] daily or 50 mg three times weekly.[9] However, results from a study involving 396 patients suggested that the mortality rate was higher in those receiving pyrimethamine 25 mg three times weekly for primary prophylaxis than in those receiving placebo.[10] Pyrimethamine with dapsone given once a week can provide effective prophylaxis but was not well tolerated.[11] Pyrimethamine with sulfadoxine, also given once weekly, has produced promising results in bone-marrow transplant recipients.[12]

1. Saba J, *et al.* Pyrimethamine plus azithromycin for treatment of acute toxoplasmic encephalitis in patients with AIDS. *Eur J Clin Microbiol Infect Dis* 1993; **12:** 853–6.
2. Fernandez-Martin J, *et al.* Pyrimethamine-clarithromycin combination therapy of acute Toxoplasma encephalitis in patients with AIDS. *Antimicrob Agents Chemother* 1991; **35:** 2049–52.
3. Morris JT, Kelly JW. Effective treatment of cerebral toxoplasmosis with doxycycline. *Am J Med* 1992; **93:** 107–8.
4. Hagberg L, *et al.* Doxycycline and pyrimethamine for toxoplasmic encephalitis. *Scand J Infect Dis* 1993; **25:** 157–60.
5. Pedrol E, *et al.* Central nervous system toxoplasmosis in AIDS patients: efficacy of an intermittent maintenance therapy. *AIDS* 1990; **4:** 511–17.
6. Podzanczer D, *et al.* Twice-weekly maintenance therapy with sulfadiazine-pyrimethamine to prevent recurrent toxoplasmic encephalitis in patients with AIDS. *Ann Intern Med* 1995; **123:** 175–80.
7. Murphy K, *et al.* Pyrimethamine alone as long-term suppressive therapy in cerebral toxoplasmosis. *Am J Med* 1994; **96:** 95–6.
8. de Gans J, *et al.* Pyrimethamine alone as maintenance therapy for central nervous system toxoplasmosis in 38 patients with AIDS. *J Acquir Immune Defic Syndr Hum Retrovirol* 1992; **5:** 137–42.
9. Leport C, *et al.* Pyrimethamine for primary prophylaxis of toxoplasmic encephalitis in patients with human immunodeficiency virus infection: a double-blind, randomized trial. *J Infect Dis* 1996; **173:** 91–7.
10. Jacobson MA. *et al.* Primary prophylaxis with pyrimethamine for toxoplasmic encephalitis in patients with advanced human immunodeficiency virus disease: results of a randomized trial. *J Infect Dis* 1994; **169:** 384–94.
11. Opravil M, *et al.* Once-weekly administration of dapsone/pyrimethamine vs. aerosolized pentamidine as combined prophylaxis for Pneumocystis carinii pneumonia and toxoplasmic encephalitis in human immunodeficiency virus-infected patients. *Clin Infect Dis* 1995; **20:** 531–41.
12. Foot ABM, *et al.* Prophylaxis of toxoplasmosis infection with pyrimethamine/sulfadoxine (Fansidar) in bone marrow transplant recipients. *Bone Marrow Transplant* 1994; **14:** 241–5.

Preparations

BP 1998: Pyrimethamine Tablets;
USP 23: Pyrimethamine Tablets; Sulfadoxine and Pyrimethamine Tablets.

Proprietary Preparations (details are given in Part 3)

Aust.: Daraprim; ***Austral.:*** Daraprim; ***Belg.:*** Daraprim; ***Canad.:*** Daraprim; ***Fr.:*** Malocide; ***Ger.:*** Daraprim; ***Irl.:*** Daraprim; ***Neth.:*** Daraprim; ***S.Afr.:*** Daraprim; ***Spain:*** Daraprim; ***Swed.:*** Daraprim†; ***Switz.:*** Daraprim; ***UK:*** Daraprim; ***USA:*** Daraprim.

Multi-ingredient: ***Aust.:*** Fansidar; ***Austral.:*** Fansidar; Maloprim; ***Belg.:*** Fansidar; Maloprim†; ***Canad.:*** Fansidar; ***Fr.:*** Fansidar; ***Ger.:*** Fansidar†; ***Irl.:*** Fansidar; Maloprim; ***Ital.:*** Metakelfin; ***Neth.:*** Fansidar†; ***Norw.:*** Fansidar†; ***S.Afr.:*** Daraclor†; Fansidar; Maloprim; ***Swed.:*** Fansidar; ***Switz.:*** Fansidar; Fansimef; ***UK:*** Fansidar; Maloprim; ***USA:*** Fansidar.

Pyronaridine Phosphate (329-c)

Malaridine Phosphate. 7-Chloro-2-methoxy-10-[3,5-bis(pyrrolidinomethyl)-4-hydroxyanilino]benzo-[*b*]-1,5-naphthyridine phosphate.

$C_{29}H_{32}ClN_5O_2,4H_3PO_4$ = 910.0.

CAS — 74847-35-1 (pyronaridine); 76748-86-2 (pyronaridine phosphate).

Pharmacopoeias. In *Chin.*

Pyronaridine is a naphthyridine derivative used in China in the treatment of vivax malaria and chloroquine-resistant falciparum malaria. Its use in Africa and in Thailand is also under investigation. Pyronaridine has been given as the phosphate by mouth or by intramuscular or intravenous injection.

References.

1. Shao B-R. A review of antimalarial drug pyronaridine. *Chin Med J* 1990; **103:** 428–34.
2. Shao B-R, *et al.* A 5-year surveillance of sensitivity in vivo of Plasmodium falciparum to pyronaridine/sulfadoxine/pyrimethamine in Diaoluo area, Hainan province. *Southeast Asian J Trop Med Public Health* 1991; **22:** 65–7.
3. Chen C, *et al.* Studies on a new antimalarial compound: pyronaridine. *Trans R Soc Trop Med Hyg* 1992; **86:** 7–10.
4. Basco LK, Le Bras J. In vitro activity of pyronaridine against African strains of Plasmodium falciparum. *Ann Trop Med Parasitol* 1992; **86:** 447–54.
5. Ringwald P, *et al.* Randomised trial of pyronaridine versus chloroquine for acute uncomplicated falciparum malaria in Africa. *Lancet* 1996; **347:** 24–8.
6. Winstanley P. Pyronaridine: a promising drug for Africa? *Lancet* 1996; **347:** 2–3.
7. Looareesuwan S, *et al.* Pyronaridine. *Lancet* 1996; **347:** 1189–90.
8. Anonymous. Pyronaridine: yet another promising antimalarial substance from China. *WHO Drug Inf* 1996; **10:** 9–10.
9. Looareesuwan S, *et al.* Clinical study of pyronaridine for the treatment of acute uncomplicated falciparum malaria in Thailand. *Am J Trop Med Hyg* 1996; **54:** 205–9.

Quinine (1398-j)

Quinine *(BAN).*

Chinina; Chininum; Quinina. (8*S*,9*R*)-6′-Methoxycinchonan-9-ol; (α*R*)-α-(6-Methoxy-4-quinolyl)-α-[(2*S*,4*S*,5*R*)-(5-vinylquinuclidin-2-yl)]methanol.

$C_{20}H_{24}N_2O_2$ = 324.4.

CAS — 130-95-0 (anhydrous quinine).

Pharmacopoeias. It. has the trihydrate.

The chief alkaloid of various species of *Cinchona* (Rubiaceae). It is an optical isomer of quinidine. **Protect** from light.

Quinine Bisulphate (1391-q)

Quinine Bisulphate *(BANM).*

Chininum Bisulfuricum; Neutral Quinine Sulphate; Quinine Acid Sulphate; Quinine Bisulfate; Quinini Bisulfas.

$C_{20}H_{24}N_2O_2,H_2SO_4,7H_2O$ = 548.6.

CAS — 549-56-4 (anhydrous quinine bisulphate).

Pharmacopoeias. In *Aust., Br.,* and *Int.*

Colourless crystals or white crystalline powder. It effloresces in dry air. Quinine bisulphate 169 mg is approximately equivalent to 100 mg of anhydrous quinine. Freely **soluble** in water; sparingly soluble in alcohol. A 1% solution has a pH of 2.8 to 3.4. **Protect** from light.

Quinine Dihydrochloride (1393-s)

Quinine Dihydrochloride *(BANM).*

Chinini Dihydrochloridum; Neutral Quinine Hydrochloride; Quinine Acid Hydrochloride; Quinini Dihydrochloridum.

$C_{20}H_{24}N_2O_2,2HCl$ = 397.3.

CAS — 60-93-5.

Pharmacopoeias. In *Aust., Br.,* and *Int.*

A white or almost white powder. The BP specifies not more than 10% of dihydroquinine dihydrochloride. Quinine dihydrochloride 122 mg is approximately equivalent to 100 mg of anhydrous quinine. Very **soluble** in water; freely soluble in alcohol. **Protect** from light.

Quinine Ethyl Carbonate (1394-w)

Euquinina; Euquinine; Quinine Etabonate.

$C_{23}H_{28}N_2O_4$ = 396.5.

CAS — 83-75-0.

Pharmacopoeias. In *Jpn.*

Quinine ethyl carbonate 122 mg is approximately equivalent to 100 mg of anhydrous quinine.

Quinine Hydrobromide (1395-e)

Quinine Hydrobromide *(BANM).*

Basic Quinine Hydrobromide; Bromhydrate de Quinine; Chinini Bromidum; Quinine Monohydrobromide.

$C_{20}H_{24}N_2O_2,HBr,H_2O$ = 423.3.

CAS — 549-49-5 (anhydrous quinine hydrobromide).

Pharmacopoeias. In *Fr.*

Quinine hydrobromide 130 mg is approximately equivalent to 100 mg of anhydrous quinine.

Quinine Hydrochloride (1396-l)

Quinine Hydrochloride *(BANM).*

Basic Quinine Hydrochloride; Chinini Hydrochloridum; Chininii Chloridum; Chininium Chloratum; Chininum Hydrochloricum; Quinine Monohydrochloride; Quinini Hydrochloridum.

$C_{20}H_{24}N_2O_2,HCl,2H_2O$ = 396.9.

CAS — 130-89-2 (anhydrous quinine hydrochloride); 6119-47-7 (quinine hydrochloride dihydrate).

Pharmacopoeias. In *Eur.* (see p.viii), *Int., Jpn,* and *Pol.*

Colourless, fine, silky needles, often grouped in clusters. Quinine hydrochloride 122 mg is approximately equivalent to 100 mg of anhydrous quinine. **Soluble** in water; freely soluble in alcohol. A 1% solution in water has a pH of 6.0 to 6.8. **Protect** from light.

Quinine Sulphate (1390-g)

Quinine Sulphate *(BANM).*

Basic Quinine Sulphate; Chinini Sulfas; Chininum Sulfuricum; Quinine Sulfate; Quinini Sulfas.

$(C_{20}H_{24}N_2O_2)_2,H_2SO_4,2H_2O$ = 782.9.

CAS — 804-63-7 (anhydrous quinine sulphate); 6119-70-6 (quinine sulphate dihydrate).

Pharmacopoeias. In *Eur.* (see p.viii), *Int., Jpn,* and *US.*

Colourless or white, odourless, fine needle-like crystals or a white or almost white crystalline powder, darkening on exposure to light. The USP specifies that the content of dihydroquinine is not more than 10% of the quinine content. Quinine sulphate 121 mg is approximately equivalent to 100 mg of anhydrous quinine. **Soluble** 1 in 500 of water and 1 in 120 of alcohol; sparingly soluble in boiling water; slightly soluble in chloroform; slightly soluble in ether; freely soluble in alcohol at 80° and in a mixture of 2 parts of chloroform and one part of dehydrated alcohol. A 1% suspension in water has a pH of 5.7 to 6.6. **Protect** from light.

Sorption. For reference to loss of quinine sulphate from solutions during membrane filtration, see Chloroquine, p.426.

Adverse Effects

Administration of quinine or its salts in usual therapeutic doses may give rise to a train of symptoms known as cinchonism, characterised in its mild form by tinnitus, impaired hearing, headache, nausea, and disturbed vision, with, in its more severe manifestations, vomiting, abdominal pain, diarrhoea, and vertigo.

Cinchonism may also occur after small doses in patients hypersensitive to quinine but urticaria and flushing of the skin with intense pruritus are the most frequent reactions seen in these patients. Other effects include fever, skin rashes, and dyspnoea. Angioedema may also occur and asthma can be precipitated. Thrombocytopenia and other blood disorders have been reported. Thrombocytopenic purpura has been associated with quinine hypersensitivity. Haemoglobinuria occurs rarely.

Other adverse effects of quinine include hypoglycaemia, hypoprothrombinaemia, and renal failure.

The main symptoms of overdosage, which can be fatal, include gastro-intestinal effects, oculotoxicity, central nervous system disturbances, and cardiotoxicity. Visual disturbances including sudden blindness are usually slowly reversible but there may be residual damage. Overdosage is discussed in detail below. Quinine can produce cardiovascular toxicity similar to that seen with quinidine including conduction disturbances, arrhythmias, anginal symptoms, and hypotension leading to cardiac arrest and circulatory failure. Severe or even fatal cardiovascular toxicity can result from rapid intravenous administration of quinine.

Large amounts of quinine can induce abortion; congenital malformations, particularly of the optic and auditory nerves, have been reported after failure to induce abortion with quinine. However, quinine should not be withheld from pregnant women with life-threatening malaria (see also under Pregnancy in Precautions, below).

Intramuscular injections of quinine can be irritant and have caused pain, focal necrosis, and abscess formation; tetanus has developed in some patients (see under Malaria in Uses and Administration, below).

Effects on the blood. Between 1966 and 1975 the Swedish Adverse Drug Reaction Committee received 43 reports of *thrombocytopenia* attributable to quinine or quinidine[1] and the Boston Collaborative Drug Surveillance Program had 11 similar reports in patients studied between 1972 and 1981.[2] The FDA in the USA subsequently received details of 2 fatalities due to quinine-induced thrombocytopenia.[3] Quinine-induced thrombocytopenia appears to be a hypersensitivity reaction and beverages containing quinine as a bitter in concentrations as low as 20 μg per mL have precipitated thrombocytopenic purpura in previously sensitised individuals.[4]

Although quinine can cause *haemolysis*, there is some doubt over the traditional view that irregular dosage with quinine predisposes patients with malaria to *blackwater fever*, a syndrome of severe haemolytic anaemia, haemoglobinuria, oliguria, and renal failure.[5] Some of the patients affected may have had glucose-6-phosphate dehydrogenase deficiency.[5] Haemolytic-uraemic syndrome[6] and pancytopenia with coagulopathy and renal impairment[7,8] have also been associated with the use of quinine.

There have also been reports of *disseminated intravascular coagulation*, including one fatality, following the use of quinine by patients with quinine hypersensitivity.[9-11] In one case[11] the hypersensitivity reaction closely mimicked septic shock.

There have been isolated reports of *agranulocytosis* due to quinine.[12]

1. Böttiger LE, *et al.* Drug-induced blood dyscrasias. *Acta Med Scand* 1979; **205:** 457–61.
2. Danielson DA, *et al.* Drug-induced blood disorders. *JAMA* 1984; **252:** 3257–60.
3. Freiman JP. Fatal quinine-induced thrombocytopenia. *Ann Intern Med* 1990; **112:** 308–9.
4. Murray JA, *et al.* Bitter lemon purpura. *Br Med J* 1979; **2:** 1551–2.
5. WHO. Severe and complicated malaria. 2nd ed. *Trans R Soc Trop Med Hyg* 1990; **84** (suppl 2): 1–65.
6. Hagley MT, *et al.* Hemolytic-uremic syndrome associated with ingestion of quinine. *Am J Nephrol* 1992; **12:** 192–5.
7. Maguire RB, *et al.* Recurrent pancytopenia, coagulopathy, and renal failure associated with multiple quinine-dependent antibodies. *Ann Intern Med* 1993; **119:** 215–17.
8. Schmitt SK, Tomford JW. Quinine-induced pancytopenia and coagulopathy. *Ann Intern Med* 1994; **120:** 90–1.
9. Spearing RL, *et al.* Quinine-induced disseminated intravascular coagulation. *Lancet* 1990; **336:** 1535–7.
10. Barr E, *et al.* Recurrent acute hypersensitivity to quinine. *Br Med J* 1990; **301:** 323.
11. Schattner A. Quinine hypersensitivity simulating sepsis. *Am J Med* 1998; **104:** 488–90.
12. Sutherland R, *et al.* Quinine-induced agranulocytosis: toxic effect of quinine bisulphate on bone marrow cultures in vitro. *Br Med J* 1977; **1:** 605–7.

Effects on the ears. Although ototoxicity such as tinnitus or deafness is known to be a possible adverse effect of quinine, reversible hearing loss may also occur. While one group of workers[1] found the reduction in auditory acuity to be greatest at higher frequencies another group[2] have found that hearing loss was generally equal across the range of frequencies tested and appeared to be related to the plasma concentration of quinine.

1. Roche RJ, *et al.* Quinine induces reversible high-tone hearing loss. *Br J Clin Pharmacol* 1990; **29:** 780–2.
2. Karlsson KK, *et al.* Audiometry as a possible indicator of quinine plasma concentration during treatment of malaria. *Trans R Soc Trop Med Hyg* 1990; **84:** 765–7.

Effects on the eyes. Oculotoxicity following overdosage with quinine is well recognised (see below), but there has also been a report of blindness in two patients occurring during supposedly routine therapy.[1]

1. Waddell K. Blindness from quinine as an antimalarial. *Trans R Soc Trop Med Hyg* 1996; **90:** 331–2.

Effects on glucose metabolism. Hypoglycaemia is now recognised to be a frequent complication encountered in falciparum malaria and it is often associated with a poor prognosis. Children, pregnant women, and patients with severe disease appear to be particularly at risk. It is important to recognise that hypoglycaemia may be the cause of coma rather than cerebral malaria. Hypoglycaemia may also be induced by antimalarial therapy; first episodes of hypoglycaemia have been detected after patients received quinine[1-3] or quinidine[4] intravenously although others have not found that quinine led to the development of hypoglycaemia.[5,6]

Quinine has also been reported to induce hypoglycaemia during treatment for leg cramps.[7]

1. White NJ, *et al.* Severe hypoglycemia and hyperinsulinemia in falciparum malaria. *N Engl J Med* 1983; **309:** 61–6.

2. Okitolonda W, *et al.* High incidence of hypoglycaemia in African patients treated with intravenous quinine for severe malaria. *Br Med J* 1987; **295:** 716–18.
3. Looareesuwan S, *et al.* Quinine and severe falciparum malaria in late pregnancy. *Lancet* 1985; **ii:** 4–8.
4. Phillips RE, *et al.* Hypoglycaemia and antimalarial drugs: quinidine and release of insulin. *Br Med J* 1986; **292:** 1319–21.
5. Taylor TE, *et al.* Blood glucose levels in Malawian children before and during the administration of intravenous quinine for severe falciparum malaria. *N Engl J Med* 1988; **319:** 1040–7.
6. Kawo NG, *et al.* The metabolic effects of quinine in children with severe and complicated Plasmodium falciparum malaria in Dar es Salaam. *Trans R Soc Trop Med Hyg* 1991; **85:** 711–13.
7. Limburg PJ, *et al.* Quinine-induced hypoglycemia. *Ann Intern Med* 1993; **119:** 218–19.

Effects on the heart. Cardiotoxicity following overdosage with quinine is well recognised, and prolongation of the QT interval has been noted with therapeutic doses. There has also been a report[1] of fatal ventricular fibrillation with QT prolongation in an elderly patient who received standard doses of quinine by slow intravenous infusion for falciparum malaria. It was noted that the patient had some prolongation of the QT interval before starting quinine and also that her free quinine concentrations were unusually high despite total quinine concentrations considered to be within the therapeutic range.

1. Bonington A, *et al.* Fatal quinine cardiotoxicity in the treatment of falciparum malaria. *Trans R Soc Trop Med Hyg* 1996; **90:** 305–7.

Effects on the kidneys. See Effects on the Blood, above.

Effects on the liver. Although hepatitis has been associated with quinidine therapy (see p.939) there appear to be few reports of hepatotoxicity due to quinine usage. Granulomatous hepatitis has been reported in 2 patients taking quinine[1,2] but the diagnosis in the first of these cases was challenged as the histological findings were considered to be more indicative of non-specific reactive hepatitis.[3] Hepatotoxicity due to quinine hypersensitivity has been reported in another patient.[4]

1. Katz B, *et al.* Quinine-induced granulomatous hepatitis. *Br Med J* 1983; **286:** 264–5.
2. Mathur S, *et al.* Quinine induced granulomatous hepatitis and vasculitis. *Br Med J* 1990; **300:** 613.
3. Nirodi NS. Quinine induced granulomatous hepatitis. *Br Med J* 1983; **286:** 647.
4. Punukollu RC, *et al.* Quinine hepatotoxicity: an underrecognized or rare phenomenon? *Arch Intern Med* 1990; **150:** 1112–13.

Effects on the skin. Urticaria, cutaneous flushing, various skin rashes, and pruritus are the commonest symptoms of hypersensitivity reactions to quinine.

Topical contact with quinine may cause contact as well as photocontact allergy, but quinine can also induce photosensitivity reactions following systemic administration.[1,2] Photosensitivity associated with quinine intake from excessive consumption of tonic water has been reported.[3] There have also been reports of eczematous dermatitis,[1] oedema and erythema,[4] and lichen planus.[4] Both phototoxic[4] and photoallergic[1] mechanisms have been suggested. Fatal cutaneous vasculitis related to quinine treatment for nocturnal cramps has been reported.[5]

For a comparison of the incidence of pruritus induced by various antimalarials, see under Chloroquine, p.427.

1. Ljunggren B, Sjövall P. Systemic quinine photosensitivity. *Arch Dermatol* 1986; **122:** 909–11.
2. Ljunggren B, *et al.* Systemic quinine photosensitivity with photoepicutaneous cross-reactivity to quinidine. *Contact Dermatitis* 1992; **26:** 1–4.
3. Wagner GH, *et al.* 'I'll have mine with a twist of lemon': quinine photosensitivity from excessive intake of tonic water. *Br J Dermatol* 1994; **131:** 734–5.
4. Ferguson J, *et al.* Quinine induced photosensitivity: clinical and experimental studies. *Br J Dermatol* 1987; **117:** 631–40.
5. Price EJ, *et al.* Quinine-induced cutaneous vasculitis. *Br J Clin Pract* 1992; **46:** 138–9.

Hypersensitivity. For reference to hypersensitivity reactions associated with quinine, see Effects on the Blood, Effects on the Liver, and Effects on the Skin, above.

Overdosage. Cinchonism may occur with therapeutic doses of quinine and symptoms include nausea, vomiting, tinnitus, deafness, headache, vasodilatation, and slightly disturbed vision. These symptoms may also occur in acute overdosage, but the visual disorders may be severe and there may be CNS disturbances and cardiotoxicity. A lethal dose or lethal plasma-quinine concentration has not been established but fatalities have been reported in adults after doses of 2 to 8 g and in children after 1 g.[1]

An analysis of 165 cases of acute quinine poisoning[2] revealed that: 21% had no symptoms, nausea with or without vomiting occurred in 47%, visual disturbances in 42%, tinnitus in 38%, other auditory disturbances in 23%, sinus tachycardia in 23%, and other ECG abnormalities in 8%. Mild impairment of consciousness was reported in 14% of the patients while 7 (4%) patients had deeper grades of coma. Of the 5 patients who died, 4 developed intractable ventricular arrhythmias and the fifth had a Jacksonian fit followed by cardiac arrest.

The effects of oculotoxicity may include blurred vision, defective colour perception, visual field constriction, and total blindness.[2,3] The onset of symptoms may vary from a few hours to a day or more after ingestion.[2,3] Suggested mechanisms for quinine's oculotoxicity include an action on the retinal vasculature to produce ischaemia or a direct toxic effect on the retina.[1] Visual loss in one group of patients[3] was associated with plasma-quinine concentrations in excess of 10 μg per mL. However, in another group plasma-quinine concentrations were considered to be an imprecise guide to predicting visual disturbances.[2] The speed and degree of visual recovery varies. Of 70 patients with visual disturbances following quinine poisoning 39 subsequently complained of a period of total blindness.[2] Permanent visual deficits remained in 19 of these but no patient had permanent bilateral blindness. All of the 31 patients who had had blurred vision recovered full visual acuity.

It is considered that the actions of quinine on the myocardium are similar to those of quinidine but that it is less potent.[1] Sinus tachycardia and minor ECG changes are the most common cardiovascular effects. Conduction abnormalities and ventricular dysrhythmias may occur with severe poisoning. Ventricular tachycardia is mostly associated with cardiogenic shock or circulatory collapse. Hypokalaemia may also occur.[1]

1. Jaeger A, *et al.* Clinical features and management of poisoning due to antimalarial drugs. *Med Toxicol* 1987; **2:** 242–73.
2. Boland ME, *et al.* Complications of quinine poisoning. *Lancet* 1985; **i:** 384–5.
3. Dyson EH, *et al.* Death and blindness due to overdose of quinine. *Br Med J* 1985; **291:** 31–3.

Treatment of Adverse Effects

In acute overdosage with quinine or its salts the stomach should be emptied by lavage if ingestion has been recent. Oral administration of activated charcoal may also be of some benefit. Other measures aimed at enhancing the elimination of quinine are largely ineffective. Treatment is mostly symptomatic with attention being given to maintaining blood pressure, respiration, and renal function, and to treating arrhythmias.

Vasodilators and stellate ganglion block have been used to prevent or reverse visual impairment but there is little evidence to support their use.

It has been suggested that as quinine has antimuscarinic effects gastric emptying may be delayed and considerable amounts of drug might be removed from the stomach beyond the usual 4 hours.[1] Others consider that gastric lavage is of doubtful value as quinine is rapidly absorbed and vomiting has often occurred before admission.[2] However, studies in healthy subjects and poisoned patients suggest that oral administration of charcoal may increase the elimination of quinine.[3,4] Other methods of increasing elimination are probably ineffective. In a study involving 16 patients with quinine poisoning forced acid diuresis, haemodialysis, haemoperfusion, or plasma exchange were all found to be ineffective in increasing quinine elimination.[5]

Stellate ganglion block has been recommended to prevent or reverse retinal damage, the rationale being that quinine-induced oculotoxicity might arise from retinal arteriolar constriction. However, clinical studies have failed to find sufficient improvement to justify its use.[6,7] There has been a report of the intravenous administration of nitrates producing beneficial responses in 2 patients.[8]

1. Boland M, Volans G. ABC of poisoning: miscellaneous drugs. *Br Med J* 1984; **289:** 1361–5.
2. Jaeger A, *et al.* Clinical features and management of poisoning due to antimalarial drugs. *Med Toxicol* 1987; **2:** 242–73.
3. Lockey D, Bateman DN. Effect of oral activated charcoal on quinine elimination. *Br J Clin Pharmacol* 1989; **27:** 92–4.
4. Prescott LF, *et al.* Treatment of quinine overdosage with repeated oral charcoal. *Br J Clin Pharmacol* 1989; **27:** 95–7.
5. Bateman DN, *et al.* Pharmacokinetics and clinical toxicity of quinine overdosage: lack of efficacy of techniques intended to enhance elimination. *Q J Med* 1985; **54:** 125–31.
6. Boland ME, *et al.* Complications of quinine poisoning. *Lancet* 1985; **i:** 384–5.
7. Dyson EH, *et al.* Quinine amblyopia: is current management appropriate? *J Toxicol Clin Toxicol* 1985–6; **23:** 571–8.
8. Moore D, *et al.* Research into quinine ocular toxicity. *Br J Ophthalmol* 1992; **76:** 703.

Precautions

Quinine and its salts are contra-indicated in patients with a history of hypersensitivity to quinine or quinidine and in patients with tinnitus or optic neuritis. They should not be used in the presence of haemolysis. They should be used with caution in patients with atrial fibrillation, cardiac conduction defects, or heart block. Quinine should be avoided in patients with myasthenia gravis as it may aggravate their condition.

Pregnancy in a patient with malaria is not generally regarded as a contra-indication to the use of quinine.

As quinine has been implicated in precipitating blackwater fever it is generally contra-indicated in patients who have already suffered an attack. Quinine may also cause haemolysis in some types of glucose-6-phosphate dehydrogenase deficiency and should be used with care.

It is important that when quinine is given intravenously it should be given by slow infusion and the patient observed closely for signs of cardiotoxicity. Blood-glucose concentrations should also be monitored. Problems that have been associated with intramuscular administration are discussed under Malaria in Uses and Administration, below.

Breast feeding. Although quinine is distributed into breast milk in small amounts[1] the American Academy of Pediatrics considers that the use of quinine is probably compatible with breast feeding.[2]

1. Phillips RE, *et al.* Quinine pharmacokinetics and toxicity in pregnant and lactating women with falciparum malaria. *Br J Clin Pharmacol* 1986; **21:** 677–83.
2. Committee on Drugs, American Academy of Pediatrics. Transfer of drugs and other chemicals into human milk. *Pediatrics* 1989; **84:** 924–36.

Liver disease. See under Pharmacokinetics, below.

Porphyria. For a discussion of the problems of prophylaxis and treatment of malaria in patients with porphyria and a comment that quinine is considered to be safe for use in such patients, see under Precautions for Chloroquine, p.428.

Pregnancy. The use of quinine in large doses as an abortifacient in the past has led to concern over its use during pregnancy but Looareesuwan *et al.*[1] could find no evidence of an oxytocic effect when it was used to treat severe falciparum malaria in women in the third trimester of pregnancy.

Congenital abnormalities including damage to the auditory and optic nerves have been seen, usually following attempted abortions, but WHO[2] consider quinine to be safe when used in normal therapeutic doses during pregnancy. Jitteriness attributed to quinine withdrawal has been reported in one infant whose mother had drunk large quantities of tonic water containing quinine during the last 17 weeks of pregnancy.[3]

As malaria infection is potentially serious during pregnancy and poses a threat to the mother and fetus, there appears to be little justification for withholding treatment in the absence of a suitable alternative. However, pregnant patients treated for malaria are at special risk from hypoglycaemia exacerbated or caused by quinine-induced hyperinsulinaemia (see under Effects on Glucose Metabolism in Adverse Effects, above) and should be managed appropriately.

1. Looareesuwan S, *et al.* Quinine and severe falciparum malaria in late pregnancy. *Lancet* 1985; **ii:** 4–8.
2. WHO. Practical chemotherapy of malaria: report of a WHO scientific group. *WHO Tech Rep Ser 805* 1990.
3. Evans ANW, *et al.* The ingestion by pregnant women of substances toxic to the foetus. *Practitioner* 1980; **224:** 315–19.

Renal impairment. See under Pharmacokinetics, below.

Interactions

There is an increased risk of inducing ventricular arrhythmias if quinine is given together with halofantrine (see p.431) or other arrhythmogenic drugs such as amiodarone, the antihistamines astemizole and terfenadine, cisapride, and the antipsychotic pimozide. There may be an increased risk of convulsions when quinine is administered with mefloquine.

For further details of interactions, see below.

As quinine shares many of the actions of quinidine, interactions seen between quinidine and other drugs (see p.939) might also occur with quinine. Both have actions on skeletal muscle and may potentiate the effects of drugs with neuromuscular-blocking activity (see under Antiarrhythmics on p.1306). Quinidine has been reported to increase serum-digoxin concentrations (see p.851) and quinine has reduced total body clearance of *digoxin* (see p.851).

Quinine can cause hypoprothrombinaemia and thereby enhance the effect of *anticoagulants*. In one report, reductions in warfarin dosage were necessary after ingestion of large amounts of tonic water containing quinine (see p.967).

For a report of quinine reducing renal clearance of *amantadine*, see p.1130, of quinine decreasing plasma concentrations of *cyclosporin*, see p.522, of quinine inhibiting the metabolism of *flecainide*, see p.869, and of quinine reducing plasma concentrations of *primaquine*, see p.435.

Drugs affecting quinine have included *cimetidine* which has been reported to reduce the clearance of quinine and prolong its elimination half-life in a study in healthy subjects; no significant effect was seen with *ranitidine*.[1] Elimination of quinine has been reported to increase in patients also receiving *rifampicin*.[2] Quinine and *chloroquine* may be antagonistic when used for falciparum malaria (see p.428).

A single-dose study in healthy subjects has suggested that blood concentrations of quinine are lower in heavy smokers than in non-smokers, potentially impairing efficacy.[3]

1. Wanwimolruk S, *et al.* Effects of cimetidine and ranitidine on the pharmacokinetics of quinine. *Br J Clin Pharmacol* 1986; **22:** 346–50.
2. Wanwimolruk S, *et al.* Marked enhancement by rifampicin and lack of effect of isoniazid on the elimination of quinine in man. *Br J Clin Pharmacol* 1995; **40:** 87–91.
3. Wanwimolruk S, *et al.* Cigarette smoking enhances the elimination of quinine. *Br J Clin Pharmacol* 1993; **36:** 610–14.

Pharmacokinetics

The pharmacokinetics of quinine are altered significantly by malaria infection, the major effects being reductions in both its apparent volume of distribution and its clearance.

Quinine is rapidly and almost completely absorbed from the gastro-intestinal tract and peak concentrations in the circulation are attained about 1 to 3 hours after oral administration of the sulphate or bisulphate. Plasma protein binding is about 70% in healthy subjects and rises to 90% or more in patients with malaria. Quinine is widely distributed throughout the body. Concentrations attained in the CSF of patients with cerebral malaria have been reported to be about 2 to 7% of those in the plasma.

Quinine is extensively metabolised in the liver and rapidly excreted mainly in the urine. Estimates of the proportion of unchanged quinine excreted in the urine vary from less than 5 to 20%. Excretion is increased in acid urine. The elimination half-life is about 11 hours in healthy subjects but may be prolonged in patients with malaria. Small amounts of quinine also appear in the bile and saliva.

Quinine crosses the placenta and is distributed into breast milk (see Breast Feeding, above).

References.

1. White NJ. Clinical pharmacokinetics of antimalarial drugs. *Clin Pharmacokinet* 1985; **10:** 187–215.
2. WHO. Severe and complicated malaria. 2nd ed. *Trans R Soc Trop Med Hyg* 1990; **84** (suppl 2): 1–65.
3. Supanaranond W, *et al.* Disposition of oral quinine in acute falciparum malaria. *Eur J Clin Pharmacol* 1991; **40:** 49–52.
4. Wanwimolruk S, *et al.* Pharmacokinetics of quinine in young and elderly subjects. *Trans R Soc Trop Med Hyg* 1991; **85:** 714–17.
5. Dyer JR, *et al.* The pharmacokinetics and pharmacodynamics of quinine in the diabetic and non-diabetic elderly. *Br J Clin Pharmacol* 1994; **38:** 205–12.
6. Sowunmi A, Salako LA. Effect of dose size on the pharmacokinetics of orally administered quinine. *Eur J Clin Pharmacol* 1996; **49:** 383–6.
7. Krishna S, White NJ. Pharmacokinetics of quinine, chloroquine and amodiaquine: clinical implications. *Clin Pharmacokinet* 1996; **30:** 263–99.
8. Boele van Hensbroek M, *et al.* Quinine pharmacokinetics in young children with severe malaria. *Am J Trop Med Hyg* 1996; **54:** 237–42.
9. Zhang H, *et al.* Evidence for involvement of human CYP3A in the 3-hydroxylation of quinine. *Br J Clin Pharmacol* 1997; **43:** 245–52.

Administration in liver disease. Reduced clearance of quinine and prolonged elimination half-life have been reported in patients with acute hepatitis B given a single intravenous dose.[1] The results suggested that quinine accumulation following multiple doses could be greater in patients with hepatitis, even once hepatic function had returned to normal. In another study[2] patients with moderate chronic liver disease were given quinine by mouth; the half-life was prolonged but total clearance was not affected.

1. Karbwang J, *et al.* The pharmacokinetics of quinine in patients with hepatitis. *Br J Clin Pharmacol* 1993; **35:** 444–6.
2. Auprayoon P, *et al.* Pharmacokinetics of quinine in chronic liver disease. *Br J Clin Pharmacol* 1995; **40:** 494–7.

Administration in renal impairment. As urinary clearance comprises only 20% of total clearance of quinine it appears that high plasma concentrations reported in patients with severe falciparum malaria and acute renal failure may be related more to the severity of the malaria and associated pharmacokinetic changes rather than to any reduction in the glomerular filtration rate (GFR).[1] There were significant changes in the pharmacokinetics of quinine in 6 patients with chronic renal failure following a single oral dose.[2] The changes included a prolonged half-life, but there was no clear relationship between severity of renal failure and the degree of impairment of quinine clearance.

1. White NJ. Clinical pharmacokinetics of antimalarial drugs. *Clin Pharmacokinet* 1985; **10:** 187–215.
2. Rimchala P, *et al.* Pharmacokinetics of quinine in patients with chronic renal failure. *Eur J Clin Pharmacol* 1996; **49:** 497–501.

Uses and Administration

Quinine is a cinchona alkaloid and a 4-methanolquinoline antimalarial which is a rapid-acting blood schizontocide with activity against *Plasmodium falciparum*, *P. vivax*, *P. ovale*, and *P. malariae*. It is active against the gametocytes of *P. malariae* and *P. vivax*, but not against mature gametocytes of *P. falciparum*. The precise mechanism of action of quinine is unclear but it may interfere with lysosome function or nucleic acid synthesis in the malaria parasite. Since it has no activity against exoerythrocytic forms, quinine does not produce a radical cure in vivax or ovale malarias. The increasing spread of resistance to chloroquine has been responsible for the re-emergence of quinine as an important drug in the treatment of falciparum malaria. Quinine is not generally used for malaria prophylaxis.

Quinine is also used to treat the protozoal infection babesiosis and for the relief of nocturnal leg cramps.

Quinine has mild analgesic and antipyretic properties and is sometimes included in preparations used for the symptomatic relief of the common cold and influenza; additional salts that have been used for this purpose include the camsylate and the gluconate.

Quinine is also used as a bitter and a flavouring agent.

For the *treatment of malaria* quinine is given by mouth, usually as the sulphate, hydrochloride, or dihydrochloride, or parenterally as the dihydrochloride; quinine ethyl carbonate is sometimes used for oral administration because, unlike other quinine salts which are intensely bitter, it is tasteless. They all contain approximately the same amount of quinine and any of them can be used when the dose is cited in terms of "quinine salt"; this is not the case for the bisulphate which contains a correspondingly smaller amount of quinine. Quinine formate is sometimes used for parenteral administration.

A course of treatment with quinine for falciparum malaria usually lasts 7 days and in uncomplicated infections treatment should preferably be given by the oral route. The usual oral dose is 600 mg of quinine salt given every 8 hours for 7 days. For children a dose of 10 mg of quinine salt per kg body-weight given every 8 hours for 7 days has been recommended.

In severe or complicated falciparum malaria or when the patient is unable to take oral medication quinine should be given parenterally by slow intravenous infusion, but this can be hazardous and patients generally need monitoring, particularly for signs of cardiotoxicity. Therapy should be changed to oral administration as soon as possible to complete the course. To obtain therapeutic concentrations rapidly with parenteral therapy, quinine is often given in an initial loading dose followed by maintenance doses. Recommended dosage regimens for intravenous administration include an initial loading dose of 20 mg of quinine dihydrochloride per kg (up to a maximum of 1.4 g) given over 4 hours with maintenance infusions being started 8 to 12 hours later. Alternatively, in intensive care units, an initial loading dose of 7 mg per kg may be given over 30 minutes followed immediately by the first of the maintenance infusions. Maintenance infusions consist of 10 mg per kg (up to a maximum of 700 mg) given over 4 hours every 8 to 12 hours. A loading dose should not be given if the patient has received quinine, quinidine, mefloquine, or halofantrine, during the previous 24 hours. If parenteral therapy is required for more than 48 hours the maintenance dose of quinine dihydrochloride should be reduced to 5 to 7 mg per kg. If intravenous infusion is not possible quinine dihydrochloride has been given intramuscularly where doses, including the loading dose, are the same as those used for intravenous administration; however, intramuscular administration can be irritant and there have been concerns regarding its safety and efficacy (see under Malaria, below).

When used for the *relief of nocturnal leg cramps*, quinine is given at night in a dose of 200 to 300 mg by mouth of the sulphate or bisulphate. Quinine benzoate has also been used.

Babesiosis. Although there is no established specific treatment for babesiosis (p.574), a combination of quinine and clindamycin has been used for *Babesia microti* infections.[1-3] Suggested doses[3] are quinine 650 mg three times daily by mouth with clindamycin 1.2 g twice daily intravenously or 600 mg three times daily by mouth; treatment is continued for 7 days. Children may be given quinine 25 mg per kg bodyweight daily plus clindamycin 20 to 40 mg per kg daily, both by mouth in 3 divided doses. Quinine with azithromycin was reported to be effective in a patient who had not responded to quinine with clindamycin.[4]

1. Wittner M, *et al.* Successful chemotherapy of transfusion babesiosis. *Ann Intern Med* 1982; **96:** 601–4.
2. Anonymous. Clindamycin and quinine treatment for Babesia microti infections. *MMWR* 1983; **32:** 65–6, 72.
3. Anonymous. Drugs for parasitic infections. *Med Lett Drugs Ther* 1998; **40:** 1–12.
4. Shaio MF, Yang KD. Response of babesiosis to a combined regimen of quinine and azithromycin. *Trans R Soc Trop Med Hyg* 1997; **91:** 214–15.

Flavouring. The Joint FAO/WHO Expert Committee on Food Additives concluded that quinine levels in soft drinks of up to 100 mg per litre (as quinine base) were not of toxicological concern.[1] However, because of the possibility of hypersensitivity reactions in some individuals, the committee recommended that consumers be informed of the presence of quinine in food or beverages.

1. FAO/WHO. Evaluation of certain food additives and contaminants: forty-first report of the joint FAO/WHO expert committee on food additives. *WHO Tech Rep Ser 837* 1993.

Malaria. Quinine has an important role in the treatment of falciparum malaria (see p.422) being used where there is chloroquine or multidrug *Plasmodium falciparum* resistance,[1-5] and also (in view of the widespread problem of *P. falciparum* resistance) where the infective species is not known, or if the infection is mixed. Ideally treatment should be with one of the quinine salts given by mouth when a dose of 600 mg of quinine salt for adults or 10 mg per kg bodyweight for children is given every 8 hours for 7 days. However, to reduce quinine-related adverse effects and thereby improve compliance, a 3-day course of quinine salt combined with either 7 days of tetracycline or a single dose of pyrimethamine-sulfadoxine (Fansidar) or clindamycin for 3 days may be considered in regions without quinine resistance. The dose of quinine salt applies to the hydrochloride, dihydrochloride, sulphate, and ethyl carbonate, but not to the bisulphate. Any quinine lost through vomiting within one hour after oral administration should be replaced by additional doses.[2]

The oral route may not provide effective treatment in severe infection and in such cases quinine should be given as the dihydrochloride by slow intravenous infusion the patient being observed closely, particularly for any signs of cardiotoxicity.[1,5] Loading doses of quinine are often used to obtain therapeutic blood concentrations as soon as possible in severely ill patients but they should not be given to patients who have received quinine, quinidine, mefloquine, or halofantrine, within the previous 24 hours.

WHO[1,5] recommends that an initial loading dose of 20 mg of quinine dihydrochloride per kg [up to a maximum of 1.4 g] be given intravenously over 4 hours followed [after 8 hours] by maintenance infusions of 10 mg per kg given over 4 hours every 8 hours (sometimes the interval may be every 12 hours). Alternatively, in intensive care units, a loading dose of 7 mg per kg body-weight may be given by intravenous infusion over 30 minutes followed immediately by the first of the maintenance infusions. The loading and maintenance doses given above were found to be necessary in Thailand where the MIC of quinine for local strains of *Plasmodium falciparum* was around 10 μg per mL. In some areas where *P. falciparum* is more sensitive to quinine a regimen consisting of a loading dose of 10 mg per kg and maintenance doses of 5 mg per kg, given at 12-hour intervals, might also produce adequate plasma concentrations.[1] A regimen suggested for young children in Africa with severe malaria consisted of a 15 mg per kg loading dose of quinine dihydrochloride given by intravenous infusion over 2 hours, followed by maintenance doses of 10 mg per kg every 12 hours.[6] This regimen was challenged however, on the basis that it might result in under-treatment of the disease.[7] In another study in African children with cerebral malaria,[8] a loading dose of quinine dihydrochloride 20 mg per kg given intravenously over the first 4 hours (followed by maintenance doses of 10 mg per kg intravenously, over 4 hours, every 8 hours for 3 days, and then orally for 4 days) was judged to be more effective than a similar regimen without a loading dose. Whichever regimen is chosen patients are transferred to oral therapy as soon as possible at a dose of 10 mg of quinine salt per kg every 8 hours and treatment continued until a total of at least 7 days of therapy has been given.[1,5] However, if patients still require parenteral therapy after 48 hours it has been suggested that maintenance doses should be reduced to 5 to 7 mg per kg.[1,5] If intravenous formulations of quinine are unavailable quinidine may be used as an alternative; for further details see under the Uses and Administration of Quinidine, p.940.

If facilities for administration by intravenous infusion, including monitoring, are not available WHO[1,5] recommends that quinine should be given by deep intramuscular injection. A loading dose of 20 mg of quinine dihydrochloride per kg may be given by injection in divided sites followed by injections of 10 mg per kg every 8 hours; a dose interval of 12 hours has also been employed.[5] Patients should be transferred to oral therapy as soon as possible. The use of the intramuscular route has been controversial because of concerns over safety and efficacy. However, some studies have demonstrated that it can safely be used in adults and children with severe infections.[9-12] Intramuscular injections of quinine can be irritant and have caused pain, focal necrosis, and abscess formation; fatal tetanus has developed in some patients.[13] It has been suggested that some such reactions may be related to the use of preparations formulated in urethane or other irritant substances.[1] Diluted solutions of quinine dihydrochloride 60 mg per mL adjusted to neutral pH appear to be less painful than the usual undiluted preparation of 300 mg per mL.[1]

If facilities do not exist to administer quinine parenterally then patients with severe malaria should receive quinine by mouth or nasogastric tube. Rectal administration has also been suggested.[14]

Quinine as formerly standardised used to contain a higher concentration of cinchona alkaloids and there might be synergy between mixtures of these alkaloids.[15] In practice no advantage has been demonstrated by such mixtures over quinine alone in the treatment of chloroquine-resistant falciparum malaria.[16]

1. WHO. Practical chemotherapy of malaria: report of a WHO scientific group. *WHO Tech Rep Ser 805* 1990.
2. WHO. *WHO model prescribing information: drugs used in parasitic diseases.* 2nd ed. Geneva: WHO, 1995.
3. Molyneux M, Fox R. Diagnosis and treatment of malaria in Britain. *Br Med J* 1993; **306:** 1175–80.
4. Anonymous. Drugs for parasitic infections. *Med Lett Drugs Ther* 1998; **40:** 1–12.
5. Gilles HM. *Management of severe and complicated malaria.* Geneva: WHO, 1991.
6. Winstanley PA, *et al.* Towards optimal regimens of parenteral quinine for young African children with cerebral malaria: unbound quinine concentrations following a simple loading dose regimen. *Trans R Soc Trop Med Hyg* 1994; **88:** 577–80.
7. White NJ. Optimal regimens of parenteral quinine. *Trans R Soc Trop Med Hyg* 1995; **89:** 462–3.
8. van der Torn M, *et al.* Loading dose of quinine in African children with cerebral malaria. *Trans R Soc Trop Med Hyg* 1998; **92:** 325–31.
9. Wattanagoon Y, *et al.* Intramuscular loading dose of quinine for falciparum malaria: pharmacokinetics and toxicity. *Br Med J* 1986; **293:** 11–13. Correction. *ibid.*; 362.
10. Mansor SM, *et al.* The safety and kinetics of intramuscular quinine in Malawian children with moderately severe falciparum malaria. *Trans R Soc Trop Med Hyg* 1990; **84:** 482–7.
11. Waller D, *et al.* The pharmacokinetic properties of intramuscular quinine in Gambian children with severe falciparum malaria. *Trans R Soc Trop Med Hyg* 1990; **84:** 488–91.
12. Schapira A, *et al.* Comparison of intramuscular and intravenous quinine for the treatment of severe and complicated malaria in children. *Trans R Soc Trop Med Hyg* 1993; **87:** 299–302.
13. Yen LM, *et al.* Role of quinine in the high mortality of intramuscular injection tetanus. *Lancet* 1994; **344:** 786–7.
14. Barennes H. Is intrarectal injectable quinine a safe alternative to intramuscular injectable quinine? *Trop Doct* 1994; **24:** 32–3.
15. Druilhe P, *et al.* Activity of a combination of three cinchona bark alkaloids against Plasmodium falciparum in vitro. *Antimicrob Agents Chemother* 1988; **32:** 250–4.
16. Bunnag D, *et al.* A combination of quinine, quinidine and cinchonine (LA 40221) in the treatment of chloroquine resistant falciparum malaria in Thailand: two double-blind trials. *Trans R Soc Trop Med Hyg* 1989; **83:** 66.

Muscle spasm. Quinine (usually as quinine sulphate or bisulphate) has traditionally been used for nocturnal cramps (p.1303) but there has been concern over its efficacy and potential for adverse effects, especially in the elderly. In the USA, for example, the FDA ruled that quinine products should no longer be used for the management of nocturnal cramps.[1,2] A meta-analysis[3] concluded that although quinine was effective in the treatment of nocturnal cramps in ambulatory patients the risk of serious adverse effects should be borne in mind. It was recommended that patients should be closely monitored while the efficacy of quinine is assessed over a period of at least 4 weeks. Some[4] have recommended that treatment be stopped every 3 months to see whether it was still needed.

Haemodialysis-induced cramp has been reported to respond to treatment with quinine.[5,6]

1. FDA. Drug products for the treatment and/or prevention of nocturnal leg muscle cramps for over-the-counter human use. *Fed Regist* 1994; **59:** 43234–52.
2. Nightingale SL. Quinine for nocturnal leg cramps. *ACP J Club* 1995; **123:** 86.
3. Man-Son-Hing M, Wells G. Meta-analysis of efficacy of quinine for treatment of nocturnal leg cramps in elderly people. *Br Med J* 1995; **310:** 13–17.
4. Anonymous. Quinine for nocturnal leg cramps? *Drug Ther Bull* 1996; **34:** 7–8.
5. Kaji DM, *et al.* Prevention of muscle cramps in haemodialysis patients by quinine sulphate. *Lancet* 1976; **ii:** 66–7.
6. Roca AO, *et al.* Dialysis leg cramps; efficacy of quinine versus vitamin E. *ASAIO J* 1992; **38:** M481–M485.

Preparations

BP 1998: Quinine Bisulphate Tablets; Quinine Sulphate Tablets;
USP 23: Quinine Sulfate Capsules; Quinine Sulfate Tablets.

Proprietary Preparations (details are given in Part 3)
Austral.: Adaquin†; Bi-Chinine†; Biquin†; Biquinate; Chinine†; Myoquin; Quinate; Quinbisul; Quinoctal; Quinsul; ***Fr.:*** Quinoforme; ***Ger.:*** Limptar N; Sagittaproct; ***Swed.:*** Kinin; ***Switz.:*** Circonyl N; ***USA:*** Formula Q†; Legatrin†; M-KYA†; Night Leg Cramp Relief; Q-Vel†; Quinamm†; Quindan†; Quiphile†.

Multi-ingredient: ***Aust.:*** Dilatol-Chinin; Iromin Chinin C; Limptar; Seltoc; Togal; ***Belg.:*** Antigrip†; Eugrippine; Latepyrine†; Spasmosedine; ***Fr.:*** Arsiquinoforme; Cequinyl; Dinacode; Gripponyl†; Hexaquine; Pholcones; Pholcones Bismuth-Quinine†; Pholcones Guaiphenesine-Quinine†; Quinimax; Quinisedine; Tussipax a l'Euquinine; ***Ger.:*** Antigrippalin†; Antiphlebin; Ascorbin-Chinin-Dragees Michallik†; Circovegetalin compositum†; Circovegetalin†; Limptar; Poikicin†; Togal; Zynedo-B†; Zynedo-K†; ***Irl.:*** Anadin; ***Ital.:*** Monotrean; ***Neth.:*** Aflukin C; ***S.Afr.:*** Cetamine; Ilvico; ***Spain:*** Brota Rectal Bals; Frikton†; ***Switz.:*** Limptar; Monotrean†; ***UK:*** Anadin; Nicobrevin; Ronpirin APCQ.

Antimigraine Drugs

This chapter reviews the management of headache, in particular, migraine, cluster headache, and tension-type headache. It also describes the drugs used mainly for migraine and cluster headache, including the ergot alkaloid ergotamine; the semisynthetic ergot alkaloids dihydroergotamine and methysergide (a potent serotonin antagonist); the serotonin antagonist pizotifen; and selective serotonin (5-HT_1) agonists such as naratriptan, rizatriptan, sumatriptan, and zolmitriptan.

The mechanisms of head pain or headache are not fully understood but may involve neurovascular changes (as in migraine and cluster headache), muscle contraction (as in tension headache), nerve lesions (neuralgias), direct head injury, infection (meningitis), or be referred (sinusitis, toothache, eye disorders). Headache is also an adverse effect of many drugs including those used to treat it. The International Headache Society has published guidelines to aid the diagnosis of the various headache types. Patients may have more than one headache disorder and require separate treatment for each.

References.

1. Headache Classification Committee of the International Headache Society. Classification and diagnostic criteria for headache disorders, cranial neuralgias and facial pain. *Cephalalgia* 1988; **8** (suppl 7): 1–96.

Analgesic-induced headache

Many substances can cause headache. Paradoxically, overuse of analgesics and other drugs used to treat headaches can induce chronic daily headache in headache-prone patients, but this does not appear to occur when they are used to treat other disorders.[1] Analgesic-induced headache is well recognised in adults, but has also been reported in children.[2] Such analgesic-induced headaches, also referred to as rebound headaches or analgesic abuse headaches, are relieved by withdrawal of the offending drug, although the primary headache may still persist. Furthermore, chronic administration of some drugs used in headache treatments, such as ergotamine (p.446) and caffeine (p.750), may lead to a state of dependency and their abrupt discontinuation can produce headache and other symptoms of withdrawal. This may then lead the patient to resume treatment to relieve the headache thereby setting up a vicious circle. Patients with analgesic-induced headache can be difficult to treat. Options for outpatient treatment include either gradual or abrupt withdrawal of the overused analgesic, sometimes together with substitution by a long-acting NSAID or intramuscular dihydroergotamine.[3] However, withdrawal symptoms may persist for up to 2 weeks and detoxification may require hospitalisation; intravenous metoclopramide and repetitive intravenous dihydroergotamine may be required to control nausea and vomiting and intractable headache, respectively. General advice on the prevention of analgesic-induced headache has included limiting the frequency of administration of analgesics and the avoidance of compound and opioid analgesics.[1,3]

1. Olesen J. Analgesic headache. *Br Med J* 1995; **310:** 479–80.
2. Symon DNK. Twelve cases of analgesic headache. *Arch Dis Child* 1998; **78:** 555–6.
3. Silberstein SD, Young WB. Analgesic rebound headache. *Drug Safety* 1995; **13:** 133–44.

Cluster headache

Cluster headache (migrainous neuralgia, histaminic cephalalgia, Horton's syndrome) is a headache of unknown aetiology that may be neurovascular in origin. Patients experience one or more short-lived attacks of intense unilateral head pain, usually at the same time every day and often at night, during cluster periods which last for several weeks. Restlessness during the attacks appears to be a characteristic feature of cluster headache. In the typical episodic form of cluster headache, cluster periods are followed by periods of remission lasting for months or years but in the more rare chronic form, patients may have cluster periods lasting for more than a year or with very short periods of remission in between. Substances such as alcohol or glyceryl trinitrate can precipitate headache attacks during cluster periods, but not during periods of remission.

The **treatment** of individual acute attacks during a cluster period is difficult because the headache is short-lived and analgesics administered by the oral route are unlikely to be absorbed fast enough to produce much benefit. Inhalation of 100% oxygen is rapid and effective in aborting attacks, but because of practical difficulties other treatments such as inhaled ergotamine or subcutaneous sumatriptan are more likely to be used. Dihydroergotamine is also effective but generally requires administration by injection and is usually reserved for use in emergency settings. Intranasal instillation of lignocaine has been reported to be effective in aborting attacks but does not appear to be widely used.

Since individual attacks are difficult to treat it is probably more effective to manage cluster headache by **prophylaxis** once a cluster period has started. Several drugs have been used to prevent attacks. Ergotamine is used for prevention in episodic cluster headache when it is given by mouth or rectally for limited periods of up to 2 weeks. It is often given for only 5 to 6 days in each week, which allows the patient to assess whether the cluster period has ended. Other drugs that have been used, either alone or with ergotamine, include verapamil, lithium carbonate, and prednisolone. Lithium may be particularly useful for the chronic form of the disorder. Methysergide and pizotifen have also been tried.

Chronic paroxysmal hemicrania is a rare variant of cluster headache in which patients experience numerous attacks every day for years. One of its features, which may be diagnostic, is its invariable response to indomethacin.

References.

1. Kudrow L. Treatment of cluster headache. *Headache Q* 1993; **4** (suppl 2): 42–7.
2. Kumar KL, Cooney TG. Headaches. *Med Clin North Am* 1995; **79:** 261–86.

Migraine

Migraine is characterised by recurrent attacks of headache which typically last 4 to 72 hours. Attacks persisting for longer than 72 hours are referred to as status migrainosus. The headache is a unilateral pulsating pain that is aggravated by movement and is usually of sufficient severity to disturb or prevent daily activities. It is frequently accompanied by nausea, vomiting, or other gastro-intestinal disturbances and there may be photophobia and phonophobia. Migraine with aura (classic migraine) is characterised by an aura consisting of visual or sensory symptoms that lasts less than an hour. The headache usually follows the aura directly, or within 1 hour, but may begin simultaneously with the aura. In addition, aura can occur without headache. Migraine without aura (common migraine) is the more common form occurring in about 75% of patients with migraine. Premonitory symptoms may occur before a migraine attack (with or without aura). Familial hemiplegic migraine is a rare syndrome in which migraine with aura may be preceded or accompanied by aphasia, confusion, and hemiparesis. Basilar migraine is another rare form of migraine with aura in which there may be disturbances of the brain stem or occipital lobes accompanied by symptoms such as impairment of consciousness, vertigo, ataxia, dysarthria, and diplopia.

Migraine is described as a neurovascular headache. Traditionally, intracranial vasoconstriction was considered responsible for the aura and extracranial vasodilatation for the headache. However, it appears that vascular events may be secondary to neurogenic changes and the liberation of vasoactive substances including serotonin (5-HT), catecholamines, histamine, kinins, neuropeptides, and prostaglandins.

There are several factors which may precipitate migraine attacks. These include anxiety, physical and emotional stress, a change in sleep pattern, bright lights, fasting, some foods, and menstruation. Migraine may also be precipitated by drugs including oral contraceptives and oestrogens, and glyceryl trinitrate. The frequency of migraine attacks can be reduced if such precipitating factors can be identified and avoided. Quiet, darkness, and sleep can ease an attack, with sleep heralding recovery.

Treatment. Simple analgesics such as aspirin and other NSAIDs or paracetamol are effective if taken at the earliest signs of an attack. Weak opioid analgesics such as codeine are sometimes included in oral compound analgesic preparations, but many consider that opioids are best avoided, especially in patients who experience frequent headaches. Other drugs used with analgesics in antimigraine preparations have included the sympathomimetic vasoconstrictor isometheptene and sedatives such as dichloralphenazone.

If the initial treatment of migraine is delayed, absorption of oral drugs may be compromised by gastric stasis and nausea and vomiting which commonly develop as the attack progresses. Antiemetics are often included in compound antimigraine preparations; those commonly used include buclizine, cyclizine, and the prokinetic drugs metoclopramide and domperidone. Prokinetic drugs also have the advantage of promoting gastric emptying and normal peristalsis. Dispersible and effervescent analgesic preparations are preferable because of their more rapid absorption. If nausea and vomiting is prominent rectal administration may be necessary.

Attacks not responding to simple analgesics or NSAIDs may be treated with specific antimigraine drugs such as the selective serotonin (5-HT_1) agonists (e.g. sumatriptan) and the ergot derivatives ergotamine and dihydroergotamine. Selective serotonin (5-HT_1) agonists are generally preferred to ergot derivatives in patients whose migraines do not respond to simple analgesics or NSAIDs. Sumatriptan was the first serotonin (5-HT_1) agonist developed and is available for oral, intranasal, or subcutaneous use. A single dose is usually administered at the first sign of a migraine attack, but it is also effective if used during the established headache phase of an attack. There is some evidence that it is not effective if administered in the aura phase of migraine with aura. Some patients experience recurrence of the headache within 24 to 48 hours, and often respond to a second dose. Other available serotonin (5-HT_1) agonists include zolmitriptan (oral preparation), naratriptan (oral), and rizatriptan (oral). These drugs have better oral bioavailability than sumatriptan, but as yet there are little comparative clinical data. If ergotamine is used it should be given at the first warning of an attack; the earlier it is given, the more effective the treatment. Since its oral bioavailability is poor and may be reduced further during a migraine attack, ergotamine has sometimes been administered in sublingual or rectal preparations or by inhaler. Ergotamine can also exacerbate nausea and vomiting necessitating antiemetics such as metoclopramide or domperidone; if nausea and vomiting becomes severe the phenothiazine antiemetics chlorpromazine or prochlorperazine may be given. Dihydroergotamine may be of use if parenteral treatment is required; it can also be given intranasally but there is less experience with this route.

Patients who rapidly develop severe migraine may be given dihydroergotamine or sumatriptan parenterally. If there is no response to these drugs dopamine antagonists such as metoclopramide, chlorpromazine, or prochlorperazine given parenterally may be effective in relieving the pain of acute migraine attacks. Prolonged attacks (status migrainosus) may require intravenous administration of dihydroergotamine with metoclopramide. Other drugs that may be given alone or in combination include prochlorperazine, chlorpromazine, corticosteroids, or pethidine. Lignocaine has been given intravenously for the emergency treatment of migraine and more recently intranasal lignocaine has been tried. The opioid agonist-antagonist butorphanol, administered by nasal spray, has been advocated, but its place in therapy, if any, remains to be established.

Prophylactic treatment should be considered for patients in whom abortive measures are ineffective or migraine attacks occur frequently, or for those with less frequent but severe or prolonged attacks. Some recommend prophylaxis if attacks occur more often than once or twice a month. Prophylaxis can reduce the severity and/or frequency of attacks but does not eliminate them completely and patients still need additional abortive or symptomatic treatment. Drugs suggested for prophylaxis have a range of actions which reflects uncertainty over the pathogenesis of migraine. It is important to give prophylactic drugs for an adequate period before assessing their efficacy. Once an optimum effect has been achieved the need for continuing prophylaxis should be reviewed at intervals of about 3 to 6 months. The main prophylactic drugs are beta blockers, pizotifen, and tricyclic antidepressants. Propranolol is considered by many to be the prophylactic drug of choice. Lethargy appears to be the most common adverse effect. Other beta blockers reported to be effective are those that, like propranolol, possess no intrinsic sympathomimetic activity and include atenolol, metoprolol, nadolol, and timolol. The potential for beta blockers to interact with some serotonin ($5-HT_1$) agonists and ergotamine should be borne in mind. Pizotifen, an antihistamine and serotonin antagonist, is one of the main alternatives to propranolol. Drowsiness and increased appetite with weight gain may be a problem, although these may be overcome to some extent by gradual increases in dose and administration at night. Tricyclic antidepressants, particularly amitriptyline, given in gradually increasing doses at night are useful for preventing migraine, especially in patients who also have depression or tension-type headache, although antimuscarinic side-effects may occur.

Other drugs have been used for the prophylaxis of migraine; of the drugs with calcium-channel blocking activity, flunarizine appears to be effective and verapamil may be useful, but evidence for the efficacy of other calcium-channel blockers such as diltiazem, nifedipine, or nimodipine is less convincing. Valproate, a gamma-aminobutyric acid (GABA) agonist, may be effective, and NSAIDs may be worth trying.

The use of methysergide, a potent serotonin antagonist, has declined because of serious side-effects, in particular retroperitoneal fibrosis. MAOIs such as phenelzine have been used occasionally but are best reserved for severe cases refractory to other prophylactic treatment. Cyproheptadine, an antihistamine and serotonin antagonist, has been used for migraine prophylaxis, particularly in children. Other drugs used for the prophylaxis of migraine have included clonidine, cyclandelate, indoramin, and feverfew and the ergot derivatives lysuride and metergoline.

References.

1. Lance JW. Treatment of migraine. *Lancet* 1992; **339:** 1207–9.
2. MacGregor EA. Prescribing for migraine. *Prescribers' J* 1993; **33:** 50–8.
3. Solomon GD. Therapeutic advances in migraine. *J Clin Pharmacol* 1993; **33:** 200–209.
4. Welch KMA. Drug therapy of migraine. *N Engl J Med* 1993; **329:** 1476–83.
5. Kumar KL, Cooney TG. Headaches. *Med Clin North Am* 1995; **79:** 261–86.
6. Goadsby PJ, Olesen J. Diagnosis and management of migraine. *Br Med J* 1996; **312:** 1279–83.
7. Capobianco DJ, *et al.* An overview of the diagnosis and pharmacologic treatment of migraine. *Mayo Clin Proc* 1996; **71:** 1055–66.
8. Pryse-Phillips WEM, *et al.* Guidelines for the diagnosis and management of migraine in clinical practice. *Can Med Assoc J* 1997; **156:** 1273–87.
9. Ferrari MD. Migraine. *Lancet* 1998; **351:** 1043–51.
10. Anonymous. Managing migraine. *Drug Ther Bull* 1998; **36:** 41–4.
11. Anonymous. New "triptans" and other drugs for migraine. *Med Lett Drugs Ther* 1998; **40:** 97–100.

Post-dural puncture headache

For the management of headache associated with lumbar puncture or spinal anaesthesia, see Post-dural Puncture Headache under Local Anaesthetics, p.1282.

Tension-type headache

Tension-type headaches, also referred to as muscle-contraction headaches, are probably the commonest form of headache. They are characterised by bilateral pain, which unlike migraine is continuous and non-pulsatile. The pain is often described by the patient as feeling like a tight band pressed around the head. Headaches of this type may be precipitated by many factors including psychosocial stress or muscular stress. Many patients also have associated symptoms of anxiety or depression. Also tension-type headaches and migraine frequently co-exist when they are often referred to as combination or mixed headaches. Some patients may only experience isolated acute attacks of tension-type headache (episodic tension-type headache), but others may develop chronic tension-type headache which is difficult to treat.

Treatment is aimed at removing the underlying causes where these can be identified. Simple massage may help if muscle contraction is a prominent component of the pain. Non-opioid analgesics, such as aspirin or other NSAIDs and paracetamol, may be tried for individual acute attacks of headache, but analgesic overuse must be avoided as this can lead to chronic headache resistant to other measures (see Analgesic-induced Headache, above). Opioids alone or in combination preparations with other analgesics should also be avoided. Antidepressants, especially tricyclics, can also be effective, particularly in patients with chronic tension-type headache or in those with associated depression; addition of a beta blocker such as propranolol may sometimes be of benefit. Hypnotics or sedatives have sometimes been used in combination preparations with analgesics in the management of tension-type headache which disrupts sleep but because of the potential for abuse they should be avoided in chronic headaches. Muscle relaxants appear to have little place in the management of tension-type headache; although some patients may respond results are generally disappointing. Other drugs that have been tried include valproate.

References.

1. Clough C. Non-migrainous headaches: classification and management. *Br Med J* 1989; **299:** 70–2.
2. Olesen J, Schoenen J, eds. *Tension-type headache: classification, mechanisms, and treatment.* New York: Raven Press, 1993.
3. Silberstein SD. Tension-type and chronic daily headache. *Neurology* 1993; **43:** 1644–9.
4. Kumar KL, Cooney TG. Headaches. *Med Clin North Am* 1995; **79:** 261–86.

Almotriptan (18584-t)

Almotriptan *(BAN, rINN).*

LAS-31416. 1-[({3-[2-(Dimethylamino)ethyl]indol-5-yl}methyl)sulfonyl]pyrrolidine; Dimethyl {2-[5-(pyrrolidin-1-ylsulfonylmethyl)indol-3-yl]ethyl}amine.

$C_{17}H_{25}N_3O_2S$ = 335.5.

CAS — 154323-57-6.

Almotriptan is a selective serotonin ($5-HT_1$) agonist with actions similar to those of sumatriptan (p.450). It is under investigation for the acute treatment of migraine attacks and has been administered orally.

Alpiropride (11925-j)

Alpiropride *(rINN).*

(±)-*N*-[(1-Allyl-2-pyrrolidinyl)methyl]-4-amino-5-(methylsulfamoyl)-*o*-anisamide.

$C_{17}H_{26}N_4O_4S$ = 382.5.

CAS — 81982-32-3.

Alpiropride is a dopamine antagonist that has been given by mouth for the treatment and prophylaxis of migraine.

Preparations

Proprietary Preparations (details are given in Part 3)
Port.: Rivistel†.

Dihydroergotamine (11340-l)

Dihydroergotamine *(BAN, rINN).*

(5′*S*,8*R*)-5′-Benzyl-9,10-dihydro-12′-hydroxy-2′-methyl-3′,6′,18-trioxoergotaman.

$C_{33}H_{37}N_5O_5$ = 583.7.

CAS — 511-12-6.

Dihydroergotamine Mesylate (1504-d)

Dihydroergotamine Mesylate *(BANM, USAN).*

Dihydroergotamine Mesilate *(rINNM)*; Dihydroergotamine Methanesulphonate; Dihydroergotamini Mesilas. (5′*S*,8*R*)-5′-Benzyl-9,10-dihydro-12′-hydroxy-2′-methyl-3′,6′,18-trioxoergotaman methanesulphonate.

$C_{33}H_{37}N_5O_5,CH_4O_3S$ = 679.8.

CAS — 6190-39-2.

Pharmacopoeias. In *Eur.* (see p.viii), *Jpn, Pol.,* and *US.*

Colourless crystals or a white or almost white or faintly red crystalline powder, with a slight odour. **Soluble** 1 in 125 of water, 1 in 90 of alcohol, 1 in 175 of chloroform, and 1 in 2600 of ether; sparingly soluble in methyl alcohol. A 0.1% solution in water has a pH of 4.4 to 5.4. **Protect** from light.

Dihydroergotamine Tartrate (1505-n)

Dihydroergotamine Tartrate *(BANM, rINNM).*

Dihydroergotamini Tartras.

$(C_{33}H_{37}N_5O_5)_2,C_4H_6O_6$ = 1317.4.

CAS — 5989-77-5.

Pharmacopoeias. In *Eur.* (see p.viii).

Colourless crystals or a white or almost white crystalline powder. Very slightly **soluble** in water; sparingly soluble in alcohol. A 0.1% suspension in water has a pH of 4.0 to 5.5. **Protect** from light.

Adverse Effects and Treatment

As for Ergotamine Tartrate, p.445, although vasoconstriction may be less pronounced and the frequency of nausea and vomiting lower with dihydroergotamine mesylate than with ergotamine tartrate. Dihydroergotamine does not appear to produce physical dependence.

Effects on the cardiovascular system. There are conflicting reports on the risk of vasospasm in patients given dihydroergotamine with heparin for thrombo-embolism prophylaxis. Vasospastic or necrotic reactions have been reported on several occasions during such therapy.[1-4] In an Austrian study of 147 290 patients given drug prophylaxis for thrombo-embolism, complications attributable to ergotism were seen in 142 of 61 092 (0.23%) who received dihydroergotamine and heparin.[5] Schlag *et al.*,[6] however, observed only one case of vasospasm in 5100 trauma patients (0.02%) given the combination. In 1989 the Swedish Adverse Drug Reactions Advisory Committee reported[7] that up to the end of September 1987 the manufacturer had received 201 reports of vasospastic reactions associated with the use of Orstanorm (dihydroergotamine + lignocaine) with heparin. Permanent damage occurred in 59% of these patients. Vasospastic reactions had occurred more frequently in patients who had undergone surgery for trauma and the prognosis for such patients was generally poorer than for others. Since the risk of permanent damage appeared to be related to treatment length the Committee recommended that this preparation should not be given for more that 7 days. The possibility of such reactions and the contra-indications of dihydroergotamine should be borne in mind when employing this form of prophylaxis (see Venous Thrombo-embolism, under Uses, below).

1. van den Berg E, *et al.* Ergotism leading to threatened limb amputation or to death in two patients given heparin-dihydroergotamine prophylaxis. *Lancet* 1982; **i:** 955–6.
2. van den Berg E, *et al.* Vascular spasm during thromboembolism prophylaxis with heparin-dihydroergotamine. *Lancet* 1982; **ii:** 268–9.
3. Monreal M, *et al.* Skin and muscle necrosis during heparin-dihydroergotamine prophylaxis. *Lancet* 1984; **ii:** 820.
4. Kilroy RA, *et al.* Vascular spasm during heparin-dihydroergotamine prophylaxis. *Clin Pharm* 1987; **6:** 575–7.
5. Gatterer R. Ergotism as complication of thromboembolic prophylaxis with heparin and dihydroergotamine. *Lancet* 1986; **ii:** 638–9.
6. Schlag G, *et al.* Risk/benefit of heparin-dihydroergotamine thromboembolic prophylaxis. *Lancet* 1986; **ii:** 1465.
7. Swedish Adverse Drug Reaction Advisory Committee. Dihydroergotamine + lidocaine – vasospasm. *Bull Swed Adverse Drug React Advisory Committee* 1989; (54): 1.

Fibrosis. For reference to fibrosis associated with the administration of dihydroergotamine, see Methysergide Maleate, p.448.

Precautions

As for Ergotamine Tartrate, p.446.

Porphyria. Dihydroergotamine has been associated with acute attacks of porphyria and is considered unsafe in patients with acute porphyria.[1]

1. Moore MR, McColl KEL. *Porphyria: drug lists.* Glasgow: Porphyria Research Unit, University of Glasgow, 1991.

Interactions

Interactions involving those ergot alkaloids used primarily in the management of migraine are discussed under ergotamine (p.446). References specific to dihydroergotamine may be found there under the headings Antibacterials and Glyceryl Trinitrate.

Pharmacokinetics

Peak plasma-dihydroergotamine concentrations have been attained within about 2 to 3 hours after oral administration, about 30 minutes after intramuscular injection, about 15 to 45 minutes after subcutaneous injection, and about 55 minutes after administration by intranasal spray. However, the bioavailability of dihydroergotamine after oral administration is very low; values ranging from less than

0.1 to 1.5% have been reported. Although dihydroergotamine is incompletely absorbed from the gastro-intestinal tract, the low bioavailability is considered to be determined primarily by extensive first-pass hepatic metabolism.

Dihydroergotamine undergoes extensive metabolism, the major metabolite, 8′-hydroxydihydroergotamine, being pharmacologically active. Plasma concentrations of this metabolite are greater than those of dihydroergotamine. A further oxidation step produces 8′,10′-dihydroxydihydroergotamine which is also pharmacologically active. Other metabolites are also formed. Most of a dose is excreted as metabolites, mainly in the bile; 5 to 10% is excreted in the urine of which only trace amounts are of unchanged drug. The elimination of dihydroergotamine is biphasic; half-lives of about 1 to 2 hours and 22 to 32 hours have been reported for the 2 phases, respectively.

References.

1. Bobik A, *et al.* Low oral bioavailability of dihydroergotamine and first-pass extraction in patients with orthostatic hypotension. *Clin Pharmacol Ther* 1981; **30:** 673–9.
2. Little PJ, *et al.* Bioavailability of dihydroergotamine in man. *Br J Clin Pharmacol* 1982; **13:** 785–90.
3. Lindblad B, *et al.* The pharmacokinetics of subcutaneous dihydroergotamine with and without a dextran 70 infusion. *Eur J Clin Pharmacol* 1983; **24:** 813–18.
4. Maurer G, Frick W. Elucidation of the structure and receptor binding studies of the major primary, metabolite of dihydroergotamine in man. *Eur J Clin Pharmacol* 1984; **26:** 463–70.
5. Müller-Schweinitzer E. Pharmacological actions of the main metabolites of dihydroergotamine. *Eur J Clin Pharmacol* 1984; **26:** 699–705.
6. Aellig WH, Rosenthaler J. Venoconstrictor effects of dihydroergotamine after intranasal and intramuscular administration. *Eur J Clin Pharmacol* 1986; **30:** 581–4.
7. de Marées H, *et al.* Relationship between the venoconstrictor activity of dihydroergotamine and its pharmacokinetics during acute and chronic oral dosing. *Eur J Clin Pharmacol* 1986; **30:** 685–9.
8. Humbert H, *et al.* Human pharmacokinetics of dihydroergotamine administered by nasal spray. *Clin Pharmacol Ther* 1996; **60:** 265–75.

Uses and Administration

Dihydroergotamine is a semisynthetic ergot alkaloid that has weaker oxytocic and vasoconstrictor effects than ergotamine (p.447). It is used in the treatment of migraine and cluster headache, and in the treatment of orthostatic hypotension. It has also been used for the prophylaxis of venous thrombo-embolism.

Dihydroergotamine is commonly used as the mesylate and is usually given by subcutaneous, intramuscular, or intravenous injection although it may be given as a nasal spray or by mouth.

For the treatment of migraine and to terminate an acute attack of cluster headache, dihydroergotamine mesylate is usually given by subcutaneous or intramuscular injection in doses of 1 mg repeated, if necessary, after 30 to 60 minutes up to a maximum daily dose of 3 mg. If a more rapid effect is desired it may be administered intravenously in doses of 0.5 mg up to a maximum daily dose of 2 mg. The total weekly dose given by any route of injection should not exceed 6 mg. The usual nasal dose of dihydroergotamine mesylate for an acute attack of migraine is 0.5 mg sprayed into each nostril as a 0.4% solution followed after 15 minutes by an additional 0.5-mg dose in each nostril. A total intranasal dose of 2 mg per attack, or 3 to 4 mg in a 24-hour period, or 12 mg in a 7-day period should not be exceeded. In some countries it is given by mouth; up to 10 mg daily has been given by mouth for the treatment of acute attacks of migraine. Lower oral doses have been given in some countries for migraine prophylaxis.

Dihydroergotamine mesylate has also been used alone or with etilefrine hydrochloride (p.867) in the treatment of orthostatic hypotension in usual doses of up to 10 mg daily by mouth in divided doses.

Dihydroergotamine mesylate has been used in conjunction with a low-dose heparin regimen in the prophylaxis of postoperative venous thrombo-embolism. A suggested dose is dihydroergotamine mesylate 500 μg with heparin 5000 units, both given subcutaneously 1 to 2 hours before surgery. This regimen has then been given every 8 to 12 hours for 5 to 14 days depending on the risk of thrombosis, but see below.

Dihydroergotamine tartrate has been used for indications similar to those of the mesylate.

Analgesic-induced headache. Dihydroergotamine may be used in the treatment of analgesic-induced headache (p.443), including symptoms of ergotamine withdrawal.

Migraine and cluster headache. Sumatriptan is often the treatment of choice to abort acute attacks of migraine (p.443) that do not respond to simple analgesic preparations; parenteral dihydroergotamine is an alternative for patients who develop severe or refractory migraine.[1,2] Dihydroergotamine is used similarly in the treatment of cluster headache (p.443) where it is given to abort individual headache attacks. Although dihydroergotamine is usually given by injection, in some countries preparations for oral or intranasal[3,4] administration are also available. In a comparative study, relief of migraine was slower after subcutaneous dihydroergotamine than after subcutaneous sumatriptan, but headache recurred less often.[5] In another study, intranasal dihydroergotamine was not as effective as subcutaneous sumatriptan.[4]

1. Scott AK. Dihydroergotamine: a review of its use in the treatment of migraine and other headaches. *Clin Neuropharmacol* 1992; **15:** 289–96.
2. Silberstein SD, Young WB. Safety and efficacy of ergotamine tartrate and dihydroergotamine in the treatment of migraine and status migrainosus. *Neurology* 1995; **45:** 577–84.
3. Ziegler D, *et al.* Dihydroergotamine nasal spray for the acute treatment of migraine. *Neurology* 1994; **44:** 447–53.
4. Touchon J, *et al.* A comparison of subcutaneous sumatriptan and dihydroergotamine nasal spray in the acute treatment of migraine. *Neurology* 1996; **47:** 361–5.
5. Winner P, *et al.* A double-blind study of subcutaneous dihydroergotamine vs subcutaneous sumatriptan in the treatment of acute migraine. *Arch Neurol* 1996; **53:** 180–4.

Orthostatic hypotension. Dihydroergotamine might be of use in patients with orthostatic hypotension (p.1040) resistant to the usual treatment. It is sometimes administered in preparations with sympathomimetics such as etilefrine. After parenteral administration of dihydroergotamine, standing blood pressure is increased, but total peripheral resistance and supine blood pressure are also increased indicating that its action is not entirely restricted to capacitance vessels.[1] It does not prevent postprandial hypotension, presumably because it does not constrict the splanchnic veins, although the administration of caffeine with dihydroergotamine may overcome this problem. The main disadvantage of dihydroergotamine, however, is that it is ineffective, or at best weakly effective, when given by mouth although there has been some evidence that oral ergotamine tartrate may be of value.

Dihydroergotamine has been suggested for use in the prevention of hypotension associated with epidural anaesthesia,[2] the usual management of which is discussed under Overdosage, Local Anaesthetics, on p.1282. It has also been tried in the management of hypotension associated with haemodialysis.[3]

1. Anonymous. Management of orthostatic hypotension. *Lancet* 1987; **i:** 197–8.
2. Mattila M, *et al.* Dihydroergotamine in the prevention of hypotension associated with extradural anaesthesia. *Br J Anaesth* 1985; **57:** 976–82.
3. Milutinovic S. Dihydroergotamin in der behandlung von patienten mit symptomatischer hypotonie während dauerhämodialyse. *Arzneimittelforschung* 1987; **37:** 554–6.

Venous thrombo-embolism. Standard prophylaxis for surgical patients at high risk of venous thrombo-embolism is usually with heparin (p.802). Dihydroergotamine can reduce venous stasis by vasoconstriction of capacitance vessels and has enhanced postoperative prophylaxis when used in association with heparin. A review[1] of studies of thrombo-embolism prophylaxis found that the addition of dihydroergotamine to heparin further reduced the incidence of deep-vein thrombosis and of fatal pulmonary embolism compared with heparin alone in patients undergoing elective orthopaedic surgery. In studies in traumatic orthopaedic surgery the rates of deep-vein thrombosis were reduced to a similar level with either mode of prophylaxis; however, these studies involved only a small number of patients. Some workers have investigated the use of dihydroergotamine with low-molecular-weight heparin fractions. In a study involving 260 patients undergoing abdominal surgery[2] and one involving 146 patients undergoing total hip replacement[3] this combination was demonstrated to be of similar efficacy to dihydroergotamine with heparin but might offer a more convenient dosing schedule. However, although dihydroergotamine might enhance the effect of heparin, a US National Institutes of Health consensus conference warned of the potential risk associated with its vasoconstrictive effects, and the contra-indications to its use.[4] In 1989 the Swedish Adverse Drug Reactions Advisory Committee recommended that dihydroergotamine with heparin should not be given for more than 7 days (see Effects on the Cardiovascular System, under Adverse Effects, above).

1. Lindblad B. Prophylaxis of postoperative thromboembolism with low dose heparin alone or in combination with dihydroergotamine: a review. *Acta Chir Scand* 1988; (suppl 543): 31–42.
2. Sasahara AA, *et al.* Low molecular weight heparin plus dihydroergotamine for prophylaxis of postoperative deep vein thrombosis. *Br J Surg* 1986; **73:** 697–700.
3. Haas S, *et al.* Prophylaxis of deep vein thrombosis in high risk patients undergoing total hip replacement with low molecular weight heparin plus dihydroergotamine. *Arzneimittelforschung* 1987; **37:** 839–43.
4. Consensus conference. Prevention of venous thrombosis and pulmonary embolism. *JAMA* 1986; **256:** 744–9.

Preparations

USP 23: Dihydroergotamine Mesylate Injection.

Proprietary Preparations (details are given in Part 3)
Aust.: Adhaegon; Detemes; Dihydergot; Divegal; Ergont; Ergovasan; ***Austral.:*** Dihydergot; ***Belg.:*** Dihydergot; Ikaran; ***Fr.:*** Dergiflux†; Dergotamine†; Ikaran; Seglor; Tamik; ***Ger.:*** Agit; Angionorm; Clavigrenin; DET MS; DET MS spezial; Dihydergot; Dihytamin; Endophleban; Ergomimet; Ergont; Ergotam; Tonopres; Verladyn; ***Ital.:*** Diidergot; Ikaran; Migranal; Seglor; ***Neth.:*** Dihydergot; ***S.Afr.:*** Dihydergot; ***Spain:*** Dihydergot; Tenuatina; ***Swed.:*** Orstanorm; ***Switz.:*** Dihydergot; Ergont†; Ergotonine; Ikaran; ***UK:*** Dihydergot†; Migranal; ***USA:*** DHE 45; Migranal.

Multi-ingredient: ***Aust.:*** Agilan; Cedanon; Defluina; Dihydergot; Effortil comp; Embolex; Hypodyn; Tonopan; Troparin compositum; Veno; Venotop; ***Belg.:*** Diergo; ***Fr.:*** Diergo; ***Ger.:*** Agit plus; Ansudoral†; Dihydergot plus; Effortil plus; Embolex NM; Ergo-Lonarid PD; Ergo-Lonarid†; Ergodystan†; Ergolefrin; Ergomimet plus; Optalidon special Noc; Venelbin; ***Norw.:*** Dihydergot; ***Spain:*** Tonopan; ***Swed.:*** Orstanorm med heparin†; ***Switz.:*** Addergit†; Dihydergot; Dihydergot plus; Effortil plus; Embolex LM†; Silentan†; Tonopan.

Eletriptan (18395-j)

Eletriptan *(BAN, rINN)*.

UK-116044. (*R*)-2-[3-(1-Methylpyrrolidin-2-ylmethyl)indol-5-yl]ethyl phenyl sulfone.

$C_{22}H_{26}N_2O_2S$ = 382.5.

CAS — 143322-58-1.

Eletriptan is a selective serotonin (5-HT_1) agonist with actions similar to those of sumatriptan (p.450). It is under investigation for the acute treatment of migraine attacks and has been given orally.

Ergotamine Tartrate (1508-b)

Ergotamine Tartrate *(BANM, rINNM)*.

Ergotamini Tartras; Ergotaminii Tartras. (5′*S*)-12′-Hydroxy-2′-methyl-5′-benzylergotaman-3′,6′,18-trione tartrate; (5′*S*)-12′-Hydroxy-2′-methyl-3′,6′,18-trioxo-5-benzylergotaman (+)-tartrate.

$(C_{33}H_{35}N_5O_5)_2,C_4H_6O_6$ = 1313.4.

CAS — 113-15-5 (ergotamine); 379-79-3 (ergotamine tartrate).

Pharmacopoeias. In *Chin., Eur.* (see p.viii), *Int., Jpn, Pol.,* and *US.*

Slightly hygroscopic colourless odourless crystals or a white or yellowish-white crystalline powder. It may contain 2 molecules of methanol of crystallisation. **Soluble** 1 in about 3200 of water, but soluble 1 in about 500 of water in the presence of a slight excess of tartaric acid; soluble 1 in 500 of alcohol; practically insoluble in ether. A 0.25% suspension in water has a pH of 4.0 to 5.5. **Store** in airtight glass containers at a temperature of 2° to 8°. Protect from light.

Stability in solution. References.

1. Kreilgård B, Kisbye J. Stability of ergotamine tartrate in aqueous solution. *Arch Pharm Chemi (Sci)* 1974; **2:** 1–13 and 38–49.

Adverse Effects

The adverse effects of ergotamine may be attributed either to its effects on the CNS, or to vasoconstriction of blood vessels and possible thrombi formation.

After therapeutic doses nausea and vomiting commonly occur as a result of the direct emetogenic effect of ergotamine; some patients may also experience abdominal pain. Weakness and muscle pains in the extremities and numbness and tingling of the fingers and toes may occur. There may occasionally be localised oedema and itching in hypersensitive patients. Treatment should be stopped if symptoms of vasoconstriction develop. Susceptible patients, especially those with severe infections, liver disease, kidney disease, or occlusive peripheral vascular disease, may show signs of acute or chronic poisoning with normal doses of ergotamine.

Symptoms of acute overdosage include nausea, vomiting, diarrhoea, extreme thirst, coldness, tingling, and itching of the skin, a rapid and weak pulse, hypotension, shock, confusion, convulsions, and unconsciousness; fatalities have been reported. Further symptoms of peripheral vasoconstriction or of cardiovascular disturbances, as seen in chronic ergotamine poisoning, may also occur but be delayed.

In chronic poisoning or ergotism, resulting from therapeutic overdosage or the use of ergotamine in susceptible patients, severe circulatory disturbances may develop. The extremities, especially the feet and legs, become numb, cold, tingling, and pale or cyanotic, with muscle pain; there may be no pulse in the affected limb. Eventually gangrene develops in the toes and sometimes the fingers. Anginal pain, tachycardia or bradycardia, and hypertension or hypotension have been reported. Myocardial infarction has occurred rarely. Pleural and peritoneal fibrosis may occur with excessive use. Chronic, intractable headache (rebound headache) may occur and is also a major withdrawal symptom following the development of ergotamine dependence (see under Precautions, below). Other adverse effects include confusion and convulsions. On rare occasions symptoms of vasoconstriction of blood vessels in the brain, eye, intestines, and kidneys occur. Anorectal ulceration sometimes leading to rectal necrosis and stenosis has been reported after excessive use of suppositories containing ergotamine.

Effects on the cardiovascular system. Reports of adverse cardiovascular effects associated with ergotamine, including mention of fatalities.

1. Joyce DA, Gubbay SS. Arterial complications of migraine treatment with methysergide and parenteral ergotamine. *Br Med J* 1982; **285:** 260–1.
2. Corrocher R, *et al.* Multiple arterial stenoses in chronic ergot toxicity. *N Engl J Med* 1984; **310:** 261.
3. Fisher PE, *et al.* Ergotamine abuse and extra-hepatic portal hypertension. *Postgrad Med J* 1985; **61:** 461–3.
4. Deviere J, *et al.* Ischemic pancreatitis and hepatitis secondary to ergotamine poisoning. *J Clin Gastroenterol* 1987; **9:** 350–2.
5. Galer BS, *et al.* Myocardial ischemia related to ergot alkaloids: a case report and literature review. *Headache* 1991; **31:** 446–50.
6. Redfield MM, *et al.* Valve disease associated with ergot alkaloid use: echocardiographic and pathologic correlations. *Ann Intern Med* 1992; **117:** 50–2.
7. Lazarides MK, *et al.* Severe facial ischaemia caused by ergotism. *J Cardiovasc Surg* 1992; **33:** 383–5.
8. Hillis W, MacIntyre PD. Drug reactions: sumatriptan and chest pain. *Lancet* 1993; **341:** 1564–5. Correction. *ibid.*; **342:** 1310.

Fibrosis. For reference to fibrosis associated with the administration of ergotamine tartrate, see Methysergide Maleate, p.448.

Treatment of Adverse Effects

Treatment of acute poisoning with ergotamine is symptomatic. Following recent ingestion the stomach should be emptied by lavage or emesis; activated charcoal may be used to reduce absorption. In chronic poisoning, withdrawal of ergotamine may be all that is required in some patients.

In both acute and chronic poisoning, attempts must be made to maintain an adequate circulation to the affected parts in order to prevent the onset of gangrene. In severe arterial vasospasm vasodilators such as sodium nitroprusside by intravenous infusion have been given; heparin and dextran 40 have also been advocated to minimise the risk of thrombosis. Analgesics may be required for severe ischaemic pain.

Sodium nitroprusside has been administered in severe ergotamine poisoning for its vasodilating and hypotensive actions; it should therefore be used with care if hypotension is a symptom of poisoning. It is usually given by intravenous infusion[1-4] although there have also been reports of intra-arterial infusion for ergotamine-induced ischaemia;[5,6] for details of precautions to be observed, see p.944.

Many other drugs have been used in the treatment of circulatory disturbances induced by ergotamine. These include captopril by mouth[7] and alprostadil by intra-arterial infusion.[8,9]

For reference to the ergotamine withdrawal syndrome see Dependence under Precautions, below.

1. Carliner NH, *et al.* Sodium nitroprusside treatment of ergotamine-induced peripheral ischemia. *JAMA* 1974; **277:** 308–9.
2. Andersen PK, *et al.* Sodium nitroprusside and epidural blockade in the treatment of ergotism. *N Engl J Med* 1977; **296:** 1271–3.
3. Eurin B, *et al.* Ergot and sodium nitroprusside. *N Engl J Med* 1978; **298:** 632–3.
4. Carr P. Self-induced myocardial infarction. *Postgrad Med J* 1981; **57:** 654–5.
5. O'Dell CW, *et al.* Sodium nitroprusside in the treatment of ergotism. *Radiology* 1977; **124:** 73–4.
6. Whitsett TL, *et al.* Nitroprusside reversal of ergotamine-induced ischemia. *Am Heart J* 1978; **96:** 700.
7. Zimran A, *et al.* Treatment with captopril for peripheral ischaemia induced by ergotamine. *Br Med J* 1984; **288:** 364.
8. Levy JM, *et al.* Prostaglandin E_1 for alleviating symptoms of ergot intoxication: a case report. *Cardiovasc Intervent Radiol* 1984; **7:** 28–30.
9. Horstmann R, *et al.* Kritische extremitätenischämie durch ergotismus: behandlung mit intraarterieller prostaglandin-E_1-infusion. *Dtsch Med Wochenschr* 1993; **118:** 1067–71.

Precautions

Ergotamine tartrate is contra-indicated in patients with severe or uncontrolled hypertension, severe or persistent sepsis, peripheral vascular disease, ischaemic heart disease, hyperthyroidism, or impaired hepatic or renal function. Ergotamine tartrate should be administered with care to patients with anaemia. It is contra-indicated in pregnancy because of its oxytocic effect (see also below). Ergotamine tartrate should be avoided in nursing mothers; the distribution of unchanged drug and metabolites into breast milk presents a risk of ergotism in the infant and repeated doses of ergotamine may impair lactation.

Patients should be warned to keep within the recommended dosage. Ergotamine dependence has occurred following regular use of ergotamine tartrate even if dosage recommendations are adhered to (see below). Some symptoms of overdosage may mimic those of migraine. Numbness or tingling of the extremities generally indicates that ergotamine should be discontinued. Ergotamine should not be administered prophylactically, as prolonged use may give rise to gangrene.

Dependence. Ergotamine dependence can develop insidiously when ergotamine tartrate is used for more than 2 days a week, even if total daily or weekly dosage recommendations are observed.[1] Individual reports indicate a state of addiction characterised by a predictable and irresistible pattern of drug usage, the development of tolerance to adverse effects, and a syndrome of withdrawal on discontinuing the drug. Ergotamine-dependent patients suffer from daily, or almost daily, migraine headaches, often referred to as 'analgesic-induced headaches' or 'rebound headaches', which are only alleviated by ergotamine. An intensifying headache in association with autonomic disturbances occurs within 24 to 48 hours of withdrawal of ergotamine and may continue for 72 hours or longer. As with other analgesic-induced headaches (p.443), supportive and symptomatic measures should be taken to treat the withdrawal syndrome.

1. Saper JR. Ergotamine dependency—a review. *Headache* 1987; **27:** 435–8.

Porphyria. Ergotamine tartrate has been associated with clinical exacerbations of porphyria and is considered unsafe in porphyric patients.[1]

1. Moore MR, McColl KEL. *Porphyria: drug lists.* Glasgow: Porphyria Research Unit, University of Glasgow, 1991.

Pregnancy. Ergotamine is contra-indicated in pregnancy because of its oxytocic effect. Jejunal atresia has been reported[1] in an infant born prematurely to a woman who had taken ergotamine tartrate 6 to 8 mg daily, as Cafergot tablets, throughout her pregnancy.

Accidental administration of ergotamine 2 mg in the form of a Cafergot suppository to a patient at 39 weeks of pregnancy caused uterine contractions and fetal tachycardia.[2] An emergency caesarean section was undertaken because of suspected placental abruption but no clear signs of retroplacental haemorrhage were found. The neonate recovered quickly after delivery and had developed normally during the next 10 years.

1. Graham JM, *et al.* Jejunal atresia associated with Cafergot ingestion during pregnancy. *Clin Pediatr (Phila)* 1983; **22:** 226–8.
2. de Groot ANJA, *et al.* Ergotamine-induced fetal stress: review of side effects of ergot alkaloids during pregnancy. *Eur J Obstet Gynecol Reprod Biol* 1993; **51:** 73–7.

Interactions

The vasoconstrictor effects of ergotamine are enhanced by sympathomimetics such as adrenaline. There is also an increased risk of peripheral vasoconstriction during concomitant administration of ergotamine and beta blockers. Administration of ergotamine with a macrolide antibiotic such as erythromycin has produced ergotism. Ergotamine should not be given until at least 6 hours after stopping a serotonin (5-HT_1) agonist such as sumatriptan, since there is an additional risk of prolonged vasospastic reactions (see also p.451).

Antibacterials. Acute reactions ranging from minor ergotism[1] to severe vasospasm[2] have been reported in patients given erythromycin in addition to ergotamine. There is also a report of acute ergotism in 2 patients receiving ergotamine tartrate and triacetyloleandomycin.[3] The theoretical possibility exists that there may be a similar interaction with azithromycin. Ergotism has also been reported in patients receiving erythromycin[4] or triacetyloleandomycin[5] in conjunction with dihydroergotamine.

1. Lagier G, *et al.* Un cas d'ergotisme mineur semblant en rapport avec une potentialisation de l'ergotamine par l'éthylsuccinate d'érythromycine. *Therapie* 1979; **34:** 515–21.
2. Ghali R, *et al.* Erythromycin-associated ergotamine intoxication: arteriographic and electrophysiologic analysis of a rare cause of severe ischemia of the lower extremities and associated ischemic neuropathy. *Ann Vasc Surg* 1993; **7:** 291–6.
3. Matthews NT, Havill JH. Ergotism with therapeutic doses of ergotamine tartrate. *N Z Med J* 1979; **89:** 476–7.
4. Leroy F, *et al.* Dihydroergotamine-erythromycin-induced ergotism. *Ann Intern Med* 1988; **109:** 249.
5. Franco A, *et al.* Ergotisme aigu par association dihydroergotamine-triacétyloléandomycine. *Nouv Presse Med* 1978; **7:** 205.

Antimigraine drugs. Arterial occlusion has been reported[1] in 2 patients taking methysergide and a high parenteral dosage of ergotamine concomitantly for cluster headache; the combination should be avoided.

For a report of gangrene in a patient taking propranolol and methysergide, see below. See also above for a comment on the risk of vasospastic reactions with serotonin (5-HT_1) agonists such as sumatriptan.

1. Joyce DA, Gubbay SS. Arterial complications of migraine treatment with methysergide and parenteral ergotamine. *Br Med J* 1982; **285:** 260–1.

Antivirals. Ergotism developed in a patient receiving treatment with ergotamine after combination antiviral treatment was started for HIV infection.[1] Symptoms initially resolved after both ritonavir and ergotamine were withdrawn and it was suggested that the ergotism might have been caused by inhibition of ergotamine metabolism by ritonavir.

1. Caballero-Granado FJ, *et al.* Ergotism related to concurrent administration of ergotamine tartrate and ritonavir in an AIDS patient. *Antimicrob Agents Chemother* 1997; **41:** 1207.

Beta blockers. Peripheral vasoconstriction was reported in a patient with migraine after addition of propranolol to regular use of Cafergot suppositories twice daily.[1] This combination has been used without complication by other workers who suggested that ergotism caused by excessive dosage of ergotamine tartrate, rather than an interaction between ergotamine and propranolol, was responsible.[2] However, arterial vasoconstriction has been reported after concomitant use of methysergide and propranolol and of oxprenolol and ergotamine.[3] Such combinations should therefore be used with caution.

1. Baumrucker JF. Drug interaction—propranolol and Cafergot. *N Engl J Med* 1973; **288:** 916–17.
2. Diamond S. Propranolol and ergotamine tartrate. *N Engl J Med* 1973; **289:** 159.
3. Venter CP, *et al.* Severe peripheral ischaemia during concomitant use of beta blockers and ergot alkaloids. *Br Med J* 1984; **289:** 288–9.

Glyceryl trinitrate. Glyceryl trinitrate has been reported to increase the oral bioavailability and plasma concentrations of dihydroergotamine in patients with orthostatic hypotension.[1]

1. Bobik A, *et al.* Low oral bioavailability of dihydroergotamine and first-pass extraction in patients with orthostatic hypotension. *Clin Pharmacol Ther* 1981; **30:** 673–9.

Tacrolimus. Ergotamine may inhibit the metabolism of tacrolimus (see p.563).

Pharmacokinetics

Absorption from the gastro-intestinal tract after administration by mouth is poor and may be further decreased by the occurrence of gastric stasis during migraine attacks. Bioavailability of ergotamine is also diminished by a high first-pass hepatic metabolism. Ergotamine has been given rectally or by inhalation in an attempt to overcome these effects with some improvement in rate and/or extent of absorption but bioavailability is still of the order of 5% or less. Absorption of sublingual ergotamine is very poor. There is considerable interindividual variation in the bioavailability of ergotamine, regardless of the route of administration. Caffeine is sometimes included in oral and rectal preparations of ergotamine with the intention of improving the latter's absorption, although whether it does so is not clear. Drugs such as metoclopramide are sometimes given with the aim of alleviating gastric stasis to improve absorption of ergotamine.

Ergotamine is metabolised extensively in the liver, the majority of metabolites being excreted in the bile. About 4% of a dose is excreted in the urine. Ergotamine or its metabolites have been detected in breast milk. Some of the metabolites are pharmacologically active. The elimination of ergotamine is biphasic; half-lives of about 2 hours and 21 hours have been reported for the 2 phases respectively.

References.

1. Schmidt R, Fanchamps A. Effect of caffeine on intestinal absorption of ergotamine in man. *Eur J Clin Pharmacol* 1974; **7:** 213–16.
2. Eadie MJ. Ergotamine pharmacokinetics in man: an editorial. *Cephalalgia* 1983; **3:** 135–8.
3. Perrin VL. Clinical pharmacokinetics of ergotamine in migraine and cluster headache. *Clin Pharmacokinet* 1985; **10:** 334–52.

Uses and Administration

Ergotamine is an alkaloid derived from ergot (p.1576). It has marked vasoconstrictor effects; it also has a powerful oxytocic action on the uterus, although less so than ergometrine (p.1575). It is used in migraine and cluster headache, and has been tried in orthostatic hypotension.

Ergotamine is commonly used as the tartrate. It is usually given by mouth, but has also been given sublingually, rectally, and by oral inhalation. It was formerly given by subcutaneous or intramuscular injection. Caffeine is sometimes given with ergotamine tartrate with the intention of improving the latter's absorption, although whether it does so is not clear. Antiemetics such as cyclizine hydrochloride are sometimes included in combination preparations with ergotamine tartrate.

Ergotamine is used in migraine unresponsive to non-opioid analgesics. However, its adverse effects limit how much it can be used and prevent its use for prophylaxis. It is most effective when administered as early as possible in a migraine attack, preferably during the prodromal phase.

The usual dose is 1 to 2 mg of ergotamine tartrate by mouth, repeated, if necessary, half an hour later. Usually not more than 6 mg should be administered in 24 hours, although some manufacturers recommend not more than 4 mg in 24 hours and others not more than 8 mg per attack. The recommended minimum interval between successive 24-hour courses is 4 days, with the additional restriction of the total weekly dose being limited to a maximum of 12 mg, although some manufacturers recommend a lower weekly limit of 8 mg. It is also recommended that patients should receive no more than 2 courses per month. Similar doses may be administered sublingually.

Ergotamine tartrate may also be administered rectally as suppositories, especially if the oral route is not effective or not practicable. The rectal dose of ergotamine tartrate is 2 mg repeated, if necessary, one hour later. Usually, not more than 4 mg should be administered in 24 hours and not more than 8 mg in a week with an interval of at least 4 days between successive 24-hour courses.

A more rapid onset of action may be achieved by oral inhalation. One dose containing 360 µg of ergotamine tartrate may be inhaled at the onset of the attack and repeated, if necessary, at 5-minute intervals. Not more than 6 inhalation doses should be taken in 24 hours and not more than 12 in a week with an interval of at least 4 days between successive 24-hour courses.

Ergotamine is used in patients with cluster headache to treat individual attacks of headache but since such attacks are short-lived oral inhalation may be preferable to oral, sublingual, or rectal routes. Doses used are similar to those given to treat migraine. It has also been used to prevent headache attacks during cluster periods, when it is usually given daily in low doses for up to 2 weeks, either by mouth or rectally (see below).

Migraine and cluster headache. Ergotamine was formerly one of the main drugs used to treat acute attacks of migraine (p.443) unresponsive to antimigraine preparations containing non-opioid analgesics, but serotonin (5-HT_1) agonists such as sumatriptan are now preferred. Since ergotamine may exacerbate the nausea and vomiting that commonly develops as a migraine attack progresses it is often necessary to give an antiemetic as well. Poor oral bioavailability may be reduced further during a migraine attack and ergotamine has sometimes been given sublingually, rectally, or by inhalation. Adverse effects limit how much ergotamine can be used for an individual attack and prevent the long-term use that would be required for migraine prophylaxis.

Ergotamine may be used similarly in cluster headache (p.443) to treat individual headaches during a cluster period. Since such attacks are short-lived administration by oral inhalation may be more effective than other routes. Ergotamine is also used in low doses given by mouth or rectally for limited periods of up to 2 weeks in the prophylaxis of cluster headache during a cluster period. Regimens that have been tried for such prophylaxis include 1 to 2 mg of ergotamine tartrate given 1 to 2 hours before an expected attack or 1 to 2 hours before bedtime for nocturnal attacks. The total maximum dose of ergotamine tartrate that may be given weekly for the prevention of cluster headache is less well established than for the treatment of migraine. Ergotamine is often given for only 5 to 6 days in each week, which allows the patient to assess whether the cluster period has ended.

References.

1. Silberstein SD, Young WB. Safety and efficacy of ergotamine tartrate and dihydroergotamine in the treatment of migraine and status migrainosus. *Neurology* 1995; **45:** 577–84.

Orthostatic hypotension. Ergotamine and dihydroergotamine might be of use in patients with orthostatic hypotension resistant to the more usual treatment (see p.1040). Ergotamine is believed[1] to be less selective than dihydroergotamine (p.445) in its actions and affects both venous capacitance and peripheral resistance.[2,3] However, the oral bioavailability of ergotamine is greater[2] than that of dihydroergotamine and there have also been some reports of successful treatment with inhaled ergotamine.[3,4]

1. Anonymous. Management of orthostatic hypotension. *Lancet* 1987; **i:** 197–8.
2. Ahmad RAS, Watson RDS. Treatment of postural hypotension: a review. *Drugs* 1990; **39:** 74–85.
3. Tonkin AL, Wing LMH. Hypotension: assessment and management. *Med J Aust* 1990; **153:** 474–85.
4. Stumpf JL, Mitrzyk B. Management of orthostatic hypotension. *Am J Hosp Pharm* 1994; **51:** 648–60.

Preparations

BP 1998: Ergotamine Injection;
USP 23: Ergotamine Tartrate and Caffeine Suppositories; Ergotamine Tartrate and Caffeine Tablets; Ergotamine Tartrate Inhalation Aerosol; Ergotamine Tartrate Injection; Ergotamine Tartrate Tablets.

Proprietary Preparations (details are given in Part 3)
Aust.: Ergokapton; Ergotartrat†; ***Austral.:*** Ergodryl Mono; ***Canad.:*** Ergomar; Gynergen†; Medihaler-Ergotamine†; ***Ger.:*** Clavigrenin akut†; ergo sanol SL†; ergo sanol spezial N; Ergo-Kranit mono; Gynergen†; Migrexa; ***Irl.:*** Lingraine; ***Ital.:*** Ergotan; Gynergen†; ***S.Afr.:*** Ergate†; ***Spain:*** Gynergeno†; ***Switz.:*** Ergosanol SL†; ***UK:*** Lingraine; Medihaler-Ergotamine; ***USA:*** Ergomar; Ergostat†.

Multi-ingredient: ***Aust.:*** Avamigran; Cafergot; Lenticor†; Medium†; Migril; Pansecoff; Synkapton; ***Austral.:*** Cafergot; Ergodryl; Migral; ***Belg.:*** Cafergot; Cafergot-PB†; Dystonal; Migril†; ***Canad.:*** Bellergal; Cafergot; Cafergot-PB; Ergodryl; Gravergol; Megral; Wigraine; ***Fr.:*** Gynergene Cafeine; Migwell; ***Ger.:*** Avamigran N; bella sanol†; Bellaravil-retard†; Bellergal†; Cafergot N; Celetil†; Circovegetalin compositum†; ergo sanol spezial†; ergo sanol†; Ergo-Kranit; Ergoffin; Migrane-Kranit spezial N†; Migranex spezial N†; Migratan S; Praecimal†; Regium†; ***Irl.:*** Cafergot; Migranat; Migril; ***Ital.:*** Bellergil; Cafergot; Distonium†; Virdex; ***Neth.:*** Cafergot; Migril†; Neo-Cranimal†; ***Norw.:*** Anervan; Cafergot; Cafergot Comp; ***S.Afr.:*** Bellergal; Cafergot; Cafergot-PB; Migril; ***Spain:*** Bellergal†; Cafergot; Cafergot-PB; Distovagal; Hemicraneal; Igril; ***Swed.:*** Anervan; Cafergot; ***Switz.:*** Bellagotin; Bellergal; Cafergot; Cafergot-PB; Ergosanol; Ergosanol a la cafeine; Ergosanol special; Ergosanol special a la cafeine; Migrexa; Migril; ***UK:*** Cafergot; Migril; ***USA:*** Bel-Phen-Ergot S; Bellergal-S; Cafatine; Cafatine-PB; Cafergot; Cafetrate; Ercaf; Folergot-DF; Migergot; Phenerbel-S; Wigraine.

Feverfew (16808-m)

Camomille (Grande); Tanaceti Parthenii Herba.

Pharmacopoeias. In *Fr.* Also in *USNF* which also describes Powdered Feverfew.

The leaves of the plant *Tanacetum parthenium* (*Chrysanthemum parthenium*) (Compositae), collected when the plant is in flower. **Protect** from light.

Adverse Effects and Precautions

Mouth ulceration and soreness have been reported following ingestion of feverfew, and may be due to sensitisation; if they occur feverfew should be discontinued. Contact dermatitis has been reported. Feverfew is reputed to have abortifacient properties and the manufacturer cautions against use in pregnancy.

Uses and Administration

Feverfew is a traditional herbal remedy used in the prophylactic treatment of migraine. Its effects have been attributed to the plant's content of sesquiterpene lactones, notably parthenolide. A preparation of the dried leaf powder, which has been standardised to provide a minimum of 0.2% parthenolide, is available in some countries. A suggested dose is 125 or 250 mg daily by mouth.

Migraine. Feverfew is a traditional herbal remedy used in the management of migraine (p.443).[1] Two double-blind studies have shown that standardised preparations of the freeze-dried powdered leaf are effective in preventing or ameliorating migraine attacks,[2,3] whereas a third did not.[4]

1. Berry M. Feverfew. *Pharm J* 1994; **253:** 806–8.
2. Johnson ES, *et al.* Efficacy of feverfew as prophylactic treatment of migraine. *Br Med J* 1985; **291:** 569–73.
3. Murphy JJ, *et al.* Randomised double-blind placebo controlled trial of feverfew in migraine prevention. *Lancet* 1988; **ii:** 189–92.
4. de Weerdt CJ, *et al.* Herbal medicines in migraine prevention: randomized double-blind placebo-controlled crossover trial of a feverfew preparation. *Phytomedicine* 1996; **3:** 225–30.

Rheumatoid arthritis. Although it has anti-inflammatory activity *in vitro*, feverfew was found to be ineffective in rheumatoid arthritis (p.2).[1]

1. Pattrick M, *et al.* Feverfew in rheumatoid arthritis: a double blind, placebo controlled study. *Ann Rheum Dis* 1989; **48:** 547–9.

Preparations

Proprietary Preparations (details are given in Part 3)
Austral.: Herbal Headache Relief; ***Canad.:*** Tanacet; ***Switz.:*** Partenelle†; ***UK:*** Tanacet.

Multi-ingredient: ***Ger.:*** Presselin Stoffwechseltee†.

Frovatriptan (1885-g)

Frovatriptan *(BAN, rINN)*.

SB-209509AX; VML-251. (6*R*)-5,6,7,8-Tetrahydro-6-methylaminocarbazole-3-carboxamide.

$C_{14}H_{17}N_3O = 243.3.$

CAS — 158747-02-5 (frovatriptan); 158930-17-7 (frovatriptan succinate monohydrate).

Frovatriptan is a serotonin (5-HT_1) agonist with actions similar to those of sumatriptan (p.450). It is under investigation for the acute treatment of migraine attacks.

Isometheptene Hydrochloride (2072-d)

Isometheptene Hydrochloride *(BANM, rINNM)*.

1,5,*N*-Trimethylhex-4-enylamine hydrochloride; 1,5-Dimethylhex-4-enyl(methyl)amine hydrochloride.

$C_9H_{19}N,HCl = 177.7.$

CAS — 503-01-5 (isometheptene); 6168-86-1 (isometheptene hydrochloride).

Isometheptene Mucate (2073-n)

Isometheptene Mucate *(BANM, rINNM)*.

Isometheptene galactarate.

$(C_9H_{19}N)_2,C_6H_{10}O_8 = 492.6.$

CAS — 7492-31-1.

Pharmacopoeias. In *Br.* and *US.*

A white crystalline powder. Very **soluble** or freely soluble in water; soluble in alcohol; slightly soluble in absolute alcohol; very slightly soluble or practically insoluble in chloroform; practically insoluble in ether. The BP specifies that a 5% solution has a pH of 5.4 to 6.6; the USP specifies a pH of 6.0 to 7.5. **Store** in airtight containers. Protect from light.

Adverse Effects and Precautions

For the adverse effects of sympathomimetics, and precautions to be observed, see p.951.

Porphyria. Isometheptene mucate has been associated with clinical exacerbations of porphyria and is considered unsafe in porphyric patients.[1]

1. Moore MR, McColl KEL. *Porphyria: drug lists.* Glasgow: Porphyria Research Unit, University of Glasgow, 1991.

Interactions

For the interactions of sympathomimetics in general, see p.951. Isometheptene has been reported to produce severe hypertensive reactions in patients receiving MAOIs.

For a report of hypertension and life-threatening complications following concomitant use of isometheptene and bromocriptine, see under Sympathomimetics, p.1134.

Uses and Administration

Isometheptene is an indirect-acting sympathomimetic (see p.951). It is included for its vasoconstrictor effect, usually as the mucate, in some analgesic combination products used to treat acute migraine attacks (p.443). Typical doses of isometheptene mucate in migraine are 130 mg at the beginning of an attack with 65 mg hourly thereafter as necessary up to a total maximum dose of 325 mg in a 12-hour period.

Isometheptene as the hydrochloride and as the mucate is also used in the management of smooth muscle spasm. Usual doses of the hydrochloride in painful muscle spasm or migraine are 75 to 100 mg by mouth 3 or 4 times daily, although higher doses have been given. It is also given by intramuscular, or occasionally subcutaneous or slow intravenous injection.

Preparations

USP 23: Isometheptene Mucate, Dichloralphenazone, and Acetaminophen Capsules.

Proprietary Preparations (details are given in Part 3)
Ital.: Octinum†; *Switz.:* Octinum.

Multi-ingredient: *Ger.:* Neopyrin-N†; *UK:* Midrid; *USA:* Isocom; Isopap; Midchlor; Midrin; Migralam; Migratine.

Methysergide Maleate (1513-n)

Methysergide Maleate *(BANM, rINNM).*

1-Methyl-D-lysergic Acid Butanolamide Maleate. *N*-[1-(Hydroxymethyl)propyl]-1-methyl-D-lysergamide hydrogen maleate; 9,10-Didehydro-*N*-[1-(hydroxymethyl)propyl]-1,6-dimethylergoline-8β-carboxamide hydrogen maleate.

$C_{21}H_{27}N_3O_2,C_4H_4O_4$ = 469.5.

CAS — 361-37-5 (methysergide); 129-49-7 (methysergide maleate).

NOTE. Methysergide is *USAN.*

Pharmacopoeias. In *Br., Swiss,* and *US.*

A white to yellowish-white or reddish-white, odourless or almost odourless, crystalline powder. Methysergide 1 mg is approximately equivalent to 1.33 mg of methysergide maleate. **Soluble** 1 in 200 of water and 1 in 165 of alcohol; practically insoluble or soluble 1 in 3400 of chloroform; practically insoluble in ether; slightly soluble in methyl alcohol. A 0.2% solution in water has a pH of 3.7 to 4.7. **Store** in airtight containers at a temperature of 2° to 8°. Protect from light.

Adverse Effects

Gastro-intestinal effects such as nausea, vomiting, and abdominal pain are common on initial treatment with methysergide maleate, as are dizziness and drowsiness. Other CNS effects reported include ataxia, insomnia, weakness, restlessness, lightheadedness, euphoria, and hallucinations. Peripheral or localised oedema, leg cramps, and weight gain have occurred and there have been occasional reports of skin rashes, loss of hair, joint and muscle pain, neutropenia, and eosinophilia. Orthostatic hypotension and tachycardia have been observed.

Arterial spasm has occurred in some patients with manifestations such as paraesthesia of the extremities and anginal pain, similar to those reported with ergotamine (p.445); if such symptoms occur methysergide should be withdrawn, although rebound headaches may be experienced if it is withdrawn suddenly. Vascular insufficiency of the lower limbs may represent arterial spasm or fibrotic changes. Retroperitoneal fibrosis, with obstruction of abdominal blood vessels and ureters, pleuropulmonary fibrosis, and fibrotic changes in heart valves have occurred in patients on long-term treatment. Methysergide must be withdrawn immediately if fibrosis occurs. Retroperitoneal fibrosis is usually reversible, but other fibrotic changes are less readily reversed.

Fibrosis. Fibrosis has been associated with the long-term administration of methysergide maleate. Graham *et al.*[1] reported on 27 patients in whom development of retroperitoneal fibrosis was attributed to daily administration of methysergide for headache. Methysergide [maleate] was given for periods of 9 to 54 months in doses ranging from 2 to 28 mg daily. Treatment was withdrawn in 13 patients; there was partial or complete regression of the symptoms, signs, and X-ray evidence of the process in all patients. Improvement usually began within a few days, in some cases with the aid of prednisone. The other 14 patients were treated by surgery; those few who continued taking methysergide had difficult postoperative courses. Cardiac murmurs occurred in 7 patients, and regressed wholly or partially in 3 after therapy was stopped. Fibrotic changes affecting the aorta, heart valves, and pulmonary tissues occurred in a few of the patients. Bana *et al.*[2] have reported the development of endocardial fibrosis indicated by cardiac murmurs in 48 patients receiving methysergide. The murmurs gradually regressed in 27 when methysergide was discontinued. Retroperitoneal fibrosis was present in 9 patients and pleuropulmonary fibrosis in 2. Fibrosis of the iliac vein has been described in one patient.[3]

Graham *et al.*[1] also noted a few cases of retroperitoneal fibrosis which appeared to be associated with the administration of ergotamine tartrate or dihydroergotamine. These two drugs have additionally been implicated in a few other cases of retroperitoneal fibrosis or other fibrotic disorders in patients taking high doses for long periods.[4-7]

1. Graham JR, *et al.* Fibrotic disorders associated with methysergide therapy for headache. *N Engl J Med* 1966; **274:** 359–68.
2. Bana DS, *et al.* Cardiac murmurs and endocardial fibrosis associated with methysergide therapy. *Am Heart J* 1974; **88:** 640–55.
3. Bucci JA, Manoharan A. Methysergide-induced retroperitoneal fibrosis: successful outcome and two new laboratory features. *Mayo Clin Proc* 1997; **72:** 1148–50.
4. Lepage-Savary D, Vallières A. Ergotamine as a possible cause of retroperitoneal fibrosis. *Clin Pharm* 1982; **1:** 179–80.
5. Damstrup L, Jensen TT. Retroperitoneal fibrosis after long-term daily use of ergotamine. *Int Urol Nephrol* 1986; **18:** 299–301.
6. Robert M, *et al.* Fibrotic processes associated with long-term ergotamine therapy. *N Engl J Med* 1984; **311:** 601 and 602.
7. Malaquin F, *et al.* Pleural and retroperitoneal fibrosis from dihydroergotamine. *N Engl J Med* 1989; **321:** 1760.

Treatment of Adverse Effects

As for Ergotamine Tartrate, p.446. Methysergide maleate should be withdrawn immediately if fibrosis develops. Corticosteroids can be used to treat fibrosis, although surgery may be required.

Precautions

As for Ergotamine Tartrate, p.446. In addition, methysergide maleate is contra-indicated in valvular heart disease, pulmonary and collagen diseases, diseases of the urinary tract, and debilitated states. It should be used with caution in patients with peptic ulcer because it may increase gastric acidity. Patients should be closely supervised and methysergide withdrawn immediately if symptoms of fibrosis or arterial spasm develop. Methysergide maleate should not be given continuously for more than 6 months and should be withdrawn gradually (see Uses, below).

Interactions

Interactions involving those ergot alkaloids used primarily in the management of migraine are discussed under ergotamine (p.446). References specific to methysergide may be found there under the headings Antimigraine Drugs and Beta Blockers.

Pharmacokinetics

Methysergide maleate is rapidly absorbed from the gastro-intestinal tract with maximum plasma concentrations being obtained within about one hour of ingestion. Methysergide undergoes extensive first-pass hepatic metabolism to methylergometrine (p.1603). Methysergide is excreted in the urine as unchanged drug and metabolites.

References.

1. Bredberg U, *et al.* Pharmacokinetics of methysergide and its metabolite methylergometrine in man. *Eur J Clin Pharmacol* 1986; **30:** 75–7.

Uses and Administration

Methysergide maleate is a semisynthetic ergot alkaloid. It is a potent serotonin antagonist and, compared with ergotamine, has only feeble vasoconstrictor and oxytocic effects. It has been used prophylactically in the management of severe recurrent migraine (p.443) and in the prevention of headache attacks during cluster periods (p.443), although its use has declined because of adverse effects. It is ineffective in the treatment of acute attacks.

Methysergide maleate is given by mouth in a dosage equivalent to 2 to 6 mg of methysergide base daily in divided doses with meals. It is suggested that treatment should be started with 1 mg at bedtime and doses increased gradually over about 2 weeks; the minimum effective dose should be used. In the USA and some other countries doses are expressed in terms of the maleate a usual dose of which is 4 to 8 mg daily. Careful and regular observation of the patient is essential because of the high incidence of side-effects and it is recommended that treatment should only be carried out under hospital supervision. If treatment still proves to be ineffective after 3 weeks, further administration is unlikely to be of benefit. Treatment should not be continued for more than 6 months, after which it should be gradually withdrawn over 2 or 3 weeks and then discontinued for at least a month for reassessment. Some consider that treatment courses should not exceed 3 months without a break.

Methysergide maleate has also been used to control diarrhoea associated with carcinoid syndrome (p.477) in high doses equivalent to 12 to 20 mg of methysergide daily.

As a serotonin antagonist, methysergide might be expected to help reverse the serotonin syndrome (p.303).

Preparations

BP 1998: Methysergide Tablets;
USP 23: Methysergide Maleate Tablets.

Proprietary Preparations (details are given in Part 3)
Austral.: Deseril; *Belg.:* Deseril; *Canad.:* Sansert; *Fr.:* Desernil; *Ger.:* Deseril; *Irl.:* Deseril; *Ital.:* Deserril; *Neth.:* Deseril; *Norw.:* Deseril†; *S.Afr.:* Deseril; *Spain:* Deseril†; *Swed.:* Sansert†; *Switz.:* Deseril; *UK:* Deseril; *USA:* Sansert.

Naratriptan Hydrochloride (17247-k)

Naratriptan Hydrochloride *(BANM, USAN, rINNM).*

GR-85548A (naratriptan hydrochloride); GR-85548X (naratriptan). *N*-Methyl-3-(1-methyl-4-piperidyl)indole-5-ethanesulfonamide hydrochloride.

$C_{17}H_{25}N_3O_2S,HCl$ = 371.9.

CAS — 121679-13-8 (naratriptan); 121679-19-4 (naratriptan hydrochloride); 143388-64-1 (naratriptan hydrochloride).

Adverse Effects and Precautions

As for Sumatriptan, p.450. Naratriptan should not be used in patients with severe hepatic impairment or severe renal impairment (creatinine clearance less than 15 mL per minute). Patients with hypersensitivity to sulphonamides may theoretically exhibit a similar reaction to naratriptan.

Interactions

As for Sumatriptan, p.451.

Pharmacokinetics

Following oral administration, peak plasma-naratriptan concentrations are observed at 2 to 3 hours, and bioavailability is reported to be 63% in men and 74% in women. Plasma protein binding is 29%. Naratriptan undergoes some hepatic metabolism by a wide range of cytochrome P450 isoenzymes. It is predominantly excreted in the urine with 50% of a dose being recovered as unchanged drug and 30% as inactive metabolites. The elimination half-life is 6 hours, and is significantly prolonged in patients with renal or hepatic impairment.

Uses and Administration

Naratriptan is a selective serotonin (5-HT_1) agonist with actions and uses similar to those of sumatriptan (p.451). It is used for the acute treatment of migraine attacks (p.443), and should be administered as soon as possible after onset of migraine headache. It should not be used prophylactically. It is given by mouth as the hydrochloride, and doses are expressed in terms of the base.

The recommended initial dose of naratriptan in the UK is 2.5 mg, and in the USA is 1 or 2.5 mg. If no response is obtained with the initial dose, a second dose should not be taken for the same attack. If symptoms recur following an initial response, the dose may be repeated after an interval of 4 hours, to a maximum of 5 mg in any 24-hour period. In patients with mild to moderate hepatic or renal impairment, the recommended maximum dose in 24 hours is 2.5 mg and a lower starting dose should be considered.

Migraine. In dose-finding studies in patients with acute migraine,[1,2] naratriptan 2.5 mg was marginally more effective than 1 mg, and both these doses were more effective than a 0.25-mg dose or placebo. There are few published details of studies comparing naratriptan with other serotonin (5-HT_1) agonists but is has been suggested that naratriptan appears to be less effective in treating a migraine attack than sumatriptan.[3] Naratriptan was effective when used to treat acute migraine over 6 months.[4]

1. Klassen A, *et al.* Naratriptan is effective and well tolerated in the acute treatment of migraine: results of a double-blind, placebo-controlled, parallel-group study. *Headache* 1997; **37:** 640–5.
2. Mathew NT, *et al.* Naratriptan is effective and well tolerated in the acute treatment of migraine: results of a double-blind, placebo-controlled, crossover study. *Neurology* 1997; **49:** 1485–90.
3. Anonymous. Managing migraine. *Drug Ther Bull* 1998; **36:** 41–4.
4. Bomhof MAM, *et al.* Tolerability and efficacy of naratriptan tablets with long-term treatment (6 months). *Cephalalgia* 1998; **18:** 33–7.

Preparations

Proprietary Preparations (details are given in Part 3)
Swed.: Naramig; ***UK:*** Naramig; ***USA:*** Amerge.

Oxetorone Fumarate (13059-b)

Oxetorone Fumarate *(USAN, rINNM).*

L-6257. 3-(6,12-Dihydrobenzofuro[3,2-*c*][1]benzoxepin-6-ylidene)-*NN*-dimethylpropylamine hydrogen fumarate.

$C_{21}H_{21}NO_2,C_4H_4O_4$ = 435.5.

CAS — 26020-55-3 (oxetorone); 34522-46-8 (oxetorone fumarate).

Oxetorone fumarate is an antihistamine and serotonin antagonist used in the treatment of migraine (p.443) and cluster headache (p.443) in doses of up to 180 mg daily by mouth. Oxetorone was reported to have induced hyperplastic changes in breast tissue and the uterine endometrium of *rodents.*

Preparations

Proprietary Preparations (details are given in Part 3)
Belg.: Nocertone; ***Fr.:*** Nocertone; ***Spain:*** Nocertone†.

Pizotifen (14855-k)

Pizotifen *(BAN, rINN).*

BC-105; Pizotyline *(USAN).* 9,10-Dihydro-4-(1-methylpiperid-in-4-ylidene)-4*H*-benzo[4,5]cyclohepta[1,2-*b*]thiophene.

$C_{19}H_{21}NS$ = 295.4.

CAS — 15574-96-6.

Pharmacopoeias. In *Chin.*

Pizotifen Malate (6157-j)

Pizotifen Malate *(BANM, rINNM).*

Pizotifen Hydrogen Malate; Pizotyline Malate. 9,10-Dihydro-4-(1-methylpiperidin-4-ylidene)-4*H*-benzo[4,5]cyclohepta[1,2-*b*]thiophene hydrogen malate.

$C_{19}H_{21}NS,C_4H_6O_5$ = 429.5.

CAS — 5189-11-7.

Pharmacopoeias. In *Br.*

A white or slightly yellowish-white, odourless or almost odourless, crystalline powder. Pizotifen 1 mg is approximately equivalent to 1.45 mg of pizotifen malate. Very slightly **soluble** in water; slightly soluble in alcohol and chloroform; sparingly soluble in methyl alcohol. **Protect** from light.

Adverse Effects and Precautions

As for the antihistamines in general, see p.397. Increased appetite and weight gain may occur with pizotifen. Drowsiness may be troublesome.

Of 47 patients with severe migraine given pizotifen 1 to 2 mg daily adverse effects were recorded in 22 patients.[1] These reactions included weight increase (15), muscle pain or cramps (3), heavy legs or restless legs (3), fluid retention (3), drowsiness (2), more frequent milder headaches (2), facial flushing (1), reduced libido (1), exacerbation of epilepsy (1), and dreaming (2). Adverse effects necessitating withdrawal from the study occurred in 11 patients.

1. Peet KMS. Use of pizotifen in severe migraine: a long-term study. *Curr Med Res Opin* 1977; **5:** 192–9.

Interactions

As for the antihistamines in general, see p.399.

Antihypertensives. Following a report[1] of loss of blood pressure control when treatment with pizotifen was started in a patient receiving debrisoquine the manufacturer suggested that since pizotifen had a similar chemical structure to the tricyclic antidepressants it might antagonise the actions of adrenergic neurone blockers in a similar manner.

1. Bailey RR. Antagonism of debrisoquine sulphate by pizotifen (Sandomigran). *N Z Med J* 1976; **1:** 449.

Pharmacokinetics

Pizotifen is well absorbed from the gastro-intestinal tract, peak plasma concentrations occurring approximately 5 hours after a single oral dose. Over 90% is bound to plasma proteins. Pizotifen undergoes extensive metabolism. Over half of a dose is excreted in the urine, chiefly as metabolites; a significant proportion is excreted in the faeces. The primary metabolite of pizotifen (*N*-glucuronide conjugate) has a long elimination half-life of about 23 hours.

Uses and Administration

Pizotifen is an antihistamine (p.399) that has strong serotonin antagonist and weak antimuscarinic properties. It also antagonises the action of tryptamine. Pizotifen is used, usually as the malate, for the prophylaxis of migraine (p.443) and for the prevention of headache attacks during cluster periods (p.443). It is not effective in treating an acute attack. Doses of pizotifen malate are expressed in terms of the equivalent amount of the base. The usual adult dose is 1.5 mg daily by mouth either in three divided doses or as a single dose at night. Gradual increase from an initial dose of 0.5 mg may help to avoid undue drowsiness. Doses in individual patients may vary from 0.5 mg up to a maximum of 4.5 mg daily. Not more than 3 mg should be given as a single dose. Doses of up to 1.5 mg daily in divided doses or up to 1 mg at night have been recommended for children.

Pizotifen hydrochloride has also been used in the management of migraine.

Abdominal migraine. The term abdominal migraine has been proposed by some workers for a syndrome in children consisting of recurrent episodes of midline abdominal pain lasting for many hours.[1,2] There is usually a family history of migraine. Patients commonly wish to lie down and try to sleep, and the pain is severe enough to disrupt normal activities. Other symptoms include pallor, anorexia, nausea, and vomiting. Sleep, and sometimes vomiting, terminate the attack.

However the existence of this syndrome is not universally recognised and is a matter of debate.[2,3] In 1988 the Headache Classification Committee of the International Headache Society[4] were unable to include abdominal migraine as a separate syndrome in their classification of headache and related conditions since they were unable to propose diagnostic criteria to differentiate it from a number of similar childhood periodic syndromes. Nonetheless, in a recent study[5] pizotifen was found to be effective for the prophylaxis of abdominal pain in children considered to have this disorder.

1. Symon DNK, Russell G. Abdominal migraine: a syndrome defined. *Cephalalgia* 1986; **6:** 223–8.
2. Symon DNK. Is there a place for "abdominal migraine" as a separate entity in the IHS classification? Yes! *Cephalalgia* 1992; **12:** 345–6.
3. Hockaday JM. Is there a place for "abdominal migraine" as a separate entity in the IHS classification? NO! *Cephalalgia* 1992; **12:** 346–8.
4. Headache Classification Committee of the International Headache Society. Classification and diagnostic criteria for headache disorders, cranial neuralgias and facial pain. *Cephalalgia* 1988; **8** (suppl 7): 1–96.
5. Symon DNK, Russell G. Double blind placebo controlled trial of pizotifen syrup in the treatment of abdominal migraine. *Arch Dis Child* 1995; **72:** 48–50.

Migraine and cluster headache. References.

1. Bellavance AJ, Meloche JP. A comparative study of naproxen sodium, pizotyline and placebo in migraine prophylaxis. *Headache* 1990; **30:** 710–15.

Preparations

BP 1998: Pizotifen Tablets.

Proprietary Preparations (details are given in Part 3)
Aust.: Sandomigran; ***Austral.:*** Sandomigran; ***Belg.:*** Mosegor†; Sandomigran; ***Canad.:*** Sandomigran; ***Fr.:*** Sanmigran; ***Ger.:*** Mosegor; Sandomigran; ***Irl.:*** Sanomigran; ***Ital.:*** Sandomigran; ***Neth.:*** Sandomigran; ***Norw.:*** Sandomigrin; ***S.Afr.:*** Sandomigran; ***Spain:*** Mosegor; Sandomigran; ***Swed.:*** Sandomigrin; ***Switz.:*** Mosegor; Sandomigran†; ***UK:*** Sanomigran.

Rizatriptan Benzoate (3685-j)

Rizatriptan Benzoate *(BANM, USAN, pINNM).*

MK-462; MK-0462. 3-[2-(Dimethylamino)ethyl]-5-(1*H*-1,2,4-triazol-1-ylmethyl)indole monobenzoate; Dimethyl{2-[5-(1*H*-1,2,4-triazol-1-ylmethyl)indol-3-yl]ethyl}amine monobenzoate.

$C_{15}H_{19}N_5,C_7H_6O_2$ = 391.5.

CAS — 144034-80-0 (rizatriptan); 145202-66-0 (rizatriptan benzoate).

Adverse Effects and Precautions

As for Sumatriptan, p.450. Rizatriptan should not be used in patients with severe hepatic or renal impairment.

Breast feeding. Studies in *rats* indicated a high distribution of rizatriptan into milk. The manufacturer recommends that infant exposure be minimised by avoiding breast feeding for 24 hours after treatment.

Interactions

As for Sumatriptan, p.451. Propranolol increases plasma-rizatriptan concentrations; it is recommended that the initial dose of rizatriptan be reduced to 5 mg in patients receiving propranolol, and that administration of the 2 drugs should be separated by at least 2 hours. In addition, the recommended maximum dose of rizatriptan in 24 hours is 10 mg in the UK and 15 mg in the USA when used with propranolol.

Pharmacokinetics

After oral administration, peak plasma-rizatriptan concentrations are obtained in about 1 to 1.5 hours or 1.6 to 2.5 hours depending on the formulation, with a bioavailability of about 40 to 45%. Food may delay the time to peak-plasma concentrations of the tablet formulation by about 1 hour. Plasma protein binding is low (14%).

Rizatriptan is metabolised, primarily by monoamine oxidase type A to the inactive indole acetic acid derivative. The active metabolite N-monodesmethyl-rizatriptan is formed to a minor degree; other minor metabolites are also produced. About 14% of an oral dose is excreted in the urine as unchanged rizatriptan, 51% as the indole acetic acid metabolite, and 1% as N-monodesmethyl-rizatriptan. The plasma half-life is about 2 to 3 hours.

References.

1. Sciberras DG, *et al.* Initial human experience with MK-462 (rizatriptan): a novel 5-HT_{1D} agonist. *Br J Clin Pharmacol* 1997; **43:** 49–54.

Uses and Administration

Rizatriptan is a selective serotonin (5-HT_1) agonist with actions and uses similar to those of sumatriptan (p.451). It is used for the acute treatment of the headache phase of migraine attacks (p.443). It should not be used prophylactically. Rizatriptan is administered as the benzoate, and doses are expressed in terms of the base.

A usual initial dose is 10 mg by mouth. If this is ineffective, a second dose should not be taken for the same attack. If the headache recurs, a further dose of 10 mg may be taken after an interval of at least 2 hours. The recommended maximum dose in 24 hours is 20 mg in the UK and 30 mg in the USA. In patients with mild to moderate hepatic or renal impairment, the dose should be reduced to 5 mg and no more than 10 mg should be taken in 24 hours. Doses may need to be reduced in patients receiving propranolol (see under Interactions, above).

Migraine. In a comparative study,[1] the efficacy of oral rizatriptan 10 or 20 mg was similar to that of oral sumatriptan 100 mg in the acute treatment of migraine. Rizatriptan 40 mg was more effective than sumatriptan 100 mg, but was associated with a higher frequency of adverse effects. In a dose-ranging study,[2] both 5-mg and 10-mg doses of rizatriptan were more effective than placebo, whereas a 2.5-mg dose was subtherapeutic. Adverse effects generally increased with increasing dosage.

1. Visser WH, *et al.* Rizatriptan vs sumatriptan in the acute treatment of migraine: a placebo-controlled, dose-ranging study. *Arch Neurol* 1996; **53:** 1132–7.
2. Gijsman H, *et al.* Double-blind, placebo-controlled, dose-finding study of rizatriptan (MK-462) in the acute treatment of migraine. *Cephalalgia* 1997; **17:** 647–51.

Preparations

Proprietary Preparations (details are given in Part 3)
UK: Maxalt; *USA:* Maxalt.

Sumatriptan Succinate (3945-a)

Sumatriptan Succinate *(BANM, USAN, rINNM).*

GR-43175C; GR-43175X (sumatriptan). 3-(2-Dimethylaminoethyl)indol-5-yl-*N*-methylmethanesulphonamide succinate.

$C_{14}H_{21}N_3O_2S,C_4H_6O_4 = 413.5.$

CAS — 103628-46-2 (sumatriptan); 103628-47-3 (sumatriptan hemisuccinate); 103628-48-4 (sumatriptan succinate).

Stability. References.

1. Fish DN, *et al.* Stability of sumatriptan succinate in extemporaneously prepared oral liquids. *Am J Health-Syst Pharm* 1997; **54:** 1619–22.

Adverse Effects

The most commonly reported adverse effects of serotonin ($5-HT_1$) agonists such as sumatriptan include dizziness, flushing, weakness, drowsiness, and fatigue. Nausea and vomiting may occur. Pain or sensations of tingling, heaviness, heat, pressure, or tightness have also been commonly reported, and can affect any part of the body including the throat and chest, and may be intense. These symptoms may be due to vasospasm, which on rare occasions has resulted in severe cardiovascular events including cardiac arrhythmias, myocardial ischaemia, or myocardial infarction. There have been isolated reports of associated cerebrovascular events in patients receiving sumatriptan. Transient increases in blood pressure may occur soon after treatment. Hypotension, bradycardia or tachycardia, and palpitations have been reported. Visual disturbances have also occurred.

Sumatriptan has occasionally been associated with minor disturbances in liver function. There have also been rare reports of seizures with sumatriptan, mainly in patients with a previous history of epilepsy or with structural lesions predisposing to seizures. Hypersensitivity reactions ranging from skin rashes to, more rarely, anaphylaxis have occurred.

Pain at the injection site is common after subcutaneous sumatriptan administration. Irritation of the nasal mucosa and throat and epistaxis have been reported after intranasal sumatriptan administration.

In a Dutch postmarketing survey[1] completed by 1187 patients who had taken sumatriptan the most common adverse reactions attributed to sumatriptan were paraesthesia (reported by 11.7% of patients), dizziness (8.1%), feeling of heaviness (8.0%), chest pain (7.9%), nausea and/or vomiting (7.3%), drowsiness/sedation (7.0%), flushing (5.1%), fatigue (4.6%), pressure in throat (3.3%), headache (3.1%), injection site reaction (3.0%), palpitations (2.8%), abdominal pain (2.6%), muscle pain (2.4%), and dyspnoea (2.2%).

1. Ottervanger JP, *et al.* Adverse reactions attributed to sumatriptan: a postmarketing study in general practice. *Eur J Clin Pharmacol* 1994; **47:** 305–9.

Effects on the cardiovascular system. About 10 months after sumatriptan injection had been made available commercially, the UK Committee on Safety of Medicines (CSM) reported that it had received 34 reports of pain or tightness in the chest and 2 reports of myocardial ischaemia associated with this injection.[1] The Netherlands Centre for Monitoring of Adverse Reactions to Drugs reported about that time that it had received 12 reports of chest or anginal pain mostly associated with oral sumatriptan.[2] A later postmarketing survey based on data from Dutch general practitioners identified chest pain in 1.3% of 1727 patients,[3] a figure considered to be lower than that seen in earlier studies, but in a subsequent questionnaire completed by 1187 of these patients 7.9% reported chest pain.[4] The Australian Adverse Drug Reactions Advisory Committee (ADRAC)[5] stated in December 1994 that they had received 114 reports of chest pain since sumatriptan had been marketed in mid 1992. Most patients had recovered quickly but 2 had died. The first developed a fatal myocardial infarction after coronary artery dissection but the causal relation between this and taking sumatriptan was unclear. The second patient who had hypertrophic obstructive cardiomyopathy developed ventricular fibrillation a few hours after the onset of chest pain and this led to fatal cardiac arrest.

One group of workers[6] who studied the effect of sumatriptan 16 mg given subcutaneously suggested that the symptoms of chest pain might be due to an effect of sumatriptan on oesophageal function, but others have argued against this suggestion.[7] ADRAC[5] considered that the reaction in the 28 reports of throat tightness they had received by December 1994 was a different reaction to that of chest pain, and probably resulted from changes in oesophageal motility.

Several reports have provided details of individual cases of the adverse cardiovascular effects of sumatriptan including arrhythmias,[8] acute myocardial infarction,[9-13] and unstable angina.[14] Most of these reports concerned subcutaneous sumatriptan administration, but 1 case of myocardial infarction occurred after oral administration.[11] Curtin *et al.* described 2 patients who developed ventricular tachycardia following subcutaneous sumatriptan.[8] In the first patient the ventricular fibrillation following immediately after the sumatriptan injection would have been fatal but for rapid treatment with DC shock. In another report[9] a 47-year-old woman experienced chest pain after each of 3 subcutaneous injections of sumatriptan 6 mg for acute attacks of cluster headache. On the third occasion the patient was admitted to hospital and was diagnosed as having an acute myocardial infarction. In this instance, the patient did not have a history of ischaemic heart disease or Prinzmetal's angina, or any predisposing conditions.

Hillis and MacIntyre[15] reviewed published reports on chest pain as well as relevant data held by the UK manufacturer and considered that the risk of myocardial ischaemia following vasoconstriction induced by sumatriptan was small. However, the contra-indications and cautions given under Precautions, below, should be observed.

1. Committee on Safety of Medicines. Sumatriptan (Imigran) and chest pain. *Current Problems 34* 1992.
2. Stricker BHC. Coronary vasospasm and sumatriptan. *Br Med J* 1992; **305:** 118.
3. Ottervanger JP, *et al.* Postmarketing study of cardiovascular adverse reactions associated with sumatriptan. *Br Med J* 1993; **307:** 1185.
4. Ottervanger JP, *et al.* Adverse reactions attributed to sumatriptan: a postmarketing study in general practice. *Eur J Clin Pharmacol* 1994; **47:** 305–9.
5. Boyd IW, Rohan AP. Sumatriptan-induced chest pain. *Lancet* 1994; **344:** 1704–5.
6. Houghton LA, *et al.* Is chest pain after sumatriptan oesophageal in origin? *Lancet* 1994; **344:** 985–6.
7. Hood S, *et al.* Sumatriptan-induced chest pain. *Lancet* 1994; **344:** 1500–1.
8. Curtin T, *et al.* Cardiorespiratory distress after sumatriptan given by injection. *Br Med J* 1992; **305:** 713–14.
9. Ottervanger JP, *et al.* Transmural myocardial infarction with sumatriptan. *Lancet* 1993; **341:** 861–2.
10. Kelly KM. Cardiac arrest following use of sumatriptan. *Neurology* 1995; **45:** 1211–13.
11. O'Connor P, Gladstone P. Oral sumatriptan-associated transmural myocardial infarction. *Neurology* 1995; **45:** 2274–6.
12. Mueller L, *et al.* Vasospasm-induced myocardial infarction with sumatriptan. *Headache* 1996; **36:** 329–31.
13. Main ML *et al.* Cardiac arrest and myocardial infarction immediately after sumatriptan injection. *Ann Intern Med* 1998; **128:** 874.
14. Walton-Shirley M, *et al.* Unstable angina pectoris associated with Imitrex therapy. *Cathet Cardiovasc Diagn* 1995; **34:** 188.
15. Hillis WS, MacIntyre PD. Drug reactions: sumatriptan and chest pain. *Lancet* 1993; **341:** 1564–5. Correction. *ibid.*; **342:** 1310.

Effects on the cerebrovascular system. Various adverse cerebrovascular effects have been reported after the use of subcutaneous sumatriptan including hemiparesis,[1] stroke,[2,3] and intracerebral haemorrhage.[4]

1. Luman W, Gray RS. Adverse reactions associated with sumatriptan. *Lancet* 1993; **341:** 1091–2.
2. Cavazos J, *et al.* Sumatriptan-induced stroke in sagittal sinus thrombosis. *Lancet* 1994; **343:** 1105–6.
3. Meschia JF, *et al.* Reversible segmental cerebral arterial vasospasm and cerebral infarction: possible association with excessive use of sumatriptan and Midrin. *Arch Neurol* 1998; **55:** 712–14.
4. Edwards KR, *et al.* Intracerebral hemorrhage associated with sumatriptan. *Headache* 1995; **35:** 309.

Effects on the oesophagus. Oesophageal constriction or throat tightness has been reported in some patients taking sumatriptan and may be due to a direct effect on the oesophagus. See Effects on the Cardiovascular System, above.

Effects on the respiratory system. See under Asthma in Precautions, below.

Hypersensitivity. Reactions to sumatriptan such as skin rashes and, more rarely, anaphylaxis are noted by the manufacturer. Published reports include a case of angioedema occurring in a patient 5 minutes after subcutaneous administration of sumatriptan,[1] and urticaria occurring 20 to 24 hours after oral or subcutaneous sumatriptan.[2]

1. Dachs R, Vitillo J. Angioedema associated with sumatriptan administration. *Am J Med* 1995; **99:** 684–5.
2. Pradalier A, *et al.* Delayed urticaria with sumatriptan. *Cephalalgia* 1996; **16:** 280–1.

Precautions

Sumatriptan and other serotonin ($5-HT_1$) agonists should only be used where there is a clear diagnosis of migraine or cluster headache and care should be taken to exclude other potentially serious neurological conditions. They should not be used prophylactically and should not be administered to patients with basilar or hemiplegic migraine.

Serotonin ($5-HT_1$) agonists are contra-indicated in patients with uncontrolled hypertension, ischaemic heart disease (coronary artery disease), a history of myocardial infarction, coronary vasospasm (Prinzmetal's angina), peripheral vascular disease, or a previous cerebrovascular accident or transient ischaemic attack. Unrecognised cardiovascular disease should be excluded before the use of serotonin ($5-HT_1$) agonists in postmenopausal women, men over 40 years of age, and those with risk factors for ischaemic heart disease (see below). If chest pain and tightness occur during use, appropriate investigations for ischaemic changes should be performed.

Drowsiness may occur following treatment with serotonin ($5-HT_1$) agonists and patients thus affected should not drive or operate machinery.

Sumatriptan should be used with caution in patients with hepatic or renal impairment, and should generally be avoided if these are severe. Sumatriptan injection should not be administered intravenously because of the increased risk of producing coronary vasospasm. Sumatriptan should also be used with caution in patients with a history of epilepsy or structural brain lesions. Patients with hypersensitivity to sulphonamides may exhibit a similar reaction to sumatriptan.

Patients with risk factors for ischaemic heart disease such as diabetes, hypertension, hypercholesterolaemia, obesity, and a strong family history of atheroma, as well as postmenopausal women, men over 40 years of age, and smokers should be given their first dose of sumatriptan under medical supervision.[1]

1. Hillis WS, MacIntyre PD. Drug reactions: sumatriptan and chest pain. *Lancet* 1993; **341:** 1564–5. Correction. *ibid.*; **342:** 1310.

Abuse. Sumatriptan may have a similar risk of misuse to that associated with analgesics and ergotamine compounds in patients with chronic headache. There have been reports[1-3] of patients using one or more daily doses of sumatriptan to control migraine. Many of the patients had a history of abuse of other antimigraine drugs and were using sumatriptan to prevent recurrence of headache. Whether misuse of sumatriptan was due to addiction or rebound headache as seen with ergotamine, remains to be determined. A postmarketing study in 952 patients receiving sumatriptan found that 36 of the patients (4%) used sumatriptan daily or more than 10 times a week. This overuse was related to poor efficacy and not to rebound headache.[4] One study[5] and an anecdotal report[6] suggest that, rather than producing euphoria or other effects associated with drugs of abuse such as morphine, sumatriptan is more likely to be associated with dysphoria and apathetic sedation.

1. Osborne MJ, *et al.* Is there a problem with long term use of sumatriptan in acute migraine? *Br Med J* 1994; **308:** 113.
2. Kaube H, *et al.* Sumatriptan. *Br Med J* 1994; **308:** 1573–4.
3. Gaist D, *et al.* Misuse of sumatriptan. *Lancet* 1994; **344:** 1090.
4. Ottervanger JP, *et al.* Pattern of sumatriptan use and overuse in general practice. *Eur J Clin Pharmacol* 1996; **50:** 353–5.
5. Sullivan JT, *et al.* Psychoactivity and abuse potential of sumatriptan. *Clin Pharmacol Ther* 1992; **52:** 635–42.
6. Bakshi R, Yan-Go FL. Prolonged marijuana-like dysphoria after subcutaneous sumatriptan. *Ann Pharmacother* 1996; **30:** 683.

Asthma. The manufacturers reviewed data from more than 75 clinical studies of sumatriptan involving 12 701 patients and reported[1] that the incidence of adverse events related to asthma did not differ between patients with or without asthma. Earlier there had been concern over the safety of sumatriptan in patients with asthma following 2 reports of bronchospasm and a report of a patient with asthma who died during a study of sumatriptan although the patient had not received sumatriptan in the month before her death.

1. Lloyd DK, Pilgrim AJ. The safety of sumatriptan in asthmatic migraineurs. *Cephalalgia* 1993; **13:** 201–4.

Breast feeding. The distribution of sumatriptan into breast milk following a 6-mg subcutaneous dose has been studied in 5 lactating mothers.[1] The mean total recovery of sumatriptan in breast milk was estimated to be 14.4 μg or 0.24% of the dose. It was calculated that on a weight adjusted basis an infant could receive a maximum of 3.5% of the maternal dose. The manufacturers have suggested that infant exposure can be minimised by avoiding breast feeding for 24 hours after treatment.

1. Wojnar-Horton RE, *et al.* Distribution and excretion of sumatriptan in human milk. *Br J Clin Pharmacol* 1996; **41:** 217–21.

Cerebrovascular disorders. A patient with a superior sagittal sinus thrombosis who presented with headache and was misdiagnosed as having migraine variant developed a cortical stroke within minutes of a second 6-mg subcutaneous injection of sumatriptan.[1] The authors of the report emphasised the importance of establishing a diagnosis of typical migraine or cluster headache before using sumatriptan and cautioned against its use in any patient who may have unstable cerebrovascular disease or raised intracranial pressure. They also pointed out that there was no clinical evidence that a second injection would relieve a headache when the initial injection had been ineffective.

1. Cavazos J, *et al.* Sumatriptan-induced stroke in sagittal sinus thrombosis. *Lancet* 1994; **343:** 1105–6.

Interactions

Sumatriptan and other serotonin (5-HT_1) agonists should not be given concurrently with ergotamine or related compounds (including methysergide) since there is an increased risk of vasospastic reactions. In addition, a delay is advised before starting a serotonin (5-HT_1) agonist in patients who have been receiving ergotamine: sumatriptan or rizatriptan should not be given until at least 24 hours, and zolmitriptan until at least 6 hours, after stopping the use of preparations containing ergotamine. Conversely, ergotamine should not be given until 6 hours after stopping these drugs (p.446). Serotonin (5-HT_1) agonists should not be given together.

It is recommended that sumatriptan or rizatriptan should not be used concurrently with, and for 2 weeks after stopping, an MAOI. The dosage of zolmitriptan should be reduced if it is used with an MAOI that inhibits monoamine oxidase type A. There is a theoretical possibility that the use of serotonin (5-HT_1) agonists with selective serotonin reuptake inhibitors may increase the risk of serotonin syndrome, but see under Antidepressants, below. It has also been suggested that sumatriptan may similarly interact with lithium.

Oral sumatriptan appeared to delay gastric emptying and might affect the absorption of co-administered drugs, as judged by its delaying effect on paracetamol absorption in migraine patients.[1]

1. Rani PU, *et al.* Sumatriptan delays paracetamol absorption in migraine patients. *Clin Drug Invest* 1996; **11:** 300–304.

Antidepressants. Sumatriptan and rizatriptan are metabolised predominantly by monoamine oxidase type A and the manufacturers advise that patients taking MAOIs, including reversible selective type A inhibitors such as moclobemide, should not be given these serotonin (5-HT_1) agonists. Clearance of zolmitriptan was decreased after administration of moclobemide; therefore, a reduced dose of zolmitriptan is advised if the drug is used concomitantly with an MAOI that inhibits monoamine oxidase type A. Selective serotonin reuptake inhibitors (SSRIs) such as fluoxetine may also interact with serotonin (5-HT_1) agonists with an increased risk of serotonin syndrome, and it has been suggested that lithium and sumatriptan may interact similarly. However, a review of the concomitant use of sumatriptan with MAOIs, SSRIs, or lithium found little evidence of an increased risk of serotonin syndrome.[1] It was concluded that most patients tolerate the combination of sumatriptan and an SSRI or lithium without incidence. However, it was suggested that the combination of sumatriptan and an MAOI should continue to be avoided until further data supporting its safety becomes available.

1. Gardner DM, Lynd LD. Sumatriptan contraindications and the serotonin syndrome. *Ann Pharmacother* 1998; **32:** 33–8.

Antimigraine drugs. The efficacy and tolerability of subcutaneous sumatriptan in the acute treatment of migraine did not appear to be affected in patients already taking dihydroergotamine orally for migraine prophylaxis.[1] However, the bioavailability of dihydroergotamine after oral administration is low and it could not be assumed that it was safe to use parenteral dihydroergotamine and sumatriptan concomitantly.[2] Note also that the concomitant use of sumatriptan and ergotamine or related compounds is considered contra-indicated (see above).

1. Henry P, *et al.* Subcutaneous sumatriptan in the acute treatment of migraine in patients using dihydroergotamine as prophylaxis. *Headache* 1993; **33:** 432–5.
2. Campbell JK. *Headache* 1993; **33:** 435 [editor's comment].

Antipsychotics. For reference to a potential interaction between sumatriptan and loxapine, see under Interactions for Chlorpromazine, p.653.

Pharmacokinetics

Sumatriptan is rapidly but incompletely absorbed following oral administration and undergoes first-pass metabolism, resulting in a low absolute bioavailability of about 14%. Peak plasma concentrations following oral administration are achieved in about 2 hours. Bioavailability is much higher (96%) following subcutaneous administration with peak concentrations occurring within 25 minutes. Bioavailability after intranasal administration is 16% relative to subcutaneous administration, with peak concentrations occurring in 1 to 1.5 hours. Plasma protein binding is low at about 14 to 21%.

The elimination half-life of sumatriptan is about 2 hours. Sumatriptan is extensively metabolised in the liver predominantly by monoamine oxidase type A and is excreted mainly in the urine as the inactive indole acetic acid derivative and its glucuronide. Sumatriptan and its metabolites also appear in the faeces. Small amounts of sumatriptan are distributed into breast milk (see above).

Reviews.

1. Scott AK. Sumatriptan clinical pharmacokinetics. *Clin Pharmacokinet* 1994; **27:** 337–44.
2. Lacey LF, *et al.* Single dose pharmacokinetics of sumatriptan in healthy volunteers. *Eur J Clin Pharmacol* 1995; **47:** 543–8.

Uses and Administration

Sumatriptan is a selective serotonin agonist which acts at 5-HT_1 receptors and produces vasoconstriction of cranial arteries. It is used for the acute treatment of migraine attacks and of cluster headache. It should not be used prophylactically. It may be administered by mouth or subcutaneously as the succinate and intranasally as the base. Doses are expressed in terms of sumatriptan base.

For the acute treatment of **migraine** sumatriptan should be administered as soon as possible after the onset of the headache phase, but efficacy is independent of the duration of the attack prior to starting treatment. If no response is obtained with the initial dose by any route, a second dose should not be given for the same attack.

The recommended initial dose by mouth in the UK is 50 mg, although some patients may require 100 mg. A 50-mg dose is considered suitable for patients with hepatic impairment. A clinical response can be expected after about 30 minutes. If there is a response but the migraine returns, further doses may be given up to a maximum of 300 mg in a 24-hour period. In the USA a lower initial dose of 25 mg is used, followed by a second dose of up to 100 mg if a satisfactory response has not been obtained after 2 hours.

When administered intranasally a clinical response can be expected in 15 minutes. The recommended initial dose of sumatriptan in the UK is 20 mg administered into one nostril (10 mg may be effective in some patients). In the USA, the recommended initial dose is 5, 10, or 20 mg administered into one nostril. If symptoms recur, a second dose may be given in the next 24 hours, at least 2 hours after the first dose. Not more than 40 mg should be used in a 24-hour period.

Sumatriptan may be self-administered by subcutaneous injection in a single dose of 6 mg when a clinical response may be expected after 10 to 15 minutes. If symptoms recur, a second dose of 6 mg may be injected at least one hour after the first dose; not more than 12 mg should be administered in a 24-hour period.

For the acute treatment of **cluster headache,** sumatriptan succinate is given by subcutaneous injection in similar doses to those used for migraine.

Migraine and cluster headache. The use of sumatriptan in the treatment of cluster headache and migraine has been reviewed.[1-5] Discussions on the overall management of these disorders may be found on p.443.

In **migraine** serotonin (5-HT_1) agonists are preferred to ergotamine for the treatment of acute attacks unresponsive to non-opioid analgesics. Sumatriptan has been shown to be effective in placebo-controlled studies when given orally in a dose of 100 mg,[6] subcutaneously in a 6-mg dose,[7,8] or intranasally in a dose of 20 mg,[9] but there are few comparative studies with other antimigraine drugs. In one study[10] sumatriptan given orally was found to be more effective than ergotamine with caffeine, but in others[11,12] it was only of similar efficacy to aspirin compounds given with metoclopramide and was associated with more adverse effects. In another study, oral sumatriptan was of similar efficacy to the NSAID tolfenamic acid.[13] Subcutaneous sumatriptan had a faster onset of action but a higher headache recurrence rate than subcutaneous dihydroergotamine in one study.[14] Subcutaneous sumatriptan was more effective than intranasal dihydroergotamine.[15] One review[5] noted that 50 to 69% of patients given sumatriptan orally, and 62 to 78% given sumatriptan intranasally, obtained relief of their headache within 2 hours, and 56 to 80% had relief within one hour when sumatriptan was given subcutaneously. About 21 to 57% of patients who initially respond to sumatriptan have a recurrence of their headache within 24 to 48 hours; this may be related in part to its short half-life. Such recurrences usually respond to a second dose[16,17] but studies indicate that if a first dose is ineffective subsequent doses for the same attack are of no benefit.[7,8,16] Sumatriptan is considered[18] to be effective when given at any time once the headache phase of migraine has started but prior administration during migraine aura appears to be of little benefit since it does not affect the aura or prevent or delay the development of headache.[19] Repeated or long-term use does not appear to be associated with reduced efficacy.[20,21]

Sumatriptan's effectiveness appears to be maintained in menses-related migraine, a condition which is considered to be less responsive to treatment than nonmenstrual migraine.[22] Experience of use in children has been reported.[23]

Subcutaneous sumatriptan has also been shown to be effective in relieving acute attacks of headache in patients with **cluster headache**. In studies about 75% of patients have obtained relief within 15 minutes of a 6-mg subcutaneous injection;[24,25] the use of higher doses was found to be of no advantage. Long term efficacy appears to be maintained[26] but the significance of the transient increase in the frequency of attacks seen in some patients remains to be determined.[27] It does not appear to be effective for the prevention of headache during cluster periods.[28]

1. Fullerton T, Gengo FM. Sumatriptan: a selective 5-hydroxytryptamine receptor agonist for the acute treatment of migraine. *Ann Pharmacother* 1992; **26:** 800–8.
2. Anonymous. Sumatriptan for migraine. *Med Lett Drugs Ther* 1992; **34:** 91–3.
3. Hsu VD. Sumatriptan: a new drug for vascular headache. *Clin Pharm* 1992; **11:** 919–29.
4. Bateman DN. Sumatriptan. *Lancet* 1993; **341:** 221–4.
5. Perry CM, Markham A. Sumatriptan: an updated review of its use in migraine. *Drugs* 1998; **55:** 889–922.
6. Goadsby PJ, *et al.* Oral sumatriptan in acute migraine. *Lancet* 1991; **338:** 782–3.
7. Cady RK, *et al.* Treatment of acute migraine with subcutaneous sumatriptan. *JAMA* 1991; **265:** 2831–21.
8. The Subcutaneous Sumatriptan International Study Group. Treatment of migraine attacks with sumatriptan. *N Engl J Med* 1991; **325:** 316–21.
9. Ryan R. Sumatriptan nasal spray for the acute treatment of migraine: results of two clinical studies. *Neurology* 1997; **49:** 1225–30.
10. The Multinational Oral Sumatriptan and Cafergot Comparative Study Group. A randomized, double-blind comparison of sumatriptan and cafergot in the acute treatment of migraine. *Eur Neurol* 1991; **31:** 314–22.
11. The Oral Sumatriptan and Aspirin plus Metoclopramide Comparative Study Group. A study to compare oral sumatriptan with oral aspirin plus oral metoclopramide in the acute treatment of migraine. *Eur Neurol* 1992; **32:** 177–84.
12. Tfelt-Hansen P, *et al.* The effectiveness of combined oral lysine acetylsalicylate and metoclopramide compared with oral sumatriptan for migraine. *Lancet* 1995; **346:** 923–6.
13. Myllylä VV, *et al.* Tolfenamic acid rapid release versus sumatriptan in the acute treatment of migraine: comparable effect in a double-blind, randomized, controlled, parallel-group study. *Headache* 1998; **38:** 201–7.
14. Winner P, *et al.* A double-blind study of subcutaneous dihydroergotamine vs subcutaneous sumatriptan in the treatment of acute migraine. *Arch Neurol* 1996; **53:** 180–4.
15. Touchon J, *et al.* A comparison of subcutaneous sumatriptan and dihydroergotamine nasal spray in the acute treatment of migraine. *Neurology* 1996; **47:** 361–5.
16. Ferrari MD, *et al.* Oral sumatriptan: effect of a second dose, and incidence and treatment of headache recurrences. *Cephalalgia* 1994; **14:** 330–8.
17. Dahlöf C. Headache recurrence after subcutaneous sumatriptan and early treatment. *Lancet* 1992; **340:** 909.

18. Ferrari MD. Sumatriptan in the treatment of migraine. *Neurology* 1993; **43** (suppl 3): S43–S47.
19. Bates D, *et al.* Sumatriptan Aura Study Group. Subcutaneous sumatriptan during the migraine aura. *Neurology* 1994; **44:** 1587–92.
20. Cady RK, *et al.* Efficacy of subcutaneous sumatriptan in repeated episodes of migraine. *Neurology* 1993; **43:** 1363–8.
21. Tansey MJB, *et al.* Long-term experience with sumatriptan in treatment of migraine. *Eur Neurol* 1993; **33:** 310–15.
22. Solbach MP, Waymer RS. Treatment of menstruation-associated migraine headache with subcutaneous sumatriptan. *Obstet Gynecol* 1993; **82:** 769–72.
23. Linder SL. Subcutaneous sumatriptan in the clinical setting: the first 50 consecutive patients with acute migraine in a pediatric neurology office practice. *Headache* 1996; **36:** 419–22.
24. The Sumatriptan Cluster Headache Study Group. Treatment of acute cluster headache with sumatriptan. *N Engl J Med* 1991; **325:** 322–6.
25. Ekbom K, *et al.* Subcutaneous sumatriptan in the acute treatment of cluster headache: a dose comparison study. *Acta Neurol Scand* 1993; **88:** 63–9.
26. Ekbom K, *et al.* Cluster headache attacks treated for up to three months with subcutaneous sumatriptan (6 mg). *Cephalalgia* 1995; **15:** 230–6.
27. Hardebo JE. Subcutaneous sumatriptan in cluster headache: a time study of the effect on pain and autonomic symptoms. *Headache* 1993; **33:** 18–21.
28. Monstad I, *et al.* Preemptive oral treatment with sumatriptan during a cluster period. *Headache* 1995; **35:** 607–13.

Preparations

Proprietary Preparations (details are given in Part 3)

Aust.: Imigran; ***Austral.:*** Imigran; ***Belg.:*** Imitrex; ***Canad.:*** Imitrex; ***Fr.:*** Imigrane; Imiject; ***Ger.:*** Imigran; ***Irl.:*** Imigran; ***Ital.:*** Imigran; Sumadol†; Sumigrene; ***Neth.:*** Imigran; ***Norw.:*** Imigran; ***S.Afr.:*** Imigran; ***Spain:*** Arcoiran; Imigran; Novelian; ***Swed.:*** Imigran; ***Switz.:*** Imigran; ***UK:*** Imigran; ***USA:*** Imitrex.

Zolmitriptan (17598-k)

Zolmitriptan *(BAN, USAN, rINN).*

311C90. (S)-4-{3-[2-(Dimethylamino)ethyl]indol-5-ylmethyl}-1,3-oxazolidin-2-one.

$C_{16}H_{21}N_3O_2 = 287.4.$

CAS — 139264-17-8.

Adverse Effects and Precautions

As for Sumatriptan, p.450. Other reported adverse effects include dry mouth and myalgia. Zolmitriptan should also be avoided in patients with Wolff-Parkinson-White syndrome or arrhythmias associated with accessory cardiac conduction pathways. The dose of zolmitriptan should be reduced in patients with moderate to severe hepatic impairment.

Hepatic impairment. A study[1] indicating that while there is no need to reduce the size of the initial dose of zolmitriptan in patients with moderate or severe hepatic impairment, accumulation may occur with repeated administration in patients with severe hepatic impairment and their total daily dosage should be reduced (see Uses and Administration, below).

1. Dixon R, *et al.* Effect of hepatic impairment on the pharmacokinetics of zolmitriptan. *J Clin Pharmacol* 1998; **38:** 694–701.

Renal impairment. Although renal clearance of zolmitriptan and its metabolites was reduced in 1 study in patients with moderate to severe renal impairment, the resulting effect was thought unlikely to be of clinical importance and adjustment of zolmitriptan dosage in patients with renal impairment was considered unnecessary.

1. Gillotin C, *et al.* No need to adjust the dose of 311C90 (zolmitriptan), a novel anti-migraine treatment in patients with renal failure not requiring dialysis. *Int J Clin Pharmacol Ther* 1997; **35:** 522–6.

Interactions

As for Sumatriptan, p.451. It is recommended that the maximum dose of zolmitriptan in 24 hours should be reduced to 7.5 mg in patients receiving an MAOI that inhibits monoamine oxidase type A. In addition, cimetidine inhibits the metabolism of zolmitriptan, and a maximum dose of 5 mg of zolmitriptan in 24 hours is recommended if these drugs are used concurrently. A similar reduction in zolmitriptan dosage is anticipated if it is given with drugs, such as fluvoxamine and ciprofloxacin, that inhibit the cytochrome P450 isoenzyme CYP1A2. Zolmitriptan should not be used within 12 hours of other serotonin (5-HT_1) agonists.

References.

1. Dixon R, *et al.* The metabolism of zolmitriptan: effects of an inducer and an inhibitor of cytochrome P450 on its pharmacokinetics in healthy volunteers. *Clin Drug Invest* 1998; **15:** 515–22.

Beta blockers. *Propranolol* increased plasma-zolmitriptan concentrations in a study in 12 healthy volunteers, but the changes were not thought to be clinically important, therefore dosage adjustment of zolmitriptan in patients taking propranolol for migraine prophylaxis was not considered necessary.[1]

1. Peck RW, *et al.* The interaction between propranolol and the novel antimigraine agent zolmitriptan (311C90). *Br J Clin Pharmacol* 1997; **44:** 595–9.

Pharmacokinetics

The absolute bioavailability of zolmitriptan following oral administration is about 40 to 50%, and peak-plasma concentrations are achieved in about 2 to 3.5 hours. Plasma protein binding is low (about 25%). Zolmitriptan undergoes hepatic metabolism, principally to the indole acetic acid, and also the *N*-oxide and *N*-desmethyl analogues. The *N*-desmethyl metabolite (183C91) was more active than the parent compound in *animal* studies, and would be expected to contribute to the therapeutic effect of zolmitriptan. The primary metabolism of zolmitriptan is mediated mainly by the cytochrome P450 isoenzyme CYP1A2 while monoamine oxidase type A is responsible for further metabolism of the *N*-desmethyl metabolite. Over 60% of a dose is excreted in the urine, mainly as the indole acetic acid, and about 30% appears in the faeces, mainly as unchanged drug. The elimination half-life is 2.5 to 3 hours, and is prolonged in patients with liver disease.

References.

1. Seaber E, *et al.* The tolerability and pharmacokinetics of the novel antimigraine compound 311C90 in healthy male volunteers. *Br J Clin Pharmacol* 1996; **41:** 141–7.
2. Dixon R, *et al.* The pharmacokinetics and effects on blood pressure of multiple doses of the novel anti-migraine drug zolmitriptan (311C90) in healthy volunteers. *Br J Clin Pharmacol* 1997; **43:** 273–81.
3. Seaber E, *et al.* The absolute bioavailability and metabolic disposition of the novel antimigraine compound zolmitriptan (311C90). *Br J Clin Pharmacol* 1997; **43:** 579–87.
4. Peck RW, *et al.* The pharmacodynamics and pharmacokinetics of the $5\text{HT}_{1B/1D}$-agonists zolmitriptan in healthy young and elderly men and women. *Clin Pharmacol Ther* 1998; **63:** 342–53.

Uses and Administration

Zolmitriptan is a selective serotonin (5-HT_1) agonist with actions and uses similar to those of sumatriptan (p.451). It is used for the acute treatment of migraine attacks (p.443). Zolmitriptan should not be used prophylactically. It should be administered as early as possible after the onset of migraine headache, but efficacy is independent of the duration of the attack before starting treatment.

The recommended initial dose in the UK is 2.5 mg. If symptoms persist or return within 24 hours, a second dose may be taken not less than 2 hours after the first dose. The maximum dose of zolmitriptan in 24 hours is 15 mg; in those with moderate or severe hepatic impairment a reduced maximum dose of 5 mg in 24 hours is recommended. If a patient does not achieve satisfactory relief with an initial dose of 2.5 mg, subsequent attacks may be treated with initial doses of 5 mg. Recommended doses in the USA are somewhat lower; the initial dose is 1.25 to 2.5 mg with a maximum dose of 10 mg in 24 hours. A single dose of less than 2.5 mg is recommended for patients with hepatic disease or impairment.

Migraine. An initial dose of zolmitriptan 2.5 mg appeared to offer the best balance of efficacy and tolerability in a dose-finding study of the treatment of acute migraine.[1] Efficacy was better after 2.5 or 5 mg than after 1 mg, but the 5-mg dose offered little additional benefit over the 2.5-mg dose and had a higher incidence of adverse effects.

Further references.[2-5]

1. Rapoport AM, *et al.* Optimizing the dose of zolmitriptan (Zomig, 311C90) for the acute treatment of migraine: a multicenter, double-blind, placebo-controlled dose range-finding study. *Neurology* 1997; **49:** 1210–18.
2. Ferrari MD. 311C90: Increasing the options for therapy with effective acute antimigraine $5\text{HT}_{1B/1D}$ receptor agonists. *Neurology* 1997; **48** (suppl 3): S21–S24.
3. Solomon GD, *et al.* Clinical efficacy and tolerability of 2.5 mg zolmitriptan for the acute treatment of migraine. *Neurology* 1997; **49:** 1219–25.
4. Anonymous. Zolmitriptan for migraine. *Med Lett Drugs Ther* 1998; **40:** 27–8.
5. The International 311C90 Long-term Study Group. The long-term tolerability and efficacy of oral zolmitriptan (Zomig, 311C90) in the acute treatment of migraine: an international study. *Headache* 1998; **38:** 173–83.

Preparations

Proprietary Preparations (details are given in Part 3)

Swed.: Zomig; ***UK:*** Zomig; ***USA:*** Zomig.

Antimuscarinics

Antimuscarinic drugs are competitive inhibitors of the actions of acetylcholine at the muscarinic receptors of autonomic effector sites innervated by parasympathetic (cholinergic postganglionic) nerves, as well as being inhibitors of the action of acetylcholine on smooth muscle lacking cholinergic innervation. They have also been described as parasympatholytic, atropinic, atropine-like, and as anticholinergic, although the latter term should encompass compounds that also have antinicotinic actions.

Antimuscarinics can be classified as tertiary amine or quaternary ammonium compounds. The naturally occurring alkaloids such as atropine, hyoscine, and hyoscyamine are tertiary amines, that is they have a tertiary nitrogen atom; semisynthetic derivatives or synthetic antimuscarinics may be either tertiary (e.g. homatropine or benzhexol) or quaternary ammonium (e.g. homatropine methobromide or ipratropium) compounds. At least 5 different pharmacologically identifiable types of **muscarinic receptor** (M_1, M_2, M_3, M_4, and M_5) have been described as have 5 different molecular forms (m_1, m_2, m_3, m_4, and m_5) of these receptors. While the traditional antimuscarinics appear to be relatively nonspecific, newer compounds like pirenzepine and telenzepine have a selective action on the M_1 receptors within ganglia supplying cholinergic postganglionic nerves to the gastro-intestinal tract. At therapeutic doses tertiary amine antimuscarinics have little effect on the actions of acetylcholine at nicotinic receptors. However, the quaternary ammonium antimuscarinics exhibit a greater degree of antinicotinic potency, and some of their side-effects at high doses are due to ganglionic blockade; excessively high doses may even produce neuromuscular block. There are also pharmacokinetic differences between tertiary amine and quaternary ammonium antimuscarinics. Quaternary ammonium compounds are less lipid soluble than tertiary amines; their gastro-intestinal absorption is poor and they do not readily pass the blood-brain barrier or conjunctiva.

Antimuscarinics can produce a wide range of effects at therapeutic doses. The **peripheral** antimuscarinic effects that are produced as the dose increases are: decreased production of secretions from the salivary, bronchial, and sweat glands; dilatation of the pupils (mydriasis) and paralysis of accommodation (cycloplegia); increased heart rate; inhibition of micturition and reduction in gastro-intestinal tone; and inhibition of gastric acid secretion. As for **central** effects, with the exception of hyoscine, which causes CNS depression at therapeutic doses, tertiary amines stimulate the medulla and higher cerebral centres producing mild central vagal excitation and respiratory stimulation. At toxic doses all tertiary amines, including hyoscine, cause stimulation of the CNS with restlessness, disorientation, hallucinations, and delirium. As the dose increases stimulation is followed by central depression and death from respiratory paralysis. Synthetic tertiary amines are less potent in their central effects than natural tertiary amines; quaternary ammonium compounds have negligible central effects.

These actions of antimuscarinics have led to their use in a variety of clinical conditions.

References.

1. Goyal RK. Muscarinic receptor subtypes: physiology and clinical implications. *N Engl J Med* 1989; **321:** 1022–9.
2. Caulfield MP. Muscarinic receptors—characterization, coupling and function. *Pharmacol Ther* 1993; **58:** 319–79.
3. Caulfield MP, Birdsall NJM. International Union of Pharmacology. XVII. Classification of muscarinic acetylcholine receptors. *Pharmacol Rev* 1998; **50:** 279–90.

Anaesthesia

Antimuscarinics, including *atropine, hyoscine,* and *glycopyrronium,* have been used pre-operatively to inhibit salivation and excessive secretions of the respiratory tract during anaesthesia (p.1220). This use is less important now that less irritating anaesthetics are used. Atropine and glycopyrronium are given to reduce intra-operative bradycardia and hypotension induced by drugs such as suxamethonium, halothane, or propofol, or following vagal stimulation. Glycopyrronium causes less tachycardia than atropine when given intravenously. When hyoscine is used as a premedicant it also provides some amnesia, sedation, and antiemesis but, unlike atropine, may cause bradycardia rather than tachycardia. Atropine or glycopyrronium is also used before, or with, anticholinesterases such as neostigmine to prevent their muscarinic adverse effects (see p.1394).

Cardiac disorders

The cardiac uses of *atropine* are discussed on p.456.

Colic pain

Antimuscarinics may relieve painful spasms of the biliary and genito-urinary systems and have been used in biliary or renal (ureteral) colic, although, as discussed on p.8, analgesics are normally used. However, an antispasmodic should be given with morphine and its derivatives in patients with biliary disorders to counteract painful spasms of the sphincter of Oddi which may be produced by the opioid. See Gastro-intestinal Disorders (below) for reference to gastro-intestinal spasm.

Dystonias

Antimuscarinics such as benzhexol have been used in the management of dystonias (p.1141). The high doses which may be required are tolerated much better by children and adolescents than by adults.

Extrapyramidal disorders

See Dystonias (above) and Parkinsonism, including drug-induced extrapyramidal disorders (below).

Eye disorders

See under Mydriasis and Cycloplegia (below).

Gastro-intestinal disorders

Antimuscarinics may relieve **visceral spasms** of the gastro-intestinal tract. They may thus be of use in relieving the pain due to smooth muscle spasm in diverticular disease (p.1169), dyspepsia (p.1169), and irritable bowel syndrome (p.1172); they are no longer considered appropriate for use in infantile colic (see above for use in other forms of colic). Antimuscarinics have also been tried in an attempt to relax the smooth muscle in oesophageal spasm (p.1174), although results are often disappointing. They should be avoided in patients with oesophageal reflux because of a tendency to relax the oesophageal sphincter. For a discussion of the management of gastro-intestinal spasm in general, including mention of the use of antimuscarinics such as *propantheline*, see p.1170.

Antimuscarinics have been used for their antisecretory effects in the treatment of **peptic ulcer disease** (p.1174), generally as adjuncts to other antiulcer drugs. *Pirenzepine*, a selective antimuscarinic, was considered to have the advantage over nonselective antimuscarinics of fewer adverse effects.

Hyoscine is one of the principal drugs used to prevent **motion sickness** (see under Nausea and Vomiting, p.1172). It may be given by mouth for short-term protection or transdermally from controlled release systems for a prolonged duration of action.

Hyperhidrosis

Antimuscarinics such as *diphemanil methylsulphate, glycopyrronium bromide,* and *hyoscine hydrobromide* have been applied topically as alternatives to aluminium salts in the treatment of hyperhidrosis (p.1074). Side-effects of antimuscarinics administered by mouth generally preclude their use by this route, although oral *propantheline* has been used successfully.

Micturition disorders

Normal micturition — awareness of the need to void urine as a result of bladder filling, postponement of urination until convenient, and the ability to empty the bladder voluntarily — is controlled by the smooth detrusor muscle of the bladder (innervated predominantly by parasympathetic nerves) and the external sphincter (sympathetic innervation). During urination parasympathetic stimulation causes the detrusor muscle to contract while reduced sympathetic tone allows the external sphincter to relax. Micturition disorders can occur through local effects on the bladder or urethra or may result through disturbances of their nervous control. They include nocturnal enuresis, urinary incontinence, and urinary retention. The terms 'neurogenic bladder' and 'neuropathic bladder' are used loosely to describe any bladder dysfunction resulting from any neurological disturbance.

Nocturnal enuresis. Involuntary discharge of urine during sleep, termed nocturnal enuresis (bed-wetting), is a normal occurrence in young children, but may persist in up to 5% by the age of 10 years. Nonpharmacological approaches to treatment include bladder retention training, motivational therapy, and behaviour modification or conditioning therapy using moisture-sensitive alarms. Drug therapy may initially produce a more rapid response, but training and the use of alarms has generally appeared to be more effective and to have a lower relapse rate. Although preparations are available to treat children as young as 5 years of age many consider drug therapy to be inappropriate for children under 7 years. Drug therapy is probably most useful for intermittent use on special occasions such as sleeping away from home or when added to treatment in children who fail to respond to nonpharmacological methods alone. The long-term use of drugs for enuresis is controversial.

The synthetic vasopressin analogue desmopressin, tricyclic antidepressants, or antimuscarinics have all been used to treat nocturnal enuresis. Administration of *desmopressin* at night can be effective in the short-term control of nocturnal enuresis and many now consider it to be the drug of choice in terms of safety. However, it should not be given when enuresis is due to polydipsia as desmopressin may provoke water intoxication and convulsions due to hyponatraemia.

Of the tricyclics most experience has been with *imipramine.* Their mechanism of action in nocturnal enuresis is unclear. It may be partly the result of their antimuscarinic and antispasmodic actions.

Antimuscarinics such as *oxybutynin* reduce uninhibited bladder contractions, but although they may be of benefit in diurnal enuresis they are rarely of benefit in nocturnal enuresis alone.

References.

1. Marcovitch H. Treating bed wetting. *Br Med J* 1993; **306:** 536.
2. Rappaport L. The treatment of nocturnal enuresis—where are we now? *Pediatrics* 1993; **92:** 465–6.
3. Mark SD, Frank JD. Nocturnal enuresis. *Br J Urol* 1995; **75:** 427–34.
4. Monda JM, Husmann DA. Primary nocturnal enuresis: a comparison among observation, imipramine, desmopressin acetate and bed-wetting alarm systems. *J Urol (Baltimore)* 1995, **154:** 745–8.

5. Burke JR, *et al.* A comparison of amitriptyline, vasopressin and amitriptyline with vasopressin in nocturnal enuresis. *Pediatr Nephrol* 1995; **9:** 438–40.
6. Tietjen DN, Husmann DA. Nocturnal enuresis: a guide to evaluation and treatment. *Mayo Clin Proc* 1996; **71:** 857–62.
7. Owens RG, Karram MM. Comparative tolerability of drug therapies used to treat incontinence and enuresis. *Drug Safety* 1998; **19:** 123–39.

Urinary incontinence and retention. Urinary incontinence is defined as an involuntary loss of urine which is objectively demonstrable and a social or hygienic problem. Nocturnal enuresis is discussed above. Depending on the cause patients may have symptoms of urinary frequency, nocturia, urgency, dribbling, or dysuria. Classifications of incontinence vary but the main types include: stress incontinence, urge incontinence, and overflow incontinence (a consequence of urinary retention). The term functional incontinence is used when the patient's condition is due to impaired mobility or mental function. It is important to determine the type and, where possible, cause of urinary incontinence before attempting treatment. Urinary-tract infections, constipation, and prostatic hyperplasia may mimic or cause the symptoms of urinary incontinence and should be excluded.

Stress incontinence is the commonest form of incontinence in women. The patient usually has urethral sphincter incompetence and loss of urine is associated with increases in intra-abdominal pressure such as may occur on standing or coughing. Treatment may be with nonpharmacological measures such as pelvic floor exercises, electrical stimulation, or biofeedback, and the use of devices such as vaginal cones; with surgery; or with drugs. Some consider that drug therapy has little part in the treatment of stress incontinence. Alpha-adrenoceptor agonists such as *ephedrine, phenylpropanolamine,* and *pseudoephedrine* have been used to increase tone in the muscles of the urethra and at the base of the bladder; they may be helpful when used prophylactically in certain stress situations, but long-term experience has been mostly disappointing. *Oestrogens* used with an alpha-adrenoceptor agonist such as phenylpropanolamine appear to be effective and this combination may be of use for postmenopausal women with mild stress incontinence; unfortunately addition of a progestogen to treatment to reduce the risk of endometrial carcinoma in women with an intact uterus might exacerbate the incontinence. The value of oestrogens used without an alpha-adrenoceptor agonist is less clear. Intra-urethral injections of *collagen* or *polytef* appear to be effective, but there are concerns over migration and granuloma formation with polytef.

In **urge incontinence**, also known as unstable bladder or detrusor instability, uninhibited contractions of the detrusor muscle occur without warning and overcome urethral sphincter resistance. Micturition occurs despite any attempt the patient might make to prevent it. Urge incontinence is the most common form of incontinence in the elderly and is often refractory to treatment. The cause is usually unknown and these cases are referred to as being due to **idiopathic detrusor instability**. When there is overt neurological disease, such as upper motor neurone lesions in spinal cord injury or multiple sclerosis, the term **detrusor hyperreflexia** is used. Reduction of excessive fluid intake and avoidance of drinks containing alcohol or caffeine may control mild symptoms of urge incontinence. Physiotherapy and behaviour therapy including bladder drill, biofeedback, hypnotherapy, acupuncture, and electrical stimulation may help. No drug treatment has been found to be universally effective. Drugs with antimuscarinic activity have been used to relax the detrusor muscle by inhibiting unstable detrusor muscle contractions but the incidence of adverse effects can be high. As these drugs can increase bladder volume they should not be used in patients with urinary retention. The antimuscarinic *oxybutynin* also has direct smooth muscle relaxant properties and is considered by some to be the most useful drug, but adverse effects are common. *Tolterodine* and *propiverine* have recently been introduced as alternatives to oxybutynin. *Flavoxate* has also been used but appears to be less effective than oxybutynin. *Propantheline,* although once widely used, is not recommended for routine use due to its low response rate and a high incidence of side-effects. Other antimuscarinics used include *dicyclomine* which also possesses antispasmodic properties. *Emepronium* was once popular but is now considered to be of limited use. *Tricyclic antidepressants* have also been used in urge incontinence because of their antimuscarinic activity but their main use has been in nocturnal enuresis and nocturia (see above). *Desmopressin* is also mainly used in nocturnal enuresis and nocturia. Evidence regarding the use of *oestrogens* is inconclusive, but they may be useful in the adjunctive treatment of postmenopausal women with symptoms of urgency, frequency, and nocturia. Surgery is reserved for intractable cases.

Urge incontinence can also be due to abnormalities in bladder sensation; the causes of **sensory urgency** are often unknown but may be due to conditions such as urinary-tract infections or interstitial cystitis. Bladder retraining techniques and antimuscarinic therapy have been suggested when no underlying disorder can be identified.

Patients with **overflow incontinence** suffer from a continuous or frequent dribbling of urine as a consequence of an overdistended bladder produced by **urinary retention**. It may result from some form of urethral blockage or may be associated with drug treatment or conditions that reduce detrusor contractions or interfere with relaxation of the urethra. Overflow incontinence is uncommon in women and most patients are elderly men with urethral blockage due to benign prostatic hyperplasia (p.1446). However, urinary retention may also occur postpartum or postoperatively. Treatment depends on the underlying condition. Catheterisation is used to relieve acute painful urinary retention or when no cause can be found. Surgical procedures or dilatation are often used to correct any mechanical outflow obstruction. Alpha-adrenoceptor blocking drugs such as *alfuzosin, doxazosin, indoramin, prazosin, tamsulosin,* and *terazosin* may be given to patients waiting for surgery or to those unfit for surgery. They decrease outflow resistance and improve bladder emptying. Patients with detrusor hypotonicity have been given parasympathomimetics such as *bethanechol, carbachol,* and *distigmine* to increase detrusor muscle contractions but there have been doubts about their efficacy. Parasympathomimetics have also been used for the management of postoperative urinary retention, but have been superseded by catheterisation.

References.

1. International Continence Society Standardization Committee. The standardization of terminology of lower urinary tract function. *Br J Obstet Gynaecol* 1990; **97** (suppl 6): 1–16.
2. Battock TM, Castleden CM. Pharmacological treatment of urinary incontinence. *Br Med Bull* 1990; **46:** 147–55.
3. Cardozo L. Urinary incontinence in women: have we anything new to offer? *Br Med J* 1991; **303:** 1453–7.
4. Anonymous. Non-surgical treatment of stress incontinence. *Lancet* 1992; **340:** 643–4.
5. Eckford SD, Keane DP. Management of detrusor instability. *Br J Hosp Med* 1993; **49:** 282–5.
6. Wise BG, Cardozo LD. Urinary urgency in women. *Br J Hosp Med* 1993; **50:** 243–50.
7. Richmond D. The incontinent woman: 2. *Br J Hosp Med* 1993; **50:** 490–2.
8. Resnick NM. Urinary incontinence. *Lancet* 1995; **346:** 94–9.
9. Chutka DS, *et al.* Urinary incontinence in the elderly population. *Mayo Clin Proc* 1996; **71:** 93–101.
10. Owens RG, Karram MM. Comparative tolerability of drug therapies used to treat incontinence and enuresis. *Drug Safety* 1998; **19:** 123–39.

Mydriasis and cycloplegia

Drugs that dilate the pupil (mydriatics) and paralyse accommodation (cycloplegics) are used topically as in the examination of the eye and other ophthalmic procedures, in the management of inflammatory conditions of the eye to treat or prevent the formation of adhesions between the lens and the iris (see Uveitis, p.1030), and in strabismus (p.1389).

Mydriasis can be achieved by paralysis of the pupillary constrictor muscles (which is how antimuscarinics act) or by stimulation of the dilator muscles (which is how sympathomimetics act). Cycloplegia results from paralysis of the ciliary muscles (antimuscarinics, but not sympathomimetics, have this effect).

Antimuscarinics used in ophthalmology vary in onset and duration of action. *Atropine* can take up to 40 minutes or more to produce mydriasis, which persists for at least 7 days; it takes 1 to 3 hours to produce cycloplegia and 6 to 12 days for recovery of accommodation. *Hyoscine* has a shorter duration of action than atropine, although the effects may still persist for 3 to 7 days. For ophthalmic procedures, antimuscarinics such as *homatropine, cyclopentolate,* or *tropicamide,* which have a more rapid onset and shorter duration of action than atropine, may be preferable. Tropicamide has the shortest duration of action with recovery occurring in up to 6 hours. The effects of cyclopentolate may last for 24 hours. Recovery following administration of homatropine may take up to 3 days. However, cycloplegia with homatropine may be incomplete and for young children who are often resistant to the action of homatropine, cyclopentolate or atropine may be preferred.

The sympathomimetic most commonly used topically is *phenylephrine* but *hydroxyamphetamine* is also used in some countries. They are often used with antimuscarinic to enhance mydriasis especially in patients who might respond poorly to antimuscarinic alone, such as those with dark irides or diabetes or those who are receiving prolonged miotic therapy. Adrenaline has been used for maintenance of mydriasis during ophthalmic surgery.

The local anaesthetic *cocaine* also has an independent mydriatic effect but because of concern over corneal toxicity it is now little used in ophthalmology.

Miosis (pupil constriction) resistant to conventional mydriatics often develops during ocular surgery, possibly due to the release of prostaglandins and other substances associated with trauma. NSAIDs are prostaglandin synthetase inhibitors and have been tried before ocular surgery to prevent or reduce intra-operative miosis. They do not possess intrinsic mydriatic properties.

Parkinsonism

Antimuscarinics are used in Parkinson's disease (idiopathic or primary parkinsonism) and drug-induced parkinsonism. Those most commonly used are the tertiary amines, *benzhexol, benztropine, orphenadrine,* and *procyclidine.* In Parkinson's disease (p.1128), antimuscarinics are generally used in the early stages when the condition is mild and tremor is the predominant symptom, as they provide little benefit in bradykinesia. They can also reduce the sialorrhoea experienced by patients with this disease but can aggravate other associated conditions such as constipation or dementia. Antimuscarinics may also be used later as adjuvant therapy to levodopa such as in patients with refractory tremor or dystonias.

Although antimuscarinics may provide relief from the extrapyramidal symptoms that occur as side-effects of antipsychotic therapy (see p.650), they do not relieve the symptoms of tardive dyskinesia and should be discontinued if it develops.

Respiratory-tract disorders

The parasympathetic nervous system is involved in regulating bronchomotor tone, with an increase in parasympathetic activity resulting in bronchoconstriction. Antimuscarinics have potent bronchodilatory activity and may be used in the management of bronchospasm. The main ones used are *ipratropium* and *oxitropium*; *atropine* and *glycopyrronium* have also been used. Ipratropium and oxitropium by inhalation are used in chronic bronchitis (p.747) and are as effective or possibly slightly more effective than $beta_2$ agonists. They are also among the bronchodilators that may be added to the existing regimen of an inhaled short-acting $beta_2$ agonist plus regular high-dose inhaled corticosteroid in severe asthma (p.745).

References.

1. Gross NJ, Skorodin MS. Role of the parasympathetic system in airway obstruction due to emphysema. *N Engl J Med* 1984; **311:** 421–5.

Rhinitis

The antimuscarinic drug ipratropium is used intranasally for the treatment of rhinitis (see p.755).

Vertigo

Antihistamines are the mainstay of the treatment of vertigo (p.401), although the antimuscarinic drug *hyoscine* is effective in the prophylaxis and treatment of vertigo and nausea associated with vestibular disorders, such as Ménière's disease (p.400). See also motion sickness under Nausea and Vomiting (p.463).

Atropine (331-w)

Atropine *(BAN)*.

(±)-Hyoscyamine. (1*R*,3*r*,5*S*,8*r*)-Tropan-3-yl (*RS*)-tropate.

$C_{17}H_{23}NO_3$ = 289.4.

CAS — 51-55-8.

Pharmacopoeias. In Swiss and US.

An alkaloid which may be obtained from solanaceous plants, or prepared by synthesis.

White needle-like crystals or white crystalline powder. **Soluble** 1 in 460 of water, 1 in 2 of alcohol, 1 in 1 of chloroform, 1 in 25 of ether, and 1 in 90 of water at 80°. A saturated solution in water is alkaline to phenolphthalein. **Store** in airtight containers. Protect from light.

Atropine Methobromide (332-e)

Atropine Methobromide *(BANM)*.

Atropine Methylbromide; Methylatropine Bromide; Methylatropini Bromidum; Methylatropinium Bromatum; Mydriasine. (1*R*,3*r*,5*S*)-8-Methyl-3-[(±)-tropoyloxy]tropanium bromide.

$C_{18}H_{26}BrNO_3$ = 384.3.

CAS — 2870-71-5.

Pharmacopoeias. In *Eur.* (see p.viii).

Colourless crystals or a white crystalline powder. Freely **soluble** in water; sparingly soluble in alcohol; practically insoluble in ether. **Protect** from light.

Atropine Methonitrate (333-l)

Atropine Methonitrate *(BANM, rINN)*.

Atrop. Methonit.; Atropini Methonitras; Methylatropine Nitrate *(USAN)*; Methylatropini Nitras. (1*R*,3*r*,5*S*)-8-Methyl-3-[(±)-tropoyloxy]tropanium nitrate.

$C_{18}H_{26}N_2O_6$ = 366.4.

CAS — 52-88-0.

Pharmacopoeias. In *Eur.* (see p.viii).

Colourless crystals or a white crystalline powder. Freely **soluble** in water; soluble in alcohol; practically insoluble in ether. Aqueous solutions are unstable; stability is enhanced in acid solutions of pH below 6. **Protect** from light.

Atropine Sulphate (335-j)

Atropine Sulphate *(BANM)*.

Atrop. Sulph.; Atropine Sulfate; Atropini Sulfas.

$(C_{17}H_{23}NO_3)_2,H_2SO_4,H_2O$ = 694.8.

CAS — 55-48-1 (anhydrous atropine sulphate); 5908-99-6 (atropine sulphate monohydrate).

NOTE. Compounded preparations of atropine sulphate and diphenoxylate hydrochloride in the proportions, by weight, 1 part to 100 parts have the British Approved Name Co-phenotrope.

ATR is a code approved by the BP for use on single unit dose eye drops containing atropine sulphate where the individual container may be too small to bear all the appropriate labelling information.

Pharmacopoeias. In *Chin., Eur.* (see p.viii), *Int., Jpn, Pol.,* and *US.*

Odourless colourless crystals or white crystalline powder. It effloresces in dry air. **Soluble** 1 in 0.5 of water, 1 in 2.5 of boiling water, 1 in 5 of alcohol, 1 in 2.5 of glycerol; practically insoluble in ether. A 2% solution in water has a pH of 4.5 to 6.2. **Store** in airtight containers. Protect from light.

Incompatibilities. Incompatibility between atropine sulphate and hydroxybenzoate preservatives has been observed,[1] resulting in a total loss of the atropine in 2 to 3 weeks.

1. Deeks T. Oral atropine sulphate mixtures. *Pharm J* 1983; **230:** 481.

Adverse Effects

The pattern of adverse effects seen with atropine and other antimuscarinics can mostly be related to their pharmacological actions at muscarinic and, at high doses, nicotinic receptors (see p.453). These effects are dose-related and are usually reversible when therapy is discontinued. The **peripheral** side-effects of atropine and other antimuscarinics are a consequence of their inhibitory effect on muscarinic receptors within the autonomic nervous system. At therapeutic doses, adverse effects include dryness of the mouth with difficulty in swallowing and talking, thirst, reduced bronchial secretions, dilatation of the pupils (mydriasis) with loss of accommodation (cycloplegia) and photophobia, flushing and dryness of the skin, transient bradycardia followed by tachycardia, with palpitations and arrhythmias, and difficulty in micturition, as well as reduction in the tone and motility of the gastro-intestinal tract leading to constipation. Some of the **central** side-effects of atropine and other tertiary antimuscarinics seen at toxic doses (see below) may also occur at therapeutic doses.

In overdosage, the peripheral effects become more pronounced and other symptoms such as hyperthermia, hypertension, increased respiratory rate, and nausea and vomiting may occur. A rash may appear on the face or upper trunk. Toxic doses also cause CNS stimulation marked by restlessness, confusion, excitement, ataxia, incoordination, paranoid and psychotic reactions, hallucinations and delirium, and occasionally seizures. However, in severe intoxication, central stimulation may give way to CNS depression, coma, circulatory and respiratory failure, and death.

There is considerable variation in susceptibility to atropine; recovery has occurred even after 1 g, whereas deaths have been reported from doses of 100 mg or less for adults and 10 mg for children.

Quaternary ammonium antimuscarinics, such as atropine methobromide or methonitrate and propantheline bromide, have some ganglion-blocking activity so that high doses may cause postural hypotension and impotence; in toxic doses non-depolarising neuromuscular block may be produced.

Systemic toxicity may be produced by the instillation of antimuscarinic eye drops, particularly in children and in the elderly. Prolonged administration of atropine to the eye may lead to local irritation, hyperaemia, oedema, and conjunctivitis. An increase in intra-ocular pressure may occur, especially in patients with angle-closure glaucoma.

Hypersensitivity to atropine is not uncommon and may occur as conjunctivitis or a skin rash.

Effects on body temperature. Atropine can cause hyperthermia as a result of inhibition of sweating. This may be attenuated by atropine's ability to dilate cutaneous blood vessels. However, there has been a report of hypothermia in a 14-year-old feverish patient following intravenous administration of atropine.[1]

For reports of fatal heat stroke in patients receiving an antimuscarinic and an antipsychotic concomitantly, see under Interactions in Benztropine, p.458.

1. Lacouture PG, *et al.* Acute hypothermia associated with atropine. *Am J Dis Child* 1983; **137:** 291–2.

Effects on the CNS. Relatively recent references to the CNS toxicity of atropine describe a toxic psychosis[1] and an increase in frequency of seizures.[2] In both instances the effects followed the administration of atropine (alone or with hyoscine hydrobromide and phenylephrine hydrochloride) as eye drops.

1. Kortabarría RP, *et al.* Toxic psychosis following cycloplegic eyedrops. *DICP Ann Pharmacother* 1990; **24:** 708–9.
2. Wright BD. Exacerbation of akinetic seizures by atropine eye drops. *Br J Ophthalmol* 1992; **76:** 179–80.

Effects on the eyes. In addition to the expected ocular effects of atropine there have been instances of acute angle-closure glaucoma in patients receiving nebulised atropine.[1]

1. Berdy GJ, *et al.* Angle closure glaucoma precipitated by aerosolized atropine. *Arch Intern Med* 1991; **151:** 1658–60.

Effects on the gastro-intestinal tract. A report of paralytic ileus in a 77-year-old man with Parkinson's disease who had been receiving atropine sulphate by mouth to control excess salivation.[1]

1. Beatson N. Atropine and paralytic ileus. *Postgrad Med J* 1982; **58:** 451–3.

Effects on the heart. Atropine sulphate to a total of 1 mg per 70 kg body-weight given intravenously to 79 patients before surgery produced arrhythmias in over 20% of patients but particularly frequently in the young.[1] Atrioventricular dissociation was the most common disturbance in adults and in children atrial rhythm disturbances were common. In another study[2] premedication including atropine or glycopyrronium given intramuscularly resulted in a significantly greater incidence of tachycardia during anaesthetic induction and intubation compared with controls who received no antimuscarinic drug. Patients who received glycopyrronium also had a higher incidence of tachycardia during surgery than the controls. No significant difference in bradycardia or extrasystoles was found in the atropine- or the glycopyrronium-treated patients. Atrial fibrillation has been reported in 2 elderly glaucoma patients following post-surgical application of atropine ointment or eye drops to the eye.[3]

1. Dauchot P, Gravenstein JS. Effects of atropine on the electrocardiogram in different age groups. *Clin Pharmacol Ther* 1971; **12:** 274–80.
2. Shipton EA, Roelofse JA. Effects on cardiac rhythm of premedication with atropine or glycopyrrolate. *S Afr Med J* 1984; **66:** 287–8.
3. Merli GJ, *et al.* Cardiac dysrhythmias associated with ophthalmic atropine. *Arch Intern Med* 1986; **146:** 45–7.

Effects on mental function. A study[1] in patients with Parkinson's disease and healthy control subjects suggested that although short-term memory was impaired in patients receiving long-term antimuscarinic therapy the effect was reversible on discontinuation.

See also under benzhexol (p.457) and under oxybutynin (p.466).

1. Van Herwaarden G, *et al.* Short-term memory in Parkinson's disease after withdrawal of long-term anticholinergic therapy. *Clin Neuropharmacol* 1993; **16:** 438–43.

Hypersensitivity. A report[1] of anaphylactic shock developing in a 38-year-old woman following an intravenous injection of atropine.

1. Aguilera L, *et al.* Anaphylactic reaction after atropine. *Anaesthesia* 1988; **43:** 955–7.

Overdosage. Reports of atropine poisoning or overdosage have included a respiratory therapist[1] who had given 10 atropine sulphate aerosol treatments in the preceding 24 hours and children who had taken overdoses of a preparation containing diphenoxylate and atropine.[2]

1. Larkin GL. Occupational atropine poisoning via aerosol. *Lancet* 1991; **337:** 917.
2. McCarron MM, *et al.* Diphenoxylate-atropine (Lomotil) overdose in children: an update (report of eight cases and review of the literature). *Pediatrics* 1991; **87:** 694–700.

Treatment of Adverse Effects

If overdoses of atropine have been taken by mouth the stomach should be emptied. Activated charcoal has also been suggested to reduce absorption. Supportive therapy should be given as required.

Physostigmine has been tried for antimuscarinic poisoning (see p.1396) but such use can be hazardous and is not generally recommended. Diazepam may be given to control marked excitement and convulsions; phenothiazines should not be given as they may exacerbate antimuscarinic effects.

Precautions

Atropine needs to be used with caution in children and the elderly (who may be more susceptible to its adverse effects), in patients with or at risk of urinary retention (including those with prostatic enlargement), and in those with paralytic ileus or pyloric stenosis. In patients with ulcerative colitis its use may lead to ileus or megacolon, and its effects on the lower oesophageal sphincter may exacerbate reflux. Caution is generally advisable in any patient with diarrhoea. It should not be given to patients with myasthenia gravis except to reduce adverse muscarinic effects of an anticholinesterase.

Atropine should not be given to patients with angle-closure glaucoma or with a narrow angle between the iris and the cornea, since it may raise intra-ocular pressure and precipitate an acute attack. Acute angle-closure glaucoma has been reported in patients receiving nebulised atropine. Some recommend that atropine eye drops should not be used in infants aged less than 3 months due to the possible association between the induced cycloplegia and the development of amblyopia. Systemic reactions have followed the absorption of atropine from eye drops; overdosage is less likely if the eye ointment is used. In the event of blurred vision, following topical administration of atropine to the eye, patients should not drive or operate machinery. Systemic administration of antimuscarinics may also cause blurred vision, dizziness, and other effects that may impair a patient's ability to perform skilled tasks such as driving.

Because of the risk of provoking hyperthermia atropine should not be given to patients, especially children, when the ambient temperature is high. It should also be used cautiously in patients with fever.

Atropine and other antimuscarinics need to be used with caution in conditions characterised by tachycardia such as thyrotoxicosis, heart failure, and in cardiac surgery, where they may further accelerate the heart rate. Care is required in patients with acute myocardial infarction, as ischaemia and infarction may be made worse, and in patients with hypertension.

Atropine may cause confusion, especially in the elderly. Reduced bronchial secretion caused by systemic administration of atropine may be associated with the formation of mucous plugs.

In the treatment of parkinsonism, increases in dosage and transfer to other forms of treatment should be gradual and antimuscarinic should not be withdrawn abruptly. Minor reactions may be controlled by reducing the dose until tolerance has developed.

Persons with Down's syndrome appear to have an increased susceptibility to some of the actions of atropine, whereas those with albinism may have a reduced susceptibility.

Interactions

The effects of atropine and other antimuscarinics may be enhanced by the concomitant administration of other drugs with antimuscarinic properties, such as amantadine, some antihistamines, phenothiazine antipsychotics, and tricyclic antidepressants. Inhibition of drug-metabolising enzymes by MAOIs may possibly enhance the effects of antimuscarinics. The reduction in gastric motility caused by antimuscarinics may affect the absorption of other drugs. Antimuscarinics and parasympathomimetics may counteract each others effects.

Pharmacokinetics

Atropine is readily absorbed from the gastro-intestinal tract; it is also absorbed from mucous membranes, the eye, and to some extent through intact skin. It is rapidly cleared from the blood and is distributed throughout the body. It crosses the blood-brain barrier. It is incompletely metabolised in the liver and is excreted in the urine as unchanged drug and metabolites. A half-life of about 4 hours has been reported. Atropine crosses the placenta and traces appear in breast milk.

Quaternary ammonium salts of atropine, such as the methonitrate, are less readily absorbed after oral administration. They are highly ionised in body fluids and being poorly soluble in lipids they do not readily cross the blood-brain barrier.

Pregnancy. Studies of the pharmacokinetics of atropine in mother and fetus in late pregnancy[1-3] indicated that atropine rapidly crosses the placenta. However, whereas peak concentrations of atropine in fetal cord blood were reached about 5 minutes after intravenous administration, the maximum effect on fetal heart rate occurred after about 25 minutes.

1. Barrier G, *et al.* La pharmacocinétique de l'atropine chez la femme enceinte et le foetus en fin de grossesse. *Anesth Analg Reanim* 1976; **33:** 795–800.
2. Onnen I, *et al.* Placental transfer of atropine at the end of pregnancy. *Eur J Clin Pharmacol* 1979; **15:** 443–6.
3. Kanto J, *et al.* Placental transfer and pharmacokinetics of atropine after a single maternal intravenous and intramuscular administration. *Acta Anaesthesiol Scand* 1981; **25:** 85–8.

Uses and Administration

Atropine is a tertiary amine antimuscarinic alkaloid with both central and peripheral actions (see p.453). It is usually given as the sulphate. It first stimulates and then depresses the CNS and has antispasmodic actions on smooth muscle and reduces secretions, especially salivary and bronchial secretions; it also reduces perspiration, but has little effect on biliary or pancreatic secretion. Atropine depresses the vagus and thereby increases the heart rate. When given by mouth atropine reduces smooth-muscle tone and diminishes gastric and intestinal motility but has little effect on gastric secretion in usual therapeutic doses. Quaternary ammonium derivatives, such as the methonitrate, have less effect on the CNS but strong ganglion-blocking activity. Atropine is used for a variety of purposes, including: in anaesthetic practice as a premedicant and to counteract the muscarinic effects of anticholinesterases such as neostigmine and other parasympathomimetics; as an antispasmodic in gastro-intestinal disorders; as an adjunct to opioid analgesics for the symptomatic relief of biliary or renal colic; to treat bradycardia; to treat or prevent bronchospasm; and in the treatment of poisoning with mushrooms that contain muscarine and in organophosphorus pesticide poisoning. Atropine is used topically as a mydriatic and cycloplegic in ophthalmology.

See below for details on dosage and administration of atropine and its derivatives.

Anaesthesia. The role of antimuscarinics in anaesthesia is discussed on p.453.

Atropine has been given as a premedicant before general anaesthesia to diminish the risk of vagal inhibition of the heart and to reduce salivary and bronchial secretions. For premedication 300 to 600 µg of atropine sulphate may be given by subcutaneous or intramuscular injection, usually 30 to 60 minutes before anaesthesia. Alternatively 300 to 600 µg of atropine sulphate may be given intravenously immediately before induction of anaesthesia. Atropine sulphate may also be given in combination with up to 10 mg morphine sulphate by subcutaneous or intramuscular injection about an hour before anaesthesia. Suitable paediatric premedication doses of atropine sulphate are: 100 µg subcutaneously for children weighing up to 3 kg; 200 µg for children weighing 7 to 9 kg; 300 µg for children weighing 12 to 16 kg; 400 µg for children weighing 20 to 27 kg; 500 µg for children weighing 32 kg; and 600 µg for children weighing 41 kg.

To counteract the muscarinic effects of anticholinesterases when they are used to reverse the effects of competitive muscle relaxants (see Neostigmine, p.1394) atropine sulphate 0.6 to 1.2 mg is given by intravenous injection before or with the anticholinesterase.

Anoxic seizures. A reflex anoxic seizure is a paroxysmal event triggered by a noxious stimulus which, by vagal stimulation, causes pronounced bradycardia or cardiac arrest and consequent relative cerebral ischaemia.[1] Certain features of the attack may lead to a misdiagnosis of epilepsy. To avoid confusion with epileptic seizures (p.335), reflex anoxic seizures have also been called white or type 2 breath holding attacks. Depending on the degree of vagal hypersensitivity or noxious stimulus attacks may occur infrequently or several times a day.

Infants and young children are mainly affected, however, the condition usually resolves by early childhood. It is generally benign and children do not suffer cardiac or cerebral damage. Treatment is seldom necessary, but atropine has been advocated to prevent vagal hypersensitivity in those children with frequent, persistent attacks. As atropine may require frequent administration with an attendant risk of overdosage, transdermal hyoscine has been tried as an alternative.[2]

1. Appleton RE. Reflex anoxic seizures. *Br Med J* 1993; **307:** 214–5.
2. Palm L, Blennow G. Transdermal anticholinergic treatment of reflex anoxic seizures. *Acta Paediatr Scand* 1985; **74:** 803–4.

Cardiac disorders. Atropine depresses the vagus and thereby increases the heart rate. It is therefore used in a variety of disorders or circumstances in which bradyarrhythmias occur. It is frequently used in sudden onset bradyarrhythmias and although it may also be employed for the initial treatment of chronic arrhythmias (p.782), cardiac pacing is generally preferred for long-term control. Examples of acute use include the prevention and treatment of arrhythmias associated with anaesthesia (see above), the treatment of other drug-induced arrhythmias, and in cardiac arrest due to asystole. Atropine sulphate has been used in the management of bradycardia of acute myocardial infarction; however, caution is required, as atropine may exacerbate ischaemia or infarction in these patients. European and US authorities have published standards and guidelines for cardiopulmonary resuscitation and emergency cardiac care, including recommendations on the use of atropine. The dosage of atropine sulphate, and the frequency at which doses are repeated, varies according to the severity of the condition. In **asystole**, the recommended adult dose of atropine in the European guidelines is 3 mg given intravenously once only, although it is stated that the evidence for benefit is equivocal;[1] in the USA the dose is 1 mg intravenously which is repeated in 3 to 5 minutes if asystole continues.[2] The European guidelines do not consider that atropine is necessary for the management of paediatric asystole.[3] In **bradycardia**, atropine is given in doses of 0.5 to 1.0 mg intravenously repeated every 3 to 5 minutes to a total dose of 0.04 mg per kg body-weight.[2] If an intravenous line cannot be established, atropine can be given via an endotracheal tube.

1. Advanced Life Support Working Group of the European Resuscitation Council. The 1998 European Resuscitation Council guidelines for adult advanced life support. *Br Med J* 1998; **316:** 1863–9.
2. Emergency Cardiac Care Committee and Subcommittees, American Heart Association. Guidelines for cardiopulmonary resuscitation and emergency cardiac care. *JAMA* 1992; **268:** 2171–2295.
3. Paediatric Life Support Working Party of the European Resuscitation Council. Guidelines for paediatric life support. *Br Med J* 1994; **308:** 1349–55.

Colic pain. Atropine has been used as an adjunct to opioid analgesics for symptomatic relief of biliary or renal colic (see p.453).

Eye disorders. Atropine is used to produce mydriasis and cycloplegia (p.454) for ophthalmic examination. Dilatation of the pupil occurs in half an hour following one local application and lasts for a week or more; marked paralysis of accommodation is obtained in 1 to 3 hours with recovery in 6 to 12 days. However, other antimuscarinics such as cyclopentolate, homatropine, or tropicamide may be preferred because they have a more rapid onset and shorter duration of action than atropine. Atropine is also used in the management of uveitis and iritis, and in strabismus. It is used in the treatment of iritis and uveitis to immobilise the ciliary muscle and iris and to prevent or break down adhesions. Because of its powerful cycloplegic action atropine is also used in the determination of refraction in children below the age of 6 and in children with convergent strabismus (p.1389).

In the treatment of **inflammatory eye disorders** such as uveitis or iritis (p.1030), the dose of atropine sulphate for adults is 1 or 2 drops of a 0.5 or 1% solution instilled into the eye(s) up to four times daily. The dose in children is 1 or 2 drops of a 0.5% solution (or one drop of a 1% solution) instilled up to three times daily. For **refraction** in adults the dose is one drop of a 1% solution of atropine sulphate; this may be instilled either twice daily for 1 or 2 days before the procedure or on a single occasion one hour before the procedure. In children the dose for refraction is 1 or 2 drops of a 0.5% solution (or one drop of a 1% solution) instilled twice daily for 1 to 3 days before the procedure, with a further dose given one hour before the procedure. An ophthalmic ointment of atropine sulphate 1% may be preferred for children under 5 years of age and particularly in infants under 3 months of age who are at increased risk of systemic effects with eye drops. Some recommend that atropine sulphate should not be used in the eyes of children younger than 3 months of age due to a possible association between the cycloplegia produced and the development of amblyopia.

Atropine borate has also been used in ophthalmic preparations.

References.

1. Stolovitch C, *et al.* Atropine cycloplegia: how many instillations does one need? *J Pediatr Ophthalmol Strabismus* 1992; **29:** 175–6.
2. Foley-Nolan A, *et al.* Atropine penalisation versus occlusion as the primary treatment for amblyopia. *Br J Ophthalmol* 1997; **81:** 54–7.

Gastro-intestinal disorders. Antimuscarinics may be used in gastro-intestinal disorders (see p.453) because of their marked inhibitory effect on gastro-intestinal motility and their antisecretory effects. Atropine (as the sulphate or quaternary derivatives such as the methobromide or methonitrate) has been used to reduce smooth-muscle tone and diminish motility, but has little effect on gastric secretion at usual therapeutic doses (about 200 µg of atropine sulphate). It has been tried as an adjunct to the treatment of gastric and duodenal ulcers and the antispasmodic action of atropine has been used to facilitate radiological examination of the gut. Atropine sulphate has also been used in the treatment of irritable bowel syndrome. Atropine oxide hydrochloride is also used for gastro-intestinal disorders.

Poisoning. Atropine is used in the management of overdosage or poisoning due to various substances with muscarinic actions. It is used to overcome the effects of accumulation of acetylcholine produced by anticholinesterase compounds including organophosphorus pesticides,[1,2] chemical warfare nerve gases,[3] and parasympathomimetics such as neostigmine. It is also used to antagonise the effects of cholinomimetic substances in the treatment of overdosage with parasympathomimetics such as bethanechol and in the treatment of poisoning with mushrooms that contain muscarine. Atropine blocks the action of these compounds at muscarinic receptors reversing bradycardia and decreasing tracheobronchial secretions, bronchoconstriction, intestinal secretions, and intestinal motility.

In the treatment of poisoning with organophosphorus pesticides or chemical warfare nerve gases atropine may be given to adults in an initial dose of 2 mg or more intramuscularly or intravenously every 10 to 30 minutes until muscarinic effects disappear or signs of atropine toxicity are seen but depending on the severity of the symptoms injections have been given as often as every 5 minutes in some centres. In moderate to severe poisoning a state of atropinisation is usually maintained for at least 2 days and continued for as long as symptoms are evident. In severely poisoned patients this may entail prolonged treatment.[4,5] As large amounts of atropine may be required it is important to use a preservative-free preparation to avoid the potential toxicity associated with administration of excess quantities of preservatives such as benzyl alcohol or chlorobutanol. Since atropine is ineffective against any nicotinic effects of these compounds a cholinesterase reactivator such as pralidoxime (p.992) may be used as an adjunct.

The use of atropine in poisoning or overdosage with other compounds having muscarinic actions is similar to that for organophosphorus pesticides but the duration of treatment necessary is usually shorter. An initial dose of 0.5 to 1 mg given subcutaneously or intravenously and repeated every 2 hours may be adequate for overdosage with cholinomimetics such as bethanechol.

1. Karalleidde L, Senanayake N. Organophosphorus insecticide poisoning. *Br J Anaesth* 1989; **63:** 736–50.
2. Lotti M. Treatment of acute organophosphate poisoning. *Med J Aust* 1991; **154:** 51–5.
3. Anonymous. Prevention and treatment of nerve gas poisoning. *Med Lett Drugs Ther* 1990; **32:** 103–5.
4. Golsousidis H, Kokkas V. Use of 19 590 mg of atropine during 24 days of treatment, after a case of unusually severe parathion poisoning. *Hum Toxicol* 1985; **4:** 339–40.
5. Afzaal S, *et al.* High dose atropine in organophosphorus poisoning. *Postgrad Med J* 1990; **66:** 70–1.

Respiratory tract disorders. Although atropine is a potent bronchodilator its use in the management of reversible airways obstruction has largely been replaced by other antimuscarinics (see p.454). It is sometimes used in combination preparations with antihistamines and decongestants for the symptomatic relief of symptoms of the common cold.

References.

1. Sur S, *et al.* A random double-blind trial of the combination of nebulized atropine methylnitrate and albuterol in nocturnal asthma. *Ann Allergy* 1990; **65:** 384–8.
2. Vichyanond P, *et al.* Efficacy of atropine methylnitrate alone and in combination with albuterol in children with asthma. *Chest* 1990; **98:** 637–42.

Preparations

BP 1998: Atropine Eye Drops; Atropine Eye Ointment; Atropine Injection; Atropine Tablets; Morphine and Atropine Injection;
USP 23: Atropine Sulfate Injection; Atropine Sulfate Ophthalmic Ointment; Atropine Sulfate Ophthalmic Solution; Atropine Sulfate Tablets; Diphenoxylate Hydrochloride and Atropine Sulfate Oral Solution; Diphenoxylate Hydrochloride and Atropine Sulfate Tablets.

Proprietary Preparations (details are given in Part 3)

Austral.: Atropt; ***Belg.:*** Stellatropine; ***Canad.:*** Atropisol; ***Fr.:*** Chibro-Atropine; Genatropine; Vitatropine†; ***Ger.:*** Atropinol; Borotropin†; Dysurgal N; Noxenur S; ***Ital.:*** Liotropina; ***S.Afr.:*** Spersatropine†; ***Switz.:*** Bellafit N; Skiatropine; ***USA:*** AtroPen; Atropisol; Ocean-A/S†; Sal-Tropine.

Multi-ingredient: ***Aust.:*** Causat; Dysurgal; Ichtho-Bellol; Lactolavol; Myocardon; Noxenur; Peribilan†; Perphyllon; ***Austral.:*** Contac; Donnagel; Donnalix; Donnatab; Neo-Diophen; ***Belg.:*** Perphyllone†; ***Canad.:*** Diban; Donnagel†; Donnatal; ***Ger.:*** Adenovasin†; afdosa-duo†; Angiocardyl N; Ansudoral†; Antisacer comp.†; Bilicombin sp†; Bronchovydrin†; Brox-Aerosol N†; Causat B12 N; Causat N; Dilaudid-Atropin; Eupond; Ichtho-Bellol; Ichtho-Bellol compositum S; Ichtho-Himbin†; Mandrogallan†; Mydrial-Atropin†; Myocardetten†; Noxenur N†; Titretta analgica B†; Tonaton N†; Ulcumel†; ***Ital.:*** Asman-Valeas†; Cardiostenol; Deltamidrina; Genatrop; ***S.Afr.:*** Allertac; Bellatard; Bellavern†; Colstat; Donnatal; Dyrosol; Famucaps; Millerspas; Telament†; Tropax†; Virobis†; ***Spain:*** Abdominol; Derbitan Antibiotico; Laxo Vian; Midriatic; Paidenur†; Rinotiazol Fenilefri†; Rubia Paver; Salvacolina NN†; Sulmetin Papaver; Sulmetin Papaverina; Tabletas Quimpe; ***Swed.:*** Dilaudid-Atropin; ***Switz.:*** Brosol; Dilaudid-Atropin; Dolopyrine; Nardyl; Spasmanodine†; Spasmosol; Viaggio; ***UK:*** Actonorm; ***USA:*** Antispasmodic Elixir; Antrocol; Arco-Lase Plus; Atrohist Plus; Atropine and Demerol; Atrosept; Barbidonna; Bellatal; Dasin†; Deconhist LA; Dolsed; Donna-Sed; Donnagel-PG†; Donnamor; Donnapine†; Donnatal; Emergent-Ez; Festalan†; Hyosophen; Kinesed†; Malatal†; Phenahist-TR; Phenchlor SHA; Prosed/DS; Relaxadon†; Ru-Tuss; Spasmophen†; Spasquid†; Stahist; Susano; Trac Tabs 2X; UAA; Uridon Modified; Urised.

Used as an adjunct in: ***Austral.:*** Lofenoxal; Lomotil; ***Belg.:*** Reasec; ***Canad.:*** Lomotil; ***Fr.:*** Diarsed; ***Ger.:*** Reasec; ***Irl.:*** Lomotil; ***Ital.:*** Reasec; ***S.Afr.:*** Dioctin†; Eldox; Lomotil; Lyspafen†; ***Spain:*** Protector; Saleton†; ***Switz.:*** Lyspafen; Reasec; ***UK:*** Diarphen; Lomotil; Lotharin; Tropergen; ***USA:*** Di-Atro†; Enlon-Plus; Logen; Lomotil; Lonox; Motofen; Neostigmine Min-I-Mix.

Belladonna (339-a)

Belladona; Belladone; Deadly Nightshade; Tollkirschen.

Pharmacopoeias. Chin., Eur. (see p.viii), and *US* include a monograph for Belladonna Herb.

Eur. also includes Prepared Belladonna Herb. and Standardised Belladonna Leaf Dry Extract

Aust. also includes Belladonna Root. *Jpn* includes only Belladonna Root.

Belladonna [*Atropa belladonna* (Solanaceae)] contains alkaloids that consist mainly of the hyoscyamine (the laevo-isomer of atropine) together with small quantities of hyoscine. The total alkaloidal content of belladonna preparations is usually calculated as hyoscyamine.

Belladonna Herb (Belladonna Leaf; Belladonnae Folium) is the dried leaves, or leaves and flowering, and occasionally fruit-bearing, tops of the plant. The Ph. Eur. specifies not less than 0.3% of total alkaloids; the USP specifies not less than 0.35% of alkaloids.

Standardised Belladonna Leaf Dry Extract (Belladonnae Folii Extractum Siccum Normatum) is produced from Belladonna Herb and contains 0.95 to 1.05% of total alkaloids.

NOTE. The BP directs that when Belladonna Herb, Belladonna Leaf, or Powdered Belladonna Herb is prescribed, Prepared Belladonna Herb be dispensed. Prepared Belladonna Herb (Belladonnae Pulvis Normatus) is belladonna herb, reduced to a powder and adjusted to contain 0.28 to 0.32% of total alkaloids.

Store in airtight containers. Protect from light.

Stability in mixtures. Atropine in belladonna preparations was unstable at alkaline pH and would quickly be degraded in mixtures with a pH above 7.[1] Such mixtures in the BPC 1973 included Aluminium Hydroxide and Belladonna Mixture, Cascara and Belladonna Mixture, and Magnesium Trisilicate and Belladonna Mixture.

1. *PSGB Lab Report P/71/9* 1971.

Adverse Effects, Treatment, and Precautions

As for Atropine Sulphate, p.455.

Interactions

As for antimuscarinics in general (see Atropine Sulphate, p.456).

Uses and Administration

Belladonna has the actions of atropine (p.455). Belladonna herb and its preparations have been used for their antimuscarinic actions in a wide range of conditions, including the relief of gastro-intestinal and urinary-tract disorders associated with smooth muscle spasm, but they are generally regarded as an outmoded form of treatment.

Belladonna liniments and plasters have been used as counter-irritants for the relief of pain but there is little evidence that they have a beneficial effect and side-effects have occurred.

Belladonna is used in homoeopathic medicine.

Preparations

BP 1998: Belladonna Dry Extract; Belladonna Tincture;
USP 23: Belladonna Extract; Belladonna Extract Tablets; Belladonna Tincture.

Proprietary Preparations (details are given in Part 3)

Aust.: Bellanorm; ***Austral.:*** Atrobel; ***Ger.:*** Belladonnysat Burger; Bellafolin†; Tremoforat; ***Ital.:*** Bellafolina†; ***USA:*** Bellafoline†.

Multi-ingredient: ***Aust.:*** Asthma 23 D; Bellasthman; Medium†; Tampositorien mit Belladonna; ***Austral.:*** Alophen†; Cold & Flu Tablets†; Medimonth†; ***Belg.:*** Alcasedine†; Asperal-B†; Baume Dalet; Boldolaxine Aloes†; Cafergot-PB†; Calmant Martou; Captol†; Cigarettes Anti-asthmatiques†; Colimax; Dystonal; Escouflaire; Eucalyptine Le Brun; Eucalyptine Pholcodine Le Brun; Folcodex; Gastrofilm; Gloceda; Glottyl†; Grains de Vals; Hemosedan; Revocyl†; Sanicolax; Sirop Toux du Larynx; Solucamphre; ***Canad.:*** Bellergal; Cafergot-PB; Cystoforce†; Rheumalan; Wigraine; ***Fr.:*** Asthmasedine†; Boldolaxine†; Bronpax; Camphopneumine Aminophylline†; Clarix; Codotussyl; Colarine†; Curibronches†; Dinacode avec codeine; Elastocapsil†; Gastropax; Gastrosedyl; Gelumaline; Grains de Vals; Gripponyl†; Humex; Intesticarbine†; Lamaline; Mucinum; Neo-Boldolaxine†; Nican†; Pecto 6†; Pectospir†; Pectovox†; Peter's Sirop; Polery; Premidan Adult†; Pulmospir†; Pulmothiol†; Sedibaine; Sirop Pectoral adulte; Suppomaline; Tuberol†; ***Ger.:*** Asthmacolat†; Baldronit forte N†; Belladonna-Strath†; Belladonna-Valobonin†; Bellaravil-retard†; Bellaravil†; Bellergal†; Dalet-Balsam; Dystomin forte†; Eukliman†; Expectorans Solucampher†; Nephros-Strath†; Opobyl†; Protitis†; Regium†; Secafobell†; Sedapon D†; Solu-Vetan NG cum Belladonna†; Tampositorien B†; Vegomed†; ***Ital.:*** Anacidase†; Antiemorroidali; Antispasmina Colica; Antispasmina Colica B†; Bellergil; Entero-V†; Enteroton Digestivo†; Enteroton Lassativo†; Epar Euchessina†; Farmospasmina Colica†; Gastrosanol†; Heparbil†; Lassatina; Menabil Complex†; Neo-Heparbil; Neutralon Con Belladonna†; Sinulene†; ***Neth.:*** Abdijsiroop (Akker-Siroop)†; Opobyl†; ***Norw.:*** Cafergot Comp; ***S.Afr.:*** Atrofed†; Belladenal†; Bellergal; Cafergot-PB; Diastat†; Peter Pote's†; Rectosan 'A'†; ***Spain:*** Alofedina; Antihemorroidal†; Bellacanfor†; Bellergal†; Boldolaxin; Broncovital; Cafergot-PB; Carminativo Juventus; Crislaxo; Digestovital; Distovagal; Dolokey; Emuliquen Antiespasmodic†; Equidan†; Iodocafedrina†; Kolotanino†; Laxante Bescansa Aloico; Laxante Richelet†; Medecitral; Menabil Complex; Pildoras Zeninas; Servetinal; Sin Mareo x 4; Super Koki†; Takata; Tanagel; ***Switz.:*** Ajaka; Aloinophen; Bellagotin; Bellergal; Bromocod N; Bronchalin; Bronchofluid; Cafergot-PB; Demo elixir pectoral; Demo sirop contre la toux; Demodon†; Dipect†; Dragees laxatives no 510; Escotussin; Lysedil; Lysedil compositum; Melior†; Neo-Codion Enfants†; Nican; Obducti laxativi vegetabiles S; Phol-Tux; Physiolax; Phytolax; Saintbois nouvelle formule; Sedovalin†; Sirop pectoral DP2; Solucamphre; Spedro; Tampositoires B†; Tavolax; Thymodrosin; ***UK:*** Aluhyde†; Bellocarb†; Bolus Eucalypti Comp; Enterosan; Opazimes; ***USA:*** B & O Supprettes No. 15A; B & O Supprettes No. 16A; Bel-Phen-Ergot S; Bellergal-S; Butibel; Cafatine-PB; Chardonna-2; Folergot-DF; Phenerbel-S; Wyanoids.

Benzhexol Hydrochloride (342-y)

Benzhexol Hydrochloride *(BANM)*.

Trihexyphenidyl Hydrochloride *(rINNM)*; Cloridrato de Triexilfenidila; Cyclodolum; Trihexyphenidyli Hydrochloridum; Trihexyphenidylium Chloratum. 1-Cyclohexyl-1-phenyl-3-piperidinopropan-1-ol hydrochloride.

$C_{20}H_{31}NO,HCl = 337.9.$

CAS — 144-11-6 (benzhexol); 52-49-3 (benzhexol hydrochloride).

Pharmacopoeias. In *Br., Chin., Fr., Int., Jpn, Pol.,* and *US.*

A white or creamy-white, odourless or almost odourless, crystalline powder. Slightly **soluble** in water; soluble in alcohol, in chloroform, and in methyl alcohol. A saturated solution in water has a pH of 5.2 to 6.2. **Store** in airtight containers.

Adverse Effects, Treatment and Precautions

As for Atropine Sulphate, p.455. In some patients, such as those with arteriosclerosis or a history of drug idiosyncrasy, benzhexol may produce severe mental disturbances, excitement, nausea, and vomiting; such patients should be allowed to develop a tolerance by starting with a small initial dose and gradually increasing it until an effective level is reached.

Abuse. Benzhexol hydrochloride has been abused for its euphoric effect[1] especially by psychiatric patients.[2] However, its abuse potential by schizophrenic patients has been questioned[3] and its unpleasant antimuscarinic effects tend to limit its repeated use.[4]

1. Crawshaw JA, Mullen PE. A study of benzhexol abuse. *Br J Psychiatry* 1984; **145:** 300–3.
2. Pullen GP, *et al.* Anticholinergic drug abuse: a common problem? *Br Med J* 1984; **289:** 612–13.
3. Goff DC, *et al.* A placebo-controlled trial of trihexyphenidyl in unmedicated patients with schizophrenia. *Am J Psychiatry* 1994; **151:** 429–31.
4. WHO. WHO expert committee on drug dependence: twenty-ninth report. *WHO Tech Rep Ser 856* 1995.

Effects on the heart. Paradoxical sinus bradycardia developed in a schizophrenic patient after receiving benzhexol for extrapyramidal side-effects due to antipsychotic medication.[1] Normal sinus rhythm was restored after benzhexol was discontinued. The patient had previously received benzhexol and suffered bradycardia which at the time was attributed to haloperidol.

1. Blumensohn R, *et al.* Bradycardia due to trihexyphenidyl hydrochloride. *Drug Intell Clin Pharm* 1986; **20:** 786–7.

Effects on mental function. Benzhexol 2 mg by mouth significantly impaired memory function compared with placebo in a study in 13 elderly patients.[1] Impairment of memory has also been observed in patients with Parkinson's disease given antimuscarinics such as benzhexol.[2] However, impairment may be reversible on discontinuation of the antimuscarinic (see Atropine, p.455).

1. Potamianos G, Kellett JM. Anti-cholinergic drugs and memory: the effects of benzhexol on memory in a group of geriatric patients. *Br J Psychiatry* 1982; **140:** 470–2.
2. Sadeh M, *et al.* Effects of anticholinergic drugs on memory in Parkinson's disease. *Arch Neurol* 1982; **39:** 666–7.

Overdosage. A 34-year-old woman developed a toxic reaction with widely dilated pupils, dry skin, and visual hallucinations within 24 hours of taking about 300 mg of benzhexol hydrochloride with suicidal intent.[1] After 3 to 4 days the hallucinations were replaced by illusions; complete recovery occurred after a week, with no special treatment.

1. Ananth JV, *et al.* Toxic psychosis induced by benzhexol hydrochloride. *Can Med Assoc J* 1970; **103:** 771.

Withdrawal. A 61-year-old woman who had taken benzhexol 6 mg daily for a year for Parkinson's disease developed encephalopathy and miosis on two occasions when treatment was abruptly withdrawn.[1] Slowly tapered withdrawal avoided these effects.

1. Johkura K, *et al.* Trihexyphenidyl withdrawal encephalopathy. *Ann Neurol* 1997; **41:** 133–4.

Interactions

As for antimuscarinics in general (see Atropine Sulphate, p.456).

Chlorpromazine. For the effect of benzhexol on plasma concentrations of chlorpromazine, see under Antiparkinsonian Drugs, p.653.

Pharmacokinetics

Benzhexol hydrochloride is well absorbed from the gastro-intestinal tract and has been stated to exert an effect within 1 hour of a dose by mouth.

Half-life. The reported half-life of benzhexol has varied according to the assay method used. Values reported when using radioreceptor and chromatographic techniques have ranged from about 1 to more than 24 hours[1] and from 10 to 29 hours,[2] respectively, but the sensitivity and specificity of these methods has been criticised.[3] With a more recently developed radio immunoassay it was found that following oral administration of benzhexol there was an initial elimination phase with an estimated half-life of 5.33 hours followed by a terminal elimination phase with an estimated half-life of 32.7 hours.

1. Burke RE, Fahn S. Pharmacokinetics of trihexyphenidyl after short-term and long-term administration to dystonic patients. *Ann Neurol* 1985; **18:** 35–40.
2. Garbarg S, *et al.* Comparaison pharmacoclinique de deux formes galéniques de trihexyphénidyle. *Encephale* 1983; **IX:** 167–74.
3. He H, *et al.* Development and application of a specific and sensitive radioimmunoassay for trihexyphenidyl to a pharmacokinetic study in humans. *J Pharm Sci* 1995; **84:** 561–7.

Uses and Administration

Benzhexol hydrochloride is a tertiary amine antimuscarinic with actions similar to those of atropine (p.456). It also has a direct antispasmodic action on smooth muscle.

Benzhexol is employed in the symptomatic treatment of parkinsonism including the alleviation of the extrapyramidal syndrome induced by drugs such as phenothiazines, but is of no value against tardive dyskinesias. It has been used in the treatment of dystonias.

In idiopathic parkinsonism, benzhexol hydrochloride is given in 3 or 4 divided doses daily before or with food. The initial dose of 1 mg daily is gradually increased over a period of several days by increments of 2 mg to 6 to 10 mg daily according to the response of the patient; for advanced cases, 12 to 15 mg or even more may be needed daily. As a rule, postencephalitic patients tolerate and require the larger doses; elderly patients may require smaller doses.

Usual doses for drug-induced extrapyramidal symptoms lie within the range of 5 to 15 mg daily, although as little as 1 mg daily may be sufficient in some cases.

Antimuscarinic treatment of parkinsonism should never be terminated suddenly and it is usual when changing from one drug to another to withdraw one in small amounts while gradually increasing the dose of the other.

Benzhexol hydrochloride may be given with other drugs used for the relief of parkinsonism, such as levodopa, but the dose of each drug may need to be reduced.

Extrapyramidal disorders. Antimuscarinics such as benzhexol can be effective when used in the management of dystonias (p.1141).[1] However, adults tolerate antimuscarinics less well than children and adolescents and for these patients it is often not possible to achieve the high doses that may be required for control.[2] Side-effects may be limited by starting with a low dose such as benzhexol 2.5 mg twice daily and increasing by 2.5 mg daily every one or two weeks to the maximum tolerable, which in some young patients might be as much as 180 mg daily.

1. Burke RE, *et al.* Torsion dystonia: a double-blind, prospective trial of high-dosage trihexyphenidyl. *Neurology* 1986; **36:** 160–4.
2. Marsden CD, Quinn NP. The dystonias. *Br Med J* 1990; **300:** 139–44.

Parkinsonism. For the use of antimuscarinics, such as benzhexol, in the symptomatic treatment of parkinsonism, see p.454.

Subacute sclerosing panencephalitis. Subacute sclerosing panencephalitis (SSPE), a late complication of measles infection, may be managed with antivirals, although results are equivocal (see p.602). A recent study[1] found that the additional of benzhexol to inosine pranobex treatment produced beneficial responses in 2 patients with SSPE-associated myoclonic seizures refractory to valproic acid. A third patient who was not receiving inosine pranobex showed no improvement in seizure control when benzhexol was added to valproic acid therapy.

1. Nunes ML, *et al.* Trihexyphenidyl and isoprinosine in the treatment of subacute sclerosing panencephalitis. *Pediatr Neurol* 1995; **13:** 153–6.

Preparations

BP 1998: Trihexyphenidyl Tablets;
USP 23: Trihexyphenidyl Hydrochloride Elixir; Trihexyphenidyl Hydrochloride Extended-release Capsules; Trihexyphenidyl Hydrochloride Tablets.

Proprietary Preparations (details are given in Part 3)
Aust.: Artane; ***Austral.:*** Artane; ***Belg.:*** Artane; ***Canad.:*** Apo-Trihex; Artane; Novo-Hexidyl; ***Fr.:*** Artane; Parkinane; ***Ger.:*** Artane; Parkopan; ***Irl.:*** Artane; ***Ital.:*** Artane; ***Neth.:*** Artane; ***Norw.:*** Peragit†; ***S.Afr.:*** Artane; ***Spain:*** Artane; ***Swed.:*** Pargitan; ***Switz.:*** Artane; ***UK:*** Artane†; Broflex; ***USA:*** Artane; Trihexy.

Multi-ingredient: ***Ger.:*** Spasman; ***Spain:*** Largatrex.

Benztropine Mesylate (344-z)

Benztropine Mesylate *(BANM)*.

Benzatropine Mesilate *(rINNM)*; Benzatropine Methanesulfonate. (1*R*,3*r*,5*S*)-3-Benzhydryloxytropane methanesulphonate.

$C_{21}H_{25}NO,CH_4O_3S = 403.5$.

CAS — 86-13-5 (benztropine); 132-17-2 (benztropine mesylate).

Pharmacopoeias. In Br. and US.

A white, odourless or almost odourless, slightly hygroscopic, crystalline powder. Very **soluble** in water; freely soluble in alcohol; very slightly soluble or practically insoluble in ether. **Store** in airtight containers.

Adverse Effects, Treatment, and Precautions

As for Atropine Sulphate, p.455. Drowsiness may be severe in some patients and patients so affected should not drive or operate machinery. Benztropine may also produce severe mental disturbances and excitement.

Effects on the heart. Paradoxical sinus bradycardia in a patient with depression and psychotic symptoms was attributed to benztropine since it persisted despite modification to other treatment and resolved only when benztropine was withdrawn.[1]

1. Voinov H, *et al.* Sinus bradycardia related to the use of benztropine mesylate. *Am J Psychiatry* 1992; **149:** 711.

Interactions

As for antimuscarinics in general (see Atropine Sulphate, p.456).

Antidepressants. A report[1] of 5 patients who developed delirium while taking an antipsychotic, a selective serotonin reuptake inhibitor (SSRI), and benztropine suggested that there might be an interaction between SSRIs and benztropine.

1. Roth A, *et al.* Delirium associated with the combination of a neuroleptic, an SSRI, and benztropine. *J Clin Psychiatry* 1994; **55:** 492–5.

Antipsychotics. Fatal heat stroke has been reported[1,2] in patients receiving benztropine and antipsychotic drugs following exposure to an ambient temperature of over 29°. Paralytic ileus, sometimes fatal, has also been documented in patients taking benztropine mesylate and antipsychotics concomitantly.[3]

1. Stadnyk AN, Glezos JD. Drug-induced heat stroke. *Can Med Assoc J* 1983; **128:** 957–9.
2. Tyndel F, Labonté R. Drug-facilitated heat stroke. *Can Med Assoc J* 1983; **129:** 680.
3. Wade LC, Ellenor GL. Combination mesoridazine- and benztropine mesylate-induced paralytic ileus: two case reports. *Drug Intell Clin Pharm* 1980; **14:** 17–22.

Uses and Administration

Benztropine mesylate is a tertiary amine antimuscarinic with actions and uses similar to those of benzhexol (p.458); it also has antihistaminic properties.

Benztropine is used for the symptomatic treatment of parkinsonism (p.454), including the alleviation of the extrapyramidal syndrome induced by drugs such as phenothiazines, but is of no value against tardive dyskinesias.

Benztropine mesylate is given by mouth or, if necessary, by intramuscular or intravenous injection.

In idiopathic parkinsonism benztropine mesylate is usually given by mouth in an initial daily dose of 0.5 to 1 mg. Its actions are cumulative, and may not be manifest for several days after beginning therapy. Patients with post-encephalitic parkinsonism often tolerate an initial dose of 2 mg. The dose may be gradually increased by 500 µg every 5 to 6 days to a maximum of 6 mg daily until the optimum dose for each individual patient is reached. Maintenance therapy may be given as a single daily dose or in divided doses 2 to 4 times daily.

In the management of drug-induced extrapyramidal disorders doses of 1 to 4 mg once or twice daily have been given orally or parenterally. Therapy may be withdrawn after one to two weeks to assess whether it is still necessary.

In emergency, benztropine mesylate may be injected intramuscularly or intravenously in a dose of 1 to 2 mg; intramuscular administration is reported to produce an effect as quickly as intravenous administration, so the latter is rarely necessary.

Benztropine has also been given as the hydrochloride.

Preparations

BP 1998: Benzatropine Injection; Benzatropine Tablets;
USP 23: Benztropine Mesylate Injection; Benztropine Mesylate Tablets.

Proprietary Preparations (details are given in Part 3)
Aust.: BETE; Cogentin; ***Austral.:*** Cogentin; ***Canad.:*** Cogentin; ***Ger.:*** Cogentinol; ***Irl.:*** Cogentin; ***Norw.:*** Cogentin; ***Swed.:*** Cogentin; ***UK:*** Cogentin; ***USA:*** Cogentin.

Biperiden (346-k)

Biperiden *(BAN, rINN)*.

1-(Bicyclo[2.2.1]hept-5-en-2-yl)-1-phenyl-3-piperidinopropan-1-ol.

$C_{21}H_{29}NO = 311.5$.

CAS — 514-65-8.

Pharmacopoeias. In *Int.* and *US.*

A white, practically odourless, crystalline powder. Practically **insoluble** in water; sparingly soluble in alcohol; freely soluble in chloroform. **Protect** from light.

Biperiden Hydrochloride (347-a)

Biperiden Hydrochloride *(BANM, rINNM)*.

Biperideni Hydrochloridum.

$C_{21}H_{29}NO,HCl = 347.9$.

CAS — 1235-82-1.

Pharmacopoeias. In *Eur.* (see p.viii), *Int., Jpn,* and *US.*

A white, almost odourless, crystalline powder. Slightly **soluble** in water, in alcohol, and in chloroform; very slightly soluble in dichloromethane; slightly soluble to practically insoluble in ether; sparingly soluble in methyl alcohol. A 0.2% solution in water has a pH of 5.0 to 6.5. **Store** in airtight containers. Protect from light.

Biperiden Lactate (348-t)

Biperiden Lactate *(BANM, rINNM)*.

$C_{21}H_{29}NO,C_3H_6O_3 = 401.5$.

CAS — 7085-45-2.

Pharmacopoeias. US includes Biperiden Lactate Injection.

Adverse Effects, Treatment, and Precautions

As for Atropine Sulphate, p.455.

Parenteral administration may be followed by slight transient hypotension. Biperiden may cause drowsiness and patients so affected should not drive or operate machinery.

Abuse. A report[1] of abuse of biperiden in psychiatric patients.

1. Pullen GP, *et al.* Anticholinergic drug abuse: a common problem? *Br Med J* 1984; **289:** 612–13.

Interactions

As for antimuscarinics in general (see Atropine Sulphate, p.456).

Pharmacokinetics

Biperiden is readily absorbed from the gastro-intestinal tract, but bioavailability is only about 30% suggesting that is undergoes extensive first-pass metabolism. Biperiden has an elimination half-life of about 20 hours.

References.

1. Hollmann M, *et al.* Biperiden effects and plasma levels in volunteers. *Eur J Clin Pharmacol* 1984; **27:** 619–21.

2. Grimaldi R, *et al.* Pharmacokinetic and pharmacodynamic studies following the intravenous and oral administration of the antiparkinsonian drug biperiden to normal subjects. *Eur J Clin Pharmacol* 1986; **29:** 735–7.

Uses and Administration

Biperiden is a tertiary amine antimuscarinic with actions and uses similar to those of benzhexol (p.458) but with more potent antinicotinic properties.

Biperiden is used in the symptomatic treatment of parkinsonism (p.454), including the alleviation of the extrapyramidal syndrome induced by drugs such as phenothiazines, but is of no value against tardive dyskinesias.

Biperiden is administered by mouth as the hydrochloride and by injection as the lactate.

In the UK, the initial dose by mouth is 1 mg of the hydrochloride twice daily, gradually increased over several days according to the needs of the patient. The usual optimum maintenance dosage varies from 3 to 12 mg daily in divided doses. The dose of the lactate given by intramuscular or slow intravenous injection is 2.5 to 5 mg as a single dose to a maximum of 20 mg in 24 hours.

In the USA, the initial dose by mouth for idiopathic parkinsonism is 2 mg of the hydrochloride three or four times daily increased according to the needs of the patient to a maximum of 16 mg in 24 hours. The dose for drug-induced extrapyramidal symptoms is 2 mg by mouth one to three times daily or 2 mg of biperiden lactate given by intramuscular or slow intravenous injection and repeated every 30 minutes if needed up to a maximum of 4 doses in 24 hours.

Preparations

USP 23: Biperiden Hydrochloride Tablets; Biperiden Lactate Injection.

Proprietary Preparations (details are given in Part 3)
Aust.: Akineton; ***Austral.:*** Akineton; ***Belg.:*** Akineton; ***Canad.:*** Akineton; ***Fr.:*** Akineton; ***Ger.:*** Akineton; Desiperiden; Norakin N; ***Irl.:*** Akineton; ***Ital.:*** Akineton; ***Neth.:*** Akineton; ***Norw.:*** Akineton; ***S.Afr.:*** Akineton; ***Spain:*** Akineton; ***Swed.:*** Akineton; ***Switz.:*** Akineton; ***UK:*** Akineton; ***USA:*** Akineton.

Bornaprine Hydrochloride (349-x)

Bornaprine Hydrochloride *(BANM, rINNM).*

3-Diethylaminopropyl 2-phenylbicyclo[2.2.1]heptane-2-carboxylate hydrochloride.

$C_{21}H_{31}NO_2,HCl$ = 365.9.

CAS — 20448-86-6 (bornaprine); 26908-91-8 (bornaprine hydrochloride).

Bornaprine hydrochloride is a quaternary ammonium antimuscarinic with actions and uses similar to those of benzhexol (p.457). It is used in the symptomatic treatment of parkinsonism (p.454), but it is claimed to be mainly effective against tremor. It is given by mouth in initial doses of 2 mg daily gradually increased to 6 to 12 mg daily according to the response of the patient.

Preparations

Proprietary Preparations (details are given in Part 3)
Aust.: Sormodren; ***Ger.:*** Sormodren; ***Irl.:*** Sormodren†; ***Ital.:*** Sormodren; ***Spain:*** Sormodren†.

Butropium Bromide (350-y)

Butropium Bromide *(rINN).*

(−)-(1*R*,3*r*,5*S*)-8-(4-Butoxybenzyl)-3-[(*S*)-tropoyloxy]tropanium bromide.

$C_{28}H_{38}BrNO_4$ = 532.5.

CAS — 29025-14-7.

Pharmacopoeias. In *Jpn.*

Butropium bromide is a quaternary ammonium antimuscarinic with peripheral effects similar to those of atropine (p.455). It has been used in the symptomatic treatment of visceral spasms in a dose of 10 mg three times daily by mouth.

Preparations

Proprietary Preparations (details are given in Part 3)
Jpn: Coliopan.

Buzepide Metiodide (351-j)

Buzepide Metiodide *(rINN).*

Diphexamide Iodomethylate; FI-6146; Metazepium Iodide; R-661. 1-(3-Carbamoyl-3,3-diphenylpropyl)-1-methylperhydroazepinium iodide.

$C_{23}H_{31}IN_2O$ = 478.4.

CAS — 15351-05-0.

Buzepide metiodide is a quaternary ammonium antimuscarinic with peripheral effects similar to those of atropine (p.455). It has been given with other compounds for upper respiratory-tract disorders and in gastro-intestinal disorders with smooth muscle spasm.

Preparations

Proprietary Preparations (details are given in Part 3)
Multi-ingredient: ***Belg.:*** Denoral; ***Fr.:*** Denoral; Vesadol; ***Ger.:*** Neutromil†; ***Ital.:*** Denoral; ***Spain:*** Senioral Comp†.

Cimetropium Bromide (1702-g)

Cimetropium Bromide *(rINN).*

DA-3177; Hyoscine-*N*-(cyclopropylmethyl) Bromide. 8-(Cyclopropylmethyl)-6β,7β-epoxy-3α-hydroxy-1αH,5αH-tropanium bromide, (−)-(*S*)-tropate.

$C_{21}H_{28}BrNO_4$ = 438.4.

CAS — 51598-60-8.

Cimetropium bromide is a quaternary ammonium antimuscarinic with peripheral effects similar to those of atropine (p.455). It has been used as an antispasmodic in the treatment of gastro-intestinal disorders (p.453) in usual doses of 50 mg two or three times daily by mouth or by rectal suppository. It has also been given intramuscularly or intravenously in doses of 5 to 10 mg.

References.

1. Gullo L, *et al.* Inhibition of caerulein-induced gall bladder emptying by cimetropium bromide in humans. *Eur J Clin Pharmacol* 1989; **37:** 483–6.
2. Dobrilla G, *et al.* Longterm treatment of irritable bowel syndrome with cimetropium bromide: a double blind placebo controlled clinical trial. *Gut* 1990; **31:** 355–8.
3. Marzio L, *et al.* Effect of cimetropium bromide on esophageal motility and transit in patients affected by primary achalasia. *Dig Dis Sci* 1994; **39:** 1389–94.

Preparations

Proprietary Preparations (details are given in Part 3)
Ital.: Alginor.

Clidinium Bromide (354-k)

Clidinium Bromide *(BAN, USAN, rINN).*

Ro-2-3773. 3-Benziloyloxy-1-methylquinuclidinium bromide.

$C_{22}H_{26}BrNO_3$ = 432.4.

CAS — 7020-55-5 (clidinium); 3485-62-9 (clidinium bromide).

Pharmacopoeias. In *US.*

A white or nearly white almost odourless crystalline powder. **Soluble** in water and in alcohol; slightly soluble in ether. **Store** in airtight containers. Protect from light.

Clidinium bromide is a quaternary ammonium antimuscarinic with peripheral effects similar to those of atropine (p.455). It is used alone or in conjunction with chlordiazepoxide in the symptomatic treatment of peptic ulcer and other gastro-intestinal disorders (p.453). The usual dose of clidinium bromide is 2.5 mg three or four times a day before meals and at bedtime; this may be increased to 5 mg four times a day if necessary.

Preparations

USP 23: Chlordiazepoxide Hydrochloride and Clidinium Bromide Capsules; Clidinium Bromide Capsules.

Proprietary Preparations (details are given in Part 3)
USA: Quarzan.

Multi-ingredient: ***Aust.:*** Librax; ***Austral.:*** Librax†; ***Belg.:*** Librax; ***Canad.:*** Apo-Chlorax; Corium; Librax; ***Fr.:*** Librax; ***Ger.:*** Librax†; ***Irl.:*** Libraxin†; ***Ital.:*** Librax; ***S.Afr.:*** Librax; ***Spain:*** Librax†; ***Swed.:*** Librax†; ***Switz.:*** Librax; ***USA:*** Clindex; Clinoxide†; Clipoxide†; Librax; Lidox.

Cyclodrine Hydrochloride (9269-d)

GT-92. 2-Diethylaminoethyl 2-(1-hydroxycyclopentyl)-2-phenylacetate hydrochloride.

$C_{19}H_{29}NO_3,HCl$ = 355.9.

CAS — 52109-93-0 (cyclodrine); 78853-39-1 (cyclodrine hydrochloride).

Cyclodrine is an analogue of cyclopentolate (p.459). It has been used as the hydrochloride in eye drops to produce mydriasis and cycloplegia.

Preparations

Proprietary Preparations (details are given in Part 3)
Ger.: Cyclopent†.

Cyclopentolate Hydrochloride

(355-a)

Cyclopentolate Hydrochloride *(BANM, rINNM).*

Cloridrato de Ciclopentolato; Cyclopentolati Hydrochloridum. 2-Dimethylaminoethyl 2-(1-hydroxycyclopentyl)-2-phenylacetate hydrochloride.

$C_{17}H_{25}NO_3,HCl$ = 327.8.

CAS — 512-15-2 (cyclopentolate); 5870-29-1 (cyclopentolate hydrochloride).

NOTE. CYC is a code approved by the BP for use on single unit doses of eye drops containing cyclopentolate hydrochloride where the individual container may be too small to bear all the appropriate labelling information. PHNCYC is a similar code approved for eye drops containing phenylephrine hydrochloride and cyclopentolate hydrochloride.

Pharmacopoeias. In *Eur.* (see p.viii), *Jpn,* and *US.*

A white crystalline powder, which develops a characteristic odour on standing. Very **soluble** in water; freely soluble in alcohol; practically insoluble in ether. A 1% solution in water has a pH of 4.5 to 5.5. **Store** at a temperature not exceeding 8° in airtight containers.

Adverse Effects, Treatment, and Precautions

As for Atropine Sulphate, p.455.

Eye drops of cyclopentolate hydrochloride may cause temporary irritation.

Of 29 male and 37 female patients who received one drop of 2% cyclopentolate eye drops in each eye, 10 developed systemic toxicity of mild to moderate severity.[1] The manifestations were: physical weakness, nausea, lightheadedness, changes in emotional attitude, unprovoked weeping, and loss of equilibrium; tachycardia was always present but changes in blood pressure were insignificant. Nine of the 10 were female and spontaneous recovery occurred within 1 hour to several days.

As with atropine, it has been recommended that cyclopentolate eye drops should not be used during the first 3 months of life because of the possible association between the cycloplegia produced and development of amblyopia. Systemic toxicity has also been reported in neonates following ocular administration of cyclopentolate.[2]

A 4.5-year-old boy with cerebral palsy and paraplegia suffered tonic-clonic seizures, facial flushing, and tachycardia 70 minutes after one drop of a 1% cyclopentolate solution was instilled into each eye to dilate his pupils.[3] The child had no prior history of convulsions and had received 1% cyclopentolate eye drops on 2 previous occasions without incident.

1. Awan KJ. Adverse systemic reactions of topical cyclopentolate hydrochloride. *Ann Ophthalmol* 1976; **8:** 695–8.
2. Bauer CR, *et al.* Systemic cyclopentolate (Cyclogyl) toxicity in the newborn infant. *J Pediatr* 1973; **92:** 501–5.
3. Fitzgerald DA, *et al.* Seizures associated with 1% cyclopentolate eyedrops. *J Paediatr Child Health* 1990; **26:** 106–7.

Abuse. A report[1] of abuse of cyclopentolate eye drops by 2 patients. One of the patients who had been instilling 200 to 400 drops of cyclopentolate into both eyes daily for about 4 months, presumably for its CNS effects, experienced intense nausea, vomiting, weakness, and tremors on withdrawal.

1. Sato EH, *et al.* Abuse of cyclopentolate hydrochloride (Cyclogyl) drops. *N Engl J Med* 1992; **326:** 1363–4.

Hypersensitivity. Two children developed hypersensitivity reactions shortly after the instillation of 1% cyclopentolate hydrochloride eye drops into each eye.[1] Both children initially had a facial rash but in one of them the rash later spread to include the arms and legs and was accompanied by mild breathlessness.

1. Jones LWJ, Hodes DT. Possible allergic reactions to cyclopentolate hydrochloride: case reports with literature review of uses and adverse reactions. *Ophthalmic Physiol Opt* 1991; **11:** 16–21.

Interactions

As for antimuscarinics in general (see Atropine Sulphate, p.456).

Uses and Administration

Cyclopentolate hydrochloride is a tertiary amine antimuscarinic with actions similar to those of atropine (p.455). It is used as eye drops to produce mydriasis and cycloplegia (p.454) for ophthalmic diagnostic procedures and also in the treatment of uveitis and iritis (p.1030). It acts more quickly than atropine and has a shorter duration of action; the maximum mydriatic effect is produced 30 to 60 minutes after instillation, and may persist for up to 24 hours; the maximum cycloplegic effect is produced within 25 to 75 minutes and accommodation recovers within 6 to 24 hours.

For diagnostic procedures, 1 drop of a 0.5% solution of cyclopentolate hydrochloride repeated after about 5 to 15 minutes is usually sufficient for adults. Higher strengths have been used. For children 1 or 2 drops of a 1% solution are instilled similarly although some recommend that strengths greater than 0.5% should not be used in infants and that cyclopentolate should not be used at all during the first 3 months of life.

In the treatment of uveitis and iritis 1 or 2 drops of a 0.5% solution of cyclopentolate hydrochloride are instilled into the eye(s) up to four times daily.

Deeply pigmented eyes are more resistant to pupillary dilatation and may require the use of a 1% solution.

Preparations

BP 1998: Cyclopentolate Eye Drops;
USP 23: Cyclopentolate Hydrochloride Ophthalmic Solution.

Proprietary Preparations (details are given in Part 3)
Austral.: Cyclogyl; ***Belg.:*** Cyclopentol; ***Canad.:*** Cyclogyl; Diopentolate; ***Fr.:*** Skiacol; ***Ger.:*** Zykolat-EDO; ***Irl.:*** Mydrilate; ***Ital.:*** Ciclolux; ***Neth.:*** Cyclogyl†; Cyclomydril†; ***S.Afr.:*** Cyclogyl; ***Spain:*** Ciclople; Cicloplejic; Cicloplejico; ***Swed.:*** Cyclogyl; ***Switz.:*** Cyclogyl; ***UK:*** Alnide†; Mydrilate; ***USA:*** Ak-Pentolate; Cyclogyl; Cylate; Pentolair.

Multi-ingredient: ***Ger.:*** Ophtomydrol†; ***S.Afr.:*** Cyclomydril; ***USA:*** Cyclomydril.

Darifenacin (17411-y)

Darifenacin *(BAN, rINN)*.

UK-88525. (S)-1-[2-(2,3-Dihydro-5-benzofuranyl)ethyl]-α,α-diphenyl-3-pyrrolidineacetamide.

$C_{28}H_{30}N_2O_2$ = 426.6.
CAS — 133099-04-4 (darifenacin); 133099-07-7 (darifenacin hydrobromide).

Darifenacin is a selective M_3 antimuscarinic under investigation in the treatment of urinary incontinence. It is also being studied in irritable bowel syndrome.

References.

1. Rosario DJ, *et al.* A pilot study of the effects of multiple doses of the M3 muscarinic receptor antagonist darifenacin on ambulatory parameters of detrusor activity in patients with detrusor instability. *Neurourol Urodyn* 1995; **14:** 464–5.

Dexetimide Hydrochloride (358-r)

Dexetimide Hydrochloride *(BANM, rINNM)*.

Dexbenzetimide Hydrochloride; R-16470. (+)-(S)-2-(1-Benzyl-4-piperidyl)-2-phenylglutarimide hydrochloride; (+)-(S)-3-(1-Benzyl-4-piperidyl)-3-phenylpiperidine-2,6-dione hydrochloride.

$C_{23}H_{26}N_2O_2$,HCl = 398.9.
CAS — 21888-98-2 (dexetimide); 21888-96-0 (dexetimide hydrochloride).

NOTE. Dexetimide is *USAN*.

Dexetimide is a tertiary antimuscarinic with actions similar to those of benzhexol (p.457). It has been used as the hydrochloride to alleviate drug-induced extrapyramidal symptoms, but like other antimuscarinics it is of no value against tardive dyskinesias. It has been given in once daily doses of 0.5 to 1 mg by mouth; it has also been given by intramuscular injection.

Preparations

Proprietary Preparations (details are given in Part 3)
Belg.: Tremblex; ***Ital.:*** Tremblex†; ***Neth.:*** Tremblex; ***Switz.:*** Tremblex†.

Dicyclomine Hydrochloride (360-z)

Dicyclomine Hydrochloride *(BANM)*.

Dicycloverine Hydrochloride *(rINNM)*; Cloridrato de Dicicloverina; Dicycloverini Hydrochloridum. 2-Diethylaminoethyl bicyclohexyl-1-carboxylate hydrochloride.

$C_{19}H_{35}NO_2$,HCl = 345.9.
CAS — 77-19-0 (dicyclomine); 67-92-5 (dicyclomine hydrochloride).

Pharmacopoeias. In *Eur.* (see p.viii) and *US.*

A white or almost white, practically odourless, crystalline powder. It exhibits polymorphism. **Soluble** 1 in 13 of water, 1 in 5 of alcohol, 1 in 2 of chloroform and of glacial acetic acid, 1 in 770 of ether; freely soluble in dichloromethane. The pH of a 1% solution is 5.0 to 5.5.

Adverse Effects, Treatment, and Precautions

As for Atropine Sulphate, p.455. Dicyclomine hydrochloride should not be given to infants younger than 6 months of age.

Reports of severe apnoea in infants aged 5 to 10 weeks associated with the administration of dicyclomine.

1. Williams J, Watkin-Jones R. Dicyclomine: worrying symptoms associated with its use in some small babies. *Br Med J* 1984; **288:** 901.
2. Edwards PDL. Dicyclomine in babies. *Br Med J* 1984; **288:** 1230.
3. Spoudeas H, Shribman S. Dicyclomine in babies. *Br Med J* 1984; **288:** 1230.

Pregnancy. For a review of the risks to the fetus of antiemetic therapy during pregnancy, with particular reference to Debendox (Bendectin: dicyclomine with doxylamine and pyridoxine), see under Antihistamines on p.398.

Interactions

As for antimuscarinics in general (see Atropine Sulphate, p.456).

Uses and Administration

Dicyclomine hydrochloride is a tertiary amine antimuscarinic with effects similar to but weaker than those of atropine (p.455); it also has a direct antispasmodic action.

Dicyclomine is used in gastro-intestinal spasm, particularly that associated with the irritable bowel syndrome. For adults, 10 to 20 mg of dicyclomine hydrochloride is given 3 times daily; in the USA, up to 40 mg four times daily has been recommended where adverse effects permit. Children aged 6 months to 2 years may be given 5 to 10 mg up to 3 or 4 times daily; doses are usually given 15 minutes before meals. Children aged 2 to 12 years may be given 10 mg three times daily.

Dicyclomine hydrochloride may be given intramuscularly in doses of 20 mg given 4 times daily to patients in whom oral therapy is temporarily impractical, but should not be used for longer than 1 to 2 days.

Preparations

BP 1998: Dicycloverine Oral Solution; Dicycloverine Tablets;
USP 23: Dicyclomine Hydrochloride Capsules; Dicyclomine Hydrochloride Injection; Dicyclomine Hydrochloride Syrup; Dicyclomine Hydrochloride Tablets.

Proprietary Preparations (details are given in Part 3)
Austral.: Merbentyl; ***Canad.:*** Bentylol; Formulex; ***Irl.:*** Diarrest; Merbentyl; ***Ital.:*** Bentyl†; ***S.Afr.:*** Clomin†; Medicyclomine; Merbentyl; ***Spain:*** Bentylol; Tarestin†; ***UK:*** Merbentyl; ***USA:*** Antispas; Bemote†; Bentyl; Byclomine; Di-Spaz; Dibent; Dilomine; Or-Tyl; Spasmoject†.

Multi-ingredient: ***Austral.:*** Infacol-C†; ***Canad.:*** Spasmo Nil; ***Irl.:*** Kolanticon; ***Ital.:*** Merankol Gel†; Merankol Pastiglie; ***S.Afr.:*** Alkalite D; Alumite; Auspastyl†; Asic; Betaclomin; Co-Gel; Dynagastrin; Gel-S†; Gelumen; Kaoneo†; Kolantyl; Medigel; Microgel; Neutragel; pH 550; Propan Gel-S; Remotrox; Rubragel-D†; ***Spain:*** Colchimax; Neocolan; ***UK:*** Diarrest; Kolanticon; ***USA:*** Byclomine with Phenobarbital†.

Diethazine Hydrochloride (361-c)

Diethazine Hydrochloride *(BANM, rINNM)*.

Diaethazinium Chloratum; Eazamine Hydrochloride; RP-2987. 10-(2-Diethylaminoethyl)phenothiazine hydrochloride.

$C_{18}H_{22}N_2S$,HCl = 334.9.
CAS — 60-91-3 (diethazine); 341-70-8 (diethazine hydrochloride).

Pharmacopoeias. In *Fr.*

Diethazine hydrochloride is an antimuscarinic with actions similar to those of ethopropazine hydrochloride (p.461), but it is more toxic and bone marrow depression may occur. It has been used in the treatment of parkinsonism.

Difemerine Hydrochloride (362-k)

Difemerine Hydrochloride *(rINNM)*.

UP-57. 2-Dimethylamino-1,1-dimethylethyl benzilate hydrochloride.

$C_{20}H_{25}NO_3$,HCl = 363.9.
CAS — 80387-96-8 (difemerine); 70280-88-5 (difemerine hydrochloride).

Difemerine hydrochloride is an antimuscarinic with effects similar to those of atropine (p.455) and was used in the symptomatic treatment of visceral spasms.

Preparations

Proprietary Preparations (details are given in Part 3)
Fr.: Luostyl†.

Dihexyverine Hydrochloride (363-a)

Dihexyverine Hydrochloride *(USAN, rINNM)*.

Dihexiverine Hydrochloride; JL-1078. 2-Piperidinoethyl bicyclohexyl-1-carboxylate hydrochloride.

$C_{20}H_{35}NO_2$,HCl = 358.0.
CAS — 561-77-3 (dihexyverine); 5588-25-0 (dihexyverine hydrochloride).

Dihexyverine hydrochloride is an antimuscarinic with effects similar to those of atropine (p.455). It is given in the symptomatic treatment of gastro-intestinal spasm in daily doses of 20 to 60 mg by mouth or 50 to 150 mg rectally. It has also been given in doses of 10 mg by intramuscular injection.

Preparations

Proprietary Preparations (details are given in Part 3)
Fr.: Spasmodex; ***Ital.:*** Seclin†.

Dimevamide (15840-a)

Dimevamide *(rINN)*.

Aminopentamide. α-[2-(Dimethylamino)propyl]-α-phenylbenzeneacetamide.

$C_{19}H_{24}N_2O$ = 296.4.
CAS — 60-46-8.

Dimevamide is a tertiary amine and has been used as an antimuscarinic.

Preparations

Proprietary Preparations (details are given in Part 3)
Multi-ingredient: ***S.Afr.:*** Kantrexil.

Diphemanil Methylsulphate (364-t)

Diphemanil Methylsulphate *(BAN)*.

Diphemanil Metilsulfate *(rINN)*; Diphemanil Methylsulfate; Diphenmethanil Methylsulphate; Vagophemanil Methylsulphate. 4-Benzhydrylidene-1,1-dimethylpiperidinium methylsulphate.

$C_{20}H_{24}N,CH_3SO_4$ = 389.5.
CAS — 62-97-5.

Diphemanil methylsulphate is a quaternary ammonium antimuscarinic with peripheral effects similar to those of atropine (p.455). It is used topically as a 2% cream or powder to treat hyperhidrosis (excessive sweating).

Diphemanil methylsulphate, given by mouth, has been investigated for the treatment of symptomatic bradycardia in infants.

References.

1. Vidal AM, *et al.* Pharmacokinetics of diphemanil methylsulphate in healthy subjects. *Eur J Clin Pharmacol* 1992; **42:** 689–91.
2. Vidal AM, *et al.* Pharmacokinetics of diphemanil methylsulphate in infants. *Eur J Clin Pharmacol* 1993; **45:** 89–91.
3. Pariente-Khayat A, *et al.* Pharmacokinetics of diphemanil methylsulphate in neonates and in premature infants. *Eur J Clin Pharmacol* 1996; **50:** 429–30.

Preparations

Proprietary Preparations (details are given in Part 3)
Austral.: Prantal; ***Ital.:*** Prantal.

Drofenine Hydrochloride (11601-k)

Drofenine Hydrochloride *(pINNM)*.

Hexahydroadiphenine Hydrochloride. 2-(Diethylamino)ethyl α-phenylcyclohexaneacetate hydrochloride.

$C_{20}H_{31}NO_2$,HCl = 353.9.
CAS — 1679-76-1 (drofenine); 548-66-3 (drofenine hydrochloride).

Pharmacopoeias. In *Belg.* and *Swiss.*

Drofenine hydrochloride is an antimuscarinic available in preparations for the treatment of visceral spasms.

Preparations

Proprietary Preparations (details are given in Part 3)

Multi-ingredient: ***Aust.:*** Spasmoplus; ***Belg.:*** Spasmo-Cibalgine; Spasmoplus; ***Ger.:*** Cibalen†; Spasmo-Cibalgin compositum S; Spasmo-Cibalgin S; ***Ital.:*** Spasmo-Cibalgina; ***Spain:*** Espasmo Cibalgina†; ***Switz.:*** Lunadon; Sonotryl; Spasmo-Cibalgin; Spasmo-Cibalgin comp.

Emepronium Bromide (365-x)

Emepronium Bromide *(BAN, rINN).*

Ethyldimethyl(1-methyl-3,3-diphenylpropyl)ammonium bromide.

$C_{20}H_{28}BrN = 362.3.$

CAS — 27892-33-7 (emepronium); 3614-30-0 (emepronium bromide).

Emepronium Carrageenate (18635-j)

Emepronium Carrageenate *(BAN).*

Adverse Effects, Treatment, and Precautions

As for Atropine Sulphate, p.455.

To avoid oesophageal ulceration, tablets of emepronium bromide should always be swallowed with an adequate volume of water, and patients should always be in the sitting or standing position while, and for 10 to 15 minutes after, taking the tablets. Emepronium is contra-indicated in patients with symptoms or signs of oesophageal obstruction or with pre-existing oesophagitis.

Buccal and oesophageal ulceration. Tablet-induced oesophageal damage is widely recognised and is related to direct mucosal injury by the medication. Emepronium bromide is one of the most frequently implicated medications in this type of mucosal injury, although it rarely results in stricture formation.[1]

1. McCord GS, Clouse RE. Pill-induced esophageal strictures: clinical features and risk factors for development. *Am J Med* 1990; **88:** 512–18.

Interactions

As for antimuscarinics in general (see Atropine Sulphate, p.456).

Pharmacokinetics

Emepronium is incompletely absorbed from the gastro-intestinal tract and is mainly excreted unchanged in the urine and faeces. It does not cross the blood-brain barrier in therapeutic doses.

Uses and Administration

Emepronium is a quaternary ammonium antimuscarinic with peripheral effects similar to those of atropine (p.455). It is used mainly in the treatment of urinary frequency and incontinence (p.454). A usual dose by mouth is 200 mg of the bromide, or its equivalent as the carrageenate, three times daily.

Preparations

Proprietary Preparations (details are given in Part 3)

Aust.: Cetiprin; ***Ger.:*** Uro-Ripirin; ***Irl.:*** Cetiprin; ***Ital.:*** Detrulisin†; ***Neth.:*** Cetiprin; ***Norw.:*** Cetiprin; ***S.Afr.:*** Cetiprin†; ***Spain:*** Hexanium; ***Swed.:*** Cetiprin; ***Switz.:*** Cetiprin.

Ethopropazine Hydrochloride (367-f)

Ethopropazine Hydrochloride *(BANM).*

Profenamine Hydrochloride *(rINNM)*; Cloridrato de Profenamina; Isothazine Hydrochloride; Profenamini Hydrochloridum; Prophenamini Chloridum. 10-(2-Diethylaminopropyl)phenothiazine hydrochloride.

$C_{19}H_{24}N_2S,HCl = 348.9.$

CAS — 522-00-9 (ethopropazine); 1094-08-2 (ethopropazine hydrochloride).

Pharmacopoeias. In *US.*

A white or slightly off-white, odourless, crystalline powder. **Soluble** in water at 40°; slightly soluble in water at 20°; soluble in alcohol and in chloroform; sparingly soluble in acetone; practically insoluble in ether. **Store** in airtight containers. Protect from light.

Adverse Effects, Treatment, and Precautions

As for Atropine Sulphate, p.455.

Drowsiness and confusion are common in patients taking ethopropazine; patients so affected should not drive or operate machinery. Ethopropazine may also cause muscle cramps, paraesthesia, and a sense of heaviness in the limbs, epigastric discomfort, and nausea.

Ethopropazine is a phenothiazine derivative—for adverse effects associated with phenothiazines, see p.649.

Breast feeding. A report[1] of ethopropazine distributed into the milk of lactating mothers.

1. Rowan JJ. Excretion of drugs in milk. *Pharm J* 1976; **217:** 184–7.

Interactions

As for antimuscarinics in general (see Atropine Sulphate, p.456).

Uses and Administration

Ethopropazine hydrochloride is a phenothiazine derivative with antimuscarinic, adrenergic-blocking, antihistaminic, local anaesthetic and ganglion-blocking properties. It has been used in the symptomatic treatment of parkinsonism (p.454), including the alleviation of the extrapyramidal syndrome induced by drugs such as other phenothiazine compounds but is of no value against tardive dyskinesias. It has been used in a usual dose of 50 mg once or twice daily by mouth initially, gradually increased to up to 500 or 600 mg daily in divided doses, according to the response of the patient.

Preparations

USP 23: Ethopropazine Hydrochloride Tablets.

Proprietary Preparations (details are given in Part 3)

Canad.: Parsitan.

Eucatropine Hydrochloride (369-n)

Eucatropine Hydrochloride *(BANM, rINNM).*

Clorhidrato de Euftalmina; Eucatropinium Chloride. 1,2,2,6-Tetramethyl-4-piperidyl mandelate hydrochloride.

$C_{17}H_{25}NO_3,HCl = 327.8.$

CAS — 100-91-4 (eucatropine); 536-93-6 (eucatropine hydrochloride).

Pharmacopoeias. In *US.*

A white odourless granular powder. Very **soluble** in water; freely soluble in alcohol and chloroform; practically insoluble in ether. **Store** in airtight containers. Protect from light.

Eucatropine hydrochloride is a tertiary amine antimuscarinic that has been used as a mydriatic. It has little or no effect on accommodation.

Preparations

USP 23: Eucatropine Hydrochloride Ophthalmic Solution.

Fentonium Bromide (370-k)

Fentonium Bromide *(rINN).*

Fa-402; Fentonii Bromidum; Ketoscilium; *N*-(4-Phenylphenacyl)-1-hyoscyaminium Bromide; Z-326. (−)-(1*R*,3*r*,5*S*)-8-(4-Phenylphenacyl)-3-[(*S*)-tropoyloxy]tropanium bromide.

$C_{31}H_{34}BrNO_4 = 564.5.$

CAS — 5868-06-4.

Fentonium bromide is a quaternary ammonium antimuscarinic with peripheral effects similar to those of atropine (p.455). It has been used to relieve visceral spasms.

Preparations

Proprietary Preparations (details are given in Part 3)

Ital.: Ulcesium†.

Multi-ingredient: ***Switz.:*** Dessertase†.

Flavoxate Hydrochloride (5233-h)

Flavoxate Hydrochloride *(BANM, USAN, rINNM).*

DW-61; NSC-114649; Rec-7-0040. 2-Piperidinoethyl 3-methyl-4-oxo-2-phenyl-4*H*-chromene-8-carboxylate hydrochloride.

$C_{24}H_{25}NO_4,HCl = 427.9.$

CAS — 15301-69-6 (flavoxate); 3717-88-2 (flavoxate hydrochloride).

Pharmacopoeias. In *Br.* and *Jpn.*

A white or almost white crystalline powder. Slightly **soluble** in water and in alcohol; sparingly soluble in dichloromethane. **Protect** from light.

Adverse Effects, Treatment, and Precautions

As for Atropine Sulphate, p.455.

Adverse effects of flavoxate hydrochloride include increased intra-ocular pressure, difficulty in ocular accommodation, and blurred vision. There may be dry mouth, gastro-intestinal disturbances and hypersensitivity reactions. Other adverse effects include headache, sedation, vertigo, dysuria, and confusion, particularly in the elderly. Tachycardia and palpitations have also been reported. Leucopenia has been reported rarely.

Interactions

As for antimuscarinics in general (see Atropine Sulphate, p.456).

Pharmacokinetics

Flavoxate is readily absorbed from the gastro-intestinal tract and rapidly metabolised, about 50 to 60% of a dose being excreted in the urine within 24 hours as methyl flavone carboxylic acid.

Uses and Administration

Flavoxate hydrochloride is described as a smooth muscle relaxant but it also has antimuscarinic effects; it is a tertiary amine. It is used for the symptomatic relief of pain, urinary frequency and incontinence associated with inflammatory disorders of the urinary tract. It is also used for the relief of vesico-urethral spasms resulting from instrumentation or surgery. A usual dose is 200 mg by mouth three times daily.

Urinary incontinence. Flavoxate is indicated mainly in the treatment of urge incontinence (p.454). Results of studies have sometimes been disappointing,[1-4] although side-effects are said to be less marked than those seen with other antimuscarinics such as oxybutynin.

1. Stanton SL. A comparison of emepronium bromide and flavoxate hydrochloride in the treatment of urinary incontinence. *J Urol (Baltimore)* 1973; **110:** 529–32.
2. Meyhoff HH, *et al.* Placebo—the drug of choice in female motor urge incontinence? *Br J Urol* 1983; **55:** 34–7.
3. Robinson JM, Brocklehurst JC. Emepronium bromide and flavoxate hydrochloride in the treatment of urinary incontinence associated with detrusor instability in elderly women. *Br J Urol* 1983; **55:** 371–6.
4. Chapple CR, *et al.* Double-blind, placebo-controlled, cross-over study of flavoxate in the treatment of idiopathic detrusor instability. *Br J Urol* 1990; **66:** 491–4.

Preparations

BP 1998: Flavoxate Tablets.

Proprietary Preparations (details are given in Part 3)

Aust.: Urispas; ***Belg.:*** Urispas; ***Canad.:*** Urispas; ***Fr.:*** Urispas; ***Ger.:*** Spasuret; ***Irl.:*** Urispas; ***Ital.:*** Genurin; ***Neth.:*** Urispas; ***S.Afr.:*** Urispas; ***Spain:*** Uronid; ***Switz.:*** Urispas; ***UK:*** Urispas; ***USA:*** Urispas.

Multi-ingredient: ***Ital.:*** Cistalgan.

Flutropium Bromide (2157-v)

Flutropium Bromide *(rINN).*

BA-598BR. (8*r*)-8-(2-Fluoroethyl)-3α-hydroxy-1α*H*,5α*H*-tropanium bromide benzilate.

$C_{24}H_{29}BrFNO_3 = 478.4.$

CAS — 63516-07-4.

Flutropium bromide is a quaternary ammonium antimuscarinic with peripheral effects similar to those of atropine (p.455). It has bronchodilator properties and has been investigated for the treatment of respiratory-tract disorders.

Glycopyrronium Bromide (371-a)

Glycopyrronium Bromide *(BAN, rINN).*

AHR-504; Glycopyrrolate *(USAN).* 3-(α-Cyclopentylmandeloyloxy)-1,1-dimethylpyrrolidinium bromide.

$C_{19}H_{28}BrNO_3 = 398.3.$

CAS — 596-51-0.

Pharmacopoeias. In *US.*

A white odourless crystalline powder. **Soluble** 1 in 4.2 of water, 1 in 30 of alcohol, 1 in 260 of chloroform, and 1 in 35 000 of ether. **Incompatible** with alkalis. **Store** in airtight containers.

Stability. Investigation of the compatibility of glycopyrronium bromide with infusion solutions and additives showed that the stability of glycopyrronium bromide is questionable above a pH of 6, owing to ester hydrolysis.[1]

1. Ingallinera TS, *et al.* Compatibility of glycopyrrolate injection with commonly used infusion solutions and additives. *Am J Hosp Pharm* 1979; **36:** 508–10. Correction. *ibid.*; 745.

Adverse Effects, Treatment, and Precautions

As for Atropine Sulphate, p.455.

Renal impairment. A comparison[1] of the pharmacokinetics of intravenous glycopyrronium in 11 uraemic and 7 control patients indicated that the renal elimination of glycopyrronium is considerably prolonged in patients with uraemia. The mean amount of a dose excreted in the urine within 3 hours of administration was 0.7% in the uraemic patients and 50% in the control patients; 24-hour excretion was 7% and 65% respectively. The authors of the study concluded that repeated or large doses of glycopyrronium should be avoided or perhaps the drug should not be used in patients with uraemia.

1. Kirvelä M, *et al.* Pharmacokinetics of glycopyrronium in uraemic patients. *Br J Anaesth* 1993; **71:** 437–9.

Interactions

As for antimuscarinics in general (see Atropine Sulphate, p.456).

Pharmacokinetics

Glycopyrronium bromide is poorly absorbed from the gastro-intestinal tract; about 10 to 25% has been stated to be absorbed following a dose by mouth. Glycopyrronium bromide penetrates the blood-brain barrier only poorly. Glycopyrronium is excreted in bile and urine.

References.

1. Kaltiala E, *et al.* The fate of intravenous [^{3}H]glycopyrrolate in man. *J Pharm Pharmacol* 1974; **26:** 352–4.
2. Ali-melkkilä TM, *et al.* Pharmacokinetics of IM glycopyrronium. *Br J Anaesth* 1990; **64:** 667–9.
3. Rautakorpi P, *et al.* Pharmacokinetics of glycopyrrolate in children. *J Clin Anesth* 1994; **6:** 217–20.

Uses and Administration

Glycopyrronium bromide is a quaternary ammonium antimuscarinic with peripheral effects similar to those of atropine (p.455). Following intramuscular administration, onset of effects is within 15 to 30 minutes; vagal blocking effects last for 2 to 3 hours and antisialagogue effects persist for up to 7 hours. Following intravenous administration, onset of action occurs within one minute.

Glycopyrronium bromide is used similarly to atropine in anaesthetic practice. It is also used in the iontophoretic treatment of hyperhidrosis and has been used as an adjunct in the treatment of peptic ulcer disease.

See below for details on dosage and administration of glycopyrronium.

Anaesthesia. Glycopyrronium bromide is given as a premedicant before general anaesthesia (see p.453) to diminish the risk of vagal inhibition of the heart and to reduce salivary and bronchial secretions. It is given in doses of 200 to 400 μg intravenously or intramuscularly before the induction of anaesthesia; alternatively, it may be given in a dose of 4 to 5 μg per kg body-weight to a maximum of 400 μg. If necessary, similar or lower doses may be given intravenously during the operation and repeated if required. A suggested dosage for premedication in children is 4 to 8 μg per kg intravenously or intramuscularly to a maximum of 200 μg.

Glycopyrronium bromide is given before or with anticholinesterases to counteract their muscarinic effects when they are used to reverse the effects of competitive muscle relaxants (see Neostigmine Methylsulphate, p.1394). The dose is glycopyrronium bromide 200 μg intravenously per 1 mg of neostigmine (or the equivalent dose of pyridostigmine); alternatively, it may be given in a dose of 10 to 15 μg per kg intravenously with neostigmine 50 μg per kg. A suggested dosage for children is 10 μg per kg intravenously with neostigmine 50 μg per kg. Glycopyrronium bromide can be administered mixed in the same syringe with the anticholinesterase, and it has been suggested that greater cardiovascular stability results from this method of administration.

Gastro-intestinal disorders. Antimuscarinics, including glycopyrronium bromide, may be used in the treatment of gastro-intestinal spasms and as an adjunct in the treatment of peptic ulcer disease, but they have only a limited role (see p.453).

As an adjunct in the treatment of peptic ulcer disease the usual initial dose of glycopyrronium bromide is 3 to 6 mg daily by mouth in divided doses adjusted according to response to a maximum of 8 mg daily; a maintenance dose of 1 mg twice daily is often adequate. Doses of 100 to 200 μg have been given by intramuscular or intravenous injection.

Hyperhidrosis. Adverse effects of antimuscarinics given orally generally preclude their use by this route for the management of hyperhidrosis (p.1074), but some, such as glycopyrronium, have been applied topically as alternatives to aluminium salts.

In studies involving 22 patients with the Frey syndrome (localised flushing and sweating on eating) glycopyrronium bromide as 1 and 2% cream or roll-on solution gave good control of symptoms;[1] patients tended to prefer the roll-on lotion as it was easier to apply. Topical hyoscine as 0.25, 1, or 3% solution or cream also gave control of sweating, but was associated with a much higher incidence of side-effects. Patients with diabetic gustatory sweating have also noted a reduction in the frequency and severity of episodes after applying glycopyrronium 0.5% cream.[2]

Glycopyrronium bromide has also been used as a 0.05% solution in the iontophoretic treatment of hyperhidrosis.

1. Hays LL, *et al.* The Frey syndrome: a simple, effective treatment. *Otolaryngol Head Neck Surg* 1982; **90:** 419–25.
2. Shaw JE, *et al.* A randomised controlled trial of topical glycopyrrolate, the first specific treatment for diabetic gustatory sweating. *Diabetologia* 1997; **40:** 299–301.

Respiratory-tract disorders. Antimuscarinics have potent bronchodilatory activity and may be used in the management of reversible airways obstruction as discussed on p.454, although glycopyrronium is not one of the main ones used.

References.

1. Schroeckenstein DC, *et al.* Twelve-hour bronchodilation in asthma with a single aerosol dose of the anticholinergic compound glycopyrrolate. *J Allergy Clin Immunol* 1988; **82:** 115–19.
2. Gilman MJ, *et al.* Comparison of aerosolized glycopyrrolate and metaproterenol in acute asthma. *Chest* 1990; **98:** 1095–8.
3. Cydulka RK, Emerman CL. Effects of combined treatment with glycopyrrolate and albuterol in acute exacerbation of chronic obstructive pulmonary disease. *Ann Emerg Med* 1995; **25:** 470–3.

Preparations

USP 23: Glycopyrrolate Injection; Glycopyrrolate Tablets.

Proprietary Preparations (details are given in Part 3)
Aust.: Robinul; ***Austral.:*** Robinul; ***Belg.:*** Robinul; ***Canad.:*** Robinul; ***Ger.:*** Robinul; ***Neth.:*** Robinul; ***Norw.:*** Robinul; ***S.Afr.:*** Robinul; ***Swed.:*** Robinul; ***Switz.:*** Robinul; ***UK:*** Robinul; ***USA:*** Robinul.

Used as an adjunct in: ***Belg.:*** Robinul-Neostigmine; ***Norw.:*** Robinul-Neostigmin; ***Swed.:*** Robinul-Neostigmin; ***Switz.:*** Robinul-Neostigmine; ***UK:*** Robinul-Neostigmine.

Homatropine (373-x)

Homatropine *(BAN)*.

(1*R*,3*r*,5*S*)-Tropan-3-yl (*RS*)-mandelate.

$C_{16}H_{21}NO_3$ = 275.3.

CAS — 87-00-3.

Homatropine Hydrobromide (374-r)

Homatropine Hydrobromide *(BANM)*.

Bromidrato de Homatropina; Homatr. Hydrobrom.; Homatropini Hydrobromidum; Homatropinium Bromide; Homatropinum Bromatum; Omatropina Bromidrato; Oxtolyltropine Hydrobromide; Tropyl Mandelate Hydrobromide.

$C_{16}H_{21}NO_3,HBr$ = 356.3.

CAS — 51-56-9.

NOTE. HOM is a code approved by the BP for use on single unit doses of eye drops containing homatropine hydrobromide where the individual container may be too small to bear all the appropriate labelling information.

Pharmacopoeias. In *Eur.* (see p.viii), *Int., Jpn, Pol.,* and *US.*

Colourless crystals or a white crystalline powder. **Soluble** 1 in 6 of water, 1 in 40 of alcohol, and 1 in 420 of chloroform; very slightly soluble to insoluble in ether. The Ph. Eur. specifies that a 5% solution in water has a pH of 5.0 to 6.5. The USP specifies that a 2% solution in water has a pH between 5.7 and 7.0. **Store** in airtight containers. Protect from light.

Homatropine Methobromide (375-f)

Homatropine Methylbromide *(BANM, rINN)*; Brometo de Metil-Homatropina; Homatropini Methylbromidum; Methylhomatropinium Bromatum; Methylhomatropinium Bromide. (1*R*,3*r*,5*S*)-3-[(±)-Mandeloyloxy]-8-methyltropanium bromide.

$C_{16}H_{21}NO_3,CH_3Br$ = 370.3.

CAS — 80-49-9.

Pharmacopoeias. In *Eur.* (see p.viii), *Int.,* and *US.*

Colourless crystals or a white odourless crystalline powder that slowly darkens on exposure to light. Very **soluble** or freely soluble in water; freely soluble or soluble in alcohol; practically insoluble in acetone and in ether. The Ph. Eur. specifies that a 5% solution in water, and the USP that a 1% solution, has a pH of 4.5 to 6.5. **Store** in airtight containers. Protect from light.

Adverse Effects, Treatment, and Precautions

As for Atropine Sulphate, p.455.

Anticholinergic toxicity (including ataxia, restlessness, excitement, hallucinations) has been reported in children[1] and the elderly[2,3] following administration of homatropine eye drops.

1. Hoefnagel D. Toxic effects of atropine and homatropine eye-drops in children. *N Engl J Med* 1961; **264:** 168–71.
2. Reid D, Fulton JD. Tachycardia precipitated by topical homatropine. *Br Med J* 1989; **299:** 795–6.
3. Tune LE, *et al.* Anticholinergic delirium caused by topical homatropine ophthalmologic solution: confirmation by anticholinergic radioreceptor assay in two cases. *J Neuropsychiatr Clin Neurosci* 1992; **4:** 195–7.

Interactions

As for antimuscarinics in general (see Atropine Sulphate, p.456).

Uses and Administration

Homatropine is a tertiary amine antimuscarinic with effects similar to those of atropine (p.455). It is used as the hydrobromide, also a tertiary amine, to produce mydriasis and cycloplegia (p.454); its actions are more rapid and of shorter duration than those of atropine, but it is less potent and has a relatively weak cycloplegic effect. In general, onset of action is between 30 and 60 minutes, and recovery within 1 to 3 days. Homatropine hydrobromide is generally used as a 1, 2, or 5% ophthalmic solution. For the determination of refraction, one or two drops may be instilled, repeated if necessary 5 or 10 minutes later. In the treatment of uveitis (p.1030), one or two drops may be instilled up to every 3 to 4 hours.

Homatropine has also been used as the quaternary ammonium methobromide derivative in the treatment of gastro-intestinal spasm and as an adjunct in peptic ulcer.

Preparations

BP 1998: Homatropine Eye Drops;
USP 23: Homatropine Hydrobromide Ophthalmic Solution; Homatropine Methylbromide Tablets.

Proprietary Preparations (details are given in Part 3)
Austral.: Homat†; ***Ital.:*** Novatropina†; ***Spain:*** Coliriocilina Homatrop; Homatrop.

Multi-ingredient: ***Austral.:*** Hycomine; ***Canad.:*** Ancatropine Infant Drops†; ***Fr.:*** Entercine†; Vagantyl†; ***Ger.:*** B_1-Neurischian†; ***Hung.:*** Neotroparin; ***Ital.:*** Distonium†; ***Spain:*** Bleukawine; Cortenema; Enterowas†; Templax†; ***Switz.:*** Supadol†; ***UK:*** APP Stomach Preparations†; ***USA:*** Codan†; Gustase Plus; Hycodan; Hydromet; Hydropane; Tussigon.

Hyoscine (11415-z)

Hyoscine *(BAN)*.

Scopolamine. (−)-(1*S*,3*s*,5*R*,6*R*,7*S*,8*s*)-6,7-Epoxy-3[(*S*)-tropoyloxy] tropane.

$C_{17}H_{21}NO_4$ = 303.4.

CAS — 51-34-3.

Hyoscine Butylbromide (376-d)

Hyoscine Butylbromide *(BANM)*.

Butylscopolamine Bromide; *N*-Butylscopolammonium Bromide; Butylscopolamonii Bromidum; Hyoscine-*N*-butyl Bromide; Hyoscini Butylbromidum; Scopolamine *N*-Butyl Bromide; Scopolamine Butylbromide. (−)-(1*S*,3*s*,5*R*,6*R*,7*S*,8*r*)-6,7-Epoxy-8-butyl-3-[(*S*)-tropoyloxy]tropanium bromide.

$C_{21}H_{30}BrNO_4$ = 440.4.

CAS — 149-64-4.

Pharmacopoeias. In *Eur.* (see p.viii) and *Jpn.*

A white or almost white, crystalline powder. Freely **soluble** in water and in dichloromethane; sparingly soluble in dehydrated alcohol. A 5% solution in water has a pH of 5.5 to 6.5.

Hyoscine Hydrobromide (377-n)

Hyoscine Hydrobromide *(BANM)*.

Bromhidrato de Escopolamina; Hyoscini Hydrobromidum; Ioscina Bromidrato; Scopolamine Bromhydrate; Scopolamine Hydrobromide; Scopolamini Hydrobromidum. (−)-(1*S*,3*s*,5*R*,6*R*,7*S*)-6,7-Epoxytropan-3-yl (*S*)-tropate hydrobromide trihydrate.

$C_{17}H_{21}NO_4,HBr,3H_2O$ = 438.3.

CAS — 114-49-8 (anhydrous hyoscine hydrobromide); 6533-68-2 (hyoscine hydrobromide trihydrate).

NOTE. HYO is a code approved by the BP for use on single unit doses of eye drops containing hyoscine hydrobromide where the individual container may be too small to bear all the appropriate labelling information.

Pharmacopoeias. In *Chin., Eur.* (see p.viii), *Jpn, Pol.,* and *US.*

Efflorescent odourless, colourless, crystals or white crystalline powder. **Soluble** 1 in 1.5 of water and 1 in 20 of alcohol; slightly soluble in chloroform; practically insoluble in ether. A 5% solution in water has a pH of 4.0 to 5.5. **Store** below 15° in well-filled airtight containers of small capacity. Protect from light.

Hyoscine Methobromide (378-h)

Hyoscine Methobromide *(BAN)*.

Epoxymethamine Bromide; Hyoscine Methylbromide; Methscopolamine Bromide; Scopolamine Methobromide; Scopolamine Methylbromide. (−)-(1*S*,3*s*,5*R*,6*R*,7*S*)-6,7-Epoxy-8-methyl-3-[(*S*)-tropoyloxy]tropanium bromide.

$C_{18}H_{24}BrNO_4$ = 398.3.

CAS — 155-41-9.

Hyoscine Methonitrate (379-m)

Hyoscine Methonitrate *(BANM)*.

Hyoscine Methylnitrate; Methscopolamine Nitrate; Methylhyoscini Nitras; Methylscopolamini Nitras; Scopolamine Methonitrate; Scopolamine Methylnitrate. (−)-(1*S*,3*s*,5*R*,6*R*,7*S*)-6,7-Epoxy-8-methyl-3-[(*S*)-tropoyloxy]tropanium nitrate.

$C_{18}H_{24}N_2O_7$ = 380.4.

CAS — 6106-46-3.

Pharmacopoeias. In *Aust.* and *It.*

Adverse Effects, Treatment, and Precautions

As for Atropine Sulphate, p.455. In contrast to atropine, hyoscine produces central depression at therapeutic doses and symptoms include drowsiness and fatigue. Toxic doses of hyoscine produce stimulation of the CNS in a similar manner to atropine. However, hyoscine does not stimulate the medullary centres and therefore does not produce the increases in respiration rate or blood pressure seen with atropine. Hyoscine may produce CNS stimulation rather than depression at therapeutic doses if used in the presence of pain without opioid analgesics; symptoms include excitement, restlessness, hallucinations, or delirium.

Patients who experience drowsiness should not drive or operate machinery. Caution has been advised in elderly patients and in patients with impaired metabolic, liver, or kidney function, as adverse CNS effects have been stated to be more likely in these patients. There have been rare reports of an increase in frequency of seizures in epileptic patients.

The quaternary derivatives, such as the butylbromide, methobromide, or methonitrate, do not readily cross the blood-brain barrier, so central effects are rare.

Effects on the eyes. ANISOCORIA. Although bilateral mydriasis has been observed concomitantly with the use of transdermal hyoscine, development of a unilateral fixed dilated pupil (anisocoria) may be due to contamination of a finger with hyoscine in applying the device, and then rubbing the eye.[1-4]

1. Chiaramonte JS. Cycloplegia from transdermal scopolamine. *N Engl J Med* 1982; **306:** 174.
2. Lepore FE. More on cycloplegia from transdermal scopolamine. *N Engl J Med* 1982; **307:** 824.
3. McCrary JA, Webb NR. Anisocoria from scopolamine patches. *JAMA* 1982; **248:** 353–4.
4. Bienia RA, *et al.* Scopolamine skin-disks and anisocoria. *Ann Intern Med* 1983; **99:** 572–3.

GLAUCOMA. A report[1] of 2 cases of angle-closure glaucoma precipitated by transdermal hyoscine.

1. Fraunfelder FT. Transdermal scopolamine precipitating narrow-angle glaucoma. *N Engl J Med* 1982; **307:** 1079.

STRABISMUS. Strabismus developed in a 4-year-old boy during treatment with transdermal hyoscine patches for drooling.[1] The strabismus resolved shortly after discontinuation of hyoscine.

1. Good WV, Crain LS. Esotropia in a child treated with a scopolamine patch for drooling. *Pediatrics* 1996; **97:** 126–7.

Effects on mental function. There have been reports of psychotic reactions associated with the transdermal administration of hyoscine.[1-3] Psychotic reactions have also occurred following instillation of hyoscine eye drops.[4]

1. Osterholm RK, Camoriano JK. Transdermal scopolamine psychosis. *JAMA* 1982; **247:** 3081.
2. Rodysill KJ, Warren JB. Transdermal scopolamine and toxic psychosis. *Ann Intern Med* 1983; **98:** 561.
3. MacEwan GW, *et al.* Psychosis due to transdermally administered scopolamine. *Can Med Assoc J* 1985; **133:** 431–2.
4. Barker DB, Solomon DA. The potential for mental status changes associated with systemic absorption of anticholinergic ophthalmic medications: concerns for the elderly. *DICP Ann Pharmacother* 1990; **24:** 847–50.

Effects on the skin. Contact dermatitis occurred in 16 men being treated for seasickness with transdermal hyoscine for 6 weeks to 15 months.[1]

1. Gordon CR, *et al.* Allergic contact dermatitis caused by transdermal hyoscine. *Br Med J* 1989; **298:** 1220–1.

Porphyria. Hyoscine butylbromide has been associated with clinical exacerbations of porphyria and is considered unsafe in porphyric patients.[1]

1. Moore MR, McColl KEL. *Porphyria: drug lists.* Glasgow: Porphyria Research Unit, University of Glasgow, 1991.

Pregnancy. A report[1] of hyoscine toxicity in a neonate born to a mother who had received a total of 1.8 mg of hyoscine in divided doses with pethidine and levorphanol prior to delivery. The neonate was lethargic, barrel chested, and had a heart rate of 200 beats per minute. Symptoms subsided following physostigmine 100 μg given intramuscularly.

1. Evens RP, Leopold JC. Scopolamine toxicity in a newborn. *Pediatrics* 1980; **66:** 329–30.

Withdrawal. Dizziness and nausea occurred three days after removal of a hyoscine transdermal delivery system. The patient had been using the transdermal patches to prevent seasickness during a 10-day cruise.[1]

1. Meyboom RHB. More on Transderm Scop patches. *N Engl J Med* 1984; **311:** 1377.

Interactions

As for antimuscarinics in general (see Atropine Sulphate, p.456).

The sedative effect of hyoscine may be enhanced by alcohol or other CNS depressants.

Pharmacokinetics

Hyoscine is readily absorbed from the gastro-intestinal tract following oral doses of the hydrobromide. It is almost entirely metabolised, probably in the liver; only a small proportion of an oral dose has been reported to be excreted unchanged in the urine. It crosses the blood-brain barrier and has been stated to cross the placenta. Hyoscine is also well absorbed following application to the skin.

The quaternary derivatives, such as the butylbromide or methobromide, are poorly absorbed from the gastro-intestinal tract and do not readily pass the blood-brain barrier.

References.

1. Ebert U, *et al.* Pharmacokinetics and pharmacodynamics of scopolamine after subcutaneous administration. *J Clin Pharmacol* 1998; **38:** 720–6.

Uses and Administration

Hyoscine is a tertiary amine antimuscarinic with central and peripheral actions (see p.453). It is a more powerful suppressant of salivation than atropine, and usually slows rather than increases heart rate, especially in low doses. Its central action differs from that of atropine in that it depresses the cerebral cortex and produces drowsiness and amnesia. Hyoscine hydrobromide is also a tertiary amine, whereas hyoscine butylbromide, hyoscine methobromide, and hyoscine methonitrate are quaternary ammonium derivatives.

Hyoscine and hyoscine hydrobromide are used in the management of motion sickness and other forms of nausea and vomiting; hyoscine hydrobromide is also given as a premedicant in anaesthesia, and to produce cycloplegia and mydriasis. Hyoscine butylbromide and other quaternary ammonium derivatives are used in conditions associated with visceral spasms. In addition, hyoscine methobromide has been employed as an adjunct in the treatment of peptic ulcer disease.

In the prevention and control of *motion sickness*, hyoscine hydrobromide 300 μg may be taken by mouth 30 minutes before a journey; followed by 300 μg every 6 hours if required up to a maximum of 3 doses in 24 hours. Children aged 4 to 10 years may be given 75 to 150 μg and those over 10 years, 150 to 300 μg. Hyoscine is also given to prevent motion sickness via a transdermal delivery system which is placed behind the ear and supplies 1 mg over 3 days. The patch should be applied 5 to 6 hours before travelling or on the preceding evening. Patches have been used in adults for the prevention of postoperative nausea and vomiting.

Hyoscine hydrobromide has also been given by intravenous, subcutaneous, or intramuscular injection for its antiemetic effect in a usual dose of 300 μg to 600 μg.

For *premedication* hyoscine hydrobromide is injected subcutaneously or intramuscularly in doses of 200 to 600 μg, usually in association with papaveretum about half to one hour before induction of general anaesthesia.

Hyoscine hydrobromide is used in the eye for its *mydriatic* and *cycloplegic* actions usually in a concentration of 0.25%. It has a faster onset and shorter duration of action than atropine although the effects may still persist for up to 3 to 7 days. It may be useful for patients who are hypersensitive to atropine.

In conditions associated with *visceral spasm*, usual doses of 20 mg of hyoscine butylbromide are administered intramuscularly or intravenously, repeated after 30 minutes if necessary; alternatively, 10 mg may be given by mouth three times daily, increased to 20 mg four times daily if necessary. Children aged 6 to 12 years may be given 10 mg three times daily by mouth.

Other hyoscine salts or derivatives that have been used include hyoscine borate, hyoscine hydrochloride, and hyoscine oxide hydrobromide.

Anaesthesia. The role of antimuscarinics, including hyoscine, in anaesthesia is discussed on p.453. For the use of hyoscine in the prevention of postoperative nausea and vomiting see below.

Anoxic seizures. For mention of the use of transdermal hyoscine as an alternative to atropine in the management of reflex anoxic seizures in children, see p.456.

Cardiac disorders. Although hyoscine is not one of the conventional therapies for heart failure (p.785) or myocardial infarction (p.791), low-dose transdermal hyoscine can increase cardiac vagal activity and thereby reduce the autonomic imbalance seen in patients with these conditions.[1-3]

1. Casadei B, *et al.* Low doses of scopolamine increase cardiac vagal tone in the acute phase of myocardial infarction. *Circulation* 1993; **88:** 353–7.
2. La Rovere MT, *et al.* Scopolamine improves autonomic balance in advanced congestive heart failure. *Circulation* 1994; **90:** 838–43.
3. Venkatesh G, *et al.* Double blind placebo controlled trial of short term transdermal scopolamine on heart rate variability in patients with chronic heart failure. *Heart* 1996; **76:** 137–43.

Colic pain. Hyoscine has been used as an adjunct to opioid analgesics for symptomatic relief of biliary or renal colic (see p.453).

Eye disorders. Hyoscine is used to produce mydriasis and cycloplegia (p.454) to facilitate examination of the eye.

Gastro-intestinal disorders. Hyoscine has been used to relieve the pain of smooth muscle spasm associated with the gastro-intestinal tract (p.453). It may be useful as an antispasmodic in endoscopy and radiological procedures of the gastro-intestinal tract.[1] Hyoscine has also been used as an adjunct in the treatment of peptic ulcer disease. Its antiemetic effect is discussed under Nausea and Vomiting, below.

1. Goei R, *et al.* Use of antispasmodic drugs in double contrast barium enema examination: glucagon or Buscopan? *Clin Radiol* 1995: **50:** 553–7.

Hyperhidrosis. Adverse effects of antimuscarinics given orally generally preclude their use by this route for the management of hyperhidrosis (p.1074), but some, such as hyoscine, have been applied topically as alternatives to aluminium salts. Hyoscine hydrobromide applied as a 3% cream was successful in reducing gustatory sweating, consisting of flushing and sweating over the right mandible during eating, in a patient who had previously undergone surgical excision of the right submandibular salivary gland.[1]

1. Bailey BMW, Pearce DE. Gustatory sweating following submandibular salivary gland removal. *Br Dent J* 1985; **158:** 17–18.

Nausea and vomiting. Early studies have established that hyoscine is an effective agent in the prevention of **motion sickness**[1,2] and is one of the principal drugs used. It may be given by mouth for short-term protection or transdermally from controlled-release systems for a prolonged duration of action.

In an attempt to maintain therapeutic blood concentrations over prolonged periods, and reduce side-effects, interest has focussed on the transdermal administration of hyoscine from controlled-release skin patches. Placebo-controlled studies have shown transdermal hyoscine to be more effective than agents such as oral dimenhydrinate or meclozine for the prophylaxis of motion sickness for periods less than 8 hours.[3,4] In a study of the prevention of longer-term sea sickness[5] transdermal hyoscine for the first 3 days of a week's exposure to heavy or moderate seas reduced nausea compared with placebo in the first 2 days. However, vomiting was greater in the active drug group 3 days after removal of the delivery system, perhaps due to a delay in adaptation to motion because of the use of hyoscine.

Although transdermal hyoscine was more effective than placebo in reducing **postoperative nausea and vomiting** in a study completed by 38 patients undergoing gynaecological surgery,[6] the effect was limited and this treatment alone was not considered to be the answer to postoperative nausea and vomiting. This was reinforced by another study[7] in 283 women that showed no difference between transdermal hyoscine and placebo in duration, frequency, or severity of postoperative nausea and vomiting. Antimuscarinics such as hyoscine have long been given as premedicants before surgery and their antiemetic action has helped to prevent postoperative nausea and vomiting associated with opioid analgesics. However, because they have a shorter duration of action than morphine slow-release transdermal patches containing hyoscine have been tried for the prophylaxis of postoperative nausea and vomiting, but results have been variable.[6-9]

The other drugs used in the management of motion sickness and postoperative nausea and vomiting are discussed on p.1172.

1. Report of study by Army, Navy, Air Force Motion Sickness Team. Evaluation of drugs for protection against motion sickness aboard transport ships. *JAMA* 1956; **160:** 755–60.
2. Wood CD, Graybiel A. Theory of antimotion sickness drug mechanisms. *Aerospace Med* 1972: **43:** 249–52.
3. Price NM, *et al.* Transdermal scopolamine in the prevention of motion sickness at sea. *Clin Pharmacol Ther* 1981; **29:** 414–19.
4. Dahl E, *et al.* Transdermal scopolamine, oral meclizine, and placebo in motion sickness. *Clin Pharmacol Ther* 1984; **36:** 116–20.
5. van Marion WF, *et al.* Influence of transdermal scopolamine on motion sickness during 7 days' exposure to heavy seas. *Clin Pharmacol Ther* 1985; **38:** 301–5.
6. Uppington J, *et al.* Transdermal hyoscine and postoperative nausea and vomiting. *Anaesthesia* 1986; **41:** 16–20.
7. Koski EMJ, *et al.* Double blind comparison of transdermal hyoscine and placebo for the prevention of postoperative nausea. *Br J Anaesth* 1990; **64:** 16–20.
8. Doyle E, *et al.* Prevention of postoperative nausea and vomiting with transdermal hyoscine in children using patient-controlled analgesia. *Br J Anaesth* 1994; **72:** 72–6.
9. Honkavaara P, *et al.* Prevention of nausea and vomiting with transdermal hyoscine in adults after middle ear surgery during general anaesthesia. *Br J Anaesth* 1994; **73:** 763–6.

Urinary incontinence. Various antimuscarinics have been used in the management of urge incontinence (p.454) but the incidence of adverse effects can be high. Results of a recent small study[1] suggested that transdermal hyoscine might be of benefit in females with detrusor instability.

1. Muskat Y, *et al.* The use of scopolamine in the treatment of detrusor instability. *J Urol (Baltimore)* 1996; **156:** 1989–90.

Vertigo. Hyoscine has a long history of use in the management of vertigo, although other drugs are now preferred (p.401). Results of a study[1] involving 30 patients with vertigo suggested that a single transdermal patch of hyoscine was a reasonable alternative to other forms of treatment for acute peripheral vertigo.

1. Rahko T, Karma P. Transdermal scopolamine for peripheral vertigo (a double-blind study). *J Laryngol Otol* 1985; **99:** 653–6.

Preparations

BP 1998: Hyoscine Butylbromide Injection; Hyoscine Butylbromide Tablets; Hyoscine Eye Drops; Hyoscine Injection; Hyoscine Tablets;
USP 23: Scopolamine Hydrobromide Injection; Scopolamine Hydrobromide Ophthalmic Ointment; Scopolamine Hydrobromide Ophthalmic Solution; Scopolamine Hydrobromide Tablets.

Proprietary Preparations (details are given in Part 3)
Aust.: Buscopan; Scopoderm; ***Austral.:*** Buscopan; Kwells; Scop†; ***Belg.:*** Buscopan; ***Canad.:*** Buscopan; Transderm-V; ***Fr.:*** Buscopan†; Genoscopolamine; Scopoderm TTS; ***Ger.:*** Boro-Scopol; BS-ratiopharm; Buscolysin; Buscopan; espa-butyl; Holopon†; Scopoderm TTS; Skopyl†; ***Irl.:*** Buscopan; Kwells; ***Ital.:*** Buscopan; Transcop; ***Neth.:*** Buscopan; Scopoderm TTS; ***Norw.:*** Buscopan; Scopoderm; ***S.Afr.:*** Buscopan; Hyospasmol; Scopex; Scopoderm TTS†; ***Spain:*** Buscapina; Vorigeno; ***Swed.:*** Buscopan; Scopoderm; ***Switz.:*** Buscopan; Scopoderm TTS; ***UK:*** Buscopan; Joy-Rides; Kwells; Scopoderm TTS; Travel Calm; ***USA:*** Pamine; Scopace; Transderm Scop.

Multi-ingredient: ***Aust.:*** Asthma; Buscopamol; Buscopan Compositum; Modiscop; ***Austral.:*** Benacine†; Contac; Donnagel; Donnalix; Donnatab; Travacalm; ***Belg.:*** Buscopan Compositum; Spasma; Tranquo-Buscopan†; ***Canad.:*** Diban; Donnagel†; Donnatal; ***Fr.:*** Algo-Buscopan†; Vagantyl†; ***Ger.:*** B_1-Neurischian†; bella sanol†; Brox-Aerosol N†; Buscopan Plus; Circovegetalin compositum†; Felsolyn N†; Ichthospasmin N†; Oragallin S; Seda-Stenocrat-N†; Spasmo-Bilicura†; ***Irl.:*** Feminax; ***Ital.:*** Buscopan Compositum; Spasmeridan; Tranquo-Buscopan†; ***S.Afr.:*** Allertac; Bellatard; Bellavern†; Buscopan Compositum; Donnatal; Dyka-D; Dykatuss†; Millerspas; Respinol; Respinol Compound; Scopex Co†; Tropax†; Virobis†; ***Spain:*** Buscapina Compositum; Buscopax†; Frenespan†; Furantoina Sedante†; Lotanal†; Midriatic; Nolotil Compositum; Oragallin Espasmolitico; PH 3 Compuesto†; Psico Blocan; Urogobens Antiespasmo; ***Swed.:*** Spasmofen; ***Switz.:*** Buscopan Compositum†; Nardyl; Viaggio; ***UK:*** Feminax; ***USA:*** AH-chew; Antispasmodic Elixir; Atrohist Plus; Barbidonna; Bellatal; DA Chewable; DA II; Dallergy; Deconhist LA; Donna-Sed; Donnagel-PG†; Donnamor; Donnapine†; Donnatal; Dura-Vent/DA; Ex-Histine; Extendryl; Histaspan-D†; Histor-D Timecelles; Hyosophen; Kinesed†; Malatal†; Mescolor; Murocoll-2; OMNIhist LA; Pannaz; Phenacon; Phenahist-TR; Phenchlor SHA; Prehist D; Relaxadon†; Rhinolar†; Ru-Tuss; Spasmophen†; Spasquid†; Stahist; Susano.

Hyoscyamine (381-x)

Hyoscyamine *(BAN)*.

(−)-Hyoscyamine; *l*-Hyoscyamine. (−)-(1*R*,3*r*,5*S*)-Tropan-3-yl (*S*)-tropate.

$C_{17}H_{23}NO_3$ = 289.4.

CAS — 101-31-5.

Pharmacopoeias. In US.

An alkaloid obtained from various solanaceous plants. It is the laevo-isomer of atropine into which it can be converted by heating or by the action of alkali. A white crystalline powder, m.p. 106° to 109°. Slightly **soluble** in water; freely soluble in alcohol, in chloroform, and in dilute acids; sparingly soluble in ether. A solution in water is alkaline to litmus. **Store** in airtight containers. Protect from light.

Hyoscyamine Hydrobromide (382-r)

Hyoscyamine Hydrobromide *(BANM)*.

Bromidrato de Hiosciamina; Hyoscyamine Bromhydrate.

$C_{17}H_{23}NO_3,HBr$ = 370.3.

CAS — 306-03-6.

Pharmacopoeias. In US.

White, odourless crystals or crystalline powder. M.p. not less than 149°. Freely **soluble** in water; soluble 1 in 2.5 of alcohol, 1 in 1.7 of chloroform, and 1 in 2300 of ether. A 5% solution in water has a pH of about 5.4. **Store** in airtight containers. Protect from light.

Hyoscyamine Sulphate (383-f)

Hyoscyamine Sulphate *(BANM)*.

Hyoscyamine Sulfate; Hyoscyamini Sulfas; Hyoscyaminum Sulfuricum; Iosciamina Solfato.

$(C_{17}H_{23}NO_3)_2,H_2SO_4,2H_2O$ = 712.8.

CAS — 620-61-1 (anhydrous hyoscyamine sulphate); 6835-16-1 (hyoscyamine sulphate dihydrate).

Pharmacopoeias. In *Eur.* (see p.viii) and US.

White, odourless crystals or deliquescent crystalline powder. M.p. not less than 200°. Ph. Eur. **solubilities** are: very soluble in water; sparingly soluble to soluble in alcohol; practically insoluble in ether. USP solubilities are: soluble 1 in 0.5 of water and 1 in 5 of alcohol; practically insoluble in ether. The Ph. Eur. specifies that a 2% solution in water has a pH of 4.5 to 6.2. The USP states that a 1% solution in water has a pH of about 5.3. **Store** in airtight containers. Protect from light.

Adverse Effects, Treatment, and Precautions

As for Atropine Sulphate, p.455.

Interactions

As for antimuscarinics in general (see Atropine Sulphate, p.456).

Uses and Administration

Hyoscyamine is a tertiary amine antimuscarinic with the actions of atropine (p.455), which is racemic hyoscyamine; hyoscyamine, the laevo-isomer, has approximately twice the potency of atropine since the dextro-isomer has only very weak antimuscarinic activity. Hyoscyamine is used mainly in the relief of conditions associated with visceral spasm. It has also been given for rhinitis and was formerly used in the treatment of parkinsonism.

Hyoscyamine is given in usual doses of 150 to 300 μg up to four times daily by mouth, but it is more usually employed as the sulphate; the hydrobromide is also used. Suggested doses of hyoscyamine sulphate are 125 to 250 μg by mouth or sublingually every four hours as needed, up to a maximum of 1.5 mg in 24 hours. Modified-release oral preparations of hyoscyamine sulphate are available in some countries; dosage is specific to a particular formulation. Hyoscyamine sulphate has also been given by injection.

Preparations

USP 23: Hyoscyamine Sulfate Elixir; Hyoscyamine Sulfate Injection; Hyoscyamine Sulfate Oral Solution; Hyoscyamine Sulfate Tablets; Hyoscyamine Tablets.

Proprietary Preparations (details are given in Part 3)
Canad.: Levsin; ***Fr.:*** Duboisine†; ***Neth.:*** Egacene Durettes; ***Norw.:*** Egazil; ***Swed.:*** Egazil; ***UK:*** Peptard†; ***USA:*** A-Spas; Anaspaz; Cystospaz; Cystospaz-M; Donnamar; ED-SPAZ; Gastrosed; Levbid; Levsin; Levsinex.

Multi-ingredient: ***Aust.:*** Normensan; ***Austral.:*** Contac; Donnagel; Donnalix; Donnatab; ***Canad.:*** Diban; Donnagel†; Donnatal; ***Ger.:*** bella sanol†; Circovegetalin compositum†; ***S.Afr.:*** Allertac; Bellatard; Bellavern†; Donnatal; Millerspas; Tropax†; ***Spain:*** Salvacolina NN†; ***Switz.:*** Bronchalin; Nardyl; Viaggio; ***USA:*** Antispasmodic Elixir; Arco-Lase Plus; Atrohist Plus; Atrosept; Barbidonna; Bellacane; Bellatal; Deconhist LA; Dolsed; Donna-Sed; Donnagel-PG†; Donnamor; Donnapine†; Donnatal; Hyosophen; Kinesed†; Kutrase; Levsin with Phenobarbitone; Malatal†; Phenahist-TR; Phenchlor SHA; Prosed/DS; Pyridium Plus†; Relaxadon†; Ru-Tuss; Spasmophen†; Spasquid†; Stahist; Susano; Trac Tabs 2X; UAA; Uridon Modified; Urimar-T; Urised; Urisedamine; Urogesic Blue.

Hyoscyamus (384-d)

Banotu; Beleño; Bilsenkraut; Giusquiamo; Henbane; Hyoscy.; Hyoscyami; Jusquiame; Jusquiame Noire; Meimendro.

Pharmacopoeias. Eur. (see p.viii) includes a monograph for Hyoscyamus Leaf and Prepared Hyoscyamus.
Chin. specifies only the seeds.

Hyoscyamus [*Hyoscyamus niger* (Solanaceae)] contains alkaloids that consist mainly of hyoscyamine (the laevo-isomer of atropine) with hyoscine in varying proportions. The total alkaloidal content of hyoscyamus preparations is usually calculated as hyoscyamine. The Ph. Eur. specifies not less than 0.05% of total alkaloids.

Hyoscyamus Leaf (Henbane Leaves; Hyoscyami Folium) is the dried leaves, or leaves, flowering tops, and occasionally fruits of the plant.

Prepared Hyoscyamus (Hyoscyami Pulvis Normatus; Prep. Hyoscy.) is hyoscyamus leaf reduced to a powder and adjusted to contain 0.05 to 0.07% of total alkaloids.

Store in airtight containers. Protect from light.

Hyoscyamus has peripheral and central effects similar to those of atropine (p.455); its preparations have been used mainly for the relief of visceral spasm. The fresh whole flowering plant (*Hyoscyamus niger*) has been used in herbal and homoeopathic medicine.

Preparations

BP 1998: Hyoscyamus Dry Extract.

Proprietary Preparations (details are given in Part 3)
Aust.: Kelosoft; ***Switz.:*** Kelosoft.

Multi-ingredient: ***Belg.:*** Escouflaire; Sanicolax; Valeria-Fordine†; ***Fr.:*** Asthmalgine; Baume Dalet; Broncorinol toux seches; Colarine†; Creme Rap; Gastrosedyl; Ideolaxyl; Laccoderme a l'huile de cade†; Sedibaine; Thiosedal; ***Ger.:*** Opobyl†; Reflex-Zonen-Salbe (RZS) (Rowo-333)†; Unguentum Lymphaticum; ***Ital.:*** Kindian†; ***Neth.:*** Opobyl†; ***Spain:*** Laxo Vian; ***Switz.:*** Baby Liberol; Dicalm†; Gouttes contre la toux "S"; Histacyl Cutane†; Keli-med; Kernosan Huile de Massage; Liberol; Sedovalin†; Sirop S contre la toux et la bronchite; ***UK:*** Onopordon Comp B.

Isopropamide Iodide (387-m)

Isopropamide Iodide *(BAN, rINN)*.

Iodeto de Isopropamida. (3-Carbamoyl-3,3-diphenylpropyl)di-isopropylmethylammonium iodide.

$C_{23}H_{33}IN_2O$ = 480.4.

CAS — 7492-32-2 (isopropamide); 71-81-8 (isopropamide iodide).

Pharmacopoeias. In US.

A white to pale yellow crystalline powder. Isopropamide iodide 1.36 mg is approximately equivalent to 1 mg of isopropamide. **Soluble** 1 in 50 of water, 1 in 10 of alcohol, and 1 in 5 of chloroform; very slightly soluble in ether. **Protect** from light.

Isopropamide iodide is a quaternary ammonium antimuscarinic with peripheral effects similar to those of atropine (p.455). It has been used as an adjunct in the treatment of peptic ulcer disease, in the relief of gastro-intestinal and urinary-tract disorders associated with smooth muscle spasm, in rhinitis, and for the relief of symptoms of colds.

Isopropamide bromide has been used similarly.

Preparations

USP 23: Isopropamide Iodide Tablets.

Proprietary Preparations (details are given in Part 3)
Belg.: Priamide; ***Ital.:*** Dipramid†.

Multi-ingredient: ***Aust.:*** Stelabid; Vesalium; ***Austral.:*** Stelabid†; ***Belg.:*** Rinomar; Vesalium; ***Canad.:*** Stelabid; ***Fr.:*** Enuretine; ***Ger.:*** Ornatos†; Stelabid†; ***Hung.:*** Bispan; Triospan; ***Irl.:***

Stelabid; *Ital.:* Fluvaleas; Iodosan Raffreddore Contact†; Raffreddoremed; Valtrax; Vesalium†; *S.Afr.:* Stelabid†; *Spain:* Ornade; Ornasec†; *Switz.:* Vesalium†.

Mecloxamine Citrate (11607-d)

Mecloxamine Citrate *(rINNM)*.

2-[1-(4-Chlorophenyl)-1-phenylethoxy]-*N*,*N*-dimethyl-1-propanamine citrate.

$C_{19}H_{24}ClNO,C_6H_8O_7 = 510.0.$

CAS — 5668-06-4 (mecloxamine); 56050-03-4 (mecloxamine citrate).

Mecloxamine citrate is reported to have antimuscarinic properties and has been used for its antiemetic action in antimigraine preparations.

Preparations

Proprietary Preparations (details are given in Part 3)
Multi-ingredient: *Aust.:* Avamigran.

Mepenzolate Bromide (390-r)

Mepenzolate Bromide *(BAN, rINN)*.

Mepenzolate Methylbromide; Mepenzolone Bromide. 3-Benziloyloxy-1,1-dimethylpiperidinium bromide.

$C_{21}H_{26}BrNO_3 = 420.3.$

CAS — 25990-43-6 (mepenzolate); 76-90-4 (mepenzolate bromide).

Pharmacopoeias. In *Jpn* and *US*.

A white or light cream-coloured powder. **Soluble** 1 in 110 of water, 1 in 120 of dehydrated alcohol, 1 in 630 of chloroform, and 1 in about 8 of methyl alcohol; practically insoluble in ether. **Store** in airtight containers.

Mepenzolate bromide is a quaternary ammonium antimuscarinic with peripheral actions similar to those of atropine (p.455). It has been used in the relief of gastro-intestinal disorders associated with smooth muscle spasm and as an adjunct in the treatment of peptic ulcer disease. It is given in doses of 25 to 50 mg three or four times daily.

Preparations

USP 23: Mepenzolate Bromide Tablets.

Proprietary Preparations (details are given in Part 3)
Belg.: Cantil†; *Swed.:* Cantil; *UK:* Cantil†; *USA:* Cantil.
Multi-ingredient: *Ital.:* Enterocantril†.

Methanthelinium Bromide (391-f)

Methanthelinium Bromide *(BAN, pINN)*.

Dixamonum Bromidum; Methantheline Bromide; MTB-51; SC-2910. Diethylmethyl[2-(xanthen-9-ylcarbonyloxy)ethyl]ammonium bromide.

$C_{21}H_{26}BrNO_3 = 420.3.$

CAS — 5818-17-7 (methanthelinium); 53-46-3 (methanthelinium bromide).

Methanthelinium bromide is a quaternary ammonium antimuscarinic with peripheral effects similar to those of atropine (p.455). It has been used as an adjunct in the treatment of peptic ulcer disease, in gastro-intestinal disorders associated with smooth muscle spasm, and in the management of urinary incontinence. A usual dose is 50 to 100 mg by mouth four times daily.

Preparations

Proprietary Preparations (details are given in Part 3)
Ger.: Vagantin; *USA:* Banthine.

Methixene Hydrochloride (392-d)

Methixene Hydrochloride *(BANM, USAN)*.

Metixene Hydrochloride *(rINNM)*; Methixene Hydrochloride Monohydrate; Metixeni Hydrochloridum; NSC-78194; SJ-1977. 9-(1-Methyl-3-piperidylmethyl)thioxanthene hydrochloride monohydrate.

$C_{20}H_{23}NS,HCl,H_2O = 363.9.$

CAS — 4969-02-2 (methixene); 1553-34-0 (anhydrous methixene hydrochloride); 7081-40-5 (methixene hydrochloride monohydrate).

Pharmacopoeias. In *Eur.* (see p.viii).

A white or almost white, crystalline or fine crystalline powder. **Soluble** in water, in alcohol, and in dichloromethane; practically insoluble in ether. A 1.8% solution in water has a pH of 4.4 to 5.8. **Protect** from light.

Methixene hydrochloride is a tertiary antimuscarinic with actions similar to those of atropine (p.455); it also has antihistaminic and direct antispasmodic properties.

It is used for the symptomatic treatment of parkinsonism (p.454), including the alleviation of the extrapyramidal syndrome induced by other drugs such as phenothiazines, but it is of no value against tardive dyskinesias. The usual dose by mouth of methixene hydrochloride is 2.5 mg three times daily initially, gradually increased according to the response of the patient to a total of 15 to 60 mg daily in divided doses.

Methixene hydrochloride has also been used in preparations to relieve gastro-intestinal spasms.

Preparations

Proprietary Preparations (details are given in Part 3)
Ger.: Metixen; Tremarit; *Irl.:* Tremonil†; *Ital.:* Tremaril; *Spain:* Tremaril†; *Swed.:* Tremoquil; *Switz.:* Tremaril†; *UK:* Tremonil†.
Multi-ingredient: *Ger.:* Spasmo-Canulase N†; *Ital.:* Canulase†; *S.Afr.:* Spasmo-Canulase; *Spain:* Espasmo Canulasa; *Switz.:* Gillazyme plus; Spasmo-Canulase.

Methylbenactyzium Bromide (8150-d)

Methylbenactyzium Bromide *(rINN)*.

Benactyzine Methobromide. Diethyl(2-hydroxyethyl)methylammonium bromide benzilate.

$C_{21}H_{28}BrNO_3 = 422.4.$

CAS — 3166-62-9.

Pharmacopoeias. In *Jpn*.

Methylbenactyzium bromide, a derivative of benactyzine (p.280), is an antimuscarinic with effects similar to those of atropine (p.455). It has been given by mouth for the treatment of gastro-intestinal spasm and nocturnal enuresis.

Preparations

Proprietary Preparations (details are given in Part 3)
Jpn: Finalin†.
Multi-ingredient: *Aust.:* Anxiolit plus; *Ital.:* Spasmodil Complex†.

Octatropine Methylbromide (393-n)

Octatropine Methylbromide *(BAN, rINN)*.

Anisotropine Methobromide; Anisotropine Methylbromide *(USAN)*. (1*R*,3*r*,5*S*)-8-Methyl-3-(2-propylvaleryloxy)tropanium bromide.

$C_{17}H_{32}BrNO_2 = 362.3.$

CAS — 80-50-2.

Pharmacopoeias. In *It.*

Octatropine methylbromide is a quaternary ammonium antimuscarinic with peripheral actions similar to those of atropine (p.455). It is used in doses of 50 mg three times daily as an adjunct in the treatment of peptic ulcer disease. It is also used in doses of 10 mg three or four times daily by mouth to relieve visceral spasms.

Preparations

Proprietary Preparations (details are given in Part 3)
Spain: Vapin.
Multi-ingredient: *Ital.:* Valpinax; *Spain:* Vapin Complex.

Orphenadrine Citrate (394-h)

Orphenadrine Citrate *(BANM, rINNM)*.

Mephenamine Citrate; Orphenadin Citrate. (*RS*)-Dimethyl[2-(2-methylbenzhydryloxy)ethyl]amine dihydrogen citrate.

$C_{18}H_{23}NO,C_6H_8O_7 = 461.5.$

CAS — 83-98-7 (orphenadrine); 4682-36-4 (orphenadrine citrate).

Pharmacopoeias. In *Br.* and *US*.

A white or almost white, odourless or almost odourless, crystalline powder. Orphenadrine citrate 100 mg is approximately equivalent to 66 mg of orphenadrine hydrochloride. Sparingly **soluble** in water; slightly soluble in alcohol; practically insoluble in chloroform and in ether. **Store** in airtight containers. Protect from light.

Orphenadrine Hydrochloride (395-m)

Orphenadrine Hydrochloride *(BANM, rINNM)*.

BS-5930; Mephenamine Hydrochloride; Orphenadin Hydrochloride. (*RS*)-Dimethyl[2-(2-methylbenzhydryloxy)ethyl]amine hydrochloride.

$C_{18}H_{23}NO,HCl = 305.8.$

CAS — 341-69-5.

Pharmacopoeias. In *Br.*

A white or almost white, odourless or almost odourless, crystalline powder. Freely **soluble** in water, in alcohol, and in chloroform; practically insoluble in ether. **Protect** from light.

Adverse Effects, Treatment, and Precautions

As for Atropine Sulphate, p.455.

Abuse. A 23-year-old schizophrenic man, whose treatment included orphenadrine 100 mg three times daily, obtained illicit supplies and increased the dose for euphoric effect.[1] On one occasion he had an epileptic convulsion after a 600-mg dose.

1. Shariatmadari ME. Orphenadrine dependence. *Br Med J* 1975; **3:** 486.

Overdosage. A report[1] of acute poisoning with orphenadrine following massive overdosage in a schizophrenic patient, who responded to intensive supportive treatment, including large doses of adrenaline, dopamine, and dobutamine to restore blood pressure following asystole. Between 1977 and 1980 twelve deaths due to orphenadrine were recorded by the National Poisons Unit at Guy's Hospital in London.

1. Clarke B, *et al.* Acute poisoning with orphenadrine. *Lancet* 1985; **i:** 1386.

Porphyria. Orphenadrine has been associated with acute attacks of porphyria and is considered unsafe in patients with acute porphyria.[1]

1. Moore MR, McColl KEL. *Porphyria: drug lists.* Glasgow: Porphyria Research Unit, University of Glasgow, 1991.

Interactions

As for antimuscarinics in general (see Atropine Sulphate, p.456).

Chlorpromazine. For the effect of orphenadrine on plasma concentrations of chlorpromazine, see under Antiparkinsonian Drugs, p.653.

Dextropropoxyphene. A suggested interaction between orphenadrine and dextropropoxyphene was open to question.[1,2]

1. Pearson RE, Salter FJ. Drug interaction? — orphenadrine with propoxyphene. *N Engl J Med* 1970; **282:** 1215.
2. Puckett WH, Visconti JA. Orphenadrine and propoxyphene (cont.). *N Engl J Med* 1970; **283:** 544.

Pharmacokinetics

Orphenadrine is readily absorbed from the gastro-intestinal tract and is almost completely metabolised to at least 8 metabolites. It is mainly excreted in the urine as metabolites and small amounts of unchanged drug.

Half-life. While the mean elimination half-life of orphenadrine in 5 healthy subjects given a single dose of the hydrochloride was found to be 15.5 hours, elimination half-lives of 30.5 and 40 hours were calculated in 2 patients who had received repeated oral administration.[1]

1. Labout JJM, *et al.* Difference between single and multiple dose pharmacokinetics of orphenadrine hydrochloride in man. *Eur J Clin Pharmacol* 1982; **21:** 343–50.

Uses and Administration

Orphenadrine, which is a congener of diphenhydramine (p.409) without sharing its soporific effect, is a tertiary amine antimuscarinic with actions and uses similar to those of benzhexol (p.458). It also has weak antihistaminic and local anaesthetic properties.

Orphenadrine is used as the hydrochloride in the symptomatic treatment of **parkinsonism**, including the alleviation of the extrapyramidal syndrome induced by drugs such as phenothiazines, but is of no value against tardive dyskinesias. The initial dose of orphenadrine hydrochloride is 150 mg daily in divided doses gradually increased by 50 mg every 2 or 3 days according to the response of the patient; the usual maintenance dose is in the range of 150 to 300 mg daily, but some patients may require a total of up to 400 mg daily. Orphenadrine hydrochloride has also been given intramuscularly.

Orphenadrine is also used as the citrate to relieve pain due to **skeletal muscle spasm**. It is sometimes given by mouth in a dose of 100 mg twice daily or by intramuscular or slow intravenous (over 5 minutes) injection in a dose of 60 mg which has been repeated every 12 hours. In the UK it was only used for the short-term treatment of such pain when it was given by injection which was generally only repeated once after 12 hours.

Since the elderly are more susceptible to the adverse effects of antimuscarinics a reduced dose is usually recommended.

Hiccup. Orphenadrine citrate has been used in some countries for the treatment of intractable hiccup. A protocol for the management of intractable hiccups may be found under Chlorpromazine, p.655.

Muscle spasm. References to the use of orphenadrine in the management of leg cramps and other painful conditions associated with skeletal muscle spasm.

1. Latta D, Turner E. An alternative to quinine in nocturnal leg cramps. *Curr Ther Res* 1989; **45:** 833–7.
2. Hunskaar S, Donnell D. Clinical and pharmacological review of the efficacy of orphenadrine and its combination with paracetamol in painful conditions. *J Int Med Res* 1991; **19:** 71–87.

Preparations

BP 1998: Orphenadrine Hydrochloride Tablets;
USP 23: Orphenadrine Citrate Injection.

Proprietary Preparations (details are given in Part 3)
Aust.: Norflex; ***Austral.:*** Disipal; Norflex; ***Belg.:*** Disipal; Norflex; ***Canad.:*** Disipal; Norflex; Orfenace; ***Fr.:*** Disipal†; ***Ger.:*** Norflex; ***Irl.:*** Disipal; ***Ital.:*** Disipal; ***Neth.:*** Disipal†; Disipaletten†; ***Norw.:*** Disipal; ***S.Afr.:*** Disipal; Norflex; ***Swed.:*** Disipal; Norflex; ***Switz.:*** Disipal†; Norflex; ***UK:*** Biorphen; Disipal; Norflex†; ***USA:*** Banflex; Flexoject; Flexon; Myolin; Myophen; Myotrol†; Norflex.

Multi-ingredient: ***Aust.:*** Dolpasse†; Neodolpasse; Norgesic; ***Austral.:*** Norgesic; ***Canad.:*** Norgesic; ***Ger.:*** Norgesic N; Silentan spezial†; ***Irl.:*** Norgesic; ***Norw.:*** Norgesic†; ***S.Afr.:*** Norflex Co; ***Swed.:*** Norgesic; ***Switz.:*** Norgesic; ***USA:*** Norgesic; Orphengesic.

Oxybutynin Hydrochloride (396-b)

Oxybutynin Hydrochloride *(BANM, rINNM).*

5058; MJ-4309-1; Oxybutynin Chloride *(USAN)*; Oxybutynini Hydrochloridum. 4-Diethylaminobut-2-ynyl α-cyclohexylmandelate hydrochloride.

$C_{22}H_{31}NO_3,HCl = 393.9.$

CAS — 5633-20-5 (oxybutynin); 1508-65-2 (oxybutynin hydrochloride).

Pharmacopoeias. In *Eur.* (see p.viii) and *US.*

A white or almost white, practically odourless, crystalline powder. Freely **soluble** in water and in alcohol; very soluble in methyl alcohol and in chloroform; soluble in acetone; slightly soluble in cyclohexane and in ether; very slightly soluble in hexane. **Protect** from light.

Adverse Effects, Treatment, and Precautions

As for Atropine Sulphate, p.455.

Animal studies have shown reproductive toxicity with high doses of oxybutynin, hence the recommendation that it should be avoided during pregnancy; caution should also be observed during breast feeding.

Effects on body temperature. A 76-year-old man taking oxybutynin hydrochloride 5 mg three times daily suffered heatstroke on a day when the ambient temperature was about 37°. He had had a similar febrile episode the previous summer while taking oxybutynin.[1]

1. Adubofour KO, *et al.* Oxybutynin-induced heatstroke in an elderly patient. *Ann Pharmacother* 1996; **30:** 144–7.

Effects on the gastro-intestinal tract. Reflux oesophagitis has been reported[1] in a 36-year-old woman with cerebral palsy and hiatus hernia who had taken oxybutynin for 5 years to prevent urinary incontinence. Symptoms of gastro-oesophageal reflux resolved when oxybutynin was discontinued.

1. Lee M, Sharifi R. Oxybutynin-induced reflux esophagitis. *DICP Ann Pharmacother* 1990; **24:** 583–5.

Effects on mental function. Oxybutynin was associated with the development of acute confusional states in 4 patients with Parkinson's disease and some cognitive impairment.[1]

1. Donnellan CA, *et al.* Oxybutynin and cognitive dysfunction. *Br Med J* 1997; **315:** 1363–4.

Night terrors. Night terrors have been reported in 5 patients taking oxybutynin.[1] Four of the patients were young children and the fifth was an elderly woman. Rechallenge was positive in 2 cases.

1. Valsecia ME, *et al.* New adverse effect of oxybutynin: "night terror". *Ann Pharmacother* 1998; **32:** 506.

Overdosage. A report[1] of a 34-year-old woman who ingested 100 mg of oxybutynin. The main symptoms were antimuscarinic effects and included drowsiness, hallucinations, dilatation of pupils, and urinary retention. Tachycardia resolved shortly after admission to hospital but ventricular ectopic beats and bigeminy persisted for over 24 hours. The patient recovered with symptomatic treatment.

1. Banerjee S, *et al.* Poisoning with oxybutynin. *Hum Exp Toxicol* 1991; **10:** 225–6.

Interactions

As for antimuscarinics in general (see Atropine Sulphate, p.456).

Itraconazole. Concomitant administration of itraconazole and oxybutynin resulted in moderate increases of serum concentrations of the latter.[1] However, concentrations of the active metabolite, *N*-desethyloxybutynin, were virtually unchanged and the interaction was considered to be of minor clinical significance.

1. Lukkari E, *et al.* Itraconazole moderately increases serum concentrations of oxybutynin but does not affect those of the active metabolite. *Eur J Clin Pharmacol* 1997; **52:** 403–6.

Pharmacokinetics

Following oral administration of oxybutynin, peak plasma concentrations are reached within one hour. It undergoes extensive first-pass metabolism and systemic bioavailability has been reported to be only 6%. A half-life of 2 to 3 hours has been reported. *N*-desethyloxybutynin is an active metabolite. Oxybutynin has been detected in breast milk. Evidence suggests that it may cross the blood-brain barrier.

References.

1. Douchamps J, *et al.* The pharmacokinetics of oxybutynin in man. *Eur J Clin Pharmacol* 1988; **35:** 515–20.
2. Pietzko A, *et al.* Influences of trospium chloride and oxybutynin on quantitative EEG in healthy volunteers. *Eur J Clin Pharmacol* 1994; **47:** 337–43.

Uses and Administration

Oxybutynin hydrochloride is a tertiary amine antimuscarinic with actions similar to those of atropine (p.455); it also has direct effects on smooth muscle. It is used for the management of urinary frequency, urgency, and incontinence in neurogenic bladder disorders and in idiopathic detrusor instability and for nocturnal enuresis, as an adjunct to nonpharmacological therapy.

Usual doses of oxybutynin hydrochloride are 5 mg two or three times daily by mouth, increased to 5 mg four times daily if required. In elderly patients lower doses of 2.5 or 3 mg twice daily initially, increased to 5 mg twice daily if necessary, may be adequate.

In children over 5 years of age, oxybutynin is used for neurogenic bladder disorders and nocturnal enuresis in an initial dose of 2.5 or 3 mg twice daily by mouth increased to 5 mg two or three times daily according to response. For nocturnal enuresis the last dose is usually given before bedtime. However, some authorities consider that drug therapy for nocturnal enuresis is not appropriate in children under 7 years of age.

Reviews.

1. Robinson TG, Castelden CM. Oxybutynin hydrochloride. *Prescribers' J* 1994; **34:** 27–30.

Nocturnal enuresis. Antimuscarinics such as oxybutynin reduce uninhibited bladder contractions but, although they may be of use in diurnal enuresis, they are rarely of benefit in nocturnal enuresis (p.453) alone. Oxybutynin did not appear to be effective in treating primary nocturnal enuresis in children with normal bladders.[1]

1. Lovering JS, *et al.* Oxybutynin efficacy in the treatment of primary enuresis. *Pediatrics* 1988; **82:** 104–6.

Urinary incontinence. The treatment of urinary incontinence, including urge incontinence, is reviewed on p.454. In addition to its antimuscarinic effect, oxybutynin has a direct antispasmodic effect which also contributes to reducing the number of uninhibited bladder contractions. It has been shown to be effective when given by mouth for urge incontinence[1-3] and some consider it to be the drug of choice.[4] However, frequent adverse effects may limit its use. Oxybutynin has also been studied in detrusor hyperreflexia[5] but, as most of these studies do not distinguish in their analyses between patients with neurogenic and non-neurogenic incontinence, its value remains to be determined. Direct instillation of oxybutynin into the bladder has also been tried in urge incontinence.[6,7]

1. Riva D, Casolati E. Oxybutynin chloride in the treatment of female idiopathic bladder instability: results from double blind treatment. *Clin Exp Obstet Gynecol* 1984; **11:** 37–42.
2. Moore KH, *et al.* Oxybutynin hydrochloride (3 mg) in the treatment of women with idiopathic detrusor instability. *Br J Urol* 1990; **66:** 479–85.
3. Tapp AJS, *et al.* The treatment of detrusor instability in post-menopausal women with oxybutynin chloride: a double blind placebo controlled study. *Br J Obstet Gynaecol* 1990; **97:** 521–6.
4. Yarker YE, *et al.* Oxybutynin: a review of its pharmacodynamic and pharmacokinetic properties, and its therapeutic use in detrusor instability. *Drugs Aging* 1995; **6:** 243–62.
5. Thüroff J, *et al.* Randomized, double-blind, multicenter trial on treatment of frequency, urgency and incontinence related to detrusor hyperactivity: oxybutynin versus propantheline versus placebo. *J Urol (Baltimore)* 1991; **145:** 813–17.
6. Weese DL, *et al.* Intravesical oxybutynin chloride: experience with 42 patients. *Urology* 1993; **41:** 527–30.
7. Szollar SM, Lee SM. Intravesical oxybutynin for spinal cord injury patients. *Spinal Cord* 1996; **34:** 284–7.

Preparations

USP 23: Oxybutynin Chloride Syrup; Oxybutynin Chloride Tablets.

Proprietary Preparations (details are given in Part 3)
Aust.: Ditropan; ***Austral.:*** Ditropan; ***Belg.:*** Ditropan; Driptane; ***Canad.:*** Ditropan; Oxybutyn; ***Fr.:*** Ditropan; Driptane; ***Ger.:*** Dridase; ***Irl.:*** Cystrin; Ditropan; ***Ital.:*** Ditropan; ***Neth.:*** Dridase; ***S.Afr.:*** Ditropan; ***Spain:*** Ditropan; ***Swed.:*** Ditropan; ***Switz.:*** Ditropan; ***UK:*** Cystrin; Ditropan; ***USA:*** Ditropan.

Oxyphencyclimine Hydrochloride (397-v)

Oxyphencyclimine Hydrochloride *(BANM, rINNM).*

1,4,5,6-Tetrahydro-1-methylpyrimidin-2-ylmethyl α-cyclohexylmandelate hydrochloride.

$C_{20}H_{28}N_2O_3,HCl = 380.9.$

CAS — 125-53-1 (oxyphencyclimine); 125-52-0 (oxyphencyclimine hydrochloride).

Oxyphencyclimine hydrochloride is a tertiary amine antimuscarinic with effects similar to those of atropine (p.455). It has been used as an adjunct in the treatment of peptic ulcer disease in usual doses of 5 to 10 mg by mouth two or three times daily. It has also been given for the relief of smooth muscle spasms in gastro-intestinal disorders.

Preparations

Proprietary Preparations (details are given in Part 3)
Belg.: Daricon†; ***Fr.:*** Manir†; ***Ital.:*** Vagogastrin†; ***Neth.:*** Daricon†; ***Swed.:*** Daricol†.

Multi-ingredient: ***Ital.:*** Gastrised†; ***S.Afr.:*** Enarax†; ***Swed.:*** Kombistrat†.

Oxyphenonium Bromide (398-g)

Oxyphenonium Bromide *(BAN, rINN).*

Oxphenonii Bromidum; Oxyphenonium Bromatum. 2-(α-Cyclohexylmandeloyloxy)ethyldiethylmethylammonium bromide.

$C_{21}H_{34}BrNO_3 = 428.4.$

CAS — 14214-84-7 (oxyphenonium); 50-10-2 (oxyphenonium bromide).

Pharmacopoeias. In *Pol.*

Oxyphenonium bromide is a quaternary ammonium antimuscarinic with peripheral effects similar to those of atropine (p.455). It has been used to relieve visceral spasms, in usual doses of 5 to 10 mg by mouth 4 times daily.

Preparations

Proprietary Preparations (details are given in Part 3)
Belg.: Antrenyl†; ***Neth.:*** Antrenyl†; ***S.Afr.:*** Spastrex; ***Switz.:*** Antrenyl†.

Penthienate Bromide (402-s)

Penthienate Bromide *(BANM).*

Penthienate Methobromide. 2-[2-Cyclopentyl-2-(2-thienyl)glycoloyloxy]ethyldiethylmethylammonium bromide.

$C_{18}H_{30}BrNO_3S = 420.4.$

CAS — 22064-27-3 (penthienate); 60-44-6 (penthienate bromide).

Penthienate bromide is a quaternary ammonium antimuscarinic with peripheral effects similar to those of atropine (p.455). It was used as an adjunct in the treatment of peptic ulcer disease and to relieve smooth muscle spasms in gastro-intestinal disorders. It has also been tried in urinary incontinence.

References.

1. Coombes GM, Millard RJ. Urinary urge incontinence: randomised crossover trials of penthienate versus placebo and propantheline. *Med J Aust* 1996; **165:** 473–6.

Preparations

Proprietary Preparations (details are given in Part 3)
Austral.: Monodral†.

Phenamazide Hydrochloride (19980-c)

Phenamacide Hydrochloride. (±)-α-Aminobenzeneacetic acid 3-methylbutyl ester hydrochloride.

$C_{13}H_{19}NO_2,HCl = 257.8.$

CAS — 84580-27-8 (phenamazide); 31031-74-0 (phenamazide hydrochloride).

Phenamazide is an antimuscarinic with actions similar to those of atropine (p.455). It has been used as the hydrochloride in the treatment of visceral spasms in doses of up to 75 mg daily in divided doses.

Preparations

Proprietary Preparations (details are given in Part 3)
Ger.: Aklonin.

Pipenzolate Bromide (404-e)

Pipenzolate Bromide *(BAN, rINN).*

Pipenzolate Methylbromide. 3-Benziloyloxy-1-ethyl-1-methylpiperidinium bromide.

$C_{22}H_{28}BrNO_3$ = 434.4.

CAS — 13473-38-6 (pipenzolate); 125-51-9 (pipenzolate bromide).

Pharmacopoeias. In *It.*

Pipenzolate bromide is a quaternary ammonium antimuscarinic with peripheral actions similar to those of atropine (p.455). It has been used as an adjunct in the treatment of gastro-intestinal disorders characterised by smooth muscle spasm.

Preparations

Proprietary Preparations (details are given in Part 3)
Austral.: Piptal†; ***Ital.:*** Piper†; Piptal†; ***UK:*** Piptal†.
Multi-ingredient: ***S.Afr.:*** Pediachol; ***UK:*** Piptalin†.

Piperidolate Hydrochloride (405-l)

Piperidolate Hydrochloride *(BANM, rINNM).*

1-Ethyl-3-piperidyl diphenylacetate hydrochloride.

$C_{21}H_{25}NO_2,HCl$ = 359.9.

CAS — 82-98-4 (piperidolate); 129-77-1 (piperidolate hydrochloride).

Piperidolate hydrochloride is a tertiary amine antimuscarinic with effects similar to those of atropine (p.455). It has been given in the symptomatic treatment of smooth muscle spasm associated with gastro-intestinal disorders.

Preparations

Proprietary Preparations (details are given in Part 3)
Multi-ingredient: ***Belg.:*** Dactil†.

Pipethanate Ethobromide (13123-t)

Pipethanate Ethobromide *(rINNM).*

Ethylpipethanate Bromide; Piperilate Ethobromide. 1-(2-Benziloyloxyethyl)-1-ethylpiperidinium bromide.

$C_{23}H_{30}BrNO_3$ = 448.4.

CAS — 4546-39-8 (pipethanate); 23182-46-9 (pipethanate ethobromide).

Pipethanate ethobromide is an antimuscarinic with actions similar to those of atropine (p.455). It has been used in the symptomatic treatment of visceral spasm in usual doses by mouth of 30 to 80 mg daily in divided doses. Pipethanate ethobromide has also been given subcutaneously, intramuscularly, or intravenously in a dose of 10 mg.

Preparations

Proprietary Preparations (details are given in Part 3)
Ital.: Spalgin; Spasmodil; ***Jpn:*** Panpurol.

Pirenzepine Hydrochloride (13129-h)

Pirenzepine Hydrochloride *(BANM, USAN, rINNM).*

LS-519 (pirenzepine); LS-519-Cl2. 5,11-Dihydro-11-(4-methylpiperazin-1-ylacetyl)pyrido[2,3-*b*][1,4]benzodiazepin-6-one dihydrochloride monohydrate.

$C_{19}H_{21}N_5O_2,2HCl,H_2O$ = 442.3.

CAS — 28797-61-7 (pirenzepine); 29868-97-1 (pirenzepine hydrochloride).

Pharmacopoeias. In *Ger.* and *It.*

Adverse Effects

Pirenzepine is an antimuscarinic and dry mouth and blurred vision have been reported. Other side-effects associated with antimuscarinics (see Atropine Sulphate, p.455) are stated to be less likely to occur because of its selective action on the gastric mucosa and poor penetration across the blood-brain barrier.

Thrombocytopenia in one patient and agranulocytosis in another was probably associated with the administration of pirenzepine.[1]

1. Stricker BHC, *et al.* Blood disorders associated with pirenzepine. *Br Med J* 1986; **293:** 1074.

Precautions

Pirenzepine is contra-indicated in patients with prostatic enlargement, and in those with paralytic ileus or pyloric stenosis. It should not be given to patients with or at risk of angle-closure glaucoma. Pirenzepine should be used with caution in patients with renal impairment, particularly those with end-stage renal failure.

Interactions

As for antimuscarinics in general (see Atropine Sulphate, p.456).

Pharmacokinetics

Pirenzepine is absorbed from the gastro-intestinal tract but the bioavailability is reported to be only about 20 to 30% being decreased to about 10 to 20% when taken with food. Very little pirenzepine is metabolised. About 10% of an oral dose is excreted unchanged in the urine, the remainder being excreted in the faeces.

Pirenzepine has an elimination half-life of about 12 hours and is only slightly (about 12%) bound to plasma proteins. Diffusion across the blood-brain barrier is poor and only minimal amounts are stated to be present in the milk of lactating women.

References.

1. Tanswell P, *et al.* Absolute bioavailability of pirenzepine in intensive care patients. *Eur J Clin Pharmacol* 1990; **38:** 265–8.

Renal impairment. The renal clearance and total plasma clearance of pirenzepine may be significantly reduced in patients with renal insufficiency,[1,2] with clearance decreasing proportionately with renal impairment. The half-life of pirenzepine is increased with reported values ranging from 14 to 20 hours.[1-3] Plasma concentrations of pirenzepine may be reduced by up to about 50% during haemodialysis.[1,3]

1. Krakamp B, *et al.* Steady-state intravenous pharmacokinetics of pirenzepine in patients with differing degrees of renal dysfunction. *Eur J Clin Pharmacol* 1989; **36:** 75–8.
2. Krakamp B, *et al.* Steady-state intravenous pharmacokinetics of pirenzepine in patients with hepatic insufficiency and combined renal- and hepatic insufficiency. *Eur J Clin Pharmacol* 1989; **36:** 71–3.
3. MacGregor T, *et al.* Oral pharmacokinetics of pirenzepine in patients with chronic renal insufficiency, failure, and maintenance haemodialysis. *Eur J Clin Pharmacol* 1990; **38:** 405–6.

Uses and Administration

Pirenzepine is a selective M_1 tertiary amine antimuscarinic which displays a preferential action on the gastric mucosa thus causing a reduction in the secretion of gastric acid; it also reduces the secretion of pepsin. At therapeutic doses it has few other antimuscarinic actions.

Pirenzepine hydrochloride has been used in the management of benign peptic ulcer disease (p.453) in a usual dose of 50 mg two or three times daily by mouth for 4 to 6 weeks.

Reviews.

1. Carmine AA, Brogden RN. Pirenzepine: a review of its pharmacodynamic and pharmacokinetic properties and therapeutic efficacy in peptic ulcer disease and other allied diseases. *Drugs* 1985; **30:** 85–126.

Preparations

Proprietary Preparations (details are given in Part 3)
Aust.: Gastrozepin; ***Canad.:*** Gastrozepin†; ***Ger.:*** durapirenz; Gastri-P; Gastricur; Gastrozepin; Pirehexal; Ulcoprotect; Ulcosafe; Ulcufort on†; Ulgescum; ***Irl.:*** Gastrozepin†; ***Ital.:*** Duogastral; Frazim; Gasteril†; Gastrol; Gastropiren; Gastrosed; Gastrozepin; Leblon†; Maghen†; Renzepin†; Ulcin; Ulcopir; Ulcosyntex†; Ulpir†; ***Neth.:*** Abrinac†; ***S.Afr.:*** Gastrozepin†; ***Spain:*** Gastrozepin†; ***Switz.:*** Gastrozepine; piren-basan; ***UK:*** Gastrozepin†.

Poldine Methylsulphate (407-j)

Poldine Methylsulphate *(BAN).*

Poldine Metilsulfate *(pINN)*; IS-499; McN-R-726-47; Poldine Methosulphate; Poldine Methylsulfate *(USAN).* 2-Benziloyloxymethyl-1,1-dimethylpyrrolidinium methylsulphate.

$C_{21}H_{26}NO_3,CH_3O_4S$ = 451.5.

CAS — 596-50-9 (poldine); 545-80-2 (poldine methylsulphate).

Pharmacopoeias. In *Br.*

A white odourless or almost odourless crystalline powder. Freely **soluble** in water; soluble in alcohol; slightly soluble in chloroform. A 1% solution in water has a pH of 5.0 to 7.0.

Poldine methylsulphate is a quaternary ammonium antimuscarinic with peripheral actions similar to those of atropine (p.455) and has been used in the management of gastro-intestinal disorders, including peptic ulcer disease.

Preparations

BP 1998: Poldine Tablets.
Proprietary Preparations (details are given in Part 3)
UK: Nacton†.

Prifinium Bromide (409-c)

Prifinium Bromide *(rINN).*

PDB; Pyrodifenium Bromide. 3-Diphenylmethylene-1,1-diethyl-2-methylpyrrolidinium bromide.

$C_{22}H_{28}BrN$ = 386.4.

CAS — 10236-81-4 (prifinium); 4630-95-9 (prifinium bromide).

Prifinium bromide is a quaternary ammonium antimuscarinic with peripheral effects similar to those of atropine (p.455). It is structurally related to diphemanil methylsulphate (p.460).

Prifinium bromide is used to relieve visceral spasms. Oral doses usually range from 45 to 120 mg daily in divided doses; higher doses have sometimes been employed. It has also been administered rectally in a dose of 60 mg three or four times daily, or by subcutaneous, intramuscular, or intravenous injection in a dose of 7.5 to 15 mg.

Preparations

Proprietary Preparations (details are given in Part 3)
Fr.: Riabal; ***Ital.:*** Riabal; ***Jpn:*** Padrin.

Procyclidine Hydrochloride (410-s)

Procyclidine Hydrochloride *(BANM, rINNM).*

Procyclidini Hydrochloridum. 1-Cyclohexyl-1-phenyl-3-(pyrrolidin-1-yl)propan-1-ol hydrochloride.

$C_{19}H_{29}NO,HCl$ = 323.9.

CAS — 77-37-2 (procyclidine); 1508-76-5 (procyclidine hydrochloride).

Pharmacopoeias. In *Br.* and *US.*

A white crystalline powder, odourless or with a characteristic odour. **Soluble** 1 in 35 of water, 1 in 9 of alcohol, 1 in 6 of chloroform, and 1 in 11 000 of ether; practically insoluble in acetone. The BP states that a 1% solution in water has a pH of 4.5 to 6.5, the USP that it has a pH between 5.0 and 6.5. **Store** in a dry place in airtight containers. Protect from light.

Adverse Effects, Treatment, and Precautions

As for Atropine Sulphate, p.455.

Abuse. A report[1] of 2 cases of abuse of procyclidine by adolescents.

1. McGucken RB, *et al.* Teenage procyclidine abuse. *Lancet* 1985; **i:** 1514.

Interactions

As for antimuscarinics in general (see Atropine Sulphate, p.456).

Pharmacokinetics

Procyclidine hydrochloride is absorbed from the gastro-intestinal tract and disappears rapidly from the tissues. Procyclidine given intravenously acts within 5 to 20 minutes and has a duration of effect of up to 4 hours.

References.

1. Whiteman PD, *et al.* Pharmacokinetics and pharmacodynamics of procyclidine in man. *Eur J Clin Pharmacol* 1985; **28:** 73–8.

Uses and Administration

Procyclidine hydrochloride is a tertiary amine antimuscarinic with actions and uses similar to those of benzhexol (p.458). It is used for the symptomatic treatment of parkinsonism (p.454), including the alleviation of the extrapyramidal syndrome induced by drugs such as phenothiazines but, is of no value against tardive dyskinesias.

The initial dose of 2.5 mg three times daily by mouth may be increased gradually by 2.5 to 5 mg every 2 or 3 days until the optimum maintenance dose, usually 20 to 30 mg daily in 3 (or occasionally 4) divided doses, is reached; daily doses of up to 60 mg have occasionally been required. In emergency, 5 to 10 mg may be given by intravenous injection; higher doses have sometimes been used. The intramuscular route has also been employed when 5 to 10 mg has been given as one injection, repeated if necessary after 20 minutes to a maximum of 20 mg daily.

Preparations

BP 1998: Procyclidine Injection; Procyclidine Tablets;
USP 23: Procyclidine Hydrochloride Tablets.

Proprietary Preparations (details are given in Part 3)
Aust.: Kemadrin; ***Austral.:*** Kemadrin; ***Belg.:*** Kemadrin; ***Canad.:*** Kemadrin; Procyclid; ***Ger.:*** Osnervan; ***Irl.:*** Kemadrin; ***Ital.:*** Kemadrin; ***Neth.:*** Kemadrin; ***Norw.:*** Kemadrin†; ***Spain:*** Kemadren; ***Swed.:*** Kemadrin; ***Switz.:*** Kemadrin; ***UK:*** Arpicolin; Kemadrin; ***USA:*** Kemadrin.

Propantheline Bromide (411-w)

Propantheline Bromide *(BAN, rINN).*

Bromuro de Propantelina; Propanthelini Bromidum. Di-isopropylmethyl[2-(xanthen-9-ylcarbonyloxy)ethyl]ammonium bromide.

$C_{23}H_{30}BrNO_3$ = 448.4.

CAS — 298-50-0 (propantheline); 50-34-0 (propantheline bromide).

Pharmacopoeias. In *Chin., Eur.* (see p.viii), *Jpn,* and *US.*

A white or yellowish-white odourless slightly hygroscopic powder or crystals. Very **soluble** in water, in alcohol, in chloroform, and in dichloromethane; practically insoluble in ether. **Store** in airtight containers.

Adverse Effects, Treatment, and Precautions

As for Atropine Sulphate, p.455.

Toxic doses of propantheline bromide may produce non-depolarising neuromuscular blocking effects with paralysis of voluntary muscle. Contact dermatitis has been reported following topical application.

Buccal and oesophageal ulceration. Severe buccal mucosal ulceration has been reported[1] in a 95-year-old woman as a result of retaining emepronium bromide tablets in her mouth, and recurred on administration of propantheline bromide tablets.

1. Huston GJ, *et al.* Anticholinergic drugs, buccal ulceration and mucosal potential difference. *Postgrad Med J* 1978; **54:** 331–2.

Interactions

As for antimuscarinics in general (see Atropine Sulphate, p.456).

Pharmacokinetics

Propantheline bromide is incompletely absorbed from the gastro-intestinal tract and bioavailability is reported to be reduced by food; it is extensively metabolised in the small intestine before absorption. Propantheline is eliminated mainly in the urine as metabolites and less than 10% as unchanged drug. The duration of action is about 6 hours.

Uses and Administration

Propantheline bromide is a quaternary ammonium antimuscarinic with peripheral effects similar to those of atropine (p.455). It has been used in the management of spasm of the gastro-intestinal tract and as an adjunct in the treatment of peptic ulcer disease (p.453). The usual initial dose is 15 mg by mouth three times daily before meals and 30 mg at bedtime; doses of up to 120 mg per day may be needed in some patients. In mild cases or elderly patients, doses of 7.5 mg three times daily may be sufficient.

Propantheline bromide has been used in the treatment of adult enuresis or urinary incontinence (p.454) in doses of 15 to 30 mg two or three times daily.

Hyperhidrosis. Some antimuscarinics, including propantheline, have been applied topically in the treatment of hyperhidrosis (p.453). Side-effects of antimuscarinics administered by mouth generally preclude their use by this route, although there is a report of oral propantheline being used successfully to control excessive sweating in 2 patients with spinal cord injuries.[1]

1. Canaday BR, Stanford RH. Propantheline bromide in the management of hyperhidrosis associated with spinal cord injury. *Ann Pharmacother* 1995; **29:** 489–92.

Preparations

BP 1998: Propantheline Tablets;
USP 23: Propantheline Bromide Tablets; Sterile Propantheline Bromide.

Proprietary Preparations (details are given in Part 3)
Austral.: Panthelinet†; Pro-Banthine; ***Belg.:*** Pro-Banthine; ***Canad.:*** Pro-Banthine; Propanthel; ***Fr.:*** Pro-Banthine; ***Ger.:*** Corrigast†; ***Irl.:*** Pro-Banthine; ***Neth.:*** Pro-Banthine; ***S.Afr.:*** Pro-Banthine†; ***Swed.:*** Ercotina; Pro-Banthine; ***Switz.:*** Ercorax Roll-on; Pro-Banthine; ***UK:*** Pro-Banthine; ***USA:*** Pro-Banthine; Probamide†.

Multi-ingredient: ***Ger.:*** Hydonan†; ***Ital.:*** Lexil.

Propiverine Hydrochloride (17897-v)

Propiverine Hydrochloride *(BANM, rINNM).*

BUP-4 (propiverine). 1-Methyl-4-piperidyl diphenylpropoxyacetate hydrochloride.

$C_{23}H_{29}NO_3,HCl$ = 403.9.

CAS — 60569-19-9 (propiverine); 54556-98-8 (propiverine hydrochloride).

Adverse Effects, Treatment, and Precautions

As for Atropine Sulphate, p.455. Hypotension and drowsiness may also occur with propiverine. Propiverine is contra-indicated in patients with hepatic or severe renal impairment. Liver enzyme values should be monitored in patients receiving long-term therapy. Skeletal retardation has occurred in the offspring of *animals* given high doses of propiverine during pregnancy and therefore its use is not recommended during pregnancy.

Interactions

As for antimuscarinics in general (see Atropine Sulphate, p.456). Hypotension may occur in patients treated with propiverine and isoniazid. Drowsiness may be enhanced by drugs with CNS-depressant properties.

Pharmacokinetics

Propiverine is absorbed from the gastro-intestinal tract and peak plasma concentrations are achieved about 2.3 hours after oral administration. It undergoes extensive first-pass metabolism and the average absolute bioavailability is reported to be about 41%. Plasma concentrations of the principal metabolite, the *N*-oxide, greatly exceed those of the parent compound. Protein binding is about 90% for propiverine and 60% for the *N*-oxide metabolite. Propiverine and its metabolites are excreted in the urine, bile, and faeces. The elimination half-life is about 20 hours.

Uses and Administration

Propiverine hydrochloride is a tertiary antimuscarinic with actions similar to those of atropine (p.455). It is used for the management of urinary frequency, urgency, and incontinence (p.454) in neurogenic bladder disorders and in idiopathic detrusor instability. Usual doses of propiverine hydrochloride are 15 mg two or three times daily by mouth, increased to 4 times daily if required. In elderly frail patients doses of 15 mg twice daily, increased to 3 times daily if necessary, may be advisable. A daily dose of 1 mg per kg body-weight should not be exceeded.

References.

1. Haustein KO, Huller G. On the pharmacokinetics and metabolism of propiverine in man. *Eur J Drug Metab Pharmacokinet* 1988; **13:** 81–90.

Preparations

Proprietary Preparations (details are given in Part 3)
Ger.: Mictonetten; Mictonorm; ***Jpn:*** BUP-4†; ***UK:*** Detrunorm.

Stramonium (413-l)

Datura; Estramonio; Inferno; Jamestown Weed; Jimson Weed; Stechapfel; Stramoine; Thornapple.

NOTE. The terms Datura, Datura Herb, and Datura Leaf have been applied to preparations of various species of the genus Datura including *Datura metel.*

Pharmacopoeias. Eur. (see p.viii) includes a monograph for Stramonium Leaf and Prepared Stramonium.

Stramonium [*Datura stramonium* (Solanaceae)] contains alkaloids that consist mainly of hyoscyamine (the laevo-isomer of atropine) together with hyoscine. The total alkaloidal content of stramonium preparations is usually calculated as hyoscyamine.

Stramonium Leaf (Stramonii Folium; Feuille de Datura) is the dried leaves or dried leaves, flowering tops and, occasionally, fruits of the plant. The Ph. Eur. specifies that it contains not less than 0.25% of total alkaloids.

Prepared Stramonium (Stramonii Pulvis Normatus; Prep. Stramon.; Poudre Titrée de Datura) is stramonium leaf reduced to a powder and adjusted to contain 0.23 to 0.27% of total alkaloids.

Store in airtight containers. Protect from light.

Adverse Effects, Treatment, and Precautions

As for Atropine Sulphate, p.455.

Abuse. Some reports[1-3] of poisoning following abuse of *Datura stramonium* or its preparations.

1. Gowdy JM. Stramonium intoxication: review of symptomatology in 212 cases. *JAMA* 1972; **221:** 585–7.
2. Shervette RE, *et al.* Jimson "Loco" weed abuse in adolescents. *Pediatrics* 1979; **63:** 520–3.
3. Anonymous. Jimson weed poisoning—Texas, New York, and California, 1994. *MMWR* 1995; **44:** 41–4.

Effects on the eyes. A report[1] of anisocoria (unequal dilatation of the pupils) in a patient following accidental entry of a piece of jimson weed *(Datura stramonium)* into the eye while gardening.

1. Savitt DL, *et al.* Anisocoria from Jimsonweed. *JAMA* 1986; **255:** 1439–40.

Uses and Administration

Stramonium has the actions of atropine (p.455). It has been given in respiratory-tract disorders with other drugs in oral and rectal dosage forms. It has also been smoked in cigarettes or burnt in powders and the fumes inhaled but the irritation produced by the fumes may aggravate bronchitis.

Stramonium has been used in homoeopathic medicine.

Preparations

Proprietary Preparations (details are given in Part 3)

Multi-ingredient: ***Austral.:*** Potassium Iodide and Stramonium Compound; ***Belg.:*** Cigarettes Anti-asthmatiques†; Escouflaire; ***Fr.:*** Dinacode avec codeine; ***Ger.:*** Asthmacolat†; ***Spain:*** Balsamo Analgesic Karmel; ***Switz.:*** Sedovalin†.

Telenzepine (3637-g)

Telenzepine *(rINN).*

4,9-Dihydro-3-methyl-[(4-methyl-1-piperazinyl)acetyl]-10*H*-thieno[3,4-*b*][1,5]-benzodiazepin-10-one.

$C_{19}H_{22}N_4O_2S$ = 370.5.

CAS — 80880-90-6.

Telenzepine is reported to be a selective M_1 antimuscarinic and has been investigated for its ability to reduce gastric acid secretion in the management of peptic ulcer disease.

References.

1. Londong W, *et al.* Telenzepine is at least 25 times more potent than pirenzepine—a dose response and comparative secretory study in man. *Gut* 1987; **28:** 888–95.
2. Simon B, *et al.* 3 mg Telenzepin nocte in der therapie der benignen ulcus-ventriculi-erkrankung: eine doppelblinde vergleichsstudie mit 300 mg ranitidin nocte. *Z Gastroenterol* 1990; **28** 90–3.

Terodiline Hydrochloride (13310-f)

Terodiline Hydrochloride *(BANM, USAN, rINNM).*

N-tert-Butyl-1-methyl-3,3-diphenylpropylamine hydrochloride.

$C_{20}H_{27}N,HCl$ = 317.9.

CAS — 15793-40-5 (terodiline); 7082-21-5 (terodiline hydrochloride).

Terodiline hydrochloride is an antimuscarinic with actions similar to those of atropine (p.455); it is also reported to possess calcium-channel blocking activity. It was formerly used for the relief of urinary incontinence. However, in 1991 the manufacturer withdrew terodiline from all countries because of its association with cardiac arrhythmias.

References.

1. Committee on Safety of Medicines. Withdrawal of terodiline (Micturin, Kabi Pharmacia Ltd). *Current Problems 32* 1991.
2. Stewart DA, *et al.* Terodiline causes polymorphic ventricular tachycardia due to reduced heart rate and prolongation of QT interval. *Eur J Clin Pharmacol* 1992; **42:** 577–80.

Preparations

Proprietary Preparations (details are given in Part 3)
Irl.: Micturin†; ***Swed.:*** Mictrol†; ***Switz.:*** Mictrol†.

Tiemonium Iodide (418-k)

Tiemonium Iodide *(BAN, rINN).*

TE-114. 4-[3-Hydroxy-3-phenyl-3-(2-thienyl)propyl]-4-methylmorpholinium iodide.

$C_{18}H_{24}INO_2S$ = 445.4.

CAS — 6252-92-2 (tiemonium); 144-12-7 (tiemonium iodide).

Tiemonium Methylsulphate (16217-m)

4-[3-Hydroxy-3-phenyl-3-(2-thienyl)propyl]-4-methylmorpholinium methylsulphate.

$C_{19}H_{27}NO_6S_2$ = 429.6.

CAS — 6504-57-0.

Tiemonium iodide and tiemonium methylsulphate are quaternary ammonium antimuscarinics with peripheral effects similar to those of atropine (p.455) and are used in the relief of visceral spasms.

Tiemonium iodide is used in a usual dose of 100 mg twice daily by mouth. A dose of 5 mg has been given by intramuscular or slow intravenous injection.

Tiemonium methylsulphate is given in a dose of 100 to 300 mg daily in divided doses by mouth. A dose of 5 mg has been given three times daily by intramuscular or slow intravenous injection. Tiemonium methylsulphate has also been given as a rectal suppository in daily doses of 20 to 40 mg.

Preparations

Proprietary Preparations (details are given in Part 3)
Belg.: Visceralgine; ***Fr.:*** Visceralgine; ***Ital.:*** Ottimal†; Visceralgina†.

Multi-ingredient: ***Belg.:*** Visceralgine Compositum; ***Fr.:*** Colchimax; Visceralgine Forte; ***Ger.:*** Coffalon.

Timepidium Bromide (13346-e)

Timepidium Bromide *(rINN)*.

SA-504. 3-[Di-(2-thienyl)methylene]-5-methoxy-1,1-dimethylpiperidinium bromide monohydrate.

$C_{17}H_{22}BrNOS_2H_2O$ = 418.4.

CAS — 35035-05-3.

Pharmacopoeias. In *Jpn.*

Timepidium bromide is a quaternary ammonium antimuscarinic with peripheral actions similar to those of atropine (p.455). It has been used for the symptomatic treatment of visceral spasms in usual doses of 30 mg three times daily by mouth. It has also been given intravenously, intramuscularly, or subcutaneously, in a dose of 7.5 mg.

Urinary metabolites of timepidium may cause a reddish coloration of the urine.

Preparations

Proprietary Preparations (details are given in Part 3)
Ital.: Mepidium†; ***Jpn:*** Sesden.

Tolterodine Tartrate (15401-a)

Tolterodine Tartrate *(BANM, rINNM)*.

Tolterodine L-Tartrate. (+)-(*R*)-2-{α-[2-(Diisopropylamino)ethyl]benzyl}-*p*-cresol tartrate.

$C_{22}H_{31}NO,C_4H_6O_6$ = 475.6.

CAS — 124937-51-5 (tolterodine).

Adverse Effects, Treatment, and Precautions

As for Atropine Sulphate, p.455. Tolterodine should be used with caution in patients with hepatic or renal impairment. *Animal* studies have shown that high doses may cause fetal toxicity, hence the recommendation that tolterodine should be avoided during pregnancy.

Interactions

As for antimuscarinics in general (see Atropine Sulphate, p.456).

There is a theoretical risk of interactions between tolterodine and other drugs metabolised by or inhibiting cytochrome P450 isoenzymes CYP2D6 or CYP3A4; the US manufacturers advise that the dose of tolterodine should not exceed 1 mg twice daily in patients receiving potent CYP3A4 inhibitors such as the macrolide antibiotics erythromycin or clarithromycin, and the antifungals ketoconazole, itraconazole, or miconazole.

Pharmacokinetics

Peak plasma concentrations of tolterodine occur 1 to 3 hours after a dose by mouth. Tolterodine is mainly metabolised by the cytochrome P450 isoenzyme CYP2D6 to the active 5-hydromethyl derivative; in a minority of poor metabolisers tolterodine is metabolised by CYP3A4 isoenzymes to its inactive N-dealkylated derivative. Tolterodine is excreted primarily in the urine with about 17% appearing in the faeces; less than 1% of a dose is excreted as unchanged drug.

References.

1. Brynne N, *et al.* Pharmacokinetics and pharmacodynamics of tolterodine in man: a new drug for the treatment of urinary bladder overactivity. *Int J Clin Pharmacol Ther* 1997; **35:** 287–95.
2. Brynne N, *et al.* Influence of CYP2D6 polymorphism on the pharmacokinetics and pharmacodynamics of tolterodine. *Clin Pharmacol Ther* 1998; **63:** 529–39.

Uses and Administration

Tolterodine tartrate is a tertiary antimuscarinic with actions similar to those of atropine (p.455); it is claimed to have a greater selectivity for the muscarinic receptors of the bladder. Tolterodine is used in the management of urinary frequency, urgency, and incontinence in detrusor instability (p.454). Usual doses of tolterodine tartrate are 2 mg twice daily by mouth although doses of 1 mg twice daily are recommended in patients with hepatic impairment or in those experiencing troublesome adverse effects or those receiving drugs that inhibit the cytochrome P450 isoenzyme CYP3A4 (see Interactions, above).

References.

1. Hills CJ, *et al.* Tolterodine. *Drugs* 1998; **55:** 813–20.
2. Anonymous. Tolterodine for overactive bladder. *Med Lett Drugs Ther* 1998; **40:** 101–102.

Preparations

Proprietary Preparations (details are given in Part 3)
Swed.: Detrusitol; ***UK:*** Detrusitol; ***USA:*** Detrol.

Tridihexethyl Chloride (421-l)

Tridihexethyl Chloride *(BAN)*.

(3-Cyclohexyl-3-hydroxy-3-phenylpropyl)triethylammonium chloride.

$C_{21}H_{36}ClNO$ = 354.0.

CAS — 60-49-1 (tridihexethyl); 4310-35-4 (tridihexethyl chloride); 125-99-5 (tridihexethyl iodide).

NOTE. Tridihexethyl Iodide is *rINN*.

Tridihexethyl chloride is a quaternary ammonium antimuscarinic with peripheral effects similar to those of atropine (p.455). It has been used as an adjunct in the treatment of peptic ulcer disease.

Preparations

Proprietary Preparations (details are given in Part 3)
USA: Pathilon.

Tropatepine Hydrochloride (13385-a)

Tropatepine Hydrochloride *(rINNM)*.

SD-1248-17. 3-(Dibenzo[*b,e*]thiepin-11(6*H*)-ylidene)tropane hydrochloride.

$C_{22}H_{23}NS,HCl$ = 370.0.

CAS — 27574-24-9 (tropatepine); 27574-25-0 (tropatepine hydrochloride).

Tropatepine hydrochloride is an antimuscarinic with actions and uses similar to those of benzhexol (p.457). It is used in the management of parkinsonism, including the alleviation of extrapyramidal symptoms induced by drugs such as phenothiazines, but it is of no value in tardive dyskinesias. Tropatepine hydrochloride is given in usual doses of 10 to 30 mg daily by mouth; it is also given intramuscularly or by slow intravenous injection in doses of 10 to 20 mg daily.

Preparations

Proprietary Preparations (details are given in Part 3)
Fr.: Lepticur.

Tropicamide (424-z)

Tropicamide *(BAN, USAN, rINN)*.

Bistropamide; Ro-1-7683; Tropicamidum. *N*-Ethyl-*N*-(4-pyridylmethyl)tropamide.

$C_{17}H_{20}N_2O_2$ = 284.4.

CAS — 1508-75-4.

NOTE. TRO is a code approved by the BP for use on single unit doses of eye drops containing tropicamide where the individual container may be too small to bear all the appropriate labelling information.

Pharmacopoeias. In *Eur.* (see p.viii), *Jpn*, and *US*.

A white or almost white, odourless or almost odourless, crystalline powder. Slightly **soluble** in water; freely soluble in alcohol, in chloroform, in dichloromethane, and in solutions of strong acids. **Store** in airtight containers. Protect from light.

Adverse Effects, Treatment, and Precautions

As for Atropine Sulphate, p.455.

References.

1. Vuori M-L, *et al.* Systemic absorption and anticholinergic activity of topically applied tropicamide. *J Ocul Pharmacol* 1994; **10:** 431–7.

Interactions

As for antimuscarinics in general (see Atropine Sulphate, p.456).

Uses and Administration

Tropicamide is a tertiary amine antimuscarinic with actions similar to those of atropine (p.455). It is used as eye drops to produce mydriasis and cycloplegia (p.454). It has a more rapid onset and a shorter duration of effect than atropine: mydriasis is produced within 20 to 40 minutes of instillation and usually lasts for about 6 hours; cycloplegia is maximal within about 30 minutes and is short-lasting, with complete recovery of accommodation normally within 6 hours. Tropicamide has been reported to be inadequate for cycloplegia in children.

To produce **mydriasis**, 1 or 2 drops of a 0.5% solution are instilled 15 to 20 minutes before examination of the eye. To produce **cycloplegia** 1 or 2 drops of a 1% solution are required, repeated after 5 minutes; a further drop may be necessary to prolong the effect after 20 to 30 minutes.

Alzheimer's disease. Tropicamide has been studied for use in the differential diagnosis of Alzheimer's disease (p.1386). Excessive pupil dilatation in response to tropicamide eye drops occurred in patients with signs and symptoms of Alzheimer's disease.[1] However, a double-blind placebo-controlled study[2] in similar patients and healthy subjects indicated that this was not a reliable diagnostic test for Alzheimer's disease.

1. Gómez-Tortosa E, *et al.* Pupil response to tropicamide in Alzheimer's disease and other neurodegenerative disorders. *Acta Neurol Scand* 1996; **94:** 104–9.
2. Graff-Radford NR, *et al.* Tropicamide eyedrops cannot be used for reliable diagnosis of Alzheimer's disease. *Mayo Clin Proc* 1997; **72:** 495–504.

Preparations

BP 1998: Tropicamide Eye Drops;
USP 23: Tropicamide Ophthalmic Solution.

Proprietary Preparations (details are given in Part 3)
Aust.: Mydriaticum; ***Austral.:*** Mydriacyl; ***Belg.:*** Mydriacyl†; Mydriaticum; Tropicol; ***Canad.:*** Diotrope; Mydriacyl; RO-Tropamide†; ***Fr.:*** Mydriaticum; ***Ger.:*** Mydriaticum; Mydrum; ***Irl.:*** Mydriacil; ***Ital.:*** Tropimil; Visumidriatic; ***Norw.:*** Mydrian; ***S.Afr.:*** Mydriacyl; Mydriaticum; ***Swed.:*** Mydriacyl; ***Switz.:*** Mydriaticum; ***UK:*** Mydriacyl; ***USA:*** Mydral; Mydriacyl; Opticyl; Tropi-Storz; Tropicacyl.

Multi-ingredient: ***Canad.:*** Diophenyl-T; ***Ital.:*** Visumidriatic Antiflogistico; Visumidriatic Fenilefrina; ***USA:*** Paremyd.

Tropine Benzilate Hydrochloride (17601-t)

Benztropeine Hydrochloride. 1α*H*,5α*H*-Tropan-3α-ol benzilate hydrochloride.

$C_{22}H_{25}NO_3,HCl$ = 387.9.

CAS — 3736-36-5 (tropine benzilate); 1674-94-8 (tropine benzilate hydrochloride).

Tropine benzilate hydrochloride is an antimuscarinic that has been used as an antispasmodic in the treatment of gastro-intestinal spasms.

Preparations

Proprietary Preparations (details are given in Part 3)
Ger.: BTE†.

Multi-ingredient: ***Aust.:*** Nealgon†.

Valethamate Bromide (425-c)

Diethylmethyl[2-(3-methyl-2-phenylvaleryloxy)ethyl]ammonium bromide.

$C_{19}H_{32}BrNO_2$ = 386.4.

CAS — 16376-74-2 (valethamate); 90-22-2 (valethamate bromide).

Valethamate bromide is a quaternary ammonium antimuscarinic with peripheral effects similar to those of atropine (p.455). It is used in the symptomatic treatment of visceral spasms. Doses of 10 to 20 mg have been given three times daily by mouth; valethamate bromide has also been given by injection and as a rectal suppository.

Preparations

Proprietary Preparations (details are given in Part 3)
Ger.: Epidosin.

Multi-ingredient: ***Spain:*** Trizima†.

Xenytropium Bromide (11617-h)

Xenytropium Bromide *(rINN)*.

N-399. 8-(*p*-Phenylbenzyl)atropinium bromide.

$C_{30}H_{34}BrNO_3$ = 536.5.

CAS — 511-55-7.

Xenytropium bromide is reported to have antimuscarinic properties; it has been given by mouth in preparations for the management of gastro-intestinal disorders.

Preparations

Proprietary Preparations (details are given in Part 3)

Multi-ingredient: ***Aust.:*** Spasmo Gallosanol; ***Ger.:*** para sanol†; Spasmo Gallo Sanol N.

Zamifenacin (15972-q)

Zamifenacin *(BAN, rINN)*.

UK-76654-2 (zamifenacin fumarate). (*R*)-3-(Diphenylmethoxy)-1-[3,4-(methylenedioxy)phenetyl]piperidene.

$C_{27}H_{29}NO_3$ = 415.5.

CAS — 127308-82-1 (zamifenacin); 127308-98-9 (zamifenacin fumarate).

Zamifenacin is an antimuscarinic with a selective action at M_3 receptors. It is under investigation for the treatment of irritable bowel syndrome and motion sickness.

References.

1. Golding JF, Stott JRR. Comparison of the effects of a selective muscarinic receptor antagonist and hyoscine (scopolamine) on motion sickness, skin conductance and heart rate. *Br J Clin Pharmacol* 1997; **43:** 633–7.

Antineoplastics and Immunosuppressants

Antineoplastic drugs (also known as cytotoxic drugs) are used in the treatment of malignant neoplasms when surgery or radiotherapy is not possible or has proved ineffective, as an adjunct to surgery or radiotherapy, or, as in leukaemia, as the initial treatment. Therapy with antineoplastics is notably successful in a few malignant conditions and may be used to palliate symptoms and prolong life in others.

The two main groups of drugs used in the treatment of malignant disease are the alkylating agents and the antimetabolites. Nitrogen mustards, ethyleneimine compounds, and alkyl sulphonates are the main **alkylating agents**. Other compounds with an alkylating action are the various nitrosoureas. Cisplatin and dacarbazine appear to act similarly.

The **antimetabolites** may be subdivided into folic acid, purine, or pyrimidine antagonists.

Several natural products, or their derivatives, are used for their actions as **mitotic inhibitors**; they include the vinca alkaloids, the derivatives of podophyllotoxin such as etoposide, taxanes such as paclitaxel, and camptothecin derivatives such as irinotecan and topotecan.

Some **antibiotics** interfere with nucleic acids and are effective as antineoplastics.

Also described in this section are **other drugs** which act by various routes to affect the growth and proliferation of malignant cells. They include: aminoglutethimide, asparaginase, hydroxyurea, mitotane, procarbazine, and tamoxifen.

In recent years considerable interest has focused on immunological approaches to the treatment of malignant disease and a number of monoclonal antibodies such as muromonab-CD3 have been, or are being, developed. The use of biological response modifiers such as interleukins continues to be the subject of investigation and attempts to develop vaccines against individual neoplasms also continue.

Glucocorticoids (see Corticosteroids, p.1015) are used in association with antineoplastics in the treatment of malignant disease, especially in acute leukaemias and lymphomas. Other agents used in antineoplastic therapy include sex hormones (p.1426) and radiopharmaceuticals (p.1422).

Adverse Effects

The acute effects of antineoplastic administration frequently include nausea and vomiting, often via a central mechanism, and sometimes extremely severe. In addition, many of these compounds are irritant or vesicant, and produce local pain, irritation, and inflammation at the administration site; extravasation may lead to ulceration and necrosis. Hypersensitivity reactions may also occur.

However, many of the adverse effects of antineoplastics are an extension of their therapeutic action, which is not selective for malignant cells but affects all rapidly-dividing cells: antineoplastic therapy is made possible only by increased sensitivity or less effective recovery of malignant cells compared with normal cells, and administration is carefully controlled and timed, and, where possible, localised, to maximise the differences.

In consequence, adverse effects may be expected from most antineoplastics in tissues where normal cell division is fairly rapid, e.g. the bone-marrow, lymphoreticular tissue, gastro-intestinal mucosa, skin, and gonads, as well as in the fetus. The effects may not manifest for days or weeks, depending both on the agents used and the rate of division in the tissue concerned, and may sometimes be cumulative. Perhaps the most common serious effect, and one which has frequently limited the doses that can be given, is bone-marrow depression. Because of their effects on the various types of white blood cell many antineoplastics also cause profound suppression of normal immunity, and patients may be at greatly increased risk of severe and disseminated infection.

The rapid destruction of large numbers of cells during antineoplastic therapy of certain highly sensitive tumours, and the consequent release of breakdown products, may also lead to problems with hyperuricaemia and acute renal failure due to uric acid nephropathy (the 'tumour lysis syndrome').

Additionally, some drugs may have specific toxicities which are not necessarily related to their therapeutic action, such as cardiotoxicity due to anthracycline antibiotics, nephrotoxicity with cisplatin, or the effects of bleomycin on the lung.

In the very long term, patients who have undergone successful antineoplastic chemotherapy may develop secondary malignancies, suggesting that antineoplastics may themselves be carcinogenic. In addition, most are potentially mutagenic and teratogenic, and administration in pregnancy, particularly in the first trimester, may lead to fetal abortion, stunting, or malformation.

Carcinogenicity. Although it is difficult to control for a possible effect of the primary disease, there is clear evidence that some antineoplastic drugs may themselves be carcinogenic.[1] Most convincingly associated with secondary malignancies are the various *alkylating agents*,[2-5] including the nitrosoureas.[6] The secondary disease appears to manifest most frequently as leukaemia,[3-8] particularly acute non-lymphoid leukaemia, although solid tumours have been reported such as bladder cancer following cyclophosphamide treatment,[9] and a variety of solid cancers after treatment for Hodgkin's disease,[10] (although radiotherapy rather than chemotherapy may be chiefly responsible for these[11]). It has been suggested by some workers that cyclophosphamide is less leukaemogenic than melphalan or busulphan,[4,12] and there is a suggestion that the risk may be particularly high with lomustine,[6] but others consider that there is little difference in carcinogenic effect between the different alkylating agents.[3]

There is little evidence of carcinogenicity associated with antimetabolites such as methotrexate, although a review by Lien and Ou suggests that they may act as co-carcinogens,[2] and immunosuppression associated with their use may allow the development of Epstein-Barr virus-related lymphoma (see below). Other drugs that have been associated with the development of secondary malignancies are procarbazine,[5,13] podophyllotoxin derivatives such as etoposide,[14-16] and, in particular, teniposide,[12] carboplatin,[17] combinations of cisplatin with doxorubicin,[4] and possibly other anthracycline-based regimens.[35] Agents such as the platinum compounds and podophyllotoxin derivatives which act as DNA topoisomerase II inhibitors have been suggested to be associated particularly with acute non-lymphoblastic leukaemias.[17]

Immunosuppression with azathioprine, cyclosporin, and corticosteroids has also been associated with the development of malignancies,[18-20] although in immunosuppressed patients the characteristic neoplasms are lymphomas and skin cancers, including Kaposi's sarcoma.[20] Infection with Epstein-Barr virus after transplantation appears to play a role in the development of lymphoproliferative disorders in immunosuppressed patients.[21-23] Skin cancer may be a particular risk in immunosuppressed patients with a history of high sun exposure.[24]

Estimates of risk have varied very widely between studies, and have been calculated in various ways, making direct comparison impossible. Pui and colleagues consider that secondary acute non-lymphoid neoplasia will occur in at least 1% of patients receiving conventional chemotherapy for childhood acute lymphoblastic leukaemia,[14,25] and Althouse and others have suggested that over 10 years between 5% and 15% of patients treated with alkylating agents will develop cancer, a substantial excess over expected figures.[26] Several factors appear to influence the risk: treatment-associated neoplasia is more likely in patients given a higher cumulative dose,[3,5,6,16,27] in splenectomised patients,[5] and in older rather than younger patients.[3,8,28] (After transplantation, however, the risk of lymphoproliferative disorders is greater in younger than in older patients.[23]) One study in patients treated for Hodgkin's disease in childhood found the risk of secondary neoplasia to be considerably greater in girls than boys.[29]

Although some studies suggest that risk is increased when chemotherapy is combined with radiotherapy,[1,8,30] others do not,[3-6] and the effect of the combination continues to be a matter of debate.[31,32]

In many cases the risk of secondary malignancy is far less than that of undertreating, or of failing to treat, the primary disease.[7,33] However, secondary malignancies may be more resistant to treatment and more aggressive than primary disease,[34] and the risk of inducing malignant neoplasia is certainly a consideration in the use of alkylating agents and immunosuppressants to treat non-malignant disease,[26] and is an increasing challenge in the design of suitable treatment regimens for primary neoplastic disease.[7]

1. Curtis RE, *et al.* Risk of leukemia associated with the first course of cancer treatment: an analysis of the surveillance, epidemiology, and end results program experience. *J Natl Cancer Inst* 1984; **72:** 531–44.
2. Lien EJ, Ou X-C. Carcinogenicity of some anticancer drugs—a survey. *J Clin Hosp Pharm* 1985; **10:** 223–42.
3. Pedersen-Bjergaard J, *et al.* Risk of therapy-related leukaemia and preleukaemia after Hodgkin's disease: relation to age, cumulative dose of alkylating agents, and time from chemotherapy. *Lancet* 1987; **ii:** 83–8.
4. Kaldor JM, *et al.* Leukemia following chemotherapy for ovarian cancer. *N Engl J Med* 1990; **322:** 1–6.
5. Kaldor JM, *et al.* Leukemia following Hodgkin's disease. *N Engl J Med* 1990; **322:** 7–13.
6. Devereux S, *et al.* Leukaemia complicating treatment for Hodgkin's disease: the experience of the British National Lymphoma Investigation. *Br Med J* 1990; **301:** 1077–80.
7. Williams CJ. Leukaemia and cancer chemotherapy. *Br Med J* 1990; **301:** 73–4.
8. Pui C-H. Myeloid neoplasia in children treated for solid tumours. *Lancet* 1990; **336:** 417–21.
9. Pedersen-Bjergaard J, *et al.* Carcinoma of the urinary bladder after treatment with cyclophosphamide for non-Hodgkin's lymphoma. *N Engl J Med* 1988; **318:** 1028–32.
10. Swerdlow AJ, *et al.* Risk of second primary cancers after Hodgkin's disease by type of treatment: analysis of 2864 patients in the British National Lymphoma Investigation. *Br Med J* 1992; **304:** 1137–43.
11. Bhatia S, *et al.* Breast cancer and other second neoplasms after childhood Hodgkin's disease. *N Engl J Med* 1996; **334:** 745–51.
12. Hawkins MM, *et al.* Epipodophyllotoxins, alkylating agents, and radiation and risk of secondary leukaemia after childhood cancer. *Br Med J* 1992; **304:** 951–8.
13. Lee IP, Dixon RL. Mutagenicity, carcinogenicity and teratogenicity of procarbazine. *Mutat Res* 1978; **55:** 1–14.
14. Pui C-H, *et al.* Secondary acute myeloid leukemia in children treated for acute lymphoid leukemia. *N Engl J Med* 1989; **321:** 136–42.
15. Meadows AT, *et al.* Potential long-term toxic effects in children treated for acute lymphoblastic leukemia. *N Engl J Med* 1989; **321:** 1830.
16. Pedersen-Bjergaard J, *et al.* Increased risk of myelodysplasia and leukaemia after etoposide, cisplatin, and bleomycin for germ-cell tumours. *Lancet* 1991; **338:** 359–63.
17. Snowden JA, *et al.* Acute promyelocytic leukaemia after treatment for seminoma with carboplatin. *Lancet* 1994; **344:** 1361.
18. Maize JC. Skin cancer in immunosuppressed patients. *JAMA* 1977; **237:** 1857–8.
19. Kinlen LJ, *et al.* Collaborative United Kingdom-Australasian study of cancer in patients treated with immunosuppressive drugs. *Br Med J* 1979; **2:** 1461–6.
20. Li PKT, *et al.* The complications of newer transplant antirejection drugs: treatment with cyclosporin A, OKT3, and FK 506. *Adverse Drug React Acute Poisoning Rev* 1990; **9:** 123–55.
21. Starzl TE, *et al.* Reversibility of lymphomas and lymphoproliferative lesions developing under cyclosporin-steroid therapy. *Lancet* 1984; **i:** 583–7.
22. Kamel OW, *et al.* Brief report: reversible lymphomas associated with Epstein-Barr virus occurring during methotrexate therapy for rheumatoid arthritis and dermatomyositis. *N Engl J Med* 1993; **328:** 1317–21.
23. Boyle GJ, *et al.* Posttransplantation lymphoproliferative disorders in pediatric thoracic organ recipients. *J Pediatr* 1997; **131:** 309–13.
24. Boyle J, *et al.* Cancer, warts, and sunshine in renal transplant patients: a case-control study. *Lancet* 1984; **i:** 702–5.
25. Pui C-H, *et al.* Potential long-term toxic effects in children treated for acute lymphoblastic leukemia. *N Engl J Med* 1989; **321:** 1830–1.
26. Althouse R, *et al.* Cyclophosphamide in chronic active hepatitis. *Br Med J* 1979; **1:** 1630–1.
27. Boice JD, *et al.* Leukemia after adjuvant chemotherapy with semustine (methyl-CCNU)—evidence of a dose-response effect. *N Engl J Med* 1986; **314:** 119–20.
28. Pedersen-Bjergaard J, Larsen SO. Incidence of acute nonlymphocytic leukemia, preleukemia, and acute myeloproliferative syndrome up to 10 years after treatment of Hodgkin's disease. *N Engl J Med* 1982; **307:** 965–71.
29. Tarbell NJ, *et al.* Sex differences in risk of second malignant tumours after Hodgkin's disease in childhood. *Lancet* 1993; **341:** 1428–32.
30. Krikorian JG, *et al.* Occurrence of non-Hodgkin's lymphoma after therapy for Hodgkin's disease. *N Engl J Med* 1979; **300:** 452–8.
31. Prosnitz LR. Leukemia after treatment of ovarian cancer or Hodgkin's disease. *N Engl J Med* 1990; **322:** 1819–20.
32. Coltman CA, Dahlberg S. Leukemia after treatment of ovarian cancer or Hodgkin's disease. *N Engl J Med* 1990; **322:** 1820.
33. Macleod AM, Catto GRD. Cancer after transplantation. *Br Med J* 1988; **297:** 4–5.
34. Neugut AI, *et al.* Poor survival of treatment-related acute nonlymphocytic leukemia. *JAMA* 1990; **264:** 1006–8.
35. Levine MN, *et al.* Randomized trial of intensive cyclophosphamide, epirubicin, and fluorouracil chemotherapy compared with cyclophosphamide, methotrexate, and fluorouracil in premenopausal women with node-positive breast cancer. *J Clin Oncol* 1998; **16:** 2651–8.

EFFECTS ON CHROMOSOMES. Visible chromosome gaps, breaks, and structural rearrangements are found in blood lymphocytes from patients who have received substantial doses of combination chemotherapy, and the changes persist for years after the end of treatment. A more sensitive, if transient, measure of genetic damage is the increased rate of sister chromatid exchange (SCE) that occurs with even quite small doses of cytotoxic drugs.[1] Evidence from a study by Palmer *et al.*[2] in patients given chlorambucil suggests that as the dose increases so the capacity of the cells to cope with induced genetic damage is progressively exceeded, and thus SCE frequency reflects cumulative toxicity throughout the course of treatment.

In patients who develop acute non-lymphocytic leukaemia following antineoplastic therapy, the most common chromosomal losses involve chromosomes 5, 7, or both; a balanced translocation involving chromosomes 11 and 16 is closely associated with treatment using topoisomerase II inhibitors.[3]

See also under Effects on Reproductive Potential, below.

1. Anonymous. Drugs that can cause cancer. *Lancet* 1984; **i:** 261–2.
2. Palmer RG, *et al.* Chlorambucil-induced chromosome damage to human lymphocytes is dose-dependent and cumulative. *Lancet* 1984; **i:** 246–9.
3. Rowley JD, *et al.* Chromosomal translocations in secondary acute myeloid leukaemia. *N Engl J Med* 1996; **334:** 601–3.

Effects on the bladder. Cyclophosphamide (p.516) and ifosfamide (p.540) are the antineoplastics most frequently associated with adverse effects on the bladder, but see also Busulphan, p.509, Chlorambucil, p.512, and Mitomycin, p.552.

Effects on the blood. BONE-MARROW DEPRESSION. Bone-marrow depression, or myelosuppression, is common to the majority of antineoplastics, and is probably the single most important dose-limiting adverse effect, although its significance has been somewhat reduced in recent years by the availability of colony-stimulating factors, and the development of techniques such as peripheral blood stem cell transfusion.

The formation and development of blood cells takes place in the bone marrow. A common progenitor, the pluripotent stem cell, gives rise to 3 major cell lines from which red cells, white cells, and platelets are derived. All the cellular elements of blood may be affected by antineoplastic therapy, resulting in pancytopenia, but in many cases the toxicity appears to be greater for particular cell types. In addition, the different cell types have very different half-lives in the circulation. White blood cells and platelets tend to have the shortest half-lives in circulation. Hence the most usual manifestation of bone-marrow depression is leucopenia with a consequent increased risk of infection, and thrombocytopenia is also fairly common. Erythrocytes have the longest life (about 120 days) and anaemia is somewhat less frequent, and may be associated with megaloblastic changes in the bone marrow.

The onset, duration, and severity of bone marrow depression vary considerably with different antineoplastics. Little or only relatively mild myelosuppression seems to occur with conventional regimens of aromatase inhibitors such as anastrozole (p.504), asparaginase (p.505), bleomycin (p.508), flutamide (p.537), formestane (p.537), mitotane (p.553), streptozocin (p.562), tamoxifen (p.563), and vincristine (p.570). Megaloblastic anaemia occurring with hydroxyurea (p.539) may be treatable by blood transfusions, if necessary, without interrupting therapy.

Many of the alkylating agents are associated with severe and sometimes irreversible bone-marrow depression, particularly at high doses. Busulphan (p.509) and the nitrosoureas such as lomustine (p.544) pose a particular problem because the nadir of white-blood cell and platelet counts may not be reached for up to 6 weeks after a dose. Although high doses of antineoplastic generally produce greater and more rapid bone-marrow toxicity, with some agents, such as thiotepa (p.567), the relationship of toxicity to dose is very variable. These drugs affect both resting and actively cycling stem cells.

Many antimetabolites are also associated with myelosuppression and some, such as cytarabine (p.525) and methotrexate (p.547), may produce megaloblastic anaemia in addition to leucopenia and thrombocytopenia. Cytarabine has a biphasic effect on granulocytes, producing an initial nadir about 7 to 9 days after a dose, and a second and more severe one after 15 to 24 days. Unlike alkylating agents, antimetabolites affect actively proliferating, but not resting, stem cells.

Of the other drugs mitomycin (p.552) and procarbazine (p.559) in particular have both been associated with prolonged, delayed myelosuppression. Recovery from the bone-marrow toxicity of mitomycin may take months and about 25% of cases do not recover. Cisplatin (p.514) and the anthracycline antibiotics (p.529) are both myelosuppressant, although other toxic effects may be more important in determining dose, but it is a problem with carboplatin (p.511).

Bone marrow depression is also a significant adverse effect of vinblastine (p.569) vindesine, and vinorelbine, although the effects of vincristine on the bone marrow are much less marked, as mentioned above. Neutropenia is common with the camptothecin derivatives irinotecan (p.543) and topotecan (p.567) and can be dose-limiting.

For further details, see under the individual monographs.

See also Effects on Immune Response, below.

Effects on body weight. Although the effects of antineoplastics on the gastro-intestinal tract (below) may lead to anorexia, malabsorption, and malnutrition, and hence to weight loss, antineoplastic therapy for breast cancer has also been associated with weight gain, sometimes dramatic.[1] Weight gain appeared to be more likely in premenopausal women, in those receiving multidrug regimens, and in those treated for longer periods of time.

1. Denmark-Wahnefried W, *et al.* Why women gain weight with adjuvant chemotherapy for breast cancer. *J Clin Oncol* 1993; **11:** 1418–29.

Effects on bones and joints. The possibility that antineoplastic chemotherapy may produce avascular necrosis of bone has been briefly reviewed in the *Lancet*.[1] Most reports were in patients being treated for lymphomas, and of these the majority of cases were in patients with Hodgkin's disease, perhaps because the chemotherapy cycle was more prolonged than in other lymphomas, and there had been a preponderance of men aged 30 to 50 years. These chemotherapy regimens mostly included corticosteroids though not in doses that would normally be expected to result in avascular necrosis, and it was suggested that administration with cytotoxics might increase the risk of this condition developing.[1] There have been reports of avascular necrosis in patients receiving antineoplastics without corticosteroids[2,3] but these are not sufficient to attribute the effect to specific drugs. A study in children receiving chemotherapy for leukaemia has suggested that the effects of chemotherapy on gastro-intestinal and renal handling of nutrients may lead to alterations in calcium and magnesium homoeostasis and hence to abnormal turnover of bone mineral.[4]

1. Anonymous. Osteonecrosis caused by combination chemotherapy. *Lancet* 1982; **i:** 433–4.
2. Obrist R, *et al.* Osteonecrosis after chemotherapy. *Lancet* 1978; **i:** 1316.
3. Harper PG, *et al.* Avascular necrosis of bone caused by combination chemotherapy without corticosteroids. *Br Med J* 1984; **288:** 267–8.
4. Atkinson SA, *et al.* Mineral homeostasis and bone mass in children treated for acute lymphoblastic leukemia. *J Pediatr* 1989; **114:** 793–800.

Effects on the cardiovascular system. THROMBO-EMBOLISM. There have been numerous reports which suggest that combination antineoplastic chemotherapy may be associated with thrombo-embolic events, including angina pectoris,[1] deep-vein thrombosis,[2,3] pulmonary embolism,[2-4] and stroke,[5] sometimes with fatal results.[3-5] Arterial thromboses have also occurred.[5,6] Patients with malignant disease are already at increased risk of thrombo-embolism, but results of a study in women with breast cancer suggest that the risk is further increased in patients receiving chemotherapy.[7] Several reports have implicated the combinations of bleomycin with a vinca alkaloid and another agent such as cisplatin or etoposide.[1,3,4,6] Such combinations are widely used for testicular cancer and have also been implicated in producing Raynaud's syndrome,[8,9] although there is no evidence of a relationship between the two forms of toxicity,[3] but reports of thrombosis are not confined to such regimens.[2,3,5] Toxic effects on vascular endothelium have been proposed as a possible mechanism for these effects;[2,6] there is also evidence that chemotherapy further elevates an already increased coagulant activity in the blood of cancer patients, an increase which can be diminished by heparin.[10]

Thrombo-embolic complications may also be associated with the indwelling catheters used to provide vascular access for antineoplastic therapy;[11] low-dose warfarin prophylaxis may reduce the risk.[12]

For a discussion of the cardiotoxicity of antineoplastics see Effects on the Heart, below.

1. Rodriguez J, *et al.* Angina pectoris following cisplatin, etoposide, and bleomycin in a patient with advanced testicular cancer. *Ann Pharmacother* 1995; **29:** 138–9.
2. Cantwell BMJ, *et al.* Thromboses and thromboemboli in patients with lymphoma during cytotoxic chemotherapy. *Br Med J* 1988; **297:** 179–80.
3. Cantwell BMJ, *et al.* Thromboembolic events during combination chemotherapy for germ cell malignancy. *Lancet* 1988; **ii:** 1086–7.
4. Hall MR, *et al.* Thromboembolic events during combination chemotherapy for germ cell malignancy. *Lancet* 1988; **ii:** 1259.
5. Wall JG, *et al.* Arterial thrombosis associated with adjuvant chemotherapy for breast carcinoma: a Cancer and Leukemia Group B study. *Am J Med* 1989; **87:** 501–4.
6. Garstin IWH, *et al.* Arterial thrombosis after treatment with bleomycin and cisplatin. *Br Med J* 1990; **300:** 1018.
7. Levine MN, *et al.* The thrombogenic effect of anticancer drug therapy in women with stage II breast cancer. *N Engl J Med* 1988; **318:** 404–7.
8. Vogelzang NJ, *et al.* Raynaud's phenomenon: a common toxicity after combination chemotherapy for testicular cancer. *Ann Intern Med* 1981; **95:** 288–92.

9. Pechère M, *et al.* Fingertip necrosis during chemotherapy with bleomycin, vincristine and methotrexate for HIV-related Kaposi's sarcoma. *Br J Dermatol* 1996; **134:** 378–9.
10. Edwards RL, *et al.* Heparin abolishes the chemotherapy-induced increase in plasma fibrinopeptide A levels. *Am J Med* 1990; **89:** 25–8.
11. Anderson AJ, *et al.* Thrombosis: the major Hickman catheter complication in patients with solid tumor. *Chest* 1989; **95:** 71–5.
12. Bern MM, *et al.* Very low doses of warfarin can prevent thrombosis in central venous catheters: a randomized prospective trial. *Ann Intern Med* 1990; **112:** 423–8.

Effects on electrolytes. Brenton and Gordon have suggested that cancer chemotherapy and its complicating opportunistic infection exposes some patients to a combination of treatments likely to produce hypomagnesaemia, including: drug-induced loss of appetite; increased gastro-intestinal magnesium loss due to vomiting and diarrhoea; impaired intestinal absorption due to drug-induced mucosal damage; and a direct magnesium-losing effect on the kidney of certain drugs such as cisplatin and some antibiotics.[1] Hypoparathyroidism and associated hypocalcaemia and hypomagnesaemia have been reported in patients receiving chemotherapy for acute leukaemias,[2] and it has been suggested that such changes in electrolyte homoeostasis may result in abnormal bone turnover (see Effects on Bones and Joints, above). Release of the contents of cells destroyed by chemotherapy is well-known to be associated with hyperuricaemia (below) but has also produced hyperphosphataemia, hyperkalaemia, and hypocalcaemia.[3,4]

Disturbances of electrolyte homoeostasis have been reported particularly with cisplatin (p.514), cyclophosphamide (p.516), and cyclosporin (p.519).

1. Brenton DP, Gordon TE. Fluid and electrolyte disorders: magnesium. *Br J Hosp Med* 1984; **32:** 60–9.
2. Freedman DB, *et al.* Hypoparathyroidism and hypocalcaemia during treatment for acute leukaemia. *Br Med J* 1982; **284:** 700–2.
3. Kanfer A, *et al.* Extreme hyperphosphataemia causing acute anuric nephrocalcinosis in lymphosarcoma. *Br Med J* 1979; **1:** 1320–1.
4. Chasty RC, Liu-Yin JA. Acute tumour lysis syndrome. *Br J Hosp Med* 1993; **49:** 488–92.

Effects on the gastro-intestinal tract. Apart from anorexia, and nausea and vomiting (see below), many antineoplastics produce gastro-intestinal disturbances. Mucosal inflammation (mucositis), notably as stomatitis and sometimes proctitis, is quite common, as are mucosal cellular changes, xerostomia, impaired absorption, and diarrhoea. In some cases gastro-intestinal damage may progress to ulceration, haemorrhage, and perforation. Antimetabolites affecting pyrimidine metabolism, such as cytarabine (p.525) and fluorouracil (p.535), and the antifolates such as methotrexate (p.547), seem to be particularly associated with severe gastro-intestinal effects, especially at high doses, but there appear to be few antineoplastics that do not cause some degree of gastro-intestinal disturbance. Irinotecan can produce both an initial transient diarrhoea related to cholinergic stimulation, and more severe prolonged diarrhoea with a delayed onset which may be dose limiting and potentially fatal. Combination with radiotherapy may increase the toxicity of some agents on the gastro-intestinal tract. The neutropenia induced by many antineoplastic regimens may lead to secondary gastro-intestinal effects, such as stomatitis and gastro-intestinal inflammation, associated with infection.

CLOSTRIDIUM DIFFICILE INFECTION. Antineoplastic therapy has occasionally been associated with the development of *Clostridium difficile*-induced gastro-intestinal disease, even in the absence of concomitant antibacterial therapy.[1] Most patients had received multiple drug regimens. Methotrexate, fluorouracil, cyclophosphamide, and doxorubicin have all been associated with a number of cases but this may simply reflect the frequency of their use. For discussion of the treatment of such disease, see Antibiotic-associated Colitis, p.123

1. Anand A, Glatt AE. Clostridium difficile infection associated with antineoplastic chemotherapy: a review. *Clin Infect Dis* 1993; **17:** 109–13.

MUCOSITIS. The suffering associated with oral mucositis is by far the worst part of treatment for many patients undergoing curative chemotherapy or bone-marrow transplantation, and for those undergoing oral radiotherapy.[1] Apart from pain and dysphagia the ulcerated mucosa provides a portal of entry for infection; loss of weight and malnutrition may further impair immune function, and if symptoms are severe enough the treatment cycle may have to be interrupted. Before the patient starts any intensive chemotherapy or local or systemic radiotherapy the oral cavity must be assessed with a view to eliminating sources of infection and chronic irritation.

1. Calman FMB, Langdon J. Oral complications of cancer. *Br Med J* 1991; **302:** 485–6.

NAUSEA AND VOMITING. Nausea and vomiting (p.1172) are common side-effects of antineoplastic therapy, and for many patients, represent a major drawback to treatment. A survey of patient perceptions of adverse effects among 99 patients receiving cancer chemotherapy found that nausea and vomiting were ranked as by far their greatest concern.[1]

Once experienced, anticipatory vomiting may occur at the sight of medical staff, or a needle. The problem may be severe enough in some cases to hinder or completely prevent further treatment.

Antineoplastic or cytotoxic drugs may induce vomiting by both a central action on the chemoreceptor trigger zone and a peripheral action on the gastro-intestinal tract. Several neurotransmitters have been implicated over the years including acetylcholine, histamine, enkephalins, dopamine, and serotonin or 5-hydroxytryptamine (5-HT). The cerebral cortex is probably responsible for anticipatory vomiting. Antineoplastics may not all induce emesis by a common pathway, but 5-HT_3-receptor mechanisms are clearly important in the pathogenesis of *acute* cisplatin-associated vomiting. This was suspected when the antiemetic metoclopramide, a dopamine antagonist, was found to have serotonin (5-HT) antagonist activity at the high doses used against cisplatin emesis and confirmed when specific 5-HT_3 antagonists such as ondansetron proved to be effective. Different mechanisms are probably involved in *delayed* emesis since 5-HT_3 antagonists are less effective.

Some patients are more susceptible to emesis than others. The emetic potential of antineoplastics also varies in terms of severity and incidence. Emetogenicity may depend to some extent on the dose, route, and schedule of administration. Some combination therapy has resulted in a higher incidence of vomiting than would be expected from the constituents. Vomiting may be *very severe* with cisplatin, dacarbazine, dactinomycin, mustine, high-dose cyclophosphamide, and streptozocin, and occurs in most patients. *Moderate* vomiting is likely with drugs such as doxorubicin and more modest doses of cyclophosphamide, as well as with high-dose methotrexate, while other agents such as the vinca alkaloids, fluorouracil, lower doses of methotrexate, chlorambucil, bleomycin, and etoposide *rarely* cause significant vomiting.

The *onset and duration* of vomiting also varies from drug to drug. With cisplatin the onset may be between 4 and 8 hours following a dose, while the duration may be up to 48 hours or occasionally even longer; a persistent feeling of nausea, and sometimes vomiting, lasting for several days may also occur, and requires prolonged antiemetic therapy. After mustine, vomiting may begin within a half to 2 hours, whereas after cyclophosphamide there may be a latent interval of 9 to 18 hours, but in both cases vomiting is generally less prolonged than with cisplatin. Acute emesis (that occurring within 24 hours of chemotherapy) has generally been easier to control than delayed emesis (that occurring more than 24 hours after chemotherapy); different mechanisms appear to be involved.

1. Coates A, *et al.* On the receiving end—patient perception of the side-effects of cancer chemotherapy. *Eur J Cancer Clin Oncol* 1983; **19:** 203–8.

Effects on the heart. The cardiotoxicity of antineoplastics has been reviewed by Von Hoff.[1] Cardiotoxicity is the major dose-limiting toxicity with anthracyclines such as doxorubicin and daunorubicin, manifesting most seriously as drug-induced cardiomyopathy, which is frequently fatal, and for which no specific treatment exists. Some of the newer anthracycline analogues were developed to be less toxic to the heart, although this is difficult to prove in controlled studies, and liposomal formulations may also prove of benefit. Cardiotoxicity has also been associated with other antineoplastics, although less frequently. High-dose cyclophosphamide may produce haemorrhagic cardiac necrosis, and congestive heart failure, sometimes delayed by up to 2 weeks, while fluorouracil has been associated with angina pectoris and myocardial infarction, perhaps due to a combination of vasospastic effects and activation of coagulation. Amsacrine has been associated with arrhythmias, sometimes fatal. Occasional reports of cardiotoxicity associated with busulphan, cisplatin, etoposide, mitomycin, and vincristine also exist.

For a discussion of the thrombo-embolic events seen with antineoplastics see Effects on the Cardiovascular System, above.

1. Von Hoff DD, *et al.* The cardiotoxicity of anticancer agents. *Semin Oncol* 1982; **9:** 23–33.

Effects on immune response. Lymphocytes are produced by stem cells in the bone marrow and at other sites, including the thymus, and are involved in humoral and cell-mediated immunity. Most antineoplastics have a depressant effect on bone marrow (see Effects on the Blood, above) and many have immunosuppressant properties although the degree of suppression varies considerably and may depend on the dose and schedule of administration used. Immunosuppression decreases the patient's resistance to infection and has also been implicated in the development of malignancies (see Carcinogenicity, above). Siber and others[1] reported that immunisation of 53 patients with Hodgkin's disease and 10 controls, using dodecavalent pneumococcal vaccine, indicated that antibody response was profoundly impaired in patients who had received intensive radiotherapy and/or chemotherapy. Some impairment persisted for at least 4 years after the completion of intensive combined therapy.

The length of time after onset of immunosuppression in transplant patients correlates with the type of infection acquired.[2] In the first few months local bacterial infections predominate. After about 1 month of immunosuppression *Aspergillus* infections become more common, while between 3 weeks and 4 months after transplantation cytomegalovirus infection (both primary and reactivated) occurs in 20 to 40% of those at risk. *Pneumocystis carinii* pneumonia is uncommon immediately after transplantation, more usually occurring after months or years. Infection in transplant patients tends to occur in or near the transplanted organ.

For a discussion on the effects of immunosuppressant therapy on the immune response and the infections associated with it, see Corticosteroids, p.1012.

1. Siber GR, *et al.* Impaired antibody response to pneumococcal vaccine after treatment for Hodgkin's disease. *N Engl J Med* 1978; **299:** 442–8.
2. Anonymous. Immunosuppressive drugs and their complications. *Drug Ther Bull* 1994; **32:** 66–70.

Effects on the kidneys. Nephrotoxicity is well-recognised as an adverse effect of cisplatin (p.514), cyclosporin (p.520), and methotrexate (p.547), but there have also been occasional reports of renal toxicity with other agents including ifosfamide (p.540), plicamycin (p.558), and semustine (p.561), as well as of haemolytic-uraemic syndrome with mitomycin and fluorouracil (p.552).

Effects on the liver. Occasional reports of hepatotoxicity exist for many antineoplastics and immunosuppressants including aminoglutethimide (p.502), azathioprine (p.506), busulphan (p.509), cyclophosphamide (p.516), dacarbazine (p.527), dactinomycin (p.527), doxorubicin (p.530), floxuridine (p.534), hydroxyurea (p.539), methotrexate (p.547), mitomycin (p.552), mitozantrone (p.553), sparfosic acid with fluorouracil (p.561), tamoxifen (p.564), and thioguanine (p.566). However, the relationship of the drug to the adverse effect is not always easy to establish.

A detailed review by Ménard and colleagues suggested that methotrexate, mercaptopurine, azathioprine, cytarabine, carmustine, streptozocin, asparaginase, and plicamycin could probably be classified as hepatotoxic. There was considered to be insufficient evidence to classify fluorouracil, cyclophosphamide, busulphan, dacarbazine, the anthracyclines, the vinca alkaloids, and the podophyllum derivatives as hepatotoxic, although this classification was not definitive.[1] Liver toxicity may not be confined to patients: Sotaniemi and others reported 3 cases of liver damage in nurses working on an oncology ward.[2]

1. Ménard DB, *et al.* Antineoplastic agents and the liver. *Gastroenterology* 1980; **78:** 142–64.
2. Sotaniemi EA, *et al.* Liver damage in nurses handling cytostatic agents. *Acta Med Scand* 1983; **214:** 181–9.

Effects on mental function. Combination chemotherapy has been associated with psychiatric morbidity (anxiety, depression, behavioural changes) in both adults[1] and children.[2] It has been pointed out that patients receiving cancer chemotherapy inevitably suffer emotional distress, associated in part with the adverse effects of treatment. Patients should be fully informed of aims and likely outcomes of treatment, and adverse effects minimised, in order to keep emotional distress to a minimum.[3]

A number of individual antineoplastics and immunosuppressants have been associated with mental symptoms including asparaginase (p.505), chlorambucil (p.513), cyclosporin (p.519), methotrexate (p.548), mitotane (p.553), and the vinca alkaloids (p.569). In many cases such symptoms can be attributed to direct central neurotoxicity (see also under Effects on the Nervous System, below).

1. Maguire GP, *et al.* Psychiatric morbidity and physical toxicity associated with adjuvant chemotherapy after mastectomy. *Br Med J* 1980; **281:** 1179–80.
2. Dolgin MJ, *et al.* Behavioral distress in pediatric patients with cancer receiving chemotherapy. *Pediatrics* 1989; **84:** 103–10.
3. Brinkley D. Emotional distress during cancer chemotherapy. *Br Med J* 1983; **286:** 663–4.

Effects on the nervous system. Neurotoxic effects have been reported for many antineoplastics, including altretamine (p.502), asparaginase (p.505), busulphan (p.509), carboplatin (p.511), carmustine (p.512), chlorambucil (p.512), cisplatin (p.514), cladribine (p.515), cyclosporin (p.519), cytarabine (p.525), etanidazole (p.532), etoposide (p.532), fludarabine (p.534), fluorouracil (p.535), hydroxyurea (p.539), ifosfamide (p.540), lomustine (p.544), methotrexate (p.547), misonidazole (p.551), mitotane (p.553), mitozantrone (p.553), mustine (p.555), paclitaxel (p.556), pentostatin (p.557), procarbazine (p.559), sparfosic acid (p.561), tacrolimus (p.562), tegafur (p.565), vinblastine (p.569), vincristine (p.570), and vindesine (p.571). In some cases these effects may be associated with particular routes such as the intrathecal. See under the individual monographs for further details. Radiotherapy can also cause damage to the nervous system so combination of the two modalities may lead to additive effects.

EFFECTS ON THE EARS. Several antineoplastics have been associated with ototoxicity,[1] including vincristine and vinblastine, but cisplatin in particular is associated with high-frequency hearing loss and tinnitus. In addition, agents such as the nitrogen mustards and bleomycin are potentially ototoxic.

1. Huang MY, Schacht J. Drug-induced ototoxicity: pathogenesis and prevention. *Med Toxicol Adverse Drug Exp* 1989; **4:** 452–67.

Effects on reproductive potential. CHROMOSOMES. If patients are fertile after treatment with antineoplastics, no significant increase has been seen in fetal chromosome damage, fetal abnormality, or the abortion rate. Several small or medium-sized studies have failed to show any increase in congenital abnormalities or miscarriage rate in the offspring of patients who have received chemotherapy,[1-4] although one study did show an increased risk of abnormal offspring in patients with Hodgkin's disease who received both chemotherapy and irradiation. Another study, while finding no overall link between chemotherapy and the incidence of congenital abnormality did suggest an increased incidence of heart defects in children born to mothers who received dactinomycin,[4] but this was not subsequently confirmed in a larger group.[5] A large case-control study carried out in Canada, and involving over 85 000 parents of children with congenital anomalies, also has failed to confirm a higher incidence of congenital abnormality in the offspring of patients treated with radiotherapy or alkylating agents.[6] However, despite these generally reassuring results, it has been suggested that women should delay conception for a year after cessation of chemotherapy to allow mature ova which might have been damaged to be eliminated.[7]

See also Effects on Chromosomes under Carcinogenicity, above.

1. Rustin GJS, *et al.* Pregnancy after cytotoxic chemotherapy for gestational trophoblastic tumours. *Br Med J* 1984; **288:** 103–6.
2. Li FP, *et al.* Offspring of patients treated for cancer in childhood. *J Natl Cancer Inst* 1979; **62:** 1193–7.
3. Holmes GE, Holmes FF. Pregnancy outcome of patients treated for Hodgkin's disease: a controlled study. *Cancer* 1978; **41:** 1317–22.
4. Green DM, *et al.* Congenital anomalies in children of patients who received chemotherapy for cancer in childhood and adolescence. *N Engl J Med* 1991; **325:** 141–6.
5. Byrne J, *et al.* Absence of birth defects in offspring of women treated with dactinomycin. *N Engl J Med* 1992; **326:** 137.
6. Dodds L, *et al.* Case-control study of congenital anomalies in children of cancer patients. *Br Med J* 1993; **307:** 164–8.
7. Walden PAM, Bagshawe KD. Pregnancies after chemotherapy for gestational trophoblastic tumours. *Lancet* 1979; **ii:** 1241.

GONADS. The effects of drugs, including cytotoxic drugs, on the gonads have been extensively reviewed by Beeley,[1] and more recently, but in less detail, by Parkinson and Bateman.[2]

Alkylating agents are believed to be the most toxic to the testis. The extent of gonadal damage depends on the dose and duration of treatment. Methotrexate appears less toxic than the alkylating agents. Doxorubicin, even in high doses, appears not to have a permanent effect on human germ cells.

Combination chemotherapy regimens as used to treat Hodgkin's disease produce complete azoospermia in all patients during treatment, usually after only 1 or 2 cycles. Mustine and procarbazine are thought to be mainly responsible for the infertility produced.

In women, cytotoxic drugs act on the ovary to produce loss of primordial follicles with failure of ovulation, oligomenorrhoea or amenorrhoea, and failure of endocrine function resulting in loss of libido and menopausal symptoms. The degree of damage and its reversibility depend partly on the drug and its dose but more on the age of the woman at the time of treatment, with older women (35 to 40 or over) being more sensitive, probably a reflection of the decrease in oocyte numbers with age.

1. Beeley L. Drug-induced sexual dysfunction and infertility. *Adverse Drug React Acute Poisoning Rev* 1984; **3:** 23–42.
2. Parkinson M, Bateman N. Disorders of sexual function caused by drugs. *Prescribers' J* 1994; **34:** 183–90.

SEXUAL FUNCTION. Loss of libido and decline in sexual performance seem to be relatively common in men receiving combination chemotherapy,[1,2] and may persist after chemotherapy has ended.[1] However, it may sometimes be difficult to distinguish the effects of chemotherapy from those of the disease and the patient's reaction to it: at least one study has shown that gonadal function is disturbed in patients with Hodgkin's disease before treatment.[2] Evidence for decreased libido in women is harder to find, but failure of endocrine function after chemotherapy may lead to loss of libido and menopausal symptoms.[3]

1. Chapman RM, *et al.* Cyclical combination chemotherapy and gonadal function: retrospective study in males. *Lancet* 1979; **i:** 285–9.
2. Chapman RM, *et al.* Male gonadal dysfunction in Hodgkin's disease: a prospective study. *JAMA* 1981; **245:** 1323–8.
3. Shalet SM. Effects of cancer chemotherapy on gonadal function of patients. *Cancer Treat Rev* 1980; **7:** 141–52.

Effects on respiratory function. Lung injury occurs in about 10% of all patients who receive bleomycin, with death in 1 to 2%. The changes in the lung are diffuse and include fibrosis of the alveolar septa, chronic pneumonitis, and enlargement of the type II alveolar lining cells with bizarre alteration of the nucleus; clinically, the reaction presents as non-productive cough and dyspnoea, often with fever, and develops over days to weeks. The reaction is dose-related, being more likely at total doses over 450 units, although it has occurred at much lower doses, and is more common in elderly patients.[1] Hypersensitivity pneumonitis, which is more amenable to treatment, has also been reported.[2]

Pulmonary damage has also been reported in association with an increasing number of antineoplastics apart from bleomycin, a subject extensively reviewed by Twohig and Matthay.[3] Among the alkylating agents cyclophosphamide has been reported to produce lung injury in less than 1% of cases, although this may be increased where it is a component of combination regimens or where it is combined with radiotherapy. Busulphan may produce lung toxicity including insidious pulmonary fibrosis in as many as 4% of patients, usually developing several years after initiation of therapy, and with increased risk the longer that therapy lasts. A few reports exist of interstitial pneumonitis and fibrosis associated with chlorambucil and melphalan, but these appear to be extremely rare. The prognosis in patients with alkylating-agent-induced fibrosis is often poor, with mortality rates of around 50%.

The antimetabolite methotrexate can produce symptoms similar to hypersensitivity pneumonitis in up to 7% of patients, sometimes with pleuritis and acute respiratory failure due to pulmonary oedema, but it is not clear whether a true hypersensitivity mechanism is involved, and symptoms are usually reversible even without discontinuing therapy. High-dose cytarabine has also been associated with pulmonary oedema, while azathioprine has been associated with a few cases of interstitial pneumonitis and fibrosis.

Other antineoplastics known to be associated with pulmonary toxicity include mitomycin (usually in less than 10% of patients though the incidence may be much higher in combination regimens); the vinca alkaloids (generally in combination, and usually producing acute respiratory failure); chlorozotocin; procarbazine; and possibly teniposide. The nitrosoureas, and particularly carmustine, have also emerged as pulmonary toxins. Carmustine has been associated with an insidious chronic pulmonary fibrosis, which in some early studies occurred in as many as 30% of patients and had a high mortality. Symptoms are associated particularly with cumulative doses in excess of about 1.4 g per square metre body-surface area, although toxicity has occurred at cumulative doses as low as 240 mg per square metre. The onset of symptoms may be very delayed: O'Driscoll and others reported fibrosis occurring up to 17 years after treatment with carmustine.[4]

1. Rosenow EC, *et al.* Pulmonary disease in the immunocompromised host. *Mayo Clin Proc* 1985; **60:** 473–87.
2. Holoye PY, *et al.* Bleomycin hypersensitivity pneumonitis. *Ann Intern Med* 1978; **88:** 47–9.
3. Twohig KJ, Matthay RA. Pulmonary effects of cytotoxic agents other than bleomycin. *Clin Chest Med* 1990; **11:** 31–54.
4. O'Driscoll BR, *et al.* Active lung fibrosis up to 17 years after chemotherapy with carmustine (BCNU) in childhood. *N Engl J Med* 1990; **323:** 378–82.

Effects on the skin. Alopecia occurs with many antineoplastics, and may be severe with doxorubicin, the nitrosoureas, taxanes, and cyclophosphamide. The alkylating agents and some antibiotic antineoplastics are often associated with hyperpigmentation, most commonly of skin, although pigmentation of nails, hair, and teeth has occurred. Some drugs, such as the taxanes, cause dystrophic changes in the nails. Certain drugs may interact with ultraviolet light or x-ray radiation to enhance its effects on the skin and may cause radiation recall, photosensitivity, or, in the case of methotrexate, reactivation of ultraviolet burns. Hypersensitivity to antineoplastics may produce cutaneous reactions including allergic rashes, angioedema, and pruritus. In addition to the above there may be local reactions to irritant and vesicant drugs following extravasation. Finally, certain drugs are associated with specific dermatological reactions: bleomycin may produce hyperkeratotic and sclerotic lesions, dactinomycin is associated with an erythematous papular or pustular rash mimicking septic emboli, fluorouracil may produce inflammation of solar keratoses, and plicamycin is associated with a distinctive flushing phenomenon.

See also Effects on the Gastro-intestinal Tract, above, and Local Toxicity, below. References may also be found under individual monographs, including to the palmar-plantar erythrodysesthesia syndrome seen with fluorouracil (p.535) and a number of other antineoplastics.

Hyperuricaemia. Overproduction of purines is a known complication of antineoplastic therapy and may result in hyperuricaemia (p.390). Hyperuricaemia is also an important part of the tumour lysis syndrome—see below.

Local toxicity. Local toxicity due to intravenous cancer chemotherapy may include local irritation, extravasation necrosis, and hypersensitivity.[1] Venous irritation, presenting as vasospasm and pain or endothelial chemical burn of the vessel, resulting in a painful, streaky, long-lasting sterile phlebitis, may be due to the drug, or, as with carmustine, due to the diluent (alcohol). Irritation and phlebitis have been reported particularly with fluorouracil, carmustine, bisantrene, and mustine.

Up to 6% of patients treated with peripheral intravenous chemotherapy may experience extravasation, usually with pain, erythema, and swelling at the site of injection. Severe necrosis requiring surgical intervention may develop, particularly with antibiotic antineoplastics such as doxorubicin. For a discussion of extravasation and its management, including those drugs most commonly associated with problems, see Extravasation, p.474.

Local hypersensitivity reactions, usually self-limiting, may occur: it is important to distinguish such reactions from extravasation. In contrast to the latter, there is no swelling at the injection site, and pain is felt as a dull ache along the course of the vein, as opposed to the stinging commonly noted following extravasation.

1. Brigden ML, Barnett JB. Local toxicity of cancer chemotherapy—practical considerations. *Can J Hosp Pharm* 1986; **39:** 96–9.

Tumour lysis syndrome. The tumour lysis syndrome represents a biochemical disturbance following massive release of cellular breakdown products from tumour cells sensitive to therapy. The amount of breakdown products is sufficient to overwhelm normal excretory and metabolic mechanisms for their clearance, and the cardinal features of the syndrome are hyperkalaemia, hyperuricaemia, and hyperphosphataemia accompanied by hypocalcaemia. Clinical symptoms may include urate nephropathy or nephrocalcinosis leading to renal impairment, and cardiac arrhythmias associated with the potassium abnormalities. The syndrome is seen particularly when bulky chemosensitive disease is present, and may be more likely in patients with pre-existing renal impairment or hyperuricaemia. The most frequent cases are in patients with Burkitt's or lymphoblastic lymphoma, or an acute leukaemia. Of patients with solid tumours, most reports have implicated those with breast cancer, small-cell lung cancer, or neuroblastoma.

References.

1. Chasty RC, Liu-Yin JA. Acute tumour lysis syndrome. *Br J Hosp Med* 1993; **49:** 488–92.
2. Kalemkerian GP, *et al.* Tumor lysis syndrome in small cell carcinoma and other solid tumors. *Am J Med* 1997; **103:** 363–7.

Treatment of Adverse Effects

Intensive supportive care may be necessary to prevent or control the adverse effects of antineoplastic therapy. Antiemetic therapy should be given to reduce, and if possible prevent, nausea and vomiting, since once experienced it may become a conditioned response, and may not respond to antiemetics. Intensive oral care is desirable to minimise the effects of stomatitis while corticosteroids, and if necessary nutritional supplements, may be of some help in patients with anorexia.

Techniques attempting to prevent the occurrence of alopecia have met with varying success (see below). Scalp tourniquets and ice-packs have been used to minimise concentrations of antineoplastics in the scalp after intravenous injection. However, such methods may allow the development of a cancer-cell sanctuary and should not be used in patients with leukaemia or other conditions with circulating malignant cells.

Of particular importance is the management of bone-marrow depression. Recent interest has focused on the use of colony-stimulating factors (see p.714 and below) to promote the formation of replacement blood elements. Active measures may be necessary to combat infection and bleeding. Transfusions of blood products may be required; granulocyte transfusions have been given for infections unresponsive to antibiotics, although their value is a matter of debate, while transfusion of blood platelets or use of growth factors such as oprelvekin (interleukin-II) may be of value in preventing thrombocytopenia-induced bleeding.

Extravasation of antineoplastics can pose serious problems and its treatment is controversial (see below). Infusion should be stopped immediately once extravasation is noticed and any drug remaining at the site aspirated if possible. Ice-packs are often applied, although warm moist soaks have been advocated for some drugs such as the vinca alkaloids, and some, but not all, centres suggest local injection of a corticosteroid. If ulceration occurs plastic surgery may be required. The value of specific antidotes is not proven.

Hyperuricaemia secondary to tumour lysis in patients with leukaemias or lymphomas can be prevented by the addition of allopurinol to treatment schedules, and by adequate hydration and, if necessary, alkalinisation of the urine. Good hydration is also important to minimise the nephrotoxic effects of drugs such as cisplatin and methotrexate.

Specific treatments exist for the toxicity of certain antineoplastics (for example the use of calcium folinate to reduce methotrexate toxicity, or mesna to control the bladder toxicity of cyclophosphamide or ifosfamide). For further details of the treatment of specific adverse effects see under the individual monographs.

Alopecia. Attempts to prevent or reduce chemotherapy-induced alopecia have relied on either restriction of scalp blood-flow with a tourniquet or the use of local hypothermia. Following early reports of benefit[1,2] a scalp tourniquet was applied 5 minutes before administration in patients receiving doxorubicin, cyclophosphamide, and vincristine or teniposide, and was left in position for 20 minutes.[3] Alopecia occurred in 12 of 37 patients so treated, but in 22 of 31 controls. However, the tourniquet was uncomfortable: 5 patients originally assigned to the tourniquet group could not tolerate it.

Several studies have investigated the use of local scalp cooling.[4-6] Of 33 patients in whom ice-packs were applied to the scalp 5 minutes before injections of doxorubicin, and left in place for 30 minutes after injection, 20 maintained good protection against hair loss over 6 to 8 months of treatment, although the benefit decreased with time and was less at higher doses.[4] The results may also depend on the degree of cooling achieved, and the drug regimen used:[5] most studies have concentrated on doxorubicin, which is a potent producer of alopecia, but which is quite rapidly cleared. Vincristine also produces alopecia which, it has been suggested, is less likely to be prevented because of the drug's more prolonged clearance from the circulation,[5] although vincristine-induced alopecia has reportedly been reduced using a tourniquet.[1] There is also concern that restricting access of the antineoplastic to the scalp may create a sanctuary for circulating malignant cells, thus precluding the use of these techniques in patients with conditions such as leukaemias.[4]

In the USA commercial distribution of cooling caps designed to produce localised scalp hypothermia was halted by the FDA in 1990 because of concerns about their effectiveness and their potential to create sanctuary sites and interfere with drug distribution elsewhere in the body. However, they continue to be available in many countries.

1. O'Brien R, *et al.* Scalp tourniquet to lessen alopecia after vincristine. *N Engl J Med* 1970; **283:** 1469.
2. Lyons AR. Prevention of hair loss by head-band during cytotoxic therapy. *Lancet* 1974; **i:** 354.
3. Pesce A, *et al.* Scalp tourniquet in the prevention of chemotherapy-induced alopecia. *N Engl J Med* 1978; **298:** 1204–5.
4. Dean JC, *et al.* Prevention of doxorubicin-induced hair loss with scalp hypothermia. *N Engl J Med* 1979; **301:** 1427–9.
5. Gregory RP, *et al.* Prevention of doxorubicin-induced alopecia by scalp hypothermia: relation to degree of cooling. *Br Med J* 1982; **284:** 1674.
6. Guy R, *et al.* Scalp cooling by thermocirculator. *Lancet* 1982; **i:** 937–8.

Bone-marrow depression. Use of granulocyte or granulocyte-macrophage colony-stimulating factors (G-CSF or GM-CSF), alone or in combination with autologous bone-marrow transplants, or peripheral blood stem-cells,[1] can markedly reduce the period of neutropenia after high-dose chemotherapy regimens.[2-4] The subject has been reviewed by Khwaja and Goldstone[6] and by Steward.[7] Whether the enhancement of neutrophil recovery seen with these colony-stimulating factors has objective benefits in terms of lower infection rates and reduced time in hospital may depend on the patients and the severity and duration of neutropenia—at present, clinical benefits are still ambiguous.[8-11] Interleukin-3, interleukin-6, and interleukin-11, have been evaluated for their ability to increase platelet numbers *in vivo* and the latter is now available as oprelvekin, which can reduce chemotherapy-induced thrombocytopenia.[17,18] Erythropoietin may be used to reduce requirements for transfusion of red cells. Interleukin-1α and macrophage colony-stimulating factor (M-CSF) have been investigated in the prevention or treatment of thrombocytopenia,[12,13] and stem cell factor is being developed for use in mobilising and transplanting peripheral stem cells.[5] Treatment with colony-stimulating factors has been generally well-tolerated and symptoms, such as fever and bone pain, controllable.[6,7] Although receptors for growth factors are present on several malignant cells lines stimulation of tumour growth does not appear to have been a problem so far. The field is still developing, with new growth factors being discovered, and their ultimate place in oncology remains to be determined. Although they are unlikely to be used with reasonably well-tolerated conventional chemotherapy because of their cost, they may permit the use of more intensive regimens. They play an integral role in mobilising peripheral stem cells to permit haematopoietic reconstitution by peripheral stem-cell (progenitor cell) transplantation.[5,14,15] Results suggest that in future combination therapy with several haematopoietic growth factors may prove more successful than use of single agents. However, the comment has been made that establishing which combinations are more efficient and effective in which circumstances may prove a logistical nightmare.[16]

1. Anonymous. Peripheral stem cells made to work. *Lancet* 1992; **339:** 648–9.
2. Fouillard L, *et al.* Recombinant human granulocyte-macrophage colony-stimulating factor plus the BEAM regimen instead of autologous bone marrow transplantation. *Lancet* 1989; **i:** 1460.
3. Gianni AM, *et al.* Granulocyte-macrophage colony-stimulating factor to harvest circulating haemopoietic stem cells for autotransplantation. *Lancet* 1989; **ii:** 580–4.
4. Sheridan WP, *et al.* Granulocyte colony-stimulating factor and neutrophil recovery after high-dose chemotherapy and autologous bone marrow transplantation. *Lancet* 1989; **ii:** 891–5.
5. Moskowitz CH, *et al.* Recombinant methionyl human stem cell factor and filgrastim for peripheral blood progenitor cell mobilization and transplantation in non-Hodgkin's lymphoma patients: results of a phase I/II trial. *Blood* 1997; **89:** 3136–47.
6. Khwaja A, Goldstone AH. Haemopoietic growth factors. *Br Med J* 1991; **302:** 1164–5.
7. Steward WP. Granulocyte and granulocyte-macrophage colony-stimulating factors. *Lancet* 1993; **342:** 153–7. Correction. *ibid.*: 679.
8. Anaissie EJ, *et al.* Randomized comparison between antibiotics alone and antibiotics plus granulocyte-macrophage colony-stimulating factor (Escherichia coli-derived) in cancer patients with fever and neutropenia. *Am J Med* 1996; **100:** 17–23.
9. Croockewit AJ, *et al.* Should hematopoietic growth factors routinely be given concurrently with cytotoxic chemotherapy? *Clin Pharmacol Ther* 1996; **59:** 1–6.
10. Hartmann LC, *et al.* Granulocyte colony-stimulating factor in severe chemotherapy-induced afebrile neutropenia. *N Engl J Med* 1997; **336:** 1776–80.
11. Pui C-H, *et al.* Human granulocyte colony-stimulating factor after induction chemotherapy in children with acute lymphoblastic leukemia. *N Engl J Med* 1997; **336:** 1781–7.
12. Smith JW, *et al.* The effects of treatment with interleukin-1α on platelet recovery after high-dose carboplatin. *N Engl J Med* 1993; **328:** 756–61.
13. Hatake K, *et al.* Macrophage colony-stimulating factor and platelet recovery after chemotherapy. *Lancet* 1993; **341:** 963.
14. Anonymous. Progenitor cell transplantation. *Drug Ther Bull* 1997; **35:** 62–4.
15. Brugger W, *et al.* Reconstitution of hematopoiesis after high-dose chemotherapy by autologous progenitor cells generated ex vivo. *N Engl J Med* 1995; **333:** 283–7.
16. Metcalf D. Hematopoietic regulators: redundancy or subtlety? *Blood* 1993; **82:** 3515–23.
17. Gordon MS, *et al.* A phase I trial of recombinant human interleukin-11 (neumega rhIL-11 growth factor) in women with breast cancer receiving chemotherapy. *Blood* 1996; **87:** 3615–24.
18. Isaacs C, *et al.* Randomized placebo-controlled study of recombinant human interleukin-11 to prevent chemotherapy-induced thrombocytopenia in patients with breast cancer receiving dose-intensive cyclophosphamide and doxorubicin. *J Clin Oncol* 1997; **15:** 3368–77.

Extravasation. Extravasation is the leakage of a vesicant or irritant drug into subcutaneous tissue during parenteral administration. This can result in ulceration and severe necrosis in some cases if not dealt with promptly. It is a particular problem with vesicant antineoplastics such as amsacrine, the anthracyclines (doxorubicin and its derivatives), carmustine, dacarbazine, dactinomycin, mitomycin, mustine, plicamycin, streptozocin, the taxanes (docetaxel and paclitaxel), and the vinca alkaloids. Carboplatin, methotrexate, mitozantrone, and the podophyllotoxin derivatives (etoposide and teniposide) are examples of irritant drugs which may also cause problems.

Measures to prevent the occurrence of extravasation include giving vesicant or irritant drugs via a central line, or peripherally via a recently sited cannula; vesicants are generally given by intravenous injection into a fast-running infusion. Glyceryl trinitrate patches may be used to dilate veins where venous access is a problem. The site of administration should be regularly checked, and the patient asked to report any untoward sensations.

If extravasation should occur the infusion should be stopped immediately and as much as possible of the infiltrating drug removed by aspiration. Beyond this, however, the management of extravasation is not well standardised and there has been disagreement as to the most appropriate course; there is little data from controlled studies and much practice is based on anecdotal reports and individual experience. Intravenous and subcutaneous injection of a corticosteroid (usually hydrocortisone) has been suggested, although some consider it ineffective or possibly even disadvantageous. Topical application of a 1% hydrocortisone cream to inflamed skin has also been suggested, and antihistamines and, if necessary, analgesics, may be given by mouth. In most cases application of a cold dressing or ice pack is appropriate. However, following extravasation of the taxanes, vinca alkaloids, or cisplatin the use of warm packs with hyaluronidase to enhance uptake from the skin has been recommended; a similar procedure has been suggested for large volume extravasations of the podophyllotoxin derivatives.

The use of specific antidotes is a particularly contentious area, since few are clinically validated and some (such as the use of sodium bicarbonate 8.4% for anthracycline extravasations) may do more harm than good. Brief infiltration of a less concentrated (2.1%) sodium bicarbonate solution, followed after a few minutes by aspiration, is still, however, advocated by some in the management of extravasations of the anthracyclines, carmustine, and plicamycin. Better accepted in the management of anthracycline and mitomycin extravasation is the topical application of dimethyl sulphoxide every 6 hours or so, sometimes alternated with hydrocortisone 1% cream. Sodium thiosulphate 3 or 4% has been used to infiltrate the site of extravasations of cisplatin, dactinomycin, or mustine.

The role of surgery is also important. It is unequivocally necessary in cases where other methods have failed to prevent evolving tissue damage, but there is some dispute as to the role of early surgery to remove drug-laden tissue and prevent the development of more serious ulceration and necrosis. Techniques of saline flushout and liposuction have been developed for removing drug and non-viable tissue while preserving overlying skin.

Some references to the management of extravasation are given below.

1. Brigden ML, Barnett JB. Local toxicity of cancer chemotherapy—practical considerations. *Can J Hosp Pharm* 1986; **39:** 96–9.
2. Dorr RT. Antidotes to vesicant chemotherapy extravasations. *Blood Rev* 1990; **4:** 41–60.
3. Stanley A. Managing complications of chemotherapy. In: Allwood M, *et al.*, eds. *The Cytotoxics Handbook*. 3rd ed. Oxford: Radcliffe Medical Press, 1997: 105–24.
4. Gault DT. Extravasation injuries. *Br J Plast Surg* 1993; **46:** 91–6.
5. Bertelli G. Prevention and management of extravasation of cytotoxic drugs. *Drug Safety* 1995; **12:** 245–55.

Mucositis. A number of drugs have been tried for the prophylaxis of mucositis caused by antineoplastic therapy, both directly and indirectly (due to neutropenia and infection).[1] Some degree of benefit has been demonstrated for sucralfate, chlorhexidine, or benzydamine in the prophylaxis of oral mucositis, and further studies were required to evaluate reports of benefit with dinoprostone, silver nitrate, betacarotene, oxpentifylline, and lozenges containing polymyxin B, tobramycin and amphotericin. However, allopurinol and granulocyte colony-stimulating factor were not considered effective for prophylaxis. Nonpharmacological treatments, including local cooling with ice chips, and low intensity helium-neon laser irradiation could also be beneficial in some circumstances. Given the number of variables involved in the development of mucositis it was thought unlikely that any one prophylactic regimen would prove suitable for all patients.

1. Verdi CJ. Cancer therapy and oral mucositis: an appraisal of drug prophylaxis. *Drug Safety* 1993; **9:** 185–95.

Nausea and vomiting. For a detailed discussion of the management of chemotherapy-induced nausea and vomiting, see p.1172.

Precautions

In view of their severe toxicity and possible carcinogenicity these drugs should generally be reserved for severe or life-threatening disease, and it is widely suggested that their use and administration should be confined to experienced staff in specialised centres.

Immunosuppression and bone-marrow depression are features of most of these drugs and their use is associated with an increased risk of infections caused by pathogenic or opportunistic micro-organisms, and a reduced capacity to cope with them. The use of live vaccines is contra-indicated in these patients, and the response to all vaccines is likely to be diminished. Those drugs which are immunosuppressant should not be given, where possible, to patients with acute infections, and dosage reduction or withdrawal should be considered if infection develops, until the infection has been controlled. For discussion of the treatment of infections in immunosuppressed patients, see p.127. Special care is necessary in debilitated patients.

Blood counts and measurement of haemoglobin concentrations should be carried out routinely to help predict the onset of bone-marrow depression. Great caution is needed when the marrow is already depressed following radiotherapy or therapy with other antineoplastics, and modification of dosage regimens may be required.

Although positive evidence of teratogenicity in humans is not available for all antineoplastic agents, pregnancy should be avoided in women receiving antineoplastics: in particular they should not be given, if possible, during the first trimester. Mothers receiving antineoplastic therapy should not breast feed. Because some regimens may result in permanent infertility in male patients the storage of semen samples before such therapy may be desirable.

Many antineoplastic drugs are vesicant or irritant. Care must be taken to avoid extravasation since severe pain and tissue damage may ensue. They must be handled with great care and contact with skin and eyes avoided; they should not be inhaled. In many countries official or professional guidelines on precautions for the safe handling of cytotoxic drugs have been issued.

For precautions specific to particular drugs, see under the individual monographs.

Administration in the elderly. Concern has been expressed by workers in a number of countries that neoplastic disorders in the elderly are undertreated because of an impression that these diseases are less aggressive, and the effects of chemotherapy more likely to be severe, in this age group.[1-3] Although there is a suggestion that haematopoietic reserve is reduced with increasing age, which might lead to greater sensitivity to myelosuppression in the elderly,[3] old people vary as much as any other group in their response to drugs,[3] and the consensus is that they should not be excluded from any form of treatment on the grounds of age alone.[4] However, there have been few studies of chemotherapy specifically in elderly patients, and selection of a suitable dosage regimen is more difficult in consequence.[2]

1. Phister JE, *et al.* Problems in the use of anticancer drugs in the elderly. *Drugs* 1989; **37:** 551–65.
2. Fentiman IS, *et al.* Cancer in the elderly: why so badly treated? *Lancet* 1990; **335:** 1020–2.
3. Gurwitz JH, Avorn J. The ambiguous relation between aging and adverse drug reactions. *Ann Intern Med* 1991; **114:** 956–66.
4. Tirelli U, *et al.* Cancer treatment and old people. *Lancet* 1991; **338:** 114.

Contraception. Immunosuppressive treatment contra-indicates the use of an intra-uterine device for contraception.[1]

1. Anonymous. Medical factors in contraceptive choice. *Drug Ther Bull* 1986; **24:** 73–6.

Down's syndrome. Results suggesting that children with Down's syndrome may tolerate myelosuppressive chemotherapy less well than other children, possibly due to abnormalities of drug metabolism, particularly of methotrexate.[1]

1. Blatt J, *et al.* Excessive chemotherapy-related myelotoxicity in children with Down syndrome and acute lymphoblastic leukaemia. *Lancet* 1986; **ii:** 914.

Handling and disposal. Many antineoplastics are potent and potentially highly toxic drugs, which must be handled with due care. In many countries official or professional guidelines are available for the handling, reconstitution, and disposal of antineoplastic agents,[1-6] and most centres or institutions in which these drugs are used will have individual handling policies based on these.[7]

Recommendations generally include:

that these drugs be reconstituted by trained personnel;

that reconstitution take place in designated areas, designed to protect personnel and the environment—for example, the use of safety cabinets;

that protective clothing be worn, including gloves, eye protection, and masks if necessary (it should be noted that gloves may vary in their resistance to penetration, depending upon their thickness, the material of which they are made, and the drug in question. Double gloving has been recommended for dealing with major spillages, and for handling amsacrine, carmustine, mustine, and thiotepa in particular[7]);

that waste should be disposed of carefully in suitable separate containers, clearly labelled as to their contents (it should be noted that the patient's body fluids and excreta may contain appreciable amounts of antineoplastic agents and it has been suggested that they and materials such as bed linen contaminated with them should also be treated as hazardous waste[8,9]);

that adequate procedures should be in place for accidental contamination due to spillages;

that staff exposure to antineoplastic agents be recorded and monitored;

that pregnant staff should avoid handling these agents if possible.

1. A Working Party of the Pharmaceutical Society of Great Britain. Guidelines for the handling of cytotoxic drugs. *Pharm J* 1983; **230:** 230–1.
2. Clinical Oncology Society of Australia. Guidelines and recommendations for safe handling of antineoplastic agents. *Med J Aust* 1983; **1:** 426–8.
3. Council on Scientific Affairs of the American Medical Association. Guidelines for handling parenteral antineoplastics. *JAMA* 1985; **253:** 1590–2.
4. Asscher W. Handling cytotoxic drugs. *Br Med J* 1986; **292:** 59–60.
5. Occupational Safety and Health Administration. OSHA work-practice guidelines for personnel dealing with cytotoxic (antineoplastic) drugs. *Am J Hosp Pharm* 1986; **43:** 1193–1204.
6. American Society of Hospital Pharmacists. ASHP technical assistance bulletin on handling cytotoxic and hazardous drugs. *Am J Hosp Pharm* 1990; **47:** 1033–49.
7. Allwood M, Wright P, eds. *The Cytotoxics Handbook.* 2nd ed. Oxford: Radcliffe Medical Press, 1993.
8. Harris J, Dodds LJ. Handling waste from patients receiving cytotoxic drugs. *Pharm J* 1985; **235:** 289–91.
9. Cass Y, Musgrave CF. Guidelines for the safe handling of excreta contaminated by cytotoxic agents. *Am J Hosp Pharm* 1992; **49:** 1957–8.

HIV infection and AIDS. Use of conventional cytotoxic therapy to treat Kaposi's sarcoma (p.496) in patients with the acquired immunodeficiency syndrome (AIDS) has resulted in unexpectedly severe myelosuppression, and there is some evidence that chemotherapy further damages the immune system, increasing the risk of opportunistic infections.[1]

1. Volberding PA. The clinical spectrum of the acquired immunodeficiency syndrome: implications for comprehensive patient care. *Ann Intern Med* 1985; **103:** 729–33.

Pregnancy. The teratogenic effects of antineoplastics on the fetus have been frequently reviewed.[1-3] The highest risk seems to be associated with alkylating agents and antimetabolites, in particular the folic-acid antagonists.[2] The incidences of spontaneous abortion and malformation are reported to reach 70% and 40% respectively with aminopterin.[2] Other agents reported to be teratogenic or potentially teratogenic include azathioprine,[2] busulphan,[1-3] chlorambucil,[1-3] cyclophosphamide,[2,3] dactinomycin,[2] fluorouracil,[1,3] mercaptopurine,[1,3] methotrexate,[2,3] mustine,[1,3] the podophyllotoxin derivatives,[2] procarbazine,[3] thiotepa,[1] vinblastine,[2,3] and vincristine.[2,3] However, in an early review Sokal and Lessmann presented evidence that some of these drugs have proved less toxic to the fetus than had been anticipated, particularly when treatment was deferred until after the first trimester.[1] Although it is wise to avoid the use of potentially teratogenic drugs during pregnancy, the risk to the mother of inadequate treatment may outweigh whatever risks exist of abnormality in the fetus.

There has also been concern that long-term occupational exposure to antineoplastics might have an adverse effect on the fetus of pregnant health-care workers: a study in 650 Finnish nurses found that women who experienced fetal loss were more than twice as likely to have had first trimester exposure to antineoplastic drugs as women who successfully gave birth.[4] These results have been criticised on the grounds that such results are not seen in cancer patients,[5,6] who presumably are exposed to much higher doses of antineoplastic agents, but are nonetheless cause for concern. Another study[7] has suggested that the rate of ectopic pregnancy may be increased in nurses occupationally exposed to antineoplastics, but the small number of ectopic pregnancies involved (15 in 734 pregnancies) means that the association with antineoplastics may be due to chance, and again, such an effect does not appear to have been reported in women treated with antineoplastic agents.

See also Effects on Reproductive Potential, above.

1. Sokal JE, Lessmann EM. Effects of cancer chemotherapeutic agents on the human fetus. *JAMA* 1960; **172:** 1765–71.
2. Ashton H. Teratogenic drugs. *Adverse Drug React Bull* 1983; (Aug): 372–5.
3. Kalter H, Warkany J. Congenital malformations. *N Engl J Med* 1983; **308:** 491–7.
4. Selevan SG, *et al.* A study of occupational exposure to antineoplastic drugs and fetal loss in nurses. *N Engl J Med* 1985; **313:** 1173–8.
5. Kalter H. Antineoplastic drugs and spontaneous abortion in nurses. *N Engl J Med* 1986; **314:** 1048–9.
6. Mulvihill JJ, Stewart KR. Antineoplastic drugs and spontaneous abortion in nurses. *N Engl J Med* 1986; **314:** 1049.
7. Saurel-Cubizolles MJ, *et al.* Ectopic pregnancy and occupational exposure to antineoplastic drugs. *Lancet* 1993; **341:** 1169–71.

Interactions

Because of their effects on the gastro-intestinal mucosa antineoplastics have the potential to interfere with the absorption of other drugs given by mouth. In addition, many antineoplastics are inhibitors of certain subtypes of cytochrome P450 and some antineoplastics are also metabolised by these enzymes, and in consequence the possibility of interactions between antineoplastics, or between antineoplastics and concomitant medication, cannot be discounted.

For details of interactions affecting specific drugs see under the individual monographs.

References.

1. Le Blanc GA, Waxman DJ. Interaction of anticancer drugs with hepatic monooxygenase enzymes. *Drug Metab Rev* 1989; **20:** 395–439.
2. Loadman PM, Bibby MC. Pharmacokinetic drug interactions with anticancer drugs. *Clin Pharmacokinet* 1994; **26:** 486–500.
3. Kivistö KT, *et al.* The role of human cytochrome P450 enzymes in the metabolism of anticancer agents: implications for drug interactions. *Br J Clin Pharmacol* 1995; **40:** 523–30.
4. Mignat C. Clinically significant drug interactions with new immunosuppressive agents. *Drug Safety* 1997; **16:** 267–78.

Effects on other drugs. For reference to the effects of antineoplastics on the duration of action of suxamethonium, see p.1321. For the effects of antineoplastic drugs on the activity of oral anticoagulants, see Warfarin, p.967, and for their effects on phenytoin, see p.356.

Action

Much of the development of cancer chemotherapy has been based on an understanding of the way in which tumour cells grow, and the way in which the drugs affect this growth.

After cell division the daughter cells enter a period of growth, $\mathbf{G_1}$, which lasts for different lengths of time in different tissues. This is followed by a period of DNA synthesis, **S**, in which the amount of chromosomal material is doubled, then a postsynthetic, or premitotic, phase, $\mathbf{G_2}$, then finally by mitotic cell division, **M**. As an alternative to re-entering the cycle, the products of cell division may enter a kinetically-dormant, nonproliferative stage, $\mathbf{G_0}$, although it is not clear if this differs fundamentally from the G_1 phase, nor what recruits such 'resting' cells back into the cell cycle.

The rate of cell division varies for different tumours; the doubling time for Burkitt's lymphoma and acute lymphoblastic leukaemia is less than 5 days, whereas the mean doubling time for seminoma is about 20 days, that for small-cell lung cancer about 50 days, and those for colon cancer and advanced breast cancer about 100 and 150 days respectively. The range of reported doubling times may also vary widely for a particular tumour type. The majority of common cancers increase very slowly in size in comparison with sensitive normal tissues, including those from which they derive, and the rate may decrease further in large tumours. This difference allows normal cells to recover more quickly than malignant ones from chemotherapy, and is the rationale behind current cyclic dosage schedules. The lethal body tumour burden is reached when the tumour cell mass approaches or exceeds 1×10^{12} cells, equivalent to about 1 kg of tissue, and representing about 40 doublings.

Cell killing by cytotoxic agents is a first order process, so a given dose or course of antineoplastic kills a fixed percentage of tumour cells rather than a fixed number. Thus an agent which killed 99% of tumour cells would leave behind 10^{10} cells from a tumour containing 10^{12} cells, but only 10^2 cells from one containing 10^4, reinforcing the importance of treating malignant neoplasms as early as possible.

Cytotoxic drugs act to damage the reproductive integrity of cells. Some are active at a particular stage of the cell cycle. The antimetabolites all act at various points to interfere with DNA synthesis, as does hydroxyurea, and are thus active against cells in S phase, while the vinca alkaloids inhibit microtubular function and act on cells in phase M. Other agents such as the alkylating agents, the anthracyclines, and cisplatin are not phase-specific, but since their actions are dependent at least in part on damaging DNA they are more effective against proliferating cells, particularly in S phase. It is now thought that many antineoplastics exert their ultimate effect by inducing cellular apoptosis (programmed cell death). Some agents, such as bleomycin or vinblastine also have the property of arresting the cycle in a particular phase, and attempts have been made to synchronise tumour cell division in this way, to maximise the number of cells in a sensitive phase when a particular agent is given. However, in practice this approach has been less successful than early experimental results suggested.

Some drugs used in the treatment of neoplasms do not attack the tumour cells directly but are given in order to increase cell vulnerability to other modalities: these include radiosensitisers (which have proved of only limited benefit to date), and photosensitisers such as porfimer sodium, which are employed in photodynamic therapy (PDT) using lasers.

Apart from attacking cell division, increased understanding of the molecular biology of tumour cells has begun to open the possibility of other approaches to the treatment of malignant neoplasms. These include inducing tumour cells to differentiate into non-malignant forms, manipulation of cellular apoptosis, inhibiting the expression of abnormal growth factors, telomerases and other oncogene products (including the use of ribozymes or of 'antisense' compounds which inhibit oncogenic messenger RNA), control of tumour growth through inhibition of angiogenesis, prevention or inhibition of metastasis, and stimulating the immune system to recognise and attack tumour cells. Gene therapy (p.1583) is another form of treatment under consideration. However, such approaches remain largely experimental at present.

References to investigational modes of cancer therapy.

1. Hobbs JR. Immunotherapy of human cancers. *Br Med J* 1989; **299:** 1177–8.
2. Thomas H, Sikora K. Biological approaches to cancer therapy. *J Int Med Res* 1989; **17:** 191–204.
3. Anonymous. Molecular targets for cancer therapy. *Lancet* 1990; **335:** 826.
4. Sutton PM. Treatment of cancer by infectious nucleic acid. *Lancet* 1991; **337:** 1553.
5. Sikora K, James N. Immune modulation and cancer. *Br Med Bull* 1991; **47:** 209–26.
6. Rew DA, Wilson GD. Advances in cell kinetics. *Br Med J* 1991; **303:** 532–3.
7. Gutierrez AA, *et al.* Gene therapy for cancer. *Lancet* 1992; **339:** 715–21.
8. Goldenberg DM. Monoclonal antibodies in cancer detection and therapy. *Am J Med* 1993; **94:** 297–312.
9. Frei E. Gene deletion: a new target for cancer chemotherapy. *Lancet* 1993; **342:** 662–4.
10. Kim S. Liposomes as carriers of cancer chemotherapy: current status and future prospects. *Drugs* 1993; **46:** 618–38.
11. Ma DDF, Doan TL. Antisense oligonucleotide therapies: are they the 'magic bullets'? *Ann Intern Med* 1994; **120:** 161–3.
12. Voest EE, *et al.* Iron-chelating agents in non-iron overload conditions. *Ann Intern Med* 1994; **120:** 490–9.
13. Sikora K. Genes, dreams, and cancer. *Br Med J* 1994; **308:** 1217–21.
14. Culver KW, *et al.* Gene therapy for solid tumors. *Br Med Bull* 1995; **51:** 192–204.
15. Kiehntopf M, *et al.* Clinical applications of ribozymes. *Lancet* 1995; **345:** 1027–31.
16. Haber DA. Telomeres, cancer, and immortality. *N Engl J Med* 1995; **332:** 955–6.
17. Skuse GR, Ludlow JW. Tumor suppressor genes in disease and therapy. *Lancet* 1995; **345:** 902–6.
18. Houghton AN. On course for a cancer vaccine. *Lancet* 1995; **345:** 1384–5.
19. Baltz JK. Vaccines in the treatment of cancer. *Am J Health-Syst Pharm* 1995; **52:** 2574–85.
20. Askari FK, McDonnell WM. Antisense-oligonucleotide therapy. *N Engl J Med* 1996; **334:** 316–18.
21. Harris AL. Antiangiogenesis for cancer therapy. *Lancet* 1997; **349** (suppl II): 13–15.
22. Shu S, *et al.* Tumor immunology. *JAMA* 1997; **278:** 1972–81.
23. Weichselbaum RR, Kufe D. Gene therapy of cancer. *Lancet* 1997; **349** (suppl II): 10–12.
24. Martin LA, *et al.* Genetic prodrug activation therapy. *Lancet* 1997; **350:** 1793–4.

Resistance

Resistance to antineoplastics is one of the greatest limitations to the use of chemotherapy in malignant disease. Resistance may be intrinsic to the tumour or may be acquired during chemotherapy, which effectively acts to select resistant cells from a heterogeneous population; the latter is one reason that relapses, or malignancies in heavily-pretreated patients, may be particularly difficult to treat.

The mechanisms of resistance in cancer cells are complex and imperfectly understood, but appear to include:

- hypoxia and imperfect drug penetration in the centre of large, solid tumours
- the small proportion of cells actively dividing and thus vulnerable to antineoplastics (particularly in slow-growing tumours)
- decreased cellular uptake or increased efflux of antineoplastic
- increased metabolic breakdown or decreased activation of antineoplastic
- increased expression of target enzymes
- metabolism via alternative biochemical pathways to those blocked by the antineoplastic
- more efficient repair of damaged DNA
- possibly the expression of genes which inhibit drug-induced apoptosis.

Several of these mechanisms may be in operation at one time. Much interest has been expressed in the potential use of drugs which can modulate or inhibit mechanisms of resistance, and in particular in compounds such as verapamil, quinidine, and cyclosporin, which have the ability to block the action of p-glycoprotein, a membrane glycoprotein which acts as an efflux pump for a range of cytotoxic substances and which is responsible for the multi-drug resistant (MDR) phenotype. However, for sustained benefit it seems likely that several agents would be required, each to overcome a different mechanism of resistance, and it would be necessary to ensure that toxicity of antineoplastics to normal cells was not also enhanced.

If the emergence of heritable resistant phenotypes is a natural part of tumour-cell biology (the Goldie-Coldman hypothesis) it implies that the larger and older the tumour, the more likely is resistance to occur. This would confirm the benefits of surgery and radiotherapy to shrink the primary tumour, and of starting chemotherapy as soon as possible after (a preferably early) diagnosis.

Reviews of antineoplastic resistance.

1. Anonymous. Multidrug resistance in cancer. *Lancet* 1989; **ii:** 1075–6.
2. Hochhauser D, Harris AL. Drug resistance. *Br Med Bull* 1991; **47:** 178–96.
3. Booser DJ, Hortobagyi GN. Anthracycline antibiotics in cancer therapy: focus on drug resistance. *Drugs* 1994; **47:** 223–58.
4. Ling V. P-Glycoprotein: its role in drug resistance. *Am J Med* 1995; **99** (suppl 6A): 31S–34S.
5. Kaye SB. Clinical drug resistance: the role of factors other than P-glycoprotein. *Am J Med* 1995; **99** (suppl 6A): 40S–44S.
6. Holmes J. Multidrug resistance as a cause of cytotoxic drug failure. *Pharm J* 1996; **257:** 294–6.

Some drugs have been reported to partially abolish multidrug resistance to antineoplastics *in vitro*.[1] These include verapamil, its enantiomers and analogues such as Ro-11-2933; other calcium channel blockers including prenylamine, diltiazem, nifedipine analogues such as nicardipine and niludipine, and bepridil; various phenothiazines and thioxanthenes including trifluoperazine and the *trans*-isomer of flupenthixol, which lacks dopamine-antagonist properties and the consequent extrapyramidal effects; structural analogues of the anthracyclines and vinca alkaloids; progesterone and other steroid hormones, as well as, to some extent, anti-oestrogens such as tamoxifen; cyclosporin and various of its nonimmunosuppressive analogues (such as SDZ-PSC-833); and various miscellaneous agents including amiodarone, quinidine, propranolol, reserpine, yohimbine, dipyridamole, erythromycin, cefoperazone, and ceftriaxone.

However, despite reported effects on resistance *in vitro* clinical results may be less impressive: studies in which verapamil was added to therapy for small cell lung cancer[2] or multiple myeloma[3] failed to demonstrate any benefit.

1. Ford JM, Hait WN. Pharmacology of drugs that alter multidrug resistance in cancer. *Pharmacol Rev* 1990; **42:** 155–99.
2. Milroy R, *et al.* A randomised clinical study of verapamil in addition to combination chemotherapy in small cell lung cancer. *Br J Cancer* 1993; **68:** 813–18.
3. Dalton WS, *et al.* A phase III randomized study of oral verapamil as a chemosensitizer to reverse drug resistance in patients with refractory myeloma: a Southwest Oncology Group Study. *Cancer* 1995; **75:** 815–20.

Choice of Antineoplastic

Role of chemotherapy

In 1994, in a consultation document on cancer chemotherapy,[1] WHO considered that 24 drugs could be considered essential for the rational management of malignant neoplasms. These were: *asparaginase* for acute lymphoblastic leukaemia; *bleomycin* for germ-cell cancers, Hodgkin's disease, and Kaposi's sarcoma, as well as for palliation of cancers of the nasopharynx; *cisplatin* for germ-cell cancers, gestational trophoblastic tumours, epithelial ovarian cancer, and small cell lung cancer, and for palliation in bladder, cervical, nasopharyngeal, oesophageal, and head and neck cancers; *cladribine* for hairy-cell leukaemia; *cyclophosphamide* for breast cancer, non-Hodgkin's lymphoma, small cell lung cancer, epithelial ovarian cancer, neuroblastoma, Ewing's sarcoma and paediatric soft tissue sarcoma, and for palliation in chronic leukaemia; *cytarabine* for acute lymphoblastic and non-lymphoblastic leukaemias and non-Hodgkin's lymphoma; *dacarbazine* for Hodgkin's disease; *dactinomycin* for gestational trophoblastic tumours, Wilms' tumour, Kaposi's sarcoma, Ewing's sarcoma, and paediatric soft tissue sarcoma; *daunorubicin* for acute non-lymphoblastic leukaemias; *doxorubicin* for Hodgkin's disease and non-Hodgkin's lymphoma, breast cancer, small cell lung cancer, neuroblastoma, Ewing's sarcoma, osteosarcoma and paediatric soft tissue sarcoma, as well as for palliation in bladder cancer and adult soft tissue sarcoma; *etoposide* for germ-cell cancers and small cell lung cancer; *fluorouracil* for malignancies of the breast, colon, and rectum, and for palliation in advanced gastro-intestinal malignancy, cervical, head and neck, and nasopharyngeal cancer; *hydroxyurea* for palliation in chronic myeloid leukaemia; *mercaptopurine* for acute lymphoblastic leukaemia; *mustine* for Hodgkin's disease; *methotrexate* for acute lymphoblastic leukaemia, gestational trophoblastic tumours, breast cancer, and osteosarcoma, and for palliation in bladder and head and neck cancers; *mitomycin* for palliation of cancer of the anus; *procarbazine* for Hodgkin's disease; *tamoxifen* for breast cancer and the palliation of endometrial cancer; *vinblastine* for germ-cell cancers, Hodgkin's disease, and Kaposi's sarcoma; and *vincristine* for acute lymphoblastic leukaemia, Hodgkin's and non-Hodgkin's lymphomas, Wilms' tumour, small cell lung cancer, neuroblastoma, Ewing's sarcoma and paediatric soft tissue sarcoma. The list also includes *calcium folinate* for use in colorectal metastases (with fluorouracil), *levamisole* as an adjuvant in colon cancer, and *prednisone* in leukaemias, lymphomas, and multiple myeloma.

Despite the real benefits achieved in selected conditions, reassessment of the role and value of chemotherapy for malignant neoplasms has led a number of oncologists to express the view that it has not lived up to its promise. Braverman suggested in 1991 that for many or most patients medical management should be confined to symptom management and enrolment in a hospice programme, with a considerable reduction in the prescription of antineoplastics and a confinement of studies to agents with novel mechanisms of action, or refinement of regimens known to be effective,[2] a view he has since re-iterated.[3] Similar views have been expressed by others during the 1980s and 90s, pointing out the failure of treatment for most common adult tumours,[4] and suggesting that widespread use of chemotherapy is not justified outside clinical trials or specialised centres.[5,6] Bailar and Smith, in a statistical review in 1986, suggested that the 'war against cancer' was being lost, and that concentration on prevention rather than treatment might produce more promising results.[7] Despite acknowledging some areas of progress, an update of this review including data up to the end of 1994 came to the same conclusion.[8] Others have also pointed out the failure to adequately address methods for cancer prevention.[9]

Such views have naturally provoked controversy, and others consider that developments in the use of adjuvant and intensive regimens, as well as the continuing development of new agents, are significant and should not be denigrated.[10-14] However, the frequent reference to the hoped-for benefits of a greatly-improved knowledge of the molecular biology of cancer, and in particular the use of biological response modifiers,[11,15] or gene therapy,[16] does seem to concede that present chemotherapeutic regimens could be improved. Whether dose intensification is one appropriate route for improvement is a matter of some debate.[17,18]

It has been suggested that perhaps attempts to destroy cancer cells are based on a false analogy between oncology and microbiology, and that a more appropriate goal would be the restoration of mechanisms of cellular control, enabling the patient to live with their cancer. Understanding of malignancy as a process, involving complex interactions between the malignant cell and its environment, in which intervention may be feasible to restore regulation of cellular growth, offers a potentially useful approach to cancer treatment. However, such an approach remains largely theoretical at present.[9,19,20]

1. WHO. Essential drugs for cancer chemotherapy. *Bull WHO* 1994; **72:** 693–8.
2. Braverman AS. Medical oncology in the 1990s. *Lancet* 1991; **337:** 901–2.
3. Braverman AS. Chemotherapeutic failure: resistance or insensitivity? *Ann Intern Med* 1993; **118:** 630–2.
4. Kearsley JH. Cytotoxic chemotherapy for common adult malignancies: the emperor's new clothes revisited? *Br Med J* 1986; **293:** 871–6.
5. Milsted RAV, *et al.* Cancer chemotherapy—what have we achieved? *Lancet* 1980; **i:** 1343–6.

6. Mead GM. Chemotherapy for solid tumours: routine treatment not yet justified. *Br Med J* 1995; **310:** 246–7.
7. Bailar JC, Smith EM. Progress against cancer? *N Engl J Med* 1986; **314:** 1226–32.
8. Bailar JC, Gornik HL. Cancer undefeated. *N Engl J Med* 1997; **336:** 1569–74.
9. Sporn MB. The war on cancer. *Lancet* 1996; **347:** 1377–81.
10. Tobias JS. Medical oncology in the 1990s. *Lancet* 1991; **337:** 1220.
11. Chabner BA, Rothenberg ML. Medical oncology in the 1990s. *Lancet* 1991; **338:** 576–7.
12. Chabner BA. Biological basis for cancer treatment. *Ann Intern Med* 1993; **118:** 633–7.
13. Cunningham D. Chemotherapy for solid tumours; important progress in treatment. *Br Med J* 1995; **310:** 247–8.
14. Kramer BS, Klausner RD. Grappling with cancer—defeatism versus the reality of progress. *N Engl J Med* 1997; **337:** 931–4.
15. Malpas JS. Oncology. *Postgrad Med J* 1990; **66:** 80–93.
16. Lemoine NR, Sikora K. Interventional genetics and cancer treatment. *Br Med J* 1993; **306:** 665–6.
17. Hryniuk W. Will increases in dose intensity improve outcome: pro. *Am J Med* 1995; **99** (suppl 6A): 69S–70S.
18. Souhami RL. Will increases in dose intensity improve outcome: con. *Am J Med* 1995; **99** (suppl 6A): 71S–76S.
19. Astrow AB. Rethinking cancer. *Lancet* 1994; **343:** 494–5.
20. Schipper H, *et al.* A new biological framework for cancer research. *Lancet* 1996; **348:** 1149–51.

Management of malignant disease

Carcinoid tumours and other secretory neoplasms. All neoplastic cells have some abnormalities of metabolism, and many secrete characteristic metabolic products. Where the substance secreted has hormonal or pharmacological properties profound clinical effects may result, particularly since secretion is generally unregulated by normal homoeostatic mechanisms. Examples of syndromes associated with such secretory neoplasms include acromegaly (p.1235) and other endocrine disorders associated with pituitary adenomas, phaeochromocytoma (p.795), carcinoid syndrome, and the various syndromes associated with pancreatic endocrine tumours.

Carcinoid syndrome. Carcinoid tumours occur mainly in the gastro-intestinal tract, although they occasionally arise in other organs with a common embryological origin. Although they are relatively common, accounting for about 30% of all small bowel tumours, symptomatic carcinoid syndrome is rare, both because the tumours vary in their behaviour depending on their embryological origin and because the liver is capable of metabolising those tumour products which are secreted into the portal circulation; only if the carcinoid tumour secretes into the systemic circulation, notably after metastasis to the liver, do symptoms occur. Tumours of embryological foregut origin, usually found in the stomach, predominantly secrete histamine or serotonin (5-HT); mid-gut tumours, with a usual primary site in the terminal ileum, are the most likely to metastasise and produce carcinoid syndrome, and predominantly secrete serotonin; hind-gut tumours, commonly benign, do not secrete active substances.

The characteristic symptoms of carcinoid syndrome include flushing of the face and upper trunk (which may be provoked by alcohol, food, or stress), secretory diarrhoea, wheezing and dyspnoea, weight loss, pellagra, painful hepatomegaly, and right-sided cardiac fibrosis, which sometimes progresses to right heart failure and death.

The management of carcinoid tumours is largely symptomatic,[1-3] although if the primary tumour has not metastasised surgical resection can be curative. Antineoplastic chemotherapy appears to be of little value, although there are occasional reports of its use,[4-6] and given the relatively slow and benign course of the disease the toxicities of intensive chemotherapy would be difficult to justify. There is some evidence that treatment with interferon alfa can stabilise the disease or occasionally produce tumour regression,[8] although some authorities remain sceptical about its value.[2] Hepatic arterial embolisation to destroy the blood supply of the tumours has produced symptomatic palliation but its effects are temporary and it has been associated with significant morbidity and mortality although better results have been seen in some recent studies.[3] Results may be better in combination with chemotherapy in selected patients.[3,7]

For symptomatic relief of carcinoid syndrome somatostatin analogues such as octreotide or lanreotide appear to be emerging as the treatment of choice.[3,9-11] Excellent results have been reported from self-administration of subcutaneous octreotide,[9] which appears to be well tolerated. Octreotide may also be useful in the perioperative management of these patients, in whom anaesthetic management is difficult.[12] However, with prolonged use some patients develop resistance even to the highest doses.[3] Since in many cases symptoms are due primarily to 5-HT release, antagonists such as cyproheptadine or the 5-HT_3 antagonist ondansetron have proved helpful in providing symptomatic relief; ketanserin and high-dose methysergide have also been tried. Fenclonine, which inhibits the conversion of tryptophan to 5-HT, can also produce symptomatic relief but its use is limited by a high incidence of adverse effects. For patients with histamine-secreting gastric carcinoid, a combination of histamine H_1- and H_2-antagonists such as cimetidine and diphenhydramine is sometimes, but not always, useful.[13-15]

Apart from such specific pharmacological therapies, antidiarrhoeals such as codeine phosphate and loperamide are sometimes helpful in controlling diarrhoea. Wheezing (bronchoconstriction) and heart failure are managed conventionally. Supplementation with nicotinamide is advisable to prevent pellagra. It is also important to avoid provocative factors such as stress, alcohol, and particular foods.[1-3]

Pancreatic endocrine tumours. Neoplasms of the pancreatic islet cells, whether benign or malignant, usually secrete clinically significant amounts of hormone; the hormone secreted, and hence the resultant clinical syndrome, depends on which of the several types of hormone-secreting islet cells is the origin of the tumour. Primary therapy for solitary islet-cell tumours is surgical resection; metastatic islet-cell carcinoma may require a combination of symptomatic drug therapy, chemotherapy, radiotherapy, and surgical debulking. In contrast to the generally gloomy prognosis in patients with cancer of the exocrine pancreas, islet-cell carcinoma often responds to chemotherapy with streptozocin, either alone[16,17] or combined with other drugs such as fluorouracil[18] or doxorubicin.[19] Chlorozotocin is also active.[19] Chemotherapy may produce significant improvements in survival.[7,16] Symptomatic control can often be achieved with somatostatin, or more usually a long-acting analogue such as octreotide.[20-23]

In patients with **insulinoma** (tumours originating in the islet beta cells) excessive insulin secretion results in hypoglycaemia. Where surgical resection is not feasible or not successful diazoxide is probably the treatment of choice to control hypoglycaemia. Although beneficial results have been achieved with octreotide,[20-23] this treatment is perhaps less successful than in some of the other islet cell neoplasms.

In **glucagonoma** the primary neoplasm derives from the alpha cell and the clinical syndrome (a characteristic skin rash known as necrolytic migratory erythema, diabetes mellitus or glucose intolerance, weight loss, and anaemia) results from excessive glucagon secretion. Surgical resection is indicated for localised disease but the majority of cases have metastasised at presentation; surgical debulking of the tumour mass may ameliorate symptoms of metastatic disease. Antineoplastic chemotherapy (see above) may however produce significant remissions. Octreotide usually decreases glucagon secretion and improves symptoms.[20,24] Zinc supplements may be useful in improving skin rash.

Another well characterised syndrome results from tumours which release vasoactive intestinal polypeptide (VIP). Such **vipomas** result in profound but intermittent secretory diarrhoea, with consequent hypokalaemia and acidosis; the syndrome is sometimes known as pancreatic cholera. Surgical resection is the treatment of choice and may be considered even in metastatic disease because of the profound systemic effects of the tumour. Metabolic imbalances should be corrected by fluid and electrolyte supplementation. Dramatic responses to octreotide therapy have also been seen,[25-28] and it may be useful for symptom control before surgery as well as for palliation in metastatic disease. Transient responses have been seen to a variety of other drugs.

Of the other pancreatic endocrine tumours **gastrinoma** is probably the commonest: it results in Zollinger-Ellison syndrome, the treatment of which is discussed on p.1176. Octreotide has been reported to be of benefit in reducing bone pain in a patient with gastrinoma metastasised to the skeleton.[29] Rarer tumours include **somatostatinoma** and **PPoma** (secreting pancreatic polypeptide) which may be treated with antineoplastic chemotherapy if surgery is infeasible.

1. Maton PN. The carcinoid syndrome. *JAMA* 1988; **260:** 1602–5.
2. Saini A, Waxman J. Management of carcinoid syndrome. *Postgrad Med J* 1991; **67:** 506–8.
3. Caplin ME, *et al.* Carcinoid tumour. *Lancet* 1998; **352:** 799–805.
4. Stathopoulos GP, *et al.* Tamoxifen in carcinoid syndrome. *N Engl J Med* 1981; **305:** 52.
5. Engstrom PF, *et al.* Streptozocin plus fluorouracil versus doxorubicin therapy for metastatic carcinoid tumor. *J Clin Oncol* 1984; **2:** 1255–9.
6. King MD, *et al.* Carcinoid syndrome: an unusual cause of diarrhoea. *Arch Dis Child* 1985; **60:** 269–271.
7. Moertel CG, *et al.* The management of patients with advanced carcinoid tumors and islet cell carcinomas. *Ann Intern Med* 1994; **120:** 302–9.
8. Öberg K, *et al.* Treatment of malignant carcinoid tumors: a randomized controlled study of streptozotocin plus 5-FU and human leukocyte interferon. *Eur J Cancer Clin Oncol* 1989; **25:** 1475–9.
9. Kvols LK, *et al.* Treatment of the malignant carcinoid syndrome: evaluation of a long-acting somatostatin analogue. *N Engl J Med* 1986; **315:** 663–6.
10. Altman AR, *et al.* Treatment of malignant carcinoid syndrome with a long-acting somatostatin analogue. *Arch Dermatol* 1989; **125:** 394–6.
11. Smith S, *et al.* Resolution of musculoskeletal symptoms in the carcinoid syndrome after treatment with the somatostatin analog octreotide. *Ann Intern Med* 1990; **112:** 66–8.
12. Veall GRQ, *et al.* Review of the anaesthetic management of 21 patients undergoing laparotomy for carcinoid syndrome. *Br J Anaesth* 1994; **72:** 335–41.
13. Roberts LJ, *et al.* Blockade of the flush associated with metastatic gastric carcinoid by combined histamine H_1 and H_2 receptor antagonists: evidence for an important role of H_2 receptors in human vasculature. *N Engl J Med* 1979; **300:** 236–8.
14. Wingert TD, *et al.* Histamine antagonists and carcinoid flush. *N Engl J Med* 1980; **302:** 234.
15. Pyles JD, *et al.* Histamine antagonists and carcinoid flush. *N Engl J Med* 1980; **302:** 234–5.
16. Broder LE, Carter SK. Pancreatic islet cell carcinoma II: results of therapy with streptozotocin in 52 patients. *Ann Intern Med* 1973; **79:** 108–18.
17. Woods SM, *et al.* Treatment of pancreatic islet cell carcinoma with streptozotocin—experience in 15 patients. *Gut* 1983; **24:** A596.
18. Moertel CG, *et al.* Streptozocin alone compared with streptozocin plus fluorouracil in the treatment of advanced islet-cell carcinoma. *N Engl J Med* 1980; **303:** 1189–94.
19. Moertel CG, *et al.* Streptozocin-doxorubicin, streptozocin-fluorouracil, or chlorozotocin in the treatment of advanced islet-cell carcinoma. *N Engl J Med* 1992; **326:** 519–23.
20. Kvols LK, *et al.* Treatment of metastatic islet cell carcinoma with a somatostatin analogue (SMS 201-995). *Ann Intern Med* 1987; **107:** 162–8.
21. Longnecker SM. Remission of symptoms of chemotherapy-refractory metastatic insulinoma using octreotide. *Drug Intell Clin Pharm* 1988; **22:** 136–8.
22. Hearn PR, *et al.* The use of SMS 201-995 (somatostatin analogue) in insulinomas: additional case report and literature review. *Horm Res* 1988; **29:** 211–13.
23. Eriksson B, *et al.* Treatment of malignant endocrine pancreatic tumors with a new long-acting somatostatin analogue, SMS 201-995. *Scand J Gastroenterol* 1988; **23:** 508–12.
24. Boden G, *et al.* Treatment of inoperable glucagonoma with the long-acting somatostatin analogue SMS 201-995. *N Engl J Med* 1986; **314:** 1686–9.
25. Clements D, Elias E. Regression of metastatic vipoma with somatostatin analogue SMS 201-995. *Lancet* 1985; **i:** 874–5.
26. Ch'ng JL, *et al.* Remission of symptoms during long term treatment of metastatic pancreatic endocrine tumours with long acting somatostatin analogue. *Br Med J* 1986; **292:** 981–2.
27. Maton PN, *et al.* Successful therapy of pancreatic cholera with the long-acting somatostatin analogue SMS 201-995. *Scand J Gastroenterol* 1986; **21:** 181–6.
28. Juby LD, *et al.* Somatostatin analogue SMS 201-995 long term therapy for vipoma. *Postgrad Med J* 1987; **63:** 287–9.
29. Burgess JR, *et al.* Effective control of bone pain by octreotide in a patient with metastatic gastrinoma. *Med J Aust* 1996; **164:** 725–7.

Gestational trophoblastic tumours. The gestational trophoblastic tumours are derived from the trophoblast, the first tissue to differentiate in the early embryo, and thus are associated with conception and pregnancy and affect women of reproductive age. They may be divided into invasive mole and choriocarcinoma; a third tumour, placental site trophoblastic tumour, comes under the broader heading of gestational trophoblastic disease, a term that also encompasses hydatidiform mole.

Choriocarcinoma arises from a mole in about 50% of cases, but may also occur after normal delivery, abortion, or ectopic pregnancy. Invasive mole is hydatidiform mole that has penetrated deeply into the uterine wall, has produced metastases, or both. All these tumours secrete human chorionic gonadotrophin (hCG), and measurement of the urinary or serum concentrations, which are generally proportional to the total tumour mass, is important in diagnosis of disease and monitoring of treatment.

The trophoblastic tumours vary in aggressiveness but some, such as choriocarcinoma, are highly invasive and rapidly fatal if untreated; however, appropriate treatment, based on the perceived risk category, can result in an excellent prognosis. Prognostic factors for increased risk include high titres of hCG, liver or brain metastases, and failure of previous single-agent chemotherapy as well as, perhaps, greater age. With current treatment, including local irradiation for metastases, virtually 100% of patients with localised disease should be cured, as are over 70% of patients with more advanced stages.

In patients with gestational trophoblastic tumours (choriocarcinoma or invasive mole) who have **low-risk** disease the treatment of choice is single-agent chemotherapy with methotrexate.[1,2] Dactinomycin or etoposide have also been used.[2-4] The vinca alkaloids, bleomycin, cisplatin, cyclophosphamide, doxorubicin, fluorouracil, hydroxyurea, and mercaptopurine also have some activity in this disease.[2,3] Various of these agents have been used in patients considered to be at high or medium risk, in a variety of combination regimens. Regimens that have been suggested for **medium-risk** patients include MAC III (methotrexate, dactinomycin, and cyclophosphamide) or the more complex EHMMAC (based on etoposide, with hydroxyurea, methotrexate, mercaptopurine, dactinomycin, vincristine, and cyclophosphamide).[2] In **high-risk** patients various modifications of the fairly toxic CHAMOMA regimen (hydroxyurea, vincristine, methotrexate, melphalan, dactinomycin, and doxorubicin) have been used, such as CHAMOCA (substituting cyclophosphamide for melphalan),[2] although there is some evidence that the MAC regimen (methotrexate, dactinomycin, chlorambucil) is just as effective as modified CHAMOMA.[5] However, given the effectiveness of etoposide-based regimens, EMA-Co (etoposide, methotrexate, dactinomycin, cyclophosphamide, and vincristine) has been said to be the current preferred treatment in high-risk patients.[4]

Brain or liver metastases are generally treated by local irradiation.

1. Bagshawe KD, *et al.* The role of low-dose methotrexate and folinic acid in gestational trophoblastic tumours (GTT). *Br J Obstet Gynaecol* 1989; **96:** 795–802.
2. WHO. Gestational trophoblastic diseases: report of a WHO scientific group. *WHO Tech Rep Ser 692* 1983.
3. Anonymous. Drugs of choice for cancer chemotherapy. *Med Lett Drugs Ther* 1997; **39:** 21–8.
4. Berkowitz RS, Goldstein DP. Chorionic tumors. *N Engl J Med* 1996; **335:** 1740–8.
5. Curry SL, *et al.* A prospective randomized comparison of methotrexate, dactinomycin, and chlorambucil versus methotrexate, dactinomycin, cyclophosphamide, doxorubicin, melphalan, hydroxyurea, and vincristine in "poor prognosis" metastatic gestational trophoblastic disease: a Gynecologic Oncology Group study. *Obstet Gynecol* 1989; **73:** 357–62.

Histiocytic syndromes. Langerhans-cell histiocytosis (histiocytosis X) encompasses a spectrum of disorders characterised by proliferation of histiocytes, with giant cell formation, granuloma, and fibrosis. It includes eosinophilic granuloma, which typically produces single destructive bone lesions; Hand-Schüller-Christian disease, in which multiple bone lesions may be linked with exophthalmos and diabetes insipidus; and the usually fatal Letterer-Siwe syndrome, in which there are bone lesions, skin infiltration, lymphadenopathy, and hepatosplenomegaly. These disorders mainly present in childhood, and are of uncertain aetiology: it is not clear whether they should be considered malignancies.

The morbidity and prognosis of Langerhans-cell histiocytosis depends upon the number of organ systems involved, and whether normal function of these organs is affected. Patients with restricted disease have a generally benign course, and single lesions often regress spontaneously; if not, topical corticosteroids, or if necessary mild systemic chemotherapy or local irradiation, have been used for skin lesions, or curettage, intralesional corticosteroids, or radiotherapy for a bone lesion.[1]

In more extensive disease the prognosis is not as good, mainly due to organ dysfunction.[1] Topical mustine has been used for multiple skin lesions.[2] Systemic chemotherapy has been widely used, because the disease tends to be progressive in these patients, but its degree of benefit is uncertain[1,3-5] and some consider it primarily of value for palliation.[5] A comparative study of the effects of vinblastine or etoposide, both of which have been widely used in moderate- to high-risk patients, was initiated in 1991.[6] Cyclosporin has also been reported to produce benefit,[7] while it has been suggested that the use of cladribine[8] or anti-CD1 monoclonal antibodies[9] may offer improved therapeutic options in the future.

1. Egeler RM, D'Angio GJ. Langerhans cell histiocytosis. *J Pediatr* 1995; **127:** 1–11.
2. Sheehan MP, *et al.* Topical nitrogen mustard: an effective treatment for cutaneous Langerhans cell histiocytosis. *J Pediatr* 1991; **119:** 317–21.
3. Broadbent V, Pritchard J. Histiocytosis X—current controversies. *Arch Dis Child* 1985; **60:** 605–7.
4. The Writing Group of the Histiocyte Society. Histiocytosis syndromes in children. *Lancet* 1987; **i:** 208–9.
5. Komp DM. Concepts in staging and clinical studies for treatment of Langerhans' cell histiocytosis. *Semin Oncol* 1991; **18:** 18–23.
6. Ladisch S, *et al.* LCH-I: a randomized trial of etoposide vs vinblastine in disseminated Langerhans cell histiocytosis. *Med Pediatr Oncol* 1994; **23:** 107–10.
7. Mahmoud HH, *et al.* Cyclosporine therapy for advanced Langerhans cell histiocytosis. *Blood* 1991; **77:** 721–5.
8. Saven A, *et al.* 2-Chlorodeoxyadenosine-induced complete remissions in Langerhans-cell histiocytosis. *Ann Intern Med* 1994; **121:** 430–2.
9. Kelly K, *et al.* CD1 antibody immunolocalisation in Langerhans' cell histiocytosis. *Lancet* 1993; **342:** 367–8.

Leukaemias, acute. The acute leukaemias are malignancies affecting haematopoietic precursor cells. They are relatively rare (about 1 to 3 cases per 100 000 of population), and of uncertain cause in the majority of cases, although radiation, carcinogenic substances, or oncogenic retroviruses have been implicated in some types, and certain individuals appear to have a genetic predisposition to these diseases.

Following the initiating event or events the progeny of the affected cell do not differentiate normally but proliferate in an uncontrolled fashion. The result is the accumulation in the blood and bone marrow of immature cell types (blasts) at the expense of normal functional blood cells.

The acute leukaemias may be broadly divided into **acute lymphoblastic leukaemia** (ALL), in which the neoplastic proliferation affects lymphoid cell lines, and the **acute non-lymphoblastic leukaemias** (ANLL), variously known as acute myeloid or acute myelogenous leukaemias (AML), which affect myeloid cell lines. These broad groups can be divided in various ways. ALL is sometimes divided morphologically into L1, L2, and L3 subtypes; alternatively, an immunophenotypic classification, which distinguishes disease of B- and T-cell lineage, may be preferred. For ANLL the French-American-British (FAB) classification is widely used. This distinguishes, by lineage and estimated degree of differentiation:

M1, ANLL without differentiation
M2, ANLL with differentiation
M3, acute promyelocytic leukaemia
M4, acute myelomonocytic leukaemia
M5, acute monocytic leukaemia
M6, erythroleukaemia
M7, megakaryocytic leukaemia.

Alternatively, the term M0 may be used for acute undifferentiated leukaemia with M1 being used for disease with minimal differentiation. Knowledge of the genotype, via cytogenetic or molecular analysis, is becoming increasingly important in the treatment of leukaemia.

Acute leukaemia usually presents with anaemia, infection (due to granulocytopenia), and bleeding (mainly due to thrombocytopenia). Onset is usually rapid with ALL, although ANLL may be preceded by myelodysplasia lasting months or years. Bone pain, and enlargement of liver, spleen and lymph nodes due to infiltration of leukaemic cells may occur. Other organs may also be affected, and various metabolic disturbances, including hyperuricaemia, hyponatraemia, and hypokalaemia may be present.

If untreated the acute leukaemias are normally fatal, usually within months. However, these malignancies are among those in which medical treatment can make a substantial difference to life expectancy, and in some cases a permanent remission may be effected.

ACUTE LYMPHOBLASTIC LEUKAEMIA. Treatment of acute lymphoblastic leukaemias may be divided into several phases: induction of remission, prevention of CNS disease, and maintenance, or consolidation or intensification therapy.

In patients classified as having standard risk, vincristine and corticosteroids form the basis of **induction of remission.**[1-3] Vincristine by intravenous injection weekly, plus prednisone or prednisolone daily by mouth can induce haematological remission in over 90% of children, and in at least 50% of adults.[2] However, it is now accepted that better remission rates and more prolonged remissions can be achieved with more intensive induction therapy. The most usual induction regimen involves addition of asparaginase and daunorubicin to vincristine and the corticosteroid. Some induction regimens include cyclophosphamide. In a randomised study Gottlieb *et al.* found that addition of daunorubicin to induction therapy with vincristine, prednisone, and asparaginase improved remission rates from 47 to 83% in similar groups of adult patients.[4] In children too, results have shown the benefit of more intensive induction, despite the greater toxicity involved.[5-8] Results from Germany indicate that by use of an intensive induction regimen, with additional treatment for children deemed at high risk of relapse, a group containing many patients with unfavourable prognostic indicators such as male sex and high white-cell count can achieve about a 60% chance of disease-free survival at 5 years, at the cost of increased toxicity.[5] The use of dexamethasone, rather than prednisolone, in the induction regimen appears to yield improved event-free survival and a lower incidence of CNS relapse.[9]

The majority of children who achieve an initial remission will subsequently relapse with meningeal involvement unless **CNS therapy** directed at the sanctuary sites in the meninges is undertaken. Standard therapy consists of a combination of cranial irradiation with intrathecal methotrexate or sometimes cytarabine.[1,2] However, such a combination does carry some risk of serious sequelae, including leucoencephalopathy, particularly when high doses of methotrexate are given. Effective prophylaxis can reduce the incidence of CNS relapse to well below 10%.[10,11] Prophylaxis with chemotherapy alone (intrathecal methotrexate, hydrocortisone or prednisolone, and cytarabine) has also been tried.[9-13] The value of CNS prophylaxis in adult acute lymphoblastic leukaemia is less well established since CNS relapse is rarer in adults but it can still occur in up to 40% of cases, and the rate of CNS relapse can be reduced by appropriate CNS prophylaxis, tailored to the patient's perceived risk.[14]

Once remission has been achieved, further chemotherapy is indicated to prevent relapse. Two strategies have been used: consolidation or intensification, and maintenance.

Consolidation or **intensification** therapy involves continuation of intensive chemotherapy regimens after the achievement of complete remission. The UKALL Trial X showed that addition of intensification therapy at 5 and 20 weeks from the beginning of induction, (using cytarabine, etoposide, thioguanine, and daunorubicin), produced 5-year disease-free survival of 71% compared with 57% in those who received only maintenance therapy.[15] Benefit was seen even in children considered at low risk of treatment failure. Results in adults have been contradictory but appear to suggest a longer duration of remission with intensive consolidation therapy.[1] **Re-induction** therapy (repeating induction therapy shortly after the induction of remission) has produced improved results in adults and children.[3]

Maintenance therapy is generally given for some 2 to 3 years after remission;[1-3] at present in the UK treatment is continued for 100 weeks from diagnosis.[16] The standard combination of drugs consists of daily mercaptopurine, weekly methotrexate, and prednisolone and vincristine monthly. Three years rather than two years of maintenance therapy is associated with a lower risk of relapse but not a markedly different survival rate.[17] Some protocols provide for periods of re-induction therapy alternating with standard maintenance,[1,8] and such intensive therapy is associated with an absolute improvement of about 4% in long-term survival.[17] It has been suggested that individualisation of methotrexate dosage to take account of the patient's ability to clear the drug can improve the outcome.[18]

It is generally agreed that patients who maintain remission for 4 years after the end of maintenance therapy are at little risk of relapse and may be regarded as effectively cured. Between 50% and 80% of children entering remission may now expect to be cured.[2,19] Age of less than 2 or greater than 10 at presentation, male sex (in part because of the risk of testicular relapse), high white-cell count, presence of a mediastinal mass, and CNS disease at presentation are all high-risk factors, probably reflecting the presence of different biological species of acute lymphoblastic leukaemia with different treatment requirements.[2,20]

Cure rates in adults have been relatively poor until recently, but with intensive chemotherapy are starting to improve, particularly in those with favourable risk factors such as T-cell or common type ALL, or age below 35 years; overall, prolonged survival or cure may be achievable in 15 to 50%,[1-3] although realistically, expected cure rates are closer to 25% in most centres.[21,22] Patients with ALL positive for the Philadelphia chromosome have the poorest prognosis.[23]

Patients who relapse after stopping treatment can usually be brought to **second remission**, often by a repeat of their original induction therapy.[1,2] However, if relapse occurs during treatment the prognosis is poor, and chemotherapy is unlikely to bring lasting benefit. Some extension of second remission may be obtained through therapy with teniposide and cytarabine; Rivera and colleagues concluded that intensive chemotherapy including teniposide and cytarabine could produce durable second remissions in about half the patients whose initial remissions had lasted 18 months or more.[24]

The role of **bone-marrow transplantation** in the treatment of acute lymphoblastic leukaemia is a matter of some controversy.[25,26] In children, bone-marrow transplantation is essentially reserved for those who relapse. Allogeneic bone-marrow transplantation has been reported to produce stable remission in up to 50% of patients,[27,28] but many authorities consider its value limited.[29-31] The value of autologous transplantation in those children without an HLA-matched donor is even less clear.[32] In adults, allogeneic bone-marrow transplantation has been compared with chemotherapy in patients in first remission: despite a lower relapse rate in the transplanted group survival rates were ultimately similar because of a greater treatment-related mortality in transplant patients.[33] It was therefore suggested that (as in children), adult patients without exceptional risk factors should have allogeneic bone-marrow transplantation (where possible) held in reserve for the management of relapse.

Some of the value of allogeneic marrow transplants seems to depend upon graft-versus-host effects,[34,35] and compromise may be necessary between antileukaemic efficacy and preventing graft-versus-host reactions; there is some evidence that methotrexate prophylaxis of graft-versus-host disease leads to a lower risk of leukaemia recurrence than cyclosporin or T-cell depletion.[36] The use of autologous bone-marrow transplantation avoids the problems of finding suitably matched donors, and of graft-versus-host disease, but may be less effective for this very reason,[34,35] and carries the risk of re-introducing malignant cells unless the bone marrow can be completely purged: the techniques available for purging are considered, at best, experimental.[37]

1. McCauley DL. Treatment of adult acute leukemia. *Clin Pharm* 1992; **11:** 767–96.
2. Juttner CA. Changing concepts in the management of leukaemia. *Med J Aust* 1989; **151:** 43–51.
3. Pui C-H, Evans WE. Acute lymphoblastic leukemia. *N Engl J Med* 1998; **339:** 605–15.
4. Gottlieb AJ, *et al.* Efficacy of daunorubicin in the therapy of adult acute lymphocytic leukemia: a prospective randomized trial by Cancer and Leukemia Group B. *Blood* 1984; **64:** 267–74.
5. Riehm H, *et al.* The Berlin childhood acute lymphoblastic leukemia therapy study, 1970-1976. *Am J Pediatr Hematol Oncol* 1980; **2:** 299–306.
6. MRC Working Party on Leukaemia in Childhood. Improvement in treatment for children with acute lymphoblastic leukaemia: The Medical Research Council UKALL Trials, 1972-84. *Lancet* 1986; **i:** 408–11.
7. Gaynon PS, *et al.* Intensive therapy for children with acute lymphoblastic leukaemia and unfavourable presenting features: early conclusions of study CCG-106 by the Childrens Cancer Study Group. *Lancet* 1988; **ii:** 921–4.
8. Rivera GK, *et al.* Improved outcome in childhood acute lymphoblastic leukaemia with reinforced early treatment and rotational combination chemotherapy. *Lancet* 1991; **337:** 61–6.
9. Veerman AJP, *et al.* Dutch Childhood Leukaemia Study Group: early results of study ALL VI (1984-88). *Haematol Blood Transfus* 1990; **33:** 473–7.
10. Anonymous. Leukaemia and the central nervous system. *Lancet* 1985; **i:** 1196–8.
11. Blaney SM, *et al.* Current pharmacological treatment approaches to central nervous system leukaemia. *Drugs* 1991; **41:** 702–16.
12. Komp DM, *et al.* CNS prophylaxis in acute lymphoblastic leukemia: comparison of two methods: a Southwest Oncology Group study. *Cancer* 1982; **50:** 1031–6.
13. Sullivan MP, *et al.* Equivalence of intrathecal chemotherapy and radiotherapy as central nervous system prophylaxis in children with acute lymphatic leukemia: a Pediatric Oncology Group study. *Blood* 1982; **60:** 948–58.
14. Cortes J, *et al.* The value of high-dose systemic chemotherapy and intrathecal therapy for central nervous system prophylaxis in different risk groups of adult acute lymphoblastic leukemia. *Blood* 1995; **86:** 2091–7.
15. Chessells JM, *et al.* Intensification of treatment and survival in all children with lymphoblastic leukaemia: results of UK Medical Research Council trial UKALL X. *Lancet* 1995; **345:** 143–8.
16. Chessells JM. Maintenance treatment and shared care in lymphoblastic leukaemia. *Arch Dis Child* 1995; **73:** 368–73.
17. Childhood ALL Collaborative Group. Duration and intensity of maintenance chemotherapy in acute lymphoblastic leukaemia: overview of 42 trials involving 12000 randomised children. *Lancet* 1996; **347:** 1783–8.
18. Evans WE, *et al.* Conventional compared with individualized chemotherapy for childhood acute lymphoblastic leukemia. *N Engl J Med* 1998; **338:** 499–505.
19. Rivera GK, *et al.* Treatment of acute lymphoblastic leukemia: 30 years' experience at St Jude Children's Research Hospital. *N Engl J Med* 1993; **329:** 1289–95.
20. Pinkel D. Current issues in the management of children with acute lymphocytic leukaemia. *Postgrad Med J* 1985; **61:** 93–102.
21. Kantarjian HM. Adult acute lymphocytic leukemia: critical review of current knowledge. *Am J Med* 1994; **97:** 176–84.
22. Ho TC, *et al.* Acute lymphocytic leukemia in adults: a retrospective study and analysis of current management options. *Mayo Clin Proc* 1994; **69:** 937–48.
23. Hoelzer D. Acute lymphoblastic leukemia—progress in children, less in adults. *N Engl J Med* 1993; **329:** 1343–4.
24. Rivera GK, *et al.* Intensive retreatment of childhood acute lymphoblastic leukemia in first bone marrow relapse: a Pediatric Oncology Group study. *N Engl J Med* 1986; **315:** 273–8.
25. Pinkel D. Allogeneic bone marrow transplantation in children with acute leukemia: a practice whose time has gone. *Leukemia* 1989; **3:** 242–4.
26. Chessells JM, *et al.* Bone marrow transplantation for high-risk childhood lymphoblastic leukaemia in first remission: experience in MRC UKALL X. *Lancet* 1992; **340:** 565–8.
27. Graham-Pole J. Treating acute lymphoblastic leukaemia after relapse: bone marrow transplantation or not? *Lancet* 1989; **ii:** 1517–18.
28. Barrett AJ, *et al.* Bone marrow transplants from HLA-identical siblings as compared with chemotherapy for children with acute lymphoblastic leukemia in a second remission. *N Engl J Med* 1994; **331:** 1253–8.
29. Chessells JM, *et al.* Bone-marrow transplantation has a limited role in prolonging second marrow remission in childhood lymphoblastic leukaemia. *Lancet* 1986; **i:** 1239–41.
30. Butturini A, *et al.* Which treatment for childhood acute lymphoblastic leukaemia in second remission? *Lancet* 1987; **i:** 429–32.
31. Darbyshire PJ, *et al.* Treatment of acute lymphoblastic leukaemia after relapse. *Lancet* 1990; **335:** 733.
32. Borgmann A, *et al.* Autologous bone-marrow transplants compared with chemotherapy for children with acute lymphoblastic leukaemia in a second remission: a matched-pair analysis. *Lancet* 1995; **346:** 873–6.
33. Zhang M-J, *et al.* Long-term follow-up of adults with acute lymphoblastic leukemia in first remission treated with chemotherapy or bone marrow transplantation. *Ann Intern Med* 1995; **123:** 428–31.
34. Gale RP, Butturini A. Autotransplants in leukaemia. *Lancet* 1989; **ii:** 315–17.
35. O'Connor NTJ. Haematology. *Postgrad Med J* 1990; **66:** 595–611.
36. International Bone Marrow Transplant Registry. Effect of methotrexate on relapse after bone-marrow transplantation for acute lymphoblastic leukaemia. *Lancet* 1989; **i:** 535–7.
37. Diagnostic and Therapeutic Technology Assessment (DATTA) Panel. Autologous bone marrow transplantation—reassessment. *JAMA* 1990; **263:** 881–7.

ACUTE NON-LYMPHOBLASTIC LEUKAEMIA. Treatment of acute non-lymphoblastic leukaemia is problematic because normal stem-cell precursors are sensitive to the agents used, and therapy aimed at myeloid leukaemic clones results in destruction of part of the normal stem-cell pool.

Induction of remission is usually possible with intensive chemotherapy. Most regimens are based on cytarabine with an anthracycline such as daunorubicin;[1-5] the first successful regimens also included thioguanine,[3,4] and some centres continue to use it, although most consider that it gives no additional advantage and have dropped it from induction protocols.[1,2] Excellent initial results with idarubicin,[6] especially in younger patients and those with very high white cell counts, make it a possible replacement for daunorubicin in combinations for induction of remission. Mitozantrone is another alternative to daunorubicin.[7] Addition of etoposide to induction protocols appears to improve results in younger patients.[8] Remission has been stated to be achievable in up to 80% of patients, but patients suffer severe neutropenia during induction and remission rate is to some extent dependent upon the standard of supportive care. Remission rates are lower in older patients (who form the majority of those with acute non-lymphoblastic leukaemia) or those with poor performance status or other risk factors. Additionally, care is required in comparisons of remission rate since one study has demonstrated that remission rate varied between 43.8 and 85.3% depending on the exclusion criteria used.[9]

As in acute lymphoblastic leukaemia (see above) there is a trend towards the use of more intensive induction regimens. Use of high-dose cytarabine (with daunorubicin and etoposide) has been reported to improve the duration of first remission and disease-free survival compared with standard doses of cytarabine.[10] Equally the timing of induction cycles may be important: intensive timing (where the second cycle was given 10 days after the first) has improved disease-free survival, despite more toxicity-related deaths, compared with the standard interval of 14 days or more.[11]

Many patients presenting with acute myeloid leukaemia are elderly, and debility or concomitant medical conditions may make intensive chemotherapy impossible: palliative treatment with oral hydroxyurea or etoposide is often given, while idarubicin or low-dose subcutaneous cytarabine may also be of benefit.[12] Good results have been reported with a combination of idarubicin and etoposide in elderly patients.[13]

Although appropriate management of patients in remission is less well established than for acute lymphoblastic leukaemia, results of intensive **consolidation** therapy with daunorubicin and high-dose cytarabine suggest that this combination may markedly improve the prospects for long-term survival, particularly in younger patients. Long-term survival rates in patients with ANLL are rarely much above 20% overall, but survival rates of about 50% of patients achieving first remission have been projected following such intensive consolidation therapy in selected groups.[2] Presumably, the theoretical advantage would be even greater if alternative, non-cross resistant drugs were used for consolidation therapy.

In contrast, routine use of **maintenance** chemotherapy does not appear to prolong duration of remission, or survival,[14,15] although absolute agreement on this point is lacking.[2,16]

CNS relapse is much less common in patients with ANLL than in acute lymphoblastic leukaemia, and in consequence prophylactic **CNS therapy** is not generally given.[2]

Because of the poorer prognosis there seems to be much wider acceptance of **bone-marrow transplantation** for acute non-lymphoblastic than acute lymphoblastic leukaemia. When performed in patients in first remission, allogeneic bone-marrow transplantation has been reported to produce a long-term survival rate of about 50%,[17-19] and similar benefits have been shown with autologous bone-marrow transplantation,[20-22] which is more readily available. However, because comparable survival rates have been achieved with chemotherapy alone,[23] some centres have reserved bone-marrow transplantation for patients who relapse and are brought to second remission.[1,19] The MRC AML10 Trial,[22] however, demonstrated benefit from autologous bone-marrow transplantation above that from intensive chemotherapy, and it was suggested that while reserving transplantation for salvage therapy in children and patients with good-risk disease was appropriate, in older patients and those with standard risk it might be better to employ the procedure in first remission.

Great interest has resulted from early results in some rare forms of acute non-lymphoblastic leukaemia in which relatively non-toxic therapy has been used for **induction of differentiation** in the leukaemic cells. Over 80% of patients with acute promyelocytic leukaemia (M3), which accounts for perhaps 10% of all adult ANLL, can achieve complete remission following treatment with tretinoin.[24] However the duration of remission is short unless consolidation, usually with an anthracycline- and cytarabine-based regimen, is given subsequently; prolonged maintenance with tretinoin has been thought unhelpful and resistance may develop, although one large study has reported benefit.[25] (The synthetic retinoid, tamibarotene (AM-80), has been used to induce remission in patients who relapsed following successful remission induction with tretinoin.[26]) The combination of tretinoin followed by chemotherapy has been shown to result in improved survival compared with chemotherapy alone.[25,27,28] Combination of tretinoin with a colony-stimulating factor may improve response.[29]

Unfortunately, these results appear to be achievable only because the characteristic chromosomal abnormalities in acute promyelocytic leukaemia result in an abnormal retinoic acid receptor. The development of agents which can effect differentiation in other forms of ANLL, and indeed in other neoplasms, seems likely to be a long and difficult task. However, in one report, the control of acute non-lymphoblastic leukaemia for several weeks following the use of a granulocyte colony-stimulating factor (filgrastim) was attributed to leukaemic cell differentiation,[30] although the benefit was temporary.

Among other experimental therapies under investigation the use of antisense oligonucleotides aimed at abnormal genes and the use of toxin-linked monoclonal antibodies are considered promising.

1. Stein RS. Advances in the therapy of acute nonlymphocytic leukemia. *Am J Med Sci* 1989; **297:** 26–34.
2. McCauley DL. Treatment of adult acute leukemia. *Clin Pharm* 1992; **11:** 767–96.
3. Gale RP, Cline MJ. High remission-induction rate in acute myeloid leukaemia. *Lancet* 1977; **i:** 497–9.
4. Rees JKH, Hayhoe FGJ. DAT (daunorubicin, cytarabine, 6-thioguanine) in acute myeloid leukaemia. *Lancet* 1978; **i:** 1360–1.
5. Rees JKH, *et al.* Principal results of the Medical Research Council's 8th acute myeloid leukaemia trial. *Lancet* 1986; **ii:** 1236–41.
6. Wiernik PH, *et al.* Cytarabine plus idarubicin or daunorubicin as induction and consolidation therapy for previously untreated adult patients with acute myeloid leukemia. *Blood* 1992; **79:** 313–19.
7. Arlin Z, *et al.* Randomized multicenter trial of cytosine arabinoside with mitoxantrone or daunorubicin in previously untreated adult patients with acute nonlymphocytic leukemia (ANLL). *Leukemia* 1990; **4:** 177–83.
8. Bishop JF, *et al.* Etoposide in acute nonlymphocytic leukemia. *Blood* 1990; **75:** 27–32.
9. The Toronto Leukemia Study Group. Results of chemotherapy for unselected patients with acute myeloblastic leukaemia: effect of exclusions on interpretation of results. *Lancet* 1986; **i:** 786–8.
10. Bishop JF, *et al.* A randomized study of high-dose cytarabine in induction in acute myeloid leukemia. *Blood* 1996; **87:** 1710–17.
11. Woods WG, *et al.* Timed sequential therapy improves postremission outcome in acute myeloid leukemia: a report from the Children's Cancer Group. *Blood* 1996; **87:** 4979–89.
12. Burnett AK, Eden OB. The treatment of acute leukaemia. *Lancet* 1997; **349:** 270–5.
13. Jackson GH, *et al.* The use of an all oral chemotherapy (idarubicin and etoposide) in the treatment of acute myeloid leukaemia in the elderly: a report of toxicity and efficacy. *Leukemia* 1997; **11:** 1193–6.
14. Sauter C, *et al.* Acute myelogenous leukaemia: maintenance chemotherapy after early consolidation treatment does not prolong survival. *Lancet* 1984; **i:** 379–82.
15. Champlin R, *et al.* Prolonged survival in acute myelogenous leukaemia without maintenance chemotherapy. *Lancet* 1984; **i:** 894–6.
16. Büchner T, *et al.* Role of chemotherapy for AML in remission. *Lancet* 1985; **i:** 1224.
17. Thomas ED, *et al.* Marrow transplantation for acute nonlymphoblastic leukaemia in first remission. *N Engl J Med* 1979; **301:** 597–9.
18. Champlin RE, *et al.* Treatment of acute myelogenous leukaemia: a prospective controlled trial of bone marrow transplantation versus consolidation chemotherapy. *Ann Intern Med* 1985; **102:** 285–91.
19. International Bone Marrow Transplant Registry. Transplant or chemotherapy in acute myelogenous leukaemia. *Lancet* 1989; **i:** 1119–22.
20. Zittoun RA, *et al.* Autologous or allogeneic bone marrow transplantation compared with intensive chemotherapy in acute myelogenous leukemia. *N Engl J Med* 1995; **332:** 217–23.
21. Ravindranath Y, *et al.* Autologous bone marrow transplantation versus intensive consolidation chemotherapy for acute myeloid leukemia in childhood. *N Engl J Med* 1996; **334:** 1428–34.
22. Burnett AK, *et al.* Randomised comparison of addition of autologous bone-marrow transplantation to intensive chemotherapy for acute myeloid leukaemia in first remission: results of MRC AML 10 trial. *Lancet* 1998; **351:** 700–8.
23. Mayer RJ, *et al.* Intensive postremission chemotherapy in adults with acute myeloid leukemia. *N Engl J Med* 1994; **331:** 896–903.
24. Warrell RP, *et al.* Acute promyelocytic leukaemia. *N Engl J Med* 1993; **329:** 177–89.
25. Tallman MS, *et al.* All trans-retinoic acid in acute promyelocytic leukemia. *N Engl J Med* 1997; **337:** 1021–8. Correction. *ibid.*; 1639.
26. Tobita T, *et al.* Treatment with a new synthetic retinoid, Am80, of acute promyelocytic leukemia relapsed from complete remission induced by all-trans retinoic acid. *Blood* 1997; **90:** 967–73.
27. Fenaux P, *et al.* Tretinoin with chemotherapy in newly diagnosed acute promyelocytic leukaemia. *Lancet* 1994; **343:** 1033.
28. Frankel SR, *et al.* All-trans retinoic acid for acute promyelocytic leukemia: results of the New York study. *Ann Intern Med* 1994; **120:** 278–86.
29. Usuki K, *et al.* Filgrastim combined with tretinoin in acute promyelocytic leukaemia. *Lancet* 1994; **343:** 803–4.
30. Cavenagh JD, *et al.* Treatment of acute myeloid leukaemia in pregnancy. *Lancet* 1995; **346:** 441–2.

Leukaemias, chronic. CHRONIC LYMPHOCYTIC LEUKAEMIA. Chronic lymphocytic leukaemia typically occurs in people over 50 years of age, and accounts for about 30% of leukaemias in the West although it is rare in the Far East. The clinical course is variable: low-risk patients, comprising about 30% of cases by the Rai classification, have a median survival of more than 10 years, while the 10% of cases classified as high risk have a median survival of 2 years; median survival in the intermediate group is about 6 years.[1]

In patients at low risk, cytotoxic therapy is not recommended unless disease-related symptoms such as fever and night sweats, bone-marrow failure, bulky disease or massive splenomegaly, recurrent bacterial infections, or progressive lymphocytosis occur.[2,3] Intermediate-risk patients with indolent disease are also not treated.

When therapy is required, it is essentially symptomatic and palliative. Continuous or intermittent chlorambucil has been most widely used, and is given until the indications for treatment are controlled or normalised;[1] response rates range from about 40 to 70%.[2] Cyclophosphamide has also been tried.[2] Although chlorambucil is usually combined with a corticosteroid (prednisone or prednisolone), there is now some doubt as to whether this has a real advantage over chlorambucil alone.[2,4] Corticosteroid therapy is, however, the treatment of choice where patients present with cytopenias due to an immune mechanism. Combination chemotherapy has been tried in some patients. However, addition of vincristine, and doxorubicin (COP or CHOP), has not been conclusively shown to be better than just chlorambucil and prednisone.[5] High-dose chlorambucil, together with prednisone, is reportedly more effective than CHOP in patients with advanced disease.[6] Similarly, a comparison of a combination of cyclophosphamide, doxorubicin, and prednisone versus fludarabine found the latter to give improved response rates in patients with advanced disease;[7] there was some evidence suggesting a potential survival advantage in previously untreated patients.

There are no established chemotherapy regimens for patients with chronic lymphocytic leukaemia once initial therapy has failed. The preferred second-line therapy is probably fludarabine,[1,2,5,8] which has produced some promising results alone and is under study in combination with chlorambucil. There are some preliminary reports of responses to cladribine.[9-11] Pentostatin has also been investigated.[1,5] In patients who fail treatment with conventional therapy, campath-1H has produced responses.[12]

Patients may require supportive care for systemic complications. Hypogammaglobulinaemia is common, and the chief cause of infections. Normal immunoglobulin may reduce the infection rate in these patients but it is not clear that it improves survival.[2] If infection occurs broad spectrum antibacterials will be required. Colony-stimulating factors and erythropoietin may be useful for associated cytopenias.

Recent results from patients given allogeneic bone-marrow transplants after chemoradiotherapy have suggested for the first time the possibility of cure in chronic lymphocytic leukaemia, but this approach is limited by the need for a suitable donor and must still be considered experimental.[1,2]

1. Foon KA, *et al.* Chronic lymphocytic leukemia: new insights into biology and therapy. *Ann Intern Med* 1990; **113:** 525–39.
2. Rozman C, Montserrat E. Chronic lymphocytic leukemia. *N Engl J Med* 1995; **333:** 1052–7. Correction. *ibid.*; 1515.
3. Cheson BD, *et al.* National Cancer Institute-sponsored working group guidelines for chronic lymphocytic leukemia: revised guidelines for diagnosis and treatment. *Blood* 1996; **87:** 4990–7.
4. Catovsky D, *et al.* CLL trials in the United Kingdom: the Medical Research Council CLL trials 1, 2 and 3. *Leukemia Lymphoma* 1991; **5** (suppl): 105–12.
5. Tefferi A, Phyliky RL. A clinical update on chronic lymphocytic leukaemia II: critical analysis of current chemotherapeutic modalities. *Mayo Clin Proc* 1992; **67:** 457–61.
6. Jaksic B, *et al.* High dose chlorambucil versus Binet's modified cyclophosphamide, doxorubicin, vincristine, and prednisone regimen in the treatment of patients with advanced B-cell chronic lymphocytic leukemia: results of an international multicenter randomized trial. *Cancer* 1997; **79:** 2107–14.
7. The French Cooperative Group on CLL, *et al.* Multicentre prospective randomised trial of fludarabine versus cyclophosphamide, doxorubicin, and prednisone (CAP) for treatment of advanced-stage chronic lymphocytic leukaemia. *Lancet* 1996; **347:** 1432–8.
8. Keating MJ, *et al.* Clinical experience with fludarabine in leukaemia. *Drugs* 1994; **47:** 39–49.
9. Juliusson G, Liliemark J. High complete remission rate from 2-chloro-2′-deoxyadenosine in previously treated patients with B-cell chronic lymphocytic leukemia: response predicted by rapid decrease of blood lymphocyte count. *J Clin Oncol* 1993; **11:** 679–89.
10. Juliusson G, Liliemark J. Complete remission of B-cell chronic lymphocytic leukaemia after oral cladribine. *Lancet* 1993; **341:** 54.
11. Delannoy A, *et al.* 2-Chlorodeoxyadenosine (CdA) for patients with previously untreated chronic lymphocytic leukemia (CLL). *Leukemia* 1995; **9:** 1130–5.
12. Osterborg A, *et al.* Phase II multicenter study of human CD52 antibody in previously treated chronic lymphocytic leukemia. *J Clin Oncol* 1997; **15:** 1567–74.

CHRONIC MYELOID LEUKAEMIA. Chronic myeloid (myelogenous) or chronic granulocytic leukaemia is a rare disease, occurring usually in older patients, and representing about a quarter of all adult leukaemias. It is associated in over 90% of cases with the presence in blood cells of an abnormal chromosome, the Philadelphia chromosome (Ph^1).[1-3] The median survival for patients with Ph^1-positive disease is about 5 to 6 years, while in Ph^1-negative disease, which carries a worse prognosis, median survival is about 25 months.[3]

During the chronic phase, which may last for several years, the patient may be asymptomatic and require no treatment. Where symptoms arise a course of palliative therapy with busulphan or hydroxyurea will usually provide relief for some time.[1-3] Both drugs can control haematological manifestations of the disease in more than 70% of patients,[3] with duration of chronic phase and overall survival perhaps somewhat better with hydroxyurea.[4] Other investigational agents which have produced some benefit in chronic phase include low-dose cytarabine[5] and homoharringtonine.[6] However, evidence from a number of recent studies[7-9] suggests that interferon alfa may be the treatment of choice. Some 70 or 80% of patients treated with interferon experience a haematological response, and about 30% seem to undergo suppression of the Ph^1-positive clone, a response associated with more prolonged survival. The optimum dosage for such therapy has yet to be determined:[3,10] although some good results have been reported with low-dose therapy[11] most reports of benefit have been with 5 million units per m^2 body-surface daily.[3] Results seem to be better in patients treated within 1 year of diagnosis.[3] Combination of interferon alfa with cytarabine produces increased suppression of the Ph^1-positive clone, and increased survival of 3 years.[12]

The onset of the subsequent transformed phase is unpredictable and may present as rapid onset of a blast cell crisis with the behaviour of an acute leukaemia, or a more gradual appearance of blast cells accompanied by gradual resistance to previous treatment (accelerated phase).[1-3] Transformation may produce lymphoblastic or myeloblastic cells and the disease may then be treated as acute lymphoblastic or non-lymphoblastic leukaemia, but cure, or even remission of long duration, is not generally possible with current chemotherapy regimens.[1-3]

In suitable patients, however, allogeneic bone-marrow transplantation may be curative, particularly when performed in the chronic phase.[13-15] Results with autologous transplantation have been less good, suggesting that some of the benefit may derive from a 'graft-versus-leukaemia' effect;[16] nonetheless, in selected patients, prolonged survival appears possible.[17] Deliberate induction of graft-versus-host disease with interferon alfa-2b and infusion of donor mononuclear cells has been used successfully to treat patients whose disease relapsed after allogeneic bone marrow transplantation.[18]

The results of bone-marrow transplantation may perhaps be improved by the use of differentiation-inducing agents to remove residual leukaemic cells: treatment with retinoic acid, cytarabine, and hexamethylene bisacetamide was reported to induce differentiation of the majority of acute myeloid blast cells *in vitro* and has been suggested as a potential post-transplantation therapy.[19] Interestingly, the retinoic acid derivative isotretinoin has been investigated in children with the juvenile form of chronic myeloid leukaemia.[20]

New treatments are badly needed to delay or control the transformed phase. Preliminary reports of a return to the chronic phase after treatment with plicamycin and hydroxyurea[21] do not seem to have led to further progress, but there have been suggestions of remission following the use of interferon alfa.[1,2] The use of antisense nucleotides directed against the abnormal genetic sequence is theoretically attractive,[22] but is difficult to achieve *in vivo*.

1. Champlin RE, Golde DW. Chronic myelogenous leukemia: recent advances. *Blood* 1985; **65:** 1039–47.
2. Juttner CA. Changing concepts in the management of leukaemia. *Med J Aust* 1989; **151:** 43–51.
3. Cortes JE, *et al.* Chronic myelogenous leukemia: a review. *Am J Med* 1996; **100:** 555–70.
4. Hehlmann R, *et al.* Randomized comparison of busulfan and hydroxyurea in chronic myelogenous leukemia: prolongation of survival by hydroxyurea. *Blood* 1993; **82:** 398–407.

5. Robertson MJ, *et al.* Hematologic remission and cytogenetic improvement after treatment of stable-phase chronic myelogenous leukemia with continuous infusion of low-dose cytarabine. *Am J Hematol* 1993; **43:** 95–102.
6. O'Brien S, *et al.* Homoharringtonine produces high hematologic and cytogenetic response rates in Philadelphia chromosome positive chronic myelogenous leukemia. *Blood* 1992; **80** (suppl 1): 358.
7. The Italian Cooperative Study Group on Chronic Myeloid Leukemia. Interferon alfa-2a as compared with conventional chemotherapy for the treatment of chronic myeloid leukemia. *N Engl J Med* 1994; **330:** 820–5.
8. Allan NC, *et al.* UK Medical Research Council randomised, multicentre trial of interferon-αn1 for chronic myeloid leukaemia: improved survival irrespective of cytogenetic response. *Lancet* 1995; **345:** 1392–7.
9. Kantarjian HM, *et al.* Prolonged survival in chronic myelogenous leukemia after cytogenetic response to interferon-α therapy. *Ann Intern Med* 1995; **122:** 254–61.
10. Talpaz M, Kantarjian H. Low-dose interferon-α in chronic myeloid leukemia. *Ann Intern Med* 1995; **122:** 728.
11. Schofield JR, *et al.* Low doses of interferon-α are as effective as higher doses in inducing remissions and prolonging survival in chronic myeloid leukemia. *Ann Intern Med* 1994; **121:** 736–44.
12. Guilhot F, *et al.* Interferon alfa-2b combined with cytarabine versus interferon alone in chronic myelogenous leukemia. *N Engl J Med* 1997; **337:** 223–9.
13. Goldman JM, *et al.* Bone marrow transplantation for patients with chronic myeloid leukemia. *N Engl J Med* 1986; **314:** 202–7.
14. Thomas ED, *et al.* Marrow transplantation for the treatment of chronic myelogenous leukemia. *Ann Intern Med* 1986; **104:** 155–63.
15. Diagnostic and Therapeutic Technology Assessment Panel. Allogeneic bone marrow transplantation for chronic myelogenous leukemia. *JAMA* 1990; **264:** 3208–11.
16. Butturini A, *et al.* Autotransplants in chronic myelogenous leukaemia: strategies and results. *Lancet* 1990; **335:** 1255–8.
17. Hansen JA, *et al.* Bone marrow transplants from unrelated donors for patients with chronic myeloid leukemia. *N Engl J Med* 1998; **338:** 962–8.
18. Porter DL, *et al.* Induction graft-versus-host disease as immunotherapy for relapsed chronic myeloid leukemia. *N Engl J Med* 1994; **330:** 100–6.
19. Hassan HT. Induced differentiation of leukaemic cells. *Lancet* 1990; **335:** 118.
20. Castleberry RP, *et al.* A pilot study of isotretinoin in the treatment of juvenile chronic myelogenous leukemia. *N Engl J Med* 1994; **331:** 1680–4.
21. Koller CA, Miller DM. Preliminary observations on the therapy of the myeloid blast phase of chronic granulocytic leukemia with plicamycin and hydroxyurea. *N Engl J Med* 1986; **315:** 1433–8.
22. Anonymous. Chronic myeloid leukaemia: potential for antisense therapy. *Lancet* 1992; **340:** 1262–3.

HAIRY-CELL LEUKAEMIA. Hairy-cell leukaemia is a rare, chronic, B-cell lymphoproliferative disorder marked by the presence of white blood cells with prominent cytoplasmic villi, pancytopenia, and splenomegaly. Splenectomy corrects pancytopenia in most patients and improves survival in some but about 80% of patients require other forms of treatment at some stage. Chlorambucil was formerly popular but was largely superseded by interferon. Interferon alfa-2a or -2b given for one year produces at least a partial response in most cases[1] but patients have a tendency to relapse once therapy is discontinued.

Excellent results have been reported with the purine analogues cladribine and pentostatin, which appear to be emerging as first-line treatments for this disease, with complete remission rates of 50% or more[2,4,5] after relatively short courses of therapy, and generally acceptable toxicity (pentostatin has produced severe toxicity at higher doses but is less toxic in the doses required for hairy-cell leukaemia). They do not appear to show cross-resistance, and cladribine has been used successfully in patients resistant to, or intolerant of, pentostatin.[3]

1. Gollard R, *et al.* The optimal management of hairy cell leukaemia. *Drugs* 1995; **49:** 921–31.
2. Kane BJ, *et al.* Pentostatin: an adenosine deaminase inhibitor for the treatment of hairy cell leukemia. *Ann Pharmacother* 1992; **26:** 939–47.
3. Saven A, Piro LD. Complete remissions in hairy cell leukemia with 2-chlorodeoxyadenosine after failure with 2'deoxycoformycin. *Ann Intern Med* 1993; **119:** 278–83.
4. Saven A, Piro L. Newer purine analogues for the treatment of hairy-cell leukemia. *N Engl J Med* 1994; **330:** 691–7.
5. Cheson BD, *et al.* Treatment of hairy cell leukemia with 2-chlorodeoxyadenosine via the group C protocol mechanism of the National Cancer Institute: a report of 979 patients. *J Clin Oncol* 1998; **16:** 3007–3015.

MYELODYSPLASIA. Myelodysplastic syndromes are low-grade neoplasms of haematopoietic stem cells characterised by anaemia, neutropenia, or thrombocytopenia in various combinations and have been described as smouldering leukaemia; progression to acute non-lymphoblastic leukaemia occurs in some patients. Patients are often elderly, and management is generally conservative. Many patients survive for a period with transfusions and antibiotic therapy alone, and there is often reluctance to introduce cytotoxic therapy. Isotretinoin or tretinoin, interferons, colony-stimulating factors, or low-dose cytarabine have been given to try to induce cellular differentiation but clinical studies are needed to provide better guidelines for the management of these patients.[1-5]

1. Larson RA. Management of myelodysplastic syndromes. *Ann Intern Med* 1985; **103:** 136–8.
2. Jacobs A. Myelodysplastic syndromes: pathogenesis, functional abnormalities, and clinical implications. *J Clin Pathol* 1985; **38:** 1201–17.
3. Oscier DG. The myelodysplastic syndromes. *Br Med J* 1997; **314:** 883–6.
4. Galton DAG. The myelodysplastic syndrome. *Br Med J* 1989; **299:** 582.
5. Provan D. Myelodysplastic syndromes. *Prescribers' J* 1997; **37:** 17–23.

Lymphomas. The malignant lymphomas are neoplastic disorders of the lymphoreticular cells. These cells are primarily located in the lymph nodes, but because of their wide distribution in the body lymphomas may arise in extranodal and extralymphatic tissues such as lung, gastro-intestinal tract, and skin.

The term covers a heterogeneous group of diseases, comprising two main subgroups: Hodgkin's disease, and the non-Hodgkin's lymphomas (NHL). The cellular origin of Hodgkin's disease is uncertain; the non-Hodgkin's lymphomas are monoclonal malignancies arising from B cells in about 80% of cases, with the remainder from cells of T lineage and from undifferentiated cells.

Management of patients with malignant lymphoma is largely determined by interpretation of histological features, and, especially for non-Hodgkin's lymphomas, by an allocation of subtype and grade. Various classification systems have been proposed for non-Hodgkin's lymphomas of which the National Cancer Institute Working Formulation is currently in wide use, although it has been suggested that improved diagnostic techniques, which are revealing new entities, and greater recognition of peripheral T-cell lymphomas, are making this system, too, obsolete.[1] Under the Working Formulation, non-Hodgkin's lymphomas are divided into *low grade*, including small lymphocytic, follicular small cleaved cell (the commonest type, occurring in about 22% of cases), and follicular mixed small cleaved and large cell lymphoma; *intermediate grade*, including follicular large cell, diffuse large cell (the next most common type, at about 20%), diffuse small cleaved cell, and diffuse mixed types; and *high grade*, including large cell immunoblastic, lymphoblastic, and small non-cleaved cell (including Burkitt's) lymphomas. More recently the International Lymphoma Study Group has proposed a revised classification for all lymphomas,[2] based on a division into B-cell, T-cell and natural killer cell, and Hodgkin's neoplasms.

1. Anonymous. Lymphoma classification—where now? *Lancet* 1992; **339:** 1084–5.
2. Harris NL, *et al.* A revised European-American classification of lymphoid neoplasms: a proposal from the International Lymphoma Study Group. *Blood* 1994; **84:** 1361–92.

HODGKIN'S DISEASE. Hodgkin's disease is a lymphoma of unknown aetiology characterised histologically by the presence of a particular type of giant cell, the Reed-Sternberg cell. It is more common in males than in females, and in the West is seen particularly in young adults and in the elderly, although the age distribution differs elsewhere.

It usually presents as painless enlargement of one or more lymph nodes, particularly in the neck or axillae. About a third of all patients also have constitutional symptoms of fever, weight loss, and night sweats, which carry adverse prognostic significance. In advanced disease, signs of organ infiltration may occur, as may infectious complications. The mass of the tumour may result in compression of vital organs.

Hodgkin's disease can be treated by radiotherapy or chemotherapy or both, and the choice of treatment depends on the volume and histological subtype of the tumour, the age of the patient, but particularly the stage of the disease. The Ann Arbor classification recognises 4 stages:

Stage I, with involvement of a single lymph node region or extralymphatic site;

Stage II, in which spread is restricted to lymph nodes and sites on one side of the diaphragm only;

Stage III, involving spread on both sides of the diaphragm with possible splenic and extralymphatic involvement;

Stage IV, where the patient has diffuse or disseminated disease in one or more extralymphatic organs or tissues.

Stages are subclassified A or B according to the absence or presence respectively of the aforementioned constitutional symptoms.[1] The more recent Cotswold staging system also includes a subclass X for patients with bulky disease.

There is some debate about the treatment of localised disease (stages I and II). Radiotherapy is probably the treatment of choice in adult patients with early disease and good prognosis, but in patients with poor prognostic characteristics the consensus appears to be that treatment should be with chemotherapy, alone or combined with radiotherapy.[1-6] The overall probability of survival in patients with early stage disease treated with radiotherapy alone is about 85 to 88%;[3,6] opinions differ as to whether results as good can be obtained with chemotherapy alone,[2,3] but combination therapy appears to improve control, although improvements in survival are small.[7] Initial treatment of early stage disease in children should probably always be with chemotherapy, as long-term adverse effects are likely to be less than with radiotherapy.[2,3]

Chemotherapy is generally considered to be the treatment of choice in advanced disease (stages III and IV). There are currently a number of 4-drug standard regimens available and the choice lies between one of these, alternating cycles of 2 different regimens, or a hybrid cycle that involves giving 7 or 8 drugs in the same course of treatment.[4] However, the single most important factor governing the outcome of chemotherapy is thought to be dose intensity of the drugs given. The earliest of the successful 4-drug regimens was combination chemotherapy with mustine, vincristine, procarbazine, and prednisone or prednisolone (MOPP) introduced by DeVita and colleagues.[8] No combination regimen has been conclusively shown to be more effective than MOPP,[1,3] but a number of MOPP-variant regimens exist which may be as effective and less toxic; these include substitution of chlorambucil for mustine (LOPP), vinblastine for vincristine (MVPP), and both of these changes in one regimen (ChlVPP). Complete remission can be achieved in 80 to 95% of patients with such regimens; although some subsequently relapse, salvage chemotherapy is reported to bring the overall cure rate to about 75%.[3] Further elaborations are possible: ChlVPP/EVA, using chlorambucil, vinblastine, procarbazine and prednisolone with etoposide, vincristine, and doxorubicin, has been reported to be superior to MVPP.[9]

An alternative to the MOPP-based regimens exists in a combination of doxorubicin, bleomycin, vinblastine, and dacarbazine (ABVD), introduced by Bonadonna and colleagues,[10] and found to be as effective as MOPP with a reduced risk of inducing sterility. It is not clear whether ABVD is in fact superior to MOPP for the treatment of Hodgkin's disease.[3,4] Better results have been reported with ABVD than with MOPP,[11] but such comparisons have been criticised in the past on the grounds that the dose-intensity of the MOPP regimen has often been suboptimal.[4] Similar objections have been raised when alternating cycles of MOPP and ABVD or ABV (without dacarbazine) were compared with MOPP alone:[12-14] it has frequently proved necessary to adjust the dosage of the MOPP regimen. However, DeVita has suggested that if alternating regimens are better tolerated it is preferable that they should be used correctly rather than using 4-drug programs poorly.[4] There is also a view gaining currency that doxorubicin-based chemotherapy, in adequate doses, is indicated in most patients with advanced Hodgkin's disease,[15] although it may be premature to dismiss MOPP based regimens.[16]

Other regimens have been tried, both for the conventional-dose salvage of refractory disease[3,17,18] and as first-line therapy,[3,19,20] but as yet none seems to have been proven much of an improvement on MOPP and ABVD-based regimens. However, high-dose salvage regimens, often combined with radiotherapy and employing bone-marrow transplantation or peripheral-blood stem-cell support appear to be curative in one-third or more of previously incurable patients.[3,4] Patients who are candidates for salvage therapy can be divided into 4 groups: those initially treated with radiotherapy who have a recurrence, in whom standard chemotherapy regimens are effective; those who never achieve complete remission with standard chemotherapy, in whom prognosis is very poor, and who are candidates for an intensive salvage regimen with autologous stem-cell or bone-marrow transplantation; those whose original remission lasted for over a year, of whom about a quarter will respond to re-treatment with standard therapy, but in whom intensive salvage regimens may be considered; and those whose remission is short, less than one year, in whom standard chemotherapy may be used to reduce tumour volume before intensive therapy and bone- marrow rescue.[4] Once again, dose intensity appears to play an important role in the success of salvage regimens: a comparison of the carmustine, etoposide, cytarabine, and melphalan (BEAM) regimen in very high doses, followed by autologous bone-marrow transplantation, found that progression-free survival was better than after treatment with the same drugs at doses which did not require bone-marrow rescue.[21] Benefit has been reported in a few patients with refractory disease given infusions of an anti-CD16/anti-CD30 monoclonal antibody.[22]

1. Mead GM, Whitehouse JMA. Clinical aspects of Hodgkin's disease. *Br Med J* 1988; **297:** 1562–4.
2. Brada M. Early stage Hodgkin's disease in adults: which is the correct treatment? *Postgrad Med J* 1989; **65:** 824–9.
3. Longo DL. The use of chemotherapy in the treatment of Hodgkin's disease. *Semin Oncol* 1990; **17:** 716–35.
4. DeVita VT, Hubbard SM. Hodgkin's disease. *N Engl J Med* 1993; **328:** 560–5.
5. Shore T, *et al.* A meta-analysis of stages I and II Hodgkin's disease. *Cancer* 1990; **65:** 1155–60.
6. Haybittle JL, *et al.* Review of British National Lymphoma Investigation studies of Hodgkin's disease and development of prognostic index. *Lancet* 1985; **i:** 967–72.
7. Specht L, *et al.* Influence of more extensive radiotherapy and adjuvant chemotherapy on long-term outcome of early-stage Hodgkin's disease: a meta-analysis of 23 randomized trials involving 3888 patients. *J Clin Oncol* 1998; **16:** 830–43.
8. DeVita VT, *et al.* Combination chemotherapy in the treatment of advanced Hodgkin's disease. *Ann Intern Med* 1970; **73:** 881–95.
9. Radford JA, *et al.* Results of a randomized trial comparing MVPP chemotherapy with a hybrid regimen, ChlVPP/EVA, in the initial treatment of Hodgkin's disease. *J Clin Oncol* 1995; **13:** 2379–85.
10. Bonadonna G, *et al.* Combination chemotherapy of Hodgkin's disease with adriamycin, bleomycin, vinblastine, and imidazole carboxamide versus MOPP. *Cancer* 1975; **36:** 252–9.
11. Canellos GP, *et al.* Chemotherapy of advanced Hodgkin's disease with MOPP, ABVD, or MOPP alternating with ABVD. *N Engl J Med* 1992; **327:** 1478–84.
12. Santoro A, *et al.* Alternating drug combinations in the treatment of advanced Hodgkin's disease. *N Engl J Med* 1982; **306:** 770–5.
13. Straus DJ, *et al.* Treatment of advanced Hodgkin's disease with chemotherapy and irradiation: controlled trial of two versus three alternating, potentially non-cross-resistant drug combinations. *Am J Med* 1984; **76:** 270–8.
14. Bonadonna G, *et al.* Alternating non-cross-resistant combination chemotherapy or MOPP in stage IV Hodgkin's disease: a report of 8-year results. *Ann Intern Med* 1986; **104:** 739–46.
15. Anonymous. Lymphoma classification—where now? *Lancet* 1992; **339:** 1084–5.
16. Aisenberg AC. MOPP, ABVD, or both to treat Hodgkin's disease. *N Engl J Med* 1993; **328:** 1045.
17. Miller AM, *et al.* All-oral chemotherapy in refractory Hodgkin's disease. *Lancet* 1991; **337:** 1408.
18. Lennard A. All-oral chemotherapy in refractory Hodgkin's disease. *Lancet* 1991; **338:** 57.
19. Diggs CH, *et al.* Treatment of advanced untreated Hodgkin's disease with SCAB—an alternative to MOPP. *Cancer* 1981; **47:** 224–8.
20. Wiernik PH, Schiffer CA. Long-term follow-up of advanced Hodgkin's disease patients treated with a combination of streptozocin, lomustine (CCNU), doxorubicin, and bleomycin (SCAB). *J Cancer Res Clin Oncol* 1988; **114:** 105–7.
21. Linch DC, *et al.* Dose intensification with autologous bone-marrow transplantation in relapsed and resistant Hodgkin's disease: results of a BNLI randomised trial. *Lancet* 1993; **341:** 1051–4.
22. Renner C, *et al.* Treatment of refractory Hodgkin's disease with an anti-CD16/CD30 bispecific antibody. *Cancer Immunol Immunother* 1997; **45:** 184–6.

MYCOSIS FUNGOIDES. Mycosis fungoides is the most important of the cutaneous T-cell lymphomas. It is considered to have 3 stages: a premycotic erythematous or patch phase, characterised by a pruritic rash resembling psoriasis, which may persist for years or even decades; an infiltrative or plaque phase, in which some patches become thickened, darker plaques with marked T-cell infiltration; and a tumour phase where lesions enlarge and ulcerate. Ultimately there may be visceral involvement or potentially fatal sepsis secondary to skin breakdown. A variant of mycosis fungoides presents as widespread pruritic erythroderma, accompanied by abnormal T-cells in the blood, and is known as the Sézary syndrome.

Treatment depends on disease stage and spread. Patients with limited and slowly progressive patch phase disease may be managed just with emollients and topical antipruritics, together with UVB irradiation,[1] given their good prognosis (median survival of up to 25 years). Others, however, have advocated the use of electron beam irradiation in the hope of producing cure.[2] In more aggressive patch phase disease, and in the plaque phase, a variety of therapies have been tried. Topical application of aqueous mustine solution produces a response in 80% of cases;[3] the effect does not appear to depend on the alkylating effect of the drug. Topical carmustine is a potential alternative,[4] and contact sensitisation with 2,4-dinitrochlorobenzene has been tried,[1] but a more common alternative is the use of methoxsalen plus ultraviolet light (PUVA). Electron beam radiation also produces responses, and some consider that it may improve survival,[2] although this is contentious.

In more advanced disease, systemic chemotherapy, usually with regimens effective in other lymphomas[5] such as COP (cyclophosphamide, vincristine, and prednisone), MOPP (mustine, vincristine, procarbazine, prednisone),[6,7] or cyclophosphamide, doxorubicin, vincristine, and etoposide,[8] may be given, and has been combined with electron beam radiotherapy.[6-8] However, despite often quite high response rates, responses are almost always of short duration, and there is little evidence that current regimens prolong survival. Nonetheless, aggressive therapy may be justified where control of symptoms can be achieved for a satisfactory period.[9]

Therapy with interferons has produced good results, especially in combination with PUVA[10,11] or extracorporeal photopheresis.[12,13] The place of agents such as cladribine, fludarabine, or temozolomide (all of which are reported to be active) in therapy remains to be determined. There is also some interest in the use of retinoids,[10] but anecdotal report of complete remission with a retinoid plus calcitriol[14] was not confirmed in 3 further patients.[15] This may have been because of the use of a different retinoid (isotretinoin rather than acitretin), but there is also a suggestion that different cutaneous T-cell lymphomas differ in sensitivity,[16,17] and some may even be encouraged to proliferate by retinoid therapy.[17] Responses have also been seen with the interleukin-2 fusion toxin denileukin diftitox.[18]

1. Lorincz AL. Cutaneous T-cell lymphoma (mycosis fungoides). *Lancet* 1996; **347:** 871–6.
2. Jones GW, Thorson B. Cutaneous T-cell lymphoma (mycosis fungoides). *Lancet* 1996; **348:** 130–1.
3. Vonderheid EC, *et al.* Long-term efficacy, curative potential and carcinogenicity of topical mechlorethamine chemotherapy in cutaneous T-cell lymphoma. *J Am Acad Dermatol* 1989; **20:** 416–28.
4. Zackheim HS, *et al.* Topical carmustine (BCNU) for cutaneous T cell lymphoma: a 15-year experience in 143 patients. *J Am Acad Dermatol* 1990; **22:** 802–10.
5. Anonymous. Drugs of choice for cancer chemotherapy. *Med Lett Drugs Ther* 1997; **39:** 21–8.
6. Hamminga L, van Vloten WA. Report of the Dutch Mycosis Fungoides Study Group. *Br J Dermatol* 1980; **102:** 477–8.
7. Sentis HJ, *et al.* Polychemotherapy in advanced mycosis fungoides. *Br J Dermatol* 1985; **112:** 232–3.
8. Kaye FJ, *et al.* A randomized trial comparing combination electron-beam radiation and chemotherapy with topical therapy in the initial treatment of mycosis fungoides. *N Engl J Med* 1989; **321:** 1784–90.
9. Young RC. Mycosis fungoides: the therapeutic search continues. *N Engl J Med* 1989; **321:** 1822–4.
10. Bunn PA, *et al.* Systemic therapy of cutaneous T-cell lymphomas (mycosis fungoides and the Sézary syndrome). *Ann Intern Med* 1994; **121:** 592–602.
11. Parry EJ, Mackie RM. Management of cutaneous T cell lymphoma. *Br Med J* 1994; **308:** 858–9.
12. Dippel E, *et al.* Extracorporeal photopheresis and interferon-α in advanced cutaneous T-cell lymphoma. *Lancet* 1997; **350:** 32–3.
13. Russell-Jones R, *et al.* Extracorporeal photopheresis in Sézary syndrome. *Lancet* 1997; **350:** 886.
14. French LE, *et al.* Remission of cutaneous T-cell lymphoma with combined calcitriol and acitretin. *Lancet* 1994; **344:** 686–7.
15. Thomsen K. Cutaneous T-cell lymphoma and calcitriol and isotretinoin treatment. *Lancet* 1995; **345:** 1583.
16. French LE, Saurat J-H. Treatment of cutaneous T-cell lymphoma by retinoids and calcitriol. *Lancet* 1995; **346:** 376.
17. Bagot M. Treatment of cutaneous T-cell lymphoma by retinoids and calcitriol. *Lancet* 1995; **346:** 376–7.
18. Saleh MN, *et al.* Antitumor activity of DAB_{389}IL-2 fusion toxin in mycosis fungoides. *J Am Acad Dermatol* 1998; **39:** 63–73.

NON-HODGKIN'S LYMPHOMAS. The non-Hodgkin's lymphomas are a heterogeneous group of malignancies which vary considerably in their behaviour, prognosis, and management.[1-7] A variety of classifications have been used, of which the National Cancer Institute Working Formulation, which identifies 10 basic types, classified as low-, intermediate-, or high- grade, is currently in wide use (see Lymphomas, above). The non-Hodgkin's lymphomas include Burkitt's lymphoma (a high-grade lymphoma), and mycosis fungoides (a cutaneous T-cell lymphoma which does not fit well into the Working Formulation classification), both of which are discussed separately.

The usual presentation of lymphomas is lymphadenopathy, which in low-grade lymphoma may develop insidiously over a long period. There may be constitutional symptoms of fever, night sweats, and weight loss. Extranodal involvement may occur, as may various symptoms due to organ compression by the tumour mass. Lymphomas of T-cell origin have a worse prognosis than B-cell lymphomas of the same type, and excess tumour bulk, involvement of bone marrow or gastro-intestinal tract, and elevated serum-lactic dehydrogenase concentrations are also adverse prognostic factors. Staging is of somewhat less importance as a determinant of treatment and prognosis than in Hodgkin's disease.

About 40% of all lymphomas seen in North America and western Europe are of *low grade*; follicular lymphoma is the commonest form.[5] They typically present in a patient aged 50 to 60, and follow a fairly chronic and indolent course, with a median survival of 7 or more years. However, they are difficult to manage, and, if advanced, rarely curable. If disease is limited, radiotherapy may achieve long-term freedom from disease, and, perhaps cure.[2,5] In more advanced disease treatment has not been shown to affect survival,[1] and is often withheld until symptoms require it. For similar reasons, when treatment is required, single agent therapy with chlorambucil or cyclophosphamide, sometimes with a corticosteroid such as prednisone or prednisolone in the initial stages, is preferred.[1,2] Patients treated with more aggressive chemotherapy tend to have remission earlier but the remissions do not last longer than those achieved more slowly with single agent therapy.[4] Nonetheless, because of the poor ultimate prognosis, particularly in younger patients, a number of protocols of intensive chemotherapy, sometimes combined with autologous bone-marrow transplantation, are under investigation:[4] they include cyclophosphamide, doxorubicin, vincristine, prednisone, and bleomycin (CHOP-Bleo);[8] prednisone, methotrexate, doxorubicin, cyclophosphamide, and etoposide, plus mustine, vincristine, procarbazine, and prednisone (ProMACE-MOPP);[9] and cyclophosphamide, doxorubicin, vincristine or teniposide, and prednisone plus interferon alfa.[10,11] These intensive regimens may also employ local radiotherapy.[8,9,12] The use of interferons as 'maintenance', has produced promising results.[13]

Patients with low-grade lymphomas who relapse can achieve second or third remissions with standard treatment, but the duration of remission tends to decrease.[4] Alternative therapies such as the use of cladribine,[14] the anti-CD20 antibody rituximab,[15,34] or toxin-linked or radiolabelled monoclonal antibodies,[16-19] offer some promise. Allogeneic bone-marrow transplantation can result in long-term remission.[20] Remission can also be achieved with myeloablative therapy followed by autologous bone-marrow transplantation.[21] The low-grade lymphomas are also at the centre of attempts to develop antitumour vaccines (see below).

Chemotherapy is the treatment of choice in late-stage *intermediate-grade* lymphoma: cure can be achieved in about half of all patients with large cell disease who enter complete remission with combined chemotherapy. However, patients with diffuse small cleaved cell and diffuse mixed large and small cell disease respond less well to chemotherapy despite the less aggressive natural history of these disorders, and in early stage disease radiotherapy may be a more appropriate treatment. Many of the regimens used for intermediate-grade lymphoma have included the vinca alkaloids and doxorubicin with alkylating agents: cyclophosphamide, vincristine, and prednisone (CVP or COP) and cyclophosphamide, doxorubicin, vincristine, and prednisone (CHOP) have been widely used. More intensive regimens such as MACOP-B (an intensive 12-week programme of cyclic methotrexate, doxorubicin, cyclophosphamide, vincristine, prednisone, and bleomycin) have come to be widely used in intermediate-grade lymphomas. However, some studies have cast doubt on the superiority of third generation regimens such as MACOP-B, m-BACOD (with dexamethasone rather than prednisone), or ProMACE-CytaBOM (prednisone, doxorubicin, cyclophosphamide, etoposide, cytarabine, bleomycin, vincristine, and methotrexate), over CHOP in the treatment of these diseases.[7,22,23]

Major difficulties are posed by the treatment of the *high-grade* lymphomas, which occur particularly in children and young adults. Doxorubicin-containing regimens such as CHOP and its derivatives are widely used;[7] combination with radiotherapy may produce better results in localised intermediate- or high-grade disease.[35] In children with lymphoblastic lymphoma, good results have been seen with protocols based on those used for high-risk acute lymphoblastic leukaemia (see above), including the use of CNS prophylaxis.[4] Good results have been seen with intensive chemotherapy using cyclophosphamide, doxorubicin, vincristine, and prednisone, with high-dose methotrexate plus folinic acid, and, in some patients, asparaginase; all patients also received CNS prophylaxis with intrathecal methotrexate alone or with cranial irradiation. Good results have also been reported from intensive chemotherapy in Burkitt's lymphoma (see below). In children or young adults who do not have lymphoblastic lymphoma, a regimen omitting continuation therapy with mercaptopurine and methotrexate, and with no radiotherapy, is adequate in most cases of locoregional disease.[24] Relapsed or refractory disease may respond to a combination of idarubicin and high-dose cytarabine, followed by maintenance with idarubicin and etoposide.[25] High-dose (myeloablative) chemotherapy and peripheral blood stem cell transfusion has increasingly come to represent standard salvage therapy in patients with relapsed chemosensitive disease.[7]

Many protocols call for more intensive therapy in lymphomas of T-cell origin, regardless of grade. Results from pentostatin and interferon alfa in these patients have been disappointing. Cutaneous T-cell lymphomas such as mycosis fungoides pose special problems; for discussion of the management of the latter, see Mycosis Fungoides, above. There is experimental evidence of benefit with a combination of cytarabine and hydroxyurea, and also with antithymocyte immunoglobulin, in T-cell lymphomas.

Bone marrow transplantation with intensive chemotherapy has been tried in patients with aggressive non-Hodgkin's lymphoma, but results have not been as favourable as with the leukaemias; a trial of early myeloablative therapy and autologous bone marrow transplantation failed to show any benefit over CHOP chemotherapy in patients slow to respond to therapy.[26] However, a more recent study comparing high-dose sequential therapy (with doxorubicin, prednisone, vincristine, cyclophosphamide, methotrexate, etoposide, melphalan, and mitozantrone), together with bone marrow and peripheral stem cell transfusion, versus MACOP-B found the sequential regimen produced higher complete response rates and event-free survival.[27] A small retrospective study has also suggested that allogeneic bone-marrow transplantation has less benefit in patients with intermediate- or high-grade lymphomas than in low-grade.[20] However, high-dose chemotherapy with radiotherapy followed by autologous bone-marrow transplantation may be superior to conventional salvage regimens such as DHAP (dexamethasone, high-dose cytarabine, and cisplatin) in the management of non-Hodgkin's lymphoma in relapse.[28,29]

Because B-cell lymphomas are associated with a particular surface immunoglobulin (the idiotype) they are also attractive candidates for immunotherapy. As well as the use of monoclonal antibodies, there has been much interest in attempting to develop vaccines against the lymphomatous clone.[30,31] Although good responses have been reported in a few patients (mostly with low-grade lymphomas) such an approach remains experimental, and is limited in lymphoma by the need to create a new vaccine for each patient.[32]

Another novel and promising approach is the use of an antisense oligonucleotide specific for *BCL-2*, a gene which is often overexpressed on tumour cells including lymphomas, and is responsible for cell resistance to apoptosis; a preliminary study[33] (although again mostly in patients with low-grade lymphomas) has demonstrated tumour regression and symptomatic improvement after *BCL-2* antisense therapy.

1. Vincent PC. The non-Hodgkin's lymphomas. *Med J Aust* 1990; **153:** 277–88.
2. O'Reilly SE, Connors JM. Non-Hodgkin's lymphoma I: characterisation and treatment. *Br Med J* 1992; **304:** 1682–6.
3. O'Reilly SE, Connors JM. Non-Hodgkin's lymphoma II: management problems. *Br Med J* 1992; **305:** 39–42.
4. Armitage JO. Treatment of non-Hodgkin's lymphoma. *N Engl J Med* 1993; **328:** 1023–30.
5. Rohatiner AZS, Lister TA. The management of follicular lymphoma. *Drugs* 1994; **47** (suppl 6): 10–18.
6. Johnson PWM. The high grade non-Hodgkin's lymphomas. *Br J Hosp Med* 1995; **53:** 14–19.
7. Martelli M, *et al.* Current guidelines for the management of aggressive non-Hodgkin's lymphoma. *Drugs* 1997; **53:** 957–72.
8. McLaughlin P, *et al.* Stage III follicular lymphoma: durable remissions with a combined chemotherapy-radiotherapy regimen. *J Clin Oncol* 1987; **5:** 867–74.
9. Young RC, *et al.* The treatment of indolent lymphomas: watchful waiting V aggressive combined modality treatment. *Semin Hematol* 1988; **25** (suppl 2): 11–16.
10. Smalley RV, *et al.* Interferon alfa combined with cytotoxic chemotherapy for patients with non-Hodgkin's lymphoma. *N Engl J Med* 1992; **327:** 1336–41.
11. Solal-Celigny P, *et al.* Recombinant interferon alfa-2b combined with a regimen containing doxorubicin in patients with advanced follicular lymphoma. *N Engl J Med* 1993; **329:** 1608–14.
12. Seymour JF, *et al.* High rate of prolonged remissions following combined modality therapy for patients with localized low-grade lymphoma. *Ann Oncol* 1996; **7:** 157–63.
13. Solal-Céligny P, *et al.* Doxorubicin-containing regimen with or without interferon alfa-2b for advanced follicular lymphomas: final analysis of survival and toxicity in the Groupe d'Etude des Lymphomes Folliculaires 86 trial. *J Clin Oncol* 1998; **16:** 2332–8.
14. Hickish T, *et al.* 2′-Chlorodeoxyadenosine: evaluation of a novel predominantly lymphocyte selective agent in lymphoid malignancies. *Br J Cancer* 1993; **67:** 139–43.
15. Maloney DG, *et al.* IDEC-C2B8: results of a phase I multiple-dose trial in patients with relapsed non-Hodgkin's lymphoma. *J Clin Oncol* 1997; **15:** 3266–74.
16. Kaminski MS, *et al.* Radioimmunotherapy of B-cell lymphoma with [^{131}I]anti-B1 (anti-CD20) antibody. *N Engl J Med* 1993; **329:** 459–65.
17. Press OW, *et al.* Radiolabeled-antibody therapy of B-cell lymphoma with autologous bone marrow support. *N Engl J Med* 1993; **329:** 1219–24.
18. Press OW, *et al.* Phase II trial of ^{131}I-B1 (anti-CD20) antibody therapy with autologous stem cell transplantation for relapsed B cell lymphomas. *Lancet* 1995; **346:** 336–40.
19. French RR, *et al.* Treatment of B-cell lymphomas with combination of bispecific antibodies and saporin. *Lancet* 1995; **346:** 223–4.
20. van Besien KW, *et al.* Allogeneic bone marrow transplantation for poor-prognosis lymphoma: response, toxicity, and survival depend on disease histology. *Am J Med* 1996; **100:** 299–307.
21. Rohatiner AZS, Lister TA. Myeloablative therapy for follicular lymphoma. *Hematol Oncol Clin North Am* 1991; **5:** 1003–12.
22. Gordon LI, *et al.* Comparison of a second-generation combination chemotherapeutic regimen (m-BACOD) with a standard regimen (CHOP) for advanced diffuse non-Hodgkin's lymphoma. *N Engl J Med* 1992; **327:** 1342–9.
23. Fisher RI, *et al.* Comparison of a standard regimen (CHOP) with three intensive chemotherapy regimens for advanced non-Hodgkin's lymphoma. *N Engl J Med* 1993; **328:** 1002–6.
24. Link MP, *et al.* Treatment of children and young adults with early-stage non-Hodgkin's lymphoma. *N Engl J Med* 1997; **337:** 1259–66.
25. Dufour P, *et al.* Idarubicin and high dose cytarabine: a new salvage treatment for refractory or relapsing non-Hodgkin's lymphoma. *Leukemia Lymphoma* 1996; **22:** 329–34.
26. Verdonck LF, *et al.* Comparison of CHOP chemotherapy with autologous bone marrow transplantation for slowly responding patients with aggressive non-Hodgkin's lymphoma. *N Engl J Med* 1995; **332:** 1045–51.
27. Gianni AL, *et al.* High-dose chemotherapy and autologous bone marrow transplantation compared with MACOP-B in aggressive B-cell lymphoma. *N Engl J Med* 1997; **336:** 1290–7.
28. Philip T, *et al.* Autologous bone marrow transplantation as compared with salvage chemotherapy in relapses of chemotherapy-sensitive non-Hodgkin's lymphoma. *N Engl J Med* 1995; **333:** 1540–5.
29. Vose JM. Treatment for non-Hodgkin's lymphoma in relapse: what are the alternatives? *N Engl J Med* 1995; **333:** 1565–6.
30. Kwak LW, *et al.* Induction of immune responses in patients with B-cell lymphoma against the surface-immunoglobulin idiotype expressed by their tumors. *N Engl J Med* 1992; **327:** 1209–15.
31. Hsu FJ, *et al.* Clinical trials of idiotypic-specific vaccine in B cell lymphomas. *Ann N Y Acad Sci* 1993; **690:** 385–7.
32. Hamblin TJ. From dendritic cells to tumour vaccines. *Lancet* 1996; **347:** 705–6.
33. Webb A, *et al.* BCL-2 antisense therapy in patients with non-Hodgkin lymphoma. *Lancet* 1997; **349:** 1137–41.
34. McLaughlin P, *et al.* Rituximab chimeric anti-CD20 monoclonal antibody therapy for relapsed indolent lymphoma: half of patients respond to a four-dose treatment program. *J Clin Oncol* 1998; **16:** 2825–33.
35. Miller TP, *et al.* Chemotherapy alone compared with chemotherapy plus radiotherapy for localized intermediate- and high-grade non-Hodgkin's lymphoma. *N Engl J Med* 1998; **339:** 21–6.

AIDS-related lymphoma. Between 3 and 10% of AIDS patients will develop non-Hodgkin's lymphoma at some stage of their illness, usually high-grade large cell lymphomas of B-cell origin, or Burkitt's lymphoma (a small non-cleaved lymphoma).[1] Unlike post-transplant lymphomas, only about 50% are associated with the presence of Epstein-Barr virus, although other factors may contribute to their development: DNA sequences associated with a novel herpesvirus also isolated from patients with Kaposi's sarcoma have been found in AIDS-related lymphomas.[2] A few patients present with localised disease, and may benefit from radiotherapy, but most have disseminated disease, often extranodal, at presentation.[1,3] Although standard dose or even intensive chemotherapy regimens have been used successfully in selected patients with AIDS-related non-Hodgkin's lymphomas,[4,5] in general this group of patients tolerates chemotherapy poorly,[5,6] and intensive regimens may even shorten their survival.[5] A low-dose modification of m-BACOD (cyclophosphamide, doxorubicin, vincristine, bleomycin, dexamethasone, and methotrexate plus folinic acid rescue, together with intrathecal cytarabine and if necessary cranial irradiation) has produced responses and survival comparable with more intensive regimens[7,8] but neutropenia and *Pneumocystis carinii* pneumonia were still a problem. The use of colony-stimulating factors with low or standard dose m-BACOD has been suggested to be helpful,[8,9] and a pilot study has suggested that a regimen of infusional cyclophosphamide, doxorubicin and etoposide is very active in producing remission.[10] However, the prognosis remains poor at present, and median survival remains only about 5 to 8 months.[1] There are currently moves to stratify patients by prognosis, with the intention of identifying those in whom more intensive therapy is appropriate.[1,3] Some workers have also investigated the use of biological response modifiers: only limited success has been reported with interleukin-2,[11] but a combination of zidovudine and interferon alfa has proved successful in inducing remission in a few patients with small non-cleaved cell lymphomas, although not in the more common large cell lymphomas.[12]

1. Schulz TF, *et al.* HIV infection and neoplasia. *Lancet* 1996; **348:** 587–91.
2. Cesarman E, *et al.* Kaposi's sarcoma-associated herpesvirus-like DNA sequences in AIDS-related body-cavity-based lymphomas. *N Engl J Med* 1995; **332:** 1186–91.
3. Denton AS, *et al.* AIDS-related lymphoma: an emerging epidemic. *Br J Hosp Med* 1996; **55:** 282–8.
4. Gisselbrecht C, *et al.* Human immunodeficiency virus-related lymphoma treatment with intensive combination chemotherapy. *Am J Med* 1993; **95:** 188–96.
5. Kaplan LD, *et al.* AIDS-associated non-Hodgkin's lymphoma in San Francisco. *JAMA* 1989; **261:** 719–24.
6. O'Reilly SE, Connors JM. Non-Hodgkin's lymphoma II: management problems. *Br Med J* 1992; **305:** 39–42.
7. Levine AM, *et al.* Low-dose chemotherapy with central nervous system prophylaxis and zidovudine maintenance in AIDS-related lymphoma. *JAMA* 1991; **266:** 84–8.
8. Kaplan LD, *et al.* Low-dose compared with standard-dose m-BACOD chemotherapy for non-Hodgkin's lymphoma associated with human immunodeficiency virus infection. *N Engl J Med* 1997; **336:** 1641–8.
9. Walsh C, *et al.* Phase I trial of m-BACOD and granulocyte macrophage colony stimulating factor in HIV-associated non-Hodgkin's lymphoma. *J Acquir Immune Defic Syndr* 1993; **6:** 265–71.
10. Sparano JA, *et al.* Infusional cyclophosphamide, doxorubicin, and etoposide in human immunodeficiency virus- and human T-cell leukemia virus type I-related non-Hodgkin's lymphoma: a highly active regimen. *Blood* 1993; **81:** 2810–15.
11. Mazza P, *et al.* Recombinant interleukin-2 in acquired immune deficiency syndrome: preliminary report in patients with lymphoma associated with HIV infection. *Eur J Haematol* 1992; **49:** 1–6.
12. Harrington WJ, *et al.* Azothymidine and interferon-α are active in AIDS-associated small non-cleaved cell lymphoma but not large-cell lymphoma. *Lancet* 1996; **348:** 833.

Burkitt's lymphoma. Burkitt's lymphoma is a small non-cleaved cell lymphoma (SNCL) of B-cell origin, which is seen particularly in children and has its peak incidence in equatorial Africa. It is associated with the Epstein-Barr virus although a causal relationship has not been proven.

The primary mode of treatment for Burkitt's lymphoma is chemotherapy. Regimens are generally based on cyclophosphamide, in various combinations with vincristine and methotrexate, doxorubicin, prednisone or prednisolone, and cytarabine.[1,2] Ifosfamide (with mesna prophylaxis) has also been tried.[2] Cytarabine and methotrexate may be given intrathecally for CNS prophylaxis.[1]

In children complete remission is common and prognosis good: probability of cure is about 80% in early disease, and even in more advanced disease comparable results can be achieved following debulking. Relapse may occur in up to 50% of all patients, but responds readily to reinduction chemotherapy if it occurs more than 3 months after remission (late relapse).[1] However, early relapse, occurring soon after remission, is associated with drug resistance and a poorer prognosis, despite the use of more aggressive regimens involving high-dose chemotherapy and autologous bone-marrow transplantation.[1] Prognosis has been somewhat less good in adults, but with the increasing use of more intensive regimens similar to those used in children, is improving. About half of all adult cases are reported to be curable with intensive chemotherapy regimens, and it is possible that even more intensive regimens coupled with bone-marrow transplantation or the use of colony-stimulating factors may improve results further.[3]

1. Ziegler JL. Burkitt's lymphoma. *N Engl J Med* 1981; **305:** 735–45.
2. Anonymous. Drugs of choice for cancer chemotherapy. *Med Lett Drugs Ther* 1997; **39:** 21–8.
3. Straus DJ, *et al.* Small non-cleaved-cell lymphoma (undifferentiated lymphoma, Burkitt's type) in American adults: results with treatment designed for acute lymphoblastic leukemia. *Am J Med* 1991; **90:** 328–37.

MALT lymphoma. Most gastric lymphomas are large cell lymphomas of B-lineage;[1] however, rarer low-grade lymphomas of mucosa-associated lymphoid tissue (MALT) also occur. The latter condition has aroused considerable recent interest because of an association with *Helicobacter pylori* infection.[1,2] The bacterium stimulates the formation of MALT in the stomach, which normally lacks organised lymphoid tissue, and there is evidence that it indirectly stimulates tumour growth.[3] Eradication of *H. pylori* infection using antibacterial and antisecretory therapy, as described in Peptic Ulcer Disease, p.1174, has been shown to result in regression of MALT lymphoma in a number of patients,[4-6] and this is now suggested to be the first line of therapy in this condition.[7] MALT lymphomas outside the stomach may also respond to antibacterials.[8]

1. Parsonnet J, *et al.* Helicobacter pylori infection and gastric lymphoma. *N Engl J Med* 1994; **330:** 1267–71.
2. Wotherspoon AC, *et al.* Helicobacter pylori-associated gastritis and primary B-cell gastric lymphoma. *Lancet* 1991; **338:** 1175–6.
3. Hussell T, *et al.* The response of cells from low-grade B-cell gastric lymphomas of mucosa-associated lymphoid tissue to Helicobacter pylori. *Lancet* 1993; **342:** 571–4.
4. Wotherspoon AC, *et al.* Regression of primary low-grade B-cell gastric lymphoma of mucosa-associated lymphoid tissue type after eradication of Helicobacter pylori. *Lancet* 1993; **342:** 575–7.
5. Wotherspoon AC, *et al.* Antibiotic treatment for low-grade gastric MALT lymphoma. *Lancet* 1994; **343:** 1503.
6. Cammarota G, *et al.* Prevention and treatment of low-grade B-cell primary gastric lymphoma by anti-H pylori therapy. *J Clin Gastroenterol* 1995; **21:** 118–22.
7. Stolte M, Eidt S. Healing gastric MALT lymphomas by eradicating H pylori? *Lancet* 1993; **342:** 568.
8. Alkan S, *et al.* Regression of salivary gland MALT lymphoma after treatment for Helicobacter pylori. *Lancet* 1996; **348:** 268–9.

Malignant effusions. The amount of interstitial fluid is normally regulated by a complex equilibrium between capillary filtration, osmotic pressure, and physical hydrostatic or hydraulic forces. Malignant neoplasms can disturb this equilibrium by obstruction of capillary or lymphatic drainage as well as causing active exudation of additional fluid following metastatic implantation. Malignant effusions are associated most often with lung, breast, and ovarian malignancies. Symptoms vary, and the fluid build-up may be asymptomatic, but pericardial effusions may progress to cardiac tamponade, while pleural effusions can produce cough, pleuritic chest pain, and dyspnoea. For brief reference to peritoneal effusions associated with malignancy (malignant ascites) see under Ascites, p.781.

The primary therapy for malignant effusions is drainage of the fluid and where possible systemic treatment of the underlying disease.[1-4] Various drugs have also been given for intracavitary sclerotherapy, including tetracycline, doxycycline, minocycline, mustine, bleomycin, cisplatin, fluorouracil, teniposide, thiotepa, radiopharmaceuticals, talc, and mepacrine. The principle involved is the instillation of an irritant agent into the pleural or pericardial cavity to promote inflammatory and fibrotic changes which result in the membranes adhering together and abolition of the space between the membranes in which fluid accumulates.[1,2]

Following drainage of the effusions the sclerosant is instilled in a small volume (20 to 50 mL) of diluent[1,2] except for talc, which is usually insufflated as a powder.[5] The patient's position must be adjusted from time to time to allow as much as possible of the cavitary membrane to come into contact with the sclerosant solution.[1] The resulting inflammation is painful and local anaesthetics or analgesics should be given.[1,6] The general consensus appears to be that tetracycline is probably the sclerosant of choice,[1,2,5,6] since adverse effects are relatively few and it is reasonably effective: the usual dose is 500 mg.[1,2] Control of effusions has been reported in about 70% of cases for one month.[5] Talc in a dose of 2 to 10 g[1,5] and mepacrine (5 instillations of 100 mg)[1] are probably both at least as effective as tetracycline but are usually associated with a higher incidence of pain and adverse effects,[1,4] and require more complex administration procedures.[1] The antineoplastics do not seem to produce any benefits over that expected from a simple irritant action[1] but some consider bleomycin a better agent for pleural effusions than a tetracycline.[7] However, a controlled study found talc slurry to be as effective as bleomycin, and suggested that talc should be preferred.[8] The ultimate therapy is surgery, but this may be associated with significant morbidity and mortality.[1,6]

1. Dhillon DP, Spiro SG. Malignant pleural effusions. *Br J Hosp Med* 1983; **29:** 506–10.
2. Press OW, Livingstone R. Management of malignant pericardial effusion and tamponade. *JAMA* 1987; **257:** 1088–92.
3. Andrews CO, Gora ML. Pleural effusions: pathophysiology and management. *Ann Pharmacother* 1994; **28:** 894–903.
4. Vaitkus PT, *et al.* Treatment of malignant pericardial effusion. *JAMA* 1994; **272:** 59–64.
5. Eselin J. Thompson DF. Talc in the treatment of malignant pleural effusion. *DICP Ann Pharmacother* 1991; **25:** 1187–9.
6. Tattersall MHN, Boyer MJ. Management of malignant pleural effusions. *Thorax* 1990; **45:** 81–2.
7. Fuller DK. Bleomycin versus doxycycline: a patient-oriented approach to pleurodesis. *Ann Pharmacother* 1993; **27:** 794.
8. Zimmer PW, *et al.* Prospective randomized trial of talc slurry vs bleomycin in pleurodesis for symptomatic malignant pleural effusions. *Chest* 1997; **112:** 430–4.

Malignant neoplasms of the bladder. Cancer of the bladder is one of the commoner cancers in Western society, and appears to be increasing in incidence. About two-thirds of all cases occur in men. It is commoner in white than in black patients, and known risk factors include smoking, exposure to aniline dyes, and schistosomiasis. Most patients present with haematuria; there may also be urinary frequency or dysuria.

Urothelial tumours fall into two major groups, superficial and invasive, with substantially different natural history, and requiring different management.[1,2]

About 80% of cases at presentation are low grade superficial tumours or carcinoma *in situ*, which remain confined to the mucosa or submucosa. The main means of treatment for superficial disease is surgery, in the form of transurethral resection, or diathermy. Preliminary results suggest that photodynamic therapy of superficial tumours using intravesical 5-aminolaevulinic acid is also a promising technique.[3] Although patients treated with standard therapy have good prospects for survival, with a 5-year survival rate of 80% or more, the rate of disease-free survival is much lower, since recurrence is common.

In an attempt to prolong remission and reduce the relapse rate various antineoplastic agents have been instilled into the bladder after resection, either prophylactically or to treat minimal residual disease.[1,2,4-6] Effective agents include doxorubicin, epirubicin, mitomycin, thiotepa, and interferon alfa. Cisplatin is reported to be active, but is associated with an unacceptably high incidence of anaphylaxis when given by the intravesical route.[1] Good results have also been reported with intravesical BCG, which is at least as effective as chemotherapy by the intravesical route, and in some studies has produced lower recurrence rates; it appears to be the agent of choice in the treatment of carcinoma *in situ*.[1,5,6] Another immunostimulant, bropirimine, is reported to be effective when given by mouth to patients with carcinoma *in situ*.[7]

Management of invasive bladder cancer is a matter of controversy,[8] but conventional therapy has revolved around radical surgery, radiotherapy, or a combination of the two. However, such conventional therapy offers a 5-year survival rate of 50% or less.[1,8] In consequence, alternatives, including the use of systemic chemotherapy before, or in combination with, cystectomy or radiotherapy, have been tried.

The optimal regimen remains to be defined but regimens incorporating cisplatin and methotrexate, such as M-VAC (methotrexate, vinblastine, doxorubicin, and cisplatin), appear to be widely used. Such therapy has produced delays in recurrence of disease, but evidence for improved survival appears to be lacking. A recent large study comparing neo-adjuvant therapy using cisplatin, methotrexate, and vinblastine, before cystectomy or radiotherapy, found this regimen to be of little benefit.[9]

Recurrent and metastatic bladder cancer also continues to pose a problem. Fortunately, recurrences in patients with superficial disease are usually not invasive or high-grade. Recurrent invasive or metastatic disease is more problematic. The chemotherapy regimens which produce the highest response rate in adjuvant treatment of invasive disease not surprisingly give the best results in these patients as well, and complete responses may occur in 30% or more of patients, but only a small proportion go on to long-term remission. Combination therapy with gemcitabine and cisplatin is under investigation in this situation.[10]

1. Raghavan D, *et al.* Biology and management of bladder cancer. *N Engl J Med* 1990; **322:** 1129–38.
2. Dawson C, Whitfield H. Urological malignancy—II: urothelial tumours. *Br Med J* 1996; **312:** 1090–4.
3. Kriegmair M, *et al.* Early clinical experience with 5-aminolevulinic acid for the photodynamic therapy of superficial bladder cancer. *Br J Urol* 1996; **77:** 667–71.
4. Batts CN. Adjuvant intravesical therapy for superficial bladder cancer. *Ann Pharmacother* 1992; **26:** 1270–6.
5. Moss JT, Kadmon D. BCG and the treatment of superficial bladder cancer. *DICP Ann Pharmacother* 1991; **25:** 1355–67.
6. Hall RR. Superficial bladder cancer. *Br Med J* 1994; **308:** 910–13.
7. Sarosdy MF, *et al.* Oral bropirimine immunotherapy of carcinoma in situ of the bladder: results of a phase II trial. *Urology* 1996; **48:** 21–7.
8. Parker CC, Huddart RA. Management of invasive bladder cancer. *Br J Hosp Med* 1996; **56:** 213–18.
9. Hall RR, *et al.* Neo-adjuvant CMV chemotherapy and cystectomy or radiotherapy in muscle invasive bladder cancer: first analysis of MRC/EORTC intercontinental trial. *Proc Am Soc Clin Oncol* 1996; **15:** 244.
10. von der Maase H, *et al.* A phase II study of gemcitabine and cisplatin in patients with transitional cell carcinoma (TCC) of the urothelium. *Proc Am Soc Clin Oncol* 1997; **16:** 324a.

Malignant neoplasms of the bone. Solid cancers frequently metastasise to the skeleton and metastatic bone disease is a common problem with cancers of the breast, prostate, and lung. Bone metastases are often responsible for cancer pain (the general management of which is discussed on p.8) and also result in immobility, bone fractures, bone-marrow failure, spinal cord compression, and hypercalcaemia.[1] The most common sites of metastasis are the spine, hip, and femur. Primary bone malignancies are rare, and are usually sarcomas (p.495). Multiple myeloma (p.494) may also produce bone involvement.

Management is essentially palliative since cure is rarely possible. External beam radiotherapy is the best treatment for localised metastatic bone pain, and radiation delivered by bone seeking isotopes such as samarium-153 or strontium-89 has also been reported to give pain relief.[1-3] Surgical fixation or stabilisation may be undertaken to treat or prevent fractures.

Bone metastases cause local osteolysis and various inhibitors of bone resorption have been tried, not only to correct hypercalcaemia of malignancy (p.1148), but also to relieve bone pain and progression of the disease. Plicamycin and gallium nitrate were formerly used in this context but have now been largely replaced by other agents such as the calcitonins, and more particularly the bisphosphonates. Although results with etidronate have conflicted,[4,5] there have been beneficial results using clodronate[6,7,15] and pamidronate,[8-12] both for bone metastases of breast cancer and in multiple myeloma; bisphosphonates should probably form part of the standard management of these conditions.[13]

Systemic antineoplastic therapy may also be given. Endocrine treatment is usually preferred for patients with breast and prostatic cancers, with response rates of up to 50% and 90% respectively, and a median duration of response of 12 to 20 months. Cytotoxic drugs may be used when endocrine treatment fails, but response rates are usually lower, and durations of response shorter.[1] Because of their bone-seeking properties, bisphosphonates are under investigation as carriers for the delivery of antineoplastics to bone.[14]

1. Dodwell D, Howell A. Treating bony metastases. *Br Med J* 1991; **303:** 429–30.
2. Aaron AD. The management of cancer metastatic to bone. *JAMA* 1994; **272:** 1206–9.
3. Nightengale B, *et al.* Strontium chloride Sr89 for treating pain from metastatic bone disease. *Am J Health-Syst Pharm* 1995; **52:** 2189–95.
4. Carey PO, Lippert MC. Treatment of painful prostatic bone metastases with oral etidronate disodium. *Urology* 1988; **32:** 403–7.
5. Smith JA. Palliation of painful bone metastases from prostate cancer using sodium etidronate: results of a randomized, prospective, double-blind, placebo-controlled study. *J Urol (Baltimore)* 1989; **141:** 85–7.
6. Elomaa I, *et al.* Treatment of skeletal disease in breast cancer: a controlled clodronate trial. *Bone* 1987; **8** (suppl 1) S53–6.
7. Lahtinen R, *et al.* Randomised, placebo-controlled multicentre trial of clodronate in multiple myeloma. *Lancet* 1992; **340:** 1049–52. Correction. *ibid.*: 1420.
8. van Holten-Verzantvoort, *et al.* Palliative pamidronate treatment in patients with bone metastases from breast cancer. *J Clin Oncol* 1993; **11:** 491–8.
9. Conte PF, *et al.* Delayed progression of bone metastases with pamidronate therapy in breast cancer patients: a randomized, multicenter phase III trial. *Ann Oncol* 1994; **5** (suppl 7): 41S–44S.

10. Berenson JR, *et al.* Efficacy of pamidronate in reducing skeletal events in patients with advanced multiple myeloma. *N Engl J Med* 1996; **332:** 488–93.
11. Hortobagyi GN, *et al.* Efficacy of pamidronate in reducing skeletal complications in patients with breast cancer and lytic bone metastases. *N Engl J Med* 1996; **335:** 1785–91.
12. Berenson JR, *et al.* Long-term pamidronate treatment of advanced multiple myeloma patients reduces skeletal events. *J Clin Oncol* 1998; **16:** 593–602.
13. Bloomfield DJ. Should bisphosphonates be part of the standard therapy of patients with multiple myeloma or bone metastases from other cancers? An evidence-based review. *J Clin Oncol* 1998; **16:** 1218–25.
14. Spencer RP. Relief of pain from osseous metastatic lesions. *Drugs* 1996; **52:** 475.
15. Diel IJ, *et al.* Reduction in new metastases in breast cancer with adjuvant clodronate treatment. *N Engl J Med* 1998; **339:** 357–63.

Malignant neoplasms of the brain. Both primary and metastatic brain tumours are relatively common and are of a wide variety of types. Most primary brain malignancies are gliomas, such as astrocytoma, ependymoma, and glioblastoma multiforme. The frequency and natural history of brain tumours differ between children and adults.Astrocytomas and medulloblastomas are among the commonest primary brain tumours in children;[1-3] in adults, apart from astroglial neoplasms, meningioma and pituitary adenoma are also relatively frequent.[1] The most frequent metastases to the brain derive from breast cancer, lung cancer, and melanoma. CNS involvement in patients with leukaemia or lymphoma is also quite common.

The symptoms of cranial neoplasms are those of local pressure and damage to the brain (such as focal seizures and visual field defects), of displacement of brain structures (like oculomotor paresis with tentorial herniation), and of raised intracranial pressure (such as impaired consciousness and papilloedema). The single most frequent symptom is headache, which is seen in about 60% of cases.

The mainstay of treatment for most brain tumours is surgery to relieve compression and cerebral oedema, establish diagnosis, and where feasible resect as much of the tumour as possible.[1,3,4] The combination of high-dose corticosteroids and computed tomography has profoundly reduced the morbidity of surgery, both for biopsy and excision.[5] For benign tumours resection may be curative and even for malignant tumours there is evidence that extensive resection prolongs survival. Radiotherapy is also widely used, alone or more often with surgery; it is the mainstay of treatment for high-grade glioma.[6]

The role of chemotherapy for primary brain malignancies is uncertain, in part because of the difficulty in finding drugs that can cross the blood-brain barrier; the nitrosoureas such as carmustine and lomustine have been the drugs most frequently used, because of their lipid solubility.[4] The PCV regimen, in which procarbazine, lomustine, and vincristine are given, is now generally preferred to single-agent nitrosoureas in the treatment of gliomas.[7]

In young children chemotherapy may be used as a stop-gap measure to delay, or reduce the frequency of, radiotherapy, which can cause neurodevelopmental damage.[1-3] Studies in children under 3 years of age given either cyclophosphamide, vincristine, cisplatin, and etoposide[8] or carboplatin, cyclophosphamide, vincristine, cisplatin, and methotrexate,[9] after surgical resection of tumour found that radiotherapy could be safely delayed in most and that a few children might never require it.

Other drugs used for chemotherapy, alone or in various combinations, include dactinomycin, doxorubicin (with cyclophosphamide), teniposide, and mustine (as part of the MOPP regimen).[1,2,4,10] Drugs such as mitolactol and temozolomide are also under investigation, as is thalidomide.

Response to the antiprogestogenic, mifepristone, has been reported in meningioma;[11] buserelin[12] and octreotide[13] have produced symptomatic relief, and interferon alfa has been reported to control the expansion of a meningioma in one case.[14] Some benefit has also been reported from the use of hydroxyurea in unresectable meningiomas.[15]

Since present regimens are far from optimal, alternatives continue to be tried. These have included local infusion of natural killer cells activated in various ways,[16,17] implantation of biodegradable polymers impregnated with carmustine (which has been shown to improve survival in patients with malignant glioma),[18] and the use of gene therapy.[19] This involves the incorporation of the herpes simplex thymidine kinase gene into tumour cells via a retrovirus; such transduced tumour cells can then activate, and be killed by, the antiviral agent ganciclovir. Following *animal* studies such a procedure is under investigation in patients with progressive brain tumours.[20,21]

The value of chemotherapy in cerebral metastatic disease seems to be limited: the primary tumour may be intrinsically resistant to chemotherapy, or metastasis may develop despite treatment of the primary tumour, which will encourage the selection of resistant species. Furthermore, although the blood-brain barrier may not be completely intact in these patients, allowing some passage of antineoplastics into the brain, drug delivery of the less lipid-soluble drugs to cerebral metastases may not be sufficient, or sufficiently consistent, to produce a response. Nonetheless there is evidence for response of cerebral metastases of some chemosensitive primary tumours.[22,23]

1. Black PM. Brain tumors. *N Engl J Med* 1991; **324:** 1471–6 and 1555–64.
2. Crist WM, Kun LE. Common solid tumors of childhood. *N Engl J Med* 1991; **324:** 461–71.
3. Pollack IF. Brain tumors in children. *N Engl J Med* 1994; **331:** 1500–7.
4. WHO. Chemotherapy of solid tumours: report of an expert committee. *WHO Tech Rep Ser 605* 1977.
5. Miller JD. Surgical excision for single cerebral metastasis? *Lancet* 1993; **341:** 1566.
6. Bliss P, Brada M. The management of gliomas. *Br J Hosp Med* 1996; **55:** 82–3.
7. Kaba SE, Kyritsis AP. Recognition and management of gliomas. *Drugs* 1997; **53:** 235–44.
8. Duffner PK, *et al.* Postoperative chemotherapy and delayed radiation in children less than three years of age with malignant brain tumors. *N Engl J Med* 1993; **328:** 1725–31.
9. Lashford LS, *et al.* An intensive multiagent chemotherapy regimen for brain tumours occurring in very young children. *Arch Dis Child* 1996; **74:** 219–23.
10. Anonymous. Drugs of choice for cancer chemotherapy. *Med Lett Drugs Ther* 1997; **39:** 21–8.
11. Lamberts SWJ, *et al.* Mifepristone (RU 486) treatment of meningiomas. *J Neurol Neurosurg Psychiatry* 1992; **55:** 486–90.
12. van Seters AP, *et al.* Symptomatic relief of meningioma by buserelin maintenance therapy. *Lancet* 1989; **i:** 564–5.
13. Rünzi MW, *et al.* Successful treatment of meningioma with octreotide. *Lancet* 1989; **i:** 1074.
14. Wöber-Bingöl C, *et al.* Interferon-alfa-2b for meningioma. *Lancet* 1995; **345:** 331.
15. Schrell UMH, *et al.* Hydroxyurea for treatment of unresectable meningiomas. *Lancet* 1996; **348:** 888–9.
16. Nitta T, *et al.* Preliminary trial of specific targeting therapy against malignant glioma. *Lancet* 1990; **335:** 368–71.
17. Jeffes EWB, *et al.* Therapy of recurrent high grade gliomas with surgery, and autologous mitogen activated IL-2 stimulated killer (MAK) lymphocytes I: enhancement of MAK lytic activity and cytokine production by PHA and clinical use of PHA. *J Neurooncol* 1993; **15:** 141–55.
18. Brem H, *et al.* Placebo-controlled trial of safety and efficacy of intraoperative controlled delivery by biodegradable polymers of chemotherapy for recurrent gliomas. *Lancet* 1995; **345:** 1008–12.
19. Jinnah HA, Friedmann T. Gene therapy and the brain. *Br Med Bull* 1995; **51:** 138–48.
20. Izquierdo M, *et al.* Human malignant brain tumor response to herpes simplex thymidine kinase (HSVtk)/ganciclovir gene therapy. *Gene Ther* 1996; **3:** 491–5.
21. Ram Z, *et al.* Therapy of malignant brain tumors by intratumoral implantation of retroviral vector-producing cells. *Nature Med* 1997; **3:** 1354–61.
22. Twelves CJ, *et al.* The response of cerebral metastases in small cell lung cancer to systemic chemotherapy. *Br J Cancer* 1990; **61:** 147–50.
23. Rustin GJS, *et al.* Weekly alternating etoposide, methotrexate, and actinomycin/vincristine and cyclophosphamide chemotherapy for the treatment of CNS metastases for choriocarcinoma. *J Clin Oncol* 1989; **7:** 900–3.

Malignant neoplasms of the breast. Cancer of the breast is the most common malignant neoplasm in women, accounting for as many as one in five of all female cancer deaths in the UK.[1] The disease is rare under the age of 25, and increases steadily in incidence with age, reaching its peak incidence in elderly women. Mothers, daughters, and sisters of women with breast cancer have an increased risk, as do women who have not borne children: the highest incidence is seen in nuns. It is an extremely heterogeneous disorder, and the clinical course is consequently very variable; such factors as patient age and menopausal status, tumour size and grade, involvement of axillary lymph nodes or skin, and presence of hormone receptors within the tumour may be a guide to the extent and aggressiveness of disease, and hence have prognostic significance for treatment.

In patients with **early disease** (stage I or II; a relatively small tumour with no or limited nodal involvement) the prognosis is fair.[3] Primary treatment has traditionally been surgical, with an increasing trend to less-extensive and less-mutilating surgery, and sometimes combined with radiotherapy, which has been shown to reduce local recurrence,[4-6] and appears to improve survival.[5,6] The most important single prognostic factor has generally been thought to be nodal status: the 10-year survival in women with node-negative disease is some 70 to 80% overall,[7,8] whereas in node-positive disease up to 60% of women relapse and may ultimately die of their disease.[7] However the size at diagnosis is also important, with an excellent prognosis for node-negative tumours less than 15 mm in size (12-year survival 94%) and a prognosis for node-positive tumours less than 15 mm which is similar to that of larger node-negative tumours (12-year survival about 80%).[8]

Adjuvant therapy with cytotoxic chemotherapy, hormonal manipulations such as ovarian ablation, tamoxifen, or gonadorelin analogues has been given to try to eradicate the micrometastases which cause relapses.[7,9,10] Overviews of a large number of trials by the Early Breast Cancer Trialists' Collaborative Group have confirmed the benefits of adjuvant therapy and attempted to determine which women derive most benefit and which regimens are most effective.

Chemotherapy or hormonal therapy has now been shown to have benefits in all women with early breast cancer, regardless of age and nodal status.[11,13,14] However, although the proportional benefit is similar in node-positive and node-negative disease, women with the latter have a much better prognosis and so their absolute reduction in risk is lower, and treatment decisions more difficult.[27]

Chemotherapy has mainly been used in premenopausal node-positive women. Most commonly, this has involved cyclophosphamide, methotrexate, and fluorouracil (CMF),[11,13] sometimes together with doxorubicin,[12] although other agents used include epirubicin, melphalan, thiotepa, and vincristine.[11] It has now been calculated that 3 to 6 months of combination chemotherapy in women aged under 50 can produce reductions in risk of recurrence and of mortality of around 35% and 27% respectively.[13] However, the benefits are not confined to this age group: in older women chemotherapy reduced the risks of recurrence and death by about 20% and 8 to 14% (depending on age) respectively.[13]

More prolonged chemotherapy has no greater benefit than treatment for 3 to 6 months, and there is some evidence that anthracycline-containing regimens produce more benefit than those without.[13] There is some recent suggestion that addition of paclitaxel to chemotherapy regimens for early breast cancer may further improve response. Reducing dose intensity results in poorer survival[15] but it is not clear that the reverse applies,[16,17] and studies of high-dose adjuvant therapy have produced conflicting results.[18] It has been suggested that the benefits of high-dose adjuvant therapy may be seen only in a subgroup of patients identifiable by molecular markers.[19]

Adjuvant chemotherapy may also be combined with adjuvant radiotherapy. A recent study, primarily in premenopausal women, found that giving chemotherapy first followed by radiotherapy produced better overall results than the reverse order.[20]

In postmenopausal women, hormonal therapy with tamoxifen has historically been preferred.[4,7,9,10,22] Its effects seem to be small in women with oestrogen-receptor negative tumours,[14] although some benefit cannot be excluded (it has been suggested[24] that 'receptor negative' tumours responding to tamoxifen may simply have very low concentrations of oestrogen receptors). However, in women with oestrogen-receptor positive tumours 5 years of tamoxifen is associated with reductions in risk of disease recurrence and death of 50% and 28% respectively.[14] Unlike chemotherapy, these results are constant regardless of age—premenopausal women also benefit from ovarian ablation,[11,21] and it has been suggested that some of the benefit of chemotherapy in younger women derives from its ablative effect on the ovaries.[9]

Combined chemotherapy and tamoxifen may offer additional benefits, although a meta-analysis[25] taking quality of life into consideration suggested that in older women such combined therapy offered little advantage; the benefit may be greater if combined therapy is restricted to those with oestrogen-receptor negative disease.[26]

Although the benefits of adjuvant therapy are now being clarified, particular problems remain in deciding on appropriate management of node-negative patients, in whom widespread use of adjuvant therapy would involve treating large numbers of patients who do not need it. Ideally, prognostic factors should be used to identify those patients at risk of relapse, who alone should receive adjuvant treatment, but at present this is not possible with any degree of accuracy.[27-29] In consequence, while some authorities favour the use of some form of adjuvant treatment in all women with early breast cancer,[29] it is generally considered that some effort should be made to identify node-negative women at higher risk, as potential candidates for treatment.[9,23,27,28]

If treatment is given, there is also little consensus as to what it should be. Tamoxifen is probably appropriate in postmenopausal node-negative women,[9,23] but opinions have differed as to whether its relatively low toxicity outweighs a possibly reduced benefit in premenopausal women.[23,27,30] There is also some uncertainty as to the appropriate duration of therapy, since there is evidence that more than 5 years of treatment is unlikely to be beneficial.[30] Adjuvant chemotherapy is not widely used in women aged over 50 in the UK, although this is not the case in the USA; it may be considered with or without tamoxifen, in premenopausal women considered at high risk.[23] A recent US study suggested that adjuvant chemotherapy produces benefit in all subgroups of women with early breast cancer, regardless of age or nodal status.[31]

As mentioned above, the primary therapy of early breast cancer has generally been considered to be surgery and/or radiotherapy. However, following good results with the use of **primary chemotherapy** to treat locally-advanced disease,[32] a number of investigators have tried initial chemotherapy in women with operable disease.[33-35] Such an approach may permit downstaging of the tumour and more conservative surgery than would otherwise be possible,[33,35] and in addition the response of the tumour to endocrine therapy or chemotherapy can be gauged directly, and an alternative regimen substituted if no response occurs.[34] Chemotherapy can achieve some regression in 70% or more of patients.[9,36,37] Such neoadjuvant chemotherapy has been suggested as a possible approach for all women, but whether it offers a benefit is unclear, since once again women who would not need chemotherapy would be exposed to it. However, regimens such as mitozantrone, methotrexate, and tamoxifen,[36] or continuous infusion of fluorouracil with intermittent cisplatin and epirubicin,[37] seem to be relatively well tolerated, and some authorities consider that primary medical therapy aimed at cure will become the norm in many patients with palpable breast cancer and likely micrometastasis.[38]

The role of chemotherapy in **advanced disease** is chiefly palliative; cure is not possible with current regimens, and median survival in metastatic disease (about 2 years from first metastasis) has not markedly improved in the past 50 years.[39] In the UK, a generally conservative approach has been advocated, with chemotherapy being used as a first-line treatment only in patients with aggressive disease, particularly where metastasis is to critical visceral sites such as the liver; in other patients an initial trial of endocrine therapy, usually with tamoxifen has been suggested, with chemotherapy reserved until metastases progress despite endocrine therapy.[40] Some newer endocrine agents including aromatase inhibitors such as anastrozole, formestane, or letrozole, or anti-oestrogens such as droloxifene or toremifene are also being tried, as is hormonal manipulation with gonadorelin analogues. Aminoglutethimide is now generally less favoured than newer hormonal drugs because of a higher incidence of adverse effects. The use of bisphosphonates may be helpful in limiting metastases to bone (see Malignant Neoplasms of Bone, above) and possibly to other sites.[49] Various chemotherapy regimens continue to be tried, often based on an anthracycline such as doxorubicin or the related mitozantrone,[41-44] and a few patients achieve complete remission. In patients with anthracycline-resistant disease the taxanes, paclitaxel and docetaxel, are favoured for second-line treatment, with vinorelbine often reserved for third-line treatment.[2] Other newer agents being tried include capecitabine, gemcitabine, idarubicin, and raltitrexed, some of which have produced promising results.[2,47] There is evidence that response rates are reduced in patients who have received previous adjuvant therapy,[42] although a salvage regimen of lonidamine, mitomycin, vinblastine, and prednisone has been reported to produce some response in anthracycline-refractory disease.[45] Higher response rates can be achieved by intensive regimens, sometimes combined with colony-stimulating factors or autologous bone-marrow transplants,[39,40,43,46] but despite preliminary evidence of disease free survival in selected patients[40] others have found no improvement in response,[48] and morbidity is considerable.[43,48] One interesting experimental approach is the use of gene therapy to add multidrug resistance genes to the patients' normal stem cells, enabling them to resist increased doses of chemotherapy,[46] but again, other forms of toxicity such as cardiotoxicity or gastro-intestinal effects then limit the dose. Another possible approach is active specific immunotherapy, with a vaccine against tumour-associated mucin antigens, or the use of monoclonal antibodies such as trastuzumab.

1. Anonymous. Consensus development conference: treatment of primary breast cancer. *Br Med J* 1986; **293:** 946–7.
2. Hortobagyi GN. Treatment of breast cancer. *N Engl J Med* 1998; **339:** 974–84.
3. Haybittle JL. Curability of breast cancer. *Br Med Bull* 1991; **47:** 319–23.
4. Early Breast Cancer Trialists' Collaborative Group. Effects of radiotherapy and surgery in early breast cancer: an overview of the randomized trials. *N Engl J Med* 1995; **333:** 1444–55. Correction. *ibid.* 1996; **334:** 1003.
5. Overgaard M, *et al.* Postoperative radiotherapy in high-risk premenopausal women with breast cancer who receive adjuvant chemotherapy. *N Engl J Med* 1997; **337:** 949–55.
6. Ragaz J, *et al.* Adjuvant radiotherapy and chemotherapy in node-positive premenopausal women with breast cancer. *N Engl J Med* 1997; **337:** 956–62.
7. Anonymous. Adjuvant chemotherapy of early breast cancer. *Med Lett Drugs Ther* 1990; **32:** 49–50.
8. Tabár L, *et al.* Breast cancer treatment and natural history: new insights from results of screening. *Lancet* 1992; **339:** 412–14.
9. Allum WH, Smith IE. Carcinoma of the breast. *Br J Hosp Med* 1995; **54:** 255–8.
10. Williams C. Adjuvant systemic therapies for breast cancer. *Prescribers' J* 1996; **36:** 125–9.
11. Early Breast Cancer Trialists' Collaborative Group. Systematic treatment of early breast cancer by hormonal, cytotoxic, or immune therapy: 133 randomised trials involving 31 000 recurrences and 24 000 deaths among 75 000 women. *Lancet* 1992; **339:** 1–15 and 71–85.
12. Bonadonna G, *et al.* Sequential or alternating doxorubicin and CMF regimens in breast cancer with more than three positive nodes: ten-year results. *JAMA* 1995; **273:** 542–7.
13. Early Breast Cancer Trialists' Collaborative Group. Polychemotherapy for early breast cancer: an overview of the randomised trials. *Lancet* 1998; **352:** 930–42.
14. Early Breast Cancer Trialists' Collaborative Group. Tamoxifen for early breast cancer: an overview of the randomised trials. *Lancet* 1998; **351:** 1451–67.
15. Wood WC, *et al.* Dose and dose intensity of adjuvant chemotherapy for stage II, node-positive breast carcinoma. *N Engl J Med* 1994; **330:**1253–9.
16. Gradishar WJ, *et al.* High-dose chemotherapy for breast cancer. *Ann Intern Med* 1996; **125:** 599–604.
17. Protheroe AS, Johnson PWM. High-dose chemotherapy with stem cell rescue for solid tumours. *Br J Hosp Med* 1996; **55:** 437–41.
18. Peters WP, *et al.* High dose chemotherapy and autologous bone marrow support as consolidation after standard-dose adjuvant therapy for high risk primary breast cancer. *J Clin Oncol* 1993; **11:** 1132–43.
19. Muss HB, *et al.* c-erb-B-2 Expression and response to adjuvant therapy in women with node-positive early breast cancer. *N Engl J Med* 1994; **330:** 1260-6.
20. Recht A, *et al.* The sequencing of chemotherapy and radiation therapy after conservative surgery for early-stage breast cancer. *N Engl J Med* 1996; **334:** 1356–61.
21. Early Breast Cancer Trialists' Collaborative Group. Ovarian ablation in early breast cancer: overview of the randomised trials. *Lancet* 1996; **348:** 1189–96.
22. Nolvadex Adjuvant Trial Organisation. Controlled trial of tamoxifen as a single adjuvant agent in the management of early breast cancer. *Br J Cancer* 1988; **57:** 608–11.
23. Richards MA, *et al.* Role of systemic treatment for primary operable breast cancer. *Br Med J* 1994; **309:** 1363–6. Correction. *ibid.*; 1497.
24. Elledge RM, Osborne CK. Oestrogen receptors and breast cancer. *Br Med J* 1997; **314:** 1843–4.
25. Gelber RD, *et al.* Adjuvant chemotherapy plus tamoxifen compared with tamoxifen alone for postmenopausal breast cancer: meta-analysis of quality-adjusted survival. *Lancet* 1996; **347:** 1066–71.
26. Pritchard KI. Postmenopausal breast cancer: is the short-term pain worth the long-term gain? *Lancet* 1996; **347:** 1057–8.
27. O'Reilly SM, Richards MA. Node negative breast cancer. *Br Med J* 1990; **300:** 346–8.
28. McGuire WL. Adjuvant therapy of node-negative breast cancer. *N Engl J Med* 1989; **320:** 525–7.
29. DeVita VT. Breast cancer therapy: exercising all our options. *N Engl J Med* 1989; **320:** 527–9.
30. Bulbrook RD. Long-term adjuvant therapy for primary breast cancer. *Br Med J* 1996; **312:** 389–90. Correction. *ibid.*; 992.
31. Fisher B, *et al.* Tamoxifen and chemotherapy for lymph node-negative, estrogen receptor-positive breast cancer. *J Natl Cancer Inst* 1997; **89:** 1673–82.
32. Jacquillat C, *et al.* Results of a conservative treatment combining induction (neoadjuvant) and consolidation chemotherapy, hormonotherapy, and external and interstitial irradiation in 98 patients with locally advanced breast cancer (IIIA - IIIB). *Cancer* 1988; **61:** 1977–82.
33. Bonadonna G, *et al.* Primary chemotherapy to avoid mastectomy in tumors with diameters of three centimeters or more. *J Natl Cancer Inst* 1990; **82:** 1539–45.
34. Forrest APM, *et al.* Primary systemic therapy for breast cancer. *Br Med Bull* 1991; **47:** 357–71.
35. Fisher B, *et al.* Effect of preoperative chemotherapy on local-regional disease in women with operable breast cancer: findings from National Surgical Adjuvant Breast and Bowel Project B-18. *J Clin Oncol* 1997; **15:** 2483–93.
36. Powles TJ, *et al.* Randomized trial of chemoendocrine therapy started before or after surgery for treatment of primary breast cancer. *J Clin Oncol* 1995; **13:** 547–52.
37. Smith IE, *et al.* High complete remission rates with primary neoadjuvant infusional chemotherapy for large early breast cancer. *J Clin Oncol* 1995; **13:** 424–9.
38. Forrest AP, *et al.* Primary treatment in breast cancer. *Br Med J* 1991; **302:** 590.
39. Antman K, Gale RP. Advanced breast cancer: high-dose chemotherapy and bone marrow autotransplants. *Ann Intern Med* 1988; **108:** 570–4.
40. Leonard RCF, *et al.* Metastatic breast cancer. *Br Med J* 1994; **309:** 1501–4.
41. Harris AL, *et al.* Comparison of short-term and continuous chemotherapy (mitozantrone) for advanced breast cancer. *Lancet* 1990; **335:** 186–90.
42. Heidemann E, *et al.* Randomized clinical trial comparing mitoxantrone with epirubicin and with doxorubicin, each combined with cyclophosphamide in the first-line treatment of patients with metastatic breast cancer. *Onkologie* 1990; **13:** 24–7.
43. Jones RB, *et al.* The Duke AFM program: intensive induction chemotherapy for metastatic breast cancer. *Cancer* 1990; **66:** 431–6.
44. Cantwell BMJ, *et al.* Epidermal growth factor receptors and doxorubicin plus ifosfamide/mesna in recurrent breast cancer. *Lancet* 1991; **337:** 1417.
45. Zaniboni A, *et al.* Mitomycin-C, vinblastine, and lonidamine as salvage treatment of advanced breast cancer: a pilot study. *Am J Clin Oncol* 1990; **13:** 520–3.
46. O'Shaughnessy JA, Cowan KH. Dose-intensive therapy for breast cancer. *JAMA* 1993; **270:** 2089–92.
47. de Valeriola D, *et al.* Breast cancer therapies in development: a review of their pharmacology and clinical potential. *Drugs* 1997; **54:** 385–413.
48. Rodenhuis S, *et al.* Randomised trial of high-dose chemotherapy and haemopoietic progenitor-cell support in operable breast cancer with extensive axillary lymph-node involvement. *Lancet* 1998; **352:** 515–21.
49. Diel IJ, *et al.* Reduction in new metastases in breast cancer with adjuvant clodronate treatment. *N Engl J Med* 1998; **339:** 357–63.

PROPHYLAXIS. Treatment with tamoxifen as part of the management of breast cancer is apparently associated with a reduced risk of developing cancer in the other breast.[1] In view of the difficulty of treating breast cancer once it develops this has led some authorities to suggest the use of prophylactic tamoxifen to prevent the development of breast cancer in women at risk.[1-3]

This proposal has proved enormously controversial.[4,5] Following pilot studies in women with family histories of breast cancer,[6] larger studies have been initiated, including one in the UK and one in the USA, but this has only served to exacerbate the controversy. Proponents of the studies suggest that in addition to potential benefits in breast cancer the actions of tamoxifen may reduce the risk of osteoporosis and cardiovascular disease.[2,5,7,8] However, critics consider the evidence for all these benefits to be dubious;[4,9,10] in addition, there are questions about the selection criteria for the studies, since determination of risk of breast cancer is inexact. Although relatively non-toxic, tamoxifen is not devoid of adverse effects. In particular there is concern about the risk of liver cancer (increased in *rats* although this has not been demonstrated in humans) and endometrial cancer.[11] The UK study was delayed because of concerns about these potential risks.

Ultimately, the value of these studies depends on clinical assessment of the potential benefits versus the potential risks,[12] but the data needed to make this assessment are still scanty. Unfortunately, the US study was terminated early because of a reduced incidence of breast cancer in women receiving the active drug, which has limited the conclusions that can be drawn.[13] Although the trends in this study were extremely favourable,[16] preliminary results from studies in the UK[17] and Italy[18] do not suggest any benefit from tamoxifen. Nonetheless, tamoxifen has been approved in the USA for short-term use in reducing the incidence of breast cancer in women at high risk.

Although studies of vitamins for the chemoprevention of cancer have largely produced disappointing results (see p.1333), other potential candidates for prophylaxis of breast cancer include newer anti-oestrogens such as droloxifene, raloxifene, and toremifene and retinoids such as fenretinide.[14]

There is also some evidence that weight gain, as measured by a high body-mass index, is associated with a greater risk of post menopausal breast cancer, and that avoidance of weight gain might be beneficial.[15]

1. Cuzick J, Baum M. Tamoxifen and contralateral breast cancer. *Lancet* 1985; **i:** 282.
2. Baum M, *et al.* Prospects for the chemoprevention of breast cancer. *Br Med Bull* 1991; **47:** 493–503.
3. Love RR. Prospects for antiestrogen chemoprevention of breast cancer. *J Natl Cancer Inst* 1990; **82:** 18–21.
4. Fugh-Berman A, Epstein S. Tamoxifen: disease prevention or disease substitution? *Lancet* 1992; **340:** 1143–5.
5. Powles TJ. The case for clinical trials of tamoxifen for prevention of breast cancer. *Lancet* 1992; **340:** 1145–7.
6. Powles TJ, *et al.* A pilot trial to evaluate the acute toxicity and feasibility of tamoxifen for prevention of breast cancer. *Br J Cancer* 1989; **60:** 126–31.
7. Cuzick J, Baum M. Prevention of breast cancer. *Lancet* 1992; **340:** 1550–1.
8. Fisher B, *et al.* Should healthy women take tamoxifen? *N Engl J Med* 1992; **327:** 1596–7.
9. Fugh-Berman A, Epstein S. Should healthy women take tamoxifen? *N Engl J Med* 1992; **327:** 1596.
10. Fugh-Berman A, Epstein SS. Tamoxifen and prevention. *Lancet* 1993; **341:** 695.
11. van Leeuwen FE, *et al.* Risk of endometrial cancer after tamoxifen treatment of breast cancer. *Lancet* 1994; **343:** 448–52.
12. Nease RF, Ross JM. The decision to enter a randomized trial of tamoxifen for the prevention of breast cancer in healthy women: an analysis of the tradeoffs. *Am J Med* 1995; **99:** 180–9.
13. Bruzzi P. Tamoxifen for the prevention of breast cancer. *Br Med J* 1998; **316:** 1181–2.
14. O'Shaughnessy JA. Chemoprevention of breast cancer. *JAMA* 1996; **275:** 1349–53.
15. Huang Z, *et al.* Dual effects of weight and weight gain on breast cancer risk. *JAMA* 1997; **278:** 1407–11.
16. Fisher B, *et al.* Tamoxifen for prevention of breast cancer: report of the National Surgical Adjuvant Breast and Bowel Project P-1 study. *J Natl Cancer Inst* 1998; **90:** 1371–88.
17. Powles T, *et al.* Interim analysis of the incidence of breast cancer in the Royal Marsden Hospital tamoxifen randomised chemoprevention trial. *Lancet* 1998; **352:** 98–101.
18. Veronesi U, *et al.* Prevention of breast cancer with tamoxifen: preliminary findings from the Italian randomised trial among hysterectomised women. *Lancet* 1998; **352:** 93–7.

MALIGNANT NEOPLASMS OF THE MALE BREAST. Although uncommon in most countries, breast cancer can occur in men; it may sometimes be associated with gynaecomastia and abnormalities of sex hormone metabolism, including those acquired through liver disease or testicular trauma. With improved treatment, prognosis is roughly equivalent to that in women, although lack of awareness of the risks may allow the disease to develop to a more advanced and less treatable stage before intervention is sought.

Treatment is similar to that for women. Primary management is surgical removal and axillary lymph node dissection. Because of the rarity of the disease large controlled trials are lacking but studies in limited numbers of men and extrapolation from results in women suggest that adjuvant drug therapy is appropriate in most patients. Opinions differ as to whether first-line adjuvant therapy should be with tamoxifen or chemotherapy. However, in advanced, metastatic disease tamoxifen appears to be the first choice treatment as the great majority of tumours are oestrogen-receptor positive. Combination chemotherapy with cyclophosphamide, methotrexate and fluorouracil (CMF) or, preferably, an anthracycline-containing regimen, can then be reserved for unresponsive or relapsing disease. Hormonal ablation by adrenalectomy or orchidectomy can produce responses in distant metastases but the former may have severe adverse effects and the latter can pose psychological problems: these therapies have become less popular since the advent of tamoxifen.

Some references to the management of male breast cancer are given below.

1. Jaiyesimi IA, *et al.* Carcinoma of the male breast. *Ann Intern Med* 1992; **117:** 771–7.
2. Nagadowska MM, Fentiman IS. Male breast cancer. *Br J Hosp Med* 1993; **49:** 104–10.

Malignant neoplasms of the cervix. Cancer of the uterine cervix is one of the most common cancers in women, accounting for about 12% of all female malignancies. It is associated with vaginal intercourse and it appears that human papilloma virus is implicated in its causation; high-risk types of the virus produce proteins (E6 and E7) which inactivate host tumour suppressor proteins and thus encourage malignant transformation. Smoking and long-term use of oral contraceptives (p.1428) are also risk factors.

Primary treatment of cervical cancer is with radiotherapy or surgery. Widespread screening has meant that in many women the disease has been detected in the early stages, when the prognosis is good:[1-3] up to 85% of women with early disease can be cured. Chemotherapy has been used in advanced disease, and may produce a response, but this is likely to be short-lived, without any overall impact on survival: its goals are essentially palliative.[3] Cisplatin is probably the most active single agent and has been used alone or in various combinations, for example with ifosfamide and bleomycin or vincristine and bleomycin.[1] Carboplatin has been substituted for cisplatin.[4] Other agents with some activity include cyclophosphamide, doxorubicin, fluorouracil, mitomycin, and vinblastine.[5] Neo-adjuvant therapy has been given before surgery or radiotherapy in order to reduce tumour size as well as treat micrometastases. However, there is a suggestion that chemotherapy (with cisplatin and epirubicin) before radiotherapy may reduce the activity of the latter,[6] and it is not clear, despite some impressive response rates, that combination chemotherapy with platinum-containing regimens improves survival when given as initial treatment for locally advanced disease.[3]

Chemoprevention of cervical cancer, by application of retinoic acid or its derivatives to cervical dysplasia, is under investigation. The use of human papilloma virus proteins E6 and E7 as targets for a therapeutic or prophylactic vaccine is also under investigation,[7] as is the use of gene therapy to supply a tumour suppressor protein (p53) directly to the tumour cells.[8]

1. Bridges J, Oram D. Management of advanced gynaecological malignancies. *Br J Hosp Med* 1993; **49:** 191–9.
2. Shaw LMA, *et al.* Cervical cancer: a two-pronged attack. *Practitioner* 1984; **228:** 555–9.
3. Cannistra SA, Niloff JM. Cancer of the uterine cervix. *N Engl J Med* 1996; **334:** 1030–8.
4. Murad AM, *et al.*. Phase II trial of bleomycin, ifosfamide, and carboplatin in metastatic cervical cancer. *J Clin Oncol* 1994; **12:** 55–9.
5. Anonymous. Drugs of choice for cancer chemotherapy. *Med Lett Drugs Ther* 1997; **39:** 21–8.
6. Tattersall MHN, *et al.* Randomized trial of epirubicin and cisplatin chemotherapy followed by pelvic radiation in locally advanced cervical cancer. *J Clin Oncol* 1995; **13:** 444–51.
7. Borysiewicz LK, *et al.* A recombinant vaccinia virus encoding human papillomavirus types 16 and 18, E6 and E7 proteins as immunotherapy for cervical cancer. *Lancet* 1996; **347:** 1523–7.
8. Hamada K, *et al.* Adenovirus-mediated transfer of a wild-type p53 gene and induction of apoptosis in cervical cancer. *Cancer Res* 1996; **56:** 3047–54.

Malignant neoplasms of the endometrium. Cancer of the endometrium is a disease primarily of postmenopausal women, and is more common in developed than developing countries. It may be associated with use of oestrogens in postmenopausal women and there is a slightly increased risk in women taking tamoxifen. The disease is insidious and symptoms of vaginal discharge, bleeding, or pain may be confused with menopausal disorders. Disease progression is relatively slow, thanks in part to the barrier formed by the muscular wall of the uterus. Endometrial hyperplasia and endometrial polyps have been regarded as precancerous lesions but their relationship with endometrial cancer is debatable.

About 80% of women with endometrial cancer present with early (Stage I) disease and almost all of these can be cured by adequate surgery combined with adjuvant radiotherapy and a progestogen.[1-3] Chemotherapy with cytotoxic agents has been tried in advanced disease, mainly for palliation, and with limited success.[1-3] The agents of choice are probably doxorubicin, cisplatin, and cyclophosphamide or ifosfamide although other agents including fluorouracil and altretamine have been tried[4] and recent results suggest paclitaxel is active.[1] Hormonal manipulation with progestogens has a long history in the management of advanced endometrial cancer, although response may depend on the hormone receptor concentration of the tumour and has not always been good.[3] Tamoxifen has also been tried (with indifferent results[3]) but there is now evidence that it can promote endometrial cancer.[5] Also under investigation is the use of gonadorelin analogues.[6]

1. Rose PG. Endometrial carcinoma. *N Engl J Med* 1996; **335:** 640–9. Correction. *ibid.* 1997; **336:** 1335.
2. Burke TW, *et al.* Treatment failure in endometrial carcinoma. *Obstet Gynecol* 1990; **75:** 96–101.
3. Bridges J, Oram D. Management of advanced gynaecological malignancies. *Br J Hosp Med* 1993; **49:** 191–9.
4. Anonymous. Drugs of choice for cancer chemotherapy. *Med Lett Drugs Ther* 1997; **39:** 21–8.
5. van Leeuwen FE, *et al.* Risk of endometrial cancer after tamoxifen treatment of breast cancer. *Lancet* 1994; **343:** 448–52.
6. Gallagher CJ, *et al.* A new treatment for endometrial cancer with gonadotrophin-releasing hormone analogue. *Br J Obstet Gynaecol* 1991; **98:** 1037–41.

Malignant neoplasms of the eye. Tumours of the orbit of the eye in adults are most commonly metastases from primary lesions elsewhere in the body, usually in the breast or lung, and local radiotherapy may be required for control of visual symptoms unresponsive to chemotherapeutic treatment of primary disease. Lymphoma and rhabdomyosarcoma are the most common primary orbital tumours. The most common primary tumour of the eye itself is ocular melanoma (conjunctival or uveal melanoma), which may be treated by surgical excision, cryotherapy, or radiotherapy;[1-3] local application of mitomycin (as 0.04% eye drops) has been reported to reduce tumour volume.[1]

In children, the most common intra-ocular tumour is retinoblastoma, which is discussed on p.495.

1. Finger PT, *et al.* Topical chemotherapy for conjunctival melanoma. *Br J Ophthalmol* 1993; **77:** 751–3.
2. Paridaens ADA, *et al.* Orbital exenteration in 95 cases of primary conjunctival malignant melanoma. *Br J Ophthalmol* 1994; **78:** 520–8.
3. Shields JA, Shields CL. Current management of posterior uveal melanoma. *Mayo Clin Proc* 1993; **68:** 1196–1200.

Malignant neoplasms of the gastro-intestinal tract. Considered as a whole (and excluding skin cancers, which are often poorly registered) the gastro-intestinal tract is the most frequent site of malignancies in the world's population, although the frequencies of the various types of gastro-intestinal cancer vary greatly from country to country. Direct exposure to various environmental carcinogens is thought to play an important role in many of these cancers. Treatment may include surgery, radiotherapy, and chemotherapy, but the prognosis in most forms of gastro-intestinal cancer is not encouraging.

Cancer of the mouth accounts for as much as 40% of head and neck cancer (see also p.489), most often as squamous cell carcinoma arising from the oropharyngeal mucosa. Incidence of oral cancer is increasing in some countries. Onset is often insidious and patients often present with advanced disease. Leukoplakia and erythroplasia of the mouth represent premalignant lesions in some cases, and require biopsy. Oral use of tobacco or betel-nut mixtures are potential risk factors, as is alcohol. The choice of treatment, in general terms, lies between radiotherapy and surgery. Response rates to chemotherapy are variable, the most active agents being cisplatin, fluorouracil, bleomycin, and methotrexate (particularly in recurrent disease). Although single-agent and combination chemotherapy has been tried as adjuvant and neo-adjuvant treatment there is no evidence of any consistent survival benefit.[1] There is some evidence that isotretinoin may be useful in preventing the development of squamous cell carcinoma in patients with leukoplakia.[2]

Oesophageal cancer, which comprises about 2% of all non-skin malignant tumours worldwide, usually develops as a growth or ulcerative lesion of the oesophagus with extensive infiltration of the mucosa and invasion of neighbouring structures. Lymphatic and blood-borne metastasis occurs at a relatively early stage. Symptoms of pain and dysphagia due to obstruction occur late and disease is usually well advanced at diagnosis. Although factors such as diet and achalasia have been suggested as possible causative factors, only smoking and alcohol have clearly been implicated. Surgery, or for some upper oesophageal lesions, radiotherapy, is again the primary treatment[3-5] although in half to two-thirds of cases disease is too advanced for anything but palliation.[3] The use of local laser therapy alone or together with photosensitisers such as porfimer sodium[6] may be helpful in relieving obstruction. Some results in patients with advanced squamous cell carcinoma of the oesophagus treated with cisplatin, vindesine, and bleomycin,[3] suggest that chemotherapy may have some clinical benefit in this subgroup of patients, and small series of radiotherapy combined with concomitant fluorouracil and cisplatin,[7] or pre- and post-operative adjuvant chemotherapy combined with resection[8] have reported prolonged survival. Another small study in patients with adenocarcinoma found that pre-operative radiotherapy and chemotherapy (with cisplatin and fluorouracil) offers an improvement in survival over surgery alone,[9] but it is not clear that such treatment is appropriate in all patients;[10] survival benefits of pre-operative chemoradiotherapy were less clear in a study in patients with squamous cell carcinoma.[11] Only about 5 to 10% of all patients with oesophageal cancer will be alive after 5 years, and there is clearly a need for improved therapy.

Cancer of the stomach is the most common non-skin cancer worldwide, with particularly high incidence in the Far East, Russia, and parts of Latin America, although the incidence is declining almost everywhere. Dietary factors are thought to play a role in the development of stomach cancer; *Helicobacter pylori* infection, and resultant gastritis, may also play an important role. Early disease is relatively asymptomatic but more advanced disease may produce discomfort or pain, anaemia, weight loss, and anorexia; obstruction, haemorrhage, and perforation may develop. Extension to the liver and pancreas, and lymphatic and blood-borne (portal) metastases may occur. As for oesophageal cancer, the overall prognosis is not good, and 5-year survival rates are only 5 to 10%. Surgery is the mainstay of treatment, but many tumours are inoperable at presentation. Persistent gastric ulcers may well be malignant and warrant biopsy and if necessary surgical intervention.[12] Whether elimination of *Helicobacter pylori* infection will prove useful in preventing the development of gastric cancer is a matter of debate.[13-16] (For the role of *Helicobacter* infection in gastric MALT lymphoma see above).

Gastric cancer has traditionally been regarded as resistant to chemotherapy, but in fact responses may be seen to therapy. Fluorouracil produces responses in about 20% of patients, and the superiority of the various combination regimens tried over fluorouracil alone is debatable.[17,18] Other agents with some activity include mitomycin, anthracyclines such as doxorubicin or epirubicin, cisplatin, and etoposide.[17-19]

Postoperative adjuvant therapy has not been shown to produce any benefit,[20,21] but there is some interest in pre-operative or neo-adjuvant therapy to reduce tumour bulk and improve resection rates in locally advanced disease;[17,19] a combination of etoposide, doxorubicin, and cisplatin is reported to be effective in this role,[22] but toxicity is high. Other regimens include cisplatin with continuous infusion of fluorouracil,[19] or cisplatin, epirubicin, and fluorouracil.[17] Immunostimulants are also under investigation.[23]

Chemotherapy has been most extensively investigated in advanced disease. Despite doubts about the superiority of combination chemotherapy over single agents fluorouracil, doxorubicin, and mitomycin (FAM) has been widely used.[18,19] More recently good results have been seen with combinations of epirubicin, cisplatin, and fluorouracil (ECF),[17,24,25] or fluorouracil, doxorubicin, and methotrexate (FAMTX).[17,19,26,27] Recent results[25] have suggested a modest improvement in survival may be possible with such chemotherapy.

Cancers of the colon and rectum are very common in developed areas such as the USA and western Europe, but rare among African and Asian populations. Dietary factors may be related to development of the disease. Intestinal polyps, particularly if large or multiple, may predispose to development of cancer. Over 50% of large bowel tumours occur in the rectum and about 20% in the sigmoid colon. There may be direct invasion of neighbouring structures and metastatic spread to the lymph nodes, and to lungs, bone, and in particular, liver. Symptoms include blood in the stools, altered bowel habit, anaemia, and weight loss; there may be local obstruction (depending on location) or perforation.

The first-line treatment for localised disease is surgery. Patients with tumours of the colon and rectum have a slightly better prognosis than most other forms of gastro-intestinal cancer, since the majority of cases are operable at the time of diagnosis,[28,29] but 50 to 60% ultimately die of recurrent disease.[28,30] Adjuvant therapy, usually based on fluorouracil, has been widely used, although some have questioned the magnitude of the benefit.[31] Some studies have suggested a benefit from combined chemotherapy and radiotherapy in rectal cancer[32] but not from chemotherapy in colonic[33] cancer, perhaps because rectal disease seems less likely to metastasise.[34] In the USA, owing to results in patients with high-risk rectal carcinoma,[34,35] it has been concluded that patients with advanced (stages B and C) rectal cancer who do not participate in clinical trials should receive adjuvant fluorouracil and radiotherapy after surgery.[36]

Various approaches have been considered to improve the efficacy of fluorouracil adjuvant therapy. Fluorouracil is only active against actively dividing cells, and there is some evidence that maximising the chances of exposure, by giving prolonged fluorouracil infusions, may improve the results of adjuvant therapy compared with bolus administration.[37] Another approach is the use of biochemical modulators such as folinic acid, or immunomodulators such as levamisole. In the USA, good results with adjuvant fluorouracil and levamisole in patients with locally-advanced (Dukes stage B2 or C) colon cancer[38,39] produced recommendations that all patients outside clinical trials with stage C disease should receive this combination.[30,36,39] Like the recommendation for the use of fluorouracil with radiotherapy in rectal carcinoma, this has not been universally adopted,[29] because of scepticism about the degree of benefit and the effects on quality of life.[40,41] Combination of fluorouracil with folinic acid improves tumour response rates in advanced disease,[42,43] and although most individual studies of the combination for adjuvant therapy have not been able to show more than minimal improvements in survival there is some evidence that this is the case.[44]

Newer agents such as raltitrexed and oxaliplatin, which have been used for palliative therapy, offer potential alternative candidates for adjuvant treatment too,[29] although the studies remain to be done. There are also reports of benefit with calcium supplementation,[45] and with cimetidine.[46] Improved survival over 5 years of follow-up has however been reported with the adjuvant use of edrecolomab, a murine monoclonal antibody directed against an epithelial cell surface glycoprotein.[47]

Another potential approach is the adjuvant use of intraportal chemotherapy directed at the liver, one of the commonest sites of metastasis for colon cancer. Although good results have been reported following intraportal infusion of mitomycin and fluorouracil,[48] it is not clear whether the benefits of this procedure were truly localised, since systemic metastases were also reduced, and the procedure remains investigational. Liver metastases may respond better to chemotherapy than metastases in other sites.[42] Adjuvant intraperitoneal chemotherapy has also been investigated.[29]

Chemotherapy is also used in the palliative management of inoperable colorectal malignancy. Combination of fluorouracil with low-dose folinic acid has been recommended as standard therapy for patients with advanced colorectal cancer, although the benefits are modest. A bimonthly schedule of high-dose folinic acid with bolus fluorouracil followed by continuous infusion may be more effective and less toxic.[65] Others suggest that protracted venous infusion of fluorouracil via an infusion pump and a central venous catheter is a valid alternative as standard therapy.[42] Combination of fluorouracil with interferon alfa,[49,50] or with interferon alfa and folinic acid,[50] has been investigated, as has combination with sparfosic acid.[30,51] The platinum derivative oxaliplatin has also been used in combination with fluorouracil and folinic acid, as well as being used alone. Results suggest that the toxicity of such therapy can be reduced, and efficacy perhaps increased, if it is timed to coincide with circadian rhythms (chronotherapy),[52] rather than being given by continuous infusion, a concept which probably applies to other regimens. Other new drugs being investigated in the treatment of advanced metastatic disease include irinotecan, which has improved survival in patients refractory to fluorouracil,[53,66] and raltitrexed, which appears to be as effective as fluorouracil but better tolerated.[42,54-56] Orally-active derivatives of fluorouracil such as capecitabine are also under investigation and look extremely promising. The taxane docetaxel has reportedly proved disappointing.[57] More exotic therapies, including anti-idiotype vaccines, gene therapy, and antisense therapy are under consideration.[42]

Also of some interest is the use of NSAIDs such as aspirin[58-61] or sulindac (which has proved of benefit in familial adenomatous polyposis[62,63]) in possibly preventing the development of colorectal cancer. Calcium supplementation may also be effective,[45] and current postmenopausal hormone replacement therapy also appears to reduce the risk of colorectal cancer.[64] Vitamin supplementation, however, does not appear to be helpful in this regard, as discussed on p.1333.

1. McAndrew PG. Oral cancer and precancer: treatment. *Br Dent J* 1990; **168:** 191–8.
2. Lippman SM, *et al.* Comparison of low-dose isotretinoin with beta carotene to prevent oral carcinogenesis. *N Engl J Med* 1993; **328:** 15–20.
3. Bancewicz J. Cancer of the oesophagus. *Br Med J* 1990; **300:** 3–4.
4. Chung SCS, *et al.* Surgical therapy for squamous-cell carcinoma of the oesophagus. *Lancet* 1994; **343:** 521–4.
5. O'Reilly S, Forastiere A. New approaches to treating oesophageal cancer. *Br Med J* 1994; **308:** 1249–50.
6. Lightdale CJ, *et al.* Photodynamic therapy with porfimer sodium versus thermal ablation therapy with Nd:YAG laser for palliation of esophageal cancer: a multicenter randomized trial. *Gastrointest Endosc* 1995; **42:** 507–12.
7. Seitz JF, *et al.* Inoperable nonmetastatic squamous cell carcinoma of the oesophagus managed by concomitant chemotherapy (5-fluorouracil and cisplatin) and radiation therapy. *Cancer* 1990; **66:** 214–19.
8. Hilgenberg AD, *et al.* Preoperative chemotherapy, surgical resection, and selective postoperative therapy for squamous cell carcinoma of the esophagus. *Ann Thorac Surg* 1988; **45:** 357–63.
9. Walsh TN, *et al.* A comparison of multimodal therapy and surgery for esophageal adenocarcinoma. *N Engl J Med* 1996; **335:** 462–7.
10. Wilke HJ, Fink U. Multimodal therapy for adenocarcinoma of the esophagus and esophagogastric junction. *N Engl J Med* 1996; **335:** 509–10.
11. Bosset J-F, *et al.* Chemoradiotherapy followed by surgery compared with surgery alone in squamous-cell cancer of the esophagus. *N Engl J Med* 1997; **337:** 161–7.
12. Thompson GB, *et al.* Adenocarcinoma of the stomach: are we making progress? *Lancet* 1993; **342:** 713–18.
13. Leon-Barua R, *et al.* Can eradication of Helicobacter pylori prevent gastric cancer? *Drugs* 1993; **46:** 341–6.
14. Goodwin CS. Gastric cancer and Helicobacter pylori: the whispering killer? *Lancet* 1993; **342:** 507–8.
15. Reed PI, *et al.* Gastric cancer and Helicobacter pylori. *Lancet* 1993; **342:** 987.
16. Kuipers EJ, *et al.* Long-term sequelae of Helicobacter pylori gastritis. *Lancet* 1995; **345:** 1525–8.
17. Ellis P, Cunningham D. Management of carcinomas of the upper gastrointestinal tract. *Br Med J* 1994; **308:** 834–8.
18. Fuchs CS, Mayer RJ. Gastric carcinoma. *N Engl J Med* 1995; **333:** 32–41.
19. Hendlisz A, Bleiberg H. Diagnosis and treatment of gastric cancer. *Drugs* 1995; **49:** 711–20.
20. Allum WH, *et al.* Adjuvant chemotherapy in operable gastric cancer: 5-year follow-up of first British Stomach Cancer Group trial. *Lancet* 1989; **i:** 571–4.
21. Hallissey MT, *et al.* The second British Stomach Cancer Group trial of adjuvant radiotherapy or chemotherapy in resectable gastric cancer: five-year follow-up. *Lancet* 1994; **343:** 1309–12.
22. Wilke H, *et al.* Neoadjuvant chemotherapy with etoposide/adriamycin/cisplatin (EAP) in locally advanced gastric cancer. *Proc Am Soc Clin Oncol* 1988; **7:** 100.
23. Nakazato H, *et al.* Efficacy of immunochemotherapy as adjuvant treatment after curative resection of gastric cancer. *Lancet* 1994; **343:** 1122–6.
24. Cunningham D, *et al.* Cisplatin, epirubicin and 5-fluorouracil (CEF) has significant activity in advanced gastric cancer. *Proc Am Soc Clin Oncol* 1990; **9:** 123.
25. Webb A, *et al.* Randomized trial comparing epirubicin, cisplatin, and fluorouracil versus fluorouracil, doxorubicin, and methotrexate in advanced esophagogastric cancer. *J Clin Oncol* 1997; **15:** 261–7.
26. Wils JA, *et al.* Sequential high-dose methotrexate and fluorouracil combined with doxorubicin—a step ahead in the treatment of advanced gastric cancer: a trial of the European Organization for Research and Treatment of Cancer Gastrointestinal Tract Cooperative Group. *J Clin Oncol* 1991; **9:** 827–31.
27. Murad A, *et al.* Modified therapy with 5 fluorouracil, doxorubicin, and methotrexate in advanced gastric cancer. *Cancer* 1993; **72:** 37–41.
28. Buyse M, *et al.* Adjuvant therapy of colorectal cancer: why we still don't know. *JAMA* 1988; **259:** 3571–7.
29. Kerr DJ, Gray R. Adjuvant chemotherapy for colorectal cancer. *Br J Hosp Med* 1996; **55:** 259–62.
30. Slevin ML, Gray R. Adjuvant therapy for cancer of the colon. *Br Med J* 1991; **302:** 1100–1.
31. Gray R, *et al.* AXIS: a suitable case for treatment. *Br J Cancer* 1991; **63:** 841–5.
32. Gastrointestinal Tumor Study Group. Prolongation of the disease-free interval in surgically treated rectal carcinoma. *N Engl J Med* 1985; **312:** 1465–72.
33. Gastrointestinal Tumor Study Group. Adjuvant therapy of colon cancer—results of a prospectively randomized trial. *N Engl J Med* 1984; **310:** 737–43.
34. Steele G. Combined-modality therapy for rectal carcinoma—the time has come. *N Engl J Med* 1991; **324:** 764–6.
35. Krook JE, *et al.* Effective surgical adjuvant therapy for high-risk rectal carcinoma. *N Engl J Med* 1991; **324:** 709–15.
36. NIH Consensus Panel. Adjuvant therapy for patients with colon and rectal cancer. *JAMA* 1990; **264:** 1444–50.
37. O'Connell MJ, *et al.* Improving adjuvant therapy for rectal cancer by combining protracted infusion fluorouracil with radiation therapy after curative surgery. *N Engl J Med* 1994; **331:** 502–7.
38. Moertel CG, *et al.* Levamisole and fluorouracil for adjuvant therapy of resected colon carcinoma. *N Engl J Med* 1990; **322:** 352–8.
39. Moertel CG, *et al.* Fluorouracil plus levamisole as effective adjuvant therapy after resection of stage III colon carcinoma: a final report. *Ann Intern Med* 1995; **122:** 321–6.
40. Steele G. Accomplishment and promise in the understanding and treatment of colorectal cancer. *Lancet* 1993; **342:** 1092–6.
41. Sagar P, Taylor B. Adjuvant therapy and quality of life. *Lancet* 1993; **341:** 376.
42. Ross PJ, Cunningham D. Chemotherapy of metastatic bowel cancer. *Br J Hosp Med* 1996; **55:** 263–6.

43. Advanced Colorectal Cancer Meta-analysis Project. Modulation of fluorouracil by leucovorin in patients with advanced colorectal cancer: evidence in terms of response rate. *J Clin Oncol* 1992; **10:** 896–903.
44. International Multicentre Pooled Analysis of Colon Cancer Trials (IMPACT) Investigators. Efficacy of adjuvant fluorouracil and folinic acid in colon cancer. *Lancet* 1995; **345:** 939–44.
45. Duris I, *et al.* Calcium chemoprevention in colorectal cancer. *Hepatogastroenterology* 1996; **43:** 152–4.
46. Matsumoto S. Cimetidine and survival with colorectal cancer. *Lancet* 1995; **346:** 115.
47. Riethmüller G, *et al.* Randomised trial of monoclonal antibody for adjuvant therapy of resected Dukes' C colorectal carcinoma. *Lancet* 1994; **343:** 1177–83.
48. Swiss Group for Clinical Cancer Research. Long-term results of single course of adjuvant intraportal chemotherapy for colorectal cancer. *Lancet* 1995; **345:** 349–53.
49. Cunningham D, *et al.* Survival after systemic therapy for metastatic colorectal cancer. *Lancet* 1995; **345:** 328–9.
50. Allegra CJ. New therapeutic strategies for patients with gastrointestinal malignancies using biochemical modulation of fluorouracil. *JAMA* 1995; **273:** 236–9.
51. Kemeny NE, *et al.* Chemotherapy for colorectal cancer. *N Engl J Med* 1994; **331:** 680.
52. Lévi F, *et al.* Randomised multicentre trial of chronotherapy with oxaliplatin, fluorouracil, and folinic acid in metastatic colorectal cancer. *Lancet* 1997; **350:** 681–6.
53. Rougier P, *et al.* Randomised trial of irinotecan versus fluorouracil by continuous infusion after fluorouracil failure in patients with metastatic colorectal cancer. *Lancet* 1998; **352:** 1407–12.
54. Cunningham D, *et al.* Tomudex (ZD1694): results of a randomised trial in advanced colorectal cancer demonstrate efficacy and reduced mucositis and leucopenia. *Eur J Cancer* 1995; **31A:** 1945–54.
55. Cunningham D, *et al.* Tomudex (ZD1694): a novel thymidylate synthase inhibitor with clinical antitumour activity in a range of solid tumours. *Ann Oncol* 1996; **7:** 179–82.
56. Mead GM. Raltitrexed, a new drug for advanced colorectal cancer. *Lancet* 1996; **347:** 1568–9.
57. Pazdur R, *et al.* Phase II trial of docetaxel (Taxotere) in metastatic colorectal carcinoma. *Ann Oncol* 1994; **5:** 468–70.
58. Paganini-Hill A. Aspirin and colorectal cancer. *Br Med J* 1993; **307:** 278–9.
59. Logan RFA, *et al.* Effect of aspirin and non-steroidal anti-inflammatory drugs on colorectal adenomas: case-control study of subjects participating in the Nottingham faecal occult blood screening programme. *Br Med J* 1993; **307:** 285–9.
60. Giovannucci E, *et al.* Aspirin use and the risk for colorectal cancer and adenoma in male health professionals. *Ann Intern Med* 1994; **121:** 241–6.
61. Giovannucci E, *et al.* Aspirin and the risk of colorectal cancer in women. *N Engl J Med* 1995; **333:** 609–14.
62. Giardiello FM, *et al.* Treatment of colonic and rectal adenomas with sulindac in familial adenomatous polyposis. *N Engl J Med* 1993; **328:** 1313–16.
63. Tonelli F, Valanzano R. Sulindac in familial adenomatous polyposis. *Lancet* 1993; **342:** 1120.
64. Grodstein F, *et al.* Postmenopausal hormone use and risk for colorectal cancer and adenoma. *Ann Intern Med* 1998; **128:** 705–12.
65. de Gramont A, *et al.* Randomized trial comparing monthly low-dose leucovorin and fluorouracil bolus with bimonthly high-dose leucovorin and fluorouracil bolus plus continuous infusion for advanced colorectal cancer: a French intergroup study. *J Clin Oncol* 1997; **15:** 808–15.
66. Cunningham D, *et al.* Randomised trial of irinotecan plus supportive care versus supportive care alone after fluorouracil failure for patients with metastatic colorectal cancer. *Lancet* 1998; **352:** 1413–18.

Malignant neoplasms of the head and neck. Cancers of the head and neck include neoplasms of lip, oral cavity, pharynx, larynx, sinuses, and salivary glands; the majority are squamous cell carcinomas. About 40% of head and neck cancers occur in the oral cavity, 25% in the larynx, 15% in the pharynx, and the remainder in other sites. Overall, cancers of the head and neck account for about 10% of all malignant neoplasms worldwide.

For discussion of the role of chemotherapy in the treatment of malignant neoplasms of the mouth, see under Malignant Neoplasms of the Gastro-intestinal Tract, above.

Despite improvements in surgery, radiotherapy, and chemotherapy for cancer of the head and neck, there has been little change in survival, which is poor in advanced disease, in part because of the frequent development of second malignant tumours,[1-4] although nasopharyngeal carcinoma has a more indolent course.[3]

Surgery and radiotherapy are the mainstays of treatment, while chemotherapy is used essentially for palliation or as adjuvant therapy. Palliative treatment in metastatic or recurrent disease is likely to be with a combination of cisplatin and fluorouracil, or with methotrexate.[2,4] Combination regimens such as cisplatin, bleomycin, and methotrexate, with or without a vinca alkaloid, produce more responses but survival is not definitively improved.[4] Good initial response rates have been seen with paclitaxel[5] and docetaxel;[6] other drugs under investigation include vinorelbine and oxaliplatin.[4]

The role of adjuvant therapy in locally advanced disease is much less clear. However, pre-operative or neoadjuvant therapy with cisplatin and fluorouracil,[3,7,8] does produce responses and may permit preservation of the larynx in advanced laryngeal squamous carcinoma.[7] It is not clear whether neoadjuvant therapy improves survival.[9] Concomitant administration of cisplatin, or cisplatin and fluorouracil, with radiotherapy does appear, however, to improve survival,[10,11,15] and for nasopharyngeal carcinoma concomitant cisplatin and radiotherapy is now considered standard in the USA.[12]

Chemoprevention is also under investigation: results indicating that isotretinoin can reduce the occurrence of second primary tumours (although not apparently the recurrence of primary disease)[13] suggest that such an approach may be helpful in the management of head and neck cancer.[14]

1. Ogden GR. Second malignant tumours in head and neck cancer. *Br Med J* 1991; **302:** 193–4.
2. Vokes EE, *et al.* Head and neck cancer. *N Engl J Med* 1993; **328:** 184–94.
3. Tobias JS. Cancer of the head and neck. *Br Med J* 1994; **308:** 961–6.
4. Catimel G. Head and neck cancer: guidelines for chemotherapy. *Drugs* 1996; **51:** 73–88.
5. Forastière A. Use of paclitaxel ('Taxol') in squamous cell carcinoma of the head and neck. *Semin Oncol* 1993; **20** (suppl 3): 56–60.
6. Dreyfuss A, *et al.* 'Taxotere' (TXTR) for advanced incurable squamous cell carcinoma of the head and neck (SCCHN). *Proc Am Soc Clin Oncol* 1994; **13:** 287.
7. The Department of Veterans Affairs Laryngeal Cancer Study Group. Induction chemotherapy plus radiation compared with surgery plus radiation in patients with advanced laryngeal cancer. *N Engl J Med* 1991; **324:** 1685–90.
8. Dreyfuss AI, *et al.* Continuous infusion high-dose leucovorin with 5-fluorouracil and cisplatin for untreated stage IV carcinoma of the head and neck. *Ann Intern Med* 1990; **112:** 167–72.
9. Tobias JS. Current role of chemotherapy in head and neck cancer. *Drugs* 1992; **43:** 333–45.
10. Merlano M, *et al.* Treatment of advanced squamous-cell carcinoma of the head and neck with alternating chemotherapy and radiotherapy. *N Engl J Med* 1992; **327:** 1115–21.
11. Al-Sarraf M. *et al.* Superiority of chemo-radiotherapy (CT-RT) vs radiotherapy (RT) in patients with locally advanced nasopharyngeal cancer. *Proc Am Soc Clin Oncol* 1996; **15:** 313.
12. Vokes EE, *et al.* Nasopharyngeal carcinoma. *Lancet* 1997; **350:** 1087–91.
13. Hong WK, *et al.* Prevention of second primary tumors with isotretinoin in squamous-cell carcinoma of the head and neck. *N Engl J Med* 1990; **323:** 795–801.
14. Meyskens FL. Coming of age—the chemoprevention of cancer. *N Engl J Med* 1990; **323:** 825–7.
15. Brizel DM, *et al.* Hyperfractionated irradiation with or without concurrent chemotherapy for locally advanced head and neck cancer. *N Engl J Med* 1998; **338:** 1798–1804.

Malignant neoplasms of the kidney. Cancer of the kidney is relatively uncommon. About 80% of such cancers in adults are renal cell carcinoma, with the remainder mostly cancer of the renal pelvis. The disease is about twice as common in men as in women. The risk may be increased by smoking or exposure to certain NSAIDs. Disease is often clinically silent; there may however be haematuria and vague pain, and renal cell carcinoma in particular may be associated with metabolic disturbances such as hypercalcaemia.

The main treatment is surgery, which can prolong survival, but metastasis is common and the majority of patients eventually relapse.[1,2] Renal cell carcinoma is largely resistant to chemotherapy with currently available antineoplastics, and hormonal therapy has also had poor success.[1,2] A review of 83 studies involving 4542 patients and over 70 different drugs found that only floxuridine and fluorouracil appeared to have even modest activity.[3] Slightly better results have been reported from treatment with interleukin-2,[4-7] although the results are still not striking. One large series[6] has reported complete responses in 10 of 149 patients with metastatic renal cell cancer, with prolonged response in 7. It should be noted that the toxicity of such treatment can be considerable,[1,4,6] and few patients are able to tolerate a full bolus dose.[6] Attempts to reduce the toxicity of treatment have included the use of continuous infusion[5,7] and the use of lower doses of interleukin-2 given by the subcutaneous route.[8] Some studies combined the use of interleukin-2 with infusion of lymphokine-activated killer cells,[4] but this does not appear to add a therapeutic benefit.[7] There has been a report of increased survival in patients given a monthly infusion of their own lymphocytes, activated *in vitro* with an autologous lymphokine mixture.[9] The interferons (mainly interferon alfa) have also produced some responses, particularly in patients who have undergone nephrectomy and with metastases mainly confined to the lung.[1] Monotherapy with interferon alfa has been shown to produce modest benefit (improvement in median survival of 2.5 months).[15] (However, interferon gamma-1b was no better than placebo in one study.[13]) Combination of interleukin-2 and interferon alfa may produce greater benefit than either alone, but again, is associated with considerable toxicity:[10,11,14] benefits of such a combination with fluorouracil were reported to be confined to the fittest patients.[8] Also under investigation is the use of interferon alfa plus isotretinoin.[12]

1. Motzer RJ, *et al.* Renal-cell carcinoma. *N Engl J Med* 1996; **335:** 865–75.
2. Dawson C, Whitfield H. Urological malignancy III: renal and testicular carcinoma. *Br Med J* 1996; **312:** 1146–8.
3. Yagoda A, *et al.* Chemotherapy for advanced renal-cell carcinoma: 1983-1993. *Semin Oncol* 1995; **22:** 42–60.
4. Rosenberg SA, *et al.* A progress report on the treatment of 157 patients with advanced cancer using lymphokine-activated killer cells and interleukin-2 or high-dose interleukin-2 alone. *N Engl J Med* 1987; **316:** 889–97.
5. West WH, *et al.* Constant-infusion recombinant interleukin-2 in adoptive immunotherapy of advanced cancer. *N Engl J Med* 1987; **316:** 898–905.
6. Rosenberg SA, *et al.* Treatment of 283 consecutive patients with metastatic melanoma or renal cell cancer using high-dose bolus interleukin 2. *JAMA* 1994; **271:** 907–13.
7. Law TM, *et al.* Phase III randomized trial of interleukin-2 with or without lymphokine-activated killer cells in the treatment of patients with advanced renal cell carcinoma. *Cancer* 1995; **76:** 824–32.
8. Joffe JK, *et al.* A phase II study of interferon-alpha, interleukin-2 and 5-fluorouracil in advanced renal carcinoma: clinical data and laboratory evidence of protease activation. *Br J Urol* 1996; **77:** 638–49.
9. Osband ME, *et al.* Effect of autolymphocyte therapy on survival and quality of life in patients with metastatic renal-cell carcinoma. *Lancet* 1990; **335:** 994–8.
10. Besana C, *et al.* Treatment of advanced renal cell cancer with sequential intravenous recombinant interleukin-2 and subcutaneous α-interferon. *Eur J Cancer* 1994; **30A**: 1292–8.
11. Négrier S, *et al.* Intensive regimen of cytokines with interleukin-2 and interferon alfa-2B in selected patients with metastatic renal carcinoma. *J Immunother* 1995; **17:** 62–8.
12. Motzer RJ, *et al.* Interferon alfa-2a and 13-cis-retinoic acid in renal cell carcinoma: antitumor activity in a phase II trial and interactions in vitro. *J Clin Oncol* 1995; **13:** 1950–7.
13. Gleave ME, *et al.* Interferon gamma-1b compared with placebo in metastatic renal-cell carcinoma. *N Engl J Med* 1998; **338:** 1265–71.
14. Negrier S, *et al.* Recombinant human interleukin-2, recombinant human interferon alfa-2a, or both in metastatic renal-cell carcinoma. *N Engl J Med* 1998; **338:** 1272–8.
15. Medical Research Council Renal Cancer Collaborators. Interferon-α and survival in metastatic renal carcinoma: early results of a randomised controlled trial. *Lancet* 1999; **353:** 14–17.

WILMS' TUMOUR. In children most cases of renal tumours are due to Wilms' tumour (nephroblastoma). This is one of the most frequent solid tumours in childhood with a peak incidence between 1 and 5 years of age and accounting for about 6% of all childhood malignancies. The usual presentation is an asymptomatic abdominal mass; abdominal pain is less frequent and haematuria occurs only in about a quarter of patients. Metastasis may occur in advanced disease, usually to the lungs and occasionally to the lymph nodes and liver.

Unlike other forms of renal cancer Wilms' tumour responds well to chemotherapy. The basis of treatment is surgery, combined with postoperative chemotherapy, and if necessary radiotherapy; precise management varies with disease stage.[1,2] In early disease, chemotherapy consists of vincristine alone or combined with dactinomycin; in more advanced disease radiotherapy, and doxorubicin and cyclophosphamide may be added.[1-3] Overall survival rates are 80 to 90%, although in metastatic disease survival is somewhat lower.[2,3] The good prognosis has been sustained despite a trend towards less-intensive treatment in many children.[3] However, in children who relapse after initial treatment survival is poor, possibly because of the development of antineoplastic resistance:[4] salvage rates of about 10 to 25% have been reported.[2]

1. Bailey CC. Childhood cancers. *Br J Hosp Med* 1984; **31:** 36–40.
2. Mehta MP, *et al.* Treatment of Wilms' tumour: current recommendations. *Drugs* 1991; **42:** 766–80.
3. D'Angio GJ, *et al.* Treatment of Wilms' tumor: results of the third National Wilms' Tumor Study. *Cancer* 1989; **64:** 349–60.
4. Groot-Loonen JJ, *et al.* How curable is relapsed Wilms' tumour? *Arch Dis Child* 1990; **65:** 968–70.

Malignant neoplasms of the liver. Primary liver cancer, in the form of hepatocellular carcinoma, is uncommon in northern Europe and America but is the most common cancer among men in large parts of Africa and Asia. The incidence in men is about 4 times that in women. Chronic infection with hepatitis B virus (and possibly hepatitis C virus) is by far the most important factor associated with development of liver cancer, although other risk factors include ingestion of foodstuffs contaminated with aflatoxins (see p.1544), alcohol, cigarette smoking, and possibly the long-term use of oral contraceptives, although this is the subject of controversy (see p.1428).

Clinical manifestations of liver cancer include increasing obstructive jaundice, pain, malaise, and the presence of an epigastric mass; there may be metastasis to the lungs, kidney, bones, brain or other sites, or invasion of local structures.

Hepatocellular carcinoma is relatively resistant to chemotherapy and radiotherapy; surgical resection, or perhaps liver transplantation, offers the only hope of cure.[1-3] Most patients present with advanced or unresectable disease; of those that present with resectable disease about 20 to 30% are alive at 5 years after surgery.[1] Survival is better in patients with small rather than large tumours: liver transplantation produced an overall survival rate of 85% at 4 years in patients with tumours less than 5 cm in diameter.[4] Screening of high risk patients to detect hepatocellular carcinoma while still small enough for surgery or intratumour injection of alcohol has been proposed.[3,5]

Chemotherapy has been tried in unresectable disease. Treatment with doxorubicin alone has been associated with a response rate of 11 to 25%, which has not been bettered by combination chemotherapy;[1] there has also been a report of response to low-dose oral tegafur.[6] Doxorubicin has also been given by intra-arterial infusion into the hepatic artery, as have fluorouracil, floxuridine, and other agents such as cisplatin and mitomycin, but there is no evidence of an improvement in survival from such an approach.[1,2,7,8] Alternative approaches include implantation of cytotoxic agents in a solid or semi-solid matrix directly into the tumour mass, intraperitoneal infusion, or isolation and perfusion of the liver to achieve locally high concentrations of the antineoplastic without systemic toxicity.[8] Chemo-embolisation, to supply an antineoplastic agent and then cut off blood supply to the tumour has been tried with variable results.[9,10]

Ultimately, prevention of the disease is clearly preferable, and screening programmes and vaccination against hepatitis B may be a more promising approach in areas where the disease is common. Interferon alfa has been reported to decrease the incidence of hepatocellular carcinoma in cirrhotic patients with hepatitis C infection.[11,14] Chemoprevention may also be a useful approach after surgical resection: use of a synthetic retinoid, polyprenoic acid, was found to reduce the development of second primary tumours after resection.[12]

The liver is a common site of metastasis for colorectal cancer. Although survival is somewhat more prolonged than for patients with hepatocellular carcinoma, resection is possible in only a small minority of such patients. However, intra-arterial infusion of floxuridine into the hepatic artery has been associated with prolongation of survival in patients with colorectal liver metastases and may have a valuable palliative role.[13]

1. Di Bisceglie AM, *et al.* Hepatocellular carcinoma. *Ann Intern Med* 1988; **108:** 390–401.
2. Dusheiko GM. Hepatocellular carcinoma associated with chronic viral hepatitis: aetiology, diagnosis and treatment. *Br Med Bull* 1990; **46:** 492–511.
3. Haydon GH, Hayes PC. Hepatocellular carcinoma. *Br J Hosp Med* 1995; **53:** 74–80.
4. Mazzaferro V, *et al.* Liver transplantation for the treatment of small hepatocellular carcinomas in patients with cirrhosis. *N Engl J Med* 1996; **334:** 693–9.
5. Dusheiko GM, *et al.* Treatment of small hepatocellular carcinomas. *Lancet* 1992; **340:** 285–8.
6. Shindo K, *et al.* Hepatocellular carcinoma response to low-dose oral tegafur. *DICP Ann Pharmacother* 1991; **25:** 1009.
7. Malik STA, Wrigley PFM. Intra-arterial hepatic chemotherapy for liver malignancy. *Br Med J* 1988; **297:** 434–5.
8. Anderson JH, *et al.* Clinical pharmacokinetic advantages of new drug delivery methods for the treatment of liver tumours. *Clin Pharmacokinet* 1994; **27:** 191–201.
9. Taguchi T. Chemo-occlusion for the treatment of liver cancer: a new technique using degradable starch microspheres. *Clin Pharmacokinet* 1994; **26:** 275–91.
10. Groupe d'Etude et de Traitement du Carcinome Hépatocellulaire. A comparison of lipiodol chemoembolization and conservative treatment for unresectable hepatocellular carcinoma. *N Engl J Med* 1995; **332:** 1256–61.
11. Imai Y, *et al.* Relation of interferon therapy and hepatocellular carcinoma in patients with chronic hepatitis C. *Ann Intern Med* 1998; **129:** 94–9.
12. Muto Y, *et al.* Prevention of second primary tumors by an acyclic retinoid, polyprenoic acid, in patients with hepatocellular carcinoma. *N Engl J Med* 1996; **334:** 1561–7.
13. Allen-Mersh TG, *et al.* Quality of life and survival with continuous hepatic-artery floxuridine infusion for colorectal liver metastases. *Lancet* 1994; **344:** 1255–60.
14. International Interferon-α Hepatocellular Carcinoma Study Group. Effect of interferon-α on progression of cirrhosis to hepatocellular carcinoma: a retrospective cohort study. *Lancet* 1998; **351:** 1535–9.

Malignant neoplasms of the lung. Lung cancer is the most common non-skin cancer in the developed countries and the second most common overall worldwide. About 20 to 25% of all lung cancers are small cell lung cancers (SCLC) derived from endocrine cells in the bronchial mucosa; the remainder, comprising chiefly squamous carcinomas (40 to 45% of cases), adenocarcinoma (25 to 30%), and large cell carcinoma (about 10%), are known collectively as non-small cell lung cancer (NSCLC). More than 80% of all lung cancers are associated with tobacco smoking, and there is some evidence that exposure to the cigarette smoke of others can increase the risk in non-smokers. Other risk factors may include occupational exposure to substances such as asbestos, and the effects of environmental toxins such as air pollutants.

Symptoms due to a lesion in a main bronchus (the most common site) include persistent cough, dyspnoea, haemoptysis, weight loss and sometimes chest pain. Metastasis is common, and may affect sites such as brain, liver, and bone; the primary tumour is often asymptomatic, with initial symptoms being those of the metastasis.

Disease staging plays an important role in determining treatment; small cell lung cancer, which is almost always a disseminated disease at diagnosis, is managed rather differently than non-small cell.

The treatment of **small cell lung cancer** is based on chemotherapy,[1-5] although combination with surgery, and perhaps radiotherapy, may be of benefit in the small proportion of patients with less-advanced disease. Around 80% of patients with small cell lung cancer respond to chemotherapy, with slightly better response in those with limited disease (confined to one hemithorax) than those with extensive disease. Despite these impressive responses, resistance and relapse almost always occur; the median survival is improved by treatment, but long-term survival is very poor, with about 10 to 20% of patients with limited disease and 5% of those with extensive disease surviving 2 years from the start of the treatment, and only about half of these survivors continuing to be alive 6 years from diagnosis.[1-6] However, the few that do survive more than 5 years rarely relapse thereafter, and may be regarded as effectively cured.

Various single agents have been reported to have activity, including cyclophosphamide, doxorubicin, vincristine, ifosfamide, etoposide, teniposide, and cisplatin or carboplatin, and various combinations of these have been tried, including cyclophosphamide, doxorubicin and vincristine, and cisplatin with etoposide, which appears to have a good index of toxicity relative to effectiveness. Among newer agents under investigation, gemcitabine is reported to be active,[7] and some good results have been reported with topotecan;[8,9] a combination of vinorelbine with paclitaxel has also been investigated.[10] There is some suggestion that in that subset of patients with normal serum sodium, alkaline phosphatase, aspartate aminotransferase, and lactate dehydrogenase, whose prognosis is considerably better than average, intensive chemotherapy, perhaps with the use of colony-stimulating factors to reduce myelosuppression, might produce further improvement,[1,5] but on the whole, evidence of the value of dose intensification is lacking.[2] Once relapse has occurred, the function of treatment is palliative, and chemotherapy may be inappropriate; if given, minimal toxicity is the most important criterion. Oral etoposide is under investigation in this regard,[5] but a comparative study of oral etoposide versus intravenous chemotherapy with standard regimens was terminated early because of the poor results with the oral treatment.[11]

In contrast to small cell disease, about 20 to 25% of patients with **non-small cell lung cancer** present with tumour localised to the lung, and the treatment of choice in such cases is surgery. More advanced disease is usually treated with radiotherapy, although in disseminated disease this is purely palliative. About 25 to 40% of patients resected for localised disease are still alive after 5 years, while 5-year survival is 4 to 8% in locally advanced disease and less than 1% in disseminated disease.[1,2] Chemotherapy has been tried in the management of metastatic or recurrent disease, as an adjuvant to surgery and/or radiotherapy in less-advanced disease, and as 'neo-adjuvant' therapy to debulk tumour and render it potentially manageable with local therapy.[12] Recent US guidelines recommend the use of platinum-based chemotherapy in patients with advanced, unresectable disease and good performance status.[13] The role of neo-adjuvant therapy is uncertain.

Cisplatin, mitomycin, vinblastine, vindesine, ifosfamide, and etoposide have been reported to have limited single-agent activity in non-small cell disease[2] and newer drugs such as paclitaxel and docetaxel, gemcitabine, or the camptothecin derivatives, such as irinotecan, as well as modifications of existing regimens, are being tried. Gene therapy with the p53 tumour suppressor gene is also under investigation.[14] It is considered that combination therapy based on a platinum compound produces the greatest benefits: cisplatin with paclitaxel, vinorelbine, or vinblastine has been recommended for first-line treatment.[13] Unfortunately, while meta-analysis indicates a survival advantage from combination regimens[15-17] it is modest, and achieved at the cost of significant toxicity.[12] Nonetheless, it can improve quality of life, and the size of the overall effect is equivalent to that seen with adjuvant chemotherapy in breast cancer; if it were possible to identify the subset of patients who respond to chemotherapy the risk-benefit ratio could be dramatically improved.[18] Also while the indications for chemotherapy in patients with advanced disease are currently limited, some authorities consider that the value of palliative chemotherapy in this group has been underestimated.[19]

Randomised studies of adjuvant chemotherapy have produced variable results,[12,20] but there has been some benefit, particularly in patients with less advanced disease. Typical adjuvant regimens have employed cyclophosphamide, doxorubicin, and cisplatin, or cisplatin and etoposide.

There is now growing evidence of a survival benefit from induction or neo-adjuvant therapy in patients with regionally-advanced but resectable (Stage IIIA) disease.[12,20,21] Such an approach may be of value in carefully selected patients until better treatments are found.

For mention of the treatment of pulmonary Kaposi's sarcoma see Kaposi's Sarcoma, under Sarcoma, below.

1. Spiro SG. Management of lung cancer. *Br Med J* 1990; **301:** 1287–8.
2. Ihde DC. Chemotherapy of lung cancer. *N Engl J Med* 1992; **327:** 1434–41.
3. Crompton G. Small cell lung cancer. *Br Med J* 1990; **300:** 209–10.
4. Hansen HH. Management of small-cell cancer of the lung. *Lancet* 1992; **339:** 846–9.
5. Rudd RM. Inoperable lung cancer. *Prescribers' J* 1996; **36:** 14–21.
6. Report of a Meeting of Physicians and Scientists at the Royal Marsden Hospital, Sutton, UK. Small-cell lung cancer. *Lancet* 1995; **345:** 1285–9.
7. Cormier Y, *et al.* Gemcitabine is an active new agent in previously untreated extensive small cell lung cancer (SCLC): a study of the National Cancer Institute of Canada Clinical Trials Group. *Ann Oncol* 1994; **5:** 283–5.
8. Schiller JH, *et al.* Phase II study of topotecan in patients with extensive-stage small-cell carcinoma of the lung: an Eastern Cooperative Oncology Group Trial. *J Clin Oncol* 1996; **14:** 2345–52.
9. Ardizzoni A, *et al.* Topotecan, a new active drug in the second-line treatment of small-cell lung cancer: a phase II study in patients with refractory and sensitive disease. *J Clin Oncol* 1997; **15:** 2090–6.
10. Iaffaioli RV, *et al.* Phase I study of vinorelbine and paclitaxel in small-cell lung cancer. *Cancer Chemother Pharmacol* 1997; **41:** 86–90.
11. Medical Research Council Lung Cancer Working Party. Comparison of oral etoposide and standard intravenous multidrug chemotherapy for small-cell lung cancer: a stopped multicentre randomised trial. *Lancet* 1996; **348:** 563–6.
12. Vokes EE, *et al.* Role of systemic therapy in advanced non-small-cell lung cancer. *Am J Med* 1990; **89:** 777–86.
13. American Society of Clinical Oncology. Clinical practice guidelines for the treatment of unresectable non-small-cell lung cancer. *J Clin Oncol* 1997; **15:** 2996–3018.
14. Roth JA, *et al.* Retrovirus-mediated wild-type p53 gene transfer to tumors of patients with lung cancer. *Nature Med* 1996; **2:** 985–91.
15. Souquet PJ, *et al.* Polychemotherapy in advanced non small cell lung cancer: a meta-analysis. *Lancet* 1993; **342:** 19–21.
16. Non-small Cell Lung Cancer Collaborative Group. Chemotherapy in non-small cell lung cancer: a meta-analysis using updated data on individual patients from 52 randomised clinical trials. *Br Med J* 1995; **311:** 899–909.
17. Lilenbaum RC, *et al.* Single agent versus combination chemotherapy in patients with advanced nonsmall cell lung carcinoma: a meta-analysis of response, toxicity, and survival. *Cancer* 1998; **82:** 116–26.
18. Carbone DP, Minna JD. Chemotherapy for non-small cell lung cancer. *Br Med J* 1995; **311:** 889–90.
19. Smith IE. Palliative chemotherapy for advanced non-small cell lung cancer. *Br Med J* 1994; **308:** 429–30.
20. Bastin KT, Curley R. Non-small-cell lung carcinoma: current and future therapeutic management. *Drugs* 1995; **49:** 362–75.
21. Rosell R, *et al.* A randomized trial comparing preoperative chemotherapy plus surgery with surgery alone in patients with non-small-cell lung cancer. *N Engl J Med* 1994; **330:** 153–8.

Malignant neoplasms of the ovary. Ovarian cancers account for about 5% of all malignancies in women; the most common form is epithelial ovarian cancer. The lethality of this disease is related to the absence of symptoms in the majority of women during its early stages: in about three-quarters of all patients disease is advanced at diagnosis and has spread to the peritoneum or beyond.[1,2] Presence of an elevated serum concentration of the antigen CA-125 may be helpful in confirming diagnosis, although it is not specific for ovarian cancer, but diagnosis may require a laparotomy.

In confirmed epithelial ovarian cancer the basis of treatment is surgical removal of womb, ovaries and fallopian tubes, and omentum, together with debulking of any remaining gross disease.[3] The use of adjuvant chemotherapy depends on disease stage.

The minority of patients who have localised disease at diagnosis have a fairly good prognosis. Patients with well differentiated early disease have a 5-year disease-free survival of some 90 to 98%; adjuvant therapy with oral melphalan has not been shown to improve survival in this group,[4] and less extensive surgery may be possible without greatly affecting survival.[5] In those subgroups with less well differentiated or more extensive localised disease postoperative chemotherapy is usually considered appropriate: in a study in patients with poorly-differentiated stage I or stage II disease (extended to the pelvis), the 5-year survival rates were 78% in those given intraperitoneal phosphorus-32 after surgery and 81% in those given melphalan.[4]

Prognosis is less good in patients with advanced disease, who presently form the majority at diagnosis. Patients with extra-pelvic disease or positive nodes who have only minimal residual disease after surgery have a 4-year survival rate of about 30%[2,5] but in patients with distant metastases or suboptimal debulking there is a less than 10% chance of long-term survival.[2] A wide range of adjuvant regimens have been tried in advanced ovarian cancer, mostly based on cisplatin, although some centres prefer carboplatin, because of its lower toxicity.[3,6] Combinations of cisplatin or carboplatin with cyclophosphamide and sometimes doxorubicin have been widely used,[2,3,6,7] while other agents that have been tried include altretamine, fluorouracil, chlorambucil, paclitaxel, etoposide, gonadorelin analogues, melphalan, treosulfan, tamoxifen, thiotepa, and ifosfamide.[3,7] Other agents under investigation include gemcitabine and topotecan,[3] and marimastat.[8]

An overview of 45 studies involving over 8000 patients failed to reach any definite conclusions about the relative benefits of differing chemotherapeutic regimens, but did suggest that immediate treatment was better than delaying until relapse, that platinum-based regimens were probably better than those without a platinum derivative, that combination regimens were better than single-agent platinum where the doses were equivalent, and that carboplatin was as effective as cisplatin.[6] It was suggested that most clinical studies have been far too small to accurately detect the modest degree of benefit that is likely to be derived. Another overview suggested that regimens of cisplatin, doxorubicin, and cyclophosphamide offered a survival advantage over cisplatin with cyclophosphamide alone,[9] but some commentators do not consider that doxorubicin-containing regimens have been demonstrated to be more effective.[2,3,10] Results of combined therapy with cisplatin and paclitaxel have been sufficiently good[11] to lead to suggestions that this should become standard therapy in advanced ovarian cancer,[10,12] but this is not yet endorsed by all.[3,10] Combination therapy with carboplatin and paclitaxel is also under investigation,[13] and carboplatin with docetaxel is being tried.

Neoadjuvant therapy with cisplatin and either doxorubicin and bleomycin, or mitozantrone, reportedly permitted surgical removal of all macroscopic disease in about half of a group of women with bulky residual disease, but the effects of such treatment on survival are not yet known.[14] However, encouraging results in women with residual lesions greater than 1 cm after primary surgery indicated that chemotherapy with cyclophosphamide and cisplatin, followed by debulking surgery and then further chemotherapy, was associated with some prolongation of disease free survival and reduction in the risk of death.[15]

The role of intraperitoneal chemotherapy in the treatment of ovarian cancer remains to be defined.[3,10] Benefit is likely to be greatest in small volume disease, as tumour penetration is limited:[3] improved efficacy and tolerability have been reported with intraperitoneal rather than intravenous cisplatin in patients with residual tumour masses of 2 cm or less after resectioning.[16]

Ovarian germ-cell cancers are much less common than epithelial ovarian cancer. Unlike epithelial ovarian cancer, most patients present with early disease, and up to 90% of patients with completely-resected early-stage disease remain disease-free. In the minority with more advanced disease, the introduction of cisplatin-based chemotherapy similar to that used in male germ-cell tumours (such as bleomycin, cisplatin and vinblastine or etoposide)[10,17] has been reported to produce a 2-year survival of 71%, and is potentially curative in a substantial number of patients.[17]

1. Berck JS. Adjuvant therapy for early-stage ovarian cancer. *N Engl J Med* 1990; **322:** 1076–8.
2. Cannistra SA. Cancer of the ovary. *N Engl J Med* 1993; **329:** 1550–9.
3. Lorigan PC, *et al.* Current drug treatment guidelines for epithelial ovarian cancer. *Drugs* 1996; **51:** 571–84.
4. Young RC, *et al.* Adjuvant therapy in stage I and stage II epithelial ovarian cancer: results of two prospective randomized trials. *N Engl J Med* 1990; **322:** 1021–7.
5. Hand R, *et al.* Staging procedures, clinical management, and survival outcome for ovarian carcinoma. *JAMA* 1993; **269:** 1119–22.
6. Advanced Ovarian Cancer Trialists Group. Chemotherapy in advanced ovarian cancer: an overview of randomised clinical trials. *Br Med J* 1991; **303:** 884–93.
7. Anonymous. Drugs of choice for cancer chemotherapy. *Med Lett Drugs Ther* 1997; **39:** 21–8.
8. Gore M, *et al.* Tumour marker levels during marimastat therapy. *Lancet* 1996; **348:** 263.
9. Fanning J, *et al.* Meta-analysis of cisplatin, doxorubicin, and cyclophosphamide versus cisplatin and cyclophosphamide chemotherapy of ovarian carcinoma. *Obstet Gynecol* 1992; **80:** 954–60.
10. NIH Consensus Development Panel on Ovarian Cancer. Ovarian cancer: screening, treatment, and follow-up. *JAMA* 1995; **273:** 491–7.
11. McGuire WP, *et al.* Cyclophosphamide and cisplatin compared with paclitaxel and cisplatin in patients with stage III and stage IV ovarian cancer. *N Engl J Med* 1996; **334:** 1–6.
12. Neijt JP. New therapy for ovarian cancer. *N Engl J Med* 1996; **334:** 50–1.
13. Bookman MA, *et al.* Carboplatin and paclitaxel in ovarian carcinoma: a phase I study of the Gynecologic Oncology Group. *J Clin Oncol* 1996; **14:** 1895–1902.
14. Lawton FG, *et al.* Neoadjuvant (cytoreductive) chemotherapy combined with intervention debulking surgery in advanced, unresected epithelial ovarian cancer. *Obstet Gynecol* 1989; **73:** 61–5.
15. van der Burg MEL, *et al.* The effect of debulking surgery after induction chemotherapy on the prognosis in advanced epithelial ovarian cancer. *N Engl J Med* 1995; **332:** 629–34.
16. Alberts DS, *et al.* Intraperitoneal cisplatin plus intravenous cyclophosphamide versus intravenous cisplatin plus intravenous cyclophosphamide for stage III ovarian cancer. *N Engl J Med* 1996; **335:** 1950–5.
17. Williams SD, *et al.*. Cisplatin, vinblastine, and bleomycin in advanced and recurrent ovarian germ-cell tumors: a trial of the Gynecologic Oncology Group. *Ann Intern Med* 1989; **111:** 22–7.

Malignant neoplasms of the pancreas. Although rare below the age of 30 the incidence of pancreatic cancer rises steadily with age; overall, malignant neoplasms of the pancreas account for about 3% of all cancers. Pancreatic adenocarcinoma is ductal in origin and metastasises early to the lymph nodes, and by the time of diagnosis more than half of all patients have liver metastases, more than a quarter have peritoneal seeding, and a third have invasion of the duodenum causing ulceration. The most frequent symptom at presentation in patients with cancer of the pancreatic head is jaundice, often with other symptoms indicative of obstruction of the bile duct. In lesions of the body of the pancreas severe and relentless pain may develop. Islet cell tumours, which are rare, can result in various metabolic derangements due to excessive hormone secretion—see Pancreatic Endocrine Tumours, under Carcinoid Tumours and Other Secretory Neoplasms, p.477.

Pancreatic cancer has a very poor prognosis; apart from a small number of patients with carcinoma of the head of the pancreas in whom potentially hazardous surgery offers some chance of a cure,[1] almost all patients with pancreatic malignancies will be dead within 2 years.[2] Although there are occasional reports of individual patients who respond to fluorouracil,[3] or combination chemotherapy regimens such as doxorubicin, methotrexate, and fluorouracil,[2] or cisplatin, doxorubicin, and fluorouracil, or epirubicin and carboplatin,[4] the results of chemotherapy are generally disappointing and often no better than no treatment at all.[5] One study has suggested that slightly better short-term survival can be achieved by combining radiotherapy with combination chemotherapy (using fluorouracil, cisplatin, and streptozocin) although the improvement was not sustained.[6] A number of newer agents are being tried in this condition, including gemcitabine,[7,8] lithium gamolenate,[9] and marimastat.[10] There are reports of response to gonadorelin analogues,[11] and markedly improved survival has now been shown in patients treated with flutamide.[12]

1. Carter DC. Clinical features and management of carcinoma of the pancreas. *Br J Hosp Med* 1995; **54:** 459–64.
2. Pyrhönen S, Valtonen M. Response to doxorubicin/methotrexate/fluorouracil in advanced adenocarcinoma of pancreas or biliary tract. *Lancet* 1990; **336:** 127.
3. Kao GD. Chemotherapy for pancreatic carcinoma. *Lancet* 1991; **337:** 177.
4. van Klaveren RJ, *et al.* Pancreatic carcinoma with polyarthritis, fat necrosis, and high serum lipase and trypsin activity. *Gut* 1990; **31:** 953–5.
5. Porta C, *et al.* Doxorubicin/methotrexate/fluorouracil in advanced pancreatic cancer. *Lancet* 1990; **336:** 1454–5.
6. Bruckner HW, *et al.* Survival after combined modality therapy for pancreatic cancer. *J Clin Gastroenterol* 1993; **16:** 199–203.
7. Carmichael J, *et al.* Phase II study of gemcitabine in patients with advanced pancreatic cancer. *Br J Cancer* 1996; **73:** 101–5.
8. Burris HA, *et al.* Improvements in survival and clinical benefit with gemcitabine as first-line therapy for patients with advanced pancreas cancer: a randomized trial. *J Clin Oncol* 1997; **15:** 2403–13.
9. Fearon KCH, *et al.* An open-label phase I/II dose escalation study of the treatment of pancreatic cancer using lithium gammalinolenate. *Anticancer Res* 1996; **16:** 867–74.
10. Millar A, *et al.* Tumour marker levels during marimastat therapy. *Lancet* 1996; **348:** 263–4.
11. Andrén-Sandberg Å. Treatment with an LHRH analogue in patients with advanced pancreatic cancer: a preliminary report. *Acta Chir Scand* 1990; **156:** 549–51.
12. Greenway BA. Effect of flutamide on survival in patients with pancreatic cancer: results of a prospective, randomised, double blind, placebo controlled trial. *Br Med J* 1998; **316:** 1935–8.

Malignant neoplasms of the prostate. Prostatic cancer is about the tenth most common malignancy worldwide and the fifth most common in developed countries: about one in ten men can be expected to develop clinically evident carcinoma of the prostate during his lifetime. The incidence rises steadily with age, but many lesions remain asymptomatic until death, or are misdiagnosed as benign prostatic hyperplasia. More than 95% of all prostate cancer is adenocarcinoma, which begins as a hard mass in the peripheral portion of the gland and infiltrates surrounding tissues slowly. Metastasis may occur in advanced disease, notably to bone. Presenting symptoms are usually those of urinary outflow obstruction, or pelvic or back pain due to bone metastases: up to 80% of patients have locally advanced or metastatic disease at presentation.[1]

Management of the minority of patients with localised disease has long been controversial. Since many patients are elderly, and disease progression relatively slow, some workers consider that no therapy is required, at least where the tumour is well differentiated and asymptomatic, or where the patient is frail. However, in medically fit patients with a life expectancy of 10 years or more radical prostatectomy or radiotherapy may be considered with curative intent.[1-8] Although radiotherapy has tended to be the preferred treatment in the UK, surgery is becoming more widely used,[6] in line with practice in the USA. Radical prostatectomy may be associated with 10-year survival rates as high as 77 to 94% depending on tumour grade.[7] Adjuvant therapy with goserelin has been reported to improve local control and survival when added to radiotherapy in patients with locally advanced disease.[9] Neoadjuvant therapy usually with a gonadorelin analogue plus an anti-androgen, is under investigation to downstage the tumour and reduce its size before surgery or radiotherapy, but its effects on long-term survival are not yet known.[5]

Since therapy for localised disease is not yet standardised, there is great controversy over the benefits of screening for early disease by detection of prostate specific antigen (PSA), and other tests;[4,10,11] those who favour such a move suggest that detection of small localised tumours offers a chance for cure, whereas others remain to be convinced.

For patients with metastatic disease cure is not possible and therapy is aimed at prolonging survival and palliating symptoms. The basis of therapy is hormonal manipulation, by orchidectomy or with drugs, since prostate cancer is dependent upon androgens.[1-4,8] About 80% of cases will respond to such therapy, but resistance eventually develops. The use of gonadorelin analogues such as goserelin or leuprorelin is as effective as orchidectomy in producing a response; because such therapy produces an initial tumour flare due to stimulation of testosterone concentrations, an anti-androgen such as cyproterone acetate or flutamide should be given with the first dose.[1] An alternative approach is the use of an anti-androgen alone: flutamide,[12] nilutamide,[13] and bicalutamide[14] have all produced some responses. Although historically oestrogens such as stilboestrol have been used in patients with prostate cancer they are now less favoured because of their greater adverse effects.[1,3] For similar reasons, ketoconazole, which has anti-androgenic properties in large doses, is of limited value.[15]

The continued use of anti-androgens such as flutamide together with ablation of testicular androgen production (by surgery or gonadorelin analogues) has the advantage of blocking the effects of adrenal androgen production as well (total or complete androgen blockade). However, meta-analysis[16] seems to indicate that this approach does not produce a better survival rate compared with conventional castration, although some debate on this point continues.[5,17]

In patients who relapse, or never respond, after hormonal therapy, addition or substitution of other hormonal agents is unlikely to be of benefit. Aminoglutethimide has been tried but is not now thought to be of value.[18] In general, second-line therapy produces responses in 30% of patients at best,[3] and responses are generally brief.[3,4] One potentially beneficial manoeuvre in patients treated with flutamide is withdrawal of the drug, as some patients experience a paradoxical response to this.[4,19] Chemotherapy with agents such as cyclophosphamide, fluorouracil, streptozocin, estramustine, cisplatin, methotrexate, and mitomycin, as well as combinations such as cyclophosphamide, methotrexate, and fluorouracil or fluorouracil, doxorubicin, and mitomycin, has failed to demonstrate a convincing survival advantage,[20,21] and although reports of benefit with various agents continue to be seen (for example with epirubicin[22] and with mitozantrone[23]) the variability of the natural history of prostatic cancer makes it difficult to demonstrate convincing advantage from treatment.[2] Newer agents such as suramin[24] are under investigation, and studies of retinoids, paclitaxel, and interferons are reported to be under way.[4] There has been a resurgence of interest in the use of chemotherapy for hormone-refractory disease, and a feeling that multimodality treatments may yet lead to improved survival.[8]

Because of the difficulties involved in managing metastatic disease there has been some interest in the concept of disease prophylaxis. Studies with finasteride, which has produced variable results in the management of existing disease, are being initiated to examine whether 5 mg daily can help reduce the incidence of prostatic cancer in men aged over 55 years.

1. Brewster SF, Gillatt DA. Advanced prostate cancer: what's new in hormonal manipulation? *Br J Hosp Med* 1993; **49:** 710–15.
2. Whitmore WF. Management of clinically localized prostatic cancer: an unresolved problem. *JAMA* 1993; **269:** 2676–7.
3. Dearnaley DP. Cancer of the prostate. *Br Med J* 1994; **308:** 780–4. Correction. *ibid.*; 975.
4. Catalona WJ. Management of cancer of the prostate. *N Engl J Med* 1994; **331:** 996–1004. Correction. *ibid.*; **332:** 335–6.
5. Garnick MB, Fair WR. Prostate cancer: emerging concepts. *Ann Intern Med* 1996; **125:** 118–25 and 205–12.
6. Clarke NW. The management of localized prostate cancer. *Br J Hosp Med* 1996; **55:** 232–3.
7. Gerber GS, *et al.* Results of radical prostatectomy in men with clinically localized prostate cancer: multi-institutional pooled analysis. *JAMA* 1996; **276:** 615–19.
8. Frydenberg M, *et al.* Prostate cancer diagnosis and management. *Lancet* 1997; **349:** 1681–7.
9. Bolla M, *et al.* Improved survival in patients with locally advanced prostate cancer treated with radiotherapy and goserelin. *N Engl J Med* 1997; **337:** 295–300.
10. Adami H-O, *et al.* Ethics of a prostate cancer screening trial. *Lancet* 1994; **343:** 958–60.
11. American College of Physicians. Screening for prostate cancer. *Ann Intern Med* 1997; **126:** 480–4.
12. Delaere KPJ, Van Thillo EL. Flutamide monotherapy as primary treatment in advanced prostatic carcinoma. *Semin Oncol* 1991; **18** (suppl 6): 13–18.
13. Decensi AU, *et al.* Monotherapy with nilutamide, a pure nonsteroidal antiandrogen, in untreated patients with metastatic carcinoma of the prostate. *J Urol (Baltimore)* 1991; **146:** 377–81.
14. Soloway MS, *et al.* Bicalutamide in the treatment of advanced prostatic carcinoma: a phase II noncomparative multicenter trial evaluating safety, efficacy and long-term endocrine effects of monotherapy. *J Urol (Baltimore)* 1995; **154:** 2110–14.
15. Mahler C, *et al.* Ketoconazole and liarozole in the treatment of advanced prostatic cancer. *Cancer* 1993; **71:** 1068–73.
16. Prostate Cancer Trialists' Collaborative Group. Maximum androgen blockade in advanced prostate cancer: an overview of 22 randomised trials with 3283 deaths in 5710 patients. *Lancet* 1995; **346:** 265–9.
17. Labrie F, Crawford D. Anti-androgens in treatment of prostate cancer. *Lancet* 1995; **346:** 1030–1.
18. Plowman PN. Aminoglutethimide: a toxic object lesson in the endocrine management of cancer. *Hum Toxicol* 1987; **6:** 187–8.
19. Figg WD, *et al.* Prostate specific antigen decline following the discontinuation of flutamide in patients with stage D2 prostate cancer. *Am J Med* 1995; **98:** 412–15.
20. Eisenberger MA, *et al.* A reevaluation of nonhormonal cytotoxic chemotherapy in the treatment of prostatic carcinoma. *J Clin Oncol* 1985; **3:** 827–41.
21. Yagoda A, Petrylak D. Cytotoxic chemotherapy for advanced hormone-resistant prostate cancer. *Cancer* 1993; **71:** 1098–1109.
22. Gasser TC. Carcinoma of the prostate. *N Engl J Med* 1991; **324:** 1893.
23. Tannock IF, *et al.* Chemotherapy with mitoxantrone plus prednisone or prednisone alone for symptomatic hormone-resistant prostate cancer: a Canadian randomized trial with palliative end points. *J Clin Oncol* 1996; **14:** 1756–64.
24. Woll PJ, *et al.* Suramin for breast and prostate cancer: a pilot study of intermittent short infusions without adaptive control. *Ann Oncol* 1994; **5:** 597–600.

Malignant neoplasms of the skin. Skin cancers are the most common malignancies among white populations but because many are not recorded the exact incidence is uncertain and they are often omitted from calculations of the relative frequency of malignancy. Most are related to solar radiation, and the incidence is greatest in those regions where light-skinned individuals are exposed to a very sunny climate. Other risk factors include immunosuppression due to drugs or HIV infection. A small but increasing proportion of all skin cancers are melanomas, arising from melanocytes (pigment cells); of the remainder, about 80% are basal cell carcinomas, the rest being mainly squamous cell carcinomas. Other cancers which may manifest in the skin include T-cell lymphomas such as mycosis fungoides (see p.482), and diseases such as Kaposi's sarcoma (see p.496).

BASAL-CELL AND SQUAMOUS-CELL CARCINOMA. The great majority of skin cancers are basal cell carcinomas, which are completely curable if diagnosed early and treated appropriately. The remainder are mainly squamous cell carcinomas which although curable when treated early have a greater risk of metastatic spread. Diagnosis of suspect lesions is by biopsy, and when the lesion is small this may take the form of excision with a 2 to 3 mm margin of normal skin, accomplishing treatment and diagnosis in a single step. Options for treatment include surgery, cryotherapy, and radiotherapy.[1-4]

Excisional surgery is suitable for all types of non-melanoma skin cancer and is a mainstay of treatment but options such as radiotherapy may be more appropriate in patients at risk of surgical complications or where tissue preservation is desirable for cosmetic reasons. Photodynamic therapy, for example with topical aminolaevulinic acid and laser light, is under investigation both for malignant disease[5] and precursor lesions.[5-8]

Chemotherapy does not have much of a role in the treatment of nonmelanoma skin cancers. Although topical fluorouracil (usually as a 5% ointment or cream) has been used for superficial basal cell carcinomas[9,10] it is not recommended because of the risk of inhibiting the surface layers of a tumour, giving the appearance of control, while permitting the growth of deeper extensions.[11] However, fluorouracil application, alone or with tretinoin, may be useful in the precursor lesions of squamous cell carcinoma such as actinic keratoses or Bowen's disease (squamous cell carcinoma *in situ*).[1,12-14] The plant product masoprocol is applied similarly in the treatment of actinic keratoses.[15] Also reported to be effective for actinic keratoses is a gel containing diclofenac in hyaluronic acid.[16] Preliminary results in patients with basal cell carcinoma, particularly of the face, have suggested that intralesional injection of interferon alfa is effective in producing tumour regression.[17] There has also been a report[18] of responses in 4 patients with multiple actinic keratoses and squamous cell carcinomas (and in 1 case a basal cell carcinoma) who were given isotretinoin with calcitriol, both by mouth. Etretinate has also been used in the prophylaxis of squamous-cell carcinoma in patients with xeroderma pigmentosum, which predisposes to skin cancer.[19]

The prognosis with appropriate treatment is good, with more or less 100% cure rates in early disease, and 70 to 75% 5-year disease free survival even with local node involvement. However, about 50% of patients will subsequently develop another skin cancer,[1] and regular monitoring to detect this as early as possible is desirable.

There has also been considerable interest in reducing the risk of skin cancer. At its most basic this includes measures to reduce exposure to solar radiation, including appropriate clothing and the use of sunscreens.[20] However, chemoprevention, using agents such as betacarotene[21] has also been investigated. Although the use of vitamins has not met with much success (see also p.1333), retinoids have been used successfully against actinic keratoses and in xeroderma pigmentosum, as mentioned above. Recent evidence suggests that a low-fat diet may reduce the incidence of actinic keratosis in patients with a history of nonmelanoma skin cancer.[22]

1. Preston DS, Stern RS. Nonmelanoma cancers of the skin. *N Engl J Med* 1992; **327:** 1649–62.
2. Marks R, Motley RJ. Skin cancer: recognition and treatment. *Drugs* 1995; **50:** 48–61.
3. Goldberg LH. Basal cell carcinoma. *Lancet* 1996; **347:** 663–7.
4. Marks R. Squamous cell carcinoma. *Lancet* 1996; **347:** 735–8.
5. Svanberg K, *et al.* Photodynamic therapy of non-melanoma malignant tumours of the skin using topical δ-amino levulinic acid sensitization and laser irradiation. *Br J Dermatol* 1994; **130:** 743–51.
6. Morton CA, *et al.* Comparison of photodynamic therapy with cryotherapy in the treatment of Bowen's disease. *Br J Dermatol* 1996; **135:** 766–71.
7. Jeffes EW, *et al.* Photodynamic therapy of actinic keratosis with topical 5-aminolevulinic acid: a pilot dose-ranging study. *Arch Dermatol* 1997; **133:** 727–32.
8. Stables GI, *et al.* Large patches of Bowen's disease treated by topical aminolaevulinic acid photodynamic therapy. *Br J Dermatol* 1997; **136:** 957–60.
9. WHO. Chemotherapy of solid tumours: report of a WHO expert committee. *WHO Tech Rep Ser 605* 1977.
10. Epstein E. Fluorouracil paste treatment of thin basal cell carcinomas. *Arch Dermatol* 1985; **121:** 207–13.
11. Mohs FE, *et al.* Tendency of fluorouracil to conceal deep foci of invasive basal cell carcinoma. *Arch Dermatol* 1978; **114:** 1021–2.
12. Goncalves JCA. Treatment of solar keratoses with a 5-fluorouracil and salicylic acid varnish. *Br J Dermatol* 1975; **92:** 85–8.
13. Robinson TA, Kligman AM. Treatment of solar keratoses of the extremities with retinoic acid and 5-fluorouracil. *Br J Dermatol* 1975; **92:** 703–6.
14. Bercovitch L. Topical chemotherapy of actinic keratoses of the upper extremity with tretinoin and 5-fluorouracil: a double-blind controlled study. *Br J Dermatol* 1987; **116:** 549–52.
15. Olsen EA, *et al.* A double-blind, vehicle-controlled study evaluating masoprocol cream in the treatment of actinic keratoses on the head and neck. *J Am Acad Dermatol* 1991; **24:** 738–43.
16. Rivers JK, McLean DI. An open study to assess the efficacy and safety of topical 3% diclofenac in a 2.5% hyaluronic acid gel for the treatment of actinic keratoses. *Arch Dermatol* 1997; **133:** 1239–42.
17. Pizarro A, Fonseca E. Treatment of basal cell carcinoma with intralesional interferon alpha-2b: evaluation of efficacy with emphasis on tumours located on "H" zone on face. *Eur J Dermatol* 1994; **4:** 287–90.
18. Majewski S, *et al.* Combination of isotretinoin and calcitriol for precancerous and cancerous skin lesions. *Lancet* 1994; **344:** 1510–11.
19. Finkelstein E, *et al.* Treatment of xeroderma pigmentosum variant with low-dose etretinate. *Br J Dermatol* 1996; **134:** 815–16.
20. Thompson SC, *et al.* Reduction of solar keratoses by regular sunscreen use. *N Engl J Med* 1993; **329:** 1147–51.
21. Greenberg ER, *et al.* A clinical trial of beta carotene to prevent basal-cell and squamous-cell cancers of the skin. *N Engl J Med* 1990; **323:** 789–95.
22. Black HS, *et al.* Effect of a low-fat diet on the incidence of actinic keratosis. *N Engl J Med* 1994; **330:** 1272–5.

MELANOMA. Although melanoma is a rare skin cancer it has been increasing in incidence in recent years. It is uncommon in dark-skinned populations and is strongly related to exposure to ultraviolet light. Melanomas are often characterised by irregularity of colour, thickness or contour; itching, enlargement, ulceration, or bleeding may occur. The risk of metastasis and long-term prognosis are related to the thickness of the lesion: lesions less than 0.75 mm thick are rarely metastatic, whereas a lesion more than 4 mm thick carries a more than 50% risk of metastasis and eventual death.[1] Surgery is the primary treatment for melanoma,[1-3] and is capable of producing cures in localised disease: the 5-year survival in early disease is about 50 to 95%, depending on subtype.[2] Prognosis is much poorer in patients with nodal metastases (overall 5-year survival of 36%), and those with advanced disease (distant metastases) have a median survival of only 6 months;[2] adjuvant therapy, including chemotherapy, is often given to patients with metastatic disease although without definitive evidence that it improves survival.[1-3]

Dacarbazine, with a response rate of 15 to 25%, is the most commonly used single agent. The orally active analogue temozolomide also produces benefit,[4] and it has been suggested,[5] may come to replace dacarbazine in the treatment of disseminated melanoma. Other cytotoxics tried in melanoma include nitrosoureas (such as carmustine, lomustine, and semustine), vindesine, and cisplatin.[1,2,5,6] Melphalan at a temperature of 39° to 41° has been given by perfusion into an isolated limb. Various combination regimens have been tried, but without marked improvement on the response rates for single agents,[2,5] and often with less effect in randomised studies than initial reports suggest.[6] Although some studies have reported improved results when tamoxifen was added to chemotherapy regimens,[7,8] others have found no benefit from such combinations.[9] Of the newer agents available docetaxel is reported to have comparable activity to other conventional agents in malignant melanoma;[10] some benefit is also reported with the nitrosourea fotemustine.[11]

Interleukin-2 has produced responses in patients with metastatic melanoma,[12,13] but complete responses are rare,[14] and toxicity is a problem although it is reduced with continuous infusion.[13,15] Interleukin-2 is also used with lymphokine-activated killer cells (LAK)[12,15] or tumour-infiltrating lymphocytes (TIL).[16,17] Response rates to LAK therapy are also of the order of 15 to 25%,[2] but may be higher with TIL.[1,16] Treatment with interferons may have benefits in selected high-risk patients as an adjuvant to surgery.[18,19] Addition of interferons to chemotherapy regimens has been reported to produce favourable results,[20] although the benefits of interferon alfa as an adjuvant to surgery have been reported to vary with age and sex.[21] However, recent results have suggested benefit from adjuvant therapy with interferon alfa-2a after resection of high-risk primary melanoma in patients without detectable nodal metastases.[27]

Immunological modulation is the basis of a number of still more experimental therapies. Monoclonal antibodies to melanoma-associated gangliosides have produced a few responses[22] but response rates have generally been low, and toxicity considerable.[13] A variety of therapeutic vaccines for melanoma are under investigation.[23,24] This is considered one of the most promising approaches, particularly to treat residual disease after the surgical removal of primary tumour and involved nodes, and has been associated with some improvements in survival compared with historical controls.[24-26] Gene therapy, involving transfer of genes to the tumour to increase its immunogenicity to the body, has also been undertaken.[23]

1. Ho VC, Sober AJ. Therapy for cutaneous melanoma: an update. *J Am Acad Dermatol* 1990; **22:** 159–76.
2. Koh HK. Cutaneous melanoma. *N Engl J Med* 1991; **325:** 171–82.
3. Hunter DC, Thomas JM. Controversies in the management of malignant melanoma. *Br J Hosp Med* 1993; **49:** 174–83.
4. Bleehen NM, *et al.* Cancer research campaign phase II trial of temozolomide in metastatic melanoma. *J Clin Oncol* 1995; **13:** 910–13.
5. Lee SM, *et al.* Melanoma: chemotherapy. *Br Med Bull* 1995; **51:** 609–30.
6. Creagan ET. Regional and systemic strategies for metastatic malignant melanoma. *Mayo Clin Proc* 1989; **64:** 852–60.
7. Cocconi G, *et al.* Treatment of metastatic malignant melanoma with dacarbazine plus tamoxifen. *N Engl J Med* 1992; **327:** 516–23.
8. McKeage MJ, *et al.* Tamoxifen and chemotherapy for refractory metastatic malignant melanoma. *N Engl J Med* 1993; **328:** 140–1.
9. Rusthoven JJ, *et al.* Randomized, double-blind, placebo-controlled trial comparing the response rates of carmustine, dacarbazine, and cisplatin with and without tamoxifen in patients with metastatic melanoma. *J Clin Oncol* 1996; **14:** 2083–90.
10. Aamdal S, *et al.* Docetaxel (Taxotere) in advanced malignant melanoma: a phase II study of the EORTC Early Clinical Trials Group. *Eur J Cancer* 1994; **30A:** 1061–4.
11. Calabresi F, *et al.* Multicenter phase II trial of the single agent fotemustine in patients with advanced malignant melanoma. *Ann Oncol* 1991; **2:** 377–8.
12. Rosenberg SA, *et al.* A progress report on the treatment of 157 patients with advanced cancer using lymphokine-activated killer cells and interleukin-2 or high-dose interleukin-2 alone. *N Engl J Med* 1987; **316:** 889–97.
13. Bridgewater JA, Gore ME. Biological response modifiers in melanoma. *Br Med Bull* 1995; **51:** 656–77.
14. Rosenberg SA, *et al.* Treatment of 283 consecutive patients with metastatic melanoma or renal cell cancer using high-dose bolus interleukin 2. *JAMA* 1994; **271:** 907–13.
15. West WH, *et al.* Constant-infusion recombinant interleukin-2 in adoptive immunotherapy of advanced cancer. *N Engl J Med* 1987; **316:** 898–905.
16. Rosenberg SA, *et al.* Use of tumor-infiltrating lymphocytes and interleukin-2 in the immunotherapy of patients with metastatic melanoma: a preliminary report. *N Engl J Med* 1988; **319:** 1676–80.
17. Rosenberg SA, *et al.* Gene transfer into humans—immunotherapy of patients with advanced melanoma, using tumor-infiltrating lymphocytes modified by retroviral gene transduction. *N Engl J Med* 1990; **323:** 570–8.
18. Creagan ET, *et al.* Randomized, surgical adjuvant clinical trial of recombinant interferon alfa-2a in selected patients with malignant melanoma. *J Clin Oncol* 1995; **13:** 2776–83.
19. Kirkwood JM, *et al.* Interferon alfa-2b adjuvant therapy of high-risk resected cutaneous melanoma: the Eastern Cooperative Oncology Group Trial EST 1684. *J Clin Oncol* 1996; **14:** 7–17.
20. Hahka-Kemppinen M, *et al.* Response of subcutaneous and cutaneous metastases of malignant melanoma to combined cytostatic plus interferon therapy. *Br J Dermatol* 1995; **132:** 973–7.
21. Cascinelli N, *et al.* Results of adjuvant interferon study in WHO melanoma programme. *Lancet* 1994; **343:** 913–14.
22. Irie RF, *et al.* Human monoclonal antibody to ganglioside GM2 for melanoma treatment. *Lancet* 1989; **i:** 786–7.
23. Hersey P. Melanoma vaccines: current status and future prospects. *Drugs* 1994; **47:** 373–82.
24. Mitchell MS. Active specific immunotherapy of melanoma. *Br Med Bull* 1995; **51:** 631–46.
25. Berd D, *et al.* Autologous hapten-modified melanoma vaccine as postsurgical adjuvant treatment after resection of nodal metastases. *J Clin Oncol* 1997; **15:** 2359–70.
26. Morton DL, *et al.* Prolongation of survival in metastatic melanoma after active specific immunotherapy with a new polyvalent melanoma vaccine. *Ann Surg* 1992; **216:** 463–82.
27. Grob JJ, *et al.* Randomised trial of interferon α-2a as adjuvant therapy in resected primary melanoma thicker than 1.5 mm without clinically detectable node metastases. *Lancet* 1998; **351:** 1905–10.

Malignant neoplasms of the testis. The great majority of testicular tumours arise from germinal cells, although a few derive from cells of the gonadal stroma or are secondary to diseases such as leukaemias or lymphomas. Testicular cancer only accounts for about 1% of all male malignancies but it is the most common cancer in young men. Increased risk of developing testicular cancer occurs in patients with a history of cryptorchidism. About 40% of all germ cell tumours of the testis are seminomas; the remainder include (in the WHO classification) embryonal carcinoma, teratocarcinoma, teratoma, and, rarely, choriocarcinoma, but other systems of classification exist, and many nonseminomatous tumours are of mixed cell types. Metastasis can occur, initially mainly to the lymph nodes but in advanced disease to distant sites such as lung, liver, brain, and bones. The leading symptom is a hard, painless swelling of the testis, but once metastasis occurs the patient may present with back pain (due to enlargement of retroperitoneal lymph nodes), cough, dyspnoea, gynaecomastia due to chorionic gonadotrophin production, or weight loss.

Surgical removal of the testis (orchidectomy) when diagnosis is confirmed is fundamental to the treatment of all types of testicular cancer, but further therapy depends upon the disease type and stage. In patients with **nonseminomatous** disease with no detectable metastases standard postorchidectomy management in the UK is surveillance.[1,2] About 20 to 30% of these patients will relapse and require chemotherapy, and in the USA standard management is to perform retroperitoneal lymph node dissection at the time of orchidectomy, thus permitting more accurate staging and removing any lymph node metastases, although at the cost of some unnecessary surgery. An alternative in patients with prognostic factors suggesting a high risk of relapse (vascular or lymphatic invasion, the presence of undifferentiated cells or absence of yolk sac elements) is to give adjuvant chemotherapy with 2 cycles of standard BEP (bleomycin, etoposide, and cisplatin), which will prevent relapse in the vast majority of cases.[1]

Where metastasis to the lymph nodes or beyond has occurred, standard therapy is now combination chemotherapy with 4 cycles of BEP, which has largely replaced the effective but more toxic PVB regimen (cisplatin, vinblastine, and bleomycin).[1-3] Over 80% of patients with metastatic disease can be cured with such a regimen.[1,4,5] In good-risk patients, 3 cycles of BEP, or 4 copies of cisplatin and etoposide alone, may be adequate.[6,7] Multiple lung metastases, large mediastinal masses, metastases to bone, liver or CNS, or high blood concentrations of tumour markers (alpha fetoprotein and chorionic gonadotrophin) are associated with a poorer prognosis;[1,2] such patients may be offered more intensive chemotherapy, for example, preceding BEP with a regimen of carboplatin, bleomycin, vincristine, and cisplatin.[1] Another approach is to follow BEP with high-dose chemotherapy (usually based on etoposide and carboplatin) and peripheral blood stem cell support.[3]

Patients who fail standard chemotherapy have a poor prognosis, with an overall survival of only 20 to 30%.[1] Various types of salvage chemotherapy have been tried, based on etoposide,[8] or cisplatin, vinblastine, and ifosfamide;[9] high-dose chemotherapy with some form of haematopoietic support may also be tried.[1,6,10]

Because almost all patients with nonseminomatous disease are likely to enjoy long-term survival there has been some concern about the long-term effects of therapy, and in particular the risk of second malignancies with etoposide.[11] It remains to be seen whether this will prove to be a problem in the longer term.

Seminoma is extremely sensitive to radiation, and radiotherapy is the treatment of choice after orchidectomy in limited disease.[1,12] About three-quarters of the patients have no metastases at diagnosis and cure rates are between 95 and 100%.[13] However, it also responds very well to chemotherapy, and more advanced or metastatic disease is usually treated with BEP or a similar regimen[1] with survival rates similar to those in nonseminomatous disease.

1. Wilkins M, Horwich A. Diagnosis and treatment of urological malignancy: the testes. *Br J Hosp Med* 1996; **55:** 199–203.
2. Read G. Modern management for testicular teratoma. *Br J Hosp Med* 1996; **56:** 218–21.
3. Welch RS, Wilkinson PM. The management of poor prognosis teratoma. *Br J Hosp Med* 1996; **56:** 222–4.
4. Report from the Medical Research Council Working Party on Testicular Tumours. Prognostic factors in advanced non-seminomatous germ-cell testicular tumours: results of a multicentre study. *Lancet* 1985; **i:** 8–11.
5. Peckham MJ, *et al.* The treatment of metastatic germ-cell testicular tumours with bleomycin, etoposide and cisplatin (BEP). *Br J Cancer* 1983; **47:** 613–19.
6. Bosl GJ, Motzer RJ. Testicular germ-cell cancer. *N Engl J Med* 1997; **337:** 242–53. Correction. *ibid.*, 1403.
7. Saxman SB, *et al.* Long-term follow-up of a phase III study of three versus four cycles of bleomycin, etoposide, and cisplatin in favorable-prognosis germ-cell tumors: the Indiana University experience. *J Clin Oncol* 1998; **16:** 702–6.
8. Cantwell BMJ, *et al.* 21-Day cycles of oral etoposide in heavily pretreated metastatic germ-cell cancer. *Lancet* 1990; **336:** 1011.
9. Loehrer PJ *et al.* Salvage therapy in recurrent germ cell cancer: ifosfamide and cisplatin plus either vinblastine or etoposide. *Ann Intern Med* 1988; **109:** 540–6. Correction. *ibid.*; 846.
10. Brown ER, *et al.* Long-term outcome of patients with relapsed and refractory germ cell tumors treated with high-dose chemotherapy and autologous bone marrow rescue. *Ann Intern Med* 1992; **117:** 124–8.
11. Boshoff C, *et al.* Treatment of good-risk, stage II, non-seminomatous testis cancer. *Lancet* 1994; **344:** 1085–6.
12. WHO. Chemotherapy of solid tumours: report of a WHO expert committee. *WHO Tech Rep Ser 605* 1977.
13. Mead GM. Testicular cancer and related neoplasms. *Br Med J* 1992; **304:** 1426–9.

Malignant neoplasms of the thymus. Thymomas are tumours of the mediastinum, arising from thymic tissue. They are rare, and most commonly present in patients between 40 and 60 years of age. Thymoma originates from the epithelium of the thymus but may also contain a lymphocyte component. The initial diagnosis may be heralded by local symptoms such as cough, chest pain, dyspnoea, and obstruction of the vena cava; syndromes such as myasthenia gravis, red cell aplasia, and hypogammaglobulinaemia may also develop.

Thymomas vary in their invasiveness but the majority of patients present with localised disease, and surgical resection remains the mainstay of therapy;[1] long-term survival in this group is 80% or more. Postoperative radiotherapy may be required, especially in more extensive or incompletely resected disease.

About a third of all patients with thymomas have invasive or metastatic disease in which resection alone is unlikely to be curative,[1] and in this group some mildly promising results have been seen with combination chemotherapy.

Although some responses have been seen with regimens such as cyclophosphamide, doxorubicin, and vincristine, or vincristine, cyclophosphamide, and lomustine, the demonstration that cisplatin had significant activity against thymoma has led to much interest in cisplatin-containing regimens such as cisplatin, doxorubicin, and cyclophosphamide.[2,3] Ifosfamide is also active as a single agent against thymoma, and has been given with cisplatin and etoposide.[1] Corticosteroids have been added to some regimens, and may be useful where the lymphocytic component of disease is marked, although whether this represents an antineoplastic effect has been questioned.[1] A report[4] of the dramatic regression of refractory thymoma in a patient given interleukin-2 is considered to warrant further investigation of the potential of this agent.[1] There is also a report of complete response to a combination of octreotide and prednisone.[5]

Radiotherapy has been tried as primary therapy in patients with unresectable disease, but is inadequate if used alone; combination with chemotherapy has been investigated.[1]

1. Loehrer PJ, *et al.* Thymomas: current experience and future directions in therapy. *Drugs* 1993; **45:** 477–87.
2. Loehrer PJ, *et al.* Chemotherapy for advanced thymoma: preliminary results of an intergroup study. *Ann Intern Med* 1990; **113:** 520–4.
3. Loehrer PJ, *et al.* Cisplatin, doxorubicin, and cyclophosphamide plus thoracic radiation therapy for limited-stage unresectable thymoma: an intergroup trial. *J Clin Oncol* 1997; **15:** 3093–9.

4. Berthaud P, *et al.* Effectiveness of interleukin-2 in invasive lymphoepithelial thymoma. *Lancet* 1990; **335:** 1590.
5. Palmieri G, *et al.* Successful treatment of a patient with a thymoma and pure red-cell aplasia with octreotide and prednisone. *N Engl J Med* 1997; **336:** 263–5.

Malignant neoplasms of the thyroid. Thyroid cancer accounts for only about 1% of all malignancies. The incidence is reportedly higher in women than men, in patients who received irradiation of the thyroid during childhood, and in populations where goitre is endemic. The natural history varies with the cell type and degree of differentiation. Well-differentiated papillary or follicular tumours, which constitute the majority of cases, are very slow to grow and metastasise, sometimes persisting for years with little change in size and extent, although they may prove more aggressive in children. In contrast medullary carcinomas, which develop from the cells responsible for calcitonin secretion, and undifferentiated (anaplastic) tumours metastasise early and follow a much more rapid and aggressive course. The well-differentiated types usually present as a thyroid nodule, although most nodules are not malignant, while with anaplastic tumours there is usually bulky disease and often difficulty in breathing due to encroachment on the tracheal lumen.

In patients with well-differentiated tumours total or partial thyroidectomy may be followed by a course of iodine-131 to destroy any residual tumour[1-3] (this is more useful in follicular than papillary tumours since only 10 to 15% of the latter take up iodine). In low-risk patients the prognosis after surgery alone is so favourable that iodine-131 is not usually recommended.[3] Thyroxine treatment should be given to suppress thyroid stimulating hormone (TSH) production, and must be continued for life, but there is some uncertainty as to whether TSH concentrations should be lowered to the bottom of the normal range or to clearly subnormal values.[1] Five-year survival of up to 70% in patients with follicular tumours and up to 90% with papillary tumours has been seen, although the naturally indolent course of these diseases makes evaluation difficult.

In patients with the more aggressive medullary cancers total thyroidectomy and neck dissection are indicated, but 5-year survival is only 30 to 40%. Resection may relieve symptoms in patients with anaplastic tumours, but cure is impossible and treatment is purely palliative. Chemotherapy has been tried in anaplastic thyroid cancer, as well as in unresponsive disease of other cell types, with limited benefit.[4-6] Most regimens seem to have included doxorubicin: treatment with doxorubicin, vincristine, and bleomycin is reportedly of benefit in some patients with anaplastic thyroid carcinoma.[1] Cisplatin also has some activity but reports differ as to the benefits of combined cisplatin and doxorubicin treatment;[4,5] one group, which failed to achieve any complete remissions with such a regimen has suggested that such responses may have occurred in patients in whom lymphoma was misconstrued as anaplastic thyroid carcinoma.[5]

1. Mazzaferri EL. Management of a solitary thyroid nodule. *N Engl J Med* 1993; **328:** 553–9.
2. Mazzaferri EL, Jhiang SM. Long-term impact of initial surgical and medical therapy on papillary and follicular thyroid cancer. *Am J Med* 1994; **97:** 418–28. Correction. *ibid.* 1995; **98:** 215.
3. Schlumberger MJ. Papillary and follicular thyroid carcinoma. *N Engl J Med* 1998; **338:** 297–306.
4. Sokal M, Harmer CL. Chemotherapy for anaplastic carcinoma of the thyroid. *Clin Oncol* 1978; **4:** 3–10.
5. Shimaoka K, *et al.* A randomized trial of adriamycin versus adriamycin plus cis-diammine-dichloroplatinum in patients with thyroid carcinoma. *Proc Am Soc Clin Oncol* 1983; **2:** 168.
6. Williams SD, *et al.* Phase II evaluation of doxorubicin plus cisplatin in advanced thyroid cancer: a Southeastern Cancer Study Group trial. *Cancer Treat Rep* 1986; **70:** 405–7.

Myeloma. Multiple myeloma (myelomatosis) is a lymphoproliferative disorder of B-cell origin, involving the development of an abnormal plasma-cell precursor. It occurs predominantly in the elderly, and accounts for only 1% or less of all malignancies. It is more common in black than in white patients and in men than in women.

The proliferation of the abnormal clone tends to suppress normal haematopoiesis, resulting in anaemia and immunosuppression, with an increased risk of serious infection. Perhaps the most characteristic complication, however, is skeletal destruction, apparently due to release of an osteoclast stimulating factor, resulting in osteoporosis, lytic lesions and fractures, and bone pain, as well as consequent hypercalcaemia. In addition, the plasma cells release large quantities of monoclonal immunoglobulins, known as paraproteins, which can produce a hyperviscosity syndrome and in some cases may interfere with platelet function. Renal failure of various causes and neurological problems due to compression are also common.

Multiple myeloma is not curable with presently-available treatment, and therapy is concerned with prolongation of survival and alleviation of symptoms.[1-6] Treatment is generally reserved for patients with overt, progressive disease, those with stable, indolent or smouldering myeloma, or benign monoclonal gammopathy, being followed carefully but not treated until progression occurs.[1-5]

In patients with overt disease, chemotherapy with the aim of inducing remission and prolonging survival, is the treatment of choice. The standard regimen has long been a combination of oral melphalan and corticosteroids, usually prednisolone or prednisone, particularly in elderly and frail patients. This regimen produces an objective response in about half of all patients, and prolongs median survival to between 19 and 39 months.[1] The contribution of corticosteroids to the regimen is controversial although their palliative effects are invaluable;[4] however, high-dose dexamethasone given alone has been reported to be effective in producing remissions.[5,7] It has been suggested that comparative trials of melphalan and prednisone, high-dose dexamethasone, and melphalan with dexamethasone are needed.[5] A combination of idarubicin and dexamethasone has also been found to be an effective induction therapy.[8]

More intensive combination regimens are also used, particularly in younger, fitter patients. A number of studies (although not all) suggest that improved response rates and longer survival can be achieved with combination regimens that add doxorubicin and carmustine to alkylating agents,[3] such as the ABCM regimen (doxorubicin, carmustine, cyclophosphamide, and melphalan),[9] or alternating combinations of vincristine, melphalan, cyclophosphamide, and prednisone with vincristine, doxorubicin, carmustine, and prednisone.[10] Other approaches include the use of the VAD regimen (vincristine, doxorubicin, and dexamethasone)[11] or high dose melphalan with or without autologous bone marrow transplantation.[12,13] However, in the longer term survival is not markedly improved, so these regimens cannot be considered curative, and some disagreement remains about the optimum induction regimen.[3-6] There has been interest in the potential of bone marrow transplantation, but allogeneic transplantation is of limited applicability (although there are intriguing reports of a graft-versus-myeloma effect[14,15]), and autologous transplantation, although better tolerated, carries the risk of re-infusing myeloma stem cells and thus guaranteeing relapse.[1-5] Peripheral blood stem cells may be preferable.[4]

Once remission has been achieved chemotherapy is often stopped as maintenance chemotherapy has not been shown convincingly to improve total duration of remissions or survival.[3,4,6] However, maintenance treatment with interferon has been reported to improve remission duration,[16-18] and appears to prolong overall and event-free survival,[19,20] although toxicity may be a problem. (Addition of interferons to initial induction therapy appears to be of little extra value.[17,18])

In patients who fail to respond to initial treatment, or who subsequently relapse, various regimens have been tried; the prognosis is better in patients who relapse after remission than in those who are resistant or relapse during induction therapy.[4,6,21] Treatment with the VAD regimen has been reported to be effective in producing a second response in some patients,[22,23] and patients with refractory disease have responded to high-dose cyclophosphamide and radiotherapy combined with autologous transfusion of peripheral blood stem cells.[24] In patients with unresponsive myeloma, high-dose corticosteroids may also sometimes produce responses.[23] Clinical resistance to the VAD regimen due to the multidrug resistance (MDR) gene can be overcome by concomitant infusion of cyclosporin,[25] although neurotoxicity may be increased;[26] however, attempts to reverse resistance with verapamil have been disappointing.[27]

Although chemotherapy aimed at the myelomatous clone will produce symptomatic relief as disease is brought under control, supportive and symptomatic care is also important, particularly initially. Radiotherapy is the treatment of choice for bone disease producing spinal cord compression, and is often effective in relieving bone pain, which may otherwise require opioid analgesics. Some bisphosphonates have been found to be effective in the management of bone symptoms.[28,29] A high fluid intake is essential in patients with renal dysfunction or hypercalcaemia (for the appropriate management of the latter, see p.1148). Vigorous antibacterial treatment may be required if infection occurs (see Infections in Immunocompromised Patients, p.127) and plasma exchange may alleviate the hyperviscosity syndrome.

1. Camba L, Durie BGM. Multiple myeloma: new treatment options. *Drugs* 1992; **44:** 170–81.
2. Dunbar CE, Nienhuis AW. Multiple myeloma: new approaches to therapy. *JAMA* 1993; **269:** 2412–16.
3. MacLennan ICM, *et al.* Multiple myeloma. *Br Med J* 1994; **308:** 1033–6.
4. Newland AC. Management of multiple myeloma. *Prescribers' J* 1994; **34:** 102–10.
5. Alexanian R, Dimopoulos M. The treatment of multiple myeloma. *N Engl J Med* 1994; **330:** 484–9.
6. Oken MM. Standard treatment of multiple myeloma. *Mayo Clin Proc* 1994; **69:** 781–6.
7. Alexanian R, *et al.* Primary dexamethasone treatment of multiple myeloma. *Blood* 1992; **80:** 887–90.
8. Cook G, *et al.* A phase I/II trial of Z-Dex (oral idarubicin and dexamethasone), an oral equivalent of VAD, as initial therapy at diagnosis or progression in multiple myeloma. *Br J Haematol* 1996; **93:** 931–4.
9. MacLennan ICM, *et al.* Combined chemotherapy with ABCM versus melphalan for treatment of myelomatosis. *Lancet* 1992; **339:** 200–5.
10. Durie BGM, *et al.* Improved survival duration with combination chemotherapy induction for multiple myeloma: a Southwest Oncology Group study. *J Clin Oncol* 1986; **4:** 1227–37.
11. Samson D, *et al.* Infusion of vincristine and doxorubicin with oral dexamethasone as first-line therapy for multiple myeloma. *Lancet* 1989; **ii:** 882–5.
12. Gore ME, *et al.* Intensive treatment of multiple myeloma and criteria for complete remission. *Lancet* 1989; **ii:** 879–82.
13. Attal M, *et al.* A prospective, randomized trial of autologous bone marrow transplantation and chemotherapy in multiple myeloma. *N Engl J Med* 1996; **335:** 91–7.
14. Verdonck LF, *et al.* Graft-versus-myeloma effect in two cases. *Lancet* 1996; **347:** 800–1.
15. Aschan J, *et al.* Graft-versus-myeloma effect. *Lancet* 1996; **348:** 346.
16. Attal M, *et al.* Maintenance treatment with recombinant alpha interferon after autologous bone marrow transplantation for aggressive myeloma in first remission after conventional induction chemotherapy. *Bone Marrow Transplant* 1991; **8:** 125–8.
17. The Nordic Myeloma Study Group. Interferon-α2b added to melphalan-prednisone for initial and maintenance therapy in multiple myeloma: a randomized, controlled trial. *Ann Intern Med* 1996; **124:** 212–22.
18. Ludwig H, *et al.* Interferon-alpha for induction and maintenance in multiple myeloma: results of two multicenter randomized trials and summary of other studies. *Ann Oncol* 1995; **6:** 467–76.
19. Browman GP, *et al.* Randomized trial of interferon maintenance in multiple myeloma: a study of the National Cancer Institute of Canada Clinical Trials Group. *J Clin Oncol* 1995; **13:** 2354–60.
20. Cunningham D, *et al.* A randomized trial of maintenance interferon following high-dose chemotherapy in multiple myeloma: long-term follow-up results. *Br J Haematol* 1998; **102:** 495–502.
21. Barlogie B, *et al.* Salvage therapy for multiple myeloma: the University of Arkansas experience. *Mayo Clin Proc* 1994; **69:** 787–95.
22. Barlogie B, *et al.* Effective treatment of advanced multiple myeloma refractory to alkylating agents. *N Engl J Med* 1984; **310:** 1353–6.
23. Alexanian R, *et al.* High-dose glucocorticoid treatment of resistant myeloma. *Ann Intern Med* 1986; **105:** 8–11.
24. Reiffers J, *et al.* Peripheral blood stem-cell transplantation in intensive treatment of multiple myeloma. *Lancet* 1989; **ii:** 1336.
25. Sonneveld P, *et al.* Modulation of multidrug-resistant multiple myeloma by cyclosporin. *Lancet* 1992; **340:** 255–9.
26. Weber DM, *et al.* Increased neurotoxicity with VAD-cyclosporin in multiple myeloma. *Lancet* 1993; **341:** 558–9.
27. Dalton WS, *et al.* A phase III randomized study of oral verapamil as a chemosensitizer to reverse drug resistance in patients with refractory myeloma. *Cancer* 1995; **75:** 815–20.
28. Lahtinen R, *et al.* Randomised, placebo-controlled multicentre trial of clodronate in multiple myeloma. *Lancet* 1992; **340:** 1049–52. Correction. *ibid.*; 1420.
29. Berenzon JR, *et al.* Long-term pamidronate treatment of advanced multiple myeloma patients reduces skeletal events. *J Clin Oncol* 1998; **16:** 593–602.

Neuroblastoma. Neuroblastoma accounts for about 7% of all childhood malignancies overall but is probably the most frequent neoplasm in the first year of life. Three-quarters of all cases present before the age of 5 years, and the use of ultrasonography has permitted the detection of some cases *in utero* although it is unclear whether all of these represent active malignancies.[1] The tumour is derived from cells of the neural crest, and may occur anywhere within the sympathetic nervous system, notably the sympathetic ganglia and the adrenal medulla. Metastasis tends to occur early, and bone marrow disease is present in about two-thirds of cases at diagnosis; other sites of metastasis include lymph nodes, liver, and skin.

Progress in the treatment of neuroblastoma over the last 20 years has increased 5-year survival to about 55% overall, although in patients with disseminated disease the gains have been modest.[2] In children with localised disease (stage I or II) surgery and radiotherapy are the appropriate treatment, and these patients (about a fifth of all cases)[2] generally enjoy good long-term survival prospects. About 90% of those with localised but unresectable disease can be cured with a course of cyclophosphamide and doxorubicin.[2]

In more advanced disease, chemotherapy, together with surgery and radiotherapy, is used extensively. Prognosis for any given stage depends in part on age, with much better results in infants (who can usually be cured regardless of stage if under one year old[2]) than in older children.[2] Various regimens have been used, many based on doxorubicin and cyclophosphamide, for example combined with cisplatin and either etoposide or teniposide; cyclophosphamide with cisplatin, and bone-marrow ablation plus autologous bone-marrow transplantation have also been used, as have a variety of other agents including dactinomycin, the vinca alkaloids, mustine, and dacarbazine. Targeted radiation, using iodine-131-labelled *m*-iodobenzylguanidine, which is actively taken up by cells synthesising catecholamines, is also employed.[3] Unfortunately, fewer than 20% of older children with stage III or IV disease have become long-term survivors;[2] although some degree of response is common, relapse often occurs within a year. New treatment strategies are urgently needed in such patients.

1. Ho PTC, *et al.* Prenatal detection of neuroblastoma: a ten-year experience from the Dana-Farber Cancer Institute and Children's Hospital. *Pediatrics* 1993; **92:** 358–64.
2. Crist WM, Kun LE. Common solid tumors of childhood. *N Engl J Med* 1991; **324:** 461–71.
3. Meller S. Targeted radiotherapy for neuroblastoma. *Arch Dis Child* 1997; **77:** 389–91.

Polycythaemia vera. Polycythaemia vera is a myeloproliferative disorder, apparently due to an abnormal stem cell clone, which results in increased red cell mass, usually with concomitant increases in white cell and platelet counts. It is a disease of later life, with a median age at presentation of about 60 years.

The cellular proliferation increases blood viscosity and volume, and the resultant circulatory disturbance may produce headache, dizziness, tinnitus, vertigo, and visual disturbances (blurring and diplopia). Patients show an increased tendency to bruising and bleeding, and the thrombotic or haemorrhagic complications may ultimately prove fatal; survival ranges from about 6 to 18 months in untreated patients. Other symptoms include pruritus, characteristically exacerbated by warmth, hyperuricaemia, and a burning sensation in the feet (erythromelalgia).

Although cure is not possible at present, appropriate management may produce prolonged survival. The initial treatment is phlebotomy to reduce the packed cell volume to normal values; one this has been achieved, appropriate maintenance therapy can be given. The maintenance treatment of choice in younger patients is periodic phlebotomy,[1] but in older patients or those who do not tolerate phlebotomy well or have high platelet counts some form of myelosuppressive therapy may be considered.

Chlorambucil, which was formerly used for this purpose, has largely been discontinued because of a high incidence of leukaemia in patients so treated,[2] and although some authorities consider busulphan to be a less leukaemogenic alternative the use of alkylating agents has come to be viewed with suspicion. (Other alkylating agents to have been tried include mitobronitol and pipobroman.) In the older age group radioactive phosphorus-32 is probably appropriate, and produces good results with few immediate adverse effects.[1] However, like the alkylating agents it is associated with an increased risk of secondary malignancies. In younger patients requiring myelosuppressive therapy the most appropriate therapy is probably hydroxyurea,[1,3,4] which has not yet been shown to be associated with leukaemogenesis, although its use in these patients has not gone on long enough for a definite conclusion. Good preliminary results have also been reported from the use of interferon alfa.[5]

Although long-term control is possible for many years with the above methods, transition ultimately occurs from the proliferative phase to a 'burnt-out' stage marked by massive splenomegaly and myelofibrosis, or to acute leukaemia. The former is managed primarily by blood transfusion, iron, and folate replacement, with splenectomy if necessary; the latter should be managed with appropriate chemotherapy but is usually extremely refractory to treatment.

Various agents may also be required for symptomatic relief in the management of polycythaemia vera. In particular, histamine H_1- and H_2-receptor antagonists, alone or in combination, may be tried for pruritus, and allopurinol is used for the management of associated hyperuricaemia.[1,4] Erythromelalgia may respond to low dose aspirin.

1. Berk PD, *et al.* Therapeutic recommendations in polycythaemia vera based on Polycythaemia Vera Study Group protocols. *Semin Hematol* 1986; **23:** 132–43.
2. Berk PD, *et al.* Increased incidence of acute leukemia in polycythemia vera associated with chlorambucil therapy. *N Engl J Med* 1981; **304:** 441–7.
3. Donovan PB, *et al.* Treatment of polycythemia vera with hydroxyurea. *Am J Hematol* 1984; **17:** 329–34.
4. Smith AG. Polycythaemia and its management. *Prescribers' J* 1994; **34:** 142–51.
5. Silver RT. Interferon-α2b: a new treatment for polycythemia vera. *Ann Intern Med* 1993; **119:** 1091–2.

Retinoblastoma. Retinoblastoma is a tumour arising in the eye which accounts for about 3% of all childhood malignancies. In 60 to 70% of cases the tumour is sporadic and non-hereditary, producing a unilateral, unifocal lesion, but in 30 to 40% there is an abnormal gene inherited: these tumours are typically bilateral, and other family members are at increased risk. The most common manifestations are leukocoria (white pupil) or strabismus (squint). Invasion of the optic nerve is considered to indicate a high risk of metastatic disease.[1]

The great majority of patients with retinoblastoma present with localised disease which can be successfully treated with cryotherapy or radiotherapy; in advanced disease enucleation may be required. Overall survival is excellent: about 90% of patients are reportedly alive and disease-free 5 to 10 years after diagnosis.[2] A study has suggested that combination of cyclosporin (which inhibits P glycoprotein) with chemotherapy can produce good remission rates without the use of radiotherapy.[3] Adjuvant chemotherapy after enucleation, may be of value in patients with optic nerve invasion.[1] Intravitreal thiotepa has been used in an attempt to salvage the remaining eye in patients with bilateral retinoblastoma who have had one eye enucleated.[4] Neoadjuvant chemotherapy with etoposide and carboplatin (a combination active in metastatic disease) has been reported to be of benefit in avoiding the need for external beam irradiation;[7] carboplatin has also been used in combination with laser hyperthermia.

Although metastatic disease is rare it is difficult to treat. Regimens similar to those used in neuroblastoma (see above) have been advocated, such as a combination of doxorubicin and cyclophosphamide with agents such as cisplatin, teniposide, and vincristine,[5] but although such combination chemotherapy may produce a response it does not appear to be curative in such advanced disease.[2,6] Intrathecal methotrexate may be combined with surgery and radiotherapy for ectopic cranial tumours.[6]

1. Hungerford J. Factors influencing metastasis in retinoblastoma. *Br J Ophthalmol* 1993; **77:** 541.
2. Crist WM, Kun LE. Common solid tumors of childhood. *N Engl J Med* 1991; **324:** 461–71.
3. Gallie BL, *et al.* Chemotherapy with focal therapy can cure intraocular retinoblastoma without radiotherapy. *Arch Ophthalmol* 1996; **114:** 1321–8.
4. Seregard S, *et al.* Intravitreal chemotherapy for recurrent retinoblastoma in an only eye. *Br J Ophthalmol* 1995; **79:** 194–5.
5. Anonymous. Drugs of choice for cancer chemotherapy. *Med Lett Drugs Ther* 1997; **39:** 21–8.
6. Kingston JE, *et al.* Ectopic intracranial retinoblastoma in childhood. *Br J Ophthalmol* 1985; **69:** 742–8.
7. Levy C, *et al.* Role of chemotherapy alone or in combination with hyperthermia in the primary treatment of intraocular retinoblastoma: preliminary results. *Br J Ophthalmol* 1998; **82:** 1154–8.

Sarcomas. The sarcomas are tumours arising from mesodermal cells which form the bone and connective tissue (as opposed to carcinomas, which arise from ectodermal and endodermal cells, and leukaemias and lymphomas which arise from the bone marrow and immune system).

Sarcomas are uncommon, and vary considerably in their sites, presentation, and prognosis. The primary malignancies of bone include osteosarcoma and Ewing's sarcoma, which most often occur in older children and adolescents, and chondrosarcoma which is most common in later life. Soft tissue sarcomas include those of fibrous tissue (fibrosarcoma), skeletal muscle (rhabdomyosarcoma), smooth muscle (leiomyosarcoma), adipose tissue (liposarcoma), and blood vessels (a group which includes Kaposi's sarcoma).

BONE SARCOMA. The commonest primary malignant tumour of bone is **osteosarcoma** (osteogenic sarcoma) which accounts for about 3 to 4% of all childhood malignancies. It is composed of malignant osteoblasts which form an osteoid matrix within which new bone formation may occur. Most osteosarcomas are aggressive high-grade malignancies which destroy overlying cortical bone and invade adjacent soft tissue, as well as spreading along the medulla. Metastasis, almost exclusively via the vascular system to the lungs and other distant sites, is usual and occurs early.

The primary therapy is surgery, with an increasing trend to more conservative, limb-sparing operations rather than amputation. However, over 80% of patients develop metastatic disease, and eventually die, without systemic treatment. Adjuvant chemotherapy has generally relied upon intensive combinations of high-dose methotrexate (plus folinic acid rescue) with doxorubicin and other agents such as cisplatin, cyclophosphamide, ifosfamide, or vincristine. An intensive, short chemotherapy regimen employing pre- and postoperative doxorubicin and cisplatin has been shown to be as effective in prolonging survival as a multi-drug regimen based on the widely used T10 protocol (pre-operative vincristine, high-dose methotrexate, and doxorubicin, and postoperative bleomycin, cyclophosphamide, dactinomycin, vincristine, methotrexate, doxorubicin, and cisplatin).[1] The use of adjuvant therapy has produced overall disease-free survival of about 60% at 5 years.[2] Patients with metastatic disease at diagnosis fare poorly, although some pulmonary metastases (the commonest site) may be resectable.[3] There has been considerable interest in the use of neoadjuvant therapy before surgery to reduce tumour burden, permit use of chemotherapy early in the course of disease, and evaluate tumour response. Intra-arterial cisplatin[2,3] or doxorubicin[3] have been employed in this way, and such neoadjuvant therapy may permit increased use of limb-sparing surgery.[3] Neoadjuvant therapy has been reported to produce fewer relapses than adjuvant therapy,[4] and is now widely employed.

Like osteosarcoma, **Ewing's sarcoma** is seen mainly in adolescents and older children. It is a round cell tumour that most commonly arises in the pelvis or the long bones of the limbs. There may be diffuse erosion of the bone and marked periosteal reaction. It spreads through the medullary cavity, and metastases to lung and other bones are common.

Unlike most bone sarcomas this is highly radiosensitive, and treatment consists of local radiotherapy with adjuvant chemotherapy. Such a protocol, employing combination chemotherapy with cyclophosphamide, vincristine, dactinomycin, and doxorubicin (VACA), has resulted in a 5-year survival rate of 65% in patients with early (non-metastatic) disease.[5] Prognosis is poorer in patients with metastatic disease, but even in this group VACA chemotherapy, or VACA combined with fluorouracil, has resulted in a 30% survival rate at 5 years, suggesting a potential for cure.[6]

Chemotherapy appears to have little place in the treatment of other bone sarcomas such as **chondrosarcoma** or **osteoclastoma**; it has been employed in high-grade **fibrosarcomas** and in **histiocytoma** but its value is uncertain.

1. Souhami RL, *et al.* Randomised trial of two regimens of chemotherapy in operable osteosarcoma: a study of the European Osteosarcoma Intergroup. *Lancet* 1997; **350:** 911–17.
2. Hudson M, *et al.* Pediatric osteosarcoma: therapeutic strategies, results, and prognostic factors derived from a 10-year experience. *J Clin Oncol* 1990; **8:** 1988–97.
3. Meyer WH, Malawer MM. Osteosarcoma: clinical features and evolving surgical and chemotherapeutic strategies. *Pediatr Clin North Am* 1991; **38:** 317–48.
4. Bacci G, *et al.* Changing pattern of relapse in osteosarcoma of the extremities treated with adjuvant and neoadjuvant chemotherapy. *J Chemother* 1995; **7:** 230–9.
5. Nesbit ME, *et al.* Multimodal therapy for the management of primary, nonmetastatic Ewing's sarcoma of bone: a long-term following of the first intergroup study. *J Clin Oncol* 1990; **8:** 1664–74.
6. Cangir A, *et al.* Ewing's sarcoma metastatic at diagnosis: results and comparisons of two intergroup Ewing's sarcoma studies. *Cancer* 1990; **66:** 887–93.

KAPOSI'S SARCOMA. Kaposi's sarcoma is a tumour of endothelial or spindle cell origin. In its classical form it manifests as red or violet cutaneous lesions of the limbs in elderly men, usually of Jewish or Mediterranean ancestry. It is also endemic in certain areas of Africa.[1] Lesions may eventually affect the whole of the skin, upper airways, gastro-intestinal tract, lungs, and lymph nodes, but in general disease is only very slowly progressive, and may require no treatment. In recent years an epidemic form of the disease has appeared in patients with disease due to HIV infection. HIV-associated Kaposi's sarcoma is more aggressive, with a greater tendency to disseminated and metastatic disease.

A novel herpesvirus has been implicated in the pathogenesis of Kaposi's sarcoma.[2,3] Whether antiviral agents will therefore prove useful in its prevention is unclear: although some evidence suggests that use of foscarnet or ganciclovir (although not aciclovir) reduces the risk of developing Kaposi's sarcoma in HIV-infected patients,[4] others have not found this to be the case.[5] However, some results in HIV-infected patients given highly active antiretroviral therapy incorporating HIV-protease inhibitors suggest that it may stabilise or regress Kaposi's sarcoma.[30,31]

Patients with the classical, non-epidemic form of Kaposi's sarcoma respond well to treatment with low-dose vinca alkaloids, given systemically or intralesionally,[6-8] or dactinomycin;[2] chemotherapy with these agents, and surgery,[8] or more often local or extended-field radiotherapy, remains the treatment of choice.[7,8] Intravenous liposomal doxorubicin,[9] or intralesional injection of interferon have been found to be effective.[10] There is also a report of the control of non-epidemic Kaposi's sarcoma by the use of dapsone in 2 patients.[11]

The epidemic form of Kaposi's sarcoma is associated with HIV infection, and seen particularly in homosexual patients. Localised disease may be managed with radiotherapy or cryotherapy, the latter being favoured for areas of thinner skin on the face or genitalia,[12] although intralesional injection of vinblastine, as for the classical form, may be effective.[12] Sclerotherapy, with intralesional injection of sodium tetradecyl sulphate, may be useful in providing local control of oral lesions.[13] Photodynamic therapy, using tin ethyletiopurpurin as the photosensitiser, has also been tried.[14] There is a report of a good response to perilesional injection of granulocyte-macrophage colony-stimulating factor,[15] and platelet factor 4, an inhibitor of the growth of vascular epithelium, has been investigated for local and systemic use.

Systemic chemotherapy is generally reserved for patients with more extensive disease or mucosal or visceral involvement. In patients with a CD4 cell count of 200 cells per μL or above, treatment with interferon alfa, in combination with zidovudine, has been advocated.[12,16,17] There has been some concern about the use and tolerability of chemotherapy in patients who are already immunosuppressed, and many of whom are receiving other myelosuppressive drugs such as zidovudine. Nonetheless, single agent chemotherapy with vincristine or vinblastine, or bleomycin has proved effective in moderately extensive disease,[12] and it is possible to give such therapy concomitantly with zidovudine without excessive toxicity.[18] For more extensive disease, for example with pulmonary involvement, the standard regimen has become bleomycin and vincristine,[12,16] with doxorubicin added (or substituted for vincristine) in the most severe and life-threatening disease.[12,17] Etoposide is also active.[12]

A number of newer agents are under investigation: particularly promising results have been reported with liposomal formulations of doxorubicin or daunorubicin.[19-22] Paclitaxel is also reported to produce some partial responses,[23] although toxicity may be a problem. Control of Kaposi's sarcoma has been reported in a few patients given high-dose intramuscular chorionic gonadotrophin,[24] but tumour regression ceased and regrowth occurred when dosage was reduced or withdrawn. Although a subsequent study (using lower doses) was discontinued due to toxicity and lack of benefit,[25] others have noted that different preparations may vary in their activity against the tumour (suggesting that it is not chorionic gonadotrophin itself but some impurity that is active) and have confirmed a benefit following intralesional injection.[26,27] Some results suggest the impurity in question may be a ribonuclease.[28] Other lines of investigation include the use of sulphated polysaccharide peptidoglycans, various other inhibitors of angiogenesis (including captopril[29]), thalidomide, and the retinoids.[12,16]

1. Ziegler JL. Endemic Kaposi's sarcoma in Africa and local volcanic soils. *Lancet* 1993; **342:** 1348–51.
2. Moore PS, Chang Y. Detection of herpesvirus-like DNA sequences in Kaposi's sarcoma in patients with and those without HIV infection. *N Engl J Med* 1995; **332:** 1181–5.
3. Foreman KE, *et al.* Propagation of a human herpesvirus from AIDS-associated Kaposi's sarcoma. *N Engl J Med* 1997; **336:** 163–71.
4. Mocroft A, *et al.* Anti-herpesvirus treatment and risk of Kaposi's sarcoma in HIV infection. *AIDS* 1996; **10:** 1101–5.
5. Costagliola D, Mary-Krause M. Can antiviral agents decrease the occurrence of Kaposi's sarcoma? *Lancet* 1995; **346:** 578.
6. Vogel CL, *et al.* Treatment of Kaposi's sarcoma with a combination of actinomycin D and vincristine: results of a randomized clinical trial. *Cancer* 1973; **31:** 1382–91.
7. De Boeck K, *et al.* Treatment for Kaposi's sarcoma in HIV-negative, non-homosexual men. *Lancet* 1991, **337:** 919.
8. Zurrida S, *et al.* Classic Kaposi's sarcoma: a review of 90 cases. *J Dermatol* 1992; **19:** 548–52.
9. Gottlieb JJ, *et al.* Treatment of classic Kaposi's sarcoma with liposomal encapsulated doxorubicin. *Lancet* 1997; **350:** 1363–4.
10. Trattner A, *et al.* The therapeutic effect of intralesional interferon in classical Kaposi's sarcoma. *Br J Dermatol* 1993; **129:** 590–3.
11. De Haas ERM, *et al.* Non-HIV-related Kaposi's sarcoma suppressed by dapsone. *Br J Dermatol* 1996; **135:** 813–14.
12. Northfelt DW. Treatment of Kaposi's sarcoma: current guidelines and future perspectives. *Drugs* 1994; **48:** 569–82.
13. Muzyka BC, Glick M. Sclerotherapy for the treatment of nodular intraoral Kaposi's sarcoma in patients with AIDS. *N Engl J Med* 1993; **328:** 210–11.
14. Allison RR, *et al.* Tin ethyl etiopurpurin-induced photodynamic therapy for the treatment of human immunodeficiency virus-associated Kaposi's sarcoma. *Curr Ther Res* 1998; **59:** 23–7.
15. Boente P, *et al.* Local peri-lesional therapy with rhGM-CSF for Kaposi's sarcoma. *Lancet* 1993; **341:** 1154.
16. Denton AS, *et al.* Management of pulmonary Kaposi's sarcoma: new perspectives. *Br J Hosp Med* 1995; **53:** 345–50.
17. Vaccher E, *et al.* HIV infection and neoplasia. *Lancet* 1996; **348:** 1317–18.
18. Brunt AM, *et al.* The safety of intravenous chemotherapy and zidovudine when treating epidemic Kaposi's sarcoma. *AIDS* 1989; **3:** 457–60.
19. Presant CA, *et al.* Liposomal daunorubicin treatment of HIV-associated Kaposi's sarcoma. *Lancet* 1993; **341:** 1242–3.
20. Hengge UR, *et al.* Liposomal doxorubicin in AIDS-related Kaposi's sarcoma. *Lancet* 1993; **342:** 497.
21. Harrison M, *et al.* Liposomal-entrapped doxorubicin: an active agent in AIDS-related Kaposi's sarcoma. *J Clin Oncol* 1995; **13:** 914–20.
22. Bergin C, *et al.* Treatment of Kaposi's sarcoma with liposomal doxorubicin. *Am J Health-Syst Pharm* 1995; **52:** 2001–4.
23. Saville MW, *et al.* Treatment of HIV-associated Kaposi's sarcoma with paclitaxel. *Lancet* 1995; **346:** 26–8.
24. Harris PJ. Treatment of Kaposi's sarcoma and other manifestations of AIDS with human chorionic gonadotropin. *Lancet* 1995; **346:** 118–19.
25. Bower M, *et al.* Human chorionic gonadotrophin for AIDS-related Kaposi's sarcoma. *Lancet* 1995; **346:** 642.
26. Gill PS, *et al.* The effects of preparations of human chorionic gonadotropin on AIDS-related Kaposi's sarcoma. *N Engl J Med* 1996; **335:** 1261–9. Correction. *ibid.* 1997; **336:** 670 and 1115.
27. Gill PS, *et al.* Intralesional human chorionic gonadotropin for Kaposi's sarcoma. *N Engl J Med* 1997; **336:** 1188.
28. Griffiths SJ, *et al.* Ribonuclease inhibits Kaposi's sarcoma. *Nature* 1997; **390:** 568.
29. Vogt B, Frey FJ. Inhibition of angiogenesis in Kaposi's sarcoma by captopril. *Lancet* 1997; **349:** 1148.
30. Aboulafia DM. Regression of acquired immunodeficiency syndrome-related pulmonary Kaposi's sarcoma after highly active antiretroviral therapy. *Mayo Clin Proc* 1998; **73:** 439–43.
31. Krischer J, *et al.* Regression of Kaposi's sarcoma during therapy with HIV-1 protease inhibitors: a prospective pilot study. *J Am Acad Dermatol* 1998; **38:** 594–8.

SOFT-TISSUE SARCOMA. **Rhabdomyosarcoma** is the commonest soft-tissue sarcoma in childhood, and is thought to arise from progenitor cells for skeletal muscle found throughout the body. The most frequent sites are the head and neck, genito-urinary tract, and extremities. The tumour spreads at an early stage into adjacent tissues and regional lymph nodes, and about 20% of patients have metastatic disease at diagnosis, most frequently in the lungs.

Effective treatment of rhabdomyosarcoma requires a combination of surgery, radiotherapy, and chemotherapy. Complete surgical excision is to be preferred, but where this is impossible wide-field irradiation should be given. However, the addition of adjuvant chemotherapy is crucial, and has resulted in improvement of 3-year survival rates to about 75% overall. Patients with primary tumours in the orbit or genito-urinary area have a better prognosis than those with tumours of the extremities, and tumours of the embryonal subtype carry a better prognosis than alveolar tumours. The agents used for adjuvant chemotherapy have varied, and include vincristine, dactinomycin, doxorubicin, cyclophosphamide, ifosfamide, and etoposide.[1] The optimal regimen remains to be determined: VAC (vincristine, dactinomycin, and cyclophosphamide) is widely used, but the evidence suggests that a combination of vincristine and dactinomycin is as effective in patients with good prognosis disease, although repetitive 'pulse' therapy with more intensive regimens may give better results in some patients with more advanced disease.[2] A meta-analysis of studies in adults with various types of **soft-tissue sarcoma** suggested that adjuvant chemotherapy based on doxorubicin improved recurrence-free survival.[3]

1. Crist WM, Kun LE. Common solid tumors of childhood. *N Engl J Med* 1991; **324:** 461–71.
2. Maurer HM, *et al.* The Intergroup Rhabdomyosarcoma Study-II. *Cancer* 1993; **71:** 1904–22.
3. Sarcoma Meta-analysis Collaboration. Adjuvant chemotherapy for localised resectable soft-tissue sarcoma of adults: meta-analysis of individual data. *Lancet* 1997; **350:** 1647–54.

Thrombocythaemia. Thrombocythaemia (thrombocytosis) is an increase in the platelet count to abnormally high levels, usually due to overproduction. It can result from myeloproliferative disorders including essential thrombocythaemia, polycythaemia vera (see p.495), and chronic myeloid leukaemia (see p.480), or be secondary to splenectomy, the stress of major surgery, inflammatory disease, connective tissue disorders, or malignancy.

Essential thrombocythaemia is a rare myeloproliferative disorder with predominantly proliferation of the megakaryocyte series. It occurs mainly during later life. There is often associated neutrophilia and iron deficiency anaemia secondary to the bleeding which is one of the most common symptoms. Other symptoms include thrombo-embolic disorders including neurological manifestations, and peptic ulceration. Splenomegaly may be present but repeated thromboses can reduce the size of the spleen.

The management of essential thrombocythaemia is controversial,[1-3] particularly in young or asymptomatic patients who may remain well for years without treatment. Antiplatelet agents may be useful, but specific therapy with antineoplastic agents or radioactive phosphorus-32 is usually reserved for symptomatic patients or those at high risk of developing thrombo-embolic complications. As in the treatment of polycythaemia vera, hydroxyurea is often preferred since the risk of inducing leukaemia is lower than with alkylating agents such as busulphan or radioactive phosphorus-32. Interferon alfa is an alternative, as is anagrelide,[4] an agent which is used specifically for the treatment of thrombocythaemia.

1. van Genderen PJJ, Michiels JJ. Primary thrombocythemia: diagnosis, clinical manifestations and management. *Ann Hematol* 1993; **67:** 57–62.
2. Tefferi A, Hoagland HC. Issues in the diagnosis and management of essential thrombocythemia. *Mayo Clin Proc* 1994; **69:** 651–5.
3. Harrison CN, *et al.* Desirability and problems of early diagnosis of essential thrombocythaemia. *Lancet* 1998; **351:** 846–7.
4. Anonymous. Anagrelide for essential thrombocythemia. *Med Lett Drugs Ther* 1997; **39:** 120.

Waldenström's macroglobulinaemia. Waldenström's macroglobulinaemia (primary macroglobulinaemia) is a lymphoproliferative (neoplastic) disorder in which the abnormal lymphocytes secrete an IgM protein resulting in increased plasma viscosity and abnormal platelet function. Patients are mainly elderly, and more often male. Although often asymptomatic, patients can present with weakness and fatigue, and may experience purpura, epistaxis and haemorrhage, visual disturbances and retinal haemorrhage, neurological disturbances, recurrent infections, and heart failure.

Asymptomatic patients require no treatment and may remain stable for some years. Where treatment is required it has usually been with the alkylating agent, chlorambucil. Plasmapheresis may be given to reduce plasma viscosity. When disease stabilises treatment may be discontinued and reinstituted on relapse. Combination chemotherapy with the M2 regimen (carmustine, cyclophosphamide, melphalan, prednisone, and vincristine) has been found to improve survival to about 6 to 10 years in these patients, compared with a reported 3 to 4 years with chlorambucil alone.[1] Responses have been reported to cladribine,[2] interferons,[3] and high-dose dexamethasone,[4] although the advantages of these agents over more conventional drugs have yet to be demonstrated.

1. Case DC, *et al.* Waldenström's macroglobulinemia: long-term results with the M-2 protocol. *Cancer Invest* 1991; **9:** 1–7.
2. Dimopoulos MA, *et al.* Treatment of Waldenström macroglobulinemia with 2-chlorodeoxyadenosine. *Ann Intern Med* 1993; **118:** 195–8.

3. De Rosa G, *et al.* Treatment of Waldenstrom's macroglobulinemia with interferon. *Haematologica* 1989; **74:** 313–15.
4. Jane SM, Salem HH. Treatment of resistant Waldenstrom's macroglobulinemia with high dose glucocorticosteroids. *Aust N Z J Med* 1988; **18:** 77–8.

Choice of Immunosuppressant

Amyloidosis. Amyloidosis refers to a group of conditions characterised by accumulation of a waxy proteinaceous infiltrate within body tissues. Various forms are known, including AL amyloidosis, in which the amyloid is derived from immunoglobulin light chains, ATTR amyloidosis, in which it is derived from transthyretin, and AA amyloidosis, which is most often secondary to chronic inflammation, such as that associated with rheumatoid arthritis and tuberculosis.[1] Amyloidosis may also be secondary to malignant disease. Familial Mediterranean fever (see p.394) is associated with AA amyloidosis.

Symptoms vary, depending on where the amyloid is deposited, and may include nephrotic syndrome and renal failure, peripheral neuropathy, carpal tunnel syndrome, restrictive cardiomyopathy leading to heart failure, gastro-intestinal bleeding, malabsorption, protein-losing enteropathy, polyarthritis, skin nodules, and macroglossia (due to deposition in the tongue).

Management depends to some extent upon the type of amyloidosis involved, and the site, but no agent or combination of agents is unequivocally effective. Colchicine is extremely effective at preventing renal deterioration in patients with familial Mediterranean fever,[2,3] but although benefit has been claimed in other forms of amyloidosis,[4-8] evidence is unconvincing.[1] Although the consensus is that colchicine cannot reverse established renal amyloid deposition and damage, occasional reports suggest that some reversal of nephropathy may be possible.[9,10]

AL amyloidosis is often associated with myeloma, and may respond to similar regimens, based on melphalan and prednisone (and sometimes also including colchicine),[4,6,7,11-13] even if overt myeloma is not present. Such combined regimens are more effective than colchicine alone in AL amyloidosis,[14] and survival has been reported to be slightly better in patients treated with melphalan and prednisone than in similar patients given these drugs with colchicine.[15] High-dose melphalan regimens appear to be of value.[16] Other cytotoxic immunosuppressants, such as chlorambucil, may be of benefit,[17-19] but corticosteroids do not appear to be of much value, and dimethyl sulphoxide, which has been suggested to be effective in dissolving subunit proteins, is of dubious value[19] and is unpleasant for patients to use because of its odour.

Symptomatic management is also important. Care must be taken to avoid digitalis toxicity when cardiac amyloid is present, as well as to avoid salt and water depletion through injudicious use of diuretics. The intractable diarrhoea that can occur due to autonomic neuropathy or infiltration of the gastro-intestinal tract may respond to octreotide.[20] Renal transplantation may be considered in end-stage renal failure due to amyloidosis, but unless amyloid production has been stopped disease is likely to recur in the new kidney. Cardiac transplantation, and subsequent chemotherapy with epirubicin, carmustine, and cyclophosphamide to suppress the underlying disease and control amyloid deposition in the graft has also been described.[21] Liver transplantation is the definitive therapy for patients with ATTR amyloidosis.[1]

1. Falk, RH, *et al.* The systemic amyloidoses. *N Engl J Med* 1997; **337:** 898–909.
2. Zemer D, *et al.* Colchicine in the prevention and treatment of the amyloidosis of familial Mediterranean fever. *N Engl J Med* 1986; **314:** 1001–5.
3. Majeed HA, *et al.* Long-term colchicine prophylaxis in children with familial Mediterranean fever (recurrent hereditary polyserositis). *J Pediatr* 1990; **116:** 997–9.
4. Benson MD. Treatment of AL amyloidosis with melphalan, prednisone, and colchicine. *Arthritis Rheum* 1986; **29:** 683–7.
5. Cohen AS, *et al.* Survival of patients with primary (AL) amyloidosis: colchicine-treated cases from 1976 to 1983 compared with cases seen in previous years (1961 to 1973). *Am J Med* 1987; **82:** 1182–90.
6. Fritz DA, *et al.* Unusual longevity in primary systemic amyloidosis: a 19-year survivor. *Am J Med* 1989; **86:** 245–8.
7. Schattner A, *et al.* Primary amyloidosis with unusual bone involvement: reversibility with melphalan, prednisone, and colchicine. *Am J Med* 1989; **86:** 347–8.
8. Kuwertz-Bröking E, *et al.* colchicine for secondary nephropathic amyloidosis in cystic fibrosis. *Lancet* 1995; **345:** 1178–9.
9. Zemer D, *et al.* Reversal of the nephrotic syndrome by colchicine in amyloidosis of familial Mediterranean fever. *Ann Intern Med* 1992; **116:** 426.
10. Fak AS, *et al.* Colchicine and secondary amyloidosis. *Ann Intern Med* 1992; **117:** 795–6.
11. Gertz MA, Kyle RA. Response of primary hepatic amyloidosis to melphalan and prednisone: a case report and review of the literature. *Mayo Clin Proc* 1986; **61:** 218–23.
12. Sheehan-Dare RA, Simmons AV. Amyloid myopathy and myeloma: response to treatment. *Postgrad Med J* 1987; **63:** 141–2.
13. Brown MP, Walls RS. Amyloidosis of immunoglobulin origin: useful treatment? *Med J Aust* 1990; **152:** 95–7.
14. Skinner M, *et al.* Treatment of 100 patients with primary amyloidosis: a randomized trial of melphalan, prednisone, and colchicine versus colchicine only. *Am J Med* 1996; **100:** 290–8.
15. Kyle RA, *et al.* A trial of three regimens for primary amyloidosis: colchicine alone, melphalan and prednisone, and melphalan, prednisone, and colchicine. *N Engl J Med* 1997; **336:** 1202–7.
16. Comenzo RL, *et al.* Advanced therapy for AL amyloidosis: iv melphalan with blood stem-cell rescue. *Arthritis Rheum* 1995; **38:** S402.
17. Ahlmen M, *et al.* Cytotoxic drug treatment of reactive amyloidosis in rheumatoid arthritis with special reference to renal insufficiency. *Clin Rheumatol* 1987; **6:** 27–38.
18. Berglund K, *et al.* Alkylating cytostatic treatment in renal amyloidosis secondary to rheumatic disease. *Ann Rheum Dis* 1987; **46:** 757–62.
19. David J, Woo P. Reactive amyloidosis. *Arch Dis Child* 1992; **67:** 258–61.
20. Yam LT, Oropilla SB. Octreotide for diarrhea in amyloidosis. *Ann Intern Med* 1991; **115:** 577.
21. Hall R, *et al.* Cardiac transplantation for AL amyloidosis. *Br Med J* 1994; **309:** 1135–7.

Asthma. Immunosuppressant drugs do not play a role in the regular management of asthma (p.745). In individual patients requiring oral corticosteroids for chronic severe asthma immunosuppressants have however been investigated for their anti-inflammatory and steroid-sparing properties. The results in the few patients treated with azathioprine have been disappointing,[1] but the evidence for benefit with methotrexate is more ambiguous.[2] At least one controlled study has failed to show any benefit of methotrexate compared with placebo when added to the therapy of steroid-dependent asthmatics,[3] but other studies suggest that the addition of low-dose (usually 15 mg weekly) methotrexate enables reduction of the steroid dose,[4-6] sometimes by up to half.[5] There is, however, some concern about the potential toxicity of methotrexate therapy, particularly to the liver.[7]

More recently, a controlled study in patients with chronic severe asthma requiring long-standing oral corticosteroid treatment found that addition of cyclosporin in an initial dose of 5 mg per kg body-weight daily to their regimen resulted in significant improvement in lung function and a reduced frequency of disease exacerbation, compared with placebo.[8] The results were interesting because of the improvement in what had been considered 'irreversible' airflow obstruction, but again, the potential toxicity of cyclosporin is a drawback.

1. Shiner RJ, Geddes DM. Treating patients with asthma who are dependent on systemic steroids. *Br Med J* 1989; **299:** 216–17.
2. Brown PH, *et al.* Steroid dependent asthma. *Br Med J* 1989; **299:** 682.
3. Erzurum SC, *et al.* Lack of benefit of methotrexate in severe, steroid-dependent asthma. *Ann Intern Med* 1991; **114:** 353–60.
4. Mullarkey MF, *et al.* Methotrexate in the treatment of corticosteroid-dependent asthma: a double-blind crossover study. *N Engl J Med* 1988; **318:** 603–7.
5. Shiner RJ, *et al.* Randomised, double-blind, placebo-controlled trial of methotrexate in steroid-dependent asthma. *Lancet* 1990; **336:** 137–40.
6. Mullarkey MF, *et al.* Long-term methotrexate treatment in corticosteroid-dependent asthma. *Ann Intern Med* 1990; **112:** 577–81.
7. Reid DJ, Segars LW. Methotrexate for the treatment of chronic corticosteroid-dependent asthma. *Clin Pharm* 1993; **12:** 762–7.
8. Alexander AG, *et al.* Trial of cyclosporin in corticosteroid-dependent chronic severe asthma. *Lancet* 1992; **339:** 324–8.

Blood disorders, non-malignant. For the use of immunosuppressants in aplastic anaemia, see p.701.

Diabetes mellitus. For a discussion of diabetes mellitus and its treatment, including the experimental use of immunosuppressants, see p.313. See also under Organ and Tissue Transplantation, below.

Gastro-intestinal disorders. INFLAMMATORY BOWEL DISEASES. A number of immunosuppressants have been tried in inflammatory bowel disease (p.1171), with some success, but the mainstays of drug therapy remain the aminosalicylates and the corticosteroids. Immunosuppressants may be valuable in some circumstances for their steroid-sparing effect.

Liver disorders, non-malignant. For a discussion of the role of immunosuppressants, and particularly azathioprine, in the management of chronic active hepatitis, see p.1019.

PRIMARY BILIARY CIRRHOSIS. Primary biliary cirrhosis is a chronic liver disease of unknown aetiology which develops due to progressive destruction of small and intermediate bile ducts within the liver, subsequently evolving to fibrosis and cirrhosis. Over 90% of patients are female, usually aged between 40 and 60 years. The disease is thought to be auto-immune in nature, perhaps triggered by a micro-organism in the environment, and most patients exhibit auto-antibodies to mitochondria. Development of such antibodies may be evident in patients with primary biliary cirrhosis before disease is clinically apparent.[1] Symptoms include pruritus, jaundice, hepatomegaly, hypercholesterolaemia leading to xanthoma formation, and in late disease portal hypertension, bleeding oesophageal varices and liver failure may develop. Impaired calcium and vitamin D absorption may result in osteomalacia or osteoporosis, and there may be accumulation of copper in the liver. Various other disorders including rheumatoid arthritis, scleroderma, renal tubular acidosis, thyroiditis, and Sjögren's syndrome may be associated with primary biliary cirrhosis.[2]

The disease is slowly progressive but no specific treatment is available. Symptomatic therapy includes the use of cholestyramine for pruritus; this and a low-fat diet help to control hypercholesterolaemia. Vitamin D and calcium supplementation will prevent osteomalacia; supplementation with vitamins K and A may also be necessary.

Because the disease is thought to have an auto-immune component various attempts have been made to modify the disease process, but to date none has proven unequivocally successful. Corticosteroids should not be used as they may exacerbate the bone disease.[2-4] Azathioprine was not found to be of much benefit at first,[5,6] although later results[7] did seem to show some evidence of improved survival and disease retardation. Other studies or reports have purported to show some benefit with chlorambucil,[8] cyclosporin,[9] or methotrexate,[10,11] but all of these pose problems of toxicity.

Trials of penicillamine, originally tried for its copper-binding properties, have mostly found it to be ineffective,[12-14] despite some good preliminary results,[15] and it too poses problems due to its adverse effects. Colchicine, although it may improve biochemical parameters has not convincingly demonstrated any clinical benefits.[3,4,16] However, there has recently been much interest in the potential role of ursodeoxycholic acid.[3,4,16] Several reports indicate marked symptomatic benefit,[17-19] and recent results suggest that it may improve survival.[20] However, its value and ultimate place in the treatment of primary biliary cirrhosis remain a matter of controversy;[21-24] it has been pointed out that only about 5% of patients treated with ursodeoxycholic acid alone achieve full remission,[22] and some workers consider that combination therapy using ursodeoxycholic acid with colchicine with or without methotrexate may prove more promising.[21,22,25]

In patients in whom disease progresses to liver failure the ultimate therapy is liver transplantation.[2] Disease can recur after transplantation,[16,26] but with little short-term adverse clinical effect.[16]

1. Metcalf JV, *et al.* Natural history of early primary biliary cirrhosis. *Lancet* 1996; **348:** 1399–1402.
2. Kaplan MM. Primary biliary cirrhosis. *N Engl J Med* 1996; **335:** 1570–80.
3. Bateson MC. New directions in biliary cirrhosis. *Br Med J* 1990; **301:** 1290–1.
4. Stavinoha MW, Soloway RD. Current therapy of chronic liver disease. *Drugs* 1990; **39:** 814–40.
5. Heathcote J, *et al.* A prospective controlled trial of azathioprine in primary biliary cirrhosis. *Gastroenterology* 1976; **70:** 656–60.
6. Crowe J, *et al.* Azathioprine in primary biliary cirrhosis: a preliminary report of an international trial. *Gastroenterology* 1980: **78:** 1005–10.
7. Christensen E, *et al.* Beneficial effect of azathioprine and prediction of prognosis in primary biliary cirrhosis: final results of an international trial. *Gastroenterology* 1985; **89:** 1084–91.
8. Hoofnagle JH, *et al.* Randomized trial of chlorambucil for primary biliary cirrhosis. *Gastroenterology* 1986; **91:** 1327–34.
9. Lombard M, *et al.* Cyclosporin A treatment in primary biliary cirrhosis: results of a long-term placebo controlled trial. *Gastroenterology* 1993; **104:** 519–26.
10. Kaplan MM, *et al.* Primary biliary cirrhosis treated with low-dose oral pulse methotrexate. *Ann Intern Med* 1988; **109:** 429–31.

11. Kaplan MM, *et al.* Sustained biochemical and histologic remission of primary biliary cirrhosis in response to medical treatment. *Ann Intern Med* 1997; **126:** 682–8.
12. Matloff DS, *et al.* A prospective trial of D-penicillamine in primary biliary cirrhosis. *N Engl J Med* 1982; **306:** 319–26.
13. Dickson ER, *et al.* Trial of penicillamine in advanced primary biliary cirrhosis. *N Engl J Med* 1985; **312:** 1011–15.
14. Neuberger J, *et al.* Double blind controlled trial of D-penicillamine in patients with primary biliary cirrhosis. *Gut* 1985; **26:** 114–19.
15. Epstein O, *et al.* D-Penicillamine treatment improves survival in primary biliary cirrhosis. *Lancet* 1981; **i:** 1275–7.
16. Neuberger J. Primary biliary cirrhosis. *Lancet* 1997; **350:** 875–9.
17. Poupon RE, *et al.* A multicenter controlled trial of ursodiol for the treatment of primary biliary cirrhosis. *N Engl J Med* 1991; **324:** 1548–54.
18. Battezzati PM, *et al.* Ursodeoxycholic acid for symptomatic primary biliary cirrhosis: preliminary analysis of a double-blind multicenter trial. *J Hepatol* 1993; **17:** 332–8.
19. Lindor KD, *et al.* Ursodeoxycholic acid delays the onset of esophageal varices in primary biliary cirrhosis. *Mayo Clin Proc* 1997; **72:** 1137–40.
20. Poupon RE, *et al.* Ursodiol for the long-term treatment of primary biliary cirrhosis. *N Engl J Med* 1994; **330:** 1342–7.
21. Kaplan MM. Primary biliary cirrhosis—a first step in prolonging survival. *N Engl J Med* 1994; **330:** 1386–7.
22. Goddard CJR, Warnes TW. Primary biliary cirrhosis: how should we evaluate new treatments? *Lancet* 1994; **343:** 1305–6.
23. Bateson MC. Evaluation of new treatment for primary biliary cirrhosis. *Lancet* 1994; **344:** 61.
24. Lim AG, Northfield TC. Ursodeoxycholic acid and primary biliary cirrhosis. *Br Med J* 1994; **309:** 491–2.
25. Ikeda T, *et al.* Effects of additional administration of colchicine in ursodeoxycholic acid-treated patients with primary biliary cirrhosis: a prospective randomized study. *J Hepatol* 1996; **24:** 88–94.
26. Anonymous. Is PBC cured by liver transplantation? *Lancet* 1991; **337:** 272–3.

Lung disorders, non-malignant. INTERSTITIAL LUNG DISEASE. Corticosteroids are the mainstay of treatment for interstitial lung disease (p.1024) but azathioprine or cyclophosphamide have occasionally proved useful steroid-sparing agents in patients with cryptogenic fibrosing alveolitis.

Neurological disorders. MULTIPLE SCLEROSIS. Immunosuppressants have been tried in the treatment of multiple sclerosis (p.620), although in some studies the benefit obtained may have been outweighed by toxicity.

MYASTHENIA GRAVIS. Patients with myasthenia gravis (p.1388) who require immunosuppression are usually treated with corticosteroids. Azathioprine is used mainly in myasthenia gravis for its corticosteroid-sparing effect but may also be of use when corticosteroids are contra-indicated or when response to corticosteroids alone is insufficient. Other immunosuppressants which have been tried similarly include cyclosporin, cyclophosphamide, and methotrexate.

Ocular disorders, non-malignant. Immunosuppressive agents have been used with some success in a variety of ocular disorders with inflammatory or immunological components. In *scleritis* and *uveitis* (see p.1029 and p.1030) necessitating treatment corticosteroids, given topically, intra-ocularly, or systemically are usually the first line of treatment, but in unresponsive disease, or in patients with unacceptable side-effects at the required dose of corticosteroids, immunosuppressants such as azathioprine, chlorambucil, cyclophosphamide, or methotrexate, may be given.[1,2] These agents are particularly valuable in the management of the ocular lesions of *Behçet's disease*, *rheumatoid arthritis*, or *Wegener's granulomatosis*,[2] (see p.1018, p.2, and p.1031, respectively). Cyclosporin is also of value in both scleritis[1] and uveitis,[2,3] and has proved useful as an alternative to cyclophosphamide or azathioprine when combined with corticosteroids in the management of both ocular and vascular symptoms of *Cogan's syndrome*[4] (p.1020). However, nephrotoxicity remains a potential problem with systemic cyclosporin,[3] and in this respect a report of response in refractory corneal ulcers secondary to rheumatic disease, oculomucocutaneous syndrome, or *Sjögren's syndrome* following treatment with 2% cyclosporin eye drops is of interest.[5]

In *Graves' ophthalmopathy,* (p.1489), immunosuppressants have been tried with equivocal results; benefit has however been reported from the use of cyclosporin with prednisone.[6,7]

1. Wakefield D, McCluskey P. Cyclosporin therapy for severe scleritis. *Br J Ophthalmol* 1989; **73:** 743–6.
2. Herman DC. Endogenous uveitis: current concepts of treatment. *Mayo Clin Proc* 1990; **65:** 671–83.
3. de Vries J, *et al.* Cyclosporin in the treatment of severe chronic idiopathic uveitis. *Br J Ophthalmol* 1990; **74:** 344–9.
4. Allen NB, *et al.* Use of immunosuppressive agents in the treatment of severe ocular and vascular manifestations of Cogan's syndrome. *Am J Med* 1990; **88:** 296–301.
5. Zierhut M, *et al.* Topical treatment of severe corneal ulcers with cyclosporin A. *Graefes Arch Clin Exp Ophthalmol* 1989; **227:** 30–5.
6. Kahaly G, *et al.* Ciclosporin and prednisone v prednisone in treatment of Graves' ophthalmopathy: a controlled, randomized and prospective study. *Eur J Clin Invest* 1986; **16:** 415–22.
7. Prummel MF, *et al.* Prednisone and cyclosporine in the treatment of severe Graves' ophthalmopathy. *N Engl J Med* 1989; **321:** 1353–9.

Organ and tissue transplantation. Although surgical techniques suitable for the removal of organs and tissues from a donor, and their engraftment into a host, have existed for many years, such grafts would not normally survive for long. The host's immune system recognises the donor cells as 'nonself' or immunologically foreign and attacks them, producing rejection. Such recognition involves proteins encoded by the major histocompatibility complex of the genes, together with a variety of other antigens, which are known collectively as the human leucocyte antigens or HLA. Macrophages take up and process these antigens, permitting T cells to become activated and resulting in the production of antibodies and cytotoxic lymphocytes which attack the graft. Only from the 1960s with the development of agents capable of attenuating or suppressing this response, did transplantation start to become a feasible mode of treatment.

The agents available vary in their mechanisms of action, and are often combined for optimum effect. The glucocorticoids act at several points in the immune cascade, including antigen recognition and production of lymphokines. Cyclosporin and newer polypeptide immunosuppressants such as tacrolimus prevent formation of cytotoxic T cells by inhibiting release of interleukin-2 from helper T cells, while polyclonal or monoclonal antilymphocyte antibodies such as antilymphocyte immunoglobulin and muromonab CD3 bind to and deplete T cell populations. Cytotoxic immunosuppressants such as azathioprine, methotrexate, or cyclophosphamide act by preventing cell division, and thus proliferation, of lymphocytes.

Immunosuppressant regimens may be divided into those aimed at prevention of rejection in the early period after transplantation; long-term maintenance prophylaxis; and treatment of acute episodes of rejection. In bone marrow transplantation, where an immunologically competent tissue is transplanted it is the donor cells which attack host tissues (graft versus host disease), and immunosuppression is required for prophylaxis of this condition.

Because of the critical nature of the early stage, when the organ or tissue must recover normal function, and perhaps to permit better long-term tolerance, initial immunosuppressant regimens tend to be intensive. Cyclosporin is the mainstay of most modern regimens, but combinations of three or four agents (triple or quadruple therapy) are common.

Since immunosuppressant therapy must in most cases be given for the lifetime of the graft, in long-term maintenance the toxicity of the drugs used, and the risks of infection and neoplasia, must be considered. Doses and numbers of agents used tend to be reduced, and in particular there is a tendency to taper or sometimes even eliminate the doses of corticosteroids used in maintenance regimens because of the potential sequelae of prolonged corticosteroid use.

The use of less intensive maintenance regimens must be balanced against the risk of an acute rejection episode, and the likelihood of its responding to therapy. High-dose corticosteroids and polyclonal or monoclonal antilymphocyte antibodies often play a role in the rescue therapy of patients with acute rejection episodes, although much depends upon the severity of the reaction, and whether such episodes have occurred previously.

The management of immunosuppression for the transplantation of particular organs is discussed in more detail below. With the use of suitable immunosuppressant regimens long-term graft survival can be obtained following transplantation of heart, kidney or liver; the transplantation of other organs such as bowel, lung, or pancreas remains more experimental. Ultimately, however, the complications of chronic rejection are likely to lead to loss of the graft: the induction of specific tolerance to the donor organ remains the goal of much research. In allogeneic bone marrow transplantation, where the aim of immunosuppression is prevention of graft versus host disease rather than rejection, immunosuppressant therapy can often be tapered off and eventually withdrawn.

Much recent interest has been aroused by the possibility of organ transplants from *animals*, genetically modified to reduce complement-mediated hyperacute rejection. It is not clear whether such xenotransplantation will require modified immunosuppressive regimens.

BONE MARROW. Bone-marrow transplantation (BMT) is used in the treatment of a variety of malignancies, notably in the acute leukaemias and lymphomas; to permit the use of very high-dose chemotherapy in the management of some solid tumours (bone marrow rescue); and to treat some other serious disorders affecting the bone marrow, such as aplastic anaemia and the haemoglobinopathies. Two types of bone-marrow transplant are in use: in one the patient's own bone marrow is harvested and subsequently re-infused after treatment (autologous BMT), while in the other the marrow is harvested from a donor (usually a sibling) whose HLA antigens are as closely matched as possible to those of the recipient (allogeneic BMT). In recent years, however, a third procedure involving collection of haematopoietic stem cells from peripheral blood (mobilised from bone marrow during recovery from chemotherapy, or by treatment with colony-stimulating factors, or both) has come to be preferred.

With autologous transplants problems of compatibility do not arise, but if abnormal cell clones are present in the marrow (as in leukaemia) they may be transferred back into the patient and cause disease relapse. Contamination is less of a problem with peripheral blood stem cells.[1] Allogeneic bone-marrow transplants require immunosuppression but it can usually be withdrawn after 6 to 12 months.[2-5] The need is for suppression of graft-versus-host disease (see below), in which the donor immune system attacks host cells, until a new immunological balance is achieved.

The patient is normally prepared by total body irradiation, or myeloablative chemotherapy with agents such as cyclophosphamide or busulphan, or more often both, in order to destroy host bone marrow cells. Bone marrow is aspirated from the donor, and infused into the recipient via an indwelling catheter or directly into a peripheral vein. Peripheral blood stem cells are collected by cell separation after mobilisation. Engraftment[5,6] and survival[7] after peripheral blood stem cell transplants may be superior to those seen with conventional autologous grafts. Another potential source of allogeneic stem cells for transplantation are those collected from placental or cord blood.[8-10]

Once bone-marrow transplantation has taken place treatment with colony-stimulating factors can speed engraftment and functional recovery and thus reduce infection and the length of hospitalisation;[2,4] such therapy should be given to all patients who do not engraft within 21 to 28 days.[4] The role of colony-stimulating factors after stem cell transplantation is less clear. Prophylactic cover with antimicrobials and normal immunoglobulins is recommended to prevent infection.[4] Ursodeoxycholic acid has been investigated for the prophylaxis of hepatic complications.[25]

In addition to such supportive care, patients who have received allogeneic transplants require immunosuppressive therapy aimed at the prevention of **graft-versus-host disease** (GVHD). GVHD is usually characterised as acute or chronic depending on the manifestations, and the time of presentation (by convention acute disease occurs within a hundred days of transplantation, and chronic disease after this time, although in practice there is considerable overlap). The organ systems primarily affected are skin, liver, and gastro-intestinal tract. Both forms are marked by maculopapular rashes, which in severe disease may progress to bullous lesions and epidermal necrolysis. Liver disease may include cholestatic jaundice (usually in the acute form) and hepatitis; symptoms may need to be distinguished from the veno-occlusive disease which sometimes complicates bone-marrow transplantation and is due to the pre-transplant conditioning regimen (the latter may respond to treatment with antithrombin III[11]). The primary symptom of gastro-intestinal GVHD is diarrhoea, often severe and painful. In patients with chronic GVHD other manifestations may include arthritis, mucositis, lung disease, and scleroderma.

Various agents have been used for the prophylaxis of graft-versus-host disease following allogeneic bone-marrow transplantation, but most modern regimens are based on cyclosporin.[2-4] Although GVHD still occurs in many cyclosporin-treated patients, morbidity is much reduced and survival improved. Combined prophylaxis using a short course of methotrexate plus cyclosporin given for 6 months after transplant has been shown to be more effective than either drug alone in preventing acute GVHD,[12,13] and is currently in wide use in many centres, but even with this regimen the incidence of acute graft-versus-host disease may be some 20 to 30%. A significantly lower incidence (roughly 10%) has been reported in patients treated with a combination of cyclosporin, methotrexate, and a corticosteroid.[14] However, a degree of acute graft-versus-host disease may be desirable in some bone-marrow transplants, since it can result in a 'graft-versus-leukaemia' effect which reduces leukaemic relapse.[2] Thus, too effective an immunosuppressant regimen may not always be desirable, and leukaemic patients given bone-marrow transplants purged of T cells, which virtually abolishes GVHD, do not have a better survival rate than those given conventional prophylaxis (engraftment too is reduced in the absence of all T cells).

Other agents which have been tried in the prophylaxis of GVHD include antithymocyte immunoglobulin, tacrolimus, and experimental agents such as anti-interleukin-2-receptor antibodies[15] or zolimomab aritox (anti-CD5 murine monoclonal antibody conjugated with ricin A chain).[4] Normal immunoglobulin, which has been recommended for the prophylaxis of cytomegalovirus infection in at-risk recipients,[4] may also reduce the incidence of GVHD,[16,17] although its use for this purpose is not widely accepted.[3] However, initial results suggesting possible benefits from oxpentifylline[18] do not seem to have been borne out by subsequent study.[19]

The main aim of therapy has been the prevention of graft-versus-host disease, and the success rate in treating the established condition has not been high.[3,4]

Corticosteroids form the basis of most treatment regimens for acute disease,[2-4] usually given in fairly high doses initially (methylprednisolone 2 to 2.5 mg per kg body-weight daily by intravenous infusion is a common regimen), and gradually tapered off. Some centres prefer to use lower doses in limited cutaneous disease and reserve higher doses for patients with systemic or severe cutaneous disease.[3,4] There is no evidence that combination with other agents improves the efficacy of corticosteroid therapy, and survival is very poor in patients who fail to respond to it.[3] Second-line agents include all of those used in prophylaxis (see above): the most commonly used salvage drug is antithymocyte immunoglobulin. Some studies have reported benefit from the use of monoclonal antibodies (such as CBL-1[20] or triple therapy with antibodies to tumour necrosis factor and CD2 plus inolimomab[21]) in established steroid-resistant GVHD. Patients with chronic,[22] and perhaps acute,[3] GVHD may respond to thalidomide; teratogenicity is unlikely to be a problem as conditioning radiotherapy results in sterility.[2] Extracorporeal phototherapy with methoxsalen and UVA has been used to treat chronic GVHD.[23] A pilot study has indicated that octreotide may be useful in some patients with gastrointestinal GVHD to control diarrhoea.[24]

1. Nemunaitis J. A comparative review of colony-stimulating factors. *Drugs* 1997; **54:** 709–29.
2. Boughton B. Bone-marrow transplantation. *Prescribers' J* 1991; **31:** 77–88.
3. Vogelsang GB, Morris LE. Prevention and management of graft-versus-host disease: practical recommendations. *Drugs* 1993; **45:** 668–76.
4. Rowe JM, *et al.* Recommended guidelines for the management of autologous and allogeneic bone marrow transplantation: a report from the Eastern Cooperative Oncology Group (ECOG). *Ann Intern Med* 1994; **120:** 143–58.
5. Duncombe A. Bone marrow and stem cell transplantation. *Br Med J* 1997; **314:** 1179–82.
6. Schmitz N, *et al.* Randomized trial of filgrastim-mobilised peripheral blood progenitor cell transplantation versus autologous bone-marrow transplantation in lymphoma patients. *Lancet* 1996; **347:** 353–7.
7. Armitage JO. Bone marrow transplantation. *N Engl J Med* 1994; **330:** 827–38.
8. Kurtzberg J, *et al.* Placental blood as a source of hematopoietic stem cells for transplantation into unrelated recipients. *N Engl J Med* 1996; **335:** 157–66.
9. Laporte J-P, *et al.* Cord-blood transplantation from an unrelated donor in an adult with chronic myelogenous leukemia. *N Engl J Med* 1996; **335:** 167–70.
10. Gluckman E, *et al.* Outcome of cord-blood transplantation from related and unrelated donors. *N Engl J Med* 1997; **337:** 373–81.
11. Morris JD, *et al.* Antithrombin-III for the treatment of chemotherapy-induced organ dysfunction following bone marrow transplantation. *Bone Marrow Transplant* 1997; **20:** 871–8.
12. Storb R, *et al.* Methotrexate and cyclosporine compared with cyclosporine alone for prophylaxis of acute graft versus host disease after marrow transplantation for leukemia. *N Engl J Med* 1986; **314:** 729–35.
13. Storb R, *et al.* Marrow transplantation for severe aplastic anemia: methotrexate alone compared with a combination of methotrexate and cyclosporine for prevention of acute graft-versus-host disease. *Blood* 1986; **68:** 119–25.
14. Chao NJ, *et al.* Cyclosporine, methotrexate, and prednisone compared with cyclosporine and prednisone for prophylaxis of acute graft-versus-host disease. *N Engl J Med* 1993; **329:** 1225–30.
15. Blaise D, *et al.* Prevention of acute graft-versus-host disease by monoclonal antibody to interleukin-2 receptors. *Lancet* 1989; **i:** 1333–4.
16. Winston DJ, *et al.* Intravenous immune globulin for prevention of cytomegalovirus infection and interstitial pneumonia after bone marrow transplantation. *Ann Intern Med* 1987; **106:** 12–18.
17. Sullivan KM, *et al.* Immunomodulatory and antimicrobial efficacy of intravenous immunoglobulin in bone marrow transplantation. *N Engl J Med* 1990; **323:** 705–12.
18. Bianco JA, *et al.* Phase I-II trial of pentoxifylline for the prevention of transplant-related toxicities following bone marrow transplantation. *Blood* 1991; **78:** 1205–11.
19. Clift RA, *et al.* A randomized controlled trial of pentoxifylline for the prevention of regimen-related toxicities in patients undergoing allogeneic marrow transplantation. *Blood* 1993; **82:** 2025–30.
20. Heslop HE, *et al.* Response of steroid-resistant graft-versus-host disease to lymphoblast antibody CBL1. *Lancet* 1995; **346:** 805–6.
21. Racadot E, *et al.* Sequential use of three monoclonal antibodies in corticosteroid-resistant acute GVHD: a multicentre pilot study including 15 patients. *Bone Marrow Transplant* 1995; **15:** 669–77.
22. Vogelsang GB, *et al.* Thalidomide for the treatment of chronic graft-versus-host disease. *N Engl J Med* 1992; **326:** 1055–8.
23. Konstantinow A, *et al.* Chronic graft-versus-host disease: successful treatment with extracorporeal photochemotherapy: a follow-up. *Br J Dermatol* 1996; **135:** 1007–8.
24. Ely P, *et al.* Use of a somatostatin analogue, octreotide acetate, in the management of acute gastrointestinal graft-versus-host disease. *Am J Med* 1991; **90:** 707–10.
25. Essell JH, *et al.* Ursodiol prophylaxis against hepatic complications of allogeneic bone marrow transplantation: a randomized, double-blind, placebo-controlled trial. *Ann Intern Med* 1998; **128:** 975–81.

HEART. Marked improvements have been seen in outcome following heart transplantation since the introduction of cyclosporin, which has resulted in a reduced incidence and severity of rejection episodes.[1-3] Formerly an experimental procedure with limited success, heart transplantation has now become an acceptable therapy of last resort in patients crippled by heart disease, and is now limited more by a lack of suitable donor organs than by doubts as to its value.[4]

Unlike renal transplantation, where haemodialysis exists as a backup therapy if graft rejection occurs, rejection of a heart graft is likely to mean death, and in consequence fairly intensive immunosuppressant therapy is the rule.[4] A typical regimen might include preoperative doses of cyclosporin and azathioprine, methylprednisolone and muromonab-CD3 during the operation, and treatment with corticosteroids, cyclosporin, azathioprine, and a short course of antithymocyte immunoglobulin or muromonab-CD3 in the immediate post-operative period.[3-5] Substituting cyclophosphamide for azathioprine for 6 weeks after transplantation is reported to reduce the development of anti-muromonab-CD3 antibodies in such a regimen.[6] Triple therapy with cyclosporin, azathioprine, and prednisone is then used for long-term maintenance, and has been shown to produce an actuarial survival at 5 years of 78%.[7] Reportedly 90% of transplanted patients are able to resume an active life.[2] Infection may be a problem in such heavily immunosuppressed patients, however, and cytomegalovirus infection is a particular problem, possibly increasing the risk of graft rejection and atherosclerosis.[8] Apart from the use of agents such as ganciclovir and cytomegalovirus immunoglobulins to control cytomegalovirus, some centres have attempted to reduce morbidity by a gradual tapering of the corticosteroid maintenance dose, with the possibility of withdrawal in selected patients.[3,5] It has been suggested that the high doses of corticosteroids employed increase the risk of cardiac adverse events in the longer term.[9] Patients may also receive diltiazem[10] or lipid lowering drugs such as pravastatin[11] or simvastatin[12] in an attempt to reduce the development of coronary artery disease in the graft, which is the major threat to long-term survival.[13] Routine therapy with lipid lowering drugs appears to improve survival compared with diet alone.[12]

Rescue or salvage therapy is required if acute rejection episodes develop despite maintenance immunosuppression. Although the exact regimen will depend upon the severity of the reaction, how often previous episodes have occurred, and how long after transplantation, moderate to severe episodes may be treated with fairly high doses of oral prednisone or intravenous methylprednisolone; muromonab-CD3, or antilymphocyte immunoglobulin if antibodies to the former are present, may be added if deterioration continues. When necessary, total lymphoid irradiation may be given.[3] Newer agents such as mycophenolate mofetil,[14] tacrolimus[15] and inolimomab[16] (an anti-interleukin-2-receptor antibody) have also been reported to be of benefit in some cases.

Improved surgical techniques and the use of cyclosporin have also made possible successful combined heart-lung transplants,[17,18] although these may require enhanced immunosuppression to prevent obliterative bronchiolitis,[19] a possible manifestation of chronic rejection.

1. Austen WG, Cosimi AB. Heart transplantation after 16 years. *N Engl J Med* 1984; **311:** 1436–8.
2. Keown PA. Emerging indications for the use of cyclosporin in organ transplantation and autoimmunity. *Drugs* 1990; **40:** 315–25.
3. McGoon MD, Frantz RP. Techniques of immunosuppression after cardiac transplantation. *Mayo Clin Proc* 1992; **67:** 586–95.
4. Wreghitt T. Cytomegalovirus infections in heart and heart-lung transplant recipients. *J Antimicrob Chemother* 1989; **23** (suppl E): 49–60.
5. Gay WA, *et al.* OKT3 monoclonal antibody in cardiac transplantation. *Ann Surg* 1988; **208:** 287–90.
6. Taylor DO, *et al.* A prospective, randomized comparison of cyclophosphamide and azathioprine for early rejection prophylaxis after cardiac transplantation: decreased sensitization to OKT3. *Transplantation* 1994; **58:** 645–9.
7. Olivari M-T, *et al.* Five-year experience with triple-drug immunosuppressive therapy in cardiac transplantation. *Circulation* 1990; **82** (suppl IV): 276–80.
8. Grattan MT, *et al.* Cytomegalovirus infection is associated with cardiac allograft rejection and atherosclerosis. *JAMA* 1989; **261:** 3561–6.
9. Mehra MR, *et al.* The prognostic impact of immunosuppression and cellular rejection on cardiac allograft vasculopathy: time for a reappraisal. *J Heart Lung Transplant* 1997; **16:** 743–51.
10. Schroeder JS, *et al.* A preliminary study of diltiazem in the prevention of coronary artery disease in heart-transplant recipients. *N Engl J Med* 1993; **328:** 164–70.
11. Kobashigawa JA, *et al.* Effect of pravastatin on outcomes after cardiac transplantation. *N Engl J Med* 1995; **333:** 621–7.
12. Wenke K, *et al.* Simvastatin reduces graft vessel disease and mortality after heart transplantation: a four-year randomized trial. *Circulation* 1997; **96:** 1398–1402.
13. Keogh AM. Coronary artery disease in cardiac transplant recipients. *Med J Aust* 1995; **163:** 212–14.
14. Kirklin JK, *et al.* Treatment of recurrent heart rejection with mycophenolate mofetil (RS-61443): initial clinical experience. *J Heart Lung Transplant* 1994; **13:** 444–50.
15. Swenson JM, *et al.* Immunosuppression switch in pediatric heart transplant recipients: cyclosporine to FK506. *J Am Coll Cardiol* 1995; **25:** 1183–8.
16. Iberer F, *et al.* Clinical experience with a monoclonal interleukin-2 receptor antibody (BT563) for rejection therapy after orthotopic heart transplantation. *Transplant Proc* 1994; **26:** 3237–9.
17. Scott J, *et al.* Heart-lung transplantation for cystic fibrosis. *Lancet* 1988; **ii:** 192–4.
18. Smyth RL, *et al.* Early experience of heart-lung transplantation. *Arch Dis Child* 1989; **64:** 1225–30.
19. Glanville AR, *et al.* Obliterative bronchiolitis after heart-lung transplantation: apparent arrest by augmented immunosuppression. *Ann Intern Med* 1987; **107:** 300–4.

KIDNEY. The transplantation of kidneys is now established as the ultimate therapy for end-stage renal disease. Although good results can be achieved with regimens based on azathioprine and a corticosteroid,[1] regimens based on cyclosporin are now widely used as first-choice immunosuppression, in the light of studies which suggested cyclosporin was superior to previous regimens in terms of graft and patient survival.[2-5] However, not all studies found cyclosporin to be significantly better,[6-8] and potential problems arise from the nephrotoxicity of cyclosporin, which may impair graft function in ways difficult to distinguish from rejection of the kidney.

As a result, there is no single generally accepted immunosuppressant regimen, and different centres have achieved good results with a variety of strategies.[9-12] Some have suggested **initial therapy** should be with azathioprine and corticosteroids, with judicious use of cyclosporin in those intolerant of such a regimen or with a history of rejection.[1] Such an approach may be appropriate where the graft is from an HLA-identical sibling, rather than a matched cadaver.[9] An alternative is the initial use of a cyclosporin regimen, often for 3 months, followed by conversion to immunosuppression with azathioprine and a corticosteroid,[13-17] which may produce better graft function than continuing cyclosporin,[15,17] without necessarily producing many more rejection episodes.[14] However, the experience of other centres[18] has suggested that continuing cy closporin, but perhaps omitting corticosteroids,[19] gives better results. Low-dose cyclosporin maintenance has also been investigated.[20] Mycophenolate mofetil has been suggested as an alternative to azathioprine in maintenance regimens.[21]

Another strategy, and one which has found favour in many institutions,[10,11] is the combination of low doses of cyclosporin, azathioprine, and prednisolone, known as triple therapy. Triple therapy is popular because it allows lower doses of nephrotoxic cyclosporin, and the eventual tapering or even elimination of corticosteroids in some patients.[9]

Triple therapy has been further extended in some centres by the addition of an initial short course of antilymphocyte or antithymocyte immunoglobulin or muromonab-CD3 (quadruple or sequential therapy).[9,10,12,22] However, such strongly immunosuppressive regimens may increase the risk of cytomegalovirus and other infections and some centres have reverted to the use of triple therapy.[22] There is some evidence that the incidence of complications is lower with antilymphocyte immunoglobulin than with muromonab-CD3.[23] The more specific anti-interleukin-2-receptor antibodies basiliximab,[24] daclizumab,[25] and inolimomab[26] have also been added to initial therapy and appear to reduce the incidence of rejection episodes without increased toxicity.

As immunosuppressant regimens have developed the role of corticosteroids has come to be questioned, mainly because of the adverse effects associated with their prolonged use.[27] Studies indicate that corticosteroid withdrawal is feasible in many patients initially receiving triple therapy,[19,28,29] although there is debate about the long-term consequences of this for graft survival.[27] Some centres go further and avoid the use of corticosteroids at all stages, preferring cyclosporin-based regimens supplemented with agents such as antithymocyte immunoglobulins or muromonab-CD3, and mycophenolate mofetil.[30] It is unclear which approach gives the best results, and whether all patients would benefit or only selected groups.

Where a **rejection** episode occurs treatment is likely to be with high-dose corticosteroids, or with agents such as antilymphocyte or antithymocyte immunoglobulins, or muromonab-CD3, which are potent and effective reversers of rejection.[9-11] Many centres prefer to reserve the antibody preparations for corticosteroid-resistant rejection.[9] Cyclosporin and azathioprine are ineffective in treating established rejection.[10] Anti-interleukin-2-receptor antibodies may be of potential benefit in reversing rejection episodes. Other agents such as tacrolimus,[31] mycophenolate mofetil,[32,33] and gusperimus,[34] have been found to be effective in reversing acute rejection episodes. There has also been evidence that asymptomatic cytomegalovirus infection may be associated with episodes of late acute rejection;[35] ganciclovir is reported to improve graft function in such circumstances. Unfortunately there is little that can be done about chronic rejection, which eventually progresses to graft failure,[11] although there is a suggestion that mycophenolate mofetil can delay this process.[36]

The results that can be achieved with existing regimens are good in the short to medium term, with a three-year **graft survival** of the order of 70 to 80%,[5,8] and a 5-year survival (using triple therapy) of about 67%.[11] However, in the longer term most grafts are eventually claimed by rejection; by 10 years, survival of first cadaveric grafts is down to about 40%, although better results are seen with grafts from siblings.[9] There is some evidence that regimens which incorporate antilymphocyte immunoglobulins into initial therapy result in better graft survival than those which do not.[40] Present regimens can clearly not be considered ideal, and studies are continuing with newer agents, such as tacrolimus, which has been reported to produce good initial results in kidney transplantation,[37] and to be an effective salvage therapy.[31] A variety of agents not conventionally regarded as immunosuppressants have also been added to conventional regimens in an attempt to increase their efficacy or reduce their toxicity. Such agents include allopurinol and prostaglandins, or the use of calcium-channel [b]ockers or fish oil[38] to reduce cyclosporin toxicity.

[As ment]ioned on p.470 the use of immunosuppressants [is ass]ociated with malignancies. As renal transplant patients are surviving for longer the risk of neoplasms developing grows.[39]

1. McGeown MG, *et al.* Ten-year results of renal transplantation with azathioprine and prednisolone as only immunosuppression. *Lancet* 1988; **i:** 983–5. Correction. *ibid.*; 1120.
2. European Multicentre Trial Group. Cyclosporin in cadaveric renal transplantation: one year follow-up of a multicentre trial. *Lancet* 1983; **ii:** 986–9.
3. Calne RY. Cyclosporin in cadaveric renal transplantation: 5-year follow-up of a multicentre trial. *Lancet* 1987; **ii:** 506–7.
4. Canadian Multicentre Transplant Study Group. A randomized clinical trial of cyclosporine in cadaveric renal transplantation. *N Engl J Med* 1983; **309:** 809–15.
5. Canadian Multicentre Transplant Study Group. A randomized clinical trial of cyclosporine in cadaveric renal transplantation: analysis at three years. *N Engl J Med* 1986; **314:** 1219–25. Correction. *ibid.*; 1652.
6. Hall BM, *et al.* Treatment of renal transplantation rejection: cyclosporin A versus conventional treatment with azathioprine, prednisone and antithymocyte immunoglobulin in primary cadaveric renal transplantation. *Med J Aust* 1985; **142:** 179–85.
7. Merion RM, *et al.* Cyclosporine: five years' experience in cadaveric renal transplantation. *N Engl J Med* 1984; **310:** 148–54.
8. Notghi A, *et al.* A comparison of cyclosporin versus azathioprine treatment in renal transplants in Edinburgh. *Scott Med J* 1989; **34:** 459–62.
9. Barry JM. Immunosuppressive drugs in renal transplantation: a review of the regimens. *Drugs* 1992; **44:** 554–66.
10. Bunn RJ. Immunosuppression after kidney transplantation. *Pharm J* 1990; **244:** 538–41.
11. Collier St J, Calne R. Practical problems in immunosuppression: kidney and liver transplants. *Prescribers' J* 1991; **31:** 122–7.
12. Suthanthiran M, Strom TB. Renal transplantation. *N Engl J Med* 1994; **331:** 365–75.
13. Hoitsma AJ, *et al.* Cyclosporin treatment with conversion after three months versus conventional immunosuppression in renal allograft recipients. *Lancet* 1987; **i:** 584–6.
14. Morris PJ, *et al.* Cyclosporin conversion versus conventional immunosuppression: long-term follow-up and histological evaluation. *Lancet* 1987; **i:** 586–91.
15. Hall BM, *et al.* Comparison of three immunosuppressive regimens in cadaver renal transplantation: long-term cyclosporine, short-term cyclosporine followed by azathioprine and prednisolone, and azathioprine and prednisolone without cyclosporine. *N Engl J Med* 1988; **318:** 1499–1507.
16. Adu D, *et al.* Conversion from cyclosporin to azathioprine/prednisolone. *Lancet* 1985; **i:** 392.
17. Hollander AAMJ, *et al.* Beneficial effects of conversion from cyclosporin to azathioprine after kidney transplantation. *Lancet* 1995; **345:** 610–14.
18. Opelz G. Conversion from cyclosporin to azathioprine after kidney transplantation. *Lancet* 1995; **345:** 1504.
19. Opelz G. Effect of the maintenance immunosuppressive drug regimen on kidney transplant outcome. *Transplantation* 1994; **58:** 443–6.
20. Dantal J, *et al.* Effect of long-term immunosuppression in kidney-graft recipients on cancer incidence: randomised comparison of two cyclosporin regimens. *Lancet* 1998; **351:** 623–8.
21. Sollinger HW, *et al.* Mycophenolate mofetil for the prevention of acute rejection in primary cadaveric renal allograft recipients. *Transplantation* 1995; **60:** 225–32.
22. Verran D, *et al.* Quadruple immunosuppression in renal allografts—the Auckland experience. *N Z Med J* 1991; **104:** 517–18.
23. Bock HA, *et al.* A randomized prospective trial of prophylactic immunosuppression with ATG-Fresenius versus OKT3 after renal transplantation. *Transplantation* 1995; **59:** 830–40.
24. Nashan B, *et al.* Randomised trial of basiliximab versus placebo for control of acute cellular rejection in renal allograft recipients. *Lancet* 1997; **350:** 1193–8. Correction. *ibid.*; 1484.
25. Vincenti F, *et al.* Interleukin-2-receptor blockade with daclizumab to prevent acute rejection in renal transplantation. *N Engl J Med* 1998; **338:** 161–5.
26. Van Gelder T, *et al.* A double-blind, placebo-controlled study of monoclonal anti-interleukin-2 receptor antibody (BT563) administration to prevent acute rejection after kidney transplantation. *Transplantation* 1995; **60:** 248–52.
27. Tarantino A, *et al.* Corticosteroids in kidney transplant recipients: safety issues and timing of discontinuation. *Drug Safety* 1995; **13:** 145–56.
28. Opelz G, *et al.* Influence of treatment with cyclosporine, azathioprine and steroids on chronic allograft failure. *Kidney Int* 1995; **48** (suppl 52): S89–S92.
29. Ratcliffe PJ, *et al.* Randomised controlled trial of steroid withdrawal in renal transplant recipients receiving triple immunosuppression. *Lancet* 1996; **348:** 643–8.
30. Birkeland SA. Steroid-free immunosuppression in renal transplantation. *Lancet* 1996; **348:** 1105–6.
31. Jordan ML, *et al.* Tacrolimus rescue therapy for renal allograft rejection—five year experience. *Transplantation* 1997; **63:** 223–8.
32. European Mycophenolate Mofetil Cooperative Study Group. Placebo-controlled study of mycophenolate mofetil combined with cyclosporin and corticosteroids for prevention of acute rejection. *Lancet* 1995; **345:** 1321–5.
33. Mycophenolate Mofetil Renal Refractory Rejection Study Group. Mycophenolate mofetil for the treatment of refractory, acute, cellular renal transplant rejection. *Transplantation* 1996; **61:** 722–9.
34. Matas AJ, *et al.* Pilot evaluation of 15-deoxyspergualin for refractory acute renal transplant rejection. *Clin Transplant* 1994; **8:** 116–19.
35. Reinke P, *et al.* Late-acute renal allograft rejection and symptomless cytomegalovirus infection. *Lancet* 1994; **344:** 1737–8.
36. Laskon DA, *et al.* The incidence of subsequent acute rejection following the treatment of refractory renal allograft rejection with mycophenolate mofetil (RS61443). *Transplantation* 1994; **57:** 640–3.
37. Starzl TE, *et al.* Kidney transplantation under FK 506. *JAMA* 1990; **264:** 63–7.
38. van der Heide JJH, *et al.* Effect of dietary fish oil on renal function and rejection in cyclosporine-treated recipients of renal transplants. *N Engl J Med* 1993; **329:** 769–73.
39. London NJ, *et al.* Risk of neoplasia in renal transplant patients. *Lancet* 1995; **346:** 403–6.
40. Szczech LA, *et al.* The effect of antilymphocyte induction therapy on renal allograft survival: a meta-analysis of individual patient-level data. *Ann Intern Med* 1998; **128:** 817–26.

LIVER. Marked improvements have occurred in the outcome and reliability of liver transplantation in recent years,[1,2] and it is now seen as a useful option in end-stage liver disease and some metabolic disorders, due both to improved immunosuppressive regimens and to better techniques for the storage and preservation of donor livers.[2,3]

Current immunosuppressive regimens generally combine cyclosporin with azathioprine and prednisolone (triple therapy) and sometimes also include a fourth drug such as antilymphocyte immunoglobulin, cyclophosphamide, or a monoclonal anti-T-cell receptor antibody such as muromonab-CD3.[1,2] Addition of an antibody to triple therapy reduces rejection rates by about half,[4] although prophylactic antiviral therapy against cytomegalovirus is advisable. Inolimomab is also reported to be effective, in combination with cyclosporin and low-dose corticosteroids,[5] or with triple therapy, where it is reported to be more effective than antilymphocyte immunoglobulin.[6] The one-year survival after liver transplantation is currently more than 80% using cyclosporin-based regimens.[1] However, even better results may be seen with tacrolimus, which is effective both for prophylaxis and reversal of established rejection episodes.[7-11] Multicentre studies[9,10] have indicated that a regimen of tacrolimus and low-dose corticosteroids is as effective as a cyclosporin-based regimen in terms of patient and graft survival, and may be associated with fewer acute rejection episodes. Although the adverse effects of tacrolimus have been reported to be troublesome,[9,12] Starzl and others consider that there is little difference in the safety profiles of tacrolimus and cyclosporin when the former is administered optimally.[13] Muromonab-CD3 is reported to be effective in patients who do develop rejection episodes.[14]

Patients with good graft function at one year go on to long-term survival, and do not usually suffer the eventual graft loss that occurs in most heart or kidney transplants.[15] In some animal species the liver can be transplanted without immunosuppression, and there is some evidence for the development of tolerance to donor livers in man,[16,17] perhaps due to exchange of immunologically competent donor cells (microchimerism) or to the effects of donor antigens secreted by the liver.[15] As in kidney transplantation (see above) the possibility of reduction or withdrawal of the corticosteroid dose, in patients with stable graft function, is being investigated.[18,19]

1. De Groen PC. Cyclosporine: a review and its specific use in liver transplantation. *Mayo Clin Proc* 1989; **64:** 680–9.
2. Starzl TE, *et al.* Liver transplantation. *N Engl J Med* 1989; **321:** 1014–22 and 1092–9.
3. Kalayoglu M, *et al.* Extended preservation of the liver for clinical transplantation. *Lancet* 1988; **i:** 617–19.
4. McVicar JP, *et al.* Induction immunosuppressive therapy is associated with a low rejection rate after liver transplantation. *Clin Transplant* 1997; **11:** 328–33.
5. Nashan B, *et al.* Immunoprophylaxis with a monoclonal anti-IL-2 receptor antibody in liver transplant patients. *Transplantation* 1996; **61:** 546–54.
6. Langrehr JM, *et al.* A prospective randomized trial comparing interleukin-2 receptor antibody versus antithymocyte globulin as part of a quadruple immunosuppressive induction therapy following orthotopic liver transplantation. *Transplantation* 1997; **63:** 1772–81.
7. Starzl TE, *et al.* FK 506 for liver, kidney, and pancreas transplantation. *Lancet* 1989; **ii:** 1000–4.
8. Macleod AM, Thomson AW. FK 506: an immunosuppressant for the 1990s? *Lancet* 1991; **337:** 25–7. Correction. *ibid.*; 928.
9. The US Multicenter FK506 Liver Study Group. A comparison of tacrolimus (FK506) and cyclosporine for immunosuppression in liver transplantation. *N Engl J Med* 1994; **331:** 1110–15.
10. European FK506 Multicentre Liver Study Group. Randomised trial comparing tacrolimus (FK506) and cyclosporin in prevention of liver allograft rejection. *Lancet* 1994; **344:** 423–8.
11. Woodle ES, *et al.* FK506 rescue therapy for hepatic allograft rejection: experience with an aggressive approach. *Clin Transplant* 1995; **9:** 45–52.
12. Moore R, Lord R. Tacrolimus (FK506) versus cyclosporin in prevention of liver allograft rejection. *Lancet* 1994; **344:** 948.
13. Starzl TE, *et al.* Randomised trialomania? The multicentre liver transplant trials of tacrolimus. *Lancet* 1995; **346:** 1346–50.
14. Haverty TP, *et al.* OKT3 monoclonal antibody treatment of steroid-resistant liver transplant rejection. *Curr Ther Res* 1994; **55:** 382–95.
15. Calne R, Davies H. Organ graft tolerance: the liver effect. *Lancet* 1994; **343:** 67–8.
16. Starzl TE, *et al.* Systemic chimerism in human female recipients of male livers. *Lancet* 1992; **340:** 876–7.
17. Ramos HC, *et al.* Weaning of immunosuppression in long-term liver transplant recipients. *Transplantation* 1995; **59:** 212–17.

18. Pedrosa MC, *et al.* Alternate-day prednisone in the maintenance immunosuppressive therapy after orthotopic liver transplantation. *Clin Transplant* 1995; **9:** 322–5.
19. Punch JD, *et al.* Corticosteroid withdrawal after liver transplantation. *Surgery* 1995; **118:** 783–8.

LUNG. Lung transplantation may be tried for end stage pulmonary disease such as pulmonary hypertension, cystic fibrosis, emphysema, and pulmonary fibrosis.[1] Immunosuppressant therapy is usually with a triple therapy regimen of cyclosporin, azathioprine, and prednisone; antilymphocyte immunoglobulin or muromonab-CD3 may be added in the early post-transplant period.[2] Regimens based on tacrolimus have also been used, and have proved useful in children receiving lung transplants.[3] High doses of intravenous corticosteroids are generally used to control acute episodes of rejection (although some doubt their efficacy[4]), and if instituted early may also be useful in preventing progression of obliterative bronchiolitis, although this is less common than after heart-lung transplantation (see under Heart, above). Inhaled cyclosporin has also been reported to be beneficial in refractory rejection.[5] Prognosis has improved with better regimens and greater experience, and survival rates of 75% or more after 1 to 2 years have been reported from some centres.[2,6] However, 5-year survival is still less than 50% and it is hoped that newer drugs such as mycophenolate mofetil and sirolimus may bring improvement in long-term survival.[7]

1. Peters SG, *et al.* Lung transplantation: selection of patients and analysis of outcome. *Mayo Clin Proc* 1997; **72:** 85–8.
2. Midthun DE, *et al.* Medical management and complications in the lung transplant recipient. *Mayo Clin Proc* 1997; **72:** 175–84.
3. Noyes BE, *et al.* Experience with pediatric lung transplantation. *J Pediatr* 1994; **124:** 261–8.
4. Kesten S, *et al.* Treatment of presumed and proven acute rejection following six months of lung transplant survival. *Am J Respir Crit Care Med* 1995; **152:** 1321–4.
5. Keenan RJ, *et al.* Efficacy of inhaled cyclosporine in lung transplant recipients with refractory rejection: correlation of intragraft cytokine gene expression with pulmonary function and histologic characteristics. *Surgery* 1995; **118:** 385–91.
6. Weinberger SE. Recent advances in pulmonary medicine. *N Engl J Med* 1993; **328:** 1462–70.
7. Briffa N, Morris RE. Immunosuppressive drugs after lung transplantation. *Br Med J* 1998; **316:** 719–20.

OTHER ORGANS. Transplantation of the *pancreas* may be considered in some diabetic patients. Pancreatic grafts have often been transplanted together with a kidney in patients with end-stage diabetic nephropathy; current one-year survival following such a transplant may be as high as 90%, with 75% of patients restored to insulin-independence,[1] but in other centres survival rates have not been as high, especially in older patients.[2] These good results are partly due to better organ preservation and surgical techniques,[3] but also depend on the use of intensive immunosuppression with regimens of antilymphocyte immunoglobulin, azathioprine, corticosteroids, and cyclosporin, with high-dose corticosteroids, muromonab-CD3, or antilymphocyte immunoglobulin being used for rejection episodes.[4] The role of tacrolimus in pancreatic transplantation remains to be determined.[5] Given the potential adverse affects of immunosuppression, some workers are not enthusiastic about the benefits of such transplantation, and it has been pointed out that evidence for a reversal of diabetic complications, other than perhaps neuropathy, is not good.[2] There is some evidence that the autoimmune destruction of pancreatic beta cells that leads to the original disease may recur in the grafted organ.[6] One possible alternative to complete pancreatic transplantation is an *islet-cell* graft, but conventional immunosuppression is not effective in preventing rejection, although a regimen containing gusperimus has been reported to maintain islet cell function in 2 patients in the short term.[7] The use of various means of encapsulating or otherwise separating donor islet cells from the host immune system is under investigation.[2] See also under Diabetes Mellitus, p.313.

Transplantation of the *small bowel* appears to be becoming more common, and somewhat more successful, despite the technical problems of transplanting a highly-immunogenic and non-sterile organ.[8-10] Registry data indicates that the use of tacrolimus has improved graft and patient survival compared with earlier cyclosporin-based immunosuppression, resulting in short-term results comparable with those of lung transplantation,[9] although the risks of the procedure are still too great to make it appropriate in patients who can be successfully maintained with total parenteral nutrition. It has been suggested that in the longer term techniques designed to produce graft-host chimerism and circumvent rejection are required.[8,10]

Transplantation of multiple organs (*cluster grafts*) have also been carried out in a few patients, with evisceration and replacement of liver, pancreas, and parts of the bowel.[11] There is some suggestion that transplantation of the liver with other organs improves host tolerance of the graft, and graft survival.[12] Immunosuppression has usually involved cyclosporin and corticosteroids, and in some cases muromonab-CD3; newer regimens may include tacrolimus.

For reference to the use of corticosteroid immunosuppression to treat graft rejection after *corneal* transplant see Corneal Graft Rejection, under Uses of Corticosteroids, p.1020.

1. Sutherland DER. Pancreas transplantation or insulin? *Lancet* 1990; **336:** 110.
2. Remuzzi G, *et al.* Pancreas and kidney/pancreas transplants: experimental medicine or real improvement? *Lancet* 1994; **343:** 27–31.
3. Perkins JD, *et al.* Pancreas transplantation at Mayo II: operative and perioperative management. *Mayo Clin Proc* 1990; **65:** 483–95.
4. Perkins JD, *et al.* Pancreas transplantation at Mayo III: multidisciplinary management. *Mayo Clin Proc* 1990; **65:** 496–508.
5. Gruessner RWG, *et al.* A multicenter analysis of the first experience with FK506 for induction and rescue therapy after pancreas transplantation. *Transplantation* 1996; **61:** 261–73.
6. Tydén G, *et al.* Recurrence of autoimmune diabetes mellitus in recipients of cadaveric pancreatic grafts. *N Engl J Med* 1996; **335:** 860–3.
7. Gores PF, *et al.* Insulin independence in type 1 diabetes after transplantation of unpurified islets from single donor with 15-deoxyspergualin. *Lancet* 1993; **341:** 19–21.
8. Woodward JM, Mayer D. The unique challenge of small intestinal transplantation. *Br J Hosp Med* 1996; **56:** 285–90.
9. Grant D, *et al.* Current results of intestinal transplantation. *Lancet* 1996; **347:** 1801–3.
10. Soin AS, Friend PJ. Recent developments in transplantation of the small intestine. *Br Med Bull* 1997; **53:** 789–97.
11. Starzl TE, *et al.* Abdominal organ cluster transplantation for the treatment of upper abdominal malignancies. *Ann Surg* 1989; **210:** 374–86.
12. Anonymous. When surgeons experiment. *Lancet* 1990; **335:** 199–200.

Renal disorders, non-malignant. Corticosteroids tend to be the first choice of treatment in most forms of glomerular kidney disease (p.1021), with immunosuppressants, usually in the form of cyclophosphamide, being reserved for more severe disease because of the potential for long-term toxicity.

Rheumatic disorders. RHEUMATOID ARTHRITIS. A variety of antirheumatic drugs including gold salts, penicillamine, hydroxychloroquine, sulphasalazine, and immunosuppressants may be given to patients with rheumatoid arthritis (p.2) in an attempt to modify the course of the disease. There is little agreement concerning the choice of such disease modifying antirheumatic drugs.

The most widely used immunosuppressant is probably low-dose methotrexate, which produced clear short-term clinical benefits in patients unresponsive to gold or penicillamine;[1-3] although doubts exist about its ability to prevent radiological disease progression,[1,4-7] this is also true for other disease modifying antirheumatic drugs.[8] There is also considerable concern about the potential toxicity, particularly to the liver, of long-term treatment.[9,10]

The role of other immunosuppressants in rheumatoid arthritis is more debatable. Azathioprine has been used, but is reported to be less effective than methotrexate,[3] although it may be useful with prednisone in rheumatoid vasculitis,[11] and cyclophosphamide[12] is generally reserved for patients with concomitant severe vasculitis, because of its long-term toxicity. Cyclosporin appears to be effective,[13,14] but nephrotoxicity has been a problem;[13] starting at low doses, and not exceeding a dose of 5 mg per kg body-weight daily may help to minimise nephrotoxic effects.[13] However, combination of cyclosporin with methotrexate has produced clinical improvement in patients who had only partial responses to methotrexate alone.[15]

1. Nordstrom DM, *et al.* Pulse methotrexate therapy in rheumatoid arthritis: a controlled prospective roentgenographic study. *Ann Intern Med* 1987; **107:** 797–801.
2. Tugwell P, *et al.* Methotrexate in rheumatoid arthritis: impact on quality of life assessed by traditional standard-item and individualized patient preference health status questionnaires. *Arch Intern Med* 1990; **150:** 59–62.
3. Jeurissen MEC, *et al.* Influence of methotrexate and azathioprine on radiologic progression in rheumatoid arthritis: a randomized, double-blind study. *Ann Intern Med* 1991; **114:** 999–1004.
4. Weinstein J. Methotrexate in rheumatoid arthritis. *Ann Intern Med* 1988; **108:** 640.
5. Nordstrom DM, *et al.* Methotrexate in rheumatoid arthritis. *Ann Intern Med* 1988; **108:** 640–1.
6. Boerbooms AMT, *et al.* Pulse methotrexate therapy in rheumatoid arthritis. *Ann Intern Med* 1988; **108:** 905.
7. Nordstrom D, *et al.* Pulse methotrexate therapy in rheumatoid arthritis. *Ann Intern Med* 1988; **108:** 905.
8. Kushner I. Does aggressive therapy of rheumatoid arthritis affect outcome. *J Rheumatol* 1989; **16:** 1–4.
9. Whiting-O'Keefe QE, *et al.* Methotrexate and histologic hepatic abnormalities: a meta-analysis. *Am J Med* 1991; **90:** 711–16.
10. Tugwell P, *et al.* Methotrexate in rheumatoid arthritis: feedback on American College of Physicians guidelines. *Ann Intern Med* 1989; **110:** 581–3.
11. Heurkens AHM, *et al.* Prednisone plus azathioprine treatment in patients with rheumatoid arthritis complicated by vasculitis. *Arch Intern Med* 1991; **151:** 2249–54.
12. Iannuzzi L, *et al.* Does drug therapy slow radiographic deterioration in rheumatoid arthritis? *N Engl J Med* 1983; **309:** 1023–8.
13. Yocum DE, *et al.* Cyclosporin A in severe, treatment-refractory rheumatoid arthritis: a randomized study. *Ann Intern Med* 1988; **109:** 863–9.
14. Tugwell P, *et al.* Low-dose cyclosporin versus placebo in patients with rheumatoid arthritis. *Lancet* 1990; **335:** 1051–5.
15. Tugwell P, *et al.* Combination therapy with cyclosporine and methotrexate in severe rheumatoid arthritis. *N Engl J Med* 1995; **333:** 137–41.

Sarcoidosis. Where drug therapy is required for sarcoidosis (p.1028), corticosteroids are the usual treatment. In patients in whom these are ineffective or poorly tolerated, cytotoxic immunosuppressants have been given, with variable results. Methotrexate has perhaps been most useful,[1,2] but other agents including azathioprine, chlorambucil, and cyclosporin, have been tried.[3]

1. Webster GF, *et al.* Methotrexate therapy in cutaneous sarcoidosis. *Ann Intern Med* 1989; **111:** 538–9.
2. Soriano FG, *et al.* Neurosarcoidosis: therapeutic success with methotrexate. *Postgrad Med J* 1990; **66:** 142–3.
3. Muthiah MM, Macfarlane JT. Current concepts in the management of sarcoidosis. *Drugs* 1990; **40:** 231–7.

Scleroderma. The term scleroderma has been used for both systemic sclerosis, a multisystem disease characterised by collagen proliferation and fibrosis throughout the body, and for localised fibrotic changes of the skin (morphea) without involvement of other organs. Systemic sclerosis is an uncommon disease which has been linked to various environmental toxins as well as to genetic factors. Vascular involvement produces Raynaud's syndrome, which usually precedes any skin changes and there may be ulceration or ischaemic changes of the digits. A long history of Raynaud's syndrome before skin changes occur suggests a more indolent course (limited cutaneous disease) as opposed to the more aggressive diffuse cutaneous form. Skin oedema is followed by thickening and tightening of the skin of hands and face, and sometimes limbs and trunk, before progressing to atrophy and contractures. There may be decreased gastro-intestinal motility, dysphagia and gastro-oesophageal reflux, arthritis, muscle weakness, and cardiac involvement. Among the most serious potential symptoms, which may result in death, are pulmonary disease and renal failure with malignant hypertension.

No treatment has been clearly demonstrated to affect the progression of disease, and much management is essentially symptomatic. Antibiotics or vaccines may be required for the prophylaxis of pulmonary and gastro-intestinal infections, while antacids, histamine H_2-receptor antagonists or proton pump inhibitors such as omeprazole, and stimulants of gastric motility may be required for the management of gastro-intestinal symptoms.[1,2] Peripheral vascular disease (p.794) requires appropriate management. The use of ACE inhibitors to manage the consequences of renal involvement has resulted in a decrease in the number of patients developing permanent renal damage.[3]

Despite the lack of conclusive evidence in its favour penicillamine, which affects the cross-linking of collagen,[4] is widely thought to be of benefit in scleroderma, and perhaps in some visceral manifestations.[1,5] If used, treatment should probably be begun early in disease and continued for several years. Penicillamine may produce severe adverse effects, however; colchicine is a possible alternative,[1] although it too can be toxic.

Corticosteroids do not appear to be of value in controlling scleroderma but may be useful for symptoms of myositis, pericarditis, and perhaps for pulmonary involvement.[1] In the latter case combination with a cytotoxic immunosuppressant such as cyclophosphamide may be of value.[6] A few reports of benefit in scleroderma with methotrexate[7] or cyclosporin[8,9] also exist, but immunosuppressant therapy remains experimental. It is probably appropriate in the early oedematous stages diffuse scleroderma, followed by an antifibrotic drug such as penicillamine or an interferon,[2,10] although the latter may be poorly tolerated.[2,11] There is a report of the treatment of scleroderma in one patient by bone-marrow ablation using cyclophosphamide followed by infusion of autologous peripheral blood stem cells.[12]

A variety of other agents have been tried in systemic sclerosis, including potassium aminobenzoate and sulphasalazine. Newer agents under investigation include thymopentin and relaxin. PUVA therapy, using methoxsalen applied topically in bath water has been reported to produce improvement of localised skin symptoms.[13]

1. Oliver GF, Winkelmann RK. The current treatment of scleroderma. *Drugs* 1989; **37:** 87–96.
2. Fine LG, *et al.* Systemic sclerosis: current pathogenetic concepts and future prospects for targeted therapy. *Lancet* 1996; **347:** 1453–8.
3. Steen VD, *et al.* Outcome of renal crisis in systemic sclerosis: relation to the availability of angiotensin converting enzyme (ACE) inhibitors. *Ann Intern Med* 1990; **113:** 352–7.
4. Herbert CM, *et al.* Biosynthesis and maturation of skin collagen in scleroderma, and effect of D-penicillamine. *Lancet* 1974; **i:** 187–92.
5. Steen VD, *et al.* D-Penicillamine therapy in progressive systemic sclerosis (scleroderma): a retrospective analysis. *Ann Intern Med* 1982; **97:** 652–9.
6. Silver RM, *et al.* Evaluation and management of scleroderma lung disease using bronchoalveolar lavage. *Am J Med* 1990; **88:** 470–6.
7. van den Hoogen FHJ, *et al.* Methotrexate treatment in scleroderma. *Am J Med* 1989; **87:** 116–17.
8. Zachariae H, *et al.* Cyclosporin A treatment of systemic sclerosis. *Br J Dermatol* 1990; **122:** 677–81.
9. Pryce DW, *et al.* Safety and efficacy of longer-term lower-dose cyclosporin A therapy. *Br J Dermatol* 1994; **130:** 681–9.
10. Isenberg DA, Black C. Raynaud's phenomenon, scleroderma, and overlap syndromes. *Br Med J* 1995; **310:** 795–8.
11. Polisson RP, *et al.* A multicenter trial of recombinant human interferon gamma in patients with systemic sclerosis: effects on cutaneous fibrosis and interleukin 2 receptor levels. *J Rheumatol* 1996; **23:** 654–8.
12. Tyndall A, *et al.* Treatment of systemic sclerosis with autologous haematopoietic stem-cell transplantation. *Lancet* 1997; **349:** 254.
13. Kerscher M, *et al.* Treatment of localised scleroderma with PUVA bath photochemotherapy. *Lancet* 1994; **343:** 1233. Correction. *ibid.*; 1580.

Skin and connective-tissue disorders, non-malignant. Immunosuppressants have been tried in various skin and connective tissue disorders, including Behçet's syndrome (p.1018), eczema (p.1073), pemphigus and pemphigoid (p.1075), polymyositis (p.1027), psoriasis (p.1075), systemic lupus erythematosus (p.1029), and the various vasculitic syndromes (p.1031). See also Scleroderma, above.

Aceglatone (12305-k)

Aceglatone *(rINN)*.

D-Glucaric acid 1,4:6,3-dilactone diacetate.

$C_{10}H_{10}O_8$ = 258.2.

CAS — 642-83-1.

Aceglatone inhibits the activity of β-glucuronidase and has an anti-inflammatory action. It has been given by mouth to prevent relapse after surgery of carcinoma of the bladder. Adverse effects have included anorexia, gastric discomfort, dry skin, and pigmentation.

Aclarubicin Hydrochloride (12318-f)

Aclarubicin Hydrochloride *(BANM, rINNM)*.

Aclacinomycin A Hydrochloride; NSC-208734 (aclarubicin). Methyl (1*R*,2*R*,4*S*)-4-(*O*-{2,6-dideoxy-4-*O*-[(2*R*,6*S*)-tetrahydro-6-methyl-5-oxopyran-2-yl]-α-L-*lyxo*-hexopyranosyl}-(1→4)-2,3,6-trideoxy-3-dimethylamino-L-*lyxo*-hexopyranosyloxy)-2-ethyl-1,2,3,4,6,11-hexahydro-2,5,7-trihydroxy-6,11-dioxonaphthacene-1-carboxylate hydrochloride.

$C_{42}H_{53}NO_{15}$,HCl = 848.3.

CAS — 57576-44-0 (aclarubicin).

NOTE. Aclarubicin is *USAN*.

Pharmacopoeias. In *Jpn*.

The hydrochloride of an anthracycline antineoplastic antibiotic isolated from *Streptomyces galilaeus*. Aclarubicin hydrochloride 1.04 mg is approximately equivalent to 1 mg of aclarubicin.

In a study of the stability of anthracycline antineoplastic agents in 4 infusion fluids—glucose injection (5%), sodium chloride injection (0.9%), lactated Ringer's injection, and a commercial infusion fluid—stability appeared to be partly related to pH; aclarubicin was most stable in sodium chloride injection, with a pH of 6.2, and any increase or decrease in pH [illegible]ared to affect stability adversely.[1]

1. [illegible]ian GK, *et al.* Stability of anthracycline antitumor [illegible]ur infusion fluids. *Am J Hosp Pharm* 1981; **38:**

Adverse Effects, Treatment, and Precautions

As for Doxorubicin Hydrochloride, p.529.

Alopecia and cardiotoxicity may be less pronounced than with other anthracyclines. Bone-marrow depression is dose-limiting, with platelet counts reaching a nadir 1 to 2 weeks after administration, while leucopenia is greatest after 2 to 3 weeks; recovery generally occurs within 4 weeks. Myelosuppression may be particularly severe in patients who have received mitomycin or a nitrosourea.

Uses and Administration

Aclarubicin is an anthracycline antibiotic with antineoplastic actions similar to those of the other anthracyclines (see Doxorubicin Hydrochloride, p.531), although it inhibits RNA synthesis more strongly than DNA synthesis. It is used as the hydrochloride in the treatment of malignant blood disorders, such as acute non-lymphoblastic leukaemia (p.479). The usual initial dose as a single agent is the equivalent of 175 to 300 mg of base per m² body-surface, given divided over 3 to 7 consecutive days, by intravenous infusion. Where appropriate and tolerated, maintenance doses of the equivalent of 25 to 100 mg of aclarubicin per m² may be given as a single infusion every 3 to 4 weeks. The total dose that can be given over the patient's life-time depends upon cardiological status but most patients have not received more than 400 mg per m². Dosages may need to be reduced when given as part of a combination regimen.

A review of the development and uses of aclarubicin.[1] Studies in patients with relapsed acute non-lymphoblastic leukaemia have confirmed the activity of aclarubicin, with reported complete remission rates of the order of 12 to 24%. Doses have varied from 10 to 30 mg per m² body-surface daily to higher doses of 75 to 120 mg per m² for 2 to 4 days; in general a total dose of about 300 mg per m² appears to be necessary to induce remission. Less information is available concerning activity in acute lymphoblastic leukaemia, but response rates have been lower than those in acute non-lymphoblastic leukaemia. Results in the malignant lymphomas have been generally disappointing. It has become apparent in the course of clinical studies that aclarubicin is not devoid of cardiotoxicity. A strikingly high incidence of ECG changes has been observed but although acute cardiotoxicity occurs the chronic cardiomyopathy classically associated with the anthracyclines appears to be a rare event. Alopecia is also rare, although gastro-intestinal disturbances and mucositis are as common or more common than with doxorubicin.

1. Warrell RP. Aclacinomycin A: clinical development of a novel anthracycline antibiotic in the haematological cancers. *Drugs Exp Clin Res* 1986; **12:** 275–82.

Preparations

Proprietary Preparations (details are given in Part 3)
Aust.: Aclaplastin; ***Fr.:*** Aclacinomycine†; ***Ger.:*** Aclaplastin; ***UK:*** Aclacin.

AG-337 (15981-p)

AG-337 is, like raltitrexed (p.560), a selective inhibitor of thymidylate synthase. It is under investigation as an antimetabolite antineoplastic.

Altretamine (1838-f)

Altretamine *(BAN, USAN, rINN)*.

Hexamethylmelamine; HMM; NSC-13875; WR-95704. 2,4,6-Tris(dimethylamino)-1,3,5-triazine; N^2,N^2,N^4,N^4,N^6,N^6-Hexamethyl-1,3,5-triazine-2,4,6-triamine.

$C_9H_{18}N_6$ = 210.3.

CAS — 645-05-6.

Pharmacopoeias. In *US*.

White crystalline powder. Practically **insoluble** in water; soluble in chloroform.

CAUTION. *Altretamine is irritant; avoid contact with skin and mucous membranes.*

Adverse Effects, Treatment, and Precautions

For a general outline see Antineoplastics, p.470, p.473, and p.474.

Bone-marrow depression is usually moderate, manifesting as leucopenia, thrombocytopenia, and anaemia. Nausea and vomiting are common and usually moderate although they may be dose-limiting. Prolonged or high-dose therapy may be associated with neurotoxicity, both peripheral (neuropathies) and central (ataxia, depression, confusion, drowsiness, and hallucinations). Other adverse effects include rashes and renal toxicity.

Interactions

Concomitant administration of altretamine with pyridoxine appears to reduce the activity of the former.

Antidepressants. Severe and potentially life-threatening orthostatic hypotension developed in 3 patients who received amitriptyline or imipramine concurrently with altretamine and in a fourth patient who took phenelzine and altretamine concurrently.[1] One patient was able to tolerate a combination of the antineoplastic with nortriptyline.

1. Bruckner HW, Schleifer SJ. Orthostatic hypotension as a complication of hexamethylmelamine antidepressant interaction. *Cancer Treat Rep* 1983; **67:** 516.

Pharmacokinetics

Altretamine is well absorbed from the gastro-intestinal tract following oral administration. It is rapidly demethylated in the liver to pentamethylmelamine and other metabolites which are excreted in urine. The plasma elimination half-life has been variously reported to be 4 to 10 hours or about 13 hours.

References.

1. Darmia G, D'Incalci M. Clinical pharmacokinetics of altretamine. *Clin Pharmacokinet* 1995; **28:** 439–48.

Uses and Administration

Altretamine is an antineoplastic agent structurally similar to the alkylating agent tretamine although its mode of action may be different. It is given by mouth in the treatment of ovarian carcinoma (p.491) and other solid tumours such as endometrial cancer (p.487). Usual doses in ovarian cancer are 260 mg per m² body-surface daily, often for 14 days out of a 28-day cycle. Lower doses are used in combination regimens.

Blood counts should be monitored regularly and therapy should be stopped if the white-cell count falls below 2000 per mm³ or the platelet count below 75 000 per mm³.

Reviews.

1. Hahn DA. Hexamethylmelamine and pentamethylmelamine: an update. *Drug Intell Clin Pharm* 1983; **17:** 418–24.
2. Hansen LA, Hughes TE. Altretamine. *DICP Ann Pharmacother* 1991; **25:** 146–52.
3. Anonymous. Altretamine for ovarian cancer. *Med Lett Drugs Ther* 1991; **33:** 76–7.
4. Lee CR, Faulds D. Altretamine: a review of its pharmacodynamic and pharmacokinetic properties, and therapeutic potential in cancer chemotherapy. *Drugs* 1995; **49:** 932–53.

Preparations

USP 23: Altretamine Capsules.

Proprietary Preparations (details are given in Part 3)
Austral.: Hexalen; ***Canad.:*** Hexalen; ***Fr.:*** Hexastat; ***Ital.:*** Hexastat; ***Neth.:*** Hexastat†; ***Norw.:*** Hexalen; Hexastat; ***Spain:*** Hexinawas; ***Swed.:*** Hexalen; ***UK:*** Hexalen; ***USA:*** Hexalen.

Aminoglutethimide (1803-e)

Aminoglutethimide *(BAN, rINN)*.

Ba-16038. 2-(4-Aminophenyl)-2-ethylglutarimide; 3-(4-Aminophenyl)-3-ethylpiperidine-2,6-dione.

$C_{13}H_{16}N_2O_2$ = 232.3.

CAS — 125-84-8.

Pharmacopoeias. In *Eur.* (see p.viii), and *US*.

A white or creamy-white, fine, crystalline powder. Very slightly **soluble** or practically insoluble in water; readily soluble in most organic solvents. It forms water-soluble salts with strong acids. The pH of a 0.1% solution in dilute methyl alcohol (1 in 20) is between 6.2 and 7.3. The USP directs that the tablets should be **stored** in airtight containers and protected from light.

Adverse Effects

Adverse effects reported with aminoglutethimide include drowsiness, lethargy, ataxia, fever, skin rashes, and gastro-intestinal disturbances; most side-effects diminish after the first 6 weeks of therapy due to enhanced metabolism of the drug. Bone-marrow depression, with leucopenia, thrombocytopenia, agranulocytosis, or severe pancytopenia has occurred rarely. Adrenal insufficiency may sometimes occur, and there have been reports of other endocrine disturbances including hypothyroidism, and virilisation. Orthostatic hypotension may occur in some patients.

Overdosage may lead to CNS depression and impairment of consciousness, electrolyte disturbances, and respiratory depression.

Effects on the liver. Aminoglutethimide has been associated with reports of cholestatic jaundice, accompanied by rash[1,2] and fever,[2] and probably due to an idiosyncratic hypersensitivity reaction.[1] It has been suggested that liver function tests should be carried out in patients receiving aminoglutethimide who develop fever and eruptions.[2]

1. Gerber SB, Miller KB. Cholestatic jaundice and aminoglutethimide. *Ann Intern Med* 1982; **97:** 138.
2. Perrault DJ, Domovitch E. Aminoglutethimide and cholestasis. *Ann Intern Med* 1984; **100:** 160.

Effects on respiratory function. Pulmonary infiltrates in a patient who developed progressive dyspnoea on commencing therapy with aminoglutethimide were found to be due to diffuse alveolar damage and haemorrhage; thrombocytopenia was present but prothrombin and bleeding times were normal. The patient's gas exchange and chest radiographs improved on discontinuation of aminoglutethimide and institution of corticosteroid therapy.[1]

1. Rodman DM, *et al.* Aminoglutethimide, alveolar damage, and hemorrhage. *Ann Intern Med* 1986; **105:** 633.

Lupus. A report of systemic lupus erythematosus induced by aminoglutethimide in one patient.[1]

1. McCraken M, *et al.* Systemic lupus erythematosus induced by aminoglutethimide. *Br Med J* 1980; **281:** 1254.

Precautions

Aminoglutethimide inhibits adrenal steroid production and the adrenal response to stress may be impaired; it has been suggested that aminoglutethimide should be temporarily withdrawn in patients who undergo shock or trauma, or develop intercurrent infection. Supplementary glucocorticoid therapy with hydrocortisone must normally be given although supplementation may not be necessary in patients with Cushing's syndrome. Some patients also require a mineralocorticoid. Blood counts and serum electrolytes should be regularly monitored during aminoglutethimide therapy and periodic monitoring of liver and thyroid function is recommended.

Aminoglutethimide should not be given during pregnancy as pseudohermaphroditism may occur in the fetus.

Aminoglutethimide may cause drowsiness: patients so affected should not drive or operate machinery.

Aminoglutethimide has been reported to produce raised serum-cholesterol concentrations in patients with breast cancer,[1,2] although not, apparently, in those with Cushing's disease.[3] However, the significance of this rise is uncertain in the context of the other biochemical changes which aminoglutethimide may provoke.[2]

1. Bonneterre J, *et al.* Aminoglutethimide-induced hypercholesterolaemia. *Lancet* 1984; **i:** 912–13.
2. Ceci G, *et al.* Aminoglutethimide and serum cholesterol. *Lancet* 1984; **ii:** 358.
3. Kasperlik-Zaluska A, Migdalska B. Aminoglutethimide and serum cholesterol. *Lancet* 1984; **ii:** 358.

Porphyria. Aminoglutethimide has been associated with clinical exacerbations of porphyria and is considered unsafe in porphyric patients.[1]

1. Moore MR, McColl KEL. *Porphyria: drug lists.* Glasgow: Porphyria Research Unit, University of Glasgow, 1991.

Interactions

The rate of metabolism of some drugs is increased by aminoglutethimide; patients receiving concomitant therapy with warfarin or other coumarin anticoagulants, with theophylline, with tamoxifen, or with oral hypoglycaemic agents, may require increased dosages of these drugs. The metabolism of dexamethasone is also accelerated, which limits its value for corticosteroid supplementation in patients receiving aminoglutethimide. Concomitant administration of diuretics may lead to hyponatraemia, while alcohol may potentiate the central effects of aminoglutethimide.

For reference to an increase in the clearance of digitoxin by aminoglutethimide, see under Digitoxin, p.849, and for reference to increased clearance of theophylline in patients given aminoglutethimide, see under Theophylline, p.769. Aminoglutethimide has also been reported to reduce serum concentrations of some progestogens (see p.1460). For the effects of aminoglutethimide on anticoagulants, see under Warfarin, p.967.

Pharmacokinetics

Aminoglutethimide is rapidly and completely absorbed following oral administration with peak plasma concentrations occurring after 1 to 2 hours. It is metabolised in the liver, primarily by acetylation to form *N*-acetylaminoglutethimide, and appears to induce its own metabolism. The half-life, which is reported to be about 13 hours after the administration of a single dose, is decreased to around 7 hours after about 2 weeks of continuous therapy. Aminoglutethimide is excreted in urine, about half a dose being excreted unchanged and the remainder as metabolites. Only about 20 to 25% of a dose is bound to plasma protein.

A report of the characterisation of 4 minor metabolites in the urine of patients undergoing therapy with aminoglutethimide.[1] These are in addition to the two major metabolites, acetylaminoglutethimide and hydroxylaminoglutethimide, and 2 minor metabolites, *p*-nitroglutethimide and formylaminoglutethimide, which have been previously reported.

1. Foster AB, *et al.* Metabolism of aminoglutethimide in humans: identification of four new urinary metabolites. *Drug Metab Dispos* 1984; **12:** 511–16.

A study of the single- and multiple-dose pharmacokinetics of aminoglutethimide in 17 patients demonstrated that the plasma half-life had a mean value of 15.5 hours after single-dose administration but fell to 8.9 hours during multiple-dose therapy.[1] This marked reduction in half-life could largely be attributed to a decrease in the volume of distribution; auto-induction of metabolism may be of less importance in decreasing half-life than has been previously suggested.

1. Lønning PE, *et al.* Single-dose and steady-state pharmacokinetics of aminoglutethimide. *Clin Pharmacokinet* 1985; **10:** 353–64.

Uses and Administration

Aminoglutethimide is an analogue of glutethimide (see p.673) and was formerly used for its weak anticonvulsant properties. Aminoglutethimide blocks the production of adrenal steroids and acts as an aromatase inhibitor to block the conversion of androgens to oestrogens (the major source of oestrogens in women without ovarian function). It has been used in the treatment of metastatic breast cancer (p.485) in post menopausal or oophorectomised women, in doses of 250 mg up to four times daily by mouth. Aminoglutethimide has also been used as palliative treatment in patients with advanced prostatic cancer (p.491) but there are doubts about its value. Replacement therapy with a corticosteroid must also be given, usually hydrocortisone 20 to 30 mg daily in divided doses (see p.1017 for a description of corticosteroid replacement therapy).

Aminoglutethimide is used in similar or higher doses in the treatment of Cushing's syndrome (p.1236); up to 2 g daily may be needed. Corticosteroid supplementation may not be required in these patients.

The *dextro*-isomer of aminoglutethimide, dexaminoglutethimide has also been investigated.

References to the effects of aminoglutethimide on adrenal steroid secretion[1] and its mechanisms of action in breast cancer.[2]

1. Vermeulen A, *et al.* Effects of aminoglutethimide on adrenal steroid secretion. *Clin Endocrinol (Oxf)* 1983; **19:** 673–82.
2. Lønning PE, Kvinnsland S. Mechanisms of action of aminoglutethimide as endocrine therapy of breast cancer. *Drugs* 1988; **35:** 685–710.

Preparations

USP 23: Aminoglutethimide Tablets.

Proprietary Preparations (details are given in Part 3)
Aust.: Orimeten; ***Austral.:*** Cytadren; ***Belg.:*** Orimeten; ***Canad.:*** Cytadren; ***Fr.:*** Orimetene; ***Ger.:*** Orimeten; Rodazol†; ***Irl.:*** Orimeten; ***Ital.:*** Orimeten; ***Neth.:*** Orimeten; ***Norw.:*** Orimeten; ***S.Afr.:*** Aminoblastin†; Orimeten; ***Spain:*** Orimeten; ***Swed.:*** Orimeten; ***Switz.:*** Orimetene; ***UK:*** Orimeten; ***USA:*** Cytadren.

5-Aminolaevulinic Acid (14918-c)

ALA; 5-ALA; δ-Aminolaevulinic Acid.

5-Aminolaevulinic acid is a naturally occurring haem precursor, which is metabolised in the body to protoporphyrin IX and then to haem. It has been used as a photosensitiser by oral or topical application, in combination with laser treatment, in the treatment of malignant neoplasms such as those of skin (p.492) and bladder (p.484), and skin disorders such as psoriasis.

5-Aminolaevulinic acid has been used as a photosensitiser in the photodynamic therapy of gastro-intestinal tumours,[1,2] in which case it has normally been given by mouth, doses of 60 mg per kg having been found effective; it has also been used topically for malignant or premalignant lesions of the skin,[3-5] in which case a 20% dispersion in a suitable cream basis has often been employed. This is also favoured in non-malignant skin conditions such as psoriasis, xeroderma pigmentosum or actinic cheilitis.[6-10] An intravesical solution has been instilled into the bladder in the management of superficial bladder cancer.[11] Photodynamic therapy using oral 5-aminolaevulinic acid as the photosensitiser has also been used to treat Barrett's oesophagus.[12]

1. Grant WE, *et al.* Photodynamic therapy of oral cancer: photosensitisation with systemic aminolaevulinic acid. *Lancet* 1993; **342:** 147–8.
2. Regula J, *et al.* Photosensitisation and photodynamic therapy of oesophageal, duodenal, and colorectal tumours using 5 aminolaevulinic acid induced protoporphyrin IX—a pilot study. *Gut* 1995; **36:** 67–75.
3. Svanberg K, *et al.* Photodynamic therapy of non-melanoma malignant tumours of the skin using topical δ-amino levulinic acid sensitization and laser irradiation. *Br J Dermatol* 1994; **130:** 743–51.
4. Morton CA, *et al.* Topical photodynamic therapy for Bowen's disease and basal cell carcinoma—an effective therapy? *Br J Dermatol* 1996; **135** (suppl 47): 22–3.
5. Jeffes EW, *et al.* Photodynamic therapy of actinic keratosis with topical 5-aminolevulinic acid: a pilot dose-ranging study. *Arch Dermatol* 1997; **133:** 727–32.
6. Wolf P, Kerl H. Photodynamic therapy in patient with xeroderma pigmentosum. *Lancet* 1991; **337:** 1613–14.
7. Boehncke W-H, *et al.* Treatment of psoriasis by topical photodynamic therapy with polychromatic light. *Lancet* 1994; **343:** 801.
8. Collins P, *et al.* Topical 5-aminolaevulinic acid photodynamic therapy for psoriasis: the light dose response. *Br J Dermatol* 1996; **135** (suppl 47): 18.
9. Stender I-M, Wulf HC. Photodynamic therapy with 5-aminolevulinic acid in the treatment of actinic cheilitis. *Br J Dermatol* 1996; **135:** 454–6.
10. Collins P, *et al.* The variable response of plaque psoriasis after a single treatment with topical 5-aminolaevulinic acid photodynamic therapy. *Br J Dermatol* 1997; **137:** 743–9.
11. Kriegmair M, *et al.* Early clinical experience with 5-aminolevulinic acid for the photodynamic therapy of superficial bladder cancer. *Br J Urol* 1996; **77:** 667–71.
12. Barr J, *et al.* Eradication of high-grade dysplasia in columnar-lined (Barrett's) oesophagus by photodynamic therapy with endogenously generated protoporphyrin IX. *Lancet* 1996; **348:** 584–5.

Amonafide (19508-z)

Amonafide *(rINN)*.

M-FA-142. 3-Amino-*N*-[2-(dimethylamino)ethyl]naphthalimide.

$C_{16}H_{17}N_3O_2$ = 283.3.
CAS — 69408-81-7.

Amonafide is under investigation as an antineoplastic.

References.

1. Evans WK, *et al.* Phase II study of amonafide: results of treatment and lessons learned from the study of an investigational agent in previously untreated patients with extensive small-cell lung cancer. *J Clin Oncol* 1990; **8:** 390–5.

Amsacrine (12374-q)

Amsacrine *(BAN, USAN, pINN)*.

Acridinyl Anisidide; *m*-AMSA; CI-880; NSC-249992. 4′-(Acridin-9-ylamino)methanesulphon-*m*-anisidide.

$C_{21}H_{19}N_3O_3S$ = 393.5.
CAS — 51264-14-3.

Incompatibility. Amsacrine is incompatible with 0.9% sodium chloride injection and with other chloride-containing solutions,[1,2] apparently because of the poor solubility of the hydrochloride salt in aqueous solution.[2] Precipitation has been reported when amsacrine was mixed with aciclovir sodium, amphotericin, aztreonam, ceftazidime, ceftriaxone sodium, cimetidine hydrochloride, frusemide, ganciclovir sodium, heparin sodium, methylprednisolone sodium succinate, or metoclopramide hydrochloride, in 5% glucose injection.[2] Amsacrine reacts with certain plastics.[1]

1. D'Arcy PF. Reactions and interactions in handling anticancer drugs. *Drug Intell Clin Pharm* 1983; **17:** 532–8.
2. Trissel LA, *et al.* Visual compatibility of amsacrine with selected drugs during simulated Y-site injection. *Am J Hosp Pharm* 1990; **47:** 2525–8.

Adverse Effects, Treatment, and Precautions

For a general outline see Antineoplastics, p.470, p.473, and p.474.

Bone-marrow depression is usually dose-limiting and may be severe. The nadir of the white cell count has been reported at about 12 days after treatment, with recovery usually by the 25th day. Pancytopenia may occur. Gastro-intestinal disturbances including severe stomatitis, grand mal seizures, renal dysfunction, and hepatotoxicity, which is usually transient but has occasionally proved fatal, have been reported. Cardiac arrhythmias may occur, especially in patients with pre-existing hypokalaemia; the risk of cardiotoxicity may be greater in patients previously treated with anthracyclines such as doxorubicin. Amsacrine is irritant: there may be phlebitis and local tissue necrosis associated especially with intravenous administration of high concentrations.

It should be given with caution to patients with liver or kidney disease, who may require dosage adjustments.

Interactions

Concomitant use of diuretics or nephrotoxic drugs such as the aminoglycosides may increase the risk of cardiotoxicity with amsacrine by precipitating hypokalaemia.

Pharmacokinetics

Amsacrine is poorly absorbed following oral administration. When given intravenously it has a reported terminal half-life of about 5 to 8 hours. It is metabolised in the liver and excreted primarily in the bile, mostly as metabolites. It is reported to be about 98% protein bound.

Uses and Administration

Amsacrine is an antineoplastic agent that appears to act by intercalation with DNA and inhibition of nucleic acid synthesis. It may also exert an action on cell membranes. Cells in G2 or S phases may be most sensitive to its actions.

It is used for the induction and maintenance of remission in adult acute leukaemias, particularly acute non-lymphoblastic leukaemia (p.479).

Amsacrine is prepared as a solution in lactic acid and dimethylacetamide, and is given, diluted in glucose injection (5%) by intravenous infusion over 1 to 1½ hours.

For the induction of remission, amsacrine may be given in a dose of 90 mg per m^2 body-surface area daily for 5 to 8 days, depending on toxicity. Courses may be repeated at 2- to 4-week intervals according to response, and the dose may be increased to 120 mg per m^2 daily in subsequent courses if tolerated. Maintenance doses of 150 mg per m^2 as a single dose or divided over 3 consecutive days have been given every 3 to 4 weeks, adjusted if necessary according to response. The granulocyte and platelet counts should be allowed to recover to more than 1500 per mm^3 and 100 000 per mm^3 respectively between courses. Dosage should be adjusted appropriately when given as part of a combination regimen.

Complete blood counts should be performed regularly, and cardiac, liver, kidney, and CNS function should be monitored. Doses should be reduced by 20 to 30% in patients with impaired hepatic or renal function.

Preparations

Proprietary Preparations (details are given in Part 3)

Austral.: Amsidyl; ***Belg.:*** Amsidine; ***Canad.:*** Amsa P-D; ***Fr.:*** Amsidine; ***Ger.:*** Amsidyl; ***Irl.:*** Amsidine; ***Neth.:*** Amsidine; ***Norw.:*** Amekrin; ***Swed.:*** Amekrin; ***Switz.:*** Amsidyl; ***UK:*** Amsidine.

Anastrozole (14549-q)

Anastrozole *(BAN, USAN, rINN).*

ICI-D1033; ZD-1033. 2,2′-Dimethyl-2,2′-[5-(1*H*-1,2,4-triazol-1-ylmethyl)-1,3-phenylene]bis(propiononitrile); α,α,α′,α′-Tetramethyl-5-(1*H*-1,2,4-triazol-1-ylmethyl)-*m*-benzenediacetonitrile.

$C_{17}H_{19}N_5$ = 293.4.

CAS — 120511-73-1.

Adverse Effects and Precautions

Anastrozole is generally well tolerated and the most frequent adverse effects are gastro-intestinal disturbances including anorexia, nausea and vomiting, and diarrhoea; asthenia; hot flushes; dizziness; drowsiness; headache; and rash. Other reported effects include hair thinning, vaginal dryness or bleeding, oedema, myalgia and arthralgia, fever, thrombophlebitis, leucopenia, and a flu-like syndrome. Abnormalities in liver enzyme values have occurred in some patients receiving anastrozole.

The use of anastrozole in contra-indicated in premenopausal women (particularly in pregnancy). It is not known whether it can be safely given to patients with moderate or severe hepatic impairment, or severe renal impairment.

Pharmacokinetics

Anastrozole is rapidly and almost completely absorbed from the gastro-intestinal tract following oral administration, with peak plasma concentrations occurring within about 2 hours. Food decreases the rate of absorption, though this is not considered clinically significant. It is metabolised in the liver, and excreted in urine, chiefly as metabolites. The terminal elimination half-life is about 50 hours, and steady-state concentrations are achieved after about 7 days in patients receiving once-daily doses.

Uses and Administration

Anastrozole is a potent and selective inhibitor of the aromatase (oestrogen synthetase) system. It is used in the treatment of breast cancer (p.485) in postmenopausal women in a dose of 1 mg daily.

References.

1. Anonymous. Anastrozole for metastatic breast cancer. *Med Lett Drugs Ther* 1996; **38:** 61–2.
2. Buzdar A, *et al.* Anastrozole, a potent and selective aromatase inhibitor, versus megestrol acetate in postmenopausal women with advanced breast cancer: results of overview analysis of two phase III trials. *J Clin Oncol* 1996; **14:** 2000–11.

Preparations

Proprietary Preparations (details are given in Part 3)

Aust.: Arimidex; ***Austral.:*** Arimidex; ***Canad.:*** Arimidex; ***Ger.:*** [illegible]imidex; ***Irl.:*** Arimidex; ***Ital.:*** Arimidex; ***Neth.:*** Arimidex; [illegible] Arimidex; ***S.Afr.:*** Arimidex; ***Swed.:*** Arimidex; ***Switz.:*** Ar[illegible]; [illegible]K: Arimidex; ***USA:*** Arimidex.

Ancitabine Hydrochloride (1824-c)

Ancitabine Hydrochloride *(rINNM).*

Ancytabine Hydrochloride; Cyclocytidine Hydrochloride; NSC-145668. 2,2′-Anhydro-(1-β-D-arabinofuranosyl)cytosine hydrochloride.

$C_9H_{11}N_3O_4,HCl$ = 261.7.

CAS — 31698-14-3 (ancitabine); 10212-25-6 (ancitabine hydrochloride).

Ancitabine hydrochloride is an antineoplastic agent which is hydrolysed slowly to cytarabine (see p.525) *in vivo.* It has been used in acute non-lymphoblastic and other leukaemias.

Antilymphocyte Immunoglobulins

(1808-c)

Antilymphocyte immunoglobulins are polyclonal antibodies to human lymphocytes produced by the purification of sera from appropriately immunised animals. Although the term antilymphocyte immunoglobulin (ALG; lymphocyte immune globulin) implies a product raised against all lymphocyte subsets, whereas antithymocyte immunoglobulin (ATG) implies specificity for T-cells (thymus lymphocytes or thymocytes), in practice the nomenclature does not seem to be used consistently, and both terms have been used for apparently similar products. Nomenclature normally includes an indication of the animal source of the immunoglobulin e.g. antilymphocyte immunoglobulin (horse), or antithymocyte immunoglobulin (rabbit).

In addition to the purified immunoglobulins the native sera (antilymphocyte serum and antithymocyte serum, sometimes referred to as lymphocytic antiserum and thymitic antiserum) have also been used as immunosuppressants.

Adverse Effects and Precautions

Antilymphocyte immunoglobulins contain foreign proteins and hypersensitivity reactions are common, although the fact that these preparations are usually given with other immunosuppressants may help to reduce the incidence of reactions. Hypersensitivity may be manifested as serum sickness or dermatological reactions including rash, pruritus, and urticaria; anaphylaxis may occur in up to 1% of patients.

Other adverse effects may include fever and chills or shivering, nausea, tachycardia, and hypotension, occurring shortly after administration. Headache, dizziness, pains in muscles and joints, gastro-intestinal disturbances, and dyspnoea have also been reported. As well as lymphocytopenia patients may experience leucopenia and thrombocytopenia, usually transient. Nephrotoxicity has been reported. Thrombophlebitis is common following intravenous administration and administration into a vein with a rapid blood flow is recommended.

Antilymphocyte preparations are contra-indicated in hypersensitive patients, and patients should be tested for sensitivity before administration.

A study[1] in renal transplant patients given an immunosuppressive regimen comprising azathioprine and prednisone, with or without antithymocyte immunoglobulin, found that those who received antithymocyte immunoglobulin were more likely to have herpesvirus infections and inverted T-cell subset ratios. Regimens containing antithymocyte immunoglobulin may also increase infection with cytomegalovirus and Epstein-Barr virus.

1. Schooley RT, *et al.* Association of herpesvirus infections with T-lymphocyte-subset alterations, glomerulopathy, and opportunistic infections after renal transplantation. *N Engl J Med* 1983; **308:** 307–13.

Uses and Administration

Antilymphocyte immunoglobulins are antibodies, raised in *animals*, which act against lymphocytes, and in particular against T-cells, to produce suppression of cell-mediated immunity.

They may be added to existing immunosuppressant regimens to treat acute rejection episodes in patients who have undergone organ or tissue transplantation. Alternatively, they may be given prophylactically as part of a combination immunosuppressant regimen with other agents such as azathioprine, corticosteroids, and cyclosporin (so-called 'quadruple' therapy). For discussion of the role of antilymphocyte immunoglobulins in transplantation, see p.498 *et seq.*

Antilymphocyte immunoglobulins have also been used in the treatment of aplastic anaemia (p.701) in patients unsuitable for bone-marrow transplantation, and have been tried in other immunological disorders. Antilymphocyte immunoglobulins have been tried in the management of T-cell lymphomas (p.482).

Different antilymphocyte preparations may vary in their activity, as may different lots of the same preparation. However, doses in transplantation have usually ranged from 10 to 30 mg of immunoglobulin per kg body-weight daily, given as a slow intravenous infusion diluted in 250 to 500 mL or more of sodium chloride injection (0.9%), or other suitable diluent. It has been recommended that the final dilution should contain no more than 1 mg of immunoglobulin per mL and be given over 4 hours or more, via an in-line filter.

Immunoglobulin raised in *goats* was considered to be consistently more potent and less toxic than that from *horses.*[1] More recently, antithymocyte immunoglobulin derived from *rabbits* has been found to be more effective than the equine product in preventing renal graft rejection.[2]

1. Mears DC, *et al.* Guidelines for the preparation and use in humans of antithymocyte globulin. *Aust J Hosp Pharm* 1985; **15:** 153–7.
2. Gaber AO, *et al.* Results of the double-blind, randomized, multicenter, phase III clinical trial of Thymoglobulin versus Algam in the treatment of acute graft rejection episodes after renal transplantation. *Transplantation* 1998; **66:** 29–37.

Preparations

Proprietary Preparations (details are given in Part 3)

Austral.: Atgam; ***Belg.:*** ATG; Lymphoglobuline; Thymoglobuline; ***Canad.:*** Atgam; ***Fr.:*** Lymphoglobuline; Thymoglobuline; ***Ger.:*** Lymphoglobulin; Pressimmun†; ***Ital.:*** Lymphoglobuline; Lymphoser†; Pressimmun†; Uman-Gal E; ***Neth.:*** Atgam†; Lymphoglobuline; ***S.Afr.:*** Lymphoglobuline; Thymoglobuline; ***Spain:*** Atgam; Linfoglobulina; Lymphoser†; ***Switz.:*** ATG; Atgam; Lymphoglobuline; Lymphoser†; Thymoglobuline; ***UK:*** Pressimmune†; ***USA:*** Atgam.

Antineoplaston A10 (18767-m)

3-Phenylacetylamino-2,6-piperidinedione.

$C_{13}H_{14}N_2O_3$ = 246.3.

Antineoplaston A10 is one of a group of peptide derivatives isolated from blood and urine that has been investigated for the treatment of breast cancer and other malignant neoplasms although its value has been questioned (see below).

A critical review of the antineoplastons.[1] Most work has been done with antineoplaston A10, which is insoluble in aqueous solutions, and its derivatives antineoplaston AS2.5 (phenylacetylglutamine), and antineoplaston AS2.1 (a 4:1 mixture of phenylacetic acid and phenylacetylglutamine), which have not been independently shown to be active against cancer.

1. Green S. Antineoplastons: an unproved cancer therapy. *JAMA* 1992; **267:** 2924–8.

Asparaginase (1823-z)

Asparaginase *(USAN).*

L-Asparaginase; L-Asparagine Amidohydrolase; MK-965; NSC-109229; Re-82-TAD-15.

CAS — 9015-68-3.

NOTE. Colaspase and crisantaspase are *BAN* for asparaginase obtained from cultures of *Escherichia coli* and *Erwinia chrysanthemi* (*E. carotovora*) respectively.

Asparaginase should be stored at 2° to 8°. **Incompatible** with rubber. The manufacturers recommend that it should not be mixed with other drugs.

Stability. Although asparaginase was routinely kept under refrigeration,[1] information from a manufacturer (Merck Sharp & Dohme) indicated that it would remain stable for 48 hours at 15° to 30°.

1. Vogenberg FR, Souney PF. Stability guidelines for routinely refrigerated drug products. *Am J Hosp Pharm* 1983; **40:** 101–2.

Pegaspargase (15343-n)

Pegaspargase *(USAN, rINN)*.

PEG-L-asparaginase. A conjugate of colaspase with a polyethylene glycol of molecular weight 5000; Monomethoxypolyethylene glycol succinimidyl L-asparaginase.

CAS — 130167-69-0.

The manufacturers of pegaspargase state that it should be stored at 2° to 8° but should not be frozen as this destroys the activity.

Units

One unit of asparaginase splits 1 μmol of ammonia from L-asparagine in 1 minute under standard conditions.

Adverse Effects

Asparaginase may produce anaphylaxis and other hypersensitivity reactions including fever, rashes, and bronchospasm, due to its protein nature; there does not appear to be cross-sensitivity between asparaginase derived from *Escherichia coli* and that from *Erwinia chrysanthemi*. Hypersensitivity to pegaspargase is less common, but about 30% of patients hypersensitive to the native enzyme experience hypersensitivity to pegaspargase treatment.

Liver disorders occur in many patients, and there may be decreased blood concentrations of fibrinogen and clotting factors, alterations in blood lipids and cholesterol, and hypoalbuminaemia. Hyperammonaemia, due to the production of ammonia from asparagine, may occur. Uraemia, and occasionally renal failure, have been reported frequently. Pancreatitis may occur and may be fatal: there may also be hyperglycaemia due to decreased insulin production, and death from ketoacidosis has occurred.

Gastro-intestinal disturbances, including nausea and vomiting, and CNS disturbances, including drowsiness, depression, coma, hallucinations, and a Parkinson-like syndrome, have also been reported. Bone-marrow depression is rare, but acute leucopenia has occurred.

Effects on the blood. Both haemorrhage[1] (including intracranial haemorrhage[2]) and thrombosis[1,3] have been reported following asparaginase therapy, but overt symptoms seem to be relatively rare, perhaps because falls in antithrombin III are counteracted by the decrease in plasma coagulation factors.[3]

1. Priest JR, *et al.* A syndrome of thrombosis and hemorrhage complicating L-asparaginase therapy for childhood acute lymphoblastic leukemia. *J Pediatr* 1982; **100:** 984–9.
2. Lederman GS. Stroke due to treatment with L-asparaginase in an adult. *N Engl J Med* 1982; **307:** 1643.
3. Pitney WR, *et al.* Antithrombin III deficiency during asparaginase therapy. *Lancet* 1980; **i:** 493–4.

Effects on body temperature. Extreme hyperpyrexia, with a temperature of 42.6°, developed in a boy following administration of asparaginase as part of a combination regimen for relapsing acute lymphocytic leukaemia. The patient was successfully treated with ice packs and intravenous dantrolene.[1]

1. Smithson WA, *et al.* Dantrolene and potentially fatal hyperthermia secondary to L-asparaginase. *Cancer Treat Rep* 1983; **67:** 318–19.

Effects on carbohydrate metabolism. Hyperglycaemia occurred in 6 of 136 children receiving asparaginase; in 2 this was accompanied by ketoacidosis and both these patients required insulin therapy.[1] The other 4 children had their blood sugar regulated by dietary means.

1. Çetin M, *et al.* Hyperglycemia, ketoacidosis and other complications of L-asparaginase in children with acute lymphoblastic leukemia. *J Med* 1994; **25:** 219–29.

Effects on mental function. In a study involving 23 patients receiving asparaginase, 14 developed changes in mental function, ranging from mild lethargy and confusion to semicoma, delusions of persecution, bizarre behaviour, and inappropriate affect.[1] Most patients had moderate to marked elevation of blood-ammonia concentrations, and changes in mental function were generally accompanied by abnormal EEG readings.

1. Moure JMB, *et al.* Electroencephalogram changes secondary to asparaginase. *Arch Neurol* 1970; **23:** 365–8.

Precautions

For reference to the precautions necessary with antineoplastic agents and immunosuppressants, see Antineoplastic Agents, p.474.

Asparaginase is contra-indicated in patients with pancreatitis. It should be avoided in pregnancy. It should be given cautiously to patients with impaired liver function. Test doses should be administered at the start of treatment to check for hypersensitivity, as described below under Uses although such tests may not always be predictive. Re-treatment with asparaginase may be associated with an increased risk of allergic reactions.

Interactions

Asparaginase has been reported to interfere with tests of thyroid function by transient reduction of concentrations of thyroxine-binding globulin. If asparaginase is given before, rather than after, methotrexate the activity of the latter may be reduced. Asparaginase is also reported to decrease the clearance of vincristine.

Pharmacokinetics

Following intravenous injection the plasma half-life of the native enzyme has varied from about 8 to 30 hours; half-lives of up to 49 hours may be seen after intramuscular dosage. The half-life of pegaspargase is reported to be about 5.7 days. Asparaginase is found in the lymph at about 20% of the concentration in plasma. There is virtually no diffusion into the CSF. Little is excreted in the urine.

Uses and Administration

Asparaginase is an enzyme which acts as an antineoplastic agent by breaking down the amino acid L-asparagine to aspartic acid and ammonia. It interferes with the growth of those malignant cells which, unlike most healthy cells, are unable to synthesise L-asparagine for their metabolism, but resistance to its action develops fairly rapidly. Its action is reportedly specific for the G_1 phase of the cell cycle.

Asparaginase is used mainly for the induction of remissions in acute lymphoblastic leukaemia (p.478), although similar regimens have also been used for high-grade lymphomas (p.482). Regimens vary but it may be given intravenously in a dose of 1000 units per kg body-weight daily for 10 days following treatment with vincristine and prednisone or prednisolone, or intramuscularly in a dose of 6000 units per m^2 body-surface given every third day for 9 doses during treatment with vincristine and prednisone or prednisolone. Alternatively, in patients hypersensitive to the native enzyme it may be given as pegaspargase, in doses of 2500 units per m^2 every 14 days, preferably by intramuscular injection although the intravenous route may also be used. In patients with a body-surface area less than 0.6 m^2 a dose of 82.5 units of pegaspargase per kg body-weight, given every 14 days, is recommended.

Asparaginase is not generally used alone as an induction agent but doses of 200 units per kg daily have been given intravenously for 28 days to adults and children. If pegaspargase is used alone doses are the same as for combination regimens. Children appear to tolerate asparaginase better than adults.

Although not entirely reliable, an intradermal test dose of about 2 units has been recommended in the USA before treatment with asparaginase, or where more than a week has elapsed between doses; the injection site is observed for at least an hour for evidence of a positive reaction. Desensitisation has been advocated if no alternative antineoplastic treatment is available. The incidence of hypersensitivity is lower in patients given pegaspargase, and a test dose is not advocated.

When administered intravenously a solution of asparaginase in Water for Injections or sodium chloride injection (0.9%) should be given over not less than 30 minutes through a running infusion of sodium chloride injection or glucose injection (5%). When given intramuscularly no more than 2 mL of a solution in sodium chloride injection should be injected at a single site.

Conjugates of asparaginase with dextrans have also been tried.

References.

1. Anonymous. Pegaspargase for acute lymphoblastic leukemia. *Med Lett Drugs Ther* 1995; **37:** 23–4.
2. Holle LM. Pegaspargase: an alternative? *Ann Pharmacother* 1997; **31:** 616–24.

Preparations

Proprietary Preparations (details are given in Part 3)
Austral.: Leunase; ***Belg.:*** Paronal; ***Canad.:*** Kidrolase; ***Fr.:*** Kidrolase; ***Ger.:*** Crasnitin†; ***Ital.:*** Crasnitin; ***Jpn:*** Leunase; ***Neth.:*** Crasnitin†; ***S.Afr.:*** Laspar; ***Swed.:*** Erwinase; ***Switz.:*** Crasnitine†; ***UK:*** Erwinase; ***USA:*** Elspar; Oncaspar.

Azacitidine (1809-k)

Azacitidine *(USAN, rINN)*.

5-Azacytidine; Ladakamycin; NSC-102816; U-18496. 4-Amino-1-β-D-ribofuranosyl-1,3,5-triazin-2(1*H*)-one.

$C_8H_{12}N_4O_5$ = 244.2.

CAS — 320-67-2.

Stability. Azacitidine is very unstable in aqueous solutions, with a 10% loss of drug in about 2 to 3 hours at room temperature in sodium chloride solution (0.9%) or lactated Ringer's injection.[1,2] It is least unstable at higher concentrations and at a pH of between about 6 and 7 in such solutions.[2] However, it is markedly less stable in glucose injection (5%), with a 90% stability time of only 0.8 hours.[2] There has been reported to be no substantial decomposition of azacitidine dissolved in lactated Ringer's injection and stored in syringes at –20°.[3]

1. Chatterji DC. Stability of azacytidine in infusion solutions: clarification of conflicting literature data. *Am J Hosp Pharm* 1982; **39:** 1638–40.
2. Cheung Y-W, *et al.* Stability of azacitidine in infusion fluids. *Am J Hosp Pharm* 1984; **41:** 1156–9.
3. den Hartigh J, *et al.* Stability of azacitidine in lactated Ringer's injection frozen in polypropylene syringes. *Am J Hosp Pharm* 1989; **46:** 2500–5.

Uses and Administration

Azacitidine is an antimetabolite antineoplastic with general properties similar to those of cytarabine (p.526). It also inhibits cellular pyrimidine synthesis. It has been used mainly in the treatment of acute non-lymphoblastic leukaemia (p.479).

Azacitidine has also been investigated for the stimulation of fetal haemoglobin production in patients with thalassaemia (p.704) and sickle-cell anaemia (p.703).

Azathioprine (1812-l)

Azathioprine *(BAN, USAN, rINN)*.

Azathioprinum; BW-57322; NSC-39084. 6-(1-Methyl-4-nitroimidazol-5-ylthio)purine.

$C_9H_7N_7O_2S$ = 277.3.

CAS — 446-86-6.

NOTE. The abbreviation AZT, which has sometimes been used for azathioprine, has also been used to denote the antiviral zidovudine.

Pharmacopoeias. In *Eur.* (see p.viii), *Int.*, *Jpn*, *Pol.*, and *US*.
US also includes Azathioprine Sodium for Injection.

A pale yellow odourless powder. Practically **insoluble** in water, alcohol, and in chloroform; sparingly soluble in dilute mineral acids; dissolves in dilute solutions of alkali hydroxides. **Store** in airtight containers. Protect from light.

Adverse Effects and Treatment

For a general outline see Antineoplastics, p.470 and p.473.

Dose-related bone-marrow depression may be manifested as leucopenia or thrombocytopenia, or less often anaemia, and may occasionally be delayed. Macrocytic, including megaloblastic, anaemia has occurred. Azathioprine has also been associated with the development of liver damage; it has been suggested that cholestatic symptoms may be due to the mercaptopurine moiety. Rarely, delayed and potentially fatal veno-occlusive liver disease has occurred.

Other side-effects associated with azathioprine include gastro-intestinal disturbances, reversible alopecia, and symptoms including rashes, muscle and joint pains, fever, rigors, pneumonitis, pancreatitis, meningitis, arrhythmias, renal dysfunction, and h potension, some or all of which may represent hypersensitivity reactions.

Solutions for injection are irritant.

References.

1. Lawson DH, *et al.* Adverse effects of azathioprine. *Adverse Drug React Acute Poisoning Rev* 1984; 3: 161–71.

Carcinogenicity. Although immunosuppression may be associated with an increased risk of certain neoplasms (see p.470) a study in 755 patients given azathioprine for inflammatory bowel disease and followed for up to 29 years failed to show any increased risk of neoplasia.[1]

1. Connell WR, *et al.* Long-term neoplasia risk after azathioprine treatment in inflammatory bowel disease. *Lancet* 1994, **343:** 1249–52.

Effects on the blood. For the view that bone-marrow depression by azathioprine may be predictable, see under Mercaptopurine, p.546. However, despite suggestions of a correlation between low thiopurine methyltransferase (TPMT) activity and an increased risk of myelotoxicity (some clinicians have suggested that all patients should be tested for TPMT activity before receiving azathioprine[1]), Boulieu and colleagues noted that intracellular concentrations of thiopurine nucleotides alone were not correlated with bone marrow depression or red or white cell counts in patients receiving azathioprine.[2]

1. Jackson AP, *et al.* Thiopurine methyltransferase levels should be measured before commencing patients on azathioprine. *Br J Dermatol* 1997; **136:** 133–4.
2. Boulieu R, *et al.* Intracellular thiopurine nucleotides and azathioprine myelotoxicity in organ transplant patients. *Br J Clin Pharmacol* 1997; **43:** 116–18.

Effects on the liver. A review[1] of drug-related hepatotoxicity noted that azathioprine has been associated with hepatocanalicular cholestasis, in which the interference with bile flow is combined with hepatocyte damage, and with several hepatic vascular disorders, including focal sinusoidal dilatation, peliosis, and veno-occlusive disease.

1. Sherlock S. The spectrum of hepatotoxicity due to drugs. *Lancet* 1986; **ii:** 440–4.

Hypersensitivity. A report of 5 patients with acute allergic reactions associated with azathioprine.[1] In 2 of these patients, who had undergone renal transplantation, the symptoms (interstitial nephritis) were initially mistaken for acute rejection episodes.

1. Parnham AP, *et al.* Acute allergic reactions associated with azathioprine. *Lancet* 1996; **348:** 542–3.

Precautions

For reference to the precautions necessary with antineoplastics and immunosuppressants, see p.474.

Azathioprine should be used with care in patients with renal or hepatic impairment, in whom reduced doses may be required. It should generally be avoided in pregnancy (see below).

Pregnancy. Despite reports of chromosomal aberrations[1] or fetal growth retardation[2] in the offspring of mothers who received azathioprine during pregnancy, there seems to be little evidence that azathioprine is teratogenic in humans.[1,3-5] Given the nature of the severe chronic conditions for which azathioprine is generally used, discontinuing therapy in patients who become pregnant may not be necessary or desirable, but it seems prudent to avoid its use where possible during pregnancy.

1. The Registration Committee of the European Dialysis and Transplant Association. Successful pregnancies in women treated by dialysis and kidney transplantation. *Br J Obstet Gynaecol* 1980; **87:** 839–45.
2. Pirson Y, *et al.* Retardation of fetal growth in patients receiving immunosuppressive therapy. *N Engl J Med* 1985; **313:** 328.
3. Hou S. Retardation of fetal growth in patients receiving immunosuppressive therapy. *N Engl J Med* 1985; **313:** 328.
4. Whittle MJ, Hanretty KP. Prescribing in pregnancy: identifying abnormalities. *Br Med J* 1986; **293:** 1485–8.
5. Alstead EM, *et al.* Pregnancy in inflammatory bowel disease (IBD) patients on azathioprine. *Gut* 1989; **30:** A718.

Interactions

The effects of azathioprine are enhanced by allopurinol and the dose of azathioprine should be reduced to one-third to one-quarter of the usual dose when allopurinol is given concomitantly.

In addition to being affected by allopurinol, azathioprine may itself affect other drugs. For reference to the effects of azathioprine on competitive neuromuscular blockade, see under Immunosuppressants on p.1307. For the effects of azathioprine on warfarin anticoagulation see p.967.

[Ph]armacokinetics

[Azathi]oprine is well absorbed from the gastro-intes[tinal tract w]hen given by mouth. After oral or intra[venous admin]istration it disappears rapidly from the circulation and is extensively metabolised to mercaptopurine (which is then further metabolised—see p.546). Both azathioprine and mercaptopurine are about 30% bound to plasma proteins. About 10% of a dose of azathioprine is reported to be split between the sulphur and the purine ring to give 1-methyl-4-nitro-5-thioimidazole. The proportion of different metabolites is reported to vary between patients. Small amounts of unchanged azathioprine and mercaptopurine are eliminated in the urine.

Although plasma concentrations of 6-thiouric acid (the inactive product of mercaptopurine, and hence of azathioprine) can be readily measured in patients who have been receiving azathioprine, they are of little value in therapeutic drug monitoring.[1] The active moieties are the thioguanine nucleotides formed intracellularly, which appear to have extremely long half-lives,[2] and mean erythrocyte concentrations of which appear to vary considerably between individuals.[2]

1. Chan GLC, *et al.* Pharmacokinetics of 6-thiouric acid and 6-mercaptopurine in renal allograft recipients after oral administration of azathioprine. *Eur J Clin Pharmacol* 1989; **36:** 265–71.
2. Chan GLC, *et al.* Azathioprine metabolism: pharmacokinetics of 6-mercaptopurine, 6-thiouric acid and 6-thioguanine nucleotides in renal transplant patients. *J Clin Pharmacol* 1990; **30:** 358–63.

Uses and Administration

Azathioprine is an immunosuppressant with similar actions to those of mercaptopurine (see p.546), to which it is converted in the body. Its effects may not be seen for several weeks after administration. It is given by mouth; in patients in whom oral administration is not feasible it may be given intravenously as azathioprine sodium, by slow intravenous injection or by infusion, diluted in glucose or sodium chloride injections.

Azathioprine is mainly used as an immunosuppressant for the prevention of rejection in organ and tissue transplantation. The dose for this purpose varies from 1 to 5 mg per kg body-weight daily and depends partly on whether other drugs, such as a corticosteroid, or radiotherapy are employed at the same time. Withdrawal of the drug, with concomitant likelihood of rejection, may be necessary if toxicity occurs.

Azathioprine is also used in a wide variety of conditions which are considered to have an auto-immune component as indicated by the references given below. Its use in conjunction with a corticosteroid (see p.1015) may allow a lower dose of both drugs to be used, thus reducing adverse effects. The usual dose of azathioprine in these conditions is in the range of 1 to 3 mg per kg body-weight daily by mouth.

Blood counts should be carried out regularly during treatment and azathioprine withdrawn or the dosage reduced at the first indication of bone-marrow depression.

Blood disorders, non-malignant. Immunosuppressants such as azathioprine are occasionally tried in auto-immune haemolytic anaemia (p.702) refractory to other treatment and may permit reduction of corticosteroid dosage. Similarly in patients with idiopathic thrombocytopenic purpura (p.1023), immunosuppressants may be tried as a last resort.

Connective-tissue and muscular disorders. Azathioprine is one of many agents tried for disease control in Behçet's syndrome (p.1018). It is used similarly in polymyositis and systemic lupus erythematosus (see p.1027 and p.1029 respectively) and in the former condition combined therapy with azathioprine and a corticosteroid has been found to be better than a corticosteroid alone for maintenance long-term.[1] However, there is also some evidence that methotrexate may be more effective in refractory polymyositis than azathioprine.[2]

1. Bunch TW. Prednisone and azathioprine for polymyositis: long-term followup. *Arthritis Rheum* 1981; **24:** 45–8.
2. Joffe MM, *et al.* Drug therapy of the idiopathic inflammatory myopathies; predictors of response to prednisone, azathioprine, and methotrexate and a comparison of their efficacy. *Am J Med* 1993; **94:** 379–87.

Inflammatory bowel disease. Various drugs have been used in inflammatory bowel disease (p.1171) as an alternative to corticosteroids and aminosalicylates. Studies with azathioprine or its metabolite mercaptopurine have appeared to indicate some benefit in Crohn's disease, particularly where complicated by fistulas, and perhaps in refractory ulcerative colitis.[1-4] The onset of any benefit from oral azathioprine may be delayed for several months, but there is some evidence that a more rapid response can be achieved with an intravenous loading dose.[5] Azathioprine also exhibits a useful steroid-sparing effect, as confirmed by a meta-analysis[4] which found azathioprine to be useful both in the treatment of active Crohn's disease and in the maintenance of remission.

1. Lennard-Jones JE. Azathioprine and 6-mercaptopurine have a role in the treatment of Crohn's disease. *Dig Dis Sci* 1981; **26:** 364–8.
2. Kirk AP, Lennard-Jones JE. Controlled trial of azathioprine in chronic ulcerative colitis. *Br Med J* 1982; **284:** 1291–2.
3. Verhave M, *et al.* Azathioprine in the treatment of children with inflammatory bowel disease. *J Pediatr* 1990; **117:** 809–14.
4. Pearson DC, *et al.* Azathioprine and 6-mercaptopurine in Crohn disease: a meta-analysis. *Ann Intern Med* 1995; **122:** 132–42.
5. Sandborn WJ, *et al.* An intravenous loading dose of azathioprine decreases the time to response in patients with Crohn's disease. *Gastroenterology* 1995; **109:** 1808–17.

Liver disorders, non-malignant. Azathioprine has been widely used in combination with corticosteroids to produce and maintain remission of chronic active hepatitis,[1-5] as discussed on p.1019, and such combination therapy, which also permits a reduction in corticosteroid dosage, is generally thought to be more effective than azathioprine alone.[2,4] However recent results suggest that many patients successfully maintained in remission for at least a year on azathioprine with a corticosteroid can subsequently be maintained on azathioprine (at a higher dose of 2 mg per kg body-weight daily) alone.[6] Results in patients with primary biliary cirrhosis (p.497) have been more equivocal, and initial studies did not indicate much benefit from azathioprine,[7,8] although a later study did seem to indicate improved survival and disease retardation.[9]

1. Stavinoha MW, Soloway RD. Current therapy of chronic liver disease. *Drugs* 1990; **39:** 814–40.
2. Giusti G, *et al.* Immunosuppressive therapy in chronic active hepatitis (CAH): a multicentric retrospective study on 867 patients. *Hepatogastroenterology* 1984; **31:** 24–9.
3. Vegnente A, *et al.* Duration of chronic active hepatitis and the development of cirrhosis. *Arch Dis Child* 1984; **59:** 330–5.
4. Stellon AJ, *et al.* Randomised controlled trial of azathioprine withdrawal in autoimmune chronic active hepatitis. *Lancet* 1985; **i:** 668–70.
5. Brunner G, Hopf U. Relapse after azathioprine withdrawal in autoimmune chronic active hepatitis. *Lancet* 1985; **i:** 1216.
6. Johnson PJ, *et al.* Azathioprine for long-term maintenance of remission in autoimmune hepatitis. *N Engl J Med* 1995; **333:** 958–63.
7. Heathcote J, *et al.* A prospective controlled trial of azathioprine in primary biliary cirrhosis. *Gastroenterology* 1976; **70:** 656–60.
8. Crowe J, *et al.* Azathioprine in primary biliary cirrhosis: a preliminary report of an international trial. *Gastroenterology* 1980: **78:** 1005–10.
9. Christensen E, *et al.* Beneficial effect of azathioprine and prediction of prognosis in primary biliary cirrhosis: final results of an international trial. *Gastroenterology* 1985; **89:** 1084–91.

Lung disorders, non-malignant. For mention of the use of azathioprine in permitting a reduction of corticosteroid dosage in patients with interstitial lung disease, see p.1024.

Neuromuscular disorders. Azathioprine may be used for its steroid-sparing properties[5] in patients who require corticosteroid treatment for myasthenia gravis (p.1388). It may also be of use when corticosteroids are contra-indicated or when response to corticosteroids alone is insufficient.[6] Azathioprine is not usually used alone because it may be several months before any beneficial effect is seen. Studies have also indicated modest benefit from azathioprine[1,2] in patients with multiple sclerosis (p.620). It has been suggested that the benefits are too slight to justify the toxicity of the required doses,[3] but it has also been pointed out that in terms of relapse reduction azathioprine appears as effective as newer treatments such as interferon beta.[4]

1. British and Dutch Multiple Sclerosis Azathioprine Trial Group. Double-masked trial of azathioprine in multiple sclerosis. *Lancet* 1988; **ii:** 179–83.
2. Ellison GW, *et al.* A placebo-controlled, randomized, double-masked, variable dosage, clinical trial of azathioprine with and without methylprednisolone in multiple sclerosis. *Neurology* 1989; **39:** 1018–26.
3. Yudkin PL, *et al.* Overview of azathioprine treatment in multiple sclerosis. *Lancet* 1991; **338:** 1051–5.
4. Palace J, Rothwell P. New treatments and azathioprine in multiple sclerosis. *Lancet* 1997; **350:** 261.
5. Mantegazza R, *et al.* Azathioprine as a single drug or in combination with steroids in the treatment of myasthenia gravis. *J Neurol* 1988; **235:** 449–53.
6. Gajdos P, *et al.* Myasthenia Gravis Clinical Study Group. A randomised clinical trial comparing prednisone and azathioprine in myasthenia gravis: results of the second interim analysis. *J Neurol Neurosurg Psychiatry* 1993; **56:** 1157–63.

Ocular disorders, non-malignant. For mention of the use of azathioprine in various disorders characterised by ocular lesions such as scleritis or uveitis, see p.498.

Organ and tissue transplantation. Azathioprine plays an important part in regimens for the prevention of graft rejection following organ transplantation. For references to its use in the transplantation of heart, kidney, liver, and lung see p.499, p.499, p.500, and p.501 respectively, while its use in pancreatic transplantation is discussed on p.501.

Psoriatic arthritis. Azathioprine may be useful for severe or progressive cases of psoriatic arthritis (see under Spondyloarthropathies, p.4) when the arthritis is not controlled by physical therapy and NSAIDs.

Rheumatoid arthritis. Azathioprine has been tried in rheumatoid arthritis (p.2) but is reported to be less effective than methotrexate,[1] and is certainly much less widely used. It may however be useful in patients with severe disease unresponsive to other drugs especially in those with extra-articular manifestations such as vasculitis.[2]

1. Jeurissen MEC, *et al.* Influence of methotrexate and azathioprine on radiologic progression in rheumatoid arthritis: a randomized, double-blind study. *Ann Intern Med* 1991; **114:** 999–1004.
2. Heurkens AHM, *et al.* Prednisone plus azathioprine treatment in patients with rheumatoid arthritis complicated by vasculitis. *Arch Intern Med* 1991; **151:** 2249–54.

Sarcoidosis. Cytotoxic immunosuppressants such as azathioprine have been tried in patients with sarcoidosis (p.1028) who do not respond to or cannot tolerate corticosteroids.

Skin disorders, non-malignant. Like other immunosuppressants, azathioprine has been tried in various refractory skin disorders, notably in pemphigus (see below). Other conditions in which it has been tried include atopic eczema,[1-3] nodular prurigo,[4] chronic actinic dermatitis,[3] pyoderma gangrenosum,[2] and erythema multiforme[2,5] (see p.1074) as well as in the skin manifestations of systemic disorders such as dermatomyositis and lupus erythematosus.

1. Lear JT, *et al.* A retrospective review of the use of azathioprine in severe atopic dermatitis. *Br J Dermatol* 1996; **135:** (suppl 47): 38.
2. Tan BB, *et al.* Azathioprine in dermatology: a survey of current practice in the UK. *Br J Dermatol* 1997; **136:** 351–5.
3. Younger IR, *et al.* Azathioprine in dermatology. *J Am Acad Dermatol* 1991; **25:** 281–6.
4. Lear JT, *et al.* Nodular prurigo responsive to azathioprine. *Br J Dermatol* 1996; **134:** 1151.
5. Schofield JK, *et al.* Recurrent erythema multiforme: clinical features and treatment in a large series of patients. *Br J Dermatol* 1993; **128:** 542–5.

PEMPHIGUS AND PEMPHIGOID. Corticosteroids are the main treatment for blistering in pemphigus and pemphigoid (p.1075). Immunosuppressive therapy, including azathioprine,[1] has been used in combination with corticosteroids to permit a reduction in corticosteroid dosage. However, it has been suggested that evidence for the steroid-sparing effect is lacking and that immunosuppressants should be reserved for patients who cannot tolerate corticosteroids or in whom they are contra-indicated.[2]

1. Aberer W, *et al.* Azathioprine in the treatment of pemphigus vulgaris: a long-term follow-up. *J Am Acad Dermatol* 1987; **16:** 527–33.
2. Bystryn J-C, Steinman NM. The adjuvant therapy of pemphigus: an update. *Arch Dermatol* 1996; **132:** 203–12.

Vasculitic syndromes. Azathioprine has been tried in a number of the vasculitic syndromes, including giant cell arteritis (p.1021), microscopic polyangiitis (p.1027), Churg-Strauss syndrome (p.1019), and Wegener's granulomatosis (p.1031). In general it is most useful in maintenance for its steroid-sparing effect. Cyclophosphamide tends to be preferred where a more aggressive regimen is required, as in some combinations for induction of remission.

Preparations

BP 1998: Azathioprine Tablets;
USP 23: Azathioprine Sodium for Injection; Azathioprine Tablets.

Proprietary Preparations (details are given in Part 3)
Aust.: Imurek; ***Austral.:*** Imuran; Thioprine; ***Belg.:*** Imuran; ***Canad.:*** Imuran; ***Fr.:*** Imurel; ***Ger.:*** Imurek; Zytrim; ***Irl.:*** Azopine; Imuran; ***Ital.:*** Imuran†; ***Neth.:*** Imuran; ***Norw.:*** Imurel; ***S.Afr.:*** Azapress; Imuran; ***Spain:*** Imurel; ***Swed.:*** Imurel; ***Switz.:*** Imurek; ***UK:*** Azamune; Berkaprine†; Immunoprin; Imuran; Oprisine; ***USA:*** Imuran.

Multi-ingredient: ***Ger.:*** Azamedac.

Basiliximab (9707-g)

Basiliximab *(rINN)*.

CAS — 179045-86-4.

Basiliximab is a chimeric murine monoclonal anti-interleukin-2 receptor (CD25) antibody. It is used in the prevention of acute graft rejection in patients undergoing organ transplantation, in conjunction with other immunosuppressants. The recommended dose is 20 mg by intravenous infusion over 20 to 30 minutes, given within 2 hours before surgery and repeated after 4 days.

References.

1. Nashan B, *et al.* Randomised trial of basiliximab versus placebo for control of acute cellular rejection in renal allograft recipients. *Lancet* 1997; **350:** 1193–8. Correction. *ibid.*; 1484.

Preparations

Proprietary Preparations (details are given in Part 3)
UK: Simulect; ***USA:*** Simulect.

Batimastat (14528-h)

Batimastat *(BAN, USAN, rINN)*.

BB-94. (2*S*,3*R*)-5-Methyl-3-{[(α*S*)-α-(methylcarbamoyl)phenethyl]carbamoyl}-2-[(2-thienylthio)methyl]hexanohydroxamic acid; (2*S*,3*R*)-*N*¹-Hydroxy-3-isobutyl-*N*⁴-[(*S*)-α-(methylcarbamoyl)phenethyl]-2-(2-thienylthiomethyl)succinamide.

$C_{23}H_{31}N_3O_4S_2$ = 477.6.

CAS — 130370-60-4.

Batimastat is an inhibitor of matrix metalloproteinases, enzymes which are thought to play a role in the metastasis of cancer cells. It has been investigated in a variety of malignant disorders.

Bicalutamide (7259-v)

Bicalutamide *(BAN, USAN, rINN)*.

ICI-176334. (*RS*)-4′-Cyano-α′,α′,α′-trifluoro-3-(4-fluorophenylsulphonyl)-2-hydroxy-2-methylpropiono-*m*-toluidide.

$C_{18}H_{14}F_4N_2O_4S$ = 430.4.

CAS — 90357-06-5.

Adverse Effects and Precautions

As for Flutamide, p.537.

Cardiovascular effects including angina, arrhythmias, and ECG changes have been reported rarely.

Although clinical experience with bicalutamide was limited, there was some evidence that it was better tolerated than either flutamide or nilutamide; in particular it appeared to be associated with a lower incidence of diarrhoea in clinical trials.[1]

1. Kaisary AV. Compliance with hormonal treatment for prostate cancer. *Br J Hosp Med* 1996; **55:** 359–66.

Pharmacokinetics

Bicalutamide is well absorbed following oral administration. It undergoes extensive metabolism in the liver, the active *R*-enantiomer predominantly by oxidation, the *S*-enantiomer primarily by glucuronidation. It is excreted as metabolites in urine and faeces. The half-life of the *R*-enantiomer is about 5.8 days, and may be prolonged still further in severe hepatic impairment. The *S*-enantiomer is cleared more rapidly. Bicalutamide is about 96% bound to plasma proteins.

Uses and Administration

Bicalutamide is a nonsteroidal anti-androgen with actions and uses similar to those of flutamide (p.537). It is used in the palliative treatment of prostatic cancer (p.491). The usual dose by mouth is 50 mg daily in combination with a gonadorelin analogue; treatment should be started at least 3 days before commencing the gonadorelin analogue to suppress any flare reaction. Bicalutamide has also been given in combination with surgical castration.

References.

1. Anonymous. Bicalutamide for prostate cancer. *Med Lett Drugs Ther* 1996; **38:** 56–7.
2. Soloway MS, *et al.* Bicalutamide in the treatment of advanced prostatic carcinoma: a phase II noncomparative multicenter trial evaluating safety, efficacy and long-term endocrine effects of monotherapy. *J Urol (Baltimore)* 1995; **154:** 2110–14.
3. Schellhammer P, *et al.* A controlled trial of bicalutamide versus flutamide, each in combination with luteinizing hormone-releasing hormone analogue therapy, in patients with advanced prostate cancer. *Urology* 1995; **45:** 745–52.
4. Schellhammer PF, *et al.* Clinical benefits of bicalutamide compared with flutamide in combined androgen blockade for patients with advanced prostatic carcinoma: final report of a double-blind, randomized, multicenter trial. *Urology* 1997; **50:** 330–6.

Preparations

Proprietary Preparations (details are given in Part 3)
Austral.: Cosudex; ***Canad.:*** Casodex; ***Ger.:*** Casodex; ***Irl.:*** Casodex; ***Ital.:*** Casodex; ***Neth.:*** Casodex; ***Norw.:*** Casodex; ***S.Afr.:*** Casodex; ***Spain:*** Casodex; ***Swed.:*** Casodex; ***Switz.:*** Casodex; ***UK:*** Casodex; ***USA:*** Casodex.

Bisantrene Hydrochloride (18846-h)

Bisantrene Hydrochloride *(USAN, rINNM)*.

ADAH; ADCA; CL-216942; NSC-337766; Orange Crush. 9,10-Anthracenedicarboxaldehyde bis(2-imidazolin-2-ylhydrazone) dihydrochloride.

$C_{22}H_{22}N_8,2HCl$ = 471.4.

CAS — 78186-34-2 (bisantrene); 71439-68-4 (bisantrene hydrochloride).

Bisantrene is a cell-cycle nonspecific antineoplastic agent which is believed to act by intercalation with DNA. It has been used as the hydrochloride in the treatment of acute non-lymphoblastic leukaemias relapsed or refractory to other therapy.

Preparations

Proprietary Preparations (details are given in Part 3)
Fr.: Zantrene†.

Bleomycin Sulphate (1815-z)

Bleomycin Sulphate *(BANM, pINNM)*.

Bleomycin Sulfate *(USAN)*; Bleomycini Sulfas.

CAS — 11056-06-7 (bleomycin); 9041-93-4 (bleomycin sulphate).

Pharmacopoeias. In *Eur.* (see p.viii), *Int.*, *Jpn*, and *US*.
Int. and *Jpn* also include Bleomycin Hydrochloride. *Chin.* includes Bleomycin Hydrochloride for Injection.

The sulphates of a mixture of basic antineoplastic glycopeptide antibiotics, obtained by the growth of *Streptomyces verticillus* or by any other means; the two principal components of the mixture are *N*¹-[3-(dimethyl-sulphonio)propyl]-bleomycinamide (bleomycin A_2) and *N*¹-4-(guanidobutyl)bleomycinamide (bleomycin B_2).

A white or yellowish white or cream-coloured amorphous very hygroscopic powder. It loses not more than 3% of its weight when dried. Very **soluble** in water; slightly soluble in dehydrated alcohol; practically insoluble in acetone and in ether. A 0.5% solution in water has a pH of 4.5 to 6.0. **Store** in airtight containers at a temperature of 2° to 8°.

Bleomycin Sulfate (USP) contains between 55% and 70% of bleomycin A_2 and between 25% and 32% of bleomycin B_2; the content of bleomycin B_4 is not more than 1%. The combined percentage of bleomycin A_2 and B_2 is not less than 85%.

The manufacturers of bleomycin suggest that it should be protected from light.

Incompatibility. Dorr and colleagues have reported a loss of bleomycin activity when bleomycin sulphate solutions were mixed with solutions of carbenicillin, cephazolin or cephalothin sodium, nafcillin sodium, benzylpenicillin sodium, methotrexate, mitomycin, hydrocortisone sodium succinate, aminophylline, ascorbic acid, or terbutaline.[1] D'Arcy has summarised the interactions of bleomycin as the chelation of divalent and trivalent cations (especially copper), inactivation by compounds containing sulfhydryl groups, and precipitation by hydrophobic anions; solutions of bleomycin should not be mixed with solutions of essential amino acids, riboflavine, dexamethasone, or frusemide.[2]

1. Dorr RT, *et al.* Bleomycin compatibility with selected intravenous medications. *J Med* 1982; **13:** 121–30.
2. D'Arcy PF. Reactions and interactions in handling anticancer drugs. *Drug Intell Clin Pharm* 1983; **17:** 532–8.

Stability. Suggestions that bleomycin sulphate solutions lost potency when stored in plastic containers, and should be stored in glass,[1,2] have not been borne out by subsequent studies. De Vroe and colleagues reported no significant loss of bleomycin from solutions diluted in either 0.9% sodium chloride or 5% glucose infusion solutions stored in glass or plastic,[3] while Stajich and others found no significant difference in bleomycin-induced cell lethality between solutions added to 5% glucose injection and stored in glass or plastic containers.[4] Other work suggests that in fact it is the diluent rather than the container which affects stability: Koberda and coworkers noted an approximately 13% loss of bleomycin at room temperature over 24 hours from solutions diluted in 5% glucose injection, whether stored in glass or plastic, whereas concentrations in 0.9% sodium chloride remained constant over this time.[5] They conclude that bleomycin should not be diluted in 5% glucose injection.

1. Benvenuto JA, *et al.* Stability and compatibility of antitumor agents in glass and plastic containers. *Am J Hosp Pharm* 1981; **38:** 1914–18.
2. Adams J, *et al.* Instability of bleomycin in plastic containers. *Am J Hosp Pharm* 1982; **39:** 1636.
3. De Vroe C, *et al.* A study on the stability of three antineoplastic drugs and on their sorption by iv delivery systems and end-line filters. *Int J Pharmaceutics* 1990; **65:** 49–56.
4. Stajich GV, *et al.* In vitro evaluation of bleomycin-induced cell lethality from plastic and glass containers. *DICP Ann Pharmacother* 1991; **25:** 14–16.
5. Koberda M, *et al.* Stability of bleomycin sulfate reconstituted in 5% dextrose injection or 0.9% sodium chloride injection stored in glass vials or polyvinyl chloride containers. *Am J Hosp Pharm* 1990; **47:** 2528–9.

Units

8910 units of bleomycin complex A_2/B_2 are contained in 5 mg of bleomycin complex in one ampoule of the first International Reference Preparation (1980). The Ph. Eur. specifies a potency of not less than 1500 international units (iu) per mg, calculated with reference to the dried substance.

These units differ from those used by the USP: Bleomycin Sulfate (USP) contains 1.5 to 2.0 units of bleomycin in each mg. Doses are expressed in terms of these units.

In some countries doses were formerly described in terms of mg-potency, where 1 mg-potency corresponded to 1 unit. In the original preparation 1 mg-potency was equivalent to 1 mg-weight but improvements in purification of the product led to a situation in which ampoules labelled as containing 15 mg (i.e. 15 units) contained far fewer mg-weight of bleomycin. Doses are therefore now given in terms of units. However, a recent change in the labelling of the commercial preparation in the UK, from units equivalent to those of the USP to units equivalent to those of the Ph. Eur., has resulted in an apparent but artefactual increase in UK doses by a factor of 1000.

Adverse Effects and Treatment

For a general outline see Antineoplastics, p.470 and p.473.

The most frequent side-effects with bleomycin involve the skin and mucous membranes and include rash, erythema, pruritus, vesiculation, hyperkeratosis, nail changes, alopecia, hyperpigmentation, striae, and stomatitis. Fever is also common, and acute anaphylactoid reactions with hyperpyrexia and cardiorespiratory collapse have been reported in about 1% of patients with lymphoma. There is little depression of the bone marrow. Local reactions and thrombophlebitis may occur at the site of parenteral administration.

The most serious delayed effect is pulmonary toxicity; interstitial pneumonitis and fibrosis occurs in about 10% of patients and produces an overall mortality rate of 1% of patients treated with bleomycin. Pulmonary toxicity is more likely in elderly patients and those given total doses greater than 400 000 international units (400 USP units).

Effects on the nails. A patient developed blistering and ulceration after injection of bleomycin into periungual warts, and many nails fell off.[1] A previous set of injections, 1 month before, had caused only mild pain. Two years later the patient still had complete loss of the nail in one finger, which had also developed Raynaud's phenomenon, and partial loss of nails on 3 other digits.

1. Czarnecki D. Bleomycin and periungual warts. *Med J Aust* 1984; **141:** 40.

Effects on respiratory function. For discussion of the effects of bleomycin on the lungs, see under the chapter introduction, p.473. For the suggestion that pulmonary toxicity may be potentiated by concomitant use of cisplatin or colony-stimulating factors, see Interactions, below.

Effects on the vascular system. Although reports of thrombo-embolic disorders and Raynaud's syndrome have been associated with use of bleomycin in combination regimens, particularly with cisplatin and the vinca alkaloids (see p.471) there is some evidence for an association of Raynaud's syndrome with the use of bleomycin alone.[1,2]

See also Effects on the Nails, above.

1. Sundstrup B. Raynaud's phenomenon after bleomycin treatment. *Med J Aust* 1978; **2:** 266.
2. Adone D, Arlet P. Bleomycin and Raynaud's phenomenon. *Ann Intern Med* 1984; **100:** 770.

Precautions

For reference to the precautions necessary with antineoplastics and immunosuppressants, see p.474.

The risk of pulmonary toxicity is increased in the ᵉˡderly, in patients with renal impairment or pulmonary infection or pre-existing impairment of pulmonary function, and in those who have received radiotherapy, particularly to the thorax. Bleomycin should be given with great caution to such patients and a reduction in dosage may well be necessary.

In view of the risk of an anaphylactoid reaction it has been suggested that patients with lymphomas should receive a test dose of 1000 or 2000 iu (1 or 2 USP units) initially.

AIDS. Cutaneous adverse effects occurred in 12 of 50 patients being treated with bleomycin for AIDS-associated Kaposi's sarcoma and increased in severity until bleomycin was withdrawn.[1] Bleomycin should be stopped in people with AIDS if cutaneous side-effects are seen, and rechallenge should be avoided. However, the incidence of side-effects did not appear to be higher in these patients than in cancer patients, and patients with AIDS seem to be less sensitive to bleomycin than to antibacterials such as co-trimoxazole and penicillins.

1. Caumes E, *et al.* Cutaneous side-effects of bleomycin in AIDS patients with Kaposi's sarcoma. *Lancet* 1990; **336:** 1593.

Diving. Since the partial pressure of oxygen in the inspired air of a scuba diver increases with increasing depth, a theoretical possibility exists of a toxic [pulmonary] reaction to oxygen in bleomycin-treated patients who subsequently go diving, and such a risk would increase with the depth and duration of each dive.[1]

1. Zanetti CL. Scuba diving and bleomycin therapy. *JAMA* 1990; **264:** 2869.

Handling and disposal. Urine produced for up to 72 hours after a dose of bleomycin should be handled wearing protective clothing.[1]

1. Harris J, Dodds LJ. Handling waste from patients receiving cytotoxic drugs. *Pharm J* 1985; **235:** 289–91.

Interactions

There may be an increased risk of pulmonary toxicity in patients given bleomycin who receive oxygen, for example as part of a general anaesthetic procedure.

Enhanced pulmonary toxicity, in some cases fatal, has been reported in patients given bleomycin and cisplatin,[1-3] presumably because cisplatin-induced renal failure led to a decrease in bleomycin elimination. It seems reasonable to assume that similar interactions might occur if bleomycin were given with other nephrotoxic agents. It has been suggested that apart from a decrease in bleomycin dosage if nephrotoxicity occurs with such a combination, administration of bleomycin by constant infusion rather than intermittent bolus might increase the therapeutic to toxic ratio.[1]

An increased incidence of pulmonary toxicity has also been reported in patients receiving bleomycin as part of the ABVD regimen (with doxorubicin, vinblastine, and dacarbazine) who were given granulocyte colony-stimulating factor to alleviate neutropenia.[4] It was suggested that the increase in neutrophil counts and stimulation of their ability to produce superoxide radicals produced by the colony-stimulating factor might be potentiating lung injury. Another case of rapidly developing and fatal pneumonitis in a patient given BEP (bleomycin, etoposide, and cisplatin) with granulocyte colony-stimulating factor has been reported;[5] however, others have queried the association.[6,7]

1. Bennett WM, *et al.* Fatal pulmonary bleomycin toxicity in cisplatin-induced acute renal failure. *Cancer Treat Rep* 1980; **64:** 921–4.
2. van Barneveld PWC, *et al.* Influence of platinum-induced renal toxicity on bleomycin-induced pulmonary toxicity in patients with disseminated testicular carcinoma. *Oncology* 1984; **41:** 4–7.
3. Brodsky A, *et al.* Stevens-Johnson syndrome, respiratory distress and acute renal failure due to synergic bleomycin-cisplatin toxicity. *J Clin Pharmacol* 1989; **29:** 821–3.
4. Matthews JH. Pulmonary toxicity of ABVD chemotherapy and G-CSF in Hodgkin's disease: possible synergy. *Lancet* 1993; **342:** 988.
5. Dirix LY, *et al.* Pulmonary toxicity and bleomycin. *Lancet* 1994; **344:** 56.
6. Bastion Y, *et al.* Possible toxicity with the association of G-CSF and bleomycin. *Lancet* 1994; **343:** 1221–2.
7. Bastion Y, Coffier B. Pulmonary toxicity of bleomycin: is G-CSF a risk factor? *Lancet* 1994; **344:** 474.

Pharmacokinetics

Bleomycin is thought to be poorly absorbed from the gastro-intestinal tract. Following parenteral administration some 60 to 70% of a dose has been reported to be excreted in urine as active drug. Most tissues, but not lung or skin, are capable of enzymic degradation of bleomycin. Bleomycin does not cross the blood-brain barrier.

Bleomycin appears to be eliminated in a biphasic manner: Alberts and colleagues reported mean initial and terminal elimination half-lives of 24 minutes and 4 hours respectively in 8 adult patients with normal renal function who received bleomycin by intravenous bolus.[1] Elimination may be more prolonged when bleomycin is given by continuous intravenous infusion, and Broughton and others reported mean initial and terminal half-lives of 1.3 and 8.9 hours in 8 patients after termination of infusion.[2] Although about 60% of a dose was eliminated in urine over 48 hours,[2] and both studies demonstrated markedly prolonged half-lives in patients with renal failure,[1,2] Broughton reported evidence that a non-renal mechanism could contribute to the elimination of bleomycin.[2] Yee and co-workers studied the disposition of bleomycin in children, with results suggesting that although the pharmacokinetics of bleomycin are the same in older children as in adults, younger children eliminate the drug significantly more rapidly.[3]

1. Alberts DS, *et al.* Bleomycin pharmacokinetics in man I: intravenous administration. *Cancer Chemother Pharmacol* 1978; **1:** 177–81.
2. Broughton A, *et al.* Clinical pharmacology of bleomycin following intravenous infusion as determined by radioimmunoassay. *Cancer* 1977; **40:** 2772–8.
3. Yee GC, *et al.* Bleomycin disposition in children with cancer. *Clin Pharmacol Ther* 1983; **33:** 668–73.

Uses and Administration

Bleomycin is an antineoplastic antibiotic which binds to DNA and causes strand scissions. It is widely used to treat malignant disease, as indicated by the cross references below; uses include squamous cell carcinomas, including those of the cervix and external genitalia, oesophagus, skin, and head and neck; Hodgkin's disease and other lymphomas; and malignant neoplasms of the testis. It has also been tried in other malignancies, including carcinoma of the bladder, lung, and thyroid, some sarcomas, including Kaposi's sarcoma, and in the treatment of malignant effusions.

Bleomycin is often used in association with other antineoplastic agents, notably with doxorubicin, vinblastine, and dacarbazine for Hodgkin's disease, and with etoposide and cisplatin in testicular tumours. Bleomycin is given by either the intramuscular, intravenous, or subcutaneous route. It may also be administered intra-arterially and has been instilled intrapleurally or intraperitoneally. If intramuscular injections are painful they may be given in a 1% solution of lignocaine.

- *Doses are calculated in terms of units of the base but the **units** used for the commercial preparation in the UK, which were formerly equivalent to those of the USP, are now international units (iu) equivalent to those of the Ph. Eur. (see Units, above). Since 1000 iu is equivalent to 1 USP unit, UK doses now appear to be 1000 times greater than those previously in use, or than those in use in the USA, and care is recommended in evaluating the literature.*

In the UK the usual dose as a single agent for **squamous cell** or **testicular tumours** is 15 000 iu (15 USP units) three times a week, or 30 000 iu twice a week, by intramuscular or intravenous injection. This may be repeated, at usual intervals of 3 to 4 weeks, up to a total cumulative dose of 500 000 iu or less (see below). Doses should be adjusted according to tolerance, and may need to be adjusted as part of combination chemotherapy. The dose should be reduced in those over 60 years of age. Continuous intravenous infusion at a rate of 15 000 iu per 24 hours for up to 10 days or 30 000 iu per 24 hours for up to 5 days may also be used. In patients with **lymphoma** a dose of 15 000 iu once or twice weekly by intramuscular injection has been suggested, to a total dose of 225 000 iu. Again, dosage should be reduced in older patients and in combination regimens if necessary. In the treatment of **malignant effusions** a solution of 60 000 iu in 100 mL of 0.9% sodium chloride solution may be instilled into the affected serous cavity. Treatment may be repeated as necessary up to the appropriate total cumulative dose for the patient's age.

In the USA recommended doses for **lymphomas** as well as **squamous cell** and **testicular** neoplasms are 250 to 500 iu per kg body-weight (0.25 to 0.5 USP units per kg), or 10 000 to 20 000 iu per m^2 body-surface (10 to 20 USP units per m^2), given once or twice weekly. A dose of 1000 or 2000 iu (1 or 2 USP units) initially, or for the first two doses, has been suggested in patients with lymphoma. In patients with Hodgkin's disease, once a 50% response has been achieved it may be maintained with 1000 iu (1 USP unit) of bleomycin daily, or 5000 iu (5 USP units) weekly.

In the UK, manufacturers suggest that a total dose of 500 000 iu (500 USP units) should not be exceeded. Total cumulative dose should not exceed 300 000 iu in those aged 60 to 69, 200 000 iu in those 70 to 79, and 100 000 iu in those 80 and over; the weekly dose should be no more than 30 000 and 15 000 iu respectively in the latter 2 groups. In the USA the recommended maximum total dose is 400 000 iu (400 USP units); it is generally agreed that patients receiving 400 000 iu or more are at increased risk of pulmonary toxicity (see Adverse Effects, above).

Doses may require adjustment when given in combination with other antineoplastic agents, or with radiotherapy. Dosage should be reduced in patients with renal impairment.

Leucoplakia. Leucoplakia is used to describe a white patch or plaque in the mouth which cannot be otherwise characterised: such lesions are of concern because they may be premalignant (see also p.487). It should be distinguished from oral hairy leucoplakia which is associated with HIV infection. Where active treatment is desirable small, easily accessible lesions can be removed surgically; for the treatment of extensive patches or those in which surgery would be difficult topical bleomycin may be dissolved in dimethyl sulphoxide and applied at a dose of 15 000 iu daily for 10 consecutive days.[1] Clinical response to this form of treatment is good and can give sustained effects on long-term follow-up.

Chemoprevention with retinoids or betacarotene is under investigation for patients with leucoplakia.[2]

1. Lamey P-J, Lewis MAO. Oral medicine in practice: white patches. *Br Dent J* 1990; **168:** 147–52.
2. Boyle P, *et al.* Oral cancer: necessity for prevention strategies. *Lancet* 1993; **342:** 1129.

Malignant effusions. Bleomycin is used for the sclerotherapy of malignant pleural effusions (p.484) and some consider it a better agent for this purpose than a tetracycline, which are often considered the sclerosants of choice.

Malignant neoplasms. Bleomycin is employed in regimens for the management of Hodgkin's disease and non-Hodgkin's lymphomas (see p.481, p.482, and p.483), for cervical cancer, gestational trophoblastic tumours, and tumours of the ovary and testis (see p.487, p.477, p.491, and p.493), and for some other malignancies including those of the gastro-intestinal tract (p.487), head and neck, (p.489), thyroid (p.494), sarcomas of bone (p.495), and Kaposi's sarcoma (p.496).

Pneumothorax. In a patient with AIDS and *Pneumocystis carinii* pneumonia who developed pneumothorax, instillation of bleomycin into each pleural cavity was successful in resolving the pneumothorax after tetracycline sclerotherapy failed to do so.[1]

1. Hnatiuk OW, *et al.* Bleomycin sclerotherapy for bilateral pneumothoraces in a patient with AIDS. *Ann Intern Med* 1990; **113:** 988–90.

Warts. A number of studies have examined the local use of bleomycin sulphate to treat warts. Shumack and Haddock reported an overall cure rate of over 99% from the injection of bleomycin into the base of 1052 warts of the common, plane, plantar, eponychial, and mosaic types[1] while Bunney and colleagues found intralesional injection of bleomycin to be superior to placebo in a double-blind study in 24 patients with 59 matched pairs of refractory warts.[2] In both these studies bleomycin was given as a 0.1% solution, usually as a 0.1 mL injection. In addition to intralesional injection, bleomycin has also been reported to be successful in clearing common warts from 6 of 7 patients when applied as a pressure-sensitive adhesive tape, although the technique failed in 2 patients with plantar warts.[3] Although most studies have reported benefit from the use of bleomycin, Munkvad and colleagues failed to find any benefit from intralesional injection of bleomycin in 62 patients with 108 warts when compared with placebo treatment.[4] These authors advise against the use of bleomycin, pointing out the potential for toxicity, but at the doses used adverse effects, other than pain at the injection site,[1,2,4] do not seem to be common; however, nail dystrophy and Raynaud's phenomenon have been reported (see under Effects on the Nails, under Adverse Effects, above).

Use of cytotoxic agents for the management of warts is usually reserved for severe or resistant cases; for discussion of other methods that may be used, see p.1076.

1. Shumack PH, Haddock MJ. Bleomycin: an effective treatment for warts. *Australas J Dermatol* 1979; **20:** 41–2.
2. Bunney MH, *et al.* The treatment of resistant warts with intralesional bleomycin: a controlled clinical trial. *Br J Dermatol* 1984; **111:** 197–207.
3. Takigawa M, *et al.* Treatment of viral warts with pressure-sensitive adhesive tape containing bleomycin sulfate. *Arch Dermatol* 1985; **121:** 1108.
4. Munkvad M, *et al.* Locally injected bleomycin in the treatment of warts. *Dermatologica* 1983; **167:** 86–9.

Preparations

USP 23: Bleomycin for Injection.

Proprietary Preparations (details are given in Part 3)
Austral.: Blenoxane; ***Canad.:*** Blenoxane; ***Ger.:*** Bleo-cell; ***Jpn:*** Bleo; Bleo-S; Oil Bleo†; ***S.Afr.:*** Blenoxane; ***UK:*** Bleo; ***USA:*** Blenoxane.

Brequinar Sodium (1739-t)

Brequinar Sodium *(USAN, rINNM)*.

DuP-785; NSC-368390. Sodium 6-fluoro-2-(2′-fluoro-4-biphenylyl)-3-methyl-4-quinolinecarboxylate.

$C_{23}H_{14}F_2NO_2Na = 397.3$.

CAS — 96187-53-0 (brequinar); 96201-88-6 (brequinar sodium).

Brequinar sodium is an inhibitor of pyrimidine metabolism with potent immunosuppressant properties which is under investigation for the prevention and treatment of rejection episodes following organ and tissue transplantation.

References.

1. Arteaga CL, *et al.* Phase I clinical and pharmacokinetic trial of brequinar sodium (DuP-785; NSC-368390). *Cancer Res* 1989; **49:** 4648–53.
2. Murphy MP, Morris RE. Brequinar sodium (Dup 785) is a highly potent antimetabolite immunosuppressant that suppresses heart allograft rejection. *Med Sci Res* 1991; **19:** 835–6.
3. Jaffee BD, *et al.* The unique immunosuppressive activity of brequinar sodium. *Transplant Proc* 1993; **25** (suppl 2): 19–22.
4. Joshi AS, *et al.* Phase I safety and pharmacokinetic studies of brequinar sodium after single ascending oral doses in stable renal, hepatic, and cardiac allograft recipients. *J Clin Pharmacol* 1997; **37:** 1121–8.

Bropirimine (18707-j)

Bropirimine *(BAN, USAN, rINN)*.

ABPP; U-54461; U-54461S. 2-Amino-5-bromo-6-phenyl-4(3*H*)-pyrimidinone.

$C_{10}H_8BrN_3O = 266.1$.

CAS — 56741-95-8.

Bropirimine is reported to have antineoplastic and antiviral actions, possibly due to the induction of interferons. It is under investigation in the management of bladder cancer (p.484).

Broxuridine (1816-c)

Broxuridine *(rINN)*.

BUDR; NSC-38297. 5-Bromo-2′-deoxyuridine; 5-Bromo-1-(2-deoxy-β-D-ribofuranosyl)pyrimidine-2,4(1*H*,3*H*)-dione.

$C_9H_{11}BrN_2O_5 = 307.1$.

CAS — 59-14-3.

Broxuridine is a thymidine analogue which acts as a radiosensitiser to enhance the effects of radiotherapy. It is also reported to possess antiviral activity.

Broxuridine has been given by intra-arterial infusion, in association with radiotherapy and other antineoplastic agents, in the treatment of tumours of the brain, head, and neck.

In a study[1] in 8 patients with malignant glioma broxuridine was given as a radiosensitiser in doses of 350 to 700 mg per m² body-surface daily. Each dose was given by intravenous infusion over 12 hours and repeated daily for up to 14 days; the course was repeated after 2 weeks. The patients underwent concomitant radiotherapy over a 7-week period. Some antitumour response was noted but overall efficacy was low, and dose-limiting myelotoxicity occurred in almost all patients; however there was evidence from bone-marrow samples of radiation enhancement by up to a factor of 2.2 at high plasma concentrations. Results suggested that intracarotid arterial infusion would be more effective than intravenous infusion providing that new technology could overcome the complications of prolonged intra-arterial administration.

1. Russo A, *et al.* Pharmacological evaluation of intravenous delivery of 5-bromodeoxyuridine to patients with brain tumors. *Cancer Res* 1984; **44:** 1702–5.

Broxuridine can be used to label DNA of tumour cells *in vivo*, enabling their cell cycle to be followed and an estimate of the potential doubling time of the tumour to be derived.[1]

1. Rew DA, Wilson GD. Advances in cell kinetics. *Br Med J* 1991; **303:** 532–3.

Busulphan (1817-k)

Busulphan *(BAN)*.

Busulfan *(rINN)*; Bussulfam; Busulfanum; CB-2041; GT-41; Myelosan; NSC-750; WR-19508. Tetramethylene di(methanesulphonate); Butane-1,4-diol di(methanesulphonate).

$C_6H_{14}O_6S_2 = 246.3$.

CAS — 55-98-1.

Pharmacopoeias. In *Chin., Eur.* (see p.viii), *Int., Jpn, Pol.,* and *US.*

A white or almost white crystalline powder. The Ph. Eur. states that it is very slightly **soluble** in water, alcohol, and in ether; freely soluble in acetone and in acetonitrile. The USP gives a solubility of 1 in 45 of acetone.

Store in airtight containers. Protect from light.

CAUTION. *Busulphan is irritant; avoid contact with skin and mucous membranes.*

Adverse Effects and Treatment

For a general outline see Antineoplastics, p.470 and p.473.

The major side-effect of busulphan is bone-marrow depression, manifest as leucopenia, thrombocytopenia, and sometimes, anaemia. The nadir of the granulocyte count usually occurs after about 10 to 30 days with recovery occurring over up to 5 months, but busulphan has sometimes caused irreversible or extremely-prolonged bone-marrow depression.

Interstitial pulmonary fibrosis, known as 'busulphan lung', and cataract formation can occur on prolonged treatment as can hyperpigmentation which may be part of a syndrome simulating Addison's disease. Gastro-intestinal disturbances are rare at usual therapeutic doses but may be dose-limiting where high doses are given before bone-marrow transplantation. Other rare adverse effects include dry skin and other skin reactions, liver damage, gynaecomastia, and, at high doses, CNS effects including convulsions.

Busulphan may result in impaired fertility and gonadal function. As with other alkylating agents, it is potentially carcinogenic and teratogenic.

Effects on the bladder. Haemorrhagic cystitis occurred in a patient who had received prolonged therapy with busulphan.[1]

1. Pode D, *et al.* Busulfan-induced hemorrhagic cystitis. *J Urol (Baltimore)* 1983; **130:** 347–8.

Effects on the liver. Jaundice in the terminal phase of chronic granulocytic leukaemia in a 31-year-old man was attributed to busulphan which had been taken for 6 years, in a report by Underwood and others.[1] Foadi and colleagues have also reported busulphan toxicity involving the liver in a patient who had taken busulphan for 54 months,[2] while hepatitis possibly associated with busulphan therapy has also been reported by Morris and Guthrie.[3] Dose-dependent veno-occlusive disease has been reported in up to about 20% of patients receiving high-dose busulphan before bone-marrow transplantation.[4]

1. Underwood JCE, *et al.* Jaundice after treatment of leukaemia with busulphan. *Br Med J* 1971; **1:** 556–7.
2. Foadi MD, *et al.* Portal hypertension in a patient with chronic myeloid leukaemia. *Postgrad Med J* 1977; **53:** 267–9.
3. Morris L, Guthrie T. Busulfan-induced hepatitis. *Am J Gastroenterol* 1988; **83:** 682–3.
4. Vassal G, *et al.* Busulfan and veno-occlusive disease of the liver. *Ann Intern Med* 1990; **112:** 881.

Effects on the nervous system. High-dose busulphan, used in conditioning regimens for bone-marrow transplantation, has been associated with the development of convulsions,[1-4] both generalised[1,3,4] and myoclonic.[2,4] As a result, the use of prophylactic antiepileptic therapy has been suggested as a component of such regimens.[1,3,4] However, some authorities do not consider the routine use of prophylactic antiepileptics justified,[5] and Fitzsimmons and colleagues have pointed out the potential for interaction between agents such as phenytoin and busulphan.[6] Careful dosage adjustment may also be required: Grigg and colleagues found phenytoin plasma concentrations to be subtherapeutic in patients who developed convulsions despite a standard prophylactic dose,[4] and the regimen was subsequently adjusted to take account of plasma concentrations. Schwarer and others have suggested the use of clobazam as an alternative to phenytoin for prophylaxis of busulphan-induced seizures.[7]

1. Marcus RE, Goldman JM. Convulsions due to high-dose busulphan. *Lancet* 1984; **ii:** 1463.
2. Martell RW, *et al.* High-dose busulfan and myoclonic epilepsy. *Ann Intern Med* 1987; **106:** 173.
3. Sureda A, *et al.* High-dose busulfan and seizures. *Ann Intern Med* 1989; **111:** 543–4.

4. Grigg AP, *et al.* Busulphan and phenytoin. *Ann Intern Med* 1989; **111:** 1049–50. Correction. *ibid.*; **112:** 313.
5. Hugh-Jones K, Shaw PJ. No convulsions in children on high-dose busulphan. *Lancet* 1985; **i:** 220.
6. Fitzsimmons WE, *et al.* Anticonvulsants and busulfan. *Ann Intern Med* 1990; **112:** 552–3.
7. Schwarer AP, *et al.* Clobazam for seizure prophylaxis during busulfan chemotherapy. *Lancet* 1995; **346:** 1238.

Effects on the skin. For the effect of radiotherapy in activating skin lesions in busulphan-treated patients, see under Precautions, below.

Precautions

For reference to the precautions necessary with antineoplastics and immunosuppressants, see p.474.

Porphyria. Busulphan was considered to be unsafe in patients with acute porphyria because it has been shown to be porphyrinogenic in *animals* or *in-vitro* systems.[1]

1. Moore MR, McColl KEL. *Porphyria: drug lists.* Glasgow: Porphyria Research Unit, University of Glasgow, 1991.

Radiotherapy. Severe cutaneous reactions occurred in patients given radiotherapy at least 30 days after combined chemotherapy with high-dose busulphan.[1]

1. Vassal G, *et al.* Radiosensitisation after busulphan. *Lancet* 1987; **i:** 571.

Interactions

Antiepileptics. For mention of the potential interactions between busulphan and phenytoin see Effects on the Nervous System, above.

Antifungals. Concomitant administration of *itraconazole* with busulphan resulted in a decrease in the clearance of the latter; fluconazole had no such effect.[1] Busulphan doses may need to be adjusted if itraconazole is given concomitantly.

1. Buggia I, *et al.* Itraconazole can increase systemic exposure to busulfan in patients given bone marrow transplantation. *Anticancer Res* 1996; **16:** 2083–8.

Pharmacokinetics

Busulphan is readily absorbed from the gastro-intestinal tract and rapidly disappears from the blood with a half-life of 2 to 3 hours. It is extensively metabolised, and excreted in the urine almost entirely as sulphur-containing metabolites. It crosses the blood-brain barrier.

Results of a study of the pharmacokinetics of high-dose busulphan in 5 patients receiving 1 mg per kg body-weight by mouth every six hours for 4 days showed that the mean elimination half-life decreased from about 3.4 hours after the first dose to about 2.3 hours after the final dose, suggesting that busulphan may induce its own metabolism.[1]

1. Hassan M, *et al.* Pharmacokinetic and metabolic studies of high-dose busulphan in adults. *Eur J Clin Pharmacol* 1989; **36:** 525–30.

Uses and Administration

Busulphan is an antineoplastic with a cell-cycle nonspecific alkylating action unlike that of the nitrogen mustards, and having a selective depressant action on bone marrow. In small doses, it depresses granulocytopoiesis and to a lesser extent thrombocytopoiesis but has little effect on lymphocytes. With larger doses, severe bone-marrow depression eventually ensues.

Because of its selective action, busulphan is used in the palliative treatment of chronic myeloid leukaemia (p.480). It provides symptomatic relief with a reduction in spleen size and a general feeling of well-being. The fall in leucocyte count is usually accompanied by a rise in the haemoglobin concentration. Permanent remission is not induced and resistance to its beneficial effects gradually develops.

Busulphan has been used in patients with polycythaemia vera (p.495) and in some patients with myelofibrosis and primary thrombocythaemia (p.496). It has also been used at high doses as part of a conditioning regimen to prepare patients for bone-marrow transplantation, a procedure discussed on p.498.

The usual dosage of busulphan in chronic myeloid [illegible]aemia is 60 μg per kg body-weight daily by [illegible] to a maximum single daily dose of 4 mg. [illegible]inued until the white-cell count has fall- [illegible] 15 000 and 25 000 per mm³. It should be discontinued earlier if the platelet count falls below 100 000 per mm³. Higher doses may be given if the response after 3 weeks is inadequate but this increases the risk of irreversible damage to the bone marrow and calls for special vigilance. Complete blood counts should be made at least every week and the trends followed closely; if haemorrhagic tendencies occur or there is a steep fall in the white cell count indicating severe bone-marrow depression, busulphan should be withdrawn until marrow function has returned.

Once an initial remission has been attained treatment is discontinued and not resumed until the white blood cell count returns to 50 000 per mm³. If this occurs within 3 months continuous maintenance treatment with 0.5 to 2 mg daily, or in some regimens more, may be given.

In patients with polycythaemia vera the usual dose is 4 to 6 mg daily, continued for 4 to 6 weeks with careful monitoring of blood counts. Further courses are given when relapse occurs, or alternatively maintenance therapy may be given at half the dose required for induction. Doses of 2 to 4 mg daily have been given for essential thrombocythaemia or myelofibrosis.

In conditioning regimens for bone-marrow transplantation busulphan has been given in usual doses of 16 mg per kg, in association with cyclophosphamide, for ablation of the recipient's bone marrow. Intravenous formulations of busulphan are under development for use in conditioning regimens.

References.

1. Buggia I, *et al.* Busulfan. *Ann Pharmacother* 1994; **28:** 1055–62.

Preparations

BP 1998: Busulfan Tablets;
USP 23: Busulfan Tablets.

Proprietary Preparations (details are given in Part 3)
Aust.: Myleran; ***Austral.:*** Myleran; ***Belg.:*** Myleran; ***Canad.:*** Myleran; ***Ger.:*** Myleran; ***Irl.:*** Myleran; ***Ital.:*** Misulban; Myleran; ***Mon.:*** Misulban†; ***Neth.:*** Myleran; ***Norw.:*** Myleran; ***S.Afr.:*** Myleran; ***Swed.:*** Myleran; ***Switz.:*** Myleran; ***UK:*** Myleran; ***USA:*** Myleran.

Campath-1H (18904-t)

Campath-1.

Campath-1H is a modified form of campath-1, a rat monoclonal antibody to the CDw52 antigen found on lymphocytes; it is genetically engineered to retain the binding site of the rodent antibody in a human antibody structure, thus reducing its immunogenicity.

Campath-1H has been tried in a few patients with lymphomas and lymphoproliferative disorders, and has orphan drug status in the treatment of chronic lymphocytic leukaemia (p.480). It has also been investigated for the prevention of graft-versus-host disease. It has also been tried with variable results in auto-immune disorders including vasculitis and rheumatoid arthritis, and multiple sclerosis.

References.

1. Hale G, *et al.* Remission induction in non-Hodgkin lymphoma with reshaped human monoclonal antibody campath-1H. *Lancet* 1988; **ii:** 1394–9.
2. Lim SH, *et al.* Differential response in a patient treated with campath-1H monoclonal antibody for refractory non-Hodgkin lymphoma. *Lancet* 1993; **341:** 432–3.
3. Poynton CH, *et al.* Adverse reactions to campath-1H monoclonal antibody. *Lancet* 1993; **341:** 1037.
4. Mathieson PW, *et al.* Monoclonal-antibody therapy in systemic vasculitis. *N Engl J Med* 1990; **323:** 250–4.
5. Lockwood CM, *et al.* Long-term remission of intractable systemic vasculitis with monoclonal antibody therapy. *Lancet* 1993; **341:** 1620–2.
6. Isaacs JD, *et al.* Monoclonal antibody therapy of chronic intraocular inflammation using campath-1H. *Br J Ophthalmol* 1995; **79:** 1054–5.
7. Weinblatt ME, *et al.* Campath-1H, a humanized monoclonal antibody, in refractory rheumatoid arthritis: an intravenous dose-escalation study. *Arthritis Rheum* 1995; **38:** 1589–94.
8. Osterborg A, *et al.* Phase II multicenter study of human CD52 antibody in previously treated chronic lymphocytic leukemia. *J Clin Oncol* 1997; **15:** 1567–74.

Capecitabine (17817-l)

Capecitabine *(USAN, rINN).*

Ro-09-1978/000. Pentyl 1-(5-deoxy-β-D-ribofuranosyl)-5-fluoro-1,2-dihydro-2-oxo-4-pyrimidinecarbamate.

$C_{15}H_{22}FN_3O_6$ = 359.4.

CAS — 154361-50-9.

Capecitabine is a prodrug that is converted to fluorouracil (p.534) in body tissues following oral administration. It is given by mouth for the treatment of metastatic breast cancer. The recommended daily dose is 2.5 g per m² body-surface, in 2 divided doses about 12 hours apart with food; doses are given for 2 weeks, followed by a 1-week rest period. Doses should be modified in subsequent cycles according to toxicity. Capecitabine is also under investigation in the treatment of other malignancies, notably colorectal cancer.

Adverse effects similar to those of fluorouracil (p.535) may be expected: diarrhoea, nausea and vomiting, stomatitis, palmar-plantar syndrome (erythema and desquamation of hands and feet), dermatitis, and bone-marrow depression have all been reported. Hyperbilirubinaemia has occurred.

References.

1. Bajetta E, *et al.* A pilot safety study of capecitabine, a new oral fluoropyrimidine, in patients with advanced neoplastic disease. *Tumori* 1996; **82:** 450–2.
2. Budman DR, *et al.* Preliminary studies of a novel oral fluoropyrimidine carbamate: capecitabine. *J Clin Oncol* 1998; **16:** 1795–1802.

Preparations

Proprietary Preparations (details are given in Part 3)
USA: Xeloda.

Caracemide (3408-c)

Caracemide *(USAN, pINN).*

NSC-253272. *N*-Acetyl-*N*,*O*-bis(methylcarbamoyl)hydroxylamine.

$C_6H_{11}N_3O_4$ = 189.2.

CAS — 81424-67-1.

Caracemide is an inhibitor of nucleic acid and protein synthesis which is under investigation as an antineoplastic.

Carbetimer (3410-w)

Carbetimer *(USAN, pINN).*

Carboxyimamidate; N-137. Maleic anhydride polymer with ethylene, reaction product with ammonia.

CAS — 82230-03-3.

Carbetimer has been investigated as an antineoplastic.

References.

1. Hanauske AR, *et al.* Phase I clinical trial of carbetimer. *Cancer Res* 1988; **48:** 5353–7.
2. Ardalan B, *et al.* Carbetimer: a re-evaluation of a drug with a novel mechanism of action. *Cancer Treat Rev* 1991; **18:** 73–83.

Carboplatin (16564-f)

Carboplatin *(BAN, USAN, rINN).*

Carboplatinum; CBDCA; JM-8; NSC-241240. *cis*-Diammine(cyclobutane-1,1-dicarboxylato)platinum.

$C_6H_{12}N_2O_4Pt$ = 371.2.

CAS — 41575-94-4.

Pharmacopoeias. In Eur. (see p.viii) and US.

A colourless crystalline powder. Sparingly **soluble** in water; very slightly soluble in alcohol and in acetone. **Incompatible** with aluminium. A 1% solution in water has a pH of 5 to 7. **Store** in airtight containers. Protect from light.

Stability. About 5% of the initial carboplatin concentration was lost over 24 hours when solutions were diluted in 0.9% sodium chloride solution and stored at 25°; lesser degrees of degradation were seen at lower sodium chloride concentrations but carboplatin was apparently stable over this period if diluted with 5% glucose injection.[1] The authors suggested that chloride-containing infusion solutions are not suitable for carboplatin, not only because of the loss of active drug but because of the possibility that conversion to cisplatin may be occurring, with a risk of increased toxicity.[1] This has been contested by the manufacturers (*Bristol-Myers, USA*), who found that only 0.5% or 0.7%, depending on formulation, of a carboplatin solution in 0.9% sodium chloride, had been converted to cisplatin after 24 hours.[2] However, the total degradation of carboplatin was not measured. In another study, Allsopp and colleagues examined the degradation kinetics of carboplatin in various solutions, and calculated the time to 5% degradation of carboplatin at 25° as 29.2 hours in 0.9% sodium chloride solution compared with 52.7 hours in water.[3] It was concluded that carboplatin should not be diluted in

0.9% sodium chloride solution when intended for continuous infusion over a prolonged period.[3]

1. Cheung Y-W, *et al.* Stability of cisplatin, iproplatin, carboplatin, and tetraplatin in commonly used intravenous solutions. *Am J Hosp Pharm* 1987; **44:** 124–30.
2. Perrone RK, *et al.* Extent of cisplatin formation in carboplatin admixtures. *Am J Hosp Pharm* 1989; **46:** 258–9.
3. Allsopp MA, *et al.* The degradation of carboplatin in aqueous solutions containing chloride or other selected nucleophiles. *Int J Pharmaceutics* 1991; **69:** 197–210.

Adverse Effects, Treatment, and Precautions

As for Cisplatin, p.514; nephrotoxicity and gastro-intestinal toxicity are less severe than with cisplatin. A reversible myelosuppression is the dose-limiting toxicity; platelet counts reach a nadir between 14 and 21 days after a dose, with recovery within 35 days, but recovery from leucopenia may be slower. Carboplatin should be given at reduced doses to patients with impaired renal function and should be avoided in those with a creatinine clearance of 20 mL per minute or less.

Analysis by the manufacturers of the adverse effects of carboplatin, in studies involving 710 patients.[1] Myelosuppression was the dose-limiting toxicity: leucopenia occurred in 55% of the evaluable patients. Leucopenia and thrombocytopenia result in symptomatic events such as infection or bleeding in a minority of patients. Anaemia was frequent (59%) and required transfusional support in about one-fifth of the patients. Nephrotoxicity and serum electrolyte loss were much less of a problem; no high-volume fluid hydration or electrolyte supplementation was given during treatment. Vomiting occurred in about half the patients, and a further 25% had nausea without vomiting. Peripheral neurotoxicity was reported in 6% of evaluable patients and clinical ototoxicity occurred in only 8 cases (about 1%). Increases in liver enzyme values have also been reported, as well as, more rarely, alopecia, skin rash, a flu-like syndrome, and local effects at the injection site.

1. Canetta R, *et al.* Carboplatin: the clinical spectrum to date. *Cancer Treat Rev* 1985; **12** (suppl A): 125–36.

Effects on the eyes. Cortical blindness developed in 2 patients with impaired renal function receiving high-dose carboplatin;[1] although 10 cases of visual disturbances in patients receiving carboplatin have been reported to the manufacturers to date, none had had sudden blindness and it was thought that the effect represented CNS toxicity in the presence of poor renal excretion. It would appear unwise to give high-dose carboplatin to patients whose glomerular filtration rate is less than 50 mL per minute.

1. O'Brien MER, *et al.* Blindness associated with high-dose carboplatin. *Lancet* 1992; **339:** 558.

Effects on the kidneys. Although carboplatin is reported to be much less nephrotoxic than cisplatin it is not devoid of adverse effects on the kidney. Salt wasting nephropathy (similar to that seen with cisplatin),[1] and decreased creatinine clearance[2] and glomerular filtration rate[3] have occurred, as has acute renal failure in 2 patients given intraperitoneal carboplatin[4] (although these patients had been heavily pretreated with cisplatin). It has been suggested that renal toxicity may be more likely at cumulative carboplatin doses of about 750 mg per square metre body-surface or more,[3] and there is some evidence to suggest that intensive hydration may ameliorate nephrotoxic effects.[2]

1. Welborn J, *et al.* Renal salt wasting and carboplatinum. *Ann Intern Med* 1988; **108:** 640.
2. Reed E, Jacob J. Carboplatin and renal dysfunction. *Ann Intern Med* 1989; **110:** 409.
3. Smit EF, *et al.* Carboplatin and renal function. *Ann Intern Med* 1989; **110:** 1034.
4. McDonald BR, *et al.* Acute renal failure associated with the use of intraperitoneal carboplatin: a report of two cases and review of the literature. *Am J Med* 1991; **90:** 386–91.

Pharmacokinetics

Following intravenous injection carboplatin exhibits a biphasic elimination and is excreted primarily in the urine, about 70% of a dose being excreted within 24 hours, almost all unchanged. Platinum slowly becomes protein bound, and is subsequently excreted with a half-life of 5 days or more; the terminal half-life of intact carboplatin is reported to be about 3 to 6 hours.

References.

1. van der Vijgh WJF. Clinical pharmacokinetics of carboplatin. *Clin Pharmacokinet* 1991; **21:** 242–61.

Uses and Administration

Carboplatin is an analogue of cisplatin with similar actions and uses (see p.515). It is used in the treatment of advanced ovarian cancers and of small-cell lung cancer, both alone and combined with other antineoplastics. It has also been tried as an alternative to cisplatin in other solid tumours.

Carboplatin is given by intravenous infusion over 15 minutes to 1 hour. In the UK an initial dose of 400 mg per m^2 body-surface has been recommended, while in the USA an initial dose of 360 mg per m^2 has been suggested. Doses should be reduced in patients with renal impairment or at risk of myelosuppression; dosage may be calculated on the basis of renal function (see Administration, below). Subsequent doses should be adjusted according to the nadir of the white-blood cell and platelet counts, and should not be given more frequently than every 4 weeks. Lower doses may be required when carboplatin is given as part of a combination regimen.

There is some disagreement about the relative advantages of carboplatin over cisplatin. Some sources have suggested that the safety advantages of carboplatin are not as marked as is suggested,[1,2] given its myelosuppressive effects, and that emesis may still be severe, especially in combination regimens.[1] It has also been pointed out that carboplatin is considerably more expensive. However, these views have been vigorously contested by others who have found carboplatin to be far better tolerated than, and of equal efficacy to, cisplatin;[3,4] some suggest that when all costs are taken into account treatment with carboplatin, which can be given to outpatients, may work out cheaper than cisplatin (for which admission is required).[4]

In a review of carboplatin, Wagstaff and colleagues[5] concluded that it was active in ovarian cancer, with similar responses to those seen with cisplatin; its activity in small-cell lung cancer, seminoma, and squamous-cell carcinomas of the head and neck seemed likely to be comparable, whereas results in gastro-intestinal and breast cancers, lymphomas and leukaemias, melanoma, mesothelioma, renal carcinoma, and sarcoma were, generally unimpressive. Another review[6] suggested that in testicular cancer, where there was a prospect of cure, cisplatin, which appeared to give better results in some studies should be preferred. However, in ovarian cancer, where treatment was largely palliative, carboplatin does have the advantage of being better tolerated.

1. Von Hoff DD. Whither carboplatin—a replacement for or an alternative to cisplatin? *J Clin Oncol* 1987; **5:** 169–71.
2. Anonymous. Cancer chemotherapy: carboplatin v cisplatin. *Drug Ther Bull* 1987; **25:** 67–8.
3. Calvert AH, *et al.* Carboplatin or cisplatin? *Lancet* 1988; **ii:** 577–8.
4. Tighe M, Goodman S. Carboplatin versus cisplatin. *Lancet* 1988; **ii:** 1372–3.
5. Wagstaff AJ, *et al.* Carboplatin: a preliminary review of its pharmacodynamic and pharmacokinetic properties and therapeutic efficacy in the treatment of cancer. *Drugs* 1989; **37:** 162–90.
6. Anonymous. Cisplatin or carboplatin for ovarian and testicular cancer? *Drug Ther Bull* 1994; **32:** 62–3.

Administration. Pharmacokinetic studies by Calvert and colleagues[1] have indicated that the dose of carboplatin to produce a desired area under the concentration-time curve (AUC) could be calculated, based on the patient's glomerular filtration rate (GFR), as:

$$\text{Dose in mg} = \text{target AUC} \times (\text{GFR} + 25)$$

It should be noted that the resultant dose is given in mg and not in mg per m^2 body-surface. This formula was found to be useful in patients with higher than normal as well as reduced GFR. Suggested target AUCs were 5 mg per mL per minute in previously treated patients and 7 mg per mL per minute in those who had not previously received chemotherapy. In combination therapy the appropriate AUC value depended on the other drugs used: an AUC of 4.5 mg per mL per minute gave acceptable results when carboplatin was combined with bleomycin and etoposide for testicular teratoma.

However, determination of GFR may be a problem: clearance of technetium-99m-labelled diethylenetriamine penta-acetic acid (DTPA) or chromium-51-labelled edetic acid is more accurate than 24-hour creatinine clearance, with the first of these more convenient than the second.[2] (It has been suggested that creatinine clearance should not be used to estimate GFR for the Calvert equation.[3]) Nonetheless, radioisotopic determination of GFR is still an elaborate procedure, and may be less accurate in children than adults.[4] Chatelut and colleagues have proposed formulae for determining clearance of carboplatin in both adults[5] and children.[4]

It has been suggested that the Calvert and Chatelut formulae are not sufficiently accurate for use in children, or in adults with very severe renal impairment. Bayesian methods are the technique of choice where serum carboplatin concentrations can be monitored.[3]

1. Calvert AH, *et al.* Carboplatin dosage: prospective evaluation of a simple formula based on renal function. *J Clin Oncol* 1989; **7:** 1748–56.
2. Millward MJ, *et al.* Carboplatin dosing based on measurement of renal function—experience at the Peter MacCallum Cancer Institute. *Aust N Z J Med* 1996; **26:** 372–9.
3. Duffull SB, Robinson BA. Clinical pharmacokinetics and dose optimisation of carboplatin. *Clin Pharmacokinet* 1997; **33:** 161–83.
4. Chatelut E, *et al.* Population pharmacokinetics of carboplatin in children. *Clin Pharmacol Ther* 1996; **59:** 436–43.
5. Chatelut E, *et al.* Prediction of carboplatin clearance from standard morphological and biological patient characteristics. *J Natl Cancer Inst* 1995; **87:** 573–80.

Malignant neoplasms. Carboplatin has been employed in chemotherapy regimens for a number of solid neoplasms, usually as an alternative to cisplatin. Such use is discussed in the introduction to this chapter for malignant neoplasms of the brain (p.485), cervix (p.487), lung (p.490), ovary (p.491), pancreas (p.491), and testis (p.493), and retinoblastoma (p.495).

Preparations

USP 23: Carboplatin for Injection.

Proprietary Preparations (details are given in Part 3)
Aust.: Carbosol; Paraplatin; ***Austral.:*** Paraplatin†; ***Belg.:*** Paraplatin; ***Canad.:*** Paraplatin; ***Fr.:*** Paraplatine; ***Ger.:*** Carboplat; Ribocarbo; ***Irl.:*** Paraplatin; ***Ital.:*** Paraplatin; ***Neth.:*** Paraplatin; ***Norw.:*** Carbosin; Paraplatin; ***S.Afr.:*** Carbosin; Paraplatin; ***Spain:*** Ercar; Nealorin; Paraplatin; Platinwas; ***Swed.:*** Paraplatin; ***Switz.:*** Paraplatine; ***UK:*** Paraplatin; ***USA:*** Paraplatin.

Carboquone (1818-a)

Carboquone (*rINN*).

Carbazilquinone. 2,5-Bis(aziridin-1-yl)-3-(2-hydroxy-1-methoxyethyl)-6-methyl-*p*-benzoquinone carbamate.

$C_{15}H_{19}N_3O_5 = 321.3.$

CAS — 24279-91-2.

Carboquone is reported to be an alkylating agent and has been used in the treatment of a variety of malignant neoplasms including those in lung (p.490), stomach (p.487), and ovary (p.491); it has also been tried in lymphomas (p.481) and in chronic myeloid leukaemia (p.480). It has been given in doses of 4 to 6 mg weekly in divided doses by the intravenous route, or 1 to 1.5 mg daily in 2 or 3 divided doses by mouth. It has also been given by the intra-arterial route. Adverse effects include bone-marrow depression, with leucopenia, thrombocytopenia, and anaemia, as well as gastro-intestinal disturbances, liver damage, interstitial pneumonitis and pulmonary fibrosis, hypersensitivity, malaise, alopecia, and proteinuria.

Preparations

Proprietary Preparations (details are given in Part 3)
Jpn: Esquinon.

Carmofur (18912-t)

Carmofur (*rINN*).

HCFU. 5-Fluoro-*N*-hexyl-3,4-dihydro-2,4-dioxo-1-(2*H*)-pyrimidinecarboxamide.

$C_{11}H_{16}FN_3O_3 = 257.3.$

CAS — 61422-45-5.

Pharmacopoeias. In *Jpn.*

Carmofur is a derivative of fluorouracil (p.534) and has similar actions. It is given by mouth in the treatment of malignant neoplasms of the gastro-intestinal tract. Carmofur has been associated with the development of neurological disorders including leucoencephalopathy.

Carmustine (1819-t)

Carmustine (*BAN, USAN, rINN*).

BCNU; BiCNU; Carmustinum; NSC-409962; WR-139021.

1,3-Bis(2-chloroethyl)-1-nitrosourea.

$C_5H_9Cl_2N_3O_2 = 214.0.$

CAS — 154-93-8.

Pharmacopoeias. In *Eur.* (see p.viii).

A yellowish, granular powder. Very slightly **soluble** in water; freely soluble in dehydrated alcohol; very soluble in ether and in dichloromethane. It melts at about 31° with decomposition. **Store** at a temperature of 2° to 8° in airtight containers. Protect from light.

Stability. The manufacturers state that carmustine must be stored at 2° to 8°. It has a melting-point of between 30.5 and 32.0° and exposure to these or higher temperatures will cause the drug to liquefy and decompose.

Solutions may be prepared by dissolving carmustine 100 mg in 3 mL of alcohol 100%, then adding 27 mL of Water for Injections to produce a solution with a pH of 5.6 to 6.0, and are then subject to approximately 6% decomposition in 3 hours, or about 8% after 6 hours, if stored at room temperature; decomposition may be reduced to about 4% in 24 hours if this solution is stored at 4° and protected from light. This solution is further diluted in 500 mL sodium chloride injection 0.9% or glucose 5% before administration; such diluted solutions are stable for 48 hours if stored at 4° and protected from light. There is some evidence that carmustine interacts with plastic giving sets and containers, although the relevance of this to clinical practice is uncertain.

A study by Colvin and colleagues has indicated that diluted solutions of carmustine undergo increased degradation in the presence of sodium bicarbonate, with only 73% of the original concentration of carmustine remaining after 90 minutes, much of the loss being in the first 15 minutes.[1]

1. Colvin M, *et al.* Stability of carmustine in the presence of sodium bicarbonate. *Am J Hosp Pharm* 1980; **37:** 677–8.

Adverse Effects and Treatment

For a general outline see Antineoplastics, p.470 and p.473. Delayed and cumulative bone-marrow depression is the most frequent and serious side-effect of carmustine. Platelets and leucocytes are mainly affected with platelet nadirs occurring at 4 to 5 weeks after administration and leucocyte nadirs at 5 to 6 weeks after administration; although thrombocytopenia is usually more severe, leucopenia may also be dose-limiting. Other side-effects reported include pulmonary fibrosis (mainly but not exclusively at high cumulative doses), renal and hepatic damage, and optic neuritis. Nausea and vomiting, beginning up to 2 hours after a dose, is common but can be reduced by prophylactic antiemetic therapy. Venous irritation may follow intravenous injection and transient hyperpigmentation has been noted after contact of a solution with the skin. Flushing of the skin and suffusion of the conjunctiva may occur following rapid intravenous infusion.

Convulsions, cerebral oedema, and various neurological symptoms have been reported in patients given carmustine-containing polymer implants; abnormalities of wound healing at the site of implantation, and an increased incidence of urinary-tract infection have also been reported.

As with other alkylating agents, carmustine is potentially carcinogenic, mutagenic, and teratogenic.

Effects on the eyes. Ocular toxicity has been reported in patients receiving carmustine,[1,2] and seems to be more likely following administration into the carotid artery,[1,2] although it was also seen following high-dose intravenous therapy. There is some evidence that the alcohol diluent used to prepare carmustine solutions may contribute to the retinopathy.[2]

1. Shingleton BJ, *et al.* Ocular toxicity associated with high-dose carmustine. *Arch Ophthalmol* 1982; **100:** 1766–72.
2. Greenberg HS, *et al.* Intra-arterial BCNU chemotherapy for treatment of malignant gliomas of the central nervous system. *J Neurosurg* 1984; **61:** 423–9.

Extravasation. For mention of the use of sodium bicarbonate as a specific antidote following carmustine extravasation, see under Treatment of Adverse Effects of Antineoplastics, p.474.

Precautions

For reference to the precautions necessary with antineoplastics and immunosuppressants, see p.474.

Handling and disposal. Carmustine has been shown to permeate latex, PVC, and rubber gloves, the degree of permeation tending to increase with time,[1,2] up to an equilibrium value.[2] The permeation rate appears not to depend solely on glove thickness and material, and may be different for different gloves made from the same material.[2] The time for initial penetration was reported to vary between 4.7 and 66.0 minutes in one study,[2] and gloves could be chosen accordingly depending on the anticipated length of exposure. Double-gloving, particularly with thicker PVC gloves, may offer some additional protection.[1]

1. Connor TH, *et al.* Permeability of latex and polyvinyl chloride gloves to carmustine. *Am J Hosp Pharm* 1984; **41:** 676–9.
2. Thomas PH, Fenton-May V. Protection offered by various gloves to carmustine exposure. *Pharm J* 1987; **238:** 775–7.

Interactions

Antineoplastics. For the suggestion that antineoplastics (such as the nitrosoureas) that undergo metabolism by cytochrome P450 may have their metabolism altered by other antineoplastics that reduce the activity of this enzyme system, see Interactions, in the chapter introduction, p.475.

Cimetidine. Reductions in white cell counts and platelet counts well below those normally attributed to treatment with carmustine alone were seen in 6 of 8 patients receiving their first course of carmustine and steroids in association with cimetidine given prophylactically.[1]

1. Selker RG, *et al.* Bone-marrow depression with cimetidine plus carmustine. *N Engl J Med* 1978; **299:** 834.

Pharmacokinetics

Following intravenous administration, carmustine is rapidly metabolised, and no intact drug is detectable after 15 minutes; metabolites have a much longer half-life and are presumed to be responsible for its activity. It is excreted in the urine; some is also excreted as carbon dioxide, via the lungs. Carmustine readily crosses the blood-brain barrier, appearing in cerebrospinal fluid in substantial concentrations almost immediately after intravenous injection. Very small amounts have been detected in the faeces.

Uses and Administration

Carmustine is a cell-cycle phase nonspecific antineoplastic belonging to the nitrosourea group of compounds, which are considered to function as alkylating agents. It has been used in the treatment of brain tumours, and in combination chemotherapy for multiple myeloma, and has been given as second-line therapy in Hodgkin's disease, and some other lymphomas. Carmustine has also been tried in a variety of other malignant neoplasms including melanoma, and in Waldenström's macroglobulinaemia and amyloidosis. The management of these conditions is discussed in the chapter introduction as indicated by the cross-references below.

Carmustine is given intravenously as a single dose of 150 to 200 mg per m^2 body-surface area or divided into doses of 75 to 100 mg per m^2 given on 2 successive days. Lower doses are given in combination therapy. Doses may be repeated every 6 weeks provided that blood counts have returned to acceptable levels, that is, platelets above 100 000 per mm^3 and leucocytes above 4 000 per mm^3. Subsequent doses must be adjusted according to the haematological response. Reconstituted solutions are further diluted with sodium chloride (0.9%) or glucose (5%) injection and infused over 1 to 2 hours.

Polymer implants containing carmustine have been developed for implantation into the brain in the localised treatment of malignant glioma. Each implant contains 7.7 mg of carmustine: up to 8 such implants are inserted into the cavity left by surgical removal of the tumour.

Administration. A study in *rats* indicated that intracranial implantation of ethylene-vinyl acetate copolymer loaded with carmustine achieved controlled release of carmustine into the implanted hemisphere for 9 days, and produced higher concentrations of carmustine in the affected hemisphere, and lower concentrations in the blood, than following intraperitoneal implantation.[1]

A subsequent multicentre study[2] in patients with recurrent malignant glioma implanted a biodegradable poly(carboxyphenoxypropane/sebacic acid)anhydride polymer (BIODEL), in the form of wafers containing 7.7 mg into the brain after resection; the maximum dose thus implanted was 8 wafers (61.6 mg). The effects of treatment were held to favour the implant; 59 of 112 patients given placebo implants were dead at 6 months, compared with 44 of 110 given carmustine implants, with a median survival of 23 and 31 weeks respectively.

1. Yang MB, *et al.* Controlled delivery of 1,3-bis(2-chloroethyl)-1-nitrosourea from ethylene-vinyl acetate copolymer. *Cancer Res* 1989; **49:** 5103–7.
2. Brem H, *et al.* Placebo-controlled trial of safety and efficacy of intraoperative controlled delivery by biodegradable polymers of chemotherapy for recurrent gliomas. *Lancet* 1995; **345:** 1008–12.

Amyloidosis. For mention of chemotherapy with epirubicin, cyclophosphamide, and carmustine to suppress amyloidosis after cardiac transplantation, see p.497.

Malignant neoplasms. Carmustine has been used in chemotherapeutic regimens for a number of malignancies. Because of its ability to pass the blood-brain barrier it has been extensively used in malignant neoplasms of the brain, the management of which is discussed further on p.485. Other conditions in which it has been employed, as discussed in the chapter introduction, include malignant melanoma (p.492), Hodgkin's disease (p.481), multiple myeloma (p.494), and Waldenström's macroglobulinaemia (see p.496).

MYCOSIS FUNGOIDES. Topical application of carmustine is a possible alternative to mustine, PUVA, or electron beam radiation in early mycosis fungoides (p.482).

The use of topical carmustine, usually as a 0.2% solution or 0.4% ointment, in mycosis fungoides was described by Zackheim and others.[1] Over a 10-year period 86 patients had been treated in this way, and complete remission was achieved in 21 of 25 with less than 10% skin involvement (stage IA), and in 11 of 21 patients in whom there was greater than 10% involvement (stage IB). Among patients with more advanced disease the degree of involvement was also predictive of response, and those with predominantly superficial lesions responded better than those with infiltrating plaque lesions. Erythema and telangiectasia were troublesome side-effects but severe cutaneous reactions were generally rare with current dosage schedules of 10 mg carmustine applied daily.[1] In a subsequent report Zackheim and colleagues reported the use of carmustine, usually 10 mg daily as a topical alcoholic solution, to treat lymphomatoid papulosis. Although all 7 patients so treated experienced a rapid reduction in the number and size of papules, prolonged lesion-free remission was not seen.[2]

1. Zackheim HS, *et al.* Topical carmustine (BCNU) for mycosis fungoides and related disorders: a 10-year experience. *J Am Acad Dermatol* 1983; **9:** 363–74.
2. Zackheim HS, *et al.* Topical carmustine therapy for lymphomatoid papulosis. *Arch Dermatol* 1985; **121:** 1410–14.

Preparations

Proprietary Preparations (details are given in Part 3)
Austral.: BiCNU; ***Belg.:*** Nitrumon; ***Canad.:*** BiCNU; ***Fr.:*** BiCNU; ***Ger.:*** Carmubris; ***Irl.:*** BiCNU; ***Ital.:*** Nitrumon†; ***Norw.:*** Becenun; ***S.Afr.:*** BiCNU; ***Spain:*** Nitrourean; ***Swed.:*** Becenun; ***UK:*** BiCNU; ***USA:*** BiCNU; Gliadel.

Chlorambucil (1820-l)

Chlorambucil *(BAN, rINN).*

CB-1348; Chlorambucilum; Chloraminophene; Chlorbutinum; NSC-3088; WR-139013. 4-[4-Bis(2-chloroethyl)aminophenyl]butyric acid.

$C_{14}H_{19}Cl_2NO_2$ = 304.2.

CAS — 305-03-3.

Pharmacopoeias. In *Eur.* (see p.viii), *Int.*, *Pol.*, and *US.*

A white or off-white crystalline or granular powder. Practically **insoluble** in water; freely soluble in alcohol; soluble 1 in 2 of acetone; soluble in dilute alkali. **Store** in airtight containers. Protect from light.

In the UK the manufacturers recommend that tablets of chlorambucil be stored at 2° to 8°.

CAUTION. *Chlorambucil is irritant; avoid contact with skin and mucous membranes.*

Adverse Effects and Treatment

For a general outline see Antineoplastics, p.470 and p.473.

A reversible progressive lymphocytopenia tends to develop during treatment with chlorambucil. Neutropenia may continue to develop up to 10 days after the last dose. Irreversible bone-marrow depression can occur particularly when the total dosage for the course approaches 6.5 mg per kg body-weight.

Other reported adverse effects include gastro-intestinal disturbances, hepatotoxicity, skin rashes (occasionally Stevens-Johnson syndrome or toxic epidermal necrolysis), peripheral neuropathy, and central neurotoxicity, including seizures. Interstitial pneumonia and pulmonary fibrosis have occurred; the latter is usually reversible but fatalities have been recorded. Chlorambucil in high doses may produce azoospermia and amenorrhoea; sterility has developed particularly when chlorambucil has been given to boys at or before puberty.

Overdosage may result in pancytopenia and in neurotoxicity, including agitation, ataxia, and grand mal seizures.

Like other alkylating agents, chlorambucil is potentially mutagenic, teratogenic, and carcinogenic, and an increased incidence of acute leukaemias and other secondary malignancies has been reported in patients who have received the drug.

Effects on the bladder. Chlorambucil-induced cystitis was reported in a 73-year-old woman given 2 mg daily for over 2 years for the treatment of lymphocytic lymphoma.[1]

1. Daoud D, *et al.* Sterile cystitis associated with chlorambucil. *Drug Intell Clin Pharm* 1977; **11:** 491.

Effects on the eyes. Visual impairment and optic atrophy in a patient who had been receiving chlorambucil for five years to control non-Hodgkin's lymphoma were thought to be due to the drug,[1] although ocular effects are extremely rare with chlorambucil.

1. Yiannakis PH, Larner AJ. Visual failure and optic atrophy associated with chlorambucil therapy. *Br Med J* 1993; **306:** 109.

Effects on mental function. CNS toxicity, manifesting as lethargy, confusion, coma, convulsions, restlessness, and hallucinations, was dose-limiting in 4 of 30 patients in a phase-I study of high-dose chlorambucil.[1]

1. Blumenreich MS, *et al.* A phase I trial of chlorambucil administered in short pulses in patients with advanced malignancies. *Cancer Invest* 1988; **6:** 371–5.

Precautions

For reference to the precautions necessary with antineoplastics and immunosuppressants, see p.474. Chlorambucil should not be administered, or should be given with great care and at reduced doses, for at least 4 weeks after treatment with radiotherapy or other antineoplastic agents unless only low doses of radiation have been given to parts remote from the bone marrow and the neutrophil and platelet counts are not depressed. The dose should be reduced if there is lymphocytic involvement of the bone marrow or if it is hypoplastic. Chlorambucil should be given with care to patients with impaired renal function; the manufacturers state that consideration should also be given to dose reduction in patients with gross hepatic dysfunction.

Handling and disposal. Urine produced for up to 48 hours after a dose of chlorambucil should be handled wearing protective clothing.[1]

1. Harris J, Dodds LJ. Handling waste from patients receiving cytotoxic drugs. *Pharm J* 1985; **235:** 289–91.

Porphyria. Chlorambucil was considered to be unsafe in patients with acute porphyria although there is conflicting experimental evidence of porphyrinogenicity.[1]

1. Moore MR, McColl KEL. *Porphyria: drug lists*. Glasgow: Porphyria Research Unit, University of Glasgow, 1991.

Pharmacokinetics

Chlorambucil is rapidly and almost completely absorbed from the gastro-intestinal tract following oral doses and is reported to have a terminal half-life in plasma of about 1.5 hours. It is extensively metabolised in the liver, primarily to active phenylacetic acid mustard, which has a slightly longer plasma half-life of about 2.5 hours, and which like chlorambucil also undergoes some spontaneous degradation to further derivatives. Chlorambucil and its metabolites are extensively protein bound. It is excreted in the urine almost entirely as metabolites with less than 1% unchanged.

Uses and Administration

Chlorambucil is an antineoplastic derived from mustine (p.555) and has a similar mode of action. It acts on lymphocytes and to a lesser extent on neutrophils and platelets. Chlorambucil is most valuable in those conditions associated with the proliferation of white blood cells, especially lymphocytes, and is used in the treatment of chronic lymphocytic leukaemia and lymphomas, including Hodgkin's disease. It is also used in Waldenström's macroglobulinaemia and has been given in hairy-cell leukaemia, carcinoma of the breast and ovary and gestational trophoblastic tumours. Although formerly widely used in the management of polycythaemia vera it has largely been superseded. Chlorambucil has immunosuppressant properties and has been given in various auto-immune disorders including amyloidosis, Behçet's syndrome, glomerular kidney disease, primary biliary cirrhosis, polymyositis, rheumatoid arthritis, sarcoidosis, and systemic lupus erythematosus.

The use of chlorambucil in these disorders is discussed further elsewhere, as indicated by the cross-references given below.

Chlorambucil is better tolerated than mustine hydrochloride and serious bone-marrow toxicity is not usually a problem with normal doses. Chlorambucil is administered by mouth in usual doses of 100 to 200 µg per kg body-weight daily (usually 4 to 10 mg as a single daily dose), for 4 to 8 weeks. A dose of 100 µg per kg daily may be adequate for the treatment of lymphosarcoma; an initial dose of 150 µg per kg daily until the total leukocyte count falls below 10 000 per mm^3 is followed by 100 µg per kg daily in chronic lymphocytic leukaemia; in Hodgkin's disease, 200 µg per kg daily is usually required. Lower doses may be given as part of a combination regimen. If lymphocytic infiltration of the bone marrow is present or if the bone marrow is hypoplastic, the daily dose should not exceed 100 µg per kg. Alternatively, chlorambucil may be given intermittently. For example, in chronic lymphocytic leukaemia it may be given in an initial dose of 400 µg per kg increased by 100 µg per kg at each 2- or 4-week dose interval until control of lymphocytosis is achieved or toxicity occurs.

Once a remission has been established the patient may receive continuous maintenance with 30 to 100 µg per kg body-weight daily. However, short intermittent courses appear to be safer and are generally preferred for maintenance.

In patients with Waldenström's macroglobulinaemia chlorambucil may be given in an initial dose of 6 to 12 mg daily by mouth until leucopenia develops. Maintenance therapy with doses of 2 to 8 mg daily may then be given indefinitely.

Total and differential white-cell counts and haemoglobin examinations are recommended each week during treatment with chlorambucil.

Amyloidosis. Chlorambucil may be of use in preserving kidney function in patients with amyloidosis,[1,2] the management of which is discussed in more detail on p.497.

1. Bergland K, *et al.* Alkylating cytostatic treatment in renal amyloidosis secondary to rheumatic disease. *Ann Rheum Dis* 1987; **46:** 757–62.
2. David J, Woo P. Reactive amyloidosis. *Arch Dis Child* 1992; **67:** 258–61.

Connective-tissue and muscular disorders. Chlorambucil has been used with corticosteroids as a steroid-sparing agent in patients with Behçet's syndrome (p.1018). It has occasionally been tried in polymyositis (p.1027). In both these conditions, the potential benefits must be weighed against the possibility of toxicity.

Kidney disorders, non-malignant. Chlorambucil has been used in some forms of glomerular kidney disease (p.1021). In minimal change nephropathy, in which cytotoxics are reserved for the most severe cases because of fears about toxicity, cyclophosphamide is generally preferred to chlorambucil because it is perceived as entailing somewhat less risk, but chlorambucil has been used with corticosteroids in patients with membranous nephropathy.[1-3]

1. Ponticelli C, *et al.* Methylprednisolone plus chlorambucil as compared with methylprednisolone alone for the treatment of idiopathic membranous nephropathy. *N Engl J Med* 1992; **327:** 599–603.
2. Reichert LJM, *et al.* Preserving renal function in patients with membranous nephropathy: daily oral chlorambucil compared with intermittent monthly pulses of cyclophosphamide. *Ann Intern Med* 1994; **121:** 328–33.
3. Ponticelli C, *et al.* A 10-year follow-up of a randomized study with methylprednisolone and chlorambucil in membranous nephropathy. *Kidney Int* 1995; **48:** 1600–4.

Liver disorders, non-malignant. No treatment has proven unequivocally successful in the management of primary biliary cirrhosis (p.497). Chlorambucil is one of a number of agents for which reports of benefit exist.[1]

1. Hoofnagle JH, *et al.* Randomized trial of chlorambucil for primary biliary cirrhosis. *Gastroenterology* 1986; **91:** 1327–34.

Malignant neoplasms. Chlorambucil is used in the management of a number of haematological malignancies including chronic lymphocytic and hairy-cell leukaemias (p.480 and p.481, although it has been superseded for the latter), Hodgkin's disease (p.481), non-Hodgkin's lymphomas (p.482), and Waldenström's macroglobulinaemia (p.496). It was formerly used in polycythaemia vera (p.495) but is now largely superseded. For mention of the use of chlorambucil in gestational trophoblastic tumours and malignant neoplasms of the ovary, see p.477 and p.491, respectively.

Ocular disorders, non-malignant. As mentioned on p.498 chlorambucil is one of the immunosuppressants that may be considered for patients with uveitis or scleritis unresponsive to corticosteroids in tolerable doses.

Rheumatoid arthritis. Chlorambucil has been used for its immunosuppressant properties in a few patients with severe rheumatoid arthritis (especially with vasculitis) who have failed to respond to other drugs. However the use of cytotoxic immunosuppressants other than methotrexate is considered debatable, as mentioned in the discussion of rheumatoid arthritis on p.2.

Sarcoidosis. Where drug therapy is required for sarcoidosis (p.1028), corticosteroids are the usual treatment. Chlorambucil is one of a number of cytotoxic immunosuppressants that have been tried, with variable results, as a second-line therapy.

Preparations

BP 1998: Chlorambucil Tablets;
USP 23: Chlorambucil Tablets.

Proprietary Preparations (details are given in Part 3)
Aust.: Leukeran; ***Austral.:*** Leukeran; ***Belg.:*** Leukeran; ***Canad.:*** Leukeran; ***Ger.:*** Leukeran; ***Irl.:*** Leukeran; ***Ital.:*** Leukeran; Linfolysin; ***Mon.:*** Chloraminophene; ***Neth.:*** Leukeran; ***Norw.:*** Leukeran; ***S.Afr.:*** Leukeran; ***Spain:*** Leukeran; ***Swed.:*** Leukeran; ***Switz.:*** Leukeran; ***UK:*** Leukeran; ***USA:*** Leukeran.

Chlorozotocin (1821-y)

DCNU; NSC-178248. 2-[3-(2-Chloroethyl)-3-nitrosoureido]-2-deoxy-D-glucopyranose.
$C_9H_{16}ClN_3O_7$ = 313.7.
CAS — 54749-90-5.

Chlorozotocin is an analogue of the antineoplastic streptozocin (p.562) and has been reported to have little diabetogenic effect. It has been tried as an antineoplastic, notably in islet cell carcinoma (p.477), in usual doses of 120 to 200 mg per m^2 body-surface intravenously every 6 weeks.

Progressive normochromic normocytic anaemia was noted in a 46-year-old woman who had been given chlorozotocin 120 mg per m^2 body-surface intravenously every 6 weeks during the previous 12 months, for the treatment of bronchoalveolar carcinoma.[1] Therapy was continued for a further 6 months, when a total dose of 2.1 g had been given. Over the following 4 to 6 weeks progressive renal failure developed from which the patient died.

1. Baker JJ, *et al.* Renal-failure anemia and nitrosourea therapy. *N Engl J Med* 1979; **301:** 662.

Chromomycin (18961-v)

CAS — 7059-24-7 (chromomycin A_3).

Chromomycin is an antibiotic complex produced by *Streptomyces griseus* and comprising chiefly chromomycin A_3 (aburamycin B; toyomycin). It is given parenterally for its antineoplastic properties in the management of malignant neoplasms. Nephrotoxicity, hypocalcaemia, liver disorders, and thrombophlebitis are among the adverse effects reported.

Cisplatin (1822-j)

Cisplatin *(BAN, USAN, rINN)*.
CDDP; Cisplatina; Cisplatinum; Cis-platinum; DDP; *cis*-DDP; NSC-119875; Peyrone's Salt; Platinum Diamminodichloride.
cis-Diamminedichloroplatinum.
$(NH_3)_2.PtCl_2$ = 300.0.
CAS — 15663-27-1.

Pharmacopoeias. In *Chin., Eur.* (see p.viii), *Int.*, and *US.*

A yellow powder or yellow or orange-yellow crystals. Slightly **soluble** in water; practically insoluble in alcohol; sparingly soluble in dimethylformamide. A 0.1% solution in 0.9% sodium chloride solution has a pH of 4.5 to 6.0 immediately after preparation.

Store in airtight containers. Protect from light.

Incompatibility. Cisplatin is rapidly degraded in the presence of bisulphite or metabisulphite,[1,2] and admixture with preparations containing these as preservatives may result in loss of activity.[2] Sodium bicarbonate may also increase the loss of cisplatin from solution, and in some cases may cause precipitation.[3] The stability of cisplatin when mixed with fluorouracil is reported to be limited, with 10% loss of cisplatin in 1.2 to 1.5 hours.[4] Mixtures with etoposide in 0.9% sodium chloride injection formed a precipitate if mannitol and potassium chloride were present as additives, but not when the diluent was 5% glucose with 0.45% sodium chloride.[5] Turbidity has been reported within 4 hours of mixing 0.1% solutions of cisplatin and thiotepa in 5% glucose.[6] Cisplatin exhibits variable incompatibility with paclitaxel, depending on the paclitaxel concentration and the temperature.[7] Cisplatin has also been reported to be incompatible with aluminium in dispensing equipment.[8]

1. Hussain AA, *et al.* Reaction of cis-platinum with sodium bisulfite. *J Pharm Sci* 1980; **69:** 364–5.
2. Garren KW, Repta AJ. Incompatibility of cisplatin and Reglan Injectable. *Int J Pharmaceutics* 1985; **24:** 91–9.

3. Hincal AA, *et al.* Cis-platin stability in aqueous parenteral vehicles. *J Parenter Drug Assoc* 1979; **33:** 107–16.
4. Stewart CF, Fleming RA. Compatibility of cisplatin and fluorouracil in 0.9% sodium chloride injection. *Am J Hosp Pharm* 1990; **47:** 1373–7.
5. Stewart CF, Hampton EM. Stability of cisplatin and etoposide in intravenous admixtures. *Am J Hosp Pharm* 1989; **46:** 1400–4.
6. Trissel LA, Martinez JF. Compatibility of thiotepa (lyophilized) with selected drugs during simulated Y-site administration. *Am J Health-Syst Pharm* 1996; **53:** 1041–5.
7. Zhang Y, *et al.* Compatibility and stability of paclitaxel combined with cisplatin and with carboplatin in infusion solutions. *Ann Pharmacother* 1997; **31:** 1465–70.
8. Ogawa GS, *et al.* Dispensing-pin problems. *Am J Hosp Pharm* 1985; **42:** 1042–5.

Stability. Decomposition of cisplatin in aqueous solutions is primarily due to reversible substitution of water for chloride, and its stability is enhanced in sodium chloride solutions because of the excess of chloride ions available.[1,2] A solution in 0.9% sodium chloride injection has been reported to lose 3% of the drug in less than one hour and to remain stable at this equilibrium value for 24 hours at room temperature.[1] Stability is decreased if exposed to intense light, but the effect of normal lighting conditions is apparently smaller.[1,2] It has been recommended that admixtures of cisplatin with mannitol and magnesium sulphate (in glucose 5% with sodium chloride 0.45%) stored at room temperature in polyvinyl chloride bags should be used within 48 hours, but may be stored for 4 days at 4° or frozen and stored at −15° for up to 30 days.[3] However, solutions containing 600 μg per mL or more of cisplatin precipitate out when refrigerated and are slow to redissolve.[1]

1. Greene RF, *et al.* Stability of cisplatin in aqueous solution. *Am J Hosp Pharm* 1979; **36:** 38–43.
2. Hincal AA, *et al.* Cis-platin stability in aqueous parenteral vehicles. *J Parenter Drug Assoc* 1979; **33:** 107–16.
3. LaFollette JM, *et al.* Stability of cisplatin admixtures in polyvinyl chloride bags. *Am J Hosp Pharm* 1985; **42:** 2652.

Adverse Effects and Treatment

For a general outline see Antineoplastics, p.470 and p.473.

Severe nausea and vomiting occur in most patients during treatment with cisplatin; nausea may persist for up to a week.

Serious toxic effects on the kidneys, bone marrow, and ears have been reported in up to about one third of patients given a single dose of cisplatin; the effects are generally dose-related and cumulative. Damage to the renal tubules may be evident during the second week after a dose of cisplatin and renal function must return to normal before further cisplatin is given. Adequate hydration, and use of osmotic diuretics such as mannitol to increase urine volume and thus decrease the urinary concentration of platinum, can reduce the incidence of nephrotoxicity. Electrolyte disturbances, particularly hypomagnesaemia and hypocalcaemia, may occur, possibly as a result of renal tubular damage. Hyperuricaemia is also seen.

Bone-marrow depression may be severe with higher doses of cisplatin. Nadirs in platelet and leucocyte counts occur between days 18 and 23 and most patients recover by day 39; anaemia is commonly seen.

Ototoxicity may be more severe in children. It can be manifest as tinnitus, loss of hearing in the high frequency range, and occasionally deafness or vestibular toxicity. Other neurological effects reported include peripheral neuropathies including optic neuritis, papilloedema, cerebral blindness, and seizures.

Anaphylactoid reactions and cardiac abnormalities have occurred.

Cisplatin is potentially mutagenic and teratogenic, and its actions are thought to resemble those of the alkylating agents which are potentially carcinogenic.

Effects on the blood. Findings suggested that cisplatin-induced anaemia probably has 2 mechanisms, the more usual being destruction of the erythroid stem-cell pool and the less usual being haemolysis.[1]

1. Rothmann SA, Weick JK. Cisplatin toxicity for erythroid precursors. *N Engl J Med* 1981; **304:** 360.

THROMBO-EMBOLISM. For discussion of thrombo-embolic events possibly associated with cisplatin-containing chemotherapy regimens see Thrombo-embolism, under Adverse Effects of Antineoplastics and Immunosuppressants, p.471.

Effects on electrolytes. In a retrospective study of 37 patients who had received cisplatin 70 mg per m^2 body-surface by intravenous injection every 3 weeks, 21 patients developed hypomagnesaemia while receiving cisplatin, which eventually returned to normal in 10 patients, and a further 8 developed hypomagnesaemia after cisplatin was withdrawn.[1] Symptomatic hypomagnesaemia requiring hospitalisation occurred in 2 patients, while inappropriate renal magnesium loss occurred in 4 patients. In a prospective study of a further 7 patients who received a standard liquid diet for 4 days before cisplatin administration, 2 developed hypomagnesaemia. Hypomagnesaemia and hypocalcaemia may be severe enough to provoke tetany in some patients,[2,3] although this has responded to electrolyte infusion without the need to interrupt chemotherapy.[2] Cisplatin therapy may also be associated with significant hypokalaemia[2] and hyponatraemia.[4,5]

See also Effects on the Kidneys, below.

1. Schilsky RL, Anderson T. Hypomagnesemia and renal magnesium wasting in patients receiving cisplatin. *Ann Intern Med* 1979; **90:** 929–31.
2. Winkler CF, *et al.* Cisplatin and renal magnesium wasting. *Ann Intern Med* 1979; **91:** 502.
3. Stuart-Harris R, *et al.* Tetany associated with cis-platin. *Lancet* 1980; **ii:** 1303.
4. Hutchison FN, *et al.* Renal salt wasting in patients treated with cisplatin. *Ann Intern Med* 1988; **108:** 21–5.
5. Mariette X, *et al.* Cisplatin and hyponatremia. *Ann Intern Med* 1988; **108:** 770–1.

Effects on the kidneys. The nephrotoxic effects of cisplatin have been reviewed by Blachley and Hill.[1] Cisplatin may produce azotaemia and acute renal failure, with tubular necrosis primarily in the distal portions of the nephron. It has been shown that most patients whose renal function is impaired by cisplatin never regain their pretreatment level of function. Selective renal wasting of magnesium is not unusual and may be commoner than azotaemia as an expression of nephrotoxicity: hypocalcaemia and hypokalaemia may result. These findings probably result from a specific membrane or transport-system defect. The nephrotoxic effects of cisplatin are cumulative, and increase with total dose and duration of treatment: adequate hydration and urine volumes greater than 2 litres daily reduce the frequency of renal insufficiency as may simultaneous infusion of mannitol, and the use of chloride-containing vehicles such as sodium chloride injection rather than glucose.[1] El-Sharkawi and others have suggested that cisplatin may mobilise lead accumulated in bone and cause temporary accumulation in the kidney, with concomitant toxicity,[2] but this has been vigorously disputed.[3-5]

See also under Effects on Electrolytes, above.

1. Blachley JD, Hill JB. Renal and electrolyte disturbances associated with cisplatin. *Ann Intern Med* 1981; **95:** 628–32.
2. El-Sharkawi AM, *et al.* Unexpected mobilisation of lead during cisplatin chemotherapy. *Lancet* 1986; **ii:** 249–50.
3. Tothill P, *et al.* Is lead mobilised by cisplatin? *Lancet* 1989; **ii:** 333.
4. Tothill P, *et al.* Mobilisation of lead by cisplatin. *Lancet* 1989; **ii:** 1342.
5. Hainsworth IR, Morgan WD. Plasma lead and cisplatin. *Lancet* 1989; **ii:** 624.

PROPHYLAXIS. Hydration with 1 to 2 litres of fluid before treatment, and infusion of cisplatin in a further 2 litres of infusion fluid containing an osmotic diuretic such as mannitol reduces the nephrotoxicity of cisplatin, but does not abolish it.

There is some evidence that sodium thiosulphate may have a protective effect. Injection of sodium thiosulphate 7.5 g per m^2 body-surface as an intravenous loading dose, followed by 2.13 g per m^2 per hour by intravenous infusion over 12 hours, reduced the incidence of nephrotoxicity associated with intraperitoneal cisplatin in 17 patients.[1] When cisplatin 90 mg per m^2 was given by instillation into the peritoneum, there was an average rise in serum creatinine of 55% above pretreatment values, whereas this rise averaged only 9% when the same dose was given with thiosulphate. As a result of the effectiveness of thiosulphate protection the dose of cisplatin could be increased to 270 mg per m^2 without evidence of nephrotoxicity. Nausea and vomiting occurred after all courses of cisplatin and was not affected by thiosulphate; myelosuppression was transient and tolerable and there was no evidence of peripheral neuropathy or hearing loss.

Glutathione (p.983) is also reported to reduce cisplatin toxicity including nephrotoxicity, as is amifostine (p.973).

1. Howell SB, *et al.* Intraperitoneal cisplatin with systemic thiosulfate protection. *Ann Intern Med* 1982; **97:** 845–51.

Effects on the nervous system. Peripheral cisplatin neurotoxicity has been reviewed by Mollman.[1] The features of cisplatin-induced peripheral neuropathy are consistent with damage predominantly to sensory fibres, with numbness, tingling, and decreased vibratory sensation and deep tendon reflexes, progressing in severe cases to disabling sensory ataxia. The toxicity is dose-dependent, with symptoms usually appearing in patients who have received cumulative doses of 300 to 600 mg per square metre body-surface, although individuals vary in susceptibility. Neuropathy is reversible but recovery may take a year or more. The pathophysiology is unknown. Peripheral neuropathy is now a dose-limiting toxicity for cisplatin and agents such as Org-2766 (a corticotrophin analogue) and amifostine have been investigated for their potential in protecting peripheral nerves.[1] Autonomic neuropathy, with, in some cases, consequent postural hypotension, has also been described following treatment with cisplatin-containing regimens.[2] Apart from ototoxicity, cisplatin has also been associated with central neurotoxicity, including focal encephalopathy, seizures, aphasia, confusion, agitation, and cortical blindness.[3-6] It has been suggested that the mechanism of focal encephalopathy may be vascular,[4] although this is uncertain. Glutathione is also under investigation for the prevention of neurotoxicity.

1. Mollman JE. Cisplatin neurotoxicity. *N Engl J Med* 1990; **322:** 126–7.
2. Richardson P, Cantwell BMJ. Autonomic neuropathy after cisplatin based chemotherapy. *Br Med J* 1990; **300:** 1466–7.
3. Gorman DJ, *et al.* Focal encephalopathy after cisplatin therapy. *Med J Aust* 1989; **150:** 399–401.
4. Lindeman G, *et al.* Cisplatin neurotoxicity. *N Engl J Med* 1990; **323:** 64–5.
5. Philip PA, *et al.* Convulsions and transient cortical blindness after cisplatin. *Br Med J* 1991; **302:** 416.
6. Higa GM, *et al.* Severe, disabling neurologic toxicity following cisplatin retreatment. *Ann Pharmacother* 1995; **29:** 134–7.

Extravasation. For discussion of the management of extravasation, including mention of the potential use of sodium thiosulphate in cisplatin extravasation, see under Treatment of the Adverse Effects of Antineoplastics, p.474.

Hypersensitivity. Anaphylactoid reactions to intravenous cisplatin generally appear within a few minutes of administration and have manifested as facial oedema, wheezing, tachycardia, and hypotension.[1] A high incidence of anaphylactoid reaction has also been seen following intravesical instillation in patients with bladder cancer,[2] but intraperitoneal or intrapleural administration does not seem to be associated with an enhanced risk of hypersensitivity,[3] although anaphylactoid reactions have occurred when cisplatin is given intraperitoneally.[4] Anaphylactoid symptoms and ischaemia of the hands accompanied severe exfoliative dermatitis in one patient on the second cycle of cisplatin-based chemotherapy;[5] she had earlier experienced exfoliative dermatitis associated with carboplatin.

1. Von Hoff DD, *et al.* Allergic reactions to cis platinum. *Lancet* 1976; **i:** 90.
2. Denis L. Anaphylactic reactions to repeated intravesical instillation with cisplatin. *Lancet* 1983; **i:** 1378–9.
3. Markman M. No increase in allergic reactions with intracavitary administration of cisplatin. *Lancet* 1984; **ii:** 1164.
4. Hebert ME, *et al.* Anaphylactoid reactions with intraperitoneal cisplatin. *Ann Pharmacother* 1995; **29:** 260–3.
5. Lee TC, *et al.* Severe exfoliative dermatitis associated with hand ischemia during cisplatin therapy. *Mayo Clin Proc* 1994; **69:** 80–2.

Nausea and vomiting. For discussion of the treatment of antineoplastic-induced nausea and vomiting, see under Nausea and Vomiting, p.1172.

Precautions

For reference to the precautions necessary with antineoplastics and immunosuppressants, see p.474.

Cisplatin is generally contra-indicated in patients with renal or hearing impairment, or bone-marrow depression. Renal and neurological function and hearing should be monitored during treatment, and regular blood counts performed. Adequate hydration and urinary output must be maintained before, and for 24 hours after, administration.

Handling and disposal. Methods for the destruction of cisplatin wastes by reduction with zinc powder under acidic conditions or by reaction with ditiocarb sodium.[1] Residue produced by the degradation of cisplatin by either method showed no mutagenicity *in vitro*.

1. Castegnaro M, *et al.*, eds. Laboratory decontamination and destruction of carcinogens in laboratory wastes: some antineoplastic agents. *IARC Scientific Publications 73*. Lyon: WHO/International Agency for Research on Cancer, 1985.

Urine produced for up to 7 days after a dose of cisplatin should be handled wearing protective clothing.[1]

1. Harris J, Dodds LJ. Handling waste from patients receiving cytotoxic drugs. *Pharm J* 1985; **235:** 289–91.

Radiotherapy. Enhanced ototoxicity has been reported in patients given cisplatin for brain tumours who had also received cranial irradiation.[1,2]

1. Granowetter L, *et al.* Enhanced cis-platinum neurotoxicity in pediatric patients with brain tumors. *J Neurooncol* 1983; **1:** 293–7.
2. Mahoney DH, *et al.* Ototoxicity with cisplatin therapy. *J Pediatr* 1983; **103:** 1006.

Interactions

The concomitant use of other nephrotoxic or ototoxic drugs may exacerbate the adverse effects of cisplatin. The effects of cisplatin on renal function may also affect the pharmacokinetics of other drugs excreted by the renal route.

Antibacterials. Although the use of cisplatin with other nephrotoxic or ototoxic drugs requires great caution, there is some evidence that aminoglycosides can be used in patients who have recently received cisplatin if appropriate supportive care is available.[1]

1. Cooper BW, *et al.* Renal dysfunction during high-dose cisplatin therapy and autologous hematopoietic stem cell transplantation: effect of aminoglycoside therapy. *Am J Med* 1993; **94:** 497–504.

Antineoplastics. The ototoxicity of cisplatin was reportedly enhanced by concomitant use of ifosfamide,[1] an agent which is not ototoxic when given alone, although it does have nephrotoxic potential, making reports of increased nephrotoxicity in patients who have received both unsurprising.[2,3]

For a report of increased toxicity with etoposide, see p.533.

1. Meyer WH, *et al.* Ifosfamide and exacerbation of cisplatin-induced hearing loss. *Lancet* 1993; **341:** 754–5.
2. Rossi R, Ehrich JHH. Partial and complete de Toni-Debré-Fanconi syndrome after ifosfamide chemotherapy of childhood malignancy. *Eur J Clin Pharmacol* 1993; **44** (suppl 1): S43–S45.
3. Martinez F, *et al.* Ifosfamide nephrotoxicity: deleterious effect of previous cisplatin administration. *Lancet* 1996; **348:** 1100–1.

Cardiovascular drugs. A patient whose renal function was unaffected by cisplatin alone developed nephrotoxicity when given cisplatin and antihypertensive therapy with frusemide, hydralazine, diazoxide, and propranolol.[1] Previous results in *animals* suggest that frusemide may aggravate cisplatin nephrotoxicity, while the other antihypertensives might have contributed to a transient fall in renal-blood flow with resultant increased renal-tubular cisplatin concentration.

1. Markman M, Trump DL. Nephrotoxicity with cisplatin and antihypertensive medications. *Ann Intern Med* 1982; **96:** 257.

Pharmacokinetics

After intravenous administration cisplatin disappears from the plasma in a biphasic manner and half-lives of 25 to 49 minutes and 58 to 73 hours have been reported for total platinum. The majority of the platinum from a dose is rapidly bound to plasma protein. Cisplatin is concentrated in the liver, kidneys, and large and small intestines. Penetration into the central nervous system appears to be poor. Excretion is mainly in the urine but is incomplete and prolonged: up to about 50% of a dose has been reported to be excreted in urine over 5 days, and platinum may be detected in tissue for several months afterwards. Cisplatin is well-absorbed following intraperitoneal administration.

A review of the pharmacokinetics of some antineoplastics, including cisplatin.[1] Most pharmacokinetic studies have measured total platinum but cisplatin is believed to be non-enzymatically transformed into 1 or more metabolites, which are protein bound; only the non-bound fraction has more than minimal cytotoxic activity. Protein-bound platinum species represent more than 90% of the dose by 2 to 4 hours after administration. Although total platinum has a bi-exponential decline with a prolonged terminal half-life of 58 to 96 hours the non-bound active form has a much more rapid decline with an initial phase half-life of 8 to 30 minutes and a terminal half-life of 40 to 48 minutes. By 4 to 5 hours, unbound cisplatin accounts for less than 2 to 3% of the total circulating platinum. Excretion is primarily renal, with an initial period of rapid output followed within 4 hours by a decline in renal clearance due to protein binding. There is evidence to suggest that the unbound drug may be actively secreted by the renal tubules. The fraction of a dose excreted in urine increases with increased length of infusion. Faecal excretion is probably insignificant, although the drug is found in bile.

1. Balis FM, *et al.* Clinical pharmacokinetics of commonly used anticancer drugs. *Clin Pharmacokinet* 1983; **8:** 202–32.

Distribution into breast milk. Platinum was found in breast milk of a patient receiving chemotherapy at a concentration of 0.9 μg per mL; the concentration in plasma was 0.8 μg per mL.[1] Although most of the platinum in breast milk is probably protein-bound the authors consider that a mother should not breast feed while receiving cisplatin chemotherapy.

1. de Vries EGE, *et al.* Excretion of platinum into breast milk. *Lancet* 1989; **i:** 497. Correction. *ibid.*; 798.

Uses and Administration

The antineoplastic cisplatin is a platinum-containing complex which may act similarly to the alkylating agents. Its antineoplastic actions are cell-cycle nonspecific and are dependent upon the *cis* configuration: the *trans* isomer is inactive. Although it causes immunosuppression, stimulation of the host immune response against the tumour has been suggested as contributing to its antineoplastic action.

Cisplatin is of value in the treatment of metastatic tumours of the testis, usually as a major component of combination chemotherapy regimens, and particularly in combination with bleomycin and etoposide. It is also used in metastatic ovarian tumours and advanced bladder cancer, and has been reported to be active against a wide range of other solid tumours, as indicated by the cross references given below.

Cisplatin is administered intravenously, not more frequently than every 3 to 4 weeks. It is usually given as a single dose of 50 to 120 mg per m^2 body-surface, or in a dose of 15 to 20 mg per m^2 daily for 5 days. In combination chemotherapy regimens, lower doses may be given. A dose of 20 mg per m^2 daily for 5 days every 3 weeks has been employed in combination chemotherapy of testicular tumours.

It is recommended by the manufacturers that the reconstituted injection is administered in 2 litres of sodium chloride 0.9% injection or in a glucose and sodium chloride solution and infused over at least 1 to 2 hours; an infusion time of 6 to 8 hours may reduce the toxicity. In practice, other regimens may be used at expert centres: for example, doses of up to 100 mg of cisplatin are reportedly dissolved in as little as 250 mL of 0.9% sodium chloride and infused over 30 minutes, provided the patient has acceptable renal function and is well hydrated. To aid diuresis and protect the kidneys, 37.5 g of mannitol is usually added to the infusion; alternatively an infusion of mannitol 10% may be given immediately before cisplatin. In order to initiate diuresis the patient is usually hydrated by the infusion of 1 to 2 litres of a suitable fluid over several hours before the administration of cisplatin. Adequate hydration must also be maintained for up to 24 hours after a dose. Renal, haematological, auditory, and neurological function should be monitored during therapy, and administration adjusted accordingly.

Cisplatin has also been administered by the intra-arterial and intraperitoneal routes, and by instillation into the bladder. It has also been investigated as a less toxic but apparently less effective cisplatin-albumin complex, as a liposomal formulation, and as an implant containing cisplatin in a protein matrix, MPI-5010.

Various analogues of cisplatin have been investigated in the hope of improved activity, fewer adverse effects, or activity following oral administration.

Action. A review of inorganic pharmacology, including cisplatin.[1] The cytotoxicity of cisplatin appears to be related to its hydrolysis in the body. The aquated form, *cis*-$Pt(NH_3)_2(H_2O)(OH)^+$, is very reactive, and can also form hydroxyl-bridged dimers and trimers. Selective killing of tumour cells is probably due to attack on the guanine- and cytosine-rich regions of DNA, producing damage which is repairable by normal cells. Platinum crosslinks between DNA strands are not now thought to be important cytotoxic events. It has also been suggested that platinum binding to guanine activates the base so that it can form abnormal base pairs, resulting in unwinding of DNA.

1. Sadler PJ. Inorganic pharmacology. *Chem Br* 1982; **18:** 182–8.

Administration. Various adjustments to the standard administration of cisplatin have been suggested in an attempt to improve effectiveness while reducing toxicity.

Hydration before and after a dose of cisplatin, together with the use of mannitol to promote diuresis, is now standard (see Uses and Administration, above). Higher doses of cisplatin (up to 200 mg per square metre body-surface area per treatment course) have been successfully given by infusion in hypertonic sodium chloride, accompanied by intensive hydration.[1,2] However, while such a regimen may limit nephrotoxicity, other toxic effects, such as peripheral neuropathy, are not prevented,[1-4] although myelosuppression may be less if the total dose is given in 2 divided doses rather than as a 5-day continuous infusion.[2]

Toxicity has been reported to be reduced when cisplatin was given by continuous intra-arterial[5] or intravenous[6] infusion, while Hrushesky and colleagues have suggested that giving cisplatin in the evening rather than the morning results in less damage to renal function, apparently because of circadian variations in urine production.[7]

An alternative way to increase the platinum dose without crippling toxicity has been suggested to be the combination of cisplatin and carboplatin.[8]

Various drugs have been investigated to reduce toxicity, including amifostine, glutathione, and thiosulphate, as discussed under Effects on the Kidney, and Effects on the Nervous System, above.

1. Ozols RF, *et al.* High-dose cisplatin in hypertonic saline. *Ann Intern Med* 1984; **100:** 19–24.
2. Gandara DR, *et al.* Cisplatin dose intensity in non-small cell lung cancer: phase II results of a day 1 and day 8 high-dose regimen. *J Natl Cancer Inst* 1989; **81:** 790–4.
3. Bagley CM, *et al.* High-dose cisplatin therapy for cancer of the ovary: neurotoxicity. *Ann Intern Med* 1985; **102:** 719.
4. Ozols RF, Young RC. High-dose cisplatin therapy for cancer of the ovary: neurotoxicity. *Ann Intern Med* 1985; **102:** 719.
5. Jacobs SC, *et al.* Intraarterial cisplatin infusion in the management of transitional cell carcinoma of the bladder. *Cancer* 1989; **64:** 388–91.
6. Salem P, *et al.* Cis-diamminedichloroplatinum (II) by 5-day continuous infusion: a new dose schedule with minimal toxicity. *Cancer* 1984; **53:** 837–40.
7. Hrushesky WJM, *et al.* Circadian time dependence of cisplatin urinary kinetics. *Clin Pharmacol Ther* 1982; **32:** 330–9.
8. Piccart MJ, *et al.* Cisplatin combined with carboplatin: a new way of intensification of platinum dose in the treatment of advanced ovarian cancer. *J Natl Cancer Inst* 1990; **82:** 703–7.

Malignant neoplasms. Cisplatin is used in the management of many solid malignancies, notably those of the bladder, ovary, and testis, as discussed on p.484, p.491, and p.493 respectively. Other malignancies where cisplatin may be employed, as discussed in the introduction to this chapter, include gestational trophoblastic tumours (p.477), non-Hodgkin's lymphomas (p.482), tumours of brain (p.485), cervix (p.487), endometrium (p.487), upper gastro-intestinal tract (p.487), head and neck (p.489), liver (p.489), lung (p.490), pancreas (though to little effect— see p.491), prostate (p.491), thymus (p.493) and thyroid (p.494), neuroblastoma (p.494), retinoblastoma (p.495), melanoma (p.492), and sarcoma of bone (p.495). It has also been employed in the treatment of malignant effusions (p.484), although it is not the treatment of choice.

Preparations

BP 1998: Cisplatin Injection;
USP 23: Cisplatin for Injection.

Proprietary Preparations (details are given in Part 3)
Aust.: Abiplatin; Platiblastin; Platinol; ***Belg.:*** Platinol; ***Canad.:*** Platinol; ***Fr.:*** Cisplatyl; ***Ger.:*** Platiblastin; Platinex; ***Ital.:*** Citoplatino; Platamine; Platinex; Pronto Platamine; ***Jpn:*** Randa; ***Neth.:*** Abiplatin†; Platinol; ***Norw.:*** Platinol; Platistin; ***S.Afr.:*** Abiplatin; Norplatin†; Platamine; Platosin; ***Spain:*** Neoplatin; Placis; Platistil; ***Swed.:*** Lederplatin; Platinol; Platistin†; ***Switz.:*** Platiblastine-S; Platinol; ***USA:*** Platinol.

Cladribine (4849-m)

Cladribine (*BAN, USAN, rINN*).

2-Chlorodeoxyadenosine; RWJ-26251; RWJ-26251-000. 2-Chloro-2′-deoxyadenosine.

$C_{10}H_{12}ClN_5O_3$ = 285.7.

CAS — 4291-63-8.

Adverse Effects, Treatment, and Precautions

For a general outline see Antineoplastics, p.470, p.473, and p.474.

Cladribine produces myelosuppression, with neutropenia, prolonged lymphopenia, and severe anaemia; thrombocytopenia is less common. Prolonged bone-marrow hypocellularity has been noted in some patients, although it is not clear if this is due to the drug or underlying disease.

Other adverse effects include fever, fatigue, malaise, mild nausea and gastro-intestinal disturbances, rashes, pruritus, purpura, headache, dizziness, cough, dyspnoea, oedema, and tachycardia. High doses of cladribine have been associated with severe renal and nervous system toxicity as well as myelosuppression. Severe neurotoxicity is rare at currently recommended doses, but confusion, neuropathy, ataxia, insomnia, and somnolence have occurred.

Uses and Administration

Cladribine is a purine antimetabolite antineoplastic which inhibits DNA synthesis and repair particularly in lymphocytes and monocytes. It is used for the treatment of lymphoid malignancies including hairy-cell leukaemia (p.481), non-Hodgkin's lymphomas (p.482) including mycosis fungoides (p.482), and chronic lymphocytic leukaemia (p.480). It has been tried in histiocytic syndromes (p.478) and in Waldenström's macroglobulinaemia (p.496).

Cladribine is given by continuous intravenous infusion; the recommended dose in hairy-cell leukaemia is 90 μg per kg body-weight or 3.6 mg per m^2 body-surface daily for 7 days. Higher doses have been given but may be associated with more severe toxicity (see above). For the treatment of chronic lymphocytic leukaemia the recommended dose is 120 μg per kg or 4.8 mg per m^2 daily for 5 consecutive days of a 28-day cycle; the infusion is given over 2 hours. Response should be determined every 2 cycles, and once maximum response has occurred a further 2 cycles of treatment are recommended, up to a maximum of 6 cycles. Patients who do not respond with a lymphocyte reduction of 50% or more after 2 cycles should not receive further therapy.

The use of cladribine by mouth in chronic lymphocytic leukaemia is under investigation.

Cladribine has also been tried in the management of multiple sclerosis (p.620).

References.

1. Piro LD, *et al.* Lasting remissions in hairy-cell leukemia induced by a single infusion of 2-chlorodeoxyadenosine. *N Engl J Med* 1990; **322:** 1117–21.
2. Piro LD. 2-Chlorodeoxyadenosine treatment of lymphoid malignancies. *Blood* 1992; **79:** 843.
3. Juliusson G, *et al.* Response to 2-chlorodeoxyadenosine in patients with B-cell chronic lymphocytic leukemia resistant to fludarabine. *N Engl J Med* 1992; **327:** 1056–61.
4. Beutler E. Cladribine (2-chlorodeoxyadenosine). *Lancet* 1992; **340:** 952–6.
5. Bryson HM, Sorkin EM. Cladribine: a review of its pharmacodynamic and pharmacokinetic properties and therapeutic potential in haematological malignancies. *Drugs* 1993; **46:** 872–94.
6. Baltz JK, Montello MJ. Cladribine for the treatment of hematologic malignancies. *Clin Pharm* 1993; **12:** 805–13.
7. Saven A, Piro LD. 2-Chlorodeoxyadenosine: a newer purine analog active in the treatment of indolent lymphoid malignancies. *Ann Intern Med* 1994; **120:** 784–91.
8. O'Brien S, *et al.* Lack of effect of 2-chlorodeoxyadenosine therapy in patients with chronic lymphocytic leukemia refractory to fludarabine therapy. *N Engl J Med* 1994; **330:** 319–22.
9. Saven A, *et al.* 2-Chlorodeoxyadenosine-induced complete remissions in Langerhans-cell histiocytosis. *Ann Intern Med* 1994; **121:** 430–2.
10. Sipe JC, *et al.* Cladribine in treatment of chronic progressive multiple sclerosis. *Lancet* 1994; **344:** 9–13.
11. Liliemark J. The clinical pharmacokinetics of cladribine. *Clin Pharmacokinet* 1997; **32:** 120–31.

Preparations

Proprietary Preparations (details are given in Part 3)
Austral.: Leustatin; ***Canad.:*** Leustatin; ***Fr.:*** Leustatine; ***Neth.:*** Leustatin; ***Swed.:*** Leustatin; ***UK:*** Leustat; ***USA:*** Leustatin.

Corynebacterium parvum (12609-w)

C. parvum; NSC-220537; *Propionibacterium acnes.*

Inactivated *Corynebacterium parvum* has been used in the treatment of malignant effusions, and has been tried as an adjuvant to cancer chemotherapy for its immunostimulant properties. It has also been used in the treatment of musculoskeletal and joint disorders.

Fever has followed intracavitary injection and abdominal pain has occurred after intraperitoneal injection. There have been reports of nephrotoxicity following intravenous use.

Preparations

Proprietary Preparations (details are given in Part 3)
Ger.: Arthrokehlan "A"; ***Ital.:*** Coparvax†; ***UK:*** Coparvax†.

Crisnatol Mesylate (4868-g)

Crisnatol Mesylate *(USAN)*.

Crisnatol Mesilate *(rINNM)*; BW-A770U (crisnatol); BW-A770U (crisnatol mesylate).

CAS — 96389-68-3 (crisnatol); 96389-69-4 (crisnatol mesylate).

Crisnatol is reported to act as a topoisomerase inhibitor and an intercalator of DNA. It is under investigation for its antineoplastic properties, notably for malignant neoplasms of the brain.

Cyclophosphamide (1825-k)

Cyclophosphamide *(BAN, rINN)*.

B-518; Ciclofosfamida; Cyclophosphamidum; Cyclophosphanum; NSC-26271; WR-138719. 2-[Bis(2-chloroethyl)amino]perhydro-1,3,2-oxazaphosphorinan 2-oxide monohydrate.

$C_7H_{15}Cl_2N_2O_2P,H_2O$ = 279.1.

CAS — 6055-19-2 (cyclophosphamide monohydrate); 50-18-0 (anhydrous cyclophosphamide).

Pharmacopoeias. In *Chin., Eur.* (see p.viii), *Int., Jpn, Pol.,* and *US.*

A white or almost white, crystalline powder. M.p. 49.5° to 53°. It liquefies upon loss of its water of crystallisation. **Soluble** in water and freely soluble in alcohol; slightly soluble in ether. The Ph. Eur. states that a freshly prepared 2% solution in water has a pH of 4.0 to 6.0. The USP requires that a 1% solution should have a pH of 3.9 to 7.1 when determined 30 minutes after preparation. Solutions deteriorate on storage. Aqueous solutions may be kept for a few hours at temperatures up to 25°. At temperatures above 30° hydrolysis occurs with removal of chlorine.

Store in airtight containers at 2° to 30°. The USP recommends that tablets should be stored at a temperature not exceeding 25°, although they will withstand brief exposure to temperatures up to 30°; it requires preparations to be protected from temperatures above 30°.

Isomerism. For the suggestion that the (−)-enantiomer of cyclophosphamide may be more active, see Action, under Uses and Administration, below.

Adverse Effects and Treatment

For a general outline see Antineoplastics, p.470 and p.473. The major dose-limiting effect is myelosuppression. After single doses the nadir of the white-cell count may occur in around 1 to 2 weeks with full recovery usually in 3 to 4 weeks. Thrombocytopenia and anaemia may occur but tend to be less common and less severe.

Excretion of active metabolites in urine after high or prolonged dosage may be responsible for cystitis, often severe and haemorrhagic, which can be life-threatening. Adequate hydration to maintain urine output or administration of mesna (see p.984) are generally recommended in an attempt to reduce urotoxicity.

Alopecia, usually reversible, occurs in about 20% of patients within 3 weeks of starting treatment at normal doses and in practically all patients given high doses. Hyperpigmentation of skin, especially that of the palms and soles, and of the nails, has been reported.

Other reported adverse effects include gastro-intestinal disturbances, hepatotoxicity, a syndrome resembling inappropriate secretion of antidiuretic hormone, disturbances of carbohydrate metabolism, gonadal suppression, occasionally resulting in sterility, interstitial pulmonary fibrosis, and, especially at high doses, cardiotoxicity.

Cyclophosphamide, in common with other alkylating agents, has carcinogenic, mutagenic, and teratogenic potential and secondary malignancies have occurred in patients given previous antineoplastic therapy including cyclophosphamide.

Effects on the bladder. Sterile haemorrhagic cystitis, believed to be secondary to renal excretion of alkylating metabolites, has occurred following high-dose infusions of cyclophosphamide, or after prolonged low-dose-administration.[1,2] The reported incidence has been as high as 40%,[3] although this has been markedly reduced since the introduction of mesna.[4] The cystitis appears to result from chronic inflammation leading to fibrosis and telangiectasia of the bladder epithelium; haemorrhage may become life-threatening if drug administration is continued.[1] Symptoms may be delayed, and have been reported to occur up to 6 months after discontinuation of the drug.[5] An increased incidence of cystitis when patients on a high-dose cyclophosphamide regimen were transferred from one brand to another has been reported,[6] apparently because one was labelled in terms of the anhydrous substance and one as the monohydrate, resulting in a 6.4% difference in the content of active substance.[7] Vigorous hydration (increasing urine output and thus diluting the excreted metabolites), or the use of mesna, may prevent the occurrence of cystitis. Where bleeding occurs, an initial trial of diathermy, and then alum instillation, should probably be made before progressing to the instillation of more toxic agents such as formaldehyde solution, or silver nitrate, or the use of more problematic non-drug techniques.[3] Prostaglandins instilled into the bladder may also be effective in controlling haemorrhagic cystitis.[8-10]

In addition to the shorter term effects, cyclophosphamide has been reported to be associated with the development of bladder carcinoma.[11-15] A history of cyclophosphamide-induced cystitis may be associated with an increased risk of bladder carcinoma[11,15] but some studies have not found a link,[13] and bladder malignancies can develop in patients who have not experienced cystitis while receiving cyclophosphamide.[12] For a discussion of the carcinogenic effects of antineoplastics, including cyclophosphamide, see p.470. For a suggestion that acetylcysteine can help prevent urothelial toxicity, see p.1054.

1. Bender RA, *et al.* Antineoplastic drugs: clinical pharmacology and therapeutic use. *Drugs* 1978; **16:** 46–87.
2. Spiers ASD, *et al.* Haemorrhagic cystitis after low-dose cyclophosphamide. *Lancet* 1983; **i:** 1213–14.
3. Bullock N, Whitaker RH. Massive bladder haemorrhage. *Br Med J* 1985; **291:** 1522–3.
4. de Kraker J. Massive bladder haemorrhage. *Br Med J* 1986; **292:** 628.
5. Armstrong B, *et al.* Delayed cystitis due to cyclophosphamide. *N Engl J Med* 1979; **300:** 45.
6. Shaw IC, *et al.* Difference in bioactivity between two preparations of cyclophosphamide. *Lancet* 1983; **i:** 709.
7. Hilgard P, *et al.* Bioactivity of cyclophosphamide preparations. *Lancet* 1983; **i:** 1436.
8. Mohiuddin J, *et al.* Treatment of cyclophosphamide-induced cystitis with prostaglandin E_2. *Ann Intern Med* 1984; **101:** 142.
9. Miller LJ, *et al.* Treatment of cyclophosphamide-induced hemorrhagic cystitis with prostaglandins. *Ann Pharmacother* 1994; **28:** 590–4.
10. Ippoliti C, *et al.* Intravesicular carboprost for the treatment of hemorrhagic cystitis after marrow transplantation. *Urology* 1995; **46:** 811–15.
11. Wall RL, Clausen KP. Carcinoma of the urinary bladder in patients receiving cyclophosphamide. *N Engl J Med* 1975; **293:** 271–3.
12. Plotz PH, *et al.* Bladder complications in patients receiving cyclophosphamide for systemic lupus erythematosus or rheumatoid arthritis. *Ann Intern Med* 1979; **91:** 221–3.
13. Pedersen-Bjergaard J, *et al.* Carcinoma of the urinary bladder after treatment with cyclophosphamide for non-Hodgkin's lymphoma. *N Engl J Med* 1988; **318:** 1028–32.
14. Travis LB, *et al.* Bladder cancer after chemotherapy for non-Hodgkin's lymphoma. *N Engl J Med* 1989; **321:** 544–5.
15. Talar-Williams C, *et al.* Cyclophosphamide-induced cystitis and bladder cancer in patients with Wegener granulomatosis. *Ann Intern Med* 1996; **124:** 477–84.

Effects on electrolytes. Water intoxication has been reported following administration of cyclophosphamide,[1-4] usually in high doses (30 to 50 mg per kg body-weight or more) although symptoms have been reported after a dose of 20 mg per kg in a patient with renal disease,[3] and in another patient with systemic lupus erythematosus but apparently normal renal function who received 10 mg per kg.[4] One case of severe hyponatraemia leading to convulsions and death has been reported.[5] Symptoms resemble the syndrome of inappropriate antidiuretic hormone secretion (SIADH)[5] but plasma concentrations of antidiuretic hormone do not appear to be raised in these patients.[3]

1. DeFronzo RA, *et al.* Water intoxication in man after cyclophosphamide therapy: time course and relation to drug activation. *Ann Intern Med* 1973; **78:** 861–9.
2. Green TP, Mirkin BL. Prevention of cyclophosphamide-induced antidiuresis by furosemide infusion. *Clin Pharmacol Ther* 1981; **29:** 634–42.
3. Bressler RB, Huston DP. Water intoxication following moderate-dose intravenous cyclophosphamide. *Arch Intern Med* 1985; **145:** 548–9.
4. McCarron MO, *et al.* Water intoxication after low dose cyclophosphamide. *Br Med J* 1995; **311:** 292.
5. Harlow PJ, *et al.* A fatal case of inappropriate ADH secretion induced by cyclophosphamide therapy. *Cancer* 1979; **44:** 896–8.

Effects on the eyes. Recurrent transient myopia was induced by intravenous bolus administration of cyclophosphamide in an adolescent with systemic lupus erythematosus, apparently due to increased hydration of the lens of the eye.[1]

1. Arranz JA, *et al.* Cyclophosphamide-induced myopia. *Ann Intern Med* 1992; **116:** 92–3.

Effects on reproductive potential. Although severe gonadal failure with transient or permanent azoospermia is common in men treated with cyclophosphamide, Masala and colleagues[1] reported that suppression of germ-cell function with intramuscular testosterone in 5 men during cyclophosphamide therapy for nephrotic syndrome was associated with a more rapid return of spermatogenesis compared with 10 patients who did not receive the androgen.

1. Masala A, *et al.* Use of testosterone to prevent cyclophosphamide-induced azoospermia. *Ann Intern Med* 1997; **126:** 292–5.

Effects on the skin. An erythematous pruritic rash, similar to the palmar-plantar syndrome but occurring on the dorsal surfaces of the hands and feet, occurred 6 days after the first high dose of cyclophosphamide in a patient being prepared for bone-marrow transplantation.[1] Previous cyclophosphamide-containing chemotherapy did not produce this reaction. The symptoms improved somewhat on treatment with triamcinolone ointment, and subsequently desquamation of the hands occurred with decreased purplish discoloration and oedema of the feet. Assier-Bonnet and colleagues also reported on 2 patients who developed Stevens-Johnson syndrome, with some features suggestive of overlapping toxic epidermal necrolysis.[2]

1. Matsuyama JR, Kwok KK. A variant of the chemotherapy-associated erythrodysesthesia syndrome related to high-dose cyclophosphamide. *DICP Ann Pharmacother* 1989; **23:** 776–9.
2. Assier-Bonnet H, *et al.* Stevens-Johnson syndrome induced by cyclophosphamide: report of two cases. *Br J Dermatol* 1996; **135:** 864–6.

Hypersensitivity. Occasional anaphylaxis has been reported with cyclophosphamide;[1] analysis of data by the Boston Collaborative Drug Surveillance Program detected only one allergic skin reaction among 210 patients given cyclophosphamide, resulting in a calculated incidence of 4.8 reactions per 1000 recipients.[2]

1. Jones JB, *et al.* Cyclophosphamide anaphylaxis. *DICP Ann Pharmacother* 1989; **23:** 88–9.
2. Bigby M, *et al.* Drug-induced cutaneous reactions: a report from the Boston Collaborative Drug Surveillance Program on 15 438 consecutive inpatients, 1975 to 1982. *JAMA* 1986; **256:** 3358–63.

Precautions

For reference to the precautions necessary with antineoplastics and immunosuppressants, see p.474.

Cyclophosphamide should not be given to patients with bone-marrow aplasia, haemorrhagic cystitis, acute systemic or urinary infection, or drug- or radiation-induced urothelial toxicity. It should be given with care to those with diabetes mellitus. Care is also needed in elderly or debilitated patients, or those with renal or hepatic failure or who have undergone adrenalectomy. Liberal fluid intake and frequent micturition are advised to reduce the risk of cystitis but care must be taken to avoid water retention and intoxication.

Cyclophosphamide has teratogenic and mutagenic potential; its use in pregnancy should be avoided where possible. Mothers taking cyclophosphamide should avoid breast feeding.

Handling and disposal. A method for the destruction of cyclophosphamide or ifosfamide using alkaline hydrolysis in the presence of dimethylformamide.[1] Residues of either drug dealt with by this method showed no mutagenicity *in vitro*. However, an alternative method exists, involving refluxing of cyclophosphamide with hydrochloric acid, neutralising, and then reacting with sodium thiosulphate. This method is effective for the degradation of cyclophosphamide, but residues from ifosfamide were still highly mutagenic *in vitro* and this second method should therefore not be used to degrade ifosfamide.

1. Castegnaro M, *et al.*, eds. Laboratory decontamination and destruction of carcinogens in laboratory wastes: some antineoplastic agents. *IARC Scientific Publications 73*. Lyon: WHO/International Agency for Research on Cancer, 1985.

Urine and faeces produced for up to 72 hours and 5 days respectively after an oral dose of cyclophosphamide should be handled wearing protective clothing.[1] As cyclophosphamide was present in sweat and saliva, protective clothing was advised for 72 hours after a dose when bathing the patient or carrying out oral procedures.

1. Harris J, Dodds LJ. Handling waste from patients receiving cytotoxic drugs. *Pharm J* 1985; **235:** 289–91.

Interactions

Since cyclophosphamide must undergo metabolism before it is active, interactions are possible with drugs which either inhibit or stimulate the enzymes responsible. There may be an increased risk of cardiotoxicity in patients who have also received doxorubicin or other cardiotoxic drugs, or have had irradiation to the area of the heart.

Allopurinol. Although the Boston Collaborative Drug Surveillance Program reported an increased incidence of bone-marrow depression in patients who received allopurinol with cyclophosphamide than in those receiving cyclophosphamide without allopurinol (15 of 26 compared with only 6 of 32),[1] a subsequent study in patients receiving combination chemotherapy, including cyclophosphamide, for lymphomas failed to find any difference in the nadirs of the platelet and white blood cell counts in cycles in which allopurinol was given concomitantly.[2] Bagley and colleagues, in a study in 26 patients receiving cyclophosphamide, found that although allopurinol pretreatment in 4 resulted in a longer cyclophosphamide half-life, urinary excretion of cyclophosphamide was unchanged.[3] Increased half-life was also seen in a study in children who had received allopurinol.[4]

1. Boston Collaborative Drug Surveillance Program. Allopurinol and cytotoxic drugs: interaction in relation to bone marrow depression. *JAMA* 1974; **227:** 1036–40.
2. Stolbach L, *et al.* Evaluation of bone marrow toxic reaction in patients treated with allopurinol. *JAMA* 1982; **247:** 334–6.
3. Bagley CM, *et al.* Clinical pharmacology of cyclophosphamide. *Cancer Res* 1973; **33:** 226–33.
4. Yule SM, *et al.* Cyclophosphamide pharmacokinetics in children. *Br J Clin Pharmacol* 1996; **41:** 13–19.

Antibacterials. Administration of chloramphenicol prior to cyclophosphamide prolonged the mean cyclophosphamide serum half-life from 7.5 to 11.5 hours and reduced the peak activity in all of 5 subjects.[1] Administration of sulphaphenazole prior to cyclophosphamide significantly inhibited the rate of biotransformation of cyclophosphamide in 2 of 7 subjects and enhanced it in 2; it remained unchanged in 3.

1. Faber OK, *et al.* The effect of chloramphenicol and sulphaphenazole on the biotransformation of cyclophosphamide in man. *Br J Clin Pharmacol* 1975; **2:** 281–5.

Anticoagulants. For reference to the interaction of cyclophosphamide with warfarin, see p.967.

Barbiturates. Although patients receiving cyclophosphamide developed higher peak plasma concentrations of active cyclophosphamide metabolites when given enzyme-inducing agents such as barbiturates, the active metabolites also disappeared rapidly.[1]

1. Bagley CM, *et al.* Clinical pharmacology of cyclophosphamide. *Cancer Res* 1973; **33:** 226–33.

Chlorpromazine. The half-life of cyclophosphamide was approximately 200% greater in 2 children who were receiving chlorpromazine concurrently than in children who were not receiving the phenothiazine.[1]

1. Yule SM, *et al.* Cyclophosphamide pharmacokinetics in children. *Br J Clin Pharmacol* 1996; **41:** 13–19.

Colony-stimulating factors. Fatal respiratory insufficiency associated with alveolar fibrosis developed in an infant given cyclophosphamide and doxorubicin followed by filgrastim.[1] Since pulmonary toxicity with cyclophosphamide is normally associated with high cumulative doses it was suggested that in this case the effects might have been exacerbated by the granulocyte colony-stimulating factor. (The pulmonary toxicity of bleomycin has also been suggested to be exacerbated by colony-stimulating factors, as discussed on p.508).

1. van Woensel JBM, *et al.* Acute respiratory insufficiency during doxorubicin, cyclophosphamide, and G-CSF therapy. *Lancet* 1994; **344:** 759–60.

Corticosteroids. Single doses of prednisone have been found to inhibit the activation of cyclophosphamide but after longer-term treatment the rate of activation has increased.[1] A study in children found that pretreatment with dexamethasone was associated with increased clearance of cyclophosphamide and a decrease in its half-life relative to children who had not received the corticosteroid.[2]

1. Faber OK, Mouridsen HT. Cyclophosphamide activation and corticosteroids. *N Engl J Med* 1974; **291:** 211.
2. Yule SM, *et al.* Cyclophosphamide pharmacokinetics in children. *Br J Clin Pharmacol* 1996; **41:** 13–19.

Digoxin. Cardiac arrhythmias during combination chemotherapy in a patient with atrial fibrillation previously well controlled with digoxin might have been due to an interaction between cyclophosphamide and digoxin.[1]

1. Echizen G, Ishizaki T. A possible drug interaction between cyclophosphamide and digoxin. *Br Med J* 1985; **291:** 1172.

NSAIDs. A report of acute life-threatening water intoxication in a patient given low-dose cyclophosphamide concomitantly with indomethacin.[1] The patient had previously received treatment with cyclophosphamide (for multiple myeloma) without significant adverse effect.

1. Webberley MJ, Murray JA. Life-threatening acute hyponatraemia induced by low dose cyclophosphamide and indomethacin. *Postgrad Med J* 1989; **65:** 950–2.

Suxamethonium. For reference to a possible interaction between cyclophosphamide and suxamethonium, see under Suxamethonium Chloride, p.1321.

Pharmacokinetics

Following oral administration, cyclophosphamide is well absorbed from the gastro-intestinal tract with a bioavailability greater than 75%. It is widely distributed in the tissues and crosses the blood-brain barrier. It undergoes activation by the mixed function oxidase systems in the liver. The initial metabolites are 4-hydroxycyclophosphamide and its acyclic tautomer, aldophosphamide, which both undergo further metabolism; aldophosphamide may undergo non-enzymatic conversion to active phosphoramide mustard. Acrolein is also produced and may be responsible for bladder toxicity. Cyclophosphamide is excreted principally in urine, as metabolites and some unchanged drug.

It crosses the placenta, and is found in breast milk.

Reviews.

1. Grochow LB, Colvin M. Clinical pharmacokinetics of cyclophosphamide. *Clin Pharmacokinet* 1979; **4:** 380–94.
2. Balis FM, *et al.* Clinical pharmacokinetics of commonly used anticancer drugs. *Clin Pharmacokinet* 1983; **8:** 202–32.
3. Moore MJ. Clinical pharmacokinetics of cyclophosphamide. *Clin Pharmacokinet* 1991; **20:** 194–208.

Absorption. Cyclophosphamide was detected in the urine of 5 patients following application to intact skin, demonstrating that cyclophosphamide can be absorbed via this route.[1] Absorption continued after the site of application had been cleaned, suggesting that cyclophosphamide had penetrated subcutaneous lipid and was slowly released to the circulation from this depot. Cyclophosphamide was also identified in the urine of 2 oncology nurses but appeared more quickly than in patients, suggesting a faster route of absorption, perhaps by inhalation of aerosols generated during dissolution of the drug.

1. Hirst M, *et al.* Occupational exposure to cyclophosphamide. *Lancet* 1984; **i:** 186–8.

Uses and Administration

Cyclophosphamide is an antineoplastic that is converted in the body to an active alkylating metabolite with properties similar to those of mustine (p.555). It also possesses marked immunosuppressant properties.

Cyclophosphamide is widely used, often in combination with other agents, in the treatment of a variety of malignant diseases as indicated by the cross-references below. It is employed for Burkitt's and other lymphomas, some leukaemias, multiple myeloma, and mycosis fungoides. It is also used in the treatment of gestational trophoblastic tumours and malignancies of the brain, breast, cervix, endometrium, lung, prostate, and ovary; in childhood malignancies such as neuroblastoma, retinoblastoma, and Wilm's tumour; and sarcomas.

The immunosuppressant properties of cyclophosphamide have been used in tissue and organ transplantation. It has also been used in the management of various disorders thought to have an auto-immune component including amyloidosis, Behçet's syndrome, glomerular kidney disease, idiopathic thrombocytopenic purpura, interstitial lung disease, polymyositis, scleroderma, systemic lupus erythematosus, and various vasculitic syndromes including the Churg-Strauss syndrome, polyarteritis nodosa, Takayasu's arteritis, and Wegener's granulomatosis.

Cyclophosphamide is usually given by mouth or intravenous injection; it is not a tissue irritant or vesicant. The dosage given depends on the malignant disease being treated, the condition of the patient including the state of the bone marrow, and the concomitant use of radiotherapy or other chemotherapy, and may vary considerably. The white cell count is usually used to guide appropriate dosing. In the UK an example of a low-dose regimen is cyclophosphamide 2 to 6 mg per kg body-weight weekly as a single intravenous dose or in divided doses by mouth; a moderate-dose regimen might be 10 to 15 mg per kg weekly as a single intravenous dose. An example of a high-dose regimen is 20 to 40 mg per kg as a single intravenous dose every 10 to 20 days, although higher doses have been used. The use of mesna is recommended with single doses of cyclophosphamide over 10 mg per kg.

In the USA, an initial dose of 40 to 50 mg per kg has been advocated for single agent therapy of malignancy, given intravenously in divided doses over 2 to 5 days. Other intravenous regimens include 3 to 5 mg per kg twice weekly or 10 to 15 mg per kg every 7 to 10 days. Alternatively, 1 to 5 mg per kg daily has been given orally.

Children have been given initial doses of 2 to 8 mg per kg daily by intravenous injection or by mouth and maintenance doses of 2 to 5 mg per kg twice weekly by mouth.

A daily oral dose of 2 to 3 mg per kg body-weight has been used in children with minimal change nephropathy leading to the nephrotic syndrome, in whom corticosteroids have been unsuccessful.

In patients who are to undergo bone-marrow transplantation very high doses of cyclophosphamide such as 60 mg per kg daily for 2 to 4 days may be given as part of the conditioning regimen.

In the BP the potency of Cyclophosphamide Injection is expressed in terms of the equivalent amount of anhydrous cyclophosphamide whereas the potency of Cyclophosphamide Tablets is given in terms of the monohydrate; the USP expresses potency in terms of anhydrous cyclophosphamide for both injection and tablets. Confusion has arisen when patients were changed from proprietary preparations in which the content was expressed as the monohydrate to one in which it was expressed as the anhydrous substance (see Effects on the Bladder, above).

Cyclophosphamide has also been given intramuscularly, intraperitoneally, and intrapleurally, as well as intra-arterially, and by local perfusion (but passage through the liver is required for its activation—see Pharmacokinetics, above). A liquid preparation of cyclophosphamide for oral use may be prepared using the powder for injection.

Regular blood counts are essential during therapy with cyclophosphamide and in general treatment should be withdrawn or delayed if leucopenia or thrombocytopenia becomes severe. Patients should be adequately hydrated and urine output maintained.

Action. There is some evidence to suggest that cyclophosphamide could be better employed if the (−)-enantiomer was used.[1] Although the toxicity of the two enantiomers is equivalent the cytotoxic activity of the (−)-enantiomer is twice as great as that of the (+)-enantiomer. The former thus has a therapeutic index approximately twice that of the latter and about 1.3 times greater than that of the racemate, implying that it would have less toxicity in clinical practice.

1. Williams K, Lee E. Importance of drug enantiomers in clinical pharmacology. *Drugs* 1985; **30:** 333–54.

Amyloidosis. Although there is no unequivocally effective treatment for amyloidosis (p.497), cyclophosphamide may reduce the decline in renal function;[1] it has also been used in combination with epirubicin and carmustine to suppress the disease in a patient who had undergone heart transplantation for cardiac amyloid.[2]

1. Berglund K, *et al.* Alternating cytostatic treatment in renal amyloidosis secondary to rheumatic disease. *Ann Rheum Dis* 1987; **46:** 757–62.
2. Hall R, *et al.* Cardiac transplantation for AL amyloidosis. *Br Med J* 1994; **309:** 1135–7.

Blood disorders, non-malignant. Cyclophosphamide has been used in patients with idiopathic thrombocytopenic purpura (p.1023), but cytotoxic immunosuppressants tend to be a treatment of last resort. Responses generally occur within 8 weeks.[1] In patients with refractory, life-threatening disease high-dose cyclophosphamide,[1] or if that is unsuccessful, combination chemotherapy including cyclophosphamide, which has produced responses in a few patients,[2] may be tried.

1. McMillan R. Therapy for adults with refractory chronic immune thrombocytopenic purpura. *Ann Intern Med* 1997; **126:** 307–14.
2. Figueroa M, *et al.* Combination chemotherapy in refractory immune thrombocytopenic purpura. *N Engl J Med* 1993; **328:** 1226–9.

Cogan's syndrome. For reference to the use of cyclophosphamide in combination with corticosteroids for Cogan's syndrome, see p.1020.

Connective tissue and muscular disorders. Cyclophosphamide is one of a number of immunosuppressants that have been tried for disease control in Behçet's syndrome (p.1018); such agents may permit a reduction in the use of corticosteroids, although they carry their own risks of toxicity. In polymyositis (p.1027), however, there is some debate about the value of cyclophosphamide as a second-line agent in corticosteroid-unresponsive disease,[1-3] and the role of immunosuppressants other than azathioprine or methotrexate is poorly defined. In patients with systemic lupus erythematosus (p.1029), cyclophosphamide has been used with some success for severe disease or disease refractory to corticosteroids alone.[4-8]

1. Oddis CV, Medsger TA. Current management of polymyositis and dermatomyositis. *Drugs* 1989; **37:** 382–90.
2. Bombardieri S, *et al.* Cyclophosphamide in severe polymyositis. *Lancet* 1989; **i:** 1138–9.
3. Bunch TW. Polymyositis: a case history approach to the differential diagnosis and treatment. *Mayo Clin Proc* 1990; **65:** 1480–97.
4. Barr WG, *et al.* Plasmapheresis and pulse cyclophosphamide in systemic lupus erythematosus. *Ann Intern Med* 1988; **108:** 152–3.
5. Sigal LH. Chronic inflammatory polyneuropathy complicating SLE: successful treatment with monthly oral pulse cyclophosphamide. *J Rheumatol* 1989; **16:** 1518–19.
6. Fricchione GL, *et al.* Electroconvulsive therapy and cyclophosphamide in combination for severe neuropsychiatric lupus with catatonia. *Am J Med* 1990; **88:** 442–3.
7. Boumpas DT, *et al.* Intermittent cyclophosphamide for the treatment of autoimmune thrombocytopenia in systemic lupus erythematosus. *Ann Intern Med* 1990; **112:** 674–7.
8. Gourley MF, *et al.* Methylprednisolone and cyclophosphamide, alone or in combination, in patients with lupus nephritis: a randomized, controlled trial. *Ann Intern Med* 1996; **125:** 549–57.

Kidney disorders, non-malignant. Cyclophosphamide is used with corticosteroids in the treatment of a number of forms of glomerular kidney disease (p.1021). In minimal change nephropathy, cyclophosphamide 2 to 3 mg per kg body-weight daily for 8 weeks may be added to a course of corticosteroid therapy in relapsing disease;[1-3] addition of cyclophosphamide to corticosteroid therapy also improves the prospect of remission in focal glomerulosclerosis. Oral cyclophosphamide helps to stabilise progressive disease in patients with membranous nephropathy[4] although intermittent intravenous pulses are reported to be ineffective.[5] Such treatment is usually reserved for those whose disease is severe and progressive enough to justify it. Cyclophosphamide has been given with methylprednisolone for rapidly progressive glomerulonephritis,[6] and has been used as part of the aggressive management of renal lesions in Goodpasture's syndrome.

1. Boulton-Jones M. Management of nephrotic syndrome. *Prescribers' J* 1993; **33:** 96–102. Correction *ibid.*; 176.
2. Melvin T, Bennett W. Management of nephrotic syndrome in childhood. *Drugs* 1991; **42:** 30–51.
3. Trompeter RS, *et al.* Long-term outcome for children with minimal-change nephrotic syndrome. *Lancet* 1985; **i:** 368–70.
4. Falk RJ, *et al.* Treatment of progressive membranous glomerulopathy: a randomized trial comparing cyclophosphamide and corticosteroids with corticosteroids alone. *Ann Intern Med* 1992; **116:** 438–45.
5. Reichert LJM, *et al.* Preserving renal function in patients with membranous nephropathy: daily oral chlorambucil compared with intermittent monthly pulses of cyclophosphamide. *Ann Intern Med* 1994; **121:** 328–33.
6. Bruns FJ, *et al.* Long-term follow-up of aggressively treated idiopathic rapidly progressive glomerulonephritis. *Am J Med* 1989; **86:** 400–6.

Liver disorders, non-malignant. For mention of the use of cyclophosphamide in autoimmune hepatitis inadequately controlled by corticosteroids and azathioprine see Chronic Active Hepatitis, p.1019.

Lung disorders, non-malignant. Cyclophosphamide may be useful in permitting a dosage reduction in the lifelong corticosteroid therapy generally considered necessary in patients with cryptogenic fibrosing alveolitis, as mentioned on p.1024.

Malignant neoplasms. Cyclophosphamide is one of the most widely used agents for the chemotherapy of malignancy, and mention of its role may be found in the discussions of the management of gestational trophoblastic tumours (p.477); chronic lymphocytic leukaemia (p.480); the non-Hodgkin's lymphomas, including AIDS-related lymphoma, Burkitt's lymphoma, and mycosis fungoides (p.482, p.483, p.483, p.482); malignancies of the brain (p.485), breast (p.485), cervix (p.487), endometrium (p.487), lung (p.490), ovary (p.491), prostate (p.491), and thymus (p.493); multiple myeloma (p.494) and Waldenström's macroglobulinaemia (p.496); Wilm's tumour, neuroblastoma, and retinoblastoma (p.489, p.494, and p.495 respectively); and sarcomas of bone (p.495) and rhabdomyosarcoma (p.496).

Neuromuscular disorders. Cyclophosphamide has been tried in myasthenia gravis (p.1388) in patients who require immunosuppressants but are intolerant of or unresponsive to corticosteroids and azathioprine. In multiple sclerosis (p.620), the benefits of immunosuppressants such as cyclophosphamide are slight, and outweighed by the toxicity of the required doses. However, moderate dose cyclophosphamide has been employed in conjunction with the 'Gorski manoeuvre' (multiple plasma exchange to reduce antibody titres, a thymic extract to recruit memory cells into division, and then 2 doses of cyclophosphamide after 24 and 48 hours).

References.

1. Currier RD, *et al.* Cyclophosphamide and plasma exchange in multiple sclerosis. *Lancet* 1991; **337:** 1034.
2. The Canadian Cooperative Multiple Sclerosis Study Group. The Canadian cooperative trial of cyclophosphamide and plasma exchange in progressive multiple sclerosis. *Lancet* 1991; **337:** 441–6.
3. Hobbs JR. Controversy in treatment of multiple sclerosis. *Lancet* 1991; **338:** 193–4.

Ocular disorders, non-malignant. Immunosuppressive agents, including cyclophosphamide, have, as mentioned on p.498 been used in scleritis and uveitis unresponsive to corticosteroids in tolerable doses. Cyclophosphamide with a corticosteroid is also reported to be of value in ocular cicatricial pemphigoid,[1] although treatment may not completely prevent cicatrisation.

1. Elder MJ, *et al.* Role of cyclophosphamide and high dose steroid in ocular cicatricial pemphigoid. *Br J Ophthalmol* 1995; **79:** 264–6.

Organ and tissue transplantation. Cyclophosphamide is used in high doses, usually with busulphan or irradiation, in conditioning regimens for bone-marrow transplantation (p.498), and has been tried as part of immunosuppressant regimens following transplantation of heart and liver grafts (p.499 and p.500, respectively).

Paraquat poisoning. Although a study by Addo and Poon-King reported that 52 of 72 patients severely poisoned with paraquat survived following treatment with an intensive regimen including cyclophosphamide and dexamethasone (together with measures to remove unabsorbed paraquat from the gut, forced diuresis, and vitamins B and C),[1] the results of this study have been criticised.[2] Only 25 of the 72 patients had their plasma-paraquat concentrations measured, and in 6 of these no paraquat was detected, indicating that insignificant amounts had been ingested, and of the 19 remaining, 12 with very high plasma-paraquat concentrations all died while it is uncertain how many of the remaining 7 would have survived without the intensive regimen.[2] However, another small study[3] has reported better results with cyclophosphamide and methylprednisolone than with supportive treatment in patients with moderate to severe paraquat poisoning; 4 of 16 given the former treatment died compared with 12 of 17 given the latter.

1. Addo E, Poon-King T. Leucocyte suppression in treatment of 72 patients with paraquat poisoning. *Lancet* 1986; **i:** 1117–20.
2. Anonymous. Cyclophosphamide for paraquat poisoning? *Lancet* 1986; **ii:** 375–6.
3. Lin J-L, *et al.* Pulse therapy with cyclophosphamide and methylprednisolone in patients with moderate to severe paraquat poisoning: a preliminary report. *Thorax* 1996; **51:** 661–3.

Pemphigus and pemphigoid. Corticosteroids are the main treatment for blistering in pemphigus and pemphigoid (p.1075). Immunosuppressive therapy, including cyclophosphamide,[1,2] has been used in combination with corticosteroids to permit a reduction in corticosteroid dosage. However, it has been suggested that evidence for the steroid-sparing effect is lacking and that immunosuppressants should be reserved for patients who cannot tolerate corticosteroids or in whom they are contra-indicated.[3]

1. Pandya AG, Sontheimer RD. Treatment of pemphigus vulgaris with pulse intravenous cyclophosphamide. *Arch Dermatol* 1992; **128:** 1626–30.
2. Itoh T, *et al.* Successful treatment of bullous pemphigoid with pulsed intravenous cyclophosphamide. *Br J Dermatol* 1996; **134:** 931–3.
3. Bystryn J-C, Steinman NM. The adjuvant therapy of pemphigus: an update. *Arch Dermatol* 1996; **132:** 203–12.

Rheumatoid arthritis. Cyclophosphamide has been used as an antirheumatic drug in rheumatoid arthritis (p.2), usually in patients with severe disease unresponsive to other drugs. It is of most value in controlling antibody-mediated systemic complications of the disease such as vasculitis[1] through inhibition of B-cell function.

1. Choy E, Kingsley G. How do second-line agents work? *Br Med Bull* 1995; **51:** 472–92.

Scleroderma. As discussed on p.501 the role of drug treatment for scleroderma is not well determined, but cyclophosphamide may perhaps be useful combined with a corticosteroid for patients with lung involvement.

Vasculitic syndromes. Treatment of the systemic vasculitides has revolved around the use of corticosteroids and cyclophosphamide. The benefits are uncertain in polyarteritis nodosa (p.1027) and Takayasu's arteritis (p.1030), but the benefits of combined therapy are generally accepted in Churg-Strauss syndrome (p.1019) and microscopic polyangiitis (p.1027), and cyclophosphamide is the mainstay of effective treatment of Wegener's granulomatosis (p.1031). A number of administration regimens are in use; in particular intermittent high-dose intravenous ('pulsed') administration is being evaluated in comparison with continuous therapy.[1]

1. Richmond R, *et al.* Optimisation of cyclophosphamide therapy in systemic vasculitis. *Clin Pharmacokinet* 1998; **34:** 79–90.

Preparations

BP 1998: Cyclophosphamide Injection; Cyclophosphamide Tablets;
USP 23: Cyclophosphamide for Injection; Cyclophosphamide Tablets.

Proprietary Preparations (details are given in Part 3)
Aust.: Endoxan; ***Austral.:*** Cycloblastin; Endoxan; ***Belg.:*** Cycloblastine; Endoxan; ***Canad.:*** Cytoxan; Procytox; ***Fr.:*** Endoxan; ***Ger.:*** Cyclo-cell; Cyclostin; Endoxan; ***Ital.:*** Endoxan; ***Neth.:*** Cycloblastine†; Endoxan; ***Norw.:*** Sendoxan; ***S.Afr.:*** Cycloblastin; Endoxan; ***Spain:*** Cicloxal; Genoxal; ***Swed.:*** Sendoxan; ***Switz.:*** Endoxan; ***UK:*** Endoxana; ***USA:*** Cytoxan; Neosar.

Cyclosporin (1882-m)

Cyclosporin *(BAN)*.

Ciclosporin *(rINN)*; 27-400; Ciclosporinum; Cyclosporin A; Cyclosporine *(USAN)*; OL-27-400. Cyclo{-[4-(*E*)-but-2-enyl-*N*,4-dimethyl-L-threonyl]-L-homoalanyl-(*N*-methylglycyl)-(*N*-methyl-L-leucyl)-L-valyl-(*N*-methyl-L-leucyl)-L-alanyl-D-alanyl-(*N*-methyl-L-leucyl)-(*N*-methyl-L-leucyl)-(*N*-methyl-L-valyl)-}.

$C_{62}H_{111}N_{11}O_{12}$ = 1202.6.

CAS — 59865-13-3.

Pharmacopoeias. In *Eur.* (see p.viii), *Jpn*, and *US*.

A substance produced by *Beauveria nivea* (=*Tolypocladium inflatum* Gams) or obtained by any other means.

A white or almost white powder; practically **insoluble** in water; freely soluble in dehydrated alcohol and in dichloromethane; soluble in alcohol, acetone, chloroform, ether, and in methyl alcohol. **Store** in airtight containers. Protect from light.

Incompatibility. The plasticiser diethylhexyl phthalate, which is a possible carcinogen, was leached from PVC containers by cyclosporin preparations.[1] Such preparations should not be given through PVC tubing nor stored in PVC containers.

1. Pearson SD, Trissel LA. Leaching of diethylhexyl phthalate from polyvinyl chloride containers by selected drugs and formulation components. *Am J Hosp Pharm* 1993; **50:** 1405–9.

Stability. Cyclosporin was stable over 72 hours following dilution in glucose 5% or glucose/amino-acid solutions and storage at room temperature in the dark; similar stability was seen following dilution in lipid emulsion, but dilutions in sodium chloride 0.9% were considered to be stable only for 8 hours.[1] In all cases miscibility in the diluent was poor and vigorous shaking was required after addition to produce even distribution of cyclosporin. An extemporaneously compounded paste produced from cyclosporin oral solution (Sandimmun) in an oral gel base was found to be stable for at least 31 days in aluminium-lined ointment tubes stored at 2° to 37°.[2]

1. McLeod HL, *et al.* Stability of cyclosporin in dextrose 5%, NaCl 0.9%, dextrose/amino acid solution, and lipid emulsion. *Ann Pharmacother* 1992; **26:** 172–5.
2. Ghnassia LT, *et al.* Stability of cyclosporine in an extemporaneously compounded paste. *Am J Health-Syst Pharm* 1995; **52:** 2204–7.

Adverse Effects and Treatment

Nephrotoxicity is the major adverse effect of cyclosporin and occurs in approximately one-third of all patients. It is related to drug-plasma concentrations and is usually reversible on reduction of the dose. In renal graft recipients episodes of nephrotoxicity may be difficult to distinguish from graft rejection. Hypertension and electrolyte disturbances, notably hyperkalaemia, have occurred.

Other adverse effects include gastro-intestinal disturbances, hepatotoxicity, hypertrichosis, facial oedema, and acne, hyperplasia of the gums, and neurotoxicity. Tremor is common, and paraesthesias or burning sensations in the extremities, hallucinations and convulsions have been reported, the latter possibly related to hypomagnesaemia in some cases. Convulsions have sometimes been associated with hypertension and fluid retention.

Anaphylactoid reactions have occurred following intravenous administration; it has been suggested that these represent a reaction to the polyethoxylated castor oil vehicle of the intravenous preparation.

There is an increased incidence of development of certain malignancies in patients receiving cyclosporin therapy.

Alopecia. Although cyclosporin is more often associated with reports of hypertrichosis, there have been cases of alopecia areata developing in patients receiving cyclosporin,[1] sometimes with complete hair loss (alopecia universalis).[2,3]

1. Davies MG, Bowers PW. Alopecia areata arising in patients receiving cyclosporin immunosuppression. *Br J Dermatol* 1995; **132:** 835–6.
2. Monti M, *et al.* Alopecia universalis in liver transplant patients treated with cyclosporin. *Br J Dermatol* 1995; **133:** 663–4.
3. Parodi A, *et al.* Alopecia universalis and cyclosporin A. *Br J Dermatol* 1996; **135:** 657.

Carcinogenicity. Like other forms of immunosuppression the use of cyclosporin is associated with an increased incidence of malignancy, notably lymphoma,[1] but also including skin cancer and Kaposi's sarcoma. The manufacturers have stated that of an estimated 5550 transplant patients who had been treated with cyclosporin by February 1984, lymphoproliferative disorders had been reported in 40, an overall incidence of 0.7%.[2] In a more recent paper Malatack and colleagues, reporting 12 cases of lymphoproliferative disorders among 132 paediatric liver graft recipients estimated the incidence at about 2.8% per year for the first 6 years after transplantation, giving a cumulative risk of nearly 20% after 7 years.[3] One wonders if these much higher figures for incidence are due to differences in the regimen, since there is evidence that the incidence of malignancy is related to dose,[2,4,5] and is greater when cyclosporin is combined with other potent immunosuppressants.[2]

It has been suggested that these lymphomas represent proliferation of B-cells under the influence of Epstein-Barr virus, a process normally prevented by the T-cells which are specifically inhibited by cyclosporin.[3,6] The resultant, usually polyclonal, lymphoproliferative tumours appear to regress on prompt excision of the affected tissue and reduction or discontinuation of the immunosuppressant regimen, in most cases without graft loss.[7] However, Malatack and colleagues stress the need for vigilance and rapid response to these conditions, since the responsive polyclonal disorder may evolve into a monoclonal, frankly malignant form; where the presentation is indistinguishable from a classic non-Hodgkins lymphoma the prognosis is much less good.[3] Interestingly, use of lower dose cyclosporin regimens appears to maintain normal elimination of Epstein-Barr virus-infected B-cells by specific T-cells,[8] and may lead to a reduced incidence of malignancy compared with earlier results.[4,5,8]

There is no clear evidence that cyclosporin is associated with an increased incidence of malignancy compared with other immunosuppressants, although Shuttleworth and colleagues found dysplastic skin lesions in 14 of 64 transplant patients receiving cyclosporin compared with 3 of 33 previous similar patients who had received azathioprine.[9] However, such comparisons are difficult, not least because many transplant patients tend to have received multiple immunosuppressant agents, and debate on the subject continues.[4,10,11]

See also under Adverse Effects of Antineoplastics and Immunosuppressants, p.470.

1. Penn I. Cancers following cyclosporine therapy. *Transplantation* 1987; **43:** 32–5.
2. Beveridge T, *et al.* Lymphomas and lymphoproliferative lesions developing under cyclosporin therapy. *Lancet* 1984; **i:** 788.
3. Malatack JJ, *et al.* Orthotopic liver transplantation, Epstein-Barr virus, cyclosporine, and lymphoproliferative disease: a growing concern. *J Pediatr* 1991; **118:** 667–75.
4. Kahan BD. Cyclosporine. *N Engl J Med* 1990; **322:** 1531.
5. Dantal J, *et al.* Effect of long-term immunosuppression in kidney-graft recipients on cancer incidence: randomised comparison of two cyclosporin regimens. *Lancet* 1998; **351:** 623–8.
6. Anonymous. Lymphoma in organ transplant recipients. *Lancet* 1984; **i:** 601–3.
7. Starzl TE, *et al.* Reversibility of lymphomas and lymphoproliferative lesions developing under cyclosporin-steroid therapy. *Lancet* 1984; **i:** 583–7.
8. Crawford DH, Edwards JMB. Immunity to Epstein-Barr virus in cyclosporin A-treated renal allograft recipients. *Lancet* 1982; **i:** 1469–70.
9. Shuttleworth D, *et al.* Epidermal dysplasia and cyclosporine therapy in renal transplant patients: a comparison with azathioprine. *Br J Dermatol* 1989; **120:** 551–4.
10. Mor F. Cyclosporine. *N Engl J Med* 1990; **322:** 1530–1.
11. Arellano F, Krupp PF. Cutaneous malignant melanoma occurring after cyclosporin A therapy. *Br J Dermatol* 1991; **124:** 611.

Dysmorphic changes. There was pronounced coarsening of facial features in 11 children who were treated with prednisone and cyclosporin for renal transplantation and followed up for more than 6 months.[1] The changes resembled those seen with phenytoin therapy.

1. Reznik VM, *et al.* Changes in facial appearance during cyclosporin treatment. *Lancet* 1987; **i:** 1405–7.

Effects on blood and vascular system. Cyclosporin treatment is associated with a variety of effects on the blood and cardiovascular system. Erythraemia[1,2] and thrombocytosis[3] have both been reported, both of which may contribute to **thrombo-embolic complications.** One retrospective study reported 17 thrombo-embolic events (pulmonary embolism, renal-vein or deep-vein thrombosis, or haemorrhoidal thrombosis) in 13 of 90 renal allograft recipients treated with cyclosporin and corticosteroids, compared with only 1 episode of superficial thrombophlebitis in 90 similar patients treated with an azathioprine-based regimen,[4] although other workers dispute that the incidence of thrombo-embolic events is any greater after cyclosporin than azathioprine,[5-7] and one group found the reverse.[8]

Marked **hyperlipidaemia** has been associated with cyclosporin therapy, with notable increases reported in low-density lipoprotein cholesterol,[9,10] and lipoprotein(a).[11] However, although accelerated atherosclerosis remains a major cause of death in transplant patients[10] the contribution of cyclosporin remains a matter of controversy, and some workers do not accept that cyclosporin has a significant effect on serum lipids and coronary risk.[12-15]

Probably the most notorious cardiovascular adverse effect of cyclosporin is **hypertension.** This may be severe,[16] and appears to be dose-related;[16,17] it is reportedly particularly common in recipients of cardiac or heart-lung grafts.[18,19] There may be an association with low serum-magnesium concentrations.[20] A variety of mechanisms have been suggested to contribute to cyclosporin-induced hypertension, including impaired sodium excretion,[21] enhanced sympathetic nervous activity,[18,22] effects on renal prostaglandin metabolism,[17] and direct damage to endothelial cells[23] with release of the potent vasoconstrictor endothelin.[24] Thus hypertension may occur independently of nephrotoxicity,[17,22] and may be difficult to treat with conventional antihypertensive regimens.[21] Occasionally, hypertension may be irreversible.[17,25] However, it should be borne in mind that, at least in patients receiving renal grafts, hypertension may occur in the post-transplant period with other immunosuppressive regimens.[16,17,19]

Other effects that have been associated with cyclosporin therapy include cases of Raynaud's syndrome,[26] the haemolytic-uraemic syndrome,[27] and thrombocytopenia,[28] or leucopenia.[29]

1. Tatman AJ, *et al.* Erythraemia in renal transplant recipients treated with cyclosporin. *Lancet* 1988; **i:** 1279.
2. Innes A, *et al.* Cyclosporin and erythraemia. *Lancet* 1988; **ii:** 285.
3. Itami N, *et al.* Thrombocytosis after cyclosporin therapy in child with nephrotic syndrome. *Lancet* 1988; **ii:** 1018.
4. Vanrenterghem Y, *et al.* Thromboembolic complications and haemostatic changes in cyclosporin-treated cadaveric kidney allograft recipients. *Lancet* 1985; **i:** 999–1002.
5. Bergentz S-E, *et al.* Venous thrombosis and cyclosporin. *Lancet* 1985; **ii:** 101–2.
6. Zazgornik J, *et al.* Venous thrombosis and cyclosporin. *Lancet* 1985; **ii:** 102.
7. Choudhury N, *et al.* Thromboembolic complications in cyclosporin-treated kidney allograft recipients. *Lancet* 1985; **ii:** 606.
8. Allen RD, *et al.* Venous thrombosis and cyclosporin. *Lancet* 1985; **ii:** 1004.
9. Luke DR, *et al.* Longitudinal study of cyclosporine and lipids in patients undergoing bone marrow transplantation. *J Clin Pharmacol* 1990; **30:** 163–9.
10. Ballantyne CM, *et al.* Effects of cyclosporine therapy on plasma lipoprotein levels. *JAMA* 1989; **262:** 53–6.
11. Webb AT, *et al.* Does cyclosporin increase lipoprotein(a) concentrations in renal transplant recipients? *Lancet* 1993; **341:** 268–70.
12. Rosman J, *et al.* Cyclosporin A has no impact on alterations of the lipid profile after renal transplantation. *Transpl Int* 1992; **5** (suppl 1): 532–5.
13. Kronenberg F, *et al.* Cyclosporin and serum lipids in renal transplant recipients. *Lancet* 1993; **341:** 765.
14. Segarra A, *et al.* Cyclosporin and serum lipids in renal transplant recipients. *Lancet* 1993; **341:** 766.
15. Hunt BJ, *et al.* Does cyclosporin affect lipoprotein(a) concentrations? *Lancet* 1994; **343:** 119–20.
16. Textor SC, *et al.* Cyclosporine-induced hypertension after transplantation. *Mayo Clin Proc* 1994; **69:** 1182–93.
17. Porter GA, *et al.* Cyclosporine-associated hypertension. *Arch Intern Med* 1990; **150:** 280–3.
18. Scherrer U, *et al.* Cyclosporine-induced sympathetic activation and hypertension after heart transplantation. *N Engl J Med* 1990; **323:** 693–9.
19. Weidle PJ, Vlasses PH. Systemic hypertension associated with cyclosporine: a review. *Drug Intell Clin Pharm* 1988; **22:** 443–51.
20. June CH, *et al.* Correlation of hypomagnesemia with the onset of cyclosporine-associated hypertension in marrow transplant patients. *Transplantation* 1986; **41:** 47–51.
21. Weinman EJ. Cyclosporine-associated hypertension. *Am J Med* 1989; **86:** 256–7.
22. Mark AL. Cyclosporine, sympathetic activity, and hypertension. *N Engl J Med* 1990; **323:** 748–50.
23. Zaal MJW, *et al.* Is cyclosporin toxic to endothelial cells? *Lancet* 1988; **ii:** 956–7.
24. Deray G, *et al.* Increased endothelin level after cyclosporine therapy. *Ann Intern Med* 1991; **114:** 809.
25. Sennesael JJ, *et al.* Hypertension and cyclosporine. *Ann Intern Med* 1986; **104:** 729.
26. Deray G, *et al.* Cyclosporin and Raynaud phenomenon. *Lancet* 1986; **ii:** 1092–3.
27. Bonser RS, *et al.* Cyclosporin-induced haemolytic uraemic syndrome in liver allograft recipient. *Lancet* 1984; **ii:** 1337.
28. Dejong DJ, Sayler DJ. Possible cyclosporine-associated thrombocytopenia. *DICP Ann Pharmacother* 1990; **24:** 1007.
29. Michel F, *et al.* Bone marrow toxicity of cyclosporin in a kidney transplant patient. *Lancet* 1986; **ii:** 394.

Effects on the gastro-intestinal tract. There have been reports[1,2] of severe non-specific colitis associated with both elevated[1] and therapeutic[2] blood or serum concentrations of cyclosporin.

1. Innes A, *et al.* Cyclosporin toxicity and colitis. *Lancet* 1988; **ii:** 957. Correction. *ibid.*; 1094.
2. Bowen JRC, Sahi S. Cyclosporin induced colitis. *Br Med J* 1993; **307:** 484.

Effects on glucose tolerance. There is some evidence that cyclosporin, particularly in high doses, may be associated with reduced insulin production,[1] impaired glucose tolerance,[2] and occasional overt diabetes mellitus,[3,4] although cyclosporin has also been tried, with some apparent benefit, in the treatment of recent-onset diabetes mellitus (for mention of the use of immunosuppressants in diabetes mellitus, see p.313). The incidence of fasting hyperglycaemia has been estimated at about 8% in cyclosporin-treated renal transplant recipients, compared with about 5% in those given an azathioprine-based regimen.[4]

1. Scott JP, Higenbottam TW. Adverse reactions and interactions of cyclosporin. *Med Toxicol* 1983; **3:** 107–27.
2. Gunnarsson R, *et al.* Deterioration in glucose metabolism in pancreatic transplant recipients given cyclosporin. *Lancet* 1983; **ii:** 571–2.

3. Bending JJ, *et al.* Diabetogenic effect of cyclosporin. *Br Med J* 1987; **294:** 401–2.
4. Yagisawa T, *et al.* Deterioration in glucose metabolism in cyclosporine-treated kidney transplant recipients and rats. *Transplant Proc* 1986; **18:** 1548–51.

Effects on the kidneys. The use of cyclosporin is associated with nephrotoxicity, characterised by fluid retention, increased serum creatinine and urea concentrations, a fall in glomerular filtration rate, and decreased sodium and potassium excretion.[1,2] Extremely high intravenous doses (21 mg per kg body-weight per 24 hours for 60 hours) have been reported to be associated with fatal acute tubular necrosis.[3] In renal graft recipients it may be difficult to distinguish nephrotoxicity from graft rejection.[1] Symptoms are usually chronic, dose-related, and reversible,[1] and increase with the duration of exposure.[2] Prolonged administration has been associated with progressive irreversible renal dysfunction in heart transplant patients,[4] despite maintenance of plasma cyclosporin concentrations below 400 ng per mL, the value above which nephrotoxicity is more frequent;[1] however, impairment of renal function has been reported to be reversible in psoriatic patients who had received low-dose cyclosporin for 5 years.[5] It has been pointed out that with current regimens, which tend to use low doses of cyclosporin, the majority of transplant and other patients receiving cyclosporin long-term tolerate the drug without evidence of progressive nephrotoxicity.[5-7]

There is some evidence that suggests that renal effects are due to a toxic metabolite,[8,9] and in consequence total cyclosporin and metabolite concentrations, as given by radioimmunoassay, may be more helpful in predicting toxicity than concentration of the parent drug alone.[8]

In addition to these chronic changes cyclosporin has also been associated with a syndrome of acute renal failure, occurring shortly after beginning treatment.[2,10] It has been proposed that this is due to arteriolar vasoconstriction secondary to inhibition of renal prostaglandin synthesis, with serious consequences in patients with clinical conditions in which prostaglandin-induced renal vasodilatation is necessary to maintain glomerular perfusion.[10] Such a mechanism would be in line with suggestions that inhibition of prostaglandin E_2 or prostacyclin synthesis may play a role in the development of chronic cyclosporin-induced nephrotoxicity.[11-13] However, endothelin has also been proposed as a causative agent,[14] and the relationship between the renal and vascular effects of cyclosporin has been a matter of some debate.[2]

For reference to means of minimising nephrotoxicity in patients receiving cyclosporin, see under Treatment of Adverse Effects, below.

1. Bennett WM, Pulliam JP. Cyclosporine nephrotoxicity. *Ann Intern Med* 1983; **99:** 851–4.
2. Scott JP, Higenbottam TW. Adverse reactions and interactions of cyclosporin. *Med Toxicol* 1988; **3:** 107–27.
3. Schechter P. Acute tubular necrosis following high-dose cyclosporine A therapy. *Eur J Clin Pharmacol* 1996; **49:** 521–3.
4. Myers BD, *et al.* Cyclosporine-associated chronic nephropathy. *N Engl J Med* 1984; **311:** 699–705.
5. Powles AV, *et al.* Renal function after 10 years' treatment with cyclosporin for psoriasis. *Br J Dermatol* 1998; **138:** 443–9.
6. Burke JF, *et al.* Long-term efficacy and safety of cyclosporine in renal-transplant recipients. *N Engl J Med* 1994; **331:** 358–63.
7. Leaker B, Cairns HS. Clinical aspects of cyclosporin nephrotoxicity. *Br J Hosp Med* 1994; **52:** 529–34.
8. Leunissen KML, *et al.* Cyclosporin metabolites and nephrotoxicity. *Lancet* 1986; **ii:** 1398.
9. Lucey MR, *et al.* Cyclosporin toxicity at therapeutic blood levels and cytochrome P-450 IIIA. *Lancet* 1990; **335:** 11–15.
10. Praga M, *et al.* Cyclosporine-induced acute renal failure in the nephrotic syndrome. *Ann Intern Med* 1987; **107:** 786–7.
11. Duarte R. Cyclosporine: renal effects and prostacyclin. *Ann Intern Med* 1985; **102:** 420.
12. Adu D, *et al.* Cyclosporine and prostaglandins. *Ann Intern Med* 1985; **103:** 303.
13. Stahl RAK, *et al.* Cyclosporine and renal prostaglandin E_2 production. *Ann Intern Med* 1985; **103:** 474.
14. Cairns HS, *et al.* Endothelin and cyclosporin nephrotoxicity. *Lancet* 1988; **ii:** 1496–7.

Effects on the nervous system. Increasing attention is being paid to the effects of cyclosporin on the central nervous system. Symptoms include tremor,[1-3] ataxia,[1-3] confusion[1,2] or agitation,[2] mental depression,[3] flushing, headache and sleep disturbances,[2] lethargy,[1,2,4] or coma[2,4] (in one case coma persisted for 44 days),[5] convulsions,[2,3,6-89] leucoencephalopathy,[2,5,6] cortical blindness,[2,6] and spasticity or paralysis of the limbs.[1,2] Convulsions have sometimes been associated with hypertension and fluid retention,[8] but this is by no means always the case.[6,7] Severe CNS toxicity has been stated to vary in incidence from 0.1% in renal transplant patients to about 1.6% in bone-marrow transplant recipients.[9] There is some evidence for an association of serious neurological effects with low total serum-cholesterol concentrations,[2] and the use of the intravenous formulation.[2] Neurotoxicity may also be associated with the concomitant administration of lipid solutions.[10] An association with hypomagnesaemia has also been proposed[3] but may just represent concomitant nephrotoxicity.[11] Convulsions may be more likely or more severe in patients with a familial history of epilepsy,[12] subclinical aluminium overload,[13] or who are given concomitant high-dose corticosteroids.[14,15] The mechanism of toxicity is unknown but may be associated with disturbance of the blood-brain barrier;[7,9,16] it has been suggested that the metabolite M-17, or possibly other metabolites, are responsible for neurotoxicity.[4] Although neurotoxicity usually manifests within a month of beginning treatment, it may be delayed, and in one case occurred only after 3 years of cyclosporin therapy.[17]

1. Atkinson K, *et al.* Cyclosporine-associated central-nervous-system toxicity after allogenic bone-marrow transplantation. *N Engl J Med* 1984; **310:** 527.
2. de Groen PC, *et al.* Central nervous system toxicity after liver transplantation: the role of cyclosporine and cholesterol. *N Engl J Med* 1987; **317:** 861–6.
3. Thompson CB, *et al.* Association between cyclosporin neurotoxicity and hypomagnesaemia. *Lancet* 1984; **ii:** 1116–20.
4. Kunzendorf U, *et al.* Cyclosporin metabolites and central-nervous-system toxicity. *Lancet* 1988; **i:** 1223.
5. Berden JHM, *et al.* Severe central-nervous-system toxicity associated with cyclosporin. *Lancet* 1985; **i:** 219–20.
6. Hughes RL. Cyclosporine-related central nervous system toxicity in cardiac transplantation. *N Engl J Med* 1990; **323:** 420–1.
7. Gottrand F, *et al.* Cyclosporine neurotoxicity. *N Engl J Med* 1991; **324:** 1744–5.
8. Joss DV, *et al.* Hypertension and convulsions in children receiving cyclosporin A. *Lancet* 1982; **i:** 906.
9. Krupp P, *et al.* Encephalopathy associated with fat embolism induced by solvent for cyclosporin. *Lancet* 1989; **i:** 168–9.
10. De Klippel N. Cyclosporin leukoencephalopathy induced by intravenous lipid solution. *Lancet* 1992; **339:** 1114.
11. Allen RD, *et al.* Cyclosporin and magnesium. *Lancet* 1985; **i:** 1283–4.
12. Velu T, *et al.* Cyclosporin-associated fatal convulsions. *Lancet* 1985; **i:** 219.
13. Nordal KP, *et al.* Aluminium overload, a predisposing condition for epileptic seizures in renal-transplant patients treated with cyclosporin. *Lancet* 1985; **ii:** 153–4.
14. Durrant S, *et al.* Cyclosporin A, methylprednisolone, and convulsions. *Lancet* 1982; **ii:** 829–30.
15. Bogaerts MA, *et al.* Cyclosporin, methylprednisolone, and convulsions. *Lancet* 1982; **ii:** 1216–17.
16. Sloane JP, *et al.* Disturbance of blood-brain barrier after bone-marrow transplantation. *Lancet* 1985; **ii:** 280–1.
17. Welge-Lüssen UC, Gerhartz HH. Late onset of neurotoxicity with cyclosporin. *Lancet* 1994; **343:** 293.

Effects on skeletal muscle. Cyclosporin has been associated with a number of reports of myopathy.[1-4] The manufacturers (*Sandoz*) have stated that 29 cases had been reported by December 1990, which appeared to be divided into cases of toxic or non-specific myopathy, or mild sensory motor neuropathy, which were generally dose-related; and rhabdomyolysis, often, but not always, associated with concomitant medication with lovastatin or colchicine.[5]

1. Noppen M, *et al.* Cyclosporine and myopathy. *Ann Intern Med* 1987; **107:** 945–6.
2. Goy J-J. Myopathy as possible side-effect of cyclosporin. *Lancet* 1989; **i:** 1446–7.
3. Grezard O, *et al.* Cyclosporin-induced muscular toxicity. *Lancet* 1990; **335:** 177.
4. Fernandez-Sola J, *et al.* Reversible cyclosporin myopathy. *Lancet* 1990; **335:** 362–3.
5. Arellano F, Krupp P. Muscular disorders associated with cyclosporin. *Lancet* 1991; **337:** 915.

Hyperplasia. Cyclosporin is well known to be associated with the development of gingival hyperplasia: one review[1] has estimated the incidence at about 30% in transplant patients, while noting that reported values in the literature range from about 7 to 70%. The mechanism is uncertain although a hypothesis has been advanced that reactive metabolites, whose formation is catalysed by cytochrome P450 in gingival cells, induce an inflammatory response and fibroblastic proliferation by causing cellular injury.[2] The presence of dental plaque may exacerbate the response,[1] and the concomitant administration of nifedipine (which can itself produce hyperplasia) may produce very much greater enlargement.[3] Enlargement is generally reversible following dosage reduction or withdrawal of cyclosporin; where this is not feasible, surgical excision is the recommended treatment.[1] However, improvement or resolution of the hypertrophy has also been reported following a course of metronidazole[4,5] or azithromycin.[6]

Enlargement of the papillae of the tongue has also occurred in association with cyclosporin.[7]

1. Brunet L, *et al.* Gingival enlargement induced by drugs. *Drug Safety* 1996; **15:** 219–31.
2. Zhou LX, *et al.* Metabolism of phenytoin by the gingiva of normal humans: the possible role of reactive metabolites of phenytoin in the initiation of gingival hyperplasia. *Clin Pharmacol Ther* 1996; **60:** 191–8.
3. Slavin J, Taylor J. Cyclosporin, nifedipine, and gingival hyperplasia. *Lancet* 1987; **ii:** 739.
4. Wong W, *et al.* Resolution of cyclosporin-induced gingival hypertrophy with metronidazole. *Lancet* 1994; **343:** 986.
5. Cecchin E, *et al.* Treatment of cyclosporine-induced gingival hypertrophy. *Ann Intern Med* 1997; **126:** 409–10.
6. Jugglà A, *et al.* The use of azithromycin for cyclosporin-induced gingival overgrowth. *Br J Dermatol* 1998; **138:** 198–9.
7. Silverberg NB, *et al.* Lingual fungiform papillae hypertrophy with cyclosporin A. *Lancet* 1996; **348:** 967.

Hypersensitivity. Anaphylactoid reactions in 5 of 21 patients given intravenous cyclosporin infusions were found to be associated with improper mixing of the cyclosporin concentrate, which has a polyethoxylated castor oil vehicle, with the infusion solution.[1] It was concluded that this had led to an initial bolus of polyethoxylated castor oil which had triggered the anaphylactic reactions. Subsequent study indicated that peak concentrations of up to 9 times the intended concentration of cyclosporin and polyethoxylated castor oil were present in the first 10 minutes of a poorly mixed infusion.[2]

1. Liau M, *et al.* High incidence of anaphylactoid reactions to iv cyclosporin A caused by improper dissolution of Cremophor EL. *Clin Pharmacol Ther* 1995; **57:** 209.
2. Liau-Chu M, *et al.* Mechanism of anaphylactoid reactions: improper preparation of high-dose intravenous cyclosporine leads to bolus infusion of Cremophor EL and cyclosporine. *Ann Pharmacother* 1997; **31:** 1287–91.

Hyperuricaemia. Cyclosporin therapy may be associated with marked hyperuricaemia,[1-3] which may lead (predominantly in male patients[1]) to episodes of severe gouty arthritis.[1-3] It has been suggested that cyclosporin specifically reduces urate clearance by the kidney independently of its effects on glomerular filtration.[4,5] Treatment of cyclosporin-induced gout may be difficult since interactions with NSAIDs may lead to enhanced kidney toxicity[5] and patients who are also receiving azathioprine may experience increased bone-marrow toxicity if given allopurinol.[6]

1. Lin H-Y, *et al.* Cyclosporine-induced hyperuricemia and gout. *N Engl J Med* 1989; **321:** 287–92.
2. Kahl LE, *et al.* Gout in the heart transplant recipient: physiologic puzzle and therapeutic challenge. *Am J Med* 1989; **87:** 289–94.
3. Burack DA, *et al.* Hyperuricemia and gout among heart transplant recipients receiving cyclosporine. *Am J Med* 1992; **92:** 141–6.
4. Noordzij TC, *et al.* Cyclosporine-induced hyperuricemia and gout. *N Engl J Med* 1990; **322:** 335.
5. Farge D, *et al.* Hyperuricemia and gouty arthritis in heart transplant recipients. *Am J Med* 1990; **88:** 553.
6. Figg WD. Cyclosporine-induced hyperuricemia and gout. *N Engl J Med* 1990; **332:** 334–5.

Overdosage. Anxiety, diarrhoea, vomiting, and perspiration, with weak and irregular pulse, occurred in a patient accidentally injected with 250 mg of cyclosporin.[1] The patient subsequently developed atrial fibrillation, which was treated with digoxin, and in the following 36 hours showed signs of slight renal insufficiency. Two days later no adverse effects were apparent. No adverse renal, hepatic, or neurological effects were seen in another patient who took 25 g of cyclosporin over 8 days.[2] There was a mild increase in blood pressure and other symptoms included burning sensations in the mouth and the extremities, dysgeusia, facial flushing, and gastro-intestinal disturbances. Symptoms resolved within 2 weeks of stopping cyclosporin.

For reference to fatal tubular necrosis in a patient who received 21 mg per kg body-weight of cyclosporin per 24 hours for 60 hours, see under Effects on the Kidneys, above.

1. Wallemacq PE, Lesne ML. Accidental massive IV administration of cyclosporine in man. *Drug Intell Clin Pharm* 1985; **19:** 29–30.
2. Baumhefner RW, *et al.* High cyclosporin overdose with favourable outcome. *Lancet* 1987; **ii:** 332.

Treatment of adverse effects. A variety of agents have been given in an attempt to ameliorate the nephrotoxic effects of cyclosporin in patients who have undergone transplantation, including calcium-channel blockers such as diltiazem, nifedipine, and verapamil (see p.856, p.922, and p.963), clonidine (see p.843), co-dergocrine,[1-3] omega-3 triglycerides,[4] and misoprostol and other prostaglandin analogues.[5,6] Although benefits have been reported with some of these drugs, hydration, careful monitoring of cyclosporin concentrations, and the use where possible of low-dose or intermittent regimens of cyclosporin appear to remain the major means of keeping nephrotoxicity to a minimum.

Reports suggest that hyperplasia of the gums may respond to a course of metronidazole or azithromycin—see above.

1. Heinrichs DA, *et al.* The effects of co-dergocrine on cyclosporin A pharmacokinetics and pharmacodynamics. *Br J Clin Pharmacol* 1987; **24:** 117–18.
2. Nussenblatt RB, *et al.* Hydergine and cyclosporin nephrotoxicity. *Lancet* 1986; **i:** 1220–1.
3. Kho TL, *et al.* Hydergine and reversibility of cyclosporin nephrotoxicity. *Lancet* 1986; **ii:** 394–5.
4. Stoof TJ, *et al.* Does fish oil protect renal function in cyclosporin-treated psoriasis patients? *Br J Dermatol* 1990; **123:** 535.
5. Moran M, *et al.* Prevention of acute graft rejection by the prostaglandin E_1 analogue misoprostol in renal-transplant recipients treated with cyclosporine and prednisone. *N Engl J Med* 1990; **322:** 1183–8.
6. Di Palo FQ, *et al.* Role of a prostaglandin E_1 analogue in the prevention of acute graft rejection by cyclosporine. *N Engl J Med* 1990; **323:** 832.

Precautions

Regular monitoring of renal and hepatic function, blood pressure, and serum electrolytes (chiefly potassium) is required in patients receiving cyclosporin. Monitoring of drug concentrations is advisable in all patients and is mandatory in transplant patients. Dosage adjustment may frequently be necessary in patients with renal impairment or other factors affecting plasma concentrations. Care is required in patients with hyperuricaemia, and intravenous formulations should be given cautiously to those who have previously received parenteral drugs formulated in polyethoxylated castor oil, or to those with a history of allergic reactions.

Cyclosporin should not be given to psoriatic patients who have untreated malignant or pre-malignant lesions of the skin, and patients who do receive cyclosporin should not be given concomitant ultraviolet irradiation and should avoid excessive sun exposure. Other malignant neoplasms are generally a contra-indication to the use of cyclosporin for non-life-threatening disease.

The commercially available oral formulations of cyclosporin differ in their bioavailability, and patients should not be transferred from one to another without appropriate monitoring.

An oral microemulsion formulation of cyclosporin, with improved bioavailability, has been made available commercially, and patients have undergone conversion from the old formulation (initially on a 1:1 basis by weight, with monitoring of resultant cyclosporin concentrations and subsequent dosage adjustment). However, Bennett and colleagues[1,2] have questioned the wisdom of such routine conversion: they reported 3 patients with biopsy-proven rejection of stable renal grafts following conversion from the old to the new formulation, despite higher trough cyclosporin concentrations. They also noted nephrotoxicity following conversion in 3 other patients. Although other physicians consider the new formulation superior,[3,4] there are some with experiences that seem to support the doubts of Bennett,[5,6] and he has pointed out[7] that the evidence suggests that the two formulations are equivalent in efficacy.

1. Bennett WM, *et al.* Which cyclosporin formulation? *Lancet* 1996; **348:** 205.
2. Olyaei AJ, *et al.* Switching between cyclosporin formulations: what are the risks? *Drug Safety* 1997; **16:** 366–73.
3. Johnston A, Holt DW. Which cyclosporin formulation? *Lancet* 1996; **348:** 1175.
4. Pollard S. Which cyclosporin formulation? *Lancet* 1996; **348:** 1175–6.
5. Filler G, Ehrich J. Which cyclosporin formulation? *Lancet* 1996; **348:** 1176–7.
6. Gennery A, *et al.* Which cyclosporin formulation? *Lancet* 1996; **348:** 1177.
7. Bennet WM. Which cyclosporin formulation? *Lancet* 1996; **348:** 1176.

Pregnancy. Although successful pregnancies have been reported in women receiving cyclosporin[1,2] the incidence of severe intra-uterine growth retardation may be increased[3-5] and some groups prefer to maintain immunosuppression with other drugs during pregnancy.[3] One case of osseous malformation, resulting in hypoplasia of the right leg has been reported in an infant born to a cyclosporin-treated mother.[6]

The American Academy of Pediatrics considers that cyclosporin is contra-indicated in breast-feeding mothers since it is transferred into breast milk.[7] However, a study[8] in the breastfed infants of 7 women receiving cyclosporin found that the amounts ingested produced undetectable blood concentrations in the infants.

1. Lewis GJ, *et al.* Successful pregnancy in a renal transplant recipient taking cyclosporin A. *Br Med J* 1983; **286:** 603.
2. Haagsma EB, *et al.* Successful pregnancy after orthotopic liver transplantation. *Obstet Gynecol* 1989; **74:** 442–3.
3. Cundy TF, *et al.* Recovery of menstruation and pregnancy after liver transplantation. *Gut* 1990; **31:** 337–8.
4. Pickrell MD, *et al.* Pregnancy after renal transplantation: severe intrauterine growth retardation during treatment with cyclosporin A. *Br Med J* 1988; **296:** 825.
5. Williams PF, *et al.* Pregnancy after renal transplantation. *Br Med J* 1988; **296:** 1400.
6. Pujals JM, *et al.* Osseous malformation in baby born to woman on cyclosporin. *Lancet* 1989; **i:** 667.
7. American Academy of Pediatrics Committee on Drugs. The transfer of drugs and other chemicals into human milk. *Pediatrics* 1994; **93:** 137–50.
8. Nyberg G, *et al.* Breast feeding during treatment with cyclosporine. *Transplantation* 1998; **65:** 253–5.

Interactions

Cyclosporin is metabolised in the liver: phenytoin, phenobarbitone, rifampicin, and other inducers of hepatic enzymes may cause lowered plasma concentrations of cyclosporin. Increased plasma concentrations have been reported following concurrent administration of ketoconazole, erythromycin, calcium-channel blockers, androgens or oestrogens, and corticosteroids. Concurrent administration of lovastatin may increase the risk of myopathy, and potassium-sparing diuretics should be avoided because of the risk of hyperkalaemia. Patients receiving cyclosporin should avoid a high dietary intake of potassium.

Care should be taken when cyclosporin is given concomitantly with other nephrotoxic drugs.

Reviews of the interactions of cyclosporin.

1. Yee GC, McGuire TR. Pharmacokinetic drug interactions with cyclosporin. *Clin Pharmacokinet* 1990; **19:** 319–32 and 400–15.
2. Lake KD, Canafax DM. Important interactions of drugs with immunosuppressive agents used in transplant recipients. *J Antimicrob Chemother* 1995; **36** (suppl B): 11–22.
3. Campana C, *et al.* Clinically significant drug interactions with cyclosporin: an update. *Clin Pharmacokinet* 1996; **30:** 141–79.

Allopurinol. A patient who had been receiving maintenance doses of cyclosporin for some years, with consistent whole-blood trough concentrations of around 130 ng per mL at doses of 175 mg twice daily experienced a rise in cyclosporin concentrations to 410 ng per mL following 2 months of treatment with allopurinol 200 mg daily.[1] Cyclosporin concentrations returned to their previous levels over several weeks following discontinuation of allopurinol, and rose again on rechallenge. Dosage of cyclosporin was then reduced.

1. Gorrie M, *et al.* Allopurinol interaction with cyclosporin. *Br Med J* 1994; **308:** 113.

Analgesics. Raised serum-cyclosporin trough concentrations, together with small increases in serum creatinine and BUN concentrations, followed the administration of *sulindac* to a previously-stabilised renal graft recipient taking an immunosuppressive regimen including cyclosporin.[1] Nephrotoxicity, in the absence of significantly raised blood-cyclosporin concentrations, has been reported in other patients given *diclofenac* concomitantly with cyclosporin.[2] In general, because of the known potential of NSAIDs to adversely affect renal function care is advised if these drugs are added to cyclosporin therapy or their dosages altered.

1. Sesin GP, *et al.* Sulindac-induced elevation of serum cyclosporine concentration. *Clin Pharm* 1989; **8:** 445–6.
2. Branthwaite JP, Nicholls A. Cyclosporin and diclofenac interaction in rheumatoid arthritis. *Lancet* 1991; **337:** 252.

Antibacterials. There are a number of reports of raised blood concentrations of cyclosporin when given with *erythromycin*,[1-4] although opinions differ on whether the mechanism represents decreased hepatic metabolism of cyclosporin, increased absorption, or a decrease in excretion or volume of distribution.[5] Similar elevations of cyclosporin concentrations have been noted following concomitant use of other macrolide antibiotics, including *clarithromycin*,[6] *miocamycin*,[7] and *roxithromycin*[8] (although in this case no dosage adjustment was required) and the structurally-related streptogramin, *pristinamycin*;[9] however, *spiramycin* does not appear to affect the pharmacokinetics of cyclosporin.[10] The manufacturers state that the tetracycline *doxycycline* is also suspected of increasing cyclosporin concentrations, but the evidence for this seems to be scant.

The manufacturers recommend caution in the concomitant use of other nephrotoxic medications (such as *nalidixic acid* or the *aminoglycosides*) with cyclosporin, but a retrospective analysis in 21 patients given cyclosporin for allogeneic bone-marrow transplant, in whom aminoglycosides were used if fever and neutropenia developed, showed no greater incidence of nephrotoxicity than in 20 autologous bone-marrow recipients who did not receive cyclosporin, suggesting that these drugs can be given together provided careful monitoring is maintained.[11]

Although a number of reports have indicated that the quinolone *ciprofloxacin* has no effect on the pharmacokinetics of cyclosporin,[12-14] there is a report of enhanced nephrotoxicity (without a change in cyclosporin concentrations) in one patient given this combination.[15] Another quinolone, *norfloxacin*, has been reported to decrease clearance and increase blood concentrations of cyclosporin in paediatric patients,[16] probably by inhibition of cyclosporin metabolism.

Increased nephrotoxicity has also been reported with concomitant use of cyclosporin and *nafcillin*,[17] although cyclosporin concentrations were not apparently increased.

The antimycobacterial antibiotic *rifampicin* has been associated with marked decreases in blood-cyclosporin concentrations when given concomitantly,[18-20] and has resulted in graft rejection.[18,20] Although it has been assumed that this effect represents induction of the hepatic metabolism of cyclosporin by rifampicin, there is some suggestion that rifampicin may decrease the absorption of cyclosporin or induce intestinal metabolism, resulting in reduced bioavailability.[21] Topical application of *rifamycin* has also been associated with a decrease in blood-cyclosporin concentrations in another patient;[22] cyclosporin concentrations rose immediately after withdrawal of rifamycin, suggesting that the effect was not due to enzyme induction. Intravenous, but not oral, therapy with *sulphonamides* and *trimethoprim* has also been associated with falls in cyclosporin concentrations to subtherapeutic values.[23,24]

1. Ptachcinski RJ, *et al.* Effect of erythromycin on cyclosporine levels. *N Engl J Med* 1985; **313:** 1416–17.
2. Martell R, *et al.* The effects of erythromycin in patients treated with cyclosporine. *Ann Intern Med* 1986; **104:** 660–1.
3. Wadhwa NK, *et al.* Interaction between erythromycin and cyclosporine in a kidney and pancreas allograft recipient. *Ther Drug Monit* 1987; **9:** 123–5.
4. Gupta SK, *et al.* Cyclosporin-erythromycin interaction in renal transplant patients. *Br J Clin Pharmacol* 1989; **27:** 475–81.
5. Ignoffo RJ, Kim LE. Erythromycin and cyclosporine drug interaction. *DICP Ann Pharmacother* 1991; **25:** 30–1.
6. Ferrari SL, *et al.* The interaction between clarithromycin and cyclosporine in kidney transplant recipients. *Transplantation* 1994; **58:** 725–7.
7. Couet W, *et al.* Effect of ponsinomycin on cyclosporin pharmacokinetics. *Eur J Clin Pharmacol* 1990; **39:** 165–7.
8. Billaud EM, *et al.* Interaction between roxithromycin and cyclosporin in heart transplant patients. *Clin Pharmacokinet* 1990; **19:** 499–502.
9. Garraffo R, *et al.* Pristinamycin increases cyclosporin blood levels. *Med Sci Res* 1987; **15:** 461.
10. Vernillet L, *et al.* Lack of effect of spiramycin on cyclosporin pharmacokinetics. *Br J Clin Pharmacol* 1989; **27:** 789–94.
11. Chandrasekar PH, Cronin SM. Nephrotoxicity in bone marrow transplant recipients receiving aminoglycoside plus cyclosporine or aminoglycoside alone. *J Antimicrob Chemother* 1991; **27:** 845–9.
12. Hooper TL, *et al.* Ciprofloxacin: a preferred treatment for legionella infections in patients receiving cyclosporin A. *J Antimicrob Chemother* 1988; **22:** 952–3.
13. Tan KKC, *et al.* Co-administration of ciprofloxacin and cyclosporin: lack of evidence for a pharmacokinetic interaction. *Br J Clin Pharmacol* 1989; **28:** 185–7.
14. Krüger HU, *et al.* Investigation of potential interaction of ciprofloxacin with cyclosporine in bone marrow transplant recipients. *Antimicrob Agents Chemother* 1990; **34:** 1048–52.
15. Elston RA, Taylor J. Possible interaction of ciprofloxacin with cyclosporin A. *J Antimicrob Chemother* 1988; **21:** 679–80.
16. McLellan RA, *et al.* Norfloxacin interferes with cyclosporine disposition in pediatric patients undergoing renal transplantation. *Clin Pharmacol Ther* 1995; **58:** 322–7.
17. Jahansouz F, *et al.* Potentiation of cyclosporine nephrotoxicity by nafcillin in lung transplant recipients. *Transplantation* 1993; **55:** 1045–8.
18. Langhoff E, Madsen S. Rapid metabolism of cyclosporin and prednisone in kidney transplant patient receiving tuberculostatic treatment. *Lancet* 1983; **ii:** 1031.
19. Daniels NJ, *et al.* Interaction between cyclosporin and rifampicin. *Lancet* 1984; **ii:** 639.
20. Allen RDM, *et al.* Cyclosporin and rifampicin in renal transplantation. *Lancet* 1985; **i:** 980.
21. Hebert MF, *et al.* Bioavailability of cyclosporine with concomitant rifampin administration is markedly less than predicted by hepatic enzyme induction. *Clin Pharmacol Ther* 1992; **52:** 453–7.
22. Renoult E, *et al.* Effect of topical rifamycin SV treatment on cyclosporin A blood levels in a renal transplant recipient. *Eur J Clin Pharmacol* 1991; **40:** 433–4.
23. Wallwork J, *et al.* Cyclosporin and intravenous sulphadimidine and trimethoprim therapy. *Lancet* 1983; **i:** 366–7.
24. Jones DK, *et al.* Serious interaction between cyclosporin A and sulphadimidine. *Br Med J* 1986; **292:** 728–9.

Antidepressants. Administration of *fluoxetine* to a patient receiving cyclosporin as part of an immunosuppressant regimen after cardiac transplantation was associated with a subsequent marked increase in cyclosporin trough blood concentrations to approximately twice their original value, necessitating a reduction in cyclosporin dosage.[1] Following subsequent withdrawal of fluoxetine, cyclosporin concentrations fell, and dosage had to be increased again. However, a study in 13 other patients receiving cyclosporin with fluoxetine failed to find any evidence that the antidepressant altered cyclosporin concentrations.[2]

1. Horton RC, Bonser RS. Interaction between cyclosporin and fluoxetine. *Br Med J* 1995; **311:** 422.
2. Strouse TB, *et al.* Fluoxetine and cyclosporine in organ transplantation: failure to detect significant drug interactions or adverse clinical events in depressed organ recipients. *Psychosomatics* 1996; **37:** 23–30.

Antiepileptics. The antiepileptics *carbamazepine*,[1,2] *phenobarbitone*,[3] and *phenytoin*,[4] which are all inducers of hepatic cytochrome P450, have been associated with a reduction in blood-cyclosporin concentrations when given concomitantly. Since cyclosporin may produce convulsions this poses a problem in treatment, but *valproate* has been successfully used in cyclosporin-treated patients without apparent interaction.[1,2]

1. Hillebrand G, *et al.* Valproate for epilepsy in renal transplant recipients receiving cyclosporine. *Transplantation* 1987; **43:** 915–16.
2. Schofield OMV, *et al.* Cyclosporin A in psoriasis: interaction with carbamazepine. *Br J Dermatol* 1990; **122:** 425–6.
3. Carstensen H, *et al.* Interaction between cyclosporin A and phenobarbitone. *Br J Clin Pharmacol* 1986; **21:** 550–1.
4. Freeman DJ, *et al.* Evaluation of cyclosporin-phenytoin interaction with observations on cyclosporin metabolites. *Br J Clin Pharmacol* 1984; **18:** 887–93.

Antifungals. The imidazole *ketoconazole* is a potent inhibitor of hepatic cytochrome P-450 and is recognised to result in markedly increased blood-cyclosporin concentrations when the two drugs are given concomitantly.[1-4] The interaction has been employed, similarly to the calcium-channel blockers (see below), to permit therapeutic blood concentrations of cyclosporin to be achieved at lower doses;[5,6] however, the procedure may result in considerable variations in cyclosporin pharmacokinetics, and has been criticised on several grounds.[7] A similar interaction appears to occur with the related drug *itraconazole*,[8] and there is a single report of such an interaction with *miconazole*.[9] However, although such an interaction has also been reported with another related drug, *fluconazole*,[10] a small study has failed to note any significant interaction;[11,12] it has been suggested that an interaction may take place only at high doses of fluconazole.[13]

Increased nephrotoxicity may occur if cyclosporin is given concomitantly with *amphotericin*,[14] while liposomal amphotericin has been reported possibly to exacerbate cyclosporin neurotoxicity.[15] There is a report of decreased cyclosporin concentrations following addition of *griseofulvin* to an immunosuppressant regimen in one patient.[16] Modest decreases have also been seen in cyclosporin concentrations when *terbinafine* was given.[17]

1. Ferguson RM, *et al.* Ketoconazole, cyclosporin metabolism, and renal transplantation. *Lancet* 1982; **ii:** 882–3.
2. Dieperink H, Møller J. Ketoconazole and cyclosporin. *Lancet* 1982; **ii:** 1217.
3. Shepard JH, *et al.* Cyclosporine-ketoconazole: a potentially dangerous drug-drug interaction. *Clin Pharm* 1986; **5:** 468.
4. Gomez DY, *et al.* The effects of ketoconazole on the intestinal metabolism and bioavailability of cyclosporine. *Clin Pharmacol Ther* 1995; **58:** 15–19.
5. First MR, *et al.* Concomitant administration of cyclosporin and ketoconazole in renal transplant recipients. *Lancet* 1989; **ii:** 1198–1201.
6. Keogh A, *et al.* Ketoconazole to reduce the need for cyclosporine after cardiac transplantation. *N Engl J Med* 1995; **333:** 628–33.
7. Frey FJ. Concomitant cyclosporin and ketoconazole. *Lancet* 1990; **335:** 109–10.
8. Kramer MR, *et al.* Cyclosporine and itraconazole interaction in heart and lung transplant recipients. *Ann Intern Med* 1990; **113:** 327–9.
9. Horton CM, *et al.* Cyclosporine interactions with miconazole and other azole-antimycotics: a case report and review of the literature. *J Heart Lung Transplant* 1992; **11:** 1127–32.
10. Collignon P, *et al.* Interaction of fluconazole with cyclosporin. *Lancet* 1989; **i:** 1262.
11. Krüger HU, *et al.* Absence of significant interaction of fluconazole with cyclosporin. *J Antimicrob Chemother* 1989; **24:** 781–6.
12. Ehninger G, *et al.* Interaction of fluconazole with cyclosporin. *Lancet* 1989; **ii:** 104–5.
13. López-Gil JA. Fluconazole-cyclosporine interaction: a dose-dependent effect? *Ann Pharmacother* 1993; **27:** 427–30.
14. Kennedy MS, *et al.* Acute renal toxicity with combined use of amphotericin B and cyclosporine after marrow transplantation. *Transplantation* 1983; **35:** 211–15.
15. Ellis ME, *et al.* Is cyclosporin neurotoxicity enhanced in the presence of liposomal amphotericin B? *J Infect* 1994; **29:** 106–7.
16. Abu-Romeh SH, *et al.* Ciclosporin A and griseofulvin: another drug interaction. *Nephron* 1991; **58:** 237.
17. Lo ACY, *et al.* The interaction of terbinafine and cyclosporine A in renal transplant patients. *Br J Clin Pharmacol* 1997; **43:** 340–1.

Antimalarials. A large rise in serum-cyclosporin concentration was seen on 2 occasions in a renal graft recipient when *chloroquine* was added to his medication for malaria prophylaxis.[1] *Quinine* has also been reported to affect cyclosporin concentrations, in this case reducing them.

1. Finielz P, *et al.* Interaction between cyclosporin and chloroquine. *Nephron* 1993; **65:** 333.

Antineoplastics. Elevated plasma-cyclosporin concentrations and an increased incidence of nephrotoxic effects and hypertension have been reported in patients receiving cyclosporin for psoriasis who had been previously treated with *methotrexate*.[1] Severe neurological toxicity has been seen in a patient on long-term cyclosporin therapy given *doxorubicin*,[2] and it has been suggested that the use of cyclosporin or its analogues such as SDZ PSC 833 to modulate resistance to antineoplastics should be approached with caution.[3] Severe renal failure has been reported when standard oral doses of cyclosporin were given after high-dose intravenous *melphalan* (used as a bone-marrow conditioning agent before allogeneic bone-marrow transplantation).[4]

For the effects of cyclosporin on the pharmacokinetics of *teniposide*, see p.566.

1. Powles AV, *et al.* Cyclosporin toxicity. *Lancet* 1990; **i:** 610.
2. Barbui T, *et al.* Neurological symptoms and coma associated with doxorubicin administration during chronic cyclosporin therapy. *Lancet* 1992; **339:** 1421.
3. Beck WT, Kuttesch JF. Neurological symptoms associated with cyclosporin plus doxorubicin. *Lancet* 1992; **340:** 496.
4. Morgernstern GR, *et al.* Cyclosporin interaction with ketoconazole and melphalan. *Lancet* 1982; **ii:** 1342.

Cardiovascular drugs. ACE INHIBITORS. Acute renal failure has been reported in 2 patients receiving cyclosporin after renal transplantation following administration of *enalapril*.[1] Renal function recovered when the ACE inhibitor was withdrawn.

1. Murray BM, *et al.* Enalapril-associated acute renal failure in renal transplants: possible role of cyclosporine. *Am J Kidney Dis* 1990; **16:** 66–9.

ANTIARRHYTHMICS. Marked rises in serum-cyclosporin concentrations despite reductions in dose have been noted in recipients of heart or heart-lung transplants following treatment with *amiodarone*.[1,2] A rise in serum cyclosporin has similarly been seen in a patient given both cyclosporin and *propafenone*.[3]

1. Mamprin F, *et al.* Amiodarone-cyclosporine interaction in cardiac transplantation. *Am Heart J* 1992; **123:** 1725–6.
2. Egami J, *et al.* Increase in cyclosporine levels due to amiodarone therapy after heart and heart-lung transplantation. *J Am Coll Cardiol* 1993; **21:** 141A.
3. Spes CH, *et al.* Ciclosporin-propafenone interaction. *Klin Wochenschr* 1990; **68:** 872.

ANTICOAGULANTS. Treatment with warfarin for deep-vein thrombosis in a patient maintained on cyclosporin 3 mg per kg body-weight daily for pure red-cell aplasia resulted in a relapse of the latter and a significant fall in cyclosporin blood concentrations.[1] Increase in the cyclosporin dose to 7 mg per kg daily restored control of the aplasia but resulted in a marked increase in prothrombin activity requiring an increase in warfarin dosage. The results suggest that each drug interferes with the activity of the other. The influence of the patient's other medications (including phenobarbitone and folic acid), if any, is unknown.

1. Snyder DS. Interaction between cyclosporine and warfarin. *Ann Intern Med* 1988; **108:** 311.

CALCIUM-CHANNEL BLOCKERS. The calcium-channel blockers *diltiazem*,[1,2] *nicardipine*,[3,4] and *verapamil*[5] have all been associated with increases in cyclosporin concentrations in blood when given concomitantly. It has been suggested that such an interaction can be made use of, permitting effective cyclosporin concentrations to be maintained at lower doses;[6] in addition, there is some evidence of mitigation of cyclosporin-induced nephrotoxicity when calcium-channel blockers are given concomitantly (see Treatment of Adverse Effects, above). However, some caution is required: one report has pointed out that diltiazem does not increase cyclosporin concentrations in all cases,[7] while others have found that concomitant administration alters the pattern of cyclosporin metabolites, and that pharmacokinetic changes are greater in female than in male patients.[8] Interestingly, *nifedipine* has not been shown to increase blood-cyclosporin concentrations,[5] although there is some evidence of a renal protective effect in transplantation (p.922). However, concomitant administration with cyclosporin may exacerbate the problem of gingival hyperplasia—see under Adverse Effects, above.

1. Brockmöller J, *et al.* Pharmacokinetic interaction between cyclosporin and diltiazem. *Eur J Clin Pharmacol* 1990; **38:** 237–42.
2. Bourge RC, *et al.* Diltiazem-cyclosporine interaction in cardiac transplant recipients: impact on cyclosporine dose and medication costs. *Am J Med* 1991; **90:** 402–4.
3. Todd P, *et al.* Nicardipine interacts with cyclosporin. *Br J Dermatol* 1989; **121:** 820.
4. Kessler M, *et al.* Influence of nicardipine on renal function and plasma cyclosporin in renal transplant patients. *Eur J Clin Pharmacol* 1989; **36:** 637–8.
5. Tortorice KL, *et al.* The effects of calcium channel blockers on cyclosporine and its metabolites in renal transplant patients. *Ther Drug Monit* 1990; **12:** 321–8.
6. Sketris IS, *et al.* Effect of calcium-channel blockers on cyclosporine clearance and use in renal transplant patients. *Ann Pharmacother* 1994; **28:** 1227–31.
7. Jones TE, Morris RG. Diltiazem does not always increase blood cyclosporin concentration. *Br J Clin Pharmacol* 1996; **42:** 642–4.
8. Bleck JS, *et al.* Diltiazem increases blood concentrations of cyclized cyclosporine metabolites resulting in different cyclosporine metabolite patterns in stable male and female renal allograft recipients. *Br J Clin Pharmacol* 1996; **41:** 551–6.

CLONIDINE. Addition of clonidine to the regimen of a 3-year-old child who had developed hypertension after a renal transplant resulted in a marked increase in whole blood cyclosporin concentrations, despite a reduction in cyclosporin dose.[1] Withdrawal of clonidine resulted in a rapid fall in cyclosporin concentrations.

1. Gilbert RD, *et al.* Interaction between clonidine and cyclosporine A. *Nephron* 1995; **71:** 105.

DIURETICS. Enhanced nephrotoxicity, without apparent change in cyclosporin blood concentrations, has been seen in individual patients following addition of *metolazone*[1] or *amiloride* with *chlorothiazide*[2] to their regimen. Severe nephrotoxicity, resulting in loss of graft function, has been seen in a renal transplant patient given *mannitol* with cyclosporin;[3] graft function recovered on withdrawal of the diuretic.

1. Christensen P, Leski M. Nephrotoxic drug interaction between metolazone and cyclosporin. *Br Med J* 1987; **294:** 578.
2. Deray G, *et al.* Enhancement of cyclosporin nephrotoxicity by diuretic therapy. *Clin Nephrol* 1989; **32:** 47.
3. Brunner FP, *et al.* Mannitol potentiates cyclosporine nephrotoxicity. *Clin Nephrol* 1986; **25** (suppl 1): 3130–6.

Colchicine. Concurrent administration of cyclosporin and colchicine may result in myopathy—see Effects on Skeletal Muscle, under Adverse Effects, above.

Corticosteroids. Cyclosporin plasma concentrations rose strikingly in 22 of 33 renal transplant patients given high-dose *methylprednisolone* for rejection episodes.[1] The mean trough plasma concentration in these patients while receiving cyclosporin maintenance therapy, together with prednisolone, was 205 ng per mL by radioimmunoassay; this rose to peaks of 482 ng per mL during or immediately after intravenous methylprednisolone injections.

For further discussions of the interaction between cyclosporin and corticosteroids, see p.1014.

1. Klintmalm G, Säwe J. High dose methylprednisolone increases plasma cyclosporin levels in renal transplant recipients. *Lancet* 1984; **i:** 731.

Dermatological drugs. Following a report of increased whole-blood cyclosporin concentrations and nephrotoxicity in a patient given *etretinate* with cyclosporin, *in-vitro* results indicated that etretinate inhibited hepatic microsomal metabolism of cyclosporin, as did *acitretin* and *isotretinoin*.[1] However, another study failed to find evidence of such an interaction *in vitro*.[2]

1. Shah IA, *et al.* The effects of retinoids and terbinafine on the human hepatic microsomal metabolism of cyclosporin. *Br J Dermatol* 1993; **129:** 395–8.
2. Webber IR, Back DJ. Effect of etretinate on cyclosporin metabolism in vitro. *Br J Dermatol* 1993; **128:** 42–4.

Gastro-intestinal drugs. Administration of *cisapride* to renal transplant recipients being treated with cyclosporin has been reported to increase peak cyclosporin concentrations and increase the speed of absorption.[1] *Cimetidine*,[2,3] *ranitidine*,[2] or *famotidine*,[3] do not appear to affect cyclosporin pharmacokinetics.

1. Finet L, *et al.* Effects of cisapride on the intestinal absorption of cyclosporine in renal transplant recipients. *Gastroenterology* 1991; **100:** A209.
2. Barri YM, *et al.* Cimetidine or ranitidine in renal transplant patients receiving cyclosporine. *Clin Transplant* 1996; **10:** 34–8.
3. Shaefer MS, *et al.* Evaluation of the pharmacokinetic interaction between cimetidine or famotidine and cyclosporine in healthy men. *Ann Pharmacother* 1995; **29:** 1088–91.

Hypoglycaemic drugs. Concurrent administration of *glibenclamide* with cyclosporin in 6 patients was associated with a mean 57% increase in the steady-state plasma concentration of cyclosporin, suggesting that dosage adjustment may become necessary when these drugs are given concomitantly.[1]

1. Islam SI, *et al.* Possible interaction between cyclosporine and glibenclamide in posttransplant diabetic patients. *Ther Drug Monit* 1996; **18:** 624–6.

Lipid regulating drugs. A study in 10 renal transplant recipients indicated that concomitant administration of cyclosporin and *probucol* markedly reduced the whole blood and plasma concentrations of the former in 9 of them, compared with administration of cyclosporin alone.[1] Concurrent administration of *bezafibrate* has been reported to result in increased blood concentrations of cyclosporin and resultant nephrotoxicity.[2] *Simvastatin* increases the unbound fraction of cyclosporin in the blood, resulting in a modest increase in apparent clearance of the immunosuppressant.[3]

Concurrent administration of cyclosporin and *lovastatin* may result in myopathy—see Effects on Skeletal Muscle, under Adverse Effects, above, and also under Lovastatin, p.1275.

1. Gallego C, *et al.* Interaction between probucol and cyclosporine in renal transplant patients. *Ann Pharmacother* 1994; **28:** 940–3.
2. Hirai M, *et al.* Elevated blood concentrations of cyclosporine and kidney failure after bezafibrate in renal graft recipient. *Ann Pharmacother* 1996; **30:** 883–4.
3. Akhlaghi F, *et al.* Effect of simvastatin on cyclosporine unbound fraction and apparent blood clearance in heart transplant recipients. *Br J Clin Pharmacol* 1997; **44:** 537–42.

Muromonab-CD3. Treatment of acute rejection of kidney grafts in 10 patients using muromonab-CD3 resulted in increases in mean trough cyclosporin concentrations, despite a reduction in cyclosporin dosage.[1] Once muromonab-CD3 was withdrawn the cyclosporin dosage had to be increased again to provide adequate concentrations.

1. Vrahnos D, *et al.* Cyclosporin levels during OKT3 treatment of acute renal allograft rejection. *Pharmacotherapy* 1991; **11:** 278.

Octreotide. A marked reduction in cyclosporin serum concentrations was seen in 10 diabetic patients with pancreatic transplants when octreotide was given concomitantly;[1] it was suggested that if these 2 drugs are given together the oral dosage of cyclosporin needs to be increased on average by 50%.

1. Landgraf R, *et al.* Effect of somatostatin analogue (SMS 201-995) on cyclosporin levels. *Transplantation* 1987; **44:** 724–5.

Sex hormones. Raised cyclosporin concentrations in blood have been seen when therapy with *danazol*,[1] *methyltestosterone*,[2] or *norethisterone*[1] was given concurrently with cyclosporin, and clinical evidence of both nephrotoxicity[1,2] and hepatotoxicity[2] has been seen. Severe hepatotoxicity and raised plasma-cyclosporin trough values also resulted when an oral contraceptive containing *levonorgestrel* and *ethinyloestradiol* was taken by a woman receiving cyclosporin;[3] she had taken the same contraceptive before beginning cyclosporin without ill-effects.

1. Ross WB, *et al.* Cyclosporin interaction with danazol and norethisterone. *Lancet* 1986; **i:** 330.
2. Møller BB, Ekelund B. Toxicity of cyclosporine during treatment with androgens. *N Engl J Med* 1985; **313:** 1416.
3. Deray G, *et al.* Oral contraceptive interaction with cyclosporin. *Lancet* 1987; **i:** 158.

Sirolimus. For the effect of cyclosporin on the pharmacokinetics of sirolimus, see p.561.

Vaccines. Efficacy of immunoprophylaxis may be expected to be diminished during cyclosporin therapy, and administration of live virus vaccines, in particular, is contra-indicated in an immunocompromised host.[1] Further, there is some evidence that antigens administered during cyclosporin therapy may induce tolerance, which might result in increased susceptibility to the diseases one wishes to protect against.

1. Grabenstein JD, Baker JR. Comment: cyclosporine and vaccination. *Drug Intell Clin Pharm* 1985; **19:** 679–80.

Vitamins. For reference to increased absorption of cyclosporin when given with a water-soluble macrogol derivative of *vitamin E*, see Absorption, under Pharmacokinetics, below.

With food. Several studies have indicated that *grapefruit juice* increases the bioavailability of oral,[1-4] but not intravenous[4] cyclosporin, resulting in marked increases in blood-cyclosporin concentrations. The effect appears to be due to inhibition of cytochrome P450 enzymes in the gut wall by flavonoids present in grapefruit juice,[3] resulting in transiently reduced cyclosporin metabolism. Although it has been suggested that the effect might be employed similarly to that of calcium-channel blockers or ketoconazole in reducing the required dose of cyclosporin,[2] others have pointed out that grapefruit juice is not standardised and its effects are variable.[5]

1. Proppe DG, *et al.* Influence of chronic ingestion of grapefruit juice on steady-state blood concentrations of cyclosporine A in renal transplant patients with stable graft function. *Br J Clin Pharmacol* 1995; **39:** 337–8.
2. Yee GC, *et al.* Effect of grapefruit juice on blood cyclosporin concentration. *Lancet* 1995; **345:** 955–6.
3. Hollander AAMJ, *et al.* The effect of grapefruit juice on cyclosporine and prednisone metabolism in transplant patients. *Clin Pharmacol Ther* 1995; **57:** 318–24.
4. Ducharme MP, *et al.* Disposition of intravenous and oral cyclosporine after administration with grapefruit juice. *Clin Pharmacol Ther* 1995; **57:** 485–91.
5. Johnston A, Holt DW. Effect of grapefruit juice on blood cyclosporin concentration. *Lancet* 1995; **346:** 122–3.

Pharmacokinetics

The pharmacokinetics of cyclosporin are variable and difficult to determine. Results vary depending on the use of a HPLC assay or a radio-immunoassay, and values obtained by the two methods are not strictly comparable.

Absorption of conventional formulations of cyclosporin from the gastro-intestinal tract is variable and incomplete. An oral microemulsion formulation with improved absorption characteristics is available and is more rapidly and completely absorbed, with peak concentrations achieved about 1.5 to 2 hours after a dose.

Cyclosporin is widely distributed throughout the body. Distribution in the blood is concentration- and temperature-dependent, with between 41 and 58% in erythrocytes and 10 to 20% in leucocytes; the remainder is found in plasma, about 90% protein-bound, mostly to lipoprotein. Because of distribution into blood cells whole blood concentrations are higher than, and not comparable with, plasma concentrations; where peak plasma concentrations are reported to be approximately 1 ng per mL (by specific HPLC assay) for each mg of oral cyclosporin, whole blood concentrations for each mg range from about 1.4 to 2.7 ng per mL. Cyclosporin is reported to cross the placenta, and to be distributed into breast milk.

Clearance from the blood is biphasic. The terminal elimination half-life of an oral dose is reported to range from about 5 to 20 hours; clearance in children is more rapid.

Cyclosporin is extensively metabolised in the liver and primarily excreted in faeces via the bile. Toxicity has been attributed to the metabolites, notably M-17 (see above). About 6% of a dose is reported to be excreted in urine, less than 0.1% unchanged.

Absorption. Ingestion of cyclosporin with food may increase its bioavailability, although the effect only appears to be significant when the meal is high in fat;[1] ingestion with food and added bile acids may also increase absorption moderately.[2] Administration with a micelle-forming macrogol derivative of vitamin E has also been reported to markedly increase cyclosporin absorption.[3,4]

Because of the problems of variable oral absorption, an oral microemulsion has been developed which offers greatly improved and more predictable bioavailability,[5-9] particularly in liver transplant patients with impaired bile flow.[5-7] It should be noted that the formulation of this microemulsion in fact includes a vitamin E compound.

However, a recent study[10] has suggested that contrary to previous assumptions, conventional formulations of cyclosporin are quite well absorbed, and that the low bioavailability is due to extensive cytochrome-mediated metabolism in the gut wall (see also Metabolism, below). If this were the case, the improved bioavailability seen with the microemulsion formulation is presumably less to do with improved absorption than with protection from such metabolism.

1. Gupta SK, *et al.* Effect of food on the pharmacokinetics of cyclosporine in healthy subjects following oral and intravenous administration. *J Clin Pharmacol* 1990; **30:** 643–53.
2. Lindholm A, *et al.* The effect of food and bile acid administration on the relative bioavailability of cyclosporin. *Br J Clin Pharmacol* 1990; **29:** 541–8.
3. Sokol RJ, *et al.* Improvement of cyclosporin absorption in children after liver transplantation by means of water-soluble vitamin E. *Lancet* 1991; **338:** 212–15.
4. Chang T, *et al.* The effect of water-soluble vitamin E on cyclosporine pharmacokinetics in healthy volunteers. *Clin Pharmacol Ther* 1996; **59:** 297–303.
5. Trull AK, *et al.* Cyclosporin absorption from microemulsion formulation in liver transplant recipient. *Lancet* 1993; **341:** 433.
6. Sketris IS, *et al.* Increased cyclosporin bioavailability from a microemulsion formulation in a liver transplant recipient. *Ann Pharmacother* 1994; **28:** 962–3.
7. Trull AK, *et al.* Absorption of cyclosporin from conventional and new microemulsion oral formulations in liver transplant recipients with external biliary diversion. *Br J Clin Pharmacol* 1995; **39:** 627–31.
8. van den Borne BEEM, *et al.* Relative bioavailability of a new oral form of cyclosporin A in patients with rheumatoid arthritis. *Br J Clin Pharmacol* 1995; **39:** 172–5.
9. Friman S, Bäckman L. A new microemulsion formulation of cyclosporin: pharmacokinetic and clinical features. *Clin Pharmacokinet* 1996; **30:** 181–93.
10. Wu C-Y, *et al.* Differentiation of absorption and first-pass gut and hepatic metabolism in humans: studies with cyclosporine. *Clin Pharmacol Ther* 1995; **58:** 492–7.

Metabolism. Evidence has been seen *in vitro*[1] and *in vivo*[2-4] that the low oral bioavailability of cyclosporin is due to first-pass metabolism in the gastro-intestinal tract rather than the liver.

1. Tjia JF, *et al.* Cyclosporin metabolism by the gastrointestinal mucosa. *Br J Clin Pharmacol* 1991; **31:** 344–6.
2. Kolars JC, *et al.* First-pass metabolism of cyclosporin by the gut. *Lancet* 1991; **338:** 1488–90.
3. Hoppu K, *et al.* Evidence for pre-hepatic metabolism of oral cyclosporine in children. *Br J Clin Pharmacol* 1991; **32:** 477–81.
4. Wu C-Y, *et al.* Differentiation of absorption and first-pass gut and hepatic metabolism in humans: studies with cyclosporine. *Clin Pharmacol Ther* 1995; **58:** 492–7.

Monitoring drug concentrations. Considerable debate has attended the necessity for therapeutic monitoring of cyclosporin concentrations and has concentrated mainly on the questions of which assay methods to use and whether to measure drug concentrations in whole blood or plasma.

Before the introduction of specific monoclonal radio-immunoassay the HPLC assay for cyclosporin had the advantage of being specific for the parent compound, and some workers suggested it to be the method of choice.[1,2] However, it is a more complex procedure, is not universally available, and is slower to perform than radio-immunoassay.[1,3-5] Specific monoclonal radio-immunoassays are now widely available; a comparative study of specific and non-specific radio-immunoassays, HPLC, and polyclonal fluorescence polarisation immunoassay (FPIA) found that the specific assays, used on whole blood samples, gave the best correlation with clinical events.[6]

Because the distribution of cyclosporin between blood cells and plasma is temperature-dependent, plasma concentrations may be twice as high at 37° as at 21°.[7] The temperature at which samples are stored and processed may therefore considerably influence results. In consequence, measurement of drug concentrations in whole blood is to be preferred.[1,3,4,8] However, many, particularly early, clinical studies have given plasma or serum concentrations, which makes comparison of literature data difficult. This problem is compounded by a considerable degree of variation between laboratories,[9,10] even when the same technique is used,[10] and by circadian variations in cyclosporin metabolism which mean that samples should be taken at the same time of day.[11]

Because of the variability in results caused by difficulties in monitoring it has proved difficult to determine precisely the cyclosporin concentrations associated with therapeutic benefit and toxicity,[1,3-5] and it has been suggested that measurement of the therapeutic concentrations is unnecessary (provided the patient's clinical condition and renal function are monitored) when low-dose cyclosporin is being given (for example, in psoriasis).[12] However, others consider that it is always critical that cyclosporin blood trough concentrations are regularly measured,[13] in addition to other monitoring, and this would seem to represent the general practice.[3-5] Lindholm[14] has suggested that trough cyclosporin concentrations, measured by a specific method in whole blood, should not be less than 150 ng per mL during the first month after renal transplantation, although lower concentrations are subsequently acceptable; trough concentrations of 250 to 300 ng per mL are recommended in the 3 months following liver transplantation.

1. Ptachcinski RJ, *et al.* Cyclosporine concentration determinations for monitoring and pharmacokinetic studies. *J Clin Pharmacol* 1986; **26:** 358–66.
2. Varghese Z, *et al.* How to measure cyclosporin. *Lancet* 1984; **i:** 1407–8.
3. Faynor SM, *et al.* Therapeutic drug monitoring of cyclosporine. *Mayo Clin Proc* 1984; **59:** 571–2.
4. Burkle WS. Cyclosporine pharmacokinetics and blood level monitoring. *Drug Intell Clin Pharm* 1985; **19:** 101–5.
5. Rodighiero V. Therapeutic drug monitoring of cyclosporin: practical applications and limitations. *Clin Pharmacokinet* 1989; **16:** 27–37.
6. Lindholm A, *et al.* A prospective study of cyclosporine concentration in relation to its therapeutic effect and toxicity after renal transplantation. *Br J Clin Pharmacol* 1990; **30:** 443–52.
7. Dieperink H. Temperature dependency of cyclosporin plasma levels. *Lancet* 1983; **i:** 416.
8. Bandini G, *et al.* Measuring cyclosporin in plasma. *Lancet* 1983; **i:** 762.
9. Moyer TP. Measurement of cyclosporine: a challenge to the professional laboratory organizations. *Ther Drug Monit* 1985; **7:** 123–4.
10. Johnston A, *et al.* The United Kingdom Cyclosporin Quality Assessment Scheme. *Ther Drug Monit* 1986; **8:** 200–4.
11. Venkataramanan R, *et al.* Diurnal variation in cyclosporine kinetics. *Ther Drug Monit* 1986; **8:** 380–1.
12. Feutren G, *et al.* Cyclosporin monitoring in psoriasis. *Lancet* 1990; **335:** 866–7.
13. Gupta AK, *et al.* Short-term changes in renal function, blood pressure, and electrolyte levels in patients receiving cyclosporine for dermatologic disorders. *Arch Intern Med* 1991; **151:** 356–62.
14. Lindholm A. Therapeutic monitoring of cyclosporin—an update. *Eur J Clin Pharmacol* 1991; **41:** 273–83.

Uses and Administration

Cyclosporin is a powerful immunosuppressant which appears to act specifically on lymphocytes, mainly helper T-cells, and inhibits the production of lymphokines including interleukin-2, resulting in a depression of cell-mediated immune response. Unlike cytotoxic immunosuppressants such as cyclophosphamide it has little effect on bone marrow.

It is used, usually combined with corticosteroids (and often with other immunosuppressants), in organ and tissue transplantation (p.498) for the prophylaxis of graft rejection, or in the management of graft rejection in patients previously treated with other immunosuppressants.

Cyclosporin has also been tried in various diseases considered to have an auto-immune component as indicated by the cross-references given below; they include asthma, aplastic anaemia, Behçet's syndrome, diabetes mellitus, glomerular kidney disease, chronic active hepatitis, neurological disorders such as multiple sclerosis and myasthenia gravis, primary biliary cirrhosis, rheumatoid arthritis, sarcoidosis, scleritis or uveitis, scleroderma, and various skin disorders, notably psoriasis and atopic dermatitis.

Cyclosporin is given by mouth as liquid-filled capsules or as an oily solution, which may be diluted with milk or fruit juice (not grapefruit) immediately before administration to improve palatability. Microemulsion formulations with improved bioavailability are available in a number of countries; patients receiving conventional oral formulations may be given the same initial dosage of a microemulsion formulation, although dosage reduction may subsequently be advisable. However, the daily dose of the microemulsion formulation is administered in 2 divided doses; this is not necessarily the case with the conventional formulation.

In **organ transplantation** the usual initial dose of either formulation is 10 to 15 mg per kg bodyweight daily, beginning 4 to 12 hours before transplantation, and continued for 1 to 2 weeks; lower initial doses may be given in combination with other immunosuppressants (e.g. in 'triple' or 'quadruple' therapy). Dosage may subsequently be reduced gradually to a daily maintenance dose of 2 to 6 mg per kg.

Kidney and liver function should be determined regularly, as well as blood or plasma concentrations of cyclosporin (for discussion of the methods used to determine concentration, see Monitoring Drug Concentrations, above). Dosage should be adjusted in patients who show signs of deterioration in renal or hepatic function.

Cyclosporin may also be given intravenously, at one-third of the oral dose, in patients in whom oral administration is not feasible. It is given by slow intravenous infusion over 2 to 6 hours, the 5% concentrate being diluted 1:20 to 1:100 in sodium chloride injection 0.9% or glucose injection 5%, to give a 0.05% to 0.25% solution of cyclosporin. Because of the risk of anaphylactoid reactions, which have been attributed to the polyethoxylated castor oil vehicle, patients should be transferred to oral therapy as soon as possible.

For the prevention of graft rejection in **bone-marrow transplantation** and prevention and treatment of graft-versus-host disease an initial dose of 3 to 5 mg per kg daily by the intravenous route has been suggested, continued for up to 2 weeks until maintenance by mouth, in doses of 12.5 mg per kg daily can be instituted. Unlike organ transplantation, in which some form of immunosuppression is required for life, cyclosporin maintenance can be gradually reduced, after at least 3 to 6 months, until it is withdrawn altogether.

In the treatment of **psoriasis**, cyclosporin may be given in doses of 2.5 to 5 mg per kg daily (a maximum of 4 mg per kg daily is recommended in the USA), in 2 divided doses by mouth, reduced once remission is achieved to the lowest effective maintenance dose. Treatment should be discontinued if there is insufficient response within 6 weeks to the maximum dose. A similar dosage range may be given for a maximum of 8 weeks in the treatment of severe **atopic dermatitis**.

In **rheumatoid arthritis** where classical second-line drugs are ineffective or unsuitable, cyclosporin may be given by mouth in initial daily doses of 2.5 mg per kg, divided into two doses, for a period of 6 or 8 weeks. If the clinical effect is insufficient dosage may then be increased to a maximum of 4 mg per kg daily; if there is no response after 3 months, treatment should then be discontinued.

For **nephrotic syndrome** secondary to glomerular kidney disease (minimal change nephropathy, focal glomerulosclerosis, or membranous nephropathy) dosage of cyclosporin depends on age and renal function. To induce remission in patients with normal renal function 5 mg per kg daily may be given to adults and 6 mg per kg daily to children, in 2 divided doses by mouth. In patients with renal impairment the initial dose should not exceed 2.5 mg per kg daily. Treatment may be discontinued if there is no response after 3 months (or 6 months in patients with membranous nephropathy). In patients who do respond, maintenance doses should be gradually reduced to the minimum effective value.

Administration. It has been suggested that calculating doses in mg per kg body-weight may not be the best way to achieve the desired blood concentrations of cyclosporin.[1] Retrospective study of 1071 renal transplant recipients indicated that blood cyclosporin concentrations were not significantly correlated with patient weight, the best prediction of trough blood concentration being given by the formula:

Blood concentration (ng/mL) = dose in mg/day x (1.34 + 0.00011 x days after transplant − 0.0049 x height in cm)

This formula appeared useful in predicting blood concentrations in prospective studies; from the seventh day after transplantation target trough concentrations could be expected to be about 0.3 times the daily cyclosporin dose in mg.

1. Bock HA, *et al.* Weight-independent dosing of cyclosporine—an alternative to the mg/kg doctrine. *Transplantation* 1994; **57:** 1484–9.

INHALATION. Aerosolised cyclosporin given by inhalation has proved effective in the management of acute graft rejection in lung transplantation.[1] Cyclosporin was administered at a dose of 100 to 300 mg daily via a nebuliser, in addition to continued systemic therapy with cyclosporin or tacrolimus, azathioprine and prednisone. Liposomal formulations are under investigation for the aerosolised administration of cyclosporin.

1. Keenan RJ, *et al.* Efficacy of inhaled cyclosporine in lung transplant recipients with refractory rejection: correlation of intragraft cytokine gene expression with pulmonary function and histologic characteristics. *Surgery* 1995; **118:** 385–91.

ORAL. A review of the newer microemulsion formulation of cyclosporin.[1] For discussion of the potential problems involved in converting from conventional to microemulsion oral formulations see under Precautions, above.

1. Noble S, Markham A. Cyclosporin: a review of the pharmacokinetic properties, clinical efficacy and tolerability of a microemulsion-based formulation (Neoral). *Drugs* 1995; **50:** 924–41.

Asthma. Cyclosporin is being considered as a potential treatment for some cases of asthma (p.745). A study involving 39 patients with severe corticosteroid-dependent asthma found that low-dose cyclosporin by mouth (an initial dose of 5 mg per kg body-weight daily) permitted a substantial reduction in the daily dosage of prednisolone, from a median of 10 to 3.5 mg daily.[1]

1. Lock SH, *et al.* Double-blind, placebo-controlled study of cyclosporin A as a corticosteroid-sparing agent in corticosteroid-dependent asthma. *Am J Respir Crit Care Med* 1996; **153:** 509–14.

Cogan's syndrome. Cyclosporin has been used in conjunction with corticosteroids for severe Cogan's syndrome with large-vessel vasculitis (p.1020).

Connective tissue and muscular disorders. Cyclosporin has been tried[1] in Behçet's syndrome (p.1018) and refractory polymyositis and dermatomyositis[2,3] (p.1027), although its role is not established in these conditions. As mentioned on p.1029, it has also been investigated for systemic lupus erythematosus, particularly lupus nephritis, but there are doubts about its value.

1. Masuda K, *et al.* Double-masked trial of cyclosporin versus colchicine and long-term open study of cyclosporin in Behçet's disease. *Lancet* 1989; **i:** 1093–6.
2. Heckmatt J, *et al.* Cyclosporin in juvenile dermatomyositis. *Lancet* 1989; **i:**1063–6.
3. Lueck CJ, *et al.* Cyclosporin in the management of polymyositis and dermatomyositis. *J Neurol Neurosurg Psychiatry* 1991; **54:** 1007–8.

Diabetes mellitus. Immunosuppressants have been used in attempts to prolong the so called 'honeymoon period' in recently diagnosed diabetics (p.313). Cyclosporin has apparently produced modest benefits in such a context,[1,2] but its overall value remains to be determined.

1. Bougneres PF, *et al.* Factors associated with early remission of type 1 diabetes in children treated with cyclosporine. *N Engl J Med* 1988; **318:** 663–70.
2. The Canadian-European Randomized Control Trial Group. Cyclosporin-induced remission of IDDM after early intervention: association of 1 yr of cyclosporin treatment with enhanced insulin secretion. *Diabetes* 1988; **37:** 1574–82.

Glaucoma. Topical cyclosporin has produced some encouraging results[1] when used as an adjunct to reduce formation of scar tissue and improve outcome of glaucoma filtering surgery (see p.1387).

1. Turaçli E, *et al.* A comparative clinical trial of mitomycin C and cyclosporin A in trabeculectomy. *Eur J Ophthalmol* 1996; **6:** 398–401.

Histiocytic syndromes. As mentioned in the discussion on p.478 cyclosporin has been reported to produce benefit in patients with advanced Langerhans-cell histiocytosis.

Inflammatory bowel disease. Cyclosporin has been tried with variable success as a second-line drug in inflammatory bowel disease (p.1171). Intravenous high-dose cyclosporin has been found to be effective in refractory ulcerative colitis,[1] and may also be useful if given by enema.[2] However, benefit in Crohn's disease is less clear. Although intravenous therapy is reportedly useful in healing refractory fistulae,[3] lower oral doses have produced disappointing results in adults and children with active Crohn's disease.[4-6]

1. Lichtiger S, *et al.* Cyclosporine in severe ulcerative colitis refractory to steroid therapy. *N Engl J Med* 1994; **330:** 1841–5.
2. Sandborn WJ, *et al.* Cyclosporine enemas for treatment-resistant, mildly to moderately active, left-sided ulcerative colitis. *Am J Gastroenterol* 1993; **88:** 640–5.
3. Hanauer SB, Smith MB. Rapid closure of Crohn's disease fistulas with continuous intravenous cyclosporin A. *Am J Gastroenterol* 1993; **88:** 646–9.
4. Feagan BG, *et al.* Low-dose cyclosporine for the treatment of Crohn's disease. *N Engl J Med* 1994; **330:** 1846–51.
5. Nicholls S, *et al.* Cyclosporin as initial treatment for Crohn's disease. *Arch Dis Child* 1994; **71:** 243–7.
6. Stange EF, *et al.* European trial of cyclosporine in chronic active Crohn's disease: a 12-month study. *Gastroenterology* 1995; **109:** 774–82.

Kidney disorders, non-malignant. Cyclosporin has been tried in a number of forms of glomerular kidney disease (p.1021) but use has been cautious because of fears about nephrotoxicity. Nonetheless, responses have been seen in patients with corticosteroid-resistant minimal change nephropathy,[1,2] focal glomerulosclerosis,[1,2] and membranous nephropathy.[3,4]

1. Nyrop M, Olgaard K. Cyclosporin A treatment of severe steroid resistant nephrotic syndrome in adults. *J Intern Med* 1990; **227:** 65–8.
2. Niaudet P, *et al.* Steroid-resistant idiopathic nephrotic syndrome and ciclosporin. *Nephron* 1991; **57:** 481.
3. Rostoker G, *et al.* Cyclosporin in idiopathic steroid-resistant membranous glomerulonephritis. *Lancet* 1989; **ii:** 975–6.
4. Cattran DC, *et al.* A controlled trial of cyclosporine in patients with progressive membranous nephropathy. *Kidney Int* 1995; **47:** 1130–5.

Lichen planus. Lichen planus is a skin disorder generally controlled with corticosteroids (see p.1075), although cyclosporin has also been used. Cyclosporin has been given successfully in relatively low doses (3 to 5 mg per kg body-weight by mouth) to produce remission of severe lichen planus,[1] but such therapy may be associated with the development of hypertension and impairment of renal function. In consequence, topical application of cyclosporin oral solution as a mouthwash for oral lichen planus has been tried with conflicting results.[2-7] One such study failed to note any benefit long-term from either cyclosporin mouthwash or corticosteroid oral paste.[7]

1. Pigatto PD, *et al.* Cyclosporin A for treatment of severe lichen planus. *Br J Dermatol* 1990; **121:** 121–3.
2. Eisen D, *et al.* Cyclosporin wash for oral lichen planus. *Lancet* 1990; **335:** 535–6.
3. Eisen D, *et al.* Effect of topical cyclosporine rinse on oral lichen planus: a double-blind analysis. *N Engl J Med* 1990; **323:** 290–4.
4. Porter SR, *et al.* The efficacy of topical cyclosporin in the management of desquamative gingivitis due to lichen planus. *Br J Dermatol* 1993; **129:** 753–5.
5. Levell NJ, *et al.* Lack of effect of cyclosporin mouthwash in oral lichen planus. *Lancet* 1991; **337:** 796–7.
6. Ho VC, Conklin RJ. Effect of topical cyclosporine rinse on oral lichen planus. *N Engl J Med* 1991; **325:** 435.
7. Sieg P, *et al.* Topical cyclosporin in oral lichen planus: a controlled, randomized prospective trial. *Br J Dermatol* 1995; **132:** 790–4.

Liver diseases, non-malignant. In chronic active hepatitis (p.1019), limited evidence[1] suggests that cyclosporin may offer an alternative therapy in patients with severe auto-immune (non-viral) disease where corticosteroids alone or with azathioprine do not suffice. In primary biliary cirrhosis, on the other hand, no form of treatment has proven unequivocally successful (see p.497); some benefit has been reported with cyclosporin,[2] but there are problems with toxicity.

1. Mistilis SP, *et al.* Cyclosporin, a new treatment for autoimmune chronic active hepatitis. *Med J Aust* 1985; **143:** 463–5.
2. Lombard M, *et al.* Cyclosporin A treatment in primary biliary cirrhosis: results of a long-term placebo controlled trial. *Gastroenterology* 1993; **104:** 519–26.

Multiple sclerosis. As noted on p.620, immunosuppressants, including cyclosporin,[1,2] have produced modest benefit in patients with multiple sclerosis. However, it has been concluded that the scanty benefits of therapy are outweighed by the toxicity of the doses required.

1. Rudge P, *et al.* Randomised double blind controlled trial of cyclosporin in multiple sclerosis. *J Neurol Neurosurg Psychiatry* 1989; **52:** 559–65.
2. The Multiple Sclerosis Study Group. Efficacy and toxicity of cyclosporine in chronic progressive multiple sclerosis: a randomized, double-blinded, placebo-controlled clinical trial. *Ann Neurol* 1990; **27:** 591–605.

Muscular dystrophies. A study in 15 boys with Duchenne muscular dystrophy (p.1025) given cyclosporin 5 mg per kg body-weight daily by mouth in divided doses, adjusted according to trough serum concentrations of cyclosporin, found that muscular force generation was improved during treatment, but declined again once treatment ceased.[1] The clinical significance, if any, of this effect remains to be established.

1. Sharma KR, *et al.* Cyclosporine increases muscular force generation in Duchenne muscular dystrophy. *Neurology* 1993; **43:** 527–32.

Myasthenia gravis. Cyclosporin may be of use as an alternative to azathioprine in the management of myasthenia gravis (p.1388) for its steroid-sparing effect[1] or when patients are intolerant of or unresponsive to corticosteroids and azathioprine. It appears to be of similar efficacy to azathioprine[2] with a more rapid effect but serious adverse effects such as nephrotoxicity may limit its use.

1. Tindall RSA, *et al.* A clinical therapeutic trial of cyclosporine in myasthenia gravis. *Ann N Y Acad Sci* 1993; **681:** 539–51.
2. Schalke BCG, *et al.* Ciclosporin A vs azathioprine in the treatment of myasthenia gravis: final results of a randomized, controlled double-blind clinical trial. *Neurology* 1988; **38** (suppl 1): 135.

Ocular disorders, non-malignant. For reference to the value of cyclosporin in the management of scleritis see p.1029, while for its use in uveitis see p.1030.

Organ and tissue transplantation. Cyclosporin has greatly improved the prospects for successful organ and tissue transplantation, and is a mainstay of regimens used to prevent rejection of solid organ grafts as well as being used for the prevention of graft-versus-host disease in bone marrow transplantation. For more detailed discussion of organ and tissue transplantation and the role of cyclosporin, see p.498.

Psoriatic arthritis. Cyclosporin is used in the management of severe refractory psoriasis (see below). One study[1] has shown that low-dose cyclosporin effectively improves not only skin lesions, but also joint complaints in psoriatic arthritis (see under Spondyloarthropathies, p.4).

1. Mahrle G, *et al.* Anti-inflammatory efficacy of low-dose cyclosporin A in psoriatic arthritis. A prospective multicentre study. *Br J Dermatol* 1996; **135:** 752–7.

Rheumatoid arthritis. Various antirheumatic drugs are used in rheumatoid arthritis (p.2) in an attempt to modify the disease process. Cyclosporin has produced responses in active disease,[1-4] and there is some evidence that it can slow radiological progression of disease[4] as well as providing symptomatic relief. There has been some concern about associated nephrotoxicity,[1] but the use of low-dose regimens may help to minimise this. Cyclosporin has also been combined with other disease-modifying antirheumatic drugs, and a combination of cyclosporin with methotrexate has reportedly produced responses in patients unresponsive to methotrexate alone.[5] International consensus recommendations exist for the use of cyclosporin in rheumatoid arthritis.[6] These suggest that the use of cyclosporin may be considered in patients who are candidates for disease-modifying antirheumatic drugs and who do not have risk factors such as malignancy, uncontrolled hypertension, renal dysfunction, cytopenias, or marked disorder of liver function. They recommend a starting dose of between 2.5 and 3.0 mg per kg body-weight daily, increased if necessary after 4 to 8 weeks, in increments of 0.5 or 1 mg per kg at 1 to 2 month intervals, up to a maximum of 5 mg per kg daily, particular care being taken at doses over 4 mg per kg daily. Once the patient's disease has been stable for at least 3 months the daily dose should be decreased monthly or bimonthly in increments of 0.5 mg per kg to the lowest effective dose. If it is only partially effective after 3 months at the maximum tolerable dose another medication should be considered instead or in addition; if there is no response to the maximum tolerable dose after 3 months, cyclosporin should be discontinued. Patients should be carefully monitored before and during therapy.

1. Yocum DE, *et al.* Cyclosporin A in severe, treatment-refractory rheumatoid arthritis: a randomized study. *Ann Intern Med* 1988; **109:** 863–9.
2. Tugwell P, *et al.* Low-dose cyclosporin versus placebo in patients with rheumatoid arthritis. *Lancet* 1990; **335:** 1051–5.
3. Landewé RBM, *et al.* A randomized, double-blind, 24-week controlled study of low-dose cyclosporine versus chloroquine for early rheumatoid arthritis. *Arthritis Rheum* 1994; **37:** 637–43.
4. Førre Ø, *et al.* Radiologic evidence of disease modification in rheumatoid arthritis patients treated with cyclosporine: results of a 48-week multicenter study comparing low-dose cyclosporine with placebo. *Arthritis Rheum* 1994; **37:** 1506–12.
5. Tugwell P, *et al.* Combination therapy with cyclosporine and methotrexate in severe rheumatoid arthritis. *N Engl J Med* 1995; **333:** 137–41.
6. Panayi GS, Tugwell P. The use of cyclosporin A microemulsion in rheumatoid arthritis: conclusions of an international review. *Br J Rheumatol* 1997; **36:** 808–11.

Sarcoidosis. Corticosteroids are the usual therapy for symptomatic sarcoidosis (p.1028), and other agents are very much second-line; cyclosporin is one of a number of immunosuppressants that have been tried with variable results.

Skin disorders, non-malignant. Cyclosporin has been tried in a variety of skin disorders. It is effective in atopic eczema (atopic dermatitis),[1-3] where it is employed as adjunctive therapy (see p.1073 for further discussion of eczema and its management). It is generally reserved for short-term treatment (up to 8 weeks) in patients with severe disease unresponsive to all conventional therapies, although reports have described long-term use in adult patients.[4-6] Short-term treatment with cyclosporin has been reported in children.[7,8] Responses have also been reported in severe eczematisation associated with Darier's disease[9] (p.1073) and in nodular prurigo.[10] Although pemphigus is usually treated with corticosteroids (see p.1075), cyclosporin has also been tried in a few patients with pemphigus vulgaris.[11] Rather better established is the use of cyclosporin to induce remission or prevent relapse in severe refractory psoriasis[12,13] (p.1075). Cyclosporin appears to improve the joint symptoms of psoriatic arthritis (see above) as well as skin symptoms.[14] There have also been reports of responses to cyclosporin in patients with pustular folliculitis[15] and pyoderma gangrenosum[16,17] (p.1076). There are also a few reports of responses to cyclosporin in patients with scleroderma, although as discussed on p.501 the use of immunosuppressants remains experimental in this condition. For reference to the use of cyclosporin in lichen planus, see above.

1. van Joost T, *et al.* Cyclosporin in atopic dermatitis: a multicentre placebo-controlled study. *Br J Dermatol* 1994; **130:** 634–40.
2. Munro CS, *et al.* Maintenance treatment with cyclosporin in atopic eczema. *Br J Dermatol* 1994; **130:** 376–80.
3. Granlund H, *et al.* Cyclosporin in atopic dermatitis: time to relapse and effect of intermittent therapy. *Br J Dermatol* 1995; **132:** 106–12.
4. Sepp N, Fritsch PO. Can cyclosporin A induce permanent remission of atopic dermatitis? *Br J Dermatol* 1993; **128:** 213–16.
5. Pryce DW, *et al.* Safety and efficacy of longer-term lower-dose cyclosporin A therapy. *Br J Dermatol* 1994; **130:** 681–9.
6. Berth-Jones J, *et al.* Long-term efficacy and safety of cyclosporin in severe adult atopic dermatitis. *Br J Dermatol* 1996; **135** (suppl 47): 26.
7. Zaki I, *et al.* Treatment of severe atopic dermatitis in childhood with cyclosporin. *Br J Dermatol* 1996; **135** (suppl 48): 21–4.
8. Berth-Jones J, *et al.* Cyclosporine in severe childhood atopic dermatitis: a multicenter study. *J Am Acad Dermatol* 1996; **34:** 1016–21.
9. Shahidullah H, *et al.* Darier's disease: severe eczematization successfully treated with cyclosporin. *Br J Dermatol* 1994; **131:** 713–16.
10. Berth-Jones J, *et al.* Nodular prurigo responds to cyclosporin. *Br J Dermatol* 1995; **132:** 795–9.
11. Luisi AF, Stoukides CA. Cyclosporine for the treatment of pemphigus vulgaris. *Ann Pharmacother* 1994; **28:** 1183–5.
12. Ellis CN, *et al.* Cyclosporine improves psoriasis in a double-blind study. *JAMA* 1986; **256:** 3110–16.
13. Laburte C, *et al.* Efficacy and safety of oral cyclosporin A (CyA; Sandimmun) for long-term treatment of chronic severe plaque psoriasis. *Br J Dermatol* 1994; **130:** 366–75.
14. Mahrle G, *et al.* Anti-inflammatory efficacy of low-dose cyclosporin A in psoriatic arthritis: a prospective multicentre study. *Br J Dermatol* 1996; **135:** 752–7.
15. Taniguchi S, *et al.* Eosinophilic pustular folliculitis responding to cyclosporin. *Br J Dermatol* 1994; **131:** 736–7.
16. Schmitt EC, *et al.* Pyoderma gangrenosum treated with low-dose cyclosporin. *Br J Dermatol* 1993; **128:** 230–1.
17. Ruzicka T. Cyclosporin in less common immune-mediated skin diseases. *Br J Dermatol* 1996; **135** (suppl 48): 40–2.

Preparations

USP 23: Cyclosporine Capsules; Cyclosporine Injection; Cyclosporine Oral Solution.

Proprietary Preparations (details are given in Part 3)
Aust.: Sandimmun; ***Austral.:*** Neoral; Sandimmun; ***Belg.:*** Neoral-Sandimmun; Sandimmun†; ***Canad.:*** Sandimmune; ***Fr.:*** Neoral; Sandimmun; ***Ger.:*** Sandimmun; ***Irl.:*** Neoral; Sandimmun; ***Ital.:*** Sandimmun; ***Neth.:*** Neoral; Sandimmune; ***Norw.:*** Sandimmun; ***S.Afr.:*** Sandimmun; ***Spain:*** Sandimmun; ***Swed.:*** Sandimmun; ***Switz.:*** Sandimmun; ***UK:*** Neoral; Sandimmun; ***USA:*** Neoral; Sandimmune.

Cytarabine (1826-a)

Cytarabine *(BAN, USAN, rINN).*

Arabinosylcytosine; Ara-C; Cytarabinum; Cytosine Arabinoside; NSC-63878 (cytarabine hydrochloride); U-19920; U-19920A (cytarabine hydrochloride); WR-28453. 1-β-D-Arabinofuranosylcytosine; 4-Amino-1-β-D-arabinofuranosylpyrimidin-2(1*H*)-one.

$C_9H_{13}N_3O_5$ = 243.2.

CAS — 147-94-4 (cytarabine); 69-74-9 (cytarabine hydrochloride).

Pharmacopoeias. In *Eur.* (see p.viii), *Int.*, *Jpn*, and *US.*
Chin. includes the hydrochloride.

An odourless white to off-white crystalline powder. Freely **soluble** in water; slightly soluble or very slightly soluble in alcohol; slightly soluble in chloroform; very slightly soluble in dichloromethane. A 1% solution in water has a pH of 4 to 6. **Store** in airtight containers. Protect from light.

Incompatibility. Although cytarabine has been stated in the literature to be incompatible with solutions of fluorouracil[1,2] and methotrexate[1] some studies have reported it to be stable for some hours when mixed with the latter.[3]

1. D'Arcy PF. Reactions and interactions in handling anticancer drugs. *Drug Intell Clin Pharm* 1983; **17:** 532–8.
2. McRae MP, King JC. Compatibility of antineoplastic, antibiotic and corticosteroid drugs in intravenous admixtures. *Am J Hosp Pharm* 1976; **33:** 1010–13.
3. Cheung Y-W, *et al.* Stability of cytarabine, methotrexate sodium, and hydrocortisone sodium succinate admixtures. *Am J Hosp Pharm* 1984; **41:** 1802–6.

Adverse Effects, Treatment, and Precautions

For general discussions see Antineoplastics, p.470, p.473, and p.474.

The major adverse effect of cytarabine is bone-marrow depression, manifest as leucopenia, particularly granulocytopenia, thrombocytopenia, and anaemia, sometimes with striking megaloblastic changes. Myelosuppression appears to be more evident after high doses and continuous infusions. Granulocytopenia is biphasic, with a nadir at 7 to 9 days after a dose and another, more severe, at 15 to 24 days. The nadir of the platelet count occurs at about 12 to 15 days. Recovery generally occurs in a further ten days.

Gastro-intestinal disturbances may occur: nausea and vomiting may be more severe when doses are given rapidly (but other adverse effects are reported to be worse when the drug is given by infusion). Other adverse effects reported include hepatic dysfunction, renal dysfunction, neurotoxicity (particularly via the intrathecal route), rashes, oral and anal ulceration, gastro-intestinal haemorrhage, oesophagitis, and conjunctivitis. A syndrome of bone and muscle pain, fever, malaise, conjunctivitis, and rash, sometimes described as 'flu-like', has been reported, which may be treated with corticosteroid therapy if severe. Anaphylactoid reactions have occurred rarely. There may be local pain, cellulitis, and thrombophlebitis at the site of injection.

High-dose therapy has been associated with particularly severe gastro-intestinal and central nervous system effects, including severe ulceration of the gastro-intestinal tract, pneumatosis cystoides leading to peritonitis, necrotising colitis and bowel necrosis, peripheral neuropathy, and cerebral and cerebellar dysfunction, with personality changes, somnolence, and coma. There may also be corneal toxicity leading to punctate keratitis and haemorrhagic conjunctivitis, sepsis, liver abscess, severe skin rash leading to desquamation, alopecia, and cardiac disorders including pericarditis and fatal cardiomyopathy. Pulmonary oedema, sometimes fatal, has occurred.

Cytarabine is teratogenic in *animals* (but see Pregnancy, below).

It should be given with care to patients with impaired liver function; dosage reduction may be necessary. In addition to blood counts, blood-uric acid should be monitored because of the risk of hyperuricaemia, and renal and hepatic function should be periodically assessed.

A detailed review of the toxicity of cytarabine.[1] The principal toxicity of standard dosage regimens is myelosuppression but bleeding complications and gastro-intestinal toxicity are also major problems at standard doses. With the high-dose regimens neurological toxicity may be dose-limiting: severe and sometimes irreversible symptoms have been seen in some 6 to 10% of patients receiving a cumulative dose of 36 g per square metre body-surface. Ocular toxicity may occur in up to 80% of patients at the highest doses. Since cytarabine toxicity is largely dose-related low-dose cytarabine is generally well tolerated, even in elderly patients, who are more susceptible: its only significant toxicity is myelosuppression.

1. Stentoft J. The toxicity of cytarabine. *Drug Safety* 1990; **5:** 7–27.

Effects on the nervous system. Although paraplegia has been reported with intrathecal cytarabine[1] (see also under Benzyl Alcohol, p.1103) and peripheral neuropathy has occurred in a patient who had received only conventional intravenous doses,[2] the majority of cases of neurotoxicity associated with cytarabine appear to be in patients given high-dose regimens.[3-7] Although some cases have manifested as demyelinating peripheral neuropathy,[3,4] including a syndrome of painful legs and involuntary movements in the toes which showed some response to carbamazepine,[3] most studies have reported in particular a syndrome of cerebellar toxicity,[5-8] with symptoms such as dysarthria, nystagmus, and ataxia. Toxicity appears to be dose-related: Lazarus and colleagues reported CNS toxicity in 4 of 43 patients given total doses of up to 48 g per m^2 body-surface of cytarabine, none of which were life-threatening or irreversible, whereas 4 of 6 given 54 g per m^2 (as 4.5 g per m^2 every 12 hours for 12 doses) developed neurotoxicity, which was fatal in one and irreversible in another.[5] However, there is some evidence that patients aged over 50,[6] and those who have recently received conventional-dose cytarabine[7] may be at increased risk, and persistent, severe cerebellar toxicity has also been reported in a patient with neither of these risk factors who had received a total dose of only 36 g per m^2 (as 3 g per m^2 every 12 hours).

1. Saleh MN, *et al.* Intrathecal cytosine arabinoside-induced acute, rapidly reversible paralysis. *Am J Med* 1989; **86:** 729–30.
2. Russell JA, Powles RL. Neuropathy due to cytosine arabinoside. *Br Med J* 1974; **4:** 652–3.
3. Malapert D, Degos JD. Jambes douloureuses et orteils instables: neuropathie induite par la cytarabine. *Rev Neurol* 1989; **145:** 869–71.
4. Nevill TJ, *et al.* Horner's syndrome and demyelinating peripheral neuropathy caused by high-dose cytosine arabinoside. *Am J Hematol* 1989; **32:** 314–15.
5. Lazarus HM, *et al.* Central nervous system toxicity of high-dose systemic cytosine arabinoside. *Cancer* 1981; **48:** 2577–82.
6. Graves T, Hooks MA. Drug-induced toxicities associated with high-dose cytosine arabinoside infusions. *Pharmacotherapy* 1989; **9:** 23–8.
7. Barnett MJ, *et al.* Neurotoxicity of high-dose cytosine arabinoside. *Prog Exp Tumor Res* 1985; **29:** 177–82.
8. Dworkin LA, *et al.* Cerebellar toxicity following high-dose cytosine arabinoside. *J Clin Oncol* 1985; **3:** 613–16.

Effects on the skin. A syndrome of pain and erythema of the palms and soles, progressing to bullae and desquamation, has been seen in patients receiving intermediate- or high-dose cytarabine.[1,2] The syndrome is similar to the palmar-plantar syndrome reported in patients receiving chemotherapy not including cytarabine,[3] although some considered the two forms of toxicity distinct.[4] Cutaneous small vessel necrotising vasculitis has been reported after high-dose therapy with cytarabine.[5]

1. Baer MR, *et al.* Palmar-plantar erythrodysesthesia and cytarabine. *Ann Intern Med* 1985; **102:** 556.
2. Peters WG, Willernze R. Palmar-plantar skin changes and cytarabine. *Ann Intern Med* 1985; **103:** 805.
3. Lokich JJ, Moore C. Chemotherapy-associated palmar-plantar erythrodysesthesia syndrome. *Ann Intern Med* 1984; **101:** 798–800.
4. Vogelzang NJ, Ratain MJ. Cancer chemotherapy and skin changes. *Ann Intern Med* 1985; **103:** 303–4.
5. Ahmed I, *et al.* Cytosine arabinoside-induced vasculitis. *Mayo Clin Proc* 1998; **73:** 239–42.

Pregnancy. Although there has been a report of limb and ear deformities in the infant of a woman given cytarabine at the estimated time of conception and at an estimated 4 to 8 weeks after conception,[1] no congenital abnormalities were noted in 17 infants, 5 therapeutic abortions, and one still-birth (following pre-eclamptic toxaemia) resulting from over 20 known cases in which cytarabine was administered during pregnancy.[2]

1. Wagner VM, *et al.* Congenital abnormalities in baby born to cytarabine treated mother. *Lancet* 1980; **ii:** 98–9.
2. Morgenstern G. Cytarabine in pregnancy. *Lancet* 1980; **ii:** 259.

Interactions

Antifungals. Cytarabine has been reported to inhibit the action of flucytosine—see p.379.

Antineoplastics. Acute pancreatitis has been reported in patients given cytarabine who had previously received asparaginase therapy.[1] Subclinical damage to the pancreas by asparaginase may have rendered it susceptible to cytarabine.

For a report of hepatic dysfunction associated with the combined use of cytarabine and daunorubicin see under Daunorubicin Hydrochloride, p.528.

Administration of cytarabine after fludarabine is reported to result in a 5-fold increase in intracellular cytarabine concentrations in leukaemic cells,[2] producing improved clinical response rates.

1. Altman AJ, *et al.* Acute pancreatitis in association with cytosine arabinoside therapy. *Cancer* 1982; **49:** 1384–6.
2. Avramis VI, *et al.* Pharmacokinetic and pharmacodynamic studies of fludarabine and cytosine arabinoside administered as loading boluses followed by continuous infusions after a phase I/II study in pediatric patients with relapsed leukemias. *Clin Cancer Res* 1998; **4:** 45–52.

Pharmacokinetics

Cytarabine is not effective by mouth due to rapid deamination in the gastro-intestinal tract; less than 20% of an oral dose is absorbed. After intravenous injection it disappears rapidly from the plasma with an initial half-life of about 10 minutes; the terminal elimination half-life ranges from 1 to 3 hours. It is converted by phosphorylation to an active form which is rapidly deaminated, mainly in the liver and the kidneys, to inactive 1-β-D-arabinofuranosyluracil (uracil arabinoside, ara-U). The majority of an intravenous dose is excreted in the urine within 24 hours, mostly as the inactive metabolite with about 10% as unchanged cytarabine.

There is only moderate diffusion of cytarabine across the blood-brain barrier following intravenous injection, but, because of low deaminase activity in the cerebrospinal fluid, concentrations achieved after continuous intravenous infusion or intrathecal injection are maintained for longer in the CSF than are those in plasma. Cytarabine also crosses the placenta.

References.

1. Ho DHW, Frei E. Clinical pharmacology of 1-β-D-arabinofuranosyl cytosine. *Clin Pharmacol Ther* 1971; **12:** 944–54.
2. van Prooijen R, *et al.* Pharmacokinetics of cytosine arabinoside in acute myeloid leukemia. *Clin Pharmacol Ther* 1977; **21:** 744–50.
3. Harris AL, *et al.* Pharmacokinetics of cytosine arabinoside in patients with acute myeloid leukaemia. *Br J Clin Pharmacol* 1979; **8:** 219–27.
4. Slevin ML, *et al.* The pharmacokinetics of subcutaneous cytosine arabinoside in patients with acute myelogenous leukaemia. *Br J Clin Pharmacol* 1981; **12:** 507–10.

Uses and Administration

Cytarabine, a pyrimidine nucleoside analogue, is an antimetabolite antineoplastic which inhibits the synthesis of deoxyribonucleic acid. Its actions are specific for the S phase of the cell cycle. It also has antiviral and immunosuppressant properties.

Cytarabine is used mainly in the treatment of acute leukaemia, especially acute non-lymphoblastic leukaemia when it is often given in association with thioguanine and an anthracycline such as doxorubicin or daunorubicin. It has also been given in the blast crisis of chronic myeloid leukaemia, and in the treatment of lymphoma, and has been tried in the management of myelodysplasia. Cross-references to these uses may be found below.

Cytarabine is given by the intravenous route. Higher doses can be tolerated when given by rapid injection rather than slow infusion, because of the rapid clearance of cytarabine, but there is little evidence of clinical advantage for either route.

For the induction of remission in adults and children with acute leukaemias a wide variety of dosage regimens have been used: 100 mg per m^2 body-surface twice daily by rapid intravenous injection, or 100 mg per m^2 daily by continuous intravenous infusion, have often been employed. These doses are generally given for 5 to 10 days, depending on therapeutic response and toxicity. Children reportedly tolerate high doses better than adults.

For maintenance 75 to 100 mg per m^2, or 1 to 1.5 mg per kg or more may be given intravenously, intramuscularly, or subcutaneously once or twice weekly; other regimens have been used.

In the treatment of refractory disease high-dose regimens have been employed, with cytarabine given in doses of up to 3 g per m^2 every 12 hours for up to 6 days. These doses should be given by intravenous infusion over at least 1 hour.

In leukaemic meningitis cytarabine has been given intrathecally, often in a dose of 10 to 30 mg per m^2 body-surface every 2 to 4 days; it has also been used prophylactically. A depot formulation of cytarabine has also been investigated in meningeal metastasis.

White cell and platelet counts should be determined regularly during treatment with cytarabine and therapy should be stopped immediately if the count falls rapidly or to low values.

Administration. LOW-DOSE THERAPY. Because of suggestions that low doses of cytarabine might induce differentiation and maturation of leukaemic cells, low-dose therapy (usually 10 mg per square metre body-surface twice daily) has been tried in patients with acute lymphoblastic[1-3] and non-lymphoblastic leukaemia,[3-5] and in the myelodysplastic syndromes.[3,6,7] Although complete remission may occur in about 16% of patients with myelodysplastic syndromes a similar proportion succumb to treatment-related mortality,[3] and remissions do not appear to be particularly long-lasting. Cytopenia may be marked even at these doses,[8] which has prompted trials of very low doses (3 to 5 mg per square metre twice daily),[2,9-11] but even these may be associated with bone-marrow suppression.[9,10] There is also some controversy about the supposed method of action,[4,11,12] and some workers consider that the effects of low-dose cytarabine *in vivo* are due not to a differentiating but a cytotoxic action.[3,4]

1. Onundarson PT, Rowe JM. Low-dose cytosine arabinoside as remission induction therapy in refractory adult acute lymphocytic leukemia. *Am J Med* 1989; **86:** 493–4.
2. Amara F, Colonna P. Low-dose cytosine arabinoside in relapsed acute lymphocytic leukemia. *Am J Med* 1990; **88:** 82–3.
3. Cheson BD, *et al.* A critical appraisal of low-dose cytosine arabinoside in patients with acute non-lymphocytic leukemia and myelodysplastic syndromes. *J Clin Oncol* 1986; **4:** 1857–64.
4. Manoharan A, *et al.* Low-dose cytarabine in acute myeloid leukaemia. *Med J Aust* 1984; **141:** 643–6.
5. Harousseau JL, *et al.* Treatment of acute non-lymphoblastic leukaemia in elderly patients. *Lancet* 1984; **ii:** 288.
6. Wisch JS, *et al.* Response of preleukemic syndromes to continuous infusion of low-dose cytarabine. *N Engl J Med* 1983; **309:** 1599–1602.
7. Miller KB, *et al.* Evaluation of low dose ARAC-C versus supportive care in the treatment of myelodysplastic syndromes: an intergroup study by the Eastern Cooperative Oncology Group and the Southwest Oncology Group. *Blood* 1988; **72** (suppl 1): 215.
8. Mufti GJ, *et al.* Low doses of cytarabine in the treatment of myelodysplastic syndrome and acute myeloid leukemia. *N Engl J Med* 1983; **309:** 1653–4.
9. Worsley A, *et al.* Very-low-dose cytarabine for myelodysplastic syndromes and acute myeloid leukaemia in the elderly. *Lancet* 1986; **i:** 966.
10. Pesce A, *et al.* Very-low-dose cytarabine for elderly patients. *Lancet* 1986; **i:** 1436.
11. Poirier O, *et al.* Pharmacokinetic data on very-low-dose cytarabine. *Lancet* 1986; **i:** 1436–7.
12. Tilly H, *et al.* Low-dose cytarabine: persistence of a clonal abnormality during complete remission of acute nonlymphocytic leukemia. *N Engl J Med* 1986; **314:** 246–7.

Leucoencephalopathy. There are anecdotal reports[1-3] of marked improvement in patients with progressive multifocal leucoencephalopathy secondary to AIDS or chemotherapy-induced immunosuppression following intravenous or intrathecal cytarabine. However, a randomised multicentre study has indicated that cytarabine was ineffective and has no role in this condition.[4]

1. O'Riordan T, *et al.* Progressive multifocal leukoencephalopathy-remission with cytarabine. *J Infect* 1990; **20:** 51–4.
2. Portegies P, *et al.* Response to cytarabine in progressive multifocal leucoencephalopathy in AIDS. *Lancet* 1991; **337:** 680–1.
3. Nicoli F, *et al.* Efficacy of cytarabine in progressive multifocal leucoencephalopathy in AIDS. *Lancet* 1992; **339:** 306.
4. Hall CD, *et al.* Failure of cytarabine in progressive multifocal leukoencephalopathy associated with human immunodeficiency virus infection. *N Engl J Med* 1998; **338:** 1345–51.

Malignant neoplasms. Cytarabine plays an important role in the treatment of the haematological malignancies. It is one of the mainstays of the treatment of acute non-lymphoblastic leukaemias, together with an anthracycline and thioguanine, (see p.479), and is used for the prophylaxis of meningeal leukaemia, as well as in regimens for consolidation, in patients with acute lymphoblastic leukaemia (p.478). It has also been investigated in chronic myeloid leukaemia and the myelodysplasias (see p.480 and p.481) as a potential differentiation-inducing agent (see also Administration, above). The other main group of diseases in which it has been employed are the lymphomas: for CNS prophylaxis in Burkitt's lymphoma and in salvage regimens for Hodgkin's disease (see p.483 and p.481), and as part of the complex regimens sometimes employed in intermediate- and high-grade non-Hodgkin's lymphomas (p.482), including those associated with AIDS (p.483).

Preparations

BP 1998: Cytarabine Injection;
USP 23: Cytarabine for Injection.

Proprietary Preparations (details are given in Part 3)
Aust.: Alexan; Cytosar; ***Austral.:*** Alexan†; Cytosar-U; ***Belg.:*** Cytosar; ***Canad.:*** Cytosar; ***Fr.:*** Aracytine; Cytarbel; ***Ger.:*** Alexan; ARA-cell; Udicil; ***Irl.:*** Cytosar; ***Ital.:*** Alexan†; Aracytin; Erpalfa; ***Jpn:*** Starasid; ***Neth.:*** Alexan†; Cytosar; ***Norw.:*** Cytosar; ***S.Afr.:*** Alexan; Cytosar; ***Swed.:*** Alexan; Arabine; Cytosar; ***Switz.:*** Alexan; Cytosar; ***UK:*** Alexan†; Cytosar; ***USA:*** Cytosar-U.

Dacarbazine (1827-t)

Dacarbazine *(BAN, USAN, rINN).*

DIC; DTIC; Imidazole Carboxamide; NSC-45388; WR-139007. 5-(3,3-Dimethyltriazeno)imidazole-4-carboxamide.

$C_6H_{10}N_6O$ = 182.2.

CAS — 4342-03-4.

Pharmacopoeias. In *Br.* and *US.*

A colourless or pale-yellow crystalline powder. Slightly **soluble** in water and in alcohol. **Store** in airtight containers at 2° to 8°. Protect from light.

CAUTION. *Dacarbazine is irritant; avoid contact with skin and mucous membranes.*

Incompatibility. Dacarbazine has been reported to be incompatible with hydrocortisone sodium succinate but not with the sodium phosphate.[1] It has been reported to be incompatible with heparin,[2] although only with concentrated dacarbazine solutions (25 mg per mL).

1. Dorr RT. Incompatibilities with parenteral anticancer drugs. *Am J Intravenous Ther* 1979; **6:** 42–52.
2. Nelson RW, *et al.* Visual incompatibility of dacarbazine and heparin. *Am J Hosp Pharm* 1987; **44:** 2028.

Stability. References to the photodegradation of dacarbazine solution.[1-3] Dacarbazine is more sensitive to direct sunlight than to artificial lighting or diffuse daylight.

1. Stevens MFG, Peatey L. Photodegradation of solutions of the antitumour drug DTIC. *J Pharm Pharmacol* 1978; **30** (suppl): 47P.
2. Horton JK, Stevens MFG. Search for drug interactions between the antitumour agent DTIC and other cytotoxic agents. *J Pharm Pharmacol* 1979; **31** (suppl): 64P.
3. Kirk B. The evaluation of a light-protecting giving set. *Intensive Therapy Clin Monit* 1987; **8:** 78–86.

Storage. The manufacturers state that following reconstitution of dacarbazine as a solution for injection the solution may be further diluted with glucose (5%) or sodium chloride (0.9%) injections, and the resulting solution may be stored at 4° for up to 24 hours. The undiluted reconstituted solution may be stored at 4° for 72 hours or at normal room temperature for up to 8 hours if suitably protected from light.

Adverse Effects, Treatment, and Precautions

For general discussions see Antineoplastics, p.470, p.473, and p.474.

Leucopenia and thrombocytopenia with dacarbazine, although usually moderate, may be severe. The nadir of the white-cell count usually occurs 21 to 25 days after a dose. Anorexia, nausea, and vomiting occur in more than 90% of patients initially but tolerance may develop after repeated doses. Other side-effects include rare but potentially fatal hepatotoxicity, skin reactions, alopecia, an influenza-like syndrome, and facial flushing and paraesthesia. There may be local pain at the injection site; extravasation produces pain and tissue damage. Anaphylaxis has occurred occasionally.

Effects on the liver. Based on experience in more than 100 patients it was reported in 1982 that the spectrum of adverse hepatic effects with dacarbazine was broader than previously documented cases of vasculitis leading to acute hepatic failure and death had suggested.[1] Necrosis may be associated with venous thrombosis or occur without signs of inflammation; granulomatous hepatitis has occurred, as has a case of acute toxic hepatitis during the first course of dacarbazine. Morphological studies suggested that dacarbazine may exert a toxic effect on the microfilamentous cytoskeleton of the hepatocytes.

1. Dancygier H, *et al.* Dacarbazine (DTIC)-induced human liver injury. *Gut* 1982; **23:** A447.

Interactions

For the effect of dacarbazine on levodopa see p.1139.

Pharmacokinetics

Dacarbazine is poorly absorbed from the gastro-intestinal tract. Following intravenous injection it is rapidly distributed with an initial plasma half-life of about 20 minutes; the terminal half-life is reported to be about 5 hours. The volume of distribution is larger than body water content, suggesting localisation in some body tissues, probably mainly the liver. Only about 5% is bound to plasma protein. It crosses the blood-brain barrier to a limited extent with concentrations in cerebrospinal fluid about 14% of those in plasma. Dacarbazine is extensively metabolised in the liver; the major metabolite appears to be 5-aminoimidazole-4-carboxamide (AIC). About half of a dose is excreted unchanged in the urine by tubular secretion.

Uses and Administration

Dacarbazine is a cell-cycle nonspecific antineoplastic which may function as an alkylating agent after it has been activated in the liver. Dacarbazine is used mainly in the treatment of metastatic malignant melanoma (p.492). It is also given to patients with Hodgkin's disease (p.481), notably in association with doxorubicin, bleomycin, and vinblastine (ABVD), and has been given in neuroblastoma (p.494), and in the treatment of soft-tissue sarcomas and other tumours.

It is given intravenously in doses of 2 to 4.5 mg per kg body-weight daily for 10 days, repeated at intervals of 4 weeks, or 250 mg per m^2 body-surface daily for 5 days, repeated at intervals of 3 weeks. For melanoma it can also be given in a dose of 850 mg per m^2 by intravenous infusion at 3-week intervals. In the treatment of Hodgkin's disease doses of 150 mg per m^2 daily for 5 days repeated every 4 weeks, or 375 mg per m^2 every 15 days have been given in association with other agents. Injections may be given over one to two minutes. In an attempt to prevent pain along the injected vein the reconstituted solution has been further diluted with up to 500 mL of glucose 5% or sodium chloride 0.9% and given by infusion over 15 to 30 minutes.

Preparations

BP 1998: Dacarbazine Injection;
USP 23: Dacarbazine for Injection.

Proprietary Preparations (details are given in Part 3)
Aust.: DTIC-Dome; ***Belg.:*** DTIC-Dome; ***Canad.:*** DTIC; ***Fr.:*** Deticene; ***Ger.:*** Deticene†; Detimedac; DTIC; ***Irl.:*** DTIC-Dome; ***Ital.:*** Deticene; ***Neth.:*** Deticene; ***S.Afr.:*** DTIC-Dome; ***Spain:*** DTIC-Dome; ***Swed.:*** DTIC; ***Switz.:*** DTIC; ***UK:*** DTIC-Dome; ***USA:*** DTIC-Dome.

Daclizumab (17621-d)

Dacliximab; Ro-24-7375.

CAS — 152923-56-3.

Daclizumab is a humanised monoclonal murine anti-interleukin-2-receptor antibody. It is used in the prevention of acute graft rejection following kidney transplantation (p.499). It is given in a dose of 1 mg per kg body-weight, at intervals of 2 weeks, for 5 doses, in combination with other immunosuppressants. Daclizumab is also under investigation for its immunosuppressant properties in other forms of transplantation and in various diseases with an autoimmune component.

Preparations

Proprietary Preparations (details are given in Part 3)
USA: Zenapax.

Dactinomycin (1802-w)

Dactinomycin *(BAN, USAN, rINN).*

Actinomycin C_1; Actinomycin D; Meractinomycin; NSC-3053.

$N^{2.1}$,$N^{2'.1'}$-(2-Amino-4,6-dimethyl-3-oxo-3*H*-phenoxazine-1,9-diyldicarbonyl)bis[threonyl-D-valylprolyl(*N*-methylglycyl)(*N*-methylvaline) 1.5–3.1-lactone].

$C_{62}H_{86}N_{12}O_{16}$ = 1255.4.

CAS — 50-76-0.

Pharmacopoeias. In *Chin., Int., Jpn, Pol.,* and *US.*

An antineoplastic antibiotic produced by the growth of *Streptomyces chrysomallus* and other species of *Streptomyces.* It is a bright red, somewhat hygroscopic, crystalline powder. It has a potency of not less than 950 and not more than 1030 μg per mg, calculated on the dried basis.

Soluble in water at 10°, slightly soluble in water at 37°, freely soluble in alcohol; very slightly soluble in ether. **Store** at a temperature not exceeding 40° in airtight containers. Protect from light.

Actinomycin C (cactinomycin; HBF-386; NSC-18268) is a mixture of dactinomycin (actinomycin D) (10%), actinomycin C_2 (45%), and actinomycin C_3 (45%).

CAUTION. *Dactinomycin is irritant; avoid contact with skin and mucous membranes.*

Dactinomycin binds to cellulose ester filters,[1] and such filtration should be avoided.[2] Although it has been suggested that significant amounts of drug may be adsorbed to glass or plastic,[3] Benvenuto and colleagues have reported that dactinomycin is compatible with glass and PVC infusion containers,[4] and administration into the tubing of a fast-running intravenous infusion is the recommended manner of administration—see Uses and Administration, below.

1. Kanke M, *et al.* Binding of selected drugs to a "treated" inline filter. *Am J Hosp Pharm* 1983; **40:** 1323–8.
2. D'Arcy PF. Reactions and interactions in handling anticancer drugs. *Drug Intell Clin Pharm* 1983; **17:** 532–8.
3. Rapp RP, *et al.* Guidelines for the administration of commonly-used intravenous drugs—1984 update. *Drug Intell Clin Pharm* 1984; **18:** 218–32.
4. Benvenuto JA, *et al.* Stability and compatibility of antitumor agents in glass and plastic containers. *Am J Hosp Pharm* 1981; **38:** 1914–18.

Adverse Effects, Treatment, and Precautions

For general discussions see Antineoplastics, p.470, p.473, and p.474.

Apart from nausea and vomiting adverse effects are often delayed, occurring days or weeks after the completion of a course of treatment. Fatalities have occurred. Bone-marrow depression and gastro-intestinal effects (including nausea and vomiting) may prove dose-limiting. Bone-marrow depression is apparent 1 to 7 days after therapy and may be manifest first as thrombocytopenia; the nadir of the platelet and white-cell counts usually occurs within 14 to 21 days, with recovery in 21 to 25 days. Other adverse effects include oral and gastro-intestinal effects such as stomatitis, diarrhoea, and proctitis; fever, malaise, hypocalcaemia, erythema, myalgia, alopecia, and kidney and liver abnormalities. Anaphylactoid reactions have occurred. Dactinomycin is very irritant and extravasation results in severe tissue damage.

The effects of radiotherapy are enhanced by dactinomycin and severe reactions may follow the concomitant use of high doses. Erythema and pigmentation of the skin may occur in areas previously irradiated.

Dactinomycin should not be given to patients with varicella, as severe and even fatal systemic disease may occur. Its use is best avoided in infants under 1 year who are reported to be highly susceptible to the toxicity of dactinomycin.

Effects on the liver. Although doses below about 50 μg per kg body-weight or 1.5 mg per m^2 body-surface area do not seem to be associated with an unacceptable degree of hepatotoxicity,[1] administration of dactinomycin as a single dose of 60 μg per kg (about 1.8 mg per m^2) every 3 weeks to children with Wilms' tumour has been associated with a high incidence of severe hepatotoxicity;[2] reduction of this dose to 45 μg per kg every 3 weeks reduced the incidence of hepatotoxicity to one similar to that seen with a standard regimen of 15 μg per kg daily for 5 successive days.[3] Other workers have not seen such a high incidence of hepatotoxicity with doses of 60 μg per kg (despite some raised liver enzyme values), but in this case the high dose was given only every 6 weeks.[4] In general, it is recommended that dactinomycin be given with caution to children with a history of antecedent liver damage, including abdominal irradiation or recent halothane anaesthesia.[1]

1. Pritchard J, *et al.* Hepatotoxicity of actinomycin-D. *Lancet* 1989; **i:** 168.
2. D'Angio GJ. Hepatotoxicity with actinomycin D. *Lancet* 1987; **ii:** 104.
3. D'Angio GJ. Hepatotoxicity and actinomycin D. *Lancet* 1990; **335:** 1290.
4. de Camargo B. Hepatotoxicity and actinomycin D. *Lancet* 1990; **335:** 1290.

Pharmacokinetics

Following intravenous administration dactinomycin is rapidly distributed with high concentrations in bone marrow and nucleated cells. It undergoes only minimal metabolism and is slowly excreted in urine and bile. The terminal plasma half-life is reported to be about 36 hours. It does not cross the blood-brain barrier but is thought to cross the placenta.

Uses and Administration

Dactinomycin is a highly toxic antibiotic with antineoplastic properties. It inhibits the proliferation of cells in a cell-cycle nonspecific way by forming a stable complex with DNA and interfering with DNA-dependent RNA synthesis. It may enhance the cytotoxic effects of radiotherapy (see also Adverse Effects, above). Dactinomycin also has immunosuppressant properties.

It has been used, usually with other drugs, in the treatment of gestational trophoblastic tumours, and other solid tumours including brain tumours, Wilm's tumour, and various sarcomas. The treatment of these conditions is discussed further in the introduction to this chapter as indicated by the cross references given below.

The usual adult dose is 500 μg intravenously, daily, for a maximum of 5 days and this course may be repeated after 3 or more weeks if there are no signs of residual toxic effects. The daily dose should not exceed 15 μg per kg body-weight, or 400 to 600 μg per m^2 body-surface. Lower doses may be given where dactinomycin is combined with other antineoplastics or with radiotherapy. Localised administration using an isolation-perfusion technique has permitted the use of higher doses, 50 μg per kg being suggested for an isolated lower extremity and 35 μg per kg for an upper extremity.

The usual dose for children is 15 μg per kg daily for 5 days; alternatively, a total of 2.5 mg per m^2 of body-surface may be given over a period of 7 days.

Great care must be taken to avoid extravasation and administration should, for preference, be into the tubing of a fast-running intravenous infusion. Platelet and white cell counts should be performed daily to detect bone-marrow depression; if either count shows a marked decrease the drug should be withheld until recovery occurs.

For reference to the use of dactinomycin in various malignant neoplasms including gestational trophoblastic tumours, tumours of brain and kidney, neuroblastoma, and bone, Kaposi's, and soft-tissue sarcomas, see p.477, p.485, p.489, p.494, p.495, p.496, and p.496 respectively.

Preparations

USP 23: Dactinomycin for Injection.

Proprietary Preparations (details are given in Part 3)
Aust.: Cosmegen; ***Austral.:*** Cosmegen; ***Belg.:*** Lyovac Cosmegen; ***Canad.:*** Cosmegen; ***Ger.:*** Lyovac Cosmegen; ***Irl.:*** Cosmegen; ***Ital.:*** Cosmegen; ***Neth.:*** Lyovac Cosmegen; ***Norw.:*** Cosmegen; ***S.Afr.:*** Cosmegen; ***Swed.:*** Cosmegen; ***Switz.:*** Cosmegen; ***UK:*** Cosmegen; ***USA:*** Cosmegen.

Daunorubicin Hydrochloride

(1828-x)

Daunorubicin Hydrochloride *(BANM, USAN, rINNM).*

Cloridrato de Daunorrubicina; Daunomycin Hydrochloride; Daunorubicini Hydrochloridum; FI-6339 (daunorubicin); NDC-0082-4155; NSC-82151; RP-13057 (daunorubicin); Rubidomycin Hydrochloride. (1S,3S)-3-Acetyl-1,2,3,4,6,11-hexahydro-3,5,12-trihydroxy-10-methoxy-6,11-dioxo-naphthacen-1-yl 3-amino-2,3,6-trideoxy-α-L-*lyxo*-pyranoside hydrochloride; (8S-*cis*)-8-Acetyl-10-[(3-amino-2,3,6-trideoxy-α-L-*lyxo*-hexopyranosyl)]oxy-7,8,9,10-tetrahydro-6,8,11-trihydroxy-1-methoxy-5,12-naphthacenedione hydrochloride.

$C_{27}H_{29}NO_{10},HCl$ = 564.0.

CAS — 20830-81-3 (daunorubicin); 23541-50-6 (daunorubicin hydrochloride).

Pharmacopoeias. In Eur. (see p.viii) and US.

The hydrochloride of an antineoplastic anthracycline antibiotic produced by *Streptomyces coeruleorubidus* or *S. peucetius*. It is manufactured by methods designed to minimise or eliminate the presence of histamine. An orange-red, hygroscopic crystalline powder. The USP states that it has a potency equivalent to 842 to 1030 µg of the base per mg, whereas the Ph. Eur. requires a content of 950 to 1030 µg of the hydrochloride per mg, calculated on the anhydrous substance.

Freely **soluble** in water and in methyl alcohol; slightly soluble in alcohol; very slightly soluble in chloroform; practically insoluble in acetone. A 0.5% solution in water has a pH of 4.5 to 6.5. **Store** at a temperature not exceeding 40° in airtight containers. Protect from light.

CAUTION. *Daunorubicin hydrochloride is irritant; avoid contact with skin and mucous membranes.*

Incompatibility. Daunorubicin is incompatible with heparin sodium,[1] and Ogawa and others[2] reported that it was incompatible with aluminium, which had been used in the design of a dispensing pin intended to aid antineoplastic drug preparation. On inspection, a solution of daunorubicin hydrochloride in contact with a part-aluminium needle darkened to ruby red, and black patches appeared on the aluminium surface after 12 to 24 hours. A similar reaction occurred with a solution of doxorubicin hydrochloride.

Daunorubicin hydrochloride solution has also been reported to be incompatible with a solution of dexamethasone sodium phosphate. The manufacturer recommends that daunorubicin hydrochloride should not be administered mixed with other drugs.

Liposomal daunorubicin should not be diluted with saline solutions as aggregation of the liposomes may result.

1. D'Arcy PF. Reactions and interactions in handling anticancer drugs. *Drug Intell Clin Pharm* 1983; **17:** 532–8.
2. Ogawa GS, *et al.* Dispensing-pin problems. *Am J Hosp Pharm* 1985; **42:** 1042–5.

Stability. In a study of the stability of anthracycline antineoplastic agents in 4 infusion fluids (glucose injection (5%), sodium chloride injection (0.9%), lactated Ringer's injection, and a commercial infusion fluid) daunorubicin hydrochloride was stable in all 4, the percentage remaining after 24 hours being 98.5%, 97.4%, 94.7%, and 95.4% respectively. Stability appeared to be partly related to pH; daunorubicin was more stable as the pH of the mixture became more acidic, with the best stability in glucose injection (5%) with a pH of 4.5.[1] Although daunorubicin solutions are degraded by light, the effect is reported not to be significant at concentrations of 500 µg per mL or above; however, below this concentration precautions should be taken to protect solutions from light, and storage should be in polyethylene or polypropylene containers to minimise adsorptive losses.[2] It has been suggested that formulation with the food colouring Scarlet GN, which absorbs light over the same spectral region as daunorubicin, would stabilise daunorubicin solutions to light.[3]

1. Poochikian GK, *et al.* Stability of anthracycline antitumor agents in four infusion fluids. *Am J Hosp Pharm* 1981; **38:** 483–6.
2. Wood MJ, *et al.* Photodegradation of doxorubicin, daunorubicin and epirubicin measured by high-performance liquid chromatography. *J Clin Pharm Ther* 1990; **15:** 291–300.
3. Thoma K, Klimek R. Photostabilization of drugs in dosage forms without protection from packaging materials. *Int J Pharmaceutics* 1991; **67:** 169–75.

Adverse Effects, Treatment, and Precautions

As for Doxorubicin, p.529.

Cardiotoxicity is more likely when the total cumulative dose of daunorubicin exceeds 550 mg per m^2 body-surface in adults, or 300 mg per m^2 in children. Liposomal formulations of daunorubicin may be associated with a reduced potential for local tissue necrosis, and possibly a reduced incidence of cardiotoxicity, although current clinical experience is limited and such toxicity remains a possibility.

Transient red discoloration of the urine may occur.

Effects on the skin. A report of the development of red-brown erythematous hyperpigmentation in a patient given a 3-day course of daunorubicin;[1] the pigmentation subsequently lightened and disappeared within 6 weeks, but recurred on subsequent re-administration of the drug.

1. Kelly TM, *et al.* Hyperpigmentation with daunorubicin therapy. *Arch Dermatol* 1984; **120:** 262–3.

Handling and disposal. For a method for the destruction of daunorubicin in wastes see under Doxorubicin Hydrochloride, p.530.

Interactions

Antineoplastics. Hepatic dysfunction was reported in 13 patients who had received daunorubicin 180 to 450 mg per m^2 body-surface.[1] Eleven of the patients had also received thioguanine, cytarabine, or vincristine, or combinations of these antineoplastics. Other studies had suggested that doxorubicin might enhance the hepatotoxicity of mercaptopurine, and a similar interaction could be involved in the possible hepatotoxicity of daunorubicin, thioguanine, cytarabine, and other antineoplastics.

1. Penta JS, *et al.* Hepatotoxicity of combination chemotherapy for acute myelocytic leukemia. *Ann Intern Med* 1977; **87:** 247–8.

Pharmacokinetics

After intravenous injection, daunorubicin is rapidly distributed into body tissues, particularly the liver, lungs, kidneys, spleen, and heart with an initial distribution half-life of about 45 minutes. It is rapidly metabolised and excreted in bile and urine as unchanged drug and metabolites. The major metabolite, daunorubicinol, has antineoplastic activity. Up to 25% of a dose is excreted in urine in an active form over several days (the elimination half-lives of daunorubicin and its major metabolite are reported to be 18.5 and 26.7 hours respectively); an estimated 40% is excreted in bile. Daunorubicin does not appear to cross the blood-brain barrier, but crosses the placenta.

The pharmacokinetics of liposomal doxorubicin are significantly different from those of the conventional drug, with a decreased uptake by normal tissues (although tumour neovasculature is reported to have increased permeability to the liposomes), and a terminal half-life of 4 to 5 hours.

Uses and Administration

Daunorubicin is an antineoplastic antibiotic closely related to doxorubicin (p.529). It forms a stable complex with DNA and interferes with the synthesis of nucleic acids. Daunorubicin is a cell-cycle non-specific agent, but its cytotoxic effects are most marked on cells in the S phase. Daunorubicin also has antibacterial and immunosuppressant properties. It is used with other antineoplastic agents to induce remissions in acute leukaemias. Daunorubicin hydrochloride is given in association with vincristine and prednisone or prednisolone in acute lymphoblastic leukaemia (see p.478) and with cytarabine and thioguanine in acute non-lymphoblastic leukaemias (see p.479). It has also been tried in some other malignancies. A liposomal formulation of daunorubicin has been developed for use in the management of Kaposi's sarcoma in patients with AIDS (see also p.496).

In combination treatment regimens for adult acute leukaemia, daunorubicin hydrochloride is usually given in doses equivalent to 30 to 45 mg of base per m^2 body-surface daily for 2 to 3 days, by injecting a solution in sodium chloride injection 0.9% into a fast-running infusion of sodium chloride or glucose. Courses may be repeated after 3 to 6 weeks. A dose equivalent to 25 mg of base per m^2 has been given intravenously once a week, in combination with vincristine and prednisone or prednisolone, to children with acute lymphoblastic leukaemia.

The total cumulative dose in adults should not exceed 550 mg per m^2; in patients who have received radiotherapy to the chest it may be advisable to limit the total dose to about 400 to 450 mg per m^2. Lower limits apply in children: a total cumulative dose of no more than 300 mg per m^2, or in children aged under 2 years 10 mg per kg body-weight, is recommended. Dosage should be reduced in patients with impaired hepatic or renal function.

In the treatment of Kaposi's sarcoma, liposomal daunorubicin is given intravenously every 2 weeks starting with a dose of 40 mg per m,[2] and continued for as long as disease control can be maintained. It is diluted with 5% glucose injection (sodium chloride 0.9% should not be used) and given over 30 to 60 minutes.

Blood counts should be determined frequently during treatment as daunorubicin has a potent effect on bone-marrow function. Electrocardiogram examination should be made at regular intervals to detect signs of cardiotoxicity.

Preparations

USP 23: Daunorubicin Hydrochloride for Injection.

Proprietary Preparations (details are given in Part 3)
Aust.: Daunoblastin; DaunoXome; ***Austral.:*** Cerubidin†; ***Belg.:*** Cerubidine; DaunoXome; ***Canad.:*** Cerubidine; ***Fr.:*** Cerubidine; ***Ger.:*** Daunoblastin; ***Ital.:*** Daunoblastina; DaunoXome; ***Neth.:*** Cerubidine; DaunoXome; ***Norw.:*** Cerubidin; ***S.Afr.:*** Cerubidin; Daunoblastin; ***Spain:*** Daunoblastina; ***Swed.:*** Cerubidin; DaunoXome; ***Switz.:*** Cerubidine; ***UK:*** Cerubidin; DaunoXome; ***USA:*** Cerubidine†; DaunoXome.

Decitabine (10963-l)

Decitabine *(BAN, USAN, rINN).*

5-Aza-2′-deoxycytidine; DAC; NSC-127716. 4-Amino-1-(2-deoxy-β-D-*erythro*-pentofuranosyl)-1,3,5-triazin-2(1*H*)-one.

$C_8H_{12}N_4O_4$ = 228.2.

CAS — 2353-33-5.

Decitabine is an antineoplastic structurally related to cytarabine (see p.525) which has been tried in the treatment of acute leukaemias and some solid tumours.

References.

1. Momparler RL, *et al.* Pilot phase I-II study on 5-aza-2′-deoxycytidine (decitabine) in patients with metastatic lung cancer. *Anticancer Drugs* 1997; **8:** 358–68.
2. Kantarjian HM, *et al.* Results of decitabine therapy in the accelerated and blastic phases of chronic myelogenous leukemia. *Leukemia* 1997; **11:** 1617–20.

Diaziquone (19066-v)

Diaziquone *(USAN, rINN).*

Aziridinylbenzoquinone; AZQ; CI-904; NSC-182986. Diethyl 2,5-bis-(1-aziridinyl)-3,6-dioxo-1,4-cyclohexadiene-1,4-dicarbamate.

$C_{16}H_{20}N_4O_6$ = 364.4.

CAS — 57998-68-2.

Diaziquone is under investigation as an antineoplastic in the treatment of malignant brain tumours. It has also been tried in some other malignancies such as leukaemia. Adverse effects include bone marrow suppression, manifesting chiefly as leucopenia and thrombocytopenia, gastro-intestinal disturbances, and alopecia. Anaphylactoid reactions have occurred.

References.

1. Castleberry RP, *et al.* Aziridinylbenzoquinone (AZQ) in the treatment of recurrent pediatric brain and other malignant solid tumours: a Pediatric Oncology Group phase II study. *Invest New Drugs* 1990; **8:** 401–6.

Didemnin B (19075-g)

NSC-325319.

$C_{57}H_{89}N_7O_{15}$ = 1112.4.

The didemnins are biologically active peptides extracted from a marine sea squirt of the genus *Trididemnum*. They possess antineoplastic and antiviral properties; didemnin B is reported to be more active than didemnin A or didemnin C and has been investigated as an antineoplastic. Nausea and vomiting are dose-limiting; myelosuppression, cardiac and renal toxicity, liver dysfunction, other gastro-intestinal disturbances, myalgia, fatigue, and phlebitis may occur. Hypersensitivity reactions, possibly due to the polyethoxylated castor oil vehicle, have been reported.

Docetaxel (14634-b)

Docetaxel *(BAN, USAN, rINN)*.

RP-56976. (2R,3S)-N-Carboxy-3-phenylisoserine, N-tert-butyl ester, 13-ester with 5β-20-epoxy-1,2α,4,7β,10β,13α-hexahydroxytax-11-en-9-one 4-acetate 2-benzoate; *tert*-Butyl {(1S,2S)-2-[(2S,5R,7S,10R,13S)-4-acetoxy-2-benzoyloxy-1,7,10-trihydroxy-9-oxo-5,20-epoxytax-11-en-13-yloxy-carbonyl]-2-hydroxy-1-phenylethyl}carbamate.

$C_{43}H_{53}NO_{14}$ = 807.9.

CAS — 114977-28-5 (anhydrous docetaxel); 148408-66-6 (docetaxel trihydrate).

Adverse Effects, Treatment, and Precautions

As for Paclitaxel, p.556. Anaemia and skin reactions are common and may be severe. Fluid retention, resulting in oedema, ascites, pleural and pericardial effusion, and weight gain, is also common, and may be cumulative; premedication with a corticosteroid can reduce fluid retention as well as the risk of hypersensitivity reactions.

Pharmacokinetics

Following intravenous administration docetaxel is rapidly distributed to body tissues. It is extensively metabolised via hepatic cytochromes of the CYP 3A group, and excreted chiefly in the faeces as metabolites. Only about 6% of a dose is excreted in urine within 7 days. The terminal elimination half-life is about 11 hours. Docetaxel is more than 95% bound to plasma proteins in the blood.

References.

1. Bruno R, *et al.* Pharmacokinetic and pharmacodynamic properties of docetaxel: results of phase I and phase II trials. *Am J Health-Syst Pharm* 1997; **54** (suppl 2): S16–S19.

Uses and Administration

Docetaxel is a semisynthetic analogue of paclitaxel (see p.556) with similar actions but a reportedly higher potency. It has been given for various malignant neoplasms, notably of breast and lung (see p.485 and p.490 respectively) in suggested initial doses of 60 to 100 mg per m^2 body-surface area every 3 weeks. It is also reported to have some effect in melanoma (see p.492) and the palliative treatment of cancers of the head and neck (see p.489), and is being tried in ovarian cancer (p.491), although it has reportedly proved disappointing in colorectal malignancies (p.487).

Docetaxel is administered by intravenous infusion. It is available in vials which contain more than the labelled amount of drug, to allow for losses due to foaming and adhesion to the container, as well as dead space, during reconstitution. Following reconstitution with the full volume of solvent provided a solution containing 10 mg docetaxel per mL is produced, a suitable volume of which should be added to 5% glucose or 0.9% sodium chloride infusion solution. The concentration of docetaxel in the final infusion should not exceed 0.9 mg per mL. Infusion is normally over 1 hour; the procedure should be completed within 4 hours of reconstitution.

Regular blood counts are required, and dosage in subsequent courses should be reduced in patients who experience severe or febrile neutropenia, or severe cutaneous reactions or peripheral neuropathy. Dosage should be reduced in hepatic impairment, and hepatic function should be monitored.

References.

1. Gelmon K. The taxoids: paclitaxel and docetaxel. *Lancet* 1994; **344:** 1267–72.
2. Anonymous. Docetaxel (Taxotere) for advanced breast cancer. *Med Lett Drugs Ther* 1996; **38:** 87–8.
3. Fulton B, Spencer CM. Docetaxel: a review of its pharmacodynamic and pharmacokinetic properties and therapeutic efficacy in the management of metastatic breast cancer. *Drugs* 1996; **51:** 1075–92.
4. Leahy M, Howell A. Docetaxel. *Br J Hosp Med* 1997; **57:** 141–4.
5. Eckardt JR. Antitumor activity of docetaxel. *Am J Health-Syst Pharm* 1997; **54** (suppl 2): S2–S6.
6. Fumoleau P. Efficacy and safety of docetaxel in clinical trials. *Am J Health-Syst Pharm* 1997; **54** (suppl 2): S19–S24.
7. Anonymous. Paclitaxel and docetaxel in breast cancer and ovarian cancer. *Drug Ther Bull* 1997; **35:** 43–6.

Preparations

Proprietary Preparations (details are given in Part 3)
Aust.: Taxotere; ***Austral.:*** Taxotere; ***Canad.:*** Taxotere; ***Fr.:*** Taxotere; ***Ger.:*** Taxotere; ***Irl.:*** Taxotere; ***Ital.:*** Taxotere; ***Neth.:*** Taxotere; ***Norw.:*** Taxotere; ***S.Afr.:*** Taxotere; ***Spain:*** Taxotere; ***Swed.:*** Taxotere; ***UK:*** Taxotere; ***USA:*** Taxotere.

Doxifluridine (19107-r)

Doxifluridine *(rINN)*.

5′-Deoxy-5-fluorouridine; 5-DFUR; FUDR; Ro-21-9738.

$C_9H_{11}FN_2O_5$ = 246.2.

CAS — 3094-09-5.

Doxifluridine is an antineoplastic which probably acts through its conversion in the body to fluorouracil (see p.534). It is given in the management of malignant neoplasms of the breast (p.485) and gastro-intestinal tract (p.487), and of other solid tumours, in doses of up to 1.2 g daily by mouth. It has also been given by the intravenous route.

Pharmacokinetics. The pharmacokinetics and metabolism of doxifluridine in patients given up to 15 g per m^2 weekly as an intravenous infusion.[1] Doxifluridine was metabolised to fluorouracil and 5,6-dihydrofluorouracil; plasma concentrations of fluorouracil were approximately 6% of those of doxifluridine.

1. Sommadossi J-P, *et al.* Kinetics and metabolism of a new fluoropyrimidine, 5′-deoxy-5-fluorouridine, in humans. *Cancer Res* 1983; **43:** 930–3.

Preparations

Proprietary Preparations (details are given in Part 3)
Jpn: Furtulon.

Doxorubicin Hydrochloride (1831-z)

Doxorubicin Hydrochloride *(BANM, rINNM)*.

Adriamycin Hydrochloride; Cloridrato de Doxorrubicina; Doxorubicini Hydrochloridum; FI-106 (doxorubicin); 3-Hydroxyacetyldaunorubicin Hydrochloride; 14-Hydroxydaunorubicin Hydrochloride; NSC-123127. 8-Hydroxyacetyl (8S,10S)-10-[(3-amino-2,3,6-trideoxy-α-L-*lyxo*-hexopyranosyl)oxy]-6,8,11-trihydroxy-1-methoxy-7,8,9,10-tetrahydronaphthacene-5,12-dione hydrochloride.

$C_{27}H_{29}NO_{11}$,HCl = 580.0.

CAS — 23214-92-8 (doxorubicin); 25316-40-9 (doxorubicin hydrochloride).

NOTE. Doxorubicin is *USAN*. In many countries the name 'Adriamycin' is a trade-mark.

Pharmacopoeias. In *Eur.* (see p.viii), *Int., Jpn, Pol.,* and *US.*

The hydrochloride of an anthracycline antineoplastic antibiotic isolated from certain strains of *Streptomyces coeruleorubidus* or *S. peucetius*. It contains not less than 98% and not more than 102% of $C_{27}H_{29}NO_{11}$,HCl, calculated on the dried basis.

An orange-red hygroscopic crystalline powder. **Soluble** in water and soluble or slightly soluble in methyl alcohol; practically insoluble in chloroform, ether, and other organic solvents. A 0.5% solution in water has a pH of 4.0 to 5.5. **Store** in airtight containers.

CAUTION. *Doxorubicin hydrochloride is irritant; avoid contact with skin and mucous membranes.*

Incompatibility. Admixture of doxorubicin hydrochloride with cephalothin sodium, dexamethasone, diazepam, or hydrocortisone sodium succinate is reported to result in immediate precipitation;[1] similarly precipitation has occurred when doxorubicin hydrochloride was mixed with frusemide or heparin sodium.[2] A mixture of fluorouracil or aminophylline with doxorubicin hydrochloride is reported to darken in colour from red to purple, indicating degradation of doxorubicin.[1] Doxorubicin reacts with aluminium, similarly to daunorubicin (see p.528) but the reaction is slow and doxorubicin can safely be injected via aluminium-hubbed needles.[3]

Liposomal doxorubicin differs in its incompatibilities from conventional formulations: whereas the latter are reportedly incompatible with allopurinol, cefepime, and ganciclovir, the liposomal formulation apparently is not. However, it was incompatible with a number of drug solutions including amphotericin B, docetaxel, gallium nitrate, hydroxyzine hydrochloride, metoclopramide hydrochloride, miconazole, mitozantrone hydrochloride, morphine sulphate and some other opioids, paclitaxel, sodium bicarbonate, and some antibacterials.[4]

1. Dorr RT. Incompatibilities with parenteral anticancer drugs. *Am J Intravenous Ther* 1979; **6:** 42–52.
2. Cohen MH, *et al.* Drug precipitation within IV tubing: a potential hazard of chemotherapy administration. *Cancer Treat Rep* 1985; **69:** 1325–6.
3. Williamson NY, *et al.* Doxorubicin hydrochloride-aluminum interaction. *Am J Hosp Pharm* 1983; **40:** 214.
4. Trissel LA, *et al.* Compatibility of doxorubicin hydrochloride liposome injection with selected other drugs during simulated Y-site administration. *Am J Health-Syst Pharm* 1997; **54:** 2708–13.

Stability. Although sensitive to light at low concentrations, doxorubicin is not subject to significant photodegradation at clinical concentrations and special precautions to protect solutions from light during administration do not appear to be necessary.[1,2] Solutions in sodium chloride solution 0.9% were reported to be stable for 24 days when stored in PVC minibags at 25° and for even longer if stored in minibags or polypropylene syringes at 4°.[3] Stability in solution seems to be partly related to pH, with doxorubicin becoming more stable at acid pH.[3-5] A fall in pH of the solution also significantly decreases the loss of doxorubicin by adsorption and precipitation onto the surface of a positively-charged in-line filter.[6]

1. Tavoloni N, *et al.* Photolytic degradation of adriamycin. *J Pharm Pharmacol* 1980; **32:** 860–2.
2. Wood MJ, *et al.* Photodegradation of doxorubicin, daunorubicin and epirubicin measured by high-performance liquid chromatography. *J Clin Pharm Ther* 1990; **15:** 291–300.
3. Wood MJ, *et al.* Stability of doxorubicin, daunorubicin and epirubicin in plastic syringes and minibags. *J Clin Pharm Ther* 1990; **15:** 279–89.
4. Poochikian GK, *et al.* Stability of anthracycline antitumor agents in four infusion fluids. *Am J Hosp Pharm* 1981; **38:** 483–6.
5. Beijnen JH, *et al.* Stability of anthracycline antitumour agents in infusion fluids. *J Parenter Sci Technol* 1985; **39:** 220–2.
6. Francomb MM, *et al.* Effect of pH on the adsorption of cytotoxic drugs to a 96 hour intravenous filter. *Pharm J* 1991; **247:** R26.

Adverse Effects and Treatment

For general discussions see Antineoplastics, p.470 and p.473.

Doxorubicin causes pronounced bone-marrow depression with leucopenia at a maximum 10 to 15 days after administration; blood counts usually recover by about 21 days after a dose.

The anthracyclines may produce cardiac toxicity, both as an acute, usually transient disturbance of cardiac function marked by ECG abnormalities and, sometimes, arrhythmias; and as a delayed, sometimes fatal, chronic congestive heart failure. Severe cardiotoxicity is more likely in adults receiving total cumulative doses of doxorubicin greater than 550 mg per m^2 body-surface area, and may occur months or even years after administration.

Gastro-intestinal disturbances including moderate or sometimes severe nausea and vomiting, stomatitis, and, more rarely, facial flushing, conjunctivitis, and lachrymation may occur. Doxorubicin is very irritant and thrombophlebitis and streaking of the skin over the vein used for injection has been reported; extravasation is serious and may produce extensive local necrosis and ulceration. Alopecia occurs in the majority of patients. The urine may be coloured red. Occasional hypersensitivity reactions may occur.

Formulations of liposomal doxorubicin may be associated with a reduced potential for local tissue necrosis, and possibly a reduced incidence of cardiotoxicity, although current clinical experience is limited, and such toxicity remains a possibility. An acute pseudo-allergic reaction may be seen on initial infusion, but generally resolves on slowing or temporarily discontinuing the infusion.

The toxicity of doxorubicin is reported to be greatly reduced by liposomal encapsulation.[1-3] Mucositis and palmar-plantar erythema however, both toxicities associated with the infusion regimen, appear to be more likely with the liposomal formulation;[3] fatal hepatotoxicity in a patient also positive for hepatitis B[4] may represent an idiosyncratic reaction.[2]

1. Sells RA, *et al.* Reduction in toxicity of doxorubicin by liposomal entrapment. *Lancet* 1987; **ii:** 624–5.
2. Coker RJ, *et al.* Hepatic toxicity of liposomal encapsulated doxorubicin. *Lancet* 1993; **341:** 756.
3. Alberts DS, Garcia DJ. Safety aspects of pegylated liposomal doxorubicin in patients with cancer. *Drugs* 1997; **54** (suppl 4): 30–5.
4. Hengge UR, *et al.* Fatal hepatic failure with liposomal doxorubicin. *Lancet* 1993; **341:** 383–4.

Effects on the heart. Cardiotoxicity has been a major factor in limiting the use of the anthracyclines, doxorubicin and daunorubicin.[1,2] Toxicity is essentially of 2 kinds: acute, usually reversible ECG changes, including a wide range of arrhythmias, and a delayed, dose-related cardiomyopathy, resulting in congestive heart failure.[1-3] The latter may be further subdivided into chronic effects, occurring up to about a year after administration, and late-onset toxicity occurring years after treatment.[2] Delayed toxicity may be fatal in as many as 60% of patients who develop it,[4] and is reported to be more likely in children and elderly patients, in those who have received prior radiotherapy to the chest, and in those given relatively-high single doses on an infrequent schedule (presumably resulting in higher peak concentrations) rather than lower, weekly doses, or continuous infusion.[1,3-5] There is reason to believe that previous cardiovascular disease may also increase the risk,[4-6] although such patients are commonly excluded from studies of anthracycline therapy.[4] Females may be at greater risk than males.[7] Concomitant administration of cyclophosphamide,[1,6] and possibly other antineoplastics with cardiotoxic potential[1] may increase the likelihood of cardiomyopathy.

The single most important determinant of cardiac toxicity appears to be cumulative dose, with the risk of toxicity becoming ever greater at cumulative doxorubicin doses above 550 mg per square metre body-surface area or daunorubicin doses of 600 mg per square metre or more.[1,4,8] However, patients vary widely in sensitivity,[2] and these values represent relatively arbitrary choices on a continuum of risk: there is no single safe dose.[4] Even at doses which produce no symptoms, subclinical myocardial damage may occur, and in children this may result in diminished cardiac reserve and heart disease in later life.[5,9,10]

The late development of cardiac toxicity is a source of some concern: although in one study the mean time to development of symptoms was 33 days after administration, with a range of 0 to 231 days,[4] several recent reports have indicated that late cardiac failure may occur up to 18 years after anthracycline therapy.[2,11,12]

Given that doxorubicin-induced cardiac failure has been reported to occur in between 0.4 and 9% of all recipients, and that the fatality rate is high, much effort has gone into ways of predicting and preventing anthracycline-induced cardiotoxicity. Non-invasive cardiac monitoring, by means of echocardiography or radionuclide angiography, may be useful in predicting the development of cardiomyopathy[1,3] (although there is a history of controversy about the value of various monitoring techniques in specifically detecting toxicity[1]) but since the majority of patients are not at risk its overall benefits are marginal.[3] Nonetheless, the Childrens Cancer Study Group[13] has issued guidelines for monitoring using ECG, echocardiography, and radionuclide angiocardiography in patients receiving anthracyclines. The role of such techniques in predicting late-onset cardiotoxicity remains to be clarified.[2]

Dexrazoxane (p.978) has been shown to protect against the cardiotoxicity of doxorubicin and other anthracyclines[20-22] and is used to reduce cardiomyopathy in women receiving doxorubicin for metastatic breast cancer. A number of other compounds have been given in an effort to reduce cardiotoxicity,[1] including digoxin,[14,15] vitamin E,[14,16] ubidecarenone,[17] carnitine,[18] acetylcysteine,[19] and corticosteroids;[15] none appears particularly effective.

Alteration of the dosage schedule to weekly rather than three-weekly dosage, or the use of continuous infusion, has also been advocated as a way of reducing cardiotoxicity,[23-25] as has administration of doxorubicin formulated in liposomes.[2]

Several anthracycline derivatives have been developed with the aim of reducing the inherent cardiotoxicity of this class of compounds, including aclarubicin (p.502), epirubicin (p.532), and mitozantrone (p.553). However, although this strategy has met with some success, almost all these compounds exhibit some degree, admittedly reduced, of cardiotoxicity.

If cardiotoxicity does develop, the result of treatment has generally been equivocal.[1] However, recent results in patients with epirubicin-induced cardiotoxicity[26] have indicated that treatment with an ACE inhibitor can improve cardiac function and survival. Study is underway to determine whether ACE inhibitors can also prevent the initial toxicity if given immediately after an anthracycline.[27]

1. Von Hoff DD, *et al.* The cardiotoxicity of anticancer agents. *Semin Oncol* 1982; **9:** 23–33.
2. Shan K, *et al.* Anthracycline-induced cardiotoxicity. *Ann Intern Med* 1996; **125:** 47–58.
3. Doroshow JH. Doxorubicin-induced cardiac toxicity. *N Engl J Med* 1991; **324:** 843–5.
4. Von Hoff DD, *et al.* Risk factors for doxorubicin-induced congestive heart failure. *Ann Intern Med* 1979; **91:** 710–17.
5. Hale JP, Lewis IJ. Anthracyclines: cardiotoxicity and its prevention. *Arch Dis Child* 1994; **71:** 457–62.
6. Minow RA, *et al.* Adriamycin cardiomyopathy—risk factors. *Cancer* 1977; **39:** 1397–1402.
7. Lipshultz SE, *et al.* Female sex and higher drug dose as risk factors for late cardiotoxic effects of doxorubicin therapy for childhood cancer. *N Engl J Med* 1995; **332:** 1738–43.
8. Von Hoff DD, *et al.* Daunomycin-induced cardiotoxicity in children and adults: a review of 110 cases. *Am J Med* 1977; **62:** 200–8.
9. Yeung ST, *et al.* Functional myocardial impairment in children treated with anthracyclines for cancer. *Lancet* 1991; **337:** 816–18.
10. Lipschultz SE, *et al.* Late cardiac effects of doxorubicin therapy for acute lymphoblastic leukemia in childhood. *N Engl J Med* 1991; **324:** 808–15.
11. Goorin AM, *et al.* Initial congestive heart failure, six to ten years after doxorubicin chemotherapy for childhood cancer. *J Pediatr* 1990; **116:** 144–7.
12. Steinherz LJ, *et al.* Cardiac toxicity 4 to 20 years after completing anthracycline therapy. *JAMA* 1991; **266:** 1672–7.
13. Steinherz LJ, *et al.* Guidelines for cardiac monitoring of children during and after anthracycline therapy: report of the Cardiology Committee of the Childrens Cancer Study Group. *Pediatrics* 1992; **89:** 942–9.
14. Whittaker JA, Al-Ismail SAD. Effect of digoxin and vitamin E in preventing cardiac damage caused by doxorubicin in acute myeloid leukaemia. *Br Med J* 1984; **288:** 283–4.
15. Gupta M, *et al.* Systolic time interval (STI) in adriamycin (ADM)-treated patients on digoxin or prednisone cardioprophylaxis. *Proc Am Assoc Cancer Res* 1976; **17:** 269.
16. Myers CE, *et al.* Adriamycin: the role of lipid peroxidation in cardiac toxicity and tumor response. *Science* 1977; **197:** 165–7.
17. Cortes EP, *et al.* Adriamycin cardiotoxicity: early detection by systolic time interval and possible prevention by coenzyme Q10. *Cancer Treat Rep* 1978; **62:** 887–91.
18. Goa KL, Brogden RN. l-Carnitine: a preliminary review of its pharmacokinetics, and its therapeutic use in ischaemic cardiac disease and primary and secondary carnitine deficiencies in relationship to its role in fatty acid metabolism. *Drugs* 1987; **34:** 1–24.
19. Dresdale AR, *et al.* Prospective randomized study of the role of N-acetyl cysteine in reversing doxorubicin-induced cardiomyopathy. *Am J Clin Oncol* 1982; **5:** 657–63.
20. Speyer JL, *et al.* Protective effect of the bispiperazinedione ICRF-187 against doxorubicin-induced cardiac toxicity in women with advanced breast cancer. *N Engl J Med* 1988; **319:** 745–52.
21. Seifert CF, *et al.* Dexrazoxane in the prevention of doxorubicin-induced cardiotoxicity. *Ann Pharmacother* 1994; **28:** 1063–72.
22. Kolaric K, *et al.* A phase II trial of cardioprotection with Cardioxane (ICRF-187) in patients with advanced breast cancer receiving 5-fluorouracil, doxorubicin and cyclophosphamide. *Oncology* 1995; **52:** 251–5.
23. Legha SS, *et al.* Reduction of doxorubicin cardiotoxicity by prolonged continuous intravenous infusion. *Ann Intern Med* 1982; **96:** 133–9.
24. Torti FM, *et al.* Reduced cardiotoxicity of doxorubicin delivered on a weekly schedule: assessment by endomyocardial biopsy. *Ann Intern Med* 1983; **99:** 745–9.
25. Lum BL, *et al.* Doxorubicin: alteration of dose scheduling as a means of reducing cardiotoxicity. *Drug Intell Clin Pharm* 1985; **19:** 259–64.
26. Jensen BV, *et al.* Treatment with angiotensin-converting-enzyme inhibitor for epirubicin-induced dilated cardiomyopathy. *Lancet* 1996; **347:** 297–9.
27. Jensen BV, *et al.* Angiotensin-converting enzyme inhibitor for epirubicin-induced dilated cardiomyopathy. *Lancet* 1996; **347:** 1485.

Effects on the liver. Hepatitis and non-specific hepatocellular damage has been reported in patients receiving doxorubicin as part of combination therapy.[1] A characteristic hepatotoxicity can also be produced by the combination of radiotherapy with doxorubicin.[2]

For mention of fatal hepatotoxicity associated with liposomal doxorubicin, see above.

1. Avilés A, *et al.* Hepatic injury during doxorubicin therapy. *Arch Pathol Lab Med* 1984; **108:** 912–13.
2. Price LA. Surviving malignant disease: medical and oncological aspects. *Br J Hosp Med* 1983; **30:** 8–12.

Treatment of adverse effects. For specific reference to treatment of the adverse effects of doxorubicin, see under Alopecia and Extravasation in the chapter introduction, p.474. For the various agents tried in an attempt to prevent cardiotoxicity, see above.

Precautions

For general discussion see Antineoplastics, p.474.

Doxorubicin is generally contra-indicated in patients with heart disease. Doses should not be repeated while there is bone-marrow depression or ulceration of the mouth. It should be given with great care in reduced doses to patients with hepatic impairment; dosage reduction may also be necessary in children and the elderly. Extravasation results in severe tissue damage and doxorubicin should not be given by intramuscular or subcutaneous injection. The adverse effects of irradiation may be enhanced by doxorubicin and skin reactions previously induced by radiotherapy may recur; the maximum cumulative dose should be reduced to no more than 400 mg per m^2 in patients who have received radiotherapy to the chest or heart.

Handling and disposal. A method for the destruction of doxorubicin or daunorubicin wastes using sulphuric acid and potassium permanganate.[1] Residues produced by degradation of daunorubicin by this method showed no mutagenicity *in vitro*; some mutagenicity was seen with high concentrations of residues from doxorubicin.

1. Castegnaro M, *et al.*, eds. Laboratory decontamination and destruction of carcinogens in laboratory wastes; some antineoplastic agents. *IARC Scientific Publications 73*. Lyon: WHO/International Agency for Research on Cancer, 1985.

Urine and faeces produced for up to 7 days after a dose of doxorubicin should be handled wearing protective clothing.[1]

1. Harris J, Dodds LJ. Handling waste from patients receiving cytotoxic drugs. *Pharm J* 1985; **235:** 289–91.

Pregnancy and lactation. Although doxorubicin has been reported not to be present in detectable amounts in amniotic fluid[1,2] it has been found in fetal tissue (liver, kidney, and lungs) at concentrations several times those in maternal plasma,[2] indicating that it does pass the placenta.

The American Academy of Pediatrics considers that doxorubicin is contra-indicated during breast feeding because of evidence that it is concentrated in human milk.[3]

1. Roboz J, *et al.* Does doxorubicin cross the placenta? *Lancet* 1979; **ii:** 1382–3.
2. D'Incalci M, *et al.* Transplacental passage of doxorubicin. *Lancet* 1983; **i:** 75.
3. American Academy of Pediatrics Committee on Drugs. The transfer of drugs and other chemicals into human milk. *Pediatrics* 1994; **93:** 137–50.

Interactions

The cumulative dose of doxorubicin should be reduced in patients who have received other cardiotoxic drugs such as daunorubicin or cyclophosphamide.

Antibacterials. Hypersensitivity reactions to doxorubicin or daunorubicin have been reported in 2 patients with recent exposure to clindamycin, one of whom had exhibited hypersensitivity to that antibiotic.[1] The possibility of cross-sensitivity between anthracyclines and clindamycin should be considered.

1. Arena FP, Sherlock S. Doxorubicin hypersensitivity and clindamycin. *Ann Intern Med* 1990; **112:** 150.

Antineoplastics. Administration of doxorubicin with or after agents such as streptozocin[1] or methotrexate,[2] which can impair hepatic function, has resulted in increased doxorubicin toxicity, possibly due to reduced hepatic clearance. A high incidence of cardiotoxicity (manifest as congestive heart failure) has been reported in patients who received doxorubicin in association with paclitaxel (which also has cardiotoxic effects).[3]

For a suggestion that doxorubicin might enhance the hepatotoxicity of mercaptopurine, see under Daunorubicin Hydrochloride, p.528 and for a report of increased neurotoxicity when doxorubicin was given with cyclosporin, see under Cyclosporin, p.522.

1. Anonymous. Two drugs may not be better than one. *JAMA* 1976; **236:** 913.
2. Robertson JH, *et al.* Toxicity of doxorubicin and methotrexate in osteogenic sarcoma. *Br Med J* 1976; **1:** 23.
3. Gianni L, *et al.* Paclitaxel by 3-hour infusion in combination with bolus doxorubicin in women with untreated metastatic breast cancer: high antitumor efficacy and cardiac effects in a dose-finding and sequence-finding study. *J Clin Oncol* 1995; **13:** 2688–99.

Pharmacokinetics

Following intravenous injection, doxorubicin is rapidly cleared from the blood, and distributed into tissues including lungs, liver, heart, spleen, and kidneys. It undergoes rapid metabolism in the liver to metabolites including the active metabolite doxorubicinol (adriamycinol). About 40 to 50% of a dose is stated to be excreted in bile within 7 days, of which about half is as unchanged drug. Only about 5% of a dose is excreted in urine within 5 days. It does not cross the blood-brain barrier but may cross the placenta and is distributed into breast milk. The disappearance of doxorubicin from the blood is triphasic: mean half-lives are 12 minutes, 3.3 hours and about 30 hours.

The pharmacokinetics of liposomal formulations are somewhat different from the conventional drug. The use of macrogols in the surface layer of the liposomes (pegylation) reduces removal of liposomes by macrophages. This results in prolonged circulation in the plasma, with relatively little tissue distribution, but tumour neovasculature is reported to permit penetration of liposomes into tumour tissue. Pharmacokinetics are reported to be biphasic with mean half-lives of 5 hours and 55 hours respectively.

References.

1. Speth PAJ, *et al.* Clinical pharmacokinetics of doxorubicin. *Clin Pharmacokinet* 1988; **15:** 15–31.
2. Rushing DA, *et al.* The disposition of doxorubicin on repeated dosing. *J Clin Pharmacol* 1993; **33:** 698–702.
3. Piscitelli SC, *et al.* Pharmacokinetics and pharmacodynamics of doxorubicin in patients with small cell lung cancer. *Clin Pharmacol Ther* 1993; **53:** 555–61.

Clearance. The clearance of doxorubicin, given as an intravenous bolus of 50 mg per square metre body-surface area as part of a combination regimen, was greater when given in the morning than in the evening, the mean terminal elimination half-lives being 12.6 and 21.7 hours respectively in a study in 18 patients.[1]

1. Canal P, *et al.* Chronopharmacokinetics of doxorubicin in patients with breast cancer. *Eur J Clin Pharmacol* 1991; **40:** 287–91.

Uses and Administration

Doxorubicin is an antineoplastic antibiotic which may act by forming a stable complex with DNA and interfering with the synthesis of nucleic acids. It is a cell-cycle nonspecific agent but is most active against cells in S phase. It also has actions on cell membranes, and immunosuppressant properties. It is an effective antineoplastic against a wide range of tumours as indicated by the cross-references given below. Doxorubicin is used, often in association with other antineoplastics, in the treatment of leukaemias, lymphomas, sarcomas, neuroblastoma, Wilms' tumour, and malignant neoplasms of the bladder, breast, lung, ovary, and thyroid. It has also been used in other tumours including those of the brain, cervix, endometrium, liver, stomach, pancreas, and thymus, in gestational trophoblastic tumours, retinoblastoma, and in myeloma. Liposomal doxorubicin is used in the management of Kaposi's sarcoma in patients with AIDS.

Doxorubicin hydrochloride is administered intravenously by injecting a solution in sodium chloride injection 0.9%, into a fast-running infusion of sodium chloride 0.9% or glucose 5% over 3 minutes or more. It is given as a single agent in doses of 60 to 75 mg per m^2 body-surface, or 1.2 to 2.4 mg per kg body-weight, as a single dose every 3 weeks; alternatively, doses of 20 to 30 mg per m^2 may be given daily for 3 days every 3 to 4 weeks, although dividing the dose in this way may increase the incidence of mucositis. A regimen of 20 mg per m^2 as a single weekly dose has also been tried and is reported to be associated with a lower incidence of cardiotoxicity.

Doses may need to be reduced if doxorubicin is given with other antineoplastics: a dose of 30 to 40 mg per m^2 every 3 weeks has been suggested. Doses should also be halved in patients with moderate liver dysfunction (serum-bilirubin concentrations of 12 to 30 μg per mL); those with severe impairment (serum bilirubin greater than 30 μg per mL) should be given a quarter of the usual dose.

The maximum total dose should not exceed 550 mg per m^2 or in patients aged over 70, 450 mg per m^2; in patients who have received radiotherapy to the chest, or other cardiotoxic drugs, it may be advisable to limit the total dose to about 400 mg per m^2.

In the management of AIDS-related Kaposi's sarcoma pegylated liposomal doxorubicin has been given intravenously in a dose of 20 mg per m^2 every 2 to 3 weeks. Treatment should be continued for at least 2 to 3 months before response is assessed. It is given by intravenous infusion over 30 minutes diluted in 250 mL of glucose 5%.

Blood counts should be made routinely during treatment with doxorubicin and electrocardiograms should be examined at regular intervals for early signs of cardiotoxicity.

Conjugates of doxorubicin with monoclonal antibodies are reported to be under investigation.

Doxorubicin has also been instilled into the bladder in the local treatment of malignant neoplasms. For this purpose 50 mL of a 1 mg per mL solution may be instilled into the bladder once a month.

Administration. Promising initial results were seen in 14 patients with inoperable lung metastases in whom local injection of doxorubicin was combined with the establishment of an electric field, encouraging migration of the electropositive drug into neoplastic tissue.[1]

Liposomal formulations of doxorubicin have been developed[2,3] and have produced some benefit in the management of epidemic Kaposi's sarcoma in patients with AIDS (see p.496). They are also under investigation in other malignancies.[4,5]

1. Nordenström BEW, *et al.* Electrochemical treatment of cancer II: effect of electrophoretic influence on adriamycin. *Am J Clin Oncol* 1990; **13:** 75–88.
2. Working PK, Dayan AD. CPMP Preclinical Expert Report: Caelyx (Stealth liposomal doxorubicin HCL). *Hum Exp Toxicol* 1996; **15:** 752–85.
3. Coukell AJ, Spencer CM. Polyethylene glycol-liposomal doxorubicin: a review of its pharmacodynamic and pharmacokinetic properties, and therapeutic efficacy in the management of AIDS-related Kaposi's sarcoma. *Drugs* 1997; **53:** 520–38.
4. Gabizon A, Martin F. Polyethylene glycol-coated (pegylated) liposomal doxorubicin: rationale for use in solid tumours. *Drugs* 1997; **54** (suppl 4): 15–21.
5. Muggia FM. Clinical efficacy and prospects for use of pegylated liposomal doxorubicin in the treatment of ovarian and breast cancers. *Drugs* 1997; **54** (suppl 4): 22–9.

Malignant neoplasms. Doxorubicin plays a major role in combination regimens for chemotherapy of solid malignancies; it is often employed for tumours of the breast and lung (see p.485 and p.490) and for Wilms' tumour and neuroblastoma or retinoblastoma in children (see p.489, p.494, and p.495) but has been used for malignancies of the bladder (p.484) and brain (p.485); for various gynaecological cancers including gestational trophoblastic tumours and those of the cervix, endometrium, and ovary (see p.477, p.487, p.487, and p.491); for cancer of the liver, stomach, and pancreas (p.489, p.487, p.491); for secretory pancreatic neoplasms (p.477), and those of prostate, thyroid, and thymus (p.491, p.494, and p.493). It is also used in the treatment of sarcomas of bone and soft-tissue (see p.495 and p.496) and liposomal doxorubicin is proving of considerable interest in patients with Kaposi's sarcoma (see p.496).

In addition, doxorubicin is a component of the ABVD regimen used to treat Hodgkin's disease (see p.481) and is used in regimens for non-Hodgkin's lymphoma (p.482) including Burkitt's lymphoma (p.483), mycosis fungoides (p.482), and the lymphomas associated with AIDS (see p.483). It has been employed in chronic lymphocytic leukaemia as part of the CHOP regimen (though with uncertain benefit—see p.480) and in myeloma (p.494).

Preparations

BP 1998: Doxorubicin Injection;
USP 23: Doxorubicin Hydrochloride for Injection; Doxorubicin Hydrochloride Injection.

Proprietary Preparations (details are given in Part 3)
Aust.: Adriblastin; Caelyx; ***Belg.:*** Adriblastina; ***Fr.:*** Adriblastine; ***Ger.:*** Adriblastin; Adrimedac; DOXO-cell; ***Ital.:*** Adriblastina; ***Neth.:*** Adriblastina; Caelyx; ***S.Afr.:*** Adriblastina; ***Spain:*** Farmiblastina; ***Swed.:*** Caelyx; ***Switz.:*** Adriblastine; ***UK:*** Caelyx; ***USA:*** Doxil; Rubex.

Droloxifene (2796-y)

Droloxifene *(USAN, rINN).*

3-Hydroxytamoxifen; K-21060E. (*E*)-α-{*p*-[2-(Dimethylamino)ethoxy]phenyl}-α′-ethyl-3-stilbenol.

$C_{26}H_{29}NO_2$ = 387.5.

CAS — 82413-20-5.

Droloxifene is a selective oestrogen receptor modulator related to tamoxifen (p.563) and with similar general properties. It has been investigated in the hormonal treatment and prophylaxis of breast cancer (see p.486) and is under study for osteoporosis.

Echinomycin (19121-t)

NSC-526417; Quinomycin A.

$C_{51}H_{64}N_{12}O_{12}S_2$ = 1101.3.

CAS — 512-64-1.

Echinomycin is an antibiotic derived from *Streptomyces echinatus* which is reported to intercalate with DNA, and which has been investigated as an antineoplastic. Nausea and vomiting may be dose-limiting; other adverse reactions include mild thrombocytopenia, liver dysfunction, fever, and hypersensitivity reactions.

References.

1. Kuhn J. Phase I evaluation of echinomycin. *Drug Intell Clin Pharm* 1985; **19:** 457–8.
2. Wadler S, *et al.* Phase II trial of echinomycin in patients with advanced or recurrent colorectal cancer. *Cancer Chemother Pharmacol* 1994; **34:** 266–9.

Edatrexate (10981-j)

Edatrexate *(USAN, rINN).*

CGP-30694. *N*-(*p*-{1-[(2,4-Diamino-6-pteridinyl)methyl]propyl}benzoyl)-L-glutamic acid.

$C_{22}H_{25}N_7O_5$ = 467.5.

CAS — 80576-83-6.

Edatrexate is an analogue of methotrexate (p.547) and has similar general properties. It is under investigation as an antineoplastic in the treatment of various malignant neoplasms. Mucositis may be dose limiting.

References.

1. Souhami RL, *et al.* Phase II study of edatrexate in stage III and IV non-small cell lung cancer. *Cancer Chemother Pharmacol* 1992; **30:** 465–8.
2. Lee JS, *et al.* Improved therapeutic index by leucovorin of edatrexate, cyclophosphamide, and cisplatin regimen for non-small cell lung cancer. *J Natl Cancer Inst* 1992; **84:** 1039–40.
3. Schornagel JH, *et al.* Randomized phase III trial of edatrexate versus methotrexate in patients with metastatic and/or recurrent squamous cell carcinoma of the head and neck: a European Organization for Research and Treatment of Cancer Head and Neck Cancer Cooperative Group study. *J Clin Oncol* 1995; **13:** 1649–55.

Edrecolomab (15646-c)

Edrecolomab *(USAN, rINN).*

17-1A Antibody; C1; Monoclonal Antibody 17-1A.

CAS — 156586-89-9.

Edrecolomab is a monoclonal antibody of murine origin directed at epithelial cell surface glycoproteins that has been used as adjuvant therapy following surgery in patients with colorectal cancer (p.487). It is given by intravenous infusion over 2 hours, in an initial dose of 500 mg, followed by 4 further doses of 100 mg at monthly intervals. The drug is of murine origin and most patients develop antibodies following administration. Hypersensitivity reactions, including anaphylactic reactions, have occurred.

It has also been tried for other malignant neoplasms including pancreatic cancer.

References.

1. Riethmüller G, *et al.* Randomised trial of monoclonal antibody for adjuvant therapy of resected Dukes' C colorectal carcinoma. *Lancet* 1994; **343:** 1177–83.
2. Riethmüller G, *et al.* Monoclonal antibody therapy for resected Dukes' C colorectal cancer: seven-year outcome of a multicenter randomized trial. *J Clin Oncol* 1998; **16:** 1788–94.

Preparations

Proprietary Preparations (details are given in Part 3)
Ger.: Panorex.

Elliptinium Acetate (18634-y)

Elliptinium Acetate *(BAN, rINN).*

HME; NSC-264137. 9-Hydroxy-2,5,11-trimethyl-6*H*,2*H*-pyrido[4,3-*b*]carbazolium acetate.

$C_{20}H_{20}N_2O_3$ = 336.4.

CAS — 58337-35-2.

Elliptinium acetate is an antineoplastic which was formerly used in the treatment of metastatic breast cancer.

Enloplatin (15005-g)

Enloplatin *(USAN, rINN).*

CL-287110. *cis*-(1,1-Cyclobutane dicarboxylato)[tetrahydro-4*H*-pyran-4,4-bis(methylamine)]platinum.

$C_{13}H_{22}N_2O_5Pt$ = 481.4.

CAS — 111523-41-2.

Enloplatin is a platinum derivative with general properties similar to those of cisplatin (p.513). It is under investigation as an antineoplastic in the treatment of a variety of malignant neoplasms.

References.

1. Weiss RB, Christian MC. New cisplatin analogues in development: a review. *Drugs* 1993; **46:** 360–77.

Enocitabine (19135-h)

Enocitabine *(rINN).*

Behenoyl Cytarabine; Behenoylcytosine Arabinoside; BH-AC; NSC-239336. *N*-(1-β-D-Arabinofuranosyl-1,2-dihydro-2-oxo-4-pyrimidinyl)docosanamide.

$C_{31}H_{55}N_3O_6$ = 565.8.

CAS — 55726-47-1.

Enocitabine is an antineoplastic that is converted in the body to cytarabine (p.525). It has been used similarly in the treatment of acute leukaemias.

Epirubicin Hydrochloride (16631-k)

Epirubicin Hydrochloride *(BANM, USAN, rINNM)*.

4′-Epiadriamycin Hydrochloride; 4′-Epidoxorubicin Hydrochloride; IMI-28; Pidorubicin Hydrochloride. (8S,10S)-10-(3-Amino-2,3,6-trideoxy-α-L-*arabino*-hexopyranosyloxy)-8-glycolloyl-7,8,9,10-tetrahydro-6,8,11-trihydroxy-1-methoxynaphthacene-5,12-dione hydrochloride.

$C_{27}H_{29}NO_{11},HCl = 580.0$.

CAS — 56420-45-2 (epirubicin); 56390-09-1 (epirubicin hydrochloride).

The manufacturers state that epirubicin is **incompatible** with heparin and with alkali.

Epirubicin was not subject to significant photodegradation at clinical concentrations,[1,2] and special precautions to protect solutions from light during administration do not appear to be necessary. However, photodegradation may be significant at lower concentrations (below 500 μg per mL).[1]

1. Wood MJ, *et al.* Photodegradation of doxorubicin, daunorubicin and epirubicin measured by high-performance liquid chromatography. *J Clin Pharm Ther* 1990; **15:** 291–300.
2. Pujol M, *et al.* Stability study of epirubicin in NaCl 0.9% injection. *Ann Pharmacother* 1997; **31:** 992–5.

Adverse Effects, Treatment, and Precautions

As for Doxorubicin Hydrochloride, p.529. Cardiotoxicity and myelotoxicity may be less than with doxorubicin. Cardiotoxicity is more likely when the cumulative dose exceeds 0.9 to 1 g per m^2 body-surface.

Effects on the heart. For the suggestion that ACE inhibitors can be used to treat anthracycline-induced (and specifically epirubicin-induced) cardiotoxicity, see under Adverse Effects of Doxorubicin, p.529.

Interactions

Cimetidine. Cimetidine increased the formation of the active metabolite of epirubicin in a study in 8 patients; there was also a substantial increase in systemic exposure to unchanged epirubicin.[1] The mechanisms and potential clinical significance of the interaction were unclear.

1. Murray LS, *et al.* The effect of cimetidine on the pharmacokinetics of epirubicin in patients with advanced breast cancer: preliminary evidence of a potentially common drug interaction. *Clin Oncol* 1998; **10:** 35–8.

Pharmacokinetics

Following intravenous administration epirubicin is rapidly and extensively distributed into body tissues, and undergoes metabolism in the liver, with the formation of epirubicinol (13-hydroxyepirubicin) and appreciable amounts of glucuronide derivatives. Epirubicin is eliminated mainly in bile, with a terminal plasma elimination half-life of about 30 to 40 hours. About 10% of a dose is recovered in urine within 48 hours. Epirubicin does not cross the blood-brain barrier.

References.

1. Morris RG, *et al.* Disposition of epirubicin and metabolites with repeated courses to cancer patients. *Eur J Clin Pharmacol* 1991; **40:** 481–7.
2. Robert J. Clinical pharmacokinetics of epirubicin. *Clin Pharmacokinet* 1994; **26:** 428–38.

Uses and Administration

Epirubicin is an anthracycline antibiotic with antineoplastic actions similar to those of doxorubicin (p.531). It has been tried, alone or in combination with other antineoplastics, in acute leukaemias, lymphomas, multiple myeloma, and in solid tumours, including cancer of the bladder, breast, cervix, ovary, prostate, and gastro-intestinal tract. Some of these uses are discussed further under Choice of Antineoplastic, as indicated by the cross-references given below.

Epirubicin hydrochloride is administered intravenously by injecting a solution in sodium chloride 0.9% or Water for Injections into a fast-running infusion of sodium chloride 0.9% or glucose 5% over 3 to 5 minutes, or by infusion over up to 30 minutes. It is given as a single agent in usual doses of 60 to 90 mg per m^2 body-surface as a single dose every 3 weeks; this dose may be divided over 2 or 3 days if desired. High-dose regimens, of 120 mg or more per m^2 every 3 weeks, or 45 mg per m^2 for 3 consecutive days every 3 weeks have been used. A regimen of 20 mg as a single weekly dose has also been tried and is reported to be associated with lower toxicity. Doses should be reduced if epirubicin is given with other antineoplastics, and should be halved in patients with moderate liver dysfunction (serum bilirubin concentrations of 14 to 30 μg per mL), while those with severe liver impairment (serum bilirubin greater than 30 μg per mL) should be given a quarter of the usual dose. Reduced doses are also recommended in those whose bone-marrow function is impaired by age or previous chemotherapy or radiotherapy.

A total cumulative dose of 0.9 to 1 g per m^2 should not generally be exceeded, because of the risk of cardiotoxicity.

Epirubicin has also been given by intravesical instillation in the local treatment of bladder cancer. Instillation of 50 mg weekly as a 0.1% solution for 8 weeks has been suggested, reduced to 30 mg weekly if chemical cystitis develops; for carcinoma in-situ, the dose may be increased, if tolerated, to 80 mg weekly. For the prophylaxis of recurrence in patients who have undergone transurethral resection, 50 mg weekly for 4 weeks, followed by 50 mg instilled once a month for 11 months is the suggested regimen.

Blood counts should be made routinely during treatment with epirubicin and cardiac function should be carefully monitored. Liver function should be assessed before and if possible during therapy.

References.

1. Plosker GL, Faulds D. Epirubicin: a review of its pharmacodynamic and pharmacokinetic properties, and therapeutic use in cancer chemotherapy. *Drugs* 1993; **45:** 788–856.
2. Coukell AJ, Faulds D. Epirubicin: an updated review of its pharmacodynamic and pharmacokinetic properties and therapeutic efficacy in the management of breast cancer. *Drugs* 1997; **53:** 453–82.

Amyloidosis. For reference to a regimen including epirubicin used to control disease in a patient with amyloidosis, see p.497.

Malignant neoplasms. Epirubicin has been used in a variety of neoplastic disorders in which the anthracyclines are active. As mentioned on p.484 it is used for the local treatment and prophylaxis of superficial bladder cancer; it has also been given in cancer of the breast (p.485), cervix (p.487), stomach (p.487), pancreas (p.491), and prostate (p.491).

Preparations

Proprietary Preparations (details are given in Part 3)
Aust.: Farmorubicin; ***Austral.:*** Pharmorubicin; ***Belg.:*** Farmorubicine; ***Canad.:*** Pharmorubicin; ***Fr.:*** Farmorubicine; ***Ger.:*** Farmorubicin; ***Irl.:*** Pharmorubicin; ***Ital.:*** Farmorubicina; ***Neth.:*** Farmorubicine; ***Norw.:*** Farmorubicin; ***S.Afr.:*** Farmorubicin; ***Spain:*** Farmorubicina; ***Swed.:*** Farmorubicin; ***Switz.:*** Farmorubicine; ***UK:*** Pharmorubicin.

Estramustine Sodium Phosphate (1832-c)

Estramustine Sodium Phosphate *(BANM, rINNM)*.

Estramustine Phosphate Sodium *(USAN)*; NSC-89199 (estramustine phosphate); Ro-21-8837/001; Ro-22-2296/000 (estramustine). Estra-1,3,5(10)-triene-3,17β-diol 3-[bis(2-chloroethyl)carbamate] 17-(disodium phosphate); Disodium 3-[bis(2-chloroethyl)-carbamoyloxy]estra-1,3,5(10)-trien-17β-yl orthophosphate.

$C_{23}H_{30}Cl_2NNa_2O_6P = 564.3$.

CAS — 2998-57-4 (estramustine); 4891-15-0 (estramustine phosphate); 52205-73-9 (estramustine sodium phosphate).

Pharmacopoeias. In Br.

A white or almost white powder. Freely **soluble** in water and in methyl alcohol; very slightly soluble in dehydrated alcohol and in chloroform. A 0.5% solution in water has a pH of 8.5 to 10.0. **Protect** from light.

Adverse Effects, Treatment, and Precautions

Oestrogenic side-effects are fairly common, and may include gynaecomastia, fluid retention, and cardiovascular effects. Gastro-intestinal disturbances, hepatic dysfunction, loss of libido, hypersensitivity reactions, and occasionally leucopenia and thrombocytopenia may occur. Estramustine is contra-indicated in patients with peptic ulceration and severe hepatic or cardiovascular disease. Diabetes mellitus may be exacerbated, and it should be given with care to patients with disorders such as congestive heart failure, epilepsy, hypertension, and migraine which may be adversely affected by additional fluid retention. Care is also required in patients with conditions predisposing to hypercalcaemia, and serum calcium should be monitored in hypercalcaemic patients.

Estramustine should not be administered concomitantly with milk products or products high in calcium, which may interfere with its absorption.

Pharmacokinetics

About 75% of a dose of estramustine sodium phosphate is absorbed from the gastro-intestinal tract. It is concentrated in prostatic tissue. The phosphate moiety appears to be lost in the gastro-intestinal tract, liver, and phosphatase-rich tissue such as the prostate and estramustine is found in the body mainly as its 17-keto analogue, estromustine. Following breakage of the carbamate linkage the oestrogenic and alkylating moieties are excreted independently.

Uses and Administration

Estramustine is a combination of oestradiol and normustine and has weaker oestrogenic activity than oestradiol and weaker antineoplastic activity than and most other alkylating agents. Estramustine phosphate is given by mouth as the disodium salt in the treatment of advanced prostatic carcinoma (see also p.491); it has been used with meglumine by intravenous injection.

The usual initial dosage by mouth is the equivalent of 560 mg of estramustine phosphate daily in divided doses; the dose may later be adjusted to between 140 mg and 1.4 g daily according to the response and gastro-intestinal tolerance. It should be given not less than 1 hour before or 2 hours after meals. In the USA a dose of 14 mg per kg body-weight or 600 mg per m^2 body-surface area, daily in divided doses, is usually employed.

References.

1. Bergenheim AT, Henriksson R. Pharmacokinetics and pharmacodynamics of estramustine phosphate. *Clin Pharmacokinet* 1998; **34:** 163–72.

Preparations

BP 1998: Estramustine Phosphate Capsules.

Proprietary Preparations (details are given in Part 3)
Aust.: Estracyt; ***Austral.:*** Estracyt; ***Belg.:*** Estracyt; ***Canad.:*** Emcyt; ***Fr.:*** Estracyt; ***Ger.:*** cellmustin; Estracyt; Multosin; ***Irl.:*** Estracyt; ***Ital.:*** Estracyt; ***Neth.:*** Estracyt; ***Norw.:*** Estracyt; ***S.Afr.:*** Estracyt; ***Spain:*** Estracyt; ***Swed.:*** Estracyt; ***Switz.:*** Estracyt; ***UK:*** Estracyt; ***USA:*** Emcyt.

Etanidazole (1798-q)

Etanidazole *(USAN, rINN)*.

NSC-301467; SR-2508. *N*-(2-Hydroxyethyl)-2-nitroimidazole-1-acetamide.

$C_7H_{10}N_4O_4 = 214.2$.

CAS — 22668-01-5.

Etanidazole is a radiosensitiser structurally related to metronidazole, and which is under investigation as an adjunct to radiotherapy in the treatment of cancer. Peripheral neuropathy may be dose-limiting.

Etoposide (1834-a)

Etoposide *(BAN, USAN, rINN)*.

EPEG; Etoposidum; NSC-141540; VP-16; VP-16-213. 4′-Demethylepipodophyllotoxin 9-[4,6-*O*-(*R*)-ethylidene-β-D-glucopyranoside]; (5S,5aR,8aS,9R)-9-(4,6-*O*-Ethylidene-β-D-glucopyranosyloxy)-5,8,8a,9-tetrahydro-5-(4-hydroxy-3,5-dimethoxyphenyl)-isobenzofuro[5,6-*f*][1,3]benzodioxol-6(5a*H*)-one.

$C_{29}H_{32}O_{13} = 588.6$.

CAS — 33419-42-0.

NOTE. The trivial name epipodophyllotoxin has occasionally been used incorrectly for this derivative.

Pharmacopoeias. In *Eur.* (see p.viii) and *US.*

A fine white, or almost white, crystalline powder. The Ph. Eur. states that it is practically **insoluble**, and the USP that it is very slightly soluble, in water; slightly soluble in alcohol, in chloroform, in dichloromethane, and in ethyl acetate; sparingly soluble in methyl alcohol. **Store** in airtight containers. Protect from light.

For reference to precipitation when mannitol or potassium chloride was added to mixtures of etoposide and cisplatin in sodium chloride injection, see Cisplatin, p.513.

Adverse Effects, Treatment, and Precautions

For general discussions see Antineoplastics, p.470, p.473, and p.474.

The dose-limiting toxicity with etoposide is myelosuppression, predominantly manifesting as leucopenia, but also thrombocytopenia, and sometimes anaemia. The nadir of the white cell count usually occurs 7 to 14 days after a dose, with recovery by about 21 days. Nausea and vomiting are common; there may also be anorexia, diarrhoea, and stomatitis. Gastro-intestinal toxicity may be more common after oral administration. Reversible alopecia may occur in about two-thirds of all patients. Peripheral or central neuropathies, including transient cortical blindness, have been reported rarely, as have hypersensitivity or anaphylactoid reactions, apnoea, fever, rashes and skin pigmentation, pruritus, and dysphagia. Disturbances of liver function have been reported, mainly at high doses. There have been occasional reports of cardiotoxicity. Local irritation and thrombophlebitis may occur at the site of injection. Care should be taken to avoid extravasation although tissue damage (possibly associated with the vehicle) is rare.

Following rapid intravenous administration hypotension may occur; etoposide should be given by infusion over at least 30 minutes. Etoposide should not be given to patients with severe hepatic dysfunction nor by intracavitary administration.

Some of the adverse effects associated with intravenous administration of etoposide may be due to the formulation of the vehicle.

There is evidence that etoposide may be associated with the development of secondary leukaemias—see p.470.

Effects on the nervous system. A report of an acute dystonic reaction in a child given etoposide as part of a combined maintenance regimen for acute lymphoblastic leukaemia;[1] the patient had been receiving the same regimen uneventfully for over a year but symptoms (which responded to diphenhydramine) recurred on rechallenge with etoposide.

1. Ascher DP, Delaney RA. Acute dystonia from etoposide. *Drug Intell Clin Pharm* 1988; **22:** 41–2.

Handling and disposal. Urine and faeces produced for up to 4 and 7 days respectively after a dose of etoposide should be handled wearing protective clothing.[1]

1. Harris J, Dodds LJ. Handling waste from patients receiving cytotoxic drugs. *Pharm J* 1985; **235:** 289–91.

Hypersensitivity. A report of a hypersensitivity reaction to etoposide and a review of 92 further reactions.[1] Hypersensitivity reactions to intravenous etoposide are characterised by one or more of: hypotension, bronchospasm, flushing, exanthema, dyspnoea, fever, chills, tachycardia, tightness in the chest, cyanosis, and hypertension. Although originally stated to be rare, some investigators have reported an incidence of up to about 50%, particularly in younger patients. (Hypersensitivity reactions to teniposide appear to be more frequent than with etoposide, perhaps because the former is formulated with polyethoxylated castor oil whereas the latter is not.) The mechanism of reactions to etoposide is uncertain but may be non-immunogenic as reducing the rate of infusion may prevent reactions, as may reducing etoposide concentration in the infusion solution. Hypersensitivity appears to have been reported less frequently with the oral formulation.

1. Hoetelmans RMW, *et al.* Hypersensitivity reactions to etoposide. *Ann Pharmacother* 1996; **30:** 367–71.

Interactions

Antineoplastics. Administration of etoposide 2 days after a dose of cisplatin was associated with a marked decrease in etoposide clearance and an increase in toxicity, compared with the same dose given 21 days after a dose of cisplatin, in a study involving 17 children.[1] There was no evidence of a persistent decrease in etoposide clearance associated with the cumulative dose of cisplatin, however.

1. Relling MV, *et al.* Etoposide pharmacokinetics and pharmacodynamics after acute and chronic exposure to cisplatin. *Clin Pharmacol Ther* 1994; **56:** 503–11.

Pharmacokinetics

Following administration by mouth absorption is variable, but on average about 50% of the dose of etoposide is absorbed. The pharmacokinetics of etoposide are subject to considerable interindividual variation. It is rapidly distributed, and concentrations in plasma fall in a biphasic manner, with a terminal half-life of 3 to 19 hours. It is extensively bound to plasma protein (about 94%). Etoposide is excreted in urine and faeces as unchanged drug and metabolites: about 45% of a dose is reported to be excreted in urine over 72 hours, two-thirds as unchanged drug. It crosses the blood-brain barrier poorly, with concentrations in CSF from 1 to 10% of those in plasma.

Metabolism. Studies *in vitro* suggested that metabolic activation of etoposide by oxidation into the *O*-quinone derivative might play an essential role in its activity against DNA.[1]

1. van Maanen JMS, *et al.* Metabolic activation of anti-tumour agent VP 16-213. *Hum Toxicol* 1986; **5:** 136.

Uses and Administration

Etoposide is a semisynthetic derivative of podophyllotoxin with antimitotic and antineoplastic properties; it inhibits DNA synthesis and is most active against cells in the late S and G_2 phases of the cell cycle.

It is used, usually in combination with other antineoplastics, in the treatment of tumours of the testis, and cancers of the lung. It has also been tried in other solid tumours including those of the brain, gastro-intestinal tract, ovary, and thymus, gestational trophoblastic tumours, and some childhood neoplasms; in lymphomas and acute leukaemias, and in the treatment of Kaposi's sarcoma associated with AIDS. These uses are discussed further under Choice of Antineoplastic, as indicated by the cross-references given below.

It is given by slow intravenous infusion over at least 30 minutes, as a solution in sodium chloride 0.9% or glucose 5% injection. In the UK the manufacturers recommend that the concentration of the infusion should not exceed 250 μg per mL, to avoid the risk of the drug crystallising out of solution, but in the USA an upper limit of 400 μg per mL is regarded as acceptable. Etoposide phosphate, a prodrug with improved solubility in water, has been developed. Intravenous doses are calculated in terms of etoposide, and are identical to those of the base, but it may be given in concentrations up to the equivalent of 20 mg etoposide per mL.

The usual dose is 50 to 120 mg of etoposide per m^2 body-surface daily for 5 days. Somewhat lower doses have been suggested in lung cancer. Alternatively, 100 mg per m^2 has been given on alternate days to a total of 300 mg per m^2. Double the dose given intravenously may be given when etoposide is taken by mouth. Courses may be repeated after 3 to 4 weeks.

Blood disorders, non-malignant. For reference to the use of combination chemotherapy, including etoposide, in a few patients with refractory idiopathic thrombocytopenic purpura, see p.1023.

Histiocytic syndromes. Systemic chemotherapy is often tried in patients with extensive Langerhans-cell histiocytosis (p.478), although its value is uncertain. Etoposide is one of the drugs widely used for this purpose.

Hypereosinophilic syndrome. Etoposide has been reported to produce clinical responses in patients with the hypereosinophilic syndrome.[1]

1. Bourrat E, *et al.* Etoposide for treating the hypereosinophilic syndrome. *Ann Intern Med* 1994; **121:** 899–900.

Malignant neoplasms. Etoposide has been used for a variety of solid tumours: in particular it is part of the BEP regimen used in the treatment of testicular cancer (see p.493), and is used with cisplatin in the treatment of lung cancer (p.490). Other solid neoplasms in which it is sometimes employed include those of the brain (p.485), stomach (p.487), ovary (p.491), and thymus (p.493), as well as in neuroblastoma (p.494), retinoblastoma (p.495), and rhabdomyosarcoma (p.496); it has also formed part of systemic regimens for disseminated Kaposi's sarcoma (see p.496), and gestational trophoblastic tumours (p.477). In patients with relapsed Hodgkin's disease etoposide-containing salvage therapy has been tried (see p.481); it is also used in intermediate- and high-grade non-Hodgkin's lymphomas, including those associated with AIDS (see p.482 and p.483 respectively), and may produce short-term responses in mycosis fungoides (p.482). Etoposide may have benefits when added to induction protocols for acute non-lymphoblastic leukaemia (p.479). For reference to the benefits of consolidation therapy in acute lymphoblastic leukaemia using a regimen containing etoposide, see p.478.

Vasculitic syndromes. For mention of the use of etoposide to induce remission in patients with Wegener's granulomatosis resistant to standard therapy with cyclophosphamide and corticosteroids, see p.1031.

Preparations

USP 23: Etoposide Capsules.

Proprietary Preparations (details are given in Part 3)

Aust.: Abiposid; Cehaposid; Exitop; Vepesid; ***Austral.:*** Etopophos; Vepesid; ***Belg.:*** Vepesid; ***Canad.:*** Vepesid; ***Fr.:*** Celltop; Etopophos; Vepeside; ***Ger.:*** Vepesid; ***Irl.:*** Vepesid; ***Ital.:*** Lastet; Vepesid; ***Jpn:*** Lastet; ***Neth.:*** Etopophos; Vepesid; ***Norw.:*** Eposin; Vepesid; ***S.Afr.:*** Vepesid; ***Spain:*** Lastet; Vepesid; ***Swed.:*** Eposin; Etopofos; Exitop; Vepesid; ***Switz.:*** Exitop†; Vepesid; ***UK:*** Etopophos; Vepesid; ***USA:*** Etopophos; Toposar; Vepesid.

Exemestane (15427-v)

Exemestane *(rINN)*.

FCE-24304. 6-Methyleneandrosta-1,4-diene-3,17-dione.

$C_{20}H_{24}O_2$ = 296.4.

CAS — 107868-30-4.

Exemestane, like the related compound formestane (p.537), is a selective inhibitor of the aromatase (oestrogen synthetase) system responsible for the production of oestrogens from androgens. It is under investigation in the endocrine therapy of breast cancer. Unlike formestane it is active when given by mouth.

Fadrozole Hydrochloride (11128-p)

Fadrozole Hydrochloride *(USAN, rINNM)*.

CGS-16949 (fadrozole); CGS-16949A. (±)-*p*-(5,6,7,8-Tetrahydroimidazo[1,5-*a*]pyridin-5-yl)benzonitrile monohydrochloride.

$C_{14}H_{13}N_3HCl$ = 259.7.

CAS — 102676-47-1 (fadrozole); 102676-96-0 (fadrozole hydrochloride).

Fadrozole hydrochloride is an inhibitor of the aromatase (oestrogen synthetase) system and is used for the endocrine therapy of breast cancer. It has been given in doses of 1 mg twice daily by mouth.

References.

1. Stein RC, *et al.* Preliminary study of the treatment of advanced breast cancer in postmenopausal women with aromatase inhibitor CGS 16949A. *Cancer Res* 1990; **50:** 1381–4.
2. Miller WR. Oestrogens and breast cancer: biological considerations. *Br Med Bull* 1990; **47:** 470–83.
3. Buzdar AU, *et al.* Fadrozole HCl (CGS-16949A) versus megestrol acetate treatment of postmenopausal patients with metastatic breast carcinoma: results of two randomized double blind controlled multiinstitutional trials. *Cancer* 1996; **77:** 2503–13.

Fenretinide (19171-g)

Fenretinide *(USAN, rINN)*.

4-Hydroxyphenylretinamide; McN-R-1967. *all-trans*-4′-Hydroxyretinanilide.

CAS — 65646-68-6.

Fenretinide is a retinoid derivative given by mouth and being studied in the treatment of breast and prostate cancer and some other malignancies. It has also been tried in oral lichen planus and leucoplakia.

A study of fenretinide for the treatment of psoriasis was discontinued before any therapeutic effect was observed as 2 of 8 patients developed night blindness and 2 developed severe toxic erythema.[1] Fenretinide is being studied for the treatment of breast cancer[2] and cutaneous malignancies but early results have been disappointing and night blindness and mucocutaneous effects have also been associated with this use.[3] However, a combination of tamoxifen and fenretinide, given intermittently, has been reported to be well tolerated.[4] As mentioned on p.486 fenretinide is a potential candidate for studies aimed at the prevention of breast cancer.

1. Kingston TP, *et al.* Visual and cutaneous toxicity during N-(4-hydroxyphenyl) retinamide therapy for psoriasis. *Clin Exp Dermatol* 1986; **11:** 624–7.
2. Baum M, *et al.* Prospects for the chemoprevention of breast cancer. *Br Med Bull* 1991; **47:** 493–503.
3. Modiano MR, *et al.* Phase II study of fenretinide (N-[4-hydroxyphenyl]retinamide) in advanced breast cancer and melanoma. *Invest New Drugs* 1990; **8:** 317–19.
4. Cobleigh MA, *et al.* Phase I/II trial of tamoxifen with or without fenretinide, an analog of vitamin A, in women with metastatic breast cancer. *J Clin Oncol* 1993; **11:** 474–7.

Floxuridine (1835-t)

Floxuridine *(USAN, rINN)*.

5-Fluorouracil Deoxyriboside; FUDR; NSC-27640; WR-138720. 2′-Deoxy-5-fluorouridine; 5-Fluoro-2′-deoxyuridine; 1-(2-Deoxy-β-D-ribofuranosyl)-5-fluoropyrimidine-2,4(1*H*,3*H*)-dione.

$C_9H_{11}FN_2O_5$ = 246.2.

CAS — 50-91-9.

Pharmacopoeias. In US.

A 2% solution in water has a pH of 4.0 to 5.5. **Store** in airtight containers. Protect from light. The USP states that reconstituted solutions of Sterile Floxuridine may be stored at 2° to 8° for not more than 2 weeks.

Adverse Effects, Treatment, and Precautions

As for Fluorouracil, p.535. Adverse reactions following intra-arterial infusion commonly include local reactions, thrombo-embolic complications, and infection, bleeding, or blockage of the catheter. Erythema, stomatitis, and gastro-intestinal disturbances are relatively common. There have also been signs of liver dysfunction.

Effects on the liver. Serious biliary toxicity has been reported in over half of all patients receiving hepatic arterial infusions of floxuridine, usually manifesting as sclerosing cholangitis or acalculous cholecystitis;[1] as a result some surgeons routinely remove the gallbladder at the time of infusion pump implantation.[2] Floxuridine infusions have also been associated with a case of fatal progressive cirrhosis of the liver in the absence of overt cholestasis.[3]

1. Sherlock S. The spectrum of hepatotoxicity due to drugs. *Lancet* 1986; **ii:** 440–4.
2. Anonymous. An implanted infusion pump for chemotherapy of liver metastases. *Med Lett Drugs Ther* 1984; **26:** 89–90.
3. Pettavel J, *et al.* Fatal liver cirrhosis associated with long-term arterial infusion of floxuridine. *Lancet* 1986; **ii:** 1162–3.

Interactions

As for Fluorouracil, p.535.

Pharmacokinetics

Floxuridine is poorly absorbed from the gastro-intestinal tract and it is usually given by injection. Floxuridine is metabolised mainly in the liver to fluorouracil following rapid injection. When given by slow infusion, usually intra-arterially, it is reported to be converted to active floxuridine monophosphate. It is excreted as carbon dioxide via the lungs; some is excreted, as unchanged drug and metabolites, in urine. Floxuridine crosses the blood-brain barrier to some extent and is found in CSF.

Uses and Administration

Floxuridine is an antineoplastic which acts as an antimetabolite similarly to fluorouracil. When it is administered by rapid injection it acts as fluorouracil, but when infused slowly, usually intra-arterially, it is converted to active floxuridine monophosphate (F-dUMP) which leads to enhanced inhibition of DNA synthesis.

Floxuridine is used in the palliative treatment of malignant neoplasms of the liver (usually due to metastasis from the gastro-intestinal tract—see Choice of Antineoplastic, p.489). It has been tried in some other solid neoplasms. Doses of 100 to 600 μg per kg body-weight daily are given by continuous arterial infusion, usually with the aid of an infusion pump, until toxicity occurs.

White-cell and platelet counts should be carried out regularly during therapy and treatment should be stopped if the white-cell count falls rapidly or falls to below 3500 per mm³, if the platelet count falls below 100 000 per mm³, or if major adverse effects occur.

Preparations

USP 23: Floxuridine for Injection.

Proprietary Preparations (details are given in Part 3)
USA: FUDR.

Fludarabine Phosphate (19183-w)

Fludarabine Phosphate *(BAN, USAN, rINNM)*.

2-F-ara-AMP; Fludarabine Monophosphate; 2-Fluoro-ara-AMP; NSC-312887. 9-β-D-Arabinofuranosyl-2-fluoroadenine 5′-dihydrogenphosphate.

$C_{10}H_{13}FN_5O_7P$ = 365.2.

CAS — 21679-14-1 (fludarabine); 75607-67-9 (fludarabine phosphate).

Adverse Effects, Treatment, and Precautions

For general discussions see Antineoplastics, p.470, p.473, and p.474.

Bone-marrow suppression from fludarabine is dose-limiting, manifesting as leucopenia, thrombocytopenia, and anaemia; the nadir of the white cell and platelet counts usually occurs after about 2 to 3 weeks. Myelosuppression can be severe and cumulative and prolonged lymphopenia with concomitant risk of opportunistic infections may occur.

Other adverse effects include cough, dyspnoea, pneumonia, gastro-intestinal disturbances, stomatitis, oedema, angina pectoris, the tumour lysis syndrome, skin rashes, haemolytic anaemia, haemorrhagic cystitis, and neurological disturbances including peripheral neuropathy, agitation, confusion, visual disturbances, and coma. High doses have been associated with progressive encephalopathy and blindness.

Dosage should be reduced in renal impairment and fludarabine should not be given if creatinine clearance is less than 30 mL per minute.

Effects on the nervous system. Progressive cerebral dysfunction due to leucoencephalopathy developed 6 months after a course of fludarabine in usual doses for chronic lymphocytic leukaemia.[1] The patient became comatose and died 8 weeks after onset of the neurological symptoms.

1. Zabernigg A, *et al.* Late-onset fatal neurological toxicity of fludarabine. *Lancet* 1994; **344:** 1780.

Graft-versus-host disease. Transfusion-associated graft-versus-host disease has been reported following administration of blood products in patients treated with fludarabine.[1] Fludarabine-treated patients should receive irradiated red cells and platelets (to inactivate any viable T-cells) if they require a transfusion.

1. Williamson LM, *et al.* Fludarabine treatment and transfusion-associated graft-versus-host disease. *Lancet* 1996; **348:** 472–3.

Interactions

Increased pulmonary toxicity has been reported in patients given concomitant therapy with fludarabine and pentostatin. Administration with cytarabine may reduce the metabolic activation of fludarabine but results in increased intracellular concentrations of cytarabine—see p.526. The therapeutic efficacy of fludarabine may also be reduced by concomitant administration of dipyridamole and other inhibitors of adenosine uptake.

Aminoglycosides. A report of severe ototoxicity when a short course of gentamicin was given to a patient who had recently completed a course of fludarabine.[1]

1. O'Brien RK, Sparling TG. Gentamicin and fludarabine ototoxicity. *Ann Pharmacother* 1995; **29:** 200–1.

Pharmacokinetics

After intravenous administration, fludarabine phosphate is rapidly dephosphorylated to fludarabine which is taken up by lymphocytes and rephosphorylated to the active triphosphate nucleotide. Peak intracellular concentrations of fludarabine triphosphate are seen about 4 hours after a dose.

Clearance of fludarabine from the plasma is triphasic with a terminal half-life of about 10 to 30 hours. Elimination is mostly via renal excretion: 60% of a dose is excreted in the urine within 24 hours. The pharmacokinetics of fludarabine exhibit considerable interindividual variation.

Uses and Administration

Fludarabine is a fluorinated nucleotide analogue of the antiviral vidarabine (p.628) which acts as a purine antagonist antimetabolite. It is used for its antineoplastic properties in the treatment of chronic lymphocytic leukaemia. Fludarabine phosphate is given by bolus injection or by intravenous infusion over 30 minutes in a usual dose of 25 mg per m² body-surface daily for five consecutive days. Courses may be repeated every 28 days.

Haematological function should be monitored regularly; the dosage may need to be reduced, or further courses delayed, if blood counts indicate severe or persistent myelosuppression. Doses should be reduced by up to 50% in patients with mild to moderate renal impairment (creatinine clearance between 30 and 70 mL per minute); the drug should not be given in more severe renal impairment.

General references.

1. Adkins JC, *et al.* Fludarabine: an update of its pharmacology and use in the treatment of haematological malignancies. *Drugs* 1997; **53:** 1005–37.

Malignant neoplasms. Fludarabine is probably the preferred second-line therapy for chronic lymphocytic leukaemia once initial treatment fails and may give better results (combined with other agents) for the initial management of advanced disease than conventional regimens (see p.480). It has also been tried in other malignancies. Listed below are some references to the use of fludarabine phosphate for the treatment of chronic lymphocytic leukaemia,[1,2] and its potential activity against a variety of other malignancies, including non-Hodgkin's lymphoma,[3,4] mycosis fungoides,[5] heavy chain disease,[6] prolymphocytic leukaemia,[7,8] hairy cell leukaemia,[9] and Waldenström's macroglobulinaemia.[10]

1. Keating MJ, *et al.* Clinical experience with fludarabine in leukaemia. *Drugs* 1994; **47** (suppl 6): 39–49.
2. French Cooperative Group on CLL, *et al.* Multicentre prospective randomised trial of fludarabine versus cyclophosphamide, doxorubicin, and prednisone (CAP) for treatment of advanced-stage chronic lymphocytic leukaemia. *Lancet* 1996; **347:** 1432–8.
3. Leiby JM, *et al.* Phase II trial of 9-β-D-arabinofuranosyl-2-fluoroadenine 5′-monophosphate in non Hodgkins lymphoma: prospective comparison of response with deoxycytidine kinase activity. *Cancer Res* 1987; **47:** 2719–22.
4. Hiddemann W, Pott-Hoeck C. Fludarabine in the management of malignant lymphomas. *Drugs* 1994; **66** (suppl 6): 50–60.
5. Kuzel TM, *et al.* Mycosis fungoides: time to define the best therapy. *J Natl Cancer Inst* 1990; **82:** 183–5.
6. Agrawal S, *et al.* First report of fludarabine in gamma-heavy chain disease. *Br J Haematol* 1994; **88:** 653–5.
7. Smith OP, Mehta AB. Fludarabine monophosphate for prolymphocytic leukaemia. *Lancet* 1990; **336:** 820.
8. Kantarjian HM, *et al.* Efficacy of fludarabine, a new adenine nucleoside analogue, in patients with prolymphocytic leukemia and the prolymphocytoid variant of chronic lymphocytic leukemia. *Am J Med* 1991; **90:** 223–8.
9. Kantarjian HM, *et al.* Fludarabine therapy in hairy cell leukemia. *Cancer* 1991; **67:** 1291–3.
10. Dimopoulos MA, *et al.* Fludarabine therapy in Waldenström's macroglobulinemia. *Am J Med* 1993; **95:** 49–52.

Preparations

Proprietary Preparations (details are given in Part 3)
Austral.: Fludara; ***Belg.:*** Fludara; ***Canad.:*** Fludara; ***Fr.:*** Fludara; ***Ital.:*** Fludara; ***Neth.:*** Fludara; ***Spain:*** Beneflur; ***Swed.:*** Fludara; ***Switz.:*** Fludara; ***UK:*** Fludara; ***USA:*** Fludara.

Fluorouracil (1836-x)

Fluorouracil *(BAN, USAN, rINN)*.

5-Fluorouracil; Fluorouracilo; Fluorouracilum; 5-FU; NSC-19893; Ro-2-9757; WR-69596. 5-Fluoropyrimidine-2,4(1*H*,3*H*)-dione.

$C_4H_3FN_2O_2$ = 130.1.

CAS — 51-21-8.

Pharmacopoeias. In *Eur.* (see p.viii), *Int.*, *Jpn*, and *US*.

A white to almost white, practically odourless, crystalline powder. Sparingly **soluble** in water; slightly soluble in alcohol; practically insoluble in chloroform and ether. A 1% solution has a pH of 4.5 to 5.0. **Store** in airtight containers. Protect from light.

CAUTION. *Fluorouracil is irritant; avoid contact with skin and mucous membranes.*

Incompatibility. Preparations of fluorouracil are alkaline, and compatibility problems may be expected with acidic drugs and preparations, or those which are unstable in the presence of alkali. Fluorouracil is reported to be incompatible with cytarabine,[1] diazepam,[2] doxorubicin[2] (and presumably other anthracyclines which are unstable at alkaline pH) and calcium folinate;[3] although it has been stated to be incompatible with methotrexate[1] a study of the long-term stability of an admixture of the 2 drugs in sodium chloride (0.9%) injection suggests otherwise.[4]

1. McRae MP, King JC. Compatibility of antineoplastic, antibiotic and corticosteroid drugs in intravenous admixtures. *Am J Hosp Pharm* 1976; **33:** 1010–13.
2. Dorr RT. Incompatibilities with parenteral anticancer drugs. *Am J Intravenous Ther* 1979; **6:** 42–52.
3. Trissel LA, *et al.* Incompatibility of fluorouracil with leucovorin calcium or levoleucovorin calcium. *Am J Health-Syst Pharm* 1995; **52:** 710–15.
4. Vincké BJ, *et al.* Extended stability of 5-fluorouracil and methotrexate solutions in PVC containers. *Int J Pharmaceutics* 1989; **54:** 181–9.

Stability. Although fluorouracil has been reported to be of limited stability when dissolved in 5% glucose injection at room temperature (10% loss from solution in 43 hours when stored in polyvinyl chloride (PVC) and in only 7 hours when stored in glass),[1] other workers have found such a solution to be stable for at least 16 weeks when stored in polyvinyl chloride at 5°.[2] Results of a study of fluorouracil and methotrexate admixtures in 0.9% sodium chloride solution suggest that extended stability (up to 13 weeks) is possible in this diluent at

5° in PVC bags.[3] When stored at room temperature in PVC, solutions of fluorouracil appear to be stable but subject to evaporative loss of water, which slowly increases their concentration.[2,3] Commercial solutions of fluorouracil for injection have been reported to be stable for 7 days at 37° in a portable infusion pump, although at 25° one brand showed evidence of precipitation.[4] Fluorouracil solutions may be incompatible with synthetic elastomers: microscopic precipitation has been reported as soon as 4 hours after placement into polyisoprene reservoirs of elastomeric infusers and in polypropylene syringes with an elastomeric joint.[5] (Some authorities have questioned the validity of this finding.[6,7])

1. Benvenuto JA, *et al.* Stability and compatibility of antitumor agents in glass and plastic containers. *Am J Hosp Pharm* 1981; **38:** 1914–18.
2. Quebbeman EJ, *et al.* Stability of fluorouracil in plastic containers used for continuous infusion at home. *Am J Hosp Pharm* 1984; **41:** 1153–6.
3. Vincké B, *et al.* Extended stability of 5-fluorouracil and methotrexate solutions in PVC containers. *Int J Pharmaceutics* 1989; **54:** 181–9.
4. Stiles ML, *et al.* Stability of fluorouracil administered through four portable infusion pumps. *Am J Hosp Pharm* 1989; **46:** 2036–40.
5. Corbrion V, *et al.* Precipitation of fluorouracil in elastomeric infusers with a polyisoprene reservoir and in polypropylene syringes with an elastomeric joint. *Am J Health-Syst Pharm* 1997; **54:** 1845–8.
6. Trissel LA. Fluorouracil precipitate. *Am J Health-Syst Pharm* 1998; **55:** 1314–15.
7. Allwood MC. Fluorouracil precipitate. *Am J Health-Syst Pharm* 1998; **55;** 1315–16.

Adverse Effects and Treatment

For general discussions see Antineoplastics, p.470 and p.473.

The toxic effects of fluorouracil may be severe and sometimes fatal. The main adverse effects are on the bone marrow and the gastro-intestinal tract. Toxicity is schedule dependent: reducing the rate of injection to a slow infusion over several hours is associated with less haematological toxicity but may increase gastro-intestinal toxicity and the palmar-plantar syndrome (erythema and painful desquamation of the hands and feet). Gastro-intestinal toxicity may also be exacerbated if fluorouracil is given with folinic acid.

Leucopenia, thrombocytopenia, stomatitis, gastro-intestinal ulceration and bleeding, severe diarrhoea, or haemorrhage from any site, are signs that treatment should be stopped. The nadir of the white-cell count may occur from 7 to 20 days after a dose, and counts usually return to normal after about 30 days. Thrombocytopenia is usually at a maximum 7 to 17 days after a dose. Anaemia may also occur. Nausea and vomiting, effects on the skin including rashes and hyperpigmentation, alopecia, ocular irritation, central neurotoxicity (notably cerebellar ataxia), and myocardial ischaemia have occurred.

Local inflammatory and photosensitivity reactions have occurred following topical use.

Effects on the eyes. Systemic fluorouracil treatment has been associated with various types of ocular toxicity including several cases of excessive lachrymation and watering of the eyes,[1] in one patient associated with symptoms suggesting fibrosis of the tear duct,[1] and possibly representing local irritation due to the presence of fluorouracil in tear fluid[2] although symptoms have not always resolved on discontinuing the drug.[1] More seriously a case of bilateral total corneal epithelial erosion has been described in a patient receiving fluorouracil.[3] Optic neuropathy, culminating in near blindness, has also occurred in a patient receiving fluorouracil as part of a combination regimen.[4] Severe ulceration and corneal abscess with hyopyon has followed local injection of fluorouracil into the eye in a diabetic patient with idiopathic band keratopathy.[5]

1. Haidak DJ, *et al.* Tear-duct fibrosis (dacryostenosis) due to 5-fluorouracil. *Ann Intern Med* 1978; **88:** 657.
2. Christophidis N, *et al.* Lacrimation and 5-fluorouracil. *Ann Intern Med* 1978; **89:** 574.
3. Hirsh A, *et al.* Bilateral total corneal epithelial erosion as a side effect of cytotoxic therapy. *Br J Ophthalmol* 1990; **74:** 638.
4. Adams JW, *et al.* Recurrent acute toxic optic neuropathy secondary to 5-FU. *Cancer Treat Rep* 1984; **68:** 565–6.
5. Hickey-Dwyer M, Wishart PK. Serious corneal complication of 5-fluorouracil. *Br J Ophthalmol* 1993; **77:** 250–1.

Effects on the heart. Life-threatening cardiotoxicity (arrhythmias, ventricular tachycardia, and cardiac arrest, secondary to transmural ischaemia) has been reported to occur in 0.55% of patients given fluorouracil,[1] although the incidence of angina and less severe cardiotoxicity associated with coronary artery spasm may be higher.[1-3] Pre-existing heart disease or mediastinal radiotherapy may increase the risk as does administration by prolonged infusion, but symptoms can also occur in patients without these risk factors.[2-4] It has been suggested that the cardiotoxicity (and neurotoxicity) of fluorouracil may be due in part to conversion of an impurity, fluoroacetaldehyde, into highly toxic fluoroacetate.[5]

1. Keefe DL, *et al.* Clinical cardiotoxicity of 5-fluorouracil. *J Clin Pharmacol* 1993; **33:** 1060–70.
2. McLachlan SA, *et al.* The spectrum of 5-fluorouracil cardiotoxicity. *Med J Aust* 1994; **161:** 207–9.
3. Anand AJ. Fluorouracil cardiotoxicity. *Ann Pharmacother* 1994; **28:** 374–8.
4. Hannaford R. Sudden death associated with 5-fluorouracil. *Med J Aust* 1994; **161:** 225.
5. Lemaire L, *et al.* Fluoroacetaldehyde as cardiotoxic impurity in fluorouracil (Roche). *Lancet* 1991; **337:** 560.

Effects on the liver. For reference to hepatotoxicity following administration of fluorouracil with sparfosic acid, see p.561.

Effects on the nervous system. Central neurotoxicity, including cerebellar ataxia, confusion, disorientation, and emotional lability is reported to occur rarely in patients receiving fluorouracil, although the incidence may be increased with high-dose or intensive regimens. Patients with disorders of pyrimidine metabolism may be at increased risk of neurotoxicity.[1-3]

See also Effects on the Heart, above.

1. Tuchman M, *et al.* Familial pyrimidinemia and pyrimidinuria associated with severe fluorouracil toxicity. *N Engl J Med* 1985; **313:** 245–9.
2. Stéphan F, *et al.* Depressed hepatic dihydropyrimidine dehydrogenase activity and fluorouracil-related toxicities. *Am J Med* 1995; **99:** 685–8.
3. Takimoto C, *et al.* Reversible 5-fluorouracil-associated encephalopathy in a dihydropyrimidine dehydrogenase (DPD) deficient patient. *Clin Pharmacol Ther* 1996; **59:** 161.

Effects on the skin. In addition to reports of fluorouracil-associated dermatitis and photosensitivity a syndrome of erythema, pain, and desquamation of the skin of palms and soles has been reported[1-4] (sometimes referred to as the 'palmar-plantar erythrodysesthesia syndrome'). Although particularly associated with administration by continuous infusion[1,2] the syndrome may also occur following bolus doses.[3,4] Symptoms generally respond to discontinuation of the drug, but addition of oral pyridoxine to chemotherapy regimens has been reported to prevent or resolve symptoms,[5] as has application of a nicotine patch in one patient.[6]

Rash and confusion developing in an elderly man with malabsorption and poor nutritional intake who received fluorouracil for a biliary-tract tumour were diagnosed as pellagra.[7] Symptoms responded to nicotinic acid therapy.

1. Lokich JJ, Moore C. Chemotherapy-associated palmar-plantar erythrodysesthesia syndrome. *Ann Intern Med* 1984; **101:** 798–800.
2. Feldman LD, Ajani JA. Fluorouracil-associated dermatitis of the hands and feet. *JAMA* 1985; **254:** 3479.
3. Atkins JN. Fluorouracil and the palmar-plantar erythrodysesthesia syndrome. *Ann Intern Med* 1985; **102:** 419.
4. Curran CF, Luce JK. Fluorouracil and palmar-plantar erythrodysesthesia. *Ann Intern Med* 1989; **111:** 858.
5. Vukelja SJ, *et al.* Pyridoxine for the palmar-plantar erythrodysesthesia syndrome. *Ann Intern Med* 1989; **111:** 688–9.
6. Kingsley EC. 5-Fluorouracil dermatitis prophylaxis with a nicotine patch. *Ann Intern Med* 1994; **120:** 813.
7. Stevens HP, *et al.* Pellagra secondary to 5-fluorouracil. *Br J Dermatol* 1993; **128:** 578–80.

Treatment of adverse effects. In some studies allopurinol reduced the myelosuppressive and gastro-intestinal toxicity of fluorouracil infusion, permitting dose escalation.[1-3] With bolus dose regimens of fluorouracil allopurinol has been less successful,[4,5] largely because the dose-limiting toxicity of such regimens tends to be neurotoxicity,[6] against which allopurinol has no protective effect.

Local application of allopurinol, as a 0.1% mouthwash to prevent mucositis,[7,8] or as a 2% cream for the palmar-plantar syndrome,[9] has proved at best of modest benefit, perhaps because of poor penetration of allopurinol into the cells or low concentrations of the enzymes required to convert it to active oxypurinol.

Modest benefit in reducing fluorouracil toxicity was also reported with high-dose uridine.[10,11] Nicotine patches or pyridoxine administration have been reported to be helpful in the prevention of the palmar-plantar syndrome (see under Effects on the Skin, above).

1. Fox RM, *et al.* Allopurinol modulation of high-dose fluorouracil toxicity. *Lancet* 1979; **i:** 677.
2. Howell SB, *et al.* Modulation of 5-fluorouracil toxicity by allopurinol in man. *Cancer* 1981; **48:** 1281–9.
3. Tsavaris N, *et al.* Concomitant administration of 4-hydroxypyrazolopyrimidine (allopurinol) and high-dose continuous infusion 5-fluorouracil. *Oncology* 1990; **47:** 70–4.
4. Campbell TN, *et al.* High-dose allopurinol modulation of 5-FU toxicity: phase 1 trial of an outpatient dose schedule. *Cancer Treat Rep* 1982; **66:** 1723–7.
5. Garewal H, Ahmann F. Allopurinol and bolus fluorouracil. *N Engl J Med* 1985; **312:** 587.
6. Woolley PV, *et al.* A controlled trial of the effect of 4-hydroxypyrazolopyrimidine (allopurinol) on the toxicity of a single bolus dose of 5-fluorouracil. *J Clin Oncol* 1985; **3:** 103–9.
7. Clark PI, Slevin ML. Allopurinol mouthwashes and 5-fluorouracil induced oral toxicity. *Eur J Surg Oncol* 1985; **11:** 267–8.
8. Van der Vliet W, *et al.* Allopurinol mouthwash for prevention of fluorouracil-induced stomatitis. *Clin Pharm* 1989; **8:** 655–8.
9. Anonymous. Allopurinol cream for 5-FU side effects. *Pharm J* 1990; **245:** 359.
10. Leyva A, *et al.* Phase 1 and pharmacokinetic studies of high-dose uridine intended for rescue from 5-fluorouracil toxicity. *Cancer Res* 1984; **44:** 5928–33.
11. van Groeningen CJ, *et al.* Reversal of 5-fluorouracil-induced myelosuppression by prolonged administration of high-dose uridine. *J Natl Cancer Inst* 1989; **81:** 157–62.

Precautions

For general discussions see Antineoplastics, p.474.

Fluorouracil should be given with care to weak or malnourished patients, to those with a history of heart disease, or to those with hepatic or renal insufficiency. Mothers should not breast feed while receiving fluorouracil.

Painful burns around the parts of the face where spectacle frames rested in a patient treated with topical fluorouracil were probably due to occlusion of the drug by the frame, increasing the absorption and irritation of the treatment.[1]

1. White MD, Solomon LM. Plastic eyeglass frames and topical fluorouracil therapy. *JAMA* 1985; **253:** 3166.

Handling and disposal. Urine and faeces produced for up to 48 hours and 5 days respectively after an oral dose of fluorouracil should be handled wearing protective clothing.[1]

1. Harris J, Dodds LJ. Handling waste from patients receiving cytotoxic drugs. *Pharm J* 1985; **235:** 289–91.

Interference with diagnostic tests. Fluorouracil could interfere with diagnostic tests of thyroid function by causing rises in total thyroxine and liothyronine due to increased globulin binding.[1]

1. Ramsay I. Drug and non-thyroid induced changes in thyroid function tests. *Postgrad Med J* 1985; **61:** 375–7.

Metabolic disorders. For reference to increased neurotoxicity in patients with a defect of pyrimidine metabolism given fluorouracil, see under Effects on the Nervous System, above.

Interactions

The actions of fluorouracil may be modified by the concomitant administration of some other drugs including allopurinol, folinic acid, methotrexate, and metronidazole.

For reference to the co-administration of fluorouracil with calcium folinate, methotrexate, sparfosic acid, and thymidine in attempts to improve its activity, see under Administration, below.

Antineoplastics. For reference to the effect of fluorouracil on the action of *paclitaxel*, see p.557. For the increased risk of haemolytic-uraemic syndrome that may be seen if fluorouracil is used with *mitomycin*, see Effects on the Kidneys, under Adverse Effects of Mitomycin, p.552.

Antiprotozoals. *Metronidazole* increased the toxicity of fluorouracil in patients with colorectal cancer, apparently by reducing the clearance of the antineoplastic. No enhanced antineoplastic effect was seen with the combination *in vitro*.[1]

1. Bardakji Z, *et al.* 5-Fluorouracil–metronidazole combination therapy in metastatic colorectal cancer. *Cancer Chemother Pharmacol* 1986; **18:** 140–4.

Antivirals. Co-administration of *interferon alfa-2b* with fluorouracil has been reported to produce a marked increase in the initial plasma concentration of fluorouracil and a decrease in fluorouracil clearance.[1]

Severe leucopenia, leading to death in some cases, has been reported in patients who received fluorouracil concomitantly with *sorivudine*, an antiviral developed for herpes zoster.[2]

1. Czejka MJ, *et al.* Clinical pharmacokinetics of 5-fluorouracil: influence of the biomodulating agents interferon, dipyridamole and folic acid alone and in combination. *Arzneimittelforschung* 1993; **43:** 387–90.
2. Yawata M. Deaths due to drug interaction. *Lancet* 1993; **342:** 1166.

Gastro-intestinal drugs. Pretreatment with *cimetidine* for 4 weeks led to increased plasma concentrations of fluorouracil following intravenous and oral administration in 6 patients.[1] The effect was probably due to a combination of hepatic enzyme inhibition and reduced hepatic blood flow. No such effect was seen following single doses of cimetidine in 5 patients or pretreatment for just 1 week in 6. Care is required in patients taking both drugs simultaneously.

1. Harvey VJ, *et al.* The influence of cimetidine on the pharmacokinetics of 5-fluorouracil. *Br J Clin Pharmacol* 1984; **18:** 421–30.

Pharmacokinetics

Absorption of fluorouracil from the gastro-intestinal tract is unpredictable and fluorouracil is usually given intravenously. Little is absorbed when fluorouracil is applied to healthy skin.

After intravenous injection fluorouracil is cleared rapidly from plasma with a mean half-life of about 16 minutes. It is distributed throughout body tissues and fluids including crossing the blood-brain barrier to appear in the cerebrospinal fluid, and disappears from the plasma within about 3 hours. Within the target cell fluorouracil is converted to 5-fluorouridine monophosphate and floxuridine monophosphate, the former undergoing conversion to the triphosphate which can be incorporated into RNA while the latter inhibits thymidylate synthetase. About 15% of an intravenous dose is excreted unchanged in the urine within 6 hours. The remainder is inactivated primarily in the liver and is catabolised via dihydropyrimidine dehydrogenase similarly to endogenous uracil. A large amount is excreted as respiratory carbon dioxide; urea and other metabolites are also produced.

The plasma concentrations of fluorouracil during continuous intravenous infusion are reported to undergo circadian variations of as much as 50% of the mean, peak concentrations occurring in the middle of the night.[1] The variation may be due to a circadian variation in the activity of the enzyme dihydropyrimidine dehydrogenase in blood,[2] but striking interpatient variations in peak concentrations of fluorouracil and peak enzyme activity suggest that any adjustment of infusion times would need to be individualised.[2]

1. Petit E, *et al.* Circadian rhythm-varying plasma concentration of 5-fluorouracil during a five-day continuous venous infusion at a constant rate in cancer patients. *Cancer Res* 1988; **48:** 1676–9.

2. Harris BE, *et al.* Relationship between dihydropyrimidine dehydrogenase activity and plasma 5-fluorouracil levels with evidence for circadian variation of enzyme activity and plasma drug levels in cancer patients receiving 5-fluorouracil by protracted continuous infusion. *Cancer Res* 1990; **50:** 197–201.

Uses and Administration

Fluorouracil, a pyrimidine analogue, is an antineoplastic that acts as an antimetabolite to uracil. After intracellular conversion to the active deoxynucleotide it interferes with the synthesis of DNA by blocking the conversion of deoxyuridylic acid to thymidylic acid by the cellular enzyme thymidylate synthetase. It can also interfere with RNA synthesis. It also has immunosuppressant properties.

Fluorouracil is used alone or in combination in the adjuvant treatment of breast and gastro-intestinal cancer, and palliation of inoperable malignant neoplasms, especially those of the gastro-intestinal tract, breast, head and neck, liver, genito-urinary system, and pancreas. Its use in these malignancies is further discussed under Choice of Antineoplastic as indicated by the cross-references given below. It is often used with cyclophosphamide and methotrexate in the combination chemotherapy of breast cancer. Fluorouracil is also sometimes combined with folinic acid, which appears to increase its activity but also its toxicity (see Administration, below).

A wide range of dosage regimens has been used. As a single agent, a usual dose by intravenous injection is 12 mg per kg body-weight daily (to a maximum of 0.8 to 1 g daily) for 3 or 4 days. If there is no evidence of toxicity, this may be followed after 1 day by 6 mg per kg on alternate days for 3 or 4 further doses. An alternative schedule is to give 15 mg per kg intravenously once a week throughout the course. The course may be repeated after 4 to 6 weeks or maintenance doses of 5 to 15 mg per kg (up to a maximum of 1 g) may be given weekly.

Fluorouracil may also be given by intravenous infusion, usual doses of 15 mg per kg daily (to a maximum of 1 g daily) being infused in 500 mL of 0.9% sodium chloride or 5% glucose injection over 4 hours and repeated on successive days until toxicity occurs or a total of 12 to 15 g has been given. Continuous infusion may also be used. The course may be repeated after 4 to 6 weeks. Fluorouracil has also been given by continuous intra-arterial infusion in doses of 5 to 7.5 mg per kg daily (regional perfusion).

As an alternative to parenteral administration fluorouracil may also be given by mouth, although the parenteral route is generally preferred. The most frequent use of oral therapy is for maintenance, in which case a dose of 15 mg per kg, to a maximum of 1 g, may be given once weekly.

A variety of regimens have also been used in combination with folinic acid. One suggested regimen is 200 mg per m^2 body-surface area of folinic acid (as calcium folinate) by slow intravenous injection followed immediately by an intravenous bolus of fluorouracil 370 mg per m^2; the treatment is given daily for 5 consecutive days, and may be repeated after 21 to 28 days. Lower doses of folinic acid (20 mg per m^2) followed by fluorouracil 425 mg per m^2 have also been used. See also under Administration, below, where the use of 2-day regimen of high-dose folinic acid and fluorouracil is discussed.

The white-cell count should be determined frequently during treatment with fluorouracil and therapy stopped immediately if the count falls rapidly or falls to below 3500 per mm^3, if the platelet count falls below 100 000 per mm^3, or if severe adverse effects occur. Doses should be reduced by up to half in patients with poor nutritional status, impaired bone-marrow, hepatic, or renal function, and within 30 days of major surgery.

Fluorouracil is used topically in the treatment of solar (actinic) keratoses and other tumours and premalignant conditions of the skin including Bowen's disease and superficial basal cell carcinomas. It is usually applied as a 1 or 5% cream or as a 1 to 5% solution in propylene glycol.

Therapeutic implants containing fluorouracil in a controlled-release protein matrix are under investigation. Such a preparation, comprising fluorouracil 3% in a collagen gel basis, together with adrenaline 0.01% to enhance local retention, has been used for the treatment of condylomata acuminata (genital warts) by intralesional intradermal injection in doses of 7.5 to 30 mg of fluorouracil, depending on the size of the lesion. A total dose of 5 mL (150 mg of fluorouracil) for the entire wart burden should not be exceeded. Doses may be repeated at weekly intervals until complete response occurs, up to a maximum of 6 doses.

Administration. Co-administration of fluorouracil with various drugs has been tried in an effort to enhance its effects. Au and colleagues found no improvement in the response-rate of colorectal cancer treated with fluorouracil and *thymidine*.[1] Pretreatment with *sparfosic acid* also had little apparent value in a study by Casper and others,[2] and when given in high doses of 1 to 2 g per m^2 body-surface prevented the use of fluorouracil in full doses because of severe toxicity. However, more promising results were reported by O'Connell and co-workers with sequential administration of sparfosate sodium, thymidine, and fluorouracil[3] and these results were particularly encouraging in patients with aggressive or highly anaplastic carcinomas.

Following an initial report from Madajewicz and others that infusion of *calcium folinate* might enhance the antineoplastic effect of fluorouracil,[4] a number of studies have examined the combination.[5] Although such combinations appear to have enhanced activity the optimal regimen has yet to be determined,[6,7] and some regimens also exhibit greater toxicity,[8] particularly gastro-intestinal, which means that lower doses of fluorouracil have to be used in many patients. Nonetheless, de Gramont and colleagues[9,10] have reported good results and modest toxicity from a regimen employing folinic acid 200 mg per m^2 body-surface area, followed by fluorouracil 400 mg per m^2 as an intravenous bolus, and then continuous infusion of fluorouracil 600 mg per m^2. This dosage is given for 2 consecutive days every two weeks and has been tried in both colorectal and gastric cancer. This regimen appeared more effective and less toxic than a monthly regimen employing low-dose folinic acid (20 mg per m^2) plus fluorouracil 425 mg per m^2 by intravenous bolus, both for 5 days every 4 weeks.[14]

Interferon alfa also appears to modify the actions of fluorouracil (see also under Interactions, above), and has been investigated in combination with fluorouracil and folinic acid.[11]

Possibly improved activity has also been reported when *methotrexate* is given before fluorouracil,[6] a relatively well-tolerated combination.[12] Meta-analysis of several studies of fluorouracil preceded by methotrexate found that the combination doubled the response rate to fluorouracil in metastatic colorectal cancer and produced some survival benefits.[13] (Combination in the reverse order, i.e. methotrexate preceded by fluorouracil, may reduce methotrexate toxicity—see p.548.)

For the administration of allopurinol and uridine with fluorouracil, see under Treatment of Adverse Effects, above.

1. Au JL-S, *et al.* Clinical pharmacological studies of concurrent infusion of 5-fluorouracil and thymidine in treatment of colorectal carcinomas. *Cancer Res* 1982; **42:** 2930–7.
2. Casper ES, *et al.* Phase 1 and clinical pharmacological evaluation of biochemical modulation of 5-fluorouracil with N-(phosphonacetyl)-L-aspartic acid. *Cancer Res* 1983; **43:** 2324–9.
3. O'Connell MJ, *et al.* Clinical trial of sequential N-phosphonacetyl-L-aspartate, thymidine, and 5-fluorouracil in advanced colorectal carcinoma. *J Clin Oncol* 1984; **2:** 1133–8.
4. Madajewicz S, *et al.* Phase I-II trial of high-dose calcium leucovorin and 5-fluorouracil in advanced colorectal cancer. *Cancer Res* 1984; **44:** 4667–9.
5. Etienne M-C, *et al.* Critical factors for optimizing the 5-fluorouracil-folinic acid association in cancer chemotherapy. *Ann Oncol* 1996; **7:** 283–9.
6. Poon MA, *et al.* Biochemical modulation of fluorouracil: evidence of significant improvement of survival and quality of life in patients with advanced colorectal carcinoma. *J Clin Oncol* 1989; **7:** 1407–18.
7. Advanced Colorectal Cancer Meta-analysis Project. Modulation of fluorouracil by leucovorin in patients with advanced colorectal cancer: evidence in terms of response rate. *J Clin Oncol* 1992; **10:** 896–903.
8. Petrelli N, *et al.* The modulation of fluorouracil with leucovorin in metastatic colorectal carcinoma: a prospective randomized phase III trial. *J Clin Oncol* 1989; **7:** 1419–26.
9. de Gramont A, *et al.* High-dose folinic acid and 5-fluorouracil bolus and continuous infusion in advanced colorectal cancer. *Eur J Cancer Clin Oncol* 1988; **24:** 1499–1503.
10. Louvet C, *et al.* High-dose folinic acid, 5-fluorouracil bolus and continuous infusion in poor-prognosis patients with advanced measurable gastric cancer. *Ann Oncol* 1991; **2:** 229–30.
11. Allegra CJ. New therapeutic strategies for patients with gastrointestinal malignancies using biochemical modulation of fluorouracil. *JAMA* 1995; **273:** 236–9.
12. Benz C, *et al.* Sequential infusions of methotrexate and 5-fluorouracil in advanced cancer: pharmacology, toxicity, and response. *Cancer Res* 1985; **45:** 3354–8.
13. Advanced Colorectal Cancer Meta-analysis Project. Meta-analysis of randomized trials testing the biochemical modulation of fluorouracil by methotrexate in metastatic colorectal cancer. *J Clin Oncol* 1994; **12:** 960–9.
14. de Gramont A, *et al.* Randomized trial comparing monthly low-dose leucovorin and fluorouracil bolus with bimonthly high-dose leucovorin and fluorouracil bolus plus continuous infusion for advanced colorectal cancer: a French Intergroup study. *J Clin Oncol* 1997; **15:** 808–15.

Darier's disease. Two patients with resistant Darier's disease (see p.1073) responded to treatment with topical fluorouracil applied as a 1% cream once daily.[1] There was complete clearance of skin lesions after three weeks of treatment.

1. Knulst AC, *et al.* Topical 5-fluorouracil in the treatment of Darier's disease. *Br J Dermatol* 1995; **133:** 463–6.

Malignant neoplasms. Fluorouracil plays an important role in the adjuvant treatment of gastro-intestinal cancer, as discussed on p.487, and is part of one of the most widely used adjuvant regimens in breast cancer (p.485). It may also be employed in the management of a wide variety of other malignancies including islet-cell tumours (p.477) and gestational trophoblastic tumours (p.477), as well as cancers of the cervix (p.487), endometrium (p.487), head and neck (p.489), kidney (p.489), liver (p.489), ovary (p.491), pancreas (p.491), and prostate (p.491), and sarcomas of bone (p.495). In addition, it is sometimes applied topically as part of the management of malignant or pre-malignant lesions of the skin (p.492) and is one of a number of agents employed as sclerosants in malignant effusions (p.484).

Ocular disorders, non-malignant. GLAUCOMA. A regimen of subconjunctival injections of fluorouracil is effective in improving the outcome of glaucoma filtering surgery[1-3] in selected patients when used as an adjunct to prevent the formation of scar tissue (see p.1387). However, in view of the increased risk of late-onset conjunctival wound leaks caution has been suggested in its use in eyes with a good prognosis.[3] Although Gandolfi and Vecchi[4] recently found that fluorouracil improved the success rate of combined glaucoma filtering surgery and cataract surgery several earlier studies had failed to demonstrate any advantage.[5,6]

Intraoperative topical application of fluorouracil has been tried as an alternative to subconjunctival injection with conflicting results.[7,8]

1. Ophir A, Ticho U. A randomized study of trabeculectomy and subconjunctival administration of fluorouracil in primary glaucomas. *Arch Ophthalmol* 1992; **110:** 1072–5.
2. Goldenfeld M, *et al.* 5-Fluorouracil in initial trabeculectomy: a prospective, randomized, multicenter study. *Ophthalmology* 1994; **101:** 1024–9.

3. The Fluorouracil Filtering Surgery Study Group. Five-year follow-up of the Fluorouracil Filtering Surgery Study. *Am J Ophthalmol* 1996; **121:** 349–66.
4. Gandolfi SA, Vecchi M. 5-Fluorouracil in combined trabeculectomy and clear-cornea phacoemulsification with posterior chamber intraocular lens implantation: a one-year randomized, controlled clinical trial. *Ophthalmology* 1997; **104:** 181–6.
5. Wong PC, *et al.* 5-Fluorouracil after primary combined filtration surgery. *Am J Ophthalmol* 1994; **117:** 149–54.
6. O'Grady JM, *et al.* Trabeculectomy, phacoemulsification, and posterior chamber lens implantation with and without 5-fluorouracil. *Am J Ophthalmol* 1993; **116:** 594–9.
7. Egbert PR, *et al.* A prospective trial of intraoperative fluorouracil during trabeculectomy in a black population. *Am J Ophthalmol* 1993; **116:** 612–16.
8. Lachkar Y, *et al.* Trabeculectomy with intraoperative sponge 5-fluorouracil in Afro-Caribbeans. *Br J Ophthalmol* 1997; **81:** 555–8.

RETINAL DETACHMENT. Subconjunctival or intravitreal injection of fluorouracil has been found useful in preventing further retinal detachment in patients who had undergone retinal re-attachment surgery for proliferative vitreoretinopathy;[1] doses were 10 mg subconjunctivally or 1 mg intravitreally, repeated up to 5 times if necessary.

1. Blumenkranz M, *et al.* 5-Fluorouracil: new applications in complicated retinal detachment for an established antimetabolite. *Ophthalmology* 1984; **91:** 122–30.

Toxoplasmosis. For mention of the use of fluorouracil with clindamycin to treat cerebral toxoplasmosis, see p.576.

Warts. Fluorouracil has been used in wart treatment as a 5% cream, which should be applied accurately to the wart daily and covered with a waterproof dressing. It is not always successful and should be used, with care, only under exceptional circumstances.[1] Some authorities have claimed success using fluorouracil without a covering in the treatment of plane warts. For a discussion of the various agents, including cytotoxics such as fluorouracil employed to produce destruction of warts, see p.1076.

Fluorouracil has also been used, as a 1% or more usually a 5% cream or solution in the treatment of genital warts (condylomata acuminata),[2-5] and has been tried as an adjuvant to laser therapy in severe papillomavirus-associated vulvar disease,[6] with variable results. A preparation of fluorouracil 3% in a collagen gel basis, together with adrenaline as a local vasoconstrictor, has been tried for the injection of genital warts.[7]

1. Anderson FE. Warts: fact and fiction. *Drugs* 1985; **30:** 368–75.
2. Adler MW, Mindel A. Genital infections. *Br Med Bull* 1985; **41:** 361–6.
3. Anonymous. Interferon for treatment of genital warts. *Med Lett Drugs Ther* 1988; **30:** 70–2.
4. Davis AJ, Emans SJ. Human papilloma virus infection in the pediatric and adolescent patient. *J Pediatr* 1989; **115:** 1–9.
5. Pride GL. Treatment of large lower genital tract condylomata acuminata with topical 5-fluorouracil. *J Reprod Med* 1990; **35:** 384–7.
6. Reid R, *et al.* Superficial laser vulvectomy IV: extended laser vaporization and adjunctive 5-fluorouracil therapy of human papillomavirus-associated vulvar disease. *Obstet Gynecol* 1990; **76:** 439–48.
7. Anonymous. Injectable gel for genital warts. *Pharm J* 1996; **257:** 13.

Preparations

BP 1998: Fluorouracil Cream; Fluorouracil Injection;
USP 23: Fluorouracil Cream; Fluorouracil Injection; Fluorouracil Topical Solution.

Proprietary Preparations (details are given in Part 3)
Austral.: Efudix†; Fluoroplex; ***Belg.:*** Efudix; Fluroblastine; ***Canad.:*** Adrucil; Efudex; Fluoroplex; ***Fr.:*** Efudix; ***Ger.:*** Actino-Hermal; Cytosafe†; Efudix; Fluroblastin; Ribofluor; ***Irl.:*** Efudix; ***Ital.:*** Efudix; ***Neth.:*** Efudix; ***Norw.:*** Flurablastin; Fluracedyl; ***S.Afr.:*** Efudix; Fluroblastin; ***Spain:*** Efudix; ***Swed.:*** Flurablastin; Fluracedyl; ***Switz.:*** Efudix; Fluroblastine†; ***UK:*** AccuSite†; Efudix; ***USA:*** Adrucil; Efudex; Fluoroplex.

Multi-ingredient: ***Ger.:*** Verrumal; ***Switz.:*** Verrumal.

Flutamide (9050-b)

Flutamide *(BAN, USAN, rINN).*

Sch-13521. α',α',α'-Trifluoro-4'-nitroisobutyro-*m*-toluidide; α,α,α-Trifluoro-2-methyl-4'-nitro-*m*-propionotoluidide.

$C_{11}H_{11}F_3N_2O_3$ = 276.2.

CAS — 13311-84-7.

Pharmacopoeias. In *US.*

A pale yellow, crystalline powder. Practically **insoluble** in water and in petroleum spirit; freely soluble in acetone, in ethyl acetate, and in methyl alcohol; soluble in chloroform and in ether. **Store** in airtight containers. Protect from light.

Adverse Effects and Precautions

The most frequently reported adverse effects with flutamide are reversible gynaecomastia or breast tenderness, sometimes accompanied by galactorrhoea. Nausea, vomiting, diarrhoea, increased appetite, and sleep disturbances may occur. There have been reports of skin reactions, including epidermal necrolysis, and of liver damage, sometimes fatal. Other adverse effects reported in patients receiving flutamide include anaemias, haemolysis, headache, dizziness, malaise, blurred vision, anxiety, depression, decreased libido, and hypertension.

Flutamide should be used with care in patients with cardiovascular disease because of the possibility of fluid retention. Periodic liver function testing is recommended: therapy should be discontinued or dosage reduced if there is evidence of hepatotoxicity.

Effects on the blood. A report of methaemoglobinaemia attributed to flutamide.[1]

1. Schott AM, *et al.* Flutamide-induced methemoglobinemia. *DICP Ann Pharmacother* 1991; **25:** 600–1.

Effects on the liver. Hart and Stricker[1] reported hepatitis developing in a 79-year-old man receiving flutamide 750 mg daily as sole therapy following a prostatectomy, but a study by Gomez and others[2] in 1091 patients receiving flutamide 250 mg three times daily as part of a regimen for prostate cancer found marked signs of liver damage only in 4, of whom only 2 had clinical evidence of liver toxicity. In the USA, the Food and Drug Administration had received 19 reports of serious hepatotoxicity associated with flutamide up to March 1991. Of these patients, 5 died from progressive liver disease.[3]

1. Hart W, Stricker BHC. Flutamide and hepatitis. *Ann Intern Med* 1989; **110:** 943–4.
2. Gomez J-L, *et al.* Incidence of liver toxicity associated with the use of flutamide in prostate cancer patients. *Am J Med* 1992; **92:** 465–70.
3. Wysowski DK, *et al.* Fatal and nonfatal hepatotoxicity associated with flutamide. *Ann Intern Med* 1993; **118:** 860–4.

Effects on the skin. A report of photosensitivity reactions in 2 patients receiving flutamide.[1]

1. Fujimoto M, *et al.* Photosensitive dermatitis induced by flutamide. *Br J Dermatol* 1996; **135:** 496–7.

Interactions

For mention of an interaction between warfarin and flutamide, see p.967.

Pharmacokinetics

Flutamide is reported to be rapidly and completely absorbed from the gastro-intestinal tract with peak plasma concentrations occurring 1 hour after a dose. It is rapidly and extensively metabolised; the major metabolite (2-hydroxyflutamide) possesses anti-androgenic properties. The half-life of the metabolite is about 6 hours. Both flutamide and 2-hydroxyflutamide are more than 90% bound to plasma proteins. Excretion is predominantly in the urine with only minor amounts appearing in the faeces.

References.

1. Radwanski E, *et al.* Single and multiple dose pharmacokinetic evaluation of flutamide in normal geriatric volunteers. *J Clin Pharmacol* 1989; **29:** 554–8.

Uses and Administration

Flutamide is a nonsteroidal compound reported to have anti-androgenic properties which appears to act by inhibiting the uptake and/or binding of androgens in target tissues. It is used, usually in combination with gonadorelin analogues, in the palliative treatment of prostatic carcinoma (p.491). The usual dose by mouth is 250 mg three times daily. When used in combination therapy the UK manufacturers recommend that flutamide treatment be started at least 3 days before the gonadorelin analogue to suppress any 'flare' reaction; however, in the USA the manufacturers recommend beginning treatment with both agents simultaneously for optimum effect.

A topical formulation of flutamide has been investigated in the treatment of acne.

Congenital adrenal hyperplasia. For mention of the use of flutamide with testolactone to block androgenic effects in congenital adrenal hyperplasia, see p.1020.

Hirsutism. Anti-androgens (usually cyproterone or spironolactone) are widely used for the drug treatment of hirsutism (p.1441). Flutamide has no particular advantage in this context;[1,2] one study has found flutamide to be more effective than spironolactone in inhibiting hirsutism,[3] but another found them to be of similar efficacy,[4] and the risk of hepatotoxicity with flutamide is a problem.[2]

1. Rittmaster RS. Hyperandrogenism—what is normal? *N Engl J Med* 1992; **327:** 194–6.
2. Rittmaster RS. Hirsutism. *Lancet* 1997; **349:** 191–5.
3. Cusan L, *et al.* Comparison of flutamide and spironolactone in the treatment of hirsutism: a randomized controlled trial. *Fertil Steril* 1994; **61:** 281–7.
4. Erenus M, *et al.* Comparison of the efficacy of spironolactone versus flutamide in the treatment of hirsutism. *Fertil Steril* 1994; **61:** 613–6.

Malignant neoplasms. Androgen blockade, which may include the use of flutamide, is used in the management of metastatic hormone-responsive prostate cancer (p.491); once the cancer begins to progress despite such therapy, discontinuation of flutamide occasionally produces paradoxical disease regression. Promising results have also followed the use of flutamide in patients with adenocarcinoma of the pancreas (p.491).

Preparations

USP 23: Flutamide Capsules.

Proprietary Preparations (details are given in Part 3)
Aust.: Fugerel; ***Austral.:*** Eulexin; Fugerel; ***Belg.:*** Eulexin; ***Canad.:*** Euflex; ***Fr.:*** Eulexine; ***Ger.:*** Apimid; Fluta-Gry; Flutamex; Fugerel; Prostogenat; Testac; Testotard; ***Irl.:*** Drogenil; ***Ital.:*** Drogenil; Eulexin; ***Neth.:*** Drogenil; Eulexin; ***Norw.:*** Eulexin; ***S.Afr.:*** Eulexin; ***Spain:*** Eulexin; Grisetin; Oncosal; Prostacur; ***Swed.:*** Eulexin; Flutacan; ***Switz.:*** Flucinome; ***UK:*** Chimax; Drogenil; ***USA:*** Eulexin.

Formestane (19307-g)

Formestane *(BAN, rINN).*

CGP-32349; 4-Hydroxyandrostenedione; 4-OHA; 4-OHAD. 4-Hydroxyandrost-4-ene-3,17-dione.

$C_{19}H_{26}O_3$ = 302.4.

CAS — 566-48-3.

Adverse Effects, Treatment, and Precautions

The most frequent adverse effects of formestane are local irritation and pain at the site of injection. Patients may experience hot flushes due to oestrogen deprivation. Other adverse effects include rashes, drowsiness, dizziness, emotional lability, oedema of the leg, thrombophlebitis, vaginal spotting or bleeding, gastro-intestinal disturbances, muscle cramps, arthralgia, and a vasovagal reaction. Hypersensitivity reactions to the drug or the formulation have occurred.

Care should be taken to avoid intravascular injection. Injection into or near the sciatic nerve may result in pain and nerve trauma. Caution is required if patients drive or operate machinery.

Effects on carbohydrate metabolism. Recurrent hypoglycaemic episodes developed in a diabetic patient previously well maintained on gliclazide following addition of formestane to treatment for metastatic breast cancer.[1] Episodic hypoglycaemia continued following dosage reduction, and eventually withdrawal, of gliclazide, suggesting that the effect was not simply an interaction with the sulphonylurea.

1. Brankin E, *et al.* Hypoglycaemia associated with formestane treatment. *Br Med J* 1997; **314:** 869.

Pharmacokinetics

Following intramuscular administration formestane is reported to form a depot which slowly releases active drug into the systemic circulation; maximum plasma concentrations occur about 30 to 48 hours after a single dose and then decline fairly rapidly over 2 to 4 days before declining more slowly, with an apparent elimination half-life of 5 to 6 days. The systemic uptake has been estimated at 20 to 25% of the dose in 14 days. Formestane is about 85% bound to plasma protein in the circulation. It is metabolised by conjugation to the inactive glucuronide: less than 1% of the dose is excreted in urine unchanged.

Uses and Administration

Formestane is an inhibitor of the aromatase (oestrogen synthetase) system which is responsible for the production of oestrogens from androgens. It is used for its anti-oestrogenic properties in the adjuvant endocrine treatment of breast cancer (p.485).

It is given by intramuscular injection, as an aqueous suspension, in doses of 250 mg every 2 weeks. Injections should be given into each buttock alternately.

Reviews.

1. Wiseman LR, McTavish D. Formestane: a review of its pharmacodynamic and pharmacokinetic properties and therapeutic potential in the management of breast cancer and prostatic cancer. *Drugs* 1993; **45:** 66–84.
2. Anonymous. Formestane for advanced breast cancer in postmenopausal women. *Drug Ther Bull* 1993; **31:** 85–7.

Preparations

Proprietary Preparations (details are given in Part 3)
Aust.: Lentaron; ***Belg.:*** Lentaron; ***Canad.:*** Lentaron; ***Fr.:*** Lentaron; ***Ger.:*** Lentaron; ***Irl.:*** Lentaron; ***Ital.:*** Lentaron; ***Neth.:*** Lentaron; ***S.Afr.:*** Lentare; ***Spain:*** Lentaron; ***Switz.:*** Lentaron; ***UK:*** Lentaron.

Fotemustine (3682-e)

Fotemustine *(BAN, rINN).*

S-10036. (±)-Diethyl {1-[3-(2-chloroethyl)-3-nitrosoureido]ethyl}phosphonate.

$C_9H_{19}ClN_3O_5P = 315.7$.

CAS — 92118-27-9.

Fotemustine is a nitrosourea derivative (see Carmustine, p.511). It is used in the treatment of disseminated malignant melanoma, particularly where cerebral metastases are present (p.492) and has been tried in primary malignancies of the brain (p.485). It is given by intravenous infusion in usual doses of 100 mg per m^2 body-surface weekly for 3 weeks to induce remission, followed after 4 to 6 weeks, if blood counts permit, by maintenance dosage with 100 mg per m^2 every 3 weeks. Regular blood counts should be taken and treatment withheld if granulocyte counts are below 2000 per mm^3 or platelet counts less than 100 000 per mm^3. Bone-marrow suppression may be delayed, with the nadir of the white-cell counts 5 or 6 weeks after administration.

References.

1. Ings RMJ, *et al.* The pharmacokinetics and metabolism of [^{14}C]-fotemustine in cancer patients. *Br J Clin Pharmacol* 1989; **28:** 238P.
2. Avril M-F, *et al.* Combination chemotherapy of dacarbazine and fotemustine in disseminated malignant melanoma: experience of the French Study Group. *Cancer Chemother Pharmacol* 1990; **27:** 81–4.

Preparations

Proprietary Preparations (details are given in Part 3)
Aust.: Muphoran; ***Fr.:*** Muphoran.

Gemcitabine Hydrochloride

(12197-g)

Gemcitabine Hydrochloride *(BANM, USAN, rINNM).*

LY-188011 (gemcitabine). 4-Amino-1-(2-deoxy-2,2-difluoro-β-D-ribofuranosyl)pyrimidin-2(1*H*)-one hydrochloride; 2′-Deoxy-2′,2′-difluorocytidine hydrochloride.

$C_9H_{11}F_2N_3O_4,HCl = 299.7$.

CAS — 95058-81-4 (gemcitabine); 122111-03-9 (gemcitabine hydrochloride).

Gemcitabine hydrochloride 1.14 mg is approximately equivalent to 1 mg of gemcitabine.

Adverse Effects, Treatment, and Precautions

As for Cytarabine, p.525, although gemcitabine maybe somewhat better tolerated, with myelotoxicity reported to be modest even at high doses. Oedema (including pulmonary oedema), hypotension, and alopecia have also been reported. Gemcitabine may produce somnolence: patients so affected should not drive or operate machinery. Severe toxicity, in the form of potentially life-threatening oesophagitis and pneumonitis has been seen in patients given radical radiotherapy to the thorax in association with gemcitabine. It should be used with caution in patients with impaired renal or hepatic function. Haemolytic-uraemic syndrome has been reported and has led to irreversible renal failure; gemcitabine should be discontinued at the first signs of microangiopathic haemolytic anaemia.

Effects on the nervous system. A report of autonomic neuropathy associated with gemcitabine therapy.[1] Symptoms resolved 4 weeks after stopping therapy.

1. Dormann AJ, *et al.* Gemcitabine-associated autonomic neuropathy. *Lancet* 1998; **351:** 644.

Pharmacokinetics

Following intravenous administration gemcitabine is rapidly cleared from the blood and metabolised by cytidine deaminase in the liver, kidney, blood, and other tissues. Clearance is approximately 30% lower in women than in men. Almost all of the dose is excreted in urine as 2′-deoxy-2′,2′-difluorouridine (dFdU), only about 1% being found in the faeces. Intracellular metabolism produces mono-, di-, and triphosphate metabolites, the latter two active. The mean terminal half-life of gemcitabine is 17 minutes; the intracellular half-life of the triphosphate is stated to range from 0.7 to 12 hours.

Uses and Administration

Gemcitabine is an analogue of cytarabine (p.525) which is metabolised intracellularly to active diphosphate and triphosphate nucleosides, which inhibit DNA synthesis and induce apoptosis. It is primarily active against cells in S-phase. It is given in the management of solid tumours including those of the lung and pancreas (see p.490 and p.491, respectively). It is also being tried in cancers of the bladder, breast, and ovary.

Gemcitabine is given intravenously as the hydrochloride; doses are calculated in terms of the base. Doses are reconstituted in sodium chloride 0.9% injection. The concentration of the infusion solution should not exceed the equivalent of 40 mg of gemcitabine per mL. The recommended initial dose is the equivalent of 1 g of gemcitabine per m^2 body-surface, by infusion over 30 minutes. The dose may be repeated at weekly intervals adjusted according to response and toxicity. In the treatment of non-small cell lung cancer, doses are given once weekly for 3 weeks, followed by a one-week rest period. In the treatment of pancreatic cancer, an initial course of up to 7 doses at weekly intervals may be given, followed after a one-week recovery period by a regimen of infusions once weekly for 3 consecutive weeks out of 4.

References.

1. Cormier Y, *et al.* Gemcitabine is an active new agent in previously untreated extensive small cell lung cancer (SCLC): a study of the National Cancer Institute of Canada Clinical Trials Group. *Ann Oncol* 1994; **5:** 283–5.
2. Casper ES, *et al.* Phase II trial of gemcitabine (2,2′-difluorodeoxycytidine) in patients with adenocarcinoma of the pancreas. *Invest New Drugs* 1994; **12:** 29–34.
3. Anonymous. Gemcitabine for lung cancer. *Drug Ther Bull* 1996; **34:** 71–2.
4. Anonymous. Gemcitabine for treatment of pancreatic cancer. *Med Lett Drugs Ther* 1996; **38:** 102.
5. Hui YF, Reitz J. Gemcitabine: a cytidine analogue active against solid tumors. *Am J Health-Syst Pharm* 1997; **54:** 162–70.
6. Noble S, Goa KL. Gemcitabine: a review of its pharmacology and clinical potential in non-small cell lung cancer and pancreatic cancer. *Drugs* 1997; **54:** 447–72.

Preparations

Proprietary Preparations (details are given in Part 3)
Aust.: Gemzar; ***Austral.:*** Gemzar; ***Fr.:*** Gemzar; ***Ger.:*** Gemzar; ***Ital.:*** Gemzar; ***Neth.:*** Gemzar; ***Norw.:*** Gemzar; ***S.Afr.:*** Gemzar; ***Spain:*** Gemzar; ***Swed.:*** Gemzar; ***UK:*** Gemzar; ***USA:*** Gemzar.

Gusperimus Hydrochloride (3060-b)

Gusperimus Hydrochloride *(rINNM).*

BMS-181173; BMY-42215-1; Deoxyspergualin Hydrochloride; 15-Deoxyspergualin Hydrochloride; Gusperimus Trihydrochloride *(USAN)*; NKT-01; NSC-356894. (±)-*N*-[({4-[(3-Aminopropyl)amino]butyl}carbamoyl)hydroxymethyl]-7-guanidinoheptanamide trihydrochloride.

$C_{17}H_{37}N_7O_3,3HCl = 496.9$.

CAS — 104317-84-2 (gusperimus); 89149-10-0 (gusperimus); 85468-01-5 (gusperimus hydrochloride).

Gusperimus is a guanidine derivative with immunosuppressant activity. It inhibits both cell-mediated and antibody-mediated immunity. It is used in the treatment of graft rejection and has been investigated in the management of graft-versus-host disease. For mention of its role in reversing acute graft rejection in kidney transplantation, see p.499, while reference is made to the use of gusperimus in islet-cell transplantation on p.501.

Gusperimus is used as the hydrochloride. A dose of 3 to 5 mg of gusperimus hydrochloride per kg body-weight daily for 7 days, given by intravenous infusion over 3 hours, has been suggested in the treatment of acute renal graft rejection. Treatment may be continued for a further 3 days if required.

Adverse effects reported with gusperimus include bone-marrow depression, numbness of face and extremities, headache, gastro-intestinal disturbances, alterations in liver enzyme values, and facial flushing. Rapid injection should be avoided as studies in *animals* suggest that excessive plasma concentrations associated with bolus administration may produce hypotension and respiratory depression.

References.

1. Amemiya H, *et al.* A novel rescue drug, 15-deoxyspergualin: first clinical trials for recurrent graft rejection in renal recipients. *Transplantation* 1990; **49:** 337–43.
2. Suzuki S, *et al.* Clinical application of 15-deoxyspergualin for treatment of acute graft rejection following renal transplantation. *Transplant Proc* 1990; **22:** 1615–17.
3. Groth CG, *et al.* Deoxyspergualin for liver graft rejection. *Lancet* 1990; **336:** 626.
4. Gores PF, *et al.* Insulin independence in type 1 diabetes after transplantation of unpurified islets from single donor with 15-deoxyspergualin. *Lancet* 1993; **341:** 19–21.
5. Matas AJ, *et al.* Pilot evaluation of 15-deoxyspergualin for refractory acute renal transplant rejection. *Clin Transplant* 1994; **8:** 116–19.
6. Chan G, *et al.* Pharmacokinetics of deoxyspergualin in repeat renal transplant patients. *Clin Pharmacol Ther* 1995; **57:** 219.

Preparations

Proprietary Preparations (details are given in Part 3)
Jpn: Spanidin.

Homoharringtonine (19300-f)

NSC-141633. Cephalotaxine 2-(methoxycarbonylmethyl)-2,6-dihydroxy-5-methylheptanoate.

$C_{29}H_{39}NO_9 = 545.6$.

Pharmacopoeias. In *Chin.*

Adverse Effects

Severe hypotension may occur, particularly after bolus injection and may be dose limiting. Tachycardia and cardiac arrhythmias, bone-marrow suppression, gastro-intestinal disturbances, alopecia, rash, myalgia, and hyperglycaemia have also been reported.

Effects on carbohydrate metabolism. Results in a patient who developed hyperglycaemia during continuous infusions of homoharringtonine indicated that the effect appeared to be due to induction of insulin resistance, and might persist for some time after therapy.[1] Hyperglycaemia associated with homoharringtonine seems to be fairly frequent, and may be more likely in adults and in those receiving doses above 5 mg per m^2 body-surface.

1. Sylvester RK, *et al.* Homoharringtonine-induced hyperglycemia. *J Clin Oncol* 1989; **7:** 392–5.

Uses and Administration

Homoharringtonine is an alkaloid derived from the tree *Cephalotaxus harringtonia*, and related species. It is thought to act at the ribosome to inhibit protein synthesis and is most active against cells in stage G_1. It has been tried as an antineoplastic in the treatment of acute non-lymphoblastic leukaemias (p.479) and other neoplastic disorders. Some benefit has also been seen in chronic myeloid leukaemia (p.480). A variety of dosage regimens have been employed. One regimen that has been recommended involves continuous infusion of homoharringtonine over 8 days, an initial dose of 3.5 mg per m^2 body-surface being given over the first 24 hours and then 6 mg per m^2 daily on days 2 to 8.

The related compounds harringtonine, isoharringtonine, and deoxyharringtonine have also been investigated.

The properties and uses of some naturally-derived antineoplastics, including homoharringtonine have been reviewed by Slichenmyer and Von Hoff.[1] Studies indicate that it is active in the treatment of acute non-lymphoblastic leukaemia, and complete remissions have been seen in a few patients. In contrast results in solid tumours have been generally disappointing, although there is some evidence to suggest that more prolonged administration (over 7 or more days) might give better results.

1. Slichenmyer WJ, Von Hoff DD. New natural products in cancer chemotherapy. *J Clin Pharmacol* 1990; **30:** 770–88.

Hydroxyurea (1839-d)

Hydroxyurea *(BAN, USAN)*.

Hydroxycarbamide *(rINN)*; NSC-32065; SQ-1089; WR-83799.

$NH_2.CO.NHOH$ = 76.05.

CAS — 127-07-1.

Pharmacopoeias. In *Br., Fr.,* and *US.*

A white to off-white, odourless or almost odourless, crystalline powder. It is hygroscopic and decomposes in the presence of moisture. Freely **soluble** in water and hot alcohol. **Store** in airtight containers in a dry atmosphere.

Adverse Effects, Treatment, and Precautions

For general discussions see Antineoplastics, p.470, p.473, and p.474.

Bone-marrow suppression, including megaloblastic changes, is the main adverse effect of hydroxyurea. The erythema caused by irradiation may be exacerbated by hydroxyurea. Other side-effects reported have included gastro-intestinal disturbances, impairment of renal function, pulmonary oedema, mild dermatological reactions, alopecia, and neurological reactions such as headache, dizziness, drowsiness, disorientation, hallucinations, and convulsions.

If anaemia occurs, it may be corrected by transfusions of whole blood without stopping therapy. Megaloblastic changes are usually self-limiting.

Hydroxyurea should be used with caution in patients with impaired renal function. The elderly may be more sensitive to the adverse effects of hydroxyurea. Pre-existing anaemia should be corrected before beginning therapy with hydroxyurea.

Effects on the liver. A report of self-limited hepatitis and a flu-like syndrome in a patient receiving hydroxyurea.[1] Symptoms recurred when the patient was rechallenged with the drug.

1. Heddle R, Calvert AF. Hydroxyurea induced hepatitis. *Med J Aust* 1980; **1:** 121.

Effects on the skin. Reports of skin reactions with hydroxyurea include one of reversible hyperpigmentation in 2 patients of African origin receiving hydroxyurea in high doses for chronic myeloid leukaemia.[1] Hyperpigmentation of the nails has also been reported.[2]

Hydroxyurea therapy may also be associated with scaly erythematous skin lesions resembling those of dermatomyositis.[3,4] Such lesions usually occur after several years of hydroxyurea treatment and the course is usually benign. However, withdrawal of hydroxyurea is obligatory if lesions become painful or ulcerated, in which case resolution may take several months. Ulceration may recur on rechallenge.[5]

1. Majumdar G, *et al.* Reversible hyperpigmentation associated with high dose hydroxyurea. *Br Med J* 1990; **300:** 1468.
2. Adams-Graves P, *et al.* Hydroxyurea in sickle cell disease. *N Engl J Med* 1996; **334:** 333–4.
3. Senet P, *et al.* Hydroxyurea-induced dermatomyositis-like eruption. *Br J Dermatol* 1995; **133:** 455–9.
4. Bahadoran P, *et al.* Pseudo-dermatomyositis induced by long-term hydroxyurea therapy: report of two cases. *Br J Dermatol* 1996; **134:** 1161–2.
5. Best PJ, *et al.* Hydroxyurea-induced leg ulceration in 14 patients. *Ann Intern Med* 1998; **128:** 29–32.

Effects on the vascular system. Acral erythema occurred in a patient given hydroxyurea as part of the treatment of chronic myeloid leukaemia.[1] Symptoms resolved on discontinuation of hydroxyurea and treatment with indomethacin, but recurred with greater severity when hydroxyurea was restarted at a lower dose.

1. Silver FS, *et al.* Acral erythema and hydroxyurea. *Ann Intern Med* 1983; **98:** 675.

Handling and disposal. Urine produced for up to 48 hours after a dose of hydroxyurea should be handled wearing protective clothing.[1]

1. Harris J, Dodds LJ. Handling waste from patients receiving cytotoxic drugs. *Pharm J* 1985; **235:** 289–91.

Pharmacokinetics

Hydroxyurea is readily absorbed from the gastro-intestinal tract and distributed throughout the body. Peak plasma concentrations are reached within 2 hours. Hydroxyurea is metabolised by the liver, and excreted in urine as urea and unchanged drug. Some is excreted as carbon dioxide via the lungs. About 80% of a dose is reported to be excreted in the urine within 12 hours. It crosses the blood-brain barrier.

Uses and Administration

Hydroxyurea is an antineoplastic that may act by inhibition of DNA synthesis. It is S-phase specific. Hydroxyurea is used, as indicated by the cross-references below, in the treatment of chronic myeloid leukaemia, in non-Hodgkin's lymphoma, and in polycythaemia vera and thrombocythaemia. Hydroxyurea has been tried, often combined with radiotherapy, in some solid malignancies such as gestational trophoblastic tumours, and its use has been advocated in tumours of the cervix, head and neck, and ovary.

Hydroxyurea has also been found to be of benefit in the haemoglobinopathies, particularly in sickle-cell disease (see below).

In the treatment of malignancies, hydroxyurea is given by mouth in a single dose of 20 to 30 mg per kg body-weight daily or in a single dose of 60 to 80 mg per kg every third day. If a beneficial effect is evident after 6 weeks, therapy may be continued indefinitely. In sickle-cell disease initial doses of 15 mg per kg daily are suggested, increased if necessary according to response and blood counts.

The haemoglobin concentration, white-cell and platelet counts, and hepatic and renal function should be determined repeatedly during treatment. Treatment should be interrupted if the white-cell count drops to 2500 per mm^3 or the platelet count to 100 000 per mm^3.

Haemoglobinopathies. Hydroxyurea is considered a promising therapy in the treatment of the haemoglobinopathies. Hydroxyurea can stimulate fetal haemoglobin production,[1,2] which in turn can reduce the tendency for haemoglobin polymerisation.[3,4] Initial studies in patients with sickle-cell disease (p.703) demonstrated responses, but not clinical benefit.[5-7] However, a more recent controlled study produced evidence that hydroxyurea in initial doses of 15 mg per kg daily, adjusted according to response and tolerance to up to 35 mg per kg daily, reduced the rate of sickle-cell crisis compared with placebo.[8] Despite some concerns about the administration of a potential carcinogen to children, preliminary studies in paediatric populations have also reported evidence of benefit.[9,10] A report in 2 adult patients has suggested that hydroxyurea might reverse splenic dysfunction.[11]

It has been suggested that combination of hydroxyurea with erythropoietin might enhance the production of fetal haemoglobin, but results from studies of the combination have been conflicting.[12,13]

There appear to have been few studies of hydroxyurea specifically in thalassaemia (p.704). However hydroxyurea in initial doses of 8.2 to 10.3 mg per kg daily by mouth, increased until toxicity occurred did produce increases in fetal haemoglobin in 3 patients, but these were not sustained.[14] There is a report of sustained responses to therapy with sodium phenylbutyrate and hydroxyurea in 2 siblings with thalassaemia major.[15]

1. Letvin NL, *et al.* Augmentation of fetal-hemoglobin production in anemic monkeys by hydroxyurea. *N Engl J Med* 1984; **310:** 869–73.
2. Veith R, *et al.* Stimulation of F-cell production in patients with sickle-cell anemia treated with cytarabine or hydroxyurea. *N Engl J Med* 1985; **313:** 1571–5.
3. Adamson JW. Hemoglobin—from F to A, and back. *N Engl J Med* 1984; **310:** 917–19.
4. Marwick C. Sickle cell problems continue to challenge medical science, but some progress is noted. *JAMA* 1990; **263:** 490, 3.
5. Rodgers GP, *et al.* Hematologic responses of patients with sickle cell disease to treatment with hydroxyurea. *N Engl J Med* 1990; **322:** 1037–45.
6. Rodgers GP. Recent approaches to the treatment of sickle cell anemia. *JAMA* 1991; **265:** 2097–2101.
7. Charache S, *et al.* Hydroxyurea: effects on hemoglobin F production in patients with sickle cell anemia. *Blood* 1992; **79:** 2555–65.
8. Charache S, *et al.* Effect of hydroxyurea on the frequency of painful crises in sickle cell anemia. *N Engl J Med* 1995; **332:** 1317–22.
9. Scott JP, *et al.* Hydroxyurea therapy in children severely affected with sickle cell disease. *J Pediatr* 1996; **128:** 820–8.
10. Jayabose S, *et al.* Clinical and hematologic effects of hydroxyurea in children with sickle cell anemia. *J Pediatr* 1996; **129:** 559–65.
11. Claster S, Vichinsky E. First report of reversal of organ dysfunction in sickle cell anemia by the use of hydroxyurea: splenic regeneration. *Blood* 1996; **88:** 1951–3.
12. Goldberg MA, *et al.* Treatment of sickle cell anemia with hydroxyurea and erythropoietin. *N Engl J Med* 1990; **323:** 366–72.
13. Rodgers GP, *et al.* Augmentation by erythropoietin of the fetal-hemoglobin response to hydroxyurea in sickle-cell disease. *N Engl J Med* 1993; **328:** 73–80.
14. Hajjar FM, Pearson HA. Pharmacologic treatment of thalassemia intermedia with hydroxyurea. *J Pediatr* 1994; **125:** 490–2.
15. Olivieri NF, *et al.* Treatment of thalassaemia major with phenylbutyrate and hydroxyurea. *Lancet* 1997; **350:** 491–2.

HIV infection and AIDS. Studies *in vitro* indicate that hydroxyurea (and other hydroxamates) act synergistically with didanosine (p.607) to suppress the replication of HIV and prevent its cytopathic effects.[1,2] A number of studies of such a combination are in progress. In 25 HIV-positive patients given didanosine 200 mg twice daily, together with hydroxyurea 15 mg per kg body-weight daily in 2 divided doses, all patients showed a drop in viral load and an increase in CD4+ lymphocyte count.[3] Viraemia was not detectable in 13 of 24 patients evaluated at 6 months and 10 of 20 patients evaluated at 1 year. In 2 of these patients who subsequently received no antiviral treatments for 1 year there was no viral rebound, although some proviral DNA was detected.[4] In another study in 6 patients, didanosine 200 mg twice daily together with hydroxyurea 250 mg four times daily (suggested to be a better regimen because of the short half-life of hydroxyurea) produced a sharp decrease in viraemia, which was maintained for up to 72 weeks.[5] A rebound occurred in 1 patient on interrupting treatment but viral replication was again suppressed when treatment was restarted. Combination of hydroxyurea with didanosine and indinavir has also been tried.[6] For further discussion of the management of HIV infection and AIDS, see p.599.

1. Lori F, *et al.* Hydroxyurea as an inhibitor of human immunodeficiency virus-type 1 replication. *Science* 1994; **266:** 801–5.
2. Malley SD, *et al.* Suppression of HIV production in resting lymphocytes by combining didanosine and hydroxamate compounds. *Lancet* 1994; **343:** 1292.
3. Vila J, *et al.* 1-year follow-up of the use of hydroxycarbamide and didanosine in HIV infection. *Lancet* 1996; **848:** 203–4.
4. Vila J, *et al.* Absence of viral rebound after treatment of HIV-infected patients with didanosine and hydroxycarbamide. *Lancet* 1997; **350:** 635–6.
5. Lori F, *et al.* Long-term suppression of HIV-1 by hydroxyurea and didanosine. *JAMA* 1997; **277:** 1437–8.
6. Lisziewicz J, *et al.* HIV-1 suppression by early treatment with hydroxyurea, didanosine, and a protease inhibitor. *Lancet* 1998; **352:** 199–200.

Malignant neoplasms. Hydroxyurea is used for palliative symptomatic relief in chronic myeloid leukaemia although, as discussed on p.480 interferon alfa may produce better results. It remains probably the most appropriate therapy for younger patients with polycythaemia vera who require myelosuppression, as discussed on p.495, and similar therapy may be used in essential thrombocythaemia (see p.496) although it is less well established. Use in other tumours has produced variable results, although its use with cytarabine for T-cell lymphomas is mentioned on p.482, possible benefit in meningioma is referred to on p.485, and it does play a role in the standard regimens for medium- and high-risk gestational trophoblastic tumours, many of which can be cured (see p.477).

Psoriasis. An immunosuppressant (usually methotrexate or cyclosporin) may be useful in patients with severe refractory psoriasis (p.1075). Hydroxyurea has also been tried, although experience is limited.

In a study[1] in 85 patients with refractory psoriasis, treatment was usually begun with hydroxyurea 1.5 g daily and adjusted according to clinical and bone-marrow response; a maintenance dose of 0.5 to 1.5 g daily was achieved in the majority. Complete or almost complete clearance of lesions occurred in 51 patients and partial clearance in a further 17; 3 patients responded initially but subsequently relapsed while on treatment. Adverse effects were seen in about half of all patients receiving hydroxyurea, and treatment was withdrawn in 16. While a fall in the blood count was usual, this was clinically significant only in 30 patients and generally responded to dose reduction or temporary interruption of treatment. Thus, hydroxyurea appeared to be an effective long-term treatment for resistant psoriasis, and its adverse effects compared favourably with those of other immunosuppressant agents that have been used, but in common with other agents relapse is frequent once the treatment is discontinued.

1. Layton AM, *et al.* Hydroxyurea in the management of therapy resistant psoriasis. *Br J Dermatol* 1989; **121:** 647–53.

Preparations

BP 1998: Hydroxycarbamide Capsules;
USP 23: Hydroxyurea Capsules.

Proprietary Preparations (details are given in Part 3)

Austral.: Hydrea; ***Belg.:*** Hydrea; ***Canad.:*** Hydrea; ***Fr.:*** Hydrea; ***Ger.:*** Litalir; Syrea; ***Irl.:*** Hydrea; ***Ital.:*** Onco-Carbide; ***Neth.:*** Hydrea; ***S.Afr.:*** Hydrea; ***Switz.:*** Litalir; ***UK:*** Hydrea; ***USA:*** Hydrea.

Idarubicin Hydrochloride (12058-a)

Idarubicin Hydrochloride *(BANM, USAN, rINNM)*.

4-Demethoxydaunorubicin Hydrochloride; IMI-30; NSC-256439 (idarubicin). (7S,9S)-9-Acetyl-7-(3-amino-2,3,6-trideoxy-α-L-*lyxo*-hexopyranosyloxy)-7,8,9,10-tetrahydro-6,9,11-trihydroxynaphthacene-5,12-dione hydrochloride.

$C_{26}H_{27}NO_9,HCl = 534.0$.

CAS — 58957-92-9 (idarubicin); 57852-57-0 (idarubicin hydrochloride).

Pharmacopoeias. In US.

A 0.5% solution has a pH between 5.0 and 6.5. **Store** in airtight containers.

Adverse Effects, Treatment, and Precautions

As for Doxorubicin Hydrochloride, p.529. A cumulative total dose limit of 400 mg per m² body-surface has been recommended for oral therapy, although it has been suggested that idarubicin may be associated with less cardiotoxicity than doxorubicin.

Pharmacokinetics

Following intravenous administration idarubicin is rapidly distributed into body tissues and extensively tissue bound, with a volume of distribution which may be in excess of 2000 litres. It is extensively metabolised, both in the liver and extrahepatically; the principal metabolite, idarubicinol (13-dihydroidarubicin) has equal antineoplastic activity. Peak concentrations of idarubicin and idarubicinol in bone marrow and nucleated blood cells are 400 (idarubicin) and 200 (idarubicinol) times greater than those in plasma; cellular concentrations of drug and metabolite decline with apparent terminal half-lives of 15 and 72 hours respectively, whereas plasma half-lives are reported to be 20 to 22 hours and about 45 hours respectively. Idarubicin is excreted in bile, and to a lesser extent in urine, as unchanged drug and metabolites.

Idarubicin is also absorbed following oral administration, but estimates of its oral bioavailability vary from about 20 to 50%.

References.

1. Robert J. Clinical pharmacokinetics of idarubicin. *Clin Pharmacokinet* 1993; **24:** 275–88.

Uses and Administration

Idarubicin is an anthracycline antibiotic with antineoplastic actions similar to those of doxorubicin (p.531). It is used as the hydrochloride, alone or in combination with other drugs, for the induction of remission in patients with acute non-lymphoblastic leukaemias. It has also been tried in acute lymphoblastic leukaemia refractory to other therapy, and in the management of various solid tumours such as breast cancer. The management of these neoplasms and the potential role of idarubicin is discussed further in the chapter introduction, as indicated by the cross-references given below.

Idarubicin hydrochloride is given by intravenous injection (reconstituted with Water for Injections in the UK, but 0.9% sodium chloride for the US preparation) into a fast-running infusion of 0.9% sodium chloride or 5% glucose over 5 to 15 minutes. The suggested dose in adult acute non-lymphoblastic leukaemia is 12 mg per m² body-surface area daily for 3 days, in combination with cytarabine. A similar dose, as a single agent, has been given in acute lymphoblastic leukaemia. An alternative dosage schedule in acute non-lymphoblastic leukaemia is 8 mg per m² given daily for 5 days. In children with acute lymphoblastic leukaemia a dose of 10 mg per m² daily for 3 days as a single agent has been suggested. When the intravenous route cannot be employed, idarubicin hydrochloride may be given by mouth. A suggested dose in adult acute non-lymphoblastic leukaemia is 30 mg per m² daily for 3 days as a single agent, or 15 to 30 mg per m² daily in combination with other drugs.

In patients with refractory late breast cancer idarubicin hydrochloride has been given by mouth in doses of 45 mg per m², as a single dose or divided over 3 consecutive days; the treatment may be repeated every 3 or 4 weeks depending on the haematological recovery.

Blood counts should be performed frequently in patients receiving idarubicin, and monitoring of cardiac, hepatic, and renal function is recommended. Doses should be reduced in patients with impaired hepatic or renal function; in patients who receive a second course of idarubicin dosage should be reduced by 25% if severe mucositis developed with the first course.

The actions and uses of idarubicin have been reviewed.[1] A study in leukaemia cells *in vitro* suggested that idarubicin was more active than a conventional anthracycline, daunorubicin, against cells with the multidrug resistance (MDR) phenotype.[2]

1. Cersosimo RJ. Idarubicin: an anthracycline antineoplastic agent. *Clin Pharm* 1992; **11:** 152–67.
2. Berman E, McBride M. Comparative cellular pharmacology of daunorubicin and idarubicin in human multidrug-resistant leukaemia cells. *Blood* 1992; **79:** 3267–73.

Malignant neoplasms. For reference to the use of idarubicin in acute non-lymphoblastic leukaemia, in malignant neoplasms of the breast, and in multiple myeloma, see under Choice of Antineoplastic, p.479, p.485, and p.494. The use of idarubicin for salvage therapy in non-Hodgkin's lymphomas is mentioned on p.482.

Preparations

USP 23: Idarubicin Hydrochloride for Injection.

Proprietary Preparations (details are given in Part 3)
Aust.: Zavedos; *Austral.:* Zavedos; *Belg.:* Zavedos; *Canad.:* Idamycin; *Fr.:* Zavedos; *Ger.:* Zavedos; *Irl.:* Zavedos; *Ital.:* Zavedos; *Neth.:* Zavedos; *Norw.:* Zavedos; *S.Afr.:* Zavedos; *Spain:* Zavedos; *Swed.:* Zavedos; *Switz.:* Zavedos; *UK:* Zavedos; *USA:* Idamycin.

Idoxifene (17090-l)

Idoxifene *(BAN, USAN, rINN)*.

CB-7432; SB-223030. (E)-1-{2-[4-(1-p-Iodophenyl-2-phenylbut-1-enyl)phenoxy]ethyl}pyrrolidine.

$C_{28}H_{30}INO = 523.4$.

CAS — 116057-75-1.

Idoxifene is an analogue of tamoxifen (p.563) with similar general properties. It is under investigation in the endocrine treatment of breast cancer and has also been investigated in the treatment of osteoporosis.

Ifosfamide (1840-c)

Ifosfamide *(BAN, USAN, rINN)*.

Iphosphamide; Isophosphamide; MJF-9325; NSC-109724; Z-4942. 3-(2-Chloroethyl)-2-(2-chloroethylamino)perhydro-1,3,2-oxazaphosphorinane 2-oxide.

$C_7H_{15}Cl_2N_2O_2P = 261.1$.

CAS — 3778-73-2.

Pharmacopoeias. In US.

A white, crystalline powder. M.p. about 40°. Freely **soluble** in water; very soluble in alcohol, methyl alcohol, isopropyl alcohol, dichloromethane, and ethyl acetate; very slightly soluble in hexanes. A 10% solution in water has a pH of between 4 and 7. Solutions deteriorate on standing. **Store** in airtight containers at a temperature not exceeding 25°.

Ifosfamide undergoes a reversible chemical re-arrangement in aqueous solution, which is sensitive to changes in pH.[1] The ratio of these compounds to one another in biological fluids may have a bearing on the toxicity and efficacy of ifosfamide.

1. Küpfer A, *et al.* Intramolecular rearrangement of ifosfamide in aqueous solutions. *Lancet* 1990; **335:** 1461.

Incompatibility. Ifosfamide appears to be compatible when mixed in solution with mesna.[1,2] However, ifosfamide appears to be incompatible with benzyl alcohol used as a preservative in Water for Injections: solutions made up with water preserved in this way became turbid, with the formation of aqueous and oily phases, at concentrations of ifosfamide greater than 60 mg per mL.[3]

1. Shaw IC, Rose JWP. Infusion of ifosphamide plus mesna. *Lancet* 1984; **i:** 1353–4.
2. Rowland CG, *et al.* Infusion of ifosfamide plus mesna. *Lancet* 1984; **ii:** 468.
3. Behme RJ, *et al.* Incompatibility of ifosfamide with benzyl-alcohol-preserved bacteriostatic water for injection. *Am J Hosp Pharm* 1988; **45:** 627–8.

Adverse Effects, Treatment, and Precautions

As for Cyclophosphamide, p.516. Toxic effects on the urinary tract may be more severe with ifosfamide and may involve the kidneys as well as the bladder. Central nervous system side-effects have been reported, especially confusion and lethargy.

Effects on the heart. Severe myocardial depression, with heart failure and ventricular arrhythmias, has been reported in patients receiving high-dose ifosfamide.[1] Symptoms were reversible with appropriate treatment in most cases although one patient died of cardiogenic shock.

1. Quezado ZMN, *et al.* High-dose ifosfamide is associated with severe, reversible cardiac dysfunction. *Ann Intern Med* 1993; **118:** 31–6.

Effects on the kidneys. In addition to its effects on the bladder ifosfamide may be associated with serious nephrotoxicity. Both proximal and distal tubular damage,[1,2] and to a lesser extent glomerular effects,[2] are seen, and the Fanconi syndrome (with development of hypophosphataemic rickets in a number of children),[2-6] and nephrogenic diabetes insipidus[1,6] may result. Progressive chronic renal failure after high-dose ifosfamide has been described.[7] Life-threatening hypokalaemia possibly due to a renal lesion has also occurred.[8] Results in *rats* suggest that generation of toxic metabolites within the kidney itself may be responsible, and that repairable renal damage occurs after the first dose, which is aggravated by repeated toxic insults.[9] This is in agreement with clinical results, since although renal damage has been seen after a single dose, perhaps representing an idiosyncratic reaction,[10,11] most cases have been in children receiving relatively high doses long-term. Renal damage appears to persist after withdrawal of ifosfamide in these patients and may be largely irreversible.[12] It has been suggested that cumulative doses of 100 g of ifosfamide per m² body-surface or more should be avoided in children in an attempt to reduce the incidence of nephrotoxicity,[13] although a subsequent review has suggested that cumulative doses above 60 g per m² are problematic, particularly in children under 5 years of age.[14]

1. Skinner R, *et al.* Nephrotoxicity after ifosfamide. *Arch Dis Child* 1990; **65:** 732–8.
2. Burk CD, *et al.* Ifosfamide-induced renal tubular dysfunction and rickets in children with Wilms tumor. *J Pediatr* 1990; **117:** 331–5.
3. Skinner R, *et al.* Hypophosphataemic rickets after ifosfamide treatment in children. *Br Med J* 1989; **298:** 1560–1.
4. Newbury-Ecob RA, Barbor PRH. Hypophosphataemic rickets after ifosfamide treatment. *Br Med J* 1989; **299:** 258.
5. Newbury-Ecob RA, *et al.* Ifosfamide-induced Fanconi syndrome. *Lancet* 1989; **i:** 1328.
6. Skinner R, *et al.* Nephrotoxicity of ifosfamide in children. *Lancet* 1989; **ii:** 159.
7. Krämer A, *et al.* Progressive renal failure in two breast cancer patients after high-dose ifosfamide. *Lancet* 1994; **334:** 1569.
8. Husband DJ, Watkin SW. Fatal hypokalaemia associated with ifosfamide/mesna chemotherapy. *Lancet* 1988; **i:** 1116.
9. Graham MI, *et al.* A proposed mechanism for isophosphamide-induced kidney toxicity. *Hum Toxicol* 1985; **4:** 545–6.
10. Heney D, *et al.* Acute ifosfamide-induced tubular toxicity. *Lancet* 1989; **ii:** 103–4.
11. Devalck C, *et al.* Acute ifosfamide-induced proximal tubular toxic reaction. *J Pediatr* 1991; **118:** 325–6.
12. Heney D, *et al.* Progressive renal toxicity due to ifosfamide. *Arch Dis Child* 1991; **66:** 966–70.
13. Skinner R, *et al.* Risk factors for ifosfamide nephrotoxicity in children. *Lancet* 1996; **348:** 578–80.
14. Loebstein R, Koren G. Ifosfamide-induced nephrotoxicity in children: critical review of predictive risk factors. *Pediatrics* 1998; **101:** 1067.

Effects on the nervous system. The administration of ifosfamide (with mesna for urothelial protection) may be associated with the development of severe encephalopathy, with EEG abnormalities, disorientation, hallucinations, catatonia, and coma; occasionally central nervous system depression has led to circulatory collapse and death.[1,2] The effect has been suggested to be due to a metabolite, perhaps chloroacetaldehyde,[3] a hypothesis with which the increased incidence of encephalopathy after oral rather than intravenous administration may agree.[4,5] Others suggest that the dechloroethylated metabolites may contribute, and in particular the *R*-enantiomer of 3-dechloroethyl-ifosfamide which is a metabolite of *S*-ifosfamide.[6] There is some uncertainty about the contributory role of mesna, if any: encephalopathy has not been seen when mesna is given with cyclophosphamide,[7] and has been seen when ifosfamide is given alone,[5] but an exacerbatory role for mesna cannot be ruled out,[8] perhaps via its chelating properties.[1,7] A nomogram has been proposed to identify patients at greatest risk of toxicity,[9,10] such as those with renal or hepatic impairment,[9] although doubts have been raised as to its general applicability,[11] and it has also been suggested that administration should be by continuous infusion over several days where possible, since this route has by far the lowest incidence of encephalopathy (7%, versus 26% with intravenous bolus and 43% with oral administration).[4] Care may also be required when giving other antineoplastics to patients who have experienced encephalopathy after ifosfamide, since a case of encephalopathy following bleomycin (not normally associated with neurotoxicity) has been reported in such a patient.[12]

Preliminary reports suggest that intravenous or oral administration of methylene blue may prevent or reverse signs of encephalopathy.[13,14] It was proposed that ifosfamide neurotoxicity was due to derangement of mitochondrial metabolism, and that the process was reversed by methylene blue.[13]

1. Meanwell CA, *et al.* Encephalopathy associated with ifosphamide/mesna therapy. *Lancet* 1985; **i:** 406–7.
2. Cantwell BMJ, Harris AL. Ifosfamide/mesna and encephalopathy. *Lancet* 1985; **i:** 752.
3. Goren MP, *et al.* Dechloroethylation of ifosfamide and neurotoxicity. *Lancet* 1986; **ii:** 1219–20.
4. Cerny T, *et al.* Ifosfamide by continuous infusion to prevent encephalopathy. *Lancet* 1990; **335:** 175.
5. Lewis LD, Meanwell CA. Ifosfamide pharmacokinetics and neurotoxicity. *Lancet* 1990; **335:** 175–6.
6. Wainer IW, *et al.* Ifosfamide stereoselective dichloroethylation [sic] and neurotoxicity. *Lancet* 1994; **343:** 982–3.
7. Osborne RJ, Slevin ML. Ifosfamide, mesna, and encephalopathy. *Lancet* 1985; **i:** 1398–9.
8. Pinkerton R, *et al.* Ifosfamide, mesna, and encephalopathy. *Lancet* 1985; **i:** 1399.
9. Meanwell CA, *et al.* Avoiding ifosfamide/mesna encephalopathy. *Lancet* 1986; **ii:** 406.
10. Perren TJ, *et al.* Encephalopathy with rapid infusion ifosfamide/mesna. *Lancet* 1987; **i:** 390–1.
11. McCallum AK. Ifosfamide/mesna encephalopathy. *Lancet* 1987; **i:** 987. Correction. *ibid.*; 1048.
12. Atherton P, *et al.* Drug-induced encephalopathy after previous ifosfamide treatment. *Lancet* 1988; **ii:** 1084.
13. Küpfer A, *et al.* Prophylaxis and reversal of ifosfamide encephalopathy with methylene-blue. *Lancet* 1994; **343:** 763–4.
14. Zuhan GB, *et al.* Methylene blue for ifosfamide-associated encephalopathy. *N Engl J Med* 1995; **332:** 1239–40.

Handling and disposal. Corlett and colleagues[1] found that ifosfamide 8% solution penetrated all of 4 brands of latex glove and one polyvinyl chloride glove, although the diffusion rate was 4 or more times slower than through cadaver skin. Permeation was greater through the polyvinyl chloride glove than the latex gloves, partly due to its lesser thickness, although permeation was not dependent on thickness alone and varied between gloves of the same brand as well as between brands. They recommended that latex gloves of a suitable brand should be worn when handling ifosfamide, and changed at least every 2 hours.

1. Corlett SA, *et al.* Permeation of ifosfamide through gloves and cadaver skin. *Pharm J* 1991; **247:** R39.

Interactions

For reference to the effects of ifosfamide on oral anticoagulants, see under Warfarin Sodium, p.967. For a report of the enhancement of cisplatin-induced ototoxicity and nephrotoxicity, see under Cisplatin, p.515.

Pharmacokinetics

Ifosfamide is normally given intravenously, although it is well absorbed from the gastro-intestinal tract. The pharmacokinetics of ifosfamide are reported to exhibit considerable interindividual variation. Although the manufacturers state that a mean terminal elimination half-life of about 15 hours has been reported following a single high-dose intravenous bolus, most studies at lower doses appear to have recorded elimination half-lives of about 4 to 8 hours. Following repeated doses (fractionated therapy) there is a decrease in the elimination half-life, apparently due to autoinduction of metabolism. It is extensively metabolised, chiefly by mixed function oxidases in the liver, to a variety of active and inactive metabolites; there is some evidence that metabolism is saturated at very high doses. It is excreted largely in urine, as unchanged drug and metabolites.

General references.

1. Wagner T. Ifosfamide clinical pharmacokinetics. *Clin Pharmacokinet* 1994; **26:** 439–56.

In a study in 20 patients receiving intravenous ifosfamide over 3 or 5 days, the median elimination half-life of ifosfamide was 3.85 hours in patients under 60 years of age compared with 6.03 hours in those over age 60;[1] this difference appeared to be due to an increased volume of distribution in the older age group. The autoinduction of metabolism typically seen with multiple doses of ifosfamide was not affected by age.

In another study the half-life of the *S*-enantiomer of ifosfamide was found to be 5.98 hours after an intravenous bolus of the racemate, compared with 7.12 hours for the *R*-enantiomer.[2]

1. Lind MJ, *et al.* The effect of age on the pharmacokinetics of ifosfamide. *Br J Clin Pharmacol* 1990; **30:** 140–3.
2. Corlett SA, *et al.* Pharmacokinetics of ifosfamide and its enantiomers following a single 1h intravenous infusion of the racemate in patients with small cell lung carcinoma. *Br J Clin Pharmacol* 1995; **39:** 452–5.

The increased clearance seen over time during a 5-day cycle of ifosfamide treatment, due to increased metabolism, was not sustained over the 21 days between cycles, but was reproducible and of similar magnitude in the subsequent cycle.[1]

1. Lewis LD. A study of 5 day fractionated ifosfamide pharmacokinetics in consecutive treatment cycles. *Br J Clin Pharmacol* 1996; **42:** 179–86.

Uses and Administration

Ifosfamide is an alkylating agent with properties similar to those of cyclophosphamide (p.517), of which it is a congener. It is used in the treatment of a variety of solid tumours including those of the cervix, endometrium, lung, ovary, testis, and thymus, as well as in sarcoma and in the treatment of Burkitt's lymphoma. For further mention of these uses see the cross-references given below.

Ifosfamide is given intravenously, either by injection as a solution diluted to less than 4%, or by infusion. It is usually given in a total dose of 8 to 12 g per m^2 body-surface divided over 3 to 5 days, although a dose of 6 g per m^2 divided over 5 days has been recommended in the USA; alternatively, courses comprising 5 to 6 g per m^2, to a maximum of 10 g, have been given as a single 24-hour infusion. Courses may be repeated at intervals of 2 to 4 weeks, depending on the blood count. Ifosfamide has also been investigated by oral administration.

Ifosfamide should be administered in association with mesna (p.984), and adequate hydration should be maintained, to avoid urological toxicity; fluid intake should not be less than 2 litres daily.

The isomeric form dexifosfamide (D-4809) is also under investigation, as is a combination of ifosfamide with methylene blue.

Malignant neoplasms. Ifosfamide has been tried in Burkitt's lymphoma as an alternative to cyclophosphamide (p.483). It is also used in a variety of solid neoplasms, including in palliative regimens for advanced cervical cancer (p.487) and endometrial cancer (p.487); in the treatment of small-cell and (with less evidence of benefit) non-small-cell lung cancer (p.490); in ovarian cancer (p.491) and second-line and salvage regimens for testicular cancer (p.493); in thymoma (p.493); in adjuvant therapy for osteosarcoma (p.495) and rhabdomyosarcoma (p.496).

Preparations

USP 23: Ifosfamide for Injection.

Proprietary Preparations (details are given in Part 3)
Aust.: Holoxan; ***Austral.:*** Holoxan; ***Belg.:*** Holoxan; ***Canad.:*** Ifex; ***Fr.:*** Holoxan; ***Ger.:*** Holoxan; IFO-cell; ***Ital.:*** Holoxan; ***Neth.:*** Holoxan; ***Norw.:*** Holoxan; ***S.Afr.:*** Holoxan; ***Spain:*** Tronoxal; ***Swed.:*** Holoxan; ***Switz.:*** Holoxan; ***UK:*** Mitoxana; ***USA:*** Ifex.

Ilmofosine (2954-e)

Ilmofosine *(USAN, rINN)*.

BM-41440. (±)-3-(Hexadecylthio)-2-(methoxymethyl)propyl hydrogen phosphate choline hydroxide inner salt.

$C_{26}H_{56}NO_5PS = 525.8$.

CAS — 83519-04-4; 89315-55-9.

Ilmofosine is a phospholipid derivative similar to miltefosine (p.551) that has been investigated for its antineoplastic properties. Gastro-intestinal disturbances may be dose-limiting.

Improsulfan Tosylate (12846-d)

Improsulfan Tosilate *(rINNM)*; NSC-140117; 864T. Iminodipropyl dimethanesulphonate 4-toluenesulphonate.

$C_8H_{19}NO_6S_2,C_7H_8O_3S = 461.6$.

CAS — 13425-98-4 (improsulfan); 32784-82-0 (improsulfan tosylate).

Improsulfan is an alkylating agent related to busulphan (p.509). It has been used as the tosylate in the management of chronic myeloid leukaemia.

Inolimomab (17632-m)

Inolimomab *(rINN)*.

BT-563.

CAS — 152981-31-2.

Inolimomab is a murine antihuman monoclonal antibody directed against the α-chain of the interleukin-2 receptor (CD25). It is under investigation for its immunosuppressant properties in the treatment and prevention of rejection episodes following organ transplantation.

References to the use of inolimomab are given below. See also under Bone Marrow and Heart Transplantation, p.498 and p.499, respectively, while for reference to its potential benefit in preventing or reversing kidney graft rejection, see p.499, and its use in liver transplantation is mentioned on p.500.

1. Otto G, *et al.* Monoclonal antibody to interleukin-2 receptor in liver graft rejection. *Lancet* 1990; **335:** 1596–7.
2. Otto G, *et al.* Monoclonal anti-CD25 for acute rejection after liver transplantation. *Lancet* 1991; **338:** 195.
3. van Gelder T, *et al.* Reversal of graft rejection with monoclonal anti-interleukin-2 receptor. *Lancet* 1992; **339:** 873.
4. Neuhaus P, *et al.* Comparison of quadruple immunosuppression after liver transplantation with ATG or IL-2 receptor antibody. *Transplantation* 1993; **55:** 1320–7.
5. Iberer F, *et al.* Clinical experience with a monoclonal interleukin-2 receptor antibody (BT 563) for rejection therapy after orthotopic heart transplantation. *Transplant Proc* 1994; **26:** 3237–9.
6. Carl S, *et al.* Effect of anti-IL-2-receptor monoclonal antibody BT563 in treatment of acute interstitial renal rejection. *Transplant Proc* 1995; **27:** 854–5.
7. Lemmens HP, *et al.* Interleukin-2 receptor antibody vs ATG for induction immunosuppression after liver transplantation: initial results of a prospective randomized trial. *Transplant Proc* 1995; **27:** 1140–1.

Interleukin-2 (16854-s)

BG-8301 (teceleukin); Epidermal Thymocyte Activating Factor; ETAF; IL-2; T-cell Growth Factor.

NOTE. The names Aldesleukin (*BAN, USAN, rINN*), Celmoleukin (*pINN*), and Teceleukin (*BAN, USAN, rINN*) are in use for modified forms of interleukin-2 produced by recombinant DNA technology.

A naturally-occurring 133-amino-acid glycoprotein with a molecular weight of about 15 000. It is available from natural sources or as a product of recombinant DNA technology (rIL-2) in a variety of slightly modified forms.

Incompatibility. Aldesleukin 33 800 units per mL in 5% glucose injection lost significant biological activity when mixed with a variety of other drugs including ganciclovir sodium, lorazepam, pentamidine isethionate, prochlorperazine edisylate, and promethazine hydrochloride.[1] However, the incompatibility was not detectable by spectrophotometric methods and only lorazepam was visually incompatible, suggesting that these methods may be invalid for assessing the compatibility of proteins.

1. Alex S, *et al.* Compatibility and activity of aldesleukin (recombinant interleukin-2) in presence of selected drugs during simulated Y-site administration: evaluation of three methods. *Am J Health-Syst Pharm* 1995; **52:** 2423–6.

Sorption. For reference to adsorption of interleukin-2 onto plastic infusion devices, see under Adverse Effects, below.

Units

100 units of human interleukin-2 are contained in one ampoule of the first International Standard Preparation (1987). The activity of interleukin-2 has also been expressed in Nutley and Cetus units: 100 international units is reportedly equivalent to about 83.3 Nutley units and to about 16.7 Cetus units. According to the manufacturers of one aldesleukin product 18 million international units of aldesleukin are equivalent to 1.1 mg of protein.

Adverse Effects, Treatment, and Precautions

Toxicity is dose-related and is often severe; fatalities have been recorded. Decreased vascular resistance and increased capillary permeability (the 'capillary leak syndrome') are common in patients given interleukin-2; fluid replacement may be necessary to treat the resultant hypovolaemia and dopamine or other pressor agents may be needed to help maintain organ perfusion. Hypotension, fluid retention and weight gain, renal abnormalities including uraemia and oliguria or anuria, dyspnoea, mild liver dysfunction, gastro-intestinal disturbances, fever and flu-like symptoms (malaise, rigors, and myalgia), rashes, anaemia and thrombocytopenia, headache, confusion, disorientation, and drowsiness are also relatively common, particularly at high doses. Cardiac disorders, including myocardial infarction, and pulmonary oedema and respiratory distress, have occurred.

Interleukin-2 should be given with great care, if at all, to patients with pre-existing cardiac or pulmonary disease; caution is also required in patients with impaired renal function who may be at increased risk of severe toxicity and interleukin-2 therapy should preferably be avoided in patients with dysfunction of any major organ or those with poor performance status. It should be avoided in patients with CNS metastases or seizure disorders. Bacterial infections should be adequately treated before beginning therapy. Interleukin-2 may exacerbate effusions from serosal surfaces.

Activity. Interleukin-2 has been shown to be adsorbed from solutions in 5% glucose or 0.9% sodium chloride onto the plastic of infusion devices,[1,2] resulting in an almost total loss of activity, and it has been suggested that the lack of toxicity seen with some interleukin-2 regimens may be due to such a loss of activity,[1,3] although this is hotly disputed.[4,5] Adsorptive losses can be prevented by formulation of interleukin-2 solutions with low concentrations of albumin (2% or less).[1,6] Some brands of interleukin-2 are formulated with albumin as part of the commercial product.[2]

1. Miles DW, *et al.* Reconstitution of interleukin 2 with albumin for infusion. *Lancet* 1990; **335:** 1602–3.
2. Vlasveld LT, *et al.* Reconstitution of interleukin-2. *Lancet* 1990; **336:** 446.
3. Miles DW, *et al.* Toxicity and reconstitution of recombinant interleukin-2 with albumin. *Lancet* 1991; **338:** 1464.
4. Hamblin T. Reconstitution of interleukin-2 with albumin for infusion. *Lancet* 1990; **336:** 251.
5. Franks CR. Reconstitution of interleukin-2. *Lancet* 1990; **336:** 445–6.
6. Lamers CHJ, *et al.* Bioavailability of interleukin-2 after reconstitution with albumin. *Lancet* 1992; **340:** 241.

Bacterial infections. The incidence of sepsis and bacteraemia is increased in patients receiving interleukin-2 via intravenous catheters,[1,2] and possibly subcutaneously,[3] although others have not found this to be the case.[4,5] The increased incidence of nonopportunistic bacterial infection may be a particular problem in patients with AIDS who are treated with interleukin-2.[6] The mechanism is uncertain, but may be related to impairment of neutrophil function by the cytokine.[7]

1. Snydman DR, *et al.* Nosocomial sepsis associated with interleukin-2. *Ann Intern Med* 1990; **112:** 102–7.
2. Shiloni E, *et al.* Interleukin-2 therapy, central venous catheters, and nosocomial sepsis. *Ann Intern Med* 1990; **112:** 882–3.
3. Jones AL, *et al.* Infectious complications of subcutaneous interleukin-2 and interferon-alpha. *Lancet* 1992; **339:** 181–2.
4. Buter J, *et al.* Infection after subcutaneous interleukin-2. *Lancet* 1992; **339:** 552.
5. Schomburg AG, *et al.* Cytokines and infection in cancer patients. *Lancet* 1992; **339:** 1061.
6. Murphy PM, *et al.* Marked disparity in incidence of bacterial infections in patients with the acquired immunodeficiency syndrome receiving interleukin-2 or interferon-γ. *Ann Intern Med* 1988; **108:** 36–41.
7. Klempner MS, *et al.* An acquired chemotactic defect in neutrophils from patients receiving interleukin-2 immunotherapy. *N Engl J Med* 1990; **322:** 959–65.

Catheter blockage. Prolonged administration of interleukin-2 via a double-lumen catheter appeared to result in fibrin deposition and capping of the catheter tip in 3 patients.[1]

1. van Schijndel RJMS, *et al.* Interleukin-2 therapy and blockage of double-lumen catheters. *Lancet* 1989; **i:** 962–3.

Effects on endocrine function. It has been suggested that patients with adrenal metastases may be particularly susceptible to adrenal haemorrhage and consequent failure during interleukin therapy.[1] Results also suggested that lack of endogenous steroid production may increase the risk of early severe interleukin-2 toxicity.[1]

Effects on thyroid function have also been reported, with the development of hypothyroidism[2-4] and goitre.[3]

1. VanderMolen LA, *et al.* Adrenal insufficiency and interleukin-2 therapy. *Ann Intern Med* 1989; **111:** 185.
2. Atkins MB, *et al.* Hypothyroidism after treatment with interleukin-2 and lymphokine-activated killer cells. *N Engl J Med* 1988; **318:** 1557–63.
3. van Liessum PA, *et al.* Hypothyroidism and goitre during interleukin-2 therapy without LAK cells. *Lancet* 1989; **i:** 224.
4. Sauter NP, *et al.* Transient thyrotoxicosis and persistent hypothyroidism due to acute autoimmune thyroiditis after interleukin-2 and interferon-α therapy for metastatic carcinoma: a case report. *Am J Med* 1992; **92:** 441–4.

Effects on the kidneys. Interleukin-2 therapy in 99 consecutive patients was associated with varying degrees of acute renal dysfunction in almost all patients.[1] The clinical syndrome of hypotension, oliguria, fluid retention, and associated azotaemia with intense tubular avidity for filtered sodium all support prerenal acute renal failure as the cause of renal dysfunction. However, renal function values returned to baseline levels within 7 days in 62% of patients and in 95% by 30 days. Patients with elevated pretreatment serum-creatinine values, particularly those aged over 60 years, and those who had previously undergone a nephrectomy, were at risk of more severe and prolonged changes in renal function, and might be particularly vulnerable to the use of indomethacin for associated fever and chills, which might potentiate renal impairment through its effects on intrarenal prostaglandin production.

1. Belldegrun A, *et al.* Effects of interleukin-2 on renal function in patients receiving immunotherapy for advanced cancer. *Ann Intern Med* 1987; **106:** 817–22.

Inflammatory bowel disease. Two patients with a history of Crohn's disease had a recurrence of the condition when given interleukin-2. It was suggested that interleukin-2 should be contra-indicated in such patients.[1]

1. Sparano JA, *et al.* Symptomatic exacerbation of Crohn disease after treatment with high-dose interleukin-2. *Ann Intern Med* 1993; **118:** 617–18.

Psoriasis. Exacerbations of psoriasis developed in 3 patients during therapy with interleukin-2 and lymphokine-activated killer cells in 2. The psoriatic symptoms remitted with topical therapy.[1]

1. Lee RE, *et al.* Interleukin 2 and psoriasis. *Arch Dermatol* 1988; **124:** 1811–15.

Interactions

Corticosteroids (which reduce some of the adverse effects of interleukin-2 administration) may also reduce its antineoplastic properties: concomitant administration should be avoided.

NSAIDs. Administration of concomitant *indomethacin* to patients receiving interleukin-2 led to more severe weight gain, oliguria, and azotaemia.[1] However, *ibuprofen* has been reported to reduce interleukin-2 toxicity, especially fever, chills, myalgia, and nausea and vomiting.[2]

See also Effects on the Kidneys, above.

1. Sosman JA, *et al.* Repetitive weekly cycles of interleukin-2 II: clinical and immunologic effects of dose, schedule, and addition of indomethacin. *J Natl Cancer Inst* 1988; **80:** 1451–61.
2. Eberlein TJ, *et al.* Ibuprofen causes reduced toxic effects of interleukin 2 administration in patients with metastatic cancer. *Arch Surg* 1989; **124:** 542–7.

Uses and Administration

Interleukin-2 is a lymphokine which stimulates the proliferation of T-lymphocytes and thus amplifies immune response to an antigen; it also has actions on B-lymphocytes, and induces the production of interferon-γ and the activation of natural killer cells.

Interleukin-2 is used in the adoptive immunotherapy of metastatic renal cell carcinoma in selected patients. It is also used in melanoma and has been tried in some other malignant neoplasms, such as thymoma, as indicated by the cross-references below.

Interleukin-2 is usually given by intravenous infusion of one of its recombinant forms, such as aldesleukin. Some preparations are formulated with albumin; if not, infusions are given in glucose 5% with an added 0.1% of albumin to protect against loss of activity.

A variety of dosage regimens have been tried. In the UK, a regimen comprising 18 million units per m^2 body-surface daily for 5 days, by continuous infusion, has been recommended for metastatic renal cell carcinoma. This is repeated after 2 to 6 days, and a further two infusions at the same intervals are given after 3 weeks; administration may be delayed or the dosage reduced if toxicity is severe. Up to 4 further 5-day infusions may be given at 4-week intervals in patients who respond.

In the USA, a suggested regimen involves infusion of 600 000 units per kg body-weight over 15 minutes, every 8 hours for 14 doses. The schedule is repeated after 9 days, toxicity permitting, and further courses may be given at intervals of at least 7 weeks in patients who respond.

Interleukin-2 has also been given with lymphokine-activated killer (LAK) cells or tumour-infiltrating lymphocytes (TIL), which are harvested from the patient, activated *ex vivo,* and then re-infused.

Interleukin-2 has also been tried in patients with HIV infection and AIDS in an attempt to restore immune response and has been given in some other infections or immune diseases.

Other interleukins are under investigation (see also p.1591). Conjugates of interleukin-2 with macrogol (PEG-IL2; pegaldesleukin) have also been investigated and liposome-encapsulated interleukin-2 has also been investigated for the treatment of brain and CNS tumours. Interleukin-2 has also been given subcutaneously (see below).

General references to interleukin-2 and its use.

1. Winkelhake JL, Gauny SS. Human recombinant interleukin-2 as an experimental therapeutic. *Pharmacol Rev* 1990; **42:** 1–28.
2. Kintzel PE, Calis KA. Recombinant interleukin-2: a biological response modifier. *Clin Pharm* 1991; **10:** 110–28.
3. Whittington R, Faulds D. Interleukin-2: a review of its pharmacological properties and therapeutic use in patients with cancer. *Drugs* 1993; **46:** 446–514.
4. Aulitzky WE, *et al.* Interleukins: clinical pharmacology and therapeutic use. *Drugs* 1994; **48:** 667–77.
5. Anderson PM, Sorenson MA. Effects of route and formulation on clinical pharmacokinetics of interleukin-2. *Clin Pharmacokinet* 1994; **27:** 19–31.

Administration. A review of polymer conjugates by Duncan and Spreafico[1] includes some discussion of the macrogol-interleukin-2 conjugate PEG-IL2. This conjugate is more soluble than interleukin-2 itself and has a much more prolonged elimination half-life (947 minutes compared with 70 to 85 minutes for the parent drug).

1. Duncan R, Spreafico F. Polymer conjugates: pharmacokinetic considerations for design and development. *Clin Pharmacokinet* 1994; **27:** 290–306.

SUBCUTANEOUS INJECTION. Interleukin-2 has been reported to be well absorbed following subcutaneous injection of doses between 12 and 18 million units daily for 5 consecutive days.[1] Administration was repeated every 8 weeks for a total of 6 cycles. It appeared to be associated with a reduced systemic exposure compared with continuous intravenous infusion, but the prolonged absorption and half-life did permit administration on a once- or twice-daily basis.

1. Piscitelli SC, *et al.* Pharmacokinetics and pharmacodynamics of subcutaneous interleukin-2 in HIV-infected patients. *Pharmacotherapy* 1996; **16:** 754–9.

HIV infection and AIDS. Interleukin-2 has been reported to partially restore the deficient proliferation response and natural killer cell activity of lymphocytes from persons with AIDS (p.599) when added *in vitro*.[1] In consequence it has been tried in doses of up to 2.5 million units by intravenous infusion over 24 hours, for 5 days a week over 4 to 8 weeks, in patients with AIDS, with some minor benefit, including elevation in the number of T4 lymphocytes and a decrease in HIV isolation.[2] Interleukin-2 has also been given in doses of up to 12 million units per square metre body-surface area daily for 5 days a week, in combination with zidovudine 200 mg every 4 hours, in patients with asymptomatic HIV infection, with a resultant increase in CD4 counts which persisted after a mean 10 months of follow-up.[3] Another pilot study[4] found that intermittent therapy, using interleukin-2 in doses of 6 to 18 million units daily for 5 days every 8 weeks was associated with increases in CD4 counts which were sustained for up to 8 months after discontinuing the drug and could be re-induced by further treatment. Side-effects were common and were more severe in patients with initial CD4 counts below 200 per mm^3. Because of concerns about the potential for increased HIV replication with interleukin-2 patients in this study also received antiretroviral drugs. However, a subsequent controlled study[5] compared the combination against antiretroviral therapy alone, and found a significant increase in CD4 count over 12 months of combined therapy, compared with a decrease in those receiving antiretroviral drugs alone; 21 of 29 patients receiving combined therapy, and 24 of 29 controls subsequently elected to receive interleukin-2 therapy, and CD4 counts were maintained at about twice their base-line value in the former group.

Interleukin-2 has been tried in patients with AIDS-associated lymphomas but only limited success has been reported (see p.483).

The macrogol conjugate PEG-IL2 has also been investigated in patients with HIV infection, and again has been associated with improvements in CD4 counts.[6] Interestingly PEG-IL2 has also proved effective in common variable immunodeficiency, a primary immunodeficiency disorder associated with B cell defects—see Hypogammaglobulinaemia, below.

1. Lifson JD, *et al.* Human recombinant interleukin-2 partly reconstitutes deficient in-vitro immune responses of lymphocytes from patients with AIDS. *Lancet* 1984; **i:** 698–702.
2. De Vita VT, *et al.* Developmental therapeutics and the acquired immunodeficiency syndrome. *Ann Intern Med* 1987; **106:** 568–81.
3. Schwartz DH, *et al.* Safety and effects of interleukin-2 plus zidovudine in asymptomatic individuals infected with human immunodeficiency virus. *J Acquir Immune Defic Syndr* 1991; **4:** 11–23.

4. Kovacs JA, *et al.* Increases in CD4 T lymphocytes with intermittent courses of interleukin-2 in patients with human immunodeficiency virus infection: a preliminary study. *N Engl J Med* 1995; **332:** 567–75.
5. Kovacs JA, *et al.* Controlled trial of interleukin-2 infusions in patients infected with the human immunodeficiency virus. *N Engl J Med* 1996; **335:** 1350–6.
6. Wood R, *et al.* Safety and efficacy of polyethylene glycol-modified interleukin-2 and zidovudine in human immunodeficiency virus type 1 infection: a phase I/II study. *J Infect Dis* 1993; **167:** 519–25.

Hypogammaglobulinaemia. Weekly subcutaneous injection of PEG-IL2, a macrogol conjugate of interleukin-2, in a patient with common variable immunodeficiency was associated with reduced rates of infection and relief of some other clinical symptoms including diarrhoea and arthralgia, as well as increased serum-immunoglobulin concentrations.[1] The B-cell defect in this condition may be due to lack of essential cytokines.

1. Cunningham-Rundles C, *et al.* Brief report: enhanced humoral immunity in common variable immunodeficiency after long-term treatment with polyethylene glycol-conjugated interleukin-2. *N Engl J Med* 1994; **331:** 918–21.

Leishmaniasis. Encouraging preliminary results were seen in 3 patients with disseminated cutaneous leishmaniasis (p.575) who received injections of interleukin-2 180 000 units into their lesions on 3 occasions at 48-hour intervals. There was an influx of T-cells and monocytes into the injected lesions, and a marked reduction in parasite numbers.[1] These results were analogous to those seen in patients with lepromatous leprosy, in whom local injection of interleukin-2 can reconstitute a cell-mediated immune response leading to an extensive reduction in bacterial load at the site of injection.[2]

1. Akuffo H, *et al.* Administration of recombinant interleukin-2 reduces the local parasite load of patients with disseminated cutaneous leishmaniasis. *J Infect Dis* 1990; **161:** 775–80.
2. Kaplan G, *et al.* The reconstitution of cell-mediated immunity in the cutaneous lesions of lepromatous leprosy by recombinant interleukin 2. *J Exp Med* 1989; **169:** 893–907.

Leprosy. See under Leishmaniasis, above.

Malignant neoplasms. For reference to the use of interleukin-2 in malignant neoplasms of the kidney and thymus, and in melanoma, see under Choice of Antineoplastic, p.489, p.493, and p.492, respectively. Although there have been a few sustained responses in otherwise untreatable cancers, such therapy has been beset by problems with severe toxicity. It has also been tried in AIDS-associated lymphomas (p.483) but again with only limited success.

For mention of the use of melatonin as an adjunct to interleukin-2 in the treatment of malignant neoplasms, see p.1599.

Viral hepatitis. Following reports from Japan suggesting that interleukin-2 might be of benefit in patients with chronic hepatitis B,[1] Bach and colleagues examined the effect of a 12-week course of interleukin-2 in 2 patients with chronic hepatitis B and 2 with non-A non-B hepatitis[2] but found that the doses used (100 000 units per kg body-weight on 3 days a week) were too toxic and, even with dosage reduction, only 2 patients completed the 12-week course. Although there was some evidence of a decrease in raised liver-enzyme values in 3 of the 4 patients this was temporary in 2, and these workers concluded that interleukin-2, at least in these doses, was not a practical therapy for chronic viral hepatitis.[2]

A more promising approach was demonstrated by Meuer and others, who gave interleukin-2 250 000 units intramuscularly 4 hours after vaccination for hepatitis B in 10 haemodialysis patients who had previously failed to respond to several attempts at hepatitis B vaccination.[3] Protective antibody titres developed in 6, and one showed seroconversion but at low titres, whereas in 8 similar patients given the vaccine alone only one showed any seroconversion, suggesting that interleukin-2 is an efficient means of inducing antigen-specific immune responses in a subgroup of immunodeficient subjects. However, another study in which local injection of 1 million units of interleukin-2 was given to 27 uraemic patients 5 minutes after hepatitis B injection failed to demonstrate any difference in seroconversion rate compared with 25 further patients given placebo.[4]

1. Onji M, *et al.* Effect of recombinant interleukin 2 on hepatitis Be antigen positive chronic hepatitis. *Gut* 1987; **28:** 1648–52.
2. Bach N, *et al.* High-dose recombinant interleukin-2 for chronic viral hepatitis. *Lancet* 1989; **ii:** 281.
3. Meuer SC, *et al.* Low-dose interleukin-2 induces systemic immune responses against HBsAg in immunodeficient non-responders to hepatitis B vaccination. *Lancet* 1989; **i:** 15–18.
4. Jungers P, *et al.* Randomised placebo-controlled trial of recombinant interleukin-2 in chronic uraemic patients who are non-responders to hepatitis B vaccine. *Lancet* 1994; **344:** 856–7.

Preparations

Proprietary Preparations (details are given in Part 3)
Aust.: Proleukin; ***Canad.:*** Proleukin; ***Fr.:*** Proleukin; ***Ger.:*** Proleukin; ***Ital.:*** Proleukin; ***Neth.:*** Proleukin; ***Spain:*** Proleukin; ***Switz.:*** Proleukin; ***UK:*** Proleukin; ***USA:*** Proleukin.

Irinotecan Hydrochloride (19006-c)

Irinotecan Hydrochloride (*BANM, USAN, rINNM*).

CPT-11 (irinotecan); U-101440E. (+)-7-Ethyl-10-hydroxycamptothecine 10-[1,4′-bipiperidine]-1′-carboxylate hydrochloride trihydrate; (*S*)-4,11-Diethyl-3,4,12,14-tetrahydro-4-hydroxy-3,14-dioxo-1*H*-pyrano[3′,4′:6′,7′]indolizino[1,2-*b*]quinolin-9-yl [1,4′-dipiperidine]-1′-carboxylate hydrochloride trihydrate.

$C_{33}H_{38}N_4O_6,HCl,3H_2O = 677.2$.

CAS — 97682-44-5 (irinotecan); 136572-09-3 (irinotecan hydrochloride trihydrate).

Adverse Effects, Treatment, and Precautions

Neutropenia and diarrhoea may be dose-limiting in patients receiving irinotecan. The nadir of the white-cell count usually occurs about 8 days after a dose, with recovery by about the 22nd day. Anaemia also occurs and, less commonly, thrombocytopenia. Gastro-intestinal disturbances are common: acute diarrhoea, occurring within 24 hours of administration, may be part of a cholinergic syndrome which can also include sweating, hypersalivation, abdominal cramps, lachrymation, and miosis. These symptoms can be controlled with atropine. However a more severe, prolonged diarrhoea may occur, beginning more than 24 hours after a dose, and can be life-threatening; prompt management with high-dose loperamide and fluid replacement is required, and irinotecan treatment should be interrupted and any further doses reduced. Other adverse effects include nausea and vomiting, weakness, alopecia, and skin reactions.

Irinotecan should not be given to patients with inflammatory bowel disease. The risk of diarrhoea may be increased in the elderly and in patients who have received radiotherapy to the abdomen or pelvis.

Pharmacokinetics

Following intravenous administration irinotecan is metabolised by carboxyesterase in body tissues to active SN-38. It exhibits biphasic or triphasic pharmacokinetics, with a terminal half-life of about 14 hours. Only about 20% of a dose is excreted in urine within 24 hours.

References.

1. Chabot GG. Clinical pharmacokinetics of irinotecan. *Clin Pharmacokinet* 1997; **33:** 245–59.

Uses and Administration

Irinotecan is a derivative of the alkaloid camptothecin, obtained from the shrub *Camptotheca acuminata*. The camptothecin derivatives are inhibitors of the enzyme topoisomerase I which inhibit nucleic acid synthesis by interfering with the coiling and uncoiling of DNA during replication. Its actions are specific for S-phase.

Irinotecan is used in the treatment of metastatic colorectal cancer refractory to standard therapy, and has been tried in the management of other solid tumours including those of the lung and ovaries.

It is given as the hydrochloride, by intravenous infusion. In the treatment of refractory colorectal malignancies one suggested dose regimen is 125 mg of irinotecan hydrochloride per m^2 body-surface infused over 90 minutes once a week for 4 weeks, followed by a 2-week rest period. Additional courses may be given if required, with doses modified according to toxicity. Another regimen requires administration of an initial dose of 350 mg per m^2 over 30 to 90 minutes repeated every 3 weeks and adjusted according to toxicity.

References,[1-7] including evidence[4,8,9] of response to irinotecan in colorectal cancer refractory to fluorouracil. (For a discussion of the management of gastro-intestinal malignancies, see p.487.)

1. Shimada Y, *et al.* Phase II study of CPT-11, a new camptothecin derivative, in metastatic colorectal cancer. *J Clin Oncol* 1993; **11:** 909–13.
2. Shimada Y, *et al.* Combination phase I study of CPT-11 (irinotecan) combined with continuous infusion of 5-fluorouracil in metastatic colorectal cancer. *Proc Am Soc Clin Oncol* 1993; **12:** 196.
3. Von Hoff DD, *et al.* Preclinical and phase I trials of topoisomerase I inhibitors. *Cancer Chemother Pharmacol* 1994; **34** (suppl): S41–S45.
4. Armand JP, *et al.* CPT-11 (irinotecan) in the treatment of colorectal cancer. *Eur J Cancer* 1995; **31A:** 1283–7.
5. Wiseman LR, Markham A. Irinotecan: a review of its pharmacological properties and clinical efficacy in the management of advanced colorectal cancer. *Drugs* 1996; **52:** 606–23.
6. Anonymous. Irinotecan for metastatic colorectal cancer. *Med Lett Drugs Ther* 1997; **39:** 8.
7. Siu LL, Rowinsky EK. A risk-benefit assessment of irinotecan in solid tumours. *Drug Safety* 1998; **18:** 395–417.
8. Rougier P, *et al.* Randomised trial of irinotecan versus fluorouracil by continuous infusion after fluorouracil failure in patients with metastatic colorectal cancer. *Lancet* 1998; **352:** 1407–12.
9. Cunningham D, *et al.* Randomised trial of irinotecan plus supportive case versus supportive care alone after fluorouracil failure for patients with metastatic colorectal cancer. *Lancet* 1998; **352:** 1413–18.

Preparations

Proprietary Preparations (details are given in Part 3)
Austral.: Camptosar; ***Fr.:*** Campto; ***Ital.:*** Campto; ***S.Afr.:*** Campto; ***UK:*** Campto; ***USA:*** Camptosar.

JM-216 (16686-s)

Bisacetoamminedichloro(cyclohexylamine)platinum IV.

$C_{10}H_{22}Cl_2N_2O_4Pt = 500.3$.

JM-216 is an analogue of cisplatin (p.513) with generally similar properties, but which is well absorbed following oral administration. It is under investigation for its antineoplastic properties.

In a review of cisplatin analogues under investigation[1] it was noted that JM-216 was active against some human cancer cell lines resistant to cisplatin. Together with reduced nephrotoxicity in *animal* studies and its oral availability these results suggested that JM-216 might be one of the most interesting platinum complexes currently under development. A subsequent review commented that [significant] nephrotoxicity, peripheral neurotoxicity, or ototoxicity had not been noted with JM-216: myelosuppression was the dose-limiting toxicity.[2]

1. Weiss RB, Christian MC. New cisplatin analogues in development: a review. *Drugs* 1993; **46:** 360–77.
2. McKeage MJ. Comparative adverse effect profiles of platinum drugs. *Drug Safety* 1995; **13:** 228–44.

Leflunomide (10839-p)

Leflunomide (*BAN, rINN*).

HWA-486. α,α,α-Trifluoro-5-methyl-4-isoxazolecarboxy-*p*-toluidide.

$C_{12}H_9F_3N_2O_2 = 270.2$.

CAS — 75706-12-6.

Leflunomide has immunosuppressant properties believed to be partly due to the action of its active metabolite A77-1726 in inhibiting pyrimidine synthesis. It is used in the treatment of rheumatoid arthritis, and has been investigated in organ and tissue transplantation and psoriasis. Adverse effects reportedly include gastro-intestinal disturbances, alopecia, hypertension, and dizziness.

Preparations

Proprietary Preparations (details are given in Part 3)
USA: Arava.

Letrozole (17432-a)

Letrozole (*BAN, USAN, rINN*).

CGS-20267. 4,4′-(1*H*-1,2,4-Triazol-1-ylmethylene)dibenzonitrile.

$C_{17}H_{11}N_5 = 285.3$.

CAS — 112809-51-5.

Letrozole is a nonsteroidal inhibitor of the aromatase (oestrogen synthetase) system, similar to anastrozole (p.504). It is used in the treatment of breast cancer (p.485). The recommended dose in postmenopausal women unresponsive to conventional anti-oestrogenic therapy is 2.5 mg daily by mouth.

Studies[1,2] and reviews.[3,4]

1. Iveson TJ, *et al.* Phase I study of oral aromatase inhibitor CGS20267 in postmenopausal patients with breast cancer. *Cancer Res* 1993; **53:** 266–70.
2. Dombernowsky P, *et al.* Letrozole, a new oral aromatase inhibitor for advanced breast cancer: double-blind randomized trial showing a dose effect and improved efficacy and tolerability compared with megestrol acetate. *J Clin Oncol* 1998; **16:** 453–61.
3. Anonymous. New aromatase inhibitors for breast cancer. *Drug Ther Bull* 1997; **35:** 55–6.
4. Anonymous. Toremifene and letrozole for advanced breast cancer. *Med Lett Drugs Ther* 1998; **40:** 43–5.

Preparations

Proprietary Preparations (details are given in Part 3)
Austral.: Femara; ***Ital.:*** Femara; ***S.Afr.:*** Femara; ***Swed.:*** Femar; ***UK:*** Femara; ***USA:*** Femara.

Lithium Gamolenate (17722-v)

EF-13; LiGLA; Lithium Gammalinolenate.

Lithium gamolenate is a derivative of gamolenic acid (p.1582) which is under investigation for its antineoplastic properties, notably in the treatment of pancreatic cancer (p.491). It has also been investigated in patients with HIV infection.

References.

1. Fearon KC, *et al.* An open-label phase I/II dose escalation study of the treatment of pancreatic cancer using lithium gammalinolenate. *Anticancer Res* 1996; **16:** 867–74.

Lobaplatin (15418-b)

Lobaplatin *(rINN)*.

D-19466. *cis*-[*trans*-1,2-Cyclobutanebis(methylamine)][(*S*)-lactato-*O*[1],*O*[1]]platinum.

$C_9H_{18}N_2O_3Pt$ = 397.3.

CAS — 135558-11-1.

Lobaplatin is an analogue of cisplatin (p.513) which is under investigation for its antineoplastic properties. Thrombocytopenia is reported to be dose-limiting. It may be active against some cancer cells resistant to cisplatin or carboplatin.

References.

1. Weiss RB, Christian MC. New cisplatin analogues in development: a review. *Drugs* 1993; **6:** 360–77.
2. Gietema JA, *et al.* A phase 1 study of 1,2-diamminomethyl-cyclobutane-platinum (II) lactate (D-19466; lobaplatin) administered daily for 5 days. *Br J Cancer* 1993; **67:** 396–401.
3. Manegold C, *et al.* Lobaplatin (D-19466) in patients with advanced non-small-cell lung cancer: a trial of the association for medical oncology (AIO) phase II study group. *Onkologie* 1996; **19:** 248–51.
4. Fiebig HH, *et al.* Phase II clinical trial of lobaplatin (D-19466) in pretreated patients with small-cell lung cancer. *Onkologie* 1996; **19:** 328–32.
5. Sternberg CN, *et al.* Lobaplatin in advanced urothelial tract tumors. *Ann Oncol* 1997; **8:** 695–6.

Lomustine (1841-k)

Lomustine *(BAN, USAN, rINN)*.

CCNU; Lomustinum; NSC-79037; RB-1509; WR-139017. 1-(2-Chloroethyl)-3-cyclohexyl-1-nitrosourea.

$C_9H_{16}ClN_3O_2$ = 233.7.

CAS — 13010-47-4.

Pharmacopoeias. In *Chin.* and *Eur.* (see p.viii).

A yellow crystalline powder. Practically **insoluble** in water; soluble in alcohol; freely soluble in acetone and in dichloromethane. **Protect** from light.

Adverse Effects, Treatment, and Precautions

As for Carmustine, p.512, although bone-marrow depression may be even more delayed with lomustine. Neurological reactions such as confusion and lethargy have been reported.

Handling and disposal. A method for the destruction of lomustine waste by reaction with hydrobromic acid in glacial acetic acid.[1] The residue produced by the degradation of lomustine by this method showed no mutagenicity. This method is not suitable for the degradation of carmustine, semustine, or PCNU.

1. Castegnaro M, *et al.*, eds. Laboratory decontamination and destruction of carcinogens in laboratory wastes: some antineoplastic agents. *IARC Scientific Publications 73.* Lyon: WHO/International Agency for Research on Cancer, 1985.

Overdosage. A patient who inadvertently received 200 mg of lomustine for 7 days instead of a single 200 mg dose developed pancytopenia and subsequent multiorgan dysfunction including liver dysfunction, abdominal pain, pulmonary toxicity with tachypnoea and hypoxaemia, and CNS toxicity leading to confusion and disorientation.[1] Although the white cell count recovered other signs of toxicity did not and the patient developed fever and hypotension and died 59 days after the initial dose of lomustine.

1. Trent KC, *et al.* Multiorgan failure associated with lomustine overdose. *Ann Pharmacother* 1995; **29:** 384–6.

Interactions

As for Carmustine, p.512.

Theophylline. Leucopenia and thrombocytopenia in a 45-year-old woman were believed to have been secondary to an interaction between theophylline and lomustine.[1]

1. Zeltzer PM, Feig SA. Theophylline-induced lomustine toxicity. *Lancet* 1979; **ii:** 960–1.

Pharmacokinetics

Lomustine is absorbed from the gastro-intestinal tract and is rapidly metabolised, with peak plasma concentrations of metabolites occurring within 6 hours of a dose by mouth. Metabolites have a prolonged plasma half-life reported to range from 16 to 48 hours. Active metabolites readily cross the blood-brain barrier and appear in the cerebrospinal fluid in concentrations higher than those in plasma. About half a dose is excreted as metabolites in the urine within 24 hours and about 75% is excreted within 4 days.

Uses and Administration

Lomustine is a nitrosourea with actions and uses similar to those of carmustine (p.512). It has been used in the treatment of brain tumours (p.485) and resistant or relapsed Hodgkin's disease and other lymphomas (p.481), and also lung cancer (p.490), malignant melanoma (p.492), and various solid tumours.

Lomustine is given by mouth to adults and children as a single dose usually of 120 to 130 mg per m^2 body-surface; division of the dose over 3 consecutive days may reduce gastro-intestinal effects. A dose of 100 mg per m^2 should be given to patients with compromised bone-marrow function. Doses are also generally reduced when lomustine is given as part of a combination regimen. Providing blood counts have returned to acceptable levels, that is, platelets above 100 000 per mm^3 and leucocytes above 4000 per mm^3, doses may be repeated every 6 to 8 weeks, and should be adjusted according to the haematological response.

Preparations

BP 1998: Lomustine Capsules.

Proprietary Preparations (details are given in Part 3)
Aust.: Lucostin†; ***Austral.:*** CeeNU; ***Belg.:*** Cecenu; ***Canad.:*** CeeNU; ***Fr.:*** Belustine; ***Ger.:*** Cecenu; Lomeblastin†; ***Ital.:*** Belustine; ***Norw.:*** Lucostine†; ***S.Afr.:*** CeeNU; ***Spain:*** Belustine; CCNU†; ***Swed.:*** Lucostine†; ***Switz.:*** CiNU†; Prava; ***UK:*** CCNU; ***USA:*** CeeNU.

Lonidamine (19416-e)

Lonidamine *(BAN, rINN)*.

AF-1890; Diclondazolic Acid. 1-(2,4-Dichlorobenzyl)indazole-3-carboxylic acid.

$C_{15}H_{10}Cl_2N_2O_2$ = 321.2.

CAS — 50264-69-2.

Lonidamine is an antineoplastic that is thought to act by inhibiting mitochondrial function in tumour cells. It may be given by mouth in the treatment of various solid neoplasms, including those of the lung, breast, prostate, and brain, in usual doses of 450 to 900 mg daily, in 3 divided doses. See also under Choice of Antineoplastic, p.485, for mention of its use in breast cancer. Myalgia is common, and may be dose-limiting. Other adverse effects include testicular pain, auditory dysfunction, gastro-intestinal disturbances, drowsiness, weakness, and conjunctivitis with photophobia, but it is reported to lack myelosuppressive effects and not to cause stomatitis or alopecia.

References.

1. Putzolu S, Taddei I. New perspectives in anticancer therapy: a review on lonidamine. *Drugs Today* 1989; **25:** 195–209.
2. De Lena M, *et al.* Revertant and potentiating activity of lonidamine in patients with ovarian cancer previously treated with platinum. *J Clin Oncol* 1997; **15:** 3208–13.

Preparations

Proprietary Preparations (details are given in Part 3)
Ital.: Doridamina.

Mafosfamide (18785-v)

Mafosfamide *(rINN)*.

(±)-2-({2-[Bis(2-chloroethyl)amino]tetrahydro-2*H*-1,3,2-oxazaphosphorin-4-yl}thio)ethanesulphonic acid *P-cis* oxide.

$C_9H_{19}Cl_2N_2O_5PS_2$ = 401.3.

CAS — 88859-04-5.

Mafosfamide is a derivative of cyclophosphamide (p.516) that has been used to treat bone marrow for transplantation.

Marimastat (17715-g)

Marimastat *(BAN, USAN, rINN)*.

BB-2516. (2*S*,3*R*)-3-{(*S*)-[2,2-Dimethyl-1-(methylcarbamoyl)propyl]carbamoyl}-2-hydroxy-5-methylhexanohydroxamic acid.

$C_{15}H_{29}N_3O_5$ = 331.4.

CAS — 154039-60-8.

Like batimastat (p.507) marimastat is an inhibitor of matrix metalloproteinases, enzymes which are thought to play a role in the metastasis of cancer cells. It is under investigation in various malignant disorders, notably in advanced pancreatic cancer. It is given by mouth.

Gore and colleagues have commented that the alterations in tumour markers reported in patients with ovarian cancer given marimastat might be artefactual;[1] however the manufacturers considered that these and further results in patients with pancreatic, prostatic, and colorectal cancers were evidence of genuine activity.[2] In healthy subjects given doses between 25 and 800 mg by mouth marimastat was reportedly well tolerated and rapidly absorbed, with peak drug concentrations achieved within 3 hours of a dose, and mean half-life of the order of 8 to 10 hours, suggesting that twice daily dosage would be appropriate.[3]

1. Gore M, *et al.* Tumour marker levels during marimastat therapy. *Lancet* 1996; **348:** 263.
2. Millar A, *et al.* Tumour marker levels during marimastat therapy. *Lancet* 1996; **348:** 263–4.
3. Millar AW, *et al.* Results of single and repeat dose studies of the oral matrix metalloproteinase inhibitor marimastat in healthy male volunteers. *Br J Clin Pharmacol* 1998; **45:** 21–6.

Masoprocol (13920-h)

Masoprocol *(USAN, rINN)*.

CHX-10; CHX-100; Mesonordihydroguaiaretic Acid; *meso*-NDGA. *meso*-4,4′-(2,3-Dimethyltetramethylene)dipyrocatechol.

CAS — 27686-84-6.

Adverse Effects and Precautions

Masoprocol may produce transient local burning following application. It frequently causes allergic contact dermatitis; masoprocol should be discontinued if this occurs. Local skin reactions such as erythema, itching, and dryness are frequent but usually resolve within a couple of weeks of stopping treatment. Contact with the eyes or mucous membranes should be avoided. Masoprocol may stain clothing and fabrics.

Uses and Administration

Masoprocol is a 5-lipoxygenase inhibitor isolated from the plant *Larrea divaricata*. It is reported to have antineoplastic activity. It is used as a 10% cream in the treatment of actinic (solar) keratoses. The cream is applied twice daily for 28 days. Masoprocol is also being studied in the treatment of basal cell epitheliomas.

Actinic keratoses. Application of a cream containing masoprocol 10% twice daily for 14 to 28 days appeared to be effective in the treatment of actinic keratoses of the head and neck but of 113 patients evaluated 25 had to discontinue treatment because of local adverse effects such as erythema, flaking, itching, burning, oedema, dryness, soreness, or bleeding.[1]

1. Olsen EA, *et al.* A double-blind, vehicle-controlled study evaluating masoprocol cream in the treatment of actinic keratoses on the head and neck. *J Am Acad Dermatol* 1991; **24:** 738–43.

Preparations

Proprietary Preparations (details are given in Part 3)
USA: Actinex.

Melphalan (1843-t)

Melphalan *(BAN, USAN, rINN)*.

CB-3025; NSC-8806 (melphalan hydrochloride); PAM; Phenylalanine Mustard; Phenylalanine Nitrogen Mustard; L-Sarcolysine; WR-19813. 4-Bis(2-chloroethyl)amino-L-phenylalanine.

$C_{13}H_{18}Cl_2N_2O_2$ = 305.2.

CAS — 148-82-3.

NOTE. Merphalan (CB-3007; NSC-14210; sarcolysine) is the racemic form of melphalan; Medphalan (CB-3026; NSC-35051) is the D-isomer of melphalan.

Pharmacopoeias. In *Br.*, *Jpn*, and *US.*

A white to buff-coloured powder, odourless or with a faint odour. It loses not more than 7% of its weight on drying.

Practically **insoluble** in water, chloroform, and ether; slightly soluble in alcohol and methyl alcohol; dissolves in dilute mineral acids. **Store** at a temperature not exceeding 25° in airtight containers. Protect from light.

Stability. A study of the stability of melphalan 40 and 400 μg per mL in infusion fluids reported that the time for a 10% loss of drug at 20° in sodium chloride injection (0.9%) was 4.5

hours, compared with 2.9 hours in lactated Ringer's injection, which has a considerably lower chloride ion content, and only 1.5 hours in glucose injection (5%).[1] At 25° the corresponding figures were 2.4, 1.5, and 0.6 hours, and at 37° they were 0.6, 0.4, and 0.3 hours. It was concluded that melphalan is sufficiently stable at 20° in sodium chloride injection to permit infusion, but that increased temperature and decreased chloride ion concentration were associated with faster degradation rates.[1] Another study recommended that solutions of melphalan be handled at temperatures above 5° for the minimum time but found that a solution containing 20 μg per mL in 0.9% sodium chloride could be stored for at least 6 months at −20° without significant deterioration.[2] A more recent study, while recommending storage at 4° from preparation of the admixture until the infusion began, considered that administration at a room temperature of 20° or below, and use of hypertonic (3%) saline as a diluent, would be sufficient to allow prolonged infusion.[3] The practicalities of such a procedure were not addressed.

1. Tabibi SE, Cradock JC. Stability of melphalan in infusion fluids. *Am J Hosp Pharm* 1984; **41:** 1380–2.
2. Bosanquet AG. Stability of melphalan solutions during preparation and storage. *J Pharm Sci* 1985; **74:** 348–51.
3. Pinguet F, *et al.* Effect of sodium chloride concentration and temperature on melphalan stability during storage and use. *Am J Hosp Pharm* 1994; **51:** 2701–4.

Adverse Effects and Treatment

For general discussions see Antineoplastics, p.470 and p.473.

The onset of neutropenia and thrombocytopenia is variable; bone-marrow depression has been reported 2 to 3 weeks after starting treatment with melphalan, with a nadir at 3 to 5 weeks, but has also occurred after only 5 days. Recovery may be prolonged.

Skin rashes and hypersensitivity reactions, including anaphylaxis, may occur. Cardiac arrest has been reported in association with such effects. Gastro-intestinal disturbances may sometimes occur, particularly at high doses where diarrhoea, vomiting, and stomatitis may become dose-limiting. Haemolytic anaemia, vasculitis, and pulmonary fibrosis have been reported. Suppression of ovarian function is common in premenopausal women; temporary or permanent sterility may occur in male patients. As with other alkylating agents, melphalan also has carcinogenic, mutagenic, and teratogenic potential.

Overdosage. A 12-month old child given melphalan 140 mg (a tenfold overdose) intravenously developed pronounced lymphopenia within 24 hours but had no other significant adverse effects until the 7th day, when neutropenia, thrombocytopenia, oral ulceration, and diarrhoea developed.[1] Bone marrow recovered within 40 days. Treatment was by vigorous hyperalimentation and close surveillance during the period of suppression and the patient has subsequently remained well 9 months afterwards, without complications.

1. Coates TD. Survival from melphalan overdose. *Lancet* 1984; **ii:** 1048.

Precautions

For general discussions see Antineoplastics, p.474.

Care is required in patients with impaired renal function. The dose of the intravenous preparation should be reduced by 50% in patients with moderate to severe renal impairment and dosage reduction should be considered when administering melphalan by mouth. High dose regimens are not recommended in patients with severe renal impairment.

Handling and disposal. Urine and faeces produced for up to 48 hours and 7 days respectively after a dose of melphalan by mouth should be handled wearing protective clothing.[1]

1. Harris J, Dodds LJ. Handling waste from patients receiving cytotoxic drugs. *Pharm J* 1985; **235:** 289–91.

Interactions

Concomitant administration of nalidixic acid with high-dose intravenous melphalan in children has resulted in fatal haemorrhagic enterocolitis.

For reference to enhanced toxicity when melphalan was given with cyclosporin, see under Cyclosporin, p.522. For the effect of interferon alfa on the pharmacokinetics of melphalan, see under Pharmacokinetics, below.

With food. The bioavailability of oral melphalan is significantly reduced, by up to 45%, by concomitant administration with food. Some recommend that melphalan should not be taken with food, and that if administration is switched from after to before food patients should be monitored for increased toxicity.[1]

1. Nathan C, Betmouni R. Melphalan: avoid with food. *Pharm J* 1996; **257:** 264.

Pharmacokinetics

Absorption of melphalan from the gastro-intestinal tract is variable; the mean bioavailability is reported to be 56% but it may range from 25 to 89%. Absorption is reduced by the presence of food (see above). Following absorption it is rapidly distributed throughout body water with a volume of distribution of about 0.5 litres per kg body-weight, and has been reported to be inactivated mainly by spontaneous hydrolysis. The terminal plasma half-life of melphalan has been reported to be of the order of 40 to 140 minutes. Melphalan is excreted in the urine, about 10% as unchanged drug. About 50 to 60% of an absorbed dose has been stated to be protein bound initially, increasing to 80 to 90% after 12 hours.

Effect of temperature. The fever caused by concomitant administration of interferon alfa with melphalan resulted in a reduction in the area under the plasma concentration-time curve (AUC) in 10 patients although the peak plasma concentration and time to peak concentration were not affected.[1] The effect was thought to represent increased chemical reactivity of melphalan at the elevated temperature.

1. Ehrsson H, *et al.* Oral melphalan pharmacokinetics: influence of interferon-induced fever. *Clin Pharmacol Ther* 1990; **47:** 86–90.

Uses and Administration

Melphalan is an antineoplastic that acts as a bifunctional alkylating agent. It is used mainly in the treatment of multiple myeloma. Melphalan has also been given to patients with carcinoma of the breast and ovary, in gestational trophoblastic tumours, Hodgkin's disease, and in polycythaemia vera and Waldenström's macroglobulinaemia, and has been administered by intra-arterial regional perfusion for malignant melanoma and soft-tissue sarcomas. See also the cross-references given below.

Melphalan is usually given by mouth; it is also administered intravenously. By mouth, it may be given as a single daily dose or in divided doses.

Numerous **conventional-dose** regimens have been tried for the treatment of multiple myeloma and there is still uncertainty as to the best schedule. Oral dosage regimens include: 150 μg per kg body-weight daily in divided doses for 4 to 7 days; or melphalan 250 μg per kg daily for 4 days; or 6 mg daily for 2 to 3 weeks. Melphalan is usually combined with corticosteroids. Courses are followed by a rest period of up to 6 weeks to allow recovery of haematological function and are then repeated, or maintenance therapy may be instituted, usually with a daily dose of 1 to 3 mg, or up to 50 μg per kg. For optimum effect, therapy is usually adjusted to produce a moderate leucopenia, with white-cell counts in the range 3000 to 3500 per mm^3.

In the treatment of breast cancer, suggested doses of melphalan by mouth are 150 μg per kg daily or 6 mg per m^2 body-surface daily for 5 days, repeated every 6 weeks. Doses of 200 μg per kg daily for 5 days every 4 to 8 weeks have been given to patients with ovarian carcinoma.

In patients with polycythaemia vera, doses of 6 to 10 mg daily for 5 to 7 days, and then 2 to 4 mg daily, have been used for remission induction; a dose of 2 to 6 mg once a week has been used for maintenance.

Melphalan therapy should be interrupted if the platelet count falls below 100 000 per mm^3 or the white-cell count below 3000 per mm^3. During administration of melphalan, frequent blood counts are essential. It should be given with great caution if the neutrophil count has recently been depressed by chemotherapy or radiotherapy.

Melphalan is also given intravenously; a single dose of 1 mg per kg, repeated in 4 weeks if the platelet and neutrophil counts permit, has been given in ovarian adenocarcinoma. It may be infused in sodium chloride injection (0.9%) or injected into the tubing of a fast-running drip; when given by infusion the time from reconstitution of the solution to completion of infusion should not exceed 1.5 hours and prolonged infusions should be carried out with several batches of solution, each freshly prepared. In multiple myeloma, the usual intravenous dose is 400 μg per kg or 16 mg per m^2, infused over 15 to 20 minutes, at 4-week intervals if toxicity permits. Dosage should be adjusted according to haematological response.

High-dose melphalan has been given intravenously in some malignancies: doses of 100 to 240 mg per m^2 have been cited in neuroblastoma, and 100 to 200 mg per m^2 in multiple myeloma, generally followed by autologous stem cell rescue, which becomes essential where doses exceed 140 mg per m^2.

Melphalan may be given by **local perfusion** in the management of melanoma and soft-tissue sarcomas. A typical dosage range for upper extremity perfusions is 0.6 to 1 mg per kg, whereas for lower extremity perfusions doses of 0.8 to 1.5 mg per kg (in melanoma) or 1.0 to 1.4 mg per kg (in sarcoma) are typically used.

The hydrochloride has also been used.

Amyloidosis. For reference to the use of melphalan in amyloidosis, see p.497.

Bone disorders, non-malignant. A patient with fibrogenesis imperfecta ossium, a progressive abnormality of bone structure leading to bone pain and fractures, responded to treatment with melphalan 10 mg and prednisolone 20 mg daily, in 7-day courses.[1]

1. Stamp TCB, *et al.* Fibrogenesis imperfecta ossium: remission with melphalan. *Lancet* 1985; **i:** 582–3.

Malignant neoplasms. The important role played by melphalan in the management of multiple myeloma is discussed on p.494. Melphalan is also used in high doses as part of salvage regimens for relapsed Hodgkin's disease (see p.481) and as part of the M2 regimen in the treatment of Waldenström's macroglobulinaemia (see p.496). Melphalan is also part of regimens that have been used for high-risk patients with gestational trophoblastic tumours (p.477), in the adjuvant chemotherapy of breast cancer (p.485), in ovarian cancer (p.491), and for local perfusion of melanoma (p.492).

Preparations

BP 1998: Melphalan Injection; Melphalan Tablets;
USP 23: Melphalan Tablets.

Proprietary Preparations (details are given in Part 3)

Aust.: Alkeran; ***Austral.:*** Alkeran; ***Belg.:*** Alkeran; ***Canad.:*** Alkeran; ***Fr.:*** Alkeran; ***Ger.:*** Alkeran; ***Irl.:*** Alkeran; ***Ital.:*** Alkeran; ***Neth.:*** Alkeran; ***Norw.:*** Alkeran; ***S.Afr.:*** Alkeran; ***Swed.:*** Alkeran; ***Switz.:*** Alkeran; ***UK:*** Alkeran; ***USA:*** Alkeran.

Menogaril (19470-k)

Menogaril *(USAN, rINN).*

NSC-269148; 7-Omen; U-52047. (2*R*,3*S*,4*R*,5*R*,6*R*,11*R*,13*R*)-4-(Dimethylamino)-3,4,5,6,11,12,13,14-octahydro-3,5,8,10,13-pentahydroxy-11-methoxy-6,13-dimethyl-2,6-epoxy-2*H*-naphthaceno[1,2-*b*]oxocin-9,16-dione; 7-(*R*)-*O*-methylnogarol.

$C_{28}H_{31}NO_{10}$ = 541.5.

CAS — 71628-96-1.

Menogaril is an anthracycline derivative related to doxorubicin (p.529) but which may not act by intercalation of DNA.

References.

1. Mazurek C, *et al.* Phase I clinical and pharmacokinetic study of menogaril (7-con-O-methylnogarol) in previously treated patients with acute leukaemia. *Invest New Drugs* 1993; **11:** 313–22.

Mercaptopurine (1844-x)

Mercaptopurine (*BAN, rINN*).

Mercaptopurinum; NSC-755; 6MP; Purinethiol; WR-2785. 6-Mercaptopurine monohydrate; Purine-6-thiol monohydrate; 1,7-Dihydro-6*H*-purine-6-thione monohydrate.

$C_5H_4N_4S,H_2O$ = 170.2.

CAS — 6112-76-1 (mercaptopurine monohydrate); 50-44-2 (anhydrous mercaptopurine).

Pharmacopoeias. In *Chin., Eur.* (see p.viii), *Jpn, Pol.*, and *US.*

A yellow, odourless or almost odourless, crystalline powder. Practically **insoluble** in water, acetone, and ether; slightly soluble in alcohol; soluble in hot alcohol and in dilute solutions of alkali; slightly soluble in M sulphuric acid. **Protect** from light.

Adverse Effects, Treatment, and Precautions

For general discussions see Antineoplastics, p.470, p.473, and p.474.

Bone-marrow depression with mercaptopurine may be delayed; hypoplasia may occur. Mercaptopurine is less toxic to the gastro-intestinal tract than the folic acid antagonists or fluorouracil but gastro-intestinal disturbances may occur. Hepatotoxicity has been reported, with cholestatic jaundice and necrosis, sometimes fatal. Gastro-intestinal and hepatic toxicity are reported to be more frequent in adults than in children, and are more likely at higher doses. Crystalluria with haematuria has been observed rarely as have skin disorders including hyperpigmentation. Fever may occur.

Mercaptopurine is potentially carcinogenic and mutagenic; an increased incidence of abortion has occurred in women given mercaptopurine during the first trimester of pregnancy.

Mercaptopurine should be used with care in patients with impaired hepatic or renal function. Hepatic function should be monitored periodically.

Effects on the blood. The degree of neutropenia in patients receiving mercaptopurine has been reported to correlate with the concentration of the metabolite thioguanine nucleotide in erythrocytes,[1] and it has been suggested that measurement of metabolite concentrations in erythrocytes permits prediction of bone-marrow toxicity,[2] both with mercaptopurine and the related drugs thioguanine and azathioprine. Higher concentrations of thioguanine nucleotides are found in patients with low levels of the enzyme thiopurine methyltransferase, which metabolises mercaptopurine via an alternative pathway, and it has been suggested that particular care is needed in such patients to avoid myelotoxicity.[3,4] However, effects on the bone marrow with this class of drugs are probably multifactorial,[5] and low activity of other enzymes such as lymphocyte 5-nucleotidase,[6] and other factors, may contribute to toxicity.

For the view that dosage should be titrated until myelotoxicity occurs, see Administration, below.

1. Lennard L, *et al.* Childhood leukaemia: a relationship between intracellular 6-mercaptopurine metabolites and neutropenia. *Br J Clin Pharmacol* 1983; **16:** 359–63.
2. Maddocks JL, *et al.* Azathioprine and severe bone marrow depression. *Lancet* 1986; **i:** 156.
3. Schütz E, *et al.* Azathioprine-induced myelosuppression in thiopurine methyltransferase deficient heart transplant recipient. *Lancet* 1993; **341:** 436.
4. Lennard L, *et al.* Congenital thiopurine methyltransferase deficiency and 6-mercaptopurine toxicity during treatment for acute lymphoblastic leukaemia. *Arch Dis Child* 1993; **69:** 577–9.
5. Soria-Royer C, *et al.* Thiopurine-methyl-transferase activity to assess azathioprine myelotoxicity in renal transplant recipients. *Lancet* 1993; **341:** 1593–4.
6. Kerstens PJSM, *et al.* 5-Nucleotidase and azathioprine-related bone-marrow toxicity. *Lancet* 1993; **342:** 1245–6.

Effects on the pancreas. Pancreatitis occurred in 13 of 396 patients treated with mercaptopurine for inflammatory bowel disease.[1] Symptoms resolved on withdrawal but recurred in 7 who were re-challenged with the mercaptopurine or azathioprine.

1. Present DH, *et al.* 6-Mercaptopurine in the management of inflammatory bowel disease: short- and long-term toxicity. *Ann Intern Med* 1989; **111:** 641–9.

-dling and disposal. Urine and faeces produced for up -urs and 5 days, respectively after a dose of mercap- hould be handled wearing protective clothing.[1]

-odds LJ. Handling waste from patients receiving cy- . *Pharm J* 1985; **235:** 289–91.

A method for the destruction of mercaptopurine or thioguanine in wastes by oxidation with potassium permanganate in sulphuric acid.[1] Residues produced by this method had no mutagenic activity.

1. Castegnaro M, *et al.*, eds. Laboratory decontamination and destruction of carcinogens in laboratory wastes: some antineoplastic agents. *IARC Scientific Publications 73.* Lyon: WHO/International Agency for Research on Cancer, 1985.

Interactions

Mercaptopurine should be given with particular caution in combination with other drugs known to be hepatotoxic. The effects of mercaptopurine are enhanced by allopurinol and the dose of mercaptopurine should be reduced to one-third to one-quarter of the usual dose when allopurinol is given concomitantly.

Allopurinol. Mercaptopurine plasma concentrations were markedly increased by allopurinol when mercaptopurine was given by mouth but not when it was given intravenously.[1] The results appear to indicate that allopurinol inhibits the first-pass metabolism of mercaptopurine.

1. Zimm S, *et al.* Inhibition of first-pass metabolism in cancer chemotherapy: interaction of 6-mercaptopurine and allopurinol. *Clin Pharmacol Ther* 1983; **34:** 810–17.

Anticoagulants. For reference to mercaptopurine diminishing the activity of warfarin, see Warfarin Sodium, p.967.

Doxorubicin. For a suggestion that doxorubicin might enhance the hepatotoxicity of mercaptopurine, see under Daunorubicin Hydrochloride, p.528.

Gastro-intestinal drugs. The enzyme thiopurine methyltransferase was inhibited by sulphasalazine and mesalazine *in vitro*, raising the possibility of an interaction in patients treated simultaneously with an aminosalicylate and mercaptopurine.[1] Myelotoxicity has been reported in a patient receiving mercaptopurine concomitantly with olsalazine.[2]

1. Szumlanski C, Weinshilboum RM. Sulfasalazine inhibition of thiopurine methyltransferase: possible mechanism for interaction with 6-mercaptopurine. *Clin Pharmacol Ther* 1995; **57:** 184.
2. Lewis LD, *et al.* Olsalazine and 6-mercaptopurine-related bone marrow suppression: a possible drug-drug interaction. *Clin Pharmacol Ther* 1997; **62:** 464–75.

Methotrexate. Concurrent administration of mercaptopurine and low-dose methotrexate by mouth resulted in an increase in mean peak plasma concentrations of mercaptopurine of 26% compared with administration of the same dose of mercaptopurine alone in a study in 14 patients with acute lymphoblastic leukaemia.[1] The effect was probably due to inhibition of the first-pass metabolism of mercaptopurine by methotrexate, which is a potent inhibitor of xanthine oxidase. Although the resultant increase in mercaptopurine concentrations was unlikely to be significant in this case, higher doses of methotrexate given concurrently with mercaptopurine might be cause for concern.

1. Balis FM, *et al.* The effect of methotrexate on the bioavailability of oral 6-mercaptopurine. *Clin Pharmacol Ther* 1987; **41:** 384–7.

Pharmacokinetics

Mercaptopurine is variably and incompletely absorbed from the gastro-intestinal tract; about 50% of an oral dose has been reported to be absorbed, but the absolute bioavailability is somewhat lower, probably due to gastro-intestinal or first-pass metabolism, and is also subject to wide interindividual variation. Once absorbed it is widely distributed throughout body water and tissues. Plasma half-lives ranging from about 20 to 90 minutes have been reported after intravenous injection and the drug is not found in plasma after about 8 hours but this is of limited significance since mercaptopurine is activated intracellularly by conversion to nucleotide derivatives which persist for much longer. It is rapidly and extensively metabolised in the liver, by methylation and oxidation as well as by the formation of inorganic sulphates. Considerable amounts are oxidised to thiouric acid by the enzyme xanthine oxidase. It is excreted in urine as metabolites and some unchanged drug; about half an oral dose has been recovered in 24 hours. A small proportion is excreted over several weeks.

Mercaptopurine crosses the blood-brain barrier to some extent and is found in the cerebrospinal fluid, but only in subtherapeutic concentrations.

Uses and Administration

Mercaptopurine is an antineoplastic that acts as an antimetabolite. It is an analogue of the natural purines hypoxanthine and adenine. After the intracellular conversion of mercaptopurine to active nucleotides, including thioinosinic acid, it appears to exhibit a variety of actions including interfering with nucleic acid synthesis. It also has immunosuppressant properties. Its actions are specific for cells in S phase.

Mercaptopurine is used, usually with other agents, in the treatment of leukaemia. It induces remissions in acute lymphoblastic and non-lymphoblastic leukaemias (p.478 and p.479, respectively) but other agents are generally preferred and mercaptopurine is chiefly employed in maintenance programmes, commonly in association with methotrexate. It may also be effective in chronic myeloid leukaemia (p.480). There is cross-resistance between mercaptopurine and thioguanine (p.566).

Mercaptopurine has been used for its immunosuppressant properties in the treatment of various autoimmune disorders such as inflammatory bowel disease but has been largely replaced by azathioprine.

Mercaptopurine is administered by mouth. The usual initial dose for children and adults is 2.5 mg per kg body-weight or 75 to 100 mg per m^2 body-surface area daily but the dosage varies according to individual response and tolerance. If there is no clinical improvement and no evidence of white-cell depression after 4 weeks, the dose may be cautiously increased up to 5 mg per kg daily. In maintenance schedules the dose may vary from 1.5 to 2.5 mg per kg daily. Blood counts should be taken at least once a week and if there is a steep fall in the white-cell count or severe bone-marrow depression the drug should be withdrawn immediately. Therapy may be resumed carefully if the white-cell count remains constant for 2 or 3 days or rises.

It has been administered intravenously as mercaptopurine sodium. Thioinosine (mercaptopurine riboside) has also been used.

Administration. There is evidence[1] that the maintenance dosage of mercaptopurine should be tailored individually to achieve an appropriate systemic exposure in children with acute lymphoblastic leukaemia (although this would involve determining mercaptopurine pharmacokinetics in each child). Improvements in survival since 1980 may be associated with changes in the prescribing of mercaptopurine which have resulted in greater cumulative doses being given;[2] some children may have been undertreated in the past because of variations in the pharmacokinetics of mercaptopurine (particularly boys, who tolerate mercaptopurine better than girls,[3] but who have a poorer prognosis).[2] The concentration of thioguanine nucleotide metabolites in the erythrocytes has been shown to be directly related to the risk of relapse in children with acute lymphoblastic leukaemia.[4] Thiopurine methyltransferase activity (which results in methylation and inactivation of mercaptopurine rather than the formation of active nucleotides) may play a substantial role in this variation,[5] but titration of the dose of mercaptopurine until myelotoxicity occurs may prevent the problem:[2] despite gaps in therapy caused by more frequent drug withdrawal, it appears to result in greater accumulation of thioguanine nucleotides in the cells.[6] See also under Effects on the Blood, above.

1. Koren G, *et al.* Systemic exposure to mercaptopurine as a prognostic factor in acute lymphocytic leukemia in children. *N Engl J Med* 1990; **323:** 17–21.
2. Hale JP, Lilleyman JS. Importance of 6-mercaptopurine dose in lymphoblastic leukaemia. *Arch Dis Child* 1991; **66:** 462–6.
3. Lilleyman JS, *et al.* Childhood lymphoblastic leukaemia: sex difference in 6-mercaptopurine utilization. *Br J Cancer* 1984; **49:** 703–7.
4. Lilleyman JS, Lennard L. Mercaptopurine metabolism and risk of relapse in childhood lymphoblastic leukaemia. *Lancet* 1994; **343:** 1188–90.
5. Lennard L, *et al.* Genetic variation in response to 6-mercaptopurine for childhood acute lymphoblastic leukaemia. *Lancet* 1990; **336:** 225–9.
6. Lennard L, *et al.* Mercaptopurine in childhood leukaemia: the effects of dose escalation on thioguanine nucleotide metabolites. *Br J Clin Pharmacol* 1996; **42:** 525–7.

Inflammatory bowel disease. Mercaptopurine has been reported to be of benefit in ulcerative colitis[1,2] and Crohn's disease,[3,4] although azathioprine has generally been preferred (see p.1171).

1. Adler DJ, Korelitz BI. The therapeutic efficacy of 6-mercaptopurine in refractory ulcerative colitis. *Am J Gastroenterol* 1990; **85:** 717–22.
2. George J, *et al.* The long-term outcome of ulcerative colitis treated with 6-mercaptopurine. *Am J Gastroenterol* 1996; **91:** 1711–14.
3. Present DH, *et al.* Treatment of Crohn's disease with 6-mercaptopurine: a long-term randomized, double-blind study. *N Engl J Med* 1980; **302:** 981–7.
4. Pearson DC, *et al.* Azathioprine and 6-mercaptopurine in Crohn disease: a meta-analysis. *Ann Intern Med* 1995; **122:** 132–42.

Polymyositis. Mercaptopurine has been tried in a few patients with polymyositis but has not been formally assessed; most experience seems to be with azathioprine (see p.1027).

Preparations

BP 1998: Mercaptopurine Tablets;
USP 23: Mercaptopurine Tablets.

Proprietary Preparations (details are given in Part 3)
Aust.: Puri-Nethol; ***Austral.:*** Puri-Nethol; ***Belg.:*** Puri-Nethol; ***Canad.:*** Puri-Nethol; ***Fr.:*** Puri-Nethol; ***Ger.:*** Mercap; Puri-Nethol; ***Irl.:*** Puri-Nethol; ***Ital.:*** Ismipur; Puri-Nethol; ***Neth.:*** Puri-Nethol; ***Norw.:*** Puri-Nethol; ***S.Afr.:*** Puri-Nethol; ***Swed.:*** Puri-Nethol; ***Switz.:*** Puri-Nethol; ***UK:*** Puri-Nethol; ***USA:*** Puri-Nethol.

Methotrexate (9550-n)

Methotrexate *(BAN, USAN, rINN).*

Amethopterin; 4-Amino-4-deoxy-10-methylpteroyl-L-glutamic Acid; 4-Amino-10-methylfolic Acid; CL-14377; α-Methopterin; Methotrexatum; Metotrexato; MTX; NSC-740; WR-19039. *N*-{4-[(2,4-Diaminopteridin-6-ylmethyl)methylamino]benzoyl}-L(+)-glutamic acid.

$C_{20}H_{22}N_8O_5$ = 454.4.

CAS — 59-05-2.

Pharmacopoeias. In *Chin., Eur.* (see p.viii), *Int., Jpn,* and *US.*

Methotrexate is a mixture of 4-amino-10-methylfolic acid and related substances; the Ph. Eur. specifies not less than 97% and the USP not less than 98% of $C_{20}H_{22}N_8O_5$, calculated on the anhydrous basis. A yellow to orange-brown crystalline powder. It contains not more than 12% of water.

Practically **insoluble** in water, alcohol, chloroform, and ether; dissolves in dilute solutions of mineral acids and of alkali hydroxides and carbonates. **Store** in airtight containers. Protect from light.

Methotrexate Sodium (1845-r)

Methotrexate Sodium *(BANM, rINNM).*

Methotrexate Disodium.

$C_{20}H_{20}N_8Na_2O_5$ = 498.4.

CAS — 7413-34-5 (methotrexate disodium); 15475-56-6 (methotrexate sodium, xNa).

Pharmacopoeias. US includes under the title Methotrexate for Injection.

CAUTION. *Methotrexate is irritant; avoid contact with skin and mucous membranes.*

Incompatibility. Methotrexate sodium has been reported to be incompatible with cytarabine, fluorouracil, and prednisolone sodium phosphate;[1] however, its incompatibility with fluorouracil has been questioned.[2] Furthermore a mixture of methotrexate sodium with cytarabine and hydrocortisone sodium succinate in various infusion fluids has been reported to be visually compatible for at least 8 hours at 25°, although precipitation did occur on storage for several days.[3]

1. McRae MP, King JC. Compatibility of antineoplastic, antibiotic and corticosteroid drugs in intravenous admixtures. *Am J Hosp Pharm* 1976; **33:** 1010–13.
2. Morrison RA, *et al.* 5-Fluorouracil and methotrexate sodium: an admixture incompatibility? *Am J Hosp Pharm* 1978; **35:** 15–18.
3. Cheung Y-W, *et al.* Stability of cytarabine, methotrexate sodium, and hydrocortisone sodium succinate admixtures. *Am J Hosp Pharm* 1984; **41:** 1802–6.

Stability to light. Methotrexate undergoes photodegradation when stored in the light in diluted solutions,[1] although undiluted commercial preparations are reported to show negligible photodegradation.[1] The bicarbonate ion catalyses this reaction and such admixtures should be avoided if possible, although they may be stable in light for 12 hours. Storage of solutions diluted in 0.9% sodium chloride injection in polyvinyl chloride bags was reported to protect against photodegradation although the length of the study was only 4 hours.[2] Photodegradation can take place under normal lighting, but is more rapid in direct sunlight, with about 11% drug loss from a 1 mg per mL solution after 7 hours; storage under normal lighting resulted in little change in drug concentration over 24 hours with a decrease of up to 12% by 48 hours.[3] Loss was greatest from unprotected polybutadiene tubing, with almost 80% drug loss in 48 hours.

1. Chatterji DC, Gallelli JF. Thermal and photolytic decomposition of methotrexate in aqueous solutions. *J Pharm Sci* 1978; **67:** 526–31.
2. Dyvik O, *et al.* Methotrexate in infusion solutions—a stability test for the hospital pharmacy. *J Clin Hosp Pharm* 1986; **11:** 343–8.
3. McElnay JC, *et al.* Stability of methotrexate and vinblastine in burette administration sets. *Int J Pharmaceutics* 1988; **47:** 239–47.

Adverse Effects

For general discussions see Antineoplastics, p.470.

The most common toxic effects of methotrexate are on the bone marrow and gastro-intestinal tract. Bone-marrow depression can occur abruptly, and leucopenia, thrombocytopenia, and anaemia may all occur. The nadir of the platelet and white-blood cell counts is usually around 5 to 10 days after a bolus dose, with recovery between about 14 to 28 days, but some sources suggest that leucocytes may exhibit an early fall and rise, followed by a second nadir and recovery, within this period. Megaloblastic anaemia has also been reported. Ulceration of the mouth and gastro-intestinal disturbances are also early signs of toxicity: stomatitis and diarrhoea are signs that treatment should be interrupted, otherwise haemorrhagic enteritis, intestinal perforation, and death may follow.

Methotrexate therapy is associated with liver damage, both acute (notably after high doses) and, more seriously, chronic (generally after long-term administration). Hepatic fibrosis and cirrhosis may develop without obvious signs of hepatotoxicity, and have led to eventual death.

Other adverse effects include renal failure and tubular necrosis following high doses, pulmonary reactions including life-threatening interstitial lung disease, skin reactions, alopecia, osteoporosis, arthralgia, myalgia, ocular irritation, and precipitation of diabetes. Neurotoxicity may be seen in 5% or more of patients: leucoencephalopathy, paresis, demyelination, and arachnoiditis are associated particularly with intrathecal administration and are more likely when cranial irradiation is also given. Intrathecal administration may also produce an acute syndrome of headache, nuchal rigidity, back pain, and fever.

Methotrexate may cause defective oogenesis and spermatogenesis, and fertility may be impaired. Like other folate inhibitors it is teratogenic, and it has been associated with fetal deaths.

Carcinogenicity. There are reports of lymphomas associated with low-dose methotrexate therapy for rheumatic disorders,[1-3] which in some cases have been associated with concomitant Epstein-Barr virus infection.[2] Transitional cell bladder cancer has also been associated with such therapy.[4] However, a retrospective analysis involving 16 263 patients with rheumatoid arthritis found no evidence of a relationship between the use of methotrexate as an antirheumatic and the development of haematological malignancy.[5] The carcinogenic risk with antimetabolites such as methotrexate has generally been considered less than with alkylating agents (p.470).

1. Zimmer-Galler I, Lie JT. Choroidal infiltrates as the initial manifestation of lymphoma in rheumatoid arthritis after treatment with low-dose methotrexate. *Mayo Clin Proc* 1994; **69:** 258–61.
2. Kamel OW, *et al.* Brief report: reversible lymphomas associated with Epstein-Barr virus occurring during methotrexate therapy for rheumatoid arthritis and dermatomyositis. *N Engl J Med* 1993; **328:** 1317–21.
3. Viraben R, *et al.* Reversible cutaneous lymphoma occurring during methotrexate therapy. *Br J Dermatol* 1996; **135:** 116–18.
4. Millard RJ, McCredie S. Bladder cancer in patients on low-dose methotrexate and corticosteroids. *Lancet* 1994; **343:** 1222–3.
5. Moder KG, *et al.* Hematologic malignancies and the use of methotrexate in rheumatoid arthritis: a retrospective study. *Am J Med* 1995; **99:** 276–81.

Effects on the blood. Although serious and sometimes fatal blood dyscrasias are a well-known consequence of high-dose methotrexate therapy the Committee on Safety of Medicines in the UK[1] stated in September 1997 that it was also aware of 83 reports of blood dyscrasias associated with low-dose methotrexate used to treat psoriasis or rheumatoid arthritis; there were 36 fatalities. Many of the cases had contributing factors such as advanced age, impaired renal function, or concomitant therapy with interacting drugs.

1. Committee on Safety Medicines/Medicines Control Agency. Blood dyscrasias and other ADRs with low-dose methotrexate. *Current Problems* 1997; **23:** 12.

MEGALOBLASTIC ANAEMIA. Megaloblastic anaemia, usually with marked macrocytosis, has been reported in mainly elderly patients receiving long-term weekly methotrexate therapy.[1,2] It has been suggested that therapy should be withdrawn if the mean corpuscular volume exceeds 106 fL.[1] Symptoms appear to be associated with folate depletion by methotrexate,[2-4] probably due to increased excretion,[5] and in one case megaloblastic anaemia developed following embarkation on a weight-reducing diet poor in folate.[3] Folate supplementation, conversely, may permit continuation of methotrexate therapy with resolution of the anaemia.[4]

1. Dodd HJ, *et al.* Megaloblastic anaemia in psoriatic patients treated with methotrexate. *Br J Dermatol* 1985; **112:** 630.
2. Dahl MGC. Folate depletion in psoriatics on methotrexate. *Br J Dermatol* 1984; **111** (suppl 26): 18.
3. Fulton RA. Megaloblastic anaemia and methotrexate treatment. *Br J Dermatol* 1986; **114:** 267–8.
4. Oxholm A, Thomsen K. Megaloblastic anaemia and methotrexate treatment. *Br J Dermatol* 1986; **114:** 268–9.
5. Duhra P, *et al.* Intestinal folate absorption in methotrexate treated psoriatic patients. *Br J Dermatol* 1988; **119:** 327–32.

Effects on the liver. Methotrexate has been associated with periportal fibrosis and cirrhosis,[1] and its potential for hepatotoxicity has been a source of some concern given its use in non-malignant disorders such as psoriasis and rheumatoid arthritis. The UK Committee on Safety of Medicines recommends liver function tests (as well as blood count and renal function tests) before beginning such therapy, repeated weekly until therapy is stabilised, and thereafter every 2 to 3 months.[2] Zachariae and others[3] found evidence of cirrhosis in 21 of 328 psoriatics on biopsy (although in 2 of these this was before methotrexate was given) and reported that patients who developed cirrhosis had received larger cumulative doses on average than the rest. They recommended liver biopsies in all patients in whom the cumulative dosage exceeded 1.5 g.[3] A similar relationship with cumulative dose was reported by Klaber and colleagues in 82 patients with severe psoriasis.[4] In the UK it has been suggested that in patients with psoriasis a biopsy should be considered after every 1.5 g cumulative dose, or if liver tests become abnormal.[1] Others, however, question the need to repeat routine biopsies.[5]

Increased risk of liver damage also appears to be associated with concomitant alcohol intake and administration of methotrexate in repeated daily doses rather than as a single weekly dose.[3,6]

A lower incidence of hepatotoxicity reported in patients with rheumatoid arthritis may be a genuine difference in susceptibility or due to improved dosage regimens and greater awareness of the risks compared with older studies in patients with psoriasis.[6] It is unclear how rapidly the lesions may progress: Zachariae and colleagues reported that 12 patients with cirrhosis continued to receive methotrexate, for lack of an alternative, and in most of these there was little or no evidence of progression.[3] Boffa and others[5] found that in 49 patients with psoriasis given multiple biopsies during methotrexate treatment only 9 showed a deterioration in histology, with improvement in 12 and no change in 28. Short of biopsy, methotrexate hepatotoxicity is also difficult to detect before the late, symptomatic stages: serum concentrations of the aminoterminal peptide of type III procollagen tend to be raised in methotrexate-treated patients with liver damage,[7,8] but assays differ in their specificity, and both false positive and false negative results occur.[8] An initial increase in serum aminotransferases in patients starting methotrexate does not seem to indicate increased risk.[9]

See also Hepatitis under Precautions, below.

1. Neuberger J. Methotrexate and liver disorders. *Prescribers' J* 1995; **35:** 158–63.
2. Committee on Safety of Medicines/Medicines Control Agency. Blood dyscrasias and other ADRs with low-dose methotrexate. *Current Problems* 1997; **23:** 12.
3. Zachariae H, *et al.* Methotrexate induced liver cirrhosis. *Br J Dermatol* 1980; **102:** 407–12.
4. Klaber MR, *et al.* Prospective study of liver biopsies in patients with psoriasis receiving methotrexate therapy. *Br J Dermatol* 1982; **107** (suppl 22): 28.
5. Boffa MJ, *et al.* Sequential liver biopsies during long-term methotrexate treatment for psoriasis: a reappraisal. *Br J Dermatol* 1995; **133:** 774–8.
6. Kevat S, *et al.* Hepatotoxicity of methotrexate in rheumatic diseases. *Med Toxicol* 1988; **3:** 197–208.
7. Mitchell D, *et al.* Serum type III procollagen peptide, dynamic liver function tests and hepatic fibrosis in psoriatic patients receiving methotrexate. *Br J Dermatol* 1990; **122:** 1–7.
8. Boffa MJ, *et al.* Serum type III procollagen aminopeptide for assessing liver damage in methotrexate-treated psoriatic patients. *Br J Dermatol* 1996; **135:** 538–44.
9. Dufour J-FJ, Kaplan MM. Methotrexate therapy and liver disease. *N Engl J Med* 1996; **335:** 898–9.

Effects on the lungs. A retrospective review[1] involving 130 patients with rheumatoid arthritis treated with methotrexate found adverse bronchopulmonary effects had occurred in 12: in 4 cases this was considered to be hypersensitivity pneumonitis, whereas in the remainder lung disease was attributed to infection. Intensive care measures were required in all 4 patients with hypersensitivity pneumonitis, despite which 2 died. One patient with infectious lung disease also required hospitalisation. The authors pointed out that pulmonary complications warranted vigilance, and methotrexate should be withdrawn in these patients at the first signs of respiratory intolerance. A multicentre case-control study which examined 29 cases of methotrexate-induced lung injury among rheumatoid arthritis patients reported a number of risk factors.[2] These included age over 60 years, pleuropulmonary disease (or to a lesser extent other extra-articular disease), previous use of other disease-modifying antirheumatic drugs, and low serum-albumin; an association with smoking, nonsedentary occupations, and diabetes mellitus was also noted.

1. Hilliquin P, *et al.* Occurrence of pulmonary complications during methotrexate therapy in rheumatoid arthritis. *Br J Rheumatol* 1996; **35:** 441–5.
2. Alarcón GS, *et al.* Risk factors for methotrexate-induced lung injury in patients with rheumatoid arthritis: a multicenter, case-control study. *Ann Intern Med* 1997; **127:** 356–64.

Effects on mental function. Children who had received intrathecal methotrexate with cranial irradiation for the prophylaxis of CNS leukaemia, had a significant intellectual deficit compared with their siblings.[1] There was no corresponding significant reduction in IQ in a group of children who had received systemic chemotherapy and radiotherapy when compared with their sibling controls. The results suggest that intrathecal methotrexate and cranial irradiation cause intellectual problems, particularly on the higher, more complex and integrated intellectual functions, and that the repercussions are greater in younger children. Subsequent results in these patients indicated that although the lowering of IQ had persisted, it had not progressed since the original study.[2]

A further study by Chessells and colleagues confirmed the adverse neurological effects of leukaemia treatment, and its effects on IQ, and did not find a reduced radiation dose to be any less toxic.[3] Neurotoxicity appeared to be greater when systemic therapy with intramuscular rather than oral methotrexate was given with CNS prophylaxis.

A study in 20 patients receiving intermittent oral methotrexate for psoriasis found no evidence of psychological impairment.[4]

1. Twaddle V, *et al.* Intellectual function after treatment for leukaemia or solid tumours. *Arch Dis Child* 1983; **58:** 949–52.
2. Twaddle V, *et al.* Intellect after malignancy. *Arch Dis Child* 1986; **61:** 700–2.
3. Chessells JM, *et al.* Neurotoxicity in lymphoblastic leukaemia: comparison of oral and intramuscular methotrexate and two doses of radiation. *Arch Dis Child* 1990; **65:** 416–22.
4. Duller P, van de Kerkhof PCM. The impact of methotrexate on psycho-organic functioning. *Br J Dermatol* 1985; **113:** 503–4.

Effects on the nervous system. Intrathecal methotrexate is associated with a spectrum of neurotoxic reactions.[1] Acute arachnoiditis and meningismus can develop within hours of administration. The incidence is dose-related and usually subsides within a few days. A subacute form of toxic reaction, characterised by varying degrees of paresis, is generally associated with multiple intrathecal injections and apparently results from prolonged elevation of methotrexate concentrations in the CSF. Paraplegia has been reported, but appears to be rare, and decreasing in incidence with improved drug preparation and monitoring of drug concentrations in CSF. There is also a more delayed syndrome, occurring months to years after treatment, and characterised by necrotising leucoencephalopathy. The syndrome may begin insidiously, and progress to dementia, confusion, ataxia, seizures, and eventual stupor. The effects are dose-related and occur particularly when intrathecal methotrexate in doses greater than 50 mg is combined with cranial irradiation and systemic methotrexate therapy. A late feature may be calcification of the necrotic brain tissue. Not all patients develop this severe encephalopathy but minor neurological injuries, presenting as mild ataxia, seizures, or perceptual disorders, have been reported in at least half the patients in some studies.

See also under Effects on Mental Function, above.

1. Goldberg ID, *et al.* Nervous system toxic effects of cancer therapy. *JAMA* 1982; **247:** 1437–41.

CEREBRAL OEDEMA. A case of acute cerebral oedema associated with haematoma in a patient given intrathecal methotrexate as part of a combination regimen has been reported by Hughes and Lane.[1] However, the attribution of the symptoms to methotrexate has been questioned.[2,3]

1. Hughes PJ, Lane RJM. Acute cerebral oedema induced by methotrexate. *Br Med J* 1989; **298:** 1315.
2. Ellis SJ. Acute cerebral oedema induced by methotrexate. *Br Med J* 1989; **299:** 122–3.
3. Enevoldson TP. Acute cerebral oedema induced by methotrexate. *Br Med J* 1989; **299:** 516.

Effects on the skin. Methotrexate therapy may be associated with erythematous rashes,[1,2] bullae,[2,3] skin ulceration and necrosis consistent with toxic epidermal necrolysis,[2,3] desquamation,[1] exacerbation of photosensitivity reactions,[4] and purpuric skin lesions due to vasculitis.[5,6] Reactivation of sunburn has also been reported.[7]

1. Doyle LA, *et al.* Erythema and desquamation after high-dose methotrexate. *Ann Intern Med* 1983; **98:** 611–12.
2. Reed KM, Sober AJ. Methotrexate-induced necrolysis. *J Am Acad Dermatol* 1983; **8:** 677–9.
3. Lawrence CM, Dahl MGC. Cutaneous necrosis associated with methotrexate treatment for psoriasis. *Br J Dermatol* 1982; **107** (suppl 22): 24.
4. Nedorost ST, *et al.* Drug-induced photosensitivity reaction. *Arch Dermatol* 1989; **125:** 433–4.
5. Marks CR, *et al.* Small-vessel vasculitis and methotrexate. *Ann Intern Med* 1984; **100:** 916.
6. Navarro M, *et al.* Leukocytoclastic vasculitis after high-dose methotrexate. *Ann Intern Med* 1986; **105:** 471–2.
7. Mallory SB, Berry DH. Severe reactivation of sunburn following methotrexate use. *Pediatrics* 1986; **78:** 514–15.

Hypersensitivity. A report of anaphylactic reactions in 2 patients given high-dose methotrexate.[1] See also under Effects on the Lungs, above.

1. Klimo P, Ibrahim E. Anaphylactic reaction to methotrexate used in high doses as an adjuvant treatment of osteogenic sarcoma. *Cancer Treat Rep* 1981; **65:** 725.

Treatment of Adverse Effects

For general guidelines, see p.473.

Folinic acid neutralises the immediate toxic effects of methotrexate on the bone marrow. It is given as calcium folinate by mouth, intramuscularly, by intravenous bolus injection, or by infusion. When overdosage is suspected the dose of calcium folinate should be at least as high as that of methotrexate and should be administered within the first hour, if possible; further doses are given as required. In patients with delayed elimination of methotrexate calcium folinate may need to be continued until methotrexate concentrations in serum fall below 0.05 μM. When average doses of methotrexate have an adverse effect, the equivalent of 6 to 12 mg of folinic acid may be given intramuscularly every 6 hours for 4 doses. See also under Calcium Folinate, p.1342.

Folinic acid is usually given in association with high-dose methotrexate regimens to prevent damage to normal tissue and this is discussed in Uses and Administration, below.

An adequate flow of alkaline urine should be maintained following high doses of methotrexate to prevent precipitation of methotrexate or its metabolites in the renal tubules; in addition to adequate hydration, the use of acetazolamide or sodium bicarbonate has been suggested.

A discussion of the selection of the appropriate route of administration for folinic acid rescue.[1] The general objective is to give folinic acid (as calcium folinate) at doses which maintain plasma concentrations of reduced folates at a level equivalent to or greater than the plasma-methotrexate concentration. In any clinical situation suggesting impaired gastro-intestinal function calcium folinate should be given by injection. Although absorption of intramuscular doses is relatively complete and rapid the intravenous route is usually preferable for other reasons, such as a reduced risk of bleeding at injection sites. In the absence of impaired gastro-intestinal function, and where there are no concomitant risk factors for methotrexate toxicity, the oral route may be used provided that methotrexate concentrations are expected to be less than 1 nmol per mL. For very high dose methotrexate regimens it is generally appropriate to begin folinic acid rescue intravenously to ensure adequate initial therapy, but the majority of the dosage regimen can generally be given orally.

1. Rodman JH, Crom WR. Selecting an administration route for leucovorin rescue. *Clin Pharm* 1989; **8:** 617,21.

Pretreatment with fluorouracil is reported to reduce the toxicity of subsequent methotrexate administration to a degree sufficient to permit high-dose methotrexate administration without the need for folinic acid rescue.[1]

For reference to the ineffectiveness of diltiazem in preventing the nephrotoxicity due to high-dose methotrexate, see Kidney Disorders, under Diltiazem Hydrochloride, p.856.

For evidence that cholestyramine might decrease serum-methotrexate concentrations, see Interactions, Lipid Regulating Drugs, below.

The acute neurotoxic effects of methotrexate have been reported to be relieved in some patients given aminophylline or theophylline, as mentioned on p.748.

1. White RM. 5-Fluorouracil modulates the toxicity of high dose methotrexate. *J Clin Pharmacol* 1995; **35:** 1156–65.

Precautions

For general discussions see p.474.

Methotrexate should be used with great care in patients with bone-marrow, hepatic, or renal impairment. It should also be used cautiously in alcoholics or those with ulcerative disorders of the gastro-intestinal tract, and in the elderly and the very young.

Regular monitoring of haematological, renal, and hepatic function is advisable. In patients receiving low-dose methotrexate for psoriasis or rheumatoid arthritis full blood counts and renal and liver function tests should be performed before starting treatment and weekly until treatment is stabilised, and every 2 to 3 months thereafter. Treatment should be avoided in significant renal impairment and should be discontinued if any abnormality of liver function is detected. Patients or their carers should report any symptoms or signs suggestive of infection, especially sore throat, or if dyspnoea or cough develop. With high-dose regimens, plasma concentrations of methotrexate should be monitored. Maintenance of an adequate flow of alkaline urine is essential (see Treatment of Adverse Effects, above). Pleural or ascitic effusions may act as a depot for methotrexate and produce enhanced toxicity.

Methotrexate is a potent teratogen and should be avoided in pregnancy.

Breast feeding. The American Academy of Pediatrics Committee on Drugs considered that the use of methotrexate in breast-feeding women was contra-indicated.[1]

1. American Academy of Pediatrics Committee on Drugs. The transfer of drugs and other chemicals into human milk. *Pediatrics* 1994; **93:** 137–50.

Down's syndrome. For the suggestion that children with Down's syndrome are less able to tolerate methotrexate, see p.475.

Handling and disposal. Methods for the destruction of methotrexate wastes by oxidation with potassium permanganate and sulphuric acid, by oxidation with aqueous alkaline potassium permanganate, or by oxidation with sodium hypochlorite.[1] The first method may also be used for dichloromethotrexate. Residues produced by the degradation of methotrexate by these methods showed no mutagenicity *in vitro*.

1. Castegnaro M, *et al.* eds. Laboratory decontamination and destruction of carcinogens in laboratory wastes: some antineoplastic agents. *IARC Scientific Publications 73*. Lyon: WHO/International Agency for Research on Cancer, 1985.

Urine and faeces produced for up to 72 hours and 7 days respectively after a dose of methotrexate should be handled wearing protective clothing.[1]

1. Harris J, Dodds LJ. Handling waste from patients receiving cytotoxic drugs. *Pharm J* 1985; **235:** 289–91.

Hepatitis. Reactivation of hepatitis B infection, with the development of hepatocellular necrosis and fulminant hepatic failure requiring liver transplantation, developed on discontinuation of low-dose methotrexate therapy in a patient with rheumatoid arthritis who was also an asymptomatic chronic hepatitis B carrier.[1] It was suggested that all patients being considered for low-dose methotrexate therapy should be screened for the presence of serum HBsAg before beginning therapy.

1. Flowers MA, *et al.* Fulminant hepatitis as a consequence of reactivation of hepatitis B virus infection after discontinuation of low-dose methotrexate therapy. *Ann Intern Med* 1990; **112:** 381–2.

Interactions

Folic acid and its derivatives may decrease the effectiveness of methotrexate, although they are often used in combination to reduce methotrexate toxicity. The effects of methotrexate may be enhanced by concurrent administration of agents which can displace it from protein binding or decrease its renal excretion, such as aminobenzoic acid, some antibacterials, many anti-inflammatory agents, diuretics, and phenytoin. Fatal toxicity has occurred in patients given NSAIDs concurrently with methotrexate. Use with other hepatotoxic or nephrotoxic agents may increase the risk of toxicity: an increased incidence of cirrhosis has been reported in patients receiving methotrexate who have an excessive alcohol intake.

Amiodarone. Ulcerated skin lesions developed in a patient maintained on methotrexate for psoriasis shortly after introduction of amiodarone.[1]

1. Reynolds NJ, *et al.* Methotrexate induced skin necrosis: a drug interaction with amiodarone? *Br Med J* 1989; **299:** 980–1.

Antibacterials. The oral *aminoglycosides* neomycin[1] and paromomycin[2] have been reported to reduce the absorption of methotrexate. Various *penicillins* have been reported to decrease the clearance of methotrexate quite markedly,[3,4] although *ceftazidime* may not.[4] Methotrexate toxicity has been reported in a patient receiving low-dose methotrexate following a course of *tetracycline*.[5] The *sulphonamides* such as sulphafurazole and sulphamethoxazole may displace methotrexate from binding sites[6] and reduce renal clearance;[7] clinical toxicity has been reported on a number of occasions when methotrexate was given concomitantly with co-trimoxazole.[8,9] Although an interaction with *chloramphenicol* has been reported in *mice*[10] there do not appear to be any reports of interaction in human subjects.

1. Shen DD, Azarnoff DL. Clinical pharmacokinetics of methotrexate. *Clin Pharmacokinet* 1978; **3:** 1–13.
2. Cohen MH, *et al.* Effect of oral prophylactic broad spectrum nonabsorbable antibiotics on the gastrointestinal absorption of nutrients and methotrexate in small cell bronchogenic carcinoma patients. *Cancer* 1976; **38:** 1556.
3. Bloom EJ, *et al.* Delayed clearance (CL) of methotrexate (MTX) associated with antibiotics and antiinflammatory agents. *Clin Res* 1986; **34:** 560A.
4. Yamamoto K, *et al.* Delayed elimination of methotrexate associated with piperacillin administration. *Ann Pharmacother* 1997; **31:** 1261–2.
5. Turck M. Successful psoriasis treatment then sudden 'cytotoxicity'. *Hosp Pract* 1984; **19:** 175–6.
6. Liegler DG, *et al.* The effect of organic acids on renal clearance of methotrexate in man. *Clin Pharmacol Ther* 1969; **10:** 849–57.
7. Ferrazzini G, *et al.* Interaction between trimethoprim-sulfamethoxazole and methotrexate in children with leukemia. *J Pediatr* 1990; **117:** 823–6.
8. Liddle BJ, Marsden JR. Drug interactions with methotrexate. *Br J Dermatol* 1989; **120:** 582–3.
9. Jeurissen ME, *et al.* Pancytopenia and methotrexate with trimethoprim-sulfamethoxazole. *Ann Intern Med* 1989; **111:** 261.
10. Dixon RL. The interaction between various drugs and methotrexate. *Toxicol Appl Pharmacol* 1968; **12:** 308.

Antiepileptics. For mention of the reduction in serum-valproate concentration produced by methotrexate see p.363.

Antineoplastics and immunosuppressants. Administration of methotrexate with other myelosuppressive or immunosuppressive agents might be expected to result in enhanced bone-marrow toxicity and immunosuppression; in addition enhanced methotrexate toxicity might be expected with nephrotoxic agents such as cisplatin which could reduce methotrexate excretion by impairing renal function. Sequential use of methotrexate and fluorouracil may result in synergistic enhancement of effect (see p.536), and equally, fluorouracil before methotrexate may reduce its toxicity (see above), but if asparaginase (p.505) is given before methotrexate the cytotoxic effect of methotrexate may be reduced. For a report of enhanced toxicity with cyclosporin in patients who have received methotrexate see p.522.

Methotrexate may increase the bioavailability of mercaptopurine by interference with first-pass metabolism (see p.546).

Antivirals. For reference to the risk when methotrexate and vidarabine are given concurrently, see under Vidarabine Phosphate, p.628.

Blood products. Enhanced toxicity was seen in 2 of 14 patients receiving methotrexate by 24-hour infusion when packed red cells were transfused immediately after the methotrexate infusion.[1] Erythrocytes act as reservoirs for methotrexate and probably resulted in the prolonged high serum-methotrexate concentrations seen in these patients. Great care should be exercised whenever packed red blood cells and methotrexate are given concurrently.

1. Yap AKL, *et al.* Methotrexate toxicity coincident with packed red cell transfusions. *Lancet* 1986; **ii:** 641.

Etretinate. An increased risk of hepatotoxicity has been reported when methotrexate and etretinate are given concurrently,[1] possibly due to increased plasma concentrations of methotrexate.[2,3]

1. Zachariae H. Dangers of methotrexate/etretinate combination therapy. *Lancet* 1988; **i:** 422.
2. Harrison PV, *et al.* Methotrexate and retinoids in combination for psoriasis. *Lancet* 1987; **ii:** 512.
3. Larsen FG, *et al.* Interaction of etretinate with methotrexate pharmacokinetics in psoriatic patients. *J Clin Pharmacol* 1990; **30:** 802–7.

Lipid regulating drugs. Serum-methotrexate concentrations were markedly reduced in 2 patients given cholestyramine to treat methotrexate toxicity;[1] methotrexate was found to be appreciably bound to cholestyramine *in vitro*.

1. Erttmann R, Landbeck G. Effect of oral cholestyramine on the elimination of high-dose methotrexate. *J Cancer Res Clin Oncol* 1985; **110:** 48–50.

Nitrous oxide. Severe unpredictable myelosuppression and stomatitis have been attributed to the use of nitrous oxide anaesthesia in patients receiving methotrexate, potentiating the effects of methotrexate on folate metabolism.[1] The effect could be reduced by the use of folinic acid rescue.

1. Goldhirsch A, *et al.* Methotrexate/nitrous-oxide toxic interaction in perioperative chemotherapy for early breast cancer. *Lancet* 1987; **ii:** 151.

NSAIDs. Severe, and in some cases fatal, aggravation of methotrexate toxicity has been reported when it was administered concomitantly with various NSAIDs including aspirin and other salicylates,[1,2] azapropazone,[3] diclofenac,[4] indomethacin,[4,5] and ketoprofen.[6] The mechanism is uncertain but may include both displacement of methotrexate from protein-binding sites or an effect of NSAIDs on the kidney resulting in reduced methotrexate excretion.[6,7] Naproxen has been reported not to affect the pharmacokinetics of methotrexate,[8] but a fatal interaction has nonetheless been reported.[9] Despite the risks, some commentators have pointed out that methotrexate and NSAIDs are frequently prescribed together in the treatment of rheumatoid arthritis,[10,11] and that provided this is done with caution, in low doses, and patients are appropriately monitored and cautioned to avoid additional 'over-the-counter' analgesics, such combinations need not be contra-indicated. A study in patients receiving low-dose methotrexate for rheumatoid arthritis suggested that flurbiprofen, ketoprofen, or piroxicam given concomitantly did not influence methotrexate clearance.[12]

1. Baker H. Intermittent high dose oral methotrexate therapy in psoriasis. *Br J Dermatol* 1970; **82:** 65–9.
2. Zuik M, Mandel MA. Methotrexate-salicylate interaction: a clinical and experimental study. *Surg Forum* 1975; **26:** 567–9.
3. Daly HM, *et al.* Methotrexate toxicity precipitated by azapropazone. *Br J Dermatol* 1986; **114:** 733–5.
4. Gabrielli A, *et al.* Methotrexate and nonsteroidal anti-inflammatory drugs. *Br Med J* 1987; **294:** 776.
5. Maiche AG. Acute renal failure due to concomitant action of methotrexate and indomethacin. *Lancet* 1986; **i:** 1390.
6. Thyss A, *et al.* Clinical and pharmacokinetic evidence of a life-threatening interaction between methotrexate and ketoprofen. *Lancet* 1986; **i:** 256–8.
7. Furst DE, *et al.* Effect of aspirin and sulindac on methotrexate clearance. *J Pharm Sci* 1990; **79:** 782–6.
8. Stewart CF, *et al.* Coadministration of naproxen and low-dose methotrexate in patients with rheumatoid arthritis. *Clin Pharmacol Ther* 1990; **47:** 540–6.
9. Singh RR, *et al.* Fatal interaction between methotrexate and naproxen. *Lancet* 1986; **i:** 1390.
10. Tully M. NSAIDs. *Pharm J* 1991; **247:** 746.
11. Zachariae H. Methotrexate and nonsteroidal anti-inflammatory drugs. *Br J Dermatol* 1992; **126:** 95.
12. Tracy TS, *et al.* Methotrexate disposition following concomitant administration of ketoprofen, piroxicam and flurbiprofen in patients with rheumatoid arthritis. *Br J Clin Pharmacol* 1994; **37:** 453–6.

Omeprazole. Elevated serum concentrations of methotrexate have been reported when it was given to a patient also receiving omeprazole.[1] The effect was not seen with subsequent cycles of methotrexate therapy once omeprazole had been discontinued.

1. Reid T, *et al.* Impact of omeprazole on the plasma clearance of methotrexate. *Cancer Chemother Pharmacol* 1993; **33:** 82–4.

Probenecid. Probenecid can result in three- or fourfold increases in serum-methotrexate concentrations when given concurrently,[1,2] presumably by inhibiting renal excretion of methotrexate.

1. Aherne GW, *et al.* Prolongation and enhancement of serum methotrexate concentrations by probenecid. *Br Med J* 1978; **1:** 1097–9.
2. Howell SB, *et al.* Effect of probenecid on cerebrospinal fluid methotrexate kinetics. *Clin Pharmacol Ther* 1979; **26:** 641–6.

With PUVA. Of a total of 94 patients with psoriasis and 38 with mycosis fungoides treated with PUVA therapy (methoxsalen and ultraviolet light) 2 psoriatics who received concomitant methotrexate and PUVA therapy developed subsequent skin cancers.[1] It was suggested that the combination of methotrexate and PUVA may be synergistic in inducing cutaneous malignancy.

1. Fitzsimons CP, *et al.* Synergistic carcinogenic potential of methotrexate and PUVA in psoriasis. *Lancet* 1983; **i:** 235–6.

With radiation. Analysis of neutrophil counts for 18 months in children with acute lymphoblastic leukaemia showed that methotrexate-induced neutropenia was significantly greater in patients given CNS irradiation and was considered to have contributed to 3 of 5 deaths during remission.[1]

For the role of cranial irradiation and intrathecal methotrexate in producing neurotoxicity, see Effects on the Nervous System, above.

1. Report to the Medical Research Council of the Working Party on Leukaemia in Childhood. Analysis of treatment in childhood leukaemia: I—predisposition to methotrexate-induced neutropenia after craniospinal irradiation. *Br Med J* 1975; **3:** 563–6.

Pharmacokinetics

When given in low doses, methotrexate is rapidly absorbed from the gastro-intestinal tract, but higher doses are less well absorbed. It is also rapidly and completely absorbed following intramuscular administration. Peak serum concentrations are achieved in 1 to 2 hours after an oral dose, and 30 to 60 minutes after an intramuscular one.

Methotrexate is distributed to tissues and extracellular fluid with a steady-state volume of distribution of 0.4 to 0.8 litres per kg body-weight; it penetrates ascitic fluid and effusions which may act as a depot and thus enhance toxicity. Clearance from plasma is reported to be triphasic, with a terminal elimination half-life of between 3 and 10 hours after low oral doses or 8 to 15 hours after high-dose parenteral therapy. It is about 50% bound to plasma protein. Methotrexate enters the cells in part by an active transport mechanism and is bound as polyglutamate conjugates: bound drug may remain in the body for several months, particularly in the liver.

Only small or insignificant amounts cross the blood-brain barrier and enter CSF following oral or parenteral administration although this may be increased by giving higher doses; however, following intrathecal doses there is significant passage into the systemic circulation.

Methotrexate has been detected in very small amounts in saliva and breast milk. It crosses the placenta.

Methotrexate does not appear to undergo significant metabolism at low doses; following high-dose therapy the 7-hydroxy metabolite has been detected. Methotrexate may be partly metabolised by the intestinal flora before absorption. It is excreted primarily in the urine, by glomerular filtration and active tubular secretion. Small amounts are excreted in bile and found in faeces; there is some evidence for enterohepatic recirculation.

Considerable interindividual variation exists in the pharmacokinetics of methotrexate: those patients in whom clearance is delayed are at increased risk of toxicity.

References.

1. Shen DD, Azarnoff DL. Clinical pharmacokinetics of methotrexate. *Clin Pharmacokinet* 1978; **3:** 1–13.
2. Balis FM, *et al.* Clinical pharmacokinetics of commonly used anticancer drugs. *Clin Pharmacokinet* 1983; **8:** 202–32.
3. Wang Y-M, Fujimoto T. Clinical pharmacokinetics of methotrexate in children. *Clin Pharmacokinet* 1984; **9:** 335–48.
4. Luyckx M, *et al.* Clinical pharmacokinetics of 6-hour infusion of high-dose methotrexate: preliminary trial of monitoring high infusion doses. *Eur J Clin Pharmacol* 1985; **28:** 457–62.
5. Wolfrom C, *et al.* Pharmacokinetic study of methotrexate, folinic acid and their serum metabolites in children treated with high-dose methotrexate and leucovorin rescue. *Eur J Clin Pharmacol* 1990; **39:** 377–83.
6. Witter FR. Clinical pharmacokinetics in the treatment of rheumatoid arthritis in pregnancy. *Clin Pharmacokinet* 1993; **25:** 444–9.
7. Bannwarth B, *et al.* Clinical pharmacokinetics of low-dose pulse methotrexate in rheumatoid arthritis. *Clin Pharmacokinet* 1996; **30:** 194–210.

Clearance. In a study[1] involving 108 children given high-dose methotrexate intravenously and intrathecally as part of the maintenance therapy of acute lymphoblastic leukaemia methotrexate clearance varied widely between individuals from 44.7 to 132.1 mL per minute per m^2. When the group was subdivided by creatinine clearance and liver function (as measured by abnormal liver-enzyme values) it became apparent that the observed interpatient variability in clearance was not totally random but was related in part to differences in renal and hepatic function. There was also some evidence that in patients with the slowest creatinine clearance and abnormal liver-enzyme values, boys may have faster methotrexate clearance than girls.

Another study in children receiving low-dose methotrexate found that the area under the plasma concentration-time curve (AUC) for methotrexate increased with increasing age, which might account for the fact that higher doses per kg body-weight have been reported to be necessary for antirheumatic activity in children than in adults.[2] The 7-hydroxy metabolite was present in high concentrations in these children but its AUC did not vary with age and it was suggested that the metabolism of methotrexate was more extensive in younger children.

1. Crom WR, *et al.* Use of the automatic interaction detector method to identify patient characteristics related to methotrexate clearance. *Clin Pharmacol Ther* 1986; **39:** 592–7.
2. Albertioni F, *et al.* Methotrexate in juvenile rheumatoid arthritis: evidence of age dependent pharmacokinetics. *Eur J Clin Pharmacol* 1995; **47:** 507–11.

Distribution. IN ERYTHROCYTES. In 5 psoriatic patients receiving their first oral dose of methotrexate, there was an initial peak in the erythrocyte concentration of methotrexate which was related to the peak in plasma concentration and was probably due to diffusion; however, after 3 to 4 days methotrexate re-appeared in significant amounts in erythrocytes despite the fact that the plasma concentration remained below the level of detection, suggesting an energy dependent uptake process. Erythrocyte concentrations of methotrexate steadily increased until a steady-state concentration was achieved after the fourth to sixth weekly dose.

1. Hendel J, Nyfors A. Pharmacokinetics of methotrexate in erythrocytes in psoriasis. *Eur J Clin Pharmacol* 1984; **27:** 607–10.

IN SALIVA. Results of a pilot study in 9 children suggested that salivary-methotrexate concentration after high intravenous doses was closely correlated with concentration in CSF, but not with plasma-methotrexate concentration.[1]

1. Baird GM, *et al.* Salivary levels of methotrexate (MTX) as an index of CSF levels in children: a pilot study. *Br J Clin Pharmacol* 1981; **11:** 112P–13P.

Uses and Administration

Methotrexate is an antineoplastic which acts as an antimetabolite of folic acid. It also has immunosuppressant properties. Within the cell, folic acid is reduced to dihydrofolic and then tetrahydrofolic acid. Methotrexate competitively inhibits the enzyme dihydrofolate reductase and prevents the formation of tetrahydrofolate which is necessary for purine and pyrimidine synthesis and consequently the formation of DNA and RNA. It is most active against cells in the S phase of the cell cycle but its actions on protein and nucleic acid synthesis slow the entry of cells into S phase and so are to some extent self-limiting. Folinic acid (the 5-formyl derivative of tetrahydrofolic acid), or the nucleoside thymidine, have been given after high doses to bypass the block in tetrahydrofolate production in normal cells and prevent the adverse effects of methotrexate. A suggested schedule for *folinic acid rescue* is described under Calcium Folinate, p.1342. (See also under Treatment of Adverse Effects, above). Methotrexate, in very high doses, followed by folinic acid rescue, has been tried in a number of malignant diseases.

Methotrexate is used in the management of acute lymphoblastic leukaemia. It is seldom used for the induction of remission but is employed in maintenance programmes and in the prophylaxis and treatment of meningeal leukaemia. It is effective in the treatment of choriocarcinoma and other trophoblastic tumours and has been used, often in association with other antineoplastics, in the treatment of a variety of malignant diseases including Burkitt's lymphoma and other non-Hodgkin's lymphomas, osteosarcoma, and tumours of the bladder, brain, breast, gastro-intestinal tract, head and neck, lung, pancreas, and prostate, and in retinoblastoma. Its use in many of these conditions is discussed in the introduction to this chapter, as indicated by the cross-references given below.

Methotrexate is of value in the treatment of psoriasis but because of the risks associated with this use, it should only be given when the disease is severe and has not responded to other forms of treatment. It is also used in rheumatoid arthritis and in bone marrow transplantation, and has been tried in other non-malignant disorders such as primary biliary cirrhosis, polymyositis, sarcoidosis, scleroderma, and Wegener's granulomatosis (see the cross-references below).

Methotrexate may be given by mouth as the base or the sodium salt, or by injection as methotrexate sodium. Doses are calculated in terms of methotrexate. The doses and regimens employed vary enormously, and may need to be adjusted according to the bone-marrow or other toxicity. Doses larger than 100 mg are usually given partly or wholly by intravenous infusion over not more than 24 hours.

A common dose for maintenance therapy of acute lymphoblastic leukaemia is 15 to 30 mg per m^2 body-surface once or twice weekly, by mouth or intramuscularly, with other agents such as mercaptopurine. Alternatively, 2.5 mg per kg body-weight may be given intravenously every 14 days. Meningeal leukaemia may be treated by the intrathecal injection of 12 mg per m^2 body-surface, or 15 mg, whichever is less, once or twice weekly; alternatively a regimen based on the age of the patient has been suggested, with children under the age of 1 year receiving 6 mg, 8 mg for those 1 year of age, 10 mg in 2-year-olds, and 12 mg in those 3 years of age or older. Similar doses have been given prophylactically to patients with lymphoblastic leukaemia, sometimes in association with intrathecal cytarabine and hydrocortisone. Methotrexate in intravenous doses of about 500 mg per m^2, followed by folinic acid rescue, may also produce effective concentrations in the CSF.

Choriocarcinoma has been treated with doses of 15 to 30 mg daily by mouth or intramuscularly for 5 days, at intervals of 1 to 2 weeks, for 3 to 5 courses. Alternatively 0.25 to 1 mg per kg body-weight up to a maximum of 60 mg has been given intramuscularly every 48 hours for 4 doses, followed by folinic acid rescue, and repeated at intervals of 7 days. Combination chemotherapy may be necessary in patients with metastases. Doses of 10 to 60 mg per m^2 have also been employed in the treatment of breast cancer, often in combination with cyclophosphamide and fluorouracil.

In advanced lymphosarcoma doses of 0.625 to 2.5 mg per kg daily have been suggested in combination with other antineoplastics. For Burkitt's lymphoma 10 to 25 mg of methotrexate may be given daily by mouth for 4 to 8 days, repeated after an interval of 7 to 10 days, while patients with mycosis fungoides may be given 2.5 to 10 mg daily by mouth to induce remission; alternatively 50 mg may be given weekly as a single dose or two divided doses, by intramuscular injection.

Very high doses, in the range 12 to 15 g per m^2 have been given by intravenous infusion, followed by folinic acid, as part of combined adjuvant therapy in patients with osteosarcoma; high-dose regimens have been tried in a variety of other malignancies, including carcinoma of the lung and of the head and neck.

Single weekly doses of 10 to 25 mg may be given by mouth or by intramuscular or intravenous injection in the treatment of psoriasis. Other, more frequent, regimens have been used but a weekly dosage regimen appears to be less hepatotoxic than a daily one. In the treatment of rheumatoid arthritis doses of 7.5 mg by mouth once weekly have been given.

It is essential that examinations of blood and tests of renal and liver function should be made before, during, and after each course of treatment with methotrexate. If there is a severe fall in the white-cell or platelet counts, methotrexate should be withdrawn. Treatment should also be withdrawn if liver function abnormalities develop.

Methotrexate has a role in the management of ectopic pregnancy (see below).

Action. Inhibition of dihydrofolate reductase by methotrexate depletes intracellular pools of reduced folate and thymidylate synthesis is thereby brought to a halt at concentrations of 1×10^{-8} M of methotrexate. Cessation of purine synthesis occurs at concentrations of methotrexate approximately tenfold greater. The lack of thymidylate or purine blocks synthesis of DNA. The polyglutamate derivatives to which methotrexate is extensively converted within the cell have an affinity for dihydrofolate reductase at least as great as the parent drug, and their inhibition is less readily reversible; in addition they inhibit other enzymes, including thymidylate synthetase and enzymes involved in purine synthesis, which are not directly affected by methotrexate. According to a review by Horton,[1] methotrexate appears to have multiple sites of action within the immune system, including stimulation of interleukin-2 production, antiproliferative effects on B and T cells, inhibition of histamine release from basophils, and inhibition of immunoglobulin production. While its antiproliferative effects are apparently related to dihydrofolate reductase inhibition, other effects may not be.[1]

Methotrexate resistance may occur by several mechanisms which are discussed by Hill,[2] and by Gorlick and others.[3] Influx of drug to the cell may be impaired by a decrease in the amount or function of the carrier that actively transports the drug. Alternatively increased amounts of dihydrofolate reductase may be produced, often by gene amplification (increased expression of the enzyme-producing gene). A third alternative is the production of variant forms of dihydrofolate reductase that are less sensitive to methotrexate. In addition, a fourth mechanism comprises decreased accumulation of active metabolites in the cell due to a reduced ability to form polyglutamates or increased polyglutamate breakdown. Results *in vitro* suggest that the first mechanism produces a relatively low order of resistance, while the second and third are associated with increasingly high orders of resistance.[2] Intrinsic resistance, as in many patients with acute non-lymphoblastic leukaemia, is often due to the fourth mechanism.[3]

1. Horton RC. Methotrexate—an immunomodulator with expanding indications. *J Clin Pharm Ther* 1990; **15:** 89–95.
2. Hill BT. Resistance of mammalian tumour cells to anticancer drugs: mechanisms and concepts relating specifically to methotrexate and vincristine. *J Antimicrob Chemother* 1986; **18** (suppl B): 61–73.
3. Gorlick R, *et al.* Intrinsic and acquired resistance to methotrexate in acute leukemia. *N Engl J Med* 1996; **335:** 1041–8.

Asthma. Various immunosuppressants, including methotrexate, have been tried for their anti-inflammatory and steroid-sparing properties in chronic asthma (p.745), but because of fears about toxicity are largely reserved for individual patients dependent upon systemic corticosteroids. Results of individual studies with methotrexate have been conflicting[1-3] but it appears that some patients may benefit from the corticosteroid-sparing effects of methotrexate.[4,5] Methotrexate therapy must be given for at least 3 months for an adequate assessment of efficacy.

1. Shiner RJ, *et al.* Methotrexate in steroid-dependent asthma: long-term results. *Allergy* 1994; **49:** 565–8.
2. Coffey MJ, *et al.* The role of methotrexate in the management of steroid-dependent asthma. *Chest* 1994; **105:** 117–21.
3. Hedman J, *et al.* Controlled trial of methotrexate in patients with severe chronic asthma. *Eur J Clin Pharmacol* 1996; **49:** 347–9.
4. Shulimzon TR, Shiner RJ. A risk-benefit assessment of methotrexate in corticosteroid-dependent asthma. *Drug Safety* 1996; **15:** 283–90.
5. Marin MG. Low-dose methotrexate spares steroid usage in steroid-dependent asthmatic patients: a meta-analysis. *Chest* 1997; **112:** 29–33.

Connective tissue and muscular disorders. Reports in a limited number of patients indicate that methotrexate given once weekly in low to moderate doses may be of benefit in patients with systemic lupus erythematosus,[1,2] with benefit reported particularly for joint[1] and mucocutaneous[2] symptoms. Benefit was also reported in 2 of 4 patients with discoid lupus erythematosus refractory to hydroxychloroquine.[3] For a discussion of the management of systemic lupus erythematosus see p.1029.

Methotrexate therapy has been investigated for its potential corticosteroid-sparing properties in polymyalgia rheumatica;[4] it is widely employed in rheumatoid arthritis (see below). Methotrexate has also been employed in polymyositis, as mentioned on p.1027.

1. Wilson K, Abeles M. A 2 year, open ended trial of methotrexate in systemic lupus erythematosus. *J Rheumatol* 1994; **21:** 1674–7.
2. Bottomley WW, Goodfield M. Methotrexate for the treatment of severe mucocutaneous lupus erythematosus. *Br J Dermatol* 1995; **133:** 311–14.
3. Bottomley WW, Goodfield MJD. Methotrexate for the treatment of discoid lupus erythematosus. *Br J Dermatol* 1995; **133:** 655–6.
4. Ferraccioli G, *et al.* Methotrexate in polymyalgia rheumatica: preliminary results of an open, randomized study. *J Rheumatol* 1996; **23:** 624–8.

Ectopic pregnancy. Ectopic pregnancy occurs when the fertilised ovum implants outside the uterus, usually in the fallopian tube itself (tubal pregnancy). The problem is increasingly encountered in some developed countries such as the USA, thanks in part to improved diagnostic techniques.[1-3] Although ectopic pregnancies may spontaneously abort early, without clinical sequelae, the potential adverse effects are serious, ranging from pelvic pain and bleeding at 5 to 6 weeks of gestation (indistinguishable from spontaneous abortion), to potentially fatal intra-abdominal haemorrhage later in the course of an otherwise asymptomatic pregnancy.[1]

Surgery remains the standard treatment.[1,2,4] The use of conservative techniques at laparoscopy can preserve subsequent fertility, where this is desirable, although such women remain at increased risk of a subsequent ectopic pregnancy. However, non-surgical methods are increasingly used.[3]

Perhaps the most experience is with the use of methotrexate, which is becoming the primary therapy in many centres.[3] Stovall and colleagues reported excellent results from a single intramuscular injection of methotrexate 50 mg per m^2 body-surface area,[5,6] this regimen replacing an earlier one of 1 mg per kg body-weight, with folinic acid rescue, repeated as required.[7] The single-dose regimen has been reported to be effective in about 90% of cases.[8] Use of methotrexate in this way appears to maintain tubal patency well, and the rate of subsequent successful pregnancies is comparable with surgery. Methotrexate has also been given in combination with oral mifepristone.[4] Methotrexate has been given successfully by local injection direct into the ectopic,[9-11] although the success rate is lower than with systemic methotrexate or surgery.[4]

Systemic methotrexate (with folinic acid rescue) has also been reported to be effective in resolving persistent ectopic pregnancy unsuccessfully treated with surgery.[12] However, surgical therapy may be indicated in those cases where cardiac activity is present,[13] since the presence of a living embryo may increase resistance to methotrexate.

The role of other agents in the management of ectopic pregnancy is less well established. Local instillation of glucose 50% into unruptured tubes is reported to be more effective than the other major alternative, prostaglandin therapy[14] (in this case with dinoprost injected into the gestational sac, sulprostone intramuscularly, and oestrogens for luteolysis). Whether glucose therapy will prove to be as effective as, and produce less tubal damage than, methotrexate remains a matter of debate.

1. Carson SA, Buster JE. Ectopic pregnancy. *N Engl J Med* 1993; **329:** 1174–81.
2. Ory SJ. New options for diagnosis and treatment of ectopic pregnancy. *JAMA* 1992; **267:** 534–7.
3. Pisarska MD, *et al.* Ectopic pregnancy. *Lancet* 1998; **351:** 1115–20.
4. Gazvani MR. Modern management of ectopic pregnancy. *Br J Hosp Med* 1996; **56:** 597–9.
5. Stovall TG, *et al.* Single-dose methotrexate for treatment of ectopic pregnancy. *Obstet Gynecol* 1991; **77:** 754–7.
6. Stovall TG, Ling FW. Single-dose methotrexate: an expanded clinical trial. *Am J Obstet Gynecol* 1993; **168:** 1759–65.
7. Stovall TG, *et al.* Methotrexate treatment of unruptured ectopic pregnancy: a report of 100 cases. *Obstet Gynecol* 1991; **77:** 749–53.
8. Thoen LRD, Creinin MD. Medical treatment of ectopic pregnancy with methotrexate. *Fertil Steril* 1997; **68:** 727–30.
9. Pansky M, *et al.* Tubal patency after local methotrexate injection for tubal pregnancy. *Lancet* 1989; **ii:** 967–8.
10. Thompson GR, *et al.* Methotrexate injection of tubal ectopic pregnancy: a logical evolution? *Med J Aust* 1991; **154:** 469–71.
11. Tulandi T, *et al.* Treatment of ectopic pregnancy by transvaginal intratubal methotrexate administration. *Obstet Gynecol* 1991; **77:** 627–30.
12. Rose PG, Cohen SM. Methotrexate therapy for persistent ectopic pregnancy after conservative laparoscopic management. *Obstet Gynecol* 1990; **76:** 947–9.
13. Brown DL, *et al.* Serial endovaginal sonography of ectopic pregnancies treated with methotrexate. *Obstet Gynecol* 1991; **77:** 406–9.
14. Lang PF, *et al.* Conservative treatment of ectopic pregnancy with local injection of hyperosmolar glucose solution or prostaglandin-$F_{2}\alpha$: a prospective randomised study. *Lancet* 1990; **336:** 78–81.

Inflammatory bowel disease. Methotrexate (given intramuscularly once weekly in a dose of 25 mg) was reported to improve symptoms and reduce corticosteroid requirements in patients with chronic active Crohn's disease.[1] A later review[2] concluded that low-dose methotrexate could be recommended for induction of remission and for its steroid-sparing effect in refractory and corticosteroid-dependent Crohn's disease, although the precise indications for its use were still unclear. Adverse effects are stated to be fewer, and relapse less common, in this group of patients with intramuscular rather than oral administration of methotrexate.[3] The value of methotrexate in ulcerative colitis is also uncertain, although benefits have been seen in some patients.[3] Thus, although corticosteroids and aminosalicylates remain the mainstays of therapy for inflammatory bowel disease (see p.1171), immunosuppressants are considered potentially useful in reducing corticosteroid doses.

1. Feagan BG, *et al.* Methotrexate for the treatment of Crohn's disease. *N Engl J Med* 1995; **332:** 292–7.
2. Egan LJ, Sandborn WJ. Methotrexate for inflammatory bowel disease: pharmacology and preliminary results. *Mayo Clin Proc* 1996; **71:** 69–80.
3. Kozarek RA. Methotrexate for refractory Crohn's disease: preliminary answers to definitive questions. *Mayo Clin Proc* 1996; **71:** 104–5.

Liver disorders, non-malignant. Like other agents used for primary biliary cirrhosis (p.497) methotrexate has been associated with biochemical improvement but evidence of clinical and in particular histological improvement is harder to demonstrate, and the toxicity of immunosuppressants such as methotrexate is problematic.

Methotrexate has reportedly proved of benefit in a few patients with idiopathic granulomatous hepatitis.[1]

1. Knox TA, *et al.* Methotrexate treatment of idiopathic granulomatous hepatitis. *Ann Intern Med* 1995; **122:** 592–5.

Malignant neoplasms. Methotrexate is extensively used in the management of malignant disease. In acute lymphoblastic leukaemia it is used for maintenance therapy, and intrathecally for prophylaxis of CNS relapse, as discussed on p.478, while it also forms part of a number of regimens used for Burkitt's and other non-Hodgkin's lymphomas (see p.483 and p.482), including those associated with AIDS (p.483). In the solid neoplasms it is an important part of curative regimens for gestational trophoblastic tumours (p.477), the adjuvant therapy of osteosarcoma (p.495) and retinoblastoma (intrathecally for ectopic cranial tumours—see p.495), and in regimens for tumours of the bladder (p.484), brain (p.485), breast (p.485), gastro-intestinal tract (p.487), head and neck (p.489), pancreas (p.491), and prostate (p.491).

Multiple sclerosis. Recent results suggest that methotrexate 7.5 mg by mouth weekly may be of benefit in slowing the progression of multiple sclerosis.[1] Although, as discussed on p.620, the results of studies of immunosuppressant therapy in this condition have tended to be disappointing, it has been pointed out that benefit was assessed differently in the methotrexate study,[2] which may have a bearing on its more favourable conclusions.

1. Goodkin DE, *et al.* Low-dose (7.5 mg) oral methotrexate reduces the rate of progression in chronic progressive multiple sclerosis. *Ann Neurol* 1995; **37:** 30–40.
2. Whitaker JN, *et al.* Clinical outcomes and documentation of partial beneficial effects of immunotherapy for multiple sclerosis. *Ann Neurol* 1995; **37:** 5–6.

Myasthenia gravis. Methotrexate has been tried in the management of myasthenia gravis (p.1388) in patients who require immunosuppression but are intolerant of or unresponsive to corticosteroids and azathioprine.

Organ and tissue transplantation. For reference to the use of methotrexate (usually with cyclosporin) in bone marrow transplantation, see p.498.

Psoriatic arthritis. Methotrexate may be useful for severe or progressive cases of psoriatic arthritis (see under Spondyloarthropathies, p.4) when the arthritis is not controlled by physical therapy and NSAIDs, although toxicity may limit long-term use in some patients.

Rheumatoid arthritis. Therapy of rheumatoid arthritis (p.2) is conventionally begun with an analgesic and an NSAID for symptomatic relief, to which a disease-modifying antirheumatic drug is subsequently added in an attempt to retard the disease process. Methotrexate or sulphasalazine tend to be the most widely used of such second-line drugs.[1] Methotrexate has also been tried in combination with cyclosporin,[2] and with hydroxychloroquine and sulphasalazine.[3]

1. Anonymous. Modifying disease in rheumatoid arthritis. *Drug Ther Bull* 1998; **36:** 3–6.
2. Tugwell P, *et al.* Combination therapy with cyclosporine and methotrexate in severe rheumatoid arthritis. *N Engl J Med* 1995; **333:** 137–41.
3. O'Dell JR, *et al.* Treatment of rheumatoid arthritis with methotrexate alone, sulfasalazine and hydroxychloroquine, or a combination of all three medications. *N Engl J Med* 1996; **334:** 1287–91.

Sarcoidosis. Where therapy is required for sarcoidosis (p.1028) corticosteroids are the first choice of drug, and other agents are very much second-line. There are however reports of benefit from the use of methotrexate,[1,2] by mouth or intramuscularly.

1. Webster GF, *et al.* Methotrexate therapy in cutaneous sarcoidosis. *Ann Intern Med* 1989; **111:** 538–9.
2. Soriano FG, *et al.* Neurosarcoidosis: therapeutic success with methotrexate. *Postgrad Med J* 1990; **66:** 142–3.

Scleroderma. Although there are a few reports of benefit with methotrexate in patients with scleroderma,[1] immunosuppressant therapy is generally considered experimental as indicated in the discussion on p.501.

1. van der Hoogen FHJ, *et al.* Methotrexate treatment in scleroderma. *Am J Med* 1989; **87:** 116–17.

Skin disorders, non-malignant. Methotrexate has been widely used in the treatment of severe refractory psoriasis.[1] As discussed on p.1075 the aim of such therapy is to bring the disease under control, enabling a return to other therapy. For use in psoriatic arthritis see above. Methotrexate is also used in conjunction with corticosteroids in the management of pemphigus and pemphigoid (see p.1075) but its value has been questioned.[2]

1. van Dooren-Greebe RJ, *et al.* Methotrexate revisited: effects of long-term treatment in psoriasis. *Br J Dermatol* 1994; **130:** 204–10.
2. Carson PJ, *et al.* Influence of treatment on the clinical course of pemphigus vulgaris. *J Am Acad Dermatol* 1996; **34:** 645–52.

Termination of pregnancy. Methotrexate has been investigated as an alternative to mifepristone in combination with misoprostol for the termination of pregnancy, a topic discussed further on p.1412. Intramuscular methotrexate followed 3 days later by intravaginal misoprostol was more effective than misoprostol alone for termination at 56 days or less;[1] the combination was reported to be less successful after 57 to 63 days' gestation.[2] Later studies[3,4] however found the combination to be safe and effective in terminating pregnancies up to 63 days' gestation; in these the misoprostol was administered up to 7 days after the methotrexate.

1. Creinin MD, Vittinghoff E. Methotrexate and misoprostol vs misoprostol alone for early abortion: a randomized controlled trial. *JAMA* 1994; **272:** 1190–5.
2. Creinin MD. Methotrexate and misoprostol for abortion at 57-63 days gestation. *Contraception* 1994; **50:** 511–15.
3. Hausknecht RU. Methotrexate and misoprostol to terminate early pregnancy. *N Engl J Med* 1995; **333:** 537–40.
4. Creinin MD, *et al.* A randomized trial comparing misoprostol three and seven days after methotrexate for early abortion. *Am J Obstet Gynecol* 1995; **173:** 1578–84.

Vasculitic syndromes. For the use of methotrexate in Wegener's granulomatosis (for which cyclophosphamide with a corticosteroid is the standard treatment), see p.1031.

Preparations

BP 1998: Methotrexate Injection; Methotrexate Tablets;
USP 23: Methotrexate for Injection; Methotrexate Injection; Methotrexate Tablets.

Proprietary Preparations (details are given in Part 3)
Aust.: Abitrexate; ***Austral.:*** Ledertrexate; Methoblastin; ***Belg.:*** Ledertrexate; ***Canad.:*** Rheumatrex; ***Fr.:*** Ledertrexate; ***Ger.:*** Farmitrexat; Lantarel; Lumexon†; Metex; MTX; ***Ital.:*** Brimexate†; ***Neth.:*** Ledertrexate; ***Norw.:*** Emthexat; ***S.Afr.:*** Abitrexate; Emthexate; Methoblastin; ***Spain:*** Emthexate; ***Swed.:*** Emthexat; Trametex†; ***UK:*** Maxtrex; ***USA:*** Abitrexate; Folex; Rheumatrex.

Miboplatin (15907-r)

Miboplatin (*rINN*).

(−)-*cis*-[(*R*)-2-(Aminomethyl)pyrrolidine](1,1-cyclobutanedicarboxylato)platinum.

$C_{11}H_{18}N_2O_4Pt$ = 437.3.

CAS — 103775-75-3.

Miboplatin is a platinum derivative which is reported to have properties similar to carboplatin (p.510) and has been used for its antineoplastic properties.

References.

1. Weiss RB, Christian MC. New cisplatin analogues in development: a review. *Drugs* 1993; **46:** 360–77.

Miltefosine (11021-x)

Miltefosine (*BAN, rINN*).

D-18506; HDPC; Hexadecylphosphocholine. [2-(Trimethylammonio)ethyl][hexadecyloxyphosphonate].

$C_{21}H_{46}NO_4P$ = 407.6.

CAS — 58066-85-6.

Miltefosine is a phospholipid derivative which is structurally related to the phospholipid components of the cell membrane and is thought to exert its antineoplastic actions by disruption of cell-membrane function. A 6% solution is applied once or twice daily as a topical antineoplastic agent for skin metastases of breast cancer. Miltefosine has also been tried by mouth for various malignant neoplasms.

Malignant neoplasms. Recurrent cutaneous breast cancer in 14 women was treated with miltefosine, applied as a 6% solution: 7 patients also received systemic chemotherapy.[1] The mean duration of treatment was 7 months and 6 patients were continuing at the time of writing. Of the 14, 7 had a partial remission, and a further 5 had either a minor response or stable disease: only in 2 did disease progress. The mean duration of response was 5 months. Local toxicity, manifest as skin dryness, atrophy, itching, or burning, was easily managed with an emollient cream.

1. Clive S, Leonard RCF. Miltefosine in recurrent cutaneous breast cancer. *Lancet* 1997; **349:** 621–2.

Preparations

Proprietary Preparations (details are given in Part 3)
Ger.: Miltex; ***Swed.:*** Miltex.

Misonidazole (12966-p)

Misonidazole (*BAN, USAN, rINN*).

NSC-261037; Ro-7-0582. 3-Methoxy-1-(2-nitroimidazol-1-yl)propan-2-ol.

$C_7H_{11}N_3O_4$ = 201.2.

CAS — 13551-87-6.

Misonidazole is structurally related to metronidazole (p.585) and shares some of the same properties. It has been given by mouth to sensitise resistant, hypoxic tumour cells to the effects of irradiation. Misonidazole may produce dose-related peripheral neuropathy, and at high doses encephalopathy. It is reported to be a teratogen *in vitro*.

References.

1. Phillips TL. Final report on the United States phase I clinical trial of the hypoxic cell radiosensitizer, misonidazole (Ro-07-0582; NSC 261037). *Cancer* 1981; **48:** 1697–1704.
2. A report from the MRC Working Party on Misonidazole for Cancer of the Cervix. The Medical Research Council trial of misonidazole in carcinoma of the uterine cervix. *Br J Radiol* 1984; **57:** 491–9.

Mitobronitol (1847-d)

Mitobronitol (*BAN, rINN*).

DBM; Dibromomannitol; NSC-94100; R-54; WR-220057. 1,6-Dibromo-1,6-dideoxy-D-mannitol.

$C_6H_{12}Br_2O_4$ = 308.0.

CAS — 488-41-5.

Pharmacopoeias. In Br.

A white or almost white crystalline solid. Slightly **soluble** in water, alcohol, and acetone; practically insoluble in chloroform. **Protect** from light.

Mitobronitol is an antineoplastic which appears to act as an alkylating agent, perhaps by epoxide formation. It has been used in the management of thrombocythaemia, both primary, and secondary to chronic myeloid leukaemia or polycythaemia vera.

The usual dose is 250 mg daily by mouth until the platelet count falls to acceptable levels. Intermittent dosage has been given for maintenance therapy, adjusted according to the blood count. Frequent examination of the blood should be performed during treatment.

Mitobronitol is well absorbed from the gastro-intestinal tract and is excreted through the liver into the bile, with reabsorption from the small intestine. It is eliminated as unchanged drug and some bromine-containing metabolites in the urine over several days.

Long-term follow-up of a cooperative study[1] involving 350 patients with polycythaemia vera and treated with mitobronitol found that of 113 patients followed for over 10 years, 68 had survived, and there were no deaths due to acute non-lymphoblastic leukaemia. Among the 168 living and 69 dead patients who had been followed for between 2 and 10 years there were 7 cases of acute non-lymphoblastic leukaemia. The frequency of this leukaemia was less than that observed with other chemotherapy regimens and it was thought possible that mitobronitol had an advantage not only over the already discarded chlorambucil but also over phosphorus-32 or busulphan in rarely inducing acute non-lymphoblastic leukaemia.

For a discussion of the usual management of polycythaemia vera, see p.495.

1. Kelemen E, *et al.* Decreasing risk of leukaemia during prolonged follow-up after mitobronitol therapy for polycythaemia vera. *Lancet* 1987; **ii:** 625.

Preparations

BP 1998: Mitobronitol Tablets.

Proprietary Preparations (details are given in Part 3)
Aust.: Myelobromol; ***UK:*** Myelobromol.

Mitoguazone Dihydrochloride (13502-q)

Mitoguazone Dihydrochloride *(rINNM)*.

Methyl-GAG; Methylglyoxal Bisguanylhydrazone (mitoguazone); MGBG; NSC-32946. 1,1′-[(Methylethanediylidene)dinitrilo]diguanidine dihydrochloride.

$C_5H_{12}N_8,2HCl = 257.1$.

CAS — 459-86-9 (mitoguazone); 7059-23-6 (mitoguazone dihydrochloride).

Mitoguazone is an antineoplastic which may exert its cytotoxic effects by its ability to inhibit polyamine biosynthesis. It has been given as the dihydrochloride monohydrate, by intravenous infusion in doses of 80 to 300 mg daily, for 3 to 5 days, in the treatment of acute non-lymphoblastic leukaemias (p.479). It may also be given by intramuscular injection. Mitoguazone has also been tried, as the dihydrochloride or the acetate, in the treatment of solid tumours, and has been investigated in patients with AIDS-related lymphomas (p.483).

Mitoguazone may produce hypoglycaemia and should be administered dissolved in glucose-containing infusion fluids; sugar may be taken by mouth if hypoglycaemia develops during infusion. Granulocytopenia and thrombocytopenia are generally mild and reversible on stopping treatment. Gastro-intestinal effects frequently occur.

References.

1. Von Hoff DD. MGBG: teaching an old drug new tricks. *Ann Oncol* 1994; **5:** 487–93.

Preparations

Proprietary Preparations (details are given in Part 3)
Fr.: Methyl-Gag†.

Mitolactol (1849-h)

Mitolactol *(rINN)*.

DBD; Dibromodulcitol; NSC-104800; WR-138743. 1,6-Dibromo-1,6-dideoxy-D-galactitol.

$C_6H_{12}Br_2O_4 = 308.0$.

CAS — 10318-26-0.

Mitolactol is an antineoplastic which may act by alkylation, probably as epoxide metabolites including dianhydrogalactitol. It has been given by mouth in the treatment of metastatic breast and cervical carcinoma, although other drugs are usually preferred (see p.485 and p.487), and has also been tried in other malignant neoplasms, notably those of the brain (p.485). Doses of 130 to 180 mg per m² body-surface have been given daily, or 300 to 530 mg per m² weekly. Blood counts should be taken regularly during treatment and mitolactol withdrawn if bone-marrow depression occurs.

In addition to myelosuppression, which is usually dose-limiting, and manifests chiefly as leucopenia and thrombocytopenia, adverse effects include gastro-intestinal disturbances, alopecia, skin rashes, grey pigmentation of the skin, dyspnoea, transient disturbances of hepatic function, elevated blood-urea nitrogen (BUN), and hypersensitivity reactions.

Mitomycin (1850-a)

Mitomycin *(BAN, USAN, rINN)*.

Mitomycin C; Mitomycine C; NSC-26980. 6-Amino-1,1a,2,8,8a,8b-hexahydro-8-hydroxymethyl-8a-methoxy-5-methylazirino[2′,3′:3,4]pyrrolo[1,2-*a*]indole-4,7-dione carbamate; (1*S*,2*S*,9*S*,9a*R*)-7-Amino-2,3,5,8,9,9a-hexahydro-9a-methoxy-6-methyl-5,8-dioxo-1,2-epimino-1-*H*-pyrrolo[1,2-*a*]indol-9-ylmethyl carbamate.

$C_{15}H_{18}N_4O_5 = 334.3$.

CAS — 50-07-7.

Pharmacopoeias. In *Fr.*, *Jpn*, and *US*.

An antineoplastic antibiotic produced by the growth of *Streptomyces caespitosus*. It has a potency of not less than 970 μg per mg.

It occurs as a blue-violet crystalline powder. Slightly **soluble** in water; soluble in acetone, methyl alcohol, butyl acetate, and cyclohexanone. A 0.5% solution in water has a pH of 6.0 to 7.5. **Store** in airtight containers. Protect from light.

Stability. Mitomycin undergoes degradation in acid solution,[1] and two studies suggest that mitomycin is much less stable in glucose 5% injection than in sodium chloride 0.9%.[2,3] These results have been queried by a manufacturer (*Bristol, USA*) whose results suggest that mitomycin is stable for 48 hours in glucose injection 5% at 25°,[4] and it is uncertain whether different manufacturers' formulations differ in stability, or, as has been suggested, that an unsuitable assay was used by the manufacturer to measure stability.[5]

1. Beijnen JH, Underberg WJM. Degradation of mitomycin C in acidic solution. *Int J Pharmaceutics* 1985; **24:** 219–29.
2. Benvenuto JA, *et al.* Stability and compatibility of antitumour agents in glass and plastic containers. *Am J Hosp Pharm* 1981; **38:** 1914–18.
3. Quebbeman EJ, *et al.* Stability of mitomycin admixtures. *Am J Hosp Pharm* 1985; **42:** 1750–4.
4. Keller JH. Stability of mitomycin admixtures. *Am J Hosp Pharm* 1986; **43:** 59,64.
5. Quebbeman EJ, Hoffman NE. Stability of mitomycin admixtures. *Am J Hosp Pharm* 1986; **43:** 64.

Adverse Effects, Treatment, and Precautions

For general discussions see Antineoplastics, p.470.

The main adverse effect of mitomycin is delayed cumulative bone-marrow suppression. Profound leucopenia and thrombocytopenia occurs after about 4 weeks with recovery in about 8 to 10 weeks after a dose. Blood counts may not recover in about one-quarter of patients. Other serious adverse effects include renal damage and pulmonary reactions; a potentially fatal haemolytic-uraemic syndrome has been reported in some patients. The incidence of renal toxicity is greatly increased if the total cumulative dose exceeds 120 mg (see also below). Gastro-intestinal toxicity, dermatitis, alopecia, fever, malaise, and rarely cardiotoxicity may also occur. Local tissue necrosis, ulceration, and cellulitis may occur following extravasation.

Mitomycin is contra-indicated in patients with impaired renal function or coagulation disorders. Renal function should be tested before beginning treatment and after each course.

Effects on the bladder. Intravesical instillation of mitomycin after resection of superficial bladder tumours has led to the development of indolent asymptomatic ulcers at the resection site which may persist for months, and must be distinguished from persistent infiltrating bladder cancer.[1,2] Severe bladder contracture resulting in intolerable urinary frequency has also occurred.[3]

See also under Effects on the Skin, below.

1. Richards B, Tolley D. Benign ulcers after bladder instillation of mitomycin C. *Lancet* 1986; **i:** 45.
2. Hetherington JW, Whelan P. Persistent ulcers after bladder instillation of mitomycin C. *Lancet* 1986; **i:** 324.
3. Wajsman Z, *et al.* Severely contracted bladder following intravesical mitomycin C therapy. *J Urol (Baltimore)* 1983; **130:** 340–1.

Effects on the kidneys. A syndrome of thrombotic microangiopathy resembling the haemolytic-uraemic syndrome has been seen in patients receiving mitomycin,[1] either alone[2,3] or more frequently combined with other drugs,[1,4-6] particularly fluorouracil[4,6] or tamoxifen.[7] Symptoms of haemolysis and renal failure may be complemented by hypertension and cardiovascular problems, pulmonary oedema and hypertension, and neurological symptoms.[1] Mitomycin dose may be significant, and Cordonnier and colleagues found that all of 25 cases they reported had received total doses of 70 mg or more.[3] Symptoms may be exacerbated if blood transfusions are given, sometimes fatally.[4] Plasma exchange has been suggested as possibly helpful,[3] although it may not relieve renal failure.[6]

1. Fields SM, Lindley CM. Thrombotic microangiopathy associated with chemotherapy: case report and review of the literature. *DICP Ann Pharmacother* 1989; **23:** 582–8.
2. Rumpf KW, *et al.* Mitomycin-induced haemolysis and renal failure. *Lancet* 1980; **ii:** 1037–8.
3. Cordonnier D, *et al.* La néphrotoxicité de la mitomycine C (à propos de 25 observations): résultats d'une enquête multicentrique organisée par la société de néphrologie. *Nephrologie* 1985; **6:** 19–26.
4. Jones BG, *et al.* Intravascular haemolysis and renal impairment after blood transfusion in two patients on long-term 5-fluorouracil and mitomycin-C. *Lancet* 1980; **i:** 1275–7.
5. Karlin DA, Stroehlein JR. Rash, nephritis, hypertension, and haemolysis in a patient on 5-fluorouracil, doxorubicin, and mitomycin C. *Lancet* 1980; **ii:** 534–5.
6. Lempert KD. Haemolysis and renal impairment syndrome in patients on 5-fluorouracil and mitomycin-C. *Lancet* 1980; **ii:** 369–70.
7. Montes A, *et al.* A toxic interaction between mitomycin C and tamoxifen causing the haemolytic uraemic syndrome. *Eur J Cancer* 1993; **29A:** 1854–7.

Effects on the liver. Hepatic veno-occlusive disease developed in 6 of 29 patients given intensive mitomycin therapy and autologous bone-marrow transplantation.[1] The effect was manifest as abdominal pain, hepatomegaly, and ascites, and liver failure was progressive and fatal in 3. A further patient, who had no symptoms, was found to have veno-occlusive disease at post mortem.

1. Lazarus HM, *et al.* Veno-occlusive disease of the liver after high-dose mitomycin C therapy and autologous bone marrow transplantation. *Cancer* 1982; **49:** 1789–95.

Effects on respiratory function. A report and brief review of mitomycin-induced pulmonary toxicity.[1] There have been reports of toxicity at total dosages as low as 40 mg of mitomycin, but the average cumulative dose associated with toxicity is 78 mg.

See also p.473. For reference to the respiratory effects of mitomycin in combination with a vinca alkaloid see Interactions, Antineoplastics, under Vinblastine Sulphate, p.569.

1. Linette DC, *et al.* Mitomycin-induced pulmonary toxicity: case report and review of the literature. *Ann Pharmacother* 1992; **26:** 481–4.

Effects on the skin. Severe eczematous symptoms in patients receiving intravesical mitomycin[1,2] appear to be due to a delayed hypersensitivity reaction,[2] which also appears to be responsible for the bladder irritation and cystitis which may follow intravesical mitomycin.[2]

1. Neild VS, *et al.* Dermatitis due to mitomycin bladder instillations. *J R Soc Med* 1984; **77:** 610–11.
2. Colver GB, *et al.* Dermatitis due to intravesical mitomycin C: a delayed-type hypersensitivity reaction? *Br J Dermatol* 1990; **122:** 217–24.

Interactions

Antineoplastics. Cardiotoxicity developed in 14 of 91 patients who received mitomycin therapy as second-line treatment for breast cancer after the failure of *doxorubicin*-containing regimens, compared with 3 of 89 similar patients whose second-line treatment did not include mitomycin.[1]

For reports of acute bronchospasm following injection of a *vinca alkaloid* in patients pretreated with mitomycin see Vinblastine Sulphate, p.569. For the increased risk of haemolytic-uraemic syndrome that may occur if mitomycin is given with *fluorouracil* or *tamoxifen* see under Effects on the Kidneys, above.

1. Buzdar AU, *et al.* Adriamycin and mitomycin C: possible synergistic cardiotoxicity. *Cancer Treat Rep* 1978; **62:** 1005–8.

Pharmacokinetics

Mitomycin disappears rapidly from the blood after intravenous injection with an initial (distribution) half-life of 17 minutes. It is widely distributed but does not appear to cross the blood-brain barrier. Mitomycin is metabolised mainly but not exclusively in the liver. The terminal half-life is about 50 minutes. Following normal doses about 10% of a dose is excreted unchanged in the urine; small amounts are also present in bile and faeces. With increasing doses metabolic pathways are saturated, and more drug is excreted unchanged in the urine.

Uses and Administration

Mitomycin is a highly toxic antibiotic with antineoplastic properties. It acts as an alkylating agent after activation *in vivo* and suppresses the synthesis of nucleic acids. It is a cell-cycle nonspecific agent, but is most active in the late G_1 and early S phases.

Mitomycin is used, with other antineoplastic agents, in the palliative treatment of gastric and pancreatic adenocarcinomas. It has also been given to patients with other solid tumours including those of the bladder, breast, cervix, eye, liver, lung, and prostate as indicated by the cross-references given below. Mitomycin has been tried in various other neoplasms including those of the gastro-intestinal tract, head and neck, in melanoma, sarcomas, and in leukaemias.

Various dosage regimens have been tried. An initial dose of 20 mg per m^2 body-surface intravenously has been suggested in the USA; subsequent doses may be repeated at intervals of 6 to 8 weeks if blood counts permit, and should be reduced according to the previous haematological response. In the UK doses are usually in the range 4 to 10 mg (60 to 150 μg per kg body-weight) given intravenously at intervals of 1 to 6 weeks, although higher doses have been given. Another suggested regimen is 2 mg per m^2 daily for 5 days, repeated after 2 days.

Doses are adjusted according to the effect on bone marrow and treatment should not be repeated until the leucocyte count is above at least 3000 per mm^3 and the platelet count above at least 75 000 per mm^3. The drug should not be given again if the nadir of the leucocyte count is below 2000 per mm^3. Dosage may need to be reduced when used in combination with other antineoplastics.

Mitomycin is also used as a bladder instillation: 10 to 40 mg is instilled one to three times a week for a total of 20 doses in the treatment of superficial bladder tumours. For the prevention of recurrent bladder tumours 20 mg may be instilled every 2 weeks, or 40 mg monthly or 3-monthly. Alternatively 4 to 10 mg may be instilled one to three times a week.

Mitomycin has been given by the intra-arterial route in the treatment of liver tumours, sometimes as an infusion of microcapsules designed to produce localised embolisation.

Malignant neoplasms. Mitomycin is used in the prevention of recurrent bladder cancer (p.484), in the palliative therapy of advanced breast cancer (p.485), in malignancies of the cervix (p.487), eye (p.487), gastro-intestinal tract (p.487), liver (p.489), non-small-cell lung cancer (p.490), and has been tried in advanced prostatic cancer (see p.491).

Ocular disorders, non-malignant. GLAUCOMA. Mitomycin,[1-4] like fluorouracil, is effective in improving the outcome of glaucoma filtering surgery in selected patients when used as an adjunct to prevent the formation of scar tissue (see p.1387). Fluorouracil is usually administered as a regimen of multiple injections but mitomycin given as a single intraoperative topical application in usual concentrations ranging from 0.2 to 0.5 mg per mL appears to be of similar efficacy.[5,6] Although good rates of success have been achieved, both drugs are associated with adverse effects and caution has been urged in their use until the long-term effects of such antiproliferative drugs are known.[7] Chronic hypotony, sometimes associated with maculopathy and irreversible visual loss, has been one of the most commonly reported adverse effects for mitomycin.

1. Shin DH, *et al.* Primary glaucoma triple procedure with or without adjunctive mitomycin: prognostic factors for filtration failure. *Ophthalmology* 1996; **103:** 1925–33.
2. Cohen JS, *et al.* A placebo-controlled, double-masked evaluation of mitomycin C in combined glaucoma and cataract procedures. *Ophthalmology* 1996; **103:** 1934–42.
3. Martini E, *et al.* Low-dosage mitomycin C as an adjunct to trabeculectomy: a prospective controlled study. *Eur J Ophthalmol* 1997; **7:** 40–8.
4. Carlson DW, *et al.* A randomized study of mitomycin augmentation in combined phacoemulsification and trabeculectomy. *Ophthalmology* 1997; **104:** 719–24.
5. Skuta GL, *et al.* Intraoperative mitomycin versus postoperative 5-fluorouracil in high-risk glaucoma filtering surgery. *Ophthalmology* 1992; **99:** 438–44.
6. Katz GJ, *et al.* Mitomycin C versus 5-fluorouracil in high-risk glaucoma filtering surgery: extended follow-up. *Ophthalmology* 1995; **102:** 1263–9.
7. Khaw PT. Antiproliferative agents and the prevention of scarring after surgery: friend or foe? *Br J Ophthalmol* 1995; **79:** 627.

PTERYGIUM. Pterygium is a degenerative condition of subconjunctival tissues that results in a vascularised overgrowth of the conjunctiva and cornea. It is cosmetically unappealing but does not usually require treatment. However, if it affects the pupillary area it can be treated surgically. Pterygium often recurs after removal. Methods used to prevent recurrence include radiotherapy or the use of eye drops containing mitomycin[1-4] or thiotepa.[5] Depigmentation of the eyelids may be a problem with topical thiotepa,[5] especially in darkly pigmented patients and most recent studies seem to have used mitomycin. Mitomycin has been applied topically to the surgical site,[3,6] or given as eye drops postoperatively.[1,2,4] The optimal concentration is uncertain; although 0.04% eye drops have been used there is some risk of adverse effects, which may be severe and sight-threatening,[7] and a 0.02% solution may be as effective, and better tolerated.[1,4,6,8] Batimastat is also under investigation for the prevention of pterygium recurrence.

1. Wong L. Ophthalmic mitomycin for preventing recurrent pterygium. *Can J Hosp Pharm* 1990; **43:** 251–2.
2. Mahar PS, Nwokora GE. Role of mitomycin C in pterygium surgery. *Br J Ophthalmol* 1993; **77:** 433–5.
3. Cano-Parra J, *et al.* Prospective trial of intraoperative mitomycin C in the treatment of primary pterygium. *Br J Ophthalmol* 1995; **79:** 439–41.
4. Rachmiel R, *et al.* Results of treatment with topical mitomycin C 0.02% following excision of primary pterygium. *Br J Ophthalmol* 1995; **79:** 233–6.
5. Meacham CT. Triethylene thiophosphoramide in the prevention of pterygium recurrence. *Am J Ophthalmol* 1962; **54:** 751.
6. Mastropasqua L, *et al.* Long term results of intraoperative mitomycin C in the treatment of recurrent pterygium. *Br J Ophthalmol* 1996; **80:** 288–91.
7. Rubinfeld RS, *et al.* Serious complications of topical mitomycin C after pterygium. *Ophthalmology* 1992; **99:** 1647–54.
8. Levartovsky S, Moskowitz Y. Application of mitomycin C 0.02% for 2 minutes at the end of pterygium surgery. *Br J Ophthalmol* 1998; **82:** 97–100.

Preparations

USP 23: Mitomycin for Injection.

Proprietary Preparations (details are given in Part 3)
Canad.: Mutamycin; ***Fr.:*** Ametycine; ***Ger.:*** Mito-medac; ***Neth.:*** Mutamycin†; ***Norw.:*** Mutamycin; ***Swed.:*** Mutamycin; ***Switz.:*** Mutamycine; ***USA:*** Mutamycin.

Mitotane (1852-x)

Mitotane *(USAN, rINN)*.

CB-313; o,p'DDD; NSC-38721; WR-13045. 1,1-Dichloro-2-(2-chlorophenyl)-2-(4-chlorophenyl)ethane.

$C_{14}H_{10}Cl_4$ = 320.0.

CAS — 53-19-0.

Pharmacopoeias. In US.

A white crystalline powder with a slight aromatic odour. Practically **insoluble** in water; soluble in alcohol, ether, petroleum spirit, and in fixed oils. **Store** in airtight containers. Protect from light.

Adverse Effects

Almost all patients given mitotane experience anorexia, nausea and vomiting, and sometimes diarrhoea, and about 40% suffer some central toxicity with dizziness, vertigo, sedation, lethargy, and mental depression. Permanent brain damage may develop with prolonged dosage. Ocular side-effects may occur including blurred vision, diplopia, lenticular opacities, and retinopathy. Other side-effects include hypersensitivity reactions, albuminuria, skin rashes, hyperpigmentation, fever, myalgia, haemorrhagic cystitis, flushing, hypertension, and orthostatic hypotension.

Precautions

Mitotane inhibits the adrenal cortex and adrenocortical insufficiency may develop during treatment; concomitant corticosteroid therapy is often required. In trauma or shock the drug should be temporarily withdrawn and corticosteroids should be given systemically. Mitotane should be given with care to patients with liver disease. Patients should not take charge of vehicles or machinery where loss of attention may lead to accidents. Behavioural and neurological assessments should be carried out regularly in patients who have been receiving treatment for 2 years or more.

Interactions

Mitotane may induce hepatic microsomal enzymes and enhance the metabolism of some other drugs, including coumarin anticoagulants.

Spironolactone. Administration of mitotane up to 3 g daily to a 65-year-old patient with Cushing's syndrome appeared to be ineffective and did not produce the side-effects usually associated with mitotane while the patient was also receiving treatment with spironolactone.[1]

1. Wortsman J, Soler NG. Mitotane: spironolactone antagonism in Cushing's syndrome. *JAMA* 1977; **238:** 2527.

Pharmacokinetics

Up to 40% of a dose of mitotane is absorbed from the gastro-intestinal tract. After daily doses of 5 to 15 g, concentrations in the blood of 7 to 90 μg per mL of unchanged drug and 29 to 54 μg per mL of metabolite have been reported. Mitotane has been detected in the blood 6 to 9 weeks after stopping treatment. It is widely distributed and appears to be stored mainly in fatty tissues. It is metabolised in the liver and other tissues and excreted as metabolites in urine and bile. From 10 to 25% of a dose has been recovered in the urine as a water-soluble metabolite.

Monitoring of mitotane and its major metabolite *o,p'*-DDE in 2 patients receiving mitotane in low doses for Cushing's disease demonstrated that there is a prolonged lag time in the plasma concentration changes in response to alterations in dosage,[1] presumably because of the lipophilicity of both compounds which leads to accumulation in adipose tissue.

1. Benecke R, *et al.* Plasma level monitoring of mitotane (o,p'-DDD) and its metabolite (o,p'-DDE) during long-term treatment of Cushing's disease with low doses. *Eur J Clin Pharmacol* 1991; **41:** 259–61.

Uses and Administration

Mitotane is an antineoplastic with a selective inhibitory action on adrenal cortex activity. It may also modify peripheral steroid metabolism. It is given in the treatment of inoperable adrenocortical tumours and has also been used in patients with Cushing's syndrome (p.1236).

The usual initial dosage is 2 to 6 g daily by mouth in 3 or 4 divided doses, adjusted to the maximum tolerated dose which may range from 2 to 16 g daily.

Luton and colleagues in a retrospective study involving 105 patients with adrenocortical carcinoma found the prognosis to be generally poor with a 5-year survival of 22% among 88 patients followed-up.[1] Surgical resection was the treatment of choice; treatment with mitotane had no effect on survival although 8 patients had transient tumour regression and it was of some benefit in controlling adrenal hypersecretion. However, van Slooten and colleagues have previously reported improved survival in patients with adrenocortical carcinoma in whom mitotane serum concentrations were above 14 μg per mL, and Haak and others,[2] writing for this group, have suggested that the unimpressive results with mitotane in Luton's study may have been due to low serum-mitotane concentrations.

1. Luton J-P, *et al.* Clinical features of adrenocortical carcinoma, prognostic factors, and the effect of mitotane therapy. *N Engl J Med* 1990; **322:** 1195–1201.
2. Haak HR, *et al.* Mitotane therapy of adrenocortical carcinoma. *N Engl J Med* 1990; **323:** 758.

Preparations

USP 23: Mitotane Tablets.

Proprietary Preparations (details are given in Part 3)
Canad.: Lysodren; ***USA:*** Lysodren.

Mitozantrone Hydrochloride

(12967-s)

Mitozantrone Hydrochloride *(BANM)*.

Mitoxantrone Hydrochloride *(USAN, rINNM)*; CL-232315; DHAD; Dihydroxyanthracenedione Dihydrochloride; Mitoxantroni Hydrochloridum; NSC-301739. 1,4-Dihydroxy-5,8-bis[2-(2-hydroxyethylamino)ethylamino]anthraquinone dihydrochloride.

$C_{22}H_{28}N_4O_6$,2HCl = 517.4.

CAS — 65271-80-9 (mitozantrone); 70476-82-3 (mitozantrone hydrochloride).

Pharmacopoeias. In Eur. (see p.viii) and US.

A dark-blue hygroscopic powder. Sparingly **soluble** in water; slightly soluble in methyl alcohol; practically insoluble in acetone, acetonitrile, or chloroform. **Store** in airtight containers.

Adverse Effects, Treatment, and Precautions

As for Doxorubicin Hydrochloride, p.529. Mitozantrone is reported to be better tolerated than doxorubicin. The nadir of the white blood cell count usually occurs about 10 days after a dose, with recovery by the 21st day. Elevation in liver enzyme values may occur; there are occasional reports of severe impairment of hepatic function in patients with leukaemia, in whom doses are generally higher and adverse effects of mitozantrone may be more frequent and severe.

Transient blue-green coloration of the urine, and occasionally the sclerae, may occur. Tissue necrosis is rare following extravasation.

Mitozantrone should not be given intrathecally: severe neurotoxicity has resulted. Care is required in patients with pre-existing heart disease, or who have had prior anthracycline treatment or radiotherapy to the chest, as they are at increased risk of cardiotoxicity; regular examinations of cardiac function should be performed in such patients and in those who receive a total cumulative dose of mitozantrone in excess of 160 mg per m^2 body-surface. Care is also required in patients with hepatic impairment.

Alopecia. Two patients receiving therapy with mitozantrone developed selective alopecia of white but not of dark hair.[1]

1. Arlin ZA, *et al.* Selective alopecia with mitoxantrone. *N Engl J Med* 1984; **310:** 1464.

Effects on the heart. Data from over 4000 patients treated with mitozantrone included 172 reports of cardiac events, including 42 cases of congestive heart failure and 66 of decreased ejection fraction.[1] Prior treatment with an anthracycline increased the risk, and congestive heart failure seemed to be more likely in patients exposed to a cumulative mitozantrone dose of 160 mg per square metre body-surface or 100 mg per square metre in those who had already received anthracyclines. In a further 78 patients, 2 developed clinical heart failure after cumulative doses of 174 and 243 mg per square metre.[2] Four of 9 other patients who received mitozantrone in doses above 100 mg per square metre showed signs of cardiotoxicity, and a further patient who had previously received doxorubicin 313 mg per square metre had a fall in stress ejection fraction after only 47 mg per square metre of mitozantrone. However, sinus bradycardia has also been reported in 2 previously untreated patients after commencing continuous infusions of mitozantrone 10 mg per square metre.[3]

1. Crossley RJ. Clinical safety and tolerance of mitoxantrone. *Semin Oncol* 1984; **11:** (suppl 1): 54–8.
2. Stuart-Harris R, *et al.* Cardiotoxicity associated with mitoxantrone. *Lancet* 1984; **ii:** 219–20.
3. Benekli M, *et al.* Mitoxantrone-induced bradycardia. *Ann Intern Med* 1997; **126:** 409.

Handling and disposal. Urine and faeces produced for up to 7 days after a dose of mitozantrone should be handled wearing protective clothing.[1]

1. Harris J, Dodds LJ. Handling waste from patients receiving cytotoxic drugs. *Pharm J* 1985; **235:** 289–91.

Hypersensitivity. A report of 3 patients with allergic-type reactions to mitozantrone, including vasculitis, facial oedema and skin rashes, and in one, breathlessness, tachypnoea, cyanosis, and unrecordable pulse and blood pressure.[1] Allergic reactions to the drug appear to be rare.

1. Taylor WB, *et al.* Allergic reactions to mitoxantrone. *Lancet* 1986; **i:** 1439.

Pharmacokinetics

Following intravenous administration mitozantrone is rapidly and extensively distributed to body tissues, and slowly excreted in urine and bile as unchanged drug and metabolites. The elimination half-life is reported to range from 5 to 18 days. Between 6 and 11% of a dose has been recovered from urine, and 13 to 25% in faeces, within 5 days of administration. It does not appear to cross the blood-brain barrier.

References.

1. Ehninger G, *et al.* Pharmacokinetics and metabolism of mitoxantrone: a review. *Clin Pharmacokinet* 1990; **18:** 365–80.

Uses and Administration

Mitozantrone is an antineoplastic structurally related to doxorubicin (p.529). Its mode of action has not been fully established but it inhibits topoisomerase II and causes DNA strand breakage, as well as intercalating with DNA. It is cell-cycle nonspecific but is most active against cells in the late S phase.

It is used in the treatment of advanced breast cancer, and of non-Hodgkin's lymphomas, alone or in combination with other agents. It may also be given to treat adult acute non-lymphoblastic leukaemias, especially in relapse, and has been used in patients with ovarian and refractory prostate cancer. The management of these malignancies is discussed in the introduction to this chapter, as indicated by the cross-references given below. Mitozantrone has also been used in the treatment of liver cancer.

In the treatment of breast cancer and lymphomas, mitozantrone is given as the hydrochloride in an initial dose equivalent to 14 mg of base per m^2 body-surface, repeated every 3 weeks, by injecting a solution diluted in sodium chloride 0.9% or glucose 5% injection into a freely-running intravenous infusion of either, over at least 3 minutes. Subsequent doses may be adjusted according to the degree of myelosuppression produced. Initial dosage may need to be reduced to 12 mg per m^2 in debilitated patients or those who have had previous chemotherapy. Doses should also probably be reduced when mitozantrone is given as part of a combination regimen: an initial dose of 10 to 12 mg per m^2 has been suggested.

In the treatment of patients with acute non-lymphoblastic leukaemia a dose of 12 mg per m^2 daily for 5 days may be given to induce remission; alternatively a similar dose may be given for 3 days in association with cytarabine.

Cardiac examinations are recommended in all patients who receive a cumulative dose of mitozantrone greater than 160 mg per m^2. Regular blood counts should be performed during treatment and courses should not be repeated until blood counts have recovered.

References.

1. Faulds D, *et al.* Mitoxantrone: a review of its pharmacodynamic and pharmacokinetic properties, and therapeutic potential in the chemotherapy of cancer. *Drugs* 1991; **41:** 400–49.

Malignant neoplasms. For reference to the use of mitozantrone in malignant neoplasms of the breast and ovary see under Choice of Antineoplastic, p.485 and p.491. For mention of its use as an alternative to daunorubicin in induction protocols for acute non-lymphoblastic leukaemias, see p.479. The use of mitozantrone in the palliative management of metastatic prostate cancer is mentioned on p.491.

Multiple sclerosis. Mitozantrone has produced some apparent benefit in patients with multiple sclerosis (p.620) but cardiotoxicity limits the dose that can be given.[1]

1. Gonsette RE. Mitoxantrone immunotherapy in multiple sclerosis. *Multiple Sclerosis* 1996; **1:** 329–32.

Preparations

USP 23: Mitoxantrone Injection.

Proprietary Preparations (details are given in Part 3)
Aust.: Novantron; ***Austral.:*** Novantrone; ***Belg.:*** Novantrone; ***Canad.:*** Novantrone; ***Fr.:*** Novantrone; ***Ger.:*** Novantron; ***Irl.:*** Novantrone; ***Ital.:*** Novantrone; ***Neth.:*** Novantrone; ***Norw.:*** Novantrone; ***S.Afr.:*** Novantrone; ***Spain:*** Novantrone; Pralifan; ***Swed.:*** Novantrone; ***Switz.:*** Novantron; ***UK:*** Novantrone; ***USA:*** Novantrone.

Mizoribine (16900-f)

Mizoribine *(rINN)*.

HE-69. 5-Hydroxy-1-β-D-ribofuranosylimidazole-4-carboxamide.

$C_9H_{13}N_3O_6$ = 259.2.

CAS — 50924-49-7.

Mizoribine is an oral immunosuppressant.

Mopidamol (12975-s)

Mopidamol *(BAN, rINN)*.

Ra-233. 2,2′,2″,2‴-(4-Piperidinopyrimido[5,4-*d*]pyrimidine-2,6-diyldinitrilo)tetraethanol.

$C_{19}H_{31}N_7O_4$ = 421.5.

CAS — 13665-88-8.

Mopidamol was formerly used as an antineoplastic. It is also a phosphodiesterase inhibitor which inhibits platelet aggregation.

Multialchilpeptide (10733-r)

CAS — 9076-25-9.

Multialchilpeptide is a complex of metamelfalan, an analogue of melphalan (p.544) with peptides. It has been used in the treatment of malignant neoplasms of the blood and lymphatic systems.

Preparations

Proprietary Preparations (details are given in Part 3)
Ital.: Peptichemio.

Muromonab-CD3 (3278-f)

Muromonab-CD3 *(USAN, rINN)*.

OKT3.

A murine monoclonal antibody comprising a purified IgG_{2a} immunoglobulin with a heavy chain having a molecular weight of about 50 000 and a light chain with a molecular weight of approximately 25 000.

Adverse Effects, Treatment, and Precautions

An acute syndrome ranging from fever, chills, gastro-intestinal disturbances, myalgia, and tremor to dyspnoea, pulmonary oedema, collapse, and cardiac arrest has occurred typically 30 to 60 minutes after the first few doses of muromonab-CD3, and is apparently due to the release of cytokines. Frequency and severity tend to decrease with successive doses, while prophylactic administration of corticosteroids may reduce initial adverse reactions (see Uses and Administration, below). Other reported effects include encephalopathy, cerebral oedema, and a syndrome resembling aseptic meningitis, with headache, fever, stiff neck, and photophobia; seizures have also occurred. Reversible impairment of renal function may also be seen.

Hypersensitivity reactions, including anaphylaxis, have occurred, and may be difficult to distinguish from the cytokine release syndrome.

As with other potent immunosuppressants, treatment with muromonab-CD3 may increase the risk of serious infections and the development of certain malignancies.

Muromonab-CD3 should not be given to patients with pre-existing fever, or in patients hypersensitive to products of murine origin. It should be avoided in patients with a history of seizures. Because fluid overload is associated with an increased risk of pulmonary oedema due to the cytokine release syndrome, muromonab-CD3 is contra-indicated in patients who have undergone a more than 3% weight gain in the week preceding therapy, or who have radiographic evidence of fluid overloading. Repeated courses of muromonab-CD3 may be less effective because of the development of antibodies to the drug.

Effects on the blood. THROMBO-EMBOLISM. Intragraft thromboses developed in 9 of 93 consecutive kidney transplant recipients given high-dose muromonab-CD3 (10 mg daily) as part of their immunosuppressive regimen.[1] In one patient the thrombosis was in the renal artery, and in 3 in the renal vein; the remainder had thromboses in the glomerular capillaries and thrombotic microangiopathy similar to that of haemolytic-uraemic syndrome. The authors suggested that muromonab-CD3 has procoagulant effects, perhaps mediated by released tumour necrosis factor; these effects had also been seen in 3 patients receiving muromonab-CD3 at conventional doses (5 mg daily). Another group[2] has also reported an apparently increased incidence of acute vascular thrombosis in patients given muromonab-CD3 at conventional doses, but in the experience of others,[3] despite evidence of activation of coagulation by the drug, treatment of acute rejection with 5 mg daily was not associated with thrombo-embolic complications.

1. Abramowicz D, *et al.* Induction of thromboses within renal grafts by high-dose prophylactic OKT3. *Lancet* 1992; **339:** 777–8.
2. Gomez E, *et al.* Main graft vessels thromboses due to conventional-dose OKT3 in renal transplantation. *Lancet* 1992; **339:** 1612–13.
3. Raasveld MHM, *et al.* Thromboembolic complications and dose of monoclonal OKT3 antibody. *Lancet* 1992; **339:** 1363–4.

Effects on the ears. Marked bilateral hearing loss developed in a patient given muromonab-CD3 to treat pancreas allograft rejection.[1] The patient also experienced fever, muscle cramps, and hypotension, and had a previous history of gradual hearing loss. The deficit in hearing had persisted on follow-up 6 months after discharge.

1. Michals M, *et al.* Hearing loss associated with muromonab-CD3 therapy. *Clin Pharm* 1988; **7:** 867–8.

Effects on the nervous system. A report of generalised seizures in 2 uraemic kidney-graft recipients following administration of muromonab-CD3.[1] Delayed graft function may result in the accumulation of uraemic toxins which combine with cytokines released by the immunosuppressant to produce the effects on the CNS.

1. Seifeldin RA, *et al.* Generalised seizures associated with the use of muromonab-CD3 in two patients after kidney transplantation. *Ann Pharmacother* 1997; **31:** 586–9.

Uses and Administration

Muromonab-CD3 is a murine monoclonal antibody to the T3 (CD3) antigen of human T-lymphocytes, which is essential to antigen recognition and response; the antibody thus specifically blocks T-cell generation and function to exert an immunosuppressant effect without affecting the bone marrow.

It is used in the treatment of acute allograft rejection in organ transplant recipients, in doses of 5 mg daily by intravenous injection for 10 to 14 days. The dose of any concomitant immunosuppressant therapy may need to be reduced. Patients should be monitored closely for 48 hours after the first dose of muromonab-CD3. The first dose may be preceded by intravenous administration of methylprednisolone sodium succinate, in a dose of 8 mg per kg, 1 to 4 hours before the first dose of muromonab-CD3. Paracetamol and antihistamines may also be given concomitantly with muromonab-CD3 to reduce early reactions.

Muromonab-CD3 has also been given experimentally as part of regimens for the prophylaxis of graft rejection. For further details of the use of muromonab-CD3 in the treatment and prophylaxis of graft rejection see p.499, p.499, p.500, and p.501.

References.

1. Todd PA, Brogden RN. Muromonab CD3: a review of its pharmacology and therapeutic potential. *Drugs* 1989; **37:** 871–99.
2. Wilde MI, Goa KL. Muromonab CD3: a reappraisal of its pharmacology and use as prophylaxis of solid organ transplant rejection. *Drugs* 1996; **51:** 865–94.
3. Burk ML, Matuszewski KA. Muromonab-CD3 and antithymocyte globulin in renal transplantation. *Ann Pharmacother* 1997; **31:** 1370–7.

Preparations

Proprietary Preparations (details are given in Part 3)
Austral.: Orthoclone OKT3; ***Belg.:*** Orthoclone OKT3; ***Canad.:*** Orthoclone OKT3; ***Fr.:*** Orthoclone OKT3; ***Ger.:*** Orthoclone OKT3; ***Ital.:*** Orthoclone OKT3; ***Neth.:*** Orthoclone OKT3; ***Norw.:*** Orthoclone OKT3; ***Swed.:*** Orthoclone OKT3; ***Switz.:*** Orthoclone OKT3; ***USA:*** Orthoclone OKT3.

Mustine Hydrochloride (1853-r)

Mustine Hydrochloride *(BANM)*.

Chlormethine Hydrochloride *(rINNM)*; Chlorethazine Hydrochloride; HN2 (mustine); Mechlorethamine Hydrochloride; Nitrogen Mustard (mustine); NSC-762; WR-147650. Bis(2-chloroethyl)methylamine hydrochloride; 2,2′-Dichloro-*N*-methyldiethylamine hydrochloride.

$C_5H_{11}Cl_2N,HCl$ = 192.5.

CAS — 51-75-2 (mustine); 55-86-7 (mustine hydrochloride).

Pharmacopoeias. In *Br., Chin., Int.,* and *US.*

A white or almost white, hygroscopic, vesicant, crystalline powder or mass. Very **soluble** in water. A 0.2% solution in water has a pH of 3 to 5. Solutions lose their activity very rapidly particularly at neutral or alkaline pH.

Store at a temperature of 8° to 15° in airtight containers. Protect from light.

CAUTION. *Mustine hydrochloride is a strong vesicant; avoid contact with skin and mucous membranes.*

Stability. A study using an assay specific for mustine[1] found that a 0.1% solution in Water for Injections or sodium chloride injection (0.9%) underwent a loss of approximately 10% when stored for 6 hours at room temperature, and of approximately 4 to 6% when stored for the same period at 4°; similar results were obtained whether the solution was stored in glass vials or plastic syringes. Solutions in 500 mL of sodium chloride or glucose (5%) injection and stored in PVC infusion bags were still less stable, with 15% and 10% degradation respectively after 6 hours at room temperature.

1. Kirk B. Stability of reconstituted Mustine Injection BP during storage. *Br J Parenter Ther* 1986; **7:** 86–92.

Adverse Effects, Treatment, and Precautions

For general discussions see Antineoplastics, p.470, p.473, and p.474.

Mustine hydrochloride is extremely toxic and its use is invariably accompanied by side-effects. Severe nausea and vomiting may commence within an hour of injection of the drug and last for some hours; antiemetics and sedatives should be given 10 to 30 minutes before a dose. It causes varying degrees of bone-marrow depression depending on the dose. In heavily pretreated patients, or when the total dose for a single course exceeds 400 µg per kg bodyweight, there is a risk of severe and possibly fatal depression with anaemia, lymphocytopenia, granulocytopenia, and thrombocytopenia with consequent haemorrhage. Depression of lymphocytes may be apparent within 24 hours of the administration of mustine hydrochloride and maximum suppression of granulocytes and platelets occurs within 7 to 21 days; haematological recovery may be adequate after 4 weeks.

Tinnitus, vertigo, deafness, headache, drowsiness, and other neurological symptoms have been reported, as have episodes of jaundice. Skin reactions to mustine hydrochloride include maculopapular rashes. There is a high incidence of hypersensitivity when topical preparations are used.

Mustine hydrochloride has a powerful vesicant action on the skin and mucous membranes and great care must be taken to avoid contact with the eyes. Thrombophlebitis is a potential hazard of mustine particularly if it is not sufficiently diluted. Extravasation of the injection causes severe irritation and even sloughing. If extravasation occurs during injection, the involved area should be infiltrated with an isotonic 4% solution of sodium thiosulphate, followed by the application of an ice compress intermittently for 6 to 12 hours. A 1% lignocaine solution may also be infiltrated.

Mustine hydrochloride may produce temporary or permanent inhibition of fertility. There is some evidence of teratogenicity and carcinogenicity.

Effects on the nervous system. Severe immediate neurotoxicity developed in 14 of 21 evaluable patients who underwent bone-marrow transplantation after preparation with cytotoxic regimens including mustine 0.3 to 2.0 mg per kg body-weight.[1] Symptoms, which developed a median of 4 days after treatment, included headache, hallucinations, confusion, convulsions, paraplegia, and tremor. Symptoms resolved in most, although in some they had not done so before their death. However, of the 13 patients who survived more than 60 days, 6, all of whom had earlier recovered from acute toxicity, developed a delayed neurotoxicity, beginning a median of 169 days after the first mustine injection and characterised by symptoms including confusion, somnolence, personality change, dementia, focal motor seizures, and hydrocephalus. Patients older than 21 years, those who had received CNS irradiation, and those treated concomitantly with other cytotoxic agents were at increased risk of neurotoxicity.

1. Sullivan KM, *et al.* Immediate and delayed neurotoxicity after mechlorethamine preparation for bone marrow transplantation. *Ann Intern Med* 1982; **97:** 182–9.

Handling and disposal. Urine produced for up to 48 hours after a dose of mustine should be handled wearing protective clothing.[1]

1. Harris J, Dodds LJ. Handling waste from patients receiving cytotoxic drugs. *Pharm J* 1985; **235:** 289–91.

The manufacturers state that unused injection solutions may be neutralised by mixing with an equal volume of a solution containing sodium thiosulphate 2.5% and sodium bicarbonate 2.5% and allowing to stand for 45 minutes. Equipment used in the preparation and administration of mustine hydrochloride solutions may be treated similarly. Alternatively a solution containing sodium carbonate 2.5% or sodium hydroxide in a mixture of industrial methylated spirit and water has been suggested for the decontamination of equipment.

Pharmacokinetics

Following intravenous injection, mustine is rapidly converted to a reactive ethyleneimmonium ion. It usually disappears from the blood in a few minutes. A very small proportion is excreted unchanged in the urine.

Uses and Administration

Mustine belongs to the group of antineoplastic drugs described as alkylating agents. It also possesses weak immunosuppressant properties.

Mustine hydrochloride is used in the treatment of advanced Hodgkin's disease, usually in conjunction with a vinca alkaloid, procarbazine, and prednisone or prednisolone (the MOPP regimen). It may also be used in other lymphomas and in tumours of the brain and neuroblastoma, as indicated by the cross-references given below. Mustine has also been tried in some other malignancies including chronic leukaemias, tumours of the breast, ovary, and lung, and in polycythaemia vera. Mustine has been used in the management of malignant effusions but is not the agent of choice.

In the MOPP regimen mustine hydrochloride has been given in doses of 6 mg per m^2 body-surface area. However, as a single agent, the usual dose of mustine hydrochloride is 400 µg per kg bodyweight, preferably as a single dose, although it may be divided into 2 or 4 equal doses on successive days. It is given by intravenous injection in a strength of 1 mg per mL in Water for Injections or sodium chloride 0.9%. Injection over 2 minutes into the tubing of a fast running intravenous infusion of sodium chloride 0.9% or glucose 5% may reduce the incidence of thrombophlebitis and the risk of extravasation.

The response should be assessed by the trend of the blood counts. Treatment with mustine may be repeated when the bone-marrow function has recovered.

Intracavitary injections of 200 to 400 µg per kg have been given in the treatment of malignant, especially pleural, effusions. In mycosis fungoides with extensive skin involvement, very dilute solutions of mustine (e.g. 200 µg per mL) have been applied topically.

Histiocytic syndromes. As discussed on p.478 the value of systemic chemotherapy for Langerhans cell histiocytosis is uncertain; however dilute solutions of mustine (200 µg per mL) have been applied topically for the cutaneous symptoms.[1]

1. Sheehan MP, *et al.* Topical nitrogen mustard: an effective treatment for cutaneous Langerhans cell histiocytosis. *J Pediatr* 1991; **119:** 317–21.

Malignant neoplasms. Mustine plays a central role in the MOPP regimen which was the first effective combination regimen to be widely used for the treatment of Hodgkin's disease, as described on p.481. By extension this and similar regimens have also been given in some forms of non-Hodgkin's lymphoma (see p.482). Topical mustine is often used in the treatment of mycosis fungoides (p.482). Because of relatively good CNS penetration mustine has also been used in the treatment of brain tumours and neuroblastoma (see p.485 and p.494 respectively).

For mention of the use of mustine as a sclerosing agent for malignant effusions, see p.484.

Preparations

BP 1998: Chlormethine Injection;
USP 23: Mechlorethamine Hydrochloride for Injection.

Proprietary Preparations (details are given in Part 3)
Aust.: Mustargen; ***Canad.:*** Mustargen; ***Fr.:*** Caryolysine; ***Switz.:*** Mustargen; ***USA:*** Mustargen.

Mycophenolate Mofetil (11701-r)

Mycophenolate Mofetil *(BANM, USAN)*.

Mycophenolate Morpholinoethyl; RS-61443. 2-Morpholinoethyl (*E*)-6-(4-hydroxy-6-methoxy-7-methyl-3-oxo-5-phthalanyl)-4-methyl-4-hexenoate.

$C_{23}H_{31}NO_7$ = 433.5.

CAS — 115007-34-6.

Adverse Effects, Treatment, and Precautions

For general discussions see Antineoplastics, p.470, p.473, and p.474.

Mycophenolate mofetil is associated with gastro-intestinal disturbances, particularly diarrhoea; gastro-intestinal haemorrhage and perforation has occurred. Leucopenia may develop; as with other immunosuppressants there is an increased risk of infection and certain malignancies in patients receiving mycophenolate mofetil. Other reported adverse effects include pain, headache, anaemia, thrombocytopenia, renal tubular necrosis, haematuria, hypertension, hyperglycaemia, disturbances of electrolytes and blood lipids, peripheral oedema, dyspnoea, cough, dizziness, insomnia, and tremor. Hypersensitivity reactions have occurred. Mycophenolate is teratogenic in *animals*.

Mycophenolate mofetil should be given with care to patients with severe renal impairment or active disorders of the gastro-intestinal tract.

Interactions

Mycophenolate mofetil may compete with other drugs that undergo active renal tubular secretion, resulting in increased concentrations of either drug. Concomitant administration with antacids, or to patients receiving cholestyramine, may result in reduced absorption of mycophenolate.

Antacids. Although concomitant administration of mycophenolate mofetil and an antacid mixture (aluminium and magnesium hydroxides) or food both resulted in reductions in peak plasma concentrations of mycophenolic acid, the differences were small compared with interindividual variation, and were not considered likely to have clinically significant effects.[1]

1. Bullingham R, *et al.* Effects of food and antacid on the pharmacokinetics of single doses of mycophenolate mofetil in rheumatoid arthritis patients. *Br J Clin Pharmacol* 1996; **41:** 513–16.

Pharmacokinetics

Mycophenolate mofetil is rapidly and extensively absorbed from the gastro-intestinal tract, and undergoes presystemic metabolism to active mycophenolic acid. It undergoes enterohepatic recirculation. Mycophenolic acid is metabolised by glucuronidation and excreted primarily in the urine; about 6% of a dose is recovered in faeces. Mycophenolic acid is 97% bound to plasma albumin. The half-life of mycophenolic acid after oral administration of mycophenolate is about 18 hours.

Mycophenolate mofetil is rapidly de-esterified in the body to active mycophenolic acid which is subsequently excreted in the urine, mostly as the inactive glucuronide conjugate,[1] clearance being reduced in patients with impaired renal function. There is some evidence that the pharmacokinetics of mycophenolate mofetil alter with prolonged administration, resulting in reduction in trough plasma concentrations over time.[2]

1. Shah J, *et al.* Pharmacokinetics of oral mycophenolate mofetil (MMF) and metabolites in renally impaired patients. *Clin Pharmacol Ther* 1995; **57:** 149.

2. Sanquer S, *et al.* Trough blood concentrations in long-term treatment with mycophenolate mofetil. *Lancet* 1998; **351:** 1557.

Uses and Administration

Mycophenolic acid is an immunosuppressant derived from *Penicillium stoloniferum*. It is a reversible inhibitor of inosine monophosphate dehydrogenase and thus inhibits purine synthesis, with potent cytostatic effects on both T- and B-lymphocytes. It has been used mainly as the morpholinoethyl derivative, mycophenolate mofetil. It is given combined with other immunosuppressants, for the treatment and prevention of graft rejection, and has also been tried in various diseases with an auto-immune or immune-mediated inflammatory component. For mention of the use of mycophenolate mofetil in heart and kidney transplantation, see p.499 and p.499 respectively.

In the prophylaxis of acute renal graft rejection mycophenolate mofetil is given by mouth in doses of 1 g twice daily; 1.5 g twice daily is recommended in the prophylaxis of cardiac graft rejection. Therapy should begin as soon as possible after transplantation, in combination with cyclosporin and corticosteroids. Patients should undergo regular blood counts; if neutropenia develops consideration should be given to interrupting mycophenolate therapy or reducing the dose.

References.

1. Ensley RD, *et al.* The use of mycophenolate mofetil (RS-61443) in human heart transplant recipients. *Transplantation* 1993; **56:** 75–82.

2. Morris RE. Commentary on new xenobiotic immunosuppressants for transplantation: where are we, how did we get here, and where are we going? *Clin Transplant* 1993; **7:** 138–46.

3. European Mycophenolate Mofetil Cooperative Study Group. Placebo-controlled study of mycophenolate mofetil combined with cyclosporin and corticosteroids for prevention of acute rejection. *Lancet* 1995; **345:** 1321–5.

4. Anonymous. Mycophenolate mofetil—a new immunosuppressant for organ transplantation. *Med Lett Drugs Ther* 1995; **37:** 84–6.

5. Fulton B, Markham A. Mycophenolate mofetil: a review of its pharmacodynamic and pharmacokinetic properties and clinical efficacy in renal transplantation. *Drugs* 1996; **51:** 278–98.

6. Lipsky JJ. Mycophenolate mofetil. *Lancet* 1996; **348:** 1357–9.

7. Hood KA, Zarembski DG. Mycophenolate mofetil: a unique immunosuppressive agent. *Am J Health-Syst Pharm* 1997; **54:** 285–94.

8. Anonymous. Mycophenolate mofetil for the transplanted kidney? *Drug Ther Bull* 1997; **35:** 38–40.

9. Simmons WD, *et al.* Preliminary risk-benefit assessment of mycophenolate mofetil in transplant rejection. *Drug Safety* 1997; **17:** 75–92.

Mycophenolate mofetil is being investigated in a number of conditions with an autoimmune component: these include IgA nephropathy (see Glomerular Kidney Disease, p.1021) and various vasculitic syndromes (see Polyarteritis Nodosa and Microscopic Polyangiitis, p.1027 and Wegener's Granulomatosis, p.1031).

Preparations

Proprietary Preparations (details are given in Part 3)

Aust.: CellCept; ***Austral.:*** CellCept; ***Belg.:*** CellCept; ***Canad.:*** CellCept; ***Fr.:*** CellCept; ***Ger.:*** CellCept; ***Irl.:*** CellCept; ***Ital.:*** CellCept; ***Neth.:*** CellCept; ***Norw.:*** CellCept; ***Spain:*** CellCept; ***Swed.:*** CellCept; ***Switz.:*** CellCept; ***UK:*** CellCept; ***USA:*** CellCept.

Nedaplatin (17044-g)

Nedaplatin *(rINN)*.

cis-Diammine(glycolato-O^1,O^2)platinum.

$C_2H_8N_2O_3Pt$ = 303.2.

CAS — 95734-82-0.

Nedaplatin is a platinum derivative with general properties similar to those of cisplatin (see p.513) although it may be associated with less nephrotoxicity. It is given by intravenous infusion over 1 hour or more, dissolved in at least 300 mL of an appropriate infusion solution, in doses of 80 to 100 mg per m² body-surface. Administration should be followed by infusion of at least 1 litre of fluid to ensure adequate hydration and reduce the risk of renal damage.

References.

1. Weiss RB, Christian MC. New cisplatin analogues in development: a review. *Drugs* 1993; **46:** 360–77.

Preparations

Proprietary Preparations (details are given in Part 3)

Jpn: Aqupla.

Nilutamide (2968-k)

Nilutamide *(BAN, USAN, rINN)*.

RU-23908. 5,5-Dimethyl-3-(α,α,α-trifluoro-4-nitro-*m*-tolyl)-imidazolidine-2,4-dione.

$C_{12}H_{10}F_3N_3O_4$ = 317.2.

CAS — 63612-50-0.

Adverse Effects and Precautions

As for Flutamide, p.537. Interstitial pneumonitis has occurred in patients receiving nilutamide, and the drug is contra-indicated in those with severe respiratory insufficiency. It should also not be given in severe hepatic impairment.

Reversible visual disturbances have been associated with the use of nilutamide.[1,2] Although some consider such visual disturbances to be mild and generally well tolerated,[3] others suggest that these, together with alcohol intolerance and, more seriously, effects on the lung, mean that other nonsteroidal anti-androgens should be preferred.[4]

1. Harnois C, *et al.* Ocular toxicity of Anandron in patients treated for prostatic cancer. *Br J Ophthalmol* 1986; **70:** 471–3.
2. Brisset JM, *et al.* Ocular toxicity of Anandron. *Br J Ophthalmol* 1987; **71:** 639.
3. Dijkman GA, *et al.* Comment: clinical experiences of visual disturbances with nilutamide. *Ann Pharmacother* 1997; **31:** 1550–1.
4. Dole EJ, Holdsworth MT. Comment: clinical experiences of visual disturbances with nilutamide. *Ann Pharmacother* 1997; **31:** 1551–2.

Interactions

Patients receiving nilutamide may exhibit intolerance to alcohol.

Uses and Administration

Nilutamide is a nonsteroidal anti-androgen which is used similarly to flutamide (p.537) in the treatment of prostatic carcinoma (p.491). It is given by mouth in usual doses of 300 mg daily, as a single dose or in divided doses, in patients who have undergone orchiectomy. Dosage may be reduced to 150 mg daily after 1 month. It has also been used in combination with a gonadorelin analogue.

References.

1. Dole EJ, Holdsworth MT. Nilutamide: an antiandrogen for the treatment of prostate cancer. *Ann Pharmacother* 1997; **31:** 65–75.

Preparations

Proprietary Preparations (details are given in Part 3)

Austral.: Anandron; ***Canad.:*** Anandron; ***Fr.:*** Anandron; ***Neth.:*** Anandron; ***Norw.:*** Anandron; ***Swed.:*** Anandron; ***USA:*** Nilandron.

Nimustine Hydrochloride (11478-q)

Nimustine Hydrochloride *(rINNM)*.

ACNU; NSC-245382; Pimustine Hydrochloride. 3-[(4-Amino-2-methylpyrimidin-5-yl)methyl]-1-(2-chloroethyl)-1-nitrosourea hydrochloride.

$C_9H_{13}ClN_6O_2,HCl$ = 309.2.

CAS — 42471-28-3 (nimustine); 55661-38-6 (nimustine hydrochloride).

Nimustine is a nitrosourea antineoplastic with actions and uses similar to those of carmustine (p.511). It is given as the hydrochloride in suggested doses of 2 to 3 mg per kg bodyweight or 90 to 100 mg per m² body-surface as a single dose by slow intravenous administration, repeated at intervals of 4 to 6 weeks depending on haematological response. Solutions for injection must be freshly prepared and protected from light.

Preparations

Proprietary Preparations (details are given in Part 3)

Ger.: ACNU; ***Jpn:*** Nidran; ***Neth.:*** ACNU; ***Switz.:*** ACNU.

Oxaliplatin (2972-y)

Oxaliplatin *(rINN)*.

[(1*R*,2*R*)-1,2-Cyclohexanediamine-*N*,*N*′][oxalato(2-)-*O*,*O*′]platinum.

$C_8H_{14}N_2O_4Pt$ = 397.3.

CAS — 61825-94-3.

Oxaliplatin is a platinum-containing complex similar to cisplatin (see p.513). It is given alone or in combination with fluorouracil in the treatment of refractory metastatic colorectal cancer. The recommended dose is 130 mg per m² body-surface by intravenous infusion over 2 to 6 hours, dissolved in 250 to 500 mL of glucose 5%. The dose may be repeated at intervals of 3 weeks if toxicity permits, reduced according to tolerance. Peripheral neuropathy may be dose-limiting. In the USA it has orphan drug status for the treatment of ovarian cancer.

References to the use of oxaliplatin in colorectal cancer.[1-6] (For further discussion of colorectal malignancy and its management see p.487.) Oxaliplatin is also under investigation in cancer of the head and neck (see p.489).

1. Lévi FA, *et al.* Chronomodulated versus fixed-infusion-rate delivery of ambulatory chemotherapy with oxaliplatin, fluorouracil and folinic acid (leucovorin) in patients with colorectal cancer metastases: a randomized multi-institutional trial. *J Natl Cancer Inst* 1994; **86:** 1608–17.
2. Diaz-Rubio E, *et al.* Multicentric phase II study with oxaliplatin (L-OHP) in 5-FU refractory patients with advanced colorectal cancer (ACC). *Proc Am Soc Clin Oncol* 1995; **14:** 209.
3. Lévi F, *et al.* Randomised multicentre trial of chronotherapy with oxaliplatin, fluorouracil, and folinic acid in metastatic colorectal cancer. *Lancet* 1997; **350:** 681–6.
4. Becouarn Y, Rougier P. Clinical efficacy of oxaliplatin monotherapy: phase II trials in advanced colorectal cancer. *Semin Oncol* 1998; **25** (suppl 5): 23–31.
5. Bleiberg H, de Gramont A. Oxaliplatin plus 5-fluorouracil: clinical experience in patients with advanced colorectal cancer. *Semin Oncol* 1998; **25** (suppl 5): 32–9.
6. Ducreux M, *et al.* Oxaliplatin for the treatment of advanced colorectal cancer: future directions. *Semin Oncol* 1998; **25** (suppl 5): 47–53.

Preparations

Proprietary Preparations (details are given in Part 3)

Fr.: Eloxatine.

P-30 Protein (10730-a)

NOTE. P-30 protein has been incorrectly stated to contain ergotamine.

P-30 protein is a ribonuclease reported to have antineoplastic properties. It is under investigation in the management of a variety of solid tumours, notably in advanced pancreatic cancer with variable results. It is also reported to have activity *in vitro* against HIV.

Paclitaxel (2453-y)

Paclitaxel *(BAN, USAN, rINN)*.

BMS-181339-01; NSC-125973; Taxol; Taxol A. (2*S*,5*R*,7*S*,10*R*,13*S*)-10,20-Bis(acetoxy)-2-benzoyloxy-1,7-dihydroxy-9-oxo-5,20-epoxytax-11-en-13-yl (3*S*)-3-benzoylamino-3-phenyl-D-lactate.

$C_{47}H_{51}NO_{14}$ = 853.9.

CAS — 33069-62-4.

NOTE. Paclitaxel has frequently been referred to as taxol, but the use of this name is now limited, as Taxol is a trademark.

Incompatibility. The vehicle for paclitaxel injection, which contains alcohol and polyethoxylated castor oil, was found to leach the plasticiser diethylhexyl phthalate from some plastic administration sets.[1,2]

For mention of the incompatibility of paclitaxel and cisplatin see p.513.

1. Trissel LA, *et al.* Compatibility of paclitaxel injection vehicle with intravenous administration and extension sets. *Am J Hosp Pharm* 1994; **51:** 2804–10.
2. Mazzo DJ, *et al.* Compatibility of docetaxel and paclitaxel in intravenous solutions with polyvinyl chloride infusion materials. *Am J Health-Syst Pharm* 1997; **54:** 566–9.

Adverse Effects, Treatment, and Precautions

Paclitaxel produces severe dose-limiting bone marrow depression, the nadir of the white cell count usually occurring after about 11 days, with recovery usually by day 15 to 21 after a dose. Myelosuppression may be less frequent and less severe when infusions are given over 3 rather than 24 hours.

Peripheral neuropathy may also be severe, and occasionally dose-limiting. Hypersensitivity reactions, with dyspnoea, hypotension, and angioedema have occurred, and patients should receive premedication with corticosteroids and histamine antagonists. Other adverse effects include alopecia, arthralgia and myalgia, gastro-intestinal disturbances, mucositis, ileus, seizures, encephalopathy, bradycardia and cardiac conduction abnormalities, chest pain, flushing, rashes, nail dystrophies, hepatic necrosis, and elevation of liver enzyme values. Extravasation may result in tissue damage.

Paclitaxel is not recommended in patients with severely impaired hepatic function. The drug is formulated in polyethoxylated castor oil and should be avoided in patients hypersensitive to this substance. Continuous cardiac monitoring should be performed in patients who have experienced previous significant conduction abnormalities while receiving paclitaxel.

Alcohol intoxication. A report of acute alcohol intoxication resulting from paclitaxel infusion;[1] it was calculated that the dose required supplied 50 mL of alcohol, or the equivalent of about 3 drinks, in the formulation.

1. Wilson DB, *et al.* Paclitaxel formulation as a cause of ethanol intoxication. *Ann Pharmacother* 1997; **31:** 873–5.

Effects on the heart. Infusion of paclitaxel has been associated with myocardial infarction,[1] sudden death[2] and symptoms suggestive of heart failure.[3] In another report sudden death 7 days after paclitaxel treatment raised the question of whether paclitaxel might have had a delayed effect.[4] There is some evidence of cellular damage to the myocardium of a patient with paclitaxel-associated cardiac symptoms.[3] The manufacturers note that severe cardiovascular events have been observed more frequently following the use of paclitaxel in patients with non-small cell lung cancer than in those with breast or ovarian carcinoma.

1. Rowinsky EK, *et al.* Cardiac disturbances during the administration of taxol. *J Clin Oncol* 1991; **9:** 1704–12.
2. Arbuck S, *et al.* A reassessment of cardiac toxicity associated with Taxol. *Proc Am Soc Clin Oncol* 1993; **12:** 138.
3. Jekunen A, *et al.* Paclitaxel-induced myocardial damage detected by electron microscopy. *Lancet* 1994; **343:** 727–8.
4. Alagaratnam TT. Sudden death 7 days after paclitaxel infusion for breast cancer. *Lancet* 1993; **342:** 1232–3.

Effects on the respiratory system. Acute bilateral interstitial pneumonitis has been reported rarely in patients receiving paclitaxel, despite premedication with corticosteroids and histamine antagonists.[1] Symptoms resolved on treatment with parenteral corticosteroids.

1. Khan A, *et al.* Paclitaxel-induced acute bilateral pneumonitis. *Ann Pharmacother* 1997; **31:** 1471–4.

Interactions

Pretreatment with cisplatin may reduce the clearance of paclitaxel, resulting in increased toxicity, and when the 2 drugs are given in combination paclitaxel should be given first; presumably such a risk may also apply if paclitaxel is given to patients who have received other nephrotoxic drugs.

Antineoplastics. For reference to enhanced cardiotoxicity when paclitaxel was given in association with *doxorubicin*, see p.530.

Pretreatment with *fluorouracil* has been reported to inhibit paclitaxel's cytotoxic action, possibly by preventing tumour cells from entering the G_2-M phases of the cell cycle.[1] The effect also occurred when the 2 drugs were given simultaneously, suggesting that combination therapy might not be appropriate.

1. Johnson KR, *et al.* 5-Fluorouracil interferes with paclitaxel cytotoxicity against human solid tumor cells. *Clin Cancer Res* 1997; **3:** 1739–45.

Pharmacokinetics

Following intravenous administration paclitaxel exhibits a biphasic decline in plasma concentrations, with a mean terminal half-life of anywhere between about 3 and 50 hours. The pharmacokinetics are non-linear. The steady-state volume of distribution is reported to range from about 200 to about 700 litres per m^2, indicating extensive extravascular distribution, tissue binding, or both. Paclitaxel is 89% or more bound to plasma protein *in vitro*. The elimination of paclitaxel has not been fully elucidated; only about 1 to 12% of a dose is reported to be excreted in urine, as unchanged drug, indicating extensive non renal clearance. Paclitaxel is metabolised in the liver, with the major metabolic pathway apparently mediated by the cytochrome P450 isoform CYP2C8, although CYP3A4 may play a minor role. High paclitaxel concentrations have been reported in bile.

References.

1. Wiernik PH, *et al.* Phase I clinical and pharmacokinetic study of Taxol. *Cancer Res* 1987; **47:** 2486–93.
2. Sonnichsen DS, Relling MV. Clinical pharmacokinetics of paclitaxel. *Clin Pharmacokinet* 1994; **27:** 256–69.
3. Walle T, *et al.* [^{3}H]-Paclitaxel disposition and metabolism in cancer patients. *Clin Pharmacol Ther* 1995; **57:** 153.
4. Sonnichsen D, *et al.* Variability in human in vitro and in-vivo metabolism of paclitaxel. *Clin Pharmacol Ther* 1995; **57:** 193.

Uses and Administration

Paclitaxel is a complex diterpene derived from the bark of the Pacific yew tree *Taxus brevifolia* (Taxaceae) or by synthesis. It induces microtubule formation and disrupts normal cell division in the G_2 and M phases of the cell cycle. It is used for its antineoplastic action against malignant neoplasms of the breast and ovary, and in advanced non-small cell lung cancer, but has also been tried in other malignancies including tumours of the head and neck, prostate, and Kaposi's sarcoma, as indicated by the cross references below.

The recommended dose for cancer of the breast or ovary is 175 mg per m^2 body-surface by intravenous infusion over 3 hours, and repeated after 3 or more weeks, depending on tolerance. A similar regimen, in combination with cisplatin, is used in the treatment of advanced non-small cell lung cancer. The dose should be reduced by 20% in subsequent courses in patients who experience severe neutropenia or peripheral neuropathy. For primary treatment of ovarian cancer a dose of 135 mg per m^2 may be given, followed by cisplatin, every 3 weeks. In the USA, a dose of 135 mg per m^2 as a single agent, repeated after 3 weeks, has also been recommended for ovarian cancer. A similar dose has been suggested for AIDS-related Kaposi's sarcoma. Alternatively, 100 mg per m^2 over 3 hours every 2 weeks may be given, especially in patients with poor performance status.

Regular blood counts should be performed on patients receiving paclitaxel, and dosage should not be repeated until the neutrophil count is greater than 1500 per mm^3 (1000 per mm^3 in patients with AIDS) and the platelet count greater than 100 000 per mm^3. Patients should be pretreated with corticosteroids and histamine antagonists.

References.

1. Rowinsky EK, *et al.* Taxol: the first of the taxanes, an important new class of antitumor agents. *Semin Oncol* 1992; **19:** 646–62.
2. Gelmon K. The taxoids: paclitaxel and docetaxel. *Lancet* 1994; **344:** 1267–72.
3. Long HJ. Paclitaxel (Taxol): a novel anticancer chemotherapeutic drug. *Mayo Clin Proc* 1994: **69:** 341–5.
4. Spencer CM, Faulds D. Paclitaxel: a review of its pharmacodynamic and pharmacokinetic properties and therapeutic potential in the treatment of cancer. *Drugs* 1994; **48:** 794–847.
5. Bailey N, Calvert H. Role of taxanes in cancer therapy. *Br J Hosp Med* 1995; **53:** 10–13.
6. Rowinsky EK, Donehower RC. Paclitaxel (Taxol). *N Engl J Med* 1995; **332:** 1004–14. Correction. *ibid.*; **333:** 75.
7. Gianni L, *et al.* Paclitaxel by 3-hour infusion in combination with bolus doxorubicin in women with untreated metastatic breast cancer: high antitumor efficacy and cardiac effects in a dose-finding and sequence-finding study. *J Clin Oncol* 1995; **13:** 2688–99.
8. Anonymous. Paclitaxel and docetaxel in breast and ovarian cancer. *Drug Ther Bull* 1997; **35:** 43–6.

Malignant neoplasms. The place of paclitaxel in antineoplastic therapy is still to be determined. It is active in ovarian cancer, where a regimen of paclitaxel with cisplatin has been suggested to be the treatment of choice in advanced disease (see p.491). It has also been given in breast cancer (p.485), and has been tried in malignancies of the head and neck (p.489), lung cancer (p.490), prostatic cancer (p.491), and Kaposi's sarcoma (p.496).

Preparations

Proprietary Preparations (details are given in Part 3)

Aust.: Taxol; ***Austral.:*** Anzatax; Taxol; ***Belg.:*** Taxol; ***Canad.:*** Taxol; ***Fr.:*** Taxol; ***Ger.:*** Taxol; ***Irl.:*** Taxol; ***Ital.:*** Taxol; ***Neth.:*** Taxol; ***Norw.:*** Taxol; ***S.Afr.:*** Taxol; Yewtaxan; ***Spain:*** Taxol; ***Swed.:*** Taxol; ***Switz.:*** Taxol; ***UK:*** Taxol; ***USA:*** Taxol.

Peldesine (17274-x)

Peldesine *(USAN, pINN)*.

BCX-34; Peldesina; Peldésine. 2-Amino-3,5-dihydro-7-(3-pyridylmethyl)-4*H*-pyrrolo[3,2-*d*]pyrimidin-4-one.

$C_{12}H_{11}N_5O$ = 241.2.

CAS — 133432-71-0.

Peldesine is an inhibitor of the enzyme purine nucleoside phosphorylase and is reported to suppress T-cell proliferation. It is under investigation in the management of cutaneous T-cell lymphomas, and has also been tried topically in psoriasis and some T-cell mediated eye disorders.

Pentostatin (16946-y)

Pentostatin *(BAN, USAN, rINN)*.

CI-825; Covidarabine; Co-vidarabine; Deoxycoformycin; 2′-Deoxycoformycin; NSC-218321; PD-81565. (*R*)-3-(2-Deoxy-β-D-*erythro*-pentofuranosyl)-3,6,7,8-tetrahydroimidazo[4,5-*d*][1,3]diazepin-8-ol; 1,2-Dideoxy-1-[(*R*)-3,6,7,8-tetrahydro-8-hydroxyimidazo[4,5-*d*][1,3]diazepin-3-yl]-D-*erythro*-pentofuranose.

$C_{11}H_{16}N_4O_4$ = 268.3.

CAS — 53910-25-1.

Adverse Effects and Precautions

The most common adverse effects in patients receiving pentostatin include myelosuppression (and in particular suppression of CD4+ lymphocyte subset), headache, abdominal pain, fever and chills, gastro-intestinal disturbances (notably diarrhoea and nausea and vomiting), hypersensitivity reactions, and hepatotoxicity. Central neurotoxicity may be manifest as tiredness, anxiety, depression, sleep disturbances, and paraesthesias: treatment should be withheld or discontinued in such patients. Impaired renal function and pulmonary toxicity (cough, dyspnoea, and pneumonia) may occur. Severe toxicity in early studies, affecting mainly the CNS, kidneys, and lungs, was associated with the use of doses higher than those currently recommended and produced some fatalities.

Other adverse effects reported with pentostatin include dry skin and rashes (sometimes severe and worsening with continued treatment), pruritus, conjunctivitis, alopecia, arthralgia and myalgia, peripheral oedema, thrombophlebitis, and cardiovascular disorders including arrhythmias, angina pectoris, and heart failure.

Pentostatin should not be given to patients with impaired renal function, or in active infection. It is teratogenic in *animals* and potentially genotoxic: men receiving pentostatin should not father children for 6 months after therapy.

Interactions

Pentostatin should not be given in association with fludarabine, as the combination may result in enhanced pulmonary toxicity.

Allopurinol. Fatal acute necrotising arteritis developed in a patient given pentostatin and allopurinol.[1] Although the hypersensitivity vasculitis may have been due to allopurinol alone there is circumstantial evidence to suggest that pentostatin may predispose patients to drug hypersensitivity and it may be wise to avoid this combination, and to observe pentostatin-treated patients closely for allergic manifestations.

1. Steinmetz JC, *et al.* Hypersensitivity vasculitis associated with 2-deoxycoformycin and allopurinol therapy. *Am J Med* 1989; **86:** 499.

Uses and Administration

Pentostatin is a potent inhibitor of the enzyme adenosine deaminase that probably exerts its cytotoxic actions through the interruption of normal purine metabolism and DNA synthesis. Lymphocytes are particularly sensitive to its actions. It enhances the antiviral and antineoplastic actions of vidarabine, which is normally rapidly metabolised by adenosine deaminase.

Pentostatin has been given in the treatment of hairy-cell leukaemia (see p.481), in usual doses of 4 mg per m^2 body-surface intravenously every other week. Hydration with 500 mL to 1 L of 5% glucose in sodium chloride 0.45% injection is recommended before administration; a further 500 mL of the hydration solution should be infused once the drug has been given.

Pentostatin has been tried in some other lymphoid malignancies, including chronic lymphocytic leukaemia (see p.480), and in T-cell non-Hodgkin's lymphomas (see p.482).

References.

1. O'Dwyer PJ, *et al.* 2′-Deoxycoformycin (pentostatin) for lymphoid malignancies: rational development of an active new drug. *Ann Intern Med* 1988; **108:** 733–43.
2. Brogden RN, Sorkin EM. Pentostatin: a review of its pharmacodynamic and pharmacokinetic properties, and therapeutic potential in lymphoproliferative disorders. *Drugs* 1993; **46:** 652–77.

Preparations

Proprietary Preparations (details are given in Part 3)

Belg.: Nipent†; ***Canad.:*** Nipent†; ***Fr.:*** Nipent; ***Ger.:*** Nipent; ***Ital.:*** Nipent; ***Spain:*** Nipent; ***UK:*** Nipent; ***USA:*** Nipent.

Peplomycin Sulphate (13092-v)

Peplomycin Sulphate *(rINNM).*

NK-631; Pepleomycin Sulphate; Peplomycin Sulfate *(USAN).* N^1-{3-[(*S*)-(α-Methylbenzyl)amino]propyl}bleomycinamide sulphate.

$C_{61}H_{88}N_{18}O_{21}S_2,H_2SO_4$ = 1571.7.

CAS — 68247-85-8 (peplomycin); 70384-29-1 (peplomycin sulphate).

Pharmacopoeias. In *Jpn.*

Peplomycin is an antineoplastic derived from bleomycin (see p.507) and with similar properties. It is given as the sulphate in the treatment of a variety of malignant neoplasms, including tumours of the head and neck, lung, prostate, and skin. The usual dose is 5 to 10 mg two to three times weekly by intravenous, intramuscular, or intra-arterial injection. A total cumulative dose of 150 mg should not be exceeded.

Preparations

Proprietary Preparations (details are given in Part 3)
Jpn: Pepleo.

Pipobroman (1857-h)

Pipobroman *(USAN, pINN).*

A-8103; NSC-25154. 1,4-Bis(3-bromopropionyl)piperazine.

$C_{10}H_{16}Br_2N_2O_2$ = 356.1.

CAS — 54-91-1.

Pipobroman is an antineoplastic which appears to act by alkylation. It has been tried in the treatment of polycythaemia vera (p.495), particularly in patients resistant to conventional therapy, and in chronic myeloid leukaemia (p.480) resistant to busulphan and radiotherapy.

The usual dose initially is 1 mg per kg body-weight by mouth daily, increased to 3 mg per kg, if necessary, according to the patient's response. Maintenance dosage is 0.1 to 0.2 μg per kg daily for polycythaemia vera.

The principal adverse effect is moderate bone-marrow depression, which may be delayed 4 weeks or more from initiation of treatment. Anaemia may be marked at higher doses and is usually accompanied by leucopenia. Thrombocytopenia and haemolysis have occurred. In the initial stages of treatment, white-cell and platelet counts should be determined on alternate days and complete blood counts once or twice weekly. Doses should be discontinued if the white-cell count is below 3000 per mm^3 or the platelet count below 150 000 per mm^3.

Preparations

Proprietary Preparations (details are given in Part 3)
Fr.: Vercyte; ***Ital.:*** Vercite; ***USA:*** Vercyte†.

Pirarubicin (2917-g)

Pirarubicin *(rINN).*

1609RB; Tepirubicin; THP-ADM; THP-doxorubicin. (8*S*,10*S*)-10-{[3-Amino-2,3,6-trideoxy-4-*O*-(2*R*-tetrahydro-2*H*-pyran-2-yl)-α-L-*lyxo*-hexopyranosyl]oxy}-8-glycoloyl-7,8,9,10-tetrahydro-6,8,11-trihydroxy-1-methoxy-5,12-naphthacenedione.

$C_{32}H_{37}NO_{12}$ = 627.6.

CAS — 72496-41-4.

Pirarubicin is an anthracycline antibiotic antineoplastic which is a structural analogue of doxorubicin (see p.529), and has similar properties. It has been given in the management of breast cancer and other solid neoplasms, and has also been tried in acute leukaemias and lymphomas.

Pirarubicin is formulated as the hydrochloride but doses are in terms of the base. A usual dose of 25 to 50 mg per m^2 body-surface every 3 to 4 weeks has been recommended in breast cancer, according to response, but other dosage regimens have been used. Doses may be given by intravenous injection over 5 to 10 minutes into a rapidly-flowing intravenous infusion. Patients should undergo regular blood counts and monitoring of cardiac function: at cumulative doses above 600 mg per m^2 ejection fraction should be checked before each course. Pirarubicin has also been given by the intra-arterial and intravesical routes.

Preparations

Proprietary Preparations (details are given in Part 3)
Aust.: Berirubin; ***Fr.:*** Theprubicine; ***Jpn:*** Therarubicin.

Piritrexim Isethionate (18894-w)

Piritrexim Isethionate *(USAN).*

Piritrexim Isetionate *(rINNM)*; BW-301U (piritrexim); NSC-351521. 2,4-Diamino-6-(2,5-dimethoxybenzyl)-5-methylpyrido[2,3-*d*]pyrimidine mono(2-hydroxyethanesulphonate).

$C_{17}H_{19}N_5O_2,C_2H_6O_4S$ = 451.5.

CAS — 72732-56-0 (piritrexim); 79483-69-5 (piritrexim isethionate).

Piritrexim is a folate antagonist with general properties similar to those of methotrexate (see p.547) and which has been tried by mouth for its antineoplastic properties, and has also been used (as the isethionate) for the treatment of opportunistic infections in immunosuppressed patients. Myelosuppression, gastro-intestinal disturbances, and hepatotoxicity have been reported.

Piritrexim isethionate has also been investigated for severe psoriasis.

Piritrexim has been tried as an alternative to methotrexate in the treatment of malignant neoplasms,[1] and in the management of psoriasis.[2-4] The use of methotrexate in psoriasis is discussed on p.1075.

1. Feun LG, *et al.* Phase II trial of piritrexim in metastatic melanoma using intermittent, low-dose administration. *J Clin Oncol* 1991; **9:** 464–7.
2. Perkins W, *et al.* Piritrexim in severe psoriasis. *Br J Dermatol* 1991; **125** (suppl 38): 26–7.
3. Guzzo C, *et al.* Treatment of psoriasis with piritrexim, a lipid-soluble folate antagonist. *Arch Dermatol* 1991; **127:** 511–14.
4. Perkins W, *et al.* A multicentre 12-week open study of a lipid-soluble folate antagonist, piritrexim in severe psoriasis. *Br J Dermatol* 1993; **129:** 584–9.

Piroxantrone Hydrochloride (6493-q)

Piroxantrone Hydrochloride *(USAN, rINNM).*

Anthrapyrazole Hydrochloride; CI-942; NSC-349174; Oxantrazole Hydrochloride; PD-111815 (piroxantrone). 5-[(3-Aminopropyl)amino]-7,10-dihydroxy-2-{2-[(2-hydroxyethyl)amino]ethyl}anthra[1,9-*cd*]pyrazol-6(2*H*)-one dihydrochloride.

$C_{21}H_{25}N_5O_4,2HCl$ = 484.4.

CAS — 91441-23-5 (piroxantrone); 105118-12-5 (piroxantrone hydrochloride).

Piroxantrone like mitozantrone (p.553) is a structural analogue of the anthracycline antibiotics. It has been investigated for its antineoplastic properties against various malignant neoplasms. Myelosuppression, which may be severe and cumulative, is dose-limiting.

References.

1. Hantel A, *et al.* Phase I study and pharmacodynamics of piroxantrone (NSC 349174), a new anthrapyrazole. *Cancer Res* 1990; **50:** 3284–8.
2. Ames MM, *et al.* Phase I and clinical pharmacological evaluation of pirozantrone hydrochloride (oxantrazole). *Cancer Res* 1990; **50:** 3905–9.
3. Ingle JN, *et al.* Evaluation of piroxantrone in women with metastatic breast cancer and failure on nonanthracycline chemotherapy. *Cancer* 1994; **74:** 1733–8.

Plicamycin (1846-f)

Plicamycin *(BAN, USAN, rINN).*

A-2371; Aureolic Acid; Mithramycin; NSC-24559; PA-144.

$C_{52}H_{76}O_{24}$ = 1085.1.

CAS — 18378-89-7.

Pharmacopoeias. In *US.*

An antineoplastic antibiotic produced by the growth of *Streptomyces argillaceus*, *S. plicatus* and *S. tanashiensis.* It is a yellow, odourless, hygroscopic, crystalline powder, with a potency of not less than 900 μg per mg, calculated on the dry basis. It loses not more than 8% of its weight when dried. Slightly **soluble** in water and methyl alcohol; very slightly soluble in alcohol; freely soluble in ethyl acetate. A 0.05% solution in water has a pH of 4.5 to 5.5. **Store** at 2° to 8° in airtight containers. Protect from light.

Adsorption. Plicamycin is bound to cellulose filters used for inline filtration of intravenous infusions,[1] with more drug likely to be lost from glucose than from sodium chloride injection at the low concentrations of drug used in therapy.

1. Butler LD, *et al.* Effect of inline filtration on the potency of low-dose drugs. *Am J Hosp Pharm* 1980; **37:** 935–41.

Incompatibility. Plicamycin readily chelates divalent cations, especially iron. Admixture with trace element solutions should be avoided.[1]

1. D'Arcy PF. Reactions and interactions in handling anticancer drugs. *Drug Intell Clin Pharm* 1983; **17:** 532–8.

Adverse Effects, Treatment, and Precautions

For general discussions see Antineoplastics, p.470, p.473, and p.474.

The major adverse effect of plicamycin is a dose-related bleeding syndrome, manifest initially as epistaxis, which may progress to haematemesis and potentially fatal haemorrhage. Effects on clotting factors in the blood are thought to contribute to this syndrome. Severe thrombocytopenia may also occur due to bone-marrow depression. Leucopenia is relatively uncommon.

Gastro-intestinal effects are common during treatment with plicamycin. Other side-effects include fever, malaise, drowsiness, lethargy and weakness, headache, depression, skin rashes, facial flushing, and reduced serum concentrations of calcium, phosphorus, and potassium. There may also be reversible impairment of renal and hepatic function.

Extravasation of plicamycin solutions may cause local irritation, cellulitis, and phlebitis. Application of moderate heat to the site of extravasation may aid dispersal of plicamycin and minimise discomfort and local irritation.

Plicamycin should only be given with great care to patients with impaired hepatic or renal function. It should not be administered to patients with thrombocytopenia or depressed bone-marrow function, coagulation disorders, or increased susceptibility to bleeding for any cause.

Although it is recommended that plicamycin be administered as an intravenous infusion over four to six hours, on the grounds that more rapid administration is associated with increased severity of gastro-intestinal toxicity, Mutch and colleagues reported that a search of the literature failed to find any evidence of improved tolerance or enhanced efficacy with infusion rather than bolus injection of plicamycin.[1]

1. Mutch RS, *et al.* Plicamycin: bolus or infusion? *DICP Ann Pharmacother* 1990; **24:** 885–6.

Effects on the kidneys. A report of reversible oliguria and deterioration of renal function occurring on 2 occasions in a patient given single doses of plicamycin.[1]

1. Benedetti RG, *et al.* Nephrotoxicity following single dose mithramycin therapy. *Am J Nephrol* 1983; **3:** 277–8.

Effects on the skin. Toxic epidermal necrolysis occurring in a 22-year-old man was attributed to treatment with plicamycin.[1]

1. Purpora D, *et al.* Toxic epidermal necrolysis after mithramycin. *N Engl J Med* 1978; **299:** 1412.

Local toxicity. Disodium edetate has been suggested as an antidote to local toxicity following extravasation of plicamycin.[1] However, there is a suggestion that the classification of plicamycin as a vesicant is inappropriate.[2]

1. MacCara ME. Extravasation: a hazard of intravenous therapy. *Drug Intell Clin Pharm* 1983; **17:** 713–17.
2. Loughner JE, Olek C. Comment; plicamycin infusion. *DICP Ann Pharmacother* 1991; **25:** 215.

Uses and Administration

Plicamycin is a highly toxic antibiotic with antineoplastic and hypocalcaemic properties. It may act by complexing with DNA in the presence of divalent cations and inhibiting synthesis of ribonucleic acid. Lowering of serum calcium concentrations has been suggested to result from antagonism of the effects of vitamin D and parathyroid hormone on osteoclasts.

Plicamycin is used in the symptomatic management of hypercalcaemia and hypercalciuria associated with malignancy if it cannot be managed by other means (see below). The usual dose is 15 to 25 μg per kg body-weight daily by slow intravenous infusion over 4 to 6 hours in a litre of glucose 5% or sodium chloride 0.9%, for 3 or 4 days if necessary. Further courses may be given at intervals of a week or more if required.

Plicamycin has also been used in the treatment of malignant neoplasms of the testis not susceptible to surgery or radiotherapy; however, other agents are usually preferred (p.493). The usual dose is 25 to 30 μg per kg daily by slow intravenous infusion for 8 to 10 doses. No more than 10 doses should be given and individual daily doses should not normally exceed 30 μg per kg, because of the increased risk of haemorrhage; however an alternative regimen employing up to 50 μg per kg on alternate days is reported to produce less toxicity. Courses may be repeated at monthly intervals.

Blood cell counts, bleeding time, prothrombin time, and hepatic and renal function should be determined frequently during treatment and for several days after, and treatment stopped if there is any sudden change.

Administration. The manufacturers recommend that plicamycin be given by infusion rather than bolus injection, as this is reportedly associated with fewer and less severe gastro-intestinal adverse effects. For a suggestion that this distinction is unjustified, see under Adverse Effects, above.

Chronic myeloid leukaemia. For mention of the use of plicamycin with hydroxyurea to treat the transformed phase of chronic myeloid leukaemia see p.480.

Hypercalcaemia. Where treatment is required for hypercalcaemia it is aimed at increasing urinary excretion of calcium and maintaining adequate hydration. Drugs that inhibit bone resorption may also be employed if hypercalcaemia is severe, particularly when it is associated with malignancy (see p.1148). Although plicamycin is effective, it is highly toxic, and the bisphosphonates and calcitonins are generally preferred. See also under Malignant Neoplasms of Bone, p.484.

Paget's disease of bone. Despite attempts to reduce toxicity through low-dose or short-term regimens (e.g. 15 μg per kg for 3 days followed by 10 μg per kg for 7 days) plicamycin remains a second- or third-line agent in the therapy of Paget's disease of bone (p.732), reserved for patients refractory to other treatment.[1,2] Nonetheless, occasional successes are reported: one patient with refractory Paget's disease had apparent cure of her symptoms after treatment with plicamycin 25 μg per kg daily for 15 doses, followed by 1500 μg weekly for about 2 months and every 2 weeks for 6 weeks.[3] She had remained asymptomatic for 18 years after treatment. However, similar regimens have been used in other patients without this degree of success.[3]

1. Stumpf JL. Pharmacologic management of Paget's disease. *Clin Pharm* 1989; **8:** 485–95.
2. Stevenson JC. Paget's disease of bone. *Prescribers' J* 1991; **31:** 98–103.
3. Ryan WG, *et al.* Apparent cure of Paget's disease of bone. *Am J Med* 1990; **89:** 825–6.

Preparations

USP 23: Plicamycin for Injection.

Proprietary Preparations (details are given in Part 3)
Fr.: Mithracine; ***Neth.:*** Mithracin†; ***Norw.:*** Mithracin; ***Switz.:*** Mithracine†; ***UK:*** Mithracin†; ***USA:*** Mithracin.

Porfimer Sodium (10687-p)

Porfimer Sodium *(BAN, USAN, rINN).*

CL-184116; Dihaematoporphyrin Ether.

CAS — 87806-31-3.

Porfimer sodium is a haematoporphyrin derivative which reportedly accumulates in malignant tissue following administration, and is then activated by laser light to release oxygen radicals within malignant cells, producing cytotoxicity. It is used in the treatment of superficial bladder, lung, and oesophageal cancer, and has been investigated in some other neoplasms including tumours of gastro-intestinal tract and cervix. Administration is by slow intravenous injection at a dose of 2 mg per kg body-weight. This is followed, 40 to 50 hours later, by activation using a laser tuned to a wavelength of 630 nm and delivered to the area of the tumour using a fibre optic guide. The tumour may subsequently be debrided surgically. A second laser treatment may be given 96 to 120 hours after the original injection. Prolonged photosensitivity, lasting several weeks, is likely in patients treated with porfimer sodium. Other reported adverse effect include constipation, abdominal pain, dysphagia, nausea and vomiting, tachycardia and atrial fibrillation, dyspnoea, pneumonia, pleural effusion, and anaemia.

Photodynamic therapy probably has the greatest potential of the various forms of light-activated treatment.[1] Because of the limited penetration of light into living tissues photodynamic therapy is best suited to the treatment of small thin lesions but it can also produce beneficial effects in advanced and recurrent tumours by reducing their bulk.[2] Although surgery is still the best treatment for early tumours photodynamic therapy has potential for the treatment of residual microscopic deposits of malignant cells left after surgery.[2,3] It is also well suited to endoscopic, laparoscopic, and percutaneous treatment and has produced encouraging results in gastric, laryngeal, oesophageal, colorectal, and bronchial tumours[3-6] (for reference to the use of photodynamic therapy to relieve obstruction in oesophageal cancer, see p.487). There is also an interesting report of cytotoxicity against leukaemic cells *in vitro* when exposure to porfimer sodium was combined with ultrasound.[7]

The main adverse effect is photosensitivity lasting 4 to 8 weeks; patients should be advised to avoid sunlight during this period[1,2] and therapy is best delayed until the darker winter months if possible.[1] The natural haem precursor 5-aminolaevulinic acid (p.503) has the advantage that photosensitivity lasts only a few hours.

1. Bown SG. New techniques in laser therapy. *Br Med J* 1998; **316:** 754–7.
2. Abulafi AM, Williams NS. Photodynamic therapy for cancer. *Br Med J* 1992; **304:** 589–90.
3. van Hillegersberg R, *et al.* Current status of photodynamic therapy in oncology. *Drugs* 1994; **48:** 510–27.
4. Wilson JHP, *et al.* Photodynamic therapy for gastrointestinal tumors. *Scand J Gastroenterol* 1991; **26** (suppl 188): 20–5.
5. Abramson AL, *et al.* Clinical effects of photodynamic therapy on recurrent laryngeal papillomas. *Arch Otolaryngol Head Neck Surg* 1992; **118:** 25–9.
6. Cortese DA, *et al.* Photodynamic therapy for early stage squamous cell carcinoma of the lung. *Mayo Clin Proc* 1997; **72:** 595–602.
7. Tachibana K, *et al.* Eliminating adult T-cell leukaemia cells with ultrasound. *Lancet* 1997; **349:** 325.

Preparations

Proprietary Preparations (details are given in Part 3)
Canad.: Photofrin; ***USA:*** Photofrin.

Porfiromycin (6442-t)

Porfiromycin *(BAN, USAN).*

Methyl Mitomycin; NSC-56410; U-14743. 6-Amino-1,1a,2,8,8a,8b-hexahydro-8-(hydroxymethyl)-8a-methoxy-1,5-dimethylazirino[2′,3′:3,4]pyrrolo[1,2-*a*]-indole-4,7-dione carbamate ester.

$C_{16}H_{20}N_4O_5$ = 348.4.

CAS — 801-52-5.

Porfiromycin is an antibiotic antineoplastic structurally related to mitomycin (p.552). It is under investigation as a radiosensitiser in the management of malignant neoplasms of the head and neck.

References.

1. Haffty BG, *et al.* Bioreductive alkylating agent porfiromycin in combination with radiation therapy for the management of squamous cell carcinoma of the head and neck. *Radiat Oncol Invest* 1997; **5:** 235–45.

Prednimustine (1859-b)

Prednimustine *(USAN, rINN).*

Leo-1031; NSC-134087. 11β,17,21-Trihydroxypregna-1,4-diene-3,20-dione 21-(4-{4-[bis(2-chloroethyl)amino]phenyl}butyrate).

$C_{35}H_{45}Cl_2NO_6$ = 646.6.

CAS — 29069-24-7.

Prednimustine is the prednisolone ester of chlorambucil, (p.512) and is used in the treatment of various malignant diseases. It has been given by mouth in doses of 200 mg daily for 3 to 5 consecutive days, repeated after an interval of at least 10 days.

Preparations

Proprietary Preparations (details are given in Part 3)
Aust.: Sterecyt†; ***Fr.:*** Stereocyt†; ***Ger.:*** Sterecyt†; ***Spain:*** Mostarina†; ***Swed.:*** Sterecyt†; ***Switz.:*** Sterecyt†.

Procarbazine Hydrochloride (1860-x)

Procarbazine Hydrochloride *(BANM, USAN, rINNM).*

Ibenzmethyzin Hydrochloride; NSC-77213; Ro-4-6467/1. *N*-Isopropyl-α-(2-methylhydrazino)-*p*-toluamide hydrochloride.

$C_{12}H_{19}N_3O,HCl$ = 257.8.

CAS — 671-16-9 (procarbazine); 366-70-1 (procarbazine hydrochloride).

Pharmacopoeias. In *Chin., Int., Jpn,* and *US.*

Procarbazine hydrochloride 116 mg is approximately equivalent to 100 mg of procarbazine. **Store** in airtight containers. Protect from light.

Adverse Effects, Treatment, and Precautions

For general discussions see Antineoplastics, p.470, p.473, and p.474.

The most common adverse effects associated with procarbazine are gastro-intestinal disturbances such as nausea and vomiting (although patients may soon become tolerant), and bone-marrow depression. Leucopenia and thrombocytopenia may be delayed with a nadir at about 4 weeks after a dose, and recovery usually within 6 weeks. Anaemia, haemolysis, and bleeding tendencies have been reported.

Neurotoxicity is also common, with central effects such as somnolence, depression, nervousness or confusion, headache, hallucinations, and dizziness, and peripheral neuropathies including paraesthesias and decreased reflexes. Lethargy, ataxia, and sleep disorders have also occurred, and tremors, convulsions, and coma have been reported.

Other side-effects reported with procarbazine include fever and myalgia, pulmonary fibrosis or pneumonitis, haematuria, urinary frequency, skin reactions including dermatitis, pruritus, and hyperpigmentation, tachycardia, orthostatic hypotension, ocular defects, infertility, and impaired liver function.

Procarbazine is a carcinogen, mutagen, and teratogen.

Procarbazine should be used with caution in patients with impaired liver or kidney function, and is contra-indicated if impairment is severe. Care is also advisable in patients with phaeochromocytoma, epilepsy, or cardiovascular or cerebrovascular disease.

Handling and disposal. Urine produced for up to 48 hours after a dose of procarbazine should be handled wearing protective clothing.[1]

1. Harris J, Dodds LJ. Handling waste from patients receiving cytotoxic drugs. *Pharm J* 1985; **235:** 289–91.

Interactions

Procarbazine is a weak MAOI and the possibility of reactions with other drugs and food, although very rare, must be borne in mind—for details of such reactions see p.304. Procarbazine may enhance the sedative effects of other CNS depressants. A disulfiram-like reaction has been reported with alcohol and the effects of antihypertensive agents may be enhanced.

Antiepileptics. Concomitant use of enzyme-inducing antiepileptics is associated with an increased risk of hypersensitivity reactions to procarbazine, possibly through a reactive intermediate generated by CYP3A isoform induction.[1] Non-enzyme-inducing antiepileptics might be more appropriate in patients with brain tumours in whom procarbazine therapy is anticipated.

1. Lehmann DF, *et al.* Anticonvulsant usage is associated with an increased risk of procarbazine hypersensitivity reactions in patients with brain tumors. *Clin Pharmacol Ther* 1997; **62:** 225–9.

Pharmacokinetics

Procarbazine is readily absorbed from the gastro-intestinal tract. It crosses the blood-brain barrier and diffuses into the cerebrospinal fluid. A plasma half-life of about 10 minutes has been reported. Procarbazine is rapidly metabolised (mainly in liver and kidneys) and only about 5% is excreted unchanged in the urine. The remainder is oxidised to *N*-isopropylterephthalamic acid and excreted in the urine, up to about 70% of a dose being excreted in 24 hours. Some of the drug is excreted as carbon dioxide and methane via the lungs. During oxidative breakdown in the body hydrogen peroxide is formed which may account for some of the drug's actions.

Uses and Administration

Procarbazine hydrochloride is an antineoplastic which appears to inhibit protein and nucleic acid synthesis and suppress mitosis. It is unrelated to the other antineoplastics and it may be effective when other drugs have become ineffective.

Its main use is the treatment of Hodgkin's disease when it is usually given in association with other drugs such as mustine, vincristine, and prednisone (the MOPP regimen). Procarbazine has also been used in the treatment of other lymphomas (including mycosis fungoides) and in some other malignant neoplasms including tumours of the brain. Management of these conditions is discussed further in the introduction to this chapter as indicated by the cross-references given below.

Doses of procarbazine hydrochloride are calculated in terms of procarbazine. In many of the combination regimens it has been given to adults and children in doses of the equivalent of procarbazine 100 mg per m^2 body-surface on days 1 to 14 of each 4- or 6-week cycle. If used as a single agent a dose equivalent to 50 mg of procarbazine by mouth daily, increased by 50 mg daily to 250 to 300 mg daily in divided doses has been suggested in the UK, while in the USA the recommended regimen is 2 to 4 mg per kg body-weight daily for the first week, subsequently increased to 4 to 6 mg per kg, doses being given to the nearest 50 mg. These doses are continued until maximum response is achieved or leucopenia, thrombocytopenia, or other signs of toxicity ensue. Maintenance doses are usually 50 to 150 mg, or 1 to 2 mg per kg, daily, until a cumulative dose of at least 6 g has been given. In children, initial daily doses of the equivalent of 50 mg per m^2 have been suggested (some sources simply suggest a dose of 50 mg), increased to 100 mg per m^2 and then adjusted according to response.

The haematological status of the patient should be determined at least every 3 or 4 days and hepatic and renal function determined weekly.

Blood disorders, non-malignant. Combination chemotherapy with regimens including procarbazine has been employed in a few patients with refractory idiopathic thrombocytopenic purpura (p.1023), and has produced prolonged remission although in most cases of the disease such aggressive therapy is difficult to justify.

Malignant neoplasms. Procarbazine is a component of the MOPP regimen which was the first combination regimen to be widely and successfully employed to treat Hodgkin's disease (see p.481). Procarbazine has also been used in the treatment of mycosis fungoides, other non-Hodgkin's lymphomas, and tumours of the brain, as discussed under Choice of Antineoplastic, p.482, p.482, and p.485.

Preparations

USP 23: Procarbazine Hydrochloride Capsules.

Proprietary Preparations (details are given in Part 3)
Aust.: Natulan; ***Austral.:*** Natulan; ***Belg.:*** Natulan; ***Canad.:*** Natulan; ***Fr.:*** Natulan; ***Ger.:*** Natulan; ***Ital.:*** Natulan; ***Neth.:*** Natulan; ***Norw.:*** Natulan; ***S.Afr.:*** Natulan; ***Spain:*** Natulan; ***Swed.:*** Natulan†; ***Switz.:*** Natulan; ***UK:*** Natulan; ***USA:*** Matulane.

Raltitrexed (11782-z)

Raltitrexed *(BAN, USAN, rINN)*.

ICI-D1694; ZD-1694. *N*-{5-[3,4-Dihydro-2-methyl-4-oxoquinazolin-6-ylmethyl(methyl)amino]-2-thenoyl}-L-glutamic acid.

$C_{21}H_{22}N_4O_6S = 458.5$.

CAS — 112887-68-0.

Adverse Effects, Treatment, and Precautions

Raltitrexed produces bone marrow depression, usually mild to moderate, with leucopenia, anaemia, and, less frequently, thrombocytopenia. The nadir of the white cell count usually occurs 7 to 14 days after a dose, with recovery by the third week. Gastro-intestinal toxicity is also common, with nausea and vomiting, diarrhoea, and anorexia: mucositis may occur. Reversible increases in liver enzyme values have occurred. Other adverse effects include weakness and malaise, fever, pain, headache, skin rashes, arthralgia, muscle cramps, weight loss, peripheral oedema, alopecia, and conjunctivitis. The use of folinic acid 25 mg per m^2 every 6 hours intravenously has been suggested in patients who develop very severe toxicity.

Raltitrexed should be given with care to patients with impaired hepatic function and should be avoided if impairment is severe. It should also be avoided in severe renal impairment and be given in reduced doses in moderate impairment of renal function. Care is also advisable in debilitated or elderly patients.

Raltitrexed is teratogenic; pregnancy should be avoided if either partner is receiving the drug. It may impair male fertility.

Interactions

Raltitrexed should not be given with folic or folinic acid which may impair its cytotoxic action. (For the deliberate use of folinic acid to counteract the effects of raltitrexed in patients with severe toxicity see above.)

Pharmacokinetics

Following intravenous administration raltitrexed exhibits triphasic pharmacokinetics, with an initial rapid decline from peak plasma concentrations followed by a slow terminal elimination phase. Raltitrexed is actively transported into cells and metabolised to active polyglutamate forms. The remainder of a dose is excreted unchanged, about 50% of a dose appearing in the urine, and about 15% in the faeces. The terminal elimination half-life is stated to be about 8 days. Clearance is markedly reduced in renal impairment.

Uses and Administration

Raltitrexed is a folate analogue that is a potent and specific inhibitor of the enzyme thymidylate synthase, which is involved in the synthesis of DNA. It is used in the treatment of advanced colorectal cancer and has also been tried in breast cancer.

The recommended initial dose is 3 mg of raltitrexed per m^2 body-surface, given by intravenous infusion over 15 minutes. Subsequent doses, which should be reduced by up to 50% depending on the severity of initial toxicity, may be given at intervals of 3 weeks provided toxicity has resolved. Doses should be reduced by 50% and repeated at 4-week intervals in patients with creatinine clearance less than 65 mL per minute; the drug should not be given if creatinine clearance is below 25 mL per minute.

A full blood count should be performed before each dose and treatment withheld if the white cell count is below 4000 per mm^3 or the platelet count less than 100 000 per mm^3. Hepatic and renal function should also be tested.

References.[1-6] Although clearly active[1-3] against colorectal cancer (p.487) raltitrexed does not seem to provide much improvement in survival-time for patients with metastatic disease.[4,5] However, it may well improve quality of life for these patients, since it is associated with less gastro-intestinal and haematological toxicity than some conventional fluorouracil regimens,[2] and is more convenient to administer.[4] Raltitrexed is also active against some other malignancies, notably of the breast[3] (p.485).

1. Jackman AL, *et al.* ZD1694 (Tomudex): a new thymidylate synthase inhibitor with activity in colorectal cancer. *Eur J Cancer* 1995; **31A:** 1277–82.
2. Cunningham D, *et al.* Tomudex (ZD 1694): results of a randomised trial in advanced colorectal cancer demonstrate efficacy and reduced mucositis and leucopenia. *Eur J Cancer* 1995; **31A:** 1945–54.
3. Cunningham D, *et al.* Tomudex (ZD1694) a novel thymidylate synthase inhibitor with clinical antitumour activity in a range of solid tumours. *Ann Oncol* 1996; **7:** 179–82.
4. Mead GM. Raltitrexed, a new drug for advanced colorectal cancer. *Lancet* 1996; **347:** 1568–9.
5. Anonymous. Raltitrexed in colorectal cancer. *Drug Ther Bull* 1996; **34:** 78–80.
6. Gunasekara NS, Faulds D. Raltitrexed: a review of its pharmacological properties and clinical efficacy in the management of advanced colorectal cancer. *Drugs* 1998; **55:** 423–35.

Preparations

Proprietary Preparations (details are given in Part 3)
Austral.: Tomudex; ***Fr.:*** Tomudex; ***Irl.:*** Tomudex; ***Ital.:*** Tomudex; ***Neth.:*** Tomudex; ***UK:*** Tomudex.

Ranimustine (3170-w)

Ranimustine *(rINN)*.

MCNU; NSC-0270516; Ranomustine. Methyl 6-[3-(2-chloroethyl)-3-nitrosoureido]-6-deoxy-α-D-glucopyranoside.

$C_{10}H_{18}ClN_3O_7 = 327.7$.

CAS — 58994-96-0.

Ranimustine is a nitrosourea derivative with general properties similar to those of carmustine (see p.511). It is used intravenously in the treatment of malignant neoplasms in usual doses of 50 to 90 mg per m^2 body-surface every 6 to 8 weeks according to haematological response.

Preparations

Proprietary Preparations (details are given in Part 3)
Jpn: Cymerin.

Razoxane (1861-r)

Razoxane *(BAN, rINN)*.

ICI-59118; ICRF-159; NSC-129943. (±)-4,4′-Propylenebis(piperazine-2,6-dione).

$C_{11}H_{16}N_4O_4 = 268.3$.

CAS — 21416-87-5.

Razoxane is an antineoplastic with inhibitory activity during the pre-mitotic and early mitotic phases of cell growth (G_2-M). It enhances the effects of radiotherapy. It has been used in association with radiotherapy in the treatment of sarcomas, including Kaposi's sarcoma. Razoxane has also been tried in other malignant diseases including acute leukaemias and non-Hodgkin's lymphomas. However, it is no longer widely employed. Razoxane was formerly used in psoriasis, but its carcinogenic properties militate against such use, as discussed below.

In the treatment of sarcomas it has generally been given by mouth in doses of 125 mg twice daily; higher doses have been given in the management of acute leukaemias and Kaposi's sarcoma. The peripheral blood count should be monitored during treatment.

The principal adverse effects of razoxane include bone-marrow depression, gastro-intestinal disturbances, skin reactions, and alopecia. It may enhance the adverse effects of radiotherapy. Razoxane therapy has been associated with the development of secondary malignancies: it is contra-indicated in the treatment of non-malignant conditions.

Cardiotoxicity. Dexrazoxane (p.978), the (+)-enantiomorph of razoxane, is reportedly effective in preventing doxorubicin-induced cardiotoxicity when given concomitantly.[1,2] It has been suggested that the beneficial effect may derive from chelation of body iron by dexrazoxane and minimising the formation of reactive hydroxyl radicals.[3]

1. Speyer JL, *et al.* Protective effect of the bispiperazinedione ICRF-187 against doxorubicin-induced cardiotoxicity in women with advanced breast cancer. *N Engl J Med* 1988; **319:** 745–52.
2. Kolaric K, *et al.* A phase II trial of cardioprotection with Cardioxane (ICRF-187) in patients with advanced breast cancer receiving 5-fluorouracil, doxorubicin and cyclophosphamide. *Oncology* 1995; **52:** 251–5.
3. Seifert CF, *et al.* Dexrazoxane in the prevention of doxorubicin-induced cardiotoxicity. *Ann Pharmacother* 1994; **28:** 1063–72.

Malignant neoplasms. Razoxane in association with radiotherapy produced partial response in 12 of 25 patients with liver metastases from gastro-intestinal or lung cancers;[1] 4 further patients had minor responses (less than 50% reduction in hepatic tumour load) and 2 had disease progression. Therapy consisted of razoxane 125 mg three times daily and then 125 mg daily for 1 month with radiotherapy on days 4 to 8. It was considered unlikely that such results could have been achieved with this dose of radiotherapy (4 Gray daily) or razoxane if either was given alone, but it remained to be seen whether responses would translate into improved long-term survival. Quality of life was excellent in most patients although 2 showed evidence of radiation hepatitis.

1. Hellmann K, *et al.* Responses of liver metastases to radiotherapy and razoxane. *J R Soc Med* 1992; **85:** 136–8.

Skin disorders, non-malignant. Razoxane was formerly used in the systemic treatment of psoriasis, and has been found to be extremely effective, with an initial response rate of 97% overall. It was found to be of use in all forms of cutaneous psoriasis and psoriatic arthropathy.[1] However, the development of acute myeloid leukaemias and other malignancies in patients given razoxane[2-5] has led to its being contra-indicated in non-malignant conditions.

For a discussion of psoriasis and its management, see p.1075.

1. Horton JJ, Wells RS. Razoxane: a review of 6 years' therapy in psoriasis. *Br J Dermatol* 1983; **109:** 669–73.
2. Horton JJ, *et al.* Epitheliomas in patients receiving razoxane therapy for psoriasis. *Br J Dermatol* 1983; **109:** 675–8.
3. Lakhani S, *et al.* Razoxane and leukaemia. *Lancet* 1984; **ii:** 288–9.
4. Caffrey EA, *et al.* Acute myeloid leukaemia after treatment with razoxane. *Br J Dermatol* 1985; **113:** 131–4.
5. Zuiable AG, *et al.* Razoxane and T-cell lymphoma. *Br J Dermatol* 1989; **121:** 149.

Preparations

Proprietary Preparations (details are given in Part 3)
UK: Razoxin.

9-*cis*-Retinoic Acid (15789-p)

Alitretinoin.

9-*cis*-Retinoic acid is a retinoid related to tretinoin (p.1093) that is under investigation by mouth in acute promyelocytic leukaemia and some other malignancies, and topically, as a 0.1% gel, in the management of Kaposi's sarcoma and other cutaneous neoplasms.

References.

1. Miller WH, *et al.* 9-cis Retinoic acid induces complete remission but does not reverse clinically acquired retinoid resistance in acute promyelocytic leukemia. *Blood* 1995; **85:** 3021–7.
2. Weber C, Dumont E. Pharmacokinetics and pharmacodynamics of 9-cis-retinoic acid in healthy men. *J Clin Pharmacol* 1997; **37:** 566–74.

Rituximab (17534-n)

Rituximab *(BAN, USAN, rINN)*.

IDEC-102; IDEC-C2B8.

CAS — 174722-31-7.

Rituximab is a chimeric monoclonal antibody to CD20 antigen used in the treatment of non-Hodgkin's lymphoma (p.482). Recommended doses are 375 mg per m^2 body-surface by intravenous infusion once weekly, for 4 doses. The first infusion is given initially at a rate of 50 mg per hour; subsequently this may be increased in increments of 50 mg per hour every 30 minutes to a maximum of 400 mg per hour, if well tolerated. Subsequent doses may be begun at a rate of 100 mg per hour, and incremented to a maximum of 400 mg per hour. Combination with chemotherapy and radiolabelled forms of rituximab have also been investigated.

Infusion of rituximab has been associated with a cytokine release syndrome of fever and rigors, usually within 2 hours of beginning therapy. Other reported symptoms include pruritus and rashes, dyspnoea, bronchospasm, angioedema, transient hypotension, and flushing. Severe cases may be associated with tumour lysis syndrome, respiratory failure, and death. Thrombocytopenia, neutropenia, and anaemia have occurred in a few patients, as have exacerbation of angina pectoris and heart failure. Patients with an extensive tumour burden, pulmonary tumour infiltration, or pulmonary insufficiency may be at increased risk of severe reactions and should be treated with caution and possibly a decreased initial infusion rate. Therapy should be interrupted in patients who develop severe symptoms and only resumed, at half the previous rate, once all signs and symptoms have resolved. Premedication with analgesics, antihistamines, and possibly corticosteroids is recommended in all patients before receiving rituximab.

References.

1. Maloney DG, *et al.* IDEC-C2B8 (rituximab) anti-CD20 monoclonal antibody therapy in patients with relapsed low-grade non-Hodgkin's lymphoma. *Blood* 1997; **90:** 2188–95.
2. McLaughlin P, *et al.* Rituximab chimeric anti-CD20 monoclonal antibody therapy for relapsed indolent lymphoma: half of patients respond to a four-dose treatment program. *J Clin Oncol* 1998; **16:** 2825–33.

Preparations

Proprietary Preparations (details are given in Part 3)
UK: Mabthera; ***USA:*** Rituxan.

Rogletimide (15076-r)

Rogletimide *(BAN, USAN, rINN).*

Pyridoglutethimide. (±)-2-Ethyl-2-(4-pyridyl)glutarimide.

$C_{12}H_{14}N_2O_2$ = 218.3.

CAS — 121840-95-7.

Rogletimide is an inhibitor of the aromatase (oestrogen synthetase) system. It has been investigated in the treatment of breast and prostate cancer.

Roquinimex (2828-v)

Roquinimex *(USAN, rINN).*

FCF-89; LS-2616. 1,2-Dihydro-4-hydroxy-*N*,1-dimethyl-2-oxo-3-quinolinecarboxanilide.

$C_{18}H_{16}N_2O_3$ = 308.3.

CAS — 84088-42-6.

Roquinimex is an immunomodulator which is reported to stimulate various immune functions including macrophage cytotoxicity. It has been investigated for its potential against various malignant neoplasms including as adjuvant therapy following bone marrow transplantation in acute leukaemia, to prolong the time to relapse. Roquinimex has also been investigated in a variety of autoimmune diseases or diseases characterised by immune abnormalities, including multiple sclerosis, rheumatoid arthritis, and AIDS.

Promising early results (in terms of halting clinical progression and reducing lesion development) have been seen in patients with *multiple sclerosis* (p.620) treated with roquinimex 2.5 mg daily by mouth.[1,2] Adverse effects reported with roquinimex include myalgia and arthralgia, gastro-intestinal disturbances, and pleuropericarditis. More recently, studies have been halted because of a possible association with myocardial infarction.

1. Karussis DM, *et al.* Treatment of secondary progressive multiple sclerosis with the immunomodulator linomide: a double-blind, placebo-controlled pilot study with monthly magnetic resonance imaging evaluation. *Neurology* 1996; **47:** 341–6.
2. Andersen O, *et al.* Linomide reduces the rate of active lesions in relapsing-remitting multiple sclerosis. *Neurology* 1996; **47:** 895–900.

Sebriplatin (17110-d)

Sebriplatin *(rINN).*

CI-973; NK-121. (+)-*cis*-(1,1-Cyclobutanedicarboxylato)[(2*R*)-2-methyl-1,4-butanediamine-*N*,*N'*]platinum.

$C_{11}H_{20}N_2O_4Pt$ = 439.4.

CAS — 110172-45-7.

Sebriplatin is an analogue of cisplatin (p.513) with generally similar properties. It has been investigated in a variety of solid neoplasms and in the treatment of acute leukaemias.

References.

1. Weiss RB, Christian MC. New cisplatin analogues in development: a review. *Drugs* 1993; **46:** 360–77.
2. Kantarjian HM, *et al.* Evaluation of CI-973, a platinum analogue, in refractory or relapsed acute leukemia. *Leukemia* 1996; **10:** 396–401.
3. Theriault RL, *et al.* A phase II study of CI-973 [SP-4-3(R)-1,1-cyclobutane-dicarboxylato (2-)] (2-methyl-1,4-butanediamine-N,N') platinum in patients with refractory advanced breast cancer. *Cancer Chemother Pharmacol* 1996; **38:** 289–91.

Semustine (1863-d)

Semustine *(USAN, rINN).*

Methyl Lomustine; Methyl-CCNU; NSC-95441; WR-220076. 1-(2-Chloroethyl)-3-(4-methylcyclohexyl)-1-nitrosourea.

$C_{10}H_{18}ClN_3O_2$ = 247.7.

CAS — 13909-09-6.

Adverse Effects, Treatment, and Precautions

As for Carmustine, p.512.

Nephrotoxicity has been reported in patients receiving high cumulative doses of semustine. Harmon and others reported severe renal damage in 6 of 17 children given semustine after radiotherapy for brain tumours; all 6 children had received a total dose above 1.5 g per m^2 body-surface area in contrast to those not so affected, who had received lower doses.[1] A decrease in kidney size was seen in 2 patients who had received lower cumulative doses. There had been no evidence during treatment that patients were losing renal function. Similarly Micetich and others reported an increased risk of renal abnormalities in patients given a cumulative dose of 1.4 g per m^2 or more.[2] Some 25% of patients given higher doses were so affected, while those given lower doses were not. Overall, however, the problem may not be particularly frequent: Nichols and Moertel considered that only 4 of 857 patients treated with semustine over 6 years might have had delayed renal insufficiency possibly related to semustine.[3]

1. Harmon WE, *et al.* Chronic renal failure in children treated with methyl-CCNU. *N Engl J Med* 1979; **300:** 1200–3.
2. Micetich KC, *et al.* Nephrotoxicity of semustine (methyl-CCNU) in patients with malignant melanoma receiving adjuvant chemotherapy. *Am J Med* 1981; **71:** 967–72.
3. Nichols WC, Moertel CG. Nephrotoxicity of methyl-CCNU. *N Engl J Med* 1979; **301:** 1181.

Pharmacokinetics

Semustine is well absorbed from the gastro-intestinal tract following oral doses, and is rapidly metabolised. The metabolites are reported to possess prolonged plasma half-lives, and cross the blood-brain barrier into the cerebrospinal fluid. It is excreted in urine as metabolites: up to 60% of a dose is excreted in this way within 48 hours. Small amounts may be excreted in faeces and via the lungs as carbon dioxide.

Uses and Administration

Semustine is a nitrosourea with actions and uses similar to those of carmustine (p.512) and lomustine (p.544). It has been given by mouth in single doses of 125 to 200 mg per m^2 body-surface, repeated every 6 weeks if blood counts recover adequately.

Malignant neoplasms. For reference to the use of semustine in melanoma, see p.492.

Sirolimus (8273-e)

Sirolimus *(BAN, USAN, rINN).*

AY-22989; AY-022989; Rapamycin; WY-090217. (3*S*,6*R*,7*E*,9*R*,10*R*,12*R*,14*S*,15*E*,17*E*,19*E*,21*S*,23*S*,26*R*,27*R*,34a*S*)-9,10,12,13,14,21,22,23,24,25,26,27,32,33,34,34a-Hexadecahydro-9,27-dihydroxy-3-{(1*R*)-2-[(1*S*,3*R*,4*R*)-4-hydroxy-3-methoxycyclohexyl]-1-methylethyl}-10,21-dimethoxy-6,8,12,14,20,26-hexamethyl-23,27-epoxy-3*H*-pyrido[2,1-c][1,4]oxaazacyclohentriacontine-1,5,11,28,29(4*H*,6*H*,31*H*)-pentone.

$C_{51}H_{79}NO_{13}$ = 914.2.

CAS — 53123-88-9.

Sirolimus is a macrolide compound obtained from *Streptomyces hygroscopicus* with potent immunosuppressant properties. It is being studied for the prevention of graft rejection in organ transplantation, and for induction of remission in some auto-immune diseases. Sirolimus is also under investigation in combination with cyclosporin.

Sirolimus has been shown to possess antifungal and antineoplastic properties. It is under investigation for gene regulation in gene therapy.

References.

1. Kahan B. Sirolimus: a new agent for clinical renal transplantation. *Transplant Proc* 1997; **29:** 48–50.
2. Ferron GM, *et al.* Population pharmacokinetics of sirolimus in kidney transplant patients. *Clin Pharmacol Ther* 1997; **61:** 416–28.

Interactions. Trough concentrations of sirolimus, and area under the concentration-time curve (AUC) were significantly higher when sirolimus and cyclosporin were administered concomitantly than when the 2 drugs were given 4 hours apart.[1]

1. Kaplan B, *et al.* The effects of relative timing of sirolimus and cyclosporine microemulsion formulation coadministration on the pharmacokinetics of each agent. *Clin Pharmacol Ther* 1998; **63:** 48–53.

Sizofiran (1796-v)

Sizofiran *(rINN).*

Schizophyllan. Poly[3→-(*O*-β-D-glucopyranosyl-(1→3)-*O*-[β-D-glucopyranosyl-(1→6)]-*O*-β-D-glucopyranosyl-(1→3)-*O*-β-D-glucopyranosyl)→1].

$(C_{24}H_{40}O_{20})_n$.

CAS — 9050-67-3.

Sizofiran is a polysaccharide obtained from cultures of the basidiomycete fungus *Schizophyllum commune*. It is reported to have antineoplastic and immunomodulating activity and is given in conjunction with radiotherapy in malignant neoplasms of the cervix (p.487). It is given by intramuscular injection in usual doses of 40 mg weekly. It has also been tried with chemotherapy or radiotherapy in other malignant neoplasms. Hypersensitivity reactions, including anaphylactoid shock, may occur.

References.

1. Fujimoto S, *et al.* Clinical outcome of postoperative adjuvant immunochemotherapy with sizofiran for patients with resectable gastric cancer: a randomised controlled study. *Eur J Cancer* 1991; **27:** 1114–18.
2. Shimizu Y, *et al.* Augmenting effect of sizofiran on the immunofunction of regional lymph nodes in cervical cancer. *Cancer* 1992; **69:** 1188–94.

Preparations

Proprietary Preparations (details are given in Part 3)
Jpn: Sonifilan.

Sobuzoxane (5512-s)

Sobuzoxane *(rINN).*

MST-16. 4,4'-Ethylenebis[1-(hydroxymethyl)-2,6-piperazinedione] bis(isobutyl carbonate).

$C_{22}H_{34}N_4O_{10}$ = 514.5.

CAS — 98631-95-9.

Sobuzoxane is an orally active inhibitor of topoisomerase II which is used for its antineoplastic properties in the treatment of non-Hodgkin's lymphomas and adult T-cell leukaemia/lymphoma. The usual dose is 1.6 g of sobuzoxane daily for five days, adjusted according to response. Courses may be repeated at intervals of 2 to 3 weeks. Adverse effects include myelosuppression, bleeding tendency, renal and hepatic dysfunction, gastro-intestinal disturbances, alopecia, headache, and fever.

Preparations

Proprietary Preparations (details are given in Part 3)
Jpn: Perazolin.

Sodium Bromebrate (13243-b)

Sodium Bromebrate *(BANM, rINNM).*

MBBA; NSC-104801; WR-149912. The sodium salt of (*E*)-3-*p*-anisoyl-3-bromoacrylic acid.

$C_{11}H_8BrNaO_4$ = 307.1.

CAS — 5711-40-0 (bromebric acid); 21739-91-3 (sodium bromebrate).

Sodium bromebrate is reported to possess antineoplastic properties and has been given in a usual initial dose of 200 mg daily by intramuscular or intravenous injection in various gynaecological neoplasms.

Sparfosic Acid (16995-f)

Sparfosic Acid *(rINN).*

PALA. *N*-Phosphonoacetyl-L-aspartic acid.

$C_6H_{10}NO_8P$ = 255.1.

CAS — 51321-79-0.

Sparfosate Sodium (12022-g)

Sparfosate Sodium *(USAN, rINNM).*

CI-882; NSC-224131; PALA Disodium. The disodium salt of sparfosic acid.

$C_6H_8NNa_2O_8P$ = 299.1.

CAS — 66569-27-5.

Adverse Effects and Precautions

Stomatitis, gastro-intestinal disturbances, and effects on the skin have occurred. Central neurotoxicity has been reported, with seizures and encephalopathy.

Care should be taken to avoid extravasation.

Transient hepatic abnormalities developed in 15 of 17 patients with a complete or partial response to combined therapy with sparfosic acid and fluorouracil,[1] comprising ascites (in 5), hyperbilirubinaemia (in 6), hypoalbuminaemia (in 12) and elevations of serum transaminase (in 7). Liver function abnormalities also developed in 12 of 27 patients who failed to respond to this regimen, but in most of these, changes were progressive. It is possible that some of these abnormalities could be related to the effects of the regimen on hepatic protein synthesis.

1. Kemeny N, *et al.* A new syndrome: ascites, hyperbilirubinemia, and hypoalbuminemia after biochemical modulation of fluorouracil with N-phosphonacetyl-L-aspartate (PALA). *Ann Intern Med* 1991; **115:** 946–51.

Uses and Administration

Sparfosic acid is an antineoplastic agent that prevents the first step of pyrimidine biosynthesis by inhibition of the enzyme aspartate transcarbamylase. When combined with fluorouracil this depletion of cellular pyrimidines results in increased incorporation of the latter into nucleic acid, and increased inhibition of protein synthesis.

It has been tried with limited success in the management of various solid tumours, but is more frequently used in combination with other agents such as fluorouracil. See also under Choice of Antineoplastic, p.487, for mention of its use in colorectal cancer.

For reference to the use of sparfosic acid to enhance the antineoplastic activity of fluorouracil, see p.536.

Streptozocin (1864-n)

Streptozocin *(USAN, rINN).*

NSC-85998; Streptozotocin; U-9889. 2-Deoxy-2-(3-methyl-3-nitrosoureido)-D-glucopyranose.

$C_8H_{15}N_3O_7$ = 265.2.

CAS — 18883-66-4.

The manufacturers recommend that it be **stored** at 2° to 8° and protected from light.

Adverse Effects, Treatment, and Precautions

For general discussions see Antineoplastics, p.470, p.473, and p.474.

Cumulative nephrotoxicity is common with streptozocin and may be severe. Fatal irreversible renal failure has been reported. Intra-arterial administration may be associated with increased risk of nephrotoxicity.

Other adverse effects include severe nausea and vomiting and alterations in liver function or occasionally severe hepatotoxicity. Myelosuppression may occur but is rarely severe. Streptozocin may affect glucose metabolism. A diabetogenic effect has been reported; hypoglycaemia attributed to the release of insulin from damaged cells has also occurred.

Streptozocin is irritant to tissues and extravasation may lead to local ulceration and necrosis.

Streptozocin should be used with extreme care in patients with pre-existing renal impairment.

Handling and disposal. Methods for the destruction of streptozocin waste by reaction with hydrobromic acid in glacial acetic acid or by oxidation with a solution of potassium permanganate in sulphuric acid.[1] Residues produced by either method were free of mutagenic activity.

1. Castegnaro M, *et al.*, eds. Laboratory decontamination and destruction of carcinogens in laboratory wastes: some antineoplastic agents. *IARC Scientific Publications 73.* Lyon: WHO/International Agency for Research on Cancer, 1985.

Interactions

Streptozocin should not be given in association with other potentially nephrotoxic drugs.

Phenytoin. A suggestion that, since phenytoin appeared to protect the beta cells of the pancreas from the cytotoxic effects of streptozocin, its concomitant use with streptozocin should be avoided in patients being treated for pancreatic tumours.[1]

1. Koranyi L, Gero L. Influence of diphenylhydantoin on the effect of streptozotocin. *Br Med J* 1979; **1:** 127.

Pharmacokinetics

Following intravenous administration streptozocin is rapidly cleared from the blood and distributed to body tissues, particularly the liver, kidneys, intestines, and pancreas. It is extensively metabolised, mainly in the liver and perhaps the kidney, and excreted principally in the urine as metabolites and a small amount of unchanged drug. Approximately 60 to 70% of an intravenous dose is excreted in urine within 24 hours. Some is also excreted via the lungs. Streptozocin itself does not cross the blood-brain barrier but its metabolites are found in the CSF.

Uses and Administration

Streptozocin is an antibiotic antineoplastic agent belonging to the nitrosoureas (see Carmustine, p.512) and is used, alone or in combination with other antineoplastic agents, mainly in the treatment of islet-cell tumours of the pancreas (p.477). It has been tried in other tumours including non-endocrine pancreatic cancer and prostate cancer (see p.491 and p.491). It has been given by intravenous injection or infusion in doses of 1 g per m^2 body-surface weekly, increased if necessary after 2 weeks to up to 1.5 g per m^2. Alternatively doses of 500 mg per m^2 may be given daily for 5 days and repeated every 4 to 6 weeks.

Streptozocin has also been given by intra-arterial infusion (but see Adverse Effects above).

Renal and hepatic function tests should be performed routinely during treatment; doses should be reduced or treatment withdrawn if renal toxicity occurs.

Preparations

Proprietary Preparations (details are given in Part 3)
Canad.: Zanosar; ***Fr.:*** Zanosar; ***Neth.:*** Zanosar†; ***USA:*** Zanosar.

Sulofenur (12231-z)

Sulofenur *(BAN, USAN, rINN).*

LY-186641. 1-(4-Chlorophenyl)-3-(indan-5-ylsulphonyl)urea.

$C_{16}H_{15}ClN_2O_3S$ = 350.8.

CAS — 110311-27-8.

Sulofenur is a sulphonylurea derivative which has been investigated for its antineoplastic properties. Methaemoglobinaemia and haemolytic anaemia may be dose-limiting.

References.

1. Hainsworth JD, *et al.* Phase I clinical study of N-[(4-chlorophenyl)amino]carbonyl-2,3-dihydro-1H-indene-5-sulfonamide (LY186641). *Cancer Res* 1989; **49:** 5217–20.
2. Mahjoubi M, *et al.* Phase II trial of LY 186641 in advanced renal cancer. *Invest New Drugs* 1993; **11:** 323–8.
3. Pratt CB, *et al.* A phase I study of sulofenur in refractory pediatric malignant solid tumors. *Invest New Drugs* 1995; **13:** 63–6.
4. Krarup-Hansen A, *et al.* Early clinical investigation of sulofenur with a daily schedule in advanced solid tumours. *Invest New Drugs* 1997; **15:** 147–51.

Tacrolimus (4992-w)

Tacrolimus *(BAN, USAN, rINN).*

FK-506; FR-900506.

(−)-(3*S*,4*R*,5*S*,8*R*,9*E*,12*S*,14*S*,15*R*,16*S*,18*R*,19*R*,26a*S*)-8-Allyl-5,6,8,11,12,13,14,15,16,17,18,19,24,25,26,26a-hexadecahydro-5,19-dihydroxy-3-{(*E*)-2-[(1*R*,3*R*,4*R*)-4-hydroxy-3-methoxycyclohexyl]-1-methylvinyl}-14,16,-dimethoxy-4,10,12,18-tetramethyl-15,19-epoxy-3*H*-pyrido[2,1-c][1,4]oxaazacyclotricosine-1,7,20,21(4*H*,23*H*)-tetrone monohydrate.

$C_{44}H_{69}NO_{12},H_2O$ = 822.0.

CAS — 104987-11-3 (anhydrous tacrolimus); 109581-93-3 (tacrolimus monohydrate).

Adverse Effects and Precautions

Tacrolimus may produce nephrotoxicity and neurotoxicity. The most common adverse effects include tremor, headache, paraesthesias, nausea and diarrhoea, hypertension, and impaired renal function. Other adverse effects include disturbances of serum electrolytes, notably hyperkalaemia; mood changes, sleep disturbances, confusion, dizziness, tinnitus, visual disturbances, and convulsions; disturbances of carbohydrate metabolism or frank diabetes mellitus; ECG changes and tachycardia, as well as hypertrophic cardiomyopathy (particularly in children); constipation, dyspepsia, and gastro-intestinal haemorrhage; dyspnoea, asthma, pleural effusions; alopecia, hirsutism, skin rash and pruritus; and arthralgia or myalgia, spasm, leg cramps, peripheral oedema, liver dysfunction, and coagulation disorders.

Tacrolimus injection is formulated with polyethoxylated castor oil: anaphylactoid reactions have occurred, and appropriate means for their management should be available in patients given the injection. Use of tacrolimus should be avoided in patients hypersensitive to macrolides. Dosage reduction may be necessary in patients with hepatic impairment. Care is also required in patients with pre-existing renal impairment, and some sources consider that dosage reduction may prove advisable in such patients. Monitoring of blood concentrations of tacrolimus is recommended in all patients. Renal and hepatic function, blood pressure and haematological and cardiac function, as well as visual function should be monitored regularly. As with other immunosuppressants, patients receiving tacrolimus are at increased risk of infection. Tacrolimus may affect visual or neurological function, and patients so affected should not drive or operate dangerous machinery.

Effects on the blood. A report of severe anaemia due to selective depression of erythropoiesis in a patient given tacrolimus.[1] Anaemia resolved when tacrolimus was replaced with cyclosporin. More generalised bone marrow suppression has also been reported.[2]

1. Winkler M, *et al.* Anaemia associated with FK 506 immunosuppression. *Lancet* 1993; **341:** 1035–6.
2. de-la-Serna-Higuera C, *et al.* Tacrolimus-induced bone marrow suppression. *Lancet* 1997; **350:** 714–15.

Effects on carbohydrate metabolism. A retrospective study involving 52 patients given primary immunosuppression with tacrolimus and corticosteroids after liver transplantation found that 7 previously non-diabetic patients required temporary insulin therapy after transplantation.[1] Insulin requirements were not changed in 4 patients with pre-existing type 1 diabetes mellitus, although 3 patients with type 2 diabetes mellitus did experience a temporary need for insulin. The effects on blood glucose did not seem to depend on the dose of tacrolimus.

1. Tabasco-Minguillan J, *et al.* Insulin requirements after liver transplantation and FK-506 immunosuppression. *Transplantation* 1993; **56:** 862–7.

Effects on the cardiovascular system. Hypertrophic cardiomyopathy, and in some cases heart failure, has been described in paediatric patients receiving tacrolimus after organ grafting (small bowel or liver).[1] Symptoms largely resolved on discontinuation or dosage reduction. A similar case had been found *post mortem* in an adult,[2] and the UK Committee on Safety of Medicines was aware of 29 reported cases worldwide as of July 1995.[3] Echocardiographic monitoring of patients receiving tacrolimus has been recommended, with dose reduction or withdrawal in those who developed hypertrophic changes.[3] However, echocardiographic abnormalities may be quite common after orthotopic liver transplantation in adults, with no obvious relationship to the use of tacrolimus.[4]

1. Atkison P, *et al.* Hypertrophic cardiomyopathy associated with tacrolimus in paediatric transplant patients. *Lancet* 1995; **345:** 894–6.
2. Natazuka T, *et al.* Immunosuppressive drugs and hypertrophic cardiomyopathy. *Lancet* 1995; **345:** 1644.
3. Committee on Safety of Medicines/Medicines Control Agency. Tacrolimus (Prograf) and hypertrophic cardiomyopathy in transplant patients. *Current Problems* 1995; **21:** 6.
4. Dollinger MM, *et al.* Tacrolimus and cardiotoxicity in adult liver transplant recipients. *Lancet* 1995; **346:** 507.

Effects on the kidney. A comparison in patients who had undergone liver transplantation suggested that nephrotoxicity was somewhat more of a problem in those receiving tacrolimus than in those given a cyclosporin-based regimen.[1] In particular intravenous administration of tacrolimus during the first week after transplantation was associated with acute renal failure in 4 of 20 patients. Furthermore, on follow-up for 1 year, glomerular filtration rate was somewhat lower in the tacrolimus-treated group.

1. Porayko MK, *et al.* Nephrotoxic effects of primary immunosuppression with FK-506 and cyclosporine regimens after liver transplantation. *Mayo Clin Proc* 1994; **69:** 105–11.

Effects on the nervous system. Severe peripheral neuropathy together with signs of cerebral dysfunction has been reported in 2 patients receiving tacrolimus.[1] Among other central effects, tacrolimus has also been associated with speech disorders, including severe dysarthria and mutism in 1 patient;[2] some degree of speech dysfunction, in the form of an apparent Norwegian accent, appeared to be permanent in this case.

1. Ayres RCS, *et al.* Peripheral neurotoxicity with tacrolimus. *Lancet* 1994; **343:** 862–3.
2. Boeve BF, *et al.* Dysarthria and apraxia of speech associated with FK-506 (tacrolimus). *Mayo Clin Proc* 1996; **71:** 969–72.

Effects on skeletal muscle. Severe acute rhabdomyolysis, leading to fatal acute renal failure, developed in an 18-month-old child given tacrolimus after bone-marrow transplantation.[1]

1. Hibi S, *et al.* Severe rhabdomyolysis associated with tacrolimus. *Lancet* 1995; **346:** 702.

Interactions

Increased nephrotoxicity may result if tacrolimus is given with other potentially nephrotoxic drugs: concomitant use with cyclosporin should be avoided for this reason. Potassium-sparing diuretics should also be avoided in patients receiving tacrolimus.

Tacrolimus is metabolised by one of the forms of cytochrome P450 (CYP3A), and drugs which inhibit this enzyme system, such as azole antifungals, bromocriptine, calcium-channel blockers, cimetidine, some corticosteroids, cyclosporin, danazol, macrolide antibacterials, and metoclopramide, may produce increased blood concentrations of tacrolimus if given concomitantly. Equally, inducers of this enzyme system (such as carbamazepine, phenobarbitone, phenytoin, and rifampicin) may reduce blood concentrations of tacrolimus.

A study[1] *in vitro* found that metabolism of tacrolimus by CYP3A in human liver microsomes was inhibited by bromocriptine, corticosterone, dexamethasone, ergotamine, erythromycin, ethinyloestradiol, josamycin, ketoconazole, miconazole, midazolam, nifedipine, omeprazole, tamoxifen, triacetyloleandomycin, and verapamil. No effect on tacrolimus metabolism was seen with aspirin, amphotericin, captopril, cefotaxime, ciprofloxacin, diclofenac, diltiazem, doxycycline, frusemide, glibenclamide, imipramine, lignocaine, paracetamol, prednisolone, progesterone, ranitidine, sulphamethoxazole, trimethoprim, or vancomycin.

1. Christians U, *et al.* Identification of drugs inhibiting the in vitro metabolism of tacrolimus by human liver microsomes. *Br J Clin Pharmacol* 1996; **41:** 187–90.

Antibacterials. Increased concentrations of tacrolimus in plasma have been reported when *erythromycin* was given concomitantly;[1] the interaction was accompanied by some evidence of nephrotoxicity. A similar interaction has been reported between tacrolimus and *clarithromycin*.[2] For reference to the effects of macrolides on tacrolimus metabolism *in vitro* see above.

Marked reduction (below measurable values) in tacrolimus concentrations has been reported in a child who was given *rifampicin* concomitantly.[3]

1. Jensen C, *et al.* Interaction between tacrolimus and erythromycin. *Lancet* 1994; **344:** 825.
2. Wolter K, *et al.* Interaction between FK 506 and clarithromycin in a renal transplant patient. *Eur J Clin Pharmacol* 1994; **47:** 207–8.
3. Furlan V, *et al.* Interactions between FK506 and rifampicin or erythromycin in pediatric liver recipients. *Transplantation* 1995; **59:** 1217–18.

Antiepileptics. For the effect of tacrolimus on phenytoin, see Phenytoin, p.356.

Antifungals. Elevated plasma-tacrolimus concentrations have been reported in patients given *clotrimazole*[1] or *fluconazole*[2] concomitantly; a reduction in the dose of tacrolimus was likely to be necessary if it were given with an azole antifungal. A study involving tacrolimus and *ketoconazole* suggested that an increase in the oral bioavailability of tacrolimus from a mean of 14 to 30% when given with the azole was probably due to decreased CYP3A4 metabolism in the gut wall, or improved absorption due to inhibition of P-glycoprotein mediated efflux, rather than an effect on hepatic metabolism.[3]

1. Mieles L, *et al.* Interaction between FK506 and clotrimazole in a liver transplant recipient. *Transplantation* 1991; **52:** 1086–7.
2. Mañez R, *et al.* Fluconazole therapy in transplant recipients receiving FK506. *Transplantation* 1994; **57:** 1521–3.
3. Floren LC, *et al.* Tacrolimus oral bioavailability doubles with coadministration of ketoconazole. *Clin Pharmacol Ther* 1997; **62:** 41–9.

Calcium-channel blockers. Dosage requirements for tacrolimus were substantially reduced in 22 liver graft recipients who also received nifedipine, compared with 28 patients who did not, in a 1-year retrospective study.[1]

1. Seifeldin RA, *et al.* Nifedipine interaction with tacrolimus in liver transplant recipients. *Ann Pharmacother* 1997; **31:** 571–5.

Danazol. Nephrotoxicity and tremors associated with elevated concentrations of tacrolimus developed in a patient given danazol concomitantly with the immunosuppressant.[1] The effect might be due to inhibition of the metabolism of tacrolimus.

1. Shapiro R, *et al.* FK 506 interaction with danazol. *Lancet* 1993; **341:** 1344–5.

Pharmacokinetics

Absorption of tacrolimus following oral administration is reported to be erratic. Oral bioavailability varies very widely, although a bioavailability of about 15 to 20% seems common. Following intravenous administration it is widely distributed to the tissues; in the blood, about 80% is bound to erythrocytes, and variations in red-cell binding account for much of the variability in pharmacokinetics. Tacrolimus is extensively metabolised by the liver and excreted, primarily in bile, almost entirely as metabolites. Some metabolism may occur in the gastro-intestinal tract. Plasma elimination half-life has been reported to vary from about 3.5 to 40.5 hours.

References.

1. Venkataramanan R, *et al.* Pharmacokinetics of FK 506: preclinical and clinical studies. *Transplant Proc* 1990; **22** (suppl 1): 52–6.
2. Lee C, *et al.* Pharmacokinetics of tacrolimus (FK506) in liver transplant patients. *Clin Pharmacol Ther* 1993; **53:** 181.
3. Gruber SA, *et al.* Pharmacokinetics of FK506 after intravenous and oral administration in patients awaiting renal transplantation. *J Clin Pharmacol* 1994; **34:** 859–64.
4. Gonschior A-K, *et al.* Measurement of blood concentrations of FK506 (tacrolimus) and its metabolites in seven liver graft patients after the first dose by hplc-MS and microparticle enzyme immunoassay (MEIA). *Br J Clin Pharmacol* 1994; **38:** 567–71.
5. Jusko WJ, *et al.* Pharmacokinetics of tacrolimus in liver transplant patients. *Clin Pharmacol Ther* 1995; **57:** 281–90.
6. Venkataramanan R, *et al.* Clinical pharmacokinetics of tacrolimus. *Clin Pharmacokinet* 1995; **29:** 404–30.

Uses and Administration

Tacrolimus is a potent macrolide immunosuppressant derived from *Streptomyces tsukubaensis*, and has actions similar to those of cyclosporin (see p.523). It is used to prevent or reverse rejection in patients receiving organ transplants, as indicated by the cross-references given below, and has been tried in a few patients with refractory auto-immune or immune-mediated disorders. In the UK the suggested initial dose in liver graft recipients is 100 to 200 µg per kg body-weight daily by mouth, in 2 divided doses. The suggested initial oral dose in kidney transplant patients is 150 to 300 µg per kg daily in 2 divided doses. Administration should begin about 6 hours after completion of liver grafting and within 24 hours of a kidney transplant. If the patient's condition does not permit oral administration, therapy may be commenced intravenously, by continuous 24-hour infusion: suggested initial doses are 10 to 50 µg per kg daily for liver transplants and 50 to 100 µg per kg daily for kidney transplants. In the USA, initial oral doses in patients with liver grafts are 100 to 150 µg per kg daily, in 2 divided doses, and in kidney grafts 200 µg per kg daily, in 2 divided doses.

Dosage should be adjusted according to whole-blood or plasma trough concentrations in individual patients: it is suggested that most patients can be satisfactorily maintained at whole-blood concentrations below 20 ng per mL. Children generally require doses 1.5 to 2 times greater than those recommended in adults to achieve the same blood concentrations.

Reviews.

1. Macleod AM, Thomson AW. FK 506: an immunosuppressant for the 1990s? *Lancet* 1991; **337:** 25–7. Correction. *ibid.*; 928.
2. Peters DH, *et al.* Tacrolimus: a review of its pharmacology, and therapeutic potential in hepatic and renal transplantation. *Drugs* 1993; **46:** 746–94.
3. Anonymous. Tacrolimus (FK506) for organ transplants. *Med Lett Drugs Ther* 1994; **36:** 82–3.
4. Hooks MA. Tacrolimus, a new immunosuppressant—a review of the literature. *Ann Pharmacother* 1994; **28:** 501–11.
5. Winkler M, Christians U. A risk-benefit assessment of tacrolimus in transplantation. *Drug Safety* 1995; **12:** 348–57.
6. Kelly PA, *et al.* Tacrolimus: a new immunosuppressive agent. *Am J Health-Syst Pharm* 1995; **52:** 1521–35.
7. Spencer CM, *et al.* Tacrolimus: an update of its pharmacology and clinical efficacy in the management of organ transplantation. *Drugs* 1997; **54:** 925–75.

Experience with tacrolimus in applications other than transplantation is extremely limited; however, there are some reports of such use, including in focal glomerulosclerosis,[1] chronic active hepatitis,[2] atopic eczema,[3-5] psoriasis,[6] and pyoderma gangrenosum.[7,8] Topical formulations of tacrolimus are reported to be under development for skin disorders such as atopic eczema.

1. McCauley J, *et al.* FK 506 in steroid-resistant focal sclerosing glomerulonephritis of childhood. *Lancet* 1990; **335:** 674.
2. Van Thiel DH, *et al.* Tacrolimus: a potential new treatment for autoimmune chronic active hepatitis: results of an open-label preliminary trial. *Am J Gastroenterol* 1995; **90:** 771–6.
3. Nakagawa H, *et al.* Tacrolimus ointment for atopic dermatitis. *Lancet* 1994; **344:** 883.
4. Aoyama H, *et al.* Successful treatment of resistant facial lesions of atopic dermatitis with 0.1% FK506 ointment. *Br J Dermatol* 1995; **133:** 494–6.
5. Ruzicka T, *et al.* A short-term trial of tacrolimus ointment for atopic dermatitis. *N Engl J Med* 1997; **337:** 816–21.
6. European FK 506 Multicentre Psoriasis Study Group. Systemic tacrolimus (FK 506) is effective for the treatment of psoriasis in a double-blind, placebo-controlled study. *Arch Dermatol* 1996; **132:** 419–23.
7. Abu-Elmagd K, *et al.* Resolution of severe pyoderma gangrenosum in a patient with streaking leukocyte factor disease after treatment with tacrolimus (FK 506). *Ann Intern Med* 1993; **119:** 595–8.
8. Schuppe H-C, *et al.* Topical tacrolimus for pyoderma gangrenosum. *Lancet* 1998; **351:** 832.

Administration. The mean dose of tacrolimus required to produce a standard trough concentration of 10 to 15 ng per mL was reported to be 96% higher in 7 black renal graft recipients than in 20 such patients of white or Asian descent.[1]

1. Andrews PA, *et al.* Racial variation in dosage requirements of tacrolimus. *Lancet* 1996; **348:** 1446.

Organ and tissue transplantation. Tacrolimus has been used both for primary immunosuppression and for the control of graft rejection. Much of the initial experience with the drug was for liver grafts, (see p.500), but it is also employed in the transplantation of heart (p.499), kidney (p.499), lung (p.501), and other organs (p.501). It has also been tried for the prophylaxis of graft-versus-host disease following bone marrow transplantation (p.498).

A few selected references to the use of tacrolimus in transplantation are given below.

1. Starzl TE, *et al.* FK 506 for liver, kidney, and pancreas transplantation. *Lancet* 1989; **ii:** 1000–4.
2. Starzl TE, *et al.* Kidney transplantation under FK 506. *JAMA* 1990; **264:** 63–7.
3. Jordan ML, *et al.* FK506 "rescue" for resistant rejection of renal allografts under primary cyclosporine immunosuppression. *Transplantation* 1994; **57:** 860–5.
4. European FK506 Multicentre Liver Study Group. Randomised trial comparing tacrolimus (FK506) and cyclosporin in prevention of liver allograft rejection. *Lancet* 1994; **344:** 423–8.
5. The US Multicenter FK506 Liver Study Group. A comparison of tacrolimus (FK506) and cyclosporine for immunosuppression in liver transplantation. *N Engl J Med* 1994; **331:** 1110–15.
6. Woodle ES, *et al.* FK 506 rescue therapy for hepatic allograft rejection: experience with an aggressive approach. *Clin Transplant* 1995; **9:** 45–52.
7. Swenson JM, *et al.* Immunosuppression switch in pediatric heart transplant recipients: cyclosporine to FK 506. *J Am Coll Cardiol* 1995; **25:** 1183–8.

Preparations

Proprietary Preparations (details are given in Part 3)
Austral.: Prograf; ***Canad.:*** Prograf; ***Fr.:*** Prograf; ***Ger.:*** Prograf; ***Irl.:*** Prograf; ***Jpn:*** Prograf; ***Spain:*** Prograf; ***Swed.:*** Prograf; ***UK:*** Prograf; ***USA:*** Prograf.

Tamoxifen Citrate (1865-h)

Tamoxifen Citrate *(BANM, USAN, rINNM)*.

ICI-46474; Tamoxifeni Citras. (*Z*)-2-[4-(1,2-Diphenylbut-1-enyl)phenoxy]ethyldimethylamine citrate.

$C_{26}H_{29}NO,C_6H_8O_7$ = 563.6.

CAS — 10540-29-1 (tamoxifen); 54965-24-1 (tamoxifen citrate).

Pharmacopoeias. In *Eur.* (see p.viii), *Int.*, and *US.*

A white or almost white polymorphic crystalline powder. Slightly or very slightly **soluble** in water and acetone; soluble in methyl alcohol; very slightly soluble in alcohol and in chloroform. **Protect** from light.

Tamoxifen citrate 15.2 mg is approximately equivalent to 10 mg of tamoxifen.

Adverse Effects and Precautions

Tamoxifen is generally well-tolerated, and the most frequent adverse effects are hot flushes and nausea and vomiting in up to 25% of patients. Other adverse effects include oedema, vaginal bleeding or discharge, pruritus vulvae, rashes, and dry skin. There may be an increased tendency to thrombo-embolism, and pulmonary embolism has occurred; alterations in blood lipids have been reported. Tumour pain and flare may be a sign of response, but hypercalcaemia, sometimes severe, has developed in patients with bony metastases. There have also been reports of dizziness, headache, depression, confusion, fatigue, hepatotoxicity, and muscle cramps. Transient thrombocytopenia and leucopenia have been reported. Blurred vision and loss of visual acuity, corneal opacities, and retinopathies have occurred.

Tamoxifen should not be given during pregnancy and should be used with caution in women with functioning ovaries; the latter may also develop menstrual irregularities and cystic ovarian swelling.

Tamoxifen is a carcinogen and teratogen in *animals*; although it has been associated with endometrial hyperplasia and malignancy, there is some debate about its carcinogenicity in man (see below). Women who develop abnormal vaginal bleeding or discharge, menstrual irregularities, or pelvic pain should undergo appropriate investigations.

Carcinogenicity. Tamoxifen appears to have a stimulant effect on the endometrium (probably by acting as a partial oestrogen agonist) and its use has been associated with the development of endometrial polyps[1] and endometriosis,[2] and an increased risk of endometrial cancer.[3-5] The risk, which increases with duration of therapy, is generally agreed to be modest, and the clinical benefit in women with breast cancer outweighs any increased risk of endometrial neoplasm.[6-8] Whether regular endometrial screening is desirable or feasible remains a moot point, since hyperplasia is not necessarily the precursor of a malignancy.[7,8] It has been suggested that colour doppler ultrasonography, which distinguishes vascularised lesions, such as polyps and carcinomas, from avascular atrophic lesions may be a useful and noninvasive diagnostic tool.[9]

However, tamoxifen has also been associated with the formation of DNA adducts in *rodents*[10] and perhaps the development of liver cancer,[11] and a theoretical risk of ovarian neoplasm in premenopausal women given tamoxifen has been proposed.[12] Together with the effects on the endometrium, this has led to concern about the use of tamoxifen for the *prevention* of breast cancer in women considered at high risk of developing the disease. For further discussion of this topic see Prophylaxis, under Malignant Neoplasms of the Breast, p.486.

1. Corley D, *et al.* Postmenopausal bleeding from unusual endometrial polyps in women on chronic tamoxifen therapy. *Obstet Gynecol* 1992; **79:** 111–16.
2. Cano A, *et al.* Tamoxifen and the uterus and endometrium. *Lancet* 1989, **i:** 376.
3. Fornander T, *et al.* Adjuvant tamoxifen in early breast cancer: occurrence of new primary cancers. *Lancet* 1989; **i:** 117–20.
4. Gusberg SB. Tamoxifen for breast cancer: associated endometrial cancer. *Cancer* 1990; **65:** 1463–4.
5. van Leeuwen FE, *et al.* Risk of endometrial cancer after tamoxifen treatment of breast cancer. *Lancet* 1994; **343:** 448–52.
6. Baum M, *et al.* Endometrial cancer during tamoxifen treatment. *Lancet* 1994; **343:** 1291.
7. Bissett D, *et al.* Gynaecological monitoring during tamoxifen therapy. *Lancet* 1994; **344:** 1244.
8. Neven P, Vergote I. Should tamoxifen users be screened for endometrial lesions? *Lancet* 1998; **351:** 155–7.
9. Aleem FA, Predanic M. Endometrial changes in patients on tamoxifen. *Lancet* 1995; **346:** 1292–3.
10. Han X, Liehr JG. Induction of covalent DNA adducts in rodents by tamoxifen. *Cancer Res* 1992; **52:** 1360–3.
11. Nayfield SG, *et al.* Potential role of tamoxifen in prevention of breast cancer. *J Natl Cancer Inst* 1991; **83:** 1450–9.
12. Spicer DV, *et al.* Ovarian cancer and long-term tamoxifen in premenopausal women. *Lancet* 1991; **337:** 1414.

Effects on the blood. Pancytopenia developed shortly after beginning tamoxifen therapy in an elderly woman, and persisted for some years;[1] the patient eventually developed very severe leucopenia and died of infection.

1. Miké V, *et al.* Fatal neutropenia associated with long-term tamoxifen therapy. *Lancet* 1994; **344:** 541–2.

Effects on the eyes. Tamoxifen has been reported to be associated with decreased visual acuity, corneal opacities and cataract, and retinopathy. The latter is sometimes progressive although in most cases it has shown improvement once the drug was discontinued.[1] A prospective study in 63 patients receiving tamoxifen 20 mg daily found evidence of decreased visual acuity, macular oedema, and retinal opacities in 4, occurring after 10 to 35 months of therapy.[2] Studies *in vitro* have suggested that cataract formation may be due to inhibition of chloride channels in the lens by tamoxifen or its hydroxy metabolite.[3]

1. Mihm LM, Barton TL. Tamoxifen-induced ocular toxicity. *Ann Pharmacother* 1994; **28:** 740–2.
2. Pavlidis NA, *et al.* Clear evidence that long-term, low-dose tamoxifen treatment can induce ocular toxicity. *Cancer* 1992; **69:** 2961–4.
3. Zhang JJ, *et al.* Tamoxifen blocks chloride channels: a possible mechanism for cataract formation. *J Clin Invest* 1994; **94:** 1690–7.

Effects on the genito-urinary system. A report of persistent nocturnal priapism in a man receiving tamoxifen 20 mg daily.[1] Symptoms abated within 24 hours of withdrawing the drug. Impotence has been reported in men receiving tamoxifen therapy, and has been attributed to a paradoxical oestrogenic effect.[2]

1. Fernando IN, Tobias JS. Priapism in patient on tamoxifen. *Lancet* 1989; **i:** 436.
2. Collinson MP, *et al.* Two case reports of tamoxifen as a cause of impotence in male subjects with carcinoma of the breast. *Breast* 1993; **2:** 48–9.

Effects on the liver. Cholestasis and increased liver enzyme values have been reported following administration of tamoxifen to a 75-year-old patient.[1] Enzyme activity rose again on rechallenge with tamoxifen. Fatal hepatocellular necrosis and agranulocytosis, possibly exacerbated by continuing to take the drug once jaundice developed, has also been reported;[2] the authors noted that 4 cases of hepatic failure (3 fatal) and 5 cases of hepatitis (1 fatal) had been reported to the Committee on Safety of Medicines in the UK. Patients taking tamoxifen may also develop steatohepatitis,[3-5] indistinguishable from alcohol-induced liver disease.

For a report of peliosis hepatis and liver haemorrhage in a patient receiving tamoxifen and warfarin, see under Interactions, below.

For reference to the development of liver cancer in *animals* given tamoxifen, see Carcinogenicity, above.

1. Blackburn AM, *et al.* Tamoxifen and liver damage. *Br Med J* 1984; **289:** 288.
2. Ching CK, *et al.* Tamoxifen-associated hepatocellular damage and agranulocytosis. *Lancet* 1992; **339:** 940.
3. Pratt DS, *et al.* Tamoxifen-induced steatohepatitis. *Ann Intern Med* 1995; **123:** 236.
4. Van Hoof M, *et al.* Tamoxifen-induced steatohepatitis. *Ann Intern Med* 1996; **124:** 855–6.
5. Ogawa Y, *et al.* Tamoxifen-induced fatty liver in patients with breast cancer. *Lancet* 1998; **351:** 725.

Effects on the ovaries. Ovarian cysts are relatively common as an adverse effect in women receiving adjuvant tamoxifen: a study[1] in 95 such women reported the development of ovarian cysts in 6 of 16 (37.5%) who were premenopausal and in 5 of 79 postmenopausal women (6.3%). In 2 of the premenopausal women the cysts were complex. Two women underwent laparotomy for persistent cysts that were found to be benign, and 1 for leiomyoma; the cysts in the other 8 women resolved after withdrawal of tamoxifen.

1. Shushan A, *et al.* Ovarian cysts in premenopausal and postmenopausal tamoxifen-treated women with breast cancer. *Am J Obstet Gynecol* 1996; **174:** 141–4.

Effects on the skin and hair. A report of purpuric leucocytoclastic vasculitis in a patient receiving tamoxifen.[1] Withdrawal of the drug resulted in complete clearance of the lesions within 2 weeks; on re-introduction purpura developed again within a few days. The results suggest that tamoxifen can produce immune-mediated vascular damage.

Another report concerned a patient with white hair who developed darkening and repigmentation of the hair after about 2½ years of tamoxifen therapy.[2] Alopecia has also been reported in women receiving tamoxifen,[3,4] (possibly exacerbated by use of gonadorelin analogues), and in older patients the follicle may not recover.[3]

1. Drago F, *et al.* Tamoxifen and purpuric vasculitis. *Ann Intern Med* 1990; **112:** 965–6.
2. Hampson JP, *et al.* Tamoxifen-induced hair colour change. *Br J Dermatol* 1995; **132:** 483–4.
3. Gately CA, Bundred NJ. Alopecia and breast disease. *Br Med J* 1997; **314:** 481.
4. Ayoub J-PM, *et al.* Tamoxifen-induced female androgenetic alopecia in a patient with breast cancer. *Ann Intern Med* 1997; **126:** 745–6.

Pregnancy. Ambiguous genitalia have been reported in an infant exposed to tamoxifen *in utero*, although no causal link was demonstrated.[1]

1. Tewari K, *et al.* Ambiguous genitalia in infant exposed to tamoxifen in utero. *Lancet* 1997; **350:** 183.

Thrombo-embolism. A case control study,[1] involving 25 cases of deep vein thrombosis or pulmonary embolism among more than 10 000 women with breast cancer, suggested that current use of tamoxifen was associated with an estimated relative risk of developing idiopathic venous thrombo-embolism of 7.1 (95% confidence interval 1.5 to 33). Past use of tamoxifen was not associated with a materially increased risk.

1. Meier CR, Jick H. Tamoxifen and risk of idiopathic venous thromboembolism. *Br J Clin Pharmacol* 1998; **45:** 608–12.

Interactions

There is a risk of increased anticoagulant effect if tamoxifen is given concomitantly with coumarin anticoagulants. Conversely, concomitant use with cytotoxic drugs may increase the risk of thromboembolic events. Tamoxifen increases the dopaminergic effect of bromocriptine.

Allopurinol. For reference to exacerbation of hepatotoxicity when tamoxifen was given concurrently with allopurinol, see under Allopurinol, p.391.

Anticoagulants. A potentially life-threatening interaction between tamoxifen and *warfarin*, with marked prolongation of prothrombin times, haematuria, and haematoma, has been reported in a number of cases.[1-3] Peliosis hepatis and fatal liver haemorrhage have been reported in a patient who was receiving tamoxifen with warfarin and a thyroxine-liothyronine preparation.[4] It has been suggested that in addition to enhancement of the effects of warfarin, competition for the same metabolic enzyme systems might reduce the activity of tamoxifen against tumours,[2] but such a suggestion remains speculative.

1. Lodwick R, *et al.* Life threatening interaction between tamoxifen and warfarin. *Br Med J* 1987; **295:** 1141.
2. Tenni P, *et al.* Life threatening interaction between tamoxifen and warfarin. *Br Med J* 1989; **298:** 93.
3. Ritchie LD, Grant SMT. Tamoxifen-warfarin interaction: the Aberdeen hospitals drug file. *Br Med J* 1989; **298:** 1253.
4. Loomus GN, *et al.* A case of peliosis hepatis in association with tamoxifen therapy. *Am J Clin Pathol* 1983; **80:** 881–3.

Antineoplastics. For mention of an increased risk of haemolytic-uraemic syndrome in patients who received therapy with tamoxifen and mitomycin see Effects on the Kidneys, under Adverse Effects of Mitomycin, p.552.

Gonadorelin analogues. Combined treatment with triptorelin and tamoxifen in *mice* inoculated with a strain of murine mammary carcinoma resulted in enhancement of tumour growth;[1] neither compound alone had an effect on the tumour, which had become hormone independent. On the basis of these results caution is advised in the use of gonadorelin analogues in combination with tamoxifen in patients with oestrogen receptor-negative tumours.

For the suggestion that concomitant use of tamoxifen and a gonadorelin analogue may exacerbate alopecia, see Effects on the Skin and Hair, above.

1. Szende B, *et al.* Adverse effect of tamoxifen with LHRH agonist on oestrogen-receptor-negative mammary carcinoma. *Lancet* 1989; **ii:** 222–3.

Immunosuppressants. For the results of a study *in vitro* suggesting that tamoxifen might inhibit the metabolism of tacrolimus, see under Interactions of Tacrolimus, p.563.

Neuromuscular blockers. For reference to prolonged neuromuscular blockade in a patient given atracurium while receiving tamoxifen, see p.1306.

With radiotherapy. Reports of radiation recall, with erythema at the site of previous radiotherapy, in patients receiving tamoxifen.[1,2]

1. Parry BR. Radiation recall induced by tamoxifen. *Lancet* 1992; **340:** 49.
2. Extermann M, *et al.* Radiation recall in a patient with breast cancer treated for tuberculosis. *Eur J Clin Pharmacol* 1995; **48:** 77–8.

Pharmacokinetics

Peak plasma concentrations of tamoxifen occur 4 to 7 hours after an oral dose. It is extensively protein bound. Plasma clearance is reported to be biphasic and the terminal half-life may be longer than 7 days. It is extensively metabolised, the major serum metabolite being *N*-desmethyltamoxifen. Several of the metabolites are stated to have similar pharmacological activity to the parent compound. Tamoxifen is excreted slowly in the faeces, mainly as conjugates. Small amounts are excreted in urine. Tamoxifen appears to undergo enterohepatic circulation.

Uses and Administration

Tamoxifen is an oestrogen antagonist with actions similar to those of clomiphene citrate (see p.1440). It may also inhibit the production or release of cellular growth factors and induce apoptosis. It is used as the citrate in the adjuvant endocrine therapy of early breast cancer and is also given for the palliative treatment of advanced disease and has been investigated for prophylaxis in women at increased risk. It has been tried in some other malignancies including tumours of the endometrium and ovary and in malignant melanoma. Tamoxifen citrate is also used to stimulate ovulation in women with anovulatory infertility. See also the cross-references below.

Tamoxifen is given by mouth as the citrate. Doses are calculated in terms of the base. In the treatment of breast cancer, usual doses are the equivalent of tamoxifen 20 mg daily, in 2 divided doses or as a single daily dose. Doses of up to 40 mg daily may be given but no additional benefit has been demonstrated. Adjuvant therapy is normally continued for several years.

In the treatment of anovulatory infertility the usual dose is the equivalent of tamoxifen 20 mg daily on days 2, 3, 4, and 5 of the menstrual cycle, increased if necessary in subsequent cycles up to 80 mg daily. In women with irregular menstruation the initial course may be begun on any day, and a second course begun at a higher dose after 45 days if there has been no response. If the patient responds by menstruation, subsequent courses may begin on day 2 of the cycle.

Tamoxifen methiodide is reported to be under investigation.

Breast disorders, non-malignant. GYNAECOMASTIA. Tamoxifen, usually in doses of 10 mg twice daily, has been reported to be effective[1-3] in relieving pain and swelling in men or pubertal boys with gynaecomastia (p.1442). Tamoxifen has been recommended as a drug of choice in patients requiring drug therapy, given for 3 months to see if a response occurs.[4]

1. Jefferys DB. Painful gynaecomastia treated with tamoxifen. *Br Med J* 1979; **1:** 1119–20.
2. Hooper PD. Puberty gynaecomastia. *J R Coll Gen Pract* 1985; **35:** 142.
3. McDermott MT, *et al.* Tamoxifen therapy for painful idiopathic gynecomastia. *South Med J* 1990; **83:** 1283–5.
4. Braunstein GD. Gynecomastia. *N Engl J Med* 1993; **328:** 490–5.

MASTALGIA. Tamoxifen 20 mg daily has been shown to be effective in patients with both cyclic and non-cyclic mastalgia,[1] and improvement has also been reported at a lower dose of 10 mg daily.[2] However, there is concern about the use of tamoxifen in otherwise healthy premenopausal women,[3-5] particularly since many patients relapse on withdrawal,[2] and it has been recommended[6,7] that tamoxifen be reserved for patients who fail to respond to other drugs (see p.1443).

1. Fentiman IS, *et al.* Double-blind controlled trial of tamoxifen therapy for mastalgia. *Lancet* 1986; **i:** 287–8.
2. Fentiman IS, *et al.* Studies of tamoxifen in women with mastalgia. *Br J Clin Pract* 1989; **43** (suppl 68): 34–6.
3. Anonymous. Tamoxifen for benign breast disease. *Lancet* 1986; **i:** 305.
4. Smallwood JA, Taylor I. Tamoxifen for mastalgia. *Lancet* 1986; **i:** 680–1.
5. Fentiman IS, *et al.* Tamoxifen for mastalgia. *Lancet* 1986; **i:** 681.
6. Gateley CA, Mansel RE. Management of the painful and nodular breast. *Br Med Bull* 1991; **47:** 284–94.
7. Anonymous. Cyclical breast pain: what works and what doesn't. *Drug Ther Bull* 1992; **30:** 1–3.

Cardiovascular disorders. Tamoxifen has been reported to have a generally favourable effect on lipid profiles in postmenopausal women,[1] and may reduce the incidence of myocardial infarction in women receiving it.[2] It has been suggested that this may represent an additional benefit in women given tamoxifen for the prophylaxis of breast cancer,[3] although others dispute the potential benefit.[4] A wider role in postmenopausal hormone replacement therapy has been suggested,[5] but concerns about toxicity would seem to be an obstacle (see also Osteoporosis, below).

1. Love RR, *et al.* Effects of tamoxifen on cardiovascular risk factors in postmenopausal women. *Ann Intern Med* 1991; **115:** 860–4.
2. McDonald CC, *et al.* Cardiac and vascular morbidity in women receiving adjuvant tamoxifen for breast cancer in a randomised trial. *Br Med J* 1995; **311:** 977–80.
3. Powles TJ. The case for clinical trials of tamoxifen for prevention of breast cancer. *Lancet* 1992; **340:** 1145–7.
4. Fugh-Berman A, Epstein S. Tamoxifen: disease prevention or disease substitution? *Lancet* 1992; **340:** 1143–5.
5. Jackson G. Postmenopausal HRT—a role for tamoxifen? *Int J Clin Pract* 1997; **51:** 267.

Disorders related to the menstrual cycle. Apart from cyclic mastalgia (see above) tamoxifen has been used in a number of cases in which disorders were linked to the hormonal changes of the menstrual cycle, including menorrhagia due to myometrial hypertrophy,[1] an auto-immune dermatitis due to post-ovulatory rises in serum progesterone,[2,3] and premenstrual migraine.[4]

1. Fraser IS. Menorrhagia due to myometrial hypertrophy: treatment with tamoxifen. *Obstet Gynecol* 1987; **70:** 505–6.
2. Wojnarowska F, *et al.* Progesterone-induced erythema multiforme. *J R Soc Med* 1985; **78:** 407–8.
3. Stephens CJM, *et al.* Autoimmune progesterone dermatitis responding to tamoxifen. *Br J Dermatol* 1989; **121:** 135–7.
4. O'Dea JPK, Davis EH. Tamoxifen in the treatment of menstrual migraine. *Neurology* 1990; **40:** 1470–1.

Infertility. Tamoxifen is reported to be as effective as clomiphene in the treatment of anovulatory infertility (p.1239) in women,[1] and may be useful in women in whom abnormal cervical mucus acts as a barrier to spermatozoa.[2] In infertile men, however, results are reportedly contradictory, with some studies reporting increase in sperm density and improved pregnancy rates while others failed to demonstrate any effect.[3]

1. Messinis IE, Nillius SJ. Comparison between tamoxifen and clomiphene for induction of ovulation. *Acta Obstet Gynecol Scand* 1982; **61:** 377–9.
2. Roumen FJME, *et al.* Treatment of infertile women with a deficient postcoital test with two antiestrogens: clomiphene and tamoxifen. *Fertil Steril* 1984; **41:** 237–43.
3. Howards SS. Treatment of male infertility. *N Engl J Med* 1995; 312–17.

Malignant neoplasms. For reference to the use of tamoxifen in malignant neoplasms of breast, endometrium, and ovary, and in melanoma, see under Choice of Antineoplastic, p.485, p.487, p.491, and p.492. The most common use of tamoxifen is for the adjuvant endocrine therapy of breast cancer, where there seems to be a clear benefit. How long such therapy should be continued, however, remains uncertain although recent results suggest that continuing therapy beyond 5 years may not increase the overall benefit. Extension of tamoxifen use to the attempted prophylaxis of breast cancer, however, has proved extremely controversial, because of fears about carcinogenicity (see p.486 and above). Nonetheless, evidence that tamoxifen can reduce short-term incidence of breast cancer in some women at increased risk has been seen, and tamoxifen has been approved for such use in the USA.

Osteoporosis. As indicated on p.731 tamoxifen has been reported to have favourable effects on bone mass,[1-3] but any general role in the prevention of osteoporosis seems unlikely given concerns about the carcinogenicity of tamoxifen. The effects are reported to be comparable in magnitude to those of calcium supplementation, and less than those of oestrogens (see also p.1437) or bisphosphonates. It has been suggested that such an effect on bone would provide an additional benefit in women receiving tamoxifen for the prophylaxis of breast cancer,[4] although others dispute the benefits.[5]

1. Love RR, *et al.* Effects of tamoxifen on bone mineral density in postmenopausal women with breast cancer. *N Engl J Med* 1992; **326:** 852–6.
2. Love RR, *et al.* Effect of tamoxifen on lumbar spine bone mineral density in postmenopausal women after 5 years. *Arch Intern Med* 1994; **154:** 2585–8.
3. Grey AB, *et al.* The effect of the antiestrogen tamoxifen on bone mineral density in normal late postmenopausal women. *Am J Med* 1995; **99:** 636–41.
4. Powles TJ. The case for clinical trials of tamoxifen for prevention of breast cancer. *Lancet* 1992; **340:** 1145–7.
5. Fugh-Berman A, Epstein S. Tamoxifen: disease prevention or disease substitution? *Lancet* 1992; **340:** 1143–5.

Preparations

BP 1998: Tamoxifen Tablets;
USP 23: Tamoxifen Citrate Tablets.

Proprietary Preparations (details are given in Part 3)
Aust.: Kessar; Nolvadex; Tamax; Tamofen; Tamoplex; ***Austral.:*** Estroxyn; Genox; Kessar; Nolvadex; Noxitem; Tamosin; Tamoxen; ***Belg.:*** Nolvadex; Tamizam; ***Canad.:*** Apo-Tamox; Nolvadex; Tamofen; Tamone; Tamoplex†; ***Fr.:*** Kessar; Lesporene†; Nolvadex; Oncotam; Tamofene; ***Ger.:*** Dignotamoxi†; duratamoxifen; Jenoxifen; Kessar; Nolvadex; Nourytam; Tamobeta; Tamofen; Tamokadin; Tamox; Tamoxasta; Tamoxigenat; Tamoximerck; Tamoxistad; Zemide; Zitazonium; ***Irl.:*** Clonoxifen; Nolgen; Nolvadex; Tamofen; Tamox; ***Ital.:*** Kessar; Ledertam; Nolvadex; ***Neth.:*** Nolvadex; ***Norw.:*** Nolvadex; Tamofen; ***S.Afr.:*** Kessar; Neophedan; Nolvadex; Tamoplex; ***Spain:*** Nolvadex; Oxeprax; ***Swed.:*** Ledertam; Nolvadex; Tamaxin; ***Switz.:*** Kessar; Nolvadex; ***UK:*** Emblon; Fentamox; Noltam†; Nolvadex; Oestrifen; Tamofen; ***USA:*** Nolvadex.

Tegafur (1866-m)

Tegafur *(BAN, USAN, rINN)*.

FT-207; Ftorafur; MJF-12264; NSC-148958; WR-220066. 5-Fluoro-1-(tetrahydro-2-furyl)uracil; 5-Fluoro-1-(tetrahydro-2-furyl)pyrimidine-2,4(1*H*,3*H*)-dione.

$C_8H_9FN_2O_3$ = 200.2.

CAS — 17902-23-7.

Pharmacopoeias. In *Jpn.*

Adverse Effects, Treatment, and Precautions

As for Fluorouracil, p.535.

Bone-marrow depression may be less severe with tegafur but gastro-intestinal toxicity is often dose-limiting and central neurotoxicity is more common.

Results in *animals* suggested that co-administration of uracil with tegafur reduced the latter's cardiotoxic and neurotoxic effects.[1]

1. Yamamoto J, *et al.* Effect of coadministration of uracil on the toxicity of tegafur. *J Pharm Sci* 1984; **73:** 212–14.

Pharmacokinetics

Tegafur is well absorbed from the gastro-intestinal tract after oral administration. Following an intravenous dose it is reported to have a prolonged plasma half-life of 6 to 16 hours, and to be slowly metabolised to fluorouracil. It crosses the blood-brain barrier and is found in the CSF.

Uses and Administration

Tegafur is an antineoplastic agent which appears to act by the release of fluorouracil (p.534) in the body. It has been used in the management of a variety of malignant neoplasms including those of the breast (p.485) and gastro-intestinal tract (p.487); it has also been given for malignancies of the liver (p.489). Tegafur is given by mouth in doses up to 1.2 g daily. It is often given in combination with uracil. Doses of 1 to 3 g per m^2 body-surface daily for 5 days have been administered intravenously.

References.

1. Uchibayashi T, *et al.* Adjuvant therapy with 5-fluoro-1-(2-tetrahydrofuryl)-2,4(1H,3H)-pyrimidinedione (UFT) and Bestatin in patients with transitional cell carcinoma of the bladder—comparison between UFT therapy alone and UFT therapy in combination with Bestatin. *Int J Clin Pharmacol Ther* 1995; **33:** 465–8.
2. Morimoto T, *et al.* Postoperative adjuvant trial comparing chemo-endocrine therapy, chemotherapy and immunotherapy for patients with stage II breast cancer: 5-year results from the Nishinihon Cooperative Study Group of Adjuvant Chemo-endocrine Therapy for Breast Cancer (ACETBC) of Japan. *Eur J Cancer* 1996; **32**A: 235–42.

Preparations

Proprietary Preparations (details are given in Part 3)
Aust.: Ftoralon; ***Ital.:*** Citofur; ***Jpn:*** Futraful; ***Spain:*** Utefos.

Multi-ingredient: ***Jpn:*** UFT; ***Spain:*** UFT.

Teloxantrone Hydrochloride (14993-b)

Teloxantrone Hydrochloride *(USAN, rINNM)*.

DuP-937; Moxantrazole Hydrochloride; NSC-355644. 7,10-Dihydroxy-2-{2-[(2-hydroxyethyl)amino]ethyl}-5-{[2-(methylamino)ethyl]amino}anthra[1,9-*cd*]pyrazol-6(2*H*)-one dihydrochloride monohydrate.

$C_{21}H_{25}N_5O_4,2HCl,H_2O$ = 502.4.

CAS — 91441-48-4 (teloxantrone); 132937-88-3 (teloxantrone hydrochloride).

Teloxantrone is an anthrapyrazole derivative with structural similarities to mitozantrone (see p.553). It is under investigation for its antineoplastic properties as the dihydrochloride.

Temoporfin (17451-r)

Temoporfin *(BAN, USAN, rINN)*.

EF-9; mTHPC. 3,3′,3″,3‴-(7,8-Dihydroporphyrin-5,10,15,20-tetrayl)tetraphenol; 7,8-Dihydro-5,10,15,20-tetrakis(3-hydroxyphenyl)porphyrin.

$C_{44}H_{32}N_4O_4$ = 680.7.

CAS — 122341-38-2.

Temoporfin is a porphyrin derivative under investigation as a photosensitiser in the photodynamic therapy of various superficial neoplasms. It is reported to require smaller light doses, and therefore shorter treatment times, than some other photosensitisers.

References.

1. Dilkes MG, *et al.* Treatment of head and neck cancer with photodynamic therapy: results after one year. *J Laryngol Otol* 1995; **109:** 1072–6.
2. Savary JF, *et al.* Photodynamic therapy for early squamous cell carcinomas of the esophagus, bronchi, and mouth with m-tetra (hydroxyphenyl) chlorin. *Arch Otolaryngol Head Neck Surg* 1997; **123:** 162–8.
3. Wierrani F, *et al.* Clinical effect of meso-tetrahydroxyphenylchlorine based photodynamic therapy in recurrent carcinoma of the ovary: preliminary results. *Br J Obstet Gynaecol* 1997; **104:** 376–8.
4. Fan KF, *et al.* Photodynamic therapy using mTHPC for malignant disease in the oral cavity. *Int J Cancer* 1997; **73:** 25–32.

Temozolomide (2543-z)

Temozolomide *(BAN, rINN)*.

CCRG-81045; M&B-39831; NSC-362856. 3,4-Dihydro-3-methyl-4-oxoimidazo[5,1-*d*][1,2,3,5]tetrazine-8-carboxamide.

$C_6H_6N_6O_2$ = 194.2.

CAS — 85622-93-1.

Temozolomide is a compound which is believed to act by spontaneous generation of the same active metabolite as dacarbazine (p.526) and might be expected to have similar properties, but can be given by mouth. It is under investigation as an antineoplastic agent particularly in the treatment of brain tumours (p.485), but also in mycosis fungoides and melanoma (p.482 and p.492 respectively). Typical dosage regimens for malignant glioma have been 150 to 200 mg per m^2 body-surface daily by mouth for 5 days, repeated every 28 days. Myelosuppression is dose limiting.

References.

1. O'Reilly SM, *et al.* Temozolomide: a new oral cytotoxic chemotherapeutic agent with promising activity against primary brain tumours. *Eur J Cancer* 1993; **29A:** 940–2. Correction. *ibid.*; 1500.
2. Bleehen NM, *et al.* Cancer research campaign phase II trial of temozolomide in metastatic melanoma. *J Clin Oncol* 1995; **13:** 910–13.
3. Bower M, *et al.* Multicentre CRC phase II trial of temozolomide in recurrent or progressive high-grade glioma. *Cancer Chemother Pharmacol* 1997; **40:** 484–8.
4. Newlands ES, *et al.* Temozolomide: a review of its discovery, chemical properties, pre-clinical development and clinical trials. *Cancer Treat Rev* 1997; **23:** 35–61.

Teniposide (1867-b)

Teniposide *(BAN, USAN, rINN)*.

ETP; NSC-122819; VM-26. (5*S*,5a*R*,8a*S*,9*R*)-5,8,8a,9-Tetrahydro-5-(4-hydroxy-3,5-dimethoxyphenyl)-9-(4,6-*O*-thenylidene-β-D-glucopyranosyloxy)isobenzofuro[5,6-*f*][1,3]benzodioxol-6(5a*H*)-one.

$C_{32}H_{32}O_{13}S$ = 656.7.

CAS — 29767-20-2.

Precipitation occurred repeatedly in preparations for infusion containing teniposide 0.2 mg per mL in either glucose 5% or sodium chloride 0.9% injection, although previously such preparations had been used uneventfully.[1] Dilution of teniposide solutions to 0.1 mg per mL or less reduced the frequency of the problem, which could not be attributed to a change in formulation and remained unexplained.

1. Strong DK, Morris LA. Precipitation of teniposide during infusion. *Am J Hosp Pharm* 1990; **47:** 512.

Adverse Effects, Treatment, and Precautions

As for Etoposide, p.532. There is some evidence that teniposide may be a more potent mutagen and carcinogen than etoposide.

Hypersensitivity. Habibi and colleagues reported the development of haemolytic anaemia and acute renal failure with tubular necrosis in a patient who developed an antibody to teniposide.[1] Anaphylactic reactions occur, and may be severe;[2,3] the frequency may be as high as 13% in neuroblastoma patients.[2] Although it has been suggested that hypersensitivity reactions might be due to the polyethoxylated castor oil in the injection vehicle,[2] studies *in vitro* suggest that it is the drug rather than the vehicle which is responsible.[3]

1. Habibi B, *et al.* Immune hemolytic anemia and renal failure due to teniposide. *N Engl J Med* 1982; **306:** 1091–3.
2. Siddall SJ, *et al.* Anaphylactic reactions to teniposide. *Lancet* 1989; **i:** 394.
3. Carstensen H, *et al.* Teniposide-induced hypersensitivity reactions in children. *Lancet* 1989; **ii:** 55.

Interactions

Antiepileptics. Clearance of teniposide was markedly increased by concomitant treatment with *phenytoin* or *phenobarbitone*; the resultant decrease in systemic exposure to the antineoplastic might reduce its efficacy, and increased dosage would be needed in patients receiving anticonvulsants to guarantee equivalent exposure.[1]

1. Baker DK, *et al.* Increased teniposide clearance with concomitant anticonvulsant therapy. *J Clin Oncol* 1992; **10:** 311–15.

Cyclosporin. Concomitant administration of cyclosporin with teniposide has been reported[1] to produce a decrease in the clearance of the latter, with increased terminal half-life, peak plasma concentrations, and toxicity.

1. Toffoli G, *et al.* Cyclosporin A as a multidrug-resistant modulator in patients with renal cell carcinoma treated with teniposide. *Br J Cancer* 1997; **75:** 715–21.

Uses and Administration

Teniposide is an antineoplastic agent with general properties similar to those of etoposide (p.532). It has been given alone or with other antineoplastic agents in the treatment of refractory acute lymphoblastic leukaemia, as well as in non-Hodgkin's lymphoma, and in various solid tumours including those of the brain and lung, neuroblastoma, and retinoblastoma. The management of these malignancies is discussed further under Choice of Antineoplastic, as indicated by the cross-references given below.

A variety of dosage regimens have been used, ranging from 30 mg per m^2 body-surface area every 5 days, to 180 mg per m^2 weekly, as a single agent. Doses of 165 mg per m^2 twice weekly for 8 or 9 doses with cytarabine, or up to 250 mg per m^2 weekly for 4 to 8 weeks with vincristine have been given in the treatment of refractory acute lymphoblastic leukaemia. Teniposide is given by slow intravenous infusion over at least 30 to 60 minutes, as a solution of up to 1 mg teniposide per mL in sodium chloride 0.9% injection or glucose 5% injection.

Malignant neoplasms. Teniposide has been used, usually with cytarabine, to produce second remissions in some patients who relapse with acute lymphoblastic leukaemia (see p.478). It has also been used as a component of intensive regimens for low-grade non-Hodgkin's lymphoma (p.482), in the treatment of brain tumours (p.485), is active in small-cell lung cancer (p.490), and may produce responses in advanced neuroblastoma (p.494) and retinoblastoma (p.495) as part of a combination regimen. Teniposide has also been employed as a sclerosing agent in malignant effusions, but is probably not the agent of choice (see p.484).

Preparations

Proprietary Preparations (details are given in Part 3)
Aust.: Vumon; ***Austral.:*** Vumon; ***Belg.:*** Vumon; ***Canad.:*** Vumon; ***Fr.:*** Vehem; ***Ital.:*** Vumon; ***Neth.:*** Vumon; ***S.Afr.:*** Vumon; ***Spain:*** Vumon; ***Swed.:*** Vumon; ***Switz.:*** Vumon†; ***USA:*** Vumon.

Testolactone (9107-v)

Testolactone *(USAN, rINN).*

1-Dehydrotestololactone; NSC-23759; SQ-9538. D-Homo-17a-oxaandrosta-1,4-diene-3,17-dione.

$C_{19}H_{24}O_3$ = 300.4.

CAS — 968-93-4.

Pharmacopoeias. In US.

A white to off-white, practically odourless, crystalline powder. **Soluble** 1 in 4050 of water; soluble in alcohol and chloroform; slightly soluble in benzyl alcohol; practically insoluble in ether and petroleum spirit. **Store** in airtight containers.

Testolactone is a derivative of testosterone (see p.1464) and it is used in the palliative treatment of malignant neoplasms of the breast in postmenopausal women (p.485). It is reported to be an aromatase inhibitor that reduces peripheral oestrogen synthesis but has no significant androgenic activity.

The usual dose is 250 mg four times daily by mouth.

It should not be given to men with breast cancer.

Peripheral neuropathies have occurred in patients receiving testolactone; gastro-intestinal disturbances, pain or oedema of the extremities, hypertension, rashes, and glossitis have also been reported.

Congenital adrenal hyperplasia. For mention of the use of testolactone with flutamide to block androgenic effects in congenital adrenal hyperplasia, see p.1020.

Precocious puberty. Encouraging results have been reported using testolactone in the treatment of 5 girls with precocious puberty (p.1241) due to the McCune-Albright syndrome.[1] Testolactone blocked the synthesis of oestrogens from androgens by virtue of its being an aromatase inhibitor. Long-term therapy (for up to 5 years) was associated with continued benefit in many patients; however, signs of puberty were not always completely suppressed, in some cases perhaps because of difficulties in maintaining the dosage regimen.[3] Encouraging results were also obtained using a combination of testolactone and spironolactone in the treatment of familial precocious puberty in boys, although neither agent was successful when used alone.[2] Again, signs of a diminished response to treatment occurred with longer-term therapy; in this case control was restored by addition of a gonadorelin analogue.[4]

1. Feuillan PP, *et al.* Treatment of precocious puberty in the McCune-Albright syndrome with the aromatase inhibitor testolactone. *N Engl J Med* 1986; **315:** 1115–19.
2. Laue L, *et al.* Treatment of familial male precocious puberty with spironolactone and testolactone. *N Engl J Med* 1989; **320:** 496–502.
3. Feuillan PP, *et al.* Long term testolactone therapy for precocious puberty in girls with the McCune-Albright syndrome. *J Clin Endocrinol Metab* 1993; **77:** 647–51.
4. Laue L, *et al.* Treatment of familial male precocious puberty with spironolactone, testolactone, and deslorelin. *J Clin Endocrinol Metab* 1993; **76:** 151–5.

Preparations

USP 23: Testolactone Tablets.

Proprietary Preparations (details are given in Part 3)
Belg.: Teslac†; ***Ger.:*** Fludestrin; ***USA:*** Teslac.

Thioguanine (1868-v)

Thioguanine *(BAN, USAN).*

Tioguanine *(rINN)*; NSC-752; 6-TG; 6-Thioguanine; WR-1141. 2-Aminopurine-6(1*H*)-thione; 2-Amino-6-mercaptopurine; 2-Aminopurine-6-thiol.

$C_5H_5N_5S$ = 167.2.

CAS — 154-42-7 (anhydrous thioguanine); 5580-03-0 (thioguanine hemihydrate).

Pharmacopoeias. In Br.

US permits anhydrous or hemihydrate.

A pale yellow, odourless or almost odourless, crystalline powder. Practically **insoluble** in water, alcohol, and chloroform; dissolves in dilute solutions of alkali hydroxides. **Store** in airtight containers.

Adverse Effects, Treatment, and Precautions

As for Mercaptopurine, p.546.

In some patients, gastro-intestinal reactions are reported to be less frequent than with mercaptopurine. Normal doses of thioguanine may be employed when it is used with allopurinol.

Effects on the blood. For the view that bone-marrow depression by thioguanine may be predictable, see under Mercaptopurine, p.546.

Effects on the liver. There have been occasional reports of hepatic veno-occlusive disease attributed to thioguanine.[1,2]

1. Gill RA, *et al.* Hepatic veno-occlusive disease caused by 6-thioguanine. *Ann Intern Med* 1982; **96:** 58–60.
2. Krivoy N, *et al.* Reversible hepatic veno-occlusive disease and 6-thioguanine. *Ann Intern Med* 1982; **96:** 788.

Handling and disposal. For reference to a method for the destruction of thioguanine in wastes, see Mercaptopurine, p.546.

Pharmacokinetics

Thioguanine is incompletely and variably absorbed from the gastro-intestinal tract; on average about 30% of a dose is absorbed following oral administration. It is rapidly activated in the body by intracellular conversion to its nucleotide, thioguanylic acid and its thioguanosine phosphate derivatives. With repeated doses increasing amounts of the nucleotide are incorporated into DNA. Very little unchanged thioguanine has been detected circulating in the blood but the half-life of the nucleotide in the tissues is prolonged. Thioguanine is inactivated primarily by methylation to aminomethylthiopurine; small amounts are deaminated to thioxanthine, and may go on to be oxidised by xanthine oxidase to thiouric acid, but inactivation is essentially independent of xanthine oxidase and is not affected by inhibition of the enzyme.

It is excreted in the urine almost entirely as metabolites; only negligible amounts of thioguanine have been detected. Thioguanine does not appear to cross the blood-brain barrier to a significant extent; very little is found in cerebrospinal fluid after normal clinical doses. It crosses the placenta.

Uses and Administration

Thioguanine is an analogue of the naturally occurring purine, guanine, and is an antineoplastic with actions and uses similar to those of mercaptopurine (p.546). It appears to cause fewer gastro-intestinal reactions but cross-resistance exists between it and mercaptopurine so that patients who do not respond to one are unlikely to respond to the other.

Thioguanine is given by mouth with other agents, usually cytarabine and an anthracycline, in the induction and maintenance of remissions in acute non-lymphoblastic leukaemia (p.479) although there is some uncertainty about its value. It has also been used in acute lymphoblastic leukaemia (p.478).

Doses up to 200 mg per m^2 body-surface daily have been given for 5 to 20 days as part of a combined induction regimen. A dose of 2 to 2.5 mg per kg body-weight daily increased after 4 weeks, if there is no response or toxicity allows, to 3 mg per kg daily may be given to adults and children in those rare cases when single agent therapy is considered appropriate.

Blood counts should be made frequently, particularly during induction and when thioguanine is given with other antineoplastic agents. Therapy should be withdrawn at the first sign of severe bone-marrow depression.

It has been administered intravenously as thioguanine sodium.

Preparations

BP 1998: Tioguanine Tablets;
USP 23: Thioguanine Tablets.

Proprietary Preparations (details are given in Part 3)
Austral.: Lanvis; ***Belg.:*** Lanvis; ***Canad.:*** Lanvis; ***Irl.:*** Lanvis; ***Neth.:*** Lanvis; ***S.Afr.:*** Lanvis; ***Swed.:*** Lanvis; ***Switz.:*** Lanvis; ***UK:*** Lanvis.

Thiotepa (1869-g)

Thiotepa *(BAN, rINN).*

NSC-6396; TESPA; Thiophosphamide; Triethylenethiophosphoramide; TSPA; WR-45312. Phosphorothioic tri(ethyleneamide); Tris(aziridin-1-yl)phosphine sulphide.

$C_6H_{12}N_3PS$ = 189.2.

CAS — 52-24-4.

Pharmacopoeias. In Br., Chin., Fr., Jpn, and US.

Fine white, odourless or almost odourless, crystalline flakes. M.p. 52° to 57°. The BP states that it is freely **soluble** in water, in alcohol, and in chloroform; USP solubilities are 1 in 13 of water, 1 in about 8 of alcohol, 1 in about 2 of chloroform, and 1 in about 4 of ether. **Store** at 2° to 8° in airtight containers. At higher temperatures it polymerises and becomes inactive. Protect from light.

Incompatibility. Lyophilised thiotepa 1 mg per mL in 5% glucose injection was incompatible when mixed with solutions of cisplatin or minocycline hydrochloride.

1. Trissel LA, Martinez JF. Compatibility of thiotepa (lyophilized) with selected drugs during simulated Y-site administration. *Am J Health-Syst Pharm* 1996; **53:** 1041–5.

Stability. A solution of a lyophilised thiotepa preparation 0.5 mg per mL in 5% glucose injection was considered to be stable (less than 10% loss of thiotepa) for 8 hours at both 4° and 23°.[1] After 24 hours losses ranged between about 10 and 17%. At a higher thiotepa concentration (5 mg per mL) thiotepa was stable for 3 days at 23° and 14 days at 4°. Another study found that solutions containing 1 or 3 mg of thiotepa per mL in 0.9% sodium chloride were stable for 24 hours at 25° and 48 hours at 8°, but solutions containing 0.5% thiotepa needed to be used immediately.[2]

1. Xu QA, *et al.* Stability of thiotepa (lyophilized) in 5% dextrose injection at 4 and 23°C. *Am J Health-Syst Pharm* 1996; **53:** 2728–30.
2. Murray KM, *et al.* Stability of thiotepa (lyophilized) in 0.9% sodium chloride injection. *Am J Health-Syst Pharm* 1997; **54:** 2588–91.

Adverse Effects, Treatment, and Precautions

For general discussions, see Antineoplastics, p.470, p.473, and p.474.

Bone-marrow depression may be delayed; the nadir of white cell and platelet counts may occur up to 30 days after therapy has been discontinued. Bone-marrow depression has been reported after intravesical as well as parenteral administration, and has occasionally been prolonged.

Gastro-intestinal disturbances, headache and dizziness, hypersensitivity reactions, and impaired fertility have also been reported. Local irritation, and occasionally frank chemical or haemorrhagic cystitis may follow intravesical instillation. Depigmentation of periorbital skin has occurred following the use of thiotepa eye drops. As with other alkylating agents, thiotepa is potentially mutagenic, teratogenic, and carcinogenic.

Thiotepa should be given with extreme care, if at all, to patients with pre-existing impairment of hepatic, renal, or bone-marrow function.

Pharmacokinetics

The absorption of thiotepa from the gastro-intestinal tract is incomplete and unreliable; variable absorption also occurs from intramuscular injection sites. Absorption through serous membranes such as the bladder and pleura occurs to some extent. Following intravenous administration it is rapidly cleared from plasma, with an elimination half-life of about 2.4 hours. It is extensively metabolised: triethylenephosphoramide (TEPA), the primary metabolite, and some of the other metabolites have cytotoxic activity and are eliminated more slowly than the parent compound. It is excreted in the urine: less than 2% of a dose is reported to be present as unchanged drug or its primary metabolite.

Uses and Administration

Thiotepa is an ethyleneimine compound whose antineoplastic effect is related to its alkylating action. It has generally been replaced by cyclophosphamide (p.517) or other drugs. It is not a vesicant and may be given by all parenteral routes, as well as directly into tumour masses.

Instillations of thiotepa may be used in the treatment of superficial tumours of the bladder (p.484) and in the control of malignant effusions (p.484). It has been given parenterally in the palliative treatment of various solid tumours, including those of breast and ovary (p.485 and p.491), and intravitreal injection has been tried in an attempt to save a remaining eye in children with retinoblastoma (p.495). It has also been given intrathecally to patients with malignant meningeal disease, and has been used, in the form of eye drops, as an adjunct to the surgical removal of pterygium, to prevent recurrence (see p.553).

Thiotepa is given in a variety of dosage schedules. In general, initial doses to suit the individual patient are followed by maintenance doses given at intervals of one to 4 weeks. Blood counts are recommended before and during administration and should continue for at least 3 weeks after stopping therapy. Thiotepa should not be given if the white cell count falls below 3000 per mm³ or the platelet count below 150 000 per mm³ and treatment should be discontinued if the white cell count falls rapidly. Dosage should be reduced in patients with lesser degrees of leucopenia.

In the treatment of bladder cancer thiotepa in doses up to 60 mg may be instilled in 30 to 60 mL of sterile water into the bladder of a patient previously dehydrated for 8 to 12 hours, and retained if possible for 2 hours. The instillation may be repeated weekly for up to 4 weeks. Similar instillations have been given at intervals of 1 to 2 weeks, for up to 8 instillations in the prophylaxis of recurrence after surgical removal of bladder cancer. Single doses of 90 mg in 100 mL of sterile water have also been used prophylactically. For malignant effusions suggested doses of up to 65 mg of thiotepa in 20 to 60 mL of sterile water may be instilled after aspiration; in the USA the usual recommended dose is 600 to 800 μg per kg body-weight, a dose similar to that suggested for injection directly into tumours. Thiotepa for local use may be mixed with solutions of procaine and adrenaline.

Intramuscular and intravenous dosage regimens vary considerably; several regimens have employed courses of 15 mg daily for 4 or 5 days. In the USA a suggested dose is 300 to 400 μg per kg given at 1- to 4-week intervals. A solution containing 1 mg per mL has been tried intrathecally in doses of up to 10 mg.

A 0.05% solution has been instilled as eye drops every 3 hours for up to 8 weeks following surgical removal of pterygium in order to reduce the likelihood of recurrence.

A dose of 60 mg weekly has been instilled into the urethra for the treatment of condylomata acuminata (genital warts). Topical application of thiotepa has also been used for condylomata.

Preparations

BP 1998: Thiotepa Injection;
USP 23: Thiotepa for Injection.

Proprietary Preparations (details are given in Part 3)
Belg.: Ledertepa; *Jpn:* Tespamin; *Neth.:* Ledertepa; *Spain:* Onco Tiotepa; *USA:* Thioplex.

Tirapazamine (17120-h)

Tirapazamine *(USAN, rINN)*.

Win-59075. 3-Amino-1,2,4-benzotriazine 1,4-dioxide.

$C_7H_6N_4O_2$ = 178.1.

CAS — 27314-97-2.

Tirapazamine is reported to be reduced in hypoxic cells to an active anion that causes DNA strand breaks. It is under investigation for its cytotoxic actions, alone or in combination with cisplatin or radiotherapy. Adverse effects reported with tirapazamine include nausea and vomiting, skin rashes, muscle cramps and fatigue; myelosuppression is said to be rare.

References.

1. Miller VA, *et al.* Phase II study of the combination of the novel bioreductive agent, tirapazamine, with cisplatin in patients with advanced non-small-cell lung cancer. *Ann Oncol* 1997; **8:** 1269–71.

Topotecan Hydrochloride (15104-s)

Topotecan Hydrochloride *(BANM, USAN, pINNM)*.

SKF-104864A; SKFS-104864-A. (*S*)-10-Dimethylaminomethyl-4-ethyl-4,9-dihydroxy-1*H*-pyrano[3′,4′:6,7]indolizino[1,2*b*]quinoline-3,14(4*H*,12*H*)-dione hydrochloride.

$C_{23}H_{23}N_3O_5$,HCl = 457.9.

CAS — 123948-87-8 (topotecan); 119413-54-6 (topotecan hydrochloride).

Topotecan hydrochloride 1.09 mg is approximately equivalent to 1 mg of topotecan.

Adverse Effects and Precautions

For general discussions, see Antineoplastics, p.470 and p.474. Neutropenia is common and is usually dose-limiting. Thrombocytopenia and anaemia are less frequent. Gastro-intestinal disturbances are also common. Other adverse effects include fatigue and weakness, alopecia, malaise, and hyperbilirubinaemia.

Topotecan should be avoided in patients with pre-existing bone-marrow depression, and the manufacturers suggest that it should not be given in severe renal or hepatic impairment. Topotecan has been reported to produce fetal death and malformations in *animals*.

Pharmacokinetics

Topotecan is widely distributed following intravenous administration. It undergoes reversible hydrolysis of the lactone ring to the inactive hydroxy acid form; only small amounts are demethylated in the liver. A significant proportion of a dose is excreted in urine. Topotecan has a terminal half-life of 2 to 3 hours.

References.

1. Herben VMM, *et al.* Clinical pharmacokinetics of topotecan. *Clin Pharmacokinet* 1996; **31:** 85–102.

Uses and Administration

Like irinotecan (p.543), topotecan is a semisynthetic derivative of the alkaloid camptothecin that exerts its antineoplastic activity by inhibition of topoisomerase I. It is used in the treatment of metastatic carcinoma of the ovary refractory to other therapy (see p.491) and may be tried in small cell lung cancer (p.490) refractory to standard therapy. Topotecan is also under investigation in the management of other malignancies.

Topotecan is given as the hydrochloride but doses are calculated in terms of the base. The recommended initial dose for ovarian cancer is the equivalent of topotecan 1.5 mg per m² body-surface, given by intravenous infusion over 30 minutes, on days 1 to 5 of a 21-day course. A minimum of 4 courses should be given, provided that the neutrophil count has recovered to over 1000 per mm³, and platelet count and haemoglobin are over 100 000 per mm³ and 9 g per 100 mL respectively.

If severe neutropenia occurs in any course the dose in the subsequent courses may be reduced by 0.25 mg per m², or a granulocyte colony-stimulating factor may be given from day 6 of the course once topotecan administration is complete. Dosage should also be reduced after severe thrombocytopenia, and in patients with impaired renal function: halving of the initial dose is recommended in those with a creatinine clearance between 20 and 39 mL per minute.

References[1-5] to the use of topotecan in various malignancies.

1. Anonymous. Topotecan hydrochloride for metastatic ovarian cancer. *Med Lett Drugs Ther* 1996; **38:** 96–7.
2. Macdonald D, et al. Phase II study of topotecan in patients with recurrent malignant glioma. *Ann Oncol* 1996; **7:** 205–7.
3. Schiller JH, *et al.* Phase II study of topotecan in patients with extensive-stage small-cell carcinoma of the lung: an Eastern Cooperative Oncology Group Trial. *J Clin Oncol* 1996; **14:** 2345–52.
4. Beran M, *et al.* Topotecan, a topoisomerase I inhibitor, is active in the treatment of myelodysplastic syndrome and chronic myelomonocytic leukemia. *Blood* 1996; **88:** 2473–9.
5. Ardizzoni A, *et al.* Topotecan, a new active drug in the second-line treatment of small-cell lung cancer: a phase II study in patients with refractory and sensitive disease. *J Clin Oncol* 1997; **15:** 2090–6.

Preparations

Proprietary Preparations (details are given in Part 3)
Austral.: Hycamtin; *Ger.:* Hycamtin; *Neth.:* Hycamtin; *Swed.:* Hycamtin; *UK:* Hycamtin; *USA:* Hycamtin.

Toremifene (2830-f)

Toremifene *(BAN, rINN)*.

FC-1157a (toremifene citrate). (*Z*)-2-[4-(4-Chloro-1,2-diphenylbut-1-enyl)phenoxy]ethyldimethylamine.

$C_{26}H_{28}ClNO$ = 406.0.

CAS — 89778-26-7 (toremifene); 89778-27-8 (toremifene citrate).

NOTE. Toremifene Citrate is *USAN*.

Adverse Effects and Precautions

As for Tamoxifen Citrate, p.563.

Uses and Administration

Toremifene is an anti-oestrogen which might be expected to have properties similar to those of tamoxifen (p.563), and is used similarly in the treatment of breast cancer (p.485). It is also under investigation for the treatment of fibrous tumours.

Toremifene is given by mouth as the citrate in doses equivalent to 60 mg of the base daily.

General references.

1. Wiseman LR, Goa KL. Toremifene: a review of its pharmacological properties and clinical efficacy in the management of advanced breast cancer. *Drugs* 1997; **54:** 141–60.
2. Anonymous. Toremifene and letrozole for advanced breast cancer. *Med Lett Drugs Ther* 1998; **40:** 43–5.

Action. Ebbs and colleagues reported that some breast tumour shrinkage occurred in 4 of 16 postmenopausal women in whom locally advanced disease had progressed while receiving tamoxifen when therapy was changed to toremifene 200 mg daily.[1] A further 4 patients had no change while the remaining 8 had disease progression. They considered that the partial success of high-dose toremifene in patients unresponsive to tamoxifen might involve a secondary action separate from its anti-oestrogenic action. However, a large multicentre study involving 648 women with metastatic breast cancer failed to note any difference in response rate and duration between toremifene 60 mg and 200 mg daily, or between these and tamoxifen 20 mg daily.[2] Overall survival and adverse effects were also comparable in the three groups, apart from an increased incidence of nausea in the high-dose toremifene group.

1. Ebbs SR, *et al.* Alternative mechanism of action of "anti-oestrogens" in breast cancer. *Lancet* 1987; **ii:** 621.
2. Hayes DF, *et al.* Randomized comparison of tamoxifen and two separate doses of toremifene in postmenopausal patients with metastatic breast cancer. *J Clin Oncol* 1995; **13:** 2556–66.

Preparations

Proprietary Preparations (details are given in Part 3)
Aust.: Fareston; *Irl.:* Fareston; *Ital.:* Fareston; *Neth.:* Fareston; *Swed.:* Fareston; *UK:* Fareston; *USA:* Fareston.

Trastuzumab (15020-v)

Trastuzumab *(rINN)*.

HER-2 Monoclonal Antibody; rhuMAb HER2.

Trastuzumab is a monoclonal antibody directed against the cell surface protein $p185^{HER2}$, produced by the HER2 gene, which is overexpressed in about one-third of all breast cancers. Trastuzumab is used in the adjuvant treatment of breast cancer. Recommended doses are 4 mg per kg body-weight initially, by intravenous infusion over 90 minutes, followed by 2 mg per kg over 30 minutes at weekly intervals. Hypersensitivity and infusion-related reactions have occurred; trastuzumab has also been associated with cardiotoxicity.

References.

1. Baselga J, *et al.* Phase II study of weekly intravenous recombinant humanized anti-p185HER2 monoclonal antibody in patients with HER2/neu-overexpressing metastatic breast cancer. *J Clin Oncol* 1996; **14:** 737–44.

Preparations

Proprietary Preparations (details are given in Part 3)
USA: Herceptin.

Treosulfan (1871-d)

Treosulfan *(BAN, rINN)*.

Dihydroxybusulphan; NSC-39069. L-Threitol 1,4-dimethanesulphonate.

$C_6H_{14}O_8S_2$ = 278.3.

CAS — 299-75-2.

Treosulfan is an antineoplastic agent related to busulphan (p.509), which is reported to act by alkylation after conversion *in vivo* to epoxide compounds. It is used palliatively or as an adjunct to surgery mainly in the treatment of ovarian cancer (p.491).

Treosulfan 1 g daily is given by mouth in 4 divided doses for 2 or 4 weeks followed by the same period without treatment. Alternatively 1.5 g daily in 3 divided doses may be given for 1 week, followed by 3 weeks without therapy. The cycle is then repeated, the dose being adjusted if necessary according to the effect on bone marrow. Lower doses should be used if treatment with other antineoplastic drugs or radiotherapy is being given concomitantly. Treosulfan may also be given intravenously in doses of 3 to 8 g per m^2 body-surface every one to three weeks. Doses larger than 3 g per m^2 should be given by infusion at a rate of 3 g per m^2 every 5 to 10 minutes. Doses up to 1.5 g per m^2 have been given intraperitoneally.

Regular blood counts should be made and treatment should be interrupted if the white-blood cell count is less than 3000 per mm^3 or the platelet count below 100 000 per mm^3. Because bone-marrow depression may be cumulative the interval between blood counts should be reduced after the second course of treatment with treosulfan.

Preparations

Proprietary Preparations (details are given in Part 3)
Ger.: Ovastat.

Trimetrexate Glucuronate (19502-s)

Trimetrexate Glucuronate *(BANM, USAN, rINNM)*.

CI-898 (trimetrexate); JB-11 (trimetrexate); NSC-352122; NSC-249008 (trimetrexate). 5-Methyl-6-(3,4,5-trimethoxyanilinomethyl)quinazolin-2,4-diyldiamine mono-D-glucuronate.

$C_{19}H_{23}N_5O_3,C_6H_{10}O_7$ = 563.6.

CAS — 52128-35-5 (trimetrexate); 82952-64-5 (trimetrexate glucuronate).

Trimetrexate glucuronate 1.53 mg is approximately equivalent to 1 mg of trimetrexate.

Incompatibility. For reference to the incompatibility of trimetrexate and foscarnet, see under Foscarnet Sodium, p.610.

Adverse Effects, Treatment, and Precautions

As for Methotrexate, p.547.

Interactions

Studies in *animals* suggest that cimetidine and imidazole antifungal drugs such as clotrimazole and ketoconazole may inhibit trimetrexate metabolism, and there is a risk of possible interactions with all drugs that affect hepatic cytochrome P450 systems.

Uses and Administration

Trimetrexate is a dihydrofolate reductase inhibitor with general properties similar to those of methotrexate (p.550). It is used in the management of *Pneumocystis carinii* pneumonia in patients with AIDS where other therapy has proved ineffective (see also p.370). It has also been tried as an antineoplastic in the management of various solid tumours.

Trimetrexate is given by intravenous infusion, as the glucuronate. A suggested schedule in *Pneumocystis carinii* pneumonia has been 45 mg per m^2 daily for 21 days, in association with folinic acid rescue for 24 days. The dosage of trimetrexate and folinic acid should be adjusted according to the results of blood tests, which should be performed at least twice a week during therapy. It has been suggested that treatment with zidovudine and other myelosuppressive drugs should be interrupted to allow full doses of trimetrexate to be given. Renal and hepatic function and haemoglobin values should also be monitored.

Doses of 8 mg per m^2 body-surface area daily for 5 days at 3-week intervals, or 150 to 220 mg per m^2 every 28 days, have been given in the management of neoplastic disease, usually in combination with folinic acid rescue.

Trimetrexate is a non-classical antifolate which is a potent inhibitor of dihydrofolate reductase but differs from methotrexate in two important aspects.[1] It is taken up avidly by most mammalian tumour cells by a process independent of the folate carrier system, and within the cell it does not undergo polyglutamylation. In consequence, cell lines resistant to methotrexate may retain sensitivity to trimetrexate, particularly where resistance is due to polyglutamylation defects, uptake defects, or low level gene amplification. Only methotrexate resistant cells with altered dihydrofolate reductase have been shown to be insensitive to trimetrexate while those with high level amplification of the dihydrofolate reductase gene are partially cross resistant. A few cell lines have shown trimetrexate resistance of unknown cause.

1. Bertino JR. Folate antagonists: toward improving the therapeutic index and development of new analogs. *J Clin Pharmacol* 1990; **30:** 291–5.

Further reviews.

1. Marshall JL, DeLap RJ. Clinical pharmacokinetics and pharmacology of trimetrexate. *Clin Pharmacokinet* 1994; **26:** 190–200.
2. Fulton B, *et al.* Trimetrexate: a review of its pharmacodynamic and pharmacokinetic properties and therapeutic potential in the treatment of Pneumocystis carinii pneumonia. *Drugs* 1995; **49:** 563–76.

Preparations

Proprietary Preparations (details are given in Part 3)
Canad.: Neutrexin; ***Fr.:*** Neutrexin; ***Irl.:*** Neutrexin; ***Ital.:*** Neutrexin; ***Swed.:*** Neutrexin; ***UK:*** Neutrexin; ***USA:*** Neutrexin.

Trofosfamide (1875-b)

Trofosfamide *(rINN)*.

A-4828; NSC-109723; Trilophosphamide; Trophosphamide; Z-4828. 3-(2-Chloroethyl)-2-[bis(2-chloroethyl)amino]tetrahydro-2*H*-1,3,2-oxazaphosphorine-2-oxide.

$C_9H_{18}Cl_3N_2O_2P$ = 323.6.

CAS — 22089-22-1.

Trofosfamide is a derivative of cyclophosphamide (see p.516) and has the same general properties. It is used in the treatment of a variety of malignant disorders in usual initial doses of 300 to 400 mg daily by mouth. Doses of 50 to 150 mg daily have been given for maintenance therapy.

Preparations

Proprietary Preparations (details are given in Part 3)
Aust.: Ixoten; ***Ger.:*** Ixoten; ***Ital.:*** Ixoten†; ***Spain:*** Genoxal Trofosfamida.

Tumour Necrosis Factor (1331-a)

TNF.

Tumour necrosis factor is a cytokine of which 2 forms have been identified with similar biological properties: TNFα or cachectin, which is produced predominantly by macrophages, and TNFβ or lymphotoxin, which is produced by lymphocytes. Various recombinant forms of TNFα, both human and mouse, are available: the names sonermin and sertenef have been used for such products.

The antitumour effects of tumour necrosis factor *in vitro* and in *animals* have prompted investigation of recombinant TNFα in the treatment of cancer either alone or in combination with other cytokines such as interleukin-2 or the interferons. However, results to date have been somewhat disappointing, and there has been great concern over the potential toxicity. Adverse effects in patients treated with tumour necrosis factor include fever, hypotension, shock, capillary leak syndrome, neurological disorders, coagulation disorders, and thrombocytopenia and leucopenia.

References.

1. Malik S, Balkwill FR. Tumour necrosis factor. *Br Med J* 1988; **296:** 1214.
2. Balkwill FR. Tumour necrosis factor. *Br Med Bull* 1989; **45:** 389–400.
3. Tracey KJ, *et al.* Cachectin/tumour necrosis factor. *Lancet* 1989; **i:** 1122–6.
4. Windebank KP. The cytokines are coming. *Arch Dis Child* 1990; **65:** 1283–5.
5. Tsuboi R, *et al.* Primary cutaneous plasmacytoma: treatment with intralesional tumour necrosis factor-α. *Br J Dermatol* 1992; **126:** 395–7.
6. Meager A. 5th International congress on tumour necrosis factor and related cytokines: scientific advances and their medical applications. *Biologicals* 1994; **22:** 291–5.
7. Hieber U, Heim ME. Tumor necrosis factor for the treatment of malignancies. *Oncology* 1994; **51:** 142–53.
8. Bazzoni F, Beutler B. The tumor necrosis factor ligand and receptor families. *N Engl J Med* 1996; **334:** 1717–25.
9. Lejeune FJ. High dose recombinant tumour necrosis factor (rTNF alpha) administered by isolation perfusion for advanced tumours of the limbs: a model for biochemotherapy of cancer. *Eur J Cancer* 1995; **31A:** 1009–16.

Units. The first International Standard for human tumour necrosis factor α, which contained 40 000 international units per ampoule, was considered unsuitable for the assay of recombinant *mouse* tumour necrosis factor α, for human tumour necrosis factor β, or for preparations of tumour necrosis factor α of modified structure.[1]

1. WHO. WHO expert committee on biological standardisation: forty-second report. *WHO Tech Rep Ser 822* 1992.

Ubenimex (16531-y)

Ubenimex *(rINN)*.

NK-421. (−)-*N*-[(2*S*,3*R*)-3-Amino-2-hydroxy-4-phenylbutyryl]-L-leucine.

$C_{16}H_{24}N_2O_4$ = 308.4.

CAS — 58970-76-6.

Ubenimex is a peptide derived from *Streptomyces olivoreticuli*. It is reported to have antineoplastic and immunostimulant properties. It is used in the adjuvant treatment of acute nonlymphoblastic leukaemia in doses of 30 mg daily by mouth. Adverse effects include gastro-intestinal and hepatic function disturbances, skin rashes, headache, and paraesthesias.

Ubenimex has been tried as an adjuvant to tegafur and uracil in the treatment of bladder cancer.[1]

1. Uchibayashi T, *et al.* Adjuvant therapy with 5-fluoro-1-(2-tetrahydrofuryl)-2,4-(1H,3H)-pyrimidinedione (UFT) and Bestatin in patients with transitional cell carcinoma of the bladder—comparison between UFT therapy alone and UFT therapy in combination with Bestatin. *Int J Clin Pharmacol Ther* 1995; **33:** 465–8.

Preparations

Proprietary Preparations (details are given in Part 3)
Jpn: Bestatin.

Uramustine (1876-v)

Uramustine *(BAN, rINN)*.

NSC-34462; U-8344; Uracil Mustard *(USAN)*. 5-Bis(2-chloroethylamino)uracil; 5-[Bis(2-chloroethyl)amino]pyrimidine-2,4(1*H*,3*H*)-dione.

$C_8H_{11}Cl_2N_3O_2$ = 252.1.

CAS — 66-75-1.

Uramustine is an antineoplastic agent derived from mustine (see p.555) and has a similar mode of action but it has largely been replaced by more effective agents. It has been given by mouth in doses of 150 μg per kg body-weight weekly, as a single dose, for 4 weeks.

Verteporfin (14529-m)

Verteporfin *(USAN, rINN)*.

Benzoporphyrin Derivative; BPD; CL-318952. *trans*-18-Ethenyl-4,4a-dihydro-3,4-bis(methoxycarbonyl)-4a,8,14,19-tetramethyl-23*H*,25*H*-benzo[*b*]porphine-9,13-dipropanoic acid monomethyl ester.

$C_{41}H_{42}N_4O_8$ = 718.8.

CAS — 129497-78-5.

Verteporfin is under investigation as a photosensitiser in the photodynamic therapy of a variety of disorders, including malignant neoplasms and age-related macular degeneration.

Vinblastine Sulphate (1878-q)

Vinblastine Sulphate *(BANM, rINNM)*.

29060-LE; NSC-49842; Sulfato de Vimblastina; Vinblastine Sulfate *(USAN)*; Vinblastini Sulfas; Vincaleukoblastine Sulphate; VLB (vinblastine).

$C_{46}H_{58}N_4O_9,H_2SO_4$ = 909.1.

CAS — 865-21-4 (vinblastine); 143-67-9 (vinblastine sulphate).

Pharmacopoeias. In *Chin., Eur.* (see p.viii), *Int., Jpn,* and *US.*

The sulphate of an alkaloid, vincaleukoblastine, extracted from *Vinca rosea* (*Catharanthus roseus*) (Apocynaceae). A white to slightly yellow, odourless, very hygroscopic, amorphous or crystalline powder. It loses not more than 15% of its weight on drying.

Freely **soluble** in water; practically insoluble in alcohol and in ether. A 0.15% solution in water has a pH of 3.5 to 5.0. **Store** at −20° in airtight containers. Protect from light.

Stability. Between about 5 and 20% of active drug was lost from solution when a solution of vinblastine sulphate 3 μg per mL in 5% glucose injection was stored for 48 hours in a range of intravenous burette giving sets, the highest loss being from cellulose propionate sets and the lowest from one made from methacrylate butadiene styrene.[1] Similarly storage in polyvinyl chloride (PVC) tubing led to a 42 to 44% loss from solution whereas only about 6% was lost over the 48 hours in polybutadiene tubing. The losses appeared to be due to drug sorption, and were therefore greater from the tubing which had a greater surface-area-to-volume ratio than the burettes.

1. McElnay JC, *et al.* Stability of methotrexate and vinblastine in burette administration sets. *Int J Pharmaceutics* 1988; **47:** 239–47.

Adverse Effects, Treatment, and Precautions

For general discussions, see Antineoplastics, p.470, p.473, and p.474.

Bone-marrow depression, especially leucopenia, is the most common adverse effect with vinblastine and tends to be dose-limiting. Maximum depression occurs 4 to 10 days after administration with recovery in a further 1 to 3 weeks. Gastro-intestinal effects including stomatitis and gastro-intestinal bleeding may occur; nausea and vomiting respond to treatment with antiemetics.

The vinca alkaloids can produce central and peripheral (including autonomic) neurotoxicity, although these effects are less frequent with vinblastine. Symptoms include malaise, dizziness, weakness, headache, depression, psychoses, paraesthesia and numbness, loss of deep tendon reflexes, ataxia, peripheral neuropathies, constipation and adynamic ileus, jaw pain, and convulsions. A routine prophylactic regimen against constipation is recommended in patients receiving high doses of vinblastine. Overdosage has caused permanent damage to the central nervous system and inappropriate intrathecal administration has proved fatal.

Other reported effects include skin reactions, alopecia, ischaemic cardiac toxicity, hypertension, dyspnoea and bronchospasm, and bone and tumour pain. A syndrome of inappropriate secretion of antidiuretic hormone has occurred at high doses, and may be relieved by fluid restriction and, if necessary, a suitable diuretic.

Vinblastine is irritant to the skin and mucous membranes and extravasation may cause necrosis, cellulitis, and sloughing. The application of warmth and local injection of hyaluronidase may be of benefit in relieving the effects of extravasation. Folinic acid has been suggested in overdosage, by analogy with vincristine.

Vinblastine should not be injected into an extremity with impaired circulation because of an increased risk of thrombosis. Intrathecal administration of the vinca alkaloids is contra-indicated because of the likelihood of severe or fatal neurotoxicity. Leucopenia may be more severe in patients with cachexia or extensive skin ulceration: vinblastine should not be used in elderly patients with these conditions. Vinblastine should be given with caution and at reduced dosage to patients with hepatic impairment.

Handling and disposal. A method for the destruction of vincristine or vinblastine wastes using sulphuric acid and potassium permanganate.[1] Residues produced by degradation of either drug by this method showed no mutagenicity *in vitro*.

1. Castegnaro M, *et al.*, eds. Laboratory decontamination and destruction of carcinogens in laboratory wastes: some antineoplastic agents. *IARC Scientific Publications 73* Lyon: WHO/International Agency for Research on Cancer, 1985.

Urine and faeces produced for up to 4 and 7 days respectively after a dose of vinblastine should be handled wearing protective clothing.[1]

1. Harris J, Dodds LJ. Handling waste from patients receiving cytotoxic drugs. *Pharm J* 1985; **235:** 289–91.

Interactions

Concurrent administration of vinblastine with drugs that inhibit cytochromes of the CYP3A subfamily may result in decreased metabolism of vinblastine and increased toxicity.

Analgesics. A report of enhanced hepatotoxicity in patients treated with interferon alfa and vinblastine who were given *paracetamol*.[1]

1. Kellokumpu-Lehtinen P, *et al.* Hepatotoxicity of paracetamol in combination with interferon and vinblastine. *Lancet* 1989; **i:** 1143.

Antibacterials. There is a report of severe vinblastine toxicity in 3 patients who received vinblastine and cyclosporin with *erythromycin*.[1] Discontinuing erythromycin produced resolution of the adverse effects, which recurred following rechallenge with erythromycin in 1 patient.

1. Tobe SW, *et al.* Vinblastine and erythromycin: an unrecognised serious drug interaction. *Cancer Chemother Pharmacol* 1995; **35:** 188–90.

Antineoplastics. Acute bronchospastic reactions following injection of a vinca alkaloid have been reported, usually in patients who have also received *mitomycin*,[1] and presenting as acute respiratory distress, cyanosis, and dyspnoea, often with the development of pulmonary infiltrates and pneumonitis.[2,3] A number of fatalities due to respiratory complications have occurred.

1. Dyke RW. Acute bronchospasm after a vinca alkaloid in patients previously treated with mitomycin. *N Engl J Med* 1984; **310:** 389.
2. Konits PH, *et al.* Possible pulmonary toxicity secondary to vinblastine. *Cancer* 1982; **50:** 2771–4.
3. Ozols RF, *et al.* MVP (mitomycin, vinblastine, and progesterone): a second-line regimen in ovarian cancer with a high incidence of pulmonary toxicity. *Cancer Treat Rep* 1983; **67:** 721–2.

Pharmacokinetics

Vinblastine is not reliably absorbed from the gastro-intestinal tract. Following intravenous administration it is rapidly cleared from the blood and distributed to tissues; it is reported to be concentrated in blood platelets. It is extensively protein bound. Vinblastine is metabolised in the liver, by cytochrome P450 isoenzymes of the CYP3A subfamily, to an active metabolite desacetylvinblastine, and is excreted in faeces via the bile, and in urine; some is excreted as unchanged drug. The terminal half-life is reported to be about 25 hours. It does not cross the blood-brain barrier in significant amounts.

Uses and Administration

Vinblastine sulphate is an antineoplastic agent which apparently acts by binding to the microtubular proteins of the spindle and arresting mitosis at the metaphase; it is thus specific for the M phase of the cell cycle. It also interferes with glutamate metabolism and possibly nucleic acid synthesis, and has some immunosuppressant activity. Significant cross-resistance with vincristine has not been reported although pleiotropic resistance may occur.

Vinblastine sulphate is mainly used, in association with other antineoplastic agents, in the combination chemotherapy of testicular cancer (although the vinblastine-containing PVB regimen has now largely been replaced by other regimens), and in the treatment of Hodgkin's disease and other lymphomas. It is also of use in the treatment of some inoperable malignant neoplasms including those of the breast, bladder, and cervix, and in non-small cell lung cancer, neuroblastoma, choriocarcinoma, and Kaposi's sarcoma; the management of these conditions is discussed under Choice of Antineoplastic, as indicated by the cross-references given below.

In carcinoma of the testis vinblastine has often been given with bleomycin and cisplatin (PVB). In the treatment of Hodgkin's disease it may be given with an alkylating agent such as cyclophosphamide or mustine, plus procarbazine and prednisone, or with doxorubicin, bleomycin, and dacarbazine (ABVD).

Vinblastine sulphate is given by intravenous injection as a solution containing 1 mg per mL in sodium chloride 0.9%. Care should be taken to avoid extravasation and the injection may be given into a freely running infusion of sodium chloride injection if preferred. One suggested dosage scheme is as follows: weekly injections starting with 100 μg per kg body-weight or 3.7 mg per m^2 body-surface, raised by increments of 50 μg per kg or 1.8 to 1.9 mg per m^2 to a maximum weekly dose of 500 μg per kg or 18.5 mg per m^2, or until the white-cell count has fallen to 3000 per mm^3. Most patients respond to 150 to 200 μg per kg or 5.5 to 7.4 mg per m^2 weekly. If a maintenance dose is required, it may be given every 7 to 14 days and should be one increment smaller than the maximum dose that the patient is able to tolerate without serious leucopenia occurring. An alternative maintenance regimen has consisted of 10 mg given once or twice a month. Doses of 300 to 400 μg per kg, sometimes divided over 2 consecutive days, may be given every 3 weeks in testicular cancer.

Children may be given vinblastine sulphate in an initial dose of 2.5 mg per m^2 body-surface intravenously, increased by 1.25 mg per m^2 weekly to a usual maximum weekly dose of 7.5 mg per m^2. Doses of up to 12.5 mg per m^2 per week have been given.

White-cell counts should be made before each injection and a repeat dose should never be given unless the count has risen to 4000 per mm^3. A dosage reduction of 50% is advised in patients with moderately severe hepatic impairment (serum bilirubin above 3 mg per 100 mL).

Blood disorders, non-malignant. The vinca alkaloids vinblastine and vincristine have been used experimentally in the treatment of various autoimmune blood disorders such as *idiopathic thrombocytopenic purpura, and autoimmune haemolytic anaemia* (p.1023 and p.702 respectively). There are also reports of the *haemolytic-uraemic syndrome/thrombotic thrombocytopenic purpura* responding to treatment with intravenous injection of vincristine,[1,2] and vincristine has been given with normal immunoglobulin in the management of a patient with life-threatening thrombocytopenia due to *sarcoidosis*.[3]

1. Gutterman LA, *et al.* The hemolytic-uremic syndrome: recovery after treatment with vincristine. *Ann Intern Med* 1983; **98:** 612–13.
2. Wolf G, *et al.* Behandlung einer thrombotisch-thrombo-zytopenischen Purpura (Morbus Moschcowitz) mit Vincristine. *Dtsch Med Wochenschr* 1995; **120:** 442–6.
3. Larner AJ. Life threatening thrombocytopenia in sarcoidosis. *Br Med J* 1990; **300:** 317–19.

Histiocytic syndromes. The value of systemic chemotherapy in patients with histiocytic syndromes (p.478) is uncertain; however, it is certainly widely used in extensive disease, vinblastine being one of the drugs often employed.[1,2]

1. Ladisch S, *et al.* LCH-1: a randomized trial of etoposide vs vinblastine in disseminated Langerhans cell histiocytosis. *Med Pediatr Oncol* 1994; **23:** 107–10.
2. The French Langerhans' Cell Histiocytosis Study Group. A multicentre retrospective survey of Langerhans' cell histiocytosis: 348 cases observed between 1983 and 1993. *Arch Dis Child* 1996; **75:** 17–24.

Malignant neoplasms. Vinblastine plays an important role in the ABVD regimen, which is an alternative to MOPP in patients with Hodgkin's disease (see p.481). It also formed part of the effective, if toxic, PVB regimen used to treat testicular cancer, although other regimens tend now to be preferred, as mentioned on p.493. The vinca alkaloids are also active in gestational trophoblastic tumours (p.477), although most regimens seem to employ vincristine rather than vinblastine, and vinblastine is also used in the adjuvant therapy of invasive bladder cancer (p.484), in the palliative care of advanced breast cancer (p.485) and cervical cancer (p.487); it has limited activity in non-small-cell lung cancer (p.490) and has been used in neuroblastoma (p.494) and in Kaposi's sarcoma (p.496).

Preparations

BP 1998: Vinblastine Injection;
USP 23: Vinblastine Sulfate for Injection.

Proprietary Preparations (details are given in Part 3)
Aust.: Velbe; ***Austral.:*** Velbe; ***Belg.:*** Velbe; ***Canad.:*** Velbe; ***Fr.:*** Velbe; ***Ger.:*** Cellblastin; Velbe; ***Ital.:*** Velbe; ***Neth.:*** Velbe; ***Norw.:*** Velbe; ***S.Afr.:*** Periblastine; ***Swed.:*** Velbe; ***Switz.:*** Velbe; ***UK:*** Velbe; ***USA:*** Alkaban; Velban.

Vincristine Sulphate (1879-p)

Vincristine Sulphate *(BANM, rINNM)*.

Compound 37231; Leurocristine Sulphate; NSC-67574; 22-Oxovincaleukoblastine Sulphate; Sulfato de Vincristina; Vincristine Sulfate *(USAN)*; Vincristini Sulfas.

$C_{46}H_{56}N_4O_{10},H_2SO_4$ = 923.0.

CAS — 57-22-7 (vincristine); 2068-78-2 (vincristine sulphate).

Pharmacopoeias. In *Chin., Eur.* (see p.viii), *Int., Jpn, Pol.,* and *US.*

The sulphate of an alkaloid, 22-oxovincaleukoblastine, obtained from *Vinca rosea* (*Catharanthus roseus*) (Apocynaceae). A white to slightly yellow, odourless, very hygroscopic, amorphous or crystalline powder. It loses not more than 12% of its weight on drying.

Freely **soluble** in water; slightly soluble in alcohol; soluble in methyl alcohol; practically insoluble in ether. A 0.1% solution in water has a pH of 3.5 to 4.5. **Store** at −20° in airtight containers. Protect from light.

Adverse Effects, Treatment, and Precautions

As for Vinblastine Sulphate, p.569.

Bone-marrow depression occurs less commonly than with vinblastine but neurological and neuromuscular effects are more severe with vincristine and are dose-limiting. Walking may be impaired and the neurological effects may not be reversed for several months after the drug is discontinued. Convulsions, often with hypertension, have occurred. Constipation is common and there may be abdominal pain. Urinary disturbances have occurred and alopecia is common.

Folinic acid has been given for the treatment of overdosage: suggested doses are as much as 100 mg of folinic acid intravenously every 3 hours for 24 hours, then every 6 hours for at least 48 hours. However, this is unlikely to be of benefit in reversing neuromuscular toxicity. For mention of the use of glutamic acid in managing the usually fatal consequences of inadvertent intrathecal administration, see below.

Because severe constipation and impaction of faeces often occur with vincristine, laxatives or enemas may be necessary to ensure regular bowel function. Vincristine should be given with caution to patients with pre-existing neuromuscular disease and is contra-indicated in patients with the demyelinating form of Charcot-Marie-Tooth syndrome (see under Effects on the Nervous System, below). Doses may need to be adjusted in patients with impaired liver function. Care should also be taken in elderly patients, who may be more susceptible to neurotoxicity.

Inadvertent intrathecal administration of vincristine results in ascending paralysis and death.[1,2] However, in one case[3] treatment immediately following the error, and consisting of removal of contaminated spinal fluid and flushing with lactated Ringer's solution and fresh frozen plasma diluted in lactated Ringer's solution, plus intravenous and oral glutamic acid, was reported successful in stabilising neurological dysfunction and preventing death. The role of glutamic acid in this case is uncertain, but a study involving 84 patients found that the administration of glutamic acid 1.5 g daily by mouth in divided doses during a 6-week induction chemotherapy course decreased vincristine-induced neurotoxicity.[4]

1. Manelis J, *et al.* Accidental intrathecal vincristine administration: report of a case. *J Neurol* 1982; **228:** 209–13.
2. Dyer C. Manslaughter convictions for making mistakes. *Br Med J* 1991; **303:** 1218.
3. Dyke RW. Treatment of inadvertent intrathecal injection of vincristine. *N Engl J Med* 1989; **321:** 1270–1.
4. Jackson DV, *et al.* Amelioration of vincristine neurotoxicity by glutamic acid. *Am J Med* 1988; **84:** 1016–22.

Effects on the nervous system. The neurotoxic effects of vincristine have been reviewed by Legha.[1] In its most typical form, neurotoxicity manifests as a mixed sensorimotor neuropathy of the distal type. The earliest symptoms are sensory changes in the form of paraesthesias, accompanied by impairment and ultimately loss of deep tendon reflexes. In more severe forms, impairment of motor function occurs with wrist drop and foot drop, ataxia and gait abnormalities, and occasionally progressive quadriparesis.

In contrast to these peripheral neuropathies which are usually associated with long-term usage there may be short-term autonomic neuropathy resulting in constipation and occasionally ileus, abdominal pain, atony of the urinary bladder (which may lead to urinary retention), postural hypotension, and rarely, impotence. There may be effects on the cranial nerves, resulting in ptosis, hoarseness (due to laryngeal nerve paralysis), or optic neuropathies. Effects on the CNS are rare, probably in part because of poor penetration into CSF, but include excessive release of antidiuretic hormone and consequent hyponatraemia.

Hallucinations have occurred[2] and effects on the special senses have been reported: both bilateral optic atrophy and blindness,[3] and profound neurological deafness (which was largely reversible on drug withdrawal)[4] have occurred. Convulsions associated with hypertension are another feature of vincristine toxicity.[5]

Toxicity is related to both the cumulative and the individual dose.[1] It usually begins in adults after receiving a total of 5 to 6 mg, and is significant by the time a cumulative dose of 15 to 20 mg is reached. If individual doses are low (less than 2 mg) or intervals between doses are longer than the usual week, patients can tolerate higher cumulative doses. Children tolerate vincristine better than adults, but the elderly are particularly prone to neurotoxicity. Patients with existing neurological disorders such as poliomyelitis or the Charcot-Marie-Tooth syndrome may be at increased risk of neurotoxicity.[6-9] It has been suggested that increased neurotoxicity may be associated with the use of ready-to-use solutions rather than reconstituted lyophilised preparations but this has not been proved.[10-14]

There is no good treatment for the effects of vincristine on the nervous system: symptoms are largely reversible once administration is interrupted, and should be managed with appropriate symptomatic care.[1] However, there is some suggestion that glutamic acid may be of benefit in treating neurotoxicity—see above. For the use of dinoprost to alleviate ileus induced by vinca alkaloids, see p.1414.

1. Legha SS. Vincristine neurotoxicity: pathophysiology and management. *Med Toxicol* 1986; **1:** 421–7.
2. Holland JF, *et al.* Vincristine treatment of advanced cancer: a cooperative study of 392 cases. *Cancer Res* 1973; **33:** 1258–64.
3. Awidi AS. Blindness and vincristine. *Ann Intern Med* 1980; **93:** 781.
4. Yousif H, *et al.* Partially reversible nerve deafness due to vincristine. *Postgrad Med J* 1990; **66:** 688–9.
5. Ito S, *et al.* Seizures and hypertension complicating vincristine therapy in children. *Clin Pharmacol Ther* 1995; **57:** 208.
6. Hogan-Dann CM, *et al.* Polyneuropathy following vincristine therapy in two patients with Charcot-Marie-Tooth syndrome. *JAMA* 1984; **252:** 2862–3.
7. Miller BR. Neurotoxicity and vincristine. *JAMA* 1985; **253:** 2045.
8. Chauncey TR, *et al.* Vincristine neurotoxicity. *JAMA* 1985; **254:** 507.
9. Griffiths JD, *et al.* Vincristine neurotoxicity in Charcot-Marie-Tooth syndrome. *Med J Aust* 1985; **143:** 305–6.
10. Arnold AM, *et al.* Acute vincristine neurotoxicity. *Lancet* 1985; **i:** 346.
11. Jalihal S, Roebuck N. Acute vincristine neurotoxicity. *Lancet* 1985; **i:** 637.
12. Davies CE, *et al.* Acute vincristine neurotoxicity. *Lancet* 1985; **i:** 637–8.
13. Warrier RP, Ducos R. Acute vincristine neurotoxicity. *Lancet* 1985; **i:** 980.
14. Gennery BA. Vincristine neurotoxicity. *Lancet* 1985; **ii:** 385.

Handling and disposal. Urine and faeces produced for up to 4 and 7 days respectively after a dose of vincristine should be handled wearing protective clothing.[1]

1. Harris J, Dodds LJ. Handling waste from patients receiving cytotoxic drugs. *Pharm J* 1985; **235:** 289–91.

For a method for the destruction of vincristine wastes, see under Vinblastine Sulphate, p.569.

Interactions

Concurrent administration of vincristine with drugs that inhibit cytochromes of the CYP3A subfamily may result in decreased metabolism of vincristine and increased toxicity. If vincristine is used in combination with asparaginase it should be given 12 to 24 hours before the enzyme: administration of asparaginase with or before vincristine may reduce vincristine clearance and increase toxicity.

Antimicrobials. Toxicity has been reported to be increased in children who received *itraconazole* and nifedipine during leukaemia treatment involving vincristine.[1] Severe neurotoxicity has occurred when *isoniazid* was added to the regimen of a patient receiving vincristine.[2]

1. Murphy JA, *et al.* Vincristine toxicity in five children with acute lymphoblastic leukaemia. *Lancet* 1995; **346:** 443.
2. Carrión C, *et al.* Possible vincristine-isoniazid interaction. *Ann Pharmacother* 1995; **29:** 201.

Pharmacokinetics

Vincristine is not reliably absorbed from the gastro-intestinal tract. After intravenous injection it disappears rapidly from the blood. It is extensively protein bound and is reported to be concentrated in blood platelets. It is metabolised in the liver and excreted primarily in the bile; about 70 to 80% of a dose is found in faeces, as unchanged drug and metabolites, while 10 to 20% appears in the urine. The terminal half-life is reported to be about 85 hours but may range from about 10 to 155 hours. Vincristine does not appear to cross the blood-brain barrier in significant amounts.

Uses and Administration

Vincristine sulphate is an antineoplastic agent which may act similarly to vinblastine (above) by arresting mitosis at the metaphase. Significant cross-resistance with vinblastine has not been reported although pleiotropic resistance may occur.

It is used principally in combination chemotherapy regimens for acute leukaemia and Hodgkin's disease and other lymphomas, including Burkitt's lymphoma. It may also be used in the treatment of Wilm's tumour, myeloma, neuroblastoma, in sarcomas including Kaposi's sarcoma and rhabdomyosarcoma and in tumours of the brain, breast, head and neck, and lung, among others. It has also been given in Waldenström's macroglobulinaemia, and in idiopathic thrombocytopenic purpura refractory to other agents. See also the cross-references given below.

Remissions are induced in acute lymphoblastic leukaemia with vincristine in association with prednisone alone or with an anthracycline or asparaginase or both. In Hodgkin's disease, vincristine may be given with mustine, procarbazine, and prednisone (MOPP), and similar regimens have been used in other lymphomas.

Vincristine sulphate is administered by intravenous injection, usually as a solution containing 1 mg per mL in sodium chloride 0.9%. Care should be taken to avoid extravasation and the injection may be given into a freely-running intravenous infusion of sodium chloride injection if preferred.

In acute leukaemia the usual weekly dose of vincristine sulphate for induction of remission in children is 2 mg per m^2 body-surface, or 50 µg per kg body-weight increasing by weekly increments of 25 µg per kg to a maximum of 150 µg per kg. Adults may be given about 1.4 mg per m^2 or 25 to 75 µg per kg weekly; a maximum weekly dose of 2 mg has been suggested (but see below). For other malignancies 25 µg per kg may be given weekly and reduced to 5 to 10 µg per kg for maintenance.

Blood counts should be carried out before giving each dose. A dose reduction of 50% is recommended in patients with moderately severe hepatic impairment (serum bilirubin above 3 mg per 100 mL).

Action. Results *in vitro* suggesting a selective action of vincristine against lymphocytes of patients with chronic lymphocytic leukaemia;[1] lymphocytes of healthy subjects were not so affected.

1. Vilpo J, *et al.* Selective toxicity of vincristine against chronic lymphocytic leukaemia in vitro. *Lancet* 1996; **347:** 1491–2.

Administration. Although a maximum single dose of 2 mg is recommended for vincristine sulphate to reduce neurotoxicity, a review by McCune and Lindley[1] has suggested that this guideline is overly rigid, since it does not take into account interindividual variations in pharmacokinetics and susceptibility to toxicity, which may be considerable.

Furthermore they considered the evidence for effectiveness of this dosage limitation to be equivocal. They suggested beginning therapy at 1.4 mg per m^2 body-surface and adjusting subsequent doses according to toxicity.

1. McCune JS, Lindley C. Appropriateness of maximum-dose guidelines for vincristine. *Am J Health-Syst Pharm* 1997; **54:** 1755–8.

Blood disorders, non-malignant. Vincristine may be employed in the treatment of refractory idiopathic thrombocytopenic purpura (p.1023), either by conventional injection or in the form of vincristine-loaded platelets, but results have been equivocal. Vincristine has also been used for life-threatening haemangioma (p.1022).

Malignant neoplasms. Vincristine is widely used in the treatment of malignant neoplasms. It is a fundamental part of potentially curative regimens for acute lymphoblastic leukaemia and Hodgkin's disease (see p.478 and p.481) and has also been used in chronic lymphocytic leukaemia (p.480) and in other non-Hodgkin's lymphomas (p.482), including AIDS-related lymphoma (p.483), Burkitt's lymphoma (p.483) and mycosis fungoides (p.482). Other haematological malignancies in which it has been tried include multiple myeloma (p.494) and Waldenström's macroglobulinaemia (see p.496). Among the solid neoplasms, vincristine is used in regimens to treat gestational trophoblastic tumours (p.477), tumours of the brain (p.485), breast (p.485), cervix (p.487), head and neck (p.489), Wilms' tumour (p.489), small-cell lung cancer (p.490), malignancies of the testis (p.493), thymoma (p.493) and thyroid cancer (p.494). It is also employed in regimens for neuroblastoma (p.494), retinoblastoma (p.495), and some sarcomas including sarcomas of bone, Kaposi's sarcoma, and rhabdomyosarcoma (see p.495, p.496, and p.496).

Preparations

BP 1998: Vincristine Injection;
USP 23: Vincristine Sulfate for Injection; Vincristine Sulfate Injection.

Proprietary Preparations (details are given in Part 3)
Aust.: Oncovin; ***Austral.:*** Oncovin; ***Belg.:*** Oncovin; ***Canad.:*** Oncovin; ***Fr.:*** Oncovin; ***Ger.:*** Cellcristin; ***Irl.:*** Oncovin; ***Neth.:*** Oncovin; ***Norw.:*** Oncovin; ***S.Afr.:*** Norcristine†; Oncovin; Pericristine; ***Spain:*** Vincrisul; ***Swed.:*** Oncovin; ***Switz.:*** Oncovin; ***UK:*** Oncovin; ***USA:*** Oncovin; Vincasar PFS.

Vindesine Sulphate (1880-n)

Vindesine Sulphate *(BANM, rINNM).*

Compound 112531 (vindesine); Desacetyl Vinblastine Amide Sulfate; LY-099094; NSC-245467; Vindesine Sulfate *(USAN)*; Vindesini Sulfas. 3-Carbamoyl-4-*O*-deacetyl-3-de(methoxycarbonyl)vincaleukoblastine.

$C_{43}H_{55}N_5O_7,H_2SO_4$ = 852.0.

CAS — 53643-48-4 (vindesine); 59917-39-4 (vindesine sulphate).

Pharmacopoeias. In *Eur.* (see p.viii).

A white or almost white, hygroscopic, amorphous substance. Freely **soluble** in water and in methyl alcohol; practically insoluble in cyclohexane. The pH of a 0.5% solution is 3.5 to 5.5. **Store** in airtight polypropylene containers with a polypropylene cap, at a temperature not exceeding −50°.

Adverse Effects, Treatment, and Precautions

As for Vinblastine Sulphate, p.569.

The main dose-limiting effect of vindesine is granulocytopenia with the nadir of the white-cell count usually occurring 3 to 5 days after a dose, with recovery after a further 4 to 5 days. Although neurotoxicity occurs it may be less severe than that seen with vincristine (see p.570). Alopecia is the most common side-effect.

Folinic acid has been suggested for the treatment of overdosage by analogy with vincristine.

Vindesine should not be given by the intrathecal route, as this may produce fatal toxicity. Care should be taken if acute abdominal pain occurs: further administration may result in paralytic ileus.

In a 10-year-old child who was accidentally given an intrathecal injection of vindesine, treatment with folinic acid and dexamethasone produced transient recovery but symptoms subsequently recurred and the patient died of progressive ascending paralysis.[1] The CNS showed changes at necropsy similar to those seen following intrathecal administration of vincristine.

1. Robbins G. Accidental intrathecal injection of vindesine. *Br Med J* 1985; **291:** 1094.

Interactions

As for Vinblastine Sulphate, p.569.

Pharmacokinetics

The pharmacokinetics of vindesine are similar to those of the other vinca alkaloids. After intravenous administration elimination from the blood is triphasic; the drug is rapidly distributed to body tissues. The terminal half-life is reported to be about 20 hours. It is metabolised primarily in the liver and excreted in bile and urine.

Uses and Administration

Vindesine sulphate is an antineoplastic agent derived from vinblastine (see p.569); like the other vinca alkaloids it causes mitotic arrest in metaphase by binding to microtubular protein. It has been tried in refractory malignant melanoma (see p.492), and in malignant neoplasms of the gastro-intestinal tract, and lung (p.487 and p.490). It has also been used in refractory leukaemias, and in malignant neoplasms of the breast.

Vindesine sulphate is given weekly by intravenous injection as a solution containing 1 mg per mL in sodium chloride injection (0.9%). Care should be taken to avoid extravasation and it may be given into a fast-running infusion of sodium chloride, glucose (5%), or glucose-saline injection. The usual starting dose for adults is 3 mg per m^2 body-surface which may be raised by increments of 500 μg per m^2 weekly providing that the granulocyte count does not fall below 1500 per mm^3, the platelet count does not fall below 100 000 per mm^3, and acute abdominal pain is not experienced; weekly doses are usually between 3 and 4 mg per m^2. Children may be given 4 mg per m^2 initially, with weekly doses usually ranging between 4 and 5 mg per m^2. Blood counts should be made before each injection. It may be necessary to reduce initial doses in patients with significantly impaired hepatic function.

Preparations

Proprietary Preparations (details are given in Part 3)
Aust.: Eldisin; ***Austral.:*** Eldisine; ***Belg.:*** Eldisine; ***Canad.:*** Eldisine; ***Fr.:*** Eldisine; ***Ger.:*** Eldisine; ***Ital.:*** Eldisine; ***Neth.:*** Eldisine; ***S.Afr.:*** Eldisine; ***Spain:*** Enison; ***Swed.:*** Eldisine; ***Switz.:*** Eldisine; ***UK:*** Eldisine.

Vinorelbine Tartrate (3773-j)

Vinorelbine Tartrate *(BANM, USAN, rINNM).*

Vinorelbine Ditartrate. 3′,4′-Didehydro-4′-deoxy-8′-norvincaleukoblastine ditartrate.

$C_{45}H_{54}N_4O_8,2C_4H_6O_6$ = 1079.1.

CAS — 71486-22-1 (vinorelbine); 125317-39-7 (vinorelbine tartrate).

Adverse Effects and Precautions

As for Vinblastine Sulphate, p.569. The nadir of the granulocyte count occurs 5 to 10 days after a dose with recovery usually after a further 7 to 14 days. The drug should be discontinued if moderate or severe neurotoxicity develops. Local pain and thrombophlebitis may be seen with repeated injection of vinorelbine.

Pharmacokinetics

As with the other vinca alkaloids, vinorelbine exhibits triphasic pharmacokinetics after intravenous injection, and has a terminal half-life of between about 28 and 44 hours. It is metabolised in the liver; deacetylvinorelbine has antineoplastic activity. Vinorelbine and its metabolites are excreted primarily in faeces via the bile but also in urine.

References.

1. Levêque D, Jehl F. Clinical pharmacokinetics of vinorelbine. *Clin Pharmacokinet* 1996; **31:** 184–97.

Uses and Administration

Vinorelbine is a semisynthetic derivative of vinblastine (see p.569) with similar general properties. It is used as the tartrate in the treatment of breast cancer and non-small cell lung cancers (see p.485 and p.490 respectively), and has been tried in other malignancies.

Vinorelbine is administered as the tartrate but doses are calculated in terms of vinorelbine. It is given by intravenous injection over 5 to 10 minutes, as a solution containing the equivalent of vinorelbine 1.5 to 3.0 mg per mL in glucose 5% or sodium chloride 0.9% injection, directly or into a freely-running intravenous infusion. It may also be given by intravenous infusion over 20 to 30 minutes after dilution in 125 mL of glucose 5% or sodium chloride 0.9%. The usual initial dose is the equivalent of vinorelbine 25 to 30 mg per m^2 body-surface weekly. Subsequent doses should be halved if granulocyte counts fall to between 1000 and 1500 per mm^3; treatment should be interrupted if counts are below 1000 per mm^3 and discontinued if granulocytopenia persists for more than 2 weeks. Doses should also be reduced in hepatic insufficiency. In the UK a dose reduction of one-third has been suggested in patients with massive liver metastases (but see also below). In the USA, the manufacturers recommend that the dose of vinorelbine be reduced by 50% in patients with bilirubin values of 2.1 to 3.0 mg per 100 mL, and by 75% in those with bilirubin greater than 3.0 mg per 100 mL.

Oral formulations of vinorelbine have been investigated.

References.

1. Toso C, Lindley C. Vinorelbine: a novel vinca alkaloid. *Am J Health-Syst Pharm* 1995; **52:** 1287–1304.
2. Jones SF, Burris HA. Vinorelbine: a new antineoplastic drug for the treatment of non-small-cell lung cancer. *Ann Pharmacother* 1996; **30:** 501–6.

Administration in hepatic impairment. Clearance of vinorelbine was markedly reduced in patients with diffuse liver metastases and hence severely altered hepatic function: a 50% dose reduction was probably appropriate in such patients even if hyperbilirubinaemia was not marked.[1] However, reduced doses were not necessary in patients with moderate liver involvement in whom liver function, as measured by lignocaine metabolism, was not markedly reduced.

1. Robieux I, *et al.* Pharmacokinetics of vinorelbine in patients with liver metastases. *Clin Pharmacol Ther* 1996; **59:** 32–40.

Preparations

Proprietary Preparations (details are given in Part 3)
Aust.: Navelbine; ***Austral.:*** Navelbine; ***Canad.:*** Navelbine; ***Fr.:*** Navelbine; ***Ger.:*** Navelbine; ***Ital.:*** Navelbine; ***Spain:*** Biovelbin; Navelbine; ***Swed.:*** Navelbine; ***Switz.:*** Navelbine; ***UK:*** Navelbine; ***USA:*** Navelbine.

Vorozole (15359-s)

Vorozole *(BAN, USAN, rINN).*

R-83842. (+)-6-[4-Chloro-α-(1,2,4-triazol-1-yl)benzyl]-1-methyl-1*H*-benzotriazole.

$C_{16}H_{13}ClN_6$ = 324.8.

CAS — 129731-10-8.

Vorozole is a nonsteroidal inhibitor of the aromatase (oestrogen synthetase) system. It has been investigated in the treatment of breast cancer.

References.

1. Goss PE, *et al.* Phase II study of vorozole (R83842), a new aromatase inhibitor, in postmenopausal women with advanced breast cancer in progression on tamoxifen. *Clin Cancer Res* 1995; **1:** 287–94.
2. Paridaens R, *et al.* Vorozole (Rivizor): an active and well tolerated new aromatase inhibitor for the treatment of advanced breast cancer patients with prior tamoxifen exposure. *Anticancer Drugs* 1998; **9:** 29–35.

Zinostatin (1881-h)

Zinostatin *(USAN, rINN)*.

Neocarzinostatin; NSC-157365 (formerly NSC-69856).

CAS — 9014-02-2.

An antineoplastic antibiotic obtained from *Streptomyces carzinostaticus*.

Zinostatin is an antibiotic with antineoplastic activity and has been used in the treatment of malignant neoplasms.

Zinostatin stimalamer (SMANCS), a conjugate of zinostatin with a styrene-maleic acid polymer, is used for the treatment of liver cancer.

Zolimomab Aritox (9389-p)

Zolimomab Aritox *(USAN, rINN)*.

CD5 T-lymphocyte Immunotoxin; H65-RTA.

CAS — 141483-72-9.

Zolimomab aritox is a conjugate of a murine monoclonal antibody against the CD5 antigen of human lymphocytes with the A chain of ricin (see p.1625). It has been investigated in the prevention and treatment of graft-versus-host disease in patients receiving bone marrow transplants (p.498). Zolimomab aritox has also been investigated in the treatment of various auto-immune diseases, or diseases considered to have an immune component, including diabetes mellitus and rheumatoid arthritis.

References.

1. Weisdorf D, *et al.* Combination graft-versus-host disease prophylaxis using immunotoxin (anti-CD5-RTA [Xomazyme-CD5]) plus methotrexate and cyclosporine or prednisone after unrelated donor marrow transplantation. *Bone Marrow Transplant* 1993; **12:** 531–6.
2. Stand V, *et al.* Effects of administration of an anti-CD5 plus immuno-conjugate in rheumatoid arthritis: results of two phase II studies. *Arthritis Rheum* 1993; **36:** 620–30.
3. Skyler JS, *et al.* Effects of an anti-CD5 immunoconjugate (CD5-plus) in recent onset type I diabetes mellitus: a preliminary investigation. *J Diabetes Complications* 1993; **7:** 224–32.
4. Olsen NJ, *et al.* A double-blind, placebo-controlled study of anti-CD5 immunoconjugate in patients with rheumatoid arthritis. *Arthritis Rheum* 1996; **39:** 1102–8.

Zorubicin Hydrochloride (14032-n)

Zorubicin Hydrochloride *(USAN, rINNM)*.

NSC-164011; RP-22050 (zorubicin). Benzoic acid (2*S*-*cis*)-{1-[4-(3-amino-2,3,6-trideoxy-α-L-*lyxo*-hexopyranosyloxy)-1,2,3,4,6,11-hexahydro-2,5,12-trihydroxy-7-methoxy-6,11-dioxonaphthacen-2-yl]ethylidene}hydrazide hydrochloride.

$C_{34}H_{35}N_3O_{10}$,HCl = 682.1.

CAS — 54083-22-6 (zorubicin); 36508-71-1 (zorubicin hydrochloride).

Zorubicin is an anthracycline antibiotic with antineoplastic actions similar to those of doxorubicin (see p.529). It has been used as the hydrochloride in the treatment of acute leukaemias.

Preparations

Proprietary Preparations (details are given in Part 3)

Fr.: Rubidazone†.

Antiprotozoals

The drugs described in this chapter are those used primarily in the treatment of parasitic protozoal infections. In addition to their use as antiprotozoals, metronidazole and related nitroimidazole derivatives are also important in the treatment of anaerobic bacterial infections. Some veterinary antiprotozoal drugs are included. Drugs used in the treatment of malaria are described in the Antimalarials chapter; some of these are also used in other protozoal infections.

The principal antiprotozoal drugs are listed in Table 1, below.

Choice of Antiprotozoal

Protozoal infections occur throughout the world and are a major cause of morbidity and mortality in some regions. The choice of treatment for the more important protozoal diseases in humans is discussed below.

Amoebic infections

The most common amoebic infection of man is amoebiasis caused by infection with the protozoan parasite *Entamoeba histolytica* and related species. Free-living amoebae can also cause disease in man, though these infections are rare. Infection with *Naegleria fowleri* results in primary amoebic meningoencephalitis while infection with *Acanthamoeba* species or leptomyxid amoebae leads to granulomatous amoebic encephalitis. *Acanthamoeba* is also a cause of keratitis.

Acanthamoeba infections. ACANTHAMOEBA KERATITIS. *Acanthamoeba* keratitis is usually associated with the wearing of soft contact lenses. It is treated by surgical debridement of the damaged corneal epithelium and prompt topical antiamoebic therapy, although an optimum regimen has yet to be determined. The antiseptic propamidine isethionate applied topically is a mainstay of treatment, and has been used in various combinations with neomycin[1,2] or a neomycin-polymyxin-gramicidin preparation,[3,4] and/or a biguanide (usually polyhexanide[2,5,6] but chlorhexidine[7] has also been proposed). Combinations of systemic itraconazole or ketoconazole with topical miconazole have also been tried with some success.[4,8] Hexamidine isethionate has been suggested[9] as an alternative to propamidine isethionate. *Acanthamoeba* keratitis in contact lens wearers should be preventable by good lens hygiene (see p.1097). Disinfection regimens recommended for lens storage cases include soaking in very hot water (70° or more) and suitable hydrogen peroxide-based solutions.[10,11]

1. Wright P, *et al.* Acanthamoeba keratitis successfully treated medically. *Br J Ophthalmol* 1985; **69:** 778–82.
2. Varga JH, *et al.* Combined treatment of Acanthamoeba keratitis with propamidine, neomycin, and polyhexamethylene biguanide. *Am J Ophthalmol* 1993; **115:** 466–70.
3. Moore MB, McCulley JP. Acanthamoeba keratitis associated with contact lenses: six consecutive cases of successful management. *Br J Ophthalmol* 1989; **73:** 271–5.
4. Asbell PA, Torres MA. Therapeutic dilemmas in external ocular diseases. *Drugs* 1991; **42:** 606–15.
5. Illingworth CD, *et al.* Acanthamoeba keratitis: risk factors and outcome. *Br J Ophthalmol* 1995; **79:** 1078–82.
6. Elder MJ, Dart JKG. Chemotherapy for acanthamoeba keratitis. *Lancet* 1995; **345:** 791–2.
7. Seal DV, *et al.* Chlorhexidine or polyhexamethylene biguanide for acanthamoeba keratitis. *Lancet* 1995; **345:** 136.
8. Anonymous. Drugs for parasitic infections. *Med Lett Drugs Ther* 1998; **40:** 1–12.
9. Perrine D, *et al.* Amoebicidal efficiencies of various diamidines against two strains of Acanthamoeba polyphaga. *Antimicrob Agents Chemother* 1995; **39:** 339–42.
10. Radford CF, *et al.* Risk factors for acanthamoeba keratitis in contact lens users: a case-control study. *Br Med J* 1995; **310:** 1567–70.
11. Gray TB, *et al.* Acanthamoeba, bacterial, and fungal contamination of contact lens storage cases. *Br J Ophthalmol* 1995; **79:** 601–5.

DISSEMINATED ACANTHAMOEBA INFECTION. Granulomatous amoebic encephalitis (GAE) is caused by infection with free-living amoebae, usually *Acanthamoeba* spp. or sometimes leptomyxid amoebae. It is an opportunistic infection occurring mainly in debilitated or immunocompromised individuals. The protozoa spread to the CNS from pulmonary or skin lesions and produce focal neurological deficits that progress over days or weeks to a diffuse meningoencephalitis. The infection is usually fatal and most cases have been diagnosed at postmortem so little is known about effective treatments.

Clinical responses to chemotherapy have been reported in a few patients[1,2] with disseminated infection, but no evidence of CNS involvement. Disseminated *Acanthamoeba* infection in an immunocompromised patient was successfully treated with intravenous pentamidine followed by maintenance therapy with oral itraconazole.[1] Skin lesions were treated topically with chlorhexidine and ketoconazole. Clinical improvement was reported in disseminated acanthamoebiasis in a patient with AIDS following treatment with intravenous pentamidine and oral flucytosine, and in an infant with HIV infection treated with fluconazole, flucytosine, and sulphadiazine.[2]

1. Slater CA, *et al.* Brief report: successful treatment of disseminated Acanthamoeba infection in an immunocompromised patient. *N Engl J Med* 1994; **331:** 85–7.
2. Murakawa GJ, *et al.* Disseminated Acanthamoeba in patients with AIDS: a report of five cases and a review of the literature. *Arch Dermatol* 1995; **131:** 1291–6.

Table 1. Classification of principal antiprotozoals.

Arsenicals, trivalent	*Nitrofurans*
Melarsoprol	Furazolidone
	Nifuratel
Arsenicals, pentavalent	Nifurtimox
Acetarsol	
Tryparsamide	*5-Nitroimidazoles*
	Metronidazole
Aromatic diamidines	Nimorazole
Pentamidine	Ornidazole
Antimony compounds	Secnidazole
Meglumine antimonate	Tinidazole
Sodium stibogluconate	*Miscellaneous*
Dichloroacetamides	Atovaquone
Diloxanide	Benznidazole
	Dehydroemetine
Halogenated hydroxyquinolines	Eflornithine
Di-iodohydroxyquinoline	Mepacrine
	Suramin

Amoebiasis. The term amoebiasis is generally applied to infections with obligate parasitic species of amoeba, principally *Entamoeba histolytica*. Other parasitic species which occasionally cause human infections include *E. polecki* (primarily a parasite of pigs and reported mainly in Papua New Guinea) and *Dientamoeba fragilis* (often found in association with the helminth *Enterobius vermicularis* and now thought to be a trichomonad).

Transmission of *E. histolytica* is by the faeco-oral route and infection results from the ingestion of cysts, usually in contaminated food and drink. The cysts transform to trophozoites in the intestines and reproduction occurs by fission of the trophozoites. Further cysts develop and are excreted in the faeces. Amoebiasis occurs throughout the world. It is more prevalent and severe in the tropics and subtropics, but is more closely related to sanitation and socio-economic status than to climate. The majority of people infected with *E. histolytica* are asymptomatic cyst passers in whom trophozoites live as commensals in the large intestine. In others, the trophozoites invade the wall of the large intestine causing ulceration and may migrate to other tissues, especially the liver, where they continue to divide and destroy tissue. Factors increasing susceptibility to tissue invasion include malnutrition, immunosuppression, and pregnancy.

The WHO has classified symptomatic amoebiasis into intestinal or extra-intestinal amoebiasis.[1] Intestinal amoebiasis comprises two main states, amoebic dysentery and non-dysenteric amoebic colitis; amoeboma, a localised form of intestinal amoebiasis, and amoebic appendicitis may also occur. Hepatic amoebiasis, the most common form of extra-intestinal amoebic disease, may present as acute non-suppurative disease or as amoebic liver abscess. Amoebic infection is a less common cause of liver abscess than bacterial infection, the management of which is discussed on p.116. Amoebiasis may also involve the skin, genito-urinary tract, or organs such as the lungs and brain.

Drugs used in the **treatment** of amoebiasis may be classified according to their site of action as follows:

- *Luminal amoebicides* acting principally in the bowel lumen have included:
  - diloxanide furoate and other dichloroacetamide derivatives;
  - di-iodohydroxyquinoline and other halogenated hydroxyquinoline derivatives;
  - acetarsol and other arsenical derivatives.

  Diloxanide furoate is still widely used as the luminal amoebicide of choice. The arsenicals are toxic and are no longer used and, although some authorities still recommend di-iodohydroxyquinoline, most oral preparations of halogenated hydroxyquinolines have been withdrawn since the association between clioquinol and subacute myelo-opticoneuropathy (SMON) was established. The antibiotics paromomycin and tetracycline have also been used.
- *Tissue* or *systemic amoebicides* acting principally in the intestinal wall and liver include the alkaloid emetine, and its synthetic derivative dehydroemetine, and the antimalarial chloroquine which acts principally in the liver.
- *Mixed amoebicides* acting at all sites of infection, that is within the intestinal lumen and in the intestinal wall and other tissues, include metronidazole and other 5-nitroimidazole derivatives. However, because of their rapid absorption from the gastro-intestinal tract, the nitroimidazoles are less effective against parasites in the lumen.

In non-endemic areas, patients with asymptomatic intestinal amoebiasis (cyst passers) are generally treated with a luminal amoebicide. The choice of drug is influenced by availability; diloxanide furoate is generally used in the UK while di-iodohydroxyquinoline or paromomycin are used in the USA.[2] Invasive amoebiasis (amoebic dysentery; hepatic amoebiasis) requires treatment with a systemically absorbed amoebicide followed by a luminal amoebicide to eradicate any surviving organisms from the lumen of the large intestine and prevent relapse. Such treatment is generally with metronidazole or tinidazole followed by a luminal amoebicide. Other treatments that have been used in seriously ill patients are emetine or dehydroemetine, together with chloroquine in hepatic amoebiasis, followed by a luminal amoebicide.[3] Needle aspiration may be beneficial if there is a large liver abscess or if rupture of the abscess is imminent.[3] Tetracycline has been added to treatment regimens in severe amoebic dysentery.[3] In acute diarrhoea of any aetiology the priority is to maintain hydration by prevention or treatment of fluid and electrolyte depletion, especially in infants and the elderly. Oral rehydration therapy is discussed under Diarrhoea on p.1168.

Drugs suggested for the treatment of *Dientamoeba fragilis* infections include di-iodohydroxyquinoline, paromomycin, or tetracycline.[2] Metronidazole has been suggested for *E. polecki* infections.[2]

1. WHO. Amoebiasis. *WHO Tech Rep Ser 421* 1969.
2. Anonymous. Drugs for parasitic infections. *Med Lett Drugs Ther* 1998; **40:** 1–12.
3. Anonymous. Protozoan intestinal infections. *WHO Drug Inf* 1988; **2:** 200–5.

Naegleria infections. PRIMARY AMOEBIC MENINGOENCEPHALITIS. Primary amoebic meningoencephalitis (PAM) is usually caused by the free-living amoeba *Naegleria fowleri*. It occurs mainly in healthy children and young adults and is usually associated with swimming in warm fresh water. The protozoa invade the CNS directly through the nasal mucosa to produce a meningoencephalitis that is usually rapidly fatal. The few cases of successful treatment that have been reported[1-3] have all involved intravenous and usually intrathecal amphotericin; some patients were also given oral rifampicin.

1. Anderson K, Jamieson A. Primary amoebic meningoencephalitis. *Lancet* 1972; **i:** 902–3.
2. Seidel JS, *et al.* Successful treatment of primary amebic meningoencephalitis. *N Engl J Med* 1982; **306:** 346–8.
3. Brown RL. Successful treatment of primary amebic meningoencephalitis. *Arch Intern Med* 1991; **151:** 1201–2.

Babesiosis

Babesiosis (piroplasmosis) is a rare infection caused by protozoa of the *Babesia* spp., which are transmitted to man by the bite of infected *Ixodes* ticks. Transmission by blood transfusion has also been reported.

Infections in North America are commonly due to *B. microti* and though often asymptomatic may produce prolonged severe illness with fever and haemolytic anaemia, particularly in patients who are asplenic, elderly, debilitated, or immunocompromised. Co-infection with *B. microti* and *Borrelia burgdorferi* (Lyme disease) has resulted in more severe symptoms. In Europe infections are principally caused by *B. divergens* or *B. bovis* and have only been described in asplenic persons, in most of whom the infection was rapidly fatal. Clinical features include severe haemolytic anaemia, jaundice, and renal failure.

There is no established specific treatment for babesiosis. For serious infections, supportive therapies include blood transfusion and haemodialysis. Exchange transfusions have been used to reduce parasitaemia. A combination of clindamycin and quinine has been used[1-3] for the treatment of *B. microti* infections. Azithromycin in combination with quinine was reported to be effective in 1 patient who had not responded to quinine plus clindamycin.[4] In *B. divergens* infections, treatment is complicated by the rapid progression of the disease. A number of antiprotozoal and antimalarial drugs have been tried with limited success although a combination of pentamidine and co-trimoxazole was successful in 1 patient,[5] and a marked reduction in parasite load was seen in 1 patient treated with pentamidine in addition to exchange transfusions.[6] Pentamidine has also been reported to produce clinical improvement in patients with *B. microti* infection[7] but the efficacy and safety of pentamidine in this self-limiting disease has been questioned.[8]

1. Wittner M, *et al.* Successful chemotherapy of transfusion babesiosis. *Ann Intern Med* 1982; **96:** 601–4.
2. Anonymous. Clindamycin and quinine treatment for Babesia microti infections. *MMWR* 1983; **32:** 65–6,72.
3. Anonymous. Drugs for parasitic infections. *Med Lett Drugs Ther* 1998; **40:** 1–12.
4. Shaio MF, Yang KD. Response of babesiosis to a combined regimen of quinine and azithromycin. *Trans R Soc Trop Med Hyg* 1997; **91:** 214–15.
5. Raoult D, *et al.* Babesiosis, pentamidine, and cotrimoxazole. *Ann Intern Med* 1987; **107:** 944.
6. Clarke CS, *et al.* Babesiosis: under-reporting or case-clustering? *Postgrad Med J* 1989; **65:** 591–3.
7. Francioli PB, *et al.* Response of babesiosis to pentamidine therapy. *Ann Intern Med* 1981; **94:** 326–30.
8. Teutsch SM, Juranek DD. Babesiosis. *Ann Intern Med* 1981; **95:** 241.

Balantidiasis

Infection with the ciliate protozoan *Balantidium coli* results from the ingestion of cysts, the commonest source of which is pigs.[1] Water-borne epidemics of balantidiasis have been reported. Most infections are asymptomatic and the organism lives in the large intestine as a luminal commensal, but those with symptomatic infections have diarrhoea. Colonic ulceration resulting in a severe dysenteric syndrome resembling amoebic dysentery may occur in some individuals, especially those who are malnourished. Treatment is with tetracycline; metronidazole or di-iodohydroxyquinoline are alternatives.[1]

1. Anonymous. Drugs for parasitic infections. *Med Lett Drugs Ther* 1998; **40:** 1–12.

Blastocystis hominis infection

There is controversy over whether the protozoan parasite *Blastocystis hominis* is a pathogen or a harmless commensal of the intestinal tract. It has increasingly been reported both in immunocompetent and immunocompromised subjects,[1] with transmission probably by the faeco-oral route. Symptoms ascribed to infection with the organism include diarrhoea and other gastro-intestinal symptoms.

Treatment is with standard antiprotozoals, especially metronidazole, but with variable success. Co-trimoxazole has been reported to eliminate *B. hominis* from the stools of all but 1 of a group of 47 otherwise healthy subjects with diarrhoea.[2]

1. Anonymous. Blastocystis hominis: commensal or pathogen? *Lancet* 1991; **337:** 521–2.
2. Schwartz E, Houston R. Effect of co-trimoxazole on stool recovery of Blastocystis hominis. *Lancet* 1992; **339:** 428–9.

Coccidiosis

Coccidiosis is a term sometimes applied to infections with protozoa of the order *Eucoccidiorida*. The predominant coccidian infections in man are caused by *Cryptosporidium* (see below), *Cyclospora cayetanensis* (see p.574), *Isospora* (see p.575), *Plasmodium* (see p.422), and *Toxoplasma* (see p.576). Coccidian protozoa, primarily *Eimeria*, cause economically important infections in domesticated animals.

Cryptosporidiosis

Cryptosporidiosis is a gastro-intestinal infection caused by species of the coccidian protozoan parasite *Cryptosporidium*. It has a worldwide distribution and occurs in many animal species as well as in man. Infection is acquired through ingestion, and perhaps inhalation, of oocysts. Infection in immunocompetent individuals usually causes a self-limiting diarrhoea lasting up to 2 weeks. In immunocompromised patients there may be profuse and persistent diarrhoea, profound weight loss, and severe abdominal pain, and the infection may be life-threatening. Crytosporidiosis is increasingly recognised as a cause of diarrhoea in patients with AIDS. Other sites of infection include the respiratory and biliary tracts.

There is currently no consistently effective specific therapy and priority should be given to maintaining hydration by prevention or treatment of fluid and electrolyte depletion, especially in infants and the elderly. Oral rehydration therapy is discussed under Diarrhoea on p.1168. Responses to paromomycin have generally been favourable, although patient numbers are small.[1-8] There have also been reports indicating improvement in immunocompromised patients given azithromycin,[9,10] hyperimmune bovine colostrum,[11-14] eflornithine,[15] normal immunoglobulin with high cryptosporidium antibody titres,[16] or letrazuril,[17,18] but again the numbers of patients involved are small. Nitazoxanide may also be effective. Responses to spiramycin have not been consistent.[19-21] Beneficial responses to octreotide have been reported in a few cases,[22,23] but a study in patients with refractory AIDS-related diarrhoea suggested that response was better in patients without identifiable pathogens.[24]

Clarithromycin and rifabutin may be useful for disease prophylaxis.[25]

1. Clezy K, *et al.* Paromomycin for the treatment of cryptosporidial diarrhoea in AIDS patients. *AIDS* 1991; **5:** 1146–7.
2. Armitage K, *et al.* Treatment of cryptosporidiosis with paromomycin: a report of five cases. *Arch Intern Med* 1992; **152:** 2497–9.
3. Danziger LH, *et al.* Treatment of cryptosporidial diarrhea in an AIDS patient with paromomycin. *Ann Pharmacother* 1993; **27:** 1460–2.
4. Fichtenbaum CJ, *et al.* Use of paromomycin for treatment of cryptosporidiosis in patients with AIDS. *Clin Infect Dis* 1993; **16:** 298–300.
5. White AC, *et al.* Paromomycin for cryptosporidiosis in AIDS: a prospective, double-blind trial. *J Infect Dis* 1994; **170:** 419–24.
6. Bissuel F, *et al.* Paromomycin: an effective treatment for cryptosporidial diarrhea in patients with AIDS. *Clin Infect Dis* 1994; **18:** 447–9.
7. Mohri H, *et al.* Case report: inhalation therapy of paromomycin is effective for respiratory infection and hypoxia by Cryptosporidium with AIDS. *Am J Med Sci* 1995; **309:** 60–2.
8. Flanigan TP, *et al.* Prospective trial of paromomycin for cryptosporidiosis in AIDS. *Am J Med* 1996; **100:** 370–2.
9. Vargas SL, *et al.* Azithromycin for treatment of severe Cryptosporidium diarrhea in two children with cancer. *J Pediatr* 1993; **123:** 154–6.
10. Bessette RE, Amsden GW. Treatment of non-HIV cryptosporidial diarrhea with azithromycin. *Ann Pharmacother* 1995; **29:** 991–3.
11. Tzipori S, *et al.* Remission of diarrhoea due to cryptosporidiosis in an immunodeficient child treated with hyperimmune bovine colostrum. *Br Med J* 1986; **293:** 1276–7.
12. Tzipori S, *et al.* Chronic cryptosporidial diarrhoea and hyperimmune cow colostrum. *Lancet* 1987; **ii:** 344–5.
13. Nord J, *et al.* Treatment with bovine hyperimmune colostrum of cryptosporidial diarrhea in AIDS patients. *AIDS* 1990; **4:** 581–4.
14. Shield J, *et al.* Bovine colostrum immunoglobulin concentrate for cryptosporidiosis in AIDS. *Arch Dis Child* 1993; **69:** 451–3.
15. Rolston KVI, *et al.* Intestinal crytosporidiosis treated with eflornithine: a prospective study among patients with AIDS. *J Acquir Immune Defic Syndr* 1989; **2:** 426–30.
16. Borowitz SM, Saulsbury FT. Treatment of chronic cryptosporidial infection with orally administered human serum immune globulin. *J Pediatr* 1991; **119:** 593–5.
17. Harris M, *et al.* A phase I study of letrazuril in AIDS-related cryptosporidiosis. *AIDS* 1994; **8:** 1109–13.
18. Loeb M, *et al.* Treatment with letrazuril of refractory cryptosporidial diarrhea complicating AIDS. *J Acquir Immune Defic Syndr Hum Retrovirol* 1995; **10:** 48–53.
19. Portnoy D, *et al.* Treatment of intestinal cryptosporidiosis with spiramycin. *Ann Intern Med* 1984; **101:** 202–4.
20. Moskovitz BL, *et al.* Spiramycin therapy for cryptosporidial diarrhoea in immunocompromised patients. *J Antimicrob Chemother* 1988; **22** (suppl B): 189–91.
21. Wittenberg DF, *et al.* Spiramycin is not effective in treating cryptosporidium diarrhea in infants: results of a double-blind randomized trial. *J Infect Dis* 1989; **159:** 131–2.
22. Cook DJ, *et al.* Somatostatin treatment for cryptosporidial diarrhea in a patient with the acquired immunodeficiency syndrome (AIDS). *Ann Intern Med* 1988; **108:** 708–9.
23. Clotet B, *et al.* Efficacy of the somatostatin analogue (SMS-201-995), Sandostatin, for cryptosporidial diarrhoea in patients with AIDS. *AIDS* 1989; **3:** 857–8.
24. Cello JP, *et al.* Effect of octreotide on refractory AIDS-associated diarrhea: a prospective, multicenter clinical trial. *Ann Intern Med* 1991; **115:** 705–10.
25. Holmberg SD, *et al.* Possible effectiveness of clarithromycin and rifabutin for cryptosporidiosis chemoprophylaxis in HIV disease. *JAMA* 1998; **279:** 384–6.

Cyclosporiasis

An organism originally described as cyanobacterium-like or coccidian-like bodies (CLB), but recently identified as the coccidian protozoan *Cyclospora cayetanensis* has been reported to be a cause of diarrhoea in both immunodeficient and immunocompetent patients. Infection results from ingestion of spores or oocysts in contaminated food or water. In immunocompetent patients, infection may be asymptomatic or cause a self-limiting diarrhoeal illness. Immunocompromised patients may develop severe or persistent symptoms. Beneficial responses have been reported in patients treated with co-trimoxazole.[1-3]

1. Pape JW, *et al.* Cyclospora infection in adults infected with HIV: clinical manifestations, treatment, and prophylaxis. *Ann Intern Med* 1994; **121:** 654–7.
2. Hoge CW, *et al.* Placebo-controlled trial of co-trimoxazole for cyclospora infections among travellers and foreign residents in Nepal. *Lancet* 1995; **345:** 691–3. Correction. *ibid.;* 1060.
3. Goodgame RW. Understanding intestinal spore-forming protozoa: cryptosporidia, microsporidia, isospora and cyclospora. *Ann Intern Med* 1996; **124:** 429–41.

Gastro-enteritis

Although bacteria and viruses are responsible for many cases of infective diarrhoea, protozoal infections are being increasingly recognised as a cause of diarrhoea, which can be severe especially in immunocompromised patients, including those with AIDS. In acute diarrhoea of any aetiology the priority is to maintain hydration by prevention or treatment of fluid and electrolyte depletion, especially in infants and the elderly. Oral rehydration is discussed under Diarrhoea on p.1168. Specific therapy with antiprotozoals may also be necessary to control enteric protozoal infections. For the management of the protozoal infections that are generally associated with diarrhoea see under amoebiasis (p.573), balantidiasis (p.574), *Blastocystis hominis* infections (p.574), cryptosporidiosis (p.574), cyclosporiasis (above), giardiasis (below), isosporiasis (p.575), and microsporidiosis (p.576).

References.

1. Guerrant RL, Bobak DA. Bacterial and protozoal gastroenteritis. *N Engl J Med* 1991; **325:** 327–40.
2. Goodgame RW. Diagnosis and treatment of gastrointestinal protozoal infections. *Curr Opin Infect Dis* 1996; **9:** 346–52.

Giardiasis

Infection with *Giardia intestinalis* (*G. lamblia*; *Lamblia intestinalis*) occurs throughout the world and is one of the commonest intestinal protozoal infections. Infection is acquired by oral ingestion of *Giardia* cysts, and transmission may be person-to-person or from contaminated drinking water or foodstuffs. Cysts are transformed in the small intestine to trophozoites which become attached to the intestinal mucosa. The trophozoites divide by binary fission, undergo encystment in the gut lumen, and are excreted in the faeces. Infected patients may have acute or chronic diarrhoea or they may be asymptomatic. In acute diarrhoea of any aetiology the priority is to maintain hydration by prevention or treatment of fluid and electrolyte depletion, especially in infants and the elderly. Oral rehydration is discussed under Diarrhoea on p.1168.

Treatment is with metronidazole or another nitroimidazole derivative. Mepacrine and furazolidone have been used but may be less well tolerated. Paromomycin has also been suggested;[1] although it is less effective than other drugs, it is not absorbed systemically and may be a useful alternative during pregnancy. Mebendazole[2] or albendazole[3] have produced beneficial results in children. Treatment may sometimes need to be repeated, possibly due to resistance,[4,5] and drug combinations such as metronidazole with mepacrine have been reported to be of value in these cases.[4]

1. Anonymous. Drugs for parasitic infections. *Med Lett Drugs Ther* 1998; **40:** 1–12.
2. Al-Waili, NSD, Hassan NU. Mebendazole in giardial infection: a comparative study with metronidazole. *J Infect Dis* 1992; **165:** 1170–1.
3. Hall A, Nahar Q. Albendazole as a treatment for infections with Giardia duodenalis in children in Bangladesh. *Trans R Soc Trop Med Hyg* 1993; **87:** 84–6.
4. Farthing MJG. Giardia comes of age: progress in epidemiology, immunology and chemotherapy. *J Antimicrob Chemother* 1992; **30:** 563–6.
5. Boreham PFL. Giardiasis and its control. *Pharm J* 1991; **247:** 271–4.

Infections in immunocompromised patients

Patients with a defective immune system are at especial risk of infection. Primary immune deficiency is rare, whereas secondary deficiency is more common: immunosuppressive therapy, cancer and its treatment, HIV infection, and splenectomy may all cause neutropenia and impaired humoral and cellular immunity in varying degrees. The risk of infection is linked to the duration and severity of neutropenia. Most protozoal infections present in a more severe form in immunocompromised patients than in immunocompetent patients. Those of particular concern in patients with HIV infection include cryptosporidiosis (above), isosporiasis (below), leishmaniasis (p.575), microsporidiosis (p.576), and toxoplasmosis (p.576).

References.

1. Canning EU. Protozoan infections. *Trans R Soc Trop Med Hyg* 1990; **84** (suppl 1): 19–24.
2. Wilson ME, *et al.* Infections in HIV-infected travelers: risks and prevention. *Ann Intern Med* 1991; **114:** 582–92.
3. Sharpstone D, Gazzard B. Gastrointestinal manifestations of HIV infection. *Lancet* 1996; **348:** 378–83.
4. Centers for Disease Control. 1997 USPHS/IDSA guidelines for the prevention of opportunistic infections in persons infected with human immunodeficiency virus. *MMWR* 1997; **46** (RR-12): 1–46.

Isosporiasis

Isosporiasis is a coccidian protozoal infection of the gastro-intestinal tract caused by *Isospora belli*. Oocysts are excreted in faeces and infection is acquired when sporulated oocysts are ingested. In immunocompetent individuals the infection is usually mild and self-limiting but in immunocompromised patients there may be severe, chronic gastro-enteritis. Treatment is usually with co-trimoxazole.[1,2] Pyrimethamine has been used successfully in individual patients with sulphonamide sensitivity.[3] In acute diarrhoea of any aetiology the priority is to maintain hydration by prevention or treatment of fluid and electrolyte depletion, especially in infants and the elderly. Oral rehydration therapy is discussed under Diarrhoea on p.1168.

Recurrence of infection is common and long-term suppressive treatment with either co-trimoxazole or pyrimethamine plus sulfadoxine has been recommended.[4]

1. WHO. *WHO model prescribing information: drugs used in parasitic diseases*. Geneva: WHO, 1995.
2. Anonymous. Drugs for parasitic infections. *Med Lett Drugs Ther* 1998; **40:** 1–12.
3. Weiss LM, *et al.* Isospora belli infection: treatment with pyrimethamine. *Ann Intern Med* 1988; **109:** 474–5.
4. Pape JW, *et al.* Treatment and prophylaxis of Isospora belli infection in patients with the acquired immunodeficiency syndrome. *N Engl J Med* 1989; **320:** 1044–7.

Leishmaniasis

Leishmaniasis is caused by parasitic protozoa of the genus *Leishmania*. It occurs throughout Africa, the Middle East, Central Asia, and the Mediterranean (Old World leishmaniasis), and throughout Central and South America (New World leishmaniasis). In endemic areas there is generally a reservoir of disease in a mammalian host, often dogs or rodents. The usual vectors are sandflies of the genus *Phlebotomus* in the Old World and *Lutzomyia* in the New World. Leishmaniasis can be categorised as cutaneous, mucosal, and visceral and ranges from self-limiting, localised, cutaneous ulcers to widely disseminated progressive disease and involvement of the reticuloendothelial system. Incubation periods can be prolonged, with clinical features not appearing until several months or even years after the primary infection.

In endemic areas an intergrated approach to controlling leishmaniasis involves case detection and treatment of patients, vector and animal reservoir control, environmental management to reduce suitable vector habitats, and personal protection against sandfly bites including the use of insect repellents and bednets.[1] Strategies aimed at controlling malaria are believed to have reduced leishmaniasis transmission dramatically.[1]

Visceral leishmaniasis of the Old World is mainly caused by *L. donovani* and *L. infantum* and of the New World by *L. chagasi*. The onset of the disease is gradual in residents of an endemic area but may present as an acute illness in non-immune visitors to the region. Many infections result in sub-clinical or self-limiting disease. Common symptoms are fever, malaise, shivering or chills, weight loss, anorexia, and discomfort in the left hypochondrium. Common clinical signs are non-tender splenomegaly with or without hepatomegaly, wasting, pallor of mucous membranes, anaemia, leucopenia, and lymphadenopathy. Continued deterioration can lead to potentially fatal secondary infection. Darkening of the skin of the face, hands, feet, and abdomen is common in endemic visceral leishmaniasis in India (kala-azar = black sickness). Rare complications can include severe acute haemolytic anaemia, acute renal damage, and severe mucosal haemorrhage. In recent years, visceral leishmaniasis has emerged as an opportunistic infection in patients with HIV or other conditions associated with reduced immunity, in whom it is particularly difficult to treat.

A small percentage of patients develop post-kala-azar dermal leishmaniasis (PKDL) following recovery from visceral leishmaniasis and such patients represent a human reservoir for the disease.

The pentavalent antimonials meglumine antimonate and sodium stibogluconate are the traditional first-line drugs for the treatment of visceral leishmaniasis.[1] Patients relapsing after the initial course of treatment may be given a further course, but there is growing evidence that responsiveness to the antimonials is declining. Four regimens have been suggested for the first-line treatment of visceral leishmaniasis due to *L. infantum* in Mediterranean countries.[2] They are: pentavalent antimonials, pentavalent antimonials plus allopurinol, liposomal amphotericin, and paromomycin alone or in combination with pentavalent antimonials. These regimens are also being evaluated in other regions and in patients with HIV infection.[3-12] Amphotericin has also been tried successfully as a second-line drug in drug-resistant infections.[13-16] Lipid complex and other non-conventional forms of amphotericin are better tolerated than conventional amphotericin, and are likely to become a useful alternative to pentavalent antimonials. Pentamidine has also been used as a second-line drug but its usefulness as alternative first-line therapy is doubtful[17] due to its toxicity, increasing failure rates, and slow disease response. Nevertheless it has been tried as an adjunct to meglumine antimonate for first-line therapy[18] and alone for long-term secondary prophylaxis in patients with HIV infection.[19] In view of the toxicity of both first- and second-line drugs and the number of treatment failures the search for alternative therapies continues. Beneficial responses to ketoconazole have been reported in some patients[20,21] but unfavourable reports have also appeared.[22,23] Another line of investigation is to boost the immune response to the parasite by adding interferon gamma to conventional treatment.[24-26]

Cutaneous leishmaniasis is caused by various species of *Leishmania* and a wide variety of clinical presentations is possible. A 'classical' lesion starts as a nodule at the site of inoculation. A crust develops centrally which may fall away exposing an ulcer which heals gradually. Satellite nodules at the edge of the lesion are common. Cutaneous leishmaniasis of the Old World is normally caused by *L. tropica*, *L. major*, or *L. aethiopica*, although cutaneous lesions due to *L. infantum* have been reported. Cutaneous leishmaniasis of the New World (American cutaneous leishmaniasis) is caused by numerous species and subspecies of *Leishmania* including *L. braziliensis*, *L. mexicana*, *L. panamensis*, and *L. peruviana*. In general New World forms tend to be more severe and longer lasting than Old World forms. The disease ranges from single, self-healing lesions which are troublesome and unsightly but not a threat to life to multiple, deep, and destructive ulcers which cause considerable disfigurement and disability.

Diffuse cutaneous leishmaniasis occurs occasionally following infection with *L. aethiopica* or members of the *L. mexicana* complex and involves dissemination of the disease from the original site of infection to distant skin sites, typically the face and exterior surfaces of the limbs. The lesions resemble lepromatous leprosy, do not heal spontaneously, and are resistant to treatment.

Another variant is leishmaniasis recidivans which is a lupoid or tuberculoid form. This chronic disease often occurs as slowly progressive, destructive and disfiguring lesions on the face which are very resistant to most forms of therapy.

There is no established treatment for cutaneous leishmaniasis. The decision to treat depends upon the site and extent of the lesions and the likelihood of dissemination. Small lesions, particularly in Old World cutaneous leishmaniasis, may be left untreated if they are not troublesome to the patient. Treatment for disfiguring or potentially disabling lesions may be local or systemic. Systemic treatment is required where there is a risk that the infecting organism may be one causing mucocutaneous leishmaniasis (see below) or where there is evidence of lymphatic spread or extensive local involvement. WHO[1] suggested that early noninflamed nodular lesions due to *L. tropica*, *L. major*, *L. mexicana*, *L. panamensis*, or *L. peruviana* may be treated with intralesional injections of mepacrine, sodium stibogluconate, or meglumine antimonate or removed by surgery and curettage. Beneficial responses have been reported with this therapy.[27,28] However, local infiltration of drugs can be difficult as well as painful. Surgical curettage may promote dissemination of the parasite.[29] Other local treatments include application of heat to bring the temperature of the lesion to about 40° which may aid healing.[30] Topical treatment with paromomycin sulphate 15% plus methylbenzethonium chloride 5% or 12% has produced promising responses;[31,32] paromomycin 12 to 15% with urea 10% was better tolerated.[33] However, not all studies have shown beneficial responses.[34,35] Systemic treatment is similar to that used for visceral leishmaniasis[1,36,37] (see above). Treatment with topical paromomycin plus systemic meglumine antimonate was promising in patients with New World infections.[38] Cutaneous leishmaniasis due to *L. aethiopica* including diffuse cutaneous leishmaniasis does not generally respond to antimonials[1] although responses to antimonials in combination with paromomycin have been reported.[39] It may also be treated with pentamidine.[1] Other drugs tried in cutaneous leishmaniasis have included berberine derivatives,[40] itraconazole,[41-43] and ketoconazole.[44-47] Variable responses to allopurinol have been reported in patients with New World infections.[48-50] Dapsone was reported to be effective in a study in patients in India[51] but not in Colombia.[52] Among the non-specific therapies tried in cutaneous leishmaniasis, topical application of the nitric oxide donor S-nitroso-N-acetylpenicillamine (SNAP)[53] and intralesional injection of hypertonic sodium chloride solution[54] have produced beneficial responses. Immunomodulation using leishmania antigens mixed with BCG,[55,56] interferon gamma,[57,58] or interleukin-2[59] has produced encouraging results.

While there has been some work on vaccines against cutaneous leishmaniasis much more needs to be done. However, leishmanisation (deliberate infection with *L. major*) has been used as a last resort in some countries when other measures have failed.

Mucocutaneous leishmaniasis of the New World (espundia) is caused by *L. braziliensis* or *L. panamensis*. In mucocutaneous leishmaniasis the primary lesions do not heal spontaneously. Metastatic spread to the mucosa may occur during the presence of the primary lesion or up to 30 years later. The nasal mucosa is always affected. Ulceration and erosion progressively destroy the soft tissue and cartilage of the oronasal/pharyngeal cavity. Mutilation is severe and secondary bacterial infection is frequent and can be fatal. Mucocutaneous leishmaniasis responds poorly to treatment and relapses are common. Initial treatment is with pentavalent antimony; failure to respond is an indication to use amphotericin or pentamidine. Nifurtimox has been reported to be effective in some cases of mucocutaneous leishmaniasis.[1] Treatment with corticosteroids may be required to control severe inflammation. Mucosal disease in Old World leishmaniasis is much less common than visceral or cutaneous forms, but treatment with antimony compounds or ketoconazole has been described.[60]

1. WHO. Control of the leishmaniases. *WHO Tech Rep Ser 793* 1990.
2. Gradoni L, *et al.* Treatment of Mediterranean visceral leishmaniasis. *Bull WHO* 1995; **73:** 191–7.
3. Mishra M, *et al.* Amphotericin versus sodium stibogluconate in first-line treatment of Indian Kala-azar. *Lancet* 1994; **344:** 1599–1600.
4. Dietze R, *et al.* Treatment of kala-azar in Brazil with Amphocil (amphotericin B cholesterol dispersion) for 5 days. *Trans R Soc Trop Med Hyg* 1995; **89:** 309–11.
5. Russo R, *et al.* Visceral leishmaniasis in HIV infected patients: treatment with high dose liposomal amphotericin B (AmBisome). *J Infect* 1996; **32:** 133–7.
6. Thakur CP, *et al.* Aminosidine plus sodium stibogluconate for the treatment of Indian kala-azar: a randomized dose-finding clinical trial. *Trans R Soc Trop Med Hyg* 1995; **89:** 219–23.
7. Scott JAG, *et al.* Aminosidine (paromomycin) in the treatment of leishmaniasis imported into the United Kingdom. *Trans R Soc Trop Med Hyg* 1992; **86:** 617–19.
8. Chunge CN, *et al.* Visceral leishmaniasis unresponsive to antimonial drugs III: successful treatment using a combination of sodium stibogluconate plus allopurinol. *Trans R Soc Trop Med Hyg* 1985; **79:** 715–18.
9. Dellamonica P, *et al.* Allopurinol for treatment of visceral leishmaniasis in patients with AIDS. *J Infect Dis* 1989; **160:** 904–5.
10. Laguna F, *et al.* Assessment of allopurinol plus meglumine antimoniate in the treatment of visceral leishmaniasis in patients infected with HIV. *J Infect* 1994; **28:** 255–9.
11. Sundar S, *et al.* Short-course, low-dose amphotericin B lipid complex therapy for visceral leishmaniasis unresponsive to antimony. *Ann Intern Med* 1997; **127:** 133–7.
12. Jha TK, *et al.* Randomised controlled trial of aminosidine (paromomycin) v sodium stibogluconate for treating visceral leishmaniasis in North Bihar, India. *Br Med J* 1998; **316:** 1200–5.
13. Davidson RN, *et al.* Liposomal amphotericin B in drug-resistant visceral leishmaniasis. *Lancet* 1991; **337:** 1061–2.
14. Mishra M, *et al.* Amphotericin versus pentamidine in antimony-unresponsive kala-azar. *Lancet* 1992; **340:** 1256–7.
15. Jha TK, *et al.* Use of amphotericin B in drug-resistant cases of visceral leishmaniasis in North Bihar, India. *Am J Trop Med Hyg* 1995; **52:** 536–8.
16. Sundar S, *et al.* Cure of antimony-unresponsive Indian visceral leishmaniasis with amphotericin B liquid complex. *J Infect Dis* 1996; **173:** 762–5.
17. Baily GG, Nandy A. Visceral leishmaniasis: more prevalent and more problematic. *J Infect* 1994; **29:** 241–7.
18. Özsoylu S. Treatment of kala azar. *Lancet* 1996; **347:** 1701.
19. Pérez-Molina JA, *et al.* Pentamidine isethionate as secondary prophylaxis against visceral leishmaniasis in HIV-positive patients. *AIDS* 1996; **10:** 237–8.
20. Wali JP, *et al.* Ketoconazole in treatment of visceral leishmaniasis. *Lancet* 1990; **336:** 810–11.
21. Wali JP, *et al.* Ketoconazole in the treatment of antimony- and pentamidine-resistant kala-azar. *J Infect Dis* 1992; **166:** 215–16.
22. Sundar S, *et al.* Ketoconazole in visceral leishmaniasis. *Lancet* 1990; **336:** 1582–3.
23. Rashid JR, *et al.* The efficacy and safety of ketoconazole in visceral leishmaniasis. *East Afr Med J* 1994; **71:** 392–5.
24. Badaro R, *et al.* Treatment of visceral leishmaniasis with pentavalent antimony and interferon gamma. *N Engl J Med* 1990; **322:** 16–21.
25. Sundar S, *et al.* Successful treatment of refractory visceral leishmaniasis in India using antimony plus interferon-γ. *J Infect Dis* 1994; **170:** 659–62.
26. Sundar S, *et al.* Immunochemotherapy for a systemic intracellular infection: accelerated response using interferon-γ in visceral leishmaniasis. *J Infect Dis* 1995; **171:** 992–6.
27. Alkhawajah AM, *et al.* Treatment of cutaneous leishmaniasis with antimony: intramuscular versus intralesional administration. *Ann Trop Med Parasitol* 1997; **91:** 899–905.
28. Aste N, *et al.* Intralesional treatment of cutaneous leishmaniasis with meglumine antimoniate. *Br J Dermatol* 1998; **138:** 370–1.
29. Moss JT, Wilson JP. Current treatment recommendations for leishmaniasis. *Ann Pharmacother* 1992; **26:** 1452–5.
30. Navin TR, *et al.* Placebo-controlled clinical trial of meglumine antimonate (Glucantime) vs localized controlled heat in the treatment of cutaneous leishmaniasis in Guatemala. *Am J Trop Med Hyg* 1990; **42:** 43–50.
31. El-On J, *et al.* Topical treatment of Old World cutaneous leishmaniasis caused by Leishmania major: a double-blind control study. *J Am Acad Dermatol* 1992; **27:** 227–31.
32. Krause G, Kroeger A. Topical treatment of American cutaneous leishmaniasis with paromomycin and methylbenzethonium chloride: a clinical study under field conditions in Ecuador. *Trans R Soc Trop Med Hyg* 1994; **88:** 92–4.
33. Bryceson ADM, *et al.* Treatment of Old World cutaneous leishmaniasis with aminosidine ointment: results of an open study in London. *Trans R Soc Trop Med Hyg* 1994; **88:** 226–8.
34. Ben Salah A, *et al.* A randomized, placebo-controlled trial in Tunisia treating cutaneous leishmaniasis with paromomycin ointment. *Am J Trop Med Hyg* 1995; **53:** 162–6.
35. Asilian A, *et al.* A randomized, placebo-controlled trial of a two week regimen of aminosidine (paromomycin) ointment for treatment of cutaneous leishmaniasis in Iran. *Am J Trop Med Hyg* 1995; **53:** 648–51.
36. Soto J, *et al.* Limited efficacy of injectable aminosidine as single-agent therapy for Colombian cutaneous leishmaniasis. *Trans R Soc Trop Med Hyg* 1994; **88:** 695–8.
37. Hepburn NC, *et al.* Aminosidine (paromomycin) versus sodium stibogluconate for the treatment of American Cutaneous leishmaniasis. *Trans R Soc Trop Med Hyg* 1994; **88:** 700–3.
38. Soto J, *et al.* Successful treatment of New World cutaneous leishmaniasis with a combination of topical paromomycin/methylbenzethonium chloride and injectable meglumine antimonate. *Clin Infect Dis* 1995; **20:** 47–51.
39. Teklemariam S, *et al.* Aminosidine and its combination with sodium stibogluconate in the treatment of diffuse cutaneous leishmaniasis caused by Leishmania aethiopica. *Trans R Soc Trop Med Hyg* 1994; **88:** 334–9.
40. Vennerstrom JL, *et al.* Berberine derivatives as antileishmanial drugs. *Antimicrob Agents Chemother* 1990; **34:** 918–21.
41. Albanese G, *et al.* Cutaneous leishmaniasis: treatment with itraconazole. *Arch Dermatol* 1989; **125:** 1540–2.
42. Pialoux G, *et al.* Cutaneous leishmaniasis in an AIDS patient: cure with itraconazole. *J Infect Dis* 1990; **162:** 1221–2.
43. Akuffo H, *et al.* The use of itraconazole in the treatment of leishmaniasis caused by Leishmania aethiopica. *Trans R Soc Trop Med Hyg* 1990; **84:** 532–4.
44. Dedet J-P, *et al.* Failure to cure Leishmania braziliensis guyanensis cutaneous leishmaniasis with oral ketoconazole. *Trans R Soc Trop Med Hyg* 1986; **80:** 176.
45. Weinrauch L, *et al.* Ketoconazole in cutaneous leishmaniasis. *Br J Dermatol* 1987; **117:** 666–7.
46. Saenz RE, *et al.* Efficacy of ketoconazole against Leishmania braziliensis panamensis cutaneous leishmaniasis. *Am J Med* 1990; **89:** 147–55.
47. Navin TR, *et al.* Placebo-controlled clinical trial of sodium stibogluconate (Pentostam) versus ketoconazole for treating cutaneous leishmaniasis in Guatemala. *J Infect Dis* 1992; **165:** 528–34.
48. Martinez S, Marr JJ. Allopurinol in the treatment of American cutaneous leishmaniasis. *N Engl J Med* 1992; **326:** 741–4.
49. Velez I, *et al.* Inefficacy of allopurinol as monotherapy for Colombian cutaneous leishmaniasis: a randomized, controlled trial. *Ann Intern Med* 1997; **126:** 232–6.
50. Martinez S, *et al.* Treatment of cutaneous leishmaniasis with allopurinol and stibogluconate. *Clin Infect Dis* 1997; **24:** 165–9.
51. Dogra J. A double-blind study on the efficacy of oral dapsone in cutaneous leishmaniasis. *Trans R Soc Trop Med Hyg* 1991; **85:** 212–13.
52. Osorio LE, *et al.* Treatment of cutaneous leishmaniasis in Colombia with dapsone. *Lancet* 1998; **351:** 498–9.
53. López-Jaramillo P, *et al.* Treatment of cutaneous leishmaniasis with nitric-oxide donor. *Lancet* 1998; **351:** 1176–7.
54. Sharquie KE. A new intralesional therapy of cutaneous leishmaniasis with hypertonic sodium chloride solution. *J Dermatol* 1995; **22:** 732–7.
55. Convit J, *et al.* Immunotherapy of localized, intermediate, and diffuse forms of American cutaneous leishmaniasis. *J Infect Dis* 1989; **160:** 104–15.
56. Sharifi I, *et al.* Randomised vaccine trial of single dose of killed Leishmania major plus BCG against anthroponotic cutaneous leishmaniasis in Bam, Iran. *Lancet* 1998; **351:** 1540–3.
57. Harms G, *et al.* A randomized trial comparing a pentavalent antimonial drug and recombinant interferon-γ in the local treatment of cutaneous leishmaniasis. *Trans R Soc Trop Med Hyg* 1991; **85:** 214–16.
58. Falcoff E, *et al.* Clinical healing of antimony-resistant cutaneous or mucocutaneous leishmaniasis following the combined administration of interferon-γ and pentavalent antimonial compounds. *Trans R Soc Trop Med Hyg* 1994; **88:** 95–7.
59. Akuffo H, *et al.* Administration of recombinant interleukin-2 reduces the local parasite load of patients with disseminated cutaneous leishmaniasis. *J Infect Dis* 1990; **161:** 775–80.
60. El-Hassan AM, *et al.* Sudanese mucosal leishmaniasis: epidemiology, clinical features, diagnosis, immune responses and treatment. *Trans R Soc Trop Med Hyg* 1995; **89:** 647–52.

Malaria

For a discussion of malaria, its prophylaxis and treatment, see p.422.

Microsporidiosis

Microsporidia are obligate intracellular spore-forming protozoal parasites. They were primarily regarded as a cause of disease in nonhuman species, but *Encephalitozoon*, *Enterocytozoon*, *Nosema*, *Pleistophora*, and *Septata* spp. are now recognised as human pathogens.[1,2] Transmission is believed to be predominantly faeco-oral although inhalation and direct inoculation also occur. Infections usually occur in immunocompromised patients. Small bowel infection with *Enterocytozoon bieneusi* is being increasingly reported in AIDS patients as a cause of chronic diarrhoea and weight loss. Other manifestations of microsporidiosis in AIDS include keratoconjunctivitis, respiratory-tract infections, renal and urinary-tract infections, peritonitis, cholangitis, granulomatous hepatitis, and disseminated myositis.

There is no established effective treatment. Metronidazole has been reported to produce a transient symptomatic response in some patients[3] but not in those with severe diarrhoea.[4] Beneficial responses have been reported with albendazole[5-8] and atovaquone.[9] Topical treatment of keratoconjunctivitis has been disappointing although there are reports of individual patients responding to topical propamidine isethionate,[10] topical fumagillin,[11,12] or oral itraconazole plus topical antibacterials.[13]

1. Muscat I. Human microsporidiosis. *J Infect* 1990; **21:** 125–9.
2. Curry A, Canning EU. Human microsporidiosis. *J Infect* 1993; **27:** 229–36.
3. Schattenkerk JKME, *et al.* Clinical significance of small-intestinal microsporidiosis in HIV-1-infected individuals. *Lancet* 1991; **337:** 895–8.
4. Blanshard C, Gazzard BG. Microsporidiosis in HIV-1-infected individuals. *Lancet* 1991; **337:** 1488–9.
5. Blanshard C, *et al.* Treatment of intestinal microsporidiosis with albendazole in patients with AIDS. *AIDS* 1992; **6:** 311–13.
6. Dieterich DT, *et al.* Treatment with albendazole for intestinal disease due to Enterocytozoon bieneusi in patients with AIDS. *J Infect Dis* 1994; **169:** 178–82.
7. Franzen C, *et al.* Intestinal microsporidiosis with Septata intestinalis in a patient with AIDS—response to albendazole. *J Infect* 1995; **31:** 237–9.
8. Dore GJ, *et al.* Disseminated microsporidiosis due to Septata intestinalis in nine patients infected with the human immunodeficiency virus: response to therapy with albendazole. *Clin Infect Dis* 1995; **21:** 70–6.
9. Anwar-Bruni DM, *et al.* Atovaquone is effective treatment for the symptoms of gastrointestinal microsporidiosis in HIV-1-infected patients. *AIDS* 1996; **10:** 619–23.
10. Metcalfe TW, *et al.* Microsporidial keratoconjunctivitis in a patient with AIDS. *Br J Ophthalmol* 1992; **76:** 177–8.
11. Diesenhouse MC, *et al.* Treatment of microsporidial keratoconjunctivitis with topical fumagillin. *Am J Ophthalmol* 1993; **115:** 293–8.
12. Garvey MJ, *et al.* Topical fumagillin in the treatment of microsporidial keratoconjunctivitis in AIDS. *Ann Pharmacother* 1995; **29:** 872–4.
13. Yee RW, *et al.* Resolution of microsporidial epithelial keratopathy in a patient with AIDS. *Ophthalmology* 1991; **98:** 196–201.

Pneumocystis carinii pneumonia

Although *Pneumocystis carinii* has been classified as a protozoan, recent evidence suggests that it is probably a fungus. For the treatment of *Pneumocystis carinii* pneumonia see p.370.

Toxoplasmosis

Toxoplasmosis is a zoonosis with a worldwide distribution caused by the protozoan parasite *Toxoplasma gondii*. There is a high incidence of *Toxoplasma* antibody, an indication of previous infection, in the general population although infection will have been diagnosed in few individuals. Sexual reproduction of *T. gondii* occurs in the gastro-intestinal tract of cats. Soil becomes contaminated from excretion of oocysts in cat faeces. Other animals such as pigs and sheep may become infected by ingestion of these oocysts and act as intermediate hosts. In man infection is acquired through contact with infected cat faeces or contaminated soil or from eating raw or undercooked meat from infected animals. Ingested oocysts rapidly transform into trophozoites which multiply in tissue macrophages. The intracellular trophozoites disseminate in the blood stream and lymphatic system to reach the brain, heart, and lungs. As immunity develops the trophozoites form latent cystic aggregates (bradyzoites), mainly in the brain, heart, and skeletal muscle, and these are subject to reactivation throughout the life of the host.

Toxoplasma infection in immunocompetent individuals is usually asymptomatic and if symptomatic infection does occur it is usually self-limiting. Very rarely myocarditis or encephalitis may occur. Patients with impaired immunity may develop serious complications such as encephalitis, chorioretinitis, myocarditis, and pneumonitis. Toxoplasmic encephalitis is the most common presentation in patients with AIDS.

Congenital toxoplasmosis is not a problem in women who have *Toxoplasma* antibody before conception, but primary toxoplasmosis during early pregnancy is serious because of the risk of transplacental transmission which may result in fetal death or congenital toxoplasmosis. Primary infection during later pregnancy can also result in congenital infection although this often only becomes symptomatic later in life. The sequelae in live-born infants with signs of infection are generally severe and include a potentially fatal syndrome in which hydrocephalus, hepatosplenomegaly with jaundice, mental retardation, and chorioretinitis may occur. Congenital disease that becomes clinically evident later in life is usually less severe, but it frequently results in ocular or neurological impairment. Infection in the pregnant woman is usually asymptomatic and antenatal screening programmes have been set up in some countries for the diagnosis of acute infections during pregnancy. However, the value and practicality of such schemes has been debated.[1-5] Ocular toxoplasmosis causes chorioretinitis and is often a result of congenital infection; patients may be asymptomatic until later in life.

Treatment. Toxoplasmosis in immunocompetent patients is not usually treated unless symptoms are severe. Currently there is no drug active against the cystic form, so any treatment is directed against the acute forms of the disease. Active toxoplasmosis in immunocompromised patients requires prompt, effective treatment. Toxoplasmosis is normally treated with pyrimethamine together with sulphadiazine.[6] Folinic acid should also be given every third day during treatment to counteract the megaloblastic anaemia associated with these drugs. Treatment is ideally continued for several weeks after clinical cure. Indefinite, usually lifelong, maintenance therapy should be given to AIDS patients. Clindamycin plus pyrimethamine has been used as an alternative in patients unable to take the sulphonamide.[7-10] Other approaches for such patients are to give pyrimethamine alone[6] or to carry out sulphadiazine desensitisation.[11] Other drug regimens which have produced encouraging results in small numbers of AIDS patients with encephalitis include pyrimethamine with clarithromycin,[12] pyrimethamine with doxycycline,[13] atovaquone,[14] clindamycin with fluorouracil,[15] clarithromycin with minocycline,[16] and azithromycin with pyrimethamine.[17]

Pyrimethamine should not be used to treat primary toxoplasmosis during the first trimester of **pregnancy** in immunocompetent patients.[6] Spiramycin has been used throughout the first trimester but, although it reduces the risk of congenital transmission, it does not readily penetrate the cerebrospinal space and does not prevent toxoplasmic encephalitis in immunodeficient mothers. After the first trimester pyrimethamine may be given with sulphadiazine and folinic acid and when there is evidence of placental or fetal infection that treatment may be alternated with courses of spiramycin until term. In **neonates** without overt disease, but born to mothers known to have become infected during pregnancy, pyrimethamine together with sulphadiazine and folinic acid are given for the first 4 weeks with further courses of treatment if the infants are subsequently shown to be infected.[6] Some workers have suggested treatment for one year initially.[5,18] Alternating courses of pyrimethamine-sulphadiazine with spiramycin has been suggested as a means of reducing the risk of bone marrow suppression and has produced good results when given throughout the first year of life. Severely infected neonates are treated with daily pyrimethamine-sulphadiazine for 6 months after which alternating monthly courses of pyrimethamine-sulphadiazine and spiramycin for at least a further 6 months have been used.[6] A corticosteroid, usually prednisolone, is added for active chorioretinitis or CNS involvement.[6]

In immunocompetent individuals **ocular toxoplasmosis** is a self-limiting disease, and requires no treatment unless visual acuity is threatened or there is a large retinal lesion with marked vitritis.[19-21] All immunocompromised patients should be treated and prolonged treatment is necessary to prevent recrudescence. The optimum drug regimen is undecided. The most commonly used regimens are pyrimethamine with sulphadiazine or pyrimethamine with clindamycin (which is concentrated in the choroid). A beneficial response has been reported with clindamycin and corticosteroid therapy.[22] The role of corticosteroids is the subject of debate. They should never be used alone since fulminant cases may occur. Spiramycin is not indicated for ocular toxoplasmosis.

Prophylaxis. Primary prophylaxis against *T. gondii* infection has been investigated in AIDS patients and recipients of organ transplants. Clindamycin[23] alone was found to be too toxic. While some studies have suggested that pyrimethamine[23-25] alone may be of value, increased mortality risk has been reported[26] and a controlled study has shown no benefit.[27] Co-trimoxazole, in regimens designed for *Pneumocystis carinii* pneumonia prophylaxis, appears to provide effective primary prophylaxis for toxoplasma encephalitis.[28] Alternatively, pyrimethamine plus dapsone may be effective.[28,29] However, pyrimethamine with dapsone was not tolerated by 30% of patients in one study.[30]

1. Anonymous. Antenatal screening for toxoplasmosis in the UK. *Lancet* 1990; **336:** 346–8. Correction. *ibid.*: 576.
2. Jeannel D, *et al.* What is known about the prevention of congenital toxoplasmosis? *Lancet* 1990; **336:** 359–61.
3. Ho-Yen DO, *et al.* Congenital toxoplasmosis and TORCH. *Lancet* 1990; **336:** 624.
4. Desmonts G. Preventing congenital toxoplasmosis. *Lancet* 1990; **336:** 1017–18.
5. Guerina NG, *et al.* Neonatal serologic screening and early treatment for congenital Toxoplasma gondii infection. *N Engl J Med* 1994; **330:** 1858–63.
6. WHO. *WHO model prescribing information: drugs used in parasitic diseases.* 2nd ed. Geneva: WHO, 1995.
7. Remington JS, Vildé JL. Clindamycin for toxoplasma encephalitis in AIDS. *Lancet* 1991; **338:** 1142–3.
8. Luft BJ, *et al.* Toxoplasmic encephalitis in patients with the acquired immunodeficiency syndrome. *N Engl J Med* 1993; **329:** 995–1000.
9. Dannemann B, *et al.* Treatment of toxoplasmic encephalitis in patients with AIDS: a randomized trial comparing pyrimethamine plus clindamycin to pyrimethamine plus sulfadiazine. *Ann Intern Med* 1992; **116:** 33–43.
10. Katlama C, *et al.* Pyrimethamine-clindamycin vs pyrimethamine-sulfadiazine as acute and long-term therapy for toxoplasmic encephalitis in patients with AIDS. *Clin Infect Dis* 1996; **22:** 268–75.
11. Tenant-Flowers M, *et al.* Sulphadiazine desensitization in patients with AIDS and cerebral toxoplasmosis. *AIDS* 1991; **5:** 311–15.
12. Fernandez-Martin J, *et al.* Pyrimethamine-clarithromycin combination for therapy of acute Toxoplasma encephalitis in patients with AIDS. *Antimicrob Agents Chemother* 1991; **35:** 2049–52.
13. Hagberg L, *et al.* Doxycycline and pyrimethamine for toxoplasmic encephalitis. *Scand J Infect Dis* 1993; **25:** 157–60.
14. Kovacs JA, *et al.* Efficacy of atovaquone in treatment of toxoplasmosis in patients with AIDS. *Lancet* 1992; **340:** 637–8.
15. Dhiver C, *et al.* 5-Fluoro-uracil–clindamycin for treatment of cerebral toxoplasmosis. *AIDS* 1993; **7:** 143–4.
16. Lacassin F, *et al.* Clarithromycin-minocycline combination as salvage therapy for toxoplasmosis in patients infected with human immunodeficiency virus. *Antimicrob Agents Chemother* 1995; **39:** 276–7.
17. Saba J, *et al.* Pyrimethamine plus azithromycin for treatment of acute toxoplasmic encephalitis in patients with AIDS. *Eur J Clin Microbiol Infect Dis* 1993; **12:** 853–6.
18. Roizen N, *et al.* Neurologic and developmental outcome in treated congenital toxoplasmosis. *Pediatrics* 1995; **95:** 11–20.
19. Rothova A. Ocular involvement in toxoplasmosis. *Br J Ophthalmol* 1993; **77:** 371–7.
20. Nussenblatt RB, Belfort R. Ocular toxoplasmosis: an old disease revisited. *JAMA* 1994; **271:** 304–7. Correction. *ibid.*; **272:** 356.
21. Hay J, Dutton GN. Toxoplasma and the eye. *Br Med J* 1995; **310:** 1021–2.
22. Djurković-Djaković O, *et al.* Short-term effects of the clindamycin-steroid regimen in the treatment of ocular toxoplasmosis. *J Chemother* 1995; **7** (suppl 4): 199–201.
23. Jacobson MA, *et al.* Toxicity of clindamycin as prophylaxis for AIDS-associated toxoplasmic encephalitis. *Lancet* 1992; **339:** 333–4.
24. Wreghitt TG, *et al.* Efficacy of pyrimethamine for the prevention of donor-acquired Toxoplasma gondii infection in heart and heart-lung transplant recipients. *Transpl Int* 1992; **5:** 197–200.
25. Murphy K, *et al.* Pyrimethamine alone as long-term suppressive therapy in cerebral toxoplasmosis. *Am J Med* 1994; **96:** 95–6.
26. Jacobson MA, *et al.* Primary prophylaxis with pyrimethamine for toxoplasmic encephalitis in patients with advanced human immunodeficiency virus disease: results of a randomized trial. *J Infect Dis* 1994; **169:** 384–94.
27. Leport C, *et al.* Pyrimethamine for primary prophylaxis of toxoplasmic encephalitis in patients with human immunodeficiency virus infection: a double-blind, randomized trial. *J Infect Dis* 1996; **173:** 91–7.
28. Centers for Disease Control. 1997 USPHS/IDSA guidelines for the prevention of opportunistic infections in persons infected with human immunodeficiency virus. *MMWR* 1997; **46** (RR-12): 1–48.
29. Podzamczer D, *et al.* Intermittent trimethoprim-sulfamethoxazole compared with dapsone-pyrimethamine for the simultaneous primary prophylaxis of Pneumocystis pneumonia and toxoplasmosis in patients infected with HIV. *Ann Intern Med* 1995; **122:** 755–61.
30. Opravil M, *et al.* Once-weekly administration of dapsone/pyrimethamine vs aerosolized pentamidine as combined prophylaxis for Pneumocystis carinii pneumonia and toxoplasmic encephalitis in human immunodeficiency virus-infected patients. *Clin Infect Dis* 1995; **20:** 531–41.

Trichomoniasis

Trichomoniasis is caused by invasion of the genito-urinary tract with the protozoan *Trichomonas vaginalis*. Transmission is primarily sexual. It is a common cause of vaginitis and vaginal discharge; some infected women are asymptomatic but should still be treated to prevent sexual transmission and symptomatic infection. Men are usually asymptomatic although it may cause urethritis. Treatment is usually with a nitroimidazole such as metronidazole when a single oral dose can be effective.[1,7] Sexual partners should be treated concomitantly. The incidence of treatment failures appears to be increasing and some at least have been due to metronidazole resistance.[2-4] Patients who do not respond to single-dose treatment may be given a more intensive course of metronidazole. Tinidazole has been widely used as an alternative to metronidazole, and may be effective in cases of metronidazole resistance.[5] One patient with metronidazole- and tinidazole-resistant infection was successfully treated with paromomycin.[6] Clotrimazole, administered intravaginally, has been suggested[1] for symptomatic relief during pregnancy, especially during the first trimester when metronidazole therapy is not recommended. However, clotrimazole is curative only about 20% of patients and definitive treatment may be required later in pregnancy.

1. WHO. *WHO model prescribing information: drugs used in sexually transmitted diseases and HIV infection.* Geneva: WHO, 1995.
2. Krajden S, *et al.* Persistent Trichomonas vaginalis infection due to a metronidazole-resistant strain. *Can Med Assoc J* 1986; **134:** 1373–4.
3. Lumsden WHR, *et al.* Treatment failure in Trichomonas vaginalis infections in females II: in-vitro estimation of the sensitivity of the organism to metronidazole. *J Antimicrob Chemother* 1988; **21:** 555–64.
4. Grossmann JH, Galask RP. Persistent vaginitis caused by metronidazole-resistant trichomonas. *Obstet Gynecol* 1990; **76:** 521–2.
5. Hamed KA, Studemeister AE. Successful response of metronidazole-resistant trichomonal vaginitis to tinidazole: a case report. *Sex Transm Dis* 1992; **19:** 339–40.
6. Nyirjesy P, *et al.* Paromomycin for nitroimidazole-resistant trichomonosis. *Lancet* 1995; **346:** 1110.
7. Centers for Disease Control. 1998 Guidelines for treatment of sexually transmitted diseases. *MMWR* 1998; **47** (RR-1): 74–5.

African trypanosomiasis

African trypanosomiasis (sleeping sickness) is caused by subspecies of the protozoan *Trypanosoma brucei*, transmitted by the bite of infected tsetse flies (*Glossina* spp.). Gambian or West African sleeping sickness is caused by *T. brucei gambiense*, carried by riverine tsetse flies, and Rhodesian or East African sleeping sickness is caused by *T. brucei rhodesiense*, carried by savannah tsetse flies. *T. brucei brucei* does not infect man. Infection can follow blood transfusion and congenital trypanosomiasis has also occurred.

Although it has proven impractical to eliminate trypanosomiasis from endemic areas, the intensity of transmission can be reduced by detection and treatment of cases and vector control including insecticide spraying of breeding sites and the use of insecticide-impregnated traps and screens.[1,2] Control of infection in domestic animals may also be beneficial.[1]

Trypanosomiasis can be divided into the early haematolymphatic stage (infection of the blood stream and lymph nodes) and the late or meningoencephalitic stage (infection of the central nervous system).[1] Trypanosomiasis due to *T. b. gambiense* develops slowly over several months or even years and the disease stages are relatively distinct. Infection with *T. b. rhodesiense* is more acute with a rapid onset of symptoms and indistinct disease stages, and if left untreated will usually lead to death in a matter of weeks or months.

The haematolymphatic phase of African trypanosomiasis is treated with suramin or pentamidine. Pentamidine may be used for treatment of *T. b. gambiense* infections, but increasing resistance makes it unsuitable for *T. b. rhodesiense* infections; suramin is used for *T. b. rhodesiense* infections and for *T. b. gambiense* infections which are resistant to pentamidine.[1] Combination therapy with pentamidine and suramin for *T. b. gambiense* infections has not been shown to reduce the incidence of relapse.[3] Eflornithine can also be effective in this phase of infection caused by *T. b. gambiense*; it is not very effective on its own against *T. b. rhodesiense.*[2]

Suramin and pentamidine penetrate the blood-brain barrier poorly and are only used in the meningoencephalitic stage as adjuncts before starting treatment with melarsoprol or eflornithine.[1] Melarsoprol, which is effective against both *T. b. gambiense* and *T. b. rhodesiense*, is usually only given to treat the meningoencephalitic stage of the infection because of its toxicity in producing potentially fatal encephalopathy.[1] However, protection against this toxicity may be provided by prophylaxis with prednisolone.[4,5] Also those patients with *T. b. gambiense* infection may be treated more safely with eflornithine than melarsoprol on its own, although its cumbersome dosage schedule limits its use by some to those patients who relapse from melarsoprol.[6] Combination therapy with melarsoprol and eflornithine was reported to be effective in one patient who had not responded to either drug alone.[7]

Other alternative treatments to melarsoprol for *T. b. gambiense* infection include a combination of tryparsamide and suramin,[8] or high doses of nifurtimox,[9,10] although tryparsamide is associated with a high risk of toxicity.

There is no established effective alternative treatment for melarsoprol-resistant *T. b. rhodesiense* although suramin given in combination with high-dose metronidazole was successful in 1 patient.[11]

Patients should be seen every 6 months for a follow-up period of at least 2 years, to ascertain if treatment has been successful.[1]

1. WHO. Epidemiology and control of African trypanosomiasis. *WHO Tech Rep Ser 739* 1986.
2. WHO. *WHO model prescribing information: drugs used in parasitic diseases.* 2nd ed. Geneva: WHO, 1995.
3. Pépin J, Khonde N. Relapses following treatment of early-stage Trypanosoma brucei gambiense sleeping sickness with a combination of pentamidine and suramin. *Trans R Soc Trop Med Hyg* 1996; **90:** 183–6.
4. Pepin J, *et al.* Trial of prednisolone for prevention of melarsoprol-induced encephalopathy in gambiense sleeping sickness. *Lancet* 1989; **i:** 1246–50.
5. Pepin J, *et al.* Risk factors for encephalopathy and mortality during melarsoprol treatment of Trypanosoma brucei gambiense sleeping sickness. *Trans R Soc Trop Med Hyg* 1995; **89:** 92–7.
6. Milord F, *et al.* Efficacy and toxicity of eflornithine for treatment of Trypanosoma brucei gambiense sleeping sickness. *Lancet* 1992; **340:** 652–5.
7. Simarro PP, Asumu PN. Gambian trypanosomiasis and synergism between melarsoprol and eflornithine: first case report. *Trans R Soc Trop Med Hyg* 1996; **90:** 315.
8. Anonymous. Drugs for parasitic infections. *Med Lett Drugs Ther* 1998; **40:** 1–12.
9. Pepin J, *et al.* An open clinical trial of nifurtimox for arseno-resistant Trypanosoma brucei gambiense sleeping sickness in central Zaire. *Trans R Soc Trop Med Hyg* 1989; **83:** 514–17.
10. Pepin J, *et al.* High-dose nifurtimox for arseno-resistant Trypanosoma brucei gambiense sleeping sickness: an open trial in central Zaire. *Trans R Soc Trop Med Hyg* 1992; **86:** 254–6.
11. Foulkes JR. Metronidazole and suramin combination in the treatment of arsenical refractory rhodesian sleeping sickness—a case study. *Trans R Soc Trop Med Hyg* 1996; **90:** 422.

American trypanosomiasis

South American trypanosomiasis (Chagas' disease) is caused by *Trypanosoma cruzi*, carried by reduviid or triatomine bugs which feed on human blood.[1] Infected bugs defaecate on the human host while feeding and metacyclic trypanosomes are shed and enter the host via skin abrasions or by direct penetration of mucous membranes such as the conjunctiva. Transmission by blood transfusion is a growing problem. Congenital infection can also occur. Control measures include case detection and treatment, vector control by insecticide applications within domestic buildings, and screening of blood donors.[1]

Infection with *T. cruzi* is found throughout South and Central America and has been recorded in Mexico and Texas; there have also been reports of transfusion-induced infection in northern USA and Canada. Three phases of the disease are recognised. In the early acute phase of infection parasites are present in the blood; this phase may be asymptomatic or there may be a swelling or chagoma at the site of infection, allergic reactions, and more rarely acute heart failure or meningoencephalitis. The acute phase may be fatal in children but patients usually survive to enter the next stage of the disease called the indeterminate phase in which infection may be present in tissue for years without clinical manifestations. Classical features of the chronic phase are cardiomyopathy, megacolon, and mega-oesophagus. Parasites are rarely found in the blood after the acute phase.

Available treatment is generally unsatisfactory but despite their toxicity, nifurtimox or benznidazole are of value especially in the acute phase; it is not known whether trypanocidal treatment during the indeterminate phase can prevent the development of chronic disease. Although it is generally felt that there is no benefit from treatment in the chronic phase, treatment during the early chronic phase was reported to be beneficial,[2] and long-term follow-up of patients who had received benznidazole showed a reduction in cardiac complications and parasitaemia.[3] The efficacy of treatment varies from country to country and may be linked to variations in the sensitivity of different strains of *T. cruzi*. Treatment is said to be successful when both parasitaemia and serological tests become negative and remain so for at least one year after the end of treatment.

Symptomatic treatment is often given, particularly in the chronic stage for cardiac and gastro-intestinal lesions. Injections of botulinum toxin have been used to treat a patient with oesophageal involvement.[4]

Allopurinol and allopurinol riboside are under investigation for the treatment of American trypanosomiasis since they have shown trypanocidal activity. Allopurinol has been reported to be as effective as nifurtimox or benznidazole in reducing parasitaemia during the indeterminate phase and to be better tolerated.[5] Allopurinol and itraconazole have both been shown to produce beneficial responses in patients with mild chronic disease.[6]

In areas where the proportion of seropositive blood donors is high, emergency blood supplies positive for *T. cruzi* can be made safe by the addition of crystal violet. The risk of transmission to transplant recipients can be reduced considerably by nifurtimox or benznidazole treatment of the donor for 2 weeks before transplantation, and of the recipient for 2 weeks after. In laboratory workers at risk of an infection after an accident, trypanocidal treatment for 8 to 10 days, started preferably on the day of the accident usually aborts the presumptive infection.

1. WHO. Control of Chagas disease: report of a WHO expert committee. *WHO Tech Rep Ser 811* 1991.
2. de Andrade ALSS, *et al.* Randomised trial of efficacy of benznidazole in treatment of early Trypanosoma cruzi infection. *Lancet* 1996; **348:** 1407–13.
3. Viotti R, *et al.* Treatment of chronic Chagas' disease with benznidazole: clinical and serologic evolution of patients with long-term follow-up. *Am Heart J* 1994; **127:** 151–62.
4. Ferrari AP, *et al.* Treatment of achalasia in Chagas' disease with botulinum toxin. *N Engl J Med* 1995; **332:** 824–5.
5. Gallerano RH, *et al.* Therapeutic efficacy of allopurinol in patients with chronic Chagas' disease. *Am J Trop Med Hyg* 1990; **43:** 159–66.
6. Sánchez G, *et al.* Treatment with allopurinol and itraconazole changes lytic activity in patients with chronic, low grade Trypanosoma cruzi infection. *Trans R Soc Trop Med Hyg* 1995; **89:** 438–9.

Acetarsol (4752-k)

Acetarsol *(BAN, rINN)*.

Acetaminohydroxyphenylarsonsäure; Acetarsone; Acetphenarsinum; Osarsolum. 3-Acetamido-4-hydroxyphenylarsonic acid.

$C_8H_{10}AsNO_5$ = 275.1.

CAS — 97-44-9.

Pharmacopoeias. Fr. includes Acetarsol Sodium.

Acetarsol, a pentavalent organic arsenical derivative, is a luminal amoebicide and also has antitrichomonal activity. Acetarsol was formerly administered orally in the treatment of intestinal amoebiasis and vaginally in the treatment of trichomoniasis, but the use of pentavalent arsenical compounds has been abandoned in favour of more effective and less toxic drugs. For the adverse effects of arsenic and their treatment, see Arsenic Trioxide, p.1550.

Acetarsol suppositories were once tried in the treatment of proctitis. Acetarsol lithium and acetarsol sodium have been included in some preparations for minor mouth infections.

Preparations

Proprietary Preparations (details are given in Part 3)
Belg.: Laryngarsol†; ***Ital.:*** Gynoplix Theraplix; ***S.Afr.:*** R.V.C.†; SVC†.

Multi-ingredient: ***Belg.:*** Sulfaryl; ***Fr.:*** Arpha†; Gynoplix†; Humex†; ***Ital.:*** Sanogyl Bianco; ***S.Afr.:*** Poly-Gynedron†; Tricho-Gynedron†.

Amprolium Hydrochloride (12372-v)

Amprolium Hydrochloride *(BANM, rINNM)*.

1-(4-Amino-2-propylpyrimidin-5-ylmethyl)-2-methylpyridinium chloride hydrochloride.

$C_{14}H_{19}ClN_4,HCl$ = 315.2.

CAS — 121-25-5 (amprolium); 137-88-2 (amprolium hydrochloride).

NOTE. Amprolium is the USP title for amprolium hydrochloride.

Pharmacopoeias. In BP(Vet). Also in Fr. and US, for veterinary use only.

A white or almost white to light yellow, odourless or almost odourless powder. BP(Vet) **solubilities** are: freely soluble in water; slightly soluble in alcohol; very slightly soluble in ether; practically insoluble in chloroform. USP solubilities are: freely soluble in water, in alcohol, in methyl alcohol, and in dimethylformamide; sparingly soluble in dehydrated alcohol; practically insoluble in acetone, in butyl alcohol, and in isopropyl alcohol.

Amprolium hydrochloride is an antiprotozoal used in veterinary practice, alone or in conjunction with other drugs such as ethopabate, for the control of coccidiosis.

Pentavalent Antimony Compounds (5010-w)

Meglumine Antimonate (792-c)

Antimony Meglumine; Meglumine Antimoniate; Protostib; RP-2168. 1-Deoxy-1-methylamino-D-glucitol antimonate.

$C_7H_{18}NO_8Sb$ = 366.0.

CAS — 133-51-7.

Sodium Stibogluconate (809-s)

Sodium Stibogluconate *(BAN, rINN)*.

Sod. Stibogluc.; Sodium Antimony Gluconate; Stibogluconat-Natrium.

CAS — 16037-91-5.

Pharmacopoeias. In Br., Chin., Int., and It.

A pentavalent antimony compound of indefinite composition containing, when dried, 30 to 34% of pentavalent antimony. It has been represented by the formula $C_6H_9Na_2O_9Sb$ but usually there are less than 2 atoms of Na for each atom of Sb.

It is a colourless, odourless or almost odourless, mostly amorphous powder. Very **soluble** in water; practically insoluble in alcohol and in ether. A solution containing 10% of pentavalent antimony has a pH of 5.0 to 5.6 after autoclaving. Solutions may be **sterilised** by autoclaving.

Adverse Effects, Treatment, and Precautions

As for Trivalent Antimony Compounds, p.98.

Adverse effects are generally less frequent and less severe with the pentavalent antimony compounds sodium stibogluconate and meglumine antimonate than with trivalent compounds such as antimony sodium tartrate. Nevertheless, similar precautions should be observed, especially in patients on high-dose therapy.

Intramuscular injections of sodium stibogluconate can be painful and intravenous administration has been associated with thrombophlebitis.

On a weight-for-weight basis children require more pentavalent antimony than adults and tolerate it better, but in both adults and children tolerance is adversely affected by impaired renal function.[1] Common side-effects are anorexia, vomiting, nausea, malaise, myalgia, headache, and lethargy. ECG changes are dose-dependent and most commonly T-wave inversion and prolonged QT interval. Renal damage is a rarely reported toxic effect. Pentavalent antimony is usually well tolerated. Serious side-effects when they occur usually involve the liver or the heart when it is prudent to interrupt the course temporarily.

1. WHO. Control of the leishmaniases. *WHO Tech Rep Ser 793* 1990.

Breast feeding. There was some distribution of antimony into breast milk following administration of sodium stibogluconate to one patient.[1] The authors considered that the amount present did not constitute a hazard and oral absorption was not detected in an *animal* study. Verschoyle[2] in commenting on the report felt more safety evaluation was required before pronouncing on the safety of antimony to breast-feeding infants.

1. Berman JD, *et al.* Concentration of Pentostam in human breast milk. *Trans R Soc Trop Med Hyg* 1989; **83:** 784–5.
2. Verschoyle RD. Comment. *Trop Dis Bull* 1990; **87:** 919.

Effects on the blood. Although thrombocytopenia is associated with leishmaniasis, there are case reports of it also being associated with sodium stibogluconate.[1,2]

1. Braconier JH, Miörner H. Recurrent episodes of thrombocytopenia during treatment with sodium stibogluconate. *J Antimicrob Chemother* 1993; **31:** 187–8.
2. Hepburn NC. Thrombocytopenia complicating sodium stibogluconate therapy for cutaneous leishmaniasis. *Trans R Soc Trop Med Hyg* 1993; **87:** 691.

Effects on the heart. The ECG was monitored during 65 courses of treatment with sodium stibogluconate in 59 Kenyan patients with leishmaniasis.[1] ECG abnormalities developed during 35 treatment courses. They were qualitatively similar to those previously described during treatment with trivalent antimonial drugs, but occurred less frequently and later during the course of treatment. The most common abnormality was inversion and/or decreased amplitude of T waves. Incidence was related to total daily dose and duration of treatment. One patient died suddenly during the 4th week of treatment with 60 mg of antimony per kg body-weight daily. Other deaths probably related to cardiac toxicity have been reported in patients receiving 60 mg per kg daily[2] and 30 mg per kg daily.[3] Guidelines[1] for monitoring during treatment with sodium stibogluconate include the recommendation that ECGs be obtained every 3 to 4 days in patients receiving 20 mg of antimony per kg daily for more than 20 days or a higher dose for more than 10 days. If Stokes-Adams attacks or ventricular tachyarrhythmias develop, sodium stibogluconate should be stopped and treatment should be instituted for the cardiac toxicity.

1. Chulay JD, *et al.* Electrocardiographic changes during treatment of leishmaniasis with pentavalent antimony (sodium stibogluconate). *Am J Trop Med Hyg* 1985; **34:** 702–9.
2. Bryceson ADM, *et al.* Visceral leishmaniasis unresponsive to antimonial drugs II: response to high dosage sodium stibogluconate or prolonged treatment with pentamidine. *Trans R Soc Trop Med Hyg* 1985; **79:** 705–14.
3. Thakur CP. Harmful effect of high stibogluconate treatment of kala-azar in India. *Trans R Soc Trop Med Hyg* 1986; **80:** 672–3.

Effects on the kidneys. Sodium stibogluconate given to 16 young men with cutaneous leishmaniasis, but otherwise healthy, for 10 days had no apparent adverse effect on glomerular or tubular renal function.[1] However, evidence of renal tubular dysfunction has been reported in patients with mucocutaneous leishmaniasis given meglumine antimonate or sodium stibogluconate for 30 days or more[2] and acute renal failure occurred in a patient with pre-existing renal impairment.[3]

1. Joliffe DS. Nephrotoxicity of pentavalent antimonials. *Lancet* 1985; **i:** 584.
2. Veiga JPR, *et al.* Renal tubular dysfunction in patients with mucocutaneous leishmaniasis treated with pentavalent antimonials. *Lancet* 1983; **ii:** 569.
3. Balzan M, Fenech F. Acute renal failure in visceral leishmaniasis treated with sodium stibogluconate. *Trans R Soc Trop Med Hyg* 1992; **86:** 515–16.

Effects on the liver. The WHO has reported that when serious side-effects occur with sodium stibogluconate they usually involve the liver or the heart.[1] There have been reports of disturbed liver function[2,3] in patients given sodium stibogluconate, although there has also been a report[4] that signs of altered liver function improved during treatment with sodium stibogluconate and may be a feature of visceral leishmaniasis.

1. WHO. Control of the leishmaniases. *WHO Tech Rep Ser 793* 1990.
2. Ballou WR, *et al.* Safety and efficacy of high-dose sodium stibogluconate therapy of American cutaneous leishmaniasis. *Lancet* 1987; **ii:** 13–16.
3. Hepburn NC, *et al.* Hepatotoxicity of sodium stibogluconate in leishmaniasis. *Lancet* 1993; **342:** 238–9.
4. Misbahuddin M, *et al.* Stibogluconate for leishmaniasis. *Lancet* 1993; **342:** 804.

Effects on the musculoskeletal system. Arthralgia is common with pentavalent antimony compounds. It is usually dose-dependent[1] but a patient has been described who experienced symptoms early in treatment.[2] Palindromic arthropathy with effusion was associated with sodium stibogluconate treatment in one patient.[3]

1. Ballou WR, *et al.* Safety and efficacy of high-dose sodium stibogluconate therapy of American cutaneous leishmaniasis. *Lancet* 1987; **ii:** 13–16.
2. Castro C, *et al.* Severe arthralgia, not related to dose, associated with pentavalent antimonial therapy for mucosal leishmaniasis. *Trans R Soc Trop Med Hyg* 1990; **84:** 362.
3. Donovan KL, *et al.* Pancreatitis and palindromic arthropathy with effusions associated with sodium stibogluconate treatment in a renal transplant recipient. *J Infect* 1990; **21:** 107–10.

Effects on the pancreas. Pancreatitis has been associated with sodium stibogluconate treatment.[1-3] Withdrawing treatment usually resulted in resolution of pancreatitis.

1. Donovan KL, *et al.* Pancreatitis and palindromic with effusions associated with sodium stibogluconate treatment in a renal transplant recipient. *J Infect* 1990; **21:** 107–10.
2. Gasser RA, *et al.* Pancreatitis induced by pentavalent antimonial agents during treatment of leishmaniasis. *Clin Infect Dis* 1994; **18:** 83–90.
3. Domingo P, *et al.* Treatment of Indian kala-azar with pentavalent antimony. *Lancet* 1995; **345:** 584–5.

Pharmacokinetics

The pentavalent antimony compounds are poorly absorbed from the gastro-intestinal tract. After intravenous administration an initial distribution phase is followed by biexponential elimination by the kidneys. The elimination half-life of the initial phase is about 1.7 hours and that of the slow terminal phase is about 33 hours. The corresponding half-lives after intramuscular administration are 2 hours and 766 hours respectively. The slow elimination phase may reflect reduction to trivalent antimony. Accumulation occurs on daily administration and maximum tissue concentrations may not be reached for 7 days or more. Antimony has been detected in breast milk (see Breast Feeding in Precautions, above).

References.

1. Rees PH, *et al.* Renal clearance of pentavalent antimony (sodium stibogluconate). *Lancet* 1980; **ii:** 226–9.
2. Chulay JD, *et al.* Pharmacokinetics of antimony during treatment of visceral leishmaniasis with sodium stibogluconate or meglumine antimoniate. *Trans R Soc Trop Med Hyg* 1988; **82:** 69–72.
3. Al Jaser M, *et al.* Pharmacokinetics of antimony in patients treated with sodium stibogluconate for cutaneous leishmaniasis. *Pharm Res* 1995; **12:** 113–16.

Uses and Administration

Pentavalent antimony, as sodium stibogluconate or meglumine antimonate, is the treatment of choice for all forms of leishmaniasis except *Leishmania aethiopica* infections.

Sodium stibogluconate is administered by intravenous or intramuscular injection as a solution containing the equivalent of 100 mg of pentavalent antimony per mL. Intravenous injections must be administered very slowly (over at least 5 minutes) and preferably through a fine needle to avoid thrombophlebitis; as with trivalent antimony compounds they should be discontinued immediately if coughing, vomiting, or substernal pain occurs. Meglumine antimonate is administered by deep intramuscular injection as a solution containing the equivalent of 85 mg of pentavalent antimony per mL. Doses are expressed in terms of the equivalent amount of pentavalent antimony. Local variations exist in treatment schedules but WHO recommends the following regimens.

In visceral leishmaniasis initial treatment is based on a daily injection of 20 mg of pentavalent antimony per kg body-weight to a maximum of 850 mg (but see below) for at least 20 days. The length of treatment varies from one endemic area to another, but is continued until no parasites are detected in consecutive splenic aspirates taken at 14-day intervals. Patients who relapse are re-treated at the same dose.

Early non-inflamed lesions of cutaneous leishmaniasis due to all forms of *Leishmania* except *L. aethiopica*, *L. amazonensis*, and *L. braziliensis* may be treated by infiltration with intralesional injections of 1 to 3 mL of sodium stibogluconate or meglumine antimonate (approximately 100 to 300 mg of pentavalent antimony), repeated once or twice if necessary at intervals of 1 to 2 days. Systemic therapy with 10 to 20 mg of pentavalent antimony per kg daily is given if the lesions are more severe and continued until a few days after clinical and parasitological cure is achieved. Cutaneous leishmaniasis due to *L. aethiopica* is not responsive to antimonials at conventional doses. In cutaneous leishmaniasis due to *L. braziliensis*, prolonged systemic treatment with 20 mg of pentavalent antimony per kg daily for a minimum of 4 weeks is indicated to prevent the later development of mucocutaneous leishmaniasis. Similar doses are required for diffuse cutaneous leishmaniasis due to *L. amazonensis* and are continued for several months after clinical improvement occurs.

In mucocutaneous leishmaniasis daily doses of 20 mg of pentavalent antimony per kg are given for a minimum of 4 weeks; if toxic effects develop or the response is poor, 10 to 15 mg per kg may be given every 12 hours. Relapses are well known and have generally been associated with inadequate or interrupted treatment; they are treated with the same drug given for at least twice as long as the original treatment. Only when that fails should alternative treatment be given.

Leishmaniasis. The main treatment for leishmaniasis (p.575) is a pentavalent antimony compound such as sodium stibogluconate. Higher doses of antimony compounds than those recommended by WHO (see above) have been tried in order to overcome the unresponsiveness of leishmaniasis to therapy. Drug-resistant strains of *Leishmania infantum* have been associated with unresponsiveness to treatment with meglumine antimonate.[1] Grogl and colleagues[2] suggested that the use of suboptimal doses may be increasing the prevalence of drug-resistant strains of the parasite. The Centers for Disease Control (CDC) in the USA recommend the use of 20 mg per kg body-weight per day of pentavalent antimony without restriction to the 850-mg maximum daily dose.[3] At this dose the most common adverse effects are musculoskeletal disorders, elevated liver enzyme values, and T-wave changes on the ECG, and the CDC recommends that the ECG, blood chemistry, and blood count should be monitored throughout therapy if resources permit. Severe cardiotoxicity is rare at 20 mg per kg per day but fatal cardiac toxicity has been reported with doses of up to 60 mg per kg per day (see under Effects on the Heart, above).

1. Faraut-Gambarelli F, *et al.* In vitro and in vivo resistance of Leishmania infantum to meglumine antimoniate: a study of 37 strains collected from patients with visceral leishmaniasis. *Antimicrob Agents Chemother* 1997; **41:** 827–30.
2. Grogl M, *et al.* Drug resistance in leishmaniasis: its implication in systemic chemotherapy of cutaneous and mucocutaneous disease. *Am J Trop Med Hyg* 1992; **47:** 117–26.
3. Herwaldt BL, Berman JD. Recommendations for treating leishmaniasis with sodium stibogluconate (Pentostam) and review of pertinent clinical studies. *Am J Trop Med Hyg* 1992; **46:** 296–306.

PROPHYLAXIS. Sodium stibogluconate or meglumine antimonate given once a month provided effective secondary prophylaxis against visceral leishmaniasis in patients with HIV infection.[1]

1. Ribera E, *et al.* Prophylaxis of visceral leishmaniasis in human immunodeficiency virus-infected patients *Am J Med* 1996; **100:** 496–501.

Preparations

BP 1998: Sodium Stibogluconate Injection.

Proprietary Preparations (details are given in Part 3)
Fr.: Glucantime; ***Ital.:*** Glucantim; ***Spain:*** Glucantime; ***UK:*** Pentostam.

Atovaquone (11117-v)

Atovaquone *(BAN, USAN, rINN).*

BW-A566C; BW-566C; BW-566C80; 566C; 566C80. 2-[*trans*-4-(4-Chlorophenyl)cyclohexyl]-3-hydroxy-1,4-naphthoquinone.

$C_{22}H_{19}O_3Cl$ = 366.8.

CAS — 95233-18-4.

Adverse Effects and Precautions

Adverse reactions to atovaquone include skin rashes, headache, fever, insomnia, and gastro-intestinal effects such as nausea, diarrhoea, and vomiting. Raised liver enzyme values, hyponatraemia, and haematological disturbances such as anaemia and neutropenia may occur occasionally. Atovaquone should be avoided in patients with gastro-intestinal disorders that may limit absorption of the drug.

Interactions

Concurrent administration of atovaquone with either metoclopramide, tetracycline, or rifampicin (and possibly also rifabutin) may result in decreases in plasma-atovaquone concentrations. Other drugs which have produced small reductions in plasma-atovaquone concentrations include aciclovir, antidiarrhoeals, benzodiazepines, cephalosporins, laxatives, opioids, and paracetamol.

Atovaquone is reported to decrease the metabolism of zidovudine resulting in moderate increases in zidovudine plasma concentrations. A decrease in the area under the time-concentration curve for didanosine has been reported when atovaquone is given concurrently. Small decreases in the plasma concentrations of co-trimoxazole have been noted in patients receiving atovaquone. There is a theoretical possibility that atovaquone could displace other highly protein-bound drugs from plasma-protein binding sites.

References.

1. Lee BL, *et al.* Atovaquone inhibits the glucuronidation and increases the plasma concentrations of zidovudine. *Clin Pharmacol Ther* 1996; **59:** 14–21.
2. Davis JD, *et al.* Atovaquone has no effect on the pharmacokinetics of phenytoin in healthy male volunteers. *Br J Clin Pharmacol* 1996; **42:** 246–8.

Pharmacokinetics

Atovaquone is poorly absorbed from the gastro-intestinal tract following administration by mouth but bioavailability can be increased by administration with food, particularly meals with a high fat content. Bioavailability is reduced in patients with AIDS. It is more than 99% bound to plasma proteins and has a reported plasma half-life of between 60 and 70 hours, thought to be due to entero-hepatic recycling. Atovaquone is excreted almost exclusively in faeces as unchanged drug.

References.

1. Hughes WT, *et al.* Safety and pharmacokinetics of 566C80, a hydroxynaphthoquinone with anti-Pneumocystis carinii activity: a phase I study in human immunodeficiency virus (HIV)-infected men. *J Infect Dis* 1991; **163:** 843–8.
2. Rolan PE, *et al.* Examination of some factors responsible for a food-induced increase in absorption of atovaquone. *Br J Clin Pharmacol* 1994; **37:** 13–20.
3. Dixon R, *et al.* Single-dose and steady-state pharmacokinetics of a novel microfluidized suspension of atovaquone in human immunodeficiency virus-seropositive patients. *Antimicrob Agents Chemother* 1996; **40:** 556–60.
4. Hussein Z, *et al.* Population pharmacokinetics of atovaquone in patients with acute malaria caused by Plasmodium falciparum. *Clin Pharmacol Ther* 1997; **61:** 518–30.
5. Rolan PE, *et al.* Disposition of atovaquone in humans. *Antimicrob Agents Chemother* 1997; **41:** 1319–21.

Uses and Administration

Atovaquone is a hydroxynaphthoquinone antiprotozoal that is also active against the fungus *Pneumocystis carinii*. It is used in the treatment of *Pneumocystis carinii* pneumonia as an alternative to co-trimoxazole in patients unable to tolerate the latter drug, and with proguanil in the treatment of malaria.

In the treatment of mild to moderate *Pneumocystis carinii* pneumonia, atovaquone is given by mouth in a dose of 750 mg with food three times daily as tablets, or twice daily as a suspension, for 21 days.

In the treatment of uncomplicated falciparum malaria, atovaquone is given in a single dose of 1 g daily in combination with proguanil hydrochloride 400 mg daily for 3 days. Children weighing 11 to 20 kg may be given one-quarter the adult dose, those weighing 21 to 30 kg may be given half the adult dose, and those weighing 31 to 40 kg may be given three-quarters the adult dose.

Reviews.

1. Haile LG, Flaherty JF. Atovaquone: a review. *Ann Pharmacother* 1993; **27:** 1488–94.
2. Artymowicz RJ, James VE. Atovaquone: a new antipneumocystis agent. *Clin Pharm* 1993; **12:** 563–70.
3. Spencer CM, Goa KL. Atovaquone: a review of its pharmacological properties and therapeutic efficacy in opportunistic infections. *Drugs* 1995; **50:** 176–96.

Malaria. Atovaquone with proguanil (Malarone) is used in the treatment of uncomplicated malaria caused by *Plasmodium falciparum* (see p.422). Atovaquone, a blood schizontocide, is associated with an unacceptably high rate of recrudescence when used alone[1,2] but is more successful in malaria when used with proguanil,[2,3] including that produced by multidrug-resistant strains.[4] Use of the combination to treat *P. ovale* and *P. malariae* malarias has also been studied.[5]

A recent study has also suggested that atovaquone-proguanil might be useful for *prophylaxis* of falciparum malaria in children in endemic areas.[6]

1. Chiodini PL, *et al.* Evaluation of atovaquone in the treatment of patients with uncomplicated Plasmodium falciparum malaria. *J Antimicrob Chemother* 1995; **36:** 1073–5.
2. Looareesuwan S, *et al.* Clinical studies of atovaquone, alone or in combination with other antimalarial drugs, for treatment of acute uncomplicated malaria in Thailand. *Am J Trop Med Hyg* 1996; **54:** 62–6.
3. Radloff PD, *et al.* Atovaquone and proguanil for Plasmodium falciparum malaria. *Lancet* 1996; **347:** 1511–14.
4. Sabchareon A, *et al.* Efficacy and pharmacokinetics of atovaquone and proguanil in children with multidrug-resistant Plasmodium falciparum malaria. *Trans R Soc Trop Med Hyg* 1998; **92:** 201–6.
5. Radloff PD, *et al.* Atovaquone plus proguanil is an effective treatment for Plasmodium ovale and P. malariae malaria. *Trans R Soc Trop Med Hyg* 1996; **90:** 682.
6. Lell B, *et al.* Randomised placebo-controlled study of atovaquone plus proguanil for malaria prophylaxis in children. *Lancet* 1998; **351:** 709–13.

Microsporidiosis. There is no established effective treatment for microsporidiosis (p.576). Beneficial responses were reported with atovaquone in a preliminary study.[1]

1. Anwar-Bruni DM, *et al.* Atovaquone is effective treatment for the symptoms of gastrointestinal microsporidiosis in HIV-1-infected patients. *AIDS* 1996; **10:** 619–23.

Pneumocystis carinii pneumonia. Atovaquone is one alternative to co-trimoxazole or pentamidine for the treatment of mild to moderate *Pneumocystis carinii* pneumonia (PCP—p.370). In open studies, a clinical response to atovaquone was reported in 78% of patients with mild to moderate PCP and in 56% of patients with severe PCP who were intolerant of or who failed to respond to both co-trimoxazole and pentamidine.[1] Comparative studies have shown atovaquone to be less effective than co-trimoxazole[2] and probably less effective than pentamidine,[3,4] but to produce fewer treatment-limiting adverse effects than either.

1. White A, *et al.* Clinical experience with atovaquone on a treatment investigational new drug protocol for Pneumocystis carinii pneumonia. *J Acquir Immune Defic Syndr Hum Retrovirol* 1995; **9:** 280–5.
2. Hughes W, *et al.* Comparison of atovaquone (566C80) with trimethoprim-sulfamethoxazole to treat Pneumocystis carinii pneumonia in patients with AIDS. *N Engl J Med* 1993; **328:** 1521–7.
3. Dohn MN, *et al.* Oral atovaquone compared with intravenous pentamidine for Pneumocystis carinii pneumonia in patients with AIDS. *Ann Intern Med* 1994; **121:** 174–80.
4. Lederman MM, van der Horst C. Atovaquone for Pneumocystis carinii pneumonia. *Ann Intern Med* 1995; **122:** 314.

Toxoplasmosis. Atovaquone has produced encouraging results[1] in AIDS patients with toxoplasmosis (p.576).

1. Kovacs JA, *et al.* Efficacy of atovaquone in treatment of toxoplasmosis in patients with AIDS. *Lancet* 1992; **340:** 637–8.

Preparations

Proprietary Preparations (details are given in Part 3)
Aust.: Wellvone; ***Austral.:*** Wellvone; ***Belg.:*** Wellvone; ***Canad.:*** Mepron; ***Fr.:*** Wellvone; ***Ger.:*** Wellvone; ***Ital.:*** Wellvone; ***Neth.:*** Wellvone; ***S.Afr.:*** Wellvone; ***Swed.:*** Wellvone; ***Switz.:*** Wellvone; ***UK:*** Wellvone; ***USA:*** Mepron.

Multi-ingredient: ***Austral.:*** Malarone; ***Swed.:*** Malarone; ***UK:*** Malarone.

Azanidazole (12411-t)

Azanidazole *(BAN, USAN, rINN).*

F-4. 4-[(*E*)-2-(1-Methyl-5-nitroimidazol-2-yl)vinyl]pyrimidin-2-ylamine.

$C_{10}H_{10}N_6O_2$ = 246.2.

CAS — 62973-76-6.

Azanidazole is a 5-nitroimidazole derivative similar to metronidazole (see p.585) and is used in the treatment of trichomoniasis.

Preparations

Proprietary Preparations (details are given in Part 3)
Ital.: Triclose.

Benznidazole (4756-r)

Benznidazole *(rINN).*

Ro-7-1051. *N*-Benzyl-2-(2-nitroimidazol-1-yl)acetamide.

$C_{12}H_{12}N_4O_3$ = 260.2.

CAS — 22994-85-0.

Adverse Effects

Nausea, vomiting, abdominal pain, peripheral neuropathy, blood dyscrasias, and severe skin reactions have been reported following the administration of benznidazole.

A study[1] involving 20 patients with chronic American trypanosomiasis given benznidazole 5 mg per kg bodyweight daily had to be stopped because of the high incidence of skin rashes and neurological symptoms.

1. Apt W, *et al.* Clinical trial of benznidazole and an immunopotentiator against Chagas disease in Chile. *Trans R Soc Trop Med Hyg* 1986; **80:** 1010.

Pharmacokinetics

Benznidazole is absorbed from the gastro-intestinal tract following administration by mouth.

Peak plasma concentrations of 2.22 to 2.81 μg per mL (average 2.54 μg per mL) of benznidazole were obtained in 6 healthy subjects 3 to 4 hours after administration of a single 100-mg dose of benznidazole by mouth.[1] The half-life of elimination ranged from 10.5 to 13.6 hours (average 12 hours). Benznidazole was about 44% bound to plasma proteins.

1. Raaflaub J, Ziegler WH. Single-dose pharmacokinetics of the trypanosomicide benznidazole in man. *Arzneimittelforschung* 1979; **29:** 1611–14.

Uses and Administration

Benznidazole is a 2-nitroimidazole derivative with antiprotozoal activity. It is of value in the treatment of South American trypanosomiasis (Chagas' disease) due to infection with *Trypanosoma cruzi*, especially the early acute stage of the disease.

Benznidazole has been given by mouth in a dose of 5 to 7 mg per kg body-weight daily in two divided doses usually for 60 days (but see below). Children have been given 10 mg per kg daily in two divided doses.

American trypanosomiasis. Available treatment for South American trypanosomiasis (p.578) is generally unsatisfactory, but benznidazole is of value especially in the acute phase. WHO[1] recommends that benznidazole should be given for 30 to 60 days but some in the USA[2] suggest courses of up to 90 days. Although treatment is usually confined to the acute phase of the disease, treatment during the early chronic phase was reported to be beneficial,[3] and long-term follow-up in patients who had received benznidazole has shown a reduction in cardiac complications and parasitaemia.[4]

1. WHO. Control of Chagas disease: report of a WHO expert committee. *WHO Tech Rep Ser 811* 1991.
2. Anonymous. Drugs for parasitic infections. *Med Lett Drugs Ther* 1998; **40:** 1–12.
3. de Andrade ALSS, *et al.* Randomised trial of efficacy of benznidazole in treatment of early Trypanosoma cruzi infection. *Lancet* 1996; **348:** 1407–13.
4. Viotti R, *et al.* Treatment of chronic Chagas' disease with benznidazole: clinical and serologic evolution of patients with long-term follow-up. *Am Heart J* 1994; **127:** 151–62.

Preparations

Proprietary Preparations (details are given in Part 3)
Arg.: Radanil; ***Braz.:*** Rochagan; ***Ecuad.:*** Ragonil.

Carnidazole (4763-x)

Carnidazole *(BAN, USAN, pINN).*

R-25831; R-28096 (carnidazole hydrochloride). *O*-Methyl [2-(2-methyl-5-nitroimidazol-1-yl)ethyl]thiocarbamate.

$C_8H_{12}N_4O_3S$ = 244.3.

CAS — 42116-76-7.

Carnidazole is a 5-nitroimidazole derivative similar to metronidazole. It is used in veterinary practice in the treatment and control of trichomoniasis in pigeons.

Clazuril (2940-v)

Clazuril *(BAN, USAN, rINN).*

R-62690. (±)-[2-Chloro-4-(4,5-dihydro-3,5-dioxo-*as*-triazin-2(3*H*)-yl)phenyl]-(*p*-chlorophenyl)acetonitrile.

$C_{17}H_{10}Cl_2N_4O_2$ = 373.2.

CAS — 101831-36-1.

Clazuril is an antiprotozoal used in veterinary practice for the control of coccidiosis in pigeons.

Clopidol (12589-f)

Clopidol *(BAN, USAN, rINN).*

Clopindol; Meticlorpindol. 3,5-Dichloro-2,6-dimethylpyridin-4-ol.

$C_7H_7Cl_2NO$ = 192.0.

CAS — 2971-90-6.

Clopidol is an antiprotozoal used in veterinary practice for the prevention of coccidiosis in poultry and rabbits either alone or in combination with methyl benzoquate (p.584).

Decoquinate (12626-e)

Decoquinate *(BAN, USAN, rINN).*

HC-1528; M&B-15497. Ethyl 6-decyloxy-7-ethoxy-4-hydroxyquinoline-3-carboxylate.

$C_{24}H_{35}NO_5$ = 417.5.

CAS — 18507-89-6.

Pharmacopoeias. In *USP* and *BP(Vet)*.

A cream to buff-coloured, odourless or almost odourless, microcrystalline powder. **Insoluble** in water; practically insoluble in alcohol; very slightly soluble in chloroform and ether. **Store** in airtight containers.

Decoquinate is an antiprotozoal used in veterinary practice for the control of coccidiosis in calves and sheep. It is also used for toxoplasmosis in sheep.

Dehydroemetine Hydrochloride (4773-f)

Dehydroemetine Hydrochloride *(BANM, rINNM).*

BT-436; 2,3-Dehydroemetine Hydrochloride; DHE; Ro-1-9334. 2,3-Didehydro-6′,7′,10,11-tetramethoxyemetan dihydrochloride; 3-Ethyl-1,6,7,11b-tetrahydro-9,10-dimethoxy-2-(1,2,3,4-tetrahydro-6,7-dimethoxy-1-isoquinolylmethyl)-4*H*-benzo[*a*]quinolizine dihydrochloride.

$C_{29}H_{38}N_2O_4,2HCl$ = 551.5.

CAS — 4914-30-1 (dehydroemetine); 2228-39-9 (dehydroemetine hydrochloride).

NOTE. The name DHE 45 has been used to denote a preparation of dihydroergotamine mesylate.

Pharmacopoeias. In *Int.*

Dehydroemetine, a synthetic derivative of emetine (p.582), is a tissue amoebicide with similar actions and uses, although probably of a lower toxicity.

Dehydroemetine should be avoided in patients with cardiac, renal, or neuromuscular disease and patients should be monitored for cardiac toxicity during treatment.

When used in the treatment of amoebiasis (p.573), dehydroemetine hydrochloride is given by intramuscular injection in a dose of 1 mg per kg body-weight daily, but no more than 60 mg daily, generally for up to 4 to 6 days (no more than 5 days in children). A dose of 0.5 mg per kg has been suggested for elderly or severely ill patients. At least 6 weeks should elapse before treatment is repeated. Following treatment with dehydroemetine, all patients should receive a luminal amoebicide to eliminate organisms from the colon. Patients with hepatic amoebiasis may be given supplementary treatment with chloroquine.

Liver fluke infections. Dehydroemetine has been given in the treatment of the liver fluke infection fascioliasis,[1] although the usual treatment is with bithionol (see p.94).

1. Farid Z, *et al.* Treatment of acute toxaemic fascioliasis. *Trans R Soc Trop Med Hyg* 1988; **82:** 299.

Diclazuril (2942-q)

Diclazuril *(BAN, USAN, rINN)*.

R-64433. (±)-4-Chlorophenyl[2,6-dichloro-4-(2,3,4,5-tetrahydro-3,5-dioxo-1,2,4-triazin-2-yl)phenyl]acetonitrile.

$C_{17}H_9Cl_3N_4O_2$ = 407.6.

CAS — 101831-37-2.

Diclazuril is an antiprotozoal that has been tried in AIDS patients for the management of coccidian diarrhoea. It has also been used in veterinary medicine.

References.

1. Kayembe K, *et al.* Diclazuril for Isospora belli infections in AIDS. *Lancet* 1989; **i:** 1397.
2. Connolly GM, *et al.* Diclazuril in the treatment of severe cryptosporidial diarrhoea in AIDS patients. *AIDS* 1990; **4:** 700–701.
3. Menichetti F, *et al.* Diclazuril for cryptosporidiosis in AIDS. *Am J Med* 1991; **90:** 271–2.

Di-iodohydroxyquinoline (4777-m)

Di-iodohydroxyquinoline *(BAN)*.

Diiodohydroxyquinoline *(rINN)*; Diiodohydroxyquin; Di-iodoxychinolinum; Diiodoxyquinoléine; Iodoquinol *(USAN)*. 5,7-Di-iodoquinolin-8-ol.

$C_9H_5I_2NO$ = 397.0.

CAS — 83-73-8.

Pharmacopoeias. In *US.*

A light yellowish to tan-coloured, microcrystalline powder, not readily wetted in water, odourless or with a slight odour. Practically **insoluble** in water; sparingly soluble in alcohol and ether.

Adverse Effects

Major concerns have been expressed about the safety of the halogenated hydroxyquinolines since the recognition of severe neurotoxicity with clioquinol. In Japan, the epidemic development of subacute myelo-opticoneuropathy (SMON) in the 1960s was associated with the ingestion of normal or high doses of clioquinol for prolonged periods and the sale of clioquinol and related hydroxyquinolines was subsequently banned in Japan. Symptoms of subacute myelo-opticoneuropathy are principally those of peripheral neuropathy, including optic atrophy, and myelopathy. Abdominal pain and diarrhoea often precede neurological symptoms such as paraesthesias in the legs progressing to paraplegia in some patients and loss of visual acuity sometimes leading to blindness. Cerebral disturbances, including confusion and retrograde amnesia, have also been reported. Although many patients improved when clioquinol was withdrawn, others had residual disablement.

It was suggested that the Japanese epidemic might have been due to genetic susceptibility, but a few similar cases of subacute myelo-opticoneuropathy have been reported from several other countries in association with clioquinol or related hydroxyquinoline derivatives, such as broxyquinoline or di-iodohydroxyquinoline.

Di-iodohydroxyquinoline has also been associated with gastro-intestinal effects such as abdominal cramps, nausea, and diarrhoea. Adverse effects which may be attributable to the iodine content of di-iodohydroxyquinoline include pruritus ani, skin eruptions, and enlargement of the thyroid gland. Fever, chills, headache, and vertigo have also occurred.

Precautions

Di-iodohydroxyquinoline is contra-indicated in patients known to be hypersensitive to iodine or halogenated hydroxyquinolines and in those with impaired kidney or liver function. It should be used with caution in thyroid disease and may interfere with determinations of protein-bound iodine for up to 6 months in tests for thyroid function. Its use is best avoided in patients with neurological disorders. Long-term use should be avoided.

The Committee on Drugs of the American Academy of Pediatrics[1] considered that there was a potential risk of toxicity to infants and children from clioquinol and di-iodohydroxyquinoline applied topically. Since alternative effective preparations are available for dermatitis the Committee recommended that products containing either of these compounds should not be used.

Also the WHO considered that the use of halogenated hydroxyquinolines for the treatment of acute diarrhoea or amoebiasis in children cannot be justified.[2] There is no evidence of their efficacy in acute diarrhoea and they have been associated with severe neurological effects. On the rare occasions when a luminal amoebicide is required other less toxic and more effective agents are available.

1. Kauffman RE, *et al.* Clioquinol (iodochlorhydroxyquin, Vioform) and iodoquinol (diiodohydroxyquin): blindness and neuropathy. *Pediatrics* 1990; **86:** 797–8.
2. WHO. The rational use of drugs in the management of acute diarrhoea in children. Geneva: WHO, 1990.

Pharmacokinetics

Di-iodohydroxyquinoline is partly and irregularly absorbed from the gastro-intestinal tract. Concern has been expressed about possible absorption following application to the skin (see above).

Uses and Administration

Di-iodohydroxyquinoline, a halogenated hydroxyquinoline, is a luminal amoebicide acting principally in the bowel lumen and is used in the treatment of intestinal amoebiasis, although a less toxic amoebicide such as diloxanide furoate is usually preferred; children should not be treated with di-iodohydroxyquinoline (see Precautions, above). It is given alone in the treatment of asymptomatic cyst-passers and in conjunction with an amoebicide that acts in the tissues, such as metronidazole, in patients with invasive amoebiasis (p.573). The usual dosage in the treatment of amoebiasis is 630 or 650 mg three times daily by mouth for 20 days.

Di-iodohydroxyquinoline has also been given in the treatment of *Dientamoeba fragilis* infections, in balantidiasis (p.574) as an alternative to tetracycline, and in *Blastocystis hominis* infections (p.574).

Di-iodohydroxyquinoline was formerly used in the treatment of acrodermatitis enteropathica; it is reported to act by enhancing zinc absorption and has now been superseded by oral zinc therapy (see p.1373).

Di-iodohydroxyquinoline is claimed to have some antibacterial and antifungal activity and has been used topically (but see under Precautions, above).

Preparations

USP 23: Iodoquinol Tablets.

Proprietary Preparations (details are given in Part 3)
Canad.: Diodoquin; ***Fr.:*** Direxiode†; ***S.Afr.:*** Floraquin†; ***USA:*** Sebaquin†; Yodoxin.

Multi-ingredient: ***Austral.:*** Floraquin; ***Canad.:*** Ovoquinol†; ***S.Afr.:*** Vagarsol; Viocort; Viodor; ***Spain:*** Floraquin†; ***USA:*** Vytone.

Diloxanide Furoate (4779-v)

Diloxanide Furoate *(BANM, rINNM)*.

4-(*N*-Methyl-2,2-dichloroacetamido)phenyl 2-furoate.

$C_{14}H_{11}Cl_2NO_4$ = 328.1.

CAS — 579-38-4 (diloxanide); 3736-81-0 (diloxanide furoate).

Pharmacopoeias. In *Br.* and *Int.*

A white or almost white, odourless or almost odourless, crystalline powder. Very slightly **soluble** in water; slightly soluble in alcohol and in ether; freely soluble in chloroform. **Protect** from light.

Adverse Effects

Flatulence is the most common adverse effect during treatment with diloxanide furoate. Vomiting, pruritus, and urticaria may occasionally occur.

Pharmacokinetics

Diloxanide furoate is hydrolysed before absorption from the gastro-intestinal tract. The resulting diloxanide is readily absorbed and excreted mainly in the urine as the glucuronide; less than 10% of a dose appears in the faeces.

Uses and Administration

Diloxanide furoate, a dichloroacetamide derivative, is a luminal amoebicide acting principally in the bowel lumen and is used in the treatment of intestinal amoebiasis (p.573). It is given alone in the treatment of asymptomatic cyst-passers and in conjunction with an amoebicide that acts in the tissues, such as metronidazole, in patients with invasive amoebiasis.

Diloxanide furoate is administered by mouth in a dosage of 500 mg three times daily for 10 days; children weighing more than 25 kg may be given 20 mg per kg body-weight daily, in divided doses, for 10 days. The course of treatment may be repeated if necessary.

Preparations

BP 1998: Diloxanide Tablets.

Proprietary Preparations (details are given in Part 3)
Austral.: Furamide†; ***Irl.:*** Furamide; ***Switz.:*** Furamid; ***UK:*** Furamide.

Multi-ingredient: ***UK:*** Entamizole†.

Dimetridazole (12662-z)

Dimetridazole *(BAN, pINN)*.

1,2-Dimethyl-5-nitroimidazole.

$C_5H_7N_3O_2$ = 141.1.

CAS — 551-92-8.

Pharmacopoeias. In *BP(Vet).*

Fr. includes Dimetridazole and Dimetridazole Mesylate for veterinary use only.

An almost white to brownish-yellow, odourless or almost odourless powder which darkens on exposure to light. Slightly **soluble** in water; sparingly soluble in alcohol; freely soluble in chloroform; slightly soluble in ether. **Protect** from light.

Dimetridazole is a 5-nitroimidazole derivative similar to metronidazole. It is used in veterinary practice for the prevention and treatment of blackhead (histomoniasis) in turkeys and other poultry and of swine dysentery, and for the prevention of hexamitiasis and trichomoniasis in game birds.

Diminazene Aceturate (4780-r)

Diminazene Aceturate *(BANM, rINNM)*.

1,3-Bis(4-amidinophenyl)triazene bis(*N*-acetylglycinate).

$C_{22}H_{29}N_9O_6$ = 515.5.

CAS — 536-71-0 (diminazene); 908-54-3 (diminazene aceturate).

NOTE. Diminazene aceturate is often referred to by its veterinary proprietary name Berenil.

Diminazene aceturate, an aromatic diamidine derivative related to pentamidine, is an antiprotozoal which has been used in veterinary medicine in the treatment of trypanosomiasis and babesiosis. It has also been tried in human infections.

Dinitolmide (12665-a)

Dinitolmide *(BAN, rINN)*.

Dinitrotoluamide; Methyldinitrobenzamide. 3,5-Dinitro-*o*-toluamide.

$C_8H_7N_3O_5$ = 225.2.

CAS — 148-01-6.

Pharmacopoeias. In *BP(Vet).*

A cream-coloured to light tan-coloured odourless or almost odourless powder. Practically **insoluble** in water; slightly soluble in alcohol, in chloroform, and in ether; soluble in acetone.

Dinitolmide is an antiprotozoal used in veterinary practice for the prevention of coccidiosis in poultry.

Eflornithine Hydrochloride (16604-j)

Eflornithine Hydrochloride *(BANM, USAN, rINNM)*.

DFMO; α-Difluoromethylornithine Hydrochloride; MDL-71782; MDL-71782A; RMI-71782. 2-(Difluoromethyl)-DL-ornithine monohydrochloride monohydrate.

$C_6H_{12}F_2N_2O_2,HCl,H_2O$ = 236.6.

CAS — 67037-37-0 (eflornithine); 96020-91-6 (eflornithine hydrochloride).

Adverse Effects and Precautions

Reported adverse effects with eflornithine include myelosuppression producing anaemia, leucopenia, and thrombocytopenia. Some patients have experienced hearing loss and alopecia. Gastro-intestinal disturbances, especially diarrhoea, can be a problem with oral administration. Seizures have occurred in about 8% of patients given eflornithine but they may have been related to the disease rather than treatment.

Effects on the ears. A study in 58 patients[1] receiving eflornithine alone or in combination with interferon alfa for the treatment of metastatic melanoma demonstrated that hearing loss at multiple frequencies was related to the cumulative dose of eflornithine and was worse in patients with pre-existing hearing deficit.

1. Croghan MK, *et al.* Dose-related α-difluoromethylornithine ototoxicity. *Am J Clin Oncol* 1991; **14:** 331–5.

Effects on the heart. Fatal cardiac arrest occurred in an AIDS patient with *Pneumocystis carinii* pneumonia during the intravenous infusion of eflornithine 100 mg per kg body-weight over 1 hour.[1] Sudden death after infusion of eflornithine had occurred in several other critically ill patients with AIDS.

1. Barbarash RA, *et al.* Alpha-difluoromethylornithine infusion and cardiac arrest. *Ann Intern Med* 1986; **105:** 141–2.

Pharmacokinetics

Eflornithine hydrochloride is absorbed from the gastro-intestinal tract. Following intravenous administration approximately 80% is excreted unchanged in the urine in 24 hours. The terminal elimination half-life is approximately 3 hours. It is distributed to the CSF.

References.

1. Haegele KD, *et al.* Kinetics of α-difluoromethylornithine: an irreversible inhibitor of ornithine decarboxylase. *Clin Pharmacol Ther* 1981; **30:** 210–17.
2. Milord F, *et al.* Eflornithine concentrations in serum and cerebrospinal fluid of 63 patients treated for Trypanosoma brucei gambiense sleeping sickness. *Trans R Soc Trop Med Hyg* 1993; **87:** 473–7.

Uses and Administration

Eflornithine hydrochloride is an antiprotozoal which acts as an irreversible inhibitor of ornithine decarboxylase, the rate-limiting enzyme in polyamine biosynthesis; trypanosomes are more susceptible to the effects of eflornithine than are humans, probably because of their slower turnover of this enzyme.

Eflornithine is used in African trypanosomiasis mainly due to *Trypanosoma brucei gambiense* and is effective in the early and more importantly in the late stage of the disease when there is central involvement. Eflornithine also has activity against *Pneumocystis carinii* and there are several reports of it being effective in patients whose pneumonia due to this organism failed to respond to standard treatment such as co-trimoxazole or pentamidine.

It is administered intravenously or by mouth, though diarrhoea can be troublesome with the latter route. In the treatment of African trypanosomiasis the usual dose is 100 mg per kg body-weight every 6 hours by intravenous infusion for at least 14 days. Some clinicians then give 300 mg per kg per day by mouth for a further 3 to 4 weeks. Dosage should be reduced in patients with impaired renal function.

Cryptosporidiosis. Eflornithine has been tried in the treatment of cryptosporidiosis (p.574) in AIDS patients.[1]

1. Rolston KVI, *et al.* Intestinal cryptosporidiosis treated with eflornithine: a prospective study among patients with AIDS. *J Acquir Immune Defic Syndr* 1989; **2:** 426–30.

Malignant neoplasms. Eflornithine has antimetabolic activity and has been studied as a potential inhibitor of malignant disease. Palliative activity was reported in patients with recurrent gliomas[1] but eflornithine given in combination with interferon gamma had no therapeutic activity in patients with advanced renal cell carcinoma, malignant melanoma, or colorectal carcinoma.[2]

1. Levin VA, *et al.* Treatment of recurrent gliomas with eflornithine. *J Natl Cancer Inst* 1992; **84:** 1432–7.
2. Zeller W, *et al.* Phase I-II study of interferon-γ and eflornithine (DFMO) in patients with advanced renal cell carcinoma, malignant melanoma and colorectal carcinoma. *Oncol Rep* 1996; **3:** 447–51.

Pneumocystis carinii pneumonia. Eflornithine has been tried in the treatment of *Pneumocystis carinii* pneumonia as a potential alternative to co-trimoxazole and pentamidine (see p.370). In a study in 31 AIDS patients who had not responded to co-trimoxazole and/or pentamidine, 21 (68%) subsequently responded to eflornithine.[1] However in an open study eflornithine was less effective than co-trimoxazole.[2]

1. Smith D, *et al.* Pneumocystis carinii pneumonia treated with eflornithine in AIDS patients resistant to conventional therapy. *AIDS* 1990; **4:** 1019–21.
2. Smith DE, *et al.* Eflornithine versus cotrimoxazole in the treatment of Pneumocystis carinii pneumonia in AIDS patients. *AIDS* 1992; **6:** 1489–93.

African trypanosomiasis. As discussed on p.577, eflornithine is effective in the treatment of *Trypanosoma brucei gambiense* infections, and is particularly valuable in providing an alternative to melarsoprol in meningoencephalitic disease. The cumbersome dosage schedule and relatively high cost may limit its use to patients who relapse after melarsoprol therapy.[1] Eflornithine 100 mg per kg body-weight intravenously every 6 hours for 7 days rather than the standard 14 days produced long-term responses in 42 of 47 patients who had previously relapsed following treatment with other regimens.[2] One patient who had relapsed following treatment with melarsoprol and eflornithine given singly was cured when the drugs were given in combination.[3] It is not effective when given alone in *T. b. rhodesiense* infections, but its use in combination with suramin is being assessed.[4,5]

1. Milord F, *et al.* Efficacy and toxicity of eflornithine for treatment of Trypanosoma brucei gambiense sleeping sickness. *Lancet* 1992; **340:** 652–5.
2. Khonde N, *et al.* A seven days course of eflornithine for relapsing Trypanosoma brucei gambiense sleeping sickness. *Trans R Soc Trop Med Hyg* 1997; **91:** 212–13.
3. Simarro PP, Asumu PN. Gambian trypanosomiasis and synergism between melarsoprol and eflornithine: first case report. *Trans R Soc Trop Med Hyg* 1996; **90:** 315.
4. WHO. *WHO model prescribing information: drugs used in parasitic diseases.* 2nd ed. Geneva: WHO, 1995.
5. Taelman H, *et al.* Combination treatment with suramin and eflornithine in late stage rhodesian trypanosomiasis: case report. *Trans R Soc Trop Med Hyg* 1996; **90:** 572–3.

Preparations

Proprietary Preparations (details are given in Part 3)
USA: Ornidyl.

Emetine Hydrochloride (4782-d)

Emetine Hydrochloride *(BANM)*.

Cloridrato de Emetina; Emet. Hydrochlor.; Emetine Dihydrochloride; Emetine Hydrochloride Heptahydrate; Emetini Chloridum; Emetini Hydrochloridum Heptahydricum; Ipecine Hydrochloride; Methylcephaëline Hydrochloride. 6′,7′,10,11-Tetramethoxyemetan dihydrochloride heptahydrate; (2*S*,3*R*,11b*S*)-3-Ethyl-1,3,4,6,7,11b-hexahydro-9,10-dimethoxy-2-[(1*R*)-1,2,3,4-tetrahydro-6,7-dimethoxy-1-isoquinolylmethyl]-2*H*-benzo[*a*]quinolizine dihydrochloride heptahydrate.

$C_{29}H_{40}N_2O_4,2HCl,7H_2O$ = 679.7.

CAS — 483-18-1 (emetine); 316-42-7 (emetine hydrochloride, anhydrous); 7083-71-8 (emetine hydrochloride, hydrate); 79300-08-6 (emetine hydrochloride, heptahydrate).

Pharmacopoeias. In *Eur.* (see p.viii), which also has a monograph for Emetine Hydrochloride Pentahydrate; *Int.* permits the heptahydrate or pentahydrate in the same monograph. *US* has a monograph for the anhydrous salt.

The dihydrochloride of an alkaloid obtained from ipecacuanha, or prepared by methylation of cephaëline (another alkaloid present in ipecacuanha), or prepared synthetically.

A white or slightly yellow odourless crystalline powder. Freely **soluble** in water and in alcohol. A 2% solution in water has a pH of 4.0 to 6.0. Solutions are **sterilised** by heating in an autoclave. **Protect** from light. In addition the USP specifies that the anhydrous form should be stored in airtight containers.

Adverse Effects

Administration of emetine hydrochloride is commonly associated with aching, tenderness, stiffness, and weakness of the muscles in the area of the injection site; there may be necrosis and abscess formation. After injection diarrhoea and nausea and vomiting, sometimes accompanied by dizziness and headache, are common. There may be generalised muscle weakness and muscular pain, especially in the neck and limbs, and, more rarely, mild sensory disturbances. Eczematous, urticarial, and purpuric skin lesions have been reported.

Cardiovascular effects are considered the most serious and include precordial pain, dyspnoea, tachycardia, and hypotension. Changes in the ECG, particularly flattening or inversion of the T-wave and prolongation of the Q-T interval, occur in many patients. Emetine accumulates in the body and large doses or prolonged administration may cause lesions of the heart, gastro-intestinal tract, kidneys, liver, and skeletal muscle. Severe acute degenerative myocarditis may occur and may give rise to sudden cardiac failure and death. In some patients cardiotoxic effects have appeared after the completion of treatment with therapeutic doses.

Emetine hydrochloride is very irritant and contact with mucous membranes should be avoided.

Precautions

Emetine is contra-indicated in cardiac, renal, or neuromuscular disease. Its use should be avoided during pregnancy and it should not be given to children, except in severe amoebic dysentery unresponsive to other drugs. It should be used with great caution in old or debilitated patients. Patients receiving emetine should be closely supervised; ECG monitoring is advisable during treatment.

Pharmacokinetics

After injection emetine hydrochloride is concentrated in the liver. Appreciable concentration occurs also in kidney, lung, and spleen. Excretion is slow and detectable concentrations may persist in urine 40 to 60 days after treatment has been discontinued. Cumulation may occur.

Uses and Administration

Emetine, an alkaloid of ipecacuanha (p.1062), is a tissue amoebicide acting principally in the bowel wall and in the liver. It has been given by deep subcutaneous or intramuscular injection in the treatment of severe invasive amoebiasis (p.573) including hepatic amoebiasis in patients who do not respond to metronidazole although dehydroemetine has tended to replace it.

Emetine was formerly administered by mouth as emetine and bismuth iodide.

Preparations

USP 23: Emetine Hydrochloride Injection.

Proprietary Preparations (details are given in Part 3)

Multi-ingredient: ***Aust.:*** Spirbon; ***Canad.:*** Cophylac; ***Fr.:*** Doudol†; ***Switz.:*** Ipeca; Rectopyrine†; Sano Tuss.

Ethopabate (12705-w)

Ethopabate *(BAN)*.

Methyl 4-acetamido-2-ethoxybenzoate.

$C_{12}H_{15}NO_4$ = 237.3.

CAS — 59-06-3.

Pharmacopoeias. In *BP(Vet)*. Also in *US* for veterinary use only.

A white or pinkish-white, odourless or almost odourless powder. Very slightly **soluble** in water; sparingly soluble in alcohol, in dichloromethane, in dioxan, in ethyl acetate, and in isopropyl alcohol; soluble in acetone, in acetonitrile, in dehydrated alcohol, in chloroform, and in methyl alcohol; slightly soluble in ether. **Protect** from light.

Ethopabate is an antiprotozoal used in veterinary practice, usually in conjunction with other drugs such as amprolium, for the control of coccidiosis.

Etofamide (4783-n)

Etofamide *(rINN)*.

Ethychlordiphene; K-430. 2,2-Dichloro-*N*-(2-ethoxyethyl)-*N*-[4-(4-nitrophenoxy)benzyl]acetamide.

$C_{19}H_{20}Cl_2N_2O_5$ = 427.3.

CAS — 25287-60-9.

Etofamide, a dichloroacetamide derivative, is a luminal amoebicide with actions and uses similar to those of diloxanide furoate (p.581).

References.

1. Pamba HO, *et al.* Comparative study of aminosidine, etophamide and nimorazole, alone or in combination, in the treatment of intestinal amoebiasis in Kenya. *Eur J Clin Pharmacol* 1990; **39:** 357–7.

Fumagillin (9454-n)

Fumagillin *(BAN)*.

4-(1,2-Epoxy-1,6-dimethylhex-4-enyl)-5-methoxy-1-oxaspiro[2.5]oct-6-yl hydrogen deca-2,4,6,8-tetraenedioate.

$C_{26}H_{34}O_7$ = 458.5.

CAS — 23110-15-8.

Fumagillin is an alicyclic antibiotic produced by certain strains of *Aspergillus fumigatus*. It has activity against Microsporidia and has been tried topically in the treatment of microsporidial keratoconjunctivitis. It was formerly given by mouth in the treatment of intestinal amoebiasis, but produced an unacceptably high frequency of adverse effects. Analogues of fumagillin have been investigated for effects on angiogenesis in solid tumours.

Microsporidiosis. As discussed on p.576, topical treatment of microsporidial keratoconjunctivitis has been disappointing. There have been several reports of successful treatment in individual patients using fumagillin topically,[1-3] usually as a solution of bicyclohexylammonium fumagillin containing the equivalent of 70 mg of fumagillin per mL.

1. Rosberger DF, *et al.* Successful treatment of microsporidial keratoconjunctivitis with topical fumagillin in a patient with AIDS. *Cornea* 1993; **12:** 261–5.
2. Diesenhouse MC, *et al.* Treatment of microsporidial keratoconjunctivitis with topical fumagillin. *Am J Ophthalmol* 1993; **115:** 293–8.
3. Garvery MJ, *et al.* Topical fumagillin in the treatment of microsporidial keratoconjunctivitis in AIDS. *Ann Pharmacother* 1995; **29:** 872–4.

Preparations

Proprietary Preparations (details are given in Part 3)
UK: Fumidil.

Furazolidone (4784-h)

Furazolidone *(BAN, rINN)*.

Nifurazolidonum. 3-(5-Nitrofurfurylideneamino)-2-oxazolidone.

$C_8H_7N_3O_5$ = 225.2.

CAS — 67-45-8.

Pharmacopoeias. In *Br., Fr., It.,* and *US.*

A yellow odourless or almost odourless crystalline powder. BP **solubilities** are: very slightly soluble in water and in alcohol; slightly soluble in chloroform; practically insoluble in ether. USP solubilities are: practically insoluble in water, in alcohol, and in carbon tetrachloride. The filtrate from a 1% suspension in water has a pH of 4.5 to 7.0. **Store** in airtight containers. Protect from light.

Adverse Effects

The most common adverse effects of furazolidone involve the gastro-intestinal tract and include nausea and vomiting. Dizziness, drowsiness, headache, and a general malaise have also been reported.

Allergic reactions, most commonly skin reactions such as rashes or angioedema, may occur. There have been instances of acute pulmonary reactions, similar to those seen with the structurally related drug nitrofurantoin, and of hepatotoxicity. Agranulocytosis has been reported rarely. Haemolytic anaemia may occur in patients with a deficiency of glucose-6-phosphate dehydrogenase given furazolidone.

Darkening of the urine has been attributed to the presence of metabolites.

Precautions

Because of the risk of haemolytic anaemia furazolidone should be used with caution in those with glucose-6-phosphate dehydrogenase deficiency and should not be given to infants under one month of age since their enzyme systems are immature.

Interactions

A disulfiram-like reaction has been reported in patients taking alcohol while on furazolidone therapy; alcohol should be avoided during and for a short period after treatment with furazolidone.

Furazolidone is an MAOI and the cautions advised for these drugs regarding the concomitant administration of other drugs, especially indirect acting sympathomimetic amines, and the consumption of food and drink containing tyramine, should be observed (see Phenelzine Sulphate, p.304). However, there appear to be no reports of hypertensive crises in patients receiving furazolidone and it has been suggested that, since furazolidone inhibits monoamine oxidase gradually over several days, the risks are small if treatment is limited to a 5-day course. Toxic psychosis has been reported in a patient receiving furazolidone and amitriptyline.

Pharmacokinetics

Although furazolidone has been considered to be largely unabsorbed when administered orally, the occurrence of systemic adverse effects and coloured metabolites in the urine suggest that this may not be the case. Rapid and extensive metabolism, possibly in the intestine, has been proposed.

Uses and Administration

Furazolidone is a nitrofuran derivative with antiprotozoal and antibacterial activity. It is active against the protozoan *Giardia intestinalis* (*Giardia lamblia*) and against a range of enteric bacteria *in vitro*, including staphylococci, enterococci, *Escherichia coli*, *Salmonella* spp., *Shigella* spp., and *Vibrio cholerae*. Furazolidone is bactericidal and appears to act by interfering with bacterial enzyme systems. Resistance is reported to be limited. It is used in the treatment of giardiasis (p.575) and cholera (p.124). It has been suggested for other bacterial gastro-intestinal infections but antibacterial therapy is regarded as unnecessary in mild and self-limiting gastroenteritis (see p.123).

Furazolidone is given by mouth in a dose of 100 mg four times daily; children may be given 1.25 mg per kg bodyweight four times daily. It is usually given for 2 to 5 days, but may be given for up to 7 days in some patients, or for up to 10 days for giardiasis.

Peptic ulcer disease. Furazolidone is not one of the main drugs used in the treatment of peptic ulceration (p.1174). However, it has been reported to possess anti-*Helicobacter* activity[1] and to have some ulcer-healing properties.[2-4]

1. Howden A, *et al.* In-vitro sensitivity of Campylobacter pyloridis to furazolidone. *Lancet* 1986; **ii:** 1035.
2. Zheng Z-T, *et al.* Double-blind short-term trial of furazolidone in peptic ulcer. *Lancet* 1985; **i:** 1048–9.
3. Zhao H-Y, *et al.* Furazolidone in peptic ulcer. *Lancet* 1985; **ii:** 276–7.
4. Segura AM, *et al.* Furazolidone, amoxycillin, bismuth triple therapy for Helicobacter pylori infection. *Aliment Pharmacol Ther* 1997; **11:** 529–32.

Preparations

USP 23: Furazolidone Oral Suspension; Furazolidone Tablets.

Proprietary Preparations (details are given in Part 3)
Ger.: Nifuran; *Ital.:* Furoxone; *S.Afr.:* Furoxone†; *USA:* Furoxone.

Multi-ingredient: *Ital.:* Ginecofuran; Tricofur†; *Spain:* Desinvag; Saleton†.

Halofuginone Hydrobromide (12813-j)

Halofuginone Hydrobromide *(BANM, USAN, rINNM)*.

RU-19110. (±)-*trans*-7-Bromo-6-chloro-3-[3-(3-hydroxy-2-piperidyl)acetonyl]quinazolin-4(3*H*)-one hydrobromide.

$C_{16}H_{17}BrClN_3O_3,HBr$ = 495.6.

CAS — 55837-20-2 (halofuginone); 64924-67-0 (halofuginone hydrobromide).

Halofuginone hydrobromide is an antiprotozoal used in veterinary practice for the prevention of coccidiosis in poultry.

Imidocarb Dipropionate (4983-s)

Imidocarb Dipropionate *(BANM, rINNM)*.

4A65 (imidocarb hydrochloride). 1,3-Bis[3-(2-imidazolin-2-yl)phenyl]urea dipropionate; 3,3′-Di-2-imidazolin-2-ylcarbanilide dipropionate; .

$C_{19}H_{20}N_6O,2C_3H_6O_2$ = 496.6.

CAS — 27885-92-3 (imidocarb); 55750-06-6 (imidocarb dipropionate); 5318-76-3 (imidocarb hydrochloride).

NOTE. Imidocarb Hydrochloride is *USAN*.

Imidocarb dipropionate is an antiprotozoal used in veterinary practice in the treatment of babesiosis in cattle. Imidocarb hydrochloride has also been used.

Isometamidium Chloride (7322-t)

Isometamidium Chloride *(rINN)*.

Isometamidium *(BAN)*. 8-[3-(*m*-Amidinophenyl)-2-triazeno]3-amino-5-ethyl-6-phenylphenanthridinium chloride.

$C_{28}H_{26}ClN_7$ = 496.0.

CAS — 34301-55-8.

Isometamidium chloride is an antiprotozoal used in veterinary practice for the control of trypanosomiasis.

Lasalocid Sodium (12890-b)

Lasalocid Sodium *(BANM, rINNM)*.

Ro-02-2985 (lasalocid). Sodium 6-[(3*R*,4*S*,5*S*,7*R*)-7-{(2*S*,3*S*,5*S*)-5-ethyl-5-[(2*R*,5*R*,6*S*)-5-ethyltetrahydro-5-hydroxy-6-methyl-2*H*-pyran-2-yl]tetrahydro-3-methyl-2-furyl}-4-hydroxy-3,5-dimethyl-6-oxononyl]-2-hydroxy-*m*-toluate.

$C_{34}H_{53}NaO_8$ = 612.8.

CAS — 11054-70-9 (lasalocid); 25999-31-9 (lasalocid); 25999-20-6 (lasalocid sodium).

NOTE. Lasalocid is *USAN*.

An antibiotic produced by *Streptomyces lasaliensis*.

Lasalocid sodium is an antiprotozoal used in veterinary practice for the prevention of coccidiosis in poultry.

Letrazuril (11010-k)

Letrazuril *(rINN)*.

(±)-[2,6-Dichloro-4-(4,5-dihydro-3,5-dioxo-*as*-triazin-2(3*H*)-yl)phenyl](*p*-fluoro-phenyl)acetonitrile.

$C_{17}H_9Cl_2FN_4O_2$ = 391.2.

CAS — 103337-74-2.

Letrazuril is an antiprotozoal which is being investigated in the treatment of cryptosporidiosis (p.574) in patients with AIDS.

References.

1. Victor GH, *et al.* Letrazuril therapy for cryptosporidiosis: clinical response and pharmacokinetics. *AIDS* 1993; **7:** 438–40.
2. Harris M, *et al.* A phase I study of letrazuril in AIDS-related cryptosporidiosis. *AIDS* 1994; **8:** 1109–13.
3. Loeb M, *et al.* Treatment with letrazuril of refractory cryptosporidial diarrhea complicating AIDS. *J Acquir Immune Defic Syndr Hum Retrovirol* 1995; **10:** 48–53.

Maduramicin (2749-g)

Maduramicin *(BAN, USAN, rINN)*.

CL-273703; Maduramicin Ammonium. Ammonium (2*R*,3*S*,4*S*,5*R*,6*S*)-tetrahydro-2-hydroxy-6-{(*R*)-1-[(2*S*,5*R*,7*S*,8*R*,9*S*)-9-hydroxy-2,8-dimethyl-2-{(2*S*,2′*R*,3′*S*,5*R*,5′*R*)-octahydro-2-methyl-3′-[(2*R*,4*S*,5*S*,6*S*)-tetrahydro-4,5-dimethoxy-6-methyl-2*H*-pyran-2-yl]oxy}-5′-[(2*S*,3*S*,5*R*,6*S*)-tetrahydro-6-hydroxy-3,5,6-trimethyl-2*H*-pyran-2-yl](2,2′-bifuran-5-yl)-1,6-dioxaspiro[4,5]dec-7-yl]ethyl}-4,5-dimethoxy-3-methyl-2*H*-pyran-2-acetate.

$C_{47}H_{80}O_{17},NH_3$ = 934.2.

CAS — 84878-61-5.

NOTE. The name maduramicin has also been used to denote the acid.

Maduramicin is an antiprotozoal used in veterinary practice for the prevention of coccidiosis in poultry.

Melarsomine (15288-w)

Melarsomine *(rINN)*.

Bis(2-aminoethyl) *p*-[(4,6-diamino-*s*-triazin-2-yl)amino]dithiobenzenearsonite.

$C_{13}H_{21}AsN_8S_2$ = 428.4.

CAS — 128470-15-5.

Melarsomine is a trivalent arsenical derivative used in veterinary practice for the control of trypanosomiasis and canine heartworm (dirofilariasis).

Melarsoprol (4788-g)

Melarsoprol *(BAN, rINN)*.

Mel B; Melarsen Oxide-BAL; RP-3854. 2-[4-(4,6-Diamino-1,3,5-triazin-2-ylamino)phenyl]-1,3,2-dithiarsolan-4-ylmethanol.

$C_{12}H_{15}AsN_6OS_2$ = 398.3.

CAS — 494-79-1.

A slightly cream-coloured or greyish cream-coloured, odourless powder containing about 18.5% of As.

Practically **insoluble** in water, in alcohol, and in ether; slowly soluble in propylene glycol but more readily soluble on warming. Solutions in propylene glycol are **sterilised** by autoclaving.

Adverse Effects and Treatment

Adverse effects are common and may be severe during the treatment of African trypanosomiasis with melarsoprol. It may be difficult to distinguish between effects of the disease, Herxheimer-type reactions resulting from the trypanocidal activity of melarsoprol, and adverse effects of the drug itself attributed to its arsenic content or to hypersensitivity. For the adverse effects of arsenic and their treatment, see Arsenic Trioxide, p.1550.

A severe febrile reaction may occur after the first injection of melarsoprol, especially in patients with large numbers of trypanosomes in their blood. It is therefore common practice to give two or three injections of suramin or pentamidine before starting melarsoprol therapy.

The greatest risk is from reactive encephalopathy which occurs in about 10% of patients treated with melarsoprol and is usually seen between the end of the first 3- or 4-day course of injections and the start of the second course. Some have attributed it to a toxic effect of melarsoprol and others to a Herxheimer-type reaction resulting from the release of antigen from trypanosomes killed in the brain; a combination of drug toxicity and host immune responses may be responsible. Encephalopathy may be sudden in onset or develop slowly. Symptoms include fever, headache, tremor, slurring of speech, convulsions, and coma; death has occurred in up to 5% of patients treated with melarsoprol. Less commonly, haemorrhagic encephalopathy may occur. The prophylactic use of corticosteroids has been suggested during treatment courses of melarsoprol (see African Trypanosomiasis, below). Treatment of reactive encephalopathy has included the use of corticosteroids, hypertonic solutions to combat cerebral oedema, anticonvulsants such as diazepam, and subcutaneous adrenaline; dimercaprol has been given on the assumption that encephalopathy resulted from arsenic poisoning, but has not generally been of benefit.

Hypersensitivity reactions to melarsoprol may occur during the second and subsequent courses of treatment. Desensitisation has been attempted by recommencing treatment with smaller and gradually increasing doses of melarsoprol; the concomitant administration of corticosteroids may help to control symptoms during this procedure. Some authorities consider that the use of small doses of melarsoprol may increase the risk of resistance.

Melarsoprol injection is very irritant and extravasation during intravenous administration should be avoided. Vomiting and abdominal colic may occur if it is injected too rapidly. Other adverse effects reported include agranulocytosis, hypertension, peripheral neuropathy, proteinuria, severe diarrhoea, myocardial damage, exfoliative dermatitis, and hepatic disturbances.

References.

1. Pepin J, *et al.* Trial of prednisolone for prevention of melarsoprol-induced encephalopathy in gambiense sleeping sickness. *Lancet* 1989; **i:** 1246–50.
2. Pepin J, Milord F. African trypanosomiasis and drug-induced encephalopathy: risk factors and pathogenesis. *Trans R Soc Trop Med Hyg* 1991; **85:** 222–4.
3. Pepin J, *et al.* Risk factors for encephalopathy and mortality during melarsoprol treatment of Trypanosoma brucei gambiense sleeping sickness. *Trans R Soc Trop Med Hyg* 1995; **89:** 92–7.

Precautions

Melarsoprol should not be administered during epidemics of influenza. Intercurrent infections such as malaria and pneumonia should be treated before melarsoprol is administered. Severe haemolytic reactions have been reported in patients with glucose-6-phosphate dehydrogenase deficiency. It may precipitate erythema nodosum when administered to patients with leprosy.

Patients should be in hospital when they are treated with melarsoprol and dosage decided after taking into account their general condition.

Treatment of pregnant women with trypanosomiasis should be deferred until after delivery. Pregnant women with meningoencephalitis may be treated with pentamidine (*T. b. gambiense*) or suramin (*T. b. rhodesiense*).

Pharmacokinetics

Melarsoprol is reported to be unreliably absorbed if given by mouth and is usually given by intravenous injection. A small amount penetrates to the CSF where it has a local trypanocidal action. It is rapidly metabolised and excreted in the faeces and urine so any prophylactic effect is short-lived.

Uses and Administration

Melarsoprol, a trivalent arsenical derivative, is a trypanocide which appears to act by inhibiting trypanosomal pyruvate kinase. It is effective in the treatment of all stages of African trypanosomiasis due to *Trypanosoma brucei gambiense* or *T. brucei rhodesiense*, but because of its toxicity its use is usually reserved for stages of the disease involving the CNS. Resistance has been reported to develop.

Patients undergoing therapy with melarsoprol should be treated in hospital. Melarsoprol is administered by intravenous injection as a 3.6% solution in propylene glycol. The injection should be given slowly, care being taken to prevent leakage into the surrounding tissues, and the patient should remain supine and fasting for at least 5 hours after the injection.

Treatment protocols vary, but in general melarsoprol is given in low doses initially, especially in children and debilitated patients, increased gradually to the maximum daily dose of 3.6 mg per kg body-weight. Doses are given daily for 3 or 4 days and the course repeated 2 or 3 times with an interval of at least 7 days between courses. Since massive destruction of parasites resulting in a Herxheimer reaction is particularly dangerous during treatment with melarsoprol, it may be preceded by several doses of suramin or pentamidine to induce the reaction beforehand.

Melarsonyl potassium is a water-soluble derivative of melarsoprol which was formerly used as an alternative to melarsoprol but was probably more toxic and less effective.

Administration. Results observed in *mice* suggest that the topical application of melarsoprol might be a practical route.[1,2]

1. Jennings FW, *et al.* Topical melarsoprol for trypanosomiasis. *Lancet* 1993; **341:** 1341–2.
2. Atouguia JM, *et al.* Successful treatment of experimental murine Trypanosoma brucei infection with topical melarsoprol gel. *Trans R Soc Trop Med Hyg* 1995; **89:** 531–3.

African trypanosomiasis. The treatment of African trypanosomiasis is discussed on p.577. Melarsoprol, which is effective against both *Trypanosoma brucei gambiense* and *T. b. rhodesiense*, is usually only given to treat the meningoencephalitic stage of the infection because of its toxicity in producing potentially fatal encephalopathy. However, protection against this toxicity may be provided by prophylaxis with prednisolone.[1,2] Combination therapy with melarsoprol and eflornithine was reported to be effective in one patient who had not responded to either drug alone.[3]

1. Pepin J, *et al.* Trial of prednisolone for prevention of melarsoprol-induced encephalopathy in gambiense sleeping sickness. *Lancet* 1989; **i:** 1246–50.
2. Pepin J, *et al.* Risk factors for encephalopathy and mortality during melarsoprol treatment of Trypanosoma brucei gambiense sleeping sickness. *Trans R Soc Trop Med Hyg* 1995; **89:** 92–7.
3. Simarro PP, Asumu PN. Gambian trypanosomiasis and synergism between melarsoprol and eflornithine: first case report. *Trans R Soc Trop Med Hyg* 1996; **90:** 315.

Preparations

Proprietary Preparations (details are given in Part 3)
Fr.: Arsobal†; ***S.Afr.:*** Arsobal.

Mepacrine Hydrochloride (1382-g)

Mepacrine Hydrochloride *(BANM, rINNM).*

Acrichinum; Acrinamine; Antimalarinae Chlorhydras; Chinacrina; Mepacrini Hydrochloridum; Quinacrine Hydrochloride. 6-Chloro-9-(4-diethylamino-1-methylbutylamino)-2-methoxyacridine dihydrochloride dihydrate.

$C_{23}H_{30}ClN_3O,2HCl,2H_2O = 508.9.$

CAS — 83-89-6 (mepacrine); 69-05-6 (mepacrine dihydrochloride, anhydrous); 6151-30-0 (mepacrine dihydrochloride, dihydrate).

Pharmacopoeias. In Aust. and It.

A bright yellow odourless crystalline powder. **Soluble** 1 in 35 of water; soluble in alcohol. A 1% solution in water has a pH of about 4.5. **Store** in airtight containers. Protect from light.

Adverse Effects

The most common adverse effects associated with mepacrine are dizziness, headache, and gastro-intestinal disturbances such as nausea and vomiting. Reversible yellow discoloration of the skin and urine may occur during long-term administration or after large doses; blue/black discoloration of the palate and nails has also been reported. Doses such as those used in the treatment of giardiasis may occasionally cause transient acute toxic psychosis and CNS stimulation. Convulsions have been reported at high doses. Ocular toxicity similar to that seen with chloroquine (see p.427) and chronic dermatoses, including severe exfoliative dermatitis and lichenoid eruptions, have also occurred after prolonged administration of mepacrine. Hepatotoxicity and aplastic anaemia occur rarely.

Effects on the blood. In endemic malarial areas mepacrine has been a significant cause of aplastic anaemia with an incidence of about 1 in 20 000.[1]

1. Eden OB. The haemopoietic system in childhood. *Br Med Bull* 1986; **42:** 191–5.

Effects on the nervous system. Two patients had convulsions a few hours after the intrapleural administration of mepacrine hydrochloride 400 mg for malignant effusions. One developed status epilepticus and died and the other was successfully treated with anticonvulsants.[1]

1. Borda I, Krant M. Convulsions following intrapleural administration of quinacrine hydrochloride. *JAMA* 1967; **201:** 1049–50.

Precautions

Mepacrine should be used with caution in elderly patients or patients with a history of psychosis, or in the presence of hepatic disease or porphyria. Mepacrine can cause exacerbation of psoriasis and should be avoided in psoriatic patients.

Interactions

Mepacrine has been reported to produce a mild disulfiram-like reaction (see p.1573) when taken with alcohol.

Theoretically, mepacrine may increase the plasma concentrations of primaquine resulting in a higher risk of toxicity, and it has been recommended that these drugs should not be used concomitantly.

Pharmacokinetics

Mepacrine is readily absorbed from the gastro-intestinal tract and widely distributed throughout the body. It accumulates in body tissues particularly the liver and is liberated slowly. It is excreted slowly mainly in the urine, and is still detectable in the urine after 2 months. Mepacrine crosses the placenta.

Intrapleural administration. Peak plasma concentrations of mepacrine far above those associated with CNS effects were rapidly attained in 3 of 4 patients following intrapleural instillation of a solution of mepacrine hydrochloride and remained at these levels for several hours.[1]

1. Björkman S, *et al.* Pharmacokinetics of quinacrine after intrapleural instillation in rabbits and man. *J Pharm Pharmacol* 1989; **41:** 160–73.

Uses and Administration

Mepacrine hydrochloride is a 9-aminoacridine antiprotozoal used mainly as an alternative to one of the nitroimidazoles in the treatment of giardiasis (p.575). It is no longer used to treat malaria.

In giardiasis, mepacrine hydrochloride is given by mouth in doses of 100 mg three times daily after food for 5 to 7 days. A second course of treatment after 2 weeks may sometimes be required. A suggested dose for children is 2 mg per kg body-weight given three times daily (maximum 300 mg daily).

Mepacrine hydrochloride has also been used locally in the treatment of some forms of cutaneous leishmaniasis, as a sterilisation technique for contraception, and in the management of malignant effusions.

Contraception. Sterilisation with intra-uterine mepacrine has been attempted as an irreversible method of contraception (p.1434). This technique produces occlusion of the fallopian tube and has been reported to be an effective nonsurgical means of female sterilisation.[1] There has been speculation about the risk of cancer from this technique but there appeared to be no evidence to confirm such a risk.[2,3] However, the method remains controversial and some authorities[4] have recommended that a full evaluation of its safety and efficacy is still needed. More recently it was reported that the Indian government had banned the use of mepacrine for sterilisation.[5]

1. Hieu DT, *et al.* 31 781 Cases of non-surgical female sterilisation with quinacrine pellets in Vietnam. *Lancet* 1993; **342:** 213–17.
2. Anonymous. Death of a study: WHO, what, and why. *Lancet* 1994; **343:** 987–8.
3. Hieu DT. Quinacrine method of family planning. *Lancet* 1994; **343:** 1040.
4. Benagiano G. Sterilisation by quinacrine. *Lancet* 1994; **344:** 689.
5. Sharma DC. Indian government bans use of quinacrine for sterilisation. *Lancet* 1998; **352:** 717.

Leishmaniasis. Mepacrine has been suggested for intralesional injection in the treatment of early noninflamed nodular lesions of cutaneous leishmaniasis (p.575) due to *Leishmania tropica*, *L. major*, *L. mexicana*, *L. panamensis*, or *L. peruviana*.[1] A suggested course of treatment is 3 intralesional injections of a 5% solution of mepacrine given at intervals of 3 to 5 days. However, local infiltration of drugs can be difficult and painful, and a number of other local and systemic treatments have been tried.

1. WHO. Control of the leishmaniases. *WHO Tech Rep Ser 793* 1990.

Malignant effusions. Intrapleural instillations of mepacrine hydrochloride have been used as sclerosants in the management of malignant pleural effusions and recurrent pneumothorax but the treatment is associated with pain and a high frequency of toxic effects and tetracycline is generally preferred (see p.484); mepacrine mesylate has been used similarly.

Preparations

Proprietary Preparations (details are given in Part 3)
USA: Atabrine†.

Multi-ingredient: ***Aust.:*** Acrisuxin; ***Ger.:*** Acrisuxin†; ***Switz.:*** Acrisuxin.

Methyl Benzoquate (12946-b)

Methyl Benzoquate *(BAN).*

Nequinate *(USAN, pINN)*; AY-20385; ICI-55052. Methyl 7-benzyloxy-6-butyl-1,4-dihydro-4-oxoquinoline-3-carboxylate.

$C_{22}H_{23}NO_4 = 365.4.$

CAS — 13997-19-8.

Methyl benzoquate is an antiprotozoal used in veterinary practice, in association with clopidol (p.580), for the prevention of coccidiosis in poultry and rabbits.

Metronidazole (16893-c)

Metronidazole *(BAN, USAN, rINN)*.

Bayer-5360; Metronidazolum; NSC-50364; RP-8823; SC-10295. 2-(2-Methyl-5-nitroimidazol-1-yl)ethanol.

$C_6H_9N_3O_3$ = 171.2.

CAS — 443-48-1.

Pharmacopoeias. In *Chin., Eur.* (see p.viii), *Int., Jpn, Pol.,* and *US.*

A white to pale yellow odourless crystalline powder or crystals. It darkens on exposure to light.

Ph. Eur. **solubilities** are: slightly soluble in water, in alcohol, in acetone, and in dichloromethane; very slightly soluble in ether. USP solubilities are: sparingly soluble in water and in alcohol; slightly soluble in chloroform and in ether. **Protect** from light.

See below for **incompatibilities**.

Metronidazole Benzoate (4757-f)

Metronidazole Benzoate *(BAN)*.

Benzoyl Metronidazole; RP-9712. 2-(2-Methyl-5-nitroimidazol-1-yl)ethyl benzoate.

$C_{13}H_{13}N_3O_4$ = 275.3.

CAS — 13182-89-3.

Pharmacopoeias. In *Eur.* (see p.viii).

A white or slightly yellowish crystalline powder or flakes. Practically **insoluble** in water; slightly soluble in alcohol; soluble in acetone; freely soluble in dichloromethane; very slightly soluble in ether. **Protect** from light.

Metronidazole Hydrochloride (4751-c)

Metronidazole Hydrochloride *(BANM, USAN)*.

SC-32642.

$C_6H_9N_3O_3,HCl$ = 207.6.

CAS — 69198-10-3.

Incompatibility. Solutions of metronidazole hydrochloride have a low pH, usually of less than 2.0, before dilution and neutralisation to produce a suitable solution for intravenous administration. These undiluted solutions react with aluminium in equipment such as needles to produce reddish-brown discoloration, and a precipitate has been reported with ready-to-use preparations of metronidazole hydrochloride, although this occurred after contact for 6 hours or more.[1,2]

Several studies have assessed the compatibility of antibiotic injections and other drugs when added to metronidazole solution for intravenous infusion.[3-7] Results have varied according to the criteria applied and the preparations and conditions used. Physical incompatibilities due to the low pH of metronidazole injections appear to be more of a problem than chemical incompatibility. Regardless of these studies, it is generally recommended that other drugs should not be added to intravenous solutions of metronidazole or its hydrochloride. Specific information on the compatibility of individual formulations may be found in the manufacturers' literature.

1. Schell KH, Copeland JR. Metronidazole hydrochloride-aluminum interaction. *Am J Hosp Pharm* 1985; **42:** 1040, 1042.
2. Struthers BJ, Parr RJ. Clarifying the metronidazole hydrochloride-aluminum interaction. *Am J Hosp Pharm* 1985; **42:** 2660.
3. Bisaillon S, Sarrazin R. Compatibility of several antibiotics or hydrocortisone when added to metronidazole solution for intravenous infusion. *J Parenter Sci Technol* 1983; **37:** 129–32.
4. Gupta VD, Stewart KR. Chemical stabilities of hydrocortisone sodium succinate and several antibiotics when mixed with metronidazole injection for intravenous infusion. *J Parenter Sci Technol* 1985; **39:** 145–8.
5. Gupta VD, *et al.* Chemical stabilities of cefamandole nafate and metronidazole when mixed together for intravenous infusion. *J Clin Hosp Pharm* 1985; **10:** 379–83.
6. Barnes AR. Chemical stabilities of cefuroxime sodium and metronidazole in an admixture for intravenous infusion. *J Clin Pharm Ther* 1990; **15:** 187–96.
7. Nahata MC, *et al.* Stability of metronidazole and ceftizoxime sodium in ready-to-use metronidazole bags stored at 4 and 25° C. *Am J Health-Syst Pharm* 1996; **53:** 1046–8.

Adverse Effects

The adverse effects of metronidazole are generally dose-related. The most common are gastro-intestinal disturbances, especially nausea and an unpleasant metallic taste. Vomiting, and diarrhoea or constipation may also occur. A furred tongue, glossitis, and stomatitis may be associated with an overgrowth of *Candida*. There have been rare reports of antibiotic-associated colitis associated with metronidazole; (it is also used in the treatment of this condition).

Weakness, dizziness, ataxia, headache, drowsiness, insomnia, and changes in mood or mental state such as depression or confusion have also been reported. Peripheral neuropathy, usually presenting as numbness or tingling in the extremities, and epileptiform seizures are serious adverse effects on the nervous system that have been associated with high doses of metronidazole or prolonged treatment.

Temporary moderate leucopenia and thrombocytopenia may occur in some patients receiving metronidazole. Skin rashes, urticaria, and pruritus occur occasionally and erythema multiforme, angioedema, and anaphylaxis have been reported rarely. Other side-effects include urethral discomfort and darkening of the urine. Raised liver enzyme values, cholestatic hepatitis, and jaundice have occasionally been reported. Thrombophlebitis may follow the intravenous administration of metronidazole.

Studies have shown metronidazole to be mutagenic in bacteria and carcinogenic in some *animals*.

Carcinogenicity and mutagenicity. Metronidazole is mutagenic in some strains of bacteria[1] and the urine of patients treated with metronidazole was found to be mutagenic in bacteria.[2] However, although increased chromosome aberrations were noted in patients following prolonged treatment with relatively high doses of metronidazole[3] no evidence of a cytogenic effect was found in a subsequent controlled study.[4] Tumours have been induced in *rats* and *mice* given metronidazole in chronic studies, but there was no appreciable increase in the incidence of cancer in a retrospective study of 771 patients in Rochester, Minnesota given metronidazole for vaginal trichomoniasis[5] nor in a similar study of 2460 patients in San Francisco.[6] However, Beard *et al.*'s study[5] of the patients in Rochester did show an excess of cases of lung cancer although all 4 women were smokers. Subsequent follow-up[7] to 1984 covering a period of 15 to 25 years still showed an excess of lung cancer cases even after allowing for smoking status. However, the follow-up also continued to show no significant increase overall in cancer-related morbidity or mortality. Further follow-up of the San Francisco patients[8] for 11 to 15 years to 1984 also showed no increase in the overall incidence of cancers nor did it confirm any increase in lung cancer.

Risks to the fetus are discussed under Pregnancy in Precautions, below.

1. Voogd CE, *et al.* The mutagenic action of nitroimidazoles I: metronidazole, nimorazole, dimetridazole and ronidazole. *Mutat Res* 1974; **26:** 483–90.
2. Speck WT, *et al.* Mutagenicity of metronidazole: presence of several active metabolites in human urine. *J Natl Cancer Inst* 1976; **56:** 283–4.
3. Mitelman F, *et al.* Chromosome aberrations and metronidazole. *Lancet* 1976; **ii:** 802.
4. Mitelman F, *et al.* No cytogenetic effect of metronidazole. *Lancet* 1980; **i:** 1249–50.
5. Beard CM, *et al.* Lack of evidence for cancer due to use of metronidazole. *N Engl J Med* 1979; **301:** 519–22.
6. Friedman GD. Cancer after metronidazole. *N Engl J Med* 1980; **302:** 519.
7. Beard CM, *et al.* Cancer after exposure to metronidazole. *Mayo Clin Proc* 1988; **63:** 147–53.
8. Friedman GD, Selby JV. Metronidazole and cancer. *JAMA* 1989; **261:** 866.

Effects on the blood. Adverse haematological effects associated with metronidazole therapy include a report of bone marrow aplasia, with leucopenia and markedly reduced erythropoiesis and granulopoiesis,[1] aplastic anaemia,[2] and the haemolytic-uraemic syndrome.[3]

1. White CM, *et al.* Bone marrow aplasia associated with metronidazole. *Br Med J* 1980; **280:** 647.
2. Raman R, *et al.* Metronidazole induced aplastic anaemia. *Clinician* 1982; **46:** 464–8.
3. Powell HR, *et al.* Haemolytic-uraemic syndrome after treatment with metronidazole. *Med J Aust* 1988; **149:** 222–3.

Effects on the ears. A review of reports of ototoxicity notified to the Australian Adverse Drug Reactions Advisory Committee revealed a number of cases of deafness associated with the use of metronidazole.[1]

1. Anonymous. Drug-induced ototoxicity. *WHO Drug Inf* 1991; **5:** 12.

Effects on the eyes. Myopia which developed in a patient after 11 days of oral metronidazole for trichomoniasis had resolved 4 days after withdrawal of treatment but recurred when she resumed treatment.[1]

Retrobulbar or optic neuritis has been reported in seven patients receiving metronidazole.[2] Dosage varied from 750 mg to 1 g daily by mouth and duration of treatment from 7 days to a year. Abnormalities included defects in colour vision, decreased vision, and scotomas. Vision improved following withdrawal of metronidazole, although there was a residual deficit in 2 patients.

1. Grinbaum A, *et al.* Transient myopia following metronidazole treatment for Trichomonas vaginalis. *JAMA* 1992; **267:** 511–12.
2. Putnam D, *et al.* Metronidazole and optic neuritis. *Am J Ophthalmol* 1991; **112:** 737.

Effects on the gastro-intestinal tract. ANTIBIOTIC-ASSOCIATED COLITIS. Reports of pseudomembranous colitis associated with the administration of metronidazole.

1. Thomson G, *et al.* Pseudomembranous colitis after treatment with metronidazole. *Br Med J* 1981; **282:** 864–5.
2. Daly JJ, Chowdary KVS. Pseudomembranous colitis secondary to metronidazole. *Dig Dis Sci* 1983; **28:** 573–4.

Effects on the liver. Severely elevated liver enzyme values, consistent with a drug-induced hepatitis, occurred in a patient given metronidazole hydrochloride 500 mg every 6 hours intravenously for 4 days. He was also receiving cefapirin sodium and tobramycin sulphate.[1] A case of reversible hepatotoxicity caused by an overdose of metronidazole 12.5 g has also been reported.[2]

1. Appleby DH, Vogtland HD. Suspected metronidazole toxicity. *Clin Pharm* 1983; **2:** 373–4.
2. Lam S, Bank S. Hepatotoxicity caused by metronidazole overdose. *Ann Intern Med* 1995; **122:** 803.

Effects on the nervous system. EFFECTS ON MENTAL FUNCTION. Although metronidazole is sometimes used to reduce colonic flora in the treatment of hepatic encephalopathy, impaired metabolism of metronidazole in such patients can result in elevated plasma concentrations and consequent toxicity. Psychosis and manic behaviour was reported in one such patient during treatment for hepatic encephalopathy with metronidazole and lactulose, although plasma-metronidazole concentrations were not found to be elevated (24 mg per mL).[1] Symptoms resolved when metronidazole was discontinued. Acute psychosis has also been reported in a patient following a 5-day course of intravenous metronidazole 1 g daily for a gynaecological disorder.[2]

1. Uhl MD, Riely CA. Metronidazole in treating portosystemic encephalopathy. *Ann Intern Med* 1996; **124:** 455.
2. Schreiber W, Spernal J. Metronidazole-induced psychotic disorder. *Am J Psychiatry* 1997; **154:** 1170–1.

PERIPHERAL NEUROPATHY. Peripheral neuropathy has been reported in patients receiving prolonged treatment with metronidazole.[1-4] Discontinuation of metronidazole or reduction of the dose usually results in complete resolution or improvement of the neuropathy but in some patients it may persist despite these measures. For reports of retrobulbar or optic neuritis associated with metronidazole see Effects on the Eyes, above.

1. Duffy LF, *et al.* Peripheral neuropathy in Crohn's disease patients treated with metronidazole. *Gastroenterology* 1985; **88:** 681–4.
2. Boyce EG, *et al.* Persistent metronidazole-induced peripheral neuropathy. *DICP Ann Pharmacother* 1990; **24:** 19–21.
3. Learned-Coughlin S. Peripheral neuropathy induced by metronidazole. *Ann Pharmacother* 1994; **28:** 536.
4. Dreger LM, *et al.* Intermittent-dose metronidazole-induced peripheral neuropathy. *Ann Pharmacother* 1998; **32:** 267–8.

Effects on the pancreas. A small number of cases of acute pancreatitis associated with metronidazole, recurrent on rechallenge, have been reported.[1,2] No cases were found in a retrospective study of about 6500 patients who had received metronidazole.[3]

1. Plotnick BH, *et al.* Metronidazole-induced pancreatitis. *Ann Intern Med* 1985; **103:** 891–2.
2. Sanford KA, *et al.* Metronidazole-associated pancreatitis. *Ann Intern Med* 1988; **109:** 756–7.
3. Friedman G, Selby JV. How often does metronidazole induce pancreatitis? *Gastroenterology* 1990; **98:** 1702–3.

Gynaecomastia. Gynaecomastia occurred in a 36-year-old man with ulcerative colitis after taking metronidazole for about a month.[1]

1. Fagan TC, *et al.* Metronidazole-induced gynecomastia. *JAMA* 1985; **254:** 3217.

Hypersensitivity. A hypersensitivity reaction with chills, fever, generalised erythema, and a maculopapular rash developed after a single dose of metronidazole in a patient who had previously developed a rash during treatment with intravaginal metronidazole.[1]

1. Knowles S, *et al.* Metronidazole hypersensitivity. *Ann Pharmacother* 1994; **28:** 325–6.

Precautions

Peripheral neuropathy, transient epileptiform seizures, and leucopenia have sometimes been associated with prolonged or intensive treatment with metronidazole (see Adverse Effects, above). Clinical and laboratory monitoring is advised in patients receiving metronidazole for more than 10 days. Doses should be reduced in patients with severe liver disease.

It is suggested that the use of metronidazole should be avoided during pregnancy, especially during the first trimester and especially high-dose regimens (see also below). Some authorities consider that women taking metronidazole should not breast feed their babies (see also below).

Patients are advised not to drink alcoholic beverages while taking metronidazole (see Interactions, below).

Breast feeding. Metronidazole is distributed into breast milk giving it a bitter taste which may impair feeding.[1] Unnecessary exposure of the infant to the drug should be avoided, and breast feeding should generally be interrupted during treatment and for 1 to 2 days afterwards.[2]

1. Rubin PC. Prescribing in pregnancy: general principles. *Br Med J* 1986; **293:** 1415–17.
2. American Academy of Pediatrics, Committee on Drugs. The transfer of drugs and other chemicals into human milk. *Pediatrics* 1994; **93:** 137–50.

Pregnancy. Metronidazole is mutagenic in bacteria and carcinogenic in *rodents*. It readily crosses the placenta to the fetus achieving similar concentrations in the placental cord and maternal plasma and its use in pregnancy is controversial. Meta-analyses of studies involving the use of metronidazole in the first trimester of pregnancy[1,2] concluded that there did not appear to be an increased risk of teratogenicity. However, in the USA the manufacturer considers metronidazole to be contra-indicated during the first trimester in patients with trichomoniasis; use for trichomoniasis during the second and third trimesters may be acceptable. For other indications the risks and benefits of treatment with metronidazole should be weighed carefully, especially in the first trimester.

1. Burtin P, *et al.* Safety of metronidazole in pregnancy: a meta-analysis. *Am J Obstet Gynecol* 1995; **172:** 525–9.
2. Caro-Patón T, *et al.* Is metronidazole teratogenic? A meta-analysis. *Br J Clin Pharmacol* 1997; **44:** 179–82.

Interactions

When given in conjunction with alcohol, metronidazole may provoke a disulfiram-like reaction in some individuals. Acute psychoses or confusion have been associated with the concomitant use of metronidazole and disulfiram.

Metronidazole is reported to impair the metabolism or excretion of several drugs including warfarin (see p.968), phenytoin (see p.356), lithium (see p.293), and fluorouracil (see p.535), with the consequent potential for an increased incidence of adverse effects. There is some evidence that phenytoin might accelerate the metabolism of metronidazole. Plasma concentrations of metronidazole are decreased by the concomitant administration of phenobarbitone, with a consequent reduction in the effectiveness of metronidazole. Cimetidine has increased plasma concentrations of metronidazole and might increase the risk of neurological side-effects. For references to some of these interactions, see below.

For incompatibilities between metronidazole and other drugs in solutions for injection, see above.

Alcohol. Metronidazole may provoke a disulfiram-like reaction in some individuals when given in conjunction with alcohol; reactions have occurred after the administration of pharmaceutical preparations formulated with alcohol, including injections, as well as after drinking alcohol.[1] Acute psychosis or confusional state was reported in 6 of 29 alcoholic patients who were also receiving disulfiram.[2]

1. Edwards DL. *et al.* Disulfiram-like reaction associated with intravenous trimethoprim-sulfamethoxazole and metronidazole. *Clin Pharm* 1986; **5:** 999–1000.
2. Rothstein E, Clancy DD. Toxicity of disulfiram combined with metronidazole. *N Engl J Med* 1969; **280:** 1006–7.

Carbamazepine. For a report of a possible interaction between metronidazole and carbamazepine, see p.341.

Cimetidine. In a study in six healthy volunteers metronidazole plasma concentrations were increased by concurrent twice-daily administration of cimetidine. The effect was presumed to be due to inhibition of cytochrome P450 isoenzymes responsible for metronidazole metabolism.[1] However, cimetidine was not found to affect the pharmacokinetics of metronidazole in a study in patients with Crohn's disease[2] nor in a single-dose study in healthy subjects.[3]

1. Gugler R, Jansen JC. Interaction between cimetidine and metronidazole. *N Engl J Med* 1983; **309:** 1518–19.
2. Eradiri O, *et al.* Interaction of metronidazole with cimetidine and phenobarbital in Crohn's disease. *Clin Pharmacol Ther* 1987; **41:** 235.
3. Loft S, *et al.* Lack of effect of cimetidine on the pharmacokinetics and metabolism of a single oral dose of metronidazole. *Eur J Clin Pharmacol* 1988; **35:** 65–8.

Disulfiram. For a report of acute psychosis or confusional state following metronidazole treatment in alcoholic patients receiving disulfiram, see under Alcohol, above.

Omeprazole. Although concentrations in plasma and saliva of metronidazole and its 'hydroxy' metabolite were unaffected by concurrent administration of omeprazole in healthy volunteers, those in gastric juice were substantially lowered, possibly as a result of a reduction in transfer from the plasma.[1] However, this may be of limited clinical significance during treatment of *Helicobacter pylori* infections.

1. Jessa MJ, *et al.* The effect of omeprazole on the pharmacokinetics of metronidazole and hydroxymetronidazole in human plasma, saliva and gastric juice. *Br J Clin Pharmacol* 1997; **44:** 245–53.

Phenobarbitone. An increase in the rate of metabolism of metronidazole, resulting in treatment failure, was reported in a patient receiving concurrent treatment with phenobarbitone.[1] In a retrospective survey of patients who had not responded to treatment with metronidazole, 80% were found to be receiving long-term phenobarbitone therapy.[2] Subsequently it was found that up to three times the usual dose was required to produce a parasitological cure of giardiasis in such patients.

1. Mead PB, *et al.* Possible alteration of metronidazole metabolism by phenobarbital. *N Engl J Med* 1982; **306:** 1490.
2. Gupte S. Phenobarbital and metabolism of metronidazole. *N Engl J Med* 1983; **308:** 529.

Phenytoin. In addition to conflicting reports on the effects of metronidazole on the metabolism of phenytoin (see p.356), increased metabolism of metronidazole was reported in 1 patient during treatment with phenytoin.[1]

1. Wheeler LA, *et al.* Use of high-pressure liquid chromatography to determine plasma levels of metronidazole and metabolites after intravenous administration. *Antimicrob Agents Chemother* 1978; **13:** 205–9.

Antimicrobial Action

Metronidazole is active against several protozoa including *Balantidium coli*, *Blastocystis hominis*, *Entamoeba histolytica*, *Giardia intestinalis* (*Giardia lamblia*), and *Trichomonas vaginalis*. Most obligate anaerobic bacteria, including *Bacteroides* and *Clostridium* spp., are sensitive *in vitro* to metronidazole. It is bactericidal. Minimum inhibitory concentrations (MICs) for susceptible anaerobic bacteria generally range from 0.1 to 8 μg per mL. It also has activity against the facultative anaerobes *Gardnerella vaginalis* and *Helicobacter pylori* and against some spirochaetes. Resistance to metronidazole has been reported and cross-resistance to other nitroimidazoles, such as tinidazole, may occur.

Metronidazole has well-established bactericidal activity against obligate anaerobic bacteria *in vitro*, including the Gram-negative organisms *Bacteroides fragilis* and other *Bacteroides* spp., *Fusobacterium* spp., and *Veillonella* spp. and the Gram-positive organisms *Clostridium difficile*, *Cl. perfringens*, and other *Clostridium* spp., *Eubacterium* spp., *Peptococcus* spp., and *Peptostreptococcus* spp.; *Propionibacterium* and *Actinomyces* spp. are often resistant.[1-6] It also has activity against the facultative anaerobe *Gardnerella vaginalis*, although its bactericidal effect is reported to be much slower than against obligate anaerobes,[7] against some strains of *Campylobacter* spp. including *C. fetus* subsp. *jejuni*,[8,9] and against *Helicobacter pylori*.[10,11]

The oxidative metabolites of metronidazole have antibacterial activity; MICs of the 'hydroxy' metabolite against anaerobic bacteria are reported to be generally within one dilution of the parent compound whereas the 'acid' metabolite is much less active.[12,13] The hydroxy metabolite has been reported to be consistently more active than metronidazole against strains of *G. vaginalis*.[14,15]

The mode of action of metronidazole is not entirely clear, but is thought to involve reduction by bacterial 'nitroreductases' to an unstable intermediate which interacts with DNA, effectively preventing further replication.[16] A number of factors affect the sensitivity of micro-organisms to metronidazole *in vitro*. Anaerobic conditions are important for optimal activity. Interactions between micro-organisms and metronidazole have been described, including inhibition of *Escherichia coli* by metronidazole in the presence of *B. fragilis* and enhancement of the rate of killing of *B. fragilis* by metronidazole in the presence of *E. coli*.

Resistance to metronidazole has developed in sensitive species. Although Tally *et al.*[17,18] observed no resistance among the *B. fragilis* group over several years, there have been occasional reports of resistance in this group[19-24] and in other *Bacteroides* spp.[25-27] now known as *Prevotella* spp. Nitroimidazole resistance in *Helicobacter pylori* has been associated with reduced response rates to standard bismuth-based triple therapy for peptic ulcer disease, but the effect on modified regimens is uncertain.[28]

1. Wüst J. Susceptibility of anaerobic bacteria to metronidazole, ornidazole, and tinidazole and routine susceptibility testing by standardized methods. *Antimicrob Agents Chemother* 1977; **11:** 631–7.
2. Dubreuil L, *et al.* Susceptibility of anaerobic bacteria from several French hospitals to three major antibiotics. *Antimicrob Agents Chemother* 1984; **25:** 764–6.
3. Hill GB, Ayers OM. Antimicrobial susceptibilities of anaerobic bacteria isolated from female genital tract infections. *Antimicrob Agents Chemother* 1985; **27:** 324–31.
4. Chow AW, *et al.* In vitro susceptibility of Clostridium difficile to new β-lactam and quinolone antibiotics. *Antimicrob Agents Chemother* 1985; **28:** 842–4.
5. Brazier JS, *et al.* Antibiotic susceptibility of clinical isolates of clostridia. *J Antimicrob Chemother* 1985; **15:** 181–5.
6. Van der Auwera P, *et al.* Comparative serum bactericidal activity against test anaerobes in volunteers receiving imipenem, clindamycin, latamoxef and metronidazole. *J Antimicrob Chemother* 1987; **19:** 205–10.
7. Ralph ED, Amatnieks YE. Metronidazole in treatment against Haemophilus vaginalis (Corynebacterium vaginale). *Antimicrob Agents Chemother* 1980; **18:** 101–4.
8. Hof H, *et al.* Comparative in vitro activities of niridazole and metronidazole against anaerobic and microaerophilic bacteria. *Antimicrob Agents Chemother* 1982; **22:** 332–3.
9. Freydière AM, *et al.* In vitro susceptibilities of 40 Campylobacter fetus subsp jejuni strains to niridazole and metronidazole. *Antimicrob Agents Chemother* 1984; **25:** 145–6.
10. Marshall BJ, *et al.* Pyloric campylobacter infection and gastroduodenal disease. *Med J Aust* 1985; **142:** 439–44.
11. Howden A, *et al.* In-vitro sensitivity of Campylobacter pyloridis to furazolidone. *Lancet* 1986; **ii:** 1035.
12. Haller I. In vitro activity of the two principal oxidative metabolites of metronidazole against Bacteroides fragilis and related species. *Antimicrob Agents Chemother* 1982; **22:** 165–6.
13. O'Keefe JP, *et al.* Activity of metronidazole and its hydroxy and acid metabolites against clinical isolates of anaerobic bacteria. *Antimicrob Agents Chemother* 1982; **22:** 426–30.
14. Ralph ED, Amatnieks YE. Relative susceptibilities of Gardnerella vaginalis (Haemophilus vaginalis), Neisseria gonorrhoeae, and Bacteroides fragilis to metronidazole and its two major metabolites. *Sex Transm Dis* 1980; **7:** 157–60.
15. Shanker S, Munro R. Sensitivity of Gardnerella vaginalis to metabolites of metronidazole and tinidazole. *Lancet* 1982; **i:** 167.
16. Ingham HR, *et al.* Interactions between micro-organisms and metronidazole. *J Antimicrob Chemother* 1982; **10:** 84–7.
17. Tally FP, *et al.* Susceptibility of the Bacteroides fragilis group in the United States in 1981. *Antimicrob Agents Chemother* 1983; **23:** 536–40.
18. Tally FP, *et al.* Nationwide study of the susceptibility of the Bacteroides fragilis group in the United States. *Antimicrob Agents Chemother* 1985; **28:** 675–7.
19. Ingham HR, *et al.* Bacteroides fragilis resistance to metronidazole after long-term therapy. *Lancet* 1978; **i:** 214.
20. Eme A, *et al.* Bacteroides fragilis resistant to metronidazole. *J Antimicrob Chemother* 1983; **12:** 523–5.
21. Lamothe F, *et al.* Bacteroides fragilis resistant to both metronidazole and imipenem. *J Antimicrob Chemother* 1986; **18:** 642–3.
22. Brogan O, *et al.* Bacteroides fragilis resistant to metronidazole, clindamycin and cefoxitin. *J Antimicrob Chemother* 1989; **23:** 660–2.
23. Hickey MM, *et al.* Metronidazole resistant Bacteroides fragilis infection of a prosthetic hip joint. *J Infect* 1990; **20:** 129–33.
24. Turner P, *et al.* Simultaneous resistance to metronidazole, co-amoxiclav, and imipenem in clinical isolate of Bacteroides fragilis. *Lancet* 1995; **345:** 1275–7.
25. Sprott MS, *et al.* Metronidazole-resistant anaerobes. *Lancet* 1983; **i:** 1220.
26. McWalter PW, Baird DR. Metronidazole-resistant anaerobes. *Lancet* 1983; **i:** 1220.
27. Sprott MS, Kearns AM. Metronidazole-resistant Bacteroides melaninogenicus. *J Antimicrob Chemother* 1988; **22:** 951–4.
28. Goddard AF, Logan RPH. Antimicrobial resistance and Helicobacter pylori. *J Antimicrob Chemother* 1996; **37:** 639–43.

Pharmacokinetics

Metronidazole is readily absorbed following administration by mouth and bioavailability approaches 100%. Peak plasma concentrations of approximately 5 and 10 μg per mL are achieved, usually within 1 to 2 hours, after single doses of 250 and 500 mg respectively. Some accumulation and consequently higher concentrations occur when multiple doses are given. Absorption may be delayed, but is not reduced overall by administration with food. Metronidazole benzoate is also given by mouth and is hydrolysed in the gastro-intestinal tract to release metronidazole, which is then absorbed.

Following the intravenous administration of metronidazole, peak steady-state plasma concentrations of about 25 μg per mL with trough concentrations of about 18 μg per mL have been reported in patients given a loading dose of 15 mg per kg body-weight followed by 7.5 mg per kg every 6 hours. The bioavailability of metronidazole from rectal suppositories is 60 to 80%; peak plasma concentrations are half those achieved with equivalent oral doses and effective concentrations occur after about 5 to 12 hours. Absorption from vaginal pessaries has been reported to be poor with a bioavailability of about 20 to 25% and gradual absorption producing peak plasma concentrations of about 2 μg per mL following a dose of 500 mg. An intravaginal gel formulation providing a dose of 37.5 mg metronidazole produced peak plasma concentrations of 0.3 μg per mL at 8 hours, with a bioavailability of 56%.

Metronidazole is widely distributed. It appears in most body tissues and fluids including bile, bone, breast milk, cerebral abscesses, cerebrospinal fluid, liver and liver abscesses, saliva, seminal fluid, and vaginal secretions, and achieves concentrations similar to those in plasma. It also crosses the placenta and rapidly enters the fetal circulation. No more than 20% is bound to plasma proteins.

Metronidazole is metabolised in the liver by side-chain oxidation and glucuronide formation. The principal oxidative metabolites are 1-(2-hydroxyethyl)-2-hydroxymethyl-5-nitroimidazole (the 'hydroxy' metabolite), which has antibacterial activity and is detected in plasma and urine, and 2-methyl-5-nitroimidazole-1-acetic acid (the 'acid' metabolite), which has virtually no antibacterial activity and is often not detected in plasma, but is excreted in urine. Small amounts of reduced metabolites, acetamide and *N*-(2-hydroxyethyl)oxamic acid (HOA), have also been detected in urine and are probably formed by the intestinal flora.

The elimination half-life of metronidazole is about 8 hours; that of the hydroxy metabolite is slightly longer. The half-life of metronidazole is reported to be longer in neonates and in patients with severe liver disease; that of the hydroxy metabolite is prolonged in patients with renal failure.

The majority of a dose of metronidazole is excreted in the urine, mainly as metabolites; a small amount appears in the faeces.

References.

1. Lau AH, *et al.* Clinical pharmacokinetics of metronidazole and other nitroimidazole anti-infectives. *Clin Pharmacokinet* 1992; **23:** 328–64.
2. Cunningham FE, *et al.* Pharmacokinetics of intravaginal metronidazole gel. *J Clin Pharmacol* 1994; **34:** 1060–5.

Hepatic impairment. There have been differing results from pharmacokinetic studies of the elimination of metronidazole in patients with liver disease. Daneshmend *et al.*[1] reported no marked difference between patients with cirrhosis or hepatosplenic schistosomiasis given a single 500-mg oral dose of metronidazole when compared with healthy subjects and suggested that, in the absence of renal impairment, dosage adjustment was not needed in patients with liver disease. However, Farrell *et al.*[2] found that elimination of metronidazole, administered intravenously, was considerably impaired in a study of 10 patients with alcoholic liver disease or chronic active hepatitis, 7 of whom had reduced creatinine clearance. Daneshmend and Roberts[3] commented that these differing results were probably due to impaired renal elimination, whereas Farrell *et al.*[4] suggested that impaired elimination of metronidazole was due to impaired hepatic metabolism rather than decreased renal clearance; other studies have shown metronidazole clearance to be normal in renal failure. Farrell *et al.* nevertheless agreed that reduction in the dosage of metronidazole is required only when liver function is very poor, particularly when renal function is impaired. A study in 10 severely ill patients with or without impaired hepatic and/or renal function[5] also suggested that liver function is a very important determinant of metronidazole elimination.

1. Daneshmend TK, *et al.* Disposition of oral metronidazole in hepatic cirrhosis and in hepatosplenic schistosomiasis. *Gut* 1982; **23:** 807–13.
2. Farrell G, *et al.* Impaired elimination of metronidazole in decompensated chronic liver disease. *Br Med J* 1983; **287:** 1845.
3. Daneshmend TK, Roberts CJC. Impaired elimination of metronidazole in decompensated chronic liver disease. *Br Med J* 1984; **288:** 405.
4. Farrell G, *et al.* Impaired elimination of metronidazole in decompensated chronic liver disease. *Br Med J* 1984, **288:** 1009.
5. Ljungberg B, *et al.* Metronidazole: pharmacokinetic observations in severely ill patients. *J Antimicrob Chemother* 1984; **14:** 275–83.

Infants and children. A single intravenous dose of 15 mg per kg body-weight has been suggested for neonates[1] which would produce therapeutic concentrations of metronidazole for around 24 hours in term neonates and 48 hours in preterm neonates. Renal and hepatic function is incompletely developed in newborn infants and consequently the elimination half-life of metronidazole is prolonged and has been reported to range from 25 to 109 hours.[1] Elimination half-life is inversely proportional to gestational age[1,2] and as the infant matures half-life is reduced to values closer to those in adults.[1,3]

1. Jager-Roman E, *et al.* Pharmacokinetics and tissue distribution of metronidazole in the newborn infant. *J Pediatr* 1982; **100:** 651–4.
2. Hall P, *et al.* Intravenous metronidazole in the newborn. *Arch Dis Child* 1983; **58:** 529–31.
3. Amon I, *et al.* Disposition kinetics of metronidazole in children. *Eur J Clin Pharmacol* 1983; **24:** 113–19.

Renal impairment. Pharmacokinetic studies have indicated that doses of metronidazole need not be altered in patients with renal insufficiency[1] although adjustments might be required in patients undergoing haemodialysis since metronidazole and its hydroxy metabolite are efficiently cleared and extensively removed in such patients.[2] However, in another study[3] the amount of metronidazole and its hydroxy metabolite cleared was found to depend on the type of dialysis membrane used; the authors concluded that dosage supplementation may be needed only for seriously ill patients undergoing haemodialysis with a membrane having high metronidazole clearance.

Routine adjustment of dosage was not considered necessary in patients undergoing peritoneal dialysis.[4] However, the potential for metabolites to accumulate was noted in patients on continuous ambulatory peritoneal dialysis[5] and it was suggested that dosage reduction may be necessary if excessive concentrations of metabolites are found to be toxic.

1. Houghton GW, *et al.* Pharmacokinetics of metronidazole in patients with varying degrees of renal failure. *Br J Clin Pharmacol* 1985; **19:** 203–9.
2. Somogyi A, *et al.* Disposition and removal of metronidazole in patients undergoing haemodialysis. *Eur J Clin Pharmacol* 1983; **25:** 683–7.
3. Lau AH, *et al.* Hemodialysis clearance of metronidazole and its metabolites. *Antimicrob Agents Chemother* 1986; **29:** 235–8.
4. Cassey JG, *et al.* Pharmacokinetics of metronidazole in patients undergoing peritoneal dialysis. *Antimicrob Agents Chemother* 1983; **24:** 950–1.
5. Guay DR, *et al.* Pharmacokinetics of metronidazole in patients undergoing continuous ambulatory peritoneal dialysis. *Antimicrob Agents Chemother* 1984; **25:** 306–10.

Uses and Administration

Metronidazole is a 5-nitroimidazole derivative with activity against anaerobic bacteria and protozoa (see Antimicrobial Action, above); it also has a radiosensitising effect on hypoxic tumour cells. Its mechanism of action is thought to involve interference with DNA by a metabolite in which the nitro group of metronidazole has been reduced.

Metronidazole is used in the treatment of susceptible protozoal infections such as amoebiasis, balantidiasis, *Blastocystis hominis* infections, giardiasis, and trichomoniasis; it has also been tried in leishmaniasis and microsporidiosis. For details of these infections and their treatment see under Choice of Antiprotozoal, p.573. Metronidazole is also used in the treatment and prophylaxis of anaerobic bacterial infections. Specific bacterial infections treated with metronidazole include bacterial vaginosis, acute necrotising ulcerative gingivitis, pelvic inflammatory disease, tetanus, and antibiotic-associated colitis. For details of these infections and their treatment see under Choice of Antibacterial, p.116.

It is used to eradicate *Helicobacter pylori* in peptic ulcer disease (in combination with other antimicrobials, and either bismuth compounds or proton pump inhibitors) and in the management of malodorous tumours and ulcers where there is anaerobic infection. It is also used in the treatment of rosacea and of dracunculiasis (guinea-worm infection) and has been given in the treatment of perianal Crohn's disease and hepatic encephalopathy, and has been tried as an adjunct to the radiotherapy of malignant neoplasms. See also below for these miscellaneous uses.

ADMINISTRATION AND DOSAGE. Metronidazole is administered by mouth in tablets or, as metronidazole benzoate, in oral suspension; the tablets are taken with or after food and the suspension at least 1 hour before food. Metronidazole is also given rectally in suppositories, applied topically as a cream or gel, or administered by intravenous infusion of metronidazole or metronidazole hydrochloride. Doses are expressed in terms of metronidazole base.

In **amoebiasis**, metronidazole acts as an amoebicide at all sites of infection with *Entamoeba histolytica*. Because of its rapid absorption it is probably less effective against parasites in the bowel lumen and is therefore used in conjunction with a luminal amoebicide such as diloxanide furoate or di-iodohydroxyquinoline in the treatment of invasive amoebiasis. Metronidazole is given in doses of 400 to 800 mg three times daily by mouth for 5 to 10 days. Children aged 1 to 3 years may be given one-quarter, those aged 3 to 7 years one-third, and those aged 7 to 10 years one-half the adult dose; alternatively 35 to 50 mg per kg body-weight daily in divided doses has been suggested. An alternative adult dose is 1.5 to 2.5 g as a single dose daily for 2 or 3 days.

In **balantidiasis** and ***Blastocystis hominis*** **infection**, metronidazole has been given in doses similar to those used in amoebiasis.

In **giardiasis**, the usual dose of metronidazole is 2 g once daily by mouth for 3 successive days. Dosage for children is proportional, as for amoebiasis (above). An alternative suggested schedule is 250 mg three times daily for 5 days for adults or 15 mg per kg daily in divided doses for children.

In **trichomoniasis**, metronidazole is given by mouth either as a single 2-g dose, as a 2-day course of 800 mg in the morning and 1.2 g in the evening, or as a 7-day course of 600 to 1 g daily in two or three divided doses. Sexual partners should be treated concomitantly. If treatment needs to be repeated an interval of 4 to 6 weeks between courses has been recommended. Vaginal preparations containing metronidazole are available for the treatment of vaginal trichomoniasis in some countries. Children with trichomoniasis may be given a 7-day course of metronidazole by mouth as follows: 1 to 3 years, 50 mg three times daily; 3 to 7 years, 100 mg twice daily, and 7 to 10 years, 100 mg three times daily. An alternative children's dose is 15 mg per kg daily in divided doses for 7 days.

Bacterial vaginosis is treated similarly to vaginal trichomoniasis with which it may co-exist; metronidazole is usually given by mouth as a single 2-g dose or as a 7-day course of 400 or 500 mg twice daily. Alternatively it may be administered locally as 5 g of a 0.75% gel once or twice daily for 5 days.

In **acute necrotising ulcerative gingivitis**, metronidazole 200 mg three times daily is given by mouth for 3 days; similar doses are used in acute dental infections. A 25% dental gel has also been used as an adjunct to the treatment of chronic periodontal infections.

For the treatment of most **anaerobic bacterial infections**, metronidazole is given by mouth in an initial dose of 800 mg followed by 400 mg every 8 hours, usually for about 7 days. A regimen of 500 mg every 8 hours is also used. When oral therapy is precluded metronidazole may be administered intravenously, 500 mg being infused as 100 mL of a 5 mg per mL solution at a rate of 5 mL per minute every 8 hours, or rectally as a 1-g suppository every 8 hours for 3 days, then every 12 hours; oral therapy should be substituted as soon as possible. Suppositories may be unsuitable for the initiation of therapy in serious infections because of the slower absorption of metronidazole. Children may be given 7.5 mg per kg every 8 hours by mouth, rectally, or by intravenous infusion. In the USA recommended adult doses of metronidazole are 7.5 mg per kg every 6 hours by mouth or 15 mg per kg by intravenous infusion followed by 7.5 mg per kg every 6 hours, doses being infused over 1 hour; by either route a total dose of 4 g in 24 hours should not be exceeded. In mixed anaerobic and aerobic infections metronidazole is given in association with the appropriate antibiotics.

For the **prevention of postoperative anaerobic bacterial infections**, especially in patients undergoing abdominal or gynaecological surgery, metronidazole is administered orally, intravenously, or rectally in doses similar to those used for the treatment of established infections, usually in combination with a beta-lactam or an aminoglycoside antibiotic. Various schedules have been employed. By mouth, 400 mg of metronidazole may be given every 8 hours in the 24 hours before surgery followed postoperatively by intravenous or rectal administration until oral therapy is possible. By intravenous infusion, 500 mg may be given shortly before operation and repeated every 8 hours, oral doses of 400 mg every 8 hours being substituted as soon as possible. By rectum, 1 g may be administered every 8 hours starting 2 hours before surgery. Children's prophylactic doses are as for treatment (above). In the USA the recommended schedule for adults undergoing colorectal surgery is metronidazole 15 mg per kg by intravenous infusion over 30 to 60 minutes, completed about 1 hour before surgery, followed by two further intravenous doses of 7.5 mg per kg infused at 6 and 12 hours after the initial dose.

In **peptic ulcer disease**, metronidazole is used in combination therapy to eradicate *Helicobacter pylori*. Typical regimens include metronidazole 400 mg three times daily with omeprazole and either amoxycillin or clarithromycin for 1 week; metronidazole 400 mg twice daily with lansoprazole and either amoxycillin or clarithromycin for 1 week; metronidazole 400 mg three times daily with tripotassium dicitratobismuthate and tetracycline for 2 weeks; and metronidazole 500 mg three times daily with ranitidine and amoxycillin for 2 weeks.

For **leg ulcers** and **pressure sores** infected with anaerobic bacteria, metronidazole 400 mg may be given three times daily by mouth for 7 days. Metronidazole is also applied topically as a 0.75% or 0.8% gel to reduce the odour associated with anaerobic infection in **fungating tumours**.

In the treatment of **rosacea** metronidazole is given by mouth or applied topically.

Administration in hepatic impairment. Since metronidazole is mainly metabolised by hepatic oxidation accumulation of metronidazole and its metabolites is likely in patients with severely impaired hepatic function. Metronidazole should therefore be administered with caution and at reduced doses to patients with severe hepatic disease, and especially hepatic encephalopathy when adverse affects of metronidazole can add to the symptoms of the disease. One-third of the usual daily dose may be administered once daily in these patients. For patients with lesser degrees of hepatic impairment, pharmacokinetic studies have not produced consistent results (see under Pharmacokinetics, above) and no recommendations about dosage reduction have been made by the manufacturers.

Administration in renal impairment. The elimination of metronidazole is largely unchanged in patients with renal impairment although metabolites may accumulate in patients with end-stage renal disease on dialysis (see under Pharmacokinetics, above). Dosage reductions are therefore not usually recommended for patients with renal impairment, although, since both metronidazole and its metabolites are removed by haemodialysis, doses need to be administered immediately after haemodialysis.

Dracunculiasis. Metronidazole may be beneficial in the management of dracunculiasis (p.93). It provides symptomatic relief and is also thought to weaken the anchorage of the worms within subcutaneous tissue, thus allowing them to be removed more quickly.

Metronidazole has been given in a variety of dosage regimens including: 400 mg three times daily for 5 days;[1] 40 mg per kg body-weight daily in three divided doses, to a maximum daily dose of 2.4 g, for 3 days;[2] 400 mg daily for 10 to 20 days.[3] A dose of 250 mg three times daily for 10 days has also been recommended.[4]

1. Padonu KO. A controlled trial of metronidazole in the treatment of dracontiasis in Nigeria. *Am J Trop Med Hyg* 1973; **22:** 42–4.
2. Kale OO. A controlled field trial of the treatment of dracontiasis with metronidazole and niridazole. *Ann Trop Med Parasitol* 1974; **68:** 91–5.
3. Muller R. Guinea worm disease: epidemiology, control, and treatment. *Bull WHO* 1979; **57:** 683–9.
4. Anonymous. Drugs for parasitic infections. *Med Lett Drugs Ther* 1998; **40:** 1–12.

Hepatic encephalopathy. The treatment of hepatic encephalopathy is discussed on p.1170. It includes the administration of an antimicrobial such as metronidazole to reduce the intestinal flora.

Inflammatory bowel disease. Metronidazole is not a standard treatment for inflammatory bowel disease (p.1171) but it has a limited role in the management of Crohn's disease,[1-4] particularly in perineal disease.[1,2] Metronidazole has also been tried in combination with ciprofloxacin in a small number of patients with active Crohn's disease.[5]

1. Bernstein LH, *et al.* Healing of perineal Crohn's disease with metronidazole. *Gastroenterology* 1980; **79:** 357–65.
2. Brandt LJ, *et al.* Metronidazole therapy for perineal Crohn's disease: a follow-up study. *Gastroenterology* 1982; **83:** 383–7.
3. Ursing B, *et al.* A comparative study of metronidazole and sulfasalazine for active Crohn's disease: the cooperative Crohn's disease study in Sweden. *Gastroenterology* 1982; **83:** 550–62.
4. Sutherland L, *et al.* Double blind, placebo controlled trial of metronidazole in Crohn's disease. *Gut* 1991; **32:** 1071–5.
5. Prantera C, *et al.* An antibiotic regimen for the treatment of active Crohn's disease: a randomized, controlled clinical trial of metronidazole plus ciprofloxacin. *Am J Gastroenterol* 1996; **91:** 328–32.

Malignant neoplasms. A review of the use of hypoxic sensitisers such as metronidazole and misonidazole as adjuncts to radiotherapy in patients with solid tumours.[1]

1. Chapman JD. Hypoxic sensitizers—implications for radiation therapy. *N Engl J Med* 1979; **301:** 1429–32.

Metabolic disorders. There are case reports[1,2] of children with methylmalonic aciduria showing clinical improvement when given metronidazole which reduced the excretion of faecal propionate and urinary methylmalonate. Metronidazole is considered to act through its antimicrobial effect on gut anaerobes that are involved in propionate production; such propionate cannot be handled by these children who are deficient in the relevant enzyme.

1. Bain MD, *et al.* Contribution of gut bacterial metabolism to human metabolic disease. *Lancet* 1988; **i:** 1078–9.
2. Koletzko B, *et al.* Antibiotic therapy for improvement of metabolic control in methylmalonic aciduria. *J Pediatr* 1990; **117:** 99–101.

Mouth disorders and infections. Cyclosporin-induced gingival hyperplasia resolved in 4 patients following treatment with metronidazole.[1]

Metronidazole is considered to be effective for the treatment of acute necrotising ulcerative gingivitis and is an alternative to penicillin in other dental infections (see Mouth Infections, p.132).

1. Wong W, *et al.* Resolution of cyclosporin-induced gingival hypertrophy with metronidazole. *Lancet* 1994; **343:** 986.

Peptic ulcer disease. The use of metronidazole is well established in regimens for eradicating *Helicobacter pylori* (see p.1174). However, the emergence of metronidazole-resistant strains of *H. pylori* has been associated with an increased rate of treatment failures with some regimens.[1-4] In populations in which the incidence of resistance is high, it may become necessary to use alternative regimens,[5] but in many populations metronidazole-containing regimens continue to produce adequate response rates.[6]

1. Buckley MJM, *et al.* Metronidazole resistance reduces efficacy of triple therapy and leads to secondary clarithromycin resistance. *Dig Dis Sci* 1997; **42:** 2111–15.
2. Lerang F, *et al.* Highly effective twice-daily triple therapies for Helicobacter pylori infection and peptic ulcer disease: does in vitro metronidazole resistance have any clinical relevance? *Am J Gastroenterol* 1997; **92:** 248–53.
3. Misiewicz JJ, *et al.* One week triple therapy for Helicobacter pylori: a multicentre comparative study. *Gut* 1997; **41:** 735–9.
4. van Zanten SV, *et al.* Adding once-daily omeprazole 20 mg to metronidazole/amoxicillin treatment for helicobacter pylori gastritis: a randomized, double-blind trial showing the importance of metronidazole resistance. *Am J Gastroenterol* 1998; **93:** 5–10.
5. Fennerty MB. Should we abandon metronidazole containing Helicobacter pylori treatment regimens? The clinical relevance of metronidazole resistance. *Am J Gastroenterol* 1998; **93:** 2–3.
6. Walt RP. Metronidazole-resistance H pylori—of questionable clinical importance. *Lancet* 1996; **348:** 489–90.

Skin disorders. Metronidazole may be effective in the management of ulceration associated with skin infections (p.142), including *pressure sores* and *fungating tumours*. Metronidazole 200 mg three times daily was reported to be successful in reducing the smell of fungating tumours.[1,2] Once-daily topical application of metronidazole has also proved effective. Treatment is supplemented by metronidazole irrigation for wound cleansing of large or deep cavities.[3,4]

In addition, several studies have indicated that metronidazole by mouth or applied topically is effective in the treatment of *rosacea*. Metronidazole 200 mg twice daily by mouth was significantly better than placebo[5] and as effective as oxytetracycline by mouth.[6] Similarly, topical application of a 1% metronidazole cream was found to be better than placebo[7,8] and as effective as oxytetracycline by mouth.[9] A 0.75% metronidazole gel also proved effective when compared with placebo in patients with acne rosacea (p.1076), although the telangiectatic component of the disease was not altered.[10]

1. Ashford RFU, *et al.* Metronidazole in smelly tumours. *Lancet* 1980; **i:** 874–5.
2. Ashford R, *et al.* Double-blind trial of metronidazole in malodorous ulcerating tumours. *Lancet* 1984; **i:** 1232–3.
3. Allwood MC, *et al.* Metronidazole topical gel. *Pharm J* 1986; **236:** 158.
4. Anonymous. Management of smelly tumours. *Lancet* 1990; **335:** 141–2.
5. Pye RJ, Burton JL. Treatment of rosacea by metronidazole. *Lancet* 1976; **i:** 1211–12.
6. Saihan EM, Burton JL. A double-blind trial of metronidazole versus oxytetracycline therapy for rosacea. *Br J Dermatol* 1980; **102:** 443–5.
7. Nielsen PG. Treatment of rosacea with 1% metronidazole cream. A double-blind study. *Br J Dermatol* 1983; **108:** 327–32.
8. Bitar A, *et al.* A double-blind randomised study of metronidazole (Flagyl®) 1% cream in the treatment of acne rosacea: a placebo-controlled study. *Drug Invest* 1990; **2:** 242–8.
9. Nielsen P. A double-blind study of 1% metronidazole cream versus systemic oxytetracycline therapy for rosacea. *Br J Dermatol* 1983; **109:** 63–5.
10. Aronson IK, *et al.* Evaluation of topical metronidazole gel in acne rosacea. *Drug Intell Clin Pharm* 1987; **21:** 346–51.

Surgical infection. Metronidazole and related nitroimidazoles are used in surgical infection prophylaxis (p.144) to reduce the rate of wound infection.

HAEMORRHOIDECTOMY. Prophylactic metronidazole reduced pain following haemorrhoidectomy in a small study.[1]

1. Carapeti EA, *et al.* Double-blind randomised controlled trial of effect of metronidazole on pain after day-case haemorrhoidectomy. *Lancet* 1998; **351:** 169–72.

African trypanosomiasis. Although there is no established alternative treatment for *Trypanosoma brucei rhodesiense* infections that are resistant to melarsoprol (see p.577), metronidazole and suramin were effective in 1 patient.[1]

1. Foulkes JR. Metronidazole and suramin combination in the treatment of arsenical refractory rhodesian sleeping sickness—a case study. *Trans R Soc Trop Med Hyg* 1996; **90:** 422.

Preparations

BP 1998: Metronidazole Gel; Metronidazole Intravenous Infusion; Metronidazole Suppositories; Metronidazole Tablets;
USP 23: Metronidazole Gel; Metronidazole Injection; Metronidazole Tablets.

Proprietary Preparations (details are given in Part 3)
Aust.: Acsacea; Anaerobex; Ariline; Elyzol; Flagyl; Oecozol; Trichex; ***Austral.:*** Flagyl; Metrogyl; Metrozine; Rozex; ***Belg.:*** Anaeromet; Flagyl; Pharmaflex; Rozex; ***Canad.:*** Flagyl; Metrocream; Metrogel; NidaGel; Noritate; Novo-Nidazol; Trikacide; ***Fr.:*** Flagyl; Rosaced; Rozagel; Rozex; ***Ger.:*** Arilin; Clont; Elyzol; Flagyl; Fossyol; Rathimed N†; Rathimed†; Tricho Cordes†; Ulcolind Metro; Vagimid; ***Irl.:*** Elyzol; Flagyl; Metrogel; Metronide; Metrotop; Rozex; ***Ital.:*** Deflamon; Flagyl; Gineflavir†; Pernyzol; Rozex; Vagilen; ***Neth.:*** Elyzol†; Flagyl; Metrogel; Rozex; ***Norw.:*** Elyzol; Flagyl; ***S.Afr.:*** Abbonidazole†; Acuzole; Ambral†; Anaerobyl†; Bemetrazole; Berazole; Clinazole†; Dynametron; Flagyl; Medamet; Metazol; Metrazole; Metrostat; Metryl†; Nabact†; Narobic; Nidatron; Rozex; Trichazole; Urometron†; Zagyl; Zobacide; Zolerol; ***Spain:*** Amotein; Flagyl; Rozex; Tricowas B; ***Swed.:*** Elyzol; Flagyl; ***Switz.:*** Arilin; Elyzol; Flagyl; Metrizol†; Metrolag†; Monasin†; Perilox; Rivozol; Rosalox; Rozex; Servizol; ***UK:*** Anabact; Elyzol; Flagyl; Metrogel; Metrolyl; Metrotop; Metrozol; Noritate; Norzol; Rozex; Vaginyl; Zadstat; Zidoval; ***USA:*** Flagyl; Metizol†; Metric†; Metro; Metrogel; Noritate; Protostat.

Multi-ingredient: ***Aust.:*** Helicocin; ***Austral.:*** Helidac; Losec Helicopak; ***Canad.:*** Flagystatin; ***Fr.:*** Rodogyl; ***Irl.:*** Flagyl Compak; ***Ital.:*** Meclon; ***Spain:*** Blastoestimulina; Rhodogil; ***UK:*** Entamizole†; Flagyl Compak; ***USA:*** Helidac.

Monensin Sodium (12973-q)

Monensin Sodium *(BANM, rINNM).*

Lilly-67314 (monensin). Sodium 4-{2-[2-ethyl-3′-methyl-5′-(tetrahydro-6-hydroxy-6-hydroxymethyl-3,5-dimethyl-2*H*-pyran-2-yl)perhydro-2,2′-bifuran-5-yl]-9-hydroxy-2,8-dimethyl-1,6-dioxaspiro[4.5]dec-7-yl}-3-methoxy-2-methylvalerate.

$C_{36}H_{61}NaO_{11}$ = 692.9.
CAS — 17090-79-8 (monensin); 22373-78-0 (monensin sodium).

NOTE. Monensin is *USAN.*

Pharmacopoeias. In US, for veterinary use only; US also has a monograph for Monensin.

An antibiotic produced by *Streptomyces cinnamonensis.*

It is an off-white to tan crystalline powder. Slightly **soluble** in water; soluble in methyl alcohol and in chloroform; practically insoluble in petroleum spirit.

Monensin sodium is an antiprotozoal used in veterinary practice for the prevention of coccidiosis in poultry and as a growth promoter for cattle. It has also been used for toxoplasmosis in sheep.

Narasin (12016-p)

Narasin *(BAN, USAN, rINN).*

Compound 79891; Lilly-79891. 2-(6-{5-[2-(5-Ethyltetrahydro-5-hydroxy-6-methylpyran-2-yl)-15-hydroxy-2,10,12-trimethyl-1,6,8-trioxadispiro[4.1.5.3]pentadec-13-en-9-yl]-2-hydroxy-1,3-dimethyl-4-oxoheptyl}tetrahydro-3,5-dimethylpyran-2-yl)butyric acid.

$C_{43}H_{72}O_{11}$ = 765.0.
CAS — 55134-13-9.

Pharmacopoeias. US includes Narasin Granular and Narasin Premix.

An antibiotic produced by *Streptomyces aureofaciens.*

Narasin is an antiprotozoal used in veterinary practice for the prevention of coccidiosis in poultry.

Nicarbazin (13007-z)

Nicarbazin *(BAN)*.

An equimolecular complex of 1,3-bis(4-nitrophenyl)urea ($C_{13}H_{10}N_4O_5$) and 4,6-dimethylpyrimidin-2-ol ($C_6H_8N_2O$).

$C_{19}H_{18}N_6O_6$ = 426.4.

CAS — 330-95-0.

Nicarbazin is an antiprotozoal used in veterinary practice for the prevention of coccidiosis in poultry.

Nifuratel (4789-q)

Nifuratel *(BAN, USAN, rINN)*.

Methylmercadone. 5-Methylthiomethyl-3-(5-nitrofurfurylideneamino)-2-oxazolidone.

$C_{10}H_{11}N_3O_5S$ = 285.3.

CAS — 4936-47-4.

Adverse Effects

Adverse effects associated with nifuratel include gastro-intestinal disturbances, peripheral neuropathy, and thrombocytopenic purpura. Allergic reactions, hepatotoxicity, blood dyscrasias, and pulmonary reactions similar to those soon with the structurally related drug nitrofurantoin have been reported rarely. Haemolytic anaemia may occur in patients with a deficiency of glucose-6-phosphate dehydrogenase given nifuratel.

Hypersensitivity. A report of contact dermatitis after only one application of nifuratel ointment in a man whose wife was undergoing treatment with nifuratel vaginal pessaries.[1]

1. Bedello PG, *et al*. Contact dermatitis from nifuratel. *Contact Dermatitis* 1983; **9:** 166.

Precautions

Nifuratel should not be given to patients with renal impairment, neuropathies, or glucose-6-phosphate dehydrogenase deficiency.

Interactions

A disulfiram-like reaction may occur in patients taking alcohol while on nifuratel therapy.

Pharmacokinetics

When taken by mouth nifuratel is absorbed from the gastro-intestinal tract. A metabolite, with activity against bacteria but not against trichomonads, is excreted in the urine.

Uses and Administration

Nifuratel is a nitrofuran derivative with a broad antimicrobial spectrum. It is active against the protozoan *Trichomonas vaginalis* and has an antibacterial spectrum similar to that of nitrofurantoin. Nifuratel has been used in the treatment of susceptible infections of the genito-urinary tract in doses of 200 to 400 mg three times daily by mouth. It has also been administered vaginally.

Preparations

Proprietary Preparations (details are given in Part 3)
Aust.: Macmiror; ***Ital.:*** Macmiror; ***Spain:*** Macmiror; ***Switz.:*** Macmiror.

Multi-ingredient: ***Fr.:*** Mycomnes; ***Ital.:*** Emorril; Macmiror Complex; ***Switz.:*** Dafnegil.

Nifursol (13015-z)

Nifursol *(BAN, USAN, pINN)*.

3,5-Dinitro-2′-(5-nitrofurfurylidene)salicylohydrazide.

$C_{12}H_7N_5O_9$ = 365.2.

CAS — 16915-70-1.

Nifursol is an antiprotozoal used in veterinary practice for the management of blackhead (histomoniasis) in poultry.

Nifurtimox (4790-d)

Nifurtimox *(BAN, rINN)*.

Bayer-2502. Tetrahydro-3-methyl-4-(5-nitrofurfurylideneamino)-1,4-thiazine 1,1-dioxide.

$C_{10}H_{13}N_3O_5S$ = 287.3.

CAS — 23256-30-6.

Pharmacopoeias. In *Fr.* and *Int.*

Adverse Effects

Adverse effects are common with nifurtimox and include gastro-intestinal effects such as anorexia with loss of weight, abdominal pain, nausea and vomiting, and effects on the nervous system, especially peripheral neuropathy. Psychoses, CNS excitement, insomnia, drowsiness, headache, myalgia, arthralgia, dizziness, and convulsions have also been reported. Skin rashes and other allergic reactions may occur.

Mutagenesis. An increase in chromosomal aberrations has been observed in children given nifurtimox.[1]

1. Gorla NB, *et al*. Thirteenfold increase of chromosomal aberrations non-randomly distributed in chagasic children treated with nifurtimox. *Mutat Res* 1989; **224:** 263–7.

Pharmacokinetics

Nifurtimox is well absorbed and rapidly metabolised following administration by mouth.

References.

1. Paulas C, *et al*. Pharmacokinetics of a nitrofuran compound, nifurtimox, in healthy volunteers. *Int J Clin Pharmacol Ther Toxicol* 1989; **27:** 454–7.
2. Gonzalez-Martin G, *et al*. The pharmacokinetics of nifurtimox in chronic renal failure. *Eur J Clin Pharmacol* 1992; **42:** 671–3.

Uses and Administration

Nifurtimox is a nitrofuran derivative with antiprotozoal activity. It is of value in the treatment of South American trypanosomiasis (Chagas' disease) due to infection by *Trypanosoma cruzi*, especially the early acute stage of the disease. It has some activity against *T. brucei gambiense*, the organism responsible for West African sleeping sickness.

Nifurtimox is given by mouth in divided doses. It is better tolerated by children than by adults. Treatment for South American trypanosomiasis is given for 60 to 120 days (but see below). Recommended doses for adults are 8 to 10 mg per kg body-weight daily. Suggested doses for children are: children of 1 to 10 years, 15 to 20 mg per kg daily for 90 days; of 11 to 16 years, 12.5 to 15 mg per kg daily for 90 days.

Leishmaniasis. As described on p.575 mucocutaneous leishmaniasis of the New World is usually treated with pentavalent antimony. Those who do not respond may be treated with amphotericin or pentamidine. Nifurtimox 10 mg per kg body-weight daily for a minimum of 4 weeks has been shown to be effective in cases of mucocutaneous leishmaniasis in Colombia and Brazil. However, toxic effects with nifurtimox are common and its role as a second-line drug or in combination with pentavalent antimony has not been established.[1]

1. WHO. Control of the leishmaniases. *WHO Tech Rep Ser 793*, 1990.

African trypanosomiasis. The meningoencephalitic stage of African trypanosomiasis (p.577) is usually treated with melarsoprol or eflornithine. Nifurtimox has been tried as an alternative in *Trypanosoma brucei gambiense* infections but higher doses than those used in South American trypanosomiasis are necessary. Pepin and colleagues[1] achieved a good initial response in 25 patients with nifurtimox 15 mg per kg body-weight per day for 60 days but 3 patients relapsed while still receiving nifurtimox and a further 12 of 19 patients who were followed up relapsed subsequently. An attempt by the same investigators to improve the response by increasing the daily dose even higher to 30 mg per kg for 30 days[2] resulted in substantial toxicity and only a modest improvement in results with 9 of 25 patients relapsing.

1. Pepin J, *et al*. An open clinical trial of nifurtimox for arseno-resistant Trypanosoma brucei gambiense sleeping sickness in central Zaire. *Trans R Soc Trop Med Hyg* 1989; **83:** 514–17.
2. Pépin J, *et al*. High-dose nifurtimox for arseno-resistant Trypanosoma brucei gambiense sleeping sickness: an open trial in central Zaire. *Trans R Soc Trop Med Hyg* 1992; **86:** 254–6.

American trypanosomiasis. The treatment of South American trypanosomiasis (p.578) is generally unsatisfactory, but nifurtimox is of value especially in the acute phase. However, there has been controversy over its ability to cure completely, that is to eradicate all parasites, in chronic disease.[1] Doses recommended by WHO[2] are 8 to 10 mg per kg body-weight daily in three divided doses for adults and 15 to 20 mg per kg daily in four divided doses for children; however up to 25 mg per kg daily has been used for the alleviation of acute meningoencephalitis.[3] WHO recommends that nifurtimox should be given for 60 to 90 days.[2,3] Some in the US[4] suggest a 90- to 120-day regimen for adults but nifurtimox is not well tolerated and the experience of other workers[1] suggests that few patients may complete the full course. Doses of 8 to 25 mg per kg daily have been given for 30 days or more in the treatment of congenital infections.[3]

1. Gutteridge WE. Existing chemotherapy and its limitations. *Br Med Bull* 1985; **41:** 162–8.
2. WHO. *WHO model prescribing information: drugs used in parasitic diseases.* 2nd ed. Geneva: WHO, 1995.
3. WHO. Control of Chagas disease: report of a WHO expert committee. *WHO Tech Rep Ser 811* 1991.
4. Anonymous. Drugs for parasitic infections. *Med Lett Drugs Ther* 1998; **40:** 1–12.

Preparations

Proprietary Preparations (details are given in Part 3)
Ger.: Lampit.

Nimorazole (4791-n)

Nimorazole *(BAN, rINN)*.

Nitrimidazine. 4-[2-(5-Nitroimidazol-1-yl)ethyl]morpholine.

$C_9H_{14}N_4O_3$ = 226.2.

CAS — 6506-37-2.

Pharmacopoeias. In *It.*

Adverse Effects and Precautions

As for Metronidazole, p.585.

Pharmacokinetics

Nimorazole is readily absorbed from the gastro-intestinal tract. Peak blood concentrations are achieved within 2 hours, and high concentrations are reported to occur in salivary and vaginal secretions. Trichomonicidal urinary concentrations are reported to persist for up to 48 hours after a dose. It is excreted in the urine together with 2 active metabolites. Unchanged drug and metabolites are also excreted in the breast milk.

Uses and Administration

Nimorazole is a 5-nitroimidazole derivative. It has antimicrobial actions and uses similar to those of metronidazole (see p.587).

In the treatment of trichomoniasis, the usual dose of nimorazole is 2 g by mouth as a single dose with a main meal repeated after about 1 month. Sexual partners should be treated concomitantly. In giardiasis or amoebiasis, nimorazole 1 g is given twice daily for 5 to 7 days; a suggested dose for children is 15 to 30 mg per kg body-weight daily.

Preparations

Proprietary Preparations (details are given in Part 3)
Aust.: Naxogin; ***Belg.:*** Naxogin; ***Fr.:*** Naxogyn; ***Ger.:*** Esclama; ***Ital.:*** Naxogin†; ***S.Afr.:*** Naxogin†.

Nitazoxanide (19580-d)

Nitazoxanide *(rINN)*.

N-(5-Nitro-2-thiazolyl)salicylamide acetate (ester).

$C_{12}H_9N_3O_5S$ = 307.3.

CAS — 55981-09-4.

Nitazoxanide is an antiprotozoal under investigation in the treatment of cryptosporidiosis in immunocompromised patients, including those with AIDS or HIV infection. It has also been used in helminth infections.

References.

1. Doumbo O, *et al*. Nitazoxanide in the treatment of cryptosporidial diarrhea and other intestinal parasitic infections associated with acquired immunodeficiency syndrome in tropical Africa. *Am J Trop Med Hyg* 1997; **56:** 637–9.
2. Cabello RR, *et al*. Nitazoxanide for the treatment of intestinal protozoan and helminthic infections in Mexico. *Trans R Soc Trop Med Hyg* 1997; **91:** 701–3.
3. Rossignol J-F, *et al*. Successful treatment of human fascioliosis with nitazoxanide. *Trans R Soc Trop Med Hyg* 1998; **92:** 103–4.
4. Abaza H, *et al*. Nitazoxanide in the treatment of patients with intestinal protozoan and helminthic infections: a report on 546 patients in Egypt. *Curr Ther Res* 1998; **59:** 116–21.

Ornidazole (4792-h)

Ornidazole *(USAN, rINN)*.

Ro-7-0207. 1-Chloro-3-(2-methyl-5-nitroimidazol-1-yl)propan-2-ol.

$C_7H_{10}ClN_3O_3$ = 219.6.

CAS — 16773-42-5.

Adverse Effects and Precautions

As for Metronidazole, p.585.

Pharmacokinetics

Ornidazole is readily absorbed from the gastro-intestinal tract and peak plasma concentrations of about 30 μg per mL have been achieved within 2 hours of a single dose of 1.5 g, falling to about 9 μg per mL after 24 hours and 2.5 μg per mL after 48 hours. After repeated oral doses of 500 mg every 12 hours, steady state peak and trough concentrations are 14 and 6 μg per mL respectively. Ornidazole is also absorbed from the vagina and peak plasma concentrations of about 5 μg per mL have been reported 12 hours after the insertion of a 500-mg vaginal pessary.

The plasma elimination half-life of ornidazole is 12 to 14 hours. Less than 15% is bound to plasma proteins. It is widely distributed in body tissues and fluids, including the cerebrospinal fluid.

Ornidazole is metabolised in the liver and is excreted in the urine, mainly as conjugates and metabolites, and to a lesser extent in the faeces. Biliary excretion may be important in the elimination of ornidazole and its metabolites.

References.

1. Schwartz DE, Jeunet F. Comparative pharmacokinetic studies of ornidazole and metronidazole in man. *Chemotherapy* 1976; **22:** 19–29.
2. Matheson I, *et al.* Plasma levels after a single oral dose of 1.5 g ornidazole. *Br J Vener Dis* 1977; **53:** 236–9.
3. Schwartz DE, *et al.* Metabolic studies of ornidazole in the rat, in the dog and in man. *Xenobiotica* 1979; **9:** 571–81.
4. Turcant A, *et al.* Pharmacokinetics of ornidazole in neonates and infants after a single intravenous infusion. *Eur J Clin Pharmacol* 1987; **32:** 111–13.
5. Martin C, *et al.* Pharmacokinetics and tissue penetration of a single dose of ornidazole (1,000 milligrams intravenously) for antibiotic prophylaxis in colorectal surgery. *Antimicrob Agents Chemother* 1990; **34:** 1921–4.
6. Bourget P, *et al.* Disposition of ornidazole and its metabolites during pregnancy. *J Antimicrob Chemother* 1995; **35:** 691–6.

Hepatic impairment. The elimination of ornidazole following a single intravenous dose of 500 mg was impaired in 10 patients with severe liver cirrhosis when compared with 10 healthy subjects; mean half-lives were 21.9 hours and 14.1 hours respectively.[1] These results suggested that the interval between doses of ornidazole should be doubled in patients with marked hepatic impairment. The need for dose adjustment was confirmed in further studies of patients with other forms of liver disease.[2,3]

1. Taburet AM, *et al.* Pharmacokinetics of ornidazole in patients with severe liver cirrhosis. *Clin Pharmacol Ther* 1986; **40:** 359–64.
2. Bourget P, *et al.* Ornidazole pharmacokinetics in several hepatic diseases. *J Pharmacol Clin* 1988; **7:** 25–32.
3. Taburet AM, *et al.* Pharmacokinetics of ornidazole in patients with acute viral hepatitis, alcoholic cirrhosis, and extrahepatic cholestasis. *Clin Pharmacol Ther* 1989; **45:** 373–9.

Renal impairment. The half-life of ornidazole administered intravenously was not prolonged in a study in patients with advanced chronic renal failure, including those on continuous ambulatory peritoneal dialysis, although total plasma clearance was halved; modification of the usual dosage is not necessary in such patients. However, ornidazole was removed by haemodialysis and ornidazole should be given after the dialysis session rather than before.[1] Others found[2] that the systemic availability and total body clearance of ornidazole is unaffected in chronic renal failure; their recommendation was that an additional dose should be given before haemodialysis to compensate for removal during that procedure.

1. Merdjan H, *et al.* Pharmacokinetics of ornidazole in patients with renal insufficiency; influence of haemodialysis and peritoneal dialysis. *Br J Clin Pharmacol* 1985; **19:** 211–17.
2. Horber FF, *et al.* High haemodialysis clearance of ornidazole in the presence of a negligible renal clearance. *Eur J Clin Pharmacol* 1989; **36:** 389–93.

Uses and Administration

Ornidazole is a 5-nitroimidazole derivative. It has the antimicrobial actions of metronidazole and is used similarly (see p.587) in the treatment of susceptible protozoal infections and also in the treatment and prophylaxis of anaerobic bacterial infections.

It is administered by mouth in tablets after food, by vaginal pessary, or intravenously. When given intravenously, solutions of ornidazole should be diluted to 5 mg or less per mL and 100 or 200 mL infused over 15 to 30 minutes.

In amoebiasis, 500 mg of ornidazole is given twice daily by mouth for 5 to 10 days; children are given 25 mg per kg body-weight daily as a single dose for 5 to 10 days. Patients with amoebic dysentery may be given 1.5 g as a single daily dose for 3 days; the children's dose is 40 mg per kg daily. In severe amoebic dysentery and amoebic liver abscess ornidazole may be given by intravenous infusion in a dose of 0.5 to 1 g initially, followed by 500 mg every 12 hours for 3 to 6 days; the children's dose is 20 to 30 mg per kg daily.

In giardiasis, 1 or 1.5 g of ornidazole is given by mouth as a single daily dose for 1 or 2 days; the children's dose is 30 or 40 mg per kg daily.

In trichomoniasis, a single dose of 1.5 g by mouth or 1 g by mouth together with 500 mg vaginally is given; 5-day courses of ornidazole 500 mg twice daily are also used. Sexual partners should be treated concomitantly. The children's dose is 25 mg per kg as a single dose.

For the treatment of anaerobic bacterial infections, ornidazole is given by intravenous infusion in an initial dose of 0.5 to 1 g, followed by 1 g daily as a single dose or in two divided doses for 5 to 10 days; oral therapy with 500 mg every 12 hours should be substituted as soon as possible. Children are given 10 mg per kg every 12 hours.

For the prevention of postoperative anaerobic bacterial infections, 1 g is given by intravenous infusion about 30 minutes before surgery.

Administration in hepatic impairment. In view of the prolonged half-life and reduced clearance of ornidazole reported in patients with hepatic dysfunction (see above), the interval between doses should be doubled in patients with severe hepatic impairment.

Administration in renal impairment. The elimination of ornidazole is reported to be largely unaltered in patients with impaired renal function (see above). Dosage adjustment is therefore usually unnecessary, although patients receiving haemodialysis should be given a supplemental dose equivalent to one-half of the usual dose before dialysis.

Preparations

Proprietary Preparations (details are given in Part 3)
Belg.: Tiberal; ***Fr.:*** Tiberal; ***Ital.:*** Tiberal; ***Spain:*** Tinerol; ***Switz.:*** Tiberal.

Pentamidine Isethionate (4794-b)

Pentamidine Isethionate *(BANM)*.

Pentamidine Isetionate *(rINNM)*; M & B-800; Pentamidine Diisetionate; Pentamidini Diisetionas; Pentamidini Isethionas. 4,4′-(Pentamethylenedioxy)dibenzamidine bis(2-hydroxyethanesulphonate).

$C_{19}H_{24}N_4O_2,2C_2H_6O_4S = 592.7.$

CAS — 100-33-4 (pentamidine); 140-64-7 (pentamidine isethionate).

Pharmacopoeias. In *Eur.* (see p.viii) and *Int.*

White or almost white powder or colourless crystals; it is hygroscopic. Pentamidine isethionate 1.74 mg is approximately equivalent to 1 mg of pentamidine. Freely **soluble** in water; sparingly soluble in alcohol; practically insoluble in dichloromethane. A 5% solution in water has a pH of 4.5 to 6.5. **Store** in airtight containers.

Incompatibility. Immediate precipitation was observed when a solution of pentamidine isethionate 3 mg per mL in glucose 5% was mixed with each of 5 cephalosporin and 1 cephamycin injections.[1]

For reference to the incompatibility of pentamidine isethionate and foscarnet, see Foscarnet Sodium, p.610.

1. Lewis JD, El-Gendy A. Cephalosporin-pentamidine isethionate incompatibilities. *Am J Health-Syst Pharm* 1996; **53:** 1461–2.

Pentamidine Mesylate (4793-m)

Pentamidine Mesylate *(BANM)*.

Pentamidine Mesilate *(rINNM)*; Pentamidine Dimethylsulphonate; Pentamidine Methanesulphonate; RP-2512. Pentamidine dimethanesulphonate.

$C_{19}H_{24}N_4O_2,2CH_3SO_3H = 532.6.$

CAS — 6823-79-6.

Pharmacopoeias. In *Int.*

A white or very faintly pink, almost odourless, granular powder. Pentamidine mesylate 1.56 mg is approximately equivalent to 1 mg of pentamidine. Slightly **soluble** in water and alcohol; practically insoluble in acetone, chloroform, and ether. A 5% solution in water has a pH of 4.5 to 6.5.

Adverse Effects

Pentamidine is a toxic drug and adverse effects are frequent and sometimes severe following parenteral administration; fatalities have been reported. Impaired renal function is common and, is usually manifest as mild and reversible raised blood urea nitrogen and serum creatinine concentrations, but acute renal failure can occur. Raised liver enzyme values and haematological disturbances such as leucopenia, anaemia, and occasionally thrombocytopenia, may occur. Hypoglycaemia, sometimes followed by hyperglycaemia and type 1 diabetes mellitus, is well documented; there have been occasional reports of acute pancreatitis.

The rapid intravenous injection of pentamidine has resulted in sudden hypotension and immediate reactions such as dizziness, headache, vomiting, breathlessness, tachycardia, and fainting. Hypotension may also occur when pentamidine is administered intramuscularly or by slow intravenous infusion. The intramuscular administration of pentamidine often causes pain, swelling, sterile abscess formation, and tissue necrosis at the site of injection. Similar damage can follow extravasation during intravenous administration.

Other adverse effects reported include hypocalcaemia, hyperkalaemia, skin rashes, the Stevens-Johnson syndrome, fever, flushing, gastro-intestinal effects such as nausea, vomiting, and taste disturbances, confusion, hallucinations, and cardiac arrhythmias.

Pentamidine is not so toxic when administered by inhalation for the prophylaxis of *Pneumocystis carinii* pneumonia. The commonest adverse effects with this route are cough and bronchoconstriction and may be controlled by a bronchodilator. Inhalation may leave a bitter taste. Pneumothorax has been reported, but may be associated with *Pneumocystis carinii* infection. There have been rare reports of adverse effects such as those observed when pentamidine is given by injection.

Adverse effects were observed in 46.8% of 404 patients given pentamidine parenterally for the treatment of *Pneumocystis carinii* pneumonia according to an analysis from the Center for Disease Control.[1] The reactions included impaired renal function (23.5% of patients), abnormal liver function (9.6%), hypoglycaemia (6.2%), haematological disturbances (4.2%), skin rashes (1.5%), and hypocalcaemia (1.2%). Local reactions at injection sites such as pain and abscess occurred in 18.3% and immediate side-effects such as hypotension in 9.6%. Nephrotoxicity was often the most serious adverse reaction although it was impossible to attribute it solely to pentamidine. Severe renal impairment occurred in 15 patients and contributed materially to 12 of 14 ensuing deaths. However elevation of blood urea nitrogen was usually relatively mild and reversible in those patients who had normal pretreatment renal function and had received no other nephrotoxic agents. One retrospective study[2] in patients with AIDS suggests that the development of nephrotoxicity or hyperkalaemia during parenteral administration is correlated with the total dose of pentamidine received and the duration of treatment but not with the initial degree of renal function. However, this study and other reports indicate that AIDS patients are especially susceptible to severe nephrotoxicity and hyperkalaemia,[3,4] and there have been instances of renal failure occurring when pentamidine is inhaled as an aerosol for its local effect.[5,6]

An evaluation of pentamidine in the treatment of 82 patients with visceral leishmaniasis further illustrates its toxicity.[7] Cardiotoxicity, manifested by tachycardia, hypotension, and ECG changes of nonspecific myocarditis, occurred in about 23% of patients. No hypoglycaemic reaction was noted, but 4 patients developed diabetes mellitus and 3 of them were found to be insulin-dependent. Other adverse reactions included gastro-intestinal effects (anorexia, nausea, vomiting, abdominal pain, or diarrhoea) in about 78%; CNS effects (headache associated with flushing, delirium, or sensory disturbances resembling pins and needles) in about 24%; mild reversible albuminuria in about 7%; and allergic manifestations (generalised urticaria, itching, and conjunctival congestion) in about 5%. One patient had severe anaphylaxis.

As reported above[1,7] pentamidine can have a range of effects on carbohydrate metabolism. Bouchard *et al.*[8] provided details of 4 patients receiving pentamidine for *Pneumocystis carinii* pneumonia who developed severe fasting hypoglycaemia followed later by hyperglycaemia and type 1 diabetes mellitus. It has been suggested that pentamidine has a toxic effect on the β-cells of the pancreatic islets and can induce an early cytolytic release of insulin and hypoglycaemia, followed by β-cell destruction, insulin deficiency, and diabetes mellitus.[8,9] Once again AIDS patients appear to be highly susceptible, the incidence of hypoglycaemia due to pentamidine being higher in this group.[10] The action on the pancreas has led to fatal acute pancreatitis;[11-13] fatal hypoglycaemia has also been reported.[14] These reports[8-12,14] involved pentamidine administered by injection; there have also been reports of pancreatitis[15,16] and diabetes mellitus[17,18] occurring in patients given pentamidine by aerosol inhalation.

Hypotension is a problem with the intravenous administration of pentamidine, but can be reduced by infusing the dose over

60 minutes when the incidence of hypotension appears to be similar to that with the intramuscular route.[19,20] Intravenous administration of pentamidine has also been associated with torsade de pointes.[21-23] It has been observed that renal toxicity is more common when pentamidine is given intramuscularly rather than intravenously to AIDS patients with diarrhoea, suggesting that fluid status might have an important role.[24]

Although there have been some reports of adverse reactions to inhaled pentamidine that are associated with the parenteral route, the main problem with the inhalation route is bronchoconstriction;[25] it can be prevented by giving a bronchodilator. Acute eosinophilic pneumonia associated with nebulised pentamidine administration has been reported in 1 patient.[26] Concern has been expressed at the risks to those who are with the patient at the time of inhalation and are exposed to nebulised pentamidine.[27-29]

1. Walzer PD, *et al.* Pneumocystis carinii pneumonia in the United States: epidemiologic, diagnostic and clinical features. *Ann Intern Med* 1974; **80:** 83–93.
2. Briceland LL, Bailie GR. Pentamidine-associated nephrotoxicity and hyperkalemia in patients with AIDS. *DICP Ann Pharmacother* 1991; **25:** 1171–4.
3. Lachaal M, Venuto RC. Nephrotoxicity and hyperkalemia in patients with acquired immunodeficiency syndrome treated with pentamidine. *Am J Med* 1989; **87:** 260–3.
4. Peltz S, Hashmi S. Pentamidine-induced severe hyperkalemia. *Am J Med* 1989; **87:** 698–9.
5. Miller RF, *et al.* Acute renal failure after nebulised pentamidine. *Lancet* 1989; **i:** 1271–2.
6. Chapelon C, *et al.* Renal insufficiency with nebulised pentamidine. *Lancet* 1989; **ii:** 1045–6.
7. Jha TK. Evaluation of diamidine compound (pentamidine isethionate) in the treatment of resistant cases of kala-azar occurring in North Bihar, India. *Trans R Soc Trop Med Hyg* 1983; **77:** 167–70.
8. Bouchard P, *et al.* Diabetes mellitus following pentamidine-induced hypoglycemia in humans. *Diabetes* 1982; **31:** 40–5.
9. Osei K, *et al.* Diabetogenic effect of pentamidine: in vitro and in vivo studies in a patient with malignant insulinoma. *Am J Med* 1984; **77:** 41–6.
10. Stahl-Bayliss CM, *et al.* Pentamidine-induced hypoglycemia in patients with the acquired immune deficiency syndrome. *Clin Pharmacol Ther* 1986; **39:** 271–5.
11. Salmeron S, *et al.* Pentamidine and pancreatitis. *Ann Intern Med* 1986; **105:** 140–1.
12. Zuger A, *et al.* Pentamidine-associated fatal acute pancreatitis. *JAMA* 1986; **256:** 2383–5.
13. Savleda J, *et al.* Probable pentamidine-induced acute pancreatitis. *Ann Pharmacother* 1994; **28:** 52–3.
14. Sattler FR, Waskin H. Pentamidine and fatal hypoglycemia. *Ann Intern Med* 1987; **107:** 789–90.
15. Herer B, *et al.* Pancreatitis associated with pentamidine by aerosol. *Br Med J* 1989; **298:** 605.
16. Hart CC. Aerosolized pentamidine and pancreatitis. *Ann Intern Med* 1989; **111:** 691.
17. Fisch A. Diabetes mellitus in a patient with AIDS after treatment with pentamidine aerosol. *Br Med J* 1990; **301:** 875.
18. Chen JP, *et al.* Diabetes after aerosolized pentamidine. *Ann Intern Med* 1991; **114:** 913–14.
19. Navin TR, Fontaine RE. Intravenous versus intramuscular administration of pentamidine. *N Engl J Med* 1984; **311:** 1701.
20. Helmick CG, Green JK. Pentamidine-associated hypotension and route of administration. *Ann Intern Med* 1985; **103:** 480.
21. Harel Y, *et al.* Pentamidine-induced torsade de pointes. *Pediatr Infect Dis J* 1993; **12:** 692–4.
22. Miller HC. Cardiac arrest after intravenous pentamidine in an infant. *Pediatr Infect Dis J* 1993; **12:** 694–6.
23. Zanetti LAF, Oliphant CM. Pentamidine-induced torsade de pointes. *Ann Pharmacother* 1994; **28:** 282–3.
24. Stehr-Green JK, Helmick CG. Pentamidine and renal toxicity. *N Engl J Med* 1985; **313:** 694–5.
25. Smith DE, *et al.* Reversible bronchoconstriction with nebulised pentamidine. *Lancet* 1988; **ii:** 905.
26. Dupon M, *et al.* Acute eosinophilic pneumonia induced by inhaled pentamidine isethionate. *Br Med J* 1993; **306:** 109.
27. McDiarmid MA, Jacobson-Kram D. Aerosolised pentamidine and public health. *Lancet* 1989; **ii:** 863–4.
28. Thomas SHL, *et al.* Aerosolised pentamidine. *Lancet* 1989; **ii:** 1284.
29. Smaldone GC, *et al.* Detection of inhaled pentamidine in health care workers. *N Engl J Med* 1991; **325:** 891–2.

Precautions

Pentamidine should be used under close supervision and great care is necessary if it is used in patients suffering from any condition likely to be exacerbated by pentamidine's adverse effects. Patients should remain supine during administration and their blood pressure should be monitored. Kidney and liver function, blood-glucose concentrations, blood counts, and other parameters indicative of developing toxicity, such as serum-calcium concentrations and the ECG, should also be assessed regularly during courses of treatment with pentamidine.

Patients with a history of asthma or smoking may be at increased risk of cough and bronchospasm during inhalation of nebulised pentamidine. Symptoms may be controlled by administering a bronchodilator before giving pentamidine. The manufacturers state that pentamidine solution should not be mixed with other drugs nor should a bronchodilator be administered in the same nebuliser. Extrapulmonary *P. carinii* infections may occur in patients receiving nebulised pentamidine and should be considered in patients with unexplained signs and symptoms. Precautions should be taken to minimise atmospheric pollution with pentamidine during nebulisation.

Interactions

The concomitant use of pentamidine with other nephrotoxic drugs (e.g. amphotericin, foscarnet) should preferably be avoided. Extreme caution is also necessary if pentamidine is given with other drugs (e.g. foscarnet) that can cause hypocalcaemia. There is an increased risk of ventricular arrhythmias if pentamidine is given with amiodarone.

Pharmacokinetics

Following intravenous administration of the isethionate, pentamidine is rapidly distributed to body tissues and this is followed by a prolonged elimination phase. Elimination half-lives of 6 hours following intravenous infusion and 9 hours following intramuscular injection have been cited, but probably represent an intermediate value, and terminal elimination half-lives of between several days and weeks have been reported. During repeated dosing accumulation is believed to occur, particularly in the liver and kidneys, and only small concentrations of pentamidine are found in the urine.

Distribution to the lung is relatively poor following administration by injection. Systemic absorption following inhalation is reported to result in peak plasma concentrations of between 5 and 10% of those observed after parenteral administration and there have been a few reports of systemic adverse effects. Particle or droplet size appears to be important in achieving adequate pulmonary distribution.

References.

1. Waalkes TP, *et al.* Pentamidine: clinical pharmacologic correlations in man and mice. *Clin Pharmacol Ther* 1970; **11:** 505–12.
2. Bernard EM, *et al.* Use of a new bioassay to study pentamidine pharmacokinetics. *J Infect Dis* 1985; **152:** 750–4.
3. O'Doherty MJ, *et al.* Differences in relative efficiency of nebulisers for pentamidine administration. *Lancet* 1988; **ii:** 1283–6.
4. Simonds AK, *et al.* Aerosolised pentamidine. *Lancet* 1989; **i:** 221–2.
5. Baskin MI, *et al.* Regional deposition of aerosolized pentamidine: effects of body position and breathing pattern. *Ann Intern Med* 1990; **113:** 677–83.
6. Bronner U, *et al.* Pentamidine concentrations in plasma, whole blood and cerebrospinal fluid during treatment of Trypanosoma gambiense in Côte d'Ivoire. *Trans R Soc Trop Med Hyg* 1991; **85:** 608–11.
7. Lidman C, *et al.* Plasma pentamidine concentrations vary between individuals with Pneumocystis carinii pneumonia and the drug is actively secreted by the kidney. *J Antimicrob Chemother* 1994; **33:** 803–10.
8. Bronner U, *et al.* Pharmacokinetics and adverse reactions after a single dose of pentamidine in patients with Trypanosoma gambiense sleeping sickness. *Br J Clin Pharmacol* 1995; **39:** 289–95.
9. Conte JE, Golden JA. intrapulmonary and systemic pharmacokinetics of aerosolized pentamidine used for prophylaxis of Pneumocystis carinii pneumonia in patients infected with the human immunodeficiency virus. *J Clin Pharmacol* 1995; **35:** 1166–73.

Renal impairment. In a study[1] of patients with normal renal function or on haemodialysis, renal clearance of pentamidine during the 24 hours after intravenous administration was 2.1% of the plasma clearance in those with normal renal function, suggesting that pentamidine elimination would be largely unaffected by renal impairment. In those with end-stage renal disease receiving haemodialysis the terminal elimination half-life following a single dose was prolonged to about 75 hours compared with 30 hours in the patients with normal renal function, but the volumes of distribution and area under the concentration-time curve were not significantly different. In patients with normal or mildly impaired renal function who had received between 12 and 21 doses the terminal elimination half-life after the final dose was about 12 days and pentamidine was still detectable in the plasma after 6 weeks. There was evidence of accumulation of pentamidine during repeated daily dosing.

1. Conte JE. Pharmacokinetics of intravenous pentamidine in patients with normal renal function or receiving hemodialysis. *J Infect Dis* 1991; **163:** 169–75.

Uses and Administration

Pentamidine, an aromatic diamidine derivative, is an antiprotozoal used in the treatment of the early stages of African trypanosomiasis, especially *Trypanosoma brucei gambiense* infections and in some forms of leishmaniasis. It is also used in the treatment and prophylaxis of pneumonia due to the fungus *Pneumocystis carinii.* It may act by several mechanisms including interference with protozoal DNA and folate transformation, and by inhibition of RNA and protein synthesis.

It has been given as the isethionate or mesylate salt, but pentamidine isethionate is the only form now available in most countries. There is considerable confusion in the literature regarding the dosage of pentamidine since it is often not clear whether doses are being expressed in terms of pentamidine base, the isethionate salt, or the mesylate salt. In general it would appear that when the isethionate is used doses are expressed in terms of pentamidine isethionate, individual doses usually being up to 4 mg per kg body-weight, whereas when the mesylate is used doses are expressed in terms of pentamidine base. Pentamidine isethionate 4 mg per kg is approximately equivalent to pentamidine base 2.3 mg per kg; pentamidine mesylate 3.6 mg per kg is approximately equivalent to pentamidine base 2.3 mg per kg.

Pentamidine isethionate is administered by deep intramuscular injection or by slow intravenous infusion over at least 60 minutes; direct intravenous injection must be avoided. Patients should be lying down during administration. The mesylate has usually been given intramuscularly.

In the treatment of early African trypanosomiasis due to *T. b. gambiense*, pentamidine isethionate 4 mg per kg may be given daily or on alternate days by intramuscular injection or intravenous infusion to a total of 7 to 10 doses. Pentamidine is not effective in trypanosomiasis with CNS involvement, but 2 injections of pentamidine may be given in late-stage *T. b. gambiense* infection before starting treatment with melarsoprol or eflornithine.

In the treatment of visceral leishmaniasis, and of mucocutaneous leishmaniasis due to *Leishmania braziliensis* or *L. aethiopica* that have not responded to antimonials, pentamidine isethionate 4 mg per kg may be given preferably intramuscularly three times a week for 5 to 25 weeks or even longer. An alternative regimen in visceral leishmaniasis is to give 3 to 4 mg per kg on alternate days to a maximum of 10 injections; the course may need to be repeated. In cutaneous leishmaniasis due to *L. aethiopica* or *L. guyanensis*, pentamidine isethionate 3 to 4 mg per kg may be given preferably intramuscularly once or twice a week until the condition resolves. A weekly dose of 3 to 4 mg per kg is also used for diffuse cutaneous leishmaniasis due to *L. aethiopica* and is given for at least 4 months.

In the treatment of *Pneumocystis carinii* pneumonia, pentamidine isethionate 4 mg per kg is given once daily for 14 days or more by intramuscular injection or preferably slow intravenous infusion. Pentamidine isethionate is administered by inhalation through a nebuliser to prevent *P. carinii* pneumonia in HIV-positive patients in a dose of 300 mg once every 4 weeks; in those who cannot tolerate this dose 150 mg every 2 weeks may be used. It has also occasionally been used by this route for treating mild to moderate infection in a dose of 600 mg daily for 3 weeks. Nebuliser design can affect the droplet size delivered and hence the amount of pentamidine reaching sites of action within the lungs. The optimal particle size is 1 to 2 microns. Precautions should be taken to minimise atmospheric pollution with pentamidine.

Administration in renal impairment. Since renal clearance accounts for only a small proportion of pentamidine elimination, dosage adjustment is not generally considered necessary for mild to moderate degrees of renal impairment. The UK manufacturer recommends dosage reductions in patients with *P. carinii* pneumonia who have a creatinine clearance of less than 10 mL per minute. In patients with life-threatening disease the recommended dose of 4 mg per kg daily should be given for 7 to 10 days and then on alternate days for the remainder of the 14-dose course. In less severe disease the suggested dose is 4 mg per kg on alternate days for 14 doses.

Amoebic infections. ACANTHAMOEBA INFECTIONS. Pentamidine was used to treat disseminated *Acanthamoeba* infection (see p.573) in 2 immunocompromised patients without evidence of CNS involvement.[1,2] It is unlikely that pentamidine would be effective in infections involving the CNS.

1. Slater CA, *et al.* Brief report: successful treatment of disseminated Acanthamoeba infection in an immunocompromised patient. *N Engl J Med* 1994; **331:** 85–7.
2. Murakawa GJ, *et al.* Disseminated Acanthamoeba in patients with AIDS: a report of five cases and a review of the literature. *Arch Dermatol* 1995; **131:** 1291–6.

Babesiosis. Pentamidine has been tried for babesiosis (p.574), but while some patients were reported to have improved others had not and the value of pentamidine in this infection was considered to be doubtful.

References.

1. Teutsch SM, Juranek DD. Babesiosis. *Ann Intern Med* 1981; **95:** 241.
2. Francioli PB, *et al.* Response of babesiosis to pentamidine therapy. *Ann Intern Med* 1981; **94:** 326–30.
3. Raoult D, *et al.* Babesiosis, pentamidine, and cotrimoxazole. *Ann Intern Med* 1987; **107:** 944.
4. Clarke CS, *et al.* Babesiosis: under-reporting or case-clustering? *Postgrad Med J* 1989; **65:** 591–3.

Leishmaniasis. Pentamidine has been used in the treatment of visceral leishmaniasis (p.575) both alone and in combination with antimonials in patients who have failed to respond to antimonials alone.[1,2] It has also been tried for long-term secondary prophylaxis in patients with HIV infection.[3] Cutaneous leishmaniasis due to *L. guyanensis* is usually treated with pentamidine to reduce the risk of dissemination;[1] lesions due to *L. aethiopica* may also respond to pentamidine, but can be left to heal spontaneously since the risk of diffuse cutaneous involvement is small.[1] Diffuse cutaneous or mucocutaneous disease which is unresponsive to antimonials may respond to pentamidine, especially when due to *L. aethiopica*.[1]

1. WHO. *WHO model prescribing information: drugs used in parasitic diseases.* 2nd ed. Geneva: WHO, 1995.
2. Baily GG, Nandy A. Visceral leishmaniasis: more prevalent and more problematic. *J Infect* 1994; **29:** 241–7.
3. Pérez-Molina JA, *et al.* Pentamidine isethionate as secondary prophylaxis against visceral leishmaniasis in HIV-positive patients. *AIDS* 1996; **10:** 237–8.

Pneumocystis carinii pneumonia. In the treatment of *Pneumocystis carinii* pneumonia (p.370) intravenous pentamidine is generally reserved for patients who do not respond to or cannot tolerate co-trimoxazole.[1,2] Combination therapy with co-trimoxazole and pentamidine is no more effective than pentamidine alone in these patients and is potentially more toxic than either drug.[3] Inhaled pentamidine is occasionally suggested for mild to moderate infection but is now generally only used for prophylaxis.

In both primary and secondary prophylaxis of *P. carinii* pneumonia in immunocompromised patients co-trimoxazole has been preferred to inhaled pentamidine. Comparative studies have shown that, in the short-term, inhaled pentamidine has been less effective than co-trimoxazole[4,5] and no more effective than the other common prophylactic drug, dapsone.[6,7] In addition, both co-trimoxazole and dapsone (given with pyrimethamine) also provide protection against toxoplasmosis and, being given systemically, against extrapulmonary *P. carinii* infections. However, inhaled pentamidine is better tolerated than either of the alternatives, and studies have suggested that in the long term the efficacy of the three drugs is comparable,[8,9] at least in patients with CD4+ T lymphocyte counts of more than 100 per μL. Increasing the dose of pentamidine from 300 mg every four weeks to 300 mg every two weeks[10,11] or 600 mg every week[12] may improve efficacy further.

1. Anonymous. Prevention and treatment of Pneumocystis carinii pneumonia in patients infected with HIV. *Drug Ther Bull* 1994; **32:** 12–15.
2. Anonymous. Drugs for parasitic infections. *Med Lett Drugs Ther* 1998; **40:** 1–12.
3. PCP Therapy Project Group. Assessment of therapy for Pneumocystis carinii pneumonia. *Am J Med* 1984; **76:** 501–8.
4. Schneider MME, *et al.* A controlled trial of aerosolized pentamidine or trimethoprim-sulfamethoxazole as primary prophylaxis against Pneumocystis carinii pneumonia in patients with human immunodeficiency virus infection. *N Engl J Med* 1992; **327:** 1836–41.
5. Hardy WD, *et al.* A controlled trial of trimethoprim-sulfamethoxazole or aerosolized pentamidine for secondary prophylaxis of Pneumocystis carinii pneumonia in patients with the acquired immunodeficiency syndrome. *N Engl J Med* 1992; **327:** 1842–8.
6. Girard P-M, *et al.* Dapsone-pyrimethamine compared with aerosolized pentamidine as primary prophylaxis against Pneumocystis carinii pneumonia and toxoplasmosis in HIV infection. *N Engl J Med* 1993; **328:** 1514–20.
7. Torres RA, *et al.* Randomized trial of dapsone and aerosolized pentamidine for the prophylaxis of Pneumocystis carinii pneumonia and toxoplasmic encephalitis. *Am J Med* 1993; **95:** 573–83.
8. Bozzette SA, *et al.* A randomized trial of three antipneumocystis agents in patients with advanced human immunodeficiency virus infection. *N Engl J Med* 1995; **332:** 693–9.
9. Rizzardi GP, *et al.* Risks and benefits of aerosolized pentamidine and cotrimoxazole in primary prophylaxis of Pneumocystis carinii pneumonia in HIV-1-infected patients: a two-year Italian multicentric randomized controlled trial. *J Infect* 1996; **32:** 123–31.
10. Kronawitter U, *et al.* Low incidence of Pneumocystis carinii pneumonia in HIV patients receiving 300 mg pentamidine aerosol every 2 weeks. *Clin Invest* 1992; **70:** 1089–91.
11. Rizzardi GP, *et al.* Better efficacy of twice-monthly than monthly aerosolised pentamidine for secondary prophylaxis of Pneumocystis carinii pneumonia in patients with AIDS: an Italian multicentric randomised controlled trial. *J Infect* 1995; **31:** 99–105.
12. Ong ELC, *et al.* Efficacy and effects on pulmonary function tests of weekly 600 mg aerosol pentamidine as prophylaxis against Pneumocystis carinii pneumonia. *Infection* 1992; **20:** 136–9.

African trypanosomiasis. The treatment of African trypanosomiasis is discussed on p.577. Pentamidine is used for the haematolymphatic phase of infections caused by *Trypanosoma brucei gambiense* and as an adjunct to other treatment for the meningoencephalitic stage of the infection.[1] It is reported to be less effective against *T. b. rhodesiense* and in some areas resistance of *T. b. gambiense* to pentamidine is increasing.[2] Pentamidine has been used in combination with suramin for *T. b. gambiense* infections but this has not been shown to be clinically superior to pentamidine alone.[3]

1. WHO. Epidemiology and control of African trypanosomiasis. *WHO Tech Rep Ser 739* 1986.
2. WHO. *WHO model prescribing information: drugs used in parasitic diseases.* 2nd ed. Geneva: WHO, 1995.
3. Pépin J, Khonde N. Relapses following treatment of early-stage Trypanosoma brucei gambiense sleeping sickness with a combination of pentamidine and suramin. *Trans R Soc Trop Med Hyg* 1996; **90:** 183–6.

Preparations

BP 1998: Pentamidine Injection.

Proprietary Preparations (details are given in Part 3)
Aust.: Pentacarinat; ***Austral.:*** Pentacarinat†; ***Belg.:*** Pentacarinat; ***Canad.:*** Pentacarinat; Pneumopent†; ***Fr.:*** Pentacarinat; ***Ger.:*** Pentacarinat; ***Irl.:*** Pentacarinat; ***Ital.:*** Pentacarinat; Pneumopent; ***Neth.:*** Pentacarinat; ***Norw.:*** Pentacarinat; ***S.Afr.:*** Pentacarinat; ***Spain:*** Pentacarinat; ***Swed.:*** Pentacarinat; ***Switz.:*** Pentacarinat; ***UK:*** Pentacarinat; ***USA:*** NebuPent; Pentacarinat; Pentam 300.

Propenidazole (3926-z)

Propenidazole *(rINN)*.

Ethyl *trans*-α-acetyl-1-methyl-5-nitroimidazole-2-acrylate.

$C_{11}H_{13}N_3O_5$ = 267.2.

CAS — 76448-31-2.

Propenidazole is used for protozoal and fungal infections of the genito-urinary tract. It has been given by mouth or by the vaginal route.

Preparations

Proprietary Preparations (details are given in Part 3)
Ital.: Naska†.

Robenidine Hydrochloride (13216-n)

Robenidine Hydrochloride *(BANM, USAN, rINNM)*.

CL-78116; Robenzidene Hydrochloride. 1,3-Bis(4-chlorobenzylideneamino)guanidine hydrochloride.

$C_{15}H_{13}Cl_2N_5,HCl$ = 370.7.

CAS — 25875-51-8 (robenidine); 25875-50-7 (robenidine hydrochloride).

Robenidine hydrochloride is an antiprotozoal used in veterinary practice for the prevention of coccidiosis in poultry and rabbits.

Ronidazole (13219-b)

Ronidazole *(BAN, USAN, pINN)*.

(1-Methyl-5-nitroimidazol-2-yl)methyl carbamate.

$C_6H_8N_4O_4$ = 200.2.

CAS — 7681-76-7.

Pharmacopoeias. In *BP(Vet).*

A white to yellowish-brown, odourless or almost odourless powder. Slightly **soluble** in water, alcohol, and chloroform; very slightly soluble in ether. **Protect** from light.

Ronidazole is a 5-nitroimidazole derivative similar to metronidazole. It has been used in veterinary practice for the treatment and control of swine dysentery and has also been added to turkey feeding stuffs.

Salinomycin Sodium (12017-s)

Salinomycin Sodium *(BANM, rINNM)*.

AHR-3096 (salinomycin); K-364 (salinomycin); K-748364A (salinomycin). Sodium (2*R*)-2-{(2*R*,5*S*,6*R*)-6-[(1*S*,2*S*,3*S*,5*R*)-5-{(2*S*,5*S*,7*R*,9*S*,10*S*,12*R*,15*R*)-2-[(2*R*,5*R*,6*S*)-5-ethyltetrahydro-5-hydroxy-6-methylpyran-2-yl]-15-hydroxy-2,10,12-trimethyl-1,6,8-trioxadispiro[4.1.5.3]pentadec-13-en-9-yl}-2-hydroxy-1,3-dimethyl-4-oxoheptyl]tetrahydro-5-methylpyran-2-yl}butyrate.

$C_{42}H_{69}NaO_{11}$ = 773.0.

CAS — 53003-10-4 (salinomycin); 55721-31-8 (salinomycin sodium).

An antibiotic produced by *Streptomyces albus.*

Salinomycin is an antiprotozoal used in veterinary practice for the prevention of coccidiosis in poultry and as a growth promoter in pigs.

Secnidazole (13227-b)

Secnidazole *(BAN, rINN)*.

PM-185184; 14539-RP; RP-14539. 1-(2-Methyl-5-nitroimidazol-1-yl)propan-2-ol.

$C_7H_{11}N_3O_3$ = 185.2.

CAS — 3366-95-8.

Secnidazole is a 5-nitroimidazole derivative with properties similar to those of metronidazole (see p.585), apart from a much longer plasma half-life of about 20 hours. It is used in the treatment of amoebiasis, giardiasis, and trichomoniasis.

Secnidazole is given by mouth, usually as a single dose of 2 g in adults or 30 mg per kg body-weight in children. In invasive (hepatic) amoebiasis a dose of 1.5 g a day is given in single or divided doses for 5 days; children may be given 30 mg per kg body-weight per day.

References.

1. Gillis JC, Wiseman LR. Secnidazole: a review of its antimicrobial activity, pharmacokinetic properties and therapeutic use in the management of protozoal infections and bacterial vaginosis. *Drugs* 1996; **51:** 621–38.

Preparations

Proprietary Preparations (details are given in Part 3)
Fr.: Flagentyl.

Sinefungin (932-l)

Sinefungin *(USAN)*.

Compound 57926. 6,9-Diamino-1-(6-amino-9*H*-purin-9-yl)-1,5,6,7,8,9,-hexadeoxy-β-D-*ribo*-decofuranuronic acid.

$C_{15}H_{23}N_7O_5$ = 381.4.

CAS — 58944-73-3.

Sinefungin is an antiprotozoal that has been produced from *Streptomyces griseolus.* There are reports of activity against *Leishmania* spp., *Plasmodium falciparum,* trypanosomes, and *Trichomonas vaginalis.* It has also been reported to possess antifungal activity.

References.

1. Trager W, *et al.* Plasmodium falciparum: antimalarial activity in culture of sinefungin and other methylation inhibitors. *Exp Parasitol* 1980; **50** (suppl 1): 83–9.
2. Nadler JP, *et al.* The effect of adenosine analogues on the in vitro growth of Trypanosoma cruzi. *Trans R Soc Trop Med Hyg* 1982; **76:** 285–7.
3. Dube DK, *et al.* Antitrypanosomal activity of sinefungin. *Am J Trop Med Hyg* 1983; **32:** 31–3.
4. Ferrante A, *et al.* A report on the amoebicidal activity in vitro of sinefungin against Entamoeba histolytica. *Trans R Soc Trop Med Hyg* 1984; **78:** 837.
5. Neal RA, *et al.* Anti-leishmanial effect of allopurinol ribonucleoside and the related compounds, allopurinol, thiopurinol, thiopurinol ribonucleoside, and of formycin B, sinefungin and the lepidine WR6026. *Trans R Soc Trop Med Hyg* 1985; **79:** 122.
6. Paolantonacci P, *et al.* Differential effect of sinefungin and its analogs on the multiplication of three Leishmania species. *Antimicrob Agents Chemother* 1985; **28:** 528–31.
7. Thong K-W, Coombs GH. The effects of inhibitors of sulphur-containing amino acid metabolism on the growth of Trichomonas vaginalis in vitro. *J Antimicrob Chemother* 1987; **19:** 429.
8. Nolan LL. Molecular target of the antileishmanial action of sinefungin. *Antimicrob Agents Chemother* 1987; **31:** 1542–8.
9. Zweygarth E, Röttcher D. Efficacy of experimental trypanocidal compounds against as multiple drug-resistant Trypanosoma brucei brucei stock in mice. *Parasitol Res* 1989; **75:** 178–82.
10. Avila JL, *et al.* Inhibitory effects of sinefungin and its cyclic analog on the multiplication of Trypanosoma cruzi isolates. *Am J Trop Med Hyg* 1993; **48:** 112–19.

Suramin (4797-q)

Antrypol; Bayer-205; Fourneau-309; Naganinum; Naganol.

The symmetrical 3″-urea of the sodium salt of 8-(3-benzamido-4-methylbenzamido)naphthalene-1,3,5-trisulphonic acid.

$C_{51}H_{34}N_6Na_6O_{23}S_6$ = 1429.2.

CAS — 145-63-1 (suramin); 129-46-4 (suramin sodium).

NOTE. Suramin Sodium is *rINN*

Pharmacopoeias. In *Fr., Int.,* and *It.*

A white, pinkish-white, or slightly cream-coloured, odourless or almost odourless, hygroscopic powder. **Soluble** 1 in less than 1 of water; very slightly soluble in alcohol; practically insoluble in chloroform and ether. Solutions deteriorate on storage and should be used immediately after preparation; solutions for injection are prepared aseptically. **Store** in a cool place in airtight containers. Protect from light.

Adverse Effects

An immediate and potentially fatal reaction, with nausea, vomiting, shock, and loss of consciousness, may follow the injection of suramin in some patients and thus it is usual practice to give a small test dose before initiating treatment. Abdominal pain, mouth ulceration, and skin reactions such as urticaria and pruritus may also occur. The risk of hypersensitivity reactions is reported to be greater when onchocerciasis is present.

Later adverse effects include paraesthesia, hyperaesthesia of the palms and soles, skin eruptions, fever, polyuria, increased thirst, raised liver enzyme values, and effects on the eye including photophobia and lachrymation. Proteinuria is common; haematuria and casts in the urine may also occur. There have been occasional reports of adrenal insufficiency.

Effects on the blood. Thrombocytopenia has been reported in patients receiving suramin, generally during treatment for AIDS or cancer.[1-4] An immune-mediated mechanism has been proposed[3] although there is evidence that multiple mechanisms may be involved.[4] Other adverse effects on the blood include neutropenia,[1,5] anaemia,[1] deterioration of pre-existing lymphocytopenia,[5] and one case of fatal myelosuppression.[5] Agranulocytosis and haemolytic anaemia have been mentioned in the literature as rare occurrences.

1. Levine AM, *et al.* Suramin antiviral therapy in the acquired immunodeficiency syndrome. *Ann Intern Med* 1986; **105:** 32–7.
2. Arlt W, *et al.* Suramin in adrenocortical cancer: limited efficacy and serious toxicity. *Clin Endocrinol (Oxf)* 1994; **41:** 299–307.
3. Seidman AD, *et al.* Immune-mediated thrombocytopenia secondary to suramin. *Cancer* 1993; **71:** 851–4.
4. Tisdale JF, *et al.* Severe thrombocytopenia in patients treated with suramin: evidence for an immune mechanism in one. *Am J Hematol* 1996; **51:** 152–7.
5. Rosen PJ, *et al.* Suramin in hormone-refractory metastatic prostate cancer: a drug with limited efficacy. *J Clin Oncol* 1996; **14:** 1626–36.

Effects on the eyes. Late effects on the eye associated with suramin include photophobia, lachrymation, and oedema. Keratopathy characterised by corneal deposits has been reported in patients receiving suramin. In a study of 114 patients receiving suramin for prostatic cancer 13 developed corneal deposits similar to those reported with chloroquine therapy after 34 to 98 days of therapy.[1] Symptoms in 10 of the 13 included lachrymation and foreign body sensation. The remaining 3 patients were asymptomatic. Shifts in refractive error were also found. Keratopathy has also been reported in patients with AIDS receiving suramin.[2] In patients treated with suramin for ocular onchocerciasis the incidence of optic atrophy was higher after 3 years than in untreated patients.[3] A prolonged inflammatory response to dying microfilariae in the optic nerve might be responsible although a direct toxic or allergic effect could not be ruled out.

1. Hemady RK, *et al.* Ocular symptoms and signs associated with suramin sodium treatment for metastatic cancer of the prostate. *Am J Ophthalmol* 1996; **121:** 291–6.
2. Teich SA, *et al.* Toxic keratopathy associated with suramin therapy. *N Engl J Med* 1986; **314:** 1455–6.
3. Thylefors B, Rolland A. The risk of optic atrophy following suramin treatment of ocular onchocerciasis. *Bull WHO* 1979; **57:** 479–80.

Effects on the kidneys. In addition to the proteinuria commonly seen during suramin therapy, there have been reports of individual cases of renal glycosuria[1] and of acute renal dysfunction.[2]

1. Awadzi K, *et al.* The chemotherapy of onchocerciasis XVIII: aspects of treatment with suramin. *Trop Med Parasitol* 1995; **46:** 19–26.
2. Figg WD, *et al.* Acute renal toxicity associated with suramin in the treatment of prostate cancer. *Cancer* 1994; **74:** 1612–14.

Effects on the nervous system. Neurological disorders reported in patients receiving suramin include paraesthesia and polyneuropathy. Severe polyneuropathy with generalised flaccid paralysis has generally been associated with serum-suramin concentrations greater than 350 µg per mL,[1,2] but motor neuropathy was reported in 8 patients with serum concentrations of 275 µg per mL.[3]

1. La Rocca RV, *et al.* Suramin-induced polyneuropathy. *Neurology* 1990; **40:** 954–60.
2. Arlt W, *et al.* Suramin in adrenocortical cancer: limited efficacy and serious toxicity. *Clin Endocrinol (Oxf)* 1994; **41:** 299–307.
3. Bitton RJ, *et al.* Pharmacologic variables associated with the development of neurologic toxicity in patients treated with suramin. *J Clin Oncol* 1995; **13:** 2223–9.

Effects on the skin. Pruritus and urticaria may occur as hypersensitivity reactions to suramin. Late skin reactions include erythematous maculopapular rashes[1] and severe reactions including erythema multiforme,[2] exfoliative dermatitis, and fatal toxic epidermal necrolysis[3,4] have been reported.

1. O'Donnell BP, *et al.* Suramin-induced skin reactions. *Arch Dermatol* 1992; **128:** 75–9.
2. Katz SK, *et al.* Erythema multiforme induced by suramin. *J Am Acad Dermatol* 1995; **32:** 292–3.
3. May E, Allolio B. Fatal toxic epidermal necrolysis during suramin therapy. *Eur J Cancer* 1991; **27:** 1338.
4. Falkson G, Rapoport BL. Lethal toxic epidermal necrolysis during suramin treatment. *Eur J Cancer* 1992; **28A:** 1294.

Precautions

Suramin should be administered under close medical supervision, and the general condition of patients improved as far as possible before treatment starts. Patients who experience a severe reaction after the first dose should never receive suramin again. It should not be used in elderly or infirm patients or in the presence of severe hepatic or renal disease. The urine should be tested before treatment starts and at weekly intervals during treatment; dosage should be reduced if moderate proteinuria develops and discontinued if it becomes severe or if casts appear in the urine.

Pregnancy. Suramin has been reported to be teratogenic in *mice* but not in *rats*.[1] WHO[2] recommends that when necessary suramin should be used in pregnant women with *T. b. rhodesiense* trypanosomiasis, even those with meningoencephalitic disease, because melarsoprol is contra-indicated; in onchocerciasis, suramin treatment should be delayed until after delivery.

1. Mercier-Parot L, Tuchmann-Duplessis H. Action abortive et tératogène d'un trypanocide, la suramine. *C R Soc Biol* 1973; **167:** 1518–22.
2. WHO. *WHO model prescribing information: drugs used in parasitic diseases.* 2nd ed. Geneva: WHO, 1995.

Pharmacokinetics

Following intravenous injection, suramin becomes bound to plasma proteins and a low concentration in plasma is maintained for months. Unbound suramin is excreted in the urine. Penetration of suramin into the cerebrospinal fluid appears to be poor.

The clinical pharmacokinetics of suramin were studied in 4 patients with AIDS given 6.2 g intravenously over 5 weeks.[1] Suramin accumulated during treatment and plasma concentrations exceeded 100 µg per mL for several weeks. After the last dose the terminal half-life of suramin ranged from 44 to 54 days. At least 99.7% was bound to plasma proteins. Renal clearance accounted for most of the elimination of suramin from the body. There appeared to be little or no metabolism of suramin.

1. Collins JM, *et al.* Clinical pharmacokinetics of suramin in patients with HTLV-III/LAV infection. *J Clin Pharmacol* 1986; **26:** 22–6.

Uses and Administration

Suramin is a trypanocide used in the treatment of African trypanosomiasis. It has also been used as an anthelmintic in the treatment of onchocerciasis.

Suramin is administered by slow intravenous injection, usually as a 10% solution. Because of the danger of severe reactions it is advisable to give a test dose before initiating treatment or to pause during injection of the first dose.

In African trypanosomiasis suramin is used mainly for the early (haematolymphatic) stages of *Trypanosoma brucei rhodesiense* infection; pentamidine may be preferred for early-stage treatment of *T. b. gambiense* infection. Suramin is not used as sole therapy for late-stage infections with CNS involvement since its penetration into the cerebrospinal fluid is not considered to be adequate. Early-stage trypanosomiasis may be treated with a dose of 5 mg per kg body-weight of suramin on day 1, 10 mg per kg on day 3, then 20 mg per kg on days 5, 11, 17, 23, and 30. Other schedules consist of 5 doses of 1 g given over 3 weeks following a test dose of 100 to 200 mg. In late-stage *T. b. rhodesiense* infection 2 or 3 injections of suramin (5, 10, and 20 mg per kg respectively) are often given before starting treatment with melarsoprol. Combined therapy with suramin and tryparsamide has been used in late-stage *T. b. gambiense* infection; suggested doses are suramin 10 mg per kg plus tryparsamide 30 mg per kg both given once every 5 days for 12 injections, repeated after one month if necessary.

Malignant neoplasms. Suramin is reported to have antineoplastic activity and has been studied in a number of malignant neoplasms, in particular hormone-resistant prostatic cancer. Hower, its clinical usefulness is hindered by dose-limiting toxicity and problems in developing a simple administration schedule.

References.

1. Stein CA, *et al.* Suramin: an anticancer drug with a unique mechanism of action. *J Clin Oncol* 1989; **7:** 499–508.
2. Kilbourn RG. Suramin: new therapeutic concepts for an old drug. *Cancer Bull* 1991; **43:** 265–7.
3. Rapoport BL, *et al.* Suramin in combination with mitomycin C in hormone-resistant prostate cancer: a phase II clinical study. *Ann Oncol* 1993; **4:** 567–73.
4. Woll PJ, *et al.* Suramin for breast and prostate cancer: a pilot study of intermittent short infusions without adaptive controls. *Ann Oncol* 1994; **5:** 597–600.
5. Arlt W, *et al.* Suramin in adrenocortical cancer: limited efficacy and serious toxicity. *Clin Endocrinol (Oxf)* 1994; **41:** 299–307.
6. Eisenberger MA, Reyno LM. Suramin. *Cancer Treat Rev* 1994; **20:** 259–73.
7. Rosen PJ, *et al.* Suramin in hormone-refractory metastatic prostate cancer: a drug with limited efficacy. *J Clin Oncol* 1996; **14:** 1626–36.

Onchocerciasis. Although suramin is the only drug in clinical use for onchocerciasis (p.95) which is effective against adult worms, its use is restricted because of the frequency of associated complications and its intrinsic toxicity. Treatment of onchocerciasis is currently based on continuous suppression of microfilariae by regular administration of ivermectin. WHO[1] advise that suramin should only be considered for the curative treatment of individuals in areas without transmission of onchocerciasis and of individuals leaving an endemic area and for severe hyperreactive onchodermatitis where symptoms are not adequately controlled with ivermectin. WHO[2] also recommends that it should not be used to treat onchocerciasis in the elderly or infirm, in patients with severe liver or renal disease, in children aged less than 10 years, in totally blind patients (unless they require relief from intensely itchy lesions), in light to moderately infected people with no symptoms and whose eyes are not at risk, or in pregnant women (who should be treated after delivery).

A total dose of 66.7 mg per kg body-weight in six incremental weekly doses has been recommended.[1,2]

1. WHO. Onchocerciasis and its control: report of a WHO expert committee. *WHO Tech Rep Ser 852* 1995.
2. WHO. *WHO model prescribing information: drugs used in parasitic diseases.* 2nd ed. Geneva: WHO, 1995.

African trypanosomiasis. Suramin is used in the treatment of the early haematolymphatic phase of African trypanosomiasis (p.577) caused by *Trypanosoma brucei rhodesiense* and for *T. b. gambiense* infections which are resistant to pentamidine.[1] In some regions suramin is used in combination with pentamidine for *T. b. gambiense* infections but it has not been shown to be clinically superior to pentamidine alone.[2] Although suramin does not produce sufficient concentrations in the CNS to produce a cure in the meningoencephalitic phase,[3] it is used to reduce the number of trypanosomes in the blood and lymph before treatment with melarsoprol.[1] A combination of suramin with tryparsamide has been suggested as an alternative to melarsoprol or eflornithine in *T. b. gambiense* infections involving the CNS.[4] Case reports have suggested that suramin in combination with metronidazole[5] or eflornithine[6] could be useful in *T. b. rhodesiense* infections.

1. WHO. *WHO model prescribing information: drugs used in parasitic diseases.* 2nd ed. Geneva: WHO, 1995.
2. Pépin J, Khonde N. Relapses following treatment of early-stage Trypanosoma brucei gambiense sleeping sickness with a combination of pentamidine and suramin. *Trans R Soc Trop Med Hyg* 1996; **90:** 183–6.
3. Jennings FW. Suramin treatment of experimental Trypanosoma brucei infection of the central nervous system. *Trans R Soc Trop Med Hyg* 1995; **89:** 677.
4. Anonymous. Drugs for parasitic infections. *Med Lett Drugs Ther* 1998; **40:** 1–12.
5. Foulkes JR. Metronidazole and suramin combination in the treatment of arsenical refractory rhodesian sleeping sickness—a case study. *Trans R Soc Trop Med Hyg* 1996; **90:** 422.
6. Taelman H, *et al.* Combination treatment with suramin and eflornithine in late stage rhodesian trypanosomiasis: case report. *Trans R Soc Trop Med Hyg* 1996; **90:** 572–3.

Preparations

Proprietary Preparations (details are given in Part 3)
Ger.: Germanin.

Teclozan (4798-p)

Teclozan (*USAN, pINN*).

NSC-107433; Win-13146. *NN′-p*-Phenylenedimethylenebis[2,2-dichloro-*N*-(2-ethoxyethyl)acetamide].

$C_{20}H_{28}Cl_4N_2O_4$ = 502.3.

CAS — 5560-78-1.

Teclozan, a dichloroacetamide derivative, is a luminal amoebicide with actions and uses similar to those of diloxanide furoate (see p.581). It has been given by mouth in the treatment of intestinal amoebiasis in one of the following dosage schedules, all supplying a total dose of 1.5 g: 500 mg every 12 hours for 3 doses; or 500 mg daily in divided doses for 3 days; or 100 mg three times daily for 5 days.

Tenonitrozole (13318-q)

Tenonitrozole *(rINN)*.

TC-109; Thenitrazole. *N*-(5-Nitrothiazol-2-yl)thiophene-2-carboxamide.

$C_8H_5N_3O_3S_2$ = 255.3.

CAS — 3810-35-3.

Tenonitrozole is an antiprotozoal given in the treatment of trichomoniasis (p.577). It is also active against *Candida albicans*. It is given by mouth in a dose of 250 mg twice daily with meals, for 4 days.

Preparations

Proprietary Preparations (details are given in Part 3)
Fr.: Atrican; ***Ital.:*** Atrican†.

Ternidazole (13573-f)

Ternidazole *(rINN)*.

2-Methyl-5-nitroimidazole-1-propanol.

$C_7H_{11}N_3O_3$ = 185.2.

CAS — 1077-93-6.

Ternidazole is a 5-nitroimidazole similar to metronidazole (p.585) and is used locally in the treatment of vaginal trichomoniasis.

Preparations

Proprietary Preparations (details are given in Part 3)
Multi-ingredient: ***Fr.:*** Tergynan.

Tilbroquinol (17008-h)

Tilbroquinol *(pINN)*.

7-Bromo-5-methylquinolin-8-ol.

$C_{10}H_8BrNO$ = 238.1.

CAS — 7175-09-9.

Tilbroquinol is a halogenated hydroxyquinoline antiprotozoal with properties similar to those of di-iodohydroxyquinoline (p.581). It has been used together with tiliquinol (see below) in the treatment of intestinal infections including amoebiasis but less toxic drugs are preferred.

A report of neurotoxicity, considered to be subacute myelo-opticoneuropathy, in a patient who had taken tilbroquinol together with tiliquinol for 4 years.[1] Hepatotoxicity has also been reported[2] with this combination.

1. Soffer M, *et al.* Oxyquinoline toxicity. *Lancet* 1983; **i:** 709.
2. Caroli-Bosc F-X, *et al.* Hépatite aiguë due à l'association de tiliquinol et tilbroquinol (Intétrix). *Gastroenterol Clin Biol* 1996; **20:** 605–6.

Preparations

Proprietary Preparations (details are given in Part 3)
Fr.: Intetrix P.
Multi-ingredient: ***Belg.:*** Intetrix; ***Fr.:*** Intetrix.

Tiliquinol (17009-m)

Tiliquinol *(rINN)*.

5-Methylquinolin-8-ol.

$C_{10}H_9NO$ = 159.2.

CAS — 5541-67-3.

Tiliquinol has been used in conjunction with tilbroquinol (see above) in the treatment of intestinal infections including amoebiasis but less toxic drugs are preferred.

Preparations

Proprietary Preparations (details are given in Part 3)
Multi-ingredient: ***Belg.:*** Intetrix; ***Fr.:*** Intetrix.

Tinidazole (4799-s)

Tinidazole *(BAN, USAN, rINN)*.

CP-12574; Tinidazolum. 1-[2-(Ethylsulphonyl)ethyl]-2-methyl-5-nitroimidazole.

$C_8H_{13}N_3O_4S$ = 247.3.

CAS — 19387-91-8.

Pharmacopoeias. In *Eur.* (see p.viii), *Jpn*, and *Pol.*

An almost white or pale yellow crystalline powder. Practically **insoluble** in water; sparingly soluble in methyl alcohol; soluble in acetone and in dichloromethane. **Protect** from light.

Adverse Effects and Precautions

As for Metronidazole, p.585.

Pregnancy and breast feeding. Tinidazole readily crosses the placenta and is distributed into breast milk. The manufacturer recommends that tinidazole should not be given during the first trimester of pregnancy, since its effects on fetal development are unknown, and also that it should not be given to mothers who are breast feeding.

Shock. An acute severe toxic reaction occurred in a healthy subject shortly after the intravenous infusion of tinidazole 1.6 g over 80 minutes.[1] He fainted for about 10 seconds and low blood pressure, nausea, and tiredness persisted for several hours. Spasms in the left arm were also experienced but no generalised convulsions. The reaction was not considered to be allergic.

1. Aase S, *et al.* Severe toxic reaction to tinidazole. *Eur J Clin Pharmacol* 1983; **24:** 425–7.

Interactions

Tinidazole may, like metronidazole, produce a disulfiram-like reaction with alcohol (see Metronidazole, p.586).

Pharmacokinetics

The pharmacokinetics of tinidazole resemble those of metronidazole although the half-life is longer.

Tinidazole is almost completely absorbed following administration by mouth and, typically, a peak plasma concentration of about 40 μg per mL is achieved 2 hours after a single 2-g dose, falling to about 10 μg per mL at 24 hours and 2.5 μg per mL at 48 hours; concentrations above 8 μg per mL are maintained by daily maintenance doses of 1 g. Comparable concentrations are achieved with equivalent intravenous doses. The plasma elimination half-life of tinidazole is 12 to 14 hours.

Tinidazole is widely distributed and concentrations similar to those in plasma have been achieved in bile, breast milk, cerebrospinal fluid, saliva, and a variety of body tissues; it crosses the placenta readily. Only 12% is reported to be bound to plasma proteins. An active hydroxy metabolite has been identified.

Unchanged drug and metabolites are excreted in the urine and, to a lesser extent, in the faeces.

References.

1. Wood BA, *et al.* The pharmacokinetics, metabolism and tissue distribution of tinidazole. *J Antimicrob Chemother* 1982; **10** (suppl A): 43–57.
2. Karhunen M. Placental transfer of metronidazole and tinidazole in early human pregnancy after a single infusion. *Br J Clin Pharmacol* 1984; **18:** 254–7.
3. Evaldson GR, *et al.* Tinidazole milk excretion and pharmacokinetics in lactating women. *Br J Clin Pharmacol* 1985; **19:** 503–7.
4. Wood SG, *et al.* Pharmacokinetics and metabolism of ^{14}C-tinidazole in humans. *J Antimicrob Chemother* 1986; **17:** 801–9.

Renal impairment. Single-dose studies indicate that the pharmacokinetics of tinidazole in patients with chronic renal failure are not significantly different from those in healthy subjects and that no modification of tinidazole dosage is necessary. However, tinidazole is rapidly removed by haemodialysis.[1,2]

1. Flouvat BL, *et al.* Pharmacokinetics of tinidazole in chronic renal failure and in patients on haemodialysis. *Br J Clin Pharmacol* 1983; **15:** 735–41.
2. Robson RA, *et al.* Tinidazole pharmacokinetics in severe renal failure. *Clin Pharmacokinet* 1984; **9:** 88–94.

Uses and Administration

Tinidazole is a 5-nitroimidazole derivative. It has the antimicrobial actions of metronidazole and is used similarly (see p.587) in the treatment of susceptible protozoal infections, in the treatment and prophylaxis of anaerobic bacterial infections, and in the eradication of *Helicobacter pylori* in peptic ulcer disease.

Tinidazole is usually administered as a single daily dose by mouth with or after food; it is also given by intravenous infusion and as vaginal pessaries.

In invasive amoebiasis, tinidazole is administered, usually in conjunction with a luminal amoebicide such as diloxanide furoate or di-iodohydroxyquinoline, in a dose of 2 g daily by mouth for 2 or 3 days; in hepatic amoebiasis 1.5 to 2 g daily may be given for 3 days or occasionally up to 6 days. Children are given 50 to 60 mg per kg body-weight daily for 3 or 5 days respectively.

A single dose of tinidazole 2 g is given by mouth in the treatment of giardiasis, trichomoniasis, and acute necrotising ulcerative gingivitis; 50 to 75 mg per kg as a single dose is suggested for children with giardiasis or trichomoniasis. It may sometimes be necessary to repeat this dose once. In trichomoniasis sexual partners should be treated concomitantly. In bacterial vaginosis a single 2-g dose is usually given, although higher cure rates have been achieved with a 2-g dose on 2 successive days.

For the treatment of most anaerobic bacterial infections tinidazole is given by mouth, usually for 5 or 6 days, in an initial dose of 2 g followed on subsequent days by 1 g daily or 500 mg twice daily. If oral therapy is not possible tinidazole may be administered intravenously, 800 mg being infused as 400 mL of a 2 mg per mL solution at a rate of 10 mL per minute; this initial dose is followed by 800 mg daily or 400 mg twice daily until oral therapy can be substituted. For the prevention of postoperative anaerobic bacterial infections 2 g is given by mouth about 12 hours before surgery. Alternatively 1.6 g is given as a single intravenous infusion before surgery or in two divided doses, one just before surgery and the other during surgery or no later than 12 hours postoperatively.

In regimens for the treatment of peptic ulcer disease, tinidazole 500 mg twice daily in combination with clarithromycin and omeprazole for 7 days has been suggested.

Administration in renal impairment. The elimination of tinidazole is largely unchanged in patients with impaired renal function (see under Pharmacokinetics, above) and dosage adjustment is therefore not generally considered necessary. However tinidazole is removed by haemodialysis, and patients may need additional doses to compensate.

Preparations

Proprietary Preparations (details are given in Part 3)
Aust.: Fasigyn; ***Austral.:*** Fasigyn; Simplotan; ***Belg.:*** Fasigyn; ***Fr.:*** Fasigyne; ***Ger.:*** Simplotan; Sorquetan; ***Ital.:*** Fasigin; Trimonase; ***Neth.:*** Fasigyn; ***Norw.:*** Fasigyn†; ***S.Afr.:*** Fasigyn; ***Spain:*** Tricolam; ***Swed.:*** Fasigyn; ***Switz.:*** Fasigyne; ***UK:*** Fasigyn.
Multi-ingredient: ***Ital.:*** Fasigin N.

Toltrazuril (18693-n)

Toltrazuril *(BAN, USAN, rINN)*.

Bay-Vi-9142. 1-Methyl-3-(4-{*p*-[(trifluoromethyl)thio]phenoxy}-*m*-tolyl)-s-triazine-2,4,6(1*H*,3*H*,5*H*)-trione.

$C_{18}H_{14}F_3N_3O_4S$ = 425.4.

CAS — 69004-03-1.

Toltrazuril is an antiprotozoal used in veterinary practice for the treatment of coccidiosis in poultry.

Tryparsamide (6000-c)

Tryparsamide *(rINN)*.

Glyphenarsine; Tryparsam.; Tryparsone. Sodium hydrogen 4-(carbamoylmethylamino)phenylarsonate hemihydrate.

$C_8H_{10}AsN_2NaO_4,\frac{1}{2}H_2O$ = 305.1.

CAS — 554-72-3 (anhydrous tryparsamide); 6159-29-1 (tryparsamide hemihydrate).

Tryparsamide, a pentavalent arsenical compound, is a trypanocide which penetrates into the cerebrospinal fluid and has been used in combination with suramin in the treatment of late-stage African trypanosomiasis due to *Trypanosoma brucei gambiense* as an alternative to melarsoprol or eflornithine (see p.577). However, because of its toxicity, especially the risk of blindness resulting from damage to the optic nerve, melarsoprol or eflornithine are preferred.

For the adverse effects of arsenic and their treatment, see Arsenic Trioxide, p.1550. Like melarsoprol, tryparsamide can cause encephalopathy.

Tryparsamide is administered in a dose of 30 mg per kg body-weight (to a maximum of 2 g), together with suramin 10 mg per kg, both given intravenously once every 5 days for 12 injections. Treatment may be repeated after one month.

Antivirals

The drugs described in this chapter are used in the treatment of viral infections or for providing protection, usually for a brief period only, against infection. Treatment has to be started early in the infection for the antiviral to be effective and inhibit the replicating virus. There is little evidence that these compounds affect latent or nonreplicating viruses. They do not provide an alternative to available immunisation for the long-term prophylaxis of infection—for details of such treatment see the chapter on Vaccines, p.1500.

Choice of Antiviral

Antiviral drugs are effective for the treatment and prophylaxis of a range of viral infections as described below. Nonspecific symptomatic and supportive treatments are also important in the management of viral infections. Those viral infections not amenable to antiviral therapy include mumps, poliomyelitis, rabies, and rubella.

Common cold

A cold is usually a mild, self-limiting respiratory infection with a range of viruses, the rhinoviruses and coronaviruses being most frequently involved. Symptoms include nasal discharge and obstruction, sneezing, sore throat, and cough; there is little or no fever. Occasionally there may be concurrent or subsequent bacterial infection of the upper respiratory tract.

The variety of causative agents makes vaccination an unlikely prospect. Not only are there different groups of viruses, but within the rhinoviruses, for example, there are many different serotypes.

Treatment of the common cold is symptomatic with analgesics, cough suppressants, and decongestants, and symptoms usually last for about a week whether or not treatment is taken. Antimicrobial therapy has consistently failed to show any benefit.[1] Antibiotics are indicated only if there is secondary bacterial infection.[2,3] Treatment with very large doses of ascorbic acid has been widely used. Such treatment has been claimed to be beneficial in preventing and treating colds and a review[4] of published findings considered that it might reduce their severity but not their incidence. Other drugs tried have included mast cell stabilisers, interferon alfa-2b, and zinc lozenges.[5] Intranasal interferons, tried for prophylaxis or treatment, have not fulfilled their early promise. Results of trials of zinc treatment have been inconsistent.

1. Rosenstein N, *et al.* The common cold—principles of judicious use of antimicrobial agents. *Pediatrics* 1998; **101** (suppl): 181–4.
2. Kaiser L, *et al.* Effects of antibiotic treatment in the subset of common-cold patients who have bacteria in nasopharyngeal secretions. *Lancet* 1996; **347:** 1507–10.
3. Wise R. Antibiotics for the uncommon cold. *Lancet* 1996; **347:** 1499.
4. Hemilä H. Dose vitamin C alleviate the symptoms of the common cold?–a review of current evidence. *Scand J Infect Dis* 1994; **26:** 1–6.
5. Mossad SB. Treatment of the common cold. *Br Med J* 1998; **317:** 33–6.

Encephalitis

Viral infections associated with encephalitis include Epstein-Barr virus infections, herpes simplex infections, HIV infection, influenza, lassa fever, measles, mumps, rubella, and varicella-zoster infections; the specific treatment of these infections, if any, is described in the appropriate section of this chapter. However, there is also a group of viruses known as encephalitis viruses that cause infections in which encephalitis is a major clinical feature.

They include the alphaviruses (arbovirus group A) Eastern, Western, and Venezualan equine viruses transmitted by mosquitoes; the flaviviruses (arbovirus group B) Japanese encephalitis virus, St Louis encephalitis virus, Murray Valley encephalitis virus, Rocio virus, and West Nile virus all transmitted by mosquitoes and the tick-borne viruses of this group, Louping ill virus, Powassan virus, and the Eastern and Western subtype viruses; and the bunyaviruses California encephalitis virus and La Crosse virus both transmitted by mosquitoes.

Encephalitis virus infections usually present with fever, headache, nausea, vomiting, and neck rigidity. Some infections progress to produce convulsions, confusion, coma, and sometimes death. Patients who recover may be left with some permanent neurological damage. There is generally no specific treatment for encephalitis virus infections and patients must be managed with vigorous supportive care. Control of mosquito and tick populations in endemic areas and minimising contact with these vectors are important means of preventing infections. Japanese encephalitis vaccine (p.1510) and tick-borne encephalitis vaccine (p.1510) are available for active immunisation of individuals at risk of infection and tick-borne encephalitis immunoglobulins (p.1510) are available in some countries for passive immunisation against infection.

Gastro-enteritis

Viral infections are an important cause of diarrhoea, especially in children and immunocompromised patients. Those causing diarrhoea and other gastro-intestinal symptoms include adenovirus, astrovirus, calicivirus, rotavirus, Norwalk virus, and related small round structured virus infections. Cytomegalovirus is an important cause of diarrhoea in AIDS (see HIV-associated Wasting and Diarrhoea, below). Rotavirus infection is recognised as the commonest cause of endemic acute diarrhoea in childhood, and is associated with severe vomiting and fever. In acute diarrhoea of any aetiology the priority is to maintain hydration by prevention or treatment of fluid and electrolyte depletion, especially in infants and the elderly (see p.1168). Antivirals are not used in the management of viral diarrhoeas. Several rotavirus vaccines are under development.

References.

1. Elliott EJ. Viral diarrhoeas in childhood. *Br Med J* 1992; **305:** 1111–12.
2. Kapikian AZ. Viral gastroenteritis. *JAMA* 1993; **269:** 627–30.

Haemorrhagic fevers

Viruses causing haemorrhagic fever form a diverse group from several viral families. They are usually transmitted via mosquitoes, ticks, or rodents.

The more important viruses responsible for haemorrhagic fevers in man include the Alphaviridae (Arbovirus Group A) causing Chikungunya, transmitted by mosquitoes; Arenaviridae causing Argentinian haemorrhagic fever, Bolivian haemorrhagic fever, and Lassa fever and transmitted by rodents; Bunyaviridae causing Crimean Congo haemorrhagic fever, haemorrhagic fever with renal syndrome, and Rift Valley fever and transmitted by ticks, rodents and insectivores, and mosquitoes respectively; Ebola and Marburg viruses of the Filoviridae; and Flaviviridae (Arbovirus Group B) causing dengue fever and yellow fever transmitted by mosquitoes, and Kyasanur forest fever and Omsk haemorrhagic fever transmitted by ticks.

As suggested by the name, fever and haemorrhage of varying severity are characteristics of these infections. Chills, headache, malaise, myalgia, and nausea usually occur and sometimes flushing and rashes. Severe vomiting, diarrhoea, and shock may occur in advanced infections. There is often some degree of renal or hepatic impairment and occasionally CNS involvement.

While tribavirin has been reported to reduce mortality in patients with Lassa fever, haemorrhagic fever with renal syndrome, and possibly Crimean Congo haemorrhagic fever, there is generally no specific antiviral treatment for haemorrhagic fever and patients must be managed symptomatically. Control of vector populations and prevention of vector contact have an important role to play (see p.1402). Guidelines for the prevention and control of dengue and yellow fevers have been produced by WHO[1-3] and related organisations.[4] National guidelines exist in some countries.[5]

Rift Valley fever vaccine and yellow fever vaccine are available for active immunisation of individuals at risk of infection; dengue fever vaccines and haemorrhagic fever with renal syndrome vaccines are under development. Crimean Congo haemorrhagic fever immunoglobulins are available in some countries for passive immunisation against the disease.

1. WHO. *Prevention and control of yellow fever in Africa.* Geneva: WHO, 1986.
2. WHO. *Monograph on dengue/dengue haemorrhagic fever.* New Delhi: WHO, 1993.
3. WHO. *Dengue haemorrhagic fever: diagnosis, treatment, prevention and control.* 2nd ed. Geneva: WHO, 1997.
4. Pan American Health Organization. *Dengue and dengue hemorrhagic fever in the Americas: Guidelines for prevention and control.* Washington, D.C.: PAHO, 1994.
5. Advisory Committee on Dangerous Pathogens. *Management and control of viral haemorrhagic fevers.* London: HMSO, 1996.

Hantavirus pulmonary syndrome

A number of hantaviruses related to the virus causing haemorrhagic fever with renal syndrome (see above) have been identified as the probable cause of an acute, severe respiratory illness which has been named hantavirus pulmonary syndrome. Its main symptoms are fever, myalgia, headache, and cough rapidly progressing to respiratory failure; the mortality rate may be about 50% and death is usually due to non-cardiogenic pulmonary oedema and acute respiratory distress syndrome. The virus is transmitted by rodents and the syndrome has mainly been described in the United States.

Treatment is primarily symptomatic including respiratory and circulatory support with the early use of cardiac inotropic drugs being particularly important. Intravenous tribavirin has been tried but preliminary data have not indicated an improvement in mortality.

References.

1. Bremner JAG. Hantavirus infections and outbreaks in 1993. *Commun Dis Rep* 1994; **4** (review 1): R5–R9.
2. Duchin JS, *et al.* Hantavirus pulmonary syndrome: a clinical description of 17 patients with a newly recognized disease. *N Engl J Med* 1994; **330:** 949–55.
3. Anonymous. Hantavirus pulmonary syndrome—northeastern United States, 1994. *JAMA* 1994; **272:** 997–8.
4. Prochoda K, *et al.* Hantavirus-associated acute respiratory failure. *N Engl J Med* 1993; **329:** 1744.
5. Khan AS, *et al.* Hantavirus pulmonary syndrome. *Lancet* 1996; **347:** 739–41.

Hepatitis

Viral hepatitis refers to infection of the liver caused by a group of hepatitis viruses. Those so far identified are designated A, B, C, D, E, and G. Other viruses such as Epstein-Barr virus and yellow fever virus may be secondary causes of hepatitis and hepatitis may also be caused by nonviral infections, many drugs and chemicals, and alcoholism.

Hepatitis viruses are endemic throughout the world. Hepatitis A and E are spread via the faecal-oral route. Hepatitis B, C, and D are transmitted in blood and blood products and by sexual contact. Hepatitis B may also be transmitted by contact with infectious body fluids. Hepatitis C probably accounts for most cases of blood-transmitted hepatitis. Hepatitis D only occurs in the presence of hepatitis B since it requires multiplication of the hepatitis B virus for its own replication.

Acute viral hepatitis results in inflammation of the liver and hepatocellular necrosis but clinical presentation varies widely from subclinical asymptomatic illness to fulminant hepatic failure. Initial symptoms may include malaise, weakness, anorexia, nausea, vomiting, fever, and abdominal pain, followed after 3 to 10 days by jaundice. In some cases the condition may progress to fulminant hepatitis with hepatic encephalopathy, coma, and death. Recovery in patients who survive usually takes a few months but some patients will have residual liver damage. Also some patients infected with the B, C, or D virus may develop chronic hepatitis which may lead to hepatocellular carcinoma or cirrhosis.

Active immunisation in individuals at risk of infection is possible for hepatitis A and B with specific vaccines or passive immunisation can be achieved using immunoglobulins.

The management of uncomplicated acute viral hepatitis is largely symptomatic although it has been suggested that an interferon might prevent the progression of acute hepatitis C to the chronic stage,[1,2] and improvements in liver function were reported in 4 patients with fulminant hepatitis A treated with interferon beta.[3]

Chronic viral hepatitis is usually treated with interferon alfa.[4,5] Prolonged therapy is necessary, and long-term remission of disease is achieved in less than half of patients treated. Relapse is common and, in patients with hepatitis C especially, may be expected in half of responding patients on cessation of treatment.[4,6,7] Response rates may be determined by the level of viraemia and the genotype.[8] In view of these rather disappointing results and the as yet unproven effect on mortality, a number of other antiviral and immunomodulating drugs are under investigation. In hepatitis B, responses to interferon alfa can be improved by pretreatment with prednisone.[9,10] Thymosin,[11] granulocyte colony-stimulating factor,[12] ursodeoxycholic acid,[13-15] and iron depletion measures[16-18] have been tried as adjuncts to conventional therapy. Alprostadil has produced beneficial responses in small numbers of patients with fulminant disease,[19] and has been reported to be effective in patients with recurrent hepatitis B following liver transplantation.[20] Treatment of hepatitis B with the nucleoside reverse transcriptase inhibitor lamivudine shows promise.[21,22] Studies with fialuridine were stopped when severe toxicity emerged.[23] In hepatitis C, tribavirin has been shown to have some activity although biochemical improvements are generally not sustained once treatment is stopped.[24,25] The use of tribavirin in combination with interferon alfa[26-28] or beta[29] is reported to improve response rates.

1. Omata M, *et al.* Resolution of acute hepatitis C after therapy with natural beta interferon. *Lancet* 1991; **338:** 914–15.
2. Esteban R. Is there a role for interferon in acute viral hepatitis? *Gut* 1993; **34** (suppl): S77–S80.
3. Yoshiba M, *et al.* Interferon for hepatitis A. *Lancet* 1994; **343:** 288–9.
4. Dusheiko G. Treatment of chronic viral hepatitis: the end of the beginning? *Br J Hosp Med* 1994; **52:** 8–11.
5. Hoofnagle JH, Lau D. Chronic viral hepatitis—benefits of current therapies. *N Engl J Med* 1996; **334:** 1470–1.
6. van der Poel CL, *et al.* Hepatitis C virus six years on. *Lancet* 1994; **344:** 1475–9.
7. Dusheiko GM, *et al.* A rational approach to the management of hepatitis C infection. *Br Med J* 1996; **312:** 357–64.
8. Main J. Hepatitis C: clinical aspects. *J Infect* 1995; **30:** 103–6.
9. Perrillo RP, *et al.* A randomized, controlled trial of interferon alfa-2b alone and after prednisone withdrawal for the treatment of chronic hepatitis B. *N Engl J Med* 1990; **323:** 295–301.
10. Fevery J, *et al.* Efficacy of interferon alfa-2b with or without prednisone withdrawal in the treatment of chronic viral hepatitis B: a prospective double-blind Belgian-Dutch study. *J Hepatol* 1990; **11:** S108–S112.
11. Sherman KE, *et al.* Hepatitis C RNA response to combined therapy with thymosin alpha-1 and interferon. *Hepatology* 1994; **20:** 207A.
12. Pardo M, *et al.* Treatment of chronic hepatitis C with cirrhosis with recombinant human granulocyte colony-stimulating factor plus recombinant interferon-alpha. *J Med Virol* 1995; **45:** 439–44.
13. Rolandi E, *et al.* Effects of ursodeoxycholic acid (UDCA) on serum liver damage indices in patients with chronic active hepatitis: a double-blind controlled study. *Eur J Clin Pharmacol* 1991; **40:** 473–6.
14. Puoti C, *et al.* Ursodeoxycholic acid and chronic hepatitis C infection. *Lancet* 1993; **341:** 1413–14.
15. Angelico M, *et al.* Recombinant interferon-α and ursodeoxycholic acid versus interferon-α alone in the treatment of chronic hepatitis C: a randomized clinical trial with long-term follow-up. *Am J Gastroenterol* 1995; **90:** 263–9.
16. Clemente MG, *et al.* Effect of iron overload on the response to recombinant interferon-alfa treatment in transfusion-dependent patients with thalassemia major and chronic hepatitis C. *J Pediatr* 1994; **125:** 123–8.
17. James DG. Treatment options for chronic hepatitis C infection. *J Antimicrob Chemother* 1995; **36:** 591–3.
18. Hayashi H, *et al.* Improvement of serum aminotransferase levels after phlebotomy in patients with chronic active hepatitis C and excess hepatic iron. *Am J Gastroenterol* 1994; **89:** 986–8.
19. Sinclair SB, *et al.* Biochemical and clinical response of fulminant viral hepatitis to administration of prostaglandin E: a preliminary report. *J Clin Invest* 1989; **84:** 1063–9.
20. Flowers M, *et al.* Prostaglandin E in the treatment of recurrent hepatitis B infection after orthotopic liver transplantation. *Transplantation* 1994; **58:** 183–92.
21. Benhamou Y, *et al.* Efficacy of lamivudine on replication of hepatitis B virus in HIV-infected patients. *Lancet* 1995; **345:** 396–7.
22. Dienstag JL, *et al.* A preliminary trial of lamivudine for chronic hepatitis B infection. *N Engl J Med* 1995; **333:** 1657–61.
23. McKenzie R, *et al.* Hepatic failure and lactic acidosis due to fialuridine (FIAU), an investigational nucleoside analogue for chronic hepatitis B. *N Engl J Med* 1995; **333:** 1099–1105.
24. Reichard O, *et al.* Ribavirin treatment for chronic hepatitis C. *Lancet* 1991; **337:** 1058–61.
25. Di Bisceglie AM, *et al.* A pilot study of ribavirin therapy for chronic hepatitis C. *Hepatology* 1992; **16:** 649–54.
26. Chemello L, *et al.* Response to ribavirin, to interferon and to a combination of both in patients with chronic hepatitis C and its relation to HCV genotypes. *J Hepatol* 1994; **21** (suppl): S12.
27. Braconier JH, *et al.* Combined alpha-interferon and ribavirin treatment in chronic hepatitis C: a pilot study. *Scand J Infect Dis* 1995; **27:** 325–9.
28. Reichard O, *et al.* Randomised, double-blind, placebo-controlled trial of interferon α-2b with and without ribavirin for chronic hepatitis C. *Lancet* 1998; **351:** 83–7.
29. Kakumu S, *et al.* A pilot study of ribavirin and interferon beta for the treatment of chronic hepatitis C. *Gastroenterology* 1993; **105:** 507–12.

Herpesvirus infections

Established herpesvirus pathogens discussed below include cytomegalovirus, Epstein-Barr virus, herpesvirus simiae, herpes simplex virus, and varicella-zoster virus. Herpesviruses 6, 7, and 8 have also emerged as potential pathogens and have been associated with a variety of disorders including childhood febrile illnesses, various malignancies including Kaposi's sarcoma, and multiple sclerosis.

Cytomegalovirus infections. Cytomegaloviruses are members of the herpesvirus group, and are widely distributed in many animal species. Infection may occur through intra-uterine or perinatal transmission, by oral contact with the saliva of infected individuals, or by sexual transmission. Transmission by blood transfusion or by transplantation of infected tissue can also occur. After infection, viral DNA becomes incorporated into the host cells and persists for the life of the individual with occasional reactivation when infectious virions appear in the saliva and urine.

Most congenitally infected infants are asymptomatic, but some infants may present with intra-uterine growth retardation, jaundice, hepatosplenomegaly, encephalitis, and thrombocytopenia. Acquired infections generally do not cause clinical symptoms though they may occasionally present as infectious mononucleosis, lymphocytosis, or lymphadenopathy. The virus is a common cause of infection in the immunocompromised, particularly transplant recipients and patients with AIDS when it commonly presents as cytomegalovirus retinitis or enteritis, and is a major cause of morbidity and mortality in these patients.

Specific **treatment** for cytomegalovirus infection is usually only given to immunocompromised patients, in whom the infection is often complicated by extensive tissue damage leading to target organ failure and secondary opportunistic infections. Relapses are likely to occur after treatment is stopped due to the latent nature of cytomegaloviruses. *Ganciclovir* is used in the treatment of severe cytomegalovirus infections in transplant recipients and patients with AIDS.[1-4] However, ganciclovir may cause neutropenia and many AIDS patients receiving zidovudine cannot tolerate the combined haematological toxicity of these two drugs, hence the administration of granulocyte-macrophage colony-stimulating factor to treat or prevent ganciclovir-induced neutropenia.[5,6] Although less experience has been gained with *foscarnet* it appears to be an alternative to ganciclovir of similar efficacy.[7,8] It does not produce myelosuppression, but nephrotoxicity and electrolyte disturbances are common. The two drugs given in combination may be more effective than monotherapy with either.[9] Other approaches to treatment have involved administration of ganciclovir in combination with cytomegalovirus immunoglobulin,[10,11] or normal immunoglobulin.[12]

Cytomegalovirus retinitis is usually treated intravenously with ganciclovir or foscarnet, this route having the additional advantage that extra-retinal and bilateral infections are also reduced. In AIDS patients, the initial induction treatment is followed by lifelong maintenance therapy, since ganciclovir and foscarnet both suppress rather than eliminate the virus.[13] Oral ganciclovir is reported to be an effective and more convenient alternative to intravenous maintenance.[14,15] Despite maintenance treatment, recurrence is considered to be almost inevitable but it usually responds to an increase in dosage.[13,16] Foscarnet therapy has been associated with improved survival in AIDS patients[7,17] although it is often tolerated less well than ganciclovir[7] and the need for long term intravenous administration poses practical problems with both drugs. *Cidofovir* is another alternative for the treatment of cytomegalovirus retinitis,[18,19] and has the advantage of intermittent administration. For patients unable to tolerate systemic therapy, intravitreal administration of ganciclovir or foscarnet may be beneficial,[20-23] although frequent administration is associated with adverse effects which include retinal detachment, intravitreal haemorrhage, and endophthalmitis. Use of a sustained release intra-ocular formulation may limit such toxicity,[24-26] though not the risk of increased bilateral and extra-ocular infection.[16] Cidofovir has also been given by intravitreal injection with promising results.[27-29]

Guidelines for the treatment of cytomegalovirus infections have been produced by the International AIDS Society in the USA.[30]

US guidelines[31] for the **prevention** of opportunistic infections, including cytomegalovirus infection, in HIV-infected patients emphasise the importance of prophylactic ophthalmic screening for early recognition of cytomegalovirus retinitis.

Primary prophylaxis of cytomegalovirus infection in high risk patients, particularly transplant recipients, has been reported using intravenous *ganciclovir*,[32-34] *foscarnet*,[35] and *cytomegalovirus immunoglobulin*.[36] Conflicting results have been reported from studies of the efficacy of oral ganciclovir for primary prophylaxis in patients with HIV infection,[37,38] although it is recommended in the US guidelines.[31] *Aciclovir* with[39] or without[40,41] cytomegalovirus immunoglobulin has been successful in preventing infection in some transplant patients, but failure of prophylaxis has been reported,[42-44] and comparison of aciclovir with ganciclovir for prophylaxis in liver-transplant recipients has found ganciclovir to be the more effective drug.[45] The US guidelines consider aciclovir to be an ineffective prophylactic in patients with HIV infection.[31] The efficacy of prophylaxis also varies with the organ transplanted.[46] Cytomegalovirus vaccines are currently in development.

1. Collaborative DHPG Treatment Study Group. Treatment of serious cytomegalovirus infections with 9-(1,3-dihydroxy-2-propoxymethyl)guanine in patients with AIDS and other immunodeficiencies. *N Engl J Med* 1986; **314:** 801–5.
2. Harris ML, Mathalone MBR. Dihydroxypropoxymethyl guanine in the treatment of AIDS related retinitis due to cytomegalovirus. *Br Med J* 1987; **294:** 92.
3. Rostoker G, *et al.* Ganciclovir for severe cytomegalovirus infection in transplant recipients. *Lancet* 1988; **ii:** 1137–8.
4. Dieterich DT, *et al.* Ganciclovir treatment of cytomegalovirus colitis in AIDS: a randomized, double-blind, placebo-controlled multicenter study. *J Infect Dis* 1993; **167:** 278–82.
5. Fouillard L, *et al.* GM-CSF and ganciclovir for cytomegalovirus infection after autologous bone-marrow transplantation. *Lancet* 1989; **ii:** 1273.
6. Grossberg HS, *et al.* GM-CSF with ganciclovir for the treatment of CMV retinitis. *N Engl J Med* 1989; **320:** 1560.
7. Studies of Ocular Complications of AIDS Research Group, in Collaboration with the AIDS Clinical Trials Group. Mortality in patients with the acquired immunodeficiency syndrome treated with either foscarnet or ganciclovir for cytomegalovirus retinitis. *N Engl J Med* 1992; **326:** 213–20.
8. Blanshard C, *et al.* Treatment of AIDS-associated gastrointestinal cytomegalovirus infection with foscarnet and ganciclovir: a randomized comparison. *J Infect Dis* 1995; **172:** 622–8.
9. Studies of Ocular Complications of AIDS Research Group, in Collaboration with the AIDS Clinical Trials Group. Combination foscarnet and ganciclovir therapy vs monotherapy for the treatment of relapsed cytomegalovirus retinitis in patients with AIDS: the Cytomegalovirus Retreatment Trial. *Arch Ophthalmol* 1996; **114:** 23–33.
10. D'Alessandro AM, *et al.* Successful treatment of severe cytomegalovirus infections with ganciclovir and CMV hyperimmune globulin in liver transplant recipients. *Transplant Proc* 1989; **21:** 3560–1.
11. Salmela K, *et al.* Ganciclovir in the treatment of severe cytomegalovirus disease in liver transplant patients. *Transplant Proc* 1990; **22:** 238–40.
12. Emanuel D, *et al.* Cytomegalovirus pneumonia after bone marrow transplantation successfully treated with the combination of ganciclovir and high-dose intravenous immune globulin. *Ann Intern Med* 1988; **109:** 777–82.
13. Dhillon B. The management of cytomegalovirus retinitis in AIDS. *Br J Ophthalmol* 1994; **78:** 66–9.

14. Oral Ganciclovir European and Australian Cooperative Study Group. Intravenous versus oral ganciclovir: European/Australian comparative study of efficacy and safety in the prevention of cytomegalovirus retinitis recurrence in patients with AIDS. *AIDS* 1995; **9:** 471–7.
15. Drew WL, *et al.* Oral ganciclovir as maintenance treatment for cytomegalovirus retinitis in patients with AIDS. *N Engl J Med* 1995; **333:** 615–20.
16. Jabs DA. Treatment of cytomegalovirus retinitis—1992. *Arch Ophthalmol* 1992; **110:** 185–7.
17. Polis MA, *et al.* Increased survival of a cohort of patients with acquired immunodeficiency syndrome and cytomegalovirus retinitis who received sodium phosphonoformate (foscarnet). *Am J Med* 1993; **94:** 175–80.
18. Lalezari JP, *et al.* Intravenous cidofovir for peripheral cytomegalovirus retinitis in patients with AIDS: a randomized, controlled trial. *Ann Intern Med* 1997; **126:** 257–63.
19. Studies of Ocular Complications of AIDS Research Group, in collaboration with the AIDS Clinical Trials Group. Parenteral cidofovir for cytomegalovirus retinitis in patients with AIDS: the HPMPC peripheral cytomegalovirus retinitis trial: a randomized, controlled trial. *Ann Intern Med* 1997; **126:** 264–74.
20. Heinemann M-H. Long-term intravitreal ganciclovir therapy for cytomegalovirus retinopathy. *Arch Ophthalmol* 1989; **107:** 1767–72.
21. Cochereau-Massin I, *et al.* Efficacy and tolerance of intravitreal ganciclovir in cytomegalovirus retinitis in acquired immune deficiency syndrome. *Ophthalmology* 1991; **98:** 1348–55.
22. Lieberman RM, *et al.* Efficacy of intravitreal foscarnet in a patient with AIDS. *N Engl J Med* 1994; **330:** 868–9.
23. Diaz-Llopis M, *et al.* High dose intravitreal foscarnet in the treatment of cytomegalovirus retinitis in AIDS. *Br J Ophthalmol* 1994; **78:** 120–4.
24. Anand R, *et al.* Control of cytomegalovirus retinitis using sustained release of intraocular gancyclovir. *Arch Ophthalmol* 1993; **111:** 223–7.
25. Akula SK, *et al.* Treatment of cytomegalovirus retinitis with intravitreal injection of liposome encapsulated ganciclovir in a patient with AIDS. *Br J Ophthalmol* 1994; **78:** 677–80.
26. Martin DF, *et al.* Treatment of cytomegalovirus retinitis with an intraocular sustained-release ganciclovir implant: a randomized controlled clinical trial. *Arch Ophthalmol* 1994; **112:** 1531–9.
27. Kirsch LS, *et al.* Phase I/II study of intravitreal cidofovir for the treatment of cytomegalovirus retinitis in patients with the acquired immunodeficiency syndrome. *Am J Ophthalmol* 1995; **119:** 466–76.
28. Kirsch LS, *et al.* Intravitreal cidofovir (HPMPC) treatment of cytomegalovirus retinitis in patients with acquired immune deficiency syndrome. *Ophthalmology* 1995; **102:** 533–43.
29. Rahhal FM, *et al.* Treatment of cytomegalovirus retinitis with intravitreous cidofovir in patients with AIDS: a preliminary report. *Ann Intern Med* 1996; **125:** 98–103.
30. Whitley RJ, *et al.* Guidelines for the treatment of cytomegalovirus diseases in patients with AIDS in the era of potent antiretroviral therapy: recommendation of an international panel. *Arch Intern Med* 1998; **158:** 957–69.
31. Centers for Disease Control. 1997 USPHS/IDSA guidelines for the prevention of opportunistic infections in persons infected with human immunodeficiency virus. *MMWR* 1997; **46** (RR-12): 22–4.
32. Goodrich JM, *et al.* Ganciclovir prophylaxis to prevent cytomegalovirus disease after allogeneic marrow transplant. *Ann Intern Med* 1993; **118:** 173–8.
33. Winston DJ, *et al.* Ganciclovir prophylaxis of cytomegalovirus infection and disease in allogeneic bone marrow transplant recipients. *Ann Intern Med* 1993; **118:** 179–84.
34. Hibberd PL, *et al.* Preemptive ganciclovir therapy to prevent cytomegalovirus disease in cytomegalovirus antibody-positive renal transplant recipients: a randomized controlled trial. *Ann Intern Med* 1995; **123:** 18–26.
35. Reusser P, *et al.* Phase I-II trial of foscarnet for prevention of cytomegalovirus infection in autologous and allogeneic marrow transplant recipients. *J Infect Dis* 1992; **166:** 473–9.
36. Wittes JT, *et al.* Meta-analysis of CMVIG studies for the prevention and treatment of CMV infection in transplant patients. *Transplant Proc* 1996; **28** (suppl 2): 17–24.
37. Spector SA, *et al.* Oral ganciclovir for the prevention of cytomegalovirus disease in persons with AIDS. *N Engl J Med* 1996; **334:** 1491–7.
38. McCarthy M. Oral ganciclovir fails to prevent CMV in HIV trial. *Lancet* 1995; **346:** 895.
39. Eisenmann D, *et al.* Prevention of cytomegalovirus disease in heart transplant recipients by prophylaxis with cytomegalovirus hyperimmune globulin plus oral acyclovir. *Transplant Proc* 1990; **22:** 2322–3.
40. Balfour HH, *et al.* A randomized, placebo-controlled trial of oral acyclovir for the prevention of cytomegalovirus disease in recipients of renal allografts. *N Engl J Med* 1989; **320:** 1381–7.
41. Prentice HG, *et al.* Impact of long-term acyclovir on cytomegalovirus infection and survival after allogeneic bone marrow transplantation. *Lancet* 1994; **343:** 749–53.
42. Bailey TC, *et al.* Failure of high-dose oral acyclovir with or without immune globulin to prevent primary cytomegalovirus disease in recipients of solid organ transplants. *Am J Med* 1993; **95:** 273–8.
43. Singh N, *et al.* High-dose acyclovir compared with short-course pre-emptive ganciclovir therapy to prevent cytomegalovirus disease in liver transplant recipients: a randomized trial. *Ann Intern Med* 1994; **120:** 375–81.
44. Boeckh M, *et al.* Failure of high-dose acyclovir to prevent cytomegalovirus disease after autologous marrow transplantation. *J Infect Dis* 1995; **172:** 939–43.
45. Winston DJ, *et al.* Randomised comparison of ganciclovir and high-dose acyclovir for long-term cytomegalovirus prophylaxis in liver-transplant recipients. *Lancet* 1995; **346:** 69–74.
46. Griffiths PD. Prophylaxis against CMV infection in transplant patients. *J Antimicrob Chemother* 1997; **39:** 299–301.

Epstein-Barr virus infections. Epstein-Barr virus (EBV) is a DNA virus of the herpesvirus group. It is ubiquitous with a worldwide distribution. Following primary exposure the individual becomes a lifelong carrier of EBV but associated disease only occurs if the normal immune mechanisms are compromised and the virus can be reactivated. EBV is the causative agent in infectious mononucleosis and is associated with several diseases including Burkitt's lymphoma, nasopharyngeal carcinoma, chronic interstitial pneumonitis in infants with AIDS, and oral hairy leukoplakia in AIDS patients. It may also be associated with Hodgkin's disease and with amyloidosis.

Infectious mononucleosis (glandular fever) is an acute, self-limiting, lymphoproliferative infection occurring mainly in adolescents and young adults, transmission usually being via close oral contact. Symptoms may last for several weeks and include sore throat, swelling of the neck, fever, sweating, chills, and anorexia. Lymphadenopathy and splenomegaly usually occur and some patients may experience hepatomegaly and jaundice. Most patients recover uneventfully with only supportive treatment although they may continue to be easily exhausted for some time. Complications may occur in a few patients and can be fatal. They include meningitis, encephalitis, seizures, hepatic necrosis, splenic rupture, haemolytic and aplastic anaemia, agranulocytosis, and thrombocytopenia. Very rarely the illness may become chronic with symptoms persisting for years and may result in death from lymphomatous disease.

There is no specific treatment for EBV infections. Aciclovir,[1-3] ganciclovir,[4] and interferons[3,5,6] are some of the drugs that have been reported to produce some clinical or immunological improvement in patients with EBV infections but this is usually reversible on stopping treatment. Corticosteroids may be useful in severe, prolonged, or complicated infections, although concern has been expressed that they might impair immunity and increase the risk of EBV-related tumours in later years.[7] Concurrent throat infection with streptococci should not be treated with amoxycillin or ampicillin since they may cause a maculopapular rash in patients with infectious mononucleosis.

1. Andersson J, *et al.* Effect of acyclovir on infectious mononucleosis: a double-blind, placebo-controlled study. *J Infect Dis* 1986; **153:** 283–90.
2. Yao QY, *et al.* The Epstein-Barr virus: host balance in acute infectious mononucleosis patients receiving acyclovir anti-viral therapy. *Int J Cancer* 1989; **43:** 61–6.
3. Drago F, *et al.* Epstein-Barr virus-related primary cutaneous amyloidosis: successful treatment with acyclovir and interferon-alpha. *Br J Dermatol* 1996; **134:** 170–4.
4. Ishida Y, *et al.* Ganciclovir for chronic active Epstein-Barr virus infection. *Lancet* 1993; **341:** 560–1.
5. Cheeseman SH, *et al.* Epstein-Barr virus infection in renal transplant recipients: effects of antithymocyte globulin and interferon. *Ann Intern Med* 1980; **93:** 39–42.
6. Fujisaki T, *et al.* Gamma-interferon for severe chronic active Epstein-Barr virus. *Ann Intern Med* 1993; **118:** 474–5.
7. Sheagren JN. Corticosteroids for treatment of mononucleosis and aphthous stomatitis. *JAMA* 1986; **256:** 1051.

Herpes simplex infections. Herpes simplex virus (HSV, herpesvirus hominis) which is distributed worldwide is most often classified into serotypes HSV-1 and HSV-2. Transmission is by direct contact with infected secretions, with HSV-1 being associated primarily with oral transmission and HSV-2 primarily with genital transmission. Symptomatic disease normally affects the skin or mucous membranes, when HSV replicates in the epithelium with subsequent lysis of infected cells and local inflammation to produce characteristic painful lesions. Viraemia occurs rarely, except in immunocompromised individuals in whom disseminated disease can develop.

HSV becomes latent within sensory nerve ganglia from where it can be reactivated by various triggers such as stress, bacterial infection, fever, irradiation (including sunlight), or menstruation. Reactivation leads to a prodromal period before the lesions emerge.

Primary infections are usually in the perioral, ocular, or genital areas, but any skin site may be involved if the skin is damaged, or in immunocompromised patients. Anorectal lesions including herpes proctitis are especially prevalent in homosexual men with AIDS. Most primary HSV-1 infections are asymptomatic but may occasionally present as acute gingivostomatitis and pharyngitis. Infections commonly recur as *herpes labialis*, also known as fever blisters or cold sores. *Ocular herpes* is also generally caused by HSV-1, and infections range in severity from superficial conjunctivitis or dendritic keratitis, to sight-threatening diseases of the inner eye such as iridocyclitis or herpetic disciform keratitis. *Genital herpes* is usually caused by HSV-2 and tends to be a more severe condition than other herpes simplex infections, especially in women. *Herpes encephalitis* and *neonatal herpes* are rare but occasionally fatal complications of herpes simplex infections.

MANAGEMENT. The most widely used antiviral for herpes simplex infections is aciclovir.[1] In clinical practice, treatment of primary herpes simplex infections, while relieving symptoms and reducing the duration of viral shedding, does not prevent recurrences. Antiviral therapy is generally more effective for primary infections than for recurrences, and should be given as early as possible during the course of an active infection, preferably within 3 days of the onset of symptoms. Aciclovir may be administered topically, orally, or intravenously depending on the severity and nature of the infection; topical treatment is generally less effective than systemic therapy and is of little value if systemic symptoms predominate. Resistance to aciclovir is emerging, mainly in immunocompromised patients.[2]

- **Herpes labialis** is a self-limiting disorder which rarely requires antiviral therapy. If it is used then such treatment should be started early in the prodromal phase. Topical preparations of antiviral drugs, including aciclovir, penciclovir, and tromantadine, are used for herpes labialis but there is conflicting evidence of their efficacy.[3-5] Oral aciclovir may suppress frequently recurrent herpes labialis,[6,7] and protect those at high risk of recurrence.[8] However, for the majority of patients careful hygiene and, if necessary, symptomatic treatment with analgesics and the use of antiseptics such as povidone-iodine to reduce secondary infection will suffice; sunscreen agents may reduce the frequency of recurrences.
- **Ocular herpes simplex infections** usually require treatment with a suitable antiviral. Aciclovir is commonly applied as an ointment. Trifluridine and vidarabine are alternatives. Ganciclovir gel might be as effective as aciclovir.[9] Carbocyclic oxetanocin G has also been shown to be effective in healing herpes simplex corneal ulceration.[10] The use of topical corticosteroids alone is contra-indicated for most forms of ocular herpes as they can increase disease severity, but a combination of a corticosteroid with an antiviral, such as prednisolone with aciclovir[11] or trifluridine[12] may be useful. Long-term treatment with oral aciclovir has been found to reduce the rate of recurrence of ocular herpes simplex disease.[13] Patients with intra-ocular infections require systemic treatment, usually with aciclovir. However, the addition of oral aciclovir to topical therapy with trifluridine and a corticosteroid was reported to be of no benefit in patients with stromal keratitis.[14]
- **Genital herpes** is usually treated with systemic aciclovir; alternatives are famciclovir and valaciclovir.[15] Topical aciclovir has been used but it is less effective. As with other herpes simplex infections, therapy of the initial infection appears to have no effect on subsequent recurrences. In patients experiencing a recognisable prodrome, a 5-day course of oral aciclovir initiated by the patient may abort the recurrence or reduce its severity.[16] In patients who do not experience a prodrome or those with frequent recurrences, continuous suppressive therapy with aciclovir should be considered;[17,18] there is less experience with famciclovir or valaciclovir.[15] There is a risk of *neonatal herpes* in the infants of mothers with genital herpes infection. Prophylactic administration of aciclovir to the mother during late pregnancy is not recommended.[15] Infants with evidence of neonatal infection should be treated with systemic aciclovir or vidarabine.[15,19]
- **Severe or disseminated herpes simplex infections**, particularly those occurring in immunocompromised patients, usually require intravenous therapy. Aciclovir is used most commonly, with foscarnet or cidofovir as alternatives for infections resistant to aciclovir.[20] Vidarabine has also been tried, but has been reported to be less effective and more toxic than foscarnet.[21] Topical trifluridine may also be of benefit for aciclovir-resistant mucocutaneous herpes simplex in patients with AIDS.[22] Immunocompromised patients with frequent or disabling recurrences may benefit from prophylactic oral aciclovir administration.[23]

Antivirals with improved bioavailability or pharmacokinetic profiles which allow less frequent dosing are being assessed for use in herpes simplex infections, as are antivirals which are effective against aciclovir-resistant strains. These include valaciclovir, cidofovir, and imiquimod.[24] Herpes simplex vaccines have also been tried but with generally disappointing results. A number of spermicides and disinfectants have shown activity against HSV *in vitro*,[25] and some such as nonoxinol-9 have been tried topically[26] for herpes simplex infections.

1. Anonymous. Drugs for non-HIV viral infections. *Med Lett Drugs Ther* 1994; **36:** 27–32.
2. Christophers J, *et al.* Survey of resistance of herpes simplex virus to aciclovir in Northwest England. *Antimicrob Agents Chemother* 1998; **42:** 868–72.
3. Anonymous. Treatment of herpes simplex labialis. *Lancet* 1990; **335:** 1501–2.
4. Ostheimer KE, *et al.* Randomized double-blind trial of tromantadine versus aciclovir in recurrent herpes orofacialis. *Arzneimittelforschung* 1989; **39:** 1152–5.
5. Diezel W, *et al.* Efficacy of tromantadine and aciclovir in the topical treatment of recurrent herpes orofacialis: comparison in a clinical trial. *Arzneimittelforschung* 1993; **43:** 491–6.
6. Rooney JF, *et al.* Oral acyclovir to suppress frequently recurrent herpes labialis: a double-blind, placebo-controlled trial. *Ann Intern Med* 1993; **118:** 268–72.
7. Worrall G. Acyclovir in recurrent herpes labialis. *Br Med J* 1996; **312:** 6.
8. Spruance SL, *et al.* Acyclovir prevents reactivation of herpes simplex labialis in skiers. *JAMA* 1988; **260:** 1597–9.
9. Hoh HB, *et al.* Randomised trial of ganciclovir and acyclovir in the treatment of herpes simplex dendritic keratitis: a multicentre study. *Br J Ophthalmol* 1996; **80:** 140–3.
10. Shiota H, *et al.* Clinical evaluation of carbocyclic oxetanocin G eyedrops in the treatment of herpes simplex corneal ulcers. *Br J Ophthalmol* 1996; **80:** 413–15.
11. Collum LMT, *et al.* Acyclovir (Zovirax) in herpetic disciform keratitis. *Br J Ophthalmol* 1983; **67:** 115–18.
12. Wilhelmus KR, *et al.* Herpetic eye disease study: a controlled trial of topical corticosteroids for herpes simplex stromal keratitis. *Ophthalmology* 1994; **101:** 1883–96.
13. Herpetic Eye Disease Study Group. Acyclovir for the prevention of recurrent herpes simplex virus eye disease. *N Engl J Med* 1998; **339:** 300–6.
14. Barron BA, *et al.* Herpetic eye disease study: a controlled trial of oral acyclovir for herpes simplex stromal keratitis. *Ophthalmology* 1994; **101:** 1871–82.
15. Centers for Disease Control. 1998 Guidelines for treatment of sexually transmitted diseases. *MMWR* 1998; **47:** 20–6.
16. Whatley JD, Thin RN. Episodic acyclovir therapy to abort recurrent attacks of genital herpes simplex infection. *J Antimicrob Chemother* 1991; **27:** 677–81.
17. Kaplowitz LG, *et al.* Prolonged continuous acyclovir treatment of normal adults with frequently recurring genital herpes simplex virus infection. *JAMA* 1991; **265:** 747–51.
18. Goldberg LH, *et al.* Long-term suppression of recurrent genital herpes with acyclovir: a 5-year benchmark. *Arch Dermatol* 1993; **129:** 582–7.
19. Whitley R, *et al.* A controlled trial comparing vidarabine with acyclovir in neonatal herpes simplex virus infection. *N Engl J Med* 1991; **324:** 444–9.
20. Centers for Disease Control. 1997 USPHS/IDSA guidelines for the prevention of opportunistic infections in persons infected with human immunodeficiency virus. *MMWR* 1997; **46** (RR-12): 24.
21. Safrin S, *et al.* A controlled trial comparing foscarnet with vidarabine for acyclovir-resistant mucocutaneous herpes simplex in the acquired immunodeficiency syndrome. *N Engl J Med* 1991; **325:** 551–5.
22. Kessler HA, *et al.* Pilot study of topical trifluridine for the treatment of acyclovir-resistant mucocutaneous herpes simplex disease in patients with AIDS (ACTG 172). *J Acquir Immune Defic Syndr Hum Retrovirol* 1996; **12:** 147–52.
23. Peters BS, *et al.* Adverse effects of drugs used in the management of opportunistic infections associated with HIV infection. *Drug Safety* 1994; **10:** 439–54.
24. Cassady KA, Whitley RJ. New therapeutic approaches to the alphaherpesvirus infections. *J Antimicrob Chemother* 1997; **39:** 119–28.
25. Jennings R, Clegg A. The inhibitory effect of spermicidal agents on replication of HSV-2 and HIV-1 in-vitro. *J Antimicrob Chemother* 1993; **32:** 71–82.
26. Friedman-Kien AE, *et al.* Treatment of recurrent genital herpes with topical alpha interferon gel combined with nonoxynol 9. *J Am Acad Dermatol* 1986; **15:** 989–94.

Herpesvirus simiae infections. *Herpesvirus simiae* (Monkey B virus, herpes B virus) is a herpesvirus that usually infects macaque monkeys, but may rarely be transmitted to man by laboratory accidents or bites or scratches from infected monkeys.

Initially there may be vesicles at the site of the bite or scratch. As the infection progresses there is increasing neurological involvement which can lead to encephalitis, coma, and death.

Aciclovir has been recommended for the prophylaxis and treatment of this infection when it should be started immediately an infection is suspected, usually intravenously for symptomatic infections or orally for those that are asymptomatic.[1] When treatment with intravenous aciclovir followed by intravenous ganciclovir was delayed in two patients until neurological symptoms had developed it was not successful.[2] Intravenous ganciclovir for one month followed by oral aciclovir has also been tried in one patient who recovered from his meningitis.[3]

1. Wansbrough-Jones MH, *et al.* Prophylaxis against B virus infection. *Br Med J* 1988; **297:** 909.
2. Holmes GP, *et al.* B virus (Herpesvirus simiae) infection in humans: epidemiologic investigation of a cluster. *Ann Intern Med* 1990; **112:** 833–9.
3. Scinicariello F, *et al.* Identification by PCR of meningitis caused by herpes B virus. *Lancet* 1993; **341:** 1660–1.

Varicella-zoster infections. Varicella-zoster virus (VZV) is a herpesvirus which causes chickenpox (varicella) and herpes zoster (zoster, shingles). The virus is easily transmitted, particularly by close contact with infected individuals. Primary infection usually results in *chickenpox*, which presents with a characteristic generalised vesicular eruption, fever, and malaise. Chickenpox is commonly a benign disease of childhood of short duration. It can occur in adults when it can be severe, and is potentially fatal in immunocompromised patients: complications include secondary bacterial skin infections, pneumonia, and neurological disorders such as encephalitis and cerebral ataxia. Reye's syndrome, which is principally associated with viral infections in childhood (see p.17), may also be a cause of encephalopathy in patients with chickenpox. Infection during early pregnancy may result rarely in fetal varicella syndrome while infection during late pregnancy may cause neonatal varicella after delivery.

Patients who recover from primary infections with varicella-zoster have lifelong immunity against chickenpox. However, a permanent latent infection of sensory nerve ganglia is established, and reactivation produces herpes zoster.

Herpes zoster is characterised by painful vesicular eruptions localised to a single dermatome of skin, and sometimes preceded by a prodromal phase with fever, malaise, and headache. Involvement of the trigeminal nerve can lead to sight-threatening ophthalmic herpes zoster. As with chickenpox, herpes zoster is more serious in immunocompromised patients and may be severe, prolonged, or disseminated. Chronic pain which persists after the rash has healed is termed postherpetic neuralgia (see p.10) and occurs in about 10% of patients who have had herpes zoster.

MANAGEMENT. Management of **chickenpox** in otherwise healthy patients is usually symptomatic using antipyretics, analgesics, and antipruritics. Antibacterials may be required for secondary infections. The value of antivirals in the treatment of chickenpox in such patients has been questioned,[1] and their use is not recommended for the treatment of uncomplicated chickenpox in otherwise healthy children.[2] However, oral aciclovir has been reported to reduce the duration and severity of symptoms when administered within 24 hours of onset of symptoms,[3-5] but not the incidence of chickenpox-associated complications.[3] It may be useful in immunocompromised patients or those who have developed complications. Intravenous therapy may be necessary in severe chickenpox.

Transmission of chickenpox to household contacts is not prevented by administration of aciclovir to the primary case[3] but there is evidence to suggest that transmission can be suppressed by administering aciclovir to susceptible contacts during the incubation period.[6,7] However, the need for such prophylactic antiviral therapy has been questioned especially in otherwise healthy children.[8]

Varicella-zoster immunoglobulins have been suggested for the prevention of chickenpox, generally in patients at high risk of developing complications such as the immunocompromised,[9] transplant recipients,[10] and in susceptible pregnant women exposed to chickenpox.[11] There have been reports of severe chickenpox occurring in patients undergoing corticosteroid therapy and some recommend administration of varicella-zoster immunoglobulin to persons exposed to the virus who have received therapeutic doses of corticosteroids within the previous 3 months;[12] others, however, have expressed concern regarding the practicality of this approach[13] and also the corticosteroid dose at which it would become necessary[14] (see also under Precautions for Corticosteroids, p.1014). Varicella-zoster vaccines[15] are available but their role in prophylaxis is not yet established.[1]

The place of antivirals in the treatment of **herpes zoster** is well established and guidelines on management have been produced.[16] Antiviral treatment can reduce the severity and duration of acute pain, minimise complications and propagation of the rash, and reduce viral shedding.[16,17] Aciclovir may be given orally or intravenously, depending upon the severity of the infection. Oral famciclovir or valaciclovir are alternatives; valaciclovir has been shown to compare favourably with aciclovir in bringing earlier resolution of pain,[18] and famciclovir has also been found to decrease pain duration.[19] Treatment should be initiated within 72 hours of the onset of the rash and is usually continued for 7 to 10 days. Amantadine has also been used in the acute phase. Nothing appears to be gained from extending the treatment period or from adding systemic corticosteroids[20] which are best avoided anyway in patients with acute infection since they can increase the risk of viral dissemination.[17] Immunocompromised patients or others at high risk of severe or disseminated varicella-zoster infections should receive intravenous aciclovir. Combined therapy with aciclovir and vidarabine may be considered in the severely immunocompromised.[17] Foscarnet may be of value in aciclovir-resistant varicella-zoster infections[21,22] although treatment failures have been reported.[23] Sorivudine has been reported to produce benefit in immunocompromised patients with recurrent cutaneously disseminated varicella-zoster infection refractory to aciclovir and to foscarnet,[24] and may be more effective than aciclovir.[25] Brivudine has displayed comparable efficacy to that of aciclovir.[26]

Ophthalmic herpes zoster may be treated with topical aciclovir, although concurrent treatment with systemic aciclovir may be needed for optimum results.[17,27] However, a study in 20 patients with AIDS suggested that ganciclovir given either alone or in combination with foscarnet was more effective than aciclovir in terms of preserving long-term visual acuity.[28] Topical corticosteroids are usually avoided during the acute phase of the infection, but may be needed if there is a substantial inflammatory component.

There has been controversy over the use of oral aciclovir to prevent postherpetic neuralgia and ocular complications. McGill and White[29] have advocated the practice, but others have questioned the evidence for its effectiveness.[30] A further view was that, despite the conflicting data, the balance of evidence favoured its use.[31]

1. Anonymous. Controversy about chickenpox. *Lancet* 1992; **340:** 639–40.
2. Committee on Infectious Diseases. The use of oral acyclovir in otherwise healthy children with varicella. *Pediatrics.* 1993; **91:** 674–6. Correction. *ibid.*: 858.
3. Balfour HH, *et al.* Acyclovir treatment of varicella in otherwise healthy children. *J Pediatr* 1990: **116:** 633–9.
4. Feder HM. Treatment of adult chickenpox with oral acyclovir. *Arch Intern Med* 1990; **150:** 2061–5.
5. Balfour HH, *et al.* Acyclovir treatment of varicella in otherwise healthy adolescents. *J Pediatr* 1992; **120:** 627–33.
6. Asano Y, *et al.* Postexposure prophylaxis of varicella in family contact by oral acyclovir. *Pediatrics* 1993; **92:** 219–22.
7. Suga S, *et al.* Effect of oral acyclovir against primary and secondary viraemia in incubation period of varicella. *Arch Dis Child* 1993; **69:** 639–42.
8. Conway SP. Effect of oral acyclovir against primary and secondary viraemia in incubation period of varicella: commentary. *Arch Dis Child* 1993; **69:** 642–3.
9. Drwal-Klein LA, O'Donovan CA. Varicella in pediatric patients. *Ann Pharmacother* 1993; **27:** 938–49.
10. Lynfield R, *et al.* Varicella in pediatric renal transplant recipients. *Pediatrics* 1992; **90:** 216–20.
11. Gilbert GL. Chickenpox during pregnancy. *Br Med J* 1993; **306:** 1079–80.
12. Rice P, *et al.* Near fatal chickenpox during prednisolone treatment. *Br Med J* 1994; **309:** 1069–70.
13. Buss P. Severe chickenpox during treatment with corticosteroids. *Br Med J* 1995; **310:** 327.
14. Burnett I. Severe chickenpox during treatment with corticosteroids. *Br Med J* 1995; **310:** 327.
15. Isaacs D, Menser M. Modern vaccines: measles, mumps, rubella, and varicella. *Lancet* 1990; **335:** 1384–7.
16. BSSI Working Group. Guidelines for the management of shingles: report of a working group of the British Society for the study of infection (BSSI). *J Infect* 1995; **30:** 193–200.
17. Nikkels AF, Piérard GE. Recognition and treatment of shingles. *Drugs* 1994; **48:** 528–48.
18. Beutner KR, *et al.* Valaciclovir compared with acyclovir for improved therapy for herpes zoster in immunocompetent adults. *Antimicrob Agents Chemother* 1995; **39:** 1546–53.
19. Tyring S, *et al.* Famciclovir for the treatment of acute herpes zoster: effects on acute disease and postherpetic neuralgia: a randomized, double-blind, placebo-controlled trial. *Ann Intern Med* 1995; **123:** 89–96.
20. Wood MJ, *et al.* A randomized trial of acyclovir for 7 days or 21 days with and without prednisolone for treatment of acute herpes zoster. *N Engl J Med* 1994; **330:** 896–900.
21. Safrin S, *et al.* Foscarnet therapy in five patients with AIDS and acyclovir-resistant varicella-zoster virus infection. *Ann Intern Med* 1991; **115:** 19–21.
22. Smith KJ, *et al.* Acyclovir-resistant varicella zoster responsive to foscarnet. *Arch Dermatol* 1991; **127:** 1069–71.
23. Bendel AE, *et al.* Failure of foscarnet in disseminated herpes zoster. *Lancet* 1993; **341:** 1342.
24. Burdge DR, *et al.* Sorivudine (BV-ara-U) for the treatment of complicated refractory varicella zoster virus infection in HIV-infected patients. *AIDS* 1995; **9:** 810–12.
25. Gnann JW, *et al.* Sorivudine versus acyclovir for treatment of dermatomal herpes zoster in human immunodeficiency virus-infected patients: results from a randomized, controlled clinical trial. *Antimicrob Agents Chemother* 1998; **42:** 1139–45.

Incompatibility. For references to the incompatibility of aciclovir and foscarnet, see Foscarnet Sodium, p.610.

Stability. References.

1. Zhang Y, *et al.* Stability of acyclovir sodium 1, 7, and 10 mg/mL in 5% dextrose injection and 0.9% sodium chloride injection. *Am J Health-Syst Pharm* 1998; **55:** 574–7.

Adverse Effects

Aciclovir is generally well tolerated. When administered intravenously as aciclovir sodium it may cause local reactions at the injection site with inflammation and phlebitis; these reactions may be associated with extravasation that leads rarely to ulceration. Renal impairment may occur in a few patients; it is usually reversible and is reported to respond to hydration and/or dosage reduction or withdrawal, but may progress to acute renal failure. The risk of renal toxicity is increased by conditions favouring deposition of aciclovir crystals in the tubules such as when the patient is poorly hydrated, has existing renal impairment, or when the drug is given at a high dosage or by rapid or bolus injection. Some patients receiving systemic aciclovir may experience transient increases in blood concentrations of urea and creatinine though this is more acute with intravenous administration.

Occasional adverse effects following systemic administration include increased serum bilirubin and liver enzymes, haematological changes, skin rashes, fever, headache, dizziness, and gastro-intestinal effects such as nausea, vomiting, and diarrhoea. Neurological effects including lethargy, somnolence, confusion, hallucinations, agitation, tremors, psychosis, convulsions, and coma have been reported in a small number of patients, particularly in those receiving intravenous aciclovir and with predisposing factors such as renal dysfunction. Accelerated diffuse hair loss has also been reported.

Topical application of aciclovir, especially to genital lesions, may sometimes produce transient stinging, burning, itching, or erythema. Eye ointments may occasionally produce transient stinging, superficial punctate keratopathy, blepharitis, or conjunctivitis.

References.

1. Bean B, *et al.* Acyclovir therapy for acute herpes zoster. *Lancet* 1982; **ii:** 118–21.
2. Arndt KA. Adverse reactions to acyclovir: topical, oral, and intravenous. *J Am Acad Dermatol* 1988; **18:** 188–90.
3. Robbins MS, *et al.* Acyclovir pH—possible cause of extravasation tissue injury. *Ann Pharmacother* 1993; **27:** 238.

Effects on the blood. There has been no evidence of bone-marrow toxicity in patients given aciclovir following bone-marrow transplantation.[1,2] However, megaloblastic haemopoiesis has been observed in the bone marrow of 3 patients given aciclovir for suspected or proven herpes simplex encephalitis.[3] There has also been a report of inhibition of human peripheral blood lymphocytes in samples taken from healthy subjects given aciclovir.[4]

1. Serota FT, *et al.* Acyclovir treatment of herpes zoster infections: use in children undergoing bone marrow transplantation. *JAMA* 1982; **247:** 2132–5.
2. Gluckman E, *et al.* Oral acyclovir prophylactic treatment of herpes simplex infection after bone marrow transplantation. *J Antimicrob Chemother* 1983; **12** (suppl B): 161–7.
3. Amos RJ, Amess JAL. Megaloblastic haemopoiesis due to acyclovir. *Lancet* 1983; **i:** 242–3.
4. Tauris P, *et al.* Evaluation of the acyclovir-induced modulation of the plaque-forming cell response of human peripheral blood lymphocytes. *J Antimicrob Chemother* 1984; **13:** 71–7.

Effects on the kidneys. Transient renal impairment occurred in 2 adequately hydrated patients following aciclovir 10 mg per kg body-weight infused over 1 hour every 8 hours.[1] In another patient[2] severe acute renal failure occurred following administration of aciclovir 5 mg per kg over 90 minutes daily for 2 days. This reaction did not appear to be related to dosage or manner of administration, but may have been idiosyncratic or immunological.[2] Acute renal failure (with no evidence of crystals) and coma developed in two elderly patients receiving high dose oral therapy (800 mg five times daily) with aciclovir.[3,4]

1. Harrington MG, *et al.* Renal impairment and acyclovir. *Lancet* 1981; **ii:** 1281.
2. Giustina A, *et al.* Low-dose acyclovir and acute renal failure. *Ann Intern Med* 1988; **108:** 312.
3. Eck P, *et al.* Acute renal failure and coma after a high dose of oral acyclovir. *N Engl J Med* 1991; **325:** 1178.
4. Johnson GL, *et al.* Acute renal failure and neurotoxicity following oral acyclovir. *Ann Pharmacother* 1994; **28:** 460–3.

Effects on the nervous system. Aciclovir was given to 143 patients in doses ranging from 0.75 to 3.6 g per m² body-surface daily by intravenous infusion for the treatment of herpesvirus infections following bone-marrow transplantation.[1] Six of the 143 developed reversible neurological symptoms including tremor, agitation, nausea, lethargy, mild disorientation, autonomic instability, hemiparaesthesia, and slurred speech. EEGs were diffusely abnormal in all 6. Symptoms improved in all patients on withdrawing aciclovir; reinstituting aciclovir in 2 produced a recurrence of symptoms. Concomitant therapy included irradiation and methotrexate intrathecally for all 6, interferon alfa for 3, and cyclosporin for 1.

There are individual case reports of neurological and, less frequently, psychiatric adverse effects in patients given intravenous aciclovir.[2-8] Neurological toxicity following oral aciclovir was possibly associated with elevated plasma concentrations in patients with end-stage renal disease.[9,10] The association between plasma-aciclovir concentrations and neurotoxicity has been difficult to establish because of a delay of 24 to 48 hours in the development of symptoms following a concentration peak.[11]

1. Wade JC, Meyers JD. Neurologic symptoms associated with parenteral acyclovir treatment after marrow transplantation. *Ann Intern Med* 1983; **98:** 921–5.
2. Vartian CV, Shlaes DM. Intravenous acyclovir and neurologic effects. *Ann Intern Med* 1983; **99:** 568.
3. Auwerx J, *et al.* Acyclovir and neurologic manifestations. *Ann Intern Med* 1983; **99:** 882–3.
4. Cohen SMZ, *et al.* Severe but reversible neurotoxicity from acyclovir. *Ann Intern Med* 1984; **100:** 920.
5. Tomson CR, *et al.* Psychiatric side-effects of acyclovir in patients with chronic renal failure. *Lancet* 1985; **ii:** 385–6.
6. Bataille P, *et al.* Psychiatric side-effects with acyclovir. *Lancet* 1985; **ii:** 724.
7. Sirota P, *et al.* Major depression with psychotic features associated with acyclovir therapy. *Drug Intell Clin Pharm* 1988; **22:** 306–8.
8. Revankar SG, *et al.* Delirium associated with acyclovir treatment in a patient with renal failure. *Clin Infect Dis* 1995; **21:** 435–6.
9. Swan SK, Bennett WM. Oral acyclovir and neurotoxicity. *Ann Intern Med* 1989; **111:** 188.
10. Mataix AL, *et al.* Oral acyclovir and neurologic adverse effects in endstage renal disease. *Ann Pharmacother* 1994; **28:** 961–2.
11. Haefeli WE, *et al.* Acyclovir-induced neurotoxicity: concentration-side effect relationship in acyclovir overdose. *Am J Med* 1993; **94:** 212–15.

Effects on the skin. A report of vesicular lesions associated with intravenous administration of aciclovir in a patient thought to have herpes simplex encephalitis.[1] The authors warned that careful evaluation is necessary to differentiate the reaction from herpetic lesions.

1. Buck ML, *et al.* Vesicular eruptions following acyclovir administration. *Ann Pharmacother* 1993; **27:** 1458–9.

Vasculitis. Aciclovir has been associated with vasculitis. In one patient[1] it was one of many drugs given which may have caused a necrotising vasculitis. In another report an immunocompromised child with chickenpox given aciclovir by infusion developed a vasculitic rash which diminished on withdrawal of the drug.[2]

1. von Schulthess GK, Sauter C. Acyclovir and herpes zoster. *N Engl J Med* 1981; **305:** 1349.
2. Platt MPW, Eden OB. Vasculitis in association with chickenpox treatment in childhood acute lymphoblastic leukaemia. *Lancet* 1982; **ii:** 763–4.

Precautions

Aciclovir should be administered with caution to patients with renal impairment and doses should be adjusted according to creatinine clearance (see under Uses and Administration, below). Parenteral administration should be by slow intravenous infusion over one hour to avoid precipitation of aciclovir in the kidney; rapid or bolus injection should be avoided and adequate hydration maintained. The risk of renal impairment is increased by the concomitant use of other nephrotoxic drugs. Intravenous aciclovir should also be used with caution in patients with underlying neurological abnormalities, with significant hypoxia, or with serious hepatic or electrolyte abnormalities.

Pregnancy and breast feeding. The incidence of congenital abnormality and spontaneous fetal loss did not appear to be greater among 312 cases of prenatal exposure to aciclovir than among the general population, and this data was supported by evidence from 145 further retrospective reports.[1] The manufacturers report that aciclovir is distributed into breast milk following oral administration. A dose of 200 mg five times daily could expose a suckling infant to 300 μg per kg body-weight daily; caution is therefore recommended when treating nursing mothers.

1. Andrews EB, *et al.* Acyclovir in Pregnancy Registry: six years' experience. *Obstet Gynecol* 1992; **79:** 7–13.

Interactions

Probenecid is reported to block the renal clearance of aciclovir. The risk of renal impairment is increased by the concomitant use of other nephrotoxic drugs.

Antivirals. Combined therapy with zidovudine and aciclovir is not generally associated with additional toxicity.[1] Overwhelming fatigue was associated with the use of aciclovir and zidovudine in one patient;[2] when each drug was given alone there was no such effect.

1. Tartaglione TA, *et al.* Pharmacokinetic evaluations of low- and high-dose zidovudine plus high-dose acyclovir in patients with symptomatic human immunodeficiency virus infection. *Antimicrob Agents Chemother* 1991; **35:** 2225–31.
2. Bach MC. Possible drug interaction during therapy with azidothymidine and acyclovir for AIDS. *N Engl J Med* 1987; **316:** 547.

Antiviral Action

Aciclovir is active against herpes simplex virus type 1 and type 2 and against varicella-zoster virus. This activity is due to intracellular conversion of aciclovir by viral thymidine kinase to the monophosphate with subsequent conversion by cellular enzymes to the diphosphate and the active triphosphate. This active form inhibits viral DNA synthesis and replication by inhibiting the herpesvirus DNA polymerase enzyme as well as being incorporated into viral DNA. This process is highly selective for infected cells. Studies in *animals* and *in vitro* show various sensitivities but demonstrate that these viruses are inhibited by concentrations of aciclovir that are readily achieved clinically. Herpes simplex virus type 1 appears to be the most susceptible, then type 2, followed by varicella-zoster virus.

The Epstein-Barr virus and cytomegalovirus are also susceptible to aciclovir to a lesser extent. However, for cytomegalovirus it does not appear to be activated by thymidine kinase and may act via a different mechanism. Epstein-Barr virus may have reduced thymidine kinase activity but its DNA polymerase is very sensitive to inhibition by aciclovir triphosphate, which may account for the partial activity.

Aciclovir has no activity against latent viruses, but there is some evidence that it inhibits latent herpes simplex virus at an early stage of reactivation.

Reviews of the antiviral activity of aciclovir.

1. Elion GB. Mechanism of action and selectivity of acyclovir. *Am J Med* 1982; **73** (suppl 1A): 7–13.
2. Elion GB. The biochemistry and mechanism of action of acyclovir. *J Antimicrob Chemother* 1983; **12** (suppl B): 9–17.
3. Collins P. The spectrum of antiviral activities of acyclovir in vitro and in vivo. *J Antimicrob Chemother* 1983; **12** (suppl B): 19–27.
4. Elion GB. Acyclovir: discovery, mechanism of action, and selectivity. *J Med Virol* 1993; **41** (suppl 1): 2–6.
5. Wagstaff AJ, *et al.* Aciclovir: a reappraisal of its antiviral activity, pharmacokinetic properties and therapeutic efficacy. *Drugs* 1994; **47:** 153–205.

Cytomegalovirus. Studies *in vitro* have shown antiviral synergy against cytomegalovirus with aciclovir and either interferon[1] or vidarabine.[2]

1. Smith CA, *et al.* Synergistic antiviral activity of acyclovir and interferon on human cytomegalovirus. *Antimicrob Agents Chemother* 1983; **24:** 325–32.
2. Spector SA, Kelley E. Inhibition of human cytomegalovirus by combined acyclovir and vidarabine. *Antimicrob Agents Chemother* 1985; **27:** 600–4.

Epstein-Barr virus. Studies on the activity of aciclovir *in vitro* against the Epstein-Barr virus have indicated that the virus does not code for its own thymidine kinase and that phosphorylation of aciclovir is not carried out by this enzyme.[1]

1. Datta AK, Pagano JS. Phosphorylation of acyclovir in vitro in activated Burkitt somatic cell hybrids. *Antimicrob Agents Chemother* 1983; **24:** 10–14.

Herpes simplex virus. In an *in-vitro* study using Vero cells, aciclovir was found to have a greater activity against herpes simplex virus (HSV) types 1 and 2 than idoxuridine, cytarabine, trifluridine, or vidarabine.[1] Another study[2] showed that for most cell lines the order of decreasing potency against HSV type 1 was brivudine, fluoroiodoaracytosine [fiacitabine], and then aciclovir, although with murine cell lines the order was brivudine, followed by aciclovir, then fluoroiodoaracytosine.

Enhanced activity has been observed with human interferon and aciclovir against HSV types 1 and 2 in Vero cells.[3,4] This enhancement may be due to interferon-induced alterations in the nucleoside metabolism of infected cells.[5] An additive effect with aciclovir and vidarabine against HSV types 1 and 2 has also been reported.[6]

1. Collins P, Bauer DJ. The activity in vitro against herpes virus of 9-(2-hydroxethoxymethyl)guanine (acycloguanosine), a new antiviral agent. *J Antimicrob Chemother* 1979; **5:** 431–6.
2. De Clercq E. Comparative efficacy of antiherpes drugs in different cell lines. *Antimicrob Agents Chemother* 1982; **21:** 661–3.
3. Stanwick TL, *et al.* Combined antiviral effect of interferon and acyclovir on herpes simplex virus types 1 and 2. *Antimicrob Agents Chemother* 1981; **19:** 672–4.
4. Hammer SM, *et al.* Alpha interferon and acyclovir treatment of herpes simplex virus in lymphoid cell cultures. *Antimicrob Agents Chemother* 1982; **21:** 634–40.
5. O'Brien WJ, *et al.* Nucleoside metabolism in herpes simplex virus-infected cells following treatment with interferon and acyclovir, a possible mechanism of synergistic antiviral activity. *Antimicrob Agents Chemother* 1990; **34:** 1178–82.
6. Schinazi RF, *et al.* Effect of combinations of acyclovir with vidarabine or its 5′-monophosphate on herpes simplex viruses in cell culture and in mice. *Antimicrob Agents Chemother* 1982; **22:** 499–507.

LATENT INFECTION. A study *in vitro*[1] in trigeminal ganglia cells of *mice* showed that aciclovir does not affect latent infections but could affect the latent virus during early stages of reactivation. Intermittent exposure *in vitro* of latently infected ganglia to aciclovir reduced the proportion of ganglia containing reactivatable herpes simplex virus. Another study in *rabbits*[2] showed that there was no evidence that aciclovir or brivudine given by mouth prevented the recurrence of viral shedding or clinical corneal disease in experimental herpes simplex keratitis; resistant viruses were not found in tears.

1. Klein RJ, *et al.* Effect of discontinuous acyclovir treatment on in vitro reactivation of herpes simplex virus from latently infected trigeminal ganglia. *Antimicrob Agents Chemother* 1983; **24:** 129–31.
2. Kaufman HE, *et al.* Oral antiviral drugs in experimental herpes simplex keratitis. *Antimicrob Agents Chemother* 1983; **24:** 888–91.

Herpesvirus 6. Human herpesvirus 6 was found to be comparatively resistant to aciclovir *in vitro*[1] with a concentration of approximately 100 μmol per mL needed to produce 50% viral inhibition. Other studies found this virus to be more susceptible to aciclovir.[2,3]

1. Russler SK, *et al.* Susceptibility of human herpesvirus 6 to acyclovir and ganciclovir. *Lancet* 1989; **ii:** 382.
2. Kikuta H, *et al.* Susceptibility of human herpesvirus 6 to acyclovir. *Lancet* 1989; **ii:** 861.
3. Agut H, *et al.* Susceptibility of human herpesvirus 6 to acyclovir and ganciclovir. *Lancet* 1989; **ii:** 626.

Varicella-zoster virus. Aciclovir and interferon alfa showed synergistic activity *in vitro* against varicella-zoster virus.[1] An additive to synergistic activity was also observed between interferon alfa and brivudine, vidarabine, or foscarnet.

1. Baba M, *et al.* Synergistic antiviral effects of antiherpes compounds and human leukocyte interferon on varicella-zoster virus in vitro. *Antimicrob Agents Chemother* 1984; **25:** 515–17.

Resistance

Herpes simplex virus develops resistance to aciclovir *in vitro* and *in vivo* by selection of mutants deficient in thymidine kinase. Other mechanisms of resistance include altered substrate specificity of thymidine kinase and reduced sensitivity of viral DNA polymerase. Resistance has also been reported with varicella-zoster virus, probably by similar mechanisms.

Although occasional treatment failures have been reported, resistance has not yet emerged as a major problem in treating herpes simplex infections. This is partly because of the low incidence of resistant mutants *in vivo* and because viruses deficient in thymidine kinase generally appear to be of diminished virulence with reduced infectivity and latency. Viruses with altered thymidine kinase appear to be of normal or slightly diminished virulence and DNA polymerase mutants are of normal virulence, apart from apparently having a reduced neurological virulence. Resistant viruses are most likely to be a problem in patients with a suppressed immune response. AIDS patients may be particularly prone to aciclovir-resistant mucocutaneous herpes simplex virus infections.

Viruses resistant to aciclovir because of absence of thymidine kinase may be cross-resistant to other antivirals phosphorylated by this enzyme, such as brivudine, idoxuridine, and ganciclovir. Viruses resistant because of altered substrate specificity of thymidine kinase may display cross-resistance to brivudine; those with altered DNA polymerase sensitivity may be resistant to brivudine and vidarabine. However, those viruses with altered enzyme specificity or sensitivity tend to have variable cross-resistance patterns and may be relatively susceptible to the aforementioned antivirals.

Reviews of the resistance of herpes simplex viruses to aciclovir[1-4] and cross-resistance to other antivirals.[2,4]

1. Field HJ. A perspective on resistance to acyclovir in herpes simplex virus. *J Antimicrob Chemother* 1983; **12** (suppl B): 129–35.
2. Crumpacker C. Resistance of herpes simplex virus to antiviral agents: is it clinically important? *Drugs* 1983; **26:** 373–7.
3. Balfour HH. Resistance of herpes simplex to acyclovir. *Ann Intern Med* 1983; **98:** 404–6.
4. Wagstaff AJ, *et al.* Aciclovir: a reappraisal of its antiviral activity, pharmacokinetic properties and therapeutic efficacy. *Drugs* 1994; **47:** 153–205.

Resistance in human infections. Aciclovir resistance is still uncommon in clinical practice,[1] although more prevalent in immunocompromised patients. Most aciclovir-resistant herpes simplex and varicella zoster infections have been reported in immunocompromised patients receiving prolonged courses of aciclovir.[2-6] Aciclovir-resistant herpes simplex strains have generally been less virulent, but aggressive disease has been reported.[5,7,8] Recurrences in these patients may respond to increases in dosage of aciclovir,[9] but alternative antivirals may be required. Since resistance is commonly due to the emergence of strains deficient in thymidine kinase, they tend to retain sensitivity to foscarnet and vidarabine, drugs which do not depend on viral thymidine kinase for activation.[5,10,11] Aciclovir-resistant varicella zoster infections have responded to increases in aciclovir dose[12] and to foscarnet.[13,14]

1. Christophers J, *et al.* Survey of resistance of herpes simplex virus to acyclovir in Northwest England. *Antimicrob Agents Chemother* 1998; **42:** 868–72.
2. Christophers J, Sutton RNP. Characterisation of acyclovir-resistant and -sensitive clinical herpes simplex virus isolates from an immunocompromised patient. *J Antimicrob Chemother* 1987; **20:** 389–98.
3. Erlich KS, *et al.* Acyclovir-resistant herpes simplex virus infections in patients with the acquired immunodeficiency syndrome. *N Engl J Med* 1989; **320:** 293–6.
4. Englund JA, *et al.* Herpes simplex virus resistant to acyclovir: a study in a tertiary care center. *Ann Intern Med* 1990; **112:** 416–22.
5. Ljungman P, *et al.* Acyclovir-resistant herpes simplex virus causing pneumonia after marrow transplantation. *J Infect Dis* 1990; **162:** 244–8.
6. Jacobson MA, *et al.* Acyclovir-resistant varicella zoster virus infection after chronic oral acyclovir therapy in patients with the acquired immunodeficiency syndrome (AIDS). *Ann Intern Med* 1990; **112:** 187–91.
7. Gateley A, *et al.* Herpes simplex virus type 2 meningoencephalitis resistant to acyclovir in a patient with AIDS. *J Infect Dis* 1990; **161:** 711–15.
8. Sacks SL, *et al.* Progressive esophagitis from acyclovir resistant herpes simplex: clinical roles for DNA polymerase mutants and viral heterogeneity? *Ann Intern Med* 1989; **111:** 893–9.
9. Modiano P, *et al.* Acyclovir-resistant chronic cutaneous herpes simplex in Wiskott-Aldrich syndrome. *Br J Dermatol* 1995; **133:** 475–8.
10. Crumpacker CS, *et al.* Resistance to antiviral drugs of herpes simplex virus isolated from a patient treated with acyclovir. *N Engl J Med* 1982; **306:** 343–6.
11. Chatis PA, *et al.* Successful treatment with foscarnet of an acyclovir-resistant mucocutaneous infection with herpes simplex virus in a patient with acquired immunodeficiency syndrome. *N Engl J Med* 1989; **320:** 297–300.
12. Linnemann CC, *et al.* Emergence of acyclovir-resistant varicella zoster virus in an AIDS patient on prolonged acyclovir therapy. *AIDS* 1990; **4:** 577–9.
13. Safrin S, *et al.* Foscarnet therapy in five patients with AIDS and acyclovir-resistant varicella-zoster virus infection. *Ann Intern Med* 1991; **115:** 19–21.
14. Smith KJ, *et al.* Acyclovir-resistant varicella zoster responsive to foscarnet. *Arch Dermatol* 1991; **127:** 1069–71.

Pharmacokinetics

The intravenous infusion of aciclovir as the sodium salt produces plasma-aciclovir concentrations that demonstrate a biphasic pattern. The infusion over one hour of a dose equivalent to 5 mg of aciclovir per kg body-weight in adults has produced steady-state plasma concentrations with a peak of 9.8 μg per mL and a trough of 0.7 μg per mL. Similar concentrations are achieved in children over 1 year following doses of 250 mg per m^2 body-surface; a dose of 10 mg per kg in neonates of up to 3 months of age has produced a peak plasma concentration of 13.8 μg per mL and a trough of 2.3 μg per mL.

Aciclovir is excreted through the kidney by both glomerular filtration and tubular secretion. The terminal or beta-phase half-life is reported to be about 2 to 3 hours for adults without renal impairment. In chronic renal failure this value is increased, and may be up to 19.5 hours in anuric patients. During haemodialysis the half-life is reduced to 5.7 hours, with 60% of a dose of aciclovir being removed in 6 hours. Most of a dose by intravenous infusion is excreted unchanged with only up to 14% appearing in the urine as the inactive metabolite 9-carboxymethoxymethylguanine. Faecal excretion may account for about 2% of a dose. There is wide distribution, including into the CSF where concentrations achieved are about 50% of those achieved in plasma. Protein binding is reported to range from 9 to 33%.

Prior administration of probenecid increases the half-life and the area under the plasma concentration-time curve of aciclovir.

About 15 to 30% of a dose of aciclovir given by mouth is considered to be absorbed from the gastro-intestinal tract. A dose of 200 mg aciclovir every 4 hours by mouth is reported to produce maximum and minimum steady-state plasma concentrations of 0.7 and 0.4 μg per mL respectively; equivalent values following 400-mg doses are 1.2 and 0.6 μg per mL. The orally active prodrugs desciclovir (p.607) and valaciclovir (p.628) have been developed to overcome this poor absorption.

Aciclovir crosses the placenta and is distributed into breast milk in concentrations approximately 3 times higher than those in maternal serum.

Absorption of aciclovir is usually slight following topical application to intact skin, although it may be increased by changes in formulation. Aciclovir is absorbed following application of a 3% ointment to the eye giving a relatively high concentration of 1.7 μg per mL in the aqueous humour but negligible amounts in the blood.

The pharmacokinetics of aciclovir given intravenously as the sodium salt in single doses of 2.5, 5, 10, and 15 mg per kg body-weight as an infusion over 1 hour to 13 patients with various malignant disorders.[1] The declining plasma concentration was considered to be well described by a two-compartment open model. At the end of the infusion the mean plasma-aciclovir concentrations were 4.52, 8.28, 14.6, and 22.7 μg per mL respectively. The mean terminal (beta) half-lives were 2.9, 2.8, 3.3, and 2.4 hours respectively. Total clearance was 239, 268, 321, and 394 mL per minute and the volumes of distribution at steady state were 44.1, 43.1, 55.9, and 53.4 litres per 1.73 m^2 body-surface respectively. Renal clearance amounted to 77.4% of total clearance and was about three times greater than the estimated creatinine clearance; 70.2% of total aciclovir was excreted in the urine over 72 hours. It was considered that elimination involved both tubular secretion and glomerular filtration. In another study,[2] probenecid 1 g given one hour before infusion of aciclovir enhanced the plasma concentrations of aciclovir in 3 patients given 5 mg per kg body-weight by intravenous infusion over one hour. Probenecid increased the mean terminal plasma half-life by 18% from 2.3 to 2.7 hours and the area under the plasma concentration-time curve by 40%. The mean 25-hour urinary excretion declined by 12.4% from 79.0 to 69.2% of the dose. Total body clearance declined by 29% from 300 to 213 mL/min per 1.73 m^2 body-surface; renal clearance declined by 32% but was still about twofold greater than the estimated creatinine clearance.

Further information on the pharmacokinetics of aciclovir can be obtained from the reviews listed below.[3-5]

1. Laskin OL, *et al.* Pharmacokinetics and tolerance of acyclovir, a new anti-herpesvirus agent, in humans. *Antimicrob Agents Chemother* 1982; **21:** 393–8.
2. Laskin OL, *et al.* Effects of probenecid on the pharmacokinetics and elimination of acyclovir in humans. *Antimicrob Agents Chemother* 1982; **21:** 804–7.
3. de Miranda P, Blum MR. Pharmacokinetics of acyclovir after intravenous and oral administration. *J Antimicrob Chemother* 1983; **12** (suppl B): 29–37.
4. Laskin OL. Clinical pharmacokinetics of acyclovir. *Clin Pharmacokinet* 1983; **8:** 187–201.
5. Wagstaff AJ, *et al.* Aciclovir: a reappraisal of its antiviral activity, pharmacokinetic properties and therapeutic efficacy. *Drugs* 1994; **47:** 153–205.

Distribution. Good intra-ocular penetration was achieved after the administration of aciclovir by mouth to 16 patients undergoing cataract extraction.[1] Patients received 5 doses of aciclovir 400 mg in the 24 hours before surgery and a mean concentration of aciclovir 3.26 μmol per litre (0.73 μg per mL) was found in aqueous humour removed during surgery. The mean concentration in plasma obtained at the same time was 8.74 μmol per litre (1.97 μg per mL). There was a significant correlation between plasma and aqueous humour concentrations.

Aciclovir 800 mg by mouth 3 times daily for 12 months was given to patients with multiple sclerosis.[2] In 3 patients the concentration of aciclovir in the CSF was 13 to 52% (mean 31%) of that in the blood, a value not as high as that found in earlier studies using short-term intravenous administration.

Peak and trough CSF-aciclovir concentrations did not differ significantly and remained stable at 1, 4, 8, and 12 months at a level sufficient to inhibit clinically herpes simplex types 1 and 2 and varicella zoster viruses.

In another study,[3] patients seropositive for HIV given intravenous aciclovir 50 mg per kg once weekly as a 3-hour infusion with oral probenecid 1 g were found to have a meningeal penetration of aciclovir of 82%.

1. Hung SO, *et al.* Pharmacokinetics of oral acyclovir (Zovirax) in the eye. *Br J Ophthalmol* 1984; **68:** 192–5.
2. Lycke J, *et al.* Acyclovir concentrations in serum and cerebrospinal fluid at steady state. *J Antimicrob Chemother* 1989; **24:** 947–54.
3. Chavanet P, *et al.* Meningeal diffusion of high doses of acyclovir given with probenecid. *J Antimicrob Chemother* 1990; **26:** 294–5.

Uses and Administration

Aciclovir is a synthetic purine nucleoside analogue structurally related to guanine. It is used mainly for the treatment of viral infections due to herpes simplex virus (types 1 and 2) and varicella-zoster virus (herpes zoster and chickenpox).

Herpes simplex infections including herpes keratitis, herpes labialis, and genital herpes respond to aciclovir given by the intravenous, oral, or topical route as soon as possible after symptoms appear. Both initial and recurrent infections can be successfully treated. Prolonged treatment can reduce the incidence of recurrence which is important in immunocompromised patients. However, when prolonged treatment is withdrawn infections may recur.

Aciclovir also improves the healing of herpes zoster lesions and reduces acute pain when given intravenously or by mouth, although studies indicate that it has little effect on postherpetic neuralgia. Beneficial effects may be more marked in immunocompromised patients.

ADMINISTRATION AND DOSAGE. Aciclovir is administered by *intravenous infusion* as the sodium salt over 1 hour. Solutions for infusion are usually prepared to give a concentration of 25 or 50 mg of aciclovir per mL; this must then be further diluted in a suitable infusion fluid such as 0.9% sodium chloride to a final concentration not greater than about 5 mg per mL (0.5% w/v). Alternatively a solution containing 25 mg per mL may be administered by injection using a controlled rate infusion pump, over 1 hour. The dose by the intravenous route is 5 mg per kg body-weight administered every 8 hours and recommended periods of treatment range from 5 to 7 days. A higher dose of 10 mg per kg every 8 hours for 10 days is given in herpes simplex encephalitis. This higher dose may also be required in varicella-zoster infections in patients whose immune response is impaired.

Oral doses of aciclovir vary according to indication. For treatment of primary herpes simplex infections, including genital herpes, the usual dose by mouth is 200 mg five times daily (usually every 4 hours while awake) for 5 to 10 days. This dose may be doubled in severely immunocompromised patients or in those with impaired absorption. For suppression of recurrent herpes simplex the dose by mouth is 800 mg daily in two to four divided doses; dosage reduction to 400 to 600 mg daily can be tried. Higher doses have also been used. Therapy should be interrupted every 6 to 12 months for reassessment of the condition. For prophylaxis of herpes simplex in immunocompromised patients, the dose is 200 to 400 mg four times daily. Chronic suppressive treatment is not suitable for mild or infrequent recurrences of herpes simplex. In such cases episodic treatment of recurrences may be more beneficial; a dose of 200 mg up to 5 times daily (every 4 hours while awake) for 5 days has been recommended preferably initiated during the prodromal period. The usual oral dose for treatment of chickenpox is 800 mg of aciclovir four or five times daily for 5 to 7 days, while for herpes zoster 800 mg five times daily may be given for 7 to 10 days.

In herpes simplex infections of the skin, including genital herpes and herpes labialis, *topical treatment* with an ointment or cream containing aciclovir 5% may be applied 5 or 6 times daily every 3 or 4 hours for periods of 5 to 10 days. In herpes simplex keratitis a 3% eye ointment may be applied 5 times daily every 4 hours until 3 days after healing.

Doses should be reduced in *renal impairment* (see below).

Children's doses. In children the 8-hourly intravenous dose is best calculated by body-surface using 250 mg per m^2 as an equivalent of 5 mg per kg and 500 mg per m^2 for 10 mg per kg. A suggested 8-hourly dose for infants and neonates is 10 mg per kg; treatment for neonatal herpes usually continues for 10 days. In the treatment of herpes simplex infections, and in the prophylaxis of herpes simplex infections in the immunocompromised, oral doses of aciclovir for children aged 2 years and over are as for adults. Children aged under 2 years are given half the adult dose. In the treatment of chickenpox, children are given 20 mg per kg body-weight, up to a maximum of 800 mg, four times daily for 5 days. Alternatively, children aged 6 years and over may be given 800 mg four times daily, those aged 2 to 5 years may be given 400 mg four times daily, and those aged under 2 years may be given 200 mg four times daily.

Reviews.

1. Richards DM, *et al.* Acyclovir: a review of its pharmacodynamic properties and therapeutic efficacy. *Drugs* 1983; **26:** 378–438.
2. Dorsky DI, Crumpacker CS. Drugs five years later: acyclovir. *Ann Intern Med* 1987; **107:** 859–74.
3. Whitley RJ, Gnann JW. Acyclovir: a decade later. *N Engl J Med* 1992; **327:** 782–9. Correction. *ibid.* 1997; **337:** 1703.
4. Anonymous. Acyclovir in general practice. *Drug Ther Bull* 1992; **30:** 101–4.
5. Wagstaff AJ, *et al.* Aciclovir: a reappraisal of its antiviral activity, pharmacokinetic properties and therapeutic efficacy. *Drugs* 1994; **47:** 153–205.
6. Welsby PD. Acyclovir: is the honeymoon coming to an end? *J Infect* 1994; **28:** 121–9.

Administration in renal impairment. Doses of aciclovir should be reduced in renal impairment and the manufacturers have given the following guidance. For *intravenous* administration the interval between infusions may be increased to 12 hours when the creatinine clearance is between 25 and 50 mL per minute or to 24 hours for 10 to 25 mL per minute. When the creatinine clearance is less than 10 mL per minute, patients on peritoneal dialysis should receive half the usual appropriate dose given once every 24 hours. Patients on haemodialysis should receive half the usual dose every 24 hours plus an extra half-dose following haemodialysis. *Oral* doses of aciclovir may be reduced to the following: for patients with a creatinine clearance of less than 10 mL per minute, 200 mg every 12 hours for herpes simplex infections or 800 mg every 12 hours for varicella-zoster infections; for patients with a creatinine clearance of between 10 and 25 mL per minute the dose of aciclovir for varicella-zoster infections should be reduced to 800 mg three times a day at intervals of 6 to 8 hours.

Some references to the use of aciclovir in patients undergoing dialysis.

1. Burgess ED, Gill MJ. Intraperitoneal administration of acyclovir in patients receiving continuous ambulatory peritoneal dialysis. *J Clin Pharmacol* 1990; **30:** 997–1000.
2. Almond MK, *et al.* Avoiding acyclovir neurotoxicity in patients with chronic renal failure undergoing haemodialysis. *Nephron* 1995; **69:** 428–32.
3. Stathoulopoulou F, *et al.* Clinical pharmacokinetics of oral acyclovir in patients on continuous ambulatory peritoneal dialysis. *Nephron* 1996; **74:** 337–41.

Erythema multiforme. Recurrent erythema multiforme (p.1074) is an uncommon disorder that in some patients is associated with herpes simplex infection. In these patients a 5-day course of oral aciclovir at the start of the infection will often be successful in preventing the subsequent skin lesions.[1] If this fails, a 6-month course of oral aciclovir may be tried, even if the association with herpes is not obvious.

1. Schofield JK, *et al.* Recurrent erythema multiforme: clinical features and treatment in a large series of patients. *Br J Dermatol* 1993; **128:** 542–5.

Herpesvirus infections. The activity of aciclovir depends on its intracellular conversion to the triphosphate (see Antiviral Action, above). Aciclovir is highly effective against replicating herpes simplex virus with lower activity against varicella zoster and herpesvirus simiae, slight activity against Epstein-Barr virus, and minimal activity against cytomegalovirus.

Aciclovir is widely used in *herpes simplex infections.*[1-9] As discussed on p.597 it is still the main treatment and, although it does not prevent the development of latent infections, prophylactic administration of aciclovir can reduce the incidence and severity of recurrences. Treatment of *varicella zoster infections* generally requires higher doses of aciclovir than those used for herpes simplex infections. Its use in herpes zoster is well established[10,11] (see p.598). Aciclovir may be useful in *chickenpox* where there are complications or the patient is immunosuppressed, but in otherwise healthy patients it is not worthwhile.[12-15] Also the value of using aciclovir to protect contacts of chickenpox is not clear and this use has been questioned.[12,16-18] For reference to aciclovir resistance in herpes simplex and varicella-zoster infections, see Resistance in Human Infections, above.

See p.598 for mention of aciclovir being tried in *herpesvirus simiae infections.*

Although aciclovir inhibits replication of *cytomegalovirus* at high concentrations it is generally of no value in the treatment of acute infections and there have been conflicting reports of it preventing infection.[19-24] For a discussion of the treatment of cytomegalovirus infections with more effective antiviral drugs, see p.596. Various antivirals, including aciclovir,[25,26] have been tried in *Epstein-Barr virus infections* (see p.597), and although some clinical improvements have been reported any reductions in viral shedding have usually been lost when treatment was stopped.

1. Whatley JD, Thin RN. Episodic acyclovir therapy to abort recurrent attacks of genital herpes simplex infection. *J Antimicrob Chemother* 1991; **27:** 677–81.
2. Kaplowitz LG, *et al.* Prolonged continuous acyclovir treatment of normal adults with frequently recurring genital herpes simplex virus infection. *JAMA* 1991; **265:** 747–51.
3. Whitley R, *et al.* A controlled trial comparing vidarabine with acyclovir in neonatal herpes simplex virus infection. *N Engl J Med* 1991; **324:** 444–9.
4. Rooney JF, *et al.* Oral acyclovir to suppress frequently recurrent herpes labialis: a double-blind, placebo-controlled trial. *Ann Intern Med* 1993; **118:** 268–72.
5. Goldberg LH, *et al.* Long-term suppression of recurrent genital herpes with acyclovir: a 5-year benchmark. *Arch Dermatol* 1993; **129:** 582–7.
6. Barron BA, *et al.* Herpetic eye disease study: a controlled trial of oral acyclovir for herpes simplex stromal keratitis. *Ophthalmology* 1994; **101:** 1871–82.
7. Schirmer M, *et al.* Acyclovir in acute oligoarticular herpetic arthritis. *Lancet* 1995; **346:** 712–13.
8. Worrall G. Acyclovir in recurrent herpes labialis. *Br Med J* 1996; **312:** 6.
9. Herpetic Eye Disease Study Group. Acyclovir for the prevention of recurrent herpes simplex virus eye disease. *N Engl J Med* 1998; **339:** 300–6.
10. Anonymous. Treatment of ocular herpes zoster. *Lancet* 1991; **338:** 1244–5.
11. Nikkels AF, Piérard GE. Recognition and treatment of shingles. *Drugs* 1994; **48:** 528–48.
12. Balfour HH, *et al.* Acyclovir treatment of varicella in otherwise healthy children. *J Pediatr* 1990; **116:** 633–9.
13. Feder HM. Treatment of adult chickenpox with oral acyclovir. *Arch Intern Med* 1990; **150:** 2061–5.
14. Balfour HH, *et al.* Acyclovir treatment of varicella in otherwise healthy adolescents. *J Pediatr* 1992; **120:** 627–33.
15. Committee on Infectious Diseases. The use of oral acyclovir in otherwise healthy children with varicella. *Pediatrics* 1993; **91:** 674–6. Correction. *ibid.*: 858.
16. Asano Y, *et al.* Postexposure prophylaxis of varicella in family contact by oral acyclovir. *Pediatrics* 1993; **92:** 219–22.
17. Suga S, *et al.* Effect of oral acyclovir against primary and secondary viraemia in incubation period of varicella. *Arch Dis Child* 1993; **69:** 639–42.
18. Conway SP. Effect of oral acyclovir against primary and secondary viraemia in incubation period of varicella: commentary. *Arch Dis Child* 1993; **69:** 642–3.
19. Balfour HH, *et al.* A randomized, placebo-controlled trial of oral acyclovir for the prevention of cytomegalovirus disease in recipients of renal allografts. *N Engl J Med* 1989; **320:** 1381–7.
20. Eisenmann D, *et al.* Prevention of cytomegalovirus disease in heart transplant recipients by prophylaxis with cytomegalovirus hyperimmune globulin plus oral acyclovir. *Transplant Proc* 1990; **22:** 2322–3.
21. Bailey TC, *et al.* Failure of high-dose oral acyclovir with or without immune globulin to prevent primary cytomegalovirus disease in recipients of solid organ transplants. *Am J Med* 1993; **95:** 273–8.
22. Prentice HG, *et al.* Impact of long-term acyclovir on cytomegalovirus infection and survival after allogeneic bone marrow transplantation. *Lancet* 1994; **343:** 749–53.
23. Singh N, *et al.* High-dose acyclovir compared with short-course preemptive ganciclovir therapy to prevent cytomegalovirus disease in liver transplant recipients: a randomized trial. *Ann Intern Med* 1994; **120:** 375–81.
24. Boeckh M, *et al.* Failure of high-dose acyclovir to prevent cytomegalovirus disease after autologous marrow transplantation. *J Infect Dis* 1995; **172:** 939–43.
25. Andersson J, *et al.* Effect of acyclovir on infectious mononucleosis: a double-blind, placebo-controlled study. *J Infect Dis* 1986; **153:** 283–90.
26. Yao QY, *et al.* The Epstein-Barr virus: host balance in acute infectious mononucleosis patients receiving acyclovir anti-viral therapy. *Int J Cancer* 1989; **43:** 61–6.

HIV infection and AIDS. Aciclovir is not active against HIV, but encouraging results were reported using aciclovir in combination with zidovudine[1,2] to treat patients with AIDS (p.599). However, a more recent study[3] found that aciclovir did not prolong the survival of patients receiving zidovudine for advanced AIDS or AIDS-related complex.

1. Cooper DA, *et al.* The efficacy and safety of zidovudine alone or as cotherapy with acyclovir for the treatment of patients with AIDS and AIDS-related complex: a double-blind, randomized trial. *AIDS* 1993; **7:** 197–207.
2. Stein DS, *et al.* The effect of the interaction of acyclovir with zidovudine on progression to AIDS and survival: analysis of data in the Multicenter AIDS Cohort Study. *Ann Intern Med* 1994; **121:** 100–8.
3. Gallant JE, *et al.* Lack of association between acyclovir use and survival in patients with advanced human immunodeficiency virus disease treated with zidovudine. *J Infect Dis* 1995; **172:** 346–52.

Preparations

BP 1998: Aciclovir Cream; Aciclovir Eye Ointment; Aciclovir Intravenous Infusion; Aciclovir Oral Suspension; Aciclovir Tablets; ***USP 23:*** Acyclovir Capsules; Acyclovir for Injection; Acyclovir Ointment; Acyclovir Oral Suspension; Acyclovir Tablets.

Proprietary Preparations (details are given in Part 3)
Aust.: Activir; Zovirax; ***Austral.:*** Acyclo-V; Zovirax; Zyclir; ***Belg.:*** Zovirax; ***Canad.:*** Avirax; Zovirax; ***Fr.:*** Activir; Zovirax; ***Ger.:*** Aci-Sanorania; Acic; Acic-Ophtal; Aciclobeta; Aciclostad; Acivir; Herpetad; Herpofug; Herpotern; Herpoviric; Mapox; Supraviran; Virax; Virupos; Viruseen; Zoliparin; Zovirax; ***Irl.:*** Clonorax; Zovirax; ***Ital.:*** Aciclin; Aciclofta1†; Aciviran†; Acyvir; Alovir; Avirase; Avix; Avyclor; Avyplus; Cevirin; Citivir; Clovix†; Cycloviran; Dravyr; Efriviral; Esavir; Neviran; Rexan; Sifiviral; Zovirax; ***Neth.:*** Zovirax; ***Norw.:*** Geavir; Zovirax; ***S.Afr.:*** Activir; Cyclivex; Zovirax; ***Spain:*** Cusiviral; Maynar; Milavir; Vipral†; Virherpes; Virmen; Zovirax; ***Swed.:*** Geavir; Zovir†; Zovirax; ***Switz.:*** Zovirax; ***UK:*** Herpetad; Soothelip; Virasorb; Virovir; Zovirax; ***USA:*** Zovirax.

Adefovir (17807-w)

Adefovir *(BAN, USAN, rINN).*

GS-0393. {[2-(6-Amino-9*H*-purin-9-yl)ethoxy]methyl}phosphonic acid; 9-[2-(Phosphonomethoxy)ethyl]adenine.

$C_8H_{12}N_5O_4P$ = 273.2.
CAS — 106941-25-7.

Adefovir Dipivoxil (17466-v)

Adefovir Dipivoxil *(BANM, USAN, rINNM).*

GS-0840. 9-[2-({Bis[(pivaloyloxy)methoxy]phosphinyl}methoxy)ethyl]adenine.

$C_{20}H_{32}N_5O_8P$ = 501.5.
CAS — 142340-99-6.

Adefovir is a nucleoside reverse transcriptase inhibitor, structurally related to adenine, with antiviral activity. The oral prodrug adefovir dipivoxil is under investigation in the treatment of HIV infection.

References.

1. Barditch-Crovo P, *et al.* Anti-human immunodeficiency virus (HIV) activity, safety, and pharmacokinetics of adefovir dipivoxil (9-[2-(bis-pivaloyloxymethyl)-phosphonylmethoxyethyl]adenine) in HIV-infected patients. *J Infect Dis* 1997; **176:** 406–13.
2. Mulato AS, *et al.* Genotypic and phenotypic characterization of human immunodeficiency virus type 1 variants isolated from AIDS patients after prolonged adefovir dipivoxil therapy. *Antimicrob Agents Chemother* 1998; **42:** 1620–8.

Afovirsen (17400-w)

Afovirsen *(rINN).*

Isis-2105.

$C_{192}H_{250}N_{57}O_{107}P_{19}S_{19}$ = 6266.1.
CAS — 151356-08-0.

Afovirsen is an antisense oligonucleotide which has been investigated for the treatment of genital warts.

References.

1. Crooke ST, *et al.* A pharmacokinetic evaluation of ^{14}C-labeled afovirsen sodium in patients with genital warts. *Clin Pharmacol Ther* 1994; **56:** 641–6.

Amprenavir (17909-c)

KVX-478; VX-478; 141W94.

$C_{25}H_{35}N_3O_6S$ = 505.6.
CAS — 161814-49-9.

Amprenavir is a protease inhibitor with antiviral activity against HIV. It is under investigation in the treatment of HIV infection and AIDS.

References.

1. Adkins JC, Faulds D. Amprenavir. *Drugs* 1998; **55:** 837–42.

Atevirdine (17287-h)

Atevirdine *(rINN).*

U-87201 (atevirdine); U-87201E (atevirdine mesylate). 1-[3-(Ethylamino)-2-pyridyl]-4-[(5-methoxyindol-2-yl)carbonyl]piperazine.

$C_{21}H_{25}N_5O_2$ = 379.5.
CAS — 136816-75-6 (atevirdine); 138540-32-6 (atevirdine mesylate).

NOTE. Atevirdine Mesylate is *USAN.*

Atevirdine is a non-nucleoside reverse transcriptase inhibitor under investigation for the treatment of HIV infection. Viral resistance emerges rapidly when atevirdine is given alone, and it would be likely to be used mainly in combination with nucleoside reverse transcriptase inhibitors.

References.

1. Campbell TB, *et al.* Inhibition of human immunodeficiency virus type 1 replication in vitro by the bisheteroarylpiperazine atevirdine (U-87201E) in combination with zidovudine or didanosine. *J Infect Dis* 1993; **168:** 318–26.
2. Morse GD, *et al.* Didanosine reduces atevirdine absorption in subjects with human immunodeficiency virus infections. *Antimicrob Agents Chemother* 1996; **40:** 767–71.
3. Been-Tiktak AMM, *et al.* Safety, tolerance, and efficacy of atevirdine in asymptomatic human immunodeficiency virus-infected individuals. *Antimicrob Agents Chemother* 1996; **40:** 2664–8.

Brivudine (12455-p)

Brivudine *(rINN).*

BVDU. (*E*)-5-(2-Bromovinyl)-2′-deoxyuridine.

$C_{11}H_{13}BrN_2O_5$ = 333.1.
CAS — 69304-47-8.

Brivudine is a nucleoside analogue effective *in vitro* against herpes simplex virus type 1 and varicella-zoster virus; other viruses including herpes simplex virus type 2 have been reported to be sensitive, but only at relatively high concentrations. The activity appears to be due, at least in part, to selective phosphorylation of brivudine by viral deoxythymidine kinase in preference to cellular kinases. There is the possibility of cross-resistance developing between brivudine and aciclovir because of some similar features in their mode of action (see p.604).

Brivudine is given by mouth in the treatment of herpes simplex (p.597) and herpes zoster (p.598) in a dose of 125 mg 4 times daily at intervals of 6 hours. It has also been used topically.

References.

1. De Clercq E. The antiviral spectrum of (E)-5-(2-bromovinyl)-2′-deoxyuridine. *J Antimicrob Chemother* 1984; **14** (suppl A): 85–95.
2. Maudgal PC, *et al.* Efficacy of bromovinyldeoxyuridine in the treatment of herpes simplex virus and varicella-zoster virus eye infections. *Antiviral Res* 1984; **4:** 281–91.
3. van Bijsterveld OP, *et al.* Bromovinyldeoxyuridine and interferon treatment in ulcerative herpetic keratitis: a double masked study. *Br J Ophthalmol* 1989; **73:** 604–7.
4. Power WJ, *et al.* Randomised double-blind trial of bromovinyldeoxyuridine (BVDU) and trifluorothymidine (TFT) in dendritic corneal ulceration. *Br J Ophthalmol* 1991; **75:** 649–51.
5. Wildiers J, De Clercq E. Oral (E)-5-(2-bromovinyl)-2′-deoxyuridine treatment of severe herpes zoster in cancer patients. *Eur J Cancer Clin Oncol* 1984; **20:** 471–6.
6. De Clercq E, *et al.* Oral (E)-5-(2-bromovinyl)-2′-deoxyuridine in severe herpes zoster. *Br Med J* 1980; **281:** 1178.
7. Maudgal PC, *et al.* Efficacy of bromovinyldeoxyuridine in the treatment of herpes simplex virus and varicella-zoster virus eye infections. *Antiviral Res* 1984; **4:** 281–91.
8. Wutzler P, *et al.* Oral brivudin vs intravenous acyclovir in the treatment of herpes zoster in immunocompromised patients: a randomized double-blind trial. *J Med Virol* 1995; **46:** 252–7.

Preparations

Proprietary Preparations (details are given in Part 3)
Ger.: Helpin.

Carbovir (9464-m)

GR-90352; NSC-614846.

Carbovir is a nucleoside reverse transcriptase inhibitor structurally related to guanosine with antiviral activity against HIV-1.

References.

1. Parker WB, *et al.* Metabolism of carbovir, a potent inhibitor of human immunodeficiency virus type 1, and its effects on cellular metabolism. *Antimicrob Agents Chemother* 1993; **37:** 1004–9.

CD4 (10526-j)

Soluble CD4.

CD4 is a receptor on the cell membrane of helper T lymphocytes, macrophages, and related cells to which the gp120 glycoprotein of HIV binds with high affinity, thereby infecting the cell. Soluble CD4 produced by recombinant DNA technology has been tried in the treatment of AIDS and AIDS-related complex on the premise that excess CD4 in the blood will compete for HIV-binding and thus reduce HIV-binding to lymphocytes. Administration has been by intravenous, intramuscular, or subcutaneous injection.

Other CD4 compounds under investigation have included CD4 linked to *Pseudomonas* exotoxin (CD4-PE-40) (developed with the aim of delivering the toxin directly to HIV-infected cells) and CD4 immunoadhesins consisting of the Fab fragment of CD4 linked to the Fc portion of immunoglobulins (developed with the aim of increasing the half-life of CD4). CD4 antibodies are under investigation in various immunologically mediated disorders (see p.1560).

Recombinant soluble CD4 was well tolerated by patients with AIDS and AIDS-related complex.[1,2] In one study doses of 30 mg daily by intramuscular injection produced a decrease in serum concentrations of HIV p24 antigen.[1] It was noted, however,[3] that isolates of HIV collected from infected patients were significantly more resistant to soluble CD4 than were laboratory strains. The use of high doses (up to 10 mg per kg body-weight daily) produced substantial reductions in viraemia in 2 of 3 patients but did not affect intracellular viral load.[4]

The treatment of AIDS with antiretroviral drugs is discussed on p.599.

1. Schooley RT, *et al.* Recombinant soluble CD4 therapy in patients with the acquired immunodeficiency syndrome (AIDS) and AIDS-related complex: a phase I–II escalating dosage trial. *Ann Intern Med* 1990; **112:** 247–53.
2. Kahn JO, *et al.* The safety and pharmacokinetics of recombinant soluble CD4 (rCD4) in subjects with the acquired immunodeficiency syndrome (AIDS) and AIDS-related complex: a phase 1 study. *Ann Intern Med* 1990; **112:** 254–61.
3. Daar ES, Ho DD. Relative resistance of primary HIV-1 isolates to neutralization by soluble CD4. *Am J Med* 1991; **90** (suppl 4A): 22–6S.
4. Schacker T, *et al.* Phase I study of high-dose, intravenous rsCD4 in subjects with advanced HIV-1 infection. *J Acquir Immune Defic Syndr Hum Retrovirol* 1995; **9:** 145–52.

Cidofovir (15028-y)

Cidofovir *(BAN, USAN, rINN).*

GS-504; GS-0504; HPMPC. {[(*S*)-2-(4-Amino-2-oxo-1(2*H*)-pyrimidinyl)-1-(hydroxymethyl)ethoxy]methyl}phosphonic acid; 1-[(*S*)-3-Hydroxy-2-(phosphonomethoxy)propyl]-cytosine.

$C_8H_{14}N_3O_6P$ = 279.2.
CAS — 113852-37-2 (anhydrous cidofovir); 149394-66-1 (anhydrous cidofovir or cidofovir dihydrate).

Stability. References.

1. Ennis RD, Dahl TC. Stability of cidofovir in 0.9% sodium chloride injection for five days. *Am J Health-Syst Pharm* 1997; **54:** 2204–6.

Adverse Effects

The most serious dose-limiting adverse effect of cidofovir is nephrotoxicity, the incidence and severity of which can be reduced by concurrent administration of probenecid and by ensuring adequate hydration. Reversible neutropenia has also occurred. Other adverse effects include nausea and vomiting, fever, asthenia, skin rash, dyspnoea, alopecia, and ocular hypotony (decreased intra-ocular pressure). Iritis or uveitis has been reported.

Effects on the kidneys. Dose-related nephrotoxicity is the most severe adverse effect of cidofovir and severe proteinuria has been reported in 13% of patients receiving it. Fanconi's syndrome associated with renal tubular damage has been reported in 2% of patients. In one such patient, Fanconi's syndrome occurred on the third injection of cidofovir and resulted in irreversible renal impairment.[1] A case of nephrogenic diabetes insipidus occurring without premonitory laboratory abnormalities has also been reported in a patient receiving cidofovir.[2]

1. Vittecoq D, *et al.* Fanconi syndrome associated with cidofovir therapy. *Antimicrob Agents Chemother* 1997; **41:** 1846.
2. Schliefer K, *et al.* Nephrogenic diabetes insipidus in a patient taking cidofovir. *Lancet* 1997; **350:** 413–14. Correction. *ibid.*; 1558.

Precautions

Cidofovir is contra-indicated in patients with renal impairment. Renal function should be measured before each dose and treatment should be interrupted or discontinued if renal function deteriorates. Patients should receive oral probenecid and prior intravenous hydration with each dose of cidofovir. Neutrophil counts should also be monitored and regular ophthalmological follow-up is recommended.

Patients with diabetes mellitus are at increased risk of ocular hypotony. Cidofovir is embryotoxic in *animals*. Cidofovir should not be administered during pregnancy and both sexes should use effective methods of contraception during and after cidofovir treatment. There is also a possibility that cidofovir may cause male infertility.

Interactions

Additive nephrotoxicity may occur if cidofovir is given with other nephrotoxic drugs including aminoglycosides, amphotericin, foscarnet, and intravenous pentamidine. The use of probenecid with cidofovir may alter the clearance of other drugs given concomitantly (see Interactions under Probenecid, p.395).

Antiviral Action

Cidofovir undergoes intracellular phosphorylation by cellular kinases to the antiviral metabolite, cidofovir diphosphate, which acts as a competitive inhibitor of viral DNA polymerase. It is active against a range of herpes viruses including cytomegalovirus, and, since its activity is not reliant on viral enzymes, may retain activity against aciclovir- and foscarnet-resistant viruses. Cross-resistance has been noted with ganciclovir *in vitro*.

References.

1. Moore MR, *et al.* Activity of (S)-1-(3-hydroxy-2-phosphonylmethoxypropyl) cytosine against human cytomegalovirus when administered as single-bolus dose and continuous infusion in in vitro cell culture perfusion system. *Antimicrob Agents Chemother* 1994; **38:** 2404–8.
2. Polis MA, *et al.* Anticytomegaloviral activity and safety of cidofovir in patients with human immunodeficiency virus infection and cytomegalovirus viruria. *Antimicrob Agents Chemother* 1995; **39:** 882–6.

Pharmacokinetics

Following intravenous administration of cidofovir, serum concentrations decline with a reported terminal half-life of about 2.6 hours (the intracellular half-life of the active diphosphate may be up to 65 hours). Cidofovir is eliminated mainly by renal excretion, both by glomerular filtration and tubular secretion. Approximately 90% of a dose is recovered unchanged from the urine within 24 hours. Concomitant administration of probenecid may reduce the excretion of cidofovir to some extent by blocking tubular secretion, although 70 to 85% has still been reported to be excreted unchanged in the urine within 24 hours.

References.

1. Cundy KC, *et al.* Clinical pharmacokinetics of cidofovir in human immunodeficiency virus-infected patients. *Antimicrob Agents Chemother* 1995; **39:** 1247–52.

Uses and Administration

Cidofovir is a nucleoside analogue which is active against herpesviruses. It is used in the treatment of cytomegalovirus retinitis (p.596) in patients with AIDS, and is being investigated for herpes simplex infections.

In the treatment of cytomegalovirus retinitis, cidofovir is given in a dose of 5 mg per kg body-weight by intravenous infusion over one hour once a week for two consecutive weeks, then once every 2 weeks. Probenecid 2 g is given by mouth 3 hours before each dose of cidofovir and further doses of probenecid 1 g at 2 and 8 hours after completion of the infusion. To ensure adequate hydration one litre of sodium chloride 0.9% is administered by intravenous infusion over one hour immediately before each infusion of cidofovir; if the additional fluid load can be tolerated, a further one litre of sodium chloride 0.9% may be infused over 1 to 3 hours, starting at the same time as (or immediately after) the cidofovir infusion. Treatment should be discontinued if renal function deteriorates during treatment (see Precautions, above).

Cidofovir has also been administered experimentally by intravitreal injection but the commercially available formulation is unsuitable for administration by this route.

An orally active prodrug of cidofovir known as cyclic-HPMPC (GS-930) is under investigation.

Reviews.

1. Lea AP, Bryson HM. Cidofovir. *Drugs* 1996; **52:** 225–30.

References.

1. Snoeck R, *et al.* A new topical treatment for resistant herpes simplex infections. *N Engl J Med* 1993; **329:** 968–9.
2. Lalezari JP, *et al.* Treatment with intravenous (S)-1-[3-hydroxy-2-(phoshonylmethoxy)propyl]-cytosine of acyclovir-resistant mucocutaneous infection with herpes simplex virus in a patient with AIDS. *J Infect Dis* 1994; **170:** 570–2.
3. Snoeck R, *et al.* Treatment of anogenital papillomavirus infections with an acyclic nucleoside phosphonate analogue. *N Engl J Med* 1995; **333:** 943–4.
4. Rahhal FM, *et al.* Treatment of cytomegalovirus retinitis with intravitreous cidofovir in patients with AIDS: a preliminary report. *Ann Intern Med* 1996; **125:** 98–103.
5. Studies of Ocular Complications of AIDS Research Group, AIDS Clinical Trials Group. Parenteral cidofovir for cytomegalovirus retinitis in patients with AIDS: the HPMPC peripheral cytomegalovirus retinitis trial: a randomized controlled trial. *Ann Intern Med* 1997; **126:** 264–74.
6. Lalezari JP, *et al.* Intravenous cidofovir for peripheral cytomegalovirus retinitis in patients with AIDS: a randomized, controlled trial. *Ann Intern Med* 1997; **126:** 257–63.

Preparations

Proprietary Preparations (details are given in Part 3)
UK: Vistide; ***USA:*** Vistide.

Delavirdine Mesylate (17191-k)

Delavirdine Mesylate *(USAN)*.

Delavirdine Mesilate *(rINNM)*; U-90152S. 1-[3-(Isopropylamino)-2-pyridyl]-4-[(5-methanesulfonamidoindol-2-yl)carbonyl]-piperazine monomethanesulfonate.

$C_{22}H_{28}N_6O_3S,CH_4O_3S$ = 552.7.

CAS — 136817-59-9 (delavirdine); 147221-93-0 (delavirdine mesylate).

Adverse Effects

The most common adverse effect of delavirdine is skin rash, usually occurring within the first 3 weeks of starting therapy and resolving in 3 to 14 days. Severe skin reactions including Stevens-Johnson syndrome have occurred.

Precautions

Delavirdine should be discontinued if a severe skin rash develops or if a rash is accompanied by fever, blistering, oral lesions, conjunctivitis, swelling, or muscle or joint aches. Delavirdine should be used with caution in patients with impaired hepatic function.

Interactions

Similarly to the HIV-protease inhibitors (see Indinavir, p.614), delavirdine is metabolised mainly by cytochrome P450 isoenzymes of the CYP3A family. Consequently it may compete with other drugs metabolised by this system, potentially resulting in toxic concentrations; co-administration of some non-sedating antihistamines, antiarrhythmics, calcium-channel blockers, cisapride, and ergot alkaloids may be particularly hazardous. Alternatively, enzyme inducers may decrease plasma concentrations of delavirdine. The absorption of delavirdine is reduced by drugs that raise gastric pH such as antacids and histamine H_2-receptor antagonists.

Other interactions with delavirdine may include:

antibacterials—plasma concentrations of both delavirdine and *clarithromycin* may be increased by concurrent administration; plasma concentrations of *rifabutin* may be increased by delavirdine; *rifabutin* and *rifampicin* may reduce delavirdine plasma concentrations

antidepressants—plasma concentrations of delavirdine may be increased by *fluoxetine*

antiepileptics—*carbamazepine, phenobarbitone*, and *phenytoin* may decrease plasma concentrations of delavirdine

antifungals—plasma concentrations of delavirdine may be increased by *ketoconazole*

antivirals—administration of delavirdine with *didanosine* may result in reduced plasma concentrations of both drugs; plasma concentrations of *indinavir* and *saquinavir* may be increased by delavirdine.

Pharmacokinetics

Delavirdine is rapidly absorbed following oral administration, peak plasma concentrations occurring after about one hour. It is about 98% bound to plasma proteins. Delavirdine is extensively metabolised by hepatic microsomal enzymes, principally by cytochrome P450 isoenzymes of the CYP3A family. It has been shown to reversibly inhibit P450 activity. Plasma half-life following the usual dosage has ranged from 2 to 11 hours. Delavirdine is excreted as metabolites in the urine and faeces. Less than 5% is excreted in the urine unchanged.

Uses and Administration

Delavirdine is a non-nucleoside reverse transcriptase inhibitor with activity against HIV-1. Viral resistance emerges rapidly when delavirdine is used alone, and it is therefore used in combination with other antiretroviral drugs in the treatment of HIV infection (p.599).

Delavirdine is given in a usual dose of 400 mg of delavirdine mesylate three times daily.

References.

1. Dueweke TJ, *et al.* U-90152, a potent inhibitor of human immunodeficiency virus type 1 replication. *Antimicrob Agents Chemother* 1993; **37:** 1127–31.
2. Davey RT, *et al.* Randomized, controlled phase I/II trial of combination therapy with delavirdine (U-90152S) and conventional nucleosides in human immunodeficiency virus type 1-infected patients. *Antimicrob Agents Chemother* 1996; **40:** 1657–64.

Preparations

Proprietary Preparations (details are given in Part 3)
Austral.: Rescriptor; ***USA:*** Rescriptor.

Desciclovir (16807-h)

Desciclovir *(USAN, rINN)*.

A-515U; BW-A515U; BW-515U; Deoxyacyclovir; 6-Deoxyacyclovir. 2-[(2-Amino-9*H*-purin-9-yl)methoxy]ethanol.

$C_8H_{11}N_5O_2$ = 209.2.

CAS — 84408-37-7.

Desciclovir is an aciclovir prodrug reported to provide higher plasma-aciclovir concentrations than aciclovir (p.602) following oral administration.

References.

1. Petty BG, *et al.* Pharmacokinetics and tolerance of desciclovir, a prodrug of acyclovir, in healthy human volunteers. *Antimicrob Agents Chemother* 1987; **31:** 1317–22.
2. Peterslund NA, *et al.* Open study of 2-amino-9-(hydroxyethoxymethyl)-9H-purine (desciclovir) in the treatment of herpes zoster. *J Antimicrob Chemother* 1987; **20:** 743–51.
3. Greenspan D, *et al.* Efficacy of desciclovir in the treatment of Epstein-Barr virus infection in oral hairy leukoplakia. *J Acquir Immune Defic Syndr* 1990; **3:** 571–8.

Didanosine (4889-e)

Didanosine *(BAN, USAN, rINN)*.

BMY-40900; DDI; ddI; ddIno; Dideoxyinosine; NSC-612049. 2′,3′-Dideoxyinosine.

$C_{10}H_{12}N_4O_3$ = 236.2.

CAS — 69655-05-6.

Adverse Effects

The most common serious adverse effects of didanosine are peripheral neuropathy and potentially fatal pancreatitis. Abnormal liver function tests may occur and hepatitis or fatal liver failure has been reported rarely. Retinal depigmentation and optic neuritis have been reported in patients receiving high doses of didanosine. Other adverse effects include nausea, vomiting, and abdominal pain (which may also be symptoms of pancreatitis), diarrhoea, headache, hyperglycaemia, myalgia, rash, hypersensitivity reactions, and hyperuricaemia.

Effects on the blood. In general, haematological abnormalities are less common in patients taking didanosine than in those taking zidovudine. However, there have been reports of thrombocytopenia associated with didanosine.[1-3]

1. Butler KM, *et al.* Dideoxyinosine in children with symptomatic human immunodeficiency virus infection. *N Engl J Med* 1991; **324:** 137–44.
2. Lor E, Liu YQ. Didanosine-associated eosinophilia with acute thrombocytopenia. *Ann Pharmacother* 1993; **27:** 23–5.
3. Herranz P, *et al.* Cutaneous vasculitis associated with didanosine. *Lancet* 1994; **344:** 680.

Effects on the eyes. Retinal lesions with atrophy of the retinal pigment epithelium at the periphery of the retina was reported in 4 children receiving didanosine doses of 270 to 540 mg per m^2 body-surface per day.[1]

1. Whitcup SM, *et al.* Retinal lesions in children treated with dideoxyinosine. *N Engl J Med* 1992; **326:** 1226–7.

Effects on glucose metabolism. Hyperglycaemia, glucose intolerance, diabetes mellitus, and hyperosmolar nonketotic diabetic syndrome have been associated with didanosine administration.[1-3] The effect may be dose-related, and has been reported in patients who subsequently developed pancreatitis (see below).[4] The manufacturer also reports cases of hypoglycaemia in patients taking didanosine.

1. Munshi MN, *et al.* Hyperosmolar nonketotic diabetic syndrome following treatment of human immunodeficiency virus infection with didanosine. *Diabetes Care* 1994; **17:** 316–17.
2. Jablonowski H, *et al.* A dose comparison study of didanosine in patients with very advanced HIV infection who are intolerant to or clinically deteriorate on zidovudine. *AIDS* 1995; **9:** 463–9.
3. Nguyen B-Y, *et al.* Five-year follow-up of a phase I study of didanosine in patients with advanced human immunodeficiency virus infection. *J Infect Dis* 1995; **171:** 1180–9.
4. Albrecht H, *et al.* Didanosine-induced disorders of glucose tolerance. *Ann Intern Med* 1993; **119:** 1050.

Effects on the liver. Fatal fulminant hepatic failure was reported[1] in a patient receiving didanosine. A further 14 cases have been noted by the manufacturer, and elevated liver enzymes have been recorded during clinical studies.[2-5]

1. Lai KK, *et al.* Fulminant hepatic failure associated with 2′,3′-dideoxyinosine (ddI). *Ann Intern Med* 1991; **115:** 283–4.
2. Dolin R, *et al.* Zidovudine compared with didanosine in patients with advanced HIV type 1 infection and little or no experience with zidovudine. *Arch Intern Med* 1995; **155:** 961–74.
3. Jablonowski H, *et al.* A dose comparison study of didanosine in patients with very advanced HIV infection who are intolerant to or clinically deteriorate on zidovudine. *AIDS* 1995; **9:** 463–9.
4. Alpha International Coordinating Committee. The Alpha trial: European/Australian randomized double-blind trial of two doses of didanosine in zidovudine-intolerant patients with symptomatic HIV disease. *AIDS* 1996; **10:** 867–80.
5. Gatell JM, *et al.* Switching from zidovudine to didanosine in patients with symptomatic HIV infection and disease progression. *J Acquir Immune Defic Syndr Hum Retrovirol* 1996; **12:** 249–58.

Effects on mental state. Recurrent mania was associated with didanosine treatment in one patient.[1]

1. Brouillette MJ, *et al.* Didanosine-induced mania in HIV infection. *Am J Psychiatry* 1994; **151:** 1839–40.

Effects on metabolism. Hyperuricaemia has been reported to be a common adverse effect during clinical studies of didanosine.[1,2] Hypokalaemia occurred during didanosine therapy in 3 patients, 2 of whom had diarrhoea.[3] There has also been a report of hypertriglyceridaemia occurring on 2 occasions in a patient given didanosine;[4] it was suggested that this hyperlipidaemic effect might be a possible aetiological factor in the development of pancreatitis. For effects on glucose metabolism, see above.

1. Cooley TP, *et al.* Once-daily administration of 2′,3′-dideoxyinosine (ddI) in patients with the acquired immunodeficiency syndrome or AIDS-related complex: results of a phase I trial. *N Engl J Med* 1990; **322:** 1340–5.
2. Montaner JSG, *et al.* Didanosine compared with continued zidovudine therapy for HIV-infected patients with 200 to 500 CD4 cells/mm^3: a double-blind, randomized, controlled trial. *Ann Intern Med* 1995; **123:** 561–71.
3. Katlama C, *et al.* Dideoxyinosine-associated hypokalaemia. *Lancet* 1991; **337:** 183.
4. Tal A, Dall L. Didanosine-induced hypertriglyceridemia. *Am J Med* 1993; **95:** 247.

Effects on the mouth. Xerostomia (dry mouth) may be a troublesome effect in patients receiving didanosine.[1,2]

1. Dodd CL, *et al.* Xerostomia associated with didanosine. *Lancet* 1992; **340:** 790.
2. Valentine C, *et al.* Xerostomia associated with didanosine. *Lancet* 1992; **340:** 1542.

Effects on the pancreas. Pancreatitis is recognised as being the most serious adverse effect of didanosine and can be fatal.[1-3] Pancreatitis appears to be dose-related, occurring in up to 13% of patients receiving 750 mg of didanosine daily.[2,4] Pancreatitis can resolve if didanosine is withdrawn[5] and cautious reintroduction of didanosine has been possible in some patients.[6] Raised amylase concentrations[3] and glucose intolerance (see above) have been reported in patients who subsequently developed pancreatitis.

1. Bouvet E, *et al.* Fatal case of 2′,3′-dideoxyinosine-associated pancreatitis. *Lancet* 1990; **336:** 1515.
2. Kahn JO, *et al.* A controlled trial comparing continued zidovudine with didanosine in human immunodeficiency virus infection. *N Engl J Med* 1992; **327:** 581–7.
3. Dolin R, *et al.* Zidovudine compared with didanosine in patients with advanced HIV-type 1 infection and little or no previous experience with zidovudine. *Arch Intern Med* 1995; **155:** 961–74.
4. Jablonowski H, *et al.* A dose comparison study of didanosine in patients with very advanced HIV infection who are intolerant to or clinically deteriorate on zidovudine. *AIDS* 1995; **9:** 463–9.
5. Nguyen B-Y, *et al.* Five-year follow-up of a phase I study of didanosine in patients with advanced human immunodeficiency virus infection. *J Infect Dis* 1995; **171:** 1180–9.
6. Butler KM, *et al.* Pancreatitis in human immunodeficiency virus-infected children receiving dideoxyinosine. *Pediatrics* 1993; **91:** 747–51.

Effects on the skin. Didanosine has been implicated in a case of the Stevens-Johnson syndrome[1] and of cutaneous vasculitis.[2]

1. Parneix-Spake A, *et al.* Didanosine as probable cause of Stevens-Johnson syndrome. *Lancet* 1992; **340:** 857–8.
2. Herranz P, *et al.* Cutaneous vasculitis associated with didanosine. *Lancet* 1994; **344:** 680.

Precautions

Patients with a history of pancreatitis and those with increased triglyceride concentrations should be observed carefully for signs of pancreatitis during treatment with didanosine. Treatment with didanosine should be interrupted in all patients who develop abdominal pain, nausea, or vomiting, or with raised serum amylase or lipase, until pancreatitis has been excluded. Once patients have recovered from pancreatitis they should only resume treatment with didanosine if it is essential and then using a low dose increased gradually if appropriate. Concomitant treatment with other drugs likely to cause pancreatitis or peripheral neuropathy (see Interactions, below) should be avoided if possible.

It may be necessary to interrupt didanosine treatment in patients who develop peripheral neuropathy; on recovery from peripheral neuropathy a reduced dose may be tolerated. Treatment should also be interrupted if uric acid concentrations are elevated.

Didanosine should be used with caution in patients with impaired renal or hepatic function, and dosage reduction may be necessary. If liver function deteriorates during treatment then didanosine should be withdrawn. Regular checks of liver function are therefore recommended.

Children should be monitored for retinal lesions and didanosine withdrawn if they occur. Monitoring should also be considered in adults.

Some tablet formulations of didanosine contain aspartame which, as a source of phenylalanine, should be taken into consideration when treating patients with phenylketonuria.

Interactions

Concurrent administration of didanosine with other drugs known to cause pancreatitis (for example intravenous pentamidine) or with drugs that may cause peripheral neuropathy (for example metronidazole, isoniazid, and vincristine) should be avoided. If co-administration is unavoidable, patients should be monitored carefully for these adverse effects.

A decrease in the area under the time-concentration curve for didanosine has been reported when *atovaquone* is given concurrently.

Since didanosine is generally taken in conjunction with an antacid (often included in the formulation), drugs which could be affected by an increased gastric pH (for example HIV-protease inhibitors, ketoconazole, fluoroquinolone antibacterials, and dapsone) should be given at least one hour before or after didanosine. Didanosine preparations containing magnesium or aluminium antacids should not be given with tetracyclines.

See also below for interactions with antivirals.

Antivirals. Increases in plasma concentrations of didanosine were reported when *ganciclovir* was given concurrently.[1,2] Changes in the pharmacokinetics of didanosine and *zidovudine* have occurred when these drugs are given together, but results of studies have not been consistent, and the effects have generally been of limited clinical significance. For further details, see under Interactions in Zidovudine, p.631.

Concurrent administration of didanosine and *delavirdine* resulted in reductions in the area under the concentration-time curve for both drugs in a single-dose study.[3] The manufacturer of delavirdine recommends that administration of these two drugs should be separated by at least 1 hour.

Absorption of some *HIV-protease inhibitors* may be reduced by the antacids in didanosine formulations and doses should be separated by at least 1 hour.

1. Trapnell CB, *et al.* Altered didanosine pharmacokinetics with concomitant oral ganciclovir. *Clin Pharmacol Ther* 1994; **55:** 193.
2. Griffy KG. Pharmacokinetics of oral ganciclovir capsules in HIV-infected persons. *AIDS* 1996; **10** (suppl 4): S3–S6.
3. Morse GD, *et al.* Single-dose pharmacokinetics of delavirdine mesylate and didanosine in patients with human immunodeficiency virus infection. *Antimicrob Agents Chemother* 1997; **41:** 169–74.

Antiviral Action

Didanosine is converted intracellularly to its active form dideoxyadenosine triphosphate. This triphosphate halts the DNA synthesis of retroviruses, including HIV, through competitive inhibition of reverse transcriptase and incorporation into viral DNA.

Resistance. Evidence for the development of didanosine-resistant HIV was reported in 36 of 64 patients with advanced HIV infection within 24 weeks of switching from zidovudine to didanosine monotherapy.[1] Patients with the didanosine resistance mutation for HIV reverse transcriptase showed a greater decline in CD4+ T cell count and increase in viral burden than those without.

1. Kozal MJ, *et al.* Didanosine resistance in HIV-infected patients switched from zidovudine to didanosine monotherapy. *Ann Intern Med* 1994; **121:** 263–8.

Pharmacokinetics

Didanosine is rapidly hydrolysed in the acid medium of the stomach and is therefore given by mouth with pH buffers or antacids. Bioavailability is reported to range from 20 to 40% depending on the formulation used; the bioavailability is substantially reduced by administration with or after food. Maximum plasma concentrations are achieved about 1 hour after oral administration. Binding to plasma proteins is reported to be less than 5%. The plasma elimination half-life ranges from 30 minutes to 4 hours.

CSF concentrations of didanosine have been about 20% of those in plasma following intravenous infusion; it has been reported not to cross the blood brain barrier following oral administration.

Didanosine is metabolised intracellularly to the active antiviral metabolite dideoxyadenosine triphosphate. Renal clearance by glomerular filtration and active tubular secretion represents about 50% of total body clearance. Didanosine is partially cleared by haemodialysis but not by peritoneal dialysis.

References.

1. Balis FM, *et al.* Clinical pharmacology of 2′,3′-dideoxyinosine in human immunodeficiency virus-infected children. *J Infect Dis* 1992; **165:** 99–104.
2. Morse GD, *et al.* Comparative pharmacokinetics of antiviral nucleoside analogues. *Clin Pharmacokinet* 1993; **24:** 101–23.
3. Mueller BU, *et al.* Clinical and pharmacokinetic evaluation of long-term therapy with didanosine in children with HIV infection. *Pediatrics* 1994; **94:** 724–31.

Pregnancy. Fetal blood concentrations of 14 and 19% of the maternal serum-didanosine concentrations have been reported.[1] There is evidence of extensive metabolism in the placenta.[2]

1. Pons JC, *et al.* Fetoplacental passage of 2′,3′-dideoxyinosine. *Lancet* 1991; **337:** 732.
2. Dancis J, *et al.* Transfer and metabolism of dideoxyinosine by the perfused human placenta. *J Acquir Immune Defic Syndr* 1993; **6:** 2–6.

Uses and Administration

Didanosine is a nucleoside reverse transcriptase inhibitor structurally related to inosine with activity against retroviruses including HIV. It is used in the treatment of HIV infection, usually in combination with other antiretroviral drugs.

Didanosine is administered by mouth, usually as buffered tablets or solution. The tablets have a bioavailability 20 to 25% greater than that of the solution. Doses should be taken at least 30 minutes before a meal. Doses for adults are: greater than 60 kg body-weight, 200 mg (tablets) or 250 mg (oral solution) every 12 hours; under 60 kg body-weight, 125 mg (tablets) or 167 mg (oral solution) every 12 hours.

Children's doses are determined by body-surface: children over 3 months of age may be given 120 mg per m^2 body-surface every 12 hours, or 90 mg per m^2 every 12 hours when didanosine is given in combination with zidovudine.

Dosage reduction may be necessary in patients with renal or hepatic impairment.

Reviews.

1. Shelton MJ, *et al.* Didanosine. *Ann Pharmacother* 1992; **26:** 660–70.
2. Faulds D, Brogden RN. Didanosine: a review of its antiviral activity, pharmacokinetic properties and therapeutic potential in human immunodeficiency virus infection. *Drugs* 1992; **44:** 94–116.
3. Lipsky JJ. Zalcitabine and didanosine. *Lancet* 1993; **341:** 30–2.
4. Perry CM, Balfour VA. Didanosine: an update on its antiviral activity, pharmacokinetic properties and therapeutic efficacy in the management of HIV disease. *Drugs* 1996; **52:** 928–62.

HIV infection and AIDS. Didanosine was found to be a useful alternative nucleoside reverse transcriptase inhibitor in patients with HIV infection who could not tolerate or no longer responded to zidovudine.[1-4] The trend in clinical practice is to use combinations of antiretroviral drugs at an earlier stage of infection (see p.599). In patients who had not received antiretroviral treatment in the past, didanosine in combination with zidovudine delayed disease progression and reduced mortality compared to zidovudine alone.[5,6] In patients who had received previous antiretroviral treatment, the benefit was less marked[5-8] but responses were better than with zidovudine plus zalcitabine.[5,6] Didanosine used in combination with hydroxyurea has produced promising preliminary results (see p.539), and combinations including didanosine and interferons are also being investigated.[9] The use of doses of up to 750 mg didanosine daily has generally failed to produce better responses than conventional doses of up to 500 mg daily.[1,10,11] Reducing the dose to 200 mg daily has been tried but responses have been variable.[12,13] Although didanosine has been detected in the CNS following intravenous administration, a higher incidence of AIDS dementia complex was reported in patients with advanced disease receiving didanosine than in those receiving zidovudine.[14] However didanosine therapy reduced pathological changes in patients with less advanced CNS disease to a similar extent to zidovudine.[15] Didanosine has also been of benefit in children with HIV infection,[16,17] and a preliminary study found that didanosine in combination with stavudine was well tolerated.[18]

1. Kahn JO, *et al.* A controlled trial comparing continued zidovudine with didanosine in human immunodeficiency virus infection. *N Engl J Med* 1992; **327:** 581–7.
2. Spruance LS, *et al.* Didanosine compared with continuation of zidovudine in HIV-infected patients with signs of clinical deterioration while receiving zidovudine: a randomized, double-blind clinical trial. *Ann Intern Med* 1994; **120:** 360–8.
3. Abrams DI, *et al.* A comparative trial of didanosine or zalcitabine after treatment with zidovudine in patients with human immunodeficiency virus infection. *N Engl J Med* 1994; **330:** 657–62.
4. Montaner JSG, *et al.* Didanosine compared with continued zidovudine therapy for HIV-infected patients with 200 to 500 CD4 cells/mm³: a double-blind, randomized, controlled trial. *Ann Intern Med* 1995; **123:** 561–71.
5. Delta Coordinating Committee. Delta: a randomised double-blind controlled trial comparing combinations of zidovudine plus didanosine or zalcitabine with zidovudine alone in HIV-infected individuals. *Lancet* 1996; **348:** 283–91.
6. Hammer SM, *et al.* A trial comparing nucleoside monotherapy with combination therapy in HIV-infected adults with CD4 cell counts from 200 to 500 per cubic millimeter. *N Engl J Med* 1996; **335:** 1081–90.
7. Graham NMH, *et al.* Survival in HIV-infected patients who have received zidovudine: comparison of combination therapy with sequential monotherapy and continued zidovudine monotherapy. *Ann Intern Med* 1996; **124:** 1031–8.
8. D'Aquila RT, *et al.* Nevirapine, zidovudine, and didanosine compared with zidovudine and didanosine in patients with HIV-1 infection: a randomized, double-blind, placebo-controlled trial. *Ann Intern Med* 1996; **124:** 1019–30.
9. Kovacs JA, *et al.* Combination therapy with didanosine and interferon-α in human immunodeficiency virus-infected patients: results of a phase I/II trial. *J Infect Dis* 1996; **173:** 840–8.
10. Jablonowski H, *et al.* A dose comparison study of didanosine in patients with very advanced HIV infection who are intolerant to or clinically deteriorate on zidovudine. *AIDS* 1995; **9:** 463–9.
11. Dolin R, *et al.* Zidovudine compared with didanosine in patients with advanced HIV type 1 infection and little or no previous experience with zidovudine. *Arch Intern Med* 1995; **155:** 961–74.
12. Alpha International Coordinating Committee. The Alpha trial: European/Australian randomized double-blind trial of two doses of didanosine in zidovudine-intolerant patients with symptomatic HIV disease. *AIDS* 1996; **10:** 867–80.
13. Gatell JM, *et al.* Switching from zidovudine to didanosine in patients with symptomatic HIV infection and disease progression. *J Acquir Immune Defic Syndr Hum Retrovirol* 1996; **12:** 249–58.
14. Portegies P, *et al.* AIDS dementia complex and didanosine. *Lancet* 1994; **344:** 759.
15. Chrétien F, *et al.* Protection of human immunodeficiency virus encephalitis by a switch from zidovudine to didanosine. *Antimicrob Agents Chemother* 1996; **40:** 278.
16. Butler KM, *et al.* Dideoxyinosine in children with symptomatic human immunodeficiency virus infection. *N Engl J Med* 1991; **324:** 137–44.
17. Blanche S, *et al.* Randomized study of two doses of didanosine in children infected with human immunodeficiency virus. *J Pediatr* 1993; **122:** 966–73.
18. Kline MW, *et al.* Combination therapy with stavudine and didanosine in children with advanced human immunodeficiency virus infection: pharmacokinetic properties, safety, and immunologic and virologic effects. *Pediatrics* 1996; **97:** 886–90.

Preparations

Proprietary Preparations (details are given in Part 3)
Aust.: Videx; ***Austral.:*** Videx; ***Belg.:*** Videx; ***Canad.:*** Videx; ***Fr.:*** Videx; ***Ger.:*** Videx; ***Irl.:*** Videx; ***Ital.:*** Videx; ***Neth.:*** Videx; ***Norw.:*** Videx; ***S.Afr.:*** Videx; ***Spain:*** Videx; ***Swed.:*** Videx; ***Switz.:*** Videx; ***UK:*** Videx; ***USA:*** Videx.

Dideoxyadenosine (19231-h)

ddA; ddAdo.

Dideoxyadenosine is a nucleoside reverse transcriptase inhibitor structurally related to adenosine with antiviral activity against HIV, but is reported to have been abandoned because of renal toxicity.

References.

1. Hartman NR, *et al.* Pharmacokinetics of 2′,3′-dideoxyadenosine and 2′,3′-dideoxyinosine in patients with severe human immunodeficiency virus infection. *Clin Pharmacol Ther* 1990; **47:** 647–54.

Ditiocarb Sodium (1054-y)

Ditiocarb Sodium *(rINN).*

DDTC; Dithiocarb Sodium; DTC; Sodium Diethyldithiocarbamate.

$C_5H_{10}NNaS_2$ = 171.3.

CAS — 148-18-5.

Ditiocarb sodium is an immunomodulating drug that has been investigated in HIV infection. It is also a chelator that has been used in the destruction of cisplatin wastes and has been suggested for use in nickel carbonyl poisoning. Disulfiram is rapidly metabolised to ditiocarb; for its further metabolism see p.1573.

Reviews.

1. Renoux G. Immunopharmacologie et pharmacologie du diethyldithiocarbamate (DTC). *J Pharmacol* 1982; **13** (suppl 1): 95–134.

HIV infection and AIDS. Ditiocarb has been tried in patients with HIV infection and AIDS with some success.[1-4] However, a study involving 1300 patients indicated a faster rate of progression to AIDS in patients receiving ditiocarb[5] and as a result of this another study, which had found no improvement in immune function, but evidence of haematological toxicity, was halted early.[6] The more usual treatment of HIV infection and AIDS is discussed on p.599.

1. Lang J-M, *et al.* Randomised, double-blind, placebo-controlled trial of ditiocarb sodium ('Imuthiol') in human immunodeficiency virus infection. *Lancet* 1988; **ii:** 702–6.
2. Lang J-M, *et al.* Immunomodulation with diethyldithiocarbamate in patients with AIDS-related complex. *Lancet* 1985; **ii:** 1066.
3. Reisinger EC, *et al.* Inhibition of HIV progression by dithiocarb. *Lancet* 1990; **335:** 679–82.
4. Hersh EM, *et al.* Ditiocarb sodium (diethyldithiocarbamate) therapy in patients with symptomatic HIV infection and AIDS: a randomized, double-blind, placebo-controlled, multicenter study. *JAMA* 1991; **265:** 1538–44.
5. HIV87 Study Group. Multicenter, randomized, placebo-controlled study of ditiocarb (Imuthiol) in human immunodeficiency virus-infected asymptomatic and minimally symptomatic patients. *AIDS Res Hum Retroviruses* 1993; **9:** 83–9.
6. Shenep JL, *et al.* Decreased counts of blood neutrophils, monocytes, and platelets in human immunodeficiency virus-infected children and young adults treated with diethyldithiocarbamate. *Antimicrob Agents Chemother* 1994; **38:** 1644–6.

1-Docosanol (15188-g)

Behenyl Alcohol; *n*-Docosanol; Docosyl Alcohol; IK-2.

$CH_3(CH_2)_{21}OH$ = 326.6.

CAS — 661-19-8.

1-Docosanol is an antiviral under investigation for the topical treatment of superficial herpes simplex infections.

Edoxudine (12706-e)

Edoxudine *(USAN, rINN).*

EDU; Ethyl Deoxyuridine; EUDR; ORF-15817; RWJ-15817. 2′-Deoxy-5-ethyluridine.

$C_{11}H_{16}N_2O_5$ = 256.3.

CAS — 15176-29-1.

Edoxudine is an antiviral active against herpes simplex. It is used topically as a 3% cream or 1.2% gel in the treatment of mucocutaneous infections and has been used at a concentration of 0.3% in ophthalmic infections.

Herpes simplex infections. Herpes simplex infections requiring antiviral therapy are usually treated with aciclovir (see p.597). In general, systemic administration is preferred to topical. However, edoxudine has been reported to preferentially inhibit herpes simplex virus type 2 *in vitro*[1] and a multicentre study[2] involving 200 patients with genital herpes found that edoxudine 3% cream applied 6 times daily for 5 days (in 103) reduced viral shedding compared with placebo (in 97); symptoms in women, but not in men, were decreased by active treatment.

1. Teh C-Z, Sacks SL. Susceptibility of recent clinical isolates of herpes simplex virus to 5-ethyl-2′-deoxyuridine: preferential inhibition of herpes simplex virus type 2. *Antimicrob Agents Chemother* 1983; **23:** 637–40.
2. Sacks SL, *et al.* Randomized, double-blind, placebo-controlled, clinic-initiated, Canadian multicenter trial of topical edoxudine 3.0% cream in the treatment of recurrent genital herpes. *J Infect Dis* 1991; **164:** 665–72.

Preparations

Proprietary Preparations (details are given in Part 3)
Canad.: Virostat; ***Ger.:*** Aedurid†; ***Switz.:*** Edurid.

Efavirenz (3463-d)

Efavirenz *(rINN).*

DMP-266; L-743726. (*S*)-6-Chloro-4-(cyclopropylethynyl)-1,4-dihydro-4-(trifluoromethyl)-2*H*-3,1-benzoxazin-2-one.

$C_{14}H_9ClF_3NO_2$ = 315.7.

Efavirenz is a non-nucleoside reverse transcriptase inhibitor with activity against HIV. It is used in the treatment of HIV infection and is usually given in combination with other antiretroviral drugs.

Preparations

Proprietary Preparations (details are given in Part 3)
USA: Sustiva.

Famciclovir (10521-s)

Famciclovir *(BAN, USAN, rINN).*

BRL-42810. 2[2-(2-Amino-9*H*-purin-9-yl)ethyl]trimethylene diacetate.

$C_{14}H_{19}N_5O_4$ = 321.3.

CAS — 104227-87-4.

Adverse Effects and Precautions

The most common adverse effects of famciclovir are headache and nausea. Other adverse effects include vomiting, dizziness, skin rash, confusion, and hallucinations. In addition, abdominal pain, fever, and, rarely, granulocytopenia and thrombocytopenia have been reported in immunocompromised patients receiving famciclovir.

Dosage should be reduced in patients with impaired renal function.

References.

1. Saltzman R, *et al.* Safety of famciclovir in patients with herpes zoster and genital herpes. *Antimicrob Agents Chemother* 1994; **38:** 2454–7.

Pharmacokinetics

Famciclovir is rapidly absorbed following oral administration. Absorption is delayed but not reduced by administration with food. It is rapidly converted to penciclovir (see p.624), peak plasma concentrations occurring within about an hour of administration, and virtually no famciclovir is detectable in the plasma or urine. Bioavailability of penciclovir is reported to be 77%. Famciclovir is principally excreted in the urine (partly by renal tubular secretion) as penciclovir and its 6-deoxy precursor: elimination is reduced in patients with impaired renal function.

References.

1. Pue MA, Benet LZ. Pharmacokinetics of famciclovir in man. *Antiviral Chem Chemother* 1993; **4** (suppl 1): 47–55.
2. Boike SC, *et al.* Pharmacokinetics of famciclovir in subjects with varying degrees of renal impairment. *Clin Pharmacol Ther* 1994; **55:** 418–26.
3. Boike SC, *et al.* Pharmacokinetics of famciclovir in subjects with chronic hepatic disease. *J Clin Pharmacol* 1994; **34:** 1199–1207.
4. Gill KS, Wood MJ. The clinical pharmacokinetics of famciclovir. *Clin Pharmacokinet* 1996; **31:** 1–8.

Uses and Administration

Famciclovir is a prodrug of the antiviral penciclovir (p.624). It is given by mouth in the treatment of herpes zoster (see Varicella-zoster Infections, p.598) and genital herpes (see Herpes Simplex Infections, p.597).

For **herpes zoster**, famciclovir is given in a dose of 250 mg three times daily, or 750 mg once daily, for 7 days (in the USA the recommended dose is 500 mg three times daily for 7 days); immunocompromised patients are given 500 mg three times daily for 10 days.

For *first episodes* of **genital herpes**, famciclovir is given in a dose of 250 mg three times daily for 5 days; immunocompromised patients are given 500 mg twice daily for 7 days. For *acute treatment of recurrent episodes of genital herpes*, 125 mg is given twice daily for 5 days; immunocompromised patients are given 500 mg twice daily for 7 days. For *suppression of recurrent episodes of genital herpes*, 250 mg is given twice daily; HIV patients may be given 500 mg twice daily. Such suppressive treatment is interrupted every 6 to 12 months in order to recognise possible changes in the natural history of the disease.

Doses of famciclovir are reduced in patients with renal impairment (see below).

General references.

1. Vere Hodge RA. Famciclovir and penciclovir: the mode of action of famciclovir including its conversion to penciclovir. *Antiviral Chem Chemother* 1993; **4:** 67–84.
2. Perry CM, Wagstaff AJ. Famciclovir: a review of its pharmacological properties and therapeutic efficacy in herpesvirus infections. *Drugs* 1995; **50:** 396–415.

Administration in renal impairment. Doses of famciclovir need to be reduced in patients with impaired renal function. For herpes zoster or an initial episode of genital herpes the UK manufacturer suggests 250 mg twice daily for patients with a creatinine clearance of 30 to 59 mL per minute, and 250 mg once daily for those with a creatinine clearance of 10 to 29 mL per minute; in patients with recurrent genital herpes, modification of dosage is only suggested for a creatinine clearance of 10 to 29 mL per minute, when the dose is 125 mg once daily for treatment of acute recurrence or twice daily for suppression. Corresponding reductions are suggested for immunocompromised patients. Patients on haemodialysis should be given doses of famciclovir immediately following dialysis.

Viral infections. Some studies of the use of famciclovir in herpes zoster,[1-3] genital herpes,[4-7] and hepatitis B.[8]

1. Degreef H, *et al.* Famciclovir, a new oral antiherpes drug: results of the first controlled clinical study demonstrating its efficacy and safety in the treatment of uncomplicated herpes zoster in immunocompetent patients. *Int J Antimicrob Agents* 1994; **4:** 241–6.
2. Tyring S, *et al.* Famciclovir for the treatment of acute herpes zoster: effects on acute disease and postherpetic neuralgia: a randomized, double-blind, placebo-controlled trial. *Ann Intern Med* 1995; **123:** 89–96.
3. Klein JL, *et al.* Famciclovir in AIDS-related acute retinal necrosis. *AIDS* 1996; **10:** 1300–1.
4. Sacks SL, *et al.* Patient-initiated, twice daily oral famciclovir for early recurrent genital herpes: a randomized, double-blind multicenter trial. *JAMA* 1996; **276:** 44–9.
5. Mertz GJ, *et al.* Oral famciclovir for suppression of recurrent genital herpes simplex virus infection in women: a multicenter, double-blind, placebo-controlled trial. *Arch Intern Med* 1997; **157:** 343–9.
6. Schacker T, *et al.* Famciclovir for the suppression of symptomatic and asymptomatic herpes simplex virus reactivation in HIV-infected persons: a double-blind, placebo-controlled trial. *Ann Intern Med* 1998; **128:** 21–8.
7. Diaz-Mitoma F, *et al.* Oral famciclovir for the suppression of recurrent genital herpes: a randomized controlled trial. *JAMA* 1998; **280:** 887–92.
8. Main J, *et al.* A double blind, placebo-controlled study to assess the effect of famciclovir on virus replication in patients with chronic hepatitis B virus infection. *J Viral Hepatitis* 1996; **3:** 211–15.

Preparations

Proprietary Preparations (details are given in Part 3)
Aust.: Famvir; ***Austral.:*** Famvir; ***Belg.:*** Famvir; ***Canad.:*** Famvir; ***Ger.:*** Famvir; ***Irl.:*** Famvir; ***Neth.:*** Famvir; ***S.Afr.:*** Famvir; ***Spain:*** Famvir; ***Swed.:*** Famvir; ***Switz.:*** Famvir; ***UK:*** Famvir; ***USA:*** Famvir.

Fiacitabine (10251-m)

Fiacitabine *(USAN, rINN).*

FIAC; Fluoroiodoaracytosine; 2′-Fluoro-5-iodo-aracytosine. 1-(2-Deoxy-2-fluoro-β-D-arabinofuranosyl)-5-iodocytosine.

$C_9H_{11}FIN_3O_4$ = 371.1.

CAS — 69123-90-6 (fiacitabine); 69124-05-6 (fiacitabine hydrochloride).

Fiacitabine is a nucleoside analogue reported to be active against various herpesviruses including herpes simplex viruses.

Fialuridine (19187-j)

Fialuridine *(USAN, rINN).*

FIAU; Fluoroiodoarauracil. 1-(2-Deoxy-2-fluoro-β-D-arabinofuranosyl)-5-iodouracil.

$C_9H_{10}FIN_2O_5$ = 372.1.

CAS — 69123-98-4.

Fialuridine is a synthetic nucleoside analogue structurally related to thymidine with activity against hepatitis B virus. Clinical studies were suspended after hepatic failure and lactic acidosis, including several fatalities, were associated with its use.

References.

1. McKenzie R, *et al.* Hepatic failure and lactic acidosis due to fialuridine (FIAU), an investigational nucleoside analogue for chronic hepatitis B. *N Engl J Med* 1995; **333:** 1099–1105.
2. Honkoop P, *et al.* Mitochondrial injury: lessons from the fialuridine trial. *Drug Safety* 1997; **17:** 1–7.

Fomivirsen (17347-r)

Fomivirsen *(rINN).*

$C_{204}H_{263}N_{63}O_{114}P_{20}S_{20}$ = 6682.4.

CAS — 144245-52-3.

Fomivirsen is an antisense oligonucleotide that is used as the sodium salt for the local treatment of cytomegalovirus retinitis in patients with AIDS.

Foscarnet Sodium (16817-b)

Foscarnet Sodium *(BAN, USAN, rINN).*

A-29622; EHB-776 (anhydrous and hexahydrate); Phosphonatoformate Trisodium; Phosphonoformate Trisodium. Trisodium phosphonatoformate hexahydrate.

$CNa_3O_5P,6H_2O$ = 300.0.

CAS — 63585-09-1 (foscarnet sodium); 34156-56-4 (foscarnet sodium hexahydrate).

Pharmacopoeias. In Br.

A white crystalline powder. **Soluble** in water; practically insoluble in alcohol. A 2% solution has a pH of 9.0 to 11.0.

Each g of monograph substance represents about 15.6 mmol of sodium and about 5.2 mmol of phosphate.

Incompatibility. Foscarnet sodium has been found to be visually incompatible with a number of commonly used injectable drugs including aciclovir sodium, ganciclovir, certain antibacterials, amphotericin, pentamidine isethionate, and trimetrexate. The manufacturer also lists incompatibilities with glucose 30% solutions and solutions containing calcium along with a range of other drugs. It is therefore recommended that foscarnet should not be infused via an intravenous line with any other drugs.

References.

1. Lor E, Takagi J. Visual compatibility of foscarnet with other injectable drugs. *Am J Hosp Pharm* 1990; **47:** 157–9.
2. Baltz JK, *et al.* Visual compatibility of foscarnet with other injectable drugs during simulated Y-site administration. *Am J Hosp Pharm* 1990; **47:** 2075–7.

Sterilisation. No reduction in foscarnet concentration or change in pH was detected following sterilisation of a solution of foscarnet sodium 12 mg per mL in 0.9% sodium chloride injection packed in glass infusion bottles with rubber stoppers by autoclaving at 121° at 30 psi for 15 minutes.[1]

1. Stolk LM, *et al.* Autoclave and long-term sterility of foscarnet sodium admixtures. *Am J Health-Syst Pharm* 1995; **52:** 103.

Adverse Effects and Treatment

Intravenous injection of foscarnet sodium may cause phlebitis at the site of injection. Foscarnet sodium can produce renal impairment and some patients have required haemodialysis. Anaemia may be common and granulocytopenia and thrombocytopenia have been reported. Foscarnet sodium may cause hypocalcaemia and other electrolyte disturbances. Some patients may experience convulsions. Other adverse effects reported include nausea, vomiting, and diarrhoea; malaise; headache, fatigue, dizziness, paraesthesia, and tremor; mood disturbances; rash; abnormal liver function tests; blood pressure and ECG changes; genital ulceration; and isolated reports of pancreatitis.

In cases of overdosage it is important to maintain hydration, and foscarnet elimination may be increased by haemodialysis.

Effects on the CNS. Convulsions may occur in up to 10% of AIDS patients receiving foscarnet and have been reported following overdoses. Contributing factors include underlying CNS pathology (HIV-related encephalopathy or other infections) and foscarnet-related electrolyte disturbances. However, seizures have been reported in patients without apparent risk factors.[1]

1. Lor E, Liu YQ. Neurologic sequelae associated with foscarnet therapy. *Ann Pharmacother* 1994; **28:** 1035–7.

Effects on electrolyte balance. Foscarnet chelates divalent metal ions and acute hypocalcaemia has been reported to occur in about 15% of patients receiving foscarnet. Other electrolyte disturbances include hypokalaemia and hypomagnesaemia (each in about 15%), hypophosphataemia (8%), and hyperphosphataemia (6%). Hypocalcaemia may cause paraesthesias and, together with hypomagnesaemia and hypokalaemia, may predispose to seizures (see Effects on the CNS, above) and cardiovascular disturbances. Administration of foscarnet in a liposomal formulation has been proposed to overcome the effects on electrolytes.[1]

1. Omar RF, *et al.* Liposomal encapsulation of foscarnet protects against hypocalcemia induced by free foscarnet. *Antimicrob Agents Chemother* 1995; **39:** 1973–8.

Effects on the kidneys. The most serious common adverse effect of foscarnet sodium is nephrotoxicity. Clinically significant increases in serum-creatinine concentrations occur in about 30% of patients, and the incidence of nephrotoxicity tends to increase with increasing dose[1] and duration of therapy.[2] Foscarnet sodium is excreted unchanged in the urine and tubulo-interstitial lesions and deposition of crystals in the glomerular capillary lumen have been implicated.[3] Acute renal failure has occurred and haemodialysis has been reported to have reduced plasma-foscarnet concentrations in one patient.[4] The risk of nephrotoxicity can be minimised by ensuring adequate hydration, the use of intermittent dosing schedules,[5] and adjusting the dose according to serum-creatinine concentrations. Nephrogenic diabetes insipidus associated with foscarnet sodium has been reported.[6,7]

1. Jacobson MA, *et al.* A dose-ranging study of daily maintenance intravenous foscarnet therapy for cytomegalovirus retinitis in AIDS. *J Infect Dis* 1993; **168:** 444–8.
2. Gaub J, *et al.* The effect of foscarnet (phosphonoformate) on human immunodeficiency virus isolation, T-cell subsets and lymphocyte function in AIDS patients. *AIDS* 1987; **1:** 27–33.
3. Beaufils H, *et al.* Foscarnet and crystals in glomerular capillary lumens. *Lancet* 1990; **336:** 755.
4. Deray G, *et al.* Foscarnet-induced acute renal failure and effectiveness of haemodialysis. *Lancet* 1987; **ii:** 216.
5. Deray G, *et al.* Prevention of foscarnet nephrotoxicity. *Ann Intern Med* 1990; **113:** 332.
6. Farese RV, *et al.* Nephrogenic diabetes insipidus associated with foscarnet treatment of cytomegalovirus retinitis. *Ann Intern Med* 1990; **112:** 955–6.
7. Conn J, *et al.* Nephrogenic diabetes insipidus associated with foscarnet—a case report. *J Antimicrob Chemother* 1996; **37:** 1180–1.

Effects on the skin and mucous membranes. A generalised pruritic macular rash was reported in a patient receiving foscarnet which subsided after the drug was withdrawn.[1]

There have been several reports of genital ulceration,[2-7] possibly related to local toxicity arising from high concentrations of foscarnet in the urine. Oral ulceration has occurred, usually in patients also presenting with genital ulceration during foscarnet treatment.[3-5] Uvular and oesophageal ulcerations have also been reported.[4,8]

1. Green ST, *et al.* Generalised cutaneous rash associated with foscarnet usage in AIDS. *J Infect* 1990; **21:** 227–8.
2. Van Der Pijl JW, *et al.* Foscarnet and penile ulceration. *Lancet* 1990; **335:** 286.
3. Gilquin J, *et al.* Genital and oral erosions induced by foscarnet. *Lancet* 1990; **335:** 287.
4. Fégueux S, *et al.* Penile ulcerations with foscarnet. *Lancet* 1990; **335:** 547.
5. Moyle G, *et al.* Penile ulcerations with foscarnet. *Lancet* 1990; **335:** 547–8.
6. Lacey HB, *et al.* Vulval ulceration associated with foscarnet. *Genitourin Med* 1992; **68:** 182.
7. Caumes E, *et al.* Foscarnet-induced vulval erosion. *J Am Acad Dermatol* 1993; **28:** 799.
8. Saint-Marc T, *et al.* Uvula and oesophageal ulcerations with foscarnet. *Lancet* 1992; **340:** 970–1.

Precautions

Foscarnet sodium should be used with caution in renal impairment and doses should be reduced if serum creatinine is raised. Serum-creatinine concentrations should be measured on alternate days throughout induction treatment; monitoring may be weekly during maintenance therapy. An adequate state of hydration must be maintained during therapy to prevent renal toxicity. Electrolytes, especially calcium and magnesium, should also be monitored. Extreme caution must be taken when co-administering other potentially nephrotoxic drugs, such as pentamidine. Care is also needed when administering foscarnet sodium with other drugs, including pentamidine, that reduce serum-calcium concentrations.

The manufacturers contra-indicate foscarnet sodium in pregnancy and during breast feeding.

Interactions

Foscarnet should not be given concurrently with other nephrotoxic drugs or with other drugs which can affect serum-calcium concentrations. Intravenous pentamidine can produce both of these effects and severe additive toxicity may result from its use in combination with foscarnet.

Ciprofloxacin. Tonic-clonic seizures associated with foscarnet administration in 2 patients receiving multiple antimicrobial drugs were thought to have been exacerbated by the concurrent administration of ciprofloxacin.[1]

1. Fan-Havard P, *et al.* Concurrent use of foscarnet and ciprofloxacin may increase the propensity for seizures. *Ann Pharmacother* 1994; **28:** 869–72.

Antiviral Action

Foscarnet inhibits replication of human herpesviruses including cytomegalovirus, herpes simplex virus types 1 and 2, herpesvirus 6 (see under Ganciclovir, p.612), Epstein-Barr virus, and varicella-zoster virus. Activity is also reported against hepatitis B virus and HIV. Foscarnet acts by inhibition of virus-specific DNA polymerases and reverse transcriptases: unlike the nucleoside reverse transcriptase inhibitors and ganciclovir, foscarnet does not require intracellular conversion to an active triphosphate.

Pharmacokinetics

The pharmacokinetics of foscarnet are complicated by the high incidence of renal function impairment during therapy and by the deposition and subsequent gradual release of foscarnet from bone. Thus the estimation of half-life depends upon the duration of foscarnet therapy and the duration of the observation period. Terminal half-lives of up to 87 hours have been reported. Plasma protein binding is about 14 to 17%. Foscarnet crosses the blood-brain barrier in variable amounts; CSF concentrations of between 0 and 300% of plasma concentrations have been reported. Foscarnet is mostly excreted unchanged in the urine.

The pharmacokinetics of foscarnet [sodium] during and after continuous intravenous infusion (0.14 to 0.19 mg per kg body-weight per minute) was studied in 13 HIV-infected male patients with lymphadenopathy or AIDS-related complex.[1] During infusion there was a wide inter- and intra-individual variation in plasma-foscarnet concentrations, which ranged from approximately 100 to 500 µmol per litre. There appeared to be a link between the degree of adverse effects experienced and plasma-foscarnet concentrations above 350 µmol per litre. Foscarnet was excreted mainly via the kidneys. It was thought that up to 20% of the cumulative intravenous dose may have been deposited in bone 7 days after the end of infusion.

A similar foscarnet pharmacokinetic study was performed in 8 AIDS patients with cytomegalovirus retinitis treated every 8 hours intermittently with 2-hour infusions.[2] This method of administration produced plasma concentrations high enough to exert an antiviral effect.

Penetration of foscarnet into the CSF is very variable. Lumbar puncture was performed in 5 patients[1] and foscarnet was found to be distributed into the CSF at concentrations of 13 to 68% of those in the plasma. Subsequent studies have shown that CSF concentrations of foscarnet would be virostatic in the majority of patients[3] attaining a mean concentration of about 25% of plasma concentrations following a single infusion[3,4] and 66% under steady state conditions.[4] Concentrations ranged from 0 to 340% and 5 to 72%:[4] Raffi *et al.*[3] found a correlation between the amount of foscarnet in the CSF and the inflammation of the meninges, and Hengge[4] with the HIV infection stage, but neither reported a correlation with plasma concentration.

1. Sjövall J, *et al.* Pharmacokinetics of foscarnet and distribution to cerebrospinal fluid after intravenous infusion in patients with human immunodeficiency virus infection. *Antimicrob Agents Chemother* 1989; **33:** 1023–31.
2. Aweeka F, *et al.* Pharmacokinetics of intermittently administered intravenous foscarnet in the treatment of acquired immunodeficiency syndrome patients with serious cytomegalovirus retinitis. *Antimicrob Agents Chemother* 1989; **33:** 742–5.
3. Raffi F, *et al.* Penetration of foscarnet into cerebrospinal fluid of AIDS patients. *Antimicrob Agents Chemother* 1993; **37:** 1777–80.
4. Hengge UR, *et al.* Foscarnet penetrates the blood-brain barrier: rationale for therapy of cytomegalovirus encephalitis. *Antimicrob Agents Chemother* 1993; **37:** 1010–14.

Uses and Administration

Foscarnet sodium is a non-nucleoside pyrophosphate analogue active against herpes viruses. It is used mainly for the treatment of cytomegalovirus (CMV) retinitis in AIDS patients and for aciclovir-resistant herpes simplex virus infections in immunocompromised patients.

Foscarnet is administered by intravenous infusion. It is usually available as an infusion containing 24 mg of foscarnet sodium per mL. This may be administered via a central vein or diluted with glucose 5% or sodium chloride 0.9% to a concentration of 12 mg per mL and administered via a peripheral vein. Hydration with 0.5 to 1 litre of sodium chloride 0.9% may be given with each infusion to reduce renal toxicity.

For the treatment of cytomegalovirus retinitis in adults with normal renal function a usual dose is 60 mg per kg body-weight infused over at least one hour every 8 hours for 2 to 3 weeks, followed by maintenance therapy with 60 mg per kg daily increasing to 90 to 120 mg per kg daily if tolerated. For the treatment of aciclovir-resistant herpes simplex virus infections in adults with normal renal function, a dose of 40 mg per kg, infused over 1 hour, every 8 hours may be given for 2 to 3 weeks or until lesions have healed.

Doses should be reduced in patients with impaired renal function (see below).

Reviews.

1. Chrisp P, Clissold SP. Foscarnet: a review of its antiviral activity, pharmacokinetic properties and therapeutic use in immunocompromised patients with cytomegalovirus retinitis. *Drugs* 1991; **41:** 104–29.
2. Wagstaff AJ, Bryson HM. Foscarnet: a reappraisal of its antiviral activity, pharmacokinetic properties and therapeutic use in immunocompromised patients with viral infections. *Drugs* 1994; **48:** 199–226.

Administration in renal impairment. For patients with varying degrees of renal impairment [based on creatinine clearance (CC)] the manufacturers of foscarnet sodium consider the following doses to be equivalent to the 60 mg per kg body-weight dose given to patients with normal renal function for the treatment of cytomegalovirus infection:

- for CC more than 1.6 mL per kg per minute, 60 mg per kg
- for CC 1.6 to 1.4 mL per kg per minute, 55 mg per kg
- for CC 1.4 to 1.2 mL per kg per minute, 49 mg per kg
- for CC 1.2 to 1.0 mL per kg per minute, 42 mg per kg
- for CC 1.0 to 0.8 mL per kg per minute, 35 mg per kg
- for CC 0.8 to 0.6 mL per kg per minute, 28 mg per kg
- for CC 0.6 to 0.4 mL per kg per minute, 21 mg per kg.

Foscarnet is not recommended for patients with less than 0.4 mL per kg per minute.

They also suggest similar proportional reductions of the dose of 40 mg per kg used to treat herpes simplex infections in patients with normal renal function.

Cytomegalovirus infections. As discussed on p.596, foscarnet is used in the treatment of severe cytomegalovirus infections in immunocompromised patients. It has been particularly useful instead of ganciclovir in patients with AIDS who require concurrent zidovudine therapy but are unable to tolerate ganciclovir (because of haematological toxicity) and appears to possess similar efficacy[1,2] (see also under Ganciclovir, p.613). It has also been tried in combination with ganciclovir in patients unresponsive to either drug alone.[3-6] One study[7] reported that a maintenance dose of 120 mg per kg body-weight of foscarnet daily was more effective and no more toxic than 90 mg per kg per day in patients with cytomegalovirus retinitis, but long-term intravenous therapy is generally poorly tolerated.[2] Beneficial responses have been reported with intravitreal injections of foscarnet 1200 µg every 48 hours for 4 doses[8] or 2400 µg every 72 hours for 6 doses, then once weekly thereafter.[9]

Foscarnet has also been investigated for primary prophylaxis of cytomegalovirus infection in bone marrow transplant recipients at high risk of infection.[10]

1. Blanshard C, *et al.* Treatment of AIDS-associated gastrointestinal cytomegalovirus infection with foscarnet and ganciclovir: a randomised comparison. *J Infect Dis* 1995; **172:** 622–8.
2. Studies of Ocular Complications of AIDS Research Group, in collaboration with the AIDS Clinical Trials Group. Mortality in patients with the acquired immunodeficiency syndrome treated with either foscarnet or ganciclovir for cytomegalovirus retinitis. *N Engl J Med* 1992; **326:** 213–20.
3. Coker RJ, *et al.* Treatment of cytomegalovirus retinitis with ganciclovir and foscarnet. *Lancet* 1991; **338:** 574–5.
4. Enting R, *et al.* Ganciclovir/foscarnet for cytomegalovirus meningoencephalitis in AIDS. *Lancet* 1992; **340:** 559–60.
5. Dieterich DT, *et al.* Concurrent use of ganciclovir and foscarnet to treat cytomegalovirus infection in AIDS patients. *J Infect Dis* 1993; **167:** 1184–8.
6. Studies of Ocular Complications of AIDS Research Group, in Collaboration with the AIDS Clinical Trials Group. Combination foscarnet and ganciclovir therapy vs monotherapy for the treatment of relapsed cytomegalovirus retinitis in patients with AIDS: the Cytomegalovirus Retreatment Trial. *Arch Ophthalmol* 1996; **114:** 23–33.
7. Jacobson MA, *et al.* A dose-ranging study of daily maintenance intravenous foscarnet therapy for cytomegalovirus retinitis in AIDS. *J Infect Dis* 1993; **168:** 444–8.
8. Lieberman RM, *et al.* Efficacy of intravitreal foscarnet in a patient with AIDS. *N Engl J Med* 1994; **330:** 868–9.
9. Diaz-Llopis M, *et al.* High dose intravitreal foscarnet in the treatment of cytomegalovirus retinitis in AIDS. *Br J Ophthalmol* 1994; **78:** 120–4.
10. Reusser P, *et al.* Phase I-II trial of foscarnet for prevention of cytomegalovirus infection in autologous and allogeneic marrow transplant recipients. *J Infect Dis* 1992; **166:** 473–9.

Herpes simplex infections. Although foscarnet is effective in the treatment of herpes simplex infections, it is usually reserved for severe infections particularly in immunocompromised patients who have failed to respond to aciclovir (see p.597).[1-3] However, although the reason was not clear, herpes simplex infections were reported in 2 patients while receiving foscarnet for cytomegalovirus retinitis.[4]

1. Erlich KS, *et al.* Foscarnet therapy for severe acyclovir-resistant herpes simplex virus type-2 infections in patients with the acquired immunodeficiency syndrome (AIDS): an uncontrolled trial. *Ann Intern Med* 1989; **110:** 710–13.
2. Safrin S, *et al.* Foscarnet therapy for acyclovir-resistant mucocutaneous herpes simplex virus infection in 26 AIDS patients: preliminary data. *J Infect Dis* 1990; **161:** 1078–84.
3. Safrin S, *et al.* A controlled trial comparing foscarnet with vidarabine for acyclovir-resistant mucocutaneous herpes simplex in the acquired immunodeficiency syndrome. *N Engl J Med* 1991; **325:** 551–5.
4. Cotte L, *et al.* Herpes simplex virus infection during foscarnet therapy. *J Infect Dis* 1992; **166:** 447–8.

HIV infection and AIDS. A multicentre study[1] comparing foscarnet with ganciclovir for cytomegalovirus retinitis in patients with AIDS was prematurely terminated following evidence that patients in the foscarnet group showed improved survival compared with those assigned to ganciclovir. Patients in the ganciclovir group received less concomitant antiretroviral therapy, in part because of additive toxicity, but it was considered that this alone was insufficient to explain the difference. Subsequent studies have supported these observations.[2-5] However, the toxicity of foscarnet at the doses necessary make it unlikely to be used to treat HIV infection (p.599).

1. Studies of Ocular Complications of AIDS Research Group, in collaboration with the AIDS Clinical Trials Group. Mortality in patients with the acquired immunodeficiency syndrome treated with either foscarnet or ganciclovir for cytomegalovirus retinitis. *N Engl J Med* 1992; **326:** 213–20.
2. Reddy MM, *et al.* Effect of foscarnet therapy on human immunodeficiency virus p24 antigen levels in AIDS patients with cytomegalovirus retinitis. *J Infect Dis* 1992; **166:** 607–10.
3. Polis MA, *et al.* Increased survival of a cohort of patients with acquired immunodeficiency syndrome and cytomegalovirus retinitis who received sodium phosphonoformate (foscarnet). *Am J Med* 1993; **94:** 175–80.
4. Fletcher CV, *et al.* Foscarnet for suppression of human immunodeficiency virus replication. *Antimicrob Agents Chemother* 1994; **38:** 604–7.
5. Kaiser L, *et al.* Foscarnet decreases human immunodeficiency virus RNA. *J Infect Dis* 1995; **172:** 225–7.

Preparations

BP 1998: Foscarnet Intravenous Infusion.

Proprietary Preparations (details are given in Part 3)
Aust.: Foscavir; ***Austral.:*** Foscavir; ***Belg.:*** Foscavir; ***Fr.:*** Foscavir; ***Ger.:*** Foscavir; Triapten; ***Ital.:*** Foscavir; Virudin; ***Neth.:*** Foscavir; ***Norw.:*** Foscavir; ***Spain:*** Foscavir; ***Swed.:*** Foscavir; ***Switz.:*** Foscavir; ***UK:*** Foscavir; ***USA:*** Foscavir.

Ganciclovir Sodium (19084-q)

Ganciclovir Sodium *(BANM, USAN, rINNM).*

BIOLF-62; BN-B759V; BW-759; BWB-759U; BW-759U; DHPG; Dihydroxypropoxymethylguanine; 9-(1,3-Dihydroxy-2-propoxymethyl)guanine; 2′-NDG; 2′-Nor-2′-deoxyguanosine; RS-21592 (all ganciclovir). 9-[2-Hydroxy-1-(hydroxymethyl)ethoxymethyl]guanine sodium.

$C_9H_{12}N_5NaO_4$ = 277.2.

CAS — 82410-32-0 (ganciclovir); 107910-75-8 (ganciclovir sodium).

Each g of monograph substance represents about 2.8 mmol of sodium.

Incompatibility. For reference to the incompatibility of ganciclovir and foscarnet, see Foscarnet Sodium, p.610.

Stability. Ganciclovir sodium solution in 0.9% sodium chloride was found to be stable when stored in polypropylene infusion-pump syringes for 12 hours at 25° and for 10 days at 4°.[1] Little variation was found in ganciclovir concentration following storage of a 2% solution at room temperature, 5°, and −8° for 10 to 24 days.[2]

1. Mulye NV, *et al.* Stability of ganciclovir sodium in an infusion-pump syringe. *Am J Hosp Pharm* 1994; **51:** 1348–9.
2. Morlet N, *et al.* High dose intravitreal ganciclovir for CMV retinitis: a shelf life and cost comparison study. *Br J Ophthalmol* 1995; **79:** 753–5.

Adverse Effects and Treatment

The most common adverse effects of ganciclovir are haematological and include neutropenia and thrombocytopenia; anaemia also occurs but less frequently. Neutropenia affects up to 40% of patients receiving ganciclovir intravenously, most commonly starting in the first or second week of ganciclovir treatment. It is usually reversible but may be prolonged or irreversible leading to potentially fatal infections. AIDS patients may be at a greater risk of neutropenia than other immunosuppressed patients. Thrombocytopenia occurs in about 20% of patients given ganciclovir intravenously. Those with iatrogenic immunosuppression may be more at risk of developing thrombocytopenia than AIDS patients. Other adverse effects occurring in about 2 to 3% of patients given intravenous ganciclovir include fever, rash, abnormal liver function tests, and increased serum-creatinine and blood-urea nitrogen concentrations. Irritation or phlebitis may occur at the site of injection due to the high pH. Less frequent adverse effects reported have included cardiovascular, CNS, gastro-intestinal, metabolic, musculoskeletal, respiratory, urogenital, and cutaneous symptoms.

The most frequent adverse effects associated with orally administered ganciclovir include neutropenia, thrombocytopenia, anaemia, gastro-intestinal disturbances, asthenia, headache, rash, pruritus, fever, abnormal liver function tests, pain, and infection.

Local adverse effects have been associated with the insertion of ocular implants containing ganciclovir.

Animal studies have suggested that there may be a risk of adverse testicular effects with permanent inhibition of spermatogenesis. Female fertility may also be affected. Such studies also suggest that ganciclovir is a potential mutagen, teratogen, and carcinogen.

Haemodialysis may be useful in reducing plasma concentrations of ganciclovir. Haematological adverse effects may be reversed in some patients by stopping treatment or reducing dosage; blood cell counts should return to normal within 2 to 7 days.

Colony-stimulating factor has been given with ganciclovir to limit its haematological toxicity.

Recombinant human granulocyte-macrophage colony-stimulating factor given intravenously at a dose of 5 μg per kg body-weight over a 4-hour period daily successfully treated ganciclovir-induced neutropenia in a patient with cytomegalovirus retinitis and bone-marrow suppression.[1]

1. Russo CL, *et al.* Treatment of neutropenia associated with dyskeratosis congenita with granulocyte-macrophage colony-stimulating factor. *Lancet* 1990; **336:** 751–2.

Precautions

Ganciclovir should be administered with caution to patients with renal impairment and doses should be adjusted according to the serum-creatinine concentration (see below under Uses and Administration). It should not be given by rapid or bolus injection and adequate hydration should be maintained during intravenous infusion. It should be given with caution to patients with pre-existing cytopenias (low blood counts) or with a history of cytopenic reactions to drugs. Monitoring of white blood cell and platelet counts should be performed every 2 days or daily during the first 14 days of intravenous ganciclovir therapy and once weekly thereafter; ganciclovir should be withdrawn if the neutrophil count falls below 500 cells per μL. Patients receiving oral ganciclovir should also be monitored regularly.

Ganciclovir is contra-indicated in pregnancy and in mothers who are breast feeding; contraception is recommended during ganciclovir treatment and, additionally for men, for 90 days thereafter.

Because of the risk of carcinogenicity and the high pH of the solution, contact with the skin and eyes should be avoided during the reconstitution of ganciclovir sodium injection.

Interactions

Zidovudine given concomitantly with ganciclovir may have an additive neutropenic effect (see Antivirals, under Interactions of Zidovudine, p.631) and should not be given during ganciclovir induction therapy, although it has been given with caution during maintenance therapy. Probenecid and other drugs that inhibit renal tubular secretion and resorption may reduce the renal clearance of ganciclovir, and so increase its plasma half-life. Drugs that inhibit rapid cell division such as myelosuppressants may have additive toxic effects if given with ganciclovir. Convulsions have been reported when ganciclovir was given concomitantly with a combination of imipenem and cilastatin.

Antivirals. As well as the additive neutropenic effect that may occur if ganciclovir is given with *zidovudine* (see above), there are reports of increased plasma concentrations of *didanosine* when given concurrently with ganciclovir (see p.608). The manufacturer reports that decreased blood concentrations of ganciclovir may occur when it is given orally 2 hours before didanosine but not when the two drugs are given at the same time.

Antiviral Action

Ganciclovir inhibits replication of human herpesviruses *in vivo* and *in vitro*. It is active against cytomegalovirus, herpes simplex virus types 1 and 2, Epstein-Barr virus, varicella-zoster virus, and herpesvirus 6. This activity is due to intracellular conversion of ganciclovir by viral thymidine kinase (in herpes simplex and varicella-zoster infected cells) or possibly by cellular deoxyguanosine kinase (in Epstein-Barr infected cells) to ganciclovir monophosphate with subsequent cellular conversion to the diphosphate and the active triphosphate. The mechanism of phosphorylation in cells infected with cytomegalovirus has yet to be determined. Ganciclovir triphosphate inhibits viral DNA synthesis by inhibiting the viral DNA polymerase enzyme as well as being incorporated into the viral DNA. This process is selective for infected cells; the concentration of ganciclovir triphosphate is reported to be tenfold higher in cytomegalovirus-infected cells than in uninfected cells.

Ganciclovir has a similar spectrum of activity to aciclovir, herpes simplex virus types 1 and 2 being the most susceptible of the herpesviruses. However, cytomegalovirus is much more susceptible to ganciclovir than aciclovir.

Cytomegalovirus. Antiviral synergy has been demonstrated against cytomegalovirus *in vitro* with ganciclovir and foscarnet,[1] and in *mice* with ganciclovir and cytomegalovirus immunoglobulin.[2]

1. Manischewitz JF, *et al.* Synergistic effect of ganciclovir and foscarnet on cytomegalovirus replication in vitro. *Antimicrob Agents Chemother* 1990; **34:** 373–5.
2. Rubin RH, *et al.* Combined antibody and ganciclovir treatment of murine cytomegalovirus-infected normal and immunosuppressed BALB/c mice. *Antimicrob Agents Chemother* 1989; **33:** 1975–9.

Herpesvirus 6. Human herpesvirus 6 was susceptible to ganciclovir,[1-4] and foscarnet[2-4] *in vitro* but was relatively resistant to aciclovir,[1-4] brivudine,[4] and zidovudine.[3]

1. Russler SK, *et al.* Susceptibility of human herpesvirus 6 to acyclovir and ganciclovir. *Lancet* 1989; **ii:** 382.
2. Agut H, *et al.* Susceptibility of human herpesvirus 6 to acyclovir and ganciclovir. *Lancet* 1989; **ii:** 626.
3. Agut H, *et al.* In vitro sensitivity of human herpesvirus-6 to antiviral drugs. *Res Virol* 1989; **140:** 219–28.
4. Burns WH, Sandford GR. Susceptibility of human herpesvirus 6 to antivirals in vitro. *J Infect Dis* 1990; **162:** 634–7.

Resistance

Resistance to ganciclovir has been demonstrated *in vitro* in herpes simplex virus, varicella-zoster virus, and cytomegalovirus. Possible mechanisms of resistance include a reduction in the phosphorylation of ganciclovir to the active form and reduced sensitivity of viral DNA polymerase. Resistance has also been reported in cytomegalovirus strains isolated from patients receiving ganciclovir for prolonged periods. Resistance in these patients was associated with clinical progression of cytomegalovirus retinitis.

Cytomegalovirus resistance to ganciclovir has been reviewed.[1]

Resistance to ganciclovir was demonstrated in cytomegalovirus strains isolated from 3 immunosuppressed patients receiving prolonged ganciclovir therapy.[2] In all 3 patients ganciclovir ultimately failed to treat cytomegalovirus disease or eradicate the virus from blood and other sites. Viral gene mutations associated with ganciclovir resistance have been identified in AIDS patients with CNS disease caused by cytomegalovirus.[3]

1. Drew WL. Cytomegalovirus resistance to antiviral therapies. *Am J Health-Syst Pharm* 1996; **53** (suppl 2): S17–S23.
2. Erice A, *et al.* Progressive disease due to ganciclovir-resistant cytomegalovirus in immunocompromised patients. *N Engl J Med* 1989; **320:** 289–93.
3. Wolf DG, *et al.* Detection of human cytomegalovirus mutations associated with ganciclovir resistance in cerebrospinal fluid of AIDS patients with central nervous system disease. *Antimicrob Agents Chemother* 1995; **39:** 2552–4.

Pharmacokinetics

Ganciclovir is poorly absorbed from the gastro-intestinal tract following oral administration and there is minimal systemic absorption after intravitreal injection. Following intravenous administration as ganciclovir sodium it is widely distributed to body tissues and fluids including intra-ocular fluid and CSF. Binding to plasma proteins is reported to be 1 to 2%. Ganciclovir is excreted unchanged in the urine. The terminal plasma half-life is approximately 2.5 to 4 hours in patients with normal renal function. In patients with renal impairment the renal clearance decreases and the half-life increases; a half-life of 28.5 hours has been reported when the serum-creatinine concentration was greater than 398 μmol per litre.

Haemodialysis has been reported to reduce ganciclovir plasma concentrations by about 50%.

References.

1. Fletcher C, *et al.* Human pharmacokinetics of the antiviral drug DHPG. *Clin Pharmacol Ther* 1986; **40:** 281–6.
2. Jacobson MA, *et al.* Human pharmacokinetics and tolerance of oral ganciclovir. *Antimicrob Agents Chemother* 1987; **31:** 1251–4.
3. Rello J, *et al.* Effect of continuous arteriovenous hemodialysis on ganciclovir pharmacokinetics. *DICP Ann Pharmacother* 1990; **24:** 544.
4. Morse GD, *et al.* Comparative pharmacokinetics of antiviral nucleoside analogues. *Clin Pharmacokinet* 1993; **24:** 101–23.
5. Trang JM, *et al.* Linear single-dose pharmacokinetics of ganciclovir in newborns with congenital cytomegalovirus infections. *Clin Pharmacol Ther* 1993; **53:** 15–21.
6. Combarnous F, *et al.* Pharmacokinetics of ganciclovir in a patient undergoing chronic haemodialysis. *Eur J Clin Pharmacol* 1994; **46:** 379–81.
7. Arevalo JF, *et al.* Intravitreous and plasma concentrations of ganciclovir and foscarnet after intravenous therapy in patients with AIDS and cytomegalovirus retinitis. *J Infect Dis* 1995; **172:** 951–6.
8. Morlet N, *et al.* High dose intravitreal ganciclovir injection provides a prolonged therapeutic intraocular concentration. *Br J Ophthalmol* 1996; **80:** 214–16.
9. Lavelle J, *et al.* Effect of food on the relative bioavailability of oral ganciclovir. *J Clin Pharmacol* 1996; **36:** 238–41.
10. Zhou X-J, *et al.* Population pharmacokinetics of ganciclovir in newborns with congenital cytomegalovirus infection. *Antimicrob Agents Chemother* 1996; **40:** 2202–5.
11. Giffy KG. Pharmacokinetics of oral ganciclovir capsules in HIV-infected persons. *AIDS* 1996; **10** (suppl 4): S3–S6.

Uses and Administration

Ganciclovir is a synthetic nucleoside analogue of guanine closely related to aciclovir, but with a greater activity against cytomegalovirus. It is used for the treatment and suppression of life- or sight-threatening cytomegalovirus infections in immunocompromised patients including those with AIDS. It has also been tried in Epstein-Barr virus and *Herpesvirus simiae* virus infections.

Ganciclovir is administered by intravenous infusion as the sodium salt over 1 hour. Solutions for infusion are usually prepared to give a concentration of 50 mg of ganciclovir per mL, then further diluted to contain not more than 10 mg per mL. Ganciclovir may also be given by mouth.

In **cytomegalovirus infections** the usual *initial* dose for *treatment* is 5 mg per kg body-weight by intravenous infusion every 12 hours for 14 to 21 days. This induction period may be followed by *maintenance* therapy to prevent recurrence or progression of the disease. The usual maintenance dosage is 5 mg per kg by intravenous infusion as a single daily dose for 7 days a week or 6 mg per kg daily for 5 days a week. If retinitis recurs or progresses a further induction course of ganciclovir may be given. AIDS patients who have received initial treatment with intravenous ganciclovir, and who have stable cytomegalovirus retinitis following at least 3 weeks of intravenous therapy, may be given ganciclovir orally in a dose of 3 g daily in 3 or 6 divided doses, with food.

For *prevention* of cytomegalovirus infection in immunocompromised patients, specifically those receiving immunosuppressive therapy following organ transplantation, ganciclovir may be given in an *initial* dose of 5 mg per kg by intravenous infusion every 12 hours for 7 to 14 days, followed by intravenous *maintenance* therapy as above. Ganciclovir prophylaxis may be given orally in a dose of 1 g three times daily with food to patients with advanced HIV infection.

Doses should be reduced in renal impairment (see below).

Intravitreal injection has been tried in cytomegalovirus retinitis for those patients unable to tolerate systemic ganciclovir and eye implants providing controlled release of ganciclovir are available.

Ganciclovir is used in some countries as a topical ophthalmic 0.15% gel for the treatment of superficial ocular **herpes simplex infections**.

General references.

1. Faulds D, Heel RC. Ganciclovir: a review of its antiviral activity, pharmacokinetic properties and therapeutic efficacy in cytomegalovirus infections. *Drugs* 1990; **39:** 597–638.
2. Markham A, Faulds D. Ganciclovir: an update of its therapeutic use in cytomegalovirus infection. *Drugs* 1994; **48:** 455–84.
3. Crumpacker CS. Ganciclovir. *N Engl J Med* 1996; **335:** 721–9.
4. Noble S, Faulds D. Ganciclovir: an update of its use in the prevention of cytomegalovirus infection and disease in transplant recipients. *Drugs* 1998; **56:** 115–46.

Administration in renal impairment. Doses of ganciclovir should be reduced in renal impairment. This may be done by reducing the dose and/or increasing the dosage interval according to serum-creatinine concentration or creatinine clearance. The following induction doses of ganciclovir have been recommended: for patients with a serum-creatinine concentration of less than 124 μmol per litre, 5 mg per kg every 12 hours; for 125 to 225 μmol per litre, 2.5 mg per kg every 12 hours; for 226 to 398 μmol per litre, 2.5 mg per kg every 24 hours; and for over 398 μmol per litre, 1.25 mg per kg every 24 hours. For dialysis patients a dose of 1.25 mg per kg every 24 hours (or in the USA, not more than 3 times each week) given shortly after the end of dialysis has been recommended. Suggested doses for patients with renal impairment receiving oral ganciclovir are: for patients with a creatinine clearance of 70 mL per minute or more, 3 g daily in 3 or 6 divided doses; for 50 to 69 mL per minute, 1500 mg daily; for 25 to 49 mL per minute, 1000 mg daily; for 10 to 24 mL per minute, 500 mg daily; and for less than 10 mL per minute, 500 mg three times a week, following haemodialysis.

Cytomegalovirus infections. Ganciclovir is used in both the treatment and prophylaxis of cytomegalovirus infections (p.596) in immunocompromised patients.

As with other herpesvirus infections, antiviral treatment tends to be suppressive rather than curative, and long-term maintenance therapy is necessary. Treatment in patients with AIDS is complicated by the additive haematological toxicity of ganciclovir and zidovudine. Clinical studies comparing ganciclovir with foscarnet for AIDS-related cytomegalovirus retinopathy have shown higher mortality rates in patients receiving ganciclovir than in those receiving foscarnet, leading to the suggestion that foscarnet may possess intrinsic antiretroviral activity. However, an alternative explanation is that fewer patients receiving ganciclovir could tolerate full doses of zidovudine and were thus receiving suboptimal therapy. If it is possible to overcome the drug-induced neutropenia by giving colony-stimulating factors concomitantly (thus enabling the use of full therapeutic doses of zidovudine) ganciclovir may remain the preferred treatment for cytomegalovirus retinitis since foscarnet is less well tolerated. The use of ganciclovir in combination with cytomegalovirus immunoglobulins or normal immunoglobulins, or with foscarnet may improve both efficacy and tolerance. An alternative has been the development of intravitreal injection techniques and intra-ocular controlled-release ganciclovir devices to avoid systemic adverse effects. A further development has been the introduction of oral preparations of ganciclovir for maintenance therapy. Cytomegalovirus infections at other sites in AIDS patients, including gastro-intestinal and pulmonary infections, respond less well to ganciclovir than does retinitis.

Ganciclovir is also valuable for prophylaxis and early treatment of cytomegalovirus infections in transplant recipients. For established infections, ganciclovir is reported to be more effective in solid organ transplant recipients than in bone marrow transplant recipients. Ganciclovir has also been tried for prevention of cytomegalovirus infection in patients with AIDS, although results are conflicting.

Treatment of congenital infections has a generally poor outcome. Prolonged treatment periods may improve the response, but the safety of extended treatment with ganciclovir in this age group has not been fully evaluated.

Epstein-Barr virus infections. Ganciclovir has been reported to produce some improvement in patients with Epstein-Barr virus (EBV) infection, although no antiviral therapy is entirely satisfactory (p.597). Evidence of the efficacy of ganciclovir is so far anecdotal, with eradication of EBV in an organ transplant recipient[1] and in a child who had relapsed after an initial response to interleukin-2 and splenectomy,[2] neither of whom had responded to aciclovir. However, it was ineffective in a second transplant recipient.[1]

1. Pirsch JD, *et al.* Treatment of severe Epstein-Barr virus-induced lymphoproliferative syndrome with ganciclovir: two cases after solid organ transplantation. *Am J Med* 1989; **86:** 241–4.
2. Ishida Y, *et al.* Ganciclovir for chronic active Epstein-Barr virus infection. *Lancet* 1993; **341:** 560–1.

Herpesvirus infections. In patients with herpes simplex keratitis, ganciclovir 0.15% gel was reported to be as effective as aciclovir 3% ointment,[1] the drug most commonly used in this infection (see p.597).

Ganciclovir was also reported to produce beneficial responses in AIDS patients with ocular varicella zoster infections.[2]

Treatment with ganciclovir was associated with a lower incidence of Kaposi's sarcoma in patients with HIV infection,[3] supporting the suggestion that a herpesvirus infection may be associated with the development of this malignancy.

1. Hoh HB, *et al.* Randomised trial of ganciclovir and acyclovir in the treatment of herpes simplex dendritic keratitis: a multicentre study. *Br J Ophthalmol* 1996; **80:** 140–3.
2. Moorthy RS, *et al.* Management of varicella zoster virus retinitis in AIDS. *Br J Ophthalmol* 1997; **81:** 189–94.
3. Mocroft A, *et al.* Anti-herpesvirus treatment and risk of Kaposi's sarcoma in HIV infection. *AIDS* 1996; **10:** 1101–5.

Malignant neoplasms. Ganciclovir is being investigated for use in gene therapy for the treatment of a variety of disorders including malignancies (for example, Malignant Neoplasms of the Brain, p.485). The target cells are genetically modified to express a gene which makes the cell susceptible to ganciclovir; the herpes simplex virus thymidine kinase gene is typically used.

Preparations

Proprietary Preparations (details are given in Part 3)
Aust.: Cymevene; ***Austral.:*** Cymevene; ***Belg.:*** Cymevene; ***Canad.:*** Cytovene; ***Fr.:*** Cymevan; Virgan; ***Ger.:*** Cymeven; ***Irl.:*** Cymevene; ***Ital.:*** Citovirax; Cymevene; ***Neth.:*** Cymevene; ***Norw.:*** Cymevene; ***S.Afr.:*** Cymevene; ***Spain:*** Cymevene; ***Swed.:*** Cymevene; ***Switz.:*** Cymevene; ***UK:*** Cymevene; Vitrasert; ***USA:*** Cytovene; Vitrasert.

GS-4104 (10747-b)

GS-4104 is an oral prodrug of GS-4071, an inhibitor of the enzyme neuraminidase (sialidase), which has a role in the infectivity and replication of influenza A and B viruses. It is under investigation for the treatment and prevention of influenza.

Ibacitabine (12854-d)

Ibacitabine (*rINN*).

Iododesoxycytidine. 2′-Deoxy-5-iodocytidine.

$C_9H_{12}IN_3O_4$ = 353.1.

CAS — 611-53-0.

Ibacitabine is an antiviral with activity against herpes simplex viruses. It is used topically at a concentration of 1% in the treatment of herpes simplex infections of the skin and mucous membranes.

Preparations

Proprietary Preparations (details are given in Part 3)
Fr.: Cuterpes; ***Ital.:*** Herpes-Gel.

Idoxuridine (1681-k)

Idoxuridine (*BAN, USAN, rINN*).

Allergan 211; GF-I115; Idoxuridina; IDU; 5-IDUR; 5-IUDR; NSC-39661; SKF-14287. 2′-Deoxy-5-iodouridine.

$C_9H_{11}IN_2O_5$ = 354.1.

CAS — 54-42-2.

Pharmacopoeias. In *Chin., Eur.* (see p.viii), *Jpn*, and *US.*

Odourless or almost odourless, colourless crystals or a white or almost white crystalline powder from which iodine vapour is liberated on heating. M.p. about 180°, with decomposition. Slightly **soluble** in water and in alcohol; practically insoluble in chloroform and in ether; dissolves in dilute solutions of alkali hydroxides. A 0.1% solution in water has a pH of 5.5 to 6.5. It has been reported that some decomposition products such as iodouracil are more toxic than idoxuridine and reduce its antiviral activity. **Store** in airtight containers. Protect from light.

Adverse Effects

Adverse effects which occur occasionally when idoxuridine is applied to the eyes include irritation, pain, conjunctivitis, oedema and inflammation of the eye or eyelids, photophobia, pruritus, and rarely, occlusion of the lachrymal duct. Hypersensitivity reactions may occur rarely. Prolonged use may damage the cornea.

Idoxuridine applied to the skin may produce irritation and hypersensitivity reactions. Excessive application of topical idoxuridine to the eyes or skin may cause punctate defects in the cornea or skin maceration.

Adverse effects after intravenous administration of idoxuridine have included bone-marrow depression and liver damage.

Idoxuridine is a potential carcinogen and teratogen.

Squamous carcinoma in one patient was associated with topical idoxuridine treatment.[1] Reference is made to one earlier similar case.

1. Koppang HS, Aas E. Squamous carcinoma induced by topical idoxuridine therapy? *Br J Dermatol* 1983; **108:** 501–3.

Precautions

Idoxuridine should be used with caution in conditions where there is deep ulceration involving the stromal layers of the cornea, as delayed healing has resulted in corneal perforation. Prolonged topical use should be avoided.

Idoxuridine's potential teratogenicity should be taken into account when treating pregnant patients or patients likely to become pregnant. Corticosteroids should be applied with caution in patients also receiving idoxuridine as they may accelerate the spread of viral infection. Boric acid preparations should not be applied to the eye in patients also receiving ocular preparations of idoxuridine as irritation ensues.

Antiviral Action

Following intracellular phosphorylation to the triphosphate, idoxuridine is incorporated into viral DNA instead of thymidine so inhibiting replication of the virus. Idoxuridine is also incorporated into mammalian DNA. Idoxuridine is active against herpes simplex and varicella zoster viruses. It has also been shown to inhibit vaccinia virus and cytomegalovirus.

Resistance to idoxuridine occurs *in vitro* and *in vivo*.

Pharmacokinetics

Penetration of idoxuridine into the cornea and skin is reported to be poor. Following systemic administration idoxuridine is rapidly metabolised to iodouracil, uracil, and iodide.

Uses and Administration

Idoxuridine is a pyrimidine nucleoside structurally related to thymidine. It has been used topically in the treatment of herpes simplex keratitis and cutaneous forms of herpes simplex and herpes zoster, but has generally been superseded by other antivirals (see Herpes Simplex Infections, p.597, and Varicella-zoster Infections, p.598).

In the treatment of herpes simplex keratitis idoxuridine has been applied as a 0.1% ophthalmic solution.

Idoxuridine 5% in dimethyl sulphoxide (to aid absorption) can be painted onto the lesions of cutaneous herpes simplex and herpes zoster four times daily for 4 days.

Preparations

BP 1998: Idoxuridine Eye Drops;
USP 23: Idoxuridine Ophthalmic Ointment; Idoxuridine Ophthalmic Solution.

Proprietary Preparations (details are given in Part 3)
Austral.: Herplex Liquifilm†; Herplex-D; Stoxil; ***Belg.:*** Virexen; Virpex†; ***Canad.:*** Herplex; ***Fr.:*** Iduviran; ***Ger.:*** Iducutit; Ophtal; Synmiol†; Virunguent; Zostrum; ***Irl.:*** Herplex-D†; Zostrum; ***Ital.:*** Cheratil†; Iducher; Iduridin; Idustatin; ***Norw.:*** Iduridin; ***S.Afr.:*** Herplex-D†; Stoxil†; ***Spain:*** Antizona; Virexen; Virucida Idu†; ***Switz.:*** Herpidu†; Virexen; Virunguent; ***UK:*** Herpid; Idoxene†; Iduridin†; Virudox†; ***USA:*** Herplex†.

Multi-ingredient: ***Austral.:*** Virasolve; ***Ger.:*** Spersidu C†; Virunguent-P; ***Ital.:*** Iducol; Idustatin; ***Switz.:*** Herpidu Chloramphenicol†; Virunguent-P†.

Imiquimod (11696-k)

Imiquimod (*USAN, rINN*).

R-837; S-26308. 4-Amino-1-isobutyl-1*H*-imidazo[4,5-*c*]quinoline.

$C_{14}H_{16}N_4$ = 240.3.

CAS — 99011-02-6.

Imiquimod is an immune response modifier used topically in the treatment of external genital and perianal warts. It is applied as a 5% cream three times a week and is left on the skin for 6 to 10 hours.

References.

1. Anonymous. Imiquimod for genital warts. *Med Lett Drugs Ther* 1997; **39:** 118–19.
2. Beutner KR, *et al.* Imiquimod, a patient-applied immune-response modifier for treatment of external genital warts. *Antimicrob Agents Chemother* 1998; **42:** 789–94.

Preparations

Proprietary Preparations (details are given in Part 3)
UK: Aldara; ***USA:*** Aldara.

Indinavir Sulphate (3883-x)

Indinavir Sulphate (*BANM, pINNM*).

Indinavir Sulfate (*USAN*); L-735524; MK-639; MK-0639. (αR,γS,2S)-α-Benzyl-2-(*tert*-butylcarbamoyl)-γ-hydroxy-*N*-[(1S,2R)-2-hydroxy-1-indanyl]-4-(3-pyridylmethyl)-1-piperazinevaleramide sulphate (1:1).

$C_{36}H_{47}N_5O_4,H_2SO_4$ = 711.9.

CAS — 150378-17-9 (indinavir); 157810-81-6 (indinavir sulphate).

Adverse Effects

The general spectrum of adverse effects associated with *indinavir and similar HIV-protease inhibitors* commonly includes nausea, vomiting, and diarrhoea (which can be severe enough to cause dehydration with its potential for adverse renal effects).

Other side-effects reported include taste disturbances, asthenia, fatigue, headache, dizziness, paraesthesia, myalgia, skin rashes, pruritus, and renal insufficiency. Lipodystrophy (redistribution of peripheral subcutaneous fat to the shoulders and abdomen) may occur.

Additional side-effects reported with *indinavir* include acid regurgitation, dyspepsia, dry mouth, hypoaesthesia, insomnia, dysuria, dry skin, and hyperpigmentation.

Additional side-effects reported with *ritonavir* include anorexia, eructation, dyspepsia, dry mouth, ulceration of the oral mucosa, throat irritation and cough, somnolence, hypoaesthesia, seizures, insomnia and anxiety, sweating, and fever.

Additional side-effects reported with *saquinavir* include ulceration of the oral mucosa, depression, somnolence, and anxiety.

Hyperglycaemia and an association with the onset or exacerbation of diabetes mellitus has also occurred in patients receiving HIV-protease inhibitors. Nephrolithiasis has been associated with *indinavir* (often resolved by withdrawal for one to three days and administration of fluids) and acute renal failure has been reported; nephrolithiasis has also possibly been associated with *saquinavir*. A possible association with Stevens-Johnson syndrome has been reported for *indinavir* and *saquinavir*. Vasodilatation has been commonly associated with *ritonavir* and syncope and orthostatic hypotension have been reported.

Allergic reactions (sometimes anaphylaxis) have been associated with *indinavir, ritonavir* and *saquinavir*. Photosensitivity and pancreatitis have occurred with *saquinavir*. Abnormal laboratory test results associated with the administration of HIV-protease inhibitors have included raised liver enzymes and bilirubin (jaundice and hepatitis have occurred), raised creatine phosphokinase, and raised blood lipids. Other abnormal results have included haematuria (indinavir and saquinavir), raised uric acid (ritonavir), and decreased free and total thyroxine (ritonavir). Effects on the blood have included acute haemolytic anaemia (indinavir and saquinavir) and reduced neutrophil counts (reduced or increased with ritonavir).

Effects on body fat. HIV-protease inhibitors have been associated with a syndrome of peripheral lipodystrophy (fat wasting), central adiposity, hyperlipidaemia, and insulin resistance.[1] Reports have included accumulation of body fat over the shoulders[2,3] and abdomen[4] in patients receiving indinavir or other HIV-protease inhibitors (although 4 of the 8 patients reported by Lo *et al.*[3] had not taken HIV-protease inhibitors). See also under Effects on the Cardiovascular System, below.

1. Carr A, *et al.* Pathogenesis of HIV-1-protease inhibitor-associated peripheral lipodystrophy, hyperlipidaemia, and insulin resistance. *Lancet* 1998; **351:** 1881–3.
2. Hengel RL, *et al.* Benign symmetric lipomatosis associated with protease inhibitors. *Lancet* 1997; **350:** 1596.
3. Lo JC, *et al.* "Buffalo hump" in men with HIV-1 infection. *Lancet* 1998; **351:** 867–70.
4. Miller KD, *et al.* Visceral abdominal-fat accumulation associated with use of indinavir. *Lancet* 1998; **351:** 871–5.

Effects on the cardiovascular system. Following the development of angina pectoris in two patients receiving HIV-protease inhibitors, raised lipid concentrations were identified in a further 41 of 124 patients receiving protease inhibitors.[1]

1. Henry K, *et al.* Severe premature coronary artery disease with protease inhibitors. *Lancet* 1998; **351:** 1328.

Effects on glucose metabolism. In the UK the Committee on Safety of Medicines (CSM)[1] reported that by May 1997 there had been more than 100 cases of hyperglycaemia, new-onset diabetes mellitus, or exacerbation of existing diabetes in patients receiving HIV-protease inhibitors.

1. Committee on Safety of Medicines/Medicines Control Agency. Protease inhibitors and hyperglycaemia. *Current Problems* 1997; **23:** 10.

Effects on the kidneys. Reports of acute interstitial nephritis associated with indinavir[1] and deterioration of renal function associated with ritonavir.[2,3]

1. Marroni M, *et al.* Acute interstitial nephritis secondary to the administration of indinavir. *Ann Pharmacother* 1998; **32:** 843–4.
2. Duong M, *et al.* Renal failure after treatment with ritonavir. *Lancet* 1996; **348:** 693–4.
3. Chugh S, *et al.* Ritonavir and renal failure. *N Engl J Med* 1997; **336:** 138.

Effects on the liver. The use of indinavir, in combinations with other antiretroviral drugs, has been associated with the development of severe hepatitis.[1,2]

1. Bräu N, *et al.* Severe hepatitis in three AIDS patients treated with indinavir. *Lancet* 1997; **349:** 924–5.
2. Matsuda J, *et al.* Severe hepatitis in patients with AIDS and haemophilia B treated with indinavir. *Lancet* 1997; **350:** 364.

Precautions

Indinavir and similar HIV-protease inhibitors are primarily metabolised in the liver which means that caution and possible dosage reduction are required in hepatic impairment; where the hepatic impairment is severe they should be avoided. Although renal excretion is a relatively minor route of elimination, adequate hydration is recommended to avoid any risk of nephrolithiasis; monitoring is advised in the presence of renal impairment. Caution is needed in diabetic patients since HIV-protease inhibitors have been associated with hyperglycaemia and the onset or exacerbation of diabetes mellitus. Caution is also needed in patients with haemophilia who may experience increased bleeding. Excessive diarrhoea may interfere with the absorption of HIV-protease inhibitors leading to subtherapeutic blood concentrations; resultant dehydration may also be a factor in renal damage (see nephrolithiasis, above).

Indinavir and similar HIV-protease inhibitors are liable to interfere with the metabolism of a large number of drugs to create a potential for hazardous and life-threatening side-effects. Other drugs, such as rifampicin, reduce the plasma concentrations of the HIV-protease inhibitors to subtherapeutic levels and are also contra-indicated. For details of these and other important interactions, see below.

Patients with a previously unsuspected *Mycobacterium avium* complex infection experienced a severe febrile syndrome with inflammatory lymphadenitis following initiation of indinavir treatment.[1] The reaction resolved with appropriate antimycobacterial therapy.

1. Race EM, *et al.* Focal mycobacterial lymphadenitis following initiation of protease-inhibitor therapy in patients with advanced HIV-1 disease. *Lancet* 1998; **351:** 252–5.

Interactions

Indinavir and similar HIV-protease inhibitors are metabolised principally by cytochrome P450 isoenzymes of the CYP3A family. They consequently *compete for the same metabolic pathways* with a wide range of drugs that are metabolised similarly, often resulting in mutually increased plasma concentrations. The extent of such interactions depends on a number of factors, including the affinity of the relevant HIV-protease inhibitor for the various cytochrome P450 isoenzymes; in the case of indinavir, CYP3A4 is reported to be the only P450 isoenzyme that plays a major role. Where significant competition for metabolism does occur, the margin between therapeutic and toxic concentrations has a major role in determining the severity of the interaction. Thus, concurrent administration of a drug with a narrow therapeutic window such as cisapride or terfenadine is contra-indicated, whereas a drug with a wider therapeutic window such as erythromycin may only require dosage reduction at its highest dose level.

Conversely, a drug that is a *significant inducer of microsomal enzymes*, particularly isoenzymes of the CYP3A family, reduce plasma concentrations of HIV-protease inhibitors. Thus, concurrent administration of a potent enzyme inducer such as rifampicin may reduce the plasma concentration of an HIV-protease inhibitor to a subtherapeutic level so that its concurrent administration is contra-indicated. Other well-known enzyme inducers such as carbamazepine, phenobarbitone, and phenytoin also possibly reduce the plasma concentrations of HIV-protease inhibitors.

In turn, HIV-protease inhibitors may *themselves induce metabolism* and may reduce plasma concentrations of other drugs such as theophylline and hormonal contraceptives.

The principal interactions that have been reported as a risk for one or more of the various HIV-protease inhibitors currently available (indinavir, nelfinavir, ritonavir, saquinavir), are listed below.

- analgesics: plasma concentrations of *dextropropoxyphene, methadone, pethidine,* and possibly some other opioid analgesics increased (risk of increased sedation and respiratory depression); plasma concentrations of *piroxicam* increased (ritonavir) (risk of toxicity)
- antiarrhythmics: plasma concentrations of many *antiarrhythmics (e.g. amiodarone, flecainide, propafenone, and quinidine)* increased (special hazard owing to the increased risk of ventricular arrhythmias)
- antibacterials: *rifampicin* reduces plasma concentrations of HIV-protease inhibitors to the extent that antiviral efficacy is lost; *rifabutin* also reduces plasma concentrations of HIV-protease inhibitors and in turn has its own plasma concentration increased to toxic levels (special risk of uveitis); plasma concentrations of *erythromycin* and *clarithromycin* increased (but only to the extent that dosage reduction may be required at their highest dose level or, in the case of clarithromycin, where there is renal impairment)
- antidepressants: plasma concentrations of *desipramine* and *fluoxetine* possibly increased (ritonavir)
- antidiabetics: plasma concentrations of *tolbutamide* possibly increased (ritonavir)
- antiepileptics: *carbamazepine, phenobarbitone,* and *phenytoin* possibly reduce plasma concentrations of HIV-protease inhibitors and in turn some HIV-protease inhibitors (e.g. ritonavir) possibly increase plasma concentrations of *carbamazepine*
- antifungals: increased plasma concentrations of HIV-protease inhibitors occur with azole antifungals such as *ketoconazole* and *itraconazole* and, in turn, plasma concentrations of these antifungals may possibly be increased (ritonavir)
- antihistamines: plasma concentrations of the non-sedating antihistamines *astemizole* and *terfenadine* increased (special hazard owing to the increased risk of ventricular arrhythmias)
- antipsychotics: plasma concentration of *clozapine* increased (ritonavir) (special hazard owing to risk associated with various aspects of toxicity) and plasma concentration of *pimozide* increased (ritonavir) (special hazard owing to increased risk of ventricular arrhythmias)
- other antivirals: all *HIV-protease inhibitors* carry the potential for mutual increases in plasma concentrations on concurrent administration (sometimes requiring avoidance or dosage reduction); plasma concentrations may be reduced with *nevirapine* and increased by *delavirdine*; *didanosine* is administered in a buffered formulation that can reduce the absorption of some HIV-protease inhibitors and, depending on the HIV-protease inhibitor used, doses of the two drugs should be separated by at least 1 hour
- anxiolytics and hypnotics: plasma concentrations of *benzodiazepines* increased (causing an increased risk of prolonged sedation and respiratory depression); among others, this is a special hazard with *midazolam*, with *triazolam*, and with *zolpidem*

- calcium-channel blockers: plasma concentrations of *calcium channel blockers* possibly increased (calling for increased vigilance and monitoring)
- cisapride: plasma concentrations of *cisapride* increased (special hazard owing to increased risk of ventricular arrhythmias)
- corticosteroids: *dexamethasone* and *prednisolone* and possibly other corticosteroids may reduce plasma concentrations of HIV-protease inhibitors and in turn corticosteroid plasma concentrations possibly increased (ritonavir)
- cyclosporin: plasma concentration of *cyclosporin* possibly increased (ritonavir) (which would be a special hazard)
- ergot alkaloids: concurrent administration with *dihydroergotamine* and *ergotamine* has been associated with severe ergotism (peripheral vasospasm and ischaemia of the extremities)
- hormonal contraceptives: plasma concentration of both *oestrogens* and *progestogens* reported to be reduced by some HIV-protease inhibitors (alternative contraceptive methods may need to be considered)
- stimulants: a fatal serotoninergic reaction possibly due to an interaction with *methylenedioxymethamphetamine* has been reported (ritonavir)
- tacrolimus: plasma concentrations of *tacrolimus* possibly increased (ritonavir and saquinavir)
- theophylline: plasma concentration of *theophylline* reduced (ritonavir).

References to the inhibition of microsomal enzymes by HIV-protease inhibitors.

1. Eagling VA, *et al.* Differential inhibition of cytochrome P450 isoforms by the protease inhibitors, ritonavir, saquinavir and indinavir. *Br J Clin Pharmacol* 1997; **44:** 190–4.
2. von Moltke LL, *et al.* Protease inhibitors as inhibitors of human cytochromes P450: high risk associated with ritonavir. *J Clin Pharmacol* 1998; **38:** 106–11.

Antiviral Action

Indinavir and similar HIV-protease inhibitors act by binding reversibly to HIV-protease thereby preventing cleavage of the viral precursor polyproteins. This results in the formation of immature viral particles incapable of infecting other cells. Viral resistance develops rapidly when HIV-protease inhibitors are given alone and therefore they are used in combination with other antiretrovirals.

Pharmacokinetics

Indinavir is rapidly absorbed following oral administration producing peak plasma concentrations in 0.8 hours. Bioavailability is about 65% following a single dose. Absorption is reduced by administration with a high-fat meal. At doses up to 1000 mg, increases in plasma concentration are proportionately greater than increases in dose. Indinavir is about 60% bound to plasma proteins. It undergoes oxidative metabolism by the CYP3A4 isoenzyme of the cytochrome P450 system and glucuronidation. The elimination half-life is 1.8 hours. Less than 20% of the absorbed dose is excreted in the urine, about half of this as unchanged drug. The remainder is excreted in the faeces.

References.

1. Yeh KC, *et al.* Single-dose pharmacokinetics of indinavir and the effect of food. *Antimicrob Agents Chemother* 1998; **42:** 332–8. Correction. *ibid.:* 1308.

Uses and Administration

Indinavir is a protease inhibitor with antiviral activity against HIV. It is used, in combination with nucleoside reverse transcriptase inhibitors, for the treatment of HIV infection (p.599).

Indinavir is given by mouth in a dose of 800 mg (as indinavir sulphate) every 8 hours. It should be given either an hour before or two hours after meals, or with a light, low-fat meal. A reduction in dose to 600 mg every 8 hours is recommended for patients with mild to moderate hepatic insufficiency due to cirrhosis. Adequate hydration should be maintained. Treatment may have to be interrupted if acute episodes of nephrolithiasis occur.

Indinavir has also been recommended as part of the chemoprophylactic regimen with zidovudine and lamivudine in patients at high risk of HIV infection following occupational percutaneous exposure (see p.601).

HIV infection and AIDS. Reviews on the use of indinavir and other HIV-protease inhibitors.

1. Moyle GJ, Barton SE. HIV-proteinase inhibitors in the management of HIV-infection. *J Antimicrob Chemother* 1996; **33:** 921–5.
2. Moyle G, Gazzard B. Current knowledge and future prospects for the use of HIV protease inhibitors. *Drugs* 1996; **51:** 701–12.
3. Barry M, *et al.* Protease inhibitors in patients with HIV disease: clinically important pharmacokinetic considerations. *Clin Pharmacokinet* 1997; **32:** 194–209.
4. Deeks SG, *et al.* HIV-1 protease inhibitors: a review for clinicians. *JAMA* 1997; **277:** 145–53.
5. Flexner C. HIV-protease inhibitors. *N Engl J Med* 1998; **338:** 1281–92.

Other viral infections. Infection with HHV-8 (a virus associated with an increased risk of developing Kaposi's sarcoma) resolved in a patient when indinavir was added to combination therapy for HIV infection.[1] Regression of progressive multifocal leucoencephalopathy (the result of a JC virus infection of the CNS) has been reported in 2 patients receiving combination antiretroviral therapy including indinavir for HIV infection.[2,3]

1. Rizzieri DA, *et al.* Clearance of HHV-8 from peripheral blood mononuclear cells with a protease inhibitor. *Lancet* 1997; **349:** 775–6.
2. Elliot B, *et al.* 2.5 Year remission of AIDS-associated progressive multifocal leukoencephalopathy with combined antiretroviral therapy. *Lancet* 1997; **349:** 850.
3. Domingo P, *et al.* Remission of progressive multifocal leucoencephalopathy after antiretroviral therapy. *Lancet* 1997; **349:** 1554–5.

Preparations

Proprietary Preparations (details are given in Part 3)
Austral.: Crixivan; ***Belg.:*** Crixivan; ***Canad.:*** Crixivan; ***Ger.:*** Crixivan; ***Irl.:*** Crixivan; ***Ital.:*** Crixivan; ***Neth.:*** Crixivan; ***S.Afr.:*** Crixivan; ***Spain:*** Crixivan; ***Swed.:*** Crixivan; ***Switz.:*** Crixivan; ***UK:*** Crixivan; ***USA:*** Crixivan.

Inosine Pranobex (12941-f)

Inosine Pranobex *(BAN, rINNM).*

Inosiplex; Isoprinosine; Methisoprinol; NP-113; NPT-10381. Inosine 2-hydroxypropyldimethylammonium 4-acetamidobenzoate (1:3).

$C_{10}H_{12}N_4O_5$:$C_{14}H_{22}N_2O_4$ (1:3) = 1115.2.

CAS — 36703-88-5.

NOTE. Inosine pranobex has sometimes been described as inosine with dimepranol and acedoben. Dimepranol is the pINN name for (±)-1-(dimethylamino)-2-propanol and acedoben is the pINN name for *p*-acetamidobenzoic acid.
Dimepranol Acedoben is *USAN.*

Adverse Effects and Precautions

Some patients have experienced transient nausea and vomiting. Metabolism of the inosine content of inosine pranobex leads to increased serum and urine concentrations of uric acid; caution is therefore recommended in treating patients with impaired renal function, gout, or hyperuricaemia.

Antiviral Action

Inosine pranobex appears to owe its activity in viral infections more to its capacity to modify or stimulate cell-mediated immune processes than to a direct action on the virus.

Inosine pranobex was found to have slight activity against some viruses *in vitro* and also some activity in *animals* infected with herpes simplex virus type 2 and influenza virus.[1] However, another study[2] showed it to lack activity in experimental model infections.

1. Chang T-W, Weinstein L. Antiviral activity of isoprinosine in vitro and in vivo. *Am J Med Sci* 1973; **265:** 143–6.
2. Glasgow LA, Galasso GJ. Isoprinosine: lack of antiviral activity in experimental model infections. *J Infect Dis* 1972; **126:** 162–9.

Pharmacokinetics

Inosine pranobex is reported to be rapidly absorbed following administration by mouth. It is also rapidly metabolised, the inosine portion of the complex yielding uric acid; the other part of the complex undergoes oxidation and glucuronidation. The metabolites are excreted in the urine.

A study of the metabolism and excretion of the components of inosine pranobex in 2 subjects.[1]

1. Nielsen P, Beckett AH. The metabolism and excretion in man of NN-dimethylamino-isopropanol and p-acetamido-benzoic acid after administration of isoprinosine. *J Pharm Pharmacol* 1981; **33:** 549–50.

Uses and Administration

Inosine pranobex has been used in the treatment of various viral infections. Preparations are available for use in herpes simplex, genital warts, and subacute sclerosing panencephalitis, although other treatments or measures are preferred. The recommended dose in mucocutaneous herpes simplex is 1 g four times daily by mouth for 7 to 14 days. A dose of 1 g three times daily is given for 14 to 28 days as an adjunct to traditional topical treatment for genital warts. In subacute sclerosing panencephalitis the dose is 50 to 100 mg per kg bodyweight daily in divided doses given every 4 hours.

Reviews.

1. Campoli-Richards DM, *et al.* Inosine pranobex: a preliminary review of its pharmacodynamic and pharmacokinetic properties, and therapeutic efficacy. *Drugs* 1986; **32:** 383–424.

Herpes simplex infections. The usual antiviral used in the treatment of herpes simplex infections is aciclovir (see p.597), and it has been shown to be more effective than inosine pranobex for genital infections.[1,2] Inosine pranobex has also been tried in herpes labialis, but with equivocal results.[3-5]

1. Mindel A, *et al.* Treatment of first-attack genital herpes—acyclovir versus inosine pranobex. *Lancet* 1987; **i:** 1171–3.
2. Mindel A, *et al.* Suppression of frequently recurring genital herpes: acyclovir v inosine pranobex. *Genitourin Med* 1989; **65:** 103–5.
3. Galli M, *et al.* Inosiplex in recurrent herpes simplex infections. *Lancet* 1982; **ii:** 331–2.
4. Galli M, *et al.* Inosiplex in recurrent herpes simplex infections. *Lancet* 1982; **ii:** 926.
5. Kalimo KOK, *et al.* Failure of oral inosiplex treatment of recurrent herpes simplex virus infections. *Arch Dermatol* 1983; **119:** 463–7.

Subacute sclerosing panencephalitis. As discussed under Measles (see p.602) inosine pranobex has been tried in the treatment of subacute sclerosing panencephalitis but the results of clinical studies have been equivocal.[1-8] The addition of benzhexol to inosine pranobex therapy produced beneficial responses in 2 of 3 patients.[9]

1. Streletz LJ, Cracco J. The effect of isoprinosine in subacute sclerosing panencephalitis (SSPE). *Ann Neurol* 1977; **1:** 183–4.
2. Huttenlocher PR, Mattson RH. Isoprinosine in subacute sclerosing panencephalitis. *Neurology* 1979; **29:** 763–71.
3. Silverberg R, *et al.* Inosiplex in the treatment of subacute sclerosing panencephalitis. *Arch Neurol* 1979; **36:** 374–5.
4. Haddad FS, Risk WS. Isoprinosine treatment in 18 patients with subacute sclerosing panencephalitis: a controlled study. *Ann Neurol* 1980; **7:** 185–8.
5. Jones CE, *et al.* Inosiplex therapy in subacute sclerosing panencephalitis: a multicentre, non-randomised study in 98 patients. *Lancet* 1982; **i:** 1034–7.
6. Anonymous. Inosiplex: antiviral, immunomodulator, or neither? *Lancet* 1982; **i:** 1052–4.
7. DuRant RH, *et al.* The influence of inosiplex treatment on the neurological disability of patients with subacute sclerosing panencephalitis. *J Pediatr* 1982; **101:** 288–93.
8. DuRant RH, Dyken PR. The effect of inosiplex on the survival of subacute sclerosing panencephalitis. *Neurology* 1983; **33:** 1053–5.
9. Nunes ML, *et al.* Trihexyphenidyl and isoprinosine in the treatment of subacute sclerosing panencephalitis. *Pediatr Neurol* 1995; **13:** 153–6.

Preparations

Proprietary Preparations (details are given in Part 3)
Belg.: Isoprinosine; ***Fr.:*** Isoprinosine; ***Ger.:*** delimmun; Isoprinosine†; ***Irl.:*** Imunovir; ***Ital.:*** Anavir†; Antib†; Aviral†; Avirin; Farviran; Isoprinosina; Isoviral†; Metivirol; Stimuzim; Virac; Viralin; Virustop; Viruxan; ***Spain:*** Bodaril; ***UK:*** Imunovir.

Interferons (11421-y)

CAS — 9008-11-1.

Proteins or glycoproteins produced in human or animal cells in response to various stimuli including exposure to viruses. They may also be produced through recombinant DNA technology. There are 3 major immunologically distinct types of interferon: interferon alfa, interferon beta, and interferon gamma.

Interferon Alfa (11419-t)

Interferon Alfa *(BAN, rINN).*

IFN-α; Interferon-α; Ro-22-8181 (interferon alfa-2a); Sch-30500 (interferon alfa-2b).

CAS — 74899-72-2 (interferon alfa); 76543-88-9 (interferon alfa-2a); 99210-65-8 (interferon alfa-2b).

NOTE. Interferon alfa was previously known as leucocyte interferon or lymphoblastoid interferon.
Interferon alfa-2a, alfa-2b, alfa-n1, and alfa-n3 are *USAN.*

Interferon alfa may be derived from leucocytes or lymphoblasts as well as through recombinant DNA technology. Subspecies of the human alfa gene may produce interferon alfa with protein variants or a mixture of proteins. The protein variants may be designated by a number (as in interferon alfa-2) which may be further qualified by a letter to indicate the amino-acid sequences at positions 23 and 34. Interferon alfa-2a has lysine at 23 and histidine at 34, interferon alfa-2b has arginine at 23 and histidine at 34, and interferon alfa-2c has arginine at both positions. In the case of a mixture of proteins an alphanumeric designation is given (as in interferon alfa-n1).

The name may be further elaborated on the label by approved sets of initials in parentheses to indicate the method of production: (rbe) indicates production from bacteria (*Es-*

cherichia coli) genetically modified by recombinant DNA technology; (lns) indicates production from cultured lymphoblasts from the Namalwa cell line that have been stimulated by a Sendai virus; (bls) indicates production from leucocytes from human blood that have been stimulated by a Sendai virus.

References to the nomenclature of interferon alfa.

1. Finter NB. The naming of cats—and alpha-interferons. *Lancet* 1996; **348:** 348–9.

Interferon Beta (11420-l)

Interferon Beta *(BAN, rINN)*.

IFN-β; Interferon-β; SH-Y-579A (interferon beta-1b).

CAS — 74899-71-1 (interferon beta); 145258-61-3 (interferon beta-1a); 145155-23-3 (interferon beta-1b); 90598-63-3 (interferon beta-1b).

NOTE. Interferon beta was previously known as fibroblast interferon.

Interferon beta-1a and Interferon beta-1b are both *USAN*.

Interferon beta may be derived from fibroblasts as well as through recombinant DNA technology. Sub-species of the human beta gene produce interferon beta with protein variants designated by a number (as in interferon beta-1). Interferon beta-1 is further qualified by a letter to indicate the amino-acid sequences at positions 1 and 17, and to indicate whether or not glycosylation is present. Interferon beta-1a has methionine at position 1 and cysteine at 17 and is glycosylated at position 80. Interferon beta-1b has serine at position 17 and is not glycosylated.

The name may be further elaborated on the label by approved sets of initials in parenthesis to indicate the method of production: (rch) indicates production from genetically engineered Chinese hamster ovary cells; (rbe) indicates production from bacteria (*Escherichia coli*) genetically modified by recombinant DNA technology.

Interferon Gamma (1683-t)

Interferon Gamma *(BAN, rINN)*.

IFN-γ; Interferon-γ.

CAS — 98059-18-8 (interferon gamma-1a); 98059-61-1 (interferon gamma-1b).

NOTE. Interferon gamma was previously known as immune interferon.

Interferon gamma-1b is *USAN* and was previously known as interferon gamma-2a.

Interferon gamma may be derived from immunologically stimulated T-lymphocytes (hence its former name of immune interferon) as well as through recombinant DNA technology. Similarly to interferon alfa, protein variants of interferon gamma are designated by a number and further qualified by a letter to indicate the amino-acid sequences at terminal positions 1 and 139. Interferon gamma-1a has at position 1 hydrogen, cysteine, tyrosine, and cysteine and at position 139 arginine, alanine, serine, glutamine, and a hydroxyl group. Interferon gamma-1b, formerly known as interferon gamma-2a, has at position 1 hydrogen and methionine and at position 139 a hydroxyl group. Interferon gamma derived through recombinant DNA technology is labelled (rbe).

Adverse Effects and Treatment

Most reports of the adverse effects of interferons have involved interferon alfa, but limited clinical experience suggests that interferons beta and gamma have similar adverse effects.

Interferons produce influenza-like symptoms with fever, chills, headache, malaise, myalgia, and arthralgia. These symptoms tend to be dose-related, are most likely to occur at the start of treatment, and mostly respond to paracetamol (but for a possible interaction with paracetamol, see Interactions, below).

Other adverse effects include nausea, vomiting, diarrhoea, anorexia with weight loss, bone marrow depression, alopecia, rash, and taste alteration. There may be signs of altered liver function and liver necrosis has been reported. Renal failure and the nephrotic syndrome have occurred and there are rare reports of interstitial nephritis. Severe hypersensitivity reactions including anaphylaxis and bronchospasm have occurred. Cardiovascular effects include hypotension or hypertension, arrhythmias, oedema, myocardial infarction, and stroke. High doses may cause electrolyte disturbances including decreased calcium concentrations. Hyperglycaemia and thyroid dysfunction have been reported as have pulmonary oedema and pneumonitis. EEG abnormalities and neurological symptoms including ataxia, paraesthesia, somnolence, dizziness, confusion, and rarely, convulsions and coma have been reported. There may be severe fatigue, depression, anxiety, depersonalisation, or emotional lability. Visual disturbances and, rarely, ischaemic retinopathy may occur. Menstrual irregularities have been reported, particularly with interferon beta.

Subcutaneous injection may produce a reaction at the injection site. The reaction is reported frequently with interferon beta, which can produce severe reactions including local necrosis.

Nasal administration may produce mucosal irritation and damage.

Reviews.

1. Vial T, Descotes J. Clinical toxicity of the interferons. *Drug Safety* 1994; **10:** 115–50.
2. Pardo M, *et al.* Risks and benefits of interferon-α in the treatment of hepatitis. *Drug Safety* 1995; **13:** 304–16.

Effects on the blood. Restoration of bone-marrow function following marrow transplantation was delayed in 3 patients given a human interferon alfa preparation.[1] Laboratory results showed an inhibition of granulocyte colony growth by human leucocyte interferon alfa. It was considered that interferon alfa was contra-indicated in patients with severe bone-marrow insufficiency and should not be given to marrow transplant patients before the graft was fully functional. However, in another 5 patients recombinant interferon alfa did not affect bone-marrow transplants, although 3 patients experienced fever and chills, 4 experienced more than a 60% reduction in absolute peripheral granulocyte counts, and 4 had a 37 to 80% reduction in absolute platelet counts.[2] Lymphocytes were increased in all patients; blood counts returned to normal when interferon therapy stopped. Interferon alfa produced a decline in CD4-positive T-lymphocytes resulting in opportunistic infections in 2 HIV-positive patients being treated for chronic hepatitis C.[3]

Other haematological effects reported to be associated with interferon alfa include immune haemolytic anaemia[4] and immune thrombocytopenia.[5,6] Haemorrhage occurred in a patient with immune thrombocytopenic purpura treated with interferon alfa,[7] and it was thought prudent to use interferons with caution, if at all, in this condition.[6,7] Thrombosis associated with interferon alfa has also been reported.[8]

1. Nissen C, *et al.* Toxicity of human leucocyte interferon preparations in human bone-marrow cultures. *Lancet* 1977; **i:** 203–4.
2. Winston DJ, *et al.* Safety and tolerance of recombinant leukocyte A interferon in bone marrow transplant recipients. *Antimicrob Agents Chemother* 1983; **23:** 846–51.
3. Pesce A, *et al.* Opportunistic infections and CD4 lymphocytopenia with interferon treatment in HIV-1 infected patients. *Lancet* 1993; **341:** 1597.
4. Akard LP, *et al.* Alpha-interferon and immune hemolytic anemia. *Ann Intern Med* 1986; **105:** 306.
5. McLaughlin P, *et al.* Immune thrombocytopenia following α-interferon therapy in patients with cancer. *JAMA* 1985; **254:** 1353–4.
6. Färkkilä M, Iivanainen M. Thrombocytopenia and interferon. *Br Med J* 1988; **296:** 642.
7. Matthey F, *et al.* Bleeding in immune thrombocytopenic purpura after alpha-interferon. *Lancet* 1990; **335:** 471–2.
8. Durand JM, *et al.* Thrombosis and recombinant interferon-α. *Am J Med* 1993; **95:** 115.

Effects on the cardiovascular system. There have been reports of cardiomyopathy[1,2] and of Raynaud's syndrome[3,4] associated with interferon alfa therapy.

1. Deyton LR, *et al.* Reversible cardiac dysfunction associated with interferon alfa therapy in AIDS patients with Kaposi's sarcoma. *N Engl J Med* 1989; **321:** 1246–9.
2. Sonnenblick M, *et al.* Reversible cardiomyopathy induced by interferon. *Br Med J* 1990; **300:** 1174–5.
3. Roy V, Newland AC. Raynaud's phenomenon and cryoglobulinaemia associated with the use of recombinant human alpha-interferon. *Lancet* 1988; **i:** 944–5.
4. Bachmeyer C, *et al.* Raynaud's phenomenon and digital necrosis induced by interferon-alpha. *Br J Dermatol* 1996; **135:** 481–3.

Effects on the endocrine system. Both hypothyroidism[1,2] and hyperthyroidism[2,3] have been associated with interferon alfa therapy. Recombinant interferon gamma was reported not to affect thyroid function.[4] The development of type 1 diabetes has been associated with interferon alfa therapy.[5-8] Exacerbation of existing type 2 diabetes has also been reported.[9,10] Reversible hypopituitarism was reported in 1 patient receiving interferon alfa.[11]

1. Fentiman IS, *et al.* Primary hypothyroidism associated with interferon therapy of breast cancer. *Lancet* 1985; **i:** 1166.
2. Burman P, *et al.* Autoimmune thyroid disease in interferon-treated patients. *Lancet* 1985; **ii:** 100–1.
3. Schultz M, *et al.* Induction of hyperthyroidism by interferon-α-2b. *Lancet* 1989; **i:** 1452.
4. Bhakri H, *et al.* Recombinant gamma interferon and autoimmune thyroid disease. *Lancet* 1985; **ii:** 457.
5. Fabris P, *et al.* Development of type 1 diabetes mellitus during interferon alfa therapy for chronic HCV hepatitis. *Lancet* 1992; **340:** 548.
6. Guerci A-P, *et al.* Onset of insulin-dependent diabetes mellitus after interferon-alfa therapy for hairy cell leukaemia. *Lancet* 1994; **343:** 1167–8.
7. Gori A, *et al.* Reversible diabetes in patient with AIDS-related Kaposi's sarcoma treated with interferon α-2a. *Lancet* 1995; **345:** 1438–9.
8. Murakami M, *et al.* Diabetes mellitus and interferon-α therapy. *Ann Intern Med* 1995; **123:** 318.
9. Campbell S, *et al.* Rapidly reversible increase in insulin requirement with interferon. *Br Med J* 1996; **313:** 92.
10. Lopes EPA, *et al.* Exacerbation of type 2 diabetes mellitus during interferon-alfa therapy for chronic hepatitis B. *Lancet* 1994; **343:** 244. Correction. *ibid.*: 680.
11. Sakane N, *et al.* Reversible hypopituitarism after interferon-alfa therapy. *Lancet* 1995; **345:** 1305.

Effects on the eyes. In a study of 43 patients with chronic hepatitis receiving interferon alfa, retinopathy developed in 11 non-diabetic patients and 3 diabetic patients after about 8 to 10 weeks of therapy.[1] None of the patients had retinopathy prior to treatment, and it was reversible in the non-diabetic patients on cessation of therapy. Visual acuity remained unchanged. Subconjunctival haemorrhage occurred in 3 of the non-diabetic patients. This and other reports of interferon-associated retinopathy have recently been reviewed.[2]

Pain in one eyeball leading to exophthalmos and complete visual loss was reported in one patient receiving interferon alfa;[3] despite withdrawal of interferon and instigation of antibiotic and corticosteroid treatment, the eyeball subsequently ruptured necessitating ophthalmectomy.

1. Hayasaka S, *et al.* Retinopathy and subconjunctival haemorrhage in patients with chronic viral hepatitis receiving interferon alfa. *Br J Ophthalmol* 1995; **79:** 150–2.
2. Hayasaka S, *et al.* Interferon associated retinopathy. *Br J Ophthalmol* 1998; **82:** 323–5.
3. Yamada H, *et al.* Acute onset of ocular complications with interferon. *Lancet* 1994; **343:** 914.

Effects on the hair. A report of marked greying of the hair in a patient beginning after 5 months of treatment with interferon alfa for metastatic malignant melanoma.[1] On completion of interferon therapy the hair regrowth returned to its normal colour.

Reversible mild to moderate alopecia has been reported by the manufacturers.

1. Fleming CJ, MacKie RM. Alpha interferon-induced hair discolouration. *Br J Dermatol* 1996; **135:** 337–8.

Effects on hearing. Sensorineural hearing loss was reported in 18 of 49 patients and tinnitus in 14 of 49 patients receiving interferons.[1] The effects were more common in those receiving interferon beta than in those receiving interferon alfa, and resolved in all patients on discontinuation of therapy.

1. Kanda Y, *et al.* Sudden hearing loss associated with interferon. *Lancet* 1994; **343:** 1134–5.

Effects on the kidneys. In a double-blind parallel-group study all of 8 renal transplant patients given, in addition to routine immunosuppression, high doses of recombinant interferon alfa (36 million units intramuscularly three times a week for 6 weeks followed by twice weekly for a further 6 weeks) had early rejection episodes which were corticosteroid resistant; 3 also had transient nephrotic syndrome.[1] All of 8 control patients, given human albumin and saline solution, also had early rejection episodes but only one was corticosteroid resistant. These adverse effects on the transplant contrasted with the absence of adverse effect on kidney transplants reported by Hirsch *et al.*[2] who gave lower doses of leucocyte interferon alfa for the prophylaxis of cytomegalovirus infections. There have been a number of other reports of nephrotic syndrome associated with interferon alfa;[3-5] in one patient this was secondary to membranoproliferative glomerulonephritis.[5] The manufacturers have noted rare reports of interstitial nephritis.

1. Kramer P, *et al.* Recombinant leucocyte interferon A induces steroid-resistant acute vascular rejection episodes in renal transplant recipients. *Lancet* 1984; **i:** 989–90.
2. Hirsch MS, *et al.* Effects of interferon-alpha on cytomegalovirus reactivation syndromes in renal-transplant recipients. *N Engl J Med* 1983; **308:** 1489–93.
3. Averbuch SD, *et al.* Acute interstitial nephritis with the nephrotic syndrome following recombinant leukocyte A interferon therapy for mycosis fungoides. *N Engl J Med* 1984; **310:** 32–5.
4. Selby P, *et al.* Nephrotic syndrome during treatment with interferon. *Br Med J* 1985; **290:** 1180.
5. Herrman J, Gabriel F. Membranoproliferative glomerulonephritis in a patient with hairy-cell leukemia treated with alpha-II interferon. *N Engl J Med* 1987; **316:** 112–13.

Effects on lipids. Reversible hypertriglyceridaemia has been associated with interferon alfa treatment for chronic hepatitis C.[1] Gemfibrozil reduced the hypertriglyceridaemia but lipid concentrations did not return to base-line values and interferon treatment had to be withdrawn.

1. Graessle D, *et al.* Alpha-interferon and reversible hypertriglyceridemia. *Ann Intern Med* 1993; **118:** 316–17.

Effects on the liver. Therapy with interferon alfa has been associated with cases of fatal liver failure,[1,2] sometimes in association with chronic hepatitis B and/or C infection.[3,4]

1. Durand JM, *et al.* Liver failure due to recombinant alpha interferon. *Lancet* 1991; **338:** 1268–9.
2. Wandl UB, *et al.* Liver failure due to recombinant alpha interferon for chronic myelogenous leukaemia. *Lancet* 1992; **339:** 123–4.

3. Marcellin P, *et al.* Fatal exacerbation of chronic hepatitis B induced by recombinant alpha-interferon. *Lancet* 1991; **338:** 828.
4. Janssen HLA, *et al.* Fatal hepatic decompensation associated with interferon alfa. *Br Med J* 1993; **306:** 107–8.

Effects on the nervous system and mental state. Neurological effects reported in 10 women with advanced breast cancer treated for up to 12 weeks with recombinant interferon alfa in doses of 20 million units daily or 50 million units three times a week included abnormal EEG patterns in all 10 patients, profound lethargy and somnolence in 6, confusion and dysphasia in 5, paraesthesia in 2, and an upper motor-neurone lesion of the legs in one.[1] These effects resolved when interferon alfa was withdrawn and all patients tolerated its reintroduction at a lower dose. Reversible EEG abnormalities were observed in a further 11 patients given interferon alfa in doses of 100 million units per m^2 body-surface daily for 7 days by continuous intravenous infusion,[2] in 3 patients given 5 to 10 million units per m^2 three times per week by subcutaneous injection,[3] and in another patient given 4 million units per m^2 daily for 6 weeks.[4] Other adverse neurological effects reported with interferon alfa include neuropsychiatric changes,[5] neuralgic amyotrophy and polyradiculopathy,[6] seizures,[7] spastic diplegia (in infants),[8] and severe neuropathy.[9] Some of these effects were observed with doses as low as 1.5 million units[7] or 3 million units daily.[5]

Depression associated with interferon therapy was successfully treated with fluoxetine in one patient thus allowing interferon therapy to be continued.[10]

Psychiatric disturbances leading to suicidal behaviour occurred in 3 patients receiving interferon; they had no history of psychiatric disorder.[11]

1. Smedley H, *et al.* Neurological effects of recombinant human interferon. *Br Med J* 1983; **286:** 262–4.
2. Rohatiner AZS, *et al.* Central nervous system toxicity of interferon. *Br J Cancer* 1983; **47:** 419–22.
3. Suter CC, *et al.* Electroencephalographic abnormalities in interferon encephalopathy: a preliminary report. *Mayo Clin Proc* 1984; **59:** 847–50.
4. Honigsberger L, *et al.* Neurological effects of recombinant human interferon. *Br Med J* 1983; **286:** 719.
5. Adams F, *et al.* Neuropsychiatric manifestations of human leukocyte interferon therapy in patients with cancer. *JAMA* 1984; **252:** 938–41.
6. Bernsen PLJA, *et al.* Neuralgic amyotrophy and polyradiculopathy during interferon therapy. *Lancet* 1985; **i:** 50.
7. Janssen HLA, *et al.* Seizures associated with low-dose α-interferon. *Lancet* 1990; **336:** 1580.
8. Barlow CF, *et al.* Spastic diplegia as a complication of interferon alfa-2a treatment of hemangiomas of infancy. *J Pediatr* 1998; **132:** 527–30.
9. Gastineau DA, *et al.* Severe neuropathy associated with low-dose recombinant interferon-alpha. *Am J Med* 1989; **87:** 116.
10. Levenson JL, Fallon HJ. Fluoxetine treatment of depression caused by interferon-α. *Am J Gastroenterol* 1993; **88:** 760–1.
11. Janssen HLA, *et al.* Suicide associated with alfa-interferon therapy for chronic viral hepatitis. *J Hepatol* 1994; **21:** 241–3.

Effects on the oral mucosa. Painful oral ulcers occurred during interferon alfa treatment[1] for chronic hepatitis in one patient and necessitated withdrawal of interferon. Oropharyngeal lichen planus was associated with interferon alfa in another patient.[2]

1. Qaseem T, *et al.* A case report of painful oral ulcerations associated with the use of alpha interferon in a patient with chronic hepatitis due to non-A non-B non-C virus. *Milit Med* 1993; **158:** 126–7.
2. Kütting B, *et al.* Oropharyngeal lichen planus associated with interferon-α treatment for mycosis fungoides: a rare side-effect in the therapy of cutaneous lymphomas. *Br J Dermatol* 1997; **137:** 836–7.

Effects on skeletal muscle. Myalgia is one of the influenza-like symptoms frequently associated with interferons. Fatal rhabdomyolysis and multiple organ failure was reported in a patient receiving high doses of interferon alfa.[1]

1. Reinhold U, *et al.* Fatal rhabdomyolysis and multiple organ failure associated with adjuvant high-dose interferon alfa in malignant melanoma. *Lancet* 1997; **349:** 540–1.

Effects on the skin. Exacerbation or development of psoriasis was reported in patients given recombinant interferon alfa.[1,2] However, no exacerbation was seen in 7 patients given interferon gamma.[3] Exacerbation of lichen planus has also been reported[4] during interferon alfa treatment (see also Effects on the Oral Mucosa, above). Cutaneous vascular lesions with punctate telangiectasias were noted in 18 of 44 patients treated with interferon alfa-2a; lesions did not appear at the injection site.[5] Severe necrotising cutaneous lesions were reported at injection sites in a patient receiving recombinant interferon beta-1b; the lesions healed when interferon alfa-n3 was substituted.[6] However, cutaneous necrosis has also been associated with interferon alfa.[7] Fatal paraneoplastic pemphigus developed in a patient receiving interferon alfa-2a.[8]

1. Quesada JR, Gutterman JU. Psoriasis and alpha-interferon. *Lancet* 1986; **i:** 1466–8.
2. Funk J, *et al.* Psoriasis induced by interferon-α. *Br J Dermatol* 1991; **125:** 463–5.
3. Schulze H-J, Mahrle G. Gamma interferon and psoriasis. *Lancet* 1986; **ii:** 926–7.
4. Protzer U, *et al.* Exacerbation of lichen planus during interferon alfa-2a therapy for chronic active hepatitis C. *Gastroenterology* 1993; **104:** 903–5.
5. Dreno B, *et al.* Alpha-interferon therapy and cutaneous vascular lesions. *Ann Intern Med* 1989; **111:** 95–6.
6. Sheremata WA, *et al.* Severe necrotizing cutaneous lesions complicating treatment with interferon beta-1b. *N Engl J Med* 1995; **332:** 1584.
7. Shinohara K. More on interferon-induced cutaneous necrosis. *N Engl J Med* 1995; **333:** 1222.
8. Kirsner RS, *et al.* Treatment with alpha interferon associated with the development of paraneoplastic pemphigus. *Br J Dermatol* 1995; **132:** 474–8.

Shock. Fatal non-cardiogenic shock occurred following the third dose of interferon alfa-2b in a patient with malignant melanoma.[1] There were similarities to a fatal reaction reported in another patient with malignant melanoma (see under Effects on Skeletal Muscle, above).

1. Carson JJ, *et al.* Fatality and interferon α for malignant melanoma. *Lancet* 1998; **352:** 1443–4.

Precautions

Interferons should be used with caution or avoided altogether in patients with depression or psychiatric disorders, epilepsy, severe renal or hepatic impairment, cardiac disorders, myelosuppression, thyroid or pulmonary disease, diabetes mellitus, coagulation disorders, or a history of these conditions. Blood counts should be monitored, particularly in patients at high risk of myelosuppression (for example those with haematological malignancies). Hepatic and renal function should be monitored during treatment with interferons. The manufacturers of interferon alfa recommended that patients should receive adequate fluids to maintain hydration. Patients with psoriasis have been reported to experience exacerbations during interferon alfa therapy. Interferons may affect the ability to drive or operate machinery.

Antibodies may develop to exogenous interferon that reduce its activity.

Auto-immune disorders. A number of disorders thought to have an auto-immune component have developed or been exacerbated during therapy with interferon alfa, including diabetes mellitus,[1] autoimmune hepatitis,[2,3] multiple sclerosis,[4,5] rheumatoid arthritis,[6] and systemic lupus erythematosus.[7]

1. Fabris P, *et al.* Development of type 1 diabetes mellitus during interferon alfa therapy for chronic HCV hepatitis. *Lancet* 1992; **340:** 548.
2. Vento S, *et al.* Hazards of interferon therapy for HBV-seronegative chronic hepatitis. *Lancet* 1989; **ii:** 926.
3. Papo T, *et al.* Autoimmune chronic hepatitis exacerbated by alpha-interferon. *Ann Intern Med* 1992; **116:** 51–3.
4. Larrey D, *et al.* Exacerbation of multiple sclerosis after the administration of recombinant human interferon alfa. *JAMA* 1989; **261:** 2065.
5. Coyle JT. Multiple sclerosis and human interferon alfa. *JAMA* 1989; **262:** 2684.
6. Chazerain P, *et al.* Rheumatoid arthritis-like disease after alpha-interferon therapy. *Ann Intern Med* 1992; **116:** 427.
7. Tolaymat A, *et al.* Systemic lupus erythematosus in a child receiving long-term interferon therapy. *J Pediatr* 1992; **120:** 429–32.

Interactions

Interactions involving interferons have not been fully evaluated, but it is known that they can inhibit hepatic oxidative metabolism and thus caution should be exercised during concomitant administration of drugs metabolised in this way. For example, interferon alfa has been reported to enhance the effect of theophylline. Drugs likely to exacerbate the effects of interferons, such as those with myelosuppressive activity, should also be used with caution.

Interferon alfa has been reported to cause increased toxicity, accumulation, and increased plasma concentrations of *vidarabine*.[1] It has also been found to inhibit *theophylline* metabolism, thus increasing plasma concentrations,[2,3] and to exhibit synergistic cytotoxicity with *zidovudine* in AIDS-associated Kaposi's sarcoma[4] and *in vitro*.[5] Interferon-induced fever has been reported to lead to an increase in the cytotoxicity of *melphalan*.[6] An increased anticoagulant effect, together with increased serum-*warfarin* concentrations, has been reported when interferon alfa therapy is introduced.[7] Three patients experienced increases in liver enzyme values when given *paracetamol* 1 g two or three times a day on three days a week to coincide with the days of administration of interferon alfa; vinblastine was also given every third week.[8] Paracetamol has also been found to enhance the antiviral effect of interferon alfa in healthy subjects.[9] Severe granulocytopenia has been reported[10] in three patients with mixed cryoglobulinaemia treated with interferon alfa-2a who also received *ACE inhibitors*. The effect was considered to be due to synergistic haematological toxicity. However, in a further report,[11] two patients developed only mild granulocytopenia that was reversible despite continued therapy, while a third patient retained a normal granulocyte count.

1. Sacks SL, *et al.* Antiviral treatment of chronic hepatitis B virus infection: pharmacokinetics and side effects of interferon and adenine arabinoside alone and in combination. *Antimicrob Agents Chemother* 1982; **21:** 93–100.
2. Williams SJ, *et al.* Inhibition of theophylline metabolism by interferon. *Lancet* 1987; **ii:** 939–41.
3. Israel BC, *et al.* Effects of interferon-α monotherapy on hepatic drug metabolism in cancer patients. *Br J Clin Pharmacol* 1993; **36:** 229–35.
4. Krown SE, *et al.* Interferon-α (IFN-α) plus zidovudine (ZDV) in AIDS-associated Kaposi's sarcoma (AIDS/KS): an ongoing phase I trial. *Proc Am Soc Clin Oncol* 1988; **7:** 1 (abstract).
5. Berman E, *et al.* Synergistic cytotoxic effect of azidothymidine and recombinant interferon alpha on normal human bone marrow progenitor cells. *Blood* 1989; **74:** 1281–6.
6. Ehrsson H, *et al.* Oral melphalan pharmacokinetics: influence of interferon-induced fever. *Clin Pharmacol Ther* 1990; **47:** 86–90.
7. Adachi Y, *et al.* Potentiation of warfarin by interferon. *Br Med J* 1995; **311:** 292.
8. Kellokumpu-Lehtinen P, *et al.* Hepatotoxicity of paracetamol in combination with interferon and vinblastine. *Lancet* 1989; **i:** 1143.
9. Hendrix CW, *et al.* Modulation of α-interferon's antiviral and clinical effects by aspirin, acetaminophen, and prednisone in healthy volunteers. *Antiviral Res* 1995; **28:** 121–31.
10. Casato M, *et al.* Granulocytopenia after combined therapy with interferon and angiotensin-converting enzyme inhibitors: evidence for a synergistic hematologic toxicity. *Am J Med* 1995; **99:** 386–91.
11. Jacquot C, *et al.* Granulocytopenia after combined therapy with interferon and angiotensin-converting enzyme inhibitors: evidence for a synergistic hematologic toxicity. *Am J Med* 1996; **101:** 235–6.

Antiviral Action

Interferons are produced by virus-infected cells and confer protection on uninfected cells of the same species. They affect many cell functions demonstrating, in addition to their antiviral activity, antiproliferative and immunoregulatory properties; interferon gamma in particular is a potent macrophage-stimulating factor. These activities are considered to be interrelated. Following binding of interferons to a specific cell-surface protein, several enzyme systems appear to be activated to block viral and possibly cellular RNA development.

Studies have shown interferons to have benefit in infections with hepatitis B virus, hepatitis C virus, herpes simplex viruses, varicella-zoster virus, cytomegalovirus, rhinoviruses, and papillomaviruses.

Pharmacokinetics

Interferons are not absorbed from the gastro-intestinal tract. More than 80% of a subcutaneous or intramuscular dose of interferon alfa is absorbed; interferon beta and interferon gamma are less well absorbed by these routes. Following intramuscular injection interferon alfa produced by recombinant techniques and from cultured leucocytes produce similar plasma concentrations, usually reaching a peak within 4 to 8 hours. Half-lives of up to 16 hours have been reported. Intravenous administration produces more rapid distribution and elimination. Interferon alfa does not readily cross the blood-brain barrier. Negligible amounts of interferons are excreted in the urine.

References to the pharmacokinetics of interferons.

1. Gutterman JU, *et al.* Recombinant leukocyte A interferon: pharmacokinetics, single-dose tolerance, and biologic effects in cancer patients. *Ann Intern Med* 1982; **96:** 549–56.
2. Bornemann LD, *et al.* Intravenous and intramuscular pharmacokinetics of recombinant leukocyte A interferon. *Eur J Clin Pharmacol* 1985; **28:** 469–71.
3. Wills RJ. Clinical pharmacokinetics of interferons. *Clin Pharmacokinet* 1990; **19:** 390–9.
4. Maasilta P, *et al.* Pharmacokinetics of inhaled recombinant and natural alpha interferon. *Lancet* 1991; **337:** 371.

Uses and Administration

The interferons have a range of activities. In addition to their action against viruses they are active against malignant neoplasms and have an immunomodulating effect. There are several interferons available: interferon alfa-2a (rbe), interferon alfa-2b (rbe), alfa-n1 (lns), and alfa-n3 (bls); interferon beta-1a and interferon beta-1b; and interferon gamma-1b (rbe).

Alfa interferons are used in chronic hepatitis B and C (alfa-2a, alfa-2b, and alfa-n1); in several malignant neoplasms including AIDS-related Kaposi's sarcoma (alfa-2a and alfa-2b), hairy-cell leukaemia (alfa-2a, alfa-2b, and alfa-n1), chronic myeloid leukaemia, (alfa-2a, alfa-2b, and alfa-n1), follicular lymphoma (alfa-2a and alfa-2b), cutaneous T-cell lymphoma (alfa-2a), carcinoid tumours (alfa-2b), melanoma (alfa-2b), myeloma (alfa-2b), and renal cell carcinoma (alfa-2a); and in condylomata acuminata (alfa-2b and alfa-n3). *Beta interferons* are used in multiple sclerosis. *Interferon gamma-1b* is used as an adjunct to antibacterial therapy in chronic granulomatous disease.

ADMINISTRATION AND DOSAGE. Dosage regimens are as follows.

- **Chronic active hepatitis B.** *Interferon alfa-2a* is given in a dose of 2.5 to 5 million units per m^2 body-surface three times a week by subcutaneous injection for 4 to 6 months. *Interferon alfa-2b* is given in doses of 5 to 10 million units three times a week for 4 to 6 months, or 5 million units daily for 4 months by subcutaneous or intramuscular injection. *Interferon alfa-n1* is given either in doses of 10 to 15 million units (to a maximum of 7.5 million units per m^2) three times a week for 12 weeks, or 5 to 10 million units (to a maximum of 5 million units per m^2) three times a week for up to 6 months by subcutaneous or intramuscular injection.
- **Chronic hepatitis C.** *Interferon alfa-2a* is given either in an initial dose of 3 to 6 million units three times a week for 6 months followed by 3 million units three times a week for an additional 6 months, or in a dose of 3 million units three times a week for 12 months, by subcutaneous or intramuscular injection. *Interferon alfa-2b* is given in a dose of 3 million units three times a week for 12 to 18 months, or for up to 24 months, by subcutaneous or intramuscular injection. *Interferon alfa-n1* is given in a dose of 3 or 5 million units three times a week for 48 weeks by subcutaneous or intramuscular injection.
- **AIDS-related Kaposi's sarcoma.** *Interferon alfa-2a* is usually given in an escalating dose of 3 million units daily for 3 days, 9 million units daily for 3 days, 18 million units daily for 3 days, and 36 million units daily, if tolerated, on days 10 to 84, by subcutaneous or intramuscular injection; thereafter the maximum tolerated dose (up to 36 million units) may be given three times a week. *Interferon alfa-2b* is given in a dose of either 10 to 20 million units daily by subcutaneous injection or 30 million units per m^2 three times a week by subcutaneous or intramuscular injection.
- **Hairy-cell leukaemia.** *Interferon alfa-2a* is given in an initial dose of 3 million units daily for 16 to 24 weeks, then the same dose three times a week by subcutaneous or intramuscular injection. *Interferon alfa-2b* is given in a dose of 2 million units per m^2 three times a week by subcutaneous or intramuscular injection. *Interferon alfa-n1* is given in an initial dose of 3 million units daily by subcutaneous or intramuscular injection, commonly for 12 to 16 weeks, then the same dose three times a week thereafter. Alternative doses of 2 million units per m^2 or 0.2 million units per m^2 of interferon alfa-n1 have also been tried.
- **Chronic myeloid leukaemia.** *Interferon alfa-2a* is given by subcutaneous or intramuscular injection in an escalating dose of 3 million units daily for 3 days, 6 million units daily for 3 days, and 9 million units daily to complete 12 weeks of treatment. Patients showing a response should continue on 9 million units daily (or a minimum of 9 million units 3 times a week) until a complete haematological response is achieved or for a maximum of 18 months. Treatment may continue in patients who achieve a complete haematological response in order to achieve a cytogenetic response. *Interferon alfa-2b* is given in a dose of 4 to 5 million units per m^2 daily by subcutaneous injection, increasing to the maximum tolerated dose to maintain remission (usually 4 to 10 million units per m^2 daily). *Interferon alfa-n1* is given in a dose of 3 million units daily for three weeks by subcutaneous injection. The dose is then adjusted to maintain a suitable leucocyte count.
- **Follicular lymphoma.** *Interferon alfa-2a* is given as an adjunct to chemotherapy in a dose of 6 million units per m^2 daily by subcutaneous or intramuscular injection on days 22 to 26 of a 28-day chemotherapy cycle. *Interferon alfa-2b* is given as an adjunct to chemotherapy in a dose of 5 million units three times a week by subcutaneous injection for 18 months.
- **Cutaneous T-cell lymphoma.** *Interferon alfa-2a* is given in an escalating dose of 3 million units daily for 3 days, 9 million units daily for 3 days, and 18 million units daily to complete 12 weeks of treatment, by subcutaneous or intramuscular injection. The maximum tolerated dose (but not exceeding 18 million units) is then given three times a week for a minimum of 12 months.
- **Carcinoid tumours.** *Interferon alfa-2b* is given in a dose of 3 to 9 million units (usually 5 million units) three times a week by subcutaneous injection. In advanced disease, 5 million units may be given daily.
- **Multiple myeloma.** *Interferon alfa-2b* is given as maintenance treatment following chemotherapy induction at a dose of 3 million units per m^2 three times a week by subcutaneous injection.
- **Melanoma.** *Interferon alfa-2b* is given in an initial dose of 20 million units per m^2 daily on 5 days each week for 4 weeks by intravenous infusion over 20 minutes, and then for maintenance 10 million units per m^2 three times a week by subcutaneous injection for 48 weeks.
- **Renal cell carcinoma.** *Interferon alfa-2a* is given in an escalating dose of 3 million units three times a week for one week, then 9 million units three times a week for one week, then 18 million units three times a week thereafter for 3 to 12 months, by subcutaneous or intramuscular injection.
- **Condylomata acuminata.** *Interferon alfa-2b* is given in a dose of 1 million units injected into each lesion three times a week for three weeks, and repeated after 12 to 16 weeks if necessary. No more than 5 lesions should be treated in each treatment course, but courses for additional lesions may run sequentially. *Interferon alfa-n3* is given in a dose of 0.25 million units per lesion twice weekly for up to 8 weeks, to a maximum of 2.5 million units in each session.
- **Multiple sclerosis.** *Interferon beta-1a* is given in a dose of 6 million units once a week by intramuscular injection or 6 million units three times a week by subcutaneous injection, depending on the preparation. *Interferon beta-1b* is given in a dose of 8 million units (250 μg) on alternate days by subcutaneous injection.
- **Chronic granulomatous disease.** *Interferon gamma-1b* is used as an adjunct to antibacterial therapy in a dose of 50 μg per m^2 (1.5 million units per m^2) three times a week by subcutaneous injection. Patients with a body-surface area of less than 0.5 m^2 should receive 1.5 μg per kg body-weight.

See below for further details of these as well as some other uses of interferons.

General reviews of interferons.

1. Baron S, *et al.* The interferons: mechanisms of action and clinical applications. *JAMA* 1991; **266:** 1375–83.
2. Finter NB, *et al.* The use of interferon-α in virus infections. *Drugs* 1991; **42:** 749–65.
3. Volz MA, Kirkpatrick CH. Interferons 1992: how much of the promise has been realised? *Drugs* 1992; **43:** 285–94.
4. Todd PA, Goa KL. Interferon gamma-1b: a review of its pharmacology and therapeutic potential in chronic granulomatous disease. *Drugs* 1992; **43:** 111–22.
5. Dorr RT. Interferon-α malignant and viral diseases: a review. *Drugs* 1993; **45:** 177–211.
6. Goodkin DE. Interferon beta-1b. *Lancet* 1994; **344:** 1057–60.
7. Haria M, Benfield P. Interferon-α-2a: a review of its pharmacological properties and therapeutic use in the management of viral hepatitis. *Drugs* 1995; **50:** 873–96.

Age-related macular degeneration. In age-related macular degeneration (senile macular degeneration), a common cause of visual impairment in the elderly, there is a gradual and progressive deterioration of central vision usually affecting both eyes. Although some encouraging results[1-4] have been obtained with systemic interferon alfa-2a or alfa-2b for the treatment of choroidal neovascularisation considered unsuitable for laser therapy, adverse effects have been common and often severe and there is doubt over long-term benefit.

1. Gillies MC, *et al.* Treatment of choroidal neovascularisation in age-related macular degeneration with interferon alfa-2a and alfa-2b. *Br J Ophthalmol* 1993; **77:** 759–65.
2. Kirkpatrick JNP, *et al.* Clinical experience with interferon alfa-2a for exudative age-related macular degeneration. *Br J Ophthalmol* 1993; **77:** 766–70.
3. Poliner LS, *et al.* Interferon alpha-2a for subfoveal neovascularization in age-related macular degeneration. *Ophthalmology* 1993; **100:** 1417–24.
4. Engler C, *et al.* Interferon alfa-2a modifies the course of subfoveal and juxtafoveal choroidal neovascularisation. *Br J Ophthalmol* 1994; **78:** 749–53.

Angiomatous disease. Encouraging responses were reported in 4 of 5 children treated with interferon alfa-2a with a variety of angiomatous diseases.[1] Regression of haemangioma size by more than 50% was achieved in 11 of 18 infants and children who received interferon alfa-2a for 1 to 5 months.[2]

1. White CW, *et al.* Treatment of childhood angiomatous diseases with recombinant interferon alfa-2a. *J Pediatr* 1991; **118:** 59–66.
2. Deb G, *et al.* Treatment of hemangiomas of infants and babies with interferon alfa-2a: preliminary results. *Int J Pediatr Hematol/Oncol* 1996; **3:** 109–13.

Behçet's syndrome. Behçet's syndrome is usually managed with corticosteroids (see p.1018). Among many other drugs that have been tried, interferon alfa-2b was reported to produce beneficial responses in 3 patients with refractory ocular symptoms.[1] Encouraging results have also been obtained in other small studies of interferon alfa-2a.[2,3]

1. Feron EJ, *et al.* Interferon-α2b for refractory ocular Behçet's disease. *Lancet* 1994; **343:** 1428.
2. Azizlerli G, *et al.* Interferon alfa-2a in the treatment of Behçet's disease. *Dermatology* 1996; **192:** 239–41.
3. Kötter I, *et al.* Treatment of ocular symptoms of Behçet's disease with interferon α_{2a}: a pilot study. *Br J Ophthalmol* 1998; **82:** 488–94.

Blood disorders. Interferon is an alternative to anagrelide or hydroxyurea in the treatment of essential *thrombocythaemia* (p.496) Recombinant interferon alfa has generally been successful in essential thrombocythaemia.[1-5] It has been administered by subcutaneous or intramuscular injection, usually with an induction course followed by maintenance therapy at a lower dose. A reduction in platelet count greater than 50% after 28 days of treatment was observed in some patients.[1,2,5] A complete response (platelet count less than 440 x 10^9 per litre) was achieved and maintained for 12 months in 71% of patients with myeloproliferative disorders and associated thrombocytosis in one study.[4] Thrombocytosis recurred on stopping maintenance therapy, although remission was obtained on re-introducing interferon. Resistance to interferon was observed in 8 patients with thrombocythaemia;[2] in 6 patients the resistance was secondary. A number of patients have withdrawn from treatment because of adverse effects.[2,4]

Another thrombocytosis-associated myeloproliferative disease in which interferon alfa has been reported to be beneficial[4-8] is *polycythaemia vera.*

Paradoxically, interferon alfa has also been tried in patients with HIV-associated *thrombocytopenia*[9] (see HIV Infection and AIDS, below).

Following case reports of interferon alfa producing improvements in patients with idiopathic *hypereosinophilic syndrome*[10,11] who had not responded to corticosteroids and hydroxyurea two small studies have shown beneficial responses to interferon alfa alone[12] and in combination with hydroxyurea.[13]

1. Giles FJ, *et al.* Alpha-interferon therapy for essential thrombocythaemia. *Lancet* 1988; **ii:** 70–2.
2. Bellucci S, *et al.* Treatment of essential thrombocythaemia by alpha 2a interferon. *Lancet* 1988; **ii:** 960–1.
3. May D, *et al.* Treatment of essential thrombocythaemia with interferon alpha-2b. *Lancet* 1989; **i:** 96.
4. Gisslinger H, *et al.* Long-term interferon therapy for thrombocytosis in myeloproliferative diseases. *Lancet* 1989; **i:** 634–7.
5. Talpaz M, *et al.* Recombinant interferon-alpha therapy of Philadelphia chromosome-negative myeloproliferative disorders with thrombocytosis. *Am J Med* 1989; **86:** 554–8.
6. Silver RT. A new treatment for polycythemia vera: recombinant interferon alfa. *Blood* 1990; **76:** 664–5.
7. Silver RT. Interferon-α2b: a new treatment for polycythemia vera. *Ann Intern Med* 1993; **119:** 1091–2.
8. Muller EW, *et al.* Long-term treatment with interferon-α 2b for severe pruritus in patients with polycythaemia vera. *Br J Haematol* 1995; **89:** 313–18.
9. Marroni M, *et al.* Interferon-α is effective in the treatment of HIV-1-related, severe, zidovudine-resistant thrombocytopenia. *Ann Intern Med* 1994; **121:** 423–9.
10. Zielinski RM, Lawrence WD. Interferon-α for the hypereosinophilic syndrome. *Ann Intern Med* 1990; **113:** 716–18.
11. Busch FW, *et al.* Alpha-interferon for the hypereosinophilic syndrome. *Ann Intern Med* 1991; **114:** 338–9.
12. Butterfield JH, Gleich GJ. Interferon-α treatment of six patients with the idiopathic hypereosinophilic syndrome. *Ann Intern Med* 1994; **121:** 648–53.
13. Coutant G, *et al.* Traitement des syndromes hyperéosinophiliques à expression myeloproliferative par l'association hydroxyurée-interféron alpha. *Ann Med Interne (Paris)* 1993; **144:** 243–50.

Chronic granulomatous disease. Interferon gamma is reported to reduce the incidence of infections in patients with chronic granulomatous disease.[1-3]

1. The International Chronic Granulomatous Disease Cooperative Study Group. A controlled trial of interferon gamma to prevent infection in chronic granulomatous disease. *N Engl J Med* 1991; **324:** 509–16.
2. Bolinger AM, Taeubel MA. Recombinant interferon gamma for treatment of chronic granulomatous disease and other disorders. *Clin Pharm* 1992; **11:** 834–50.
3. Todd PA, Goa KL. Interferon gamma-1b: a review of its pharmacology and therapeutic potential in chronic granulomatous disease. *Drugs* 1992; **43:** 111–22.

Common cold. The management of the common cold is discussed on p.595. Despite the early promise[1-5] of intranasal interferon alfa for prophylaxis, later studies found it to be of no value for prophylaxis[6,7] or treatment.[8] Interferon beta was also reported to provide ineffective prophylaxis.[9]

1. Higgins PG, *et al.* Intranasal interferon as protection against experimental respiratory coronavirus infection in volunteers. *Antimicrob Agents Chemother* 1983; **24:** 713–15.
2. Farr BM, *et al.* Intranasal interferon-α2 for prevention of natural rhinovirus colds. *Antimicrob Agents Chemother* 1984; **26:** 31–4.

3. Tyrrell DA. The efficacy and tolerance of intranasal interferons: studies at the common cold unit. *J Antimicrob Chemother* 1986; **18** (suppl B): 153–6.
4. Douglas RM, *et al.* Prophylactic efficacy of intranasal alpha$_2$-interferon against rhinovirus infections in the family setting. *N Engl J Med* 1986; **314:** 65–70.
5. Hayden FG, *et al.* Prevention of natural colds by contact prophylaxis with intranasal alpha$_2$-interferon. *N Engl J Med* 1986; **314:** 71–5.
6. Monto AS, *et al.* Ineffectiveness of postexposure prophylaxis of rhinovirus infection with low-dose intranasal alpha 2b interferon in families. *Antimicrob Agents Chemother* 1989; **33:** 387–90.
7. Tannock GA, *et al.* A study of intranasally administered interferon A (rIFN-α2A) for the seasonal prophylaxis of natural viral infections of the upper respiratory tract in healthy volunteers. *Epidemiol Infect* 1988; **101:** 611–21.
8. Hayden FG, *et al.* Intranasal recombinant alfa-2b interferon treatment of naturally occurring common colds. *Antimicrob Agents Chemother* 1988; **32:** 224–30.
9. Sperber SJ, *et al.* Ineffectiveness of recombinant interferon-β_{serine} nasal drops for prophylaxis of natural colds. *J Infect Dis* 1989; **160:** 700–5.

Hepatitis. Interferon alfa is the main drug used in the treatment of chronic viral hepatitis (p.595).

Two meta-analyses[1,2] have confirmed the value of interferon alfa in chronic hepatitis B. Benefits appear to be greatest in patients with high aminotransferase concentrations and with a history of acute hepatitis.[1] It has been reported that about 40% of patients with chronic hepatitis C respond to interferon alfa.[3] Response is generally rapid, without the transient rise in serum alanine aminotransferase which is seen during treatment of hepatitis B, and it is suggested that treatment should be discontinued in patients who do not respond within 12 to 16 weeks.

While long-term remissions may be achieved following interferon therapy for hepatitis B,[4,5] prolonged therapy is required and relapse is frequent; relapse of hepatitis C may occur in half of responding patients on cessation of treatment,[6-8] but sustained responses have been reported.[9] In addition, it has been noted that about 70% of those who relapse may respond to further interferon treatment,[3] and more sustained responses may be achieved with prolonged courses of treatment.[10,11] There is also some evidence that interferon alfa may reduce the incidence of hepatocellular carcinoma in chronic active hepatitis C with cirrhosis.[12] Interferon beta has also been tried in hepatitis C.[13] In addition interferon alfa[14] and beta[15] may decrease the risk of chronic hepatitis C developing after acute infections.

The use of interferon alfa or beta in combination with tribavirin for hepatitis C is reported to improve response rates.[16-20]

A recent study has indicated that interferon alfa can benefit some patients with chronic hepatitis D.[21]

Although antivirals are generally not required in uncomplicated acute hepatitis, improvements in liver function were reported in 4 patients with fulminant hepatitis A treated with interferon beta.[22]

1. Krogsgaard K, *et al.* The treatment effect of alpha interferon in chronic hepatitis B is independent of pre-treatment variables: results based on individual patient data from 10 clinical controlled trials. *J Hepatol* 1994; **21:** 646–55.
2. Wong DKH, *et al.* Effect of alpha-interferon treatment in patients with hepatitis B e antigen-positive chronic hepatitis B: a meta-analysis. *Ann Intern Med* 1993; **119:** 312–23.
3. Davis GL. Interferon treatment of chronic hepatitis C. *Am J Med* 1994; **96** (suppl 1A): 41S–46S.
4. Korenman J, *et al.* Long-term remission of chronic hepatitis B after alpha-interferon therapy. *Ann Intern Med* 1991; **114:** 629–34.
5. Wong JB, *et al.* Cost-effectiveness of interferon-α2b treatment for hepatitis B e antigen-positive chronic hepatitis B. *Ann Intern Med* 1995; **122:** 664–75.
6. Dusheiko G. Treatment of chronic viral hepatitis: the end of the beginning? *Br J Hosp Med* 1994; **52:** 8–11.
7. van der Poel CL, *et al.* Hepatitis C virus six years on. *Lancet* 1994; **344:** 1475–9.
8. Dusheiko GM, *et al.* A rational approach to the management of hepatitis C infection. *Br Med J* 1996; **312:** 357–64.
9. Marcellin P, *et al.* Long-term histologic improvement and loss of detectable intrahepatic HCV RNA in patients with chronic hepatitis C and sustained response to interferon-α therapy. *Ann Intern Med* 1997; **127:** 875–81.
10. Reichard O, *et al.* Two-year biochemical, virological, and histological follow-up in patients with chronic hepatitis C responding in a sustained fashion to interferon alfa-2b treatment. *Hepatology* 1995; **21:** 918–22.
11. Poynard T, *et al.* A comparison of three interferon alfa-2b regimens for the long-term treatment of chronic non-A, non-B hepatitis. *N Engl J Med* 1995; **332:** 1457–62.
12. Nishiguchi S, *et al.* Randomised trial of effects of interferon-α on incidence of hepatocellular carcinoma in chronic active hepatitis C with cirrhosis. *Lancet* 1995; **346:** 1051–5.
13. Frosi A, *et al.* Interferon-alpha andbeta in chronic hepatitis C: efficacy and tolerability: a comparative pilot study. *Clin Drug Invest* 1995; **9:** 226–31.
14. Esteban R. Is there a role for interferon in acute viral hepatitis? *Gut* 1993; **34** (suppl 1): S77–S80.
15. Omata M, *et al.* Resolution of acute hepatitis C after therapy with natural beta interferon. *Lancet* 1991; **338:** 914–15.
16. Kakumu S, *et al.* A pilot study of ribavirin and interferon beta for the treatment of chronic hepatitis C. *Gastroenterology* 1993; **105:** 507–12.
17. Chemello L, *et al.* Response to ribavirin, to interferon and to a combination of both in patients with chronic hepatitis C and its relation to HCV genotypes. *J Hepatol* 1994; **21:** (suppl): S12.
18. Braconier JH, *et al.* Combined alpha-interferon and ribavirin treatment in chronic hepatitis C: a pilot study. *Scand J Infect Dis* 1995; **27:** 325–9.
19. Reichard O, *et al.* Randomised, double-blind, placebo-controlled trial of interferon α-2b with and without ribavirin for chronic hepatitis C. *Lancet* 1998; **351:** 83–7.
20. Poynard T, *et al.* Randomised trial of interferon α2b plus ribavirin for 48 weeks or for 24 weeks versus interferon α2b plus placebo for 48 weeks for treatment of chronic infection with hepatitis C virus. *Lancet* 1998; **352:** 1426–32.
21. Farci P, *et al.* Treatment of chronic hepatitis D with interferon alfa-2a. *N Engl J Med* 1994; **330:** 88–94.
22. Yoshiba M, *et al.* Interferon for hepatitis A. *Lancet* 1994; **343:** 288–9.

Herpes simplex infections. Although herpes simplex infections are commonly treated with aciclovir (see p.597), beneficial responses to interferon alfa, applied topically, have been reported in genital herpes[1-4] and, in combination with trifluridine[5,6] or brivudine,[7] in herpes keratitis. Similarly there are case reports of improvement in herpes labialis with interferon alfa in combination with trifluridine in 3 patients resistant to aciclovir, 2 of whom were also resistant to foscarnet.[8] Interferon beta has also been tried in a small number of patients for the treatment of labial and genital herpes.[9] However, in a comparative study[10] intramuscular interferon alfa was not superior to topical aciclovir either in treating first-episode genital herpes or in altering the frequency of recurrences.

1. Friedman-Kien AE, *et al.* Treatment of recurrent genital herpes with topical alpha interferon gel combined with nonoxynol 9. *J Am Acad Dermatol* 1986; **15:** 989–94.
2. Sacks SL, *et al.* Randomized, double-blind, placebo-controlled, patient-initiated study of topical high- and low-dose interferon-α with nonoxynol-9 in the treatment of recurrent genital herpes. *J Infect Dis* 1990; **161:** 692–8.
3. Shupack J, *et al.* Topical alpha-interferon in recurrent genital herpes simplex infection. *Dermatologica* 1990; **181:** 134–8.
4. Syed TA, *et al.* Human leukocyte interferon-alpha in cream for the management of genital herpes in Asian women: a placebo-controlled, double-blind study. *J Mol Med* 1995; **73:** 141–4.
5. de Koning EWJ, *et al.* Combination therapy for dendritic keratitis with human leucocyte interferon and trifluorothymidine. *Br J Ophthalmol* 1982; **66:** 509–12.
6. Sundmacher R, *et al.* Combination therapy for dendritic keratitis: high-titer α-interferon and trifluridine. *Arch Ophthalmol* 1984; **102:** 554–5.
7. van Bijsterveld OP, *et al.* Bromovinyldeoxyuridine and interferon treatment in ulcerative herpetic keratitis: a double masked study. *Br J Ophthalmol* 1989; **73:** 604–7.
8. Birch CJ, *et al.* Clinical effects and in vitro studies of trifluorothymidine combined with interferon-α for treatment of drug-resistant andsensitive herpes simplex virus infections. *J Infect Dis* 1992; **166:** 108–12.
9. Glezerman M, *et al.* Placebo-controlled trial of topical interferon in labial and genital herpes. *Lancet* 1988; **i:** 150–2.
10. Levin MJ, *et al.* Comparison of intramuscular recombinant alpha interferon (rIFN-2A) with topical acyclovir for the treatment of first-episode herpes genitalis and prevention of recurrences. *Antimicrob Agents Chemother* 1989; **33:** 649–52.

HIV infection and AIDS. The effects of interferons on the progression of AIDS have been mixed.[1-5] Combinations of interferon alfa with antiretroviral reverse transcriptase inhibitors have produced variable responses,[6-10] with some investigators reporting enhanced[6,10] or synergistic[7] antiretroviral effects, though often at doses associated with a high incidence of adverse effects.

Interferons have been tried with some success in the management of Kaposi's sarcoma and mycobacterial infections in patients with AIDS (see below).

Promising results have been reported with interferon alfa in patients with HIV-associated thrombocytopenia,[11] although interferons have been reported to induce immune thrombocytopenia, and there has been a report of bleeding in a patient with idiopathic thrombocytopenic purpura (see Effects on the Blood under Adverse Effects, above).

The management of HIV infection and AIDS is discussed on p.599.

1. Lane HC, *et al.* Interferon-α in patients with asymptomatic human immunodeficiency virus (HIV) infection: a randomized placebo-controlled trial. *Ann Intern Med* 1990; **112:** 805–11.
2. Brook MG, *et al.* Anti-HIV effects of alpha-interferon. *Lancet* 1989; **i:** 42.
3. Ellis ME, *et al.* An open study of interferon in HIV-antibody-positive men. *AIDS* 1989; **3:** 851–3.
4. Puppo F, *et al.* Low doses of alpha-interferon for the treatment of AIDS-related syndromes: a preliminary study. *Int J Immunother* 1988; **4:** 165–8.
5. Frissen PHJ, *et al.* High-dose interferon-α2a exerts potent activity against human immunodeficiency virus type 1 not associated with antitumor activity in subjects with Kaposi's sarcoma. *J Infect Dis* 1997; **176:** 811–14.
6. Berglund O, *et al.* Combined treatment of symptomatic human immunodeficiency virus type 1 infection with native interferon-α and zidovudine. *J Infect Dis* 1991; **163:** 710–15.
7. Mildvan D, *et al.* Synergy, activity and tolerability of zidovudine and interferon-alpha in patients with symptomatic HIV-1 infection: ACTG 068. *Antiviral Ther* 1996; **1:** 77–88.
8. Kovacs JA, *et al.* Combination therapy with didanosine and interferon-α in human immunodeficiency virus-infected patients: results of a phase I/II trial. *J Infect Dis* 1996; **173:** 840–8.
9. Bissuel F, *et al.* Tolerance of a triple combination therapy with zidovudine, didanosine and interferon-α in seven HIV-infected patients. *AIDS* 1995; **9:** 1285.
10. Fischl MA, *et al.* Safety and antiviral activity of combination therapy with zidovudine, zalcitabine, and two doses of interferon-α_{2a} in patients with HIV: AIDS Clinical Trials Group Study 197. *J Acquir Immune Defic Syndr Hum Retrovirol* 1997; **16:** 247–53.
11. Marroni M, *et al.* Interferon-α is effective in the treatment of HIV-1-related, severe, zidovudine-resistant thrombocytopenia. *Ann Intern Med* 1994; **121:** 423–9.

Inflammatory bowel disease. Interferon alfa is one of many drugs that have been tried in inflammatory bowel disease (p.1171). One recent study[1] found that clinical remission was achieved in 26 of 28 patients with ulcerative colitis after 6 to 12 months of treatment with interferon alfa-2a. Partial remission was reported in 2 of 5 patients with Crohn's disease[2] who received interferon alfa, but in another study in 12 patients[3] interferon alfa was of no benefit. Aminosalicylates and corticosteroids remain the mainstays of drug treatment at present.

1. Sümer N, Palabiyikoğlu M. Induction of remission by interferon-α in patients with chronic active ulcerative colitis. *Eur J Gastroenterol Hepatol* 1995; **7:** 597–602.
2. Davidsen B, *et al.* Tolerability of interferon alpha-2b, a possible new treatment of active Crohn's disease. *Aliment Pharmacol Ther* 1995; **9:** 75–9.
3. Gasché C, *et al.* Prospective evaluation of interferon-α in treatment of chronic active Crohn's disease. *Dig Dis Sci* 1995; **40:** 800–4.

Juvenile osteopetrosis. Interferon gamma has been tried in the treatment of juvenile osteopetrosis (p.1024). A study[1] in 14 patients found that interferon gamma-1b increased bone resorption. In 11 who received this treatment for 18 months there was stabilisation or improvement in clinical condition and a reduction in the frequency of serious infection.

1. Key LL, *et al.* Long-term treatment of osteopetrosis with recombinant human interferon gamma. *N Engl J Med* 1995; **332:** 1594–9.

Kaposi's sarcoma. The various treatments used for Kaposi's sarcoma are discussed on p.496. Interferon alfa has been used in AIDS-related Kaposi's sarcoma[1-9] and in patients with the classical, nonepidemic form.[10-12] There have been several small studies of interferon alfa in patients with immunodeficiency- or AIDS-related Kaposi's sarcoma.[1-3] Results have been mixed. From a review of published studies, Krown[4] concluded that the best responses to interferon alfa were achieved in asymptomatic patients with relatively high CD4+ T lymphocyte counts (200 cells per μL or better) and no prior opportunistic infections. However, the adverse effects which occur at the doses required limit the tolerability of long-term administration.

Interferons have also been tried in AIDS-related Kaposi's sarcoma in combination with other drugs including antineoplastics (with disappointing results)[5] and zidovudine (complete or partial tumour response and/or evidence of antiviral effects in some patients).[6-9] Low doses of interferons in combination with zidovudine have been reported to be the favoured treatment for AIDS-associated Kaposi's sarcoma.[5]

1. de Wit R, *et al.* Clinical and virological effects of high-dose recombinant interferon-α in disseminated AIDS-related Kaposi's sarcoma. *Lancet* 1988; **ii:** 1214–17.
2. Lane HC, *et al.* Anti-retroviral effects of interferon-α in AIDS-associated Kaposi's sarcoma. *Lancet* 1988; **ii:** 1218–22.
3. Sulis E, *et al.* Interferon administered intralesionally in skin and oral cavity lesions in heterosexual drug addicted patients with AIDS-related Kaposi's sarcoma. *Eur J Cancer Clin Oncol* 1989; **25:** 759–61.
4. Krown SE. Interferon and other biologic agents for the treatment of Kaposi's sarcoma. *Hematol Oncol Clin North Am* 1991; **5:** 311–22.
5. Northfelt DW. Treatment of Kaposi's sarcoma: current guidelines and future perspectives. *Drugs* 1994; **48:** 569–82.
6. Kovacs JA, *et al.* Combined zidovudine and interferon-α therapy in patients with Kaposi sarcoma and the acquired immunodeficiency syndrome (AIDS). *Ann Intern Med* 1989; **111:** 280–7.
7. Brockmeyer NH, *et al.* Regression of Kaposi's sarcoma and improvement of performance status by a combined interferon β and zidovudine therapy in AIDS patients. *J Invest Dermatol* 1989; **92:** 776.
8. Krown SE, *et al.* Interferon-α with zidovudine: safety, tolerance, and clinical and virologic effects in patients with Kaposi sarcoma associated with the acquired immunodeficiency syndrome (AIDS). *Ann Intern Med* 1990; **112:** 812–21.
9. Edlin BR, *et al.* Interferon-alpha plus zidovudine in HIV infection. *Lancet* 1989; **i:** 156.
10. Trattner A, *et al.* The therapeutic effect of intralesional interferon in classical Kaposi's sarcoma. *Br J Dermatol* 1993; **129:** 590–3.
11. Killeen RB, Marsh RD. α-Interferon for Kaposi's sarcoma in HIV-negative, non-homosexual man. *Lancet* 1991; **337:** 309–10.
12. Shimizu S, *et al.* Classic (non-AIDS-related) Kaposi's sarcoma in a Japanese patient, successfully treated with alpha-2b-interferon. *Br J Dermatol* 1995; **133:** 332–4.

Leishmaniasis. Interferon gamma has been tried both systemically and locally as an adjunct to standard treatment of leishmaniasis (see p.575) with encouraging results. In a review of the use of interferon gamma in non-viral infections,[1] Murray concluded that interferon gamma was effective when combined with antimony compounds for treatment failures in visceral leishmaniasis and could enhance the response to initial therapy in untreated patients. For cutaneous infections, intralesional interferon gamma has been shown to be effective[2] but less so than intralesional antimony compounds.[3] Subcutaneous administration of interferon gamma with antimony given intravenously was no more effective than antimony alone when administered as a short course over 10 days.[4] However, encouraging responses have been reported in patients who have failed to respond to antimony compounds alone.[5]

1. Murray HW. Interferon-gamma and host antimicrobial defense: current and future clinical applications. *Am J Med* 1994; **97:** 459–67.
2. Harms G, *et al.* Effects of intradermal gamma-interferon in cutaneous leishmaniasis. *Lancet* 1989; **i:** 1287–92.
3. Harms G, *et al.* A randomized trial comparing a pentavalent antimonial drug and recombinant interferon-γ in the local treatment of cutaneous leishmaniasis. *Trans R Soc Trop Med Hyg* 1991; **85:** 214–16.
4. Arana BA, *et al.* Efficacy of a short course (10 days) of high-dose meglumine antimonate with or without interferon-γ in treating cutaneous leishmaniasis in Guatemala. *Clin Infect Dis* 1994; **18:** 381–4.
5. Falcoff E, *et al.* Clinical healing of antimony-resistant cutaneous or mucocutaneous leishmaniasis following the combined administration of interferon-γ and pentavalent antimonial compounds. *Trans R Soc Trop Med Hyg* 1994; **88:** 95–7.

Malignant neoplasms. Many reports have been published on the effects of interferons on various neoplasms; most have involved interferon alfa.

Interferons have become established in the treatment of a few malignant disorders, notably hairy-cell leukaemia,[1-5] Kaposi's sarcoma (see above), and chronic myeloid leukaemia,[6-11] where interferon alfa may be regarded as the treatment of choice. Alfa interferons may improve the duration of remission in multiple myeloma,[12-14] but not necessarily survival.[14,15] Combination therapy including interferons has also been used in non-Hodgkin's lymphoma[16,17] and renal cell carcinoma, where response to interferon alfa in combination with interleukin-2 has been promising, but toxicity high.[18,19] (Interferon alfa alone produces very modest benefit.[34]) Beneficial responses have also been reported in a number of other neoplasms including melanoma;[20-22] carcinoid tumours[23] (although some authorities were sceptical about its value[24]); myelodysplasia; cutaneous T cell lymphomas including mycosis fungoides;[25,26] and in one reported case of meningioma.[27] Interferons have been administered locally as an adjunct to surgery for superficial bladder tumours and intralesionally in basal cell carcinoma[28,29] and also for keloid scars.[30,31] Combination of interferon alfa with fluorouracil has been tried in inoperable colorectal cancer but may not be more beneficial than fluorouracil alone.[32] Interferon alfa in combination with zidovudine has produced encouraging results in adult T-cell leukaemia-lymphoma.[33]

For further discussion of malignant neoplasms and their treatment, including the use of interferons, see under Choice of Antineoplastic, p.476.

1. Quesada JR, *et al.* Alpha interferon for induction of remission in hairy-cell leukemia. *N Engl J Med* 1984; **310:** 15–18.
2. Janssen JTP, *et al.* Treatment of hairy-cell leukaemia with recombinant human α_2-interferon. *Lancet* 1984; **i:** 1025–6.
3. Pagnucco G, *et al.* Human lymphoblastoid interferon in the treatment of hairy cell leukaemia. *Int J Immunother* 1988; **4:** 169–75.
4. Gibson J, *et al.* Clinical response of hairy-cell leukaemia to interferon-α: results of an Australian study. *Med J Aust* 1988; **149:** 293–6.
5. Holmes R, *et al.* Treatment of hairy cell leukemia with increasing doses of recombinant alpha A interferon. *Aust N Z J Med* 1988; **18:** 557–62.
6. The Italian Cooperative Study Group on Chronic Myeloid Leukemia. Interferon alfa-2a as compared with conventional chemotherapy for the treatment of chronic myeloid leukemia. *N Engl J Med* 1994; **330:** 820–5.
7. Allan NC, *et al.* UK Medical Research Council randomised, multicentre trial of interferon-αnl for chronic myeloid leukaemia: improved survival irrespective of cytogenetic response. *Lancet* 1995; **345:** 1392–7.
8. Kantarjian HM, *et al.* Prolonged survival in chronic myelogenous leukemia after cytogenetic response to interferon-α therapy. *Ann Intern Med* 1995; **122:** 254–61.
9. Schofield JR, *et al.* Low doses of interferon-α are as effective as higher doses in inducing remissions and prolonging survival in chronic myeloid leukemia. *Ann Intern Med* 1994; **121:** 736–44.
10. Talpaz M, Kantarjian H. Low-dose interferon-α in chronic myeloid leukemia. *Ann Intern Med* 1995; **122:** 728.
11. Mahon F-X, *et al.* Response to IFNα in myelogenous leukaemia. *Lancet* 1996; **347:** 57–8.
12. Mandelli F, *et al.* Maintenance treatment with recombinant interferon alfa-2b in patients with multiple myeloma responding to conventional induction chemotherapy. *N Engl J Med* 1990; **322:** 1430–4.
13. Ludwig H, *et al.* Interferon-alpha for induction and maintenance in multiple myeloma: results of two multicenter randomized trials and summary of other studies. *Ann Oncol* 1995; **6:** 467–76.
14. Nordic Myeloma Study Group. Interferon-α2b added to melphalan-prednisone for initial and maintenance therapy in multiple myeloma: a randomized, controlled trial. *Ann Intern Med* 1996; **124:** 212–22.
15. Österborg A, *et al.* Natural interferon-α in combination with melphalan/prednisone versus melphalan/prednisone in the treatment of multiple myeloma stages II and III: a randomized study from the myeloma group of central Sweden. *Blood* 1993; **81:** 1428–34.
16. Smalley RV, *et al.* Interferon alfa combined with cytotoxic chemotherapy for patients with non-Hodgkin's lymphoma. *N Engl J Med* 1992; **327:** 1336–41.
17. Solal-Celigny P, *et al.* Recombinant interferon alfa-2b combined with a regimen containing doxorubicin in patients with advanced follicular lymphoma. *N Engl J Med* 1993; **329:** 1608–14.
18. Besana C, *et al.* Treatment of advanced renal cell cancer with sequential intravenous recombinant interleukin-2 and subcutaneous α-interferon. *Eur J Cancer* 1994; **30A** 1292–8.
19. Négrier S, *et al.* Intensive regimen of cytokines with interleukin-2 and interferon alfa-2b in selected patients with metastatic renal carcinoma. *J Immunother* 1995; **17:** 62–8.
20. Hahka-Kemppinen M, *et al.* Response of subcutaneous and cutaneous metastases of malignant melanoma to combined cytostatic plus interferon therapy. *Br J Dermatol* 1995; **132:** 973–7.
21. Cascinelli N, *et al.* Results of adjuvant interferon study in WHO melanoma programme. *Lancet* 1994; **343:** 913–14.
22. Grob JJ, *et al.* Randomised trial of interferon α-2a as adjuvant therapy in resected primary melanoma thicker than 1.5 mm without clinically detectable node metastases. *Lancet* 1998; **351:** 1905–10.
23. Öberg K, *et al.* Treatment of malignant carcinoid tumors: a randomized controlled study of streptozocin plus 5-FU and human leukocyte interferon. *Eur J Cancer Clin Oncol* 1989; **25:** 1475–9.
24. Saini A, Waxman J. Management of carcinoid syndrome. *Postgrad Med J* 1991; **67:** 506–8.
25. Parry EJ, Mackie RM. Management of cutaneous T cell lymphoma. *Br Med J* 1994; **308:** 858–9.
26. Horikoshi T, *et al.* A patient with plaque-stage mycosis fungoides has successfully been treated with long-term administration of IFN-γ and has been in complete remission for more than 6 years. *Br J Dermatol* 1996; **134:** 130–3.
27. Wöber-Bingöl Ç, *et al.* Interferon-alfa-2b for meningioma. *Lancet* 1995; **345:** 331.
28. Pizarro A, Fonseca E. Treatment of basal cell carcinoma with intralesional interferon alpha-2b: evaluation of efficacy with emphasis on tumours located on "H" zone on face. *Eur J Dermatol* 1994; **4:** 287–90.
29. LeGrice P, *et al.* Treatment of basal cell carcinoma with intralesional interferon alpha-2A. *N Z Med J* 1995; **108:** 206–7.
30. Granstein RD, *et al.* A controlled trial of intralesional recombinant interferon-γ in the treatment of keloidal scarring. *Arch Dermatol* 1990; **126:** 1295–1302.
31. Larrabee WF, *et al.* Intralesional interferon gamma treatment for keloids and hypertrophic scars. *Arch Otolaryngol Head Neck Surg* 1990; **116:** 1159–62.
32. Moser R, *et al.* 5-Fluorouracil and folinic acid with or without alpha-2c interferon in the treatment of metastatic colorectal cancer: preliminary results of a multicenter prospective randomized phase-III trial. *Onkologie* 1995; **18:** 131–5.
33. Gill PS, *et al.* Treatment of adult T-cell leukemia-lymphoma with a combination of interferon alfa and zidovudine. *N Engl J Med* 1995; **332:** 1744–8.
34. Medical Research Council Renal Cancer Collaborators. Interferon-α and survival in metastatic renal carcinoma: early results of a randomised controlled study. *Lancet* 1999; **353:** 14–17.

Multiple sclerosis. Multiple sclerosis (MS) is characterised by patches of demyelination that can be scattered throughout the white matter of the CNS, but are usually localised in the brain stem, periventricular areas, the optic nerve, and the cervical spinal cord. The cause is unknown but may have an immunological basis. Symptoms may vary according to the areas affected but typically include weakness, paraesthesias, vision loss, incoordination, and bladder dysfunction. Most patients improve to some degree after the initial attack but the course and severity of the disease are unpredictable. In many patients the disease follows a relapsing-remitting course in which there are recurrent exacerbations followed by relatively long periods of remission. In some patients the disease is described as relapsing-progressive when there is little or no improvement after each exacerbation and disability slowly increases. In a few patients the disease progresses rapidly without remission and leads to early disability and death.

The evaluation of therapy for any disease such as MS that has spontaneous remissions is difficult. Until recently there has been little convincing evidence that any treatment affects the outcome of the disease.[1-3] Treatment has therefore largely been **symptomatic** and aimed at the management of spasticity, pain, fatigue, and bladder dysfunction. Baclofen, dantrolene, and diazepam are the usual drugs given for spasticity (see p.1303). There has also been a suggestion that the synthetic cannabinoid nabilone may improve spasticity.[4] Patients with MS can suffer from a number of different types of pain, including pain from spasticity, and therapy must be individualised for each specific pain syndrome[5] (see p.4). Paraesthesia and dysaesthesia, which can be common, may respond to tricyclic antidepressants or antiepileptics. Amantadine may alleviate fatigue associated with MS.[6] Treatment of bladder dysfunction may include an alpha blocker such as phenoxybenzamine and appropriate parasympathomimetic or antimuscarinic therapy to control bladder contractions[1] (see Urinary Incontinence and Retention, p.454). Fampridine has been reported to produce improvement in walking, dexterity, and vision, possibly as a result of its potassium-channel blocking activity.[7-9] 3,4-Diaminopyridine has also been reported to produce beneficial symptomatic responses.[10]

A wide range of drugs with immunological actions have been tried in the **treatment** of MS itself with the aim of improving recovery from acute attacks, preventing or decreasing the number of relapses, and halting the progressive stage of the disease.

Short-term courses of *corticotrophin* have long been used to hasten recovery from acute exacerbations although there is no effect on the degree of recovery nor on the overall course of the disease;[2,3] successive treatments may be less beneficial.[11,12] Oral *corticosteroids* such as prednisolone or prednisone have been widely used to achieve the same effect, but there is a trend towards the use of high-dose intravenous methylprednisolone.[1-3] Some[3,12,13] recommend the use of high-dose oral or intravenous methylprednisolone (the latter followed by a tapering course of oral prednisone). Also, there have been signs that corticosteroids given to patients with acute optic neuritis might reduce the rate of development of MS,[14] but a recent study using methylprednisolone in patients with chronic progressive disease found that initial improvement was not sustained.[15]

There is promise too with *interferon* therapy. Many early studies using interferons were conducted before the immunoregulatory effects of interferons were understood, but they did demonstrate that natural interferon beta could reduce exacerbations by inhibiting interferon gamma which in itself appeared to act as a disease activator. Natural interferon alfa alone was found to produce little or no benefit.[16] Subsequent studies in patients with relapsing-remitting disease have used recombinant interferon beta and patients treated with interferon *beta-1b* have obtained a reduction in the rate and severity of exacerbations;[17,18] there was also evidence from magnetic resonance imaging[19] of reduced disease activity and burden. Encouraging results have also been obtained in patients with secondary progressive disease.[20] Similar results in relapsing-remitting disease have been obtained with interferon *beta-1a*.[21,22] However, the effect of interferon beta on the progression of disability remains to be determined. Concern has been expressed over the detection of neutralising antibodies against interferon in up to 36% of patients.[23,24] Guidelines for the use of interferon beta in selected patients in specialist centres have been proposed.[25]

Results of a study[26,47] of *glatiramer* have shown that it can reduce the number of relapses and may produce some improvements in neurological disability. These benefits are produced in a different way from those gained with interferon beta-1b leading to expectations of a study of treatment with both drugs. Intermittent intravenous *immunoglobulin* might also be able to reduce the frequency of exacerbations and slow disease progression without producing troublesome adverse effects.[27,28]

Although some studies have shown modest benefits with *immunosuppressants*, the general conclusions of large controlled studies have tended to be that any slight benefits of existing therapies with immunosuppressants such as azathioprine, cyclophosphamide, or cyclosporin are outweighed by the toxicity of the doses required to have an effect.[29-35] However, it has been pointed out that in terms of relapse reduction azathioprine appeared to be as effective as newer treatments such as interferon beta.[36] A study with cladribine suggested that it might provide some benefit at well-tolerated doses,[37] and low-dose methotrexate might also slow progression of chronic disease and provide a relatively non-toxic treatment option.[38] Benefit has been reported with *roquinimex* (but see p.561).

Other immunological approaches under evaluation include the use of monoclonal antibodies such as CD4 antibodies, altered peptide ligands from myelin basic protein, and T-cell vaccination.[39] Combined total lymphoid irradiation with low-dose corticosteroid therapy has also been investigated and may slow progression of disease.[40]

A review of the relationship between *dietary fat* and MS concluded that the role of lipids remained to be proven.[41] Some studies found a reduction of severity and duration of relapse in patients taking linoleic acid supplements (as sunflower oil)[42] while another reported benefit in patients who limited their intake of dietary saturated fatty acids and supplemented their diet with polyunsaturated fatty acids.[43] Despite a lack of firm evidence many patients with MS practice dietary modification and take supplements of omega-6 group polyunsaturated acids, sunflower oil, evening primrose oil, fish oils, and omega-3 fatty acids.[41]

The use of *hyperbaric oxygen* therapy in MS has been a matter of debate for many years and continues to be controversial. Some workers have reported benefit, especially in bladder and bowel function or in cerebellar function.[44] Others have been unable to substantiate any useful long-term effect[45] and a review of the many therapeutic options available in MS concluded that there was no convincing evidence that hyperbaric oxygen therapy was successful.[46]

1. Ebers GC. Treatment of multiple sclerosis. *Lancet* 1994; **343:** 275–9.
2. van Oosten BW, *et al.* Multiple sclerosis therapy: a practical guide. *Drugs* 1995; **49:** 200–12.
3. Weinstock-Guttman B, Cohen JA. Newer versus older treatments for relapsing-remitting multiple sclerosis. *Drug Safety* 1996; **14:** 121–30.
4. Martyn CN, *et al.* Nabilone in the treatment of multiple sclerosis. *Lancet* 1995; **345:** 579.
5. Moulin DE, *et al.* Pain syndromes in multiple sclerosis. *Neurology* 1988; **38:** 1830–4.
6. Kemp BA, Gora ML. Amantadine and fatigue of multiple sclerosis. *Ann Pharmacother* 1993; **27:** 893–5.
7. Bever CT, *et al.* The effects of 4-aminopyridine in multiple sclerosis patients: results of a randomised, placebo-controlled, double-blind, concentration-controlled, crossover trial. *Neurology* 1994; **44:** 1054–9.
8. Van Diemen HAM, *et al.* 4-Aminopyridine in patients with multiple sclerosis: dosage and serum level related to efficacy and safety. *Clin Neuropharmacol* 1993; **16:** 195–204.
9. Schwid SR, *et al.* Quantitative assessment of sustained-release 4-aminopyridine for symptomatic treatment of multiple sclerosis. *Neurology* 1997; **48:** 817–21.
10. Bever CT, *et al.* Treatment with oral 3,4 diaminopyridine improves leg strength in multiple sclerosis patients: results of a randomized, double-blind, placebo-controlled, crossover trial. *Neurology* 1996; **47:** 1457–62.

11. Weiner HL, Hafler DA. Immunotherapy of multiple sclerosis. *Ann Neurol* 1988; **23:** 211–22.
12. Carter JL, Rodriguez M. Immunosuppressive treatment of multiple sclerosis. *Mayo Clin Proc* 1989; **64:** 664–9.
13. Barnes D, *et al.* Randomised trial of oral and intravenous methylprednisolone in acute relapses of multiple sclerosis. *Lancet* 1997; **349:** 902–6.
14. Beck RW, *et al.* The effect of corticosteroids for acute optic neuritis on the subsequent development of multiple sclerosis. *N Engl J Med* 1993; **329:** 1764–9.
15. Cazzato G, *et al.* Double-blind, placebo-controlled, randomized, crossover trial of high-dose methylprednisolone in patients with chronic progressive form of multiple sclerosis. *Eur Neurol* 1995; **35:** 193–8.
16. Panitch HS. Interferons in multiple sclerosis: a review of the evidence. *Drugs* 1992; **44:** 946–62.
17. The IFNB Multiple Sclerosis Study Group. Interferon beta-1b is effective in relapsing-remitting multiple sclerosis I: clinical results of a multicenter, randomized, double-blind, placebo-controlled trial. *Neurology* 1993; **43:** 655–61.
18. The IFNB Multiple Sclerosis Study Group and the University of British Columbia MS/MRI Analysis Group. Interferon beta-1b in the treatment of multiple sclerosis: final outcome of the randomised controlled trial. *Neurology* 1995; **45:** 1277–85.
19. Paty DW, *et al.* Interferon beta-1b is effective in relapsing-remitting multiple sclerosis II: MRI analysis results of a multicenter, randomized, double-blind, placebo-controlled trial. *Neurology* 1993; **43:** 662–7.
20. European Study Group on Interferon β-1b in Secondary Progressive MS. Placebo-controlled multicentre randomised trial of interferon β-1b in secondary progressive multiple sclerosis. *Lancet* 1998; **352:** 1491–7.
21. Jacobs LD, *et al.* Intramuscular interferon beta-1a for disease progression in relapsing multiple sclerosis. *Ann Neurol* 1996; **39:** 285–94.
22. PRISMS Study Group. Randomised double-blind placebo-controlled study of interferon β-1a in relapsing/remitting multiple sclerosis. *Lancet* 1998; **352:** 1498–1504.
23. IFNB Multiple Sclerosis Study Group, University of British Columbia MS/MRI Analysis Group. Neutralizing antibodies during treatment of multiple sclerosis with interferon beta-1b: experience during the first three years. *Neurology* 1996; **47:** 889–94.
24. Paty DW, *et al.* Guidelines for physicians with patients on IFNB-1b: the use of an assay for neutralizing antibodies (NAB). *Neurology* 1996; **47:** 865–6.
25. Gonsette RE. Guidance on new therapies in multiple sclerosis patients. *Lancet* 1996; **348:** 136.
26. Johnson KP, *et al.* Copolymer 1 reduces relapse rate and improves disability in relapsing-remitting multiple sclerosis: results of a phase III multicenter, double-blind, placebo-controlled trial. *Neurology* 1995; **45:** 1268–76.
27. Achiron A, *et al.* Intravenous immunoglobulin treatment in multiple sclerosis. *Isr J Med Sci* 1995; **31:** 7–9.
28. Fazekas F, *et al.* Randomised placebo-controlled trial of monthly intravenous immunoglobulin therapy in relapsing-remitting multiple sclerosis. *Lancet* 1997; **349:** 589–93.
29. British and Dutch Multiple Sclerosis Azathioprine Trial Group. Double-masked trial of azathioprine in multiple sclerosis. *Lancet* 1988; **ii:** 179–83.
30. The Multiple Sclerosis Study Group. Efficacy and toxicity of cyclosporine in chronic progressive multiple sclerosis: a randomized, double-blinded, placebo-controlled clinical trial. *Ann Neurol* 1990; **27:** 591–605.
31. Ellison GW, *et al.* A placebo-controlled, randomized, double-masked, variable dosage, clinical trial of azathioprine with and without methylprednisolone in multiple sclerosis. *Neurology* 1989; **39:** 1018–26.
32. Rudge P, *et al.* Randomised double blind controlled trial of cyclosporin in multiple sclerosis. *J Neurol Neurosurg Psychiatry* 1989; **52:** 559–65.
33. Currier RD, *et al.* Cyclophosphamide and plasma exchange in multiple sclerosis. *Lancet* 1991; **337:** 1034.
34. Yudkin PL, *et al.* Overview of azathioprine treatment in multiple sclerosis. *Lancet* 1991; **338:** 1051–5.
35. The Canadian Cooperative Multiple Sclerosis Study Group. The Canadian cooperative trial of cyclophosphamide and plasma exchange in progressive multiple sclerosis. *Lancet* 1991; **337:** 441–6.
36. Palace J, Rothwell P. New treatments and azathioprine in multiple sclerosis. *Lancet* 1997; **350:** 261.
37. Sipe JC, *et al.* Cladribine in treatment of chronic progressive multiple sclerosis. *Lancet* 1994; **344:** 9–13.
38. Goodkin DE, *et al.* Low-dose (7.5 mg) oral methotrexate reduces the rate of progression in chronic progressive multiple sclerosis. *Ann Neurol* 1995; **37:** 30–40.
39. Medaer R, *et al.* Depletion of myelin-basic-protein autoreactive T cells by T-cell vaccination: pilot trial in multiple sclerosis. *Lancet* 1995; **346:** 807–8.
40. Cook SD, *et al.* Combination total lymphoid irradiation and low-dose corticosteroid therapy for progressive multiple sclerosis. *Acta Neurol Scand* 1995; **91:** 22–7.
41. Anonymous. Lipids and multiple sclerosis. *Lancet* 1990; **336:** 25–6.
42. Millar JHD, *et al.* Double-blind trial of linoleate supplementation of the diet in multiple sclerosis. *Br Med J* 1973; **1:** 765–8.
43. Swank RL, Dugan BB. Effect of low saturated fat diet in early and late cases of multiple sclerosis. *Lancet* 1990; **336:** 37–9.
44. James PB, Webster CJ. Long-term results of hyperbaric oxygen therapy in multiple sclerosis. *Lancet* 1989; **ii:** 327.
45. Kindwall EP, *et al.* Treatment of multiple sclerosis with hyperbaric oxygen: results of a national registry. *Arch Neurol* 1991; **48:** 195–9.
46. Webb HE. Multiple sclerosis: therapeutic pessimism. *Br Med J* 1992; **304:** 1260–1.
47. Johnson KP, *et al.* Extended use of glatiramer acetate (Copaxone) is well tolerated and maintains its clinical effect of multiple sclerosis relapse rate and degree of disability. *Neurology* 1998; **50:** 701–8.

Mycobacterial infections. Interferon gamma injected into lesions of patients with leprosy was reported to stimulate an immune response similar to that of a delayed hypersensitivity reaction and to reduce the intralesional bacterial count.[1,2]

Experience with interferons for opportunistic mycobacterial infections in patients with AIDS is limited. Interferon gamma given in conjunction with antimycobacterials produced beneficial responses in 3 patients with *Mycobacterium avium* complex infections, but produced no response or only a transient response in 3 others who received interferon gamma alone.[3,4]

Beneficial responses have also been reported following treatment with interferons alfa[5] and gamma[6] as adjuncts to antimycobacterial therapy in HIV-negative patients with mycobacterial infections which had not responded to conventional therapy.

A study of 5 patients with multidrug-resistant tuberculosis[7] suggested that inhaled interferon gamma may be a useful adjunct in patients not responding to conventional therapy alone.

For discussion of these infections and their standard treatment, see under Leprosy, p.128, Opportunistic Mycobacterial Infections, p.133, and Tuberculosis, p.146.

1. Nathan CF, *et al.* Local and systemic effects of intradermal recombinant interferon-γ in patients with lepromatous leprosy. *N Engl J Med* 1986; **315:** 6–15.
2. Kaplan G, *et al.* Effect of multiple interferon γ injections on the disposal of Mycobacterium leprae. *Proc Natl Acad Sci U S A* 1989; **86:** 8073–7.
3. Squires KE, *et al.* Interferon-γ and Mycobacterium avium-intracellulare infection. *J Infect Dis* 1989; **159:** 599–600.
4. Squires KE, *et al.* Interferon-γ treatment for Mycobacterium avium-intracellulare complex bacillemia in patients with AIDS. *J Infect Dis* 1992; **166:** 686–7.
5. Maziarz RT, *et al.* Reversal of infection with Mycobacterium avium intracellulare by treatment with alpha-interferon in a patient with hairy cell leukemia. *Ann Intern Med* 1988; **109:** 292–4.
6. Holland SM, *et al.* Treatment of refractory disseminated nontuberculous mycobacterial infection with interferon gamma: a preliminary report. *N Engl J Med* 1994; **330:** 1348–55.
7. Condos R, *et al.* Treatment of multidrug-resistant pulmonary tuberculosis with interferon-γ via aerosol. *Lancet* 1997; **349:** 1513–15.

Skin disorders. Interferons have been tried in skin disorders in which IgE levels are raised. Subcutaneous interferon gamma improved eczema and reduced serum-IgE concentration in one patient, but the condition gradually returned within a week of stopping treatment.[1] In two studies[2,3] subcutaneous interferon gamma given to patients with severe atopic dermatitis and raised serum-IgE concentrations resulted in improvement of the skin condition; IgE concentrations were reduced in one study[2] but remained high in the other.[3] Subcutaneous interferon alfa, however, was unsuccessful in 2 patients with very severe atopic dermatitis; serum-IgE concentrations and severity of the skin condition remained unaffected.[4] Interferon alfa has been tried in subacute cutaneous lupus erythematosus[5,6] and discoid lupus erythematosus.[6] Although marked improvement generally occurred, the condition tended to recur within several weeks of stopping treatment. For discussion of the conventional treatment of eczema, see p.1073 and of lupus erythematosus, see Systemic Lupus Erythematosus, p.1029.

There have been reports[7,8] of the successful use of interferon alfa to control the symptoms of urticaria associated with mastocytosis (p.763).

Interferons have also been proposed for antifibrotic therapy in the management of diffuse scleroderma (see p.501). A multicentre study of interferon gamma in scleroderma[9] found that cutaneous symptoms might be improved but that treatment was associated with an unacceptable incidence of adverse effects. Interferon gamma has also been tried in eosinophilic pustular folliculitis.[10]

Interferons have also been used for the treatment of warts (see below).

Interferon alfa has improved symptoms such as pruritus in patients with polycythaemia vera. For reference to the use of interferon alfa-2b in polycythaemia vera, see Blood Disorders, above.

1. Souillet G, *et al.* Alpha-interferon treatment of patient with hyper IgE syndrome. *Lancet* 1989; **i:** 1384.
2. Reinhold U, *et al.* Recombinant interferon-γ in severe atopic dermatitis. *Lancet* 1990; **335:** 1282.
3. Boguniewicz M, *et al.* Recombinant gamma interferon in treatment of patients with atopic dermatitis and elevated IgE levels. *Am J Med* 1990; **88:** 365–70.
4. MacKie RM. Interferon-α for atopic dermatitis. *Lancet* 1990; **335:** 1282–3.
5. Nicolas J-F, Thivolet J. Interferon alfa therapy in severe unresponsive subacute cutaneous lupus erythematosus. *N Engl J Med* 1989; **321:** 1550–1.
6. Thivolet J, *et al.* Recombinant interferon α2a is effective in the treatment of discoid and subacute cutaneous lupus erythematosus. *Br J Dermatol* 1990; **122:** 405–9.
7. Kolde G, *et al.* Treatment of urticaria pigmentosa using interferon alpha. *Br J Dermatol* 1995; **133:** 91–4.
8. Lippert U, Henz BM. Long-term effect of interferon alpha treatment in mastocytosis. *Br J Dermatol* 1996; **134:** 1164–5.
9. Polisson RP, *et al.* A multicenter trial of recombinant human interferon gamma in patients with systemic sclerosis: effects on cutaneous fibrosis and interleukin 2 receptor levels. *J Rheumatol* 1996; **23:** 654–8.
10. Fushimi M, *et al.* Eosinophilic pustular folliculitis effectively treated with recombinant interferon-γ: suppression of mRNA expression of interleukin 5 in peripheral blood mononuclear cells. *Br J Dermatol* 1996; **134:** 766–72.

Varicella-zoster infections. Interferons alfa, beta, and gamma have been tried in varicella-zoster infections by a variety of routes of administration although the standard treatment is with aciclovir and related antivirals (see p.598) which are preferred since they produce fewer adverse effects.

References.

1. Merigan TC, *et al.* Human leukocyte interferon for the treatment of herpes zoster in patients with cancer. *N Engl J Med* 1978; **298:** 981–7.
2. Arvin AM, *et al.* Human leukocyte interferon for the treatment of varicella in children with cancer. *N Engl J Med* 1982; **306:** 761–5.
3. Duschet P, *et al.* Treatment of herpes zoster: recombinant alpha interferon versus acyclovir. *Int J Dermatol* 1988; **27:** 193–7.

Warts. Various interferons by various routes have been tried in the treatment of anogenital warts (condylomata acuminata) (p.1076). *Intralesional* injection has been used to ensure relatively high concentrations of interferon in the wart but the occurrence of systemic adverse effects demonstrated that there is absorption from this site. Eron and colleagues[1] reported complete responses in 36% of patients receiving intralesional interferon alfa-2b compared with 17% receiving placebo, and a corresponding overall reduction in the affected area of 62.4% compared with 1.2%. However, follow-up was not sufficiently long to comment on relapse rates. Reichman and colleagues[2] found similar responses using interferons alfa-2b, alfa-n1, or beta in patients with refractory warts, with complete responses in 47% of patients receiving intralesional interferons compared with 22% of patients receiving placebo. A study[3] evaluating two different doses of intralesional interferon beta given three times a week for three weeks reported complete responses in 63% of lesions injected with 1 million units compared with 38% of lesions injected with 33 000 units. Good responses have also been reported in patients with both refractory and recurrent warts treated with intralesional interferon alfa-n3.[4] Relapses were delayed and fewer warts recurred in patients who had received interferon rather than placebo. Intralesional interferon alfa-2b given in combination with podophyllum was more effective that podophyllum alone,[5] although about 66% of patients in each group subsequently relapsed. *Topical* application of interferon alfa has also been reported to be more effective than podophyllotoxin.[6,7] Theoretically, *systemic* administration should have advantages in controlling subclinical infections and reducing relapses. However, responses to subcutaneous interferon alfa have generally been disappointing[8-10] although Panici and colleagues[11] obtained responses comparable with cauterisation and a reduction in relapse rates with either subcutaneous or intramuscular interferon alfa-2b. Information on the use of systemic interferons as an adjunct to conventional therapy is scarce but a study in 97 patients[12] with recurrent warts found no difference in either response or relapse rates in patients receiving cryotherapy with subcutaneous interferon alfa or cryotherapy alone. A study comparing subcutaneous interferon alfa, beta, and gamma in combination with cryotherapy found no significant difference in response rate, although patients receiving interferon beta or gamma developed new warts at a lower frequency.[13]

1. Eron LJ, *et al.* Interferon therapy for condylomata acuminata. *N Engl J Med* 1986; **315:** 1059–64.
2. Reichman RC, *et al.* Treatment of condyloma acuminatum with three different interferons administered intralesionally: a double-blind, placebo-controlled trial. *Ann Intern Med* 1988; **108:** 675–9.
3. Monsonego J, *et al.* Randomised double-blind trial of recombinant interferon-beta for condyloma acuminatum. *Genitourin Med* 1996; **72:** 111–14.
4. Friedman-Kien AE, *et al.* Natural interferon alfa for treatment of condylomata acuminata. *JAMA* 1988; **259:** 533–8.
5. Douglas JM, *et al.* A randomized trial of combination therapy with intralesional interferon α_{2b} and podophyllin versus podophyllin alone for the therapy of anogenital warts. *J Infect Dis* 1990; **162:** 52–9.
6. Syed TA, *et al.* Human leukocyte interferon-alpha versus podophyllotoxin in cream for the treatment of genital warts in males: a placebo-controlled, double-blind, comparative study. *Dermatology* 1995; **191:** 129–32.
7. Syed TA, *et al.* Management of genital warts in women with human leukocyte interferon-α vs podophyllotoxin in cream: a placebo-controlled, double-blind, comparative study. *J Mol Med* 1995; **73:** 255–8.
8. Reichman RC, *et al.* Treatment of condyloma acuminatum with three different interferon-α preparations administered parenterally: a double-blind, placebo-controlled trial. *J Infect Dis* 1990; **162:** 1270–6.
9. Condylomata International Collaborative Study Group. Recurrent condylomata acuminata treated with recombinant interferon alfa-2a: a multicenter double-blind placebo-controlled clinical trial. *JAMA* 1991; **265:** 2684–7.
10. Condylomata International Collaborative Study Group. Recurrent condylomata acuminata treated with recombinant interferon alpha-2a: a multicenter double-blind placebo-controlled clinical trial. *Acta Derm Venereol (Stockh)* 1993; **73:** 223–6.
11. Panici PB, *et al.* Randomized clinical trial comparing systemic interferon with diathermocoagulation in primary multiple and widespread anogenital condyloma. *Obstet Gynecol* 1989; **74:** 393–7.
12. Eron LJ, *et al.* Recurrence of condylomata acuminata following cryotherapy is not prevented by systemically administered interferon. *Genitourin Med* 1993; **69:** 91–3.
13. Bonnez W, *et al.* A randomized, double-blind, placebo-controlled trial of systemically administered interferon-α, -β, or -γ in combination with cryotherapy for the treatment of condyloma acuminatum. *J Infect Dis* 1995; **171:** 1081–9.

Preparations

Proprietary Preparations (details are given in Part 3)
Aust.: Berofor; Imufor; Imukin; Intron A; Roferon-A; Wellferon; ***Austral.:*** Betaferon; Imukin; Intron A; Roferon-A; ***Belg.:*** Berofor†; Betaferon; Intron A; Roferon-A; ***Canad.:*** Betaseron; Intron A; Roferon-A; Wellferon; ***Fr.:*** Betaferon; Imukin; Introna; Laroferon; Roferon-A; Viraferon; ***Ger.:*** Berofor†; Betaferon; Cellferon; Fiblaferon; Glucoferon†; Imukin; Intron A; Polyferon†; Roferon-A; ***Irl.:*** Betaferon; Immukin; Intron A; Roferon-A; ***Ital.:*** Alfaferone; Alfater; Avonex; Betaferon; Betantrone; Betron R; Biaferone; Cilferon-A; Frone; Gammakine; Haimaferone; Humoferon; Imukin; Intron A; Isiferone; Naferon; Roferon-A; Serobif; Wellferon; ***Jpn:*** Feron; OIF; ***Neth.:*** Avonex; Betaferon; Immukine; Intron A; Roferon-A; ***Norw.:*** Betaferon; Imukin; Introna; Roceron; ***S.Afr.:*** Betaferon; Intron A; Roferon-A; ***Spain:*** Betaferon; Frone; Imukin; Intron A; Roferon-A; Viraferon; Wellferon; ***Swed.:*** Avonex; Imukin; Introna; Roferon-A; Wellferon; ***Switz.:*** Betaferon; Imukin; Intron A; Roferon-A; Wellferon; ***UK:*** Avonex; Betaferon; Immukin; Intron A; Rebif; Roferon-A; Viraferon; Wellferon; ***USA:*** Actimmune; Alferon N; Avonex; Betaseron; Infergen; Intron A; Roferon-A.

Multi-ingredient: *USA:* Rebetron.

Lamivudine (15566-c)

Lamivudine *(BAN, USAN, rINN).*

3TC; (−)-2′-Deoxy-3′-thiacytidine; GR-109714X. (−)-1-[(2*R*,5*S*)-2-(Hydroxymethyl)-1,3-oxathiolan-5-yl]cytosine.

$C_8H_{11}N_3O_3S$ = 229.3.

CAS — 131086-21-0; 134678-17-4.

Adverse Effects

Adverse effects commonly associated with lamivudine include abdominal pain, nausea, vomiting, diarrhoea, headache, fever, rash, malaise, insomnia, cough, nasal symptoms, and musculoskeletal pain. Peripheral neuropathy and pancreatitis have been reported rarely. Neutropenia and anaemia (when given in combination with zidovudine), thrombocytopenia, and increases in liver enzymes and serum amylase have occurred.

Effects on the hair. Hair loss was associated with lamivudine treatment in 5 patients.[1]

1. Fong IW. Hair loss associated with lamivudine. *Lancet* 1994; **344:** 1702.

Effects on the nails. Paronychia was reported in 12 HIV-infected patients receiving lamivudine.[1]

1. Zerboni R, *et al.* Lamivudine-induced paronychia. *Lancet* 1998; **351:** 1256.

Effects on the nervous system. Exacerbation of peripheral neuropathy was reported in one patient following substitution of lamivudine for zalcitabine.[1]

1. Cupler EJ, Dalakas MC. Exacerbation of peripheral neuropathy by lamivudine. *Lancet* 1995; **345:** 460–1.

Hypersensitivity. Angioedema, urticaria, and anaphylactoid reaction occurred in a patient 30 minutes after receiving the first dose of lamivudine.[1]

1. Kainer MA, Mijch A. Anaphylactoid reaction, angioedema, and urticaria associated with lamivudine. *Lancet* 1996; **348:** 1519.

Precautions

Lamivudine therapy should be stopped in patients who develop abdominal pain, nausea, or vomiting or with abnormal biochemical test results until pancreatitis has been excluded. Dosage reduction may be necessary in patients with impaired renal function. In patients with chronic hepatitis B, there is a risk of rebound hepatitis when lamivudine is discontinued, and liver function should be monitored in such patients. The possibility of HIV infection should be excluded before beginning lamivudine therapy for hepatitis B, since the lower doses used to treat the latter may permit the development of lamivudine resistant strains of HIV.

Interactions

The renal excretion of lamivudine may be inhibited by concomitant administration of other drugs mainly eliminated by active renal secretion, for example trimethoprim. Usual prophylactic doses of trimethoprim are unlikely to necessitate reductions in lamivudine dosage unless the patient has impaired renal function, but the co-administration of lamivudine with the high therapeutic doses of trimethoprim used in *Pneumocystis carinii* pneumonia and toxoplasmosis should be avoided.

Antiviral Action

Lamivudine is converted intracellularly in stages to the triphosphate. This triphosphate halts the DNA synthesis of retroviruses, including HIV, through competitive inhibition of reverse transcriptase and incorporation into viral DNA. Lamivudine is also active against hepatitis B virus. Resistance to lamivudine has been reported in isolates of HIV and hepatitis B virus.

References.

1. Coates JAV, *et al.* (−)-2′-Deoxy-3′-thiacytidine is a potent, highly selective inhibitor of human immunodeficiency virus type 1 and type 2 replication in vitro. *Antimicrob Agents Chemother* 1992; **36:** 733–9.
2. Bartholomew MM, *et al.* Hepatitis-B-virus resistance to lamivudine given for recurrent infection after orthotopic liver transplantation. *Lancet* 1997; **349:** 20–2.

Pharmacokinetics

Lamivudine is rapidly absorbed following oral administration and peak plasma concentrations are achieved in about one hour. Absorption is delayed, but not reduced by ingestion with food. Bioavailability is between 80 and 87%. Binding to plasma protein is reported to be less than 36%. Lamivudine crosses the blood-brain barrier with a ratio of CSF to serum concentrations of about 0.12. It crosses the placenta and is distributed into breast milk.

Lamivudine is metabolised intracellularly to the active antiviral triphosphate. Hepatic metabolism is low and it is cleared mainly by renal excretion. An elimination half-life of 5 to 7 hours has been reported following a single dose.

References.

1. Yuen GJ, *et al.* Pharmacokinetics, absolute bioavailability, and absorption characteristics of lamivudine. *J Clin Pharmacol* 1995; **35:** 1174–80.
2. Heald AE, *et al.* Pharmacokinetics of lamivudine in human immunodeficiency virus-infected patients with renal dysfunction. *Antimicrob Agents Chemother* 1996; **40:** 1514–19.
3. Johnson MA, *et al.* Single dose pharmacokinetics of lamivudine in subjects with impaired renal function and the effect of haemodialysis. *Br J Clin Pharmacol* 1998; **46:** 21–7.

Uses and Administration

Lamivudine is a nucleoside reverse transcriptase inhibitor structurally related to cytosine with activity against retroviruses including HIV. It is used, usually in combination with zidovudine, in the treatment of HIV infection. It is also used for the treatment of hepatitis B.

For HIV infection, the recommended dose of lamivudine for adults is 150 mg by mouth twice daily. A suggested dose for children aged between 3 months and 12 years is 4 mg per kg body-weight twice daily to a maximum of 150 mg twice daily.

For chronic hepatitis B the recommended dose is 100 mg once daily by mouth; in patients with concomitant HIV and hepatitis B infection the dosage regimen appropriate for HIV should be used.

Reduction of dosage is recommended for patients with impaired renal function.

Reviews.

1. Perry CM, Faulds D. Lamivudine: a review of its antiviral activity, pharmacokinetic properties and therapeutic efficacy in the management of HIV infection. *Drugs* 1997; **53:** 657–80.

Hepatitis. Lamivudine is one of the more promising antiviral drugs being tried as an alternative to interferon alfa in the treatment of chronic hepatitis B (p.595). In a preliminary study, lamivudine 100 or 300 mg daily reduced hepatitis B virus DNA to low or undetectable levels.[1] In a 1-year double-blind study involving about 350 patients with chronic hepatitis B, lamivudine 100 mg daily was associated with substantial histological improvement in many patients; a dose of 25 mg daily was less effective.[2] Relapses have been reported once treatment with lamivudine is stopped, and one case of reactivation of hepatitis B infection has been observed.[3] Lamivudine may also be effective in preventing re-infection with hepatitis B in patients who have received liver transplants.[4]

1. Dienstag JL, *et al.* A preliminary trial of lamivudine for chronic hepatitis B infection. *N Engl J Med* 1995; **333:** 1657–61.
2. Lai C-L, *et al.* A one-year trial of lamivudine for chronic hepatitis B. *N Engl J Med* 1998; **339:** 61–8.
3. Honkoop P, *et al.* Hepatitis B reactivation after lamivudine. *Lancet* 1995; **346:** 1156–7.
4. Grellier L, *et al.* Lamivudine prophylaxis against reinfection in liver transplantation for hepatitis B cirrhosis. *Lancet* 1996; **348:** 1212–15. Correction. *ibid.* 1997; **349:** 364.

HIV infection and AIDS. Lamivudine is a potent inhibitor of HIV-1 and HIV-2 *in vitro*, including variants resistant to zidovudine.[1] Resistance emerges rapidly when lamivudine is given alone to patients with HIV infections,[2] although sustained responses have been reported despite the emergence of resistance.[3] Combination therapy with lamivudine and zidovudine delays, and may even reverse, the emergence of zidovudine resistance and produces a sustained synergistic antiretroviral effect,[4] but HIV strains resistant to both lamivudine and zidovudine may arise during combination therapy.[5] As discussed on p.599 combination therapy at an early stage of HIV infection is likely to become standard therapy and treatment with lamivudine plus zidovudine has produced better responses than either drug alone in antiretroviral-naive patients,[6,7] and has produced additional responses in antiretroviral-experienced patients,[8,9] with little additional toxicity. The addition of lamivudine to existing antiretroviral therapy has been reported to slow the progression of the disease and improve survival.[10]

Lamivudine is also used in prophylactic regimens following occupational exposure to HIV infection (see p.601).

1. Anonymous. Lamivudine: impressive benefits in combination with zidovudine. *WHO Drug Inf* 1996; **10:** 5–7.
2. Wainberg MA, *et al.* Development of HIV-1 resistance to (−)2′-deoxy-3′-thiacytidine in patients with AIDS or advanced AIDS-related complex. *AIDS* 1995; **9:** 351–7.
3. Ingrand D, *et al.* Phase I/II study of 3TC (lamivudine) in HIV-positive, asymptomatic or mild AIDS-related complex patients: sustained reduction in viral markers. *AIDS* 1995; **9:** 1323–9.
4. Larder BA, *et al.* Potential mechanism for sustained antiretroviral efficacy of AZT-3TC combination therapy. *Science* 1995; **269:** 696–9.
5. Miller V, *et al.* Dual resistance to zidovudine and lamivudine in patients treated with zidovudine-lamivudine combination therapy: association with therapeutic failure. *J Infect Dis* 1998; **177:** 1521–32.
6. Eron JJ, *et al.* Treatment with lamivudine, zidovudine, or both in HIV-positive patients with 200 to 500 CD4+ cells per cubic millimeter. *N Engl J Med* 1995; **333:** 1662–9.
7. Katlama C, *et al.* Safety and efficacy of lamivudine-zidovudine combination therapy in antiretroviral-naive patients: a randomized controlled comparison with zidovudine monotherapy. *JAMA* 1996; **276:** 118–25.
8. Staszewski S, *et al.* Safety and efficacy of lamivudine-zidovudine combination therapy in zidovudine-experienced patients: a randomized controlled comparison with zidovudine monotherapy. *JAMA* 1996; **276:** 111–17.
9. Bartlett JA, *et al.* Lamivudine plus zidovudine compared with zalcitabine plus zidovudine in patients with HIV infection: a randomized, double-blind, placebo-controlled trial. *Ann Intern Med* 1996; **125:** 161–72.
10. CAESAR Coordinating Committee. Randomised trial of addition of lamivudine or lamivudine plus loviride to zidovudine-containing regimens for patients with HIV-1 infection: the CAESAR trial. *Lancet* 1997; **349:** 1413–21.

Preparations

Proprietary Preparations (details are given in Part 3)
Austral.: 3TC; ***Fr.:*** Epivir; ***Ger.:*** Epivir; ***Ital.:*** Epivir; ***Neth.:*** Epivir; ***Spain:*** Epivir; ***Swed.:*** Epivir; ***Switz.:*** 3TC; ***UK:*** Epivir.

Multi-ingredient: *UK:* Combivir; *USA:* Combivir.

Lobucavir (17834-y)

Lobucavir *(USAN, rINN).*

BMS-180194; SQ-34514. 9-[(1*R*,2*R*,3*S*)-2,3-Bis(hydroxymethyl)cyclobutyl]guanine.

$C_{11}H_{15}N_5O_3$ = 265.3.

CAS — 127759-89-1.

Lobucavir is a nucleoside analogue with antiviral activity and is under investigation for the treatment of herpesvirus and hepatitis B infections.

Loviride (17434-x)

Loviride *(BAN, rINN).*

R-89439. (±)-2-(6-Acetyl-*m*-toluidino)-2-(2,6-dichlorophenyl)acetamide; N^2-(6-Acetyl-*m*-tolyl)-DL-2-(2,6-dichlorophenyl)glycinamide.

$C_{17}H_{16}Cl_2N_2O_2$ = 351.2.

CAS — 147362-57-0.

Loviride is a non-nucleoside reverse transcriptase inhibitor under investigation for the treatment of HIV infection. Viral resistance emerges rapidly when loviride is given alone, and it would be likely to be used mainly in combination with nucleoside reverse transcriptase inhibitors.

References.

1. CAESAR Coordinating Committee. Randomised trial of addition of lamivudine or lamivudine plus loviride to zidovudine-containing regimens for patients with HIV-1 infection: the CAESAR trial. *Lancet* 1997; **349:** 1413–21.

Moroxydine Hydrochloride (12979-y)

Moroxydine Hydrochloride *(BANM, rINNM).*

Abitilguanide Hydrochloride; ABOB. 1-(Morpholinoformimidoyl)guanidine hydrochloride.

$C_6H_{13}N_5O,HCl = 207.7.$

CAS — 3731-59-7 (moroxydine); 3160-91-6 (moroxydine hydrochloride).

Moroxydine hydrochloride has been given by mouth in the treatment of herpes simplex and varicella-zoster infections. It has also been used topically.

It is included as an ingredient in preparations for the treatment of cold and influenza symptoms.

Preparations

Proprietary Preparations (details are given in Part 3)
Belg.: Virustat†; ***Fr.:*** Virustat†.

Multi-ingredient: ***Belg.:*** Assur†; ***Fr.:*** Assur†; ***S.Afr.:*** Corenza C; Virobis†.

Nelfinavir Mesylate (17721-b)

Nelfinavir Mesylate *(BANM, USAN).*

Nelfinavir Mesilate *(rINNM)*; AG-1343 (nelfinavir or nelfinavir mesylate). 3S[2(2S*,3S*),3α,4aβ,8aβ]-*N*-(1,1-Dimethylethyl)decahydro-2-2-hydroxy-3-[(3-hydroxy-2-methylbenzoyl)amino]-4-(phenylthio)butyl-3-isoquinolinecarboxamide monomethanesulphonate; (3S,4aS,8aS)-*N-tert*-Butyldecahydro-2-[(2R,3R)-3-(3-hydroxy-o-toluamido)-2-hydroxy-4-(phenylthio)butyl]isoquinoline-3-carboxamide monomethanesulphonate.

$C_{32}H_{45}N_3O_4S,CH_4O_3S = 663.9.$

CAS — 159989-64-7 (nelfinavir); 159989-65-8 (nelfinavir mesylate).

NOTE. Do not confuse nelfinavir with nevirapine (p.623).

Adverse Effects and Precautions

As for HIV-protease inhibitors in general (see Indinavir Sulphate, p.614).

Interactions

As for HIV-protease inhibitors in general (see Indinavir Sulphate, p.614). Nelfinavir is reported to be metabolised in part by cytochrome P450 isoenzymes of the CYP3A family and to be unlikely to inhibit other cytochrome P450 isoforms at concentrations in the therapeutic range.

Pharmacokinetics

Nelfinavir is absorbed from the gastro-intestinal tract and peak plasma concentrations occur in 2 to 4 hours. Absorption is enhanced by administration with food. Nelfinavir is extensively bound to plasma proteins (98%). It is distributed into breast milk. Nelfinavir is metabolised by oxidation by cytochrome P450 isoenzymes including CYP3A. The major oxidative metabolite has *in-vitro* antiviral activity equal to that of nelfinavir. The terminal half-life is 3.5 to 5 hours. Nelfinavir is excreted in the faeces mainly as metabolites. Only about 1 to 2% is excreted in the urine.

Uses and Administration

Nelfinavir is a protease inhibitor with antiviral activity against HIV (see Antiviral Action, p.615). It is used, in combination with nucleoside reverse transcriptase inhibitors, for the treatment of HIV infection (p.599).

Nelfinavir is given by mouth (as the mesylate) in a dose of 750 mg three times daily with food. Children aged 2 to 13 years may be given 20 to 30 mg per kg body-weight three times daily.

Reviews (for reviews of HIV-protease inhibitors in general, see Indinavir, p.615).

1. Perry C, Benfield P. Nelfinavir. *Drugs* 1997; **54:** 81–7.
2. Jarvis B, Faulds D. Nelfinavir: a review of its therapeutic efficacy in HIV infection. *Drugs* 1998; **56:** 147–67.

Preparations

Proprietary Preparations (details are given in Part 3)
UK: Viracept; ***USA:*** Viracept.

Netivudine (14532-r)

Netivudine *(BAN, rINN).*

BW-882C; BW-882C87; 882C; 882C87. 1-β-D-Arabinofuranosyl-5-prop-1-ynyluracil.

$C_{12}H_{14}N_2O_6 = 282.2.$

CAS — 84558-93-0.

Netivudine is a synthetic nucleoside analogue structurally related to thymidine, with activity against varicella-zoster virus. Netivudine is being studied for the treatment of herpes zoster although concerns have been expressed over its toxicity following long-term administration to *rodents*.

References.

1. Easterbrook P, Wood MJ. Successors to acyclovir. *J Antimicrob Chemother* 1994; **34:** 307–11.
2. Peck RW, *et al.* Pharmacokinetics and tolerability of single oral doses of 882C87, a potent, new anti-varicella-zoster virus agent, in healthy volunteers. *Antimicrob Agents Chemother* 1995; **39:** 20–7.
3. Peck RW, *et al.* The bioavailability and disposition of 1-(β-D-arabinofuranosyl)-5-(1-propynyl)uracil (882C87), a potent, new anti-varicella zoster virus agent. *Br J Clin Pharmacol* 1995; **39:** 143–9.
4. Peck RW, *et al.* Multiple dose netivudine, a potent anti-varicella zoster virus agent, in healthy elderly volunteers and patients with shingles. *J Antimicrob Chemother* 1996; **37:** 583–97.
5. Fillastre JP, *et al.* Pharmacokinetics of netivudine, a potent anti-varicella zoster virus drug, in patients with renal impairment. *J Antimicrob Chemother* 1996; **37:** 965–74.
6. Söltz-Szöts J, *et al.* A randomised controlled trial of acyclovir versus netivudine for treatment of herpes zoster. *J Antimicrob Chemother* 1998; **41:** 549–56.

Nevirapine (14530-t)

Nevirapine *(BAN, USAN, rINN).*

BI-RG-587; BIRG-0587. 11-Cyclopropyl-5,11-dihydro-4-methyl-6*H*-dipyrido[3,2-*b*:2′,3′-e]-[1,4]diazepin-6-one.

$C_{15}H_{14}N_4O = 266.3.$

CAS — 129618-40-2.

NOTE. Do not confuse nevirapine with nelfinavir (p.623).

Adverse Effects

The most common adverse effect of nevirapine is skin rash, usually occurring within the first 6 weeks of starting therapy. Severe and life-threatening skin reactions have occurred, including Stevens-Johnson syndrome and, more rarely, toxic epidermal necrolysis. Other common adverse effects include nausea, fatigue, fever, drowsiness, and headache. Abnormalities in liver function tests are also common, and hepatitis has occurred.

Effects on the skin. References.

1. Warren KJ, *et al.* Nevirapine-associated Stevens-Johnson syndrome. *Lancet* 1998; **351:** 567.
2. Barner A, Myers M. Nevirapine and rashes. *Lancet* 1998; **351:** 1133.

Precautions

Nevirapine should be discontinued if a severe skin rash develops or if a rash is accompanied by fever, blistering, oral lesions, conjunctivitis, swelling, muscle or joint aches, or general malaise. Dose escalation should not be attempted in patients developing any rash during the first 14 days of treatment until the rash has resolved. Liver function should be monitored and treatment interrupted if moderate or severe abnormalities occur; nevirapine may be restarted at the initial dose if liver function returns to normal, but should be permanently discontinued if abnormalities recur. Nevirapine should be used with caution in patients with renal or hepatic insufficiency and not at all in those with renal or hepatic failure.

Interactions

Similarly to the HIV-protease inhibitors (see Indinavir, p.614), nevirapine is metabolised mainly by cytochrome P450 isoenzymes of the CYP3A family. Consequently it may compete with other drugs metabolised by this system (possibly resulting in mutually increased plasma concentrations) or enzyme inducers may decrease plasma concentrations of nevirapine; nevirapine itself acts as a mild to moderate enzyme inducer and may thus reduce plasma concentrations of other drugs.

Drugs that may be affected by nevirapine include:

antifungals—plasma concentrations of *ketoconazole* reduced and those of nevirapine increased;

antivirals—plasma concentrations of the HIV-protease inhibitors *indinavir* and *saquinavir* reduced;

hormonal contraceptives—plasma concentrations of *oral contraceptives* and other *hormonal contraceptives* reduced (thus reducing the contraceptive effect).

Drugs found to increase plasma concentrations of nevirapine when given concomitantly have included *cimetidine* and *macrolide antibiotics*; drugs found to decrease plasma concentrations of nevirapine have included *rifabutin* and *rifampicin*.

Pharmacokinetics

Nevirapine is readily absorbed following oral administration and absorption is not affected by food. Peak plasma concentrations occur up to 4 hours after a single dose. Nevirapine is about 60% bound to plasma proteins. Concentrations in the CNS are about 45% of those in plasma. Nevirapine crosses the placenta and is distributed into breast milk. It is extensively metabolised by hepatic microsomal enzymes, principally by cytochrome P450 isoenzymes of the CYP3A family. Autoinduction of these enzymes results in a 1.5- to 2-fold increase in apparent oral clearance after 2 to 4 weeks' administration of usual doses, and a decrease in terminal half-life from 45 hours to 25 to 30 hours over the same period. Nevirapine is mainly excreted in the urine as glucuronide conjugates of the hydroxylated metabolites.

References.

1. Cheeseman SH, *et al.* Pharmacokinetics of nevirapine: initial single-rising-dose study in humans. *Antimicrob Agents Chemother* 1993; **37:** 178–82.

Uses and Administration

Nevirapine is a non-nucleoside reverse transcriptase inhibitor with activity against HIV-1. It is used in the treatment of HIV infection (p.599). Viral resistance emerges rapidly when nevirapine is used alone, and it is used in combination with other antiretroviral drugs.

Nevirapine is given in a dose of 200 mg daily for the first 14 days, then increased to 200 mg twice daily provided that no rash is present.

References.

1. Merluzzi VJ, *et al.* Inhibition of HIV-1 replication by a nonnucleoside reverse transcriptase inhibitor. *Science* 1990; **250:** 1411–13.
2. Richman D, *et al.* BI-RG-587 is active against zidovudine-resistant human immunodeficiency virus type 1 and synergistic with zidovudine. *Antimicrob Agents Chemother* 1991; **35:** 305–8.
3. Cheeseman SH, *et al.* Phase I/II evaluation of nevirapine alone and in combination with zidovudine for infection with human immunodeficiency virus. *J Acquir Immune Defic Syndr* 1995; **8:** 141–51.
4. Havlir D, *et al.* A pilot study to evaluate the development of resistance to nevirapine in asymptomatic human immunodeficiency virus-infected patients with CD4 cell counts of >500/mm³: AIDS Clinical Trials Group Protocol 208. *J Infect Dis* 1995; **172:** 1379–83.
5. Carr A, *et al.* A controlled trial of nevirapine plus zidovudine versus zidovudine alone in p24 antigenaemic HIV-infected patients. *AIDS* 1996; **10:** 635–41.
6. D'Aquila RT, *et al.* Nevirapine, zidovudine, and didanosine compared with zidovudine and didanosine in patients with HIV-1 infection: a randomized, double-blind, placebo-controlled trial. *Ann Intern Med* 1996; **124:** 1019–30.

Preparations

Proprietary Preparations (details are given in Part 3)
Austral.: Viramune; ***UK:*** Viramune; ***USA:*** Viramune.

Penciclovir (3035-m)

Penciclovir (*BAN, USAN, rINN*).

BRL-39123. 9-[4-Hydroxy-3-(hydroxymethyl)butyl]guanine.

$C_{10}H_{15}N_5O_3$ = 253.3.

CAS — 39809-25-1.

Adverse Effects and Precautions

Penciclovir applied topically may cause transient stinging, burning, and numbness.

For the effects of systemic administration, see Famciclovir, p.609.

Antiviral Action

Penciclovir has antiviral activity similar to that of aciclovir. It is active *in vitro* and *in vivo* against herpes simplex virus types 1 and 2 and against varicella-zoster virus. This activity is due to intracellular conversion by virus-induced thymidine kinase into penciclovir triphosphate, which inhibits replication of viral DNA and persists in infected cells for more than 12 hours. It also has activity against Epstein-Barr virus and hepatitis B virus.

References.

1. Weinberg A, *et al.* In vitro activities of penciclovir and acyclovir against herpes simplex virus types 1 and 2. *Antimicrob Agents Chemother* 1992; **36:** 2037–8.
2. Vere-Hodge RA. Famciclovir and penciclovir: the mode of action of famciclovir including its conversion to penciclovir. *Antiviral Chem Chemother* 1993; **4:** 67–84.
3. Boyd MR, *et al.* Penciclovir: a review of its spectrum of activity, selectivity, and cross-resistance pattern. *Antiviral Chem Chemother* 1993; **4** (suppl 1): 3–11.
4. Bacon TH, Boyd MR. Activity of penciclovir against Epstein-Barr virus. *Antimicrob Agents Chemother* 1995; **39:** 1599–1602.
5. Lin E, *et al.* The guanine nucleoside analog penciclovir is active against chronic duck hepatitis B virus infection in vivo. *Antimicrob Agents Chemother* 1996; **40:** 413–18.
6. Korba BE, Boyd MR. Penciclovir is a selective inhibitor of hepatitis B virus replication in cultured human hepatoblastoma cells. *Antimicrob Agents Chemother* 1996; **40:** 1282–4.

Pharmacokinetics

Penciclovir is poorly absorbed from the gastro-intestinal tract. For systemic use it is usually administered orally as the prodrug famciclovir which is rapidly converted to penciclovir, producing peak plasma concentrations proportional to the dose (over the range 125 to 750 mg) after 45 minutes to 1 hour. The plasma elimination half-life is approximately 2 hours. The intracellular half-life of the triphosphate is more prolonged. Penciclovir is less than 20% bound to plasma proteins. Penciclovir is mainly excreted unchanged in the urine.

References.

1. Fowles SE, *et al.* The tolerance to and pharmacokinetics of penciclovir (BRL39123A), a novel antiherpes agent, administered by intravenous infusion to healthy subjects. *Eur J Clin Pharmacol* 1992; **43:** 513–16.
2. Pue MA, *et al.* Linear pharmacokinetics of penciclovir following administration of single oral doses of famciclovir 125, 250, 500 and 750 mg to healthy volunteers. *J Antimicrob Chemother* 1994; **33:** 119–27.

Uses and Administration

Penciclovir is a nucleoside analogue structurally related to guanine which is active against herpesviruses. It is applied topically as a 1% cream in the treatment of herpes labialis (see Herpes Simplex Infections, p.597).

For systemic use, penciclovir is administered by mouth as the prodrug famciclovir (see p.609). Intravenous administration of penciclovir is being investigated.

References.

1. Spruance SL, *et al.* Penciclovir cream for the treatment of herpes simplex labialis: a randomized, multicenter, double-blind, placebo-controlled trial. *JAMA* 1997; **277:** 1374–9.

Preparations

Proprietary Preparations (details are given in Part 3)
Austral.: Vectavir; ***Belg.:*** Vectavir; ***Ger.:*** Vectavir; ***Neth.:*** Famvir; ***Swed.:*** Vectavir; ***UK:*** Vectavir.

Peptide T (3160-p)

D-Ala-peptide-T-amide.

Peptide T is an octapeptide segment of the envelope glycoprotein of human immunodeficiency virus. It has been investigated for the treatment of HIV infection and HIV-associated neurological disorders. Peptide T has also been tried in the treatment of psoriasis.

References.

1. Wetterberg L, *et al.* Peptide T in treatment of AIDS. *Lancet* 1987; **i:** 159.
2. Bridge TP, *et al.* Improvement in AIDS patients on peptide T. *Lancet* 1989; **ii:** 226–7.
3. Poizot-Martin I, *et al.* Are CD4 antibodies and peptide T new treatments for psoriasis? *Lancet* 1991; **337:** 1477.
4. Farbar EM, *et al.* Peptide T improves psoriasis when infused into lesions in nanogram amounts. *J Am Acad Dermatol* 1991; **25:** 658–64.

Pirodavir (14650-b)

Pirodavir (*BAN, USAN, rINN*).

R-77975. Ethyl 4-{2-[1-(6-methylpyridazin-3-yl)-4-piperidyl]ethoxy}benzoate.

$C_{21}H_{27}N_3O_3$ = 369.5.

CAS — 124436-59-5.

Pirodavir is an antiviral reported to be active against rhinoviruses.

References.

1. Andries K, *et al.* In vitro activity of pirodavir (R 77975), a substituted phenoxypyridazinamine with broad-spectrum antipicornaviral activity. *Antimicrob Agents Chemother* 1992; **36:** 100–7.
2. Hayden FG, *et al.* Safety and efficacy of intranasal pirodavir (R77975) in experimental rhinovirus infection. *Antimicrob Agents Chemother* 1992; **36:** 727–32.
3. Hayden FG, *et al.* Intranasal pirodavir (R77, 975) treatment of rhinovirus colds. *Antimicrob Agents Chemother* 1995; **39:** 290–4.

Poly I.poly C12U (3322-w)

Poly(I):poly(C_{12},U).

Poly I.poly C12U is a synthetic mismatched polymer of double-stranded RNA with antiviral and immunomodulatory activity. It is widely known as Ampligen which is a trade-mark. It is under investigation in the treatment of AIDS and HIV infection, and also in renal cell carcinoma, chronic fatigue syndrome, and melanoma.

For a reference to the enhancement by poly I.poly C12U of zidovudine's anti-HIV activity *in vitro* see Microbiological Interactions, under Antiviral Action of Zidovudine, p.632.

References.

1. Carter WA, *et al.* Clinical, immunological, and virological effects of Ampligen, a mismatched double-stranded RNA, in patients with AIDS or AIDS-related complex. *Lancet* 1987; **i:** 1286–92.
2. Thompson KA, *et al.* Results of a double-blind placebo-controlled study of the double-stranded RNA drug polyI:polyC12U in the treatment of HIV infection. *Eur J Clin Microbiol Infect Dis* 1996; **15:** 580–7.

Propagermanium (14652-g)

Propagermanium (*rINN*).

Propagermanium is an immunomodulator which has been used in chronic hepatitis B infections. Acute exacerbation of hepatitis, including some fatalities, has been reported in patients receiving propagermanium.

Preparations

Proprietary Preparations (details are given in Part 3)
Jpn: Serocion.

Rimantadine Hydrochloride (1686-f)

Rimantadine Hydrochloride (*BANM, USAN, rINNM*).

EXP-126. (*RS*)-1-(Adamantan-1-yl)ethylamine hydrochloride; α-Methyl-1-adamantanemethylamine hydrochloride.

$C_{12}H_{21}N,HCl$ = 215.8.

CAS — 13392-28-4 (rimantadine); 1501-84-4 (rimantadine hydrochloride).

Adverse Effects and Precautions

The incidence and severity of adverse effects associated with rimantadine appear to be low. Those reported include gastro-intestinal disturbances such as nausea, vomiting, and anorexia and CNS effects such as headache, insomnia, nightmares, nervousness, lightheadedness, and concentration difficulties. It should be given with caution to patients with epilepsy. Doses are reduced in renal or hepatic failure; reduced doses have also been used in the elderly.

A double-blind placebo-controlled study was performed in healthy subjects to compare the relative toxicities of equal doses of rimantadine hydrochloride and amantadine hydrochloride.[1] Both drugs were well tolerated at doses of 200 mg daily for 4.5 days, but rimantadine was significantly better tolerated than amantadine at a dosage of 300 mg daily.

In a study to evaluate the safety of long-term rimantadine hydrochloride for elderly, chronically ill individuals during an influenza A epidemic,[2] a significantly greater proportion of patients taking rimantadine developed anxiety and/or nausea compared with those taking placebo. There was also a significantly greater number of days in which anxiety, nausea, confusion, depression, or vomiting were reported. Most of these side-effects lasted less than 9 days and were seldom severe except in 2 patients who withdrew from the study because of insomnia, anxiety, or both and a third who suffered a generalised convulsion. In a larger study[3] the incidence of these symptoms was similar in treatment and placebo groups.

Observations of seizures in two patients receiving influenza prophylaxis with rimantadine hydrochloride emphasised that chronically ill and elderly patients prone to seizures (especially those who may have had antiepileptic therapy withdrawn) may be at risk of developing seizures.[4] A precautionary measure of reducing the rimantadine hydrochloride dosage to 100 mg daily together with temporary re-introduction of antiepileptics was suggested.

1. Hayden FG, *et al.* Comparative toxicity of amantadine hydrochloride and rimantadine hydrochloride in healthy adults. *Antimicrob Agents Chemother* 1981; **19:** 226–33.
2. Patriarca PA, *et al.* Safety of prolonged administration of rimantadine hydrochloride in the prophylaxis of influenza A virus infections in nursing homes. *Antimicrob Agents Chemother* 1984; **26:** 101–3.
3. Monto AS, *et al.* Safety and efficacy of long-term use of rimantadine for prophylaxis of type A influenza in nursing homes. *Antimicrob Agents Chemother* 1995; **39:** 2224–8.
4. Bentley DW, *et al.* Rimantadine and seizures. *Ann Intern Med* 1989; **110:** 323–4.

Antiviral Action

Rimantadine hydrochloride inhibits influenza A viruses, probably at an early stage of replication.

Resistance to rimantadine can easily be induced in influenza A virus *in vitro* and *in vivo*. Transmission of rimantadine-resistant influenza A virus has been found among household contacts, and young children treated for established influenza A infection may excrete resistant virus within a week of beginning treatment.

Rimantadine is active *in vitro* against influenza A virus.[1-5] It has been reported to be more effective than amantadine against this virus in concentrations similar to those achieved clinically in the serum, although tissue studies suggested that it might be more toxic than amantadine at certain concentrations.[3] Rimantadine hydrochloride plus tribavirin demonstrated an enhanced antiviral effect *in vitro* against influenza A virus[4] and an additive or synergistic effect was observed with interferon alfa and either rimantadine hydrochloride or tribavirin.[5]

1. Galegov GA, *et al.* Rimantadine inhibits reproduction of influenza virus A/USSR/77. *Lancet* 1979; **i:** 269–70.
2. Koff WC, Knight V. Effect of rimantadine on influenza virus replication. *Proc Soc Exp Biol Med* 1979; **160:** 246–53.
3. Burlington DB, *et al.* Anti-influenza A virus activity of amantadine hydrochloride and rimantadine hydrochloride in ferret tracheal ciliated epithelium. *Antimicrob Agents Chemother* 1982; **21:** 794–9.
4. Hayden FG, *et al.* Enhancement of activity against influenza viruses by combinations of antiviral agents. *Antimicrob Agents Chemother* 1980; **18:** 536–41.
5. Hayden FG, *et al.* Combined interferon-α_2, rimantadine hydrochloride, and ribavirin inhibition of influenza virus replication in vitro. *Antimicrob Agents Chemother* 1984; **25:** 53–7. Correction. *ibid.*; 787.

References to rimantadine resistance in influenza A virus.

1. Hall CB, *et al.* Children with influenza A infection: treatment with rimantadine. *Pediatrics* 1987; **80:** 275–82.
2. Belshe RB, *et al.* Genetic basis of resistance to rimantadine emerging during treatment of influenza virus infection. *J Virol* 1988; **62:** 1508–12.
3. Belshe RB, *et al.* Resistance of influenza A virus to amantadine and rimantadine: results of one decade of surveillance. *J Infect Dis* 1989; **159:** 430–5.
4. Hayden FG, *et al.* Emergence and apparent transmission of rimantadine-resistant influenza A virus in families. *N Engl J Med* 1989; **321:** 1696–1702.

Pharmacokinetics

Rimantadine hydrochloride is well, but slowly, absorbed from the gastro-intestinal tract. Maximum plasma concentrations are reached 3 to 6 hours after administration. It has a long plasma half-life; reported figures range from 24 to 36 hours. Protein binding of rimantadine is about 40%. The elimination half-life following a single dose is 13 to 65 hours in healthy subjects. It is extensively metabolised with less than 25% of a dose being excreted unchanged in the urine; about 75% is excreted as hydroxylated metabolites over 72 hours. In renal failure or severe hepatic dysfunction, the half-life approximately doubles, necessitating a dosage reduction.

References to the pharmacokinetics of rimantadine.

1. Wills RJ, *et al.* Rimantadine pharmacokinetics after single and multiple doses. *Antimicrob Agents Chemother* 1987; **31:** 826–8.
2. Anderson EL, *et al.* Pharmacokinetics of a single dose of rimantadine in young adults and children. *Antimicrob Agents Chemother* 1987; **31:** 1140–2.

Uses and Administration

Rimantadine hydrochloride is used similarly to amantadine hydrochloride (p.1129) in the prophylaxis and treatment of influenza A infections (p.601). It is given in usual doses of 200 mg daily by mouth in divided doses. A suggested dose for children is 5 mg per kg body-weight daily, up to a maximum of 150 mg; in elderly patients or those with renal failure or severe hepatic dysfunction the suggested daily dose is 100 mg.

References.

1. Anonymous. Rimantadine for prevention and treatment of influenza. *Med Lett Drugs Ther* 1993; **35:** 109–10.
2. Wintermeyer SM, Nahata MC. Rimantadine: a clinical perspective. *Ann Pharmacother* 1995; **29:** 299–310.

Preparations

Proprietary Preparations (details are given in Part 3)
Fr.: Roflual†; ***USA:*** Flumadine.

Ritonavir (17872-t)

Ritonavir *(BAN, USAN, rINN).*

A-84538; Abbott-84538; ABJ-538. 5-Thiazolylmethyl {(αS)-α-[(1S,3S)-1-hydroxy-3-((2S)-2-{3-[(2-isopropyl-4-thiazolyl)methyl]-3-methylureido}-3-methylbutyramido)-4-phenylbutyl]phenethyl}carbamate; N^1-[(1S,3S,4S)-1-Benzyl-3-hydroxy-5-phenyl-4-(1,3-thiazol-5-ylmethoxycarbonylamino)pentyl]-N^2-{[(2-isopropyl-1,3-thiazol-4-yl)methyl](methyl)carbamoyl}-L-valinamide.

$C_{37}H_{48}N_6O_5S_2$ = 720.9.

CAS — 155213-67-5.

Adverse Effects and Precautions

As for HIV-protease inhibitors in general (see Indinavir Sulphate, p.614). Vasodilatation has been commonly associated with ritonavir, and syncope and orthostatic hypotension have been reported.

Interactions

As for HIV-protease inhibitors in general (see Indinavir Sulphate, p.614). Ritonavir is reported to have a high affinity for several cytochrome P450 isoenzymes with the following ranked order:

CYP3A>CYP2D6>CYP2C9.

Oral liquid formulations of ritonavir contain alcohol and concurrent administration with disulfiram or metronidazole should be avoided.

Pharmacokinetics

Ritonavir is absorbed following oral administration and peak plasma concentrations occur in about 2 to 4 hours. Absorption is enhanced when ritonavir is taken with food, and is dose-related. Protein binding is reported to be about 98% and penetration into the CNS is minimal. Ritonavir is extensively metabolised in the liver principally by isoenzymes CYP3A and CYP2D6 of the cytochrome P450 system. The major metabolite has antiviral activity, but concentrations in plasma are low. Ritonavir is mainly excreted in the faeces, with a half-life of 3 to 5 hours.

References.

1. Hsu A, *et al.* Multiple-dose pharmacokinetics of ritonavir in human immunodeficiency virus-infected subjects. *Antimicrob Agents Chemother* 1997; **41:** 898–905.

Uses and Administration

Ritonavir is a protease inhibitor with antiviral activity against HIV (see Antiviral Action, p.615). It is used in combination with nucleoside reverse transcriptase inhibitors for the treatment of HIV infection (p.599).

Ritonavir is given by mouth in a dose of 600 mg twice daily with food. In order to minimise nausea, ritonavir may be started at a dose of 300 mg twice daily increasing to 600 mg twice daily over a period of 4 days. In addition the nucleoside reverse transcriptase inhibitor may be introduced up to 2 weeks after the initiation of ritonavir therapy. Children may be given an initial dose of 250 mg per m^2 body-surface twice daily increasing by 50 mg per m^2 twice daily at 2- or 3-day intervals up to 400 mg per m^2 twice daily, but not exceeding 600 mg twice daily.

Reviews (for reviews of HIV-protease inhibitors in general, see Indinavir, p.615).

1. Lea AP, Faulds D. Ritonavir. *Drugs* 1996; **52:** 541–6.

Other viral infections. Intractable molluscum contagiosum, a viral skin infection, resolved when a patient was given ritonavir for treatment of HIV infection.[1]

1. Hicks CB, *et al.* Resolution of intractable molluscum contagiosum in a human immunodeficiency virus-infected patient after institution of antiretroviral therapy with ritonavir. *Clin Infect Dis* 1997; **24:** 1023–5.

Preparations

Proprietary Preparations (details are given in Part 3)
Austral.: Norvir; ***Ital.:*** Norvir; ***Neth.:*** Norvir; ***Spain:*** Norvir; ***Swed.:*** Norvir; ***Switz.:*** Norvir; ***UK:*** Norvir; ***USA:*** Norvir.

Saquinavir Mesylate (17244-j)

Saquinavir Mesylate *(BANM, USAN).*

Saquinavir Mesilate *(rINNM)*; Ro-31-8959/003; Ro-31-8959 (saquinavir). (S)-N-[(αS)-α-{(1R)-2-[(3S,4aS,8aS)-3-(*tert*-Butylcarbamoyl)octahydro-2(1H)-isoquinolyl]-1-hydroxyethyl}phenethyl]-2-quinaldamido-succinamide methanesulfonate.

$C_{38}H_{50}N_6O_5,CH_4O_3S$ = 766.9.

CAS — 127779-20-8 (saquinavir); 149845-06-7 (saquinavir mesylate).

Adverse Effects and Precautions

As for HIV-protease inhibitors in general (see Indinavir Sulphate, p.614). A possible association with Stevens-Johnson syndrome has been reported for saquinavir. Sources in the USA have reported photosensitivity. Possible nephrolithiasis and pancreatitis have also been reported.

Bioavailability of saquinavir is reported to be low owing to a combination of incomplete absorption and extensive first-pass metabolism; it may therefore be particularly susceptible to malabsorption (e.g. in the presence of diarrhoea).

Interactions

As for HIV-protease inhibitors in general (see Indinavir Sulphate, p.614).

An interaction with warfarin has also been reported (see p.968).

Saquinavir is reported to be metabolised by the cytochrome P450 system, with the specific isoenzyme CYP3A4 responsible for more than 90% of the hepatic metabolism; it is not a strong inhibitor of CYP3A.

Pharmacokinetics

Saquinavir is absorbed to a limited extent (about 30%) following oral administration and undergoes extensive first-pass hepatic metabolism, resulting in a bioavailability of 4% when taken with food. Bioavailability is substantially less when saquinavir is taken in the fasting state. Plasma concentrations are reported to be higher in HIV-infected patients than in healthy subjects. Saquinavir is about 98% bound to plasma proteins and extensively distributed into the tissues, although CNS concentrations are reported to be negligible. It is rapidly metabolised by the cytochrome P450 system (specifically the isoenzyme CYP3A4) to a number of inactive monohydroxylated and dihydroxylated compounds. It is excreted predominantly in the faeces with a reported terminal elimination half-life of 13.2 hours.

Uses and Administration

Saquinavir is a protease inhibitor with antiviral activity against HIV (see Antiviral Action, p.615). It is used, in combination with nucleoside reverse transcriptase inhibitors, for the treatment of HIV infection (p.599).

The recommended dose is 600 mg of saquinavir (as the mesylate) by mouth three times daily, within two hours after a meal.

Reviews (for reviews of HIV-protease inhibitors in general, see Indinavir, p.615).

1. Noble S, Faulds D. Saquinavir: a review of its pharmacology and clinical potential in the management of HIV infection. *Drugs* 1996; **52:** 93–112.
2. Moyle G. Saquinavir in the management of HIV infection. *Br J Hosp Med* 1997; **57:** 560–4.
3. Vella S, Floridia M. Saquinavir: clinical pharmacology and efficacy. *Clin Pharmacokinet* 1998; **34:** 189–201.

Administration. A soft gelatin capsule formulation of saquinavir has been developed to overcome some of the problems associated with the low bioavailability of the conventional formulation.[1]

1. Perry CM, Noble S. Saquinavir soft-gel capsule formulation: a review of its use in patients with HIV infection. *Drugs* 1998; **55:** 461–86.

HIV infection and AIDS. References.

1. Kitchen VS, *et al.* Safety and activity of saquinavir in HIV infection. *Lancet* 1995; **345:** 952–5.
2. Schapiro JM, *et al.* The effect of high-dose saquinavir on viral load and CD4+ T-cell counts in HIV-infected patients. *Ann Intern Med* 1996; **124:** 1039–50.
3. Collier AC, *et al.* Treatment of human immunodeficiency virus infection with saquinavir, zidovudine, and zalcitabine. *N Engl J Med* 1996; **334:** 1011–17.

Preparations

Proprietary Preparations (details are given in Part 3)
Austral.: Invirase; ***Canad.:*** Invirase; ***Ger.:*** Invirase; ***Irl.:*** Invirase; ***Ital.:*** Invirase; ***Neth.:*** Invirase; ***S.Afr.:*** Invirase; ***Spain:*** Invirase; ***Swed.:*** Invirase; ***Switz.:*** Invirase; ***UK:*** Invirase; ***USA:*** Fortovase; Invirase.

Sorivudine (18871-m)

Sorivudine *(BAN, USAN, rINN).*

Bromovinylarauracil; BV-araU; BVAU; SQ-32756; YN-72. (E)-1-β-D-Arabinofuranosyl-5-(2-bromovinyl)uracil.

$C_{11}H_{13}BrN_2O_6$ = 349.1.

CAS — 77181-69-2.

Sorivudine is a synthetic thymidine derivative with antiviral activity against varicella-zoster virus. It is being investigated for the treatment of herpes zoster but has been withdrawn from the market in Japan following the deaths of patients receiving fluorouracil concomitantly.

References.

1. Hiraoka A, *et al.* Clinical effect of BV-araU on varicella-zoster virus infection in immunocompromised patients with haematological malignancies. *J Antimicrob Chemother* 1991; **27:** 361–7.
2. Yawata M. Deaths due to drug interaction. *Lancet* 1993; **342:** 1166.
3. Burdge DR, *et al.* Sorivudine (BV-ara-U) for the treatment of complicated refractory varicella zoster virus infection in HIV-infected patients. *AIDS* 1995; **9:** 810–12.
4. Gnann JW, *et al.* Sorivudine versus acyclovir for treatment of dermatomal herpes zoster in human immunodeficiency virus-infected patients: results from a randomized, controlled clinical trial. *Antimicrob Agents Chemother* 1998; **42:** 1139–45.

Stavudine (15405-f)

Stavudine *(BAN, USAN, pINN).*

BMY-27857; d4T. 1-(2,3-Dideoxy-β-D-*glycero*-pent-2-enofuranosyl)thymine.

$C_{10}H_{12}N_2O_4$ = 224.2.

CAS — 3056-17-5.

Adverse Effects

Stavudine produces dose-related peripheral neuropathy. Raised liver enzyme concentrations may also occur during treatment. Pancreatitis has been reported rarely, but fatalities have occurred.

Other adverse effects noted in patients taking stavudine have included asthenia, chest pain, hypersensitivity reactions, and an influenza-like syndrome; dizziness, headache, and insomnia; abdominal pain, anorexia, constipation, diarrhoea, nausea, and vomiting; neutropenia and thrombocytopenia; arthralgia and myalgia; mood changes; dyspnoea; pruritus and rashes; and lymphadenopathy and neoplasms.

Precautions

Stavudine should be used with caution in patients with a history of peripheral neuropathy and treatment suspended if peripheral neuropathy develops; if symptoms resolve on withdrawal stavudine may be resumed at half the previous dose. A similar strategy should be adopted if liver enzymes are raised significantly. Patients with a history of pancreatitis should also be observed carefully for signs of pancreatitis during treatment with stavudine. Concomitant treatment with other drugs likely to cause peripheral neuropathy or pancreatitis (see Interactions, below) should be avoided if possible. Stavudine should be used with caution in patients with renal impairment.

Interactions

The intracellular activation of stavudine and hence its antiviral effect may be inhibited by zidovudine and doxorubicin.

Concurrent administration of stavudine with other drugs known to cause pancreatitis (e.g. intravenous pentamidine) or peripheral neuropathy (e.g. metronidazole, isoniazid, and vincristine) should be avoided if possible.

Antiviral Action

Stavudine is converted intracellularly in stages to the triphosphate. This triphosphate halts the DNA synthesis of retroviruses, including HIV, through competitive inhibition of reverse transcriptase and incorporation into viral DNA.

Pharmacokinetics

Stavudine is absorbed rapidly following oral administration with a reported bioavailability of about 86%. Administration with food delays but does not reduce absorption. Stavudine crosses the blood-brain barrier producing a CSF:plasma ratio of about 0.4 after 4 hours. It is metabolised intracellularly to the active antiviral triphosphate. The elimination half-life is reported to be about 1 to 1.5 hours following single doses. The intracellular half-life of stavudine triphosphate has been estimated to be 3.5 hours *in vitro*. About 40% of the administered dose is excreted in the urine at between 6 and 24 hours after administration. Stavudine is removed by haemodialysis.

References.

1. Dudley MN, *et al.* Pharmacokinetics of stavudine in patients with AIDS or AIDS-related complex. *J Infect Dis* 1992; **166:** 480–5.
2. Cretton EM, *et al.* In vitro and in vivo disposition and metabolism of 3′-deoxy-2′,3′-didehydrothymidine. *Antimicrob Agents Chemother* 1993; **37:** 1816–25.
3. Seifert RD, *et al.* Pharmacokinetics of co-administered didanosine and stavudine in HIV-seropositive male patients. *Br J Clin Pharmacol* 1994; **38:** 405–10.
4. Horton CM, *et al.* Population pharmacokinetics of stavudine (d4T) in patients with AIDS or advanced AIDS-related complex. *Antimicrob Agents Chemother* 1995; **39:** 2309–15.
5. Schaad HJ, *et al.* Pharmacokinetics and safety of a single dose of stavudine (d4T) in patients with severe hepatic impairment. *Antimicrob Agents Chemother* 1997; **41:** 2793–6.
6. Rana KZ, Dudley MN. Clinical pharmacokinetics of stavudine. *Clin Pharmacokinet* 1997; **33:** 276–84.

Uses and Administration

Stavudine is a nucleoside reverse transcriptase inhibitor related to thymidine with activity against retroviruses including HIV. It is used either alone or in combination with other antiretroviral drugs in the treatment of HIV infection (p.599). The recommended doses are stavudine 40 mg every 12 hours by mouth for a patient weighing 60 kg or more or 30 mg every 12 hours for patients weighing less than 60 kg. A recommended dose in children over 3 months of age and weighing less than 30 kg is 1 mg per kg body-weight every 12 hours; children weighing more than 30 kg may be given the adult dose. Dosage reduction is recommended for patients with renal impairment.

References.

1. Kline MW, *et al.* A phase I/II evaluation of stavudine (d4T) in children with human immunodeficiency virus infection. *Pediatrics* 1995; **96:** 247–52.
2. Kline MW, *et al.* Combination therapy with stavudine and didanosine in children with advanced human immunodeficiency virus infection: pharmacokinetic properties, safety, and immunologic and virologic effects. *Pediatrics* 1996; **97:** 886–90.
3. Lea AP, Faulds D. Stavudine: a review of its pharmacodynamic and pharmacokinetic properties and clinical potential in HIV infection. *Drugs* 1996; **51:** 846–64.
4. Spruance SL, *et al.* Clinical efficacy of monotherapy with stavudine compared with zidovudine in HIV-infected, zidovudine-experienced patients: a randomized, double-blind, controlled trial. *Ann Intern Med* 1997; **126:** 355–63.
5. Kline MW, *et al.* A randomized comparative trial of stavudine (d4T) versus zidovudine (ZDV, AZT) in children with human immunodeficiency virus infection. *Pediatrics* 1998; **101:** 214–20.

Preparations

Proprietary Preparations (details are given in Part 3)
Austral.: Zerit; ***Canad.:*** Zerit; ***Fr.:*** Zerit; ***Ger.:*** Zerit; ***Irl.:*** Zerit; ***Ital.:*** Zerit; ***Neth.:*** Zerit; ***Spain:*** Zerit; ***Swed.:*** Zerit; ***Switz.:*** Zerit; ***UK:*** Zerit; ***USA:*** Zerit.

Tribavirin (1685-r)

Tribavirin *(BAN)*.

Ribavirin *(USAN, rINN)*; ICN-1229. 1-β-D-Ribofuranosyl-1*H*-1,2,4-triazole-3-carboxamide.

$C_8H_{12}N_4O_5$ = 244.2.

CAS — 36791-04-5.

Pharmacopoeias. In Br. and US.

A white crystalline powder. Freely **soluble** in water; slightly soluble in alcohol and in dehydrated alcohol. **Store** in airtight containers. Protect from light. A 2% solution has a pH of 4.0 to 6.5.

Adverse Effects and Precautions

When given by inhalation tribavirin has sometimes led to deterioration in pulmonary function, bacterial pneumonia, and pneumothorax, to adverse effects on the cardiovascular system (including a fall in blood pressure and cardiac arrest), and to anaemia and reticulocytosis. Conjunctivitis and skin rash have also occurred. Precipitation of inhaled tribavirin and consequent accumulation of fluid in the tubing has occurred in ventilating equipment being used during the period of treatment.

Patients have experienced increased serum-bilirubin concentrations when given tribavirin by mouth or intravenous injection. Other effects that have been reported include gastro-intestinal and CNS disturbances, and anaemia and reticulocytosis.

Tribavirin has been reported to be teratogenic in *animals* and is contra-indicated in pregnancy or in those who may become pregnant.

Reports and discussions on the safety of tribavirin aerosol and precautions to reduce occupational exposure.

1. Harrison R, *et al.* Assessing exposure of health-care personnel to aerosols of ribavirin—California. *MMWR* 1988; **37:** 560–3.
2. Guglielmo BJ, *et al.* The exposure of health care workers to ribavirin aerosol. *JAMA* 1989; **261:** 1880–1.
3. Harkness MJ. The exposure of health care workers to ribavirin aerosol. *JAMA* 1989; **262:** 1947.
4. Marks MI, *et al.* The exposure of health care workers to ribavirin aerosol. *JAMA* 1989; **262:** 1947–8.
5. Guglielmo J, *et al.* The exposure of health care workers to ribavirin aerosol. *JAMA* 1989; **262:** 1948.
6. Bradley JS, *et al.* The exposure of health care workers to ribavirin aerosol. *JAMA* 1989; **262:** 1948.
7. Fackler JC, *et al.* Precautions in the use of ribavirin at the children's hospital. *N Engl J Med* 1990; **322:** 634.

Report of damage to a nurse's soft contact lenses following intermittent occupational exposure to tribavirin over a period of one month.[1]

1. Diamond SA, Dupuis LL. Contact lens damage due to ribavirin exposure. *DICP Ann Pharmacother* 1989; **23:** 428–9.

Antiviral Action

Tribavirin inhibits a wide variety of viruses *in vitro* and in *animal* models. However, this activity has not necessarily correlated with activity against human infections. Tribavirin is phosphorylated but its mode of action is still unclear; it may act at several sites, including cellular enzymes, to interfere with viral nucleic acid synthesis. The mono- and triphosphate derivatives are believed to be responsible for the antiviral activity of the compound. Susceptible DNA viruses include herpes viruses, adenoviruses, and poxviruses. Susceptible RNA viruses include Lassa virus, members of the bunyaviridae group, influenza, parainfluenza, measles, mumps, and respiratory syncytial viruses, and human immunodeficiency virus (HIV).

Microbiological interactions. The combination of tribavirin and *rimantadine* resulted in an enhanced antiviral effect *in vitro* against influenza A viruses compared with the effects of either drug alone,[1] and an additive or synergistic effect was observed *in vitro* with *interferon alfa* and either tribavirin or rimantadine.[2] Tribavirin and *zidovudine* inhibited each others' antiviral activity *in vitro*.[3]

1. Hayden FG, *et al.* Enhancement of activity against influenza viruses by combinations of antiviral agents. *Antimicrob Agents Chemother* 1980; **18:** 536–41.
2. Hayden FG, *et al.* Combined interferon-α_2, rimantadine hydrochloride, and ribavirin inhibition of influenza virus replication in vitro. *Antimicrob Agents Chemother* 1984; **25:** 53–7. Correction. *ibid.*; 787.
3. Vogt MW, *et al.* Ribavirin antagonizes the effect of azidothymidine on HIV replication. *Science* 1987; **235:** 1376–9.

Pharmacokinetics

Tribavirin is rapidly but incompletely absorbed following oral administration and peak blood concentrations have been reported within 1 to 2 hours. Bioavailability following oral administration is less than 50%. Tribavirin is also absorbed from the respiratory tract following inhalation. Tribavirin crosses the blood-brain barrier and at steady state concentrations in the CNS are 70% or more of those in the plasma. Accumulation occurs in the red blood cells. Tribavirin undergoes phosphorylation by cellular enzymes to the mono-, di-, and triphosphate derivatives. Distribution and elimination is triphasic. The β-phase half-life is about 2 hours, and the terminal elimination half-life is reported to be 20 to 50 hours depending on the sampling time. There is evidence of first-pass metabolism following oral administration. Renal elimination accounts for about 30 to 40% of the total and hepatic metabolism is also an important route of elimination. Insignificant amounts of the drug are removed by haemodialysis. Tribavirin is still detectable in the plasma for up to 4 weeks after cessation of therapy.

References.

1. Austin RK, *et al.* Sensitive radioimmunoassay for the broad-spectrum antiviral agent ribavirin. *Antimicrob Agents Chemother* 1983; **24:** 696–701.
2. Crumpacker C, *et al.* Ribavirin enters cerebrospinal fluid. *Lancet* 1986; **ii:** 45–6.
3. Laskin OL, *et al.* Ribavirin disposition in high-risk patients for acquired immunodeficiency syndrome. *Clin Pharmacol Ther* 1987; **41:** 546–55.
4. Roberts RB, *et al.* Ribavirin pharmacodynamics in high-risk patients for acquired immunodeficiency syndrome. *Clin Pharmacol Ther* 1987; **42:** 365–73.
5. Paroni R, *et al.* Pharmacokinetics of ribavirin and urinary excretion of the major metabolite 1,2,4-triazole-3-carboxamide in normal volunteers. *Int J Clin Pharmacol Ther Toxicol* 1989; **27:** 302–7.
6. Kramer TH, *et al.* Hemodialysis clearance of intravenously administered ribavirin. *Antimicrob Agents Chemother* 1990; **34:** 489–90.
7. Connor E, *et al.* Safety, tolerance, and pharmacokinetics of systemic ribavirin in children with human immunodeficiency virus infection. *Antimicrob Agents Chemother* 1993; **37:** 532–9.

Uses and Administration

Tribavirin is a synthetic nucleoside analogue structurally related to guanine. It is administered by aerosol in the treatment of respiratory syncytial viral infections; this route appears to give better results than the oral route although its efficacy by any route is questionable. Tribavirin has been tried in other infections including Lassa and other haemorrhagic fevers, measles, hepatitis, and influenza. It is used in combination with interferon alfa-2b in the treatment of chronic hepatitis C unresponsive to interferon alone.

Preparations of tribavirin are available for administration to infants and children with severe respiratory syncytial infections via a small particle aerosol generator. Solutions containing 20 mg per mL are used; over a 12- to 18-hour period 300 mL, representing 6 g of tribavirin, are delivered by aerosol at an average concentration of 190 μg per litre of air. Treatment is for 3 to 7 days.

For the treatment of chronic hepatitis C refractory to interferon alone, tribavirin is given daily by mouth in doses of 400 mg (in patients up to 75 kg bodyweight) or 600 mg (in patients over 75 kg) in the morning, and 600 mg in the evening (regardless of weight). Treatment is continued for 6 months, in combination with interferon alfa-2b 3 million units by subcutaneous injection 3 times a week.

Haemorrhagic fevers. The treatment of haemorrhagic fevers (p.595) is primarily symptomatic. However, tribavirin has been reported to reduce mortality in patients with Lassa fever,[1] haemorrhagic fever with renal syndrome,[2] and possibly Crimean-Congo haemorrhagic fever.[3] Tribavirin has also been tried in the related hantavirus pulmonary syndrome,[4,5] but preliminary results did not indicate an improvement in mortality.[6]

For treatment of *Lassa fever*, tribavirin has been given intravenously in a suggested dose of 2 g initially, then 1 g every 6 hours for 4 days, then 500 mg every 8 hours for 6 days.[1] Treatment is most effective if instituted within 6 days of the onset of fever. For prophylaxis, a dose of tribavirin 600 mg by mouth 4 times daily for 10 days has been suggested for adults,[7] although this was considered to be excessive by other commentators[8] who suggested that oral doses of 1000 mg daily (following an intravenous loading dose for those in whom the start of prophylaxis is delayed) might be suitable.

1. McCormick JB, *et al.* Lassa fever: effective therapy with ribavirin. *N Engl J Med* 1986; **314:** 20–6.
2. Huggins JW, *et al.* Prospective, double-blind, concurrent, placebo-controlled clinical trial of intravenous ribavirin therapy of hemorrhagic fever with renal syndrome. *J Infect Dis* 1991; **164:** 1119–27.
3. Fisher-Hoch SP, *et al.* Crimean Congo-haemorrhagic fever treated with oral ribavirin. *Lancet* 1995; **346:** 472–5.
4. Anonymous. Hantavirus pulmonary syndrome—northeastern United States, 1994. *JAMA* 1994; **272:** 997–8.
5. Prochoda K, *et al.* Hantavirus-associated acute respiratory failure. *N Engl J Med* 1993; **329:** 1744.
6. Khan AS, *et al.* Hantavirus pulmonary syndrome. *Lancet* 1996; **347:** 739–41.
7. Holmes GP, *et al.* Lassa fever in the United States: investigation of a case and new guidelines for management. *N Engl J Med* 1990; **323:** 1120–23.
8. Johnson KM, Monath TP. Imported Lassa fever—reexamining the algorithms. *N Engl J Med* 1990; **323:** 1139–41.

Hepatitis. Tribavirin may be used for the treatment of chronic hepatitis C (p.595). Responses to tribavirin have been reported although liver enzymes returned to pretreatment concentrations once treatment was stopped.[1,2] Tribavirin used in combination with interferon was more effective than either drug alone.[3-7]

1. Reichard O, *et al.* Ribavirin treatment for chronic hepatitis C. *Lancet* 1991; **337:** 1058–61.
2. Di Bisceglie AM, *et al.* A pilot study of ribavirin therapy for chronic hepatitis C. *Hepatology* 1992; **16:** 649–54.
3. Kakumu S, *et al.* A pilot study of ribavirin and interferon beta for the treatment of chronic hepatitis C. *Gastroenterology* 1993; **105:** 507–12.
4. Chemello L, *et al.* Response to ribavirin, to interferon and to a combination of both in patients with chronic hepatitis C and its relation to HCV genotypes. *J Hepatol* 1994; **21** (suppl): S12.
5. Braconier JH, *et al.* Combined alpha-interferon and ribavirin treatment in chronic hepatitis C: a pilot study. *Scand J Infect Dis* 1995; **27:** 325–9.
6. Reichard O, *et al.* Randomised, double-blind, placebo-controlled trial of interferon α-2b with and without ribavirin for chronic hepatitis C. *Lancet* 1998; **351:** 83–7.
7. Poynard T, *et al.* Randomised trial of interferon α2b plus ribavirin for 48 weeks or for 24 weeks versus interferon α2b plus placebo for 48 weeks for treatment of chronic infection with hepatitis C virus. *Lancet* 1998; **352:** 1426–32.

Influenza. The treatment of influenza is usually symptomatic and supportive (see p.601). Studies have generally shown tribavirin aerosol inhalation to have limited efficacy in the treatment of both influenza A and B;[1,2] one study found no benefit from tribavirin aerosol during an influenza B epidemic.[3]

1. Bell M, *et al.* Nebulised ribavirin for influenza B viral pneumonia in a ventilated immunocompromised adult. *Lancet* 1988; **ii:** 1084–5.
2. Rodriguez WJ, *et al.* Efficacy and safety of aerosolized ribavirin in young children hospitalized with influenza: a double-blind, multicenter, placebo-controlled trial. *J Pediatr* 1994; **125:** 129–35.
3. Bernstein DI, *et al.* Ribavirin small-particle-aerosol treatment of influenza B virus infection. *Antimicrob Agents Chemother* 1988; **32:** 761–4.

Measles. There appears to be no good evidence for antivirals being effective in the complications of measles (p.602). Anecdotal reports of tribavirin in patients with severe and disseminated measles infection suggest that it may be effective, particularly in immunocompromised patients.[1,2] However, it has not been shown to be useful in subacute sclerosing panencephalitis.[3]

1. Gururangan S, *et al.* Ribavirin response in measles pneumonia. *J Infect* 1990; **20:** 219–21.
2. Forni AL, *et al.* Severe measles pneumonitis in adults: evaluation of clinical characteristics and therapy with intravenous ribavirin. *Clin Infect Dis* 1994; **19:** 454–62.
3. Ogle JW, *et al.* Oral ribavirin therapy for subacute sclerosing panencephalitis. *J Infect Dis* 1989; **159:** 748–50.

Respiratory syncytial virus infections. The treatment of respiratory syncytial virus (RSV) infections (p.602) is largely supportive. Tribavirin administered by aerosol has been shown to have beneficial effects in infants with lower respiratory-tract infections.[1-7] However, apart from one study[8] which has been criticised on methodological grounds,[9] there is no convincing evidence that tribavirin reduced the duration of hospital stay, mortality, or oxygen requirement.[10,11] The American Academy of Pediatrics has modified its recommendations[12] for use of tribavirin in the treatment of RSV infection in infants and children at high risk of developing severe or complicated disease to make tribavirin treatment discretionary.[13] In the UK, tribavirin is less frequently used and some[14] have restricted its use to patients with RSV and cystic fibrosis, severe immunodeficiency, congenital heart disease and pulmonary hypertension, and patients with bronchopulmonary dysplasia and pre-existing oxygen dependence.

1. Hall CB, *et al.* Aerosolized ribavirin treatment of infants with respiratory syncytial viral infection: a randomized double-blind study. *N Engl J Med* 1983; **308:** 1443–7.
2. Hall CB, *et al.* Ribavirin treatment of respiratory syncytial viral infection in infants with underlying cardiopulmonary disease. *JAMA* 1985; **254:** 3047–51.
3. Gelfand EW, *et al.* Ribavirin treatment of viral pneumonitis in severe combined immunodeficiency disease. *Lancet* 1983; **ii:** 732–3.
4. Taber LH, *et al.* Ribavirin aerosol treatment of bronchiolitis associated with respiratory syncytial virus infection in infants. *Pediatrics* 1983; **72:** 613–18.
5. Barry W, *et al.* Ribavirin aerosol for acute bronchiolitis. *Arch Dis Child* 1986; **61:** 593–7.
6. Groothuis JR, *et al.* Early ribavirin treatment of respiratory syncytial viral infection in high-risk children. *J Pediatr* 1990; **117:** 792–8.
7. Englund JA, *et al.* High-dose, short-duration ribavirin aerosol therapy in children with suspected respiratory syncytial virus infection. *J Pediatr* 1990; **117:** 313–20.
8. Smith DW, *et al.* A controlled trial of aerosolized ribavirin in infants receiving mechanical ventilation for severe respiratory syncytial virus infection. *N Engl J Med* 1991; **325:** 24–9.
9. Moler FW, *et al.* Ribavirin for severe RSV infection. *N Engl J Med* 1991; **325:** 1884–5.
10. Moler FW, *et al.* Effectiveness of ribavirin in otherwise well infants with respiratory syncytial virus-associated respiratory failure. *J Pediatr* 1996; **128:** 422–8.
11. Wheeler JG, *et al.* Historical cohort evaluation of ribavirin efficacy in respiratory syncytial virus infection. *Pediatr Infect Dis J* 1993; **12:** 209–13.
12. American Academy of Pediatrics, Committee on Infectious Diseases. Use of ribavirin in the treatment of respiratory syncytial virus infection. *Pediatrics* 1993; **92:** 501–4.
13. American Academy of Pediatrics, Committee on Infectious Diseases. Reassessment of the indications for ribavirin therapy in respiratory syncytial virus infections. *Pediatrics* 1996; **97:** 137–40.
14. Rakshi K, Couriel JM. Management of acute bronchiolitis. *Arch Dis Child* 1994; **71:** 463–9.

Preparations

BP 1998: Tribavirin Solution for Nebulisation;
USP 23: Ribavirin for Inhalation Solution.

Proprietary Preparations (details are given in Part 3)
Austral.: Virazide; ***Belg.:*** Virazole; ***Canad.:*** Virazole; ***Ger.:*** Virazole†; ***Irl.:*** Virazole†; ***Ital.:*** Viramid; Virazide†; ***Neth.:*** Virazole†; ***Spain:*** Virazid; ***Swed.:*** Virazole; ***Switz.:*** Virazole†; ***UK:*** Virazid; ***USA:*** Virazole.

Multi-ingredient: ***USA:*** Rebetron.

Trichosanthin (2467-t)

Compound Q; GLQ-223 (a purified form of trichosanthin).

Trichosanthin is a polypeptide extracted from the tuber of the Chinese cucumber, *Tricosanthes kirilowii* (Cucurbitaceae). It is under investigation in the treatment of AIDS and is used in China as an abortifacient.

Trichosanthin has been given to patients with AIDS, AIDS-related complex, or HIV infection.[1,2] It was generally given by intravenous injection. In one study[1] it was also given by intramuscular injection but that route was abandoned due to the occurrence of pain and necrosis at the injection site. A common adverse effect on intravenous administration was a flu-like syndrome with headache, myalgias, fever, and arthralgia and was generally mild to moderate,[3] although neurological effects progressing to coma with fatalities have been reported.[1,2] Improvements in surrogate markers for HIV infection have been reported including increases in CD4+ T lymphocyte counts in patients with moderate disease[3] and in patients failing to respond to reverse transcriptase inhibitors.[4]

1. Byers VS, *et al.* A phase I/II study of trichosanthin treatment of HIV disease. *AIDS* 1990; **4:** 1189–96.
2. Kahn JO, *et al.* The safety and pharmacokinetics of GLQ223 in subjects with AIDS and AIDS-related complex: a phase I study. *AIDS* 1990; **4:** 1197–1204.
3. Kahn JO, *et al.* Safety, activity, and pharmacokinetics of GLQ223 in patients with AIDS and AIDS-related complex. *Antimicrob Agents Chemother* 1994; **38:** 260–7.
4. Byers VS, *et al.* A phase II study of effect of addition of trichosanthin to zidovudine in patients with HIV disease and failing antiretroviral agents. *AIDS Res Hum Retroviruses* 1994; **10:** 413–20.

Trifluridine (1688-n)

Trifluridine *(USAN, rINN).*

F_3TDR; F_3T; NSC-75520; Trifluorothymidine. ααα-Trifluorothymidine; 2′-Deoxy-5-trifluoromethyluridine.

$C_{10}H_{11}F_3N_2O_5$ = 296.2.

CAS — 70-00-8.

Pharmacopoeias. In *US.*

A white odourless powder appearing under the microscope as rodlike crystals. **Store** in airtight containers. Protect from light.

Adverse Effects

Adverse effects occurring after the use of trifluridine in the eyes are similar to those for idoxuridine (p.613) but have been reported to occur less frequently.

References.

1. Udell IJ. Trifluridine-associated conjunctival cicatrization. *Am J Ophthalmol* 1985; **99:** 363–4.

Antiviral Action

Trifluridine acts similarly to idoxuridine to interfere with viral DNA synthesis following phosphorylation. It is reported to be active against herpes simplex viruses, some adenoviruses, vaccinia viruses, and cytomegalovirus. Like idoxuridine it is incorporated into mammalian DNA.

Pharmacokinetics

Trifluridine is absorbed through the cornea following ocular administration and penetration may be increased in the presence of damage or inflammation. Systemic absorption does not appear to follow ocular administration.

Uses and Administration

Trifluridine is a pyrimidine nucleoside structurally related to thymidine. It is used in the treatment of primary keratoconjunctivitis and recurrent epithelial keratitis due to herpes simplex viruses. One drop of a 1% ophthalmic solution is instilled into the eye every 2 hours up to a maximum of 9 times daily until complete re-epithelialisation has occurred. Treatment is then reduced to one drop every 4 hours to a minimum of 5 drops a day for a further 7 days.

Reviews.

1. Heidelberger C, King DH. Trifluorothymidine. *Pharmacol Ther* 1979; **6:** 427–42.
2. Carmine AA, *et al.* Trifluridine: a review of its antiviral activity and therapeutic use in the topical treatment of viral eye infections. *Drugs* 1982; **23:** 329–53.

Herpes simplex infections. Trifluridine may be used as an alternative to topical aciclovir in ocular herpes simplex infections (p.597). It has been used in combination with a corticosteroid for herpes simplex stromal keratitis.[1]

Trifluridine produced varied improvement when applied topically in combination with interferon alfa in 3 AIDS patients with mucocutaneous herpes unresponsive to aciclovir (and to foscarnet in 2).[2] A pilot study in AIDS patients indicated that topical trifluridine alone might be of benefit for aciclovir-resistant mucocutaneous herpes simplex.[3]

1. Wilhelmus KR, *et al.* Herpetic eye disease study: a controlled trial of topical corticosteroids for herpes simplex stromal keratitis. *Ophthalmology* 1994; **101:** 1883–96.
2. Birch CJ, *et al.* Clinical effects and in vitro studies of trifluorothymidine combined with interferon-α for treatment of drug-resistant and -sensitive herpes simplex virus infections. *J Infect Dis* 1992; **166:** 108–12.
3. Kessler HA, *et al.* Pilot study of topical trifluridine for the treatment of acyclovir-resistant mucocutaneous herpes simplex disease in patients with AIDS (ACTG 172). *J Acquir Immune Defic Syndr Hum Retrovirol* 1996; **12:** 147–52.

Preparations

Proprietary Preparations (details are given in Part 3)
Belg.: TFT Ophtiole; ***Canad.:*** Viroptic; ***Fr.:*** Virophta; ***Ger.:*** TFT; Triflumann; ***Ital.:*** Triherpine; ***Neth.:*** TFT Ophtiole; ***S.Afr.:*** TFT; ***Spain:*** Aflomin†; Viromidin; ***Switz.:*** Triherpine; ***USA:*** Viroptic.

Tromantadine Hydrochloride (1689-h)

Tromantadine Hydrochloride *(rINNM)*.

D-41. *N*-1-Adamantyl-2-(2-dimethylaminoethoxy)acetamide hydrochloride; 2-(2-Dimethylaminoethoxy)-*N*-(tricyclo[3.3.1.1[3,7]]dec-1-yl)acetamide hydrochloride.

$C_{16}H_{28}N_2O_2,HCl = 316.9.$

CAS — 53783-83-8 (tromantadine); 41544-24-5 (tromantadine hydrochloride).

Adverse Effects

Contact dermatitis has been reported following the topical use of tromantadine hydrochloride.

References.

1. Fanta D, Mischer P. Contact dermatitis from tromantadine hydrochloride. *Contact Dermatitis* 1976; **2:** 282–4.
2. Lembo G, *et al.* Allergic dermatitis from Viruserol ointment probably due to tromantadine hydrochloride. *Contact Dermatitis* 1984; **10:** 317.

Uses and Administration

Tromantadine hydrochloride is a derivative of amantadine (see p.1129) used for its antiviral activity. It is applied at a concentration of 1% in the treatment of herpes simplex infections of the skin and mucous membranes and of varicella-zoster skin infections although aciclovir is generally preferred (see p.596).

Preparations

Proprietary Preparations (details are given in Part 3)
Aust.: Viru-Merz; ***Belg.:*** Viru-Merz; ***Ger.:*** Viru-Merz; ***Ital.:*** Viruserol; ***Neth.:*** Viru-Merz; ***Spain:*** Viru-Serol; ***Switz.:*** Viru-Merz Serol.

Valaciclovir Hydrochloride (17334-c)

Valaciclovir Hydrochloride *(BANM, rINNM)*.

256U87 (valaciclovir); Valacyclovir Hydrochloride *(USAN)*. L-Valine, ester with 9-[(2-hydroxyethoxy)methyl]guanine hydrochloride.

$C_{13}H_{20}N_6O_4,HCl = 360.8.$

CAS — 124832-26-4 (valaciclovir); 124832-27-5 (valaciclovir hydrochloride);.

Adverse Effects and Precautions

As for aciclovir (p.603), since valaciclovir is a prodrug of aciclovir. The most commonly reported adverse effects with valaciclovir are nausea and headache. Haemolytic uraemic syndrome and thrombocytopenia purpura have been reported in severely immunocompromised patients receiving high doses of valaciclovir, but an association with valaciclovir has not been established.

Valaciclovir should be used with caution in patients with impaired renal function.

Pharmacokinetics

Valaciclovir is readily absorbed from the gastro-intestinal tract following oral administration, and is rapidly converted to aciclovir and valine by first-pass intestinal and/or hepatic metabolism. The bioavailability of aciclovir following valaciclovir administration is reported to be 54% and peak concentrations of aciclovir are achieved after 1.5 hours. Valaciclovir is eliminated principally as aciclovir (see p.604); less than 1% of a dose of valaciclovir is excreted unchanged in the urine.

References.

1. Weller S, *et al.* Pharmacokinetics of the acyclovir pro-drug valaciclovir after escalating single- and multiple-dose administration to normal volunteers. *Clin Pharmacol Ther* 1993; **54:** 595–605.
2. Rolan P. Pharmacokinetics of new antiherpetic agents. *Clin Pharmacokinet* 1995; **29:** 333–40.
3. Soul-Lawton J, *et al.* Absolute bioavailability and metabolic disposition of valaciclovir, the L-valyl ester of acyclovir, following oral administration to humans. *Antimicrob Agents Chemother* 1995; **39:** 2759–64.
4. Wang LH, *et al.* Pharmacokinetics and safety of multiple-dose valaciclovir in geriatric volunteers with and without concomitant diuretic therapy. *Antimicrob Agents Chemother* 1996; **40:** 80–5.

Uses and Administration

Valaciclovir is a prodrug of the antiviral aciclovir (p.605) that is used in the treatment of herpes zoster (p.598) and herpes simplex infections (p.597) of the skin and mucous membranes, including genital herpes. It is given by mouth as the hydrochloride; doses are expressed in terms of valaciclovir.

For herpes zoster the dose is 1 g three times daily for 7 days. For treatment of herpes simplex infections, 500 mg is given twice daily for 5 days for recurrent episodes or for up to 10 days for a first episode; in the USA the recommended dose for a first episode of genital herpes is 1 g twice daily for 10 days. For the suppression of herpes simplex infection a dose of 500 mg daily, usually in 2 divided doses, is recommended. This should be doubled to 500 mg twice daily in immunocompromised patients.

Doses of valaciclovir may need to be reduced in patients with impaired renal function. The following dosage reductions are suggested by the UK manufacturer: for herpes zoster in patients with a creatinine clearance (CC) of 15 to 30 mL per minute, 1 g twice daily and for those with a CC of less than 15 mL per minute, 1 g daily; for treatment of herpes simplex infections in patients with a CC of 15 to 30 mL per minute, no modification, but for those with a CC of less than 15 mL per minute, 500 mg daily. For the suppression of herpes simplex, usual doses are halved in patients with a CC below 15 mL per minute, to 250 mg daily in immunocompetent and 500 mg daily in immunocompromised patients.

References.

1. Jacobson MA, *et al.* Phase I trial of valaciclovir, the L-valyl ester of acyclovir, in patients with advanced human immunodeficiency virus disease. *Antimicrob Agents Chemother* 1994; **38:** 1534–40.
2. Beutner KR, *et al.* Valaciclovir compared with acyclovir for improved therapy for herpes zoster in immunocompetent adults. *Antimicrob Agents Chemother* 1995; **39:** 1546–53.
3. Perry CM, Faulds D. Valaciclovir: a review of its antiviral activity, pharmacokinetic properties and therapeutic efficacy in herpesvirus infections. *Drugs* 1996; **52:** 754–72.

Preparations

Proprietary Preparations (details are given in Part 3)
Aust.: Valtrex; ***Austral.:*** Valtrex; ***Canad.:*** Valtrex; ***Fr.:*** Zelitrex; ***Ger.:*** Valtrex; ***Irl.:*** Valtrex; ***Neth.:*** Zelitrex; ***Norw.:*** Valtrex; ***S.Afr.:*** Zelitrex; ***Spain:*** Valtrex; ***Swed.:*** Valtrex; ***Switz.:*** Valtrex; ***UK:*** Valtrex; ***USA:*** Valtrex.

Valganciclovir (11001-c)

Valganciclovir *(rINN)*.

L-Valine, ester with 9-[2-hydroxy-1-(hydroxymethyl)ethoxymethyl]guanine.

$C_{14}H_{22}N_6O_5 = 354.4.$

Valganciclovir is a prodrug of the antiviral ganciclovir (p.611) under investigation for the treatment of cytomegalovirus infections.

Vidarabine (17027-v)

Vidarabine *(BAN, USAN, rINN)*.

Adenine Arabinoside; Ara-A; CI-673. 9-β-D-Arabinofuranosyladenine monohydrate.

$C_{10}H_{13}N_5O_4,H_2O = 285.3.$

CAS — 5536-17-4 (anhydrous vidarabine); 24356-66-9 (vidarabine monohydrate).

Pharmacopoeias. In US.

A purine nucleoside obtained from *Streptomyces antibioticus*. It is a white to off-white powder. Very slightly **soluble** in water; slightly soluble in dimethylformamide. **Store** in airtight containers.

Vidarabine Phosphate (1690-a)

Vidarabine Phosphate *(BANM, USAN, rINNM)*.

Ara-AMP; Arabinosyladenine Monophosphate; CI-808; Vidarabine 5′-Monophosphate. 9-β-D-Arabinofuranosyladenine 5′-(dihydrogen phosphate).

$C_{10}H_{14}N_5O_7P = 347.2.$

CAS — 29984-33-6 (vidarabine phosphate); 71002-10-3 (vidarabine sodium phosphate).

References to the stability of vidarabine phosphate.

1. Hong W-H, Szulczewski DH. Stability of vidarabine-5′-phosphate in aqueous solutions. *J Parenter Sci Technol* 1984; **38:** 60–4.
2. Kwee MSL, Stolk LML. Formulation of a stable vidarabine phosphate injection. *Pharm Weekbl (Sci)* 1984; **6:** 101–4.
3. Patel SD, Yalkowsky SH. Development of an intravenous formulation for the antiviral drug 9-(β-D-arabinofuranosyl)-adenine. *J Parenter Sci Technol* 1987; **41:** 15–20.

Adverse Effects

Adverse effects which may occur when vidarabine is applied to the eyes include irritation, pain, superficial punctate keratitis, photophobia, lachrymation, and occlusion of the lachrymal duct.

Following intravenous administration of vidarabine the most common adverse effects are gastro-intestinal disturbances including nausea, vomiting, diarrhoea, anorexia, and weight loss. Encephalopathic changes have also occurred. CNS disturbances include tremor, dizziness, hallucinations, confusion, psychosis, ataxia, and weakness. Haematological changes induced by vidarabine have included decreases in haemoglobin concentrations or haematocrit, leucopenia, thrombocytopenia, and a decrease in reticulocyte count.

Other side-effects occurring occasionally after intravenous administration of vidarabine have included malaise, pruritus, rash, haematemesis, thrombophlebitis and pain at the site of injection, elevation in bilirubin concentrations, and abnormal liver enzyme values.

Vidarabine has been reported to be teratogenic, carcinogenic, and mutagenic in some species of *animals*.

Reversible adverse effects in patients with herpesvirus infections treated with intravenous vidarabine in daily doses ranging from 10 to 30 mg per kg body-weight included nausea and vomiting, weight loss, weakness (often with impaired movement), megaloblastosis in erythroid series in bone marrow, tremors 5 to 7 days after the start of therapy (in one patient an abnormal EEG indicated toxic metabolic encephalopathy) and thrombophlebitis at the site of injection.[1] The incidence of side-effects appeared to be dose-related. A similar range of adverse effects was observed in patients with chronic hepatitis B treated with vidarabine (most of whom also received interferon alfa concomitantly).[2] These included gastro-intestinal symptoms, weakness or fatigue, myalgia, reversible granulocytopenia and thrombocytopenia, jaw pain, tremor, ataxia, difficulty in walking, and neurological effects with EEG changes mimicking metabolic encephalopathy. The patient with the most severe neurological effects also had a transient compromise in renal function. It was felt that close monitoring of liver function, renal function, neurological status, and haematologic values should be undertaken during treatment with vidarabine.

Fatal neurological toxicity has been associated with vidarabine sodium phosphate therapy in a cancer patient with normal renal function[3] and there have been other reports of vidarabine neurotoxicity (some fatal) wherein liver dysfunction was considered a possible risk factor.[4,5] In patients with chronic hepatitis B, the neurological toxicity of vidarabine phosphate (including myalgia and peripheral neuropathy) was associated with the duration of treatment and it was suggested that the total dose should not exceed 300 mg per kg body-weight in any one course of treatment.[6] It has also been suggested that tremor or any other mild form of neurotoxicity should be considered an indication for withdrawal of vidarabine as more serious life-threatening events could rapidly follow.[7]

1. Ross AH, *et al.* Toxicity of adenine arabinoside in humans. *J Infect Dis* 1979; **133:** A192–8.
2. Sacks SL, *et al.* Toxicity of vidarabine. *JAMA* 1979; **241:** 28–9.
3. Van Etta L, *et al.* Fatal vidarabine toxicity in a patient with normal renal function. *JAMA* 1981; **246:** 1703–5.
4. Vilter RW. Vidarabine-associated encephalopathy and myoclonus. *Antimicrob Agents Chemother* 1986; **29:** 933–5.
5. Quinn JP, *et al.* Neurotoxicity associated with vidarabine therapy. *Curr Ther Res* 1987; **41:** 706–12.
6. Lok ASF, *et al.* Neurotoxicity associated with adenine arabinoside monophosphate in the treatment of chronic hepatitis B virus infection. *J Antimicrob Chemother* 1984; **14:** 93–9.
7. Burdge DR, *et al.* Neurotoxic effects during vidarabine therapy for herpes zoster. *Can Med Assoc J* 1985; **132:** 392–5.

Precautions

When given parenterally, the dose of vidarabine may need to be reduced in renal impairment because of the slower rate of excretion of the metabolite hypoxanthine arabinoside. Caution may be required in impaired liver function. Blood counts should be carried out during treatment.

For reference to liver dysfunction increasing the risk of vidarabine-associated neurotoxicity and for a suggestion that vidarabine should be withdrawn if signs of neurotoxicity develop, see above.

Interactions

Two patients receiving *allopurinol* developed severe neurotoxicity on the fourth day of concomitant vidarabine treatment.[1] This may have been due to inhibition of xanthine oxidase by allopurinol causing an increase in concentrations of the vidarabine metabolite hypoxanthine arabinoside. Homocysteine deficiency produced by vidarabine may be a risk when *methotrexate* is also given.[2] Vidarabine may possibly cause an increase in serum-*theophylline* concentrations.[3]

1. Friedman HM, Grasela T. Adenine arabinoside and allopurinol—possible adverse drug interaction. *N Engl J Med* 1981; **304:** 423.
2. Cantoni GL, *et al.* Methionine biosynthesis and vidarabine therapy. *N Engl J Med* 1982; **307:** 1079.
3. Gannon R, *et al.* Possible interaction between vidarabine and theophylline. *Ann Intern Med* 1984; **101:** 148–9.

Antiviral Action

Vidarabine appears to act by interfering in the early stages of viral DNA synthesis, but several mechanisms may be involved. It is phosphorylated intracellularly to the triphosphate which inhibits among other enzymes viral DNA polymerase; it may also be incorporated into the viral DNA.

Following administration, vidarabine is rapidly converted to hypoxanthine arabinoside which also appears to interfere with viral DNA synthesis but is reported to have less antiviral activity than the parent compound.

The activity of vidarabine *in vitro* and *in vivo* is limited to DNA viruses such as herpes simplex virus types 1 and 2, varicella-zoster virus, cytomegalovirus, and Epstein-Barr and vaccinia viruses; with few exceptions it does not inhibit RNA viruses.

Microbiological interactions. Combinations of vidarabine or vidarabine phosphate with aciclovir produced an additive effect *in vitro* against herpes simplex virus type 1 and type 2 without increasing drug toxicity.[1] These results were further substantiated in *mice*, but some adverse effects were noted at high dosages, particularly for combinations with vidarabine. Vidarabine and aciclovir were found to be synergistic *in vitro* against human cytomegalovirus;[2] vidarabine and interferon alfa showed synergy *in vitro* against varicella-zoster virus.[3]

1. Schinazi RF, *et al*. Effect of combinations of acyclovir with vidarabine or its 5′-monophosphate on herpes simplex viruses in cell culture and in mice. *Antimicrob Agents Chemother* 1982; **22:** 499–507.
2. Spector SA, Kelley E. Inhibition of human cytomegalovirus by combined acyclovir and vidarabine. *Antimicrob Agents Chemother* 1985; **27:** 600–4.
3. Baba M, *et al*. Synergistic antiviral effects of antiherpes compounds and human leukocyte interferon on varicella-zoster virus in vitro. *Antimicrob Agents Chemother* 1984; **25:** 515–17.

Pharmacokinetics

Following intravenous administration vidarabine is rapidly metabolised, principally by deamination to hypoxanthine arabinoside (arabinosyl hypoxanthine). Peak plasma concentrations of 3 to 6 μg and 0.2 to 0.4 μg per mL have been obtained for hypoxanthine arabinoside and vidarabine respectively at the end of a 12-hour infusion of vidarabine 10 mg per kg body-weight. The plasma half-life for hypoxanthine arabinoside appears to be about 3.3 to 3.5 hours.

Hypoxanthine arabinoside is widely distributed in tissues. It diffuses into the cerebrospinal fluid to give concentrations about one-third of those in plasma.

Excretion is principally through the kidney with about 40 to 53% of a dose appearing in the urine as hypoxanthine arabinoside within 24 hours and 1 to 3% as unchanged drug.

Systemic absorption does not occur following application of vidarabine to the eye; trace amounts of hypoxanthine arabinoside (and vidarabine, if the cornea is damaged) may be found in the aqueous humour.

References.

1. Buchanan RA, *et al*. Plasma levels and urinary excretion of vidarabine after repeated dosing. *Clin Pharmacol Ther* 1980; **27:** 690–6.
2. Aronoff GR, *et al*. Hypoxanthine-arabinoside pharmacokinetics after adenine arabinoside administration to a patient with renal failure. *Antimicrob Agents Chemother* 1980; **18:** 212–14.
3. Whitley RJ, *et al*. Pharmacology, tolerance, and antiviral activity of vidarabine monophosphate in humans. *Antimicrob Agents Chemother* 1980; **18:** 709–15.
4. Shope TC, *et al*. Pharmacokinetics of vidarabine in the treatment of infants and children with infections due to herpesviruses. *J Infect Dis* 1983; **148:** 721–5.

Uses and Administration

Vidarabine is a purine nucleoside that has been used in the treatment of herpes simplex and varicella-zoster infections although aciclovir is generally preferred.

Vidarabine is administered topically in the treatment of herpes simplex keratitis as a 3% ophthalmic ointment and can be used when there has been no response to treatment with other antivirals or when ocular toxicity or hypersensitivity to other drugs has occurred. The ointment is applied 5 times daily every 3 hours until corneal re-epithelialisation has occurred, then twice daily for a further 7 days to prevent recurrence. If there is no improvement within 7 days or if complete healing has not occurred within 21 days, other forms of therapy should be considered.

Vidarabine was formerly used intravenously in the treatment of severe and disseminated herpes simplex infections and herpes zoster but aciclovir is preferred.

Creutzfeldt-Jakob disease. A report of a woman with pathologically proven Creutzfeldt-Jakob disease that was repeatedly suppressed for more than 6 months with vidarabine.[1]

1. Furlow TW, *et al*. Repeated suppression of Creutzfeldt-Jakob disease with vidarabine. *Lancet* 1982; **ii:** 564–5.

Herpes simplex infections. Although vidarabine has been shown to be moderately effective in the treatment of disseminated herpes simplex infections, aciclovir or foscarnet are generally preferred (see p.597). Topically applied vidarabine was reported to be as effective as idoxuridine[1,2] or trifluridine[3,4] in early studies in herpes keratitis. In neonatal herpes simplex infection, vidarabine 15 mg per kg bodyweight daily by intravenous infusion was shown to reduce mortality and neurological morbidity in infants with disseminated and CNS disease[5,6] and had beneficial effects in infants with localised disease.[5] Increasing the dose to 30 mg per kg per day did not improve the response;[6] nevertheless this was the dose used in a comparative study with aciclovir 30 mg per kg per day which showed no differences in either morbidity or mortality between treatments.[7] Responses to topical vidarabine in genital herpes[8] and herpes labialis,[9] and to intravenous vidarabine in herpes infections in immunocompromised patients[10,11] have generally been disappointing.

1. Pavan-Langston D. Clinical evaluation of adenine arabinoside and idoxuridine in the treatment of ocular herpes simplex. *Am J Ophthalmol* 1975; **80:** 495–502.
2. Pavan-Langston D, Buchanan RA. Vidarabine therapy of simple and IDU-complicated herpetic keratitis. *Trans Am Acad Ophthalmol Otolaryngol* 1976; **81:** 813–25.
3. Travers JP, Patterson A. A controlled trial of adenine arabinoside and trifluorothymidine in herpetic keratitis. *J Int Med Res* 1978; **6:** 102–4.
4. van Bijsterveld OP, Post H. Trifluorothymidine versus adenine arabinoside in the treatment of herpes simplex keratitis. *Br J Ophthalmol* 1980; **64:** 33–6.
5. Whitley RJ, *et al*. Vidarabine therapy of neonatal herpes simplex virus infection. *Pediatrics* 1980; **66:** 495–501.
6. Whitley RJ, *et al*. Neonatal herpes simplex virus infection: follow-up evaluation of vidarabine therapy. *Pediatrics* 1983; **72:** 778–85.
7. Whitley R, *et al*. A controlled trial comparing vidarabine with acyclovir in neonatal herpes simplex virus infection. *N Engl J Med* 1991; **324:** 444–9.
8. Eron LJ, *et al*. Topically applied vidarabine sodium phosphate in genital herpes infection. *J Antimicrob Chemother* 1988; **21:** 801–5.
9. Spruance SL, *et al*. Ineffectiveness of topical adenine arabinoside 5′-monophosphate in the treatment of recurrent herpes simplex labialis. *N Engl J Med* 1979; **300:** 1180–4.
10. Shepp DH, Farber BF. Ineffectiveness of vidarabine in mucocutaneous herpes simplex virus infection. *Lancet* 1990; **335:** 1344.
11. Safrin S, *et al*. A controlled trial comparing foscarnet with vidarabine for acyclovir-resistant mucocutaneous herpes simplex in the acquired immunodeficiency syndrome. *N Engl J Med* 1991; **325:** 551–5.

Varicella-zoster infections. The usual treatment for severe or disseminated herpes zoster is intravenous aciclovir (see p.598) but combined therapy with aciclovir and vidarabine may be considered in severely immunocompromised patients.[1] In a study in 73 immunocompromised patients[2] with disseminated herpes zoster the intravenous administration of vidarabine 10 mg per kg body-weight per day or aciclovir 30 mg per kg per day produced similar responses, except that patients who received aciclovir required a shorter period in hospital.

1. Nikkels AF, Piérard GE. Recognition and treatment of shingles. *Drugs* 1994; **48:** 528–48.
2. Whitley RJ, *et al*. Disseminated herpes zoster in the immunocompromised host: a comparative trial of acyclovir and vidarabine. *J Infect Dis* 1992; **165:** 450–5.

Preparations

USP 23: Vidarabine Concentrate for Injection; Vidarabine Ophthalmic Ointment.

Proprietary Preparations (details are given in Part 3)
Austral.: Vira-A; ***Canad.:*** Vira-A†; ***Fr.:*** Vira-A†; Vira-MP; ***Irl.:*** Vira-A†; ***Jpn:*** Arasena-A; ***Spain:*** Vira-A†; ***USA:*** Vira-A.

Zalcitabine (1731-e)

Zalcitabine *(BAN, USAN, rINN)*.

DDC; ddC; ddCyd; Dideoxycytidine; NSC-606170; Ro-24-2027; Ro-24-2027/000. 2′,3′-Dideoxycytidine.

$C_9H_{13}N_3O_3$ = 211.2.

CAS — 7481-89-2.

Pharmacopoeias. In US.

A white to off-white, crystalline powder. **Soluble** in water and in methyl alcohol; sparingly soluble in alcohol, in acetonitrile, in chloroform, and in dichloromethane; slightly soluble in cyclohexane. **Store** in airtight containers. Protect from light.

CAUTION. *Avoid exposure to the skin and inhalation of zalcitabine powder.*

Adverse Effects

The most serious adverse effects of zalcitabine are peripheral neuropathy which can affect up to one third of patients and pancreatitis which is rare, affecting less than 1% of patients, but which can be fatal. Other severe adverse effects include oral and oesophageal ulceration, hypersensitivity reactions, cardiomyopathy and congestive heart failure, lactic acidosis and severe hepatomegaly with steatosis (both potentially life-threatening), and hepatic failure.

Other adverse effects noted in patients taking zalcitabine have included asthenia, chest pain, fatigue, and fever; dizziness, headache, and insomnia; abdominal pain, anorexia, constipation, diarrhoea, dysphagia, nausea, and vomiting; anaemia, leucopenia, neutropenia, and thrombocytopenia; raised liver enzyme values; arthralgia and myalgia; mood changes; dyspnoea and pharyngitis; pruritus and rashes; hearing and visual disturbances; hyperuricaemia; and renal disorders.

Precautions

Zalcitabine should be interrupted or discontinued if peripheral neuropathy develops. Neuropathy is usually slowly reversible if treatment is stopped promptly but may be irreversible if treatment is continued after symptoms develop. Zalcitabine should be avoided in patients who already have peripheral neuropathy. It should be used with caution in patients at risk of developing peripheral neuropathy (especially those with a low CD4+ cell count) and in those receiving other drugs that may cause peripheral neuropathy (see Interactions, below).

Treatment should be interrupted in patients who develop abdominal pain, nausea, or vomiting or with abnormal biochemical test results until pancreatitis has been excluded. Zalcitabine should be discontinued permanently if pancreatitis develops. Patients with a history of pancreatitis or of raised serum amylase should be monitored closely. Zalcitabine should not be administered with other drugs known to cause pancreatitis (see Interactions, below).

Zalcitabine should be used with caution in patients with impaired hepatic function and treatment interrupted or discontinued if hepatic function deteriorates or there are signs of hepatic damage or unexplained lactic acidosis. It should be used with caution in patients with impaired renal function, and dosage reductions may be necessary. It should also be used with caution in patients with cardiomyopathy or congestive heart failure.

Complete blood count and biochemical tests should be carried out before treatment starts and at regular intervals throughout therapy.

Interactions

Zalcitabine should not be administered with other drugs known to cause pancreatitis (for example intravenous pentamidine). Caution is necessary when zalcitabine is given with other drugs that may cause peripheral neuropathy such as other nucleoside reverse transcriptase inhibitors, metronidazole, isoniazid (the clearance of which may also be affected—see p.219), and vincristine.

The absorption of zalcitabine is reduced by about 25% when administered concurrently with aluminium- or magnesium-containing antacids.

The administration of either cimetidine, probenecid, or trimethoprim can reduce the renal excretion of zalcitabine, resulting in elevated plasma concentrations. Renal excretion of zalcitabine may also be reduced by concurrent administration of amphotericin, aminoglycosides, or foscarnet, potentially increasing its toxicity.

Antiviral Action

Zalcitabine is converted intracellularly in stages to the triphosphate. This triphosphate halts the DNA synthesis of retroviruses, including HIV, through competitive inhibition of reverse transcriptase and incorporation into viral DNA.

References.

1. Jeffries DJ. The antiviral activity of dideoxycytidine. *J Antimicrob Chemother* 1989; **23** (suppl A): 29–34.

Pharmacokinetics

Zalcitabine is absorbed from the gastro-intestinal tract with a bioavailability of greater than 80%. The rate of absorption is reduced by administration with food. Peak plasma concentrations in the fasting state are achieved in about 1 hour. Zalcitabine crosses the blood-brain barrier producing CSF concentrations ranging from 9 to 37% of those in plasma. Binding to plasma proteins is negligible. The plasma elimination half-life is about 2 hours.

Zalcitabine is metabolised intracellularly to the active antiviral triphosphate. It does not appear to undergo any substantial hepatic metabolism and is excreted mainly in the urine.

References.

1. Morse GD, *et al.* Comparative pharmacokinetics of antiviral nucleoside analogues. *Clin Pharmacokinet* 1993; **24:** 101–23.
2. Devineni D, Gallo JM. Zalcitabine: clinical pharmacokinetics and efficacy. *Clin Pharmacokinet* 1995; **28:** 351–60.
3. Chadwick EG, *et al.* Phase I evaluation of zalcitabine administered to human immunodeficiency virus-infected children. *J Infect Dis* 1995; **172:** 1475–9.
4. Bazunga M, *et al.* The effects of renal impairment on the pharmacokinetics of zalcitabine. *J Clin Pharmacol* 1998; **38:** 28–33.

Uses and Administration

Zalcitabine is a nucleoside reverse transcriptase inhibitor derived from cytidine with activity against retroviruses including HIV. It is used in the treatment of HIV infection, usually in combination with other antiretroviral drugs.

Zalcitabine is given by mouth in a dose of 0.75 mg every 8 hours. Suggested doses for patients with impaired renal function are: creatinine clearance 10 to 40 mL per minute, 0.75 mg every 12 hours; creatinine clearance less than 10 mL per minute, 0.75 mg every 24 hours.

Reviews.

1. Whittington R, Brodgen RN. Zalcitabine: a review of its pharmacology and clinical potential in acquired immunodeficiency syndrome (AIDS). *Drugs* 1992; **44:** 656–83.
2. Lipsky JJ. Zalcitabine and didanosine. *Lancet* 1993; **341:** 30–2.
3. Shelton MJ, *et al.* Zalcitabine. *Ann Pharmacother* 1993; **27:** 480–9.
4. Adkins JC, *et al.* Zalcitabine: an update of its pharmacodynamic and pharmacokinetic properties and clinical efficacy in the management of HIV infection. *Drugs* 1997; **53:** 1054–80.

HIV infection and AIDS. Zalcitabine has been used as an alternative antiretroviral drug to treat HIV infection in patients intolerant of or unresponsive to zidovudine, although it has not been shown to have any great advantage over zidovudine in patients with advanced disease[1,2] and may be less well tolerated.[3] Alternating schedules of zalcitabine and zidovudine[4-6] were tried in an attempt to minimise the toxicities of both drugs. In patients who had ceased to respond to zidovudine, zalcitabine was reported to produce a response similar to that with didanosine.[7]

Zalcitabine is now usually used together with other antiretroviral drugs. Combination therapy with zalcitabine and zidovudine was superior to zidovudine alone in delaying disease progression and in prolonging life in patients who had not previously received antiretroviral therapy.[8,9] Combination therapy has been less successful in patients who have previously received zidovudine than in zidovudine-naive patients,[10] and zalcitabine with zidovudine was reported to be less effective than combinations of zidovudine with didanosine[8,9] or lamivudine.[11] Preliminary studies of zalcitabine with zidovudine and the HIV-protease inhibitor saquinavir have shown favourable responses.[12]

For a general discussion on the management of HIV infection and AIDS, see p.599.

1. Fischl MA, *et al.* Zalcitabine compared with zidovudine in patients with advanced HIV-1 infection who received previous zidovudine therapy. *Ann Intern Med* 1993; **118:** 762–9.
2. Fischl MA, *et al.* Combination and monotherapy with zidovudine and zalcitabine in patients with advanced HIV disease. *Ann Intern Med* 1995; **122:** 24–32.
3. Bozzette SA, *et al.* Health status and function with zidovudine or zalcitabine as initial therapy for AIDS: a randomized controlled trial. *JAMA* 1995; **273:** 295–301.
4. Yarchoan R, *et al.* Phase I studies of 2′,3′-dideoxycytidine in severe human immunodeficiency virus infection as a single agent and alternating with zidovudine (AZT). *Lancet* 1988; **i:** 76–81.
5. Pizzo PA, *et al.* Dideoxycytidine alone and in an alternating schedule with zidovudine in children with symptomatic human immunodeficiency virus infection. *J Pediatr* 1990; **117:** 799–808.
6. Skowron G, *et al.* Alternating and intermittent regimens of zidovudine and dideoxycytidine in patients with AIDS or AIDS-related complex. *Ann Intern Med* 1993; **118:** 321–30.
7. Abrams DI, *et al.* A comparative trial of didanosine or zalcitabine after treatment with zidovudine in patients with human immunodeficiency virus infection. *N Engl J Med* 1994; **330:** 657–62.
8. Delta Coordinating Committee. Delta: a randomised double-blind controlled trial comparing combinations of zidovudine plus didanosine or zalcitabine with zidovudine alone in HIV-infected individuals. *Lancet* 1996; **348:** 283–91.
9. Hammer SM, *et al.* A trial comparing nucleoside monotherapy with combination therapy in HIV-infected adults with CD4 cell counts from 200 to 500 per cubic millimeter. *N Engl J Med* 1996; **335:** 1081–90.
10. Saravolatz LD, *et al.* Zidovudine alone or in combination with didanosine or zalcitabine in HIV-infected patients with the acquired immunodeficiency syndrome or fewer than 200 CD4 cells per cubic millimeter. *N Engl J Med* 1996; **335:** 1099–1106.
11. Bartlett JA, *et al.* Lamivudine plus zidovudine compared with zalcitabine plus zidovudine in patients with HIV infection: a randomized, double-blind, placebo-controlled trial. *Ann Intern Med* 1996; **125:** 161–72.
12. Collier AC, *et al.* Treatment of human immunodeficiency virus infection with saquinavir, zidovudine, and zalcitabine. *N Engl J Med* 1996; **334:** 1011–17.

Preparations

Proprietary Preparations (details are given in Part 3)

Aust.: Hivid; ***Austral.:*** Hivid; ***Belg.:*** Hivid; ***Canad.:*** Hivid; ***Fr.:*** Hivid; ***Ger.:*** Hivid; ***Irl.:*** Hivid; ***Ital.:*** Hivid; ***Neth.:*** Hivid; ***Norw.:*** Hivid; ***S.Afr.:*** Hivid; ***Spain:*** Hivid; ***Swed.:*** Hivid; ***Switz.:*** Hivid; ***UK:*** Hivid; ***USA:*** Hivid.

Zanamivir (17658-y)

Zanamivir *(BAN, USAN, rINN).*

GG-167; GR-121167X; 4-Guanidino-2,4-dideoxy-2,3-dehydro-*N*-acetylneuraminic Acid. 5-Acetamido-2,6-anhydro-3,4,5-trideoxy-4-guanidino-D-*glycero*-D-*galacto*-non-2-enonic acid.

$C_{12}H_{20}N_4O_7$ = 332.3.

CAS — 139110-80-8.

Zanamivir is an inhibitor of the enzyme neuraminidase (sialidase), which has a role in the infectivity and replication of influenza A and B viruses. It is under investigation for the prophylaxis and treatment of influenza.

References.

1. Hayden FG, *et al.* Safety and efficacy of the neuraminidase inhibitor GG167 in experimental human influenza. *JAMA* 1996; **275:** 295–9.
2. Hayden FG, *et al.* Efficacy and safety of the neuraminidase inhibitor zanamivir in the treatment of influenzavirus infection. *N Engl J Med* 1997; **337:** 874–80.
3. Waghorn SL, Goa KL. Zanamivir. *Drugs* 1998; **55:** 721–5.

Zidovudine (18797-s)

Zidovudine *(BAN, USAN, rINN).*

Azidodeoxythymidine; Azidothymidine; AZT; BW-A509U; BW-509U; Compound-S; Zidovudinum. 3′-Azido-3′-deoxythymidine.

$C_{10}H_{13}N_5O_4$ = 267.2.

CAS — 30516-87-1.

NOTE. The abbreviation AZT has also been used for azathioprine.

Pharmacopoeias. In *Eur.* (see p.viii) and *US.*

A white to yellowish or brownish powder. Sparingly **soluble** in water; freely soluble in alcohol; soluble in dehydrated alcohol. It shows polymorphism. **Store** in airtight containers. Protect from light.

Adverse Effects

The commonest serious adverse effects reported with zidovudine are anaemia and leucopenia, mainly neutropenia, occurring within a few weeks of starting treatment. This haematological toxicity occurs most commonly in those with pre-existing haematological abnormalities and is usually reversed by discontinuing treatment but it can be severe enough to require blood transfusion.

Other frequently reported adverse effects include asthenia, fever, and malaise; headache, insomnia, myopathy, and paraesthesia; abdominal pain, anorexia, dyspepsia, nausea, and vomiting; myalgia; and rashes. Lactic acidosis and severe hepatomegaly with steatosis have been reported as rare but potentially fatal occurrences in patients taking zidovudine. Pancreatitis, convulsions, and pigmentation of nails, skin, and oral mucosa have occurred.

Zidovudine is reported to be carcinogenic in *mice* and *rats.*

Adverse effects with zidovudine tend to be dose-related and reversible. The more advanced the state of the disease being treated, the greater the risk of zidovudine toxicity.

Some references to the incidence and range of adverse effects are given below.

1. Richman DD, *et al.* The toxicity of azidothymidine (AZT) in the treatment of patients with AIDS and AIDS-related complex: a double-blind, placebo-controlled trial. *N Engl J Med* 1987; **317:** 192–7.
2. Gelmon K, *et al.* Nature, time course and dose dependence of zidovudine-related side effects: results from the Multicenter Canadian Azidothymidine Trial. *AIDS* 1989; **3:** 555–61.
3. Fischl MA, *et al.* The safety and efficacy of zidovudine (AZT) in the treatment of subjects with mildly symptomatic human immunodeficiency virus type 1 (HIV) infection: a double-blind, placebo-controlled trial. *Ann Intern Med* 1990; **112:** 727–37.
4. McKinney RE, *et al.* Safety and tolerance of intermittent intravenous and oral zidovudine therapy in human immunodeficiency virus-infected pediatric patients. *J Pediatr* 1990; **116:** 640–7.
5. Koch MA, *et al.* Toxic effects of zidovudine in asymptomatic human immunodeficiency-virus-infected individuals with CD4+ cell counts of 0.5×10^9/L or less: detailed and updated results from protocol 019 of the AIDS Clinical Trials Group. *Arch Intern Med* 1992; **152:** 2286–92.

Effects on the blood. Adverse haematological effects reported with zidovudine may be severe and include anaemia with erythroid aplasia or hypoplasia, and neutropenia.[1-5] Although these effects may be reversed by stopping treatment,[5] they may persist for weeks after zidovudine has been withdrawn[2,3] and blood transfusions may be required in some patients.[1-4] One study indicated that zidovudine-induced neutropenia only significantly increased the risk of bacterial infection in patients whose polymorphonuclear cell count fell below 500 per μL.[6] The effects of zidovudine on the platelet count are considered to be complex, but patients with thrombocytopenia appeared not to be at risk during treatment.[7]

Recombinant erythropoietin has been used in an attempt to reduce blood-transfusion requirements in zidovudine-induced anaemia,[8,9] although the proportion of patients who derive benefit may be limited and some have reported it to have no effect.[10] Similarly granulocyte-macrophage colony-stimulating factor has been reported to improve the neutrophil count in some but not all patients.[11] Lithium carbonate has granulopoietic properties and has been tried, with mixed results, in zidovudine-induced neutropenia.[12-14] Lithium has also been given with vitamin B_{12} and folate to zidovudine recipients.[15]

1. Forester G. Profound cytopenia secondary to azidothymidine. *N Engl J Med* 1987; **317:** 772.
2. Gill PS, *et al.* Azidothymidine associated with bone marrow failure in the acquired immunodeficiency syndrome (AIDS). *Ann Intern Med* 1987; **107:** 502–5.
3. Mir N, Costello C. Zidovudine and bone marrow. *Lancet* 1988; **ii:** 1195–6.
4. Walker RE, *et al.* Anemia and erythropoiesis in patients with the acquired immunodeficiency syndrome (AIDS) and Kaposi sarcoma treated with zidovudine. *Ann Intern Med* 1988; **108:** 372–6.
5. Cohen H, *et al.* Reversible zidovudine-induced pure red-cell aplasia. *AIDS* 1989; **3:** 177–8.
6. Shaunak S, Bartlett JA. Zidovudine-induced neutropenia: are we too cautious? *Lancet* 1989; **ii:** 91–2.
7. Flegg PJ, *et al.* Effect of zidovudine on platelet count. *Br Med J* 1989; **298:** 1074–5.
8. Fischl M, *et al.* Recombinant human erythropoietin for patients with AIDS treated with zidovudine. *N Engl J Med* 1990; **322:** 1488–93.
9. Henry DH, *et al.* Recombinant human erythropoietin in the treatment of anemia associated with human immunodeficiency virus (HIV) infection and zidovudine therapy: overview of four clinical trials. *Ann Intern Med* 1992; **117:** 739–48.
10. Shepp DH, *et al.* Erythropoietin for zidovudine-induced anemia. *N Engl J Med* 1990; **323:** 1069–70.
11. Hewitt RG, *et al.* Pharmacokinetics and pharmacodynamics of granulocyte-macrophage colony-stimulating factor and zidovudine in patients with AIDS and severe AIDS-related complex. *Antimicrob Agents Chemother* 1993; **37:** 512–22.
12. Herbert V, *et al.* Lithium for zidovudine-induced neutropenia in AIDS. *JAMA* 1988; **260:** 3588.
13. Roberts DE, *et al.* Effect of lithium carbonate on zidovudine-associated neutropenia in the acquired immunodeficiency syndrome. *Am J Med* 1988; **85:** 428–31.
14. Worthington M. Lack of effect of lithium carbonate on zidovudine-associated neutropenia in patients with AIDS. *J Infect Dis* 1990; **162:** 777–8.
15. Herbert V, *et al.* Lithium for zidovudine-induced neutropenia in AIDS. *JAMA* 1989; **262:** 776.

Effects on the CNS. Reports of adverse effects on the CNS associated with zidovudine include mania,[1,2] seizures[3,4] (following an overdose in one patient),[5] psychogenic panic,[6] and Wernicke's encephalopathy,[7] mostly involving one or two patients in each case. CNS toxicity, thought to be zidovudine-related, contributed to the death of an AIDS patient.[8]

1. Maxwell S, *et al.* Manic syndrome associated with zidovudine treatment. *JAMA* 1988; **259:** 3406–7.
2. Wright JM, *et al.* Zidovudine-related mania. *Med J Aust* 1989; **150:** 339–40.
3. Harris PJ, Caceres CA. Azidothymidine in the treatment of AIDS. *N Engl J Med* 1988; **318:** 250.
4. D'Silva M, *et al.* Seizure associated with zidovudine. *Lancet* 1995; **346:** 452.
5. Routy JP, *et al.* Seizure after zidovudine overdose. *Lancet* 1989; **i:** 384–5.

6. Levitt AJ, Lippert GP. Psychogenic panic after zidovudine therapy—the therapeutic benefit of an N of 1 trial. *Can Med Assoc J* 1990; **142:** 341–2.
7. Davtyan DG, Vinters HV. Wernicke's encephalopathy in AIDS patient treated with zidovudine. *Lancet* 1987; **i:** 919–20.
8. Hagler DN, Frame PT. Azidothymidine neurotoxicity. *Lancet* 1986; **ii:** 1392–3.

Effects on the liver. The development of acute cholestatic hepatitis necessitated the withdrawal of zidovudine in one patient who was later unable to tolerate its re-institution.[1] Zidovudine also had to be withdrawn in 3 patients after abnormal liver-function values occurred;[2] it was reinstated in 2 patients without further liver changes. Reversible increases in liver enzymes and rashes were also reported in 2 patients receiving prophylaxis with zidovudine and zalcitabine following exposure to HIV.[3] There has been a report of iron deposition in the liver of patients receiving blood transfusions for zidovudine-related anaemia.[4]

Fatal hepatic dysfunction associated with steatosis in the liver was reported in 6 patients with HIV infections, who were either receiving zidovudine or had previously done so.[5] Five of these 6 patients also developed metabolic acidosis.

1. Dubin G, Braffman MN. Zidovudine-induced hepatotoxicity. *Ann Intern Med* 1989; **110:** 85–6.
2. Melamed AJ, *et al.* Possible zidovudine-induced hepatotoxicity. *JAMA* 1987; **258:** 2063.
3. Henry K, *et al.* Hepatotoxicity and rash associated with zidovudine and zalcitabine chemoprophylaxis. *Ann Intern Med* 1996; **124:** 855.
4. Lindley R, *et al.* Iron deposition in liver in zidovudine-related transfusion-dependent anaemia. *Lancet* 1989; **ii:** 681.
5. Freiman JP, *et al.* Hepatomegaly with severe steatosis in HIV-seropositive patients. *AIDS* 1993; **7:** 379–85.

Effects on the metabolism. Lactic acidosis sometimes in association with myopathy[1] or hepatotoxicity (see above) has been reported with zidovudine treatment. However, lactic acidosis has also been reported in 7 patients with HIV infection with no apparent cause:[2] 4 patients were receiving zidovudine, 1 ganciclovir, and 1 clofazimine. The disorder in these patients resembled Reye's syndrome and it is not clear whether the acidosis was induced by zidovudine or the HIV infection.

1. Gopinath R, *et al.* Chronic lactic acidosis in a patient with acquired immunodeficiency syndrome and mitochondrial myopathy: biochemical studies. *J Am Soc Nephrol* 1992; **3:** 1212–19.
2. Chattha G, *et al.* Lactic acidosis complicating the acquired immunodeficiency syndrome. *Ann Intern Med* 1993; **118:** 37–9.

Effects on the musculoskeletal system. Myalgia can occur in patients taking zidovudine; so too can other adverse muscle effects although it has sometimes been difficult to determine whether the effects were caused by the drug or the underlying HIV infection.[1-3] Dalakas *et al.* considered zidovudine-induced myopathy to be a distinct condition characterised by the presence of abnormal mitochondria in muscle-biopsy specimens;[2] this view is supported by the fact that the myopathy readily responded to the withdrawal of zidovudine or to treatment with corticosteroids or other anti-inflammatory drugs.[1-3] However, myopathy in patients receiving zidovudine is practically indistinguishable from that induced by HIV infection.[4]

Arthralgia involving the knees, elbows, ankles, and wrists was associated with zidovudine therapy in 1 patient.[5]

1. Gertner E, *et al.* Zidovudine-associated myopathy. *Am J Med* 1989; **86:** 814–18.
2. Dalakas MC, *et al.* Mitochondrial myopathy caused by long-term zidovudine therapy. *N Engl J Med* 1990; **322:** 1098–1105.
3. Till M, MacDonell KB. Myopathy with human immunodeficiency virus type 1 (HIV-1) infection: HIV-1 or zidovudine? *Ann Intern Med* 1990; **113:** 492–4.
4. Simpson DM, *et al.* Myopathies associated with human immunodeficiency virus and zidovudine: can their effects be distinguished? *Neurology* 1993; **43:** 971–6.
5. Murphy D, *et al.* Zidovudine related arthropathy. *Br Med J* 1994; **309:** 97.

Effects on the nails. Bluish or brownish discoloration of fingernails and/or toenails has been reported in a number of patients receiving zidovudine.[1-5] Dark-skinned patients appear to be most commonly affected.[2,4] Occasionally the abnormal pigmentation also involves the skin.[3,5] It has been pointed out that discoloration of nails has occurred in HIV-infected patients without exposure to zidovudine.[6]

1. Furth PA, Kazakis AM. Nail pigmentation changes associated with azidothymidine (zidovudine). *N Engl J Med* 1987; **107:** 350.
2. Vaiopoulos G, *et al.* Nail pigmentation and azidothymidine. *Ann Intern Med* 1988; **108:** 777.
3. Merenich JA, *et al.* Azidothymidine-induced hyperpigmentation mimicking primary adrenal insufficiency. *Am J Med* 1989; **86:** 469–70.
4. Don PC, *et al.* Nail dyschromia associated with zidovudine. *Ann Intern Med* 1990; **112:** 145–6.
5. Bendick C, *et al.* Azidothymidine-induced hyperpigmentation of skin and nails. *Arch Dermatol* 1989; **125:** 1285–6.
6. Chandrasekar PH. Nail discoloration and human immunodeficiency virus infection. *Am J Med* 1989; **86:** 506–7.

Precautions

Zidovudine should be used with care in patients with anaemia or bone-marrow suppression. Dosage adjustments may be necessary and it has been recommended that it should not be used if the neutrophil count or haemoglobin value is abnormally low. Care is also required in the elderly and in patients with reduced kidney or liver function who may require reductions in dose. Patients will risk factors for liver disease should be monitored during treatment. Zidovudine treatment should be stopped if there is a rapid increase in aminotransferase concentrations, progressive hepatomegaly, or metabolic or lactic acidosis of unknown aetiology. It should not be given to neonates with hyperbilirubinaemia requiring treatment other than phototherapy or with markedly increased aminotransferase concentrations.

Because of the haematological toxicity of zidovudine it is recommended that, in patients with advanced symptomatic HIV disease taking oral zidovudine, blood tests should be carried out at least every 2 weeks for the first 3 months of treatment and at least monthly thereafter; blood tests should be performed at least every week in those receiving intravenous zidovudine. In patients with early HIV infection blood tests may be performed less frequently (e.g. every 1 to 3 months).

Interference with laboratory tests. Raised urinary thymine concentrations in neonates, due to maternal zidovudine treatment, could produce erroneous results in screening tests for inborn errors of metabolism.[1]

1. Sewell AC. Zidovudine and confusion in urinary metabolic screening. *Lancet* 1998; **352:** 1227.

Pregnancy. Administration of zidovudine to pregnant women with HIV infection from 14 weeks of gestation until delivery, and subsequently to the neonate, has been shown to reduce vertical transmission of the infection (see under Uses and Administration, below). However, studies have shown that zidovudine can be fetotoxic in *animals* when given early in pregnancy, and the long-term consequences for the infant are as yet unknown. The manufacturer therefore recommends that zidovudine should not generally be administered before 14 weeks of gestation.

Interactions

Care should be taken during concomitant therapy with zidovudine and drugs that are myelosuppressive or nephrotoxic. Drugs that undergo glucuronidation may delay the metabolism of zidovudine but few of these appear to produce clinically important increases in zidovudine plasma concentrations. Increased toxicity and decreased antiretroviral activity has been reported when zidovudine is given with some other antiviral drugs, and pharmacokinetic interactions have been reported with a number of anti-infective drugs used commonly in patients with HIV infection. See below for further details of interactions.

An assessment *in vitro*[1] of the inhibition of zidovudine glucuronidation to an inactive glucuronide form indicated that such inhibition might be of more clinical significance with concomitant fluconazole or valproic acid than with atovaquone or methadone.

1. Trapnell CB, *et al.* Glucuronidation of 3′-azido-3′-deoxythymidine (zidovudine) by human liver microsomes: relevance to clinical pharmacokinetic interactions with atovaquone, fluconazole, methadone, and valproic acid. *Antimicrob Agents Chemother* 1998; **42:** 1592–6.

Analgesics. There may be an increased risk of haemotoxicity during concomitant use of zidovudine and *NSAIDs*.

Antibacterials. Studies have indicated that the absorption zidovudine could be reduced by concurrent administration of *clarithromycin*.[1] The manufacturers recommend administering zidovudine and clarithromycin 2 hours apart since this has been shown to have no overall effect on the bioavailability of zidovudine.[2] Administration of *rifampicin* to patients taking zidovudine has been reported to reduce the area under the curve, probably by inducing glucuronidation.[3] *Rifabutin* has not been shown to have a marked effect on zidovudine clearance.[4] *Trimethoprim* has been reported to decrease the renal clearance of zidovudine by up to 60%[5,6] with a consequent increase in plasma concentrations, although it was only thought likely to be of clinical significance in patients with impaired liver function.[6]

For a report of reduced *pyrazinamide* concentrations in patients receiving zidovudine, see p.241.

1. Polis MA, *et al.* Clarithromycin lowers plasma zidovudine levels in persons with human immunodeficiency virus infection. *Antimicrob Agents Chemother* 1997; **41:** 1709–14.
2. Vance E, *et al.* Pharmacokinetics of clarithromycin and zidovudine in patients with AIDS. *Antimicrob Agents Chemother* 1995; **39:** 1355–60.
3. Burger DM, *et al.* Pharmacokinetic interaction between rifampin and zidovudine. *Antimicrob Agents Chemother* 1993; **37:** 1426–31.
4. Narang PK, Sale M. Population based assessment of rifabutin effect on zidovudine disposition in AIDS patients. *Clin Pharmacol Ther* 1993; **53:** 219.
5. Chatton JY, *et al.* Trimethoprim, alone or in combination with sulphamethoxazole, decreases the renal excretion of zidovudine and its glucuronide. *Br J Clin Pharmacol* 1992; **34:** 551–4.
6. Lee BL, *et al.* Zidovudine, trimethoprim, and dapsone pharmacokinetic interactions in patients with human immunodeficiency virus infection. *Antimicrob Agents Chemother* 1996; **40:** 1231–6.

Antifungals. Administration of *fluconazole* in combination with zidovudine produced higher zidovudine serum concentrations, increases in the area under the serum concentration-time curve and prolonged terminal half-life compared with zidovudine alone in a study in 12 patients.[1] Studies *in vitro* suggested that fluconazole could inhibit the glucuronidation of zidovudine; inhibition was also seen with *amphotericin*, *ketoconazole*, and *miconazole*, but not with *flucytosine* or *itraconazole*.[2]

1. Sahai J, *et al.* Effect of fluconazole on zidovudine pharmacokinetics in patients infected with human immunodeficiency virus. *J Infect Dis* 1994; **169:** 103–7.
2. Sampol E, *et al.* Comparative effects of antifungal agents on zidovudine glucuronidation by human liver microsomes. *Br J Clin Pharmacol* 1995; **40:** 83–6.

Antivirals. Studies *in vitro* showed that *tribavirin* and zidovudine inhibited each other's anti-HIV activity[1] and that *interferon alfa* and zidovudine had a synergistic cytotoxicity to bone-marrow progenitor cells.[2] Combined therapy with zidovudine and *aciclovir* is not generally associated with additional toxicity[3] but severe fatigue and lethargy were reported in one patient receiving aciclovir with zidovudine; this did not occur when either drug was given alone.[4] Severe haematological toxicity occurred when zidovudine was added to *ganciclovir* therapy in AIDS patients with cytomegalovirus retinitis, necessitating substantial dosage reductions or withdrawal of zidovudine in the majority of patients;[5,6] this additive toxicity with ganciclovir may be one reason why patients receiving zidovudine and ganciclovir do less well than those receiving zidovudine and foscarnet. Evidence of a pharmacokinetic interaction between zidovudine and *didanosine* has been conflicting, with reports of no effect,[7] increased,[8] and decreased[9] plasma concentrations of zidovudine. Small reductions in didanosine plasma concentrations have been reported in patients also receiving zidovudine.[10] However all changes have generally been small and are likely to be of limited clinical significance. Exposure to zidovudine (as measured by peak plasma concentrations and area under the concentration-time curve) was reduced in HIV patients given *ritonavir* concomitantly, whereas the pharmacokinetics of ritonavir were not affected by zidovudine;[11] the clinical relevance of this was not known.

1. Vogt MW, *et al.* Ribavirin antagonizes the effect of azidothymidine on HIV replication. *Science* 1987; **235:** 1376–9.
2. Berman E, *et al.* Synergistic cytotoxic effect of azidothymidine and recombinant interferon alpha on normal human bone marrow progenitor cells. *Blood* 1989; **74:** 1281–6.
3. Tartaglione TA, *et al.* Pharmacokinetic evaluations of low- and high-dose zidovudine plus high-dose acyclovir in patients with symptomatic human immunodeficiency virus infection. *Antimicrob Agents Chemother* 1991; **35:** 2225–31.
4. Bach MC. Possible drug interaction during therapy with azidothymidine and acyclovir for AIDS. *N Engl J Med* 1987; **316:** 547.
5. Millar AB, *et al.* Treatment of cytomegalovirus retinitis with zidovudine and ganciclovir in patients with AIDS: outcome and toxicity. *Genitourin Med* 1990; **66:** 156–8.
6. Hochster H, *et al.* Toxicity of combined ganciclovir and zidovudine for cytomegalovirus disease associated with AIDS: an AIDS Clinical Trials Group study. *Ann Intern Med* 1990; **113:** 111–17.
7. Collier AC, *et al.* Combination therapy with zidovudine and didanosine compared with zidovudine alone in HIV-1 infection. *Ann Intern Med* 1993; **119:** 786–93.
8. Barry M, *et al.* Pharmacokinetics of zidovudine and dideoxyinosine alone and in combination in patients with the acquired immunodeficiency syndrome. *Br J Clin Pharmacol* 1994; **37:** 421–6.
9. Burger DM, *et al.* Pharmacokinetic interaction study of zidovudine and didanosine. *J Drug Dev* 1994; **6:** 187–94.
10. Gibb D, *et al.* Pharmacokinetics of zidovudine and dideoxyinosine alone and in combination in children with HIV infection. *Br J Clin Pharmacol* 1995; **39:** 527–30.
11. Cato A, *et al.* Multidose pharmacokinetics of ritonavir and zidovudine in human immunodeficiency virus-infected patients. *Antimicrob Agents Chemother* 1998; **42:** 1788–93.

Atovaquone. Administration of atovaquone in combination with zidovudine produced moderate increases in the zidovudine plasma concentration and area under the plasma concentration-time curve, probably by inhibition of glucuronidation.[1]

1. Lee BL, *et al.* Atovaquone inhibits the glucuronidation and increases the plasma concentrations of zidovudine. *Clin Pharmacol Ther* 1996; **59:** 14–21.

Paracetamol. Severe hepatotoxicity developed in one patient taking zidovudine and co-trimoxazole following paracetamol administration.[1] However neither short-term[2] nor long-term[3] studies (the latter also in one patient) have shown any alteration of zidovudine elimination in patients taking zidovudine and paracetamol.

1. Shriner K, Goetz MB. Severe hepatotoxicity in a patient receiving both acetaminophen and zidovudine. *Am J Med* 1992; **93:** 94–6.
2. Sattler FR, *et al.* Acetaminophen does not impair clearance of zidovudine. *Ann Intern Med* 1991; **114:** 937–40.
3. Burger DM, *et al.* Pharmacokinetics of zidovudine and acetaminophen in a patient on chronic acetaminophen therapy. *Ann Pharmacother* 1994; **28:** 327–30.

Valproate. Administration of valproic acid to 6 patients receiving zidovudine produced increases in zidovudine plasma concentrations and the area under the plasma concentration-time curve.[1] The evidence suggested that this was due to reduced glucuronidation of zidovudine.

1. Lertora JJL, *et al.* Pharmacokinetic interaction between zidovudine and valproic acid in patients infected with human immunodeficiency virus. *Clin Pharmacol Ther* 1994; **56:** 272–8.

Antiviral Action

Zidovudine is converted intracellularly in stages to the triphosphate via thymidine kinase and other kinases. This triphosphate halts the DNA synthesis of retroviruses, including HIV, through competitive inhibition of reverse transcriptase and incorporation into viral DNA. It has also been shown to possess activity against Epstein-Barr virus and Gram-negative bacteria *in vitro*.

Zidovudine-resistant strains of HIV emerge rapidly during zidovudine therapy which might be responsible for the lack of benefit with long-term therapy. Cross resistance to other nucleoside reverse transcriptase inhibitors has been recognised occasionally.

Microbiological interactions. The anti-HIV activity of zidovudine has been enhanced *in vitro* by a number of drugs including dextran sulphate,[1] granulocyte-macrophage colony-stimulating factor,[2,3] hydroxyurea,[4] foscarnet,[5,6] poly I.poly C12U,[7] carbovir,[8] castanospermine,[9] zalcitabine,[10] and didanosine.[11] Antiviral synergy was demonstrated against HIV *in vitro* with a combination of zidovudine, soluble CD4, and interferon alfa.[12] Interferon alfa also enhanced the activity of zidovudine in cells acutely and persistently infected with HIV.[13] Zidovudine blocked the HIV replication-enhancing effect of tumour necrosis factor.[14]

For a report of zidovudine and tribavirin mutually inhibiting each other's antiviral activity *in vitro*, see Antivirals, under Interactions, above.

1. Ueno R, Kuno S. Dextran sulphate, a potent anti-HIV agent in vitro having synergism with zidovudine. *Lancet* 1987; **i:** 1379.
2. Hammer SM, Gillis JM. Synergistic activity of granulocyte-macrophage colony-stimulating factor and 3′-azido-3′-deoxythymidine against human immunodeficiency virus in vitro. *Antimicrob Agents Chemother* 1987; **31:** 1046–50.
3. Perno C-F, *et al.* Replication of human immunodeficiency virus in monocytes: granulocyte/macrophage colony-stimulating factor (GM-CSF) potentiates viral production yet enhances the antiviral effect mediated by 3′-azido-2′3′-dideoxythymidine (AZT) and other dideoxynucleoside congeners of thymidine. *J Exp Med* 1989; **169:** 933–51.
4. Palmer S, Cox S. Increased activity of the combination of 3′-azido-3′-deoxythymidine and 2′-deoxy-3′-thiacytidine in the presence of hydroxyurea. *Antimicrob Agents Chemother* 1997; **41:** 460–4.
5. Eriksson BFH, Schinazi RF. Combinations of 3′-azido-3′-deoxythymidine (zidovudine) and phosphonoformate (foscarnet) against human immunodeficiency virus type 1 and cytomegalovirus replication in vitro. *Antimicrob Agents Chemother* 1989; **33:** 663–9.
6. Koshida R, *et al.* Inhibition of human immunodeficiency virus in vitro by combination of 3′-azido-3′-deoxythymidine and foscarnet. *Antimicrob Agents Chemother* 1989; **33:** 778–80.
7. Mitchell WM, *et al.* Mismatched double-stranded RNA (ampligen) reduces concentration of zidovudine (azidothymidine) required for in-vitro inhibition of human immunodeficiency virus. *Lancet* 1987; **i:** 890–2.
8. Smith MS, *et al.* Evaluation of synergy between carbovir and 3′-azido-2′3′-deoxythymidine for inhibition of human immunodeficiency virus type 1. *Antimicrob Agents Chemother* 1993; **37:** 144–7.
9. Johnson VA, *et al.* Synergistic inhibition of human immunodeficiency virus type 1 and type 2 replication in vitro by castanospermine and 3′-azido-3′-deoxythymidine. *Antimicrob Agents Chemother* 1989; **33:** 53–7.
10. Spector SA, *et al.* Human immunodeficiency virus inhibition is prolonged by 3′-azido-3′-deoxythymidine alternating with 2′,3′-dideoxycytidine compared with 3′-azido-3′-deoxythymidine alone. *Antimicrob Agents Chemother* 1989; **33:** 920–3.
11. Dornsife RE, *et al.* Anti-human immunodeficiency virus synergism by zidovudine (3′-azidothymidine) and didanosine (dideoxyinosine) contrasts with their additive inhibition of normal human marrow progenitor cells. *Antimicrob Agents Chemother* 1991; **35:** 322–8.
12. Johnson VA, *et al.* Three-drug synergistic inhibition of HIV-1 replication in vitro by zidovudine, recombinant soluble CD4, and recombinant interferon-alpha A. *J Infect Dis* 1990; **161:** 1059–67.
13. Pincus SH, Wehrly K. AZT demonstrates anti-HIV-1 activity in persistently infected cell lines: implications for combination chemotherapy and immunotherapy. *J Infect Dis* 1990; **162:** 1233–8.
14. Michihiko S, *et al.* Augmentation of in-vitro HIV replication in peripheral blood mononuclear cells of AIDS and ARC patients by tumour necrosis factor. *Lancet* 1989; **i:** 1206–7.

Resistance. The emergence of zidovudine-resistant HIV strains in patients receiving long-term therapy with zidovudine has been recognised since 1989.[1,2] The emergence of drug resistance is associated with the duration[3] of treatment with zidovudine, but not the dose,[4] and is attributed to a high frequency of mutations in the HIV reverse transcriptase gene.[3,5] Development of high-level resistance to zidovudine in patients with advanced HIV infection is associated with rapid disease progression and death.[6] Primary infection with zidovudine-resistant HIV strains has been recorded,[7] as has zidovudine resistance in patients receiving other nucleoside reverse transcriptase inhibitors,[8,9] although it is possible that these patients had unrecorded exposure to zidovudine.[8] Emerging resistance to zidovudine is believed to be a factor in the loss of effect of long-term therapy. Changing to an alternative antiretroviral drug, commonly didanosine, can be beneficial in patients who have progressive disease during zidovudine treatment and cross resistance with other nucleoside reverse transcriptase inhibitors has not been regarded as a problem in clinical practice,[1,2,10,11] although there is some evidence of cross resistance.[10,12] The use of combination therapy with two or more drugs may delay the emergence of resistant strains and improve the duration of the clinical response. However, analysis of data from the Delta trial[13] showed no delay in the emergence of zidovudine resistance when used in combinations with didanosine or zalcitabine although antiviral activity was apparently not impaired.

1. Larder BA, *et al.* HIV with reduced sensitivity to zidovudine (AZT) isolated during prolonged therapy. *Science* 1989; **243:** 1731–4.
2. Rooke R, *et al.* Isolation of drug-resistant variants of HIV-1 from patients on long-term zidovudine therapy. *AIDS* 1989; **3:** 411–15.
3. Japour AJ, *et al.* Prevalence and clinical significance of zidovudine resistance mutations in human immunodeficiency virus isolated from patients after long-term zidovudine treatment. *J Infect Dis* 1995; **171:** 1172–9.
4. Richman DD, *et al.* Effect of stage of disease and drug dose on zidovudine susceptibilities of isolates of human immunodeficiency virus. *J Acquir Immune Defic Syndr* 1990; **3:** 743–6.
5. Loveday C, *et al.* HIV-1 RNA serum-load and resistant viral genotypes during early zidovudine therapy. *Lancet* 1995; **345:** 820–4.
6. D'Aquila RT, *et al.* Zidovudine resistance and HIV-1 disease progression during antiretroviral therapy. *Ann Intern Med* 1995; **122:** 401–8.
7. Erice A, *et al.* Brief report: primary infection with zidovudine-resistant human immunodeficiency virus type 1. *N Engl J Med* 1993; **328:** 1163–5.
8. Lin P-F, *et al.* Genotypic and phenotypic analysis of human immunodeficiency virus type 1 isolates from patients on prolonged stavudine therapy. *J Infect Dis* 1994; **170:** 1157–64.
9. Demeter LM, *et al.* Development of zidovudine resistance mutations in patients receiving prolonged didanosine monotherapy. *J Infect Dis* 1995; **172:** 1480–5.
10. Rooke R, *et al.* Biological comparison of wild-type and zidovudine-resistant isolates of human immunodeficiency virus type 1 from the same subjects: susceptibility and resistance to other drugs. *Antimicrob Agents Chemother* 1991; **35:** 988–91.
11. Hussan RN, *et al.* High-level resistance to zidovudine but not to zalcitabine or didanosine in human immunodeficiency virus from children receiving antiretroviral therapy. *J Pediatr* 1993; **123:** 9–16.
12. Mayers DL, *et al.* Dideoxynucleoside resistance emerges with prolonged zidovudine monotherapy. *Antimicrob Agents Chemother* 1994; **38:** 307–14.
13. Brun-Vézinet F, *et al.* HIV-1 viral load, phenotype, and resistance in a subset of drug-naive participants from the Delta trial. *Lancet* 1997; **350:** 983–90.

Pharmacokinetics

Zidovudine is rapidly absorbed from the gastro-intestinal tract and undergoes first-pass hepatic metabolism with a bioavailability of about 60 to 70%. Peak plasma concentrations occur after about 1 hour. Absorption is delayed by administration with food, but bioavailability is probably unaffected. It crosses the blood-brain barrier producing CSF to plasma ratios of about 0.5. It crosses the placenta and is distributed into breast milk. Plasma protein binding is reported to be 34 to 38%. The plasma half-life is about 1 hour.

Zidovudine is metabolised intracellularly to the antiviral triphosphate. It is also metabolised in the liver mainly to the inactive glucuronide and is excreted in the urine as unchanged drug and metabolite. As there is some tubular secretion, probenecid can delay excretion.

Reviews.

1. Acosta EP, *et al.* Clinical pharmacokinetics of zidovudine: an update. *Clin Pharmacokinet* 1996; **30:** 251–62.

Bioavailability. Absorption of oral zidovudine was delayed or reduced when the dose was taken with a meal compared with when taken after an overnight fast.[1-3] It was suggested that to achieve high peak plasma concentrations of zidovudine, it should be taken on an empty stomach. The bioavailability in HIV-positive patients is reported to be erratic[4,5] but not greatly reduced by diarrhoea.[5]

1. Unadkat JD, *et al.* Pharmacokinetics of oral zidovudine (azidothymidine) in patients with AIDS when administered with and without a high-fat meal. *AIDS* 1990; **4:** 229–32.
2. Lotterer E, *et al.* Decreased and variable systemic availability of zidovudine in patients with AIDS if administered with a meal. *Eur J Clin Pharmacol* 1991; **40:** 305–8.
3. Ruhnke M, *et al.* Effects of standard breakfast on pharmacokinetics of oral zidovudine in patients with AIDS. *Antimicrob Agents Chemother* 1993; **37:** 2153–8.
4. Macnab KA, *et al.* Erratic zidovudine bioavailable in HIV seropositive patients. *J Antimicrob Chemother* 1993; **31:** 421–8.
5. Zorza G, *et al.* Absorption of zidovudine in patients with diarrhoea. *Eur J Clin Pharmacol* 1993; **44:** 501–3.

Neonates. The pharmacokinetics of zidovudine in infants more than 14 days old are reported to be similar to those in adults. Following maternal administration the half-life of zidovudine in 7 neonates has been reported to be extended to a mean of 13 hours.[1] In infants receiving zidovudine, those under 14 days of age had lower total clearance, longer terminal half-life (about 3 hours), and higher bioavailability than older infants.[2] Zidovudine clearance was low and the half-life prolonged to about 7 hours in premature infants.[3]

1. O'Sullivan MJ, *et al.* The pharmacokinetics and safety of zidovudine in the third trimester of pregnancy for women infected with human immunodeficiency virus and their infants: phase 1 Acquired Immunodeficiency Syndrome Clinical Trials Group Study (protocol 082). *Am J Obstet Gynecol* 1993; **168:** 1510–16.
2. Boucher FD, *et al.* Phase 1 evaluation of zidovudine administered to infants exposed at birth to the human immunodeficiency virus. *J Pediatr* 1993; **122:** 137–44.
3. Mirochnick M, *et al.* Zidovudine pharmacokinetics in premature infants exposed to human immunodeficiency virus. *Antimicrob Agents Chemother* 1998; **42:** 808–12.

Pregnancy. In a study in 3 pregnant women with HIV infection,[1] the area under the concentration-time curve was reduced and the clearance of an oral dose increased during pregnancy when compared with up to 4 weeks postpartum. These results differed from those reported from another study which reported no differences during or after pregnancy.[2] This latter study, however, used values obtained no later than 48 hours postpartum for comparison, at which time it is unlikely that physiological functions would have returned to the nonpregnant state. Zidovudine and its glucuronide metabolite cross the placenta reaching concentrations in the fetal blood similar to those in maternal blood.[3,4] However, concentrations of zidovudine in the fetal CNS have been reported to be below those required to exert an anti-HIV effect.[5]

1. Watts DH, *et al.* Pharmacokinetic disposition of zidovudine during pregnancy. *J Infect Dis* 1991; **163:** 226–32.
2. O'Sullivan MJ, *et al.* The pharmacokinetics and safety of zidovudine in the third trimester of pregnancy for women infected with human immunodeficiency virus and their infants: phase 1 Acquired Immunodeficiency Syndrome Clinical Trials Group Study (protocol 082). *Am J Obstet Gynecol* 1993; **168:** 1510–16.
3. Gillet JY, *et al.* Fetoplacental passage of zidovudine. *Lancet* 1989; **ii:** 269–70.
4. Chavanet P, *et al.* Perinatal pharmacokinetics of zidovudine. *N Engl J Med* 1989; **321:** 1548–9.
5. Lyman WD, *et al.* Zidovudine concentrations in human fetal tissue: implications for perinatal AIDS. *Lancet* 1990; **335:** 1280–1.

Uses and Administration

Zidovudine is a nucleoside reverse transcriptase inhibitor structurally similar to thymidine. It has activity against retroviruses including HIV and is used in the management of HIV infection and AIDS. Treatment options for patients with HIV infection are changing rapidly with a trend towards initiating therapy with combinations of antiretroviral drugs at an early stage in the infection. Until recently zidovudine was given as monotherapy to those who had developed AIDS or AIDS-related complex and to symptomatic patients with early HIV infection (with blood CD4+ cell counts of less than 500 per mm^3) or to asymptomatic patients with CD4+ cell counts of less than 200 per mm^3 or 200 to 500 per mm^3 and rapidly falling. There is now support for the initiation of therapy in all patients with CD4+ cell counts below 500 per mm^3 unless the disease is stable and viral RNA levels remain low. It may also be considered for any patient with high viral RNA levels and/or rapidly declining CD4+ cell counts.

The optimum dose of zidovudine has yet to be established and there is a general trend towards the use of lower doses. Oral doses of 500 or 600 mg daily in two to six divided doses have been commonly used. An alternative regimen is 1000 mg daily in two divided doses.

For the prevention of maternal-fetal HIV transmission, zidovudine may be given after the fourteenth week of pregnancy until the beginning of labour in a dose of 100 mg five times daily by mouth. During labour and delivery, zidovudine is given by intravenous infusion of 2 mg per kg body-weight over 1 hour, then 1 mg per kg per hour until the umbilical cord is clamped. When a caesarean section is planned the intravenous infusion is started 4 hours before the operation. The newborn infant is given 2 mg per kg orally every 6 hours starting within 12 hours after birth and continuing for 6 weeks.

Zidovudine may be given by intravenous infusion of a solution containing 2 to 4 mg per mL over 1 hour for short term management of patients unable to take it by mouth. A suggested dose is 1 to 2 mg per kg body-weight every 4 hours, equivalent to an oral dose of 1.5 or 3 mg per kg every 4 hours.

The optimum dosage for children may vary from patient to patient, but a starting dose for children over 3 months of age of zidovudine 180 mg per m^2 body-surface every 6 hours (to a maximum of 200 mg every 6 hours) by mouth has been suggested. An equivalent dose by intravenous infusion would be 120 mg per m^2. Doses used have ranged from 120 to 180 mg per m^2 by mouth or 80 to 160 mg per m^2 by intravenous infusion, all given every 6 hours.

Blood tests should be carried out regularly as described under Precautions, above. If the white cell count or haemoglobin level fall, the dose should be reduced until there is evidence of recovery or treatment may be interrupted if toxicity is severe. Dosage adjustments may also be necessary in patients with renal or hepatic impairment.

Reviews.

1. Wilde MI, Langtry HD. Zidovudine: an update of its pharmacodynamic and pharmacokinetic properties, and therapeutic efficacy. *Drugs* 1993; **46:** 515–78.

Administration and dosage. A number of studies have been performed to determine the optimal dosage regimen of zidovudine and as a result there has been a general trend to use lower doses for both prophylaxis and treatment of HIV infection and AIDS. Doses studied in patients with AIDS have ranged from 400 to 1500 mg daily in a variety of divided-dose regimens.[1,2] These studies found that low-dose regimens were as effective as higher doses in terms of prolongation of survival and were better tolerated. Similar results were found in patients with AIDS-related complex[3] and asymptomatic HIV infection,[4] and it was concluded that doses above 400 to 600 mg daily[5,6] offered no clinical advantage. Although zidovudine should ideally be administered every 4 hours owing to its short half-life, patients have been reported to take it in three or even two daily doses,[7] and there is preliminary evidence that efficacy is unaffected.[8] Modified-release formulations are under development which may allow less frequent dosing while maintaining zidovudine plasma concentrations.

Dosage reduction or interruption of treatment may be necessary in patients who develop haematological toxicity. Alternative strategies to reduce toxicity have included intermittent therapy, administering zidovudine for 4 weeks out of every 6,[9] and alternating zidovudine with other antiretroviral drugs,[10] although the use of zidovudine in combination with other antiretrovirals may offset this problem.

1. Fischl MA, *et al.* A randomized controlled trial of a reduced daily dose of zidovudine in patients with the acquired immunodeficiency syndrome. *N Engl J Med* 1990; **323:** 1009–14.
2. Nordic Medical Research Councils' HIV Therapy Group. Double blind dose-response study of zidovudine in AIDS and advanced HIV infection. *Br Med J* 1992; **304:** 13–17.
3. Collier AC, *et al.* A pilot study of low-dose zidovudine in human immunodeficiency virus infection. *N Engl J Med* 1990; **323:** 1015–21.
4. Volberding PA, *et al.* Zidovudine in asymptomatic human immunodeficiency virus infection: a controlled trial in persons with fewer than 500 CD4-positive cells per cubic millimeter. *N Engl J Med* 1990; **322:** 941–9.
5. Gøtzshe PC. Zidovudine dosage. *Br Med J* 1993; **307:** 682–3.
6. McLeod GX, Hammer SM. Zidovudine: five years later. *Ann Intern Med* 1992; **117:** 487–501.
7. Clumeck N. Current use of anti-HIV drugs in AIDS. *J Antimicrob Chemother* 1993; **32** (suppl A): 133–8.
8. Shepp DH, *et al.* A comparative trial of zidovudine administered every four versus every twelve hours for the treatment of advanced HIV disease. *J Acquir Immune Defic Syndr Hum Retrovirol* 1997; **15:** 283–8.
9. Williams IG, *et al.* Intermittent zidovudine regimen in patients with symptomatic HIV infection and previous haematological toxicity. *Antiviral Chem Chemother* 1993; **4:** 139–43.
10. Skowron G, *et al.* Alternating and intermittent regimens of zidovudine and dideoxycytidine in patients with AIDS or AIDS-related complex. *Ann Intern Med* 1993; **118:** 321–30.

HIV infection and AIDS. As discussed on p.599, the use of antiretroviral drugs in HIV infection has changed following studies which indicated that combination therapy could improve response. Monotherapy with zidovudine reduced the incidence of opportunistic infections and mortality in patients with AIDS or ARC. Benefit might also be seen in other features of AIDS such as dementia (see HIV-associated Neurological Complications, below). Unfortunately such benefit was found to be transient[1-4] and treatment during the early stages of HIV infection, while delaying disease progression,[5-10] failed to produce improvements in long-term outcome or the quality of life;[8,10-12] in addition there are concerns about resistance.[13,14]

Therapy with a combination of zidovudine and other antiretroviral drugs given early in the infection might improve efficacy, minimise toxicity, and delay drug resistance. Results from the Delta study[15] and the US AIDS Clinical Trial Group 175 (ACTG 175) study[16] showed combination therapy to be more effective than monotherapy in antiretroviral-naive patients and led to immediate changes in clinical practice. In patients who had not received zidovudine before, both studies showed substantial reductions in mortality at 30 months in patients treated with zidovudine plus either didanosine or zalcitabine compared with those receiving zidovudine alone. ACTG 175 showed that didanosine alone was as effective as the combinations and superior to zidovudine alone. Smaller studies have reported similarly beneficial responses with zidovudine in combination with other nucleoside reverse transcriptase inhibitors,[17,18] although a study in patients with advanced HIV infection failed to show a benefit over zidovudine monotherapy.[19] Resistance to both zidovudine and lamivudine has developed during combination therapy.[20] In patients who had already received zidovudine therapy the use of combination therapy is not generally as effective as in zidovudine-naive patients,[15,16,19] although some improvements have been reported.[21-25] Triple therapy with zidovudine combined with another reverse transcriptase inhibitor and an HIV-protease inhibitor has been found to reduce viral loads more effectively than monotherapy or two-drug combination therapy.[26,27]

1. Fischl MA, *et al.* The efficacy of azidothymidine (AZT) in the treatment of patients with AIDS and AIDS-related complex: a double-blind, placebo-controlled trial. *N Engl J Med* 1987; **317:** 185–91.
2. Dournon E, *et al.* Effects of zidovudine in 365 consecutive patients with AIDS or AIDS-related complex. *Lancet* 1988; **ii:** 1297–1302.
3. Lundgren JD, *et al.* Comparison of long-term prognosis of patients with AIDS treated and not treated with zidovudine. *JAMA* 1994; **271:** 1088–92.
4. Kinloch-de Loës S, Perneger TV. Primary HIV infection: follow-up of patients initially randomized to zidovudine or placebo. *J Infect* 1997; **35:** 111–16.
5. Graham NMH, *et al.* The effects on survival of early treatment of human immunodeficiency virus infection. *N Engl J Med* 1992; **326:** 1037–42.
6. Fischl MA, *et al.* The safety and efficacy of zidovudine (AZT) in the treatment of subjects with mildly symptomatic human immunodeficiency virus type 1 (HIV) infection: a double-blind, placebo-controlled trial. *Ann Intern Med* 1990; **112:** 727–37.
7. Volberding PA, *et al.* Zidovudine in asymptomatic human immunodeficiency virus infection: a controlled trial in persons with fewer than 500 CD4-positive cells per cubic millimeter. *N Engl J Med* 1990; **322:** 941–9.
8. Hamilton JD, *et al.* A controlled trial of early versus late treatment with zidovudine in symptomatic human immunodeficiency virus infection. *N Engl J Med* 1992; **326:** 437–43.
9. Cooper DA, *et al.* Zidovudine in persons with asymptomatic HIV infection and CD4+ cell counts greater than 400 per cubic millimeter. *N Engl J Med* 1993; **329:** 297–303.
10. Concorde Coordinating Committee. Concorde: MRC/ANRS randomised double-blind controlled trial of immediate and deferred zidovudine in symptom-free HIV infection. *Lancet* 1994; **343:** 871–81.
11. Volberding PA, *et al.* The duration of zidovudine benefit in persons with asymptomatic HIV infection: prolonged evaluation of protocol 019 of the AIDS clinical trials group. *JAMA* 1994; **272:** 437–42.
12. Lenderking WR, *et al.* Evaluation of the quality of life associated with zidovudine treatment in asymptomatic human immunodeficiency virus infection *N Engl J Med* 1994; **330:** 738–43.
13. Ogino MT, *et al.* Development and significance of zidovudine resistance in children infected with human immunodeficiency virus. *J Pediatr* 1993; **123:** 1–8.
14. Husson RN, *et al.* High-level resistance to zidovudine but not to zalcitabine or didanosine in human immunodeficiency virus from children receiving antiretroviral therapy. *J Pediatr* 1993; **123:** 9–16.
15. Delta Coordinating Committee. Delta: a randomised double-blind controlled trial comparing combinations of zidovudine plus didanosine or zalcitabine with zidovudine alone in HIV-infected individuals. *Lancet* 1996; **348:** 283–91.
16. Hammer SM, *et al.* A trial comparing nucleoside monotherapy with combination therapy in HIV-infected adults with CD4 cell counts from 200 to 500 per cubic millimeter. *N Engl J Med* 1996; **335:** 1081–90.
17. Eron JJ, *et al.* Treatment with lamivudine, zidovudine, or both in HIV-positive with 200 to 500 CD4+ cells per cubic millimeter. *N Engl J Med* 1995; **333:** 1662–9.
18. Katlama C, *et al.* Safety and efficacy of lamivudine-zidovudine combination therapy in antiretroviral-naive patients: a randomized controlled comparison with zidovudine monotherapy. *JAMA* 1996; **276:** 118–25.
19. Saravolatz LD, *et al.* Zidovudine alone or in combination with didanosine or zalcitabine in HIV-infected patients with the acquired immunodeficiency syndrome or fewer than 200 CD4 cells per cubic millimeter. *N Engl J Med* 1996; **335:** 1099–1106.
20. Miller V, *et al.* Dual resistance to zidovudine and lamivudine in patients treated with zidovudine-lamivudine combination therapy: association with therapy failure. *J Infect Dis* 1998; **177:** 1521–32.
21. Bartlett JA, *et al.* Lamivudine plus zidovudine compared with zalcitabine plus zidovudine in patients with HIV infection: a randomized, double-blind, placebo-controlled trial. *Ann Intern Med* 1996; **125:** 161–72.
22. Staszewski S, *et al.* Safety and efficacy of lamivudine-zidovudine combination therapy in zidovudine-experienced patients: a randomized controlled comparison with zidovudine monotherapy. *JAMA* 1996; **276:** 111–17.
23. D'Aquila RT, *et al.* Nevirapine, zidovudine, and didanosine compared with zidovudine and didanosine in patients with HIV-1 infection: a randomized, double-blind, placebo-controlled trial. *Ann Intern Med* 1996; **124:** 1019–30.
24. Collier AC, *et al.* Treatment of human immunodeficiency virus infection with saquinavir, zidovudine, and zalcitabine. *N Engl J Med* 1996; **334:** 101–17.
25. Graham NMH, *et al.* Survival in HIV-infected patients who have received zidovudine: comparison of combination therapy with sequential monotherapy and continued zidovudine monotherapy. *Ann Intern Med* 1996; **124:** 1031–8.
26. Hammer SM, *et al.* A controlled trial of two nucleoside analogues plus indinavir in persons with human immunodeficiency virus infection and CD4 cell counts of 200 per cubic millimeter or less. *N Engl J Med* 1997; **337:** 725–33.
27. Gulick RM, *et al.* Treatment with indinavir, zidovudine, and lamivudine in adults with human immunodeficiency virus infection and prior antiretroviral therapy. *N Engl J Med* 1997; **337:** 734–9.

HIV-ASSOCIATED MALIGNANCIES. As discussed on p.496, zidovudine in combination with interferons has been advocated for the management of Kaposi's sarcoma in HIV-infected patients with a CD4+ count of 200 cells per μL or above.[1-5]

In patients with AIDS-associated non-Hodgkin's lymphoma, zidovudine in combination with interferon alfa[6] and with methotrexate[7] has been reported to produce beneficial responses in small numbers of patients.

1. Northfelt DW. Treatment of Kaposi's sarcoma: current guidelines and future perspectives. *Drugs* 1994; **48:** 569–82.
2. Kovacs JA, *et al.* Combined zidovudine and interferon-α therapy in patients with Kaposi sarcoma and the acquired immunodeficiency syndrome (AIDS). *Ann Intern Med* 1989; **111:** 280–7.
3. Brockmeyer NH, *et al.* Regression of Kaposi's sarcoma and improvement of performance status by a combined interferon β and zidovudine therapy in AIDS patients. *J Invest Dermatol* 1989; **92:** 776.
4. Krown SE, *et al.* Interferon-α with zidovudine: safety, tolerance, and clinical and virologic effects in patients with Kaposi sarcoma associated with the acquired immunodeficiency syndrome (AIDS). *Ann Intern Med* 1990; **112:** 812–21.
5. Edlin BR, *et al.* Interferon-alpha plus zidovudine in HIV infection. *Lancet* 1989; **i:** 156.
6. Harrington WJ, *et al.* Azothymidine and interferon-α are active in AIDS-associated small non-cleaved cell lymphoma but not large-cell lymphoma. *Lancet* 1996; **348:** 833.
7. Tosi P, *et al.* 3′-Azido-3′-deoxythymidine + methotrexate as a novel antineoplastic combination in the treatment of human immunodeficiency virus-related non-Hodgkin's lymphomas. *Blood* 1997; **89:** 419–25.

HIV-ASSOCIATED NEUROLOGICAL COMPLICATIONS. Dementia is one of the complications associated with HIV infection and AIDS (see p.600). In a retrospective study of AIDS patients it was noted that the incidence of dementia fell after the institution of zidovudine therapy.[1] Despite criticisms of this study,[2] others have also noted an improvement in AIDS-related neurological disorders with zidovudine.[3-7] The improvement was sustained for up to 18 months in one patient.[3] Zidovudine given intrathecally for AIDS-related dementia produced improvement in 3 patients, with minimal toxicity,[8] but no improvement was observed in a further patient given zidovudine intrathecally and intravenously.[9]

1. Portegies P, *et al.* Declining incidence of AIDS dementia complex after introduction of zidovudine treatment. *Br Med J* 1989; **299:** 819–21. Correction. *ibid.*; 1141.
2. Morriss R, House A. Zidovudine in AIDS dementia complex. *Br Med J* 1989; **299:** 1218.
3. Yarchoan R, *et al.* Long-term administration of 3′-azido-2′,3′-dideoxythymidine to patients with AIDS-related neurological disease. *Ann Neurol* 1988; **23** (suppl): S82–7.
4. Schmitt FA, *et al.* Neuropsychological outcome of zidovudine (AZT) treatment of patients with AIDS and AIDS-related complex. *N Engl J Med* 1988; **319:** 1573–8.
5. Conway B, *et al.* Human immunodeficiency virus-associated progressive multifocal leukoencephalopathy: apparent response to 3′-azido-3′-deoxythymidine. *Rev Infect Dis* 1990; **12:** 479–82.
6. Chiesi A, *et al.* Epidemiology of AIDS dementia complex in Europe. *J Acquir Immune Defic Syndr Hum Retrovirol* 1996; **11:** 39–44.
7. Evers S, *et al.* Impact of antiretroviral treatment on AIDS dementia: a longitudinal prospective event-related potential study. *J Acquir Immune Defic Syndr Hum Retrovirol* 1998; **17:** 143–8.
8. Routy JP, *et al.* Intrathecal zidovudine for AIDS dementia. *Lancet* 1990; **336:** 248.
9. Lucht F, *et al.* Intrathecal zidovudine for AIDS dementia. *Lancet* 1990; **336:** 813.

HIV infection prophylaxis. Antiretroviral drugs are becoming more widely accepted for chemoprophylaxis after exposure to HIV infection. Zidovudine is commonly used in combination with other antiretroviral drugs, such as lamivudine and an HIV-protease inhibitor, after occupational exposure with a high risk of infection. For suggested regimens, see p.601.

Zidovudine has also been shown to be of value in reducing vertical transmission from mother to infant.[1] A typical dosage regimen is given under Uses and Administration, above, but the effectiveness of lower doses is being assessed. Abbreviated regimens, even begun as late as the first 48 hours of life, do seem still to be of benefit.[2]

1. Sperling RS, *et al.* Maternal viral load, zidovudine treatment, and the risk of transmission of human immunodeficiency virus type 1 from mother to infant. *N Engl J Med* 1996; **335:** 1621–9.
2. Wade NA, *et al.* Abbreviated regimens of zidovudine prophylaxis and perinatal transmission of the human immunodeficiency virus. *N Engl J Med* 1998; **339:** 1409–14.

Preparations

USP 23: Zidovudine Capsules; Zidovudine Injection; Zidovudine Oral Solution.

Proprietary Preparations (details are given in Part 3)
Aust.: Retrovir; ***Austral.:*** Retrovir; ***Belg.:*** Retrovir; ***Canad.:*** Novo-AZT; Retrovir; ***Fr.:*** Retrovir; ***Ger.:*** Retrovir; ***Irl.:*** Retrovir; ***Ital.:*** Retrovir; ***Neth.:*** Retrovir; ***Norw.:*** Retrovir; ***S.Afr.:*** Retrovir; ***Spain:*** Retrovir; ***Swed.:*** Retrovir; ***Switz.:*** Retrovir; ***UK:*** Retrovir; ***USA:*** Retrovir.

Multi-ingredient: ***UK:*** Combivir; ***USA:*** Combivir.

Anxiolytic Sedatives Hypnotics and Antipsychotics

The drugs in this chapter include those used in the management of anxiety disorders (anxiolytic sedatives, formerly called minor tranquillisers), those used to produce sleep (hypnotics), and drugs used in the treatment of psychoses (antipsychotics, formerly called major tranquillisers). The term neuroleptic is sometimes used to describe those antipsychotics that have effects on the extrapyramidal system. There is no sharp distinction between anxiolytics and hypnotics; the difference in action is mainly one of degree and the same drug or group of drugs can have both effects, larger doses being necessary to produce a state of sleep.

The benzodiazepines (typified by Diazepam, p.661) have replaced the barbiturates (typified by Amylobarbitone, p.641) and related sedatives as the major group of drugs used as anxiolytics and hypnotics. Some benzodiazepines are also used for their muscle relaxant and anticonvulsant properties. Newer anxiolytics include buspirone (p.643), a drug with antiserotonin properties.

The antipsychotics (typified by Chlorpromazine, p.649) include the butyrophenones, the diphenylbutylpiperidines, the indole derivatives, the phenothiazines, and the thioxanthenes. Some antipsychotics such as clozapine (p.657), risperidone (p.690), olanzapine (p.683), quetiapine (p.690), and amisulpride (p.641) are often referred to as atypical antipsychotics because of their reduced tendency to cause the extrapyramidal effects typical of antipsychotics.

General references.

1. WHO. Evaluation of methods for the treatment of mental disorders. *WHO Tech Rep Ser 812* 1991.

Anxiety disorders

Anxiety is an emotional condition characterised by feelings such as apprehension and fear accompanied by physical symptoms such as tachycardia, increased respiration, sweating, and tremor. It is a normal emotion but when it is severe and disabling it becomes pathological.

Anxiety disorders are difficult to define and various classifications exist. In **acute stress disorder** anxiety is associated with a recent extremely stressful event such as bereavement. Such anxiety is likely to resolve within a few weeks but in **generalised anxiety disorders** there is persistent pervasive anxiety usually lasting 6 months or more. Symptoms include motor tension, autonomic hyperactivity, irritability, and loss of concentration.

The first step in the management of anxiety that cannot be attributed to an underlying disease is the use of psychological treatments. Such therapy can be effective in most types of anxiety. If unsuccessful, short-term treatment with a *benzodiazepine* may be considered. Although benzodiazepines can exert an effect very rapidly, possibly even after the first dose,[1] their use is limited as they can cause serious problems of dependence (see under Dependence and Withdrawal in Diazepam, p.661). In the UK the Committee on Safety of Medicines has recommended that benzodiazepines should only be used for the short-term relief (two to four weeks only) of anxiety that is severe, disabling, or subjecting the individual to unacceptable distress and is occurring alone or in association with insomnia or short-term psychosomatic, organic, or psychotic illness.[2] These recommendations are similar to those of the Royal College of Psychiatrists in the UK.[3] Tolerance may develop to the anxiolytic effects of benzodiazepines although this appears to be less likely than tolerance to the psychomotor effects. In general, there are no distinct advantages for any one benzodiazepine in the treatment of anxiety disorders.[4]

Buspirone, an azaspirodecanedione, appears to have similar efficacy to the benzodiazepines although it might have a slow onset of action. Advantages over the benzodiazepines are reported to be lack of euphoriant effect, less sedation, and a lower potential for dependence. Its efficacy is reduced in patients who have had previous extensive use of benzodiazepines.[5,6] Experience with buspirone is still, however, relatively limited.

Other drugs used as alternatives to the benzodiazepines for the treatment of anxiety disorders include the *tricyclic antidepressants*.[6,7] Some consider them preferable to benzodiazepines for the treatment of generalised anxiety disorders, especially when medium or long-term therapy is necessary or when depression is also present.[5,8] It may be several weeks before their effects are apparent, therefore combined therapy with benzodiazepines may be required initially. *Selective serotonin reuptake inhibitors* (SSRIs) have been used as alternatives to the tricyclics.

Benefits of *beta blockers* in the treatment of anxiety do not appear to be particularly great and they are probably most useful for the control of the physical symptoms of anxiety such as tremor, tachycardia, and palpitations.[9] *Antihistamines* such as *hydroxyzine* have also been sometimes used in anxious patients.[5,10] However, there appears to be little evidence of their efficacy[5] and the use of antihistamines solely for their sedative effect in anxiety is not considered appropriate. *Antipsychotics* have been used by some in anxiety but ideally should be reserved for anxiety associated with psychotic disorders or primary anxiety refractory to other treatment.[10]

Panic attacks are severe, sudden, unexpected, recurrent exacerbations of anxiety. During an attack there is a feeling of fear, terror, and impending doom or even death accompanied by autonomic symptoms. If behavioural or cognitive therapy fails in the management of panic disorders drug therapy can then be tried but it may need to be prolonged as there is a high rate of relapse on discontinuation.[11] *Tricyclic antidepressants* or *SSRIs* can reduce the frequency of attacks and can often prevent them completely but there is no consensus on which are the treatment of choice.[12-14] *MAOIs* such as *phenelzine* are effective and may be useful in patients unresponsive to tricyclics and SSRIs.[14] Other antidepressants are being evaluated in panic attacks. It may take several weeks before the effects of antidepressants are seen and initially there may be an increase in anxiety and the frequency of panic attacks. *Benzodiazepines* are sometimes used as adjunct therapy until antidepressants exert their full effect.[10,14] Short courses of benzodiazepines may also be of use in patients who cannot tolerate or who are refractory to antidepressants[10,12] but any benefit may be outweighed by the risk of dependence.[13] There is little evidence to support the use of *beta blockers*, but they may control physical symptoms. Other drugs that might produce beneficial effects in some patients include *valproic acid*[12,14] and possibly *clonidine*.[15]

Phobic disorders consist of an irrational or exaggerated fear of, and a wish to avoid, specific objects, activities, or situations. As there is a strong link between **agoraphobia** and panic attacks (see above) it is treated similarly. Simple or specific phobias are usually unresponsive to pharmacotherapy and respond better to behaviour therapy. *MAOIs* such as *phenelzine* appear to be effective in social phobias and can improve anticipatory anxiety and functional disability;[10,11,16-18] encouraging results have also been obtained with *moclobemide*.[16,18] SSRIs such as paroxetine are also considered to be effective. Other drugs which have been reported[16,17,19,20] to be of some benefit include *clonazepam*. *Beta blockers* may help to reduce the physical symptoms in performance anxiety.[9-11,17,19]

Obsessive-compulsive disorder is associated with intrusive, recurrent, obsessional thoughts and/or repetitive compulsive behaviour (e.g. hand washing) performed in a ritualistic manner. A combination of pharmacological, behavioural, and psychosocial methods appears to have the most successful long-term outcome in the treatment of obsessive-compulsive disorder.[21] The only drugs that have been found to be effective when used alone in obsessive-compulsive disorders are antidepressants which inhibit reuptake of serotonin.[22-24] Of these, efficacy has best been demonstrated for *clomipramine* and the SSRIs *fluoxetine* and *fluvoxamine*[24,25] but generally there is no strong opinion on which to use first.[24-26] Their effect appears to be independent of their antidepressant activity.[22] Few patients respond completely but many improve to some degree.[21] It may take 4 to 6 weeks before any response is obtained and up to about 12 weeks to achieve an optimal effect.[10,24,26] If one serotonin reuptake inhibitor fails then another can be tried.[24] The optimum duration of treatment remains to be determined. Some suggest therapy for at least a year or longer[21,26,27] but many patients relapse when drug therapy is withdrawn and prolonged therapy may be necessary. Initial studies suggest that patients may be maintained on reduced dosage.[28] Gradual withdrawal over several months may be more successful if patients are also receiving behavioural therapy.[21] Drugs such as *buspirone* and some *antipsychotics* have also been tried as adjuncts when patients are refractory to serotonin reuptake inhibitors and behavioural therapy but results have been variable.[21,22,24,27] *Benzodiazepines* have been tried as alternatives to serotonin reuptake inhibitors but they are considered to be unsuitable because of the problems associated with prolonged therapy.[27]

Post-traumatic stress disorder anxiety is precipitated when a patient recalls and re-experiences a traumatic experience. Patients may also suffer from negative symptoms such as avoidance, alienation, emotional numbness, and social withdrawal. The main treatment is psychotherapy.[11,29] Drug therapy is largely aimed at accompanying symptoms of anxiety or depression.[11] *Tricyclic antidepressants* and *MAOIs* may also help to reduce traumatic recollections and nightmares and to repress flashbacks.[29] Negative symptoms are usually resistant to pharmacotherapy. A minimum of 8 weeks of treatment is considered necessary to judge the efficacy of treatment.[29] *Antiepileptics* such as *carbamazepine* and *sodium valproate* appear to improve symptoms of hyper-reactivity, violent behaviour, and angry outbursts but only a small number of patients have been studied.

Anxiety may be present with other disorders such as depression in **mixed anxiety and depressive disorders** the management of which is discussed under Depression on p.271.

1. Ashton H. Guidelines for the rational use of benzodiazepines: when and what to use. *Drugs* 1994; **48:** 25–40.
2. Committee on Safety of Medicines. Benzodiazepines, dependence and withdrawal symptoms. *Current Problems 21* 1988.
3. Royal College of Psychiatrists. Benzodiazepines and dependence: a college statement. *Bull R Coll Psychiatrists* 1988; **12:** 107–8.
4. Shader RI, Greenblatt DJ. Benzodiazepines in anxiety disorders. *N Engl J Med* 1993; **328:** 1398–1405.
5. Lader M. Treatment of anxiety. *Br Med J* 1994; **309:** 321–4.
6. Nutt DJ. The psychopharmacology of anxiety. *Br J Hosp Med* 1996; **55:** 187–91.
7. Schweizer E. The role of antidepressants in the treatment of generalized anxiety disorder (GAD). *Eur Neuropsychopharmacol* 1993; **3** (special issue): 213–4.
8. Lader M, *et al.* Royal College of Psychiatrists. Guidelines for the management of patients with generalised anxiety. *Psychiatr Bull* 1992; **16:** 560–5.
9. Tyrer P. Current status of β-blocking drugs in the treatment of anxiety disorders. *Drugs* 1988; **36:** 773–83.
10. Brown CS, *et al.* A practical update on anxiety disorders and their pharmacologic treatment. *Arch Intern Med* 1991; **151:** 873–84.
11. Michels R, Marzuk PM. Progress in psychiatry. *N Engl J Med* 1993; **329:** 628–38.
12. Johnson MR, *et al.* Panic disorder: pathophysiology and drug treatment. *Drugs* 1995; **49:**328—44.
13. Anonymous. Stopping panic attacks. *Drug Ther Bull* 1997; **35:** 58–62.
14. Bennett JA, *et al.* A risk-benefit assessment of pharmacological treatments for panic disorder. *Drug Safety* 1998; **18:** 419–30.
15. Puzantian T, Hart LL. Clonidine in panic disorder. *Ann Pharmacother* 1993; **27:** 1351–3.

16. Liebowitz MR. Pharmacotherapy of social phobia. *J Clin Psychiatry* 1993; **54** (suppl): 31–5.
17. den Boer JA. Social phobia: epidemiology, recognition, and treatment. *Br Med J* 1997; **315:** 796–800.
18. Hale AS. Anxiety. *Br Med J* 1997; **314:** 1886–9.
19. Healy D. Social phobia in primary care. *Prim Care Psychiatry* 1995; **1:** 31–8.
20. Stein MB. How shy is too shy? *Lancet* 1996; **347:** 1131–2.
21. Rasmussen SA, *et al.* Current issues in the pharmacologic management of obsessive compulsive disorder. *J Clin Psychiatry* 1993; **54** (suppl): 4–9.
22. Black JL. Obsessive compulsive disorder: a clinical update. *Mayo Clin Proc* 1992; **67:** 266–75.
23. Piccinelli M, *et al.* Efficacy of drug treatment in obsessive-compulsive disorder: a meta-analytic review. *Br J Psychiatry* 1995; **166:** 424–43.
24. Carpenter LL, *et al.* A risk-benefit assessment of drugs used in the management of obsessive-compulsive disorder. *Drug Safety* 1996; **15:** 116–34.
25. Anonymous. Selective serotonin reuptake inhibitors in obsessive-compulsive disorder. *Drug Ther Bull* 1995; **33:** 47–8.
26. March JS, *et al.* Expert Consensus Guideline Series: treatment of obsessive-compulsive disorder. *J Clin Psychiatry* 1997; **58** (suppl 4): 1–73.
27. Zohar J, *et al.* Current concepts in the pharmacological treatment of obsessive-compulsive disorder. *Drugs* 1992; **43:** 210–18.
28. Mundo E, *et al.* Long-term pharmacotherapy of obsessive-compulsive disorder: a double-blind controlled study. *J Clin Psychopharmacol* 1997; **17:** 4–10.
29. McIvor RJ, Turner SW. Drug treatment in post-traumatic stress disorder. *Br J Hosp Med* 1995; **53:** 501–6.

Extrapyramidal disorders

Ballism. Ballism, sometimes called hemiballism or hemiballismus because it is usually unilateral, consists of involuntary flinging movements of the upper extremities and most often results from acute vascular infarction or haemorrhage of the subthalamic nucleus. It often improves spontaneously but dopamine-blocking antipsychotics such as haloperidol or dopamine-depleting drugs such as tetrabenazine may be needed to control severe symptoms. Surgery may be necessary in severe cases.

Chorea. Chorea is characterised by brief involuntary muscle contractions and an inability to sustain voluntary contractions. It may be related to neurological abnormalities in the caudate nucleus and putamen of the striatum as well as other basal ganglia structures. Overactivity of dopaminergic nigrostriatal pathways and depletion of gamma-aminobutyric acid (GABA) and acetylcholine may also play a part. Chorea may be an adverse effect of some drugs, including antipsychotics, levodopa, and oral contraceptives; it may also be a symptom of a number of underlying disorders such as systemic lupus erythematosus.

Huntington's chorea (Huntington's disease, progressive hereditary chorea) is an autosomal dominantly inherited disease characterised by chorea, behavioural disturbances, and a progressive decline in cognitive function culminating in dementia and death. Symptoms usually appear in mid-life, with death following after about 15 years, although there are also juvenile-onset forms. Westphal variant, a form commonest in children, tends to be characterised more by rigidity than by chorea.

Sydenham's chorea (St Vitus' dance; Chorea Minor) is an acute, usually self-limiting disorder with an autoimmune basis, characterised by chorea and behavioural disturbances. It commonly occurs about 6 months after rheumatic fever but is now rare since the incidence of rheumatic fever has declined. It may also arise during pregnancy (chorea gravidarum).

Treatment of chorea is symptomatic only and does not alter the progressive decline of Huntington's chorea; Sydenham's chorea resolves spontaneously within weeks or months but antibiotic prophylaxis to prevent recurrence of rheumatic fever (p.140) has been recommended. Other forms of chorea may resolve with treatment of the underlying disorder or withdrawal of any causative drug.

Tetrabenazine has been used effectively in chorea, although not all patients respond, and it may produce depression. The mode of action is thought to involve depletion of striatal dopamine. *Reserpine*, which has a similar action and effects, has also been used.

Phenothiazines such as *chlorpromazine, fluphenazine,* and *thioridazine* have dopamine-receptor blocking activity and have also been used to treat chorea. Other antipsychotics with a similar mode of action that have been used include *haloperidol, pimozide, sulpiride,* and *tiapride*. Adverse effects such as tardive dyskinesias may limit the use of antipsychotics, and some suggest that the minimum dose possible should be administered; attempts to control choreiform movements completely are not recommended. In addition to improving chorea, antipsychotics may also be of value in controlling the behavioural symptoms associated with Huntington's chorea; anxiolytics and antidepressants may also be used.

Other drugs that have been tried with some degree of success in a limited number of patients include *carbamazepine*. The use of drugs to increase GABA activity has been of little value. Implantation of porcine fetal neural cells is being studied.

Levodopa, the metabolic precursor of dopamine, generally exacerbates the symptoms of Huntington's chorea and this effect was used diagnostically to identify patients who had not yet developed the symptoms of Huntington's chorea by provoking chorea. However, this test which was both distressing and inaccurate has been abandoned. The identification of a gene marker for Huntington's chorea now makes it possible to identify carriers of the abnormal gene.

References.

1. Marsden CD. Basal ganglia disease. *Lancet* 1982; **ii:** 1141–6.
2. Kremer B, *et al.* A worldwide study of the Huntington's disease mutation: the sensitivity and specificity of measuring CAG repeats. *N Engl J Med* 1994; **330:** 1401–6.

Tics. Tics may manifest as sudden, involuntary, brief, isolated, repetitive movements which may be simple (e.g. eye blinking, nose twitching, or head jerking) or complex (e.g. touching, jumping, or kicking); they may also be sensory in nature or may present in a vocal or phonic way and may range from simple clearing of the throat to more complex symptoms such as echolalia (involuntary repetition of others speech) or coprolalia (involuntary and inappropriate swearing). Symptoms can usually be suppressed voluntarily and may increase with stress and decrease with distraction. Some tics persist during sleep. The most common cause is **Tourette's syndrome** (Gilles de la Tourette's syndrome), in which behavioural disturbances accompany the tics. It is mainly a genetic disorder with an onset during childhood but may also be precipitated by various substances (e.g. antipsychotics), trauma, or viral encephalitis.

Most patients' symptoms wax and wane and behavioural therapy and reassurance may be sufficient to resolve mild tics. Drug treatment may be necessary when tics are severe enough to cause discomfort or embarrassment. Dopamine blockers, usually pimozide or haloperidol, often decrease the frequency and severity of tics and may improve any accompanying behavioural disturbances. Superiority of either drug in terms of efficacy or adverse effects has not been clearly demonstrated. It is usually recommended that doses are titrated to as low as possible bearing in mind that optimum treatment does not necessarily lead to the complete control of symptoms. The risk of developing serious adverse effects such as tardive dyskinesia with these drugs should be balanced against the perceived benefits of treatment. Medication can often be discontinued after a few years. Alternative drugs may be required for those unresponsive to or intolerant of haloperidol or pimozide. Other drugs that are also used in the management of tics and/or behavioural aspects of Tourette's syndrome include clonidine and sulpiride; clonazepam, fluphenazine, risperidone, and tiapride have also been tried. For drugs used in the treatment of comorbid disorders commonly associated with Tourette's syndrome, such as obsessive-compulsive disorder and attention deficit hyperactivity disorder, see above and p.1476 respectively. Nicotine has been reported to produce benefit when used alone or with haloperidol in patients whose symptoms were not satisfactorily controlled with haloperidol.

References.

1. Sandor P. Clinical management of Tourette's syndrome and associated disorders. *Can J Psychiatry* 1995; **40:** 577–83.
2. Peterson BS. Considerations of natural history and pathophysiology in the psychopharmacology of Tourette's syndrome. *J Clin Psychiatry* 1996; **57** (suppl 9): 24–34.
3. Robertson MM, Stern JS. Gilles de la Tourette syndrome. *Br J Hosp Med* 1997; **58:** 253–6.

Hypochondriasis

Hypochondriasis (hypochondriacal neurosis) is a morbid preoccupation with one's health characterised by a fear or belief that normal bodily sensations are indicative of serious disease. It persists despite medical reassurance and management is difficult. If hypochondriasis is associated with a psychiatric disorder, treatment is aimed at the primary condition.

Pimozide is used in the management of monosymptomatic hypochondriacal psychoses. Most often reported is its use in patients with delusions of parasitic infestation. A retrospective study of 282 patients revealed that 66 had been treated with pimozide: 44 of these responded and 16 did not; 6 were lost to follow-up.[1] The response varied from total disappearance of the delusion to some improvement. As a rule relapse occurred on stopping treatment but control could be re-established on starting again. A few patients had prolonged remissions. An earlier double-blind study in 11 patients also supports this use of pimozide.[2] It has also been reported that pimozide often reduces or abolishes symptoms in patients with delusions of venereal disease.[3]

1. Lyell A. Delusions of parasitosis. *Br J Dermatol* 1983; **108:** 485–99.
2. Hamann K, Avnstorp C. Delusions of infestation treated by pimozide: a double-blind crossover clinical study. *Acta Derm Venereol (Stockh)* 1982; **62:** 55–8.
3. Goldmeier D. ABC of sexually transmitted diseases: psychosexual problems. *Br Med J* 1984; **288:** 704–5.

Psychoses

Psychoses and psychotic disorders are terms that have been used to describe a collection of severe psychiatric disorders in which the patient has disordered thinking and loses contact with reality due to delusions and/or hallucinations. There may be accompanying mood or behavioural disturbances. *Organic psychoses* arise from organic brain disease produced by toxic insults, metabolic disturbances, infections, or structural abnormalities and may be acute (delirium) or chronic (dementia) in nature.

Disturbed behaviour. Drug therapy is sometimes indicated for the immediate control of severely disturbed, agitated, or violent behaviour associated with a variety of conditions such as toxic delirium, brain damage, mania (p.273), or other psychotic disorders. Antipsychotics and benzodiazepines, either alone or in combination, are commonly used for disturbed behaviour. There is little agreement as to the best antipsychotic for these indications, selection depending mainly on the condition of the patient and the adverse effect profile of the drug. The high-potency butyrophenone haloperidol is commonly used for **acutely disturbed behaviour**. Benzodiazepines such as diazepam and lorazepam are valuable sedatives for the disturbed or delirious patient. A combination of haloperidol and lorazepam allows the use of lower doses of each drug and has been advocated by some workers.

Several drugs have been used or tried as alternatives to antipsychotics for the management of disturbed behaviour. Those drugs that have had some success in the control of symptoms such as agitation, aggression, rage, or violent behaviour include beta blockers, lithium, carbamazepine, and valproate. Buspirone and antidepressants such as the selective serotonin reuptake inhibitors and trazodone may also be useful. Naltrexone has produced some benefit in patients with self-injurious behaviour.

Antipsychotics appear to be modestly effective for the control of behavioural symptoms associated with chronic conditions such as senile **dementia** or Alzheimer's disease (p.1386). However, much concern has been expressed with regard to overuse and the risk of toxicity. Antipsychotics can themselves precipitate confusion or exacerbate dementia and may hasten cognitive decline. Excessive sedation resulting from their use may increase the risk of falls, incontinence, and drowsiness, and interfere with the performance of motor skills. Elderly patients with dementia, especially Lewy-body dementia, are reported to be highly susceptible to the extrapyramidal adverse effects of antipsychotics and the reaction can be life-threatening. Antipsychotics are used only after careful consideration of the causes of disturbed behaviour and the benefits and risks of antipsychotic treatment. Very low doses are given at first and increased gradually according to clinical response and development of side-effects; the necessity for continued use is reviewed periodically. Again, there is no agreement over the choice of antipsychotic. Atypical antipsychotics, which may be less likely to produce extrapyramidal symptoms, are less well studied than conventional antipsychotics in patients with dementia and any advantage remains to be determined. The sedative drug, chlormethiazole, may be a useful alternative to antipsychotics for the control of agitated behaviour in elderly patients, generally causing fewer side-effects; respiratory depression, excessive sedation, and dependence may, however, be a problem. Benzodiazepines are not generally indicated for the management of elderly demented patients because of the risks of dependence with continued use, disinhibiting effects, and the special problems of these drugs in old people (see the Elderly, under Diazepam, p.662). They are not as effective as antipsychotics in reducing behavioural problems, but may be useful in short courses for the management of severe anxiety disorders, or given as required for patients who only have rare episodes of agitation.

The use of antipsychotics in the control of **disturbed behaviour in children** is controversial and can probably be justified only in severe cases resistant to other therapy. Autistic and mentally retarded children are among those who may require antipsychotics on a short-term basis. Some workers suggest the use of high-potency antipsychotics such as haloperidol on the grounds that they are less likely to cause sedation or impair arousal, cognitive function, and learning; others appear to favour a drug such as thioridazine which carries a lower risk of dystonic reactions. The tendency of antipsychotics to lower the seizure threshold is an important consideration in autistic children who are at a higher than normal risk of seizure disorders.

Antipsychotics and benzodiazepines have been used to control the symptoms of **drug-induced delirium**.

Benzodiazepines are favoured for palliative treatment of agitation and restlessness in patients with **terminal restlessness** since antipsychotics may exacerbate the existing tendency to myoclonus and convulsions in these patients and may not produce adequate sedation in the terminal phase.

Deviant sexual behaviour including paraphilias is rare in women therefore treatment is focussed largely towards men and consists mainly of psychotherapy and the use of libido-suppressing drugs such as the anti-androgens. The use of such pharmacotherapy is controversial and involves not only medical but legal issues. Drugs used for their anti-androgenic action include cyproterone and medroxyprogesterone. Gonadorelin analogues have also been tried for suppression of libido. Medroxyprogesterone has also been used for the control of intrusive disinhibited sexual behaviour in elderly men with dementia. There have been some case reports of fluoxetine being used with some success in the control of fantasies associated with various paraphilias. The butyrophenone antipsychotic benperidol is used in some countries for the management of sexual deviations but its value is not established. In general few well-controlled blinded studies have been conducted into the pharmacological treatment of sexual offenders and there is no evidence that drug treatment reduces the recidivism rate.

1. Schneider LS, *et al.* A metaanalysis of controlled trials of neuroleptic treatment in dementia. *J Am Geriatr Soc* 1990; **38:** 553–63.
2. Anonymous. Management of behavioural emergencies. *Drug Ther Bull* 1991; **29:** 62–4. Correction. *ibid.*; 80.
3. Fish DN. Treatment of delirium in the critically ill patient. *Clin Pharm* 1991; **10:** 456–66.
4. Druckenbrod RW, *et al.* As-needed dosing of antipsychotic drugs: limitations and guidelines for use in the elderly agitated patient. *Ann Pharmacother* 1993; **27:** 645–8.
5. Richer M, Crismon ML. Pharmacotherapy of sexual offenders. *Ann Pharmacother* 1993; **27:** 316–19.
6. Yeager BF, *et al.* Management of the behavioral manifestations of dementia. *Arch Intern Med* 1995; **155:** 250–60.
7. Carter GL, *et al.* Drug-induced delirium: incidence, management and prevention. *Drug Safety* 1996; **15:** 291–301.
8. Pabis DJ, Stanislav SW. Pharmacotherapy of aggressive behaviour. *Ann Pharmacother* 1996; **30:** 278–87.
9. Connor DF, Steingard RJ. A clinical approach to the pharmacotherapy of aggression in children and adolescents. *Ann N Y Acad Sci* 1996; **794:** 290–307.
10. American Psychiatric Association. Practice guideline for the treatment of patients with Alzheimer's disease and other dementias of late life. *Am J Psychiatry* 1997; **154** (suppl): 1–39.
11. McShane R, *et al.* Do neuroleptic drugs hasten cognitive decline in dementia: prospective study with necropsy follow up. *Br Med J* 1997; **314:** 266–70.
12. Burke AL. Palliative care: an update on "terminal restlessness". *Med J Aust* 1997; **166:** 39–42.
13. Fava M. Psychopharmacologic treatment of pathologic aggression. *Psychiatr Clin North Am* 1997; **20:** 427–51.
14. Bradford JMW. Treatment of men with paraphilia. *N Engl J Med* 1998; **338:** 464–5.

Mania. The treatment of acute attacks of mania including mention of the role of antipsychotics is described under Manic Depression, p.273.

Schizophrenia. Schizophrenia may be a group of related syndromes rather than a single disorder. The predominant clinical features of acute schizophrenia syndrome can be divided into psychotic features such as delusions and hallucinations, and disorganised features including disorganised speech, thought, and behaviour (together often known as 'positive' symptoms). The main features of the chronic syndrome are apathy, lack of drive, and social withdrawal (so-called 'negative' symptoms). The pathophysiological mechanism of schizophrenia is unclear and several hypotheses have been proposed. Since standard antipsychotics used in the treatment of schizophrenia block dopamine D_2 receptors in the midbrain it has been suggested that dopaminergic system overactivity may be involved. However, the efficacy of atypical antipsychotics such as clozapine (see below), which is a relatively weak dopamine D_2 inhibitor, has raised the possibility that an imbalance of other neurotransmitters such as serotonin may also be involved. For a more detailed discussion of the pharmacological actions of the various antipsychotics with regard to the pathophysiology and treatment of schizophrenia, see under Chlorpromazine, p.654.

Most commonly schizophrenia begins in adolescence and many patients develop a chronic illness with repeated relapses.

Treatment of schizophrenia consists mainly of a combination of social therapy and antipsychotics. Drug treatment needs to be started promptly for best outcome. Negative symptoms tend to respond less well to drug therapy than do positive symptoms.

Following the initial control of schizophrenia with antipsychotics it is not possible to identify patients who will remain relapse-free without further treatment and the question of whether maintenance therapy should be given to all patients remains to be answered. For many of those who receive maintenance treatment, such treatment appears to postpone rather than prevent relapse. The Royal College of Psychiatrists in the UK has issued advice for those considering the use of higher than normally recommended doses of antipsychotics (see under Administration in the Uses and Administration of Chlorpromazine, p.655).

Although differing widely in weight-for-weight potency, there is little difference in the efficacy of most standard antipsychotics. Choice of drug depends on past treatment and on the risk of adverse effects. A useful generalisation is that low-potency antipsychotics are sedative and strongly antimuscarinic and anti-adrenergic but are less likely to cause acute extrapyramidal symptoms than the high-potency drugs which exhibit a reversed pattern of adverse effects. Sedative and antimuscarinic effects usually diminish with continued use, although sedative effects may be useful for behavioural control in acute illness. Children and young adults are particularly prone to develop acute dystonias; elderly patients are particularly sensitive to the effects of antipsychotics and may be more likely to develop parkinsonism or tardive dyskinesia and are more sensitive to antimuscarinic and anti-adrenergic effects. It should be remembered that there is much interindividual variation in response to antipsychotics, and choosing the most appropriate one may require a trial of antipsychotics from different chemical groups and careful adjustment of dosage. The use of more than one antipsychotic at the same time is not recommended. Drugs commonly used include *phenothiazines* such as chlorpromazine, fluphenazine, thioridazine, and trifluoperazine and the *butyrophenones* such as droperidol and haloperidol.

The *diphenylbutylpiperidines*, such as pimozide, appear to be more effective than other standard antipsychotics against negative symptoms of schizophrenia. The *thioxanthene*, flupenthixol, and the *substituted benzamide*, sulpiride, have activating and antidepressant properties at low doses and are also recommended for patients with predominantly negative symptoms. Compared with standard antipsychotics, extrapyramidal disorders appear to be less of a problem with sulpiride and some newer *atypical antipsychotics* such as clozapine, risperidone, olanzapine, quetiapine, and amisulpride. Clozapine appears to be more effective than standard antipsychotics in the management of negative symptoms and has been shown to be effective in the treatment of refractory schizophrenia. It also appears to be helpful in reducing aggressive behaviour. However, it can cause potentially fatal agranulocytosis and is reserved for use in patients unresponsive to or intolerant of standard antipsychotic and adjunct therapy. Although the other atypical antipsychotics appear to be as effective as standard antipsychotics data on whether they are more effective against negative symptoms and on their efficacy in the treatment of refractory disease is limited.

The addition of a *benzodiazepine* to the initial treatment of acute episodes of schizophrenia can provide a useful extra sedative and anxiolytic effect. It may also allow a smaller dose of antipsychotic to be used and thereby reduce the likelihood of extrapyramidal effects.

About 30% of patients may have little or no response to standard antipsychotics while many others have only a partial response. In the treatment of such resistant schizophrenia consideration should first be given to patient compliance which is a major problem in schizophrenic patients; it may be a result of adverse effects or because the patient experiences a relapse while on medication and is unable to maintain treatment. If non-compliance is due to adverse effects then options for treatment include reduction of the dose, use of an alternative antipsychotic, and/or use of antimuscarinics.

The use of *antimuscarinics* for the treatment or prophylaxis of antipsychotic-induced extrapyramidal side-effects has been widely debated (see Extrapyramidal Disorders on p.650). They are particularly effective in the management of acute dystonic reactions but efficacy in parkinsonism may be minimal and little benefit has been demonstrated in akathisia. Fears that the long-term use of antimuscarinics increases the risk of tardive dyskinesia appear to be unfounded, although they may worsen the condition and should be discontinued if it develops. However, the side-effects of antimuscarinics may be troublesome and may be additive with the antimuscarinic actions of the antipsychotic. Antimuscarinics also have euphoric effects. Routine administration of prophylactic antimuscarinics is therefore not indicated with the possible exception of short-term use in patients at high risk of developing dystonias, or in patients with a previous history of drug-induced dystonias. Antimuscarinics may be given on a short-term basis to treat dystonias.

Maintenance therapy with regular injections of *long-acting depot antipsychotics* is also used to overcome non-compliance. It is particularly useful for schizophrenics living in the community, and may also be advantageous for patients who respond poorly to therapy because of increased first-pass metabolism or intestinal malabsorption. Concern over the possibility of increased extrapyramidal effects and other adverse effects with depot antipsychotics has not been substantiated.

If patients are still unresponsive following the use of the above measures then the use of adjunctive drugs or electroconvulsive therapy is considered. Addition of *lithium* to antipsychotic treatment may be worthwhile in some patients who fail to respond to an antipsychotic alone, although there is the danger of an interaction (see p.294).

The value of treatment of depressive symptoms of schizophrenia with *antidepressants* is not established but the addition of antidepressants such as the tricyclics is considered worth a trial for depression occurring during the recovery phase after an acute episode of psychosis.

Carbamazepine has produced modest benefit in some patients with refractory schizophrenia, the main effect being a reduction in accompanying symptoms such as excitement, impulsivity, and aggression, but concomitant administration of carbamazepine and haloperidol has also resulted in reduced haloperidol concentrations and clinical deterioration in a few patients.

Propranolol in high doses has been reported to be beneficial in refractory schizophrenia but several controlled studies of adjunctive use have found slight or no benefit.

However, it may be of use as an adjunct in patients who develop akathisia unresponsive to antimuscarinics.

References.

1. Glazer WM, Kane JM. Depot neuroleptic therapy: an underutilized treatment option. *J Clin Psychiatry* 1992; **53:** 426–33.
2. Davis JM, *et al.* Depot antipsychotic drugs: place in therapy. *Drugs* 1994; **47:** 741–73.
3. Barnes TRE, Curson DA. Long term depot antipsychotics: a risk-benefit assessment. *Drug Safety* 1994; **10:** 464–79.
4. Zaleon CR, Guthrie SK. Antipsychotic drug use in older adults. *Am J Hosp Pharm* 1994; **51:** 2917–43.
5. Carpenter WT, Buchanan RW. Schizophrenia. *N Engl J Med* 1994; **330:** 681–90.
6. Anonymous. The drug treatment of patients with schizophrenia. *Drug Ther Bull* 1995; **33:** 81–6.
7. Kane JM, McGlashan TH. Treatment of schizophrenia. *Lancet* 1995; **346:** 820–5.
8. Johns CA, Thompson JW. Adjunctive treatments in schizophrenia: pharmacotherapies and electroconvulsive therapy. *Schizophr Bull* 1995; **21:** 607–19.
9. Kane JM. Schizophrenia. *N Engl J Med* 1996; **334:** 34–41.
10. Cunningham Owens DG. Adverse effects of antipsychotic agents: do newer agents offer advantages? *Drugs* 1996; **51:** 895–930.
11. Fleischhacker WW, Hummer M. Drug treatment of schizophrenia in the 1990s: achievements and future possibilities in optimising outcomes. *Drugs* 1997; **53:** 915–29.
12. Buckley PF. New dimensions in the pharmacologic treatment of schizophrenia and related psychoses. *J Clin Pharmacol* 1997; **37:** 363–78. Correction. *ibid.* 1998; **38:** 27.
13. American Academy of Child and Adolescent Psychiatry. Practice parameters for the assessment and treatment of children and adolescents with schizophrenia. *J Am Acad Child Adolesc Psychiatry* 1997; **36** (suppl): 177S–193S.
14. American Psychiatric Association. Practice guideline for the treatment of patients with schizophrenia. *Am J Psychiatry* 1997; **154** (suppl): 1–63.

Sedation

Sedatives reduce excitement and anxiety. They may be used before or during various medical procedures to alleviate fear and produce a state of calmness in the patient. The optimum degree of sedation required depends on the particular procedure. A practical aim for situations requiring **conscious sedation**, for example in *dentistry*, may be the reduction or abolition of physiological and psychological responses to the stress without loss of consciousness, cooperation, or protective reflexes. A greater degree of sedation may be required for patients in *intensive care* and some consider that patients should be maintained asleep but easily rousable. The difference between sedatives and hypnotics is mainly dose related. The same drug or group of drugs can have both effects, larger doses being necessary for a hypnotic effect, that is to produce a state of sleep.

The use of sedatives in premedication for anaesthesia is discussed on p.1220.

Dental sedation. Intravenous *midazolam* has largely superseded *diazepam* for sedation in dental procedures. Although it has no analgesic activity, concomitant use of analgesics is rarely required. However, midazolam needs to be given slowly in small increments as its sedative end-point is reached much more abruptly than with diazepam. Midazolam has a rapid onset of action and produces good anterograde amnesia, but the response in children may be poor. Full recovery can take several hours. Concurrent administration of benzodiazepines such as midazolam with opioid analgesics to supplement sedation and provide postoperative analgesia is not recommended because of the possibility of respiratory depression.

Nitrous oxide is a powerful analgesic and sedative, well tolerated by children, and relatively safe and simple to use but there is some concern over its long-term effect on dental staff. It also requires a certain amount of patient cooperation.

Oral sedatives may also be used to provide dental sedation and are particularly useful to ensure that the patient has a restful night prior to the procedure. Those drugs used include the benzodiazepines *diazepam, lorazepam,* and *temazepam,* and the antihistamines *promethazine* and *trimeprazine*.

Endoscopy. Although endoscopy can be performed without sedation some form of premedication is usually employed. Routine sedation for endoscopy is a matter of debate. While some workers[1] found that sedation did little to improve patient comfort in procedures such as fibreoptic bronchoscopy and considered it should not be used routinely, others have reported good results.[2] Concern has been expressed that often there may be a failure to distinguish between the need for analgesia and the need for sedation in such procedures.[3]

Benzodiazepines are commonly used for intravenous sedation during endoscopy.[4,5] *Midazolam* is preferred because of its shorter duration of action than diazepam,[6] although *diazepam* is still used in some centres. Since hypoventilation and oxygen desaturation may occur with benzodiazepines and the procedure itself can lower oxygen saturation, some recommend the administration of prophylactic nasal oxygen in patients at risk of cardiorespiratory failure.[4,7]

Opioid analgesics such as *morphine* and *pethidine* have also been given but they have largely been replaced by the newer shorter-acting opioids, for example *fentanyl*, which are considered to have faster recovery times.[4] Combination of a benzodiazepine with an opioid analgesic is not advocated in the UK because of the increased risk of cardiorespiratory effects.[4,6] However, in the USA, benzodiazepines are often given with opioids, including pethidine,[8] since such combinations may reduce gagging and increase patient tolerance.

The use of *topical anaesthetics* such as *lignocaine* should probably be reserved for those who prefer to undergo endoscopy without sedation as topical anaesthesia appears to serve little useful function in patients premedicated with benzodiazepines or opioids.[4] There appears to be no practical difference between individual topical anaesthetics. Sprays are safer and may be more effective than lozenges but even when using a spray it is difficult to anaesthetise the oropharyngeal region effectively.

1. Hatton MQF, *et al.* Does sedation help in fibreoptic bronchoscopy? *Br Med J* 1994; **309:** 1206–7.
2. Williams TJ. Sedation in fibreoptic bronchoscopy. *Br Med J* 1995; **310:** 872.
3. Sutherland FWH. Sedation in fibreoptic bronchoscopy. *Br Med J* 1995; **310:** 872.
4. Bell GD. Review article: premedication and intravenous sedation for upper gastrointestinal endoscopy. *Aliment Pharmacol Ther* 1990; **4:** 103–22.
5. Daneshmend TK, *et al.* Sedation for upper gastrointestinal endoscopy: results of a nationwide survey. *Gut* 1991: **32:** 12–15.
6. The Royal College of Surgeons of England Commission on the Provision of Surgical Services. *Report of the working party on guidelines for sedation by non-anaesthetists.* London: Royal College of Surgeons, 1993.
7. Charlton JE. Monitoring and supplemental oxygen during endoscopy. *Br Med J* 1995; **310:** 886–7.
8. Arrowsmith JB, *et al.* Results from the American Society for Gastrointestinal Endoscopy/US Food and Drug Administration collaborative study on complication rates and drug use during gastrointestinal endoscopy. *Gastrointest Endosc* 1991; **37:** 421–7.

Intensive care. Most patients admitted to an intensive care unit require analgesia, sedation, or both during at least part of their stay. The required level of sedation may vary but in general many consider patients should be maintained asleep but easily rousable. Most sedatives and analgesics are administered parenterally. Continuous intravenous infusion avoids peaks and troughs of analgesia and sedation associated with intermittent intramuscular or intravenous administration. *Opioid analgesics*, which have both sedative and analgesic properties, are commonly administered for sedation and are appropriate for any patient in whom pain is anticipated although special care is required in those not artificially ventilated. In the artificially ventilated patient the antitussive action of the opioids may help toleration of a tracheal tube. *Morphine* is a suitable opioid in many situations in intensive care but has a slow onset of action. If prolonged sedation is required analgesia can be obtained by a loading dose followed by a continuous infusion. *Pethidine* has a rapid onset of action and may be a useful alternative to morphine but there is the potential risk of toxicity due to accumulation of its neurotoxic metabolite. *Fentanyl* has a short duration of action after single doses as a result of redistribution in the body. However, it has an elimination half-life longer than morphine and consequently following repeated administration it is not a short-acting drug and therefore offers little advantage over morphine. *Alfentanil* has a short duration of action and has provided satisfactory sedation in patients requiring overnight sedation but does not appear to offer any advantage over pethidine. However, elimination and duration of action have been prolonged in some patients. It may be suitable for use at the start and end of prolonged periods of sedation to produce a rapid effect and to decrease the risk of prolonged respiratory depression respectively.

If sufficient analgesia is achieved, not all patients require sedatives, particularly after the first 24 to 48 hours but most will require a balanced combination of analgesics and sedatives to relieve pain and anxiety. It is inappropriate to use high doses of opioids to achieve deep sedation and it is also inappropriate to use sedatives alone for patients who are in pain.

Benzodiazepines such as *diazepam* induce sleep and reduce anxiety and muscle tone. Although they produce profound amnesia they often fail to achieve satisfactory sedation and doses that do achieve sedation often interfere with verbal contact with the patient. All benzodiazepines tend to produce cardiovascular and respiratory depression and care is required if they are used with opioids. Infusion of diazepam is inappropriate as it has a long elimination half-life and an active metabolite. Administration is best as a loading dose with maintenance doses every 12 to 24 hours but recovery can take several days if large doses are used. *Midazolam* has a rapid onset and short duration of action but it may be difficult to detect clinical differences between midazolam and diazepam when administered in repeated doses. Other benzodiazepines used include *flunitrazepam* and *lorazepam*.

Barbiturates such as *thiopentone* are occasionally used in severe head injury to control raised intracranial pressure (p.796) in patients refractory to other therapy.

Propofol is used successfully for sedation in adults in intensive care and weaning times in propofol sedated patients on mechanical ventilation have been demonstrated to be shorter than those seem with midazolam. However, propofol is not recommended for use in children because of adverse effects (see p.1229).

Flumazenil is a specific benzodiazepine antagonist and some suggest that it may be of use to assist the return of spontaneous respiration and consciousness in patients receiving benzodiazepines. Multiple doses may be required as it has a short duration of action.

Sedation and analgesia for **neonates** in intensive care is a subject of debate. Many of the regimens used appear to be similar to those used in adults or modifications of existing regimens for paediatric sedation. Drugs commonly used include benzodiazepines such as diazepam or midazolam and opioids such as fentanyl or morphine. However, there has been some concern over a report of encephalopathy associated with the prolonged use of midazolam with fentanyl for sedation in infants under intensive care (see under Effects on the Nervous System, p.662). As mentioned above, propofol is not recommended for children in intensive care.

References.

1. Aitkenhead AR. Analgesia and sedation in intensive care. *Br J Anaesth* 1989; **63:** 196–206.
2. Wolf AR. Neonatal sedation: more art than science. *Lancet* 1994; **344:** 628–9.
3. Barker DP, Rutter N. Neonatal sedation. *Lancet* 1994; **344:** 1362.
4. Wagner BKJ, O'Hara DA. Pharmacokinetics and pharmacodynamics of sedatives and analgesics in the treatment of agitated critically ill patients. *Clin Pharmacokinet* 1997; **33:** 426–53.

Sleep disorders

The exact function of sleep is uncertain but it is believed to be involved in energy conservation and total body restoration and recuperation. Initially there is a period of light sleep (stages 1 and 2) followed by deep sleep (stages 3 and 4); this latter period is also known as slow-wave sleep. After stage 4, about 90 minutes after first falling asleep, there is a period of rapid eye movement (REM) sleep during which most dreams occur and EEG traces show high frequency waves. During a period of sleep there are several cycles of stages 1 to 4 followed by REM sleep, with periods of non-REM sleep becoming shorter and periods of REM sleep longer. It is the slow-wave sleep that is considered to be the more restorative. Most healthy adults sleep for single periods of between 7 to 9 hours a day. In old age there is less slow-wave sleep and sleep becomes more fragmented.

Sleep disorders include insomnia (see below) and hypersomnia in which the timing, length, and quality of sleep is altered, and parasomnias (see below) in which abnormal events occur during sleep. The treatment of hypersomnia such as narcolepsy is discussed on p.1476.

Insomnia. Insomnia and its management have been the subject of many reviews and discussions.[1-10] Insomnia is the inability to achieve or maintain sleep and is the most common of the sleep disorders. It often leaves sufferers feeling unrefreshed by sleep and may lead to impaired daytime performance. It is a symptom of various conditions and may be transient (lasting 2 to 3 days), short-term (lasting up to 3 weeks), or long-term (lasting longer than 3 weeks). Transient insomnia may occur in those who normally sleep well and may be due to an alteration in the conditions that surround sleep, for example noise, or to an unusual pattern of rest as in shift work or travelling between time zones. It may also be associated with acute disorders. Short-term insomnia is often related to an emotional problem or more serious medical illness such as acute pain and may recur. Chronic insomnia may be attributed to an underlying psychiatric disorder, especially depression, to alcohol or drug abuse, to excessive caffeine intake, or to cat napping, or physical causes such as pain, pruritus, or dyspnoea. Management of insomnia requires resolution of any stressful precipitant or identification and treatment of any underlying causes with an emphasis on non-pharmacological measures. Such measures may involve counselling, behavioural therapy, development of relaxation techniques, and avoidance of stimulant substances. Hypnotic drugs should ideally be reserved for short courses in the acutely distressed patient; they should be avoided in the elderly, and their use is rarely justified in children. Generally hypnotics should be given at the lowest effective dose for as short a period as possible. In transient insomnia one or two doses of a short-acting hypnotic may be indicated whereas in short-term insomnia intermittent doses of a short-acting hypnotic given for no more than 3 weeks may be appropriate. Routine use of hypnotics is undesirable. Tolerance can develop rapidly with continuous use and withdrawal following long-term use can lead to rebound insomnia and a withdrawal syndrome.

Benzodiazepines are generally regarded as the hypnotics of choice. They all hasten sleep onset, decrease nocturnal awakenings, increase total sleeping time, and often impart a sense of deep and refreshing sleep. Anxiolytic and muscle relaxant actions add to the hypnotic effect. Slow-wave sleep and REM sleep are, however, reduced and the extra sleeping time is largely made up of relatively light sleep.

Tolerance to the hypnotic effects develops rapidly, sleep latency and pattern returning to pretreatment levels within a few weeks of starting treatment. Long-acting benzodiazepines accumulate in the body to a greater extent than ones with a shorter half-life. Although this might be expected to increase the frequency of daytime sedation and impairment of performance (so-called hangover effects) after a hypnotic dose, such a straightforward relationship has not always been observed in practice.[11] Rebound insomnia, that is worsening of sleep disturbance beyond pretreatment levels on drug discontinuation, is more likely with short- and intermediate-acting benzodiazepines than with longer-acting ones. It is not always easy to distinguish between rebound and withdrawal symptoms (see p.661). Broken sleep with vivid dreams and increased REM sleep may persist for some weeks after benzodiazepine withdrawal. Rebound and withdrawal symptoms develop particularly rapidly with the very short-acting drug triazolam; patients have reported early-morning waking and daytime anxiety while receiving treatment. Anterograde amnesia is also more common with short-acting drugs such as triazolam; 'traveller's amnesia' has been used to describe amnesia in persons taking benzodiazepines for sleep disturbances resulting from jet lag.[12]

In 1988, because of the recognition of the hazard of dependence with benzodiazepines, the UK Committee on Safety of Medicines (CSM) recommended that they be used to treat insomnia only when it is severe, disabling, or subjecting the individual to extreme distress.[13] They should be given in the lowest dose which controls symptoms (if possible, intermittently), should not be continued beyond 4 weeks, and should be withdrawn by gradual tapering of the dose to zero. A short-acting benzodiazepine is generally used when residual sedation is undesirable or, when necessary, in elderly patients. Subsequently the EU Committee on Proprietary Medicinal Products (EU CPMP) has recommended that the treatment period should be limited to 2 weeks when brotizolam, midazolam, or triazolam are used.[14] Longer-acting benzodiazepines are indicated when early waking is a problem and possibly when an anxiolytic effect is needed during the day or when some impairment of psychomotor function is acceptable.

Zopiclone is a *cyclopyrrolone* with a similar pharmacological and pharmacokinetic profile to that of the short-acting benzodiazepines. It is claimed to initiate sleep rapidly, without reduction of total REM sleep, and then sustain it with preservation of normal slow-wave sleep. Its short duration of action may result in early-morning wakening and daytime anxiety. Although experience with zopiclone is limited, the CSM consider that it has the same potential for adverse psychiatric reactions, including dependence, as benzodiazepines.[15] It should be reserved for patients with severe sleep disturbance and its duration of use limited to 4 weeks. *Zolpidem* is an *imidazopyridine* which, like zopiclone, has a short duration of hypnotic action and appears to have little effect on the stages of sleep. Early morning wakening and daytime anxiety may occur as for zopiclone. Experience with the drug is, however, relatively limited. The EU CPMP has recommended that treatment with zolpidem should be limited to a maximum of 4 weeks.[14]

Chloral hydrate is an effective hypnotic although tolerance develops and gastric irritation and skin rashes may occur. It is dangerous in overdosage and as with all hypnotics can cause dependence. Derivatives of chloral hydrate which are used as hypnotics include chloral betaine, dichloralphenazone, and triclofos; dichloralphenazone and triclofos may cause less gastric irritation than chloral hydrate. Chloral hydrate and its derivatives have been used as alternatives to benzodiazepines in the elderly although there is no convincing evidence of any special value in these patients. They used to be considered useful hypnotics for children but the use of hypnotics in children is rarely justified.

Chlormethiazole has also been used as an alternative to benzodiazepines in the elderly. Nasal and conjunctival irritation may be troublesome, and again the danger of overdosage and risk of dependence should be considered.

Barbiturates are no longer recommended as hypnotics because of their adverse effects. The CSM[16] has advised that barbiturates should only be used for insomnia that is severe and intractable when there are compelling reasons to and then only in patients already taking barbiturates. It was also advised that attempts should be made to wean patients off barbiturate hypnotics. Compounds such as ethchlorvynol, glutethimide, and methaqualone are similarly not recommended.

Antihistamines have hypnotic properties and some including diphenhydramine, doxylamine, promethazine, and trimeprazine are marketed for insomnia. They may cause troublesome antimuscarinic effects and those with longer half-lives may cause hangover effects. Some are used at night to provide sedation and alleviate the itching of eczema, particularly in children.

Antidepressants and *antipsychotics* with sedative effects are indicated only when insomnia is a symptom of an underlying psychiatric disorder.

Alcohol is not recommended because it has a short weak hypnotic action and rebound excitation can result in early morning insomnia. Its diuretic effects can interrupt sleep and chronic use can lead to rapid development of tolerance and addiction and disturb sleep patterns and cause further insomnia.

Tryptophan, sometimes in the form of dietary supplements, has enjoyed some popularity in the treatment of insomnia. Its efficacy is difficult to substantiate and, since the publication of reports linking tryptophan with the eosinophilic-myalgia syndrome, preparations indicated for insomnia have been withdrawn from the market in many countries.

Melatonin, a hormone believed to be involved in the maintenance of circadian rhythms, is being studied in the treatment of insomnias such as those due to jet lag[17] or other disorders (where it might act by resetting the body clock) and in the elderly.

1. Gillin JC, Byerley WF. The diagnosis and management of insomnia. *N Engl J Med* 1990; **322:** 239–48.
2. Hauri PJ, Esther MS. Insomnia. *Mayo Clin Proc* 1990; **65:** 869–82.
3. Morgan K. Hypnotics in the elderly: what cause for concern? *Drugs* 1990; **40:** 688–96.
4. Maczaj M. Pharmacological treatment of insomnia. *Drugs* 1993; **45:** 44–55.
5. National Medical Advisory Committee. The management of anxiety and insomnia. A report by the National Medical Advisory Committee. Edinburgh: HMSO 1994.
6. Mendelson WB, Jain B. An assessment of short-acting hypnotics. *Drug Safety* 1995; **13:** 257–70.
7. NIH Technology Assessment Panel. Integration of behavioural and relaxation approaches into the treatment of chronic pain and insomnia. *JAMA* 1996; **276:** 313–18.
8. Anonymous. Hypnotic drugs. *Med Lett Drugs Ther* 1996; **38:** 59–61.
9. Kupfer DJ, Reynolds CF. Management of insomnia. *N Engl J Med* 1997; **336:** 341–6.
10. Ashton CH. Management of insomnia. *Prescribers' J* 1997; **37:** 1–10.
11. Greenblatt DJ, *et al.* Neurochemical and pharmacokinetic correlates of the clinical action of benzodiazepine hypnotic drugs. *Am J Med* 1990; **88** (suppl 3A): 18S–24S.
12. Meyboom RHB. Benzodiazepines and pilot error. *Br Med J* 1991; **302:** 1274–5.
13. Committee on Safety of Medicines. Benzodiazepines, dependence and withdrawal symptoms. *Current Problems 21* 1988.
14. Anonymous. Short-acting hypnotics: a comparative assessment. *WHO Drug Inf* 1993; **7:** 125–6.
15. Committee on Safety of Medicines. Zopiclone (Zimovane) and neuro-psychiatric reactions. *Current Problems 30* 1990.
16. Committee on Safety of Medicines/Medicines Control Agency. Barbiturate hypnotics: avoid whenever possible. *Current Problems* 1996; **22:** 7.
17. Waterhouse J, *et al.* Jet lag. *Lancet* 1997; **350:** 1611–16.

Parasomnias. Parasomnias are motor or autonomic disturbances that occur during sleep or are exaggerated by sleep. Some of the main parasomnias include nightmares, night terrors, sleepwalking (somnambulism), restless legs syndrome, periodic movements in sleep, nocturnal enuresis (p.453), bruxism (teeth grinding), head banging, and aggression during sleep. Parasomnias are common but rarely require treatment with drugs other than the symptomatic treatment of sleep-related medical problems. The management of some parasomnias is discussed briefly below.

The **restless legs syndrome** is characterised by an unpleasant creeping sensation deep in the legs with an irresistible urge to move them. The disorder is intermittent and begins during relaxation in the evenings and in bed. The aetiology of this condition is obscure and treatment has been largely empirical. Although there have been reports of efficacy with a wide range of treatments few have been well studied but levodopa, bromocriptine, carbamazepine, clonazepam, and clonidine are amongst those drugs shown in controlled studies to produce beneficial effects. Many patients with restless legs syndrome also suffer from **periodic movements in sleep**, another condition of obscure aetiology, which is characterised by repetitive periodic leg and foot jerking during sleep. Treatments tried are similar to those for the restless legs syndrome; clonazepam and levodopa are amongst the drugs shown to be of benefit.

Some other parasomnias have responded to treatment with benzodiazepines. These include bruxism, head banging, aggression during sleep, night terrors, and sleep walking.

1. Parkes JD. The parasomnias. *Lancet* 1986; **ii:** 1021–5.
2. Kales A, *et al.* Sleep disorders: insomnia, sleepwalking, night terrors, nightmares, and enuresis. *Ann Intern Med* 1987; **106:** 582–92.
3. Krueger BR. Restless leg syndrome and periodic movements of sleep. *Mayo Clin Proc* 1990; **65:** 999–1006.
4. Montplaisir J, *et al.* The treatment of the restless leg syndrome with or without periodic leg movements in sleep. *Sleep* 1992; **15:** 391–5.
5. Silber MH. Restless legs syndrome. *Mayo Clin Proc* 1997; **72:** 261–4.

Abecarnil (9339-r)

Abecarnil *(rINN)*.

Isopropyl-6-benzyloxy-4-methoxymethyl-β-carboline-3-carboxylate; ZK-112119.

CAS — 111841-85-1.

Abecarnil is a beta-carboline compound reported to be a partial agonist at benzodiazepine receptors. It is being studied for its anxiolytic and anticonvulsant actions in anxiety disorders and alcohol withdrawal syndrome.

References.

1. Krause W, *et al.* Pharmacokinetics and acute toleration of the β-carboline derivative abecarnil in man. *Arzneimittelforschung* 1990; **40:** 529–32.
2. Karara AH, *et al.* Pharmacokinetics of abecarnil in patients with renal insufficiency. *Clin Pharmacol Ther* 1996; **59:** 520–8.
3. Lydiard RB, *et al.* Abecarnil Work Group. A double-blind evaluation of the safety and efficacy of abecarnil, alprazolam, and placebo in outpatients with generalized anxiety disorder. *J Clin Psychiatry* 1997; **58** (suppl 11): 11–18.
4. Pollack MH, *et al.* Abecarnil for the treatment of generalized anxiety disorder: a placebo-controlled comparison of two dosage ranges of abecarnil and buspirone. *J Clin Psychiatry* 1997; **58** (suppl 11): 19–23.
5. Anton RF, *et al.* A double-blind comparison of abecarnil and diazepam in the treatment of uncomplicated alcohol withdrawal. *Psychopharmacology (Berl)* 1997; **131:** 123–9.

Acamprosate Calcium (10919-p)

Acamprosate Calcium *(BANM, rINNM).*

The calcium salt of 3-acetamido-1-propanesulphonic acid.

$C_{10}H_{20}CaN_2O_8S_2$ = 400.5.

CAS — 77337-76-9 (acamprosate); 77337-73-6 (acamprosate calcium).

Adverse Effects

The main adverse effect of acamprosate is a dosage-related diarrhoea; nausea, vomiting, and abdominal pain occur less frequently. Other adverse effects have included pruritus, and occasionally a maculopapular rash; bullous skin reactions have occurred rarely. Fluctuations in libido have also been reported.

Effects on the skin. A case of erythema multiforme in a woman with cirrhosis of the liver has been attributed to administration of acamprosate[1] although both the diagnosis and any association with acamprosate has been seriously challenged.[2]

1. Fortier-Beaulieu M, *et al.* Possible association of erythema multiforme with acamprosate. *Lancet* 1992; **339:** 991.
2. Potgieter AS, Opsomer L. Acamprosate as cause of erythema multiforme contested. *Lancet* 1992; **340:** 856–7.

Precautions

Acamprosate is contra-indicated in patients with renal or severe hepatic impairment. It should not be used during pregnancy or breast feeding.

Renal impairment. It is considered[1] likely that accumulation of acamprosate would occur with prolonged administration of therapeutic doses to patients with renal impairment. It has been reported that the mean maximum concentration of acamprosate after a single 666-mg dose was 813 ng per mL in 12 patients with moderate or severe renal impairment compared with 198 ng per mL in 6 healthy subjects; values for the plasma elimination half-life were 47 and 18 hours respectively. There appears to be a linear correlation between creatinine clearance and the plasma elimination half-life.

1. Wilde MI, Wagstaff AJ. Acamprosate: a review of its pharmacology and clinical potential in the management of alcohol dependence after detoxification. *Drugs* 1997; **53:** 1038–53.

Pharmacokinetics

Absorption of acamprosate from the gastro-intestinal tract is slow but sustained and is subject to considerable interindividual variation. Steady-state concentrations are achieved after 7 days' administration. Bioavailability is reduced by administration with food. Acamprosate is not protein bound and although it is hydrophilic it is reported to cross the blood-brain barrier. Acamprosate does not appear to be metabolised and is excreted unchanged in the urine. The apparent half-life after oral administration has been reported to be 13 hours.

Uses and Administration

Acamprosate has a chemical structure similar to that of gamma-aminobutyric acid (GABA) (p.1582). It is given by mouth to prevent relapse in alcoholics who have been weaned off alcohol. The usual dose for patients weighing 60 kg or more is 666 mg given three times daily; for patients less than 60 kg a dose of 666 mg may be given at breakfast followed by 333 mg at midday and 333 mg at night. Treatment should be started as soon as possible after alcohol withdrawal and maintained, even if the patient relapses, for the recommended period of 1 year.

Alcohol dependence. Acamprosate is considered to be of use as an adjunct to psychotherapy in maintaining abstinence after alcohol withdrawal in patients with alcohol dependence (p.1099). Reviews[1,2] of placebo-controlled studies conclude that acamprosate helps to prevent relapse and increase the number of drink-free days during a 1-year course of treatment and possibly for up to one year thereafter. Efficacy appears to be dose related but its effects in promoting abstinence may wane during treatment. Use with disulfiram may improve results but published data on concomitant use is relatively limited. Several mechanisms have been proposed to account for acamprosate's action including inhibition of neuronal hyperexcitability by antagonising excitatory amino acids such as glutamate.

1. Wilde MI, Wagstaff AJ. Acamprosate: a review of its pharmacology and clinical potential in the management of alcohol dependence after detoxification. *Drugs* 1997; **53:** 1038–53.
2. Anonymous. Acamprosate for alcohol dependence? *Drug Ther Bull* 1997; **35:** 70–2.

Preparations

Proprietary Preparations (details are given in Part 3)
Aust.: Campral; ***Fr.:*** Aotal; ***Ger.:*** Campral; ***Irl.:*** Campral; ***Neth.:*** Campral; ***Spain:*** Campral; ***Swed.:*** Campral; ***Switz.:*** Campral; ***UK:*** Campral.

Acepromazine (18320-a)

Acepromazine *(BAN, rINN).*

10-(3-Dimethylaminopropyl)phenothiazin-2-yl methyl ketone.

$C_{19}H_{22}N_2OS$ = 326.5.

CAS — 61-00-7.

Acepromazine Maleate (7001-h)

Acepromazine Maleate *(BANM, USAN, rINNM).*

Acetylpromazine Maleate. 10-(3-Dimethylaminopropyl)phenothiazin-2-yl methyl ketone hydrogen maleate.

$C_{19}H_{22}N_2OS,C_4H_4O_4$ = 442.5.

CAS — 3598-37-6.

Pharmacopoeias. In *US* for veterinary use only. Also in *BP(Vet).*

A yellow odourless or almost odourless crystalline powder. Acepromazine maleate 13.5 mg is approximately equivalent to 10 mg of acepromazine.

Soluble in water and in alcohol; freely soluble in chloroform; slightly soluble in ether. The BP(Vet) specifies that a 1% solution in water has a pH of 4.0 to 4.5; the USP specifies 4.0 to 5.5. **Protect** from light.

Acepromazine is a phenothiazine with general properties similar to those of chlorpromazine (p.649). It has been given by mouth in preparations for the management of insomnia. It is also used as the maleate in veterinary medicine.

Preparations

Proprietary Preparations (details are given in Part 3)
Fr.: Plegicil†.
Multi-ingredient: ***Fr.:*** Noctran.

Aceprometazine (12302-j)

Aceprometazine *(rINN).*

16-64 CB. 10-(2-Dimethylaminopropyl)phenothiazin-2-yl methyl ketone.

$C_{19}H_{22}N_2OS$ = 326.5.

CAS — 13461-01-3.

Aceprometazine is a phenothiazine with general properties similar to those of chlorpromazine (p.649). It is available usually as the maleate in preparations for the management of insomnia.

Preparations

Proprietary Preparations (details are given in Part 3)
Multi-ingredient: ***Fr.:*** Mepronizine; Noctran.

Acetophenazine Maleate (7002-m)

Acetophenazine Maleate *(USAN, rINNM).*

Acephenazine Maleate; Acetophenazine Dimaleate; NSC-70600; Sch-6673. 10-{3-[4-(2-Hydroxyethyl)piperazin-1-yl]propyl}phenothiazin-2-yl methyl ketone dimaleate.

$C_{23}H_{29}N_3O_2S,2C_4H_4O_4$ = 643.7.

CAS — 2751-68-0 (acetophenazine); 5714-00-1 (acetophenazine maleate).

Acetophenazine maleate is a phenothiazine with general properties similar to those of chlorpromazine (p.649). It has a piperazine side-chain.

It has been given by mouth for the treatment of psychoses.

Preparations

Proprietary Preparations (details are given in Part 3)
USA: Tindal†.

Acetylglycinamide-Chloral Hydrate (4002-h)

AGAC; AGAK.

$C_6H_{11}Cl_3N_2O_4$ = 281.5.

A complex of chloral hydrate and *N*-acetylglycinamide.

Acetylglycinamide-chloral hydrate is a derivative of chloral hydrate (p.645) which has been given by mouth as a hypnotic and sedative.

Preparations

Proprietary Preparations (details are given in Part 3)
Swed.: Ansopal†.

Adinazolam Mesylate (12327-d)

Adinazolam Mesylate *(BANM, USAN).*

Adinazolam Mesilate *(rINNM)*; U-41123 (adinazolam); U-41123F (adinazolam mesylate). 8-Chloro-1-(dimethylaminomethyl)-6-phenyl-4*H*-1,2,4-triazolo[4,3-*a*][1,4]benzodiazepine methanesulphonate.

$C_{19}H_{18}ClN_5,CH_4O_3S$ = 447.9.

CAS — 37115-32-5 (adinazolam); 57938-82-6 (adinazolam mesylate).

Adinazolam is a short-acting benzodiazepine structurally related to alprazolam (p.640) and is reported to have similar properties. It has been studied in the management of anxiety disorders and depression. It is also reported to exert a uricosuric effect.

References.

1. Fleishaker JC, *et al.* Clinical pharmacology of adinazolam and N-desmethyladinazolam mesylate after single oral doses of each compound in healthy volunteers. *Clin Pharmacol Ther* 1990; **48:** 652–64.
2. Davidson JRT, *et al.* Adinazolam sustained-release treatment of panic disorder: a double-blind study. *J Clin Psychopharmacol* 1994; **14:** 255–63.
3. Golden PL, *et al.* Effect of probenecid on the pharmacokinetics and pharmacodynamics of adinazolam in humans. *Clin Pharmacol Ther* 1994; **56:** 133–41.
4. Carter CS, *et al.* Adinazolam-SR in panic disorder with agoraphobia: relationship of daily dose to efficacy. *J Clin Psychiatry* 1995; **56:** 202–10.

Allobarbitone (4003-m)

Allobarbital *(USAN, rINN)*; Diallylbarbitone; Diallylbarbituric Acid; Diallylmalonylurea; Diallymalum; NSC-9324. 5,5-Diallylbarbituric acid.

$C_{10}H_{12}N_2O_3$ = 208.2.

CAS — 52-43-7.

Pharmacopoeias. In *Aust.*

Allobarbitone is a barbiturate with general properties similar to those of amylobarbitone (p.641). It was formerly used in combination preparations for the treatment of sleep disorders and pain.

Preparations

Proprietary Preparations (details are given in Part 3)
Multi-ingredient: ***Ger.:*** Sediomed S†.

Alpidem (1676-x)

Alpidem *(BAN, USAN, rINN).*

SL-80.0342-00. 2-(6-Chloro-2-*p*-chlorophenylimidazo[1,2-*a*]pyridin-3-yl)-*N,N*-dipropylacetamide.

$C_{21}H_{23}Cl_2N_3O$ = 404.3.

CAS — 82626-01-5.

Alpidem is an imidazopyridine derivative that was given by mouth for its anxiolytic properties but it was withdrawn from the market following reports of hepatic dysfunction.

Preparations

Proprietary Preparations (details are given in Part 3)
Fr.: Ananxyl†.

Alprazolam (7003-b)

Alprazolam *(BAN, USAN, rINN).*

Alprazolamum; U-31889. 8-Chloro-1-methyl-6-phenyl-4*H*-1,2,4-triazolo[4,3-*a*][1,4]benzodiazepine.

$C_{17}H_{13}ClN_4$ = 308.8.

CAS — 28981-97-7 (alprazolam).

Pharmacopoeias. In *Eur.* (see p.viii) and *US.*

A white to off-white crystalline powder. It exhibits polymorphism. Ph. Eur. **solubilities**: practically insoluble in water; sparingly soluble in alcohol and in acetone; freely soluble in dichloromethane. USP solubilities: practically insoluble in water; soluble in alcohol; sparingly soluble in acetone; freely soluble in chloroform; slightly soluble in ethyl acetate. **Protect** from light.

CAUTION. *The USP advises that care should be taken to prevent inhaling particles of alprazolam and exposing the skin to it.*

Dependence and Withdrawal

As for Diazepam, p.661.

Adverse Effects, Treatment, and Precautions

As for Diazepam, p.661.

Abuse. Report of the abuse of alprazolam by patients receiving methadone maintenance therapy for opioid dependence.[1] Ingestion of high doses of alprazolam after taking methadone produced a 'high' without pronounced sedation. Alprazolam was also being reportedly abused by nonopioid-drug abusers. The usual urine toxicology screens for benzodiazepines often give false-negative results for alprazolam because of the extremely low concentrations of metabolites excreted, making abuse difficult to detect.

1. Weddington WW, Carney AC. Alprazolam abuse during methadone maintenance therapy. *JAMA* 1987; **257:** 3363.

Effects on the liver. Abnormal liver enzyme values occurred on 2 occasions when alprazolam was added to the treatment regimen of a patient receiving phenelzine for depression.[1] It was not possible to say if this was due to alprazolam alone or a synergistic effect with phenelzine.

1. Roy-Byrne P, *et al.* Alprazolam-related hepatotoxicity. *Lancet* 1983; **ii:** 786–7.

Effects on the skin. PHOTOSENSITIVITY. A report of photosensitivity in one patient positive to rechallenge with alprazolam.[1]

1. Kanwar AJ, *et al.* Photosensitivity due to alprazolam. *Dermatologica* 1990; **181:** 75.

Porphyria. Alprazolam was considered to be unsafe in patients with acute porphyria because it has been shown to be porphyrinogenic in *animals* or *in-vitro* systems.[1]

1. Moore MR, McColl KEL. *Porphyria: drug lists.* Glasgow: Porphyria Research Unit, University of Glasgow, 1991.

Interactions

As for Diazepam, p.663.

Pharmacokinetics

Alprazolam is well absorbed from the gastro-intestinal tract following oral administration, with peak plasma concentrations being achieved within 1 to 2 hours of a dose. The mean half-life in plasma is 11 to 15 hours. Alprazolam is 70 to 80% bound to plasma protein. It is metabolised in the liver primarily to α-hydroxyalprazolam, which is reported to be approximately half as active as the parent compound, and to an inactive benzophenone; plasma concentrations of metabolites are very low. It is excreted in urine as unchanged drug and metabolites.

References to the pharmacokinetics of alprazolam.

1. Greenblatt DJ, Wright CE. Clinical pharmacokinetics of alprazolam: therapeutic implications. *Clin Pharmacokinet* 1993; **24:** 453–71.
2. Wright CE, *et al.* Pharmacokinetics and psychomotor performance of alprazolam: concentration-effect relationship. *J Clin Pharmacol* 1997; **37:** 321–9.
3. Kaplan GB, *et al.* Single-dose pharmacokinetics and pharmacodynamics of alprazolam in elderly and young subjects. *J Clin Pharmacol* 1998; **38:** 14–21.

Administration in hepatic impairment. A study of the effect of alcoholic liver disease on alprazolam pharmacokinetics.[1] Alprazolam 1 mg by mouth was absorbed more slowly in 17 patients with alcoholic cirrhosis but no ascites than in 17 healthy subjects; the peak alprazolam concentrations in the 2 groups were achieved at a mean of 3.34 hours and 1.47 hours respectively, and the mean elimination half-lives were 19.7 hours and 11.4 hours. However, there were no significant differences in the maximum plasma concentrations achieved. The results indicate that alprazolam, in common with other benzodiazepines which undergo oxidative metabolism, would accumulate to a greater extent in patients with alcoholic liver disease than in healthy subjects; the daily dose of alprazolam may need to be reduced by half in this population.

1. Juhl RP, *et al.* Alprazolam pharmacokinetics in alcoholic liver disease. *J Clin Pharmacol* 1984; **24:** 113–19.

Distribution into breast milk. From a study[1] of the distribution of alprazolam into breast milk in 8 lactating women it was estimated that the average daily dose of alprazolam ingested by a breast-fed infant would range from 0.3 to 5 μg per kg body-weight or about 3% of a maternal dose.

1. Oo CY, *et al.* Pharmacokinetics in lactating women: prediction of alprazolam transfer into milk. *Br J Clin Pharmacol* 1995; **40:** 231–6.

Uses and Administration

Alprazolam is a short-acting benzodiazepine with general properties similar to those of diazepam (p.666). It is used in the treatment of anxiety disorders in doses of 0.25 to 0.5 mg three times daily by mouth, increased where necessary to a total daily dose of 3 or 4 mg. In elderly or debilitated patients an initial dose of 0.25 mg twice or three times daily has been suggested.

Doses of up to 10 mg of alprazolam daily have been used in the treatment of panic attacks.

Anxiety disorders. The management of anxiety disorders, including the use of benzodiazepines, is discussed on p.635.

References.

1. Cross-National Collaborative Panic Study, Second Phase Investigators. Drug treatment of panic disorder: comparative efficacy of alprazolam, imipramine, and placebo. *Br J Psychiatry* 1992; **160:** 191–202.
2. Lepola UM, *et al.* Three-year follow-up of patients with panic disorder after short-term treatment with alprazolam and imipramine. *Int Clin Psychopharmacol* 1993; **8:** 115–18.
3. Pollack MH, *et al.* Long-term outcome after acute treatment with alprazolam or clonazepam for panic disorder. *J Clin Psychopharmacol* 1993; **13:** 257–63.
4. Woodman CL, *et al.* Predictors of response to alprazolam and placebo in patients with panic disorder. *J Affective Disord* 1994; **30:** 5–13.

Depression. Benzodiazepines are not usually considered appropriate for treatment of depression (p.271) but some drugs such as alprazolam have been tried for this indication.[1]

1. Rudorfer MV, Potter WZ. Antidepressants: a comparative review of the clinical pharmacology and therapeutic use of the 'newer' versus the 'older' drugs. *Drugs* 1989; **37:** 713–38.

Premenstrual syndrome. Alprazolam has been reported to have produced a marginal to good response in the premenstrual syndrome[1-3] (p.1456) but the role of benzodiazepines is limited by their adverse effects. If benzodiazepines are selected it is recommended that in order to reduce the risk of dependence and withdrawal symptoms they should be carefully restricted to the luteal phase in selected patients.[4] Withdrawal symptoms may be more severe after short-acting drugs such as alprazolam. Antidepressant drugs such as selective serotonin reuptake inhibitors may be preferred.

1. Smith S, *et al.* Treatment of premenstrual syndrome with alprazolam: results of a double-blind, placebo-controlled, randomized crossover clinical trial. *Obstet Gynecol* 1987; **70:** 37–43.
2. Harrison WM, *et al.* Treatment of premenstrual dysphoria with alprazolam: a controlled study. *Arch Gen Psychiatry* 1990; **47:** 270–5.
3. Freeman EW, *et al.* A double-blind trial of oral progesterone, alprazolam, and placebo in treatment of severe premenstrual syndrome. *JAMA* 1995; **274:** 51–7.
4. Mortola JF. A risk-benefit appraisal of drugs used in the management of premenstrual syndrome. *Drug Safety* 1994; **10:** 160–9.

Preparations

USP 23: Alprazolam Tablets.

Proprietary Preparations (details are given in Part 3)
Aust.: Xanor; ***Austral.:*** Kalma; Ralozam; Xanax; ***Belg.:*** Alpraz; Xanax; ***Canad.:*** Novo-Alprazol; Nu-Alpraz; Xanax; ***Fr.:*** Xanax; ***Ger.:*** Cassadan; Esparon; Tafil; Xanax; ***Irl.:*** Alprox; Gerax; Xanax; ***Ital.:*** Frontal; Mialin; Valeans; Xanax; ***Neth.:*** Xanax; ***Norw.:*** Xanor; ***S.Afr.:*** Alzam; Azor; Panix; Xanor; Zopax; ***Spain:*** Trankimazin; ***Swed.:*** Alpralid†; Xanor; ***Switz.:*** Xanax; ***UK:*** Xanax; ***USA:*** Xanax.

Amisulpride (1759-d)

Amisulpride *(BAN, rINN).*

DAN-216. 4-Amino-*N*-[(1-ethyl-2-pyrrolidinyl)methyl]-5-(ethylsulphonyl)-2-methoxybenzamide; *(RS)*-4-Amino-*N*-[(1-ethylpyrrolidin-2-yl)methyl]-5-(ethylsulfonyl)-*o*-anisamide.

$C_{17}H_{27}N_3O_4S$ = 369.5.

CAS — 71675-85-9.

Adverse Effects, Treatment, and Precautions

As for Sulpiride, p.692.

Overdosage. The effects of overdosage of amisulpride in 2 patients have been reported.[1] The first patient who had taken about 3 g of amisulpride and an unknown amount of dothiepin was found to have had a blood-amisulpride concentration of 9.63 μg per mL. The patient experienced generalised convulsions, which resolved spontaneously, followed by coma, motor restlessness, tachycardia, and slight prolongation of the QT interval. The patient was treated with gastric lavage and had recovered within 48 hours. The second patient who had been found dead had a blood-amisulpride concentration of 41.7 μg per mL.

1. Tracqui A, *et al.* Amisulpride poisoning: a report on two cases. *Hum Exp Toxicol* 1995; **14:** 294–8.

Interactions

As for Chlorpromazine, p.652.

Pharmacokinetics

Amisulpride is absorbed from the gastro-intestinal tract but bioavailability is reported to be only about 43 to 48%. An initial peak plasma concentrations has been reported to occur one hour after oral administration and a second higher one after 3 to 4 hours. Plasma protein binding is reported to be low. Metabolism is limited and most of a dose appearing in the urine and faeces is unchanged drug. The terminal elimination half-life is about 12 hours.

Uses and Administration

Amisulpride is a substituted benzamide atypical antipsychotic with general properties similar to those of sulpiride (p.692). It is reported to have a high affinity for dopamine D_2 and D_3 receptors. Amisulpride is used mainly in the management of psychoses such as schizophrenia (p.637) but has also been tried in depression (p.271).

For acute psychotic episodes daily doses of between 400 and 800 mg may be given by mouth in 2 divided doses, increased if necessary to 1200 mg daily. For patients with predominantly negative symptoms daily doses between 50 and 300 mg are recommended. Daily doses of up to 300 mg may be administered once daily. For patients with renal impairment the UK manufacturer has recommended that the dose should be reduced to half the normal dose for patients with a creatinine clearance (CC) of between 30 and 60 mL per minute and to one-third in patients with a CC between 10 and 30 mL per minute. Amisulpride has also been given by intramuscular injection in doses of up to 800 mg daily.

References.

1. Boyer P, *et al.* Treatment of negative symptoms in schizophrenia with amisulpride. *Br J Psychiatry* 1995; **166:** 68–72.
2. Möller H-J, *et al.* Improvement of acute exacerbations of schizophrenia with amisulpride: a comparison with haloperidol. *Psychopharmacology (Berl)* 1997; **132:** 396–401.
3. Loo H, *et al.* Amisulpride versus placebo in the medium-term treatment of the negative symptoms of schizophrenia. *Br J Psychiatry* 1997; **170:** 18–22.
4. Lecrubier Y, *et al.* Amisulpride Study Group. Amisulpride versus imipramine and placebo in dysthymia and major depression. *J Affective Disord* 1997; **43:** 95–103.
5. Smeraldi E. Amisulpride versus fluoxetine in patients with dysthymia or major depression in partial remission: a double-blind, comparative study. *J Affective Disord* 1998; **48:** 47–56.

Preparations

Proprietary Preparations (details are given in Part 3)
Aust.: Deniban; ***Fr.:*** Solian; ***Ital.:*** Deniban; Sulamid; ***UK:*** Solian.

Amylobarbitone (4005-v)

Amylobarbitone *(BAN).*

Amobarbital *(rINN)*; Amobarbitalum; Pentymalum. 5-Ethyl-5-isopentylbarbituric acid.

$C_{11}H_{18}N_2O_3$ = 226.3.

CAS — 57-43-2.

Pharmacopoeias. In *Chin., Eur.* (see p.viii), and *Jpn.*

A white crystalline powder.

Very slightly **soluble** in water; freely soluble in alcohol and in ether; soluble in dichloromethane. Forms water-soluble compounds with aqueous solutions of alkali hydroxides and carbonates and with ammonia.

Amylobarbitone Sodium (4006-g)

Amylobarbitone Sodium *(BANM).*

Amobarbital Sodium *(rINNM)*; Amobarbitalum Natricum; Barbamylum; Pentymalnatrium; Sodium Amobarbital; Soluble Amylobarbitone. Sodium 5-ethyl-5-isopentylbarbiturate.

$C_{11}H_{17}N_2NaO_3$ = 248.3.

CAS — 64-43-7.

Pharmacopoeias. In *Chin., Eur.* (see p.viii), and *US.*

Jpn includes Amobarbital Sodium for Injection.

A white, odourless, hygroscopic, friable, granular powder. Very **soluble** in carbon dioxide-free water, sometimes leaving a small insoluble residue; practically insoluble in chloroform and in ether. The Ph. Eur. states freely soluble, and the USP soluble in alcohol. Solutions decompose on standing; decomposition is accelerated by heat. The Ph. Eur. specifies that a 10% solution in water has a pH of not more than 11.0; the USP specifies a pH between 9.6 and 10.4. **Store** in airtight containers.

Amylobarbitone may be precipitated from preparations containing amylobarbitone sodium, depending on the concentration and pH. Amylobarbitone sodium has, therefore, been reported to be **incompatible** with many other drugs, particularly acids and acidic salts.

Dependence and Withdrawal

The development of dependence is a high risk with amylobarbitone and other barbiturates and may occur after regular use even in therapeutic doses for short periods. Barbiturates should not therefore be discontinued abruptly, but should be withdrawn by gradual reduction of the dose over a period of days or weeks. A long-acting barbiturate such as phenobarbitone may be substituted for a short- or intermediate-acting one, followed by gradual reduction of the phenobarbitone dose.

Withdrawal symptoms are similar to those of alcohol withdrawal and are characterised after several hours by apprehension and weakness, followed by anxiety, headache, dizziness, irritability, tremors, nausea and vomiting, abdominal cramps, insomnia, distortion in visual perception, muscle twitching, and tachycardia. Orthostatic hypotension and convulsions may develop after a day or two, sometimes leading to status epilepticus. Hallucinations and delirium tremens may develop after several days followed by coma before the symptoms disappear or death occurs.

Adverse Effects

Drowsiness, sedation, and ataxia are the most frequent adverse effects of amylobarbitone and other barbiturates and are a consequence of dose-related CNS depression. Other adverse effects include respiratory depression, headache, gastro-intestinal disturbances, skin reactions, confusion, and memory defects. Paradoxical excitement and irritability may occur, particularly in children, the elderly, and patients in acute pain. Hypersensitivity reactions occur rarely and include skin rashes (erythema multiforme and exfoliative dermatitis, sometimes fatal, have been reported), hepatitis and cholestasis, and photosensitivity. Blood disorders, including megaloblastic anaemia after chronic use of barbiturates, have also occurred occasionally.

Neonatal intoxication, drug dependence, and symptoms resembling vitamin-K deficiency have been reported in infants born to mothers who received barbiturates during pregnancy. Congenital malformations have been reported in children of women who took barbiturates during pregnancy, but the causal role is a matter of some debate.

Nystagmus, miosis, slurred speech, and ataxia may occur with excessive doses of barbiturates. The toxic effects of overdosage result from profound central depression and include coma, respiratory and cardiovascular depression, with hypotension and shock leading to renal failure and death. Hypothermia may occur with subsequent pyrexia on recovery. Erythematous or haemorrhagic blisters reportedly occur in about 6% of patients, but are not characteristic solely of barbiturate poisoning.

Solutions of the sodium salts of barbiturates are extremely alkaline, and necrosis has followed subcutaneous injection. Intravenous injection may be hazardous; hypotension, shock, laryngospasm, and apnoea have occurred particularly after rapid administration. Gangrene has resulted from intra-arterial injection into an extremity.

Barbiturates are abused for their euphoriant effects.

Overdosage. A detailed review of drug-induced stupor and coma, including that caused by barbiturates.[1]

1. Ashton CH, *et al.* Drug-induced stupor and coma: some physical signs and their pharmacological basis. *Adverse Drug React Acute Poisoning Rev* 1989; **8:** 1–59.

Treatment of Adverse Effects

Following recent ingestion of an overdose of a barbiturate the stomach may be emptied by lavage. Oral administration of activated charcoal may be useful. Patients should be managed with intensive supportive therapy, with particular attention being paid to the maintenance of cardiovascular, respiratory, and renal functions, and to the maintenance of the electrolyte balance.

The value of measures aimed at the active removal of barbiturates is questionable, except perhaps for charcoal haemoperfusion which can be life-saving in the most severe cases.

Precautions

Amylobarbitone and other barbiturates are best avoided in elderly and debilitated patients, young adults, in children, and in those with mental depression.

Amylobarbitone is contra-indicated in patients with pulmonary insufficiency, sleep apnoea, pre-existing CNS depression or coma, and severe hepatic impairment, and should be given with caution to those with renal insufficiency. Barbiturates given to patients in pain may provoke a paradoxical excitatory reaction, unless an analgesic is given concomitantly. With continued administration, tolerance develops to the sedative or hypnotic effects of the barbiturates to a greater extent than to their lethal effects. Barbiturates may cause drowsiness; affected patients should not drive or operate machinery.

See under Adverse Effects, above, for the hazards of administration of barbiturates during pregnancy. Small amounts of barbiturates are distributed into breast milk; they should not, therefore, be given to nursing mothers.

Dependence readily develops after use of barbiturates with a **withdrawal syndrome** on abrupt discontinuation (see under Dependence and Withdrawal, above).

Porphyria. Barbiturates including amylobarbitone have been associated with acute attacks of porphyria and are considered unsafe in patients with acute porphyria.[1]

1. Moore MR, McColl KEL. *Porphyria: drug lists.* Glasgow: Porphyria Research Unit, University of Glasgow, 1991.

Interactions

Sedation or respiratory depression may be enhanced by drugs with CNS-depressant properties; in particular alcohol should be avoided. Barbiturates generally induce liver enzymes, and thus increase the rate of metabolism, and decrease the activity, of many other drugs as well as endogenous substances. Continued use may result in induction of their own metabolism. MAOIs may prolong the CNS depressant effects of some barbiturates, probably by inhibition of their metabolism. However, MAOIs like other antidepressants also reduce the convulsive threshold and thereby antagonise the anticonvulsant action of barbiturates. For some further interactions involving barbiturates see under Phenobarbitone, p.351.

Pharmacokinetics

Amylobarbitone is readily absorbed from the gastro-intestinal tract and following absorption some 60% is bound to plasma proteins. It has a half-life of about 20 to 25 hours which is considerably extended in neonates. It crosses the placenta and small amounts are distributed into breast milk. Amylobarbitone is metabolised in the liver; up to about 50% is excreted in the urine as 3′-hydroxyamylobarbitone and up to about 30% as *N*-hydroxyamylobarbitone, less than 1% appearing unchanged; up to about 5% is excreted in the faeces.

Uses and Administration

Amylobarbitone is a barbiturate that has been used as a hypnotic and sedative. Its use can no longer be recommended because of its adverse effects and risk of dependence, although continued use may occasionally be considered necessary for severe intractable insomnia (p.638) in patients already taking it. The usual dose by mouth at bedtime was 100 to 200 mg of the base or 60 to 200 mg of the sodium salt. A more rapid onset of effect was obtained with the sodium salt.

Barbiturates with a longer action such as phenobarbitone (p.350) are still used in epilepsy and those with a shorter action such as methohexitone (p.1227) or thiopentone (p.1233) for anaesthesia.

Cerebrovascular disorders. For reference to the use of barbiturate-induced coma in the management of patients with cerebral ischaemia, see p.1234.

Epilepsy. Amylobarbitone sodium in the assessment of memory function prior to surgery for temporal lobe epilepsy.[1]

1. Jack CR, *et al.* Selective posterior cerebral artery injection of Amytal: new method of preoperative memory testing. *Mayo Clin Proc* 1989; **64:** 965–75.

Preparations

USP 23: Amobarbital Sodium for Injection; Secobarbital Sodium and Amobarbital Sodium Capsules.

Proprietary Preparations (details are given in Part 3)
Austral.: Amytal†; Neur-Amyl; ***Canad.:*** Amytal; ***Irl.:*** Sodium Amytal; ***Spain:*** Isoamitil Sedante†; ***UK:*** Amytal; Sodium Amytal; ***USA:*** Amytal.

Multi-ingredient: ***Belg.:*** Bellanox; Octonox; ***Canad.:*** Amesec†; Tuinal; ***Fr.:*** Tensophoril†; ***Ger.:*** Ansudoral†; Metrotonin†; ***Irl.:*** Tuinal; ***S.Afr.:*** Amaphil†; Amesec†; Daral†; Fabasma; Medikasma; Panasma; Repasma; Tuinal†; ***UK:*** Hypercal-B†; Tuinal; ***USA:*** Ephedrine and Amytal†; Tuinal.

Aprobarbital (4007-q)

Aprobarbital *(rINN)*.

Allylisopropylmalonylurea; Allypropymal; Aprobarbitone. 5-Allyl-5-isopropylbarbituric acid.

$C_{10}H_{14}N_2O_3$ = 210.2.

CAS — 77-02-1.

Aprobarbital is a barbiturate with general properties similar to those of amylobarbitone (p.641). It has been given by mouth for insomnia (p.638) in doses of 40 to 160 mg at night and as a sedative in usual doses of 40 mg three times daily, but barbiturates are no longer considered appropriate for such purposes. Aprobarbital sodium was also formerly used.

Preparations

Proprietary Preparations (details are given in Part 3)
USA: Alurate.

Multi-ingredient: ***Ger.:*** Nervinum Stada†; Nervisal†; Nervolitan†; Resedorm†.

Azaperone (12412-x)

Azaperone *(BAN, USAN, rINN)*.

R-1929. 4′-Fluoro-4-[4-(2-pyridyl)piperazin-1-yl]butyrophenone.

$C_{19}H_{22}FN_3O$ = 327.4.

CAS — 1649-18-9.

Pharmacopoeias. In *US* for veterinary use only. Also in *BP(Vet)*.

A white to yellowish-white microcrystalline powder. M.p. 90° to 95°. Practically **insoluble** in water; soluble in alcohol; freely soluble in chloroform; sparingly soluble in ether. **Protect** from light.

Azaperone is a butyrophenone antipsychotic used as a tranquilliser in veterinary practice.

A temporary acceptable daily intake had been established for azaperone taking into account its sedative effect in humans.[1] Further genotoxicity and carcinogenicity studies were requested as was a study of its effects on reproduction and fertility in the male.

1. FAO/WHO. Evaluation of certain veterinary drug residues in food: forty-third report of the joint FAO/WHO expert committee on food additives. *WHO Tech Rep Ser 855* 1995.

Barbitone (4009-s)

Barbitone *(BAN)*.

Barbital *(rINN)*; Barbitalum; Diemalum; Diethylmalonylurea. 5,5-Diethylbarbituric acid.

$C_8H_{12}N_2O_3$ = 184.2.

CAS — 57-44-3.

Pharmacopoeias. In *Eur.* (see p.viii), *Jpn*, and *Pol.*

A white, crystalline powder or colourless crystals. Slightly **soluble** in water; soluble in boiling water, in alcohol, and in ether. It forms water-soluble compounds with alkali hydroxides and carbonates and with ammonia.

Barbitone Sodium (4010-h)

Barbitone Sodium *(BANM)*.

Barbital Sodium *(rINN)*; Barbitalum Natricum; Diemalnatrium; Soluble Barbitone. Sodium 5,5-diethylbarbiturate.

$C_8H_{11}N_2NaO_3$ = 206.2.

CAS — 144-02-5.

Pharmacopoeias. In *Aust., Pol.,* and *Swiss.*

Barbitone is a barbiturate with general properties similar to those of amylobarbitone (p.641). It was formerly used for its hypnotic and sedative properties.

Preparations

Proprietary Preparations (details are given in Part 3)
Ger.: nervo OPT mono†.

Multi-ingredient: ***Ger.:*** Baldronit cum Nitro†; Baldronit forte N†; Nervo.opt†; Pronervon N†; ***Ital.:*** Megal†.

Benperidol (7006-q)

Benperidol *(BAN, USAN, rINN)*.

Benperidolum; Benzperidol; CB-8089; McN-JR-4584; R-4584. 1-{1-[3-(4-Fluorobenzoyl)propyl]-4-piperidyl}benzimidazolin-2-one.

$C_{22}H_{24}FN_3O_2$ = 381.4.

CAS — 2062-84-2.

Pharmacopoeias. In *Eur.* (see p.viii).

A white or almost white powder. It exhibits polymorphism. Practically **insoluble** in water; slightly soluble in alcohol; soluble in dichloromethane; freely soluble in dimethylformamide. **Protect** from light.

Benperidol is a butyrophenone with general properties similar to those of haloperidol (p.673). Doses of 0.25 to 1.5 mg daily in divided doses are given by mouth in the management of deviant sexual behaviour. Elderly or debilitated patients may require reduced doses of benperidol.

In some countries benperidol is given by mouth or parenterally for the treatment of psychotic conditions (p.636).

Pharmacokinetics. References.

1. Furlanut M, *et al.* Pharmacokinetics of benperidol in volunteers after oral administration. *Int J Clin Pharmacol Res* 1988; **8:** 13–16.

Deviant sexual behaviour. Results of a double-blind placebo-controlled crossover study demonstrated no difference between the effect of benperidol 1.25 mg daily, chlorpromazine 125 mg daily, or placebo, on sexual drive and arousal in 12 paedophilic sexual offenders, except for a lower frequency of sexual thoughts with benperidol.[1] The effects of benperidol are unlikely to be sufficient to control severe forms of antisocial sexually deviant behaviour. The management of deviant sexual behaviour is discussed under Disturbed Behaviour on p.636.

1. Tennent G, *et al.* The control of deviant sexual behaviour by drugs: a double-blind controlled study of benperidol, chlorpromazine, and placebo. *Arch Sex Behav* 1974; **3:** 261–71.

Preparations

Proprietary Preparations (details are given in Part 3)
Belg.: Frenactil; ***Ger.:*** Glianimon; ***Irl.:*** Anquil; ***Ital.:*** Psicoben†; ***Neth.:*** Frenactil; ***UK:*** Anquil.

Bentazepam (12429-g)

Bentazepam *(USAN, rINN)*.

CI-718; QM-6008. 1,3,6,7,8,9-Hexahydro-5-phenyl-2*H*-[1]benzothieno[2,3-e]-1,4-diazepin-2-one.

$C_{17}H_{16}N_2OS$ = 296.4.

CAS — 29462-18-8.

Bentazepam is a benzodiazepine with general properties similar to those of diazepam (p.661). It is given by mouth in the treatment of anxiety disorders (p.635) and insomnia (p.638).

Effects on the liver. Severe chronic active hepatitis has been reported in a 65-year-old man who had received long-term treatment with bentazepam.[1]

1. Andrade RJ, *et al.* Bentazepam-associated chronic liver disease. *Lancet* 1994; **343:** 860.

Preparations

Proprietary Preparations (details are given in Part 3)
Spain: Tiadipona.

Brallobarbital (5149-g)

Brallobarbital *(rINN)*.

UCB-5033. 5-Allyl-5-(2-bromoallyl)barbituric acid.

$C_{10}H_{11}BrN_2O_3$ = 287.1.

CAS — 561-86-4.

Brallobarbital is a barbiturate with general properties similar to those of amylobarbitone (p.641). It has been used in preparations for the management of insomnia but barbiturates are no longer considered appropriate for such a purpose. Brallobarbital calcium has been used similarly.

Preparations

Proprietary Preparations (details are given in Part 3)
Multi-ingredient: ***Belg.:*** Bellanox; Vesparax; ***Ger.:*** Vesparax†; ***Ital.:*** Vesparax†; ***Neth.:*** Vesparax; ***S.Afr.:*** Vesparax; ***Spain:*** Somatarax.

Bromazepam (7008-s)

Bromazepam *(BAN, USAN, rINN)*.

Bromazepamum; Ro-5-3350. 7-Bromo-1,3-dihydro-5-(2-pyridyl)-1,4-benzodiazepin-2-one.

$C_{14}H_{10}BrN_3O$ = 316.2.

CAS — 1812-30-2.

Pharmacopoeias. In *Eur.* (see p.viii) and *Jpn.*

A white or yellowish crystalline powder. Practically **insoluble** in water; sparingly soluble in alcohol and in dichloromethane. **Protect** from light.

Dependence and Withdrawal, Adverse Effects, Treatment, and Precautions

As for Diazepam, p.661.

Interactions

As for Diazepam, p.663.

Pharmacokinetics

Bromazepam is well absorbed from the gastro-intestinal tract following oral administration and peak plasma concentrations are achieved within 1 to 4 hours. It is highly bound to plasma proteins. Reported values for the mean plasma elimination half-life have ranged from about 12 to 32 hours. It is excreted mainly in the urine in the form of inactive conjugated metabolites.

References.

1. Kaplan SA, *et al.* Biopharmaceutical and clinical pharmacokinetic profile of bromazepam. *J Pharmacokinet Biopharm* 1976; **4:** 1–16.
2. Ochs HR, *et al.* Bromazepam pharmacokinetics: influence of age, gender, oral contraceptives, cimetidine, and propranolol. *Clin Pharmacol Ther* 1987; **41:** 562–70.

Uses and Administration

Bromazepam is a benzodiazepine with general properties similar to those of diazepam (p.666). It is used in the treatment of anxiety disorders (p.635) and insomnia (p.638). A usual dose for anxiety is 3 to 18 mg daily in divided doses by mouth. Higher doses have occasionally been given. Doses should be reduced by at least half in elderly patients.

References.

1. Erb T, *et al.* Preoperative anxiolysis with minimal sedation in elderly patients: bromazepam or clorazepate-dipotassium? *Acta Anaesthesiol Scand* 1998; **42:** 97–101.

Preparations

Proprietary Preparations (details are given in Part 3)
Aust.: Lexotanil; ***Austral.:*** Lexotan; ***Belg.:*** Bromidem; Lexotan; ***Canad.:*** Lectopam; ***Fr.:*** Lexomil; ***Ger.:*** Bromazanil; Bromazep; durazanil; Gityl 6; Lexostad; Lexotanil; neo OPT; Normoc; ***Irl.:*** Lexotan; ***Ital.:*** Compendium; Lexotan; ***Neth.:*** Lexotanil; ***S.Afr.:*** Brazepam; Bromaze; Brozam†; Lexotan; ***Spain:*** Lexatin; ***Switz.:*** Lexotanil; ***UK:*** Lexotan.
Multi-ingredient: ***Ital.:*** Lexil.

Bromisoval (4013-v)

Bromisoval *(rINN)*.

Bromisovalerylurea; Bromisovalum; Bromvalerylurea; Bromvaletone; Bromylum. *N*-(2-Bromo-3-methylbutyryl)urea.

$C_6H_{11}BrN_2O_2$ = 223.1.

CAS — 496-67-3.

Pharmacopoeias. In *Aust., Jpn,* and *Neth.*

Bromisoval has actions and uses similar to those of carbromal (p.645).

Preparations

Proprietary Preparations (details are given in Part 3)
Multi-ingredient: ***Aust.:*** Seduan†; ***Ger.:*** Sekundal†; Steno-Valocordin†.

Bromperidol (7009-w)

Bromperidol *(BAN, USAN, rINN)*.

Bromperidolum; R-11333. 4-[4-(*p*-Bromophenyl)-4-hydroxypiperidino]-4′-fluorobutyrophenone.

$C_{21}H_{23}BrFNO_2$ = 420.3.

CAS — 10457-90-6.

Pharmacopoeias. In *Eur.* (see p.viii).

A white or almost white powder. Practically **insoluble** in water; slightly soluble in alcohol; sparingly soluble in methyl alcohol and in dichloromethane. **Protect** from light.

Bromperidol Decanoate (16551-k)

Bromperidol Decanoate *(BANM, USAN, rINNM)*.

R-46541.

$C_{31}H_{41}BrFNO_3$ = 574.6.

CAS — 75067-66-2.

Bromperidol is a butyrophenone with general properties similar to those of haloperidol (p.673). It is given in the treatment of schizophrenia (p.637) and other psychoses. Some bromperidol preparations are prepared with the aid of lactic acid and may be stated to contain bromperidol lactate. However, doses are expressed in terms of the equivalent amount of bromperidol. A usual dose is 1 to 15 mg daily by mouth, although up to 80 mg daily has been given. Elderly patients may require reduced doses of bromperidol. Bromperidol may also be administered by intramuscular or intravenous injection.

The long-acting decanoate ester may be used for patients requiring long-term therapy with bromperidol. A usual dose, given by deep intramuscular injection, is the equivalent of up to 300 mg of bromperidol every 4 weeks.

References.

1. Benfield P, *et al.* Bromperidol: a preliminary review of its pharmacodynamic and pharmacokinetic properties, and therapeutic efficacy in psychoses. *Drugs* 1988; **35:** 670–84.
2. Parent M, *et al.* Long-term treatment of chronic psychotics with bromperidol decanoate: clinical and pharmacokinetic evaluation. *Curr Ther Res* 1983; **34:** 1–6.
3. McLaren S, *et al.* Positive and negative symptoms, depression and social disability in chronic schizophrenia: a comparative trial of bromperidol and fluphenazine decanoates. *Int J Clin Psychopharmacol* 1992; **7:** 67–72.

Preparations

Proprietary Preparations (details are given in Part 3)
Belg.: Impromen; ***Ger.:*** Impromen; Tesoprel; ***Ital.:*** Impromen; ***Neth.:*** Impromen.

Brotizolam (12458-e)

Brotizolam *(BAN, USAN, rINN)*.

We-941; We-941-BS. 2-Bromo-4-(2-chlorophenyl)-9-methyl-6*H*-thieno[3,2-*f*][1,2,4]triazolo[4,3-*a*][1,4]diazepine.

$C_{15}H_{10}BrClN_4S$ = 393.7.

CAS — 57801-81-7.

Dependence and Withdrawal, Adverse Effects, Treatment, and Precautions

As for Diazepam, p.661.

Abuse. Reference to abuse of brotizolam in Germany and Hong Kong.[1]

1. WHO. WHO expert committee on drug dependence: twenty-ninth report. *WHO Tech Rep Ser 856* 1995.

Interactions

As for Diazepam, p.663.

Pharmacokinetics

Brotizolam is rapidly absorbed from the gastro-intestinal tract and is almost completely metabolised. The two major hydroxylated metabolites are excreted in urine as glucuronide or sulphate conjugates. The elimination half-life of the parent drug is reported to range from 3.6 to 7.9 hours and the major metabolites probably have similar half-lives to brotizolam itself. The oral bioavailability of brotizolam is reported to be about 70%.

References.

1. Bechtel WD. Pharmacokinetics and metabolism of brotizolam in humans. *Br J Clin Pharmacol* 1983; **16:** 279S–283S.
2. Jochemsen R, *et al.* Pharmacokinetics of brotizolam in healthy subjects following intravenous and oral administration. *Br J Clin Pharmacol* 1983; **16:** 285S–290S.

Uses and Administration

Brotizolam is a short-acting benzodiazepine with general properties similar to those of diazepam (p.666). It is given by mouth for the short-term management of insomnia (p.638) in usual doses of 250 μg at night. The suggested dose for elderly and debilitated patients is 125 μg.

Reviews and references of the actions and uses of brotizolam.

1. Langley MS, Clissold SP. Brotizolam: a review of its pharmacodynamic and pharmacokinetic properties, and therapeutic efficacy as an hypnotic. *Drugs* 1988; **35:** 104–22.
2. *Br J Clin Pharmacol* 1983; **16** (suppl 2): 200S–440S.

Preparations

Proprietary Preparations (details are given in Part 3)
Aust.: Lendorm; ***Belg.:*** Lendormin; ***Ger.:*** Lendormin; ***Ital.:*** Lendormin; Nimbisan; ***Jpn:*** Lendormin; ***Neth.:*** Lendormin; ***S.Afr.:*** Lendormin; ***Spain:*** Sintonal; ***Switz.:*** Lendormine.

Buspirone Hydrochloride (12471-p)

Buspirone Hydrochloride *(BANM, USAN, rINNM)*.

MJ-9022-1. 8-[4-(4-Pyrimidin-2-ylpiperazin-1-yl)butyl]-8-azaspiro[4.5]decane-7,9-dione hydrochloride.

$C_{21}H_{31}N_5O_2,HCl$ = 422.0.

CAS — 36505-84-7 (buspirone); 33386-08-2 (buspirone hydrochloride).

Pharmacopoeias. In *US.*

A white crystalline powder. Very **soluble** in water; sparingly soluble in alcohol and in acetonitrile; very slightly soluble in ethyl acetate; freely soluble in dichloromethane and in methyl alcohol. **Store** in airtight containers at a temperature between 15° and 30°. Protect from light.

Dependence and Adverse Effects

Dizziness, nausea, headache, nervousness, light-headedness, excitement, paraesthesias, sleep disturbances, chest pain, tinnitus, sore throat, and nasal congestion are amongst the most frequent adverse effects reported following the use of buspirone hydrochloride. Other adverse effects have included tachycardia, palpitations, drowsiness, confusion, dry mouth, fatigue, and sweating. A syndrome of restlessness appearing shortly after the start of treatment has been reported in a small number of patients given buspirone. Buspirone is reported to produce less sedation, and to have a lower potential for dependence, than the benzodiazepines.

Mild acute hypertension and panic were reported on two occasions after the addition of single 10-mg doses of buspirone to therapy with tricyclic antidepressants in a 40-year-old man with panic disorder. Adrenergic or serotonin dysfunction were postulated as possible mechanisms for the reaction.[1,2] Psychotic reactions associated with buspirone treatment have also been reported in a few patients.[3] There have also been isolated reports of mania.[4]

1. Chignon JM, Lepine JP. Panic and hypertension associated with single dose of buspirone. *Lancet* 1989; **ii:** 46–7.
2. Norman TR, Judd FK. Panic attacks, buspirone, and serotonin function. *Lancet* 1989; **ii:** 615.
3. Friedman R. Possible induction of psychosis by buspirone. *Am J Psychiatry* 1991; **148:** 1606.
4. Price WA, Bielefeld M. Buspirone-induced mania. *J Clin Psychopharmacol* 1989; **9:** 150–1.

Extrapyramidal disorders. There have been isolated reports of exacerbation or precipitation of movement disorders[1-4] associated with the use of buspirone. However, buspirone has also been reported to have been of benefit in some patients with tardive dyskinesia (see under Uses and Administration, below).

1. Hammerstad JP, *et al.* Buspirone in Parkinson's disease. *Clin Neuropharmacol* 1986; **9:** 556–60.
2. Strauss A. Oral dyskinesia associated with buspirone use in an elderly woman. *J Clin Psychiatry* 1988; **49:** 322–3.
3. Ritchie EC, *et al.* Acute generalized myoclonus following buspirone administration. *J Clin Psychiatry* 1988; **49:** 242–3.
4. LeWitt PA, *et al.* Persistent movement disorders induced by buspirone. *Mov Disord* 1993; **8:** 331–4.

Precautions

Buspirone hydrochloride should be used with caution in patients with renal or hepatic disease and is contra-indicated if the disease is severe. Buspirone should be avoided during pregnancy and breast feeding. It should not be used in patients with epilepsy. It does not exhibit cross-tolerance with benzodiazepines and will not block symptoms of their withdrawal; benzodiazepines should, therefore, be gradually withdrawn before commencing treatment with buspirone. Buspirone may impair the patient's ability to drive or operate machinery.

Diagnosis and testing. Buspirone may interfere with diagnostic assays of urinary catecholamines.[1]

1. Cook FJ, *et al.* Effect of buspirone on urinary catecholamine assays. *N Engl J Med* 1995; **332:** 401.

Hepatic impairment. The mean peak plasma-buspirone concentration was about 16 times higher in 12 cirrhotic patients given a single dose of buspirone by mouth than in 12 control subjects.[1] The elimination half-life in patients with cirrhosis was prolonged about twofold. A secondary peak concentration was seen in some subjects of each group. This peak occurred between 4 and 24 hours after drug administration in the cirrhotics and between 2 and 8 hours after administration in controls. The multiple-dose pharmacokinetics of buspirone and its metabolite 1-(2-pyrimidinyl)-piperazine were studied in a further 12 patients with hepatic impairment and 12 healthy subjects.[2] Data from this study suggested that there was accumulation of buspirone and its metabolite but that plasma concentrations appeared to reach steady state after 3 days regardless of the state of liver function. The area under the curve and mean maximum concentration for buspirone were both higher in patients with hepatic impairment than in healthy subjects, but there were no significant differences for these parameters for its metabolites. Specific dosing recommendations could not be made for patients with hepatic impairment because of the high intra- and inter-subject variations in plasma-buspirone concentrations. Caution was advised when using buspirone in patients with liver disease.

1. Dalhoff K, *et al.* Buspirone pharmacokinetics in patients with cirrhosis. *Br J Clin Pharmacol* 1987; **24:** 547–50.
2. Barbhaiya RH, *et al.* Disposition kinetics of buspirone in patients with renal or hepatic impairment after administration of single and multiple doses. *Eur J Clin Pharmacol* 1994; **46:** 41–7.

Renal impairment. The pharmacokinetics of buspirone and its metabolite 1-(2-pyrimidinyl)-piperazine (1-PP) have been compared in patients with renal impairment and healthy subjects following single and multiple dose administration.[1,2] The data suggested that there was accumulation of buspirone and its metabolite following repeated administration but that plasma concentrations appeared to reach steady state after 3 days regardless of the state of renal function. At steady state both the area under the curve and maximum concentrations for buspirone and its metabolite were greater in patients with renal failure than in healthy subjects. Specific dosing recommendations could not be made for patients with renal impairment because of the high intra- and inter-subject variations in buspirone plasma concentrations following repeated administration. Buspirone should be given with caution to patients with renal impairment.

1-PP, but not buspirone, was removed by haemodialysis.[1]

1. Caccia S, *et al.* Clinical pharmacokinetics of oral buspirone in patients with impaired renal function. *Clin Pharmacokinet* 1988; **14:** 171–7.
2. Barbhaiya RH, *et al.* Disposition kinetics of buspirone in patients with renal or hepatic impairment after administration of single and multiple doses. *Eur J Clin Pharmacol* 1994; **46:** 41–7.

Interactions

The sedative effects of buspirone are enhanced by the simultaneous administration of alcohol or other CNS depressants. Because of reports of increased blood pressure in patients receiving buspirone hydrochloride with an MAOI, the manufacturers of buspirone recommend that it should not be given with an MAOI.

Pretreatment with *erythromycin* or *itraconazole* in healthy subjects given buspirone resulted in mild to moderate side-effects associated with large increases in peak plasma concentrations and the area under the curve for buspirone.[1] Increases in peak plasma concentrations and the area under the curve for buspirone have also been seen in healthy subjects pretreated with *diltiazem* or *verapamil*.[2] The effect was probably due to inhibition of first-pass metabolism of buspirone usually mediated by the cytochrome P450 isozyme CYP3A4. Buspirone should be used with caution in patients taking inhibitors of CYP3A4; the dose of buspirone may need to be greatly reduced during concomitant administration with potent inhibitors of CYP3A4.

1. Kivistö KT, *et al.* Plasma buspirone concentrations are greatly increased by erythromycin and itraconazole. *Clin Pharmacol Ther* 1997; **62:** 348–54.
2. Lamberg TS, *et al.* Effects of verapamil and diltiazem on the pharmacokinetics and pharmacodynamics of buspirone. *Clin Pharmacol Ther* 1998; **63:** 640–5.

Antipsychotics. For the effect of buspirone on serum concentrations of *haloperidol*, see under Chlorpromazine, p.653.

Rifampicin. Pretreatment with *rifampicin* greatly reduced plasma concentrations of buspirone in a study involving 10 healthy subjects.[1] A reduced anxiolytic effect could be expected if buspirone is used with rifampicin or other potent inducers of the cytochrome P450 isozyme CYP3A4.

1. Lamberg TS, *et al.* Concentrations and effects of buspirone are considerably reduced by rifampicin. *Br J Clin Pharmacol* 1998; **45:** 381–5.

Pharmacokinetics

Buspirone hydrochloride is rapidly absorbed from the gastro-intestinal tract reaching peak plasma concentrations within 40 to 90 minutes after administration by mouth. Systemic bioavailability is low because of extensive first-pass metabolism, but may be increased on administration with food as this delays absorption from the gastro-intestinal tract and thereby reduces presystemic clearance. Buspirone is about 95% bound to plasma proteins. Metabolism in the liver is extensive; hydroxylation yields several inactive metabolites and oxidative dealkylation produces 1-(2-pyrimidinyl)-piperazine which is reported to be about 25% as potent as the parent drug in one model of anxiolytic activity. The elimination half-life of buspirone is usually about 2 to 3 hours but half-lives of up to 11 hours have been reported. Buspirone is excreted mainly as metabolites in the urine, and also in the faeces.

Uses and Administration

Buspirone hydrochloride is an azaspirodecanedione anxiolytic. It is reported to be largely lacking in sedative, anticonvulsant, and muscle relaxant actions.

Buspirone hydrochloride is given, in initial doses of 5 mg two or three times daily, in the short-term management of anxiety disorders. The dose may be increased in increments of 5 mg at 2- to 3-day intervals if required. The recommended maximum daily dose, to be administered in divided doses, is 45 mg in the UK and 60 mg in the USA.

General reviews.

1. Fulton B, Brogden RN. Buspirone: an updated review of its clinical pharmacology and therapeutic applications. *CNS Drugs* 1997; **7:** 68–88.

Action. Buspirone has dopaminergic, noradrenergic, and serotonin-modulating properties[1] and its anxiolytic effects appear to be related to its action on serotonin (5-hydroxytryptamine, 5-HT) neurotransmission. Buspirone, and the newer drugs gepirone and ipsapirone, are partial agonists at 5-HT_{1A} receptors.[1,2] While such drugs may inhibit serotonin neurotransmission (most likely via 5-HT_{1A} autoreceptor stimulation), they may also have postsynaptic 5-HT_{1A} agonist activity and thus facilitate serotonin neurotransmission.[1] To complicate matters further, 5-HT_{1A} partial agonists have demonstrated both anxiolytic and anxiogenic properties in *animal* models of anxiety. Clinical studies have, however, shown that buspirone is effective in the treatment of generalised anxiety.[1,2]

Clinical studies with buspirone and gepirone suggest that 5-HT_{1A} partial agonists may be useful in the treatment of depression, possibly by downregulation of either 5-HT_{1A} or 5-HT_2 receptors or both.[1] There is some suggestion that buspirone has an anti-aggressive action in humans; it is unclear whether this is mediated via dopaminergic or serotonergic mechanisms.

Buspirone also has characteristics of both a dopamine agonist and antagonist; this may result in stimulation of both growth hormone and prolactin secretion.[3]

1. Glitz DA, Pohl R. 5-HT_{1A} partial agonists: what is their future? *Drugs* 1991; **41:** 11–18.
2. Marsden CA. The pharmacology of new anxiolytics acting on 5-HT neurones. *Postgrad Med J* 1990; **66** (suppl 2): S2–S6.
3. Meltzer HY, *et al.* The effect of buspirone on prolactin and growth hormone secretion in man. *Arch Gen Psychiatry* 1983; **40:** 1099–1102.

Anxiety disorders. Buspirone has been shown to be as effective as the benzodiazepines in the short-term treatment of generalised anxiety disorder (p.635) and to be less likely to cause sedation or psychomotor and cognitive impairment. It also appears to have a lower propensity for interaction with alcohol and a lower risk of abuse and dependence. However, its usefulness may be limited by a relatively slow response to treatment, which some commentators consider may take up to 2 to 4 weeks to appear. Its efficacy may be reduced in patients who have recently taken benzodiazepines. It appears to be ineffective in panic disorders and convincing efficacy in other anxiety disorders remains to be determined.

References.

1. Caven P. Drugs in focus: 5. buspirone. *Prescribers' J* 1992; **32:** 200–204.
2. Deakin JFW. A review of clinical efficacy of 5-HT_{1A} agonists in anxiety and depression. *J Psychopharmacol* 1993; **7:** 283–9.
3. Pecknold JC. A risk-benefit assessment of buspirone in the treatment of anxiety disorders. *Drug Safety* 1997; **16:** 118–32.
4. Fulton B, Brogden RN. Buspirone: an updated review of its clinical pharmacology and therapeutic applications. *CNS Drugs* 1997; **7:** 68–88.

Bruxism. Bruxism, which developed in a 20-year old woman during treatment with paroxetine, was successfully controlled by concomitant therapy with buspirone.[1]

1. Romanelli F, *et al.* Possible paroxetine-induced bruxism. *Ann Pharmacother* 1996; **30:** 1246–7.

Cerebellar ataxias. In general the management of cerebellar ataxias is mainly supportive; buspirone has improved some symptoms of ataxia in a small study of patients with cerebellar cortical activity.[1]

1. Trouillas P, *et al.* Buspirone, a $5\text{-hydroxytryptamine}_{1A}$ agonist, is active in cerebellar ataxia: results of a double-blind drug placebo study in patients with cerebellar cortical atrophy. *Arch Neurol* 1997; **54:** 749–52.

Disturbed behaviour. Buspirone has been tried in various disorders for the control of symptoms such as agitation, aggression, and disruptive behaviour (see Disturbed Behaviour, p.636) but evidence of efficacy is limited. Nonetheless, in the management of dementia, some[1] consider that it might be worth trying in nonpsychotic patients with disturbed behaviour, especially those with mild symptoms or those intolerant or unresponsive to antipsychotics.

1. American Psychiatric Association. Practice guideline for the treatment of patients with Alzheimer's disease and other dementias of late life. *Am J Psychiatry* 1997; **154** (suppl): 1–39.

Extrapyramidal disorders. Although there have been reports[1,2] that buspirone may improve symptoms of drug-induced dyskinesia, drugs with dopaminergic actions have mostly exacerbated symptoms and there are a few reports of extrapyramidal disorders with buspirone (see under Adverse Effects, above). The management of drug-induced extrapyramidal effects is discussed under Extrapyramidal Disorders on p.650.

1. Moss LE, *et al.* Buspirone in the treatment of tardive dyskinesia. *J Clin Psychopharmacol* 1993; **13:** 204–9.
2. Bonifati V, *et al.* Buspirone in levodopa-induced dyskinesias. *Clin Neuropharmacol* 1994; **17:** 73–82.

Tourette's syndrome. Report[1] of a 42-year-old patient with Tourette's syndrome (p.636) refractory to antipsychotics who had a 70% reduction in tic severity during treatment with buspirone 30 mg daily. Worsening of symptoms was noted during the period in which buspirone was discontinued.

1. Dursun SM, *et al.* Buspirone treatment of Tourette's syndrome. *Lancet* 1995; **345:** 1366–7.

Withdrawal syndromes. ALCOHOL. Despite an early study[1] suggesting that buspirone could reduce alcohol craving in alcohol dependent patients, later studies[2-4] have overall failed to confirm that buspirone improves abstinence or reduces alcohol consumption. Although some studies[3,5] have found that buspirone may improve certain psychopathological symptoms in these patients, others[4] have found no such benefit.

The management of alcohol withdrawal and abstinence is discussed on p.1099.

1. Bruno F. Buspirone in the treatment of alcoholic patients. *Psychopathology* 1989; **22** (suppl 1): 49–59.
2. George DT, *et al.* Buspirone does not promote long term abstinence in alcoholics. *Clin Pharmacol Ther* 1995; **57:** 161.
3. Malec E, *et al.* Buspirone in the treatment of alcohol dependence: a placebo-controlled trial. *Alcohol Clin Exp Res* 1996; **20:** 307–12.
4. Malcolm R, *et al.* A placebo-controlled trial of buspirone in anxious inpatient alcoholics. *Alcohol Clin Exp Res* 1992; **16:** 1007–13.
5. Kranzler HR, *et al.* Buspirone treatment of anxious alcoholics: a placebo-controlled trial. *Arch Gen Psychiatry* 1994; **51:** 720–31.

NICOTINE. Buspirone has produced conflicting results[1-4] in the management of smoking cessation (p.1608). Although some studies suggest that in the short-term buspirone can increase the numbers of patients who are able to cease smoking, it does not necessarily decrease withdrawal symptoms.

1. West R, *et al.* Effect of buspirone on cigarette withdrawal symptoms and short-term abstinence rates in a smokers clinic. *Psychopharmacology (Berl)* 1991; **104:** 91–6.
2. Hilleman DE, *et al.* Effect of buspirone on withdrawal symptoms associated with smoking cessation. *Arch Intern Med* 1992; **152:** 350–2.
3. Hilleman DE, *et al.* Comparison of fixed-dose transdermal nicotine, tapered-dose transdermal nicotine, and buspirone in smoking cessation. *J Clin Pharmacol* 1994; **34:** 222–4.
4. Schneider NG, *et al.* Efficacy of buspirone in smoking cessation: a placebo-controlled trial. *Clin Pharmacol Ther* 1996; **60:** 568–75.

Preparations

USP 23: Buspirone Hydrochloride Tablets.

Proprietary Preparations (details are given in Part 3)
Aust.: Buspar; ***Austral.:*** Buspar; ***Belg.:*** Buspar; ***Canad.:*** Buspar; ***Fr.:*** Buspar; ***Ger.:*** Bespar; ***Irl.:*** Buspar; ***Ital.:*** Axoren; Buspar; Buspimen; ***Neth.:*** Buspar; ***Norw.:*** Buspar; ***S.Afr.:*** Buspar; Pasrin; ***Spain:*** Ansial†; Buspar; Buspisal; Effiplen; Narol; ***Swed.:*** Buspar; ***Switz.:*** Buspar; ***UK:*** Buspar; ***USA:*** Buspar.

Butalbital (4014-g)

Butalbital *(USAN, rINN)*.

Alisobumalum; Allylbarbital; Allylbarbituric Acid; Itobarbital; Tetrallobarbital. 5-Allyl-5-isobutylbarbituric acid.

$C_{11}H_{16}N_2O_3$ = 224.3.

CAS — *77-26-9.*

NOTE. The name Butalbital has also been applied to talbutal, the *S*-butyl analogue, which was formerly used as a hypnotic and sedative.

Compounded preparations of butalbital, paracetamol (acetaminophen), and caffeine in USP 23 may be represented by the name Co-bucafAPAP.

Pharmacopoeias. In US.

A white odourless crystalline powder. Slightly **soluble** in cold water; soluble in boiling water; freely soluble in alcohol, in chloroform, and in ether; soluble in aqueous solutions of alkali hydroxides and carbonates. A saturated solution is acid to litmus.

Butalbital is a barbiturate with general properties similar to those of amylobarbitone (p.641). It has been used mainly in combination with analgesics, in the treatment of occasional tension-type headaches (p.444), but other treatments are generally preferred. Doses that have been given by mouth range from 50 to 100 mg up to every 4 hours with a maximum of 300 mg in 24 hours.

Preparations

USP 23: Butalbital and Aspirin Tablets; Butalbital, Acetaminophen, and Caffeine Capsules; Butalbital, Acetaminophen, and Caffeine Tablets; Butalbital, Aspirin, and Caffeine Capsules; Butalbital, Aspirin, and Caffeine Tablets; Butalbital, Aspirin, Caffeine, and Codeine Phosphate Capsules.

Proprietary Preparations (details are given in Part 3)

Multi-ingredient: ***Belg.:*** Cafergot-PB†; ***Canad.:*** Fiorinal; Fiorinal C; Tecnal; Tecnal C; ***Ital.:*** Optalidon; ***Norw.:*** Cafergot Comp; ***S.Afr.:*** Cafergot-PB; ***Spain:*** Cafergot-PB; ***Switz.:*** Cafergot-PB; ***USA:*** Amaphen; Amaphen with Codeine; Anoquan; Arcet; Axotal†; Bucet; Bupap; Endolor; Esgic-Plus; Femcet; Fiorgen PF†; Fioricet; Fioricet with Codeine; Fiorinal; Fiorinal with Codeine; Fiorpap; Fiortal; Isocet; Isollyl Improved†; Lanorinal; Margesic; Marnal; Medigesic; Pacaps; Phrenilin; Prominol; Pyridium Plus†; Repan; Repan CF; Sedapap-10; Tencet; Tencon; Triad; Triaprin†; Two-Dyne†.

Butobarbitone (4015-q)

Butobarbitone *(BAN).*

Butethal; Butobarbital; Butobarbitalum. 5-Butyl-5-ethylbarbituric acid.

$C_{10}H_{16}N_2O_3$ = 212.2.

CAS — 77-28-1.

NOTE. Butobarbitone should be distinguished from Butabarbitone, which is Secbutobarbitone (p.692).

Pharmacopoeias. In *Aust., Belg., Fr., It., Neth.,* and *Port.*

Dependence and Withdrawal, Adverse Effects, Treatment, and Precautions

As for Amylobarbitone, p.641.

Interactions

As for Amylobarbitone, p.642.

Antibacterials. Results suggesting that *metronidazole* alters the metabolism of butobarbitone when taken concomitantly.[1]

1. Al Sharifi MA, *et al.* The effect of anti-amoebic drug therapy on the metabolism of butobarbitone. *J Pharm Pharmacol* 1982; **34:** 126–7.

Pharmacokinetics

Butobarbitone is metabolised in the liver mainly by hydroxylation; small amounts are excreted in the urine as unchanged drug. It has been reported to have a half-life of about 40 to 55 hours and to be about 26% bound to plasma proteins.

Uses and Administration

Butobarbitone is a barbiturate with general properties similar to those of amylobarbitone (p.642). Its use can no longer be recommended because of the risk of its adverse effects and of dependence, although continued use may occasionally be considered necessary for severe intractable insomnia (p.638) in patients already taking it. It is given by mouth in usual doses of 100 to 200 mg at night.

Preparations

Proprietary Preparations (details are given in Part 3)

Austral.: Soneryl†; ***Irl.:*** Soneryl†; ***S.Afr.:*** Soneryl†; ***UK:*** Soneryl.

Multi-ingredient: ***Belg.:*** Theophylline Sedative Bruneau†; ***Canad.:*** Ancatropine Infant Drops†; ***Fr.:*** Hypnasmine; ***USA:*** Axocet.

Calcium Bromolactobionate (12504-n)

Calcium bromide lactobionate hexahydrate.

$Ca(C_{12}H_{21}O_{12})_2,CaBr_2,6H_2O$ = 1062.6.

CAS — 33659-28-8 (anhydrous calcium bromolactobionate).

Calcium bromolactobionate has sedative properties and has been given by mouth and intravenous injection in the treatment of insomnia and nervous disorders. The use of bromides is generally deprecated.

Preparations

Proprietary Preparations (details are given in Part 3)

Fr.: Calcibronat; ***Ital.:*** Calcibronat.

Multi-ingredient: ***Fr.:*** Assagix.

Camazepam (7012-v)

Camazepam *(rINN).*

SB-5833. 7-Chloro-2,3-dihydro-1-methyl-2-oxo-5-phenyl-1*H*-1,4-benzodiazepin-3-yl dimethylcarbamate.

$C_{19}H_{18}ClN_3O_3$ = 371.8.

CAS — 36104-80-0.

Camazepam is a benzodiazepine with general properties similar to those of diazepam (p.661). It is given by mouth for the treatment of anxiety disorders (p.635) and insomnia (p.638).

Preparations

Proprietary Preparations (details are given in Part 3)

Ital.: Albego†; ***Spain:*** Albego; ***Switz.:*** Albego†.

Captodiame Hydrochloride (7013-g)

Captodiame Hydrochloride *(BANM, pINNM).*

Captodiamine Hydrochloride. 2-(4-Butylthiobenzhydrylthio)ethyldimethylamine hydrochloride.

$C_{21}H_{29}NS_2,HCl$ = 396.1.

CAS — 486-17-9 (captodiame); 904-04-1 (captodiame hydrochloride).

Captodiame hydrochloride has been given in doses of 50 mg three times daily by mouth for the treatment of anxiety disorders (p.635).

Preparations

Proprietary Preparations (details are given in Part 3)

Fr.: Covatine.

Carbromal (4018-w)

Carbromal *(BAN, rINN).*

Bromodiethylacetylurea; Karbromal. *N*-(2-Bromo-2-ethylbutyryl)urea.

$C_7H_{13}BrN_2O_2$ = 237.1.

CAS — 77-65-6.

Pharmacopoeias. In *Aust.* and *Belg.*

Carbromal is a bromureide with general properties similar to those of the barbiturates (see Amylobarbitone, p.641). It was formerly used for its hypnotic and sedative properties. Chronic use of carbromal could result in symptoms resembling bromism (see Potassium Bromide, p.1620).

Porphyria. Carbromal has been associated with acute attacks of porphyria and is considered unsafe in patients with acute porphyria.[1]

1. Moore MR, McColl KEL. *Porphyria: drug lists.* Glasgow: Porphyria Research Unit, University of Glasgow, 1991.

Preparations

Proprietary Preparations (details are given in Part 3)

Multi-ingredient: ***Aust.:*** Seduan†; ***Ger.:*** Betadorm†; Plantival plus†; Sekundal†; Somnium forte†.

Carpipramine Hydrochloride (7015-p)

Carpipramine Hydrochloride *(rINNM).*

PZ-1511. 1-[3-(10,11-Dihydro-5*H*-dibenz[*b,f*]azepin-5-yl)propyl]-4-piperidinopiperidine-4-carboxamide dihydrochloride monohydrate.

$C_{28}H_{38}N_4O,2HCl,H_2O$ = 537.6.

CAS — 5942-95-0 (carpipramine); 7075-03-8 (anhydrous carpipramine hydrochloride).

Carpipramine is structurally related both to imipramine (p.289) and to butyrophenones such as haloperidol (p.673). It has been used in the management of anxiety disorders (p.635) and psychoses such as schizophrenia (p.637). Carpipramine is given as the hydrochloride in a usual dose equivalent to 50 mg of the base three times daily by mouth, with a range of 50 to 400 mg daily.

Preparations

Proprietary Preparations (details are given in Part 3)

Fr.: Prazinil.

Chloral Betaine (4019-e)

Chloral Betaine *(BAN, USAN).*

Cloral Betaine *(rINN)*; Compound 5107. An adduct of chloral hydrate and betaine.

$C_7H_{12}Cl_3NO_3,H_2O$ = 282.5.

CAS — 2218-68-0.

Chloral betaine rapidly dissociates in the stomach to release chloral hydrate and has actions and uses similar to those of chloral hydrate (below). It is given by mouth in the short-term management of insomnia (p.638).

Chloral betaine is available as tablets containing 707 mg (approximately equivalent to 414 mg of chloral hydrate). The usual hypnotic dose is one or two tablets taken at night with water or milk. The maximum daily dose is five tablets (equivalent to about 2 g of chloral hydrate).

Preparations

Proprietary Preparations (details are given in Part 3)

Irl.: Welldorm†; ***UK:*** Welldorm.

Chloral Hydrate (4020-b)

Chloral Hydrate *(BAN).*

Chlorali Hydras. 2,2,2-Trichloroethane-1,1-diol.

$C_2H_3Cl_3O_2$ = 165.4.

CAS — 302-17-0.

Pharmacopoeias. In *Chin., Eur.* (see p.viii), *Jpn, Pol.,* and *US.*

Colourless, transparent or white crystals with a pungent odour. It volatilises slowly on exposure to air and melts at about 55°. **Soluble** 1 in 0.25 of water, 1 in 1.3 of alcohol, 1 in 2 of chloroform, and 1 in 1.5 of ether; very soluble in olive oil. A 10% solution has a pH of 3.5 to 5.5. **Store** in airtight containers.

Incompatible with alkalis, alkaline earths, alkali carbonates, soluble barbiturates, borax, tannin, iodides, oxidising agents, permanganates, and alcohol (chloral alcoholate may crystallise out). It forms a liquid mixture when triturated with many organic compounds, such as camphor, menthol, phenazone, phenol, thymol, and quinine salts.

Dependence and Withdrawal, Adverse Effects, and Treatment

Chloral hydrate has an unpleasant taste and is corrosive to skin and mucous membranes unless well diluted. The most frequent adverse effect is gastric irritation; abdominal distension and flatulence may also occur. CNS effects such as drowsiness, light-headedness, ataxia, headache, and paradoxical excitement, hallucinations, nightmares, delirium, and confusion (sometimes with paranoia) occur occasionally. Hypersensitivity reactions include skin rashes. Ketonuria may occur.

The effects of acute overdosage resemble acute barbiturate intoxication (see Amylobarbitone, p.642). In addition the irritant effect may cause initial vomiting, and gastric necrosis leading to strictures. Cardiac arrhythmias have been reported. Jaundice may follow liver damage, and albuminuria may follow kidney damage.

Tolerance may develop and dependence may occur. Features of dependence and withdrawal are similar to those of barbiturates (see Amylobarbitone, p.641).

Adverse effects should be managed in a similar way to those of barbiturates (see Amylobarbitone, p.642).

In a drug surveillance programme,[1] 1618 patients received chloral hydrate as a hypnotic, usually in doses of 0.5 to 1 g. In 1130 patients evaluated, side-effects, which were reversible, occurred in 2.3% of patients and included gastro-intestinal symptoms (10 patients), CNS depression (20), and skin rash (5). In 1 patient the prothrombin time was increased; in 1 patient hepatic encephalopathy seemed to worsen; and bradycardia developed in 1 patient.

In a Boston Collaborative Drug Surveillance Program side-effects occurred in approximately 2% of 5435 patients who received chloral hydrate.[2] Three reactions were described as life-threatening.

1. Shapiro S, *et al.* Clinical effects of hypnotics II: an epidemiologic study. *JAMA* 1969; **209:** 2016–20.
2. Miller RR, Greenblatt DJ. Clinical effects of chloral hydrate in hospitalized medical patients. *J Clin Pharmacol* 1979; **19:** 669–74.

Carcinogenicity. Chloral hydrate has been widely used as a sedative, especially in children. Concern over warnings that chloral hydrate was carcinogenic in rodents[1] has prompted some experts, including the American Academy of Pediatrics, to review the relative risks of the medical use of this agent.[2,3] The original warnings appear to have been based in part on the assumption that chloral hydrate was a reactive metabolite of trichloroethylene and was responsible for its carcinogenicity but there is evidence to suggest that the carcinogenicity of trichloroethylene is due to a reactive intermediate epoxide metabolite. Studies *in vitro* indicate that choral hydrate can damage chromosomes in some mammalian test systems but there have been no studies of the carcinogenicity of chloral hydrate in humans. Some long-term studies in *mice* have linked chloral hydrate with the development of hepatic adenomas or carcinomas. However, it was noted that chloral hydrate was not the only sedative that had been shown to be a carcinogen in experimental animals. The American Academy of Pediatrics considered chloral hydrate to be an effective sedative with a low incidence of acute toxicity when administered orally in the recommended dosage for short-term sedation and although the information on carcinogenicity was of concern it was not sufficient to justify the risk associated with the use of less familiar sedatives. There was no evidence in infants or children demonstrating that any of the available alternatives were safer or more effective. However, the use of repetitive dosing with chloral hydrate to maintain prolonged sedation in neonates and other children was of concern because of the potential for accumulation of drug metabolites and resultant toxicity.

1. Smith MT. Chloral hydrate warning. *Science* 1990; **250:** 359.
2. Steinberg AD. Should chloral hydrate be banned? *Pediatrics* 1993; **92:** 442–6.
3. American Academy of Pediatrics Committee on Drugs and Committee on Environmental Health. Use of chloral hydrate for sedation in children. *Pediatrics* 1993; **92:** 471–3.

Effects on the CNS. Report[1] of a 2-year-old child who experienced the first of 2 seizures 60 minutes after receiving chloral hydrate 70 mg per kg body-weight for sedation.

1. Muñoz M, *et al.* Seizures caused by chloral hydrate sedative doses. *J Pediatr* 1997; **131:** 787–8.

Hyperbilirubinaemia. Small retrospective studies[1] have suggested that prolonged administration of chloral hydrate in neonates may be associated with the development of hyperbilirubinaemia. This may possibly be related to the prolonged half-life of the metabolite trichloroethanol in neonates.

1. Lambert GH, *et al.* Direct hyperbilirubinemia associated with chloral hydrate administration in the newborn. *Pediatrics* 1990; **86:** 277–81.

Overdosage. Of 76 cases of chloral hydrate poisoning reported to the UK National Poisons Information Service, 47 were severe.[1] Of 39 adults, 12 had cardiac arrhythmias including 5 with cardiac arrest. Antiarrhythmic drugs were recommended unless obviously contra-indicated. Haemoperfusion through charcoal or haemodialysis was recommended for patients in prolonged coma. Cardiac arrhythmias and CNS depression were also major features of 12 cases of chloral hydrate overdosage reported from Australia.[2] Lignocaine was not always successful in controlling arrhythmias, but propranolol was successful in all 7 patients in whom it was used. It was noted that resistant arrhythmias, particularly ventricular fibrillation, ventricular tachycardia, and supraventricular tachycardia were the usual cause of death in patients who had taken an overdosage of chloral hydrate. Although there had been no controlled studies of antiarrhythmic therapy in overdosage with chloral hydrate, the successful use of beta blockers appeared to be a recurring feature in reports in the literature.

Administration of flumazenil produced an increased level of consciousness, pupillary dilatation, and return of respiratory rate and blood pressure towards normal in a patient who had taken an overdosage of chloral hydrate.[3]

1. Wiseman HM, Hampel G. Cardiac arrhythmias due to chloral hydrate poisoning. *Br Med J* 1978; **2:** 960.
2. Graham SR, *et al.* Overdose with chloral hydrate: a pharmacological and therapeutic review. *Med J Aust* 1988; **149:** 686–8.
3. Donovan KL, Fisher DJ. Reversal of chloral hydrate overdose with flumazenil. *Br Med J* 1989; **298:** 1253.

Precautions

Chloral hydrate should not be used in patients with marked hepatic or renal impairment or severe cardiac disease and oral administration is best avoided in the presence of gastritis. It should be used with caution in patients susceptible to porphyria or, as with all sedatives, in those with respiratory insufficiency.

Chloral hydrate may cause drowsiness; affected patients should not drive or operate machinery. Prolonged administration and abrupt withdrawal of chloral hydrate should be avoided to prevent precipitation of withdrawal symptoms. Repeated administration in infants and children may lead to accumulation of metabolites and thereby increase the risk of adverse effects.

Chloral hydrate may interfere with tests for urinary glucose or 17-hydroxycorticosteroids.

Neonates. The half-life of trichloroethanol, an active metabolite of chloral hydrate, is prolonged in neonates;[1] values of up to 66 hours have been reported in some studies. Short-term sedation in the neonate with single oral doses of 25 to 50 mg per kg body-weight of chloral hydrate is considered[1] to be probably relatively safe, but repeated administration carries the risk of accumulation of metabolites which may result in serious toxicity. Toxic reactions may occur even after the drug has been discontinued since the metabolites may accumulate for several days.

1. Jacqz-Aigrain E, Burtin P. Clinical pharmacokinetics of sedatives in neonates. *Clin Pharmacokinet* 1996; **31:** 423–43.

Obstructive sleep apnoea. Children with obstructive sleep apnoea could be at risk from life-threatening respiratory obstruction if chloral hydrate is used for sedation. Details of 2 such children who suffered respiratory failure following sedation with chloral hydrate for lung function studies have been reported by Biban *et al.*[1]

1. Biban P, *et al.* Adverse effect of chloral hydrate in two young children with obstructive sleep apnea. *Pediatrics* 1993; **92:** 461–3.

Interactions

The sedative effects of chloral hydrate are enhanced by the simultaneous administration of depressants of the CNS such as alcohol (the 'Mickey Finn' of detective fiction), barbiturates, and other sedatives.

Chloral hydrate may enhance the effects of coumarin anticoagulants (see Warfarin, p.968). A hypermetabolic state, apparently due to displacement of thyroid hormones from their binding proteins, has been reported in patients given an intravenous dose of frusemide subsequent to chloral hydrate.

Pharmacokinetics

Chloral hydrate is rapidly absorbed from the gastro-intestinal tract and starts to act within 30 minutes of oral administration. It is widely distributed throughout the body. It is rapidly metabolised to trichloroethanol and trichloroacetic acid (p.1639) in the erythrocytes, liver, and other tissues and excreted partly in the urine as trichloroethanol and its glucuronide (urochloralic acid) and as trichloroacetic acid. Some is also excreted in the bile.

Trichloroethanol is the active metabolite, and passes into the cerebrospinal fluid, into breast milk, and across the placenta. The half-life of trichloroethanol in plasma is reported to range from about 7 to 11 hours but is considerably prolonged in the neonate.

Uses and Administration

Chloral hydrate is a hypnotic and sedative with properties similar to those of the barbiturates. It is used in the short-term management of insomnia (p.638) and has been used as a sedative for premedication (p.1220). In the USA some authorities consider chloral hydrate to be the drug of choice for sedation of children before diagnostic, dental, or medical procedures (but see under Carcinogenicity above).

Externally, chloral hydrate has a rubefacient action and has been employed as a counter-irritant.

Chloral hydrate is administered by mouth as an oral liquid or as gelatin capsules with chloral hydrate dissolved in a suitable vehicle. It has also been dissolved in a bland fixed oil and given by enema or as suppositories.

It should not be given as tablets because of the risk of damage to the mucous membrane of the alimentary tract.

The usual hypnotic dose by mouth is 0.5 to 2 g at night and as a sedative 250 mg can be given three times daily, to a maximum single or daily dose of 2 g. Oral dosage forms should be taken well diluted or with plenty of water or milk. Children may be given 30 to 50 mg per kg body-weight to a maximum single dose of 1 g as a hypnotic. A suggested sedative dose for premedication in children is 25 to 50 mg per kg to a maximum single dose of 1 g.

A reduction in dosage may be appropriate in frail elderly patients.

Derivatives of chloral hydrate, such as acetylglycinamide-chloral hydrate, chloral betaine, chloralose, chlorhexadol, and dichloralphenazone, which break down in the body to yield chloral hydrate, have been used similarly.

References.

1. McCarver-May DG, *et al.* Comparison of chloral hydrate and midazolam for sedation of neonates for neuroimaging studies. *J Pediatr* 1996; **128:** 573–6.
2. Napoli KL, *et al.* Safety and efficacy of chloral hydrate sedation in children undergoing echocardiography. *J Pediatr* 1996; **129:** 287–91.

Preparations

BP 1998: Chloral Mixture; Paediatric Chloral Elixir;
USP 23: Chloral Hydrate Capsules; Chloral Hydrate Syrup.

Proprietary Preparations (details are given in Part 3)

Aust.: Chloraldurat; ***Austral.:*** Chloralix†; Dormel†; Elix-Nocte†; Noctec†; ***Ger.:*** Chloraldurat; ***Irl.:*** Welldorm†; ***Neth.:*** Chloraldurat; ***Switz.:*** Chloraldurat; Medianox; ***UK:*** Noctec†; Welldorm; ***USA:*** Aquachloral.

Multi-ingredient: ***Belg.:*** Babygencal; Dentophar; Dermophil Indien†; Sedemol†; Sulfa-Sedemol†; Synthol; ***Canad.:*** Analgesic Balm; ***Fr.:*** Bain de Bouche Bancaud†; Bain de Bouche Lipha†; Buccawalter; Dolodent; Lini-Bombe; Oxy-thymoline†; Sirop Teyssedre†; Stom-Antiba†; Synthol; Tuberol†; ***Ger.:*** Leukona-Sedativ-Bad; ***Spain:*** Curacallos Pedykur†; Dentol Topico; Synthol†; ***Switz.:*** Histacyl Cutane†; Nervifene; Stix†; Synthol†.

Chloralose (4022-g)

Chloralose *(rINN)*.

Alphachloralose; Chloralosane; α-Chloralose; Glucochloral. *(R)*-1,2-*O*-(2,2,2-Trichloroethylidene)-α-D-glucofuranose.

$C_8H_{11}Cl_3O_6$ = 309.5.

CAS — 15879-93-3.

Chloralose has general properties similar to those of chloral hydrate (p.645), of which it is a derivative. It was formerly used for its hypnotic properties.

Chloralose is also used as a rodenticide.

Chlordiazepoxide (7017-w)

Chlordiazepoxide *(BAN, rINN)*.

Chlordiazepoxidum; Methaminodiazepoxide. 7-Chloro-2-methylamino-5-phenyl-3*H*-1,4-benzodiazepine 4-oxide.

$C_{16}H_{14}ClN_3O$ = 299.8.

CAS — 58-25-3.

Pharmacopoeias. In *Chin., Eur.* (see p.viii), *Jpn, Pol.,* and *US.*

An almost white or light yellow, practically odourless, crystalline powder, sensitive to sunlight. Chlordiazepoxide 1 mg is approximately equivalent to 1.1 mg of chlordiazepoxide hydrochloride. Practically **insoluble** in water; soluble 1 in 50 of alcohol, 1 in 6250 of chloroform, and 1 in 130 of ether. **Store** in airtight containers. Protect from light.

Chlordiazepoxide or chlordiazepoxide hydrochloride is reported to be **incompatible** with benzquinamide hydrochloride and with pentazocine lactate.

Chlordiazepoxide Hydrochloride (7018-e)

Chlordiazepoxide Hydrochloride *(BANM, USAN, rINNM)*.

Chlordiazepoxidi Hydrochloridum; Methaminodiazepoxide Hydrochloride; NSC-115748; Ro-5-0690.

$C_{16}H_{14}ClN_3O,HCl$ = 336.2.

CAS — 438-41-5.

Pharmacopoeias. In *Eur.* (see p.viii), *Pol.,* and *US.*

An odourless white or slightly yellow crystalline powder, sensitive to sunlight.

Soluble in water; sparingly soluble in alcohol; practically insoluble in ether and in petroleum spirit. **Store** in airtight containers. Protect from light.

For **incompatibilities** of chlordiazepoxide hydrochloride see under Chlordiazepoxide, above.

Dependence and Withdrawal

As for Diazepam, p.661.

For the purpose of withdrawal regimens, 15 mg of chlordiazepoxide is considered roughly equivalent to 5 mg of diazepam.

Adverse Effects and Treatment

As for Diazepam, p.661.

Precautions

As for Diazepam, p.662.

Hepatic impairment. A report of progressive drowsiness beginning after 20 days of administration of chlordiazepoxide to a woman with cirrhosis and hepatitis.[1] One week after discontinuing the drug, the patient could not be roused and full consciousness was not regained for another week. Accumulation of active metabolites of chlordiazepoxide may have been responsible for the prolonged stupor.

1. Barton K, *et al.* Chlordiazepoxide metabolite accumulation in liver disease. *Med Toxicol* 1989; **4:** 73–6.

Porphyria. Chlordiazepoxide has been associated with acute attacks of porphyria and is considered unsafe in patients with acute porphyria.[1]

1. Moore MR, McColl KEL. *Porphyria: drug lists.* Glasgow: Porphyria Research Unit, University of Glasgow, 1991.

Interactions

As for Diazepam, p.663.

Pharmacokinetics

Absorption of chlordiazepoxide is almost complete after oral administration. Absorption after intramuscular injection may be slow and erratic depending on the site of injection. Chlordiazepoxide is extensively bound (about 96%) to plasma proteins. Reported values for the elimination half-life of chlordiazepoxide have ranged from about 5 to 30 hours, but its main active metabolite desmethyldiazepam (nordazepam, p.682) has a half-life of several days. Other pharmacologically active metabolites of chlordiazepoxide include desmethylchlordiazepoxide, demoxepam, and oxazepam (p.683). Chlordiazepoxide passes into the CSF and breast milk, and crosses the placenta. Unchanged drug and metabolites are excreted in the urine, mainly as conjugated metabolites.

A detailed review of the pharmacokinetics of chlordiazepoxide.[1]

1. Greenblatt DJ, *et al.* Clinical pharmacokinetics of chlordiazepoxide. *Clin Pharmacokinet* 1978; **3:** 381–94.

Uses and Administration

Chlordiazepoxide is a benzodiazepine with general properties similar to those of diazepam (p.666). It is used in the treatment of anxiety disorders (p.635) and insomnia (p.638). Chlordiazepoxide is also used in muscle spasm (p.1303), in alcohol withdrawal syndromes (p.1099), and for premedication (p.1220).

Chlordiazepoxide is administered by mouth as the hydrochloride and sometimes as the base. It may also be administered by deep intramuscular or slow intravenous injection as the hydrochloride. Doses are expressed in terms of the base or the hydrochloride.

The usual dose by mouth of either the base or the hydrochloride for the treatment of anxiety is up to 30 mg daily in divided doses; in severe conditions up to 100 mg daily has been given. For acute or severe anxiety an initial dose of 50 to 100 mg of the hydrochloride has been given by injection, followed if necessary by 25 to 50 mg three or four times daily. For relief of muscle spasm a dose of 10 to 30 mg daily in divided doses is recommended, and 10 to 30 mg may be given before retiring for insomnia associated with anxiety.

For the control of the acute symptoms of alcohol withdrawal chlordiazepoxide or chlordiazepoxide hydrochloride may be given by mouth in a dose of 25 to 100 mg repeated as needed up to a maximum of 300 mg daily. For severe symptoms treatment may be initiated by injection of 50 to 100 mg, repeated if necessary after 2 to 4 hours.

Chlordiazepoxide hydrochloride has also been given intramuscularly in a dose of 50 to 100 mg as an anaesthetic premedicant one hour before surgery.

Elderly and debilitated patients should be given one-half or less of the usual adult dose.

Preparations formulated for intramuscular use are stated to be unsuitable for intravenous administration due to the formation of air bubbles in the solvent.

Preparations

BP 1998: Chlordiazepoxide Capsules; Chlordiazepoxide Hydrochloride Tablets;
USP 23: Chlordiazepoxide and Amitriptyline Hydrochloride Tablets; Chlordiazepoxide Hydrochloride and Clidinium Bromide Capsules; Chlordiazepoxide Hydrochloride Capsules; Chlordiazepoxide Hydrochloride for Injection; Chlordiazepoxide Tablets.

Proprietary Preparations (details are given in Part 3)

Austral.: Librium†; ***Belg.:*** Librium†; ***Canad.:*** Librium†; Novo-Poxide; Solium†; ***Fr.:*** Librium†; ***Ger.:*** Librium†; Multum; Radepur; ***Irl.:*** Librium; ***Ital.:*** Benzodiapin†; Librium; Psicofar; Psicoterina†; Reliberan; Seren Vita†; Seren†; ***Neth.:*** Librium†; ***S.Afr.:*** Librium; ***Spain:*** Huberplex; Normide†; Omnalio; ***Swed.:*** Librium†; ***Switz.:*** Librium†; ***UK:*** Librium; Tropium; ***USA:*** Libritabs; Librium; Mitran; Reposans.

Multi-ingredient: ***Aust.:*** Librax; Limbitrol; Pantrop; ***Austral.:*** Librax†; ***Belg.:*** Librax; Limbitrol; ***Canad.:*** Apo-Chlorax; Corium; Librax; ***Fr.:*** Librax; ***Ger.:*** Librax†; Limbatril; Pantrop†; ***Irl.:*** Libraxin†; Limbitrol†; ***Ital.:*** Diapatol; Librax; Limbitryl; Sedans; ***Neth.:*** Limbitrol†; ***S.Afr.:*** Librax; Limbitrol; ***Spain:*** Librax†; Psico Blocan; Relaxedans; Templax†; ***Swed.:*** Librax†; ***Switz.:*** Librax; Limbitrol; ***UK:*** Limbitrol†; ***USA:*** Clindex; Clinoxide†; Clipoxide†; Librax; Lidox; Limbitrol; Menrium†.

Chlorhexadol (4023-q)

Chlorhexadol *(BAN)*.

Chloralodol *(rINN)*; Chloralodolum. 2-Methyl-4-(2,2,2-trichloro-1-hydroxyethoxy)pentan-2-ol.

$C_8H_{15}Cl_3O_3$ = 265.6.

CAS — 3563-58-4.

Chlorhexadol has the general properties of chloral hydrate (p.645), but is reported to cause less gastric irritation. It was formerly given by mouth as a hypnotic.

The symbol † denotes a preparation no longer actively marketed

Chlormethiazole (18200-w)

Chlormethiazole *(BAN)*.

Clomethiazole *(rINN)*. 5-(2-Chloroethyl)-4-methyl-1,3-thiazole.

C_6H_8ClNS = 161.7.

CAS — 533-45-9.

Pharmacopoeias. In *Br.*

A colourless to slightly yellowish-brown liquid with a characteristic odour. Slightly **soluble** in water; miscible with alcohol, with chloroform, and with ether. A 0.5% solution in water has a pH of 5.5 to 7.0.

Store at a temperature of 2° to 8°.

Chlormethiazole Edisylate (4024-p)

Chlormethiazole Edisylate *(BANM)*.

Clomethiazole Edisilate *(rINNM)*; Chlormethiazole Ethanedisulphonate. 5-(2-Chloroethyl)-4-methylthiazole ethane-1,2-disulphonate.

$(C_6H_8ClNS)_2,C_2H_6O_6S_2$ = 513.5.

CAS — 1867-58-9.

Pharmacopoeias. In *Br.* and *Pol.*

A white crystalline powder with a characteristic odour. Freely **soluble** in water; soluble in alcohol; practically insoluble in ether.

Incompatibility. Several studies have demonstrated that chlormethiazole edisylate may permeate through or be sorbed onto plastics used in intravenous infusion bags or giving sets.[1-4] The drug may also react with and soften the plastic.[1] The UK manufacturers of chlormethiazole edisylate have suggested that thrombophlebitis, fever, and headache reported in young children during prolonged infusions may have been due to reaction with plastic giving sets and silastic cannulae and recommend the use of a motor-driven glass syringe in preference to a plastic drip set in small children. If a plastic drip set is used in older patients it should be changed at least every 24 hours. In all cases, teflon intravenous cannulas should be used.

1. Lingam S, *et al.* Problems with intravenous chlormethiazole (Heminevrin) in status epilepticus. *Br Med J* 1980; **280:** 155–6.
2. Tsuei SE, *et al.* Sorption of chlormethiazole by intravenous infusion giving sets. *Eur J Clin Pharmacol* 1980; **18:** 333–8.
3. Kowaluk EA, *et al.* Dynamics of clomethiazole edisylate interaction with plastic infusion systems. *J Pharm Sci* 1984; **73:** 43–7.
4. Lee MG. Sorption of four drugs to polyvinyl chloride and polybutadiene intravenous administration sets. *Am J Hosp Pharm* 1986; **43:** 1945–50.

Dependence and Withdrawal

Dependence may develop, particularly with prolonged use of higher than recommended doses of chlormethiazole. Features of dependence and withdrawal are similar to those of barbiturates (see Amylobarbitone, p.641).

Adverse Effects and Treatment

Chlormethiazole may produce nasal irritation, sneezing, and conjunctival irritation sometimes associated with a headache. Nasopharyngeal or bronchial secretions may be increased. Skin rashes and urticaria have also occurred and in rare cases bullous eruptions have been reported. Gastro-intestinal disturbances including nausea and vomiting, have been reported following oral administration. Chlormethiazole may cause excessive drowsiness particularly in high doses; paradoxical excitation or confusion may occur rarely. Anaphylaxis has been reported rarely with chlormethiazole. Tachycardia and a transient fall in blood pressure, related to the rate of infusion, may follow intravenous dosage, and rapid infusion has resulted in hypotension and apnoea. Phlebitis or thrombophlebitis may occur after intravenous infusion.

Excessive doses may produce coma, respiratory depression, hypotension, and hypothermia; pneumonia may follow increased respiratory secretion.

Adverse effects should be managed in a similar way to those of barbiturates (see Amylobarbitone, p.642).

Effects on the heart. Cardiac arrest in 2 chronic alcoholics might have been associated with chlormethiazole infusion.[1]

1. McInnes GT, *et al.* Cardiac arrest following chlormethiazole infusion in chronic alcoholics. *Postgrad Med J* 1980; **56:** 742–3.

Overdosage. A report of chlormethiazole poisoning on 16 occasions in 13 patients, some of whom had also taken other drugs and alcohol.[1] There was increased salivation on 7 occasions; otherwise the clinical features were those of barbiturate poisoning. The highest plasma-chlormethiazole concentration was 36 μg per mL, with the highest value in a conscious patient 11.5 μg per mL. All the patients survived following intensive supportive treatment as for barbiturate poisoning.

1. Illingworth RN, *et al.* Severe poisoning with chlormethiazole. *Br Med J* 1979; **2:** 902–3.

Parotitis. Acute bilateral parotitis has been reported in a patient given chlormethiazole.[1] The swelling disappeared after withdrawal of chlormethiazole and recurred on rechallenge.

1. Bosch X, *et al.* Parotitis induced by chlormethiazole. *Br Med J* 1994; **309:** 1620.

Precautions

Chlormethiazole is contra-indicated in patients with acute pulmonary insufficiency, and should be given with care to patients with chronic pulmonary insufficiency, or renal, liver, cerebral, or cardiac disease. When given parenterally, dose supervision is necessary and facilities to maintain the airway should be at hand. Paradoxical worsening of epilepsy may occur in the Lennox Gastaut syndrome.

Chlormethiazole may cause drowsiness; affected patients should not drive or operate machinery.

Administration. Facilities for intubation and resuscitation must be available when chlormethiazole is given intravenously and care should be taken to ensure that the patient's airway is maintained since there is a risk of mechanical obstruction during deep sedation. With intravenous administration it is important to adjust the dosage to the patient's response. With too high a rate of infusion sleep induced with chlormethiazole may lapse into deep unconsciousness and patients must be kept under close and constant observation. Rapid infusion may cause transient apnoea and hypotension and special care is needed in patients susceptible to cerebral or cardiac complications, including the elderly. With prolonged infusion there is a risk of electrolyte imbalance due to the water load involved with the glucose vehicle. Recovery can be considerably delayed after prolonged infusion.

Hepatic impairment. Studies in 8 patients with advanced cirrhosis of the liver and in 6 healthy men showed that the amount of unmetabolised chlormethiazole reaching the circulation after an oral dose was about 10 times higher in the patients than in the controls.[1] Low concentrations in the controls were related to extensive first-pass metabolism in the liver.

1. Pentikäinen PJ, *et al.* Pharmacokinetics of chlormethiazole in healthy volunteers and patients with cirrhosis of the liver. *Eur J Clin Pharmacol* 1980; **17:** 275–84.

Pregnancy. Reports of neonates being adversely affected by chlormethiazole given to their mothers for toxaemia of pregnancy.[1,2] Effects included sedation, hypotonia, and apnoea. In one report[1] it was suggested that the effects might have been due to a synergistic interaction between chlormethiazole and diazoxide as these drugs were given to most of the mothers with affected infants.

1. Johnson RA. Adverse neonatal reaction to maternal administration of intravenous chlormethiazole and diazoxide. *Br Med J* 1976; **1:** 943.
2. Wood C, Renou P. Sleepy and hypotonic neonates. *Med J Aust* 1978; **2:** 73.

Interactions

The sedative effects of chlormethiazole are enhanced by the simultaneous administration of CNS depressants such as alcohol, barbiturates, other hypnotics and sedatives, and antipsychotics.

Alcohol. Comment on the dangers of concomitant ingestion of chlormethiazole and alcohol.[1] Although chlormethiazole is a popular choice for the treatment of alcohol withdrawal symptoms, if it is given long-term, alcoholics readily transfer dependency to it, often while continuing to abuse alcohol. The outcome of such combined abuse is often severe self-poisoning with deep coma and potentially fatal respiratory depression.

1. McInnes GT. Chlormethiazole and alcohol: a lethal cocktail. *Br Med J* 1987; **294:** 592.

Beta blockers. Sinus bradycardia developed in an 84-year-old woman taking *propranolol* for hypertension 3 hours after she took a second dose of chlormethiazole 192 mg.[1] Her pulse rate increased on discontinuation of propranolol and chlormethiazole and later stabilised when she took propranolol with haloperidol.

1. Adverse Drug Reactions Advisory Committee (Australia). *Med J Aust* 1979; **2:** 553.

Diazoxide. For a report of severe adverse reactions in neonates born to mothers given chlormethiazole and diazoxide, see Pregnancy under Precautions, above.

Histamine H_2-receptor antagonists. A study of the pharmacokinetics of chlormethiazole edisylate 1 g by mouth in 8 healthy subjects, before and after administration of *cimetidine* 1 g daily for 1 week, demonstrated that mean clearance of chlormethiazole was reduced to 69% of its original value by cimetidine therapy.[1] This was associated with an increase in the mean peak plasma concentration of the hypnotic from 2.664 to 4.507 μg per mL and an increase in the mean elimination half-life from 2.33 to 3.63 hours. After the original dose of chlormethiazole subjects slept for 30 to 60 minutes, whereas following cimetidine treatment, most slept for at least 2 hours.

Ranitidine did not significantly affect the pharmacokinetics of chlormethiazole in a study in 7 healthy subjects.[2]

1. Shaw G, *et al*. Cimetidine impairs the elimination of chlormethiazole. *Eur J Clin Pharmacol* 1981; **21:** 83–5.
2. Mashford ML, *et al*. Ranitidine does not affect chlormethiazole or indocyanine green disposition. *Clin Pharmacol Ther* 1983; **34:** 231–3.

Pharmacokinetics

Chlormethiazole is rapidly absorbed from the gastro-intestinal tract, peak plasma concentrations appearing about 15 to 90 minutes after oral administration depending on the formulation used. It is widely distributed in the body and is reported to be 65% bound to plasma proteins. Chlormethiazole is extensively metabolised, probably by first-pass metabolism in the liver with only small amounts appearing unchanged in the urine. The elimination half-life has been reported to be about 4 hours but this may be increased to 8 hours or longer in the elderly or in patients with hepatic impairment. Chlormethiazole crosses the placenta and has been detected in breast milk.

Uses and Administration

Chlormethiazole is a hypnotic and sedative with anticonvulsant effects. It is used in disturbances of behaviour (p.636) such as agitation and restlessness, particularly of geriatric patients, in the short-term management of severe insomnia (p.638) in the elderly, and in the treatment of acute alcohol withdrawal symptoms (p.1099). It is one of the drugs used for the control of status epilepticus (p.337), usually to prevent recurrence of seizures once they have been brought under control with a benzodiazepine. It has been used for the initial control of impending or actual eclampsia (p.338) but magnesium sulphate is generally the preferred treatment now. It was also used as a sedative in regional anaesthesia.

Chlormethiazole as Heminevrin (*Astra*) is commonly used as capsules containing 192 mg of chlormethiazole base, as syrup containing 250 mg of edisylate in 5 mL, or as a 0.8% intravenous infusion of the edisylate; tablets containing 500 mg of edisylate have been available in some countries. As a result of differences in the bioavailability of these preparations, 500 mg of the edisylate in the tablets is considered therapeutically equivalent to 192 mg of the base in the capsules, but it is also equivalent to only 250 mg (5 mL) of the edisylate in the syrup, i.e. one tablet or one capsule or 5 mL of syrup are all equivalent in their effects.

When chlormethiazole edisylate is administered by intravenous infusion, a loading dose is generally given to produce the desired effect, followed by a maintenance infusion. The precise dose will vary from patient to patient and close supervision is essential to avoid overdosage (see also Administration, above). Rapid reversal of sedative effects usually occurs after stopping the infusion, but recovery may be considerably delayed after large and prolonged dosage. See under Incompatibility, above, for reference to the incompatibility of chlormethiazole with plastic infusion bags and administration sets.

The usual hypnotic dose of chlormethiazole for **insomnia** is 1 or 2 capsules (192 or 384 mg of the base) or the equivalent. For **daytime sedation** 1 capsule (192 mg of the base), or the equivalent dose as one of the other dosage forms, may be given three times daily.

Various chlormethiazole regimens have been suggested for the treatment of **alcohol withdrawal**, usually starting with 9 to 12 capsules, or the equivalent, divided into 3 or 4 doses, on the first day, and gradually reducing the dosage over the following 5 days. Treatment should be carried out in hospital or in specialist centres, and administration for longer than 9 days is not recommended because of the risk of dependence (see above).

For acute alcohol withdrawal symptoms, including delirium tremens, where oral therapy is insufficiently rapid or not practicable, an infusion of chlormethiazole edisylate 0.8% is given at an initial rate of 3.0 to 7.5 mL per minute until shallow sleep is induced from which the patient can easily be awakened and reduced thereafter to a usual rate of 0.5 to 1.0 mL per minute to maintain shallow sleep and adequate spontaneous respiration. Urgent deep sedation is obtained with an initial infusion of 40 to 100 mL given over 3 to 5 minutes and then reduced to a maintenance rate as before.

In **status epilepticus**, an infusion of 5 to 15 mL per minute of the 0.8% solution up to a total of 40 to 100 mL will usually stop convulsions; thereafter a slower maintenance infusion may be required depending on the patient's response (usual rate 0.5 to 1.0 mL per minute). In the management of status epilepticus in children a suggested initial infusion rate is 0.01 mL of the 0.8% solution per kg body-weight per minute, adjusted upwards according to response until seizures are abolished or drowsiness occurs. The dose is then gradually reduced once seizures have been absent for about 2 days.

For impending **eclampsia** an initial infusion of chlormethiazole edisylate 0.8% solution at the rate of 0.5 to 0.75 mL per minute during labour has been suggested with a maintenance rate of 0.5 mL per minute for 12 hours following delivery. Chlormethiazole edisylate 0.8% solution is also used to control or prevent the recurrence of eclamptic seizures. While seizures are occurring an infusion of 5 to 10 mL per minute is given until the seizures stop and then decreased to a maintenance rate of 0.5 to 1.0 mL per minute, adjusted according to response. If the infusion is started while a patient is not having a seizure chlormethiazole edisylate is given at an initial infusion rate of 3 to 5 mL per minute until deep sedation is obtained; maintenance rates are then as before.

Higher rates of infusion were required when chlormethiazole was used as a sedative during **regional anaesthesia**; the patient was premedicated with a drug such as atropine to prevent nasal congestion and upper airway mucus secretion. An initial infusion rate of 25 mL per minute of the 0.8% solution for 1 to 2 minutes induced unconsciousness. This was followed by a maintenance dose of 1 to 4 mL per minute, according to response.

Porphyria. Chlormethiazole is one of the drugs that has been used for seizure prophylaxis in patients with porphyria (p.339) who continue to experience convulsions while in remission.

Stroke. Chlormethiazole is being studied as a neuroprotective drug in the acute management of patients with stroke.[1]

1. Wahlgren NG. Clomethiazole Acute Study Collaborative Group. The Clomethiazole Acute Stroke Study (CLASS): efficacy results in a subgroup of 545 patients with total anterior circulation syndrome. *Stroke* 1998; **29:** 287.

Withdrawal syndromes. OPIOID ANALGESICS. For a discussion of the management of opioid withdrawal symptoms, including mention of the use of chlormethiazole, see p.67.

Preparations

BP 1998: Clomethiazole Capsules; Clomethiazole Intravenous Infusion; Clomethiazole Oral Solution.

Proprietary Preparations (details are given in Part 3)
Aust.: Distraneurin; ***Austral.:*** Hemineurin; ***Belg.:*** Distraneurine; ***Fr.:*** Hemineurine†; ***Ger.:*** Distraneurin; ***Irl.:*** Heminevrin; ***Neth.:*** Distraneurine; ***Norw.:*** Heminevrin; ***S.Afr.:*** Heminevrin; ***Spain:*** Distraneurine; ***Swed.:*** Heminevrin; ***Switz.:*** Distraneurin; Hemineurine†; ***UK:*** Heminevrin.

Chlormezanone (7019-l)

Chlormezanone (*BAN, rINN*).

Chlormethazanone; Chlormezanonum. 2-(4-Chlorophenyl)-3-methylperhydro-1,3-thiazin-4-one 1,1-dioxide.

$C_{11}H_{12}ClNO_3S$ = 273.7.

CAS — 80-77-3.

Dependence and Withdrawal, Adverse Effects, and Treatment

Drowsiness and dizziness are the most common adverse effects following administration of chlormezanone. Other reported side-effects include CNS effects such as lightheadedness, headache, lethargy, confusion, excitement, and depression; nausea, skin rashes, flushing of the skin, dryness of the mouth, visual disturbances, and difficulties in micturition have also been noted. Very rarely, cholestatic jaundice and potentially serious skin disorders such as fixed drug eruptions, erythema multiforme, or toxic epidermal necrolysis have occurred.

Dependence similar to that of barbiturates (see Amylobarbitone, p.641), may develop with high or prolonged dosage.

Adverse effects should be managed in a similar way to those of barbiturates (see Amylobarbitone, p.642).

Effects on the blood. A brief report of immune thrombocytopenia in a patient receiving chlormezanone.[1]

1. Finney RD, Apps J. Trancopal (chlormezanone) and thrombocytopenia. *Br Med J* 1985; **290:** 1112.

Effects on the skin. Chlormezanone was responsible for 5 of 86 cases of fixed drug eruption detected in a Finnish hospital from 1971 to 1980.[1] In the period from 1981 to 1985 chlormezanone was responsible for 1 out of 77 such eruptions.[2] In a case control study[3] comparing drug use in 245 patients hospitalised because of toxic epidermal necrolysis or Stevens-Johnson syndrome and 1147 controls, 13 patients and one control were found to have taken chlormezanone. From these figures a high crude relative risk of 62 was calculated; the excess risk was estimated to be 1.7 cases per million users per week.

1. Kauppinen K, Stubb S. Fixed eruptions: causative drugs and challenge tests. *Br J Dermatol* 1985; **112:** 575–8.
2. Stubb S, *et al*. Fixed drug eruptions: 77 cases from 1981 to 1985. *Br J Dermatol* 1989; **120:** 583.
3. Roujeau J-C, *et al*. Medication use and the risk of Stevens-Johnson syndrome or toxic epidermal necrolysis. *N Engl J Med* 1995; **333:** 1600–7.

Overdosage. Reports of non-fatal overdosage with chlormezanone.[1-3]

1. Armstrong D, *et al*. Chlormezanone poisoning. *Br Med J* 1983; **286:** 845–6.
2. Kirkham BW, Edelman JB. Overdose of chlormezanone: a new clinical picture. *Br Med J* 1986; **292:** 732.
3. Paillassou-Vakanas B, *et al*. Intoxication aiguë par la chlormézanone: 204 observations du Centre Anti-Poisons de Paris. *J Toxicol Clin Exp* 1987; **7:** 123–5.

Precautions

Chlormezanone should be used with caution in patients with hepatic or renal insufficiency. Chlormezanone should also be used with caution in those with impaired respiratory function, and should be avoided in patients with acute pulmonary insufficiency and respiratory depression.

Chlormezanone may cause drowsiness; affected patients should not drive or operate machinery. These effects are enhanced by the simultaneous administration of other CNS depressants including alcohol.

Porphyria. Chlormezanone has been associated with clinical exacerbations of porphyria and is considered unsafe in porphyric patients.[1]

1. Moore MR, McColl KEL. *Porphyria: drug lists*. Glasgow: Porphyria Research Unit, University of Glasgow, 1991.

Interactions

As with other CNS depressants (see Diazepam, p.663) enhanced sedation or respiratory and cardiovascular depression may occur if chlormezanone is given with alcohol or other drugs that have CNS depressant properties.

Pharmacokinetics

Chlormezanone is absorbed from the gastro-intestinal tract, with peak plasma concentrations being obtained 1 to 2 hours after ingestion. A plasma half-life of 24 hours has been cited.

Chlormezanone appears to be metabolised by hydrolysis then oxidation and conjugation, and is excreted in the urine, mainly as metabolites and conjugates.

Uses and Administration

Chlormezanone has been used in the treatment of anxiety disorders (p.635) but was withdrawn from use in many countries following reports of serious skin reactions (see above). It was also used in conditions associated with painful muscle spasm (p.1303), often in compound preparations with analgesics; its mechanism of action is not clear but is probably related to its sedative effect. A usual dose by mouth for the treatment of anxiety was 200 mg three or four times daily, or a single dose of 400 mg at night. The latter dose was also used for the short-term treatment of insomnia. Half the normal adult dose, or less, was recommended for elderly patients.

Preparations

Proprietary Preparations (details are given in Part 3)
Aust.: Trancopal†; ***Belg.:*** Lyseen New†; Trancopal†; ***Fr.:*** Alinam†; Trancopal†; ***Ger.:*** Muskel Trancopal†; ***Irl.:*** Trancopal†; ***Neth.:*** Trancopal†; ***Norw.:*** Trancopal†; ***Swed.:*** Trancopal†; ***Switz.:*** Myoflex†; Trancopal†; ***UK:*** Trancopal†; ***USA:*** Trancopal†.

Multi-ingredient: ***Aust.:*** Trancopal compositum†; ***Fr.:*** Trancogesic†; ***Ger.:*** Muskel Trancopal compositum†; Muskel Trancopal cum codeino†; ***Irl.:*** Lobak†; Rowacylat†; ***Ital.:*** Clormetadone†; Condol†; Eblimon†; Flexipyrin†; Tiopirin†; ***Norw.:*** Lobac†; ***S.Afr.:*** Arcanaflex; Besenol; Betaflex; Lobak; Myoflex; Rexachlor; Spasmoflex; ***Spain:*** Lumbaxol Para; ***Swed.:*** Lobac†; ***Switz.:*** Trancopal compositum†; ***UK:*** Lobak†.

Chlorproethazine Hydrochloride (7020-v)

Chlorproethazine Hydrochloride *(rINNM)*.

RP-4909 (chlorproethazine). 3-(2-Chlorophenothiazin-10-yl)-*NN*-diethylpropylamine hydrochloride.

$C_{19}H_{23}ClN_2S,HCl = 383.4$.

CAS — 84-01-5 (chlorproethazine); 4611-02-3 (chlorproethazine hydrochloride).

Chlorproethazine is a phenothiazine derivative differing chemically from chlorpromazine by the substitution of a diethyl for a dimethyl group. It has general properties similar to those of chlorpromazine (below) but is used mainly as a muscle relaxant in the management of muscle spasm (p.1303). Although exposure of the skin to phenothiazines has been associated with sensitivity reactions, chlorproethazine hydrochloride has been applied topically in an ointment, with the warning to avoid direct exposure to sunlight. It has also been given by mouth or by intramuscular or slow intravenous injection.

Preparations

Proprietary Preparations (details are given in Part 3)
Fr.: Neuriplege†.

Multi-ingredient: ***Fr.:*** Neuriplege.

Chlorpromazine (7021-g)

Chlorpromazine *(BAN, rINN)*.

3-(2-Chlorophenothiazin-10-yl)propyldimethylamine.

$C_{17}H_{19}ClN_2S = 318.9$.

CAS — 50-53-3.

Pharmacopoeias. In *Br.* and *US.*

A white or creamy-white powder or waxy solid; odourless or with an amine-like odour. It darkens on prolonged exposure to light. M.p. 56° to 58°. Chlorpromazine 100 mg is approximately equivalent to 111 mg of chlorpromazine hydrochloride.

BP **solubilities** are: practically insoluble in water; very soluble in chloroform; freely soluble in alcohol and in ether. USP solubilities are: practically insoluble in water; soluble 1 in 3 of alcohol, 1 in 2 of chloroform, and 1 in 3 of ether; freely soluble in dilute mineral acids; practically insoluble in dilute alkali hydroxides. **Store** in airtight containers. Protect from light.

Chlorpromazine Embonate (7022-q)

Chlorpromazine Embonate *(BANM, rINNM)*.

Chlorpromazine Pamoate. Chlorpromazine 4,4′-methylenebis(3-hydroxy-2-naphthoate).

$(C_{17}H_{19}ClN_2S)_2,C_{23}H_{16}O_6 = 1026.1$.

Chlorpromazine hydrochloride 100 mg is approximately equivalent to 144 mg of chlorpromazine embonate.

Chlorpromazine Hydrochloride (7023-p)

Chlorpromazine Hydrochloride *(BANM, rINNM)*.

Aminazine; Chlorpromazini Hydrochloridum; Cloridrato de Clorpromazina.

$C_{17}H_{19}ClN_2S,HCl = 355.3$.

CAS — 69-09-0.

Pharmacopoeias. In *Chin., Eur.* (see p.viii), *Int., Jpn, Pol.,* and *US.*

An odourless white or creamy-white crystalline powder. It decomposes and darkens on exposure to air and light.

Soluble 1 in 1 of water and 1 in 1.5 of alcohol and of chloroform; practically insoluble in ether. A freshly prepared 10% solution in water has a pH of 3.5 to 4.5. **Store** in airtight containers. Protect from light.

Incompatibility has been reported between chlorpromazine hydrochloride injection and several other compounds; precipitation of chlorpromazine base from solution is particularly likely if the final pH is increased. Compounds reported to be incompatible with chlorpromazine hydrochloride include aminophylline, amphotericin, aztreonam, some barbiturates, chloramphenicol sodium succinate, chlorothiazide sodium, cimetidine hydrochloride, dimenhydrinate, heparin sodium, morphine sulphate (when preserved with chlorocresol), some penicillins, ranitidine hydrochloride, and remifentanil.

For a warning about incompatibility between chlorpromazine solution (Thorazine) and carbamazepine suspension (Tegretol), see p.339.

CAUTION. Owing to the risk of contact sensitisation, pharmacists, nurses, and other health workers should avoid direct contact with chlorpromazine; tablets should not be crushed and solutions should be handled with care.

Dilution. Solutions containing 2.5% of chlorpromazine hydrochloride could be diluted to 100 mL with 0.9% sodium chloride solution provided the pH of the saline solution was such that the pH of the dilution did not exceed the critical range of pH 6.7 to 6.8.[1] With saline of pH 7.0 or 7.2, the final solution had a pH of 6.4.

1. D'Arcy PF, Thompson KM. Stability of chlorpromazine hydrochloride added to intravenous infusion fluids. *Pharm J* 1973; **210:** 28.

Sorption. There was a 41% loss of chlorpromazine hydrochloride from solution when infused for 7 hours via a plastic infusion set (cellulose propionate burette with polyvinyl chloride tubing), and a 79% loss after infusion for 1 hour from a glass syringe through silastic tubing.[1] Loss was negligible after infusion for 1 hour from a system comprising a glass syringe with polyethylene tubing.

1. Kowaluk EA, *et al.* Interactions between drugs and intravenous delivery systems. *Am J Hosp Pharm* 1982; **39:** 460–7.

Adverse Effects

Chlorpromazine produces in general a lesser degree of central depression than the barbiturates or benzodiazepines, and tolerance to its initial sedative effects develops fairly quickly in most patients. Chlorpromazine has antimuscarinic properties and may cause adverse effects such as dry mouth, constipation, difficulty with micturition, blurred vision, and mydriasis. Tachycardia, ECG changes (particularly Q- and T-wave abnormalities), and, rarely, cardiac arrhythmias may occur after administration of chlorpromazine; hypotension (usually orthostatic) is common. Other adverse effects include delirium, agitation and, rarely, catatonic-like states, insomnia, nightmares, depression, miosis, EEG changes and convulsions, nasal congestion, minor abnormalities in liver function tests, inhibition of ejaculation, impotence, and priapism.

Hypersensitivity reactions include urticaria, exfoliative dermatitis, erythema multiforme, and contact sensitivity. A syndrome resembling systemic lupus erythematosus has been reported. Jaundice has occurred, and probably has an immunological origin. Prolonged therapy may lead to deposition of pigment in the skin, or more frequently the eyes; corneal and lens opacities have been observed. Pigmentary retinopathy has occurred only rarely with chlorpromazine. Photosensitivity reactions are more common with chlorpromazine than with other antipsychotics.

Various haematological disorders, including haemolytic anaemia, aplastic anaemia, thrombocytopenic purpura, leucocytosis, and a potentially fatal agranulocytosis have occasionally been reported; they may be manifestations of a hypersensitivity reaction. Most cases of agranulocytosis have occurred within 4 to 10 weeks of starting treatment, and symptoms such as sore throat or fever should be watched for and white cell counts instituted should they appear. Mild leucopenia has been stated to occur in up to 30% of patients on prolonged high dosage.

Extrapyramidal dysfunction and resultant disorders include acute dystonia, a parkinsonism-like syndrome, and akathisia; late effects include tardive dyskinesia and perioral tremor. The neuroleptic malignant syndrome may also occur.

Chlorpromazine alters endocrine and metabolic functions. Patients have experienced amenorrhoea, galactorrhoea, gynaecomastia, weight gain, and hyperglycaemia and altered glucose tolerance. Body temperature regulation is impaired and may result in hypo- or hyperthermia depending on environment.

There have been isolated reports of sudden death with chlorpromazine; possible causes include cardiac arrhythmias or aspiration and asphyxia due to suppression of the cough and gag reflexes.

Pain and irritation at the injection site may occur on injection. Nodule formation may occur after intramuscular administration. Phenothiazines do not cause dependence of the type encountered with barbiturates or benzodiazepines. However, withdrawal symptoms have been seen following the abrupt withdrawal from patients receiving prolonged and/or high-dose maintenance therapy.

Carcinogenicity. See Effects on Endocrine Function, below.

Convulsions. Treatment with antipsychotics can result in EEG abnormalities and lowered seizure threshold.[1,2] Seizures can be induced particularly in patients with a history of epilepsy or drug-induced seizures, abnormal EEG, previous electroconvulsive therapy, or pre-existing CNS abnormalities. The risk appears to be greatest at the start of antipsychotic therapy, or with high doses, or abrupt increases of dose, or with the use of more than one antipsychotic. The incidence of antipsychotic-induced convulsions is, however, probably less than 1%.

Phenothiazines with an aliphatic side-chain such as chlorpromazine, promazine, and fluopromazine appear to present a higher risk than those with a piperazine or piperidine moiety. Despite conflicting evidence, haloperidol appears to carry a relatively low risk of seizures. In general, the epileptic potential has been correlated with the propensity of the neuroleptic to cause sedation. The following drugs have been suggested when antipsychotic therapy is considered necessary in patients at risk of seizures or being treated for epilepsy: fluphenazine, haloperidol, molindone, pimozide, and thioridazine. Antipsychotic dosage should be increased slowly and the possibility of interactions with antiepileptic therapy considered (see under Interactions, below).

The atypical antipsychotic clozapine appears to be associated with a particularly high risk of seizures (see p.658).

1. Cold JA, *et al.* Seizure activity associated with antipsychotic therapy. *DICP Ann Pharmacother* 1990; **24:** 601–6.
2. Zaccara G, *et al.* Clinical features, pathogenesis and management of drug-induced seizures. *Drug Safety* 1990; **5:** 109–51.

Effects on the blood. The UK Committee on Safety of Medicines provided data on the reports it had received between July 1963 and January 1993 on agranulocytosis and neutropenia.[1] Several groups of drugs were commonly implicated, among them phenothiazines for which there were 87 reports of agranulocytosis (42 fatal) and 33 of neutropenia (22 fatal). The most frequently implicated phenothiazines were chlorpromazine with 51 reports of agranulocytosis (26 fatal) and 12 of neutropenia (2 fatal) and thioridazine with 20 reports of agranulocytosis (9 fatal) and 10 of neutropenia (0 fatal).

1. Committee on Safety of Medicines/Medicines Control Agency. Drug-induced neutropenia and agranulocytosis. *Current Problems* 1993; **19:** 10–11.

Effects on the cardiovascular system. DiGiacomo has reviewed the adverse cardiovascular effects of psychotropic drugs.[1] Orthostatic hypotension is a common problem in patients taking such medication and is particularly pronounced with low-potency antipsychotics. T-wave changes have also been reported with low-potency antipsychotics; they are usually benign and reversible, and subject to diurnal fluctuations. Low-potency antipsychotics, particularly *thioridazine, mesoridazine*, and the high-potency drug *pimozide*, prolong the QT interval in a similar manner to class I antiarrhythmics such as quinidine or procainamide; their use is therefore contra-indicated in patients taking such antiarrhythmics. Thioridazine is most frequently discussed in case reports of psychotropic drug-induced torsade de pointes; *chlorpromazine* and *pimozide* have also been implicated. Torsade de pointes has also been reported following overdosage with the high-potency antipsychotic *haloperidol*.[2-4] There are also isolated reports of cardiac arrhythmias following rapid neuroleptisation with high doses of haloperidol.[5,6] *Melperone*, a butyrophenone antipsychotic related to haloperidol, has been reported to have class III electrophysiologic and antiarrhythmic activity.[7,8]

1. DiGiacomo J. Cardiovascular effects of psychotropic drugs. *Cardiovasc Rev Rep* 1989; **10:** 31–2, 39–41, and 47.
2. Zee-Cheng C-S, *et al.* Haloperidol and torsades de pointes. *Ann Intern Med* 1985; **102:** 418.
3. Henderson RA, *et al.* Life-threatening ventricular arrhythmia (torsades de pointes) after haloperidol overdose. *Hum Exp Toxicol* 1991; **10:** 59–62.
4. Wilt JL, *et al.* Torsade de pointes associated with the use of intravenous haloperidol. *Ann Intern Med* 1993; **119:** 391–4.
5. Mehta D, *et al.* Cardiac arrhythmia and haloperidol. *Am J Psychiatry* 1979; **136:** 1468–9.
6. Bett JHN, Holt GW. Malignant ventricular tachyarrhythmia and haloperidol. *Br Med J* 1983; **287:** 1264.

7. Møgelvang JC, *et al.* Antiarrhythmic properties of a neuroleptic butyrophenone, melperone, in acute myocardial infarction. *Acta Med Scand* 1980; **208:** 61–4.
8. Hui WKK, *et al.* Melperone: electrophysiologic and antiarrhythmic activity in humans. *J Cardiovasc Pharmacol* 1990; **15:** 144–9.

Effects on endocrine function. Via their ability to block central dopamine-D_2 receptors, antipsychotics can alter the secretion of prolactin, growth hormone, and thyrotrophin from the anterior pituitary.[1] Therapeutic doses of antipsychotics increase serum-prolactin concentrations in psychotic patients; this effect occurs at lower doses and after shorter latent periods than the antipsychotic effects. Serum-prolactin levels decline to normal values within 2 to 4 days after cessation of oral antipsychotic therapy. However, raised prolactin concentrations have not always been observed after long-term use, prompting suggestions that tolerance may develop to the hyperprolactinaemic effect.

Although long-term antipsychotic treatment increases the incidence of mammary tumours in the *rat*, studies[2,3] have found little or no evidence that chronic use of antipsychotics in humans alters the risk of breast cancer among women with schizophrenia. Fears that pituitary abnormalities, including pituitary tumours,[4] might develop in patients on long-term phenothiazine therapy have not been confirmed.[5,6]

Antipsychotics can in some circumstances reduce both basal and stimulated growth-hormone secretion but attempts to use them to treat dysfunctions in growth-hormone regulation have not been successful.[1] Although a number of clinical studies show that acute administration of antipsychotics increased both basal and stimulated thyrotrophin secretion, the majority of studies find either no change or only a small increase in thyrotrophin secretion following long-term use.

One small study has suggested that thioridazine may be more likely than other antipsychotics to decrease serum concentrations of testosterone or luteinising hormone in men.[7] However, concentrations were within the normal range in most patients taking antipsychotics.[7]

See also Effects on Fluid and Electrolyte Homoeostasis, below and Effects on Sexual Function, below.

1. Gunnet JW, Moore KE. Neuroleptics and neuroendocrine function. *Ann Rev Pharmacol Toxicol* 1988; **28:** 347–66.
2. Mortensen PB. The incidence of cancer in schizophrenic patients. *J Epidemiol Community Health* 1989; **43:** 43–7.
3. Mortensen PB. The occurrence of cancer in first admitted schizophrenic patients. *Schizophr Res* 1994; **12:** 185–94.
4. Asplund K, *et al.* Phenothiazine drugs and pituitary tumors. *Ann Intern Med* 1982; **96:** 533.
5. Rosenblatt S, *et al.* Chronic phenothiazine therapy does not increase sellar size. *Lancet* 1978; **ii:** 319–20.
6. Lilford VA, *et al.* Long-term phenothiazine treatment does not cause pituitary tumours. *Br J Psychiatry* 1984; **144:** 421–4.
7. Brown WA, *et al.* Differential effects of neuroleptic agents on the pituitary-gonadal axis in men. *Arch Gen Psychiatry* 1981; **38:** 1270–2.

Effects on the eyes. Phenothiazines may induce a pigmentary retinopathy which is dependent on both the dose and the duration of treatment.[1] Those phenothiazine derivatives with piperidine side-chains such as thioridazine have a higher risk of inducing retinal toxicity than other phenothiazine derivatives, with relatively few cases reported for those with aliphatic side-chains such as chlorpromazine; the piperazine group does not appear to exert direct ocular toxicity.[2] The retinopathy may present either acutely, with sudden loss of vision associated with retinal oedema and hyperaemia of the optic disc, or chronically, with a fine pigment scatter appearing in the central area of the fundus, extending peripherally but sparing the macula. Chronic paracentral and pericentral scotomas may be found. Although pigmentary disturbances may progress after withdrawal of thioridazine, they are not always paralleled by deterioration in visual function; long-term follow-up may be required to document stability or progression of the disease.[3] Some cases have led to progressive chorioretinopathy.[3] The critical ocular toxic dose of thioridazine is reported to be 800 mg daily and the UK manufacturers recommend that a daily dose of 600 mg should not usually be exceeded. However, there is a report of pigmentary retinopathy in a patient who received long-term thioridazine in daily doses not exceeding 400 mg; the total dose was 752 g.[4]

Pigmentation may also occur in the cornea, lens, and conjunctiva following administration of phenothiazines. It may occur in association with pigmentary changes in the skin and is dose-related. In a study of 100 Malaysian patients, ocular pigmentation was observed in slightly more than half of those who had received a total dose of chlorpromazine of 100 to 299 g and in 13 of 15 who had received 300 to 599 g.[5] All those who had received more than 600 g of chlorpromazine or thioridazine had ocular pigmentation. Cataract formation, mainly of an anterior polar variety, has been observed rarely, mainly in patients on chlorpromazine. It does not appear to be dose-related.[2]

A patient who had received fortnightly injections of fluphenazine for 10 years to an estimated total dose of 3.25 g, developed bilateral maculopathy following unprotected exposure of less than 2-minute's duration to a welding arc.[6] It was postulated that accumulation of phenothiazine in the retinal epithelium sensitised the patient to photic damage.

1. Spiteri MA, James DG. Adverse ocular reactions to drugs. *Postgrad Med J* 1983; **59:** 343–9.
2. Crombie AL. Drugs causing eye problems. *Prescribers' J* 1981; **21:** 222–7.
3. Marmor MF. Is thioridazine retinopathy progressive? Relationship of pigmentary changes to visual function. *Br J Ophthalmol* 1990; **74:** 739–42.
4. Lam RW, Remick RA. Pigmentary retinopathy associated with low-dose thioridazine treatment. *Can Med Assoc J* 1985; **132:** 737.
5. Ngen CC, Singh P. Long-term phenothiazine administration and the eye in 100 Malaysians. *Br J Psychiatry* 1988; **152:** 278–81.
6. Power WJ, *et al.* Welding arc maculopathy and fluphenazine. *Br J Ophthalmol* 1991; **75:** 433–5.

Effects on fluid and electrolyte homoeostasis. There have been occasional reports of water intoxication in patients taking antipsychotics. A review[1] of hyponatraemia and the syndrome of inappropriate antidiuretic hormone secretion associated with psychotropics summarised 20 such reports for antipsychotics in the literature. The drugs implicated were thioridazine (8 patients), haloperidol (3), chlorpromazine (2), trifluoperazine (2), fluphenazine (2), flupenthixol (1), thiothixene (1), and clozapine (1). The majority of reports did not permit clear conclusions and, particularly in the cases of prolonged treatment, the role of the medication was unclear. However, at least 3 of the cases were well documented and supported the view that antipsychotics could cause hyponatraemia.

One report not considered by the above review described water retention and peripheral oedema associated with chlorpromazine.[2] A small controlled study[3] found that 5 of the 10 evaluated patients who are receiving haloperidol decanoate had impaired fluid homoeostasis.

1. Spigset O, Hedenmalm K. Hyponatraemia and the syndrome of inappropriate antidiuretic hormone secretion (SIADH) induced by psychotropic drugs. *Drug Safety* 1995; **12:** 209–25.
2. Witz L, *et al.* Chlorpromazine induced fluid retention masquerading as idiopathic oedema. *Br Med J* 1987; **294:** 807–8.
3. Rider JM, *et al.* Water handling in patients receiving haloperidol decanoate. *Ann Pharmacother* 1995; **29:** 663–6.

Effects on lipid metabolism. There are scant data implicating phenothiazines as a cause of elevated cholesterol and decreased high-density lipoprotein concentrations.[1] The possibility of such effects should nevertheless be considered in dyslipidaemic patients treated with these drugs.

1. Henkin Y, *et al.* Secondary dyslipidemia: inadvertent effects of drugs in clinical practice. *JAMA* 1992; **267:** 961–8.

Effects on the liver. Chlorpromazine and other phenothiazines may cause hepatocanalicular cholestasis in which cholestasis is associated with features of hepatocyte damage, often suggesting immunological liver injury.[1] Only a small number of patients taking the drug are affected and the onset is usually in the first 4 weeks of therapy. The phenothiazine or one of its metabolites may induce alteration in the liver-cell membrane so that it becomes antigenic; there is also good evidence that direct hepatotoxicity may be related to the production of free drug radical. There may be an individual idiosyncrasy in the metabolism of chlorpromazine and in the production of these radicals. One study has suggested that patients who have poor sulphoxidation status combined with unimpaired hydroxylation capacity may be most likely to develop jaundice with chlorpromazine.[2]

A preliminary study[3] showing a high incidence of gallstones in psychiatric inpatients in Japan found a correlation between the presence of gallstones and the duration of illness and use of antipsychotics. It was speculated that gallstones could be a consequence of phenothiazine-induced cholestasis.

1. Sherlock S. The spectrum of hepatotoxicity due to drugs. *Lancet* 1986; **ii:** 440–4.
2. Watson RGP, *et al.* A proposed mechanism for chlorpromazine jaundice—defective hepatic sulphoxidation combined with rapid hydroxylation. *J Hepatol* 1988; **7:** 72–8.
3. Fukuzako H, *et al.* Ultrasonography detected a higher incidence of gallstones in psychiatric inpatients. *Acta Psychiatr Scand* 1991; **84:** 83–5.

Effects on sexual function. The phenothiazines can cause both impotence and ejaculatory dysfunction.[1] Thioridazine has been frequently implicated, and in an early report 60% of 57 male patients taking the drug reported sexual dysfunction compared with 25% of 64 men taking other antipsychotics.[2] There are also several reports of priapism with phenothiazines;[1,3,4] alpha-adrenoceptor blocking properties of these compounds may be partly responsible. Priapism has also been reported with clozapine.[5] Male sexual dysfunction, including priapism, has been reported only rarely with other antipsychotics such as the butyrophenones, diphenylbutylpiperidines, and thioxanthenes.[6] The effects of antipsychotics on female sexual function are less well studied. Orgasmic dysfunction has been reported with thioridazine, trifluoperazine, and fluphenazine.[7]

The effects of antipsychotic-induced hyperprolactinaemia (see Effects on Endocrine Function, above) on sexual function are described on p.1238.

1. Beeley L. Drug-induced sexual dysfunction and infertility. *Adverse Drug React Acute Poisoning Rev* 1984; **3:** 23–42.
2. Kotin J, *et al.* Thioridazine and sexual dysfunction. *Am J Psychiatry* 1976; **133:** 82–5.
3. Baños JE, *et al.* Drug-induced priapism: its aetiology, incidence and treatment. *Med Toxicol* 1989; **4:** 46–58.
4. Chan J, *et al.* Perphenazine-induced priapism. *DICP Ann Pharmacother* 1990; **24:** 246–9.
5. Patel AG, *et al.* Priapism associated with psychotropic drugs. *Br J Hosp Med* 1996; **55:** 315–19.
6. Fabian J-L. Psychotropic medications and priapism. *Am J Psychiatry* 1993, **150:** 349–50.
7. Segraves RT. Psychiatric drugs and inhibited female orgasm. *J Sex Marital Ther* 1988; **14:** 202–7.

Effects on the skin. DEPOT INJECTION. Of 217 patients who received a combined total of 2354 depot antipsychotic injections 42 (19.4%) had local problems at the site of injection; 18 (8.3%) experienced chronic complications and 30 (13.8%) acute reactions.[1] Acute problems reported included unusual pain (31 episodes), bleeding or haematoma (21), clinically important leakage of drug from injection site (19), acute inflammatory indurations (11), and transient nodules (2). Complications were more common in patients receiving concentrated preparations, higher doses, weekly injections, haloperidol decanoate or zuclopenthixol decanoate, and injection volumes greater than 1 mL and in those treated for more than 5 years. Chronic reactions were more common in patients aged over 50 years.

1. Hay J. Complications at site of injection of depot neuroleptics. *Br Med J* 1995; **311:** 421.

PHOTOSENSITIVITY. Testing in 7 subjects taking chlorpromazine revealed that photosensitivity reactions manifested primarily as immediate erythema and that sensitivity was primarily to light in the long ultraviolet (UVA) and visible wavebands. Sensitivity to UVB was normal.[1]

See also Effects on the Eyes, above.

1. Ferguson J, *et al.* Further clinical and investigative studies of chlorpromazine phototoxicity. *Br J Dermatol* 1986; **115** (suppl 30): 35.

PIGMENTATION. The pigment found in the skin of patients treated with chlorpromazine was considered[1] to be a chlorpromazine-melanin polymer formed in a light-catalysed anaerobic reaction. Hydrogen chloride liberated during the reaction could account for the skin irritation. Intracutaneous injection of a preparation of the polymer into 2 volunteers produced a bluish-purple discoloration which faded in 3 days.

1. Huang CL, Sands FL. Effect of ultraviolet irradiation on chlorpromazine II: anaerobic condition. *J Pharm Sci* 1967; **56:** 259–64.

Extrapyramidal disorders. Antipsychotics and a number of other drugs, including antiemetics such as metoclopramide and some antidepressants, can produce a range of involuntary movement disorders involving the extrapyramidal motor system including parkinsonism and the dyskinesias akathisia, acute dystonias, and chronic tardive dyskinesias.[1-4] Such reactions are a major problem in the clinical management of patients receiving antipsychotics. Reactions of this type can occur with any antipsychotic, but (excluding tardive dyskinesia) are particularly prominent during treatment with high-potency drugs such as the tricyclic piperazines and butyrophenones. Clozapine carries a low risk of extrapyramidal effects and is therefore described as an atypical antipsychotic. Other atypical antipsychotics include risperidone, olanzapine, quetiapine, and amisulpride. Although the incidence of tardive dyskinesia does appear to be minimal with clozapine, claims for other atypical antipsychotics requires confirmation.

A prospective study has examined the risk of acute extrapyramidal reactions occurring in the first few months of therapy with prochlorperazine (a drug with a high propensity to cause extrapyramidal reactions).[5] Fifty-seven of 2811 patients reported adverse effects, 16 of which involved the extrapyramidal system. There were 4 dystonic-dyskinesic reactions (an incidence of 1 in 464 and 1 in 707 for patients aged under and over 30 years respectively), 9 reports of parkinsonism (under 60 years, 1 in 1555; over 60 years, 1 in 159), and 3 reports of akathisia (1 in 562).

One explanation of extrapyramidal disorders is an imbalance between dopaminergic and cholinergic systems in the brain. However, this simple model fails to explain the co-existence of a variety of extrapyramidal effects, and several alternative mechanisms have been proposed.[2,6] Hypotheses based on interactions between different dopamine receptor types may help to explain the decreased tendency of some antipsychotic drugs to induce these reactions (see Action under Uses and Administration, below).

Akathisia is a condition of mental and motor restlessness in which there is an urge to move about constantly and an inability to sit or stand still. It is the most common motor side-effect of treatment with antipsychotics. Acute akathisia is dose-dependent, usually develops within a few days of beginning treatment or following a rapid increase in dose, and usually improves if the drug is stopped or the dose reduced. *Antimuscarinics* appear to provide only limited benefit, although success may be more likely in patients with concomitant parkinsonism. A low dose of a *beta blocker* such as *propranolol* or a *benzodiazepine* may be helpful. Improvement has also been reported with *clonidine* and *amantadine* but the usefulness of these drugs may be limited by side-effects or development of tolerance respectively. The tardive form, like tardive dyskinesia (see below) which appears after several months of treatment, does not respond to antimuscarinics, and is difficult to treat.

Acute **dystonic reactions**, which mainly affect the muscles of the face, neck, and trunk and include jaw clenching (trismus), torticollis, and oculogyric crisis are reported to occur in up to 10% of patients taking antipsychotics. Laryngeal dystonia is rare, but potentially fatal.[7] Dystonias usually occur within the first few days of treatment or after a dosage increase but may also develop on withdrawal. They are transitory, and are most common in children and young adults. Dystonic reactions may be controlled by the administration of *antimuscarinics* or *diphenhydramine*. *Benzodiazepines* such as *diazepam* can also be used. Prophylactic administration of antimuscarinics can prevent the development of dystonias, but routine use is not recommended as not all patients require them and tardive dyskinesia may be unmasked or worsened (see below); such a strategy should probably be reserved for short-term use in those at high risk of developing dystonic reactions, such as young adults starting treatment with high-potency antipsychotics or in patients with a previous history of drug-induced dystonias.[8,9] Some patients may develop tardive dystonia. A range of drugs has been tried in this condition but without consistent benefit.[10]

Parkinsonism, often indistinguishable from idiopathic Parkinson's disease (p.1128), may develop during therapy with antipsychotics, usually after the first few weeks or months of treatment. It is generally stated to be more common in adults and the elderly, although a retrospective study with haloperidol found an inverse relationship between drug-induced parkinsonism and age.[11] This parkinsonism is generally reversible on drug withdrawal or dose reduction, and may sometimes disappear gradually despite continued drug therapy. *Antimuscarinic* drugs have been used for treatment. However, they are often minimally effective and commonly cause adverse effects. Routine use for prophylaxis is not recommended because of the risk of unmasking or exacerbating tardive dyskinesia (see below).

The central feature of **tardive dyskinesia** is orofacial dyskinesia characterised by protrusion of the tongue (fly catching), lipsmacking, sucking, lateral chewing, and pouting of the lips and cheeks. The trunk and limbs also become involved with choreiform movements such as repetitive 'piano-playing' hand movements, shoulder shrugging, foot tapping, or rocking movements. The prevalence of tardive dyskinesia among those receiving antipsychotics varies widely but up to 60% of patients may develop symptoms. In most cases the condition is mild and not progressive and tends to wax and wane. Although tardive dyskinesia usually develops after many years of antipsychotic therapy no clear correlation has been shown between development of the condition and the length of drug treatment or the type and class of drug. However, administration of *clozapine* does not appear to be associated with development of the condition and in some cases has resulted in improvement of established tardive dyskinesia (see Schizophrenia under Clozapine, p.660). Symptoms of tardive dyskinesia often develop after discontinuation of the antipsychotic or after dose reduction. Factors predisposing to the development of tardive dyskinesia include old age, female sex, affective disorder, schizophrenia characterised by negative symptoms, and organic brain damage.

Various mechanisms have been suggested for the development of tardive dyskinesia including dopaminergic overactivity, imbalance between dopaminergic and cholinergic activity, supersensitivity of postsynaptic dopamine receptors, presynaptic catecholaminergic hyperfunction, and alterations of the gamma-aminobutyric acid (GABA) system. These proposals have led to trials with antidopaminergics, noradrenergic antagonists, cholinergic drugs, and GABAergic drugs as well as attempts to reverse postsynaptic supersensitivity with dopamine. Although many drugs have been tried in the treatment of tardive dyskinesia there have been relatively few double-blind studies. Reviews of tardive dyskinesia[12,13] have concluded that there appeared to be no reliable or safe treatment. Overall, standard antipsychotics appeared to be the most effective in masking symptoms of tardive dyskinesia but tolerance may develop and a worsening of the underlying pathophysiology by antipsychotics had to be assumed on theoretical grounds. Other drugs with antidopaminergic actions which were probably of comparable efficacy included *reserpine, oxypertine, tetrabenazine,* and *metirosine*. The next most effective drugs were considered to be noradrenergic antagonists such as *clonidine*; some encouraging results had also been obtained with GABAergic drugs such as the *benzodiazepines, baclofen, progabide, valproate*, and *vigabatrin*. However, the efficacy of cholinergics could not be confirmed. Dopaminergics and antimuscarinics mostly exacerbated symptoms but others[9] had commented that there was no convincing evidence that long-term administration of antimuscarinics increased the risk of developing the condition. Other drugs whose value is unclear include *vitamin E* and the calcium-channel blockers such as *nifedipine*.

In view of the unsatisfactory management of tardive dyskinesia, emphasis is placed on its prevention. Antipsychotics should be prescribed only when clearly indicated, should be given in the minimum dose, and continued only when there is evidence of benefit. Although drug holidays have been suggested for reducing the risk of tardive dyskinesia, the limited evidence indicates that interruptions in drug treatment may increase the risk of both persistent dyskinesia and psychotic relapse. Increasing the dose of antipsychotic generally improves the condition, but only temporarily. Options in the management of tardive dyskinesia include withdrawal of antimuscarinic therapy, and either withdrawal of the antipsychotic or reduction of the dosage to the minimum required or transfer to an atypical antipsychotic. Success is most likely in younger patients. Stopping the drug usually worsens the condition although symptoms often diminish or disappear over a period of weeks or sometimes a year or so. During withdrawal drugs such as *diazepam* or *clonazepam* may be given to alleviate symptoms. Although standard antipsychotics are effective their routine use to suppress symptoms is not recommended but they may be required for acute distressing or life-threatening reactions or in chronic tardive dyskinesia unresponsive to other treatment. In extremely severe resistant cases some have used an antipsychotic with *valproate* or *carbamazepine* or *reserpine* with *metirosine*.

1. Committee on Safety of Medicines/Medicines Control Agency. Drug-induced extrapyramidal reactions. *Current Problems* 1994; **20:** 15–16.
2. Ebadi M, Srinivasam SK. Pathogenesis, prevention, and treatment of neuroleptic-induced movement disorders. *Pharmacol Rev* 1995; **47:** 575–604.
3. Holloman LC, Marder SR. Management of acute extrapyramidal effects induced by antipsychotic drugs. *Am J Health-Syst Pharm* 1997; **54:** 2461–77.
4. Jiménez-Jiménez FJ, *et al.* Drug-induced movement disorders. *Drug Safety* 1997; **16:** 180–204.
5. Bateman DN, *et al.* Extrapyramidal reactions to metoclopramide and prochlorperazine. *Q J Med* 1989; **71:** 307–11.
6. Ereshefsky L, *et al.* Pathophysiologic basis for schizophrenia and the efficacy of antipsychotics. *Clin Pharm* 1990; **9:** 682–707.
7. Koek RJ, Pi EH. Acute laryngeal dystonic reactions to neuroleptics. *Psychosomatics* 1989; **30:** 359–64.
8. WHO. Prophylactic use of anticholinergics in patients on long-term neuroleptic treatment: a consensus statement. *Br J Psychiatry* 1990; **156:** 412.
9. Barnes TRE. Comment on the WHO consensus statement. *Br J Psychiatry* 1990; **156:** 413–14.
10. Raja M. Managing antipsychotic-induced acute and tardive dystonia. *Drug Safety* 1998; **19:** 57–72.
11. Moleman P, *et al.* Relationship between age and incidence of parkinsonism in psychiatric patients treated with haloperidol. *Am J Psychiatry* 1986; **143:** 232–4.
12. Haag H, *et al.*, eds. Tardive Dyskinesia. *WHO Expert Series on Biological Psychiatry Volume 1.* Seattle: Hogrefe & Huber, 1992.
13. Egan MF, *et al.* Treatment of tardive dyskinesia. *Schizophr Bull* 1997; **23:** 583–609.

Neuroleptic malignant syndrome. The neuroleptic malignant syndrome (NMS) is a potentially fatal reaction to a number of drugs including antipsychotics and dopamine antagonists such as metoclopramide. The clinical features of the classic syndrome are usually considered to include hyperthermia, severe extrapyramidal symptoms including muscular rigidity, autonomic dysfunction, and altered levels of consciousness. Skeletal muscle damage may occur and resulting myoglobinuria may lead to renal failure. However, there appears to be no universal criteria for the diagnosis of the syndrome. The relationship between NMS and catatonia is unclear. Some believe the classic syndrome to be the extreme of a range of effects associated with antipsychotics and have introduced the concept of milder variants or incomplete forms. Others consider it be a rare idiosyncratic reaction and suggest that the term neuroleptic malignant syndrome should be reserved for the full blown reaction. Consequently estimates of the incidence vary greatly and recent estimates have ranged from 0.02 to 2.5%. The mortality rate has been substantial and although it has decreased over the years with improved diagnosis and management, this may also be due to the detection and inclusion of the milder or incomplete variants. Factors which possibly predispose to development of NMS include dehydration, pre-existing organic brain disease, and a history of a previous episode; young males have also been reported to be particularly susceptible.

The pathogenesis of NMS is still unclear. It may be the result of central dopamine-receptor blockade although peripheral mechanisms such as sustained muscular contraction and vasomotor paralysis may be partly responsible for the hyperthermia. Blockade of dopaminergic receptors in the corpus striatum is thought to cause muscular contraction and rigidity generating heat while blockade of dopaminergic receptors in the hypothalamus leads to impaired heat dissipation. A syndrome resembling NMS has been seen following withdrawal of treatment with dopamine agonists such as levodopa (see p.1138). Symptoms develop rapidly over 24 to 72 hours and may occur days to months after initiation of antipsychotic medication or increase in dosage. There appears, however, to be no consistent correlation with dosage or duration of therapy. Symptoms may last for up to 14 days after cessation of oral antipsychotics, or for up to 4 weeks after cessation of depot preparations. Although a particular risk of development of NMS has been suggested for various antipsychotics, standard doses of all antipsychotics are capable of inducing the condition. Depot preparations may, however, be associated with prolonged recovery from the syndrome if it develops, and hence a higher mortality rate. Concomitant administration of lithium carbonate or antimuscarinics may increase the likelihood of developing the syndrome.

Antipsychotic medication should be withdrawn immediately the diagnosis of the classic syndrome is made, followed by symptomatic and supportive therapy including cooling measures, correction of dehydration, and treatment of cardiovascular, respiratory, and renal complications. Whether antipsychotics should be withdrawn from patients with mild attacks and how they should be managed is a matter of debate. The efficacy of specific drug therapy remains to be proven and justification for use is based mainly on case reports. *Dantrolene* was first used because of its effectiveness in malignant hyperthermia. It has a direct action on skeletal muscle and may be particularly effective for the reversal of hyperthermia of muscle origin. In contrast, dopaminergic agonists may resolve hyperthermia of central origin, restoring dopaminergic transmission and hence alleviating extrapyramidal symptoms. There have been isolated reports of success with *amantadine* and *levodopa* but *bromocriptine* is generally preferred. Any underlying psychosis may, however, be aggravated by dopaminergic drugs. In view of the differing modes of action of dantrolene and dopaminergics a combination of the two might be useful but any advantage remains to be demonstrated. *Antimuscarinics* are generally considered to be of little use and may aggravate the associated hyperthermia. *Benzodiazepines* may be used for sedation in agitated patients and may be of use against concomitant catatonia. Electroconvulsive therapy may be an alternative in refractory cases of NMS or when catatonic symptoms are present. Re-introduction of antipsychotic therapy may be possible but is not always successful and extreme caution is advised. It has been recommended that a gap of at least 5 to 14 days should be left after resolution of the symptoms before attempting re-introduction.

References.

1. Wells AJ, *et al.* Neuroleptic rechallenge after neuroleptic malignant syndrome: case report and literature review. *Drug Intell Clin Pharm* 1988; **22:** 475–80.
2. Bristow MF, Kohen D. How "malignant" is the neuroleptic malignant syndrome? *Br Med J* 1993; **307:** 1223–4.
3. Kornhuber J, Weller M. Neuroleptic malignant syndrome. *Curr Opin Neurol* 1994; **7:** 353–7.
4. Velamoor VR, *et al.* Management of suspected neuroleptic malignant syndrome. *Can J Psychiatry* 1995; **40:** 545–50.
5. Ebadi M, Srinivasan SK. Pathogenesis, prevention, and treatment of neuroleptic-induced movement disorders. *Pharmacol Rev* 1995; **47:** 575–604.
6. Bristow MF, Kohen D. Neuroleptic malignant syndrome. *Br J Hosp Med* 1996; **55:** 517–20.
7. Velamoor VR. Neuroleptic malignant syndrome: recognition, prevention and management. *Drug Safety* 1998; **19:** 73–82.

Withdrawal. Abrupt discontinuation of an antipsychotic may be accompanied by withdrawal symptoms, the most common of which are nausea, vomiting, anorexia, diarrhoea, rhinorrhoea, sweating, myalgias, paraesthesias, insomnia, restlessness, anxiety, and agitation.[1] Patients may also experience vertigo, alternate feelings of warmth and coldness, and tremor. Symptoms generally begin within 1 to 4 days of withdrawal and abate within 7 to 14 days. They are more severe and frequent when antimuscarinics are discontinued simultaneously.

1. Dilsaver SC. Withdrawal phenomena associated with antidepressant and antipsychotic agents. *Drug Safety* 1994; **10:** 103–14.

Treatment of Adverse Effects

Following recent ingestion of an overdose of chlorpromazine the stomach may be emptied by lavage and activated charcoal administered. Patients should be managed with intensive symptomatic and supportive therapy. Dialysis is of little or no value in poisoning by phenothiazines.

If a vasoconstrictor is considered necessary in the management of phenothiazine-induced hypotension the use of adrenaline or other sympathomimetics with high beta-adrenergic agonist properties should be avoided since the alpha-blocking effects of phenothiazines may impair the usual alpha-mediated vasoconstriction of these drugs, resulting in unopposed beta-adrenergic stimulation and increased hypotension.

The treatment of neuroleptic malignant syndrome and the difficulties of treating extrapyramidal side-effects, especially tardive dyskinesia, are discussed above.

Precautions

Chlorpromazine and other phenothiazines are contra-indicated in patients with pre-existing CNS depression or coma, bone-marrow suppression, phaeochromocytoma, or prolactin-dependent tumours. They should be used with caution or not at all in patients with impaired liver, kidney, cardiovascular, cerebrovascular, and respiratory function and in those with angle-closure glaucoma, parkinsonism, diabetes mellitus, hypothyroidism, myasthenia gravis, paralytic ileus, prostatic hyperplasia, or urinary retention. Care is required in patients with epilepsy or a history of seizures as phenothiazines may lower the seizure threshold. Debilitated patients may be more prone to the adverse effects of phenothiazines as may the elderly, especially those with dementia.

The sedative effects of phenothiazines are most marked during the first few days of administration; affected patients should not drive or operate machinery.

Phenothiazine effects on the vomiting centre may mask the symptoms of overdosage of other drugs, or of disorders such as gastro-intestinal obstruction. Administration at extremes of temperature may be hazardous since body temperature regulation is impaired by phenothiazines.

Regular eye examinations are advisable for patients receiving long-term phenothiazine therapy and avoidance of undue exposure to direct sunlight is recommended. Phenothiazines should be used with caution in the presence of acute infection or leucopenia. Blood counts are advised if the patient develops an unexplained infection.

Phenothiazines are generally not recommended late in pregnancy; such use may be associated with intoxication of the neonate. Chlorpromazine may prolong labour and should be withheld until the cervix is dilated 3 to 4 cm. For other possible risks of phenothiazine administration during pregnancy, see below.

Patients should remain supine for at least 30 minutes after parenteral administration of chlorpromazine; blood pressure should be monitored.

Abrupt withdrawal of phenothiazine therapy is best avoided.

AIDS. Isolated reports[1,2] have suggested that patients with AIDS may be particularly susceptible to antipsychotic-induced extrapyramidal effects.

1. Hollander H, *et al.* Extrapyramidal symptoms in AIDS patients given low-dose metoclopramide or chlorpromazine. *Lancet* 1985; **ii:** 1186.
2. Edelstein H, Knight RT. Severe parkinsonism in two AIDS patients taking prochlorperazine. *Lancet* 1987; **ii:** 341–2.

Asthma. Findings of a retrospective case-control study[1] appear to indicate that asthmatic patients who receive antipsychotics are at an increased risk of death or near death from asthma.

1. Joseph KS, *et al.* Increased morbidity and mortality related to asthma among asthmatic patients who use major tranquillisers. *Br Med J* 1996; **312:** 79–82.

The elderly. The risk of *hip fracture* has been reported to be increased in elderly patients given antipsychotics. In a study of the relationship between psychotropic drug use and the risk of hip fractures in patients over 65 years of age, 1021 cases and 5606 control subjects were assessed. Current users of antipsychotics had a twofold increase in the risk of hip fractures.[1] The effect was dose-related and the increased risk was similar for chlorpromazine, haloperidol, and thioridazine. It was suggested that antipsychotic-induced sedation or orthostatic hypotension could increase the risk of falls in elderly persons. A study in 12 schizophrenic patients receiving antipsychotics plus other drugs such as antimuscarinics or benzodiazepines has suggested that long-term treatment with antipsychotics may decrease bone mineralisation.[2] A later study suggested that any increased risk of falls might be due to an effect of antipsychotics on balance as thioridazine was found to increase sway in elderly but not young subjects.[3]

There is some evidence[7,8] to suggest that the use of antipsychotics to manage behavioural complications of *dementia* may increase the rate of cognitive decline. Elderly patients with dementia, especially Lewy-body dementia, are reported to be highly susceptible to the extrapyramidal adverse effects of antipsychotic drugs,[4,5] and the reaction can be extremely serious, even fatal. If these drugs are to be used in elderly patients with dementia, then very low doses should be employed, and special care should be taken if the dementia is suspected to be of the Lewy-body type since sudden life-threatening deterioration may occur.[6] Depot preparations should not be used and since dopamine D_2 receptors may be involved, it has been suggested that consideration could be given to using an antipsychotic such as clozapine that does not principally antagonise those receptors,[5] although it too is not without its problems.

For further discussion of the problems associated with the use of antipsychotics in disturbed behaviour in the elderly, see p.636.

1. Ray WA, *et al.* Psychotropic drug use and the risk of hip fracture. *N Engl J Med* 1987; **316:** 363–9.
2. Higuchi T, *et al.* Certain neuroleptics reduce bone mineralization in schizophrenic patients. *Neuropsychobiology* 1987; **18:** 185–8.
3. Liu Y, *et al.* Comparative clinical effects of thioridazine (THD) on fall risk on young and elderly subjects. *Clin Pharmacol Ther* 1995; **57:** 200.
4. McKeith I, *et al.* Neuroleptic sensitivity in patients with senile dementia of Lewy body type. *Br Med J* 1992; **305:** 673–8.
5. Piggott MA, *et al.* DRD2 Ser311/Cys311 polymorphism in schizophrenia. *Lancet* 1994; **343:** 1044–5.
6. Committee on Safety of Medicines/Medicines Control Agency. Neuroleptic sensitivity in patients with dementia. *Current Problems* 1994; **20:** 6.
7. McShane R, *et al.* Do neuroleptic drugs hasten cognitive decline in dementia? Prospective study with necropsy follow up. *Br Med J* 1997; **314:** 266–70.
8. Holmes C, *et al.* Do neuroleptic drugs hasten cognitive decline in dementia? Carriers of apolipoprotein E ε4 allele seem particularly susceptible to their effects. *Br Med J* 1997; **314:** 1411.

Epilepsy. See Convulsions under Adverse Effects, above.

Folic acid deficiency. Concentrations of folate in serum and erythrocytes were reduced in 15 patients receiving long-term treatment with chlorpromazine or thioridazine.[1] All the patients showed significant induction of hepatic microsomal enzymes. It was suggested that folate deficiency due to the induction of microsomal enzymes might subsequently limit enzyme induction and hence reduce drug metabolism and could thereby lead to symptoms of toxicity in patients apparently stabilised for a number of years. The dietary intake of patients on long-term treatment with enzyme-inducing drugs might be inadequate.

1. Labadarios D, *et al.* The effects of chronic drug administration on hepatic enzyme induction and folate metabolism. *Br J Clin Pharmacol* 1978; **5:** 167–73.

Hypoparathyroidism. There have been rare reports[1,2] of acute dystonic reactions associated with the use of phenothiazines in patients with untreated hypoparathyroidism. Caution was recommended in giving phenothiazine derivatives to patients with hypoparathyroidism and it was suggested that any acute reaction to such a drug should prompt investigation for some form of latent tetany.

1. Schaaf M, Payne CA. Dystonic reactions to prochlorperazine in hypoparathyroidism. *N Engl J Med* 1966; **275:** 991–5.
2. Gur H, *et al.* Acute dystonic reaction to methotrimeprazine in hypoparathyroidism. *Ann Pharmacother* 1996; **30:** 957–9.

Pregnancy and breast feeding. A review[1] of the use of phenothiazines in pregnancy and during breast feeding concluded that there was no clear evidence that these drugs caused a significant increase in fetal malformations. Nevertheless it was considered advisable that if pregnant patients required such treatment, then a single phenothiazine should be used and that the choice should be for one of the established drugs. Use during labour could be effective in controlling nausea and vomiting, but the effects of interactions should be considered as should the possibility of lethargy and extrapyramidal effects in the neonate due to slow elimination. It was also considered that there were no major problems related to use during breast feeding.

1. McElhatton PR. The use of phenothiazines during pregnancy and lactation. *Reprod Toxicol* 1992; **6:** 475–90.

Interactions

The most common interactions encountered with phenothiazines are adverse effects resulting from concomitant administration of drugs with similar pharmacological actions. When given with other drugs that produce orthostatic hypotension dosage adjustments may be necessary. However, it should be noted that phenothiazines have been reported to reduce the antihypertensive action of guanethidine and other adrenergic neurone blockers. As many phenothiazines possess antimuscarinic actions they may potentiate the adverse effects of other drugs with antimuscarinic actions, including tricyclic antidepressants and the antimuscarinic antiparkinsonian drugs that may be given to treat phenothiazine-induced extrapyramidal effects. In theory, antipsychotics with dopamine-blocking activity and dopaminergic drugs such as those used to treat parkinsonism may be mutually antagonistic. Concomitant administration of metoclopramide may increase the risk of antipsychotic-induced extrapyramidal effects.

There is an increased risk of arrhythmias when antipsychotics are used with drugs which prolong the QT interval including certain antiarrhythmics, antihistamines, antimalarials, and cisapride. There is also an increased risk of arrhythmia when tricyclic antidepressants are used with antipsychotics which prolong the QT interval. Because of an increased risk of seizures the US manufacturers recommend discontinuation of chlorpromazine before the use of metrizamide for radiographic procedures. Symptoms of CNS depression may be enhanced by other drugs with CNS-depressant properties including alcohol, general anaesthetics, hypnotics, anxiolytics, and opioids.

Most interactions with antipsychotics are as a result of additive pharmacological effects.[1] Since tolerance develops to many of these side-effects, interactions are likely to be most important in the early stages of combination therapy.

1. Livingston MG. Interactions that matter: 11 antipsychotic drugs. *Prescribers' J* 1987; **27** (Dec): 26–9.

Alcohol. Akathisia and dystonia occurred after consumption of alcohol by patients taking antipsychotics.[1] Alcohol might lower the threshold of resistance to neurotoxic side-effects.

1. Lutz EG. Neuroleptic-induced akathisia and dystonia triggered by alcohol. *JAMA* 1976; **236:** 2422–3.

Antacids. Studies in 6 patients showed that chlorpromazine plasma concentrations were significantly lower after administration of chlorpromazine with an aluminium hydroxide and magnesium trisilicate antacid gel (Gelusil) than after chlorpromazine alone.[1] *In-vitro* studies indicated that chlorpromazine was highly bound to the gel.

1. Fann WE, *et al.* Chlorpromazine: effects of antacids on its gastrointestinal absorption. *J Clin Pharmacol* 1973; **13:** 388–90.

Antiarrhythmics. There is an increased risk of arrhythmias when antipsychotics are given with other drugs which prolong the QT interval. It has been recommended that the concomitant use of pimozide, sertindole, or thioridazine with antiarrhythmics (especially amiodarone, disopyramide, procainamide, and quinidine) should be avoided. Concomitant use of haloperidol and amiodarone is also not recommended. A study[1] in healthy subjects has suggested that quinidine might increase plasma concentrations of haloperidol.

For a report of sudden cardiorespiratory arrest and death in a patient taking eproxindine and flupenthixol, see under Eproxindine, p.865.

1. Young D, *et al.* Effect of quinidine on the interconversion kinetics between haloperidol and reduced haloperidol in humans: implications for the involvement of cytochrome P450IID6. *Eur J Clin Pharmacol* 1993; **44:** 433–8.

Antibacterials. Seven schizophrenic patients whose antitubercular therapy included *rifampicin* (in addition to isoniazid, and in some cases also ethambutol) had lower serum concentrations of haloperidol compared with tuberculotic schizophrenic patients receiving no antimycobacterials and with non-tuberculotic schizophrenics.[1] Pharmacokinetic studies involving some of these patients indicated accelerated haloperidol clearance in the presence of rifampicin. Abnormally high serum-haloperidol concentrations were observed in 3 of 18 patients treated with isoniazid alone.

Black galactorrhoea occurred in a patient receiving concomitant therapy with *minocycline*, perphenazine, amitriptyline hydrochloride, and diphenhydramine hydrochloride.[2] Simultaneous occurrence of phenothiazine-induced galactorrhoea and tetracycline-induced pigmentation was considered responsible.

Sudden cardiac deaths have been reported[3] in patients given *clarithromycin* and pimozide. The manufacturer of pimozide has recommended that pimozide should not be used with macrolide antibacterials.

1. Takeda M, *et al.* Serum haloperidol levels of schizophrenics receiving treatment for tuberculosis. *Clin Neuropharmacol* 1986; **9:** 386–97.
2. Basler RSW, Lynch PJ. Black galactorrhea as a consequence of minocycline and phenothiazine therapy. *Arch Dermatol* 1985; **121:** 417–18.
3. Flockhart DA, *et al.* A metabolic interaction between clarithromycin and pimozide may result in cardiac toxicity. *Clin Pharmacol Ther* 1996; **59:** 189.

Anticoagulants. For reference to the effects of some antipsychotics on the activity of anticoagulants, see under Warfarin, p.968.

Antidepressants. Interactions between antipsychotics and *tricyclic antidepressants* are generally of two forms: either additive pharmacological effects such as antimuscarinic effects or hypotension, or pharmacokinetic interactions. Although not commonly reported in the literature additive antimuscarinic activity may be a significant risk especially in the elderly. Careful drug selection might help to prevent the development of serious adverse effects. Mutual inhibition of liver enzymes concerned with the metabolism of both the antipsychotic and the tricyclic antidepressant might result in increased plasma concentrations of either drug. In one study[1] addition of nortriptyline to chlorpromazine therapy produced an increase in plasma concentrations of chlorpromazine but this resulted in a paradoxical increase in agitation and tension.

There is an increased risk of arrhythmias when tricyclic antidepressants are given with other drugs which prolong the QT interval. It has been recommended that the concomitant use of pimozide, sertindole, or thioridazine with tricyclic antidepressants should be avoided.

Increased serum concentrations of haloperidol have occurred in patients given haloperidol with *fluoxetine*[2] or *fluvoxamine*[3] and isolated reports[4-9] of extrapyramidal symptoms, psychoneuromotor syndrome, stupor, bradycardia, and urinary retention associated with concomitant use of fluoxetine and antipsychotics suggest that fluoxetine might exacerbate the adverse effects of antipsychotics or produce additive toxicity. Similar CNS effects have been noted in volunteers given perphenazine and *paroxetine*.[10] There has also been an isolated report of a patient who complained of amenorrhoea and galactorrhoea after fluvoxamine was added to loxapine therapy.[11]

Combinations of antipsychotics and lithium should be used with care. Lithium can reduce plasma-chlorpromazine concentrations and there is a report of ventricular fibrillation on withdrawal of lithium from concomitant therapy with chlorpromazine. Chlorpromazine has also been reported to enhance the excretion of lithium. Neurotoxic or extrapyramidal symptoms have been reported rarely in patients taking antipsychotics and lithium; these may be atypical cases of lithium toxicity or neuroleptic malignant syndrome. The above issues are discussed in detail, and references given, on p.294.

There have been occasional reports of sexual disinhibition in patients taking *tryptophan* with phenothiazines.

1. Loga S, *et al.* Interaction of chlorpromazine and nortriptyline in patients with schizophrenia. *Clin Pharmacokinet* 1981; **6:** 454–62.
2. Goff DC, *et al.* Elevation of plasma concentrations of haloperidol after the addition of fluoxetine. *Am J Psychiatry* 1991; **148:** 790–2.
3. Daniel DG, *et al.* Coadministration of fluvoxamine increases serum concentrations of haloperidol. *J Clin Psychopharmacol* 1994; **14:** 340–3.
4. Tate JL. Extrapyramidal symptoms in a patient taking haloperidol and fluoxetine. *Am J Psychiatry* 1989; **146:** 399–400.
5. Ahmed I, *et al.* Possible interaction between fluoxetine and pimozide causing sinus bradycardia. *Can J Psychiatry* 1993; **38:** 62–3.
6. Ketai R. Interaction between fluoxetine and neuroleptics. *Am J Psychiatry* 1993; **150:** 836–7.
7. Hansen-Grant S, *et al.* Fluoxetine-pimozide interaction. *Am J Psychiatry* 1993; **150:** 1751–2.
8. D'Souza DC, *et al.* Precipitation of a psychoneuromotor syndrome by fluoxetine in a haloperidol-treated schizophrenic patient. *J Clin Psychopharmacol* 1994; **14:** 361–3.
9. Benazzi F. Urinary retention with fluoxetine-haloperidol combination in a young patient. *Can J Psychiatry* 1996; **41:** 606–7.
10. Özdemir V, *et al.* Paroxetine potentiates the central nervous system side effects of perphenazine: contribution of cytochrome P4502D6 inhibition in vivo. *Clin Pharmacol Ther* 1997; **62:** 334–47.
11. Jeffries J, *et al.* Amenorrhea and galactorrhea associated with fluvoxamine in a loxapine-treated patient. *J Clin Psychopharmacol* 1992; **12:** 296–7.

Antidiabetic drugs. Since chlorpromazine may cause hyperglycaemia or impair glucose tolerance the dose of oral hypoglycaemics or of insulin may need to be increased in diabetics.

Antiepileptics. *Carbamazepine, phenobarbitone*, and *phenytoin* are potent enzyme inducers and concomitant administration may decrease plasma concentrations of antipsychotics or their active metabolites.[1-5] The clinical effect of any interaction has not been consistent; worsening, improvement, or no change in psychotic symptoms have all been noted. Delirium has been reported in one patient given haloperidol and carbamazepine.[6] One case report[7] has suggested that phenytoin might also exacerbate neuroleptic-induced dyskinesia. Care should be taken when withdrawing enzyme-inducing anticonvulsants as this may result in a rise in antipsychotic serum concentrations.[8]

The effect of antipsychotics on antiepileptic concentrations is discussed on p.341 (carbamazepine) and p.356 (phenytoin). It should also be remembered that antipsychotics may lower the seizure threshold.

1. Loga S, *et al.* Interactions of orphenadrine and phenobarbitone with chlorpromazine: plasma concentrations and effects in man. *Br J Clin Pharmacol* 1975; **2:** 197–208.
2. Linnoila M, *et al.* Effect of anticonvulsants on plasma haloperidol and thioridazine levels. *Am J Psychiatry* 1980; **137:** 819–21.
3. Jann MW, *et al.* Effects of carbamazepine on plasma haloperidol levels. *J Clin Psychopharmacol* 1985; **5:** 106–9.
4. Arana GW, *et al.* Does carbamazepine-induced reduction of plasma haloperidol levels worsen psychotic symptoms? *Am J Psychiatry* 1986; **143:** 650–1.
5. Ereshefsky L, *et al.* Thiothixene pharmacokinetic interactions: a study of hepatic enzyme inducers, clearance inhibitors, and demographic variables. *J Clin Psychopharmacol* 1991; **11:** 296–301.
6. Kanter GL, *et al.* Case report of a possible interaction between neuroleptics and carbamazepine. *Am J Psychiatry* 1984; **141:** 1101–2.
7. DeVeaugh-Geiss J. Aggravation of tardive dyskinesia by phenytoin. *N Engl J Med* 1978; **298:** 457–8.
8. Jann MW, *et al.* Clinical implications of increased antipsychotic plasma concentrations upon anticonvulsant cessation. *Psychiatry Res* 1989; **28:** 153–9.

Antihistamines. For the effect of a preparation containing chlorpheniramine maleate and phenylpropanolamine hydrochloride on thioridazine, see Sympathomimetics (below). There is an increased risk of arrhythmias when antipsychotics are given with other drugs which prolong the QT interval. It has been recommended that the concomitant use of pimozide, sertindole, or thioridazine with antihistamines such as astemizole or terfenadine should be avoided.

Antihypertensives. For discussion of the interaction between phenothiazines and drugs with hypotensive properties, see Interactions, above. For a report of chlorpromazine enhancing the hyperglycaemic effect of diazoxide, see p.848. For reports of hypertension or dementia in patients given methyldopa and antipsychotics, see p.905.

Antimalarials. Pretreatment with single doses of chloroquine sulphate, amodiaquine hydrochloride, or sulfadoxine with pyrimethamine increased the plasma concentrations of chlorpromazine and 7-hydroxychlorpromazine, but not of chlorpromazine sulphoxide, in schizophrenic patients maintained on chlorpromazine.[1] The raised plasma concentrations appeared to be associated with a greater level of sedation.

There is an increased risk of arrhythmias when antipsychotics are given with other drugs which prolong the QT interval. It has been recommended that the concomitant use of antipsychotics, and pimozide in particular, with antimalarials such as halofantrine, mefloquine, or quinine should be avoided. For the possible effects of the use of quinidine with antipsychotics see Antiarrhythmics, above.

1. Makanjuola ROA, *et al.* Effects of antimalarial agents on plasma levels of chlorpromazine and its metabolites in schizophrenic patients. *Trop Geogr Med* 1988; **40:** 31–3.

Antimigraine drugs. A report[1] of a patient receiving loxapine who had a dystonic reaction within 15 minutes of subcutaneous administration of *sumatriptan* suggests that these two drugs might interact or potentiate each other's adverse effects. However, the patient had a previous history of dystonic reactions associated with haloperidol treatment and was receiving benztropine prophylactically. Furthermore, the dose of loxapine had been increased 2 days before the event and this may have predisposed the patient to developing a dystonic reaction.

1. Garcia G, *et al.* Dystonic reaction associated with sumatriptan. *Ann Pharmacother* 1994; **28:** 1199.

Antiparkinsonian drugs. Antiparkinsonian drugs are sometimes given with antipsychotics for the management of antipsychotic-induced side-effects including extrapyramidal disorders (see under Adverse Effects, above). Theoretically, dopaminergics such as *levodopa* and *bromocriptine* might induce or exacerbate psychotic symptoms. A study in 18 subjects and review of the literature suggested that bromocriptine can be used safely in patients at risk of psychotic illness provided they are clinically stable and maintained on antipsychotics.[1] Conversely, antipsychotics might antagonise the effects of dopaminergics; diminished therapeutic effects of levodopa have been noted with several antipsychotics (see p.1139) and thioridazine has been reported to oppose the prolactin-lowering action of bromocriptine (see p.1134).

Additive antimuscarinic side-effects are obviously a risk when antimuscarinic antiparkinsonian drugs are given with antipsychotics. Although these are generally mild, serious reactions have occurred. *Benzhexol*[2] and *orphenadrine*[3] have both been reported to decrease plasma concentrations of chlorpromazine, possibly by interfering with absorption from the gastro-intestinal tract. Reports suggesting that antimuscarinics may antagonise the antipsychotic effects of antipsychotics at the neurotransmitter level require substantiating.

1. Perovich RM, *et al.* The behavioral toxicity of bromocriptine in patients with psychiatric illness. *J Clin Psychopharmacol* 1989; **9:** 417–22.
2. Rivera-Calimlim L, *et al.* Effects of mode of management on plasma chlorpromazine in psychiatric patients. *Clin Pharmacol Ther* 1973; **14:** 978–86.
3. Loga S, *et al.* Interactions of orphenadrine and phenobarbitone with chlorpromazine: plasma concentrations and effects in man. *Br J Clin Pharmacol* 1975; **2:** 197–208.

Antivirals. *Ritonavir* may increase the area under the concentration-time curve of some antipsychotics. The increases expected for clozapine and pimozide were considered by the manufacturer of ritonavir to be large enough to recommend that these antipsychotics should not be used with ritonavir. Other antipsychotics predicted to have moderate increases included chlorpromazine, haloperidol, perphenazine, risperidone, and thioridazine and it was recommended that monitoring of drug concentrations and/or adverse effects were required when used with ritonavir.

Beta blockers. When given together, chlorpromazine and propranolol may mutually inhibit the liver metabolism of the other drug. *Propranolol* has been reported to increase plasma concentrations of chlorpromazine[1] and thioridazine,[2,3] and *pindolol* to increase plasma-thioridazine concentrations.[4] Neither beta blocker tested had a significant effect on haloperidol concentrations,[3,4] although there is a report of severe hypotension or cardiopulmonary arrest occurring on 3 occasions in a schizophrenic patient given haloperidol and propranolol concomitantly.[5] The clinical significance of antipsychotic-beta blocker interactions is unclear.

For the effect of chlorpromazine on propranolol, see under Beta Blockers, p.830.

There is an increased risk of arrhythmias when antipsychotics are given with other drugs which prolong the QT interval. The concomitant use of antipsychotics, and pimozide in particular, with *sotalol* should be avoided.

1. Peet M, *et al.* Pharmacokinetic interaction between propranolol and chlorpromazine in schizophrenic patients. *Lancet* 1980; **ii:** 978.
2. Silver JM, *et al.* Elevation of thioridazine plasma levels by propranolol. *Am J Psychiatry* 1986; **143:** 1290–2.
3. Greendyke RM, Kanter DR. Plasma propranolol levels and their effect on plasma thioridazine and haloperidol concentrations. *J Clin Psychopharmacol* 1987; **7:** 178–82.
4. Greendyke RM, Gulya A. Effect of pindolol administration on serum levels of thioridazine, haloperidol, phenytoin, and phenobarbital. *J Clin Psychiatry* 1988; **49:** 105–7.
5. Alexander HE, *et al.* Hypotension and cardiopulmonary arrest associated with concurrent haloperidol and propranolol therapy. *JAMA* 1984; **252:** 87–8.

Buspirone. The manufacturers have reported that concomitant administration of haloperidol and buspirone has resulted in increased serum haloperidol concentrations. However, while Goff *et al.*[1] found the mean rise in serum-haloperidol concentrations to be 26%, that observed by Huang *et al.*[2] was not statistically significant.

1. Goff DC, *et al.* An open trial of buspirone added to neuroleptics in schizophrenic patients. *J Clin Psychopharmacol* 1991; **11:** 193–7.
2. Huang HF, *et al.* Lack of pharmacokinetic interaction between buspirone and haloperidol in patients with schizophrenia. *J Clin Pharmacol* 1996; **36:** 963–9.

Cimetidine. Despite expectations that cimetidine might reduce the metabolism of chlorpromazine, mean steady-state plasma concentrations of chlorpromazine fell rather than rose in 8 patients given cimetidine for 7 days in addition to regular chlorpromazine therapy.[1] The explanation was probably that cimetidine interfered with chlorpromazine absorption. Byrne and O'Shea[2] however, reported excessive sedation, necessitating a reduction in chlorpromazine dosage, after addition of cimetidine to the drug therapy of 2 chronic schizophrenics.

1. Howes CA, *et al.* Reduced steady-state plasma concentrations of chlorpromazine and indomethacin in patients receiving cimetidine. *Eur J Clin Pharmacol* 1983; **24:** 99–102.
2. Byrne A, O'Shea B. Adverse interaction between cimetidine and chlorpromazine in two cases of chronic schizophrenia. *Br J Psychiatry* 1989; **155:** 413–15.

Cocaine. The risk of antipsychotic-induced dystonic reactions may be increased in cocaine abusers. Dystonia occurred in 6 of 7 cocaine abusers treated with haloperidol.[1]

1. Kumor K, *et al.* Haloperidol-induced dystonia in cocaine addicts. *Lancet* 1986; **ii:** 1341–2.

Desferrioxamine. Loss of consciousness lasting 48 to 72 hours occurred in 2 patients given prochlorperazine during desferrioxamine therapy.[1] Prochlorperazine may enhance the removal of transition metals from brain cells by desferrioxamine.

1. Blake DR, *et al.* Cerebral and ocular toxicity induced by desferrioxamine. *Q J Med* 1985; **56:** 345–55.

Disulfiram. A psychotic patient, previously maintained with plasma-perphenazine concentrations of 2 to 3 nmol per mL on a dose of 8 mg twice daily by mouth was readmitted with subtherapeutic plasma-perphenazine concentrations of less than 1 nmol per mL, despite unchanged dosage, following concomitant disulfiram therapy.[1] The concentration of the sulphoxide metabolite of perphenazine was much increased. Following a change from oral to intramuscular perphenazine therapy there was a substantial clinical improvement associated with a return to therapeutic plasma concentrations of perphenazine and a fall in concentration of the metabolite. Disulfiram appears to greatly enhance biotransformation of perphenazine given by mouth to inactive metabolites, but parenteral administration avoids the 'first-pass' effect in the liver.

1. Hansen LB, Larsen N-E. Metabolic interaction between perphenazine and disulfiram. *Lancet* 1982; **ii:** 1472.

General anaesthetics. A schizophrenic patient without a history of epilepsy who was receiving chlorpromazine by mouth and flupenthixol depot injection had a convulsive seizure when given *enflurane* anaesthesia.[1]

1. Vohra SB. Convulsions after enflurane in a schizophrenic patient receiving neuroleptics. *Can J Anaesth* 1994; **41:** 420–2.

Naltrexone. Two patients maintained on thioridazine experienced intense sleepiness and lethargy after receiving 2 doses of naltrexone.[1]

1. Maany I, *et al.* Interaction between thioridazine and naltrexone. *Am J Psychiatry* 1987; **144:** 966.

NSAIDs. A report of severe drowsiness and confusion in patients given haloperidol with *indomethacin.*[1]

1. Bird HA, *et al.* Drowsiness due to haloperidol/indomethacin in combination. *Lancet* 1983; **i:** 830–1.

Opioid analgesics. For reference to the effects of phenothiazines on *pethidine*, see p.77.

Piperazine. Caution has been advised when giving piperazine to patients receiving phenothiazines because of the possibility that piperazine might enhance their adverse effects. There has been an isolated report[1] of convulsions associated with the use of chlorpromazine in a child who had received piperazine several days earlier. Subsequent *animal*[1-3] studies produced conflicting evidence for an interaction but one worker[3] concluded that an interaction would only be clinically significant when high concentrations of piperazine were reached in the body.

1. Boulos BM, Davis LE. Hazard of simultaneous administration of phenothiazine and piperazine. *N Engl J Med* 1969; **280:** 1245–6.
2. Armbrecht BH. Reaction between piperazine and chlorpromazine. *N Engl J Med* 1970; **282:** 1490–1.
3. Sturman G. Interaction between piperazine and chlorpromazine. *Br J Pharmacol* 1974; **50:** 153–5.

Sympathomimetics. For reference to the possible interaction between phenothiazines and *adrenaline*, see Treatment of Adverse Effects, above.

A 27-year-old woman with schizophrenia and T-wave abnormality of the heart,[1] receiving thioridazine 100 mg daily with procyclidine 2.5 mg twice daily, died from ventricular fibrillation within 2 hours of taking a single dose of a preparation reported to contain chlorpheniramine maleate 4 mg with phenylpropanolamine hydrochloride 50 mg (Contac C), concurrently with thioridazine.

1. Chouinard G, *et al.* Death attributed to ventricular arrhythmia induced by thioridazine in combination with a single Contac C capsule. *Can Med Assoc J* 1978; **119:** 729–31.

Tobacco smoking. Smoking has been shown to decrease the incidence of chlorpromazine-induced sedation[1,2] and orthostatic hypotension.[2] Studies indicate that the clearance of chlorpromazine,[3] fluphenazine,[4] thiothixene,[5] and haloperidol[6] may be increased in patients who smoke. It has been suggested that some of the components of smoke may act as liver-enzyme inducers. The clinical significance of this effect is unclear but the possible need to use increased doses in smokers should be borne in mind.

1. Swett C. Drowsiness due to chlorpromazine in relation to cigarette smoking: a report from the Boston Collaborative Drug Surveillance Program. *Arch Gen Psychiatry* 1974; **31:** 211–13.
2. Pantuck EJ, *et al.* Cigarette smoking and chlorpromazine disposition and actions. *Clin Pharmacol Ther* 1982; **31:** 533–8.
3. Chetty M, *et al.* Smoking and body weight influence the clearance of chlorpromazine. *Eur J Clin Pharmacol* 1994; **46:** 523–6.
4. Ereshefsky L, *et al.* Effects of smoking on fluphenazine clearance in psychiatric inpatients. *Biol Psychiatry* 1985; **20:** 329–32.
5. Ereshefsky L, *et al.* Thiothixene pharmacokinetic interactions: a study of hepatic enzyme inducers, clearance inhibitors, and demographic variables. *J Clin Psychopharmacol* 1991; **11:** 296–301.
6. Jann MW, *et al.* Effects of smoking on haloperidol and reduced haloperidol plasma concentrations and haloperidol clearance. *Psychopharmacology (Berl)* 1986; **90:** 468–70.

Vitamins. Administration of ascorbic acid, for vitamin C deficiency, to a patient receiving fluphenazine for manic depression was associated with a fall in serum concentrations of fluphenazine and a deterioration of behaviour.[1]

1. Dysken MW, *et al.* Drug interaction between ascorbic acid and fluphenazine. *JAMA* 1979; **241:** 2008.

Xanthine-containing beverages. Studies *in vitro* have shown precipitation of some antipsychotics from solution by addition of coffee and tea.[1,2] However, in a study of 16 patients taking antipsychotics no correlation could be found between plasma-antipsychotic concentrations or behaviour and tea or coffee consumption.[3]

1. Kulhanek F, *et al.* Precipitation of antipsychotic drugs in interaction with coffee or tea. *Lancet* 1979; **ii:** 1130.
2. Lasswell WL, *et al.* In vitro interaction of neuroleptics and tricyclic antidepressants with coffee, tea, and gallotannic acid. *J Pharm Sci* 1984; **73:** 1056–8.
3. Bowen S, *et al.* Effect of coffee and tea on blood levels and efficacy of antipsychotic drugs. *Lancet* 1981; **i:** 1217–18.

Pharmacokinetics

Chlorpromazine is readily, although sometimes erratically, absorbed from the gastro-intestinal tract; peak plasma concentrations are attained 2 to 4 hours after ingestion. It is subject to considerable first-pass metabolism in the gut wall and is also extensively metabolised in the liver and is excreted in the urine and bile in the form of numerous active and inactive metabolites; there is some evidence of enterohepatic recycling. Owing to the first-pass effect, plasma concentrations following oral administration are much lower than those following intramuscular administration. Moreover, there is very wide intersubject variation in plasma concentrations of chlorpromazine; no simple correlation has been found between plasma concentrations of chlorpromazine and its metabolites, and their therapeutic effect (see Administration under Uses and Administration, below). Paths of metabolism of chlorpromazine include hydroxylation and conjugation with glucuronic acid, *N*-oxidation, oxidation of a sulphur atom, and dealkylation. Although the plasma half-life of chlorpromazine itself has been reported to be about 30 hours, elimination of the metabolites may be very prolonged. There is limited evidence that chlorpromazine induces its own metabolism.

Chlorpromazine is very extensively bound (about 95 to 98%) to plasma proteins. It is widely distributed in the body and crosses the blood-brain barrier to achieve higher concentrations in the brain than in the plasma. Chlorpromazine and its metabolites also cross the placental barrier and are distributed into milk.

References.

1. Yeung PK-F, *et al.* Pharmacokinetics of chlorpromazine and key metabolites. *Eur J Clin Pharmacol* 1993; **45:** 563–9.

Administration in children. References to chlorpromazine pharmacokinetics in children.

1. Rivera-Calimlim L, *et al.* Plasma chlorpromazine concentrations in children with behavioral disorders and mental illness. *Clin Pharmacol Ther* 1979; **26:** 114–21.
2. Furlanut M, *et al.* Chlorpromazine disposition in relation to age in children. *Clin Pharmacokinet* 1990; **18:** 329–31.

Administration in ethnic groups. Studies with haloperidol and chlorpromazine indicate that some noncaucasian ethnic groups may require lower doses of antipsychotics than whites, possibly due to pharmacokinetic differences or increased sensitivity.[1,2]

1. Wood AJJ, Zhou HH. Ethnic differences in drug disposition and responsiveness. *Clin Pharmacokinet* 1991; **20:** 350–73.
2. Jibiki I, *et al.* Effective clinical response at low plasma levels of haloperidol in Japanese schizophrenics with acute psychotic state. *Jpn J Psychiatry Neurol* 1993; **47:** 627–9.

Metabolism. A review of the metabolism of antipsychotic drugs.[1]

1. Caccia S, Garattini S. Formation of active metabolites of psychotropic drugs: an updated review of their significance. *Clin Pharmacokinet* 1990; **18:** 434–59.

Uses and Administration

Chlorpromazine has a wide range of activity arising from its depressant actions on the CNS and its alpha-adrenergic blocking and antimuscarinic activities. It is a dopamine inhibitor and stimulates the release of prolactin. The turnover of dopamine in the brain is also increased. There is some evidence that the antagonism of central dopaminergic function, especially at the D_2-dopaminergic receptor, is related to therapeutic effect in psychotic conditions.

Chlorpromazine possesses sedative properties but patients usually develop tolerance rapidly to the sedation. It has antiemetic, serotonin-blocking, and weak antihistaminic properties and slight ganglion-blocking activity. It inhibits the heat-regulating centre so that the patient tends to acquire the temperature of the surroundings (poikilothermy). Chlorpromazine can relax skeletal muscle.

Chlorpromazine is widely used in the management of psychotic conditions. It is used in acute and chronic schizophrenia (p.637) and reduces the manic phase of manic depression (p.273). It is used to control severely disturbed, agitated, or violent behaviour (p.636) and is sometimes given in other psychiatric conditions and as an adjunct for the short-term treatment of severe anxiety (but see also p.635).

Chlorpromazine is an antiemetic and is used to control nausea and vomiting (p.1172) and is useful in palliative care. It does not appear to be of benefit in motion sickness.

Chlorpromazine is effective in the alleviation of intractable hiccup (below).

Chlorpromazine was formerly given in conjunction with pethidine and sometimes promethazine in a form of neuroleptanalgesia (p.1220). However, such a combination was associated with considerable adverse effects and other drugs are now usually preferred for this procedure. Chlorpromazine was also given to reduce pre-operative anxiety.

Chlorpromazine has also been used as an adjunct in the treatment of tetanus (p.145 and p.1304) and to control symptoms in acute intermittent porphyria (p.983).

Chlorpromazine is administered as the hydrochloride by mouth or injection, as the embonate by mouth in doses equivalent to those of the hydrochloride, and as the base rectally by suppository.

Dosage varies both with the individual and with the purpose for which the drug is being used. In most patients oral treatment may be used from the start, commencing with a dosage of 25 to 50 mg of the hydrochloride, or its equivalent as the embonate, three times daily and increasing as necessary; daily doses of 75 mg may be given as a single dose at night. Lower doses (10 to 25 mg every 4 to 6 hours) may be sufficient in some cases, particularly for control of nausea and vomiting. Maintenance doses, when required, usually range from 25 to 100 mg three times daily, although psychotic patients may require daily doses of up to 1 g or more.

For parenteral use, deep intramuscular injection is preferable, but diluted solutions have sometimes been given by slow intravenous infusion for indications such as tetanus, severe intractable hiccup, or nausea and vomiting associated with surgery. Subcutaneous injection is contra-indicated. After injection of chlorpromazine, patients should remain in the supine position for at least 30 minutes. The usual dose by intramuscular injection is 25 to 50 mg repeated as required.

If intractable hiccup does not respond to 25 to 50 mg three or four times daily by mouth for 2 to 3 days then 25 to 50 mg may be administered intramuscularly and if this fails 25 to 50 mg in 500 to 1000 mL of 0.9% sodium chloride intravenous infusion should be given by slow intravenous infusion, with the patient supine, and careful monitoring of the blood pressure.

If the oral and parenteral routes are not suitable chlorpromazine may be administered rectally as suppositories containing 100 mg of chlorpromazine base; this is stated to have an effect comparable with 40 to 50 mg of the hydrochloride by mouth or 20 to 25 mg intramuscularly. Up to 4 suppositories may be given in 24 hours.

Initial doses of chlorpromazine of one-third to one-half the normal adult dose have been recommended for elderly and debilitated patients; doses should be increased more gradually.

Children aged 1 to 12 years may be given chlorpromazine hydrochloride in a dose of 500 μg per kg body-weight every 4 to 6 hours by mouth or every 6 to 8 hours by intramuscular injection but for psychiatric indications the oral dose for children aged over 5 years is usually one-third to one-half the adult dose. Daily doses should not normally exceed 40 mg of chlorpromazine hydrochloride for children aged 1 to 5 years or 75 mg for children over 5 years of age. Suppositories containing 25 mg of chlorpromazine base are available in some countries for use in children.

Action. The therapeutic effects of antipsychotics appear to be mediated, at least in part, by interference with dopamine transmission in the brain. Chlorpromazine, thioridazine, and thioxanthene derivatives have relatively equal affinity for D_1 or D_2 receptors, although their metabolites tend to be more potent as D_2 blockers.[1] Butyrophenones and diphenylbutylpiperidines are relatively selective for D_2 receptors, and the substituted benzamides such as sulpiride and remoxipride are highly D_2-specific. Clozapine is a relatively weak inhibitor of D_2 receptors but its actions are complex and it has a high affinity for a number of different receptors including serotonin$_2$ (5-HT_2) receptors.[2] Risperidone has a high affinity both for 5-HT_2 and D_2 receptors.[2]

The traditional hypothesis of the action of antipsychotics has been that blockade of D_2 receptors in the limbic and cortical regions is responsible for the antipsychotic effects, and that extrapyramidal motor side-effects result from blockade of D_2 receptors in the striatum (a typical motor region of the basal ganglia).[3] Modification of prolactin secretion results from blockade of D_2 receptors in the anterior pituitary. However, this hypothesis cannot satisfactorily account for the pharmacological profiles of atypical antipsychotics such as clozapine, remoxipride, risperidone, and sulpiride. Their mode of action or reasons for their relative lack of extrapyramidal effects still remain largely unclear.[2]

Unlike phenothiazines and butyrophenones, the diphenylbutylpiperidines are potent calcium antagonists. This action may explain the ability of this group of drugs to relieve the negative symptoms of schizophrenia.[4]

Division of antipsychotics into low- and high-potency agents is discussed under Administration, below. For reference to the actions of antipsychotics on neuroendocrine function, see Effects on Endocrine Function under Adverse Effects, above.

1. Ereshefsky L, *et al.* Pathophysiologic basis for schizophrenia and the efficacy of antipsychotics. *Clin Pharm* 1990; **9:** 682–707.
2. Kerwin RW. The new atypical antipsychotics: a lack of extrapyramidal side-effects and new routes in schizophrenia research. *Br J Psychiatry* 1994; **164:** 141–8.
3. Anonymous. Now we understand antipsychotics? *Lancet* 1990; **336:** 1222–3.
4. Snyder SH. Drug and neurotransmitter receptors: new perspectives with clinical relevance. *JAMA* 1989; **261:** 3126–9.

Administration. The traditional antipsychotics are often divided into **low-potency** drugs (phenothiazines with an aliphatic or piperidine side-chain or thioxanthenes with an aliphatic side-chain) or **high-potency** drugs (butyrophenones, diphenylbutylpiperidines, and phenothiazines or thioxanthenes with a piperazine side-chain). At doses with equipotent antipsychotic activity, the low-potency drugs are more prone to cause sedation and antimuscarinic or α-adrenergic-blocking effects than the high-potency drugs, but are associated with a lower incidence of extrapyramidal effects, with the exception of tardive dyskinesia which is equally likely to occur with all conventional antipsychotics.

Equivalent doses of antipsychotics quoted in the literature have varied considerably. In the UK the following daily doses of oral antipsychotics have been suggested to have approximately equipotent antipsychotic activity for doses up to the maximum licensed doses: chlorpromazine hydrochloride 100 mg, clozapine 50 mg, haloperidol 2 to 3 mg, loxapine 10 to 20 mg, pimozide 2 mg, risperidone 0.5 to 1 mg, sulpiride 200 mg, thioridazine 100 mg, and trifluoperazine 5 mg. In specialist psychiatric units where very high doses are required the equivalent dose of haloperidol might be up to 10 mg. It should be noted that all patients receiving pimozide require an annual ECG and all those receiving more than 16 mg of pimozide daily require periodic ECGs (see p.686). Suggested equipotent doses of intramuscular depot antipsychotics are: flupenthixol decanoate 40 mg every 2 weeks, fluphenazine decanoate 25 mg every 2 weeks, haloperidol (as the decanoate) 100 mg every 4 weeks, pipothiazine palmitate 50 mg every 4 weeks, and zuclopenthixol decanoate 200 mg every 2 weeks.

Baldessarini and colleagues[1] have commented that high doses of antipsychotics (greater than the equivalent of 600 mg of chlorpromazine daily) are generally not necessary for the treatment (both initial and maintenance) of psychotic disorders, and may be associated with an increased risk of side-effects as well as with a diminished clinical response. However, if high doses of antipsychotics have to be used, then doses should be increased gradually with caution and under the supervision of a specialist and facilities for emergency resuscitation should be available. The Royal College of Psychiatrists in the UK has issued advice for those considering the use of high doses of antipsychotics.[2] When patients have failed to respond to recommended doses of two different antipsychotics the diagnosis, patient compliance, and the duration of treatment already given should be reviewed before increasing the dose. Alternative approaches to treatment including the use of adjuvant therapy and newer antipsychotics such as clozapine should also be considered. Contra-indications to high-dose therapy such as cardiac disease and hepatic and renal impairment and other risk factors such as obesity and old age should be borne in mind. It is advised that an ECG should be carried out to exclude QT prolongation and repeated every 1 to 3 months while the dose remains high. The dose should be reduced if a prolonged QT interval develops. Regular checks on pulse, blood pressure, temperature, and hydration are also advised. If possible dosage should be increased gradually at intervals of at least one week. The College considered that the use of high-dose therapy was to be considered as a limited course. The patient should be reviewed regularly and the dose reduced back to accepted levels after 3 months if there had been no improvement.

The existence of a therapeutic range (or therapeutic window) has not been demonstrated for most antipsychotics (with the possible exception of haloperidol[3]), and plasma concentrations of these drugs must be interpreted with caution.[1,3] Many factors make it difficult to establish a meaningful correlation between dose, plasma concentrations, and clinical improvement. These include incomplete absorption, first-pass effect, enzyme induction, the presence of active and inactive metabolites, ethnic group, smoking, and factors occurring at the receptor level.[3]

1. Baldessarini RJ, *et al.* Significance of neuroleptic dose and plasma level in the pharmacological treatment of psychoses. *Arch Gen Psychiatry* 1988; **45:** 77–91.
2. The Royal College of Psychiatrists. Consensus statement on the use of high dose antipsychotic medication. *Council Report CR26* London: Royal College of Psychiatrists, October 1993. Also in: Thompson C. Royal College of Psychiatrists' Consensus Panel. The use of high-dose antipsychotic medication. *Br J Psychiatry* 1994; **164:** 448–58.
3. Sramek JJ, *et al.* Neuroleptic plasma concentrations and clinical response: in search of a therapeutic window. *Drug Intell Clin Pharm* 1988; **22:** 373–80.

ADMINISTRATION IN CHILDREN. The American Academy of Pediatrics reappraised the use of the sedative mixture containing chlorpromazine, promethazine, and pethidine known as lytic cocktail or DPT and recommended that other sedatives/analgesics should be considered.[1]

1. Committee on Drugs, American Academy of Pediatrics. Reappraisal of lytic cocktail/Demerol, Phenergan, and Thorazine (DPT) for sedation of children. *Pediatrics* 1995; **95:** 598–602.

Alcohol withdrawal syndrome. For advice against the use of antipsychotics for alcohol withdrawal, see p.1099.

Chorea. For a discussion of the management of various choreas, including mention of the use of phenothiazines such as chlorpromazine, see p.636.

Dyspnoea. It has been shown that in healthy subjects an oral dose of 25 mg of chlorpromazine hydrochloride can reduce exercise-induced breathlessness without affecting ventilation or causing sedation.[1] Some workers[2] have reported that in patients with advanced cancer and dyspnoea unresponsive to other measures chlorpromazine relieves air hunger and, if required, can be used to sedate dying patients who have unrelieved distress. It is recommended that initial doses should be small; 12.5 mg by slow intravenous injection or 25 mg by suppository may be given. For a discussion of the management of dyspnoea, see p.70.

1. O'Neill PA, *et al.* Chlorpromazine—a specific effect on breathlessness? *Br J Clin Pharmacol* 1985; **19:** 793–7.
2. Walsh D. Dyspnoea in advanced cancer. *Lancet* 1993; **342:** 450–1.

Dystonia. Antipsychotics such as phenothiazines, haloperidol, or pimozide are sometimes useful in the treatment of idiopathic dystonia in patients who have failed to respond to other drugs.[1] However, they often act non-specifically, damping down excessive movements by causing a degree of drug-induced parkinsonism and there is the risk of adding drug-induced extrapyramidal disorders to the dystonia being treated (see Extrapyramidal Disorders under Adverse Effects, above).

For a discussion of the management of dystonias, see under Levodopa on p.1141.

1. Marsden CD, Quinn NP. The dystonias. *Br Med J* 1990; **300:** 139–44.

Eclampsia and pre-eclampsia. Drug combinations known as lytic cocktails have been used in many countries for the management of pre-eclampsia and imminent eclampsia. The cocktail has usually consisted of a combination of chlorpromazine, pethidine, and/or promethazine.[1] However, phenothiazines are not generally recommended late in pregnancy. The more usual treatment of pre-eclampsia and eclampsia is primarily aimed at reducing hypertension (see Hypertension in Pregnancy, under Hypertension, p.788); the management of eclampsia, which is the convulsive phase, is discussed on p.338.

1. WHO. The hypertensive disorders of pregnancy. *WHO Tech Rep Ser 758* 1987.

Headache. The phenothiazines chlorpromazine and prochlorperazine have been used in migraine to control severe nausea and vomiting unresponsive to antiemetics such as metoclopramide and domperidone.

Some phenothiazines have also been effective in relieving the pain of migraine attacks.[1-6] As mentioned on p.443, dihydroergotamine or sumatriptan are the preferred drugs in patients who require parenteral treatment for severe or refractory migraine, but if there is no response dopamine antagonists such as metoclopramide, chlorpromazine, or prochlorperazine may be tried. Some phenothiazines have been tried in the management of other types of headache including cluster headache and tension-type headache.[3,7]

1. Lane PL, *et al.* Comparative efficacy of chlorpromazine and meperidine with dimenhydrinate in migraine headache. *Ann Emerg Med* 1989; **18:** 360–5.
2. Bell R, *et al.* A comparative trial of three agents in the treatment of acute migraine headache. *Ann Emerg Med* 1990; **19:** 1079–82.
3. Jones J, *et al.* Randomized double-blind trial of intravenous prochlorperazine for the treatment of acute headache. *JAMA* 1989; **261:** 1174–6.
4. Stiell IG, *et al.* Methotrimeprazine versus meperidine and dimenhydrinate in the treatment of severe migraine: a randomized, controlled trial. *Ann Emerg Med* 1991; **20:** 1201–5.
5. Jones EB, *et al.* Safety and efficacy of rectal prochlorperazine for the treatment of migraine in the emergency department. *Ann Emerg Med* 1994; **24:** 237–41.
6. Coppola M, *et al.* Randomized, placebo-controlled evaluation of prochlorperazine versus metoclopramide for emergency department treatment of migraine headache. *Ann Emerg Med* 1995; **26:** 541–6.
7. Caviness VS, O'Brien P. Cluster headache: response to chlorpromazine. *Headache* 1980; **20:** 128–31.

Hiccup. A hiccup is an involuntary spasmodic contraction of the diaphragm which causes a sudden inspiration of air which is then checked abruptly by closure of the glottis. Hiccups often have a simple cause such as gastric distension and usually resolve spontaneously or respond to simple measures. Intractable hiccups may stem from a serious underlying cause such as brain disorders, metabolic or endocrine disturbances, CNS infections, and oesophageal or other gastro-intestinal disorders. Other precipitants include anaesthesia or drug therapy.

Treatment of intractable hiccups should initially be aimed at controlling or removing the underlying cause including the relief of gastric distension or oesophageal obstruction.[1,2] Measures which raise carbon dioxide pressure such as breath holding, rebreathing, or alteration of normal respiratory rhythm can be effective. Stimulation of the pharynx can also interrupt hiccups and may explain the action of a host of remedies such as sipping iced water, gargling, and swallowing granulated sugar. Many drugs have been tried in the treatment of hiccups but evidence of efficacy is largely from anecdotal reports or uncontrolled studies. However, Williamson and Macintyre[3] formulated the following treatment protocol for intractable hiccups from a review of the early literature and their own experience:

correct any metabolic abnormality, then granulated sugar should be swallowed dry; if this is successful the sugar should be repeated if hiccups recur. If not effective, pass nasogastric tube, decompress stomach, then irritate pharynx; if successful, repeat if hiccups recur. If not successful, give chlorpromazine 25 to 50 mg intravenously; repeat up to 3 times if necessary; if parenteral therapy is effective maintain on chlorpromazine by mouth for 10 days (some manufacturers recommend the use of oral therapy first and if symptoms persist for 2 to 3 days they then recommend one dose by the intramuscular route followed if necessary by a slow intravenous infusion of a dilute solution—see under Uses and Administration, above). If hiccups are not controlled by chlorpromazine give metoclopramide 10 mg intravenously and if successful maintain on metoclopramide by mouth for 10 days. If metoclopramide is not effective give quinidine 200 mg by mouth 4 times daily; if this fails consider left phrenic nerve block and crush.

In a later discussion Howard[1] noted that chlorpromazine was still the most consistently effective drug while haloperidol was also considered to be of value. Other phenothiazine compounds which are still used for intractable hiccup include perphenazine and promazine. Howard also considered that metoclopramide, clonazepam, carbamazepine, phenytoin, and valproic acid might be of value, especially in neurogenic hiccups. More recent reports had described some beneficial results with amitriptyline, nifedipine, amantadine, and baclofen.

Other methods which have been used in the treatment of hiccups include swallowing a solution of lignocaine.

1. Howard RS. Persistent hiccups: if excluding or treating any underlying pathology fails try chlorpromazine. *Br Med J* 1992; **305:** 1237–8.
2. Rousseau P. Hiccups. *South Med J* 1995; **88:** 175–81.
3. Williamson BWA, Macintyre IMC. Management of intractable hiccup. *Br Med J* 1977; **2:** 501–3.

Lesch-Nyhan syndrome. The Lesch-Nyhan syndrome is an inherited disorder caused by a complete deficiency of hypoxanthine-guanine phosphoribosyl transferase, an enzyme involved in purine metabolism. It is characterised by hyperuricaemia, spasticity, choreoathetosis, self-mutilation, and mental retardation. The hyperuricaemia can be controlled by drugs such as allopurinol (see p.390) but there appears to be no effective treatment for the neurological deficits. It has been suggested that the behavioral problems might be associated with alterations in the brain's dopamine system. There have been rare reports of improvement in self-mutilation in patients given antipsychotics.

1. Nyhan WL, Wong DF. New approaches to understanding Lesch-Nyhan disease. *N Engl J Med* 1996; **334:** 1602–4.

Mania. Patients suffering from acute mania (p.273) are usually treated with antipsychotics as they produce rapid control of symptoms. Typical drugs used include chlorpromazine, droperidol, or haloperidol.

Migraine. See under Headache, above.

Nausea and vomiting. Most antipsychotics, with the notable exception of thioridazine, have antiemetic properties and have been used in the prevention and treatment of nausea and vomiting arising from a variety of causes such as radiation sickness, malignancy, and emesis caused by drugs, including antineoplastics and opioid analgesics. For a discussion on the management of nausea and vomiting, see p.1172. Reference to the risk to the fetus of antiemetic therapy with phenothiazines during pregnancy can be found under Precautions, above.

Neonatal opioid dependence. In a discussion of neonatal opioid withdrawal (p.67), Rivers[1] observed that, although opioids, diazepam, and phenobarbitone were widely used in the USA for the management of this condition, chlorpromazine has tended to be the preferred treatment in the UK. He suggested the following dosage schedule: chlorpromazine is begun with a loading dose of 3 mg per kg body-weight, followed by a total maintenance dose of 3 mg per kg by mouth daily, divided into 4 or 6 doses. This dose is increased by 3 mg per kg daily if withdrawal is becoming increasingly severe, until control is achieved; occasionally as much as 15 mg per kg daily is required. Once the baby's condition is stable reduction in chlorpromazine dosage by 2 mg per kg every third day is attempted. Complications of phenothiazine usage have been notably absent, although rarely seizures may occur.

1. Rivers RPA. Neonatal opiate withdrawal. *Arch Dis Child* 1986; **61:** 1236–9.

Postherpetic neuralgia. Antipsychotics have been used in conjunction with antidepressants in the treatment of postherpetic neuralgia (p.10) but are best avoided; their efficacy has not been confirmed and adverse effects are especially common in the elderly.[1]

1. Robertson DRC, George CF. Treatment of post herpetic neuralgia in the elderly. *Br Med Bull* 1990; **46:** 113–23.

Taste disorders. Disturbances of the sense of taste may be broadly divided into either loss or distortion of taste. Loss of taste may be either complete (ageusia) or partial (hypogeusia). Distortion of taste (dysgeusia) may occur as aliageusia in which stimuli such as food or drink produce an inappropriate taste or as phantogeusia in which an unpleasant taste is not associated with an external stimuli and is sometimes referred to as a gustatory hallucination. Taste disturbances have many causes including infections, metabolic or nutritional disturbances, radiation, CNS disorders, neoplasms, drug therapy, or may occur as a consequence of normal aging.[1] Management primarily consists of treatment of any underlying disorder. Withdrawal of offending drug therapy is commonly associated with resolution but occasionally effects persist and may require treatment.[2] Zinc or vitamin therapy has been used but there is insufficient evidence to indicate that they are effective[1,3] for taste disturbances secondary to drug therapy or medical conditions that do not involve low zinc or vitamin concentrations. Phantogeusia might be linked to excessive activity of dopaminergic receptors as it has been reported[4] to respond to short-term treatment with small doses of drugs such as haloperidol, thioridazine, or pimozide.

1. Schiffman SS. Taste and smell losses in normal aging and disease. *JAMA* 1997; **278:** 1357–62.
2. Henkin RI. Drug-induced taste and smell disorders: incidence, mechanisms and management related primarily to treatment of sensory receptor dysfunction. *Drug Safety* 1994; **11:** 318–77.
3. Heyneman CA. Zinc deficiency and taste disorders. *Ann Pharmacother* 1996; **30:** 186–7.
4. Henkin RI. Salty and bitter taste. *JAMA* 1991; **265:** 2253.

Preparations

BP 1998: Chlorpromazine Injection; Chlorpromazine Oral Solution; Chlorpromazine Suppositories; Chlorpromazine Tablets;
USP 23: Chlorpromazine Hydrochloride Injection; Chlorpromazine Hydrochloride Oral Concentrate; Chlorpromazine Hydrochloride Syrup; Chlorpromazine Hydrochloride Tablets; Chlorpromazine Suppositories.

Proprietary Preparations (details are given in Part 3)
Aust.: Largactil; ***Austral.:*** Largactil; ***Belg.:*** Largactil; ***Canad.:*** Chlorpromanyl; Largactil; ***Fr.:*** Largactil; ***Ger.:*** Propaphenin; ***Irl.:*** Clonazine; Largactil; ***Ital.:*** Largactil; Prozin; ***Neth.:*** Largactil; ***Norw.:*** Largactil; ***S.Afr.:*** Amazin†; Largactil; ***Spain:*** Largactil; ***Swed.:*** Hibernal; ***Switz.:*** Chlorazin; Largactil; ***UK:*** Chloractil; Largactil; ***USA:*** Ormazine†; Thorazine.

Multi-ingredient: ***Spain:*** Diminex Balsamico; Juven Tos†; Largatrex.

Chlorprothixene (7024-s)

Chlorprothixene *(BAN, USAN, rINN).*

N-714; Ro-4-0403. (*Z*)-3-(2-Chlorothioxanthen-9-ylidene)-*NN*-dimethylpropylamine.

$C_{18}H_{18}ClNS$ = 315.9.

CAS — 113-59-7.

Pharmacopoeias. In US.

A yellow, crystalline powder with a slight amine-like odour. **Soluble** 1 in 1700 of water, 1 in 29 of alcohol, 1 in 18 of acetone, 1 in 2 of chloroform, and 1 in 14 of ether. **Store** in airtight containers. Protect from light.

Chlorprothixene Hydrochloride (18327-h)

Chlorprothixene Hydrochloride *(BANM, rINNM).*

Chlorprothixeni Hydrochloridum.

$C_{18}H_{19}Cl_2NS$ = 352.3.

Pharmacopoeias. In *Eur.* (see p.viii).

A white or almost white, crystalline powder. **Soluble** in water and in alcohol; slightly soluble in dichloromethane. A 1% solution in water has a pH of 4.4 to 5.2. **Protect** from light.

Chlorprothixene Mesylate (17494-s)

Chlorprothixene Mesylate *(BANM).*

Chlorprothixene Mesilate *(rINNM)*; Chlorprothixenium Mesylicum.

$C_{19}H_{22}ClNO_3S_2,H_2O$ = 430.0.

Adverse Effects, Treatment, and Precautions

As for Chlorpromazine, p.649.

Effects on the liver. A 59-year-old man receiving chlorprothixene (for the second time) for acute mania developed severe obstructive jaundice within a few days; he was also taking chlorpropamide, digoxin, and diuretics.[1] Chlorprothixene was considered the most likely cause of the jaundice, though chlorpropamide could not be excluded.

1. Ruddock DGS, Hoenig J. Chlorprothixene and obstructive jaundice. *Br Med J* 1973; **1:** 231.

Interactions

As for Chlorpromazine, p.652.

Pharmacokinetics

For an account of the pharmacokinetics of a thioxanthene, see Flupenthixol, p.671.

Distribution into breast milk. Chlorprothixene and its sulphoxide metabolite were concentrated in the breast milk of 2 mothers receiving chlorprothixene 200 mg daily but it was calculated that the amount supplied to the nursing infant was only 0.1% of the maternal dose per kg body-weight.[1]

1. Matheson I, *et al.* Presence of chlorprothixene and its metabolites in breast milk. *Eur J Clin Pharmacol* 1984; **27:** 611–13.

Metabolism. Studies on the metabolism of chlorprothixene in *animals* and man.[1] In addition to the major metabolite chlorprothixene-sulphoxide, 2 further urinary metabolites were identified, namely *N*-desmethylchlorprothixene-sulphoxide and chlorprothixene-sulphoxide-*N*-oxide.

1. Raaflaub J. Zum metabolismus des chlorprothixen. *Arzneimittelforschung* 1967; **17:** 1393–5.

Uses and Administration

Chlorprothixene is a thioxanthene antipsychotic with general properties similar to those of the phenothiazine, chlorpromazine (p.654). It is used mainly in the treatment of psychoses (p.636). Some preparations of chlorprothixene are prepared with the aid of hydrochloric and/or lactic acid and may be stated to contain chlorprothixene hydrochloride or chlorprothixene lactate. Chlorprothixene acetate, chlorprothixene mesylate, and chlorprothixene citrate have also been used. Doses are usually expressed in terms of the equivalent amount of chlorprothixene. A usual initial dose by mouth for the treatment of psychoses is 15 to 50 mg three or four times daily, increased according to response; doses of up to 600 mg or more daily have been given in severe or resistant conditions. It may also be given intramuscularly in doses of 25 to 100 mg up to four times daily. Chlorprothixene should be used in reduced dosage for elderly or debilitated patients.

Preparations

USP 23: Chlorprothixene Injection; Chlorprothixene Oral Suspension; Chlorprothixene Tablets.

Proprietary Preparations (details are given in Part 3)
Aust.: Truxal; Truxaletten; ***Belg.:*** Truxal†; Truxalettes†; ***Ger.:*** Taractan†; Truxal; Truxaletten†; ***Ital.:*** Taractan†; ***Neth.:*** Truxal; ***Norw.:*** Truxal; ***Swed.:*** Truxal; ***Switz.:*** Truxal; Truxaletten; ***USA:*** Taractan†.

Multi-ingredient: ***S.Afr.:*** Silgastrin-T†; ***USA:*** Taractan†.

Cinolazepam (9402-l)

Cinolazepam *(rINN).*

OX-373. 7-Chloro-5-(2-fluorophenyl)-2,3-dihydro-3-hydroxy-2-oxo-1*H*-1,4-benzodiazepine-1-propionitrile.

$C_{18}H_{13}ClFN_3O_2$ = 357.8.

CAS — 75696-02-5.

Cinolazepam is a benzodiazepine derivative with general properties similar to those of diazepam (p.661).

References.

1. Saletu B, *et al.* Short-term sleep laboratory studies with cinolazepam in situational insomnia induced by traffic noise. *Int J Clin Pharmacol Res* 1987; **7:** 407–18.

Preparations

Proprietary Preparations (details are given in Part 3)
Aust.: Gerodorm.

Clobazam (7025-w)

Clobazam *(BAN, USAN, rINN).*

H-4723; HR-376; LM-2717. 7-Chloro-1,5-dihydro-1-methyl-5-phenyl-1,5-benzodiazepine-2,4(3*H*)-dione.

$C_{16}H_{13}ClN_2O_2$ = 300.7.

CAS — 22316-47-8.

Pharmacopoeias. In Br.

A white crystalline powder. Very slightly **soluble** in water; soluble in alcohol and in methyl alcohol. A 1% suspension in water has a pH of 5.5 to 7.5.

Dependence and Withdrawal, Adverse Effects, Treatment, and Precautions

As for Diazepam, p.661.

Effects on menstruation. Occasionally the use of clobazam before menstruation for catamenial epilepsy appeared to delay the period.[1]

1. Feely M. Prescribing anticonvulsant drugs 3: clonazepam and clobazam. *Prescribers' J* 1989; **29:** 111–15.

Effects on the skin. Report[1] of toxic epidermal necrolysis which developed in light-exposed areas in a patient being treated with clobazam.

1. Redondo P, *et al.* Photo-induced toxic epidermal necrolysis caused by clobazam. *Br J Dermatol* 1996; **135:** 999–1002.

Porphyria. Clobazam was considered to be unsafe in patients with acute porphyria although there is conflicting experimental evidence of porphyrinogenicity.[1]

1. Moore MR, McColl KEL. *Porphyria: drug lists* Glasgow: Porphyria Research Unit, University of Glasgow, 1991.

Interactions

As for Diazepam, p.663.

Pharmacokinetics

Clobazam is well absorbed from the gastro-intestinal tract and peak plasma concentrations have been reached 1 to 4 hours after oral administration. It is about 85% bound to plasma proteins. Clobazam is highly lipophilic and rapidly crosses the blood-brain barrier. It is metabolised in the liver by demethylation and hydroxylation but unlike the 1,4-benzodiazepines such as diazepam, clobazam, a 1,5-benzodiazepine, is hydroxylated at the 4-position rather than the 3-position (see also under Diazepam, p.666). Clobazam is excreted unchanged and as metabolites mainly in the urine. Mean half-lives of 18 hours and 42 hours have been reported for clobazam and its main active metabolite *N*-desmethylclobazam, respectively.

References.

1. Greenblatt DJ, *et al.* Clinical pharmacokinetics of the newer benzodiazepines. *Clin Pharmacokinet* 1983; **8:** 233–52.
2. Ochs HR, *et al.* Single and multiple dose kinetics of clobazam, and clinical effects during multiple dosage. *Eur J Clin Pharmacol* 1984; **26:** 499–503.

Uses and Administration

Clobazam is a long-acting 1,5-benzodiazepine with uses similar to those of diazepam (a 1,4-benzodiazepine; see p.666). The usual dose for the short-term treatment of anxiety (p.635) is 20 to 30 mg daily given in divided doses or as a single dose at night; in severe conditions up to 60 mg daily has been given. Similar daily doses have been given as adjunctive therapy in the management of epilepsy.

Doses of 10 to 20 mg daily have been suggested in elderly or debilitated patients; in children aged 3 years or over not more than half the recommended adult dose may be given.

Epilepsy. Benzodiazepines are sometimes employed in the management of epilepsy (p.335), but their long-term use is limited by problems of sedation, dependence, and tolerance to the antiepileptic effects.

Clobazam, along with clonazepam, is one of the benzodiazepines most commonly used as an oral antiepileptic. Sedation appears to be less of a problem with clobazam than with clonazepam, and this advantage may make it more appropriate as adjunctive therapy for adults.[1] Clobazam is active against partial and generalised seizures in epilepsy of widely differing aetiology in patients of all ages but is usually only indicated for adjunctive therapy. Intermittent therapy with clobazam has been used successfully in women with catamenial epilepsy (seizures associated with menstruation). Short-term therapy may also be useful for patients whose epileptic attacks occur in clusters or as cover for special events. Clobazam has also been tried with some success in children with refractory epilepsy.[2,3]

1. Feely M. Prescribing anticonvulsant drugs 3: clonazepam and clobazam. *Prescribers' J* 1989; **29:** 111–15.
2. Munn R, Farrell K. Open study of clobazam in refractory epilepsy. *Pediatr Neurol* 1993; **9:** 465–9.
3. Sheth RD, *et al.* Clobazam for intractable pediatric epilepsy. *J Child Neurol* 1995; **10:** 205–8.

Phantom limb pain. There has been a mention[1] of the complete relief of phantom limb pain (p.10) refractory to other therapy in an elderly patient given clobazam 10 mg three times daily.

1. Rice-Oxley CP. The limited list: clobazam for phantom limb pain. *Br Med J* 1986; **293:** 1309.

Preparations

BP 1998: Clobazam Capsules.

Proprietary Preparations (details are given in Part 3)
Aust.: Frisium; ***Austral.:*** Frisium; ***Belg.:*** Frisium; ***Canad.:*** Frisium; ***Fr.:*** Urbanyl; ***Ger.:*** Frisium; ***Irl.:*** Frisium; ***Ital.:*** Frisium; ***Neth.:*** Frisium; Urbadan†; ***S.Afr.:*** Urbanol; ***Spain:*** Clarmyl; Clopax†; Noiafren; ***Switz.:*** Urbanyl; ***UK:*** Frisium.

Clocapramine Hydrochloride (12582-z)

Clocapramine Hydrochloride *(rINNM)*.

Chlorcarpipramine Hydrochloride; Y-4153. 1′-[3-(3-Chloro-10,11-dihydro-5*H*-dibenz[*b,f*]azepin-5-yl)propyl][1,4′-bipiperidine]-4′-carboxamide dihydrochloride monohydrate.

$C_{28}H_{37}ClN_4O,2HCl,H_2O$ = 572.0.

CAS — 47739-98-0 (clocapramine); 28058-62-0 (clocapramine hydrochloride).

Pharmacopoeias. In *Jpn.*

Clocapramine is a chlorinated derivative of carpipramine (p.645). The hydrochloride has been given by mouth in the treatment of schizophrenia.

References.

1. Yamagami S. A crossover study of clocapramine and haloperidol in chronic schizophrenia. *J Int Med Res* 1985; **13:** 301–10.
2. Yamagami S, *et al.* A single-blind study of clocapramine and sulpiride in hospitalized chronic schizophrenic patients. *Drugs Exp Clin Res* 1988; **14:** 707–13.

Clorazepic Acid (17899-q)

Clorazepic Acid *(BAN)*.

7-Chloro-2,3-dihydro-2,2-dihydroxy-5-phenyl-1*H*-1,4-benzodiazepine-3-carboxylic acid.

$C_{16}H_{13}ClN_2O_4$ = 332.7.

CAS — 20432-69-3.

Clorazepate Monopotassium (7029-j)

Clorazepate Monopotassium *(USAN)*.

Abbott-39083; 4311-CB. Potassium 7-chloro-2,3-dihydro-2-oxo-5-phenyl-1*H*-1,4-benzodiazepine-3-carboxylate.

$C_{16}H_{10}ClKN_2O_3$ = 352.8.

CAS — 5991-71-9.

Potassium Clorazepate (7030-q)

Potassium Clorazepate *(BANM)*.

Dipotassium Clorazepate *(rINN)*; Abbott-35616; AH-3232; 4306-CB; Clorazepate Dipotassium *(USAN)*; Dikalii Clorazepas. Compound of Potassium 7-chloro-2,3-dihydro-2-oxo-5-phenyl-1*H*-1,4-benzodiazepine-3-carboxylate with potassium hydroxide.

$C_{16}H_{11}ClK_2N_2O_4$ = 408.9.

CAS — 57109-90-7.

Pharmacopoeias. In *Eur.* (see p.viii) and *US.*

A white or light yellow, crystalline powder which darkens on exposure to light. Solutions in water or in alcohol are unstable and should be used immediately. Ph. Eur. **solubilities** are: freely soluble or very soluble in water; very slightly soluble in alcohol; practically insoluble in dichloromethane. USP solubilities are: soluble in water, but may precipitate from solution on standing; slightly soluble in alcohol and in isopropyl alcohol; practically insoluble in acetone, in chloroform, in dichloromethane, and in ether. **Store** under nitrogen in airtight containers. Protect from light.

Dependence and Withdrawal, Adverse Effects, Treatment, and Precautions

As for Diazepam, p.661.

Effects on the liver. A report of jaundice and hepatic necrosis associated with clorazepate administration.[1]

1. Parker JLW. Potassium clorazepate (Tranxene)-induced jaundice. *Postgrad Med J* 1979; **55:** 908–910.

Effects on the nervous system. For reference to extrapyramidal disorders associated with administration of clorazepate, see Diazepam, p.662.

Porphyria. Clorazepate was considered to be unsafe in patients with acute porphyria because it has been shown to be porphyrinogenic in *animals* or *in-vitro* systems.[1]

1. Moore MR, McColl KEL. *Porphyria: drug lists.* Glasgow: Porphyria Research Unit, University of Glasgow, 1991.

Interactions

As for Diazepam, p.663.

Pharmacokinetics

Clorazepate is decarboxylated rapidly at the low pH in the stomach to form desmethyldiazepam (nordazepam, see p.682), which is quickly absorbed.

References to the pharmacokinetics of potassium clorazepate.

1. Ochs HR, *et al.* Comparative single-dose kinetics of oxazolam, prazepam, and clorazepate: three precursors of desmethyldiazepam. *J Clin Pharmacol* 1984; **24:** 446–51.
2. Bertler Å, *et al.* Intramuscular bioavailability of chlorazepate as compared to diazepam. *Eur J Clin Pharmacol* 1985; **28:** 229–30.

Uses and Administration

Clorazepate is a long-acting benzodiazepine with general properties similar to those of diazepam (p.666). It is mainly used in the short-term treatment of anxiety disorders (p.635), as an adjunct in the management of epilepsy, and in alcohol withdrawal syndrome (p.1099).

Potassium clorazepate is usually given by mouth but preparations for intravenous or intramuscular administration are also available in some countries. In the UK, a usual dose of 15 mg of potassium clorazepate (the dipotassium salt) by mouth has been given as a single dose at night for the treatment of anxiety; alternatively a dose of 7.5 mg may be given up to three times daily. In the USA rather higher doses have been recommended; 15 to 60 mg of potassium clorazepate may be given daily, in divided doses or as a single dose at night. Up to 90 mg has been given daily in divided doses in the management of epilepsy or alcohol withdrawal syndrome.

Reduced doses should be given in elderly or debilitated patients.

Preparations

Proprietary Preparations (details are given in Part 3)
Aust.: Tranxilium; ***Austral.:*** Tranxene; ***Belg.:*** Tranxene; Uni-Tranxene; ***Canad.:*** Novo-Clopate; Tranxene; ***Fr.:*** Tranxene; ***Ger.:*** Tranxilium; ***Irl.:*** Tranxene; ***Ital.:*** Transene; ***Neth.:*** Tranxene; ***S.Afr.:*** Tranxene; ***Spain:*** Nansius; Tranxilium; ***Swed.:*** Tranxilen†; ***Switz.:*** Tranxilium; ***UK:*** Tranxene; ***USA:*** Clorazecaps†; Clorazetabs†; Gen-Xene; Tranxene.

Multi-ingredient: ***Fr.:*** Noctran; ***Spain:*** Dorken.

Clothiapine (7031-p)

Clothiapine *(BAN, USAN)*.

Clotiapine *(rINN)*; HF-2159. 2-Chloro-11-(4-methylpiperazin-1-yl)dibenzo[*b,f*][1,4]thiazepine.

$C_{18}H_{18}ClN_3S$ = 343.9.

CAS — 2058-52-8.

Clothiapine is a dibenzothiazepine antipsychotic with general properties similar to those of the phenothiazines (see Chlorpromazine, p.649). It is used in a variety of psychiatric disorders including schizophrenia (p.637), mania (p.273), and anxiety (p.635). It is given by mouth in doses of 10 to 200 mg daily in divided doses; doses of up to 360 mg daily have been given in severe or resistant psychoses. It may also be given by slow intravenous or deep intramuscular injection.

Preparations

Proprietary Preparations (details are given in Part 3)
Belg.: Etumine; ***Ital.:*** Entumin; ***S.Afr.:*** Etomine; ***Spain:*** Etumina; ***Switz.:*** Entumine.

Clotiazepam (12592-k)

Clotiazepam *(rINN)*.

Y-6047. 5-(2-Chlorophenyl)-7-ethyl-1,3-dihydro-1-methyl-2*H*-thieno[2,3-e]-1,4-diazepin-2-one.

$C_{16}H_{15}ClN_2OS$ = 318.8.

CAS — 33671-46-4.

Pharmacopoeias. In *Jpn.*

Dependence and Withdrawal, Adverse Effects, Treatment, and Precautions

As for Diazepam, p.661.

Effects on the liver. Development of hepatitis in a 65-year-old woman was attributed to clotiazepam administration commenced 7 months earlier.[1] The patient took triazolam and lorazepam without any apparent effect on the liver, and it was speculated that the hepatotoxic effect of clotiazepam was related to the thiophene ring present in the chemical structure.

1. Habersetzer F, *et al.* Clotiazepam-induced acute hepatitis. *J Hepatol* 1989; **9:** 256–9.

Porphyria. Clotiazepam was considered to be unsafe in patients with acute porphyria because it has been shown to be porphyrinogenic in *animals* or *in-vitro* systems.[1]

1. Moore MR, McColl KEL. *Porphyria: drug lists.* Glasgow: Porphyria Research Unit, University of Glasgow, 1991.

Interactions

As for Diazepam, p.663.

Pharmacokinetics

After oral administration of a single dose, peak plasma concentrations have been obtained after 0.5 to 1.5 hours.[1,2] The elimination half-life has varied between about 4 and 18 hours[1-3] and protein binding appears to be more than 99%.[1] Hydroxyclotiazepam and desmethylclotiazepam are reported to be the major active metabolites of clotiazepam.[1] The lack of difference in systemic availability between the sublingual and oral routes suggests that there is little hepatic first-pass metabolism of clotiazepam.[2] Although the volume of distribution and clearance were decreased in 10 patients with cirrhosis when compared with controls, the elimination half-life was not significantly different between the groups.[4] Chronic renal insufficiency had no effect on the pharmacokinetics of clotiazepam.[4]

1. Arendt R, *et al.* Electron capture GLC analysis of the thienodiazepine clotiazepam. *Arzneimittelforschung* 1982; **32:** 453–5.
2. Benvenuti C, *et al.* The pharmacokinetics of clotiazepam after oral and sublingual administration to volunteers. *Eur J Clin Pharmacol* 1989; **37:** 617–19.
3. Ochs HR, *et al.* Disposition of clotiazepam: influence of age, sex, oral contraceptives, cimetidine, isoniazid and ethanol. *Eur J Clin Pharmacol* 1984; **26:** 55–9.
4. Ochs HR, *et al.* Effect of cirrhosis and renal failure on the kinetics of clotiazepam. *Eur J Clin Pharmacol* 1986; **30:** 89–92.

Uses and Administration

Clotiazepam is a short-acting thienodiazepine with general properties similar to those of diazepam (p.666). A usual daily dose for anxiety disorders (p.635) is 5 to 15 mg by mouth given in divided doses but up to 60 mg daily has been used. For insomnia (p.638) up to 20 mg has been given as a single dose at night.

References.

1. Jibiki I, *et al.* Beneficial effect of high-dose clotiazepam on intractable auditory hallucinations in chronic schizophrenic patients. *Eur J Clin Pharmacol* 1994; **46:** 367–9.

Preparations

Proprietary Preparations (details are given in Part 3)
Belg.: Clozan; ***Fr.:*** Veratran; ***Ger.:*** Trecalmo; ***Ital.:*** Rizen; Tienor; ***Jpn:*** Rize; ***Spain:*** Distensan.

Cloxazolam (7032-s)

Cloxazolam *(rINN)*.

CS-370. 10-Chloro-11b-(2-chlorophenyl)-2,3,7,11b-tetrahydro-oxazolo[3,2-*d*][1,4]benzodiazepin-6(5*H*)-one.

$C_{17}H_{14}Cl_2N_2O_2$ = 349.2.

CAS — 24166-13-0.

Pharmacopoeias. In *Jpn.*

Cloxazolam is a long-acting benzodiazepine with general properties similar to those of diazepam (p.661). It is given by mouth in doses of up to 12 mg daily in divided doses for the short-term treatment of anxiety disorders (p.635). A dose of 100 μg per kg body-weight may be used for premedication (p.1220).

Preparations

Proprietary Preparations (details are given in Part 3)
Aust.: Olcadil; ***Belg.:*** Akton; ***Jpn:*** Sepazon; ***Switz.:*** Lubalix.

Clozapine (12595-x)

Clozapine *(BAN, USAN, rINN)*.

Clozapinum; HF-1854. 8-Chloro-11-(4-methylpiperazin-1-yl)-5*H*-dibenzo[*b,e*][1,4]diazepine.

$C_{18}H_{19}ClN_4$ = 326.8.

CAS — 5786-21-0.

Pharmacopoeias. In *Eur.* (see p.viii).

A yellow crystalline powder. Practically **insoluble** in water; soluble in alcohol; freely soluble in dichloromethane. It dissolves in dilute acetic acid.

A suspension of clozapine 100 mg in 5 mL, made by crushing clozapine tablets and suspending the powder in a syrup-based mixture containing carboxymethylcellulose preserved with methyl hydroxybenzoate and propyl hydroxybenzoate (Guy's

Hospital paediatric base formula), was considered to be stable for at least 18 days after preparation.[1]

1. Ramuth S, *et al.* A liquid clozapine preparation for oral administration in hospital. *Pharm J* 1996; **257:** 190–1.

Adverse Effects and Treatment

As for Chlorpromazine, p.649 but antimuscarinic effects may be more pronounced.

Clozapine can cause reversible neutropenia which may progress to a potentially fatal agranulocytosis; strict monitoring of white blood-cell counts is essential (see Precautions, below). Eosinophilia may also occur.

Extrapyramidal disorders, including tardive dyskinesia appear to be rare with clozapine. Clozapine has little effect on prolactin secretion. Clozapine appears to carry a greater epileptic potential than chlorpromazine but a comparable risk of cardiovascular effects such as tachycardia and orthostatic hypotension. In rare cases circulatory collapse with cardiac and respiratory arrest has occurred. Hypertension and isolated cases of myocarditis or pericarditis have also been reported.

Additional side-effects of clozapine include dizziness, hypersalivation (particularly at night), headache, nausea, vomiting, anxiety, confusion, fatigue, and transient fever which must be distinguished from the signs of impending agranulocytosis. There have also been rare reports of dysphagia, thromboembolism, acute pancreatitis, hepatitis and cholestatic jaundice, and very rarely fulminant hepatic necrosis. Isolated cases of acute interstitial nephritis have been reported. Many of the adverse effects of clozapine are most common at the beginning of therapy and may be minimised by gradual increase in dosage.

Convulsions. As with other antipsychotics (see Chlorpromazine, p.649), clozapine can lower the seizure threshold and cause EEG abnormalities, although treatment with clozapine appears to be associated with a higher frequency of seizures. A review[1] of 1418 patients treated with clozapine in the USA between 1972 and 1988 found that 41 had experienced generalized tonic-clonic seizures. It was considered that the risk of clozapine-induced seizures was dose-related. The seizure frequency was calculated to be 1% at a dosage less than 300 mg daily, 2.7% at 300 to 599 mg daily, and 4.4% with a dosage of 600 mg or more daily. Six of the patients had been taking other drugs reported to lower the seizure threshold. Therapy with clozapine was continued in 31 of the 41 patients by reducing the total daily dose of clozapine; antiepileptic drug therapy was initiated in about half of the patients. The UK Committee on Safety of Medicines[2] considered that although the epileptogenic effect of clozapine was claimed to be dose-related, the metabolism and plasma concentrations of clozapine were highly variable and data from 8 cases reported to the Committee suggest that convulsions may possibly be related to high plasma concentrations in susceptible individuals. A low initial dosage followed by careful increases according to response and downward titration thereafter to a maintenance dose was recommended to avoid convulsions in susceptible individuals.

1. Devinsky O, *et al.* Clozapine-related seizures. *Neurology* 1991; **41:** 369–71.
2. Committee on Safety of Medicines. Convulsions may occur in patients receiving clozapine (Clozaril®, Sandoz). *Current Problems 31* 1991.

Effects on the blood. Clozapine can cause reversible neutropenia which, if the drug is not withdrawn immediately, may progress to a potentially fatal agranulocytosis. Particular concern over this side-effect dates from 1975 when 17 cases of neutropenia or agranulocytosis, 8 of them fatal, were reported in Finland;[1] the calculated incidence[2] of agranulocytosis or severe granulocytopenia during this Finnish epidemic was 7.1 per 1000. These reports led to the withdrawal of clozapine in some countries or to restrictions in its use and intense haematological monitoring in others. Following studies demonstrating the efficacy of clozapine in severely ill schizophrenic patients unresponsive to adequate therapy with standard antipsychotics, the drug became available in the UK and USA in 1990 with strict procedures for monitoring of white blood-cell counts. The UK Committee on Safety of Medicines provided data on the reports it had received between July 1963 and January 1993 on agranulocytosis and neutropenia.[3] Clozapine was one of the individual drugs most frequently implicated with 14 reports of agranulocytosis (one fatal) and 119 of neutropenia (none fatal). Various estimates of the incidence of clozapine-associated agranulocytosis have been made; analysis of data from 11 555 patients who had received clozapine in the USA[4] showed a cumulative incidence of agranulocytosis of 8.0 per 1000 at 1 year and 9.1 per 1000 at 1½ years with the risk being increased in elderly patients. The majority of cases of agranulocytosis occurred within 3 months of the start of treatment with the risk peaking in the third month. The manufacturers report a lower incidence of agranulocytosis of 4.8 per 1000 patients for the first 6 months[5] and an annual rate of 0.8 per 1000 patients during the next 2.5 years. These figures were based on data on 56 000 patients in the USA who had received clozapine up to the end of March 1993. Analysis of data[6] on 6316 patients registered in the UK and Ireland between January 1990 and July 1994 to receive (although not necessarily given) clozapine produced a cumulative incidence of agranulocytosis of 0.7% during the first year and 0.8% over the whole study period. Most cases of agranulocytosis and neutropenia occurred during the first 6 to 18 weeks of treatment. The incidence of agranulocytosis (0.07%) and neutropenia (0.7%) seen during the second year of therapy was of the same order of magnitude noted for some phenothiazine antipsychotics.

These data[6] and comparable data from the USA[7] were considered to indicate that mandatory haematological monitoring helped to reduce the risks of clozapine-induced neutropenia and agranulocytosis and associated deaths.

Predisposing factors for development of agranulocytosis have not been identified, apart from a possible excess of cases in female patients and an increased risk with increasing age. Furthermore, both agranulocytosis and neutropenia do not appear to be dose-related effects with clozapine. A postulated higher incidence of agranulocytosis in patients of Jewish background may be related to genetic factors.[8] Although evidence generally points to an immune mechanism for clozapine-induced agranulocytosis the possibility of a direct toxicity cannot be discounted.[9,10] Africans and Afro-Caribbeans appear to be at increased risk of developing neutropenia[6] and it has been noted[11] that many patients from these ethnic groups are currently already excluded from treatment with clozapine because their normal white-cell and neutrophil counts are below the recommended range for treatment (see below).

Evidence would suggest that development of clozapine-induced leucopenia or granulocytopenia precludes treatment with clozapine at any future date; of 9 patients re-treated all again developed leucopenia or agranulocytosis.[12] In the USA patients who have had clozapine withdrawn because of moderate leucopenia (judged to be when counts fall to 2000 to 3000 per mm³) are considered eligible for a return to clozapine treatment when this count returns to normal; such patients are considered to have a 5- or 6-fold greater risk of agranulocytosis.[5]

1. Idänpään-Heikkilä J, *et al.* Agranulocytosis during treatment with clozapine. *Eur J Clin Pharmacol* 1977; **11:** 193–8.
2. Anderman B, Griffith RW. Clozapine-induced agranulocytosis: a situation report up to August 1976. *Eur J Clin Pharmacol* 1977; **11:** 199–201.
3. Committee on Safety of Medicines/Medicines Control Agency. Drug-induced neutropenia and agranulocytosis. *Current Problems* 1993; **19:** 10–11.
4. Alvir JMJ, *et al.* Clozapine-induced agranulocytosis: incidence and risk factors in the United States. *N Engl J Med* 1993; **329:** 162–7.
5. Finkel MJ, Arellano F. White-blood-cell monitoring and clozapine. *Lancet* 1995; **346:** 849.
6. Atkin K, *et al.* Neutropenia and agranulocytosis in patients receiving clozapine in the UK and Ireland. *Br J Psychiatry* 1996; **169:** 483–8.
7. Honigfeld G. Effects of the clozapine national registry system on incidence of deaths related to agranulocytosis. *Psychiatr Serv* 1996; **47:** 52–6.
8. Leiberman JA, *et al.* HLA-B38, DR4, DQw3 and clozapine-induced agranulocytosis in Jewish patients with schizophrenia. *Arch Gen Psychiatry* 1990; **47:** 945–8.
9. Gerson SL, *et al.* Polypharmacy in fatal clozapine-associated agranulocytosis. *Lancet* 1991; **338:** 262–3.
10. Hoffbrand AV, *et al.* Mechanisms of clozapine-induced agranulocytosis. *Drug Safety* 1992; **7** (suppl 1): 1–60.
11. Fisher N, Baigent B. Treatment with clozapine: black patients' low white cell counts currently mean that they cannot be treated. *Br Med J* 1996; **313:** 1262.
12. Safferman AZ, *et al.* Rechallenge in clozapine-induced agranulocytosis. *Lancet* 1992; **339:** 1296–7.

Effects on the cardiovascular system. The UK Committee on Safety of Medicines (CSM)[1] issued a warning in November 1993 of the risk of myocarditis with clozapine. Three patients who died while taking clozapine had evidence of myocarditis. The CSM had also received one other report of myocarditis and one of cardiomyopathy associated with clozapine. The Australian Adverse Drug Reactions Advisory Committee subsequently reported another 5 cases of clozapine-associated myocarditis in November 1994.[2] As myocarditis can be difficult to diagnose and confirmation is not always possible, the CSM recommended that if there was a high clinical suspicion of myocarditis, antipsychotic medication should be stopped. Presenting features might include heart failure, arrhythmia, or symptoms mimicking myocardial infarction or pericarditis. Some studies[3] have suggested that serious cardiovascular effects might occur more frequently and might be more severe in healthy subjects than in patients with schizophrenia. The manufacturers had requested that for the purpose of pharmacokinetic studies, clozapine should not be given to healthy subjects. There have been isolated reports[4,5] of paradoxical hypertension in patients receiving clozapine. Concomitant administration of atenolol has controlled the hypertension and allowed therapy with clozapine to be continued.

A small preliminary study[6] has suggested that serum triglyceride concentrations may be higher in patients taking clozapine than in those treated with conventional antipsychotics.

For further details of effects of clozapine on the cardiovascular system, see Benzodiazepines under Interactions, below.

1. Committee on Safety of Medicines/Medicines Control Agency. Myocarditis with antipsychotics: recent cases with clozapine (Clozaril). *Current Problems* 1993; **19:** 9–10.
2. Adverse Drug Reactions Advisory Committee. Clozapine and myocarditis. *Aust Adverse Drug React Bull* 1994; **13** (Nov): 14–15.
3. Pokorny R, *et al.* Normal volunteers should not be used for bioavailability or bioequivalence studies of clozapine. *Pharm Res* 1994; **11:** 1221.
4. Gupta S. Paradoxical hypertension associated with clozapine. *Am J Psychiatry* 1994; **151:** 148.
5. Ennis LM, Parker RM. Paradoxical hypertension associated with clozapine. *Med J Aust* 1997; **166:** 278.
6. Ghaeli P, Dufresne RL. Serum triglyceride levels in patients treated with clozapine. *Am J Health-Syst Pharm* 1996; **53:** 2079–81.

Effects on fluid and electrolyte homoeostasis. Hyponatraemia has been reported to be associated with clozapine in one patient.[1] It was emphasised that hyponatraemia should be excluded as a possible trigger when considering the epileptogenic potential of clozapine. For a discussion of reports of hyponatraemia associated with antipsychotics, see p.650.

1. Ogilvie AD, Croy MF. Clozapine and hyponatraemia. *Lancet* 1992; **340:** 672.

Effects on the pancreas. There have been isolated reports of pancreatitis associated with clozapine.[1,2] Pancreatitis has also been reported[3] following overdosage with clozapine.

1. Martin A. Acute pancreatitis associated with clozapine use. *Am J Psychiatry* 1992; **149:** 714.
2. Frankenburg FR, Kando J. Eosinophilia, clozapine, and pancreatitis. *Lancet* 1992; **340:** 251.
3. Jubert P, *et al.* Clozapine-related pancreatitis. *Ann Intern Med* 1994; **121:** 722–3.

Neuroleptic malignant syndrome. A review of the literature[1] suggested that clozapine may produce fewer extrapyramidal effects and a lower rise in creatine kinase concentrations than conventional antipsychotics. The incidence of neuroleptic malignant syndrome with clozapine appeared to be similar to that with conventional antipsychotics but further study was required to confirm this.

1. Sachdev P, *et al.* Clozapine-induced neuroleptic malignant syndrome: a review and report of new cases. *J Clin Psychopharmacol* 1995; **15:** 365–71.

Withdrawal. A report[1] of 3 patients who experienced delirium with psychotic symptoms shortly after discontinuation of clozapine. One of the patients had developed symptoms within 24 hours despite gradual withdrawal of clozapine over a 2-week period. All the patients responded rapidly to resumption of low doses of clozapine.

1. Stanilla JK, *et al.* Clozapine withdrawal resulting in delirium with psychosis: a report of three cases. *J Clin Psychiatry* 1997; **58:** 252–5.

Precautions

As for Chlorpromazine, p.652.

Clozapine should not be given to patients with uncontrolled epilepsy, alcoholic or toxic psychoses, drug intoxication, or a history of circulatory collapse. It is contra-indicated in patients with bone-marrow suppression, myeloproliferative disorders, or any abnormalities of white blood-cell count or differential blood count. It is also contra-indicated in patients with a history of drug-induced neutropenia or agranulocytosis. It should not be used concurrently with drugs which carry a high risk of bone-marrow suppression (see Interactions, below).

A white blood-cell count and a differential blood count must be performed before starting clozapine therapy and regularly throughout treatment. Treatment should not be started if the white blood-cell count is less than 3500 per mm³ or if there is an abnormal differential count. In the UK, monitoring is performed at weekly intervals for the first 18 weeks and then at least every 2 weeks for the first year of treatment; if the neutrophil count has remained stable during that period then monitoring can be changed to every 4 weeks. In the USA blood counts are monitored weekly for the first 6 months and then every 2 weeks thereafter. Monitoring should continue for 4 weeks after discontinuation. Clozapine should be withdrawn immediately if the white blood-cell count falls below 3000 per mm^3 and/or the absolute neutrophil count drops below 1500 per mm^3. Repeat blood counts and more intense monitoring are required for counts just above these values. The patient should report the development of any infection or signs such as fever, sore throat, or flu-like symptoms which suggest infection.

Because of an increased risk of collapse due to hypotension associated with initial titration of dosage of clozapine it is recommended that treatment should be initiated under close medical supervision. On planned withdrawal the dose of clozapine should be reduced gradually over a 1- to 2-week period in order to avoid the risk of rebound psychosis. If abrupt withdrawal is necessary (see above) then patients should be observed carefully.

Interactions

As for Chlorpromazine, p.652.

Clozapine may enhance the central effects of MAOIs.

Clozapine should not be used concurrently with drugs which carry a high risk of bone-marrow suppression including carbamazepine, co-trimoxazole, chloramphenicol, penicillamine, sulphonamides, antineoplastics, or pyrazolone analgesics such as azapropazone. Long-acting depot antipsychotics should not be used with clozapine as they cannot be withdrawn rapidly should neutropenia occur.

Concomitant administration of phenytoin or other enzyme-inducing drugs may accelerate the metabolism of clozapine and reduce its plasma concentrations. The metabolism of clozapine is mediated mainly by the cytochrome P450 isozyme CYP1A2. Concomitant administration of drugs which inhibit or act as a substrate to this isozyme may affect plasma concentrations of clozapine.

References.

1. Taylor D. Pharmacokinetic interactions involving clozapine. *Br J Psychiatry* 1997; **171:** 109–12.

Antibacterials. A patient with schizophrenia controlled with clozapine therapy had a tonic-clonic seizure 7 days after starting treatment with *erythromycin*.[1] It appeared that erythromycin had inhibited the metabolism of clozapine and raised its serum concentrations.

1. Funderburg LG, *et al.* Seizure following addition of erythromycin to clozapine treatment. *Am J Psychiatry* 1994; **151:** 1840–1.

Antidepressants. Rises in serum concentrations of clozapine have been found in patients receiving clozapine after addition of *fluoxetine*[1] or *fluvoxamine*[2] to therapy. There has been an isolated report[3] of a patient who developed myoclonic jerks 79 days after fluoxetine was added to treatment with clozapine and lorazepam although some[4] doubt whether the effects were entirely due to an interaction. For reference to neurological reactions in patients receiving *lithium* concomitantly with clozapine, see p.294.

1. Centorrino F, *et al.* Serum concentrations of clozapine and its major metabolites: effects of cotreatment with fluoxetine or valproate. *Am J Psychiatry* 1994; **151:** 123–5.
2. Jerling M, *et al.* Fluvoxamine inhibition and carbamazepine induction of the metabolism of clozapine: evidence from a therapeutic drug monitoring service. *Ther Drug Monit* 1994; **16:** 368–74.
3. Kingsbury SJ, Puckett KM. Effects of fluoxetine on serum clozapine levels. *Am J Psychiatry* 1995; **152:** 473.
4. Baldessarini RJ, *et al.* Effects of fluoxetine on serum clozapine levels. *Am J Psychiatry* 1995; **152:** 473–4.

Antiepileptics. Concomitant administration of *phenytoin* or other *enzyme-inducing antiepileptics* may accelerate the metabolism of clozapine and reduce its plasma concentrations. Studies have found that addition of *sodium valproate* to clozapine therapy may increase[1] or decrease[2] plasma concentrations of clozapine. Although no increase in clozapine-related adverse effects or loss of control of psychotic symptoms were reported in these studies there has been a report[3] of a patient who experienced sedation, confusion, slurring of speech and other functional impairment after valproate was given with clozapine.

See also under Benzodiazepines, below.

1. Centorrino F, *et al.* Serum concentrations of clozapine and its major metabolites: effects of cotreatment with fluoxetine or valproate. *Am J Psychiatry* 1994; **151:** 123–5.
2. Finley P, Warner D. Potential impact of valproic acid therapy on clozapine disposition. *Biol Psychiatry* 1994; **36:** 487–8.
3. Costello LE, Suppes T. A clinically significant interaction between clozapine and valproate. *J Clin Psychopharmacol* 1995; **15:** 139–41.

Antipsychotics. Clinical improvement produced by concomitant treatment with *risperidone* in a patient with schizoaffective disorder partially controlled by clozapine was associated with a 74% rise in serum-clozapine concentrations over a 2-week period.[1] Although no adverse effects had occurred in this patient the potential for serious adverse effects with elevated clozapine concentrations required caution if these drugs were used together.

1. Tyson SC, *et al.* Pharmacokinetic interaction between risperidone and clozapine. *Am J Psychiatry* 1995; **152:** 1401–2.

Antivirals. HIV-protease inhibitors such as *ritonavir* can increase plasma concentrations of clozapine with a resultant increase in the risk of toxicity; concomitant use is not recommended.

Benzodiazepines. Concern has been expressed over reports of cardiorespiratory collapse in patients taking both clozapine and benzodiazepines.[1,2] In response, the manufacturers of clozapine have outlined similar cases reported to them in the USA since February 1990.[3] Of 7 cases of respiratory arrest or depression only 2 (including that described by Friedman *et al.*) involved recent use of a benzodiazepine; among 26 cases of orthostatic hypotension with syncope reported during the first year the drug was marketed, only 8 included recent benzodiazepine use. The manufacturers concluded that an increased risk of such reactions in patients taking both drugs simultaneously is possible but not established, and advised caution when initiating clozapine therapy in patients taking benzodiazepines.

Hypersalivation associated with clozapine and benzodiazepines may be exacerbated when these drugs are used together. One patient[4] experienced increased hypersalivation, salivary thickening, and distension of the parotid glands when clonazepam was added to treatment with clozapine. Adverse effects reported in 5 other patients given clozapine and benzodiazepines together included hypersalivation, sedation, ataxia, and symptoms of delirium.[5,6]

1. Sassim N, Grohmann R. Adverse drug reactions with clozapine and simultaneous application of benzodiazepines. *Pharmacopsychiatry* 1988; **21:** 306–7.
2. Friedman LJ, *et al.* Clozapine—a novel antipsychotic agent. *N Engl J Med* 1991; **325:** 518.
3. Finkel MJ, Schwimmer JL. Clozapine—a novel antipsychotic agent. *N Engl J Med* 1991; **325:** 518–19.
4. Martin SD. Drug-induced parotid swelling. *Br J Hosp Med* 1993; **50:** 426.
5. Cobb CD, *et al.* Possible interaction between clozapine and lorazepam. *Am J Psychiatry* 1991; **148:** 1606–7.
6. Jackson CW, *et al.* Delirium associated with clozapine and benzodiazepine combinations. *Ann Clin Psychiatry* 1995; **7:** 139–41.

Histamine H_2-receptor antagonists. A patient stabilised on clozapine developed increased serum clozapine concentrations and signs of clozapine toxicity after starting treatment with *cimetidine*.[1] Cimetidine was withdrawn and ranitidine substituted without recurrence of toxicity.

1. Szymanski S, *et al.* A case report of cimetidine-induced clozapine toxicity. *J Clin Psychiatry* 1991; **52:** 21–2.

Pharmacokinetics

Although clozapine is well absorbed from the gastro-intestinal tract, its bioavailability is limited to about 50% by first-pass metabolism. Peak plasma concentrations are achieved an average of about 2.5 hours after administration by mouth. Clozapine is about 95% bound to plasma proteins and has a mean terminal elimination half-life of approximately 12 hours at steady state. It is almost completely metabolised; routes of metabolism include *N*-demethylation, hydroxylation, and *N*-oxidation. The metabolism of clozapine is mediated mainly by the cytochrome P450 isozyme CYP1A2. Metabolites and trace amounts of unchanged drug are excreted mainly in the urine and also in the faeces. There is wide interindividual variation in plasma concentrations of clozapine and no simple correlation has been found between plasma concentrations and therapeutic effect.

References.

1. Jann MW, *et al.* Pharmacokinetics and pharmacodynamics of clozapine. *Clin Pharmacokinet* 1993; **24:** 161–76.
2. Lin S-K, *et al.* Disposition of clozapine and desmethylclozapine in schizophrenic patients. *J Clin Pharmacol* 1994; **34:** 318–24.
3. Freeman DJ, Oyewumi LK. Will routine therapeutic drug monitoring have a place in clozapine therapy? *Clin Pharmacokinet* 1997; **32:** 93–100.
4. Olesen OV. Therapeutic drug monitoring of clozapine treatment: therapeutic threshold value for serum clozapine concentrations. *Clin Pharmacokinet* 1998; **34:** 497–502.

Uses and Administration

Clozapine is a dibenzodiazepine derivative described as an atypical antipsychotic. It has relatively weak dopamine receptor-blocking activity at D_1, D_2, D_3, and D_5 receptors but has a high affinity for the D_4 receptor. It causes only a minimal increase in prolactin secretion. Clozapine possesses alpha-adrenergic blocking, antimuscarinic, antihistamine, antiserotonergic, and sedative properties.

Clozapine is used for the management of schizophrenia; because of the risk of agranulocytosis, it is reserved for patients who fail to respond to, or who experience severe extrapyramidal side-effects with, standard antipsychotics. Clozapine use must be accompanied by strict procedures for the monitoring of white blood-cell counts (see Precautions, above).

To minimise the incidence of adverse effects, clozapine therapy should be introduced gradually, beginning with low doses and increasing according to response. The usual dose by mouth on the first day is 12.5 mg once or twice daily followed by 25 mg once or twice daily on the second day. The daily dosage may be increased in increments of 25 to 50 mg to achieve a daily dose of up to 300 mg within 14 to 21 days; subsequent increments of 50 to 100 mg may be made once or twice weekly. Most patients respond to 200 to 450 mg daily; a daily dosage of 900 mg should not be exceeded. The total daily dose is given in divided doses; a larger proportion may be given at night. Once a therapeutic response has been obtained, a gradual reduction of dosage to a maintenance dose of 150 to 300 mg daily may be possible. Daily maintenance doses of 200 mg or less may be given as a single dose in the evening. If clozapine is to be withdrawn this should be done gradually over a 1- to 2-week period. However, immediate discontinuation with careful observation is essential if neutropenia develops (see Precautions, above).

Elderly patients may require lower doses of clozapine and it is recommended that treatment should be initiated with a dose of 12.5 mg on the first day and that subsequent dose increments should be restricted to 25 mg per day.

Patients with a history of epilepsy and those suffering from cardiovascular, renal, or hepatic disorders should receive a dose of 12.5 mg on the first day and subsequent dosage increases should be made slowly and in small increments. If seizures occur treatment should be suspended for 24 hours and resumed at a lower dose.

For patients who are restarting treatment after an interval of more than 2 days 12.5 mg may be given once or twice daily on the first day. If that dose is well tolerated it may be possible to increase the dosage more quickly than on initiation. However, patients who experienced respiratory or cardiac arrest with initial dosing should be re-titrated with extreme caution after even 24 hours discontinuation.

It is recommended that therapy with conventional antipsychotics should be withdrawn gradually before treatment with clozapine is started.

Clozapine has been given by intramuscular injection.

General references to clozapine.

1. Fitton A, Heel RC. Clozapine: a review of its pharmacological properties, and therapeutic use in schizophrenia. *Drugs* 1990; **40:** 722–47.
2. Anonymous. Clozapine and loxapine for schizophrenia. *Drug Ther Bull* 1991; **29:** 41–2. Correction. *ibid.*; 52.
3. Baldessarini RJ, Frankenburg FR. Clozapine: a novel antipsychotic agent. *N Engl J Med* 1991; **324:** 746–54.
4. Anonymous. Update on clozapine. *Med Lett Drugs Ther* 1993; **35:** 16–18.
5. Hirsch SR, Puri BK. Clozapine: progress in treating refractory schizophrenia. *Br Med J* 1993; **306:** 1427–8.
6. Kerwin RW. The new atypical antipsychotics: a lack of extrapyramidal side-effects and new routes in schizophrenia research. *Br J Psychiatry* 1994; **164:** 141–8.
7. Taylor D. Clozapine—five years on. *Pharm J* 1995; **254:** 260–3.

8. Pickar D. Prospects for pharmacotherapy of schizophrenia. *Lancet* 1995; **345:** 557–62.
9. Kerwin RW. Clozapine: back to the future for schizophrenia research. *Lancet* 1995; **345:** 1063–4.

Action. For discussion of the mode of action of antipsychotic drugs, see Chlorpromazine, p.654. Reference is made in that discussion to the traditional hypothesis that antipsychotic agents work through inhibition of dopamine D_2-receptors, but that this hypothesis fails to explain the activity of the atypical antipsychotics such as clozapine. How clozapine produces its antipsychotic activity is not clear; its actions are complex having a high affinity for a number of different receptors.[1]

1. Kerwin RW. The new atypical antipsychotics: a lack of extrapyramidal side-effects and new routes in schizophrenia research. *Br J Psychiatry* 1994; **164:** 141–8.

Disturbed behaviour. For mention that atypical antipsychotics such as clozapine might be more appropriate than conventional antipsychotics for elderly patients with dementia, see the Elderly in Precautions for Chlorpromazine, p.652. For further discussion of the management of disturbed behaviour, see p.636.

Parkinsonism. A review[1] of the use of clozapine in patients with Parkinson's disease (p.1128) concluded that from the data available clozapine appears to be of potential use as an alternative for the treatment of psychosis in these patients. Most patients given clozapine had shown resolution or improvement in psychosis without worsening of their parkinsonian symptoms. Adverse effects had been mild with daily doses lower than 100 mg and sedation had been the most frequent problem. However, there has been a report[2] of a patient with parkinsonism who experienced worsening of psychotic symptoms when her dose of clozapine was increased. There has also been a sudden return of psychosis in a patient with parkinsonism whose psychosis was successfully treated with clozapine for 5 years.[3]

Although some neurologists consider clozapine to be the antipsychotic of choice for the treatment of psychosis in patients with Parkinson's disease, the reviewers[1] considered that there was little evidence to support this. There appeared to be no comparative studies with standard antipsychotics. Many studies of the efficacy of clozapine had been flawed and the only double-blind study published had yielded the least favourable results. Because of this and the need for extensive monitoring, it was considered that the decision to use clozapine should be made on an individual basis.

Clozapine has also been tried in the treatment of the symptoms of Parkinson's disease and appears to produce some beneficial effects, especially on tremor and the frequency of 'on-off' periods.[1]

1. Pfeiffer C, Wagner ML. Clozapine therapy for Parkinson's disease and other movement disorders. *Am J Hosp Pharm* 1994; **51:** 3047–53.
2. Auzou P, *et al.* Worsening of psychotic symptoms by clozapine in Parkinson's disease. *Lancet* 1994; **344:** 955.
3. Greene P. Clozapine therapeutic plunge in patient with Parkinson's disease. *Lancet* 1995; **345:** 1172–3.

Schizophrenia. Clozapine is an effective antipsychotic for the management of schizophrenia (p.637) but its use is limited by its blood toxicity. Its effectiveness and superiority over conventional antipsychotics was demonstrated by Kane *et al.* in a multicentre study.[1] Patients refractory to at least 3 different antipsychotics and who failed to improve after a single-blind trial of haloperidol, were randomised, double-blind, to treatment for 6 weeks with either clozapine, up to 900 mg daily, or chlorpromazine hydrochloride up to 1800 mg daily with benztropine mesylate up to 6 mg daily. Of the 267 patients included in the evaluation, 5 of 141 (4%) improved with chlorpromazine and benztropine, and 38 of 126 (30%) improved with clozapine. Clozapine was superior to chlorpromazine in the treatment of negative as well as positive symptoms. Reviews[2] of clozapine indicate that these findings have been well replicated both in subsequent studies and in clinical practice. However, further research is required to determine an appropriate duration of clozapine administration that constitutes an adequate trial of therapy. Although a study by Meltzer *et al.*[3] identified new responders to clozapine up to 12 months after initiation of therapy other studies have indicated that if improvement was not seen within the first 6 to 24 weeks, it was unlikely to occur.[2,4]

Clozapine has shown consistent clinical benefit in schizophrenic patients with persistent aggressive or violent behaviour.[2] Whether this is due to a sedative effect, a specific antiaggressive action, or just reflects an overall improvement in psychosis remains to be determined.

Clozapine also appears to reduce suicidality in patients with refractory chronic schizophrenia.[5] The reported suicide rate of 0.05% per year in 6300 patients in the UK given clozapine since 1990 was considered to be tenfold less than expected.[6]

Clozapine has been advocated for use in schizophrenic patients with moderate to severe tardive dyskinesia. It is still unclear whether clozapine can itself cause tardive dyskinesia but some patients with established tardive dyskinesia have experienced improvement in their symptoms when using clozapine.[7,8]

1. Kane J, *et al.* Clozapine for the treatment-resistant schizophrenic: a double-blind comparison with chlorpromazine. *Arch Gen Psychiatry* 1988; **45:** 789–96.
2. Buckley PF. New dimensions in the pharmacologic treatment of schizophrenia and related psychoses. *J Clin Pharmacol* 1997; **37:** 363–78. Correction. *ibid.* 1998; **38:** 27.
3. Meltzer HY, *et al.* A prospective study of clozapine in treatment-resistant schizophrenic patients I: preliminary report. *Psychopharmacology (Berl)* 1989; **99:** S68–S72.
4. Conley RR, *et al.* Time to clozapine response in a standardized trial. *Am J Psychiatry* 1997; **154:** 1243–7.
5. Meltzer HY, Okayli G. Reduction of suicidality during clozapine treatment of neuroleptic-resistant schizophrenia: impact on risk-benefit assessment. *Am J Psychiatry* 1995; **152:** 183–90.
6. Kerwin RW. Clozapine: back to the future for schizophrenia research. *Lancet* 1995; **345:** 1063–4.
7. Tamminga CA, *et al.* Clozapine in tardive dyskinesia: observations from human and animal model studies. *J Clin Psychiatry* 1994; **55** (suppl B): 102–106.
8. Nair C, *et al.* Dose-related effects of clozapine on tardive dyskinesia among "treatment-refractory" patients with schizophrenia. *Biol Psychiatry* 1996; **39:** 529–30.

Preparations

Proprietary Preparations (details are given in Part 3)
Aust.: Leponex; ***Austral.:*** Clozaril; ***Belg.:*** Leponex; ***Canad.:*** Clozaril; ***Fr.:*** Leponex; ***Ger.:*** Leponex; ***Irl.:*** Clozaril; ***Ital.:*** Leponex; ***Neth.:*** Leponex; ***Norw.:*** Leponex; ***S.Afr.:*** Leponex; ***Spain:*** Leponex; ***Swed.:*** Leponex; ***Switz.:*** Leponex; ***UK:*** Clozaril; ***USA:*** Clozaril.

Cyamemazine (7033-w)

Cyamemazine *(rINN)*.

Cyamepromazine; RP-7204. 10-(3-Dimethylamino-2-methylpropyl)phenothiazine-2-carbonitrile.

$C_{19}H_{21}N_3S$ = 323.5.

CAS — 3546-03-0.

Cyamemazine is a phenothiazine with general properties similar to those of chlorpromazine (p.649). It is available as a preparation for the management of a variety of psychiatric disorders including anxiety disorders (p.635) and aggressive behaviour (p.636).

Cyamemazine is given by mouth as the base or the tartrate and by injection as the base; all doses are expressed in terms of the equivalent amount of cyamemazine. Doses of cyamemazine have ranged from 25 to 600 mg daily by mouth, depending on the individual and the condition being treated; the daily dosage is given in 2 portions with the larger amount at night. Doses given by intramuscular injection have ranged from 25 to 200 mg daily.

Cyamemazine should be given in reduced dosage to elderly patients; the parenteral route is not recommended for the elderly.

Preparations

Proprietary Preparations (details are given in Part 3)
Fr.: Tercian.

Multi-ingredient: ***Ger.:*** Neutromil†.

Cyclobarbitone (4025-s)

Cyclobarbitone *(BAN)*.

Cyclobarbital *(rINN)*; Ciclobarbital; Cyclobarbitalum; Ethylhexabital; Hexemalum. 5-(Cyclohex-1-enyl)-5-ethylbarbituric acid.

$C_{12}H_{16}N_2O_3$ = 236.3.

CAS — 52-31-3.

NOTE. The name ciclobarbital has sometimes been applied to hexobarbitone.

Pharmacopoeias. In *Aust.*

Cyclobarbitone Calcium (4026-w)

Cyclobarbitone Calcium *(BANM)*.

Cyclobarbital Calcium *(rINNM)*; Ciclobarbital Calcium; Cyclobarbitalum Calcicum; Hexemalcalcium. Calcium 5-(cyclohex-1-enyl)-5-ethylbarbiturate.

$(C_{12}H_{15}N_2O_3)_2Ca$ = 510.6.

CAS — 5897-20-1.

Pharmacopoeias. In *Aust., Belg., Fr., It., Neth., Pol.,* and *Port.*

Cyclobarbitone is a barbiturate with general properties similar to those of amylobarbitone (p.641). The calcium salt has been used as a hypnotic.

Preparations

Proprietary Preparations (details are given in Part 3)
Ger.: Somnupan C†.

Multi-ingredient: ***Belg.:*** Domidorm; ***Ger.:*** Itridal†.

Delorazepam (12552-s)

Delorazepam *(pINN)*.

Chlordesmethyldiazepam; Clordesmethyldiazepam. 7-Chloro-5-(2-chlorophenyl)-1,3-dihydro-2*H*-1,4-benzodiazepin-2-one.

$C_{15}H_{10}Cl_2N_2O$ = 305.2.

CAS — 2894-67-9.

Delorazepam is a long-acting benzodiazepine with general properties similar to those of diazepam (p.661). It is used in the short-term treatment of anxiety disorders (p.635) in doses of 0.5 to 2 mg given 2 or 3 times daily by mouth. A dose of 0.5 to 2 mg has been used at night for insomnia (p.638). It may also be given by intramuscular injection for premedication, for anxiety disorders, and in the management of epilepsy.

Administration in hepatic or renal impairment. The pharmacokinetics of total delorazepam were unchanged in patients with renal failure undergoing haemodialysis compared with controls.[1] However, the apparent volume of distribution of unbound drug was smaller and the clearance slower. The volume of distribution and clearance of unchanged drug was also reduced in patients with liver disease[2] and delorazepam should therefore be used with caution in patients with hepatic impairment.

1. Sennesael J, *et al.* Pharmacokinetics of intravenous and oral chlordesmethyldiazepam in patients on regular haemodialysis. *Eur J Clin Pharmacol* 1991; **41:** 65–8.
2. Bareggi SR, *et al.* Effects of liver disease on the pharmacokinetics of intravenous and oral chlordesmethyldiazepam. *Eur J Clin Pharmacol* 1995; **48:** 265–8.

Preparations

Proprietary Preparations (details are given in Part 3)
Ital.: En; ***Switz.:*** Briantum†.

Detomidine Hydrochloride (18627-j)

Detomidine Hydrochloride *(BAN, USAN, rINNM)*.

MPV-253-AII. 4-(2,3-Dimethylbenzyl)imidazole monohydrochloride.

$C_{12}H_{14}N_2,HCl$ = 222.7.

CAS — 90038-01-0 (detomidine hydrochloride); 76631-46-4 (detomidine).

Detomidine is an α_2-adrenoceptor agonist with sedative, muscle relaxant, and analgesic properties. It is used as the hydrochloride in veterinary medicine.

Dexmedetomidine (6469-q)

Dexmedetomidine *(BAN, USAN, rINN)*.

MPV-1440. (*S*)-4-[1-(2,3-Xylyl)ethyl]imidazole.

$C_{13}H_{16}N_2$ = 200.3.

CAS — 113775-47-6.

Dexmedetomidine is a selective alpha$_2$-adrenergic receptor agonist with anxiolytic, analgesic, and sedative properties. It is under investigation as a premedicant and adjunct to general anaesthesia. The racemate, medetomidine (p.677), is used as the hydrochloride in veterinary medicine.

References.

1. Aho MS. Effect of intravenously administered dexmedetomidine on pain after laparoscopic tubal ligation. *Anesth Analg* 1991; **73:** 112–18.
2. Aantaa R, *et al.* A comparison of dexmedetomidine, an alpha$_2$-adrenoceptor agonist, and midazolam as im premedication for minor gynaecological surgery. *Br J Anaesth* 1991; **67:** 402–9.
3. Peden CJ, Prys-Roberts C. Dexmedetomidine—a powerful new adjunct to anaesthesia? *Br J Anaesth* 1992; **68:** 123–5.
4. Scheinin B, *et al.* Dexmedetomidine attenuates sympathoadrenal responses to tracheal intubation and reduces the need for thiopentone and peroperative fentanyl. *Br J Anaesth* 1992; **68:** 126–31.
5. Jaakola M-L, *et al.* Dexmedetomidine reduces intraocular pressure, intubation responses and anaesthetic requirements in patients undergoing ophthalmic surgery. *Br J Anaesth* 1992; **68:** 570–5.
6. Scheinin H, *et al.* Pharmacodynamics and pharmacokinetics of intramuscular dexmedetomidine. *Clin Pharmacol Ther* 1992; **52:** 537–46.
7. Aho M, *et al.* Comparison of dexmedetomidine and midazolam sedation and antagonism of dexmedetomidine with atipamezole. *J Clin Anesth* 1993; **5:** 194–203.
8. Virkkilä M, *et al.* Dexmedetomidine as intramuscular premedication in outpatient cataract surgery: a placebo-controlled dose-ranging study. *Anaesthesia* 1993; **48:** 482–7.
9. Kivistö KT, *et al.* Pharmacokinetics and pharmacodynamics of transdermal dexmedetomidine. *Eur J Clin Pharmacol* 1994; **46:** 345–9.

Diazepam (7036-y)

Diazepam *(BAN, USAN, rINN)*.

Diazepamum; LA-III; NSC-77518; Ro-5-2807; Wy-3467.
7-Chloro-1,3-dihydro-1-methyl-5-phenyl-2*H*-1,4-benzodiazepin-2-one.

$C_{16}H_{13}ClN_2O = 284.7$.

CAS — 439-14-5.

Pharmacopoeias. In *Chin., Eur.* (see p.viii), *Int., Jpn, Pol.,* and *US.*

A white, almost white, or yellow, almost odourless, crystalline powder. Ph. Eur. **solubilities** are: very slightly soluble in water and soluble in alcohol. USP solubilities are: soluble 1 in 333 of water, 1 in 16 of alcohol, 1 in 2 of chloroform, and 1 in 39 of ether.

Store in airtight containers. Protect from light.

Dilution. Great care should be observed on dilution of diazepam injections for administration by infusion because of problems of precipitation. The manufacturer's directions should be followed regarding diluent and concentration of diazepam and all solutions should be freshly prepared.

Incompatibility. Incompatibility has been reported between diazepam and several other drugs. The manufacturers of diazepam injection advise against its admixture with other drugs.

Sorption. Substantial adsorption of diazepam onto some plastics may cause problems when administering the drug by continuous intravenous infusion. More than 50% of diazepam in solution may be adsorbed onto the walls of polyvinyl chloride infusion bags and their use should, therefore, be avoided. Administration sets should contain the minimum amount of polyvinyl chloride tubing and should not contain a cellulose propionate volume-control chamber. Suitable materials for infusion containers, syringes, and administration sets when administering diazepam include glass, polyolefin, polypropylene, and polyethylene.

References.

1. Cloyd JC, *et al.* Availability of diazepam from plastic containers. *Am J Hosp Pharm* 1980; **37:** 492–6.
2. Parker WA, MacCara ME. Compatibility of diazepam with intravenous fluid containers and administration sets. *Am J Hosp Pharm* 1980; **37:** 496–500.
3. Kowaluk EA, *et al.* Interactions between drugs and intravenous delivery systems. *Am J Hosp Pharm* 1982; **39:** 460–7.
4. Kowaluk EA, *et al.* Factors affecting the availability of diazepam stored in plastic bags and administered through intravenous sets. *Am J Hosp Pharm* 1983; **40:** 417–23.
5. Martens HJ, *et al.* Sorption of various drugs in polyvinyl chloride, glass, and polyethylene-lined infusion containers. *Am J Hosp Pharm* 1990; **47:** 369–73.

Dependence and Withdrawal

The development of dependence is common after regular use of diazepam or other benzodiazepines, even in therapeutic doses for short periods. Dependence is particularly likely in patients with a history of alcohol or drug abuse and in patients with marked personality disorders. Benzodiazepines should not therefore be discontinued abruptly after regular use for even a few weeks, but should be withdrawn by gradual reduction of the dose over a period of weeks or months. The extent to which tolerance occurs has been debated but appears to involve psychomotor performance more often than anxiolytic effects. Drug-seeking behaviour is uncommon with therapeutic doses of benzodiazepines. High doses of diazepam and other benzodiazepines, injected intravenously, have been abused for their euphoriant effects.

Benzodiazepine withdrawal syndrome. Development of dependence to benzodiazepines cannot be predicted but risk factors include high dosage, regular continuous use, the use of benzodiazepines with a short half-life, use in patients with dependent personality characteristics or a history of drug or alcohol dependence, and the development of tolerance.

The mechanism of benzodiazepine dependence is unclear. One possible mechanism is a relative deficiency of functional aminobutyric acid (GABA) activity resulting from down-regulation of GABA receptors.

Symptoms of benzodiazepine withdrawal include anxiety, depression, impaired concentration, insomnia, headache, dizziness, tinnitus, loss of appetite, tremor, perspiration, irritability, perceptual disturbances such as hypersensitivity to visual and auditory stimuli and abnormal taste, nausea, vomiting, abdominal cramps, palpitations, mild systolic hypertension, tachycardia, and orthostatic hypotension. Rare and more serious symptoms include muscle twitching, confusional or paranoid psychosis, convulsions, hallucinations, and a state resembling delirium tremens.

Symptoms typical of withdrawal have been observed despite continued use of benzodiazepines and have been attributed either to the development of tolerance or, as in the case of very short-acting agents such as triazolam, to rapid benzodiazepine elimination. Pseudowithdrawal has been reported in patients who believed incorrectly that their dose of benzodiazepine was being reduced. Benzodiazepine withdrawal can theoretically be distinguished from these reactions and from rebound phenomena (return of original symptoms at greater than pretreatment severity) by the differing time course. A withdrawal syndrome is characterised by its onset, by the development of new symptoms, and by a peak in intensity followed by resolution. Onset of withdrawal symptoms depends on the half-life of the drug and its active metabolites. Symptoms can begin within a few hours after withdrawal of a short-acting benzodiazepine, but may not develop for up to 3 weeks after stopping a longer-acting benzodiazepine. Resolution of symptoms may take several days or months. The dependence induced by short- and long-acting benzodiazepines appears to be qualitatively similar although withdrawal symptoms may be more severe with short-acting benzodiazepines.

With increased awareness of the problems of benzodiazepine dependence, emphasis has been placed on prevention by proper use and careful patient selection. Withdrawal from long-term benzodiazepine use should generally be encouraged. Since abrupt withdrawal of benzodiazepines may result in severe withdrawal symptoms dosage should be tapered. The patient should have professional and family support and behavioural therapy may be helpful. Withdrawal in a specialist centre may be required for some patients. There are no comparative studies of the efficacy of various withdrawal schedules and in practice the protocol should be titrated against the response of the patient. Clinicians often favour transferring the patient to an equivalent dose of diazepam given at night. Time required for withdrawal can vary from about 4 weeks to a year or longer. The daily dosage of diazepam, for example, can be reduced in steps of 0.5 to 2.5 mg at fortnightly intervals. If troublesome abstinence effects occur the dose should be held level for a longer period before further reduction; increased dosage should be avoided if possible. It is better to reduce too slowly than too quickly. In many cases the rate of withdrawal is best decided by the patient. The following approximate dosage equivalents to diazepam 5 mg have been recommended in the UK to help in a withdrawal programme that involves substituting an equivalent dose of diazepam: chlordiazepoxide 15 mg, loprazolam 0.5 to 1 mg, lorazepam 500 µg, lormetazepam 0.5 to 1 mg, nitrazepam 5 mg, oxazepam 15 mg, and temazepam 10 mg.

Adjuvant therapy should generally be avoided although a beta blocker may be given for prominent sympathetic overactivity and an antidepressant for clinical depression. Antipsychotic drugs may aggravate symptoms.

Symptoms gradually improve after withdrawal but postwithdrawal syndromes lasting for several weeks or months have been described. Continued support may be required for the first year after withdrawal to prevent relapse.

1. DoH. *Drug misuse and dependence: guidelines on clinical management.* London: HMSO, 1991.
2. Marriott S, Tyrer P. Benzodiazepine dependence: avoidance and withdrawal. *Drug Safety* 1993; **9:** 93–103.
3. Pétursson H. The benzodiazepine withdrawal syndrome. *Addiction* 1994; **89:** 1455–59.
4. Ashton H. The treatment of benzodiazepine dependence. *Addiction* 1994; **89:** 1535–41.

Adverse Effects

Drowsiness, sedation, and ataxia are the most frequent adverse effects of diazepam use. They generally decrease on continued administration and are a consequence of CNS depression. Less frequent effects include vertigo, headache, confusion, mental depression (but see Effects on Mental Function, below), slurred speech or dysarthria, changes in libido, tremor, visual disturbances, urinary retention or incontinence, gastro-intestinal disturbances, changes in salivation, and amnesia. Some patients may experience a paradoxical excitation which may lead to hostility, aggression, and disinhibition. Jaundice, blood disorders, and hypersensitivity reactions have been reported rarely. Respiratory depression and hypotension occasionally occur with high dosage and parenteral administration.

Pain and thrombophlebitis may occur with some intravenous formulations of diazepam.

Overdosage can produce CNS depression and coma or paradoxical excitation. However, fatalities are rare when taken alone.

Use of diazepam in the first trimester of pregnancy has occasionally been associated with congenital malformations in the infant but no clear relationship has been established. This topic is reviewed under Pregnancy and Breast Feeding, below. Administration of diazepam in late pregnancy has been associated with intoxication of the neonate.

In a report[1] of 2 patients who developed rhabdomyolysis secondary to hyponatraemia it was suggested that the use of benzodiazepines might have contributed to the rhabdomyolysis. These 2 patients brought the number of reported cases of rhabdomyolysis associated with hyponatraemia to 8, and of these, 5 had received benzodiazepines.

1. Fernández-Real JM, *et al.* Hyponatremia and benzodiazepines result in rhabdomyolysis. *Ann Pharmacother* 1994; **28:** 1200–1.

Carcinogenicity. In an evaluation[1] of the carcinogenic potential of several benzodiazepines the International Agency for Research on Cancer concluded that there was sufficient evidence from human studies that diazepam did not produce breast cancer and that there was inadequate data to support its potential carcinogenicity at other sites. For most other benzodiazepines the lack of human studies meant that the carcinogenic risk to humans was not classifiable. However, there appeared to be sufficient evidence of carcinogenicity in *animal* studies for oxazepam to be classified as possibly carcinogenic in humans. There was also limited evidence of carcinogenicity in *animal* studies for doxefazepam.

1. IARC/WHO. Some pharmaceutical drugs. *IARC monographs on the evaluation of carcinogenic risks to humans volume 66* 1996.

Effects on body temperature. Studies in healthy subjects[1,2] indicate that benzodiazepines can reduce body temperature. After a single dose of diazepam 10 mg by mouth in 11 subjects body temperature on exposure to cold fell to a mean of 36.93°, compared with 37.08° on exposure without the drug.[1] An 86-year-old woman developed hypothermia[3] after administration of nitrazepam 5 mg. After recovery she was mistakenly given another 5-mg dose of nitrazepam and again developed hypothermia.

Hypothermia has been reported in the neonates of mothers given benzodiazepines during the late stages of pregnancy.

1. Martin SM. The effect of diazepam on body temperature change in humans during cold exposure. *J Clin Pharmacol* 1985; **25:** 611–13.
2. Matsukawa T, *et al.* I.M. midazolam as premedication produces a concentration-dependent decrease in core temperature in male volunteers. *Br J Anaesth* 1997; **78:** 396–9.
3. Impallomeni M, Ezzat R. Hypothermia associated with nitrazepam administration. *Br Med J* 1976; **1:** 223–4.

Effects on endocrine function. Galactorrhoea with normal serum-prolactin concentrations has been noted in 4 women taking benzodiazepines.[1] Gynaecomastia has been reported in one man taking up to 140 mg diazepam daily[2] and in 5 men taking diazepam in doses of up to 30 mg daily.[3] Again, there was no change in prolactin concentrations but serum-oestradiol concentrations were raised in the group of 5 men.

Raised plasma-testosterone concentrations were observed in men taking diazepam 10 to 20 mg daily for 2 weeks.[4]

1. Kleinberg DL, *et al.* Galactorrhea: a study of 235 cases, including 48 with pituitary tumors. *N Engl J Med* 1977; **296:** 589–600.
2. Moerck HJ, Magelund G. Gynaecomastia and diazepam abuse. *Lancet* 1979; **i:** 1344–5.
3. Bergman D, *et al.* Increased oestradiol in diazepam related gynaecomastia. *Lancet* 1981; **ii:** 1225–6.
4. Argüelles AE, Rosner J. Diazepam and plasma-testosterone levels. *Lancet* 1975; **ii:** 607.

Effects on the eyes. Brown opacification of the lens occurred in a married couple who took diazepam 5 mg or more daily by mouth over several years.[1]

1. Pau H. Braune scheibenförmige einlagerungen in die linse nach langzeitgabe von diazepam (Valium). *Klin Monatsbl Augenheilkd* 1985; **187:** 219–20.

Effects on the liver. Reports of cholestatic jaundice[1] in one patient and focal hepatic necrosis with intracellular cholestasis[2] in another associated with the administration of diazepam.

1. Jick H, *et al.* Drug-induced liver disease. *J Clin Pharmacol* 1981; **21:** 359–64.
2. Tedesco FJ, Mills LR. Diazepam (Valium) hepatitis. *Dig Dis Sci* 1982; **27:** 470–2.

Effects on mental function. The effects of benzodiazepines on psychomotor performance accumulated from laboratory tests have been reviewed in detail by Woods *et al.*[1] The results of such tests are not easily extrapolated to the clinical situation.

Concern has been expressed as to the possible effects of long-term benzodiazepine use on the brain. Of the many studies of possible impairment of psychological function few have clinical significance. Golombok *et al.*[2] have carried out a detailed study using a variety of neuropsychological tests on 50 chronic benzodiazepine users, 34 chronic users who had withdrawn from medication for at least 6 months, and 61 control subjects. They found that patients taking high doses of benzodiazepines for long periods of time perform poorly on tasks involving visual-spatial ability and sustained attention. There was no evidence of impairment in global measures of intellectual functioning such as memory, flexibility, and simple reaction time. The authors could draw no conclusions as to the effect of benzodiazepine withdrawal on these changes. A few studies have examined the effect of benzodiazepine use on brain morphology. A study of 17 long-term users indicated a dose-dependent increase in ventricle size.[3]

Sexual fantasies have been reported in women sedated with intravenous diazepam or midazolam.[4] These appear to be dose-related.[5]

Mental depression is generally considered to be one of the less frequent adverse effects of benzodiazepines. However Patten and Love[6] consider that there is no good support for the view that benzodiazepines can cause depression.

Adverse effects of alprazolam on behaviour have been reviewed by Cole and Kando.[7]

1. Woods JH, *et al.* Abuse liability of benzodiazepines. *Pharmacol Rev* 1987; **39:** 251–413.
2. Golombok S, *et al.* Cognitive impairment in long-term benzodiazepine users. *Psychol Med* 1988; **18:** 365–74.
3. Schmauss C, Krieg J-C. Enlargement of cerebrospinal fluid spaces in long-term benzodiazepine abusers. *Psychol Med* 1987; **17:** 869–73.
4. Dundee JW. Fantasies during benzodiazepine sedation in women. *Br J Clin Pharmacol* 1990; **30:** 311P.
5. Brahams D. Benzodiazepine sedation and allegations of sexual assault. *Lancet* 1989; **i:** 1339–40.
6. Patten SB, Love EJ. Drug-induced depression: incidence, avoidance and management. *Drug Safety* 1994; **10:** 203–19.
7. Cole JO, Kando JC. Adverse behavioral events reported in patients taking alprazolam and other benzodiazepines. *J Clin Psychiatry* 1993; **54** (suppl): 49–61.

Effects on the nervous system. There are a few isolated reports of extrapyramidal symptoms in patients taking benzodiazepines.[1-4] Benzodiazepines have been used with limited success to treat such symptoms induced by antipsychotics (see Chlorpromazine, p.650).

1. Rosenbaum AH, De La Fuente JR. Benzodiazepines and tardive dyskinesia. *Lancet* 1979; **ii:** 900.
2. Sandyk R. Orofacial dyskinesias associated with lorazepam therapy. *Clin Pharm* 1986; **5:** 419–21.
3. Stolarek IH, Ford MJ. Acute dystonia induced by midazolam and abolished by flumazenil. *Br Med J* 1990; **300:** 614.
4. Joseph AB, Wroblewski BA. Paradoxical akathisia caused by clonazepam, clorazepate and lorazepam in patients with traumatic encephalopathy and seizure disorders: a subtype of benzodiazepine-induced disinhibition? *Behav Neurol* 1993; **6:** 221–3.

ENCEPHALOPATHY. Prolonged use of midazolam with fentanyl has been associated with encephalopathy in infants sedated under intensive care.[1]

1. Bergman I, *et al.* Reversible neurologic abnormalities associated with prolonged intravenous midazolam and fentanyl administration. *J Pediatr* 1991; **119:** 644–9.

Effects on sexual function. Benzodiazepines have no direct effects on erection or ejaculation but their sedative effect may reduce sexual arousal and lead to impotence in some patients. Conversely sexual performance may be improved where it is impaired by anxiety.[1] Increased libido and orgasmic function has been reported in 2 women after withdrawal of long-term benzodiazepine use.[2]

1. Beeley L. Drug-induced sexual dysfunction and infertility. *Adverse Drug React Acute Poisoning Rev* 1984; **3:** 23–42.
2. Nutt D, *et al.* Increased sexual function in benzodiazepine withdrawal. *Lancet* 1986; **ii:** 1101–2.

Effects on the skin. Analysis by the Boston Collaborative Drug Surveillance Program of data on 15 438 patients hospitalised between 1975 and 1982 detected 2 allergic skin reactions attributed to diazepam among 4707 recipients of the drug.[1] A reaction rate of 0.4 per 1000 recipients was calculated from these figures.

1. Bigby M, *et al.* Drug-induced cutaneous reactions. *JAMA* 1986; **256:** 3358–63.

Hypersensitivity. Hypersensitivity reactions including anaphylaxis are very rare following administration of diazepam. Reactions have been attributed to the polyethoxylated castor oil (p.1326) vehicle used for some parenteral formulations.[1] There is also a report of a type I hypersensitivity reaction to a lipid emulsion formulation of diazepam.[2]

See also under Effects on the Skin, above.

1. Hüttel MS, *et al.* Complement-mediated reactions to diazepam with Cremophor as solvent (Stesolid MR). *Br J Anaesth* 1980; **52:** 77–9.
2. Deardon DJ, Bird GLA. Acute (type 1) hypersensitivity to iv Diazemuls. *Br J Anaesth* 1987; **59:** 391.

Local reactions. Ischaemia and gangrene have been reported after accidental intra-arterial injection of diazepam.[1,2] Clinical signs may not occur until several days after the event. Pain and thrombophlebitis after intravenous administration may be similarly delayed. Local reactions after intravenous injection have been attributed to the vehicle, and have been observed more often when diazepam is given as a solution in propylene glycol than in polyethoxylated castor oil.[3] An emulsion of diazepam in soya oil and water has been associated with a lower incidence of local reactions.[3] Pain and phlebitis may also be caused by precipitation of diazepam at the site of infusion.[4] Arterial spasm experienced by one patient given diazepam intravenously was probably due to pressure from a cuff on the arm being inflated causing extravasation of diazepam out of the vein and into the radial artery.[5]

Local irritation has also been observed after rectal administration of diazepam.[6]

For a report of the exacerbation of diazepam-induced thrombophlebitis by penicillamine, see below.

1. Gould JDM, Lingam S. Hazards of intra-arterial diazepam. *Br Med J* 1977; **2:** 298–9.
2. Rees M, Dormandy J. Accidental intra-arterial injection of diazepam. *Br Med J* 1980; **281:** 289–90.
3. Olesen AS, Hüttel MS. Local reactions to iv diazepam in three different formulations. *Br J Anaesth* 1980; **52:** 609–11.
4. Hussey EK, *et al.* Correlation of delayed peak concentration with infusion-site irritation following diazepam administration. *DICP Ann Pharmacother* 1990; **24:** 678–80.
5. Ng Wing Tin L, *et al.* Arterial spasm after administration of diazepam. *Br J Anaesth* 1994; **72:** 139.
6. Hansen HC, *et al.* Local irritation after administration of diazepam in a rectal solution. *Br J Anaesth* 1989; **63:** 287–9.

Overdosage. Impairment of consciousness is fairly rapid in poisoning by benzodiazepines.[1] Deep coma or other manifestations of severe depression of brainstem vital functions are rare; more common is a sleep-like state from which the patient can be temporarily raised by appropriate stimuli. There is usually little or no respiratory depression, and cardiac rate and rhythm remain normal in the absence of anoxia or severe hypotension. Since tolerance to benzodiazepines develops rapidly consciousness is often regained while concentrations of drug in the blood are higher than those which induced coma. Anxiety and insomnia can occur during recovery from acute overdosage while a full-blown withdrawal syndrome, possibly with major convulsions, can occur in patients who have previously been chronic users.

During the years 1980 to 1989, 1576 fatal poisonings in Britain were attributed to benzodiazepines.[2] Of these, 891 were linked to overdosage with benzodiazepines alone and another 591 to overdosage combined with alcohol. A comparison of these mortality statistics with prescribing data for the same period, to calculate a toxicity index of deaths per million prescriptions, suggested that there were differences between the relative toxicities of individual benzodiazepines in overdosage. A later study of another 303 cases of benzodiazepine poisoning[3] supported these findings of differences in toxicity as well as pointing to the relative safety of the benzodiazepines in overdosage.

1. Ashton CH, *et al.* Drug-induced stupor and coma: some physical signs and their pharmacological basis. *Adverse Drug React Acute Poisoning Rev* 1989; **8:** 1–59.
2. Serfaty M, Masterton G. Fatal poisonings attributed to benzodiazepines in Britain during the 1980s. *Br J Psychiatry* 1993; **163:** 386–93.
3. Buckley NA, *et al.* Relative toxicity of benzodiazepines in overdose. *Br Med J* 1995; **310:** 219–21.

Treatment of Adverse Effects

Following recent ingestion of an overdose of diazepam the stomach may be emptied by lavage. Treatment is generally symptomatic and supportive. The specific benzodiazepine antagonist, flumazenil, may be used in the differential diagnosis of unclear cases of overdose but expert advice is essential since serious adverse effects may occur in patients dependent on benzodiazepines (see p.981).

Precautions

Diazepam should be avoided in patients with pre-existing CNS depression or coma, acute pulmonary insufficiency, or sleep apnoea, and used with care in those with chronic pulmonary insufficiency. Diazepam should be given with care to elderly or debilitated patients who may be more prone to adverse effects. Caution is required in patients with muscle weakness, or impaired liver or kidney function. The sedative effects of diazepam are most marked during the first few days of administration; affected patients should not drive or operate machinery. Monitoring of cardiorespiratory function is generally recommended when benzodiazepines are used for deep sedation.

Diazepam is not appropriate for the treatment of chronic psychosis or for phobic or obsessional states. Diazepam-induced disinhibition may precipitate suicide or aggressive behaviour and it should not, therefore, be used alone to treat depression or anxiety associated with depression; it should also be used with care in patients with personality disorders. Caution is required in patients with organic brain changes particularly arteriosclerosis. In cases of bereavement, psychological adjustment may be inhibited by diazepam.

Many manufacturers of diazepam and other benzodiazepines advise against their use in patients with glaucoma, but the rationale for this contra-indication is unclear.

For warnings on benzodiazepines during pregnancy and breast feeding, see below.

Dependence characterised by a withdrawal syndrome may develop after regular use of diazepam, even in therapeutic doses for short periods (see above); because of its dependence liability, diazepam should be used with caution in patients with a history of alcohol or drug addiction.

Since hypotension and apnoea may occur when diazepam is given intravenously it has been recommended that this route should only be used when facilities for reversing respiratory depression with mechanical ventilation are available. Patients should remain supine and under medical supervision for at least one hour after intravenous injection. Intravenous infusion should only be undertaken in specialist centres with intensive care facilities where close and constant supervision can be undertaken.

Administration. INTRAVENOUS. A warning[1] that prolonged use of high-dose intravenous infusions of diazepam preparations containing benzyl alcohol can result in benzyl alcohol poisoning.

1. López-Herce J, *et al.* Benzyl alcohol poisoning following diazepam intravenous infusion. *Ann Pharmacother* 1995; **29:** 632.

Cardiovascular disorders. See under Respiratory System Disorders, below.

Driving. Experimental studies of simulated driving and actual driving behaviour have indicated that single or repeated therapeutic doses of most benzodiazepines tested may adversely affect parameters of performance in healthy subjects.[1] Epidemiological studies have not provided a clear indication as to whether, or to what extent, benzodiazepines contribute to the risk of driving accidents. However, recent studies[2,3] have found an increased risk. A large case-control cohort study[2] in elderly drivers suggested that the risk of accidents was increased in those who took longer-acting benzodiazepines. Another study,[3] suggested that, for users of benzodiazepines or zopiclone as a group, the increased risk was greatest in younger drivers and was increased by alcohol consumption. Patients affected by drowsiness while taking benzodiazepines should not drive or operate machinery. Drowsiness often becomes less troublesome with continued use of these drugs.

1. Woods JH, *et al.* Abuse liability of benzodiazepines. *Pharmacol Rev* 1987; **39:** 251–413.
2. Hemmelgarn B, *et al.* Benzodiazepine use and the risk of motor vehicle crash in the elderly. *JAMA* 1997; **278:** 27–31.
3. Barbone F, *et al.* Association of road-traffic accidents with benzodiazepine use. *Lancet* 1998; **352:** 1331–6.

The elderly. As for many other drugs, old age may alter the distribution, elimination, and clearance of benzodiazepines.[1,2] Metabolic clearance appears to be reduced in the elderly for benzodiazepines metabolised principally by oxidation but not for those biotransformed by glucuronide conjugation or nitroreduction. Prolonged half-life in the elderly may be a result of this decrease in clearance or of an increase in the volume of distribution. The clinical consequence of these changes depends on factors such as dosage schedule and extent of first-pass extraction by the liver.

Irrespective of pharmacokinetic changes, old people may exhibit increased sensitivity to acute doses of benzodiazepines.[1-3] Impairment of memory, cognitive function, and psychomotor performance and behaviour disinhibition may be more common than with younger patients.[4] Long-term use commonly exacerbates underlying dementia in elderly patients.[4]

The upshot of the pharmacokinetic and pharmacodynamic changes of benzodiazepines in the elderly is that adverse effects may be more frequent in these patients and lower doses are commonly required. An epidemiological study of persons 65 years and older found an increased rate of hip fracture among current users of long-acting benzodiazepines (*chlordiazepoxide, clorazepate, diazepam,* and *flurazepam*) but not among users of short-acting drugs (*alprazolam, bromazepam, lorazepam, oxazepam,* and *triazolam*).[5] However, preliminary results of a later meta-analysis[6] of studies in the literature found no association between the use of benzodiazepines or other sedatives or hypnotics and falls or fractures in the elderly. Nonetheless, if administration of a benzodiazepine is considered necessary in elderly patients, a short-acting drug is to be preferred. It should also be remembered that old people are at increased risk of sleep-related breathing disorders, such as sleep apnoea and the use of hypnotics such as benzodiazepines should be avoided in these patients (see Respiratory System Disorders, below).

1. Greenblatt DJ, *et al.* Implications of altered drug disposition in elderly: studies of benzodiazepines. *J Clin Pharmacol* 1989; **29:** 866–72.
2. Greenblatt DJ, *et al.* Clinical pharmacokinetics of anxiolytics and hypnotics in the elderly: therapeutic considerations. *Clin Pharmacokinet* 1991; **21:** 165–77 and 262–73.
3. Swift CG. Pharmacodynamics: changes in homeostatic mechanisms, receptor and target organ sensitivity in the elderly. *Br Med Bull* 1990; **46:** 36–52.
4. Juergens SM. Problems with benzodiazepines in elderly patients. *Mayo Clin Proc* 1993; **68:** 818–20.
5. Ray WA, *et al.* Benzodiazepines of long and short elimination half-life and the risk of hip fracture. *JAMA* 1989; **262:** 3303–7.
6. Liu BA, *et al.* Benzodiazepines and falls in the elderly: a meta-analysis. *Clin Pharmacol Ther* 1995; **57:** 200.

Gout. A 40-year-old Chinese man with a history of gout had acute attacks on 5 occasions after taking nitrazepam 10 mg;[1] attacks were also precipitated by diazepam 5 mg, chlordiazepoxide 15 mg, and by methaqualone with diphenhydramine.

1. Leng CO. Drug-precipitated acute attacks of gout. *Br Med J* 1975; **2:** 561.

Hepatic impairment. Studies of the pharmacokinetics of diazepam in patients with liver disorders suggest that oxidative metabolism is impaired resulting in a prolonged half-life and reduced clearance.[1-3] A reduction in dosage was generally required.

1. Branch RA, *et al.* Intravenous administration of diazepam in patients with chronic liver disease. *Gut* 1976; **17:** 975–83.
2. Klotz U, *et al.* Disposition of diazepam and its major metabolite desmethyldiazepam in patients with liver disease. *Clin Pharmacol Ther* 1977; **21:** 430–6.
3. Ochs HR, *et al.* Repeated diazepam dosing in cirrhotic patients: cumulation and sedation. *Clin Pharmacol Ther* 1983; **33:** 471–6.

High-altitude disorders. Sleep may be impaired at high altitude due to frequent arousals associated with pronounced oxygen desaturation and periodic breathing. Traditional advice has been that sedatives should not be given at high altitude.[1] It has been argued that since diazepam, and possibly other sedatives blunt the hypoxic ventilatory response, sleep hypoxaemia might be exacerbated. A recent small study[2] has suggested that small doses of a short-acting benzodiazepine, such as temazepam, might actually improve the subjective quality of sleep and reduce episodes of arterial desaturation without changing mean oxygen saturation. However the possibility of an interaction between acetazolamide taken for prophylaxis or treatment of acute mountain sickness and the benzodiazepine should be borne in mind; ventilatory depression in a mountain climber with acute mountain sickness was considered to be due to the potentiation of triazolam by acetazolamide.[3]

1. Sutton JR, *et al.* Insomnia, sedation, and high altitude cerebral oedema. *Lancet* 1979; **i:** 165.
2. Dubowitz G. Effect of temazepam on oxygen saturation and sleep quality at high altitude: randomised placebo controlled crossover trial. *Br Med J* 1998; **316:** 587–9.
3. Masuyama S, *et al.* 'Ondine's curse': side effect of acetazolamide? *Am J Med* 1989; **86:** 637.

Nervous system disorders. Benzodiazepines can reduce cerebral perfusion pressure and blood oxygenation and may produce irreversible neurological damage in patients with head injuries and should therefore be administered with great care. Their use should be avoided for the control of seizures in patients with head injuries or other acute neurological lesions as these patients can be managed effectively with phenytoin.

References.

1. Eldridge PR, Punt JAG. Risks associated with giving benzodiazepines to patients with acute neurological injuries. *Br Med J* 1990; **300:** 1189–90.
2. Papazian L, *et al.* Effect of bolus doses of midazolam on intracranial pressure and cerebral perfusion pressure in patients with severe head injury. *Br J Anaesth* 1993; **71:** 267–71.

EPILEPSY. There have been rare reports of benzodiazepines producing paradoxical exacerbation of seizures in patients with epilepsy.[1,2]

1. Prior PF, *et al.* Intravenous diazepam. *Lancet* 1971; **2:** 434–5.
2. Tassinari CA, *et al.* A paradoxical effect: status epilepticus induced by benzodiazepines (Valium and Mogadon). *Electroencephalogr Clin Neurophysiol* 1971; **31:** 182.

Porphyria. Diazepam was considered to be unsafe in patients with acute porphyria although there is conflicting evidence of porphyrinogenicity.[1] Intravenous diazepam had been used successfully to control status epilepticus occurring after the acute porphyric attack. For a discussion of the management of seizures associated with acute porphyric attacks, see p.339.

1. Moore MR, McColl KEL. *Porphyria: drug lists.* Glasgow: Porphyria Research Unit, University of Glasgow, 1991.

Pregnancy and breast feeding. Benzodiazepines have been widely used in pregnant patients and the reports and studies of such use have been reviewed.[1] The early reports, usually involving diazepam and chlordiazepoxide, of some fetal malformations including facial clefts and cardiac abnormalities, were not supported by later reports. Use of benzodiazepines in the third trimester and during labour seems to be associated in some infants with the neonatal withdrawal symptoms or the floppy infant syndrome. Also a small number exposed *in utero* to benzodiazepines have shown slow development in the early years but by 4 years of age most had developed normally, and for those that had not it was not possible to prove a cause-effect relationship with benzodiazepine exposure. In a recent meta-analysis[4] of benzodiazepine use during the first trimester of pregnancy pooled data from cohort studies showed no apparent association between benzodiazepine use and the risk of major malformations or oral cleft alone. There was, however, a small but significantly increased risk of oral cleft according to data from case-control studies. Although benzodiazepines did not appear to be a major human teratogen use of ultrasonography was advised to rule out visible forms of cleft lip. The Committee on Safety of Medicines (CSM) in the UK has recommended[2] that if benzodiazepines are prescribed to women of childbearing potential they should be advised to contact the physician regarding discontinuation of the drug if they intend to become, or suspect that they are, pregnant. In the reviewer's opinion[1] the limited distribution into breast milk did not constitute a hazard to the breast-feeding infant but the infant should be monitored for sedation and the inability to suckle. It has been suggested[3] that if a benzodiazepine must be used during breast feeding it would be preferable to use a short-acting drug with minimal distribution into breast milk and inactive metabolite; oxazepam, lorazepam, alprazolam, or midazolam might be suitable. However the American Academy of Pediatrics Committee considered that use by nursing mothers for long periods was a cause for concern[5] and the CSM has recommended[2] that benzodiazepines should not be given to lactating mothers.

1. McElhatton PR. The effects of benzodiazepine use during pregnancy and lactation. *Reprod Toxicol* 1994; **8:** 461–75.
2. Committee on Safety of Medicines/Medicines Control Agency. Reminder: avoid benzodiazepines in pregnancy and lactation. *Current Problems* 1997; **23:** 10.
3. Chisholm CA, Kuller JA. A guide to the safety of CNS-active agents during breastfeeding. *Drug Safety* 1997; **17:** 127–42.
4. Dolovich LR, *et al.* Benzodiazepine use in pregnancy and major malformations or oral cleft: meta-analysis of cohort and case-control studies. *Br Med J* 1998; **317:** 839–43.
5. American Academy of Pediatrics Committee on Drugs. The transfer of drugs and other chemicals into human milk. *Pediatrics* 1994; **93:** 137–50.

Renal impairment. Although plasma protein binding of diazepam was reduced in 8 patients with advanced renal failure, the clearance of unbound drug after a single intravenous dose was not significantly changed.[1]

See also under Flurazepam, p.672.

1. Ochs HR, *et al.* Diazepam kinetics in patients with renal insufficiency or hyperthyroidism. *Br J Clin Pharmacol* 1981; **12:** 829–32.

Respiratory system disorders. Benzodiazepines may affect the control of ventilation during sleep and may worsen sleep apnoea or other sleep-related breathing disorders especially in patients with chronic obstructive pulmonary disease or cardiac failure.[1] Risk factors for sleep apnoea, which often goes undiagnosed, include old age, obesity, male sex, postmenopausal status in women, and a history of heavy snoring. Although benzodiazepines may reduce sleep fragmentation, their long-term use may result in conversion from partial to complete obstructive sleep apnoea in heavy snorers or in short repetitive central sleep apnoea in patients with recent myocardial infarction.

1. Guilleminault C. Benzodiazepines, breathing, and sleep. *Am J Med* 1990; **88** (suppl 3A): 25S–28S.

Interactions

Enhanced sedation or respiratory and cardiovascular depression may occur if diazepam or other benzodiazepines are given with other drugs that have CNS-depressant properties; these include alcohol, antidepressants, antihistamines, antipsychotics, general anaesthetics, other hypnotics or sedatives, and opioid analgesics. The sedative effect of benzodiazepines may also be enhanced by cisapride. Similar effects may be produced by concomitant administration with drugs which interfere with the metabolism of benzodiazepines. Drugs which have been reported to alter the pharmacokinetics of benzodiazepines are discussed in detail below but few of these interactions are likely to be of clinical significance. Benzodiazepines such as diazepam which are metabolised primarily by hepatic microsomal oxidation may be more susceptible to pharmacokinetic changes than those eliminated primarily by glucuronide conjugation.

Analgesics. The peak plasma concentration of oxazepam was significantly decreased during treatment with *diflunisal* in 6 healthy subjects, while the renal clearance of the glucuronide metabolite was reduced and its mean elimination half-life increased from 10 to 13 hours.[1] Diflunisal also displaced oxazepam from plasma protein binding sites *in vitro*. *Aspirin* shortened the time to induce anaesthesia with midazolam in 78 patients also possibly due to competition for plasma protein binding sites.[2] *Paracetamol* produced no significant change in plasma concentrations of diazepam or its major metabolite and only marginal changes in urine concentrations in 4 healthy subjects.[3]

Benzodiazepines such as diazepam, lorazepam, and midazolam may be used with opioid analgesics in anaesthetic or analgesic regimens. An additive sedative effect is to be expected[4] but there are also reports of severe respiratory depression with midazolam and *fentanyl*[5] or sudden hypotension with midazolam and fentanyl[6] or *sufentanil*.[7] The clearance of midazolam appears to be reduced by fentanyl,[8] possibly as a result of competitive inhibition of metabolism by the cytochrome P450 isozyme CYP3A. Careful monitoring is therefore required during concomitant administration of midazolam with these opioids and the dose of both drugs may need to be reduced. Synergistic potentiation of the induction of anaesthesia has been reported between midazolam and fentanyl,[9] but one study has suggested that midazolam can diminish the analgesic effects of sufentanil.[10] Pretreatment with *morphine* or *pethidine* has decreased the rate of oral absorption of diazepam. This has been attributed to the effect of opioid analgesics on gastro-intestinal motility.[11]

Dextropropoxyphene prolonged the half-life and reduced the clearance of alprazolam but not diazepam or lorazepam in healthy subjects.[12]

1. Van Hecken AM, *et al.* The influence of diflunisal on the pharmacokinetics of oxazepam. *Br J Clin Pharmacol* 1985; **20:** 225–34.
2. Dundee JW, *et al.* Aspirin and probenecid pretreatment influences the potency of thiopentone and the onset of action of midazolam. *Eur J Anaesthesiol* 1986; **3:** 247–51.
3. Mulley BA, *et al.* Interactions between diazepam and paracetamol. *J Clin Pharm* 1978; **3:** 25–35.
4. Tverskoy M, *et al.* Midazolam-morphine sedative interaction in patients. *Anesth Analg* 1989; **68:** 282–5.
5. Yaster M, *et al.* Midazolam-fentanyl intravenous sedation in children: case report of respiratory arrest. *Pediatrics* 1990; **86:** 463–7.
6. Burtin P, *et al.* Hypotension with midazolam and fentanyl in the newborn. *Lancet* 1991; **337:** 1545–6.
7. West JM, *et al.* Sudden hypotension associated with midazolam and sufentanil. *Anesth Analg* 1987; **66:** 693–4.
8. Hase I, *et al.* I.V. fentanyl decreases the clearance of midazolam. *Br J Anaesth* 1997; **79:** 740–3.
9. Ben-Shlomo I, *et al.* Midazolam acts synergistically with fentanyl for induction of anaesthesia. *Br J Anaesth* 1990; **64:** 45–7.
10. Luger TJ, Morawetz RF. Clinical evidence for a midazolam-sufentanil interaction in patients with major trauma. *Clin Pharmacol Ther* 1991; **49:** 133.
11. Gamble JAS, *et al.* Some pharmacological factors influencing the absorption of diazepam following oral administration. *Br J Anaesth* 1976; **48:** 1181–5.
12. Abernethy DR, *et al.* Interaction of propoxyphene with diazepam, alprazolam and lorazepam. *Br J Clin Pharmacol* 1985; **19:** 51–7.

Antiarrhythmics. An interaction between clonazepam and existing therapy with amiodarone was suspected in a 78-year-old man who experienced symptoms of benzodiazepine toxicity 2 months after starting with clonazepam 0.5 mg given at bedtime for restless leg syndrome;[1] symptoms resolved on withdrawal of clonazepam.

1. Witt DM, *et al.* Amiodarone-clonazepam interaction. *Ann Pharmacother* 1993; **27:** 1463–4.

Antibacterials. Both *erythromycin*[1] and *triacetyloleandomycin*[2] have been reported to inhibit the hepatic metabolism of triazolam in healthy subjects. Peak plasma-triazolam concentrations were increased, half-life prolonged, and clearance reduced. Triacetyloleandomycin prolonged the psychomotor impairment and amnesia produced by triazolam.[2] Loss of consciousness following erythromycin infusion in a child premedicated with midazolam was attributed to a similar interaction,[3] and increases in peak plasma concentrations of midazolam with profound and prolonged sedation have been reported following administration of erythromycin.[4] Concomitant administration of midazolam and erythromycin should be avoided or the dose of midazolam reduced by 50 to 75%. *Roxithromycin* has also been reported[5] to have some effects on the pharmacokinetics and pharmacodynamics of midazolam but it was considered that these changes were probably not clinically relevant. However, it was recommended that as a precaution the lowest possible effective dose of midazolam should be used when given with roxithromycin. In another study[6] *azithromycin* did not appear to have any effect on the metabolism or psychomotor effects of midazolam.

There is an isolated report of significant rises in steady-state blood-midazolam concentration coinciding with administration of *ciprofloxacin*.[7] Also ciprofloxacin has been reported to reduce diazepam clearance and prolong its terminal half-life,[8] although psychometric tests did not show any changes in diazepam's pharmacodynamics. However, ciprofloxacin appears to have no effect on the pharmacokinetics or pharmacodynamics of temazepam.[9]

Isoniazid has been reported to increase the half-life of a single dose of diazepam[10] and triazolam[11] but not of oxazepam[11] in healthy subjects. In contrast, *rifampicin* has decreased the half-life of diazepam[12] and midazolam[13] while *ethambutol* has no effect on diazepam pharmacokinetics.[10] In patients receiving therapy for tuberculosis with a combination of isoniazid, rifampicin, and ethambutol the half-life of a single diazepam dose was shortened and its clearance increased.[10] Thus the enzyme-inducing effect of rifampicin appears to predominate over the enzyme-inhibiting effect of isoniazid.

1. Phillips JP, *et al.* A pharmacokinetic drug interaction between erythromycin and triazolam. *J Clin Psychopharmacol* 1986; **6:** 297–9.
2. Warot D, *et al.* Troleandomycin-triazolam interaction in healthy volunteers: pharmacokinetic and psychometric evaluation. *Eur J Clin Pharmacol* 1987; **32:** 389–93.
3. Hiller A, *et al.* Unconsciousness associated with midazolam and erythromycin. *Br J Anaesth* 1990; **65:** 826–8.
4. Olkkola KT, *et al.* A potentially hazardous interaction between erythromycin and midazolam. *Clin Pharmacol Ther* 1993; **53:** 298–305.
5. Backman JT, *et al.* A pharmacokinetic interaction between roxithromycin and midazolam. *Eur J Clin Pharmacol* 1994; **46:** 551–5.
6. Mattila MJ, *et al.* Azithromycin does not alter the effects of oral midazolam on human performance. *Eur J Clin Pharmacol* 1994; **47:** 49–52.
7. Orko R, *et al.* Intravenous infusion of midazolam, propofol and vecuronium in a patient with severe tetanus. *Acta Anaesthesiol Scand* 1988; **32:** 590–2.
8. Kamali F, *et al.* The influence of steady-state ciprofloxacin on the pharmacokinetics and pharmacodynamics of a single dose of diazepam in healthy volunteers. *Eur J Clin Pharmacol* 1993; **44:** 365–7.
9. Kamali F, *et al.* The influence of ciprofloxacin on the pharmacokinetics and pharmacodynamics of a single dose of temazepam in the young and elderly. *J Clin Pharm Ther* 1994; **19:** 105–9.
10. Ochs HR, *et al.* Diazepam interaction with antituberculous drugs. *Clin Pharmacol Ther* 1981; **29:** 671–8.
11. Ochs HR, *et al.* Differential effect of isoniazid on triazolam oxidation and oxazepam conjugation. *Br J Clin Pharmacol* 1983; **16:** 743–6.
12. Brockmeyer N, *et al.* The metabolism of diazepam following different enzyme inducing agents. *Br J Clin Pharmacol* 1985; **19:** 544P.
13. Backman JT, *et al.* Rifampin drastically reduces plasma concentrations and effects of oral midazolam. *Clin Pharmacol Ther* 1996; **59:** 7–13.

Anticoagulants. Reduced plasma binding of diazepam and desmethyldiazepam and increases in the free concentrations without changes in the total blood or plasma concentrations occurred immediately following *heparin* intravenously.[1]

Benzodiazepines do not usually interact with oral anticoagulants although there have been rare reports of altered anticoagulant activity.

1. Routledge PA, *et al.* Diazepam and N-desmethyldiazepam redistribution after heparin. *Clin Pharmacol Ther* 1980; **27:** 528–32.

Antidepressants. It has been recommended that the dosage of alprazolam should be reduced when given with *fluvoxamine* as concomitant administration has resulted in doubling of plasma-alprazolam concentrations.[1] Since plasma concentrations of bromazepam[2] and of diazepam[3] also appear to be affected by fluvoxamine it has been suggested that patients taking fluvoxamine who require a benzodiazepine should preferentially receive a benzodiazepine such as lorazepam which has a different metabolic pathway.[3] Small studies suggest that *fluoxetine* can also increase plasma concentrations of alprazolam.[4,5] Fluoxetine appears to have a similar effect on diazepam but plasma concentrations of diazepam's active metabolite desmethyldiazepam are reduced and it is considered that the overall effect is likely to be minor.[6] The potential for a clinically significant interaction with *sertraline, paroxetine,* or *citalopram* is considered to be less.[7]

The manufacturers have reported that alprazolam may increase the steady-state plasma concentrations of *imipramine* and *desipramine*, although the clinical significance of such changes is unknown. For a suggestion that benzodiazepines may increase the oxidation of *amineptine* to a toxic metabolite, see under Effects on the Liver in Adverse Effects of Amitriptyline, p.274.

Concomitant administration of *nefazodone* has been reported to result in raised concentrations of alprazolam and triazolam, increased sedation, and impairment of psychomotor performance.[8,9] Nefazodone may inhibit the oxidative metabolism of alprazolam and triazolam. No interaction was reported with lorazepam which is primarily eliminated by conjunction.

For reference to an isolated report of hypothermia after administration of diazepam and *lithium*, see p.294.

There have been occasional reports of sexual disinhibition in patients taking *tryptophan* with benzodiazepines.

1. Fleishaker JC, Hulst LK. A pharmacokinetic and pharmacodynamic evaluation of the combined administration of alprazolam and fluvoxamine. *Eur J Clin Pharmacol* 1994; **46:** 35–9.
2. Van Harten J, *et al.* Influence of multiple-dose administration of fluvoxamine on the pharmacokinetics of the benzodiazepines bromazepam and lorazepam: a randomized crossover study. *Eur Neuropsychopharmacol* 1992; **2:** 381.
3. Perucca E, *et al.* Inhibition of diazepam metabolism by fluvoxamine: a pharmacokinetic study in normal volunteers. *Clin Pharmacol Ther* 1994; **56:** 471–6.
4. Lasher TA, *et al.* Pharmacokinetic pharmacodynamic evaluation of the combined administration of alprazolam and fluoxetine. *Psychopharmacology (Berl)* 1991; **104:** 323–7.
5. Greenblatt DJ, *et al.* Fluoxetine impairs clearance of alprazolam but not of clonazepam. *Clin Pharmacol Ther* 1992; **52:** 479–86.
6. Lemberger L, *et al.* The effect of fluoxetine on the pharmacokinetics and psychomotor responses of diazepam. *Clin Pharmacol Ther* 1988; **43:** 412–19.
7. Sproule BA, *et al.* Selective serotonin reuptake inhibitors and CNS drug interactions: a critical review of the evidence. *Clin Pharmacokinet* 1997; **33:** 454–71.
8. Greene DS, *et al.* Coadministration of nefazodone (NEF) and benzodiazepines I: pharmacokinetic assessment. *Clin Pharmacol Ther* 1994; **55:** 141.
9. Kroboth P, *et al.* Coadministration of nefazodone and benzodiazepines II: pharmacodynamic assessment. *Clin Pharmacol Ther* 1994; **55:** 142.

Antiepileptics. *Carbamazepine, phenobarbitone,* and *phenytoin* are all inducers of hepatic drug-metabolising enzymes. Therefore, in patients receiving long-term therapy with these drugs the metabolism of benzodiazepines may be enhanced. Interactions between benzodiazepines and these antiepileptics are further discussed on p.342 (carbamazepine) and p.356 (phenytoin).

Sodium valproate has been reported to displace diazepam from plasma-protein binding sites.[1] Sporadic reports exist of adverse effects when valproate is given with clonazepam[2,3] with the development of drowsiness and, more seriously, absence status epilepticus, but the existence of an interaction is considered to be unproven.[4] Drowsiness has also been reported when valproate was given with nitrazepam.[5] Concomitant administration of semisodium valproate and lorazepam has resulted in raised concentrations of lorazepam due to inhibition of glucuronidation of lorazepam.[6]

1. Dhillon S, Richens A. Valproic acid and diazepam interaction in vivo. *Br J Clin Pharmacol* 1982; **13:** 553–60.
2. Watson WA. Interaction between clonazepam and sodium valproate. *N Engl J Med* 1979; **300:** 678.
3. Browne TR. Interaction between clonazepam and sodium valproate. *N Engl J Med* 1979; **300:** 679.
4. Levy RH, Koch KM. Drug interactions with valproic acid. *Drugs* 1982; **24:** 543–56.
5. Jeavons PM, *et al.* Treatment of generalised epilepsies of childhood and adolescence with sodium valproate (Epilim). *Dev Med Child Neurol* 1977; **19:** 9–25.
6. Samara EE, *et al.* Effect of valproate on the pharmacokinetics and pharmacodynamics of lorazepam. *J Clin Pharmacol* 1997; **37:** 442–50.

Antifungals. Both a single dose and multiple doses of *ketoconazole* decreased the clearance of a single intravenous injection of chlordiazepoxide.[1] Ketoconazole was considered to inhibit at least one subset of the hepatic mixed-function oxidase system. Studies[2-4] have shown that ketoconazole and *itraconazole* can produce marked pharmacokinetic interactions with midazolam or triazolam and greatly increase the intensity and duration of action of these benzodiazepines. One study[5] indicated that the risk of interaction persists for several days after cessation of itraconazole therapy. It is recommended that the concomitant use of these antifungals and benzodiazepines should be avoided or that the dose of the benzodiazepine should be greatly reduced. One group of workers[2] found that the area under the plasma concentration-time curve for midazolam was increased by 15 times by ketoconazole and by 10 times by itraconazole while peak plasma concentrations of midazolam were increased fourfold and threefold respectively. They also found[3] that the area under the curve for triazolam was increased by 22 times by ketoconazole and by 27 times by itraconazole; peak plasma concentrations of triazolam were increased about threefold by both antifungals. A similar but less pronounced interaction occurs between *fluconazole* and midazolam[6] or triazolam;[7] nonetheless the dosage of the benzodiazepine should be reduced during concomitant use.

1. Brown MW, *et al.* Effect of ketoconazole on hepatic oxidative drug metabolism. *Clin Pharmacol Ther* 1985; **37:** 290–7.
2. Olkkola KT, *et al.* Midazolam should be avoided in patients receiving the systemic antimycotics ketoconazole or itraconazole. *Clin Pharmacol Ther* 1994; **55:** 481–5.
3. Varhe A, *et al.* Oral triazolam is potentially hazardous to patients receiving systemic antimycotics ketoconazole or itraconazole. *Clin Pharmacol Ther* 1994; **56:** 601–7.
4. Greenblatt DJ, *et al.* Interaction of triazolam and ketoconazole. *Lancet* 1995; **345:** 191.
5. Neuvonen PJ, *et al.* The effect of ingestion time interval on the interaction between itraconazole and triazolam. *Clin Pharmacol Ther* 1996; **60:** 326–31.
6. Ahonen J, *et al.* Effect of route of administration of fluconazole on the interaction between fluconazole and midazolam. *Eur J Clin Pharmacol* 1997; **51:** 415–19.
7. Varhe A, *et al.* Effect of fluconazole dose on the extent of fluconazole-triazolam interaction. *Br J Clin Pharmacol* 1996; **42:** 465–70.

Antihistamines. A suggestion[1] that a reduction in temazepam metabolism caused by *diphenhydramine* may have contributed to perinatal death after ingestion of these drugs by the mother.

1. Kargas GA, *et al.* Perinatal mortality due to interaction of diphenhydramine and temazepam. *N Engl J Med* 1985; **313:** 1417–18.

Antivirals. *Delavirdine* and HIV-protease inhibitors such as *indinavir, nelfinavir,* and *ritonavir* may inhibit the hepatic microsomal systems involved in the metabolism of some benzodiazepines. Concomitant administration requires monitoring and dosage adjustments for the benzodiazepine or should be avoided. Benzodiazepines which should not be used concomitantly with HIV-protease inhibitors include alprazolam, clorazepate, diazepam, estazolam, flurazepam, midazolam, and triazolam.

Beta blockers. A clear pattern of interactions between benzodiazepines and beta blockers has not emerged. *Propranolol* may inhibit the metabolism of diazepam[1,2] and bromazepam,[3] and *metoprolol* inhibit the metabolism of diazepam[1,4] or bromazepam[5] to some extent although in many cases the effect on pharmacokinetics and pharmacodynamics is unlikely to be of clinical significance. No significant pharmacokinetic interaction has been observed between propranolol and alprazolam,[2] lorazepam,[2] or oxazepam,[6] although the rate of alprazolam absorption may be decreased.[2] Similarly no pharmacokinetic interaction has been observed between *atenolol* and diazepam,[1] *labetalol* and oxazepam,[6] or metoprolol and lorazepam.[5]

1. Hawksworth G, *et al.* Diazepam/β-adrenoceptor antagonist interactions. *Br J Clin Pharmacol* 1984; **17:** 69S–76S.
2. Ochs HR, *et al.* Propranolol interactions with diazepam, lorazepam, and alprazolam. *Clin Pharmacol Ther* 1984; **36:** 451–5.
3. Ochs HR, *et al.* Bromazepam pharmacokinetics: influence of age, gender, oral contraceptives, cimetidine, and propranolol. *Clin Pharmacol Ther* 1987; **41:** 562–70.
4. Klotz U, Reimann IW. Pharmacokinetic and pharmacodynamic interaction study of diazepam and metoprolol. *Eur J Clin Pharmacol* 1984; **26:** 223–6.
5. Scott AK, *et al.* Interaction of metoprolol with lorazepam and bromazepam. *Eur J Clin Pharmacol* 1991; **40:** 405–9.
6. Sonne J, *et al.* Single dose pharmacokinetics and pharmacodynamics of oral oxazepam during concomitant administration of propranolol and labetalol. *Br J Clin Pharmacol* 1990; **29:** 33–7.

Calcium-channel blockers. Peak plasma concentrations of midazolam were doubled and the elimination half-life of midazolam prolonged when midazolam was given to healthy subjects receiving *diltiazem* or *verapamil*.[1] A similar interaction has been demonstrated between diltiazem and triazolam.[2,3] Concomitant administration should be avoided or the dose of these benzodiazepines reduced.

1. Backman JT, *et al.* Dose of midazolam should be reduced during diltiazem and verapamil treatments. *Br J Clin Pharmacol* 1994; **37:** 221–5.
2. Varhe A, *et al.* Diltiazem enhances the effects of triazolam by inhibiting its metabolism. *Clin Pharmacol Ther* 1996; **59:** 369–75.
3. Kosuge K, *et al.* Enhanced effect of triazolam with diltiazem. *Br J Clin Pharmacol* 1997; **43:** 367–72.

Clonidine. Anxiety was reduced and sedation was enhanced when *clonidine* was given with flunitrazepam for premedication.[1]

1. Kulka PJ, *et al.* Sedative and anxiolytic interactions of clonidine and benzodiazepines. *Br J Anaesth* 1994; **72** (suppl 1): 81.

Clozapine. For reports of cardiorespiratory collapse and other adverse effects in patients taking benzodiazepines and clozapine, see p.659.

Cyclosporin. *In-vitro* studies suggested that cyclosporin could inhibit the metabolism of midazolam.[1] However, blood-cyclosporin concentrations in patients given cyclosporin to prevent graft rejection were considered too low to result in such an interaction.

1. Li G, *et al.* Is cyclosporin A an inhibitor of drug metabolism? *Br J Clin Pharmacol* 1990; **30:** 71–7.

Digoxin. For the effects of alprazolam and diazepam on digoxin pharmacokinetics, see p.851.

Disulfiram. Evidence from healthy and alcoholic subjects suggests that chronic treatment with disulfiram can inhibit the metabolism of chlordiazepoxide and diazepam leading to a prolonged half-life and reduced clearance; there was little effect on the disposition of oxazepam.[1] No significant pharmacokinetic interaction was observed between disulfiram and alprazolam in alcoholic patients.[2] Temazepam toxicity, attributed to concomitant administration of disulfiram and temazepam has been reported.[3]

See also under Disulfiram, p.1573.

1. MacLeod SM, *et al.* Interaction of disulfiram with benzodiazepines. *Clin Pharmacol Ther* 1978; **24:** 583–9.
2. Diquet B, *et al.* Lack of interaction between disulfiram and alprazolam in alcoholic patients. *Eur J Clin Pharmacol* 1990; **38:** 157–60.
3. Hardman M, *et al.* Temazepam toxicity precipitated by disulfiram. *Lancet* 1994; **344:** 1231–2.

Gastro-intestinal drugs. *Antacids* have variable effects on the absorption of benzodiazepines[1-6] but any resulting interaction is unlikely to be of major clinical significance.

Several studies, usually involving single doses of diazepam given to healthy subjects, have demonstrated that *cimetidine* can inhibit the hepatic metabolism of diazepam.[7-10] The clearance of diazepam has generally been decreased and the half-life prolonged. Some studies have also demonstrated impaired metabolic clearance of the major metabolite, desmethyldiazepam (nordazepam). Cimetidine has also been reported to inhibit the metabolism of other benzodiazepines (generally those metabolised by oxidation) including adinazolam,[11] alprazolam,[12,13] bromazepam,[14] chlordiazepoxide,[15] clobazam,[16,17] flurazepam,[18] midazolam,[19] nitrazepam,[20] and triazolam.[12,13] Cimetidine does not appear to inhibit the hepatic metabolism of lorazepam,[18] oxazepam,[18] or temazepam.[21] The clinical significance of these interactions between cimetidine and benzodiazepines remains dubious. Studies which have assessed the effect of cimetidine on the pharmacology as well as the pharmacokinetics of benzodiazepines have found little effect on cognitive function or degree of sedation.

Most studies have failed to demonstrate an effect of *ranitidine* on the hepatic metabolism of diazepam,[22-25] although Fee *et al.*[26] reported an increase in the bioavailability of a single dose of midazolam given by mouth, and considered that an effect on hepatic clearance was more likely than an effect on absorption. The results of Fee *et al.* were consistent with those of another study which demonstrated an enhanced sedative effect of midazolam in patients pretreated with ranitidine.[27] Ranitidine has been reported to have no effect on the pharmacokinetics of lorazepam[23] or on the sedative effect of temazepam[27] but has increased the bioavailability of triazolam.[28]

Famotidine[10] or *nizatidine*[25] do not appear to inhibit the hepatic metabolism of diazepam.

Oral diazepam was absorbed more rapidly after the intravenous administration of *metoclopramide*.[29] Enhanced motility of the gastro-intestinal tract was implicated. *Cisapride* may also accelerate the absorption of diazepam.[30]

Studies of continuous *omeprazole* administration on the pharmacokinetics of a single intravenous dose of diazepam in healthy subjects indicate inhibition of diazepam metabolism in a similar manner to cimetidine.[31,32] Omeprazole decreases the clearance and prolongs the elimination half-life of diazepam; in addition both the formation and elimination of desmethyldiazepam appear to be decreased. The effects may be greater in rapid than in slow metabolisers of omeprazole[33] and vary between ethnic groups.[34] The clinical significance of the interaction remains to be established. *Lansoprazole*[35] and *pantoprazole*[36] have been reported not to affect the pharmacokinetics of diazepam.

1. Nair SG, *et al.* The influence of three antacids on the absorption and clinical action of oral diazepam. *Br J Anaesth* 1976; **48:** 1175–80.
2. Greenblatt DJ, *et al.* Diazepam absorption: effect of antacids and food. *Clin Pharmacol Ther* 1978; **24:** 600–9.
3. Greenblatt DJ, *et al.* Influence of magnesium and aluminum hydroxide mixture on chlordiazepoxide absorption. *Clin Pharmacol Ther* 1976; **19:** 234–9.
4. Shader RI, *et al.* Impaired absorption of desmethyldiazepam from clorazepate by magnesium aluminum hydroxide. *Clin Pharmacol Ther* 1978; **24:** 308–15.
5. Chun AHC, *et al.* Effect of antacids on absorption of clorazepate. *Clin Pharmacol Ther* 1977; **22:** 329–35.
6. Shader RI, *et al.* Steady-state plasma desmethyldiazepam during long-term clorazepate use: effect of antacids. *Clin Pharmacol Ther* 1982; **31:** 180–3.
7. Klotz U, Reimann I. Delayed clearance of diazepam due to cimetidine. *N Engl J Med* 1980; **302:** 1012–14.
8. Gough PA, *et al.* Influence of cimetidine on oral diazepam elimination with measurement of subsequent cognitive change. *Br J Clin Pharmacol* 1982; **14:** 739–42.
9. Greenblatt DJ, *et al.* Clinical importance of the interaction of diazepam and cimetidine. *N Engl J Med* 1984; **310:** 1639–43.
10. Locniskar A, *et al.* Interaction of diazepam with famotidine and cimetidine, two H_2-receptor antagonists. *J Clin Pharmacol* 1986; **26:** 299–303.
11. Hulhoven R, *et al.* Influence of repeated administration of cimetidine on the pharmacokinetics and pharmacodynamics of adinazolam in healthy subjects. *Eur J Clin Pharmacol* 1988; **35:** 59–64.
12. Abernethy DR, *et al.* Interaction of cimetidine with the triazolobenzodiazepines alprazolam and triazolam. *Psychopharmacology (Berl)* 1983; **80:** 275–8.
13. Pourbaix S, *et al.* Pharmacokinetic consequences of long term coadministration of cimetidine and triazolobenzodiazepines, alprazolam and triazolam, in healthy subjects. *Int J Clin Pharmacol Ther Toxicol* 1985; **23:** 447–51.
14. Ochs HR, *et al.* Bromazepam pharmacokinetics: influence of age, gender, oral contraceptives, cimetidine, and propranolol. *Clin Pharmacol Ther* 1987; **41:** 562–70.
15. Desmond PV, *et al.* Cimetidine impairs elimination of chlordiazepoxide (Librium) in man. *Ann Intern Med* 1980; **93:** 266–8.
16. Grigoleit H-G, *et al.* Pharmacokinetic aspects of the interaction between clobazam and cimetidine. *Eur J Clin Pharmacol* 1983; **25:** 139–42.
17. Pullar T, *et al.* The effect of cimetidine on the single dose pharmacokinetics of oral clobazam and N-desmethylclobazam. *Br J Clin Pharmacol* 1987; **23:** 317–21.
18. Greenblatt DJ, *et al.* Interaction of cimetidine with oxazepam, lorazepam, and flurazepam. *J Clin Pharmacol* 1984; **24:** 187–93.
19. Sanders LD, *et al.* Interaction of H2-receptor antagonists and benzodiazepine sedation: a double-blind placebo-controlled investigation of the effects of cimetidine and ranitidine on recovery after intravenous midazolam. *Anaesthesia* 1993; **48:** 286–92.
20. Ochs HR, *et al.* Cimetidine impairs nitrazepam clearance. *Clin Pharmacol Ther* 1983; **34:** 227–30.
21. Greenblatt DJ, *et al.* Noninteraction of temazepam and cimetidine. *J Pharm Sci* 1984; **73:** 399–401.
22. Klotz U, *et al.* Effect of ranitidine on the steady state pharmacokinetics of diazepam. *Eur J Clin Pharmacol* 1983; **24:** 357–60.
23. Abernethy DR, *et al.* Ranitidine does not impair oxidative or conjugative metabolism: noninteraction with antipyrine, diazepam, and lorazepam. *Clin Pharmacol Ther* 1984; **35:** 188–92.
24. Fee JPH, *et al.* Diazepam disposition following cimetidine or ranitidine. *Br J Clin Pharmacol* 1984; **17:** 617P–18P.
25. Klotz U, *et al.* Nocturnal doses of ranitidine and nizatidine do not affect the disposition of diazepam. *J Clin Pharmacol* 1987; **27:** 210–12.
26. Fee JPH, *et al.* Cimetidine and ranitidine increase midazolam bioavailability. *Clin Pharmacol Ther* 1987; **41:** 80–4.
27. Wilson CM, *et al.* Effect of pretreatment with ranitidine on the hypnotic action of single doses of midazolam, temazepam and zopiclone. *Br J Anaesth* 1986; **58:** 483–6.
28. Vanderveen RP, *et al.* Effect of ranitidine on the disposition of orally and intravenously administered triazolam. *Clin Pharm* 1991; **10:** 539–43.
29. Gamble JAS, *et al.* Some pharmacological factors influencing the absorption of diazepam following oral administration. *Br J Anaesth* 1976; **48:** 1181–5.
30. Bateman DN. The action of cisapride on gastric emptying and the pharmacokinetics of oral diazepam. *Eur J Clin Pharmacol* 1986; **30:** 205–8.
31. Gugler R, Jensen JC. Omeprazole inhibits elimination of diazepam. *Lancet* 1984; **i:** 969.
32. Andersson T, *et al.* Effect of omeprazole and cimetidine on plasma diazepam levels. *Eur J Clin Pharmacol* 1990; **39:** 51–4.
33. Andersson T, *et al.* Effect of omeprazole treatment on diazepam plasma levels in slow versus normal rapid metabolizers of omeprazole. *Clin Pharmacol Ther* 1990; **47:** 79–85.
34. Caraco Y, *et al.* Interethnic difference in omeprazole's inhibition of diazepam metabolism. *Clin Pharmacol Ther* 1995; **58:** 62–72.
35. Lefebvre RA, *et al.* Influence of lansoprazole treatment on diazepam plasma concentrations. *Clin Pharmacol Ther* 1992; **52:** 458–63.
36. Gugler R, *et al.* Lack of pharmacokinetic interaction of pantoprazole with diazepam in man. *Br J Clin Pharmacol* 1996; **42:** 249–52.

General anaesthetics. A synergistic interaction has been demonstrated for the hypnotic effects of midazolam and *thiopentone*.[1] Although midazolam failed to produce anaesthesia at the doses used, the drug caused a twofold increase in the anaesthetic potency of thiopentone. Similar synergistic interactions have been observed between midazolam and both *methohexitone*[2] and *propofol*.[3,4] The interaction between midazolam and propofol could not be explained solely by alteration in free-plasma concentration of either drug.[5] Midazolam has also been reported to be able to produce a marked reduction in the concentration of halothane required for anaesthesia.[6]

1. Short TG, *et al.* Hypnotic and anaesthetic action of thiopentone and midazolam alone and in combination. *Br J Anaesth* 1991; **66:** 13–19.
2. Tverskoy M, *et al.* Midazolam acts synergistically with methohexitone for induction of anaesthesia. *Br J Anaesth* 1989; **63:** 109–12.
3. McClune S, *et al.* Synergistic interaction between midazolam and propofol. *Br J Anaesth* 1992; **69:** 240–5.
4. Short TG, Chui PT. Propofol and midazolam act synergistically in combination. *Br J Anaesth* 1991; **67:** 539–45.
5. Teh J, *et al.* Pharmacokinetic interactions between midazolam and propofol: an infusion study. *Br J Anaesth* 1994; **72:** 62–5.
6. Inagaki Y, *et al.* Anesthetic interaction between midazolam and halothane in humans. *Anesth Analg* 1993; **76:** 613–7.

Grapefruit juice. Grapefruit juice has been reported to be able to increase the bioavailability of oral midazolam[1] or triazolam[2] and to raise peak plasma concentrations.

1. Kupferschmidt HHT, *et al.* Interaction between grapefruit juice and midazolam in humans. *Clin Pharmacol Ther* 1995; **58:** 20–8.
2. Hukkinen SK, *et al.* Plasma concentrations of triazolam are increased by concomitant ingestion of grapefruit juice. *Clin Pharmacol Ther* 1995; **58:** 127–31.

Kava. A patient whose medication included alprazolam, cimetidine, and terazosin became lethargic and disoriented after starting to take kava.[1] An interaction between kava and the benzodiazepine was suspected.

1. Almeida JC, Grimsley EW. Coma from the health food store: interaction between kava and alprazolam. *Ann Intern Med* 1996; **125:** 940–1.

Levodopa. For reference to the effects of benzodiazepines on levodopa, see p.1139.

Neuromuscular blockers. For reference to the effect of diazepam on neuromuscular blockade, see p.1306.

Oral contraceptives. Some studies with alprazolam,[1] chlordiazepoxide,[2] and diazepam[3] have supported suggestions that oral contraceptives may inhibit the biotransformation of benzodiazepines metabolised by oxidation, although no significant pharmacokinetic alterations have been observed with clotiazepam,[4] or triazolam.[1] The biotransformation of benzodiazepines metabolised by conjugation, such as lorazepam, oxazepam, or temazepam, may be enhanced[1,2] or unchanged.[5] No consistent correlation has been observed between the above pharmacokinetic changes and clinical effects. Ellinwood *et al.*[6] observed that psychomotor impairment due to oral diazepam was greater during the menstrual pause than during the 21-daily oral contraceptive cycle. This may have been due to an effect of oral contraceptives on diazepam absorption. As part of their pharmacokinetic study, Kroboth *et al.*,[7] noted that women taking oral contraceptives appeared to be more sensitive to psychomotor impairment following single oral doses of alprazolam, lorazepam, or triazolam, than controls. The effects of temazepam were minimal in both groups. Alterations in sedative or amnesic effect could not be established with any certainty.

1. Stoehr GP, *et al.* Effect of oral contraceptives on triazolam, temazepam, alprazolam, and lorazepam kinetics. *Clin Pharmacol Ther* 1984; **36:** 683–90.
2. Patwardhan RV, *et al.* Differential effects of oral contraceptive steroids on the metabolism of benzodiazepines. *Hepatology* 1983; **3:** 248–53.
3. Abernethy DR, *et al.* Impairment of diazepam metabolism by low-dose estrogen-containing oral-contraceptive steroids. *N Engl J Med* 1982; **306:** 791–2.
4. Ochs HR, *et al.* Disposition of clotiazepam: influence of age, sex, oral contraceptives, cimetidine, isoniazid and ethanol. *Eur J Clin Pharmacol* 1984; **26:** 55–9.
5. Abernethy DR, *et al.* Lorazepam and oxazepam kinetics in women on low-dose oral contraceptives. *Clin Pharmacol Ther* 1983; **33:** 628–32.
6. Ellinwood EH, *et al.* Effects of oral contraceptives on diazepam-induced psychomotor impairment. *Clin Pharmacol Ther* 1984; **35:** 360–6.
7. Kroboth PD, *et al.* Pharmacodynamic evaluation of the benzodiazepine-oral contraceptive interaction. *Clin Pharmacol Ther* 1985; **38:** 525–32.

Penicillamine. Phlebitis associated with intravenous diazepam resolved with local heat but recurred on two separate occasions after oral penicillamine.[1]

1. Brandstetter RD, *et al.* Exacerbation of intravenous diazepam-induced phlebitis by oral penicillamine. *Br Med J* 1981; **283:** 525.

Probenecid. Probenecid increased the half-life of intravenous lorazepam in 9 healthy subjects.[1] Probenecid was considered to impair glucuronide formation selectively and thus the clearance of drugs like lorazepam. Probenecid has also shortened the time to induce anaesthesia with midazolam in 46 patients.[2] The effect was considered to be due to competition for plasma protein binding sites. It has been suggested that the initial dose of adinazolam should be reduced and subsequent dosage monitored when it is administered with probenecid.[3] A study[3] in 16 subjects had indicated that probenecid could potentiate the psychomotor effects of adinazolam. This appeared to be mainly due to inhibition of the renal clearance of *N*-desmethyladinazolam. Probenecid has also been reported[4] to reduce the clearance of nitrazepam but not of temazepam.

1. Abernethy DR, *et al.* Probenecid inhibition of acetaminophen and lorazepam glucuronidation. *Clin Pharmacol Ther* 1984; **35:** 224.
2. Dundee JW, *et al.* Aspirin and probenecid pretreatment influences the potency of thiopentone and the onset of action of midazolam. *Eur J Anaesthesiol* 1986; **3:** 247–51.
3. Golden PL, *et al.* Effects of probenecid on the pharmacokinetics and pharmacodynamics of adinazolam in humans. *Clin Pharmacol Ther* 1994; **56:** 133–41.
4. Brockmeyer NH, *et al.* Comparative effects of rifampin and/or probenecid on the pharmacokinetics of temazepam and nitrazepam. *Int J Clin Pharmacol Ther Toxicol* 1990; **28:** 387–93.

Smooth muscle relaxants. Intracavernosal *papaverine* produced prolonged erection in 2 patients who had been given intravenous diazepam as an anxiolytic before the papaverine injection.[1]

1. Vale JA, *et al.* Papaverine, benzodiazepines, and prolonged erections. *Lancet* 1991; **337:** 1552.

Tobacco smoking. The Boston Collaborative Drug Surveillance Program reported drowsiness as a side-effect of diazepam or chlordiazepoxide less frequently in smokers than non smokers.[1] Pharmacokinetic studies have, however, been divided between those indicating that smoking induces the hepatic metabolism of benzodiazepines and those showing no effect on benzodiazepine pharmacokinetics.[2] Hence, diminished end-organ responsiveness may in part account for the observed clinical effects. Concomitant consumption of large amounts of xanthine-containing beverages may decrease any enzyme-inducing effects of smoking.[3]

1. Boston Collaborative Drug Surveillance Program, Boston University Medical Center. Clinical depression of the central nervous system due to diazepam and chlordiazepoxide in relation to cigarette smoking and age. *N Engl J Med* 1973; **288:** 277–80.
2. Miller LG. Cigarettes and drug therapy: pharmacokinetic and pharmacodynamic considerations. *Clin Pharm* 1990; **9:** 125–35.
3. Downing RW, Rickels K. Coffee consumption, cigarette smoking and reporting of drowsiness in anxious patients treated with benzodiazepines or placebo. *Acta Psychiatr Scand* 1981; **64:** 398–408.

Xanthines. There are reports of *aminophylline* given intravenously reversing the sedation from intravenous diazepam,[1-3] although not always completely[2] nor as effectively as flumazenil.[4] Blockade of adenosine receptors by aminophylline has been postulated as the mechanism of this interaction.[3,5]

Xanthine-containing beverages may be expected to decrease the incidence of benzodiazepine-induced drowsiness because of their CNS-stimulating effects and their ability to induce hepatic drug-metabolising enzymes. However, decreased drowsiness has only sometimes been observed and the actions of xanthines may themselves be decreased by concomitant heavy tobacco smoking.[6,7]

1. Arvidsson SB, *et al.* Aminophylline antagonises diazepam sedation. *Lancet* 1982; **ii:** 1467.

2. Kleindienst G, Usinger P. Diazepam sedation is not antagonised completely by aminophylline. *Lancet* 1984; **i:** 113.
3. Niemand D, *et al.* Aminophylline inhibition of diazepam sedation: is adenosine blockade of GABA-receptors the mechanism? *Lancet* 1984: **i:** 463–4.
4. Sibai AN, *et al.* Comparison of flumazenil with aminophylline to antagonise midazolam in elderly patients. *Br J Anaesth* 1991; **66:** 591–5.
5. Henauer SA, *et al.* Theophylline antagonises diazepam-induced psychomotor impairment. *Eur J Clin Pharmacol* 1983; **25:** 743–7.
6. Downing RW, Rickels K. Coffee consumption, cigarette smoking and reporting of drowsiness in anxious patients treated with benzodiazepines or placebo. *Acta Psychiatr Scand* 1981; **64:** 398–408.
7. Ghoneim MM, *et al.* Pharmacokinetic and pharmacodynamic interactions between caffeine and diazepam. *J Clin Psychopharmacol* 1986; **6:** 75–80.

Pharmacokinetics

Diazepam is readily and completely absorbed from the gastro-intestinal tract, peak plasma concentrations occurring within about 0.5 to 2 hours of oral administration. Diazepam is rapidly absorbed after administration as a rectal solution; peak plasma concentrations are achieved after about 10 to 30 minutes but are lower than those after intravenous administration. Absorption may be erratic following intramuscular administration and lower peak plasma concentrations may be obtained compared with those following oral administration. Diazepam is highly lipid soluble and crosses the blood-brain barrier; these properties qualify it for intravenous use in short-term anaesthetic procedures, since it acts promptly on the brain, and its initial effects decrease rapidly as it is redistributed into fat depots and tissues.

Diazepam has a biphasic half-life with an initial rapid distribution phase followed by a prolonged terminal elimination phase of 1 or 2 days; its action is further prolonged by the even longer half-life of 2 to 5 days of its principal active metabolite, desmethyldiazepam (nordazepam). Diazepam and desmethyldiazepam accumulate on repeated administration and the relative proportion of desmethyldiazepam in the body increases on long-term administration. No simple correlation has been found between plasma concentrations of diazepam or its metabolites and their therapeutic effect.

Diazepam is extensively metabolised in the liver and, in addition to desmethyldiazepam, its active metabolites include oxazepam, and temazepam. It is excreted in the urine, mainly in the form of its metabolites, either free or in conjugated form. Diazepam is extensively bound to plasma proteins (98 to 99%).

The plasma half-life of diazepam and/or its metabolites is prolonged in neonates, in the elderly, and in patients with liver disease. In addition to crossing the blood-brain barrier, diazepam and its metabolites also cross the placental barrier and are distributed into breast milk.

Reviews of the pharmacokinetics of benzodiazepines.

1. Bailey L, *et al.* Clinical pharmacokinetics of benzodiazepines. *J Clin Pharmacol* 1994; **34:** 804–11.

For reference to the altered pharmacokinetics of diazepam in patients with impaired liver and kidney function and in the elderly, see under Precautions, above.

Absorption and plasma concentrations. In a study of 36 patients who had received diazepam 2 to 30 mg daily for periods from one month to 10 years, plasma-diazepam concentrations were directly related to dose and inversely related to age.[1] Most of the patients were also receiving other drugs. There was a close association between the plasma concentrations of diazepam and its metabolite desmethyldiazepam and both concentrations were independent of the duration of therapy. Plasma-diazepam concentration ranges were 0.02 to 1.01 μg per mL, and plasma-desmethyldiazepam concentration ranges were 0.055 to 1.765 μg per mL. A similar study by Greenblatt *et al.*[2] has reached the same general conclusions.

1. Rutherford DM, *et al.* Plasma concentrations of diazepam and desmethyldiazepam during chronic diazepam therapy. *Br J Clin Pharmacol* 1978; **6:** 69–73.
2. Greenblatt DJ, *et al.* Plasma diazepam and desmethyldiazepam concentrations during long-term diazepam therapy. *Br J Clin Pharmacol* 1981; **1:** 35–40.

INTRAVENOUS. In a crossover study in 8 subjects plasma-diazepam concentrations were significantly higher when diazepam was injected intravenously as a solution (Valium) than when injected in an emulsion formulation (Diazemuls).[1] This difference could not, however, be confirmed by Naylor and Burlingham.[2]

1. Fee JPH, *et al.* Bioavailability of intravenous diazepam. *Lancet* 1984; **ii:** 813.
2. Naylor HC, Burlingham AN. Pharmacokinetics of diazepam emulsion. *Lancet* 1985; **i:** 518–19.

RECTAL. In 6 *adults* given diazepam 10 mg by mouth or as a solution (Valium injection) by rectum, mean bioavailability was 76 and 81% respectively compared with the same dose by intravenous injection.[1] Bioavailability was lower with suppositories than with the solution given rectally.

In a study involving 13 epileptic *children,* administration of diazepam as a rectal solution (Valium injection) to 9, in doses of 200 to 700 μg per kg body-weight, produced peak serum concentrations within 30 minutes in all but one case.[2] In contrast, doses of 300 to 600 μg per kg as suppositories resulted in peaks only after 60 to 120 minutes or more in another group of 9 children. Although the mean dose was higher in the group given suppositories, mean serum concentration 10 minutes after administration was higher in the group given the rectal solution.

The rectal solution was considered to be more suitable than the suppositories for emergency use in a convulsing child. In a similar study, Sonander *et al.* concluded that a rectal solution was also more suitable than suppositories for the anaesthetic premedication of children.[3]

1. Dhillon S, *et al.* Bioavailability of diazepam after intravenous, oral and rectal administration in adult epileptic patients. *Br J Clin Pharmacol* 1982; **13:** 427–32.
2. Dhillon S, *et al.* Rectal absorption of diazepam in epileptic children. *Arch Dis Child* 1982; **57:** 264–7.
3. Sonander H, *et al.* Effects of the rectal administration of diazepam. *Br J Anaesth* 1985; **57:** 578–80.

Biliary excretion. In a study in 4 patients who had undergone biliary surgery,[1] biliary excretion of diazepam was insufficient to account for an enterohepatic circulation of the drug.

1. Eustace PW, *et al.* Biliary excretion of diazepam in man. *Br J Anaesth* 1975; **47:** 983–5.

Metabolism. Most benzodiazepines are highly lipophilic compounds requiring biotransformation before excretion from the body and many form active metabolites that affect the duration of action. The benzodiazepines may be classified as long-, intermediate-, or short-acting compounds.[1]

Long-acting benzodiazepines are either N_1-desalkyl derivatives (*delorazepam* and *nordazepam*) or are oxidised in the liver to N_1-desalkyl derivatives (benzodiazepines so oxidised include *chlordiazepoxide, clobazam, clorazepate, cloxazolam, diazepam, flurazepam, halazepam, ketazolam, medazepam, oxazolam, pinazepam, prazepam,* and *quazepam*). Clorazepate and prazepam may be considered as prodrugs since the metabolite is the expected active principle. Both parent drug and metabolites contribute to the activity of the other long-acting drugs. Further biotransformation of N_1-desalkylated metabolites proceeds much more slowly than for the parent drug and they therefore accumulate in the body after a few days of treatment. The rate-limiting step of their metabolism (with the exception of the 1,5-derivatives) is C3-hydroxylation to the pharmacologically active oxazepam or its 2′-halogenated analogues.

Intermediate-acting benzodiazepines are 7-nitrobenzodiazepines such as *clonazepam, flunitrazepam,* and *nitrazepam* which are metabolised by nitroreduction with no important known active metabolites. The metabolites of long- and intermediate-acting benzodiazepines require conjugation before excretion in the urine.

Short-acting benzodiazepines include the C3-hydroxylated benzodiazepines such as *lorazepam, lormetazepam, oxazepam,* and *temazepam* which undergo rapid conjugation with glucuronic acid to water-soluble inactive metabolites that are excreted in the urine, and drugs such as *alprazolam, brotizolam, estazolam, etizolam, midazolam, tofisopam,* and *triazolam* which require oxidation involving aliphatic hydroxylation before subsequent conjugation. Although these hydroxylated metabolites may retain pharmacological activity they are unlikely to contribute significantly to the clinical activity because of their negligible plasma concentrations and rapid inactivation by glucuronidation.

Drug-metabolising capacity is influenced by many factors including genetics, age, sex, endocrine and nutritional status, smoking, disease, and concurrent drug therapy. This results in wide interindividual variation in both parent drug concentrations and metabolite-to-parent drug ratios.

1. Caccia S, Garattini S. Formation of active metabolites of psychotropic drugs: an updated review of their significance. *Clin Pharmacokinet* 1990; **18:** 434–59.

Pregnancy and breast feeding. DIFFUSION ACROSS THE PLACENTA. Passage of diazepam across the placenta depends in part on the relative degrees of protein binding in mother and fetus, which in turn is influenced by factors such as stage of pregnancy and plasma concentrations of free fatty acids in mother and fetus.[1-6] Adverse effects may persist in the neonate for several days after birth because of immature drug-metabolising enzymes. Competition between diazepam and bilirubin for protein binding sites could result in hyperbilirubinaemia in the neonate.[7]

See also under Precautions, above.

1. Lee JN, *et al.* Serum protein binding of diazepam in maternal and foetal serum during pregnancy. *Br J Clin Pharmacol* 1982; **14:** 551–4.
2. Kuhnz W, Nau H. Differences in in vitro binding of diazepam and N-desmethyldiazepam to maternal and fetal plasma proteins at birth: relation to free fatty acid concentration and other parameters. *Clin Pharmacol Ther* 1983; **34:** 220–6.
3. Kanto J, *et al.* Accumulation of diazepam and N-demethyldiazepam in the fetal blood during the labour. *Ann Clin Res* 1973; **5:** 375–9.
4. Nau H, *et al.* Decreased serum protein binding of diazepam and its major metabolite in the neonate during the first postnatal week related to increased free fatty acid levels. *Br J Clin Pharmacol* 1984; **17:** 92–8.
5. Ridd MJ, *et al.* The disposition and placental transfer of diazepam in cesarean section. *Clin Pharmacol Ther* 1989; **45:** 506–12.
6. Idänpään-Heikkilä J, *et al.* Placental transfer and fetal metabolism of diazepam-C^{14} in early human pregnancy. *Clin Pharmacol Ther* 1971; **12:** 293.
7. Notarianni LJ. Plasma protein binding of drugs in pregnancy and in neonates. *Clin Pharmacokinet* 1990; **18:** 20–36.

DISTRIBUTION INTO BREAST MILK. Studies measuring concentrations of diazepam and desmethyldiazepam transferred from mother to infant via breast milk.[1,2]

See also under Precautions, above.

1. Erkkola R, Kanto J. Diazepam and breast-feeding. *Lancet* 1972; **i:** 1235–6.
2. Brandt R. Passage of diazepam and desmethyldiazepam into breast milk. *Arzneimittelforschung* 1976; **26:** 454–7.

Uses and Administration

Diazepam is a long-acting benzodiazepine with anticonvulsant, anxiolytic, sedative, muscle relaxant, and amnesic properties. Its actions are mediated by enhancement of the activity of aminobutyric acid (GABA), a major inhibitory neurotransmitter in the brain. It is used in the treatment of severe anxiety disorders, as a hypnotic in the short-term management of insomnia, as a sedative and premedicant, as an anticonvulsant particularly in the management of status epilepticus and febrile convulsions, in the control of muscle spasm as in tetanus, and in the management of alcohol withdrawal symptoms.

Diazepam is **administered** orally, rectally, and parenterally with the risk of dependence very much influencing the dose and duration of treatment. Doses should be the lowest that can control symptoms and courses of treatment should be short, not normally exceeding 4 weeks, with diazepam being withdrawn gradually (see above). Elderly and debilitated patients should be given not more that one-half the usual adult dose. Dosage reduction may also be required in patients with liver or kidney dysfunction.

Oral administration is appropriate for many indications and modified-release formulations are available in some countries. Rectal administration may be by suppository or rectal solution; the rectal solution may have better absorption characteristics. Diazepam is also given by deep intramuscular or slow intravenous injection, although absorption following intramuscular injection may be erratic and provides lower blood concentrations than those following oral administration. Intravenous injection should be carried out slowly into a large vein of the antecubital fossa at a recommended rate of no more than 1 mL of a 0.5% solution (5 mg) per minute. It is advisable to keep the patient in the supine position and under medical supervision for at least an hour after administration. Diazepam may be administered by continuous intravenous infusion; because of the risk of precipitation of diazepam, solutions should be freshly prepared following the manufacturer's directions regarding diluent and concentration of diazepam. Diazepam is substantially adsorbed onto some plastics (see under Sorption, above). Facilities for resuscitation should always be available when diazepam is given intravenously.

Diazepam may be given for **severe anxiety** in oral doses of 2 mg three times daily to a maximum of 30 mg daily. A wider dose range of 4 to 40 mg daily in divided doses is used in the USA with children over 6 months of age receiving up to 10 mg daily. Diazepam may be given by the rectal route as a rectal solution in an adult dose of 500 μg per kg body-weight repeated after 12 hours if necessary or as suppositories in a dose of 10 to 30 mg. Diazepam may sometimes have to be given by intramuscular or intravenous injection when a dose of up to 10 mg may be given, repeated if necessary after 4 hours.

The benzodiazepines have a limited role in **insomnia** (p.638) and diazepam is used for the short-term management of insomnia associated with anxiety in a dose of 5 to 15 mg by mouth at bedtime. Doses of 1 to 5 mg at bedtime have been used in children to control **night terrors** and **sleepwalking**.

Diazepam may be given for **premedication** (p.1220) before general anaesthesia or to provide sedative cover for minor surgical or investigative procedures (p.638). Doses by mouth are in the range of 5 to 20 mg; a rectal dose of 10 mg as a rectal solution may also be suitable. When given by intravenous injection the dose is usually 100 to 200 μg per kg body-weight. Some regard the perioperative use of diazepam in children undesirable since its effect and onset of action are unreliable and paradoxical effects may occur.

Diazepam is used in a variety of **seizures** (p.335). It is given by mouth as an adjunct in some types of epilepsy in daily divided doses ranging from 2 to 60 mg. For febrile convulsions, status epilepticus, and convulsions due to poisoning administration of a rectal solution may be appropriate; suppositories are not suitable because absorption is too slow. Recommended doses for the rectal solution differ. Some recommend a dose of 500 μg per kg body-weight for adults and children over 10 kg, repeated every 12 hours if necessary, but if convulsions are not controlled by the first dose the use of other anticonvulsive measures is recommended. Others recommend a dose of 10 mg for adults and children over 3 years of age and 5 mg for children 1 to 3 years of age, doses being repeated after 5 minutes if necessary. Alternatively diazepam may be given intravenously in an adult dose of 10 to 20 mg given at a rate of 5 mg per minute and repeated if necessary after 30 to 60 minutes. Other schedules involve administering smaller amounts more frequently or giving diazepam intramuscularly, though again absorption may be too slow. Once the seizures have been controlled, a slow intravenous infusion providing up to 3 mg per kg over 24 hours has been administered to protect against recurrence. Doses by intravenous or intramuscular injection in children are within the range of 200 to 300 μg per kg; alternatively 1 mg may be given for each year of age.

Diazepam may be given by mouth in daily divided doses of 2 to 15 mg to alleviate **muscle spasm** increased in severe spastic disorders, such as cerebral palsy, up to 60 mg daily in adults or up to 40 mg daily in children. If given by intramuscular or slow intravenous injection the dose is 10 mg repeated if necessary after 4 hours. Larger doses are used in tetanus in adults and children with 100 to 300 μg per kg body-weight being given every 1 to 4 hours by intravenous injection. Alternatively 3 to 10 mg per kg may be given over 24 hours by continuous intravenous infusion or by nasoduodenal tube using a suitable liquid oral dose form. Diazepam may also be given by the rectal route as a rectal solution in a dose of 500 μg per kg body-weight for adults and children over 10 kg in weight, repeated every 12 hours if necessary.

Symptoms of the **alcohol withdrawal syndrome** (p.1099) may be controlled by diazepam given by mouth in a dose of 5 to 20 mg, repeated if required after 2 to 4 hours; another approach is to give 10 mg three or four times on the first day with 5 mg three or four times on the next day as required. Diazepam may need to be given by injection if the symptoms are severe and if delirium tremens has developed; 10 mg by intramuscular or intravenous injection may be adequate, although some patients may require higher doses.

Reviews.

1. Ashton H. Guidelines for the rational use of benzodiazepines: when and what to use. *Drugs* 1994; **48:** 25–40.

Action. Aminobutyric acid (GABA) is the major inhibitory neurotransmitter in the brain. GABA's functions within the CNS include involvement in sleep induction and in the control of neuronal excitability, epilepsy, anxiety, memory, and hypnosis.[1] Two subtypes of GABA receptors have been identified: A and B. Benzodiazepines interact with $GABA_A$ receptors to produce their sedative, hypnotic, anxiolytic, anticonvulsant, and antinociceptive effects. The $GABA_A$ receptors within the CNS are composed of different subunits, 4 of which have been described: α, β, γ, and δ. These subunits combine to form macromolecular complexes which include a chloride ion channel and regions to which GABA and benzodiazepines bind, as well as binding sites for other substances. The different types of subunit comprising the $GABA_A$ receptor determine its activity. The presence of a γ subunit confers benzodiazepine sensitivity and it is the type of α subunit(s) present that determines whether the benzodiazepine activity is mainly anxiolytic or mainly sedative. Two types of benzodiazepine receptor are suggested: type I, found throughout the brain and in large concentrations in the cerebellum and type II found mainly in the cerebral cortex, spinal cord, and hippocampus. It is the benzodiazepine type I receptors that are thought to be responsible for the anxiolytic actions of benzodiazepines. The possibility of different types of GABA receptor associated with different functions remains to be fully exploited with the development of a benzodiazepine specially selected for its anxiolytic effect and lacking sedative and muscle relaxant activity. The 1–5 benzodiazepines such as clobazam are examples of compounds possessing a certain degree of selectivity, being less sedating, although having muscle relaxant activity.

1. Goodchild CS. GABA receptors and benzodiazepines. *Br J Anaesth* 1993; **71:** 127–33.

Anxiety disorders. For a discussion of the management of anxiety disorders including the use of benzodiazepines, see p.635.

References.

1. Shader RI, Greenblatt DJ. Benzodiazepines in anxiety disorders. *N Engl J Med* 1993; **328:** 1398–1405.
2. Norman TR, *et al.* Benzodiazepines in anxiety disorders: managing therapeutics and dependence. *Med J Aust* 1997; **167:** 490–5.

Cardiac arrhythmias. Although not considered to be an antiarrhythmic, diazepam has been tried with good effect in treating the cardiotoxicity of chloroquine poisoning (see p.427). However, diazepam has been reported to possess both antiarrhythmic and pro-arrhythmic properties, possibly depending on the dose.[1]

1. Kumagai K, *et al.* Antiarrhythmic and proarrhythmic properties of diazepam demonstrated by electrophysiological study in humans. *Clin Cardiol* 1991; **14:** 397–401.

Chloroquine poisoning. For reference to the possible use of diazepam to decrease the cardiotoxic effects of chloroquine, see p.427.

Conversion and dissociative disorders. Conversion and dissociative disorders (formerly known as hysteria) are characterised by physical symptoms that occur in the absence of organic disease. Medication has no part to play in the treatment of these disorders unless they are secondary to conditions such as depression or anxiety disorders requiring treatment in their own right.

There have been suggestions that sedatives such as diazepam or midazolam may be used to confirm the diagnosis of hysterical paralysis.[1,2] The test tends to exacerbate organic disease while psychiatric dysfunction may improve.

1. Ellis SJ. Diazepam as a truth drug. *Lancet* 1990; **336:** 752–3.
2. Keating JJ, *et al.* Hysterical paralysis. *Lancet* 1990; **336:** 1506–7.

Disturbed behaviour. For a discussion of the management of behaviour disturbances associated with various psychotic disorders, and the value of benzodiazepines, see p.636. Benzodiazepines are considered to be useful in palliative care for the relief of terminal restlessness. A suggested dose for diazepam is 5 to 10 mg given slowly as a rectal solution and repeated every 8 to 12 hours.

Dyspnoea. Benzodiazepines such as diazepam have been tried in the treatment of dyspnoea (p.70) in the belief that reduction of an elevated respiratory drive may alleviate respiratory distress but benefits observed in some patients have not been confirmed and administration to patients with any form of respiratory depression or pulmonary insufficiency may be hazardous (see under Precautions above). However, benzodiazepines may be of use in patients with advanced cancer who have rapid shallow respiration. A daily dose of 5 to 10 mg has been suggested for diazepam.

Eclampsia and pre-eclampsia. Diazepam has been used for the initial control of impending or actual eclampsia but, as mentioned on p.338, magnesium sulphate is generally the preferred treatment now.

Epilepsy and other convulsive disorders. Some benzodiazepines such as diazepam are used for the control of status epilepticus (p.337), including status epilepticus in patients with porphyria (p.339), and for febrile convulsions (p.338); diazepam has also been used in eclampsia (see above) and for neonatal seizures (p.338). Benzodiazepines such as clobazam and clonazepam may be employed in the management of epilepsy (p.335), but their long-term use is limited by problems of sedation, dependence, and tolerance to the antiepileptic effects.

References.

1. Rosman NP, *et al.* A controlled trial of diazepam administered during febrile illnesses to prevent recurrence of febrile seizures. *N Engl J Med* 1993; **329:** 79–84.
2. Somerville ER, Antony JH. Position statement on the use of rectal diazepam in epilepsy. *Med J Aust* 1995; **163:** 268–9.
3. Uhari M, *et al.* Effect of acetaminophen and low intermittent doses of diazepam on prevention of recurrences of febrile seizures. *J Pediatr* 1995; **126:** 991–5.

Extrapyramidal disorders. For reference to the use of benzodiazepines in the treatment of neuroleptic-induced extrapyramidal disorders, see Chlorpromazine, p.650.

Irritable bowel syndrome. Although some benzodiazepines have been used in the management of irritable bowel syndrome (p.1172) there is no evidence to support their use in this condition.

Muscle spasm. Diazepam and other benzodiazepines may be used for the relief of muscle spasm (p.1303) of various aetiologies including that secondary to muscle or joint inflammation or trauma, such as in low back pain (p.10), or resulting from **spasticity** (p.1303), **dystonias**, **stiff-man syndrome** (see below), **cerebral palsy**, **poisoning**, or **tetanus** (p.1304). High doses are often required and treatment may be limited by adverse effects or by risk of dependence.

STIFF-MAN SYNDROME. Stiff-man syndrome is a rare condition characterised by painful intermittent spasms and rigidity of the axial and limb muscles. Its exact cause is unknown but there is some evidence to implicate auto-antibodies against one of the enzymes involved in the synthesis of the neurotransmitter gamma-aminobutyric acid. It is frequently associated with auto-immune diseases and type 1 diabetes mellitus. Patients typically respond to benzodiazepines and this may be of use in the differential diagnosis of the syndrome. Diazepam has been the mainstay of treatment but clonazepam may also be of use, especially in familial startle disease, a rare congenital form of stiff-man syndrome. Although rigidity and spasms in stiff-man syndrome are not completely resolved by diazepam the degree of improvement can be sufficient to restore the functional level to near normal. However, large doses are often required and sedation might be a limiting factor in some patients. Other drugs which have been used when diazepam is ineffective or poorly tolerated include baclofen or sodium valproate but benefit may be less evident. There have been isolated anecdotal reports of improvement with vigabatrin. Although corticosteroids may be of benefit the chronic nature of the disorder and the high incidence of type 1 diabetes mellitus make their use undesirable. Other attempts at immunomodulation such as plasmapheresis have yielded results and evidence of the efficacy of immunoglobulins is largely limited to anecdotal reports and uncontrolled studies.

1. Toro C, *et al.* Stiff-man syndrome. *Semin Neurol* 1994; **14:** 154–8.
2. Gerhardt CL. Stiff-man syndrome revisited. *South Med J* 1995; **88:** 805–808.

Nausea and vomiting. Benzodiazepines, particularly lorazepam, have been used as adjuncts in the management of nausea and vomiting induced by cancer chemotherapy (p.1172).

Parasomnias. Parasomnias (p.639) rarely require treatment other than the symptomatic treatment of sleep-related medical problems. A number of parasomnias such as restless leg syndrome, sleepwalking, and night terrors have been reported to respond to benzodiazepines. Although the muscle relaxant and anxiolytic action of a benzodiazepine can be helpful in bruxism (teeth grinding) it has been recommended that they should only be prescribed on a short-term basis during the acute phase.

References.

1. Schenck CH, Mahowald MW. Long-term, nightly benzodiazepine treatment of injurious parasomnias and other disorders of disrupted nocturnal sleep in 170 adults. *Am J Med* 1996; **100:** 333–7.

Premenstrual syndrome. For mention of the limited role of benzodiazepines in the management of premenstrual syndrome, see p.1456.

Schizophrenia. Benzodiazepines may be useful adjuncts to antipsychotics in the initial management of schizophrenia (p.637).

Vertigo. Although intravenous diazepam has been used to abort acute attacks of vertigo of peripheral origin (p.401), it can prolong compensation and recovery from vestibular lesions.[1]

1. Rascol O, *et al.* Antivertigo medications and drug-induced vertigo: a pharmacological review. *Drugs* 1995; **50:** 777–91.

Withdrawal syndromes. The benzodiazepines are used in the management of symptoms of alcohol withdrawal (p.1099) and of opioid withdrawal (p.67).

Preparations

BP 1998: Diazepam Capsules; Diazepam Injection; Diazepam Oral Solution; Diazepam Rectal Solution; Diazepam Tablets;
USP 23: Diazepam Capsules; Diazepam Extended-release Capsules; Diazepam Injection; Diazepam Tablets.

Proprietary Preparations (details are given in Part 3)
Aust.: Gewacalm; Psychopax; Stesolid; Umbrium; Valium; ***Austral.:*** Antenex; Diazemuls; Ducene; Valium; ***Belg.:*** Valium; ***Canad.:*** Diazemuls; Novo-Dipam; Valium; Vivol; ***Fr.:*** Novazam; Valium; ***Ger.:*** Diazemuls†; Diazep; duradiazepam†; Faustan; Lamra; Mandro-Zep†; Neurolytril†; Stesolid; Tranquase; Tranquo†; Valaxona†; Valiquid; Valium; ***Irl.:*** Anxicalm; Atensine†; Calmigen†; Diazemuls; Stesolid; Valium; ***Ital.:*** Aliseum; Ansiolin; Diazemuls; Eridan; Noan; Tranquirit; Valitran†; Valium; Vatran; ***Neth.:*** Diazemuls†; Stesolid†; Valium; ***Norw.:*** Stesolid; Valium; Vival; ***S.Afr.:*** Benzopin; Betapam; Diaquel; Doval; Dynapam†; Ethipam†; Pax; Scriptopam†; Valium; ***Spain:*** Aneurol; Asparine B6 Tranq; Calmaven; Complutine; Diaceplex; Diaceplex Simple; Dicepin B6; Drenian; Gobanal; Pacium; Podium; Sico Relax; Stesolid; Valium; Vincosedan; ***Swed.:*** Apozepam; Stesolid; Valium; ***Switz.:*** Paceum; Psychopax; Stesolid; Valium; ***UK:*** Atensine†; Dialar; Diazemuls; Rimapam; Solis†; Stesolid; Tensium; Valclair; Valium; ***USA:*** Dizac; T-Quil†; Valium; Valrelease†; Zetran†.

Multi-ingredient: ***Aust.:*** Acordin; Betamed; Harmomed; ***Ger.:*** Elthon†; Valocordin-Diazepam; ***Ital.:*** Gamibetal Plus; Gastrausil D†; Gefarnax†; Spasen Somatico; Spasmeridan; Spasmomen Somatico; Valpinax; Valtrax; ***Spain:*** Ansium; Edym Sedante; Pertranquil; Tepazepan; Tropargal; ***Switz.:*** Silentan†; ***USA:*** Emergent-Ez.

Dichloralphenazone (4028-l)

Dichloralphenazone *(BAN).*
$C_{15}H_{18}Cl_6N_2O_5$ = 519.0.
CAS — 480-30-8.
Pharmacopoeias. In US.

A white microcrystalline powder with a slight odour characteristic of chloral hydrate.

Freely **soluble** in water, in alcohol, and in chloroform; soluble in dilute acids. It is decomposed by dilute alkalis liberating chloroform.

In aqueous solution it dissociates into chloral hydrate and phenazone.

Dichloralphenazone dissociates on administration to form chloral hydrate and phenazone. It has the general properties of chloral hydrate (p.645), although it is less likely to cause gastric irritation after administration by mouth. Phenazone-induced skin eruptions may, however, occur (see p.78). Dichloralphenazone is used in some countries in combination preparations mainly for the treatment of tension and vascular headaches.

Porphyria. Dichloralphenazone has been associated with acute attacks of porphyria and is considered unsafe in patients with acute porphyria.[1]

1. Moore MR, McColl KEL. *Porphyria: drug lists.* Glasgow: Porphyria Research Unit, University of Glasgow, 1991.

Preparations

USP 23: Isometheptene Mucate, Dichloralphenazone, and Acetaminophen Capsules.

Proprietary Preparations (details are given in Part 3)

Multi-ingredient: ***USA:*** Isocom; Isopap; Midchlor; Midrin; Migratine.

Difebarbamate (13412-v)

Difebarbamate *(rINN).*
1,3-Bis(3-butoxy-2-hydroxypropyl)-5-ethyl-5-phenylbarbituric acid dicarbamate ester.
$C_{28}H_{42}N_4O_9$ = 578.7.
CAS — 15687-09-9.

Difebarbamate is a barbiturate with general properties similar to those of amylobarbitone (p.641). Tetrabamate, a complex of difebarbamate, febarbamate, and phenobarbitone has been used in the management of anxiety disorders. However, barbiturates are not considered appropriate in the management of these conditions.

Preparations

Proprietary Preparations (details are given in Part 3)

Multi-ingredient: ***Fr.:*** Atrium; ***Switz.:*** Atrium.

Dixyrazine (7037-j)

UCB-3412. 2-(2-{4-[2-Methyl-3-(phenothiazin-10-yl)propyl]piperazin-1-yl}ethoxy)ethanol.
$C_{24}H_{33}N_3O_2S$ = 427.6.
CAS — 2470-73-7.

Dixyrazine is a phenothiazine with general properties similar to those of chlorpromazine (p.649). It has a piperazine side-chain. It is given by mouth for its antipsychotic, antiemetic, and sedative properties in doses ranging from 20 to 150 mg daily. Dixyrazine has also been given by injection.

References.

1. Larsson S, *et al.* Premedication with intramuscular dixyrazine (Esucos®): a controlled double-blind comparison with morphine-scopolamine and placebo. *Acta Anaesthesiol Scand* 1988; **32:** 131–4.
2. Karlsson E, *et al.* The effects of prophylactic dixyrazine on postoperative vomiting after two different anaesthetic methods for squint surgery in children. *Acta Anaesthesiol Scand* 1993; **37:** 45–8.
3. Oikkonen M, *et al.* Dixyrazine premedication for cataract surgery: a comparison with diazepam. *Acta Anaesthesiol Scand* 1994; **38:** 214–17.
4. Feet PO, Götestam KG. Increased antipanic efficacy in combined treatment with clomipramine and dixyrazine. *Acta Psychiatr Scand* 1994; **89:** 230–4.
5. Oikkonen M, *et al.* CSF concentrations and clinical effects following intravenous dixyrazine premedication. *Eur J Clin Pharmacol* 1995; **47:** 445–7.

Porphyria. Dixyrazine was considered to be unsafe in patients with acute porphyria because it has been shown to be porphyrinogenic in *animals* or *in-vitro* systems.[1]

1. Moore MR, McColl KEL. *Porphyria: drug lists.* Glasgow: Porphyria Research Unit, University of Glasgow, 1991.

Preparations

Proprietary Preparations (details are given in Part 3)
Aust.: Esucos; ***Belg.:*** Esucos; ***Ger.:*** Esucos†; ***Ital.:*** Esucos; ***Norw.:*** Esucos; ***S.Afr.:*** Esucos†; ***Swed.:*** Esucos.

Multi-ingredient: ***Spain:*** Vertigum.

Droperidol (7038-z)

Droperidol *(BAN, USAN, rINN).*
Droperidolum; McN-JR-4749; R-4749. 1-{1-[3-(4-Fluorobenzoyl)propyl]-1,2,3,6-tetrahydro-4-pyridyl}-benzimidazolin-2-one.
$C_{22}H_{22}FN_3O_2$ = 379.4.
CAS — 548-73-2.
Pharmacopoeias. In *Eur.* (see p.viii), *Jpn,* and *US.*

A white to light tan amorphous or microcrystalline powder. It exhibits polymorphism. Ph. Eur. **solubilities** are: practically insoluble in water; sparingly soluble in alcohol; freely soluble in dichloromethane and in dimethylformamide. USP solubilities are: practically insoluble in water; soluble 1 in 140 of alcohol, 1 in 4 of chloroform, and 1 in 500 of ether. **Store** at 8° to 15° under an atmosphere of nitrogen in airtight containers. Protect from light.

Incompatibility. Droperidol has been reported to be incompatible with nafcillin sodium,[1] fluorouracil, folinic acid, frusemide, heparin, methotrexate,[2] cefmetazole sodium,[3] and some barbiturates. Most of these incompatibilities are probably a result of pH changes.

1. Jeglun EL, *et al.* Nafcillin sodium incompatibility with acidic solutions. *Am J Hosp Pharm* 1981; **38:** 462, 464.
2. Cohen MH, *et al.* Drug precipitation within iv tubing: a potential hazard of chemotherapy administration. *Cancer Treat Rep* 1985; **69:** 1325–6.
3. Hutchings SR, *et al.* Compatibility of cefmetazole sodium with commonly used drugs during Y-site delivery. *Am J Health-Syst Pharm* 1996; **53:** 2185–8.

Stability. Although droperidol appeared to be stable for 7 days in glucose injection, sodium chloride injection, or lactated Ringer's injection stored in glass bottles there was some loss due to sorption when mixtures in lactated Ringer's injection were stored in polyvinyl chloride bags.[1]

1. Ray JB, *et al.* Droperidol stability in intravenous admixtures. *Am J Hosp Pharm* 1983; **40:** 94–7.

Adverse Effects and Treatment

As for Chlorpromazine, p.649.

Precautions

As for Chlorpromazine, p.652.

Droperidol has a longer duration of action than short-acting opioid analgesics such as fentanyl, therefore, during concurrent use, repeat doses of droperidol must not be given when only the opioid analgesic is required, since this would lead to accumulation of droperidol and overdosage.

Because of reports of sudden death following the use of high doses of droperidol in patients at risk for cardiac arrhythmias, the US manufacturer has recommended that droperidol should not be used in the treatment of alcohol withdrawal or in other situations where high doses are likely to be needed in patients at risk of arrhythmias.

Interactions

As for Chlorpromazine, p.652.

Pharmacokinetics

For a detailed account of the pharmacokinetics of a butyrophenone, see Haloperidol, p.674.

Droperidol has been reported to have an initial plasma half-life of 10 minutes and a terminal plasma half-life of about 2 hours. It is extensively bound to plasma proteins. Droperidol is extensively metabolised and is mainly excreted in the urine. Some also appears in the faeces, possibly via biliary excretion.

References.

1. Cressman WA, *et al.* Absorption, metabolism and excretion of droperidol by human subjects following intramuscular and intravenous administration. *Anesthesiology* 1973; **38:** 363–9.
2. Grunwald Z, *et al.* The pharmacokinetics of droperidol in anaesthetized children. *Anesth Analg* 1993; **76:** 1238–42.

Uses and Administration

Droperidol is a butyrophenone with general properties similar to those of haloperidol (p.674). The duration of action of droperidol has been reported to last about 2 to 4 hours although alteration of alertness may last 12 hours or longer. Droperidol is used as a premedicant (p.1220), as an adjunct in anaesthesia, as an antiemetic (p.1172), and for the control of agitated patients in acute psychoses (p.636) and in mania (p.273). It has also been used in conjunction with an opioid analgesic such as fentanyl citrate to maintain a patient in a state of neuroleptanalgesia (p.1220) in which they are calm and indifferent to the surroundings and able to cooperate with the surgeon. The longer duration of action of droperidol must be kept in mind when using it in association with such opioid analgesics.

Droperidol is administered by mouth or by injection. Preparations of droperidol for injection are prepared with the aid of lactic or tartaric acid and may be stated to contain droperidol lactate or droperidol tartrate respectively. However, doses are expressed in terms of the equivalent amount of droperidol. A recommended dose for the control of **agitation**, such as in acute mania, is 5 to 20 mg by mouth, up to 10 mg intramuscularly, or 5 to 15 mg intravenously. Parenteral doses may be repeated every 4 to 6 hours, and oral doses every 4 to 8 hours if necessary. Children may be given 0.5 to 1 mg daily intramuscularly or orally.

For **premedication** up to 10 mg of droperidol may be administered intramuscularly or by mouth 30 to 60 minutes pre-operatively. The intravenous route has also been used. In the UK the recommended dose for premedication in children is 0.2 to 0.5 mg per kg body-weight by intramuscular injection or 0.3 to 0.6 mg per kg by mouth. In the USA, doses of 0.088 to 0.165 mg per kg (by the intramuscular or intravenous routes) have been suggested for premedication in children. An intravenous dose of droperidol 5 to 15 mg has been recommended for use in **neuroleptanalgesia**. A suggested dose for children is 0.2 to 0.3 mg per kg body-weight intravenously. Droperidol has been given, usually by the intravenous route, as an adjunct to **general anaesthesia**; typical doses are 15 to 20 mg at induction and 1.25 to 2.5 mg for maintenance. A dose of 2.5 to 5 mg has been given by intramuscular or slow intravenous injection when additional sedation is required during regional anaesthesia.

For the prevention of postoperative **nausea and vomiting** a dose of 5 mg intramuscularly or intravenously may be given. Droperidol has been used in cancer chemotherapy, a typical regimen was 1 to 10 mg (by intramuscular or intravenous injection)

30 minutes before commencement of antineoplastic therapy, followed by a continuous intravenous infusion of 1 to 3 mg per hour or 1 to 5 mg by intramuscular or intravenous injection every 1 to 6 hours as required. As an antiemetic, children may be given doses between 0.020 and 0.075 mg per kg intramuscularly or intravenously.

Droperidol should be used in reduced dosage in the elderly.

Nausea and vomiting. It has been reported[1] that doses of droperidol as low as 0.25 mg given intravenously are effective for the management of postoperative nausea and vomiting.

Addition of droperidol in doses of 0.05 or 0.1 mg per 1 mg of morphine has been used successfully to control nausea and vomiting associated with morphine in patient-controlled analgesia (p.7).[2-5] However, one group of workers[6] found that postoperative administration of a bolus dose of droperidol 1.25 mg intravenously before the start of patient-controlled analgesia and addition of droperidol 0.16 mg per 1 mg of morphine to the analgesic infusion were of similar efficacy. The use of a technique combining a bolus dose of droperidol and droperidol added to the analgesic infusion was not recommended as it appeared to increase sedation.

1. Millar JM. Nausea and vomiting after general anaesthesia. *Lancet* 1989; **i:** 1400.
2. Williams OA, *et al.* Addition of droperidol to patient-controlled analgesia: effect on nausea and vomiting. *Br J Anaesth* 1993; **70:** 479P.
3. Sharma SK, Davies MW. Patient-controlled analgesia with a mixture of morphine and droperidol. *Br J Anaesth* 1993; **71:** 435–6.
4. Bishop L, *et al.* Droperidol with patient-controlled analgesia. *Int J Pharm Pract* 1993; **2:** 160–2.
5. Barrow PM, *et al.* Influence of droperidol on nausea and vomiting during patient-controlled analgesia. *Br J Anaesth* 1994; **72:** 460–1.
6. Gan TJ, *et al.* Comparison of different methods of administering droperidol in patient-controlled analgesia in the prevention of postoperative nausea and vomiting. *Anesth Analg* 1995; **80:** 81–5.

Preparations

USP 23: Droperidol Injection.

Proprietary Preparations (details are given in Part 3)
Aust.: Dehydrobenzperidol; ***Austral.:*** Droleptan; ***Belg.:*** Dehydrobenzperidol; ***Canad.:*** Inapsine; ***Fr.:*** Droleptan; ***Ger.:*** Dehydrobenzperidol; ***Irl.:*** Droleptan; ***Ital.:*** Sintodian; ***Neth.:*** Dehydrobenzperidol; ***Norw.:*** Dridol; ***S.Afr.:*** Inapsin; Paxical; ***Spain:*** Dehidrobenzperidol; ***Swed.:*** Dridol; ***Switz.:*** Dehydrobenzperidol; ***UK:*** Droleptan; ***USA:*** Inapsine.

Multi-ingredient: ***Aust.:*** Thalamonal; ***Belg.:*** Thalamonal; ***Canad.:*** Innovar†; ***Ger.:*** Thalamonal; ***Ital.:*** Leptofen; ***Neth.:*** Thalamonal; ***Swed.:*** Leptanal comp†; ***Switz.:*** Thalamonal†; ***UK:*** Thalamonal†; ***USA:*** Innovar.

Eltoprazine (3678-z)

Eltoprazine *(rINN)*.

DU-28853. 1-(1,4-Benzodioxan-5-yl)piperazine.

$C_{12}H_{16}N_2O_2$ = 220.3.

CAS — 98224-03-4.

Eltoprazine is a serotonin agonist with a selective action at the 5-HT_{1AB} receptors that is reported to inhibit aggression without causing sedation or motor impairment. It is under investigation in the treatment of behaviour disorders.

References.

1. Verhoeven WMA, *et al.* Eltoprazine in mentally retarded self-injuring patients. *Lancet* 1992; **340:** 1037–8.
2. Tiihonen J, *et al.* Eltoprazine for aggression in schizophrenia and mental retardation. *Lancet* 1993; **341:** 307.
3. Kohen D. Eltoprazine for aggression in mental handicap. *Lancet* 1993; **341:** 628–9.

Enciprazine Hydrochloride (4972-g)

Enciprazine Hydrochloride *(BANM, USAN, rINNM)*.

Wy-48624 (enciprazine or enciprazine hydrochloride). 1-(4-*o*-Methoxyphenylpiperazin-1-yl)-3-(3,4,5-trimethoxyphenoxy)-propan-2-ol dihydrochloride.

$C_{23}H_{32}N_2O_6,2HCl$ = 505.4.

CAS — 68576-86-3 (enciprazine); 68576-88-5 (enciprazine hydrochloride).

Enciprazine hydrochloride has been studied for its anxiolytic potential.

References.

1. Scheibe G, *et al.* Pilot study on the therapeutic efficacy, clinical safety, and dosage finding of enciprazine in out-patients with anxious and anxious-depressive syndromes. *Arzneimittelforschung* 1990; **40:** 644–6.
2. Schweizer E, *et al.* A placebo-controlled study of enciprazine in the treatment of generalized anxiety disorder: a preliminary report *Psychopharmacol Bull* 1990; **26:** 215–17.

Estazolam (4030-g)

Estazolam *(USAN, rINN)*.

Abbott-47631; D-40TA. 8-Chloro-6-phenyl-4*H*-1,2,4-triazolo[4,3-*a*]-1,4-benzodiazepine.

$C_{16}H_{11}ClN_4$ = 294.7.

CAS — 29975-16-4.

Pharmacopoeias. In *Chin.* and *Jpn.*

Dependence and Withdrawal, Adverse Effects, Treatment, and Precautions

As for Diazepam, p.661.

Interactions

As for Diazepam, p.663.

Pharmacokinetics

Peak plasma concentrations of estazolam are reached on average within 2 hours of administration by mouth. A high proportion of estazolam is protein bound (about 93%). Reported mean elimination half-lives have generally been in the range of 10 to 24 hours. Estazolam is extensively metabolised, mainly to 4-hydroxyestazolam and 1-oxoestazolam which are considered inactive. These metabolites are excreted, either free or conjugated in the urine with small amounts detected in the faeces. Only a small proportion of a dose is excreted as unchanged drug.

Uses and Administration

Estazolam is a short-acting benzodiazepine with general properties similar to those of diazepam (p.666). It is given by mouth as a hypnotic in the short-term management of insomnia (p.638) in usual doses of 1 to 2 mg at night. Small or debilitated elderly patients may be given 0.5-mg doses.

General references.

1. Roth T, ed. Critical issues in the management of insomnia: investigators' report on estazolam. *Am J Med* 1990; **88** (suppl 3A): 1S–48S.
2. Anonymous. Estazolam—a new benzodiazepine hypnotic. *Med Lett Drugs Ther* 1991; **33:** 91–2.
3. Vogel GW, Morris D. The effects of estazolam on sleep, performance, and memory: a long-term sleep laboratory study of elderly insomniacs. *J Clin Pharmacol* 1992; **32:** 647–51.

Preparations

Proprietary Preparations (details are given in Part 3)
Canad.: Prosom†; ***Fr.:*** Nuctalon; ***Ital.:*** Esilgan; ***Jpn:*** Eurodin; ***USA:*** Prosom.

Ethchlorvynol (4031-q)

Ethchlorvynol *(BAN, rINN)*.

β-Chlorovinyl Ethyl Ethynyl Carbinol; *E*-Ethchlorvynol. 1-Chloro-3-ethylpent-1-en-4-yn-3-ol.

C_7H_9ClO = 144.6.

CAS — 113-18-8.

Pharmacopoeias. In *US.*

A colourless to yellow, slightly viscous liquid with a characteristic pungent odour. Wt per mL about 1.072 g. It darkens on exposure to air and light.

Immiscible with water; miscible with most organic solvents. **Store** in airtight containers of glass or polyethylene, using polyethylene-lined closures. Protect from light.

Dependence and Withdrawal

Prolonged use of ethchlorvynol may lead to dependence similar to that with barbiturates (see Amylobarbitone, p.641).

Adverse Effects

Side-effects of ethchlorvynol include gastro-intestinal disturbances including unpleasant after-taste, dizziness, headache, unwanted sedation and other symptoms of CNS depression such as ataxia, facial numbness, blurred vision, and hypotension. Hypersensitivity reactions include skin rashes, urticaria, and occasionally, thrombocytopenia and cholestatic jaundice. Idiosyncratic reactions include excitement, severe muscular weakness, and syncope without marked hypotension.

Acute overdosage is characterised by prolonged deep coma, respiratory depression, hypothermia, hypotension, and relative bradycardia. Pancytopenia and nystagmus has occurred.

Pulmonary oedema has followed abuse by intravenous injection.

Treatment of Adverse Effects

As for the barbiturates (see Amylobarbitone, p.642).

Haemoperfusion may be of value in the treatment of severe poisoning with ethchlorvynol.

Precautions

Ethchlorvynol should be used with caution in patients with hepatic or renal impairment or with mental depression, in patients in severe uncontrolled pain, and as with all sedatives, in those with impaired respiratory function. It may cause drowsiness; affected patients should not drive or operate machinery.

Excessively rapid absorption of ethchlorvynol in some patients has been reported to produce giddiness and ataxia; this may be reduced by administration with food.

Porphyria. Ethchlorvynol has been associated with acute attacks of porphyria and is considered unsafe in patients with acute porphyria.[1]

1. Moore MR, McColl KEL. *Porphyria: drug lists.* Glasgow: Porphyria Research Unit, University of Glasgow, 1991.

Interactions

The effect of ethchlorvynol may be enhanced by alcohol, barbiturates, and other CNS depressants. It has been reported to decrease the effects of coumarin anticoagulants.

Tricyclic antidepressants. The US manufacturers state that transient delirium has been reported with the concomitant use of ethchlorvynol and amitriptyline but details of such an interaction do not appear to have been published in the literature.

Pharmacokinetics

Ethchlorvynol is readily absorbed from the gastro-intestinal tract, peak plasma concentrations usually occurring within 2 hours of ingestion. It is widely distributed in body tissues and is extensively metabolised in the liver, and possibly to some extent in the kidneys. It has a biphasic plasma half-life with a rapid initial phase and a terminal phase reported to last from 10 to 20 hours. Ethchlorvynol and is excreted mainly in the urine as metabolites and their conjugates. Ethchlorvynol crosses the placenta.

Uses and Administration

Ethchlorvynol is a hypnotic and sedative with some anticonvulsant and muscle relaxant properties. It is given by mouth for the short-term management of insomnia (p.638); use for periods of up to one week have been recommended. Ethchlorvynol has, however, been largely superseded by other drugs. The usual hypnotic dose is 0.5 g at night but doses ranging from 0.2 to 1 g have been given. Administration with food has been recommended—see Precautions, above.

Preparations

USP 23: Ethchlorvynol Capsules.

Proprietary Preparations (details are given in Part 3)
Canad.: Placidyl†; ***USA:*** Placidyl.

Ethyl Loflazepate (15319-n)

Ethyl Loflazepate *(rINN)*.

CM-6912. Ethyl 7-chloro-5-(2-fluorophenyl)-2,3-dihydro-2-oxo-1*H*-1,4-benzodiazepine-3-carboxylate.

$C_{18}H_{14}ClFN_2O_3$ = 360.8.

CAS — 29177-84-2.

Ethyl loflazepate is a long-acting benzodiazepine derivative with general properties similar to those of diazepam (p.661). It is used in the short-term treatment of anxiety disorders (p.635) in usual doses of 1 to 3 mg daily by mouth in a single dose or in divided doses.

Preparations

Proprietary Preparations (details are given in Part 3)
Belg.: Victan; ***Fr.:*** Victan; ***Ital.:*** Victan†; ***Jpn:*** Meilax.

Etifoxin Hydrochloride (19158-s)

Etifoxin Hydrochloride *(BANM)*.

Etifoxine Hydrochloride *(rINNM)*; Hoe-36801. 6-Chloro-4-methyl-4-phenyl-3,1-benzoxazin-2-yl(ethyl)amine hydrochloride.

$C_{17}H_{17}ClN_2O,HCl$ = 337.2.

CAS — 21715-46-8 (etifoxin); 56776-32-0 (etifoxin hydrochloride).

Etifoxin hydrochloride is an anxiolytic (p.635) given by mouth in usual doses of 150 or 200 mg daily for up to 30 days.

Preparations

Proprietary Preparations (details are given in Part 3)
Fr.: Stresam.

Etizolam (16639-h)

Etizolam *(rINN)*.

AHR-3219; Y-7131. 4-(2-Chlorophenyl)-2-ethyl-9-methyl-6*H*-thieno[3,2-*f*]-s-triazolo[4,3-*a*][1,4]diazepine.

$C_{17}H_{15}ClN_4S$ = 342.8.

CAS — 40054-69-1.

Etizolam is a short-acting benzodiazepine derivative with general properties similar to those of diazepam (p.661). It is given by mouth for the short-term treatment of insomnia (p.638) and anxiety disorders (p.635) in doses of up to 3 mg daily in divided doses or as a single dose at night.

Preparations

Proprietary Preparations (details are given in Part 3)
Ital.: Depas; Pasaden; ***Jpn:*** Depas.

Etodroxizine (12718-z)

Etodroxizine (rINN).

2-{2-[2-(4-p-Chlorobenzhydrylpiperazin-1-yl)ethoxy]ethoxy}ethanol.

$C_{23}H_{31}ClN_2O_3$ = 419.0.

CAS — 17692-34-1.

Etodroxizine was formerly used as the base or the maleate as a hypnotic and for the relief of hypersensitivity disorders.

Preparations

Proprietary Preparations (details are given in Part 3)
S.Afr.: Indunox†.

Multi-ingredient: *Ger.:* Vesparax†.

Febarbamate (12728-k)

Febarbamate (rINN).

Go-560. 1-(3-Butoxy-2-carbamoyloxypropyl)-5-ethyl-5-phenylbarbituric acid.

$C_{20}H_{27}N_3O_6$ = 405.4.

CAS — 13246-02-1.

Febarbamate is a barbiturate with general properties similar to those of amylobarbitone (p.641). It has been used in the management of anxiety (p.635), insomnia (p.638), and alcohol withdrawal symptoms (p.1099). However, barbiturates are no longer considered appropriate in the management of these conditions.

Tetrabamate, a complex of febarbamate, difebarbamate, and phenobarbitone has been used similarly.

Preparations

Proprietary Preparations (details are given in Part 3)
Spain: G Tril; *Switz.:* Tymium†.

Multi-ingredient: *Fr.:* Atrium; *Switz.:* Atrium.

Fluanisone (7040-s)

Fluanisone (BAN, rINN).

Haloanisone; MD-2028; R-2028; R-2167. 4'-Fluoro-4-[4-(2-methoxyphenyl)piperazin-1-yl]butyrophenone.

$C_{21}H_{25}FN_2O_2$ = 356.4.

CAS — 1480-19-9.

Pharmacopoeias. In BP(Vet).

A white or almost white to buff-coloured, odourless or almost odourless, crystals or powder. M.p. 72° to 76°. Practically **insoluble** in water; freely soluble in chloroform, in alcohol, in ether, and in dilute solutions of organic acids. **Protect** from light.

Fluanisone is a butyrophenone with general properties similar to those of haloperidol (p.673). It has been used in the management of agitated states in psychiatric patients and as anaesthetic premedication.

Fluanisone is used in veterinary medicine for neuroleptanalgesia.

Preparations

Proprietary Preparations (details are given in Part 3)
Belg.: Sedalande†; *Fr.:* Sedalande†; *Ger.:* Sedalande†; *Switz.:* Sedalande†.

Fludiazepam (16810-x)

Fludiazepam (rINN).

ID-540. 7-Chloro-5-(2-fluorophenyl)-1,3-dihydro-1-methyl-2H-1,4-benzodiazepin-2-one.

$C_{16}H_{12}ClFN_2O$ = 302.7.

CAS — 3900-31-0.

Pharmacopoeias. In Jpn.

Fludiazepam is a short-acting benzodiazepine with general properties similar to those of diazepam (p.661). It is given by mouth in the short-term treatment of anxiety disorders (p.635).

Preparations

Proprietary Preparations (details are given in Part 3)
Jpn: Erispan.

Flunitrazepam (4034-w)

Flunitrazepam (BAN, USAN, rINN).

Flunitrazepamum; Ro-5-4200. 5-(2-Fluorophenyl)-1,3-dihydro-1-methyl-7-nitro-1,4-benzodiazepin-2-one.

$C_{16}H_{12}FN_3O_3$ = 313.3.

CAS — 1622-62-4.

Pharmacopoeias. In Eur. (see p.viii) and Jpn.

A white or yellowish crystalline powder. Practically **insoluble** in water; slightly soluble in alcohol and ether; soluble in acetone. **Protect** from light.

Dependence and Withdrawal, Adverse Effects, Treatment, and Precautions

As for Diazepam, p.661.

Abuse. A WHO review[1] concluded that flunitrazepam had a moderate abuse potential which might be higher than that of other benzodiazepines. It was reported that there was current evidence of widespread abuse of flunitrazepam among drug abusers, particularly among those who used opioids or cocaine.

Flunitrazepam has also been misused as a sedative in sexual assaults[2] or so called 'date rapes'.

1. WHO expert committee on drug dependence: twenty-ninth report. *WHO Tech Rep Ser 856* 1995.
2. Simmons MM, Cupp MJ. Use and abuse of flunitrazepam. *Ann Pharmacother* 1998; **32:** 117–19.

Local reactions. Of 43 patients given a single intravenous dose of flunitrazepam 1 to 2 mg two had local thrombosis 7 to 10 days later.[1] The incidence was lower than in those given diazepam [in solution]. Mikkelsen *et al.*,[2] however, found little difference in the incidence of local reactions after intravenous administration of flunitrazepam and diazepam.

1. Hegarty JE, Dundee JW. Sequelae after the intravenous injection of three benzodiazepines—diazepam, lorazepam, and flunitrazepam. *Br Med J* 1977; **2:** 1384–5.
2. Mikkelsen H, *et al.* Local reactions after iv injections of diazepam, flunitrazepam and isotonic saline. *Br J Anaesth* 1980; **52:** 817–19.

Porphyria. Flunitrazepam has been associated with clinical exacerbations of porphyria and is considered unsafe in porphyric patients.[1]

1. Moore MR, McColl KEL. *Porphyria: drug lists.* Glasgow: Porphyria Research Unit, University of Glasgow, 1991.

Interactions

As for Diazepam, p.663.

Pharmacokinetics

Flunitrazepam is readily absorbed from the gastro-intestinal tract. About 77 to 80% is bound to plasma proteins. It is extensively metabolised in the liver and excreted mainly in the urine as metabolites (free or conjugated). Its principal metabolites are 7-aminoflunitrazepam and *N*-desmethylflunitrazepam; *N*-desmethylflunitrazepam is reported to be pharmacologically active. The elimination half-life of flunitrazepam is reported to be between 16 and 35 hours. Flunitrazepam crosses the placental barrier and is distributed into breast milk.

References to the pharmacokinetics of flunitrazepam.

1. Davis PJ, Cook DR. Clinical pharmacokinetics of the newer intravenous anaesthetic agents. *Clin Pharmacokinet* 1986; **11:** 18–35.

Pregnancy and breast feeding. Concentrations of flunitrazepam in umbilical-vein and umbilical-artery plasma were lower than those in maternal venous plasma about 11 to 15 hours after administration of flunitrazepam 1 mg to 14 pregnant women; concentrations in amniotic fluid were lower still.[1] Concentrations in breast milk the morning after a single evening 2-mg dose were considered to be too low to produce clinical effects in breast-fed infants, although accumulation in the milk might occur after repeated administration.[1]

1. Kanto J, *et al.* Placental transfer and breast milk levels of flunitrazepam. *Curr Ther Res* 1979; **26:** 539–46.

Uses and Administration

Flunitrazepam is a short-acting benzodiazepine with general properties similar to those of diazepam (p.666). It is used in the short-term management of insomnia (p.638), as a premedicant in surgical procedures, and for induction of anaesthesia (p.1220).

A usual dose for insomnia is 0.5 to 1 mg by mouth at night; up to 2 mg may be given if necessary. In elderly or debilitated patients the initial dose should not exceed 0.5 mg at night; up to 1 mg may be given if necessary. A dose of 1 to 2 mg (0.015 to 0.030 mg per kg body-weight) has been given intramuscularly for premedication or by slow intravenous injection for induction of general anaesthesia.

Preparations

Proprietary Preparations (details are given in Part 3)
Aust.: Rohypnol; Somnubene; *Austral.:* Hypnodorm; Rohypnol; *Belg.:* Hypnocalm†; Rohypnol; *Fr.:* Narcozep†; Noriel†; Rohypnol; *Ger.:* Flunimerck; Fluninoc; Rohypnol; *Irl.:* Rohypnol; *Ital.:* Darkene; Roipnol; Valsera; *Neth.:* Rohypnol; *Norw.:* Flunipam; Flutraz; Rohypnol; *S.Afr.:* Hypnor; Insom; Rohypnol; *Spain:* Rohipnol; *Swed.:* Flupam; Fluscand; Rohypnol; *Switz.:* Rohypnol; *UK:* Rohypnol.

Fluopromazine (7041-w)

Fluopromazine (BAN).

Triflupromazine (rINN). NN-Dimethyl-3-(2-trifluoromethylphenothiazin-10-yl)propylamine.

$C_{18}H_{19}F_3N_2S$ = 352.4.

CAS — 146-54-3.

Pharmacopoeias. In US.

A pale amber viscous oily liquid which crystallises into large irregular crystals during prolonged storage. Practically **insoluble** in water. **Store** in airtight containers. Protect from light.

Fluopromazine Hydrochloride (7042-e)

Fluopromazine Hydrochloride (BANM).

Triflupromazine Hydrochloride (rINNM).

$C_{18}H_{19}F_3N_2S,HCl$ = 388.9.

CAS — 1098-60-8.

Pharmacopoeias. In US.

A white to pale tan crystalline powder with a slight characteristic odour.

Soluble 1 in less than 1 of water and of alcohol and 1 in 1.7 of chloroform; soluble in acetone; practically insoluble in ether. **Protect** from light.

Fluopromazine hydrochloride is a phenothiazine with general properties similar to those of chlorpromazine (p.649). It is used mainly in the management of psychoses (p.636) and the control of nausea and vomiting (p.1172). Fluopromazine hydrochloride is usually given by injection but in some countries preparations are available for administration by mouth.

In the management of psychosis, the usual dose is 60 to 150 mg daily by intramuscular injection. For the control of nausea and vomiting 5 to 15 mg is given intramuscularly and repeated after 4 hours if necessary up to a maximum of 60 mg daily; a dose of 1 mg to a maximum total daily dose of 3 mg may be given intravenously.

A suggested intramuscular dose for children over 2½ years of age is 0.2 to 0.25 mg per kg body-weight daily up to a maximum of 10 mg daily.

Reduced doses should be used in elderly or debilitated patients.

Preparations

USP 23: Triflupromazine Hydrochloride Injection; Triflupromazine Hydrochloride Tablets; Triflupromazine Oral Suspension.

Proprietary Preparations (details are given in Part 3)
Aust.: Psyquil; *Belg.:* Siquil†; *Ger.:* Psyquil; *Neth.:* Siquil; *Switz.:* Psyquil†; *USA:* Vesprin.

Multi-ingredient: *Ger.:* Psyquil compositum†.

Flupenthixol Decanoate (7044-y)

Flupenthixol Decanoate (BANM).

Flupentixol Decanoate (rINNM); (Z)-Flupenthixol Decanoate; cis-Flupenthixol Decanoate. (Z)-2-{4-[3-(2-Trifluoromethylthioxanthen-9-ylidene)propyl]piperazin-1-yl}ethyl decanoate.

$C_{33}H_{43}F_3N_2O_2S$ = 588.8.

CAS — 2709-56-0 (flupenthixol); 30909-51-4 (flupenthixol decanoate).

Pharmacopoeias. In Br.

A yellow viscous oil. Very slightly **soluble** in water; soluble in alcohol; freely soluble in chloroform and in ether. **Store** at a temperature below −15° and protect from light.

Flupenthixol Hydrochloride (7045-j)

Flupenthixol Hydrochloride (BANM).

Flupentixol Hydrochloride (rINNM); Flupenthixol Dihydrochloride; LC-44 (flupenthixol); N-7009 (flupenthixol). 2-{4-[3-(2-Trifluoromethylthioxanthen-9-ylidene)propyl]piperazin-1-yl}ethanol dihydrochloride.

$C_{23}H_{25}F_3N_2OS,2HCl$ = 507.4.

CAS — 2413-38-9.

Stability. References.

1. Enever RP, *et al.* Flupenthixol dihydrochloride decomposition in aqueous solution. *J Pharm Sci* 1979; **68:** 169–71.
2. Li Wan Po A, Irwin WJ. The photochemical stability of cis- and trans-isomers of tricyclic neuroleptic drugs. *J Pharm Pharmacol* 1980; **32:** 25–9.

Adverse Effects and Treatment

As for Chlorpromazine, p.649. Flupenthixol is less likely to cause sedation, but extrapyramidal disorders are more frequent.

Sudden death. A report of sudden death in 3 patients who had received depot injections of flupenthixol decanoate.[1]

1. Turbott J, Smeeton WMI. Sudden death and flupenthixol decanoate. *Aust N Z J Psychiatry* 1984; **18:** 91–4.

Precautions

As for Chlorpromazine, p.652.

Flupenthixol is not recommended in states of excitement or overactivity, including mania.

Porphyria. Flupenthixol was considered to be unsafe in patients with acute porphyria because it has been shown to be porphyrinogenic in *animals* or *in-vitro* systems.[1]

1. Moore MR, McColl KEL. *Porphyria: drug lists.* Glasgow: Porphyria Research Unit, University of Glasgow, 1991.

Interactions

As for Chlorpromazine, p.652.

Pharmacokinetics

Flupenthixol is readily absorbed from the gastro-intestinal tract and is probably subject to first-pass metabolism in the gut wall. It is also extensively metabolised in the liver and is excreted in the urine and faeces in the form of numerous metabolites; there is evidence of enterohepatic recycling. Owing to the first-pass effect, plasma concentrations following oral administration are much lower than those following estimated equivalent doses of the intramuscular depot preparation. Moreover, there is very wide intersubject variation in plasma concentrations of flupenthixol, but in practice, no simple correlation has been found between plasma concentrations of flupenthixol and its metabolites, and the therapeutic effect. Paths of metabolism of flupenthixol include sulphoxidation, side-chain *N*-dealkylation, and glucuronic acid conjugation. It is widely distributed in the body, and crosses the blood-brain barrier. Flupenthixol passes the placental barrier and small amounts have been detected in breast milk.

The decanoate ester of flupenthixol is very slowly absorbed from the site of intramuscular injection and is therefore suitable for depot injection. It is gradually released into the blood stream where it is rapidly hydrolysed to flupenthixol.

References.

1. Jørgensen A, Gottfries CG. Pharmacokinetic studies on flupenthixol and flupenthixol decanoate in man using tritium labelled compounds. *Psychopharmacologia* 1972; **27:** 1–10.
2. Jørgensen A. Pharmacokinetic studies on flupenthixol decanoate, a depot neuroleptic of the thioxanthene group. *Drug Metab Rev* 1978; **8:** 235–49.

Uses and Administration

Flupenthixol is a thioxanthene antipsychotic with general properties similar to those of the phenothiazine, chlorpromazine (p.654). It has a piperazine side-chain. Flupenthixol is used mainly in the treatment of schizophrenia (p.637) and other psychoses. Unlike chlorpromazine, a certain activating effect has been ascribed to flupenthixol and, accordingly, it is not indicated in overactive, including manic, patients. Flupenthixol has also been used for its antidepressant properties.

Flupenthixol is administered as the hydrochloride by mouth or as the longer-acting decanoate ester by deep intramuscular injection.

The usual initial dose of the hydrochloride for the treatment of **psychoses** is the equivalent of 3 to 9 mg of flupenthixol twice daily adjusted according to the response; the maximum recommended dose is a total of 18 mg daily. The initial dose in elderly and debilitated patients may need to be reduced to a quarter or a half of the normal starting dose. The long-acting decanoate preparation available in the UK contains flupenthixol as the *cis(Z)*-isomer (see Action, below) and doses are expressed in terms of the amount of *cis(Z)*-flupenthixol decanoate. It should be given by deep intramuscular injection in an initial test dose of 20 mg, as 1 mL of a 2% oily solution. Then after at least 7 days and according to the patient's response, this may be followed by doses of 20 to 40 mg at intervals of 2 to 4 weeks. Shorter dosage intervals or greater amounts may be required according to the patient's response. The initial dose in elderly and debilitated patients may need to be reduced to a quarter or a half of the normal starting dose. If doses greater than 40 mg are considered necessary they should be divided between 2 separate injection sites. Another means of reducing the volume of fluid to be injected in patients requiring high-dose therapy with flupenthixol decanoate is to give an injection containing 100 or 200 mg of the decanoate per mL (10 or 20%). The usual maintenance dose is between 50 mg every 4 weeks and 300 mg every 2 weeks but doses of up to 400 mg weekly have been given in severe or resistant conditions.

Flupenthixol has also been given as the hydrochloride by mouth, for the treatment of mild to moderate **depression**, with or without anxiety. The usual initial dose, expressed in terms of the equivalent amount of flupenthixol, is 1 mg (0.5 mg in the elderly) daily, increased after 1 week to 2 mg (1 mg in the elderly) and then to a maximum of 3 mg (2 mg in the elderly) daily in divided doses. The last dose of the day should be given no later than 4 p.m. and if no effect has been noted within 1 week of administration of the maximum dose, the treatment should be withdrawn.

Action. Patients with acute schizophrenic illnesses taking α-flupenthixol [(*Z*)-flupenthixol or *cis*-flupenthixol] improved more after 3 weeks than patients who were taking equal doses of β-flupenthixol [(*E*)-flupenthixol or *trans*-flupenthixol] or a placebo.[1] The α-isomer had more effect on the positive symptoms of the disease; this difference was less apparent for the negative symptoms. The difference in activity between the isomers was attributed to the greater dopamine-receptor blocking activity of the α-isomer rather than to differences in distribution.[2]

1. Johnstone EC, *et al.* Mechanism of the antipsychotic effect in the treatment of acute schizophrenia. *Lancet* 1978; **i:** 848–51.
2. Crow TJ, Johnstone EC. Mechanism of action of neuroleptic drugs. *Lancet* 1978; **i:** 1050.

Cocaine withdrawal. Depot flupenthixol decanoate has produced some promising results as an aid in reducing cocaine usage (see p.1291).

References.

1. Gawin FH, *et al.* Flupentixol-induced aversion to crack cocaine. *N Engl J Med* 1996; **334:** 1340–1.

Depression. Depression and its management is discussed on p.271. Flupenthixol is not one of the drugs usually considered for first-line treatment of depression but there are some small studies[1,2] claiming favourable antidepressant efficacy for flupenthixol compared with other drugs.

1. Hamilton BA, *et al.* Flupenthixol and fluvoxamine in mild to moderate depression: a comparison in general practice. *Pharmatherapeutica* 1989; **5:** 292–7.
2. Dwivedi VS, *et al.* Depression in general practice: a comparison of flupenthixol dihydrochloride and dothiepin hydrochloride. *Curr Med Res Opin* 1990; **12:** 191–7.

Preparations

BP 1998: Flupentixol Injection.

Proprietary Preparations (details are given in Part 3)

Aust.: Fluanxol; ***Austral.:*** Fluanxol; ***Belg.:*** Fluanxol; ***Canad.:*** Fluanxol; ***Fr.:*** Fluanxol; ***Ger.:*** Fluanxol; ***Irl.:*** Depixol; Fluanxol; ***Neth.:*** Fluanxol; ***Norw.:*** Fluanxol; ***S.Afr.:*** Fluanxol; ***Swed.:*** Fluanxol; ***Switz.:*** Fluanxol; ***UK:*** Depixol; Fluanxol.

Multi-ingredient: ***Aust.:*** Deanxit; ***Belg.:*** Deanxit; ***Ger.:*** Benpon†; ***Ital.:*** Deanxit; ***Spain:*** Deanxit; ***Switz.:*** Deanxit.

Fluphenazine Decanoate (7046-z)

Fluphenazine Decanoate *(BANM, rINNM).*

Fluphenazini Decanoas. 2-{4-[3-(2-Trifluoromethylphenothiazin-10-yl)propyl]piperazin-1-yl}ethyl decanoate.

$C_{32}H_{44}F_3N_3O_2S$ = 591.8.

CAS — 69-23-8 (fluphenazine); 5002-47-1 (fluphenazine decanoate).

Pharmacopoeias. In *Chin., Eur.* (see p.viii), *Int.,* and *US.*

A pale yellow viscous liquid or a yellow solid. Fluphenazine decanoate 12.5 mg is approximately equivalent to 10.75 mg of fluphenazine hydrochloride. Practically **insoluble** in water; very soluble in dehydrated alcohol, in ether, and in dichloromethane; freely soluble in methyl alcohol. **Store** in airtight containers. Protect from light.

Fluphenazine Enanthate (7047-c)

Fluphenazine Enanthate *(BANM).*

Fluphenazine Enantate *(rINNM);* Fluphenazine Heptanoate; Fluphenazini Enantas. 2-{4-[3-(2-Trifluoromethylphenothiazin-10-yl)propyl]piperazin-1-yl}ethyl heptanoate.

$C_{29}H_{38}F_3N_3O_2S$ = 549.7.

CAS — 2746-81-8.

Pharmacopoeias. In *Eur.* (see p.viii), *Int., Jpn,* and *US.*

A pale yellow to yellow-orange, clear to slightly turbid, viscous liquid or a yellow solid. Fluphenazine enanthate 12.5 mg is approximately equivalent to 11.6 mg of fluphenazine hydrochloride.

Ph. Eur. **solubilities** are: practically insoluble in water; very soluble in dehydrated alcohol, in dichloromethane, and in ether; freely soluble in methyl alcohol. USP solubilities are: insoluble in water; soluble 1 in less than 1 of alcohol and of chloroform and 1 in 2 of ether. Stable in air at room temperature but unstable in strong light. **Store** in airtight containers. Protect from light.

Fluphenazine Hydrochloride (7048-k)

Fluphenazine Hydrochloride *(BANM, rINNM).*

Fluphenazini Hydrochloridum. 2-{4-[3-(2-Trifluoromethylphenothiazin-10-yl)propyl]piperazin-1-yl}ethanol dihydrochloride.

$C_{22}H_{26}F_3N_3OS,2HCl$ = 510.4.

CAS — 146-56-5.

Pharmacopoeias. In *Chin., Eur.* (see p.viii), *Int., Pol.,* and *US.*

A white or almost white, odourless crystalline powder.

Ph. Eur. **solubilities** are: freely soluble in water; slightly soluble in alcohol and in dichloromethane; practically insoluble in ether. USP solubilities are: soluble 1 in 1.4 of water and 1 in 6.7 of alcohol; slightly soluble in chloroform and in acetone; practically insoluble in ether. A 5% solution in water has a pH of 1.9 to 2.4.

Store in airtight containers. Protect from light.

Adverse Effects and Treatment

As for Chlorpromazine, p.649. Fluphenazine is less likely to cause sedation, hypotension, or antimuscarinic effects but is associated with a higher incidence of extrapyramidal effects.

An important incidence of akinesia, involuntary movement, autonomic disturbances, and drowsiness may occur in the first few hours following injection of fluphenazine decanoate and in the first 2 days following injection of fluphenazine enanthate.[1]

1. Curry SH, *et al.* Unwanted effects of fluphenazine enanthate and decanoate. *Lancet* 1979; **i:** 331–2.

Convulsions. For mention of fluphenazine as one of the antipsychotics suitable for patients at risk of seizures, see p.649.

Effects on the liver. A patient given 3 injections of a depot antipsychotic containing fluphenazine decanoate over a 2-week period subsequently developed jaundice, beginning 17 days after the first dose.[1] The patient developed indicators of severe liver toxicity, with extreme hyperbilirubinaemia and raised liver enzyme values, and remained very ill for the next 4 months. The patient was found to exhibit cross-sensitivity to haloperidol but not to flupenthixol.

See also under Chlorpromazine, p.650.

1. Kennedy P. Liver cross-sensitivity to antipsychotic drugs. *Br J Psychiatry* 1983; **143:** 312.

Overdosage. A patient who took about 30 fluphenazine hydrochloride 2.5-mg tablets was treated with gastric lavage.[1] Twenty hours after hospital admission he experienced difficulty in breathing due to spasm of the respiratory muscles; other very severe extrapyramidal side-effects were also present. Muscle spasm was controlled by diazepam.

There were few ill-effects in a patient given intramuscular fluphenazine decanoate 50 mg every 4 hours, instead of the intended 4 weeks, to a total of 1050 mg.[2] About three weeks after the period of overdosage the patient had some degree of hypothermia and tachycardia, and after a further week parkinsonian signs appeared. No specific treatment was given.

1. Ladhani FM. Severe extrapyramidal manifestations following fluphenazine overdose. *Med J Aust* 1974; **2:** 26.
2. Cheung HK, Yu ECS. Effect of 1050 mg fluphenazine decanoate given intramuscularly over six days. *Br Med J* 1983; **286:** 1016–17.

Precautions

As for Chlorpromazine, p.652. Fluphenazine may exacerbate depression; depot injections are therefore contra-indicated in severely depressed patients.

Pregnancy. Nasal congestion with severe rhinorrhoea, respiratory distress, vomiting, and extrapyramidal symptoms occurred in a neonate delivered to a mother who had received fluphenazine hydrochloride 10 to 20 mg daily throughout pregnancy.[1] Respiratory symptoms appeared to respond to pseudoephedrine.

1. Nath SP, *et al.* Severe rhinorrhea and respiratory distress in a neonate exposed to fluphenazine hydrochloride prenatally. *Ann Pharmacother* 1996; **30:** 35–7.

Interactions

As for Chlorpromazine, p.652.

Pharmacokinetics

For an account of the pharmacokinetics of a phenothiazine, see Chlorpromazine, p.654.

Fluphenazine decanoate and fluphenazine enanthate are very slowly absorbed from the site of subcutaneous or intramuscular injection. They both gradually release fluphenazine into the body and are therefore suitable for use as depot injections.

The plasma half-life of fluphenazine after a single dose was 14.7 hours in 1 patient given the hydrochloride by mouth and 14.9 and 15.3 hours in 2 patients given the hydrochloride by intramuscular injection.[1] The half-life was 3.6 and 3.7 days in 2 patients given the enanthate intramuscularly and 9.6 and 6.8 days in 2 patients given the decanoate intramuscularly. Peak plasma-fluphenazine concentrations occurred earlier in patients given fluphenazine decanoate compared with those who received the enanthate. Fluphenazine sulphoxide and 7-hydroxyfluphenazine were identified in the urine and faeces.

1. Curry SH, *et al.* Kinetics of fluphenazine after fluphenazine dihydrochloride, enanthate and decanoate administration to man. *Br J Clin Pharmacol* 1979; **7:** 325–31.

Further references to the pharmacokinetics of fluphenazine.

1. Wistedt B, *et al.* Slow decline of plasma drug and prolactin levels after discontinuation of chronic treatment with depot neuroleptics. *Lancet* 1981; **i:** 1163.
2. Midha KK, *et al.* Kinetics of oral fluphenazine disposition in humans by GC-MS. *Eur J Clin Pharmacol* 1983; **25:** 709–11.
3. Marder SR, *et al.* Plasma levels of parent drug and metabolites in patients receiving oral and depot fluphenazine. *Psychopharmacol Bull* 1989; **25:** 479–82.

Uses and Administration

Fluphenazine is a phenothiazine with general properties similar to those of chlorpromazine (p.654). It has a piperazine side-chain. Fluphenazine is used in the treatment of a variety of psychiatric disorders including schizophrenia (p.637), mania (p.273), severe anxiety (p.635), and behavioural disturbances (p.636). Fluphenazine is administered as the hydrochloride usually by mouth or sometimes by intramuscular injection; longer-acting decanoate or enanthate esters of fluphenazine are given by intramuscular or sometimes subcutaneous injection.

The usual initial dose of the hydrochloride for the treatment of schizophrenia, mania, and other psychoses is 2.5 to 10 mg daily in two to three divided doses; the dose is then increased according to response up to a usual maximum of 20 mg daily (10 mg daily in the elderly), although up to 40 mg has occasionally been given. Dosage may subsequently be reduced to a usual maintenance dose of 1 to 5 mg daily. Treatment is sometimes started with an initial intramuscular injection of 1.25 mg of the hydrochloride adjusted thereafter according to response. The usual initial intramuscular daily dose is 2.5 to 10 mg given in divided doses every 6 to 8 hours. In general the required parenteral doses of fluphenazine hydrochloride have been found to be approximately one-third to one-half of those given by mouth.

The long-acting decanoate or enanthate esters of fluphenazine are usually given by deep intramuscular injection and are used mainly for the maintenance treatment of patients with schizophrenia or other chronic psychoses. The onset of action is usually within 1 to 3 days of injection and significant effects on psychosis are usually evident within 2 to 4 days. An initial dose of fluphenazine decanoate or enanthate 12.5 mg (6.25 mg in the elderly) is given intramuscularly to assess the extrapyramidal effects. A dose of 25 mg may then be given every 2 weeks with subsequent adjustments in the amounts and the dosage interval according to the patient's response; the amounts required may range from 12.5 to 100 mg and the intervals required may range from 2 weeks to 5 or 6 weeks. If doses greater than 50 mg are considered necessary cautious increments should be made in steps of 12.5 mg. Some studies suggest that certain patients can be adequately maintained on doses of 5 to 10 mg (see Schizophrenia, below).

Fluphenazine hydrochloride has also been given by mouth in doses of 1 mg twice daily, increased if necessary to 2 mg twice daily, for severe anxiety or behavioural disturbances.

Chorea. For a discussion of the management of various choreas, including mention of the use of phenothiazines such as fluphenazine, see p.636.

References.

1. Terrence CF. Fluphenazine decanoate is the treatment of chorea: a double-blind study. *Curr Ther Res* 1976; **20:** 177–83.

Schizophrenia. References[1-3] to fluphenazine in schizophrenia (p.637) indicating that low doses may be effective in some patients.

1. Kane JM, *et al.* Low-dose neuroleptic treatment of outpatient schizophrenics: I preliminary results for relapse rates. *Arch Gen Psychiatry* 1983; **40:** 893–6.
2. Marder SR, *et al.* Low- and conventional-dose maintenance therapy with fluphenazine decanoate: two-year outcome. *Arch Gen Psychiatry* 1987; **44:** 581–21.
3. Hogarty GE, *et al.* Dose of fluphenazine, familial expressed emotion, and outcome in schizophrenia: results of a two-year controlled study. *Arch Gen Psychiatry* 1988; **45:** 797–805.

Tourette's syndrome. Tourette's syndrome (p.636) is a disorder characterised by motor and vocal tics and behavioural disturbances. Many patients do not require medication since their symptoms are not impairing. When treatment is needed dopamine antagonists such as the antipsychotics haloperidol or pimozide are most commonly used but fluphenazine has been tried[1] as an alternative.

1. Singer HS, *et al.* Haloperidol, fluphenazine and clonidine in tourette syndrome: controversies in treatment. *Pediatr Neurosci* 1985–86; **12:** 71–4.

Preparations

BP 1998: Fluphenazine Decanoate Injection; Fluphenazine Tablets;
USP 23: Fluphenazine Decanoate Injection; Fluphenazine Enanthate Injection; Fluphenazine Hydrochloride Elixir; Fluphenazine Hydrochloride Injection; Fluphenazine Hydrochloride Oral Solution; Fluphenazine Hydrochloride Tablets.

Proprietary Preparations (details are given in Part 3)
Aust.: Dapotum; ***Austral.:*** Anatensol; Modecate; ***Belg.:*** Anatensol†; Moditen†; Sevinol; ***Canad.:*** Modecate; Moditen; ***Fr.:*** Modecate; Moditen; ***Ger.:*** Dapotum; Lyogen; Lyorodin; Omca; ***Irl.:*** Modecate; Moditen; ***Ital.:*** Anatensol; Moditen Depot; ***Neth.:*** Anatensol; Moditen†; ***Norw.:*** Pacinol†; Siqualone; ***S.Afr.:*** Decafen; Fludecate; Modecate; Modecate Acutum; ***Spain:*** Modecate; ***Swed.:*** Pacinol; Siqualone; ***Switz.:*** Dapotum; Lyogen†; Moditen†; ***UK:*** Decazate†; Modecate; Moditen; ***USA:*** Permitil; Prolixin.

Multi-ingredient: ***Belg.:*** Celestamine-F†; ***Fr.:*** Motival; ***Ger.:*** Omca Nacht†; ***Irl.:*** Motipress; Motival; ***Ital.:*** Dominans; ***S.Afr.:*** Mendrome†; Motival; ***UK:*** Motipress; Motival.

Flurazepam (11384-n)

Flurazepam *(BAN, rINN).*

7-Chloro-1-(2-diethylaminoethyl)-5-(2-fluorophenyl)-1,3-dihydro-1,4-benzodiazepin-2-one.

$C_{21}H_{23}ClFN_3O$ = 387.9.

CAS — 17617-23-1.

Pharmacopoeias. In *Jpn.*

Flurazepam Monohydrochloride (4035-e)

Flurazepam Monohydrochloride *(BANM, rINNM).*

Flurazepami Monohydrochloridum.

$C_{21}H_{23}ClFN_3O,HCl$ = 424.3.

CAS — 36105-20-1.

Pharmacopoeias. In *Eur.* (see p.viii) and *Jpn.*

A white or almost white crystalline powder. Flurazepam monohydrochloride 32.8 mg is approximately equivalent to 30 mg of flurazepam. Very **soluble** in water; freely soluble in alcohol; practically insoluble in ether. A 5% solution in water has a pH of 5.0 to 6.0. **Protect** from light.

Flurazepam Dihydrochloride (4036-l)

Flurazepam Dihydrochloride *(BANM, rINNM).*

Flurazepam Hydrochloride *(USAN)*; NSC-78559; Ro-5-6901.

$C_{21}H_{23}ClFN_3O,2HCl$ = 460.8.

CAS — 1172-18-5.

Pharmacopoeias. In *US.*

An off-white to yellow, odourless or almost odourless, crystalline powder. Flurazepam dihydrochloride 30 mg is approximately equivalent to 25.3 mg of flurazepam. **Soluble** 1 in 2 of water, 1 in 4 of alcohol, 1 in 90 of chloroform, 1 in 3 of methyl alcohol, 1 in 69 of isopropyl alcohol, and 1 in 5000 of ether and of petroleum spirit. A solution in water is acid to litmus. **Store** in airtight containers. Protect from light.

Dependence and Withdrawal, Adverse Effects, Treatment, and Precautions

As for Diazepam, p.661.

Effects on the liver. Reports of cholestatic jaundice following the use of flurazepam.[1,2]

1. Fang MH, *et al.* Cholestatic jaundice associated with flurazepam hydrochloride. *Ann Intern Med* 1978; **89:** 363–4.
2. Reynolds R, *et al.* Cholestatic jaundice induced by flurazepam hydrochloride. *Can Med Assoc J* 1981; **124:** 893–4.

Effects on taste. Flurazepam had been reported to cause dysgeusia.[1]

1. Willoughby JMT. Drug-induced abnormalities of taste sensation. *Adverse Drug React Bull* 1983 (June): 368–71.

Porphyria. Flurazepam has been associated with clinical exacerbations of porphyria and is considered unsafe in porphyric patients.[1]

1. Moore MR, McColl KEL. *Porphyria: drug lists.* Glasgow: Porphyria Research Unit, University of Glasgow, 1991.

Renal impairment. Five patients on maintenance haemodialysis developed encephalopathy attributed to flurazepam and diazepam.[1]

1. Taclob L, Needle M. Drug-induced encephalopathy in patients on maintenance haemodialysis. *Lancet* 1976; **ii:** 704–5.

Interactions

As for Diazepam, p.663.

Pharmacokinetics

Flurazepam is readily absorbed from the gastro-intestinal tract. It undergoes extensive first-pass metabolism and is excreted in the urine, chiefly as conjugated metabolites. The major active metabolite is *N*-desalkylflurazepam, which is reported to have a half-life ranging from 47 to 100 hours or more.

Metabolism. The metabolism of flurazepam was studied in 4 healthy male volunteers given 30 mg daily for 2 weeks.[1] A hydroxyethyl metabolite was present in the blood shortly after administration. The *N*-desalkyl metabolite, the major metabolite in the blood, had a half-life ranging from 47 to 100 hours. Steady-state concentrations were reached after 7 to 10 days and were approximately 5 to 6 times greater than those observed on day 1. There has been a study in 3 patients indicating that some metabolism of flurazepam may occur in the small bowel mucosa.[2]

1. Kaplan SA, *et al.* Blood level profile in man following chronic oral administration of flurazepam hydrochloride. *J Pharm Sci* 1973; **62:** 1932–5.
2. Mahon WA, *et al.* Metabolism of flurazepam by the small intestine. *Clin Pharmacol Ther* 1977; **22:** 228–33.

Uses and Administration

Flurazepam is a long-acting benzodiazepine with general properties similar to those of diazepam (p.666). It is used as a hypnotic in the short-term management of insomnia (p.638). In the USA flurazepam is given in doses of 15 to 30 mg of the dihydrochloride by mouth at night. In the UK it is given as the monohydrochloride in doses equivalent to 15 to 30 mg of flurazepam at night. A maximum initial dose of 15 mg has been suggested in the UK and the USA for elderly or debilitated patients.

Preparations

BP 1998: Flurazepam Capsules;
USP 23: Flurazepam Hydrochloride Capsules.

Proprietary Preparations (details are given in Part 3)
Aust.: Staurodorm†; ***Austral.:*** Dalmane†; ***Belg.:*** Staurodorm; ***Canad.:*** Dalmane; Novo-Flupam; Somnol; ***Ger.:*** Dalmadorm; Staurodorm Neu; ***Irl.:*** Dalmane; Irdal†; ***Ital.:*** Dalmadorm; Felison; Flunox; Midorm AR†; Remdue; Valdorm; ***Neth.:*** Dalmadorm; ***S.Afr.:*** Dalmadorm; ***Spain:*** Dormodor; ***Switz.:*** Dalmadorm; ***UK:*** Dalmane; ***USA:*** Dalmane.

Fluspirilene (7049-a)

Fluspirilene *(BAN, USAN, rINN).*

McN-JR-6218; R-6218. 8-[4,4-Bis(4-fluorophenyl)butyl]-1-phenyl-1,3,8-triazaspiro[4.5]decan-4-one.

$C_{29}H_{31}F_2N_3O$ = 475.6.

CAS — 1841-19-6.

Adverse Effects, Treatment, and Precautions

As for Chlorpromazine, p.649. Fluspirilene is less likely to cause sedation. With prolonged use subcutaneous nodules may occur at the injection site.

References.

1. McCreadie RG, *et al.* Probable toxic necrosis after prolonged fluspirilene administration. *Br Med J* 1979; **1:** 523–4.

Pharmacokinetics

Fluspirilene is slowly absorbed after intramuscular injection of a microcrystalline aqueous suspension, detectable blood concentrations being reached within 4 hours of injection. It is rapidly metabolised on release from the injection site and the main metabolite, which is 4,4-bis(4-fluorophenyl)butyric acid obtained by *N*-dealkylation, is excreted in the urine. The elimination half-life of fluspirilene is reported to be approximately 3 weeks.

Uses and Administration

Fluspirilene is a diphenylbutylpiperidine antipsychotic and has general properties similar to those of the phenothiazine, chlorpromazine (p.654). It is given by deep intramuscular injection for the treatment of schizophrenia (p.637).

Fluspirilene has a duration of action which lasts for about a week, with a range of 5 to 15 days. A usual initial dose is 2 mg weekly by deep intramuscular injection, increased by 1 to 2 mg weekly according to the patient's response. The usual maintenance dose is 2 to 10 mg weekly; doses in excess of 15 mg weekly are not usually recommended.

Elderly patients may be given a quarter to half the usual adult initial dose.

Preparations

Proprietary Preparations (details are given in Part 3)
Belg.: Imap; ***Canad.:*** Imap; ***Ger.:*** Imap; ***Irl.:*** Redeptin; ***Neth.:*** Imap; ***Norw.:*** Imap; ***Switz.:*** Imap; ***UK:*** Redeptin†.

Flutoprazepam (19191-w)

Flutoprazepam *(rINN)*.

KB-509. 7-Chloro-1-(cyclopropylmethyl)-5-(2-fluorophenyl)-1,3-dihydro-2*H*-1,4-benzodiazepin-2-one.

$C_{19}H_{16}ClFN_2O$ = 342.8.

CAS — 25967-29-7.

Flutoprazepam is a benzodiazepine with general properties similar to those of diazepam (p.661).

References.

1. Realini R, *et al.* Flutoprazepam in the treatment of generalized anxiety disorders: a dose-ranging study. *Curr Ther Res* 1990; **47:** 860–8.

Preparations

Proprietary Preparations (details are given in Part 3)
Jpn: Restas†.

Gepirone Hydrochloride (19247-w)

Gepirone Hydrochloride *(USAN, rINNM)*.

BMY-13805-1; MJ-13805-1. 3,3-Dimethyl-*N*-{4-[4-(2-pyrimidinyl)-1-piperazinyl]butyl}glutarimide hydrochloride.

$C_{19}H_{29}N_5O_2,HCl$ = 395.9.

CAS — 83928-76-1 (gepirone); 83928-66-9 (gepirone hydrochloride).

Gepirone is structurally related to buspirone (p.643). It is being investigated as the hydrochloride for the treatment of anxiety disorders and depression.

Gepirone is a partial agonist at serotonin (hydroxytryptamine, 5-HT) receptors of the 5-HT_{1A} subtype. For reference to the actions and potential uses of such drugs, see Buspirone Hydrochloride, p.644.

References.

1. Feiger AD. A double-blind comparison of gepirone extended release, imipramine, and placebo in the treatment of outpatient major depression. *Psychopharmacol Bull* 1996; **32:** 659–65.
2. Rickels K, *et al.* Gepirone and diazepam in generalized anxiety disorder: a placebo-controlled trial. *J Clin Psychopharmacol* 1997; **17:** 272–7.

Glutethimide (4037-y)

Glutethimide *(BAN, rINN)*.

Glutethimidum; Glutetimide. 2-Ethyl-2-phenylglutarimide; 3-Ethyl-3-phenylpiperidine-2,6-dione.

$C_{13}H_{15}NO_2$ = 217.3.

CAS — 77-21-4.

Pharmacopoeias. In *Eur.* (see p.viii) and *US.*

Colourless crystals or white or almost white crystalline powder. M.p. 86° to 89°.

Ph. Eur. **solubilities** are: practically insoluble in water; freely soluble in alcohol; soluble in ether; very soluble in dichloromethane. USP solubilities are: practically insoluble in water; soluble in alcohol and in methyl alcohol; freely soluble in acetone, in chloroform, in ether, and in ethyl acetate. A saturated solution in water is acid to litmus. **Protect** from light.

Dependence and Withdrawal

As for the barbiturates (see Amylobarbitone, p.641).

Adverse Effects

Side-effects of glutethimide include nausea, headache, blurred vision, unwanted sedation and other CNS effects such as ataxia, impaired memory, and paradoxical excitement, and occasional skin rashes. Acute hypersensitivity reactions, blood disorders, and exfoliative dermatitis have been reported in rare instances.

Overdosage with glutethimide produces symptoms similar to those of barbiturate overdosage; respiratory depression is usually less severe, and circulatory failure more severe than with the barbiturates (see Amylobarbitone, p.642). There are considerable fluctuations in the depth of coma and wakefulness. Antimuscarinic effects such as mydriasis, dryness of the mouth, paralytic ileus, and urinary bladder atony often occur. Irregular absorption and storage in fat depots may complicate treatment.

Overdosage. A detailed review of acute poisoning with glutethimide and other drugs acting on the CNS.[1]

1. Ashton CH, *et al.* Drug-induced stupor and coma: some physical signs and their pharmacological basis. *Adverse Drug React Acute Poisoning Rev* 1989; **8:** 1–59.

Treatment of Adverse Effects

As for the barbiturates, (see Amylobarbitone, p.642).

Precautions

Glutethimide should be used with care in patients with renal impairment and, as with all sedatives, in patients with impaired respiratory function. Because of its antimuscarinic actions it should be given with great care to patients with conditions such as angle-closure glaucoma, prostatic hyperplasia or urinary tract obstruction, pyloroduodenal obstruction, or cardiac arrhythmias.

Glutethimide may cause drowsiness; affected patients should not drive or operate machinery.

Abuse. A warning of the hazards associated with the abuse of glutethimide in a combination with codeine termed 'loads'.[1]

1. Sramek JJ, Khajawall A. "Loads". *N Engl J Med* 1981; **305:** 231.

Porphyria. Glutethimide has been associated with acute attacks of porphyria and is considered unsafe in patients with acute porphyria.[1]

1. Moore MR, McColl KEL. *Porphyria: drug lists.* Glasgow: Porphyria Research Unit, University of Glasgow, 1991.

Interactions

The sedative effects of glutethimide are enhanced by the simultaneous administration of CNS depressants such as alcohol, barbiturates, and other sedatives; absorption of glutethimide is also markedly enhanced by concomitant administration of alcohol. Glutethimide induces microsomal hepatic enzymes, and it can thus cause increased metabolism of coumarin anticoagulants and other drugs, with reduced effect. Chronic administration of glutethimide may also enhance vitamin D metabolism.

Pharmacokinetics

Glutethimide is irregularly absorbed from the gastro-intestinal tract and extensively metabolised in the liver. It has a biphasic plasma half-life; half-lives of up to 22 hours have been reported for the terminal phase. Glutethimide is excreted in urine, almost entirely as metabolites, with less than 2% of unchanged drug. Up to 2% of a dose has been reported to be present in the faeces. Glutethimide is reported to be about 50% bound to plasma proteins. It is highly lipid-soluble and may be stored in adipose tissue. It crosses the placental barrier and traces are found in breast milk.

Uses and Administration

Glutethimide is a piperidinedione hypnotic and sedative. It has been reported to act in about 30 minutes to induce sleep lasting 4 to 8 hours. It has been given by mouth for the short-term management of insomnia (p.638) in usual doses of 250 to 500 mg at night but has been superseded by other drugs.

Preparations

USP 23: Glutethimide Capsules; Glutethimide Tablets.

Halazepam (7050-e)

Halazepam *(BAN, USAN, rINN)*.

Sch-12041. 7-Chloro-1,3-dihydro-5-phenyl-1-(2,2,2-trifluoroethyl)-1,4-benzodiazepin-2-one.

$C_{17}H_{12}ClF_3N_2O$ = 352.7.

CAS — 23092-17-3.

Halazepam is a benzodiazepine with general properties similar to those of diazepam (p.661). It is given by mouth for the short-term treatment of anxiety disorders (p.635).

References.

1. Greenblatt DJ, *et al.* Halazepam, another precursor of desmethyldiazepam. *Lancet* 1982; **i:** 1358–9.

Preparations

Proprietary Preparations (details are given in Part 3)
Belg.: Pacinone†; ***Ital.:*** Paxipam; ***Neth.:*** Pacinone†; ***Spain:*** Alapryl; ***USA:*** Paxipam†.

Haloperidol (18332-f)

Haloperidol *(BAN, USAN, rINN)*.

Aloperidolo; Haloperidolum; McN-JR-1625; R-1625. 4-[4-(4-Chlorophenyl)-4-hydroxypiperidino]-4′-fluorobutyrophenone.

$C_{21}H_{23}ClFNO_2$ = 375.9.

CAS — 52-86-8.

Pharmacopoeias. In *Chin., Eur.* (see p.viii), *Int., Jpn, Pol.,* and *US.*

A white to faintly yellowish amorphous or microcrystalline powder.

Soluble 1 in more than 10 000 of water, 1 in 60 of alcohol, 1 in 15 of chloroform, and 1 in 200 of ether; slightly soluble in dichloromethane and in methyl alcohol. A saturated solution is neutral to litmus. **Store** in airtight containers. Protect from light.

Dilution. See Incompatibility, below.

Incompatibility. Formation of a precipitate was observed after dilution of haloperidol (as the lactate) in sodium chloride 0.9% injection when the final haloperidol concentration was 1.0 mg per mL or higher.[1]

Undiluted haloperidol (5 mg per mL) injection has been reported to be incompatible with heparin sodium (diluted in sodium chloride 0.9% or glucose 5% injection),[2] sodium nitroprusside (diluted in glucose 5%),[1] cefmetazole sodium,[3] and diphenhydramine.[4] A mixture of equal volumes of sargramostim 10 μg per mL and haloperidol (as the lactate) 0.2 mg per mL resulted in a precipitate at 4 hours.[5]

1. Outman WR, Monolakis J. Visual compatibility of haloperidol lactate with 0.9% sodium chloride injection or injectable critical-care drugs during simulated Y-site injection. *Am J Hosp Pharm* 1991; **48:** 1539–41.
2. Solomon DA, Nasinnyk KK. Compatibility of haloperidol lactate and heparin sodium. *Am J Hosp Pharm* 1982; **39:** 843–4.
3. Hutchings SR, *et al.* Compatibility of cefmetazole sodium with commonly used drugs during Y-site delivery. *Am J Health-Syst Pharm* 1996; **53:** 2185–8.
4. Ukhun IA. Compatibility of haloperidol and diphenhydramine in a hypodermic syringe. *Ann Pharmacother* 1995; **29:** 1168–9.
5. Trissel LA, *et al.* Visual compatibility of sargramostim with selected antineoplastic agents, anti-infectives, or other drugs during simulated Y-site injection. *Am J Hosp Pharm* 1992; **49:** 402–6.

Solubilisation. A study of haloperidol solubilisation in oils by aliphatic acids, and an evaluation *in vitro* of haloperidol release from solutions including oleic or linoleic acid.[1]

1. Radd BL, *et al.* Development of haloperidol in oil injection formulations. *J Parenter Sci Technol* 1985; **39:** 48–51.

Stability. Mention that a combination of the stabilisers benzyl alcohol and vanillin could protect haloperidol from photodegradation.[1]

1. Thoma K, Klimek R. Photostabilisation of drugs in dosage forms without protection from packaging materials. *Int J Pharmaceutics* 1991; **67:** 169–75.

Haloperidol Decanoate (7051-l)

Haloperidol Decanoate *(BANM, USAN, rINNM)*.

R-13672.

$C_{31}H_{41}ClFNO_3$ = 530.1.

CAS — 74050-97-8.

Adverse Effects and Treatment

As for Chlorpromazine, p.649. Haloperidol is less likely to cause sedation, hypotension, or antimuscarinic effects, but is associated with a higher incidence of extrapyramidal effects.

Convulsions. For mention of haloperidol as one of the antipsychotics suitable for patients at risk of seizures, see p.649.

Effects on the liver. Liver dysfunction with jaundice and eosinophilia developed in a 15-year-old male 4 weeks after administration of haloperidol and benztropine mesylate.[1] This treatment was discontinued 2 weeks later but some symptoms lasted for 28 months. The reaction was suggestive of a drug-induced hypersensitivity reaction and haloperidol was the most likely cause. Haloperidol-induced liver injury was considered to be rare.

1. Dincsoy HP, Saelinger DA. Haloperidol-induced chronic cholestatic liver disease. *Gastroenterology* 1982; **83:** 694–700.

Overdosage. Symptoms of haloperidol overdosage in children have ranged from the expected, such as drowsiness, restlessness, confusion, marked extrapyramidal symptoms, and hypothermia,[1,2] to unexpected reactions such as bradycardia (possibly secondary to hypothermia)[1] and an episode of severe, delayed hypertension.[3]

Torsade de pointes has followed overdosage in adults (for references, see Effects on the Cardiovascular System under Chlorpromazine, p.649).

1. Scialli JVK, Thornton WE. Toxic reactions from a haloperidol overdose in two children: thermal and cardiac manifestations. *JAMA* 1978; **239:** 48–9.
2. Sinaniotis CA, *et al.* Acute haloperidol poisoning in children. *J Pediatr* 1978; **93:** 1038–9.
3. Cummingham DG, Challapalli M. Hypertension in acute haloperidol poisoning. *J Pediatr* 1979; **95:** 489–90.

Retroperitoneal fibrosis. Obstructive uropathy was noted in a 45-year-old woman who had received haloperidol 5 to 15 mg daily for 8 years.[1] Benztropine was also taken during that time, and in the previous 5 years she had taken chlorpromazine and fluphenazine. A diagnosis of retroperitoneal fibrosis was made and was tentatively associated with long-term antipsychotic therapy.

1. Jeffries JJ, *et al.* Retroperitoneal fibrosis and haloperidol. *Am J Psychiatry* 1982; **139:** 1524–5.

Toxic encephalopathy. A report[1] of possible toxic encephalopathy following the use of high intravenous doses of haloperidol. The patient, who had a history of bipolar disorder and cerebrovascular accident, had been given increasing intravenous doses of haloperidol (up to 270 mg daily) to control post-surgical agitation. The encephalopathy had resolved 8 days after discontinuation of haloperidol.

1. Maxa JL, *et al.* Possible toxic encephalopathy following high-dose intravenous haloperidol. *Ann Pharmacother* 1997; **31:** 736–7.

Precautions

As for Chlorpromazine, p.652.

Severe dystonic reactions have followed the use of haloperidol, particularly in children and adolescents. It should therefore be used with extreme care in children. Haloperidol may also cause severe extrapyramidal reactions in patients with hyperthyroidism.

Porphyria. Haloperidol was considered to be unsafe in patients with acute porphyria although there is conflicting experimental evidence of porphyrinogenicity.[1]

1. Moore MR, McColl KEL. *Porphyria: drug lists.* Glasgow: Porphyria Research Unit, University of Glasgow, 1991.

Interactions

As for Chlorpromazine, p.652.

Haloperidol must be used with extreme caution in patients receiving lithium; an encephalopathic syndrome has been reported following their concomitant use (see p.294).

Pharmacokinetics

Haloperidol is readily absorbed from the gastro-intestinal tract. It is metabolised in the liver and is excreted in the urine and, via the bile, in the faeces; there is evidence of enterohepatic recycling. Owing to the first-pass effect of metabolism in the liver, plasma concentrations following oral administration are lower than those following intramuscular administration. Moreover, there is wide intersubject variation in plasma concentrations of haloperidol, but in practice, no strong correlation has been found between plasma concentrations of haloperidol and its therapeutic effect. Paths of metabolism of haloperidol include oxidative *N*-dealkylation and reduction of the ketone group to form an alcohol known as reduced haloperidol. Haloperidol has been reported to have a plasma elimination half-life ranging from about 12 to 38 hours after oral administration. Haloperidol is about 92% bound to plasma proteins. It is widely distributed in the body and crosses the blood-brain barrier. Haloperidol is distributed into breast milk.

The decanoate ester of haloperidol is very slowly absorbed from the site of injection and is therefore suitable for depot injection. It is gradually released into the bloodstream where it is rapidly hydrolysed to haloperidol.

The clinical significance of the reduced metabolite of haloperidol has been much debated.[1,2] Its activity appears to be substantially less than that of the parent drug but there is some evidence for re-oxidation of reduced haloperidol to haloperidol.[1-3] Some studies suggest that non-responders to haloperidol have elevated ratios of reduced haloperidol to haloperidol in the plasma, although other workers have reported contrary findings.[2] Pyridinium metabolites resulting from oxidation of haloperidol have been detected in the urine and there is concern that they may be neurotoxic in a manner similar to MPTP (p.1128), a compound which can induce irreversible parkinsonism.[4]

Measurement of concentrations of haloperidol or reduced haloperidol in scalp hair has been suggested as a useful means of monitoring compliance.[5,6] Evidence for the existence of any relationship between plasma concentrations of haloperidol and therapeutic effect in schizophrenia has been discussed.[7]

1. Sramek JJ, *et al.* Neuroleptic plasma concentrations and clinical response: in search of a therapeutic window. *Drug Intell Clin Pharm* 1988; **22:** 373–80.
2. Froemming JS, *et al.* Pharmacokinetics of haloperidol. *Clin Pharmacokinet* 1989; **17:** 396–423.
3. Chakraborty BS, *et al.* Interconversion between haloperidol and reduced haloperidol in healthy volunteers. *Eur J Clin Pharmacol* 1989; **37:** 45–8.
4. Eyles DW, *et al.* Quantitative analysis of two pyridinium metabolites of haloperidol in patients with schizophrenia. *Clin Pharmacol Ther* 1994; **56:** 512–20.
5. Uematsu T, *et al.* Human scalp hair as evidence of individual dosage history of haloperidol: method and retrospective study. *Eur J Clin Pharmacol* 1989; **37:** 239–44.
6. Matsuno H, *et al.* The measurement of haloperidol and reduced haloperidol in hair as an index of dosage history. *Br J Clin Pharmacol* 1990; **29:** 187–94.
7. Ulrich S, *et al.* The relationship between serum concentration and therapeutic effect of haloperidol in patients with acute schizophrenia. *Clin Pharmacokinet* 1998; **34:** 227–63.

Administration in ethnic groups. For reference to ethnic differences in the disposition of haloperidol, see Chlorpromazine, p.654.

Uses and Administration

Haloperidol is a butyrophenone with general properties similar to those of the phenothiazine, chlorpromazine (p.654). Haloperidol is an antipsychotic with actions most closely resembling those of phenothiazines with a piperazine side chain.

Haloperidol is used in the treatment of various psychoses including schizophrenia (p.637) and mania (p.273), and in behaviour disturbances (p.636), in Tourette's syndrome and severe tics (p.636), in intractable hiccups (p.655), and in severe anxiety (p.635). Haloperidol has also been used for its antiemetic effect in the management of nausea and vomiting of various causes (p.1172).

Haloperidol is usually given by mouth or injection as the base or intramuscularly as the long-acting decanoate ester. Some haloperidol preparations are prepared with the aid of lactic acid and may be stated to contain haloperidol lactate. Doses are expressed in terms of the equivalent amount of haloperidol.

The usual initial dose by mouth for the treatment of psychoses and associated behaviour disorders is 0.5 to 5 mg twice or three times daily. In severe or resistant psychoses doses of up to 100 mg daily may be required; rarely doses of up to 200 mg daily have been used. The dose should be reduced gradually according to response. Maintenance doses as low as 3 to 10 mg daily may be sufficient. A suggested initial dose for children by mouth is 0.025 to 0.05 mg per kg body-weight daily in two divided doses, increased cautiously, if necessary; a maximum daily dose of 10 mg has been suggested in the UK but in the USA the suggested maximum daily dose is 0.15 mg per kg as the manufacturer has stated that there is little evidence of behaviour improvement with daily doses of more than 6 mg.

For the control of acute psychotic conditions haloperidol may be given intramuscularly in doses of 2 to 10 mg; subsequent doses may be given hourly until symptoms are controlled although dosage intervals of 4 to 8 hours may be adequate. Up to 30 mg intramuscularly may be required for the emergency control of very severely disturbed patients. The intravenous route may be used.

In patients already stabilised on an oral dose of haloperidol and requiring long-term therapy the long-acting decanoate ester may be given by deep intramuscular injection. The usual initial dose is the equivalent of 10 to 20 times the total daily dose of haloperidol by mouth, up to a maximum of 100 mg; if more than 100 mg is required for an initial dose the excess should be given after 3 to 7 days. Subsequent doses, usually given every 4 weeks, may be increased to up to 300 mg or more, according to the patient's requirements, both dose and dose interval being adjusted as required.

In the management of nausea and vomiting haloperidol has been given in usual doses of 0.5 to 2 mg daily by intramuscular injection.

A starting dose of 0.5 to 1.5 mg three times daily by mouth has been suggested for the management of Tourette's syndrome and severe tics. Up to about 10 mg daily may be needed in Tourette's syndrome, although requirements vary considerably and the dose must be very carefully adjusted to obtain the optimum response.

For intractable hiccups a suggested oral dose is 1.5 mg given three times daily by mouth adjusted according to response; alternatively 3 to 15 mg may be given daily by intramuscular or intravenous injection in divided doses.

A dose of 0.5 mg twice daily by mouth has been used as adjunctive treatment in the short-term management of severe anxiety disorders.

Haloperidol should be used in reduced dosage in elderly or debilitated patients; doses at the lower end of the scale are also advised for adolescents.

Ballism. Dopamine-blocking antipsychotics such as haloperidol may sometimes be needed for the management of patients with ballism (p.636) when symptoms are severe.

Chorea. For a discussion of the management of various choreas, including mention of the use of haloperidol, see p.636.

References.

1. Kukla LF, *et al.* Systemic lupus erythematosus presenting as chorea. *Arch Dis Child* 1978; **53:** 345–7.
2. Donaldson JO. Control of chorea gravidarum with haloperidol. *Obstet Gynecol* 1982; **59:** 381–2.

Dystonia. Antipsychotics such as phenothiazines, haloperidol, or pimozide are sometimes useful in the treatment of idiopathic dystonia in patients who have failed to respond to other drugs.[1] However, they often act non-specifically and there is the risk of adding drug-induced extrapyramidal disorders to the dystonia being treated (see Extrapyramidal Disorders under Adverse Effects of Chlorpromazine, p.650).

For a discussion of the management of dystonias, see under Levodopa on p.1141.

1. Marsden CD, Quinn NP. The dystonias. *Br Med J* 1990; **300:** 139–44.

Sneezing. Report[1] of a patient whose intractable sneezing was controlled by haloperidol given in doses of up to 5 mg twice daily. Symptoms recurred when treatment was stopped after 5 weeks but responded again to 5 mg three times daily. On gradual reduction of dosage over 6 months the patient experienced no recurrence and had remained symptom-free after 6 months without medication.

1. Davison K. Pharmacological treatment for intractable sneezing. *Br Med J* 1982; **284:** 1163–4.

Stuttering. Stuttering (stammering) is a disorder which affects the fluency of speech. Developmental stuttering usually occurs in early childhood and is more common in boys than girls. While stuttering may cease in some children after only a few months it may become a chronic condition in others. Stuttering which starts during adulthood is rarer and may be the result of a neurological insult. While stuttering may be greatly improved with intensive speech training the effectiveness of other forms of management such as hypnosis, psychotherapy, counselling, and drug therapy has been largely unconvincing.[1] Although many drugs have been used to treat stuttering a review of the literature[2] indicated that there were few adequate studies of their efficacy. Haloperidol was considered to be the most well studied drug and its efficacy had been demonstrated by several double-blind placebo-controlled studies. However, most patients needed to continue taking haloperidol to maintain improvement but few did so because of its adverse effects. Double-blind studies have on the whole failed to confirm reports of benefit for drugs such as bethanechol, beta blockers, and calcium-channel blockers although isolated patients may have marked improvement. Other drugs which are being studied and which might be of benefit include clomipramine.

1. Andrews G, *et al.* Stuttering. *JAMA* 1988; **260:** 1445.
2. Brady JP, *et al.* The pharmacology of stuttering: a critical review. *Am J Psychiatry* 1991; **148:** 1309–16.

Taste disorders. For reference to the use of haloperidol in the treatment of taste disorders, see Chlorpromazine, p.656.

Tourette's syndrome. Tourette's syndrome (p.636) is a disorder characterised by motor and vocal tics and behavioural disturbances. Many patients with Tourette's syndrome do not require medication but when treatment is needed dopamine antagonists such as the antipsychotics haloperidol or pimozide are most commonly used. They often decrease the frequency and severity of tics and may improve any accompanying behavioural disturbances. However, superiority of either drug in terms of efficacy or adverse effects has not been clearly demonstrated.[1,2] Because of the potential for acute and long-term adverse effects it is usually recommended that doses are titrated to as low as possible; the aim of treatment is not necessarily to control symptoms completely. Medication can often be discontinued after a few years.

1. Shapiro E, *et al.* Controlled study of haloperidol, pimozide, and placebo for the treatment of Gilles de la Tourette's syndrome. *Arch Gen Psychiatry* 1989; **46:** 722–30.
2. Sallee FR, *et al.* Relative efficacy of haloperidol and pimozide in children and adolescents with Tourette's disorder. *Am J Psychiatry* 1997; **154:** 1057–62.

Preparations

BP 1998: Haloperidol Capsules; Haloperidol Injection; Haloperidol Oral Solution; Haloperidol Tablets; Strong Haloperidol Oral Solution;
USP 23: Haloperidol Injection; Haloperidol Oral Solution; Haloperidol Tablets.

Proprietary Preparations (details are given in Part 3)
Aust.: Haldol; ***Austral.:*** Haldol; Serenace; ***Belg.:*** Haldol; ***Canad.:*** Haldol; Novo-Peridol; Peridol; ***Fr.:*** Haldol; ***Ger.:*** Buteridol; dura-peridol†; Elaubat†; Haldol; Haloper; Sigaperidol; ***Irl.:*** Haldol; Serenace; ***Ital.:*** Bioperidolo; Haldol; Serenase; ***Neth.:*** Haldol; ***Norw.:*** Haldol; ***S.Afr.:*** Cereen; Serenace; ***Swed.:*** Haldol; ***Switz.:*** Haldol; Sigaperidol; ***UK:*** Dozic; Haldol; Serenace; ***USA:*** Haldol; Halperon†.

Multi-ingredient: ***Aust.:*** Vesalium; ***Belg.:*** Vesalium; ***Fr.:*** Vesadol; ***Ital.:*** Vesalium†; ***Switz.:*** Vesalium†.

Haloxazolam (19283-j)

Haloxazolam *(rINN)*.

10-Bromo-11b-(2-fluorophenyl)-2,3,7,11b-tetrahydrooxazolo[3,2-*d*][1,4]benzodiazepin-6(5*H*)-one.

$C_{17}H_{14}BrFN_2O_2$ = 377.2.

CAS — 59128-97-1.

Pharmacopoeias. In *Jpn.*

Haloxazolam is a benzodiazepine with general properties similar to those of diazepam (p.661). It is given by mouth as a hypnotic in the short-term management of insomnia (p.638).

Preparations

Proprietary Preparations (details are given in Part 3)
Jpn: Somelin.

Hexapropymate (4039-z)

Hexapropymate *(BAN, rINN)*.

L-2103; Propinylcyclohexanol Carbamate. 1-(Prop-2-ynyl)cyclohexyl carbamate.

$C_{10}H_{15}NO_2$ = 181.2.

CAS — 358-52-1.

Hexapropymate is a carbamate derivative formerly used as a hypnotic.

Overdosage. References.

1. Gustafsson LL, *et al.* Hexapropymate self-poisoning causes severe and long-lasting clinical symptoms. *Med Toxicol Adverse Drug Exp* 1989; **4:** 295–301.

Porphyria. Hexapropymate was considered to be unsafe in patients with acute porphyria because it has been shown to be porphyrinogenic in *animals* or *in-vitro* systems.[1]

1. Moore MR, McColl KEL. *Porphyria: drug lists.* Glasgow: Porphyria Research Unit, University of Glasgow, 1991.

Preparations

Proprietary Preparations (details are given in Part 3)
Belg.: Merinax†.

Hexobarbitone (4040-p)

Hexobarbitone *(BAN)*.

Hexobarbital *(rINN)*; Enhexymalum; Enimal; Hexobarbitalum; Methexenyl; Methyl-cyclohexenylmethyl-barbitursäure; Methylhexabarbital. 5-(Cyclohex-1-enyl)-1,5-dimethylbarbituric acid.

$C_{12}H_{16}N_2O_3$ = 236.3.

CAS — 56-29-1.

NOTE. The name ciclobarbital (see Cyclobarbitone, p.660) has sometimes been applied to hexobarbitone.

Pharmacopoeias. In *Eur.* (see p.viii).

A white crystalline powder. Very slightly **soluble** in water; sparingly soluble in alcohol and in ether. Forms water-soluble compounds with alkali hydroxides and carbonates and with ammonia.

Hexobarbitone Sodium (4041-s)

Hexobarbitone Sodium *(BANM)*.

Hexobarbital Sodium *(rINNM)*; Enhexymalnatrium; Hexenalum; Hexobarbitalum Natricum; Sodium Hexobarbital; Soluble Hexobarbitone. Sodium 5-(cyclohex-1-enyl)-1,5-dimethylbarbiturate.

$C_{12}H_{15}N_2NaO_3$ = 258.2.

CAS — 50-09-9.

Pharmacopoeias. In *Aust.* and *Pol.*

Hexobarbitone is a barbiturate with the general properties of amylobarbitone (p.641). It has been used as a hypnotic and sedative.

Homofenazine Hydrochloride (7052-y)

Homofenazine Hydrochloride *(rINNM)*.

D-775 (homofenazine); HFZ (homofenazine). 2-{Hexahydro-4-[3-(2-trifluoromethylphenothiazin-10-yl)propyl]-1,4-diazepin-1-yl}ethanol dihydrochloride.

$C_{23}H_{28}F_3N_3OS,2HCl$ = 524.5.

CAS — 3833-99-6 (homofenazine); 1256-01-5 (homofenazine hydrochloride).

Homofenazine hydrochloride is a phenothiazine with general properties similar to those of chlorpromazine (p.649). It has been used in the management of neuropsychiatric disorders.

Preparations

Proprietary Preparations (details are given in Part 3)
Belg.: Pasaden†.

Multi-ingredient: ***Aust.:*** Pelvichthol; ***Ger.:*** Seda-ildamen†.

Ibomal (4042-w)

Bromoaprobarbitone; Isopropyl-bromallyl-barbitursäure; Propallylonal. 5-(2-Bromoallyl)-5-isopropylbarbituric acid.

$C_{10}H_{13}BrN_2O_3$ = 289.1.

CAS — 545-93-7.

Ibomal is a barbiturate with general properties similar to those of amylobarbitone (p.641). It was formerly used as a hypnotic.

Preparations

Proprietary Preparations (details are given in Part 3)
Ger.: Noctal†.

Ipsapirone Hydrochloride (19356-z)

Ipsapirone Hydrochloride *(BANM, USAN, rINNM)*.

Bay-q-7821; TVX-Q-7821. 2-[4-(4-Pyrimidin-2-ylpiperazin-1-yl)butyl]-1,2-benzothiazol-3(2*H*)-one 1,1-dioxide hydrochloride.

$C_{19}H_{23}N_5O_3S,HCl$ = 437.9.

CAS — 95847-70-4 (ipsapirone); 92589-98-5 (ipsapirone hydrochloride).

Ipsapirone is structurally related to buspirone (p.643). It is under investigation as the hydrochloride for the treatment of anxiety disorders and depression.

Ipsapirone is a partial agonist at serotonin (hydroxytryptamine, 5-HT) receptors of the 5-HT_{1A} subtype. For reference to the actions and potential uses of such drugs, see Buspirone Hydrochloride, p.644.

References.

1. Cutler NR, *et al.* A double-blind, placebo-controlled study comparing the efficacy and safety of ipsapirone versus lorazepam in patients with generalized anxiety disorder: a prospective multicenter trial. *J Clin Psychopharmacol* 1993; **13:** 429–37.
2. Fuhr U, *et al.* Absorption of ipsapirone along the human gastrointestinal tract. *Br J Clin Pharmacol* 1994; **38:** 83–6.
3. Mandos LA, *et al.* Placebo-controlled comparison of the clinical effects of rapid discontinuation of ipsapirone and lorazepam after 8 weeks of treatment for generalized anxiety disorder. *Int Clin Psychopharmacol* 1995; **10:** 251–6.

Ketazolam (7055-c)

Ketazolam *(BAN, USAN, rINN)*.

U-28774. 11-Chloro-8,12b-dihydro-2,8-dimethyl-12b-phenyl-4*H*-[1,3]oxazino[3,2-*d*][1,4]benzodiazepine-4,7(6*H*)-dione.

$C_{20}H_{17}ClN_2O_3$ = 368.8.

CAS — 27223-35-4.

Ketazolam is a long-acting benzodiazepine with general properties similar to those of diazepam (p.661). It is given by mouth in the short-term treatment of anxiety (p.635) in usual doses of 15 to 60 mg daily, either in divided doses or as a single dose at night.

References.

1. Angelini G, *et al.* Ketazolam, a new long-acting benzodiazepine, in the treatment of anxious patients: a multicenter study of 2,056 patients. *Curr Ther Res* 1989; **45:** 294–304.

Preparations

Proprietary Preparations (details are given in Part 3)
Belg.: Solatran; Unakalm; ***Canad.:*** Loftran†; ***Ger.:*** Contamex†; ***Ital.:*** Anseren; ***Neth.:*** Unakalm; ***S.Afr.:*** Solatran; ***Spain:*** Marcen; Sedotime; ***Switz.:*** Solatran.

Loprazolam Mesylate (18341-d)

Loprazolam Mesylate *(BANM)*.

Loprazolam Mesilate *(rINNM)*; HR-158; Loprazolam Methanesulphonate; RU-31158. 6-(2-Chlorophenyl)-2,4-dihydro-2-(4-methylpiperazin-1-ylmethylene)-8-nitroimidazo[1,2-*a*][1,4]benzodiazepin-1-one methanesulphonate monohydrate.

$C_{23}H_{21}ClN_6O_3,CH_4O_3S,H_2O$ = 579.0.

CAS — 61197-73-7 (loprazolam); 70111-54-5 (anhydrous loprazolam mesylate).

Pharmacopoeias. In *Br.*

A yellow crystalline powder. Slightly **soluble** in water, in alcohol, and in chloroform; very slightly soluble in ether.

Dependence and Withdrawal, Adverse Effects, Treatment, and Precautions

As for Diazepam, p.661.

Porphyria. Loprazolam was considered to be unsafe in patients with acute porphyria because it has been shown to be porphyrinogenic in *animals* and *in-vitro* systems.[1]

1. Moore MR, McColl KEL. *Porphyria: drug lists.* Glasgow: Porphyria Research Unit, University of Glasgow, 1991.

Withdrawal. For the purpose of withdrawal regimens, 0.5 to 1 mg of loprazolam is considered roughly equivalent to 5 mg of diazepam.

Interactions

As for Diazepam, p.663.

Pharmacokinetics

A review of the pharmacokinetics of loprazolam.[1] After oral administration, peak plasma concentrations are achieved in about 1 to 2 hours. The elimination half-life has varied from 4 to 15 hours and appears to be prolonged in elderly patients to some extent. Loprazolam is reported to be approximately 80% bound to plasma proteins and has been detected in breast milk. The major pathway of metabolism in humans is *N*-oxidation of the piperazine ring. Loprazolam and its metabolites are excreted in the urine and faeces. In some studies, a secondary peak in plasma-loprazolam concentrations has been observed; this could be a result of enterohepatic recycling.

1. Garzone PD, Kroboth PD. Pharmacokinetics of the newer benzodiazepines. *Clin Pharmacokinet* 1989; **16:** 337–64.

Uses and Administration

Loprazolam is an intermediate-acting benzodiazepine with general properties similar to those of diazepam (p.666).

Loprazolam mesylate is usually used for its hypnotic properties in the short-term management of insomnia (p.638), in usual doses equivalent to 1 mg of loprazolam at night. Dosage may be increased to up to 2 mg if necessary. A starting dose of 0.5 mg increased to a maximum of 1 mg may be appropriate for elderly or debilitated patients.

Reviews.

1. Clark BG, *et al.* Loprazolam: a preliminary review of its pharmacodynamic and pharmacokinetic properties and therapeutic efficacy in insomnia. *Drugs* 1986; **31:** 500–16.

Preparations

BP 1998: Loprazolam Tablets.

Proprietary Preparations (details are given in Part 3)
Belg.: Dormonoct; ***Fr.:*** Havlane; ***Ger.:*** Sonin; ***Irl.:*** Dormonoct; ***Neth.:*** Dormonoct; ***S.Afr.:*** Dormonoct; ***Spain:*** Somnovit; ***UK:*** Dormonoct†.

Lorazepam (7060-y)

Lorazepam *(BAN, USAN, rINN)*.

Lorazepamum; Wy-4036. 7-Chloro-5-(2-chlorophenyl)-1,3-dihydro-3-hydroxy-1,4-benzodiazepin-2-one.

$C_{15}H_{10}Cl_2N_2O_2$ = 321.2.

CAS — 846-49-1.

Pharmacopoeias. In *Eur.* (see p.viii), *Jpn*, and *US.*

A white or almost white, almost odourless crystalline powder. It exhibits polymorphism. Practically **insoluble** in water; sparingly soluble in alcohol; slightly soluble in chloroform; sparingly or slightly soluble in dichloromethane. **Store** in airtight containers. Protect from light.

Incompatibility. Visual incompatibility has been noted with lorazepam and sargramostim[1] or aztreonam.[2]

1. Trissel LA, *et al.* Visual compatibility of sargramostim with selected antineoplastic agents, anti-infectives, or other drugs during simulated Y-site injection. *Am J Hosp Pharm* 1992; **49:** 402–6.
2. Trissel LA, Martinez JF. Compatibility of aztreonam with selected drugs during simulated Y-site administration. *Am J Health-Syst Pharm* 1995; **52:** 1086–90.

Solubility. The solubility of lorazepam in fluids for intravenous administration (water, glucose injection, lactated Ringer's injection, and sodium chloride injection) was greatest in glucose injection (5%) at 62 μg per mL and lowest in sodium chloride injection (0.9%) at 27 μg per mL;[1] these differences in solubility appeared to be pH related. Commercial injections are reported to contain polyethylene glycol in propylene glycol to overcome this poor solubility. However, precipitation has been noted[2] in solutions prepared by dilution of lorazepam injection with sodium chloride injection (0.9%) to a concentration of 500 μg per mL. One group of workers[3] have reported that they had overcome such problems with precipitation by using glucose injection (5%) as a diluent and by avoiding final concentrations of lorazepam between 0.08 mg per mL and 1 mg per mL. It was suggested that the propylene glycol in the mixture might account for the unusual concentration effect.

1. Newton DW, *et al.* Lorazepam solubility in and sorption from intravenous admixture solutions. *Am J Hosp Pharm* 1983; **40:** 424–7.
2. Boullata JI, *et al.* Precipitation of lorazepam infusion. *Ann Pharmacother* 1996; **30:** 1037–8.
3. Volles DF, *et al.* More on usability of lorazepam admixtures for continuous infusion. *Am J Health-Syst Pharm* 1996; **53:** 2753–4.

Sorption. Significant loss of lorazepam has been reported from solutions stored in polyvinyl chloride[1] or polypropylene[2] giving equipment; polyolefin[3] or glass[4] equipment appears to be more suitable.

1. Hoey LL, *et al.* Lorazepam stability in parenteral solutions for continuous intravenous administration. *Ann Pharmacother* 1996; **30:** 343–6.
2. Stiles ML, *et al.* Stability of deferoxamine mesylate, floxuridine, fluorouracil, hydromorphone hydrochloride, lorazepam, and midazolam hydrochloride in polypropylene infusion-pump syringes. *Am J Health-Syst Pharm* 1996; **53:** 1583–8.
3. Trissel LA, Pearson SD. Storage of lorazepam in three injectable solutions in polyvinyl chloride and polyolefin bags. *Am J Hosp Pharm* 1994; **51:** 368–72.
4. Martens HJ, *et al.* Sorption of various drugs in polyvinyl chloride, glass, and polyethylene-lined infusion containers. *Am J Hosp Pharm* 1990; **47:** 369–73.

Dependence and Withdrawal

As for Diazepam, p.661.

For the purpose of withdrawal regimens, 0.5 mg of lorazepam may be considered roughly equivalent to 5 mg of diazepam.

Adverse Effects, Treatment, and Precautions

As for Diazepam, p.661. Pain and a sensation of burning have occurred following injection of lorazepam.

There have been reports of toxicity, presumed to be due to polyethylene glycol[1] or propylene glycol,[2] following prolonged parenteral administration of lorazepam; polyethylene glycol in propylene glycol is included as a solubiliser in lorazepam solutions. Diarrhoea in an infant given large enteral doses of lorazepam or diazepam solutions may have been due to the combined osmotic effect of polyethylene glycol and propylene glycol in these preparations.[3]

1. Laine GA, *et al.* Polyethylene glycol nephrotoxicity secondary to prolonged high-dose intravenous lorazepam. *Ann Pharmacother* 1995; **29:** 1110–4.
2. Seay RE, *et al.* Possible toxicity from propylene glycol in lorazepam infusion. *Ann Pharmacother* 1997; **31:** 647–8. Woycik CL, Walker PC. Correction and comment: possible toxicity from propylene glycol in injectable drug preparations. *ibid.*: 1413.
3. Marshall JD, *et al.* Diarrhea associated with enteral benzodiazepine solutions. *J Pediatr* 1995; **126:** 657–9.

Effects on the blood. A case of pancytopenia associated with administration of lorazepam by mouth;[1] only five instances of thrombocytopenia and none of leucopenia had been reported to the Committee on Safety of Medicines or the UK manufacturers over the previous 13 years.

1. El-Sayed S, Symonds RP. Lorazepam induced pancytopenia. *Br Med J* 1988; **296:** 1332.

Effects on fluid and electrolyte homoeostasis. Inappropriate secretion of antidiuretic hormone related to ingestion of lorazepam was considered to be the cause of hyponatraemia in an 81-year-old woman.[1]

1. Engel WR, Grau A. Inappropriate secretion of antidiuretic hormone associated with lorazepam. *Br Med J* 1988; **297:** 858.

Effects on the nervous system. For reference to extrapyramidal disorders associated with administration of lorazepam, see Diazepam, p.662.

Hepatic impairment. Although the elimination half-life of lorazepam was increased in 13 patients with alcoholic cirrhosis compared with 11 control subjects, this was not associated with an impairment in systemic plasma clearance.[1] With the exception of a modest decrease in the extent of plasma protein binding, acute viral hepatitis had no effect on the disposition kinetics of lorazepam.

1. Kraus JW, *et al.* Effects of aging and liver disease on disposition of lorazepam. *Clin Pharmacol Ther* 1978; **24:** 411–19.

Local reactions. Of 40 patients given a single intravenous dose of lorazepam 4 mg three had local thrombosis 2 to 3 days later and 6 had local thrombosis 7 to 10 days later.[1] The incidence was lower than in those given diazepam [in solution].

1. Hegarty JE, Dundee JW. Sequelae after the intravenous injection of three benzodiazepines—diazepam, lorazepam, and flunitrazepam. *Br Med J* 1977; **2:** 1384–5.

Old age. For discussion of the need for reduced dosage of benzodiazepines in elderly patients, including mention of lorazepam, see Diazepam, p.662.

Interactions

As for Diazepam, p.663.

Pharmacokinetics

Lorazepam is readily absorbed from the gastro-intestinal tract following oral administration, with a bioavailability of about 90%; peak plasma concentrations are reported to occur about 2 hours after an oral dose. The absorption profile after intramuscular injection is similar to that after administration by mouth.

Lorazepam is about 85% bound to plasma protein. It crosses the blood-brain barrier and the placenta; it is also distributed into breast milk. Lorazepam is metabolised in the liver to the inactive glucuronide, and excreted in urine. The elimination half-life has been reported to range from about 10 to 20 hours.

References.

1. Greenblatt DJ. Clinical pharmacokinetics of oxazepam and lorazepam. *Clin Pharmacokinet* 1981; **6:** 89–105.

Administration in children. References to the pharmacokinetics of lorazepam in children.

1. Relling MV, *et al.* Lorazepam pharmacodynamics and pharmacokinetics in children. *J Pediatr* 1989; **114:** 641–6.

Administration in the neonate. References to slow elimination of lorazepam by neonates.

1. Cummings AJ, Whitelaw AGL. A study of conjugation and drug elimination in the human neonate. *Br J Clin Pharmacol* 1981; **12:** 511–15.
2. McDermott CA, *et al.* Pharmacokinetics of lorazepam in critically ill neonates with seizures. *J Pediatr* 1992; **120:** 479–83.
3. Reiter PD, Stiles AD. Lorazepam toxicity in a premature infant. *Ann Pharmacother* 1993; **27:** 727–9.

Distribution. Evidence that lorazepam undergoes enterohepatic recirculation, with possible first-pass metabolism and at least one other currently unknown hepatic route of elimination.[1]

1. Herman RJ, *et al.* Disposition of lorazepam in human beings: enterohepatic recirculation and first-pass effect. *Clin Pharmacol Ther* 1989; **46:** 18–25.

BREAST MILK. Free lorazepam concentrations in the breast milk of 4 lactating mothers who had received lorazepam 3.5 mg by mouth as premedication, ranged from 8 to 9 ng per mL four hours after the dose.[1] This represented approximately 15 to 26% of the concentration in plasma, and was probably sufficiently low to cause no adverse effects in breast-fed infants.

1. Summerfield RJ, Nielsen MS. Excretion of lorazepam into breast milk. *Br J Anaesth* 1985; **57:** 1042–3.

CSF. In a study involving 6 healthy subjects, peak plasma-lorazepam concentrations were reached 5 minutes after the end of a one-minute intravenous injection.[1] CNS effects, as measured by EEG activity, did not reach a maximum until 30 minutes after injection; they declined to base-line values slowly over 5 to 8 hours in a similar manner to plasma concentrations. In contrast, CNS effects of diazepam were maximal immediately after the injection. They also declined more rapidly than lorazepam, but again in a similar way to plasma concentrations. Studies in *mice* suggested that the slow onset of action of lorazepam that has been reported by some is at least partly explained by a delay in passage from systemic blood into brain tissue.

1. Greenblatt DJ, *et al.* Kinetic and dynamic study of intravenous lorazepam; comparison with intravenous diazepam. *J Pharmacol Exp Ther* 1989; **250:** 134–40.

Uses and Administration

Lorazepam is a short-acting benzodiazepine with general properties similar to those of diazepam (p.666). It is used in the treatment of anxiety disorders (p.635), as a hypnotic in the short-term management of insomnia (p.638), and as an anticonvulsant in the management of status epilepticus (p.337). When used in the treatment of status epilepticus lorazepam has a prolonged antiepileptic action. It is also used for its sedative and amnestic properties in premedication and in antiemetic regimens for the control of nausea and vomiting associated with cancer chemotherapy (p.1172).

Lorazepam is usually administered by mouth or by injection as the base although the pivalate is available for oral administration in some countries. Sublingual tablets are used in some countries in doses similar to those for standard tablets. The intramuscular route is usually only used when oral or intravenous administration is not possible. Injections should usually be diluted before administration; intravenous injections should be given at a rate of not more than 2 mg per minute into a large vein.

The usual dose of lorazepam by mouth for the treatment of **anxiety disorders** is 1 to 6 mg daily in 2 to 3 divided doses with the largest dose taken at night; up to 10 mg daily has been given. A dose of 0.025 to 0.03 mg per kg body-weight may be given by injection every 6 hours for acute anxiety. A single oral dose of 1 to 4 mg at bedtime may be given for **insomnia** associated with anxiety.

For **premedication** adults may be given a dose of 2 to 3 mg by mouth the night before the operation followed if necessary the next morning by a smaller dose. Alternatively, 2 to 4 mg may be given 1 to 2 hours before an operation. A dose of 0.05 mg per kg may be administered 30 to 45 minutes before the operation if given intravenously or 1 to 1½ hours before if given intramuscularly. Children aged 5 to 13 years of age may be given 0.5 to 2.5 mg (0.05 mg per kg body-weight) by mouth at least one hour before surgery.

In the management of **status epilepticus** 4 mg may be given as a single intravenous dose; half this amount has been suggested as a dose in children. A dose of 1 to 2 mg of lorazepam by mouth given with dexamethasone prior to chemotherapy has been suggested for prevention of acute symptoms in patients at increased risk of **emesis**.

Lorazepam should be given in reduced dosage to elderly or debilitated patients; one-half the usual adult dose, or less, may be sufficient.

Disturbed behaviour. For a discussion of the management of behaviour disturbances associated with various psychotic disorders and the value of benzodiazepines, see p.636.

References.

1. Bieniek SA, *et al.* A double-blind study of lorazepam versus the combination of haloperidol and lorazepam in managing agitation. *Pharmacotherapy* 1998; **18:** 57–62.

Premedication and sedation. Lorazepam is used as a premedicant (p.1220) and as a sedative for therapeutic and investigative procedures such as dental treatment (p.638) and endoscopy (p.638).

References.

1. Maltias F, *et al.* A randomized, double-blind, placebo-controlled study of lorazepam as premedication for bronchoscopy. *Chest* 1996; **109:** 1195–8.

Withdrawal syndromes. Lorazepam has been used in the management of symptoms of alcohol withdrawal (p.1099).

Preparations

BP 1998: Lorazepam Injection; Lorazepam Tablets;
USP 23: Lorazepam Injection; Lorazepam Oral Concentrate; Lorazepam Tablets.

Proprietary Preparations (details are given in Part 3)

Aust.: Ergocalm; Merlit; Punktyl†; Temesta; ***Austral.:*** Ativan; ***Belg.:*** Lauracalm†; Loridem; Serenase; Temesta; Vigiten; ***Canad.:*** Ativan; Novo-Lorazem; Nu-Loraz; ***Fr.:*** Temesta; ***Ger.:*** duralozam; Laubeel; Pro Dorm; Punktyl; Somagerol; Tavor; Tolid; ***Irl.:*** Ativan; ***Ital.:*** Control; Lorans; Quait; Tavor; ***Neth.:*** Temesta;

S.Afr.: Ativan; Tran-Qil; Tranqipam; *Spain:* Divial; Donix; Idalprem; Orfidal; Piralone; Placinoral; Sedizepan; *Swed.:* Temesta; *Switz.:* Lorasifar; Sedazin†; Temesta; *UK:* Ativan; *USA:* Ativan; Loraz†.

Multi-ingredient: *Aust.:* Somnium; *Switz.:* Somnium.

Lormetazepam (4077-r)

Lormetazepam *(BAN, USAN, rINN).*

Wy-4082. (*RS*)-7-Chloro-5-(2-chlorophenyl)-1,3-dihydro-3-hydroxy-1-methyl-1,4-benzodiazepin-2-one.

$C_{16}H_{12}Cl_2N_2O_2$ = 335.2.

CAS — 848-75-9.

Pharmacopoeias. In Br.

A white crystalline powder. Practically **insoluble** in water; soluble in alcohol and in methyl alcohol. **Protect** from light.

Dependence and Withdrawal, Adverse Effects, Treatment, and Precautions

As for Diazepam, p.661.

Withdrawal. For the purpose of withdrawal regimens, 0.5 to 1 mg of lormetazepam is considered roughly equivalent to 5 mg of diazepam.

Interactions

As for Diazepam, p.663.

Pharmacokinetics

Lormetazepam is rapidly absorbed from the gastro-intestinal tract and metabolised to the inactive glucuronide. The terminal half-life is reported to be about 11 hours.

A brief review of the pharmacokinetics of lormetazepam.[1]

1. Greenblatt DJ, *et al.* Clinical pharmacokinetics of the newer benzodiazepines. *Clin Pharmacokinet* 1983; **8:** 233–52.

Uses and Administration

Lormetazepam is a short-acting benzodiazepine with general properties similar to those of diazepam (p.666). It is mainly used as a hypnotic in the short-term management of insomnia (p.638) in usual doses of 0.5 to 1.5 mg by mouth at night. A dose of 0.5 mg is recommended for elderly or debilitated patients. Lormetazepam is also used in some countries for premedication (p.1220).

Preparations

BP 1998: Lormetazepam Tablets.

Proprietary Preparations (details are given in Part 3)
Aust.: Noctamid; *Belg.:* Loramet; Noctamid; Stilaze; *Fr.:* Noctamide; *Ger.:* Ergocalm; Loretam; Noctamid; Repocal†; *Irl.:* Loramet; Noctamid; *Ital.:* Minias; Noctamid†; *Neth.:* Loramet; Noctamid; *S.Afr.:* Loramet; Noctamid; *Spain:* Loramet; Noctamid; Sedobrina; *Switz.:* Loramet; Noctamid.

Loxapine (7061-j)

Loxapine *(BAN, USAN, rINN).*

CL-62362; Oxilapine; SUM-3170. 2-Chloro-11-(4-methylpiperazin-1-yl)dibenz[*b,f*][1,4]oxazepine.

$C_{18}H_{18}ClN_3O$ = 327.8.

CAS — 1977-10-2.

Loxapine Hydrochloride (3843-l)

Loxapine Hydrochloride *(BANM, rINNM).*

$C_{18}H_{18}ClN_3O,HCl$ = 364.3.

Loxapine hydrochloride 28 mg is approximately equivalent to 25 mg of loxapine.

Loxapine Succinate (7062-z)

Loxapine Succinate *(BANM, USAN, rINNM).*

CL-71563.

$C_{18}H_{18}ClN_3O,C_4H_6O_4$ = 445.9.

CAS — 27833-64-3.

Pharmacopoeias. In US.

A white to yellowish, odourless, crystalline powder. Loxapine succinate 34 mg is equivalent to 25 mg of loxapine. **Store** in airtight containers.

Adverse Effects, Treatment, and Precautions

As for Chlorpromazine, p.649.

The incidence of extrapyramidal symptoms and of sedation may be intermediate between that of chlorpromazine and of phenothiazines with a piperazine side-chain.

Other side-effects reported include nausea and vomiting, seborrhoea, dyspnoea, ptosis, headache, paraesthesia, flush, weight gain or loss, and polydipsia.

Abuse. A report of 3 cases of loxapine succinate abuse.[1]

1. Sperry L, *et al.* Loxapine abuse. *N Engl J Med* 1984; **310:** 598.

Effects on carbohydrate metabolism. Reversible non-ketotic hyperglycaemia, coma, and delirium, developed in a patient receiving loxapine 150 mg daily in addition to lithium therapy.[1] Symptoms improved following discontinuation of loxapine, but subsequently recurred when the patient was given amoxapine. The causative agent may have been 7-hydroxyamoxapine, a common metabolite of both amoxapine and loxapine.

1. Tollefson G, Lesar T. Nonketotic hyperglycemia associated with loxapine and amoxapine: case report. *J Clin Psychiatry* 1983; **44:** 347–8.

Mania. A patient, initially diagnosed as suffering from schizophrenia, developed manic symptoms after receiving loxapine.[1] The diagnosis was revised to schizoaffective disorder but it was suspected that loxapine had a role in the emergence of the affective symptoms. As loxapine shares common metabolites with the antidepressant amoxapine it was suggested that an antidepressant effect might have been instrumental in the production of manic symptoms.

1. Gojer JAC. Possible manic side-effects of loxapine. *Can J Psychiatry* 1992; **37:** 669–70.

Overdosage. An 8-year-old child was treated with activated charcoal within 30 minutes of being given 375 mg of loxapine by accident.[1] The child became drowsy and was asleep but arousable one hour after ingestion. The degree of sedation appeared to reach peak after 3.75 hours and the child was discharged about 20 hours postingestion.

1. Tarricone NW. Loxitane overdose. *Pediatrics* 1998; **101:** 496.

Porphyria. Loxapine was considered to be unsafe in patients with acute porphyria because it has been shown to be porphyrinogenic in *animals* or *in-vitro* systems.[1]

1. Moore MR, McColl KEL. *Porphyria: drug lists.* Glasgow: Porphyria Research Unit, University of Glasgow, 1991.

Interactions

As for Chlorpromazine, p.652.

Pharmacokinetics

Loxapine is readily absorbed from the gastro-intestinal tract. It is very rapidly and extensively metabolised and there is evidence for a first-pass effect. It is mainly excreted in the urine, in the form of its conjugated metabolites, with smaller amounts appearing in the faeces as unconjugated metabolites; a substantial proportion of a dose is excreted in the first 24 hours. The major metabolites of loxapine are the active 7- and 8-hydroxyloxapine, which are conjugated to the glucuronide or sulphate; other metabolites include hydroxyloxapine-*N*-oxide, loxapine-*N*-oxide, and hydroxydesmethylloxapine (hydroxyamoxapine). Loxapine is widely distributed and *animal* studies have indicated that it crosses the placenta and is distributed into breast milk.

Uses and Administration

Loxapine is a dibenzoxazepine with general properties similar to those of the phenothiazine, chlorpromazine (p.654). It is given by mouth as the hydrochloride or the succinate and by intramuscular injection as the hydrochloride in the treatment of psychoses, but doses are expressed in terms of the base.

The usual dose by mouth is 20 to 50 mg daily initially, in 2 divided doses, increased according to requirements over the next 7 to 10 days to 60 to 100 mg daily or more in 2 to 4 divided doses; the maximum recommended dose is 250 mg daily. Maintenance doses are usually in the range of 20 to 100 mg daily. For the control of acute conditions it is given by intramuscular injection in doses of 12.5 to 50 mg at intervals of 4 to 6 hours or longer.

Reduced dosage may be required in elderly patients.

Disturbed behaviour. For a discussion of the use and limitations of antipsychotics in patients with disturbed behaviour, see p.636. References to the use of loxapine in the management of disturbed behaviour are given below.

1. Carlyle W, *et al.* Aggression in the demented patient: a double-blind study of loxapine versus haloperidol. *Int J Clin Psychopharmacol* 1993; **8:** 103–8.

Schizophrenia. A brief review of loxapine[1] concluded that suggestions that loxapine was particularly effective in patients with paranoid schizophrenia had not been confirmed. The use of antipsychotics in the management of schizophrenia is discussed on p.637.

1. Anonymous. Clozapine and loxapine for schizophrenia. *Drug Ther Bull* 1991; **29:** 41–2.

Preparations

USP 23: Loxapine Capsules.

Proprietary Preparations (details are given in Part 3)
Belg.: Loxapac; *Canad.:* Loxapac; *Fr.:* Loxapac; *Irl.:* Loxapac; *Ital.:* Loxapac†; *Neth.:* Loxapac†; *Spain:* Desconex; Loxapac†; *UK:* Loxapac; *USA:* Loxitane.

Magnesium Aspartate Hydrobromide (11439-d)

Magnesium L-aspartate hydrobromide trihydrate.

Magnesium aspartate hydrobromide has been used as a sedative but the use of bromides is generally deprecated.

Preparations

Proprietary Preparations (details are given in Part 3)
Ger.: Vernelan.

Medazepam (7064-k)

Medazepam *(BAN, rINN).*

Ro-5-4556 (medazepam hydrochloride). 7-Chloro-2,3-dihydro-1-methyl-5-phenyl-1*H*-1,4-benzodiazepine.

$C_{16}H_{15}ClN_2$ = 270.8.

CAS — 2898-12-6 (medazepam); 2898-11-5 (medazepam hydrochloride).

NOTE. Medazepam Hydrochloride is *USAN.*

Pharmacopoeias. In Jpn.

Medazepam is a long-acting benzodiazepine with properties similar to those of diazepam (p.661). It is given by mouth for the treatment of anxiety disorders (p.635) and disturbed behaviour (p.636).

A usual dose is 10 to 20 mg daily in divided doses; in severe conditions up to 60 mg daily has been given. Elderly and debilitated patients should not be given more than half the normal adult dose.

Preparations

Proprietary Preparations (details are given in Part 3)
Ger.: Rudotel; *Irl.:* Nobrium†; *Ital.:* Lerisum†; Nobrium†; *Neth.:* Nobrium†; *Switz.:* Nobrium†; *UK:* Nobrium†.

Multi-ingredient: *Ital.:* Debrum; Tranquirax†; *Spain:* Nobritol.

Medetomidine Hydrochloride (2813-r)

Medetomidine Hydrochloride *(BANM, USAN, rINNM).*

MPV-785. (±)-4-[1-(2,3-Xylyl)ethyl]imidazole monohydrochloride.

$C_{13}H_{16}N_2,HCl$ = 236.7.

CAS — 86347-15-1 (medetomidine hydrochloride); 86347-14-0 (medetomidine).

Medetomidine is an α_2-adrenoceptor agonist with sedative, muscle relaxant, and analgesic properties. It is used as the hydrochloride in veterinary medicine.

Dexmedetomidine (p.660) is under investigation as a premedicant and adjunct to general anaesthesia.

Melperone Hydrochloride (7150-z)

Melperone Hydrochloride *(BANM, rINNM).*

FG-5111; Flubuperone Hydrochloride; Methylperone Hydrochloride. 4′-Fluoro-4-(4-methylpiperidino)butyrophenone hydrochloride.

$C_{16}H_{22}FNO,HCl$ = 299.8.

CAS — 3575-80-2 (melperone); 1622-79-3 (melperone hydrochloride).

Melperone is a butyrophenone with general properties similar to those of haloperidol (p.673). It is given by mouth or by intramuscular injection for the management of psychoses such as schizophrenia (p.637) and in disturbed behaviour (p.636). A usual dose by mouth as the hydrochloride is up to 400 mg daily in divided doses. In acute conditions it may be given intramuscularly in doses of 25 to 100 mg repeated to a usual maximum of 200 mg daily.

Cardiac arrhythmias. Melperone has been reported to have class III electrophysiologic and antiarrhythmic activity[1,2] but its clinical use would be limited by a high incidence of adverse effects.[2] For a discussion of the cardiovascular effects of antipsychotics in general, see under Chlorpromazine, p.649.

1. Møgelvang JC, *et al.* Antiarrhythmic properties of a neuroleptic butyrophenone, melperone, in acute myocardial infarction. *Acta Med Scand* 1980; **208:** 61–4.
2. Hui WKK, *et al.* Melperone: electrophysiologic and antiarrhythmic activity in humans. *J Cardiovasc Pharmacol* 1990; **15:** 144–9.

Pharmacokinetics. References.

1. Köppel C, *et al.* Gas chromatographic-mass spectrometric study of urinary metabolism of melperone. *J Chromatogr Biomed Appl* 1988; **427:** 144–50.

Preparations

Proprietary Preparations (details are given in Part 3)
Aust.: Buronil; Neuril†; ***Belg.:*** Buronil; ***Ger.:*** Eunerpan; ***Norw.:*** Buronil; ***Swed.:*** Buronil.

Mephenoxalone (7065-a)

Mephenoxalone *(rINN)*.

AHR-233; Methoxadone; OM-518. 5-(2-Methoxyphenoxymethyl)oxazolidin-2-one.

$C_{11}H_{13}NO_4$ = 223.2.

CAS — 70-07-5.

Mephenoxalone has actions similar to those of meprobamate (below). It is given by mouth in a dose of 500 mg three times daily for the treatment of anxiety disorders (p.635) and as a muscle relaxant in the treatment of muscle spasm (p.1303).

Preparations

Proprietary Preparations (details are given in Part 3)
Neth.: Dorsiflex; ***Switz.:*** Control.

Multi-ingredient: ***Switz.:*** Dorsilon.

Meprobamate (7066-t)

Meprobamate *(BAN, rINN)*.

Meprobamatum; Meprotanum. 2-Methyl-2-propyltrimethylene dicarbamate.

$C_9H_{18}N_2O_4$ = 218.3.

CAS — 57-53-4.

Pharmacopoeias. In *Chin., Eur.* (see p.viii), and *US.*

A white or almost white, crystalline or amorphous powder with a characteristic odour.

Ph. Eur. **solubilities** are: slightly soluble in water and in ether; freely soluble in alcohol. USP solubilities are: slightly soluble in water; freely soluble in acetone and in alcohol; practically insoluble or insoluble in ether. **Store** in airtight containers.

Dependence and Withdrawal

As for the barbiturates (see Amylobarbitone, p.641).

Adverse Effects

Drowsiness is the most frequent side-effect of meprobamate. Other effects include nausea, vomiting, diarrhoea, paraesthesia, weakness, and central effects such as headache, paradoxical excitement, dizziness, ataxia, and disturbances of vision. There may be hypotension, tachycardia, and cardiac arrhythmias. Hypersensitivity reactions occur occasionally. These may be limited to skin rashes, urticaria, and purpura or may be more severe with angioedema, bronchospasm, or anuria. Erythema multiforme and exfoliative or bullous dermatitis have been reported.

Blood disorders including agranulocytosis, eosinophilia, leucopenia, thrombocytopenia, and aplastic anaemia have occasionally been reported.

Overdosage with meprobamate produces symptoms similar to those of barbiturate overdosage (see Amylobarbitone, p.642).

Treatment of Adverse Effects

As for the barbiturates (see Amylobarbitone, p.642).

Gastric bezoars consisting of undissolved meprobamate tablets may need to be removed.

Overdosage. Two children aged 2 and 2.5 years recovered with conservative management alone following overdosage of meprobamate with bendrofluazide despite measured plasma-meprobamate concentrations of 170 and 158 µg per mL respectively.[1] Despite previous recommendations that haemoperfusion should be considered at plasma-meprobamate concentrations above 100 µg per mL, recent experience with adults has suggested that haemoperfusion should normally only be considered at plasma concentrations above 200 µg per mL.

1. Dennison J, *et al.* Meprobamate overdosage. *Hum Toxicol* 1985; **4:** 215–17.

Precautions

Meprobamate should be used with caution in patients with impaired hepatic or renal function, mental depression, muscle weakness, and, as with all sedatives, in patients with impaired respiratory function. Meprobamate may induce seizures in patients with a history of epilepsy.

Meprobamate may cause drowsiness; affected patients should not drive or operate machinery.

The use of meprobamate should be avoided in breast feeding mothers as concentrations in milk may exceed maternal plasma concentrations fourfold and may cause drowsiness in the infant.

Porphyria. Meprobamate has been associated with acute attacks of porphyria and is considered unsafe in patients with acute porphyria.[1]

1. Moore MR, McColl KEL. *Porphyria: drug lists.* Glasgow: Porphyria Research Unit, University of Glasgow, 1991.

Pregnancy. Studies on the use of meprobamate during pregnancy.

1. Milkovich L, van den Berg BJ. Effects of prenatal meprobamate and chlordiazepoxide hydrochloride on human embryonic and fetal development. *N Engl J Med* 1974; **291:** 1268–71.
2. Crombie DL, *et al.* Fetal effects of tranquilizers in pregnancy. *N Engl J Med* 1975; **293:** 198–9.
3. Hartz SC, *et al.* Antenatal exposure to meprobamate and chlordiazepoxide in relation to malformations, mental development, and childhood mortality. *N Engl J Med* 1975; **292:** 726–8.

Interactions

The sedative effects of meprobamate are enhanced by CNS depressants including alcohol. Meprobamate is capable of inducing hepatic microsomal enzyme systems involved in drug metabolism: the metabolism of other drugs may be enhanced if given concurrently.

Pharmacokinetics

Meprobamate is readily absorbed from the gastro-intestinal tract and peak plasma concentrations occur 1 to 3 hours after ingestion. Meprobamate is widely distributed. It is extensively metabolised in the liver and is excreted in the urine mainly as an inactive hydroxylated metabolite and its glucuronide conjugate. About 10% of a dose is excreted unchanged. Meprobamate has a half-life reported to range from about 6 to 17 hours, although this may be prolonged after chronic administration.

It diffuses across the placenta and appears in breast milk at concentrations of up to 4 times those in the maternal plasma.

Uses and Administration

Meprobamate is a carbamate with hypnotic, sedative, and some muscle relaxant properties, although in therapeutic doses its sedative effect rather than a direct action may be responsible for muscle relaxation. It has been used in the treatment of anxiety disorders (p.635) and also for the short-term management of insomnia (p.638) but has largely been superseded by other drugs. Meprobamate has sometimes been used, alone or in combination with an analgesic, in the management of muscle spasm (p.1303) and painful musculoskeletal disorders but such use is no longer considered appropriate.

The usual anxiolytic dose is 400 mg by mouth three or four times daily to a maximum of 2.4 g daily. In elderly patients, no more than half the usual adult dose has been suggested.

Preparations

USP 23: Meprobamate Oral Suspension; Meprobamate Tablets.

Proprietary Preparations (details are given in Part 3)
Aust.: Cyrpon; Epikur; Microbamat; Miltaun; Pertranquil; ***Austral.:*** Equanil; ***Belg.:*** Pertranquil; Procalmadiol; Quanamet†; Reposo-Mono; Sanobamat; ***Canad.:*** Equanil; Novo-Mepro; ***Fr.:*** Equanil; Norgagil; Novalm; ***Ger.:*** Exphobin N†; Urbilat†; Visano N; ***Irl.:*** Equanil†; ***Ital.:*** Quanil; Stensolo†; ***S.Afr.:*** Equanil; Meprepose†; Xeramax; ***Spain:*** Ansiowas†; Dapaz; Meprospan†; Miltown†; Oasil Simes; ***Swed.:*** Restenil; ***Switz.:*** Meprodil; ***UK:*** Equanil; Meprate; ***USA:*** Equanil; MB-Tab; Meprospan†; Miltown; Neuramate.

Multi-ingredient: ***Aust.:*** Lenticor†; Medium†; Seda-baxacor†; ***Belg.:*** Spasmosedine; ***Canad.:*** 282 Mep; Equagesic; ***Fr.:*** Kaologeais; Mepronizine; Palpipax; Precyclan; Vasocalm†; ***Ger.:*** Coritrat†; Dormilfo N†; para sanol†; Pentaneural†; Regium†; Seda Baxacor†; Sedapon D†; Tonamyl†; ***Irl.:*** Equagesic†; ***Ital.:*** Distonium†; Gastrised†; ***Norw.:*** Anervan; ***S.Afr.:*** Acugesil; Ban Pain; Briscopyn; Dimiprol; End Pain†; Equagesic; Go-Pain; Maxadol Forte; Megapyn; Meprogesic; Mepromol; Nopyn; Painagon; Painrite; PMB†; Pynmed; Salterpyn; Scriptogesic†; Spectrapain Forte; Stilpane; Stopayne; Supragesic; Synaleve; Tenston; Trinagesic; Vacudol Forte; Xerogesic; ***Spain:*** Oasil Relax†; ***Swed.:*** Anervan; ***UK:*** Equagesic; Paxidal; ***USA:*** Deprol†; Epromate; Equagesic; Equazine M; Micrainin; PMB.

Mesoridazine Besylate (7067-x)

Mesoridazine Besylate *(BANM)*.

Mesoridazine Besilate *(rINNM)*; Mesoridazine Benzenesulphonate; Mesuridazine Benzenesulphonate; NC-123 (mesoridazine); TPS-23 (mesoridazine). 10-[2-(1-Methyl-2-piperidyl)ethyl]-2-(methylsulphinyl)phenothiazine benzenesulphonate.

$C_{21}H_{26}N_2OS_2,C_6H_6O_3S$ = 544.8.

CAS — 5588-33-0 (mesoridazine); 32672-69-8 (mesoridazine besylate).

NOTE. Mesoridazine is *USAN.*

Pharmacopoeias. In *US.*

A white to pale yellow, almost odourless powder. **Soluble** 1 in 1 of water, 1 in 11 of alcohol, 1 in 3 of chloroform, and 1 in 6300 of ether; freely soluble in methyl alcohol. A freshly prepared 1% solution in water has a pH of between 4.2 and 5.7.

Store in airtight containers. Protect from light.

Adverse Effects, Treatment, and Precautions

As for Chlorpromazine, p.649.

Interactions

As for Chlorpromazine, p.652.

Pharmacokinetics

For an account of the pharmacokinetics of a phenothiazine, see Chlorpromazine, p.654.

Mesoridazine is a metabolite of thioridazine (p.695).

Uses and Administration

Mesoridazine is a phenothiazine with general properties similar to those of chlorpromazine (p.654). It has a piperidine side-chain and is a metabolite of thioridazine (p.695). It is used in the treatment of various psychoses, including schizophrenia (p.637), in behaviour disturbances (p.636), and in severe anxiety (p.635).

Mesoridazine is usually given as the besylate but the doses are expressed in terms of the base. The usual initial dose for the treatment of schizophrenia or other psychoses is 50 mg three times daily by mouth; doses may be adjusted to 100 to 400 mg daily according to response. Doses ranging from 75 to 300 mg daily by mouth are used in the management of behavioural disorders. Mesoridazine has been given in doses of 30 to 150 mg daily for the management of anxiety.

Mesoridazine may be given intramuscularly in an initial dose of 25 mg repeated after 30 to 60 minutes if necessary; up to 200 mg daily has been given.

Dosage reduction is recommended for elderly patients.

Reviews.

1. Gershon S, *et al.* Mesoridazine—a pharmacodynamic and pharmacokinetic profile. *J Clin Psychiatry* 1981; **42:** 463–9.

Preparations

USP 23: Mesoridazine Besylate Injection; Mesoridazine Besylate Oral Solution; Mesoridazine Besylate Tablets.

Proprietary Preparations (details are given in Part 3)
Canad.: Serentil; ***USA:*** Serentil.

Metaclazepam Hydrochloride (19474-r)

Metaclazepam Hydrochloride *(rINNM)*.

Brometazepam Hydrochloride; Ka-2547 (metaclazepam); KC-2547 (metaclazepam). 7-Bromo-5-(2-chlorophenyl)-2,3-dihydro-2-(methoxymethyl)-1-methyl-1*H*-1,4-benzodiazepine hydrochloride.

$C_{18}H_{18}BrClN_2O,HCl$ = 430.2.

CAS — 65517-27-3 (metaclazepam).

Metaclazepam is a short-acting benzodiazepine with general properties similar to those of diazepam (p.661). Metaclazepam hydrochloride has been given by mouth for the treatment of anxiety disorders (p.635) in a usual dose of 15 mg daily in divided doses.

Preparations

Proprietary Preparations (details are given in Part 3)
Aust.: Talis†; ***Ger.:*** Talis.

Methaqualone (4045-y)

Methaqualone *(BAN, USAN, rINN)*.

CI-705; CN-38703; Methachalonum; Methaqualonum; QZ-2; R-148; TR-495. 2-Methyl-3-o-tolylquinazolin-4-(3*H*)-one.

$C_{16}H_{14}N_2O$ = 250.3.

CAS — 72-44-6 (methaqualone); 340-56-7 (methaqualone hydrochloride).

Pharmacopoeias. In *Eur.* (see p.viii).

A white or almost white, crystalline powder. Very slightly **soluble** in water; soluble in alcohol; sparingly soluble in ether; dissolves in dilute sulphuric acid. **Protect** from light.

Methaqualone is a quinazoline derivative with hypnotic and sedative properties. It has been given by mouth in the short-term management of insomnia but the use of methaqualone for this purpose is no longer considered appropriate. It was also given with diphenhydramine for an enhanced effect.

Methaqualone has been withdrawn from the market in many countries because of problems with abuse.

Adverse effects and symptoms of overdosage are similar to those of barbiturates (see Amylobarbitone, p.642) although cardiac and respiratory depression reportedly occur less frequently.

Preparations

Proprietary Preparations (details are given in Part 3)
Ger.: Normi-Nox†; ***Spain:*** Pallidan.

Multi-ingredient: ***Switz.:*** Motolon†; Toquilone compositum.

Methotrimeprazine (7068-r)

Methotrimeprazine (*BAN, USAN*).

Levomepromazine (*rINN*); CL-36467; CL-39743; RP-7044; SKF-5116. (−)-*NN*-Dimethyl-3-(2-methoxyphenothiazin-10-yl)-2-methylpropylamine; 3-(2-Methoxyphenothiazin-10-yl)-2-methylpropyldimethylamine.

$C_{19}H_{24}N_2OS$ = 328.5.

CAS — 60-99-1.

Pharmacopoeias. In *US.* Also in *BP(Vet)*.

A fine white or slightly cream-coloured odourless or almost odourless crystalline powder. Practically **insoluble** in water; sparingly to slightly soluble in alcohol but freely soluble in boiling alcohol; sparingly soluble in methyl alcohol; freely soluble in chloroform and in ether. **Protect** from light.

Methotrimeprazine Hydrochloride (7069-f)

Methotrimeprazine Hydrochloride (*BANM*).

Levomepromazine Hydrochloride (*rINNM*); Levomepromazini Hydrochloridum.

$C_{19}H_{24}N_2OS,HCl$ = 364.9.

CAS — 4185-80-2.

Pharmacopoeias. In *Eur.* (see p.viii).

A white or very slightly yellow, slightly hygroscopic crystalline powder. It deteriorates on exposure to air and light. Methotrimeprazine hydrochloride 1.11 g is approximately equivalent to 1 g of methotrimeprazine. Freely **soluble** in water and in alcohol; practically insoluble in ether. **Store** in airtight containers. Protect from light.

Methotrimeprazine hydrochloride is reported to be **incompatible** with alkaline solutions.

Methotrimeprazine Maleate (7070-z)

Methotrimeprazine Maleate (*BANM*).

Levomepromazine Maleate (*rINNM*); Levomepromazini Maleas; Methotrimeprazine Hydrogen Maleate.

$C_{19}H_{24}N_2OS,C_4H_4O_4$ = 444.5.

CAS — 7104-38-3.

Pharmacopoeias. In *Eur.* (see p.viii), *Jpn*, and *Pol.*

A white or slightly yellow crystalline powder. It deteriorates when exposed to air and light. Methotrimeprazine maleate 1.35 g is approximately equivalent to 1 g of methotrimeprazine. Slightly **soluble** in water and in alcohol; practically insoluble in ether; sparingly soluble in dichloromethane. The supernatant of a 2% dispersion in water has a pH of 3.5 to 5.5. **Protect** from light.

Adverse Effects, Treatment, and Precautions

As for Chlorpromazine, p.649, although it may be more sedating. See also the sedating antihistamines, p.397.

Methotrimeprazine may cause severe postural hypotension therefore patients receiving large initial doses, patients over 50 years of age, or those receiving injections should be kept lying down.

Interactions

As for Chlorpromazine, p.652.

Antidepressants. Although MAOIs have been used with phenothiazines without untoward effects the concomitant use of methotrimeprazine and MAOIs should probably be avoided as this combination has been implicated in 2 fatalities.[1,2]

1. Barsa JA, Saunders JC. A comparative study of tranylcypromine and pargyline. *Psychopharmacologia* 1964; **6:** 295–8.
2. McQueen EG. New Zealand committee on adverse drug reactions: fourteenth annual report 1979. *N Z Med J* 1980; **91:** 226–9.

Pharmacokinetics

For an account of the pharmacokinetics of a phenothiazine, see Chlorpromazine, p.654.

In a study involving a total of 5 psychiatric patients peak plasma concentrations of methotrimeprazine were noted 1 to 4 hours after administration by mouth and 30 to 90 minutes after injection into the gluteal muscle.[1] About 50% of orally administered drug reached the systemic circulation. Although the metabolite methotrimeprazine sulphoxide could not be detected after a single intramuscular injection it was found in concentrations higher than unmetabolised methotrimeprazine after single and multiple oral dosage, both substances reaching a steady state in the plasma within 7 days of starting multiple dose oral therapy. Fluctuations in plasma concentration during multiple dose oral therapy indicated that until the correlation between acute side-effects and peak plasma concentration of methotrimeprazine had been further studied the total daily dose should be divided into 2 or 3 portions when larger doses of methotrimeprazine were given by mouth.

1. Dahl SG. Pharmacokinetics of methotrimeprazine after single and multiple doses. *Clin Pharmacol Ther* 1976; **19:** 435–42.

Half-life. In 8 psychiatric patients given methotrimeprazine 50 to 350 mg daily the plasma half-life showed wide variation, from 16.5 to 77.8 hours, and did not correlate with the dose given.[1]

1. Dahl SG, *et al.* Pharmacokinetics and relative bioavailability of levomepromazine after repeated administration of tablets and syrup. *Eur J Clin Pharmacol* 1977; **11:** 305–310.

Uses and Administration

Methotrimeprazine is a phenothiazine with pharmacological activity similar to that of both chlorpromazine (p.654) and promethazine (p.417). It has the histamine-antagonist properties of the antihistamines together with CNS effects resembling those of chlorpromazine. It is also reported to have analgesic activity. It is used in the treatment of various psychoses including schizophrenia (p.637), as an analgesic for moderate to severe pain usually in non-ambulatory patients, and for premedication (p.1220). It is also used for the control of symptoms such as restlessness, agitation, and vomiting and as an adjunct to opioid analgesia in terminally ill patients.

Methotrimeprazine is also used in veterinary medicine.

Methotrimeprazine is given by mouth as the maleate or by injection as the hydrochloride; the embonate has also been used.

The usual initial dose for the treatment of schizophrenia is 25 to 50 mg daily by mouth; the daily dosage is usually divided into 3 portions with a larger portion taken at night. Doses of 100 to 200 mg have been given to patients in bed increased gradually up to 1 g daily if necessary. Children are very susceptible to the hypotensive and sedative effects of methotrimeprazine: a suggested dose for a 10-year-old is 12.5 to 25 mg of the maleate daily in divided doses by mouth; a dose of 37.5 mg daily should not be exceeded.

As an adjunct to analgesics in the management of severe terminal pain, methotrimeprazine maleate is given by mouth in a dose of 12.5 to 50 mg every 4 to 8 hours. Alternatively 12.5 to 25 mg of methotrimeprazine hydrochloride may be given intramuscularly every 6 to 8 hours but patients should remain in bed for at least the first few doses; doses of up to 50 mg have been given for severe agitation. Methotrimeprazine hydrochloride may also be given intravenously in similar doses following dilution with an equal volume of sodium chloride 0.9% injection. Alternatively it may be given, suitably diluted with sodium chloride 0.9% injection, by continuous subcutaneous infusion via a syringe driver, in doses ranging from a total of 25 to 200 mg daily although lower doses of 5 to 25 mg may also be effective against nausea and vomiting and produce less sedation. Experience with parenteral administration of methotrimeprazine hydrochloride in children is limited but a dose of 0.35 to 3 mg per kg body-weight daily has been suggested.

A dose of 10 to 20 mg of methotrimeprazine hydrochloride given intramuscularly every 4 to 6 hours adjusted as required has been used for the control of acute pain. If used for postoperative analgesia an initial intramuscular dose of 2.5 to 7.5 mg has been given.

Methotrimeprazine hydrochloride has also been given as a premedicant in doses ranging from 2 to 20 mg administered intramuscularly 45 minutes to 3 hours prior to surgical procedures.

Care is required in elderly patients because of the risk of severe hypotension; if methotrimeprazine is given to such patients reduced doses may be necessary.

Pain. As methotrimeprazine appears to possess intrinsic analgesic activity in addition to its antiemetic and antipsychotic actions it has been used for the symptomatic control of restlessness and vomiting and as an adjunct to opioid analgesics in pain control (p.4) in terminally ill patients.

References.

1. Oliver DJ. The use of methotrimeprazine in terminal care. *Br J Clin Pract* 1985; **39:** 339–40.
2. Patt RB, *et al.* The neuroleptics as adjuvant analgesics. *J Pain Symptom Manage* 1994; **9:** 446–53.

HEADACHE. Similarly to chlorpromazine (p.655) and prochlorperazine (p.688), methotrimeprazine[1] has been effective in relieving the pain of severe migraine attacks.

1. Stiell IG, *et al.* Methotrimeprazine versus meperidine and dimenhydrinate in the treatment of severe migraine: a randomized, controlled trial. *Ann Emerg Med* 1991; **20:** 1201–5.

Preparations

USP 23: Methotrimeprazine Injection.

Proprietary Preparations (details are given in Part 3)
Aust.: Nozinan; ***Belg.:*** Nozinan; ***Canad.:*** Novo-Meprazine; Nozinan; ***Fr.:*** Nozinan; ***Ger.:*** Neurocil; Tisercin; ***Irl.:*** Nozinan; ***Ital.:*** Nozinan; ***Neth.:*** Nozinan; ***Norw.:*** Nozinan; Veractil†; ***Spain:*** Sinogan; ***Swed.:*** Nozinan; ***Switz.:*** Minozinan; Nozinan; ***UK:*** Nozinan; ***USA:*** Levoprome.

Methylpentynol (4048-c)

Methylpentynol (*BAN, rINN*).

Meparfynol; Methylparafynol. 3-Methylpent-1-yn-3-ol.

$C_6H_{10}O$ = 98.14.

CAS — 77-75-8.

Methylpentynol is a hypnotic and sedative. It has been given by mouth as a hypnotic in the short-term management of insomnia (p.638) in usual doses of 0.5 to 1 g at night. It has also been used as a sedative in doses of 0.25 to 0.5 g.

Preparations

Proprietary Preparations (details are given in Part 3)
Switz.: Oblivon.

Mexazolam (16895-a)

Mexazolam (*rINN*).

CS-386; Methylcloxazolam. 10-Chloro-11b-(2-chlorophenyl)-2,3,7,11b-tetrahydro-3-methyloxazolo[3,2-*d*][1,4]benzodiazepin-6(5*H*)-one.

$C_{18}H_{16}Cl_2N_2O_2$ = 363.2.

CAS — 31868-18-5.

Mexazolam is a benzodiazepine with general properties similar to those of diazepam (p.661). It is given by mouth for its anxiolytic and sedative properties.

Preparations

Proprietary Preparations (details are given in Part 3)
Jpn: Melex.

Midazolam (13499-v)

Midazolam (*BAN, rINN*).

Midazolamum; Ro-21-3971. 8-Chloro-6-(2-fluorophenyl)-1-methyl-4*H*-imidazo[1,5-*a*][1,4]benzodiazepine.

$C_{18}H_{13}ClFN_3$ = 325.8.

CAS — 59467-70-8.

Pharmacopoeias. In *Eur.* (see p.viii).

A white or yellowish crystalline powder. Practically **insoluble** in water; freely soluble in alcohol and in acetone; soluble in methyl alcohol. **Protect** from light.

Midazolam Hydrochloride (12958-p)

Midazolam Hydrochloride (*BANM, USAN, rINNM*).

Ro-21-3981/003.

$C_{18}H_{13}ClFN_3,HCl$ = 362.2.

CAS — 59467-96-8.

Incompatibility. The visual compatibility of midazolam hydrochloride with a range of drugs was studied over a period of 4 hours.[1] A white precipitate was formed immediately with dimenhydrinate, pentobarbitone sodium, perphenazine, prochlorperazine edisylate, and ranitidine hydrochloride. Similar incompatibility has been reported[2,3] with frusemide, thiopentone, and parenteral nutrition solutions. Other workers[4] have reported that a precipitate is formed with midazolam hydrochloride if the resultant mixture has a pH of 5 or more.

1. Forman JK, Souney PF. Visual compatibility of midazolam hydrochloride with common preoperative injectable medications. *Am J Hosp Pharm* 1987; **44:** 2298–9.
2. Chiu MF, Schwartz ML. Visual compatibility of injectable drugs used in the intensive care unit. *Am J Health-Syst Pharm* 1997; **54:** 64–5.

3. Trissel LA, *et al.* Compatibility of parenteral nutrient solutions with selected drugs during simulated Y-site administration. *Am J Health-Syst Pharm* 1997; **54:** 1295–300.
4. Swart EL, *et al.* Compatibility of midazolam hydrochloride and lorazepam with selected drugs during simulated Y-site administration. *Am J Health-Syst Pharm* 1995; **52:** 2020–2.

Stability. The manufacturers have stated that solutions of midazolam hydrochloride in sodium chloride 0.9% or glucose 5% are stable at room temperature for up to 24 hours. However, Pramar *et al.*[1] have reported that similar solutions containing midazolam hydrochloride equivalent to 0.5 mg per mL of the base were stable for 36 days when stored in glass bottles at temperatures of 4 to 6°, 24 to 26°, and 39 to 41°. Other workers[2] found that a solution containing midazolam hydrochloride equivalent to 1 mg per mL of the base in sodium chloride 0.9% was stable for at least 10 days when stored in PVC bags. The manufacturer advises against admixture with Hartmann's solution as the potency of midazolam is reduced.

1. Pramar YV, *et al.* Stability of midazolam hydrochloride in syringes and i.v. fluids. *Am J Health-Syst Pharm* 1997; **54:** 913–15.
2. McMullin ST, *et al.* Stability of midazolam hydrochloride in polyvinyl chloride bags under fluorescent light. *Am J Health-Syst Pharm* 1995; **52:** 2018–20.

Midazolam Maleate (15125-j)

Midazolam Maleate *(BANM, USAN, rINNM).*

Ro-21-3981/001.

$C_{18}H_{13}ClFN_3,C_4H_4O_4$ = 441.8.

CAS — 59467-94-6.

Dependence and Withdrawal, Adverse Effects, Treatment, and Precautions

As for Diazepam, p.661. There have been reports of life-threatening adverse respiratory and cardiovascular events occurring after intravenous administration of midazolam; when giving midazolam by this route the precautions given below should be observed to lessen the risk of such reactions. Pain, tenderness, and thrombophlebitis have occurred following injection of midazolam. Hiccups have been reported.

There has been concern over reports of death due to respiratory depression, hypotension, or cardiac arrest in patients given intravenous midazolam for conscious sedation.[1] Within about 6 months of its introduction in the USA in May 1986, 13 fatalities due to cardiorespiratory depression had been reported, although higher doses were used initially than in the UK. By January 1988, 66 deaths had been reported, although in November 1987 the adult dosage recommendation had been reduced to 0.07 mg per kg body-weight and to 0.05 mg per kg for elderly patients. Fatalities have also occurred in the UK [where the dose is 0.07 mg per kg, reduced in the elderly], 4 deaths having been reported to the CSM by November 1987.

While it appears that midazolam and diazepam produce very similar degrees of hypoventilation and oxygen desaturation when used in equivalent doses,[2] the sedative end-point does appear to be reached more abruptly with midazolam.[3] Facilities for resuscitation should always be available when intravenous midazolam is used, and respiratory and cardiac function monitored continuously. The dose of midazolam should be carefully titrated against the response of the patient and the manufacturer's recommendations concerning speed of administration be observed. Particular care, including a reduction in midazolam dosage, is required in patients also receiving opioid analgesics, in the elderly and children, and in patients with compromised cardiorespiratory function. The availability of the benzodiazepine antagonist, flumazenil, should not be an encouragement to use larger doses of midazolam.[1]

Since endoscopy of the upper gastro-intestinal tract can itself reduce oxygen saturation, some workers have advocated the prophylactic administration of nasal oxygen during this procedure for those patients at particular risk as outlined above.

1. Anonymous. Midazolam—is antagonism justified? *Lancet* 1988; **ii:** 140–2.
2. Bell GD. Review article: premedication and intravenous sedation for upper gastrointestinal endoscopy. *Aliment Pharmacol Ther* 1990; **4:** 103–22.
3. Ryder W, Wright PA. Dental sedation: a review. *Br Dent J* 1988; **165:** 207–16.

Children and neonates. Administration of an intravenous bolus injection of midazolam to children already receiving intravenous morphine after cardiac surgery produced an undesirable transient fall in cardiac output.[1] It was suggested that for patients already receiving other drugs which provide sedation the use of midazolam in the early postoperative period should be limited to a continuous infusion. Others[2] have similarly recommended that bolus intravenous administration of midazolam should be avoided in neonates due to the occurrence of hypotension. The initial dosage of midazolam used for continuous intravenous sedation may need to be reduced in critically ill children under 3 years of age since the plasma clearance of midazolam appears to be reduced in these patients.[3]

1. Shekerdemian L, *et al.* Cardiovascular effects of intravenous midazolam after open heart surgery. *Arch Dis Child* 1997; **76:** 57–61.
2. Jacqz-Aigrain E, Burtin P. Clinical pharmacokinetics of sedatives in neonates. *Clin Pharmacokinet* 1996; **31:** 423–43.
3. Hughes J, *et al.* Steady-state plasma concentrations of midazolam in critically ill infants and children. *Ann Pharmacother* 1996; **30:** 27–30.

Hepatic impairment. For the precautions to be observed in patients with impaired liver function, see under Pharmacokinetics, below.

Renal impairment. Five patients with severe renal impairment experienced prolonged sedation when given midazolam; this was attributed to accumulation of conjugated metabolites.[1]

1. Bauer TM, *et al.* Prolonged sedation due to accumulation of conjugated metabolites of midazolam. *Lancet* 1995; **346:** 145–7.

Dependence. Details have been reported[1] of 2 children who developed withdrawal symptoms following discontinuation of midazolam, which had been used for sedation during mechanical ventilation.

1. van Engelen BGM, *et al.* Benzodiazepine withdrawal reaction in two children following discontinuation of sedation with midazolam. *Ann Pharmacother* 1993; **27:** 579–81.

Effects on mental function. For discussion of the adverse effects of benzodiazepines on mental function, including reports of sexual fantasies in women sedated with intravenous midazolam, see Diazepam, p.661.

Effects on the nervous system. For reference to acute dystonia associated with administration of midazolam, see Diazepam, p.662.

ENCEPHALOPATHY. For a report of prolonged use of midazolam with fentanyl being associated with encephalopathy in infants sedated under intensive care, see Diazepam, p.662.

MYOCLONUS. Myoclonic twitching of all four limbs was noted[1] in 6 of 102 neonates who received a continuous intravenous infusion of midazolam at a rate of 30 to 60 μg per kg body-weight per hour. Myoclonus ceased a few hours after discontinuing the infusion and never recurred. No ictal activity was detected in EEGs recorded during the myoclonus.

1. Magny JF, *et al.* Midazolam and myoclonus in neonate. *Eur J Pediatr* 1994; **153:** 389–90.

Interactions

As for Diazepam, p.663.

Pharmacokinetics

Absorption of midazolam is rapid, peak plasma concentrations being achieved within 20 to 60 minutes of administration depending on the route. Extensive first-pass metabolism results in a low systemic bioavailability after oral administration. Bioavailability is higher, but variable, after intramuscular injection; figures of more than 90% are often cited.

Midazolam is lipophilic at physiological pH. It crosses the placenta. Midazolam is extensively (about 96%) bound to plasma proteins.

Midazolam usually has a short elimination half-life of about 2 hours although half-lives longer than 7 hours have been reported in some patients. The half-life of midazolam is prolonged in neonates, in the elderly, and in patients with liver disorders.

Midazolam is metabolised in the liver. The major metabolite, 1-hydroxymethylmidazolam, is less active than midazolam; its half-life is similar to that of midazolam. Midazolam metabolites are excreted in the urine, mainly as glucuronide conjugates.

Reviews of the pharmacokinetics of midazolam.

1. Garzone PD, Kroboth PD. Pharmacokinetics of the newer benzodiazepines. *Clin Pharmacokinet* 1989; **16:** 337–64.

Administration. ADMINISTRATION IN CHILDREN. A study of the pharmacokinetics of midazolam in children.[1] Bioavailability of a dose of 0.15 mg per kg body-weight was 100, 87, 27, and 18% after administration by the intravenous, intramuscular, oral, and rectal routes respectively. The oral bioavailability was reduced to 16 and 15% after increasing the dose to 0.45 and 1.00 mg per kg respectively. There was bioequivalence between the 0.15 mg per kg intramuscular dose and the 0.45 mg per kg oral dose from 45 to 120 minutes after administration. Absorption from the rectal route gave lower serum-midazolam concentrations than the oral route at the 0.15 mg per kg dose. Midazolam appears to be absorbed rapidly when given by the intranasal route to children with mean maximum plasma concentrations being achieved within about 12 minutes;[2-4] values of 30% and 55% have been reported for the bioavailability[3,4] but methods to optimise nasal delivery have resulted in higher bioavailability in studies in adults (see below). A study comparing intranasal, intravenous, and rectal administration of midazolam to children found that plasma concentrations from 45 minutes after intranasal and intravenous administration were similar; those following rectal administration were consistently less than after these other 2 routes.[2] Possible reasons were loss of midazolam due to first-pass metabolism during rectal administration or that the wide interindividual variations in rectal pH had influenced absorption of midazolam.

Another study has investigated the relationship between intravenous dose and plasma-midazolam concentrations in children.[5]

See also Children and Neonates under Precautions, above.

1. Payne K, *et al.* The pharmacokinetics of midazolam in paediatric patients. *Eur J Clin Pharmacol* 1989; **37:** 267–72.
2. Malinovsky J-M, *et al.* Plasma concentrations of midazolam after iv, nasal or rectal administration in children. *Br J Anaesth* 1993; **70:** 617–20.
3. Rey E, *et al.* Pharmacokinetics of midazolam in children: comparative study of intranasal and intravenous administration. *Eur J Clin Pharmacol* 1991; **41:** 355–7.
4. Kauffman RE, *et al.* Intranasal absorption of midazolam. *Clin Pharmacol Ther* 1995; **57:** 209.
5. Tolia V, *et al.* Pharmacokinetic and pharmacodynamic study of midazolam in children during esophagogastroduodenoscopy. *J Pediatr* 1991; **119:** 467–71.

ADMINISTRATION IN LIVER DISORDERS. The pharmacokinetics of midazolam in patients with advanced cirrhosis of the liver were characterised by an increase in oral systemic bioavailability[1] and by a decrease in clearance with consequent prolongation of elimination half-life.[1,2] Dosage may need to be reduced. Metabolism of midazolam has been demonstrated, however, in the anhepatic period of liver transplantation indicating extrahepatic metabolism (see below).

1. Pentikäinen PJ, *et al.* Pharmacokinetics of midazolam following intravenous and oral administration in patients with chronic liver disease and in healthy subjects. *J Clin Pharmacol* 1989; **29:** 272–7.
2. MacGilchrist AJ, *et al.* Pharmacokinetics and pharmacodynamics of intravenous midazolam in patients with severe alcoholic cirrhosis. *Gut* 1986; **27:** 190–5.

ADMINISTRATION IN THE NEONATE. References to the pharmacokinetics of midazolam in neonates. See also Children and Neonates under Precautions, above.

1. Jacqz-Aigrain E, *et al.* Pharmacokinetics of midazolam in critically ill neonates. *Eur J Clin Pharmacol* 1990; **39:** 191–2.
2. Jacqz-Aigrain E, *et al.* Pharmacokinetics of midazolam during continuous infusion in critically ill neonates. *Eur J Clin Pharmacol* 1992; **42:** 329–32.
3. Burtin P, *et al.* Population pharmacokinetics of midazolam in neonates. *Clin Pharmacol Ther* 1994; **56:** 615–25.

INTRANASAL ADMINISTRATION. Plasma concentrations of midazolam sufficient to induce conscious sedation are rapidly attained following intranasal administration.[1] Although bioavailability of up to 55% had previously been obtained in children following intranasal administration (see above) slow administration and other methods to optimise nasal delivery had resulted in a bioavailability of 83% in adults.[2] Similar techniques should be developed for use in children.

1. Burstein AH, *et al.* Pharmacokinetics and pharmacodynamics of midazolam after intranasal administration. *J Clin Pharmacol* 1997; **37:** 711–18.
2. Björkman S, *et al.* Pharmacokinetics of midazolam given as an intranasal spray to adult surgical patients. *Br J Anaesth* 1997; **79:** 575–80.

Distribution into breast milk. Midazolam could not be detected in breast milk from 11 mothers the morning after either the first or the fifth nightly 15-mg hypnotic dose by mouth.[1] Additional investigations in 2 mothers demonstrated that midazolam and its hydroxy-metabolite disappeared rapidly from milk with undetectable concentrations at 4 hours. The mean milk to plasma ratio for midazolam was 0.15 in 6 paired samples.

1. Matheson I, *et al.* Midazolam and nitrazepam in the maternity ward: milk concentrations and clinical effects. *Br J Clin Pharmacol* 1990; **30:** 787–93.

Half-life. Data collected from seven studies involving 90 participants has suggested that the prolonged midazolam half-lives reported in a small number of patients are secondary to increases in the volume of distribution and not a result of alterations in clearance and metabolism.[1]

1. Wills RJ, *et al.* Increased volume of distribution prolongs midazolam half-life. *Br J Clin Pharmacol* 1990; **29:** 269–72.

Metabolism. For a discussion of the metabolism of benzodiazepines, see Diazepam, p.666. Midazolam appears to be metabolised by at least 3 different cytochrome P450 enzymes which are found in the liver and in the kidney.[1] Variations in the activity of these enzymes might account for some of the interindividual differences in pharmacokinetics and pharmacodynamics seen with midazolam.[2] However, a study[3] in patients undergoing liver transplantation has indicated that the small intestine is a significant site for the first-pass metabolism of midazolam, metabolism presumably being catalysed by the cytochrome P450 isozyme CYP3A4 found in intestinal mucosa.

1. Wandel C, *et al.* Midazolam is metabolized by at least three different cytochrome P450 enzymes. *Br J Anaesth* 1994; **73:** 658–61.
2. Lown KS, *et al.* The erythromycin breath test predicts the clearance of midazolam. *Clin Pharmacol Ther* 1995; **57:** 16–24.
3. Paine MF, *et al.* First-pass metabolism of midazolam by the human intestine. *Clin Pharmacol Ther* 1996; **60:** 14–24.

Uses and Administration

Midazolam is a short-acting benzodiazepine with general properties similar to those of diazepam (p.666), except that it has a more potent amnesic action. It is mainly used for premedication and sedation and for induction of general anaesthesia. When midazolam is used as a premedicant or for conscious sedation, onset of sedation occurs at about 15 minutes after intramuscular injection reaching a peak at 30 to 60 minutes, and within 3 to 5 minutes after intravenous injection. When given intravenously as an anaesthetic induction agent, anaesthesia is induced in about 2.0 to 2.5 minutes. Onset of action is more rapid when premedication with an opioid analgesic has been given. Since the sedative end-point is reached abruptly with intravenous midazolam, dosage must be titrated carefully against the response of the patient and respiratory and cardiac function should be monitored continuously. Facilities for resuscitation should always be available. It is advisable to keep the patient supine during intravenous administration and throughout the procedure.

Midazolam is used as the hydrochloride for parenteral and rectal administration and as the maleate for oral administration; all doses are given in terms of the base. Lower doses of midazolam may be adequate when it is used in conjunction with opioid analgesics.

Midazolam may be given for **premedication** before general anaesthesia or to provide sedative cover for minor surgical or investigative procedures. A usual total sedative dose for dental and minor surgical and other procedures ranges from 2.5 to 7.5 mg (about 0.07 mg per kg body-weight) intravenously; an initial dose of 2 mg over 30 seconds has been suggested, with further incremental doses of 0.5 to 1.0 mg at intervals of 2 minutes if required until the desired end-point is reached. In the USA a suggested initial dose is up to 2.5 mg given intravenously over at least 2 minutes and repeated if necessary after an additional 2 or more minutes to a maximum total dose of 5 mg.

Midazolam is given intramuscularly as a premedicant about 30 to 60 minutes before surgery. The usual dose is about 5 mg; doses range from 0.07 to 0.1 mg per kg. The oral and rectal routes are used for premedication in some countries.

The usual dose of midazolam for **induction of anaesthesia** (p.1220) is about 0.2 mg per kg by slow intravenous injection in premedicated patients and at least 0.3 mg per kg in those who have not received a premedicant. In the USA further incremental doses of midazolam of approximately 25% of the induction dose have been given as a component of the regimens used for the maintenance of anaesthesia during short surgical procedures. A dose of 0.15 mg per kg has been recommended for the induction of anaesthesia in children over 7 years of age.

Patients in **intensive care** who require continuous sedation (p.638) can be given midazolam by intravenous infusion. An initial loading dose of 0.03 to 0.3 mg per kg may be given by intravenous infusion over 5 minutes to induce sedation. The maintenance dose required varies considerably but a dose of between 0.03 to 0.2 mg per kg per hour has been suggested. Sedation can also be achieved by giving intermittent intravenous bolus injections of midazolam; doses of 1 to 2 mg may be given, and repeated, until the desired level of sedation has been reached. The dosage should be reduced or the loading dose omitted for patients with hypovolaemia, vasoconstriction, or hypothermia. The need for continuous administration should be reassessed on a daily basis to reduce the risk of accumulation and prolonged recovery. Abrupt withdrawal should be avoided after prolonged administration.

Midazolam maleate is also given by mouth for the short-term management of **insomnia**; the usual dose is the equivalent of midazolam 7.5 to 15 mg at night.

Midazolam should be given in reduced doses to elderly and debilitated patients.

Administration. The rectal,[1] intranasal,[1-4] and sublingual[1,5] routes have all been proposed as alternatives to parenteral administration of midazolam.

One group of workers reported that intranasal midazolam caused intense burning, irritation, and lachrymation on instillation into the nares and they now used a nasal spray containing lignocaine before administering midazolam to children.[6] The use of midazolam spray intranasally in adults would be impractical and uncomfortable because of the large volume required. It has therefore been tried as a nebulised solution.[7]

1. Wong L, McQueen KD. Midazolam routes of administration. *DICP Ann Pharmacother* 1991; **25:** 476–7.
2. Theroux MC, *et al.* Efficacy of intranasal midazolam in facilitating suturing of lacerations in preschool children in the emergency department. *Pediatrics* 1993; **91:** 624–7.
3. Louon A, *et al.* Sedation with nasal ketamine and midazolam for cryotherapy in retinopathy of prematurity. *Br J Ophthalmol* 1993; **77:** 529–30.
4. Bates BA, *et al.* A comparison of intranasal sufentanil and midazolam to intramuscular meperidine, promethazine, and chlorpromazine for conscious sedation in children. *Ann Emerg Med* 1994; **24:** 646–51.
5. Karl HLO, *et al.* Transmucosal administration of midazolam for premedication of pediatric patients: comparison of the nasal and sublingual routes. *Anesthesiology* 1993; **78:** 885–91.
6. Lugo RA, *et al.* Complications of intranasal midazolam. *Pediatrics* 1993; **92:** 638.
7. Hodgson PE, *et al.* Administration of nebulized intranasal midazolam to healthy adult volunteers: a pilot study. *Br J Anaesth* 1994; **73:** 719P.

INTRATHECAL. See Pain, below.

Conversion and dissociative disorders. For reference to the use of midazolam in the diagnosis of conversion disorders, such as hysterical paralysis, see p.667.

Dyspnoea. Midazolam has been suggested[1] as an alternative to chlorpromazine in patients with advanced cancer and intractable dyspnoea (p.70) to relieve air hunger and to sedate dying patients who have unrelieved distress. Suggested[2] initial doses are 2.5 to 5 mg subcutaneously or 10 mg administered by infusion over a period of 24 hours, increased as necessary.

1. Walsh D. Dyspnoea in advanced cancer. *Lancet* 1993; **342:** 450–1.
2. Davis CL. ABC of palliative care: breathlessness, cough, and other respiratory problems. *Br Med J* 1997; **315:** 931–4.

Hiccup. A protocol for the management of intractable hiccups may be found under Chlorpromazine, p.655. Midazolam given intravenously or subcutaneously has been reported[1] to have been effective in 2 patients with metastatic cancer who had hiccups unresponsive to conventional treatment. However, it has been noted[1,2] that benzodiazepines such as midazolam may exacerbate or precipitate hiccups.

1. Wilcock A, Twycross R. Midazolam for intractable hiccup. *J Pain Symptom Manage* 1996; **12:** 59–61.
2. Rousseau P. Hiccups. *South Med J* 1995; **88:** 175–81.

Insomnia. For discussion of the management of insomnia including limitations on the use of benzodiazepines and a recommendation that the period of treatment with midazolam should be limited to 2 weeks, see p.638.

References.

1. Monti JM, *et al.* The effect of midazolam on transient insomnia. *Eur J Clin Pharmacol* 1993; **44:** 525–7.

Pain. The conventional use of benzodiazepines in pain management is as muscle relaxants to relieve pain associated with skeletal muscle spasm (see under Analgesics and Analgesic Adjuvants, p.5). Midazolam is being studied[1-4] for use as an intrathecal analgesic but efficacy has been inconsistent.

1. Cripps TP, Goodchild CS. Intrathecal midazolam and the stress response to upper abdominal surgery. *Clin J Pain* 1988; **4:** 125–8.
2. Serrao JM, *et al.* Intrathecal midazolam for the treatment of chronic mechanical low back pain: a controlled comparison with epidural steroid in a pilot study. *Pain* 1992; **48:** 5–12.
3. Baaijens PFJ, *et al.* Intrathecal midazolam for the treatment of chronic mechanical low back pain: a randomized double-blind placebo-controlled study. *Br J Anaesth* 1995; **74** (suppl 1): 143.
4. Valentine JMJ, *et al.* The effect of intrathecal midazolam on post-operative pain. *Eur J Anaesthesiol* 1996; **13:** 589–93.

Premedication and sedation. Midazolam is used as a premedicant (p.1220) and as a sedative for therapeutic and investigative procedures such as dental treatment (p.638) and endoscopy. It is also used to provide continuous sedation in patients in intensive care (p.638). Midazolam is usually given intravenously for sedation but other routes have also been tried (see Administration, above).

References.

1. Sandler ES, *et al.* Midazolam versus fentanyl as premedication for painful procedures in children with cancer. *Pediatrics* 1992; **89:** 631–4.
2. Stenhammar L, *et al.* Intravenous midazolam in small bowel biopsy. *Arch Dis Child* 1994; **71:** 558.
3. Jacqz-Aigrain E, *et al.* Placebo-controlled trial of midazolam sedation in mechanically ventilated newborn babies. *Lancet* 1994; **344:** 646–50.
4. Mitchell V, *et al.* Comparison of midazolam with trimeprazine as an oral premedicant for paediatric anaesthesia. *Br J Anaesth* 1995; **74** (suppl 1): 94–5.
5. McCarver-May DG, *et al.* Comparison of chloral hydrate and midazolam for sedation of neonates for neuroimaging studies. *J Pediatr* 1996; **128:** 573–6.
6. Zedie N, *et al.* Comparison of intranasal midazolam and sufentanil premedication in pediatric outpatients. *Clin Pharmacol Ther* 1996; **59:** 341–8.

ENDOSCOPY. Intravenous benzodiazepines such as diazepam or midazolam are often the preferred drugs for sedation in patients undergoing endoscopy (p.638). They are sometimes used in conjunction with opioid analgesics for sedation.[1]

A reduced dose of midazolam was required for endoscopy when it was given as a bolus intravenous injection rather than as a slow intravenous titration. A study in 788 patients undergoing endoscopy found that a mean dose of 4.65 mg of midazolam given as a bolus intravenous injection was safe and effective in patients under 70 years of age whereas a mean dose of 1.89 mg was sufficient for patients over 70 years of age.[2] Furthermore, topical pharyngeal anaesthesia was not required with these doses of midazolam.

1. Bahal-O'Mara N, *et al.* Sedation with meperidine and midazolam in pediatric patients undergoing endoscopy. *Eur J Clin Pharmacol* 1994; **47:** 319–23.
2. Smith MR, *et al.* Small bolus injections of intravenous midazolam for upper gastrointestinal endoscopy: a study of 788 consecutive cases. *Br J Clin Pharmacol* 1993; **36:** 573–8.

Status epilepticus. Benzodiazepines such as diazepam or lorazepam given parenterally are often tried first to control status epilepticus (p.337). Midazolam may be of use as an alternative when intravenous access is difficult as effective concentrations of midazolam can be obtained after intramuscular injection.[1] Intravenous midazolam has been used in some centres[2] for status epilepticus refractory to diazepam, lorazepam, or phenytoin but reviews of the literature[3] reveal that evidence of efficacy is limited mainly to uncontrolled studies and anecdotal reports. The use of intranasal midazolam for the management of seizures in children is being studied.[4,5]

1. Bauer J, Elger CE. Management of status epilepticus in adults. *CNS Drugs* 1994; **1:** 26–44.
2. Bebin M, Bleck TP. New anticonvulsant drugs: focus on flunarizine, fosphenytoin, midazolam and stiripentol. *Drugs* 1994; **48:** 153–71.
3. Denzel D, Burstein AH. Midazolam in refractory status epilepticus. *Ann Pharmacother* 1996; **30:** 1481–3.
4. Wallace SJ. Nasal benzodiazepines for management of acute childhood seizures? *Lancet* 1997; **349:** 222.
5. Lahat E, *et al.* Intranasal midazolam for childhood seizures. *Lancet* 1998; **352:** 620.

Preparations

BP 1998: Midazolam Injection.

Proprietary Preparations (details are given in Part 3)
Aust.: Dormicum; ***Austral.:*** Hypnovel; ***Belg.:*** Dormicum; ***Canad.:*** Versed; ***Fr.:*** Hypnovel; ***Ger.:*** Dormicum; ***Irl.:*** Hypnovel; ***Ital.:*** Ipnovel; ***Neth.:*** Dormicum; ***Norw.:*** Dormicum; ***S.Afr.:*** Dormicum; ***Spain:*** Dormicum; ***Swed.:*** Dormicum; ***Switz.:*** Dormicum; ***UK:*** Hypnovel; ***USA:*** Versed.

Molindone Hydrochloride (7072-k)

Molindone Hydrochloride *(BANM, USAN, rINNM)*.

EN-1733A. 3-Ethyl-1,5,6,7-tetrahydro-2-methyl-5-(morpholinomethyl)indol-4-one hydrochloride.

$C_{16}H_{24}N_2O_2$,HCl = 312.8.

CAS — 7416-34-4 (molindone); 15622-65-8 (molindone hydrochloride).

Pharmacopoeias. In US.

A 1% solution in water has a pH between 4.0 and 5.0. **Store** in airtight containers. Protect from light.

Adverse Effects, Treatment, and Precautions

As for Chlorpromazine, p.649. Molindone hydrochloride is less likely to cause hypotension than chlorpromazine and extrapyramidal effects may be frequent but less severe. The incidence of sedation is intermediate between that of chlorpromazine and of phenothiazines with a piperazine side-chain. Weight gain or loss may occur.

Convulsions. For mention of molindone as one of the antipsychotics suitable for patients at risk of seizures, see p.649.

Effects on the liver. A report of hepatotoxicity, associated with a flu-like syndrome, in a patient given molindone.[1] Symptoms and liver-enzyme values returned to normal on discontinuation of the drug and recurred on rechallenge with low doses. The effect was probably due to a hypersensitivity reaction.

1. Bhatia SC, *et al.* Molindone and hepatotoxicity. *Drug Intell Clin Pharm* 1985; **19:** 744–6.

Interactions

As for Chlorpromazine, p.652.

Pharmacokinetics

Molindone is readily absorbed from the gastro-intestinal tract, peak concentrations of unchanged molindone being obtained within about 1.5 hours of administration. It is rapidly and extensively metabolised and a large number of metabolites have been identified. It is excreted in the urine and faeces almost entirely in the form of its metabolites. The pharmacological effect from a single dose by mouth is reported to last for 24 to 36 hours.

References.

1. Zetin M, *et al*. Bioavailability of oral and intramuscular molindone hydrochloride in schizophrenic patients. *Clin Ther* 1985; **7**: 169–75.

Uses and Administration

Molindone is an indole derivative with general properties similar to those of the phenothiazine, chlorpromazine (p.654). It is given as the hydrochloride by mouth for the treatment of psychoses including schizophrenia (p.637).

The usual dose of molindone hydrochloride by mouth is 50 to 75 mg daily initially, increased within 3 or 4 days to 100 mg daily; in severe or resistant conditions doses of up to 225 mg daily may be required. The maintenance dosage can range from 15 to 225 mg daily according to severity of symptoms. The daily dosage is usually divided into 3 to 4 portions.

Molindone should be given in reduced dosage to elderly or debilitated patients.

Preparations

USP 23: Molindone Hydrochloride Tablets.

Proprietary Preparations (details are given in Part 3)
USA: Moban.

Moperone Hydrochloride (7073-a)

Moperone Hydrochloride *(rINNM)*.

Methylperidol Hydrochloride; R-1658 (moperone). 4′-Fluoro-4-(4-hydroxy-4-*p*-tolylpiperidino)butyrophenone hydrochloride.

$C_{22}H_{26}FNO_2$,HCl = 391.9.

CAS — 1050-79-9 (moperone); 3871-82-7 (moperone hydrochloride).

Moperone is a butyrophenone with general properties similar to those of haloperidol (p.673). It has been given by mouth for the treatment of psychoses.

Preparations

Proprietary Preparations (details are given in Part 3)
Swed.: Luvatren†; ***Switz.:*** Luvatren†.

Multi-ingredient: ***Spain:*** Sedalium†.

Mosapramine (15295-s)

Mosapramine *(rINN)*.

Clospipramine; Y-516. (±)-1′-[3-(3-Chloro-10,11-dihydro-5*H*-dibenz[*b,f*]azepin-5-yl)propyl]hexahydrospiro[imidazo[1,2-*a*]pyridine-3(2*H*),4′-piperidin]-2-one.

$C_{28}H_{35}ClN_4O$ = 479.1.

CAS — 89419-40-9.

Mosapramine is an antipsychotic.

References.

1. Ishigooka J, *et al*. Pilot study of plasma concentrations of mosapramine, a new iminodibenzyl antipsychotic agent, after multiple oral administration in schizophrenic patients. *Curr Ther Res* 1994; **55**: 331–42.

Nemonapride (10985-a)

Nemonapride *(rINN)*.

(±)-*cis*-*N*-(1-Benzyl-2-methyl-3-pyrrolidinyl)-5-chloro-4-(methylamino)-*o*-anisamide.

$C_{21}H_{26}ClN_3O_2$ = 387.9.

CAS — 93664-94-9.

Nemonapride is a substituted benzamide antipsychotic with general properties similar to those of sulpiride (p.692). It is given by mouth in the treatment of schizophrenia.

References.

1. Satoh K, *et al*. Effects of nemonapride on positive and negative symptoms of schizophrenia. *Int Clin Psychopharmacol* 1996; **11**: 279–81.

Preparations

Proprietary Preparations (details are given in Part 3)
Jpn: Emilace.

Nimetazepam (13018-a)

Nimetazepam *(rINN)*.

Menifazepam; S-1530. 1,3-Dihydro-1-methyl-7-nitro-5-phenyl-1,4-benzodiazepin-2-one.

$C_{16}H_{13}N_3O_3$ = 295.3.

CAS — 2011-67-8.

Nimetazepam is a benzodiazepine with the general properties of diazepam (p.661). It is given by mouth for the short-term management of insomnia.

Preparations

Proprietary Preparations (details are given in Part 3)
Jpn: Erimin.

Nitrazepam (4054-j)

Nitrazepam *(BAN, USAN, rINN)*.

Nitrazepamum; NSC-58775; Ro-4-5360; Ro-5-3059. 1,3-Dihydro-7-nitro-5-phenyl-2*H*-1,4-benzodiazepin-2-one.

$C_{15}H_{11}N_3O_3$ = 281.3.

CAS — 146-22-5.

Pharmacopoeias. In *Chin., Eur.* (see p.viii), *Int., Jpn,* and *Pol.*

A yellow, crystalline powder. Practically **insoluble** in water; slightly soluble in alcohol and in ether. **Protect** from light.

Dependence and Withdrawal

As for Diazepam, p.661.

For the purpose of withdrawal regimens, 5 mg of nitrazepam may be considered roughly equivalent to 5 mg of diazepam.

Adverse Effects and Treatment

As for Diazepam, p.661.

Effects on the digestive system. Two children given nitrazepam as part of their antiepileptic therapy developed drooling, eating difficulty, and aspiration pneumonia; symptoms improved in one patient when the dosage of nitrazepam was reduced.[1] Manometric studies indicated that the onset of normal cricopharyngeal relaxation in swallowing was delayed in these patients until after hypopharyngeal contraction, resulting in impaired swallowing and spillover of material into the trachea. Other workers[2] have found similar effects on swallowing and cricopharyngeal relaxation in children given nitrazepam. Murphy *et al.*[3] reported the deaths of six epileptic children under 5 years of age treated with nitrazepam. Three of the deaths were unexpected, and in view of the previous reports of swallowing difficulties and aspiration, they recommended that the use of nitrazepam in young children be restricted to those in whom seizure control fails to improve with other antiepileptics. They also recommended that the dose should be less than 0.8 mg per kg body-weight daily.

1. Wyllie E. *et al*. The mechanism of nitrazepam-induced drooling and aspiration. *N Engl J Med* 1986; **314**: 35–8.
2. Lim HCN, *et al*. Nitrazepam-induced cricopharyngeal dysphagia, abnormal esophageal peristalsis and associated bronchospasm: probable cause of nitrazepam-related sudden death. *Brain Dev* 1992; **14**: 309–14.
3. Murphy JV, *et al*. Deaths in young children receiving nitrazepam. *J Pediatr* 1987; **111**: 145–7.

Precautions

As for Diazepam, p.662.

Porphyria. Nitrazepam has been associated with clinical exacerbations of porphyria and is considered unsafe in porphyric patients.[1]

1. Moore MR, McColl KEL. *Porphyria: drug lists*. Glasgow: Porphyria Research Unit, University of Glasgow, 1991.

Interactions

As for Diazepam, p.663.

Pharmacokinetics

Nitrazepam is fairly readily absorbed from the gastro-intestinal tract, although there is some individual variation. It is extensively bound to plasma proteins. It crosses the blood-brain and the placental barriers and traces are found in breast milk. Nitrazepam is metabolised in the liver, mainly by nitroreduction followed by acetylation; none of the metabolites possess significant activity. It is excreted in the urine in the form of its metabolites (free or conjugated) with only small amounts of a dose appearing unchanged. Up to about 20% of an oral dose is found in the faeces. Mean elimination half-lives of 24 to 30 hours have been reported.

Administration in hepatic impairment. A study of the pharmacokinetics of intravenous nitrazepam in 12 patients with cirrhosis of the liver compared with 9 healthy subjects aged 22 to 49 years and 8 healthy elderly subjects aged 67 to 76 years.[1] The mean elimination half-life of nitrazepam was 26 hours in young and 38 hours in elderly subjects, the difference, which was not significant, being chiefly due to the greater volume of distribution in elderly subjects. Although there was also no significant difference between young and elderly subjects in percentage of unbound nitrazepam (13.0 and 13.9% respectively) there was a substantially higher unbound fraction in the patients with cirrhosis, the mean value being 18.9%, and clearance of unbound nitrazepam was reduced relative to healthy subjects.

1. Jochemsen R, *et al*. Effect of age and liver cirrhosis on the pharmacokinetics of nitrazepam. *Br J Clin Pharmacol* 1983; **15**: 295–302.

Distribution into breast milk. A mean milk-to-plasma ratio of 0.27 was obtained after administration of nitrazepam 5 mg for 5 nights to 9 puerperal women.[1] The degree of nitrazepam accumulation in milk over the study period was similar to that in plasma.

1. Matheson I, *et al*. Midazolam and nitrazepam in the maternity ward: milk concentrations and clinical effects. *Br J Clin Pharmacol* 1990; **30**: 787–93.

Metabolism. Although the acetylation of the reduced metabolite of nitrazepam has been reported to be controlled by acetylator phenotype,[1] Swift *et al.*[2] observed no significant differences between either half-life or residual effects of nitrazepam in slow and fast acetylators.

1. Karim AKMB, Price Evans DA. Polymorphic acetylation of nitrazepam. *J Med Genet* 1976; **13**: 17–19.
2. Swift CG, *et al*. Acetylator phenotype, nitrazepam plasma concentrations and residual effects. *Br J Clin Pharmacol* 1980; **9**: 312P–313P.

Uses and Administration

Nitrazepam is an intermediate-acting benzodiazepine with general properties similar to those of diazepam (p.666). It is used as a hypnotic in the short-term management of insomnia (p.638) and is reported to act in 30 to 60 minutes to produce sleep lasting for 6 to 8 hours. Nitrazepam has also been used in epilepsy, notably for infantile spasms (as for example in West's syndrome).

The usual dose for insomnia is 5 mg at night, although 10 mg may be required. Elderly or debilitated patients should not be given more than half of the normal adult dose.

Epilepsy. Benzodiazepines are sometimes employed in the management of epilepsy (p.335), but their long-term use is limited by problems of sedation, dependence, and tolerance to the antiepileptic effects. Nitrazepam has perhaps been most useful in the treatment of infantile spasms (as for example in West's syndrome) and the so-called infantile myoclonic seizures. There has been concern, however, over swallowing difficulties with subsequent aspiration associated with the use of nitrazepam in young children (see Effects on the Digestive System under Adverse Effects, above).

Preparations

BP 1998: Nitrazepam Capsules; Nitrazepam Oral Suspension; Nitrazepam Tablets.

Proprietary Preparations (details are given in Part 3)
Aust.: Mogadon; ***Austral.:*** Alodorm; Mogadon; ***Belg.:*** Mogadon; ***Canad.:*** Mogadon; ***Fr.:*** Mogadon; ***Ger.:*** Dormo-Puren; Eatan N; Imeson; Mogadan†; Nitrazep; Novanox; Radedorm; Somnibel N†; ***Irl.:*** Dormigen†; Mogadon; Nitrados†; Somnite; ***Ital.:*** Ipersed†; Mitidin†; Mogadon; Tri†; ***Neth.:*** Mogadon; ***Norw.:*** Apodorm; Mogadon; ***S.Afr.:*** Arem; Mogadon; Ormodon; Paxadorm; Protraz†; Somnipar; ***Spain:*** Mogadon†; Nitrazepan; Pelson; Serenade; ***Swed.:*** Apodorm; Mogadon; ***Switz.:*** Imeson†; Mogadon; ***UK:*** Mogadon; Remnos; Somnite; Surem†; Unisomnia.

Multi-ingredient: ***Spain:*** Pelsonfilina†.

Nordazepam (7035-l)

Nordazepam *(rINN)*.

A-101; Demethyldiazepam; Desmethyldiazepam; *N*-Desmethyldiazepam; Nordiazepam; Ro-5-2180. 7-Chloro-1,3-dihydro-5-phenyl-2*H*-1,4-benzodiazepin-2-one.

$C_{15}H_{11}ClN_2O$ = 270.7.

CAS — 1088-11-5.

Nordazepam is a long-acting benzodiazepine with the general properties of diazepam (p.661). It is the principal active metabolite of a number of benzodiazepines and has a half-life of 2 to 5 days. It is given by mouth in doses of up to 15 mg daily for the treatment of anxiety disorders (p.635) and insomnia (p.638).

Porphyria. Nordazepam was considered to be unsafe in patients with acute porphyria because it has been shown to be porphyrinogenic in *animals* or *in-vitro* systems.[1]

1. Moore MR, McColl KEL. *Porphyria: drug lists*. Glasgow: Porphyria Research Unit, University of Glasgow, 1991.

Preparations

Proprietary Preparations (details are given in Part 3)
Aust.: Stilny; ***Belg.:*** Calmday; Stilny†; ***Fr.:*** Nordaz; Praxadium†; ***Ger.:*** Tranxilium N; ***Ital.:*** Madar; ***Neth.:*** Calmday; ***Switz.:*** Veges-an.

Olanzapine (16785-l)

Olanzapine *(BAN, USAN, rINN).*

LY-170053. 2-Methyl-4-(4-methyl-1-piperazinyl)-10*H*-thieno[2,3-*b*][1,5]benzodiazepine.

$C_{17}H_{20}N_4S = 312.4$.

CAS — 132539-06-1.

Adverse Effects and Treatment

As for Chlorpromazine, p.649. The most frequent adverse effects with olanzapine are somnolence and weight gain. Olanzapine has been associated with a low incidence of extrapyramidal symptoms including tardive dyskinesia. Hyperprolactinaemia may occur but is usually asymptomatic. Other adverse effects include increased appetite, peripheral oedema, and rarely elevated creatine kinase concentrations.

References.

1. Beasley CM, *et al.* Safety of olanzapine. *J Clin Psychiatry* 1997; **58** (suppl 10): 13–17.

Precautions

As for Chlorpromazine, p.652.

Interactions

As for Chlorpromazine, p.652. The metabolism of olanzapine is mediated to some extent by the cytochrome P450 isozyme CYP1A2. Concomitant administration of drugs which inhibit or act as a substrate to this isozyme may affect plasma concentrations of olanzapine.

The clearance of olanzapine is increased by tobacco smoking.

Pharmacokinetics

Olanzapine is well absorbed from the gastro-intestinal tract but undergoes considerable first-pass metabolism. Peak plasma concentrations are achieved about 5 to 8 hours after oral administration. Olanzapine is about 93% bound to plasma proteins. It is extensively metabolised in the liver primarily by direct glucuronidation and by oxidation mediated through the cytochrome P450 isozymes CYP1A2 and to a lesser extent CYP2D6. The two major metabolites 10-*N*-glucuronide and 4′-*N*-desmethyl olanzapine appear to be inactive. About 57% of a dose is excreted in the urine, mainly as metabolites and about 30% appears in the faeces. The plasma elimination half-life has been variously reported to be about 30 to 38 hours; half-lives tend to be longer in female than in male patients.

Uses and Administration

Olanzapine is a thienobenzodiazepine atypical antipsychotic. It has affinity for dopamine (D_1, D_2, and D_4), histamine (H_1), serotonin (5-HT_2), muscarinic (M_1), and adrenergic (α_1) receptors.

Olanzapine is used for the management of schizophrenia.

A usual initial dose is 10 mg daily as a single dose; thereafter dosage adjustments of 5 mg daily may be made according to response at intervals of not less than one week to within the range of 5 to 20 mg daily. It is recommended that doses of 15 mg or more daily should be given only after clinical reassessment. Metabolism might be slower in female, elderly, or non-smoking patients; if more than one of these factors is present a lower initial dose and a more gradual dose escalation should be considered. A starting dose of 5 mg daily may be necessary for patients with renal impairment; for patients with moderate hepatic insufficiency the starting dose should be 5 mg, and only increased with caution.

References.

1. Fulton B, Goa KL. Olanzapine: a review of its pharmacological properties and therapeutic efficacy in the management of schizophrenia and related psychoses. *Drugs* 1997; **53:** 281–98.
2. Reus VI. Olanzapine: a novel atypical neuroleptic agent. *Lancet* 1997; **349:** 1264–5. Correction. *ibid.*; **350:** 372.
3. Hale AS. Olanzapine. *Br J Hosp Med* 1997; **58:** 442–5.
4. Anonymous. Olanzapine, sertindole and schizophrenia. *Drug Ther Bull* 1997; **35:** 81–3.
5. Kando JC, *et al.* Olanzapine: a new antipsychotic agent with efficacy in the management of schizophrenia. *Ann Pharmacother* 1997; **31:** 1325–34.
6. Bever KA, Perry PJ. Olanzapine: a serotonin–dopamine-receptor antagonist for antipsychotic therapy. *Am J Health-Syst Pharm* 1998; **55:** 1003–16.

Parkinsonism. Olanzapine is associated with a relatively low incidence of extrapyramidal disorders and is therefore being studied for use in the treatment of drug-induced psychosis in patients with Parkinson's disease (p.1128).

References.

1. Wolters EC, *et al.* Olanzapine in the treatment of dopaminomimetic psychosis in patients with Parkinson's disease. *Neurology* 1996; **47:** 1085–7.

Schizophrenia. Studies suggest that olanzapine is as effective as haloperidol against positive symptoms of schizophrenia (p.637) and more effective against negative symptoms in the short-term and possibly in the long-term.[1-4] Quality of life has also been judged to be greater in patients treated with olanzapine.[5] In comparative studies extrapyramidal symptoms have been less frequent with olanzapine than haloperidol and fewer patients have discontinued treatment with olanzapine. There are few published comparisons with other atypical antipsychotics but one study[6] has suggested that response of negative symptoms might be greater than with risperidone; patients in this study were also more likely to maintain their initial response with olanzapine and less likely to experience extrapyramidal effects although risperidone had been given in doses higher than usually used clinically. Olanzapine's efficacy in the treatment of patients with refractory schizophrenia remains to be determined.

1. Beasley CM, *et al.* Olanzapine HGAD Study Group. Olanzapine versus placebo and haloperidol: acute phase results of the North American double-blind olanzapine trial. *Neuropsychopharmacology* 1996; **14:** 111–23.
2. Beasley C, *et al.* Olanzapine versus haloperidol: long-term results of the multi-center international trial. *Eur Neuropsychopharmacol* 1996; **6** (suppl 3): 59.
3. Beasley CM, *et al.* Olanzapine versus haloperidol: acute phase results of the international double-blind olanzapine trial. *Eur Neuropsychopharmacol* 1997; **7:** 125–37.
4. Tollefson GD, *et al.* Olanzapine versus haloperidol in the treatment of schizophrenia and schizoaffective and schizophreniform disorders: results of an international collaborative trial. *Am J Psychiatry* 1997; **154:** 457–65.
5. Hamilton SH, *et al.* Olanzapine versus placebo and haloperidol: quality of life and efficacy results of the North American double-blind trial. *Neuropsychopharmacology* 1998; **18:** 41–9.
6. Tran PV, *et al.* Double-blind comparison of olanzapine versus risperidone in the treatment of schizophrenia and other psychotic disorders. *J Clin Psychopharmacol* 1997; **17:** 407–18.

Preparations

Proprietary Preparations (details are given in Part 3)
Austral.: Zyprexa; ***Ger.:*** Zyprexa; ***Irl.:*** Zyprexa; ***Neth.:*** Zyprexa; ***Norw.:*** Zyprexa; ***S.Afr.:*** Zyprexa; ***Spain:*** Zyprexa; ***Swed.:*** Zyprexa; ***UK:*** Zyprexa; ***USA:*** Zyprexa.

Oxazepam (7076-r)

Oxazepam *(BAN, USAN, rINN).*

Oxazepamum; Wy-3498. 7-Chloro-1,3-dihydro-3-hydroxy-5-phenyl-1,4-benzodiazepin-2-one.

$C_{15}H_{11}ClN_2O_2 = 286.7$.

CAS — 604-75-1.

Pharmacopoeias. In Eur. (see p.viii), *Pol.*, and *US*.

A white to pale yellow, almost odourless crystalline powder. Practically **insoluble** in water; soluble 1 in 220 of alcohol, 1 in 270 of chloroform, and 1 in 2200 of ether; slightly soluble in dichloromethane. A 2% suspension in water has a pH of 4.8 to 7.0. **Protect** from light.

Dependence and Withdrawal, Adverse Effects, Treatment, and Precautions

As for Diazepam, p.661.

Hepatic impairment. Seven patients with acute viral hepatitis, 6 with cirrhosis of the liver, and 16 age-matched healthy control subjects received a single dose of oxazepam 15 or 45 mg by mouth.[1] Urinary excretion rates and plasma elimination patterns were unaltered in patients with acute and chronic parenchymal liver disease. Oxazepam 15 mg was also administered three times daily by mouth for 2 weeks to 2 healthy subjects and to 2 patients with cirrhosis and did not appear to accumulate in any of the four.

1. Shull HJ, *et al.* Normal disposition of oxazepam in acute viral hepatitis and cirrhosis. *Ann Intern Med* 1976; **84:** 420–5.

Porphyria. Oxazepam was considered to be unsafe in patients with acute porphyria although there is conflicting experimental evidence of porphyrinogenicity.[1]

1. Moore MR, McColl KEL. *Porphyria: drug lists.* Glasgow: Porphyria Research Unit, University of Glasgow, 1991.

Renal impairment. Pharmacokinetic studies suggesting that, in general, the dosage of oxazepam does not need adjusting in patients with renal impairment.[1-3]

1. Murray TG, *et al.* Renal disease, age, and oxazepam kinetics. *Clin Pharmacol Ther* 1981; **30:** 805–9.
2. Busch U, *et al.* Pharmacokinetics of oxazepam following multiple administration in volunteers and patients with chronic renal disease. *Arzneimittelforschung* 1981; **31:** 1507–11.
3. Greenblatt DJ, *et al.* Multiple-dose kinetics and dialyzability of oxazepam in renal insufficiency. *Nephron* 1983; **34:** 234–8.

Thyroid disorders. There was a reduction in half-life and an increase in the apparent oral clearance of oxazepam in 7 hyperthyroid patients.[1] In 6 hypothyroid patients there was no overall change in oxazepam elimination, although 5 of the 6 complained of drowsiness despite a relatively low dose (15 mg).

1. Scott AK, *et al.* Oxazepam pharmacokinetics in thyroid disease. *Br J Clin Pharmacol* 1984; **17:** 49–53.

Withdrawal. For the purpose of withdrawal regimens, 15 mg of oxazepam is considered roughly equivalent to 5 mg of diazepam.

Interactions

As for Diazepam, p.663.

Pharmacokinetics

Oxazepam is well absorbed from the gastro-intestinal tract and reaches peak plasma concentrations about 2 to 3 hours after ingestion. It crosses the placenta and has been detected in breast milk. Oxazepam is extensively bound to plasma proteins and has been reported to have an elimination half-life ranging from about 4 to 15 hours. It is largely metabolised to the inactive glucuronide which is excreted in the urine.

Pregnancy. DIFFUSION ACROSS THE PLACENTA. A study on the placental passage of oxazepam and its metabolism in 12 women given a single dose of oxazepam 25 mg during labour.[1] Oxazepam was readily absorbed and peak plasma concentrations were in the same range as those reported in healthy males and non-pregnant females given the same dose although the plasma half-life (range 5.3 to 7.8 hours in 8 subjects studied) was shorter than that reported for non-pregnant subjects. Oxazepam was detected in the umbilical vein of all 12 patients with the ratio between umbilical to maternal vein concentration of oxazepam reaching a value of about 1.35 and remaining constant beyond a dose-delivery time of 3 hours. All of the babies had a normal Apgar score value. The oxazepam plasma half-life in the newborns was about 3 to 4 times that in the mothers although in 3 the plasma concentration of oxazepam conjugate rose during the first 6 to 10 hours after delivery indicating the ability of the neonate to conjugate oxazepam.

1. Tomson G, *et al.* Placental passage of oxazepam and its metabolism in mother and newborn. *Clin Pharmacol Ther* 1979; **25:** 74–81.

Uses and Administration

Oxazepam is a short-acting benzodiazepine with general properties similar to those of diazepam (p.666). It is used in the short-term management of anxiety disorders (p.635) and insomnia (p.638) associated with anxiety. Oxazepam is also used for the control of symptoms associated with alcohol withdrawal (p.1099). Oxazepam is usually administered as the base but the hemisuccinate has been used in some multi-ingredient preparations.

The usual dose of oxazepam for the treatment of anxiety or for control of symptoms of alcohol withdrawal is 15 to 30 mg three or four times daily by mouth. A suggested initial dose for elderly or debilitated patients is 10 mg three times daily increased if necessary up to 10 to 20 mg three or four times daily. Oxazepam 15 to 25 mg may be given one hour before retiring for the treatment of insomnia associated with anxiety; up to 50 mg may occasionally be necessary.

Preparations

BP 1998: Oxazepam Tablets;
USP 23: Oxazepam Capsules; Oxazepam Tablets.

Proprietary Preparations (details are given in Part 3)
Aust.: Adumbran; Anxiolit; Oxahexal; Praxiten; ***Austral.:*** Alepam; Benzotran†; Murelax; Serepax; ***Belg.:*** Seresta; Tranquo;

Canad.: Novoxapam; Serax; ***Fr.:*** Seresta; ***Ger.:*** Adumbran; Antoderin†; Azutranquil†; durazepam; Mirfudorm; Noctazepam; Norkotral N†; oxa; Oxa-Puren†; Praxiten; Sigacalm; Uskan; ***Ital.:*** Adumbran†; Limbial; Oxapam; Quilibrex†; Serpax; ***Neth.:*** Seresta; ***Norw.:*** Alopam; Serepax; Sobril; ***S.Afr.:*** Medopam; Noripam†; Oxaline; Purata; Serepax; ***Spain:*** Adumbran; Aplakil†; Psiquiwas†; Sobile†; ***Swed.:*** Alopam†; Oxascand; Serepax; Sobril; ***Switz.:*** Anxiolit; Seresta; Uskan; ***USA:*** Serax; Zaxopam†.

Multi-ingredient: ***Aust.:*** Anxiocard†; Anxiolit plus; Persumbran†; ***Belg.:*** Tranquo-Buscopan†; ***Ger.:*** Persumbran†; ***Ital.:*** Persumbrax; Tranquo-Buscopan†; ***Spain:*** Buscopax†; Novo Aerofil Sedante; Pankreoflat Sedante†; Suxidina.

Oxazolam (7077-f)

Oxazolam *(rINN)*.

Oxazolazepam. 10-Chloro-2,3,7,11b-tetrahydro-2-methyl-11b-phenyloxazolo[3,2-*d*][1,4]benzodiazepin-6(5*H*)-one.

$C_{18}H_{17}ClN_2O_2$ = 328.8.

CAS — 24143-17-7.

Pharmacopoeias. In *Jpn.*

Oxazolam is a long-acting benzodiazepine with general properties similar to those of diazepam (p.661). It is given by mouth for the short-term treatment of anxiety disorders.

Oxazolam has also been used as a premedicant in general anaesthesia.

References.

1. Ochs HR, *et al.* Comparative single-dose kinetics of oxazolam, prazepam, and clorazepate: three precursors of desmethyldiazepam. *J Clin Pharmacol* 1984; **24:** 446–51.

Preparations

Proprietary Preparations (details are given in Part 3)
Ger.: Tranquit†; ***Jpn:*** Serenal.

Oxypertine (7078-d)

Oxypertine *(BAN, USAN, rINN)*.

Win-18501-2. 5,6-Dimethoxy-2-methyl-3-[2-(4-phenylpiperazin-1-yl)ethyl]indole.

$C_{23}H_{29}N_3O_2$ = 379.5.

CAS — 153-87-7 (oxypertine); 40523-01-1 (oxypertine hydrochloride).

Adverse Effects, Treatment, and Precautions

As for Chlorpromazine, p.649. It is claimed to cause fewer sedative, antimuscarinic, and, possibly, extrapyramidal effects. In low doses oxypertine may produce agitation and hyperactivity. Photophobia may occur occasionally.

Interactions

As for Chlorpromazine, p.652.

Some sources have recommended that since oxypertine has been observed in *animal* studies to release small amounts of catecholamines it should be avoided in patients taking MAOIs.

Uses and Administration

Oxypertine is an indole derivative with general properties similar to those of the phenothiazine, chlorpromazine (p.654). Low doses may cause agitation and hyperactivity while high doses produce sedation. It is used in the treatment of various psychoses including schizophrenia (p.637), mania (p.273), and disturbed behaviour (p.636), and in severe anxiety (p.635). Oxypertine is given by mouth in the treatment of psychoses and associated disorders initially in doses of 80 to 120 mg daily in divided doses adjusted according to response up to a maximum of 300 mg daily.

Doses of 10 mg three or four times daily have been used as adjunctive treatment in the short-term management of severe anxiety disorders. The maximum recommended dose is 60 mg daily.

Oxypertine should be given in reduced dosage to elderly patients.

Preparations

Proprietary Preparations (details are given in Part 3)
Ger.: Forit†; ***Irl.:*** Integrin†; ***UK:*** Integrin†.

Paraldehyde (4055-z)

Paracetaldehyde; Paraldehydum. The trimer of acetaldehyde; 2,4,6-Trimethyl-1,3,5-trioxane.

$(C_2H_4O)_3$ = 132.2.

CAS — 123-63-7.

Pharmacopoeias. In *Eur.* (see p.viii) and *US.*

A clear colourless or slightly yellow liquid with a strong characteristic odour. The Ph. Eur. specifies that it may contain a suitable amount of an antioxidant; the USP permits a suitable stabiliser. Relative density 0.991 to 0.996. The Ph. Eur. gives the f.p. as 10° to 13°, and requires that not more than 10% distils below 123° and not less than 95% below 126°. The USP gives a congealing temperature of not lower than 11° and states that it distils completely between 120° and 126°.

Soluble 1 in 10 of water v/v, but only 1 in 17 of boiling water v/v; miscible with alcohol, with chloroform, with ether, and with volatile oils. **Store** in small well-filled airtight containers; the Ph. Eur. specifies a storage temperature of 8° to 15° and the USP a temperature not exceeding 25°. Protect from light. The USP specifies that it must not be used more than 24 hours after opening the container.

Because of its solvent action upon rubber, polystyrene, and styrene-acrylonitrile copolymer, paraldehyde should not be administered in plastic syringes made with these materials.

At low temperature it solidifies to form a crystalline mass. If it solidifies, the whole should be liquefied before use.

CAUTION. *Paraldehyde decomposes on storage, particularly after the container has been opened. The administration of partly decomposed paraldehyde is dangerous. It must not be used if it has a brownish colour or a sharp penetrating odour of acetic acid.*

Incompatibility. An evaluation of the compatibility of paraldehyde with plastic syringes and needle hubs concluded that, if possible, all-glass syringes should be used with paraldehyde.[1] Needles with plastic hubs could be used. Polypropylene syringes with rubber-tipped plastic plungers (Plastipak), or glass syringes with natural rubber-tipped plastic plungers (Glaspak) were acceptable only for the immediate administration or measurement of paraldehyde doses.

1. Johnson CE, Vigoreaux JA. Compatibility of paraldehyde with plastic syringes and needle hubs. *Am J Hosp Pharm* 1984; **41:** 306–8.

Dependence and Withdrawal

Prolonged use of paraldehyde may lead to dependence, especially in alcoholics. Features of dependence and withdrawal are similar to those of barbiturates (see Amylobarbitone, p.641).

Adverse Effects and Treatment

Paraldehyde decomposes on storage and deaths from corrosive poisoning have followed the use of such material. Paraldehyde has an unpleasant taste and imparts a smell to the breath; it may cause skin rashes.

Oral and rectal administration of paraldehyde may cause gastric or rectal irritation. Intramuscular administration is painful and associated with tissue necrosis, sterile abscesses, and nerve damage. Intravenous administration is extremely hazardous since it may cause pulmonary oedema and haemorrhage, hypotension and cardiac dilatation, and circulatory collapse; thrombophlebitis is also associated with intravenous use.

Overdosage results in rapid laboured breathing owing to damage to the lungs and to acidosis. Nausea and vomiting may follow an overdose by mouth. Respiratory depression and coma as well as hepatic and renal damage may occur.

Adverse effects should be managed in a similar way to those of barbiturates (see Amylobarbitone, p.642).

Precautions

Paraldehyde should not be given to patients with gastric disorders and it should be used with caution, if at all, in patients with bronchopulmonary disease or hepatic impairment. It should not be given rectally in the presence of colitis. Old paraldehyde must never be used.

Paraldehyde must be well diluted before oral or rectal administration; if it is deemed essential to give paraldehyde intravenously it must be well diluted and given very slowly with extreme caution (see also Adverse Effects, above and Uses, below). Intramuscular injections may be given undiluted but care should be taken to avoid nerve damage. Plastic syringes should be avoided (see Incompatibility, above).

Interactions

The sedative effects of paraldehyde are enhanced by simultaneous administration of CNS depressants such as alcohol, barbiturates, and other sedatives. Studies in *animals* suggest that disulfiram may enhance the activity of paraldehyde.

Pharmacokinetics

Paraldehyde is generally absorbed readily, although absorption is reported to be slower after rectal than after oral or intramuscular administration. It is widely distributed and has a reported half-life of 4 to 10 hours. About 80% of a dose is metabolised in the liver probably to acetaldehyde, which is oxidised by aldehyde dehydrogenase to acetic acid. Unmetabolised drug is largely excreted unchanged through the lungs; only small amounts appear in the urine. It crosses the placental barrier.

Uses and Administration

Paraldehyde is a hypnotic and sedative with antiepileptic effects. However, because of the hazards associated with its administration, its tendency to react with plastic, and the risks associated with its deterioration, it has largely been superseded by other drugs. It is still occasionally used to control status epilepticus (p.337) resistant to conventional treatment. It causes little respiratory depression and is therefore useful where facilities for resuscitation are poor. A usual dose for adults is 5 to 10 mL administered rectally as a 10% solution in sodium chloride 0.9% solution or diluted with 1 or 2 parts of oil. Doses of 5 to 10 mL are also occasionally given intramuscularly up to a maximum of 20 mL daily with not more than 5 mL being given at any one site. Paraldehyde has been given by slow intravenous infusion in specialist centres with intensive care facilities but this method of administration is not usually recommended; it must be diluted to a 4% solution in normal saline before administration.

Paraldehyde has been given by mouth; it should always be well diluted to avoid gastric irritation.

Preparations

BP 1998: Paraldehyde Injection.

Proprietary Preparations (details are given in Part 3)
USA: Paral.

Penfluridol (7080-k)

Penfluridol *(BAN, USAN, rINN)*.

McN-JR-16341; R-16341. 4-(4-Chloro-3-trifluoromethylphenyl)-1-[3-(*p,p'*-difluorobenzhydryl)propyl]piperidin-4-ol.

$C_{28}H_{27}ClF_5NO$ = 524.0.

CAS — 26864-56-2.

Pharmacopoeias. In *Chin.*

Adverse Effects, Treatment, and Precautions

As for Chlorpromazine, p.649.

Interactions

As for Chlorpromazine, p.652.

Pharmacokinetics

Although penfluridol is absorbed from the gastro-intestinal tract, peak plasma concentrations are not achieved until about 12 hours after a dose by mouth. The initial peak plasma concentration is followed by a rapid decrease over the next 36 hours, probably due to tissue redistribution, followed by a slower decline over the next 120 hours. Penfluridol, accordingly, has a very long duration of action possibly partly related to its storage in, and slow release from, adipose tissue.

There is evidence of enterohepatic recycling, and penfluridol is excreted mainly as the *N*-dealkylated metabolite in the faeces and urine.

Uses and Administration

Penfluridol is a diphenylbutylpiperidine antipsychotic and shares the general properties of the phenothiazine, chlorpromazine (p.654). Following administration by mouth it has a prolonged duration of action which lasts for about a week. It is used in the treatment of various psychoses including schizophrenia (p.637).

The usual dose of penfluridol for the treatment of chronic psychoses is 20 to 60 mg weekly by mouth. Doses of up to 250 mg once a week may be required in severe or resistant conditions.

Malaria. Penfluridol has been reported to increase the susceptibility of mefloquine-resistant *Plasmodium falciparum* isolates *in vitro.*[1] The treatment of malaria is discussed on p.422.

1. Oduola AMJ, *et al.* Reversal of mefloquine resistance with penfluridol in isolates of Plasmodium falciparum from south-west Nigeria. *Trans R Soc Trop Med Hyg* 1993; **87:** 81–3.

Preparations

Proprietary Preparations (details are given in Part 3)
Aust.: Semap; ***Belg.:*** Semap; ***Fr.:*** Semap; ***Neth.:*** Semap; ***Switz.:*** Semap.

Pentobarbitone (4056-c)

Pentobarbitone *(BAN)*.

Pentobarbital *(rINN)*; Aethaminalum; Mebubarbital; Mebumal; Pentobarbitalum. 5-Ethyl-5-(1-methylbutyl)barbituric acid.

$C_{11}H_{18}N_2O_3$ = 226.3.

CAS — 76-74-4.

Pharmacopoeias. In *Eur.* (see p.viii) and *US.*

Almost odourless, colourless crystals or a white or almost white crystalline powder.

Very slightly **soluble** in water and in carbon tetrachloride; freely soluble in absolute alcohol; soluble 1 in 4.5 of alcohol, 1 in 4 of chloroform, and 1 in 10 of ether; very soluble in acetone and in methyl alcohol. It forms water-soluble compounds with alkali hydroxides or carbonates, and with ammonia. **Store** in airtight containers.

Pentobarbitone Calcium (4057-k)

Pentobarbitone Calcium *(BANM)*.

Pentobarbital Calcium *(rINNM)*. Calcium 5-ethyl-5-(1-methylbutyl)barbiturate.

$(C_{11}H_{17}N_2O_3)_2Ca$ = 490.6.

Pentobarbitone Sodium (4058-a)

Pentobarbitone Sodium *(BANM)*.

Pentobarbital Sodium *(rINNM)*; Aethaminalum-Natrium; Ethaminal Sodium; Mebumalnatrium; Pentobarbitalum Natricum; Sodium Pentobarbital; Soluble Pentobarbitone. Sodium 5-ethyl-5-(1-methylbutyl)barbiturate.

$C_{11}H_{17}N_2NaO_3$ = 248.3.

CAS — 57-33-0.

Pharmacopoeias. In *Eur.* (see p.viii) and *US.*

A white, hygroscopic, crystalline powder or granules, odourless or with a slight characteristic odour. Very **soluble** in water; practically insoluble in ether; freely soluble in alcohol. The Ph. Eur. states that a 10% solution in water has a pH of 9.6 to 11.0 when freshly prepared while the USP states that such a solution has a pH between 9.8 and 11.0. Solutions decompose on standing, the decomposition being accelerated at higher temperatures. **Store** in airtight containers.

Pentobarbitone may be precipitated from preparations containing pentobarbitone sodium, depending on the concentration and pH. Pentobarbitone sodium has, therefore, been reported to be **incompatible** with many other drugs particularly acids and acidic salts.

Dependence and Withdrawal, Adverse Effects, Treatment, and Precautions

As for Amylobarbitone, p.641.

Interactions

As for Amylobarbitone, p.642.

Pharmacokinetics

Following oral or rectal administration pentobarbitone is well absorbed from the gastro-intestinal tract, and is reported to be approximately 60 to 70% bound to plasma protein. The elimination half-life appears to be dose dependent and reported values have ranged from 15 to 50 hours. It is metabolised in the liver, mainly by hydroxylation, and excreted in the urine mainly as metabolites.

Uses and Administration

Pentobarbitone is a barbiturate that has been used as a hypnotic and sedative. It has general properties and uses similar to those of amylobarbitone (p.642). It has been used as a sedative and in the short-term management of insomnia (p.638) but barbiturates are not considered appropriate for such purposes. Pentobarbitone sodium, administered by deep intramuscular or slow intravenous injection, has been used for premedication in anaesthetic procedures (p.1220) but the use of barbiturates for pre-operative sedation has been replaced by other drugs. Pentobarbitone is usually administered as the sodium salt although pentobarbitone and its calcium salt have also been used.

A usual dose of pentobarbitone sodium given at night for insomnia is 100 mg by mouth or up to 200 mg rectally. A dose of 20 mg of the sodium salt has been given by mouth 3 or 4 times daily as a sedative.

Cerebrovascular disorders. For reference to the use of barbiturate-induced coma in the management of patients with cerebral ischaemia, see p.1234. See also p.796 for reference to the use of barbiturates in the management of raised intracranial pressure.

Status epilepticus. Anaesthesia in conjunction with assisted ventilation may be instituted to control refractory tonic-clonic status epilepticus (p.337). A short-acting barbiturate such as thiopentone is usually used, but pentobarbitone has been used similarly.

Preparations

BP 1998: Pentobarbital Tablets;
USP 23: Pentobarbital Elixir; Pentobarbital Sodium Capsules; Pentobarbital Sodium Injection.

Proprietary Preparations (details are given in Part 3)
Austral.: Carbrital†; ***Canad.:*** Nembutal; Nova Rectal; ***Ger.:*** Medinox Mono†; Neodorm†; ***S.Afr.:*** Sopental†; ***USA:*** Nembutal.

Multi-ingredient: ***Canad.:*** Cafergot-PB; ***Ger.:*** Omca Nacht†; ***USA:*** Cafatine-PB.

Perazine Dimalonate (7081-a)

P-725 (perazine); Pemazine Dimalonate. 10-[3-(4-Methylpiperazin-1-yl)propyl]phenothiazine dimalonate.

$C_{20}H_{25}N_3S,2C_3H_4O_4$ = 547.6.

CAS — 84-97-9 (perazine); 14777-25-4 (perazine dimalonate).

Pharmacopoeias. In *Pol.*

Perazine dimalonate is a phenothiazine with general properties similar to those of chlorpromazine (p.649). It has a piperazine side-chain. It is given by mouth for the treatment of psychotic conditions in usual doses equivalent to 25 to 600 mg of the base daily; up to 1000 mg daily has been given in resistant cases. It may also be given intramuscularly.

Adverse effects. A report of 5 patients receiving perazine dimalonate who developed acute axonal neuropathies of superficial nerve fibres after exposure to sunlight.[1]

1. Roelcke U, *et al.* Acute neuropathy in perazine-treated patients after sun exposure. *Lancet* 1992; **340:** 729–30.

Preparations

Proprietary Preparations (details are given in Part 3)
Ger.: Taxilan; ***Neth.:*** Taxilan.

Pericyazine (7082-t)

Pericyazine *(BAN)*.

Periciazine *(pINN)*; Propericiazine; RP-8909; SKF-20716. 10-[3-(4-Hydroxypiperidino)propyl]phenothiazine-2-carbonitrile; 1-[3-(2-Cyanophenothiazin-10-yl)propyl]piperidin-4-ol.

$C_{21}H_{23}N_3OS$ = 365.5.

CAS — 2622-26-6.

Adverse Effects, Treatment, and Precautions

As for Chlorpromazine, p.649. Sedation and orthostatic hypotension may be marked.

Interactions

As for Chlorpromazine, p.652.

Pharmacokinetics

For an account of the pharmacokinetics of a phenothiazine, see Chlorpromazine, p.654.

Uses and Administration

Pericyazine is a phenothiazine with general properties similar to those of chlorpromazine (p.654). It has a piperidine side-chain. It is used in the treatment of various psychoses including schizophrenia (p.637) and disturbed behaviour (p.636), and in severe anxiety (p.635).

Pericyazine is usually given as the base but the mesylate and tartrate have also been used.

The usual dose for the treatment of severe anxiety, agitation, aggression, or impulsive behaviour is 15 to 30 mg daily given in 2 portions, the larger amount in the evening. In schizophrenia and severe psychoses initial doses of 75 mg daily have been given in divided doses, increased if necessary, at weekly intervals by steps of 25 mg, to up to 300 mg daily. It has also been given by intramuscular injection.

A suggested initial daily dose by mouth for schizophrenia or behaviour disorders in children over one year of age is 0.5 mg for a child of 10 kg body-weight; for heavier children this initial dose may be increased by 1 mg for each additional 5 kg of body-weight, to a maximum total of 10 mg daily. Thereafter the dose may be gradually increased according to response but the daily maintenance dose should not exceed twice the initial dose.

Elderly subjects should be given reduced doses.

Preparations

Proprietary Preparations (details are given in Part 3)
Aust.: Neuleptil; ***Austral.:*** Neulactil; ***Belg.:*** Neuleptil; ***Canad.:*** Neuleptil; ***Fr.:*** Neuleptil; ***Ger.:*** Aolept†; ***Irl.:*** Neulactil; ***Ital.:*** Neuleptil; ***Neth.:*** Neuleptil; ***Norw.:*** Neulactil; ***S.Afr.:*** Neulactil; ***Spain:*** Nemactil; ***Swed.:*** Neulactil†; ***Switz.:*** Neuleptil; ***UK:*** Neulactil.

Perphenazine (7084-r)

Perphenazine *(BAN, rINN)*.

Perphenazinum. 2-{4-[3-(2-Chlorophenothiazin-10-yl)propyl]piperazin-1-yl}ethanol.

$C_{21}H_{26}ClN_3OS$ = 404.0.

CAS — 58-39-9.

Pharmacopoeias. In *Chin., Eur.* (see p.viii), *Jpn, Pol.,* and *US. Jpn* also includes the maleate.

A white to creamy- or yellowish-white odourless crystalline powder.

Ph. Eur. **solubilities** are: practically insoluble in water; soluble in alcohol; sparingly soluble in ether; freely soluble in dichloromethane; dissolves in dilute solutions of hydrochloric acid. USP solubilities are: practically insoluble in water; soluble 1 in 7 of alcohol and 1 in 13 of acetone; freely soluble in chloroform.

Store in airtight containers. Protect from light.

Incompatibility. Perphenazine has been reported to be incompatible with cefoperazone sodium[1] and with midazolam hydrochloride (see p.679).

1. Gasca M, *et al.* Visual compatibility of perphenazine with various antimicrobials during simulated Y-site injection. *Am J Hosp Pharm* 1987; **44:** 574–5.

Perphenazine Decanoate (15578-x)

Perphenazine Decanoate *(BANM, rINNM)*.

2-{4-[3-(2-Chlorophenothiazin-10-yl)propyl]piperazin-1-yl}ethyl decanoate.

$C_{31}H_{44}ClN_3O_2S$ = 558.2.

Perphenazine decanoate 108.2 mg is approximately equivalent to 78.3 mg of perphenazine.

Perphenazine Enanthate (18340-f)

Perphenazine Enanthate *(BANM)*.

Perphenazine Enantate *(rINNM)*; Perphenazine Heptanoate. 2-{4-[3-(2-Chlorophenothiazin-10-yl)propyl]piperazin-1-yl}ethyl heptanoate.

$C_{28}H_{38}ClN_3O_2S$ = 516.1.

CAS — 17528-28-8.

Perphenazine enanthate 100 mg is approximately equivalent to 78.3 mg of perphenazine.

Adverse Effects, Treatment, and Precautions

As for Chlorpromazine, p.649. Perphenazine has been associated with a lower frequency of sedation, but a higher incidence of extrapyramidal symptoms.

Interactions

As for Chlorpromazine, p.652.

Pharmacokinetics

For an account of the pharmacokinetics of a phenothiazine, see Chlorpromazine, p.654.

Perphenazine decanoate and perphenazine enanthate are slowly absorbed from the site of intramuscular injection. They gradually release perphenazine into the body and are therefore suitable for use as depot injections.

Perphenazine 5 or 6 mg administered intravenously had a plasma half-life from 8.4 to 12.3 hours in a study of 4 schizophrenic patients and 4 healthy subjects.[1] Considerable fluctuations in plasma-perphenazine concentrations were observed 3 to 5 hours after administration before the exponential elimination phase. A dose of 6 mg by mouth in 4 healthy subjects failed to produce a detectable plasma concentration and only low plasma concentrations of its sulphoxide metabolite could be detected; this was attributed to a marked first-pass effect. Systemic availability was variable and poor in 4 schizophrenic patients given perphenazine 12 mg three times daily. However, it was considered that oral therapy should be on an 8-hour dosage regimen. Intramuscular injection of perphenazine enanthate 50 or 100 mg every 2 weeks gave plasma-perphenazine concentrations similar to those after continuous oral administration but with a high initial absorption within 2 to 3 days associated with the most serious neurological and sedative side-effects.

1. Hansen CE, *et al.* Clinical pharmacokinetic studies of perphenazine. *Br J Clin Pharmacol* 1976; **3:** 915–23.

Distribution into breast milk. The distribution of perphenazine into breast milk was studied[1] in a mother who was receiving perphenazine 24 mg daily, later reduced to 16 mg daily, by mouth. Breast feeding was started after it was estimated that a breast-fed infant would ingest about 0.1% of a maternal dose. Treatment with perphenazine lasted for 3.5 months and during this period the child thrived normally and no drug-induced symptoms were seen.

1. Olesen OV, *et al.* Perphenazine in breast milk and serum. *Am J Psychiatry* 1990; **147:** 1378–9.

Metabolism. In a study in 12 healthy subjects there was a clear difference in the disposition of a single oral dose of perphenazine between poor and extensive hydroxylators of debrisoquine.[1]

1. Dahl-Puustinen M-L, *et al.* Disposition of perphenazine is related to polymorphic debrisoquin hydroxylation in human beings. *Clin Pharmacol Ther* 1989; **46:** 78–81.

Uses and Administration

Perphenazine is a phenothiazine with general properties similar to those of chlorpromazine (p.654). It has a piperazine side-chain. It is used in the treatment of various psychoses including schizophrenia (p.637) and mania (p.273) as well as disturbed behaviour (p.636) and severe anxiety (p.635). Perphenazine is also used for the management of postoperative or chemotherapy-induced nausea and vomiting (p.1172) and for the treatment of intractable hiccup (p.655).

Perphenazine is usually given as the base by mouth or sometimes by intramuscular or intravenous injection. Long-acting decanoate or enanthate esters of perphenazine, available in some countries, are given by intramuscular injection.

The usual initial dose for the treatment of schizophrenia, mania, and other psychoses is 4 to 8 mg three times daily by mouth. The dose is adjusted according to response up to a usual maximum of 24 mg daily but up to 64 mg daily has occasionally been used. Similar doses have been used for the management of severe agitated or violent behaviour or in severe anxiety. Perphenazine has sometimes been used in combination with tricyclic antidepressants such as amitriptyline in the treatment of anxiety with depression.

For the control of nausea and vomiting the usual dose by mouth is 4 mg three times daily but up to 8 mg three times daily may be required.

Perphenazine may be given by intramuscular injection for control of acute psychotic symptoms or for severe nausea and vomiting. An initial dose of 5 or 10 mg is followed, if necessary, by 5 mg every 6 hours to a maximum of 15 to 30 mg daily.

Perphenazine, diluted to a concentration of 0.5 mg per mL in sodium chloride 0.9% solution, is occasionally given by intravenous injection in divided doses, not more than 1 mg being administered every 1 to 2 minutes or by continuous infusion at a rate not greater than 1 mg per minute; the maximum intravenous dose is 5 mg. The intravenous route of administration is usually reserved for the control of severe vomiting or intractable hiccup.

The long-acting decanoate or enanthate esters of perphenazine are administered by deep intramuscular injection in doses ranging from approximately 50 to 300 mg of ester given at intervals of 2 to 4 weeks.

Elderly subjects should be given reduced doses of perphenazine or its esters but it should be noted that perphenazine is not indicated for the management of agitation and restlessness in the elderly.

Preparations

BP 1998: Perphenazine Tablets;
USP 23: Perphenazine and Amitriptyline Hydrochloride Tablets; Perphenazine Injection; Perphenazine Oral Solution; Perphenazine Syrup; Perphenazine Tablets.

Proprietary Preparations (details are given in Part 3)

Aust.: Decentan; ***Austral.:*** Trilafon†; ***Belg.:*** Trilafon; ***Canad.:*** Trilafon; ***Fr.:*** Trilifan; ***Ger.:*** Decentan; ***Irl.:*** Fentazin; ***Ital.:*** Trilafon; ***Neth.:*** Trilafon; ***Norw.:*** Trilafon; ***S.Afr.:*** Trilafon; ***Spain:*** Decentan; ***Swed.:*** Trilafon; ***Switz.:*** Trilafon; ***UK:*** Fentazin; ***USA:*** Trilafon.

Multi-ingredient: ***Austral.:*** Mutabon D; ***Canad.:*** Elavil Plus; Etrafon; PMS-Levazine; Triavil; ***Ger.:*** Longopax†; ***Irl.:*** Triptafen; ***Ital.:*** Mutabon; ***Neth.:*** Mutabon A/D/F†; ***S.Afr.:*** Etrafon; ***Spain:*** Deprelio; Mutabase; Norfenazin; ***UK:*** Triptafen; ***USA:*** Etrafon; Triavil.

Phenprobamate (7086-d)

Phenprobamate *(BAN, rINN).*

MH-532; Proformiphen. 3-Phenylpropyl carbamate.

$C_{10}H_{13}NO_2$ = 179.2.

CAS — 673-31-4.

Phenprobamate is a carbamate with general properties similar to those of meprobamate (p.678). It has been used for its an anxiolytic and muscle relaxant actions.

Preparations

Proprietary Preparations (details are given in Part 3)

Multi-ingredient: ***Aust.:*** Myo-Prolixan†; ***Ger.:*** Dolo-Prolixan†; ***Switz.:*** Dolo-Prolixan.

Pimozide (7087-n)

Pimozide *(BAN, USAN, rINN).*

McN-JR-6238; Pimozidum; R-6238. 1-{1-[4,4-Bis(4-fluorophenyl)butyl]-4-piperidyl}benzimidazolin-2-one; 1-{1-[3-(4,4′-Difluorobenzhydryl)propyl]-4-piperidyl}benzimidazolin-2-one.

$C_{28}H_{29}F_2N_3O$ = 461.5.

CAS — 2062-78-4.

Pharmacopoeias. In *Eur.* (see p.viii), *Pol.*, and *US.*

A white or almost white crystalline powder. Ph. Eur. **solubilities** are: practically insoluble in water; slightly soluble in alcohol; soluble in dichloromethane; sparingly soluble in methyl alcohol. USP solubilities are: insoluble in water; soluble 1 in 1000 of alcohol, ether, and methyl alcohol, 1 in 100 of acetone, and 1 in 10 of chloroform; very slightly soluble in 0.1N hydrochloric acid. **Store** in airtight containers. Protect from light.

Adverse Effects, Treatment, and Precautions

As for Chlorpromazine, p.649.

Extrapyramidal symptoms may be more common than those associated with chlorpromazine, whereas pimozide may be less likely to cause sedation, hypotension, or antimuscarinic effects.

In view of reports of ventricular arrhythmias and other ECG abnormalities such as prolongation of the QT interval and T-wave changes associated with the use of pimozide, an ECG should be performed prior to treatment and repeated annually or earlier if indicated. In the UK, periodic assessment of cardiac function is recommended for patients receiving more than 16 mg daily. If repolarisation changes appear or arrhythmias develop, the need for continuing treatment with pimozide should be reviewed; at the very least dose reduction and close supervision are advised. Pimozide is contra-indicated in patients with pre-existing prolongation of the QT interval and in patients with a history of cardiac arrhythmias. Electrolyte disturbances such as hypokalaemia in patients receiving pimozide may lead to cardiotoxicity.

Effects on the cardiovascular system. The Committee on Safety of Medicines (CSM) in the UK has received reports of ventricular arrhythmias and other ECG abnormalities such as prolongation of the QT interval and T-wave changes associated with the use of pimozide.[1,2] In August 1990 they had received 13 reports of sudden unexpected death since 1971; many of these patients had no evidence of pre-existing cardiac disease, and 7 were aged between 17 and 30 years of age. Five of the 13 were also taking other antipsychotics. In ten cases, the dose of pimozide was greater than 20 mg daily, and in many of the patients for whom information was available the dose had been increased rapidly, possibly resulting in substantial tissue accumulation. By February 1995 the CSM had received a total of 40 reports (16 fatal) of serious cardiac reactions most of which involved arrhythmias.

See also under Chlorpromazine, p.649.

1. Committee on Safety of Medicines. Cardiotoxic effects of pimozide. *Current Problems 29* 1990.
2. Committee on Safety of Medicines/Medicines Control Agency. Cardiac arrhythmias with pimozide (Orap). *Current Problems* 1995; **21:** 2.

Interactions

As for Chlorpromazine, p.652. The risk of arrhythmias with pimozide may be increased by other drugs which prolong the QT interval and by the HIV-protease inhibitor ritonavir which raises plasma concentrations of pimozide; concomitant use should be avoided. Concomitant use should also be avoided with drugs which induce electrolyte disturbances and with macrolide antibacterials.

Pharmacokinetics

Following oral administration, more than half of a dose of pimozide is reported to be absorbed. It undergoes significant first-pass metabolism. Peak plasma concentrations have been reported after 4 to 12 hours and there is a considerable interindividual variation in the concentrations achieved. Pimozide is metabolised in the liver mainly by *N*-dealkylation and excreted in the urine and faeces, both unchanged and in the form of metabolites. Pimozide has a long terminal half-life generally considered to be approximately 55 hours, although half-lives of up to 150 hours have been noted in some patients.

Uses and Administration

Pimozide is a member of the diphenylbutylpiperidine group of antipsychotics, which are structurally similar to the butyrophenones. It is a long-acting antipsychotic with general properties similar to those of the phenothiazine, chlorpromazine (p.654), although it also has some calcium-blocking activity.

Pimozide is given by mouth in the management of psychoses including schizophrenia, paranoid states, and monosymptomatic hypochondria (p.636) and in Tourette's syndrome. An ECG should be performed in all patients before starting treatment with pimozide (see Adverse Effects, Treatment, and Precautions, above). For schizophrenia, treatment is usually initiated with a dose of 2 mg daily adjusted thereafter according to response in increments of 2 to 4 mg at intervals of not less than one week. A maximum daily dose of 20 mg should not be exceeded. It is usually given as a single daily dose.

In monosymptomatic hypochondria and paranoid psychoses the initial dose is 4 mg daily adjusted as above to a maximum daily dose of 16 mg.

For the treatment of Tourette's syndrome an initial dose of 1 to 2 mg daily is recommended, increased to a maximum of 10 mg daily, or 200 μg per kg body-weight, daily.

Pimozide should be given in reduced dosage to elderly patients.

Chorea. Antipsychotics have some action against choreiform movements as well as being of use to control the behavioural disturbances of Huntington's chorea. For a discussion of the management of various choreas, including mention of the use of pimozide, see p.636.

References.

1. Shannon KM, Fenichel GM. Pimozide treatment of Sydenham's chorea. *Neurology* 1990; **40:** 186.

Dystonia. Antipsychotics such as phenothiazines, haloperidol, or pimozide are sometimes useful in the treatment of idiopathic dystonia in patients who have failed to respond to other drugs.[1] In very severe dystonia combination therapy may be required. Pimozide in gradually increasing doses up to 12 mg daily with tetrabenazine and benzhexol is sometimes effective. However, antipsychotics often act non-specifically and there is the risk of adding drug-induced extrapyramidal disorders to the dystonia being treated (see Extrapyramidal Disorders under Adverse Effects of Chlorpromazine, p.650). For a discussion of the management of dystonias, see under Levodopa on p.1141.

1. Marsden CD, Quinn NP. The dystonias. *Br Med J* 1990; **300:** 139–44.

Schizophrenia. Pimozide and other diphenylbutylpiperidine antipsychotics may improve the negative as well as the positive symptoms of schizophrenia (p.637). In a study designed to clarify the relation between categorisation within the broad class of functional psychosis and drug treatment response, pimozide was very effective in relieving the combination of the symptoms of hallucinations, delusions, incoherence of speech, and incongruity of affect irrespective of whether or not these features were associated with elevation or depression of mood.[1] However, no effect was observed with pimozide on elevation or depression of mood or on negative symptoms, although all these sets of symptoms improved during the course of the study.

1. Johnstone EC, *et al.* The Northwick Park "functional" psychosis study: diagnosis and treatment response. *Lancet* 1988: **ii:** 119–25.

Taste disorders. For reference to the use of pimozide in the treatment of taste disorders, see Chlorpromazine, p.656.

Tourette's syndrome. Tourette's syndrome (p.636) is a disorder characterised by motor and vocal tics and behavioural disturbances. Many patients with Tourette's syndrome do not require medication but when treatment is needed dopamine antagonists such as the antipsychotics haloperidol or pimozide[1,2] are most commonly used. They often decrease the frequency and severity of tics and may improve any accompanying behavioural disturbances. However, superiority of either drug in terms of efficacy or adverse effects has not been clearly demonstrated. Because of the potential for acute and long-term adverse effects it is usually recommended that doses are titrated to as low as possible; the aim of treatment is not necessarily to control symptoms completely. Medication can often be discontinued after a few years.

1. Shapiro E, *et al.* Controlled study of haloperidol, pimozide, and placebo for the treatment of Gilles de la Tourette's syndrome. *Arch Gen Psychiatry* 1989; **46:** 722–30.
2. Sallee FR, *et al.* Relative efficacy of haloperidol and pimozide in children and adolescents with Tourette's disorder. *Am J Psychiatry* 1997; **154:** 1057–62.

Preparations

USP 23: Pimozide Tablets.

Proprietary Preparations (details are given in Part 3)
Aust.: Orap; ***Austral.:*** Orap; ***Belg.:*** Orap; ***Canad.:*** Orap; ***Fr.:*** Orap; ***Ger.:*** Antalon; Orap; ***Irl.:*** Orap; ***Ital.:*** Orap; ***Neth.:*** Orap; ***Norw.:*** Orap; ***S.Afr.:*** Orap; ***Spain:*** Orap; ***Swed.:*** Orap; ***Switz.:*** Orap; ***UK:*** Orap; ***USA:*** Orap.

Pinazepam (7088-h)

Pinazepam *(rINN).*

7-Chloro-1,3-dihydro-5-phenyl-1-(prop-2-ynyl)-2*H*-1,4-benzodiazepin-2-one.

$C_{18}H_{13}ClN_2O$ = 308.8.

CAS — 52463-83-9.

Pinazepam is a long-acting benzodiazepine with general properties similar to those of diazepam (p.661). It is given by mouth in doses of 5 to 20 mg daily in divided doses for the short-term treatment of anxiety disorders (p.635) and insomnia (p.638).

Preparations

Proprietary Preparations (details are given in Part 3)
Ital.: Domar; ***Spain:*** Duna.

Pipamperone Hydrochloride (7090-t)

Pipamperone Hydrochloride *(BANM, rINNM).*

Floropipamide Hydrochloride; R-3345 (pipamperone). 1-[3-(4-Fluorobenzoyl)propyl]-4-piperidinopiperidine-4-carboxamide dihydrochloride.

$C_{21}H_{30}FN_3O_2,2HCl$ = 448.4.

CAS — 1893-33-0 (pipamperone); 2448-68-2 (pipamperone hydrochloride).

NOTE. Pipamperone is *USAN.*

Pipamperone hydrochloride 1.2 mg is approximately equivalent to 1 mg of pipamperone.

Pipamperone is a butyrophenone with general properties similar to those of haloperidol (p.673). It is given by mouth as the hydrochloride for the treatment of psychoses. Starting doses equivalent to 20 mg of the base have been given daily, increased gradually thereafter according to response; doses of 360 mg or more have been given daily in divided doses.

Preparations

Proprietary Preparations (details are given in Part 3)
Belg.: Dipiperon; ***Fr.:*** Dipiperon; ***Ger.:*** Dipiperon; ***Ital.:*** Piperonil; ***Neth.:*** Dipiperon; ***Switz.:*** Dipiperon.

Pipothiazine (7092-r)

Pipothiazine *(BAN).*

Pipotiazine *(rINN)*; RP-19366. 10-{3-[4-(2-Hydroxyethyl)piperidino]propyl}-*NN*-dimethylphenothiazine-2-sulphonamide; 2-{4-[3-(2-Dimethylsulphamoylphenothiazin-10-yl)propyl]piperazin-1-yl}ethanol.

$C_{24}H_{33}N_3O_3S_2$ = 475.7.

CAS — 39860-99-6.

Pipothiazine Palmitate (7093-f)

Pipothiazine Palmitate *(BANM).*

Pipotiazine Palmitate *(USAN, rINNM)*; IL-19552; RP-19552.

$C_{40}H_{63}N_3O_4S_2$ = 714.1.

CAS — 37517-26-3.

Adverse Effects, Treatment, and Precautions

As for Chlorpromazine, p.649.

Manic symptoms developed in a schizophrenic patient following administration of pipothiazine palmitate. Symptoms recurred on subsequent rechallenge.[1] The possible mania-inducing or antidepressant effects of pipothiazine should be investigated further.

1. Singh AN, Maguire J. Pipothiazine palmitate induced mania. *Br Med J* 1984; **289:** 734.

Pharmacokinetics

For an account of the pharmacokinetics of a phenothiazine, see Chlorpromazine, p.654.

Pipothiazine palmitate is very slowly absorbed from the site of intramuscular injection. It gradually releases pipothiazine into the body and is therefore suitable for use as a depot injection.

References.

1. De Schepper PJ, *et al.* Pipotiazine pharmacokinetics after po and iv administration in man: correlation between blood levels and effect on the handwriting area. *Arzneimittelforschung* 1979; **29:** 1056–62.
2. Blanc M, *et al.* Pharmacocinetique de l'ester palmitique de pipotiazine, après administration intramusculaire chez des malades schizophrènes. *Therapie* 1986, **41:** 27–30.

Uses and Administration

Pipothiazine is a phenothiazine with general properties similar to those of chlorpromazine (p.654). It has a piperidine side-chain. It is used in the treatment of schizophrenia (p.637) and other psychoses.

A usual oral dose of pipothiazine for the treatment of psychoses is 10 to 20 mg daily in a single dose; in severe psychoses higher doses have been given for brief periods. In acute conditions treatment is sometimes started with intramuscular injections of 10 to 20 mg daily in one or two injections.

The long-acting palmitate ester of pipothiazine is given by deep intramuscular injection. An initial test dose of 25 mg is followed by a further 25 to 50 mg after 4 to 7 days. The dosage is then adjusted in increments of 25 to 50 mg according to response at intervals of 4 weeks. Usual maintenance doses of 50 to 100 mg are given at average intervals of 4 weeks; the maximum recommended dose is 200 mg.

Pipothiazine should be given in reduced dosage to elderly patients; a starting dose of 5 to 10 mg has been suggested for pipothiazine palmitate intramuscular injections.

Preparations

Proprietary Preparations (details are given in Part 3)
Belg.: Piportil; ***Canad.:*** Piportil L4; ***Fr.:*** Piportil; ***Irl.:*** Piportil; ***Neth.:*** Piportil; ***Norw.:*** Piportyl†; ***S.Afr.:*** Piportil; ***Spain:*** Lonseren; ***Switz.:*** Piportil; ***UK:*** Piportil.

Prazepam (7095-n)

Prazepam *(BAN, USAN, rINN).*

W-4020. 7-Chloro-1-(cyclopropylmethyl)-1,3-dihydro-5-phenyl-2*H*-1,4-benzodiazepin-2-one.

$C_{19}H_{17}ClN_2O$ = 324.8.

CAS — 2955-38-6.

Pharmacopoeias. In *Jpn* and *US.*

A white to off-white crystalline powder. **Soluble** in alcohol, chloroform, and dilute mineral acids; freely soluble in acetone. **Store** in airtight containers. Protect from light.

Dependence and Withdrawal, Adverse Effects, Treatment, and Precautions

As for Diazepam, p.661.

Porphyria. Prazepam was considered to be unsafe in patients with acute porphyria because it has been shown to be porphyrinogenic in *animals* or *in-vitro* systems.[1]

1. Moore MR, McColl KEL. *Porphyria: drug lists.* Glasgow: Porphyria Research Unit, University of Glasgow, 1991.

Interactions

As for Diazepam, p.663.

Pharmacokinetics

After oral administration, prazepam undergoes extensive first-pass metabolism in the liver to oxazepam (p.683) and desmethyldiazepam (nordazepam, p.682). Desmethyldiazepam is largely responsible for the pharmacological activity of prazepam. Peak plasma concentrations of desmethyldiazepam are reached within about 6 hours after oral administration of prazepam although considerable individual variation has been reported.

References.

1. Ochs HR, *et al.* Comparative single-dose kinetics of oxazolam, prazepam, and clorazepate: three precursors of desmethyldiazepam. *J Clin Pharmacol* 1984; **24:** 446–51.

Distribution into breast milk. The ratio of desmethyldiazepam in plasma to that in breast milk of 5 lactating women given prazepam 20 mg three times daily for 3 days was 9.6 from measurements 12 hours after the last dose.[1] It was estimated that a breast-fed infant of a mother on continuous prazepam therapy would ingest the equivalent of about 4% of the daily maternal dose.

1. Brodie RR, *et al.* Concentrations of N-descyclopropylmethylprazepam in whole-blood, plasma, and milk after administration of prazepam to humans. *Biopharm Drug Dispos* 1981; **2:** 59–68.

Uses and Administration

Prazepam is a long-acting benzodiazepine with general properties similar to those of diazepam (p.666). The usual dose by mouth for the short-term treatment of anxiety disorders (p.635) is 30 mg daily as a single nightly dose or in divided doses; in severe conditions up to 60 mg daily has been given. In elderly or debilitated patients, treatment should be initiated with a daily dose of 10 to 15 mg.

Preparations

USP 23: Prazepam Capsules; Prazepam Tablets.

Proprietary Preparations (details are given in Part 3)
Aust.: Demetrin; ***Belg.:*** Lysanxia; ***Fr.:*** Lysanxia; ***Ger.:*** Demetrin; Mono Demetrin; ***Irl.:*** Centrax; ***Ital.:*** Prazene; Trepidan; ***Neth.:*** Reapam; ***S.Afr.:*** Demetrin; ***Spain:*** Demetrin†; ***Switz.:*** Demetrin; ***USA:*** Centrax†.

Prochlorperazine (7096-h)

Prochlorperazine *(BAN, rINN).*

Chlormeprazine; Prochlorpemazine. 2-Chloro-10-[3-(4-methylpiperazin-1-yl)propyl]phenothiazine.

$C_{20}H_{24}ClN_3S$ = 373.9.

CAS — 58-38-8.

Pharmacopoeias. In *US.*

A clear, pale yellow, viscous liquid, sensitive to light. Very slightly **soluble** in water; freely soluble in alcohol, chloroform, and in ether. **Store** in airtight containers. Protect from light.

Prochlorperazine Edisylate (7097-m)

Prochlorperazine Edisylate *(BANM).*

Prochlorperazine Edisilate *(rINNM)*; Chlormeprazine Edisylate; Prochlorpemazine Edisylate; Prochlorperazine Ethanedisulphonate. Prochlorperazine ethane-1,2-disulphonate.

$C_{20}H_{24}ClN_3S,C_2H_6O_6S_2$ = 564.1.

CAS — 1257-78-9.

Pharmacopoeias. In *US.*

A white to very light yellow odourless crystalline powder. Prochlorperazine edisylate 7.5 mg is approximately equivalent to 5 mg of prochlorperazine.

Soluble 1 in 2 of water and 1 in 1500 of alcohol; practically insoluble in chloroform and in ether. Solutions in water are acid to litmus. **Store** in airtight containers. Protect from light.

Incompatibility. See under Prochlorperazine Mesylate, below.

Prochlorperazine Maleate (7098-b)

Prochlorperazine Maleate *(BANM, rINNM).*

Chlormeprazine Maleate; Prochlorpemazine Maleate; Prochlorperazine Dihydrogen Maleate; Prochlorperazine Dimaleate; Prochlorperazini Maleas.

$C_{20}H_{24}ClN_3S,2C_4H_4O_4$ = 606.1.

CAS — 84-02-6.

Pharmacopoeias. In *Eur.* (see p.viii), *Jpn, Pol.,* and *US.*

A white or pale yellow, almost odourless, crystalline powder. Prochlorperazine maleate 8 mg is approximately equivalent to 5 mg of prochlorperazine.

The Ph. Eur. states that it is very slightly **soluble** in water and in alcohol, and practically insoluble in ether. The USP states that it is practically insoluble in water; soluble 1 in 1200 of alcohol; slightly soluble in warm chloroform. A freshly prepared saturated solution in water has a pH of 3.0 to 4.0. **Store** in airtight containers. Protect from light.

Prochlorperazine Mesylate (7099-v)

Prochlorperazine Mesylate *(BANM).*

Prochlorperazine Mesilate *(rINNM)*; Chlormeprazine Mesylate; Prochlorpemazine Mesylate; Prochlorperazine Dimethanesulphonate; Prochlorperazine Methanesulphonate; Prochlorperazini Mesylas.

$C_{20}H_{24}ClN_3S,2CH_3SO_3H$ = 566.2.

CAS — 5132-55-8.

Pharmacopoeias. In *Br.*

A white or almost white, odourless or almost odourless, powder. Prochlorperazine mesylate 7.6 mg is approximately equivalent to 5 mg of prochlorperazine.

Very **soluble** in water; sparingly soluble in alcohol; slightly soluble in chloroform; practically insoluble in ether. A 2% solution in water has a pH of 2.0 to 3.0. **Protect** from light.

Incompatibility. Incompatibility has been reported between the edisylate or mesylate salts of prochlorperazine and several other compounds: these include aminophylline, amphotericin, ampicillin sodium, aztreonam, some barbiturates, benzylpenicillin salts, calcium gluconate, cefmetazole sodium, cephalothin sodium, chloramphenicol sodium succinate, chlorothiazide sodium, dimenhydrinate, heparin sodium, hydrocortisone sodium succinate, midazolam hydrochloride, and some sulphonamides. Incompatibility between prochlorperazine edisylate and morphine sulphate has been attributed to phenol present in some formulations of the opioid.[1,2] Incompatibility has been reported on dilution of prochlorperazine edisylate injection with sodium chloride injection containing methyl hydroxybenzoate and propyl hydroxybenzoate as preservatives.[3] The problem did not occur with unpreserved sodium chloride or when benzyl alcohol was used as preservative. Prochlorperazine mesylate syrup has been reported to be incompatible with magnesium trisilicate mixture.[4]

1. Stevenson JG, Patriarca C. Incompatibility of morphine sulfate and prochlorperazine edisylate in syringes. *Am J Hosp Pharm* 1985: **42:** 2651.

2. Zuber DEL. Compatibility of morphine sulfate injection and prochlorperazine edisylate injection. *Am J Hosp Pharm* 1987; **44:** 67.
3. Jett S, *et al.* Prochlorperazine edisylate incompatibility. *Am J Hosp Pharm* 1983; **40:** 210.
4. Greig JR. Stemetil syrup and magnesium trisilicate. *Pharm J* 1986; **237:** 504.

Adverse Effects, Treatment, and Precautions

As for Chlorpromazine, p.649. Prochlorperazine may cause less sedation and autonomic effects but extrapyramidal effects may be more frequent.

Severe dystonic reactions have followed the use of prochlorperazine, particularly in children and adolescents. It should therefore be used with extreme care in children.

Transient numbness of the gum and tongue has occurred after the use of buccal tablets of prochlorperazine maleate.

Effects on the cardiovascular system. Hypertension has been reported[1] in some patients given prochlorperazine intravenously for prophylaxis of cisplatin-induced nausea and vomiting.

1. Roche H, *et al.* Hypertension and intravenous antidopaminergic drugs. *N Engl J Med* 1985; **312:** 1125–6.

Effects on the mouth. Reports of ulceration and soreness of the lip and tongue associated with administration of prochlorperazine maleate oral tablets.[1,2] The erosive cheilitis resolved after withdrawal of prochlorperazine and recurred on rechallenge.

1. Duxbury AJ, *et al.* Erosive cheilitis related to prochlorperazine maleate. *Br Dent J* 1982; **153:** 271–2.
2. Reilly GD, Wood ML. Prochlorperazine—an unusual cause of lip ulceration. *Acta Derm Venereol (Stockh)* 1984; **64:** 270–1.

Interactions

As for Chlorpromazine, p.652.

Pharmacokinetics

For an account of the pharmacokinetics of a phenothiazine, see Chlorpromazine, p.654.

A study of the pharmacokinetics of prochlorperazine in 8 healthy subjects following doses of 6.25 and 12.5 mg intravenously, and 25 mg by mouth.[1] There was a marked interindividual variation in pharmacokinetics following intravenous administration but no evidence of dose-dependent pharmacokinetics; mean terminal half-lives were 6.8 hours for the higher and 6.9 hours for the lower dose. The apparent volume of distribution was very high and plasma clearance values were apparently greater than liver plasma flow, suggesting that the liver may not be the only site of metabolism. After oral administration prochlorperazine concentrations were detectable in only 4 of the 8 subjects due in part to a low bioavailability but also to the lack of sensitivity of the high-pressure liquid chromatographic assay used. The time to peak plasma concentration varied from 1.5 to 5 hours, and the peak concentrations varied from 1.6 to 7.6 ng per mL. Bioavailability was estimated to range from 0 to 16%. A low bioavailability due to high first-pass metabolism would be expected because of the high plasma clearance of prochlorperazine.

1. Taylor WB, Bateman DN. Preliminary studies of the pharmacokinetics and pharmacodynamics of prochlorperazine in healthy volunteers. *Br J Clin Pharmacol* 1987; **23:** 137–42.

Buccal administration. Comparative studies of the bioavailability of buccal and oral prochlorperazine maleate.[1] Both single- and multiple-dose studies indicated that bioavailability was greater after buccal administration. Doses of 3 mg twice daily by the buccal route and 5 mg three times daily by mouth produced similar steady-state plasma-prochlorperazine concentrations.

1. Hessell PG, *et al.* A comparison of the availability of prochlorperazine following im buccal and oral administration. *Int J Pharmaceutics* 1989; **52:** 159–64.

Uses and Administration

Prochlorperazine is a phenothiazine antipsychotic with general properties similar to those of chlorpromazine (p.654). It has a piperazine side-chain. Prochlorperazine and its salts are widely used in the prevention and treatment of nausea and vomiting (below) including that associated with migraine or drug-induced emesis. They are also used for the short-term symptomatic relief of vertigo (p.401) as occurs in Ménière's disease (p.400) or labyrinthitis and in the management of schizophrenia (p.637), mania (p.273), and other psychoses. Prochlorperazine has been used as an adjunct in the short-term management of severe anxiety (p.635).

Prochlorperazine base is generally administered by the rectal route and prochlorperazine maleate by the oral or buccal routes, while prochlorperazine edisylate and mesylate are given orally or parenterally.

Depending on the country or the manufacturer, doses of prochlorperazine are expressed either as the base or the salt. Most doses in the UK, including the rectal doses, are expressed in terms of the maleate or mesylate, while most doses in the USA are apparently expressed in terms of the base. As a result there is a disparity in the dosage recommendations for these countries, with the doses in the USA apparently tending to be higher.

For the prevention of **nausea and vomiting** in the UK, the usual dose by mouth is 5 to 10 mg of the maleate or mesylate two or three times daily. Similar doses may be given by the rectal route. The following initial doses are recommended for the treatment of nausea and vomiting: 20 mg of the maleate or mesylate by mouth, 12.5 mg of the mesylate by deep intramuscular injection, or the equivalent of prochlorperazine maleate 25 mg as suppositories; further doses, preferably by mouth, are given if necessary. The recommended buccal dose of prochlorperazine maleate for the management of nausea and vomiting is 3 to 6 mg twice daily. In the USA the dose by mouth for the control of nausea and vomiting is the equivalent of 5 to 10 mg of the base (as edisylate or maleate) given 3 or 4 times daily; alternatively the equivalent of 10 mg twice daily or 15 mg daily may be taken as modified-release capsules. The recommended intramuscular dosage is the equivalent of 5 to 10 mg of the base (as edisylate) given every 3 to 4 hours if necessary, up to a total of 40 mg of the base daily. The rectal dose is 25 mg of the base given twice daily. In the management of severe nausea and vomiting the equivalent of 2.5 to 10 mg of prochlorperazine may be given by slow intravenous injection or infusion at a rate not exceeding 5 mg per minute.

Prochlorperazine is used in the UK in the treatment of **vertigo** including that due to Ménière's disease. It is given by mouth in doses of 15 to 30 mg of the maleate daily in divided doses; after several weeks the dose may be gradually reduced to 5 to 10 mg daily. The recommended buccal dose of prochlorperazine maleate for the treatment of vertigo due to Ménière's disease is 3 to 6 mg twice daily.

For treatment of **psychoses** in the UK, prochlorperazine maleate or mesylate may be given by mouth in a dose of 12.5 mg twice daily for 7 days adjusted gradually to 75 to 100 mg daily according to response; some patients may be maintained on doses of 25 to 50 mg daily. The equivalent of prochlorperazine maleate 25 mg two or three times daily may be given by the rectal route or 12.5 to 25 mg of the mesylate two or three times daily by deep intramuscular injection.

In the USA prochlorperazine is given for the treatment of psychoses as the maleate or edisylate in usual initial doses equivalent to 5 to 10 mg of the base 3 to 4 times daily by mouth adjusted according to response up to a maximum of 150 mg of base daily. In severe disturbances it may be given by deep intramuscular injection as the edisylate in doses equivalent to 10 to 20 mg of base and repeated every 2 to 6 hours if necessary.

Doses of 5 to 10 mg of the maleate (or, in the USA, the equivalent of 5 mg of the base) up to 3 or 4 times daily have been used for short-term adjunctive management of **severe anxiety disorders**. A modified-release preparation may be given in doses similar to those used in nausea and vomiting.

There are similar discrepancies with **children's doses**; owing to the risk of severe extrapyramidal reactions, prochlorperazine should be administered with extreme caution in children: in particular it is not recommended for those weighing less than 10 kg. Where the use of prochlorperazine in children is unavoidable, UK sources have suggested 250 μg of the maleate or mesylate per kg body-weight, given two or three times daily by mouth; the intramuscular or rectal routes are considered unsuitable. In contrast, in the USA oral, rectal, and intramuscular routes have all been advocated. The usual oral or rectal antiemetic dose ranges up to 7.5 mg of the base or its equivalent daily in children weighing 10 to 13 kg; in children 14 to 17 kg, up to 10 mg daily; from 18 to 39 kg, up to 15 mg daily. Higher doses have been given for psychoses. The suggested intramuscular dose for children in the USA is the equivalent of about 130 μg of base per kg given as a single deep intramuscular injection of the edisylate.

Reduced dosage may be required in elderly patients.

Administration. BUCCAL. A buccal formulation of prochlorperazine maleate has been developed with the aim of avoiding first-pass metabolism as well as poor absorption due to gastric stasis or vomiting and hence increase the bioavailability.[1] A buccal dose of 3 mg twice daily has been reported to be pharmacokinetically equivalent to an oral dose of 5 mg three times daily (see under Pharmacokinetics, above). However, a regimen of three 6-mg doses of buccal prochlorperazine [maleate] was considered ineffective in preventing the emetic sequelae of minor gynaecological surgery.[2] Although in another study a single 6-mg pre-operative dose did appear to reduce the incidence of nausea and vomiting in patients undergoing minor gynaecological surgery or breast-biopsy the need for antiemetic therapy for patients in this study was questioned.[3] In a study of the management of nausea and vomiting associated with postoperative patient-controlled analgesia prochlorperazine given by the buccal route was found to be as effective as intramuscular administration and more acceptable to patients.[4]

1. Anonymous. Prochlorperazine in new forms: Buccastem and Stemetil EFF. *Drug Ther Bull* 1988; **26:** 87.
2. Madej TH, *et al.* A placebo controlled study to assess the efficacy and acceptability of buccal prochlorperazine given perioperatively. *Br J Clin Pharmacol* 1988; **26:** 222P–223P.
3. Patterson KW, *et al.* Use of buccal prochlorperazine in the prevention of postoperative sickness. *Br J Anaesth* 1991; **67:** 213P–214P.
4. Nguyen TPN, *et al.* A comparison of Buccastem to intramuscular prochlorperazine in post-operative nausea and vomiting when using PCA. *Pharm J* 1994; **253** (suppl): R13.

INTRAVENOUS. See under Nausea and Vomiting, below.

Headache. The phenothiazines prochlorperazine and chlorpromazine have been used in migraine to control severe nausea and vomiting unresponsive to antiemetics such as metoclopramide and domperidone.

Some phenothiazines, including prochlorperazine, have also been effective in relieving the pain of migraine attacks.[1-4] As mentioned on p.443, dihydroergotamine or sumatriptan are the preferred drugs in patients who require parenteral treatment for severe or refractory migraine, but if there is no response dopamine antagonists such as metoclopramide, chlorpromazine, or prochlorperazine may be tried. In comparative studies[3,4] prochlorperazine appears to have been more effective in relieving migraine headache and nausea and vomiting than metoclopramide when these drugs were given parenterally.

For further references to the use of phenothiazines in the management of headache including migraine, see under Chlorpromazine, p.655.

1. Jones J, *et al.* Randomized double-blind trial of intravenous prochlorperazine for the treatment of acute headache. *JAMA* 1989; **261:** 1174–6.
2. Jones EB, *et al.* Safety and efficacy of rectal prochlorperazine for the treatment of migraine in the emergency department. *Ann Emerg Med* 1994; **24:** 237–41.
3. Coppola M, *et al.* Randomized, placebo-controlled evaluation of prochlorperazine versus metoclopramide for emergency department treatment of migraine headache. *Ann Emerg Med* 1995; **26:** 541–6.
4. Jones J, *et al.* Intramuscular prochlorperazine versus metoclopramide as single-agent therapy for the treatment of acute migraine headache. *Am J Emerg Med* 1996; **14:** 262–4.

Nausea and vomiting. The management of nausea and vomiting, including the use of phenothiazines, is discussed on p.1172.

The US manufacturers of prochlorperazine recommend that intravenous doses (expressed in terms of the base) should not exceed 10 mg per dose or 40 mg per day. However, there are several studies claiming increased antiemetic efficacy and relatively few side-effects with higher doses given by slow intravenous infusion.[1-3] Examples of regimens tried are: up to 40 mg infused over 20 minutes for 3 doses;[1] single doses of up to 1.2 mg per kg body-weight over 20 minutes although doses over 0.8 mg per kg were considered more likely to be associated with major side-effects;[2] a dose of 40 mg given over 20 minutes followed by 80 mg over 8 hours.[3] Adverse effects most commonly associated with such doses appear to be hypotension, drowsiness, and dry mouth; few major extrapyramidal reactions were noted.

For reference to the use of prochlorperazine administered by the buccal route for the control of nausea and vomiting, see Administration: Buccal, above.

1. Carr BI, *et al.* High doses of prochlorperazine for cisplatin-induced emesis: a prospective, random, dose-response study. *Cancer* 1987; **60:** 2165–9.
2. Olver IN, *et al.* A dose finding study of prochlorperazine as an antiemetic for cancer chemotherapy. *Eur J Cancer Clin Oncol* 1989; **25:** 1457–61.
3. Akhtar SS, *et al.* A double-blind randomized cross-over comparison of high-dose prochlorperazine with high-dose metoclopramide for cisplatin-induced emesis. *Oncology* 1991; **48:** 226–9.

Preparations

BP 1998: Prochlorperazine Injection; Prochlorperazine Oral Solution; Prochlorperazine Tablets;
USP 23: Prochlorperazine Edisylate Injection; Prochlorperazine Maleate Tablets; Prochlorperazine Oral Solution; Prochlorperazine Suppositories.

Proprietary Preparations (details are given in Part 3)
Austral.: Anti-Naus†; Stemetil; ***Canad.:*** Nu-Prochlor; Stemetil; ***Irl.:*** Buccastem; Stemetil; Vertigon†; ***Ital.:*** Stemetil; ***Neth.:*** Stemetil; ***Norw.:*** Stemetil; ***S.Afr.:*** Mitil; Scripto-Metic; Stemetil; ***Swed.:*** Stemetil; ***UK:*** Buccastem; Proziere; Stemetil; Vertigon†; ***USA:*** Compazine.

Multi-ingredient: ***Ital.:*** Difmetre.

Prolonium Bromide (14253-j)

(2-Hydroxytrimethylene)bis(trimethylammonium bromide).
$C_9H_{24}Br_2N_2O$ = 336.1.

NOTE. Prolonium Iodide is *rINNM*.

Prolonium bromide was formerly used for its hypnotic and sedative properties.

Prolonium iodide (p.1496) has been used as a source of iodine as part of the treatment of thyroid storm and for the pre-operative management of hyperthyroidism.

Preparations

Proprietary Preparations (details are given in Part 3)
Multi-ingredient: ***Ital.:*** Brolumin†.

Promazine Embonate (7100-v)

Promazine Embonate *(BANM, rINNM).*
Promazine Pamoate.
$(C_{17}H_{20}N_2S)_2,C_{23}H_{16}O_6$ = 957.2.
CAS — 58-40-2 (promazine).

Promazine embonate 1.5 g is approximately equivalent to 1 g of promazine hydrochloride.

Promazine Hydrochloride (7101-g)

Promazine Hydrochloride *(BANM, rINNM).*
Promazini Hydrochloridum; Propazinum. *NN*-Dimethyl-3-phenothiazin-10-ylpropylammonium chloride.
$C_{17}H_{20}N_2S,HCl$ = 320.9.
CAS — 53-60-1.
Pharmacopoeias. In *Eur.* (see p.viii), *Pol.*, and *US.*

A white or slightly yellow, almost odourless, slightly hygroscopic, crystalline powder. It oxidises upon prolonged exposure to air and acquires a pink or blue colour.

Very **soluble** or soluble 1 in 3 of water; very soluble in alcohol and in dichloromethane; freely soluble in chloroform. A 5% solution in water has a pH of 4.2 to 5.2. **Store** in airtight containers. Protect from light.

Incompatibility has been reported between promazine hydrochloride and several other compounds: these include aminophylline, some barbiturates, benzylpenicillin potassium, chloramphenicol sodium succinate, chlortetracycline, chlorothiazide sodium, dimenhydrinate, heparin, hydrocortisone sodium succinate, nafcillin sodium, phenytoin sodium, prednisolone sodium phosphate, and sodium bicarbonate. The UK manufacturers of promazine hydrochloride injection recommend that it should not be mixed with other injections with the exception of pethidine hydrochloride injection.

Sorption. A study of drug loss from intravenous delivery systems.[1] There was an 11% loss of promazine hydrochloride from solution when infused for 7 hours via a plastic infusion set, and a 59% loss after infusion for one hour from a glass syringe through silastic tubing. Loss was negligible after infusion for one hour from a system comprising a glass syringe with polyethylene tubing.

1. Kowaluk EA, *et al.* Interactions between drugs and intravenous delivery systems. *Am J Hosp Pharm* 1982; **39:** 460–7.

Stability. A study of the stability of promazine diluted to a 0.1% infusion in sodium chloride solution (0.9%) or glucose (5%) found that solutions in glucose (5%) remained stable for up to 6 days at 4°, and at room temperature, provided they were stored in the dark.[1] However, with saline as the diluent deterioration of the promazine was observed 24 hours after preparation, even when stored in the dark, and after 8 hours when exposed to light. Temperature had no effect on degradation rate.

1. Tebbett IR, *et al.* Stability of promazine as an intravenous infusion. *Pharm J* 1986; **237:** 172–4.

Adverse Effects, Treatment, and Precautions

As for Chlorpromazine, p.649.

Pregnancy and the neonate. An increased incidence of neonatal jaundice coincided with the increased use of promazine.[1] A decrease in the incidence of jaundice was noted 3 months after the total withdrawal of the drug from the hospital although restriction of its use during labour had no impact.

1. John E. Promazine and neonatal hyperbilirubinaemia. *Med J Aust* 1975; **2:** 342–4.

Interactions

As for Chlorpromazine, p.652.

Pharmacokinetics

For an account of the pharmacokinetics of a phenothiazine, see Chlorpromazine, p.654.

Uses and Administration

Promazine is a phenothiazine with general properties similar to those of chlorpromazine (p.654). It has relatively weak antipsychotic activity and is not generally used for the management of psychoses. Its main indications are for the short-term management of agitated or disturbed behaviour (p.636), alleviation of nausea and vomiting (p.1172) particularly in labour or post-operatively, and relief of intractable hiccup (p.655). Promazine is given by mouth or intramuscularly as the hydrochloride. It is also given as the embonate by mouth, in doses equivalent to those of the hydrochloride. Promazine hydrochloride has also been given by slow intravenous injection, in concentrations not exceeding 25 mg per mL.

For the treatment of agitated behaviour, promazine is given in doses of 100 to 200 mg of the hydrochloride four times daily by mouth or 50 mg by intramuscular injection repeated if necessary after 6 to 8 hours. It has also been given by slow intravenous injection for severely agitated hospitalised patients in doses similar to those given by the intramuscular route. A dose of 50 mg by intramuscular injection has been given for the control of nausea and vomiting; it has also been given by mouth for this indication. For intractable hiccup 50 mg is given by intramuscular injection repeated if necessary with doses up to 100 mg every 4 hours.

Promazine should be given in reduced dosage to elderly or debilitated subjects; 25 mg by mouth of the hydrochloride initially, increasing, if necessary, to 50 mg four times daily has been suggested for the control of agitation and restlessness; for intramuscular injection a dose of 25 mg may be sufficient.

Preparations

BP 1998: Promazine Injection; Promazine Tablets;
USP 23: Promazine Hydrochloride Injection; Promazine Hydrochloride Oral Solution; Promazine Hydrochloride Syrup; Promazine Hydrochloride Tablets.

Proprietary Preparations (details are given in Part 3)
Austral.: Sparine; ***Belg.:*** Prazine; ***Ger.:*** Protactyl; Sinophenin; ***Irl.:*** Sparine; ***Ital.:*** Talofen; ***S.Afr.:*** Sparine; ***Switz.:*** Prazine; ***UK:*** Sparine; ***USA:*** Prozine; Sparine.

Prothipendyl Hydrochloride (7102-q)

Prothipendyl Hydrochloride *(BANM, rINNM).*
D-206; Phrenotropin. *NN*-Dimethyl-3-(pyrido[3,2-*b*][1,4]benzothiazin-10-yl)propylamine hydrochloride monohydrate.
$C_{16}H_{19}N_3S,HCl,H_2O$ = 339.9.
CAS — 303-69-5 (prothipendyl); 1225-65-6 (anhydrous prothipendyl hydrochloride).

Prothipendyl is an azaphenothiazine with general properties similar to those of chlorpromazine (p.649). It is given by mouth as the hydrochloride in doses of 40 to 80 mg two to four times daily for the treatment of psychoses and agitation, and as an adjunct to analgesics in the treatment of severe pain. Prothipendyl hydrochloride may also be given by injection.

Preparations

Proprietary Preparations (details are given in Part 3)
Aust.: Dominal; ***Belg.:*** Dominal; ***Ger.:*** Dominal.
Multi-ingredient: ***Belg.:*** Domidorm; ***Ger.:*** Itridal†.

Proxibarbal (4064-c)

Proxibarbal *(rINN).*
HH-184; Proxibarbital. 5-Allyl-5-(2-hydroxypropyl)barbituric acid.
$C_{10}H_{14}N_2O_4$ = 226.2.
CAS — 2537-29-3.
Pharmacopoeias. In *Pol.*

Proxibarbal is a barbiturate with general properties similar to those of amylobarbitone (p.641). It has been given by mouth as a sedative in the management of anxiety disorders. It has also been used in the treatment of headache. However, barbiturates are not considered appropriate in the management of these conditions. Proxibarbal has been associated with severe hypersensitivity-induced thrombocytopenia.

Preparations

Proprietary Preparations (details are given in Part 3)
Fr.: Centralgol; ***Ger.:*** Axeen†; ***Switz.:*** Axeen†.

Pyrithyldione (4065-k)

Pyrithyldione *(rINN).*
Didropyridinum; Nu-903. 3,3-Diethylpyridine-2,4(1*H*,3*H*)-dione.
$C_9H_{13}NO_2$ = 167.2.
CAS — 77-04-3.

Pyrithyldione has been given in preparations with diphenhydramine in the short-term management of insomnia but there have been reports of agranulocytosis associated with the use of this combination.

Preparations

Proprietary Preparations (details are given in Part 3)
Multi-ingredient: ***Belg.:*** Dormen; ***Ital.:*** Hibersulfan†; ***Spain:*** Sonodor.

Quazepam (13196-y)

Quazepam *(BAN, USAN, rINN).*
Sch-16134. 7-Chloro-5-(2-fluorophenyl)-1,3-dihydro-1-(2,2,2-trifluoroethyl)-1,4-benzodiazepine-2-thione.
$C_{17}H_{11}ClF_4N_2S$ = 386.8.
CAS — 36735-22-5.
Pharmacopoeias. In *US.*

Off-white to yellowish powder.

Dependence and Withdrawal, Adverse Effects, Treatment, and Precautions

As for Diazepam, p.661.

Interactions

As for Diazepam, p.663.

Pharmacokinetics

Quazepam is readily absorbed from the gastro-intestinal tract after administration by mouth, peak plasma concentrations being reached in about 2 hours. It is metabolised extensively in the liver. The principal active metabolites are 2-oxoquazepam and *N*-desalkyl-2-oxoquazepam (*N*-desalkylflurazepam) which have elimination half-lives of about 39 and 73 hours respectively compared with a half-life of 39 hours for quazepam. Further hydroxylation occurs and quazepam is excreted in urine and faeces mainly as conjugated metabolites.

Quazepam and its two active metabolites are more than 95% bound to plasma proteins. Quazepam and its metabolites have been detected in breast milk.

Uses and Administration

Quazepam is a long-acting benzodiazepine with general properties similar to those of diazepam (p.666). It is given by mouth as a hypnotic in the short-term management of insomnia (p.638), in an initial dose of 15 mg at night; in elderly or debilitated patients and some other patients this can be reduced to 7.5 mg.

Reviews of the actions and uses of quazepam.

1. Kales A. Quazepam: hypnotic efficacy and side effects. *Pharmacotherapy* 1990; **10:** 1–12.
2. Anonymous. Quazepam: a new hypnotic. *Med Lett Drugs Ther* 1990; **32:** 39–40.

Preparations

USP 23: Quazepam Tablets.

Proprietary Preparations (details are given in Part 3)
Ital.: Oniria†; Quazium; ***S.Afr.:*** Dorme; ***Spain:*** Quiedorm; ***USA:*** Doral.

Quetiapine Fumarate (17253-z)

Quetiapine Fumarate (*BANM, USAN, pINNM*).
ICI-204636; ZD-5077; ZM-204636. 2-[2-(4-Dibenzo[*b,f*][1,4]thiazepin-11-yl-1-piperazinyl)ethoxy]ethanol fumarate (2:1) salt.
$(C_{21}H_{25}N_3O_2S)_2,C_4H_4O_4$ = 883.1.
CAS — 111974-69-7 (quetiapine); 111974-72-2 (quetiapine fumarate).

Adverse Effects and Treatment

As for Chlorpromazine, p.649. The most frequent adverse effect with quetiapine has been somnolence. Quetiapine has been associated with a low incidence of extrapyramidal symptoms. Rises in prolactin concentrations may be less than with chlorpromazine. Other adverse effects have included mild asthenia, anxiety, myalgia, rhinitis, dyspepsia, rises in plasma-triglyceride and cholesterol concentrations, and reduced plasma-thyroid hormone concentrations. Asymptomatic changes in the lens of the eye have occurred in patients during long-term treatment with quetiapine; cataracts have developed in *dogs* during chronic dosing studies.

Precautions

As for Chlorpromazine, p.652. In the USA it is recommended that patients should have an eye examination to detect cataract formation before starting therapy with quetiapine and every 6 months during treatment.

Interactions

As for Chlorpromazine, p.652. The clearance of quetiapine is increased by concomitant administration with thioridazine.

CYP3A4 is the main isozyme responsible for cytochrome P450 mediated metabolism of quetiapine and caution is advised when quetiapine is administered with potent inhibitors of CYP3A4 such as erythromycin, fluconazole, itraconazole, and ketoconazole.

Pharmacokinetics

Quetiapine is well absorbed following oral administration and widely distributed throughout the body. It is about 83% bound to plasma proteins. Quetiapine is extensively metabolised in the liver by sulphoxidation mediated mainly by the cytochrome P450 isozyme CYP3A4 and by oxidation. It is excreted mainly as inactive metabolites, about 73% of a dose appearing in the urine and about 20% in the faeces. The elimination half-life has been reported to be about 6 to 7 hours.

Uses and Administration

Quetiapine fumarate is a dibenzothiazepine atypical antipsychotic. It is reported to have affinity for serotonin (5-HT_2), dopamine (D_2), histaminergic (H_1), and adrenergic (α_1 and α_2) receptors.

Quetiapine fumarate is given by mouth in the treatment of schizophrenia. The usual initial dose is the equivalent of 25 mg of the base twice daily on day one, 50 mg twice daily on day two, 100 mg twice daily on day three, and 150 mg twice daily on day four. The dosage is then adjusted according to response to a usual range of 300 to 450 mg daily given in 2 divided doses, although 150 mg daily may be adequate for some patients. The maximum recommended dose is 750 mg daily. Quetiapine should be given in reduced doses to the elderly or patients with impaired hepatic or renal function; a recommended starting dose is 25 mg daily increased in steps of 25 to 50 mg daily according to response.

References.

1. Anonymous. Quetiapine for schizophrenia. *Med Lett Drugs Ther* 1997; **39:** 117–18.

Schizophrenia. Short-term studies[1-3] have indicated that quetiapine is effective in the management of schizophrenia (p.637); it appears to be of comparable efficacy to haloperidol or chlorpromazine and has been associated with a lower incidence of extrapyramidal symptoms. However, its effect against negative symptoms has been less consistent than against positive symptoms.[1]

1. Small JG, *et al.* Quetiapine in patients with schizophrenia: a high- and low-dose double-blind comparison with placebo. *Arch Gen Psychiatry* 1997; **54:** 549–57.
2. Arvanitis LA, *et al.* Seroquel Trial 13 Study Group. Multiple fixed doses of "Seroquel" (quetiapine) in patients with acute exacerbation of schizophrenia: a comparison with haloperidol and placebo. *Biol Psychiatry* 1997; **42:** 233–46.
3. Peuskens J, Link CGG. A comparison of quetiapine and chlorpromazine in the treatment of schizophrenia. *Acta Psychiatr Scand* 1997; **96:** 265–73.

Preparations

Proprietary Preparations (details are given in Part 3)
UK: Seroquel; ***USA:*** Seroquel.

Quinalbarbitone (4066-a)

Secobarbital (*rINN*); Meballymal; Secobarbitalum; Secobarbitone. 5-Allyl-5-(1-methylbutyl)barbituric acid.
$C_{12}H_{18}N_2O_3$ = 238.3.
CAS — 76-73-3.
Pharmacopoeias. In US.

A white odourless amorphous or crystalline powder. Very slightly **soluble** in water; freely soluble in alcohol, ether, and solutions of fixed alkali hydroxides and carbonates; soluble in chloroform; soluble 1 in 8.5 of 0.5N sodium hydroxide. A saturated solution in water has a pH of about 5.6. **Store** in airtight containers.

Quinalbarbitone Sodium (4067-t)

Quinalbarbitone Sodium (*BAN*).
Secobarbital Sodium (*rINNM*); Meballymalnatrium; Secobarbitalum Natricum; Secobarbitone Sodium. Sodium 5-allyl-5-(1-methylbutyl)barbiturate.
$C_{12}H_{17}N_2NaO_3$ = 260.3.
CAS — 309-43-3.
Pharmacopoeias. In *Aust., Belg., Chin., Fr., It., Neth., Port., Swiss,* and *US.*

A white odourless hygroscopic powder. Very **soluble** in water; soluble in alcohol; practically insoluble in ether. A 10% solution in water has a pH between 9.7 and 10.5. Solutions decompose on standing, the process being accelerated at higher temperatures. **Store** in airtight containers.

Quinalbarbitone may be precipitated from preparations containing quinalbarbitone sodium depending on the concentration and pH. Quinalbarbitone sodium has, therefore, been reported to be **incompatible** with many other drugs, particularly acids and acidic salts.

Dependence and Withdrawal, Adverse Effects, Treatment, and Precautions

As for Amylobarbitone, p.641.

Exposure to quinalbarbitone sodium among 6 workers in the pharmaceutical industry resulted in absorption of substantial amounts of the drug, with blood concentrations approaching those expected after a therapeutic dose.[1] There continued to be evidence of absorption, despite protective masks to reduce inhalation, and it appeared that substantial absorption was taking place through the skin.

1. Baxter PJ, *et al.* Exposure to quinalbarbitone sodium in pharmaceutical workers. *Br Med J* 1986; **292:** 660–1.

Porphyria. Quinalbarbitone has been associated with clinical exacerbations of porphyria and is considered unsafe in porphyric patients.[1]

1. Moore MR, McColl KEL. *Porphyria: drug lists.* Glasgow: Porphyria Research Unit, University of Glasgow, 1991.

Interactions

As for Amylobarbitone, p.642.

Pharmacokinetics

Quinalbarbitone is well absorbed from the gastro-intestinal tract following oral doses and is reported to be about 46 to 70% bound to plasma proteins. The mean elimination half-life is reported to be 28 hours. It is metabolised in the liver, mainly by hydroxylation, and excreted in urine as metabolites and a small amount of unchanged drug.

Uses and Administration

Quinalbarbitone is a barbiturate that has been used as a hypnotic and sedative. It has general properties similar to those of amylobarbitone (p.642). As a hypnotic in the short-term management of insomnia (p.638) it was usually given by mouth in a dose of 100 mg of the sodium salt at night. However barbiturates are no longer considered appropriate for use in the management of insomnia.

Quinalbarbitone sodium has also been given by mouth or by intramuscular or intravenous injection for premedication in anaesthetic procedures (p.1220) but the use of barbiturates for pre-operative sedation has been replaced by other drugs.

Preparations

USP 23: Secobarbital Elixir; Secobarbital Sodium and Amobarbital Sodium Capsules; Secobarbital Sodium Capsules; Secobarbital Sodium for Injection; Secobarbital Sodium Injection.

Proprietary Preparations (details are given in Part 3)
Canad.: Seconal; ***Irl.:*** Seconal; ***S.Afr.:*** Seconal; ***UK:*** Seconal; ***USA:*** Seconal.

Multi-ingredient: ***Belg.:*** Bellanox; Octonox; Vesparax; ***Canad.:*** Tuinal; ***Ger.:*** Vesparax†; ***Irl.:*** Tuinal; ***Ital.:*** Neo Gratusminal†; Vesparax†; ***Neth.:*** Vesparax; ***S.Afr.:*** Tuinal†; Vesparax; ***Spain:*** Somatarax; ***UK:*** Tuinal; ***USA:*** Tuinal.

Raclopride (2420-b)

Raclopride (*BAN, rINN*).
A-40664 (raclopride tartrate); FLA-870. (S)-3,5-Dichloro-N-(1-ethylpyrrolidin-2-ylmethyl)-2-hydroxy-6-methoxybenzamide.
$C_{15}H_{20}Cl_2N_2O_3$ = 347.2.
CAS — 84225-95-6 (raclopride); 98185-20-7 (raclopride tartrate).

Raclopride is a substituted benzamide related to sulpiride (p.692). It has been investigated for the treatment of psychoses. Since it binds selectively and with high affinity to D_2 dopaminergic receptors raclopride labelled with C-11 has been tried as a tracer in computerised tomographic studies of neurological disorders associated with dysfunction of brain D_2 dopaminergic receptors.

Remoxipride Hydrochloride (497-s)

Remoxipride Hydrochloride (*BANM, USAN, rINNM*).
A-33547 (remoxipride); FLA-731 (remoxipride). (S)-3-Bromo-N-(1-ethylpyrrolidin-2-ylmethyl)-2,6-dimethoxybenzamide hydrochloride monohydrate.
$C_{16}H_{23}BrN_2O_3,HCl,H_2O$ = 425.7.
CAS — 80125-14-0 (remoxipride); 73220-03-8 (anhydrous remoxipride hydrochloride); 117591-79-4 (remoxipride hydrochloride monohydrate).

NOTE. Remoxipride is *USAN.*

Remoxipride is a substituted benzamide with general properties similar to those of sulpiride (p.692). It is described as an atypical antipsychotic. Remoxipride has been given by mouth or intramuscularly for the treatment of schizophrenia and other psychoses but was withdrawn in some countries by the manufacturer following reports of aplastic anaemia associated with its use. However, it is still available from the manufacturer for the compassionate treatment of psychoses in individual patients intolerant of other antipsychotics.

Effects on the blood. By November 1993 the UK Committee on Safety of Medicines had received 8 reports (5 in the UK) of aplastic anaemia associated with remoxipride treatment.[1] The UK patients, one of whom died, had received a dose of 150 to 600 mg daily for between 3 and 8 months. The committee recommended that treatment with remoxipride should only be initiated by psychiatrists in patients who are intolerant of other antipsychotics. They also recommended that it should not be given to patients with a history of blood disorders and that blood counts should be determined before treatment, every week for the first 6 months of treatment, and monthly thereafter. Patients or their carers should be advised to seek immediate medical attention if bruising, bleeding, fever, or a sore throat develops during treatment. Treatment should be stopped immediately if there is any evidence of a blood disorder.

1. Committee on Safety of Medicines/Medicines Control Agency. Stop press: remoxipride (Roxiam)-aplastic anaemia. *Current Problems* 1993; **19:** 9.

Preparations

Proprietary Preparations (details are given in Part 3)
Aust.: Roxiam; ***Neth.:*** Roxiam†; ***Swed.:*** Roxiam†; ***UK:*** Roxiam†.

Risperidone (5648-h)

Risperidone (*BAN, USAN, rINN*).
R-64766. 3-{2-[4-(6-Fluoro-1,2-benzisoxazol-3-yl)piperidino]ethyl}-6,7,8,9-tetrahydro-2-methylpyrido[1,2-*a*]pyrimidin-4-one.
$C_{23}H_{27}FN_4O_2$ = 410.5.
CAS — 106266-06-2.

Adverse Effects, Treatment, and Precautions

As for Chlorpromazine, p.649. Risperidone is reported to be less likely to cause sedation or extrapyramidal effects (see also Uses and Administration, below) but agitation may occur more frequently. Dyspepsia, nausea, abdominal pain, anxiety, concentration difficulties, headache, dizziness, fatigue, and rhinitis have also been reported. In addition to orthostatic hypotension hypertension has been reported infrequently.

Effects on the liver. A report of 2 cases of hepatotoxicity associated with risperidone.[1] An idiosyncratic reaction to risperidone was suspected in another patient who developed hepatotoxicity after receiving only 2 doses of risperidone.[2]

1. Fuller MA, *et al.* Risperidone-associated hepatotoxicity. *J Clin Psychopharmacol* 1996; **16:** 84–5.
2. Phillips EJ, *et al.* Rapid onset of risperidone-induced hepatotoxicity. *Ann Pharmacother* 1998; **32:** 843.

Effects on the skin. A patient with schizoaffective disorder developed facial and periorbital oedema 2 weeks after her dose had reached 6 mg daily.[1] The oedema subsequently subsided after the dose was halved but recurred shortly after it became necessary to increase her dose to 6 mg. She had previously had a similar reaction to lithium and there was also a family history of angioedema.

1. Cooney C, Nagy A. Angio-oedema associated with risperidone. *Br Med J* 1995; **311:** 1204.

Mania. There has been a report[1] that all of 6 patients with bipolar schizoaffective disorder displayed the onset of, or an increase in, manic symptoms shortly after initiation of treatment with risperidone. Symptoms resolved in some patients without the use of mood-stabilising drugs but others required the addition of valproate to treatment. It was considered that it was more likely that risperidone precipitated or exacerbated symptoms of mania rather than this being a coincidental worsening of the patients' symptoms.

1. Dwight MM, *et al.* Antidepressant activity and mania associated with risperidone treatment of schizoaffective disorder. *Lancet* 1994; **344:** 554–5.

Neuroleptic malignant syndrome. Reports and discussions of 11 cases of neuroleptic malignant syndrome associated with risperidone.[1,2]

For a discussion of neuroleptic malignant syndrome associated with the use of antipsychotics and its treatment, see Chlorpromazine p.651.

1. Sharma R, *et al.* Risperidone-induced neuroleptic malignant syndrome. *Ann Pharmacother* 1996; **30:** 775–8.
2. Tarsy D. Risperidone and neuroleptic malignant syndrome. *JAMA* 1996; **275:** 446.

Overdosage. Report[1] of a 3½-year-old child who developed extrapyramidal symptoms after accidental ingestion of a single 4-mg tablet of risperidone. The child was initially treated with gastric lavage and activated charcoal and sorbitol; extrapyramidal symptoms responded to treatment with diphenhydramine and the child recovered completely. The need to monitor for and treat hypotension following overdosage with risperidone was highlighted in a report[2] of a 15-year-old girl who took 40 mg of risperidone.

1. Cheslik TA, Erramouspe J. Extrapyramidal symptoms following accidental ingestion of risperidone in a child. *Ann Pharmacother* 1996; **30:** 360–3.
2. Himstreet JE, Daya M. Hypotension and orthostasis following a risperidone overdose. *Ann Pharmacother* 1998; **32:** 267.

Interactions

As for Chlorpromazine, p.652.

Clozapine. For a report suggesting that risperidone might increase plasma concentrations of clozapine, see p.659.

Pharmacokinetics

Risperidone is readily absorbed after oral doses, peak plasma concentrations being reached within 1 to 2 hours. It is extensively metabolised in the liver by hydroxylation to its main active metabolite, 9-hydroxyrisperidone; oxidative *N*-dealkylation is a minor metabolic pathway. Hydroxylation is mediated by the cytochrome P450 isozyme CYP2D6 and is the subject of genetic polymorphism. Excretion is mainly in the urine and to a lesser extent, in the faeces. Risperidone and 9-hydroxyrisperidone are about 88% and 77% bound to plasma proteins, respectively.

Metabolism. Although the hydroxylation of risperidone is subject to debrisoquine-type genetic polymorphism this is considered to have little clinical consequence as the pharmacokinetics and effects of the active antipsychotic fraction (risperidone plus 9-hydroxyrisperidone) has been reported to vary little between extensive and poor metabolisers.[1] A mean value of 19.5 hours has been reported for the terminal elimination half-life of the active fraction following oral administration of risperidone.[1]

1. Huang M-L, *et al.* Pharmacokinetics of the novel antipsychotic agent risperidone and the prolactin response in healthy subjects. *Clin Pharmacol Ther* 1993; **54:** 257–68.

Uses and Administration

Risperidone is a benzisoxazole antipsychotic, reported to be an antagonist at dopamine D_2 and serotonin (5-HT_2), adrenergic (α_1 and α_2), and histamine (H_1) receptors. It is described as an atypical antipsychotic. It is given by mouth for the treatment of schizophrenia and other psychoses.

Risperidone may be given in 1 or 2 divided doses daily. The usual initial daily dose of risperidone is 2 mg on the first day, 4 mg on the second day, and 6 mg on the third day. Further dosage adjustment may be needed and should generally be made at intervals of not less than one week; usual maintenance doses are 4 to 8 mg daily. Extrapyramidal symptoms may be more likely with doses above 10 mg daily. The maximum recommended dose is 16 mg daily.

An initial dose of 0.5 mg twice daily slowly increased in steps of 0.5 mg twice daily to a dose of 1 to 2 mg twice daily is suggested for the elderly and for patients with renal or hepatic impairment.

Action. Risperidone is described as an atypical antipsychotic but its atypicality is not fully translated into clinical practice. Although it does have a lower propensity to produce parkinsonism, dystonias and akathisias have been reported.[1] The traditional hypothesis is that antipsychotics work through inhibition of dopamine D_2 receptors and that extrapyramidal motor side-effects result from blockade of D_2 receptors in the striatum (see p.654). Like clozapine, risperidone has a high affinity for 5-HT_2 receptors and like haloperidol it has a high affinity for dopamine D_2 receptors. Risperidone also binds to alpha-adrenergic and histamine H_1 sites. It is unclear whether risperidone's antipsychotic effect is due to activity at dopamine D_2 receptors or at another site. It has been suggested[1] that other potent effects of risperidone may be counterbalancing the D_2 activity to produce its atypicality.

1. Kerwin RW. The new atypical antipsychotics: a lack of extrapyramidal side-effects and new routes in schizophrenia research. *Br J Psychiatry* 1994; **164:** 141–8.

AIDS. Risperidone has been used successfully to control AIDS-related psychosis in 4 patients who also had manic symptoms.[1] No extrapyramidal symptoms were reported during treatment. For a report suggesting that risperidone can induce or exacerbate manic symptoms in patients with schizoaffective disorders, see under Mania in Adverse Effects, above.

1. Singh AN, Catalan J. Risperidone in HIV-related manic psychosis. *Lancet* 1994; **344:** 1029–30.

Anxiety disorders. Although there have been anecdotal reports[1,2] of improvement following the addition of risperidone to treatment in patients with obsessive-compulsive disorder refractory to conventional treatment there has also been a report[3] of a patient whose obsessive-compulsive behaviour recurred when he was treated with risperidone for tardive dyskinesia.

1. Jacobsen FM. Risperidone in the treatment of affective illness and obsessive-compulsive disorder. *J Clin Psychiatry* 1995; **56:** 423–9.
2. McDougle CJ, *et al.* Risperidone addition in fluvoxamine-refractory obsessive-compulsive disorder: three cases. *J Clin Psychiatry* 1995; **56:** 526–8.
3. Remington G, Adams M. Risperidone and obsessive-compulsive symptoms. *J Clin Psychopharmacol* 1994; **14:** 358–9.

Dementia. Risperidone has been used for the management of behavioural disturbances in patients with dementia (p.636). Although there have been anecdotal reports[1] of efficacy in patients with Lewy-body dementia other reports[2] suggest that these patients are likely to be just as sensitive to risperidone as to standard antipsychotics (see the Elderly in Precautions for Chlorpromazine, p.652).

1. Allen RL, *et al.* Risperidone for psychotic and behavioural symptoms in Lewy body dementia. *Lancet* 1995; **346:** 185.
2. McKeith IG, *et al.* Neuroleptic sensitivity to risperidone in Lewy body dementia. *Lancet* 1995; **346:** 699.

Dystonias. Antipsychotics are sometimes useful in the treatment of idiopathic dystonia in patients who have failed to respond to treatment with levodopa or antimuscarinics, but with classic antipsychotics there is the risk of adding drug-induced extrapyramidal effects to the dystonia. Risperidone has been reported to be of benefit in 5 patients with idiopathic segmental dystonia partly insensitive to haloperidol.[1] For a discussion of the management of dystonias, see under Levodopa on p.1141.

1. Zuddas A, Cianchetti C. Efficacy of risperidone in idiopathic segmental dystonia. *Lancet* 1996; **347:** 127–8.

Parkinsonism. Psychosis occurs in patients with parkinsonism both as a complication of disease progression and due to the effects of pharmacotherapy. Such psychosis is initially managed by adjusting the antiparkinsonian therapy but patients who do not respond to such measures may require treatment with antipsychotics. Standard antipsychotics can induce extrapyramidal effects and can therefore exacerbate symptoms of parkinsonism. There have been anecdotal reports of the use of risperidone as an antipsychotic in a small number of patients with Parkinson's disease (p.1128). While one group[1] of workers found that risperidone ameliorated levodopa-induced hallucinations without worsening of extrapyramidal symptoms, another group[2] reported that patients with Parkinson's disease given risperidone had substantial worsening of their symptoms.

1. Meco G, *et al.* Risperidone for hallucinations in levodopa-treated Parkinson's disease patients. *Lancet* 1994; **343:** 1370–1.
2. Ford B, *et al.* Risperidone in Parkinson's disease. *Lancet* 1994; **344:** 681.

Schizophrenia. The use of risperidone for the management of schizophrenia (p.637) has been reviewed.[1-5] Features for which risperidone has been promoted have included a relatively low incidence of extrapyramidal effects and efficacy against both positive and negative symptoms of schizophrenia. Most studies have compared risperidone with haloperidol but, of these, some of the major studies[6-8] have been criticised for potential methodological flaws[1,9] and it is difficult to determine any difference in efficacy including effect on negative symptoms. The production of extrapyramidal effects appears to be dose dependent for risperidone.[10] Overall the incidence for risperidone appears to be similar to that for placebo but at doses of more than 10 mg it appears to approach that associated with haloperidol. In the few comparative studies with other atypical antipsychotics risperidone has appeared to be of similar efficacy to clozapine.[11] For a comparative study with olanzapine, see p.683. However, there appears to be no published data of long-term efficacy for risperidone in schizophrenia or for prevention of relapse. There is also insufficient evidence to indicate that risperidone is effective for treatment-resistant or poorly responsive patients.

1. Livingston MG. Risperidone. *Lancet* 1994; **343:** 457–60.
2. Grant S, Fitton A. Risperidone: a review of its pharmacology and therapeutic potential in the treatment of schizophrenia. *Drugs* 1994; **48:** 253–73.
3. Curtis VA, Kerwin RW. A risk-benefit assessment of risperidone in schizophrenia. *Drug Safety* 1995; **12:** 139–45.
4. Cardoni AA. Risperidone: review and assessment of its role in the treatment of schizophrenia. *Ann Pharmacother* 1995; **29:** 610–18.
5. Buckley PF. New dimensions in the pharmacologic treatment of schizophrenia and related psychoses. *J Clin Pharmacol* 1997; **37:** 363–78. Correction. *ibid.* 1998; **38:** 27.
6. Chouinard G, *et al.* A Canadian multicenter placebo-controlled study of fixed doses of risperidone and haloperidol in the treatment of chronic schizophrenic patients. *J Clin Psychopharmacol* 1993; **13:** 25–40.
7. Marder SR, Meibach RC. Risperidone in the treatment of schizophrenia. *Am J Psychiatry* 1994; **151:** 825–35.
8. Peuskens J, *et al.* Risperidone Study Group. Risperidone in the treatment of patients with chronic schizophrenia: a multi-national, multi-centre, double-blind, parallel-group study versus haloperidol. *Br J Psychiatry* 1995; **166:** 712–26.
9. Musser WS, Kirisci L. Critique of the Canadian multicenter placebo-controlled study of risperidone and haloperidol. *J Clin Psychopharmacol* 1995; **15:** 226–8.
10. Owens DGC. Extrapyramidal side effects and tolerability of risperidone: a review. *J Clin Psychiatry* 1994; **55** (suppl 5): 29–35.
11. Klieser E, *et al.* Randomized, double-blind, controlled trial of risperidone versus clozapine in patients with chronic schizophrenia. *J Clin Psychopharmacol* 1995; **15** (suppl 1): 45S–51S.

Tourette's syndrome. When treatment is required for tics and behavioural disturbances in Tourette's syndrome (p.636) haloperidol or pimozide are commonly used but risperidone has also been tried.[1]

1. Bruun RD, Budman CL. Risperidone as a treatment for Tourette's syndrome. *J Clin Psychiatry* 1996; **57:** 29–31.

Preparations

Proprietary Preparations (details are given in Part 3)
Aust.: Belivon; Risperdal; Rispolin; ***Austral.:*** Risperdal; ***Belg.:*** Risperdal; ***Canad.:*** Risperdal; ***Fr.:*** Risperdal; ***Ger.:*** Risperdal; ***Irl.:*** Risperdal; ***Ital.:*** Belivon; Risperdal; ***Neth.:*** Risperdal; ***Norw.:*** Risperdal; ***S.Afr.:*** Risperdal; ***Spain:*** Risperdal; ***Swed.:*** Risperdal; ***Switz.:*** Risperdal; ***UK:*** Risperdal; ***USA:*** Risperdal.

Ritanserin (18677-n)

Ritanserin *(BAN, USAN, rINN).*

R-55667. 6-{2-[4-(4,4′-Difluorobenzhydrylidene)piperidino]ethyl}-7-methyl[1,3]thiazolo[3,2-*a*]pyrimidin-5-one.

$C_{27}H_{25}F_2N_3OS$ = 477.6.

CAS — 87051-43-2.

Ritanserin is a serotonin antagonist which has been studied in a variety of disorders including anxiety disorders, depression, and schizophrenia. It is reported to have little sedative action.

Action. Ritanserin is a relatively selective antagonist at serotonin (5-hydroxytryptamine, 5-HT) receptors of the 5-HT_2 subtype, although it also has appreciable affinity for 5-HT_{1C} receptors.[1] Unlike ketanserin (p.895), it does not block α_1-adrenergic receptors. Ritanserin has anxiolytic activity; it also hastens the onset of slow-wave sleep although sleep may be impaired on withdrawal.

Ritanserin may interfere with platelet function[2,3] and has been reported to have no significant effect on blood pressure, blood flow, or heart rate in patients with hypertension.[2,4] Features characteristic of class III antiarrhythmic activity have also been noted.[2]

1. Marsden CA. The pharmacology of new anxiolytics acting on 5-HT neurones. *Postgrad Med J* 1990; **66** (suppl 2): S2–S6.
2. Stott DJ, *et al.* The effects of the $5HT_2$ antagonist ritanserin on blood pressure and serotonin-induced platelet aggregation in patients with untreated essential hypertension. *Eur J Clin Pharmacol* 1988; **35:** 123–9.
3. Wagner B, *et al.* Effect of ritanserin, a 5-hydroxytryptamine$_2$-receptor antagonist, on platelet function and thrombin generation at the site of plug formation in vivo. *Clin Pharmacol Ther* 1990; **48:** 419–23.
4. Chau NP, *et al.* Comparative haemodynamic effects of ketanserin and ritanserin in the proximal and distal upper limb circulations of hypertensive patients. *Eur J Clin Pharmacol* 1989; **37:** 215–20.

Alcohol dependence. Despite some encouraging preliminary data[1] suggesting that ritanserin might influence the desire to drink alcohol, subsequent studies[2] have failed to support a role for ritanserin in reducing alcohol intake in patients with alcohol dependence (p.1099).

1. Meert TF. Ritanserin and alcohol abuse and dependence. *Alcohol Alcohol* 1994; **2** (suppl): 523–30.
2. Johnson BA, *et al.* Ritanserin Study Group. Ritanserin in the treatment of alcohol dependence—a multi-center clinical trial. *Psychopharmacology (Berl)* 1996; **128:** 206–15.

Schizophrenia. Ritanserin has produced some beneficial effects when tried in small numbers of patients with schizophrenia.[1,2] For a discussion of the treatment of schizophrenia, see p.637.

1. Duinkerke SJ, *et al.* Ritanserin, a selective 5-$HT_{2/1C}$ antagonist, and negative symptoms in schizophrenia: a placebo-controlled double-blind trial. *Br J Psychiatry* 1993; **163:** 451–5.
2. Weisel F-A, *et al.* An open clinical and biochemical study of ritanserin in acute patients with schizophrenia. *Psychopharmacology (Berl)* 1994; **114:** 31–8.

Romifidine (5670-d)

Romifidine *(BAN, rINN).*

STH-2130. 2-Bromo-6-fluoro-*N*-(1-imidazolin-2-yl)aniline.

$C_9H_9BrFN_3$ = 258.1.

CAS — 65896-16-4.

Romifidine is an α_2-adrenoceptor agonist with sedative, muscle relaxant, and analgesic properties and is used in veterinary medicine.

Secbutobarbitone (4068-x)

Secbutobarbitone *(BAN).*

Secbutabarbital *(rINN)*; Butabarbital; Butabarbitone. 5-sec-Butyl-5-ethylbarbituric acid.

$C_{10}H_{16}N_2O_3$ = 212.2.

CAS — 125-40-6.

NOTE. Butabarbitone should be distinguished from Butobarbitone (p.645).

Pharmacopoeias. In *US.*

A white, odourless, crystalline powder.

Very slightly **soluble** in water; soluble in alcohol, in chloroform, in ether, and in aqueous solutions of alkali hydroxides and carbonates. **Store** in airtight containers.

Secbutobarbitone Sodium (4069-r)

Secbutobarbitone Sodium *(BANM).*

Secbutabarbital Sodium *(rINNM)*; Butabarbital Sodium; Secumalnatrium; Sodium Butabarbital. Sodium 5-*sec*-butyl-5-ethylbarbiturate.

$C_{10}H_{15}N_2NaO_3$ = 234.2.

CAS — 143-81-7.

Pharmacopoeias. In *US.*

A white powder. **Soluble** 1 in 2 of water, and 1 in 7 of alcohol; 1 in 7000 of chloroform; practically insoluble in ether. A 10% solution in water has a pH of between 10.0 and 11.2. **Store** in airtight containers.

Secbutobarbitone is a barbiturate with general properties similar to those of amylobarbitone (p.641). It was used as a hypnotic and sedative although barbiturates are no longer considered appropriate for such purposes. For the short-term management of insomnia (p.638) it was usually given as the sodium salt in doses of 50 to 100 mg by mouth at night; as a sedative 15 to 30 mg has been given 3 or 4 times daily. Similar doses have been given of secbutobarbitone base.

Preparations

USP 23: Butabarbital Sodium Capsules; Butabarbital Sodium Elixir; Butabarbital Sodium Tablets.

Proprietary Preparations (details are given in Part 3)
Canad.: Butisol; ***USA:*** Butisol.

Multi-ingredient: ***Ger.:*** Dormilfo N†; Nervolitan†; Resedorm†; ***USA:*** Butibel.

Sertindole (11056-p)

Sertindole *(BAN, USAN, rINN).*

Lu-23-174. 1-(2-{4-[5-Chloro-1-(*p*-fluorophenyl)indol-3-yl]piperidino}ethyl)-2-imidazolidinone.

$C_{24}H_{26}ClFN_4O$ = 440.9.

CAS — 106516-24-9.

Adverse Effects, Treatment, and Precautions

As for Chlorpromazine, p.649. Sertindole is associated with a low incidence of extrapyramidal symptoms and does not appear to cause sedation. Prolactin elevation may be less frequent. Other adverse effects have included peripheral oedema, rhinitis, dyspnoea, and paraesthesia.

Sertindole should not be given to patients with uncorrected hypokalaemia or hypomagnesaemia. It was also recommended that blood pressure should be monitored during dose titration and in early maintenance therapy.

Since sertindole has been associated with prolongation of the QT interval, usually during the first 3 to 6 weeks of treatment, it was recommended that patients should have an ECG before the start of therapy and periodically during treatment. Patients with pre-existing prolongation of the QT interval should not be given sertindole and sertindole should be discontinued if such prolongation occurs during treatment.

- *Marketing of sertindole was suspended in the UK in December 1998 because of cardiac arrhythmias and sudden cardiac deaths associated with its use.*

Effects on the cardiovascular system. The manufacturer has stated that in clinical studies prolongation of the QT interval had been seen in 24 of 1446 (1.66%) patients given sertindole. The effect did not correlate with plasma concentrations of sertindole and/or its metabolites. In evidence presented to the FDA it has been reported that of 1st June 1996 there had been 27 deaths, 16 due to adverse cardiac events, among the 2194 patients given sertindole in clinical studies.[1] However, in practice there have been no reports of torsade de pointes or other life-threatening arrhythmias in patients receiving sertindole[2] and opinion on the clinical implications of the QT prolongation is divided.[1] Nonetheless, monitoring of the QT interval is considered necessary.

1. Barnett AA. Safety concerns over antipsychotic drug, sertindole. *Lancet* 1996; **348:** 256.
2. Anonymous. Olanzapine, sertindole and schizophrenia. *Drug Ther Bull* 1997; **35:** 81–3.

Interactions

As for Chlorpromazine, p.652. The risk of arrhythmias with sertindole may be increased by other drugs which prolong the QT interval and concomitant use should be avoided. Concomitant use should also be avoided with drugs which produce electrolyte disturbances.

Sertindole is extensively metabolised by the cytochrome P450 isozymes CYP2D6 and CYP3A. Ketoconazole and itraconazole are potent inhibitors of CYP3A and their use with sertindole is contra-indicated. Minor increases in sertindole plasma concentrations have been noted in patients also given macrolide antibacterials or calcium-channel blockers which also inhibit CYP3A. Fluoxetine and paroxetine, potent inhibitors of CYP2D6, have increased plasma concentrations of sertindole by a factor of 2 to 3 and lower maintenance doses of sertindole may be required during concomitant treatment.

Pharmacokinetics

Sertindole is slowly absorbed with peak concentrations occurring about 10 hours after oral administration. It is about 99.5% bound to plasma proteins and readily crosses the placenta. Sertindole is extensively metabolised in the liver by the cytochrome P450 isozymes CYP2D6 and CYP3A. There is moderate intersubject variation in the pharmacokinetics of sertindole due to polymorphism in the isozyme CYP2D6. Poor metabolisers, deficient in this isozyme, may have plasma concentrations of sertindole 2 to 3 times higher than other patients. The two major metabolites identified, dehydrosertindole and norsertindole, appear to be inactive. Sertindole and its metabolites are excreted slowly, mainly in the faeces with a minor amount appearing in the urine. The mean terminal half-life is about 3 days.

References.

1. Wong SL, *et al.* Pharmacokinetics of sertindole in healthy young and elderly male and female subjects. *Clin Pharmacol Ther* 1997; **62:** 157–64.

Uses and Administration

Sertindole is an atypical antipsychotic that is an antagonist at central dopamine (D_2), serotonin (5-HT_2), and adrenergic (α_1) receptors. It was used in the treatment of schizophrenia (p.637) but marketing was suspended in the UK in December 1998 because of cardiac arrhythmias and sudden cardiac deaths associated with its use.

Sertindole was given by mouth in an initial dose of 4 mg daily, increased gradually by 4 mg every 4 to 5 days to a usual maintenance dose of 12 to 20 mg given once daily. The maximum dose was 24 mg daily. Slower dose titration and lower maintenance doses were advisable for the elderly and patients with hepatic impairment.

References.

1. van Kammen DP, *et al.* A randomized, controlled, dose-ranging trial of sertindole in patients with schizophrenia. *Psychopharmacology (Berl)* 1996; **124:** 168–75.
2. Zimbroff DL, *et al.* Sertindole Study Group. Controlled, dose-response study of sertindole and haloperidol in the treatment of schizophrenia. *Am J Psychiatry* 1997; **154:** 782–91.
3. Anonymous. Olanzapine, sertindole and schizophrenia. *Drug Ther Bull* 1997; **35:** 81–3.

Preparations

Proprietary Preparations (details are given in Part 3)
Irl.: Serdolect†; ***Neth.:*** Serdolect†; ***UK:*** Serdolect†.

Sulpiride (7107-l)

Sulpiride *(BAN, USAN, rINN).*

Sulpiridum. *N*-(1-Ethylpyrrolidin-2-ylmethyl)-2-methoxy-5-sulphamoylbenzamide.

$C_{15}H_{23}N_3O_4S$ = 341.4.

CAS — 15676-16-1 (sulpiride); 23672-07-3 (levosulpiride).

NOTE. Levosulpiride is *pINN.*

Pharmacopoeias. In *Eur.* (see p.viii) and *Jpn.*

A white or almost white crystalline powder. Practically **insoluble** in water; slightly soluble in alcohol and in dichloromethane; sparingly soluble in methyl alcohol. It dissolves in dilute solutions of mineral acids and in alkali hydroxides.

Adverse Effects, Treatment, and Precautions

As for Chlorpromazine, p.649.

Sleep disturbances, overstimulation, and agitation may occur. Extrapyramidal effects appear to occur as frequently as for chlorpromazine but have usually been mild. Whether sulpiride is less likely to cause tardive dyskinesia remains to be established. Sulpiride is less likely to cause sedation than chlorpromazine and antimuscarinic effects are minimal. Cardiovascular effects such as hypotension are generally rare although they may occur with overdosage.

Sulpiride should be given with care to manic or hypomanic patients in whom it may exacerbate symptoms.

Sulpiride may be distributed into breast milk in relatively large amounts and some recommend that its use should be avoided in mothers wishing to breast feed.

Effects on the cardiovascular system. Sulpiride 100 mg by mouth caused an attack of hypertension in 6 of 26 hypertensive patients; in 4 it induced a rise in urinary excretion of vanillylmandelic acid and catecholamines.[1] A transient rise in blood pressure and catecholamines after administration of sulpiride occurred in 3 patients who were found to have a phaeochromocytoma; another patient probably had a phaeochromocytoma. The means by which sulpiride provoked hypertension were not known but appeared to be due to a noradrenergic effect. Sulpiride should be avoided during the treatment of phaeochromocytoma, and prescribed with great care in hypertensive patients.

1. Corvol P, *et al.* Poussées hypertensives déclenchées par le sulpiride. *Sem Hop Paris* 1974; **50:** 1265–9.

Porphyria. Sulpiride was considered to be unsafe in patients with acute porphyria because it has been shown to be porphyrinogenic in *animals* or *in-vitro* systems.[1]

1. Moore MR, McColl KEL. *Porphyria: drug lists.* Glasgow: Porphyria Research Unit, University of Glasgow, 1991.

Renal impairment. For the precautions to be observed in patients with impaired renal function, see under Uses and Administration, below.

Interactions

As for Chlorpromazine, p.652

When sulpiride was given concomitantly with therapeutic doses of *sucralfate*, or of an *antacid* containing aluminium and magnesium hydroxides, in 6 healthy subjects the mean oral bioavailability of sulpiride was reduced by 40 and 32% respectively.[1] When sulpiride was given 2 hours after the antacid or sucralfate (each in 2 subjects) the reduction in bioavailability was about 25%. This interaction was expected to be clinically significant and it was recommended that if used concurrently sulpiride should be given before, rather than with or after, sucralfate or antacids.

1. Gouda MW, *et al.* Effect of sucralfate and antacids on the bioavailability of sulpiride in humans. *Int J Pharmaceutics* 1984; **22:** 257–63.

Pharmacokinetics

Sulpiride is slowly absorbed from the gastro-intestinal tract; bioavailability is low and subject to inter-individual variation. It is rapidly distributed to the tissues but passage across the blood-brain barrier is poor. Sulpiride is less than 40% bound to plasma proteins and is reported to have a plasma half-life of about 6 to 9 hours. It is excreted in the urine, chiefly as unchanged drug. Sulpiride is distributed into breast milk.

References.

1. Wiesel F-A, *et al.* The pharmacokinetics of intravenous and oral sulpiride in healthy human subjects. *Eur J Clin Pharmacol* 1980; **17:** 385–91.
2. Bressolle F, *et al.* Sulpiride pharmacokinetics in humans after intramuscular administration at three dose levels. *J Pharm Sci* 1984; **73:** 1128–36.
3. Bressolle F, *et al.* Absolute bioavailability, rate of absorption, and dose proportionality of sulpiride in humans. *J Pharm Sci* 1992; **81:** 26–32.

Distribution into breast milk. On the fifth day after starting administration of D-sulpiride, DL-sulpiride, or L-sulpiride in a dose of 50 mg twice daily, mean concentrations of sulpiride in breast milk were 840 ng, 850 ng, and 810 ng per mL respectively.[1]

1. Polatti F. Sulpiride isomers and milk secretion in puerperium. *Clin Exp Obstet Gynecol* 1982; **9:** 144–7.

Uses and Administration

Sulpiride is a substituted benzamide antipsychotic which is reported to be a selective antagonist of central dopamine (D_2, D_3, and D_4) receptors. It is also claimed to have mood elevating properties.

Sulpiride is mainly used in the treatment of psychoses such as schizophrenia (p.637). It has also been given in the management of Tourette's syndrome, anxiety disorders (p.635), vertigo (p.401), and benign peptic ulceration. Levosulpiride, the L-isomer of sulpiride, has been used similarly to sulpiride.

In the treatment of schizophrenia initial doses of 200 to 400 mg of sulpiride are given twice daily by mouth, increased if necessary up to a maximum of 1.2 g twice daily in patients with mainly positive symptoms. Doses at the lower end of the range have a greater alerting effect and patients with predominantly negative symptoms usually respond to doses below 800 mg daily. Sulpiride is also given in some countries by intramuscular injection, in doses ranging from 200 to 800 mg daily. A daily dose of 3 to 5 mg per kg body-weight may be given by mouth to children over 14 years of age.

Sulpiride should be given in reduced doses to elderly patients.

Reviews.

1. Caley CF, Weber SS. Sulpiride: an antipsychotic with selective dopaminergic antagonist properties. *Ann Pharmacother* 1995; **29:** 152–60.
2. Mauri MC, *et al.* A risk-benefit assessment of sulpiride in the treatment of schizophrenia. *Drug Safety* 1996; **14:** 288–98.

Administration in renal impairment. A single intravenous dose of sulpiride 100 mg was administered to 6 healthy subjects with normal renal function (creatinine clearance greater than 90 mL per minute) and to three groups of 6 patients each with creatinine clearances in the ranges 30 to 60, 10 to 30, and less than 10 mL per minute.[1] There was a progressive diminution in the rate of elimination and an increase in half-life with decreasing renal function. The mean plasma elimination half-lives were 5.90, 11.02, 19.27, and 25.96 hours in the four groups respectively. It was suggested that in patients with renal impairment or in the elderly, the dosage of sulpiride be reduced by 35 to 70% or the dosage interval increased by a factor of 1.5 to 3.

1. Bressolle F, *et al.* Pharmacokinetics of sulpiride after intravenous administration in patients with impaired renal function. *Clin Pharmacokinet* 1989; **17:** 367–73.

Chorea. Antipsychotics have some action against choreiform movements as well as being of use to control the behavioural disturbances of Huntington's chorea. Although sulpiride was found to have produced an overall reduction in abnormal movements in 11 patients with Huntington's chorea when compared with placebo in a double-blind study[1] there was generally no accompanying functional improvement and patients with mild disease tended to worsen when taking sulpiride. For a discussion of the management of various choreas, see p.636.

1. Quinn N, Marsden CD. A double blind trial of sulpiride in Huntington's disease and tardive dyskinesia. *J Neurol Neurosurg Psychiatry* 1984; **47:** 844–7.

Gastro-intestinal disorders. Although sulpiride is used in some countries as an adjunct in the treatment of peptic ulcer disease (p.1174) it is not among the more usual drugs used for this indication. Intramuscular administration of sulpiride (the racemic substance) or its L-isomer (levosulpiride) has been found to decrease serum-gastrin concentration without effecting basal or stimulated gastric acidity.[1] In contrast, the D-isomer significantly decreases gastric acid secretion without affecting serum-gastrin concentrations. The paradoxical response observed after D-sulpiride is similar to the action of dopamine and it is possible that the D-isomer has partial agonist actions. It has been suggested[1] that these results might explain the contradictory responses that have been reported following sulpiride treatment of peptic ulceration. There is a study which suggests that addition of oral sulpiride to cimetidine therapy, while not altering the rate of ulcer healing, might decrease the rate of relapse.[2]

Several studies have claimed efficacy for sulpiride[3] or levosulpiride[4-8] in a variety of other gastro-intestinal disorders, including irritable colon (p.1172), gastro-intestinal motility disorders (p.1168), and nausea and vomiting (p.1172), but they are not among the drugs usually considered for use in these conditions.

1. Caldara R, *et al.* Effect of sulpiride isomers on gastric acid and gastrin secretion in healthy man. *Eur J Clin Pharmacol* 1983; **25:** 319–22.
2. Tatsuta M, *et al.* Deduction of duodenal ulcer recurrence by healing with cimetidine plus sulpiride. *Gut* 1986; **27:** 1512–15.
3. Lanfranchi GA, *et al.* Inhibition of postprandial colonic motility by sulpiride in patients with irritable colon. *Eur J Clin Pharmacol* 1983; **24:** 769–72.
4. Zanoboni A, *et al.* Antiemetic efficacy and safety of L-sulpiride in patients with digestive and other disorders. *Curr Ther Res* 1987; **41:** 903–14.
5. De Jong J, *et al.* A randomized crossover clinical study on the effectiveness of L-sulpiride in the prevention of nausea and emesis induced by antiblastic chemotherapy. *Curr Ther Res* 1989; **46:** 974–9.
6. Pustorino S, *et al.* Effects of levo-sulpiride on the kinetics of gallbladder emptying and duodenal-gastric reflux in patients with idiopathic alkaline gastritis. *Curr Ther Res* 1989; **46:** 1110–18.
7. De Rossi S, *et al.* (−)Sulpiride in the radiologic examination of the gastrointestinal tract. *Curr Ther Res* 1990; **47:** 707–16.
8. Schiraldi GF, *et al.* Efficacy and safety of levosulpiride versus metoclopramide in patients with emesis induced by high doses of salmon calcitonin. *Curr Ther Res* 1993; **53:** 42–7.

Lactation. Drug therapy has been used occasionally to stimulate lactation in breast-feeding mothers, although mechanical stimulation of the nipple remains the primary method. Dopamine antagonists such as sulpiride can produce modest increases in breast milk production[1-3] although metoclopramide has been more widely used (see p.1240). However, there is concern about the presence of these drugs in breast milk. As sulpiride appears in breast milk in relatively large amounts and may be associated with adverse effects in the infant it has been recommended that it should not be used to enhance milk production.[4]

1. Aono T, *et al.* Effect of sulpiride on poor puerperal lactation. *Am J Obstet Gynecol* 1982; **143:** 927–32.
2. Ylikorkala O, *et al.* Sulpiride improves inadequate lactation. *Br Med J* 1982; **285:** 249–51.
3. Ylikorkala O, *et al.* Treatment of inadequate lactation with oral sulpiride and buccal oxytocin. *Obstet Gynecol* 1984; **63:** 57–60
4. Pons G, *et al.* Excretion of psychoactive drugs into breast milk: pharmacokinetic principles and recommendations. *Clin Pharmacokinet* 1994; **27:** 270–89.

Tourette's syndrome. When treatment is needed for tics and behavioural disturbances in Tourette's syndrome (p.636) dopamine antagonists such as the antipsychotics haloperidol or pimozide are most commonly used but sulpiride has also been tried.[1]

1. Robertson MM, *et al.* Management of Gilles de la Tourette syndrome using sulpiride. *Clin Neuropharmacol* 1990; **13:** 229–35.

Preparations

Proprietary Preparations (details are given in Part 3)
Aust.: Dogmatil; Meresa; ***Belg.:*** Dogmatil; ***Fr.:*** Aiglonyl; Dogmatil; Synedil; ***Ger.:*** Arminol; Desisulpid; Dogmatil; Meresa; Neogama; Sulp; ***Irl.:*** Dolmatil; ***Ital.:*** Championyl; Confidan†; Dobren; Equilid; Eusulpid†; Isnamide†; Levobren; Levopraid; Normum; Quiridil; ***Neth.:*** Dogmatil; ***S.Afr.:*** Depex; Eglonyl; Espiride; ***Spain:*** Digton; Dixibon†; Dogmatil; Guastil; Lebopride; Mirbanil†; Psicocen; Tepavil; ***Switz.:*** Dogmatil; ***UK:*** Dolmatil; Sulparex; Sulpitil.

Multi-ingredient: ***Spain:*** Ansium; Dogmagel†; Roter Complex; Sirodina; Tepazepan.

Sultopride Hydrochloride (7108-y)

Sultopride Hydrochloride *(rINNM).*

LIN-1418. *N*-(1-Ethylpyrrolidin-2-ylmethyl)-5-ethylsulphonyl-2-methoxybenzamide hydrochloride.

$C_{17}H_{26}N_2O_4S,HCl = 390.9.$

CAS — 53583-79-2 (sultopride); 23694-17-9 (sultopride hydrochloride).

Sultopride is a substituted benzamide with general properties similar to those of sulpiride (p.692). It is used in the emergency management of agitation in psychotic or aggressive patients (p.636) and in psychoses such as schizophrenia (p.637). It is given as the hydrochloride but doses are expressed in terms of the base. For acute agitation it may be given in doses of 400 to 800 mg daily by mouth or intramuscularly. In psychoses daily doses of 400 to 1600 mg have been given by mouth or intramuscularly. For chronically aggressive patients, maintenance doses of sultopride 400 to 600 mg daily may be given.

Ventricular arrhythmias, including torsade de pointes, have been reported. It has been recommended that sultopride should not be used in patients with bradycardia.

Porphyria. Sultopride was considered to be unsafe in patients with acute porphyria because it has been shown to be porphyrinogenic in *animals* or *in-vitro* systems.[1]

1. Moore MR, McColl KEL. *Porphyria: drug lists.* Glasgow: Porphyria Research Unit, University of Glasgow, 1991.

Preparations

Proprietary Preparations (details are given in Part 3)
Belg.: Barnetil; ***Fr.:*** Barnetil; ***Ital.:*** Barnotil.

Suriclone (13291-l)

Suriclone *(BAN, rINN).*

31264-RP; RP-31264. *(RS)*-6-(7-Chloro-1,8-naphthyridin-2-yl)-2,3,6,7-tetrahydro-7-oxo-5*H*-[1,4]dithi-ino[2,3-*c*]pyrrol-5-yl 4-methylpiperazine-1-carboxylate.

$C_{20}H_{20}ClN_5O_3S_2 = 478.0.$

CAS — 53813-83-5.

Suriclone is a cyclopyrrolone structurally related to zopiclone (p.699) and reported to possess similar properties. It has been tried as an anxiolytic.

References.

1. Saletu B, *et al.* Sleep laboratory studies on single dose effects of suriclone. *Br J Clin Pharmacol* 1990; **30:** 703–10.
2. Ansseau M, *et al.* Controlled comparison of the efficacy and safety of four doses of suriclone, diazepam, and placebo in generalized anxiety disorder. *Psychopharmacology (Berl)* 1991; **104:** 439–443.
3. Saletu B, *et al.* Pharmacokinetic anddynamic studies with a new anxiolytic, suriclone, utilizing EEG mapping and psychometry. *Br J Clin Pharmacol* 1994; **37:** 145–56.

Tandospirone Citrate (10442-w)

Tandospirone Citrate *(BANM, USAN, rINNM).*

Metanopirone Citrate; SM-3997 (tandospirone); SM-3997 (tandospirone citrate). (1R*,2S*,3R*,4S*)-*N*-{4-[4-(2-Pyrimidinyl)-1-piperazinyl]butyl}-2,3-norbornanedicarboximide citrate.

$C_{21}H_{29}N_5O_2,C_6H_8O_7 = 575.6.$

CAS — 87760-53-0 (tandospirone); 112457-95-1 (tandospirone citrate).

Tandospirone is structurally related to buspirone (p.643). It is used as the citrate as an anxiolytic.

Tandospirone is a partial agonist at serotonin (5-hydroxytryptamine, 5-HT) receptors of the $5\text{-}HT_{1A}$ subtype. For reference to the actions and potential uses of such drugs, see Buspirone Hydrochloride, p.644.

Temazepam (4072-c)

Temazepam *(BAN, USAN, rINN).*

ER-115; 3-Hydroxydiazepam; K-3917; Ro-5-5345; Temazepamum; Wy-3917. 7-Chloro-1,3-dihydro-3-hydroxy-1-methyl-5-phenyl-1,4-benzodiazepin-2-one.

$C_{16}H_{13}ClN_2O_2 = 300.7.$

CAS — 846-50-4.

Pharmacopoeias. In *Eur.* (see p.viii), *Pol.*, and *US.*

A white or almost white crystalline powder. Practically **insoluble** to very slightly soluble in water; sparingly soluble in alcohol; freely soluble in dichloromethane. **Protect** from light.

Dependence and Withdrawal, Adverse Effects, Treatment, and Precautions

As for Diazepam, p.661.

Abuse. Liquid-filled temazepam capsules (known on the street as 'eggs') were widely abused on the illicit drugs market, the liquid gel lending itself to intravenous administration.[1] This formulation was, therefore, replaced in the UK by tablets and semi-solid gel-filled capsules. The manufacturer of one such capsule formulation considers that the gel is difficult to inject even after heating or diluting in various solvents.[2] In spite of this there is evidence of abuse of these capsules[3] and there are reports of ischaemia, in some cases necessitating amputation.[4,5] The contents have also been subject to intra-arterial abuse.[6,7] The tablets may be also liable to abuse; there has been a report of death following intravenous injection of a solution containing crushed temazepam tablets.[8] The manufacturers of a temazepam elixir consider that, because of its viscosity and its low strength relative to the liquid in the capsules, it has a low potential for intravenous abuse.[9] Nonetheless, there have been reports[3] of some drug abusers injecting large quantities of diluted elixir to obtain an effect.

1. Farrell M, Strang J. Misuse of temazepam. *Br Med J* 1988; **297:** 1402.
2. Launchbury AP. Temazepam abuse. *Pharm J* 1990; **244:** 749.
3. Ruben SM, Morrison CL. Temazepam misuse in a group of injecting drug users. *Br J Addict* 1992; **87:** 1387–92.
4. Blair SD, *et al.* Leg ischaemia secondary to non-medical injection of temazepam. *Lancet* 1991; **338:** 1393–4.
5. Fox R, *et al.* Misuse of temazepam. *Br Med J* 1992; **305:** 253.
6. Scott RN, *et al.* Intra-arterial temazepam. *Br Med J* 1992; **304:** 1630.
7. Adiseshiah M, *et al.* Intra-arterial temazepam. *Br Med J* 1992; **304:** 1630.
8. Vella EJ, Edwards CW. Death from pulmonary microembolization after intravenous injection of temazepam. *Br Med J* 1993; **307:** 26.
9. Drake J, Ballard R. Misuse of temazepam. *Br Med J* 1988; **297:** 1402.

Effects on the skin. Generalised lichenoid drug eruption that had persisted for 5 months in an elderly patient receiving therapy including temazepam resolved within 10 days of discontinuing the benzodiazepine.[1]

1. Norris P, Sounex TS. Generalised lichenoid drug eruption associated with temazepam. *Br Med J* 1986; **293:** 510.

Hepatic impairment. In a study of 15 cirrhotic patients and 16 healthy subjects, liver disease had no significant effect on the pharmacokinetic parameters or pattern of elimination of temazepam.[1]

1. Ghabrial H, *et al.* The effects of age and chronic liver disease on the elimination of temazepam. *Eur J Clin Pharmacol* 1986; **30:** 93–7.

Withdrawal. For the purpose of withdrawal regimens, 10 mg of temazepam may be considered roughly equivalent to 5 mg of diazepam.

Interactions

As for Diazepam, p.663.

Pharmacokinetics

Temazepam is fairly readily absorbed from the gastro-intestinal tract, although the exact rate of absorption depends on the formulation. It is about 96% bound to plasma protein. Mean elimination half-lives of about 8 to 15 hours or longer have been reported. It is excreted in the urine in the form of its inactive glucuronide conjugate together with small amounts of the demethylated derivative, oxazepam, also in conjugated form.

A study of the effects of age and sex on the pharmacokinetics of temazepam.[1] The elimination half-life was significantly longer at 16.8 hours among 17 women given temazepam 30 mg compared with 12.3 hours among 15 men. The total clearance was also lower among women. After correction for differences in protein binding, unbound clearance was still lower in women than men but there was no significant effect of age on this parameter. Time to peak plasma concentration and volume of distribution were not affected by the age or sex of the subjects.

1. Divoll M, *et al.* Effect of age and gender on disposition of temazepam. *J Pharm Sci* 1981; **70:** 1104–7.

Absorption and plasma concentration. Various oral temazepam formulations have been available worldwide. These included powder-filled hard gelatin capsules, liquid-filled soft gelatin capsules, semi-solid gel-filled soft gelatin capsules, and an elixir. There has been considerable debate over the comparative absorption profiles of temazepam from these formulations which have, in some cases, been modified over the years. It should be noted that pharmacokinetic studies of temazepam do not always clearly state the formulation used and that there are as yet few studies on the newer formulations, particularly the gel-filled capsules.

Temazepam 30 mg was given as a premedicant to 80 patients undergoing surgery in the form of capsules [type not stated] or elixir.[1] Mean peak plasma concentrations of about 800 ng per mL occurred 30 minutes after administration of either formulation although there was wide interindividual variation in plasma concentrations. The evidence corresponded with previous suggestions that a plasma concentration of about 250 ng or more per mL was required to ensure sedation. The presence or absence of anxiety did not influence the absorption of the preparations.

1. Hosie HE, Nimmo WS. Temazepam absorption in patients before surgery. *Br J Anaesth* 1991; **66:** 20–4.

Distribution. BREAST MILK. Temazepam was detected in breast milk in one of 10 lactating mothers given temazepam as a bedtime sedative;[1] temazepam was given in a dose of 10 to 20 mg and milk concentrations were measured about 15 hours after a dose.

1. Lebedevs TH, *et al.* Excretion of temazepam in breast milk. *Br J Clin Pharmacol* 1992; **33:** 204–6.

CSF. A study in 13 male patients demonstrating a correlation between the unbound concentration of temazepam in plasma and the amount of temazepam detected in CSF.[1] The mean CSF to total plasma temazepam concentration ratio was 5.2.

1. Badcock NR. Plasma and cerebrospinal fluid concentrations of temazepam following oral drug administration. *Eur J Clin Pharmacol* 1990; **38:** 153–5.

Metabolism. References.

1. Locniskar A, Greenblatt DJ. Oxidative versus conjugative biotransformation of temazepam. *Biopharm Drug Dispos* 1990; **11:** 499–506.

Uses and Administration

Temazepam is a short-acting benzodiazepine with general properties similar to those of diazepam (p.666). It is used as a hypnotic in the short-term management of insomnia (p.638) and for premedication before surgical or investigative procedures (p.1220).

A usual dose for insomnia is 10 to 20 mg by mouth at night; exceptionally, doses up to 40 mg may be required. For premedication the usual dose is 20 to 40 mg by mouth given half to one hour beforehand. Children may be given temazepam in a dose of 1 mg per kg body-weight as premedication to a maximum total dose of 30 mg.

Temazepam should be given in reduced dosage to elderly or debilitated patients; one-half the usual adult dose, or less, may be sufficient.

Administration. For reference to the various formulations of oral temazepam that have been used, see Abuse under Dependence, Adverse Effects, Treatment, and Precautions, above.

Administration in the elderly. In one small study[1] a dose of temazepam of 7.5 mg was found to be adequate for the short-term management of insomnia in elderly patients.

1. Vgontzas AN, *et al.* Temazepam 7.5 mg: effects on sleep in elderly insomniacs. *Eur J Clin Pharmacol* 1994; **46:** 209–13.

Preparations

BP 1998: Temazepam Oral Solution;
USP 23: Temazepam Capsules.

Proprietary Preparations (details are given in Part 3)
Aust.: Levanxol; Remestan; ***Austral.:*** Euhypnos; Nomapam; Normison; Temaze; Temtabs; ***Belg.:*** Euhypnos; Levanxol; Normison; Temador; ***Canad.:*** Restoril; ***Fr.:*** Normison; ***Ger.:*** Neodorm SP; Norkotral Tema; Planum; Pronervon T; Remestan; Temazep; ***Irl.:*** Euhypnos; Normison; Nortem; Temazine; Tenox; ***Ital.:*** Euipnos; Normison; ***Neth.:*** Normison; ***S.Afr.:*** Euhypnos†; Levanxol†; Normison; Z-Pam; ***Spain:*** Dasuen†; ***Switz.:*** Normison; Planum; ***UK:*** Euhypnos; Normison; ***USA:*** Restoril; Temaz†.

Tetrabenazine (7109-j)

Tetrabenazine *(BAN, rINN)*.

Ro-1-9569. 1,3,4,6,7,11b-Hexahydro-3-isobutyl-9,10-dimethoxybenzo-[*a*]quinolizin-2-one.

$C_{19}H_{27}NO_3$ = 317.4.

CAS — 58-46-8.

Adverse Effects

Drowsiness is the most frequent side-effect of tetrabenazine. Orthostatic hypotension, symptoms of extrapyramidal dysfunction, gastro-intestinal disturbances, and depression may also occur. Overdosage has produced sedation, sweating, hypotension, and hypothermia.

Extrapyramidal effects. Dysphagia and choking were associated with tetrabenazine in the treatment of Huntington's chorea.[1] Fatal pneumonia, probably as a consequence of aspiration, had also been reported.

1. Snaith RP, Warren H de B. Treatment of Huntington's chorea with tetrabenazine. *Lancet* 1974; **i:** 413–14.

Neuroleptic malignant syndrome. A report of neuroleptic malignant syndrome following the use of tetrabenazine and metirosine in a patient with Huntington's chorea.[1]

1. Burke RE, *et al.* Neuroleptic malignant syndrome caused by dopamine-depleting drugs in a patient with Huntington disease. *Neurology* 1981; **31:** 1022–6.

Overdosage. A patient who swallowed approximately 1 g (40 tablets) of tetrabenazine became drowsy 2 hours later and marked sweating occurred.[1] Her state of consciousness improved after 24 hours and she talked rationally and gained full control of micturition after 72 hours.

1. Kidd DW, McLellan DL. Self-poisoning with tetrabenazine. *Br J Clin Pract* 1972; **26:** 179–80.

Precautions

Tetrabenazine may exacerbate the symptoms of parkinsonism. It may cause drowsiness; affected patients should not drive or operate machinery.

Interactions

Tetrabenazine has been reported to block the action of reserpine. It may also diminish the effects of levodopa and exacerbate the symptoms of parkinsonism. Use of tetrabenazine immediately following a course of an MAOI has been reported to lead to a state of confusion, restlessness, and disorientation; tetrabenazine should probably not be given with, or within 14 days of discontinuation of, such therapy.

Pharmacokinetics

Absorption of tetrabenazine is poor and erratic following oral administration. It appears to be extensively metabolised by first-pass metabolism. Its major metabolite, hydroxytetrabenazine, which is formed by reduction, is reported to be as active as the parent compound. It is excreted in the urine mainly in the form of metabolites.

Uses and Administration

Tetrabenazine is used in the management of movement disorders including chorea (p.636), ballism (p.636), dystonias (p.1141), and similar symptoms of CNS dysfunction.

Although a starting dose of 25 mg three times daily by mouth has been suggested, some authorities consider a dose of 12.5 mg twice daily to be more appropriate as it is less likely to cause excessive sedation. The dose may be gradually increased according to response up to a maximum of 200 mg daily. If the patient does not respond within 7 days of receiving the maximum dose further treatment with tetrabenazine is unlikely to be of benefit. An initial starting dose of 12.5 mg daily has been suggested for elderly patients.

Extrapyramidal disorders. In a long-term study[1] of the use of tetrabenazine in 400 patients with various movement disorders, those disorders which appeared to respond best to tetrabenazine included tardive dyskinesia, tardive dystonia, and Huntington's disease but benefit was also obtained in some patients with idiopathic dystonia, segmental myoclonus, and Tourette's syndrome. Others have commented that in severe dystonia unresponsive to other drugs a combination of tetrabenazine with benzhexol and pimozide is sometimes effective.[2]

1. Jankovic J, Beach J. Long-term effects of tetrabenazine in hyperkinetic movement disorders. *Neurology* 1997; **48:** 358–62.
2. Marsden CD, Quinn NP. The dystonias. *Br Med J* 1990; **300:** 139–44.

Preparations

Proprietary Preparations (details are given in Part 3)
Austral.: Nitoman; ***Irl.:*** Nitoman†; ***Norw.:*** Nitoman†; ***UK:*** Nitoman†.

Tetrazepam (13314-m)

Tetrazepam *(pINN)*.

CB-4261. 7-Chloro-5-(cyclohex-1-enyl)-1,3-dihydro-1-methyl-2*H*-1,4-benzodiazepin-2-one.

$C_{16}H_{17}ClN_2O$ = 288.8.

CAS — 10379-14-3.

Tetrazepam is a benzodiazepine with general properties similar to those of diazepam (p.661). It is used for its muscle relaxant properties in the treatment of muscle spasm (p.1303). The usual initial dose is 25 to 50 mg by mouth, increased if necessary to 150 mg or more daily.

Pharmacokinetics. Pharmacokinetic studies of tetrazepam.

1. Bun H, *et al.* Plasma levels and pharmacokinetics of single and multiple dose of tetrazepam in healthy volunteers. *Arzneimittelforschung* 1987; **37:** 199–202.

Porphyria. Tetrazepam was considered to be unsafe in patients with acute porphyria because it has been shown to be porphyrinogenic in *animals* or *in-vitro* systems.[1]

1. Moore M, McColl KEL. *Porphyria: drug lists*. Glasgow: Porphyria Research Unit, University of Glasgow, 1991.

Preparations

Proprietary Preparations (details are given in Part 3)
Aust.: Myolastan; ***Belg.:*** Myolastan; ***Fr.:*** Myolastan; ***Ger.:*** Mobiforton; Musapam; Musaril; Muskelat; Myospasmal; Rilex; Tepam; Tethexal; Tetra-saar; Tetramdura; Tetrazep; ***Spain:*** Myolastan.

Thioproperazine Mesylate (7113-w)

Thioproperazine Mesylate *(BANM)*.

Thioproperazine Mesilate *(rINNM)*; RP-7843; SKF-5883; Thioproperazine Dimethanesulphonate; Thioproperazine Methanesulphonate. *NN*-Dimethyl-10-[3-(4-methylpiperazin-1-yl)propyl]phenothiazine-2-sulphonamide dimethanesulphonate.

$C_{22}H_{30}N_4O_2S_2,2CH_4O_3S = 638.8$.

CAS — 316-81-4 (thioproperazine); 2347-80-0 (thioproperazine mesylate).

Pharmacopoeias. In *Fr.*

Thioproperazine is a phenothiazine with general properties similar to those of chlorpromazine (p.649). It has a piperazine side-chain. It is used in the treatment of schizophrenia (p.637), mania (p.273), and other psychoses. Thioproperazine is given as the mesylate in initial doses of the equivalent of 5 mg of thioproperazine daily, increased as necessary; the usual effective dosage is 30 to 40 mg daily. In severe or resistant cases doses of 90 mg or more daily have been given.

Preparations

Proprietary Preparations (details are given in Part 3)
Belg.: Majeptil; ***Canad.:*** Majeptil; ***Fr.:*** Majeptil; ***Spain:*** Majeptil.

Thioridazine (7114-e)

Thioridazine *(BAN, USAN, rINN)*.

TP-21. 10-[2-(1-Methyl-2-piperidyl)ethyl]-2-methylthiophenothiazine.

$C_{21}H_{26}N_2S_2 = 370.6$.

CAS — 50-52-2.

Pharmacopoeias. In *Br., Fr., Swiss,* and *US.*

A white or slightly yellow crystalline or micronised powder; odourless or with a faint odour. Thioridazine 100 mg is approximately equivalent to 110 mg of thioridazine hydrochloride. Practically **insoluble** in water; freely soluble in dehydrated alcohol and in ether; very soluble in chloroform. **Protect** from light.

Thioridazine Hydrochloride (7115-l)

Thioridazine Hydrochloride *(BANM, rINNM)*.

Thioridazini Hydrochloridum.

$C_{21}H_{26}N_2S_2,HCl = 407.0$.

CAS — 130-61-0.

Pharmacopoeias. In *Eur.* (see p.viii), *Jpn, Pol.,* and *US.*

A white to slightly yellow crystalline powder with a slight odour.

Freely **soluble** in water, in chloroform, and in methyl alcohol; soluble in alcohol; practically insoluble in ether. A 1% solution in water has a pH of 4.2 to 5.2. **Store** in airtight containers. Protect from light.

Incompatibility. For a warning about incompatibility between thioridazine hydrochloride solution (Mellaril) and carbamazepine suspension (Tegretol), see p.339.

Adverse Effects and Treatment

As for Chlorpromazine, p.649.

Thioridazine has been associated with a higher incidence of antimuscarinic effects, but lower incidence of extrapyramidal symptoms than chlorpromazine. It may also be less sedating. However, it is more likely to induce hypotension and there is possibly an increased risk of cardiotoxicity and prolongation of the QT interval. Sexual dysfunction also appears to be more frequent with thioridazine.

Pigmentary retinopathy characterised by diminution of visual acuity, brownish colouring of vision, and impairment of night vision has been observed particularly in patients taking large doses.

Convulsions. For mention of thioridazine as one of the antipsychotics suitable for patients at risk of seizures, see p.649.

Hypersensitivity. Pruritus and erythematous rash on the genitals of a woman following sexual intercourse were found to be due to thioridazine present in the seminal fluid of her husband, who was receiving 100 mg daily at night.[1]

1. Sell MB. Sensitization to thioridazine through sexual intercourse. *Am J Psychiatry* 1985; **142:** 271–2.

Overdosage. Rhabdomyolysis has been reported in a patient after overdosage with thioridazine.[1] Twenty-four hours after taking 9.4 g of thioridazine the patient presented with difficulty in moving and speaking. On examination he had swelling and tenderness over his upper arms, thighs, and calves. Ataxia and transient dysarthria were attributed to generalised muscle weakness. Other effects were consistent with antimuscarinic effects of thioridazine. He had no signs of neuroleptic malignant syndrome but his urine contained myoglobin. The patient was treated with gastric lavage, activated charcoal, and rehydration. Serum biochemistry returned to normal over one week and the muscle tenderness and weakness disappeared.

1. Nankivell BJ, *et al.* Rhabdomyolysis induced by thioridazine. *Br Med J* 1994; **309:** 378.

Precautions

As for Chlorpromazine, p.652.

Porphyria. Thioridazine has been associated with clinical exacerbations of porphyria and is considered unsafe in porphyric patients.[1]

1. Moore MR, McColl KEL. *Porphyria: drug lists*. Glasgow: Porphyria Research Unit, University of Glasgow, 1991.

Interactions

As for Chlorpromazine, p.652. Concomitant use of thioridazine with other drugs which prolong the QT interval should be avoided.

Pharmacokinetics

The pharmacokinetics of thioridazine appear to be generally similar to those of chlorpromazine (p.654). The principal active metabolite of thioridazine is mesoridazine (p.678); the metabolite, sulforidazine, also has some activity. Thioridazine and its active metabolites are reported to be highly bound to plasma proteins. The plasma half-life of thioridazine has been estimated to range from about 6 to over 40 hours.

References.

1. Mårtensson E, Roos B-E. Serum levels of thioridazine in psychiatric patients and healthy volunteers. *Eur J Clin Pharmacol* 1973; **6:** 181–6.
2. Axelsson R, Mårtensson E. Serum concentration and elimination from serum of thioridazine in psychiatric patients. *Curr Ther Res* 1976; **19:** 242–65.

Metabolism. In 10 psychiatric patients stabilised on thioridazine, therapy was replaced by equipotent doses of the side-chain sulphoxide (mesoridazine) and side-chain sulphone (sulforidazine) metabolites of thioridazine.[1] Both metabolites were shown to have an antipsychotic effect, the dose of each required being about two-thirds that of thioridazine. The serum half-lives were thioridazine 21 hours, mesoridazine 16 hours, and sulforidazine 13 hours. Apathy, depression, and restlessness gradually developed during treatment with the 2 metabolites and they could not be used for any length of time. Extrapyramidal symptoms, hypersalivation, and drowsiness were more common with the metabolites; 2 patients had epileptic seizures, and one receiving sulforidazine developed probable cholestatic jaundice.

There is some evidence that the metabolism of thioridazine is influenced by debrisoquine hydroxylation phenotype.[2] A single-dose study in 19 healthy male subjects demonstrated slower formation of mesoridazine, and hence higher serum-thioridazine concentrations in poor debrisoquine hydroxylators compared with extensive hydroxylators. Formation of thioridazine ring-sulphoxide appeared to be compensatorily increased in slow hydroxylators. The clinical importance of these findings requires evaluation.

1. Axelsson R. On the serum concentrations and antipsychotic effects of thioridazine, thioridazine side-chain sulfoxide and thioridazine side-chain sulfone, in chronic psychotic patients. *Curr Ther Res* 1977; **21:** 587–605.
2. von Bahr C, *et al.* Plasma levels of thioridazine and metabolites are influenced by the debrisoquin hydroxylation phenotype. *Clin Pharmacol Ther* 1991; **49:** 234–40.

Uses and Administration

Thioridazine is a phenothiazine with general properties similar to those of chlorpromazine (p.654). It has a piperidine side-chain and, unlike chlorpromazine, has little antiemetic activity. Thioridazine is used in a variety of psychiatric disorders including schizophrenia (p.637), mania (p.273), severe anxiety (p.635), and behaviour disturbances (p.636).

Thioridazine is administered by mouth as the hydrochloride or the base, but doses are normally given in terms of the hydrochloride. In the UK, oral suspensions contain 25 mg of thioridazine base (approximately equivalent to 27.5 mg of thioridazine hydrochloride) per unit dosage, or 100 mg of thioridazine base (approximately equivalent to 110 mg of thioridazine hydrochloride) per unit dosage, whereas other oral liquid preparations contain 27.5 mg of thioridazine hydrochloride per unit dosage and the tablets contain 10, 25, 50 or 100 mg of thioridazine hydrochloride.

The usual dosage range for the treatment of schizophrenia, mania, and other psychoses, is 150 to 600 mg of the hydrochloride daily, and may be given in divided doses. Doses of up to 800 mg daily should only be given for periods of up to 4 weeks under close supervision. Doses of 75 to 200 mg daily have been used for the short-term management of agitated or violent behaviour, and doses of 30 to 100 mg daily for severe anxiety, agitation, and restlessness in the elderly.

Thioridazine is sometimes indicated for children with severe behavioural disorders. A dose equivalent to 1 mg of the hydrochloride per kg bodyweight daily has been suggested for children aged 1 to 5 years. Children over 5 years of age may be given 75 to 150 mg daily, although up to 300 mg daily may be occasionally required. Thioridazine should be given in reduced dosage to elderly patients; dosage increases should be more gradual.

Chorea. Antipsychotics, including thioridazine, have some action against choreiform movements as well as being of use to control the behavioural disturbances of Huntington's chorea (p.636).

Taste disorders. For reference to the use of thioridazine in the treatment of taste disorders, see Chlorpromazine, p.656.

Preparations

BP 1998: Thioridazine Oral Solution; Thioridazine Oral Suspension; Thioridazine Tablets;
USP 23: Thioridazine Hydrochloride Oral Solution; Thioridazine Hydrochloride Tablets; Thioridazine Oral Suspension.

Proprietary Preparations (details are given in Part 3)
Aust.: Melleretten; Melleril; ***Austral.:*** Aldazine; Melleril; ***Belg.:*** Melleril; ***Canad.:*** Mellaril; Novo-Ridazine; ***Fr.:*** Melleril; ***Ger.:*** Melleretten; Melleril; ***Irl.:*** Melleril; Melzine; Thiozine; ***Ital.:*** Mellerette; Melleril; ***Neth.:*** Melleretten; Melleril; ***Norw.:*** Melleril; ***S.Afr.:*** Melleril; Ridazine; ***Spain:*** Meleril; ***Swed.:*** Mallorol; ***Switz.:*** Mellerettes; Melleril; ***UK:*** Melleril; Rideril; ***USA:*** Mellaril.

Multi-ingredient: ***Ital.:*** Visergil; ***Spain:*** Visergil.

Thiothixene (7116-y)

Thiothixene *(BAN, USAN)*.

Tiotixene *(rINN)*; NSC-108165; P-4657B. *(Z)-NN*-Dimethyl-9-[3-(4-methylpiperazin-1-yl)propylidene]thioxanthene-2-sulphonamide.

$C_{23}H_{29}N_3O_2S_2 = 443.6$.

CAS — 5591-45-7; 3313-26-6 (Z-isomer).

Pharmacopoeias. In *US.*

A white to tan-coloured almost odourless crystalline powder. Thiothixene 1 mg is approximately equivalent to 1.25 mg of thiothixene hydrochloride (dihydrate) or to 1.16 mg of the anhydrous hydrochloride. Practically **insoluble** in water; soluble 1 in 110 of dehydrated alcohol, 1 in 2 of chloroform, and 1 in 120 of ether; slightly soluble in acetone and in methyl alcohol. **Store** in airtight containers. Protect from light.

Thiothixene Hydrochloride (7117-j)

Thiothixene Hydrochloride *(BANM, USAN)*.

Tiotixene Hydrochloride *(rINNM)*; CP-12252-1.

$C_{23}H_{29}N_3O_2S_2,2HCl,2H_2O = 552.6$.

CAS — 58513-59-0 (anhydrous); 49746-04-5 (anhydrous, Z-isomer); 22189-31-7 (dihydrate); 49746-09-0 (dihydrate, Z-isomer).

Pharmacopoeias. In *US,* which permits both the dihydrate and the anhydrous form ($C_{23}H_{29}N_3O_2S_2,2HCl = 516.5$).

A white or almost white crystalline powder with a slight odour. **Soluble** 1 in 8 of water, 1 in 270 of dehydrated alcohol, and 1 in 280 of chloroform; practically insoluble in acetone and ether. **Store** in airtight containers. Protect from light.

A combination of the stabilisers hydroxyquinoline sulphate and vanillin could protect thiothixene from photodegradation.[1]

1. Thoma K, Klimek R. Photostabilization of drugs in dosage forms without protection from packaging materials. *Int J Pharmaceutics* 1991; **67:** 169–75.

Adverse Effects, Treatment, and Precautions

As for Chlorpromazine, p.649. Thiothixene is less likely to cause sedation but extrapyramidal disorders are more frequent.

Interactions

As for Chlorpromazine, p.652.

Pharmacokinetics

For an account of the pharmacokinetics of a thioxanthene, see Flupenthixol, p.671.

In 15 adequately controlled schizophrenic patients receiving thiothixene 15 to 60 mg daily in 2, 3, or 4 divided doses by mouth, plasma concentrations were found to be in the relatively narrow range of 10 to 22.5 ng per mL 126 to 150 minutes after the last daily dose despite the fourfold difference in dosage.[1] Investigations in a further 5 patients indicated that peak plasma concentrations were obtained about 1 to 3 hours after a dose, indicating rapid absorption with an absorption half-time of about 30 minutes. There was an early plasma half-life of about 210 minutes and a late half-life of about 34 hours; resurgence of drug concentrations in some subjects might have been due to enterohepatic recycling.

1. Hobbs DC, *et al.* Pharmacokinetics of thiothixene in man. *Clin Pharmacol Ther* 1974; **16:** 473–8.

Metabolism. A study[1] indicating that thiothixene may induce its own metabolism.

1. Bergling R, *et al.* Plasma levels and clinical effects of thioridazine and thiothixene. *J Clin Pharmacol* 1975; **15:** 178–86.

Uses and Administration

Thiothixene is a thioxanthene antipsychotic with general properties similar to those of the phenothiazine, chlorpromazine (p.654). It has a piperazine side-chain. It is used in the treatment of various psychoses including schizophrenia (p.637). Thiothixene is given by mouth as the base or hydrochloride and sometimes intramuscularly as the hydrochloride. Doses are expressed in terms of the base.

The usual initial dose is 2 mg three times daily by mouth (or 5 mg twice daily in more severe conditions) gradually increasing to 20 to 30 mg daily if necessary; once-daily dosage may be adequate. In severe or resistant psychoses doses of up to 60 mg daily may be given. The usual initial intramuscular dose is 4 mg two to four times daily increased if necessary to a maximum of 30 mg daily.

Thiothixene should be given in reduced dosage to elderly patients.

Preparations

USP 23: Thiothixene Capsules; Thiothixene Hydrochloride for Injection; Thiothixene Hydrochloride Injection; Thiothixene Hydrochloride Oral Solution.

Proprietary Preparations (details are given in Part 3)
Austral.: Navane; ***Canad.:*** Navane; ***Ger.:*** Orbinamon†; ***Neth.:*** Navane; ***Swed.:*** Navane†; ***USA:*** Navane.

Tiapride Hydrochloride (13339-l)

Tiapride Hydrochloride *(BAN, rINNM).*

FLO-1347. *N*-(2-Diethylaminoethyl)-2-methoxy-5-methylsulphonylbenzamide hydrochloride.

$C_{15}H_{24}N_2O_4S,HCl$ = 364.9.

CAS — 51012-32-9 (tiapride); 51012-33-0 (tiapride hydrochloride).

Adverse Effects, Treatment, and Precautions

As for Chlorpromazine, p.649.

Interactions

As for Chlorpromazine, p.652.

Pharmacokinetics

Tiapride is rapidly absorbed following oral administration and excreted largely unchanged in the urine. The plasma half-life is reported to range from 3 to 4 hours.

A study of the steady-state pharmacokinetics of tiapride in 5 elderly patients with tardive dyskinesia, and in 2 patients with Huntington's chorea.[1] All patients received tiapride 100 mg three times daily by mouth for 7 days. The mean peak plasma concentration of tiapride was 1.47 μg per mL, achieved a mean of 1.4 hours after dosing, and the mean elimination half-life was 3.8 hours. These values did not differ significantly from those previously reported in younger healthy subjects, although renal clearance was slightly lower in these patients. About half of the dose of tiapride was excreted unchanged by the kidney; a metabolite, probably *N*-monodesethyltiapride was detected in the urine but its identity was not confirmed.

1. Roos RAC, *et al.* Pharmacokinetics of tiapride in patients with tardive dyskinesia and Huntington's disease. *Eur J Clin Pharmacol* 1986; **31:** 191–4.

Uses and Administration

Tiapride is a substituted benzamide with general properties similar to those of sulpiride (p.693).

It is mainly used in the management of behaviour disorders and to treat dyskinesias. It is usually given as tiapride hydrochloride with doses expressed in terms of the equivalent amount of tiapride. Doses of 200 to 400 mg daily by mouth have usually been given, although higher daily doses have been used, in particular in the management of dyskinesias. Tiapride hydrochloride has also been given by intramuscular or intravenous injection.

Disturbed behaviour. For a discussion of the management of disturbed behaviour including limitations on the use of antipsychotics, see p.636.

References.

1. Gutzmann H, *et al.* Measuring the efficacy of psychopharmacological treatment of psychomotoric restlessness in dementia: clinical evaluation of tiapride. *Pharmacopsychiatry* 1997; **30:** 6–11.

Extrapyramidal disorders. For reference to the use of tiapride in suppressing the adverse effects of levodopa on respiration, see p.1138.

Tiapride has been tried in the treatment of antipsychotic-induced tardive dyskinesia, but as with all antipsychotics improvement may only be short-term. For a discussion of the management of tardive dyskinesias covering the use of antipsychotics, see Extrapyramidal Disorders under the Adverse Effects of Chlorpromazine on p.650.

Tiapride has also been tried in the treatment of Tourette's syndrome (p.636).

CHOREA. Antipsychotics have some action against choreiform movements as well as being of use to control the behavioural disturbances of Huntington's chorea. For a discussion of the management of various choreas, see p.636. Disappointing results were reported in a crossover study of tiapride 100 mg three times daily, compared with placebo, in 22 patients with Huntington's chorea.[1] However, tiapride in doses of 3 g daily by mouth was superior to placebo in relieving the symptoms of Huntington's chorea in a crossover study completed by 23 patients.[2] Treatment with high-dose tiapride was generally well-tolerated, although associated with a higher incidence of sedation and extrapyramidal signs than placebo.

1. Roos RAC, *et al.* Tiapride in the treatment of Huntington's chorea. *Acta Neurol Scand* 1982; **65:** 45–50.
2. Deroover J, *et al.* Tiapride versus placebo: a double-blind comparative study in the management of Huntington's chorea. *Curr Med Res Opin* 1984; **9:** 329–38.

Withdrawal syndromes. ALCOHOL. A review[1] concluded that the role of tiapride in acute alcohol withdrawal (p.1099) is likely to be limited as patients at risk of severe reactions would still require adjunct therapy for the control of hallucinations and seizures. Following detoxification tiapride may help to alleviate distress, improve abstinence and drinking behaviour, and facilitate reintegration within society.[2] However, the potential risk of tardive dyskinesias at the dosage used (300 mg daily) still needed to be evaluated and patients would require medical supervision.[1]

1. Peters DH, Faulds D. Tiapride: a review of its pharmacology and therapeutic potential in the management of alcohol dependence syndrome. *Drugs* 1994; **47:** 1010–32.
2. Shaw GK, *et al.* Tiapride in the prevention of relapse in recently detoxified alcoholics. *Br J Psychiatry* 1994; **165:** 515–23.

Preparations

Proprietary Preparations (details are given in Part 3)
Aust.: Delpral; ***Belg.:*** Tiapridal; ***Fr.:*** Equilium; Tiapridal; ***Ger.:*** Tiapridex; ***Ital.:*** Italprid; Luxoben; Sereprile; ***Neth.:*** Tiapridal; ***Spain:*** Porfanil†; Tiaprizal; ***Switz.:*** Tiapridal.

Timiperone (17010-t)

Timiperone *(rINN).*

DD-3480. 4′-Fluoro-4-[4-(2-thioxo-1-benzimidazolinyl)piperidino]butyrophenone.

$C_{22}H_{24}FN_3OS$ = 397.5.

CAS — 57648-21-2.

Timiperone is a butyrophenone with general properties similar to those of haloperidol (p.673). It has been used by mouth in the treatment of schizophrenia. Timiperone has also been given by injection.

Preparations

Proprietary Preparations (details are given in Part 3)
Jpn: Tolopelon†.

Tofisopam (7118-z)

Tofisopam *(rINN).*

EGYT-341; Tofizopam. 1-(3,4-Dimethoxyphenyl)-5-ethyl-7,8-dimethoxy-4-methyl-5*H*-2,3-benzodiazepine.

$C_{22}H_{26}N_2O_4$ = 382.5.

CAS — 22345-47-7.

Pharmacopoeias. In *Jpn.*

Tofisopam is a 2,3-benzodiazepine related structurally to the 1,4-benzodiazepines such as diazepam (p.661) and sharing some of the same actions. It is reported, however, to be largely lacking in the sedative, anticonvulsant, and muscle relaxant properties of the conventional benzodiazepines.

In the short-term treatment of anxiety disorders (p.635) it has been given in a usual dose of 150 mg daily by mouth in divided doses.

Tofisopam should be given in reduced dosage to elderly patients.

References.

1. Bond A, Lader M. A comparison of the psychotropic profiles of tofisopam and diazepam. *Eur J Clin Pharmacol* 1982; **22:** 137–42.

Preparations

Proprietary Preparations (details are given in Part 3)
Fr.: Seriel†; ***Hung.:*** Grandaxin; ***Jpn:*** Grandaxin†.

Triazolam (4073-k)

Triazolam *(BAN, USAN, rINN).*

Clorazolam; U-33030. 8-Chloro-6-(2-chlorophenyl)-1-methyl-4*H*-[1,2,4]triazolo[4,3-*a*][1,4]benzodiazepine.

$C_{17}H_{12}Cl_2N_4$ = 343.2.

CAS — 28911-01-5.

Pharmacopoeias. In *US.*

A white to off-white, practically odourless, crystalline powder. Practically **insoluble** in water and in ether; soluble 1 in 1000 of alcohol, 1 in 25 of chloroform, and 1 in 600 of 0.1N hydrochloric acid.

Dependence and Withdrawal, Adverse Effects, and Treatment

As for Diazepam, p.661.

Effects on the liver. A 44-year-old man developed severe pruritus with jaundice which subsequently proved fatal. Liver histology showed intense cholestasis. Triazolam was considered to be the most likely precipitant.[1]

1. Cobden I, *et al.* Fatal intrahepatic cholestasis associated with triazolam. *Postgrad Med J* 1981; **57:** 730–1.

Effects on mental function. The effects of triazolam on mental function have been controversial since van der Kroef first described in 1979 a range of symptoms including anxiety, amnesia, depersonalisation and derealisation, depression, paranoia, and severe suicidal tendencies that he had observed in 25 patients and attributed to the administration of triazolam.[1] This led to suspension of triazolam in the Netherlands (re-approved in 1990) and removal of the 1-mg tablet from other markets. Continued reporting of similar symptoms of cognitive impairment with triazolam resulted in discontinuation of the 500-μg dosage form in several countries in 1987 and 1988 and in a gradual reduction of recommended dosage from 1 mg at night down to 125 to 250 μg at night. Triazolam was withdrawn from the UK[2] and some other markets in 1991. Opinion still remains divided over the adverse effects of triazolam, the main issues being its propensity to cause side-effects relative to other benzodiazepines and whether its risk-benefit ratio is acceptable to justify its continued use.[3,4] Bixler *et al.*[5] have reviewed spontaneous adverse effects reported to the USA Food and Drug Administration for triazolam, temazepam, and flurazepam. Daytime sedation was noted with all three, but triazolam caused more agitation, confusion, hallucinations, and amnesia. Such effects occurred frequently with the 250-μg dose as well as with the 500-μg dose. Similar results were obtained after analysis of reports for triazolam and temazepam in the first 7 years of marketing, although the possibility that selection factors were producing higher reporting rates for triazolam could not be entirely excluded.[6] Adam and Oswald[7] gave triazolam 500 μg, lormetazepam 2 mg, or placebo, to groups of 40 patients for 25 nights and observed the greatest frequency of daytime anxiety, panic, derealisation, and paranoia with triazolam. Bixler *et al.*[8] found a greater total number of reports of memory impairment or amnesia after nightly administration of triazolam 500 μg compared with temazepam 30 mg. Triazolam also impaired delayed, but not immediate, memory recall. Similar cases of memory impairment occurring with triazolam at doses of 125 and 250 μg have reportedly been submitted to the UK Committee on Safety of Medicines.[2] The emergence of daytime symptoms after more than a few days' treatment with triazolam could be attributed to rebound or withdrawal phenomena occurring as a result of rapid elimination of the drug.

As regards the risk-benefit ratio of triazolam some workers have questioned the hypnotic efficacy of the drug at a dose of 250 μg and consider that reduction of the dose has decreased efficacy more than side-effects.[3]

In defence of triazolam, the FDA and the manufacturers (Upjohn) have considered epidemiological studies which, unlike the FDA spontaneous reporting scheme, have been unable to demonstrate a substantial difference in its adverse effects compared with other benzodiazepines except, perhaps, in the incidence of amnesia.[9] Retrospective studies[10,11] claiming similar findings have been the subject of criticism.[12-14] Other workers have cited studies indicating benefit of triazolam 250 μg for the treatment of insomnia.[15] A recent review by the US Institute of Medicine found that triazolam was safe when given in a dose of 250 μg daily for 7 to 10 days but called for studies of lower doses and of long-term use.[16]

Triazolam (and alprazolam) are inhibitors of platelet-activating factor (PAF) *in vitro*. It has been suggested that some of the adverse effects of triazolam, particularly effects such as skin blistering, pharyngitis, glossitis, vasculitis, asthma, and facial oedema may be withdrawal effects derived from PAF mechanisms.[17] This hypothesis has, however, been criticised.[18-22]

1. Van der Kroef C. Reactions to triazolam. *Lancet* 1979; **ii:** 526.
2. Anonymous. The sudden withdrawal of triazolam—reasons and consequences. *Drug Ther Bull* 1991; **29:** 89–90.
3. O'Donovan MC, McGuffin P. Short acting benzodiazepines. *Br Med J* 1993; **306:** 945–6.
4. Ghaeli P, *et al.* Triazolam treatment controversy. *Ann Pharmacother* 1994; **28:** 1038–40.
5. Bixler EO, *et al.* Adverse reactions to benzodiazepine hypnotics: spontaneous reporting system. *Pharmacology* 1987; **35:** 286–300.
6. Wysowski DK, Barash D. Adverse behavioral reactions attributed to triazolam in the Food and Drug Administration's spontaneous reporting system. *Arch Intern Med* 1991; **151:** 2003–8.
7. Adam K, Oswald I. Can a rapidly-eliminated hypnotic cause daytime anxiety? *Pharmacopsychiatry* 1989; **22:** 115–19.
8. Bixler EO, *et al.* Next-day memory impairment with triazolam use. *Lancet* 1991; **337:** 827–31.
9. Drucker RF, MacLeod N. Benzodiazepines. *Pharm J* 1989; **243:** 508.
10. Hindmarch I, *et al.* Adverse events after triazolam substitution. *Lancet* 1993; **341:** 55.
11. Rothschild AJ, *et al.* Triazolam and disinhibition. *Lancet* 1993; **341:** 186.
12. Hawley CJ, *et al.* Adverse events after triazolam substitution. *Lancet* 1993; **341:** 567.
13. Vela-Buena A. Adverse events after triazolam substitution. *Lancet* 1993; **341:** 567.
14. Kales A, *et al.* Adverse events after triazolam substitution. *Lancet* 1993; **341:** 567–8.
15. Gillin JC, Byerley WF. Diagnosis and management of insomnia. *N Engl J Med* 1990; **323:** 487.
16. Ault A. FDA advisers find no major Halcion dangers. *Lancet* 1997; **350:** 1760.
17. Adam K, Oswald I. Possible mechanism for adverse reactions to triazolam. *Lancet* 1991; **338:** 1157.
18. Roberts N, Barnes P. Triazolam and PAF. *Lancet* 1991; **338:** 1459.
19. Lenox RH. Triazolam and PAF. *Lancet* 1991; **338:** 1459–60.
20. Jonas JM. Triazolam and PAF inhibition. *Lancet* 1992; **339:** 57.
21. Kempe ER, Blank B. Triazolam and PAF inhibition. *Lancet* 1992; **339:** 57.
22. Adam A, Oswald I. Triazolam and platelet-aggregating factor. *Lancet* 1992; **339:** 186–7.

Effects on the skin. Evidence presented by Adam and Oswald for triazolam-induced PAF inhibition (see references cited in Effects on Mental Function, above) include reports of blistering, oedema, and vasculitis.

Precautions

As for Diazepam, p.662.

Hepatic impairment. Cirrhosis decreased the apparent oral clearance of triazolam to an extent depending on the severity of the liver disease.[1] An initial dose of 125 μg was suggested for patients with severe liver dysfunction. It was suggested that the relative lack of effect that mild to moderate cirrhosis had on the metabolism of oral triazolam might be due to some first-pass metabolism occurring in the intestinal wall.[2]

1. Kroboth PD, *et al.* Nighttime dosing of triazolam in patients with liver disease and normal subjects: kinetics and daytime effects. *J Clin Pharmacol* 1987; **27:** 555–60.
2. Robin DW, *et al.* Triazolam in cirrhosis: pharmacokinetics and pharmacodynamics. *Clin Pharmacol Ther* 1993; **54:** 630–7.

Renal impairment. Peak plasma-triazolam concentrations were lower in 11 dialysis patients compared with 11 controls.[1] It was postulated that a relatively high basal gastric acid secretion in dialysis patients could result in hydrolysis and opening of the ring structure of triazolam effectively reducing its systemic availability. Administration of an antacid could reverse this effect. Renal failure had no other effect on the pharmacokinetics of triazolam which could probably be administered in usual doses.

1. Kroboth PD, *et al.* Effects of end stage renal disease and aluminium hydroxide on triazolam pharmacokinetics. *Br J Clin Pharmacol* 1985; **19:** 839–42.

Interactions

As for Diazepam, p.663.

Pharmacokinetics

Triazolam is rapidly and nearly completely absorbed from the gastro-intestinal tract, peak plasma concentrations being achieved within 2 hours of administration by mouth. Triazolam has a plasma elimination half-life ranging from 1.5 to 5.5 hours. It is reported to be about 89% bound to plasma proteins. Hydroxylation of triazolam in the liver is mediated by the cytochrome P450 isozyme CYP3A4. Triazolam is excreted in the urine mainly in the form of its conjugated metabolites with only small amounts appearing unchanged.

Reviews of the pharmacokinetics of triazolam.

1. Garzone PD, Kroboth PD. Pharmacokinetics of the newer benzodiazepines. *Clin Pharmacokinet* 1989; **16:** 337–64.

Uses and Administration

Triazolam is a short-acting benzodiazepine with general properties similar to those of diazepam (p.666). It is used as a hypnotic in the short-term management of insomnia (p.638) in doses of 125 to 250 μg at night; initial doses of 125 μg at night have been suggested for elderly subjects, increased to 250 μg only if necessary. Doses of up to 500 μg at night have been used for resistant cases; however, these may be associated with an increased risk of severe adverse effects (see Effects on Mental Function, above).

Preparations

USP 23: Triazolam Tablets.

Proprietary Preparations (details are given in Part 3)

Aust.: Halcion; ***Austral.:*** Halcion; ***Belg.:*** Halcion; ***Canad.:*** Apo-Triazo; Halcion; Novo-Triolam; Nu-Triazo†; ***Fr.:*** Halcion; ***Ger.:*** Halcion; ***Irl.:*** Halcion; Trilam; ***Ital.:*** Halcion; Songar; ***Neth.:*** Halcion; ***S.Afr.:*** Halcion; ***Spain:*** Halcion; Novodorm†; ***Swed.:*** Dumozolam†; Halcion; ***Switz.:*** Halcion; ***USA:*** Halcion.

Triclofos Sodium (4074-a)

Triclofos Sodium *(BANM, USAN, pINNM).*

Sch-10159; Sodium Triclofos. Sodium 2,2,2-trichloroethyl hydrogen orthophosphate.

$C_2H_3Cl_3NaO_4P$ = 251.4.

CAS — 306-52-5 (triclofos); 7246-20-0 (triclofos sodium).

Pharmacopoeias. In *Br.* and *Jpn.*

A white or almost white, odourless or almost odourless, hygroscopic powder. Freely **soluble** in water; slightly soluble in alcohol; practically insoluble in ether. A 2% solution in water has a pH of 3.0 to 4.5.

Dependence and Withdrawal, Adverse Effects, Treatment, and Precautions

As for Chloral Hydrate, p.645 but causes fewer gastro-intestinal disturbances.

Triclofos sodium is not corrosive to skin and mucous membranes.

Interactions

As for Chloral Hydrate, p.646.

Pharmacokinetics

Triclofos sodium is rapidly hydrolysed to trichloroethanol. For the distribution and fate of trichloroethanol, see Chloral Hydrate, p.646.

Uses and Administration

Triclofos sodium has hypnotic and sedative actions similar to those of chloral hydrate (p.646) but it is more palatable and relatively free from the tendency to cause gastric irritation. It is given by mouth in the short-term management of insomnia (p.638).

The usual adult dose as a hypnotic is 1 g (therapeutically equivalent to about 600 mg of chloral hydrate) at night, but up to 2 g may be necessary in some patients. A suggested hypnotic dose for children up to 1 year of age is 25 to 30 mg per kg body-weight; children aged 1 to 5 years may be given single doses of 250 to 500 mg, and children aged 6 to 12 years may be given single doses of 0.5 to 1 g.

Preparations

BP 1998: Triclofos Oral Solution.

Proprietary Preparations (details are given in Part 3)

Irl.: Tricloryl; ***S.Afr.:*** Tricloryl†.

Trifluoperazine Hydrochloride

(7120-s)

Trifluoperazine Hydrochloride *(BANM, rINNM).*

Trifluoperazini Hydrochloridum; Triphthazinum. 10-[3-(4-Methylpiperazin-1-yl)propyl]-2-trifluoromethylphenothiazine dihydrochloride.

$C_{21}H_{24}F_3N_3S,2HCl$ = 480.4.

CAS — 117-89-5 (trifluoperazine); 440-17-5 (trifluoperazine hydrochloride).

Pharmacopoeias. In *Chin., Eur.* (see p.viii), *Pol.,* and *US.*

A white to pale yellow, almost odourless, hygroscopic, crystalline powder. Trifluoperazine 1 mg is approximately equivalent to 1.2 mg of trifluoperazine hydrochloride. **Soluble** 1 in 3.5 of water, 1 in 11 of alcohol, and 1 in 100 of chloroform; practically insoluble in ether. The Ph. Eur. states that a 10% solution in water has a pH of 1.6 to 2.5. The USP states that a 5% solution in water has a pH between 1.7 and 2.6. **Store** in airtight containers. Protect from light.

Adverse Effects, Treatment, and Precautions

As for Chlorpromazine, p.649. Trifluoperazine is less likely to cause sedation, hypotension, hypothermia, or antimuscarinic effects but is associated with a higher incidence of extrapyramidal effects particularly when the daily dose exceeds 6 mg.

Interactions

As for Chlorpromazine, p.652.

Pharmacokinetics

For an account of the pharmacokinetics of a phenothiazine, see Chlorpromazine, p.654.

A study of the pharmacokinetics of trifluoperazine as a single 5-mg dose by mouth in 5 healthy subjects.[1] Peak plasma concentrations of trifluoperazine were reached from 1.5 to 4.5 hours after ingestion and varied widely between subjects, ranging from 0.53 to 3.09 ng per mL. Elimination of trifluoperazine was multiphasic; the mean elimination half-life was estimated to be 5.1 hours over the period from 4.5 to 12 hours after ingestion, while the mean apparent terminal elimination half-life was estimated to be 12.5 hours.

1. Midha KK, *et al.* Kinetics of oral trifluoperazine disposition in man. *Br J Clin Pharmacol* 1983; **15:** 380–2.

Uses and Administration

Trifluoperazine is a phenothiazine antipsychotic with general properties similar to those of chlorpromazine (p.654). It has a piperazine side-chain.

Trifluoperazine is used in the treatment of a variety of psychiatric disorders including schizophrenia (p.637), severe anxiety (p.635), and disturbed behaviour (p.636). It is also used for the control of nausea and vomiting (p.1172). Trifluoperazine is given as the hydrochloride but its doses are expressed in terms of the base.

The usual initial dose for the treatment of schizophrenia and other psychoses is 2 to 5 mg twice daily, gradually increased to a usual range of 15 to 20 mg daily; in severe or resistant psychoses daily doses of 40 mg or more have been given. For the control of acute psychotic symptoms it may be given by deep intramuscular injection in a dose of 1 to 2 mg, repeated if necessary at intervals of not less than every 4 hours; more than 6 mg daily is rarely required. The initial dose for use in children is up to 5 mg daily by mouth in divided doses adjusted according to age, body-weight, and response, or 1 mg given once or twice daily by intramuscular injection.

For the control of nausea and vomiting the usual adult dose by mouth is 1 or 2 mg twice daily; up to 6 mg daily may be given in divided doses. Children aged 3 to 5 years may be given up to 1 mg daily in divided doses; this may be increased to a maximum of 4 mg daily in children aged 6 to 12 years.

When used as an adjunct in the short-term management of severe anxiety disorders doses are similar to those used for the control of nausea and vomiting.

A modified-release preparation of trifluoperazine hydrochloride is also available; the total daily dosage, as given above, may be administered in a single dose by mouth.

Trifluoperazine should be given in reduced dosage to elderly or debilitated patients.

Preparations

BP 1998: Trifluoperazine Tablets;
USP 23: Trifluoperazine Hydrochloride Injection; Trifluoperazine Hydrochloride Syrup; Trifluoperazine Hydrochloride Tablets.

Proprietary Preparations (details are given in Part 3)
Aust.: Jatroneural; ***Austral.:*** Stelazine; ***Canad.:*** Novo-Flurazine; Stelazine; Terfluzine; ***Fr.:*** Terfluzine; ***Ger.:*** Jatroneural; ***Irl.:*** Stelazine; ***Ital.:*** Modalina; ***Neth.:*** Terfluzine; ***S.Afr.:*** Stelazine; ***Spain:*** Eskazine; ***UK:*** Stelazine; ***USA:*** Stelazine.

Multi-ingredient: ***Aust.:*** Jatrosom†; Stelabid; ***Austral.:*** Parstelin†; Stelabid†; ***Canad.:*** Stelabid; ***Ger.:*** Stelabid†; ***Irl.:*** Parstelin; Stelabid; ***Ital.:*** Parmodalin; ***S.Afr.:*** Stelabid†; ***UK:*** Parstelin.

Trifluperidol (7121-w)

Trifluperidol *(BAN, USAN, rINN).*

McN-JR-2498; R-2498. 4′-Fluoro-4-[4-hydroxy-4-(3-trifluoromethylphenyl)piperidino]butyrophenone.

$C_{22}H_{23}F_4NO_2$ = 409.4.

CAS — 749-13-3.

Trifluperidol Hydrochloride (7122-e)

Trifluperidol Hydrochloride *(BANM, rINNM).*

$C_{22}H_{23}F_4NO_2,HCl$ = 445.9.

CAS — 2062-77-3.

Trifluperidol hydrochloride 1 mg is approximately equivalent to 0.92 mg of trifluperidol.

Trifluperidol is a butyrophenone with general properties similar to those of haloperidol (p.673), and is used in the treatment of psychoses including schizophrenia (p.637). It is given by mouth as the hydrochloride but doses have been expressed in terms of the equivalent amount of the base or as the amount of hydrochloride.

A usual initial dose is 500 μg of trifluperidol hydrochloride or base daily increased if necessary to a total dose of 6 mg daily. Elderly or debilitated patients may require reduced doses of trifluperidol.

Preparations

Proprietary Preparations (details are given in Part 3)
Belg.: Triperidol†; ***Fr.:*** Triperidol; ***Ger.:*** Triperidol; ***Ital.:*** Psicoperidol†; ***UK:*** Triperidol.

Valnoctamide (7125-j)

Valnoctamide *(USAN, rINN).*

McN-X-181; NSC-32363. 2-Ethyl-3-methylvaleramide.

$C_8H_{17}NO$ = 143.2.

CAS — 4171-13-5.

Valnoctamide, an isomer of valpromide (p.361), is given by mouth for anxiety disorders (p.635) in doses ranging from 400 to 600 mg daily in divided doses.

References.

1. Bialer M, *et al.* Pharmacokinetics of a valpromide isomer, valnoctamide, in healthy subjects. *Eur J Clin Pharmacol* 1990; **38:** 289–91.
2. Barel S, *et al.* Stereoselective pharmacokinetic analysis of valnoctamide in healthy subjects and in patients with epilepsy. *Clin Pharmacol Ther* 1997; **61:** 442–9.

Interactions. For a discussion of the potential interaction between carbamazepine and valnoctamide, see p.341.

Preparations

Proprietary Preparations (details are given in Part 3)
Ital.: Nirvanil; ***Switz.:*** Nirvanil†.

Veralipride (17026-b)

Veralipride *(rINN).*

N-[(1-Allyl-2-pyrrolidinyl)methyl]-5-sulphamoyl-2-veratramide.

$C_{17}H_{25}N_3O_5S$ = 383.5.

CAS — 66644-81-3.

Veralipride is a substituted benzamide antipsychotic. It has been used in the treatment of cardiovascular and psychological symptoms associated with the menopause; the usual dose by mouth is 100 mg daily for 20 days repeated at intervals of 7 to 10 days.

Menopausal disorders. Hormone replacement therapy (HRT) with oestrogens is the mainstay of treatment for acute symptoms associated with the menopause (see p.1437). When HRT is considered to be unsuitable a variety of other drugs including veralipride have been tried.[1]

1. Young RL, *et al.* Management of menopause when estrogen cannot be used. *Drugs* 1990; **40:** 220–30.

Porphyria. Veralipride was considered to be unsafe in patients with acute porphyria because it has been shown to be porphyrinogenic in *animals* or *in-vitro* systems.[1]

1. Moore MR, McColl KEL. *Porphyria: drug lists.* Glasgow: Porphyria Research Unit, University of Glasgow, 1991.

Preparations

Proprietary Preparations (details are given in Part 3)
Belg.: Agreal; ***Fr.:*** Agreal; ***Ital.:*** Agradil; Veralipril; ***Spain:*** Agreal; Faltium.

Vinylbitone (4076-x)

Vinylbitone *(BAN).*

Vinylbital *(rINN)*; Butyvinal; JD-96; Vinymalum. 5-(1-Methylbutyl)-5-vinylbarbituric acid.

$C_{11}H_{16}N_2O_3$ = 224.3.

CAS — 2430-49-1.

Vinylbitone is a barbiturate with general properties similar to those of amylobarbitone (p.641). It was used as a hypnotic.

Preparations

Proprietary Preparations (details are given in Part 3)
Fr.: Optanox†; Suppoptanox†; ***Ger.:*** Speda†.

Zaleplon (17862-k)

Zaleplon *(USAN, rINN).*

CL-284846. 3′-(3-Cyanopyrazolo[1,5-*a*]pyrimidin-7-yl)-*N*-ethylacetanilide.

$C_{17}H_{15}N_5O$ = 305.3.

CAS — 151319-34-5.

Zaleplon is being studied as a sedative and hypnotic.

References.

1. Beer B, *et al.* A placebo-controlled evaluation of single, escalating doses of CL 284,846, a non-benzodiazepine hypnotic. *J Clin Pharmacol* 1994; **34:** 335–44.

Ziprasidone (17144-w)

Ziprasidone *(BAN, rINN).*

CP-88059 (ziprasidone hydrochloride). 5-{2-[4-(1,2-Benzisothiazol-3-yl)-1-piperazinyl]ethyl}-6-chloro-2-indolinone.

$C_{21}H_{21}ClN_4OS$ = 412.9.

CAS — 146939-27-7 (ziprasidone); 138982-67-9 (ziprasidone hydrochloride).

NOTE. Ziprasidone Hydrochloride is *USAN.*

Ziprasidone is an atypical antipsychotic used for the treatment of schizophrenia (p.637). Like other atypical antipsychotics it appears to be associated with a low incidence of extrapyramidal adverse effects. It is reported to have affinity for serotonin ($5-HT_2$) and dopamine (D_2) receptors.

References.

1. Arató M, *et al.* Ziprasidone: efficacy in the prevention of relapse and in the long-term treatment of negative symptoms of chronic schizophrenia. *Eur Neuropsychopharmacol* 1997; **7** (suppl 2): S214.
2. Goff DC, *et al.* An exploratory haloperidol-controlled dose-finding study of ziprasidone in hospitalized patients with schizophrenia or schizoaffective disorder. *J Clin Psychopharmacol* 1998; **18:** 296–304.

Zolazepam Hydrochloride (18695-m)

Zolazepam Hydrochloride *(BANM, USAN, pINN).*

CI-716. 4-(2-Fluorophenyl)-1,6,7,8-tetrahydro-1,3,8-trimethylpyrazolo[3,4-e][1,4]diazepin-7-one monohydrochloride.

$C_{15}H_{15}FN_4O.HCl$ = 322.8.

CAS — 31352-82-6 (zolazepam); 33754-49-3 (zolazepam hydrochloride).

Pharmacopoeias. In US for veterinary use only.

A white to off-white crystalline powder. Freely **soluble** in water and in 0.1N hydrochloric acid; slightly soluble in chloroform; practically insoluble in ether; soluble in methyl alcohol. A 10% solution in water has a pH of 1.5 to 3.5. **Store** in airtight containers.

Zolazepam hydrochloride is a benzodiazepine with general properties similar to those of diazepam (p.666). It is used with tiletamine (p.1234) for general anaesthesia in veterinary medicine.

Zolpidem Tartrate (1667-t)

Zolpidem Tartrate *(BANM, USAN, rINNM).*

SL-80.0750 (zolpidem); SL-80.0750-23N; Zolpidemi Tartras. *N,N*-Dimethyl-2-(6-methyl-2-*p*-tolylimidazo[1,2-*a*]pyridin-3-yl)acetamide hemitartrate.

$(C_{19}H_{21}N_3O)_2,C_4H_6O_6$ = 764.9.

CAS — 82626-48-0 (zolpidem); 99294-93-6 (zolpidem tartrate).

Pharmacopoeias. In *Eur.* (see p.viii).

A white or almost white hygroscopic crystalline powder. Slightly **soluble** in water; practically insoluble in dichloromethane; sparingly soluble in methyl alcohol. **Store** in airtight containers. Protect from light.

Dependence and Withdrawal, Adverse Effects, Treatment, and Precautions

As for Diazepam, p.661.

Psychotic and/or amnesic[1-3] effects and tolerance and withdrawal symptoms[3,4] have been reported in some patients taking zolpidem. Chronic abuse has also been reported in a patient with depression who obtained a stimulant effect when taking large doses of zolpidem.[3]

1. Ansseau M, *et al.* Psychotic reactions to zolpidem. *Lancet* 1992; **339:** 809.
2. Iruela LM, *et al.* Zolpidem-induced macropsia in anorexic woman. *Lancet* 1993: **342:** 443–4.
3. Gericke CA, Ludolph AC. Chronic abuse of zolpidem. *JAMA* 1994; **272:** 1721–2.
4. Cavallaro R, *et al.* Tolerance and withdrawal with zolpidem. *Lancet* 1993; **342:** 374–5.

Overdosage. A retrospective analysis of 344 cases of acute overdosage with zolpidem reported to the Paris Poison Center and the manufacturers Synthelabo has been published.[1] For those patients whose details were available the ingested dose had ranged from 10 to 1400 mg. Drowsiness which occurred in 89 patients was the most common adverse effect reported. Adverse effects also considered to be associated with zolpidem overdosage included coma in 4 patients and vomiting in 7. Recovery was usually rapid when overdosage involved only zolpidem. It was recommended that patients who had ingested more than 100 mg of zolpidem should undergo gastric lavage and should be monitored for at least 12 hours. Although it has been shown that flumazenil[2] can effectively antagonise the CNS effects of zolpidem the authors of this analysis[1] found that in general it was not required.

1. Garnier R, *et al.* Acute zolpidem poisoning—analysis of 344 cases. *J Toxicol Clin Toxicol* 1994; **32:** 391–404.
2. Patat A, *et al.* Flumazenil antagonizes the central effects of zolpidem, an imidazopyridine hypnotic. *Clin Pharmacol Ther* 1994; **56:** 430–6.

Interactions

As for Diazepam, p.663.

Antivirals. HIV-protease inhibitors such as *ritonavir* can increase plasma concentrations of zolpidem with a risk of extreme sedation and respiratory depression; concomitant administration is not recommended.

Paroxetine. A 16-year-old girl who had been taking paroxetine 20 mg daily for 3 days began to hallucinate and became disorientated one hour after taking zolpidem 10 mg at night. The delirium cleared spontaneously 4 hours later without treatment.[1] When questioned, at least one other of the author's patients receiving this combination reported transient visual hallucinations.

1. Katz SE. Possible paroxetine-zolpidem interaction. *Am J Psychiatry* 1995; **152:** 1689.

Rifampicin. Concomitant administration of rifampicin reduced the hypnotic effect of zolpidem in a study in 8 healthy female subjects.[1] The area under the curve for zolpidem was reduced by 73% after administration of rifampicin and the peak plasma concentration by 58%. The elimination half-life of zolpidem was reduced from 2.5 to 1.6 hours. Similar effects could be expected with other potent inducers of the cytochrome P450 isozyme CYP3A4 such as carbamazepine and phenytoin.

1. Villikka K, *et al.* Rifampin reduces plasma concentrations and effects of zolpidem. *Clin Pharmacol Ther* 1997; **62:** 629–34.

Pharmacokinetics

Zolpidem is rapidly absorbed from the gastro-intestinal tract, peak plasma concentrations being reached within 3 hours. Zolpidem undergoes first-pass metabolism and an absolute bioavailability of about 70% has been reported. Zolpidem has an elimination half-life of about 2.5 hours and is approximately 92% bound to plasma proteins. The inactive metabolites of zolpidem are excreted in the urine and faeces.

References.

1. Salvà P, Costa J. Clinical pharmacokinetics and pharmacodynamics of zolpidem: therapeutic implications. *Clin Pharmacokinet* 1995; **29:** 142–53.

Distribution into breast milk. In 5 lactating women given a 20-mg dose of zolpidem, the amount of drug excreted in breast milk after 3 hours ranged between 0.76 and 3.88 μg, which represented 0.004 to 0.019% of the administered dose.[1] No detectable (below 0.5 ng per mL) zolpidem was found in subsequent milk samples.

1. Pons G, *et al.* Zolpidem excretion in breast milk. *Eur J Clin Pharmacol* 1989; **37:** 245–8.

Uses and Administration

Zolpidem tartrate is an imidazopyridine which is reported to have similar sedative properties to the benzodiazepines (see Diazepam, p.666), but minimal anxiolytic, muscle relaxant, and anticonvulsant properties. It is used as a hypnotic in the short-term management of insomnia (p.638). Zolpidem has a rapid onset of action. The usual dose by mouth is 10 mg taken immediately before retiring. In elderly or debilitated patients or patients with hepatic impairment, treatment should be initiated with a dose of 5 mg at night.

Zolpidem is an imidazopyridine with strong sedative actions, but only minor anxiolytic, muscle relaxant, or anticonvulsant properties. Some degree of amnesia has been reported. Zolpidem appears to act by binding to the benzodiazepine receptor component of the GABA receptor complex. It has, however, a selective affinity for the subtype of benzodiazepine receptors prevalent in the cerebellum (BZ1- or ω_1-receptors) as opposed to those more commonly found in the spinal cord (BZ2- or ω_2-receptors) or in the peripheral tissues (BZ3- or ω_3-receptors). Zolpidem has a rapid onset and short duration of hypnotic action and at usual doses decreases time to sleep onset and increases duration of sleep with little apparent effect on sleep stages. Reviews agree that clinical studies have shown zolpidem to have hypnotic activity superior to placebo and generally similar to comparative benzodiazepines. Although it does not appear to produce rebound insomnia to any great extent, there appears to be little evidence that zolpidem offers any advantage over short-acting benzodiazepines in terms of residual effects the next day, or its potential to induce tolerance or withdrawal symptoms or dependence (see also under Dependence and Withdrawal, Adverse Effects, Treatment, and Precautions, above).

References.

1. Langtry HD, Benfield P. Zolpidem: a review of its pharmacodynamic and pharmacokinetic properties and therapeutic potential. *Drugs* 1990; **40:** 291–313.
2. Wheatley D. Prescribing short-acting hypnosedatives: current recommendations from a safety perspective. *Drug Safety* 1992; **7:** 106–15.
3. Anonymous. Zolpidem for insomnia. *Med Lett Drugs Ther* 1993; **35:** 35–6.
4. Hoehns JD, Perry PJ. Zolpidem: a nonbenzodiazepine hypnotic for treatment of insomnia. *Clin Pharm* 1993; **12:** 814–28.
5. Anonymous. Zolpidem—a hypnotic with a difference? *Drug Ther Bull* 1995; **33:** 37–9.
6. Lobo BL, Greene WL. Zolpidem: distinct from triazolam? *Ann Pharmacother* 1997; **31:** 625–32.
7. Nowell PD, *et al.* Benzodiazepines and zolpidem for chronic insomnia: a meta-analysis of treatment efficacy. *JAMA* 1997; **278:** 2170–7.

Catatonia. Anecdotal reports[1,2] suggesting that zolpidem may be a useful test in the diagnosis of catatonia.

1. Thomas P, *et al.* Test for catatonia with zolpidem. *Lancet* 1997; **349:** 702.
2. Zaw ZF, Bates GDL. Replication of zolpidem test for catatonia in an adolescent. *Lancet* 1997; **349:** 1914.

Parkinson's disease. Although preliminary findings[1] in 10 patients suggest that zolpidem may improve symptoms of Parkinson's disease concern has been expressed[2] over the risk of falls associated with zolpidem-induced drowsiness and the serious consequences for these patients.

1. Daniele A, *et al.* Zolpidem in Parkinson's disease. *Lancet* 1997; **349:** 1222–3.
2. Lavoisy J, Marsac J. Zolpidem in Parkinson's disease. *Lancet* 1997; **350:** 74.

Preparations

Proprietary Preparations (details are given in Part 3)

Aust.: Ivadal; Stilnox; ***Belg.:*** Stilnoct; ***Fr.:*** Ivadal; Stilnox; ***Ger.:*** Bikalm; Stilnox; ***Irl.:*** Stilnoct; ***Ital.:*** Ivadal; Niotal; Stilnox; ***Neth.:*** Stilnoct; ***Norw.:*** Stilnoct; ***Spain:*** Cedrol; Dalparan; Stilnox; ***Swed.:*** Stilnoct; ***Switz.:*** Stilnox; ***UK:*** Stilnoct; ***USA:*** Ambien.

Zopiclone (14031-d)

Zopiclone *(BAN, rINN)*.

27267-RP; Zopiclonum. 6-(5-Chloro-2-pyridyl)-6,7-dihydro-7-oxo-5*H*-pyrrolo[3,4-*b*]pyrazin-5-yl 4-methylpiperazine-1-carboxylate.

$C_{17}H_{17}ClN_6O_3$ = 388.8.

CAS — 43200-80-2.

Pharmacopoeias. In *Eur.* (see p.viii).

A white or slightly yellow powder. Practically **insoluble** in water and in alcohol; sparingly soluble in acetone; freely soluble in dichloromethane. It dissolves in dilute mineral acids. **Protect** from light.

Dependence and Withdrawal, Adverse Effects, Treatment, and Precautions

As for Diazepam, p.661.

A bitter or metallic taste in the mouth has been reported.

Zopiclone is contra-indicated in severe hepatic insufficiency.

In a French postmarketing survey[1] of 20 513 patients treated with zopiclone the most commonly reported adverse events were bitter taste (3.6%), dry mouth (1.6%), difficulty arising in the morning (1.3%), sleepiness (0.5%), nausea (0.5%) and nightmares (0.5%). The UK Committee on Safety of Medicines (CSM) had received 122 reports of adverse reactions to zopiclone over a period of about one year since the product's introduction in November 1989.[2] A fifth of these were neuropsychiatric reactions, a proportion similar to that found with other hypnotics. Many of these reactions were potentially serious and involved hallucinations (3 auditory and 2 visual), amnesia (4) and behavioural disturbances (10, including 3 cases of aggression). Most reactions started immediately or shortly after the first dose and improved rapidly on stopping the drug. Three patients had difficulty in stopping treatment, 2 because of withdrawal symptoms and one due to repeated rebound insomnia. The CSM considered that, although differing structurally from the benzodiazepines, zopiclone has the same potential for adverse psychiatric reactions, including dependence. Like benzodiazepines it should be reserved for patients with severe sleep disturbance and its duration of use limited to 28 days. As with all hypnotics, care should be taken in the elderly, those who have a history of previous psychiatric illness, or who are prone to drug abuse.

1. Allain H, *et al.* Postmarketing surveillance of zopiclone in insomnia: analysis of 20,513 cases. *Sleep* 1991; **14:** 408–13.
2. Committee on Safety of Medicines. Zopiclone (Zimovane) and neuro-psychiatric reactions. *Current Problems 30* 1990.

Administration. Results in 9 healthy subjects given zopiclone indicated a significant delay in onset of action when the drug was taken in the supine, as opposed to the standing, position; this was associated with a prolongation of more than 20 minutes in the lag time before absorption began.[1] In order to obtain a rapid and complete hypnotic effect from zopiclone the tablet should be swallowed in the standing position.

1. Channer KS, *et al.* The effect of posture at the time of administration on the central depressant effects of the new hypnotic zopiclone. *Br J Clin Pharmacol* 1984; **18:** 879–86.

Dependence. Reports[1,2] of zopiclone dependence and associated withdrawal symptoms on dosage reduction or cessation of use.

1. Jones IR, Sullivan G. Physical dependence on zopiclone: case reports. *Br Med J* 1998; **316:** 117.
2. Sikdar S. Physical dependence on zopiclone. *Br Med J* 1998; **317:** 146.

Driving. For reference to the increased risk of road-traffic accidents for drivers taking zopiclone, see p.662.

Hepatic impairment. A study of the pharmacokinetics of zopiclone in cirrhosis.[1] Zopiclone was given in a dose of 7.5 mg to 7 cirrhotic patients and 8 healthy subjects; a further 2 cirrhotic patients received 3.75 mg. Mean peak plasma concentrations were similar in healthy subjects and those with hepatic impairment following equivalent doses but time to peak plasma concentration was significantly delayed in cirrhotics at 4 hours as compared with 2 hours in the healthy subjects. Elimination was greatly prolonged in cirrhotic patients, in whom the mean plasma half-life was 8.53 compared with 3.50 hours. The CNS-depressant effects of zopiclone were delayed in the cirrhotic patients in a way consistent with the pharmacokinetic changes. There was also some evidence of an increased response in these patients. Caution should be exercised in administering zopiclone to patients with severe hepatic disease.

1. Parker G, Roberts CJC. Plasma concentrations and central nervous system effects of the new hypnotic agent zopiclone in patients with chronic liver disease. *Br J Clin Pharmacol* 1983; **16:** 259–65.

Overdosage. Consciousness was rapidly regained after intravenous flumazenil administration in a patient who had taken an overdosage of zopiclone.[1]

1. Ahmad Z, *et al.* Diagnostic utility of flumazenil in coma with suspected poisoning. *Br Med J* 1991; **302:** 292.

Interactions

As for Diazepam, p.663.

Erythromycin. In a study in healthy subjects erythromycin increased the rate of absorption of zopiclone and prolonged its elimination.[1]

1. Aranko K, *et al.* The effect of erythromycin on the pharmacokinetics and pharmacodynamics of zopiclone. *Br J Clin Pharmacol* 1994; **38:** 363–7.

Rifampicin. Concomitant administration of rifampicin or other potent inducers of the cytochrome P450 isozyme CYP3A4 such as carbamazepine or phenytoin, is likely to reduce the effects of zopiclone. In a study[1] in 8 healthy subjects concomitant administration of rifampicin was associated with an 82% reduction in the area under the curve for zopiclone. The peak plasma concentration of zopiclone was reduced from 76.9 to 22.5 ng per mL and the elimination half-life from 3.8 to 2.3 hours.

1. Villikka K, *et al.* Concentrations and effects of zopiclone are greatly reduced by rifampicin. *Br J Clin Pharmacol* 1997; **43:** 471–4.

Pharmacokinetics

Zopiclone is rapidly absorbed following administration by mouth and widely distributed. It has an elimination half-life of 3.5 to 6.5 hours and is reported to be about 45 to 80% bound to plasma proteins. Zopiclone is extensively metabolised in the liver; the 2 major metabolites, the less active zopiclone *N*-oxide and the inactive *N*-desmethylzopiclone are excreted mainly in the urine. About 50% of a dose is converted by decarboxylation to inactive metabolites which are partly eliminated via the lungs as carbon dioxide. Only about 5% of a dose appears unchanged in the urine and about 16% appears in the faeces. Excretion of zopiclone in the saliva may explain reports of a bitter taste. It is also distributed into breast milk.

Reviews.

1. Fernandez C, *et al.* Clinical pharmacokinetics of zopiclone. *Clin Pharmacokinet* 1995; **29:** 431–41.

Distribution into breast milk. Zopiclone was distributed into breast milk in 12 lactating women in concentrations approximately half those in plasma.[1] The calculated dose that would be received by a neonate was 1.5 μg per kg bodyweight, corresponding to 1.2% of the maternal dose.

1. Matheson I, *et al.* The excretion of zopiclone into breast milk. *Br J Clin Pharmacol* 1990; **30:** 267–71.

Uses and Administration

Zopiclone is a cyclopyrrolone which is reported to have similar sedative, anxiolytic, muscle relaxant, amnesic, and anticonvulsant properties to those of the benzodiazepines (see Diazepam, p.666). Like diazepam, its actions are mediated by enhancement of the activity of aminobutyric acid (GABA) in the brain. Zopiclone is reported to bind to the benzodiazepine receptor component of the GABA receptor complex but at a different site to the benzodiazepines.

Zopiclone is used as a hypnotic in the short-term management of insomnia (p.638). The usual dose is 7.5 mg by mouth at night. In elderly patients and in those with renal insufficiency or mild to moderate hepatic insufficiency, treatment should be initiated with a dose of 3.75 mg at night.

Zopiclone has a similar pharmacological and pharmacokinetic profile to the short-acting benzodiazepines. It is claimed to initiate sleep rapidly, without reduction of total rapid-eye-movement (REM) sleep, and then sustain it with preservation of normal slow-wave sleep. It is generally considered to be as effective as an hypnotic as the benzodiazepines.[1,2] Rebound insomnia has occurred but does not appear to be common. Residual effects the next day may be less pronounced after zopiclone than after short-acting benzodiazepines but there appears to be little evidence that zopiclone offers any clinical advantage in terms of its potential to induce tolerance, withdrawal symptoms, or dependence. For recommendations of the UK Committee on Safety of Medicines concerning its use as a hypnotic, see under Dependence and Withdrawal, Adverse Effects, Treatment, and Precautions, above.

1. Hallstrom CO. Zopiclone. *Prescribers' J* 1994; **34:** 115–19.
2. Noble S, *et al.* Zopiclone: an update of its pharmacology, clinical efficacy and tolerability in the treatment of insomnia. *Drugs* 1998; **55:** 277–302.

Preparations

Proprietary Preparations (details are given in Part 3)

Aust.: Imovane; ***Austral.:*** Imovane; ***Belg.:*** Imovane; ***Canad.:*** Imovane; Rhovane; ***Fr.:*** Imovane; ***Ger.:*** Ximovan; ***Irl.:*** Zimovane; ***Ital.:*** Imovane; ***Neth.:*** Imovane; ***Norw.:*** Imovane; ***S.Afr.:*** Imovane; ***Spain:*** Datolan; Limovan; Siaten; ***Swed.:*** Imovane; ***Switz.:*** Imovane; ***UK:*** Zileze; Zimovane.

Zotepine (2479-d)

Zotepine *(rINN)*.

2-[(8-Chlorodibenzo[*b,f*]-thiepin-10-yl)oxy]-*N,N*-dimethylethylamine.

$C_{18}H_{18}ClNOS$ = 331.9.

CAS — 26615-21-4.

Adverse Effects and Precautions

As for Chlorpromazine, p.649.

Zotepine is contra-indicated in patients with a personal or close family history of epilepsy. It has uricosuric properties and should not be given to patients with acute gout or a history of nephrolithiasis. Since zotepine can prolong the QT interval it is recommended that an ECG is performed before starting treatment. Patients with pre-existing prolongation of the QT interval should not be given zotepine. A reduced dosage is recommended in the elderly or in those with renal or hepatic impairment. Weekly monitoring of liver function is recommended for at least the first 3 months of therapy in patients with hepatic impairment.

Interactions

As for Chlorpromazine, p.652.

The risk of arrhythmias with zotepine may be increased by use with other drugs that prolong the QT interval. Concomitant administration of zotepine with fluoxetine or diazepam may lead to increased plasma concentrations of zotepine.

Pharmacokinetics

Zotepine is absorbed from the gastro-intestinal tract and peak plasma concentrations have been achieved 2 to 3 hours after oral administration. It undergoes extensive first-pass metabolism to the equipotent metabolite norzotepine and inactive metabolites. CYP1A2 and CYP3A4 are the major cytochrome P450 isozymes involved in the metabolism of zotepine. Protein binding of zotepine and norzotepine is 97%. Zotepine is excreted mainly in the urine and faeces as metabolites and has an elimination half-life of about 14 hours.

Uses and Administration

Zotepine is an atypical antipsychotic that is an antagonist at central dopamine (D_1 and D_2) receptors; it also binds to serotonin (5-HT_2), adrenergic (α_1), and histamine (H_1) receptors and inhibits noradrenaline reuptake. It is given by mouth in the treatment of schizophrenia (p.637) in an initial dose of 25 mg three times daily increased at intervals of 4 days according to response to a maximum dose of 100 mg three times daily. There is an appreciable increase in the incidence of seizures at total daily doses above the recommended maximum of 300 mg. For elderly patients or those with renal or hepatic insufficiency the recommended starting dose is 25 mg given twice daily increased gradually up to a maximum of 75 mg twice daily.

References.

1. Barnas C, *et al.* Zotepine in the treatment of schizophrenic patients with prevailingly negative symptoms: a double-blind trial vs. haloperidol. *Int Clin Psychopharmacol* 1992; **7:** 23–7.
2. Petit M, *et al.* A comparison of an atypical and typical antipsychotic, zotepine versus haloperidol in patients with acute exacerbation of schizophrenia: a parallel-group double-blind trial. *Psychopharmacol Bull* 1996; **32:** 81–7.
3. Meyer-Lindenberg A, *et al.* Improvement of cognitive function in schizophrenic patients receiving clozapine or zotepine: results from a double-blind study. *Pharmacopsychiatry* 1997; **30:** 35–42.

Preparations

Proprietary Preparations (details are given in Part 3)

Aust.: Nipolept; ***Ger.:*** Nipolept; ***Jpn:*** Lodopin; ***UK:*** Zoleptil.

Zuclopenthixol (12014-g)

Zuclopenthixol *(BAN, rINN)*.

AY-62021 (clopenthixol); Z-Clopenthixol; *cis*-Clopenthixol; α-Clopenthixol; N-746 (clopenthixol); NSC-64087 (clopenthixol). (*Z*)-2-{4-[3-(2-Chloro-10*H*-dibenzo[*b,e*]thiin-10-ylidene)propyl]piperazin-1-yl}ethanol.

$C_{22}H_{25}ClN_2OS$ = 401.0.

CAS — 53772-83-1 (zuclopenthixol); 982-24-1 (clopenthixol).

NOTE. Clopenthixol (the racemic mixture) is *BAN* and *USAN*.

Zuclopenthixol Acetate (14093-j)

Zuclopenthixol Acetate *(BANM, rINNM)*.

$C_{24}H_{27}ClN_2O_2S$ = 443.0.

CAS — 85721-05-7.

Pharmacopoeias. In *Br.*

A yellowish, viscous oil. Very slightly **soluble** in water; very soluble in alcohol, in dichloromethane, and in ether. **Store** at a temperature not exceeding −20° and protect from light.

Zuclopenthixol Decanoate (7027-l)

Zuclopenthixol Decanoate *(BANM, rINNM)*.

$C_{32}H_{43}ClN_2O_2S$ = 555.2.

CAS — 64053-00-5.

Pharmacopoeias. In *Br.*

A yellow viscous oil. Very slightly **soluble** in water; very soluble in alcohol, in dichloromethane, and in ether. **Store** at a temperature not exceeding −20° and protect from light.

Zuclopenthixol Hydrochloride (7028-y)

Zuclopenthixol Hydrochloride *(BANM, rINNM)*.

Zuclopenthixol dihydrochloride.

$C_{22}H_{25}ClN_2OS,2HCl$ = 473.9.

CAS — 633-59-0.

Pharmacopoeias. In *Br.*

An off-white granular powder. Zuclopenthixol hydrochloride 11.8 mg is approximately equivalent to 10 mg of zuclopenthixol. Very **soluble** in water; sparingly soluble in alcohol; slightly soluble in chloroform; very slightly soluble in ether. A 1% solution has a pH of 2.0 to 3.0. **Protect** from light.

Stability. References.

1. Li Wan Po A, Irwin WJ. The photochemical stability of cis- and trans-isomers of tricyclic neuroleptic drugs. *J Pharm Pharmacol* 1980; **32:** 25–9.

Adverse Effects, Treatment, and Precautions

As for Chlorpromazine, p.649. Zuclopenthixol is less likely to cause sedation. It should not be used in apathetic or withdrawn states.

Interactions

As for Chlorpromazine, p.652.

Pharmacokinetics

For an account of the pharmacokinetics of a thioxanthene, see Flupenthixol, p.671. Following intramuscular injection the acetate and decanoate esters of zuclopenthixol are hydrolysed to release zuclopenthixol. Zuclopenthixol acetate has a relatively quick onset of action after injection, and has a duration of action of 2 to 3 days; it is, therefore, useful for the control of acute psychotic symptoms while avoiding repeated injections. The decanoate has a much longer duration of action and is a suitable depot preparation for maintenance treatment.

Metaboliser phenotype. Determination of metaboliser phenotype with regard to cytochrome P450 isozyme CYP2D6 appeared to be of limited value in patients receiving zuclopenthixol as interindividual variation appeared to be the main factor affecting dose to serum concentration ratios.[1]

1. Linnet K, Wiborg O. Influence of Cyp2D6 genetic polymorphism on ratios of steady-state serum concentration to dose of the neuroleptic zuclopenthixol. *Ther Drug Monit* 1996; **18:** 629–34.

Uses and Administration

Zuclopenthixol is a thioxanthene of high potency with general properties similar to the phenothiazine, chlorpromazine (p.654). It has a piperazine side-chain.

Zuclopenthixol is used for the treatment of schizophrenia (p.637), mania (p.273), and other psychoses. It may be particularly suitable for agitated or aggressive patients who may become over-excited with flupenthixol. Zuclopenthixol is administered as the hydrochloride, usually by mouth; doses are expressed in terms of the base. Zuclopenthixol acetate and zuclopenthixol decanoate are given by deep intramuscular injection; doses are expressed in terms of the ester. The acetate ester has an onset of action shortly after injection and a duration of action of 2 to 3 days; it is used for the initial treatment of acute psychoses and for exacerbations of chronic psychoses. The longer-acting decanoate ester is used for the maintenance treatment of chronic psychoses.

The usual initial oral dose of the hydrochloride for the treatment of psychoses is the equivalent of 20 to 30 mg of the base daily in divided doses; in severe or resistant schizophrenia up to 150 mg daily has been given. The usual maintenance dose is 20 to 50 mg daily. It has also been given intramuscularly.

The usual dose of zuclopenthixol acetate is 50 to 150 mg by deep intramuscular injection repeated, if necessary, after 2 or 3 days. Some patients may need an additional injection between 1 and 2 days after the first dose. Zuclopenthixol acetate is not intended for maintenance treatment; not more than four injections should be given in a course of treatment and the total dose should not exceed 400 mg. When maintenance therapy is required, zuclopenthixol hydrochloride by mouth may be introduced 2 to 3 days after the last injection of zuclopenthixol acetate, or intramuscular injections of the decanoate (see below) commenced with the last injection of the acetate.

The long-acting decanoate should be given by deep intramuscular injection; treatment is usually initiated with a test dose of 100 mg as 0.5 mL of a 20% oily solution. According to the patient's response over the following 1 to 4 weeks, this may be followed by a dose of 100 to 200 mg or more; thereafter, doses usually range from 200 to 400 mg every 2 to 4 weeks. Shorter dosage intervals or greater amounts may be required according to the patient's response. If doses greater than 400 mg are considered necessary they should be divided between 2 separate injection sites or, alternatively, given as a 50% oily solution. The maximum recommended dose of zuclopenthixol decanoate is 600 mg a week.

Elderly or debilitated patients should be given reduced doses of zuclopenthixol. The manufacturers recommend that for the acetate ester, half the normal recommended dose should be used for patients with hepatic impairment; a dosage reduction is considered not to be necessary in patients with renal impairment but where there is renal failure half the normal dosage is recommended.

Preparations

BP 1998: Zuclopenthixol Acetate Injection; Zuclopenthixol Decanoate Injection; Zuclopenthixol Tablets.

Proprietary Preparations (details are given in Part 3)

Aust.: Cisordinol; ***Austral.:*** Clopixol; ***Belg.:*** Clopixol; ***Canad.:*** Clopixol; ***Fr.:*** Clopixol; ***Ger.:*** Ciatyl; Sedanxol†; ***Irl.:*** Clopixol; ***Ital.:*** Clopixol; Sordinol; ***Neth.:*** Cisordinol; ***Norw.:*** Cisordinol; ***S.Afr.:*** Clopixol; ***Spain:*** Cisordinol; Clopixol; ***Swed.:*** Cisordinol; ***Switz.:*** Clopixol; ***UK:*** Clopixol.

Blood Products Plasma Expanders and Haemostatics

This chapter describes the management of blood disorders including anaemias, haemorrhagic disorders, and neutropenia and includes blood, blood products and substitutes, colloid plasma expanders (crystalloids are included under Electrolytes, p.1147), haemostatic drugs, and erythropoietin and other colony-stimulating factors.

Anaemias

Anaemia is usually understood to mean a lowering of haemoglobin concentration, red cell count, or packed cell volume to below 'normal' values, but the criteria for normality are difficult to establish. WHO's suggested definition of anaemia in populations living at around sea level is a haemoglobin concentration below 13 g per 100 mL in adult men and below 12 g per 100 mL in women; children would be considered anaemic below 12 g per 100 mL if aged 6 to 14 years, or below 11 g per 100 mL if aged 6 months to 6 years. However, because of individual variation, some apparently normal individuals have blood haemoglobin concentrations below these values, while others may be above these values and still be effectively anaemic.

Reduction in overall haemoglobin concentrations may be due just to fewer red cells with the cells retaining normal amounts of haemoglobin (normochromic anaemia), or the amount of haemoglobin in the cells may be reduced (hypochromic anaemia). Red cells themselves may be reduced in size (microcytic), enlarged (macrocytic), or normal in size (normocytic).

The immediate cause of anaemia may be decreased red-cell production (due to defective proliferation and/or maturation of red cells from their precursors in bone marrow), increased red-cell destruction (i.e. haemolysis), or loss of red cells from the circulation due to haemorrhage, either occult or overt. These conditions may occur due to underlying disease, nutritional deficiency, congenital disorders, or toxicity due to drugs or other substances and the cause must always be sought before an appropriate treatment can be determined.

The symptoms of anaemia are as variable as its causes but may include fatigue, pallor, dyspnoea, palpitations, headache, faintness or lightheadedness, tinnitus, anorexia and gastro-intestinal disturbances, and loss of libido; tachycardia, heart failure, and retinal haemorrhage may occur in severe anaemia.

The treatment of anaemia depends upon its type and cause. Some of the principal types are classified in Table 1, below, and their management is discussed in more detail under the relevant headings.

Table 1. Types of anaemias.

Classification	Anaemia	Mean cell volume	Haemoglobin	Associated with
Microcytic	Iron-deficiency anaemia	Decreased (or normal in early stages)	Hypochromic	Blood loss, malabsorption, inadequate iron intake
	Hereditary sideroblastic anaemia	Decreased	Hypochromic	
	Thalassaemias	Decreased	Hypochromic	
Macrocytic	Megaloblastic anaemia	Increased	Normochromic	Vitamin B_{12} deficiency, folate deficiency (including drug induced)
	Acquired sideroblastic anaemia	Increased	Hypochromic	Alcoholism, drug or other toxicity
Normocytic	Normocytic-normochromic anaemia	Normal	Normochromic	Anaemia of chronic disorders, bone-marrow disorders (including aplastic anaemia), malignancy, renal failure, endocrine disorders, prematurity
Haemolytic	Haemolytic anaemia	Increased		Immune disorders, drug toxicity, hereditary disorders
	Sickle-cell anaemia			

Aplastic anaemia

Aplastic anaemia is characterised by pancytopenia and hypoplasia of the bone marrow, with less than 25% of the marrow occupied by haematopoietic cells but without evident fibrosis or malignant infiltration. It is relatively rare, although it may be somewhat more common in the Far East, is predominantly seen in younger adults, and is slightly more frequent in men than women. Some forms, such as Fanconi's anaemia, are inherited but most are acquired from various causes, including the effects of cytotoxic drugs or radiation, idiosyncratic reactions to other drugs, viral infections such as hepatitis C, or auto-immune reactions. In about 50% of cases aplastic anaemia is classified as idiopathic. All cell lines are affected and patients consequently develop thrombocytopenia and neutropenia as well as anaemia, and symptoms include bleeding syndromes and infections as well as typical symptoms of anaemia.

Although spontaneous recovery has occurred, untreated aplastic anaemia is usually fatal. Management may be divided into supportive care and attempts to restore bone-marrow function and has been the subject of guidelines and reviews.[1-3]

Supportive care. Supportive care involves the prevention and treatment of infection (see Infections in Immunocompromised Patients, p.127), the control of haemorrhage with platelet concentrates, and where necessary, infusions of red blood cells (with platelets to prevent haemorrhage) for anaemia. Transfusions should be minimised in candidates for bone-marrow transplant (see below).

Restoration of bone-marrow function. In patients aged under 40 years with severe disease and with a suitable HLA-matched donor, bone-marrow transplantation has been considered the treatment of choice. Ideally this should be performed early before the patient has received too many transfusions, which increase the risk of rejection, and before infection develops. Transfusion of cord blood from an HLA-identical sibling can also produce permanent engraftment, and may be associated with less acute graft-versus-host disease than bone marrow.[1]

In patients unsuitable for bone-marrow transplantation, or where a suitable donor is not available, treatment with immunosuppressants may be tried. About 50% of patients are reported to respond to a course of equine antilymphocyte or antithymocyte immunoglobulin, although response may be slow; if there is no sign of response after about 4 months a second course (usually of a rabbit-derived product) may produce benefit in some.[4] Cyclosporin may be of benefit in non-responders to antilymphocyte immunoglobulins;[4,5] combined immunosuppression with antilymphocyte immunoglobulins, methylprednisolone, and cyclosporin produces better response rates than regimens without cyclosporin,[6] but the combined regimen has not yet been shown to produce improved survival.[1] Androgens may also be added to a second course of immunosuppressants.[1] Good response rates have been reported from combined regimens including a granulocyte colony-stimulating factor.[7]

Overall, the results of immunosuppression seem to be comparable to those of bone-marrow transplantation, except perhaps in children,[4] who generally respond less well to immunosuppressants. Responses are often partial, but this may be sufficient to free the patient from dependency on transfusions and intensive antibiotic cover, and is considered well worth achieving. Some groups have preferred immunosuppression for initial therapy even in patients suitable for transplantation, reserving the transplant for salvage in non-responders or relapse.[8] Such an approach has been reported to result in a 5-year survival of some 80%, but there is concern that patients treated with immunosuppression retain some underlying defect in marrow function, as many patients subsequently develop leukaemias or myelodysplasias.[9,10]

In moderate disease, or where immunosuppression fails, a trial of an anabolic steroid such as oxymetholone may be considered, although responses are likely to be disappointing.[4] Other drugs that have been tried include normal immunoglobulins, although it has been suggested that responses are uncommon.[9] The availability of recombinant haematopoietic growth factors has led to trials of colony-stimulating factors in a few patients,[11-13] but although some responses have occurred during therapy there is no evidence of sustained remission. The use of colony-stimulating factors alone has been criticised[14] on the grounds that such treatment delays bone-marrow transplantation or immunosuppressive therapy and thus reduces the chance of a successful outcome. They may, however, have a role in conjunction with immunosuppressive therapy (see above).

1. Bacigalupo A. Guidelines for the treatment of severe aplastic anemia. *Haematologica* 1994; **79:** 438–44.
2. Young NS. Aplastic anaemia. *Lancet* 1995; **346:** 228–32.
3. Marsh JCW, Gordon-Smith EC. Treatment options in severe aplastic anaemia. *Lancet* 1998; **351:** 1830–1.
4. Webb DKH, *et al.* Acquired aplastic anaemia: still a serious disease. *Arch Dis Child* 1991; **66:** 858–61.
5. Werner EJ, *et al.* Immunosuppressive therapy versus bone marrow transplantation for children with aplastic anemia. *Pediatrics* 1989; **83:** 61–5.
6. Frickhofen N, *et al.* Treatment of aplastic anemia with antilymphocyte globulin and methylprednisolone with or without cyclosporine. *N Engl J Med* 1991; **324:** 1297–1304.

7. Bacigalupo A, *et al.* Antilymphocyte globulin, cyclosporin, and granulocyte colony-stimulating factor in patients with acquired severe aplastic anemia (SAA): a pilot study of the EBMT SAA Working Party. *Blood* 1995; **85:** 1348–53.
8. Crump M, *et al.* Treatment of adults with severe aplastic anemia: primary therapy with antithymocyte globulin (ATG) and rescue of ATG failures with bone marrow transplantation. *Am J Med* 1992; **92:** 596–602.
9. Moore MAS, Castro-Malaspina H. Immunosuppression in aplastic anemia—postponing the inevitable? *N Engl J Med* 1991; **324:** 1358–60.
10. Socié G, *et al.* Malignant tumors occurring after treatment of aplastic anemia. *N Engl J Med* 1993; **329:** 1152–7.
11. Vadhan-Raj S, *et al.* Stimulation of myelopoiesis in patients with aplastic anemia by recombinant human granulocyte-macrophage colony-stimulating factor. *N Engl J Med* 1988; **319:** 1628–34.
12. Kurzrock R, *et al.* Very low doses of GM-CSF administered alone or with erythropoietin in aplastic anemia. *Am J Med* 1992; **93:** 41–8.
13. Geissler K, *et al.* Effect of interleukin-3 on responsiveness to granulocyte-colony-stimulating factor in severe aplastic anemia. *Ann Intern Med* 1992; **117:** 223–5.
14. Marsh JCW, *et al.* Haemopoietic growth factors in aplastic anaemia: a cautionary note. *Lancet* 1994; **344:** 172–3.

Haemoglobinopathies

Haemoglobinopathies are clinical abnormalities due to altered structure, function, or production of haemoglobin. Human haemoglobins are tetramers, constructed of 4 globin chains each enfolding an iron-containing haem moiety: two of these globins are of the 'α-like' types (globins α or ζ) and two are 'non-α' (types β, γ, δ, or ε). The normal major adult haemoglobin, haemoglobin A, comprises two α and two β chains, while the predominant fetal haemoglobin, haemoglobin F (also present in minute amounts in normal adults), is composed of two α and two γ globins. The erythroblast inherits two genes for the production of α globin and one for β globin production from each parent, and a mutation in a single α gene will therefore affect only 25% of the haemoglobin produced, whereas a single β mutation will affect 50%: the β-haemoglobinopathies, due to defective β globin production, are therefore more likely to produce symptoms, and the most widespread forms are the β-thalassaemias and sickle-cell disease, which are discussed below.

Haemolytic anaemia

The normal life span of an erythrocyte is about 120 days; a haemolytic state is defined as a reduction in this mean life span due to premature destruction of red cells, either intravascularly, or more commonly after sequestration by the spleen or liver. Healthy bone marrow can compensate for even quite severe haemolysis by increased erythropoiesis; however, if the red cell survival-time is less than 15 days, or if the bone marrow is abnormal, or there is a deficiency of folate, iron, or other necessary nutrients, then compensation will be inadequate and haemolytic anaemia will result. In addition to typical symptoms of anaemia (above) patients frequently exhibit jaundice and splenomegaly, while the increased erythropoiesis results in reticulocytosis (elevated counts of immature red cells).

Haemolytic anaemias may be either congenital or acquired. The congenital disorders include those due to membrane defects in the erythrocyte such as spherocytosis or elliptocytosis; those due to enzyme defects (including the various forms of glucose-6-phosphate dehydrogenase deficiency); and those due to haemoglobin defects (haemoglobinopathies) including sickle-cell disease and β-thalassaemia (below).

The acquired haemolytic anaemias arise from numerous causes but may be divided into immune and non-immune types. The immune types include some drug-induced haemolytic anaemias (including those produced by penicillins, rifampicin, and methyldopa); auto-immune haemolytic anaemia (further classified into warm or cold depending on the temperature at which the red cell antibodies are most active); and haemolytic disease of the newborn (see p.1503). The non-immune types include haemolysis due to infections such as malaria; chemically-induced haemolysis (due to a direct effect on the red cell rather than an immunologically-mediated one, and including the effects of toxins such as copper and arsenic as well as some snake venoms, and drugs such as amphotericin, dapsone, and sulphasalazine); and the effects of mechanical trauma.

Treatment. The appropriate treatment of haemolytic anaemia depends on the underlying cause, although general supportive measures (bed rest, transfusion if haemodynamic abnormalities make it necessary, and supplementation with folate) will be similar in all poorly-compensated patients. Well compensated haemolysis may require no treatment at all, though clearly elucidation and, where possible, removal of the cause is desirable.

Hereditary haemolytic disorders such as spherocytosis mostly respond well to splenectomy, although milder forms may not require treatment. In patients with glucose-6-phosphate dehydrogenase deficiency, treatment consists essentially of avoidance of drugs or foodstuffs likely to provoke haemolysis.

Acquired haemolytic anaemia is best treated by identification and where possible elimination of any underlying cause. Most drug-induced haemolytic anaemias respond rapidly to discontinuation of the offending substance.

Auto-immune haemolytic anaemias require treatment aimed at maintaining the patient and controlling haemolysis. Although treatment may need to be prolonged, in many patients with idiopathic disease antibodies eventually disappear or decrease to insignificant titres after months or years. The auto-immune haemolytic anaemias may be secondary to other disorders including leukaemias, lymphomas, and systemic lupus erythematosus; correction of the underlying disease often results in marked improvement of accompanying haemolysis.

In patients with warm auto-immune haemolytic anaemia initial treatment is with corticosteroids. A typical initial dose is prednisone or prednisolone 80 mg by mouth daily; higher doses are rarely required. The initial dose may be reduced over 2 to 4 weeks to 20 mg daily; thereafter, the dose may be decreased more slowly and cautiously to the minimum necessary to control symptoms. If oral therapy is inappropriate hydrocortisone has been given intravenously. If symptoms do not respond to tolerable doses of corticosteroids splenectomy should be considered. Alternative approaches include the use of vinblastine- or vincristine-loaded platelets,[1] or intravenous infusions of high-dose normal immunoglobulin.[2,3] Immunosuppressants such as azathioprine may be considered in patients refractory to other therapy; responses are reportedly variable, but they sometimes permit reduction of corticosteroid maintenance doses. Transfusion is problematic in these patients because of the difficulty in establishing compatibility between patient and donor.[4,5] Nonetheless, transfusion may be life-saving in acute disease, and the least incompatible blood should be used.

In patients with cold auto-immune haemolytic anaemias such as cold haemagglutinin disease it is additionally important to keep the patient warm. Corticosteroids and splenectomy are generally of no benefit in these patients (although there may be a responsive subgroup[6]), but treatment with chlorambucil 2 to 4 mg daily by mouth may produce a response. Blood transfusion should be avoided if possible, and if given it should be preferably via a warming coil and infused slowly.

1. Ahn YS, *et al.* Treatment of autoimmune hemolytic anemia with vinca-loaded platelets. *JAMA* 1983; **249:** 2189–94.
2. Mitchell CA, *et al.* High dose intravenous gammaglobulin in Coombs positive hemolytic anemia. *Aust N Z J Med* 1987; **17:** 290–4.
3. Blanchette VS, *et al.* Role of intravenous immunoglobulin G in autoimmune hematologic disorders. *Semin Hematol* 1992; **29:** 72–82.
4. Salama A, *et al.* Red blood cell transfusion in warm-type autoimmune hemolytic anemia. *Lancet* 1992; **340:** 1515–17.
5. Garratty G, Petz LD. Transfusing patients with autoimmune haemolytic anaemia. *Lancet* 1993; **341:** 1220.
6. Silberstein LE, *et al.* Cold hemagglutinin disease associated with IgG cold-reactive antibody. *Ann Intern Med* 1987; **106:** 238–42.

Iron-deficiency anaemia

The iron content of the body is normally kept constant by regulation of the amount absorbed to balance the amount lost. If loss is increased, and/or intake inadequate, a negative iron-balance may lead by degrees to depletion of body iron stores, iron deficiency, and eventually to anaemia. Iron requirements are increased during infancy, puberty, pregnancy, and during menstruation, and iron-deficiency anaemias are most common in women and children; the most common cause in adult males and postmenopausal women is blood loss, usually from the gastro-intestinal tract.

Iron deficiency usually results in a microcytic, hypochromic anaemia, but, the diagnosis of iron deficiency should be confirmed, if there is any doubt, by measurement of serum ferritin or total iron binding capacity (transferrin). Iron therapy can begin once deficiency is confirmed, but the underlying cause of the deficiency should still be sought.

Treatment. The prevention and control of iron-deficiency anaemias has been reviewed.[1-3] Almost all iron-deficiency anaemias respond readily to treatment with iron. The treatment of choice is oral administration of a ferrous salt (ferrous iron is better absorbed than ferric iron). Many iron compounds have been used for this purpose, but do not offer any real advantage over the simple ferrous fumarate, gluconate, or sulphate salts. The usual adult dose is sufficient of these salts to supply about 100 to 200 mg of elemental iron daily (for the elemental iron content of various iron salts see p.1347). A rise in haemoglobin concentration of about 0.1 g or more per 100 mL daily is considered a positive response. Haemoglobin response is greatest in the first few weeks of therapy and is proportional to the severity of the original anaemia. Once haemoglobin concentrations have risen to the normal range, iron therapy should be continued for a further 3 months to aid replenishment of iron stores.

Oral iron has been given with agents such as ascorbic acid which enhances iron absorption significantly if given in large enough doses, but such combinations increase the cost of therapy and may increase the incidence of adverse effects. Modified-release preparations have been used in patients intolerant to ordinary formulations of iron but some consider them therapeutically ineffective.

Failure to respond to oral iron after about 3 weeks of therapy may be indicative of non-compliance, continued blood loss with inadequate replacement of iron, malabsorption, wrong diagnosis, or other complicating factors, and the treatment should be reassessed.

Parenteral iron therapy is rarely indicated, may produce severe adverse effects, and should be reserved for patients who are genuinely intolerant of oral iron, persistently non-compliant, who have gastro-intestinal disorders exacerbated by oral iron therapy, continuing blood loss too severe for oral treatment to provide sufficient iron, or for those unable to absorb iron adequately from the gastro-intestinal tract. The most common parenteral forms are iron sorbitol (given intramuscularly) and iron dextran (given intravenously, in which case the complete iron requirement may be given as a single infusion, or intramuscularly).

Exceptionally, in patients with profound anaemia, blood transfusion may be necessary to restore dangerously low concentrations of haemoglobin. This may be the case, for example, in elderly patients with long-standing iron deficiency leading to heart failure. However, transfusion should always be avoided if possible.

Prophylaxis. Prophylaxis may be desirable in some groups at risk of iron deficiency and consequent anaemia, and may include therapy with oral iron supplements, measures to improve dietary iron intake, fortification of food staples, or control of infection.

Therapy with prophylactic iron supplements is justifiable in pregnancy where there are risk factors for deficiency, but the practice of universal supplementation is less widespread than formerly, and some authorities consider that it should be reserved for documented deficiency.[4-6] The US Preventive Services Task Force has reviewed the subject of iron supplementation during pregnancy,[7] and concluded that there was insufficient evidence for or against routine supplementation.[8]

Iron supplementation is accepted in menorrhagia, after gastrectomy, and in the management of low birth-weight infants such as the premature. Iron deficiency in infants and children may result in developmental delay,[9-12] reversible with iron supplements,[13] and WHO has suggested supplementation in pre-school children;[1] however, this does not seem to be the practice in developed countries, although there is some suggestion that screening would be valuable to identify iron-deficient children in this age group.[12,14,15]

The usual prophylactic dose in adults is sufficient of a ferrous salt to provide about 60 to 100 mg of elemental iron daily. Doses of around 1 mg per kg body-weight of elemental iron daily have been suggested for prophylaxis in children.

Dietary measures, such as addition of vitamin-C-rich foods, or other enhancers of iron absorption including iron in the form of haem (found in meat or fish) to the diet, and control of parasitic infections such as hookworm (which are responsible for considerable occult blood loss), are particularly important for the general community in developing countries. Fortification of food staples poses technical problems as iron salts react with food components and may produce rancidity or other undesirable changes on storage. Nonetheless, wheat flour, bread, and milk products are often so fortified, and consideration has been given to fortification of salt, sugar, rice, and fish sauce.

1. De Maeyer EM, *et al. Preventing and controlling iron deficiency anaemia through primary health care: a guide for health administrators and programme managers.* Geneva: WHO, 1989.
2. Chipping P. Management of iron deficiency anaemia. *Prescribers' J* 1990; **30:** 65–71.
3. Frewin R, *et al.* ABC of clinical haematology. Iron deficiency anaemia. *Br Med J* 1997; **314:** 360–3.
4. Hibbard BM. Iron and folate supplements during pregnancy: supplementation is valuable only in selected patients. *Br Med J* 1988; **297:** 1324 and 1326.
5. Horn E. Iron and folate supplements during pregnancy: supplementing everyone treats those at risk and is cost effective. *Br Med J* 1988; **297:** 1325 and 1327.
6. Chamberlain G. Medical problems in pregnancy—II. *Br Med J* 1991; **302:** 1327–30.
7. US Preventive Services Task Force. Routine iron supplementation during pregnancy: review article. *JAMA* 1993; **270:** 2848–54.
8. US Preventive Services Task Force. Routine iron supplementation during pregnancy: policy statement. *JAMA* 1993; **870:** 2846–8.
9. Walter T, *et al.* Iron deficiency anemia: adverse effects on infant psychomotor development. *Pediatrics* 1989; **84:** 7–17.
10. Filer LJ. Iron needs during rapid growth and mental development. *J Pediatr* 1990; **117:** S143–6.
11. Lozoff B, *et al.* Long-term developmental outcome of infants with iron deficiency. *N Engl J Med* 1991; **325:** 687–94.
12. Booth IW, Aukett MA. Iron deficiency anaemia in infancy and early childhood. *Arch Dis Child* 1997; **76:** 549–54.
13. Idjradinata P, Pollitt E. Reversal of developmental delays in iron-deficient anaemic infants treated with iron. *Lancet* 1993; **341:** 1–4.
14. James J, *et al.* Preventing iron deficiency in preschool children by implementing an educational and screening programme in an inner city practice. *Br Med J* 1989; **299:** 838–40.
15. James J, *et al.* Treatment of iron deficiency anaemia with iron in children. *Lancet* 1993; **341:** 572.

Megaloblastic anaemia

The megaloblastic anaemias are characterised by macrocytosis (an increased mean cell volume) and the production of distinctive morphological changes and abnormal maturation in developing haematopoietic cells in the bone marrow: white cell and platelet lines are affected as well as erythroid precursors, and in severe cases anaemia may be associated with leucopenia and thrombocytopenia. Megaloblastic anaemia is a consequence of impaired DNA biosynthesis in the bone marrow, usually due to a deficiency of vitamin B_{12} (cobalamins) or folate, both of which are essential for this process. Although the haematological symptoms of B_{12} deficiency and folate deficiency are similar it is important to distinguish between them with appropriate diagnostic tests since the use of folate alone in B_{12}-deficient megaloblastic anaemia may improve haematological symptoms without preventing aggravation of accompanying neurological symptoms, and may lead to severe nervous system sequelae such as subacute combined degeneration of the spinal cord. Where it is desirable to commence therapy immediately, combined treatment for both deficiencies may be begun once suitable samples have been taken to permit diagnosis of the deficiency, and the patient converted to the appropriate treatment once the cause of the anaemia is known.

Vitamin B_{12} deficiency anaemia. Vitamin B_{12} deficiency and its associated symptoms may be due to malabsorption (including following gastrectomy), dietary deficiency (mainly in strict vegetarians), competition with intestinal bacteria or parasites, or to the effect of drugs such as nitrous oxide. In populations of northern European origin pernicious anaemia, in which atrophy of the gastric mucosa results in a lack of the intrinsic factor essential for B_{12} absorption, is the most frequent cause. Owing to large body stores of the vitamin it may take several years for signs of deficiency to manifest once the defect in absorption occurs.

In addition to megaloblastic anaemia, vitamin B_{12} deficiency may result in neurological damage, including peripheral neuropathy and effects on mental function ranging from mild neurosis to dementia.

TREATMENT. The treatment is with vitamin B_{12}, almost always by the intramuscular or sometimes the deep subcutaneous route since in most patients absorption from the gastro-intestinal tract is inadequate. Hydroxocobalamin is generally preferred to cyanocobalamin since it need be given less often. Regimens may vary, but hydroxocobalamin 1 mg every few days for 6 to 8 doses will restore normal body stores of the vitamin. The haematological response to therapy is rapid, with improvement in most parameters and symptoms beginning within 48 hours. Neurological abnormalities may take much longer to respond, and may not do so completely.

PROPHYLAXIS. Where the defect in B_{12} handling is irreversible, as in pernicious anaemia, maintenance therapy must continue for life to prevent a recurrence of the deficiency. Therapy must also be given prophylactically after total gastrectomy or total ileal resection, or where gastro-intestinal surgery is shown to have impaired absorption of the vitamin. Typically, injection of hydroxocobalamin 1 mg every 3 months is used. In patients in whom injection is not possible, 1 mg may be given daily by mouth, since a few micrograms may be absorbed by passive diffusion. In patients whose diet supplies inadequate B_{12}, deficiency may be prevented, in the absence of other causes, by much lower oral doses given as a supplement; up to 0.15 mg (150 μg) of cyanocobalamin daily has been recommended.

Folate-deficiency anaemia. Deficiency of folate may be due to inadequate diet, or malabsorption syndromes (as in coeliac disease or sprue), to increased utilisation (as in pregnancy, one of the most common causes of megaloblastic anaemia, or the increased haematopoiesis of haemolytic syndromes), to increased urinary loss or loss due to haemodialysis, or to an adverse effect of alcohol, antiepileptics, or other drugs.

The clinical features of folate-deficient megaloblastic anaemia are similar to those of disease due to vitamin-B_{12} deficiency except that the accompanying severe neuropathy does not occur, and deficiency may develop much more rapidly. Deficiency may also be associated with neural tube defects (p.1341) if it occurs in pregnancy.

TREATMENT. Once folate deficiency has been established the usual treatment in the UK is folic acid 5 mg by mouth daily. Lower doses of 0.25 to 1.0 mg are suggested in the USA. It is customary to continue therapy for at least 4 months, the period of time necessary for complete red-cell replacement. In patients with malabsorption, therapy may require higher doses, up to 15 mg of folic acid daily. As in B_{12}-deficiency anaemia, the response to therapy is rapid.

PROPHYLAXIS. Long-term maintenance is rarely needed, except in a few patients in whom the underlying cause of folate deficiency cannot be treated (for example in some severe haemolytic syndromes). Doses of 5 mg daily or even weekly have been suggested for prophylaxis in patients undergoing dialysis or with chronic haemolytic states, depending on the diet and rate of haemolysis; doses of 0.4 to 0.8 mg daily are recommended in the USA.

For primary prophylaxis of megaloblastic anaemia in pregnancy, folic acid is given in the UK in usual doses of 0.2 to 0.5 mg daily, often in combination with a ferrous iron salt for prophylaxis of iron deficiency. In the USA, doses of up to, but not more than, 1 mg daily are suggested.

Drugs which act as inhibitors of dihydrofolate reductase, such as methotrexate, may produce severe megaloblastic anaemia which cannot be reversed by therapy with folic acid. The adverse effects of such drugs may be largely prevented or reversed by therapy with folinic acid, which can be incorporated into folate metabolism without the need for reduction by the inhibited enzyme. For details of such 'folinic acid rescue', see under Folinic Acid, p.1342.

General references.

1. Hoffbrand V, Provan D. ABC of clinical haematology: macrocytic anaemias. *Br Med J* 1997; **314:** 430–33.

Normocytic-normochromic anaemia

Anaemias in which red-cell size and cellular haemoglobin are not significantly different from normal (normocytic-normochromic anaemias) form a substantial proportion of all cases. Such anaemias are usually secondary to another disease and include the anaemia of chronic disorders (associated with chronic infection such as tuberculosis, malignancy, inflammatory disorders such as inflammatory bowel disease, polymyalgia rheumatica, rheumatoid arthritis, and systemic lupus erythematosus), anaemia of renal failure, anaemia of prematurity, anaemia associated with endocrine disorders such as hypothyroidism or hypopituitarism, and anaemias associated with primary bone-marrow failure (including aplastic anaemia, above, pure red-cell aplasia, marrow fibrosis or infiltration as in myelodysplasia or leukaemia, and marrow failure associated with AIDS). Iron-deficiency anaemia, which is usually classified as microcytic and hypochromic may in fact be neither, particularly in the early stages, and should be differentiated from anaemia of chronic disease. The latter is also accompanied by changes in iron metabolism, notably sequestration of iron in reticuloendothelial cells: plasma iron is low but in contrast to iron deficiency the total iron binding capacity is reduced and serum ferritin is often increased.

The **treatment** of most of these anaemias is essentially that of the underlying disease. Blood transfusion has been given when anaemia is severe. In patients with anaemia of renal failure, which is due at least in part to decreased erythropoietin production by the damaged kidney, regular subcutaneous or intravenous injection of recombinant human erythropoietins (epoetin alfa or epoetin beta) can completely reverse the anaemia. Erythropoietins have been investigated in patients with the anaemia of chronic disease and some other normocytic-normochromic anaemias.

Sickle-cell disease

Sickle-cell disease is a haemoglobinopathy (above) in which a structural abnormality in the β globin chain results in the formation of an abnormal haemoglobin, haemoglobin S, that polymerises in the deoxygenated state, making the red cell less flexible and, when present in sufficient amounts, deforming it into a sickle shape. Normal haemoglobins may be incorporated into the polymer although some, such as fetal haemoglobin (haemoglobin F), do not participate and if present in sufficient amounts reduce sickling.

The heterozygous form, sickle-cell trait, is generally asymptomatic except in conditions of extreme anoxia, although characteristic abnormalities of renal function (inadequate concentration of the urine) may be present. As with thalassaemia trait (below) it is more common in populations of tropical origin, and has been postulated to offer a degree of protection against malaria. In the homozygous form a varying degree of haemolytic anaemia is present, accompanied by increased erythropoiesis. In addition to shortened survival, the decreased flexibility of the deformed erythrocytes can lead to occlusion of the microvasculature, and sickle-cell crisis. The latter may manifest as excruciating pain due to infarction of the blood supply to the bones, or infarction of other organs including lung, liver, kidney, penis (leading to priapism), and brain (stroke). Occasionally a large proportion of red cell mass may become trapped in spleen or liver (sequestration crisis) with death due to gross anaemia. Chronic complications include skin ulceration, renal failure, retinal detachment, and increased susceptibility to infection.

Treatment. The treatment of sickle-cell disease is essentially symptomatic.[1] Young children should receive prophylactic penicillin, and possibly pneumococcal vaccine, to reduce the risk of infection (see Spleen Disorders, p.143). Infection should be treated early, and folate supplementation given if necessary since the increased erythropoiesis resulting from chronic haemolysis may increase folate requirements.

Sickle-cell crisis requires hospitalisation, with the use of large volumes of intravenous fluids for dehydration, analgesia including opioids for pain, and antibiotics to treat any concurrent infection. The management of pain in sickle-cell crisis is discussed further on p.11. Oxygen should be given if the patient is hypoxaemic. Where crisis affects a vital organ with life-threatening or potentially disabling consequences partial exchange transfusion should be carried out promptly, as no other therapy exists. Where rapid enlargement of spleen or liver indicates a sequestration crisis, transfusion is also important to avoid fatal anaemia.

Maintenance transfusion is rarely indicated, although it may be given to patients who have already had a stroke; measures to avoid iron overload such as phlebotomy or desferrioxamine chelation are necessary in patients receiving regular transfusions.

Research into specific therapy for sickling has recently produced promising results.[2] Because haemoglobin F is known to protect against sickling, considerable interest has centred on attempts to stimulate fetal haemoglobin production. Most studies have used hydroxyurea. Initial trials showed some elevation in mean fetal haemoglobin concentrations, but responses were very variable. However, a subsequent randomised controlled study in 299 patients[3] reported that treatment with hydroxyurea caused a 44% reduction in the median annual rate of painful crises. The beneficial effects did not become evident for several months. Beneficial effects have also been reported in initial studies in children.[4,5] However, the potential toxicity of long-term treatment with hydroxyurea (especially in children) remains a concern. A combination of hydroxyurea with erythropoietin has been reported to increase fetal haemoglobin concentrations further in one study,[6] although not in another using a different dosage regimen.[7] A short-chain fatty acid, butyric acid, that has a low order of toxicity, has been reported to stimulate fetal haemoglobin in patients with sickle-cell disease when it was given by infusion as arginine butyrate.[8]

As in thalassaemia (below), bone-marrow transplantation is potentially curative in a small minority of patients, but the indications for transplantation are much less well established, and its use and benefits remain a matter for debate.[9-11]

1. Davies SC, Oni L. Management of patients with sickle cell disease. *Br Med J* 1997; **315:** 656–60.
2. Bunn HF. Pathogenesis and treatment of sickle cell disease. *N Engl J Med* 1997; **337:** 762–9.
3. Charache S, *et al.* Effect of hydroxyurea on the frequency of painful crises in sickle cell anemia. *N Engl J Med* 1995; **332:** 1317–22.
4. Scott JP, *et al.* Hydroxyurea therapy in children severely affected with sickle cell disease. *J Pediatr* 1996; **128:** 820–8.
5. Ferster A, *et al.* Hydroxyurea for treatment of severe sickle cell anemia: a pediatric clinical trial. *Blood* 1996; **88:** 1960–4.
6. Rodgers GP, *et al.* Augmentation by erythropoietin of the fetal-hemoglobin response to hydroxyurea in sickle cell disease. *N Engl J Med* 1993; **328:** 73–80.
7. Goldberg MA, *et al.* Treatment of sickle cell anemia with hydroxyurea and erythropoietin. *N Engl J Med* 1990; **323:** 366–72.
8. Perrine SP, *et al.* A short-term trial of butyrate to stimulate fetal-globin-gene expression in the β-globin disorders. *N Engl J Med* 1993; **328:** 81–6.
9. Davies SC, Roberts IAG. Bone marrow transplant for sickle cell disease—an update. *Arch Dis Child* 1996; **75:** 3–6.
10. Walters MC, *et al.* Bone marrow transplantation for sickle cell disease. *N Engl J Med* 1996; **335:** 369–76.
11. Platt OS, Guinan EC. Bone marrow transplantation in sickle cell anemia—the dilemma of choice. *N Engl J Med* 1996; **335:** 426–8.

Sideroblastic anaemia

The sideroblastic anaemias are characterised by a population of hypochromic red cells in the presence of increased serum-iron concentrations, and abnormal erythroid precursors, known as ring sideroblasts, in the bone marrow. They are associated with abnormalities in porphyrin biosynthesis leading to diminished production of haem, and increased cellular iron uptake. Sideroblastic anaemias may be of various types, and are classified as acquired or hereditary.

Acquired sideroblastic anaemia. Acquired sideroblastic anaemia may either be idiopathic, or secondary to either a drug or toxin (such as alcohol, isoniazid, chloramphenicol, or lead) or to a disease (including hypothyroidism, rheumatoid arthritis, haemolytic or megaloblastic anaemias, leukaemias, and lymphomas). The treatment of the secondary forms is essentially the treatment of the underlying disease or removal of the precipitating cause. The anaemia is usually mild and often macrocytic.

Patients with idiopathic disease usually have only mild anaemia, and most require no treatment. Although rarely suffering from vitamin B_6 deficiency a few patients will respond at least partially to high doses of pyridoxine by mouth, up to 400 mg daily, and a trial is considered worthwhile in all patients. If patients become symptomatic, transfusion may be required, but should be kept to a minimum because of the problems of iron overload. All patients with sideroblastic anaemia must have their serum-iron and -ferritin concentrations regularly monitored, and be given desferrioxamine by regular bolus injection when there is evidence of iron overload.

Hereditary sideroblastic anaemia. The hereditary forms of the disease appear to be sex-linked, and almost always manifest themselves in males. The anaemia may be more severe than in acquired sideroblastic anaemia, and is usually microcytic.

A trial of pyridoxine, as in the acquired form, is considered worthwhile as some forms are responsive, but in many cases there is no benefit. Some patients develop gradually increasing iron loads, and may eventually develop haemosiderosis; to prevent this, regular venesection or the use of desferrioxamine are indicated if there is evidence of iron accumulation.

Disturbed mitochondrial iron metabolism is believed to be involved in sideroblastic anaemia. Ubidecarenone, a coenzyme in electron transport in the mitochondria, has been tried in few patients with refractory sideroblastic anaemia (mostly idiopathic), but results have not been encouraging.

β-Thalassaemia

β-Thalassaemia is a haemoglobinopathy (above) that is due to a deficiency in β globin production accompanied by normal production of α globin chains that, in the absence of sufficient partner chains, are insoluble and precipitate out in erythrocytes and erythroid precursors as large cellular inclusions. These interfere with red-cell maturation resulting in ineffective haematopoiesis, retard the passage of red cells from the bone marrow, and create a tendency for those red cells which do mature to be trapped and destroyed in the spleen. The condition is therefore characterised by a hypochromic, microcytic anaemia accompanied by haemolysis. In the heterozygous form, where only one of the β globin genes is affected (known as thalassaemia trait or thalassaemia minor) the anaemia is mild and clinically insignificant. There is some evidence that patients with this form of the disease experience a degree of protection from malaria, which may account for the more frequent distribution of the trait in the populations of areas such as the Mediterranean, parts of Africa, and Asia.

The more severe forms of the disease (known as thalassaemia intermedia if haemoglobin levels are high enough not to require regular transfusion, or thalassaemia major in transfusion-dependent patients) occur in homozygous patients who inherit a defective β globin gene from both parents. Severe anaemia develops in the first year of life as fetal haemoglobin production (which does not involve a β globin) is replaced by the production of adult haemoglobin. The anaemia stimulates erythropoietin production, and if not corrected massive proliferation of red cell precursors develops within, and eventually beyond, the bone marrow, resulting in recurrent bone fractures, deformity of the skull due to expansion of the marrow spaces, and compression of vital structures such as the spinal cord with consequent paresis. Other symptoms include splenomegaly and hypersplenism (resulting in neutropenia and thrombocytopenia), increased susceptibility to infection, and hypermetabolism which may lead to folate deficiency because of the increased folate requirement. If untreated, death in patients with thalassaemia major usually occurs by the 2nd or 3rd year.

Treatment. The mainstay of treatment for severe β-thalassaemia has been regular blood transfusion to correct the anaemia. Transfusions should be begun as early as possible in life once it is clear that anaemia is severe enough to warrant them. Transfusion of washed or frozen red cells every 6 to 8 weeks is usually required, to maintain haemoglobin values of between 9 and 14 g per 100 mL; a sudden increase in transfusion requirements is a sign of hypersplenism, which may be an indication for splenectomy although this should be avoided if possible below the age of 5 because of the increased risk of infection. For a discussion of antibacterial prophylaxis in splenectomised patients, see Spleen Disorders, p.143.

If anaemia is corrected by transfusion, growth and development proceed fairly normally in thalassaemic children. However, because the body lacks a mechanism for the excretion of excess iron repeated transfusion invariably results in iron overload, leading eventually to haemochromatosis. The consequences of haemochromatosis include mild liver dysfunction, endocrine dysfunction (failure of the adolescent growth spurt, hypogonadism, sometimes diabetes and hypothyroidism), and particularly heart disease (pericarditis, heart failure, and arrhythmias). If unchecked, the iron build-up usually leads to death (mainly through heart failure or arrhythmia) by the time patients reach their mid-20s. The accumulation of iron can be retarded by the use of the chelating agent desferrioxamine. This has been shown to improve survival in thalassaemic children given regular systemic therapy,[1-3] the greatest increase in iron excretion being seen in patients given the drug by continuous subcutaneous infusion rather than intramuscular bolus. There is some suggestion that intensive desferrioxamine therapy can improve impaired organ function,[4-7] but it is considered preferable to begin chelation therapy as early as possible (in practice usually at 2 to 3 years of age) to try to prevent organ damage developing in the first place. Better iron excretion is achieved if patients are given ascorbic acid 100 to 200 mg daily in addition to desferrioxamine. Patients with thalassaemia may have increased folate requirements and folate supplementation may also be necessary. Although it is not yet certain how much chelation therapy will prolong survival the fact that a nearly normal iron balance can be achieved long term[4] seems hopeful. Deferiprone has been investigated as an oral alternative to desferrioxamine,[8,9] but may not be effective in the longer term.[10]

In addition to the essentially symptomatic treatment of thalassaemia a very few patients may be candidates for bone-marrow transplantation where suitable facilities and compatible donors exist; if transplantation is carried out before organ damage is marked, successfully transplanted patients are apparently cured and can lead a normal life.[11-13] Gene therapy is also under investigation.

An alternative approach, using azacitidine or, particularly, hydroxyurea, in an attempt to stimulate fetal haemoglobin production and 'mop up' some of the excess α globin chains, has been tried experimentally but results have been mixed. Results of an initial study in patients given butyric acid (as an arginine butyrate infusion) for the same purpose appeared more promising[14] although a subsequent study failed to show any benefit.[15]

1. Zurlo MG, *et al.* Survival and causes of death in thalassaemia major. *Lancet* 1989; **ii:** 27–30.
2. Ehlers KH, *et al.* Prolonged survival in patients with beta-thalassemia major treated with deferoxamine. *J Pediatr* 1991; **118:** 540–5.
3. Olivieri NF, *et al.* Survival in medically treated patients with homozygous β-thalassemia. *N Engl J Med* 1994; **331:** 574–8.
4. Hoffbrand AV, *et al.* Improvement in iron status and liver function in patients with transfusional iron overload with long-term subcutaneous desferrioxamine. *Lancet* 1979; **i:** 947–9.
5. Maurer HS, *et al.* A prospective evaluation of iron chelation therapy in children with severe β-thalassemia: a six-year study. *Am J Dis Child* 1988; **142:** 287–92.
6. Freeman AP, *et al.* Early left ventricular dysfunction and chelation therapy in thalassemia major. *Ann Intern Med* 1983; **99:** 450–4.
7. Marcus RE, *et al.* Desferrioxamine to improve cardiac function in iron-overloaded patients with thalassaemia major. *Lancet* 1984; **i:** 392–3.
8. Olivieri NF, *et al.* Iron-chelation therapy with oral deferiprone in patients with thalassemia major. *N Engl J Med* 1995; **332:** 918–22.
9. Nathan DG. An orally active iron chelator. *N Engl J Med* 1995; **332:** 953–4.
10. Olivieri NF, *et al.* Long-term safety and effectiveness of iron-chelation therapy with deferiprone for thalassemia major. *N Engl J Med* 1998; **339:** 417–23.
11. Lucarelli G. Bone marrow transplantation for severe thalassaemia 1: the view from Pesaro. *Br J Haematol* 1991; **78:** 300–1.
12. Weatherall DJ. Bone marrow transplantation for severe thalassaemia 2: to be or not to be. *Br J Haematol* 1991; **78:** 301–3.
13. Lucarelli G, *et al.* Marrow transplantation in patients with thalassemia responsive to iron chelation therapy. *N Engl J Med* 1993; **329:** 840–4.
14. Perrine SP, *et al.* A short-term trial of butyrate to stimulate fetal-globin-gene expression in the β-globin disorders. *N Engl J Med* 1993; **328:** 81–6.
15. Sher GD, *et al.* Extended therapy with intravenous arginine butyrate in patients with β-hemoglobinopathies. *N Engl J Med* 1995; **332:** 1606–10.

Haemostasis

Haemostasis is the physiological response that occurs when blood vessels are damaged. It results in coagulation (formation of a blood clot) and thus arrests bleeding. The initial response is the formation of a plug of platelets which adhere both to the injured tissue and to each other. The vessel injury together with factors released by the platelets trigger a series of reactions (the coagulation 'cascade') mediated by proteins circulating in the plasma (blood clotting factors). This results in formation of an insoluble fibrin clot that reinforces the initial platelet plug. Regulatory mechanisms come into operation to prevent widespread coagulation. Lysis of the clot (fibrinolysis) then occurs when wound healing and tissue repair are underway.

The main haemostatic mechanisms are thus platelet aggregation, coagulation, regulation of coagulation, and fibrinolysis and these, together with the site of action of some antiplatelet, anticoagulant, thrombolytic, and antifibrinolytic drugs, are discussed below.

Platelet aggregation. Platelets usually circulate in plasma in an inactive form. Contact with damaged endothelium causes them to become activated and to adhere to the site of injury. This adhesion is partly mediated by binding of von Willebrand factor, a plasma protein that also acts as a carrier for factor VIII, to a glycoprotein (termed GPIb) on the platelet membrane surface. Substances are secreted by the activated platelets which cause further platelet aggregation (adenosine diphosphate and thromboxane A_2) and vasoconstriction (serotonin and thromboxane A_2). Thromboxane A_2 secreted by platelets is derived from arachidonic acid. The enzyme cyclo-oxygenase is required for the synthesis of thromboxane A_2 and this enzyme is inhibited by the antiplatelet drugs aspirin and sulphinpyrazone. Aspirin binds irreversibly to the enzyme and therefore the antiplatelet effect lasts for the lifetime of the platelet. Sulphinpyrazone is a reversible inhibitor of the enzyme. In addition to their action in forming the initial haemostatic plug, platelets are also involved in coagulation by providing a surface on which interactions between clotting factors take place, resulting in more efficient coagulation.

Coagulation. The series of reactions that results in formation of a fibrin clot may be conveniently considered as two pathways, the *intrinsic* pathway (initiated within the blood) and the *extrinsic* pathway (initiated by substances extraneous to the blood). While this distinction is useful for understanding *in-vitro* coagulation and is the basis for tests that are specific for each pathway (see below), the mechanism of *in-vivo* coagulation is not so segregated and factors appearing in one pathway are also necessary for reactions in the other pathway. The intrinsic and extrinsic pathways of coagulation and the *in-vivo* pathways are discussed further below and are represented in summary form in Figures 1 and 2, respectively. Factors circulate in the blood in an inactive form and are activated by cleavage of peptide bonds. The numerals attached to the factors reflect the order in which they were discovered and not their importance or position in the chain of reaction. The letter 'a' after a factor name or number denotes the activated form. Factors involved in blood coagulation are listed in Table 2. Once the coagulation cascade is initiated, activated factors act in positive feedback mechanisms to amplify the activation steps thus producing rapid coagulation. Cofactors are necessary as they increase the speed of the reactions. Other components necessary for coagulation are calcium ions and a membrane surface. Calcium ions are required for nearly all the reactions. Many of the activation steps, notably those involving factors VII, IX, and X, take place on a membrane surface provided by tissue factor or platelets. Factors bind to phospholipids on the membrane surface.

The *extrinsic* pathway is initiated when *tissue factor* (factor III) is released from damaged tissue. This forms a complex with *factor VII* and factor VIIa and directly activates *factor X*. The *intrinsic* pathway is initiated when blood comes into contact with a negatively charged surface. *Factor XII* interacts with high molecular weight kininogen (Fitzgerald factor) and prekallikrein (Fletcher factor) to produce *kallikrein* which activates factor XII. The active factor XIIa then activates *factor XI* which in turn activates *factor IX*. Factor IXa, together with activated *factor VIII* (VIIIa) as a cofactor, converts *factor X* to factor Xa. The extrinsic and intrinsic pathways therefore converge with the activation of factor X. Factor Xa, together with activated *factor V* (Va) as a cofactor, converts prothrombin to thrombin with the subsequent formation of a *fibrin* gel which is stabilised by *factor XIIIa* to form a stable clot.

The dependence on calcium ions of many steps in the coagulation cascade allows coagulation *in vitro* to be blocked by the addition of calcium chelating agents, such as sodium citrate, to collected blood. When collected blood is tested for coagulation function, addition of calcium ions allows clotting to proceed. Tests of coagulation function include activated partial thromboplastin time (APTT), which is a measure of the activity of the intrinsic system, prothrombin time (PT), a measure of the activity of the extrinsic system, and thrombin clotting time, which measures the conversion of fibrinogen to fibrin.

The factors involved in initiating the *in-vitro intrinsic* pathway, that is prekallikrein, factor XII, and possibly factor XI are probably not important in *in-vivo* blood coagulation as deficiency of any of these factors is not associated with a serious bleeding disorder. The important step in initiating the clotting cascade *in vivo* is release of *tissue factor* (factor III) from damaged tissue. As has already been mentioned, tissue factor forms a complex with *factor VII* and factor VIIa which activates *factor X*. Factor Xa activates *prothrombin* resulting in formation of a *fibrin clot* which occurs as described above under the *in-vitro* systems. To enhance coagulation, various positive feedback mechanisms and other clotting factors operate to increase production of activated factors VII and X. For example, formation of factor VIIa is amplified by factor VIIa itself and by factor Xa. Formation of factor Xa is amplified by factor IXa produced by the action of thrombin on factor XI.

Regulation of coagulation. The process of blood coagulation is regulated to ensure that it remains localised at the site of injury and does not result in more widespread clotting. This is achieved by dilution of clotting factors in flowing blood, by rapid hepatic clearance of many activated factors or products, and by natural anticoagulant mechanisms which include antithrombin III, protein C, and protein S (see Figure 2). *Antithrombin III* inhibits the serine protease clotting factors, that is, thrombin, IXa, Xa, XIa, and XIIa. Antithrombin III is activated by binding to glycosaminoglycans, such as heparan glycosaminoglycan and dermatan sulphate, present in vascular endothelium. Heparin and low-molecular-weight heparins act as anticoagulants by binding antithrombin III at a specific binding site and enhancing its inhibitory effect on the serine protease clotting factors. At therapeutic doses of heparin the factors inhibited are thrombin and factor Xa. Low-dose heparin, such as that given for the prophylaxis of thrombo-embolism, inhibits factor Xa. Very high doses of heparin have a direct inhibitory effect on antithrombin III. Heparinoids which lack the specific binding site for antithrombin III do not have the anticoagulant properties of heparin. Low-molecular-weight heparins have a higher ratio of anti-factor-Xa to antithrombin activity than heparin and therefore mainly inhibit factor Xa.

Proteins C and S are both vitamin K-dependent plasma proteins. Protein C circulates in plasma in an inactive form. It is activated by contact with thrombin that is bound to thrombomodulin, a receptor located on the surface of endothelial cells. Activated protein C inhibits factors Va and VIIIa and therefore slows blood clotting. Protein S acts as a cofactor in this inhibition. Vitamin K is essential for the activities of factors II, VII, IX, and X. It is also essential for the activity of proteins C and S. These factors contain glutamic acid residues that undergo carboxylation in the liver, a reaction requiring reduced vitamin K as a cofactor. This carboxylation step allows the factors to bind calcium, a reaction necessary for their function in the clotting cascade.

Table 2. Proteins involved in blood coagulation and in fibrinolysis.

	Proteins	Synonyms
Blood coagulation	Factor I	Fibrinogen
	Factor II*	Prothrombin
	Factor III	Tissue thromboplastin; tissue factor
	Factor IV	Calcium ion
	Factor V	Ac-globulin; labile factor; proaccelerin
	Factor VI (unassigned)	
	Factor VII*	Proconvertin; SPCA; stable factor
	Factor VIII	Antihaemophilic factor; AHF
	Factor IX*	Christmas factor; plasma thromboplastin component; PTC
	Factor X*	Stuart factor; Stuart-Prower factor
	Factor XI	Plasma thromboplastin antecedent; PTA
	Factor XII	Hageman factor
	Factor XIII	Fibrin stabilising factor; FSF
	von Willebrand factor	Factor VIII-related antigen; vWF
	High molecular weight kininogen	HMWK; Fitzgerald factor
	Prekallikrein	Fletcher factor
Fibrinolysis	Plasminogen	
	Prourokinase	
	Tissue plasminogen activator	tPA
	Antithrombin III	Major antithrombin; AT-III; Heparin cofactor
	Protein C*	Autoprothrombin
	Protein S*	
	α_2-Antiplasmin	

* denotes vitamin K-dependent factor

Figure 1. Simplified representation of *in-vitro* coagulation.

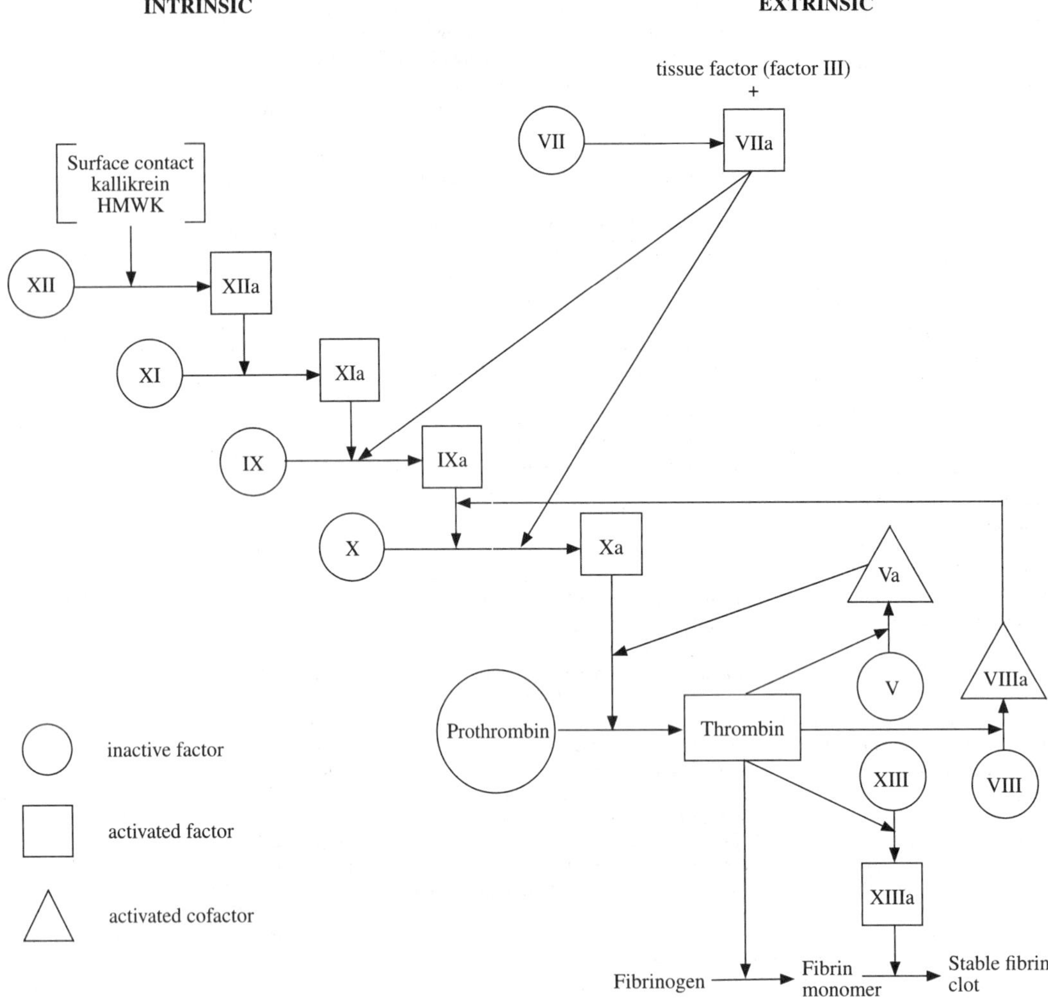

Deficiency of vitamin K or the use of oral anticoagulants (which are vitamin K antagonists) therefore impairs the function of these clotting factors. Oral anticoagulants have no effect on circulating clotting factors and thus the time required before the anticoagulant effect is seen depends on the individual clearance rate of the factor.

Fibrinolysis is the mechanism of clot dissolution. It is mediated by *plasminogen* which circulates in plasma in an inactive form; conversion to its active form, *plasmin*, occurs when plasminogen binds to fibrin in the presence of a *plasminogen activator* (see Figure 2). Plasmin, a *proteolytic enzyme*, digests fibrin clots and hydrolyses other proteins, including factors II, V, VIII, and XII. As fibrin is lysed, plasmin is released which is inhibited by α_2-antiplasmin to prevent a systemic lytic state developing. There are two types of plasminogen activator, *tissue plasminogen activator* (tPA) which originates from the endothelium, and *urokinase*, which is activated from prourokinase. Activators of prourokinase include plasmin. Tissue plasminogen activator bound to fibrin activates plasminogen much more rapidly than circulating plasminogen, and therefore the fibrinolytic action of tissue plasminogen activator is fibrin specific. Urokinase does not bind to fibrin, and therefore its fibrinolytic action is not fibrin specific, although it is activated by plasmin that is bound to fibrin. *In vivo*, fibrinolysis is almost entirely due to the activity of tissue plasminogen activator. The two types of plasminogen activator with their different modes of action provide the basis for the specificity of **thrombolytics** (the so-called 'clot specific' effect) which act by promoting the conversion of plasminogen to plasmin. The tissue plasminogen activators alteplase and duteplase are fibrin-specific thrombolytics, and streptokinase and urokinase are fibrin-nonspecific. The **antifibrinolytic drugs** aminocaproic acid and tranexamic acid act primarily by blocking the binding of plasminogen and plasmin to fibrin thereby preventing the breakdown of fibrin clots. Aprotinin, an inhibitor of proteolytic enzymes, acts as a **haemostatic** by inhibiting the action of plasmin and therefore preventing the breakdown of fibrin clots. Other drugs acting as haemostatics include batroxobin, which is reported to promote the production of fibrin from fibrinogen and ethamsylate which has a stabilising effect on the capillary wall. Drugs such as oxidised cellulose, calcium alginate, collagen, and gelatin act by providing a physical meshwork within which clotting can occur. Adrenaline acid tartrate, adrenalone hydrochloride, and noradrenaline acid tartrate produce haemostasis by causing vasoconstriction. Drugs with astringent properties such as alum, ferric chloride, silver nitrate, and trichloroacetic acid are also used for haemostasis. The use of haemostatics may be considered when bleeding cannot be controlled by direct measures such as the application of pressure, suture or ligation, or electrocoagulation.

Dysfunction of the haemostatic mechanisms or the systems regulating haemostasis produces haemorrhagic (below) or thrombo-embolic (p.801) disorders.

General references.

1. Furie B, Furie BC. Molecular and cellular biology of blood coagulation. *N Engl J Med* 1992; **326:** 800–806.

Disseminated intravascular coagulation

Disseminated intravascular coagulation (DIC) is an acute or chronic syndrome resulting from an underlying condition that causes pathological stimulation of coagulation at some point in the coagulation pathway (above); thrombin generation triggered by uncontrolled tissue factor is probably the predominant factor in most cases. Causes include obstetric emergencies (placental abruption, eclampsia), infection (notably Gram-negative septicaemia), neoplasms, trauma (head injury, burns), venomous snake bites, transfusion of incompatible blood, liver disease, and various vascular causes.

Stimulation of coagulation leads to microvascular thrombosis that produces widespread tissue ischaemia and may lead to ischaemia of major organs. Simultaneously, secondary activation of the fibrinolytic system and consumption of coagulation factors produces bleeding, which is often the predominant manifestation. Symptoms are therefore very variable and include those of bleeding, such as spontaneous bruising, prolonged bleeding from intravenous puncture sites, and gastrointestinal and pulmonary haemorrhage, and those of thrombosis, such as acute renal failure, venous thrombo-embolism, skin necrosis, liver failure, cerebral infarction, acute respiratory distress, and coma. Some cases may be asymptomatic.

Treatment of DIC is aimed primarily at the underlying cause since the condition will not resolve until the underlying trigger is removed. Recovery is often fairly

Figure 2. Simplified representation of *in-vivo* coagulation and fibrinolysis

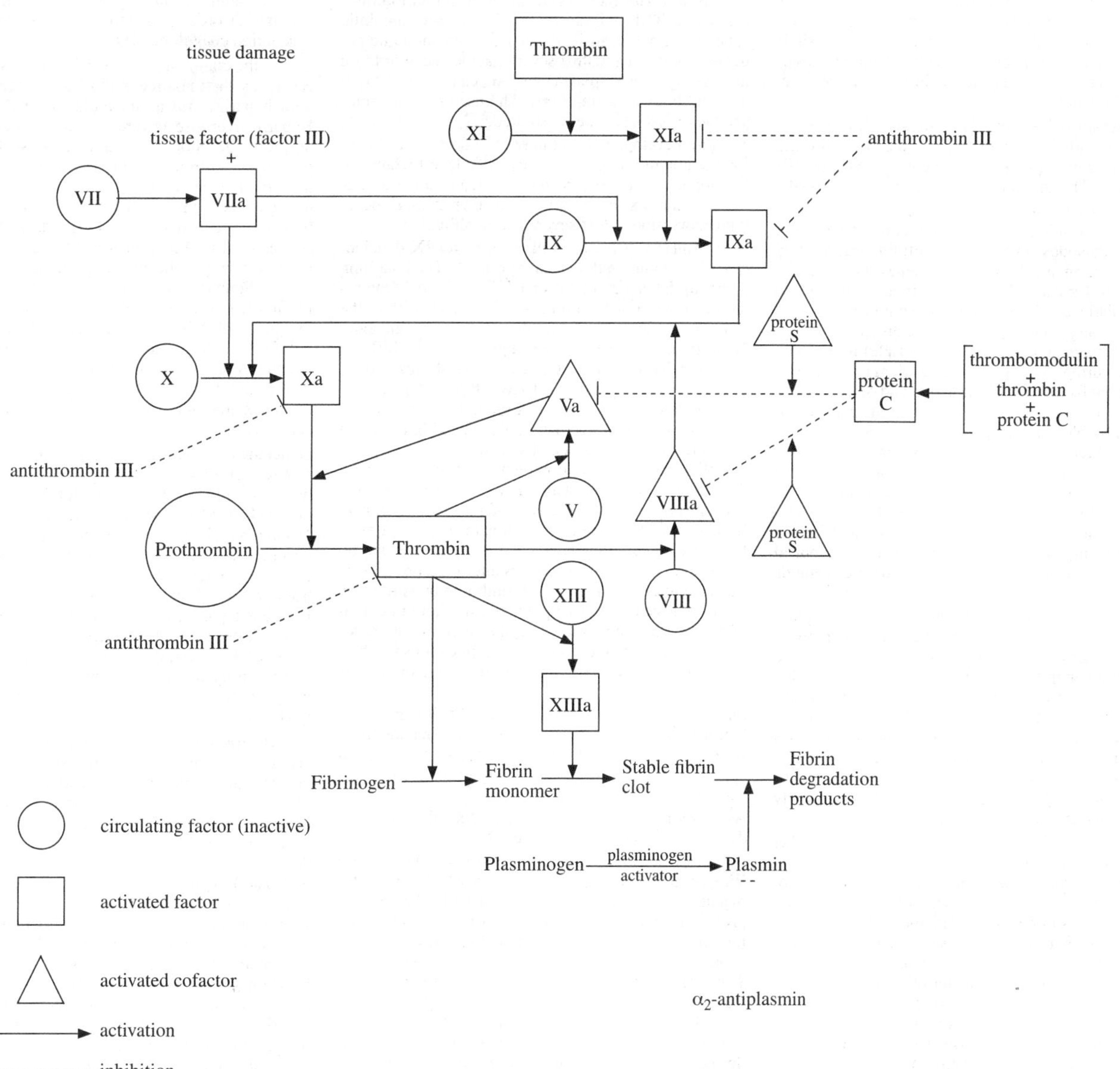

rapid once treatment is instituted. Supportive therapy to ensure adequate hydration and tissue oxygenation is also vital. These measures may be sufficient in patients with asymptomatic DIC. Most patients with symptomatic DIC also require administration of plasma and other blood components including platelets and cryoprecipitate as necessary to replace coagulation factors and arrest bleeding. Heparin has been used in the management of DIC with the aim of switching off the coagulatory mechanisms. Although benefit has been shown with some underlying causes, heparin may worsen bleeding and its use in DIC is considered by some to be controversial. Where bleeding is the main clinical problem, heparin should only be given if replacement of coagulation factors fails to stop the bleeding. Where the risk of bleeding is relatively minor and thrombosis predominates, heparin may be appropriate. Other measures that have been tried in limited numbers of patients include administration of a low-molecular-weight heparin, a thrombin inhibitor such as antithrombin III, and protein C.

General references.

1. Rubin RN, Colman RW. Disseminated intravascular coagulation: approach to treatment. *Drugs* 1992; **44:** 963–71.
2. Baglin T. Disseminated intravascular coagulation: diagnosis and treatment. *Br Med J* 1996; **312:** 683–7.
3. Frewin R, *et al.* ABC of clinical haematology. Haematological emergencies. *Br Med J* 1997; **314:** 1333–6.
4. de Jonge E, *et al.* Current drug treatment strategies for disseminated intravascular coagulation. *Drugs* 1998; **55:** 767–77.

Haemorrhagic disorders

Haemorrhage is bleeding from any part of the vascular system. The mechanisms responsible for haemostasis and its control, that is, platelet aggregation, blood coagulation, and fibrinolysis, are described under Haemostasis, above. Dysfunction of any of these systems may produce a haemorrhagic disorder, as discussed below. The dysfunction may be an inherited disorder or it may be acquired as a result of disease or a medical or surgical procedure. The management of haemorrhage is also an important part of the management of conditions such as peptic ulcer disease (p.1174), portal hypertension (p.1576), postpartum haemorrhage (p.1575), and haemorrhagic stroke (p.799).

- **Inherited haemorrhagic disorders.** Inherited disorders which lead to abnormal bleeding include platelet and vascular disorders, and disturbances in clotting factors. Inherited *platelet disorders* are rare; they include

- Bernard-Soulier syndrome (a lack of platelet GPIb receptor)
- thrombasthenia (defective glycoproteins IIb and IIIa)
- storage pool disease (lack of platelet ADP)

Disorders of *vascular function* include

- hereditary telangiectasia.

The most common inherited haemorrhagic disorders are due to absent, reduced, or malfunctioning *clotting factors*. The most important are

- **haemophilia A**
- **haemophilia B**
- **von Willebrand's disease**

Hereditary deficiency of all the clotting factors (other than calcium and thromboplastin) has been described although the incidence and clinical significance varies.

HAEMOPHILIA A (classical haemophilia, factor VIII deficiency) is the most common of the serious hereditary bleeding disorders. It is an X-linked recessive disorder and therefore with rare exceptions males are affected and females are carriers. The condition is due to deficiency of factor VIII; severity of bleeding is related to the residual factor level. The condition is severe when there is no detectable factor VIII activity, moderate when the factor VIII concentration is 2 to 5% of normal, and mild when the factor concentration is greater than 5%. Clots are slow to form and break up easily, and bleeding following trauma or surgery may continue for days or weeks. In moderate and severe haemophilia A bleeding may occur into major joints producing long-term joint destruction, a major cause of morbidity in haemophilia. Other frequent sites of bleeding are large muscles and renal and intestinal tracts. CNS haemorrhage may also occur, especially after trauma.

Treatment of bleeding episodes depends on the severity of the haemophilia.[1-4] Patients with mild haemophilia may be satisfactorily treated with desmopressin which produces an increase in factor VIII and von Willebrand factor. Desmopressin also stimulates release of plasminogen activator, and an antifibrinolytic agent, such as tranexamic acid, may be given at the same time to inhibit the enhanced fibrinolytic activity. Desmopressin is usually given intravenously; it can be given intranasally, but the factor VIII response is less predictable than with the injection.[5]

Desmopressin is ineffective in patients with more severe haemophilia A, and treatment of bleeding episodes in these patients requires replacement with a factor VIII preparation. The amount of factor given depends on the severity of bleeding.

In addition to administration of factor VIII to treat bleeding episodes, prophylactic administration may also be given in situations where haemorrhage may be anticipated, for example following trauma, and before surgery. Patients with haemophilia should also not be given intramuscular injections (because of potential muscle damage and bleeding into muscle) unless they are given during a period when the patient is covered by replacement factor. Dental extraction and other oral surgical procedures are examples of situations that may be followed by bleeding lasting days and weeks. Oral secretions which can cause clot lysis contribute to this bleeding. Patients undergoing dental or oral surgery should be given factor VIII and an antifibrinolytic agent, usually tranexamic acid, before the procedure. The antifibrinolytic agent should be continued for five days following the procedure. Fibrin glue[6] and topical aminocaproic acid[7] or tranexamic acid[8] are methods that have also been used.

An alternative method of management has been practised in Sweden since 1958 where continuous prophylaxis with factor VIII is given to patients with severe haemophilia with the aim of preventing arthropathy. Therapy is started at 1 to 2 years of age and the factor VIII concentration is maintained at a level of at least 1% of normal. Patients who began receiving prophylaxis before the age of two have had almost no bleeding episodes and joints have remained normal for up to 11 years of follow-up.[9,10] This approach has subsequently been adopted in a number of other countries.

There are various factor VIII preparations available that vary in activity and source.[11] Most products were previously derived from pooled donor plasma and were associated with transmission of viruses including HIV (leading to the subsequent development of AIDS), hepatitis B, and other hepatitis viruses. The introduction of products treated with heat or chemicals together with efforts to screen the donor material from which factor VIII is obtained seem to have overcome problems with transmission of HIV and hepatitis B, although there is concern that non-lipid-enveloped viruses such as human parvovirus B19 and hepatitis A may still be transmitted. It is recommended that patients not already immune should be vaccinated against hepatitis A and B. Factor VIII produced by recombinant DNA technology may avoid the dangers of possible viral transmission (but see under Factor VIII, Transmission of Infections, p.721) and is therefore the factor VIII preparation of choice. There are some reports[12,13] that high-purity factor VIII preparations slow the decline in CD4 count in HIV-positive patients, although the evidence is conflicting.[14]

A complication of replacement therapy in haemophilia is the development of antibodies to factor VIII. Antibodies are more likely to develop in young patients with severe haemophilia, but on rare occasions can also arise in patients with mild haemophilia. An incidence of 10 to 15% is frequently cited, although prospective studies are lacking and it has been suggested that this is an underestimate.[15]

A number of strategies have been developed to overcome the resulting resistance to treatment.[1-3,16] Continued treatment with factor VIII may produce a clinical response and a decline in antibody formation in patients with a low antibody titre. Porcine factor VIII may be useful at least in the short term, although with longer use antibodies to the porcine material can develop in turn. Other strategies to reverse inhibition are the use of factor VIII inhibitor bypassing fraction; the use of recombinant factor VIIa which bypasses the factor VIII-dependent step in the coagulation cascade; routine infusion of small doses of factor VIII; and concurrent administration of factor VIII, intravenous normal immunoglobulin, and cyclophosphamide.[16] Immunosuppressive therapy (cyclophosphamide, vincristine, prednisone) with factor VIII has been found to eliminate factor VIII inhibitor in 11 of 12 non-haemophilic patients but only transiently in 1 of 5 haemophilic patients.[17] In patients with a severe haemorrhage or those undergoing surgery plasmapheresis can be used to reduce antibody concentrations. The use of tissue factor and factor Xa is also being studied.[2]

A future development that may provide a clinical cure for haemophilia is gene therapy.[18,19] Gene therapy for haemophilia A and B is being investigated and successful treatment has been carried out in an *animal* model with conversion to less severe haemophilia.

HAEMOPHILIA B (Christmas disease, factor IX deficiency) is less common than haemophilia A. The condition is due to deficiency of factor IX. The clinical features are identical to haemophilia A. Treatment follows the same principles as haemophilia A, bleeding episodes being treated with factor IX replacement.[1,2] Mild or moderate disease may be treated with fresh frozen plasma. Factor IX preparations derived from plasma, however, contain other clotting factors in addition to factor IX (such as the activated factors IX, X, and XII) and are therefore potentially associated with thrombo-embolic complications (mainly in patients with liver disease). Antifibrinolytic drugs, which may sometimes be used concurrently, increase the risk of thrombo-embolism further, and should be used with care. Highly purified factor IX preparations have been developed which do not contain other clotting factors and therefore may be expected to avoid this risk of thrombo-embolism. It has been suggested that these preparations should be used when very large amounts of replacement factor are required, or the risk of thrombotic complications is otherwise high.[2,4] Recently, a recombinant factor IX has been introduced.

Inhibitors to factor IX can be produced although the incidence is lower than the inhibition seen in haemophilia A. As in patients with haemophilia A, vaccination against hepatitis B is recommended for all haemophiliacs not already immune.

As mentioned under haemophilia A, gene therapy is under investigation as a possible clinical cure.

VON WILLEBRAND'S DISEASE is due to deficiency of von Willebrand factor, a plasma protein which stimulates platelet aggregation and acts as a carrier for factor VIII, protecting it from premature destruction. Deficiency therefore slows clotting by reducing the platelet response to injury and reducing levels of factor VIII. There are many different types, and severity ranges from severe haemorrhagic disease to asymptomatic disease. Bleeding episodes in patients with mild to moderate forms of the disease may be managed with desmopressin which increases levels of von Willebrand factor and factor VIII.[1,2,20,21] However, some forms of von Willebrand's disease do not respond to desmopressin therapy and in these patients, and in those with more severe disease, factor VIII concentrates are used; the very highly purified factor VIII preparations or recombinant forms should not be used as they do not contain appreciable amounts of von Willebrand factor and are thus ineffective. Cryoprecipitate (obtained from a very small donor pool to reduce the risk of transmission of infection) may also be used. Antifibrinolytic drugs may be used in open bleeding and in dental or oral surgery as for haemophilia A. A recombinant activated factor VII preparation has been developed that may also be used.

OTHER INHERITED DISORDERS. *Factor XI deficiency* is quite common in Jews of Eastern European origin. Spontaneous bleeding is rare. Bleeding following trauma or surgery is generally mild and infusion of fresh frozen plasma is usually sufficient to maintain haemostasis. A factor XI concentrate is available.

Inherited deficiencies of other clotting factors are rare. Concentrates of factors II, VII, and X are available. Fresh frozen plasma or cryoprecipitate may be used in factor XIII deficiency.

- **Acquired haemorrhagic disorders.** Bleeding disorders sometimes arise due to disturbances in either clotting factors or platelets or to vascular wall defects occurring as a result of a disease or a medical or surgical procedure. Disturbances and defects may also be drug induced. In some conditions, including renal and liver disease, cardiopulmonary bypass procedures, or following massive blood transfusion, disturbances in many of the homoeostatic mechanisms occur simultaneously producing complex haemorrhagic disorders, sometimes referred to as complex acquired coagulopathies.

One of the commoner causes of haemorrhagic disorder caused by **disturbance of clotting factors** is overdose with heparin, oral anticoagulants, or thrombolytics. Heparin overdose is rarely accompanied by serious haemorrhage. Stopping treatment is usually sufficient; protamine sulphate, which reverses the action of heparin, may be given. Bleeding in patients on oral anticoagulants is more difficult to control as the patient remains anticoagulated for several days after treatment is stopped. Local measures maybe sufficient, although in life-threatening haemorrhage administration of phytomenadione (vitamin K_1), a concentrate of factors II, IX, and X, or fresh frozen plasma may be necessary (see Treatment of Adverse Effects under Warfarin Sodium, p.965). Overdose with a thrombolytic agent, such as streptokinase or urokinase, may be managed with an antifibrinolytic agent (for example aminocaproic acid or tranexamic acid), aprotinin, and packed red blood cells.

Deficiencies in clotting factors may occur in several diseases. Disorders producing a deficiency of vitamin K will lead to reduced levels of clotting factors (see also under Haemostasis, above). Vitamin K deficiency due to impaired absorption, metabolism, or synthesis may occur in small bowel disease, biliary obstruction, or liver disease. Vitamin K deficiency in neonates produces haemorrhagic disease of the newborn (p.1372). Vitamin K deficiency is treated by administration of vitamin K, although this is not always effective in patients with liver diseases. Rarely, deficiencies in clotting factors may be caused by the development of antibodies against a particular factor; factor VIII is the factor most frequently affected.

Disturbances in platelet function can give rise to a haemorrhagic disorder.[22] Sometimes the bleeding disorder is due to abnormally functioning platelets such as occurs in renal failure or following the administration of some drugs (for example, aspirin and high doses of beta-lactam antibiotics). More often the bleeding disorder is due to a reduction is the number of platelets, that is, **thrombocytopenia**. Thrombocytopenia may occur in a wide range of disorders and can result from decreased production, increased destruction, or abnormal splenic sequestration of platelets. Decreased platelet production may occur in bone marrow diseases such as leukaemias and aplastic anaemia, chronic alcohol toxicity, and some viral illnesses. Decreased platelet production also occurs following bone marrow transplantation. Some drugs, for example thiazide diuretics and many antineoplastics, also reduce platelet production. Increased destruction of platelets occurs in many disorders including idiopathic thrombocytopenic purpura (p.1023), neonatal alloimmune thrombocytopenia, sepsis, disseminated intravascular coagulation (above), and thrombotic thrombocytopenic purpura and haemolytic uraemic syndrome (see Thrombotic Microangiopathies, p.726). Many drugs also cause increased platelet destruction; they include aminosalicylic acid, cimetidine, digitalis, frusemide, heparin, methyldopa, paracetamol, and sulphonamides. Thrombocytopenia as a result of abnormal splenic sequestration may occur in hypersplenism from any cause. Thrombocytopenia also occurs in a few very rare congenital abnormalities such as Fanconi's anaemia and the Wiskott-Aldrich syndrome.

In thrombocytopenia, the severity of bleeding depends on the platelet count; clotting is impaired following surgery or trauma and spontaneous bleeding may occasionally occur when the platelet count is less than 50×10^9 per litre. Treatment is management of the underlying disorder where appropriate or discontinuation of therapy with the offending drug. If surgery is contemplated or haemorrhage occurs and the platelet count is less than 50×10^9 per litre or a platelet abnormality is manifested by a prolonged bleeding time, platelet transfusion may be given. Patients requiring long-term treatment may develop antibodies to HLA with repeated transfusions from random donors, which results in impaired responsiveness to subsequent transfusion; these patients should receive platelets obtained from a single donor for each transfusion. When thrombocytopenia is a result of increased platelet destruction, the condition is usually refractory to platelet transfusion. Interleukin-11 (oprelvekin) has recently been introduced for the treatment of thrombocytopenia. Other haematopoietic growth factors under investigation include interleukin-3 and -6, and thrombopoietin.

Complex acquired coagulopathies can arise in many surgical settings, such as cardiopulmonary bypass procedures and liver transplantation, as well as in association with, or following, infection, massive blood transfusion, prolonged hypotension, and renal failure.

In renal failure the bleeding tendency is related to the degree and duration of uraemia. The bleeding defect is the result of platelet dysfunction and clotting factor deficiencies. There may also be mild thrombocytopenia. Correction of anaemia and dialysis seems to improve the bleeding disorder. If bleeding occurs desmopressin and conjugated oestrogens may be used. Cryoprecipitate and platelet transfusions may be necessary in life-threatening haemorrhage.

In liver disease the haemorrhagic disorder is a result of impaired synthesis of clotting factors, thrombocytopenia, and impaired clearance of activated clotting factors. Desmopressin has been used to control bleeding episodes. Patients undergoing liver transplantation frequently develop a bleeding disorder as a result of the procedure itself as well as from the existing haemostatic defect. Small studies on the use of aprotinin in liver transplant patients have generally shown reductions in blood loss.

Various drugs including desmopressin, epoprostenol, tranexamic acid, aminocaproic acid, aprotinin, and nafamostat have been investigated for their effect on blood loss in patients undergoing surgery. Most of the investigations have been in surgery which involves cardiopulmonary bypass, a procedure that may be complicated by a postperfusion syndrome which includes impairment of haemostasis and pulmonary dysfunction. Aprotinin is the only agent that has shown a consistent effect in decreasing perioperative blood loss,[23] perhaps due to preservation of platelet function mediated by inhibition of plasmin. Desmopressin may be effective in those patients with excessive bleeding after cardiac surgery.[24]

1. WHO/World Federation of Haemophilia. Prevention and control of haemophilia: memorandum from a joint WHO/WFH meeting. *Bull WHO* 1991; **69:** 17–26.
2. Seremetis SV, Aledort LM. Congenital bleeding disorders: rational treatment options. *Drugs* 1993; **45:** 541–7.
3. Hoyer LW. Hemophilia A. *N Engl J Med* 1994; **330:** 38–47.
4. Berntorp E, *et al.* Modern treatment of haemophilia. *Bull WHO* 1995; **73:** 691–701.
5. Rose EH, Aledort LM. Nasal spray desmopressin (DDAVP) for mild hemophilia A and von Willebrand disease. *Ann Intern Med* 1991; **114:** 563–8.
6. Baudo F, *et al.* Management of oral bleeding in haemophilic patients. *Lancet* 1988; **ii:** 1082.
7. Casdorph DL. Topical aminocaproic acid in hemophiliac patients undergoing dental extraction. *DICP Ann Pharmacother* 1990; **24:** 160–1.
8. Sindet-Pedersen S, *et al.* Management of oral bleeding in haemophilic patients. *Lancet* 1988; **ii:** 566.
9. Nilsson IM, *et al.* Twenty-five years' experience of prophylactic treatment in severe haemophilia A and B. *J Intern Med* 1992; **232:** 25–32.
10. Aledort LM. Prophylaxis: the next haemophilia treatment. *J Intern Med* 1992; **232:** 1–2.
11. United Kingdom Haemophilia Centre Directors Organisation Executive Committee. Guidelines on therapeutic products to treat haemophilia and other hereditary coagulation disorders. *Haemophilia* 1997; **3:** 63–77.
12. Hilgartner MW, *et al.* Purity of factor VIII concentrates and serial CD4 counts. *Lancet* 1993; **341:** 1373–4.
13. Seremetis SV, *et al.* Three-year randomised study of high-purity or intermediate-purity factor VIII concentrates in symptom-free HIV-seropositive haemophiliacs: effects on immune status. *Lancet* 1993; **342:** 700–703.
14. Schwarz HP, *et al.* High-purity factor concentrates in prevention of AIDS. *Lancet* 1994; **343:** 478–9.
15. Ehrenforth S, *et al.* Incidence of development of factor VIII and factor IX inhibitors in haemophiliacs. *Lancet* 1992; **339:** 594–8.
16. Anonymous. Anti-factor-VIII inhibitors in haemophilia. *Lancet* 1989; **ii:** 363–4.
17. Lian EC-Y, *et al.* Combination immunosuppressive therapy after factor VIII infusion for acquired factor VIII inhibitor. *Ann Intern Med* 1989; **110:** 774–8.
18. Lozier JN, Brinkhous KM. Gene therapy and the hemophilias. *JAMA* 1994; **271:** 47–51.
19. Brownlee GG. Prospects for gene therapy of haemophilia A and B. *Br Med Bull* 1995; **51:** 91–105.
20. Scott JP, Montgomery RR. Therapy of von Willebrand disease. *Semin Thromb Hemost* 1993; **19:** 37–47.
21. Castaman G, Rodeghiero F. Current management of von Willebrand's disease. *Drugs* 1995; **50:** 602–14.
22. Liesner RJ, Machin SJ. ABC of clinical haematology: platelet disorders. *Br Med J* 1997; **314:** 809–12.
23. Royston D. Perioperative bleeding. *Lancet* 1993; **341:** 1629.
24. Cattaneo M, Mannucci PM. Desmopressin and blood loss after cardiac surgery. *Lancet* 1993; **342:** 812.

Neonatal intraventricular haemorrhage

Intraventricular haemorrhage, also referred to as periventricular or periventricular-intraventricular haemorrhage, is bleeding from vessels in or around the ventricles of the brain. It is the major cause of death in very-low-birthweight neonates and affects up to 60% of neonates weighing less than 1500 g. Intraventricular haemorrhage is rare in neonates over 32 weeks' gestation, since the vessels which bleed involute early in the third trimester. Intraventricular haemorrhage usually develops within the first three days of life. The haemorrhage may be graded from 1 to 4 according to severity, the higher numbered grades being the most severe and most likely to produce the long-term consequences of impaired motor and mental function. The aetiology is probably multifactorial and may include fluctuations in cerebral blood flow due to failure of autoregulatory mechanisms and tissue damage caused by oxygen free-radicals.

Once intraventricular haemorrhage has occurred **treatment** is supportive and includes correction of anaemia, hypotension, and acidaemia. As intraventricular haemorrhage is a major risk factor for impaired motor and mental development **prevention** is very important. Numerous interventions aim to reduce its incidence and include prevention of premature births, avoidance of hypercapnia, correction of major haemodynamic disturbances, and correction of coagulation abnormalities. Various drugs have also been tried including corticosteroids, ethamsylate, indomethacin, pancuronium, phenobarbitone, vitamin E, and vitamin K. Some of these drugs have been administered to the mother antenatally since the development of intraventricular haemorrhage may be related to perinatal events.

Administration of corticosteroids to pregnant women at risk of preterm delivery is recommended to prevent neonatal respiratory distress syndrome (p.1025). Antenatal administration of corticosteroids also appears to reduce the incidence of intraventricular haemorrhage.[1] A review of data from 12 controlled studies[2] showed that the risk of intraventricular haemorrhage was reduced by between 10 and 80%. Avoidance of neonatal hypotension has been suggested as a mechanism for the beneficial effect of corticosteroids.[3]

Ethamsylate limits capillary bleeding through its action on hyaluronic acid and initial studies showed a reduction in intraventricular haemorrhage. A subsequent study[4] showed little evidence of benefit on short-term follow-up, although confidence intervals were wide. The results of long-term follow-up are awaited.

Indomethacin may reduce cerebral blood flow as a result of vasoconstriction, reduce oxygen free-radical damage, and accelerate maturation of blood vessels around the ventricles. Early studies produced conflicting results but a later larger multicentre study[5] showed a reduction in both incidence and severity although there was an unusually large number of neonates with severe intraventricular haemorrhage in the control group.[6] A concern with the use of indomethacin is the possibility that it may produce cerebral ischaemia due to its vasoconstrictor action and therefore increase the risk of developmental handicaps.[6] A review[7] of studies of prophylactic indomethacin concluded that more studies of possible adverse effects and long-term outcome are needed before indomethacin can be recommended for routine use. However, follow-up[8] at 3 years of age of the infants included in the multicentre study reported no adverse effects on cognitive or motor development.

Pancuronium reduces non-synchronous respiration and therefore stabilises both cerebral and arterial blood flow velocity and some studies have shown a reduction in intraventricular haemorrhage in mechanically-ventilated neonates (p.1303). However, other studies have produced conflicting results.

Phenobarbitone was also suggested to act by stabilising fluctuations in cerebral blood flow, and studies of administration to neonates show similarly inconsistent results with many failing to show any benefit. Initial studies of antenatal phenobarbitone were more promising with a decrease in severity of haemorrhage being reported.[9] However, a larger randomised study[10] in 610 women failed to show any effect of antenatal phenobarbitone on incidence or severity of intraventricular haemorrhage. A concern with the use of phenobarbitone in the perinatal period is that it may lower Apgar scores and produce respiratory depression.

Vitamin E protects polyunsaturated fatty acids and thus membranes from oxidation. As oxygen free-radical damage may contribute to the development of intraventricular haemorrhage vitamin E may have a role in its prevention. Results have been conflicting. Some studies have shown a reduction in incidence of intraventricular haemorrhage and a review of studies suggested vitamin E may be useful in the smallest, most susceptible neonates.[11] However, larger studies and studies to assess long-term outcome are needed.

The activity of vitamin K-dependent coagulation factors is reduced in neonates and thus antenatal administration of vitamin K to mothers has been tried as a means of preventing intraventricular haemorrhage. However, results of studies have not been promising. Most trials have been too small to produce conclusive results and a recent larger randomised controlled study[12] in 139 mothers failed to find any benefit from vitamin K prophylaxis.

Plasma volume expansion using fresh frozen plasma or a plasma substitute has also been thought to reduce intraventricular haemorrhage by stabilising the circulation, but a prospective multicentre study found no evidence of reduction in haemorrhage[13] or subsequent death and disability[14] following the use of plasma or gelatin as volume expanders.

1. NIH Consensus Development Panel. Effect of corticosteroids for fetal maturation on perinatal outcomes. *JAMA* 1995; **273:** 413–18.
2. Crowley P, *et al.* The effect of corticosteroid administration before preterm delivery: an overview of the evidence from controlled trials. *Br J Obstet Gynaecol* 1990; **97:** 11–25.
3. Garland JS, *et al.* Effect of maternal glucocorticoid exposure on risk of severe intraventricular hemorrhage in surfactant-treated preterm infants. *J Pediatr* 1995; **126:** 272–9.
4. The EC Ethamsylate Trial Group. The EC randomised controlled trial of prophylactic ethamsylate for very preterm neonates: early mortality and morbidity. *Arch Dis Child* 1994; **70:** F201–F205.
5. Ment LR, *et al.* Low-dose indomethacin and prevention of intraventricular haemorrhage: a multicenter randomized trial. *Pediatrics* 1994; **93:** 543–50.
6. Volpe JJ. Brain injury caused by intraventricular hemorrhage: is indomethacin the silver bullet for prevention? *Pediatrics* 1994; **93:** 673–6.
7. Fowlie PW. Prophylactic indomethacin: systematic review and meta-analysis. *Arch Dis Child* 1996; **74:** F81–F87.
8. Ment LR, *et al.* Neurodevelopment outcome at 36 months' corrected age of preterm infants in the multicenter indomethacin intraventricular hemorrhage prevention trial. *Pediatrics* 1996; **98:** 714–18.
9. Barnes ER, Thompson DF. Antenatal phenobarbital to prevent or minimize intraventricular hemorrhage in the low-birthweight neonate. *Ann Pharmacother* 1993; **27:** 49–52.
10. Shankaran S, *et al.* The effect of antenatal phenobarbital therapy on neonatal intracranial hemorrhage in preterm infants. *N Engl J Med* 1997; **337:** 466–71.
11. Poland RL. Vitamin E for prevention of perinatal intracranial hemorrhage. *Pediatrics* 1990; **85:** 865–7.
12. Thorp JA, *et al.* Antepartum vitamin K and phenobarbital for preventing intraventricular hemorrhage in the premature newborn: a randomized, double-blind, placebo-controlled trial. *Obstet Gynecol* 1994; **83:** 70–6.
13. The Northern Neonatal Nursing Initiative Trial Group. A randomized trial comparing the effect of prophylactic intravenous fresh frozen plasma, gelatin or glucose on early mortality and morbidity in preterm babies. *Eur J Pediatr* 1996; **155:** 580–8.
14. Northern Neonatal Nursing Initiative Trial Group. Randomized trial of prophylactic early fresh-frozen plasma or gelatin or glucose in preterm babies: outcome at 2 years. *Lancet* 1996; **348:** 229–32.

Neutropenia

A circulating neutrophil count below 1.5×10^9 per litre is usually regarded as abnormal and neutrophil counts below 0.5×10^9 per litre are associated with increased risk of infections. Neutropenia may be a result of reduced production, increased peripheral destruction, or increased peripheral pooling of neutrophils, and can be inherited or acquired.

Inherited forms of neutropenia are rare and include congenital agranulocytosis (Kostmann's syndrome: severe persistent neutropenia with frequent and severe infections that start in infancy) and cyclic neutropenia (fluctuating periods of neutropenia accompanied by fever, mouth ulceration, and serious infection).

Before the development of colony-stimulating factors various treatments including plasma, glucocorticoids, androgens, and lithium were tried in patients with severe congenital neutropenias with the aim of stimulating neutrophil production. However, none was particularly effective. Granulocyte colony-stimulating factors have been shown to reduce the incidence of severe infections and have improved substantially the quality of life of patients with congenital neutropenias although there are some concerns over their safety.

There are many causes of **acquired** neutropenia. Drugs are a common cause, either by direct toxicity to the bone marrow, or by immune-mediated marrow suppression or peripheral destruction. Drugs that cause dose-related direct toxicity include cytotoxic and immunosuppressive drugs, flucytosine, ganciclovir, and zidovudine. Drugs that appear to cause neutropenia by immune-mediated mechanisms include sulphur-containing drugs such as captopril, cotrimoxazole, and some antithyroid drugs, clozapine, penicillins, and cephalosporins. Patients with drug-induced neutropenia usually present with fever of sudden onset, sore throat, mouth ulcers, headache, and malaise. This condition is also known as agranulocytosis. Other causes of acquired neutropenia include serious bacterial and viral infections and radiotherapy, neoplasms that invade bone marrow, and some autoimmune disorders.

The management of acquired neutropenia includes the treatment of any contributory condition. Drug-induced neutropenia is usually managed by withdrawal of the offending drug. In idiosyncratic reactions readministration of the implicated drug should be avoided, since abrupt neutropenia will usually be precipitated. Administration of colony-stimulating factors can be used to manage drug-induced neutropenia.

In all neutropenic patients onset of fever is indicative of serious infection and is treated immediately with empirical antibacterial therapy as described on p.127.

General references.

1. Anonymous. Drug-induced agranulocytosis. *Drug Ther Bull* 1997; **35:** 49–52.

Albumin (1215-j)

Human Albumin Solution (Ph. Eur.) (Albumin Solution (BP 1998); Albumin; Human Albumin; Albumini Humani Solutio) is an aqueous solution of protein obtained from plasma. It is prepared as a concentrated solution containing 15 to 25% of total protein or as an isotonic solution containing 3.5 to 5% of total protein; not less than 95% of the total protein is albumin. A suitable stabiliser, such as sodium caprylate or *N*-acetyltryptophan or a combination of the two, may be added but no antimicrobial preservative is added. It contains not more than 160 mmol of sodium per litre. Albumin solution intended for administration to patients undergoing dialysis or to premature infants contains not more than 200 μg of aluminium per litre. The solution is sterilised by filtration and distributed aseptically into containers which are sealed to exclude micro-organisms and maintained at 59.5° to 60.5° for not less than 10 hours. Finally, the containers are incubated for not less than 14 days at 30° to 32° or for not less than 4 weeks at 20° to 25° and examined visually for signs of microbial contamination. It should be protected from light.

Albumin Human (USP 23) is a sterile preparation, suitable for intravenous use, of serum albumin obtained by fractionating material (blood, plasma, serum, or placentas) from healthy human donors, the source material being tested for the absence of hepatitis B surface antigen. It contains 4, 5, 20, or 25% of serum albumin and not less than 96% of the total protein is albumin. It may contain sodium acetyltryptophanate with or without sodium caprylate as a stabilising agent; it contains no added antimicrobial agent. It contains 130 to 160 mmol of sodium per litre.

Adverse Effects and Precautions

Adverse reactions to albumin infusion occur rarely and include nausea and vomiting, increased salivation, and febrile reactions. Allergic reactions, including severe anaphylactic shock, are possible. Rapid increases in circulatory volume can cause vascular overload, haemodilution, and pulmonary oedema. Solutions containing albumin 20% or 25% are hyperosmotic and draw fluid from the extravascular compartment. Heating to about 60° in the presence of a stabiliser during preparation has reduced the risk of transmitting some viral infections.

Infusion of albumin solutions is contra-indicated in patients with severe anaemia or heart failure. They should be given with caution to patients with hypertension or low cardiac reserve. Dehydrated patients may require additional fluids. Injured or postoperative patients should be observed carefully following the administration of albumin as the rise in blood pressure may result in bleeding from previously undetected sites.

Volume expansion with albumin (a colloid) has been widely used in critically ill patients, although its use has never been formally tested in large controlled studies. A systematic review based on available studies up to March 1998 (relatively small, old trials that recorded only a small number of deaths) suggested that albumin was of no benefit in critically ill patients with hypovolaemia, burns, or hypoalbuminaemia, and that it might be linked to increased mortality.[1] The authors of the review stressed that these results should be treated with caution but nevertheless called for an urgent reconsideration of the use of albumin in critically ill patients. The review has been severely criticised[2] and while practitioners recognise that albumin has probably been overused in the past more studies are required to define the effect of albumin on mortality.[3,4] On a broader level, debate continues about the relative merits and risks of such colloid solutions, compared with those of crystalloids such as glucose or sodium chloride solutions, in the management of hypovolaemia and shock (p.798).

1. Cochrane Injuries Group Albumin Reviewers. Human albumin administration in critically ill patients: systematic review of randomised controlled trials. *Br Med J* 1998; **317:** 235–40.
2. Various. Human albumin administration in critically ill patients. *Br Med J* 1998; **317:** 882–6. [Letters.]
3. Tomlin M. Albumin usage in the critically ill. *Pharm J* 1998; **261:** 193.
4. McClelland B. Albumin: don't confuse us with the facts. *Br Med J* 1998; **317:** 829–30.

Aluminium toxicity. Albumin solutions may contain appreciable amounts of aluminium. Marked increases in plasma aluminium concentrations have been demonstrated in patients receiving large volumes by infusion and accumulation of aluminium may occur in patients with impaired renal function.[1-3] In the UK albumin solutions with an aluminium content of less than 200 μg per litre are available for use in patients undergoing dialysis and premature infants.

1. Milliner DS, *et al.* Inadvertent aluminum administration during plasma exchange due to aluminum contamination of albumin-replacement solutions. *N Engl J Med* 1985; **312:** 165–7.
2. Maher ER, *et al.* Accumulation of aluminium in chronic renal failure due to administration of albumin replacement solutions. *Br Med J* 1986; **292:** 306.
3. Maharaj D, *et al.* Aluminium bone disease in patients receiving plasma exchange with contaminated albumin. *Br Med J* 1987; **295:** 693–6.

Dilution. A reminder that, if concentrated albumin solutions are diluted before administration, a suitable solution such as sodium chloride 0.9% or glucose 5% must be used. Albumin 25% that was erroneously diluted with water to produce a hypo-osmolar albumin 5% solution has produced severe haemolysis and renal failure in patients undergoing plasmapheresis.[1,2]

1. Steinmuller DR. A dangerous error in the dilution of 25 percent albumin. *N Engl J Med* 1998; **338:** 1226.
2. Pierce LR, *et al.* Hemolysis and renal failure associated with use of sterile water for injection to dilute 25% human albumin solution. *Am J Health-Syst Pharm* 1998; **55:** 1057,1062, 1070.

Transmission of infections. Following concern that the use of placentas as a source for albumin may carry a potential risk of transmission of viral and subviral particles, notably Creutzfeldt-Jakob disease, *Pasteur-Mérieux* (one of the largest producers of blood products) has withdrawn all products containing albumin derived from placental blood.[1] The agent responsible for Creutzfeldt-Jakob disease might be contained in placentas from women who have been treated with growth hormone derived from cadaver pituitaries.

Ph. Eur. does not specify placentas as a source of albumin.

The production of blood products (including albumin) using plasma from UK donors is being phased out due to the possible risk of transmission of Creutzfeldt-Jakob disease.

1. Anonymous. Placental-derived albumin preparations withdrawn. *WHO Drug Inf* 1994; **8:** 29–30.

Uses and Administration

Albumin is the major protein involved in maintaining colloid osmotic pressure in the blood. It also binds a number of endogenous and exogenous substances including bilirubin, steroid hormones, and many, mainly acidic, drugs.

Albumin solutions are used for plasma volume replacement and to restore colloid osmotic pressure in acute hypovolaemic shock (p.798), burns, and severe acute albumin loss and as an exchange fluid in therapeutic plasmapheresis. Concentrated albumin solutions are used in neonatal hyperbilirubinaemia associated with haemolytic disease of the newborn (p.1503). They have also been suggested for short-term management of hypoproteinaemia in hepatic disease and in diuretic-resistant patients with nephrotic syndrome but are of little value in chronic hypoproteinaemias. Albumin preparations labelled with technetium-99m are used as radiopharmaceuticals in heart and lung scanning (p.1425) and air-filled albumin microspheres are available for enhancing cardiac ultrasound imaging.

Albumin solutions are usually available as 4.5% or 5% solutions, which are iso-osmotic with plasma, and as 20% or 25% solutions which, being hyperosmotic with respect to plasma, cause a movement of fluid from the extravascular to the intravascular compartment. These concentrated solutions may be used undiluted or may be diluted with a suitable solution, commonly sodium chloride 0.9% or glucose 5%. Adequate hydration should be maintained in patients receiving hyperosmotic solutions of albumin.

The amount of albumin solution administered will depend upon the clinical condition of the patient and the response to treatment. The following doses have been suggested: in acute hypovolaemic shock an initial dose of 25 g of albumin for adults (for example, 500 mL of a 5% solution or 100 mL of a 25% solution) and up to about 1 g per kg body-weight for children; in hypoproteinaemia a maximum daily dose of 2 g per kg; and in neonatal hyperbilirubinaemia a dose of 1 g per kg before exchange transfusion (albumin, in a dose of 1.5 to 2.5 g per 100 mL of blood, may also be added to the exchange transfusion).

A suggested rate of infusion is 1 to 2 mL per minute (5% solution) or 1 mL per minute (25% solution) although high rates may be needed in the treatment of shock.

Albumin solutions should not be used for parenteral nutrition.

References.

1. Erstad BL, *et al.* The use of albumin in clinical practice. *Arch Intern Med* 1991; **151:** 901–11.
2. McClelland DBL. Human albumin solutions. In Contreras M, ed. *ABC of transfusion*. 2nd ed. London: BMJ Publishing Group, 1992: 35–7.
3. McClelland DB. Human albumin solutions. *Prescribers' J* 1992; **32:** 157–61.
4. Tomlin M. Albumin usage on intensive care. *Pharm J* 1997; **259:** 856–9. Comment including corrections—Dash C, *et al. ibid.* 1998; **260:** 88–9.

Preparations

Ph. Eur.: Human Albumin Solution;
USP 23: Albumin Human.

Proprietary Preparations (details are given in Part 3)
Austral.: Albumex; NSA; ***Belg.:*** Albuman; ***Canad.:*** Plasbumin; ***Ger.:*** Humanalbin; Rhodalbumin†; ***Irl.:*** Albuminar; ***Ital.:*** Albital; Albuman; Albuminar†; Albutein; Endalbumin; Seralbuman; ***Norw.:*** Infosan; ***S.Afr.:*** Albusol; ***Swed.:*** Albumer†; Albuminar†; Infoson†; ***Switz.:*** Albuman; Biseko†; ***UK:*** Albuminar; Albutein; Buminate†; Zenalb; ***USA:*** Albumarc; Albuminar; Albunex; Albutein; Buminate; Plasbumin.

Aminaphthone (12357-g)

Aminaftone; Aminaphtone; Aminonaphthone. 2-Hydroxy-3-methylnaphtho-1,4-hydroquinone 2-(4-aminobenzoate); 3-Methylnaphthalene-1,2,4-triol 2-(4-aminobenzoate).

$C_{18}H_{15}NO_4$ = 309.3.

CAS — 14748-94-8.

Aminaphthone is a haemostatic. Daily doses of 150 to 225 mg by mouth have been employed.

Preparations

Proprietary Preparations (details are given in Part 3)
Ital.: Capillarema; ***Spain:*** Capilarema.

Aminocaproic Acid (1712-p)

Aminocaproic Acid *(BAN, USAN, rINN).*

Acidum Aminocaproicum; CL-10304; CY-116; EACA; Epsilon Aminocaproic Acid; JD-177; NSC-26154. 6-Aminohexanoic acid.

$C_6H_{13}NO_2$ = 131.2.

CAS — 60-32-2.

Pharmacopoeias. In *Eur.* (see p.viii), *Pol.*, and *US.*

Odourless or almost odourless, colourless crystals or white crystalline powder. **Soluble** 1 in 3 of water; slightly soluble in alcohol; practically insoluble in chloroform and in ether; soluble 1 in 450 of methyl alcohol; freely soluble in acids and in alkalis. A 20% solution in water has a pH of 7.5 to 8.0. **Store** in airtight containers.

Adverse Effects

Adverse effects associated with the administration of aminocaproic acid include dose-related gastro-intestinal disturbances, dizziness, tinnitus, headache, nasal and conjunctival congestion, and skin rashes. Aminocaproic acid may cause muscle damage. This has usually occurred with high doses given for prolonged periods; renal failure may develop. Thrombotic complications have been reported, although they are usually a consequence of inappropriate use. If aminocaproic acid is given by rapid intravenous administration it can produce hypotension, bradycardia, and arrhythmias. There have been reports of a few patients suffering from convulsions, dry ejaculation, or cardiac and hepatic damage.

Effects on the blood. Very high doses of aminocaproic acid (36 g or more daily) have been given intravenously in the management of subarachnoid haemorrhage. One study[1] reported rebleeding and excessive intra-operative bleeding in patients with subarachnoid haemorrhage receiving aminocaproic acid and suggested that this was due to an antiplatelet effect of the aminocaproic acid. However, a comment on this report[2] pointed out that any antiplatelet effect was independent of its antifibrinolytic action and that this effect could only aggravate rebleeding, if it occurs, rather than initiating it.

1. Glick R, *et al.* High dose ε-aminocaproic acid prolongs the bleeding time and increases rebleeding and intraoperative hemorrhage in patients with subarachnoid hemorrhage. *Neurosurgery* 1981; **9:** 398–401.
2. Kassell NF. Comment. *Neurosurgery* 1981; **9:** 401.

Effects on the muscles. There have been a number of cases of reversible myopathy reported with aminocaproic acid.[1-4] In presenting their case, Brown *et al.*[1] reviewed the other 18 cases that had then been reported. Daily doses ranged from 10 to 49 g and treatment lasted for about one month to 90 days. Five of the 19 were reported to have had myoglobinuria and 3 of the 19 acute reversible tubular necrosis. Vanneste and van Wijngaarden[2] also reviewed 9 of the reported cases when they reported their patient who had experienced myopathy and myoglobinuria after 6 weeks' treatment with aminocaproic acid 26 to 36 g daily. They considered that the myopathy was most probably due to a direct dose-critical toxic effect on the muscle fibre. In a further case report, Van Renterghem *et al.*[3] suggested that aminocaproic acid induced a defect in aerobic energy provision.

1. Brown JA, *et al.* Myopathy induced by epsilon-aminocaproic acid. *J Neurosurg* 1982; **57:** 130–4.
2. Vanneste JAL, van Wijngaarden GK. Epsilon-aminocaproic acid myopathy. *Eur Neurol* 1982; **21:** 242–8.
3. Van Renterghem D, *et al.* Epsilon amino caproic acid myopathy: additional features. *Clin Neurol Neurosurg* 1984; **86:** 153–7.
4. Seymour BD, Rubinger M. Rhabdomyolysis induced by epsilon-aminocaproic acid. *Ann Pharmacother* 1997; **31:** 56–8.

Precautions

As for Tranexamic Acid, p.728.

The range of adverse effects that have been noted with aminocaproic acid indicates caution in patients with renal or cardiac disorders. Should treatment be prolonged, it is advisable to monitor creatine phosphokinase values for signs of muscle damage.

Pharmacokinetics

Aminocaproic acid is readily absorbed when given by mouth and peak plasma concentrations are reached within 2 hours. It is widely distributed and is rapidly excreted in the urine, mainly unchanged, with a terminal elimination half-life of approximately 2 hours.

Uses and Administration

Aminocaproic acid is an antifibrinolytic (p.704) used similarly to tranexamic acid (p.728) in the treatment and prophylaxis of haemorrhage associated with excessive fibrinolysis. It has also been used in the prophylaxis of hereditary angioedema (p.729).

A plasma concentration of about 130 μg per mL is considered to be necessary for effective inhibition of fibrinolysis and the recommended dosage schedules are aimed at producing and maintaining this concentration for as long as is necessary. For the treatment and prophylaxis of haemorrhage, aminocaproic acid may be administered by mouth in an initial dose of 4 to 5 g, followed by 1 to 1.25 g every hour. Alternatively the same dose may be given intravenously as a 2% solution; the initial dose (4 to 5 g) should be given over one hour followed by a continuous infusion of 1 g per hour. Up to 8 hours' treatment is often sufficient. Should treatment need to be extended, then the maximum dose over 24 hours should not normally exceed 24 g. Care is required when aminocaproic acid is used in patients with renal disturbances and dosage should be reduced.

Preparations

USP 23: Aminocaproic Acid Injection; Aminocaproic Acid Syrup; Aminocaproic Acid Tablets.

Proprietary Preparations (details are given in Part 3)
Austral.: Amicar; ***Canad.:*** Amicar; ***Fr.:*** Hemocaprol†; Hexalense; ***Ital.:*** Capracid†; Caprolisin; ***S.Afr.:*** Amicar; ***Spain:*** Caproamin; Hemocaprol†; ***USA:*** Amicar.

Multi-ingredient: ***Ital.:*** Ekuba†; ***Spain:*** Caprofides Hemostatico.

Aminomethylbenzoic Acid (1713-s)

PAMBA. 4-Aminomethylbenzoic acid.

$C_8H_9NO_2$ = 151.2.

CAS — 56-91-7.

Pharmacopoeias. In *Chin.* which specifies the monohydrate.

Aminomethylbenzoic acid is an antifibrinolytic (p.704) with similar actions and uses to tranexamic acid (p.728). It is given by mouth, by intramuscular injection, or intravenously by slow injection or infusion.

Preparations

Proprietary Preparations (details are given in Part 3)
Aust.: Gumbix; ***Ger.:*** Gumbix; Pamba.

Antithrombin III (1216-z)

Antithrombin III *(BAN, rINN).*

Antithrombin III Human; AT-III; Heparin Cofactor; Heparin Cofactor I; Major Antithrombin.

CAS — 52014-67-2.

Human Antithrombin III Concentrate, Freeze-dried (Ph. Eur.) (Antithrombinum III Humanum Densatum Cryodesiccatum; Antithrombin III Concentrate (BP 1998)) is prepared from human plasma obtained from healthy donors who must, as far as can be ascertained, be free from detectable agents of infection transmissible by transfusion of blood or blood derivatives. The method of preparation includes a step or steps that have been shown to remove or to inactivate known agents of infection. The antithrombin III concentrate is passed through a bacteria-retentive filter, distributed into sterile containers, and immediately frozen. The preparation is freeze-dried and the containers sealed under vacuum or in an atmosphere of inert gas. No antimicrobial preservative is added but a suitable stabiliser (such as albumin) may be added. When reconstituted in the volume of solvent stated on the label, the resulting solution contains not less than 25 units of antithrombin III per mL. The dried product should be protected from light.

Units

The potency of antithrombin III is expressed in international units and preparations may be assayed using the first International Standard for antithrombin III concentrate (1990).

Uses and Administration

Antithrombin III is a protein in plasma; it is the major inhibitor of thrombin and other activated clotting factors including factors IX, X, XI, and XII (p.704), and is the cofactor through which heparin (p.881) exerts its effect. Genetic and acquired deficiency of antithrombin III occurs and is associated with susceptibility to thrombo-embolic disorders.

Antithrombin III is administered intravenously in the management of acute thrombotic episodes and for prophylaxis during surgery and pregnancy in patients with antithrombin III deficiency. The aim of therapy is to restore plasma-antithrombin III concentrations to at least 80% of normal. The dose, frequency of administration, and duration of therapy are individualised for each patient taking into account the patient's pretreatment concentration and presence of active coagulation. A usual initial dose is about 30 to 50 international units per kg bodyweight.

Reviews of antithrombin III.

1. Rosenberg RD, ed. Role of antithrombin III in coagulation disorders: state-of-the-art review. *Am J Med* 1989; **87** (3B): 1S–67S.
2. Harper PL. The clinical use of antithrombin concentrate in septicaemia. *Br J Hosp Med* 1994; **52:** 571–4.

Venous thrombo-embolism. Antithrombin III is one of several drugs that has been used for prophylaxis of venous thrombo-embolism (p.802) in patients at risk (such as those undergoing surgery). In one study prophylaxis with antithrombin III, 3000 units 2 hours before surgery and 2000 units daily for 5 days thereafter, and heparin, 5000 units every 12 hours beginning 2 hours before surgery and continuing for 5 days, effectively reduced the risk of venous thrombosis after total knee arthroplasty.[1]

1. Francis CW, *et al.* Prevention of venous thrombosis after total knee arthroplasty. *J Bone Joint Surg (Am)* 1990; **72-A:** 976–82.

Preparations

Ph. Eur.: Freeze-dried Human Antithrombin III Concentrate.

Proprietary Preparations (details are given in Part 3)
Aust.: Atenativ; Athimbin HS; Thrombhibin; ***Canad.:*** Thrombate; ***Ger.:*** Atenativ; Kybernin; ***Ital.:*** Kybernin P; ***Neth.:*** Atenativ; ***Norw.:*** Atenativ; ***Spain:*** Atenativ; Kybernin P; ***Swed.:*** Atenativ; ***Switz.:*** Atenativ; Kybernin; ***UK:*** Kybernin P; ***USA:*** ATnativ.

Aprotinin (1714-w)

Aprotinin *(BAN, USAN, rINN).*

Aprotininum; Bayer A-128; Riker 52G; RP-9921.

CAS — 9087-70-1.

Pharmacopoeias. In *Chin.* and *Eur.* (see p.viii).

A single-chain polypeptide derived from bovine tissues consisting of 58 amino-acid residues and having a molecular weight of about 6500.

A clear colourless solution or an almost white hygroscopic powder. When presented as a liquid (Aprotinin Concentrated Solution) it contains not less than 3 Ph. Eur. units per mg calculated with reference to the dry residue and not less than 15 Ph. Eur. units per mL. When presented as a solid it contains not less than 3 Ph. Eur. units per mg calculated with reference to the dried substance. The solid is **soluble** in water and in solutions isotonic with blood; practically insoluble in organic solvents.

Store in airtight containers. Protect from light. Aprotinin is reported to be **incompatible** with corticosteroids, heparin, tetracyclines, and nutrient solutions containing amino acids or fat emulsions.

Units

The potency of aprotinin is expressed in terms of kallikrein (kallidinogenase) inactivator units (KIU) or of trypsin inactivation (Ph. Eur. units). One KIU is contained in 140 ng of aprotinin. One Ph. Eur. unit is approximately equivalent to 1800 KIU.

Potency has also been expressed in terms of plasmin inactivation (antiplasmin units).

Adverse Effects and Precautions

Aprotinin is usually well tolerated. Side-effects that have been observed include bronchospasm, gastro-intestinal disturbances, skin rashes, and tachycardia; most of these effects are considered to be hypersensitivity reactions. Anaphylaxis has occasionally occurred as has local thrombophlebitis.

After one year's successful treatment of a diabetic patient with aprotinin and insulin given subcutaneously,[1] loss of effect from the aprotinin was accompanied by development of lipohypertrophy; this was not seen during prior or subsequent use of insulin alone. On continuing treatment glomerulonephritis was detected. It was suggested that development of antibodies against aprotinin might explain these effects.

1. Boag F, *et al.* Lipohypertrophy and glomerulonephritis after the use of aprotinin in an insulin-dependent diabetic. *N Engl J Med* 1985; **312:** 245–6.

Disseminated intravascular coagulation. Disseminated intravascular coagulation resulting in death has been reported in a patient following the use of intraoperative autotransfusion and aprotinin during surgery.[1] Activation of the clotting system occurs during autotransfusion although this usually causes no systemic adverse effects. While there were other possible causes, it was suggested that aprotinin could have contributed to deposition of fibrin microthrombi in the microvasculature and prevented subsequent fibrinolysis.

1. Milne AA, *et al.* Disseminated intravascular coagulation after aortic aneurysm repair, intraoperative salvage autotransfusion, and aprotinin. *Lancet* 1994; **344:** 470–1.

Effects on the respiratory system. Acute respiratory distress syndrome developed in a 24-year-old male two hours after the start of an intravenous infusion of aprotinin for bleeding following tonsillectomy.[1] Mechanical ventilation was required for 4 days.

1. Vucicevic Z, Suskovic T. Acute respiratory distress syndrome after aprotinin infusion. *Ann Pharmacother* 1997; **31:** 429–32.

Hypersensitivity. In a study by Freeman *et al.*[1] two of 136 courses of aprotinin led to acute allergic reactions; one patient experienced acute anaphylaxis, the other an acute urticarial reaction. Such patients might be detected by challenging their reactivity using aprotinin eye drops as an alternative to intradermal testing. However, LaFerla and Murray[2] reported a severe anaphylactic reaction in one patient after the intravenous administration of aprotinin despite negative ocular sensitivity tests. Repeat administration of aprotinin (two months after the initial dose) has produced anaphylactic shock in a 3-year-old boy.[3] In a study[4] of 248 re-exposures to aprotinin in 240 patients undergoing cardiac surgery, there were 7 cases of anaphylactic reactions ranging from mild to severe with a higher incidence of reactions occurring in those patients re-exposed within 6 months of the previous dose. It has been suggested that re-exposure should be avoided for at least 6 months,[4] that a test dose be used in all patients,[4] and that histamine H_1- and H_2-receptor antagonists should be administered before re-exposure to aprotinin to ameliorate severe anaphylactic reactions.[4,5]

1. Freeman JG, *et al.* Serial use of aprotinin and incidence of allergic reactions. *Curr Med Res Opin* 1983; **8:** 559–61.
2. LaFerla GA, Murray WR. Anaphylactic reaction to aprotinin despite negative ocular sensitivity tests. *Br Med J* 1984; **289:** 1176–7.
3. Wüthrich B, *et al.* IgE-mediated anaphylactic reaction to aprotinin during anaesthesia. *Lancet* 1992; **340:** 173–4.
4. Dietrich W, *et al.* Prevalence of anaphylactic reactions to aprotinin: analysis of two hundred forty-eight reexposures to aprotinin in heart operations. *J Thorac Cardiovasc Surg* 1997: **113:** 194–201.
5. Lamparter-Schummert B, *et al.* Aprotinin re-exposure in patients undergoing repeat cardiac surgery: effect of prophylaxis with H1- and H2-receptor antagonists. *Br J Anaesth* 1995; **74** (suppl 2): 3.

Surgery. Although aprotinin appears to prolong the activated clotting time it is recommended that, until the risks of thromboses associated with the use of aprotinin for surgery have been determined, heparin should be given in usual doses when used with aprotinin.[1,2]

1. Hunt BJ, Yacoub M. Aprotinin and cardiac surgery. *Br Med J* 1991; **303:** 660–1.
2. Hunt BJ, Murkin JM. Heparin resistance after aprotinin. *Lancet* 1993; **341:** 126.

Interactions

For comment on the use of aprotinin with heparin, see under Surgery, above.

For potentiation of the activity of neuromuscular blockers by aprotinin, see p.1306.

Pharmacokinetics

Aprotinin, being a polypeptide, is inactivated in the gastro-intestinal tract. It is excreted in the urine as inactive degradation products. The terminal elimination half-life is about 7 to 10 hours.

Renal impairment. The terminal elimination half-life of aprotinin was reported as 13.3 and 14.9 hours, respectively, in two patients with chronic renal impairment given aprotinin by intravenous infusion over 30 minutes.[1]

1. Müller FO, *et al.* Pharmacokinetics of aprotinin in two patients with chronic renal impairment. *Br J Clin Pharmacol* 1996; **41:** 619–20.

Uses and Administration

Aprotinin is a haemostatic (p.704). It is an inhibitor of proteolytic enzymes including chymotrypsin, kallikrein (kallidinogenase), plasmin, and trypsin.

Aprotinin is used in the treatment of haemorrhage associated with raised plasma concentrations of plasmin. It is also used to reduce blood loss and transfusion requirements in patients at high risk of major blood loss during and following open heart surgery with extracorporeal circulation. Aprotinin has been tried in the management of pancreatitis (p.1613) because of the postulated role of proteolytic enzymes in this condition. It has also been tried in shock (p.798). Aprotinin is applied topically as a component of fibrin glues (p.722).

In the treatment of haemorrhage, 500 000 to 1 000 000 KIU of aprotinin are given by slow intravenous injection or infusion at a maximum rate of 100 000 KIU per minute with the patient in the supine position. This may be followed by 200 000 KIU every hour until the haemorrhage is controlled.

In open heart surgery, an intravenous loading dose of 2 000 000 KIU is given after induction of anaesthesia but before incision, or re-opening of the wound. It is recommended that because of the risk of hypersensitivity reactions the first 50 000 KIU of the loading dose should be administered over several minutes, the remainder being given over 20 minutes. Alternatively, a test dose of 10 000 KIU may be given at least 10 minutes before the loading dose. The loading dose is followed by a continuous infusion of 500 000 KIU per hour until skin closure at the end of the operation. An additional dose of 2 000 000 KIU is added to the prime volume of the oxygenator. In patients with septic endocarditis, a dose of 3 000 000 KIU is added to the prime volume of the oxygenator and the continuous infusion may be continued into the early postoperative period.

Haemorrhagic disorders. Aprotinin is indicated in the treatment of life-threatening haemorrhage caused by raised plasma concentrations of plasmin. It is used alone, or with tranexamic acid or aminocaproic acid, in the treatment of severe bleeding arising from overdosage with thrombolytics.

It is also used to reduce blood loss in patients undergoing surgery, including that involving cardiopulmonary bypass.[1-3] (See also Complex Acquired Coagulopathies under Haemorrhagic Disorders, p.707.)

Cardiac surgery may be complicated by a postperfusion syndrome which includes impairment of haemostasis and pulmonary dysfunction. This syndrome has been interpreted as a 'whole-body inflammatory response'. The beneficial effect of aprotinin on haemostasis during cardiopulmonary bypass has been attributed, not to an antifibrinolytic action, but to a preservation of platelet function, possibly mediated by inhibition of plasmin.[2-7] Administration of aprotinin has reduced blood loss and transfusion requirements in patients undergoing both primary and repeat cardiac surgery.[1,8,9] The usual dosage regimen is given under Uses and Administration, above. In addition, 500 000 KIU may be added to each litre of whole blood given during the operation.[5,6]

A slightly different dosage regimen has been used in a group of patients undergoing heart-valve replacement for infective endocarditis.[10] Other workers have investigated the use of reduced dosage regimens omitting the loading dose, including the administration of aprotinin in the priming volume alone.[11-15]

Encouraging reductions in blood loss have been obtained in some patients undergoing liver transplantation,[16,17] peripheral vascular surgery,[18] orthopaedic surgery,[19] and lung transplantation,[20] but it has been advised that until risks such as postoperative thrombo-embolic disease and loss of graft patency have been investigated aprotinin should be used with caution.[21]

Aprotinin has been tried with a low-dose regimen of tranexamic acid in the prevention of rebleeding in patients with subarachnoid haemorrhage[22] (p.799). Results suggested a reduced risk of rebleeding, without the increased incidence of ischaemic complications observed after treatment with conventional doses of tranexamic acid alone.

Aprotinin is a component of fibrin glues (p.722), also known as fibrin sealants or tissue glues, that are applied topically in the control of bleeding or as a suture system. The other components of these glues include fibrinogen, factor XIII, and other plasma proteins, mixed with calcium thrombin immediately prior to use.

1. Davis R, Whittington R. Aprotinin: a review of its pharmacology and therapeutic efficacy in reducing blood loss associated with cardiac surgery. *Drugs* 1995; **49:** 954–83.
2. Robert S, *et al.* Aprotinin. *Ann Pharmacother* 1996; **30:** 372–80.
3. Dobkowski WB, Murkin JM. A risk-benefit assessment of aprotinin in cardiac surgical procedures. *Drug Safety* 1998; **18:** 21–41.
4. Anonymous. Can drugs reduce surgical blood loss? *Lancet* 1988; **i:** 155–6.
5. van Oeveren W, *et al.* Effects of aprotinin on hemostatic mechanisms during cardiopulmonary bypass. *Ann Thorac Surg* 1987; **44:** 640–5.
6. Royston D, *et al.* Effect of aprotinin on need for blood transfusion after repeat open-heart surgery. *Lancet* 1987; **ii:** 1289–91.
7. van Oeveren W, *et al.* Platelet preservation by aprotinin during cardiopulmonary bypass. *Lancet* 1988; **i:** 644.
8. Bidstrup BP, *et al.* Aprotinin therapy in cardiac operations: a report on use in 41 cardiac centers in the United Kingdom. *Ann Thorac Surg* 1993; **55:** 971–6.
9. Laupacis A, Fergusson D. Drugs to minimize perioperative blood loss in cardiac surgery: meta-analyses using perioperative blood transfusion as the outcome. *Anesth Analg* 1997; **85:** 1258–67.
10. Bidstrup BP, *et al.* Effect of aprotinin on need for blood transfusion in patients with septic endocarditis having open-heart surgery. *Lancet* 1988; **i:** 366–7.
11. Carrel T, *et al.* Low-dose aprotinin for reduction of blood loss after cardiopulmonary bypass. *Lancet* 1991; **337:** 673.
12. Vandenvelde C, *et al.* Low-dose aprotinin for reduction of blood loss after cardiopulmonary bypass. *Lancet* 1991; **337:** 1157–8.
13. Locatelli A, *et al.* Aprotinin in cardiac surgery. *Lancet* 1991; **338:** 254.
14. Bailey CR, Wielogorski AK. Randomised placebo controlled double blind study of two low dose aprotinin regimens in cardiac surgery. *Br Heart J* 1994; **71:** 349–53.
15. Levy JH, *et al.* A multicenter, double-blind, placebo-controlled trial of aprotinin for reducing blood loss and the requirement for donor-blood transfusion in patients undergoing repeat coronary artery bypass graftings. *Circulation* 1995; **92:** 2236–44.
16. Mallett SV, *et al.* Aprotinin and reduction of blood loss and transfusion requirements in orthotopic liver transplantation. *Lancet* 1990; **336:** 886–7.
17. Neuhaus P, *et al.* Effect of aprotinin on intraoperative bleeding and fibrinolysis in liver transplantation. *Lancet* 1989; **ii:** 924–5.
18. Thompson JF, *et al.* Aprotinin in peripheral vascular surgery. *Lancet* 1990; **335:** 911.
19. Janssens M, *et al.* High-dose aprotinin reduces blood loss in patients undergoing total hip replacement surgery. *Anesthesiology* 1994; **80:** 23–9.
20. Jaquiss RDB, *et al.* Use of aprotinin in pediatric lung transplantation. *J Heart Lung Transplant* 1995; **14:** 302–7.
21. Hunt BJ, Yacoub M. Aprotinin and cardiac surgery. *Br Med J* 1991; **303:** 660–1.
22. Spallone A, *et al.* Low-dose tranexamic acid combined with aprotinin in the pre-operative management of ruptured intracranial aneurysms. *Neurochirurgia (Stuttg)* 1987; **30:** 172–6.

Preparations

BP 1998: Aprotinin Injection;
Ph. Eur.: Fibrin Sealant Kit.

Proprietary Preparations (details are given in Part 3)
Aust.: Pantinol; Trasylol; ***Austral.:*** Trasylol; ***Belg.:*** Iniprol; Trasylol; ***Canad.:*** Trasylol; ***Fr.:*** Antagosan; Iniprol†; Trasylol; ***Ger.:*** Antagosan; Trasylol; ***Irl.:*** Trasylol†; ***Ital.:*** Antagosan; Fase; Inibil†; Iniprol†; Kir Richter; Midran†; Trasylol; ***Neth.:*** Trasylol; ***S.Afr.:*** Midran†; Trasylol; ***Swed.:*** Trasylol; ***Switz.:*** Trasylol; ***UK:*** Trasylol; ***USA:*** Trasylol.

Multi-ingredient: ***Aust.:*** Beriplast; TachoComb; Tissucol; Tissucol Duo Quick; ***Belg.:*** Tissucol; ***Canad.:*** Tisseel†; ***Fr.:*** Biocol; ***Ger.:*** Beriplast; TachoComb; Tissucol Duo S; Tissucol Fibrinkleber tiefgefroren; Tissucol-Kit; ***Irl.:*** Tisseel; ***Ital.:*** Tissucol; ***Spain:*** Tissucol; ***Swed.:*** Tisseel Duo Quick; ***Switz.:*** Tissucol; ***UK:*** Tisseel.

Batroxobin (12419-b)

Batroxobin (*rINN*).

CAS — 9039-61-6 (batroxobin); 9001-13-2 (haemocoagulase).

Batroxobin is an enzyme obtained from the venom of the viper *Bothrops atrox*. It has also been obtained from *Bothrops moojeni* and a similar preparation is derived from *Bothrops jararaca*. The name haemocoagulase (hemocoagulase) is used for a preparation of batroxobin with a factor-X activator.

Batroxobin is reported to act on fibrinogen to produce a fibrin monomer that can be converted by thrombin to a fibrin clot. It is used both as a haemostatic (p.704) and, in larger doses, to induce a hypofibrinogen state in the management of thrombo-embolic disorders (p.801). When used as a haemostatic it is usually given with a factor-X activator as haemocoagulase. Administration of batroxobin may be by parenteral routes or by local application.

Preparations

Proprietary Preparations (details are given in Part 3)
Aust.: Defibrase; Reptilase; ***Fr.:*** Reptilase; ***Ger.:*** Defibrase†; Reptilase†; ***Ital.:*** Botropase; Reptilase; ***Spain:*** Reptilase; ***Switz.:*** Defibrase†.

Blood (1212-e)

Whole Blood (USP 23) (ACD Whole Blood; CPD Whole Blood; CPDA-1 Whole Blood; Heparin Whole Blood) is blood which has been withdrawn aseptically from suitable human donors. It contains acid citrate dextrose, citrate phosphate dextrose, citrate phosphate dextrose with adenine, or heparin sodium as an anticoagulant. It may consist of blood from which the antihaemophilic factor has been removed, in which case it is termed 'Modified'. It should be stored in hermetically-sealed sterile containers at 1° to 6° (with a range of not more than 2°) except during transport when the temperature may be 1° to 10°. The expiration date is not later than 48 hours after withdrawal (heparin anticoagulant), not later than 21 days after withdrawal (acid citrate dextrose or citrate phosphate dextrose), or not later than 35 days after withdrawal (citrate phosphate dextrose with adenine).

Adverse Effects

The rapid transfusion of large volumes of whole blood may overload the circulation and cause pulmonary oedema. Repeated transfusions of blood, as in thalassaemia, may lead to iron overload. Transfusion of very large volumes of citrated blood can lead to hypocalcaemia which is not usually a problem unless there is impaired liver function or hypothermia. Hyperkalaemia may occur but on its own is rarely clinically significant. Hypothermia may result from rapid transfusion of large volumes of cooled blood and may, in combination with hypocalcaemia, hyperkalaemia, and resultant acidosis, lead to cardiac toxicity. Disseminated intravascular coagulation may also occur in patients receiving large-volume transfusions.

The transfusion of incompatible blood causes haemolysis, possibly with renal failure. Pyrexia, rigors, and urticaria may be due to antibodies towards a number of blood components. Severe allergic reactions and anaphylaxis may occur.

Transmission of infections. The use of blood, blood components, or blood products has been associated with the transmission of viruses, most notably transmission of the hepatitis B virus and HIV; other reports of transmission include cytomegalovirus, hepatitis C and possibly other hepatitis viruses, HTLV-I and -II, and the agent causing Creutzfeldt-Jakob disease. Transmission of bacterial and parasitic diseases is also possible including syphilis, Chagas' disease, and malaria.

The main methods of minimising the risk of transmission of infection are by rigorous selection of blood donors and by microbiological screening tests. Contamination during collection and processing is minimised by using closed systems and by strict aseptic technique. Some organisms cannot survive storage under refrigeration, for example staphylococci, while others, like malaria parasites, can survive storage in blood at 4° for at least a week. Treatment of blood products with heat or chemicals can inactivate some organisms including some viruses, in particular HIV-I, but blood and blood components cannot be treated in either of these ways. Patients receiving multiple transfusions of pooled plasma products are at increased risk of contracting infections and can be offered immunological protection, for example hepatitis B vaccine.

Reviews.

1. Contreras M, Mollison PL. Immunological complications of transfusion. In: Contreras M, ed. *ABC of transfusion.* 2nd ed. London: BMJ Publishing Group, 1992: 41–4.
2. Barbara JAJ, Contreras M. Infectious complications of blood transfusion: bacteria and parasites. In: Contreras M. ed. *ABC of transfusion.* 2nd ed. London: BMJ Publishing Group, 1992: 45–8.
3. Barbara JAJ, Contreras M. Infectious complications of blood transfusion: viruses. In: Contreras M. ed. *ABC of transfusion.* 2nd ed. London: BMJ Publishing Group, 1992: 49–52.
4. Donaldson MDJ, *et al.* Massive blood transfusion. *Br J Anaesth* 1992; **69:** 621–30.

Creutzfeldt-Jakob disease. While there is no proof that transmission of Creutzfeldt-Jakob disease by blood or blood products has occurred, it is recognised that there is a need for further assessment of the potential risk of transmission of new variant Creutzfeldt-Jakob disease by such products.[1] As precautionary measures, production of blood products using plasma from UK donors has been phased out and in some countries (including the UK) leucocytes are removed from donated blood (a procedure that early evidence suggests may remove infectivity).

Concern at the risk of transmitting Creutzfeldt-Jakob disease by albumin prepared from placental blood has lead to restriction on this source of albumin (see p.710).

1. Barbara J, Flanagan P. Blood transfusion risk: protecting against the unknown. *Br Med J* 1998; **316:** 717–18.

Effects on leucocytes. A study of 50 patients in an intensive care unit found that 45 of them developed leucocytosis following transfusion of packed red blood cells.[1] The leucocytosis, which was accounted for by neutrophils, occurred immediately after transfusion and persisted for 12 hours.

1. Fenwick JC, *et al.* Blood transfusion as a cause of leucocytosis in critically ill patients. *Lancet* 1994; **344:** 855–6.

Effects on the lungs. A rare but life-threatening complication of transfusion of blood or other plasma-containing products is acute lung injury.[1] The symptoms, which usually develop 1 to 6 hours after the start of infusion, are those of acute respiratory distress syndrome but usually resolve within about 2 to 4 days with vigorous supportive therapy. The presence of HLA-specific antileucocyte antibodies in plasma from multiparous female donors appears to play a role in initiating the reaction.

1. Popovsky MA, *et al.* Transfusion-related acute lung injury: a neglected, serious complication of hemotherapy. *Transfusion* 1992; **32:** 589–92.

Graft-versus-host disease. Acute graft-versus-host disease (p.498) has been reported in both immunocompromised and apparently immunocompetent patients following blood transfusion.[1-4] The reaction can be severe and fatal. Symptoms include fever, rash, hepatomegaly and abnormal liver function tests, diarrhoea, and pronounced pancytopenia. Infusion of products containing viable lymphocytes appears to be responsible and patients considered to be at risk may be given products depleted of viable lymphocytes by irradiation. Risk factors are incompletely defined. High-risk groups include bone marrow transplant recipients, patients with congenital immunodeficiencies, and possibly also premature infants undergoing exchange transfusions and patients receiving intensive chemotherapy for Hodgkin's disease. Immunocompetent patients who share an HLA haplotype with HLA-homozygous blood donors also appear to be at increased risk. A study in Japan[5] found that fresh and consanguineous blood transfusion was a major risk factor and that others were cardiovascular surgery, cancer, and being male.

1. Anonymous. Transfusions and graft-versus-host disease. *Lancet* 1989; **i:** 529–30.
2. Anderson KC, Weinstein HJ. Transfusion-associated graft-versus-host disease. *N Engl J Med* 1990; **323:** 315–21.
3. Webb DKH. Irradiation in the prevention of transfusion associated graft-versus-host disease. *Arch Dis Child* 1995; **73:** 388–9.
4. Williamson LM. Transfusion associated graft versus host disease and its prevention. *Heart* 1998; **80:** 211–12.
5. Takahashi K, *et al.* Analysis of risk factors for post-transfusion graft-versus-host disease in Japan. *Lancet* 1994; **343:** 700–2.

Malignant neoplasms. Blood transfusion is reported to have immunosuppressant effects, and several retrospective studies have suggested that perioperative blood transfusion in patients undergoing surgical resection of their tumours may be associated with an increased rate of tumour recurrence and decreased long-term survival.[1-5] This has been supported by experimental animal data.[6] However, the association has not been found in other studies[7,8] and at present there is insufficient data from prospective studies on which to base clinical recommendations.

Blood transfusion have also been associated with increased risk of non-Hodgkin's lymphoma in some studies, although it has been pointed out[9] that confounding factors could account for both the positive and negative associations that have been reported.

1. Burrows L, Tartter P. Effect of blood transfusions on colonic malignancy recurrence rate. *Lancet* 1982; **ii:** 662.
2. Blumberg N, *et al.* Relation between recurrence of cancer of the colon and blood transfusion. *Br Med J* 1985; **290:** 1037–9.
3. Blumberg N, *et al.* Association between transfusion of whole blood and recurrence of cancer. *Br Med J* 1986; **293;** 530–3.
4. Jackson RM, Rice DH. Blood transfusions and recurrence in head and neck cancer. *Ann Otol Rhinol Laryngol* 1989; **98:** 171–3.
5. Blumberg N, *et al.* The relationship of blood transfusion, tumor staging, and cancer recurrence. *Transfusion* 1990; **30:** 291–4.
6. Waymack JP, Chance WT. Effect of blood transfusions on immune function: IV effect on tumor growth. *J Surg Oncol* 1988; **39:** 159–64.
7. Blair SD, Janvrin SB. Relation between cancer of the colon and blood transfusion. *Br Med J* 1985; **290:** 1516–17.
8. Frankish PD, *et al.* Relation between cancer of the colon and blood transfusion. *Br Med J* 1985; **290:** 1827.
9. Alexander FE. Blood transfusion and risk of non-Hodgkin lymphoma. *Lancet* 1997; **350:** 1414–15.

Precautions

Whole blood should generally not be transfused unless the ABO and Rh groups of the patient's and the donor's blood have been verified and a compatibility check made between the patient's serum and the donor's red cells (see under Blood Groups, below).

The Rh group of the recipient should always be determined and ideally all patients should be transfused with blood of homologous Rh groups.

To reduce the possibility of cardiac arrest from cardiac hypothermia when large volumes are used or the blood is transfused rapidly, and to minimise postoperative shivering, stored blood should be carefully warmed to about 37° before transfusion.

Whole blood should not be given to patients with chronic anaemia who have a normal or elevated plasma volume.

Drugs should *not* be added to blood.

Transfusion of blood from donors who have recently been receiving drug treatment may be hazardous to the recipient.

Suggested guidelines[1] for accepting blood from donors who have been receiving drugs.

1. Ferner RE, *et al.* Drugs in donated blood. *Lancet* 1989; **ii:** 93–4.

Blood groups. The chief blood group systems are the ABO system and the Rhesus system.

In simple terms red blood cells carry on their surface genetically determined antigens. A person with antigen A, B, A plus B, or neither is classified as group A, B, AB, or O respectively. Such persons will have, in their serum, antibodies to B, A, neither, or both respectively—anti-B (β), anti-A (α), or anti-B plus anti-A (α + β). Administration of blood containing red cells from a person of group A to a person with anti-A results in agglutination or possibly haemolysis. For the determination of the ABO group the agglutinogens of the red cells and the agglutinins of the serum are determined by testing against known standards.

In the Rhesus system many persons carry an antigen (Rh-positive) which stimulates antibody formation in Rh-negative persons; subsequent exposure to Rh-positive blood causes haemolysis.

Many variants of these systems, and other systems, are recognised.

Uses and Administration

Blood is a complex fluid with many functions including the maintenance of hydration of the tissues, maintenance of body temperature, and the transport within the body of gases, ions, nutrients, hormones, enzymes, antibodies, waste products of metabolism, and drugs.

The main components of blood are plasma, red blood cells, white blood cells (leucocytes), and platelets. The leucocytes are classified according to their morphological appearance into granulocytes, lymphocytes, and monocytes. The granulocytes are further classified as neutrophils, eosinophils, and basophils, according to the characteristics of their granules. The term polymorphonuclear leucocytes can be applied to granulocytes in general but applies in particular to neutrophils. Serum is the fluid which remains once blood or plasma has clotted; it is in effect plasma with fibrinogen removed.

Whole blood is used as a source of red cell concentrates, clotting factors, platelets, plasma and plasma fractions, and immunoglobulins, each of which has specific indications for use. Because of the risks involved in transfusing whole blood and the need for economy in its use, the appropriate blood component should be used whenever possible.

Whole blood may be used where replacement of plasma proteins as well as red blood cells is needed, for example following acute blood loss during surgery and severe haemorrhage. It may also be used to supplement the circulation during cardiac bypass surgery.

The amount of whole blood transfused and the rate at which it is given depend upon the patient's age and general condition, upon the state of their circulatory system, and upon the therapeutic indication for transfusion.

The expression 'unit of blood' generally represents a volume of about 510 mL, including anticoagulant. For blood preparations a unit generally refers to the quantity of a blood component obtained from 1 unit of whole blood. Specific units of activity are used for some blood components.

The haemoglobin concentration of the blood of the average adult is raised by about 1 g per 100 mL by the transfusion of 1 unit of whole blood.

Reviews of uses of blood and blood components.

1. Contreras M, ed. *ABC of transfusion*. 2nd ed. London: BMJ Publishing Group, 1992.
2. Donaldson MDJ, *et al.* Massive blood transfusion. *Br J Anaesth* 1992; **69:** 621–30.
3. British Committee for Standards in Haematology Blood Transfusion Task Force. Guidelines for administration of blood products: transfusion of infants and neonates. *Transfus Med* 1994; **4:** 63–9.

Autologous blood transfusion. Reviews, discussions, and comments on autologous blood transfusion, the procedure of a patient acting as his own blood donor, the blood usually being collected shortly before elective surgery or salvaged during the surgical procedure.

1. Popovsky MA, *et al.* Intraoperative autologous transfusion. *Mayo Clin Proc* 1985; **60:** 125–34.
2. Council on Scientific Affairs. Autologous blood transfusions. *JAMA* 1986; **256:** 2378–80.
3. Kay LA. The need for autologous blood transfusion. *Br Med J* 1987; **294:** 137–9.
4. The National Blood Resource Education Program Expert Panel. The use of autologous blood. *JAMA* 1990; **263:** 414–17.
5. Lee D, Napier JAF. Autologous transfusion. *Br Med J* 1990; **300:** 737–40.
6. Page RJE, Wilson IH. Autologous transfusion. *Br Med J* 1990; **300:** 1139.
7. British Committee for Standards in Haematology Blood Transfusion Task Force. Guidelines for autologous transfusion I: pre-operative autologous donation. *Transfus Med* 1993; **3:** 307–16.
8. Contreras M, Chapman CE. Autologous transfusion and reducing allogeneic blood exposure. *Arch Dis Child* 1994; **71:** 105–7.
9. British Committee for Standards in Haematology Blood Transfusion Task Force. Guidelines for autologous transfusion II: perioperative haemodilution and cell salvage. *Br J Anaesth* 1997; **78:** 768–71.

Preparations

USP 23: Whole Blood.

Calcium Alginate (1715-e)

E404.

CAS — 9005-35-0.

The calcium salt of alginic acid, a polyuronic acid composed of residues of D-mannuronic and L-guluronic acids. It may be obtained from seaweeds, mainly species of *Laminaria*.

Practically **insoluble** in water and organic solvents; soluble in solutions of sodium citrate.

Calcium alginate is used as an absorbable haemostatic (p.704) and for the promotion of wound healing (p.1076); it is also used in the form of a mixed calcium-sodium salt of alginic acid as a fibre made into a dressing or packing material. Calcium ions in the calcium alginate fibres are exchanged for sodium ions in the blood and exudate to form a hydrophilic gel.

Alginic acid and its calcium and sodium salts are widely used in the food industry.

References.

1. Thomas S, Tucker CA. Sorbsan in the management of leg ulcers. *Pharm J* 1989; **243:** 706–9.
2. Anonymous. Scalpel and seaweed, nurse. *Lancet* 1990; **336:** 914.
3. Henderson NJ, *et al.* A randomised trial of calcium alginate swabs to control blood loss in 3–5-year-old children. *Br Dent J* 1998; **184:** 187–90. Correction. *ibid.*; 526.

Preparations

Proprietary Preparations (details are given in Part 3)
Austral.: Kaltostat; Sorbsan; *Fr.:* Algoderm†; Algosteril; Coalgan; Ouate Hemostatique U.S.†; Sorbsan; Stop Hemo; Trophiderm; *Irl.:* Kaltostat; *Ital.:* Kaltostat; Sorbsan; *S.Afr.:* Kaltostat; *Switz.:* Stop Hemo; *UK:* Algistat; Algosteril; Comfeel Seasorb; Kaltoclude†; Kaltostat; Sorbsan; Stop Hemo; *USA:* Kaltostat.

Multi-ingredient: *Austral.:* Kaltocarb; *UK:* Comfeel Plus; Kaltocarb.

Carbazochrome (1716-l)

Carbazochrome *(rINN)*.

Adrenochrome Monosemicarbazone. 3-Hydroxy-1-methyl-5,6-indolinedione semicarbazone.

$C_{10}H_{12}N_4O_3$ = 236.2.

CAS — 69-81-8 (carbazochrome); 13051-01-9 (carbazochrome salicylate); 51460-26-5 (carbazochrome sodium sulphonate).

Pharmacopoeias. Jpn includes Carbazochrome Sodium Sulphonate ($C_{10}H_{11}N_4NaO_5S.3H_2O$ = 376.3).

Carbazochrome, an oxidation product of adrenaline, has been given as a haemostatic (p.704) by mouth and by injection; it appears to be given as the dihydrate. It has also been used as the salicylate and the sodium sulphonate.

Preparations

Proprietary Preparations (details are given in Part 3)
Belg.: Adrenoxyl†; *Fr.:* Adrenoxyl†; *Ger.:* Adrenoxyl; *Ital.:* Adona; *Jpn:* Adona; Blockel†; *Spain:* Cromoxin†.

Multi-ingredient: *Ital.:* Fleboside; *Spain:* Cromoxin K; Cromoxin Perfus Fortific†; Flebeside; Perfus Multivitaminico; Quercetol Hemostatico; Quercetol K.

Oxidised Cellulose (1719-z)

Cellulosic Acid; Oxidized Cellulose.

CAS — 9032-53-5.

Pharmacopoeias. In *It.* and *US.*

US also includes Oxidized Regenerated Cellulose.

A sterile polyanhydroglucuronic acid, prepared by the oxidation of a suitable form of cellulose. It occurs as creamy-white gauze, lint, or knitted material, with a faint charred odour. It contains not less than 16% and not more than 24% of carboxyl groups, calculated with reference to the dried substance. Oxidized Regenerated Cellulose (USP 23) contains 18 to 24% of carboxyl groups calculated with reference to the dried substance.

Soluble in aqueous solutions of alkali hydroxides; practically insoluble in acids and in water. **Store** at a temperature not exceeding 8°. Protect from light.

Adverse Effects and Precautions

Foreign body reactions may occur after the use of oxidised cellulose or oxidised regenerated cellulose. Headache, burning, and stinging have been reported and sneezing has been noted after use in epistaxis. Oxidised cellulose swells on contact with a bleeding surface; this could result in tissue necrosis, nerve damage, obstruction, or vascular stenosis if packed closely, especially into bony cavities, or if wrapped tightly around blood vessels. To minimise such complications the removal of excess material should be considered after haemostasis is achieved, and oxidised cellulose should always be removed after use near the spinal cord or optic nerve. Oxidised cellulose should not be used in packing or implantation in fractures since it may interfere with bone regeneration or cause cyst formation. It should not be used as a surface dressing, except for immediate control of haemorrhage, as it inhibits epithelialisation.

Oxidised cellulose should be used as the dry material as moistening will reduce its ability to absorb blood. Silver nitrate or other escharotic chemicals should not be applied prior to use as cauterisation might inhibit absorption of oxidised cellulose. Thrombin is inactivated by the low pH of oxidised cellulose; it is recommended that oxidised cellulose should not be impregnated with other haemostatics or antibacterial agents.

Uses and Administration

Oxidised cellulose and oxidised regenerated cellulose are absorbable haemostatics. When applied to a bleeding surface, they swell to form a gelatinous mass which aids in the formation of a clot. It is gradually absorbed by the tissues, usually within 2 to 7 days. Complete absorption of large amounts of such material may take 6 weeks or more. These materials also have a weak bactericidal action. They are employed in surgery as adjuncts in the control of moderate bleeding where suturing or ligation is impracticable or ineffective; they should not be used to control haemorrhage from large arteries. The gauze, lint, or knitted material should be laid on the bleeding surface or held firmly against the tissues until haemostasis is achieved; removal should then be considered (see Adverse Effects and Precautions, above). Oxidised cellulose should be used as the dry material as moistening will reduce its ability to absorb blood.

Haemostasis and the various agents used as haemostatics are discussed on p.704.

Preparations

Proprietary Preparations (details are given in Part 3)
Fr.: Interceed; Sorbacel†; Surgicel; *Ger.:* Interceed; Tabotamp; *Ital.:* Tabotamp; *UK:* Interceed; Oxycel; Surgicel; *USA:* Interceed (TC7); Oxycel; Surgicel.

Colony-stimulating Factors (18987-z)

Colony-stimulating factors are glycoprotein growth factors that promote the proliferation and differentiation of haematopoietic precursors.

Sorption. Since solutions of colony-stimulating factors may be adsorbed onto glass or plastic materials, manufacturers caution that, if dilution is necessary, solutions should not be diluted to concentrations below the recommended minimum concentration and addition of albumin solution may be necessary with some colony-stimulating factors.

Adverse Effects

The main adverse effects of granulocyte colony-stimulating factors during short-term treatment are musculoskeletal pain and dysuria. Hypersensitivity reactions have been reported rarely. In patients receiving long-term treatment the most frequent adverse effects are bone pain and musculoskeletal pain. Other side-effects include splenic enlargement, thrombocytopenia, anaemia, epistaxis, headache, diarrhoea, and cutaneous vasculitis. There have been reports of pulmonary infiltrates leading to respiratory failure or acute respiratory distress syndrome.

Granulocyte-macrophage colony-stimulating factors may cause transient hypotension and flushing, bone pain and musculoskeletal pain, fever and chills, dyspnoea, rash, fatigue, and gastro-intestinal effects. Antibodies have been detected. Anaphylactic reactions, pleural and pericardial effusion, and cardiac rhythm abnormalities have been reported rarely.

Colony-stimulating factors are fetotoxic in *animal* studies.

General references.

1. Vial T, Descotes J. Clinical toxicity of cytokines used as haemopoietic growth factors. *Drug Safety* 1995; **13:** 371–406.

Antibodies. Antibodies have been reported in patients following administration of granulocyte-macrophage colony-stimulating factors produced in yeast[1] or in *Escherichia coli*.[2] Such factors are nonglycosylated or only partially glycosylated. A study[2] in 20 nonimmunocompromised patients given *E. coli*-derived granulocyte-macrophage colony-stimulating factors found that antibodies that were associated with reduced biological effectiveness developed in 95% of the patients. Only one of 8 immunocompromised patients given the colony-stimulating factor developed antibodies.

1. Gribben JG, *et al.* Development of antibodies to unprotected glycosylation sites on recombinant human GM-CSF. *Lancet* 1990; **335:** 434–7.
2. Ragnhammar P, *et al.* Induction of anti-recombinant human granulocyte-macrophage colony-stimulating factor (Escherichia coli-derived) antibodies and clinical effects in nonimmunocompromised patients. *Blood* 1994; **84:** 4078–87.

Disseminated intravascular coagulation. Long-term treatment with granulocyte colony-stimulating factor in a seven-year-old boy with HIV infection and zidovudine-induced neutropenia produced evidence of disseminated intravascular coagulation on two occasions.[1]

1. Mueller BU, *et al.* Disseminated intravascular coagulation associated with granulocyte colony-stimulating factor therapy in a child with human immunodeficiency virus infection. *J Pediatr* 1995; **126:** 749–52.

Effects on the bones. Bone mineral loss and osteoporosis have been reported in children with severe congenital neutropenia receiving granulocyte colony-stimulating factor for long periods.[1,2] However, the role of granulocyte colony-stimulating factor in producing this effect is uncertain since bone mineral loss may be a feature of the underlying disease.

1. Bishop NJ, *et al.* Osteoporosis in severe congenital neutropenia treated with granulocyte colony-stimulating factor. *Br J Haematol* 1995; **89:** 927–8.
2. Yakisan E, *et al.* High incidence of significant bone loss in patients with severe congenital neutropenia (Kostmann's syndrome). *J Pediatr* 1997; **131:** 592–7.

Effects on the eyes. Subretinal haemorrhage resulting in irreversible loss of vision in one eye occurred in a 4-year-old girl who received filgrastim and nartograstim for chemotherapy-induced neutropenia and for mobilising peripheral blood stem cells.[1] It was postulated that the colony-stimulating factor reactivated a primary ocular inflammation probably caused by an infection.

1. Matsumura T, *et al.* Subretinal haemorrhage after granulocyte colony-stimulating factor. *Lancet* 1997; **350:** 336. Correction. *ibid.*; 1406.

Effects on the lungs. There have been reports of exacerbation of chemotherapy-induced pulmonary toxicity in patients receiving granulocyte colony-stimulating factor in conjunction with bleomycin[1,2] and cyclophosphamide.[3] The patients were also receiving other antineoplastics. However, analysis of two randomised controlled studies failed to show increased pulmonary toxicity when granulocyte colony-stimulating factor was added to bleomycin therapy[4,5] and it has been suggested[5] that confounding factors, including the concomitant use of other antineoplastics, may account for the increased pulmonary toxicity.

1. Matthews JH. Pulmonary toxicity of ABVD chemotherapy and G-CSF in Hodgkin's disease: possible synergy. *Lancet* 1993; **342:** 988.
2. Dirix LY, *et al.* Pulmonary toxicity and bleomycin. *Lancet* 1994; **344:** 56.
3. van Woensel JBM, *et al.* Acute respiratory insufficiency during doxorubicin, cyclophosphamide, and G-CSF therapy. *Lancet* 1994; **344:** 759–60.
4. Bastion Y, *et al.* Possible toxicity with the association of G-CSF and bleomycin. *Lancet* 1994; **343:** 1221–2.
5. Bastion Y, Coiffier B. Pulmonary toxicity of bleomycin: is G-CSF a risk factor? *Lancet* 1994; **344:** 474.

Effects on the skin. Skin reactions may occur in patients given granulocyte-macrophage colony-stimulating factors. In a study in women with inflammatory breast cancer, a pruritic skin reaction developed at the subcutaneous injection site in all seven given granulocyte-macrophage colony-stimulating factor.[1] Exacerbation of psoriasis[2] and precipitation or exacerbation of neutrophilic dermatoses including Sweet's syndrome[3,4] and pyoderma gangrenosum[5] have been reported following administration of granulocyte colony-stimulating factor.

1. Steger GG, *et al.* Cutaneous reactions to GM-CSF in inflammatory breast cancer. *N Engl J Med* 1992; **327:** 286.
2. Kavanaugh A. Flare of psoriasis and psoriatic arthritis following treatment with granulocyte colony-stimulating factor. *Am J Med* 1996; **101:** 567.
3. Petit T, *et al.* Lymphoedema-area-restricted Sweet syndrome during G-CSF treatment. *Lancet* 1996; **347:** 690.
4. Garty BZ, *et al.* Sweet syndrome associated with G-CSF treatment in a child with glycogen storage disease type Ib. *Pediatrics* 1996; **97:** 401–3.
5. Johnson ML, Grimwood RE. Leukocyte colony-stimulating factors: a review of associated neutrophilic dermatoses and vasculitides. *Arch Dermatol* 1994; **130:** 77–81.

Effects on the thyroid. Reversible thyroid dysfunction has been reported in patients with pre-existing thyroid antibodies during treatment with granulocyte-macrophage colony-stimulating factor,[1] but not with granulocyte colony-stimulating factor.[2] However, clinical hypothyroidism has been reported in a patient with no history of thyroid dysfunction or thyroid antibodies during treatment with granulocyte colony-stimulating factor.[3]

1. Hoekman K, *et al.* Reversible thyroid dysfunction during treatment with GM-CSF. *Lancet* 1991; **338:** 541–2.
2. van Hoef MEHM, Howell A. Risk of thyroid dysfunction during treatment with G-CSF. *Lancet* 1992; **340:** 1169–70.
3. de Luis DA, Romero E. Reversible thyroid dysfunction with filgrastim. *Lancet* 1996; **348:** 1595–6.

Hypoalbuminaemia. In a series of 9 patients given prolonged treatment with granulocyte-macrophage colony-stimulating factor for myelodysplasia or aplastic anaemia, 4 developed hypoalbuminaemia that was symptomatic in 2 of the patients.[1]

1. Kaczmarski RS, Mufti GJ. Hypoalbuminaemia after prolonged treatment with recombinant granulocyte macrophage colony stimulating factor. *Br Med J* 1990; **301:** 1312–13.

Inflammatory disorders. Reactivation of various inflammatory disorders including rheumatoid arthritis[1] and pseudogout[2] has been reported following administration of colony-stimulating factors. For further reports of reactivation of sites of inflammation, see under Effects on the Eyes and Effects on the Skin, above.

1. Vildarsson B, *et al.* Reactivation of rheumatoid arthritis and development of leukocytoclastic vasculitis in a patient receiving granulocyte colony-stimulating factor for Felty's syndrome. *Am J Med* 1995; **98:** 589–91.
2. Sandor V, *et al.* Exacerbation of pseudogout by granulocyte colony-stimulating factor. *Ann Intern Med* 1996; **125:** 781.

Precautions

Since granulocyte colony-stimulating factors and granulocyte-macrophage colony-stimulating factors can promote growth of myeloid cells *in vitro* their use in myeloid malignancies has been contra-indicated, although recently they have been used in some patients with myeloid diseases without stimulation of malignant cells. However, caution is required when they are used in patients with any pre-malignant or malignant myeloid condition. Colony-stimulating factors should not be used from 24 hours before until 24 hours after cytotoxic chemotherapy or radiotherapy due to the sensitivity of rapidly dividing myeloid cells.

Granulocyte-macrophage colony-stimulating factors should be used with caution in patients with pulmonary disease as they may be predisposed to dyspnoea. Treatment should be withdrawn in patients who develop signs of pulmonary infiltrates. Caution is also necessary when colony-stimulating factors are used in patients with fluid retention or heart failure as they may aggravate fluid retention.

The complete blood count should be monitored regularly during therapy with colony-stimulating factors. Bone density should be monitored in patients with osteoporosis who are receiving long-term treatment with filgrastim.

For precautions to be taken in the preparation of solutions of colony-stimulating factors, see under Sorption, above.

Uses and Administration

Colony-stimulating factors or haematopoietic growth factors are naturally occurring glycoprotein growth factors (cytokines) that promote the proliferation and differentiation of haematopoietic precursors. Many colony-stimulating factors have been identified that stimulate development of different cell lines. Some of these factors have been produced by recombinant DNA technology and are used clinically. Erythropoietin, granulocyte colony-stimulating factors (G-CSF), and granulocyte-macrophage colony-stimulating factors (GM-CSF) are the most extensively studied. Information on erythropoietin is given on p.717. Details of granulocyte and granulocyte-macrophage colony-stimulating factors are given below. Other factors under investigation include macrophage colony-stimulating factors, such as mirimostim, thrombopoietin (p.728) (for the treatment of thrombocytopenia), interleukin-3 (p.724), interleukin-11 (oprelvekin) (p.725), and ancestim (stem cell factor).

- Granulocyte-macrophage colony-stimulating factors stimulate the development of white blood cells, particularly granulocytes, macrophages, and monocytes. They include molgramostim (p.725) and sargramostim (p.727).
- Granulocyte colony-stimulating factors stimulate the development of granulocytes. They include filgrastim (p.723), lenograstim (p.724), and nartograstim (p.725).

Both types are used to treat or prevent neutropenia (p.709) in patients receiving myelosuppressive cancer chemotherapy, to reduce the period of neutropenia in patients undergoing bone marrow transplantation (p.474), and to mobilise autologous peripheral blood progenitor cells as an alternative to bone marrow transplantation. They are also under investigation in many other neutropenic disorders, in aplastic anaemia (p.701), as adjuncts in the treatment of infections, and in the management of skin ulcers and wounds. Granulocyte colony-stimulating factors are also used in chronic neutropenia (congenital, cyclic, or idiopathic). Granulocyte-macrophage colony-stimulating factors are also used to reduce ganciclovir-induced neutropenia (p.611).

Dosage details are given under the individual drug monographs.

General references.

1. Metcalf D. Peptide regulatory factors: haemopoietic growth factors 1. *Lancet* 1989; **i:** 825–7.
2. Metcalf D. Peptide regulatory factors: haemopoietic growth factors 2: clinical applications. *Lancet* 1989; **i:** 885–7.
3. Groopman JE, *et al.* Hematopoietic growth factors: biology and clinical applications. *N Engl J Med* 1989; **321:** 1449–59.
4. Lieschke GJ, Burgess AW. Granulocyte colony-stimulating factor and granulocyte-macrophage colony-stimulating factor. *N Engl J Med* 1992; **327:** 28–35.
5. Lieschke GJ, Burgess AW. Granulocyte colony-stimulating factor and granulocyte-macrophage colony-stimulating factor. *N Engl J Med* 1992; **327:** 99–106.
6. Rowe JM, Rapoport AP. Hemopoietic growth factors: a review. *J Clin Pharmacol* 1992; **32:** 486–501.
7. Steward WP. Granulocyte and granulocyte-macrophage colony-stimulating factors. *Lancet* 1993; **342:** 153–7.
8. Hann IM. The use of haemopoietic growth factors in blood disorders. *Arch Dis Child* 1994; **71:** 543–7.
9. Stross P, Bunch C. Drugs in focus: colony-stimulating factors (filgrastim, lenograstim, molgramostim). *Prescribers' J* 1994; **34:** 119–24.
10. American Society of Clinical Oncology. Recommendations for the use of hematopoietic colony-stimulating factors: evidence-based, clinical practice guidelines. *J Clin Oncol* 1994; **12:** 2471–2508.
11. American Society of Clinical Oncology. Update of recommendations for the use of hematopoietic colony-stimulating factors: evidence-based clinical practice guidelines. *J Clin Oncol* 1996; **14:** 1957–60.
12. Nemunaitis J. A comparative review of colony-stimulating factors. *Drugs* 1997; **54:** 709–29.

Blood disorders. APLASTIC ANAEMIA. Colony-stimulating factors have been tried in a few patients with aplastic anaemia (p.701).

CHRONIC NEUTROPENIA. References.

1. Bonilla MA, *et al.* Long-term safety of treatment with recombinant human granulocyte colony-stimulating factor (r-metHuG-CSF) in patients with severe congenital neutropenias. *Br J Haematol* 1994; **88:** 723–30.

DRUG-INDUCED NEUTROPENIA. Granulocyte-macrophage colony-stimulating factor is used in the management of ganciclovir-induced neutropenia. Granulocyte colony-stimulating factor has been tried in patients with neutropenia induced by a wide range of other drugs.[1-6]

1. Gerson SL, *et al.* Granulocyte colony-stimulating factor for clozapine-induced agranulocytosis. *Lancet* 1992; **340:** 1097.
2. Wyatt S, *et al.* Filgrastim for mesalazine-associated neutropenia. *Lancet* 1993; **341:** 1476.
3. Teitelbaum AH, *et al.* Filgrastim (r-met HuG-CSF) reversal of drug-induced agranulocytosis. *Am J Med* 1993; **95:** 245–6.
4. Geibig CB, Marks LW. Treatment of clozapine- and molindone-induced agranulocytosis with granulocyte colony-stimulating factor. *Ann Pharmacother* 1993; **27:** 1190–2.
5. Chia HM, *et al.* Filgrastim for low-dose, captopril-induced agranulocytosis. *Lancet* 1993; **342:** 304.
6. Gales BJ, Gales MA. Granulocyte-colony stimulating factor for sulfasalazine-induced agranulocytosis. *Ann Pharmacother* 1993; **27:** 1052–4.

NEONATAL NEUTROPENIA. Short-term administration of colony-stimulating factors has been tried in a few preterm neonates with neutropenia and severe infections and increases in neutrophil counts have been reported in some,[1,2] though not in others.[3] Colony-stimulating factors have also been tried with mixed results in neonates with the rare condition of alloimmune neutropenia.[4-6]

1. Bedford Russell AR, *et al.* Granulocyte colony stimulating factor treatment for neonatal neutropenia. *Arch Dis Child* 1995; **72:** F53–F54.
2. Carr R, Modi N. Haemopoietic colony stimulating factors for preterm neonates. *Arch Dis Child* 1997; **76:** F128–F133.
3. Schibler KR, *et al.* A randomized, placebo-controlled trial of granulocyte colony-stimulating factor administration to newborn infants with neutropenia and clinical signs of early-onset sepsis. *Pediatrics* 1998; **102:** 6–13.
4. Gilmore MM, *et al.* Treatment of alloimmune neonatal neutropenia with granulocyte colony-stimulating factor. *J Pediatr* 1994; **125:** 948–51.
5. Bedu A, *et al.* Failure of granulocyte colony-stimulating factor in alloimmune neonatal neutropenia. *J Pediatr* 1995; **127:** 508.
6. Rodwell RL, *et al.* Granulocyte colony stimulating factor treatment for alloimmune neonatal neutropenia. *Arch Dis Child* 1996; **75:** F57–F58.

Infections. It has been suggested[1] that colony-stimulating factors may be useful as adjuncts to antibacterial or antifungal therapy in patients with severe infections and defects in phagocytic cell function. Such defects may occur in patients with diabetes mellitus (p.313) or AIDS (p.599). Addition of granulocyte colony-stimulating factor to conventional therapy improved clinical outcome of foot infection in a small study in diabetic patients[2] and 3 of 4 patients with AIDS and resistant oral candidiasis responded to treatment with granulocyte-macrophage colony-stimulating factor.[3] A controlled study in 258 patients with advanced HIV infection found that prophylactic administration of granulocyte colony-stimulating factor reduced the incidence of severe neutropenia and also suggested that the incidence and duration of bacterial infections was reduced.[4]

Colony-stimulating factors have also been tried as an adjunct to conventional therapy in chronic viral hepatitis (p.595).

1. Khwaja A, Linch DC. Haemopoietic growth factors in the treatment of infection in non-neutropenic patients. *J Antimicrob Chemother* 1994; **33:** 679–83.
2. Gough A, *et al.* Randomised placebo-controlled trial of granulocyte-colony stimulating factor in diabetic foot infection. *Lancet* 1997; **350:** 855–9.
3. Capetti A, *et al.* Employment of recombination human granulocyte-macrophage colony stimulating factor in oesophageal candidiasis in AIDS patients. *AIDS* 1995; **9:** 1378–9.
4. Kuritzkes DP, *et al.* Filgrastim prevents severe neutropenia and reduces infective morbidity in patients with advanced HIV infection: results of a randomized, multicenter, controlled trial. *AIDS* 1998; **12:** 65–74.

Wounds and ulcers. Molgramostim modifies several mechanisms involved in wound healing and is being investigated in non-healing wounds and ulcers (p.1076). It has been tried as an incubation solution for skin grafts,[1] and by perilesional injection[2,3] and topical application.[4]

1. Pojda Z, Struzyna J. Treatment of non-healing ulcers with rhGM-CSF and skin grafts. *Lancet* 1994; **343:** 1100.
2. Marques da Costa R, *et al.* Quick healing of leg ulcers after molgramostim. *Lancet* 1994; **344:** 481–2.
3. Wheeler G, Brodie GN. GM-CSF and wound healing. *Med J Aust* 1998; **168:** 580.
4. Pieters RC, *et al.* Molgramostim to treat SS-sickle cell leg ulcers. *Lancet* 1995; **345:** 528.

Cotarnine Chloride (12611-b)

Cotarnine Hydrochloride; Cotarninium Chloratum. 7,8-Dihydro-4-methoxy-6-methyl-1,3-dioxolo[4,5-g]isoquinolinium chloride dihydrate.

$C_{12}H_{14}ClNO_3,2H_2O = 291.7.$

CAS — 82-54-2 (cotarnine); 10018-19-6 (cotarnine chloride).

Cotarnine chloride is a haemostatic that has been given by mouth.

Dextran 1 (14124-v)

Dextran 1 *(BAN, rINN).*

Dextranum 1.

CAS — 9004-54-0 (dextran).

Dextran 1 consists of dextrans (glucose polymers) of weight average molecular weight about 1000 that are derived from the dextrans produced by the fermentation of sucrose by means of a certain strain of *Leuconostoc mesenteroides* (NCTC No. 10817).

Uses and Administration

Dextran 1 is used to prevent severe anaphylactic reactions to infusions of dextran. It is reported to occupy the binding sites of dextran-reactive antibodies and so prevent the formation of large immune complexes with higher molecular weight dextrans.

Dextran 1 is given in usual doses of 20 mL of a solution containing 150 mg per mL by intravenous injection about 1 to 2 minutes before the infusion of the higher molecular weight dextran; the interval should not exceed 15 minutes. A suggested dose for children is 0.3 mL per kg body-weight. The dose of dextran 1 should be repeated if further infusions of dextran are required more than 48 hours after the initial dose.

Two large multicentre studies (involving about 29 200 and 34 950 patients) have suggested that dextran 1 prevented anaphylactic reactions by hapten inhibition in a dose-dependent way.[1,2] It did not reduce the incidence of mild reactions, which are not generally mediated by antibodies. Another large study[3] comparing the effects of giving dextran 1 either 2 minutes before injection of dextran 40 or 70 or mixed with the injection, was discontinued after the occurrence of 2 severe reactions in the admixture group. A comparison[4] of severe anaphylactic reactions to dextran infusion during the period 1983 to 1992 (when prophylaxis with dextran 1 was used) with reactions reported during the period 1975 to 1979 (no prophylaxis) found that the use of dextran 1 was associated with a 35-fold reduction in severe anaphylactic reactions to dextran infusion.

There were 21, 20, and 2 adverse reactions to dextran 1 in the first 3 studies respectively, including nausea, skin reactions, bradycardia, and hypotension. Apart from one patient, reactions to dextran 1 were mild and were considered to be of minor clinical importance. In the fourth study, side-effects to dextran 1 were reported in approximately one case per 100 000 doses.

1. Ljungström K-G, *et al.* Prevention of dextran-induced anaphylactic reactions by hapten inhibition I: a Scandinavian multicenter study on the effects of 10 mL dextran 1.15% administered before dextran 70 or dextran 40. *Acta Chir Scand* 1983; **149:** 341–8.
2. Renck H, *et al.* Prevention of dextran-induced anaphylactic reactions by hapten inhibition III: Scandinavian multicenter study on the effects of 20 mL dextran 1.15%, administered before dextran 70 or dextran 40. *Acta Chir Scand* 1983; **149:** 355–60.
3. Renck H, *et al.* Prevention of dextran-induced anaphylactic reactions by hapten inhibition II: a comparison of the effects of 20 mL dextran 1.15%, administered either admixed to or before dextran 70 or dextran 40. *Acta Chir Scand* 1983; **149:** 349–53.
4. Ljungström K-G. Hapten inhibition of dextran reactions. Ten years' experience with dextran 1. *Br J Anaesth* 1995; **74** (suppl 1): 127.

Preparations

Proprietary Preparations (details are given in Part 3)
Aust.: Praedex; Promit; ***Austral.:*** Promit; ***Canad.:*** Promit†; ***Fr.:*** Promit; ***Ger.:*** Promit; ***Norw.:*** Promiten; ***Swed.:*** Promiten; ***Switz.:*** Promit; ***USA:*** Promit.

Dextran 40 (251-w)

Dextran 40 *(BAN, USAN, rINN).*

Dextranum 40; LMD; LMWD; Low-molecular-weight Dextran; LVD.

CAS — 9004-54-0 (dextran).

Pharmacopoeias. In *Chin., Jpn,* and *Pol.*

Eur. (see p.viii) and *Jpn* describe Dextran 40 for Injection.

Dextran 40 consists of dextrans (glucose polymers) of weight average molecular weight about 40 000 that are derived from the dextrans produced by the fermentation of sucrose by means of a certain strain or substrains of *Leuconostoc mesenteroides.*

A white or almost white powder. Very **soluble** in water; very slightly soluble in alcohol; slightly soluble in ether.

Incompatibilities may arise from the slightly acid pH of dextran 40 preparations.

Adverse Effects, Treatment, and Precautions

As for Dextran 70, p.717.

Rapid renal excretion of dextran 40 in patients with reduced urine flow can result in high urinary concentrations which increase urinary viscosity and may cause oliguria or acute renal failure. Therefore, infusions of dextran 40 are contra-indicated in renal disease with oliguria; should anuria or oliguria occur during treatment dextran 40 should be withdrawn. Dehydration should preferably be corrected before administration of dextran 40. Dextran 40 can cause capillary oozing of wound surfaces.

Effects on the kidneys. Acute renal failure has been associated with dextran 40[1-3] and less frequently with dextran 70.[1] The mechanism of the effect is still unclear[2-5] but low-molecular-weight dextran has been cited[1] as a common cause of drug-induced acute renal failure. Dextran should be withheld if the urine output falls during administration and diuresis induced with diuretics and a high fluid intake. Plasmapheresis has been used successfully to remove dextran from the circulation.[2]

1. Feest TG. Low molecular weight dextran: a continuing cause of acute renal failure. *Br Med J* 1976; **2:** 1300.
2. Moran M, Kapsner C. Acute renal failure associated with elevated plasma oncotic pressure. *N Engl J Med* 1987; **317:** 150–3.
3. Druml W, *et al.* Dextran-40, acute renal failure, and elevated plasma oncotic pressure. *N Engl J Med* 1988; **318:** 252–3.
4. Stein HD. Dextran-40, acute renal failure, and elevated plasma oncotic pressure. *N Engl J Med* 1988; **318;** 253.
5. Moran M, Kapsner C. Dextran-40, acute renal failure, and elevated plasma oncotic pressure. *N Engl J Med* 1988; **318:** 253–4.

Effects on the lungs. In a study[1] of 45 women undergoing gynaecological surgery, 25 received 400 to 500 mL of a 10% solution of dextran 40 intraperitoneally for prevention of adhesions. After 5 to 7 days, 12 of the dextran group and none of the controls had a pleural effusion visible on chest X-ray. The effusions were small to moderate, asymptomatic, and resolved without treatment.

1. Adoni A, *et al.* Postoperative pleural effusion caused by dextran. *Int J Gynaecol Obstet* 1980; **18:** 243–74.

Hypersensitivity. For reports of anaphylactic reactions associated with administration of dextran 40, see Dextran 70, below, and Dextran 1, above.

Pharmacokinetics

After intravenous infusion of dextran 40, about 70% is excreted unchanged in the urine within 24 hours. The dextran not excreted is slowly metabolised to glucose. A small amount is excreted into the gastro-intestinal tract and eliminated in the faeces.

Uses and Administration

Dextran 40 is a plasma volume expander used in the management of hypovolaemic shock (p.798). As a 10% solution dextran 40 exerts a slightly higher colloidal osmotic pressure than plasma proteins and thus produces a greater expansion of plasma volume than dextrans of a higher molecular weight, although the expansion may have a shorter duration because of more rapid renal excretion. Dextran 40 also reduces blood viscosity and inhibits sludging or aggregation of red blood cells. It is used in the prophylaxis and treatment of postoperative thrombo-embolic disorders, in conditions where improved circulatory flow is required, and as a priming solution during extracorporeal circulation.

Dextran 40 is given by intravenous infusion as a 10% solution in sodium chloride 0.9% or glucose 5%. Doses depend on the clinical condition of the patient.

In shock, a maximum of 20 mL per kg body-weight during the first 24 hours has been recommended; the first 10 mL per kg may be given by rapid intravenous infusion. Doses of up to 10 mL per kg may be given daily thereafter for up to 5 days. Dehydration should preferably be corrected before dextran 40 is administered.

In the treatment of thrombo-embolic disorders a suggested regimen is 500 to 1000 mL over 4 to 6 hours on the first day, then 500 mL over 4 to 6 hours on the next and subsequent alternate days for not more than 10 days.

For prophylaxis of postoperative thrombo-embolic disorders, 500 mL over 4 to 6 hours may be given during or at the end of surgery and the dose repeated on the next day; treatment may be continued in high risk patients on alternate days for up to 10 days.

Infants may be given up to 5 mL per kg body-weight and children up to 10 mL per kg.

A dose of 10 to 20 mL per kg has been added to extracorporeal perfusion fluids.

Dextran 40 is also an ingredient of artificial tears.

Stroke. Haemodilution with dextran 40 has been tried in patients with acute ischaemic stroke (p.799) in an attempt to improve reperfusion of the brain by lowering blood viscosity. However, two large controlled studies[1,2] have been unable to confirm a beneficial effect of venesection and replacement of the blood volume with dextran 40.

1. Scandinavian Stroke Study Group. Multicenter trial of hemodilution in acute ischemic stroke I: results in the total patient population. *Stroke* 1987; **18:** 691–9.
2. Italian Acute Stroke Study Group. Haemodilution in acute stroke: results of the Italian haemodilution trial. *Lancet* 1988; **i:** 318–20.

Surgical procedures. Pre-operative hypervolaemic haemodilution with 5% dextran 40 1500 mL and Ringer's lactate 1500 mL was used[1] to avoid the need for blood transfusions during major surgery in 16 patients. However, there was evidence of depressed cardiac function and pulmonary overload[2] and this technique could not be recommended for patients with a compromised cardiovascular system[1] and should be restricted to those for whom no alternative measures were available.

1. Trouwborst A, *et al.* Acute hypervolaemic haemodilution to avoid blood transfusion during major surgery. *Lancet* 1990; **336:** 1295–7. Correction. *ibid.* 1991; **337:** 504.
2. Inaba S, *et al.* Hypervolaemic haemodilution before major surgery. *Lancet* 1991; **337:** 729–30.

Venous thrombo-embolism. Dextran 40 is only one of a variety of drugs that have been used for the prophylaxis of thrombo-embolic disorders (p.802) resulting from surgical operations. In hip replacement surgery, Harris *et al.*[1] showed that warfarin and dextran 40 gave similar protection whereas in general surgery, Gruber *et al.*[2] found that heparin was better than dextran 40 in preventing deep-vein thrombosis and Francis *et al.*[3] found that dextran 40 was considerably less effective than a combination of antithrombin III and heparin in total knee arthroplasty.

1. Harris WH, *et al.* Prevention of venous thromboembolism following total hip replacement: warfarin vs dextran 40. *JAMA* 1972; **220:** 1319–22.
2. Gruber UF, *et al.* Prevention of postoperative thromboembolism by dextran 40, low doses of heparin, or xantinol nicotinate. *Lancet* 1977; **i:** 207–10.
3. Francis CW, *et al.* Prevention of venous thrombosis after total knee arthroplasty: comparison of antithrombin III and low-dose heparin with dextran. *J Bone Joint Surg (Am)* 1990; **72-A;** 976–82.

Preparations

BP 1998: Dextran 40 Intravenous Infusion.

Proprietary Preparations (details are given in Part 3)
Aust.: Elorheo; Laevodex; Onkovertin N; Rheofusin; Rheomacrodex; ***Austral.:*** Rheomacrodex; ***Canad.:*** Gentran 40; Rheomacrodex; ***Fr.:*** Plasmacair; Rheomacrodex; ***Ger.:*** Infukoll M 40; Longasteril 40; Onkovertin N; Parenteral D 40†; Rheofusin†; Rheomacrodex; Thomaedex 40; ***Irl.:*** Rheomacrodex†; ***Ital.:*** Eudextran; Plander R; Rheomacrodex†; Solplex 40; ***Jpn:*** Saviosol†; ***Norw.:*** Rheomacrodex; ***S.Afr.:*** Rheomacrodex; ***Spain:*** Fisiodex 40†; Rheomacrodex; ***Swed.:*** Perfadex; Rheomacrodex; ***Switz.:*** Rheomacrodex; ***UK:*** Gentran 40; Lomodex 40†; Rheomacrodex; ***USA:*** Gentran 40; Rheomacrodex.

Multi-ingredient: ***Canad.:*** Ocutears.

Dextran 60 (16294-c)

Pharmacopoeias. Eur. (see p.viii) describes Dextran 60 for Injection.

Dextran 60 consists of dextrans (glucose polymers) of weight average molecular weight about 60 000 that are derived from the dextrans produced by the fermentation of sucrose by means of a certain strain or substrains of *Leuconostoc mesenteroides.*

A white or almost white powder. Very **soluble** in water; very slightly soluble in alcohol; slightly soluble in ether.

Incompatibilities may arise from the slightly acid pH of dextran 60 preparations.

Dextran 60 is a plasma volume expander with actions and uses similar to dextran 70 (see below). It is given by intravenous infusion as a 3% or 6% solution in sodium chloride 0.9% or a mixture of electrolytes.

Dextran 60 is also used topically for dry eyes.

Preparations

Proprietary Preparations (details are given in Part 3)
Aust.: Laevodex; Macrodex; Onkovertin; ***Fr.:*** Dialens; Hemodex; ***Ger.:*** Macrodex; Onkovertin; Thomaedex 60; ***Norw.:*** Plasmodex; ***Swed.:*** Plasmodex; ***Switz.:*** Dialens.

Dextran 70 (252-e)

Dextran 70 *(BAN, USAN, rINN).*
Dextranum 70; Polyglucin (dextran).
CAS — 9004-54-0 (dextran).
Pharmacopoeias. In *Chin., Jpn,* and *Pol.*
Eur. (see p.viii) and *Jpn* describe Dextran 70 for Injection.

Dextran 70 consists of dextrans (glucose polymers) of weight average molecular weight about 70 000 that are derived from the dextrans produced by the fermentation of sucrose by means of a certain strain or substrains of *Leuconostoc mesenteroides.*

A white or almost white powder. Very **soluble** in water; very slightly soluble in alcohol; slightly soluble in ether.

Incompatibilities may arise from the slightly acid pH of dextran 70 preparations.

Crystals may form in solutions of dextran if they are stored at low temperatures. These may be redissolved by warming for a short time.

Adverse Effects and Treatment

Infusions of dextrans may occasionally produce hypersensitivity reactions such as fever, nasal congestion, joint pains, urticaria, hypotension, and bronchospasm. Severe anaphylactic reactions occur rarely and may be fatal. Dextran-reactive antibodies may arise in response to dietary or bacterial polysaccharides in patients who have not previously received dextran. Nausea and vomiting have also been reported. These reactions are treated symptomatically after withdrawal of the dextran. Dextran 40 can cause renal impairment as a result of increased urinary viscosity; capillary oozing has also been associated with its use.

Dextran 1 (p.716) may be used to block the formation of dextran-reactive antibodies and hence the hypersensitivity reactions.

Effects on the blood. Disseminated intravascular coagulation and acute respiratory distress syndrome developed following hysteroscopy during which 1200 mL of dextran 70 was used to dilate the uterus.[1] The large volume used was considered to have contributed to the reaction by increasing the systemic absorption of the dextran solution.

1. Jedeikin R, *et al.* Disseminated intravascular coagulopathy and adult respiratory distress syndrome: life-threatening complications of hysteroscopy. *Am J Obstet Gynecol* 1990; **162:** 44–5.

Effects on the kidneys. For a report of acute renal failure associated with administration of dextran 70, see Dextran 40, above.

Hypersensitivity. In a retrospective study of allergic reactions to dextran 40 and dextran 70 reported in Sweden from 1970 to 1979,[1] there were 478 reports of reactions, 458 of which were considered to be due to dextran, out of 1 365 266 infusions given. There was a male to female ratio of 1.5 to 1 for all reactions and a ratio of 3 to 1 for the most severe reactions. The mean age of the patients was higher in those with severe reactions. Of the 28 fatal reactions, 27 occurred within 5 minutes of the start of the infusion and 25 when less than 25 mL had been infused. Three of the fatal reactions occurred after a test dose of only 0.5 to 1.0 mL and it was strongly recommended that such test doses should not be used.

An anaphylactic reaction has also been reported[2] more than 75 minutes after intraperitoneal instillation. After successful symptomatic treatment symptoms recurred 20 minutes later, due to slow absorption of dextran from the peritoneal cavity. No further reaction occurred after removal of 200 mL of intraperitoneal fluid by culdocentesis.

Anaphylactoid reactions following BCG vaccination have been attributed to hypersensitivity to dextran included in the formulation.[3,4]

The use of dextran 1 for the prevention of hypersensitivity reactions is discussed under that monograph (p.716).

1. Ljungström K-G, *et al.* Adverse reactions to dextran in Sweden 1970–1979. *Acta Chir Scand* 1983; **149:** 253–62.
2. Borten M, *et al.* Recurrent anaphylactic reaction to intraperitoneal dextran 75 used for prevention of postsurgical adhesions. *Obstet Gynecol* 1983; **61:** 755–7.
3. Rudin C, *et al.* Anaphylactoid reaction to BCG vaccination. *Lancet* 1991; **337:** 377.
4. Pönnighaus JM, *et al.* Hypersensitivity to dextran in BCG vaccine. *Lancet* 1991; **337:** 1039.

Precautions

Dextran infusions produce a progressive dilution of oxygen-carrying capacity, coagulation factors, and plasma proteins and may overload the circulation. They are therefore contra-indicated in patients with severe heart failure, bleeding disorders such as hypofibrinogenaemia or thrombocytopenia, or renal failure and should be administered with caution to patients with impaired renal function, haemorrhage, chronic liver disease, or those at risk of developing pulmonary oedema or heart failure. Central venous pressure should be monitored during the initial period of infusion to detect fluid overload. Also patients should be watched closely during the early part of the infusion period, and the infusion stopped immediately if signs of anaphylactic reactions appear. Infusions should also be stopped if there are signs of oliguria or renal failure. The haematocrit should not be allowed to fall below 30% and all patients should be observed for early signs of bleeding complications. The bleeding time may be increased especially in patients receiving large volumes of dextrans. Deficiency of coagulation factors should be corrected and fluid and electrolyte balance maintained. Dehydration should be corrected before or at least during dextran infusions, in order to maintain an adequate urine flow.

The anticoagulant effect of heparin may be enhanced by dextran.

The higher molecular weight dextrans may interfere with blood grouping and cross matching of blood, while the lower molecular weight dextrans may interfere with some methods. Therefore, whenever possible, a sample of blood should be collected before giving the dextran infusion and kept frozen in case such tests become necessary.

The presence of dextran may interfere with the determination of glucose, bilirubin, or protein in blood or urine.

Pharmacokinetics

After intravenous infusion dextrans with a molecular weight of less than 50 000 are excreted unchanged by the kidney. Dextrans with a molecular weight greater than 50 000 are slowly metabolised to glucose. Small amounts of dextrans are excreted into the gastro-intestinal tract and eliminated in the faeces.

About 50% of dextran 70 is excreted unchanged in the urine within 24 hours.

Uses and Administration

Dextran 70 is a plasma volume expander used in the management of hypovolaemic shock (p.798). As a 6% solution dextran 70 exerts a colloidal osmotic pressure similar to that of plasma proteins and thus produces less expansion of plasma volume than dextrans of a lower molecular weight, although the expansion may have a longer duration because of less rapid renal excretion. Dextran 70 also reduces blood viscosity and inhibits sludging or aggregation of red blood cells. It is used in the prophylaxis of postoperative thrombo-embolic disorders (p.802).

Dextran 70 is given by intravenous infusion as a 6% solution in sodium chloride 0.9% or glucose 5%.

Doses depend on the severity of the plasma loss and on the degree of haemoconcentration.

In shock, the usual initial dose for rapid expansion of plasma volume is 500 to 1000 mL infused at a rate of 20 to 40 mL per minute. A suggested maximum dose is 20 mL per kg body-weight during the first 24-hour period and 10 mL per kg per day thereafter; treatment should not continue for longer than 3 days. Patients may also require administration of blood, coagulation factors, and electrolytes.

For the prophylaxis of pulmonary embolism or venous thrombosis in moderate- to high-risk patients undergoing surgery a dose of 500 to 1000 mL may be given over 4 to 6 hours either during or immediately following surgery. A dose of 500 mL should be given on the next day and in high-risk patients on subsequent alternate days for up to two weeks after the operation.

A 32% solution of dextran 70 has been instilled into the uterus in a dose of 50 to 100 mL as a rinsing and dilatation fluid to aid hysteroscopy.

Dextran 70 is also an ingredient of artificial tears.

Preparations

BP 1998: Dextran 70 Intravenous Infusion.

Proprietary Preparations (details are given in Part 3)
Austral.: Hyskon; Macrodex; ***Canad.:*** Gentran 70; Hyskon; Macrodex; ***Ger.:*** Hyskon; Longasteril 70; ***Irl.:*** Hyskon†; Macrodex†; ***Ital.:*** Macrodex†; Plander; Solplex 70; ***Norw.:*** Macrodex; ***S.Afr.:*** Macrodex; ***Spain:*** Fisiodex 70†; Macrodex; ***Swed.:*** Hyskon; Macrodex; ***Switz.:*** Macrodex; ***UK:*** Gentran 70; Hyskon; ***Ital.:*** Lomodex 70†; Macrodex; ***USA:*** Gentran 70; Hyskon; Macrodex.

Multi-ingredient: ***Austral.:*** Poly-Tears; Tears Naturale; ***Belg.:*** Lacrystat; Tears Naturale; ***Canad.:*** Aquasite; Bion Tears; Tears Naturale; ***Ger.:*** Isopto Naturale; ***Irl.:*** Tears Naturale; ***Ital.:*** Dacriosol; ***Neth.:*** Duratears†; ***S.Afr.:*** Tears Naturale; ***Spain:*** Dacrolux; Tears Humectante; ***Switz.:*** Tears Naturale; ***UK:*** Tears Naturale; ***USA:*** Aquasite; Bion Tears; LubriTears; Moisture Drops; Nature's Tears; Ocucoat; Tears Naturale; Tears Renewed.

Dextran 75 (14125-g)

Dextran 75 *(BAN, USAN, rINN).*
Dextranum 75.
CAS — 9004-54-0 (dextran).

Dextran 75 consists of dextrans (glucose polymers) of weight average molecular weight about 75 000 that are derived from the dextrans produced by the fermentation of sucrose by means of a certain strain of *Leuconostoc mesenteroides.*

Dextran 75 is a plasma volume expander with actions and uses similar to dextran 70 (p.717). It is given by intravenous infusion as a 6% solution in sodium chloride 0.9% or glucose 5%.

Preparations

Proprietary Preparations (details are given in Part 3)
USA: Gentran 75.

Dextran 110 (253-l)

Dextran 110 *(BAN, rINN).*
Dextranum 110.
CAS — 9004-54-0 (dextran).
Pharmacopoeias. Br. describes Dextran 110 Intravenous Infusion.

Dextran 110 consists of dextrans (glucose polymers) of weight average molecular weight about 110 000 that are derived from the dextrans produced by the fermentation of sucrose by means of a certain strain of *Leuconostoc mesenteroides.*

Dextran 110 is a plasma volume expander with actions and uses similar to dextran 70 (p.717). It has been given by intravenous infusion as a 6% solution.

Preparations

BP 1998: Dextran 110 Intravenous Infusion.

Proprietary Preparations (details are given in Part 3)
UK: Dextraven†.

Epoetins (16635-r)

BI-71.052 (epoetin gamma); BM-06.019 (epoetin beta); EPO (epoetin alfa); EPOCH (epoetin beta).
CAS — 113427-24-0 (epoetin alfa); 122312-54-3 (epoetin beta); 130455-76-4 (epoetin gamma).
Pharmacopoeias. Eur. (see p.viii) includes Erythropoietin Concentrated Solution.

Erythropoietin is a glycosylated protein hormone and a haematopoietic growth factor produced primarily in the kidneys. Erythropoietin for clinical use is produced by recombinant DNA technology and the name epoetin is often applied to such material. **Epoetin alfa** *(BAN, USAN, rINN)*, **epoetin beta** *(BAN, USAN, rINN)*, and **epoetin gamma** *(BAN, rINN)* are recombinant human erythropoietins derived from a cloned human erythropoietin gene. All have the same 165 amino acid sequence but differ in the glycosylation pattern.

Erythropoietin Concentrated Solution (Ph. Eur.) is a clear or slightly turbid colourless solution, containing 0.5 to 10 mg per mL of glycoproteins indistinguishable from naturally occurring erythropoietin in terms of amino acid sequence and glycosylation pattern. It has a potency of not less than 100 000 units per mg of active substance. **Store** in airtight containers below −20° and avoid repeated freezing and thawing.

Stability. Proprietary preparations of recombinant human erythropoietin contain albumin or amino acids for stability. Administration to neonates may necessitate making very dilute solutions. A study of the stability of epoetin alfa in various intravenous fluids[1] found that a minimum of 0.05% protein was required to prevent loss of drug from solutions containing epoetin alfa 0.1 units per mL. In another study,[2] 0.0125% albumin was sufficient to prevent loss of drug from a solution containing epoetin alfa 100 units per mL.

1. Ohls RK, Christensen RD. Stability of human recombinant epoetin alfa in commonly used neonatal intravenous solutions. *Ann Pharmacother* 1996; **30:** 466–8.
2. Widness JA, Schmidt RL. Comment: epoetin alfa loss with Nacl 0.9% dilution. *Ann Pharmacother* 1996; **30:** 1501–2.

Adverse Effects

Headache, hypertension, and seizures have been reported in patients treated with recombinant human erythropoietin particularly in those with poor renal function. These adverse effects are probably associated with haemodynamic changes produced by the increase in haematocrit. In patients with normal or low blood pressure there have been isolated reports of hypertensive crisis with encephalopathy-like symptoms, including headache and confusion, and generalised seizures. Other adverse effects include thrombosis at vascular access sites and clotting in the dialyser, transient increases in the platelet count, flu-like symptoms including chills and myalgia, hyperkalaemia, and skin rashes. There have been rare reports of anaphylactoid reactions.

General references.

1. Macdougall IC. Adverse reactions profile: erythropoietin in chronic renal failure. *Prescribers' J* 1992; **32:** 40–4.

Effects on the blood. Changes in rheological properties of the blood following recombinant human erythropoietin therapy were attributed to high red cell aggregation, possibly due to hyperfibrinogenaemia.[1] The increased viscosity could have contributed to an early kidney graft thrombosis in 1 patient[2] and a delay in the onset of graft function in 7 others.[3] Preoperative haemodilution was suggested as a possible solution.[3]

1. Koppensteiner R, *et al.* Changes in determinants of blood rheology during treatment with haemodialysis and recombinant human erythropoietin. *Br Med J* 1990; **300:** 1626–7.
2. Zaoui P, *et al.* Early thrombosis in kidney grafted into patient treated with erythropoietin. *Lancet* 1988; **ii:** 956.
3. Wahlberg J, *et al.* Haemodilution in renal transplantation in patients on erythropoietin. *Lancet* 1988; **ii:** 1418.

Effects on electrolytes. Hyperkalaemia and hyperphosphataemia may occur in patients receiving recombinant human erythropoietin. However, hypophosphataemia has also been reported in cirrhotic patients given erythropoietin prior to autologous blood donation.[1]

1. Kajikawa M, *et al.* Recombinant human erythropoietin and hypophosphatemia in patients with cirrhosis. *Lancet* 1993; **341:** 503–4.

Effects on mental function. Visual hallucinations occurred in 4 patients during treatment with recombinant human erythropoietin, stopped when treatment was withdrawn, and re-occurred in 2 patients when erythropoietin was reinstituted.[1] Commenting on these and a further 7 cases,[2] the manufacturers considered the reaction to be extremely rare and that the contribution of concurrent medication could not be discounted. In two groups of dialysis patients treated with recombinant human erythropoietin, 15 of 134 and 2 of 103 experienced visual hallucinations.[3] Increasing age appeared to be a risk factor.

1. Steinberg H. Erythropoietin and visual hallucinations. *N Engl J Med* 1991; **325:** 285.
2. Stead RB. Erythropoietin and visual hallucinations. *N Engl J Med* 1991; **325:** 285.
3. Steinberg H, *et al.* Erythropoietin and visual hallucinations in patients on dialysis. *Psychosomatics* 1996; **37:** 556–63.

Effects on the skin. Skin rashes may occur during treatment with recombinant human erythropoietin.

Pseudoporphyria cutanea tarda, a photosensitivity disorder, has been reported in two children undergoing peritoneal dialysis and receiving erythropoietin.[1] However, it was pointed out that this disorder has occurred in adults undergoing dialysis and the children were also receiving other potentially photosensitising drugs.

1. Harvey E, *et al.* Pseudoporphyria cutanea tarda: two case reports on children receiving peritoneal dialysis and erythropoietin therapy. *J Pediatr* 1992; **121:** 749–52.

Effects on the spleen. Aggravation of splenomegaly was reported in 2 patients with myeloproliferative disorders following administration of recombinant human erythropoietin.[1] Splenic infarction has been reported in a patient with aplastic anaemia treated with erythropoietin.[2]

1. Iki S, *et al.* Adverse effect of erythropoietin in myeloproliferative disorders. *Lancet* 1991; **337:** 187–8.
2. Imashuku S, *et al.* Splenic infarction after erythropoietin therapy. *Lancet* 1993; **342:** 182–3.

Effects of subcutaneous injection. More pain at the injection site was experienced by patients given subcutaneous injections of epoetin alfa than in those given epoetin beta.[1,2] It was suggested that different excipients in the two formulations could be responsible.[1,2]

1. Frenken LAM, *et al.* Assessment of pain after subcutaneous injection of erythropoietin in patients receiving haemodialysis. *Br Med J* 1991; **303:** 288.
2. Lui SF, *et al.* Pain after subcutaneous injection of erythropoietin. *Br Med J* 1991; **303:** 856.

Treatment of adverse effects. Venesection successfully reduced the blood pressure in 4 patients with life-threatening hypertension unresponsive to antihypertensive therapy associated with recombinant human erythropoietin treatment.[1]

1. Fahal IH, *et al.* Phlebotomy for erythropoietin-associated malignant hypertension. *Lancet* 1991; **337:** 1227.

Precautions

Recombinant human erythropoietin should be used with caution in patients with hypertension, a history of seizures, thrombocytosis, chronic liver failure, ischaemic vascular disease, or in patients with malignant tumours. Hypertension should be well controlled before treatment is started and the blood pressure monitored during treatment.

Response to recombinant human erythropoietin may be diminished by iron deficiency, infection or inflammatory disorders, haemolysis, or aluminium intoxication. Anaemia due to folic acid and vitamin B_{12} deficiencies should also be eliminated. Patients undergoing dialysis may require increased doses of heparin in view of the increase in packed cell volume.

Platelet counts and serum-potassium concentrations should be monitored regularly.

Dosage must be carefully controlled to avoid too fast an increase in haematocrit and recommended haematocrit levels should not be exceeded due to the increased risk of thrombotic events.

A study[1] involving 1233 patients undergoing haemodialysis and suffering from congestive heart failure or ischaemic heart disease found that erythropoietin in doses sufficient to increase haematocrit to 42% (within the normal range) was associated with lack of benefit and a trend towards increased mortality when compared with administration in doses sufficient to maintain a lower haematocrit of around 30%. However, these results are difficult to interpret, since within each group, increased haematocrit was associated with lower mortality, despite the between-group differences. The possibility that intravenous iron supplementation might have contributed to these adverse results was considered, but commentators suggested that until further data was available aiming for a haematocrit of 33 to 36%, and using intravenous iron supplementation where necessary, was still appropriate.[2]

1. Besarab A, *et al.* The effects of normal as compared with low hematocrit values in patients with cardiac disease who are receiving hemodialysis and epoetin. *N Engl J Med* 1998; **339:** 584–90.
2. Adamson JW, Eschbach JW. Erythropoietin for end-stage renal disease. *N Engl J Med* 1998; **339:** 625–7.

Abuse. Comments on the dangers of the abuse of recombinant human erythropoietin by athletes as an alternative to 'blood doping'.[1-4] Haematocrit may continue to rise for several days after administration of recombinant human erythropoietin, possibly reaching dangerously high levels. Lack of medical supervision and fluid loss during endurance events increase the risk of serious adverse consequences of changes in blood viscosity produced by such misuse.

1. Scott WC. The abuse of erythropoietin to enhance athletic performance. *JAMA* 1990; **264:** 1660.
2. Adamson JW, Vapnek D. Recombinant erythropoietin to improve athletic performance. *N Engl J Med* 1991; **324:** 698–9.
3. Kennedy M. Drugs and athletes—an update. *Adverse Drug React Bull* 1994; **169:** 639–42.
4. MacAuley D. Drugs in sport. *Br Med J* 1996; **313:** 211–15.

Resistance. Many factors may contribute to a poor response to recombinant human erythropoietin (see above). A study in patients with anaemia of end-stage renal disease[1] found that inadequate dialysis was associated with a reduced response to erythropoietin treatment. Antibodies to recombinant human erythropoietin have also been reported.[2] Delayed clinical response to recombinant human erythropoietin in 1 patient[3] could have been due to an inherited subclinical pyruvate kinase deficiency.

1. Ifudu O, *et al.* The intensity of hemodialysis and the response to erythropoietin in patients with end-stage renal disease. *N Engl J Med* 1996; **334:** 420–5.
2. Peces R, *et al.* Antibodies against recombinant human erythropoietin in a patient with erythropoietin-resistant anemia. *N Engl J Med* 1996; **335:** 523–4.
3. Zachée P, *et al.* Pyruvate kinase deficiency and delayed clinical response to recombinant human erythropoietin treatment. *Lancet* 1989; **i:** 1327–8.

Pharmacokinetics

Epoetin alfa and epoetin beta exhibit some differences in their pharmacokinetics, possibly due to differences in glycosylation and in the formulation of the commercial preparations.

Epoetin alfa is slowly and incompletely absorbed following subcutaneous injection, and a bioavailability of about 10 to 50% relative to intravenous administration has been reported. Peak concentrations following epoetin alfa intravenously are attained within 15 minutes, and within 4 to 24 hours following subcutaneous injection.

The elimination half-life of epoetin alfa following intravenous administration has been reported to be 4 to 16 hours in patients with chronic renal failure; the half-life is generally less in patients with normal renal function. An estimated elimination half-life of about 24 hours has been reported for epoetin alfa given subcutaneously.

Epoetin beta is similarly slowly and incompletely absorbed after subcutaneous injection, and its absolute bioavailability has been reported to be 23 to 42%. Peak serum concentrations are attained within 12 to 28 hours of subcutaneous administration. An elimination half-life of 4 to 12 hours has been reported following intravenous administration and a terminal half-life of 13 to 28 hours following subcutaneous administration.

References.

1. Macdougall IC, *et al.* Clinical pharmacokinetics of epoetin (recombinant human erythropoietin). *Clin Pharmacokinet* 1991; **20:** 99–113.
2. Halstenson CE, *et al.* Comparative pharmacokinetics and pharmacodynamics of epoetin alfa and epoetin beta. *Clin Pharmacol Ther* 1991; **50:** 702–12.
3. Gladziwa U, *et al.* Pharmacokinetics of epoetin (recombinant human erythropoietin) after long term therapy in patients undergoing haemodialysis and haemofiltration. *Clin Pharmacokinet* 1993; **25:** 145–53.
4. Brown MS, *et al.* Single-dose pharmacokinetics of recombinant human erythropoietin in preterm infants after intravenous and subcutaneous administration. *J Pediatr* 1993; **122:** 655–7.
5. Montini G, *et al.* Pharmacokinetics and hematologic response to subcutaneous administration of recombinant human erythropoietin in children undergoing long-term peritoneal dialysis: a multicenter study. *J Pediatr* 1993; **122:** 297–302.

Uses and Administration

Erythropoietin is a glycosylated protein hormone and a haematopoietic growth factor. It is secreted primarily by the kidneys, although a small amount is produced in extrarenal sites such as the liver. Erythropoietin regulates erythropoiesis by stimulating the differentiation and proliferation of erythroid precursors, stimulating the release of reticulocytes into the circulation, and stimulating the synthesis of cellular haemoglobin. The release of erythropoietin is promoted by hypoxia or anaemia, and up to 1000 times the normal serum-erythropoietin concentration may be reached under these conditions; this response may be impaired in some disease states such as chronic renal failure. The haematological response to erythropoietin is reduced if there is an inadequate supply of iron.

Epoetin alfa and epoetin beta are recombinant human erythropoietins available for clinical use that have the same pharmacological actions as endogenous erythropoietin. They are used in the management of anaemia associated with chronic renal failure in dialysis and predialysis patients; they may reduce or obviate the need for blood transfusions in these patients. They are also used in the management of chemotherapy-induced anaemia in patients with non-myeloid malignant disease. Epoetin alfa is used in zidovudine-related anaemia in HIV-positive patients. Epoetin beta is used in the management of anaemia of prematurity. Recombinant human erythropoietin is also being evaluated in the management of other types of normocytic-normochromic anaemias, including that associated with inflammatory disorders such as rheumatoid arthritis. In all patients, iron status should be monitored and supplementation provided if necessary.

Epoetin alfa and epoetin beta may also be used in patients with moderate anaemia (but no iron deficiency) before elective surgery to increase the yield of blood collected for autologous blood transfusion. Epoetin alfa may also be used in such patients to reduce the need for allogeneic blood transfusion.

In the management of **anaemia of chronic renal failure** epoetin alfa or epoetin beta may be given subcutaneously or intravenously. The aim of treatment is to increase the haemoglobin concentration to 10 to 12 g per 100 mL or to increase the haematocrit to 30 to 36%. The rate of rise in haemoglobin should be gradual to minimise side-effects such as hypertension; a rate not exceeding 2 g per 100 mL per month is suggested.

Epoetin alfa may be given subcutaneously or by intravenous injection over at least 1 minute; slow intravenous injection over 5 minutes may be used in patients who experience flu-like symptoms as side-effects. In predialysis and haemodialysis patients, a recommended initial dose of epoetin alfa is 50 international units per kg body-weight three times weekly; a higher initial dose of 50 to 100 units per kg three times weekly has been suggested in the USA. Doses may be increased at 4-week intervals in increments of 25 units per kg three times weekly until the target is reached. In patients on peritoneal dialysis an initial dose of 50 units per kg given subcutaneously twice a week is recommended. Once the target is reached doses may need to be adjusted, and even decreased, for maintenance therapy.

The usual total weekly maintenance dose of epoetin alfa in predialysis patients is 50 to 100 units per kg given in three divided doses, and in haemodialysis patients it is about 100 to 300 units per kg given in three divided doses. In predialysis patients a total weekly dose of 600 units per kg should not be exceeded. In patients on peritoneal dialysis, the usual total weekly maintenance dose is 50 to 100 units per kg given subcutaneously in two divided doses.

In children, epoetin alfa may be given intravenously to those on haemodialysis at an initial dose of 50 units per kg three times weekly. The dose may be increased at 4-week intervals in increments of 25 units per kg three times weekly until a target haemoglobin concentration of 9.5 to 11.0 g per 100 mL is reached; the usual total weekly maintenance dose given in three divided doses is: 225 to 450 units per kg for those weighing less than 10 kg; 180 to 450 units per kg for those weighing 10 to 30 kg; and 90 to 300 units per kg for those weighing over 30 kg.

Epoetin beta is used similarly in the management of anaemia of chronic renal failure in dialysis and predialysis patients. It may be given subcutaneously, by intravenous injection over 2 minutes, or by intravenous infusion. The following dosages may be used in adults and children. For subcutaneous injection the initial dose is 60 units per kg once a week for 4 weeks; alternatively, the total weekly dose may be given in daily doses or three times a week. For intravenous injection the initial dose is 40 units per kg three times weekly for 4 weeks. The dose may then be increased to 80 units per kg three times weekly. Thereafter the dose of epoetin beta may be increased at 4-week intervals (if the increase in haemoglobin concentration is less than 1 g per 100 mL per month) in increments of 20 units per kg three times weekly for intravenous administration or 60 units per kg per week for subcutaneous administration until a target haemoglobin concentration of 10 to 12 g per 100 mL is reached. A total weekly dose of 720 units per kg of epoetin beta should not be exceeded. For maintenance, the dose is halved initially and then adjusted every 1 to 2 weeks according to response.

In patients with **non-myeloid malignant disease** receiving chemotherapy, epoetin alfa or epoetin beta may be given by subcutaneous injection in an initial dose of 150 units per kg three times weekly. The dose may be increased after 4 or 8 weeks, if necessary, to 300 units per kg three times weekly. If the response is still inadequate after 4 weeks at this higher dose, treatment should be discontinued. As an alternative regimen, the total weekly dose of epoetin beta may be divided into 7 daily doses.

To increase the yield of **autologous blood**, epoetin alfa or epoetin beta may be used in conjunction with iron supplementation. The dose depends on the volume of blood required for collection and on factors such as the patient's whole blood volume and haematocrit. Suggested regimens are: epoetin alfa 600 units per kg given intravenously twice a week starting 3 weeks before surgery; or up to 800 units per kg of epoetin beta intravenously or up to 600 units per kg subcutaneously twice a week for 4 weeks before surgery. To reduce the need for allogeneic blood transfusion epoetin alfa may be given in a dose of 600 units per kg subcutaneously once a week starting 3 weeks before surgery or 300 units per kg subcutaneously daily starting 10 days before surgery.

In **HIV-positive patients** on zidovudine therapy, epoetin alfa may be beneficial if the endogenous serum-erythropoietin concentration is 500 milliunits or less per mL. Epoetin alfa is given by subcutaneous or intravenous injection in an initial dose of 100 units per kg three times weekly. The dose may be increased every 4 to 8 weeks by 50 to 100 units per kg three times weekly according to response. However, patients are unlikely to benefit from doses above 300 units per kg three times weekly if lower doses have failed to elicit a satisfactory response.

In the management of **anaemia of prematurity** epoetin beta is given subcutaneously in a dose of 250 units per kg three times a week. Treatment should be started as early as possible and continued for six weeks.

General references.

1. Markham A, Bryson HM. Epoetin alfa: a review of its pharmacodynamic and pharmacokinetic properties and therapeutic use in nonrenal applications. *Drugs* 1995; **49:** 232–54.
2. Dunn CJ, Markham A. Epoetin beta: a review of its pharmacological properties and clinical use in the management of anaemia associated with chronic renal failure. *Drugs* 1996; **51:** 299–318.

Administration to neonates. Recombinant human erythropoietin may be given to neonates for anaemia of prematurity. It is usually administered by subcutaneous injection. Administration by intravenous infusion in total parenteral nutrition solutions produced satisfactory results in a group of 20 neonates.[1]

For a warning about diluting recombinant human erythropoietin solutions, see under Stability, above.

1. Ohls RK, *et al.* Pharmacokinetics and effectiveness of recombinant erythropoietin administered to preterm infants by continuous infusion in total parenteral nutrition solution. *J Pediatr* 1996; **128:** 518–23.

Anaemias. Epoetins are used in normocytic-normochromic anaemias (p.703) associated with low endogenous erythropoietin concentrations.

Clinical studies have shown the effectiveness of epoetins in correcting the anaemia of end-stage renal disease in patients maintained by haemodialysis,[1,2] and they are also effective in anaemia in predialysis patients. Although several factors contribute to the aetiology of the anaemia, including blood loss associated with dialysis, the main cause is inadequate production of erythropoietin in the kidney. Consistently good results have been obtained with epoetins not only for correction of anaemia but also for quality of life and exercise capacity[3,4] and for improvements in haemostatic[5] and cardiorespiratory function.[6] Guidelines have been introduced for their use in chronic renal failure.[7]

Over 90% of patients with renal anaemia respond to treatment with epoetins.[8] Many factors may contribute to a poor response (see Precautions, above) and the patient should always be investigated and the cause corrected where possible.[8,9]

Epoetins may be administered intravenously or subcutaneously. Epoetin given subcutaneously produces lower but more sustained plasma concentrations and comparative studies have shown that total weekly maintenance doses are reduced by between 23% and 52% with subcutaneous rather than intravenous administration.[10,11] The subcutaneous route is thus preferred especially in patients not on haemodialysis. The frequency of administration may also be important in maximising the response to treatment;[12] daily subcutaneous administration has been reported to give a better response than the same total weekly dose given two or three times a week.[2] Intraperitoneal administration has also been investigated.[13]

Epoetins are also used to treat anaemias from other causes. Epoetins may be used for zidovudine-induced anaemia in AIDS patients, in chemotherapy-induced anaemia in patients with non-myeloid malignant disease, and in anaemia of prematurity.[14-22] Epoetins have a potential application for other anaemias associated with impaired or insufficient erythropoietin production, such as anaemias in infants with bronchopulmonary dysplasia[23,24] and infants with haemolytic disease of the newborn,[25,26] postpartum anaemia,[27,28] and in arthritis[29-31] and inflammatory bowel disease.[32-34]

1. Winearls C. Treatment of anaemia in renal failure. *Prescribers' J* 1992; **32:** 238–44.
2. De Marchi S, *et al.* Erythropoietin and the anemia of chronic diseases. *Clin Exp Rheumatol* 1993; **11:** 429–44.
3. Canadian Erythropoietin Study Group. Association between recombinant human erythropoietin and quality of life and exercise capacity of patients receiving haemodialysis. *Br Med J* 1990; **300:** 573–8.
4. Evans RW, *et al.* The quality of life of hemodialysis recipients treated with recombinant human erythropoietin. *JAMA* 1990; **263:** 825–30.
5. Moia M, *et al.* Improvement in the haemostatic defect of uraemia after treatment with recombinant human erythropoietin. *Lancet* 1987; **ii:** 1227–9.
6. Macdougall IC, *et al.* Long-term cardiorespiratory effects of amelioration of renal anaemia by erythropoietin. *Lancet* 1990; **335:** 489–93. Correction. *ibid.*; 614.
7. National Kidney Foundation. NKF-DOQI clinical practice guidelines for the treatment of anemia of chronic renal failure. *Am J Kidney Dis* 1997; **30** (suppl 3): S192–S240.
8. Macdougall IC. Poor response to erythropoietin. *Br Med J* 1995; **310:** 1424–5.
9. Koury MJ. Investigating erythropoietin resistance. *N Engl J Med* 1993; **328:** 205–6.
10. Zachée P. Controversies in selection of epoetin dosages: issues and answers. *Drugs* 1995; **49:** 536–47.
11. Kaufman JS, *et al.* Subcutaneous compared with intravenous epoetin in patients receiving hemodialysis. *N Engl J Med* 1998; **339:** 578–83.
12. Abraham PA, *et al.* Controversies in determination of epoetin (recombinant human erythropoietin) dosages. *Clin Pharmacokinet* 1992; **22:** 409–15.
13. Taylor CA, *et al.* Clinical pharmacokinetics during continuous ambulatory peritoneal dialysis. *Clin Pharmacokinet* 1996; **31:** 293–308.
14. Bechensteen AG, *et al.* Erythropoietin, protein, and iron supplementation and the prevention of anaemia of prematurity. *Arch Dis Child* 1993; **69:** 19–23.
15. Maier RF, *et al.* The effect of epoetin beta (recombinant human erythropoietin) on the need for transfusion in very-low-birth-weight infants. *N Engl J Med* 1994; **330:** 1173–8.
16. Strauss RG. Erythropoietin and neonatal anemia. *N Engl J Med* 1994; **330:** 1227–8.
17. Shannon KM, *et al.* Recombinant human erythropoietin stimulates erythropoiesis and reduces erythrocyte transfusions in very low birth weight preterm infants. *Pediatrics* 1995; **95:** 1–8.
18. Wilimas JA, Crist WM. Erythropoietin—not yet a standard treatment for anemia of prematurity. *Pediatrics* 1995; **95:** 9–10.
19. Wandstrat TL, Kaplan B. Use of erythropoietin in premature neonates: controversies and the future. *Ann Pharmacother* 1995; **29:** 166–73.
20. Williamson P, *et al.* Blood transfusions and human recombinant erythropoietin in premature newborn infants. *Arch Dis Child* 1996; **75:** F65–F68.
21. Ohls RK, *et al.* The effect of erythropoietin on the transfusion requirements of preterm infants weighing 750 grams or less: a randomized, double-blind, placebo-controlled study. *J Pediatr* 1997; **131:** 661–5.
22. Strauss RG. Recombinant erythropoietin for the anemia of prematurity: still a promise, not a panacea. *J Pediatr* 1997; **131:** 653–5.
23. Ohls RK, *et al.* A randomized, double-blind, placebo-controlled trial of recombinant erythropoietin in treatment of the anemia of bronchopulmonary dysplasia. *J Pediatr* 1993; **123:** 996–1000.
24. Al-Kharfy T, *et al.* Erythropoietin therapy in neonates at risk of having bronchopulmonary dysplasia and requiring multiple transfusions. *J Pediatr* 1996; **129:** 89–96.
25. Ohls RK, *et al.* Recombinant erythropoietin as treatment for the late hyporegenerative anemia of Rh hemolytic disease. *Pediatrics* 1992; **90:** 678–80.
26. Scaradavou A, *et al.* Suppression of erythropoiesis by intrauterine transfusions in hemolytic disease of the newborn: use of erythropoietin to treat the late anemia. *J Pediatr* 1993; **123:** 279–84.
27. Huch A, *et al.* Recombinant human erythropoietin in the treatment of postpartum anemia. *Obstet Gynecol* 1992; **80:** 127–31.
28. Breymann C, *et al.* Use of recombinant human erythropoietin in combination with parenteral iron in the treatment of postpartum anaemia. *Eur J Clin Invest* 1996; **26:** 123–30.
29. Pincus T, *et al.* Multicenter study of recombinant human erythropoietin in correction of anemia in rheumatoid arthritis. *Am J Med* 1990; **89:** 161–8.
30. Murphy EA, *et al.* Study of erythropoietin in treatment of anaemia in patients with rheumatoid arthritis. *Br Med J* 1994; **309:** 1337–8.
31. Peeters HRM, *et al.* Effect of recombinant human erythropoietin on anaemia and disease activity in patients with rheumatoid arthritis and anaemia of chronic disease: a randomised placebo controlled double blind 52 weeks clinical trial. *Ann Rheum Dis* 1996; **55:** 739–44.

32. Schreiber S, *et al.* Recombinant erythropoietin for the treatment of anemia in inflammatory bowel disease. *N Engl J Med* 1996; **334:** 619–23.
33. Gasché C, *et al.* Intravenous iron and erythropoietin for anemia associated with Crohn disease: a randomized, controlled trial. *Ann Intern Med* 1997; **126:** 782–7.
34. Dohil R, *et al.* Recombinant human erythropoietin for treatment of anemia for chronic disease in children with Crohn's disease. *J Pediatr* 1998; **132:** 155–9.

Surgery. Concern over the safety of blood transfusions and the need to conserve blood supplies has led to interest in methods of reducing blood use in surgery. Recombinant human erythropoietin has been used to increase the number of units harvested for autologous transfusion[1-4] and to reduce transfusion requirements.[4-6] It has also been used as an alternative to blood transfusions.[7,8]

1. Goodnough LT, *et al.* Increased preoperative collection of autologous blood with recombinant human erythropoietin therapy. *N Engl J Med* 1989; **321:** 1163–8.
2. Graf H, *et al.* Recombinant human erythropoietin as adjuvant treatment for autologous blood donation. *Br Med J* 1990; **300:** 1627–8.
3. Tasaki T, *et al.* Recombinant human erythropoietin for autologous blood donation: effects on perioperative red-blood-cell and serum erythropoietin production. *Lancet* 1992; **339:** 773–5.
4. Goodnough LT. The role of recombinant growth factors in transfusion medicine. *Br J Anaesth* 1993; **70:** 80–6.
5. Canadian Orthopedic Perioperative Erythropoietin Study Group. Effectiveness of perioperative recombinant human erythropoietin in elective hip replacement. *Lancet* 1993; **341:** 1227–32.
6. Biesma DH, *et al.* Lower homologous blood requirement in autologous blood donors after treatment with recombinant human erythropoietin. *Lancet* 1994; **344:** 367–70.
7. Green D, Handley E. Erythropoietin for anemia in Jehovah's Witnesses. *Ann Intern Med* 1990; **113:** 720–1.
8. Busuttil D, Copplestone A. Management of blood loss in Jehovah's Witnesses. *Br Med J* 1995; **311:** 1115–16.

Preparations

Proprietary Preparations (details are given in Part 3)
Aust.: Culat; Erypo; Recormon; ***Austral.:*** Eprex; ***Belg.:*** Eprex; Recormon; ***Canad.:*** Eprex; ***Fr.:*** Eprex; Recormon; ***Ger.:*** Erypo; Recormon; ***Irl.:*** Eprex; Recormon; ***Ital.:*** Epoxitin; Eprex; Eritrogen; Globuren; ***Jpn:*** Epogin; Espo; ***Neth.:*** Eprex; Recormon†; ***Norw.:*** Eprex; Recormon; ***S.Afr.:*** Eprex; Recormon; ***Spain:*** Epopen; Eprex; Erantin; ***Swed.:*** Eprex; NeoRecormon; ***Switz.:*** Eprex; Recormon; ***UK:*** Eprex; NeoRecormon; Recormon; ***USA:*** Epogen; Procrit.

Ethamsylate (1720-p)

Ethamsylate *(BAN, USAN)*.
Etamsilate *(rINN)*; Cyclonamine; E-141; Etamsylatum; MD-141. Diethylammonium 2,5-dihydroxybenzenesulphonate.
$C_{10}H_{17}NO_5S = 263.3$.
CAS — 2624-44-4.
Pharmacopoeias. In *Chin., Eur.* (see p.viii), and *Pol.*

A white of almost white, crystalline powder. It shows polymorphism. Very **soluble** in water; soluble in alcohol; freely soluble in methyl alcohol; practically insoluble in dichloromethane. A 10% solution in water has a pH of 4.5 to 5.6. **Store** in airtight containers. Protect from light.

Adverse Effects and Precautions

Nausea, headache, and skin rash have occurred after administration of ethamsylate. Transient hypotension has been reported following intravenous injection.

Pharmacokinetics

Ethamsylate is absorbed from the gastro-intestinal tract. It is excreted unchanged, mainly in the urine. Ethamsylate is distributed into breast milk.

Placental transfer. Ethamsylate 500 mg by mouth failed to produce adequate fetal or maternal plasma concentrations in 5 patients in labour.[1] The same dose given intramuscularly to 7 mothers produced concentrations in cord blood that were considered to be within the therapeutic range.

1. Harrison RF, Matthews T. Intrapartum ethamsylate. *Lancet* 1984; **ii:** 296.

Uses and Administration

Ethamsylate is a haemostatic (p.704) that appears to maintain the stability of the capillary wall and correct abnormal platelet adhesion. It is given for the prophylaxis and control of haemorrhages from small blood vessels.

For short-term blood loss in menorrhagia a dose of 500 mg is given by mouth four times daily during menstruation. For the prophylaxis and treatment of periventricular haemorrhage in low birth-weight neonates 12.5 mg per kg body-weight is given by intramuscular or intravenous injection every 6 hours. For the control of haemorrhage following surgery ethamsylate may be given to adults by mouth, or by intramuscular or intravenous injection in a dose of 250 to 500 mg; this dose may be repeated every 4 to 6 hours as necessary.

Haemorrhagic disorders. NEONATAL INTRAVENTRICULAR HAEMORRHAGE. Ethamsylate is one of several drugs that have been tried in the prevention of intraventricular haemorrhage in very low birth-weight infants (p.709). In a multicentre, placebo-controlled, double-blind study,[1] ethamsylate was given in an initial dose of 12.5 mg per kg body-weight intravenously or intramuscularly within 1 hour of delivery, followed by the same dose intravenously every 6 hours for 4 days to a total dose of 200 mg per kg. Of 330 infants who had had no evidence of haemorrhage soon after delivery, the incidence of haemorrhage in the 162 who received ethamsylate was reduced, particularly the more extensive grades when compared with the 168 who received placebo. Of a further 30 infants with evidence of periventricular haemorrhage before treatment, 21 were given ethamsylate and 9 placebo; treatment with ethamsylate limited the extension of bleeding. There was also a reduction in patent ductus arteriosus in the treated infants. However, a recent study using the same dosage regimen,[2] showed little benefit on short-term follow-up. It was considered that the study size may have been too small and the drug administered too late; the initial dose was given within four hours of birth whereas, in the previous study, treatment was started within one hour of birth. The results of long-term follow-up are awaited.

1. Benson JWT, *et al.* Multicentre trial of ethamsylate for prevention of periventricular haemorrhage in very low birthweight infants. *Lancet* 1986; **ii:** 1297–1300.
2. The EC Ethamsylate Trial Group. The EC randomised controlled trial of prophylactic ethamsylate for very preterm neonates: early mortality and morbidity. *Arch Dis Child* 1994; **70:** F201–F205.

Menorrhagia. When administered during menstruation to women with idiopathic menorrhagia (p.1461), ethamsylate was as effective as mefenamic acid in reducing uterine blood loss in 1 study,[1] but was ineffective in another.[2]

1. Chamberlain G, *et al.* A comparative study of ethamsylate and mefenamic acid in dysfunctional uterine bleeding. *Br J Obstet Gynaecol* 1991; **98:** 707–11.
2. Bonnar J, Sheppard BL. Treatment of menorrhagia during menstruation: randomised controlled trial of ethamsylate, mefenamic acid, and tranexamic acid. *Br Med J* 1996; **313:** 579–82.

Preparations

Proprietary Preparations (details are given in Part 3)
Belg.: Dicynone; ***Fr.:*** Dicynone; ***Ger.:*** Altodor†; ***Irl.:*** Dicynene; ***Ital.:*** Dicynone; Eselin; ***Jpn:*** Aglumin†; ***Spain:*** Dicinone; Hemo 141; ***Switz.:*** Dicynone; ***UK:*** Dicynene.

Multi-ingredient: ***Ital.:*** Transil†.

Factor VII (10819-b)

Proconvertin; SPCA; Stable Factor.

NOTE. The name Eptacog Alfa (Activated) *(BAN, rINN)* is in use for a recombinant factor VIIa.

Human Coagulation Factor VII, Freeze-dried (Ph. Eur.) (Factor VII Coagulationis Humanus Cryodesiccatus; Dried Factor VII Fraction (BP 1998)) contains the single-chain glycoprotein factor VII and may also contain small amounts of the activated form, the two-chain derivative factor VIIa, as well as coagulation factors II, IX, and X, and protein C and protein S. It is prepared from human plasma obtained from blood from healthy donors who must, as far as can be ascertained, be free from detectable agents of infection transmissible by plasma-derived products. The method of preparation is designed to minimise activation of any coagulation factor and includes a step or steps that have been shown to remove or inactivate known agents of infection. The factor VII fraction is dissolved in a suitable liquid, passed through a bacteria-retentive filter, distributed aseptically into the final containers, and immediately frozen. The preparation is freeze-dried and the containers sealed under vacuum or under an inert gas. Heparin, antithrombin, and other auxiliary substances such as a stabiliser may be added. No antimicrobial preservative is added. The potency of the preparation is not less than 2 international units of factor VII per mg of protein before the addition of any protein stabiliser. When reconstituted as stated on the label the resulting solution contains not less than 15 international units per mL. The dried product should be protected from light.

Units

The potency of factor VIIa (activated factor VII) is expressed in international units and preparations may be assayed using the first International Standard for blood coagulation factor VIIa concentrate (1993).

Adverse Effects and Precautions

Administration of factor VIIa (activated factor VII) may be associated with minor skin reactions, nausea, fever, headache, malaise, diaphoresis, and changes in blood pressure. Factor VIIa should be used with caution in patients with conditions associated with circulating tissue factor, such as advanced atherosclerosis, crush injury, or septicaemia, since there is a risk of precipitating thrombosis or disseminated intravascular coagulation.

Uses and Administration

Factor VII may be used as replacement therapy in patients with rare genetic deficiencies of factor VII. Factor VIIa (activated factor VII) is used to treat serious bleeding episodes and to prevent bleeding associated with surgery in patients with haemophilia A or haemophilia B (p.707) who have developed antibodies to factor VIII or factor IX, respectively. It may also be useful in patients with von Willebrand's disease. Factor VIIa is given by intravenous injection in a dose of 3000 to 6000 units per kg body-weight. The dose and frequency of administration depend on the type and severity of haemorrhage.

References.

1. Macik BG, *et al.* Safety and initial clinical efficacy of three dose levels of recombinant activated factor VII (rFVIIa): results of a phase I study. *Blood Coag Fibrinol* 1993; **4:** 521–7.

Preparations

Ph. Eur.: Freeze-dried Human Coagulation Factor VII.

Proprietary Preparations (details are given in Part 3)
Fr.: Acset; NovoSeven; ***Ger.:*** NovoSeven; ***Irl.:*** NovoSeven; ***Ital.:*** NovoSeven; Provertin-UM TIM 3; ***Neth.:*** NovoSeven; ***Norw.:*** NovoSeven; ***Spain:*** NovoSeven; ***Swed.:*** NovoSeven; ***Switz.:*** NovoSeven; ***UK:*** NovoSeven.

Factor VIII (1225-c)

AHF; Antihaemophilic Factor.

NOTE. The names Moroctocog Alfa *(rINN)* and Octocog Alfa *(BAN, rINN)* are in use for recombinant factor VIII.

Factor VIII is prepared from human plasma as described below. It may also be prepared using recombinant DNA technology.

Human Coagulation Factor VIII, Freeze-dried (Ph. Eur.) (Factor VIII Coagulationis Humani Cryodesiccatus; Dried Factor VIII Fraction (BP 1998); Dried Human Antihaemophilic Fraction) contains the glycoprotein coagulation factor VIII together with varying amounts of von Willebrand factor, depending on the method of preparation. It is prepared by fractionation of human plasma obtained from blood from healthy donors who must, as far as can be ascertained, be free from detectable agents of infection transmissible by plasma-derived products. The method of preparation includes a step or steps that have been shown to remove or inactivate known agents of infection. The antihaemophilic fraction is dissolved in an appropriate liquid, passed through a bacteria-retentive filter, distributed aseptically into the final containers, and immediately frozen. The preparation is freeze-dried and the containers sealed under vacuum or under an inert gas. No antimicrobial preservative is added. A wide range of preparations is available varying in respect of activity and degree of purification. The potency of the preparation is not less than 1 international unit of factor VIII:C per mg of total protein before the addition of any protein stabiliser. When reconstituted as stated on the label the resulting solution contains not less than 20 international units of factor VIII:C per mL. The dried product should be protected from light.

Antihemophilic Factor (USP 23) is a sterile freeze-dried powder containing factor VIII fraction prepared from units of human venous plasma that have been tested for the absence of hepatitis B surface antigen, obtained from whole-blood donors and pooled; it may contain heparin sodium or sodium citrate. It contains not less than 100 units per g of protein. Unless otherwise specified it should be stored at 2° to 8° in hermetically-sealed containers. It should be used within 4 hours of reconstitution and should be administered with equipment that includes a filter.

Cryoprecipitated Antihemophilic Factor (USP 23) is a sterile frozen concentrate of human antihaemophilic factor prepared from the cryoprotein fraction, rich in factor VIII, of human venous plasma obtained from suitable whole-blood donors from a single unit of plasma derived from whole blood or by plasmapheresis, collected and processed in a closed system. It contains no preservative. It has an average potency of not less than 80 units per container. It should be stored at or below −18° in hermetically-sealed containers. It should be thawed to 20° to 37° before use; this liquid should be stored at room temperature and used within 6 hours of thawing; it should also be used within 4 hours of opening the container and administered with equipment that includes a filter.

Units

The potency of factor VIII is expressed in international units and preparations may be assayed using the fifth International Standard for blood coagulation factor VIII:C concentrate, human (1994).

Adverse Effects and Precautions

Allergic reactions may sometimes follow the use of factor VIII preparations and chills, urticaria, and fever experienced by some patients may be allergic manifestations. Headache may occur. There is the possibility of intravascular haemolysis in patients with blood groups A, B, or AB receiving high doses or frequently repeated doses of factor VIII preparations due to the content of blood group isoagglutinins, also massive doses of some preparations may produce hyperfibrinogenaemia; such risks should be reduced with more highly purified preparations.

Factor VIII preparations have been associated with the transmission of some viral infections, including hepatitis B and C, and more notably transmission of HIV leading to the subsequent development of AIDS. Strenuous efforts are now undertaken to screen the donor material from which factor VIII material is obtained and new methods of manufacture have also been introduced with the aim of inactivating any viruses present. Vaccination against hepatitis B is recommended for patients not already immune.

Some patients develop antibodies to factor VIII and, although large doses of preparations of both factor VIII and factor IX or porcine or highly purified factor VIII concentrates may be effective in the management of such patients, some patients remain resistant to treatment.

Effects on blood platelets. Thrombocytopenia was associated with administration of porcine factor VIII concentrate in 2 patients.[1] Platelet aggregation was noted in addition in one patient. Platelet counts improved when treatment with factor VIII was withdrawn.

1. Green D, Tuite GF. Declining platelet counts and platelet aggregation during porcine VIII:C infusions. *Am J Med* 1989; **86:** 222–4.

Transmission of infections. Treatment with heat or chemicals together with efforts to screen the donor material from which factor VIII and other clotting factors are obtained seem to have overcome problems with transmission of HIV and hepatitis B and C, although there is concern that non-lipid-enveloped viruses, such as human parvovirus B19 and hepatitis A, may still be transmitted. A solvent-detergent-treated factor VIII product[1-4] and a similar factor IX product[4] have been associated with recent reports of hepatitis A in patients with haemophilia and vaccination against hepatitis A has been recommended for patients treated with these factor preparations. Plasma-derived factor VIII preparations may carry a risk of transmission of Creutzfeldt-Jakob disease (see under Blood, p.713). It has been pointed out[5] that, since recombinant factor VIII is prepared from mammalian cell lines, there is a theoretical risk of transmission of infection with recombinant preparations.

1. Prowse C. Hepatitis A virus infection: no conclusive link to factor VIII. *Br Med J* 1993; **307:** 561–2.
2. Thomas DP. Viral contamination of blood products. *Lancet* 1994; **343:** 1583–4.
3. Colvin BT. Viral contamination of blood products. *Lancet* 1994; **344:** 405.
4. Anonymous. Hepatitis A among persons with hemophilia who received clotting factor concentrate—United States, September-December 1995. *JAMA* 1996; **275:** 427–8.
5. Foster PR, *et al.* Hepatitis C and haemophilia. *Br Med J* 1995; **311:** 754–5.

Pharmacokinetics

References.

1. Messori A, *et al.* Clinical pharmacokinetics of factor VIII in patients with classic haemophilia. *Clin Pharmacokinet* 1987; **13:** 365–80.
2. Björkman S, *et al.* Pharmacokinetics of factor VIII in humans: obtaining clinically relevant data from comparative studies. *Clin Pharmacokinet* 1992; **22:** 385–95.

Uses and Administration

Factor VIII is used as replacement therapy in patients with haemophilia A, a genetic deficiency of factor VIII. For a discussion of inherited bleeding disorders and their management, see p.707.

Preparations of factor VIII are used to control bleeding episodes in the treatment of patients with haemophilia A and to prevent bleeding episodes in such patients undergoing dental and surgical procedures. They may also be used for long-term prophylaxis in patients with severe haemophilia A.

Preparations of factor VIII are given by slow intravenous infusion. The dosage of factor VIII should be determined for each patient and will vary with the circumstances involving bleeding or type of surgery to be performed. In adults, a dose of 1 unit per kg body-weight has been reported to raise the plasma concentration of factor VIII by about 2% (of normal). A suggested formula to calculate, approximately, the dose required for a given effect is:

units = wt (kg) × 0.5 × % desired increase (of normal)

It is suggested that for mild to moderate haemorrhage the plasma concentration of factor VIII should be raised to 20 to 30% of normal, usually achieved with a single dose of 10 to 15 units per kg body-weight; for more serious haemorrhage or minor surgery it should be raised to 30 to 50% of normal, achieved with a usual initial dose of 15 to 25 units per kg followed by 10 to 15 units per kg every 8 to 12 hours if required; and that for severe haemorrhage or major surgery an increase to 80 to 100% of normal may be necessary, achieved with a usual initial dose of 40 to 50 units per kg followed by 20 to 25 units per kg every 8 to 12 hours.

In patients with inhibitory antibodies to human factor VIII, porcine factor VIII preparation is used in doses of 25 to 100 units per kg depending upon the severity of the haemorrhage.

In addition to standard factor VIII concentrates that also contain von Willebrand's factor, several highly purified preparations, including recombinant factor VIII, are available commercially. An alternative source of clotting factors is cryoprecipitate which contains factor VIII, factor XIII, von Willebrand's factor, fibrinogen, and fibronectin. Standard factor VIII concentrates or cryoprecipitate may be used in the management of von Willebrand's disease, but commercial very highly purified preparations do not contain appreciable amounts of von Willebrand's factor and are thus ineffective.

Administration. Surgical prophylaxis or significant haemorrhage in patients with haemophilia A is usually managed with injections of Factor VIII given intravenously every 8 to 12 hours. Continuous intravenous infusion prevents wide fluctuations in Factor VIII plasma concentrations and has been used successfully following major surgery in patients with haemophilia.[1-3]

1. Bona RD, *et al.* The use of continuous infusion of factor concentrates in the treatment of hemophilia. *Am J Hematol* 1989; **32:** 8–13.
2. Martinowitz U, *et al.* Adjusted dose continuous infusion of factor VIII in patients with haemophilia A. *Br J Haematol* 1992; **82:** 729–34.
3. Hawkins TE, *et al.* Treatment of haemophilia A by continuous factor VIII infusion. *Aust N Z J Med* 1995; **25:** 37–9.

Preparations

Ph. Eur.: Freeze-dried Human Coagulation Factor VIII;
USP 23: Antihemophilic Factor; Cryoprecipitated Antihemophilic Factor.

Proprietary Preparations (details are given in Part 3)
Aust.: Beriate; Koate; Kogenate; Kryobulin s-TIM 3; Monoclate-P; ***Austral.:*** AHF; Kogenate; Recombinate; ***Belg.:*** Recombinate; ***Canad.:*** Koate-HP; Kogenate; ***Fr.:*** Hemofil M; Kogenate; Recombinate; ***Ger.:*** Alpha VIII†; Beriate; Bioclate; Haemate; Haemoctin SDH; Helixate; Hemofil; Immunate STIM; Koate†; Kogenate; Monoclate-P; Octavi; Profilate; Recombinate; ***Irl.:*** Kogenate; Monoclate-P; ***Ital.:*** Alphanate; Emoclot DI; Haemate; Hemofil M; Immunate STIM; Koate-HS; Kogenate; Kryobulin TIM 3-I; Liocrio†; Profilate HT†; Recombinate; Uman-Cry DI†; Vueffe; ***Neth.:*** Haemate; Helixate; Kogenate; ***Norw.:*** Kogenate; Octavi; Octonativ-M; ***S.Afr.:*** Haemosolvate; ***Spain:*** Beriate P; Bioclate; Criostat SD 2; Fanhdi; Haemate†; Helixate; Hemofil M; Kogenate; Kryobulin TIM 3; Monoclate-P; Recombinate; ***Swed.:*** Beriate; Haemate; Helixate; Hemofil M; Immunate; Koate†; Kogenate; Kryobulin†; Monoclate-P; Octavi†; Octonativ-M; Profilate†; Recombinate; ***Switz.:*** Haemate HS; Hyate:C; Immunate STIM plus; Kogenate; Kryobuline S-TIM 3; Premofil M; Recombinate; ***UK:*** Alpha VIII; Alphanate; Bioclate; Haemate P; Helixate; Hemofil HT; Hemofil M; Hyate:C; Kogenate; Kryobulin†; Monoclate-P; Recombinate; Replenate; ***USA:*** Alphanate; Bioclate; Helixate; Hemofil M; Humate-P; Hyate:C; Koate-HP; Koate-HS†; Kogenate; Monoclate-P; Profilate HP†; Recombinate.

Factor VIII Inhibitor Bypassing Fraction

(19165-p)

Activated Prothrombin Complex Concentrate; Anti-inhibitor Coagulant Complex.

Preparations with factor VIII inhibitor bypassing activity are prepared from human plasma.

Adverse Effects and Precautions

Allergic reactions may follow the administration of preparations having factor VIII inhibitor bypassing activity. Rapid infusion may cause headache, flushing, and changes in blood pressure and pulse rate.

It should not be given if disseminated intravascular coagulation is suspected or if there are signs of fibrinolysis. It should be used with caution in patients with liver disease.

As with other plasma-derived products, there is a risk of transmission of infection.

Uses and Administration

Preparations with factor VIII inhibitor bypassing activity are used in patients with haemophilia A (p.707) who have antibodies to factor VIII and in patients with acquired antibodies to factor VIII. The dose is administered intravenously and depends on the preparation used.

Preparations

Proprietary Preparations (details are given in Part 3)
Aust.: Feiba S-TIM 4; ***Belg.:*** Autoplex T; Feiba S-TIM 4; ***Canad.:*** Feiba; ***Ger.:*** Autoplex; Feiba S-TIM 4; ***Ital.:*** Feiba; ***Spain:*** Autoplex T; Feiba TIM 4; ***Swed.:*** Autoplex; Feiba; ***Switz.:*** Feiba; ***UK:*** Anti-inhibitor Coagulant Complex; Autoplex; Feiba; ***USA:*** Autoplex T; Feiba.

Factor IX (1227-a)

Christmas Factor; Plasma Thromboplastin Component; PTC.

NOTE. The name Nonacog Alfa *(rINN)* is in use for recombinant factor IX.

Factor IX is prepared from human plasma as described below. It may also be prepared using recombinant DNA technology.

Human Coagulation Factor IX, Freeze-dried (Ph. Eur.) (Factor IX Coagulationis Humanus Cryodesiccatus; Dried Factor IX Fraction (BP 1998)) is prepared from human plasma obtained from healthy donors who must, as far as can be ascertained, be free from detectable agents of infection transmissible by plasma-derived products. The method of preparation is designed to maintain functional integrity of factor IX, to minimise activation of any coagulation factor, and includes a step or steps that have been shown to remove or inactivate known agents of infection. The factor IX fraction is dissolved in a suitable liquid, passed through a bacteria-retentive filter, distributed aseptically into the final containers, and immediately frozen. The preparation is freeze-dried and the containers are sealed under vacuum or under an inert gas. Heparin, antithrombin, or other auxiliary substances such as a stabiliser may be included. No antimicrobial preservative is added. The potency of the preparation is not less than 50 international units of factor IX per mg of total protein before the addition of any protein stabiliser. When reconstituted as stated on the label the resulting solution contains not less than 20 international units per mL. The dried product should be protected from light.

Human Prothrombin Complex, Freeze-dried (Ph. Eur.) (Prothrombinum Multiplex Humanum Cryodesiccatum; Dried Prothrombin complex (BP 1998)) contains factor IX together with variable amounts of clotting factors II, VII, and X. It is prepared by fractionation of human plasma obtained from blood from healthy donors who must, as far as can be ascertained, be free from detectable agents of infection transmissible by plasma-derived products. The method of preparation is designed in particular to minimise thrombogenicity and includes a step or steps that have been shown to remove or inactivate known agents of infection. The prothrombin complex fraction is dissolved in a suitable liquid, sterilised by filtration, distributed aseptically into final containers, and immediately frozen. The preparation is freeze-dried and the containers are sealed under vacuum or under an inert gas. No antimicrobial preservative is added. Heparin, antithrombin, and other auxiliary substances such as a stabiliser may be added. The potency of the preparation is not less than 0.6 international units of factor IX per mg of total protein before the addition of any protein stabiliser. When reconstituted as stated on the label the resulting solution contains not less than 20 international units of factor IX per mL. The dried product should be protected from light. The reconstituted solution should be used immediately after reconstitution and on one occasion only. If solution is not complete or if it is turbid the fraction should not be used.

Factor IX Complex (USP 23) is a sterile freeze-dried powder consisting of partially purified factor IX fraction, as well as concentrated factor II, VII, and X fractions of venous plasma obtained from healthy human donors. It contains no preservatives. It should be stored at 2° to 8° in hermetically-sealed containers. It should be used within 4 hours after reconstitution and administered with equipment that includes a filter.

Units

The activity of factor IX is expressed in terms of international units and preparations may be assayed using the second International Standard for blood coagulation factor IX concentrate (1994).

Adverse Effects and Precautions

Allergic reactions may follow the administration of factor IX preparations and there may be chills, fever, and urticaria. Other adverse effects include nausea and vomiting, headache, and flushing particularly following rapid administration. Intravascular coagulation and thrombosis have been reported, mainly in patients with liver disease, and factor IX should be used with care in patients at risk of thrombo-embolism or disseminated intravascular coagulation. The risk should be less with more highly purified preparations.

As with other plasma derivatives there is a possibility of transmitting viral infection, although selection of donors and heat or chemical treatments of products are used to minimise the risk. Vaccination against hepatitis B is recommended for patients not already immune.

Antibodies to Factor IX may develop rarely.

Effects on blood coagulation. Some factor IX preparations derived from plasma contain other clotting factors in addition to factor IX (such as the activated factors IX, X and XII) and administration of these preparations is therefore potentially associated with thrombo-embolic complications. Reports of thrombosis[1] and intravascular coagulation[2,3] have been associated with the use of these factor IX preparations mainly in patients with liver disease. Machin and Miller[4] have reported deep vein thrombosis associated with postoperative factor IX administration in a patient with normal hepatic function. Highly purified factor IX preparations which do not contain other clotting factors may be expected to avoid this risk of thrombo-embolism.

1. Blatt PM, *et al.* Thrombogenic materials in prothrombin complex concentrates. *Ann Intern Med* 1974; **81:** 766–70.
2. Gazzard BG, *et al.* Coagulation factor concentrate in the treatment of the haemorrhagic diathesis of fulminant hepatic failure. *Gut* 1974; **15:** 993–8.
3. Cederbaum AI, *et al.* Intravascular coagulation with use of human prothrombin complex concentrates. *Ann Intern Med* 1976; **84:** 683–7.
4. Machin SJ, Miller BR. Thrombosis and factor-IX concentrates. *Lancet* 1978; **i:** 1367.

Effects on the heart. Myocardial infarction has occurred in patients receiving factor IX concentrates[1-3] and may be associated with the large doses employed.[4]

1. Fuerth JH, Mahrer P. Myocardial infarction after factor IX therapy. *JAMA* 1981; **245:** 1455–6.
2. Schimpf K, *et al.* Myocardial infarction complicating activated prothrombin complex concentrate substitution in patient with haemophilia A. *Lancet* 1982; **ii:** 1043.
3. Gruppo RA, *et al.* Fatal myocardial necrosis associated with prothrombin-complex-concentrate therapy in hemophilia A. *N Engl J Med* 1983; **309:** 242–3.
4. Lusher JM. Myocardial necrosis after therapy with prothrombin-complex concentrate. *N Engl J Med* 1984; **310:** 464.

Transmission of infections. For a report of hepatitis A in a patient receiving a solvent-detergent-treated factor IX preparation, see under Adverse Effects and Precautions of Factor VIII, p.721.

Uses and Administration

Factor IX is used as replacement therapy in patients with haemophilia B (Christmas disease), a genetic deficiency of factor IX (p.707). There are two forms of factor IX preparation derived from plasma; one is of high purity, the other is rich in other clotting factors. Preparations that contain other factors as well as factor IX may sometimes be useful for the treatment of bleeding due to deficiencies of factors II, VII, and X, as well as IX, and in the preparation of such patients for surgery.

Factor IX is given by slow intravenous infusion. In patients with factor IX deficiency the dosage should be determined for each patient and will vary with the preparation used and the circumstances of bleeding or type of surgery to be performed. Suggested target factor IX concentrations vary considerably.

Factor IX concentrates may also be used for immediate reversal of coumarin anticoagulants.

Factor IX preparations have been used in the management of patients with haemophilia A (p.707) who have antibodies to factor VIII.

A recombinant factor IX preparation is also available.

Preparations

Ph. Eur.: Freeze-dried Human Coagulation Factor IX; Freeze-dried Human Prothrombin Complex;
USP 23: Factor IX Complex.

Proprietary Preparations (details are given in Part 3)
Aust.: Bebulin S-TIM 4; Beriplex; Immunine; PPSB Konzentrat hepatitissicher†; Prothromplex S-TIM 4; ***Canad.:*** Bebulin†; Immunine†; ***Fr.:*** C P P A Humain†; PPSB†; ***Ger.:*** Alphanine; Berinin; Beriplex; Immunine STIM; Medactin (PPSB)†; Mononine; Nanotiv†; Octanyne; PPSB-Komplex†; PPSB-Tropon†; Preconativ†; Profilnine†; Prothromplex S-TIM 4; ***Irl.:*** Mononine; ***Ital.:*** Aimafix; Alphanine; Bebulin TIM 3; Haimaplex†; Immunine STIM; Mononine; Preconativ†; Protromplex TIM 3; Uman-Complex-IX-VI†; ***Norw.:*** Nanotiv; Octanyne; ***S.Afr.:*** Bebulin TIM 4†; Haemosolvex; Prothromplex-T TIM 4; ***Spain:*** Bebulin TIM 4; Mononine; Proplex T; ***Swed.:*** Immunine; Mononine; Nanotiv; Preconativ†; Prothromplex TIM 4†; ***Switz.:*** Bebuline S-TIM 4†; Immunine; Prothromplex Total S-TIM 4; ***UK:*** Alphanine; Beriplex PN; Mononine; Proplex; Prothromplex; Replenine; ***USA:*** Alphanine; Benefix; Konyne 80; Mononine; Profilnine; Proplex T.

Factor XIII (1228-t)

Fibrin-stabilising Factor; FSF.

Factor XIII is used as replacement therapy in patients with a genetic deficiency of factor XIII (p.707). Dosage of factor XIII is based on the degree of deficiency and the condition of the patient.

Cryoprecipitate is also used as a source of factor XIII.

Factor XIII is also a component of fibrin glues (see Fibrin, p.722).

Inflammatory bowel disease. Some patients with inflammatory bowel disease (p.1171) may be deficient in factor XIII, possibly due to increased intestinal blood loss seen in severe ulcerative colitis or increased mucosal deposition of factor XIII in Crohn's disease. Factor XIII concentrate given intravenously has produced beneficial results in 12 patients with active ulcerative colitis resistant to conventional therapy with corticosteroids and mesalazine[1] and has also been associated with healing of intractable fistulae in 3 of 4 patients with Crohn's disease.[2]

1. Lorenz R, *et al.* Factor XIII substitution in ulcerative colitis. *Lancet* 1995; **345:** 449–50.
2. Oshitani N, *et al.* Treatment of Crohn's disease fistulas with coagulation factor XIII. *Lancet* 1996: **347:** 119–20.

Preparations

Ph. Eur.: Fibrin Sealant Kit.

Proprietary Preparations (details are given in Part 3)
Aust.: Fibrogammin; ***Ger.:*** Fibrogammin; ***UK:*** Fibrogammin P.

Multi-ingredient: ***Aust.:*** Beriplast; Tissucol; Tissucol Duo Quick; ***Canad.:*** Tisseel†; ***Fr.:*** Biocol; ***Ger.:*** Beriplast; Tissucol Duo S; Tissucol Fibrinkleber tiefgefroren; Tissucol-Kit; ***Irl.:*** Tisseel; ***Spain:*** Tissucol; ***Swed.:*** Tisseel Duo Quick; ***Switz.:*** Tissucol; ***UK:*** Tisseel.

Fibrin (1229-x)

Human Fibrin Foam (BPC 1973) is a dry artificial sterile sponge of human fibrin. It is prepared by clotting with human thrombin a foam of a solution of human fibrinogen. The clotted foam is dried from the frozen state, cut into strips, and sterilised by heating at 130° for 3 hours. It should be stored below 25° in sterile containers sealed to exclude micro-organisms and moisture and be protected from light.

Fibrin Sealant Kit (Ph. Eur.) (Fibrini Glutinum; Fibrin Sealant Kit (BP 1998)) is composed of two components, a fibrinogen concentrate containing human fibrinogen and human factor XIII, and a human thrombin preparation. The kit may also contain other ingredients, such as human fibronectin, aprotinin, and human albumin. The human constituents are obtained from plasma for fractionation and the method of preparation includes a step or steps that have been shown to remove or inactivate known agents of infection. The constituents are passed through a bacteria-retentive filter and distributed aseptically into sterile containers. The containers are sealed under vacuum or filled with oxygen-free nitrogen or other suitable inert gas before sealing. No antimicrobial preservative is added. When reconstituted in the volume of solvent stated on the label, the fibrinogen concentrate contains not less than 60 g per litre of clottable protein and not less than 10 international units of factor XIII per mL; the activity of the thrombin preparation varies over a wide range (approximately 4 to 500 international units per mL). **Protect** from light.

Uses and Administration

Fibrin foam has been used in conjunction with thrombin as a haemostatic (p.704) in surgery at sites where bleeding cannot easily be controlled by the commoner methods of haemostasis.

Fibrin of animal origin, normally bovine, is also used.

Fibrin glue is prepared by mixing solutions containing fibrinogen, factor XIII, and often other clotting components with thrombin and calcium ions usually, with the addition of aprotinin to inhibit fibrinolysis. It is used to control haemorrhage during surgical procedures or as a spray to bleeding surfaces.

References to the use of fibrin glue.

1. Larson PO. Topical hemostatic agents for dermatologic surgery. *J Dermatol Surg Oncol* 1988; **14:** 623–32.
2. Narakas A. The use of fibrin glue in repair of peripheral nerves. *Orthop Clin North Am* 1988; **19:** 187–99.
3. Baudo F, *et al.* Management of oral bleeding in haemophilic patients. *Lancet* 1988; **ii:** 1082.
4. Kram HB, *et al.* Fibrin glue achieves hemostasis in patients with coagulation disorders. *Arch Surg* 1989; **124:** 385–7.
5. Lagoutte FM, *et al.* A fibrin sealant for perforated and preperforated corneal ulcers. *Br J Ophthalmol* 1989; **73:** 757–61.
6. Malviya VK, Deppe G. Control of intraoperative hemorrhage in gynecology with the use of fibrin glue. *Obstet Gynecol* 1989; **73:** 284–6.
7. Gibble JW, Ness PM. Fibrin glue: the perfect operative sealant? *Transfusion* 1990; **30:** 741–7.
8. Matar AF, *et al.* Use of biological glue to control pulmonary air leaks. *Thorax* 1990; **45:** 670–4.
9. Atrah HI. Fibrin glue. *Br Med J* 1994; **308:** 933–4.
10. Rutgeerts P, *et al.* Randomised trial of single and repeated fibrin glue compared with injection of polidocanol in treatment of bleeding peptic ulcer. *Lancet* 1997; **350:** 692–6.

Preparations

Proprietary Preparations (details are given in Part 3)
Ital.: Hemofibrine Spugna; Zimospuma.

Multi-ingredient: ***Aust.:*** Tissucol; Tissucol Duo Quick; ***Belg.:*** Tissucol; ***Canad.:*** Tisseel†; ***Fr.:*** Biocol; ***Ger.:*** Beriplast; Tissucol Duo S; Tissucol Fibrinkleber tiefgefroren; Tissucol-Kit; ***Irl.:*** Tisseel; ***Spain:*** Tissucol; ***Swed.:*** Tisseel Duo Quick; ***Switz.:*** Tissucol; ***UK:*** Tisseel.

Fibrinogen (1230-y)

Factor I.

Human Fibrinogen, Freeze-dried (Ph. Eur.) (Fibrinogenum Humanum Cryodesiccatum; Dried Fibrinogen (BP 1998)) contains the soluble constituent of human plasma that is transformed to fibrin on addition of thrombin. It is obtained from plasma for fractionation and the method of preparation includes a step or steps that have been shown to remove or inactivate known agents of infection. Stabilisers, including protein such as human albumin, salts, and buffers may be added. No antimicrobial preservative is added. When dissolved in the volume of solvent stated on the label, the solution contains not less than 10 g per litre of fibrinogen. **Protect** from light.

Fibrinogen has been used to control haemorrhage associated with low blood-fibrinogen concentration in afibrinogenaemia or hypofibrinogenaemia but the use of plasma or cryoprecipitate is usually preferred. It has also been used in disseminated intravascular coagulation (p.706). Fibrinogen is a component of fibrin glue (see Fibrin, above).

Fibrinogen labelled with radionuclides has also been used in diagnostic procedures.

Preparations

Ph. Eur.: Fibrin Sealant Kit; Freeze-dried Human Fibrinogen.

Proprietary Preparations (details are given in Part 3)
Aust.: Haemocomplettan; ***Ger.:*** Haemocomplettan; ***Ital.:*** Fibrinomer; Uman-Fibrin; ***Switz.:*** Haemocomplettan; ***UK:*** Haemocomplettan P.

Multi-ingredient: ***Aust.:*** Beriplast; TachoComb; Tissucol; Tissucol Duo Quick; ***Canad.:*** Tisseel†; ***Fr.:*** Biocol; ***Ger.:*** Beriplast; Ristofact†; TachoComb; Tissucol Duo S; Tissucol Fibrinkleber tiefgefroren; Tissucol-Kit; ***Spain:*** Tissucol; ***Swed.:*** Tisseel Duo Quick; ***Switz.:*** Tissucol; ***UK:*** Tisseel.

Filgrastim (14677-z)

Filgrastim *(BAN, USAN, rINN)*.

r-metHuG-CSF. A recombinant human granulocyte colony-stimulating factor.

CAS — 121181-53-1.

Solutions of filgrastim must not be diluted with sodium chloride solutions as precipitation will occur. Solutions should not be diluted below the recommended minimum concentration (2 μg per mL), and albumin must be added to give a final concentration of 2 mg per mL to solutions that are diluted to concentrations below 15 μg of filgrastim per mL (see also p.714).

Incompatibilities. References.

1. Trissel LA, Martinez JF. Compatibility of filgrastim with selected drugs during simulated Y-site administration. *Am J Hosp Pharm* 1994; **51:** 1907–13.

Adverse Effects and Precautions

As for Colony-stimulating Factors, p.714.

Preparations of filgrastim may contain sorbitol as an excipient; care is advisable in patients with hereditary fructose intolerance.

Uses and Administration

Filgrastim is a granulocyte colony-stimulating factor (p.715). It is used to treat or prevent neutropenia in patients receiving myelosuppressive cancer chemotherapy and to reduce the period of neutropenia in patients undergoing bone marrow transplantation (p.474). It is also used to mobilise autologous peripheral blood progenitor cells for an alternative to bone marrow transplantation, and in the management of chronic neutropenia (congenital, cyclic, or idiopathic).

As an adjunct to antineoplastic therapy, filgrastim is given in a dose of 5 μg per kg body-weight daily (or 0.5 million units per kg daily) starting not less than 24 hours after the last dose of antineoplastic. It can be given as a single daily subcutaneous injection, as a continuous intravenous or subcutaneous infusion, or as a daily intravenous infusion over 15 to 30 minutes. Treatment is continued until the neutrophil count has stabilised within the normal range which may take up to 14 days or more.

The initial dose following bone marrow transplantation is 10 μg per kg daily given by intravenous infusion over 30 minutes or 4 hours or continuous intravenous or subcutaneous infusion over 24 hours and this is adjusted according to the response.

For mobilisation of peripheral blood progenitor cells, a dose of 10 μg per kg daily of filgrastim may be given subcutaneously as a single daily injection or by continuous infusion; if given after myelosuppressive chemotherapy this dose is halved to 5 μg per kg daily by subcutaneous injection.

In patients with congenital neutropenia the recommended initial dose is 12 μg per kg daily and in patients with idiopathic or cyclic neutropenia the recommended initial dose is 5 μg per kg daily. In these forms of neutropenia the dose is given subcutaneously in single or divided doses and should be adjusted according to response.

The doses described above may also be given to children.

References.

1. Frampton JE, *et al.* Filgrastim: a review of its pharmacological properties and therapeutic efficacy in neutropenia. *Drugs* 1994; **48:** 731–60.

Preparations

Proprietary Preparations (details are given in Part 3)

Aust.: Neupogen; ***Austral.:*** Neupogen; ***Belg.:*** Neupogen; ***Canad.:*** Neupogen; ***Fr.:*** Neupogen; ***Ger.:*** Neupogen; ***Irl.:*** Neupogen; ***Ital.:*** Granulokine; Neupogen; ***Jpn:*** Gran; ***Neth.:*** Neupogen; ***Norw.:*** Neupogen; ***S.Afr.:*** Neupogen; ***Spain:*** Granulokine; Neupogen; ***Swed.:*** Neupogen; ***Switz.:*** Neupogen; ***UK:*** Neupogen; ***USA:*** Neupogen.

Gelatin (5425-w)

Gelatina.

Pharmacopoeias. In *Chin., Eur.* (see p.viii), *Int., Jpn,* and *Pol.* Also in *USNF.*

Gelatin is a purified protein obtained either by partial acid hydrolysis (type A) or by partial alkaline hydrolysis (type B) of animal collagen or it may be a mixture of types A and B.

Light amber to faintly yellow translucent sheets, shreds, flakes, powder, or granules with a slight odour.

Gelatin swells and softens when immersed in cold water, gradually absorbing 5 to 10 times its weight of water; on heating this gives a colloidal solution and on subsequent cooling forms a more or less firm gel. **Soluble** in a hot mixture of glycerol and water and in 6N acetic acid; practically insoluble in alcohol, chloroform, fixed and volatile oils, and ether. **Store** in airtight containers.

Gelatins are usually graded by jelly strength, expressed as 'Bloom strength' or 'Bloom rating'.

The gelatin described in some pharmacopoeias is not necessarily suitable for preparations for parenteral use or for other special purposes.

Incompatibilities. A white precipitate was formed immediately when vancomycin injection was administered through a giving set containing modified fluid gelatin solution.[1]

1. Taylor A, Hornbrey P. Incompatibility of vancomycin and gelatin plasma expanders. *Pharm J* 1991; **246:** 466.

Adverse Effects

Hypersensitivity reactions including anaphylactic reactions have occurred after the infusion of gelatin or its derivatives. Rapid infusion of gelatin derivatives may directly stimulate the release of histamine and other vasoactive substances.

For adverse reactions associated with the topical use of gelatin, see Haemostasis under Uses and Administration, below.

Effects on the kidneys. Acute renal failure developed in a patient undergoing aortobifemoral graft surgery who received modified fluid gelatin, blood transfusion, and diuretics following a fall in urine output.[1,2] The conclusion that gelatin was the most likely cause of the renal failure was contested[3-5] on the basis of previous experience and other major contributory factors such as diminished intravascular volume and reduced organ perfusion.

1. Hussain SF, Drew PJT. Acute renal failure after infusion of gelatins. *Br Med J* 1989; **299:** 1137–8.
2. Drew PJT, Hussain SF. Acute renal failure after infusion of gelatin. *Br Med J* 1989; **299:** 1400. Correction. *ibid.*; 1531.
3. Frazer RS, Macmillan RR. Acute renal failure after infusion of gelatin. *Br Med J* 1989; **299:** 1399.
4. Fawcett WJ. Acute renal failure after infusion of gelatin. *Br Med J* 1989; **299:** 1399.
5. Wilkins RG. Acute renal failure after infusion of gelatin. *Br Med J* 1989; **299:** 1399–1400.

Hypersensitivity. Ten severe anaphylactoid reactions to an infusion of a modified fluid gelatin were reported over a period of 3 years.[1]

For reports of fatal reactions in asthmatic patients following administration of gelatin derivatives, see Polygeline, p.727.

1. Blanloeil Y, *et al.* Accidents anaphylactoïdes sévères après perfusion d'une gélatine fluide modifiée en solution équilibrée *Therapie* 1983; **38:** 539–46.

Precautions

Precautions that should be observed with plasma expanders are described under Dextran 70, p.717, and these should be considered when gelatin and gelatin derivatives are used for this purpose. There does not appear to be any interference with blood grouping and cross matching of blood.

Pharmacokinetics

Following infusion of modified fluid gelatin (succinylated gelatin), 75% of the dose is excreted in the urine in 24 hours. The half-life is about 4 hours.

Uses and Administration

Gelatin is a protein that has both clinical and pharmaceutical uses.

Gelatin is used as a haemostatic in surgical procedures as an absorbable film or sponge and can absorb many times its weight of blood. It is also employed as a plasma volume expander similarly to the dextrans in hypovolaemic shock (p.798). A 4% solution of a modified fluid gelatin (succinylated gelatin) has been infused in doses of 500 to 1000 mL. It may also be used in the form of a gelatin derived polymer, see Polygeline, p.727.

Gelatin rods may be employed to temporarily block tear outflow in the diagnosis of dry eye (p.1470).

Gelatin is used in the preparation of pastes, pastilles, suppositories, tablets, and hard and soft capsule shells. It is also used for the microencapsulation of drugs and other industrial materials. It has been used as a vehicle for injections; Pitkin's Menstruum, which consists of gelatin, glucose, and acetic acid, has been used in a modified form for heparin while hydrolysed gelatin has been used for corticotrophin. Gelatin is an ingredient of preparations used for the protection of stoma and lesions.

Haemostasis. Gelatin acts as a haemostatic (p.704) by providing a physical meshwork within which clotting can occur. Gelatin powder may be applied dry to wound beds and may be most useful when mixed with saline or thrombin and applied to bone. Gelatin sponge can be applied dry or soaked in saline or thrombin solutions. When applied to skin wounds the gelatin liquefies within 2 to 5 days; when implanted into tissues it is absorbed within 4 to 6 weeks. Adverse reactions include an increased incidence of infection, compression of surrounding tissue due to fluid absorption, granuloma formation, and fibrosis. Generally, gelatin sponges cause little tissue reaction and can be applied to bone, dura, and pleural tissue.

References.

1. Larson PO. Topical hemostatic agents for dermatologic surgery. *J Dermatol Surg Oncol* 1988; **14:** 623–32.

Neonatal intraventricular haemorrhage. Plasma volume expansion in preterm neonates has been thought to help prevent neonatal intraventricular haemorrhage (p.709). However, a study using plasma or gelatin as plasma volume expanders,[1,2] found no evidence of a decreased risk of such haemorrhage or subsequent death or disability.

1. The Northern Neonatal Nursing Initiative Trial Group. A randomized trial comparing the effect of prophylactic intravenous fresh frozen plasma, gelatin or glucose on early mortality and morbidity in preterm babies. *Eur J Pediatr* 1996; **155:** 580–8.
2. Northern Neonatal Nursing Initiative Trial Group. Randomised trial of prophylactic early fresh-frozen plasma or gelatin or glucose in preterm babies: outcome at 2 years. *Lancet* 1996; **348:** 229–32.

Preparations

USP 23: Absorbable Gelatin Film; Absorbable Gelatin Sponge.

Proprietary Preparations (details are given in Part 3)

Aust.: Gelofusin; Spongostan; ***Austral.:*** Gel-Caps†; Gelfilm; Gelfoam; ***Belg.:*** Gelfoam; Gelofusine; Geloplasma; Willospon; ***Canad.:*** Gelfilm; Gelfoam; ***Fr.:*** Epiphane; Gel-Phan; Gelodiet; Gelofusine; Hexaphane; Orangel; ***Ger.:*** Gelafundin; Gelafusal-N in Ringeracetat; Gelaspon; Gelastypt D; Marbagelan†; Thomaegelin; ***Ital.:*** Eufusin; Spongostan; ***Neth.:*** Clinispon†; Gelfilm; Gelfoam; Geloplasma†; Willospon; ***S.Afr.:*** Gelfoam†; Spongostan†; ***Spain:*** Espongostan; Geloplasma; ***Switz.:*** Gelfoam; Physiogel; Plasmagelan†; ***UK:*** Geloflex; Gelofusine; Sterispon†; ***USA:*** Gelfilm; Gelfoam.

Multi-ingredient: ***Aust.:*** Gelacet; ***Austral.:*** Orabase; Orahesive; Stomahesive; ***Canad.:*** Orabase; Orahesive; ***Fr.:*** Plasmagel; Plasmion; Rectopanbiline; Sureskin; Totephan; ***Ger.:*** Gelacet N; Gerontamin; ***Irl.:*** Orabase; ***Ital.:*** Solecin; ***Switz.:*** Gelacet; Varihesive Hydroactive; ***UK:*** Orabase; Orahesive; Stomahesive; Varihesive; ***USA:*** Dome-Paste.

Haemoglobin (12812-y)

Haemoglobin has the property of reversible oxygenation and is the respiratory pigment of blood. Solutions of haemoglobin or modified haemoglobin have been investigated as blood substitutes.

The structure of haemoglobin gives a non-linear oxygen dissociation curve; almost maximum oxygen saturation occurs in normal arterial blood without the need for oxygen-enriched air. Thus the use of haemoglobin solutions for emergency use appears logical. Initial *animal* experiments with haemoglobin from haemolysed erythrocytes resulted in serious renal damage but haemoglobin is not itself nephrotoxic and the development of stroma-free haemoglobin solutions reduced this toxicity. However, once released from the erythrocytes, haemoglobin loses its ability to hold 2,3-diphosphoglycerate, which is essential for the delivery of oxygen, and haemoglobin, being a small molecule, is rapidly excreted by the kidneys. Various methods have been tried to overcome these problems; addition of pyridoxine 5-phosphate and formation of crosslinked haemoglobin restore the oxygen affinity to that of whole blood and polymerisation or microencapsulation in a lipid membrane extend the half-life. Polymerisation has the added advantages that this process is virucidal and also lowers the osmolality of the solution permitting higher concentrations to be used. There are, however, reservations concerning haemoglobin solutions as blood substitutes; blood itself must be available for their production, although expired blood may be employed and there is also concern about impairment of immune mechanisms. The recent production of recombinant human haemoglobin may overcome these problems.

References.

1. Anonymous. Blood substitutes: has the right solution been found? *Lancet* 1986; **i:** 717–18.
2. Urbaniak SJ. Artificial blood. *Br Med J* 1991; **303:** 1348–50.
3. Odling-Smee W. Red cell substitutes. In: Contreras M, ed. *ABC of transfusion*. 2nd ed. London: BMJ Publishing Group, 1992: 57–9.
4. Jones JA. Red blood cell substitutes: current status. *Br J Anaesth* 1995; **74:** 697–703.
5. Mallick A, Bodenham AR. Modified haemoglobins as oxygen-transporting blood substitutes. *Br J Hosp Med* 1996; **55:** 443–8.

Hetastarch (255-j)

Hetastarch *(BAN, USAN)*.

HES; Hydroxyethyl Starch. 2-Hydroxyethyl ether starch.

CAS — 9005-27-0.

NOTE. Pentastarch, which is also known as 2-hydroxyethyl ether starch, differs from hetastarch in having a lower degree of etherification.

Hetastarch is a starch that is composed of more than 90% of amylopectin and that has been etherified to the extent that an average of 7 to 8 of the hydroxy groups in each 10 D-glucopyranose units of starch polymer have been converted into OCH_2CH_2OH groups. Hetastarch as normally used has weight average molecular weight of about 450 000.

Incompatibilities. Hetastarch is incompatible with many compounds including a number of injectable antibiotics.

References.

1. Wohlford JG, Fowler MD. Visual compatibility of hetastarch with injectable critical-care drugs. *Am J Hosp Pharm* 1989; **46:** 995–6.
2. Wohlford JG, *et al.* More information on the visual compatibility of hetastarch with injectable critical-care drugs. *Am J Hosp Pharm* 1990; **47:** 297–8.

Adverse Effects and Precautions

Hypersensitivity reactions including anaphylactic reactions have occurred after infusion of hetastarch.

Precautions that should be observed with plasma expanders are described under Dextran 70, p.717 and these should be considered when hetastarch is used. There does not appear to be any interference with blood grouping and cross matching of blood.

Complement activation. Complement activation was greater following polygeline administration than a preparation of hetastarch.[1]

1. Watkins J, *et al.* Complement activation by polystarch and gelatine volume expanders. *Lancet* 1990; **335:** 233.

Effects on the blood. Coagulopathy and haemorrhage has been reported in neurosurgical patients,[1,2] in a patient with coagulation defects,[3] and in a Jehovah's Witness[4] in whom large volumes of hetastarch solution were used during major orthopaedic surgery. It was suggested that hetastarch should probably be avoided in neurosurgical patients in whom the prevention of intracranial haemorrhage is critical, and in patients with a pre-existing bleeding disorder.

1. Syrington BE. Hetastarch and bleeding complications. *Ann Intern Med* 1986; **105:** 627–8.
2. Damon L, *et al.* Intracranial bleeding during treatment with hydroxyethyl starch. *N Engl J Med* 1987; **317:** 964–5.
3. Abramson N. Plasma expanders and bleeding. *Ann Intern Med* 1988; **108:** 307.
4. Lockwood DNJ, *et al.* A severe coagulopathy following volume replacement with hydroxyethyl starch in a Jehovah's Witness. *Anaesthesia* 1988; **43:** 391–3.

Effects on the kidneys. Osmotic-nephrosis-like lesions found at biopsy in some transplanted kidneys have been attributed to use of hydroxyethyl ether starch solutions in the donor patient.[1] Such use has also been reported to impair immediate graft function.[2] However, another study[3] found no association between the use of these solutions in the donor patient and osmotic-nephrosis-like lesions or delayed graft function.

1. Legendre CH, *et al.* Hydroxyethylstarch and osmotic-nephrosis-like lesions in kidney transplantation. *Lancet* 1993; **342:** 248–9.
2. Cittanova ML, *et al.* Effect of hydroxethylstarch in brain-dead kidney donors on renal function in kidney-transplant recipients. *Lancet* 1996; **348:** 1620–22.
3. Coronel B, *et al.* Hydroxyethylstarch and renal function in kidney transplant recipients. *Lancet* 1997; **349:** 884.

Effects on the skin. Pruritus has been reported after infusion of hydroxyethyl ether starches. In a review[1] of hydroxyethyl ether starch administration, severe pruritus developed in 32% of patients. It occurred, usually on the trunk, in 3 days to 15 weeks after hydroxyethyl ether starch administration and the mean duration was nearly 9 weeks. Prolonged pruritus lasting more than 2 years has been reported.[2] The reaction is dose dependent and usually refractory to treatment. There are individual reports of response to capsaicin.[3] Hydroxyethyl ether starches have been shown to accumulate in the skin. Marked and persistent periocular swelling developed in a patient following 15 daily infusions of hetastarch.[4] Abnormal accumulation of hetastarch was found in the periocular tissues.

1. Gall H, *et al.* Persistierender pruritus nach hydroxyäthylstärke-infusionen. *Hautarzt* 1993; **44:** 713–16.
2. Cox NH, Popple AW. Persistent erythema and pruritus, with a confluent histiocytic skin infiltrate, following the use of a hydroxyethylstarch plasma expander. *Br J Dermatol* 1996; **134:** 353–7.
3. Szeimies R-M, *et al.* Successful treatment of hydroxyethyl starch-induced pruritus with topical capsaicin. *Br J Dermatol* 1994; **131:** 380–2.
4. Kiehl P, *et al.* Decreased activity of acid α-glucosidase in a patient with persistent periocular swelling after infusions of hydroxyethyl starch. *Br J Dermatol* 1998; **138:** 672–77.

Pharmacokinetics

After intravenous infusion of hetastarch, the molecules with a molecular weight of less than 50 000 are readily excreted unchanged by the kidney. About 40% of a dose is excreted in the urine in 24 hours. Larger molecular weight fractions are metabolised and eliminated more slowly.

References.

1. Mishler JM, *et al.* Changes in the molecular composition of circulating hydroxyethyl starch following consecutive daily infusions in man. *Br J Clin Pharmacol* 1979; **7:** 505–9.
2. Mishler JM, *et al.* Post-transfusion survival of hydroxyethyl starch 450/0.70 in man: a long-term study. *J Clin Pathol* 1980; **33:** 155–9.
3. Yacobi A, *et al.* Pharmacokinetics of hydroxyethyl starch in normal subjects. *J Clin Pharmacol* 1982; **22:** 206–12.

Uses and Administration

Hetastarch is a plasma volume expander used in the management of hypovolaemic shock (p.798). As a 6% solution hetastarch exerts a similar colloidal osmotic pressure to human albumin, and when given by intravenous infusion it produces an expansion of plasma volume slightly in excess of the infused volume. The effects last for 24 to 36 hours.

Hetastarch is given intravenously as a 6% solution in sodium chloride 0.9%. The dose and rate of infusion depend on the amount of fluid lost and degree of haemoconcentration but in shock it is usually between 500 to 1000 mL; more than 1500 mL or 20 mL per kg body-weight per day is not usually required. The rate of infusion may approach 20 mL per kg per hour in patients with acute haemorrhagic shock; slower rates are recommended in burns or septic shock.

Hetastarch increases the erythrocyte sedimentation rate when added to whole blood. It is therefore used in leucopheresis procedures to increase the yield of granulocytes. Doses of 250 to 700 mL may be added to venous blood in the ratio 1 part to at least 8 parts of whole blood in such procedures. Up to 2 such procedures per week and a total of 7 to 10 have been reported to be safe.

Hetastarch has also been used in extracorporeal perfusion fluids.

Various preparations of 2-hydroxyethyl starch are available. Some correspond to hetastarch or are close to it in having a slightly lower degree of etherification and lower average molecular weight, for example hexastarch. Pentastarch (p.725) has an even lower degree of etherification.

References.

1. Nakasato SK. Evaluation of hetastarch. *Clin Pharm* 1982; **1:** 509–14.
2. Hulse JD, Yacobi A. Hetastarch: an overview of the colloid and its metabolism. *Drug Intell Clin Pharm* 1983; **17:** 334–41.

Preparations

Proprietary Preparations (details are given in Part 3)

Aust.: Elohast; Expafusin; Expahes; Plasmasteril; Varihes; ***Belg.:*** Elohaes; Plasmasteril; ***Canad.:*** Hespan†; ***Fr.:*** Elohes; ***Ger.:*** Elohast†; Expafusin; Infukoll HES; Onkohas†; Plasmafusin HES; Plasmasteril; ***Ital.:*** Hespan†; ***Jpn:*** Hespander; ***Spain:*** Expafusin; ***Switz.:*** Elohast; Expahes; Plasmasteril; Varihes; ***UK:*** Elohaes; Elohes; Hespan; ***USA:*** Hespan.

Interleukin-3 (16855-w)

Interleukin-3 (IL-3) is a cytokine that acts as a colony-stimulating factor (p.714). It is under investigation in the management of myelosuppression associated with cancer chemotherapy and following bone marrow transplantation. A fusion molecule with granulocyte-macrophage colony-stimulating factor, known as milodistim (PIXY-321), is also under investigation.

References.

1. Albin N, *et al.* In vivo effects of GM-CSF and IL-3 on hematopoietic cell recovery in bone marrow and blood after autologous transplantation with mafosfamide-purged marrow in lymphoid malignancies. *Bone Marrow Transplant* 1994; **14:** 253–9.
2. Dercksen MW, *et al.* Hypotension induced by interleukin-3 in patients on angiotensin-converting enzyme inhibitors. *Lancet* 1995; **345:** 448.
3. Huhn RD, *et al.* Pharmacodynamics of daily subcutaneous recombinant human interleukin-3 in normal volunteers. *Clin Pharmacol Ther* 1995; **57:** 32–41.

Lenograstim (15280-h)

Lenograstim *(BAN, USAN, rINN)*.

rG-CSF. A recombinant human granulocyte colony- stimulating factor.

CAS — 135968-09-1.

Adverse Effects and Precautions

As for Colony-stimulating Factors, p.714.

Uses and Administration

Lenograstim is a granulocyte colony-stimulating factor (p.715). It is used to treat or prevent neutropenia in patients receiving myelosuppressive cancer chemotherapy and to reduce the period of neutropenia in patients undergoing bone marrow transplantation (p.474). It is also used to mobilise autologous peripheral blood progenitor cells for an alternative to bone marrow transplantation.

Lenograstim may be given in a dose of 150 μg per m^2 body-surface daily to patients following bone marrow transplantation and also to patients established on antineoplastic therapy although the route of administration differs; intravenous infusion over 30 minutes is used post transplant and the subcutaneous route is used for patients on antineoplastics. Treatment is given until the neutrophil count has stabilised within the normal range, but a maximum treatment period of 28 consecutive days should not be exceeded.

For mobilisation of peripheral blood progenitor cells after cytotoxic chemotherapy a dose of 150 μg per m^2 daily may be administered by subcutaneous injection starting the day after completion of chemotherapy. When used alone, or in healthy donors, a dose of 10 μg per kg body-weight daily is given subcutaneously for 4 to 6 days.

References.

1. Frampton JE, *et al.* Lenograstim: a review of its pharmacological properties and therapeutic efficacy in neutropenia and related clinical settings. *Drugs* 1995; **49:** 767–93.

Preparations

Proprietary Preparations (details are given in Part 3)

Aust.: Granocyte; ***Austral.:*** Granocyte; ***Belg.:*** Granocyte; ***Fr.:*** Granocyte; ***Ger.:*** Granocyte; ***Irl.:*** Granocyte; ***Ital.:*** Granocyte; Myelostim; ***Jpn:*** Neutrogin; ***Neth.:*** Granocyte; ***Norw.:*** Granocyte; ***Spain:*** Euprotin; Granocyte; ***Swed.:*** Granocyte; ***Switz.:*** Granocyte; ***UK:*** Granocyte.

Leucocytes (1244-t)

Preparations of leucocytes contain granulocytes with a variable content of red blood cells, lymphocytes, and platelets. Depending on the method of collection they may also contain dextran or hetastarch.

Adverse Effects and Precautions

Leucocyte transfusions may cause severe transfusion reactions and fever. As with other blood products, there is a risk of transmission of infection. Severe lung reactions including fluid overload with pulmonary oedema are a particular problem in patients with active pulmonary infections.

Red blood cell compatibility testing is necessary because of the content of red blood cells. Graft-versus-host disease may occur in immunosuppressed recipients, and may be avoided by irradiating the product before administration.

Uses and Administration

Transfusion of leucocytes has been used in patients with severe granulocytopenia and infection which has not been controlled by treatment with appropriate antimicrobial agents for 48 to 72 hours. Transfusion of $1x10^{10}$ granulocytes daily has been suggested as an effective dose. Daily transfusions for at least 3 to 4 days are usually advised. Hydrocortisone and chlorpheniramine may be given intravenously before transfusion to reduce the severity of adverse reactions.

References.

1. Hows JM, Brozović B. Platelet and granulocyte transfusions. In: Contreras M, ed. *ABC of transfusion.* 2nd ed. London: BMJ Publishing Group, 1992: 14–17.
2. Papadopoulos EB, *et al.* Infusions of donor leukocytes to treat Epstein-Barr virus-associated lymphoproliferative disorders after allogeneic bone marrow transplantation. *N Engl J Med* 1994; **330:** 1185–91.
3. Kumar L. Donor leucocyte infusions for relapse in chronic myelogenous leukaemia. *Lancet* 1994; **344:** 1101–2.

Metacresolsulphonic Acid-Formaldehyde

(1723-e)

m-Cresolsulphonic acid-formaldehyde condensation product; Dicresulene polymer; Polycresolsulfonate. Dihydroxydimethyldiphenylmethanedisulphonic acid polymer; Methylenebis(hydroxytoluenesulphonic acid) polymer.

$(C_{15}H_{16}O_8S_2)_n$.
CAS — 9011-02-3.

Preparations of metacresolsulphonic acid-formaldehyde are highly acidic and are used as topical haemostatics and antiseptics. There are a number of vaginal preparations.

Preparations

Proprietary Preparations (details are given in Part 3)
Aust.: Albothyl†; ***Belg.:*** Lotagen; ***Fr.:*** Negatol; ***Ger.:*** Albothyl; Dermidot†; ***Ital.:*** Negaderm†; Negatol; ***Norw.:*** Nelex†; ***S.Afr.:*** Nelex; ***Spain:*** Negatol; ***Swed.:*** Nelex; ***Switz.:*** Negatol; Negatol Dental.

Molgramostim (15057-a)

Molgramostim *(BAN, USAN, rINN).*

Sch-39300. A recombinant human granulocyte-macrophage colony- stimulating factor; Colony-stimulating factor 2 (human clone pHG_{25} protein moiety reduced).

CAS — 99283-10-0.

Solutions should not be diluted below the recommended minimum concentration of 7 µg per mL.

Adverse Effects and Precautions

As for Colony-stimulating Factors, p.714.

Uses and Administration

Molgramostim is a granulocyte-macrophage colony-stimulating factor (p.715). It is used to treat or prevent neutropenia in patients receiving myelosuppressive cancer chemotherapy and to reduce the period of neutropenia in patients undergoing bone marrow transplantation (p.474). It is also used to reduce ganciclovir-induced neutropenia (p.611).

As an adjunct to antineoplastic therapy, molgramostim is given by subcutaneous injection, starting 24 hours after the last dose of antineoplastic, in a dose of 5 to 10 µg per kg body-weight daily. Treatment should be continued for 7 to 10 days.

Following bone marrow transplantation, molgramostim may be given by intravenous infusion over 4 to 6 hours in a dose of 10 µg per kg daily. Treatment should be initiated the day after bone marrow transplantation and continued for up to 30 days depending on the neutrophil count.

For the management of ganciclovir-induced neutropenia, molgramostim may be given by subcutaneous injection in a dose of 5 µg per kg daily. After 5 doses have been given the dose of molgramostim should be adjusted according to the neutrophil count.

The maximum dose for any indication should not exceed 10 µg per kg daily.

Preparations

Proprietary Preparations (details are given in Part 3)
Aust.: Leucomax; ***Belg.:*** Leucomax; ***Fr.:*** Leucomax; ***Ger.:*** Leucomax; ***Irl.:*** Leucomax; ***Ital.:*** Leucomax; Mielogen; ***Neth.:*** Leucomax; ***Norw.:*** Leucomax; ***S.Afr.:*** Leucomax; ***Spain:*** Leucomax; ***Swed.:*** Leucomax; ***Switz.:*** Leucomax; ***UK:*** Leucomax.

Naftazone (1724-l)

Naftazone *(BAN, rINN).*

1,2-Naphthoquinone 2-semicarbazone.

$C_{11}H_9N_3O_2$ = 215.2.
CAS — 15687-37-3.

Naftazone is a haemostatic (p.704) used in venous insufficiency and in capillary haemorrhage. It is given by mouth in doses of 5 to 10 mg three times a day. It was formerly given by injection.

Preparations

Proprietary Preparations (details are given in Part 3)
Belg.: Karbinone†; Mediaven; ***Fr.:*** Etioven; ***Spain:*** Metorene; ***Switz.:*** Mediaven.

Nartograstim (15909-d)

Nartograstim *(rINN).*

A recombinant human granulocyte colony- stimulating factor; N-L-Methionyl-1-L-alanine-3-L-threonine-4-L-tyrosine-5-L-arginine-17-L-serine colony-stimulating factor (human clone 1034).

CAS — 134088-74-7.

Nartograstim is a granulocyte colony-stimulating factor (p.714) given by intravenous or subcutaneous injection in the management of neutropenia.

Preparations

Proprietary Preparations (details are given in Part 3)
Jpn: Neu-Up.

Oprelvekin (9779-f)

Oprelvekin *(USAN, rINN).*

$C_{854}H_{1411}N_{253}O_{235}S_2$ = 19047.0.
CAS — 145941-26-0.

Adverse Effects and Precautions

Fluid retention may occur producing oedema and dyspnoea; caution is required when giving oprelvekin to patients with a history or signs of heart failure. Fluid balance and electrolytes should be monitored in patients receiving long-term diuretic therapy. Transient atrial arrhythmias have occasionally been reported. Other adverse effects include exfoliative dermatitis, mild blurred vision, and conjunctival injection.

Fetotoxicity has been reported in *animals.*

Uses and Administration

Oprelvekin, a recombinant human interleukin-11, is a platelet growth factor that stimulates the proliferation and maturation of megakaryocytes and thus increases the production of platelets. Oprelvekin is given by subcutaneous injection in a dose of 50 µg per kg body-weight daily to prevent severe antineoplastic-induced thrombocytopenia in patients with non-myeloid malignancies.

References.

1. Tepler I, *et al.* A randomized placebo-controlled trial of recombinant human interleukin-11 in cancer patients with severe thrombocytopenia due to chemotherapy. *Blood* 1996; **87:** 3607–14.
2. Isaacs C, *et al.* Randomized placebo-controlled study of recombinant human interleukin-11 to prevent chemotherapy-induced thrombocytopenia in patients with breast cancer receiving dose-intensive cyclophosphamide and doxorubicin. *J Clin Oncol* 1997; **15:** 3368–77.

Preparations

Proprietary Preparations (details are given in Part 3)
USA: Neumega.

Oxypolygelatin (5446-z)

Oxypolygelatin is a polymer derived from gelatin (p.723). It is used as a 5.5% solution as a plasma volume expander. There have been reports of anaphylaxis.

Preparations

Proprietary Preparations (details are given in Part 3)
Aust.: Gelifundol; ***Ger.:*** Gelifundol; ***S.Afr.:*** Gelifundol; ***Switz.:*** Gelifundol.

Pentastarch (10365-y)

Pentastarch *(BAN, USAN).*

ASL-607. 2-Hydroxyethyl ether starch.

CAS — 9005-27-0.

NOTE. Hetastarch, which is also known as 2-hydroxyethyl ether starch, differs from pentastarch in having a higher degree of etherification.

Pentastarch is a starch in which more than 90% of the amylopectin has been etherified to the extent that an average of 4 or 5 of the hydroxy groups in each 10 D-glucopyranose unit of the starch polymer have been converted to OCH_2CH_2OH groups. Pentastarch as normally used has weight average molecular weight of about 250 000.

Adverse Effects and Precautions

As for Hetastarch, p.724.

Pharmacokinetics

After intravenous infusion of pentastarch, the molecules with a molecular weight of less than 50 000 are readily excreted unchanged by the kidney. About 70% of a dose is excreted in the urine in 24 hours and about 80% within a week.

Uses and Administration

Pentastarch is a plasma volume expander with actions and uses similar to those of hetastarch (p.724). Intravenous infusion produces an expansion of plasma volume of about 1.5 times the infused volume. The effects last for 18 to 24 hours. Pentastarch is used in the management of hypovolaemic shock (p.798) and in leucopheresis.

In shock, pentastarch is given as a 10% solution in sodium chloride 0.9%. The dose and rate of infusion depend upon the amount of fluid lost and degree of haemoconcentration. In general, the usual dose is 500 to 2000 mL; more than 2000 mL or 28 mL per kg body-weight per day is not usually required. In acute haemorrhagic shock, an infusion rate of approximately 20 mL per kg per hour has been suggested.

Starches similar to pentastarch that have a weight average molecular weight of 200 000 and an average of 4 to 5.5 hydroxy groups etherified are also employed as plasma volume expanders; concentrations used are 3, 6, and 10%.

In leucopheresis, doses of 250 to 700 mL of pentastarch 10% may be added to venous blood in the ratio of 1 part to at least 8 parts of whole blood.

Administration in children. A 6% solution of a low molecular weight hydroxyethyl starch (average molecular weight 200 000) was considered effective and safe when compared with human albumin in the management of volume replacement in children under 3 years of age undergoing cardiac surgery.[1]

1. Boldt J, *et al.* Volume replacement with hydroxyethyl starch solutions in children. *Br J Anaesth* 1993; **70:** 661–5.

Stroke. Haemodilution with pentastarch has been tried in patients with acute ischaemic stroke (p.799) in an attempt to improve reperfusion of the brain by lowering blood viscosity. However, one study was terminated early when an excess mortality was noted in the haemodilution group.[1] The early fatalities occurred almost exclusively in patients with severe strokes; cerebral oedema was the main cause of death within one week of the onset of symptoms. Among the survivors neurological recovery was better among those who received haemodilution.

1. Hemodilution in Stroke Study Group. Hypervolemic hemodilution treatment of stroke: results of a randomized multicenter trial using pentastarch. *Stroke* 1989; **20:** 317–23.

Preparations

Proprietary Preparations (details are given in Part 3)
Aust.: HAES; Isohes; Osmohes; ***Belg.:*** HAES-steril; ***Canad.:*** Pentaspan; ***Fr.:*** Hesteril; Lomol†; ***Ger.:*** Haemofusin; HAES-steril; Hemohes; Rheohes; ***Norw.:*** HAES-steril; ***S.Afr.:*** HAES-steril; ***Swed.:*** HAES-steril; Hemohes; ***Switz.:*** HAES-steril; Hemohes; Isohes; ***UK:*** HAES-steril; Pentaspan; ***USA:*** Pentaspan.

Plasma (1245-x)

Human Plasma for Fractionation (Ph. Eur.) (Plasma Humanum ad Separationem; Plasma for Fractionation (BP 1998)) is plasma separated from whole blood or collected in an apheresis procedure; it is intended for the manufacture of blood derivatives.

Adverse Effects and Precautions

As for Blood, p.713, though with a low risk of transmitting cell-associated viruses. However, the production of blood products using plasma from UK donors is being phased out due to the possible risk of transmission of Creutzfeldt-Jakob disease.

Uses and Administration

Fresh frozen plasma contains useful amounts of clotting factors. It should be reserved for patients with proven abnormalities in blood coagulation (see Haemorrhagic Disorders, p.707). Indications include congenital deficiencies in clotting factors for which specific concentrates are unavailable, severe multiple clotting factor deficiencies for example in patients with liver disease, rapid reversal of the action of coumarin anticoagulants, and disseminated intravascular coagulation. It may be used following massive blood transfusion when there is evidence of coagulation deficiency but its value for routine prophylaxis against abnormal bleeding tendencies in patients receiving massive blood transfusions is contentious except where clotting abnormalities have been confirmed. It has also been used in the treatment of thrombotic thrombocytopenic purpura and as a source of plasma proteins.

The amount of fresh frozen plasma transfused depends on the required level of clotting factors. A unit of fresh frozen plasma refers to the quantity of plasma obtained from 1 unit of whole blood; this generally represents a volume of about 250 mL, including anticoagulant.

Fresh frozen plasma should not be used as a volume expander or as a nutritional source.

Therapeutic plasma exchange or plasmapheresis (the terms are commonly used synonymously) which involves the removal of blood, anticoagulation, centrifugation, and the return to the patient of the cellular components suspended in a suitable vehicle such as albumin solutions or sodium chloride 0.9% is used in a wide variety of disorders.

Plasma is used for the production of various blood products including albumin, antithrombin III, blood clotting factors, immunoglobulins, and platelets. Other preparations include cryoprecipitate depleted plasma from which approximately half the fibrinogen, factor VIII, and fibronectin has been removed, and single donor plasma which is not frozen. A solvent-detergent-treated plasma preparation is available.

References.

1. McClure G. The use of plasma in the neonatal period. *Arch Dis Child* 1991; **66:** 373–5.
2. Thomson A, *et al.* Use and abuse of fresh frozen plasma. *Br J Anaesth* 1992; **68:** 237–8.
3. Cohen H, *et al.* Plasma, plasma products, and indications for their use. In: Contreras M, ed. *ABC of transfusion*. 2nd ed. London; BMJ Publishing Group, 1992: 31–4.
4. British Committee for Standards in Haematology, Working Party of the Blood Transfusion Task Force. Guidelines for the use of fresh frozen plasma. *Transfus Med* 1992; **2:** 57–63.
5. Cohen H. Avoiding the misuse of fresh frozen plasma. *Br Med J* 1993; **307:** 395–6.
6. Fresh-frozen Plasma, Cryoprecipitate, and Platelets Administration Practice Guidelines Development Task Force of the College of American Pathologists. Practice parameter for the use of fresh-frozen plasma, cryoprecipitate, and platelets. *JAMA* 1994; **271:** 777–81.

Hereditary angioedema. For a mention of fresh frozen plasma being used in hereditary angioedema, see p.729.

Neonatal intraventricular haemorrhage. Plasma volume expansion in preterm neonates has been thought to help prevent neonatal intraventricular haemorrhage (p.709). However, a study using plasma or gelatin as plasma volume expanders,[1,2] found no evidence of a decreased risk of such haemorrhage or subsequent death or disability.

1. The Northern Neonatal Nursing Initiative Trial Group. A randomized trial comparing the effect of prophylactic intravenous fresh frozen plasma, gelatin or glucose on early mortality and morbidity in preterm babies. *Eur J Pediatr* 1996; **155:** 580–8.
2. Northern Neonatal Nursing Initiative Trial Group. Randomised trial of prophylactic early fresh-frozen plasma or gelatin or glucose in preterm babies: outcome at 2 years. *Lancet* 1996; **348:** 229–32.

Plasma exchange. Therapeutic plasma exchange or plasmapheresis has been tried in a number of disorders, including many with an immunological basis, when conventional treatment has not been successful. The aim is removal or reduction of those constituents of plasma causing or aggravating a disease or replacement of deficient plasma factors if the deficiency is the cause of the disorder. Volume and frequency of plasma exchange is determined by the pathophysiology of the undesirable plasma constituent. For example, removal of antibody usually requires exchange of 1.5 times the estimated plasma volume (3 to 4 litres) repeated daily or on alternate days until the desired reduction is obtained. Technological developments, such as the use of specific adsorbents and the use of multiple filters with different pore sizes, may enable removal of only the desired constituent and avoid removal and subsequent replacement of total plasma.

References.

1. Urbaniak SJ, Robinson EA. Therapeutic apheresis. In: Contreras M, ed. *ABC of transfusion*. 2nd ed. London: BMJ Publishing Group, 1992: 53–6.
2. Robinson EA. Apheresis in the 1990s. *Br Med J* 1993; **307:** 578–9.

Thrombotic microangiopathies. Thrombotic thrombocytopenic purpura and haemolytic-uraemic syndrome are both syndromes characterised by intravascular platelet clumping.[1,2] Thrombocytopenia also occurs and fragmentation of erythrocytes, partly caused by the red cells passing through areas of the microvasculature occluded by the platelet aggregation, leads to microvascular haemolytic anaemia.

In **thrombotic thrombocytopenic purpura** (TTP) the platelet aggregation is extensive and obstructs the vessels of various organs producing ischaemia or even infarction. The central nervous system, notably the brain, is often the area predominantly affected although some degree of renal involvement may occur in over 50% of cases. It is an uncommon disorder; adult women, in whom the condition presents as a chronic relapsing illness, are slightly more frequently affected.

In **haemolytic-uraemic syndrome** (HUS) the platelet aggregation is relatively less widespread and less severe and mainly affects the renal microvasculature although extra-renal manifestations may also occur. The primary consequences of HUS are hypertension and acute renal insufficiency or ultimately, if untreated, renal failure. Most cases of HUS occur in early childhood and follow a diarrhoeal illness caused by *Shigella dysenteriae* or *Escherichia coli*. The condition is though becoming increasingly recognised in adults, particularly the elderly. Some cases may be drug induced. With appropriate symptomatic therapy HUS is typically a self-limiting disease with spontaneous recovery although fatalities have been known.

The **management** of both syndromes follows similar lines. In HUS, or TTP with renal symptoms, special attention needs to be directed towards the prevention of renal failure. If hypovolaemia has occurred due to preceding diarrhoeal illness it should be corrected,[2] and as oliguria is common crystalloids and frusemide intravenously should be given to induce a diuresis. This will usually maintain renal function and, if performed early enough, avoid the need for dialysis;[2,3] if renal failure is already established haemodialysis will need to be started. Severe anaemia requires blood transfusion.[2] Hypertension can usually be controlled by conventional means.[2]

Specific therapies for both conditions include the administration of fresh frozen plasma.[2,4] The mechanism of action is unclear, as is the optimum dose although amounts in the region of 1 litre daily are suggested. An alternative to direct infusion of plasma is plasma exchange (plasmapheresis).[2] A comparison of plasma infusion with plasma exchange[5] found no difference in outcome when similar plasma volumes were delivered. Plasma exchange may be the preferred method in patients with impaired renal function and fluid overload, and in oliguric patients with HUS may be the only way of administering enough plasma.

Antiplatelet therapy and corticosteroids are often given, although neither have been subject to detailed investigation. Improved outcome with antiplatelet drugs has been noted in patients with TTP but not in those with HUS;[2] however, the failures in the latter case may have been due to late administration. Some reports have described improved outcome in both syndromes with corticosteroids.[6]

Other drugs may also be used. Administration of epoprostenol may be tried[2] in order to inhibit platelet-endothelial interactions and to help promote diuresis but again has not been subject to controlled studies; anecdotal evidence presents both favourable[7,8] and negative[9,10] results. Alteplase has been used successfully in one patient with HUS.[11] Improved outcome has been reported with vincristine,[12,13] or normal immunoglobulin[14] as part of the overall management strategy. In chronic relapsing forms of the disorder immunosuppressants may be tried.[2] Splenectomy may also be considered.[4]

1. Moake JL. Haemolytic-uraemic syndrome: basic science. *Lancet* 1994; **343:** 393–7.
2. Neild GH. Haemolytic-uraemic syndrome in practice. *Lancet* 1994; **343:** 398–401. Correction. *ibid.*; 552.
3. Rousseau E, *et al.* Decreased necessity for dialysis with loop diuretic therapy in hemolytic uremic syndrome. *Clin Nephrol* 1990; **34:** 22–5.
4. Gillis S. The thrombocytopenic purpuras: recognition and management. *Drugs* 1996; **51:** 942–53.
5. Novitzky N, *et al.* The treatment of thrombotic thrombocytopenic purpura: plasma infusion or exchange? *Br J Haematol* 1994; **87:** 317–20.
6. Bell WR, *et al.* Improved survival in thrombotic thrombocytopenic purpura-hemolytic uremic syndrome: clinical experience in 108 patients. *N Engl J Med* 1991; **325:** 398–403.
7. Fitzgerald GA, *et al.* Intravenous prostacyclin in thrombotic thrombocytopenic purpura. *Ann Intern Med* 1981; **95:** 319–22.
8. Payton CD, *et al.* Successful treatment of thrombotic thrombocytopenic purpura by epoprostenol infusion. *Lancet* 1985; **i:** 927–8.
9. Budd GT, *et al.* Prostacyclin therapy of thrombotic thrombocytopenic purpura. *Lancet* 1980: **ii:** 915.
10. Johnson JE, *et al.* Ineffective epoprostenol therapy for thrombotic thrombocytopenic purpura. *JAMA* 1983; **250:** 3089–91.
11. Kruez W, *et al.* Successful treatment of haemolytic-uraemic syndrome with recombinant tissue-type plasminogen activator. *Lancet* 1993; **341:** 1665–6.
12. Gutterman LA, *et al.* The hemolytic-uremic syndrome: recovery after treatment with vincristine. *Ann Intern Med* 1983; **98:** 612–13.
13. Wolf G, *et al.* Behandlung einer thrombotisch-thrombo-zytopenischen purpura (morbus Moschcowitz) mit vincristin. *Dtsch Med Wochenschr* 1995; **120:** 442–6.
14. Sheth KJ, *et al.* High-dose intravenous gamma globulin infusions in hemolytic-uremic syndrome: a preliminary report. *Am J Dis Child* 1990: **144:** 268–70.

Preparations

Proprietary Preparations (details are given in Part 3)
Aust.: Octaplas; ***Ger.:*** Octaplas; ***UK:*** Octaplas.

Plasma Protein Fraction (1248-d)

Plasma Protein Fraction (USP 23) is a sterile preparation of serum albumin and globulin obtained by fractionating material (blood, plasma, or serum) from healthy human donors, the source material being tested for the absence of hepatitis B surface antigen. It contains 5% of protein; not less than 83% of the total protein is albumin; not more than 17% is alpha and beta globulins; not more than 1% has the electrophoretic properties of gamma globulin. It contains sodium acetyltryptophanate with or without sodium caprylate as a stabilising agent but no antimicrobial preservative. It contains 130 to 160 mmol of sodium per litre, and not more than 2 mmol of potassium per litre.

Uses and Administration

Plasma protein fraction consists mainly of albumin with a small proportion of globulins. It has properties and uses similar to those of other albumin solutions (p.710). It is administered intravenously as a solution containing 4 to 5% of total protein. The amount of plasma protein fraction administered will depend upon the clinical condition of the patient. For most indications an initial infusion of up to 500 mL for adults has been suggested at a rate not normally exceeding 10 mL per minute. Patients with normal blood volume may require slower rates of administration to prevent excessive volume expansion. In hypoproteinaemia administration of 1.0 to 1.5 litres of a 5% solution will provide 50 to 75 g of protein. A suggested dose in infants and small children for shock with dehydration is up to 33 mL per kg body-weight administered at a rate of up to 5 to 10 mL per minute.

As with other albumin solutions, plasma protein fraction should not be used for parenteral nutrition.

It does not contain blood-clotting factors.

Preparations

USP 23: Plasma Protein Fraction.

Proprietary Preparations (details are given in Part 3)
Aust.: Biseko; ***Canad.:*** Plasmanate; ***Ger.:*** Biseko; Serumar†; ***Ital.:*** Haimaserum; Plasmaviral; PPS; Uman-Serum; ***S.Afr.:*** Bioplasma FDP; ***UK:*** Plasmatein†; ***USA:*** Plasma-Plex; Plasmanate; Plasmatein; Protenate.

Platelets (1221-l)

Platelet Concentrate (USP 23) contains the platelets taken from plasma obtained by whole blood collection, plasmapheresis, or plateletpheresis from a single suitable human donor. The platelets are suspended in a specified volume (20 to 30 mL, or 30 to 50 mL) of the original plasma. The suspension contains not less than 5.5×10^{10} platelets per unit in not less than 75% of the units tested. It should be stored in hermetically-sealed sterile containers at 20° to 24° (30 to 50 mL volume), or at 1° to 6° (20 to 30 mL volume) except during transport when the temperature may be 1° to 10°. The expiration time is not more than 72 hours from the time of collection of the source material. Continuous gentle agitation must be maintained if stored at 20° to 24°. The suspension must be used within 4 hours of opening the container.

Adverse Effects and Precautions

Transmission of infection has been associated with the transfusion of blood products including platelets (p.713). Since platelets are stored at room temperature there is increased risk of bacterial infection following transfusion. Transfusion reactions including fever and urticaria are not uncommon. Recipients of multiple transfusions of platelet concentrates from random donors may develop antibodies to HLA which result in impaired responsiveness to subsequent transfusions. Platelet concentrates prepared from RhD-positive donors should generally not be given to RhD-negative women of child-bearing potential. Ideally platelet concentrates should also be ABO-compatible with the recipient.

ABO compatibility. A discussion[1] of ABO incompatibility and platelet transfusions concluded that, while ABO compatibility is desirable, it is better to transfuse incompatible platelets than none at all. However, acute haemolysis has occurred[2] after transfusion of platelet concentrate with high-titre anti-A. Increased use of single-donor, machine-harvested material from panels of regular platelet donors should make screening for high-titre isoagglutinins more practical.[1]

1. Anonymous. ABO incompatibility and platelet transfusion. *Lancet* 1990; **335:** 142–3.
2. Murphy MF, *et al.* Acute haemolysis after ABO-incompatible platelet transfusion. *Lancet* 1990; **335:** 974–5.

HLA antibodies. Platelets obtained from single donors have been used in patients receiving multiple transfusions of platelet concentrates to reduce the formation of antibodies to HLA. Leucocyte-depleted platelets and UVB-irradiated platelets have also been tried. A study[1] in 530 patients found that the incidence of platelet refractoriness was reduced from 13% of those patients receiving pooled platelet concentrates to 3% and 5% of those receiving leucocyte-depleted and UVB-irradiated platelets, respectively.

1. The Trial to Reduce Alloimmunization to Platelets Study Group. Leukocyte reduction and ultraviolet B irradiation of platelets to prevent alloimmunization and refractoriness to platelet transfusions. *N Engl J Med* 1997; **337:** 1861–9.

Uses and Administration

Blood platelets assist in the clotting process (p.704) by aggregation to form a platelet thrombus and by participating in the formation of thromboplastin.

Transfusions of platelet concentrates are given to patients with thrombocytopenic haemorrhage (see p.707). They are also given prophylactically to reduce the frequency of haemorrhage in thrombocytopenia associated with the chemotherapy of neoplastic disease.

References.

1. Hows JM, Brozović B. Platelet and granulocyte transfusions. In: Contreras M, ed. *ABC of transfusion*. 2nd ed. London: BMJ Publishing Group, 1992: 14–17.
2. Fresh-frozen Plasma, Cryoprecipitate, and Platelets Administration Practice Guidelines Development Task Force of the College of American Pathologists. Practice parameter for the use of fresh-frozen plasma, cryoprecipitate, and platelets. *JAMA* 1994; **271:** 777–81.

Preparations

USP 23: Platelet Concentrate.

Polygeline (5449-a)

Polygeline *(BAN, pINN).*

Polygelinum.

CAS — 9015-56-9.

Polygeline is a polymer prepared by cross-linking polypeptides derived from denatured gelatin with a di-isocyanate to form urea bridges.

Intravenous preparations of polygeline contain calcium ions and are incompatible with citrated blood.

Adverse Effects

As for Gelatin, p.723.

Complement activation. For a report of complement activation by polygeline, see Hetastarch, p.724.

Hypersensitivity. Fatal reactions following polygeline infusion have been reported in 2 patients with bronchial asthma.[1,2] In both cases, the patients were undergoing epidural analgesia with bupivacaine. Polygeline was administered to correct hypotension which had not responded to Hartmann's solution. Both patients developed refractory bronchospasm and cardiac arrhythmias and died despite intensive resuscitation attempts. One patient also developed focal seizures.[2]

The manufacturer recommends that prophylaxis with histamine H_1 or H_2 receptor antagonists should be given to patients with known allergic conditions such as asthma. Similar advice has recently been offered by Lorenz *et al.*[3] for patients undergoing anaesthesia and receiving polygeline following their findings of an increased incidence of severe histamine-related reactions in such patients.

1. Freeman MK. Fatal reaction to haemaccel. *Anaesthesia* 1979; **34:** 341–3.
2. Barratt S, Purcell GJ. Refractory bronchospasm following "Haemaccel" infusion and bupivacaine epidural anaesthesia. *Anaesth Intensive Care* 1988; **16:** 208–11.
3. Lorenz W, *et al.* Incidence and clinical importance of perioperative histamine release: randomised study of volume loading and antihistamines after induction of anaesthesia. *Lancet* 1994; **343:** 933–40.

Precautions

Precautions that should be observed with plasma expanders are described under Dextran 70, p.717, and these should be considered when polygeline is used for this purpose.

Preparations containing calcium ions should be used with caution in patients being treated with cardiac glycosides.

Renal impairment. In a study[1] in 52 patients with normal or impaired renal function given 500 mL of polygeline 3.5% about 50% of the dose was excreted in the urine within 48 hours in those with normal renal function. Excretion was not impaired in those with a glomerular filtration rate (GFR) of 31 to 90 mL per minute, slightly reduced in those with a GFR of 11 to 30 mL, reduced to 27% in 48 hours in those with a GFR of 2 to 10 mL, and to 9.3% in 48 hours in those with a GFR of 0.5 to 2 mL. The mean half-life of the elimination phase was 505 minutes in those with adequate renal function, increasing to 985 minutes in those with end-stage renal failure. Polygeline 500 mL of 3.5% solution could be given twice weekly for 1 to 2 months even in patients with total anuria.

1. Köhler H, *et al.* Elimination of hexamethylene diisocyanate cross-linked polypeptides in patients with normal or impaired renal function. *Eur J Clin Pharmacol* 1978; **14:** 405–12.

Pharmacokinetics

Like gelatin, polygeline is excreted mainly in the urine.

Uses and Administration

Polygeline is a plasma volume expander used as a 3.5% solution with electrolytes in the management of hypovolaemic shock (p.798). The rate of infusion depends on the condition of the patient and does not normally exceed 500 mL in 60 minutes although it may be greater in emergencies. Initial doses for hypovolaemic shock usually consist of 500 to 1000 mL; up to 1500 mL of blood loss can be replaced by polygeline alone. Patients losing greater volumes of blood will require blood transfusion as well as plasma expanders.

Polygeline is also used in extracorporeal perfusion fluids, as a perfusion fluid for isolated organs, as fluid replacement in plasma exchange, and as a carrier solution for insulin. For plasma exchange, up to 2 litres of polygeline may be given as sole replacement fluid.

Preparations

Proprietary Preparations (details are given in Part 3)
Aust.: Haemaccel; ***Austral.:*** Haemaccel; ***Belg.:*** Haemaccel; ***Fr.:*** Haemaccel; ***Ger.:*** Haemaccel; ***Irl.:*** Haemaccel; ***Ital.:*** Emagel; Gelplex; ***Neth.:*** Haemaccel; ***Norw.:*** Haemaccel; ***S.Afr.:*** Haemaccel; ***Swed.:*** Haemaccel; ***Switz.:*** Haemaccel; ***UK:*** Haemaccel.

Protein C (247-j)

Protein C is an endogenous inhibitor of blood coagulation that is under investigation in thrombo-embolic disorders.

References.

1. Rintala E, *et al.* Protein C in the treatment of coagulopathy in meningococcal disease. *Lancet* 1996; **347:** 1767.
2. Smith OP, *et al.* Use of protein-C concentrate, heparin, and haemodiafiltration in meningococcus-induced purpura fulminans. *Lancet* 1997; **350:** 1590–3.

Red Blood Cells (1218-k)

Red Blood Cells (USP 23) is the remaining red blood cells of whole human blood from suitable donors, from which plasma has been removed. It is prepared not later than 21 days after the blood has been withdrawn except that the period may be 35 days if the anticoagulant used was acid citrate dextrose adenine solution. If intended for extended manufacturer's storage at or below −65° it contains a portion of the plasma sufficient to ensure cell preservation, or a cryophylactic substance. It should be stored in hermetically-sealed sterile containers; store if unfrozen at 1° to 6° (with a range of not more than 2°) except during transport when the temperature may be 1° to 10°. The expiration date of unfrozen Red Blood Cells is not later than that of the whole human blood from which it is derived if plasma has not been removed, unless the hermetic seal is broken, in which case it should be used within 24 hours. The expiration date of frozen Red Blood Cells is not later than 3 years after the date of collection of the source blood when stored at or below -65° and not later than 24 hours after removal from -65° provided that it is then stored at the temperature for unfrozen Red Blood Cells. Red Blood Cells should be administered using equipment incorporating a filter.

Adverse Effects and Precautions

As for Blood, p.713.

Patients with sickle-cell anaemia frequently require repeated transfusions of red blood cells. Alloimmunisation is a common problem in these patients. Alloantibodies were detected in 32 of 107 black patients with sickle-cell anaemia who had received red cell transfusions compared with 1 of 19 non black patients who had received transfusions for other chronic anaemias.[1] The incidence of antibody formation was related to the number of transfusions received. An analysis of the red-cell phenotypes suggested that the high rate of alloimmunisation among patients with sickle-cell anaemia could be due to racial differences between donors and recipients.

1. Vichinsky EP, *et al.* Alloimmunization in sickle cell anemia and transfusion of racially unmatched blood. *N Engl J Med* 1990; **322:** 1617–21.

Uses and Administration

Transfusions of red blood cells are given for the treatment of severe anaemia without hypovolaemia (p.701).

Red blood cells are also used for exchange transfusion in babies with haemolytic disease of the newborn (p.1503). Red cells may be used with volume expanders for acute blood loss of less than half of the blood volume; if more than half of the blood volume has been lost, whole blood should be used.

Other red blood cell products are available. Concentrated red cells in an optimal additive solution containing sodium chloride, adenine, glucose, and mannitol has reduced viscosity and an extended shelf-life. Leucocyte depleted red cells may be used in patients who have developed antibodies to previous transfusions or in whom development of antibodies is undesirable. Frozen, thawed, and washed red cell concentrates in which plasma proteins are removed in addition to leucocytes and platelets may be used in patients with rare antibodies.

References.

1. Davies SC, Brozović M. Transfusion of red cells. In: Contreras M, ed. *ABC of transfusion*. 2nd ed. London: BMJ Publishing Group, 1992: 9–13.
2. Flanagan P. Red cell transfusions including autologous transfusion. *Prescribers' J* 1992; **32:** 15–21.
3. Welch HG, *et al.* Prudent strategies for elective red blood cell transfusion. *Ann Intern Med* 1992; **116:** 393–402.
4. American College of Physicians. Practice strategies for elective red blood cell transfusion. *Ann Intern Med* 1992; **116:** 403–6.
5. Royal College of Physicians of Edinburgh. Consensus statement on red cell transfusion. *Br J Anaesth* 1994; **73:** 857–9.

Preparations

USP 23: Red Blood Cells.

Sargramostim (14745-e)

Sargramostim *(BAN, USAN, rINN).*

BI-61.012; rhu GM-CSF. A recombinant human granulocyte-macrophage colony-stimulating factor; 23-L-Leucinecolony-stimulating factor 2 (human clone pHG_{25} protein moiety).

CAS — 123774-72-1.

Pharmacopoeias. In *US.*

Sargramostim is a glycosylated protein produced by recombinant DNA synthesis in yeast culture. It consists of 127 amino acids. **Store** in sealed containers at a temperature of −20° or below.

Albumin must be added to give a final concentration of 1 mg per mL to solutions for injection that are diluted to concentrations below 10 μg of sargramostim per mL.

Adverse Effects and Precautions

As for Colony-stimulating Factors, p.714.

Uses and Administration

Sargramostim is a granulocyte-macrophage colony-stimulating factor (p.715). It is used to treat or prevent neutropenia in patients receiving myelosuppressive cancer chemotherapy and to reduce the period of neutropenia in patients undergoing bone marrow transplantation (p.474). It is also used to mobilise autologous peripheral blood progenitor cells for an alternative to bone marrow transplantation.

As an adjunct to antineoplastic therapy, sargramostim is given by intravenous infusion over 4 hours in a dose of 250 μg per m^2 body-surface area daily for up to 42 days as required.

Following bone marrow transplantation, sargramostim may be given in a dose of 250 μg per m^2 daily by intravenous infusion over 2 hours. The dose may be increased to 500 μg per m^2 daily if engraftment is delayed.

For mobilisation of peripheral blood progenitor cells a dose of 250 μg per m^2 daily is given by continuous intravenous infusion over 24 hours or by subcutaneous injection.

Preparations

USP 23: Sargramostim for Injection.

Proprietary Preparations (details are given in Part 3)
Aust.: Interberin; ***USA:*** Leukine; Prokine†.

Thrombin (1250-k)

Factor IIa.

CAS — 9002-04-4.

Thrombin (USP 23) is a sterile, freeze-dried powder derived from bovine plasma containing the protein substance prepared from prothrombin through interaction with added thromboplastin in the presence of calcium. It is capable, without the addition of other substances, of causing the clotting of whole blood, plasma, or a solution of fibrinogen. It should be stored at 2° to 8°. Once reconstituted, solutions should be used within a few hours of preparation. The label should state that the prepared solution should not be injected into or otherwise allowed to enter large blood vessels.

Adverse Effects and Precautions

Hypersensitivity reactions, including anaphylaxis, have occurred rarely. Thrombin solutions must not be injected into blood vessels.

Effects on the blood. Repeated exposure to thrombin preparations of bovine origin has led to the development of antibodies to bovine thrombin and factor V with cross-reactivity, in some cases, to human factors.[1-3] The presence of inhibitors to human factors may produce bleeding abnormalities and interfere with clotting measurements.

1. Rapaport SI, *et al.* Clinical significance of antibodies to bovine and human thrombin and factor V after surgical use of bovine thrombin. *Am J Clin Pathol* 1992; **97:** 84–91.
2. Bänninger H, *et al.* Fibrin glue in surgery: frequent development of inhibitors of bovine thrombin and human factor V. *Br J Haematol* 1993; **85:** 528–32.
3. Ortel TL, *et al.* Topical thrombin and acquired coagulation factor inhibitors: clinical spectrum and laboratory diagnosis. *Am J Hematol* 1994; **45:** 128–35.

Uses and Administration

Thrombin is a protein substance produced *in vivo* from prothrombin that converts soluble fibrinogen into insoluble fibrin thus producing coagulation (p.704).

Thrombin of either human or bovine origin is applied topically to control bleeding from capillaries and small venules. It is applied directly to the bleeding surface either as a solution or dry powder. It may also be used in conjunction with absorbable gelatin sponge during surgical procedures.

Thrombin is a component of fibrin glue (p.722).

Preparations

Ph. Eur.: Fibrin Sealant Kit;
USP 23: Thrombin.

Proprietary Preparations (details are given in Part 3)
Austral.: Thrombinar†; Thrombostat; ***Canad.:*** Thrombostat; ***Ger.:*** Thrombocoll; Topostasin†; ***Ital.:*** Topostasin†; Zimotrombina; ***USA:*** Thrombinar; Thrombogen; Thrombostat.

Multi-ingredient: ***Aust.:*** Beriplast; TachoComb; Tissucol; Tissucol Duo Quick; ***Belg.:*** Tissucol; ***Canad.:*** Tisseel†; ***Fr.:*** Biocol; ***Ger.:*** Beriplast; TachoComb; Tissucol Duo S; Tissucol Fibrinkleber tiefgefroren; Tissucol-Kit; ***Irl.:*** Tisseel; ***Ital.:*** Kanatrombina†; Tissucol; ***S.Afr.:*** Tisseel; ***Spain:*** Tissucol; ***Swed.:*** Tisseel Duo Quick; ***Switz.:*** Tissucol; ***UK:*** Tisseel.

Thromboplastin (1251-a)

Cytozyme; Thrombokinase.

Preparations of thromboplastin have been used as haemostatics.

A preparation of thromboplastin derived from rabbit brain is employed in the determination of the prothrombin time for the control of anticoagulant therapy (for further details see under Warfarin Sodium, p.969).

The term factor III is used to denote tissue thromboplastin that is released from damaged tissue and initiates coagulation (p.704). The term thromboplastin may also be applied to other related substances with similar activity. Commercial preparations may contain tissue extracts comprising a variety of such substances.

Preparations

Proprietary Preparations (details are given in Part 3)
Fr.: Hemostatique Erce†.

Thrombopoietin (17553-b)

Thrombopoietin is a naturally occurring colony-stimulating factor (p.714) that regulates thrombopoiesis. Recombinant thrombopoietin is under investigation for the management of thrombocytopenia in patients receiving myelosuppressive chemotherapy. A form of recombinant thrombopoietin conjugated with polyethylene glycol (PEG-megakaryocyte growth and development factor, PEG-MGDF) has also been investigated.

References.

1. Basser RL, *et al.* Thrombopoietic effects of pegylated recombinant human megakaryocyte growth and development factor (PEG-rHuMGDF) in patients with advanced cancer. *Lancet* 1996; **348:** 1279–81.
2. Fanucchi M, *et al.* Effects of polyethylene glycol-conjugated recombinant human megakaryocyte growth and development factor on platelet counts after chemotherapy for lung cancer. *N Engl J Med* 1997; **336:** 404–9.
3. Vadhan-Raj S, *et al.* Stimulation of megakaryocyte and platelet production by a single dose of recombinant human thrombopoietin in patients with cancer. *Ann Intern Med* 1997; **126:** 673–81.
4. Kaushansky K. Thrombopoietin: platelets on demand? *Ann Intern Med* 1997; **126:** 731–3.
5. Kaushansky K. Thrombopoietin. *N Engl J Med* 1998; **339:** 746–54.

Tranexamic Acid (1726-j)

Tranexamic Acid *(BAN, USAN, rINN).*

Acidum Tranexamicum; AMCA; *trans*-AMCHA; CL-65336.

trans-4-(Aminomethyl)cyclohexanecarboxylic acid.

$C_8H_{15}NO_2$ = 157.2.

CAS — 1197-18-8.

Pharmacopoeias. In *Chin., Eur.* (see p.viii), and *Jpn.*

A white crystalline powder. Freely **soluble** in water and in glacial acetic acid; practically insoluble in alcohol and in ether. A 5% solution in water has a pH of 6.5 to 8.0. Solutions of tranexamic acid are **incompatible** with benzylpenicillin.

Adverse Effects

Tranexamic acid appears to be well tolerated. It can produce dose-related gastro-intestinal disturbances. Hypotension has occurred, particularly after rapid intravenous administration. Thrombotic complications have been reported in patients receiving tranexamic acid, but these are usually a consequence of its inappropriate use (see under Precautions, below). Manufacturers of tranexamic acid report that there have been a few instances of transient disturbance of colour vision associated with its use.

A patient undergoing regular peritoneal dialysis for Epstein's syndrome developed ligneous conjunctivitis, gingival hyperplasia, and peritoneal protein loss associated with the use of tranexamic acid.[1]

1. Diamond JP, *et al.* Tranexamic acid-associated ligneous conjunctivitis with gingival and peritoneal lesions. *Br J Ophthalmol* 1991; **75:** 753–4.

Effects on the skin. A widespread, patchy rash with associated blisters, considered on skin biopsy to be a fixed-drug eruption, occurred in a 33-year-old woman.[1] Tranexamic acid that she had taken for eight years and that had been well tolerated was identified as the causative agent. Desensitisation was attempted but was unsuccessful. Tranexamic acid was also suspected as being the cause of a fixed-drug eruption in a 36-year-old woman.[2] Pruritic, vesicle-bullous lesions appeared within a few hours of commencing treatment with tranexamic acid and the lesions resolved completely three days after discontinuing therapy even though other drug treatment was continued.

1. Kavanagh GM, *et al.* Tranexamic acid (Cyklokapron®)-induced fixed-drug eruption. *Br J Dermatol* 1993; **128:** 229–30.
2. Carrión-Carrión C, *et al.* Bullous eruption induced by tranexamic acid. *Ann Pharmacother* 1994; **28:** 1305–6.

Precautions

Tranexamic acid should not be used in patients with active intravascular clotting because of the risk of thrombosis. Patients with a predisposition to thrombosis are also at risk if given antifibrinolytic therapy. Haemorrhage due to disseminated intravascular coagulation should therefore not be treated with antifibrinolytic compounds unless the condition is predominantly due to disturbances in fibrinolytic mechanisms; tranexamic acid has been used when the latter conditions are met, but with careful monitoring and anticoagulant cover.

Lysis of existing extravascular clots may be inhibited in patients receiving tranexamic acid. Clots in the renal system can lead to intrarenal obstruction, so caution is required in the treatment of patients with haematuria. Doses of tranexamic acid should be reduced in patients with renal impairment (see Uses and Administration, below). The manufacturers recommend that regular eye examinations and liver function tests should be performed if tranexamic acid is used long term.

Some studies have suggested that tranexamic acid when given to patients following a subarachnoid haemorrhage increases the incidence of cerebral ischaemic complications (see Haemorrhagic Disorders under Uses, below).

Rapid intravenous administration may be associated with adverse effects (see above).

Interactions

Drugs with actions on haemostasis should be given with caution to patients on antifibrinolytic therapy. The potential for thrombus formation may be increased by oestrogens, for example, or the action of the antifibrinolytic antagonised by compounds such as the thrombolytics.

Pharmacokinetics

Tranexamic acid is absorbed from the gastro-intestinal tract with peak plasma concentrations occurring after about 3 hours. Bioavailability is about 30 to 50%. Tranexamic acid is widely distributed throughout the body and has very low protein binding. It diffuses across the placenta and is distributed into breast milk. Tranexamic acid has a plasma elimination half-life of about 2 hours. It is excreted in the urine mainly as unchanged drug.

References.

1. Andersson L, *et al.* Role of urokinase and tissue activator in sustaining bleeding and the management thereof with EACA and AMCA. *Ann N Y Acad Sci* 1968; **146:** 642–56.
2. Kullander S, Nilsson IM. Human placental transfer of an antifibrinolytic agent (AMCA). *Acta Obstet Gynecol Scand* 1970; **49:** 241–2.
3. Pilbrant Å, *et al.* Pharmacokinetics and bioavailability of tranexamic acid. *Eur J Clin Pharmacol* 1981; **20:** 65–72.

Uses and Administration

Tranexamic acid is an antifibrinolytic drug (p.704) which inhibits breakdown of fibrin clots. It acts primarily by blocking the binding of plasminogen and plasmin to fibrin; direct inhibition of plasmin occurs only to a limited degree. Tranexamic acid is used in the treatment and prophylaxis of haemorrhage associated with excessive fibrinolysis. It is also used in the prophylaxis of hereditary angioedema.

Tranexamic acid is given by mouth and by slow intravenous injection or continuous infusion. Administration by injection is usually changed to oral administration after a few days. Alternatively, an initial intravenous injection may be followed by continuous infusion. Oral doses are 1 to 1.5 g (or 15 to 25 mg per kg body-weight) 2 to 4 times daily. When given by slow intravenous injection doses are 0.5 to 1 g (or 10 to 15 mg per kg) 3 times daily. Tranexamic acid is administered by continuous infusion at a rate of 25 to 50 mg per kg daily. These doses are used in the short term for haemorrhage. Tranexamic acid is given for prolonged periods in hereditary angioedema in doses of 1 to 1.5 g by mouth 2 or 3 times a day.

Children may be given doses of 25 mg per kg by mouth or 10 mg per kg intravenously usually administered 2 or 3 times daily.

Reduced doses suggested by the UK manufacturer for patients with renal impairment and having serum-creatinine concentrations of 120 to 250, 250 to 500, and greater than 500 nmol per mL are: oral doses of 25 mg per kg twice daily, 25 mg per kg once daily, and 12.5 mg per kg once daily, respectively; intravenous doses of 10 mg per kg twice daily, 10 mg per kg once daily, and 5 mg per kg once daily, respectively.

Solutions of tranexamic acid have been applied topically, for example as a bladder irrigation or mouthwash.

Haemorrhagic disorders. Tranexamic acid, aminocaproic acid, and aminomethylbenzoic acid are structurally related synthetic antifibrinolytic drugs that block the binding of plasminogen and plasmin to fibrin, thereby preventing dissolution of the haemostatic plug. Tranexamic acid is also a direct, but weak, inhibitor of plasmin.[1,2] A plasma concentration of tranexamic acid of 5 to 10 μg per mL has been considered necessary for effective inhibition of fibrinolysis.[1]

Antifibrinolytics are used to control haemorrhage which is considered to be caused by excessive fibrinolysis. Antifibrinolytic therapy may also be indicated in the prevention of rebleeding in some haemorrhagic conditions, the rationale being to retard dissolution of the haemostatic plug formed in response to vascular injury.[1,2]

In haemorrhage caused by a congenital or acquired deficiency of blood coagulation factors (p.707), haemostatic drugs have a secondary role and may be useful in reducing requirements of factor concentrates.[2] The most established use of antifibrinolytic agents in these conditions is in the prophylaxis of bleeding after dental procedures in haemophiliacs.[1,2] A standard regimen is the intravenous administration of tranexamic acid 10 mg per kg body-weight given pre-operatively with factor VIII or factor IX. Tranexamic acid is continued postoperatively in a dose of 25 mg per kg 3 or 4 times daily by mouth for up to 8 days. Some workers have found that local treatment with a 4.8% solution of tranexamic acid as a mouthwash is a useful addition to systemic therapy.[3] A similar approach using tranexamic acid mouthwashes has been used to reduce the risk of bleeding after oral surgery in patients on anticoagulant therapy.[4] Treatment with tranexamic acid may prove beneficial in patients with other congenital bleeding disorders such as α_2-antiplasmin deficiency.[5,6] Aminocaproic acid has been tried in a few patients with hereditary haemorrhagic telangiectasia with mixed results.[7,8] Benefit from treatment with aminocaproic acid or tranexamic acid has been reported in coagulopathies with thrombocytopenia[9,10] and acute promyelocytic leukaemia.[11]

Tranexamic acid and aminocaproic acid have each been used in an attempt to prevent rebleeding in patients with subarachnoid haemorrhage (p.799), particularly if surgery is to be delayed. However, while rebleeding may be reduced, there can be an increase in the incidence of ischaemic complications resulting in little overall improvement in outcome.[1] Paradoxically, rebleeding has been noted in patients given high doses of aminocaproic acid after subarachnoid haemorrhage (see Adverse Effects, Effects on the Blood, under Aminocaproic Acid, p.711). Possible methods of overcoming the ischaemic complications have included the administration of agents such as nimodipine[12] or nicardipine[13] or the use of aprotinin with a low-dose regimen of tranexamic acid.[14]

Tranexamic acid has been used to control haemorrhage of gastro-intestinal origin. Henry and O'Connell[15] carried out a meta-analysis of 6 studies, involving a total of 1267 patients given tranexamic acid for acute upper gastro-intestinal haemorrhage. Treatment with tranexamic acid was associated with a 20 to 30% decrease in the rate of rebleeding, a 30 to 40% decrease in the need for surgery, and a 40% decrease in mortality. However, the validity of the results of one study included in the analysis have been disputed.[16,17] The management of bleeding associated with peptic ulcer disease and varices is discussed on p.1174 and p.1576, respectively.[16]

Tranexamic acid or aminocaproic acid have been suggested to control bleeding in many other conditions. These include haemorrhage after surgical or other procedures including prostatectomy, bladder surgery, and cervical conisation, perioperative blood loss in cardiac surgery, and other conditions associated with excessive fibrinolysis such as menorrhagia (see below), epistaxis, and abruptio placentae.

1. Verstraete M. Clinical application of inhibitors of fibrinolysis. *Drugs* 1985; **29:** 236–61.
2. Verstraete M. Haemostatic drugs. In: Bloom AL, Thomas DP, eds. *Haemostasis and thrombosis.* 2nd ed. London: Churchill Livingstone, 1987: 607–17.
3. Sindet-Pedersen S, *et al.* Management of oral bleeding in haemophilic patients. *Lancet* 1988; **ii:** 566.
4. Sindet-Pedersen S, *et al.* Hemostatic effect of tranexamic acid mouthwash in anticoagulant-treated patients undergoing oral surgery. *N Engl J Med* 1989; **320:** 840–3.
5. Koie K, *et al.* α_2-Plasmin-inhibitor deficiency (Miyasato disease). *Lancet* 1978; **ii:** 1334–6.
6. Kettle P, Mayne EE. A bleeding disorder due to deficiency of α_2-antiplasmin. *J Clin Pathol* 1985; **38:** 428–9.
7. Saba HI, *et al.* Brief report: treatment of bleeding in hereditary hemorrhagic telangiectasia with aminocaproic acid. *N Engl J Med* 1994; **330:** 1789–90.
8. Korzenik JR, *et al.* Treatment of bleeding in hereditary hemorrhagic telangiectasia with aminocaproic acid. *N Engl J Med* 1994; **331:** 1236.
9. Warrell RP, Kempin SJ. Treatment of severe coagulopathy in the Kasabach-Merritt syndrome with aminocaproic acid and cryoprecipitate. *N Engl J Med* 1985; **313:** 309–12.
10. Poon M-C, *et al.* Epsilon-aminocaproic acid in the reversal of consumptive coagulopathy with platelet sequestration in a vascular malformation of Klippel-Trenaunay syndrome. *Am J Med* 1989; **87:** 211–13.
11. Avvisati G, *et al.* Tranexamic acid for control of haemorrhage in acute promyelocytic leukaemia. *Lancet* 1989; **ii:** 122–4.
12. van Gijn J. Subarachnoid haemorrhage. *Lancet* 1992; **339:** 653–5.
13. Beck DW, *et al.* Combination of aminocaproic acid and nicardipine in treatment of aneurysmal subarachnoid hemorrhage. *Stroke* 1988; **19:** 63–7.
14. Spallone A, *et al.* Low-dose tranexamic acid combined with aprotinin in the pre-operative management of ruptured intracranial aneurysms. *Neurochirurgia (Stuttg)* 1987; **30:** 172–6.
15. Henry DA, O'Connell DL. Effects of fibrinolytic inhibitors on mortality from upper gastrointestinal haemorrhage. *Br Med J* 1989; **298:** 1142–6.
16. Brown C, Rees WDW. Drug treatment for acute upper gastrointestinal bleeding. *Br Med J* 1992; **304:** 135–6.
17. Barer D. Drug treatment for acute upper gastrointestinal bleeding. *Br Med J* 1992; **304:** 383.

Hereditary angioedema. Hereditary angioedema, formerly known as hereditary angioneurotic oedema, is a rare autosomal dominant disease caused by either a deficiency of complement C1 esterase inhibitor or, more rarely, a lack of functioning inhibitor.[1,2] The disease presents as episodic attacks of oedema, usually of the extremities and face, and often involving the mucosa of the gastro-intestinal tract producing abdominal pain. A non-pruritic rash may also occur. A few patients develop life-threatening laryngeal oedema. Attacks generally last about 1 to 3 days and may occur as frequently as weekly or there may be years between attacks. The first attack may occur at any age although initial presentation in childhood is most common. Trauma, especially dental surgery, illness, and emotional stress may provoke an attack although often there is no precipitating factor.

Treatment of the acute attack is essentially supportive. If laryngeal oedema is present adrenaline, antihistamines, and corticosteroids may be given (as for Anaphylactic Shock, p.816) even though patients with hereditary angioedema often fail to respond adequately to these. The mainstay of treatment of an acute attack is replacement therapy with complement C1 esterase inhibitor. Fresh frozen plasma has been used although there is a risk of initially exacerbating the oedema due to the presence of other complements in the plasma. Tracheostomy or tracheal intubation may be necessary.

Once the acute attack has subsided most patients will not require further treatment, but those who experience life-threatening attacks, repeated episodes of swelling around the face or neck, or incapacitating attacks require long-term prophylactic therapy. A synthetic androgen (danazol or stanozolol) or an antifibrinolytic (aminocaproic acid or tranexamic acid) is effective for long-term prophylaxis. Danazol and stanozolol raise serum concentrations of C1 esterase inhibitor possibly by enhancing its synthesis in the liver. Aminocaproic acid and tranexamic acid may act by inhibiting plasmin activation. A synthetic androgen is often preferred, with an antifibrinolytic being reserved for patients refractory to or intolerant of androgens. An antifibrinolytic may be preferred in premenopausal women. A combination of an androgen and an antifibrinolytic may be used. These drugs may also be used for short-term prophylaxis in situations expected to provoke an attack, such as surgery involving the head, neck, or respiratory track. Prophylaxis should be started a few days before the procedure. Fresh frozen plasma has also been used in situations likely to precipitate an attack.

1. Sim TC, Grant JA. Hereditary angioedema: its diagnostic and management perspectives. *Am J Med* 1990; **88:** 656–64.
2. Orphan NA, Kolski GB. Angioedema and C1 inhibitor deficiency. *Ann Allergy* 1992; **69:** 167–72.

Menorrhagia. Tranexamic acid may be considered in women with menorrhagia (p.1461) who are anaemic, or for whom NSAIDs are ineffective. It is effective in reducing uterine blood loss in such women when administered during menstruation.[1-3] A recent comparative trial[1] found tranexamic acid to be more effective than the NSAID mefenamic acid, a commonly used treatment for the condition. It is also more effective than cyclical norethisterone,[2] (although less so than a progesterone-releasing intrauterine device[3]).

1. Bonnar J, Sheppard BL. Treatment of menorrhagia during menstruation: randomised controlled trial of ethamsylate, mefenamic acid, and tranexamic acid. *Br Med J* 1996; **313:** 579–82.
2. Preston JT, *et al.* Comparative study of tranexamic acid and norethisterone in the treatment of ovulatory menorrhagia. *Br J Obstet Gynaecol* 1995; **102:** 401–406.
3. Milsom I, *et al.* A comparison of flurbiprofen, tranexamic acid, and a levonorgestrel-releasing intrauterine contraceptive device in the treatment of idiopathic menorrhagia. *Am J Obstet Gynecol* 1991; **164:** 879–83.

Preparations

BP 1998: Tranexamic Acid Injection; Tranexamic Acid Tablets.

Proprietary Preparations (details are given in Part 3)
Aust.: Cyklokapron; ***Austral.:*** Cyklokapron; ***Belg.:*** Exacyl; ***Canad.:*** Cyklokapron; ***Fr.:*** Exacyl; ***Ger.:*** Anvitoff; Cyklokapron; Ugurol; ***Irl.:*** Cyklokapron; ***Ital.:*** Amcacid†; Tranex; Ugurol; ***Jpn:*** Transamin; ***Neth.:*** Cyklokapron; ***Norw.:*** Cyklokapron; ***S.Afr.:*** Cyklokapron; ***Spain:*** Amchafibrin; ***Swed.:*** Cyklo-F; Cyklokapron; ***Switz.:*** Anvitoff; Cyklokapron; ***UK:*** Cyklokapron; ***USA:*** Cyklokapron.

Multi-ingredient: ***Ital.:*** Transil†; ***Spain:*** Caprofides Hemostatico†.

Bone Modulating Drugs

The processes of bone turnover, and the regulation of body calcium, are intimately connected. The concentration of calcium in plasma is normally kept within a narrow range (p.1147) by regulation of the absorption and excretion of calcium, and also by modulation of the normal resorption and formation of bone and hence the movement of calcium to and from the skeletal reservoir. The endogenous substances, parathyroid hormone, calcitonin, and vitamin D, are involved in the regulation of calcium homoeostasis.

Calcitonins and the bisphosphonates inhibit bone resorption and thus have a hypocalcaemic effect. They are therefore used in the treatment of conditions associated with increased bone resorption, such as osteoporosis and Paget's disease of bone, and in the management of hypercalcaemia, especially that associated with malignancy (p.1148). Bisphosphonates have a high affinity for bone and radioactively labelled bisphosphonates are used as bone scanning agents. Gallium nitrate also inhibits bone resorption, and is used for Paget's disease of bone and hypercalcaemia of malignancy.

Parathyroid hormone, which has a hypercalcaemic effect, is under investigation to promote bone formation. It was formerly used in the differential diagnosis of hypoparathyroidism and pseudohypoparathyroidism, but has been replaced by teriparatide, the synthetic 1-34 amino-acid fragment of human parathyroid hormone.

Sodium fluoride and sodium monofluorophosphate are inorganic fluoride salts which can promote bone formation when given in appropriate doses.

Bone and Bone Disease

The skeleton acts as mechanical support and protection to softer tissues and organs. It is also important in electrolyte homoeostasis, acting as a reservoir of certain ions and minerals such as calcium, phosphorus, and magnesium.

Bone has two components: an organic matrix, called **osteoid**, consisting mainly of collagen; and a mineral phase deposited through the matrix comprising about 70% of the skeletal mass, and composed chiefly of hydroxyapatite (a complex crystalline salt of calcium and phosphate). Two structural forms are known in mature bone, namely cortical (lamellar) bone, which has a dense, continuous structure, and trabecular (cancellous) bone, which has a 'spongy' structure of linked plates and is associated with high bone turnover and growth. The peripheral or appendicular parts of the skeleton are predominantly cortical bone, while the axial or central parts, such as the spine and pelvis, contain substantial amounts of trabecular bone.

Bone is a dynamic tissue: once new bone has been laid down it is subject to a continual process of formation and resorption called **remodelling**. Remodelling takes place along bone surfaces and is carried out by bone cells (osteoclasts and osteoblasts) that originate in the marrow and share common origins with blood cells. Stimulated by physical or chemical signals, **osteoclasts** dig a cavity into the bone (bone resorption); they are then replaced by **osteoblasts** that synthesise new osteoid to fill the cavity (bone formation) and may help to promote its subsequent mineralisation. The actions of these two types of bone cell are closely linked, and agents that suppress resorption ultimately decrease bone formation too. However, at any given time there is a deficit in potential bone mass, the **remodelling space**, which represents sites of bone resorption that have not yet been filled in. Any stimulus that affects bone turnover by altering the recruitment of osteoblasts and osteoclasts to remodelling will result in an increase or decrease in the remodelling space, until a new steady state is achieved, and this will be seen as a decrease or increase in bone mass.

Bone also contains **osteocytes**, which are cells derived from osteoblasts thought to be involved in the movement of minerals.

Bone cells are controlled by systemic hormones including parathyroid hormone, 1,25-dihydroxycholecalciferol (calcitriol), and calcitonin and local regulators such as bone morphogenetic proteins and interleukin-1; vitamin K is also thought to have a role, and bone cells are affected by other hormones including corticosteroids and sex hormones.

Bone diseases may be due to defects in the production of osteoid or its mineralisation, or to an imbalance in resorption and formation of bone. Some diseases of bone are described next.

Ectopic ossification

Ectopic ossification[1] (heterotopic ossification) is a condition in which mature bone develops in non-skeletal tissues, commonly the connective tissue of muscles. It occurs following local trauma, for example after joint dislocation or surgery such as total hip replacement, and also after neurological damage such as severe head or spinal cord injuries. Ectopic bone formation usually starts about 2 weeks after the injury, though symptoms which include localised pain, swelling, and restriction of movement, may not appear for 8 to 10 weeks. A congenital form of ectopic ossification, myositis ossificans progressiva, also occurs but is rare.

Ectopic ossification should be distinguished from the calcification of soft tissue which may occur in connective-tissue disorders or in parathyroid disorders due to high circulating concentrations of calcium and or phosphate; in these conditions calcification occurs without bone formation.

Treatment of established ectopic bone is limited to surgical resection. Patients at high risk of ectopic bone formation should therefore receive prophylaxis with radiotherapy, physiotherapy, or drug therapy. While prophylaxis does not always prevent the development of ectopic ossification, it can decrease its occurrence and severity. Prophylactic measures should be begun as early as possible and for orthopaedic surgery may be started before the operation. Prophylaxis is also required if mature ectopic bone is to be surgically excised in order to minimise the rate of recurrence. Bisphosphonates that inhibit the mineralisation of the deposited bone such as etidronate have been advocated[2] but they do not prevent the formation of the osteoid matrix. Also when etidronate is discontinued, some mineralisation can occur resulting in delayed ectopic ossification though it is usually less severe. More promising are the NSAIDs such as aspirin, ibuprofen, or indomethacin; these appear to significantly reduce the incidence of ectopic bone formation,[3,4] possibly by inhibiting the synthesis of osteoactive prostaglandins.

1. Singer BR. Heterotopic ossification. *Br J Hosp Med* 1993; **49:** 247–55.
2. Finerman GAM, Stover SL. Heterotopic ossification following hip replacement or spinal cord injury: two clinical studies with EHDP. *Metab Bone Dis Relat Res* 1981; **4 & 5:** 337–42.
3. Schmidt SA, *et al.* The use of indomethacin to prevent the formation of heterotopic bone after total hip replacement: a randomized, double-blind clinical trial. *J Bone Joint Surg (Am)* 1988; **70A:** 834–8.
4. Pagnani MJ, *et al.* Effect of aspirin on heterotopic ossification after total hip arthroplasty in men who have osteoarthrosis. *J Bone Joint Surg (Am)* 1991; **73A:** 924–9.

Malignant neoplasms of the bone

The bisphosphonates and calcitonins have been used to control bone pain and osteolysis in patients with malignant neoplasms of the bone (p.484), as well as to control the hypercalcaemia that often accompanies malignant disease (p.1148).

Osteogenesis imperfecta

Osteogenesis imperfecta (brittle bone syndrome) is a heterogeneous congenital disorder of connective tissue characterised by bone fragility, osteopenia, short stature, joint laxity, teeth defects, and hearing abnormalities. It may be classified into 4 forms, which vary in clinical severity.

Orthopaedic treatment and physical activity programmes form the basis of therapy: at present there is no accepted drug therapy. Beneficial effects have been reported with calcitonins,[1,2] bisphosphonates,[3,4,8] and growth hormone.[5,6] Bisphosphonates may also be useful for associated immobilisation hypercalcaemia.[7] Bone-marrow transplantation and the potential of antisense gene therapy are being investigated.[6]

1. Castells S, *et al.* Therapy of osteogenesis imperfecta with synthetic salmon calcitonin. *J Pediatr* 1979; **95:** 807–11.
2. Nishi Y, *et al.* Effect of long-term calcitonin therapy by injection and nasal spray on the incidence of fractures in osteogenesis imperfecta. *J Pediatr* 1992; **121:** 477–80.
3. Bembi B, *et al.* Intravenous pamidronate treatment in osteogenesis imperfecta. *J Pediatr* 1997; **131:** 622–5.
4. Shaw NJ. Bisphosphonates in osteogenesis imperfecta. *Arch Dis Child* 1997; **77:** 92–3.
5. Antoniazzi F, *et al.* Growth hormone treatment in osteogenesis imperfecta with quantitative defect of type I collagen synthesis. *J Pediatr* 1996; **129:** 432–9.
6. Marini JC, Gerber NL. Osteogenesis imperfecta: rehabilitation and prospects for gene therapy. *JAMA* 1997; **277:** 746–50.
7. Williams CJC, *et al.* Hypercalcaemia in osteogenesis imperfecta treated with pamidronate. *Arch Dis Child* 1997; **76:** 169–70.
8. Glorieux FH, *et al.*. Cyclic administration of pamidronate in children with severe osteogenesis imperfecta. *N Engl J Med* 1998; **339:** 947–52.

Osteomalacia

Osteomalacia occurs when there is impaired mineralisation of the bone matrix resulting in 'soft' bones. Patients usually present with bone pain and muscle weakness and may have subclinical fractures. **Rickets** refers to defective mineralisation of growing bone and is therefore restricted to children; it is associated with retarded growth, skeletal deformities, teeth defects, and muscle hypotonia.

Inadequate bone mineralisation is usually caused by vitamin D deficiency or its abnormal metabolism, but may also be due to phosphate depletion, calcium deficiency, or a primary disorder of bone matrix such as hypophosphatasia in which a deficiency of alkaline phosphatase results in an increase in pyrophosphate, an inhibitor of bone mineralisation. Some drugs including various antiepileptics (p.353), etidronate, and aluminium salts, can interfere with bone mineralisation and cause osteomalacia. Osteomalacia also occurs in renal osteodystrophy associated with chronic renal failure (see below).

Several hereditary disorders are associated with the development of rickets including vitamin D-pseudodeficiency rickets (vitamin D-dependent rickets), in which there is impaired synthesis of 1,25-dihydroxycholecalciferol (Type I) or receptor resistance to 1,25-dihydroxycholecalciferol (Type II), and X-linked hypophosphataemic rickets.[1]

Treatment of osteomalacia and rickets is primarily aimed at correcting any underlying deficiency. Vitamin D substances, calcium, or phosphate supplements can be given by mouth as appropriate but doses require careful individual adjustment to maintain calcium and phosphate concentrations within normal limits. A variety of forms or analogues of vitamin D are available. For the treatment of simple nutritional deficiencies cholecalciferol or ergocalciferol are generally preferred. If malabsorption is suspected, larger doses or parenteral administration may be necessary, but where large doses are required it may be preferable to use one of the more potent forms of vitamin D such as calcitriol.

Type I vitamin D-pseudodeficiency rickets requires replacement therapy with calcitriol. In Type II disease, resistance to calcitriol treatment may be so extreme that only very large supplements of calcium may be effective.[1,2] X-linked hypophosphataemic rickets is considered to be best treated with combined phosphate supplementation and calcitriol.[1,3] There has also been some interest in the use of growth hormone in children with hypophosphataemic rickets.[4] A form of hypophosphataemic rickets, rickets of prematurity (p.1160), may occur in small, premature infants fed exclusively on breast milk, and phosphate supplementation with concomitant calcium and vitamin D has been suggested in such cases.

1. Glorieux FH. Rickets, the continuing challenge. *N Engl J Med* 1991; **325:** 1875–7.
2. Hochberg Z, *et al.* Calcium therapy for calcitriol-resistant rickets. *J Pediatr* 1992; **121:** 803–8.
3. Verge CF, *et al.* Effects of therapy in X-linked hypophosphatemic rickets. *N Engl J Med* 1991; **325:** 1843–8.
4. Shaw NJ, *et al.* Growth hormone and hypophosphataemic rickets. *Arch Dis Child* 1995; **72:** 543–4.

Osteoporosis

Osteoporosis has been defined as a disease characterised by low bone mass and microarchitectural deterioration of bone tissue, leading to enhanced bone fragility and risk of fracture.[1] Primary fracture sites are the long bones (distal forearm and neck of the femur) and the vertebrae. Bone is continuously removed by osteoclasts (bone resorption) and replaced by osteoblasts (bone formation) in a process of remodelling (see above). Although bone formation outstrips resorption in youth, accumulated small deficits from remodelling result in a gradual loss of bone mass after the third decade. Primary osteoporosis is therefore usually an age-related disease. It can affect both sexes, though women are at greater risk because bone loss is accelerated, to a variable degree, after the menopause. Osteoporosis can also be secondary to a number of diseases and drugs.[2,3] For example, bone loss can be increased by disorders such as thyrotoxicosis, hypogonadism, Cushing's syndrome, hypoparathyroidism, and rheumatoid arthritis, or by drugs such as corticosteroids (p.1011) and heparin (p.880). Also, immobility, especially in younger patients, can result in osteoblastic failure with an increase in osteoclastic resorption and the development of osteoporosis. Other risk factors for osteoporosis include smoking, high alcohol intake, physical inactivity, thin body type, early menopause, and a family history of osteoporosis.[2,3]

Patients are usually asymptomatic until fractures occur, and up to half of vertebral fractures may also be asymptomatic. Fractures may result in pain, deformity (kyphosis, loss of height), and disability. Currently, the most reliable method of assessing osteoporosis and fracture risk is measurement of bone mass density (BMD), usually by dual energy X-ray absorptiometry.[1] Based on measurement of BMD, WHO have defined osteoporosis as a BMD 2.5 standard deviations or more below the young adult mean, and severe osteoporosis (established osteoporosis) as this BMD in the presence of one or more fragility fractures.[1] Present evidence is insufficient to support widespread screening for osteoporosis,[4] but measurement of BMD should be considered in those thought to be at risk of osteoporosis, particularly if the result is likely to affect treatment decisions.[3] A number of different approaches to the management of osteoporosis have been suggested, including changes in life-style, interventions to reduce falls, the use of drugs to decrease bone resorption such as calcium, oestrogens, calcitonins, and bisphosphonates, and the administration of pharmacological agents to stimulate bone formation, such as sodium fluoride.[3,5-12] Because bone remodelling is a coupled process decreases in resorption ultimately reduce the rate of bone formation, and antiresorptive drugs can therefore only produce modest increases in bone mass. Trials with such agents must be sufficiently prolonged to determine whether an increase in bone mass represents more than just a constriction in the remodelling space.[13] Moreover, experience with fluoride indicates that increases in BMD do not always equate to decreases in fracture risk. Thus, there is also a need to show that drugs decrease fracture rate; currently there are few trials with fracture rates as primary end-points. In addition, the optimum timing and duration of drug therapy to optimise the benefits on bone and minimise the risks is not known, particularly for the prevention of primary osteoporosis.

Prevention is the most effective method of dealing with osteoporosis as once bone mass has decreased it is difficult to replace. Optimising peak bone mass is therefore important; regular moderate weight-bearing exercise and adequate dietary calcium during growth[14,15] have been advocated. After the third decade of life, interventions should be aimed at reducing the rate of bone loss. This includes life-style modifications such as avoiding smoking,[16] moderation of alcohol intake, improving diet to ensure an adequate calcium (p.1156) and vitamin D (p.1367) intake, and regular weight-bearing exercise.[17,18] Secondary causes of osteoporosis should be identified and treated as appropriate.[3] Antiresorptive drugs may be considered.

In *postmenopausal women*, hormone replacement therapy (HRT) (p.1437) slows or eliminates postmenopausal bone loss at all skeletal sites. Many observational studies and a few randomised trials have shown that this reduces the risk of fractures. Efficacy is dependent on dose, but the duration of therapy for maximum benefit is unknown. It has been suggested that HRT may need to be continued indefinitely, since there is evidence that the risk of fracture returns to base-line after 10 or more years without HRT. However, the potential value of long-term HRT must be balanced against the potential risks, particularly breast cancer. It is generally considered that HRT is indicated in women with risk factors for osteoporosis. In women with no risk factors for osteoporosis and without menopausal symptoms, use of HRT is more controversial. In these women it may be appropriate to start HRT several years after the menopause.

Alternatives to HRT for the prevention of postmenopausal osteoporosis include the bisphosphonates alendronate and etidronate, tibolone, and raloxifene. Risedronate is another bisphosphonate under investigation for this indication. There is good evidence that these drugs prevent loss of bone mineral density in postmenopausal women. However, as yet there is little experience of the long-term use of these drugs (beyond 2 to 5 years). In postmenopausal women, the effects of calcium supplementation (about 1 g of calcium daily by mouth) have been conflicting; some studies have reported a reduction in bone loss[19-21] but others have found calcium supplements to be of little benefit.[22] However, a subsequent meta-analysis[23] found that increasing calcium intake by diet or supplements potentiated the effect of oestrogens and calcitonins on bone, confirming that an adequate intake of calcium is important when antiresorptive drugs are being used.

The use of calcitonins as prophylactic drugs has been limited by the necessity for parenteral administration. However, intranasal spray formulations of salcatonin have been developed and oral formulations are under investigation.

A number of other drugs have been reported to have favourable effects on bone mass in postmenopausal women including thiazide diuretics,[24] tamoxifen,[25] intermittent teriparatide,[26] diclofenac,[27] and potassium bicarbonate.[28] However, their role, if any, in the prevention of osteoporosis has not yet been determined.

Treatment. In patients with osteoporosis with or without fragility fractures (established osteoporosis), treatment involves supportive therapy and interventions to prevent further bone loss and reduce the risk of fractures.[3,5-12] Supportive therapy in the acute phase of a fracture includes pain relief, physiotherapy, and appropriate orthopaedic management of fracture of long bones; surgery is required for the majority of hip fractures.[10] Life-style modifications and drugs to prevent further bone loss and fractures are similar to those outlined above. In the elderly, interventions to reduce the risk of falls may be important,[29] and measures to protect the patient should falls occur may also be considered.[30]

In *postmenopausal women* with established osteoporosis, HRT increases bone mass and reduces the incidence of fractures. Alternatively, the bisphosphonates such as alendronate and etidronate may be used. Both of these drugs have been shown to increase bone mass and decrease fracture rate in established osteoporosis. Calcitonins may also have a role. It has been suggested that, in particular, the analgesic effects of calcitonins may be advantageous in patients with acute pain due to osteoporotic fractures.

Results of studies using the vitamin D substance calcitriol for the treatment of osteoporosis have been conflicting; although some have reported an increase in spinal bone density[31] and a reduction in the rate of new vertebral fractures,[32] others have found no significant effects.[33]

Vitamin D supplements have shown beneficial effects in the elderly, and it is considered that they may have a particular role in frail or housebound individuals, who are at high risk of vitamin D deficiency and resulting hyperparathyroidism.[9,10,12]

Postmenopausal osteoporosis has also been treated with agents that promote bone formation. Fluoride stimulates osteoblasts and increases the density of trabecular bone and has been administered as sodium fluoride or sodium monofluorophosphate. However, increases in BMD with fluoride have not always resulted in decreased fracture rate, and may even be associated with increased bone fragility; thus, the role of fluoride remains unclear.[9,11,12] Anabolic steroids have been tried but have considerable adverse effects. Other drugs that have been investigated for postmenopausal osteoporosis include teriparatide,[34] mecasermin,[35] and ipriflavone.[36]

There is less evidence to guide decisions on the management of osteoporosis in *men*[37-39] than in postmenopausal women. In hypogonadal men with osteoporosis, testosterone replacement therapy should be used.[39] In eugonadal men, there are concerns regarding the potential long-term adverse effects of exogenous testosterone. Therefore, in men with idiopathic osteoporosis, bisphosphonates may be the treatment of choice.[39] Calcium and vitamin D supplements did not affect the rate of bone mineral loss in healthy men with adequate diets.[40] However, there is some evidence that, as for women, elderly men may benefit from vitamin D supplements and calcium.[41] Other drugs that have been reported to have favourable effects on BMD in men include thiazides[42] and parathyroid hormone.[43]

1. WHO. Assessment of fracture risk and its application to screening for postmenopausal osteoporosis. *WHO Tech Rep Ser 843* 1994.
2. Dempster DW, Lindsay R. Pathogenesis of osteoporosis. *Lancet* 1993; **341:** 797–801.
3. Peel N, Eastell R. Osteoporosis. *Br Med J* 1995; **310:** 989–92.
4. Marshall D, *et al.* Meta-analysis of how well measures of bone mineral density predict occurrence of osteoporotic fractures. *Br Med J* 1996; **312:** 1254–9.
5. Riggs BL, Melton LJ. The prevention and treatment of osteoporosis. *N Engl J Med* 1992; **327:** 620–7.
6. Lindsay R. Prevention and treatment of osteoporosis. *Lancet* 1993; **341:** 801–5.
7. Conference Report. Consensus Development Conference: diagnosis, prophylaxis, and treatment of osteoporosis. *Am J Med* 1993; **94:** 646–50.
8. Khosla S, Riggs BL. Treatment options for osteoporosis. *Mayo Clin Proc* 1995; **70:** 978–82.
9. Anonymous. Managing osteoporosis. *Drug Ther Bull* 1996; **34:** 45–8.
10. Compston JE. Osteoporosis: management of established disease. *Prescribers' J* 1997; **37:** 119–24.
11. Gibaldi M. Prevention and treatment of osteoporosis: does the future belong to hormone replacement therapy? *J Clin Pharmacol* 1997; **37:** 1087–99.
12. Eastell R. Treatment of postmenopausal osteoporosis. *N Engl J Med* 1998; **338:** 736–46.
13. Heaney RP. Interpreting trials of bone-active agents. *Am J Med* 1995; **98:** 329–30.
14. Johnston CC, *et al.* Calcium supplementation and increases in bone mineral density in children. *N Engl J Med* 1992; **327:** 82–7.
15. Lloyd T, *et al.* Calcium supplementation and bone mineral density in adolescent girls. *JAMA* 1993; **270:** 841–4.
16. Law MR, Hackshaw AK. A meta-analysis of cigarette smoking, bone mineral density and risk of hip fracture: recognition of a major effect. *Br Med J* 1997; **315:** 841–6.
17. Nelson ME, *et al.* Effects of high intensity strength training on multiple risk factors for osteoporotic fractures: a randomized controlled trial. *JAMA* 1994; **272:** 1909–14.
18. Gregg EW, *et al.* Physical activity and osteoporotic fracture risk in older women. *Ann Intern Med* 1998; **129:** 81–8.
19. Reid IR, *et al.* Effect of calcium supplementation on bone loss in postmenopausal women. *N Engl J Med* 1993; **328:** 460–4. Correction. *ibid.*; **329:** 1281.
20. Aloia JF, *et al.* Calcium supplementation with and without hormone replacement therapy to prevent postmenopausal bone loss. *Ann Intern Med* 1994; **120:** 97–103.
21. Reid IR, *et al.* Long-term effects of calcium supplementation on bone loss and fractures in postmenopausal women: a randomized controlled trial. *Am J Med* 1995; **98:** 331–5.
22. Riis B, *et al.* Does calcium supplementation prevent postmenopausal bone loss? *N Engl J Med* 1987; **316:** 173–7.
23. Nieves JW, *et al.* Calcium potentiates the effects of estrogen and calcitonin on bone mass: review and analysis. *Am J Clin Nutr* 1998; **67:** 18–24.
24. Cauley JA, *et al.* Effects of thiazide diuretic therapy on bone mass, fractures, and falls. *Ann Intern Med* 1993; **118:** 666–73.
25. Love RR, *et al.* Effects of tamoxifen on bone mineral density in postmenopausal women with breast cancer. *N Engl J Med* 1992; **326:** 852–6.
26. Finkelstein JS, *et al.* Parathyroid hormone for the prevention of bone loss induced by estrogen deficiency. *N Engl J Med* 1994; **331:** 1618–23.
27. Bell NH, *et al.* Diclofenac sodium inhibits bone resorption in postmenopausal women. *Am J Med* 1994; **96:** 349–53.

28. Sebastian A, *et al.* Improved mineral balance and skeletal metabolism in postmenopausal women treated with potassium bicarbonate. *N Engl J Med* 1994; **330:** 1776–81.
29. Dargent-Molina P, *et al.* Fall-related factors and risk of hip fracture: the EPIDOS prospective study. *Lancet* 1996; **348:** 145–9.
30. Lauritzen JB, *et al.* Effect of external hip protectors on hip fractures. *Lancet* 1993; **341:** 11–13.
31. Gallagher JC, Goldgar D. Treatment of postmenopausal osteoporosis with high doses of synthetic calcitriol: a randomized controlled study. *Ann Intern Med* 1990; **113:** 649–55.
32. Tilyard MW, *et al.* Treatment of postmenopausal osteoporosis with calcitriol or calcium. *N Engl J Med* 1992; **326:** 357–62.
33. Ott SM, Chesnut CH. Calcitriol treatment is not effective in postmenopausal osteoporosis. *Ann Intern Med* 1989; **110:** 267–74.
34. Reeve J, *et al.* Treatment of osteoporosis with human parathyroid peptide and observations on effect of sodium fluoride. *Br Med J* 1990; **301:** 314–18. Correction. *ibid.*; 477.
35. Ebeling PR, *et al.* Short-term effects of recombinant human insulin-like growth factor I on bone turnover in normal women. *J Clin Endocrinol Metab* 1993; **77:** 1384–7.
36. Agnusdei D, *et al.* Effects of ipriflavone on bone mass and bone remodeling in patients with established postmenopausal osteoporosis. *Curr Ther Res* 1992; **51:** 82–91.
37. Anderson DC. Osteoporosis in men. *Br Med J* 1992; **305:** 489–90.
38. Seeman E. The dilemma of osteoporosis in men. *Am J Med* 1995; **98** (suppl 2A): 76S–88S.
39. Eastell R, *et al.* Management of male osteoporosis: report of the UK Consensus Group. *Q J Med* 1998; **91:** 71–92.
40. Orwoll ES, *et al.* The rate of bone mineral loss in normal men and the effects of calcium and cholecalciferol supplementation. *Ann Intern Med* 1990; **112:** 29–34.
41. Dawson-Hughes B, *et al.* Effect of calcium and vitamin D supplementation on bone density in men and women 65 years of age and older. *N Engl J Med* 1997; **337:** 670–6.
42. Wasnich R, *et al.* Effect of thiazide on rates of bone mineral loss: a longitudinal study. *Br Med J* 1990; **301:** 1303–5. Correction. *ibid.* 1991; **302:** 218.
43. Slovik DM, *et al.* Restoration of spinal bone in osteoporotic men by treatment with human parathyroid hormone (1–34) and 1,25-dihydroxyvitamin D. *J Bone Miner Res* 1986; **1:** 377–81.

Paget's disease of bone

Paget's disease of bone (osteitis deformans) is characterised by excessive and disorganised bone resorption and formation. It may affect one or more bones, usually the cranium, spine, clavicles, pelvis, or long bones, but in most patients the majority of the skeleton is uninvolved. Paget's disease occurs in about 3 to 4% of the population over 40 years of age and its frequency increases with age. Patients are often asymptomatic. However, some patients may present with musculoskeletal and bone pain or with bone weakness and deformity that can result in fractures. Other complications include hearing loss, nerve compression especially of the spinal cord, and, in severe disease, heart failure due to increased skeletal vascularity.

Patients who are asymptomatic and in whom the sites of disease are associated with little or no risk of complications do not require any treatment. Bone or articular pain may be treated with NSAIDs or paracetamol. Drug therapy with agents that reduce bone resorption,[1-6] such as the calcitonins and bisphosphonates, is indicated if bone pain is persistent or to prevent further progression of the disease, especially if complications such as spinal-cord compression are present or there is a risk of such complications. Such treatment is suppressive and while osteolytic lesions may be healed, the underlying disorder is not cured. Drug therapy is guided by monitoring biochemical improvement in disease activity.

Calcitonins improve the symptoms of Paget's disease and can heal osteolytic lesions, though complete healing may take several years.[3] Doses are usually administered parenterally by subcutaneous or intramuscular injection either daily or 2 to 3 times a week; the subcutaneous route is favoured for self-administration. Intranasal formulations have been developed and may be more convenient. Calcitonins, particularly those from animal sources, frequently elicit an antibody response and some patients develop resistance to therapy; this can often be overcome by changing to a calcitonin from a different species.[2]

Bisphosphonates also give symptomatic relief and heal osteolytic lesions. In contrast to the short-lived effects of calcitonins, disease activity may be reduced for several months, or years, after therapy has ceased; therefore, bisphosphonates have largely superseded the calcitonins.[5] Initial experience was with disodium etidronate, which has the advantage that it may be given by mouth but unfortunately it also impairs bone mineralisation and can cause osteomalacia especially with high doses or prolonged use. Other bisphosphonates that have less effect on bone mineralisation, such as clodronate, pamidronate, alendronate, and tiludronate are also effective in Paget's disease of bone and are preferred where available.[6]

Concomitant administration of a calcitonin with a bisphosphonate has been reported to induce a better response than either drug given alone,[7] but some workers consider that such combinations should be reserved for patients only partially responsive to a single agent.[4] Others suggest that a calcitonin may be useful in the first few weeks of bisphosphonate therapy for more rapid relief of bone pain.[6] When administered consecutively, results have been conflicting.[8,9]

Plicamycin (mithramycin), a cytotoxic antibiotic with particular activity against osteoclasts, is highly effective in the treatment of Paget's disease of bone when administered daily by intravenous infusion for 5 to 10 days. However, it is associated with severe toxicity and is therefore now avoided or reserved for patients refractory to other drugs.[1,3,10]

Studies with gallium nitrate,[11] another inhibitor of bone resorption, have indicated beneficial effects in the treatment of Paget's disease of bone.

In selected patients, orthopaedic surgery such as hip replacement or correction of a bone deformity may be appropriate. Drug therapy with a calcitonin or bisphosphonate is usually given 1 to 3 months before surgery in order to reduce bone vascularity (thus minimising blood loss during the operation) and also to prevent development of postoperative hypercalcaemia of immobilisation.

1. Stumpf JL. Pharmacologic management of Paget's disease. *Clin Pharm* 1989; **8:** 485–95.
2. Hosking DJ. Advances in the management of Paget's disease of bone. *Drugs* 1990; **40:** 829–40.
3. Stevenson JC. Paget's disease of bone. *Prescribers' J* 1991; **31:** 98–103.
4. Gennari C, *et al.* Management of osteoporosis and Paget's disease: an appraisal of the risks and benefits of drug treatment. *Drug Safety* 1994; **11:** 179–95.
5. Hosking D, *et al.* Paget's disease of bone: diagnosis and management. *Br Med J* 1996; **312:** 491–4.
6. Delmas PD, Meunier PJ. The management of Paget's disease of bone. *N Engl J Med* 1997; **336:** 558–66.
7. O'Donoghue DJ, Hosking DJ. Biochemical response to combination of disodium etidronate with calcitonin in Paget's disease. *Bone* 1987; **8:** 219–25.
8. Perry HM, *et al.* Alternate calcitonin and etidronate disodium therapy for Paget's bone disease. *Arch Intern Med* 1984; **144:** 929–33.
9. Rico H, *et al.* Biochemical assessment of acute and chronic treatment of Paget's bone disease with calcitonin and calcium with and without biphosphonate. *Bone* 1988; **9:** 63–6.
10. Ryan WG, *et al.* Apparent cure of Paget's disease of bone. *Am J Med* 1990; **89:** 825–6.
11. Bockman RS, *et al.* A multicenter trial of low dose gallium nitrate in patients with advanced Paget's disease of bone. *J Clin Endocrinol Metab* 1995; **80:** 595–602.

Renal osteodystrophy

Renal osteodystrophy is a complex condition associated with chronic renal failure which involves the development of osteitis fibrosa (hyperparathyroid bone disease) and osteomalacia.[1,2] Osteosclerosis, osteoporosis, and adynamic bone disease (suppression of remodelling) may also occur.[3] Treatment includes correction of hyperphosphataemia, by diet and if necessary oral phosphate binders, and the use of calcitriol or alfacalcidol to control hypocalcaemia and secondary hyperparathyroidism. Unresponsive patients may require parathyroidectomy.

Vitamin D is metabolised in the kidney to its most active form, 1,25-dihydroxycholecalciferol, and during renal disease a reduction in the synthesis of this metabolite results in reduced intestinal absorption of calcium, and thus hypocalcaemia. In addition, a reduction in the renal excretion of phosphate leads to hyperphosphataemia which exacerbates these changes and increases the risk of soft tissue and vascular calcification.

The result is inadequate bone mineralisation with the development of osteomalacia (see above) and excessive production of parathyroid hormone, resulting in secondary hyperparathyroidism (see below). Hyperparathyroidism increases bone turnover and leads to osteitis fibrosa, a condition characterised by an abundance of osteoclasts, osteoblasts, and osteocytes, and the deposition of fibrous tissue in the bone marrow.

In patients with chronic renal failure (p.1152) on dialysis, the accumulation of aluminium from either the dialysis water supply or from the use of aluminium-containing phosphate binders may also have adverse effects on bone (see Aluminium Hydroxide, p.1177) and is associated with the development of osteomalacia and adynamic bone disease.

Most patients are asymptomatic at presentation and **treatment** is aimed at controlling the plasma concentrations of calcium, phosphate, and parathyroid hormone.[2] Severe hyperphosphataemia should be corrected first to reduce the risk of metastatic calcification which may be aggravated by the use of vitamin D compounds which increase calcium absorption.

Hyperphosphataemia is initially controlled with a low-phosphate diet but many patients, especially those on dialysis, also need an oral phosphate binder to complex with dietary phosphate in the gastro-intestinal tract and reduce its absorption.[2,4]

Calcium salts such as the carbonate or acetate are effective phosphate binders[5,6] and have been found to suppress hyperparathyroidism; 2.5 to 17 g of calcium carbonate daily is given in divided doses with meals, the dosage being adjusted individually based on the dietary intake of phosphate and the plasma-phosphate concentration. Calcium salts also raise plasma-calcium concentrations and reduce acidosis but hypercalcaemia can occur;[7,8] the use of dialysis fluids with a lower calcium content has been suggested for these patients.[2,9]

Alternatively, aluminium hydroxide may be given but relatively large doses are required and as mentioned above, aluminium accumulation can lead to osteomalacia and adynamic bone disease in patients with impaired renal function. Long-term use is not generally recommended,[2] and alternative agents are probably preferable. Other compounds that have been reported to be effective phosphate binders include sucralfate[10,11] (an aluminium-containing compound) and magnesium carbonate.[12]

Vitamin D compounds that do not require renal hydroxylation such as calcitriol (1,25-dihydroxycholecalciferol) or its synthetic analogue, alfacalcidol, are the drugs of choice for correcting the *hypocalcaemia* and also contribute to the control of *secondary hyperparathyroidism*;[2] calcium supplements may also occasionally be required. Administration of alfacalcidol in the early stages of renal failure, before dialysis is required, has also been reported to improve subclinical bone disease.[13] Calcitriol or its analogues are administered by mouth; the dose is adjusted according to response but must be carefully monitored as the dose required for adequate suppression of parathyroid hormone secretion may be close to that which causes hypercalcaemia. It has also been recommended that a close watch should be kept on renal function since deterioration may be accelerated by calcitriol, an effect that may be independent of any induced hypercalcaemia.[14] Patients unresponsive to drug treatment or who develop hypercalcaemia (which may itself accelerate the decline in renal function) may require sub-total parathyroidectomy.[1,2] Alternatively, the administration of calcitriol as intermittent intravenous infusions (3 times a week during haemodialysis) has been reported to be effective in reducing plasma concentrations of parathyroid hormone and ameliorating osteitis fibrosa in some patients with moderate to severe secondary hyperparathyroidism due to chronic renal failure who had failed to respond adequately to oral calcitriol.[15]

Patients with *adynamic bone disease* related to aluminium retention require removal of aluminium from the body; desferrioxamine has been used to mobilise aluminium before haemodialysis.[16] Use of aluminium-containing phosphate binders is clearly undesirable in such patients, and it has also been suggested that vitamin D compounds should not be given because they decrease the proliferation of osteoblasts.[3]

1. Malluche HH, Faugere M-C. Renal osteodystrophy. *N Engl J Med* 1989; **321:** 317–19.
2. Gower P. Prevention of bone disease in chronic renal failure. *Prescribers' J* 1992; **32:** 245–51.
3. Hruska KA, Teitelbaum SL. Renal osteodystrophy. *N Engl J Med* 1995; **333:** 166–74.
4. Coburn JW, Salusky IB. Control of serum phosphorus in uremia. *N Engl J Med* 1989; **320:** 1140–42.
5. Mak RHK, *et al.* Suppression of secondary hyperparathyroidism in children with chronic renal failure by high dose phosphate binders: calcium carbonate versus aluminium hydroxide. *Br Med J* 1985; **291:** 623–7.
6. Slatopolsky E, *et al.* Calcium carbonate as a phosphate binder in patients with chronic renal failure undergoing dialysis. *N Engl J Med* 1986; **315:** 157–61.
7. Stein HD, *et al.* Calcium carbonate as a phosphate binder. *N Engl J Med* 1987; **316:** 109–10.
8. Raine AEG, Oliver DO. Management of hyperphosphataemia in renal dialysis patients. *Lancet* 1987; **i:** 633–4.
9. Slatopolsky E, *et al.* Calcium carbonate as a phosphate binder. *N Engl J Med* 1987; **316:** 110.
10. Leung ACT, *et al.* Aluminium hydroxide versus sucralfate as a phosphate binder in uraemia. *Br Med J* 1983; **286:** 1379–81.

11. Vucelić B, *et al.* Changes in serum phosphorus, calcium and alkaline phosphatase due to sucralfate. *Int J Clin Pharmacol Ther Toxicol* 1986; **24:** 93–6.
12. O'Donovan R, *et al.* Substitution of aluminium salts by magnesium salts in control of dialysis hyperphosphataemia. *Lancet* 1986; **i:** 880–2.
13. Hamdy NAT, *et al.* Effect of alfacalcidol on natural course of renal bone disease in mild to moderate renal failure. *Br Med J* 1995; **310:** 358–63.
14. Chan JCM, *et al.* A prospective, double-blind study of growth failure in children with chronic renal insufficiency and the effectiveness of treatment with calcitriol versus dihydrotachysterol. *J Pediatr* 1994; **124:** 520–8.
15. Andress DL, *et al.* Intravenous calcitriol in the treatment of refractory osteitis fibrosa of chronic renal failure. *N Engl J Med* 1989; **321:** 274–9.
16. McCarthy JT, *et al.* Clinical experience with desferrioxamine in dialysis patients with aluminium toxicity. *Q J Med* 1990; **74:** 257–76.

Rickets

See Osteomalacia, above.

Parathyroid Disorders

Parathyroid hormone, secreted by the parathyroid gland, maintains concentrations of ionised calcium in extracellular fluid within normal limits. It acts directly on the kidney to enhance renal reabsorption of calcium, to increase phosphate excretion, and to promote the conversion of vitamin D to its active metabolite, 1,25-dihydroxycholecalciferol, which in turn, enhances calcium absorption from the gastrointestinal tract. Parathyroid hormone also acts on bone, to accelerate bone resorption and the release of calcium and phosphate into the extracellular fluid. Secretion of parathyroid hormone is primarily regulated by the extracellular concentration of ionised calcium; hypocalcaemia stimulates secretion whereas hypercalcaemia has an inhibitory effect. 1,25-Dihydroxycholecalciferol can also suppress parathyroid hormone secretion.

Disorders of parathyroid hormone secretion cause a disruption of calcium homoeostasis and in the long-term, may result in bone disease.

Hyperparathyroidism

Primary hyperparathyroidism is a disorder of parathyroid hormone hypersecretion usually caused by adenomas or hyperplasia of the parathyroid glands. Patients are commonly asymptomatic but may have signs of hypercalcaemia (p.1148); nephrolithiasis may also be present. Secondary hyperparathyroidism occurs in response to hypocalcaemia as in chronic renal failure (p.1152) and if prolonged may progress to autonomous hypersecretion by the parathyroid gland (tertiary hyperparathyroidism).

Severe hypercalcaemia requires immediate treatment, but is rare in primary hyperparathyroidism. In the long-term, the treatment of choice for primary and tertiary hyperparathyroidism is usually surgical parathyroidectomy[1] but in patients with asymptomatic primary hyperparathyroidism no therapy may be necessary.[2] The treatment of secondary hyperparathyroidism is usually aimed at the underlying cause of the hypocalcaemia; for example, for the treatment of secondary hyperparathyroidism associated with chronic renal disease, see Renal Osteodystrophy, above.

Drug treatment in primary hyperparathyroidism appears to play only a modest role. Oral phosphate supplements have been given in the short-term to alleviate hypercalciuria and hypercalcaemia.[3] Bisphosphonates can be used in the acute management of hypercalcaemia, but seem to be of little benefit in the long-term treatment of hyperparathyroidism.[4] Oestrogens have been reported to reduce the rate of bone turnover and plasma-concentrations of calcium in postmenopausal women with primary hyperparathyroidism,[5,6] but any long-term benefits are uncertain.[7] Calcium receptor agonists (calcimimetics) are under development for hyperparathyroidism.[8]

1. Scott-Coombes DM, Lynn JA. Surgical treatment of parathyroid disease. *Br J Hosp Med* 1997; **57:** 488–91.
2. Consensus Development Conference Panel. Diagnosis and management of asymptomatic primary hyperparathyroidism: consensus development conference statement. *Ann Intern Med* 1991; **114:** 593–7.
3. Anonymous. Medical management of primary hyperparathyroidism. *Lancet* 1984; **ii:** 727–8.
4. Al Zahrani A, Levine MA. Primary hyperparathyroidism. *Lancet* 1997; **349:** 1233–8.
5. Marcus R, *et al.* Conjugated estrogens in the treatment of postmenopausal women with hyperparathyroidism. *Ann Intern Med* 1984; **100:** 633–40.
6. Selby PL, Peacock M. Ethinyl estradiol and norethindrone in the treatment of primary hyperparathyroidism in postmenopausal women. *N Engl J Med* 1986; **314:** 1481–5.
7. Coe FL, *et al.* Is estrogen preferable to surgery for postmenopausal women with primary hyperparathyroidism? *N Engl J Med* 1986; **314:** 1508–9.
8. Silverberg SJ, *et al.* Short-term inhibition of parathyroid hormone secretion by a calcium-receptor agonist in patients with primary hyperparathyroidism. *N Engl J Med* 1997; **337:** 1506–10.

Hypoparathyroidism

Hypoparathyroidism occurs when there is a deficiency of parathyroid hormone secretion due to lack of parathyroid gland development or destruction of the gland, for example by autoimmune disease or surgical removal. Other factors that may lead to a deficiency in parathyroid hormone include hypomagnesaemia and parathyroid adenomas. Where the deficiency results from resistance to parathyroid hormone the condition is termed pseudohypoparathyroidism. Parathyroid hormone, as teriparatide, is used in the differential diagnosis of hypoparathyroidism and pseudohypoparathyroidism. Hypoparathyroidism leads to hypocalcaemia and hyperphosphataemia, though in some patients these may not become significant until there is an increased calcium demand as in pregnancy.

Treatment is aimed at correcting the hypocalcaemia (p.1148); in patients with hypocalcaemic tetany the parenteral administration of calcium salts may be necessary. In the long-term, treatment is usually with oral vitamin D compounds which increase the intestinal absorption of calcium; calcium supplements may be required if dietary calcium is inadequate. Calcium concentrations and renal function require careful monitoring, especially since the lack of parathyroid hormone results in an increase in the renal excretion of calcium and the risk of nephrolithiasis. Beneficial effects on plasma-calcium concentrations have been reported following the use of thiazide diuretics to reduce the urinary excretion of calcium.[1,2] However, these effects tended to be modest and thiazide diuretics have not been found to be effective in all patients with hypoparathyroidism;[3] adverse effects such as metabolic alkalosis may also be a problem.[4]

Teriparatide also has potential in the treatment of hypoparathyroidism. In one study,[5] it maintained serum calcium in the normal range and decreased urine calcium excretion. Good results have been reported following transplantation of parathyroid cells depleted of antigen-bearing cells in a few patients with postsurgical hypoparathyroidism.[6,7] It was considered that this might prove a promising technique in the future.

1. Porter RH, *et al.* Treatment of hypoparathyroid patients with chlorthalidone. *N Engl J Med* 1978; **298:** 577–81.
2. Newman GH, *et al.* Effect of bendrofluazide on calcium reabsorption in hypoparathyroidism. *Eur J Clin Pharmacol* 1984; **27:** 41–6.
3. Gertner JM, Genel M. Chlorthalidone for hypoparathyroidism. *N Engl J Med* 1978; **298:** 1478.
4. Barzel US. Chlorthalidone for hypoparathyroidism. *N Engl J Med* 1978; **298:** 1478.
5. Winer KK, *et al.* Synthetic human parathyroid hormone 1-34 vs calcitriol and calcium in the treatment of hypoparathyroidism: results of a short-term randomized crossover trial. *JAMA* 1996; **276:** 631–6.
6. Decker GAG, *et al.* Allotransplantation of parathyroid cells. *Lancet* 1995; **345:** 124. Correction. *ibid.*; 464.
7. Hasse C, *et al.* Parathyroid allotransplantation without immunosuppression. *Lancet* 1997; **350:** 1296–7.

Alendronic Acid (4537-w)

Alendronic Acid *(BAN, rINN).*

AHButBP; Aminohydroxybutylidene Diphosphonic Acid. 4-Amino-1-hydroxybutane-1,1-diylbis(phosphonic acid).

$C_4H_{13}NO_7P_2$ = 249.1.

CAS — 66376-36-1.

Alendronate Sodium (19721-x)

Alendronate Sodium *(BANM, USAN, rINNM).*

G-704650; L-670452; MK-0217; MK-217. Monosodium alendronate; Sodium trihydrogen (4-amino-1-hydroxybutylidene)diphosphonate trihydrate.

$C_4H_{12}NNaO_7P_2,3H_2O$ = 325.1.

CAS — 121268-17-5.

Alendronate sodium 1.3 mg is approximately equivalent to 1 mg of alendronic acid.

Adverse Effects and Precautions

As for the bisphosphonates in general, p.734. Abdominal pain has been reported to be the most frequent adverse effect, but is usually mild and self-limiting. Peptic ulceration has been reported. Severe oesophageal reactions such as oesophagitis, erosions, and ulceration have occurred (see below); patients should be advised to stop taking the tablets and seek medical attention if they develop symptoms such as dysphagia, new or worsening heartburn, pain on swallowing, or retrosternal pain.

Alendronate should not be given to patients with abnormalities of the oesophagus or other factors that might delay oesophageal emptying, or those unable to stand or sit upright for at least 30 minutes. It should be used with caution in patients with upper gastro-intestinal abnormalities. To minimise the risk of oesophageal reactions, patients should be instructed to swallow alendronate tablets whole with plenty of water (not less than 200 mL), in an upright position (standing or sitting). Tablets should be taken on rising for the day, on an empty stomach, at least 30 minutes before breakfast and any other oral medication; patients should remain upright after taking the tablets, and should not lie down before eating the first meal of the day. Alendronate should not be taken at bedtime, or before getting up for the day. Hypocalcaemia should be corrected before starting alendronate therapy.

Effects on the oesophagus. Between September 1995 and March 1996 the UK Committee on Safety of Medicines (CSM) had received 10 reports of adverse effects on the oesophagus in patients receiving alendronate sodium.[1] Of these 4 were of oesophageal reflux, 4 of oesophagitis, and 2 of oesophageal ulceration. As of March 1996, worldwide an estimated 475 000 patients had received alendronate and 199 patients had oesophageal reactions reported to the manufacturer, of which 51 were serious or severe.[2] Endoscopic findings included erosions, ulcerations, exudative inflammation, and thickening of the oesophagus. Bleeding was rare, and oesophageal perforation was not reported. Most oesophageal reactions occurred within 1 week to 2 months of starting alendronate therapy. Recovery occurred when alendronate was stopped; however, it was considered important that patients be followed up for the possible development of strictures.[2] In about 60% of the cases where the information was available, alendronate had not been taken in accordance with the precautions for use (see above).

The CSM subsequently noted[3] that it had continued to receive reports of reactions; by July 1998 there had been 97 reports in the UK, in 1 case associated with a fatality. It was estimated that 1 to 2% of patients might experience oesophageal reactions even when following the precautions for use. Some have reported a much higher incidence of unacceptable upper gastro-intestinal symptoms in clinical practice.[4]

1. Committee on Safety of Medicines/Medicines Control Agency. Oesophageal reactions with alendronate sodium (Fosamax). *Current Problems* 1996; **22:** 5.
2. de Groen PC, *et al.* Esophagitis associated with the use of alendronate. *N Engl J Med* 1996; **335:** 1016–21.
3. Committee on Safety of Medicines/Medicines Control Agency. Reminder: severe oesophageal reactions with alendronate sodium (Fosamax). *Current Problems* 1998; **24:** 13.
4. Kelly R, Taggart H. Incidence of gastrointestinal side effects due to alendronate is high in clinical practice. *Br Med J* 1997; **315:** 1235.

Interactions

As for the bisphosphonates in general, p.735.

Pharmacokinetics

Like other bisphosphonates, alendronate is poorly absorbed following oral administration. Absorption is decreased by food, especially by products containing calcium or other polyvalent cations. Bioavailability is about 0.4% when administered half an hour before food, reduced from 0.7% in the fasting state; absorption is negligible when taken up to 2 hours after a meal. About half of the absorbed portion is excreted in the urine; the remainder is sequestered to bone for a prolonged period. Bisphosphonates do not appear to be metabolised.

References.

1. Gertz BJ, *et al.* Studies of the oral bioavailability of alendronate. *Clin Pharmacol Ther* 1995; **58:** 288–98.

Uses and Administration

Alendronate is an aminobisphosphonate with general properties similar to those of the other bisphosphonates (p.735). It is a potent inhibitor of bone resorption and is used as the sodium salt in osteoporosis and Paget's disease of bone. It has also been given in the treatment of bone metastases and hypercalcaemia of malignancy.

Alendronate sodium is given by mouth, and the specific instructions for its administration (see above) should be followed to minimise adverse effects and permit adequate absorption. Doses are expressed in terms of alendronic acid. The usual dosage for the treatment of osteoporosis in postmenopausal women is 10 mg daily; 5 mg daily may be given for prophylaxis. In adults with Paget's disease of bone the usual dose is 40 mg daily for 6 months; treatment may be repeated if necessary after an interval of a further 6 months.

Alendronic acid has also been given by intravenous infusion.

Malignant neoplasms of the bone. Bisphosphonates have been reported to be of benefit in some patients with malignancies of bone (p.484) both to reduce bone pain and osteolysis and to bring hypercalcaemia under control. An open study with alendronate given intravenously suggested that it might be useful in such circumstances,[1] while a randomised dose-response study[2] found that single intravenous doses of alendronate 5 mg or more effectively lowered serum-calcium concentrations in patients with hypercalcaemia of malignancy.

1. Attardo-Parrinello G, *et al.* Effects of a new aminodiphosphonate (aminohydroxybutylidene diphosphonate) in patients with osteolytic lesions from metastases and myelomatosis: comparison with dichloromethylene diphosphonate. *Arch Intern Med* 1987; **147:** 1629–33.
2. Nussbaum SR, *et al.* Dose-response study of alendronate sodium for the treatment of cancer-associated hypercalcemia. *J Clin Oncol* 1993; **11:** 1618–23.

Osteoporosis. Alendronate may be used for the prevention and treatment of osteoporosis (p.731). In randomised controlled trials of up to 3 years duration, alendronate increased bone mass density of the spine, hip, and total body in postmenopausal women with osteoporosis,[1-3] those with osteoporosis and existing vertebral fractures,[4,8] and those without osteoporosis.[5,6] Where incidence of vertebral fracture was the primary end-point, alendronate reduced the incidence of vertebral and nonvertebral fractures.[4,8] In postmenopausal women without osteoporosis, alendronate increases bone mass density, but not quite to the same extent as hormone replacement therapy.[5]

Alendronate also increases bone mass density in men and women receiving oral corticosteroids at doses equivalent to at least 7.5 mg prednisone daily.[7]

1. Chesnut CH, *et al.* Alendronate treatment of the postmenopausal osteoporotic woman: effect of multiple dosages on bone mass and bone remodeling. *Am J Med* 1995; **99:** 144–52.
2. Liberman UA, *et al.* Effect of oral alendronate on bone mineral density and the incidence of fractures in postmenopausal osteoporosis. *N Engl J Med* 1995; **333:** 1437–43.
3. Tucci JR, *et al.* Effect of three years of oral alendronate treatment in postmenopausal women with osteoporosis. *Am J Med* 1996; **101:** 488–501.
4. Black DM, *et al.* Randomised trial of effect of alendronate on risk of fracture in women with existing vertebral fractures. *Lancet* 1996; **348:** 1535–41.
5. Hosking D, *et al.* Prevention of bone loss with alendronate in postmenopausal women under 60 years of age. *N Engl J Med* 1998; **338:** 485–92.
6. McClung M, *et al.* Alendronate prevents postmenopausal bone loss in women without osteoporosis: a double-blind, randomized, controlled trial. *Ann Intern Med* 1998; **128:** 253–61.
7. Saag KG, *et al.* Alendronate for the prevention and treatment of glucocorticoid-induced osteoporosis. *N Engl J Med* 1998; **339:** 292–9.
8. Ensrud KE, *et al.* Treatment with alendronate prevents fractures in women at highest risk: results from the Fracture Intervention Trial. *Arch Intern Med* 1997; **157:** 2617–24.

Paget's disease of bone. Bisphosphonates may be indicated to control the excessive and disorganised resorption and formation of bone that occurs in Paget's disease of bone (p.732). Some references to the use of alendronate in this condition are given below.

1. Adami S, *et al.* Effects of two oral doses of alendronate in the treatment of Paget's disease of bone. *Bone* 1994; **15:** 415–17.
2. Reid LR, *et al.* Biochemical and radiologic improvement in Paget's disease of bone treated with alendronate: a randomized, placebo-controlled trial. *Am J Med* 1996; **101:** 341–8.
3. Siris E, *et al.* Comparative study of alendronate versus etidronate for the treatment of Paget's disease of bone. *J Clin Endocrinol Metab* 1996; **81:** 961–7.

Preparations

Proprietary Preparations (details are given in Part 3)
Aust.: Fosamax; ***Austral.:*** Fosamax; ***Belg.:*** Fosamax; ***Canad.:*** Fosamax; ***Ger.:*** Fosamax; ***Irl.:*** Fosamax; ***Ital.:*** Adronat; Alendros; Dronal; Fosamax; ***Neth.:*** Fosamax; ***Norw.:*** Fosamax; ***S.Afr.:*** Fosamax; ***Spain:*** Fosamax; ***Swed.:*** Fosamax; ***Switz.:*** Fosamax; ***UK:*** Fosamax.

Bisphosphonates (3267-t)

Biphosphonates; Diphosphonates.

Bisphosphonates are analogues of pyrophosphate, in which the central oxygen atom is replaced by a carbon atom with two further substituents—see Figure 1, below. Like pyrophosphate they have a strong affinity for bone. The bisphosphonates are used chiefly for their antiresorptive and hypocalcaemic properties (see Uses and Administration, below). Bisphosphonates included in this chapter are: Alendronic Acid, p.733, Clodronic Acid, p.737, Etidronic Acid, p.738, Ibandronic Acid, p.739, Medronic Acid, p.740, Neridronic Acid, p.740, Oxidronic Acid, p.740, Pamidronic Acid, p.740, Risedronic Acid, p.741, and Tiludronic Acid, p.744.

Adverse Effects and Precautions

Bisphosphonates may cause gastro-intestinal disturbances including abdominal pain, nausea and vomiting, and diarrhoea or constipation. Existing gastro-intestinal problems may be exacerbated, and oral bisphosphonates should generally be given with care or avoided if acute upper gastro-intestinal inflammation is present. Abdominal pain may be more frequent with aminobisphosphonates such as alendronate and oesophagitis has occurred.

Disturbances in serum electrolytes may occur, most commonly hypocalcaemia and hypophosphataemia. Bisphosphonates may cause musculoskeletal pain and headache. Hypersensitivity reactions have occurred, but rarely; angioedema, rashes, and pruritus have been reported. Other rare adverse effects include blood disorders such as leucopenia and disturbances in liver enzyme values.

Transient fever and influenza-like symptoms are common with infusions of ibandronate and pamidronate. There may be local reactions, including thrombophlebitis, following parenteral administration.

Impairment of renal function has been reported with bisphosphonates, particularly when given parenterally. As a result their use should generally be avoided in patients with moderate to severe renal insufficiency and they should be used with care in those with lesser degrees of renal impairment.

Etidronate interferes with bone mineralisation, especially at higher doses, which can result in osteomalacia and an increased incidence of fracture. Etidronate should be discontinued if a fracture occurs, until healing is complete. It has also been associated with a flare in bone pain in some patients with Paget's disease. Impaired mineralisation is much less marked at usual doses of other bisphosphonates.

Overdosage with bisphosphonates would be likely to result in symptoms of hypocalcaemia; if necessary, parenteral infusion of a calcium salt could be given. Administration of milk or antacids, to bind the bisphosphonate and minimise absorption, has been suggested for oral overdosage.

There is no clinical experience with bisphosphonates in pregnancy and they are generally contra-indicated; bisphosphonates have been associated with skeletal abnormalities in the fetus when given to pregnant *animals.*

Reviews.

1. Adami S, Zamberlan N. Adverse effects of bisphosphonates: a comparative review. *Drug Safety* 1996; **14:** 158–70.

Effects on the eyes. There have been a few reports of ocular effects associated with nitrogen-containing bisphosphonates. Although adverse ocular reactions to pamidronate appeared to be rare, the manufacturers were aware of 23 cases up to September 1993 which were possibly associated with the drug.[1] The reactions included anterior uveitis in 7 patients and unilateral episcleritis or scleritis in 3. In one previously reported case,[2] bilateral iritis was associated with risedronate and subsequently pamidronate in a patient who had earlier received etidronate without ill-effect.

1. Macarol V, Fraunfelder FT. Pamidronate disodium and possible ocular adverse drug reactions. *Am J Ophthalmol* 1994; **118:** 220–4.
2. Siris ES. Bisphosphonates and iritis. *Lancet* 1993; **341:** 436–7.

Effects on the kidneys. Renal failure was associated with the intravenous administration of etidronate to 2 patients with hypercalcaemia of malignancy.[1] One had been given a high dose (1 g) by short intravenous infusion on two successive days and the other had an elevated serum-creatinine concentration before administration. A third patient given clodronate also developed renal failure but had a slightly raised serum-creatinine concentration before administration. Kanis *et al.*[2] commented that with smaller doses of bisphosphonates (up to 300 mg daily) by intravenous infusion over 2 to 3 hours they had not seen renal impairment in more than 40 patients treated with disodium etidronate or disodium clodronate. They noted a trend towards raised creatinine concentrations which was reversed when etidronate infusions were discontinued. Hasling *et al.*[3] found increased serum-creatinine concentrations after the first infusion of etidronate when compared with placebo, but not after subsequent infusions.

1. Bounameaux HM, *et al.* Renal failure associated with intravenous diphosphonates. *Lancet* 1983; **i:** 471.
2. Kanis JA, *et al.* Effects of intravenous diphosphonates on renal function. *Lancet* 1983; **i:** 1328.
3. Hasling C, *et al.* Etidronate disodium for treating hypercalcaemia of malignancy: a double blind placebo-controlled study. *Eur J Clin Invest* 1986; **16:** 433–7.

Figure 1. The comparative structures of the bisphosphonates.

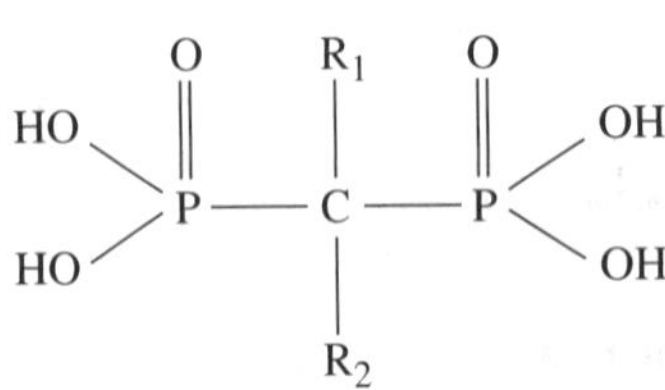

Generic structure of a bisphosphonate

Pyrophosphate

R_1	R_2	Name
$C_3H_6.NH_2$	OH	Alendronic Acid
Cl	Cl	Clodronic Acid
CH_3	OH	Etidronic Acid
$C_2H_4.NCH_3.C_5H_{11}$	OH	Ibandronic Acid
H	H	Medronic Acid
$C_5H_{10}.NH_2$	OH	Neridronic Acid
H	OH	Oxidronic Acid
$C_2H_4.NH_2$	OH	Pamidronic Acid
$CH_2.C_5H_4N$	OH	Risedronic Acid
$S.C_6H_4Cl$	H	Tiludronic Acid

Effects on the respiratory system. Bronchospasm has been induced by bisphosphonates in two patients who were aspirin-sensitive asthmatics. The first patient complained of shortness of breath and wheezing 10 minutes after the start of an infusion of clodronate while the second developed similar symptoms 2 days after the start of cyclical therapy with etidronate by mouth. Oral rechallenge in both patients resulted in a fall in the forced expiratory values at 1 second (FEV_1).[1] The reaction in these 2 patients was not considered to be immune-mediated.

1. Rolla G, *et al.* Bisphosphonate-induced bronchoconstriction in aspirin-sensitive asthma. *Lancet* 1994; **343:** 426–7.

Hypersensitivity. Bisphosphonates may rarely cause hypersensitivity reactions such as angioedema, urticaria, and pruritus. Published reports include a severe allergic reaction to sodium medronate in the form of a radiopharmaceutical,[1] and mild skin rashes in two patients given pamidronate by mouth.[2] There has also been a report of erythroderma with lesions of the mucous membranes being associated with clodronate administration in one patient,[3] and severe epidermal necrosis may have been associated with tiludronate in another.[4] A possibly drug-related rash has also been reported in a patient receiving alendronate.[5]

1. Elliott AT, *et al.* Severe reaction to diphosphonate: implications for treatment of Paget's disease. *Br Med J* 1988; **297:** 592–3.
2. Mautalen CA, *et al.* Side effects of disodium aminohydroxypropylidenediphosphonate (APD) during treatment of bone diseases. *Br Med J* 1984; **288:** 828–9.
3. Pajus I, *et al.* Erythroderma after clodronate treatment. *Br Med J* 1993; **307:** 484.
4. Roux C, *et al.* Long-lasting dermatological lesions after tiludronate therapy. *Calcif Tissue Int* 1992; **50:** 378–80.
5. Chesnut CH, *et al.* Alendronate treatment of the postmenopausal osteoporotic woman: effect of multiple dosages on bone mass and bone remodeling. *Am J Med* 1995; **99:** 144–52.

Interactions

The bisphosphonates are not well absorbed from the gastro-intestinal tract, and administration with food further impairs their absorption.

Compounds containing aluminium, calcium, iron, or magnesium, including antacids and mineral supplements and some osmotic laxatives, can also impair the absorption of bisphosphonates given by mouth.

It has been suggested that the administration of bisphosphonates with NSAIDs may result in an increased incidence of gastro-intestinal and renal adverse effects.

There may be additive hypocalcaemic effects with aminoglycosides.

Aminoglycosides. A report of a patient who developed persisting severe hypocalcaemia after treatment with clodronate and netilmicin. Bisphosphonates and aminoglycosides can induce hypocalcaemia by different mechanisms and care should be taken when administering them simultaneously.[1]

1. Pedersen-Bjergaard U, Myhre J. Severe hypocalcaemia after treatment with diphosphonate and aminoglycoside. *Br Med J* 1991; **302:** 295. Correction. *ibid.*; 791.

Pharmacokinetics

The bisphosphonates are poorly absorbed following oral administration, with bioavailabilities in the fasting state ranging from about 0.7% (alendronate; risedronate) to up to 6% (etidronate; tiludronate). Absorption is reduced by food, especially by products containing calcium or other polyvalent cations. They have a high affinity for bone, with about 50% of an absorbed dose bound to ossified tissues and retained in the body for prolonged periods. Excretion is in the urine, as unchanged drug; they do not appear to be metabolised.

Uses and Administration

The bisphosphonates inhibit bone resorption and thus have a hypocalcaemic effect. They are pyrophosphate analogues which have a high affinity for the hydroxyapatite of bone, and which inhibit bone resorption by osteoclasts; because of the coupling of resorption and formation this results in an overall reduction in remodelling and bone turnover (see Bone and Bone Disease, p.730). Their antiresorptive potency varies widely. The bisphosphonates also inhibit the formation and dissolution of hydroxyapatite crystals and thus have the potential to interfere with bone mineralisation. The degree to which the bisphosphonates inhibit mineralisation in clinical practice varies; disodium etidronate is the most potent inhibitor of those now in general clinical use.

Because bone resorption increases plasma-calcium concentrations, the bisphosphonates are used as adjuncts to the treatment of severe hypercalcaemia, especially when associated with malignancy. They are also used in disorders associated with excessive bone resorption and turnover, such as Paget's disease of bone and osteoporosis, as well as in the management of bone metastases. Etidronate has been used in the prevention and treatment of ectopic ossification.

Because of the affinity of bisphosphonates for bone, complexes labelled with radioactive technetium-99m (see p.1425) have been used diagnostically as bone scanning agents.

Bisphosphonates have been given by intravenous infusion or by mouth. In the latter case food should be avoided for a suitable period before and after administration, especially products with a high calcium content such as milk.

Reviews.

1. Compston JE. The therapeutic use of bisphosphonates. *Br Med J* 1994; **309:** 711–15.
2. Rosen CJ, Kessenich CR. Comparative clinical pharmacology and therapeutic use of bisphosphonates in metabolic bone diseases. *Drugs* 1996; **51:** 537–51.

Ectopic ossification. The only treatment for established ectopic ossification (p.730) is surgery, but drugs have been used for prophylaxis or prevention of recurrence. Bisphosphonates that are potent inhibitors of mineralisation such as etidronate have been advocated for this purpose, but they do not prevent the formation of the osteoid matrix and delayed mineralisation may occur once they are withdrawn.

Hypercalcaemia. In patients with severe symptomatic hypercalcaemia restoration and maintenance of adequate hydration and urine flow is essential, and helps to reduce plasma-calcium concentrations by promoting calcium diuresis. In hypercalcaemia of malignancy (p.1148) therapy with inhibitors of bone resorption such as the bisphosphonates may also be considered, and some have suggested that pamidronate is the drug of choice for this purpose. Although sustained, the action of bisphosphonates is not particularly rapid; they may be combined with a calcitonin where both rapid and prolonged diminution of plasma-calcium concentration is desired.

Hyperparathyroidism. Bisphosphonates have been used to inhibit bone resorption in the treatment of hypercalcaemia associated with hyperparathyroidism (p.733), but seem to be of little benefit for long-term treatment.

Malignant neoplasms of the bone. Bisphosphonates have been reported to be of benefit in some patients with malignancies of bone (p.484) both to help control bone pain and osteolysis and to manage the attendant hypercalcaemia. There is some evidence that bisphosphonates may retard the progression of malignant bone disease.

Osteogenesis imperfecta. Bisphosphonates have been tried in osteogenesis imperfecta (p.730), but orthopaedic treatment and physical activity programmes form the basis of therapy.

Osteoporosis. Bisphosphonates are used in the prevention and treatment of postmenopausal and corticosteroid-induced osteoporosis (p.731). Both alendronate and etidronate have been shown to be effective in terms of effect on bone mass density. There is less evidence for a consequent reduction in fracture rates, although this has been shown for alendronate in postmenopausal osteoporosis (see p.734). Alendronate is given continuously, whereas etidronate is given intermittently, alternating with a calcium supplement; both drugs are administered orally. Although there is less evidence for their efficacy in men with idiopathic osteoporosis, some consider bisphosphonates are the preferred treatment for this condition.

Paget's disease of bone. Paget's disease of bone (p.732) is characterised by excessive and disorganised bone resorption and formation. Not all patients require treatment, and pain can be managed in some with NSAIDs or paracetamol. Bisphosphonates may be indicated if bone pain is persistent or to prevent further progression of the disease particularly if there is a risk of complications.

Reflex sympathetic dystrophy. Osteoporosis is one of the features of reflex sympathetic dystrophy (see under Sympathetic Pain Syndromes, p.11) and preliminary data indicate that bisphosphonates may be of benefit in controlling associated pain in some patients.[1]

1. Schott GD. Bisphosphonates for pain relief in reflex sympathetic dystrophy? *Lancet* 1997; **350:** 1117. Correction. *ibid.* 1998; **351:** 682.

Calcitonins (12106-w)

Calcitonin (Human) (11091-e)

Calcitonin-human; Human Calcitonin.

$C_{151}H_{226}N_{40}O_{45}S_3,3HCl$ = 3527.2.

Pharmacopoeias. In *Swiss.*

A synthetic polypeptide comprising 32 amino acids in the same linear sequence as in naturally occurring human calcitonin.

Calcitonin (Pork) (8053-f)

Calcitonin (Pork) *(BANM).*

CAS — 12321-44-7.

NOTE. The synonym thyrocalcitonin and the CAS number 9007-12-9 have been used for calcitonin that is often of pork origin.

Pharmacopoeias. In *Br.* and *It.*

A polypeptide hormone obtained from pork thyroid. The BP specifies not less than 60 units per mg calculated with reference to the dried substance. Trace amounts of thyroid hormones may be present. The BP limits are not more than 20 ng of liothyronine and not more than 50 ng of thyroxine per unit of calcitonin.

A white or almost white powder. **Soluble** in water; practically insoluble in alcohol, in acetone, in chloroform, and in ether; sparingly soluble in solutions of mineral acids. It dissolves in solutions of alkali hydroxides. **Store** at a temperature not exceeding 25°. Protect from light. The BP states that under these conditions it may be expected to retain its potency for not less than 2 years.

Elcatonin (19126-n)

Elcatonin *(rINN).*

[Aminosuberic Acid 1,7]-eel Calcitonin; [$Asu^{1,7}$]-E-CT; Carbocalcitonin. 1-Butyric acid-7-(L-2-aminobutyric acid)-26-L-aspartic acid-27-L-valine-29-L-alaninecalcitonin (salmon).

$C_{148}H_{244}N_{42}O_{47}$ = 3363.8.

CAS — 60731-46-6.

A synthetic analogue of eel calcitonin.

Salcatonin (8054-d)

Salcatonin *(BAN).*

Calcitonin (Salmon); Calcitonin-salmon; Calcitoninum Salmonis; Salmon Calcitonin; SCT-1.

$C_{145}H_{240}N_{44}O_{48}S_2$ = 3431.9.

CAS — 47931-85-1.

NOTE. There may be some confusion between the terms Salcatonin and Calcitonin (Salmon) (Salmon Calcitonin; Calcitonin-salmon) although in practice these names appear to be used for the same substance.

Salcatonin *(BAN)* is defined as a *component* of natural salmon calcitonin. The BP defines Salcatonin and Calcitonin (Salmon) as a synthetic polypeptide having the structure determined for salmon calcitonin I.

In the USA, Calcitonin *(USAN)* includes calcitonin (human) and calcitonin (salmon). Salcatonin is there understood to be a synthetic polypeptide structurally similar to natural salmon calcitonin (Calcitonin Salmon (Synthesis)). The US manufacturers use Calcitonin-salmon for a synthetic polypeptide with the same structure as calcitonin of salmon origin.

Pharmacopoeias. In *Eur.* (see p.viii).

A synthetic polypeptide having the structure of salmon calcitonin I. Ph. Eur. specifies not less than 4000 units per mg calculated with reference to the peptide content.

A white or almost white, light powder. Freely **soluble** in water. **Store** at 2° to 8°. Protect from light. For the **incompatibility** of calcitonins with the plastic of intravenous giving sets, see under Interactions, below.

Units

0.8 units of calcitonin, porcine, are contained in one ampoule of the second International Standard Preparation (1991).

128 units of calcitonin, salmon, are contained in approximately 20 μg of freeze-dried purified synthetic salmon calcitonin, with mannitol 2 mg in one ampoule of the second International Standard Preparation (1989).

17.5 units of calcitonin, human, are contained in one ampoule of the second International Standard Preparation (1991).

There is also a first International Standard Preparation (1989) of elcatonin.

Potency of calcitonins is estimated by comparing the hypocalcaemic effect, in *rats,* with that of the standard preparation, and is expressed in international or MRC units which are considered to be equivalent. One manufacturer states that 100 international units by this assay is equivalent to 1 mg of porcine or human calcitonin, and to 25 μg of salmon calcitonin although other, slightly different, equivalencies have been cited for other preparations. However, although 1 unit of pork calcitonin, 1 unit of salmon calcitonin, and 1 unit of human calcitonin should give the same response in men this is not necessarily the case. Clinically, doses of pork and salmon calcitonin are expressed in units whereas those of human calcitonin can be expressed by weight, probably a reflection of its purity. Doses of calcitonin considered approximately equivalent in practice are 80 units of pork calcitonin, 50 units of salmon calcitonin, and 0.5 mg of human calcitonin (see Uses and Administration, below).

Adverse Effects, Treatment, and Precautions

Calcitonins may cause nausea, vomiting, flushing, and tingling of the hands. These reactions are dose dependent, usually transient, and occur more often with intravenous administration. Other adverse effects have included skin rash, an unpleasant taste, abdominal pain, urinary frequency, and tremor. A diabetogenic effect has been reported rarely. Inflammatory reactions at the injection site have been reported with some calcitonins, and rhinitis and other local reactions have been reported with nasal formulations. Transient hypocalcaemia may occur after injections of calcitonin.

Circulating antibodies may develop after several months of use but resistance does not necessarily follow (see also below). In patients with a history of allergy, a skin test has been advised prior to administration as hypersensitivity reactions, including anaphylaxis, have occurred.

Calcitonin has inhibited lactation in *animals*.

Nausea and vomiting may be reduced by administration at bedtime or by prior administration of an antiemetic.

Calcitonin (pork) may contain trace amounts of thyroid hormones (for limits, see above), but clinical effects are unlikely in most patients.

Antibody formation. Long-term treatment with heterologous calcitonins may lead to the formation of neutralising antibodies. This appears to be common in patients given pork or salmon calcitonin. Human calcitonin is less immunogenic than pork or salmon, but a study[1] has also detected antibodies to human calcitonin in 1 of 33 women with postmenopausal osteoporosis after 6 months of therapy.

The degree to which such antibodies affect therapeutic activity is uncertain. Some studies have suggested a significant loss of therapeutic activity in patients who developed neutralising antibodies to salmon calcitonin,[2] or a restoration in activity following a switch from salmon to human calcitonin in such patients;[3] equally, others have presented evidence that the activity of salmon calcitonin was not reduced by the development of antibodies to the drug.[4]

1. Grauer A, *et al.* Formation of neutralizing antibodies after treatment with human calcitonin. *Am J Med* 1993; **95:** 439–42.
2. Grauer A, *et al.* In vitro detection of neutralizing antibodies after treatment of Paget's disease of bone with nasal salmon calcitonin. *J Bone Miner Res* 1990; **5:** 387–91.
3. Muff R, *et al.* Efficacy of intranasal human calcitonin in patients with Paget's disease refractory to salmon calcitonin. *Am J Med* 1990; **89:** 181–4.
4. Reginster JY, *et al.* Influence of specific anti-salmon calcitonin antibodies on biological effectiveness of nasal salmon calcitonin in Paget's disease of bone. *Scand J Rheumatol* 1990; **19:** 83–6.

Effect on glucose metabolism. A single subcutaneous injection of salmon calcitonin has been reported to increase blood-glucose concentrations,[1] but long-term treatment with calcitonins was considered unlikely to cause diabetes.[2] Nevertheless, deterioration in diabetic control has been noted in a patient given calcitonin (pork)[3] and postprandial release of insulin was abolished by intravenous salmon calcitonin in 8 patients with duodenal ulcers.[4]

1. Gattereau A, *et al.* Hyperglycaemic effect of synthetic salmon calcitonin. *Lancet* 1977; **ii:** 1076–7.
2. Evans IMA, *et al.* Hyperglycaemic effect of synthetic salmon calcitonin. *Lancet* 1978; **i:** 280.
3. Thomas DW, *et al.* Deterioration in diabetic control during calcitonin therapy. *Med J Aust* 1979; **2:** 699–70.
4. Jonderko K. Effect of calcitonin on gastric emptying in patients with an active duodenal ulcer. *Gut* 1989; **30:** 430–5.

Gynaecomastia. A 62-year-old man developed painful gynaecomastia on two occasions following treatment with salcatonin administered by subcutaneous injection.[1]

1. Vankrunkelsven PJ, Thijs MM. Salcatonin and gynaecomastia. *Lancet* 1994; **344:** 482.

Renal impairment. Calcitonins are metabolised mainly in the kidneys and pharmacokinetic studies (see below) have indicated that the dosage of calcitonins may need to be reduced in patients with renal insufficiency, but there have been no specific guidelines.

Interactions

There is a theoretical possibility that dosage adjustments may be required in patients receiving cardiac glycosides who are given injections of calcitonin, because of the effects of the latter on serum calcium.

Like some other peptide drugs, calcitonin may be adsorbed onto the plastic of intravenous giving sets; it has been suggested that solutions for intravenous infusion should contain some protein to prevent the sorption and consequent loss of potency.

Pharmacokinetics

Calcitonins are rapidly inactivated when given by mouth. After injection, calcitonins are quickly metabolised, primarily in the kidneys but also in blood and peripheral tissues. The inactive metabolites and a small proportion of unchanged drug are excreted in the urine. The half-life of human calcitonin is stated to be 60 minutes and that of salmon calcitonin about 70 to 90 minutes.

Calcitonins are also absorbed through the nasal and rectal mucosa. Although figures have varied widely, about 3% of a nasally administered dose of salmon calcitonin is reported to be bioavailable compared with the same dose administered by intramuscular injection, with peak plasma concentrations occurring after about 30 to 40 minutes compared with 15 to 25 minutes after the parenteral dose.

Following the subcutaneous injection of 19.9 μg of synthetic salmon-calcitonin in 16 healthy subjects,[1] absorption was rapid with an absorption half-life of 23.4 minutes. The maximum mean plasma concentration was 384 pg per mL at 60 minutes after which excretion was fairly rapid with an elimination half-life of 87 minutes. These results and those from previously reported investigations of salmon, human, and porcine calcitonin could not easily be compared, especially since different assay methods had been used. Nevertheless it was concluded that bioavailability from subcutaneous and intramuscular injection sites was good; that dosage may need to be adjusted in renal insufficiency because of low metabolic clearance rate; and that the higher potency of salcatonin is due to higher intrinsic activity at the receptor site rather than to pharmacokinetic differences. The US manufacturers have cited a half-life of 1.02 hours after a single subcutaneous injection of human calcitonin 0.5 mg. The plasma elimination half-life of elcatonin was about 4.8 hours following intramuscular injection in healthy subjects.[2]

Calcitonins are absorbed following intranasal or rectal administration. Peak plasma concentrations of salmon calcitonin were achieved 20 to 60 minutes after administration by nasal spray in doses ranging from 200 to 400 units.[3] In another study[4] salmon calcitonin 200 units, repeated once after 3 hours, was given by nasal spray or suppository to healthy subjects. Absorption was prompt and the total amount absorbed was similar with either route. However, whereas intranasal administration produced low peaks with salcatonin still detectable in the blood after 3 to 5 hours, rectal administration produced peak plasma concentrations about 6 to 8 times higher than intranasal administration but salcatonin was undetectable within 2 hours; plasma concentrations were lower than those found after injection. Another group of workers[5] found human calcitonin to be poorly absorbed when given intranasally to healthy subjects. Absorption from nasal powder or spray solutions was improved by the presence of the surfactants dihydrofusinate or glycocholate.

Investigations carried out in 4 osteoporotic patients[6] suggested that the rectal administration of salcatonin could provide 65% of the bioavailability of intramuscular administration.

1. Nüesch E, Schmidt R. Comparative pharmacokinetics of calcitonins. In: Pecile A, ed. *Calcitonin international congress series no. 540*. Amsterdam: Excerpta Medica, 1980: 352–64.
2. Sergre G, *et al.* Pharmacokinetics of carbocalcitonin in humans. *Clin Trials J* 1986; **23** (suppl 1): 23–8.
3. Kurose H, *et al.* Intranasal absorption of salmon calcitonin. *Calcif Tissue Int* 1987; **41:** 249–51.
4. Buclin T, *et al.* The effect of rectal and nasal administration of salmon calcitonin in normal subjects. *Calcif Tissue Int* 1987; **41:** 252–8.
5. Pontiroli AE, *et al.* Nasal administration of glucagon and human calcitonin to healthy subjects: a comparison of powders and spray solutions and of different enhancing agents. *Eur J Clin Pharmacol* 1989; **37:** 427–30.
6. Gennari C, *et al.* Pharmacodynamic activity of synthetic salmon calcitonin in osteoporotic patients: comparison between rectal and intramuscular administration: pilot study. *Curr Ther Res* 1993; **53:** 301–8.

Uses and Administration

Calcitonin is a hormone produced by mammalian thyroid parafollicular cells or the ultimobranchial gland in non-mammalian vertebrates. In man its secretion and biosynthesis are regulated by the plasma-calcium concentration. It has a hypocalcaemic action that is due primarily to inhibition of osteoclastic bone resorption; of less importance is a direct effect on the kidneys resulting in increased urinary excretion of calcium and phosphorus. Calcitonin contains 32 amino acids; the sequence varies according to the species. Naturally occurring porcine calcitonin, synthetic salmon calcitonin (salcatonin), and synthetic human calcitonin are in clinical use; salcatonin is the most potent. Elcatonin, a synthetic derivative of eel calcitonin, is available in some countries.

Calcitonins are used in the treatment of diseases characterised by high bone turnover such as Paget's disease of bone. They are also given as an adjunct in the treatment of severe hypercalcaemia, especially that associated with malignancy. Some calcitonins are used in the management of osteoporosis and osteolysis and bone pain due to malignancies of bone. Beneficial effects have also been reported with calcitonins in the treatment of other diseases of bone such as osteogenesis imperfecta and congenital hyperphosphatasia (juvenile Paget's disease of bone).

Calcitonins are generally administered by subcutaneous or intramuscular injection; some have been given intranasally, rectally, or by intravenous infusion.

In **Paget's disease of bone** the usual dose range for calcitonin (pork) by subcutaneous or intramuscular injection is 80 units three times weekly to 160 units daily in single or divided doses; patients with bone pain or nerve compression syndromes may be given 80 or 160 units daily for 3 to 6 months. For salcatonin the range is 50 units three times weekly to 100 units daily in single or divided doses by subcutaneous or intramuscular injection. Human calcitonin is usually given by subcutaneous or intramuscular injection in a dose range of 0.5 mg two or three times weekly to 0.5 mg daily; severe cases may require up to 1 mg daily.

As an adjunct to the treatment of **hypercalcaemia**, calcitonins have a rapid effect which is greatest in patients with an increased bone turnover. Calcitonin (pork) may be given in a dose of 4 units per kg bodyweight daily by intramuscular or subcutaneous injection according to the patient's needs. In severe hypercalcaemia larger doses of calcitonin may be more conveniently administered as the more potent salcatonin. Salcatonin may be given by subcutaneous or intramuscular injection in a dose of 5 to 10 units per kg daily or up to 400 units every 6 or 8 hours. Doses greater than 8 units per kg every 6 hours are considered to have no additional benefit. In the emergency treatment of hypercalcaemic crisis, salcatonin has also been given intravenously: a suggested dose is 5 to 10 units per kg daily, diluted in 500 mL of sodium chloride 0.9% and given by slow intravenous infusion over at least 6 hours (see also under Administration below for the problems of intravenous administration). Human calcitonin is also given intravenously for acute hypercalcaemia, a dose of 0.5 mg by slow intravenous infusion every 6 hours being recommended.

Salcatonin is used in the treatment of **postmenopausal osteoporosis** in a dose of 100 units daily or every other day by subcutaneous or intramuscular injection, or 200 units daily intranasally by nasal spray, alternating nostrils each day. Supplementary calcium (equivalent to at least 600 mg of elemental calcium daily) and, if necessary, vitamin D (400 units daily) should also be given.

Salcatonin has also been used for the control of **bone pain due to malignant neoplasms**. The usual dose by intramuscular or subcutaneous injection is 200 units every 6 hours or 400 units every 12 hours for up to 48 hours. The treatment course may be repeated as appropriate.

Oral formulations of salcatonin are under investigation.

Action. Calcitonins are used primarily for their action on bone and the kidney to maintain calcium homoeostasis and to inhibit bone resorption in disorders of bone turnover. Calcitonins also appear to have some central analgesic activity[1] which perhaps plays a role in the marked relief they may bring to bone pain.[2]

In addition, calcitonins have been found to reduce gastric[3] and pancreatic secretions[4] and to delay gastric emptying.[5]

1. Fraioli F, *et al.* Subarachnoid injection of salmon calcitonin induces analgesia in man. *Eur J Pharmacol* 1982; **78:** 381–2.
2. Mannarini M, *et al.* Analgesic effect of salmon calcitonin suppositories in patients with bone pain. *Curr Ther Res* 1994; **55:** 1079–83.
3. Hotz J, *et al.* Inhibition of human gastric secretion by intragastrically administered calcitonin. *Digestion* 1980; **20:** 180–9.
4. Beglinger C, *et al.* Effect of calcitonin and calcitonin gene-related peptide on pancreatic functions in man. *Gut* 1988; **29:** 243–8.
5. Jonderko K. Effect of calcitonin on gastric emptying in patients with an active duodenal ulcer. *Gut* 1989; **30:** 430–5.

Administration. Calcitonins have poor oral bioavailability and administration is usually by subcutaneous or intramuscular injection. To improve patient acceptability, especially in diseases requiring long-term drug therapy such as osteoporosis or Paget's disease of bone, alternative methods of administration have been investigated.

Salcatonin has proved effective when given intranasally in usual doses of 50 to 200 units daily (for references, see Osteoporosis below), and intranasal products for osteoporosis are available. Suppositories containing 300 units of salcatonin have been used in the management of hypercalcaemia; one suppository being administered three times a day (total daily dose of 900 units).[1,2] Daily doses of 100 units of salcatonin by suppository have been tried in postmenopausal osteoporosis[3] and in patients with bone pain.[4]

Calcitonins have been given by intravenous infusion, but this is rarely necessary and may cause more side-effects. If intravenous administration is essential, it has been suggested[5] that some protein must be present in the solution to prevent adsorption onto the plastic of the giving set. However, in practice this does not seem to be the case; in the UK, manufacturer's recommendations are for dilution with normal saline, while acknowledging that such dilution results in a loss of potency, and dosage is adjusted accordingly. Presumably dilution with a protein-containing solution would allow lower doses to be used. The manufacturers do specify that solutions for infusion should be prepared immediately before use and that glass or hard plastic containers should not be used.

1. Thiébaud D, *et al.* Effectiveness of salmon calcitonin administered as suppositories in tumor-induced hypercalcemia. *Am J Med* 1987; **82:** 745–50.
2. Thiébaud D, *et al.* Fast and effective treatment of malignant hypercalcemia: combination of suppositories of calcitonin and a single infusion of 3-amino 1-hydroxypropylidene-1-bisphosphonate. *Arch Intern Med* 1990; **150:** 2125–8.
3. Gonnelli S, *et al.* Effect of rectal salmon calcitonin treatment on bone mass and bone turnover in patients with established postmenopausal osteoporosis: a 1-year crossover study. *Curr Ther Res* 1993; **54:** 458–65.
4. Mannarini M, *et al.* Analgesic effect of salmon calcitonin suppositories in patients with bone pain. *Curr Ther Res* 1994; **55:** 1079–83.
5. Stevenson JC. Current management of malignant hypercalcaemia. *Drugs* 1988; **36:** 229–38.

Hypercalcaemia. Calcitonins can be used in the management of moderate to severe symptomatic hypercalcaemia (p.1148) in addition to rehydration and diuresis. Because of their rapid effect, they may be particularly useful in life-threatening hypercalcaemia. However, although they have a rapid effect it is usually short-lived; calcitonins are therefore generally given as an adjunct with other therapy such as a bisphosphonate. References to the use of calcitonins for hypercalcaemia are given below.

1. Ralston SH, *et al.* Treatment of cancer associated hypercalcaemia with combined aminohydroxypropylidene diphosphonate and calcitonin. *Br Med J* 1986; **292:** 1549–50.
2. Thiébaud D, *et al.* Effectiveness of salmon calcitonin administered as suppositories in tumor-induced hypercalcemia. *Am J Med* 1987; **82:** 745–50.
3. Thiébaud D, *et al.* Fast and effective treatment of malignant hypercalcemia: combination of suppositories of calcitonin and a single infusion as 3-amino 1-hydroxypropylidene-1-bisphosphonate. *Arch Intern Med* 1990; **150:** 2125–8.
4. Kaul S, Sockalosky JJ. Human synthetic calcitonin therapy for hypercalcemia of immobilization. *J Pediatr* 1995; **126:** 825–7.

Hyperphosphatasia. Hyperphosphatasia, also known as juvenile Paget's disease, is a rare hereditary disorder that has been treated successfully with calcitonin. Bone turnover was reduced by administration of human calcitonin in a boy presenting at 5 years of age with a history of repeated fractures and progressive bone deformity.[1] Calcitonin was considered beneficial, especially if started before gross deformities have developed, and long-term therapy has been highly successful.[2]

1. Woodhouse NJY, *et al.* Paget's disease in a 5-year-old: acute response to human calcitonin. *Br Med J* 1972; **4:** 267–9.
2. Stevenson JC, Evans IMA. Pharmacology and therapeutic use of calcitonin. *Drugs* 1981; **21:** 257–72.

Malignant neoplasms of the bone. Calcitonins may be useful adjuvants in the treatment of malignant disease involving the bone (p.484), not only to correct hypercalcaemia of malignancy, but also to relieve bone pain and osteolysis. The analgesic properties of calcitonins (see Action, above) may play some part in this, although relief of bone pain has also been seen with bisphosphonates, suggesting that if such actions are of significance, they are not the sole reason for pain relief. References to the use of calcitonins for bone metastases are given below.

1. Roth A, Kolarić K. Analgetic activity of calcitonin in patients with painful osteolytic metastases of breast cancer. *Oncology* 1986; **43:** 283–7.
2. Blomqvist C, *et al.* Evaluation of salmon calcitonin treatment in bone metastases from breast cancer—a controlled trial. *Bone* 1988; **9:** 45–51.
3. Gennari C, *et al.* Salmon calcitonin treatment in bone metastases. *Curr Ther Res* 1989; **45:** 804–12.

Osteogenesis imperfecta. There have been reports[1,2] of beneficial effects with calcitonins in the treatment of osteogenesis imperfecta (p.730).

1. Castells S, *et al.* Therapy of osteogenesis imperfecta with synthetic salmon calcitonin. *J Pediatr* 1979; **95:** 807–11.
2. Nishi Y, *et al.* Effect of long-term calcitonin therapy by injection and nasal spray on the incidence of fractures in osteogenesis imperfecta. *J Pediatr* 1992; **121:** 477–80.

Osteoporosis. Calcitonins are used in the prevention and treatment of osteoporosis (p.731). In postmenopausal osteoporosis they are usually second-line agents. However, they may be particularly useful in women with high-turnover osteoporosis, and in those with bone pain due to vertebral crush fractures. References to the use of calcitonins for postmenopausal osteoporosis[1-8] and corticosteroid-induced osteoporosis[9-12] are given below.

1. Reginster JY, *et al.* 1-Year controlled randomised trial of prevention of early postmenopausal bone loss by intranasal calcitonin. *Lancet* 1987; **ii:** 1481–3.
2. MacIntyre I, *et al.* Calcitonin for prevention of postmenopausal bone loss. *Lancet* 1988; **i:** 900–2.
3. Pun KK, Chan LWL. Analgesic effect of intranasal salmon calcitonin in the treatment of osteoporotic vertebral fractures. *Clin Ther* 1989; **11:** 205–9.
4. Overgaard K, *et al.* Effect of salcatonin given intranasally on early postmenopausal bone loss. *Br Med J* 1989; **299:** 477–9.
5. Overgaard K, *et al.* Discontinuous calcitonin treatment of established osteoporosis—effects of withdrawal of treatment. *Am J Med* 1990; **89:** 1–6.
6. Overgaard K, *et al.* Effect of salcatonin given intranasally on bone mass and fracture rates in established osteoporosis: a dose response study. *Br Med J* 1992; **305:** 556–61.
7. Reginster JY, *et al.* A 5-year controlled randomized study of prevention of postmenopausal trabecular bone loss with nasal salmon calcitonin and calcium. *Eur J Clin Invest* 1994; **24:** 565–9.
8. Reginster JY, *et al.* A double-blind, placebo-controlled, dose-finding trial of intermittent nasal salmon calcitonin for prevention of postmenopausal lumbar spine bone loss. *Am J Med* 1995; **98:** 452–8.
9. Ringe J-D, Welzel D. Salmon calcitonin in the therapy of corticoid-induced osteoporosis. *Eur J Clin Pharmacol* 1987; **33:** 35–9.
10. Rizzato G, *et al.* Administration of salmon calcitonin nasal spray for long-term treatment of corticosteroid-induced osteoporosis, a preliminary report. *Curr Ther Res* 1989; **45:** 761–6.
11. Nishioka T, *et al.* Nasal administration of salmon calcitonin for prevention of glucocorticoid-induced osteoporosis in children with nephrosis. *J Pediatr* 1991; **118:** 703–7.
12. Adachi JD, *et al.* Salmon calcitonin nasal spray in the prevention of corticosteroid-induced osteoporosis. *Br J Rheumatol* 1997; **36:** 255–9.

Paget's disease of bone. Patients with Paget's disease of bone (p.732) may require no treatment or just analgesics alone, but calcitonins may be indicated if bone pain is persistent or to prevent further progression of the disease. However, the bisphosphonates have largely superseded the calcitonins in this role. References to the use of calcitonins for Paget's disease of bone are given below.

1. Nagant de Deuxchaisnes C, *et al.* New modes of administration of salmon calcitonin in Paget's disease. *Clin Orthop* 1987; **217:** 56–71.
2. Muff R, *et al.* Efficacy of intranasal human calcitonin in patients with Paget's disease refractory to salmon calcitonin. *Am J Med* 1990; **89:** 181–4.

Pain. In addition to bone pain associated with malignancy and with bone disorders such as Paget's disease, calcitonins may also have other analgesic properties (see under Action, above). References to beneficial results in various painful syndromes are given below. For a full discussion on pain and its management, see p.4.

1. Ricevuti G. Effects of human calcitonin on pain in the treatment of Tietze's syndrome. *Clin Ther* 1985; **7:** 669–73.
2. Patti F, *et al.* Calcitonin and migraine. *Headache* 1986; **26:** 172–4.
3. Micieli G, *et al.* Effectiveness of salmon calcitonin nasal spray preparation in migraine treatment. *Headache* 1988; **28:** 196–200.
4. Mannerini M, *et al.* Analgesic effect of salmon calcitonin suppositories in patients with bone pain. *Curr Ther Res* 1994; **55:** 1079–83.

Preparations

BP 1998: Calcitonin (Pork) Injection; Calcitonin (Salmon) Injection.

Proprietary Preparations (details are given in Part 3)

Aust.: Casalm; Cibacalcin; Elcimen; Ucecal; ***Austral.:*** Calcitare; Calsynar; Cibacalcin; Miacalcic; ***Belg.:*** Calsynar; Cibacalcine; Miacalcic; ***Canad.:*** Calcimar; Caltine; ***Fr.:*** Calcitar; Calsyn; Cibacalcine; Miacalcic; Staporos†; ***Ger.:*** Azucalcit; Calci; Calcimonta; Calcitonin L†; Calcitonin S†; Calsynar; Calsynar Lyo; Calsynar Lyo S†; Casalm; Cibacalcin; Karil; Osteos; Ostostabil; ***Irl.:*** Calcitare; Calsynar; ***Ital.:*** Aima-Calcin; Biocalcin; Calciben; Calcinil; Calciosint; Calcioton; Calcitar; Calcitonina-Sandoz; Calco; Carbicalcin; Catonin; Cibacalcin; Eptacalcin†; Ipocalcin; Isi-Calcin; Miacalcic; Miadenil; Osteocalcin; Osteotonina; Osteovis; Porostenina; Prontocalcin†; Quosten; Rulicalcin; Salcatyn†; Salmocalcin; Salmofar; Sical; Sintocalcin; Stalcin; Staporos†; Steocin; Tonocalcin; Turbocalcin; ***Jpn:*** Calcitoran; Elcitonin; ***Neth.:*** Calsynar†; Cibacalcin; ***Norw.:*** Calcitare†; Miacalcic; ***S.Afr.:*** Miacalcic; ***Spain:*** Bionocalcin; Calogen; Calsynar; Carbicalcin; Cibacalcina; Diatin; Kalsimin; Miacalcic; Oseototal; Osteobion; Sical; Tonocaltin; Ucecal; ***Swed.:*** Cibacalcin; Miacalcic; ***Switz.:*** Cibacalcine; Miacalcic; ***UK:*** Calcitare; Calsynar; Miacalcic; ***USA:*** Calcimar; Cibacalcin†; Miacalcin; Osteocalcin.

Clodronic Acid (3273-k)

Clodronic Acid *(BAN, USAN, rINN).*

(Dichloromethylene)diphosphonic acid.

$CH_4Cl_2O_6P_2$ = 244.9.

CAS — 10596-23-3.

Disodium Clodronate (12673-a)

BM-06.011; Cl_2 MBP; Cl_2MDP; Clodronate Disodium; Clodronate Sodium; Dichloromethane Diphosphonate Disodium; Dichloromethylene Diphosphonate Disodium; Sodium Clodronate *(BANM).* Disodium (dichloromethylene)diphosphonate tetrahydrate.

$CH_2Cl_2Na_2O_6P_2,4H_2O$ = 360.9.

CAS — 22560-50-5.

124.9 mg of disodium clodronate tetrahydrate is approximately equivalent to 100 mg of anhydrous substance.

Adverse Effects and Precautions

As for the bisphosphonates in general, p.734. Gastro-intestinal symptoms following oral dosage may be reduced by giving the drug in divided doses rather than as a single daily dose. Reversible increases in liver enzyme values and moderate leucopenia have been seen in a few patients. Monitoring of liver function and white cell counts is advised during intravenous administration. Disodium clodronate has precipitated bronchospasm, even in patients with no history of asthma. Transient proteinuria has been reported immediately after intravenous infusion.

Carcinogenicity. Early reports of a possible association between disodium clodronate and leukaemia, including a man who developed acute myeloblastic leukaemia after receiving clodronate for 6 months,[1] have not been substantiated; this particular patient had been exposed to benzene over many years.

1. Delmas PD, *et al.* Long term effects of dichloromethylene diphosphonate in Paget's disease of bone. *J Clin Endocrinol Metab* 1982; **54:** 837–44.

Effects on the respiratory system. For a report of bronchospasm in an aspirin-sensitive asthmatic, induced by an infusion of clodronate, see p.735.

Hypersensitivity. Allergic reactions to bisphosphonates are rare. Erythroderma has been associated with clodronate administration in one patient, see p.735.

Renal impairment. For mention of renal failure developing in a patient with slightly raised serum-creatinine concentrations who subsequently received an intravenous infusion of clodronate, see Effects on the Kidneys, p.734. The manufacturers recommend that intravenous infusion of clodronate be avoided in patients with moderate to severe renal failure (serum creatinine greater than 440 μmol (50 mg) per litre) and that the oral dosage form be avoided in patients with a creatinine clearance below 10 mL per minute and the dosage halved in patients with creatinine clearance between 10 and 30 mL per minute.

Interactions

As for the bisphosphonates in general, p.735.

Aminoglycosides. A report of a patient who developed persisting severe hypocalcaemia after treatment with clodronate and netilmicin. Bisphosphonates and aminoglycosides can induce hypocalcaemia by different mechanisms and care should be taken when administering them simultaneously.[1]

1. Pedersen-Bjergaard U, Myhre J. Severe hypocalcaemia after treatment with diphosphonate and aminoglycoside. *Br Med J* 1991; **302:** 295. Correction. *ibid.*; 791.

Pharmacokinetics

Disodium clodronate is poorly absorbed from the gastro-intestinal tract and absorption is reduced by food, especially products containing calcium or other polyvalent cations; bioavailability is only 1 to 4%. Following absorption or intravenous administration it is cleared rapidly from the blood with a reported plasma half-life of only about 2 hours, but has a high affinity for bone. Over 70% of an intravenous dose is excreted unchanged in the urine within 24 hours the remainder being sequestered in bone tissue. Disodium clodronate is not metabolised.

References.

1. Conrad KA, Lee SM. Clodronate kinetics and dynamics. *Clin Pharmacol Ther* 1981; **30:** 114–20.
2. Yakatan GJ, *et al.* Clodronate kinetics and bioavailability. *Clin Pharmacol Ther* 1982; **31:** 402–10.

Bioavailability. Enhanced bioavailability tablets of disodium clodronate are available in some countries, the licensed dose of which is 35% less than the dose of the standard formulation (see below). However, an open, randomised, crossover study in 88 volunteers found that a 1040 mg dose of the new formulation provided only 52% of the bioavailable dose of 1600 mg of the standard capsule formulation.[1]

1. Lapham G, *et al.* Bioavailability of two clodronate formulations. *Br J Hosp Med* 1996; **56:** 231–3.

Uses and Administration

Clodronate is a bisphosphonate with general properties similar to those of the other bisphosphonates (p.735). It inhibits bone resorption, but appears to have less effect on bone mineralisation than etidronate at comparable doses.

Disodium clodronate is used as an adjunct in the treatment of severe hypercalcaemia, especially when associated with malignancy. In addition, it is used in the treatment of osteolytic bone metastases.

It is administered by slow intravenous infusion or by mouth, as a single daily dose or in 2 divided doses; food should be avoided for at least 1 hour before or after oral administration. Doses are expressed in terms of the anhydrous substance. Disodium clodronate is available in capsules of 400 mg and standard tablets of 800 mg. Tablets of disodium clodronate 520 mg are also available in some countries, and have a greater bioavailability than the capsules or standard tablets; one such tablet of disodium clodronate 520 mg is approximately equivalent to two capsules each containing disodium clodronate 400 mg or one 800-mg standard tablet (but see Bioavailability, above).

In the management of osteolytic lesions, hypercalcaemia, and bone pain associated with skeletal metastases in patients with breast cancer or multiple myeloma, disodium clodronate 1.6 g daily has been given by mouth as capsules or standard tablets, and may be increased if necessary to a maximum of 3.2 g daily. Alternatively a dose of 1.04 g daily, increased if necessary up to 2.08 g daily, may be given as enhanced bioavailability tablets.

In hypercalcaemia of malignancy disodium clodronate is given by intravenous infusion over not less than 2 hours in a dose of 300 mg daily on successive days until normocalcaemia is achieved; duration of treatment should not exceed 10 days. Alternatively, it may be given as a single intravenous infusion of 1.5 g in 500 mL of infusion solution administered over a period of 4 hours. Once serum-calcium concentrations have been reduced to an acceptable level, maintenance therapy may be given by mouth in similar doses to those used for initial oral treatment of metastases.

General references.

1. Plosker GL, Goa KL. Clodronate: a review of its pharmacological properties and therapeutic efficacy in resorptive bone disease. *Drugs* 1994; **47:** 945–82.

Hypercalcaemia. Treatment with bisphosphonates may be considered in patients with moderate to severe symptomatic hypercalcaemia of malignancy (p.1148) in addition to rehydration and diuresis. References to the use of disodium clodronate for hypercalcaemia are given below.

1. Urwin GH, *et al.* Treatment of the hypercalcaemia of malignancy with intravenous clodronate. *Bone* 1987; **8** (suppl 1): S43–S51.
2. Ralston SH, *et al.* Comparison of three intravenous bisphosphonates in cancer-associated hypercalcaemia. *Lancet* 1989; **ii:** 1180–2.
3. Rostom AY. Clodronate as outpatient treatment for hypercalcaemia. *Lancet* 1990; **336:** 1390.
4. O'Rourke NP, *et al.* Effective treatment of malignant hypercalcaemia with a single intravenous infusion of clodronate. *Br J Cancer* 1993; **67:** 560–3.

Hyperparathyroidism. Bisphosphonates have been used to inhibit bone resorption in the treatment of hypercalcaemia associated with hyperparathyroidism (p.733) but seem to be of little benefit for long-term treatment. References to the use of clodronate in hyperparathyroidism are given below.

1. Shane E, *et al.* Effects of dichloromethylene diphosphonate on serum and urinary calcium in primary hyperparathyroidism. *Ann Intern Med* 1981; **95:** 23–7.
2. Douglas DL, *et al.* Drug treatment of primary hyperparathyroidism: use of clodronate disodium. *Br Med J* 1983; **286:** 587–90.
3. Hamdy NAT, *et al.* Clodronate in the medical management of hyperparathyroidism. *Bone* 1987; **8** (suppl 1): 869–77.

Malignant neoplasms of the bone. Bisphosphonates have been reported to be of benefit in some patients with malignancies of bone (p.484), to control bone pain and osteolysis as well as the attendant hypercalcaemia. There is some evidence that bisphosphonates may retard the progression of malignant bone disease. References to the use of disodium clodronate in patients with malignancies of bone are given below.

1. Elomaa I, *et al.* Treatment of skeletal disease in breast cancer: a controlled clodronate trial. *Bone* 1987; **8** (suppl 1): S53–S56.
2. Lahtinen R, *et al.* Randomised, placebo-controlled multicentre trial of clodronate in multiple myeloma. *Lancet* 1992; **340:** 1049–52. Correction. *ibid.*; 1420.
3. Diel IJ, *et al.* Reduction in new metastases in breast cancer with adjuvant clodronate treatment. *N Engl J Med* 1998; **339:** 357–63.

Osteoporosis. Bisphosphonates are used in the prevention and treatment of osteoporosis (p.731).

Paget's disease of bone. Patients with Paget's disease of bone (p.732) may require no treatment or just analgesics, but bisphosphonates may be indicated if bone pain is persistent or to prevent further progression of the disease. References to the use of disodium clodronate for Paget's disease of bone are given below.

1. Yates AJP, *et al.* Intravenous clodronate in the treatment and retreatment of Paget's disease of bone. *Lancet* 1985; **i:** 1474–7.
2. Gray RES, *et al.* Duration of effect of oral diphosphonate therapy in Paget's disease of bone. *Q J Med* 1987; **64:** 755–67.

Preparations

Proprietary Preparations (details are given in Part 3)

Aust.: Ascredar; Bonefos; Lodronat; Lytos; ***Austral.:*** Bonefos; ***Belg.:*** Bonefos; Ostac; ***Canad.:*** Bonefos; Ostac; ***Fr.:*** Clastoban; Lytos; ***Ger.:*** Bonefos; Ostac; ***Irl.:*** Bonefos; Loron; ***Ital.:*** Clasteon; Difosfonal; Ossiten; ***Neth.:*** Ostac; ***Norw.:*** Bonefos; Ostac; ***S.Afr.:*** Ostac; ***Spain:*** Bonefos; Mebonat; ***Swed.:*** Bonefos; Ostac; ***Switz.:*** Bonefos; Ostac; ***UK:*** Bonefos; Loron.

Etidronic Acid (3274-a)

Etidronic Acid *(BAN, USAN, rINN).*

1-Hydroxyethylidenedi(phosphonic acid).

$C_2H_8O_7P_2$ = 206.0.

CAS — 2809-21-4.

Disodium Etidronate (12674-t)

Disodium Etidronate *(BANM).*

EHDP; Etidronate Disodium *(USAN).* Disodium dihydrogen (1-hydroxyethylidene)diphosphonate.

$C_2H_6Na_2O_7P_2$ = 250.0.

CAS — 7414-83-7.

NOTE. Other etidronic acid sodium salts are designated as etidronate monosodium, etidronate trisodium, and etidronate tetrasodium. The name sodium etidronate is used only where the salt cannot be identified more precisely.

Pharmacopoeias. In US.

Store in airtight containers. A 1% solution has a pH of 4.2 to 5.2.

Adverse Effects and Precautions

As for the bisphosphonates in general, p.734. Unlike the newer bisphosphonates etidronate produces marked impairment of bone mineralisation at high therapeutic doses. An increase in bone pain has been reported in patients with Paget's disease. Impairment of bone mineralisation may result in osteomalacia and fractures have been reported. Disodium etidronate should be discontinued if a fracture occurs until healing is complete. Hyperphosphataemia may occur, usually at high doses, but generally resolves 2 to 4 weeks after therapy. Transient loss or alteration of taste has been reported mainly during and after intravenous infusion.

Effects on the gastro-intestinal tract. Oral etidronate was not associated with an increased incidence of upper gastro-intestinal problems in a retrospective cohort study.[1] There was also no evidence of an increased incidence of gastro-intestinal effects when given with NSAIDs or corticosteroids.

1. van Staa T, *et al.* Upper gastrointestinal adverse events and cyclical etidronate. *Am J Med* 1997; **103:** 462–7.

Effects on the respiratory system. For a report of bronchospasm induced by etidronate in an aspirin-sensitive asthmatic, see p.735.

Hypersensitivity. Allergic reactions to bisphosphonates do occur but appear to be rare (see p.735).

Renal impairment. Bisphosphonates are excreted by the kidneys, thus caution is advised in patients with impaired renal function. When given by intravenous infusion for the treatment of hypercalcaemia of malignancy they have been reported to affect renal function adversely; hypercalcaemia or malignancy may also have contributed. For reports of renal failure associated with etidronate administration see Effects on the Kidneys, p.734.

The manufacturers have recommended that disodium etidronate should not be given intravenously to patients with serum-creatinine concentrations greater than 440 μmol (50 mg) per litre, and that doses may need to be reduced in patients with serum creatinine concentrations between 220 and 440 μmol (25 to 50 mg) per litre.

Interactions

As for the bisphosphonates in general, p.735.

For a lack of apparent interaction between cyclical etidronate and corticosteroids or NSAIDs see under Effects on the Gastro-intestinal Tract, above.

Pharmacokinetics

Following administration by mouth, absorption is variable and appears to be dose dependent. At usual dosage ranges about 1 to 6% of a dose of disodium etidronate is absorbed. Absorption is reduced by food, especially by products containing calcium or other polyvalent cations. Disodium etidronate is rapidly cleared from the blood and has been reported to have a plasma half-life of 1 to 6 hours. It is not metabolised. About 50% is excreted in the urine within 24 hours, the remainder being chemically adsorbed on bone and slowly eliminated. The half-life of disodium etidronate in bone exceeds 90 days. Unabsorbed disodium etidronate is excreted in the faeces.

Uses and Administration

Etidronate is a bisphosphonate with general properties similar to those of the other bisphosphonates (p.735). It inhibits the growth and dissolution of hydroxyapatite crystals in bone and may also directly impair osteoclast activity. It diminishes bone resorption and thus reduces bone turnover.

Disodium etidronate is used as an adjunct in the treatment of severe hypercalcaemia, especially when associated with malignancy. It is also given in bone disorders in which excessive bone resorption is a problem, such as Paget's disease of bone and osteoporosis. In addition, it may be used for the prevention and treatment of ectopic (heterotopic) ossification and the management of malignancies of bone. A chelate of etidronate with radioactive technetium-99m (p.1425) is used diagnostically as a bone scanning agent.

Disodium etidronate is administered by intravenous infusion over at least 2 hours, or by mouth, usually as a single daily dose. Food should be avoided for 2 hours before and after oral administration.

In the treatment of **Paget's disease**, disodium etidronate is given by mouth in a usual initial dose of 5 mg per kg body-weight daily for not more than 6 months. Doses above 10 mg per kg daily should be reserved for severe disease and should not be given for more than 3 months at a time. The maximum dose is 20 mg per kg daily. The response to disodium etidronate may be slow in onset and may continue for several months after cessation of therapy. Therefore, further treatment should only be given after a drug-free interval of at least 3 months and after evidence of relapse; it should not be continued for more than the duration of the initial treatment.

In the treatment of **hypercalcaemia of malignancy** the recommended dose of disodium etidronate by slow intravenous infusion is 7.5 mg per kg body-weight daily for 3 successive days. This daily dose should be diluted in at least 250 mL of 0.9% sodium chloride and infused over at least 2 hours. There should be at least a 7-day interval between courses of treatment. Once serum-calcium concentrations have been reduced to an acceptable level, maintenance therapy with disodium etidronate 20 mg per kg daily by mouth for 30 days may be started on the day following the last intravenous dose; treatment may be extended to a maximum of 90 days.

For the prevention and treatment of **ectopic ossification** complicating hip replacement disodium etidronate has been given by mouth in a dose of 20 mg per kg daily for one month before and 3 months after the operation. For ectopic ossification due to spinal cord injury it has been given in a dose of 20 mg per kg daily for 2 weeks followed by 10 mg per kg daily for 10 weeks.

For the treatment of **osteoporosis**, the prevention of bone loss in postmenopausal women, and the prevention and treatment of corticosteroid-induced osteoporosis, etidronate is given in an intermittent or cyclical regimen with a calcium salt; disodium etidronate 400 mg is given by mouth daily for 14 days followed by the equivalent of 500 mg of elemental calcium by mouth for 76 days. Treatment has continued for 3 years in most patients; the optimum duration of treatment has not been established.

Ectopic ossification. Bisphosphonates that inhibit bone mineralisation such as disodium etidronate have been used to prevent ectopic ossification (p.730).[1]

1. Finerman GAM, Stover SL. Heterotopic ossification following hip replacement or spinal cord injury: two clinical studies with EHDP. *Metab Bone Dis Relat Res* 1981; **4 & 5:** 337–42.

Hypercalcaemia. Treatment with bisphosphonates may be considered in patients with moderate to severe symptomatic hypercalcaemia of malignancy (p.1148) in addition to rehydration and diuresis. References to the use of disodium etidronate for hypercalcaemia are given below.

1. Hasling C, *et al.* Etidronate disodium for treating hypercalcaemia of malignancy: a double blind, placebo-controlled study. *Eur J Clin Invest* 1986; **16:** 433–7.
2. Ringenberg QS, Ritch PS. Efficacy of oral administration of etidronate disodium in maintaining normal serum calcium levels in previously hypercalcemic cancer patients. *Clin Ther* 1987; **9:** 318–25.
3. Ralston SH, *et al.* Comparison of three intravenous bisphosphonates in cancer-associated hypercalcaemia. *Lancet* 1989; **ii:** 1180–2.
4. Singer FR, *et al.* Treatment of hypercalcaemia of malignancy with intravenous etidronate: a controlled, multicenter study. *Arch Intern Med* 1991; **151:** 471–6.

Hyperparathyroidism. Bisphosphonates have been used to inhibit bone resorption in the treatment of hypercalcaemia associated with hyperparathyroidism (p.733) but seem to be of little benefit in long-term treatment. References to the use of etidronate in hyperparathyroidism are given below.

1. Licata AA, O'Hanlon E. Treatment of hyperparathyroidism with etidronate disodium. *JAMA* 1983; **249:** 2063–4.

Malignant neoplasms of the bone. Bisphosphonates have been reported to be of benefit in some patients with malignancies of bone (p.484), to control bone pain and osteolysis as well as the attendant hypercalcaemia. References to the use of disodium etidronate in patients with malignancies of bone are given below.

1. Carey PO, Lippert MC. Treatment of painful prostatic bone metastases with oral etidronate disodium. *Urology* 1988; **32:** 403–7.
2. Smith JA. Palliation of painful bone metastases from prostate cancer using sodium etidronate: results of a randomized, prospective, double-blind, placebo-controlled study. *J Urol (Baltimore)* 1989; **141:** 85–7.

Osteoporosis. Bisphosphonates are used in the prevention and treatment of osteoporosis (p.731). For the treatment of postmenopausal osteoporosis, disodium etidronate is given in an intermittent or cyclical regimen;[1-4] additive effects with oestrogen have been described.[5,6] Similar cyclical regimens are used in the prevention of early postmenopausal bone loss.[7,8] Etidronate is also effective in both men and women for the prevention and treatment of corticosteroid-induced osteoporosis.[9-11] There is some interest in the use of etidronate to treat idiopathic vertebral osteoporosis in men.[12]

1. Storm T, *et al.* Effect of intermittent cyclical etidronate therapy on bone mass and fracture rate in women with postmenopausal osteoporosis. *N Engl J Med* 1990; **322:** 1265–71.
2. Watts NB, *et al.* Intermittent cyclical etidronate treatment of postmenopausal osteoporosis. *N Engl J Med* 1990; **323:** 73–9.
3. Harris ST, *et al.* Four-year study of intermittent cyclic etidronate treatment of postmenopausal osteoporosis: three years of blinded therapy followed by one year of open therapy. *Am J Med* 1993; **95:** 557–67.
4. Miller PD, *et al.* Cyclical etidronate in the treatment of postmenopausal osteoporosis: efficacy and safety after seven years of treatment. *Am J Med* 1997; **103:** 468–76.
5. Wimalawansa SJ. Combined therapy with estrogen and etidronate has an additive effect on bone mineral density in the hip and vertebrae: four-year randomized study. *Am J Med* 1995; **99:** 36–42.
6. Wimalawansa SJ. A four-year randomized controlled trial of hormone replacement and bisphosphonate, alone or in combination, in women with postmenopausal osteoporosis. *Am J Med* 1998; **104:** 219–26.
7. Herd RJM, *et al.* The prevention of early postmenopausal bone loss by cyclical etidronate therapy: a 2-year, double-blind, placebo-controlled study. *Am J Med* 1997; **103:** 92–9.
8. Meunier PJ, *et al.* Prevention of early postmenopausal bone loss with cyclical etidronate therapy. *J Clin Endocrinol Metab* 1997; **82:** 2784–91.
9. Struys A, *et al.* Cyclical etidronate reverses bone loss of the spine and proximal femur in patients with established corticosteroid-induced osteoporosis. *Am J Med* 1995; **99:** 235–42.
10. Adachi JD, *et al.* Intermittent etidronate therapy to prevent corticosteroid-induced osteoporosis. *N Engl J Med* 1997; **337:** 382–7.
11. Pitt P, *et al.* A double blind placebo controlled study to determine the effects of intermittent cyclical etidronate on bone mineral density in patients on long term oral corticosteroid treatment. *Thorax* 1998; **53:** 351–6.
12. Anderson FH, *et al.* Effect of intermittent cyclical disodium etidronate therapy on bone mineral density in men with vertebral fractures. *Age Ageing* 1997; **26:** 359–65.

Paget's disease of bone. Patients with Paget's disease of bone (p.732) may require no treatment or just analgesics, but bisphosphonates may be indicated if bone pain is persistent or to prevent further progression of the disease. References to the use of disodium etidronate for Paget's disease of bone are given below.

1. Johnston CC, *et al.* Review of fracture experience during treatment of Paget's disease of bone with etidronate disodium (EHDP). *Clin Orthop* 1983; **172:** 186–94.
2. Preston CJ, *et al.* Effective short term treatment of Paget's disease with oral etidronate. *Br Med J* 1986; **292:** 79–80.
3. Gibbs CJ, *et al.* Osteomalacia in Paget's disease treated with short term, high dose sodium etidronate. *Br Med J* 1986; **292:** 1227–9.
4. Perry HM, *et al.* Alternate calcitonin and etidronate disodium therapy for Paget's bone disease. *Arch Intern Med* 1984; **144:** 929–33.

Preparations

USP 23: Etidronate Disodium Tablets.

Proprietary Preparations (details are given in Part 3)
Aust.: Didronel; ***Austral.:*** Didronel; ***Belg.:*** Didronel; Osteodidronel; ***Canad.:*** Didronel; ***Fr.:*** Didronel; ***Ger.:*** Didronel; Diphos; ***Irl.:*** Didronel; ***Ital.:*** Etidron; ***Neth.:*** Didronel†; ***Norw.:*** Didronate; ***S.Afr.:*** Didronel; ***Spain:*** Difosfen; Osteum; ***Swed.:*** Didronate; ***Switz.:*** Didronel; ***UK:*** Didronel; ***USA:*** Didronel.

Multi-ingredient: ***Austral.:*** Didrocal; ***Canad.:*** Didrocal; ***Ital.:*** Didro-Kit; ***Neth.:*** Didrokit; ***UK:*** Didronel PMO.

Gallium Nitrate (12780-r)

Gallium Nitrate *(USAN)*.

NSC-15200; WR-135675.

$Ga(NO_3)_3,9H_2O = 417.9$.

CAS — 13494-90-1 (anhydrous gallium nitrate); 135886-70-3 (gallium nitrate nonahydrate).

Adverse Effects, Treatment, and Precautions

Gallium nitrate may produce serious nephrotoxicity, especially when given as a brief intravenous infusion; administration by continuous infusion, with adequate hydration, may reduce the incidence of renal damage. It should be given with great care and in reduced doses, if at all, to patients with existing renal dysfunction.

Gastro-intestinal disturbances, rashes, metallic taste, visual and auditory disturbances, anaemia, hypophosphataemia, and hypocalcaemia have also been reported.

Although it has been suggested, given the chemical similarity of gallium to aluminium, that repeated administration, particularly in the presence of renal impairment, might lead to severe neurotoxicity,[1] studies in *rats* do not provide any evidence of central neurological abnormalities.[2]

1. Altmann P, Cunningham J. Hazards of gallium for the treatment of Paget's disease of bone. *Lancet* 1990; **335:** 477.
2. Matkovic V, *et al.* Hazards of gallium for Paget's disease of bone. *Lancet* 1990; **335:** 1099.

Uses and Administration

Gallium nitrate is an inorganic metallic salt with hypocalcaemic properties. It acts to decrease bone resorption by osteoclasts, with a lesser and probably indirect increase in bone formation, and a consequent decline in serum calcium.

Gallium nitrate is used in the treatment of hypercalcaemia associated with malignant neoplasms and has been investigated in other disorders associated with abnormally enhanced bone turnover, such as Paget's disease of bone. For the treatment of hypercalcaemia of malignancy doses of 100 to 200 mg per m^2 body-surface area may be given daily for up to 5 days, diluted in 1 litre of sodium chloride 0.9% or glucose 5% injection and infused intravenously over 24 hours. Treatment may be repeated after 2 to 4 weeks, if necessary. Adequate hydration before and during treatment is essential: a urinary output of at least 2 litres daily should be maintained, and renal function should be regularly monitored.

Gallium nitrate has been tried, with limited benefit, as an antineoplastic in the management of lymphomas and some solid neoplasms.

Hypercalcaemia. References to the use of gallium nitrate in hypercalcaemia of malignancy (p.1148).

1. Warrell RP, *et al.* Gallium nitrate for treatment of refractory hypercalcemia from parathyroid carcinoma. *Ann Intern Med* 1987; **107:** 683–6.
2. Warrell RP, *et al.* Gallium nitrate for acute treatment of cancer-related hypercalcemia: a randomized, double-blind comparison to calcitonin. *Ann Intern Med* 1988; **108:** 669–74.
3. Warrell RP, *et al.* A randomized double-blind study of gallium nitrate compared with etidronate for acute control of cancer-related hypercalcemia. *J Clin Oncol* 1991; **9:** 1467–75.

Paget's disease of bone. Beneficial results[1] were reported when gallium nitrate was given subcutaneously in doses of 0.25 or 0.5 mg per kg body-weight daily for 14 days to patients with advanced Paget's disease of bone (p.732). In this pilot multicentre study 14 days of gallium nitrate injections were followed by 4 weeks off medication and the cycle repeated once.

1. Bockman RS, *et al.* A multicenter trial of low dose gallium nitrate in patients with advanced Paget's disease of bone. *J Clin Endocrinol Metab* 1995; **80:** 595–602.

Preparations

Proprietary Preparations (details are given in Part 3)
USA: Ganite.

Ibandronic Acid (17608-m)

Ibandronic Acid *(BAN, rINN)*.

BM-21.0955. [1-Hydroxy-3-(methylpentylamino)propylidene]diphosphonic acid.

$C_9H_{23}NO_7P_2 = 319.2$.

CAS — 114084-78-5.

Sodium Ibandronate (17801-b)

Sodium Ibandronate *(BANM, rINNM)*.

Ibandronate Sodium.

Ibandronate is a bisphosphonate (p.734) which is a potent inhibitor of bone resorption. It is used as the sodium salt in hypercalcaemia of malignancy and is under investigation in various disorders of increased bone turnover.

Sodium ibandronate is administered by intravenous infusion over 2 hours. The dose is expressed in term of ibandronic acid. For hypercalcaemia of malignancy, a single dose of the equivalent of 2 to 4 mg ibandronic acid is usually administered, up to a maximum of 6 mg.

The most common adverse effect is fever and influenza-like symptoms.

Hypercalcaemia. Treatment with bisphosphonates may be considered in patients with moderate to severe symptomatic hypercalcaemia of malignancy (p.1148) in addition to rehydration and diuresis. References to the use of ibandronate for hypercalcaemia are given below.

1. Pecherstorfer M, *et al.* Randomized phase II trial comparing different doses of the bisphosphonate ibandronate in the treatment of hypercalcemia of malignancy. *J Clin Oncol* 1996; **14:** 268–76.

Osteoporosis. Bisphosphonates may be used for the prevention and treatment of osteoporosis (p.731). References to the use of ibandronate for osteoporosis are given below.

1. Thiébaud D, *et al.* Three monthly intravenous injections of ibandronate in the treatment of postmenopausal osteoporosis. *Am J Med* 1997; **103:** 298–307.

Preparations

Proprietary Preparations (details are given in Part 3)
Ger.: Bondronat; ***Swed.:*** Bondronat.

Imidazole Oxoglurate (3906-e)

Imidazole Cetoglutarate; Imidazole α-Ketoglutarate; Imidazole 2-Oxoglutarate.

Imidazole oxoglurate is used in the treatment of bone disorders and disorders of calcium metabolism; it is also used for its reported effects on platelet aggregation in the treatment of thrombotic disorders.

Preparations

Proprietary Preparations (details are given in Part 3)
Spain: Retencal.

Ipriflavone (7310-z)

Ipriflavone *(rINN).*

FL-113. 7-Isopropoxyisoflavone.

$C_{18}H_{16}O_3$ = 280.3.

CAS — 35212-22-7.

Ipriflavone is a synthetic isoflavonoid that inhibits resorption of bone and is available in some countries for the treatment of osteoporosis (p.731). It is given by mouth in a dose of 200 mg three times daily.

References.

1. Agnusdei D, *et al.* Metabolic and clinical effects of ipriflavone in established post-menopausal osteoporosis. *Drugs Exp Clin Res* 1989; **15:** 97–104.
2. Hyodo T, *et al.* A study of the effects of ipriflavone administration on hemodialysis patients with renal osteodystrophy: preliminary report. *Nephron* 1991; **58:** 114–15.
3. Agnusdei D, *et al.* Effects of ipriflavone on bone mass and bone remodeling in patients with established postmenopausal osteoporosis. *Curr Ther Res* 1992; **51:** 82–91.

Preparations

Proprietary Preparations (details are given in Part 3)
Ital.: Iprosten; Osteofix; ***Jpn:*** Osten.

Medronic Acid (3279-d)

Medronic Acid *(BAN, USAN, pINN).*

Methylenebis(phosphonic acid).

$CH_6O_6P_2$ = 176.0.

CAS — 1984-15-2.

Disodium Medronate (9425-t)

Disodium Medronate *(BANM).*

Disodium Methylene Diphosphonate; MDP; Medronate Disodium *(USAN).* Disodium dihydrogen methylenediphosphonate.

$CH_4Na_2O_6P_2$ = 220.0.

CAS — 25681-89-4.

Medronate is a bisphosphonate with general properties similar to those of the other bisphosphonates (p.734). Like other members of the class it has a strong affinity for bone, and a complex of disodium medronate and stannous chloride or fluoride labelled with radioactive technetium-99m (p.1425) is used diagnostically as a bone scanning agent; it is given intravenously.

Hypersensitivity. For reference to a severe allergic reaction attributed to the sodium medronate component of a radiopharmaceutical, see under Adverse Effects and Precautions of Bisphosphonates, p.735.

Neridronic Acid (4536-s)

Neridronic Acid *(rINN).*

AHDP; AHHexBP; Aminohexane Diphosphonate. (6-Amino-1-hydroxyhexylidene)diphosphonic acid.

$C_6H_{17}NO_7P_2$ = 277.1.

CAS — 79778-41-9.

Neridronic acid is a bisphosphonate with similar properties to those of the bisphosphonates in general (p.734). It inhibits bone resorption and has been given intravenously or by mouth as a neridronate salt in the treatment of malignant hypercalcaemia and diseases associated with excessive bone turnover such as Paget's disease of bone.

Bisphosphonates are widely used in the treatment of Paget's disease of bone (p.732) and hypercalcaemia of malignancy (p.1148).

References to the use of neridronate in these conditions are given below.

1. Delmas PD, *et al.* Beneficial effects of aminohexane diphosphonate in patients with Paget's disease of bone resistant to sodium etidronate. *Am J Med* 1987; **83:** 276–82.
2. O'Rourke NP, *et al.* Treatment of malignant hypercalcaemia with aminohexane bisphosphonate (neridronate). *Br J Cancer* 1994; **69:** 914–17.

Oxidronic Acid (3280-c)

Oxidronic Acid *(BAN, USAN, pINN).*

(Hydroxymethylene)diphosphonic acid.

$CH_6O_7P_2$ = 192.0.

CAS — 15468-10-7.

Disodium Oxidronate (2544-c)

HMDP; Oxidronate Disodium; Oxidronate Sodium; Sodium Oxidronate *(BANM).* Disodium (hydroxymethylene)diphosphonate.

$CH_4Na_2O_7P_2$ = 236.0.

CAS — 14255-61-9.

Oxidronate is a bisphosphonate with general properties similar to those of the other bisphosphonates (p.734). Like other members of the class it has a strong affinity for bone, and a chelate of oxidronate with radioactive technetium-99m (p.1425) is used diagnostically as a bone scanning agent; it is given intravenously.

Pamidronic Acid (3392-n)

Pamidronic Acid *(BAN, rINN).*

Aminohydroxypropylidenebisphosphonate; APD. 3-Amino-1-hydroxypropylidenebis(phosphonic acid).

$C_3H_{11}NO_7P_2$ = 235.1.

CAS — 40391-99-9.

Disodium Pamidronate (12672-k)

Disodium Pamidronate *(BANM).*

Aminohydroxypropylidenebisphosphonate Disodium; CGP-23339A; CGP-23339AE; Disodium Aminohydroxypropylidenediphosphonate; Pamidronate Disodium *(USAN).* Disodium 3-amino-1-hydroxypropylidenebisphosphonate pentahydrate.

$C_3H_9NNa_2O_7P_2,5H_2O$ = 369.1.

CAS — 109552-15-0 (disodium pamidronate pentahydrate); 57248-88-1 (anhydrous disodium pamidronate).

Pharmacopoeias. In Br.

A white crystalline powder. **Soluble** in water and in 2M sodium hydroxide; sparingly soluble in 0.1M hydrochloric acid; practically insoluble in organic solvents. A 1% solution has a pH of 7.8 to 8.8.

Adverse Effects and Precautions

As for the bisphosphonates in general, p.734.

Fever and influenza-like symptoms (sometimes accompanied by malaise, rigors, fatigue, and flushes) are common during treatment with disodium pamidronate but generally resolve spontaneously. Severe local reactions and thrombophlebitis have followed administration as a bolus injection. Rare CNS effects include agitation, confusion, dizziness, somnolence, and insomnia. Seizures have been precipitated in a few patients. In addition to hypocalcaemia and hypophosphataemia (which are common), hypomagnesaemia, and rarely hypernatraemia, and hyperkalaemia or hypokalaemia have occurred. Hypotension and hypertension have been reported.

Pamidronate should be used with caution in those with cardiac disease because of the potential for fluid overload. Serum electrolytes, calcium and phosphate should be monitored during therapy. Patients should be warned against driving or operating machinery after treatment if somnolence or dizziness occur. Pamidronate should not be administered by bolus injection.

Bone mineralisation. Although pamidronate appears to be a less potent inhibitor of bone mineralisation than etidronate, mineralisation defects of bone have been reported in patients with Paget's disease of bone receiving pamidronate.[1] The resultant osteomalacia was not associated with any adverse clinical effects.

1. Adamson BB, *et al.* Mineralisation defects with pamidronate therapy for Paget's disease. *Lancet* 1993; **342:** 1459–60.

Effects on the eyes. Although adverse ocular reactions to pamidronate appeared to be rare, the manufacturers were aware of 23 cases up to September 1993 which were possibly associated with the drug.[1] The reactions included anterior uveitis in 7 patients and unilateral episcleritis or scleritis in 3. See also Effects on the Eyes under Bisphosphonates, p.734.

1. Macarol V, Fraunfelder FT. Pamidronate disodium and possible ocular adverse drug reactions. *Am J Ophthalmol* 1994; **118:** 220–4.

Effects on the gastro-intestinal tract. The tolerability of pamidronate administered *by mouth* may depend to some extent on the particular formulation. Gastro-intestinal disturbances (in 21.8%) and haematological abnormalities (in 9.4%) were the predominant side-effects associated with oral pamidronate in an open study of elderly patients.[1] Oesophagitis, noted earlier by Lufkin *et al.*[2] in 4 of 49 patients given a different formulation, was not reported by Spivacow *et al.*[1]

1. Spivacow FR, *et al.* Tolerability of oral pamidronate in elderly patients with osteoporosis and other metabolic bone diseases. *Curr Ther Res* 1996; **57:** 123–30.
2. Lufkin EG, *et al.* Pamidronate: an unrecognised problem in gastrointestinal tolerability. *Osteoporosis Int* 1994; **4:** 320–2.

Hypersensitivity. Allergic reactions to bisphosphonates are rare. Rash and pruritus occasionally follow pamidronate infusion. Mild skin rashes have also been reported in some patients taking pamidronate by mouth, as mentioned under Adverse Effects and Precautions of Bisphosphonates, p.735.

Renal impairment. Like other bisphosphonates (see Effects on the Kidneys, p.734), pamidronate may cause adverse renal effects. The manufacturer notes there have been isolated cases of haematuria, acute renal failure, and deterioration of pre-existing renal disease. Therefore, it is recommended that renal function be monitored during long-term pamidronate therapy, especially in patients with pre-existing renal disease or a predisposition to renal impairment.

Pharmacokinetic studies suggest that no dosage reduction is required in patients with renal impairment.[1] However, the UK manufacturer currently recommends that the rate of infusion be reduced to a maximum of 20 mg per hour in patients with established or suspected renal impairment.

1. Berenson JR, *et al.* Pharmacokinetics of pamidronate disodium in patients with cancer with normal or impaired renal function. *J Clin Pharmacol* 1997; **37:** 285–90.

Interactions

As for the bisphosphonates in general, p.735.

Pharmacokinetics

After intravenous administration of disodium pamidronate, about 20 to 55% of the dose is excreted in the urine unchanged within 72 hours, while the remainder is mainly adsorbed onto bone and only very slowly eliminated. Renal clearance is slower in patients with severe renal impairment and infusion rates may need to be reduced (see above).

Disodium pamidronate is poorly absorbed (about 1 to 3%) from the gastro-intestinal tract.

Uses and Administration

Pamidronate is an aminobisphosphonate with general properties similar to those of the other bisphosphonates (p.735). It inhibits bone resorption, but appears to have less effect on bone mineralisation than etidronate at comparable doses.

Disodium pamidronate is used as an adjunct in the treatment of severe hypercalcaemia, especially when associated with malignancy. It is also used in the treatment of osteolytic lesions and bone pain in multiple myeloma or bone metastases associated with breast cancer. It may also be of benefit in bone disorders associated with excessive bone resorption, including Paget's disease of bone.

Disodium pamidronate is administered by slow intravenous infusion. The UK manufacturer recommends infusion at a rate not exceeding 60 mg per hour (or not exceeding 20 mg per hour in patients with renal impairment) and at a concentration not exceeding 60 mg per 250 mL of sodium chloride 0.9%. In the USA, the recommended concentration of infusion and its rate of administration vary depending on the indication.

In **hypercalcaemia of malignancy** disodium pamidronate is administered by slow intravenous infusion in a total dose of 15 to 90 mg according to the initial plasma-calcium concentration. In the UK, the total dose is given as a single infusion or in divided doses over 2 to 4 days. In the USA, the total dose is given as a single infusion, doses of 60 mg being given over at least 4 hours, and 90 mg over 24 hours. Plasma-calcium concentrations generally start declining 24 to 48 hours after administration of pamidronate with normalisation within 3 to 7 days. Treatment may be repeated if normocalcaemia is not achieved within this time or if hypercalcaemia recurs.

In patients with **osteolytic lesions and bone pain** of multiple myeloma or bone metastases associated with breast cancer, disodium pamidronate may be given in doses of 90 mg by intravenous infusion every 3 to 4 weeks.

In the treatment of **Paget's disease** a suggested dosage regimen in the UK is 30 mg by slow infusion once a week for 6 weeks (total dose 180 mg), or 30 mg in the first week then 60 mg every other week for 6 weeks (total dose 210 mg). These courses may be repeated every 6 months, and the total dose increased if necessary up to a maximum of 360 mg. Alternatively, in the USA 30 mg by infusion over 4 hours, repeated on consecutive days to a total dose of 90 mg has been suggested. This course is repeated when clinically indicated.

Disodium pamidronate has also been given by mouth.

General references.

1. Fitton A, McTavish D. Pamidronate: a review of its pharmacological properties and therapeutic efficacy in resorptive bone disease. *Drugs* 1991; **41:** 289–318. Correction. *ibid.* 1992; **43:** 145.
2. Anonymous. Pamidronate. *Med Lett Drugs Ther* 1992; **34:** 1–2.
3. Kellihan MJ, Mangino PD. Pamidronate. *Ann Pharmacother* 1992; **26:** 1262–9.

Gaucher disease. Treatment with oral disodium pamidronate in doses of 600 mg daily in adults,[1] and 150 to 300 mg daily in children,[2] or intravenous disodium pamidronate in doses of 45 mg every 3 weeks,[3] has been reported to improve bone lesions of Gaucher disease (p.1544) in a few patients.

1. Harinck HIJ, *et al.* Regression of bone lesions in Gaucher's disease during treatment with aminohydroxypropylidene bisphosphonate. *Lancet* 1984; **ii:** 513.
2. Samuel R, *et al.* Aminohydroxy propylidine bisphosphonate (APD) treatment improves the clinical skeletal manifestations of Gaucher's disease. *Pediatrics* 1994; **94:** 385–9.
3. Ciana G, *et al.* Short-term effects of pamidronate in patients with Gaucher's disease and severe skeletal involvement. *N Engl J Med* 1997; **337:** 712.

Hypercalcaemia. In patients with moderate to severe symptomatic hypercalcaemia of malignancy (p.1148) treatment with bisphosphonates may be considered in addition to rehydration and diuresis. References to the use of disodium pamidronate for hypercalcaemia are given below.

1. Ralston SH, *et al.* Comparison of aminohydroxypropylidene diphosphonate, mithramycin, and corticosteroids/calcitonin in treatment of cancer-associated hypercalcaemia. *Lancet* 1985; **ii:** 907–10.
2. Thiébaud D, *et al.* Oral versus intravenous AHPrBP (APD) in the treatment of hypercalcemia of malignancy. *Bone* 1986; **7:** 247–53.
3. Cantwell BMJ, Harris AL. Effect of single high dose infusions of aminohydroxypropylidene diphosphonate on hypercalcaemia caused by cancer. *Br Med J* 1987; **294:** 467–9.
4. Morton AR, *et al.* Single dose versus daily intravenous aminohydroxypropylidene biphosphonate (APD) for the hypercalcaemia of malignancy. *Br Med J* 1988; **296:** 811–14.
5. Davis JRE, Heath DA. Comparison of different dose regimes of aminohydroxypropylidene-1,1-bisphosphonate (APD) in hypercalcaemia of malignancy. *Br J Clin Pharmacol* 1989; **28:** 269–74.
6. Gurney H, *et al.* Renal phosphate threshold and response to pamidronate in humoral hypercalcaemia of malignancy. *Lancet* 1989; **ii:** 241–4.
7. Ralston SH, *et al.* Comparison of three intravenous bisphosphonates in cancer-associated hypercalcaemia. *Lancet* 1989; **ii:** 1180–2.
8. Gallacher SJ, *et al.* Immobilization-related hypercalcaemia—a possible novel mechanism and response to pamidronate. *Postgrad Med J* 1990; **66:** 918–22.
9. Nussbaum SR, *et al.* Single-dose intravenous therapy with pamidronate for the treatment of hypercalcaemia of malignancy: comparison of 30-, 60-, and 90-mg dosages. *Am J Med* 1993; **95:** 297–304.
10. Kutluk MT, *et al.* Childhood cancer and hypercalcemia: report of a case treated with pamidronate. *J Pediatr* 1997; **130:** 828–31.

Malignant neoplasms of the bone. Bisphosphonates have been reported to be of benefit in some patients with malignancies of bone (p.484), to control bone pain and osteolysis, as well as the attendant hypercalcaemia. There is some evidence that bisphosphonates might be able to retard the progression of malignant bone disease. References to the use of disodium pamidronate in patients with malignancies of bone are given below.

1. van Holten-Verzantvoort AT, *et al.* Reduced morbidity from skeletal metastases in breast cancer patients during long-term bisphosphonate (APD) treatment. *Lancet* 1987; **ii:** 983–5.
2. Morton AR, *et al.* Sclerosis of lytic bone metastases after disodium aminohydroxypropylidene bisphosphonate (APD) in patients with breast carcinoma. *Br Med J* 1988; **297:** 772–3.
3. Coleman RE, *et al.* Treatment of bone metastases from breast cancer with (3-amino-1-hydroxypropylidene)-1,1-bisphosphonate (APD). *Br J Cancer* 1988; **58:** 621–5.
4. Pelger RCM, *et al.* Short-term metabolic effects of pamidronate in patients with prostatic carcinoma and bone metastases. *Lancet* 1989; **ii:** 865.
5. Man Z, *et al.* Use of pamidronate for multiple myeloma osteolytic lesions. *Lancet* 1990; **335:** 663.
6. van Holten-Verzantvoort AT, *et al.* Palliative pamidronate treatment in patients with bone metastases from breast cancer. *J Clin Oncol* 1993; **11:** 491–8.
7. Berenson JR, *et al.* Efficacy of pamidronate in reducing skeletal events in patients with advanced multiple myeloma. *N Engl J Med* 1996; **334:** 488–93.
8. Conte PF, *et al.* Delayed progression of bone metastases with pamidronate therapy in breast cancer patients: a randomized, multicenter phase III trial. *Ann Oncol* 1994; **5** (suppl 7): 41S-44S.
9. Hortobagyi GN, *et al.* Efficacy of pamidronate in reducing skeletal complications in patients with breast cancer and lytic bone metastases. *N Engl J Med* 1996; **335:** 1785–91.

Osteogenesis imperfecta. Pamidronate has produced some benefit in children with osteogenesis imperfecta (p.730).

Paget's disease of bone. Patients with Paget's disease of bone (p.732) may require no treatment or just analgesics, but bisphosphonates may be indicated if bone pain is persistent or to prevent further progression of the disease. References to the use of disodium pamidronate in Paget's disease are given below.[1-6] Bisphosphonates have also been given in other bone diseases with a similar pathology, particularly increased osteoclastic resorption. For example, pamidronate has had beneficial effects in patients with fibrous dysplasia of bone, a rare congenital disease leading to osteolytic lesions.[7]

1. Mautalen CA, *et al.* Efficacy of the bisphosphonate APD in the control of Paget's bone disease. *Bone* 1985; **6:** 429–32.
2. Cantrill JA, *et al.* Low dose intravenous 3-amino-1-hydroxypropylidene-1,1-bisphosphonate (APD) for the treatment of Paget's disease of bone. *Ann Rheum Dis* 1986; **45:** 1012–18.
3. Harinck HIJ, *et al.* Paget's disease of bone: early and late responses to three different modes of treatment with aminohydroxypropylidene bisphosphonate (APD). *Br Med J* 1987; **295:** 1301–5.
4. Anderson DC, Cantrill JC. Treatment of Paget's disease of bone. *Br Med J* 1988; **296:** 291.
5. Drake S, *et al.* Pamidronate sodium and calcitonin-resistant Paget's disease: immediate response in a patient. *Arch Intern Med* 1989; **149:** 401–3.
6. Crisp AJ. Pamidronate for Paget's disease of the bone. *Br J Hosp Med* 1995; **53:** 66–8.
7. Liens D, *et al.* Long-term effects of intravenous pamidronate in fibrous dysplasia of bone. *Lancet* 1994; **343:** 953–4.

Rheumatoid arthritis. Intravenous[1] and oral[2] administration of pamidronate has reportedly produced some modification of disease in a few patients with rheumatoid arthritis (p.2), but at present such a use is strictly investigational. Continuous oral pamidronate therapy was shown to be effective in preserving and increasing bone mass in a 3-year randomised controlled trial involving 105 patients with rheumatoid arthritis.[3]

1. Eggelmeijer F, *et al.* Clinical and biochemical response to single infusion of pamidronate in patients with active rheumatoid arthritis: a double blind placebo controlled study. *J Rheumatol* 1994: **21:** 2016–20.
2. Maccagno A, *et al.* Double blind radiological assessment of continuous oral pamidronic acid in patients with rheumatoid arthritis. *Scand J Rheumatol* 1994; **23:** 211–14.
3. Eggelmeijer F, *et al.* Increased bone mass with pamidronate treatment in rheumatoid arthritis: results of a three-year randomized, double-blind trial. *Arthritis Rheum* 1996; **39:** 396–402.

Preparations

BP 1998: Disodium Pamidronate Intravenous Infusion.

Proprietary Preparations (details are given in Part 3)
Aust.: Aredia; ***Austral.:*** Aredia; ***Belg.:*** Aredia; ***Canad.:*** Aredia; ***Fr.:*** Aredia; ***Ger.:*** Aredia; ***Irl.:*** Aredia; ***Ital.:*** Aredia; ***Neth.:*** Aredia; ***Norw.:*** Aredia; ***S.Afr.:*** Aredia; ***Swed.:*** Aredia; ***Switz.:*** Aredia; ***UK:*** Aredia; ***USA:*** Aredia.

Parathyroid Hormone (8051-x)

Parathyrin; PTH.
CAS — 9002-64-6.

Parathyroid hormone is a single-chain polypeptide isolated from the parathyroid glands. It contains 84 amino acids and in man the first (N-terminal) 34 appear to be responsible for the hormonal activity. The amino-acid sequence varies according to the source.

Endogenous parathyroid hormone is involved in the maintenance of plasma-calcium concentrations having a hypercalcaemic effect through its actions on bone, kidney, and indirectly on the gastro-intestinal tract (see also under Parathyroid Disorders, p.733).

Exogenous parathyroid hormone was formerly used in acute hypoparathyroidism with tetany. It has also been used in the differential diagnosis of hypoparathyroidism and pseudohypoparathyroidism.

Synthetic preparations of the first 34 amino acids of human and bovine parathyroid hormones (PTH 1-34; teriparatide) are now used for diagnostic purposes, and are under investigation for the treatment of osteoporosis (see Teriparatide Acetate, p.744).

Risedronic Acid (10591-d)

Risedronic Acid *(BAN, rINN).*
[1-Hydroxy-2-(3-pyridinyl)ethylidene]diphosphonic acid.
$C_7H_{11}NO_7P_2$ = 283.1.
CAS — 105462-24-6.

Sodium Risedronate (3406-j)

Sodium Risedronate *(rINNM).*
Monosodium Risedronate; NE-58095; Risedronate Sodium *(BANM, USAN).* Sodium trihydrogen [1-hydroxy-2-(3-pyridyl)ethylidene]diphosphonate.
$C_7H_{10}NNaO_7P_2$ = 305.1.
CAS — 115436-72-1.

Adverse Effects and Precautions

As for the bisphosphonates in general, p.734. The most frequent adverse effects are gastro-intestinal. To minimise the risk of gastro-intestinal effects patients should be instructed to swallow risedronate tablets with plenty of water (at least 200 mL), in an upright position (standing or sitting). Tablets should be taken on rising for the day, on an empty stomach, at least 30 minutes before breakfast and any other oral medication; patients should remain upright after taking the tablets, and should not lie down for at least 30 minutes. Hypocalcaemia should be corrected before beginning risedronate therapy.

Interactions

As for the bisphosphonates in general, p.735.

Pharmacokinetics

Like other bisphosphonates, risedronate is poorly absorbed after oral administration. Absorption is reduced by food, especially by products containing calcium or other polyvalent cations. The mean bioavailability is 0.63% in the fasting state, and is reduced by 30% when administered 1 hour before breakfast, and by 55% when administered half an hour before breakfast. Unabsorbed drug is eliminated unchanged in the faeces. Risedronate is not metabolised, and 50% of the absorbed dose is excreted unchanged in the urine within 24 hours. The remainder of the absorbed dose is apparently sequestered to bone for a prolonged period.

Uses and Administration

Risedronate is a bisphosphonate with similar properties to those of the bisphosphonates in general (p.735). It inhibits bone resorption and is used as the sodium salt in Paget's disease of bone and is under investigation for osteoporosis.

Sodium risedronate is given by mouth, and the specific instructions for its administration (see above) should be followed to minimise gastro-intestinal adverse effects and permit adequate absorption. The recommended dosage for Paget's disease of bone is 30 mg once daily for 2 months. Treatment may be repeated if necessary after an interval of a further 2 months.

Some references to the use of risedronate for osteolysis in malignant disease (p.484), for Paget's disease of bone (p.732), for primary hyperparathyroidism (p.733), and for the prevention of postmenopausal osteoporosis (p.731).

1. Roux C, *et al.* Biologic, histologic and densitometric effects of oral risedronate on bone in patients with multiple myeloma. *Bone* 1994; **15:** 41–9.
2. Brown JP, *et al.* Risedronate in Paget's disease: preliminary results of a multicenter study. *Semin Arthritis Rheum* 1994; **23:** 272.
3. Reasner CA, *et al.* Acute changes in calcium homeostasis during treatment of primary hyperparathyroidism with risedronate. *J Clin Endocrinol Metab* 1993; **77:** 1067–71.
4. Delmas PD, *et al.* Bisphosphonate risedronate prevents bone loss in women with artificial menopause due to chemotherapy of breast cancer: a double-blind, placebo-controlled study. *J Clin Oncol* 1997; **15:** 955–62.
5. Mortensen L, *et al.* Risedronate increases bone mass in early postmenopausal population: two years of treatment plus one year of follow-up. *J Clin Endocrinol Metab* 1998; **83:** 396–402.

Preparations

Proprietary Preparations (details are given in Part 3)
USA: Actonel.

Sodium Fluoride (7733-z)

Natrii Fluoridum; Natrium Fluoratum.

NaF = 41.99.

CAS — 7681-49-4.

Pharmacopoeias. In *Eur.* (see p.viii), *Pol.*, and *US.*

A white odourless powder or colourless crystals. Sodium fluoride 2.2 mg is approximately equivalent to 1 mg of fluoride. Each g provides approximately 23.8 mmol of sodium and fluoride. **Soluble** 1 in 25 of water; practically insoluble in alcohol.

Adverse Effects and Treatment

In the controlled amounts recommended for fluoridation of drinking water and at the recommended doses employed in dentistry for caries prophylaxis, sodium fluoride has not been shown to have significant side-effects.

In acute poisoning, sodium fluoride taken by mouth is corrosive, forming hydrofluoric acid in the stomach. Effects include hypocalcaemia, hyperkalaemia, tremors, hyperreflexia, paraesthesia, tetany, convulsions, cardiac arrhythmias, shock, respiratory arrest, and cardiac failure. Death may occur within 2 to 4 hours. Although there is much interindividual variation, a single oral dose of 5 to 10 g of sodium fluoride would be considered lethal in an untreated adult by most authorities. However, dangerous poisoning has been reported after oral doses of less than 1 g, and the minimum dose that can cause possibly fatal toxicity has been suggested to be 5 mg per kg bodyweight.

Treatment of acute poisoning involves gastric lavage with lime water or a weak solution of another calcium salt to precipitate fluoride, maintenance of high urine output, slow intravenous injections of calcium gluconate 10% for hypocalcaemia and tetany, and symptomatic and supportive measures. Magnesium sulphate, or aluminium hydroxide may also reduce fluoride absorption. Haemodialysis may be considered.

Chronic fluoride poisoning may result in skeletal fluorosis, manifestations of which include increased density and coarsened trabeculation of bone and calcification in ligaments, tendons, and muscle insertions. Clinical signs are bone pain, stiffness, limited movement, and in severe cases, crippling deformities. Prolonged excessive intake by children during the period of tooth development before eruption can result in dental fluorosis characterised by mottled enamel. At fluoride concentrations in drinking water of 1 to 2 ppm (1 to 2 mg per litre) dental fluorosis is mild with white opaque flecks on the teeth. At higher concentrations, enamel defects become more severe with brown to black staining and the teeth have a pitted corroded appearance.

The fluoridation of water has been a subject of considerable controversy. Suggestions that it increases the incidence of thyroid disorders, chromosome aberrations, and cancer have not been substantiated.

Reviews of the toxic effects of fluoride salts.

1. Fluorine and Fluorides. *Environmental Health Criteria 36.* Geneva: WHO 1984.
2. Whitford GM. The physiological and toxicological characteristics of fluoride. *J Dent Res* 1990; **69** (Spec Iss): 539–49.

Carcinogenicity. Based on comparisons of cancer mortality rates for communities residing in fluoridated and non-fluoridated cities, Yiamouyiannis and Burk[1] alleged that artificial fluoridation of water might be associated with an increased risk of cancer. Re-examination of their data by others failed to confirm this relationship nor did further studies in a number of countries.[2] In Great Britain, the Working Party on Fluoridation of Water and Cancer[3] found nothing which could lead them to conclude that either fluoride occurring naturally in water, or fluoride added to water supplies, was capable of inducing cancer, or of increasing the mortality from cancer. In this respect, fluoridation of drinking water was considered safe. Further study in *animal* models by the USA National Toxicology Programme[4] found no evidence of carcinogenicity in female *rats* or in *mice* of either sex. A small number of osteosarcomas was found in male *rats* in the medium- and high-dose groups, although the association between sodium fluoride administration and the tumour was uncertain.

1. Yiamouyiannis J, Burk D. Fluoridation and cancer: age-dependence of cancer mortality related to artificial fluoridation. *Fluoride* 1977; **10:** 102–25S.
2. Clemmesen J. The alleged association between artificial fluoridation of water supplies and cancer: a review. *Bull WHO* 1983; **61:** 871–83.
3. DHSS. *Fluoridation of water and cancer: a review of the epidemiological evidence: report of the working party.* London: HMSO, 1985.
4. Public Health Service report on fluoride benefits and risks. *JAMA* 1991; **266:** 1061–2, 1066–7.

Effects on bone and joints. Exacerbation of rheumatoid arthritis in a 68-year-old woman was attributed to sodium fluoride given in a dose equivalent to 22 mg of fluorine daily for osteoporosis.[1] An increased risk of hip fracture in the elderly has been suggested as being associated with fluoridated water,[2] although another study[3] reported that this association was confined to fluoride concentrations of more than 0.11 mg per litre. Use of fluoride, particularly in doses of 40 mg or more daily, may be associated with a peripheral pain syndrome, usually manifested as bone pain in the distal lower limbs, but sometimes involving the upper limbs and axial skeletal. The cause is uncertain: both stress fractures and increased bone growth at the site of pain have been proposed.[4] For comment on the influence of therapeutic doses of fluoride on the incidence of fractures, see below under Osteoporosis in Uses and Administration.

1. Duell PB, Chesnut CH. Exacerbation of rheumatoid arthritis by sodium fluoride treatment of osteoporosis. *Arch Intern Med* 1991; **151:** 783–4.
2. Danielson C, *et al.* Hip fractures and fluoridation in Utah's elderly population. *JAMA* 1992; **268:** 746–8
3. Jacqmin-Gadda H, *et al.* Fluorine concentration in drinking water and fractures in the elderly. *JAMA* 1995; **273:** 775–6.
4. Jones G, Sambrook PN. Drug-induced disorders of bone metabolism: incidence, management and avoidance. *Drug Safety* 1994; **10:** 480–9.

Effects on the kidneys. Nephrotoxicity has been associated with high plasma concentrations of fluoride during anaesthesia with fluorine-containing anaesthetics such as methoxyflurane (p.1228). Elevated fluoride ion concentrations have also been noted in the plasma of patients receiving enflurane or isoflurane, although no clinical effect on renal function was found (see p.1222 and p.1225).

Fluorosis. Discussions of chronic fluorosis.[1,2] In temperate climates, teeth seem not to be affected if fluoride concentrations in drinking water are not greatly above 1 ppm; fluorosis affecting bone has not been detected at concentrations of 4 to 8 ppm in temperate regions, although it can occur at concentrations of more than 6 ppm in tropical areas.[3] Swallowing of fluoridated toothpaste by infants may be related to fluorosis of permanent incisors.[4]

1. Anonymous. Chronic fluorosis. *Br Med J* 1981; **282:** 253–4.
2. Mason JO. A message to health professionals about fluorosis. *JAMA* 1991; **265:** 2939.
3. WHO. Fluorides and oral health: report of a WHO expert committee on oral health status and fluoride use. *WHO Tech Rep Ser 846* 1994.
4. Rock WP, Sabieha AM. The relationship between reported toothpaste usage in infancy and fluorosis of permanent incisors. *Br Dent J* 1997; **183:** 165–70.

Hypersensitivity. Rash and other hypersensitivity reactions have been reported following use of oral sodium fluoride preparations including fluoride-containing toothpastes and drinking water.[1]

1. Mummery RV. Claimed fluoride allergy. *Br Dent J* 1984; **157:** 48.

Overdosage. References.

1. McIvor ME. Acute fluoride toxicity: pathophysiology and management. *Drug Safety* 1990; **5:** 79–85.
2. Gessner BD, *et al.* Acute fluoride poisoning from a public water system. *N Engl J Med* 1994; **330:** 95–9.
3. Arnow PM, *et al.* An outbreak of fatal fluoride intoxication in a long-term hemodialysis unit. *Ann Intern Med* 1994; **121:** 339–44.

Precautions

When considering fluoride supplementation, allowance should be made for fluorides ingested from other sources; fluoride supplements in children are not generally recommended when the fluoride content of drinking water is over 0.7 ppm (0.6 ppm in the USA) (see also Uses and Administration, below). Care should be taken to prevent children swallowing excessive fluoride after topical application to teeth.

Patients with impaired renal function may be particularly susceptible to fluorosis. Regular dialysis with fluoridated water may result in additional fluoride absorption; a maximum concentration of 0.2 ppm of fluoride in the dialysate has been recommended. Dialysis patients not using deionised water are at risk from changes in the fluoride content of the water supply.

Interactions

Aluminium, calcium, and magnesium salts may decrease the absorption of fluoride.

Pharmacokinetics

Sodium fluoride and other soluble fluorides are readily absorbed from the gastro-intestinal tract. Inhaled fluorides (from industrial fumes and dusts) are absorbed through the lungs. Fluoride is deposited predominantly in the bones and teeth. It is principally excreted in the urine but small amounts may also be excreted in faeces and sweat. It readily crosses the placenta and is present in saliva, nails, and hair. There is some evidence of distribution into breast milk.

Uses and Administration

Sodium fluoride is used to prevent dental caries and may be used to increase bone density in osteoporosis (see below).

For **dental caries prophylaxis**, sodium fluoride is used as an adjunct to diet and oral hygiene. It may render the enamel of teeth more resistant to acid, promote remineralisation, or reduce microbial acid production. Fluoride may be administered through fluoridation of the public water supply to achieve a usual fluoride concentration of 1 ppm in temperate regions. The concentration may vary from 0.6 to 1.2 ppm depending on the climatic temperature with the lower concentrations being used in hotter regions where more water is likely to be consumed. Fluoridation of salt at a minimum concentration of 200 mg fluoride per kg is an alternative.

Alternatively, sodium fluoride may be administered as an oral supplement to children considered to be at high risk of caries. The daily dosage should be adjusted for the fluoride content of the drinking water, for fluorides ingested from other sources such as the diet, and for the age of the child. Guidelines have recently been amended in the USA and the UK. In both countries it is suggested that, where the drinking water contains less than 0.3 ppm of fluoride, children aged 6 months to 3 years may be given sodium fluoride 0.55 mg (equivalent to 0.25 mg of fluoride) daily; those aged 3 to 6 years, 1.1 mg (equivalent to 0.5 mg of fluoride) daily; and those aged 6 years and over, 2.2 mg (equivalent to 1 mg of fluoride) daily. Supplements are not recommended for infants under 6 months of age. When drinking water contains 0.3 to 0.7 ppm (0.3 to 0.6 ppm in the USA) of fluoride lower doses should be considered. Specifically, it is recommended that no additional fluoride should be given to children less than 3 years of age and for older children the above doses should be halved. If the water contains more than 0.7 ppm (0.6 ppm in the USA) of fluoride, supplementation is not recommended. Tablets should be sucked or chewed before swallowing since the topical action of fluoride on enamel and plaque is considered to be more important than the systemic effect. The value of giving fluoride during pregnancy, to benefit the child, is not established. Dental benefits from the use of dietary fluoride supplements by adults are unsubstantiated.

After tooth eruption, local fluoride application is effective. Daily mouth-rinses of sodium fluoride 0.05% (about 225 ppm fluoride) or weekly to monthly mouth-rinses of sodium fluoride 0.2% (900 ppm) may be used, but are not recommended for children aged under 6 years because they are unable to effectively spit the rinse out after use. Fluoridated toothpastes are now widely available and are a convenient source of fluoride. The maximum fluoride level in toothpastes is sodium fluoride 0.32% (about 1500 ppm fluoride). Low-dose formulations for children under 7 years of age usually contain sodium fluoride 0.11% (500 ppm), and their use should be supervised to avoid excessive use or ingestion. Sodium fluoride has also been applied topically as a varnish or 2% (about 9090 ppm fluoride) solution under professional supervision. Alternatively, sodium fluoride solutions or gels acidified with phosphoric acid and commonly known as acidulated phosphate fluoride preparations may be used. These preparations are considered to increase the fluoride uptake by the enamel and protect the enamel from demineralisation. For maximum benefit, eating, drinking, or rinsing should be avoided for at least 30 minutes after topical fluoride application.

Other fluoride compounds used in oral hygiene products and toothpastes include aluminium fluoride, ammonium fluoride, calcium fluoride (p.1556), olaflur (p.1610), potassium fluoride, sodium monofluorophosphate (p.743), sodium silicofluoride (p.1631), and stannous fluoride (p.1632). Other fluorides used in the fluoridation of water supplies include sodium silicofluoride.

Sodium fluoride has also been used, like some other fluoride compounds, in rodenticides and insecticides.

Human requirements. In the USA dietary reference intakes have been set for fluoride. These propose an adequate intake (AI) for dental caries prevention to be 3.8 mg daily in adult men and 3.1 mg in women;[1] lower values are suggested in children and adolescents, depending on age.

1. Standing Committee on the Scientific Evaluation of Dietary Reference Intakes of the Food and Nutrition Board. *Dietary Reference Intakes for calcium, phosphorus, magnesium, vitamin D, and fluoride*. Washington, DC: National Academy Press, 1997.

Dental caries prophylaxis. References.

1. WHO. Fluorides and oral health: report of a WHO expert committee on oral health status and fluoride use. *WHO Tech Rep Ser 846* 1994.
2. Lewis DW, *et al.* Periodic health examination, 1995 update: 2: prevention of dental caries. *Can Med Assoc J* 1995; **152:** 836–46.
3. American Academy of Pediatrics, Committee on Nutrition. Fluoride supplementation for children: interim policy recommendations. *Pediatrics* 1995; **95:** 777.
4. Holt RD, *et al.* British Society of Paediatric Dentistry: a policy document on fluoride dietary supplements and fluoride toothpastes for children. *Int J Paediatr Dent* 1996; **6:** 139–42.
5. Anonymous. Fluoride supplement dosage: a statement by the British Dental Association, the British Society of Paediatric Dentistry and the British Association for the Study of Community Dentistry. *Br Dent J* 1997; **182:** 6–7.

Osteoporosis. Fluoride has been used in the treatment of osteoporosis (p.731) to improve bone strength by inducing subclinical fluorosis. The predominant effect of fluoride on the skeleton is to stimulate osteoblasts and increase trabecular bone mass. Because antiresorptive drugs cannot restore lost bone mass, this is potentially valuable in the treatment of osteoporosis. However, too much fluoride can increase bone fragility, and the overall effect of sodium fluoride on the incidence of fracture has not been established.

A controlled study in patients with postmenopausal osteoporosis[1] found that sodium fluoride 75 mg daily with a calcium supplement increased trabecular bone mass of the spine but did not reduce the incidence of vertebral fractures. Patients given sodium fluoride also had a higher incidence of nonvertebral fractures. An extension and reanalysis of the study,[2] however, showed gradual increases in bone mass observed in patients receiving lower doses of sodium fluoride (down to about 40 mg daily) were associated with a decrease in the incidence of fractures. A previous study[3] had reported a beneficial effect in vertebral fracture rate in patients with primary osteoporosis and at least one vertebral crush fracture. In this study sodium fluoride was given in a daily dose of 50 mg; calcium and vitamin D were also given. Interim analysis of a subsequent study using a slow-release formulation of sodium fluoride 50 mg daily taken intermittently with a regular calcium supplement showed a decrease in vertebral fractures of 50% at 2.5 years.[4] At 4 years the beneficial effect was sustained, the main effect being seen in a reduced incidence of new vertebral fractures;[5] no reduction was seen in the incidence of recurrent fractures but this study found no evidence of an increase in nonvertebral fractures. Some consider that low-dose fluoride can be of benefit in established postmenopausal osteoporosis, but the therapeutic window is narrow, and calcium and vitamin D must be given concomitantly to meet the calcium demand and avoid resorption of established bone.[6] A further double-blind study failed to demonstrate a reduction in vertebral fracture rates in women with osteoporosis treated with fluoride, and calcium and vitamin D compared with women who received only calcium and vitamin D.[7] This was despite a significant increase in bone mass density of the spine in the fluoride-treated groups. Fluoride regimens consisted of 50 mg enteric-coated sodium fluoride daily, or 150 or 200 mg sodium monofluorophosphate daily.

For the administration of fluoride in the form of monofluorophosphate to patients with osteoporosis, see below.

1. Riggs BL, *et al.* Effect of fluoride treatment on the fracture rate in postmenopausal women with osteoporosis. *N Engl J Med* 1990; **322:** 802–9.
2. Riggs BL, *et al.* Clinical trial of fluoride therapy in postmenopausal osteoporotic women: extended observations and additional analysis. *J Bone Miner Res* 1994; **9:** 265–75.
3. Mamelle N, *et al.* Risk-benefit ratio of sodium fluoride treatment in primary vertebral osteoporosis. *Lancet* 1988; **ii:** 361–5.
4. Pak CYC, *et al.* Slow-release sodium fluoride in the management of postmenopausal osteoporosis: a randomized controlled trial. *Ann Intern Med* 1994; **120:** 625–32.
5. Pak CYC, *et al.* Treatment of postmenopausal osteoporosis with slow-release sodium fluoride: final report of a randomized controlled trial. *Ann Intern Med* 1995; **123:** 401–8.
6. Anonymous. New drugs for osteoporosis. *Med Lett Drugs Ther* 1996; **38:** 1–3.
7. Meunier PJ, *et al.* Fluoride salts are no better at preventing new vertebral fractures than calcium-vitamin D in postmenopausal osteoporosis. *Osteoporosis Int* 1998; **8:** 4–12.

Preparations

USP 23: Sodium Fluoride and Acidulated Phosphate Topical Solution; Sodium Fluoride and Phosphoric Acid Gel; Sodium Fluoride and Phosphoric Acid Topical Solution; Sodium Fluoride Oral Solution; Sodium Fluoride Tablets.

Proprietary Preparations (details are given in Part 3)
Aust.: Duraphat; Fluodont; Osteofluor†; Zymafluor; ***Austral.:*** Denta-Mint Topical Fluoride Solution; Floran Effervescent†; Fluor; Flurets; Hi-Fluor†; Orofluor; Phos-Flur; ***Belg.:*** Fluodontyl†; Fluogel†; Procal; Zymafluor†; ***Canad.:*** Duraflor; Fluor-A-Day; Fluorinse; Fluoritabs; Fluorosol; Fluotic; Gel "7"†; Karidium; Oral-B Anti-Cavity Dental Rinse; Oro-NaF; PDF†; Pedi-Dent; Solu-Flur; ***Fr.:*** Fluodontyl; Fluogum; Fluoplexe; Fluor-In†; Fluorex; Osteofluor; Rumafluor†; Sanogyl; Zymafluor; ***Ger.:*** Duraphat; Fluoretten; Koreberon; Ospur F; Ossin; Zymafluor; ***Irl.:*** Fluorite 200†; Reach Junior Fluoride; ***Ital.:*** Fluodent; Fluordent; Fluorigard; Fluorvitin; Oral-B Collutorio Protezione Anti-Carie Fluorinse; Oralsan; Sensifluor; Zymafluor; ***Neth.:*** Dagra Fluor; Fluortabletjes†; Zymafluor; ***Norw.:*** Duraphat; Fluor-Retard†; Fluorette; Flux; ***S.Afr.:*** Denti Gum F†; Fluorogum†; Listerfluor; Zymafluor; ***Spain:*** Fluodontyl; Fluor; Fluor-Kin; Fluoran†; ***Swed.:*** Dentan; Duraphat; Fludent; Fluorette; Top dent fluor; ***Switz.:*** Fluortop; Flurexal†; Ossin; Ossofluor; Osteopor-F†; Zymafluor; ***UK:*** En-De-Kay; Fluor-A-Day; Fluorigard; Oral-B Fluoride†; Zymafluor†; ***USA:*** ACT; Fluorigard; Fluorinse; Fluoritab; Flura; Karidium; Karigel; Karigel-N; Listermint with Fluoride†; Luride; Minute-Gel; MouthKote F/R; Pediaflor; Pharmaflur; Phos-Flur; Point-Two; Prevident; Thera-Flur.

Multi-ingredient: ***Aust.:*** Ossiplex; ***Austral.:*** Macleans Sensitive; Oral-B Sensitive; ***Belg.:*** Calcigenol Simple†; Calcigenol Vitamine†; Fluocaril†; Neocalcigenol Forte†; Neocalcigenol†; Sedemol†; Sulfa-Sedemol†; ***Canad.:*** Cepacol with Fluoride; Oral-B Anti-Bacterial with Fluoride; Poly-Vi-Flor; Sensodyne-F; Tri-Vi-Flor; Tri-Vi-Sol with Fluoride; ***Fr.:*** Fluocaril Bi-Fluore; Fluogel; Fluopate; Fluoselgine; Sanoformine; Sanogyl; Sanogyl Fluo; Sanogyl Junior; ***Ger.:*** Calcipot F†; D-Fluoretten; Elmex; Fluor-Gel†; Fluor-Vigantoletten; Multifluorid; Natabec F; Ossiplex; Zymafluor D; Zymafluor-Calcium†; ***Irl.:*** Listermint with Fluoride; ***Ital.:*** Aqua Emoform; AZ Junior; Broxo al Fluoro; Carefluor†; Clorexident Ortodontico; Dentosan Ortodontico Collutorio; Eburdent F; Ekuba†; Elmex; Eudent con Glysan; Fluocaril Bi-Fluore; Fluorvitburck†; Merfluan Sali Dentali; Oral-B Collutorio per la Protezione di Denti e Gengive; Ossiplex; Otofluor; Plax; Pronto Emoform; Tetrafluor; Valda F3; ***Neth.:*** Davitamon AD Fluor†; ***S.Afr.:*** Denti Gum CF†; ***Spain:*** Necthar Cal†; Normosedin†; Vitagama Fluor; ***Switz.:*** Elmex; Emoform†; ***UK:*** Dentyl pH; Listermint with Fluoride Mouthwash; Macleans Mouthguard; Reach†; Saliva Orthana; ***USA:*** Adeflor M; Apatate with Fluoride; Cari-Tab†; Florical; Florvite; Mulvidren-F Softab; Poly-Vi-Flor; Polytabs-F; Sensitivity Protection Crest; Soluvite; Tri Vit with Fluoride; Tri-Flor-Vite with Fluoride; Tri-Vi-Flor; Trivitamin Fluoride Drops; Vi-Daylin/F.

Sodium Monofluorophosphate

(7735-k)

MFP Sodium; Natrii Monofluorophosphas; Sodium Fluorophosphate. Disodium phosphorofluoridate.

Na_2PO_3F = 143.9.

CAS — 10163-15-2.

Pharmacopoeias. In US.

A white to slightly grey odourless powder. Freely **soluble** in water. A 2% solution in water has a pH of 6.5 to 8.0.

Sodium monofluorophosphate has similar actions to sodium fluoride (p.742) and is used similarly in toothpastes for the prevention of dental caries. It may be given by mouth in the management of osteoporosis.

Toothpastes may contain up to 1.14% of sodium monofluorophosphate, equivalent to about 1500 ppm of fluoride. Low-dose formulations for children under 7 years of age typically contain sodium monofluorophosphate 0.38% (500 ppm fluoride), and their use should be supervised to avoid excessive use or ingestion.

Other monofluorophosphate salts permitted for use in oral hygiene products and dentifrices include ammonium monofluorophosphate, calcium monofluorophosphate, and potassium monofluorophosphate.

Osteoporosis. Preliminary evidence from small studies suggested that fluoride in the form of sodium monofluorophosphate 100 mg twice daily improved bone mineral density in women with osteoporosis (p.731) when combined with calcium[1] or calcium and vitamin D.[2] A potential decrease in vertebral fractures was noted in 1 study,[1] but an increase in stress microfractures in the other.[2] No decrease in vertebral fracture rates was found in women receiving fluoride plus calcium and vitamin D compared with those receiving calcium and vitamin D alone in a subsequent large 2-year study.[3] This was despite a significant increase in bone mass density in the fluoride-treated group. Fluoride regimens included sodium monofluorophosphate 150 or 200 mg daily or enteric-coated sodium fluoride 50 mg daily (see also p.743). In contrast, a further 4-year study found a decrease in vertebral fracture rates in women with moderate osteoporosis treated with sodium monofluorophosphate 156 mg daily plus calcium compared with those receiving calcium alone.[4]

1. Bröll H, *et al.* Effect of sodium monofluorophosphate and calcium on bone density and fracture rate in osteoporosis. *Lancet* 1990; **336:** 1446–7.
2. Delmas PD, *et al.* Treatment of vertebral osteoporosis with disodium monofluorophosphate: comparison with sodium fluoride. *J Bone Miner Res* 1990; **5** (suppl 1): S143–7.
3. Meunier PJ, *et al.* Fluoride salts are no better at preventing new vertebral fractures than calcium-vitamin D in postmenopausal osteoporosis. *Osteoporosis Int* 1998; **8:** 4–12.
4. Reginster JY, *et al.* The effect of sodium monofluorophosphate plus calcium on vertebral fracture rate in postmenopausal women with moderate osteoporosis: a randomized, controlled trial. *Ann Intern Med* 1998; **129:** 1–8.

Preparations

Proprietary Preparations (details are given in Part 3)
Austral.: Nicodent†; ***Ger.:*** Mono-Tridin; ***Ital.:*** Neo-Emoform; Oralsan.

Multi-ingredient: ***Aust.:*** Fluocalcic; ***Austral.:*** Thermodent; ***Belg.:*** Fluocalcic; Fluocaril†; ***Canad.:*** Sensodyne-F; Topol Gel with Fluoride†; Topol with Fluoride†; Viadent; ***Fr.:*** Architex; Fluocalcic; Fluocaril Bi-Fluore; Fluorocalciforte; Sanogyl; Sanogyl Fluo; Sanogyl Junior; ***Ger.:*** Tridin; ***Ital.:*** Aqua Emoform; Broxo al Fluoro; Carefluor†; Cepacol; Eudent con Glysan; Fluocaril Bi-Fluore; Neo-Stomygen; Periogard; Pronto Emoform; Sanogyl Bianco; Tetrafluor; ***Switz.:*** Emoform-F au fluor; Fluo-calc; ***USA:*** Optimoist; Promise†; Sensodyne-F.

Teriparatide Acetate (3640-n)

Teriparatide Acetate (*USAN, rINNM*).

hPTH 1-34 (teriparatide); LY-333334 (teriparatide).

$C_{181}H_{291}N_{55}O_{51}S_2,xH_2O,yC_2H_4O_2$.

CAS — 52232-67-4 (teriparatide); 99294-94-7 (teriparatide acetate).

Units

The potency of teriparatide acetate is expressed in terms of units of human parathyroid hormone activity.

The first International Reference Preparation (1981) of parathyroid hormone, human, for immunoassay contains 0.1 unit in approximately 100 ng of freeze-dried purified hormone.

Adverse Effects

Gastro-intestinal disturbances, a metallic taste, tingling of the extremities, and pain at the site of injection have occasionally been associated with the intravenous infusion of teriparatide acetate. It is a peptide and the possibility of systemic hypersensitivity reactions should be borne in mind. Hypercalcaemia may develop.

Uses and Administration

Teriparatide is a synthetic polypeptide that consists of the 1-34 amino-acid biologically active N-terminal region of human parathyroid hormone (p.741). Teriparatide acetate is given by intravenous infusion in the differential diagnosis of hypoparathyroidism and pseudohypoparathyroidism; in adults a dose of 200 units is infused over 10 minutes. A suggested dose for children greater than 3 years of age is 3 units per kg body-weight to a maximum of 200 units.

Teriparatide is under investigation as a potential stimulant of bone formation in patients with osteoporosis (see below).

Hypoparathyroidism. Hypoparathyroidism is characterised by a deficiency in endogenous parathyroid hormone, whereas pseudohypoparathyroidism is characterised by resistance to the effects of parathyroid hormone (see p.733). Teriparatide acetate is used *diagnostically* to distinguish between these 2 conditions.[1] A synthetic 1-38 fragment of human parathyroid hormone (1-38 hPTH) has been used similarly.[2] Teriparatide has also been used to *treat* hypoparathyroidism.[3]

1. Mallette LE. Synthetic human parathyroid hormone 1-34 fragment for diagnostic testing. *Ann Intern Med* 1988; **109:** 800–4.
2. Kruse K, Kracht U. A simplified diagnostic test in hypoparathyroidism and pseudohypoparathyroidism type I with synthetic 1-38 fragment of human parathyroid hormone. *Eur J Pediatr* 1987; **146:** 373–7.
3. Winer KK, *et al.* Synthetic human parathyroid hormone 1-34 vs calcitriol and calcium in the treatment of hypoparathyroidism. *JAMA* 1996; **276:** 631–6.

Osteoporosis. Parathyroid hormone is capable of stimulating both formation and resorption of bone; at low doses the former effect predominates and may avoid the development of hypercalcaemia. These different actions appear to be modulated by different signalling pathways in the osteoblast, and there is much interest in developing a hormone fragment or analogue which would stimulate bone formation but not resorption.[1] Parathyroid hormone appears to have less effect on cortical than trabecular bone, suggesting that, although it may be helpful in preventing vertebral fractures, its impact on fractures of the proximal femur may be more limited. However, combination with an antiresorptive agent such as oestrogen or a bisphosphonate, the currently preferred treatments for osteoporosis (p.731), might protect other parts of the skeleton. References[2-8] to the use of teriparatide and other synthetic parathyroid hormone fragments in osteoporosis are given below.

1. Bonn D. Parathyroid hormone for osteoporosis. *Lancet* 1996; **347:** 50.
2. Slovik DM, *et al.* Restoration of spinal bone in osteoporotic men by treatment with human parathyroid hormone (1-34) and 1,25-dihydroxyvitamin D. *J Bone Miner Res* 1986; **1:** 377–81.
3. Rittinghaus EF, *et al.* Increase of vertebral density in osteoporosis: combination therapy with 1-38 hPTH and calcitonin nasal spray. *Acta Endocrinol (Copenh)* 1988; **117** (suppl 287): 167–8.
4. Reeve J, *et al.* Treatment of osteoporosis with human parathyroid peptide and observations on effect of sodium fluoride. *Br Med J* 1990; **301:** 314–18. Correction. *ibid.*; 477.
5. Finkelstein JS, *et al.* Parathyroid hormone for the prevention of bone loss induced by estrogen deficiency. *N Engl J Med* 1994; **331:** 1618–23.
6. Hodsman AB, *et al.* A randomized controlled trial to compare the efficacy of cyclical parathyroid hormone versus cyclical parathyroid hormone and sequential calcitonin to improve bone mass in postmenopausal women with osteoporosis. *J Clin Endocrinol Metab* 1997; **82:** 620–8.
7. Lindsay R, *et al.* Randomised controlled study of effect of parathyroid hormone on vertebral-bone mass and fracture incidence among postmenopausal women on oestrogen with osteoporosis. *Lancet* 1997; **350:** 550–5.
8. Finkelstein JS, *et al.* Prevention of estrogen deficiency-related bone loss with human parathyroid hormone-(1-34): a randomized controlled trial. *JAMA* 1998; **280:** 1067–73.

Preparations

Proprietary Preparations (details are given in Part 3)
USA: Parathar.

Tiludronic Acid (10451-e)

Tiludronic Acid (*BAN, rINN*).

ME-3737; SR-41319. {[(*p*-Chlorophenyl)thio]methylene}diphosphonic acid.

$C_7H_9ClO_6P_2S$ = 318.6.

CAS — 89987-06-4.

Disodium Tiludronate (17782-k)

Disodium Tiludronate (*BANM, rINNM*).

SR-41319B; Tiludronate Disodium (*USAN*). Disodium dihydrogen {[(*p*-chlorophenyl)thio]methylene}diphosphonate hemihydrate.

$C_7H_7ClNa_2O_6P_2S,\frac{1}{2}H_2O$ = 371.6.

CAS — 149845-07-8 (anhydrous disodium tiludronate); 155453-10-4 (disodium tiludronate hemihydrate).

Adverse Effects and Precautions

As for the bisphosphonates in general, p.734.

Effects on the skin. As with other bisphosphonates, tiludronate has been associated with rash and pruritus. For reference to a case of massive epidermal necrosis possibly associated with tiludronate, see Hypersensitivity, under Bisphosphonates, p.735.

Interactions

As for the bisphosphonates in general, p.735. Indomethacin may increase the bioavailability of tiludronate two to fourfold if taken concomitantly; diclofenac does not appear to have this effect. Aspirin may decrease the bioavailability of tiludronate by 50%.

Pharmacokinetics

Like other bisphosphonates tiludronate is poorly absorbed following oral administration. Absorption is reduced by food, especially by products containing calcium or other polyvalent cations. Following oral administration the bioavailability of tiludronate is about 6% in the fasting state, and is reduced by about 90% when administered within 2 hours of food. About half of the absorbed portion of tiludronate is bound to bone, and only very slowly excreted; the remainder is excreted unchanged in the urine.

Uses and Administration

Tiludronate is a bisphosphonate with similar properties to those of the bisphosphonates in general (p.735). It inhibits bone resorption and is used for Paget's disease of bone and has been tried in postmenopausal osteoporosis.

It is given by mouth as disodium tiludronate, but doses are expressed in terms of the equivalent amount of tiludronic acid. To ensure adequate absorption doses should be taken, together with plenty of water (at least 200 mL), at least 2 hours before or after meals. In Paget's disease of bone the usual dose is 400 mg once daily for 3 months, and this may be repeated if necessary after an interval of at least 3 months.

Some references to the use of tiludronate in Paget's disease of bone (p.732), and for the management of osteoporosis (p.731).

1. Audran M, *et al.* Treatment of Paget's disease of bone with (4-chloro-phenyl)thiomethylene bisphosphonate. *Clin Rheumatol* 1989; **8:** 71–9.
2. Reginster JY, *et al.* Prevention of postmenopausal bone loss by tiludronate. *Lancet* 1989; **ii:** 1469–71.
3. Reginster JY, *et al.* Paget's disease of bone treated with a five day course of oral tiludronate. *Ann Rheum Dis* 1993; **52:** 54–7.
4. Chesnut CH. Tiludronate: development as an osteoporosis therapy. *Bone* 1995; **17** (suppl 5): 517S–19S.
5. McClung MR, *et al.* Tiludronate therapy for Paget's disease of bone. *Bone* 1995; **17** (suppl 5): 493S–6S.
6. Roux C, *et al.* Comparative prospective, double-blind, multicenter study of the efficacy of tiludronate and etidronate in the treatment of Paget's disease of bone. *Arthritis Rheum* 1995; **38:** 851–8.
7. Anonymous. Tiludronate for Paget's disease of bone. *Med Lett Drugs Ther* 1997; **39:** 65–6.
8. Fraser WD, *et al.* A double-blind, multicentre, placebo-controlled study of tiludronate in Paget's disease of bone. *Postgrad Med J* 1997; **73:** 496–502.

Preparations

Proprietary Preparations (details are given in Part 3)
Aust.: Skelid; ***Belg.:*** Skelid; ***Fr.:*** Skelid; ***Ger.:*** Skelid; ***Neth.:*** Skelid; ***Swed.:*** Skelid; ***Switz.:*** Skelid; ***UK:*** Skelid; ***USA:*** Skelid.

Bronchodilators and Anti-asthma Drugs

This chapter includes many of those drugs used for their bronchodilator or anti-inflammatory properties in the management of reversible airways obstruction, as occurs in asthma and in some patients with chronic obstructive pulmonary disease.

The main bronchodilators discussed in this chapter are the sympathomimetic beta agonists (stimulants of beta-adrenoceptors), and the xanthines, primarily theophylline. The antimuscarinic bronchodilators ipratropium and oxitropium are also included. The major class of anti-inflammatory drugs, the corticosteroids, are discussed separately, on p.1010; other drugs considered to act on the processes of airway inflammation and which are included in this section include sodium cromoglycate and its analogues, and the various drugs that act on leukotriene synthesis and receptor binding, on platelet-activating factor (PAF), or on other aspects of the inflammatory cascade.

Anti-asthma Drug Groups

Antimuscarinics. The parasympathetic nervous system plays a role in the regulation of bronchomotor tone, and antimuscarinic drugs have bronchodilator properties. The quaternary ammonium compounds ipratropium bromide (p.754) and oxitropium bromide (p.757) are the main antimuscarinic bronchodilators in current use; as well as reduced CNS effects they have less effect on mucociliary clearance than drugs such as atropine, which can produce accumulation of viscid lower airway secretions and a risk of mucus plugging in these patients. An antimuscarinic may be the bronchodilator of choice in the management of chronic obstructive pulmonary disease; in patients with asthma they are usually reserved for addition to the therapy of those who cannot be managed with beta agonists and corticosteroids.

Beta agonists. The sympathetic nervous system plays a role in the regulation of bronchomotor tone and $beta_2$-adrenoceptors in bronchial smooth muscle produce bronchodilatation when stimulated. This makes selective agonists of $beta_2$-adrenoceptors ($beta_2$ agonists), of which salbutamol (p.758) is the paradigmatic example, first-line drugs in the management of asthma. They are also widely employed in the management of chronic obstructive pulmonary disease, although other bronchodilators may be preferred or used in addition.

Corticosteroids. Corticosteroids are widely employed for their anti-inflammatory (glucocorticoid) properties in the management of asthma, and may be beneficial in some patients with chronic obstructive pulmonary disease. Because of the potential adverse effects associated with prolonged systemic corticosteroid therapy, inhalation of corticosteroids with reduced systemic activity is widely employed; oral corticosteroids are preferably only employed in short courses, and at relatively low doses, to gain control of the disease. The actions and uses of the corticosteroids are discussed in much greater detail in the section beginning on p.1010.

Cromoglycate and nedocromil. The role of the mast cell in initiating an inflammatory cascade has long been recognised as important, and the best established of the mast cell stabilisers are sodium cromoglycate and nedocromil sodium. These compounds inhibit mast cell degranulation in response to antigens or other stimuli, and hence prevent the release of histamine, leukotrienes, and other inflammatory mediators. They are generally well tolerated and guidelines for the treatment of asthma mention their use for prophylactic therapy as an alternative, or a supplement, to corticosteroids, particularly in children. However, it is generally felt that the corticosteroids are more effective.

Leukotriene inhibitors and antagonists. Leukotrienes appear to play an important role in the inflammatory process of asthma, and a number of drugs attempt to modify or inhibit this action. Leukotriene synthesis may be prevented by blockade of the enzyme 5-lipoxygenase with inhibitors such as zileuton; indirect inhibition by targeting 5-lipoxygenase activating protein (FLAP) is also under investigation. Alternatively, leukotriene antagonists may be used to blockade specific receptors (usually those of leukotriene D_4) and prevent their activation; montelukast, pranlukast, and zafirlukast act this way. The role of such drugs in the prophylactic management of asthma is not yet clearly established.

PAF inhibitors. The role of platelet-activating factor (PAF) in the inflammatory cascade has been examined, and a number of PAF antagonists such as apafant have been tried in asthma, but results to date have been rather disappointing.

Xanthines. Xanthines are drugs with complex actions which include, in varying degrees, relaxation of bronchial smooth muscle and relief of bronchospasm, as well as stimulant effects on respiration. Theophylline (p.765) and its derivatives have long been used for their bronchodilator properties in the management of asthma and chronic obstructive pulmonary disease, but the narrow therapeutic range and the propensity for interactions with other drugs make theophylline a difficult drug to use, and it tends to be reserved for combination therapy in patients who cannot be managed with other bronchodilators (such as the $beta_2$ agonists) alone.

Management of Reversible Airways Obstruction

Asthma

Asthma is a chronic inflammatory disease in which the patient suffers episodes of reversible airways obstruction due to bronchial hyperresponsiveness; in a few patients, inflammation may lead to irreversible obstruction. It is a common disorder occurring in up to 5% of the adult population and perhaps up to 10% of children.[1] Fatalities can occur and mortality rates are reported to be increasing.[1,2]

The aetiology of asthma is poorly understood, but resistance to airflow is increased by a number of factors, including constriction of the airway smooth muscle, the presence of excessive secretions within the airway lumen, and shedding and thickening of the airway epithelium.[3] Asthma may be described as extrinsic when it is associated with exposure to a specific allergen such as pollen or house-dust mite, or to a non-specific stimulus such as a chemical irritant or exercise. It may be described as intrinsic when no external precipitating factor is identifiable.

The principal symptom of asthma is dyspnoea (breathlessness). Wheezing, cough, and chest tightness are often present[1,2] and nocturnal awakening tends to be a common feature.[2,4] In an acute attack, the respiratory rate is rapid and tachycardia is common. The peak expiratory flow (PEF), maximal mid-expiratory flow (MMEF), and forced expiratory volume in the first second (FEV_1) are all decreased in asthma, and in a severe asthmatic attack the PEF and FEV_1 are generally less than 50% of predicted values with a MMEF of 10 to 30% of predicted value. Life-threatening features include exhaustion, cyanosis, bradycardia, hypotension, confusion, and coma.[5]

Management of asthma. As asthma is a chronic disease, management involves prophylactic measures to reduce inflammation and airway resistance and to maintain airflow, as well as specific regimens for the treatment of acute attacks. Measurements of lung function play an important part in determining treatment and patients are encouraged to monitor their own disease by using a simple peak flow meter to measure PEF and adjust their therapy accordingly.

The standard drugs employed in the management of asthma are the $beta_2$ agonists and corticosteroids.[1,2,5,6] Therapy is preferably administered by inhalation to deliver the drugs to the desired site of action. This permits smaller dosages than would be required with oral administration, with a consequent reduction in side-effects. Spacing devices can be fitted to some metered-dose inhalers to act as reservoirs for the drug to make it easier for the patient (especially if a child) to inhale each dose. There is a general trend towards the use of metered-dose inhalers with spacer devices rather than nebulisers,[8] although the choice of spacer and the method of use may substantially affect drug delivery.[9,10] A large volume spacer device is recommended for the inhalation of high doses of corticosteroids to reduce oropharyngeal deposition and systemic absorption.[5]

$Beta_2$ agonists relax the bronchial smooth muscle to produce bronchodilatation by selectively stimulating $beta_2$-adrenergic receptors. Short-acting $beta_2$ agonists such as salbutamol or terbutaline are the initial drugs of choice; if inhaled, they can have an almost immediate bronchodilating effect.

The epidemics of increased asthma mortality associated with inhaled beta agonists (see p.753) receded some time ago and since then the way in which these compounds is used has changed. Doses have fallen and selective agonists are preferred (nonselective beta agonists such as isoprenaline no longer have a role), and there has been a change from regular administration to administration as required. Regular administration of $beta_2$ agonists, including 'long-acting' $beta_2$ agonists such as salmeterol xinafoate,[7] is reserved for patients who have already progressed to anti-inflammatory prophylactic treatment.

Corticosteroids are used for their anti-inflammatory properties and to reduce bronchial hyperresponsiveness; they must be taken regularly to achieve maximum benefit. Corticosteroid therapy is recommended both for acute attacks and chronic asthma prophylaxis. Although the use of corticosteroids for the treatment of acute asthma attacks has been questioned,[11] meta-analysis suggests that they do speed the resolution of exacerbations and reduce the rate of relapse.[12]

In addition, *xanthines* such as aminophylline or theophylline, and *antimuscarinics* such as ipratropium bromide or oxitropium bromide may be given for their bronchodilating properties; there is disagreement concerning xanthine administration in addition to bronchodilating therapy with $beta_2$ agonists for the management of acute severe asthma (see below). *Cromoglycate or nedocromil* may be used as an alternative to corticosteroids for the prophylaxis of less severe asthma or in conjunction with other therapy. *Anti-leukotrienes* such as zafirlukast and zileuton are now becoming available as another alternative.[6]

Chronic asthma. Advice for patients with chronic asthma includes avoidance of smoking, of allergens such as pollen, and of bronchoconstricting drugs such as beta blockers. Patients who have had asthma induced by aspirin and NSAIDs should also avoid these drugs. Skin testing to determine allergen sensitivity may be advisable. US guidelines[6] suggest consideration of immunotherapy to desensitise patients with poorly controlled disease unavoidably exposed to a precipitating allergen, but evidence of benefit from this approach is ambiguous, particularly for multiple allergen immunotherapy, and the potential adverse effects make it controversial; UK guidelines do not recommend immunotherapy for asthma management.[5] Gastro-oesophageal reflux is another potential exacerbating factor: acid suppressive therapy with omeprazole has been shown to reduce asthma symptoms.[15]

Drug therapy for chronic asthma is managed by a stepwise approach depending on the severity of the disease at presentation and its subsequent progression. Guidelines have been issued in the UK by the British Thoracic Society,[5] and subsequently updated;[8] guidelines in the USA have also been recently re-issued and are broadly similar.[6] These guidelines provide for a progressive approach, but now emphasise the importance of obtaining initial control, with the early use of anti-inflammatory drugs, and subsequently 'stepping-down' therapy as far as possible. Treatment strategies for the management of asthma in infants and young children are similar to those outlined for adults and older children though some modifications are usually made.[5,6,8] Some, but not all, authorities prefer to employ cromoglycate or nedocromil before trying low-dose inhaled corticosteroids in mild asthma in children; current guidelines permit initiation of prophylactic therapy with either option.[6,8] Specially adapted or modified inhalation devices are available to enable children to achieve a correct technique when using inhaled drug therapy,[5,8] but alternative routes of delivery such as oral administration or nebulisation may be necessary for some infants and small children.[16]

The recommendations for **adults and children over 5 years of age** with chronic asthma are as follows.

- Patients requiring only occasional relief from symptoms may be adequately managed with an inhaled short-acting $beta_2$ agonist such as salbutamol or terbutaline taken when needed, provided this is not more than once daily (Step 1; mild to intermittent asthma).

- If the $beta_2$ agonist is required more than once a day then regular inhalation of a corticosteroid such as beclomethasone dipropionate or budesonide (100 to 400 μg twice daily) or fluticasone (50 to 200 μg twice daily) should be added. *Alternatively* cromoglycate or nedocromil could be started with a change to inhaled corticosteroids if this fails to provide control (Step 2; mild persistent asthma).

At this stage, US guidelines permit consideration of sustained-release oral theophylline, or in patients over 12 years of age, the use of zafirlukast or zileuton.

- If adequate control is not achieved, the inhaled corticosteroid dose can be increased to 800 to 2000 μg of beclomethasone or budesonide, or 400 to 1000 μg of fluticasone, daily given via a large volume spacer. *Alternatively*, inhaled corticosteroids at lower doses may be supplemented by a long-acting inhaled $beta_2$ agonist such as salmeterol xinafoate (Step 3; moderate persistent asthma).

At this stage there are slight differences of emphasis between US and UK guidelines. *In the USA*, modified-release oral theophylline or a modified-release oral $beta_2$ agonist preparation may be considered as an alternative to an inhaled long-acting $beta_2$ agonist, and if necessary such long-acting bronchodilators may be combined with high-dose inhaled corticosteroids. *In the UK*, although oral theophylline and cromoglycate or nedocromil may be added to lower doses of inhaled corticosteroids, combination of the latter at high doses with regular bronchodilators is considered as the next step:

- treatment with high-dose inhaled corticosteroids and inhaled $beta_2$ agonists is supplemented with one or more of the following bronchodilating drugs: inhaled long-acting $beta_2$ agonists, modified-release oral theophylline, inhaled antimuscarinics, oral modified-release $beta_2$ agonists, and high doses of inhaled bronchodilators; cromoglycate or nedocromil may also be given (UK Step 4).
- If further control is needed, then a corticosteroid such as prednisolone may also be given by mouth in single daily doses (UK Step 5; US Step 4; severe persistent asthma).

A short 'rescue' course of oral prednisolone 30 to 60 mg may also be needed at any time and at any step for an acute exacerbation.

Treatment should be reviewed every 3 to 6 months and if the asthma is adequately controlled a stepwise reduction in treatment may be considered.

The UK recommendations for the management of chronic asthma in **children under 5 years of age**[8] are as follows.

- The first step involves the use of a short-acting $beta_2$ agonist as required, but not more than once daily (Step 1).
- Should that not provide control, then cromoglycate may be added in a dose of 20 mg three or four times daily as an inhaled powder or 10 mg three times daily via a metered dose inhaler if a large volume spacer is used. *Alternatively*, or if there is no control after 4 to 6 weeks cromoglycate may be replaced by inhaled beclomethasone or budesonide in doses up to 400 μg daily, or fluticasone up to 200 μg daily (Step 2).

The dose of inhaled corticosteroid may be doubled initially for stabilisation, or a short course of prednisolone may be added at a dose of 1 to 2 mg per kg body-weight daily for those under 1 year of age and 20 mg daily for those aged 1 to 5 years, for five days. (Recent evidence suggests that lower doses of prednisolone [0.5 mg per kg daily] may be as effective.[37])

- If further control is necessary, then the dose of inhaled beclomethasone or budesonide is increased to 800 μg daily, or that of fluticasone to 500 μg daily, given via a large volume spacer. *In addition* a short course of prednisolone should be considered, as should the addition of an inhaled long-acting $beta_2$ agonist twice daily or a modified-release oral xanthine (Step 3).
- Further increasing the inhaled corticosteroid dose is then recommended; again a short course of prednisolone should be considered, as should the addition of an inhaled long-acting $beta_2$ agonist or a modified-release oral xanthine. Addition of a nebulised $beta_2$ agonist should also be considered (Step 4).

Acute severe asthma (status asthmaticus). An acute attack of severe asthma is potentially life-threatening and treatment should be instituted as soon as possible. Acute severe attacks require admission to hospital. UK guidelines suggest the following regimen for the hospital management of **adults**.[5,8]

- Initially, oxygen should be given at the highest concentration available (40 to 60%) with a high flow-rate.
- High doses of inhaled $beta_2$ agonists, such as salbutamol 5 mg or terbutaline 10 mg, should be administered via a nebuliser with oxygen or compressed air, or if neither of these is available, by multiple actuations of a metered-dose inhaler into a large spacer device.
- High doses of systemic corticosteroids are also required: for example, prednisolone 30 to 60 mg by mouth or hydrocortisone 200 mg intravenously, or both.
- If life-threatening features are present, ipratropium bromide (0.5 mg) can be added to the nebuliser and aminophylline (250 mg over 20 minutes) or a $beta_2$ agonist (salbutamol or terbutaline 250 μg over 10 minutes) may be given intravenously. However, aminophylline should not be given to patients already taking oral xanthines.
- Subsequently, oxygen therapy should be continued as should corticosteroid treatment (prednisolone 30 to 60 mg daily by mouth or hydrocortisone 200 mg every 6 hours intravenously).
- Nebulised $beta_2$ agonists may be given every 4 hours, but if the patient's condition has not improved after 15 to 30 minutes, the nebulised $beta_2$ agonist should be given more frequently (up to every 15 minutes) and ipratropium bromide (0.5 mg every 6 hours) added.
- If progress is still unsatisfactory, then an infusion of aminophylline (0.5 to 0.9 mg per kg body-weight per hour, monitoring blood concentrations if continued for more than 24 hours), salbutamol (5 μg per minute), or terbutaline (1.5 to 5.0 μg per minute) may be required.
- Patients who deteriorate further with drowsiness, unconsciousness, or respiratory arrest need intermittent positive pressure ventilation.

Once lung function is stabilised the patient can be discharged taking oral prednisolone, inhaled corticosteroids, inhaled or nebulised $beta_2$ agonists as required, and oral theophylline, long-acting $beta_2$ agonists, or inhaled ipratropium bromide as necessary.

UK guidelines suggest the following regimen for **children**.

- Immediate treatment involves the administration of oxygen, nebulised $beta_2$ agonists, and oral prednisolone (1 to 2 mg per kg daily, to a maximum of 20 mg daily in children aged 1 to 5 years, or 40 mg daily in those aged 5 to 15 years).
- If life-threatening features are present, nebulised ipratropium bromide (0.125 to 0.25 mg), intravenous hydrocortisone (100 mg every 6 hours), and intravenous aminophylline (5 mg per kg over 20 minutes then 1 mg per kg per hour) can be given. Aminophylline should not be used in children at home.

Subsequent management follows a similar routine to that in adults.[8] (Although the guidelines do not suggest the use of intravenous $beta_2$ agonists in children, a recent study has suggested that intravenous salbutamol may be of benefit.[18])

In the USA guidelines for acute severe asthma are slightly different.[6] Although subcutaneous adrenaline or terbutaline has been employed in the management of acute severe asthma, the guidelines now suggest that the parenteral use of $beta_2$ agonists is an unproven treatment. Moreover, in contrast to the UK the intravenous administration of xanthines is not recommended. In compiling the UK guidelines the British Thoracic Society has taken the view that although most patients on maximal doses of nebulised $beta_2$ agonists derive no additional benefit from intravenous aminophylline, some could obtain more rapid and effective bronchodilatation; intravenous aminophylline was therefore recommended for patients with severe or unresponsive acute asthma attacks.[5] In contrast, the most recent US guidelines issued by the National Asthma Education and Prevention Program do not recommend the use of xanthines as they are considered to offer no benefit over the optimal use of inhaled $beta_2$ agonists.[6] In consequence, in the US guidelines patients who cannot be managed with oxygen, inhaled $beta_2$ agonists and antimuscarinics, and systemic corticosteroids are suggested as candidates for intubation and mechanical ventilation. The UK guidelines acknowledge that not all studies have demonstrated additional benefit with the use of ipratropium, and the benefit it provides has also been questioned in a recent study,[17] although other recent results appear to confirm its value.[13,14]

Investigational therapy. A number of other therapeutic approaches for the management of asthma are currently under investigation.[19] Immunomodulators such as methotrexate, cyclosporin, and gold have been used for their anti-inflammatory, immunosuppressant, and steroid-sparing properties: their use must be balanced against their potentially serious adverse effects and they are therefore reserved for individual patients with chronic severe asthma dependent on systemic corticosteroid therapy.[19-21]

Interestingly, frusemide administered by oral inhalation has been found to protect against bronchoconstriction induced by exercise[22] and external stimuli[23,24] (though not always against direct challenges such as methacholine or histamine) and can inhibit certain types of induced cough; any clinical application has yet to be determined.[19]

Results of clinical studies of magnesium in asthma have been conflicting, both with intravenous magnesium sulphate,[25-27] and by inhalation.[28] There has been some interest in heparin given by inhalation,[29] and nebulised lignocaine may be of some benefit;[30] intravenous lignocaine or oral mexiletine have been shown to block reflex bronchoconstriction.[31]

At a molecular level, bronchodilatation involves an increase in intracellular cyclic adenosine monophosphate (cAMP) and a reduction in the cytosolic calcium ion concentration. Selective phosphodiesterase inhibitors such as zardaverine have been used to inhibit the breakdown of cAMP[16] and calcium-channel blockers such as nifedipine have been tried but are not very effective.[19] Potassium channel activators such as cromakalim[32] have also been developed which relax airway smooth muscle.[19] Other studies have concentrated on antagonising the various mediators of asthma using platelet-activating factor (PAF) antagonists, thromboxane inhibitors, and leukotriene antagonists, for example zafirlukast, or inhibitors of leukotriene synthesis such as zileuton. Although clearly effective[33,34] the role of zileuton and zafirlukast, and other drugs of this type, has yet to be determined.[6,35] Infiltration of inflammatory cells into tissues may be suppressed by cell adhesion blockers and these are also under investigation for an application in asthma.[19]

In patients with acute severe asthma, in whom respiratory muscle fatigue can lead to ventilatory failure, use of helium-oxygen mixture, which has a lower density than air and can reduce turbulent flow and respiratory work, may be beneficial.[36]

1. Jain P, Golish JA. Clinical management of asthma in the 1990s: current therapy and new directions. *Drugs* 1996; **52** (suppl 6): 1–11.
2. McFadden ER, Gilbert IA. Asthma. *N Engl J Med* 1992; **327:** 1928–37. Correction. *ibid.* 1993; **328:** 1640–1.
3. Barnes PJ. Pathophysiology of asthma. *Br J Clin Pharmacol* 1996; **42:** 3–10.
4. Catterall JR, Shapiro CM. Nocturnal asthma. *Br Med J* 1993; **306:** 1189–92.
5. British Thoracic Society, *et al.* Guidelines on the management of asthma. *Thorax* 1993; **48** (suppl): S1–S24. Correction. *ibid.* 1994; **49:** 386. (Summary published in *Br Med J* 1993; **306:** 776–82. Correction. *ibid.* **307:** 1054.)
6. National Asthma Education and Prevention Program. *Expert Panel Report 2: guidelines for the diagnosis and management of asthma.* Bethesda: National Heart, Lung, and Blood Institute, 1997.
7. Boulet L-P. Long- versus short-acting β_2-agonists: implications for drug therapy. *Drugs* 1994; **47:** 207–22.
8. British Thoracic Society, *et al.* The British guidelines on asthma management: 1995 review and position statement. *Thorax* 1997; **52** (suppl 1): S1–S21.
9. Bisgaard H. Drug delivery from inhaler devices. *Br Med J* 1996; **313:** 895–6. Correction. *ibid.* 1997; **314:** 990.
10. O'Callaghan C, Barry P. Spacer devices in the treatment of asthma. *Br Med J* 1997; **314:** 1061–2.
11. McFadden ER, Hejal R. Asthma. *Lancet* 1995; **345:** 1215–20.
12. Rowe BH, *et al.* Effectiveness of steroid therapy in acute exacerbations of asthma: a meta-analysis. *Am J Emerg Med* 1992; **10:** 301–10.
13. Qureshi F, *et al.* Effect of nebulized ipratropium on the hospitalization rates of children with asthma. *N Engl J Med* 1998; **339:** 1030–5.
14. Brophy C, *et al.* How long should Atrovent be given in acute asthma ? *Thorax* 1998; **53:** 363–7.

15. Harding SM, *et al.* Asthma and gastroesophageal reflux: acid suppressive therapy improves asthma outcome. *Am J Med* 1996; **100:** 395–405.
16. Warner JO, *et al.* Asthma: a follow up statement from an international paediatric asthma consensus group. *Arch Dis Child* 1992; **67:** 240–8.
17. McFadden ER, *et al.* The influence of parasympatholytics on the resolution of acute attacks of asthma. *Am J Med* 1997; **102:** 7–13.
18. Browne GJ, *et al.* Randomised trial of intravenous salbutamol in early management of acute severe asthma in children. *Lancet* 1997; **349:** 301–5.
19. Barnes PJ. New therapeutic approaches. *Br Med Bull* 1991; **48:** 231–47.
20. Kon OM, Barnes N. Immunosuppressive treatment in asthma. *Br J Hosp Med* 1997; **57:** 383–6.
21. Shulimzon TR, Shiner RJ. A risk-benefit assessment of methotrexate in corticosteroid-dependent asthma. *Drug Safety* 1996; **15:** 283–90.
22. Munyard P, *et al.* Inhaled frusemide and exercise-induced bronchoconstriction in children with asthma. *Thorax* 1995; **50:** 677–9.
23. Bianco S, *et al.* Protective effect of inhaled furosemide on allergen-induced early and late asthmatic reactions. *N Engl J Med* 1989; **321:** 1069–73.
24. Seidenberg J, *et al.* Inhaled frusemide against cold air induced bronchoconstriction in asthmatic children. *Arch Dis Child* 1992; **67:** 214–17.
25. Skobeloff EM, *et al.* Intravenous magnesium sulfate for the treatment of acute asthma in the emergency department. *JAMA* 1989; **262:** 1210–13.
26. Green SM, Rothrock SG. Intravenous magnesium for acute asthma: failure to decrease emergency treatment duration or need for hospitalization. *Ann Emerg Med* 1992; **21:** 260–5.
27. Ciarallo L, *et al.* Intravenous magnesium therapy for moderate to severe pediatric asthma: results of a randomized, placebo-controlled trial. *J Pediatr* 1996; **129:** 809–14.
28. Hill J, Britton J. Dose-response relationship and time-course of the effect of inhaled magnesium sulphate on airflow in normal and asthmatic subjects. *Br J Clin Pharmacol* 1995; **40:** 539–44.
29. Diamant Z, *et al.* Effect of inhaled heparin on allergen-induced early and late asthmatic responses in patients with atopic asthma. *Am J Respir Crit Care Med* 1996; **153:** 1790–5.
30. Hunt LW, *et al.* Effect of nebulized lidocaine on severe glucocorticoid-dependent asthma. *Mayo Clin Proc* 1996; **71:** 361–8.
31. Groeben H, *et al.* Intravenous lidocaine and oral mexiletine block reflex bronchoconstriction in asthmatic subjects. *Am J Respir Crit Care Med* 1996; **154:** 885–8.
32. Williams AJ, *et al.* Attenuation of nocturnal asthma by cromakalim. *Lancet* 1990; **336:** 334–6.
33. Israel E, *et al.* Effect of treatment with zileuton, a 5-lipoxygenase inhibitor, in patients with asthma: a randomized controlled trial. *JAMA* 1996; **275:** 931–6.
34. Suissa S, *et al.* Effectiveness of the leukotriene receptor antagonist zafirlukast for mild-to-moderate asthma: a randomized, double-blind, placebo-controlled trial. *Ann Intern Med* 1997; **126:** 177–83.
35. Larsen JS, Jackson SK. Antileukotriene therapy for asthma. *Am J Health-Syst Pharm* 1996; **53:** 2821–30.
36. Kudukis TM, *et al.* Inhaled helium-oxygen revisited: effect of inhaled helium-oxygen during the treatment of status asthmaticus in children. *J Pediatr* 1997; **130:** 217–24.
37. Langton Hewer S, *et al.* Prednisolone in acute childhood asthma: clinical responses to three dosages. *Respir Med* 1998; **92:** 541–6.

Chronic obstructive pulmonary disease

Chronic obstructive pulmonary disease (COPD, chronic obstructive lung disease, chronic obstructive airways disease) covers a range of disorders of progressive airflow limitation including chronic bronchitis and emphysema. Unlike asthma, the obstruction of airflow, indicated by an abnormal decline in the forced expiratory volume in one second (FEV_1), is more or less continuous and largely irreversible. Chronic obstructive pulmonary disease is a common disorder, frequently associated with cigarette smoking; infections, environmental pollution, and occupational dust exposure may also have an aetiological role.

In *chronic bronchitis* there is enlargement of the mucous glands and an increase in the number of goblet cells within the bronchial mucosa which leads to an increase in mucus production and thickening of the bronchial wall. Patients suffer from a chronic productive cough with excessive sputum production. They may also experience dyspnoea, bronchospasm, and frequent respiratory tract infections. In severe cases (chronic obstructive bronchitis, small airways disease), irreversible narrowing of the airways leads to a disabling condition in which there is cyanosis, hypoxia, hypercapnia, and right-sided heart failure (cor pulmonale, see below); such patients have been described as 'blue bloaters'.

Emphysema is an abnormal permanent enlargement of air spaces distal to the terminal bronchioles accompanied by destruction of the alveolar wall and without obvious fibrosis. There is excessive airway collapse upon expiration and irreversible airways obstruction. Dyspnoea is a prominent symptom; a productive cough, wheezing, recurrent respiratory infection, and a marked loss of weight may also be noted. Patients may hyperventilate to maintain oxygen levels in the blood and have been called 'pink puffers' in contrast to the 'blue bloaters' of the classic bronchitic presentation. Rarely, emphysema can be caused by a hereditary deficiency of $alpha_1$ antitrypsin ($alpha_1$-proteinase inhibitor), see p.1546.

Patients with severe COPD can develop *cor pulmonale* (heart disease secondary to disease of the lungs and respiratory system) with pulmonary hypertension, right ventricular hypertrophy, and right heart failure.[1] Cor pulmonale is more often associated with chronic bronchitis than with emphysema.

Management of COPD. Although consensus is less general than for asthma, guidelines for the treatment of COPD have been issued in a number of countries.[2-6] The most important therapeutic intervention is persuading those patients who smoke to stop; psychological support and possibly adjunctive drug therapy may be required (see Smoking Cessation, p.1608). Prevention of respiratory infection should be considered, and influenza and pneumococcal vaccination are recommended,[4,6-8] although the value of pneumococcal vaccination in these patients has not been unequivocally established.[6,7]

Drug treatment is primarily symptomatic and palliative using bronchodilators, corticosteroids, and oxygen therapy. Purulent sputum indicates a respiratory infection (see under Exacerbations, below).

First-line drug therapy for the treatment of COPD consists of bronchodilators to alleviate bronchospasm and any reversible component of the airways obstruction. Either an inhaled *antimuscarinic*, such as ipratropium bromide, or a short-acting *$beta_2$ agonist*, is suggested as the initial bronchodilator.[2-6] UK guidelines recommend beginning with a $beta_2$ agonist, because of their more rapid action,[2] but there is some suggestion that antimuscarinics are slightly more effective than $beta_2$ agonists in this group of patients.[4,7] Patients vary in their responsiveness and a $beta_2$ agonist should be tried in those who do not respond well to an antimuscarinic, and vice versa.[5] Some patients benefit further from combined therapy;[2,3,11] US guidelines suggest addition of an inhaled short-acting $beta_2$ agonist to ipratropium, on an 'as needed' basis.[4] The role of longer-acting $beta_2$ agonists such as salmeterol has yet to be clearly established, but some consider that they may have a role in maintenance, particularly in the prevention of nocturnal symptoms.[6] A *xanthine* such as theophylline by mouth may also be considered and has been given in addition to inhaled agents.[2-6,11] Theophylline has been reported to improve respiratory muscle function in patients with COPD and may have positive cardiac inotropic effects which could be of value in cor pulmonale.

Meta-analysis suggests that only about 10% of COPD patients receiving optimal bronchodilator therapy exhibit a substantial further response to oral *corticosteroids*.[12] It has been recommended that all patients with COPD should receive a trial of prednisolone 40 mg daily by mouth for 2 weeks; an increase in FEV_1 of more than 15% from base-line is considered evidence of responsiveness.[6] Inhaled corticosteroids may be tried for maintenance, but only about half of those responsive to oral corticosteroids respond to the inhalational route.[13,14,15] However, some groups have reported a reduced rate of exacerbations in patients treated with inhaled corticosteroids,[16] although this remains contentious.[9,10]

In patients with severe COPD and persistent hypoxaemia, supplemental *oxygen* provided on an almost continuous long-term basis at home has been found to improve survival and alleviate complications such as cor pulmonale, polycythaemia and neuropsychological impairment.[17,18] Guidelines recommend the institution of oxygen therapy in patients whose resting PaO_2 is less than 55 mmHg (about 7.3 kPa), or whose arterial oxygen saturation is less than about 90%.[2-4,6] Non-invasive nocturnal ventilation (via a mask) may be of benefit in some patients.[7,19]

The use of *mucolytics* or *expectorants* is controversial,[3,6] although Swiss guidelines suggest that acetylcysteine may be of benefit in selected patients;[6] initially promising results with dornase alfa have not been borne out in later study.[8] However, improved pulmonary function has been reported in patients given aerosolised surfactant.[20]

Exacerbations. Patients with COPD frequently suffer exacerbations of their symptoms. Treatment options are similar to those for the chronic condition and include physiotherapy, maximal bronchodilators, systemic corticosteroids, and oxygen as necessary, together with appropriate management of any associated cardiovascular disorder.[21] The use of *antibiotics* for acute exacerbations has long been controversial, but meta-analysis suggests that a modest benefit exists,[22] mainly in patients with more severe disease, and guidelines suggest their use on an empirical basis where signs of infection are present;[2,4,5] it has been suggested that in patients with only mild exacerbations they can be withheld until the patient deteriorates or fails to improve.[6] The use of prophylactic antibiotic cover for those with recurrent acute exacerbations is even more controversial, but US guidelines suggest that prolonged courses of antibiotic may be appropriate, particularly in winter.[4] Oxygen therapy is required in patients with hypoxia; the goal is to maintain oxygen saturation above 90% but prevent increasing CO_2 retention. Relatively low oxygen concentrations (beginning at about 25%) are advised in these generally hypercapnic patients, as high concentrations may impair ventilation and respiratory drive, but some consider the risks of oxygen administration to have been overstated.[21] *Respiratory stimulants* such as doxapram are of limited use but have been given in the short term for temporary arousal.[21] Despite intensive therapy, some patients progress to respiratory muscle fatigue and require ventilatory support.

1. Palevsky HI, Fishman AP. Chronic cor pulmonale: etiology and management. *JAMA* 1990; **263:** 2347–53.
2. British Thoracic Society. BTS Guidelines for the management of chronic obstructive pulmonary disease. *Thorax* 1997; **52** (suppl 5): S1–S28.
3. Canadian Thoracic Society Workshop Group. Guidelines for the assessment and management of chronic obstructive pulmonary disease. *Can Med Assoc J* 1992; **147:** 420–8.
4. American Thoracic Society. Standards for the diagnosis and care of patients with chronic obstructive pulmonary disease. *Am J Respir Crit Care Med* 1995; **152** (suppl): S77–S120.
5. Siafakas NM, *et al.* ERS consensus statement: optimal assessment and management of chronic obstructive pulmonary disease (COPD). *Eur Respir J* 1995; **8:** 1398–1420.
6. Leuenberger P, *et al.* Management 1997 of chronic obstructive pulmonary disease. *Schweiz Med Wochenschr* 1997; **127:** 766–82.
7. Chapman KR. Therapeutic approaches to chronic obstructive pulmonary disease: an emerging consensus. *Am J Med* 1996; **100** (suppl 1A): 5S–10S.
8. Fiel SB. Chronic obstructive pulmonary disease: mortality and mortality reduction. *Drugs* 1996; **52** (suppl 2): 55–61.
9. Morice A. Fluticasone propionate for chronic obstructive pulmonary disease. *Lancet* 1998; **351:** 1890.
10. Efthimiou J, *et al.* Fluticasone propionate for chronic obstructive pulmonary disease. *Lancet* 1998; **351:** 1890–1.
11. Karpel JP, *et al.* A comparison of inhaled ipratropium, oral theophylline plus inhaled beta-agonist, and the combination of all three in patients with COPD. *Chest* 1994; **105:** 1089–94.
12. Callahan CM, *et al.* Oral corticosteroid therapy for patients with stable chronic obstructive pulmonary disease. *Ann Intern Med* 1991; **114:** 216–23.
13. Shim CS, Williams MH. Aerosol beclomethasone in patients with steroid-responsive chronic obstructive pulmonary disease. *Am J Med* 1985; **78:** 655–8.
14. Weir DC, *et al.* Corticosteroid trials in non-asthmatic chronic airflow obstruction: a comparison of oral prednisolone and inhaled beclomethasone dipropionate. *Thorax* 1990; **45:** 112–17.
15. Jackevicius CA, Chapman KR. Prevalence of inhaled corticosteroid use among patients with chronic obstructive pulmonary disease: a survey. *Ann Pharmacother* 1997; **31:** 160–4.
16. Paggiaro PL, *et al.* Multicentre randomised placebo-controlled trial of inhaled fluticasone propionate in patients with chronic obstructive pulmonary disease. *Lancet* 1998; **351:** 773–80. Correction. *ibid.*; 1968.
17. Medical Research Council Working Party. Long-term domiciliary oxygen therapy in chronic hypoxic cor pulmonale complicating chronic bronchitis and emphysema. *Lancet* 1981; **i:** 681–6.
18. Nocturnal Oxygen Therapy Trial Group. Continuous or nocturnal oxygen therapy in hypoxemic chronic obstructive lung disease: a clinical trial. *Ann Intern Med* 1980; **93:** 391–8.
19. Elliott MW. Non-invasive ventilation in chronic obstructive pulmonary disease. *Br J Hosp Med* 1997; **57:** 83–6.
20. Anzueto A, *et al.* Effects of aerosolized surfactant in patients with stable chronic bronchitis: a prospective randomized controlled trial. *JAMA* 1997; **278:** 1426–31.
21. Schmidt GA, Hall JB. Acute on chronic respiratory failure: assessment and management of patients with COPD in the emergent setting. *JAMA* 1989; **261:** 3444–53.
22. Saint S, *et al.* Antibiotics in chronic obstructive pulmonary disease exacerbations: a meta-analysis. *JAMA* 1995; **273:** 957–60.

Aminophylline (3873-a)

Aminophylline (BAN, pINN).

Aminofilina; Aminophyllinum; Euphyllinum; Metaphyllin; Theophyllaminum; Theophylline and Ethylenediamine; Theophylline Ethylenediamine Compound; Theophyllinum et Ethylenediaminum. A mixture of theophylline and ethylenediamine (2:1), its composition approximately corresponding to the formula.

$(C_7H_8N_4O_2)_2,C_2H_4(NH_2)_2$ = 420.4.

CAS — 317-34-0 (anhydrous aminophylline).

Pharmacopoeias. In *Eur.* (see p.viii), *Int.*, and *US*. Some pharmacopoeias include anhydrous and hydrated aminophylline in one monograph.

White or slightly yellowish granules or powder, odourless or with a slight ammoniacal odour. It is a stable mixture or combination of theophylline and ethylenediamine containing between 84.0% and 87.4% of anhydrous theophylline and 13.5% to 15.0% of anhydrous ethylenediamine.

Freely **soluble** in water (the solution may become cloudy in the presence of carbon dioxide); practically insoluble in alcohol and in ether. Solutions are alkaline to litmus and should not be allowed to come into contact with metals. In moist air it gradually loses ethylenediamine and absorbs carbon dioxide with the liberation of theophylline. **Store** in airtight containers. Protect from light.

Aminophylline Hydrate (628-b)

Aminophylline Hydrate (BANM, pINNM).

$(C_7H_8N_4O_2)_2,C_2H_4(NH_2)_2,2H_2O$ = 456.5.

CAS — 49746-06-7 (aminophylline dihydrate).

Pharmacopoeias. In *Chin.*, *Eur.* (see p.viii), *Jpn*, *Pol.*, and *US*. Some pharmacopoeias include anhydrous and hydrated aminophylline in one monograph. Some pharmacopoeias do not specify the hydration state.

A white or slightly yellowish powder or granular powder. It is odourless or has a slight ammoniacal odour. It is a stable mixture or combination of theophylline and ethylenediamine containing between 84.0% and 87.4% of theophylline and 13.5% to 15.0% of ethylenediamine, calculated as the anhydrous substances, with water of hydration. Aminophylline hydrate 1.09 mg is approximately equivalent to 1 mg of aminophylline.

Freely **soluble** in water (the solution may become cloudy due to the presence of carbon dioxide); practically insoluble in alcohol and in ether. Solutions are alkaline to litmus and should not be allowed to come into contact with metals. **Store** in well-filled airtight containers. Protect from light.

Incompatibility. Solutions of aminophylline are alkaline and if the pH falls below 8 crystals of theophylline will deposit.[1] Drugs known to be unstable in alkaline solutions should not be mixed with aminophylline nor should drugs that will lower the pH below the critical value. The addition of aminophylline to glucose injection has been reported to raise the pH by over 4 units to pH 7.7 to 10.45. At this pH insulin and erythromycin gluceptate are incompatible. Other examples of drugs incompatible with aminophylline include amiodarone,[2] benzylpenicillin potassium,[1] cisatracurium,[3] dobutamine,[4] tetracycline hydrochloride,[1] verapamil hydrochloride,[5] warfarin sodium,[6] and vitamin B and C injection.[1] One study has found that although ceftazidime was incompatible with aminophylline in infusion fluids, it was adequately stable for intermittent Y-site infusion over a 2-hour period.[7] Infusion fluids containing cefuroxime and aminophylline have been reported to be stable for up to 4 hours.[8] Solutions containing ceftriaxone sodium and aminophylline were found to be generally unstable if stored for 24 hours with degradation of ceftriaxone and some loss of aminophylline.[9]

1. Edward M. pH—an important factor in the compatibility of additives in intravenous therapy. *Am J Hosp Pharm* 1967; **24:** 440–9.
2. Hasegawa GR, Eder JF. Visual compatibility of amiodarone hydrochloride injection with other injectable drugs. *Am J Hosp Pharm* 1984; **41:** 1379–80.
3. Trissel LA, *et al.* Compatibility of cisatracurium besylate with selected drugs during simulated Y-site administration. *Am J Health-Syst Pharm* 1997; **54:** 1735–41.
4. Hasegawa GR, Eder JF. Visual compatibility of dobutamine hydrochloride with other injectable drugs. *Am J Hosp Pharm* 1984; **41:** 949–51.
5. Johnson CE, *et al.* Compatibility of aminophylline and verapamil in intravenous admixtures. *Am J Hosp Pharm* 1989; **46:** 97–100.
6. Bahal SM, *et al.* Visual compatibility of warfarin sodium injection with selected medications and solutions. *Am J Health-Syst Pharm* 1997; **54:** 2599–600.
7. Pleasants RA, *et al.* Compatibility of ceftazidime and aminophylline admixtures for different methods of intravenous infusion. *Ann Pharmacother* 1992; **26:** 1221–6.
8. Stewart JT, *et al.* Stability of cefuroxime sodium and aminophylline or theophylline. *Am J Hosp Pharm* 1994; **51:** 809–11.
9. Parrish MA, *et al.* Stability of ceftriaxone sodium and aminophylline or theophylline in intravenous admixtures. *Am J Hosp Pharm* 1994; **51:** 92–4.

Stability. References to the stability of aminophylline in parenteral nutrition solutions.

1. Kirk B, Sprake JM. Stability of aminophylline: a study of its stability in simple and complex neonatal parenteral nutrition solutions. *Br J Intraven Ther* 1982; **3** (Nov): 4–8.
2. Niemiec PW, *et al.* Stability of aminophylline injection in three parenteral nutrient solutions. *Am J Hosp Pharm* 1983; **40:** 428–32.
3. Kirkpatrick AE, *et al.* Effect of retrograde aminophylline administration on calcium and phosphate solubility in neonatal total parenteral nutrient solutions. *Am J Hosp Pharm* 1989; **46:** 2496–2500.

Adverse Effects, Treatment, and Precautions

As for Theophylline, p.765. Hypersensitivity has been associated with the ethylenediamine content.

Interactions

As for Theophylline, p.767.

Pharmacokinetics

Aminophylline, a complex of theophylline with ethylenediamine, readily liberates theophylline in the body. The pharmacokinetics of theophylline are discussed on p.771.

Studies in healthy subjects suggested that ethylenediamine does not affect the pharmacokinetics of theophylline after oral or intravenous administration.[1,2]

1. Aslaksen A, *et al.* Comparative pharmacokinetics of theophylline and aminophylline in man. *Br J Clin Pharmacol* 1981; **11:** 269–73.
2. Caldwell J, *et al.* Theophylline pharmacokinetics after intravenous infusion with ethylenediamine or sodium glycinate. *Br J Clin Pharmacol* 1986; **22:** 351–5.

Uses and Administration

Aminophylline has the actions and uses of theophylline (see p.772) and is used similarly as a bronchodilator in the management of asthma (p.745) and chronic obstructive pulmonary disease (p.747). It was formerly used for its diuretic action in heart failure but has been superseded by more effective drugs (see p.785). However, it may have a role in patients with heart failure and obstructive airways disease though care is needed in those with increased myocardial excitability. Aminophylline is usually preferred to theophylline when greater solubility in water is required, particularly in intravenous formulations.

Aminophylline may be given in the anhydrous form or as the dihydrate. Doses appear to be usually expressed as aminophylline hydrate though some pharmacopoeias label aminophylline preparations with respect to their anhydrous aminophylline content.

As the pharmacokinetics of theophylline are affected by a number of factors including age, smoking, disease, diet, and drug interactions, the dose of aminophylline must be carefully individualised and serum-theophylline concentrations monitored (see under Uses and Administration of Theophylline, p.772).

In the management of acute severe bronchospasm, aminophylline may be administered intravenously by slow injection or infusion. To reduce adverse effects, the rate of intravenous administration of aminophylline should not exceed 25 mg per minute. In patients who have not been taking aminophylline, theophylline, or other xanthine-containing medication, 250 to 500 mg of aminophylline (25 mg per mL) may be given by slow intravenous injection over 20 minutes. When administered by infusion, a suggested loading dose is 5 mg per kg, given over 20 to 30 minutes, followed by a maintenance dose of 0.5 mg per kg per hour. Older patients and those with cor pulmonale, heart failure, or liver disease may require lower maintenance doses; smokers often need higher maintenance doses (see Precautions under Theophylline, p.767). A loading dose may not be considered necessary unless the patient's condition is deteriorating. Children (also not currently on xanthine medication) may be given the same loading dose per kg as adults; suggested maintenance doses are 1 mg per kg per hour for children aged 6 months to 9 years and 0.8 mg per kg per hour for children aged 10 to 16 years. Some authorities suggest that the maintenance doses should be slightly higher for the first 12 hours of the infusion in both adults and children.

Intravenous aminophylline is best avoided in patients already taking theophylline, aminophylline, or other xanthine-containing medication but, if considered necessary, the serum-theophylline concentration should first be assessed and the initial loading dose should be calculated on the basis that each 0.5 mg per kg of aminophylline will increase serum theophylline concentration by 1 μg per mL.

In the treatment of acute bronchospasm that does not require intravenous therapy, aminophylline has been given by mouth in conventional dosage forms; modified-release preparations are not suitable. Doses used have generally ranged from 100 to 300 mg three or four times daily after food.

In the management of chronic bronchospasm aminophylline may be given by mouth as conventional or as modified-release preparations. The modified-release products are generally preferred and a usual dose is aminophylline hydrate 225 to 450 mg twice daily by mouth. Therapy should be initiated with the lower dose and increased as necessary. Elderly patients may require lower doses. Retitration of the dosage may be required if the patient is changed from one modified-release preparation to another as the bioavailability of modified-release aminophylline preparations may vary. Children (over 3 years) have been given modified-release aminophylline hydrate in doses of 12 mg per kg body-weight daily, increased after 1 week to 24 mg per kg daily, in 2 divided doses.

Intramuscular administration of aminophylline causes intense local pain and is not recommended.

Aminophylline has also been used as the hydrochloride.

Administration. RECTAL ADMINISTRATION. Absorption from aminophylline suppositories is erratic and this dose form has been associated with toxicity, hence the warnings that suppositories should not be used especially in children. In the UK suppositories are no longer readily available and one hospital wishing to use the rectal route for apnoea in premature infants achieved therapeutic plasma-theophylline concentrations with a specially formulated rectal gel.[1]

1. Cooney S, *et al.* Rectal aminophylline gel in treatment of apnoea in premature newborn babies. *Lancet* 1991; **337:** 1351.

Methotrexate neurotoxicity. Aminophylline by intravenous infusion or theophylline by mouth relieved the acute neurotoxicity of methotrexate (p.547) in some children[1] possibly through an anti-adenosine effect.

1. Bernini JC, *et al.* Aminophylline for methotrexate-induced neurotoxicity. *Lancet* 1995; **345:** 544–7.

Reduction of body fat. Discussion of the cosmetic use of aminophylline cream to remove fat ('cellulite') from the thighs.[1]

1. Dickinson BI, Gora-Harper ML. Aminophylline for cellulite removal. *Ann Pharmacother* 1996; **30:** 292–3.

Preparations

BP 1998: Aminophylline Injection; Aminophylline Tablets;
USP 23: Aminophylline Delayed-release Tablets; Aminophylline Enema; Aminophylline Injection; Aminophylline Oral Solution; Aminophylline Suppositories; Aminophylline Tablets.

Proprietary Preparations (details are given in Part 3)
Aust.: Euphyllin; Mundiphyllin; ***Austral.:*** Cardophyllin†; ***Belg.:*** Euphyllin; ***Canad.:*** Phyllocontin; ***Fr.:*** Planphylline; ***Ger.:*** Afonilum; duraphyllin†; Euphyllin 0.48†; Euphyllin CR†; Euphyllin†; Phyllotemp; ***Irl.:*** Clonofilin; Phyllocontin; ***Ital.:*** Aminomal; Euphyllina; Tefamin; ***Neth.:*** Euphyllin; ***S.Afr.:*** Asmalline†; Peterphyllin; Phyllocontin; ***Spain:*** Eufilina; ***Switz.:*** Escophylline; Euphyllin; Phyllotemp; ***UK:*** Amnivent; Norphyllin SR; Pecram; Phyllocontin; ***USA:*** Phyllocontin; Truphylline.

Multi-ingredient: ***Aust.:*** Asthma-Hilfe; Euphyllin-Calcium; Limptar; Myocardon; ***Canad.:*** Amesec†; ***Fr.:*** Campho-Pneumine Aminophylline†; ***Ger.:*** Limptar; Myocardetten†; ***Ital.:*** Aminomal con Antiasmatico†; Asmarectal†; ***S.Afr.:*** Amaphil†; Amesec†; Daral†; Diphenamill; Efcod†; Fabasma; Lotussin Expectorant; Medikasma; Nutrated†; Panasma; Peterphyllin Co.†; Repasma; ***Spain:*** Angiosedante; Bronquiasmol†; Codefilona†; Eufipulmo†; Lasa Antiasmatico; Navarrofilina†; ***Switz.:*** Limptar; ***USA:*** Emergent-Ez; Mudrane; Mudrane GG; Mudrane GG-2; Mudrane-2†.

Amlexanox (2893-j)

Amlexanox *(USAN, rINN)*.

AA-673; Amoxanox; CHX-3673. 2-Amino-7-isopropyl-5-oxo-5*H*-[1]benzopyrano[2,3-*b*]pyridine-3-carboxylic acid.

$C_{16}H_{14}N_2O_4$ = 298.3.

CAS — 68302-57-8.

Amlexanox has a stabilising action on mast cells resembling that of sodium cromoglycate and is also a leukotriene inhibitor. It is administered by mouth in the management of asthma (p.745) and for allergic rhinitis (p.400); a dose of 25 or 50 mg three times daily has been cited. Amlexanox is also given as a metered-dose nasal spray for allergic rhinitis.

Amlexanox is also applied as a 5% oral paste four times daily in the management of aphthous ulcers (p.1172).

Preparations

Proprietary Preparations (details are given in Part 3)
Jpn: Solfa; ***USA:*** Aphthasol.

Apafant (3658-e)

Apafant *(rINN)*.

WEB-2086. 4-{3-[4-(*o*-Chlorophenyl)-9-methyl-6*H*-thieno[3,2-*f*]-*s*-triazolo[4,3-*a*][1,4]diazepin-2-yl]propionyl}morpholine.

$C_{22}H_{22}ClN_5O_2S$ = 456.0.

CAS — 105219-56-5.

Apafant is a platelet-activating factor antagonist that has been investigated for the management or prophylactic control of asthma. It has been tried in other conditions, including acute pancreatitis.

References.

1. Lohmann HF, *et al.* Idiopathic thrombocytopenia treated with PAF-acether antagonist WEB 2086. *Lancet* 1988; **ii:** 1147.
2. Adamus WS, *et al.* Safety, tolerability, and pharmacological activity of multiple doses of the new platelet activating factor antagonist WEB 2086 in human subjects. *Clin Pharmacol Ther* 1989; **45:** 270–6.
3. Giers G, *et al.* PAF-acether-antagonist WEB 2086 for treatment of chronic idiopathic thrombocytopenia. *Lancet* 1990; **336:** 191–2.
4. Brecht HM, *et al.* Pharmacodynamics, pharmacokinetics and safety profile of the new platelet-activating factor antagonist apafant in man. *Arzneimittelforschung* 1991; **41:** 51–9.

Asthma. In a study involving 106 patients with stable atopic asthma, apafant 40 mg by mouth three times daily was no more effective than placebo in reducing the requirement for inhaled corticosteroids.[1] It was concluded that these negative results, at a dose known to produce active concentrations in the airways, cast doubt upon the role of platelet-activating factor in the pathogenesis of asthma (p.745).

1. Spence DPS, *et al.* The effect of the orally active platelet-activating factor antagonist WEB 2086 in the treatment of asthma. *Am J Respir Crit Care Med* 1994; **149:** 1142–8.

Bambuterol Hydrochloride (18825-x)

Bambuterol Hydrochloride *(BANM, rINNM)*.

KWD-2183. (*RS*)-5-(2-*tert*-Butylamino-1-hydroxyethyl)-*m*-phenylene bis(dimethylcarbamate) hydrochloride.

$C_{18}H_{29}N_3O_5,HCl$ = 403.9.

CAS — 81732-65-2 (bambuterol); 81732-46-9 (bambuterol monohydrochloride).

Pharmacopoeias. In *Eur.* (see p.viii).

A white or almost white crystalline powder. It exhibits polymorphism. Freely **soluble** in water; soluble in alcohol.

Adverse Effects and Precautions

As for Salbutamol Sulphate, p.758.

Bambuterol is not recommended for patients with severely impaired liver function as its metabolism would be unpredictable. It is unsuitable for the relief of acute bronchospasm or in patients with unstable respiratory disease.

Interactions

As for Salbutamol Sulphate, p.759. Bambuterol inhibits plasma cholinesterases and can prolong the action of drugs such as suxamethonium (see Sympathomimetics, under Suxamethonium, p.1321) that are inactivated by these enzymes.

Pharmacokinetics

Nearly 20% of a dose of bambuterol is absorbed from the gastro-intestinal tract following oral administration. It is slowly metabolised in the body to its active metabolite, terbutaline, peak terbutaline concentrations are reported to occur about 4 to 7 hours after a dose of bambuterol as tablets. The slow rate at which metabolism occurs determines the prolonged duration of action of bambuterol of at least 24 hours. Hydrolysis of bambuterol to terbutaline and carbamic acid leads to inhibition of plasma-cholinesterase activity that can be correlated with plasma concentrations of terbutaline. For the metabolism and excretion of terbutaline, see p.764.

References.

1. Sitar DS, *et al.* Pharmacokinetics and pharmacodynamics of bambuterol, a long-acting bronchodilator pro-drug of terbutaline, in young and elderly patients with asthma. *Clin Pharmacol Ther* 1992; **52:** 297–306.
2. Sitar DS. Clinical pharmacokinetics of bambuterol. *Clin Pharmacokinet* 1996; **31:** 246–56.
3. Nyberg L, *et al.* Pharmacokinetics of bambuterol in healthy subjects. *Br J Clin Pharmacol* 1998; **45:** 471–8.

Uses and Administration

Bambuterol is an inactive prodrug of terbutaline (see p.764), a direct-acting sympathomimetic with predominantly beta-adrenergic activity and a selective action on $beta_2$ receptors ($beta_2$ agonist). It has similar actions and uses to those of salbutamol, p.759, except that it has a more prolonged duration of action (at least 24 hours). Bambuterol hydrochloride is used as a long-acting bronchodilator for persistent reversible airways obstruction in conditions such as asthma (p.745) The usual dose is 10 to 20 mg by mouth once daily at bedtime; starting doses should be halved in patients with moderately or severely impaired renal function.

References.

1. Fugleholm AM, *et al.* Therapeutic equivalence between bambuterol, 10 mg once daily, and terbutaline controlled release, 5 mg twice daily, in mild to moderate asthma. *Eur Respir J* 1993; **6:** 1474–8.
2. Gunn SD, *et al.* Comparison of the efficacy, tolerability and patient acceptability of once-daily bambuterol tablets against twice-daily controlled release salbutamol in nocturnal asthma. *Eur J Clin Pharmacol* 1995; **48:** 23–8.

Preparations

Proprietary Preparations (details are given in Part 3)
Aust.: Bambec; ***Ger.:*** Bambec; ***Ital.:*** Bambec; ***Norw.:*** Bambec; ***Spain:*** Bambec; ***Swed.:*** Bambec; ***Switz.:*** Bambec; ***UK:*** Bambec.

Bamifylline Hydrochloride (629-v)

Bamifylline Hydrochloride *(BANM, USAN, rINNM)*.

AC-3810; BAX-2739Z; 8102-CB; CB-8102. 8-Benzyl-7-[2-(*N*-ethyl-*N*-2-hydroxyethylamino)ethyl]theophylline hydrochloride.

$C_{20}H_{27}N_5O_3,HCl$ = 421.9.

CAS — 2016-63-9 (bamifylline); 20684-06-4 (bamifylline hydrochloride).

Bamifylline hydrochloride is a xanthine derivative which is used for its bronchodilator properties similarly to theophylline (see p.772). It is reported to lack central stimulant effects, and mild sedation may possibly occur. It is well absorbed following oral administration and is given by mouth in doses of 600 or 900 mg twice daily. It is also given rectally as suppositories, and by intramuscular injection, or intravenous injection (over 3 to 4 minutes) or infusion.

References to the pharmacokinetics of bamifylline.

1. Schiantarelli P, *et al.* Evidence of pulmonary tropism of bamifylline and its main active metabolite. *Arzneimittelforschung* 1989; **39:** 215–19.
2. Segre G, *et al.* Pharmacokinetics of bamifylline during chronic therapy. *Arzneimittelforschung* 1990; **40:** 450–2.

Preparations

Proprietary Preparations (details are given in Part 3)
Belg.: Trentadil; ***Fr.:*** Trentadil; ***Ital.:*** Bamifix; Briofil; ***Switz.:*** Bami-med†.

Bepafant (9366-n)

Bepafant *(rINN)*.

WEB-2170. 4-{[6-(*o*-Chlorophenyl)-8,9-dihydro-1-methyl-4*H*,7*H*-cyclopenta[4,5]thieno-[3,2-*f*]-*s*-triazolo[4,3-*a*][1,4]diazepin-8-yl]carbonyl}morpholine.

$C_{23}H_{22}ClN_5O_2S$ = 468.0.

CAS — 114776-28-2.

Bepafant is a platelet-activating factor antagonist that has been investigated in inflammatory and allergic conditions.

Bitolterol Mesylate (12447-p)

Bitolterol Mesylate *(BANM, USAN)*.

Bitolterol Mesilate *(rINNM)*; Win-32784. 4-[2-(*tert*-Butylamino)-1-hydroxyethyl]-*o*-phenylene di-*p*-toluate methanesulphonate.

$C_{28}H_{31}NO_5,CH_4O_3S$ = 557.7.

CAS — 30392-40-6 (bitolterol); 30392-41-7 (bitolterol mesylate).

Bitolterol is an inactive prodrug which is hydrolysed in the body to colterol, a direct-acting sympathomimetic with predominantly beta-adrenergic activity and a selective action on $beta_2$ receptors ($beta_2$ agonist). It has similar properties to those of salbutamol, p.758.

It is used as a bronchodilator in the management of diseases with reversible airways obstruction such as asthma (p.745) or in some patients with chronic obstructive pulmonary disease (p.747); administration by inhalation results in the rapid onset of bronchodilatation (2 to 4 minutes) with a duration of action of 5 or more hours.

Bitolterol is given by inhalation via a metered-dose aerosol supplying 370 µg of bitolterol mesylate per inhalation. For the relief of bronchospasm the usual adult dose is 2 inhalations (740 µg) followed by a third inhalation (370 µg) if required. For the prevention of bronchospasm the usual adult dose is 2 inhalations (740 µg) every 8 hours. Maximum doses have been stated to be 3 inhalations (1110 µg) every 6 hours or 2 inhalations (740 µg) every 4 hours.

Alternatively, a 0.2% inhalation solution of bitolterol mesylate may be given by nebulisation.

Preparations

Proprietary Preparations (details are given in Part 3)
Ital.: Asmalene; Tolbet†; ***USA:*** Tornalate.

Broxaterol (18872-b)

Broxaterol *(rINN)*.

Z-1170. (±)-3-Bromo-α-[(*tert*-butylamino)methyl]-5-isoxazolemethanol.

$C_9H_{15}BrN_2O_2$ = 263.1.

CAS — 76596-57-1.

Broxaterol is a direct-acting sympathomimetic with predominantly selective beta-adrenergic activity on $beta_2$ receptors ($beta_2$ agonist). It has similar properties to those of salbutamol (see p.758). It has been given as a bronchodilator by mouth and by inhalation.

References.

1. Casali L, *et al.* A comparison of the bronchodilator effects of broxaterol and salbutamol. *Int J Clin Pharmacol Ther Toxicol* 1988; **26:** 93–7.
2. Robuschi M, *et al.* Dose-response curve of the bronchodilating effect of broxaterol inhaled by patients with reversible airway obstruction. *Curr Ther Res* 1988; **43:** 725–33.
3. Ziment I. Broxaterol: therapeutic trials and safety profile. *Respiration* 1989; **55** (suppl 2): 28–40.
4. Robuschi M, *et al.* The protective effect of transdermal broxaterol on exercise-induced bronchoconstriction. *Eur J Clin Pharmacol* 1995; **47:** 465–6.

Bufylline (630-r)

Bufylline *(BAN)*.

Ambuphylline *(USAN)*; Theophylline-aminoisobutanol. 2-Amino-2-methylpropan-1-ol theophyllinate.

$C_{11}H_{19}N_5O_3$ = 269.3.

CAS — 5634-34-4.

Bufylline is a theophylline derivative (see p.772), which has been used for its bronchodilator effects as an ingredient of preparations promoted for respiratory-tract disorders. The ethiodide has also been used.

Preparations

Proprietary Preparations (details are given in Part 3)
Ital.: Dilcovit†.

Multi-ingredient: ***Ger.:*** Ditenate†; ***S.Afr.:*** Nethaprin Dospan; Nethaprin Expectorant.

Caffeine (621-x)

Caffeine *(BAN)*.

Anhydrous Caffeine; Caféine; Coffeinum; Guaranine; Methyltheobromine; Théine. 1,3,7-Trimethylpurine-2,6(3*H*,1*H*)-dione; 1,3,7-Trimethylxanthine; 7-Methyltheophylline.

$C_8H_{10}N_4O_2$ = 194.2.

CAS — 58-08-2.

NOTE. Compounded preparations of butalbital, paracetamol (acetaminophen), and caffeine in USP 23 may be represented by the name Co-bucafAPAP.

Pharmacopoeias. In *Eur.* (see p.viii), *Int., Jpn, Pol.,* and *US.* Some pharmacopoeias include caffeine and caffeine hydrate under one monograph.

Odourless silky white crystals, usually matted together, or a white crystalline powder. It sublimes readily. Sparingly **soluble** in water; freely soluble in boiling water and in chloroform; slightly or sparingly soluble in alcohol; slightly soluble in ether. It dissolves in concentrated solutions of alkali benzoates or salicylates. Solutions in water are neutral to litmus.

Caffeine Citrate (626-h)

Caffeine Citrate *(BANM)*.

Citrated Caffeine; Coffeinum Citricum.

$C_8H_{10}N_4O_2,C_6H_8O_7$ = 386.3.

CAS — 69-22-7.

Pharmacopoeias. In *Aust.*

Caffeine Hydrate (622-r)

Caffeine Hydrate *(BANM)*.

Caffeine Monohydrate; Coffeinum Monohydricum.

$C_8H_{10}N_4O_2,H_2O$ = 212.2.

CAS — 5743-12-4.

Pharmacopoeias. In *Chin., Eur.* (see p.viii), *Int., Jpn, Pol.,* and *US.* Some pharmacopoeias include caffeine and caffeine hydrate under one monograph.

Odourless silky white crystals, usually matted together, or a white crystalline powder. It effloresces in air and sublimes readily. **Soluble** 1 in 50 of water, 1 in 75 of alcohol, 1 in 6 of chloroform, and 1 in 600 of ether; freely soluble in boiling water. It dissolves in concentrated solutions of alkali benzoates or salicylates. Solutions in water are neutral to litmus. **Store** in airtight containers.

Stability. References to the stability of caffeine and caffeine citrate.

1. Eisenberg MG, Kang N. Stability of citrated caffeine solutions for injectable and enteral use. *Am J Hosp Pharm* 1984; **41:** 2405–6.
2. Nahata MC, *et al.* Stability of caffeine injection in intravenous admixtures and parenteral nutrition solutions. *DICP Ann Pharmacother* 1989; **23:** 466–7.
3. Hopkin C, *et al.* Stability study of caffeine citrate. *Br J Pharm Pract* 1990; **12:** 133.
4. Donnelly RF, Tirona RG. Stability of citrated caffeine injectable solution in glass vials. *Am J Hosp Pharm* 1994; **51:** 512–14.

Adverse Effects, Treatment, and Precautions

As for Theophylline, p.765.

Prolonged high intake of caffeine may lead to tolerance to some of the pharmacological actions and physical signs of withdrawal including irritability, lethargy, and headache may occur if intake is discontinued abruptly.

General references.

1. Wills S. Drugs and substance misuse: caffeine. *Pharm J* 1994; **252:** 822–4.

Effects on the heart. For a discussion of the effects of coffee drinking on cardiovascular risk factors, see under Xanthine-containing Beverages, p.1645.

Effects on mental function. A report of 6 cases of excessive daytime sleepiness associated with high caffeine intake.[1]

1. Regestein QR. Pathologic sleepiness induced by caffeine. *Am J Med* 1989; **87:** 586–8.

Gastro-oesophageal reflux disease. Theophylline derivatives tend to relax the lower oesophageal sphincter and increase gastric acid secretion. For a report of increased gastro-oesophageal reflux in neonates receiving caffeine, see Gastro-oesophageal Reflux Disease under Precautions in Theophylline, p.767.

Overdosage. Reports and reviews of caffeine toxicity.

1. Kulkarni PB, Dorand RD. Caffeine toxicity in a neonate. *Pediatrics* 1979; **64:** 254–5.
2. Banner W, Czajka PA. Acute caffeine overdose in the neonate. *Am J Dis Child* 1980; **134:** 495–8.
3. Zimmerman PM, *et al.* Caffeine intoxication: a near fatality. *Ann Emerg Med* 1985; **14:** 1227–9.
4. Dalvi RR. Acute and chronic toxicity of caffeine: a review. *Vet Hum Toxicol* 1986; **28:** 144–50.
5. Rivenes SM, *et al.* Intentional caffeine poisoning in an infant. *Pediatrics* 1997; **99:** 736–8.

Pregnancy. In the USA, the Food and Drug Administration has advised pregnant women to limit their intake of caffeine and caffeine-containing beverages to a minimum, but this recommendation was based largely on animal studies and the effect of caffeine on the human fetus and fetal loss during pregnancy is controversial.[1] Although one recent study found no evidence that moderate caffeine use (less than 300 mg daily) increased the risk of spontaneous abortion,[2] another study has reported conflicting results[3] leading one commentator to conclude that the safety of caffeine consumption during pregnancy remains unresolved.[1] There is some evidence for an effect on fetal growth, but again it is not clear that this applies generally: a prospective population-based study in the UK found that a decreased birth weight with increased caffeine intake was only significant in smokers.[4] The authors of this study concurred that a reduction in caffeine intake during pregnancy would be prudent, together with stopping smoking. An association between high maternal caffeine intake during pregnancy and an increased risk of the sudden infant death syndrome has also been reported.[5]

1. Eskenazi B. Caffeine during pregnancy: grounds for concern? *JAMA* 1993; **270;** 2973–4.
2. Mills JL, *et al.* Moderate caffeine use and the risk of spontaneous abortion and intrauterine growth retardation. *JAMA* 1993; **269:** 593–7.
3. Infante-Rivard C, *et al.* Fetal loss associated with caffeine intake before and during pregnancy. *JAMA* 1993; **270:** 2940–3.
4. Cook DG, *et al.* Relation of caffeine intake and blood caffeine concentrations during pregnancy to fetal growth: prospective population based study. *Br Med J* 1996; **313:** 1358–62.
5. Ford RPK, *et al.* Heavy caffeine intake in pregnancy and sudden infant death syndrome. *Arch Dis Child* 1998; **78:** 9–13.

Sport. The International Olympic Committee has banned the use of large amounts of caffeine by athletes but smaller amounts, compatible with a moderate intake of coffee or soft drinks, are permitted.[1] The concentration of caffeine in the urine should not exceed 12 μg per mL.[2] However, because of the marked interindividual variation in urine-caffeine concentrations, even a modest caffeine intake equivalent to 3 to 6 cups of coffee daily, may give a urine concentration in excess of the permissible limit.[3]

1. Anonymous. Drugs in the Olympics. *Med Lett Drugs Ther* 1984; **26:** 65–6.
2. MacAuley D. Drugs in sport. *Br Med J* 1996; **313:** 211–15.
3. Birkett DJ, Miners JO. Caffeine renal clearance and urine caffeine concentrations during steady state dosing: implications for monitoring caffeine intake during sports events. *Br J Clin Pharmacol* 1991; **31:** 405–8.

Withdrawal. Headache is a recognised symptom of caffeine withdrawal and even subjects who drink moderate amounts of coffee can develop headaches lasting 1 to 6 days when switched to a decaffeinated brand.[1] It has also been suggested that postoperative headache could be attributed to caffeine withdrawal as fasting patients are required to abstain from drinking tea or coffee before surgical procedures. Several studies[2-4] have found a positive association between postoperative headache and daily caffeine consumption, although there have also been negative findings.[5] A prospective study suggested that prophylactic intravenous administration of caffeine on the day of surgery reduced the likelihood of postoperative headache in patients at risk of caffeine withdrawal.[6]

1. van Dusseldorp M, Katan MB. Headache caused by caffeine withdrawal among moderate coffee drinkers switched from ordinary to decaffeinated coffee: a 12 week double blind trial. *Br Med J* 1990; **300:** 1558–9.
2. Galletly DC, *et al.* Does caffeine withdrawal contribute to postanaesthetic morbidity? *Lancet* 1989; **i:** 1335.
3. Weber JG, *et al.* Perioperative ingestion of caffeine and postoperative headache. *Mayo Clin Proc* 1993; **68:** 842–5.
4. Nikolajsen L, *et al.* Effect of previous frequency of headache, duration of fasting and caffeine abstinence on perioperative headache. *Br J Anaesth* 1994; **72:** 295–7.
5. Verhoeff FH, Millar JM. Does caffeine contribute to postoperative morbidity? *Lancet* 1990; **336:** 632.
6. Weber JG, *et al.* Prophylactic intravenous administration of caffeine and recovery after ambulatory surgical procedures. *Mayo Clin Proc* 1997; **72:** 621–6.

Interactions

Like theophylline (see p.767) caffeine undergoes extensive metabolism by hepatic microsomal cytochrome P450, and is subject to numerous interactions with other drugs and substances which enhance or reduce its metabolic clearance.

Alcohol. In a study of 8 healthy subjects given alcohol by mouth in a dose of 2.2 mL per kg body-weight, caffeine 150 mg by mouth did not antagonise the central effects of alcohol and, instead, a synergistic interaction occurred which further increased reaction time. The common practice of drinking coffee after drinking alcohol in order to sober up is not supported by these results.[1] Another study[2] found that some antagonism of the central effects of alcohol was produced by caffeine, although there was no reversal of subjective sensations of drunkenness; however the dose of caffeine in this study (400 mg) was considerably higher.

1. Oborne DJ, Rogers Y. Interactions of alcohol and caffeine on human reaction time. *Aviat Space Environ Med* 1983; **54:** 528–34.
2. Azcona O, *et al.* Evaluation of the central effects of alcohol and caffeine interaction. *Br J Clin Pharmacol* 1995; **40:** 393–400.

Antiarrhythmics. In 7 healthy subjects and 5 patients with cardiac arrhythmias, *mexiletine* in a single dose of 200 mg and a dose of 600 mg daily respectively, reduced the elimination of caffeine by 30 to 50%.[1] *Lignocaine, flecainide,* and *tocainide* had no effect on caffeine elimination in healthy subjects.[1]

1. Joeres R, Richter E. Mexiletine and caffeine elimination. *N Engl J Med* 1987; **317:** 117.

Antibacterials. Caffeine elimination half-life has been reported to be increased and clearance decreased by the concomitant administration of *ciprofloxacin,*[1-3] *enoxacin,*[2,3] and *pipemidic acid;*[2,3] *lomefloxacin,*[4] *norfloxacin,*[2,3] and *ofloxacin*[2,3] had little or no effect on these parameters. Enoxacin had the greatest inhibitory effect on caffeine clearance.[2,3]

1. Healy DP, *et al.* Interaction between oral ciprofloxacin and caffeine in normal volunteers. *Antimicrob Agents Chemother* 1989; **33:** 474–8.
2. Harder S, *et al.* Ciprofloxacin-caffeine: a drug interaction established using in vivo and in vitro investigations. *Am J Med* 1989; **87** (suppl 5A): 89–91S.
3. Barnett G, *et al.* Pharmacokinetic determination of relative potency of quinolone inhibition of caffeine disposition. *Eur J Clin Pharmacol* 1990; **39:** 63–9.
4. Healy DP, *et al.* Lack of interaction between lomefloxacin and caffeine in normal volunteers. *Antimicrob Agents Chemother* 1991; **35:** 660–4.

Antiepileptics. The mean clearance of caffeine was increased and its half-life decreased in epileptic patients taking *phenytoin* compared with healthy controls, resulting in lower plasma-caffeine concentrations. Treatment with *carbamazepine* or *valproic acid* had no effect on the pharmacokinetics of caffeine.[1]

1. Wietholtz H, *et al.* Effects of phenytoin, carbamazepine, and valproic acid on caffeine metabolism. *Eur J Clin Pharmacol* 1989; **36:** 401–6.

Antifungals. In a single-dose study in healthy subjects, *terbinafine* 500 mg by mouth decreased the clearance and increased the elimination half-life of caffeine 3 mg per kg body-weight given intravenously. *Ketoconazole* 400 mg by mouth did not prolong the elimination of caffeine to a significant extent.[1]

1. Wahlländer A, Paumgartner G. Effect of ketoconazole and terbinafine on the pharmacokinetics of caffeine in healthy volunteers. *Eur J Clin Pharmacol* 1989; **37:** 279–83.

Antigout drugs. In a study in 2 healthy subjects, the plasma half-life of caffeine was essentially unchanged by 7 days' treatment with *allopurinol* 300 mg or 600 mg daily by mouth. However, allopurinol caused a specific, dose-dependent inhibition of the conversion of 1-methylxanthine to 1-methyluric acid.[1]

1. Grant DM, *et al.* Effect of allopurinol on caffeine disposition in man. *Br J Clin Pharmacol* 1986; **21:** 454–8.

Gastro-intestinal drugs. *Cimetidine* 1 g daily by mouth reduced the systemic clearance of caffeine and prolonged its elimination half-life in 5 healthy subjects. Although the steady-state plasma-caffeine concentration would increase by approximately 70%, it was thought unlikely that this would produce adverse clinical effects.[1] However, in contrast a study in 11 children given cimetidine in doses of 11 to 36 mg per kg body-weight daily for gastritis found no evidence that it altered the metabolism of a dose of ^{13}C-labelled caffeine.[2]

1. Broughton LJ, Rogers HJ. Decreased systemic clearance of caffeine due to cimetidine. *Br J Clin Pharmacol* 1981; **12:** 155–9.
2. Parker AC, *et al.* Lack of inhibitory effect of cimetidine on caffeine metabolism in children using the caffeine breath test. *Br J Clin Pharmacol* 1997; **43:** 467–70.

Idrocilamide. In 4 healthy subjects, the muscle relaxant idrocilamide inhibited the biotransformation of caffeine and increased its half-life 9 times. Partial or total avoidance of caffeine-containing products was recommended when idrocilamide was being taken.[1]

1. Brazier JL, *et al.* Inhibition by idrocilamide of the disposition of caffeine. *Eur J Clin Pharmacol* 1980; **17:** 37–43.

Lithium. For mention of the effect of caffeine on serum-lithium concentrations see p.294.

Oral contraceptives. The clearance of caffeine has been reported to be reduced and its elimination half-life increased in women taking oral contraceptives.[1-3] This interaction was thought to be due to impairment of hepatic metabolism of caffeine by sex hormones and could result in increased accumulation of caffeine.

1. Patwardhan RV, *et al.* Impaired elimination of caffeine by oral contraceptive steroids. *J Lab Clin Med* 1980; **95:** 603–8.
2. Abernethy DR, Todd EL. Impairment of caffeine clearance by chronic use of low-dose oestrogen-containing oral contraceptives. *Eur J Clin Pharmacol* 1985; **28:** 425–8.
3. Balogh A, *et al.* Influence of ethinylestradiol-containing combination oral contraceptives with gestodene or levonorgestrel on caffeine elimination. *Eur J Clin Pharmacol* 1995; **48:** 161–6.

Sympathomimetics. Administration of caffeine 400 mg with *phenylpropanolamine* 75 mg, both given orally as modified-release preparations, produced greater plasma-caffeine concentrations in healthy subjects than administration of caffeine alone. Greater increases in blood pressure and more reports of physical side-effects occurred after the combination than after either drug alone.[1]

1. Lake CR, *et al.* Phenylpropanolamine increases plasma caffeine levels. *Clin Pharmacol Ther* 1990; **47:** 675–85.

Theophylline. For the effect of caffeine on the metabolism and elimination of theophylline, see under Interactions in Theophylline, p.769.

Pharmacokinetics

Caffeine is absorbed readily after oral administration and is widely distributed throughout the body. It is also absorbed through the skin. Absorption following rectal administration by suppository may be slow and erratic. Absorption following intramuscular injection may be slower than after oral administration. Caffeine passes readily into the central nervous system and into saliva; low concentrations are also present in breast milk. Caffeine crosses the placenta.

In adults, caffeine is metabolised almost completely in the liver via oxidation, demethylation, and acetylation, and is excreted in the urine as 1-methyluric acid, 1-methylxanthine, 7-methylxanthine, 1,7-dimethylxanthine (paraxanthine), 5-acetylamino-6-formylamino-3-methyluracil (AFMU), and other metabolites with only about 1% unchanged. Neonates have a greatly reduced capacity to metabolise caffeine and it is largely excreted unchanged in the urine until hepatic metabolism becomes significantly developed, usually by about 6 months of age. Elimination half-lives are approximately 3 to 7 hours in adults but may be in excess of 100 hours in neonates.

Breast feeding. Studies examining the transfer of caffeine into breast milk after doses of 35 to 336 mg of caffeine by mouth have recorded peak maternal plasma concentrations of 2.4 to 4.7 μg per mL, peak maternal saliva concentrations of 1.2 to 9.2 μg per mL, and peak breast-milk concentrations of 1.4 to 7.2 μg per mL. At these concentrations in breast milk, the calculated daily caffeine ingestion by breast-fed infants ranged from 1.3 to 3.1 mg, which was not thought to present a hazard, although irritability and a poor sleeping pattern have been reported.[1-4]

1. Tyrala EE, Dodson WE. Caffeine secretion into breast milk. *Arch Dis Child* 1979; **54:** 787–800.
2. Hildebrandt R, *et al.* Transfer of caffeine to breast milk. *Br J Clin Pharmacol* 1983; **15:** 612P.
3. Sagraves R, *et al.* Pharmacokinetics of caffeine in human breast milk after a single oral dose of caffeine. *Drug Intell Clin Pharm* 1984; **18:** 507.
4. Berlin CM, *et al.* Disposition of dietary caffeine in milk, saliva, and plasma of lactating women. *Pediatrics* 1984; **73:** 59–63.

Metabolism and excretion. The metabolism of caffeine has been shown to be dose dependent[1,2] with clearance decreasing as the dose is increased suggesting saturable metabolism. Four- to five-fold differences in plasma half-lives of caffeine are common among healthy people. The plasma half-life of caffeine is decreased by smoking[3] and by exercise,[4] and is increased by liver disease such as cirrhosis and viral hepatitis,[3,5] and in pregnancy.[3] The plasma half-life of caffeine is not affected by old age[6] or obesity.[7] Drug interactions also affect the pharmacokinetics of caffeine (see above).

1. Cheng WSC, *et al.* Dose-dependent pharmacokinetics of caffeine in humans: relevance as a test of quantitative liver function. *Clin Pharmacol Ther* 1990; **47:** 516–24.
2. Denaro CP, *et al.* Dose-dependency of caffeine metabolism with repeated dosing. *Clin Pharmacol Ther* 1990; **48:** 277–85.
3. Kalow W. Variability of caffeine metabolism in humans. *Arzneimittelforschung* 1985; **35:** 319–24.
4. Collomp K, *et al.* Effects of moderate exercise on the pharmacokinetics of caffeine. *Eur J Clin Pharmacol* 1991; **40:** 279–82.
5. Scott NR, *et al.* The pharmacokinetics of caffeine and its dimethylxanthine metabolites in patients with chronic liver disease. *Br J Clin Pharmacol* 1989; **27:** 205–13.
6. Blanchard J, Sawers SJA. Comparative pharmacokinetics of caffeine in young and elderly men. *J Pharmacokinet Biopharm* 1983; **11:** 109–26.
7. Abernethy DR, *et al.* Caffeine disposition in obesity. *Br J Clin Pharmacol* 1985; **20:** 61–6.

Uses and Administration

Caffeine is a methylxanthine which like theophylline (p.772) has a variety of actions: it inhibits the enzyme phosphodiesterase and has an antagonistic effect at central adenosine receptors. It is a potent stimulant of the CNS, particularly the higher centres, and it can produce a condition of wakefulness and increased mental activity. Its bronchodilating properties are weaker than those of theophylline, but it may stimulate the respiratory centre, increasing the rate and depth of respiration. Its stimulant action on the medullary vasomotor centre and its positive inotropic action on the myocardium are compensated for by its peripheral vasodilator effect on the arterioles, so that there is usually little effect on blood pressure. Caffeine facilitates the performance of muscular work and increases the total work which can be performed by a muscle. The diuretic action of caffeine is weaker than that of theophylline.

Caffeine is used as a mild CNS stimulant in usual doses of up to about 200 mg by mouth. It is also frequently included in oral analgesic preparations with aspirin, paracetamol, or codeine in unit doses of about 15 to 65 mg but its clinical benefit is debated (see Pain, below). It is sometimes given with ergotamine in preparations for the treatment of migraine.

Caffeine has also been used in the treatment of neonatal apnoea.

Caffeine citrate has been used similarly. Caffeine and sodium benzoate and caffeine and sodium salicylate are readily soluble in water and have been used for the administration of caffeine by injection, as has caffeine citrate. Caffeine and sodium iodide (iodocaffeine) was formerly used in a similar manner.

Beverages of coffee, tea, and cola provide active doses of caffeine (see p.1645).

Asthma. Caffeine's bronchodilating activity is about 40% that of theophylline[1] and doses of 5 or 10 mg per kg bodyweight by mouth have been shown to produce an effect.[2,3] Because of its weak action other treatments are generally recommended in asthma (see p.745).

1. Gong H, *et al.* Bronchodilator effects of caffeine in coffee: a dose-response study of asthmatic subjects. *Chest* 1986; **89:** 335–42.
2. Bukowskyj M, Nakatsu K. The bronchodilator effect of caffeine in adult asthmatics. *Am Rev Respir Dis* 1987; **135:** 173–5.
3. Becker AB, *et al.* The bronchodilator effects and pharmacokinetics of caffeine in asthma. *N Engl J Med* 1984; **310:** 743–6.

Diagnosis and testing. Caffeine excretion assessed by measuring its urinary metabolites or by the exhalation of labelled CO_2 in breath following administration of ^{13}C- or ^{14}C-labelled caffeine has been used to develop liver function tests and to determine the activity of specific enzymes such as xanthine oxidase, P450 cytochromes, and polymorphic *N*-acetyltransferase.[1]

Caffeine administered orally has been used to assess acetylator status by determining the metabolic ratio of the metabolites 5-acetylamino-6-formylamino-1-methyluracil (AFMU) to 1-methylxanthine in urine,[2] but some have questioned its value.[3]

1. Kalow W, Tang B-K. The use of caffeine for enzyme assays: a critical appraisal. *Clin Pharmacol Ther* 1993; **53:** 503–14.
2. Hildebrand M, Seifert W. Determination of acetylator phenotype in caucasians with caffeine. *Eur J Clin Pharmacol* 1989; **37:** 525–6.
3. Notarianni LJ, *et al.* Caffeine as a metabolic probe: NAT2 phenotyping. *Br J Clin Pharmacol* 1996; **41:** 169–73.

ECT. In 6 patients whose seizure duration was declining despite maximal ECT stimulation, pretreatment with caffeine 250 to 750 mg, given by intravenous injection over 60 seconds as caffeine and sodium benzoate, resulted in lengthening of seizures by an average of 107% and clinical improvement of depression.[1] Status epilepticus has been reported in a patient on theophylline therapy during ECT (see p.767).

1. Hinkle PE, *et al.* Use of caffeine to lengthen seizures in ECT. *Am J Psychiatry* 1987; **144:** 1143–8.

Hypoglycaemia. Caffeine has proved of benefit in augmenting warning symptoms and physiological responses to experimentally-induced hypoglycaemia in diabetic patients,[1] and has been suggested as a potentially useful treatment for diabetics who have difficulty in recognising the onset of hypoglycaemia.

1. Debrah K, *et al.* Effect of caffeine on recognition of and physiological responses to hypoglycaemia in insulin-dependent diabetes. *Lancet* 1996; **347:** 19–24.

Neonatal apnoea. Xanthines are useful in the treatment of neonatal apnoea as discussed under Theophylline, p.773, with caffeine having several advantages over theophylline, including a wider therapeutic index, fewer peripheral adverse effects and a more useful half-life.

Orthostatic hypotension. Caffeine has been of benefit in the treatment of orthostatic hypotension due to autonomic failure in some patients, especially for postprandial hypotension.[1-3] However, efficacy has only been demonstrated in mild cases and it is usually ineffective in severe cases.[4] It may be considered in patients who have failed to respond to conventional drug therapy, which usually begins with fludrocortisone, as discussed on p.1040.

1. Onrot J, *et al.* Hemodynamic and humoral effects of caffeine in autonomic failure. *N Engl J Med* 1985; **313:** 549–54.
2. Hoeldtke RD, *et al.* Treatment of orthostatic hypotension with dihydroergotamine and caffeine. *Ann Intern Med* 1986; **105:** 168–73.
3. Tonkin AL. Postural hypotension. *Med J Aust* 1995; **162:** 436–8.
4. Mathias CJ. Orthostatic hypotension. *Prescribers' J* 1995; **35:** 124–32.

Pain. Caffeine has been widely used in analgesic preparations to enhance the effects of both non-opioid and opioid analgesics but is of debatable benefit (see under Analgesics and Analgesic Adjuvants, p.5). Some investigators have failed to show that caffeine offers any benefit[1,2] but others have shown that the adjuvant use of caffeine can increase analgesic activity.[3-7] A meta-analysis of 10 studies comparing paracetamol plus caffeine with paracetamol alone in women with postpartum uterine cramp found any benefit of the combination to be minimal.[8]

Whether caffeine enhances the gastro-intestinal absorption of ergotamine is not clear.

In the UK it is generally recommended that caffeine-containing analgesic preparations should not be used not only because of doubts about caffeine enhancing the analgesic effect but because it can add to gastro-intestinal adverse effects and in large doses can itself cause headache.

1. Winter L, *et al.* A double-blind, comparative evaluation of acetaminophen, caffeine, and the combination of acetaminophen and caffeine in outpatients with post-operative oral surgery pain. *Curr Ther Res* 1983; **33:** 115–22.
2. Sawynok J. Pharmacological rationale for the clinical use of caffeine. *Drugs* 1995; **49:** 37–50.
3. Laska EM, *et al.* Caffeine as an analgesic adjuvant. *JAMA* 1984; **251:** 1711–18.
4. Rubin A, Winter L. A double-blind randomized study of an aspirin/caffeine combination versus acetaminophen/aspirin combination versus acetaminophen versus placebo in patients with moderate to severe post-partum pain. *J Int Med Res* 1984; **12:** 338–45.
5. Schachtel BP, *et al.* Caffeine as an analgesic adjuvant: a double-blind study comparing aspirin with caffeine to aspirin and placebo in patients with sore throat. *Arch Intern Med* 1991; **151:** 733–7.
6. Migliardi JR, *et al.* Caffeine as an analgesic adjuvant in tension headache. *Clin Pharmacol Ther* 1994; **56:** 576–86.
7. Kraetsch HG, *et al.* Analgesic effects of propyphenazone in comparison to its combination with caffeine. *Eur J Clin Pharmacol* 1996; **49:** 377–82.
8. Zhang WY, Li Wan Po A. Analgesic efficacy of paracetamol and its combination with codeine and caffeine in surgical pain—a meta-analysis. *J Clin Pharm Ther* 1996; **21:** 261–82.

POST-DURAL HEADACHE. Intravenous caffeine sodium benzoate may relieve post-dural headache (p.1282) which persists despite conservative therapy.

Preparations

BP 1998: Aspirin and Caffeine Tablets;
USP 23: Acetaminophen and Caffeine Capsules; Acetaminophen and Caffeine Tablets; Acetaminophen, Aspirin, and Caffeine Capsules; Acetaminophen, Aspirin, and Caffeine Tablets; Aspirin, Caffeine, and Dihydrocodeine Bitartrate Capsules; Aspirin, Codeine Phosphate, and Caffeine Capsules; Aspirin, Codeine Phosphate, and Caffeine Tablets; Butalbital, Acetaminophen, and Caffeine Capsules; Butalbital, Acetaminophen, and Caffeine Tablets; Butalbital, Aspirin, and Caffeine Capsules; Butalbital, Aspirin, and Caffeine Tablets; Butalbital, Aspirin, Caffeine, and Codeine Phosphate Capsules; Caffeine and Sodium Benzoate Injection; Ergotamine Tartrate and Caffeine Suppositories; Ergotamine Tartrate and Caffeine Tablets; Propoxyphene Hydrochloride, Aspirin, and Caffeine Capsules.

Proprietary Preparations (details are given in Part 3)
Austral.: No Doz; ***Canad.:*** Wake-Up Tablets; ***Fr.:*** Percutafeine; ***Ger.:*** Autonic; Percoffedrinol N; ***S.Afr.:*** Doxypol†; Universal Concentration Tablets; Xeramax; ***Spain:*** Durvitan; Prolert; ***UK:*** Pro-Plus; ***USA:*** Caffedrine; Coffee Break†; NoDoz; Quick Pep; Spray-n-Wake; Tirend†; Vivarin.

Multi-ingredient: numerous preparations are listed in Part 3.

Carbuterol Hydrochloride (2046-r)

Carbuterol Hydrochloride *(BANM, USAN, rINNM).*

SKF-40383; SKF-40383-A. [5-(2-*tert*-Butylamino-1-hydroxyethyl)-2-hydroxyphenyl]urea hydrochloride.

$C_{13}H_{21}N_3O_3,HCl = 303.8.$

CAS — 34866-47-2 (carbuterol); 34866-46-1 (carbuterol hydrochloride).

Carbuterol hydrochloride is a direct-acting sympathomimetic with predominantly beta-adrenergic activity and a selective action on $beta_2$ receptors ($beta_2$ agonist). It has properties similar to those of salbutamol (see p.758). It has been used as a bronchodilator.

Preparations

Proprietary Preparations (details are given in Part 3)
Ger.: Pirem†; ***Ital.:*** Bronsecur†; Dynavent†; ***Spain:*** Risprant†.

Choline Theophyllinate (631-f)

Choline Theophyllinate *(BAN, rINN).*

Oxtriphylline; Theophylline Cholinate.

$C_{12}H_{21}N_5O_3 = 283.3.$

CAS — 4499-40-5.

Pharmacopoeias. In *Br., Chin.,* and *US.*

A white crystalline powder, odourless or with a faint amine-like odour. It contains between 41.9% and 43.6% of anhydrous choline and between 61.7% and 65.5% of anhydrous theophylline. Choline theophyllinate 1.57 mg is approximately equivalent in theophylline content to 1 mg of anhydrous theophylline. **Soluble** 1 in 1 of water; very slightly soluble in chloroform and in ether; the BP states that it is soluble, and the USP freely soluble, in alcohol. A 1% solution in water has a pH of about 10.3. **Store** at a temperature not exceeding 25° in airtight containers. Protect from light.

Adverse Effects, Treatment, and Precautions

As for Theophylline, p.765.

Interactions

As for Theophylline, p.767.

Pharmacokinetics

Choline theophyllinate is readily absorbed from the gastro-intestinal tract and liberates theophylline in the body. The pharmacokinetics of theophylline are discussed on p.771.

Uses and Administration

Choline theophyllinate is a theophylline salt which is used as a bronchodilator for the same purposes as theophylline.

The usual dosage for adults is 0.4 to 1.2 g daily by mouth, in 3 or 4 divided doses, preferably after food to reduce gastro-intestinal side-effects. Low doses should be given initially and gradually increased according to clinical response and serum-theophylline concentrations (see Uses and Administration of Theophylline, p.772). A suggested dosage for children aged 3 to 6 years is 62.5 to 125 mg three times daily and for children aged over 6 years, 300 to 400 mg daily in divided doses.

Preparations

BP 1998: Choline Theophyllinate Tablets;
USP 23: Oxtriphylline Delayed-release Tablets; Oxtriphylline Extended-release Tablets; Oxtriphylline Oral Solution; Oxtriphylline Tablets.

Proprietary Preparations (details are given in Part 3)
Austral.: Brondecon-PD; Choledyl†; ***Belg.:*** Sabidal†; ***Canad.:*** Choledyl; Novo-Triphyl; ***Ger.:*** Brontheo†; Euspirax; ***Irl.:*** Choledyl; ***Ital.:*** Sabidal SR†; Teofilcolina†; ***Norw.:*** Teovent; ***S.Afr.:*** Choledyl; ***Spain:*** Choledyl†; ***Swed.:*** Teovent; ***UK:*** Choledyl†; Sabidal SR†; ***USA:*** Choledyl.

Multi-ingredient: ***Austral.:*** Brondecon Expectorant; ***Canad.:*** Choledyl Expectorant; ***Ger.:*** Euspirax comp†; ***Ital.:*** Teofilcolina Sedativa†; ***Spain:*** Dimayon; Tilfilin; ***USA:*** Brondecon†.

Clenbuterol Hydrochloride (2047-f)

Clenbuterol Hydrochloride *(BANM, rINNM).*

NAB-365 (clenbuterol). 1-(4-Amino-3,5-dichlorophenyl)-2-*tert*-butylaminoethanol hydrochloride.

$C_{12}H_{18}Cl_2N_2O,HCl = 313.7$.

CAS — 37148-27-9 (clenbuterol); 21898-19-1 (clenbuterol hydrochloride).

NOTE. Clenbuterol has been referred to as angel dust; this name has also been used to describe illicit phencyclidine.

Clenbuterol hydrochloride is a direct-acting sympathomimetic with predominantly beta-adrenergic activity and a selective action on $beta_2$ receptors ($beta_2$ agonist). It has properties similar to those of salbutamol (see p.758). It is used as a bronchodilator in the management of reversible airways obstruction, as in asthma (p.745) and in certain patients with chronic obstructive pulmonary disease (p.747). A usual dose is 20 μg twice daily by mouth; doses of up to 40 μg twice daily have occasionally been employed. Clenbuterol hydrochloride is also given by inhalation in usual doses of 20 μg three times daily.

Abuse. Clenbuterol has been used illicitly in animal feeds in an attempt to promote weight gain and to increase muscle to lipid mass. Adverse effects typical of sympathomimetic activity have been attributed to such misuse both in farmers perpetrating such acts[1] and in innocent persons consuming meat products from affected animals.[2-4] Clenbuterol has been abused by sportsmen for its anabolic effects,[5] although it is doubtful that it leads to enhanced performance.[6]

1. Dawson J. β Agonists put meat in the limelight again. *Br Med J* 1990; **301:** 1238–9.
2. Martínez-Navarro JF. Food poisoning related to consumption of illicit β-agonist in liver. *Lancet* 1990; **336:** 1311.
3. Maistro S, *et al.* Beta blockers to prevent clenbuterol poisoning. *Lancet* 1995; **346:** 180.
4. Brambilla G, *et al.* Food poisoning following consumption of clenbuterol-treated veal in Italy. *JAMA* 1997; **278:** 635.
5. Anonymous. Muscling in on clenbuterol. *Lancet* 1992; **340:** 403.
6. Spann C, Winter ME. Effect of clenbuterol on athletic performance. *Ann Pharmacother* 1995; **29:** 75–7.

Preparations

Proprietary Preparations (details are given in Part 3)
Aust.: Spiropent; ***Ger.:*** Contraspasmin; Spiropent; ***Ital.:*** Broncodil; Clenasma; Clenbutol†; Contrasmina; Monores; Prontovent; Spiropent; ***Spain:*** Spiropent; Ventolase.

Multi-ingredient: ***Aust.:*** Mucospas; ***Ger.:*** Spasmo-Mucosolvan.

Diprophylline (633-n)

Diprophylline *(BAN, rINN).*

Dihydroxypropyltheophyllinum; Diprophyllinum; Dyphylline; Glyphyllinum; Hyphylline. 7-(2,3-Dihydroxypropyl)-1,3-dimethylxanthine; 7-(2,3-Dihydroxypropyl)theophylline.

$C_{10}H_{14}N_4O_4 = 254.2$.

CAS — 479-18-5.

Pharmacopoeias. In *Chin., Eur.* (see p.viii), *Pol.,* and *US.*

A white odourless amorphous or crystalline powder. Freely **soluble** in water; sparingly or slightly soluble in alcohol; sparingly soluble in chloroform; practically insoluble in ether. A 1% solution in water has a pH of 5.0 to 7.5.

Store in airtight containers. Protect from light.

Adverse Effects, Treatment, and Precautions

As for Theophylline, p.765. Diprophylline is primarily excreted unchanged in the urine and should therefore be used with caution in patients with renal impairment; however, unlike theophylline, plasma concentrations of diprophylline are not greatly affected by liver function or hepatic enzyme activity.

Interactions

Since diprophylline does not undergo metabolism by hepatic microsomal cytochrome P450 it does not exhibit the numerous interactions seen with theophylline (p.767). However, the possibility of synergistic effects should be borne in mind if it is prescribed concomitantly with other xanthines.

Probenecid. Probenecid has been reported to decrease the clearance of diprophylline thus prolonging its half-life.[1-3]

1. May DC, Jarboe CH. Inhibition of clearance of dyphylline by probenecid. *N Engl J Med* 1981; **304:** 791.
2. May DC, Jarboe CH. Effect of probenecid on dyphylline elimination. *Clin Pharmacol Ther* 1983; **33:** 822–5.
3. Acara M, *et al.* Probenecid inhibition of the renal excretion of dyphylline in chicken, rat and man. *J Pharm Pharmacol* 1987; **39:** 526–30.

Pharmacokinetics

Diprophylline is rapidly absorbed from the gastro-intestinal tract and from the site of intramuscular injections. Diprophylline does not liberate theophylline in the body and is largely excreted unchanged in the urine with an elimination half-life of approximately 2 hours.

Breast feeding. In a study of 20 lactating women given diprophylline by intramuscular injection,[1] diprophylline was found to concentrate in breast milk, with a milk to serum concentration ratio of approximately 2. However, it was felt that the quantity of diprophylline a breast-feeding infant would ingest was unlikely to produce any pharmacological action unless the child was very sensitive.

1. Jarboe CH, *et al.* Dyphylline elimination kinetics in lactating women: blood to milk transfer. *J Clin Pharmacol* 1981; **21:** 405–10.

Uses and Administration

Diprophylline is a theophylline derivative which is used similarly to theophylline as a bronchodilator (see p.772).

The usual dose of diprophylline by mouth is up to 15 mg per kg body-weight every 6 hours. It has also been given intramuscularly in doses of 250 to 500 mg every 6 hours as required.

Improvements in measurements of lung function after diprophylline in doses of 15 and 20 mg per kg body-weight by mouth were only one-third to one-half those obtained after theophylline 6 mg per kg by mouth.[1]

1. Furukawa CT, *et al.* Diphylline versus theophylline: a double-blind comparative evaluation. *J Clin Pharmacol* 1983; **23:** 414–18.

Preparations

USP 23: Dyphylline and Guaifenesin Elixir; Dyphylline and Guaifenesin Tablets; Dyphylline Elixir; Dyphylline Injection; Dyphylline Tablets.

Proprietary Preparations (details are given in Part 3)
Aust.: Austrophyllin; Isophyllen; Neothyllin; ***Ital.:*** Difillin†; Katasma; Neutrafillina†; ***Switz.:*** Prophyllen†; ***USA:*** Dilor; Dyflex†; Lufyllin; Neothylline†.

Multi-ingredient: ***Aust.:*** Laevostrophan compositum; Neobiphyllin†; ***Fr.:*** Ozothine a la Diprophylline; ***Ger.:*** Cor-Neo-Nervacit-S†; Coropar†; durasklerat†; Neobiphyllin; Neobiphyllin-Clys; Older†; Ozothin; Purostrophyll†; Spasdilat N†; Theo-Lanicor†; Theokombetin†; ***Irl.:*** Leotuss†; ***Ital.:*** Cort-Inal; Katasma Balsamico†; Ozopulmin Diprofillina†; Sobrepin Respiro†; ***Spain:*** Alergical Expect; Bronsal; Difilina Asmorax; Espectona Compositum†; Fluidin Mucolitico; Juven Tos†; Novofilin; Ozopulmin Antiasmatico†; ***Switz.:*** Astho-Med; Brosol; Neo-Biphyllin; Neo-Biphyllin Special†; ***UK:*** Noradran; ***USA:*** Dilor-G; Dyflex-G; Dyline GG; Dyphylline-GG; Lufyllin-EPG; Lufyllin-GG; Neothylline-GG†; Thylline-GG†.

Doxofylline (1737-k)

Doxofylline *(USAN, rINN).*

ABC 12/3. 7-(1,3-Dioxolan-2-ylmethyl)theophylline.

$C_{11}H_{14}N_4O_4 = 266.3$.

CAS — 69975-86-6.

Doxofylline is a theophylline derivative which is used as a bronchodilator similarly to theophylline (see p.772). It is given by mouth in doses of up to 1200 mg daily. It may also be given by slow intravenous injection.

Pharmacokinetics. The mean elimination half-life of doxofylline following intravenous administration of 100 mg to 6 patients with chronic bronchitis was 1.83 hours. The mean elimination half-life following oral administration of 400 mg twice daily for 5 days in 8 patients with chronic bronchitis was 7.01 hours.[1] A regimen of 400 mg twice daily has been reported to produce acceptable plasma profiles in patients with hepatic impairment.[2]

1. Bologna E, *et al.* Oral and intravenous pharmacokinetic profiles of doxofylline in patients with chronic bronchitis. *J Int Med Res* 1990; **18:** 282–8.
2. Harning R, *et al.* The pharmacokinetics of Maxivent (doxofylline) in subjects with hepatic impairment. *Clin Pharmacol Ther* 1995; **57:** 169.

Preparations

Proprietary Preparations (details are given in Part 3)
Ital.: Ansimar.

Eformoterol Fumarate (19193-l)

Eformoterol Fumarate *(BANM).*

Formoterol Fumarate *(rINNM)*; BD-40A (eformoterol); CGP-25827A (eformoterol). (±)-2′-Hydroxy-5′-[(*RS*)-1-hydroxy-2-{[(*RS*)-*p*-methoxy-α-methylphenethyl]amino}ethyl]formanilide fumarate.

$(C_{19}H_{24}N_2O_4)_2,C_4H_4O_4 = 804.9$.

CAS — 73573-87-2 (eformoterol); 43229-80-7 (eformoterol fumarate).

Pharmacopoeias. In *Jpn.*

Eformoterol is a direct-acting sympathomimetic with predominantly beta-adrenoceptor stimulant activity specific to $beta_2$ receptors ($beta_2$ agonist). It has properties similar to those of salbutamol, p.758, but like salmeterol (p.761) it has a prolonged duration of action of up to 12 hours; it is therefore not considered suitable for the symptomatic relief of acute attacks of bronchospasm. It is used when the regular administration of a long-acting $beta_2$ agonist is required for management of reversible airways obstruction, as in chronic asthma (p.745) or in some patients with chronic obstructive pulmonary disease (p.747).

Eformoterol is given as the fumarate. A usual dose is 12 or 24 μg of eformoterol fumarate twice daily by inhalation from a metered-dose aerosol or inhalational capsules. Doses of 80 μg have been given twice daily by mouth.

References.

1. Faulds D, *et al.* Formoterol: a review of its pharmacological properties and therapeutic potential in reversible obstructive airways disease. *Drugs* 1991; **42:** 115–37.
2. Kesten S, *et al.* Sustained improvement in asthma with long-term use of formoterol fumarate. *Ann Allergy* 1992; **69:** 415–20.
3. Newnham DM, *et al.* Bronchodilator subsensitivity after chronic dosing with eformoterol in patients with asthma. *Am J Med* 1994; **97:** 29–37.
4. Tan KS, *et al.* Systemic corticosteroid rapidly reverses formoterol-induced tachyphylaxis in asthmatic patients. *Br J Clin Pharmacol* 1996; **42:** 265P.
5. van Noord JA, *et al.* Salmeterol versus formoterol in patients with moderately severe asthma: onset and duration of action. *Eur Respir J* 1996; **9:** 1684–8.
6. van der Molen T, *et al.* Effects of the long acting β agonist formoterol on asthma control in asthmatic patients using inhaled corticosteroids. *Thorax* 1996; **52:** 535–9.
7. Pauwels RA, *et al.* Effect of inhaled formoterol and budesonide on exacerbations of asthma. *N Engl J Med* 1997; **337:** 1405–11. Correction. *ibid.* 1998; **338:** 139.
8. Bartow RA, Brogden RN. Formoterol: an update of its pharmacological properties and therapeutic efficacy in the management of asthma. *Drugs* 1998; **55:** 303–22.

Preparations

Proprietary Preparations (details are given in Part 3)
Aust.: Foradil; ***Austral.:*** Foradile; ***Fr.:*** Foradil; ***Irl.:*** Foradil; Oxis; ***Ital.:*** Eolus; Foradil; ***Jpn:*** Atock; ***Neth.:*** Foradil; Oxis; ***S.Afr.:*** Foradil; ***Spain:*** Foradil; Neblik; ***Swed.:*** Foradil; Oxis; ***Switz.:*** Foradil; ***UK:*** Foradil; Oxis.

Enprofylline (16624-a)

Enprofylline *(USAN, rINN).*

D-4028; 3-Propylxanthine. 3,7-Dihydro-3-propyl-1*H*-purine-2,6-dione.

$C_8H_{10}N_4O_2 = 194.2$.

CAS — 41078-02-8.

Enprofylline is a theophylline derivative that has been investigated for its bronchodilating properties which are similar to those of theophylline (see p.772), although it is reported to have practically no adenosine-antagonist activity.

Theophylline or aminophylline is normally employed if a xanthine is to be used in the treatment of asthma (p.745). However, studies comparing the efficacy of enprofylline and theophylline in asthmatic patients have indicated that enprofylline is a more potent bronchodilator.[1-3] A plasma concentration ratio of enprofylline to theophylline of about 1:4 has induced a similar degree of bronchodilatation.[2] Enprofylline is considered to have no CNS-stimulating activity; side-effects such as headache and nausea have been reported.[1-3]

1. Laursen LC, *et al.* Maximally effective plasma concentrations of enprofylline and theophylline during constant infusion. *Br J Clin Pharmacol* 1984; **18:** 591–5.
2. Laursen LC, *et al.* Comparison of oral enprofylline and theophylline in asthmatic patients. *Eur J Clin Pharmacol* 1984; **26:** 707–9.
3. Riska H, *et al.* Comparison of intravenous enprofylline and theophylline in the treatment of acute asthma. *Curr Ther Res* 1989; **45:** 907–13.

Pharmacokinetic references.

1. Tegnér K, *et al.* Protein binding of enprofylline. *Eur J Clin Pharmacol* 1983; **25:** 703–8.
2. Lunell E, *et al.* Absorption of enprofylline from the gastrointestinal tract in healthy subjects. *Eur J Clin Pharmacol* 1984; **27:** 329–33.
3. Lunell E, Borgå O. Pharmacokinetics of enprofylline in healthy elderly subjects. *Eur J Clin Pharmacol* 1987; **32:** 67–70.
4. Hultqvist C, Borgå O. Enprofylline pharmacokinetics in children with asthma. *Eur J Clin Pharmacol* 1987; **32:** 533–5.
5. Laursen LC, *et al.* Transfer of enprofylline into breast milk. *Ther Drug Monit* 1988; **10:** 150–2.
6. Laursen LC, *et al.* Distribution of enprofylline and theophylline between plasma and cerebrospinal fluid. *Ther Drug Monit* 1989; **11:** 162–4.

Etamiphylline Camsylate (634-h)

Etamiphylline Camsylate *(BANM)*.

Etamiphylline Camsilate *(rINNM)*; Diétamiphylline Camphosulfonate; Etamphyllin Camsylate. 7-(2-Diethylaminoethyl)-1,3-dimethylxanthine camphor-10-sulphonate; 7-(2-Diethylaminoethyl)theophylline camphor-10-sulphonate.

$C_{23}H_{37}N_5O_6S$ = 511.6.

CAS — 314-35-2 (etamiphylline); 19326-29-5 (etamiphylline camsylate).

Pharmacopoeias. In Br.

A white or almost white powder with a faint camphoraceous odour. Very **soluble** in water; soluble in alcohol and in chloroform; very slightly soluble in ether. A 10% solution in water has a pH of 3.9 to 5.4.

Etamiphylline camsylate is a theophylline derivative which has been used as a bronchodilator similarly to theophylline (see p.772). Etamiphylline does not liberate theophylline in the body.

Etamiphylline, etamiphylline dehydrocholate, and etamiphylline methiodide have also been used.

From a study of 27 asthmatic children given etamiphylline or theophylline 6.96 mg per kg body-weight, or placebo by mouth, it was concluded that the bronchodilator effect of oral etamiphylline is weaker than that of theophylline, possibly in part due to its poor bioavailability.[1]

1. Vazquez C, *et al.* Poor bronchodilator effect of oral etamiphylline in asthmatic children. *Lancet* 1984; **i:** 914.

Preparations

BP 1998: Etamiphylline Injection; Etamiphylline Suppositories.

Proprietary Preparations (details are given in Part 3)
Spain: Boifilina†; Solufilina Simple; Solufina.

Multi-ingredient: ***Aust.:*** Longtussin; ***Ital.:*** Spasmodil Complex†; ***Spain:*** Solufilina Sedante; ***Switz.:*** Neo-Biphyllin Special†.

Ethylnoradrenaline Hydrochloride (2060-t)

Ethylnorepinephrine Hydrochloride. 2-Amino-1-(3,4-dihydroxyphenyl)butan-1-ol hydrochloride.

$C_{10}H_{15}NO_3$,HCl = 233.7.

CAS — 536-24-3 (ethylnoradrenaline); 3198-07-0 (ethylnoradrenaline hydrochloride).

Ethylnoradrenaline is a sympathomimetic with predominantly beta-adrenergic activity. Its actions are similar to those of isoprenaline (see p.892) but it is reportedly less potent. It was formerly used as a bronchodilator.

Preparations

Proprietary Preparations (details are given in Part 3)
USA: Bronkephrine†.

Etofylline (635-m)

Etofylline *(BAN, rINN)*.

Aethophyllinum; Etofyllinum; Hydroxyaethyltheophyllinum; Hydroxyéthylthéophylline; Oxyetophylline. 7-(2-Hydroxyethyl)-1,3-dimethylxanthine; 3,7-Dihydro-7-(2-hydroxyethyl)-1,3-dimethyl-1*H*-purine-2,6-dione; 7-(2-Hydroxyethyl)theophylline.

$C_9H_{12}N_4O_3$ = 224.2.

CAS — 519-37-9.

Pharmacopoeias. In *Eur.* (see p.viii).

A white crystalline powder. **Soluble** in water; slightly soluble in alcohol. **Protect** from light.

Etofylline is a theophylline derivative used as a bronchodilator and for its cardiovascular effects similarly to theophylline (see p.772). It does not liberate theophylline in the body.

Etofylline nicotinate is also used.

Preparations

Proprietary Preparations (details are given in Part 3)
S.Afr.: Theostat; ***Spain:*** De Oxin†; ***Switz.:*** Dilaphylline†.

Multi-ingredient: ***Aust.:*** Alpha-Apoplectal; Apoplectal; Coroverlan; Instenon; Peripherin; Perphyllon; ***Belg.:*** Perphyllone†; ***Ger.:*** Alpha-Apoplectal†; Asthmacolat†; Card-Instenon†; Cordalin-Strophanthin†; Coroverlan; Coroverlan-Digoxin†; Eucard†; Eucebral-N; Instenon†; Keldrin†; Lioftal s. T.†; Peripherin†; Poikiloton†; Theo-Talusin†; Toramin N†; Venotrulan Compositum†; ***Ital.:*** Teostellarid†; ***S.Afr.:*** Actophlem; Alcophyllex; D-Tussin; Dilinct; Solphyllex; Solphyllin; Theophen; Theophen Comp; ***Spain:*** Flebo Stop; Lipostabil Forte†; Vasperdil; ***Switz.:*** Dilaphylline†; Symfona†; Theo-Talusin.

Fenoterol Hydrobromide (2063-f)

Fenoterol Hydrobromide *(BANM, rINNM)*.

Fenoteroli Hydrobromidum; TH-1165a. 1-(3,5-Dihydroxyphenyl)-2-(4-hydroxy-α-methylphenethylamino)ethanol hydrobromide.

$C_{17}H_{21}NO_4$,HBr = 384.3.

CAS — 13392-18-2 (fenoterol); 1944-12-3 (fenoterol hydrobromide).

NOTE. Fenoterol is *USAN*.

Pharmacopoeias. In *Eur.* (see p.viii) and *Pol.*

A white crystalline powder. **Soluble** in water and in alcohol; practically insoluble in ether. A 4% solution in water has a pH of 4.2 to 5.2. **Protect** from light.

Adverse Effects and Precautions

As for Salbutamol Sulphate, p.758.

Increased mortality. Since the introduction of metered-dose aerosols of beta agonists there have been two reported epidemics of increased morbidity and mortality in asthmatic patients associated with their use. The first occurred in the 1960s and was linked with the use of high-dose isoprenaline inhalers.[1] The use of isoprenaline was subsequently largely discontinued in favour of more selective beta$_2$ agonists.

The second epidemic occurred in New Zealand in the late 1970s and 1980s and was associated with the use of fenoterol.[1-5] When use of fenoterol fell in New Zealand, so too did the asthma mortality rate.[5] Heavy or regular use of fenoterol was implicated.[6,7] Fenoterol was also implicated in increased asthma morbidity and mortality in a study in Canada,[7] as was salbutamol, and recent results from Japan also suggested a relation between asthma deaths and excessive use of beta agonists, particularly fenoterol.[8] However, an analysis of the New Zealand deaths could not identify such a risk with beta agonists other than fenoterol.[5]

There is still debate about this second epidemic. The individual case control studies, including the one from Canada,[7] showed an increased morbidity and mortality in patients taking fenoterol, but a meta-analysis of the accumulated data to 1992 suggested that the increase in mortality in the patients taking beta$_2$ agonists was slight and only significant when administration was by nebulisation.[9] Also a working party of the UK Committee on Safety of Medicines considered[10] that a causal link between asthma mortality and beta-agonist use could neither be confirmed nor refuted.

Not surprisingly there are different views on the cause of the increased asthma mortality. The cardiotoxicity of the beta agonist might have to be considered, although evidence for such an effect is felt by some to be slight.[11] The severity of the asthma might have been a factor in two different ways. One hypothesis is that patients used more fenoterol because they had severe asthma and were already at increased risk of dying.[12] Another proposes that heavy beta-agonist use led to an increase in asthma severity[13] which could be explained by a down regulation of beta receptors.[14]

This may appear to be only of historical interest since mortality rates have fallen and current recommendations for the use of short-acting beta$_2$ agonists, which are generally more selective than fenoterol, are for them to be taken as required rather than on a regular basis; indeed increasing use of such drugs is seen as an indication to amend the treatment schedule. Moreover, the dose of fenoterol has been reduced in recent years. However, controversy over regular use of beta$_2$ agonists continues to be fed by conflicting studies of their benefit.[15,16] It is possible that some benefit exists in more severe disease, and current recommendations for asthma treatment do permit the regular use of long-acting beta$_2$ agonists in severe chronic asthma. It is not clear to what extent the same concerns, particularly of downregulation of beta receptors, apply to such therapy.[17] A recent case-control study found no evidence that salmeterol was associated with an increased risk of near-fatal asthma.[18]

1. Pearce N, *et al.* Beta agonists and asthma mortality: déjà vu. *Clin Exp Allergy* 1991; **21:** 401–10.
2. Crane J, *et al.* Prescribed fenoterol and death from asthma in New Zealand, 1981-83: case-control study. *Lancet* 1989; **i:** 917–22.
3. Pearce N, *et al.* Case-control study of prescribed fenoterol and death from asthma in New Zealand, 1977–81. *Thorax* 1990; **45:** 170–5.
4. Grainger J, *et al.* Prescribed fenoterol and death from asthma in New Zealand, 1981–7: a further case-control study. *Thorax* 1991; **46:** 105–111.
5. Pearce N, *et al.* End of the New Zealand asthma mortality epidemic. *Lancet* 1995; **345:** 41–4.
6. Sears MR, *et al.* Regular inhaled beta-agonist treatment in bronchial asthma. *Lancet* 1990; **336:** 1391–6.
7. Spitzer WO, *et al.* The use of β-agonists and the risk of death and near death from asthma. *N Engl J Med* 1992; **326:** 501–6.
8. Beasley R, *et al.* β-agonist therapy and asthma mortality in Japan. *Lancet* 1998; **351:** 1406–7.
9. Mullen M, *et al.* The association between β-agonist use and death from asthma: a meta-analytic integration of case control studies. *JAMA* 1993; **270:** 1842–5.
10. Committee on Safety of Medicines. Beta-agonist use in asthma: report from the CSM Working Party. *Current Problems 33* 1992.
11. Sears MR, Taylor DR. The β$_2$-agonist controversy: observations, explanations and relationship to asthma epidemiology. *Drug Safety* 1994; **11:** 259–83.
12. Fuller RW. Use of β$_2$ agonists in asthma: much ado about nothing? *Br Med J* 1994; **309:** 795–6.
13. Sears MR. Asthma deaths in New Zealand. *Lancet* 1995; **345:** 655–6.
14. Tattersfield AE. Use of β$_2$ agonists in asthma: much ado about nothing? *Br Med J* 1994; **309:** 794–6.
15. Chapman KR, *et al.* Regular vs as-needed inhaled salbutamol in asthma control. *Lancet* 1994; **343:** 1379–82.
16. Drazen JM, *et al.* Comparison of regularly scheduled with as-needed use of albuterol in mild asthma. *N Engl J Med* 1996; **335:** 841–7.
17. Lipworth BJ. Airway subsensitivity with long-acting β$_2$-agonists: is there cause for concern? *Drug Safety* 1997; **16:** 295–308.
18. Williams C, *et al.* Case-control study of salmeterol and near-fatal attacks of asthma. *Thorax* 1998; **53:** 7–13.

Pulmonary oedema. Pulmonary oedema has occurred in women given beta agonists, including fenoterol,[1] for premature labour. The risk factors, the most important of which is fluid overload, are discussed under Ritodrine, on p.1625.

1. Hawker F. Pulmonary oedema associated with β$_2$-sympathomimetic treatment of premature labour. *Anaesth Intensive Care* 1984; **12:** 143–51.

Interactions

As for Salbutamol Sulphate, p.759.

Pharmacokinetics

Fenoterol is incompletely absorbed from the gastrointestinal tract and is also subject to extensive first-pass metabolism by sulphate conjugation. It is excreted in the urine and bile almost entirely as the inactive sulphate conjugate.

References.

1. Rominger KL, Pollmann W. Vergleichende pharmacokinetik von fenoterol-hydrobromid bei ratte, hund und mensch. *Arzneimittelforschung* 1972; **22:** 1190–6.
2. Hildebrandt R, *et al.* Pharmacokinetics of fenoterol in pregnant and nonpregnant women. *Eur J Clin Pharmacol* 1993; **45:** 275–7.

Uses and Administration

Fenoterol is a direct-acting sympathomimetic with beta-adrenoceptor stimulant activity largely selective for beta$_2$ receptors (beta$_2$ agonist). It has actions and uses similar to those of salbutamol (see p.759) and is used as a bronchodilator in the management of reversible airways obstruction, as occurs in asthma (p.745) and in some patients with chronic obstructive pulmonary disease (p.747). Following inhalation, fenoterol acts rapidly (2 to 3 minutes) and has a duration of action of about 6 to 8 hours.

In the management of reversible airways obstruction, fenoterol hydrobromide is administered by inhalation in a dose of 1 or 2 inhalations of 100 μg up to three times daily; children over the age of 6 years will only normally require one inhalation (100 μg) up to three times daily. If symptoms are not adequately controlled with this low-dose inhaler then a high-dose inhaler administering 200 μg per inhalation may be employed in adults; 1 or 2 inhalations of 200 μg may be given up to 3 times daily. The dose should not exceed 400 μg every six hours or 1.6 mg in a 24-hour period; this high dose inhaler is not recommended for children under 16 years of age.

Fenoterol hydrobromide may be given as a nebulised solution; the recommended dose for inhalation by this route has varied considerably from 0.2 to 2 mg.

Fenoterol hydrobromide has also been used similarly to salbutamol in the management of premature labour (see p.760). A suggested dose, by intravenous infusion, has been 0.5 to 3 μg per minute, continued until contractions are suppressed, and followed by oral administration of 5 mg every 3 to 6 hours.

An aerosol inhalation containing both fenoterol hydrobromide and ipratropium bromide is also available.

Preparations

Proprietary Preparations (details are given in Part 3)
Aust.: Berotec; ***Austral.:*** Berotec; ***Belg.:*** Berotec; ***Canad.:*** Berotec; ***Fr.:*** Berotec; ***Ger.:*** Aruterol†; Berotec; Partusisten; ***Irl.:*** Berotec; ***Ital.:*** Dosberotec; ***Neth.:*** Berotec; Partusisten; ***Norw.:*** Berotec; ***S.Afr.:*** Berotec; Fensol†; ***Spain:*** Avantol†; Berotec; ***Swed.:*** Berotec; ***Switz.:*** Berotec; Partusisten; ***UK:*** Berotec.

Multi-ingredient: ***Aust.:*** Arelcant; Berodual; Berodualin; Ditec; ***Belg.:*** Duovent; ***Canad.:*** Duovent; ***Fr.:*** Bronchodual; ***Ger.:*** Berodual; Berotec solvens; Ditec; ***Irl.:*** Duovent; ***Ital.:*** Duovent; Iprafen; ***Neth.:*** Berodual; ***S.Afr.:*** Duovent; ***Spain:*** Berodual; Crismol; ***Switz.:*** Berodual; ***UK:*** Duovent.

Ginkgolides (3033-n)

Ginkgolides A, B, and C (BN-52020, BN-52021, and BN-52022 respectively) are isolated from *Ginkgo biloba* (Ginkgoaceae) (see also p.1584).

The ginkgolides are terpenoid molecules with platelet-activating factor (PAF) antagonist properties. They have been investigated as BN-52063, a mixture of ginkgolides A, B, and C, for asthma and other inflammatory and allergic disorders and also in immune disorders such as endotoxic shock and graft rejection; ginkgolide B, which has the most potent PAF antagonist properties, has been investigated in similar conditions administered alone.

Other ginkgolides, including ginkgolide M (BN-52023) and ginkgolide J (BN-52024) have also been identified.

References.

1. Braquet P. The ginkgolides: potent platelet- activating factor antagonists isolated from Ginkgo biloba L: chemistry, pharmacology and clinical applications. *Drugs Of The Future* 1987; **12:** 643–99.
2. Chung KF, *et al.* Effect of a ginkgolide mixture (BN 52063) in antagonising skin and platelet responses to platelet activating factor in man. *Lancet* 1987; **i:** 248–51.
3. Roberts NM, *et al.* Effect of a PAF antagonist, BN52063, on PAF-induced bronchoconstriction in normal subjects. *Br J Clin Pharmacol* 1988; **26:** 65–72.

Heptaminol Acephyllinate (636-b)

Acéfyllinate d'Heptaminol; Acefyllinum Heptaminolum; Heptaminol Theophylline Ethanoate; Heptaminol Theophylline-7-acetate. The 6-amino-2-methylheptan-2-ol salt of theophyllin-7-ylacetic acid.

$C_8H_{19}NO,C_9H_{10}N_4O_4$ = 383.4.

CAS — 5152-72-7; 10075-18-0.

Pharmacopoeias. In Fr.

Heptaminol acephyllinate is a derivative of theophylline (p.765) that has been used similarly for its bronchodilator and cardiovascular effects.

Preparations

Proprietary Preparations (details are given in Part 3)
Fr.: Corophylline†; ***Ger.:*** Theo-Heptylon†; ***Switz.:*** Cariamyl†.

Multi-ingredient: ***Fr.:*** Sureptil; ***Ger.:*** Theo-Hexanicit†; ***Ital.:*** Sureptil†; ***Spain:*** Clinadil Compositum; Diclamina.

Hexoprenaline Hydrochloride (2065-n)

Hexoprenaline Hydrochloride *(BANM, rINNM).*

ST-1512. *N,N'*-Hexamethylenebis[4-(2-amino-1-hydroxyethyl)pyrocatechol] dihydrochloride; *N,N'*-Hexamethylenebis[2-amino-1-(3,4-dihydroxyphenyl)ethanol] dihydrochloride.

$C_{22}H_{32}N_2O_6,2HCl$ = 493.4.

CAS — 3215-70-1 (hexoprenaline); 4323-43-7 (hexoprenaline dihydrochloride).

Hexoprenaline Sulphate (2066-h)

Hexoprenaline Sulphate *(BANM, rINNM).*

Hexoprenaline Sulfate *(USAN).* (±)-α,α'-[Hexamethylenebis(iminomethylene)]-bis[3,4-dihydroxybenzyl alcohol] sulfate (1:1).

$C_{22}H_{32}N_2O_6,H_2SO_4$ = 518.6.

CAS — 32266-10-7.

Hexoprenaline is a direct-acting sympathomimetic with predominantly beta-adrenergic activity selective to beta$_2$ receptors (beta$_2$ agonist). It has properties similar to those of salbutamol (see p.758) and is used as a bronchodilator in the treatment of reversible airways obstruction as occurs with asthma (p.745) and in some patients with chronic obstructive pulmonary disease (p.747). It has sometimes been used similarly to salbutamol in the management of premature labour, see p.760.

Hexoprenaline is usually administered as the hydrochloride or sulphate.

For bronchodilatation, usual doses of the salts are 0.5 to 1 mg three times daily by mouth or 200 to 400 μg by inhalation three to four times daily. Hexoprenaline salts have also been given parenterally.

In the management of premature labour an intravenous infusion of hexoprenaline sulphate can be given at an initial rate of about 0.1 to 0.3 μg per minute. Infusion may be preceded by slow intravenous injection of 10 μg as a loading dose over 5 to 10 minutes.

Preparations

Proprietary Preparations (details are given in Part 3)
Aust.: Gynipral; Ipradol; ***Ger.:*** Etoscol†; Tokolysan†; ***Ital.:*** Tocolysan†; ***S.Afr.:*** Ipradol; ***Spain:*** Ipradol; ***Switz.:*** Gynipral; Ipradol†.

Ibudilast (19376-t)

Ibudilast *(rINN).*

KC-404. 1-(2-Isopropylpyrazolo[1,5-*a*]pyridin-3-yl)-2-methyl-1-propanone.

$C_{14}H_{18}N_2O$ = 230.3.

CAS — 50847-11-5.

Ibudilast is an orally active leukotriene antagonist and platelet-activating factor antagonist. It is administered by mouth in the management of asthma (p.745) in a dose of 10 mg twice daily.

Ibudilast has also been promoted for a variety of cerebrovascular disorders in doses of 10 mg three times daily.

Preparations

Proprietary Preparations (details are given in Part 3)
Jpn: Ketas.

Ipratropium Bromide (386-h)

Ipratropium Bromide *(BAN, USAN, rINN).*

Ipratropii Bromidum; Sch-1000; Sch-1000-Br-monohydrate. (1*R*,3*r*,5*S*,8*r*)-8-Isopropyl-3-[(±)-tropoyloxy]tropanium bromide monohydrate.

$C_{20}H_{30}BrNO_3,H_2O$ = 430.4.

CAS — 22254-24-6 (anhydrous ipratropium bromide); 66985-17-9 (ipratropium bromide monohydrate).

Pharmacopoeias. In *Eur.* (see p.viii) and *Jpn.*

White or almost white crystalline powder; **soluble** in water; slightly soluble in alcohol; freely soluble in methyl alcohol. The pH of a 1% solution in water is 5.0 to 7.5.

Stability. In a study[1] of the stability of admixtures of ipratropium and salbutamol nebuliser solutions equal ratio mixtures were found to retain more than 90% of their initial concentrations after storage for 5 days at 4° or 22° in the dark or at 22° under continuous fluorescent lighting.

1. Jacobson GA, Peterson GM. Stability of ipratropium bromide and salbutamol nebuliser admixtures. *Int J Pharm Pract* 1995; **3:** 169–73.

Adverse Effects, Treatment, and Precautions

As for Atropine Sulphate, p.455.

Paradoxical bronchospasm and acute angle-closure glaucoma have sometimes been associated with the administration of nebulised ipratropium bromide.

Buccal ulceration. A report[1] of inflammation and ulceration of the buccal mucosa associated with the use of an ipratropium bromide inhaler.

1. Spencer PA. Buccal ulceration with ipratropium bromide. *Br Med J* 1986; **292:** 380.

Effects on the eyes. Although short-term studies in patients with angle-closure glaucoma and normal subjects indicate that inhalation of ipratropium alone has no effect on intraocular pressure, accommodation, or pupil diameter[1,2] there has been a report[3] of a patient with a history of glaucoma who developed angle-closure glaucoma after receiving ipratropium using a metered dose inhaler and nebulised salbutamol together. Angle-closure glaucoma,[4-6] pupillary dilatation,[6,7] and anisocoria[8] have been reported in patients receiving *nebulised* ipratropium, usually with salbutamol, through a poorly fitting face mask. The antimuscarinic effects of ipratropium can lead to impaired drainage of aqueous humour in the eyes of patients predisposed to angle-closure glaucoma; co-administration of salbutamol may intensify this problem by increasing the production of aqueous humour.[5] Studies[9,10] suggest that patients with a history of angle-closure glaucoma might be at an increased risk of developing glaucoma when nebulised ipratropium and salbutamol are used together.

1. Scheufler G. Ophthalmotonometry, pupil diameter and visual accommodation following repeated administration of Sch 1000 MDI in patients with glaucoma. *Postgrad Med J* 1975; **51** (suppl 7): 132.
2. Thumm HW. Ophthalmic effects of high doses of Sch 1000 MDI in healthy volunteers and patients with glaucoma. *Postgrad Med J* 1975; **51** (suppl 7): 132–3.
3. Hall SK. Acute angle-closure glaucoma as a complication of combined β-agonist and ipratropium bromide therapy in the emergency department. *Ann Emerg Med* 1994; **23:** 884–7.
4. Packe GE, *et al.* Nebulised ipratropium bromide and salbutamol causing closed-angle glaucoma. *Lancet* 1984; **ii:** 691.
5. Shah P, *et al.* Acute angle closure glaucoma associated with nebulised ipratropium bromide and salbutamol. *Br Med J* 1992; **304:** 40–1.
6. Mulpeter KM, *et al.* Ocular hazards of nebulized bronchodilators. *Postgrad Med J* 1992; **68:** 132–3.
7. Roberts TE, Pearson DJ. Wide eyed and breathless. *Br Med J* 1989; **299:** 1348.
8. Lust K, Livingstone I. Nebulizer-induced anisocoria. *Ann Intern Med* 1998; **128:** 327.
9. Watson WTA, *et al.* Effect of nebulized ipratropium bromide on intraocular pressures in children. *Chest* 1994; **105:** 1439–41.
10. Kalra L, Bone MF. The effect of nebulized bronchodilator therapy on intraocular pressures in patients with glaucoma. *Chest* 1988; **93:** 739–41.

Effects on the gastro-intestinal tract. Paralytic ileus developed shortly after initiation of ipratropium therapy in 2 patients, apparently due to the inadvertent swallowing of the drug during inhalation.[1,2] Both patients also had other predisposing factors for paralytic ileus (cystic fibrosis,[1] spastic diplegia[2]).

1. Mulherin D, FitzGerald MX. Meconium ileus equivalent in association with nebulised ipratropium bromide in cystic fibrosis. *Lancet* 1990; **355:** 552.
2. Markus HS. Paralytic ileus associated with ipratropium. *Lancet* 1990; **355:** 1224.

Effects on the respiratory tract. Antimuscarinic agents typically inhibit mucociliary clearance and inhibit secretions of the nose, mouth, pharynx, and bronchi. However, inhaled ipratropium bromide has virtually no effect on sputum viscosity or volume and, in contrast to atropine, it does not affect mucociliary function in the respiratory tract.[1,2]

1. Gross NJ. Ipratropium bromide. *N Engl J Med* 1988; **319:** 486–94.
2. Mann KV, *et al.* Use of ipratropium bromide in obstructive lung disease. *Clin Pharm* 1988; **7:** 670–80.

BRONCHOSPASM. Paradoxical bronchoconstriction occurring after the use of ipratropium was reported in 3 patients.[1] The authors of a further report[2] of paradoxical bronchoconstriction following nebulisation therapy with salbutamol and ipratropium suggested that this adverse effect may have been caused by benzalkonium chloride present in the nebuliser solutions. Nebuliser solutions of ipratropium in some countries contain benzalkonium chloride as a preservative. Solutions available in the UK are preservative-free but the manufacturers still recommend that the first doses of ipratropium nebuliser solution should be inhaled under medical supervision.

1. Connolly CK. Adverse reaction to ipratropium bromide. *Br Med J* 1982; **285:** 934–5.
2. Boucher M, *et al.* Possible associations of benzalkonium chloride in nebulizer solutions with respiratory arrest. *Ann Pharmacother* 1992; **26:** 772–4.

Effects on the urinary tract. Treatment with nebulised ipratropium bromide has resulted in urinary retention in elderly men especially those with prostatic hyperplasia.[1,2]

1. Lozewicz S. Bladder outflow obstruction induced by ipratropium bromide. *Postgrad Med J* 1989; **65:** 260–1.
2. Pras E, *et al.* Urinary retention associated with ipratropium bromide. *DICP Ann Pharmacother* 1991; **25:** 939–40.

Interactions

For interactions associated with antimuscarinics in general, see Atropine Sulphate, p.456. However, these interactions are not usually seen with antimuscarinics, such as ipratropium, given by inhalation.

Salbutamol. For reference to nebulised salbutamol exacerbating the adverse effects of nebulised ipratropium in patients predisposed to angle-closure glaucoma, see under Effects on the Eyes, above.

Pharmacokinetics

Following inhalation, only a small amount of ipratropium reaches the systemic circulation. Some ipratropium is inadvertently swallowed but it is poorly absorbed from the gastro-intestinal tract. Ipratropium and its metabolites are eliminated in the urine and faeces.

References.

1. Ensing K, *et al.* Pharmacokinetics of ipratropium bromide after single dose inhalation and oral and intravenous administration. *Eur J Clin Pharmacol* 1989; **36:** 189–94.

Uses and Administration

Ipratropium bromide is a quaternary ammonium antimuscarinic with peripheral effects similar to those of atropine (p.455). It is used by inhalation as a bronchodilator in the treatment of reversible airways obstruction, as in asthma (p.745) and in some patients with chronic obstructive pulmonary disease (p.747). The usual dose by inhalation is 20 or 40 μg three or four times daily; single doses of up to 80 μg may be required. In children aged 6 to 12 years the usual dose is 20 or 40 μg three times daily, and below 6 years the usual dose is 20 μg three times daily.

Ipratropium bromide may also be administered by inhalation as a nebulised solution in doses of 100 to 500 μg up to 4 times daily. In children aged 3 to 14 years the usual dose by nebuliser is 100 to 500 μg up to 3 times daily.

Ipratropium bromide, given intranasally, is also used in the management of rhinorrhoea associated with rhinitis. A dose of 42 μg is administered into each nostril by metered-dose nasal spray 2 or 3 times daily.

Rhinitis. Ipratropium bromide is used intranasally for the treatment of rhinorrhoea in allergic and non-allergic rhinitis (p.400). It has also relieved rhinorrhoea and sneezing associated with the common cold.

References.

1. Georgitis JW, *et al.* Ipratropium bromide nasal spray in non-allergic rhinitis: efficacy, nasal cytological response and patient evaluation on quality of life. *Clin Exp Allergy* 1994; **24:** 1049–55.
2. Hayden FG, *et al.* Effectiveness and safety of intranasal ipratropium bromide in common colds: a randomized, double-blind, placebo-controlled trial. *Ann Intern Med* 1996; **125:** 89–97.

Preparations

BP 1998: Ipratropium Pressurised Inhalation.

Proprietary Preparations (details are given in Part 3)
Aust.: Atronase; Atrovent; Itrop; ***Austral.:*** Atrovent; Ipratin; ***Belg.:*** Atronase; Atrovent; ***Canad.:*** Apo-Ipravent; Atrovent; Novo-Ipramide; ***Fr.:*** Atrovent; ***Ger.:*** Arutropid†; Atrovent; Itrop; ***Irl.:*** Atrovent; Rinatec; ***Ital.:*** Atem; Atrovent; Rinovagos; ***Neth.:*** Atrovent; ***Norw.:*** Atrovent; ***S.Afr.:*** Atronase†; Atrovent; Ipvent; ***Spain:*** Atrovent; Disne Asmol; Narilet; Rinoberen†; ***Swed.:*** Atrovent; ***Switz.:*** Atrovent; Itrop†; Rhinovent; ***UK:*** Atrovent; Respontin; Rinatec; Tropiovent; ***USA:*** Atrovent.

Multi-ingredient: ***Aust.:*** Arelcant; Berodual; Berodualin; Combivent; Di-Promal; ***Belg.:*** Duovent; ***Canad.:*** Combivent; Duovent; ***Fr.:*** Bronchodual; Combivent; ***Ger.:*** Berodual; ***Irl.:*** Combivent; Duovent; ***Ital.:*** Breva; Duovent; Iprafen; ***Neth.:*** Berodual; ***S.Afr.:*** Combivent; Duovent; ***Spain:*** Berodual; Crismol; ***Switz.:*** Berodual; Dospir; ***UK:*** Combivent; Duovent; ***USA:*** Combivent.

Isoetharine Hydrochloride (2070-r)

Isoetharine Hydrochloride *(BANM).*

Isoetarine Hydrochloride *(rINNM)*; Etyprenaline Hydrochloride; *N*-Isopropylethylnoradrenaline Hydrochloride. 1-(3,4-Dihydroxyphenyl)-2-isopropylaminobutan-1-ol hydrochloride.

$C_{13}H_{21}NO_3,HCl = 275.8.$

CAS — 530-08-5 (isoetharine); 50-96-4 (isoetharine hydrochloride); 2576-92-3 (isoetharine hydrochloride).

NOTE. Isoetharine is *USAN.*

Pharmacopoeias. In US.

A white to off-white odourless crystalline solid. **Soluble** in water; sparingly soluble in alcohol; practically insoluble in ether. A 1% solution in water has a pH of 4.0 to 5.6. **Store** in airtight containers.

Isoetharine Mesylate (2071-f)

Isoetharine Mesylate *(BANM).*

Isoetarine Mesilate *(rINNM)*; Isoetharine Methanesulphonate; *N*-Isopropylethylnoradrenaline Mesylate; Win-3406 (isoetharine).

$C_{13}H_{21}NO_3,CH_4O_3S = 335.4.$

CAS — 7279-75-6.

NOTE. Isoetharine is *USAN.*

Pharmacopoeias. In US.

White or practically white odourless crystals. Freely **soluble** in water; soluble in alcohol; practically insoluble in acetone and ether. A 1% solution in water has a pH of 4.5 to 5.5. **Store** in airtight containers.

Adverse Effects and Precautions

For the adverse effects and precautions pertaining to a non-selective beta agonist see under Isoprenaline Sulphate, p.892.

Abnormal coloration. Pink sputum mimicking haemoptysis occurred in many patients using isoetharine inhalation solution and could be alarming. The effect appeared to be due to oxidation of the drug when the preparation's antoxidant was diluted by water and sputum.[1]

1. Hooper PL, *et al.* Pseudohemoptysis from isoetharine. *N Engl J Med* 1983; **308:** 1602.

Effects on the respiratory system. Paradoxical bronchoconstriction in an asthmatic patient following the use of nebulised isoetharine appeared to be caused by sodium bisulphite present as a preservative.[1]

1. Koepke JW, *et al.* Dose-dependent bronchospasm from sulfites in isoetharine. *JAMA* 1984; **251:** 2982–3.

Uses and Administration

Isoetharine is a sympathomimetic with predominantly beta-adrenergic activity. Its actions are reportedly similar to those of isoprenaline (see p.892) but it has less $beta_1$-stimulant effect. It has been used as a bronchodilator in the management of reversible airways obstruction.

Isoetharine is given by inhalation, as a nebulised solution of the hydrochloride in strengths up to 0.25%; a 1% solution can be administered by a hand nebuliser. Alternatively, it may be given as an aerosol inhalation of the mesylate, as one or two inhalations of 340 μg. Isoetharine has also been given by mouth.

Preparations

USP 23: Isoetharine Inalation Solution; Isoetharine Mesylate Inhalation Aerosol.

Proprietary Preparations (details are given in Part 3)
Ger.: Asthmalitan†; ***UK:*** Numotac†; ***USA:*** Beta-2; Bronkometer; Bronkosol.

Ketotifen Fumarate (7724-j)

Ketotifen Fumarate *(BANM, USAN, rINNM).*

HC-20511 (ketotifen). 4-(1-Methylpiperidin-4-ylidene)-4*H*-benzo[4,5]cyclohepta-[1,2-*b*]thiophen-10(9*H*)-one hydrogen fumarate.

$C_{19}H_{19}NOS,C_4H_4O_4 = 425.5.$

CAS — 34580-13-7 (ketotifen); 34580-14-8 (ketotifen fumarate).

Ketotifen fumarate 1.38 mg is approximately equivalent to 1 mg of ketotifen. The manufacturers have stated that it is readily **soluble** in water.

Adverse Effects, Treatment, and Precautions

As for the antihistamines in general, p.397; drowsiness may be a problem, and dry mouth and dizziness may occur. Increased appetite and weight gain, and CNS stimulation, have been reported.

For precautions to be observed in asthmatic patients, see Sodium Cromoglycate (p.762); existing anti-asthma treatment should be continued for at least 2 weeks after starting ketotifen therapy. It should not be used for the treatment of acute asthma attacks.

Sedation, tiredness, weight gain, and dry mouth were the most common side-effects in postmarketing surveillance of ketotifen involving 19 252 patients, 8291 of whom were studied for 1 year.[1] Other frequently reported side-effects, definitely or probably related to the drug, were dizziness, nausea, and headache; exacerbation of asthma, bronchospasm, and status asthmaticus occurred in some patients while receiving ketotifen.

1. Maclay WP, *et al.* Postmarketing surveillance: practical experience with ketotifen. *Br Med J* 1984; **288:** 911–14.

Overdosage. Eight patients aged 6 to 34 years have been reported on[1] following overdoses of ketotifen in doses stated to range from 10 to 120 mg. Plasma concentrations of ketotifen base in 4 patients were 5 to 122 ng per mL (therapeutic range 1 to 4 ng per mL). Symptoms included drowsiness, confusion, dyspnoea, bradycardia or tachycardia, disorientation, and convulsions. Gastric lavage was performed in 6, and all 8 recovered within 12 hours after supportive treatment.

In an overview of 21 cases of overdosage (including those reported by Jefferys and Volans) the manufacturers stated that no serious signs or symptoms had been reported with doses below 20 mg, and there had been no fatalities.[2] The most serious effects reported had included unconsciousness, convulsions, bradycardia and tachycardia, and a severe hypotensive reaction. Management is essentially supportive and symptomatic.

1. Jefferys DB, Volans GN. Ketotifen overdose: surveillance of the toxicity of a new drug. *Br Med J* 1981; **282:** 1755–6.
2. Le Blaye I, *et al.* Acute ketotifen overdosage: a review of present clinical experience. *Drug Safety* 1992; **7:** 387–92.

Interactions

A reversible fall in the platelet count has been observed in a few patients receiving ketotifen concomitantly with oral antidiabetics and it has been suggested that this combination should therefore be avoided. Since ketotifen has the properties of the antihistamines, it may potentiate the effects of other CNS depressant drugs such as alcohol, antihistamines, hypnotics, and sedatives. For the interactions of antihistamines in general, see p.399.

Pharmacokinetics

Ketotifen fumarate is almost completely absorbed from the gastro-intestinal tract following oral administration, but bioavailability is reported to be only about 50% due to hepatic first-pass metabolism. Peak plasma concentrations occur 2 to 4 hours after a dose by mouth. It is mainly excreted in the urine as inactive metabolites with a small amount of unchanged drug; the terminal elimination half-life is about 21 hours.

Uses and Administration

Ketotifen has the properties of the antihistamines (p.399) in addition to a stabilising action on mast cells analogous to that of sodium cromoglycate. It is given orally as the fumarate in the prophylactic management of asthma, when it may take several weeks to exert its full effect; it should not be used to treat acute asthma attacks. Ketotifen is also used in the treatment of allergic conditions such as rhinitis (see p.400) and conjunctivitis.

Ketotifen fumarate is taken by mouth in doses equivalent to 1 mg of ketotifen twice daily with food, increased if necessary to the equivalent of 2 mg twice daily; 0.5 to 1 mg at night may be preferable for the first few days of treatment if drowsiness is likely to be a problem. Children over 2 or 3 years may be given the equivalent of 1 mg of ketotifen twice daily. A dose equivalent to 0.5 mg twice daily has been suggested for children between 6 months and 3 years of age.

General references.

1. Craps LP. Immunologic and therapeutic aspects of ketotifen. *J Allergy Clin Immunol* 1985; **76:** 389–93.
2. Grant SM, *et al.* Ketotifen: a review of its pharmacodynamic and pharmacokinetic properties, and therapeutic use in asthma and allergic disorders. *Drugs* 1990; **40:** 412–48. Corrections. *ibid.* 1991; **41:** 192.

Action. In a review of the pharmacology of ketotifen Greenwood[1] concluded that its anti-allergic action could be dissociated from, and was not dependent on, its antihistaminic properties. Morley *et al.*[2] discussed the anti-allergic activity of ketotifen in terms of its effect on responses to platelet-activating factor (PAF). However, the significance of PAF in the pathogenesis of asthma has been questioned.

1. Greenwood C. The pharmacology of ketotifen. *Chest* 1982; **82** (suppl): 45S–8S.
2. Morley J, *et al.* Effects of ketotifen upon responses to platelet activating factor: a basis for asthma prophylaxis. *Ann Allergy* 1986; **56:** 335–40.

Asthma. Results of studies on the effectiveness of ketotifen in the treatment of asthma (p.745) have been conflicting; although some have found it effective in reducing symptoms[1-5] and in enabling a reduction in concomitant anti-asthmatic drug therapy,[2,5,6] others have reported no significant benefits.[7,8] A study in children described as 'preasthmatic' – that is, being at high risk of developing asthma – suggested that long-term therapy with ketotifen decreased the risk of asthma onset.[9]

Although doubts exist about the efficacy of ketotifen in the management of chronic asthma, guidelines by the British Thoracic Society suggest that it may be of some help in very young children intolerant of other drugs.[10]

1. Paterson JW, *et al.* Evaluation of ketotifen (HC20-511) in bronchial asthma. *Eur J Clin Pharmacol* 1983; **25:** 187–93.
2. Tinkelman DG, *et al.* A multicenter trial of the prophylactic effect of ketotifen, theophylline, and placebo in atopic asthma. *J Allergy Clin Immunol* 1985; **76:** 487–97.
3. El Hefny A, *et al.* Ketotifen in the treatment of infants and young children with wheezy bronchitis and bronchial asthma. *J Int Med Res* 1986; **14:** 267–73.
4. Miraglia Del Giudice M, *et al.* Study of the efficacy of ketotifen treatment in asthmatic children under 3 years of age. *Curr Ther Res* 1986; **40:** 685–93.
5. Rackham A, *et al.* A Canadian multicenter study with Zaditen (ketotifen) in the treatment of bronchial asthma in children aged 5 to 17 years. *J Allergy Clin Immunol* 1989; **84:** 286–96.
6. Kasuya S, Izumi S. Steroid-sparing effect of ketotifen in steroid-dependent asthmatics: a long period evaluation in 12 patients. *Pharmatherapeutica* 1988; **5:** 177–82.
7. White MP, *et al.* Ketotifen in the young asthmatic—a double-blind placebo-controlled trial. *J Int Med Res* 1988; **16:** 107–13.
8. Volovitz B, *et al.* Efficacy and safety of ketotifen in young children with asthma. *J Allergy Clin Immunol* 1988; **81:** 526 30.
9. Bustos GJ, *et al.* Prevention of asthma with ketotifen in preasthmatic children: a three-year follow-up study. *Clin Exp Allergy* 1995; **25:** 568–73.
10. British Thoracic Society, *et al.* The British guidelines on asthma management: 1995 review and position statement. *Thorax* 1997; **52** (suppl 1): S1–S21.

Food allergy. Ketotifen has been tried in the prophylaxis of food allergy reactions (p.400). However, results have been conflicting,[1,2] and avoidance of the food allergen remains the mainstay of therapy.

1. Sogn D. Medications and their use in the treatment of adverse reactions to foods. *J Allergy Clin Immunol* 1986; **78:** 238–43.
2. Molkhou P, Dupont C. Ketotifen in prevention and therapy of food allergy. *Ann Allergy* 1987; **59:** 187–93.

Inflammatory bowel disease. Ketotifen has been reported to decrease mucosal damage in *animal* models of colitis,[1] and it has been suggested that its potential for the treatment of inflammatory bowel disease (p.1171) should be explored.

1. Eliakim R, *et al.* Ketotifen effectively prevents mucosal damage in experimental colitis. *Gut* 1992; **33:** 1498–1503.

Urticaria. Antihistamines are widely used in the treatment of urticaria (see p.1076) and ketotifen has sometimes been used.[1,2]

1. Kamide R, *et al.* Clinical evaluation of ketotifen for chronic urticaria: multicenter double-blind comparative study with clemastine. *Ann Allergy* 1989; **62:** 322–5.
2. Edge JA, Osborne JP. Terbutaline and ketotifen in cold urticaria in a child. *J R Soc Med* 1989; **82:** 439–40.

Preparations

Proprietary Preparations (details are given in Part 3)
Aust.: Zaditen; ***Belg.:*** Zaditen; ***Canad.:*** Zaditen; ***Fr.:*** Zaditen; ***Ger.:*** Airvitess; Astifat; Ketof; Zaditen; Zatofug; ***Irl.:*** Zaditen; ***Ital.:*** Allerkif†; Totifen†; Zaditen; ***Jpn:*** Zaditen; ***Neth.:*** Zaditen; ***S.Afr.:*** Zaditen; ***Spain:*** Globofil†; Ketasma; Zasten; ***Switz.:*** Zaditen; ***UK:*** Zaditen.

Lodoxamide Trometamol (12899-y)

Lodoxamide Trometamol *(BANM, rINNM).*

Lodoxamide Tromethamine *(USAN)*; U-42585 (lodoxamide); U-42718 (lodoxamide ethyl); U-42585E (lodoxamide trometamol). *N,N'*-(2-Chloro-5-cyano-*m*-phenylene)dioxamic acid compound with trometamol.

$C_{11}H_6ClN_3O_6,2C_4H_{11}NO_3$ = 553.9.

CAS — 53882-12-5 (lodoxamide); 53882-13-6 (lodoxamide ethyl); 63610-09-3 (lodoxamide trometamol).

NOTE. Lodoxamide Ethyl is also *USAN.*

Adverse Effects

The application of lodoxamide eye drops may cause local irritation. Reported effects include burning or stinging, and itching. Flushing and dizziness have also been reported.

Uses and Administration

Lodoxamide has a stabilising action on mast cells resembling that of sodium cromoglycate (p.762). It has been given by mouth, generally as the ethyl ester, or by aerosol inhalation, generally as the trometamol salt, in studies of its prophylactic effect in the treatment of asthma, but has not proved to be of benefit.

Lodoxamide trometamol has, however, been found to be effective when employed as eye drops for allergic conjunctivitis (p.399), particularly vernal keratoconjunctivitis; a concentration equivalent to 0.1% of lodoxamide is used, one or two drops usually being instilled into the eye four times daily.

Conjunctivitis. Lodoxamide is an effective treatment for vernal keratoconjunctivitis.[1,2] Although there have been suggestions that it may be more effective than sodium cromoglycate for this purpose (see p.763) well-constructed comparative studies are lacking.[2]

1. Anonymous. Lodoxamide for vernal keratoconjunctivitis. *Med Lett Drugs Ther* 1994; **36:** 26.
2. Lee S, Allard TRFK. Lodoxamide in vernal keratoconjunctivitis. *Ann Pharmacother* 1996; **30:** 535–7.

Preparations

Proprietary Preparations (details are given in Part 3)
Austral.: Lomide; ***Belg.:*** Alomide; ***Canad.:*** Alomide; ***Fr.:*** Almide; ***Irl.:*** Alomide; ***Ital.:*** Alomide; ***S.Afr.:*** Alomide; ***UK:*** Alomide; ***USA:*** Alomide.

Montelukast (1153-c)

Montelukast *(BAN, rINN).*

MK-0476; Montélukast. 1-[({(*R*)-*m*-[(*E*)2-(7-Chloro-2-quinolyl)vinyl]-α-[*o*-(1-hydroxy-1-methylethyl)phenethyl]benzyl}thio)methyl]cyclopropaneacetic acid.

$C_{35}H_{36}ClNO_3S$ = 586.2.

CAS — 158966-92-8 (montelukast); 151767-02-1 (montelukast sodium).

NOTE. Montelukast sodium is *USAN.*

Montelukast is a specific leukotriene receptor antagonist with actions similar to those of zafirlukast (see p.774) although it is reported to have a longer duration of action. It is used as the sodium salt in the management of asthma (p.745), in doses equivalent to 10 mg of montelukast once daily at bedtime; children aged 6 to 14 years may be given the equivalent of 5 mg at bedtime. It should not be used to treat an acute attack.

References.

1. Reiss TF, *et al.* Effects of montelukast (MK-0476), a new potent cysteinyl leukotriene (LTD_4) receptor antagonist, in patients with chronic asthma. *J Allergy Clin Immunol* 1996; **98:** 528–34.
2. Reiss TF, *et al.* Effects of montelukast (MK-0476), a potent cysteinyl leukotriene receptor antagonist, on bronchodilation in asthmatic subjects treated with and without inhaled corticosteroids. *Thorax* 1997; **52:** 45–8.
3. De Lepeleire I, *et al.* Montelukast causes prolonged, potent leukotriene D_4-receptor antagonism in the airways of patients with asthma. *Clin Pharmacol Ther* 1997; **61:** 83–92.
4. Knorr B, *et al.* Montelukast for chronic asthma in 6- to 14-year-old children: a randomized, double-blind trial. *JAMA* 1998; **279:** 1181–6.
5. Leff JA, *et al.* Montelukast, a leukotriene-receptor antagonist, for the treatment of mild asthma and exercise-induced bronchoconstriction. *N Engl J Med* 1998; **339:** 147–52.
6. Anonymous. Montelukast for persistent asthma. *Med Lett Drugs Ther* 1998; **40:** 71–3.
7. Markham A, Faulds D. Montelukast. *Drugs* 1998; **56:** 251–6.

Preparations

Proprietary Preparations (details are given in Part 3)
UK: Singulair; ***USA:*** Singulair.

Nedocromil Sodium (18666-r)

Nedocromil Sodium *(BANM, USAN, rINNM).*

FPL-59002 (nedocromil); FPL-59002KC (nedocromil calcium); FPL-59002KP (nedocromil sodium). Disodium 9-ethyl-6,9-dihydro-4,6-dioxo-10-propyl-4*H*-pyrano[3,2-g]quinoline-2,8-dicarboxylate.

$C_{19}H_{15}NNa_2O_7$ = 415.3.

CAS — 69049-73-6 (nedocromil); 69049-74-7 (nedocromil sodium); 101626-68-0 (nedocromil calcium).

NOTE. Nedocromil Calcium is also *USAN.*

Adverse Effects and Precautions

Nedocromil sodium is generally well tolerated, side-effects being mild and transient. Headache, nausea, abdominal discomfort, and a bitter taste have been reported. Increased bronchospasm has occurred in a few patients.

It should not be used for the treatment of acute asthma attacks. The general cautions described under sodium cromoglycate (p.762) also apply.

A recent review of nedocromil sodium commented that its adverse effects profile is similar to that of sodium cromoglycate and salbutamol.[1] Adverse effects were infrequent, mild, and short-lived. The most common effect appeared to be an unpleasant or bitter taste which seemed to be experienced by 12 to 13% of patients, although less than 1% of patients discontinued treatment because of it. Other adverse effects included cough (in 7%), headache (6%), sore throat (5.7%), nausea (4%), and vomiting (1.7%).

1. Brogden RN, Sorkin EM. Nedocromil sodium: an updated review of its pharmacological properties and therapeutic efficacy in asthma. *Drugs* 1993; **45:** 693–715.

Pharmacokinetics

Nedocromil sodium is poorly absorbed from the gastro-intestinal tract. About 5% of the inhaled dose is absorbed from the lungs and is excreted unchanged in the urine and bile. The half-life is stated to range from about 1.5 to 3.3 hours.

The extent of absorption or bioavailability of nedocromil sodium after inhalation in healthy subjects was 7 to 9% of the dose, including 2 to 3% oral absorption and 5 to 6% absorption from the respiratory tract.[1] Following inhalation of nedocromil sodium 4 mg the mean peak plasma concentration was 3.3 ng per mL in healthy subjects and 2.8 ng per mL in asthmatic patients, with peak values being reached at approximately 20 and 40 minutes respectively. The mean total urinary excretion after 24 hours following a single dose was 5.4% of the dose in healthy subjects and 2.3% in asthmatics.

1. Neale MG, *et al.* The pharmacokinetics of nedocromil sodium, a new drug for the treatment of reversible obstructive airways disease, in human volunteers and patients with reversible obstructive airways disease. *Br J Clin Pharmacol* 1987; **24:** 493–501.

Uses and Administration

Nedocromil sodium has a stabilising action on mast cells resembling that of sodium cromoglycate (p.762) and is used similarly in the management of chronic asthma. It is not effective in an established asthma attack and should not be used to treat an acute attack.

Nedocromil sodium is administered by metered-dose aerosol inhalation. The usual dose is 4 mg inhaled four times daily which may be decreased to 4 mg twice daily once control of symptoms is achieved. Clinical improvement usually occurs within 2 to 4 weeks of beginning therapy.

Nedocromil sodium is also used topically in the treatment of allergic conjunctivitis and allergic rhinitis. For allergic conjunctivitis it is given as a 2% solution, one drop being instilled into each eye twice daily. This may be increased to 4 times daily if necessary, which is the usual dose in vernal keratoconjunctivitis. In allergic rhinitis nedocromil sodium is used as a 1% nasal spray: one spray is given into each nostril 4 times a day.

General references.

1. Busse WW, *et al.* International symposium on nedocromil sodium. *Drugs* 1989; **37** (suppl 1): 1–137.
2. Brogden RN, Sorkein EM. Nedocromil sodium: an updated review of its pharmacological properties and therapeutic efficacy in asthma. *Drugs* 1993; **45:** 693–715.
3. Parish RC, Miller LJ. Nedocromil sodium. *Ann Pharmacother* 1993; **27:** 599–606.

Asthma. Nedocromil sodium can inhibit asthmatic responses provoked by allergen challenge and attenuate allergen-induced bronchial hyperresponsiveness.[1] It is generally considered to be an alternative to sodium cromoglycate in the management of asthma (p.745).

Nedocromil has been shown to improve symptoms and reduce bronchodilator intake in adults[2] and children[3] with asthma and it has been suggested that nedocromil might be more effective than cromoglycate,[4,5] though results have been inconsistent.[6]

1. Holgate ST. Clinical evaluation of nedocromil sodium in asthma. *Eur J Respir Dis* 1986; **69** (suppl 147): 149–59.
2. Fairfax AJ, Allbeson M. A double-blind group comparative trial of nedocromil sodium and placebo in the management of bronchial asthma. *J Int Med Res* 1988; **16:** 216–24.
3. Armenio L, *et al.* Double blind, placebo controlled study of nedocromil sodium in asthma. *Arch Dis Child* 1993; **68:** 193–7.
4. Crimi N, *et al.* Comparative study of the effects of nedocromil sodium (4 mg) and sodium cromoglycate (10 mg) on adenosine-induced bronchoconstriction in asthmatic subjects. *Clin Allergy* 1988; **18:** 367–74.
5. Lal S, *et al.* Nedocromil sodium is more effective than cromolyn sodium for the treatment of chronic reversible obstructive airway disease. *Chest* 1993; **104:** 438–47.
6. Brogden RN, Sorkin EM. Nedocromil sodium: an updated review of its pharmacological properties and therapeutic efficacy in asthma. *Drugs* 1993; **45:** 693–715.

Cough. For references to the use of sodium cromoglycate or nedocromil sodium in the management of cough induced by ACE inhibitor therapy, see Cough, p.763. The references indicate a positive response to sodium cromoglycate but not to nedocromil sodium.

Rhinitis and conjunctivitis. Many drugs, including nedocromil,[1,2] are employed in the management of allergic rhinitis (p.400) and conjunctivitis (p.399). For the suggestion that nedocromil may be more effective than cromoglycate in the management of vernal keratoconjunctivitis see Rhinitis and Conjunctivitis, p.763.

1. Ruhno J, *et al.* Intranasal nedocromil sodium in the treatment of ragweed-allergic rhinitis. *J Allergy Clin Immunol* 1988; **81:** 570–4.
2. Sipilä P, *et al.* Double-blind comparison of nedocromil sodium (1% nasal spray) and placebo in rhinitis caused by birch pollen. *Clin Otolaryngol* 1987; **12:** 365–70.

Preparations

Proprietary Preparations (details are given in Part 3)
Aust.: Tilade; Tilarin; Tilavist; ***Austral.:*** Tilade; ***Canad.:*** Tilade; ***Fr.:*** Tilade; Tilavist; ***Ger.:*** Halamid; Irtan; Tilade; ***Irl.:*** Tilade; Tilavist; ***Ital.:*** Kovilen; Kovinal; Tilade; Tilarin; Tilavist; ***Neth.:*** Tilade; Tilavist; ***S.Afr.:*** Tilade; ***Spain:*** Brionil; Cetimil; Ildor; Tilad; Tilavist; ***Swed.:*** Tilavist; ***Switz.:*** Tilade; Tilarin; Tilavist; ***UK:*** Rapitil; Tilade; Tilarin; ***USA:*** Tilade.

Multi-ingredient: ***Ital.:*** Zarent.

Orciprenaline Sulphate (2091-m)

Orciprenaline Sulphate *(BANM, rINNM).*

Metaproterenol Sulfate *(USAN)*; Metaproterenol Sulphate; Orciprenalini Sulfas; Th-152. 1-(3,5-Dihydroxyphenyl)-2-isopropylaminoethanol sulphate; *N*-Isopropyl-*N*(β,3,5-trihydroxyphenethyl)ammonium sulphate.

$(C_{11}H_{17}NO_3)_2,H_2SO_4$ = 520.6.

CAS — 586-06-1 (orciprenaline); 5874-97-5 (orciprenaline sulphate).

Pharmacopoeias. In *Eur.* (see p.viii), *Jpn, Pol.,* and *US.*

A white to off-white, odourless or almost odourless, hygroscopic, crystalline powder. Freely **soluble** in water and in alcohol; practically insoluble in dichloromethane and in ether. A 10% solution in water has a pH of 4.0 to 5.5. **Store** in airtight containers. Protect from light.

Adverse Effects and Precautions

For the adverse effects and precautions pertaining to a non-selective beta agonist see Isoprenaline Sulphate, p.892.

Interactions

As for Isoprenaline Sulphate, p.892.

Pharmacokinetics

Following oral administration orciprenaline is absorbed from the gastro-intestinal tract and undergoes extensive first-pass metabolism in the liver; about 40% of an oral dose is reported to reach the circulation unchanged. It is excreted in the urine primarily as metabolites.

Uses and Administration

Orciprenaline sulphate is a direct-acting sympathomimetic with predominantly beta-adrenoceptor stimulant activity. It has actions and uses similar to those of salbutamol (see p.759) but is less selective for $beta_2$-adrenergic receptors.

Orciprenaline sulphate is used as a bronchodilator in the management of reversible airways obstruction, as occurs in asthma (p.745) and in some patients with chronic obstructive pulmonary disease (p.747). However, more selective beta$_2$ agonists such as salbutamol or terbutaline are now generally preferred. Following inhalation, the onset of action is usually within 5 to 30 minutes and can last up to 6 hours, though there is wide variation.

A usual adult dose for the relief of bronchospasm is 1 or 2 inhalations of orciprenaline sulphate 750 μg from a metered-dose aerosol, repeated if required after not less than 30 minutes, up to a maximum of 12 inhalations (9 mg) in 24 hours. A suggested maximum dose within a 24-hour period for children is: under 6 years, up to 4 inhalations; 6 to 12 years, up to 8 inhalations.

Orciprenaline sulphate has also been inhaled in 5% solution from a hand nebuliser, the usual adult dose being 10 inhalations. If the solution is used with any other nebulising device such as an intermittent positive pressure breathing (IPPB) apparatus the adult dose is 0.2 to 0.3 mL of a 5% solution diluted up to about 2.5 mL with sterile water or physiological saline (i.e. dilution to a 0.4 to 0.6% solution) administered not more often than every 4 hours. Unit-dose vials containing a prediluted solution of orciprenaline sulphate 0.4% and 0.6% are also available for nebulisation by an IPPB device.

In the chronic management of reversible airways obstruction, orciprenaline sulphate may be given by mouth in a dose of 20 mg four times daily. A suggested dose for children is: up to 1 year, 5 to 10 mg three times daily; 1 to 3 years, 5 to 10 mg four times daily; 3 to 12 years, 10 mg four times daily to 20 mg three times daily.

Orciprenaline sulphate has also been used for its cardiovascular effects in the treatment of bradycardia of various types, notably in AV heart block and sinus bradycardia. In such cases doses of up to 240 mg daily by mouth in divided doses, or 250 to 500 μg by slow intravenous injection have been given; orciprenaline sulphate may also be given by intravenous infusion, or intramuscular or subcutaneous injection.

Preparations

BP 1998: Orciprenaline Tablets;
USP 23: Metaproterenol Sulfate Inhalation Aerosol; Metaproterenol Sulfate Inhalation Solution; Metaproterenol Sulfate Syrup; Metaproterenol Sulfate Tablets.

Proprietary Preparations (details are given in Part 3)
Aust.: Alupent; ***Austral.:*** Alupent; ***Belg.:*** Alupent; ***Canad.:*** Alupent; ***Fr.:*** Alupent; ***Ger.:*** Alupent; ***Irl.:*** Alupent; ***Ital.:*** Alupent; ***Neth.:*** Alupent†; ***S.Afr.:*** Alupent; ***Spain:*** Alupent; ***Switz.:*** Alupent; ***UK:*** Alupent; ***USA:*** Alupent; Metaprel; Prometa.

Multi-ingredient: ***Ger.:*** Abiadin†; ***Irl.:*** Alupent Expectorant; ***Ital.:*** Bisolpent†; Silomat Compositum†; Tussiprene†; ***S.Afr.:*** Adco-Linctopent; Bisolpent†; Bisolvon Linctus DA; Bronkese Compound; Flemeze; Silomat DA; ***Spain:*** Lomisat Compositum†; ***Swed.:*** Silomat Compositum†.

Oxitropium Bromide (13065-h)

Oxitropium Bromide *(BAN, rINN)*.

BA-253. 6,7-Epoxy-8-ethyl-3-[(*S*)-tropoyloxy]tropanium bromide; (3*s*,6*R*,7*S*,8*r*)-8-Ethyl-3-[(*S*)-tropoyloxy]-6,7-epoxytropanium bromide.

$C_{19}H_{26}BrNO_4$ = 412.3.

CAS — 30286-75-0.

Oxitropium bromide is a quaternary ammonium antimuscarinic with peripheral actions similar to those of atropine (p.455). It is used similarly to ipratropium bromide (p.754), to which it is structurally related, as a bronchodilator in the treatment of reversible airways obstruction. Doses of 200 μg by inhalation from a metered-dose aerosol are given 2 to 3 times daily. *Animal* studies have shown reproductive toxicity with high doses of oxitropium, hence the manufacturer's recommendation that it should not be used during pregnancy.

Administration and dosage. Oxitropium bromide is usually administered by inhalation from an aerosol (see above). The optimal dosage of oxitropium bromide given as a nebulised solution in studies of patients with chronic obstructive pulmonary disease has been reported[1] to be in the range of 1000 to 2000 μg.

1. Stappaerts I, *et al.* Dose-response study of oxitropium bromide inhaled as a nebulised solution. *Eur J Clin Pharmacol* 1994; **46:** 305–7.

Preparations

Proprietary Preparations (details are given in Part 3)
Aust.: Oxivent; ***Belg.:*** Oxivent; ***Fr.:*** Tersigat; ***Ger.:*** Ventilat; ***Irl.:*** Oxivent; ***Ital.:*** Oxivent; ***UK:*** Oxivent.

Pemirolast Potassium (11030-r)

Pemirolast Potassium *(USAN, rINNM)*.

BMY-26517. Potassium 9-methyl-3-(1*H*-tetrazol-5-yl)-4*H*-pyrido[1,2-*a*]-pyrimidin-4-one.

$C_{10}H_7KN_6O$ = 266.3.

CAS — 69372-19-6 (pemirolast); 100299-08-9 (pemirolast potassium).

Pemirolast potassium has mast cell stabilising properties like sodium cromoglycate (p.762) and may also be a leukotriene inhibitor. It is used in the treatment of chronic asthma (p.745). The suggested dose is 10 mg by mouth twice daily. It has no bronchodilator properties and should not be used for the treatment of acute attacks. Pemirolast potassium is also one of many drugs used in the treatment of allergic rhinitis (p.400), when a suggested dose is 5 mg by mouth twice daily.

References.

1. Tinkelman DG, Berkowitz RB. A pilot study of pemirolast in patients with seasonal allergic rhinitis. *Ann Allergy* 1991; **66:** 162–5.
2. Hasegawa T, *et al.* Kinetic interaction between theophylline and a newly developed anti-allergic drug, pemirolast potassium. *Eur J Clin Pharmacol* 1994; **46:** 55–8.

Preparations

Proprietary Preparations (details are given in Part 3)
Jpn: Alegysal.

Picumast (2498-m)

Picumast *(BAN, rINN)*.

BM-15100 (picumast dihydrochloride). 7-[3-(4-*p*-Chlorobenzylpiperazin-1-yl)propoxy]-3,4-dimethylcoumarin.

$C_{25}H_{29}ClN_2O_3$ = 441.0.

CAS — 39577-19-0 (picumast); 39577-20-3 (picumast dihydrochloride).

Picumast is an anti-allergic compound that has been investigated in the management of asthma and allergic rhinitis.

A series of articles concerning the anti-allergic activity of picumast and its use in asthma and allergic rhinitis.[1]

1. Ulmer WT. Antiallergic drug: picumast dihydrochloride. *Arzneimittelforschung* 1989; **39:** 1307–76.

Pirbuterol Acetate (3776-k)

Pirbuterol Acetate *(BANM, USAN, rINNM)*.

CP-24314-14. 2-*tert*-Butylamino-1-(5-hydroxy-6-hydroxymethyl-2-pyridyl)ethanol acetate.

$C_{12}H_{20}N_2O_3,C_2H_4O_2$ = 300.4.

CAS — 38677-81-5 (pirbuterol); 65652-44-0 (pirbuterol acetate).

Pirbuterol Hydrochloride (13127-d)

Pirbuterol Hydrochloride *(BANM, USAN, rINNM)*.

CP-24314-1; Pyrbuterol Hydrochloride. 2-*tert*-Butylamino-1-(5-hydroxy-6-hydroxymethyl-2-pyridyl)ethanol dihydrochloride.

$C_{12}H_{20}N_2O_3,2HCl$ = 313.2.

CAS — 38029-10-6.

Pirbuterol is a direct-acting sympathomimetic with predominantly beta-adrenoceptor stimulant activity and a selective action on beta$_2$ receptors (beta$_2$ agonist). It has properties similar to those of salbutamol (see p.758).

Pirbuterol is used for its bronchodilating properties. It is given as the acetate or hydrochloride in the management of reversible airways obstruction, as in asthma (p.745) and in some patients with chronic obstructive pulmonary disease (p.747). Following inhalation, pirbuterol exerts an effect within 10 minutes which is reported to last at least 5 hours. With oral administration a significant effect may not be seen for up to one hour, but the duration of action may be 6 hours or more.

Pirbuterol is given by inhalation as the acetate via a metered-dose aerosol in a usual dose equivalent to pirbuterol 200 to 400 μg (1 to 2 inhalations) as required but not more often than every four hours. It may also be given by mouth in usual doses of pirbuterol 10 or 15 mg three or four times daily, as the hydrochloride.

Preparations

Proprietary Preparations (details are given in Part 3)
Aust.: Exirel; ***Belg.:*** Spirolair; ***Canad.:*** Maxair; ***Fr.:*** Maxair†; ***Ger.:*** Zeisin; ***Switz.:*** Maxair; ***UK:*** Exirel†; ***USA:*** Maxair.

Pranlukast (16795-j)

Pranlukast *(BAN, rINN)*.

ONO-1078. *N*-[4-Oxo-2-(1*H*-tetrazol-5-yl)-4*H*-1-benzopyran-8-yl]-*p*-(4-phenylbutoxy)benzamide.

$C_{27}H_{23}N_5O_4$ = 481.5.

CAS — 103177-37-3.

Pranlukast is a selective antagonist of the leukotriene D_4 receptor with similar properties to zafirlukast (p.774). It is used in the management of asthma.

References.

1. Tamaoki J, *et al.* Leukotriene antagonist prevents exacerbation of asthma during reduction of high-dose inhaled corticosteroid. *Am J Respir Crit Care Med* 1997; **155:** 1235–40.
2. Barnes NC, *et al.* Pranlukast, a novel leukotriene receptor antagonist: results of the first European, placebo-controlled, multicentre clinical study in asthma. *Thorax* 1997; **52:** 523–7.
3. Grossman J, *et al.* Results of the first US double-blind, placebo-controlled, multicenter clinical study in asthma with pranlukast, a novel leukotriene receptor antagonist. *J Asthma* 1997; **34:** 321–8.

Procaterol Hydrochloride (13171-b)

Procaterol Hydrochloride *(BANM, USAN, rINNM)*.

CI-888; OPC-2009. (±)-*erythro*-8-Hydroxy-5-(1-hydroxy-2-isopropylaminobutyl)quinolin-2(1*H*)-one hydrochloride; (±)-8-Hydroxy-5-[(1*R**,2*S**)-1-hydroxy-2-isopropylaminobutyl]-2-quinolone hydrochloride.

$C_{16}H_{22}N_2O_3,HCl$ = 326.8.

CAS — 72332-33-3 (procaterol); 59828-07-8 (procaterol hydrochloride).

NOTE. The commercial substance is the hemihydrate ($C_{16}H_{22}N_2O_3,HCl,\frac{1}{2}H_2O$ = 335.8).

Pharmacopoeias. In *Jpn.*

Procaterol hydrochloride is a direct-acting sympathomimetic with predominantly beta-adrenoceptor stimulant activity selective to beta$_2$ receptors (beta$_2$ agonist). It has properties similar to those of salbutamol (p.758). It is used as a bronchodilator in the management of reversible airways obstruction, as in asthma (p.745) or in some patients with chronic obstructive pulmonary disease (p.747). Administration by oral inhalation produces an effect within 5 minutes and the effect can last up to 8 hours.

To relieve bronchospasm, 10 to 20 μg of procaterol hydrochloride is given by inhalation from a metered-dose aerosol. A recommended dose for maintenance therapy is 10 to 20 μg inhaled 3 times daily. An inhalation solution containing 100 μg per mL has been given via a nebuliser in usual doses of 30 to 50 μg. Procaterol hydrochloride can also be given by mouth in doses of 50 μg once or twice daily.

Preparations

Proprietary Preparations (details are given in Part 3)
Canad.: Pro-Air†; ***Ger.:*** Onsukil†; ***Ital.:*** Masacin†; Procadil; Propulm; ***Jpn:*** Meptin; ***S.Afr.:*** Normalin†; ***Spain:*** Brodiwas†; Onsukil; Promaxol.

Proxyphylline (640-d)

Proxyphylline *(BAN, rINN)*.

Proxyphyllinum. 7-(2-Hydroxypropyl)-1,3-dimethylxanthine; (*RS*)-1,3-Dimethyl-7-(2-hydroxypropyl)purine-2,6(3*H*,1*H*)-dione; 7-(2-Hydroxypropyl)theophylline.

$C_{10}H_{14}N_4O_3$ = 238.2.

CAS — 603-00-9.

Pharmacopoeias. In *Eur.* (see p.viii).

A white crystalline powder. Very **soluble** in water; soluble in alcohol. **Protect** from light.

Proxyphylline is a theophylline derivative which is used as a bronchodilator and for its cardiovascular properties similarly to theophylline (see p.772). Proxyphylline is readily absorbed from the gastro-intestinal tract and it does not liberate theophylline in the body.

Preparations

Proprietary Preparations (details are given in Part 3)
Ger.: Proxy-Retardoral†.

Multi-ingredient: ***Aust.:*** Asthma Efeum†; Neobiphyllin†; Omega; ***Ger.:*** Adenopurin†; Antihypertonicum S; Dr. Boether Bronchitten forte N†; Keldrin†; Neobiphyllin; Neobiphyllin-Clys; Poikiloton†; Solamin†; Theo-Lanicor†; Theokal†; ***Spain:*** Novofilin; ***Switz.:*** Neo-Biphyllin; Neo-Biphyllin Special†.

Pyridofylline (641-n)

Pyridofylline *(rINN)*.

Pyridophylline; Pyridoxine *O*-(Theophyllin-7-ylethyl)sulphate. 3-Hydroxy-4,5-bis(hydroxymethyl)-2-methylpyridine 2-(theophyllin-7-yl)ethyl sulphate.

$C_{17}H_{23}N_5O_9S$ = 473.5.

CAS — 53403-97-7.

Pyridofylline is a theophylline derivative with actions and uses similar to those of theophylline (see p.772).

Preparations

Proprietary Preparations (details are given in Part 3)
Multi-ingredient: ***Spain:*** Aletor Compositum.

Repirinast (2921-h)

Repirinast *(USAN, rINN)*.

MY-5116. Isopentyl 5,6-dihydro-7,8-dimethyl-4,5-dioxo-4*H*-pyrano[3,2-*c*]quinoline-2-carboxylate.

$C_{20}H_{21}NO_5$ = 355.4.

CAS — 73080-51-0.

Repirinast is an orally active anti-allergic with a stabilising action on mast cells resembling that of sodium cromoglycate (p.762). It has been given by mouth in the management of asthma (p.745).

References.

1. Takagi K, *et al.* Lack of effect of repirinast on the pharmacokinetics of theophylline in asthmatic patients. *Eur J Clin Pharmacol* 1989; **37:** 301–3.
2. Patel PC, *et al.* The effect of repirinast on airway responsiveness to methacholine and allergen. *J Allergy Clin Immunol* 1992; **90:** 782–8.

Preparations

Proprietary Preparations (details are given in Part 3)
Jpn: Romet†.

Reproterol Hydrochloride (2101-l)

Reproterol Hydrochloride *(BANM, USAN, rINNM)*.

D-1959 (reproterol); W-2946M. 7-{3-[(3,5,β-Trihydroxyphenethyl)amino]propyl}theophylline hydrochloride.

$C_{18}H_{23}N_5O_5,HCl$ = 425.9.

CAS — 54063-54-6 (reproterol); 13055-82-8 (reproterol hydrochloride).

Reproterol is a direct-acting sympathomimetic with predominantly beta-adrenergic activity and a selective action on $beta_2$ receptors ($beta_2$ agonist). It has properties similar to those of salbutamol (p.758).

Reproterol hydrochloride is used as a bronchodilator in the management of reversible airways obstruction, as in asthma (p.745) and in some patients with chronic obstructive pulmonary disease (p.747).

For the relief of acute attacks of bronchospasm the usual dose of reproterol hydrochloride is 1 or 2 inhalations of 500 μg from a metered-dose aerosol repeated every 3 to 6 hours as required. For chronic use and prophylaxis of bronchospasm, inhalation of 1 mg three times daily has been employed. For children of 6 to 12 years of age the suggested dose is one inhalation of 500 μg every 3 to 6 hours for acute attacks or three times daily for prophylaxis. It can also be given by mouth (adult doses are 10 to 20 mg three times daily), and by slow intravenous injection.

Preparations

Proprietary Preparations (details are given in Part 3)
Aust.: Bronchospasmin; ***Ger.:*** Bronchospasmin; ***Ital.:*** Broncospasmine; Reprol†; Sanasma†; ***Spain:*** Broncospasmin; Epiferol†; Gensasmol†; ***Switz.:*** Bronchospasmine; ***UK:*** Bronchodil.

Multi-ingredient: ***Aust.:*** Aarane; Allergospasmin; ***Ger.:*** Aarane; Allergospasmin; Asthmocupin†; ***Switz.:*** Aarane; Allergospasmine.

Rimiterol Hydrobromide (2102-y)

Rimiterol Hydrobromide *(BANM, USAN, rINNM)*.

R-798; WG-253. *erythro*-3,4-Dihydroxy-α-(2-piperidyl)benzyl alcohol hydrobromide; *erythro*-(3,4-Dihydroxyphenyl) (2-piperidyl)methanol hydrobromide.

$C_{12}H_{17}NO_3,HBr$ = 304.2.

CAS — 32953-89-2 (rimiterol); 31842-61-2 (rimiterol hydrobromide).

Adverse Effects and Precautions

As for Salbutamol Sulphate, p.758.

Interactions

As for Salbutamol Sulphate, p.759.

Pharmacokinetics

Rimiterol is readily absorbed from the gastro-intestinal tract. It is subject not only to extensive first-pass metabolism by sulphate and glucuronide conjugation, but also to metabolism by catechol-*O*-methyltransferase and therefore has a very short plasma half-life of less than 5 minutes. Rimiterol also appears to be metabolised by catechol-*O*-methyltransferase in the lungs. It is excreted in both the urine and the bile.

Uses and Administration

Rimiterol is a direct-acting sympathomimetic with predominantly beta-adrenergic activity and a selective action on $beta_2$ receptors ($beta_2$ agonist). It has actions and uses similar to those of salbutamol (p.759).

Rimiterol hydrobromide is used as a bronchodilator for the relief of acute bronchospasm in the management of disorders involving reversible airways obstruction such as asthma (p.745) and in certain patients with chronic obstructive pulmonary disease (p.747). The usual dose is 1 to 3 inhalations of 200 μg from a metered-dose aerosol as required. This treatment dose should not be repeated in less than 30 minutes. No more than 8 treatments should be taken in any 24-hour period.

Preparations

Proprietary Preparations (details are given in Part 3)
Belg.: Pulmadil; ***Neth.:*** Pulmadil; ***S.Afr.:*** Pulmadil†; ***UK:*** Pulmadil†.

Salbutamol (2104-z)

Salbutamol *(BAN, rINN)*.

AH-3365; Albuterol *(USAN)*; Salbutamolum; Sch-13949W. 2-*tert*-Butylamino-1-(4-hydroxy-3-hydroxymethylphenyl)ethanol.

$C_{13}H_{21}NO_3$ = 239.3.

CAS — 18559-94-9.

Pharmacopoeias. In *Eur.* (see p.viii), *Int.*, and *US.*

A white or almost white, crystalline powder. Sparingly **soluble** in water; soluble in alcohol; slightly soluble in ether. **Protect** from light.

Salbutamol Sulphate (2105-c)

Salbutamol Sulphate *(BANM, rINNM)*.

Albuterol Sulfate *(USAN)*; Salbutamol Hemisulphate; Salbutamoli Sulfas.

$(C_{13}H_{21}NO_3)_2,H_2SO_4$ = 576.7.

CAS — 51022-70-9.

Pharmacopoeias. In *Chin., Eur.* (see p.viii), *Int., Jpn, Pol.*, and *US.*

A white or almost white crystalline powder. Salbutamol sulphate 1.2 mg is approximately equivalent to 1 mg of salbutamol. Freely **soluble** in water; slightly soluble in alcohol, chloroform, and ether; very slightly soluble in dichloromethane. **Protect** from light.

Adverse Effects

Salbutamol may cause fine tremor of skeletal muscle (particularly the hands), palpitations, and muscle cramps. Tachycardia, tenseness, headaches, and peripheral vasodilatation have been reported after large doses, as has potentially serious hypokalaemia. Hypersensitivity reactions have occurred, including paradoxical bronchospasm, angioedema, urticaria, hypotension, and collapse.

The high doses of salbutamol used intravenously to delay premature labour have been associated with nausea and vomiting, and with severe adverse cardiac and metabolic effects and pulmonary oedema.

For details of the adverse effects of sympathomimetics in general, including distinction between alpha, $beta_1$, and $beta_2$ agonist effects, see p.951.

Effects on electrolytes and metabolism. Salbutamol, in common with other $beta_2$-agonists, may have effects on the electrolyte balance and on metabolism. In general the most prominent effects that may be encountered are *hypokalaemia* and *hyperglycaemia*. Not all studies have demonstrated such metabolic effects and the degree of effect will often be dependent upon the dose and route of salbutamol employed. The effects are usually reversible but may, nevertheless, lead to precautions in the use of salbutamol. Hypokalaemia may be potentiated by concomitant therapy with corticosteroids, diuretics, or xanthines; potassium concentrations should be monitored in severe asthma, where such concomitant therapy is required. Additionally, the induced hypokalaemia may provoke arrhythmias, particularly in patients receiving digoxin.

Effects on the eyes. Salbutamol and to a greater extent ritodrine have been implicated in retinopathy in the premature infant when used for premature labour.[1]

For reports of glaucoma precipitated by the combined administration of ipratropium bromide and salbutamol via a nebuliser, see Ipratropium Bromide, p.754.

1. Michie CA, *et al.* Do maternal β-sympathomimetics influence the development of retinopathy in the premature infant? *Arch Dis Child* 1994; **71:** F149.

Effects on the heart. Adverse cardiac effects with salbutamol have mainly been tachycardia due to increased sympathetic effects on the cardiovascular system. Such tachycardia has sometimes occurred in persons using inhalers[1] as well as following parenteral therapy.[2] It has been suggested that the increased metabolic demand produced by tachycardia, especially following oral β_2 agonists, might predispose to heart failure or angina in some older patients.[6]

Enhanced or additional cardiac arrhythmias have been reported in patients receiving modified-release salbutamol or terbutaline.[3] The decreased vagal (parasympathetic) stimulation, and consequently increased sympathetic dominance of cardiac function, together with a tendency to decreased baroreflex sensitivity, that may occur with $beta_2$ agonist inhalation are similar to the risk factors which predispose to ventricular tachyarrhythmias.[4] However, no clinically significant arrhythmias were seen in a study of patients given high-dose inhaled salbutamol or fenoterol.[5] As discussed under Effects on Electrolytes and Metabolism above, hypokalaemia induced by salbutamol may also lead to arrhythmias.

1. Collier JG, *et al.* Salbutamol aerosol causes a tachycardia due to the inhaled rather than the swallowed fraction. *Br J Clin Pharmacol* 1980; **9:** 273–4.
2. Johnson AJ, *et al.* Metabolic and cardiotoxic effects of salbutamol. *Br Med J* 1977; **1:** 772–3.
3. Al-Hillawi AH, *et al.* Incidence of cardiac arrhythmias in patients taking slow release salbutamol and slow release terbutaline for asthma. *Br Med J* 1984; **288:** 367.
4. Jartti T, *et al.* The acute effects of inhaled salbutamol on the beat-to-beat variability of heart rate and blood pressure assessed by spectral analysis. *Br J Clin Pharmacol* 1997; **43:** 421–8.
5. Newhouse MT, *et al.* Cardiovascular safety of high doses of inhaled fenoterol and albuterol in acute severe asthma. *Chest* 1996; **110:** 595–603.
6. Jenne JW. Can oral β_2 agonists cause heart failure? *Lancet* 1998; **352:** 1081–2.

Effects on mental function. Visual hallucinations lasting for an hour have been reported[1] following administration of nebulised salbutamol to an elderly patient. At the time of the report the manufacturers were aware of 3 cases of hallucinations in children given oral salbutamol but no such reaction had been previously reported in adults given recommended doses.

1. Khanna PB, Davies R. Hallucinations associated with the administration of salbutamol via a nebuliser. *Br Med J* 1986; **292:** 1430.

Effects on the muscles. A report on the nature and incidence of side-effects of salbutamol in 50 patients with chronic airflow obstruction who had been taking 4 mg three times daily for a year. The incidence of side-effects was: finger tremor 42%, palpitation 20%, muscle cramp 46%, and other symptoms 6%.[1]

1. Palmer KNV. Muscle cramp and oral salbutamol. *Br Med J* 1978; **2:** 833.

Effects on the respiratory system. Paradoxical bronchoconstriction has occasionally been reported following bronchodilating therapy with nebulised solutions of salbutamol and ipratropium bromide (see under Ipratropium Bromide, p.754). It has been suggested that the preservatives present in these nebuliser solutions could be responsible. In addition, regular use of salbutamol (as opposed to use on an as-needed basis) has been shown to increase airway hyperresponsiveness to various stimuli. These effects may be due specifically to the *S*-enantiomer, and it has been suggested that accumulation of this enantiomer due to stereospecific metabolism lies behind the phenomenon of tolerance (see below).

The increased risk of pulmonary oedema associated with salbutamol is mentioned under Pulmonary Oedema, below.

Increased mortality. Most of the recent attention on the increased incidence of morbidity and mortality that has occurred in asthmatic patients has concentrated on fenoterol, but salbutamol has been implicated.[1] The debate on the relevance of beta agonist therapy to this increased morbidity and mortality is discussed under Fenoterol on p.753.

1. Spitzer WO, *et al.* The use of β-agonists and the risk of death or near death from asthma. *N Engl J Med* 1992; **326:** 501–6.

Overdosage. Reports of overdosage with salbutamol[1-4] have generally only described the features that may be expected such as tachycardia, CNS stimulation, tremor, hypokalaemia, and hyperglycaemia. Symptomatic treatment of the adverse effects has proved successful. The plasma-potassium concentration and pulse rate have been found to correlate with the plasma concentration of salbutamol.[5]

1. Morrison GW, Farebrother MJB. Overdose of salbutamol. *Lancet* 1973; **ii:** 681.
2. O'Brien IAD, *et al.* Hypokalaemia due to salbutamol overdosage. *Br Med J* 1981; **282:** 1515–16.
3. Prior JG, *et al.* Self-poisoning with oral salbutamol. *Br Med J* 1981; **282:** 1932.
4. Connell JMC, *et al.* Metabolic consequences of salbutamol poisoning reversed by propranolol. *Br Med J* 1982; **285:** 779.
5. Lewis LD, *et al.* A study of self poisoning with oral salbutamol—laboratory and clinical features. *Hum Exp Toxicol* 1993; **12:** 397–401. Correction. *ibid.* 1994; **13:** 371.

Pregnancy. Most adverse effects associated with salbutamol in pregnancy relate to the cardiovascular and metabolic effects of the very high doses given by intravenous infusion in attempts to delay premature labour (see also under Pulmonary Oedema, below). Thus myocardial ischaemia on stopping an infusion[1] and unifocal ventricular ectopics associated with the hypokalaemic response to intravenous salbutamol[2] have been reported. A further report concerned congestive heart failure in a hypertensive woman.[3] Metabolic acidosis following salbutamol infusions in diabetic women has also been reported.[4,5]

1. Whitehead MI, *et al.* Myocardial ischaemia after withdrawal of salbutamol for pre-term labour. *Lancet* 1979; **ii:** 904.
2. Chew WC, Lew LC. Ventricular ectopics after salbutamol infusion for preterm labour. *Lancet* 1979; **ii:** 1383–4.
3. Whitehead MI, *et al.* Acute congestive cardiac failure in a hypertensive woman receiving salbutamol for premature labour. *Br Med J* 1980; **280:** 1221–2.

4. Chapman MG. Salbutamol-induced acidosis in pregnant diabetics. *Br Med J* 1977; **1:** 639–40.
5. Thomas DJB, *et al.* Salbutamol-induced diabetic ketoacidosis. *Br Med J* 1977; **2:** 438.

Pulmonary oedema. Pulmonary oedema has occurred in women given $beta_2$ agonists, including salbutamol,[1,2] for premature labour. The risk factors, the most important of which is fluid overload, are discussed under Precautions, below.

1. Hawker F. Pulmonary oedema associated with β_2-sympathomimetic treatment of premature labour. *Anaesth Intensive Care* 1984; **12:** 143–51.
2. Pisani RJ, Rosenow EC. Pulmonary edema associated with tocolytic therapy. *Ann Intern Med* 1989; **110:** 714–18.

Tolerance. Studies suggest that regular inhalation of a $beta_2$ agonist, although it continues to produce bronchodilatation, increases airway hyperresponsiveness and may reduce the protective effect against bronchoconstriction provoked by stimuli such as bradykinin, methacholine, or allergen.[1-6] Such tolerance is considered another argument against regular use of these agents.[1] There is some evidence that for salbutamol the effect may be due to the *S*(+)-enantiomer,[7] which unlike the *R*(−)-enantiomer does not possess bronchodilating activity: stereoselective metabolism[8,9] means that regular use of the racemate could lead to accumulation of the *S*-enantiomer, which provides a possible mechanism for the effect.

1. Cockcroft DW, *et al.* Regular inhaled salbutamol and airway responsiveness to allergen. *Lancet* 1993; **342:** 833–7.
2. O'Connor BJ, *et al.* Tolerance to the nonbronchodilator effects of inhaled β_2-agonists in asthma. *N Engl J Med* 1992; **327:** 1204–8.
3. Cheung D, *et al.* Long-term effects of a long-acting β_2-adrenoceptor agonist, salmeterol, on airway hyperresponsiveness in patients with mild asthma. *N Engl J Med* 1992; **327:** 1198–1203.
4. Cockcroft DW, *et al.* Regular use of inhaled albuterol and the allergen-induced late asthmatic response. *J Allergy Clin Immunol* 1995; **96:** 44–9.
5. Inman MD, O'Byrne PM. The effect of regular inhaled albuterol on exercise-induced bronchoconstriction. *Am J Respir Crit Care Med* 1996; **153:** 65–9.
6. Crowther SD, *et al.* Varied effects of regular salbutamol on airway responsiveness to inhaled spasmogens. *Lancet* 1997; **350:** 1450.
7. Perrin-Fayolle M. Salbutamol in the treatment of asthma. *Lancet* 1995; **346:** 1101.
8. Boulton DW, Fawcett JP. Enantioselective disposition of salbutamol in man following oral and intravenous administration. *Br J Clin Pharmacol* 1996; **41:** 35–40.
9. Eaton EA, *et al.* Stereoselective sulphate conjugation of salbutamol by human lung and bronchial epithelial cells. *Br J Clin Pharmacol* 1996; **41:** 201–6.

Precautions

Salbutamol and other $beta_2$ agonists should be given with caution in hyperthyroidism, myocardial insufficiency, arrhythmias, susceptibility to QT-interval prolongation, hypertension, and diabetes mellitus (especially on intravenous administration where blood glucose should be monitored since ketoacidosis has been reported).

In *severe asthma* particular caution is also required to avoid inducing hypokalaemia as this effect may be potentiated by hypoxia or by concomitant administration of other anti-asthma drugs (see under Interactions, below); $beta_2$ agonists such as salbutamol are not appropriate for use alone in the treatment of severe asthma (see under Asthma, p.745).

In *women being treated for premature labour* the risk of pulmonary oedema means that the patient's state of hydration and cardiac and respiratory function should be monitored very carefully; the volume of infusion fluid should be kept to the minimum (normally using glucose 5% as the diluent and avoiding sodium chloride), and $beta_2$-agonist therapy should be discontinued immediately and diuretic therapy instituted if it occurs (bearing in mind the risk of hypokalaemia with potassium-depleting diuretics). Other risk factors for pulmonary oedema include multiple pregnancy and cardiac disease, which is a specific contra-indication; where cardiac disease is suspected assessment by a physician experienced in cardiology is needed. Eclampsia and severe pre-eclampsia are also contra-indications, with special care needed in mild to moderate pre-eclampsia. Other contra-indications include intra-uterine infection, intra-uterine fetal death, antepartum haemorrhage (which requires immediate delivery), placenta praevia, and cord compression; $beta_2$ agonists should not be used for threatened abortion. See also Uses and Administration, below.

For details of the precautions to be observed with sympathomimetics in general, see p.951.

Abuse. Salbutamol inhalers have been subject to abuse, particularly by children and young adults.[1-5] This has occurred in both asthmatic and non-asthmatic individuals and has been thought to be for the effect of sympathetic stimulation and for the effect of the fluorocarbon propellants. The introduction of fluorocarbon-free inhalers should reduce the latter motivation, although not the former.

1. Brennan PO. Inhaled salbutamol: a new form of drug abuse? *Lancet* 1983; **ii:** 1030–1.
2. Thompson PJ, *et al.* Addiction to aerosol treatment: the asthmatic alternative to glue sniffing. *Br Med J* 1983; **287:** 1515–16.
3. Brennan PO. Addiction to aerosol treatment. *Br Med J* 1983; **287:** 1877.
4. Wickramasinghe H, Liebeschuetz HJ. Addiction to aerosol treatment. *Br Med J* 1983; **287:** 1877.
5. O'Callaghan C, Milner AD. Aerosol treatment abuse. *Arch Dis Child* 1988; **63:** 70.

Pregnancy. Inhalation has particular advantages as a means of administration of $beta_2$ agonists during pregnancy because the therapeutic action can be achieved without the need for plasma concentrations liable to have a pharmacological effect on the fetus.

Interactions

As mentioned under Effects on Electrolytes, above, concomitant administration of salbutamol and other $beta_2$ agonists with corticosteroids, diuretics, or xanthines increases the risk of hypokalaemia, and monitoring of potassium concentrations is recommended in severe asthma, where such combination therapy is the rule. For an outline of interactions associated with sympathomimetics in general, see p.951.

Antidepressants. For an apparent interaction between terbutaline and *toloxatone*, a reversible inhibitor of monoamine oxidase type A (RIMA) see Sympathomimetics, under Interactions of Moclobemide, p.299.

Cardiac glycosides. Hypokalaemia produced by $beta_2$ agonists may also result in an increased susceptibility to digitalis-induced arrhythmias although salbutamol intravenously and by mouth can also decrease serum concentrations of *digoxin* (see Sympathomimetics, p.852).

Corticosteroids. Corticosteroids and $beta_2$ agonists may both produce falls in plasma potassium concentrations; there is evidence that such falls can be exacerbated by concomitant administration.[1] The possibility of enhanced hyperglycaemic effects from such a combination should also be borne in mind.

1. Taylor DR, *et al.* Interaction between corticosteroid and beta-agonist drugs: biochemical and cardiovascular effects in normal subjects. *Chest* 1992; **102:** 519–24.

Diuretics. Hypokalaemia is known to be a possible side-effect during treatment with $beta_2$ agonists such as salbutamol or terbutaline, and this may be enhanced during concomitant diuretic therapy;[1,2] in addition the arrhythmogenic potential of this interaction may be clinically important in patients with ischaemic heart disease.[1]

1. Lipworth BJ, *et al.* Prior treatment with diuretic augments the hypokalemic and electrocardiographic effects of inhaled albuterol. *Am J Med* 1989; **86:** 653–7.
2. Newnham DM, *et al.* The effects of frusemide and triamterene on the hypokalaemic and electrocardiographic responses to inhaled terbutaline. *Br J Clin Pharmacol* 1991; **32:** 630–2.

Muscle relaxants. Salbutamol given intravenously has been reported to enhance the neuromuscular blockade produced by *pancuronium* and by *vecuronium*, see p.1307.

Sympathomimetics. Patients receiving *salmeterol* may require salbutamol to control an acute attack of bronchospasm. One study indicated that the effects might be additive,[1] but another demonstrated that patients receiving salmeterol had reduced sensitivity to salbutamol and might need higher doses of the latter for acute relief.[2]

1. Smyth ET, *et al.* Interaction and dose equivalence of salbutamol and salmeterol in patients with asthma. *Br Med J* 1993; **306:** 543–5.
2. Grove A, Lipworth BJ. Bronchodilator subsensitivity to salbutamol after twice daily salmeterol in asthmatic patients. *Lancet* 1995; **346:** 201–6.

Xanthines. An enhanced hypokalaemic effect may occur during coadministration of salbutamol with *theophylline*.[1,2] See also under terbutaline (p.764) and Sympathomimetics, under Interactions for theophylline (p.770) for the potentiation of other effects.

1. Whyte KF, *et al.* Salbutamol induced hypokalaemia: the effect of theophylline alone and in combination with adrenaline. *Br J Clin Pharmacol* 1988; **25:** 571–8.
2. Kolski GB, *et al.* Hypokalemia and respiratory arrest in an infant with status asthmaticus. *J Pediatr* 1988; **112:** 304–7.

Pharmacokinetics

Salbutamol is readily absorbed from the gastro-intestinal tract. It is subject to first-pass metabolism in the liver and possibly in the gut wall; the main metabolite is an inactive sulphate conjugate. It is rapidly excreted in the urine as metabolites and unchanged drug; there is some excretion in the faeces. Salbutamol does not appear to be metabolised in the lung, therefore its ultimate metabolism and excretion following inhalation depends upon the delivery method used, which determines the proportion of inhaled salbutamol relative to the proportion inadvertently swallowed. It has been suggested that the majority of an inhaled dose is swallowed and absorbed from the gut.

The plasma half-life of salbutamol has been estimated to range from 4 to 6 hours.

General references.

1. Walker SR, *et al.* The clinical pharmacology of oral and inhaled salbutamol. *Clin Pharmacol Ther* 1972; **13:** 861–7.
2. Hetzel MR, Clark TJH. Comparison of intravenous and aerosol salbutamol. *Br Med J* 1976; **2:** 919.
3. Lin C, *et al.* Isolation and identification of the major metabolite of albuterol in human urine. *Drug Metab Dispos* 1977; **5:** 234–8.
4. Morgan DJ, *et al.* Pharmacokinetics of intravenous and oral salbutamol and its sulphate conjugate. *Br J Clin Pharmacol* 1986; **22:** 587–93.
5. Lipworth BJ, *et al.* Single dose and steady-state pharmacokinetics of 4 mg and 8 mg oral salbutamol controlled-release in patients with bronchial asthma. *Eur J Clin Pharmacol* 1989; **37:** 49–52.
6. Rey E, *et al.* Pharmacokinetics of intravenous salbutamol in renal insufficiency and its biological effects. *Eur J Clin Pharmacol* 1989; **37:** 387–9.
7. Hindle M, Chrystyn H. Determination of the relative bioavailability of salbutamol to the lung following inhalation. *Br J Clin Pharmacol* 1992; **34:** 311–15.
8. Milliez JM, *et al.* Pharmacokinetics of salbutamol in the pregnant woman after subcutaneous administration with a portable pump. *Obstet Gynecol* 1992; **80:** 182–5.

Stereoselectivity. For reference to the stereoselective metabolism of salbutamol see Tolerance, under Adverse Effects, above. The *R*(−)-enantiomer of salbutamol (levosalbutamol) is preferentially metabolised and is therefore cleared from the body more rapidly than the *S*(+)-enantiomer, which largely lacks bronchodilator activity but may be implicated in some of the adverse effects of salbutamol. Some further references are given below.

1. Pacifici GM, *et al.* Interindividual variability in the rate of salbutamol sulphation in the human lung. *Eur J Clin Pharmacol* 1996 **49:** 299–303.
2. Boulton DW, *et al.* Transplacental distribution of salbutamol enantiomers at Caesarian section. *Br J Clin Pharmacol* 1997; **44:** 587–90.
3. Lipworth BJ, *et al.* Pharmacokinetics and extrapulmonary β_2 adrenoceptor activity of nebulised racemic salbutamol and its R and S isomers in healthy volunteers. *Thorax* 1997; **52:** 849–52.

Uses and Administration

Salbutamol is a direct-acting sympathomimetic with predominantly beta-adrenergic activity and a selective action on $beta_2$ receptors ($beta_2$ agonist). This preference for $beta_2$ receptor stimulation results in its bronchodilating action being more prominent than its effect on the heart.

Salbutamol and salbutamol sulphate are used as bronchodilators in the management of reversible airways obstruction, as in asthma and in some patients with chronic obstructive pulmonary disease. Salbutamol also decreases uterine contractility and may be given as the sulphate to arrest premature labour (below).

Administration by inhalation results in the rapid onset (within 5 to 15 minutes) of bronchodilatation which lasts for about 3 to 6 hours. Following administration by mouth, the onset of action is within 30 minutes, with a peak effect between 2 to 3 hours after the dose, and a duration of action of up to 8 hours; modified-release preparations have a duration of action of up to 12 hours.

Salbutamol is used as the base in aerosol inhalers and as the sulphate in other preparations. The dosage is expressed in terms of salbutamol base.

For the relief of acute **bronchospasm**, 1 or 2 inhalations of salbutamol 100 μg may be given from a metered-dose aerosol as required. Two inhalations may also be given just prior to exertion for the prophylaxis of exercise-induced bronchospasm. Current UK guidelines for the treatment of asthma (see p.745) recommend that if patients with chronic asthma need more than one dose of inhaled beta$_2$ agonist daily, then the next step is additional treatment with a corticosteroid or cromoglycate or nedocromil. However, if salbutamol were to be taken more than once daily the doses recommended by the manufacturers are 100 or 200 μg up to every 4 to 6 hours or 3 or 4 times daily. The dose for children is 100 μg which has been given up to 3 or 4 times daily.

Although salbutamol is generally inhaled in aerosol form, inhalation of the sulphate in other formulations of dry powder, such as inhalation capsules or foil blisters on a disc, may be employed by patients who experience difficulty in using the aerosol. Owing to differences in the relative bioavailability to the lungs between the dry powder systems and the inhalation aerosol a 200-μg dose (expressed in terms of salbutamol) from an inhalation capsule or disc is approximately equivalent in activity to a 100-μg dose from an aerosol and the recommended doses are therefore twice those suggested for the aerosol.

When inhalation is ineffective, salbutamol may be given by mouth in a dose of 2 to 4 mg three or four times daily as the sulphate; some patients may require doses of up to 8 mg three or four times daily, but such increased doses are unlikely to be tolerated or to provide much extra benefit. Elderly patients should be given the lower doses initially. A dose of 1 to 2 mg three or four times daily is suggested for children aged 2 to 6 years or 2 mg three of four times daily for older children. Modified-release tablets are also available; a usual adult dose is 8 mg twice daily.

In more severe or unresponsive asthma salbutamol sulphate may be given intermittently via a nebuliser in doses of 2.5 to 5 mg of salbutamol repeated up to 4 times daily; higher doses have been used. Single-dose units or a concentrated solution of salbutamol 0.5% are available for this method of administration. Continuous administration via a nebuliser is also possible, usually at a rate of 1 to 2 mg of salbutamol per hour as a 0.005 to 0.01% solution in sodium chloride 0.9%. The efficacy of nebulised salbutamol in infants under 18 months of age is uncertain. Adequate oxygenation is essential to avoid hypoxaemia.

In emergency situations where delivery via a nebuliser is not available 2 inhalations of salbutamol 100 μg can be repeated 10 to 20 times by multiple actuations of a metered-dose inhaler, preferably into a large spacer device.

In the management of a severe attack of bronchospasm a slow intravenous injection of salbutamol 250 μg as a solution containing 50 μg per mL as the sulphate may be required; alternatively salbutamol sulphate may be given by intravenous infusion of a solution containing 5 mg in 500 mL (10 μg per mL) at a usual rate of 3 to 20 μg per minute according to the patient's need; higher dosages have been used in patients with respiratory failure.

Salbutamol sulphate can also be given for bronchospasm by subcutaneous or intramuscular injection in doses of salbutamol 500 μg every 4 hours as required.

For the arrest of uncomplicated **premature labour** between 24 and 33 weeks of gestation salbutamol sulphate is given by intravenous infusion preferably with the aid of a syringe pump when the concentration should be 200 μg of salbutamol per mL, glucose 5% having been used for dilution. If no syringe pump is available then the infusion should be with a more dilute solution of 20 μg per mL with glucose 5% being used once more as the diluent. The same dose is employed as with the syringe pump. The manufacturer's recommended initial rate of infusion is 10 μg per minute increased at intervals of 10 minutes until there is a response; the rate is then increased slowly until contractions cease. The usual effective dose is 10 to 45 μg per minute. The infusion should be maintained at the rate at which contractions cease for one hour, then reduced by decrements of 50% at intervals of 6 hours. Prolonged therapy should be avoided as the risks to the mother (see Precautions, above) increase after 48 hours, and furthermore myometrial response is reduced.

The maternal pulse should be monitored throughout the infusion and the rate adjusted to avoid a maternal heart rate of more than 135 to 140 beats per minute. A close watch should also be kept on the patient's state of hydration since fluid overload is considered to be a key risk factor for pulmonary oedema.

Salbutamol may subsequently be given by mouth in a dose of 4 mg three or four times daily but such usage is no longer recommended by authorities in the UK, given the problems with prolonged therapy already mentioned.

Action. In *dogs* and *guinea-pigs R*(−)-salbutamol was much more potent than *S*(+)-salbutamol on beta-adrenergic receptors. Both *R*(−)- and *S*(+)-salbutamol showed high selectivity for beta-adrenergic receptors in bronchial muscle compared with cardiac muscle, in this way resembling racemic salbutamol.[1] The *S*-enantiomer has been reported to have no significant effects at extrapulmonary beta$_2$-receptors in healthy subjects.[2]

For the suggestion that the *S*(+)-enantiomer may play a role in some of the adverse effects associated with salbutamol, see Tolerance, under Adverse Effects, above. The *R*(−)-enantiomer levosalbutamol (levalbuterol) is being tried as an alternative to racemic salbutamol.

1. Brittain RT, *et al.* Some observations on the β-adrenoceptor agonist properties of the isomers of salbutamol. *Br J Pharmacol* 1973; **48:** 144–7.
2. Clark DJ, *et al.* Extrapulmonary β$_2$-adrenoceptor activity of nebulised racemic salbutamol and its R and S isomers. *Br J Clin Pharmacol* 1997; **43:** 529P–30P.

Administration. Beta$_2$-adrenoceptor stimulants (beta$_2$ agonists) are used extensively in the management of reversible airways obstruction. A common, effective, and convenient method of administration is by a pressurised aerosol inhaler. With this route of administration relief is provided rapidly and fewer systemic side-effects are likely to occur than with oral administration. It is important that patients using these inhalers employ the correct technique which involves coordinating actuation of the aerosol with inhalation. If patients have difficulty with correct technique, alternatives are available. Spacing devices may be used with inhalers. These are added on to the inhaler and reduce the velocity of the aerosol; also more propellant may evaporate before inhalation allowing a greater proportion of the drug to reach the lungs, and coordination of actuation of the aerosol and inhalation is less important. Inhalers of dry powder are also available and are actuated by the patient's inspiration and thus avoid entirely the need for coordination of actuation and inhalation; however, inhalation of the dry powder has occasionally caused irritation of the throat or coughing. The oral route can be employed although generally a form of inhaled therapy as described above is preferable. A variety of formulations intended for oral administration is commercially available and often includes modified-release formulations. Nebulisation of these drugs is an alternative method of delivery and this may be used in the management of severe acute attacks as may parenteral therapy.

Asthma. Short-acting beta$_2$ agonists such as salbutamol form the initial therapy of chronic as well as acute asthma (p.745). High doses are used in acute asthma and current recommendations for chronic asthma are for low doses to be inhaled as required rather than regularly. Should the patient find that more than one dose is required daily, then that should be a sign for additional treatment with other anti-asthma drugs. It has been reported that regular salbutamol provided better control than taking it as required,[1] but others have not found this to be the case;[2] any benefit might be proportional to the severity of disease,[3] and whether regular use of short-acting beta$_2$ agonists helps patients with severe asthma requires more study.[4] The discussion on p.753 on the increased mortality that has been observed in asthma patients and the connection with asthma therapy includes a view that regular administration might have contributed to the increased mortality.

1. Chapman KR, *et al.* Regular vs as-needed inhaled salbutamol in asthma control. *Lancet* 1994; **343:** 1379–82.
2. Drazen JM, *et al.* Comparison of regularly scheduled with as-needed use of albuterol in mild asthma. *N Engl J Med* 1996; **335:** 841–7.
3. O'Byrne PM, Kerstjens HAM. Inhaled β$_2$-agonists in the treatment of asthma. *N Engl J Med* 1996; **335:** 886–8.
4. Anonymous. Using β$_2$-stimulants in asthma. *Drug Ther Bull* 1997; **35:** 1–4.

Bronchiolitis. Acute bronchiolitis (inflammation of the bronchioles associated with viral respiratory tract infection, usually due to respiratory syncytial virus—see p.602) is a poorly defined respiratory condition seen in children. The diagnostic criteria, and the usual management, vary considerably from country to country. Beta$_2$ agonists such as salbutamol are widely prescribed in the USA, but not in the UK, and attempts to establish their benefits have produced conflicting results.[1] Modest benefit (but no difference in hospital admission rate) has been reported from one meta-analysis of bronchodilator therapy in general,[2] but a meta-analysis of beta$_2$ agonists therapy in bronchiolitis did not show it to be effective.[5] A comparative study has suggested that nebulised adrenaline is more effective than salbutamol,[3] and a recent study in hospitalised children found no benefit from nebulised salbutamol in terms of improved oxygenation or length of hospital stay.[4]

1. Everard ML. Acute bronchiolitis—a perennial problem. *Lancet* 1996; **348:** 279–80.
2. Kellner JD, *et al.* Efficacy of bronchodilator therapy in bronchiolitis: a meta-analysis. *Arch Pediatr Adolesc Med* 1996; **150:** 1166–72.
3. Reijonen T, *et al.* The clinical efficacy of nebulized racemic epinephrine and albuterol in acute bronchiolitis. *Arch Pediatr Adolesc Med* 1995; **149:** 686–92.
4. Dobson JV, *et al.* The use of albuterol in hospitalized infants with bronchiolitis. *Pediatrics* 1998; **101:** 361–8.
5. Flores G, Horwitz RI. Efficacy of β$_2$-agonists in bronchiolitis: a reappraisal and meta-analysis. *Pediatrics* 1997; **100:** 233–9.

Chronic obstructive pulmonary disease. Salbutamol and other beta$_2$ agonist bronchodilators form part of the first-line treatment of chronic obstructive pulmonary disease, although, as discussed on p.747, there is some evidence that an inhaled quaternary ammonium antimuscarinic, such as ipratropium bromide, may have slight advantages compared with a beta$_2$ agonist.

Cough. For a study indicating that inhaled salbutamol was ineffective in the treatment of children with recurrent cough, see under Beclomethasone, p.1033.

Hyperkalaemia. The treatment of hyperkalaemia (p.1149) is usually with calcium to reverse cardiac toxicity, and insulin and sodium bicarbonate to promote intracellular potassium uptake. Salbutamol can also lower plasma-potassium concentrations by promoting intracellular uptake,[2,4] and this effect has been used in treating mild hyperkalaemia associated with chronic disorders such as renal failure[3,5] and hyperkalaemic periodic paralysis.[1] However, such use is controversial: some clinicians prefer to avoid the use of beta$_2$ agonists because of fears that large doses may induce cardiac arrhythmias.[6]

1. Wang P, Clausen T. Treatment of attacks in hyperkalaemic familial periodic paralysis by inhalation of salbutamol. *Lancet* 1976; **i:** 221–3.
2. Bushe C. Salbutamol for hyperkalaemia. *Lancet* 1983; **ii:** 797.
3. Allon M, *et al.* Nebulized albuterol for acute hyperkalemia in patients on hemodialysis. *Ann Intern Med* 1989; **110:** 426–9.
4. Anonymous. Hyperkalaemia—silent and deadly. *Lancet* 1989; **i:** 1240.
5. McClure RJ, *et al.* Treatment of hyperkalaemia using intravenous and nebulised salbutamol. *Arch Dis Child* 1994; **70:** 126–8.
6. Halperin ML. Kamel KS. Potassium. *Lancet* 1998; **352:** 135–40.

Premature labour. Premature labour (preterm labour) is the onset of labour before the expected date, resulting in delivery of an immature infant. Conventionally the definition has included women giving birth before 37 weeks gestation but in practice most problems arise with births before 34 weeks or when the baby's birth-weight is less than 1.5 kg.[1]

A diagnosis of premature labour is not always easy to make and evidence of cervical change should usually be present in addition to uterine activity.[2,3] Once a diagnosis has been established, a decision must be made as to whether labour should be allowed to continue or whether drug therapy to inhibit uterine contractions (tocolysis) is indicated. It may not be considered appropriate to stop labour in some women. However, in patients of less than about 28 to 32 weeks gestation without complications, attempts to stop labour are usually worth trying, if only in the short-term, to allow emergency treatment such as corticosteroids to be given to the mother to enhance the maturation of the fetal respiratory system and to enable the patient to be transferred to a specialised unit for preterm delivery.[1-4] Tocolysis is rarely considered necessary after 34 weeks gestation, provided adequate neonatal support facilities are available.[3]

The commonest tocolytic agents are the beta-adrenoceptor agonists that relax the smooth muscle of the uterus by stimulation of beta$_2$-adrenoceptors.[3] Nonselective agonists, for example orciprenaline and isoxsuprine, have largely been replaced by beta-adrenoceptor stimulants that have a more selective action on the beta$_2$ receptors (beta$_2$ agonists) such as ritodrine and salbutamol.[3] These can postpone labour for a few days and the preferred route for starting treatment is intravenous infusion.[3] Oral maintenance therapy with beta$_2$ agonists after successful treatment of an episode of acute premature labour produces no further benefit.[5] There is little evidence that beta$_2$ agonists significantly reduce perinatal mortality rates.[6] The patient may experience adverse cardiovascular and metabolic effects and, in particular, pulmonary oedema has been reported in some women given $beta_2$ agonists intravenously to suppress labour (see p.1625). It is therefore essential that the patient's heart rate and state of hydration are carefully monitored throughout administration. In the event of caesarean section beta blockers may be needed to combat an increased tendency to uterine bleeding.

Magnesium salts have been given intravenously and by mouth as tocolytic agents, though their precise mode of action is unclear.[3] An intravenous infusion of magnesium sulphate can be given for the initial suppression of uterine contractions and is considered to have similar efficacy to treatment with a $beta_2$-agonist.[7,8] It has, however, been suggested that tocolytic use of magnesium may be associated with increased paediatric mortality—see p.1159. Plasma-magnesium concentrations should be monitored during therapy.[3]

Prostaglandins have a role in the induction of labour as mediators of uterine contractions and cervical softening and dilatation. Cyclo-oxygenase (prostaglandin-synthetase) inhibitors such as indomethacin have therefore been given by mouth or rectally to inhibit premature labour.[3] Although this treatment is as effective as ritodrine,[9,10] a number of adverse effects on the fetus have been reported, such as transient constriction of the ductus arteriosus,[11,12] pulmonary hypertension,[10] bronchopulmonary dysplasia,[13] oligohydramnios (a deficiency in amniotic fluid volume),[10,12] and fatal renal toxicity.[14] A retrospective study suggested that antenatal indomethacin therapy for premature labour increased the risk of serious neonatal complications in infants born at or before 30 weeks' gestation,[15] though conflicting results have also been reported.[9] Indomethacin is therefore generally reserved as a second line agent or given in conjunction with intravenous tocolytic therapy for an additive effect in patients at very early gestation (less than 28 weeks).[3] Sulindac, a cyclo-oxygenase inhibitor which seems to have little placental transfer, may reduce the incidence of fetal side-effects.[16] More recently it has been argued that the enzyme isoform cyclo-oxygenase-2 is associated with labour, while cyclo-oxygenase-1 is responsible for constant prostaglandin synthesis in body tissues. The selective cyclo-oxygenase-2 inhibitor nimesulide is under investigation for its potential in the prevention of premature labour.[17]

Other tocolytic agents under investigation are the calcium-channel blockers. These suppress the influx of calcium ions across the cell membrane resulting in a reduction in the intracellular concentration of free calcium which inhibits smooth muscle contraction.[3] Initial studies with nifedipine administered by mouth or sublingually have been promising; it appears to be at least as effective as a $beta_2$ agonist in suppressing premature labour and may have fewer adverse effects.[18,19] Similar results have been reported with nicardipine.[20] Beneficial preliminary results have also been reported following the application of patches of the nitric oxide donor glyceryl trinitrate to the abdomen which resulted in uterine relaxation.[21] The oxytocin antagonist atosiban has also been reported to be effective.[22]

The use of alcohol or progestogens as tocolytic agents is now obsolete.[1,3]

1. Chamberlain G. Preterm labour. *Br Med J* 1991; **303:** 44–8.
2. Steer PJ. Premature labour. *Arch Dis Child* 1991; **66:** 1167–70.
3. Johnson P. Suppression of preterm labour: current concepts. *Drugs* 1993; **45:** 684–92.
4. Report of a Joint Working Group of the British Association of Perinatal Medicine and the Research Unit of the Royal College of Physicians. Development of audit measures and guidelines for good practice in the management of neonatal respiratory distress syndrome. *Arch Dis Child* 1992; **67:** 1221–7.
5. Macones GA, *et al.* Efficacy of oral beta-agonist maintenance therapy in preterm labor: a meta-analysis. *Obstet Gynecol* 1995; **85:** 313–17.
6. The Canadian Preterm Labor Investigators Group. Treatment of preterm labor with the beta-adrenergic agonist ritodrine. *N Engl J Med* 1992; **327:** 308–12.
7. Wilkins IA, *et al.* Efficacy and side effects of magnesium sulfate and ritodrine as tocolytic agents. *Am J Obstet Gynecol* 1988; **159:** 685–9.
8. Ridgway LE, *et al.* A prospective randomized comparison of oral terbutaline and magnesium oxide for the maintenance of tocolysis. *Am J Obstet Gynecol* 1990; **163:** 879–82.
9. Morales WJ, *et al.* Efficacy and safety of indomethacin versus ritodrine in the management of preterm labor: a randomized study. *Obstet Gynecol* 1989; **74:** 567–72.
10. Besinger RE, *et al.* Randomized comparative trial of indomethacin and ritodrine for the long-term treatment of preterm labor. *Am J Obstet Gynecol* 1991; **164:** 981–8.
11. Moise KJ, *et al.* Indomethacin in the treatment of premature labor: effects on the fetal ductus arteriosus. *N Engl J Med* 1988; **319:** 327–31.
12. Hallak M, *et al.* Indomethacin for preterm labor: fetal toxicity in dizygotic twin gestation. *Obstet Gynecol* 1991; **78:** 911–13.
13. Eronen M, *et al.* Increased incidence of bronchopulmonary dysplasia after antenatal administration of indomethacin to prevent preterm labor. *J Pediatr* 1994; **124:** 782–8.
14. Van der Heijden BJ, *et al.* Persistent anuria, neonatal death, and renal microcystic lesions after prenatal exposure to indomethacin. *Am J Obstet Gynecol* 1994; **171:** 617–23.
15. Norton ME, *et al.* Neonatal complications after the administration of indomethacin for preterm labor. *N Engl J Med* 1993; **329:** 1602–7.
16. Carlan SJ, *et al.* Randomized comparative trial of indomethacin and sulindac for the treatment of refractory preterm labor. *Obstet Gynecol* 1992; **79:** 223–8.
17. Sawdy R, *et al.* Use of cyclo-oxygenase type-2-selective non-steroidal anti-inflammatory agent to prevent preterm delivery. *Lancet* 1997; **350:** 265–6.
18. Read MK, Wellby DE. The use of a calcium antagonist (nifedipine) to suppress preterm labour. *Br J Obstet Gynaecol* 1986; **93:** 933–7.
19. Ferguson JE, *et al.* A comparison of tocolysis with nifedipine or ritodrine: analysis of efficacy and maternal, fetal, and neonatal outcome. *Am J Obstet Gynecol* 1990; **163:** 105–11.
20. Jannet D, *et al.* Nicardipine versus salbutamol in the treatment of premature labor: a prospective randomized study. *Eur J Obstet Gynecol Reprod Biol* 1997; **73:** 11–16.
21. Lees C, *et al.* Arrest of preterm labour and prolongation of gestation with glyceryl trinitrate, a nitric oxide donor. *Lancet* 1994; **343:** 1325–6.
22. Goodwin TM, *et al.* Dose ranging study of the oxytocin antagonist atosiban in the treatment of preterm labor. *Obstet Gynecol* 1996; **88:** 331–6.

Proctalgia fugax. Inhalation of salbutamol from a metered-dose inhaler at the beginning of an attack has been shown to reduce the duration of pain in patients with proctalgia fugax.[1]

1. Eckardt VF, *et al.* Treatment of proctalgia fugax with salbutamol inhalation. *Am J Gastroenterol* 1996; **91:** 686–9.

Preparations

BP 1998: Salbutamol Injection; Salbutamol Pressurised Inhalation; Salbutamol Tablets;
USP 23: Albuterol Tablets.

Proprietary Preparations (details are given in Part 3)
Aust.: Astec; Epaq; Sultanol; Zaperin; ***Austral.:*** Asmol; Respax; Respolin; Ventolin; ***Belg.:*** Airomir; Salomol†; Ventolin; ***Canad.:*** Apo-Salvent; Asmavent; Novo-Salmol; Ventodisk; Ventolin; Volmax†; ***Fr.:*** Eolene†; Salbumol; Spreor; Ventodisks; Ventoline; ***Ger.:*** Apsomol; Arubendol; Asthma-Spray; Broncho Inhalat; Broncho Spray; Epaq; Loftan; Salbu; Salbuhexal; Salbulair; Salmundin; Salvent; Sultanol; Volmac; ***Irl.:*** Aerolin; Airomir; Gerivent; Salomol; Steri-Neb Salamol; Ventamol; Ventodisks; Ventolin; ***Ital.:*** Aerotec; Broncovaleas; Salbufax; Salbutard; Ventolin; Volmax; ***Neth.:*** Aerolin; Airomir; Ventolin; ***Norw.:*** Airomir; Salbuvent; Ventoline; ***S.Afr.:*** Abbutamol†; Airomir; Asthavent; Breatheze; Bronchospray; Salbulin; Venteze; Ventimax; Ventodisk; Ventolin; Viavent; Volmax; ***Spain:*** Buto Asma; Dipulmin; Emican; Ventadur; Ventolin; ***Swed.:*** Airomir; Buventol; Inspiryl; Ventoline; ***Switz.:*** Airomir; Asmaxen†; Butohaler; Butovent; Ecovent; Servitamol; Ventodisk; Ventolin; Volmax; ***UK:*** Aerolin; Airomir; Asmasal; Asmaven; Cyclocaps†; Libetist; Maxivent; Rimasal; Salamol; Salbulin; Salbuvent†; Ventodisks; Ventolin; Volmax; ***USA:*** Airet; Proventil; Ventolin; Volmax.

Multi-ingredient: ***Aust.:*** Combivent; Di-Promal; Duospirel; Ventide; ***Canad.:*** Combivent; ***Fr.:*** Combivent; Ventide†; ***Irl.:*** Combivent; ***Ital.:*** Breva; Clenil Compositum; Perventil†; Ventolin Espettorante; Ventolin Flogo; Zarent; ***S.Afr.:*** Combivent; ***Spain:*** Aerosoma†; Butosol; Respiroma; ***Switz.:*** Dospir; Ventolin plus†; ***UK:*** Aerocrom; Combivent; Ventide; ***USA:*** Combivent.

Salmeterol Xinafoate (18680-t)

Salmeterol Xinafoate *(BANM, USAN, rINNM).*

GR-33343G; Salmaterol Xinafoate; Salmeterol 1-Hydroxy-2-naphthoate. (*RS*)-5-{1-Hydroxy-2-[6-(4-phenylbutoxy)hexylamino]ethyl}salicyl alcohol 1-hydroxy-2-naphthoate.

$C_{25}H_{37}NO_4,C_{11}H_8O_3 = 603.7.$

CAS — 89365-50-4 (salmeterol); 94749-08-3 (salmeterol xinafoate).

Adverse Effects and Precautions

As for Salbutamol Sulphate, p.758. Inhalation of salmeterol may be associated with paradoxical bronchospasm.

Salmeterol is not appropriate for the treatment of acute bronchospasm or for patients whose asthma is deteriorating.

Effects on the respiratory system. Transient paradoxical bronchoconstriction with breathlessness, wheeze, or cough has been reported in 6 asthmatic patients following inhalation of salmeterol from a metered-dose aerosol but not after inhalation of the dry powder formulation by diskhaler.[1] The fluorocarbon propellants in the metered-dose aerosol were suspected as the irritants causing bronchoconstriction.

1. Wilkinson JRW, *et al.* Paradoxical bronchoconstriction in asthmatic patients after salmeterol by metered dose inhaler. *Br Med J* 1992; **305:** 931–2.

Effects on the skin. A case has been reported in which an urticarial rash was demonstrated to be associated with inhaled salmeterol and in which the propellant as a cause was excluded. Although many urticarial reactions and a variety of rashes had been attributed to beta-agonist therapy their reproducibility had not always been documented.[1]

1. Hatton MQF, *et al.* Salmeterol rash. *Lancet* 1991; **337:** 1169–70.

Tolerance. As with other $beta_2$ agonists (see p.759) there is evidence that regular use of salmeterol produces tachyphylaxis to its protective effect against bronchoconstriction, as provoked by stimuli such as allergen, methacholine, or exercise.[1-4] This is perhaps more of a concern with salmeterol, since, unlike the short-acting $beta_2$ agonists, its use on a regular basis is recommended. However, there is little evidence at present that symptomatic relief, that is, bronchodilator effect in patients who develop bronchospasm, is significantly reduced by regular use of $beta_2$ agonists, or that patients using salmeterol are at increased risk of severe (near fatal) attacks,[5] despite a suggestion that receptor downregulation induced by regular salmeterol might mean that patients required higher doses of inhaled salbutamol to attain relief from an acute asthma attack[6] (see also Sympathomimetics, under Interactions of Salbutamol, p.759).

1. Cheung D, *et al.* Long-term effects of a long-acting β_2-adrenoceptor agonist, salmeterol, on airway hyperresponsiveness in patients with mild asthma. *N Engl J Med* 1992; **327:** 1198–1203.
2. Bhagat R, *et al.* Rapid onset of tolerance to the bronchoprotective effect of salmeterol. *Chest* 1995; **108:** 1235–9.
3. Booth H, *et al.* Salmeterol tachyphylaxis in steroid treated asthmatic subjects. *Thorax* 1996; **51:** 1100–4.
4. Simons FER, *et al.* Tolerance to the bronchoprotective effect of salmeterol in adolescents with exercise-induced asthma using concurrent inhaled glucocorticoid treatment. *Pediatrics* 1997; **99:** 655–9.
5. Williams C, *et al.* Case-control study of salmeterol and near-fatal attacks of asthma. *Thorax* 1998; **53:** 7–13.
6. Lipworth B, Grove A. Bronchodilation subsensitivity to salbutamol after salmeterol. *Lancet* 1995; **346:** 968–9.

Interactions

As for Salbutamol Sulphate, p.759.

For a study suggesting a decreased effect of salbutamol in patients receiving salmeterol, as well as a report of additive effects, see p.759.

Pharmacokinetics

The manufacturers report that at therapeutic inhalation doses plasma concentrations of salmeterol are negligible.

Uses and Administration

Salmeterol is a direct-acting sympathomimetic with beta-adrenoceptor stimulant activity and a selective action on $beta_2$ receptors ($beta_2$ agonist). It has actions and uses similar to those of salbutamol (p.759).

When given by oral inhalation, salmeterol acts as a bronchodilator. The onset of action is about 10 to 20 minutes but the full effect may not be apparent until after regular administration of several doses. Salmeterol is therefore not suitable for the symptomatic relief of an acute attack of bronchospasm. However, it is long-acting with a duration of action of about 12 hours and is indicated where the regular administration of a long-acting $beta_2$ agonist is required for persistent reversible airways obstruction, as in chronic asthma or in some patients with chronic obstructive pulmonary disease. It may be useful in protecting against nocturnal and exercise-induced asthma attacks.

Salmeterol is employed in the form of the xinafoate (1-hydroxy-2-naphthoate); doses are expressed in terms of the equivalent amount of salmeterol.

The usual dose is two inhalations of salmeterol 25 μg twice daily from a metered-dose aerosol; if necessary, up to 100 μg may be inhaled twice daily. Alternatively, a dry powder inhalation of 50 μg, or if necessary 100 μg, twice daily may be used. Children of 4 years and over may be given 50 μg of salmeterol twice daily by inhalation.

Reviews.

1. Brogden RN, Faulds D. Salmeterol xinafoate: a review of its pharmacological properties and therapeutic potential in reversible obstructive airways disease. *Drugs* 1991; **42:** 895–912.
2. Meyer JM, *et al.* Salmeterol: a novel, long-acting $beta_2$-agonist. *Ann Pharmacother* 1993; **27:** 1478–87.
3. Bennett J, Tattersfield A. Drugs in focus: 15. Salmeterol. *Prescribers' J* 1995; **35:** 84–8.
4. Adkins JC, McTavish D. Salmeterol: a review of its pharmacological properties and clinical efficacy in the management of children with asthma. *Drugs* 1997; **54:** 331–54.

Asthma. Salmeterol is a long-acting $beta_2$ agonist (duration of action about 12 hours). Guidelines on the management of asthma, see p.745, generally recommend that the use of salmeterol be reserved for patients with chronic asthma who have already progressed to inhaled corticosteroids; it is not a substitute for corticosteroids. It may also be useful in controlling persistent nocturnal asthma or preventing exercise-induced attacks.

References.

1. Twentyman OP, *et al.* Protection against allergen-induced asthma by salmeterol. *Lancet* 1990; **336:** 1338–42.

2. Fitzpatrick MF, *et al.* Salmeterol in nocturnal asthma: a double blind, placebo controlled trial of a long acting inhaled β_2 agonist. *Br Med J* 1990; **301:** 1365–8.
3. Pearlman DS, *et al.* A comparison of salmeterol with albuterol in the treatment of mild-to-moderate asthma. *N Engl J Med* 1992; **327:** 1420–5.
4. Green CP, Price JF. Prevention of exercise induced asthma by inhaled salmeterol xinafoate. *Arch Dis Child* 1992; **67:** 1014–17.
5. Smyth ET, *et al.* Interaction and dose equivalence of salbutamol and salmeterol in patients with asthma. *Br Med J* 1993; **306:** 543–5.
6. Castle W, *et al.* Serevent nationwide surveillance study: comparison of salmeterol with salbutamol in asthmatic patients who require regular bronchodilator treatment. *Br Med J* 1993; **306:** 1034–7.
7. D'Alonzo GE, *et al.* Salmeterol xinafoate as maintenance therapy compared with albuterol in patients with asthma. *JAMA* 1994; **271:** 1412–16.
8. Greening AP, *et al.* Added salmeterol versus higher-dose corticosteroid in asthma patients with symptoms on existing inhaled corticosteroid. *Lancet* 1994; **344:** 219–24.
9. Mann RD. Results of prescription event monitoring study of salmeterol. *Br Med J* 1994; **309:** 1018.
10. Woolcock A, *et al.* Comparison of addition of salmeterol to inhaled steroids with doubling of the dose of inhaled steroids. *Am J Respir Crit Care Med* 1996; **153:** 1481–8.
11. Wilding P, *et al.* Effect of long term treatment with salmeterol on asthma control: a double blind, randomised crossover study. *Br Med J* 1997; **314:** 1441–6.

Chronic obstructive pulmonary disease. Short-acting beta$_2$ agonists are used as bronchodilators in patients with chronic obstructive pulmonary disease (see p.747), although there is some evidence to suggest that an antimuscarinic might be preferable. However the role, if any, of long-acting beta$_2$ agonists such as salmeterol, remains to be clearly established. Improvement in lung function and symptoms has been seen in such patients following regular treatment with inhaled salmeterol,[1] and some consider that long-acting beta$_2$ agonists may have a role in maintenance, particularly for nocturnal symptoms.[2]

1. Boyd G, *et al.* An evaluation of salmeterol in the treatment of chronic obstructive pulmonary disease (COPD). *Eur Respir J* 1997; **10:** 815–21.
2. Leuenberger P, *et al.* Management 1997 of chronic obstructive pulmonary disease. *Schweiz Med Wochenschr* 1997; **127:** 766–82.

Preparations

Proprietary Preparations (details are given in Part 3)
Aust.: Serevent; ***Austral.:*** Serevent; ***Belg.:*** Serevent; ***Canad.:*** Serevent; ***Fr.:*** Serevent; ***Ger.:*** Aeromax; Serevent; ***Irl.:*** Serevent; ***Ital.:*** Arial; Salmetedur; Serevent; ***Neth.:*** Serevent; ***Norw.:*** Serevent; ***S.Afr.:*** Serevent; ***Spain:*** Beglan; Betamican; Inaspir; Serevent; ***Swed.:*** Serevent; ***Switz.:*** Serevent; ***UK:*** Serevent; ***USA:*** Serevent.

Seratrodast (17446-n)

Seratrodast (*USAN, rINN*).

A-73001; AA-2414; Abbott-73001; ABT-001. (±)-2,4,5-Trimethyl-3,6-dioxo-ζ-phenyl-1,4-cyclohexadiene-1-heptanoic acid.

$C_{22}H_{26}O_4$ = 354.4.

CAS — 112665-43-7; 103186-19-2.

Seratrodast is a thromboxane A$_2$-antagonist that is reported to reduce airway hyperresponsiveness. It is given by mouth in the prophylactic management of asthma (p.745), in single doses of 80 mg in the evening after food.

Adverse effects include gastro-intestinal disturbances, drowsiness, headache, and palpitations; the drug should be withdrawn if hypersensitivity reactions such as rashes and pruritus occur, or if there is elevation of liver enzyme values. Seratrodast should be used with care in patients with pre-existing hepatic impairment. It is not suitable for the treatment of an acute asthmatic attack.

Preparations

Proprietary Preparations (details are given in Part 3)
Jpn: Bronica.

Sodium Cromoglycate (7721-e)

Sodium Cromoglycate (*BANM*).

Sodium Cromoglicate (*rINNM*); Cromolyn Sodium (*USAN*); Disodium Cromoglycate; FPL-670; Natrii Cromoglicas. Disodium 4,4′-dioxo-5,5′-(2-hydroxytrimethylenedioxy)di(4*H*-chromene-2-carboxylate).

$C_{23}H_{14}Na_2O_{11}$ = 512.3.

CAS — 16110-51-3 (cromoglycic acid); 15826-37-6 (sodium cromoglycate).

Pharmacopoeias. In *Chin., Eur.* (see p.viii), *Int., Jpn,* and *US.*

A white or almost white, odourless, hygroscopic, crystalline powder, tasteless at first with a slightly bitter after-taste. **Soluble** in water; practically insoluble in alcohol, in chloroform, and in ether. **Store** in airtight containers. Protect from light.

Adverse Effects

Sodium cromoglycate is generally well tolerated and side-effects are often transient.

Inhalation may cause transient bronchospasm, wheezing, cough, nasal congestion, and irritation of the throat. Nausea, headache, dizziness, an unpleasant taste, and joint pain and swelling have been reported. Other reactions, which have sometimes occurred after treatment for several weeks or months, include aggravation of existing asthma, urticaria, rashes, pulmonary infiltrates with eosinophilia, dysuria, and urinary frequency. Severe reactions such as bronchospasm, laryngeal oedema, angioedema, and anaphylaxis have been reported rarely; these have sometimes been referred to as pseudo-allergic.

Intranasal use of sodium cromoglycate may cause transient irritation of the nasal mucosa, sneezing, and occasionally epistaxis. Nausea, skin rashes, and joint pains have occurred when it is taken by mouth. Transient burning and stinging have occasionally been reported following use of sodium cromoglycate eye drops.

Formulation. Some of the adverse effects reported with sodium cromoglycate may be due to its formulation: there is a view that some of the irritant effects reported on inhalation may be due to the use of dry powder inhalers. It has also been suggested that in some patients receiving sodium cromoglycate via a nebuliser, hypotonicity of the nebuliser solution may induce bronchospasm,[1] although others consider this debatable.[2] In the UK a high viscosity preparation of sodium cromoglycate containing hypromellose was withdrawn by the manufacturer due to an unacceptable incidence of ocular adverse effects.[3]

1. Chin TW, Nussbaum E. Detrimental effect of hypotonic cromolyn sodium. *J Pediatr* 1992; **120:** 641–3.
2. Rachelefsky GS, *et al.* Detrimental effects of hypotonic cromolyn sodium. *J Pediatr* 1992; **121:** 992.
3. Anonymous. *Pharm J* 1989; **243:** 411.

Precautions

Although sodium cromoglycate is used in the prophylaxis of asthma it has no role in the treatment of acute asthmatic attacks. Withdrawal of sodium cromoglycate may lead to recurrence of the symptoms of asthma. Should withdrawal be necessary it has been suggested that the dose be reduced gradually over a period of one week; patients in whom sodium cromoglycate therapy has permitted a reduction of corticosteroid dosage may require restoration of full steroid cover.

Systemic corticosteroid therapy that has been reduced or discontinued in asthmatic patients may need to be reinstated if symptoms increase, during periods of stress such as infection, illness, trauma, or severe antigen challenge, or where airways obstruction impairs inhalation of sodium cromoglycate.

Nausea, bloating, abdominal cramps, and flatulence developed in a 24-year-old lactase-deficient woman 2 hours after the use of Intal (sodium cromoglycate) via a turbo-haler for exercise-induced asthma.[1] These symptoms recurred on rechallenge and were attributed to ingestion of lactose contained within the Intal capsules.

1. Brandstetter RD, *et al.* Lactose intolerance associated with Intal capsules. *N Engl J Med* 1986; **315:** 1613–14.

Pharmacokinetics

Sodium cromoglycate is poorly absorbed from the gastro-intestinal tract, with a reported bioavailability of only 1%. It has been reported that following inhalation as a fine powder only 8 to 10% of a dose is deposited in the lungs from where it is rapidly absorbed and excreted unchanged in the urine and bile. Less than 7% of an intranasal dose appears to be absorbed. The majority of an inhaled or an intranasal dose is swallowed and excreted unchanged in the faeces. Approximately 0.03% of an ophthalmic dose is reported to be absorbed. The elimination half-life has been reported to be about 20 to 60 minutes following intravenous administration, but the elimination half-life following oral administration or inhalation is longer, being stated to be about 80 minutes.

The existence of a relationship between plasma concentrations of sodium cromoglycate and its protective effect in asthma has been investigated. Patel *et al.*[1] assessed the protective effect of sodium cromoglycate in patients with exercise-induced asthma following 2, 10, and 20 mg by aerosol and 12 mg by nebuliser. They concluded that, although measurement of plasma concentration allowed comparison of different methods of inhalation, plasma concentration was almost certainly not related directly to protective effect. In a study in asthmatic children given sodium cromoglycate by dry-powder inhalation, Yahav *et al.*[2] found both blood concentration and clinical response to be correlated with inhalation technique.

1. Patel KR, *et al.* Plasma concentrations of sodium cromoglycate given by nebulisation and metered dose inhalers in patients with exercise-induced asthma: relationship to protective effect. *Br J Clin Pharmacol* 1986; **21:** 231–3.
2. Yahav Y, *et al.* Sodium cromoglycate in asthma: correlation between response and serum concentrations. *Arch Dis Child* 1988; **63:** 592–7.

Uses and Administration

Sodium cromoglycate is used for the prevention of allergic reactions. Although its precise mode of action remains uncertain, it is believed to act primarily by preventing release of mediators of inflammation from sensitised mast cells through stabilisation of mast-cell membranes. It has no intrinsic antihistaminic action and has generally been considered to possess no bronchodilator activity.

Sodium cromoglycate can prevent the asthmatic response to a variety of allergic and non-allergic stimuli. It is used in the management of chronic asthma for patients who cannot be managed with inhaled beta$_2$ agonists alone; it is not used for acute attacks including acute severe asthma (status asthmaticus).

Sodium cromoglycate is also used in the prophylaxis and treatment of seasonal and perennial allergic rhinitis and allergic conditions of the eye including acute and chronic allergic conjunctivitis and vernal keratoconjunctivitis. It has been given by mouth for the prevention of food allergies, in conjunction with dietary restriction, and is also used in the treatment of mastocytosis.

It is important that the regular administration of sodium cromoglycate is maintained both in the prophylactic control of asthma and in the management of other allergic conditions. Beneficial effects may take several weeks to become established.

In the prophylaxis of asthma, sodium cromoglycate is administered by inhalation either as a dry powder, or as a nebulised solution, or from a metered aerosol. The usual dose as dry powder or nebulised solution is 20 mg by inhalation 4 times daily increased, if necessary, to 6 or, for the powder, even to 8 times daily. Once the asthma has been stabilised it may be possible to reduce the dosage. The usual dose by aerosol in the UK is 10 mg four times daily, increased to 6 to 8 times daily if necessary; it may be possible to reduce the dosage to 5 mg four times daily once the asthma has been stabilised. Doses are administered from metered aerosols providing units of 5 mg. However, aerosols providing units of about 1 mg are also available in some countries and doses of about 2 mg four times daily have been used. The adequacy of this low dosage has been questioned (see under Administration, below) and in the UK the manufacturers have discontinued the 1-mg aerosol.

Inhalation of sodium cromoglycate may cause bronchospasm but incorporation of a beta$_2$ agonist such as salbutamol into the inhalation preparation is not recommended as the inhalation is liable to be used inappropriately for relief of bronchospasm rather than for its prophylactic effect. Separate inhalation of the beta$_2$ agonist a few minutes beforehand is preferable.

For the prophylaxis of allergic rhinitis, approximately 2.5 or 5 mg as a 2 or 4% solution is administered as drops or spray into each nostril up to 6 times daily or 10 mg of sodium cromoglycate as powder may be given by nasal insufflation into each nostril up to 4 times daily. Prophylactic treatment for seasonal allergic rhinitis should begin 2 to 3 weeks before exposure to the offending allergen and should continue throughout the season. In allergic eye conditions sodium cromoglycate is applied as drops of 2 or 4%, or as a 4% eye ointment; eye drops are generally applied 4 to 6 times daily and eye ointment is applied 2 to 3 times daily.

In food allergy and in mastocytosis, sodium cromoglycate may be given by mouth in doses of 200 mg four times daily before meals either as capsules or as an oral solution prepared by dissolving the contents of the capsules in water; children over 2 years may be given 100 mg four times daily. If satisfactory control is not achieved within 2 to 3 weeks the dosage may be doubled, but should not exceed 40 mg per kg body-weight daily; a reduction in dosage may be possible once symptoms have been controlled.

Action. Sodium cromoglycate has a range of actions at cellular level. It is known as a mast-cell stabiliser and such an action inhibits the release of histamine and other inflammatory mediators from sensitised mast cells. Other actions that have been reported include a direct effect on airway nerves[1,2] and antagonism of substance P,[3] which ties up with its inhibition of the effects of platelet activating factor (PAF).[4,5] However, sodium cromoglycate is viewed clinically as an anti-inflammatory, and it is still the view, at least of the manufacturers, that sodium cromoglycate's activity in asthma is due to mast-cell stabilisation.[6]

There have been a few reports[7-9] of sodium cromoglycate producing bronchodilatation. However, in practice other drugs with accepted bronchodilating activity are used for this effect in asthma treatment schedules, see p.745.

1. Barnes PJ. Asthma as an axon reflex. *Lancet* 1986; **i:** 242–5.
2. Dixon M, *et al.* The effects of sodium cromoglycate on lung irritant receptors and left ventricular cardiac receptors in the anaesthetized dog. *Br J Pharmacol* 1979; **67:** 569–74.
3. Page C. Sodium cromoglycate, a tachykinin antagonist? *Lancet* 1994; **343:** 70.
4. Morley J, *et al.* The platelet in asthma. *Lancet* 1984; **ii:** 1142–4.
5. Morley J. PAF and airway hyperreactivity: prospects for novel prophylactic anti-asthma drugs. In: *PAF, Platelets, and Asthma*, Basel, Birkhäuser Verlag, 1987: 87–95.
6. Edwards AM, Norris AA. Cromoglycate and asthma. *Lancet* 1994; **343:** 426.
7. Horn CR, *et al.* Bronchodilator effect of disodium cromoglycate administered as a dry powder in exercise induced asthma. *Br J Clin Pharmacol* 1984; **18:** 798–801.
8. Weiner P, *et al.* Bronchodilating effect of cromolyn sodium in asthmatic patients at rest and following exercise. *Ann Allergy* 1984; **53:** 186–8.
9. Yuksel B, Greenough A. Bronchodilator effect of nebulized sodium cromoglycate in children born prematurely. *Eur Respir J* 1993; **6:** 387–90.

Administration. The effectiveness of sodium cromoglycate 2 mg four times daily by metered-dose aerosol inhaler has been established in a number of controlled studies in adults and children with asthma.[1-5] Latimer *et al.*[6] found sodium cromoglycate 2 mg by inhalation from a metered-dose aerosol to be as effective as 20 mg inhaled as powder. However, the tenfold difference in dosage has been questioned.[7] Other workers have found 2 mg by aerosol to be less effective than 20 mg as powder,[8,9] and Tullett *et al.*[10] suggested that an aerosol supplying 5 mg per metered dose would be preferable. In a comparison of single-dose pretreatment from metered-dose inhalers, sodium cromoglycate 10 mg (2 × 5 mg puffs) was as effective as beclomethasone dipropionate 200 μg in inhibiting bronchial responsiveness to histamine.[11]

While several strengths of aerosol are available, current practice in the UK is to use aerosols delivering 5 mg per puff. Doses from these aerosols are 10 mg four times daily, increased to 8 times daily if necessary and reduced if possible to 5 mg four times daily once the asthma has been stabilised.

Care is also required if inhaled sodium cromoglycate is given via a spacer device; evidence suggests that these may greatly influence the amount of drug delivered, reducing it to one-third of the dose delivered by inhaler actuation in some cases.[12]

1. Geller-Bernstein C, Levin S. Sodium cromoglycate pressurised aerosol in childhood asthma. *Curr Ther Res* 1983; **34:** 345–9.
2. Wheatley D. Sodium cromoglycate in aerosol form in regular users of bronchodilator drugs. *Curr Med Res Opin* 1983; **8:** 333–7.
3. Rubin AE, *et al.* The treatment of asthma in adults using sodium cromoglycate pressurized aerosol: a double-blind controlled trial. *Curr Med Res Opin* 1983; **8:** 553–8.
4. Blumenthal MN, *et al.* A multicenter evaluation of the clinical benefits of cromolyn sodium aerosol by metered-dose inhaler in the treatment of asthma. *J Allergy Clin Immunol* 1988; **81:** 681–7.
5. Selcow JE, *et al.* Clinical benefits of cromolyn sodium aerosol (MDI) in the treatment of asthma in children. *Ann Allergy* 1989; **62:** 195–9.
6. Latimer KM, *et al.* Inhibition by sodium cromoglycate of bronchoconstriction stimulated by respiratory heat loss: comparison of pressurised aerosol and powder. *Thorax* 1984; **39:** 277–81.
7. Anonymous. Sodium cromoglycate aerosol. *Drug Ther Bull* 1982; **20:** 27.
8. Robson RA, *et al.* Sodium cromoglycate: spincaps or metered dose aerosol. *Br J Clin Pharmacol* 1981; **11:** 383–4.
9. Bar-Yishay E, *et al.* Duration of action of sodium cromoglycate on exercise induced asthma: comparison of 2 formulations. *Arch Dis Child* 1983; **58:** 624–7.
10. Tullett WM, *et al.* Dose-response effect of sodium cromoglycate pressurised aerosol in exercise induced asthma. *Thorax* 1985; **40:** 41–4.
11. Cockcroft DW, Murdock KY. Comparative effects of inhaled salbutamol, sodium cromoglycate, and beclomethasone dipropionate on allergen-induced early asthmatic responses, late asthmatic responses, and increased bronchial responsiveness to histamine. *J Allergy Clin Immunol* 1987; **79:** 734–40.
12. Barry PW, O'Callaghan C. Inhalational drug delivery from seven different spacer devices. *Thorax* 1996; **51:** 835–40.

Asthma. Sodium cromoglycate is used as a prophylactic agent in the management of chronic asthma (p.745), but in practice inhaled corticosteroids are generally preferred in patients who cannot be managed with occasional use of an inhaled beta$_2$ agonist alone, and in whom regular prophylactic treatment is therefore considered to be indicated. Even in children, in whom cromoglycate has tended to be more widely used, the trend appears to be towards greater use of inhaled corticosteroids. However, guidelines still specify the use of cromoglycate or nedocromil as a valid alternative to inhaled corticosteroids in some circumstances. Response to treatment with nebulised sodium cromoglycate was found to be age related in a study of children under 2 years of age with recurrent or persistent wheezy bronchitis and a history of allergic symptoms.[1] It was effective in children of 12 to 24 months of age but not in those below 12 months. Similarly, Furfaro *et al.*[2] found nebulised sodium cromoglycate to be no more effective than placebo in the treatment of a group of 31 infants with persistent wheezing aged under 1 year, and Tasche and colleagues[3] found that long-term inhalation therapy was ineffective in children aged 1 to 4 years.

1. Geller-Bernstein C, Levin S. Nebulised sodium cromoglycate in the treatment of wheezy bronchitis in infants and young children. *Respiration* 1982; **43:** 294–8.
2. Furfaro S, *et al.* Efficacy of cromoglycate in persistently wheezing infants. *Arch Dis Child* 1994; **71:** 331–4.
3. Tasche MJA, *et al.* Randomised placebo-controlled trial of inhaled sodium cromoglycate in 1-4-year-old children with moderate asthma. *Lancet* 1997; **350:** 1060–4. Correction. *ibid.* 1998; **351:** 376.

Cogan's syndrome. Cogan's syndrome is a disease characterised by non-syphilitic interstitial keratitis and audiovestibular symptoms, with diverse systemic manifestations. There may also be ocular symptoms. The management of Cogan's syndrome is discussed briefly on p.1020. Corticosteroids have been tried as has sodium cromoglycate for the ocular symptoms. Carter and Nabarro[1] reported the successful use of sodium cromoglycate eye drops to improve blurred vision in a patient with Cogan's syndrome of 18 years' duration. Sodium cromoglycate capsules [by mouth] also reduced the frequency of fever attacks in this patient.

1. Carter F, Nabarro J. Cromoglycate for Cogan's syndrome. *Lancet* 1987; **i:** 858.

Cough. Sodium cromoglycate has been used with modest success by aerosol inhalation to suppress the cough associated with ACE inhibitor therapy in some patients.[1,2] However, Puolijoki and Rekiaro[3] did not find inhalation of nedocromil sodium to be helpful in the treatment of ACE inhibitor induced cough in 6 diabetic patients. For further discussion of this topic, see p.805.

1. Keogh A. Sodium cromoglycate prophylaxis for angiotensin-converting enzyme inhibitor cough. *Lancet* 1993; **341:** 560.
2. Hargreaves MR, Benson MK. Inhaled sodium cromoglycate in angiotensin-converting enzyme inhibitor cough. *Lancet* 1995; **345:** 13–16.
3. Puolijoki H, Rekiaro M. Lack of effect of nedocromil sodium in ACE-inhibitor-induced cough. *Lancet* 1995; **345:** 394.

Food allergy. Oral sodium cromoglycate has been used in the prophylaxis of food allergy reactions (p.400). However, efficacy has not been unequivocally established.

Gastro-intestinal disorders. DIARRHOEA. Improvement has been noted in diarrhoea thought to be associated with food allergy (above) following oral administration of sodium cromoglycate.[1,2]

1. Bolin TD. Use of oral sodium cromoglycate in persistent diarrhoea. *Gut* 1980; **21:** 848–50.
2. Stefanini GF, *et al.* Efficacy of oral disodium cromoglycate in patients with irritable bowel syndrome and positive skin prick tests to foods. *Lancet* 1986; **i:** 207–8.

INFLAMMATORY BOWEL DISEASE. Although sodium cromoglycate has been tried rectally[1] and orally[2] in the management of inflammatory bowel disease (p.1171), given the variable and often negative results there is little interest in its use, and other agents are generally preferred.

1. Grace RH, *et al.* Comparative trial of sodium cromoglycate enemas with prednisolone enemas in the treatment of ulcerative colitis. *Gut* 1987; **28:** 88–92.
2. Binder V, *et al.* Disodium cromoglycate in the treatment of ulcerative colitis and Crohn's disease. *Gut* 1981; **22:** 55–60.

MOUTH ULCERATION. For discussion of mouth ulceration and its management, including reference to equivocal results from the use of topical sodium cromoglycate, see p.1172.

Mastocytosis. Mastocytosis is a condition characterised by abnormal proliferation of mast cells and their accumulation in body tissues.[1] It occurs in cutaneous or systemic forms, the former most often manifesting as urticaria pigmentosa, the latter involving diverse organs and tissues including the bones, liver, spleen, lymph nodes, haematopoietic system, gastro-intestinal tract, and also the skin.

Treatment is aimed at relieving symptoms and does not alter the course of the disease. A combination of H$_1$ and H$_2$-antagonist antihistamines is widely used to control cutaneous and gastro-intestinal symptoms, while antimuscarinics may be useful for diarrhoea.[1] Patients should carry adrenaline for self-injection in the event of severe attacks.

Sodium cromoglycate has been tried in systemic mastocytosis in doses of 100 to 200 mg four times daily by mouth, generally with favourable results. In a study of 5 patients sodium cromoglycate 100 mg four times daily relieved the symptoms of systemic mastocytosis in the skin, gastro-intestinal tract, and central nervous system when compared with placebo.[2] Of 4 patients who received a total of 18 courses of treatment, lasting from 1 to 10 months, marked improvement was seen in 3, but patients relapsed within 2 to 3 weeks of stopping sodium cromoglycate treatment. In a comparative study in 6 patients sodium cromoglycate 200 mg four times daily was indistinguishable from chlorpheniramine 4 mg plus cimetidine 300 mg four times daily in relieving overall symptoms of systemic mastocytosis.[3] However, individual symptoms responded to varying degrees: 3 of 4 patients obtained greater relief from nausea and one patient experienced a dramatic relief from bone pain with sodium cromoglycate while 5 of 6 had less pruritus and 4 of 6 had less urticaria with the combined antihistamines. A much higher dose of 100 mg per kg body-weight daily by mouth in divided doses was used with some success in a 5-year-old boy with systemic mastocytosis after lower doses had proved ineffective.[4]

1. Golkar L, Bernhard JD. Mastocytosis. *Lancet* 1997; **349:** 1379–85.
2. Soter NA, *et al.* Oral disodium cromoglycate in the treatment of systemic mastocytosis. *N Engl J Med* 1979; **301:** 465–9.
3. Frieri M, *et al.* Comparison of the therapeutic efficacy of cromolyn sodium with that of combined chlorpheniramine and cimetidine in systemic mastocytosis. *Am J Med* 1985; **78:** 9–14.
4. Businco L, *et al.* Systemic mastocytosis in a 5-year-old child: successful treatment with disodium cromoglycate. *Clin Allergy* 1984; **14:** 147–52.

Rhinitis and conjunctivitis. Many drugs, including sodium cromoglycate, are employed in the management of allergic rhinitis (p.400) and conjunctivitis (p.399). There is some evidence that nedocromil[1] or lodoxamide[2] may be more effective than cromoglycate in the management of vernal keratoconjunctivitis.

1. El Hennawi M. A double-blind placebo controlled group comparative study of ophthalmic sodium cromoglycate and nedocromil sodium in the treatment of vernal keratoconjunctivitis. *Br J Ophthalmol* 1994; **78:** 365–9.
2. Leonardi A, *et al.* Effect of lodoxamide and disodium cromoglycate on tear eosinophil cationic protein in vernal keratoconjunctivitis. *Br J Ophthalmol* 1997; **81:** 23–6.

Preparations

BP 1998: Sodium Cromoglicate Powder for Inhalation;
USP 23: Cromolyn Sodium for Inhalation; Cromolyn Sodium Inhalation Solution; Cromolyn Sodium Nasal Solution; Cromolyn Sodium Ophthalmic Solution.

Proprietary Preparations (details are given in Part 3)

Aust.: Allercrom†; Cromal; Cromoglin; Intal; Lomusol; Opticrom; Vividrin; ***Austral.:*** Cromeze; Intal; Opticrom; Rynacrom; Vistacrom†; ***Belg.:*** Lomudal; Lomusol; Opticrom; Vividrin; ***Canad.:*** Intal; Nalcrom; Opticrom; Rynacrom; Vistacrom; ***Fr.:*** Alerion†; Cromoptic; Intercron; Lomudal; Lomusol; Nalcron; Opticron; ***Ger.:*** acecromol; Allergocrom; Colimune; Crom-Ophtal; Cromo; Cromo Pur; Cromoglicin; Cromoglicin-ratiopharm†; Cromohexal; Cromol; Cromolind; Cromolyn; Diffusyl; Dispacromil; DNCG; duracroman; Esirhinol†; Flui-DNCG; Intal; Logomed Heuschnupfen-Spray; Lomupren; Nasivin gegen Heuschnupfen†; Opticrom; Otriven H; Pentatop; Prothanon Cromo; Pulbil; Sofro†; Stadaglicin†; Vividrin; ***Irl.:*** Cromogen; Hay-Crom; Intal; Nalcrom; Opticrom; Rynacrom; Steri-Neb Cromogen; Vividrin; ***Ital.:*** Cromantal; Cromosan; Cronacol; Frenal; Frenal Rinologico; Gaster; Gastrofrenal; Glicacil; Lomudal; Lomuspray; Nalcrom; Sificrom; ***Mon.:*** Cromedil; ***Neth.:*** Lomudal; Lomusol; Nalcrom; Opticrom; Vividrin; ***Norw.:*** Lecrolyn; Lomudal; ***S.Afr.:*** Cromogen; Cromohexal; Hay-Crom; Kiddicrom; Lomudal; Nalcrom; Opticrom; Rynacrom; Vistacrom; Vividrin; ***Spain:*** Cromo Asma; Cusicrom; Frenal; Gastrofrenal; Intal; Nalcrom; Nebulasma; Nebulcrom; Oralcrom; Poledin; Rinofrenal; ***Swed.:*** Lecrolyn; Lomudal; Pollyferm; Rinil; ***Switz.:*** Cromodyn; Cromosol Ophta; Intal Nasal†; Lomudal; Lomusol; Nalcrom; Novacrom†; Opticrom; ***UK:*** Brol-eze; Clariteyes; Cromogen; Cusilyn†; Hay-Crom; Intal; Nalcrom; Opticrom; Optrex Hayfever Allergy Eye Drops; Rynacrom; Vividrin; Viz-On; ***USA:*** Crolom; Gastrocrom; Intal; Nasalcrom; Opticrom.

Multi-ingredient: ***Aust.:*** Aarane; Allergospasmin; Ditec; Lomusol comp; ***Belg.:*** Lomusol plus Xylometazoline; ***Ger.:*** Aarane; Allergospasmin; Asthmocupin†; Ditec; Intal compositum†; Lomupren compositum; Vividrin comp; ***Irl.:*** Rynacrom Compound; ***Ital.:*** Cromozil; Frenal Compositum†; Rinofrenal; Visuglican; ***Neth.:*** Cromovist†; Lomudal Compositum†; ***S.Afr.:***

Lomudal Comp†; **Spain:** Cromoftol; Frenal Compositum; Rinofrenal Plus; **Switz.:** Aarane; Allergospasmine; Lomusol-X; **UK:** Aerocrom; Intal Compound†; Resiston One; Rynacrom Compound.

Suplatast Tosylate (11884-r)

Suplatast Tosilate (*rINN*); IPD-1151T; Suplatastum Tosilas. (±)-(2-{[*p*-(3-Ethoxy-2-hydroxypropoxy)phenyl]carbamoyl}-ethyl)dimethylsulphonium *p*-toluenesulphonate; (3-{[4-(3-Ethoxy-2-hydroxypropoxy)phenyl]amino}-3-oxopropyl)dimethylsulphonium *p*-toluenesulphonate.

$C_{23}H_{33}NO_7S_2$ = 499.6.

CAS — 94055-76-2.

Suplatast tosylate is an anti-allergic given by mouth in the prophylactic management of asthma and other allergic conditions.

Terbutaline Sulphate (2107-a)

Terbutaline Sulphate (*BANM, rINNM*).

KWD-2019; Terbutaline Sulfate (*USAN*); Terbutalini Sulfas. 2-*tert*-Butylamino-1-(3,5-dihydroxyphenyl)ethanol sulphate.

$(C_{12}H_{19}NO_3)_2,H_2SO_4$ = 548.6.

CAS — 23031-25-6 (terbutaline); 23031-32-5 (terbutaline sulphate).

Pharmacopoeias. In *Eur.* (see p.viii), *Jpn*, and *US*.

A white to greyish-white crystalline powder; odourless or with a faint odour of acetic acid. It exhibits polymorphism. Freely **soluble** in water; slightly soluble in alcohol and in methyl alcohol; practically insoluble in chloroform and ether. **Store** at 15° to 30° in airtight containers. Protect from light.

Adverse Effects and Precautions

As for Salbutamol Sulphate, p.758.

Overdosage. An overdose of terbutaline due to transcutaneous absorption has been reported following inappropriate topical application to skin infected with tinea.[1] Transcutaneous absorption should be considered especially when children with facial eczema or dermatitis are given terbutaline via a nebuliser and mask.

1. Ingrams GJ, Morgan FB. Transcutaneous overdose of terbutaline. *Br Med J* 1993; **307:** 484.

Pulmonary oedema. Pulmonary oedema has occurred in women given $beta_2$ agonists, including terbutaline, for premature labour.[1] The risk factors, the most important of which is fluid overload, are discussed under Precautions for Salbutamol, p.759.

1. Hawker F. Pulmonary oedema associated with β_2-sympathomimetic treatment of premature labour. *Anaesth Intensive Care* 1984; **12:** 143–51.

Tolerance. As with other $beta_2$ agonists (see p.759) there is some evidence[1] that tolerance may develop to terbutaline when it is used regularly.

1. O'Connor BJ, *et al.* Tolerance to the nonbronchodilator effects of inhaled β_2-agonists in asthma. *N Engl J Med* 1992; **327:** 1204–8.

Interactions

As for Salbutamol Sulphate, p.759.

Xanthines. The metabolic and cardiovascular responses to terbutaline infusion were significantly enhanced following administration of *theophylline* in a study in 7 healthy subjects; in particular the fall in serum potassium was greater when both drugs were given.[1] Careful monitoring of serum potassium is recommended in severe asthma where theophylline and $beta_2$-agonists may be given together.

Terbutaline conversely has an effect on theophylline. Terbutaline can reduce serum-theophylline concentrations by increasing its systemic clearance. This may, or may not, have clinical implications, as improved clinical scores have still occurred with combined therapy despite the theophylline concentration being lower than when used alone; if respiratory symptoms persist, an increase in dosage may be contemplated while monitoring theophylline side-effects and concentration.[2]

1. Smith SR, Kendall MJ. Potentiation of the adverse effects of intravenous terbutaline by oral theophylline. *Br J Clin Pharmacol* 1986; **21:** 451–3.
2. Garty M, *et al.* Increased theophylline clearance in asthmatic patients due to terbutaline. *Eur J Clin Pharmacol* 1989; **36:** 25–8.

Pharmacokinetics

Terbutaline is variably absorbed from the gastro-intestinal tract and about 60% of the absorbed dose undergoes first-pass metabolism by sulphate (and some glucuronide) conjugation in the liver and the gut wall. It is accordingly excreted in the urine partly as the inactive conjugates and partly as unchanged terbutaline, the ratio depending upon the route of administration. The half-life is reported to be about 3 to 4 hours. There is some placental transfer. Traces are distributed into breast milk.

Terbutaline, like many other sympathomimetics, exists in two stereoisometric forms but only the (−)-enantiomer of terbutaline is pharmacologically active. Pharmacokinetic studies have been conducted on the two enantiomers and on the racemate.

The oral bioavailability of (−)-terbutaline was 14.8% which was similar to that of the racemate; the bioavailability of (+)-terbutaline was much lower at 7.5%. The difference in bioavailability between the two enantiomers was mainly due to a difference in absorption (about 75% and 50% respectively) although a small difference in subsequent first-pass metabolism also occurred, with the (+)-isomer undergoing slightly more metabolism. It appeared that the (+)-isomer governed the elimination behaviour, both first-pass metabolism and renal clearance, of the racemate whereas the (−)-isomer determined the absorption.[1]

Other studies have also demonstrated stereoselective sulphate conjugation of terbutaline with sulphation of the (+)-enantiomer being double that of the (−)-enantiomer.[2] The primary site of terbutaline sulphation for both enantiomers appears to be in the gut and is significantly correlated with the activity of catechol sulphotransferase.[3]

1. Borgström L, *et al.* Pharmacokinetic evaluation in man of terbutaline given as separate enantiomers and as the racemate. *Br J Clin Pharmacol* 1989; **27:** 49–56.
2. Walle T, Walle UK. Stereoselective sulphate conjugation of racemic terbutaline by human liver cytosol. *Br J Clin Pharmacol* 1990; **30:** 127–33.
3. Pacifici GM, *et al.* (+) and (−) terbutaline are sulphated at a higher rate in human intestine than in the liver. *Eur J Clin Pharmacol* 1993; **45:** 483–7.

Uses and Administration

Terbutaline sulphate is a direct-acting sympathomimetic with predominantly beta-adrenergic activity and a selective action on $beta_2$ receptors ($beta_2$ agonist). It has actions and uses similar to those of salbutamol (see p.759).

Terbutaline is given as the sulphate for its bronchodilating properties in reversible airways obstruction, as occurs in asthma (p.745) and in some patients with chronic obstructive pulmonary disease (p.747). It also decreases uterine contractility and may be used to arrest premature labour (see p.760).

After inhalation, the bronchodilating effect of terbutaline usually begins within 5 minutes and lasts for about 3 to 4 hours. The onset of action following oral administration is about 30 minutes and its duration is up to 8 hours; the maximum effect occurs 2 to 3 hours after the dose.

To relieve **acute bronchospasm**, 1 or 2 inhalations of terbutaline sulphate 250 μg can be taken as required from a metered-dose aerosol. Current UK guidelines for the treatment of asthma (see p.745) recommend that if patients with chronic asthma need more than one dose of inhaled $beta_2$ agonist daily, then the next step is additional treatment with a corticosteroid or with cromoglycate or nedocromil. However, if terbutaline sulphate were to be taken more than once daily the doses recommended by the manufacturers are 250 or 500 μg every 4 to 6 hours, to a maximum of 8 inhalations in 24 hours. These doses are suitable, in general, for both adults and children. Alternatively, a breath-actuated metered-dose powder inhaler delivering 500 μg of terbutaline sulphate per inhalation may be used. One inhalation of 500 μg is taken when required up to a maximum of 4 inhalations in 24 hours.

When inhalation is ineffective, terbutaline sulphate may be given by mouth; for adults the usual initial dose is 2.5 or 3 mg three times daily increased to 5 mg three times daily as necessary. Children's doses may be calculated on the basis of body-weight; a dose of 75 μg per kg three times daily is suggested. A usual dose in children over 7 years of age is 2.5 mg two or three times daily. Modified-release tablets are also available; the usual adult dose is 7.5 mg twice daily.

Severe or unresponsive bronchospasm may require the administration of terbutaline sulphate intermittently via a nebuliser. A usual dose is 2 to 5 mg for children and 5 to 10 mg for adults inhaled 2 to 4 times daily. Single-dose units or a suitable dilution of a concentrated solution containing terbutaline sulphate 1% are used for this purpose. For continuous administration, a suitable adult dose is 1 to 2 mg of terbutaline sulphate per hour given as a 0.01% nebuliser solution in sodium chloride 0.9%. In emergency situations, where delivery via a nebuliser is not possible, up to 10 mg of terbutaline sulphate can be given by multiple actuations of a metered-dose inhaler, preferably into a large spacer device. In children over 5 years of age, inhalation from a metered-dose inhaler has been as effective as the same dose given by nebulisation.

In the treatment of severe forms of bronchospasm, terbutaline sulphate may be given by subcutaneous, intramuscular, or slow intravenous injection; a dose of 250 to 500 μg may be given up to four times daily. A suggested dose by injection for children over 2 years of age is 10 μg per kg body-weight to a maximum total dose of 300 μg. Terbutaline sulphate may also be given by intravenous infusion, as a solution containing 3 to 5 μg per mL at a rate of 0.5 to 1 mL per minute for adults.

Terbutaline sulphate is also used to arrest uncomplicated **premature labour** between 24 and 33 weeks of gestation. It is given by intravenous infusion in glucose 5%, preferably by syringe pump when the concentration is 100 μg per mL. If no syringe pump is available then the concentration of the infusion should be 10 μg per mL. The recommended initial rate of infusion is 5 μg per minute increased by 2.5 μg per minute at intervals of 20 minutes until contractions stop. Usually, a rate of up to 10 μg per minute is sufficient; rates in excess of 20 μg per minute should not be used and if that maximum rate does not delay labour then the infusion should be stopped. The maternal pulse should be monitored throughout the infusion which should be adjusted to avoid a maternal heart rate of more than 135 to 140 beats per minute. A close watch should also be kept on the patient's state of hydration since fluid overload is considered to be a key risk factor for pulmonary oedema. Once contractions have ceased and the infusion has been given for one hour, the dose may be decreased by 2.5 μg per minute at 20-minute intervals to the lowest maintenance dose that produces continued suppression of contractions. After a further 12 hours, oral maintenance therapy with 5 mg three times daily may be started. However, such usage is no longer recommended by authorities in the UK as the risks to the mother (see Precautions under Salbutamol, p.759) increase after 48 hours, and furthermore myometrial response is reduced. Subcutaneous doses of 250 μg four times daily have been given for a few days before oral treatment was commenced.

Hypoglycaemia. Administration of terbutaline 5 mg by mouth at night reduced the risk of nocturnal hypoglycaemia in a study in patients with type 1 diabetes.[1]

1. Saleh TY, Cryer PE. Alamine and terbutaline in the prevention of nocturnal hypoglycemia in IDDM. *Diabetes Care* 1997; **20:** 1231–6.

Systemic capillary leak syndrome. Systemic capillary leak syndrome is a rare disorder marked by shifts of plasma from the intravascular to the extracellular space, and is often fatal. Acute attacks are treated with intravenous fluid resuscitation, but there is some anecdotal evidence that treatment with terbutaline combined with aminophylline, both by mouth, may be useful in preventing further attacks.[1,2] Infusion of epoprostenol has also been employed in acute management.[3]

1. Droder RM, *et al.* Control of systemic capillary leak syndrome with aminophylline and terbutaline. *Am J Med* 1992; **92:** 523–6.
2. Amoura Z, *et al.* Systemic capillary leak syndrome: report on 13 patients with special focus on course and treatment. *Am J Med* 1997; **103:** 514–19.
3. Fellows IW, *et al.* Epoprostenol in systemic capillary leak syndrome. *Lancet* 1988; **ii:** 1143.

Urticaria. Patients with various types of urticaria unresponsive to conventional therapy with antihistamines (see p.1076) have obtained benefit from treatment with a combination of terbutaline and ketotifen; the urticarias have included chronic idiopathic urticaria,[1] dermographism,[1] and cold urticaria.[1,2] Terbutaline on its own was relatively ineffective and the mechanism of the combination was believed to be due to a stabilising effect on mast cells.[1]

1. Saihan EM. Ketotifen and terbutaline in urticaria. *Br J Dermatol* 1981; **104:** 205–6.
2. Edge JA, Osborne JP. Terbutaline and ketotifen in cold urticaria in a child. *J R Soc Med* 1989; **82:** 439–40.

Preparations

BP 1998: Terbutaline Tablets;
USP 23: Terbutaline Sulfate Inhalation Aerosol; Terbutaline Sulfate Injection; Terbutaline Sulfate Tablets.

Proprietary Preparations (details are given in Part 3)
Aust.: Bricanyl; ***Austral.:*** Bricanyl; ***Belg.:*** Bricanyl; ***Canad.:*** Bricanyl; ***Fr.:*** Bricanyl; ***Ger.:*** Aerodur; Arubendol; Asthmo-Kranit Mono; Asthmoprotect; Bricanyl; Butaliret; Butalitab; Contimit; Terbufortont†; Terbul; Terbuturmant; ***Irl.:*** Bricanyl; ***Ital.:*** Terbasmin†; ***Neth.:*** Bricanyl; ***Norw.:*** Bricanyl; ***S.Afr.:*** Bricanyl; ***Spain:*** Tedipulmo; Terbasmin; ***Swed.:*** Bricanyl; Respirol†; ***Switz.:*** Bricanyl; ***UK:*** Bricanyl; Monovent; ***USA:*** Brethaire; Brethine; Bricanyl.

Multi-ingredient: ***Aust.:*** Bricanyl comp; Eudur; ***Ger.:*** Bricanyl comp; Eudur; ***Irl.:*** Bricanyl Expectorant; ***S.Afr.:*** Bronchoped; ***Spain:*** Terbasmin Expectorante; ***Switz.:*** Eudur†.

Theobromine (643-m)

Theobromine *(BAN)*.

Santheose; Theobrominum. 3,7-Dihydro-3,7-dimethylpurine-2,6(1*H*)-dione; 3,7-Dimethylxanthine.

$C_7H_8N_4O_2$ = 180.2.

CAS — 83-67-0.

Pharmacopoeias. In *Eur.* (see p.viii) and *Pol.*

A white powder. Very slightly **soluble** in water and in alcohol; practically insoluble in ether; slightly soluble in aqueous ammonia. It dissolves in dilute solutions of alkali hydroxides and in mineral acids.

Theobromine has the general properties of the other xanthines (see Theophylline, p.772). It has a weaker activity than theophylline or caffeine and has practically no stimulant effect on the central nervous system. Large doses can cause nausea and vomiting. Theobromine has been used for its bronchodilating properties and in the treatment of cardiovascular disorders. Theobromine and calcium salicylate (theosalicin), theobromine and sodium acetate, and theobromine and sodium salicylate (themisalum, theobromsal) have all been used similarly to theobromine.

Theobromine is the chief xanthine in the beverage cocoa. It is also present in chocolate and in small amounts in tea. Theobroma oil may contain up to 2% theobromine.

The pharmacokinetics and metabolic disposition of theobromine following a single dose by mouth (as theobromine sodium acetate 10 mg per kg body-weight) in 6 healthy subjects.[1]

1. Tarka SM, *et al.* Theobromine kinetics and metabolic disposition. *Clin Pharmacol Ther* 1983; **34:** 546–55.

Preparations

Proprietary Preparations (details are given in Part 3)

Multi-ingredient: ***Aust.:*** Asthma-Hilfe; Theo-Lanicor; ***Belg.:*** Do-Do†; ***Fr.:*** Gripponyl†; ***Ger.:*** Angiocardyl N; Circovegetalin compositum†; Circovegetalin†; Colomba N†; Dynamol†; Eupond; Par-Isalon†; Spasdilat N†; Theo-Lanicor†; ***S.Afr.:*** Atrofed†; ***Spain:*** Propyre T.

Theophylline (647-q)

Theophylline *(BAN)*.

Anhydrous Theophylline; Teofillina; Theophyllinum. 3,7-Dihydro-1,3-dimethylpurine-2,6(1*H*)-dione; 1,3-Dimethylxanthine.

$C_7H_8N_4O_2$ = 180.2.

CAS — 58-55-9.

Pharmacopoeias. In *Eur.* (see p.viii), *Jpn, Pol.,* and *US.* Some pharmacopoeias include anhydrous and hydrated theophylline in one monograph.

A white odourless crystalline powder. Slightly **soluble** in water, more soluble in hot water; sparingly soluble in alcohol, in chloroform, and in ether. Dissolves in solutions of alkali hydroxides, in ammonia, and in mineral acids.

Theophylline Hydrate (648-p)

Theophylline Hydrate *(BANM)*.

Theophylline Monohydrate; Theophyllinum Monohydricum.

$C_7H_8N_4O_2,H_2O$ = 198.2.

CAS — 5967-84-0.

Pharmacopoeias. In *Chin., Eur.* (see p.viii), *Pol.,* and *US.* Some pharmacopoeias include anhydrous and hydrated theophylline in one monograph.

A white odourless crystalline powder. Theophylline hydrate 1.1 mg is approximately equivalent to 1 mg of theophylline. Slightly **soluble** in water, more soluble in hot water; sparingly soluble in alcohol, in chloroform, and in ether. Dissolves in solutions of alkali hydroxides, in ammonia, and in mineral acids.

Stability. Alcohol-free theophylline liquid repackaged in clear or amber polypropylene oral syringes could be stored at room temperature under continuous fluorescent lighting for at least 180 days without significant change in the concentration of theophylline.[1] However, it was recommended that solutions be protected from light because of the potential for discoloration.

1. Johnson CE, Drabik BT. Stability of alcohol-free theophylline liquid repackaged in plastic oral syringes. *Am J Hosp Pharm* 1989; **46:** 980–1.

Adverse Effects

The side-effects commonly encountered with theophylline and its derivatives irrespective of the route of administration, are gastro-intestinal irritation and stimulation of the CNS. Serum concentrations of theophylline greater than 20 µg per mL are associated with an increased risk of adverse effects (but see below).

Theophylline may cause nausea, vomiting, abdominal pain, diarrhoea, other gastro-intestinal disturbances, insomnia, headache, anxiety, restlessness, dizziness, tremor, and palpitations. Overdosage may also lead to agitation, diuresis and repeated vomiting (sometimes haematemesis) and consequent dehydration, cardiac arrhythmias including tachycardia, hypotension, electrolyte disturbances including profound hypokalaemia, hyperglycaemia, metabolic acidosis, convulsions, and death. Severe toxicity may not be preceded by milder symptoms. Convulsions, cardiac arrhythmias, and hypotension may follow intravenous injection, particularly if the injection is too rapid, and sudden deaths have been reported; the drug is too irritant for intramuscular use. Proctitis may follow repeated administration of suppositories.

The accepted therapeutic range for serum concentrations of theophylline has long been 10 to 20 µg per mL. Adverse effects occur relatively frequently within this range: they are uncommon at concentrations of 5 to 10 µg per mL but begin to become more frequent at 15 µg per mL or above, and are greatly increased in frequency and severity at serum concentrations greater than 20 µg per mL.[1-3] As a result, and given recent appreciation that theophylline has beneficial effects at serum concentrations below 10 µg per mL, some now consider that 5 to 15 µg per mL is a more appropriate therapeutic range for which to aim.[3]

The severity of toxicity is generally correlated with age, underlying disease, and serum-theophylline concentration, but a distinction has been made between acute and chronic theophylline intoxication; symptoms appear to occur at a lower theophylline concentration in chronic toxicity than following acute ingestion of large amounts.[1,2,4] Young infants and the elderly (over 60 years) appear to be at particular risk from chronic intoxication with theophylline.[5,6] Common clinical manifestations of theophylline toxicity following overdosage of aminophylline or theophylline include nausea, vomiting, diarrhoea, agitation, tremor, hypertonicity, hyperventilation, supraventricular and ventricular arrhythmias, hypotension, and seizures. Metabolic disturbances such as hypokalaemia, hyperglycaemia, hypophosphataemia, hypercalcaemia, metabolic acidosis, and respiratory alkalosis often occur.[1-3] Other toxic effects reported include dementia,[7] toxic psychosis,[8] symptoms of acute pancreatitis,[9] rhabdomyolysis[10-12] with associated renal failure,[10] and acute compartment syndrome.[13]

Serious toxic symptoms may not be preceded by minor symptoms. In acute intoxication with sustained-release preparations the onset of major toxic symptoms may be delayed for up to 24 hours[1] and prolonged monitoring of such patients is required. Patients have recovered despite serum-theophylline concentrations in excess of 200 µg per mL[11,13] but fatalities have occurred with much lower serum concentrations.[9,14,15] Mortality in severe poisoning may be as high as 10%.

1. Dawson AH, Whyte IM. The assessment and treatment of theophylline poisoning. *Med J Aust* 1989; **151:** 689–93.
2. Minton NA, Henry JA. Acute and chronic human toxicity of theophylline. *Hum Exp Toxicol* 1996; **15:** 471–81.
3. Hardy CC, Smith J. Adverse reactions profile: theophylline and aminophylline. *Prescribers' J* 1997; **37:** 96–101.
4. Olson KR, *et al.* Theophylline overdose: acute single ingestion versus chronic repeated overmedication. *Am J Emerg Med* 1985; **3:** 386–94.
5. Shannon M, Lovejoy FH. Effect of acute versus chronic intoxication on clinical features of theophylline poisoning in children. *J Pediatr* 1992; **121:** 125–30.
6. Shannon M. Predictors of major toxicity after theophylline overdose. *Ann Intern Med* 1993; **119:** 1161–7.
7. Drummond I. Aminophylline toxicity in the elderly. *Br Med J* 1982; **285:** 779–80.
8. Wasser WG, *et al.* Theophylline madness. *Ann Intern Med* 1981; **95:** 191.
9. Burgan THS, *et al.* Fatal overdose of theophylline simulating acute pancreatitis. *Br Med J* 1982; **284:** 939–40.
10. Macdonald JB, *et al.* Rhabdomyolysis and acute renal failure after theophylline overdose. *Lancet* 1985; **i:** 932–3.
11. Rumpf KW, *et al.* Rhabdomyolysis after theophylline overdose. *Lancet* 1985; **i:** 1451–2.
12. Modi KB, *et al.* Theophylline poisoning and rhabdomyolysis. *Lancet* 1985; **ii:** 160–1.
13. Lloyd DM, *et al.* Acute compartment syndrome secondary to theophylline overdose. *Lancet* 1990; **ii:** 312.
14. Whyte KF, Addis GJ. Toxicity of salbutamol and theophylline together. *Lancet* 1983; **ii:** 618–19.
15. Davies RJ, Hawkey CJ. Fatal theophylline toxicity precipitated by in situ pulmonary artery thrombosis. *Postgrad Med J* 1989; **65:** 49–50.

Effects on carbohydrate metabolism. Hyperglycaemia is a frequent feature of theophylline intoxication, and like hypokalaemia is thought to be mediated by catecholamines,[1,2] whose release from the adrenal medulla is induced by theophylline. Whether the effects on blood glucose are significant at more modest serum concentrations of theophylline is unclear, although in 29 preterm infants, mean plasma-glucose concentrations were significantly higher after treatment with intravenous aminophylline and oral theophylline than in those not treated. Two of 15 treated infants developed clinically significant hyperglycaemia and glycosuria. It was recommended that plasma-glucose concentrations be monitored in preterm infants receiving theophylline.[3]

1. Kearney TE, *et al.* Theophylline toxicity and the beta-adrenergic system. *Ann Intern Med* 1985; **102:** 766–9.
2. Shannon M. Hypokalemia, hyperglycemia and plasma catecholamine activity after severe theophylline intoxication. *J Toxicol Clin Toxicol* 1994; **32:** 41–7.
3. Srinivasan G, *et al.* Plasma glucose changes in preterm infants during oral theophylline therapy. *J Pediatr* 1983; **103:** 473–6.

Effects on electrolytes. Hypokalaemia is a common metabolic disturbance in theophylline intoxication (see above) but it has also been reported[1] in patients with plasma-theophylline concentrations within the therapeutic range. It is considered to be secondary to theophylline-induced adrenal catecholamine release, with stimulation of muscle cell membrane Na^+/K^+ ATPase and cellular influx of potassium ions.[2] It is recommended[1] that plasma-potassium is monitored during intravenous theophylline therapy particularly if other drugs predisposing to hypokalaemia are also administered (see also under Interactions, below). Hypophosphataemia[1,3] and hyponatraemia[1] can also occur at therapeutic plasma-theophylline concentrations. Hypomagnesaemia[4] and hypercalcaemia[5] have occurred in theophylline overdose.

1. Zantvoort FA, *et al.* Theophylline and serum electrolytes. *Ann Intern Med* 1986; **104:** 134–5.
2. Minton NA, Henry JA. Acute and chronic human toxicity of theophylline. *Hum Exp Toxicol* 1996; **15:** 471–81.
3. Laaban J-P, *et al.* Hypophosphatemia complicating management of acute severe asthma. *Ann Intern Med* 1990; **112:** 68–9.
4. Hall KW, *et al.* Metabolic abnormalities associated with intentional theophylline overdose. *Ann Intern Med* 1984; **101:** 457–62.
5. McPherson ML, *et al.* Theophylline-induced hypercalcemia. *Ann Intern Med* 1986; **105:** 52–4.

Effects on the gastro-intestinal tract. Gastro-intestinal adverse effects are among the most common effects experienced with theophylline and patients may suffer nausea and vomiting, diarrhoea, pain, and bleeding. For reports of increased gastro-oesophageal reflux in patients receiving theophylline, see Gastro-oesophageal Reflux Disease under Precautions, below.

NECROTISING ENTEROCOLITIS. Although there have been reports of necrotising enterocolitis in neonates associated with oral theophylline and aminophylline administration,[1,2] a study of 275 infants concluded that theophylline did not significantly contribute to its development.[3] It has been suggested that the high osmolality of liquid feeds and drugs including oral theophylline preparations may be involved in the aetiology of necrotising enterocolitis.[4]

1. Robinson MJ, *et al.* Xanthines and necrotising enterocolitis. *Arch Dis Child* 1980; **55:** 494–5.
2. Williams AJ. Xanthines and necrotising enterocolitis. *Arch Dis Child* 1980; **55:** 973–4.
3. Davis JM, *et al.* Role of theophylline in pathogenesis of necrotizing enterocolitis. *J Pediatr* 1986; **109:** 344–7.
4. Watkinson M, *et al.* Hyperosmolar preparations for neonates. *Pharm J* 1987; **241:** 488.

OESOPHAGEAL ULCERATION. Oesophageal erosion and ulceration have been reported in patients taking theophylline[1] or aminophylline[2] tablets while recumbent and without any accompanying fluid.

1. Enzenauer RW, *et al.* Esophageal ulceration associated with oral theophylline. *N Engl J Med* 1984; **310:** 261.
2. Stoller JL. Oesophageal ulceration and theophylline. *Lancet* 1985; **ii:** 328–9.

Effects on the heart. ARRHYTHMIAS. Theophylline or aminophylline can precipitate sinus tachycardia and supraventricular and ventricular premature contractions at therapeutic serum-theophylline concentrations[1] and in overdose.[2,3] Multifocal atrial tachycardia has also been associated with both theophylline overdose[2] and serum-theophylline concentrations within the generally accepted range of 10 to 20 μg per mL.[4] Combined administration of theophylline with beta-adrenoceptor stimulants by mouth is associated with a significant increase in the mean heart rate.[5,6]

1. Josephson GW, *et al.* Cardiac dysrhythmias during the treatment of acute asthma: a comparison of two treatment regimens by a double blind protocol. *Chest* 1980; **78:** 429–35.
2. Greenberg A, *et al.* Severe theophylline toxicity: role of conservative measures, antiarrhythmic agents, and charcoal hemoperfusion. *Am J Med* 1984; **76:** 854–60.
3. Minton NA, Henry JA. Acute and chronic human toxicity of theophylline. *Hum Exp Toxicol* 1996; **15:** 471–81.
4. Levine JH, *et al.* Multifocal atrial tachycardia: a toxic effect of theophylline. *Lancet* 1985; **i:** 12–14.
5. Coleman JJ, *et al.* Cardiac arrhythmias during the combined use of β-adrenergic agonist drugs and theophylline. *Chest* 1986; **90:** 45–51.
6. Conradson T-B, *et al.* Arrhythmogenicity from combined bronchodilator therapy in patients with obstructive lung disease and concomitant ischemic heart disease. *Chest* 1987; **91:** 5–9.

Effects on mental function. As mentioned in the general discussion on toxicity above theophylline toxicity has been associated with reports of dementia and toxic psychosis, as well as the more common adverse effects of anxiety and restlessness.

LEARNING AND BEHAVIOUR PROBLEMS. Several small studies[1-3] have suggested that theophylline may be associated with learning and behaviour problems in children, especially those with a low IQ. However, the FDA has concluded[4] that such studies provide insufficient evidence to support an adverse effect of theophylline on learning behaviour or school performance. Other studies have found no marked behavioural side-effects that could be attributed to theophylline.[5,6] Additionally, academic achievement generally appeared to be unaffected by either asthma or by treatment with appropriate doses of theophylline.[7]

1. Furukawa CT, *et al.* Learning and behaviour problems associated with theophylline therapy. *Lancet* 1984; **i:** 621.
2. Springer C, *et al.* Clinical, physiologic, and psychologic comparison of treatment by cromolyn or theophylline in childhood asthma. *J Allergy Clin Immunol* 1985; **76:** 64–9.
3. Schlieper A, *et al.* Effect of therapeutic plasma concentrations of theophylline on behavior, cognitive processing, and affect in children with asthma. *J Pediatr* 1991; **118:** 449–55.
4. Anonymous. Theophylline and school performance. *FDA Drug Bull* 1988; **18:** 32–3.
5. Bender B, Milgrom H. Theophylline-induced behavior change in children: an objective evaluation of parents' perceptions. *JAMA* 1992; **267:** 2621–4.
6. Bender BG, *et al.* Neuropsychological behavioral changes in asthmatic children treated with beclomethasone dipropionate versus theophylline. *Pediatrics* 1998; **101:** 355–60.
7. Lindgren S, *et al.* Does asthma or treatment with theophylline limit children's academic performance? *N Engl J Med* 1992; **327:** 926–30.

Effects on the nervous system. CONVULSIONS. Theophylline toxicity has frequently been associated with convulsions. The risk appears to vary with the type of poisoning: patients with acute toxicity following a single overdose are at much lower risk of seizures unless serum theophylline concentrations are greater than 60 μg per mL;[1] Olson and colleagues considered that seizures were most likely in patients with peak concentrations above 100 μg per mL.[2] In contrast, in patients suffering from chronic overdosage, the risk of seizures is much greater, even at much lower serum-theophylline concentrations.[1,2] Seizure activity in chronic toxicity has been reported at serum concentrations just above or even within the therapeutic range,[3] and elderly patients or those with previous brain injury or neurological disease may be at increased risk,[2-4] although some have questioned the association.[1] The outcome of seizures appears to be variable: death and severe neurological deficit have occurred,[2,3] but other series have recorded recovery without serious morbidity.[4]

1. Paloucek FP, Rodvold KA. Evaluation of theophylline overdoses and toxicities. *Ann Emerg Med* 1988; **17:** 135–44.
2. Olson KR, *et al.* Theophylline overdose: acute single ingestion versus chronic repeated overmedication. *Am J Emerg Med* 1985; **3:** 386–94.
3. Bahls FH, *et al.* Theophylline-associated seizures with "therapeutic" or low toxic serum concentrations: risk factors for serious outcome in adults. *Neurology* 1991; **41:** 1309–12.
4. Covelli HD, *et al.* Predisposing factors to apparent theophylline-induced seizures. *Ann Allergy* 1985; **54:** 411–15.

PAIN. A report of facial myofascial pain associated with oral theophylline therapy.[1]

1. Townend J. Myofascial pain from theophylline. *Br Dent J* 1989; **166:** 438.

Effects on the skin. For reports of cutaneous reactions to theophylline and aminophylline, see under Hypersensitivity, below.

Effects on the urinary tract. Although diuresis is more commonly seen, urinary retention has been reported in male patients during therapy with aminophylline[1] or theophylline.[2]

1. Owens GR, Tannenbaum R. Theophylline-induced urinary retention. *Ann Intern Med* 1981; **94:** 212–13.
2. Prakash M, Washburne JD. Theophylline and urinary retention. *Ann Intern Med* 1981; **94:** 823.

RENAL FAILURE. For a report of rhabdomyolysis-induced acute renal failure occurring after aminophylline overdose, see the general discussion on toxicity, above.

Gynaecomastia. Gynaecomastia occurred in a 61-year-old man after one to two months of oral theophylline therapy and resolved within one month of discontinuation.[1]

1. Dardick KR. Gynecomastia associated with theophylline. *J Fam Pract* 1984; **18:** 141–2.

Hypersensitivity. Hypersensitivity reactions have been reported following oral or intravenous administration of aminophylline. Reactions include erythematous rash with pruritus,[1,2] erythroderma,[2] and exfoliative dermatitis.[3] Aminophylline can produce both type I (immediate) and type IV (delayed) hypersensitivity reactions, the latter being due to the ethylenediamine component and can be confirmed by skin patch tests.[1-3] If hypersensitivity to ethylenediamine is confirmed it is recommended that aminophylline is avoided and treatment continued with theophylline or another theophylline salt.[1,3,4] Hypersensitivity reactions to theophylline have been reported rarely but type I reactions have occurred.[4] An erythematous, maculopapular rash has been reported[5] during treatment with a modified-release theophylline preparation which did not occur when another modified-release theophylline product was given.

1. Hardy C, *et al.* Allergy to aminophylline. *Br Med J* 1983; **286:** 2051–2.
2. Mohsenifar Z, *et al.* Two cases of allergy to aminophylline. *Ann Allergy* 1982; **49:** 281–2.
3. Nierenberg DW, Glazener FS. Aminophylline-induced exfoliative dermatitis: cause and implications. *West J Med* 1982; **137:** 328–31.
4. Gibb WRG. Delayed-type hypersensitivity to theophylline/aminophylline. *Lancet* 1985; **i:** 49.
5. Mendel S, *et al.* Dermatologic reaction to a sustained-release theophylline product. *Clin Pharm* 1985; **4:** 334–5.

Hyperuricaemia. In a study of 112 asthmatic patients receiving modified-release theophylline 200 to 400 mg 12-hourly, there was a significant correlation of serum-uric-acid concentrations and serum-theophylline concentrations.[1] Gout has been reported in a woman receiving theophylline and aminophylline;[2] her serum-uric acid concentration was increased while receiving the xanthines, but subsequently fell when they were discontinued, and rose again when treatment was resumed.

1. Morita Y, *et al.* Theophylline increases serum uric acid levels. *J Allergy Clin Immunol* 1984; **74:** 707–12.
2. Toda K, *et al.* Gout due to xanthine derivatives. *Br J Rheumatol* 1997; **36:** 1131–2.

Withdrawal syndromes. Episodes of apnoea beginning 28 hours after birth and increasing in frequency and severity over the next 4 days occurred in a neonate whose mother had taken aminophylline and theophylline throughout pregnancy. Measurement of serum-theophylline concentration showed the increasing apnoea was coincident with falling theophylline concentration and administration of theophylline to the infant resulted in resolution of apnoea; treatment was discontinued after 4 months.[1]

Worsening asthma control may occur in patients who have been receiving theophylline when the drug is withdrawn; there is some evidence of a rebound deterioration in lung function due to the development of tolerance.[2]

1. Horowitz DA, *et al.* Apnea associated with theophylline withdrawal in a term neonate. *Am J Dis Child* 1982; **136:** 73–4.
2. Bennett JA, *et al.* The airway effects of stopping regular oral theophylline in patients with asthma. *Br J Clin Pharmacol* 1998; **45:** 402–4.

Treatment of Adverse Effects

After theophylline or aminophylline overdosage by mouth the stomach should be emptied by emesis or lavage. Elimination may be enhanced by repeated oral doses of activated charcoal (see below). An osmotic laxative may also be given, especially if modified-release preparations have been taken. Treatment is symptomatic and supportive. Serum-theophylline concentrations should be monitored and if modified-release preparations have been taken monitoring should be prolonged. Metabolic abnormalities, particularly hypokalaemia, should be corrected; hypokalaemia may be so severe as to require intravenous infusion of potassium under ECG monitoring. In the non-asthmatic patient extreme tachycardia, hypokalaemia, and hyperglycaemia may be reversed by beta blockers (see also below). Convulsions should be controlled by the intravenous administration of diazepam. Charcoal haemoperfusion or haemodialysis may be required.

Reviews discussing the treatment of theophylline overdosage.[1-3]

1. Gaudreault P, Guay J. Theophylline poisoning: pharmacological considerations and clinical management. *Med Toxicol* 1986; **1:** 169–91.
2. Dawson AH, Whyte IM. The assessment and treatment of theophylline poisoning. *Med J Aust* 1989; **151:** 689–93.
3. Skinner MH. Adverse reactions and interactions with theophylline. *Drug Safety* 1990; **5:** 275–85.

Activated charcoal. Oral activated charcoal has been shown to reduce the gastro-intestinal absorption of aminophylline,[1] and repeated oral doses of activated charcoal enhance the clearance, and decrease the serum half-life of theophylline.[2,3] The decrease in theophylline serum half-life is affected by the activated charcoal dosage regimen used[4] and the surface area of the activated charcoal.[5] Work in *animals* has suggested that although the serum half-life of theophylline is decreased, the time for serum-theophylline concentrations to fall below toxic levels is not affected,[6] but nonetheless, in cases of overdosage with oral theophylline preparations the use of repeated oral activated charcoal has resulted in a reduction of serum-theophylline concentrations and resolution of signs of toxicity.[3,7]

The use of repeated oral doses of activated charcoal for theophylline poisoning has been suggested where haemoperfusion is unavailable[7,8] since activated charcoal is at least as effective as haemodialysis and, in some cases, has given clearances approaching those obtained with haemoperfusion.[9] However, administration of activated charcoal may be difficult in severely poisoned patients because of protracted vomiting which can be difficult to control. Ranitidine with or without droperidol has been used successfully to control theophylline-induced vomiting,[10] as has ondansetron: the $5HT_3$-antagonists may be more effective than haloperidol or metoclopramide.[11,12]

The addition of sorbitol to an oral regimen of multiple doses of activated charcoal has been reported[13] to decrease serum-theophylline concentrations to a greater extent than activated charcoal alone, but another study[14] found sorbitol produced no further significant lowering of serum-theophylline concentration compared with charcoal alone and excessive doses of sorbitol have been reported to cause hypernatraemia.[15]

It is generally recommended that the initial treatment of aminophylline or theophylline overdosage should consist of emesis or lavage and the administration of activated charcoal. However, in a recent study of simulated overdosage in volunteers neither emesis nor lavage prevented theophylline absorption whereas activated charcoal considerably reduced absorption.[16]

1. Neuvonen PJ, *et al.* Comparison of activated charcoal and ipecac syrup in prevention of drug absorption. *Eur J Clin Pharmacol* 1983; **24:** 557–62.
2. Berlinger WG, *et al.* Enhancement of theophylline clearance by oral activated charcoal. *Clin Pharmacol Ther* 1983; **33:** 351–4.
3. Mahutte CK, *et al.* Increased serum theophylline clearance with orally administered activated charcoal. *Am Rev Respir Dis* 1983; **128:** 820–2.
4. Park GD, *et al.* Effects of size and frequency of oral doses of charcoal on theophylline clearance. *Clin Pharmacol Ther* 1983; **34:** 663–6.
5. Park GD, *et al.* Effect of the surface area of activated charcoal on theophylline clearance. *J Clin Pharmacol* 1984; **24:** 289–92.
6. Brashear RE, Aronoff CR. Activated charcoal in theophylline intoxication. *J Clin Pharmacol* 1985; **25:** 460.
7. Gal P, *et al.* Oral activated charcoal to enhance theophylline elimination in an acute overdose. *JAMA* 1984; **251:** 3130–1.
8. Whyte KF, Addis GJ. Treatment of theophylline poisoning. *Br Med J* 1984; **288:** 1835.
9. Heath A, Knudsen K. Role of extracorporeal drug removal in acute theophylline poisoning: a review. *Med Toxicol* 1987; **2:** 294–308.
10. Amitai Y, *et al.* Repetitive oral activated charcoal and control of emesis in severe theophylline toxicity. *Ann Intern Med* 1986; **105:** 386–7.
11. Sage TA, *et al.* Ondansetron in the treatment of intractable nausea associated with theophylline toxicity. *Ann Pharmacother* 1993; **27:** 584–5. Correction. *ibid.*: 1408.
12. Brown SGA, Prentice DA. Ondansetron in the treatment of theophylline overdose. *Med J Aust* 1992; **156:** 512.
13. Goldberg MJ, *et al.* The effect of sorbitol and activated charcoal on serum theophylline concentrations after slow-release theophylline. *Clin Pharmacol Ther* 1987; **41:** 108–11.
14. Al-Shareef AH, *et al.* The effects of charcoal and sorbitol (alone and in combination) on plasma theophylline concentrations after a sustained-release formulation. *Hum Exp Toxicol* 1990; **9:** 179–82.
15. Gazda-Smith E, Synhavsky A. Hypernatremia following treatment of theophylline toxicity with activated charcoal and sorbitol. *Arch Intern Med* 1990; **150:** 689 and 692.
16. Minton NA, *et al.* Prevention of drug absorption in simulated theophylline overdose. *Hum Exp Toxicol* 1995; **14:** 170–4.

Beta blockers. During the infusion of propranolol in 2 non-asthmatic patients with hyperglycaemia, hypokalaemia, tachycardia, and hypotension following theophylline overdose, plasma glucose fell, plasma potassium increased, the pulse rate fell, and blood pressure rose. It was suggested that beta-adrenergic blockade may be of benefit in the management of the metabolic changes of theophylline poisoning following overdosage of aminophylline or theophylline, especially in the non-asthmatic patient, and possibly also in the asthmatic patient with severe hypokalaemia or cardiac arrhythmias if mechanical ventilation was available.[1,2] However, propranolol reduces the clearance of theophylline (see under Interactions, below) and it has been suggested that a water-soluble beta blocker may be more appropriate.[3]

1. Kearney TE, *et al.* Theophylline toxicity and the beta-adrenergic system. *Ann Intern Med* 1985; **102:** 766–9.
2. Amin DN, Henry JA. Propranolol administration in theophylline overdose. *Lancet* 1985; **i:** 520–1.
3. Farrar KT, Dunn AM. Beta-blockers in treatment of theophylline overdose. *Lancet* 1985; **i:** 983.

Endoscopy. Absorption is delayed following overdosage with modified-release oral preparations of aminophylline or theophylline and may be further prolonged by the formation of tablet aggregates, or bezoars, in the stomach.[1-3] Of 11 patients admitted with overdosage, one vomited a bezoar, 2 had bezoars removed at gastroscopy, and in one a bezoar was found at necropsy.[3] If bezoar formation occurs gastric lavage and activated charcoal will have little if any effect and the patient may appear to stabilise before experiencing increasing serum-theophylline concentration and clinical deterioration;[1,2] fatalities have been reported.[1] Endoscopy should be considered in cases of modified-release theophylline overdosage in which clinical signs and serial concentration measurements suggest continuing drug absorption.[2]

1. Coupe M. Self-poisoning with sustained-release aminophylline: a mechanism for observed secondary rise in serum theophylline. *Hum Toxicol* 1986; **5:** 341–2.
2. Cereda J-M, *et al.* Endoscopic removal of pharmacobezoar of slow release theophylline. *Br Med J* 1986; **293:** 1143.
3. Smith WDF. Endoscopic removal of a pharmacobezoar of slow release theophylline. *Br Med J* 1987; **294:** 125.

Haemodialysis and haemoperfusion. A review of extracorporeal theophylline removal techniques following overdosage of aminophylline or theophylline.[1] Neither peritoneal dialysis nor exchange transfusion produced a significant increase in the total body clearance of theophylline, whereas haemodialysis could be expected to double clearance, and haemoperfusion results in 4 to 6 fold increases in clearance. Charcoal haemoperfusion should be considered if the plasma-theophylline concentration exceeds 100 μg per mL in an acute intoxication, or 60 μg per mL in chronic overdose (40 μg per mL if there is significant respiratory or heart failure, or liver disease) though plasma concentrations alone should not determine its use (see under Adverse Effects, above). If there is intractable vomiting, arrhythmias, or seizures charcoal haemoperfusion should be commenced without delay. In most patients a 4-hour haemoperfusion allows significant clinical improvement, but treatment should continue until plasma concentrations are below 15 μg per mL. Plasma concentrations should be followed at least every 4 hours for the first 12 hours post-perfusion, as rebound increases have been noted on terminating perfusion. Haemodialysis may rarely be an alternative if haemoperfusion is not available, or in series with haemoperfusion if significant rhabdomyolysis is present.

1. Heath A, Knudsen K. Role of extracorporeal drug removal in acute theophylline poisoning: a review. *Med Toxicol* 1987; **2:** 294–308.

Precautions

Theophylline or aminophylline should be given with caution to patients with peptic ulceration, hyperthyroidism, hypertension, cardiac arrhythmias or other cardiovascular disease, or epilepsy, as these conditions may be exacerbated. Theophylline or aminophylline should also be given with caution to patients with heart failure, hepatic dysfunction or chronic alcoholism, acute febrile illness, and to neonates and the elderly, since in all of these circumstances theophylline clearance may be decreased, resulting in increases in serum-theophylline concentrations and serum half-life. Many drugs either increase or decrease serum concentrations and half-life of theophylline when given concomitantly; for details see under Interactions, below.

Intravenous injections of theophylline or aminophylline must be administered very slowly to prevent dangerous central nervous system and cardiovascular side-effects resulting from the direct stimulant effect.

Dosage requirements of theophylline vary widely between subjects; in view of the many factors affecting theophylline pharmacokinetics, serum concentration monitoring is necessary to ensure concentrations are within the therapeutic range.

Patients should not be transferred from one modified-release theophylline or aminophylline preparation to another without clinical assessment and the measurement of serum-theophylline concentrations because of bioavailability differences.

Acute respiratory illness. A reduction in theophylline clearance has been noted in patients presenting with acute respiratory illness[1] and appears to be associated with the severity of the underlying pulmonary disease and the rate of change in the patient's condition.[2] Caution has been advised in administering theophylline to patients with chronic obstructive pulmonary disease with acute exacerbations of a concomitant respiratory illness such as pneumonia since these patients appear most likely to exhibit altered theophylline metabolism.[2]

Similarly, a decrease in theophylline clearance and an increase in the incidence of adverse effects has been reported during acute viral infections such as influenza in children receiving theophylline therapy for chronic asthma.[3,4] Influenza vaccination has also been reported to reduce theophylline clearance (see Interactions, below). The mechanism by which theophylline metabolism is reduced in these patients may be related to increased interferon production during the acute febrile response. A dosage reduction of one half has been recommended[5] in children receiving chronic theophylline therapy who are febrile for more than 24 hours. Further dose adjustments should be based on serum-theophylline concentrations until the patients have recovered from their acute illness and are restabilised on their usual dosage. However, conflicting results have been reported and in one controlled study, respiratory syncytial virus infection was found to have no significant effect on theophylline disposition in children.[6]

1. Vozeh S, *et al.* Changes in theophylline clearance during acute illness. *JAMA* 1978; **240:** 1882–4.
2. Richer M, Lam YWF. Hypoxia, arterial pH and theophylline disposition. *Clin Pharmacokinet* 1993; **25:** 283–99.
3. Chang KC, *et al.* Altered theophylline pharmacokinetics during acute respiratory viral illness. *Lancet* 1978; **i:** 1132–3.
4. Kraemer MJ, *et al.* Altered theophylline clearance during an influenza B outbreak. *Pediatrics* 1982; **69:** 476–80.
5. American Academy of Pediatrics Committee on Drugs. Precautions concerning the use of theophylline. *Pediatrics* 1992; **89:** 781–3.
6. Muslow HA, *et al.* Lack of effect of respiratory syncytial virus infection on theophylline disposition in children. *J Pediatr* 1992; **121:** 466–71.

Age. For the effects of age on the metabolism and excretion of theophylline see under Pharmacokinetics, below. Dosage regimens for infants are discussed under Administration in Infants, in Uses and Administration, below.

Cystic fibrosis. Increased theophylline clearance has been noted in patients with cystic fibrosis,[1,2] although others have found clearance values similar to those in normal and asthmatic children.[3]

1. Isles A, *et al.* Theophylline disposition in cystic fibrosis. *Am Rev Respir Dis* 1983; **127:** 417–21.
2. Saccar C, *et al.* Pharmacokinetics of theophylline and its metabolites in cystic fibrosis. *J Clin Pharmacol* 1985; **25:** 468.
3. Georgitis JW, *et al.* Oral theophylline disposition in cystic fibrosis. *Ann Allergy* 1982; **48:** 175–7.

ECT. A 71-year-old woman with no history of seizures and with a serum-theophylline concentration slightly above the normal range (22.6 μg per mL) developed status epilepticus during electroconvulsive therapy.[1]

1. Peters SG, *et al.* Status epilepticus as a complication of concurrent electroconvulsive and theophylline therapy. *Mayo Clin Proc* 1984; **59:** 568–70.

Gastro-oesophageal reflux disease. Theophylline and theophylline derivatives have a relaxing influence on the lower oesophageal sphincter and can increase gastric acid secretion and increased episodes of gastro-oesophageal reflux have been reported in adults[1] and infants[2] receiving theophylline[1,2] or caffeine.[2]

1. Ekström T, Tibbling L. Influence of theophylline on gastro-oesophageal reflux and asthma. *Eur J Clin Pharmacol* 1988; **35:** 353–6.
2. Vandenplas Y, *et al.* Influence of xanthines on gastroesophageal reflux in infants at risk for sudden infant death syndrome. *Pediatrics* 1986; **77:** 807–10.

Gender. For reference to differences in theophylline pharmacokinetics between men and women and to the influence of the menstrual cycle, see under Pharmacokinetics, below.

Interference with theophylline assays. In a review of drug interferences in therapeutic drug monitoring, the following drugs were reported to interfere with the assay of theophylline by high pressure liquid chromatography: acetazolamide, caffeine, some cephalosporins and penicillins, chloramphenicol, dimenhydrinate, diprophylline, paracetamol, procainamide, salicylates, some sulphonamides, theobromine, and trisulphapyrimidines.[1] Metronidazole was also found to cause interference.[2] Measurement of plasma-theophylline concentrations by spectrophotometric methods, had been reported to be affected by the presence of allopurinol, barbiturates, caffeine, carbamazepine, cephazolin, chlordiazepoxide, dicoumarol, diprophylline, frusemide, gentamicin, hydrochlorothiazide, hydroxyzine, methyclothiazide, morphine, nitrofurantoin, oxazepam, oxyphenbutazone, paracetamol, phenacetin, phenylbutazone, phenytoin, probenecid, procainamide, salicylates, some sulphonamides, tetracycline, theobromine, thiamine, thiopentone, and warfarin.[1] Enzyme immunoassay techniques are more specific and only caffeine and theobromine had been reported to interfere with substrate-labelled fluorescent immunoassays.

1. Yosselson-Superstine S. Drug interferences with plasma assays in therapeutic drug monitoring. *Clin Pharmacokinet* 1984; **9:** 67–87.
2. Garfinkel D, *et al.* Metronidazole interferes with theophylline measurements. *Ann Intern Med* 1987; **106:** 171.

Obesity. Data suggesting that the difference in volume of distribution for theophylline based on ideal body-weight and total body-weight increases as the degree of obesity increases. The clinical importance of this difference on dosage calculations may be apparent only in morbidly obese patients.[1]

1. Visram N, *et al.* Theophylline loading dose in obese patients. *Clin Pharm* 1987; **6:** 188–9.

Porphyria. Theophylline has been associated with acute attacks of porphyria and is considered unsafe in patients with acute porphyria.[1]

1. Moore MR, McColl KEL. *Porphyria: drug lists.* Glasgow: Porphyria Research Unit, University of Glasgow, 1991.

Pregnancy and breast feeding. It has been recommended[1] that serum-theophylline concentrations are measured at monthly intervals throughout pregnancy and one and four weeks after delivery since the pharmacokinetics of theophylline may be altered. An increase in the volume of distribution of theophylline, a decrease in plasma-protein binding, and a continuing decrease in clearance throughout pregnancy have been noted in some patients, especially during the later part of pregnancy,[2-4] but other studies have noted an increase in theophylline clearance during pregnancy.[1,5] Some studies have found that after delivery there is a return of clearance values to those existing before pregnancy,[2] while others have not.[4]

Toxic concentrations of theophylline should not occur in breast-fed infants whose mothers are given appropriate doses of theophylline;[6] less than 1% of the total theophylline eliminated by breast-feeding women was found in breast milk.

1. Rubin PC. Prescribing in pregnancy: general principles. *Br Med J* 1986; **293:** 1415–17.
2. Carter BL, *et al.* Theophylline clearance during pregnancy. *Obstet Gynecol* 1986; **68:** 555–9.
3. Frederiksen MC, *et al.* Theophylline pharmacokinetics in pregnancy. *Clin Pharmacol Ther* 1986; **40:** 321–8.
4. Gardner MJ, *et al.* Longitudinal effects of pregnancy on the pharmacokinetics of theophylline. *Eur J Clin Pharmacol* 1987; **31:** 289–95.
5. Romero R, *et al.* Pharmacokinetics of intravenous theophylline in pregnant patients at term. *Am J Perinatol* 1983; **1:** 31–5.
6. Stec GP, *et al.* Kinetics of theophylline transfer to breast milk. *Clin Pharmacol Ther* 1980; **28:** 404–8.

Renal impairment. Theophylline is eliminated mainly by hepatic metabolism and usual doses of aminophylline or theophylline can be given to patients with renal impairment. In patients undergoing haemodialysis the clearance of theophylline is increased and its elimination half-life reduced; mean values of 84.8 and 83 mL per minute and 2.5 and 2.3 hours respectively have been reported.[1,2] Haemodialysis removes up to 40% of a dose of theophylline.[1] Peritoneal dialysis has little effect on the pharmacokinetics of theophylline removing about 3.2% of a dose.[1]

1. Lee C-SC, *et al.* Comparative pharmacokinetics of theophylline in peritoneal dialysis and hemodialysis. *J Clin Pharmacol* 1983; **23:** 274–80.
2. Anderson JR, *et al.* Effects of hemodialysis on theophylline kinetics. *J Clin Pharmacol* 1983; **23:** 428–32.

Interactions

The toxic effects of theophylline, aminophylline, and other xanthines are additive. Concomitant use with other xanthine medications should therefore be avoided; if intravenous aminophylline is to be given for acute bronchospasm in patients who have been taking maintenance xanthine therapy, serum-theophylline concentrations should be measured first and the initial dose reduced as appropriate (see under Uses and Administration, below).

Theophylline clearance may be reduced by interaction with other drugs including allopurinol, some antiarrhythmics, cimetidine, disulfiram, fluvoxamine, interferon alfa, macrolide antibiotics and quinolones, oral contraceptives, thiabendazole, and viloxazine, necessitating dosage reduction. Phenytoin and some other anticonvulsants, the antiviral ritonavir, rifampicin, sulphinpyrazone, and cigarette smoking may increase theophylline clearance, necessitating an increase in dose or dosing frequency.

Xanthines can potentiate hypokalaemia caused by hypoxia or associated with the administration of $beta_2$-adrenoceptor stimulants ($beta_2$ agonists), corticosteroids, and diuretics. There is a risk of synergistic toxicity if theophylline is given concomitantly with halothane or ketamine, and it may antagonise the effects of adenosine and of non-depolarising muscle relaxants; lithium elimination may be enhanced with a consequent loss of effect. The interaction between theophylline and beta blockers is complex (see below) but concomitant administration tends to be avoided on pharmacological grounds since beta blockers produce bronchospasm.

Theophylline is metabolised by several isozymes of hepatic cytochrome P450, of which the most important seems to be CYP1A2.[1] Numerous drugs affect the metabolic clearance of theophylline and aminophylline,[2] but the variability in theophylline pharmacokinetics makes the clinical significance of these interactions difficult to predict. It has been recommended that concurrent administration of drugs that inhibit theophylline metabolism should be avoided but, if unavoidable, the dose of theophylline should be decreased by one half and subsequently adjusted based on serum-theophylline monitoring.[3] Even when introducing concurrent medication for which no interaction is suspected, a check on the serum-theophylline concentration within 24 hours of beginning the new drug has been advised.[3]

Theophylline reduces liver plasma flow[4] and may therefore prolong the half-life and increase steady-state levels of hepatically eliminated drugs but it is claimed to have no effect on antipyrine clearance.[5]

1. Ha HR, *et al.* Metabolism of theophylline by cDNA-expressed human cytochromes P-450. *Br J Clin Pharmacol* 1995; **39:** 321–6.
2. Upton RA. Pharmacokinetic interactions between theophylline and other medication. *Clin Pharmacokinet* 1991; **20:** 66–80 (part I) and 135–50 (part II).
3. American Academy of Pediatrics Committee on Drugs. Precautions concerning the use of theophylline. *Pediatrics* 1992; **89:** 781–3.
4. Onrot J, *et al.* Reduction of liver plasma flow by caffeine and theophylline. *Clin Pharmacol Ther* 1986; **40:** 506–10.
5. Døssing M, *et al.* Effect of theophylline and salbutamol on hepatic drug metabolism. *Hum Toxicol* 1989; **8:** 225–8.

Antiarrhythmics. An increase in serum-theophylline concentration from 93.2 to 194.2 μmol per litre with symptoms of tachycardia, nervousness, and tremors occurred in a patient 9 days after starting *amiodarone* therapy.[1] Elevated theophylline concentrations and/or decreased clearance have also been reported following addition of *mexiletine* to theophylline therapy.[2-6] Amiodarone and mexiletine probably interact with theophylline through inhibition of its hepatic metabolism. *Tocainide* has also been found to impair theophylline metabolism resulting in a reduction in theophylline clearance but the effect was substantially smaller than that of mexiletine.[7] In one patient stabilised on theophylline therapy, an increase in the plasma-theophylline concentration with subsequent toxicity was noted following the initiation of treatment with *propafenone.*[8] See also under Calcium-channel Blockers, below.

1. Soto J, *et al.* Possible theophylline-amiodarone interaction. *DICP Ann Pharmacother* 1990; **24:** 1115.
2. Stanley R, *et al.* Mexiletine-theophylline interaction. *Am J Med* 1989; **86:** 733–4.
3. Ueno K, *et al.* Interaction between theophylline and mexiletine. *DICP Ann Pharmacother* 1990; **24:** 471–2.
4. Hurwitz A, *et al.* Mexiletine effects on theophylline disposition. *Clin Pharmacol Ther* 1991; **50:** 299–307.
5. Loi C-M, *et al.* Inhibition of theophylline metabolism by mexiletine in young male and female nonsmokers. *Clin Pharmacol Ther* 1991; **49:** 571–80.
6. Ueno K, *et al.* Mechanism of interaction between theophylline and mexiletine. *DICP Ann Pharmacother* 1991; **25:** 727–30.
7. Loi C-M, *et al.* The effect of tocainide on theophylline metabolism. *Br J Clin Pharmacol* 1993; **35:** 437–40.
8. Lee BL, Dohrmann ML. Theophylline toxicity after propafenone treatment: evidence for drug interaction. *Clin Pharmacol Ther* 1992; **51:** 353–5.

Antibacterials. IMIPENEM. Seizures have been reported in three patients receiving theophylline who were given imipenem,[1] although serum concentrations of theophylline were not affected.

1. Semel JD, Allen N. Seizures in patients simultaneously receiving theophylline and imipenem or ciprofloxacin or metronidazole. *South Med J* 1991; **84:** 465–8.

ISONIAZID. Isoniazid inhibits oxidative enzymes in the liver and has been found to impair the elimination of theophylline. Both clearance and volume of distribution of theophylline were reduced with an increase in serum-theophylline concentrations in healthy subjects after 14 days' pretreatment with isoniazid[1] and theophylline toxicity has been reported[2] in a patient one month after adding theophylline to isoniazid therapy.

1. Samigun, *et al.* Lowering of theophylline clearance by isoniazid in slow and rapid acetylators. *Br J Clin Pharmacol* 1990; **29:** 570–3.
2. Torrent J, *et al.* Theophylline-isoniazid interaction. *DICP Ann Pharmacother* 1989; **23:** 143–5.

MACROLIDES. There are conflicting reports of the effect of *erythromycin* on the pharmacokinetics of theophylline. Significant decreases in the clearance of theophylline and prolonged elimination half-life have been reported[1-3] but other studies have found no interaction.[4,5] It has also been noted that the serum concentrations and bioavailability of erythromycin may be reduced by theophylline.[6,7] The clearance of theophylline is also markedly decreased by the concomitant administration of *triacetyloleandomycin,*[8-10] but there have been reports that for clinical purposes the pharmacokinetics of theophylline do not seem to be significantly altered by *dirithromycin,*[11,12] *josamycin,*[9,13] *midecamycin,*[10] *miocamycin,*[14,15] *rokitamycin,*[16] *roxithromycin,*[17] or *spiramycin.*[18] *Clarithromycin* also seems unlikely to have a significant effect in most patients, but in a few theophylline dosage may need to be adjusted.[19,20]

1. Zarowitz BJM, *et al.* Effect of erythromycin base on theophylline kinetics. *Clin Pharmacol Ther* 1981; **29:** 601–5.
2. Renton KW, *et al.* Depression of theophylline elimination by erythromycin. *Clin Pharmacol Ther* 1981; **30:** 422–6.
3. May DC, *et al.* The effects of erythromycin on theophylline elimination in normal males. *J Clin Pharmacol* 1982; **22:** 125–30.
4. Maddux MS, *et al.* The effect of erythromycin on theophylline pharmacokinetics at steady state. *Chest* 1982; **81:** 563–5.
5. Hildebrandt R, *et al.* Lack of clinically important interaction between erythromycin and theophylline. *Eur J Clin Pharmacol* 1984; **26:** 485–9.
6. Iliopoulou A, *et al.* Pharmacokinetic interaction between theophylline and erythromycin. *Br J Clin Pharmacol* 1982; **14:** 495–9.
7. Paulsen O, *et al.* The interaction of erythromycin with theophylline. *Eur J Clin Pharmacol* 1987; **32:** 493–8.
8. Weinberger M, *et al.* Inhibition of theophylline clearance by troleandomycin. *J Allergy Clin Immunol* 1977; **59:** 228–31.
9. Brazier JL, *et al.* Retard d'élimination de la théophylline dû à la troléandomycine: absence d'effet de la josamycine. *Therapie* 1980; **35:** 545–9.
10. Lavarenne J, *et al.* Influence d'un nouveau macrolide, la midécamycine, sur les taux sanguins de théophylline. *Therapie* 1981; **36:** 451–6.
11. Bachmann K, *et al.* Changes in the steady-state pharmacokinetics of theophylline during treatment with dirithromycin. *J Clin Pharmacol* 1990; **30:** 1001–5.
12. Bachmann K, *et al.* Steady-state pharmacokinetics of theophylline in COPD patients treated with dirithromycin. *J Clin Pharmacol* 1993; **33:** 861–5.
13. Ruff F, *et al.* Macrolide et théophylline: absence d'interaction josamycine-théophylline. *Nouv Presse Med* 1981; **10:** 175.
14. Principi N, *et al.* Effect of miocamycin on theophylline kinetics in children. *Eur J Clin Pharmacol* 1987; **31:** 701–4.
15. Couet W, *et al.* Lack of effect of ponsinomycin on the plasma pharmacokinetics of theophylline. *Eur J Clin Pharmacol* 1989; **37:** 101–4.
16. Ishioka T. Effect of a new macrolide antibiotic, 3″-O-propionyl-leucomycin A_5 (rokitamycin) on serum concentrations of theophylline and digoxin in the elderly. *Acta Ther* 1987; **13:** 17–24.
17. Saint-Salvi B, *et al.* A study of the interaction of roxithromycin with theophylline and carbamazine. *J Antimicrob Chemother* 1987; **20** (suppl B): 121–9.
18. Debruyne D, *et al.* Spiramycin has no effect on serum theophylline in asthmatic patients. *Eur J Clin Pharmacol* 1986; **30:** 505–7.
19. Bachand RT. Comparative study of clarithromycin and ampicillin in the treatment of patients with acute bacterial exacerbations of chronic bronchitis. *J Antimicrob Chemother* 1991; **27** (suppl A): 91–100.
20. Gillum JG, *et al.* Effect of combination therapy with ciprofloxacin and clarithromycin on theophylline pharmacokinetics in healthy volunteers. *Antimicrob Agents Chemother* 1996; **40:** 1715–16.

QUINOLONES. The fluoroquinolone antibacterials vary in their ability to interact with theophylline. *Enoxacin* shows the strongest interaction and has been reported[1] to cause serious nausea and vomiting, tachycardia, and headaches, associated with unexpectedly high plasma-theophylline concentrations in patients with respiratory-tract infections. Studies,[2-5] mainly in healthy subjects, have found that enoxacin decreases theophylline clearance by up to 74%[3] with an increase in the elimination half-life and serum-theophylline concentration. A 50% decrease in theophylline clearance has been reported with *grepafloxacin.*[6]

Ciprofloxacin[2,7-9] and *pefloxacin*[2] interact with theophylline to a lesser extent than enoxacin, decreasing theophylline clearance by about 30%. Eight clinically important interactions between ciprofloxacin and theophylline had been reported to the UK Committee on Safety of Medicines[10] including 1 death. A ciprofloxacin-induced seizure has been reported[11] which may have been due to the combined inhibitory effects of the 2 drugs on GABA binding. It has been recommended that ciprofloxacin should not be used in patients treated with theophylline.[10]

Norfloxacin[4,12-14] and *ofloxacin*[4,12,15] have been reported to have minor effects on the pharmacokinetics of theophylline. Although their effects were usually considered not to be clinically significant, the US Food and Drug Administration had received 9 reports of theophylline toxicity associated with concomitant norfloxacin administration, including 1 death.[16] *Fleroxacin,*[17] *flumequine,*[18] and *lomefloxacin*[9,19,20] have been reported to have no significant effect on the pharmacokinetics of theophylline.

The mechanism of interaction involves a reduction in the metabolic clearance of theophylline due to inhibition of hepatic microsomal enzymes. However, the exact mechanism is unknown and it is difficult to predict which patients will be at risk. Extreme caution should be used when giving quinolones in conjunction with theophylline, particularly in the elderly[16] and it may be advisable to prescribe a non-interacting fluoroquinolone, although theophylline concentrations should still be monitored.

Of the non-fluorinated quinolones, *nalidixic acid*[2] has been reported not to affect theophylline clearance whereas *pipemidic acid* has markedly inhibited theophylline clearance.[20]

1. Wijnands WJA, *et al.* Enoxacin raises plasma theophylline concentrations. *Lancet* 1984; **ii:** 108–9.
2. Wijnands WJA, *et al.* The influence of quinolone derivatives on theophylline clearance. *Br J Clin Pharmacol* 1986; **22:** 677–83.
3. Beckmann J, *et al.* Enoxacin—a potent inhibitor of theophylline metabolism. *Eur J Clin Pharmacol* 1987; **33:** 227–30.
4. Sano M, *et al.* Inhibitory effect of enoxacin, ofloxacin and norfloxacin on renal excretion of theophylline in humans. *Eur J Clin Pharmacol* 1989; **36:** 323–4.
5. Koup JR, *et al.* Theophylline dosage adjustment during enoxacin coadministration. *Antimicrob Agents Chemother* 1990; **34:** 803–7.
6. Efthymiopoulos C, *et al.* Theophylline and warfarin interaction studies with grepafloxacin. *Clin Pharmacokinet* 1997; **33** (suppl 1): 39–46.
7. Nix DE, *et al.* Effect of multiple dose oral ciprofloxacin on the pharmacokinetics of theophylline and indocyanine green. *J Antimicrob Chemother* 1987; **19:** 263–9.
8. Schwartz J, *et al.* Impact of ciprofloxacin on theophylline clearance and steady-state concentrations in serum. *Antimicrob Agents Chemother* 1988; **32:** 75–7.
9. Robson RA, *et al.* Comparative effects of ciprofloxacin and lomefloxacin on the oxidative metabolism of theophylline. *Br J Clin Pharmacol* 1990; **29:** 491–3.
10. Bem JL, Mann RD. Danger of interaction between ciprofloxacin and theophylline. *Br Med J* 1988; **296:** 1131.
11. Karki SD, *et al.* Seizure with ciprofloxacin and theophylline combined therapy. *DICP Ann Pharmacother* 1990; **24:** 595–6.
12. Sano M, *et al.* Comparative pharmacokinetics of theophylline following two fluoroquinolones co-administration. *Eur J Clin Pharmacol* 1987; **32:** 431–2.
13. Ho G, *et al.* Evaluation of the effect of norfloxacin on the pharmacokinetics of theophylline. *Clin Pharmacol Ther* 1988; **44:** 35–8.
14. Davis RL, *et al.* Effect of norfloxacin on theophylline metabolism. *Antimicrob Agents Chemother* 1989; **33:** 212–14.
15. Gregoire SL, *et al.* Inhibition of theophylline clearance by coadministered ofloxacin without alteration of theophylline effects. *Antimicrob Agents Chemother* 1987; **31:** 375–8.
16. Grasela TH, Dreis MW. An evaluation of the quinolone-theophylline interaction using the Food and Drug Administration spontaneous reporting system. *Arch Intern Med* 1992; **152:** 617–21.
17. Parent M, *et al.* Safety of fleroxacin coadministered with theophylline to young and elderly volunteers. *Antimicrob Agents Chemother* 1990; **34:** 1249–53.
18. Lacarelle B, *et al.* The quinolone, flumequine, has no effect on theophylline pharmacokinetics. *Eur J Clin Pharmacol* 1994; **46:** 477–8.
19. LeBel M, *et al.* Influence of lomefloxacin on the pharmacokinetics of theophylline. *Antimicrob Agents Chemother* 1990: **34:** 1254–6.
20. Staib AH, *et al.* Interaction of quinolones with the theophylline metabolism in man: investigations with lomefloxacin and pipemidic acid. *Int J Clin Pharmacol Ther Toxicol* 1989; **27:** 289–93.

RIFAMPICIN. Rifampicin induces hepatic oxidative enzymes and a dose of 600 mg daily by mouth for 6 to 14 days has been shown to increase mean plasma-theophylline clearance by 25 to 82% due to enhancement of hepatic theophylline metabolism. This increase in clearance is sufficient to cause clinical effects in some patients,[1-4] including children.[5]

1. Straughn AB, *et al.* Effect of rifampin on theophylline disposition. *Ther Drug Monit* 1984; **6:** 153–6.
2. Robson RA, *et al.* Theophylline-rifampicin interaction: non-selective induction of theophylline metabolic pathways. *Br J Clin Pharmacol* 1984; **18:** 445–8.
3. Boyce EG, *et al.* The effect of rifampin on theophylline kinetics. *J Clin Pharmacol* 1986; **26:** 696–9.
4. Adebayo GE, *et al.* Attenuation of rifampicin-induced theophylline metabolism by diltiazem/rifampicin coadministration in healthy volunteers. *Eur J Clin Pharmacol* 1989; **37:** 127–31.
5. Brocks DR, *et al.* Theophylline-rifampin interaction in a pediatric patient. *Clin Pharm* 1986; **5:** 602–4.

TETRACYCLINES. *Tetracycline* weakly inhibited theophylline clearance after 5 days of therapy in 5 non-smoking adults with chronic obstructive airways disease[1] and theophylline toxicity has been reported[2] in a patient given a 10-day course of tetracycline during theophylline therapy. *Doxycycline* has been reported not to have any significant effect on theophylline pharmacokinetics in healthy subjects.[3]

1. Gotz VP, Ryerson GG. Evaluation of tetracycline on theophylline disposition in patients with chronic obstructive airways disease. *Drug Intell Clin Pharm* 1986; **20:** 694–7.
2. McCormack JP, *et al.* Theophylline toxicity induced by tetracycline. *Clin Pharm* 1990; **9:** 546–9.
3. Jonkman JHG, *et al.* No influence of doxycycline on theophylline pharmacokinetics. *Ther Drug Monit* 1985; **7:** 92–4.

Antidepressants. Significantly reduced clearance and increased plasma concentrations of theophylline have been reported during concomitant administration of *viloxazine* and theophylline.[1,2] The dosage of theophylline should be decreased and its plasma concentrations monitored when viloxazine is also prescribed.[2] The interaction probably involves competition between the two drugs for hepatic microsomal enzymes.

Concomitant administration of *fluvoxamine* has also been associated with a significant reduction in theophylline clearance[3] and theophylline toxicity has been described in patients when fluvoxamine was added to their therapy.[4,5] This interaction which is due to potent liver enzyme inhibition[6] has been the subject of a warning by the UK Committee on Safety of Medicines[7] in which they issued the standard advice of avoiding the two drugs if at all possible and, where they could not be avoided, of giving half the dose of theophylline and monitoring plasma concentrations.

For a mention of the effect of theophylline on the renal clearance of *lithium*, see Xanthines, under Interactions of Lithium, p.294.

1. Thomson AH, *et al.* Theophylline toxicity following coadministration of viloxazine. *Ther Drug Monit* 1988; **10:** 359–60.
2. Perault MC, *et al.* A study of the interaction of viloxazine with theophylline. *Ther Drug Monit* 1989; **11:** 520–2.
3. Donaldson KM, *et al.* The effect [of] fluvoxamine at steady state on the pharmacokinetics of theophylline after a single dose in healthy male volunteers. *Br J Clin Pharmacol* 1994; **37:** 492P.
4. Sperber AD. Toxic interaction between fluvoxamine and sustained release theophylline in an 11-year-old boy. *Drug Safety* 1991; **6:** 460–2.
5. Thomson AH, *et al.* Interaction between fluvoxamine and theophylline. *Pharm J* 1992; **249:** 137.
6. Rasmussen BB, *et al.* Selective serotonin reuptake inhibitors and theophylline metabolism in human liver microsomes: potent inhibition by fluvoxamine. *Br J Clin Pharmacol* 1995; **39:** 151–9.
7. Committee on Safety of Medicines/Medicines Control Agency. Fluvoxamine increases plasma theophylline levels. *Current Problems* 1994; **20:** 12.

Antiepileptics. *Phenytoin* markedly decreases the elimination half-life and increases the clearance of theophylline, probably due to hepatic enzyme induction, at therapeutic serum-phenytoin concentrations,[1-3] at subtherapeutic phenytoin concentrations,[2,4] and even in heavy smokers.[2] A preliminary report suggested that the serum concentration of phenytoin may be decreased simultaneously,[5] perhaps due to enzyme induction by theophylline[5] or reduced phenytoin absorption.[6] The interaction between phenytoin and theophylline has been reported to occur within 5 to 14 days of commencing concomitant therapy, and theophylline clearance has increased by up to 350%, and reductions in serum half-life have ranged from 25 to 70% of initial values.[3,4]

Carbamazepine has also been observed to increase theophylline elimination. In one patient, theophylline serum half-life was decreased by approximately 24 to 60%, and clearance was increased by about 35 to 100% when carbamazepine was given concomitantly.[2] In an 11-year-old girl theophylline-serum half-life was almost halved with loss of asthma control after 3 weeks of concurrent carbamazepine therapy.[7] In turn, theophylline has been reported to reduce the half-life of carbamazepine—see p.342.

Although *phenobarbitone* was not found to have a significant effect on the pharmacokinetics of a single dose of theophylline given intravenously,[8] enhanced theophylline clearance has been seen in patients after longer periods of treatment with phenobarbitone.[9,10] The magnitude of the changes in theophylline elimination appears to be smaller with phenobarbitone than phenytoin. *Pentobarbitone* in high doses has also been reported to increase theophylline metabolism.[11] A more recent study[12] has also shown that therapeutic doses of pentobarbitone (100 mg daily) increase plasma clearance of theophylline by a mean of 40%, although this was subject to marked interindividual variations. Renal clearance was not affected, suggesting hepatic enzyme induction as the probable mechanism.

1. Marquis J-F, *et al.* Phenytoin-theophylline interaction. *N Engl J Med* 1982; **307:** 1189–90.
2. Reed RC, Schwartz HJ. Phenytoin-theophylline-quinidine interaction. *N Engl J Med* 1983; **308:** 724–5.
3. Sklar SJ, Wagner JC. Enhanced theophylline clearance secondary to phenytoin therapy. *Drug Intell Clin Pharm* 1985; **19:** 34–6.
4. Miller M, *et al.* Influence of phenytoin on theophylline clearance. *Clin Pharmacol Ther* 1984; **35:** 666–9.
5. Taylor JW, *et al.* The interaction of phenytoin and theophylline. *Drug Intell Clin Pharm* 1980; **14:** 638.
6. Hendeles L, *et al.* Decreased oral phenytoin absorption following concurrent theophylline administration. *J Allergy Clin Immunol* 1979; **63:** 156.
7. Rosenberry KR, *et al.* Reduced theophylline half-life induced by carbamazepine therapy. *J Pediatr* 1983; **102:** 472–4.
8. Piafsky KM, *et al.* Effect of phenobarbital on the disposition of intravenous theophylline. *Clin Pharmacol Ther* 1977; **22:** 336–9.
9. Jusko WJ, *et al.* Factors affecting theophylline clearances: age, tobacco, marijuana, cirrhosis, congestive heart failure, obesity, oral contraceptives, benzodiazepines, barbiturates, and ethanol. *J Pharm Sci* 1979; **68:** 1358–66.
10. Saccar CL, *et al.* The effect of phenobarbital on theophylline disposition in children with asthma. *J Allergy Clin Immunol* 1985; **75:** 716–19.
11. Gibson GA, *et al.* Influence of high-dose phenobarbital on theophylline pharmacokinetics: a case report. *Ther Drug Monit* 1985; **7:** 181–4.
12. Dahlqvist R, *et al.* Induction of theophylline metabolism by pentobarbital. *Ther Drug Monit* 1989; **11:** 408–10.

Antifungals. There have been reports that *ketoconazole* does not appear significantly to alter the pharmacokinetics of theophylline.[1,2] The manufacturer of *fluconazole* has, however, stated that plasma clearance of theophylline may be decreased by fluconazole. A 16% reduction in theophylline clearance has been reported[3] following oral fluconazole administration but fluconazole was considered to have only a minor inhibitory effect on theophylline metabolism and theophylline disposition was not significantly affected. A similar degree of inhibition has been seen in theophylline metabolism when *terbinafine* was given concomitantly.[4]

1. Brown MW, *et al.* Effect of ketoconazole on hepatic oxidative drug metabolism. *Clin Pharmacol Ther* 1985; **37:** 290–7.
2. Heusner JJ, *et al.* Effect of chronically administered ketoconazole on the elimination of theophylline in man. *Drug Intell Clin Pharm* 1987; **21:** 514–17.
3. Konishi H, *et al.* Effect of fluconazole on theophylline disposition in humans. *Eur J Clin Pharmacol* 1994; **46:** 309–12.
4. Trépanier EF, *et al.* Effect of terbinafine on theophylline pharmacokinetics in healthy volunteers. *Antimicrob Agents Chemother* 1998; **42:** 695–7.

Antigout drugs. *Allopurinol* 300 mg by mouth daily for 7 days was found to have no effect on the pharmacokinetics of theophylline following a single intravenous dose of aminophylline[1,2] or following theophylline given by mouth to steady state.[1] However, allopurinol 600 mg by mouth daily for 28 days has been found to inhibit the metabolism of theophylline,[3] increasing the mean half-life by 25% after 14 days and 29% after 28 days and there has been a report of allopurinol increasing peak plasma-theophylline concentrations by 38% in one patient within 2 days of concomitant administration.[4]

Probenecid[5] has been reported to have no effect on the hepatic metabolism or total body clearance of theophylline in a single-dose study in healthy subjects.

Sulphinpyrazone[6] 800 mg daily for 7 days increased the total plasma clearance of theophylline by 22% in healthy subjects due to selective induction of certain cytochrome P-450 enzymes.

1. Grygiel JJ, *et al.* Effects of allopurinol on theophylline metabolism and clearance. *Clin Pharmacol Ther* 1979; **26:** 660–7.
2. Vozeh S, *et al.* Influence of allopurinol on theophylline disposition in adults. *Clin Pharmacol Ther* 1980; **27:** 194–7.
3. Manfredi RL, Vesell ES. Inhibition of theophylline metabolism by long-term allopurinol administration. *Clin Pharmacol Ther* 1981; **29:** 224–9.
4. Barry M, Feely J. Allopurinol influences aminophenazone elimination. *Clin Pharmacokinet* 1990; **19:** 167–9.
5. Chen TWD, Patton TF. Effect of probenecid on the pharmacokinetics of aminophylline. *Drug Intell Clin Pharm* 1983; **17:** 465–6.
6. Birkett DJ, *et al.* Evidence for a dual action of sulphinpyrazone on drug metabolism in man: theophylline-sulphinpyrazone interaction. *Br J Clin Pharmacol* 1983; **15:** 567–9.

Antineoplastics. There has been a report of increased clearance of theophylline in 3 patients receiving *aminoglutethimide*.[1]

For reference to a possible interaction between theophylline and *lomustine*, see Lomustine, p.544.

1. Lønning PE, *et al.* Effect of aminoglutethimide on antipyrine, theophylline, and digitoxin disposition in breast cancer. *Clin Pharmacol Ther* 1984; **36:** 796–802.

Antivirals. Serum-theophylline concentrations and half-life increased in a 62-year-old woman after 4 days of concomitant treatment with *vidarabine*. Inhibition of xanthine oxidase by a vidarabine metabolite was suspected.[1]

A single injection of recombinant human *interferon-alfa* reduced theophylline clearance by 33 to 81% in 8 of 9 subjects, resulting in a 1.5 to sixfold increase in the theophylline elimination half-life.[2] Injection of interferon-alfa once daily for 3 days in 11 healthy subjects also reduced theophylline clearance and increased elimination half-life,[3] but the magnitude of the changes were of a similar order to normal intra-individual variation and the interaction was considered of minor clinical significance.

The manufacturers of *ritonavir* state that it substantially increases the clearance of theophylline; theophylline dosage may need to be increased to maintain efficacy.

1. Gannon R, *et al.* Possible interaction between vidarabine and theophylline. *Ann Intern Med* 1984; **101:** 148.
2. Williams SJ, *et al.* Inhibition of theophylline metabolism by interferon. *Lancet* 1987; **ii:** 939–41.
3. Jonkman JHG, *et al.* Effects of α-interferon on theophylline pharmacokinetics and metabolism. *Br J Clin Pharmacol* 1989; **27:** 795–802.

Benzodiazepines. For reference to the antagonism of benzodiazepine sedation by aminophylline, see Xanthines, under Interactions of Diazepam, p.665.

Beta blockers. *Propranolol* reduced theophylline clearance by 36% in healthy subjects given aminophylline intravenously. *Metoprolol* did not reduce clearance in the group as a whole, but a reduction was noted in some smokers whose theophylline clearance was initially high.[1] Propranolol is thought to exert a dose-dependent selective inhibitory effect on the separate forms of cytochrome P450 involved in theophylline demethylation and 8-hydroxylation.[2] The less lipophilic beta blockers *atenolol*[3,4] and *nadolol*[4] had no significant effect on the pharmacokinetics of theophylline.

In general, however, beta blockers should be avoided in patients taking theophylline as they can dangerously exacerbate bronchospasm in patients with a history of asthma or chronic obstructive pulmonary disease.

1. Conrad KA, Nyman DW. Effects of metoprolol and propranolol on theophylline elimination. *Clin Pharmacol Ther* 1980; **28:** 463–7.
2. Miners JO, *et al.* Selectivity and dose-dependency of the inhibitory effect of propranolol on theophylline metabolism in man. *Br J Clin Pharmacol* 1985; **20:** 219–23.
3. Cerasa LA, *et al.* Lack of effect of atenolol on the pharmacokinetics of theophylline. *Br J Clin Pharmacol* 1988; **26:** 800–2.
4. Corsi CM, *et al.* Lack of effect of atenolol and nadolol on the metabolism of theophylline. *Br J Clin Pharmacol* 1990; **29:** 265–8.

Caffeine. Abstention from dietary methylxanthines by healthy subjects has resulted in faster elimination of theophylline.[1] While Monks *et al.* reported that the addition of extra caffeine to the diet did not alter theophylline disposition,[2] other studies in healthy subjects have indicated that the ingestion of moderate amounts of caffeine (120 to 900 mg daily), which could be consumed by drinking several cups of coffee a day, can have a pronounced influence on the pharmacokinetics of theophylline.[3,4] In these latter studies the mean theophylline clearance was reduced by 23% and 29% with a corresponding increase in the elimination half-lives.

1. Monks TJ, *et al.* Influence of methylxanthine-containing foods on theophylline metabolism and kinetics. *Clin Pharmacol Ther* 1979; **26:** 513–24.
2. Monks TJ, *et al.* The effect of increased caffeine intake on the metabolism and pharmacokinetics of theophylline in man. *Biopharm Drug Dispos* 1981; **2:** 31–7.
3. Jonkman JHG, *et al.* The influence of caffeine on the steady-state pharmacokinetics of theophylline. *Clin Pharmacol Ther* 1991; **49:** 248–55.
4. Sato J, *et al.* Influence of usual intake of dietary caffeine on single-dose kinetics of theophylline in healthy human subjects. *Eur J Clin Pharmacol* 1993; **44:** 295–8.

Calcium-channel blockers. *Verapamil* has been reported[1] to decrease the clearance of theophylline by a mean of 14% in healthy subjects and although this was not considered to be clinically significant, symptoms of theophylline toxicity, associated with near doubling of the serum-theophylline concentration have occurred in a 76-year-old woman taking theophylline after 6 days of therapy with verapamil.[2] Studies in healthy subjects and asthmatic patients have produced conflicting results of the effect of *nifedipine* on the pharmacokinetics of theophylline. Reduced clearance[1] and an increase in the volume of distribution[3,4] of theophylline have been reported and both decreased[4] and increased[5] serum-theophylline concentrations; theophylline toxicity has been reported.[6,7] However, most studies have concluded that the effects of nifedipine are unlikely to be of clinical importance.[1,4,5,8]

Diltiazem has been reported[5] to cause an increase in serum-theophylline concentration and *felodipine*[9] a decrease in serum-theophylline concentration; neither of these effects were considered to be clinically significant.

1. Robson RA, *et al.* Selective inhibitory effects of nifedipine and verapamil on oxidative metabolism: effects on theophylline. *Br J Clin Pharmacol* 1988; **25:** 397–400.
2. Burnakis TG, *et al.* Increased serum theophylline concentrations secondary to oral verapamil. *Clin Pharm* 1983; **2:** 458–61.
3. Jackson SHD, *et al.* The interaction between iv theophylline and chronic oral dosing with slow release nifedipine in volunteers. *Br J Clin Pharmacol* 1986; **21:** 389–92.
4. Adebayo GI, Mabadeje AFB. Effect of nifedipine on antipyrine and theophylline disposition. *Biopharm Drug Dispos* 1990; **11:** 157–64.
5. Smith SR, *et al.* The influence of nifedipine and diltiazem on serum theophylline concentration-time profiles. *J Clin Pharm Ther* 1989; **14:** 403–8.
6. Parrillo SJ, Venditto M. Elevated theophylline blood levels from institution of nifedipine therapy. *Ann Emerg Med* 1984; **13:** 216–17.
7. Harrod CS. Theophylline toxicity and nifedipine. *Ann Intern Med* 1987; **106:** 480.
8. Spedini C, Lombardi C. Long-term treatment with oral nifedipine plus theophylline in the management of chronic bronchial asthma. *Eur J Clin Pharmacol* 1986; **31:** 105–6.
9. Bratel T, *et al.* Felodipine reduces the absorption of theophylline in man. *Eur J Clin Pharmacol* 1989; **36:** 481–5.

Cannabis. A search of the literature[1] revealed 2 studies, both published in the 1970s, that showed that marijuana smoking increased the clearance of theophylline.

1. Brown D. Influence on theophylline clearance. *Pharm J* 1994; **253:** 595.

Corticosteroids. In 3 patients with acute severe asthma given aminophylline intravenously, serum-theophylline concentrations rose rapidly from the therapeutic range to between 40 and 50 μg per mL when *hydrocortisone* was given intravenously.[1] In studies in healthy subjects, no significant changes in serum-theophylline concentrations were noted after the concomitant administration of hydrocortisone, *methylprednisolone*,[2] or *prednisone*[3] although there was a trend towards increased theophylline clearance during corticosteroid therapy.[2,3] In pre-term neonates, exposure to *betamethasone in utero* stimulated the hepatic metabolism of theophylline,[4,5] but did not affect dosage requirements.

The possibility that adverse effects such as hypokalaemia may be potentiated by concomitant administration of theophylline and corticosteroids should be borne in mind.

1. Buchanan N, *et al.* Asthma—a possible interaction between hydrocortisone and theophylline. *S Afr Med J* 1979; 56: 1147–8.
2. Leavengood DC, *et al.* The effect of corticosteroids on theophylline metabolism. *Ann Allergy* 1983; **50:** 249–51.

3. Anderson JL, *et al.* Potential pharmacokinetic interaction between theophylline and prednisone. *Clin Pharm* 1984; **3:** 187–9.
4. Jager-Roman E, *et al.* Increased theophylline metabolism in premature infants after prenatal betamethasone administration. *Dev Pharmacol Ther* 1982; **5:** 127–35.
5. Baird-Lambert J, *et al.* Theophylline metabolism in preterm neonates during the first weeks of life. *Dev Pharmacol Ther* 1984; **7:** 239–44.

Disulfiram. In a study involving 20 recovering alcoholic patients, disulfiram decreased the plasma clearance and prolonged the elimination half-life of theophylline in a dose-dependent manner when administered concomitantly.[1] It was concluded that disulfiram exerts a dose-dependent inhibitory effect on the hepatic metabolism of theophylline and that, in order to minimise the risk of toxicity, the dosage of theophylline may need to be reduced by up to 50% during co-administration.

1. Loi C-M, *et al.* Dose-dependent inhibition of theophylline metabolism by disulfiram in recovering alcoholics. *Clin Pharmacol Ther* 1989; **45:** 476–86.

Diuretics. Although increased mean serum-theophylline concentrations were noted in 10 patients receiving continuous intravenous aminophylline infusions after intravenous injection of *frusemide*,[1] in 8 patients with chronic stable asthma, mean peak serum-theophylline concentrations were reduced from 12.14 μg per mL with placebo to 7.16 μg per mL when frusemide was given. Reduced concentrations were noted for up to 6 hours after frusemide administration.[2] Decreased theophylline concentrations were also noted in 4 neonates receiving oral or intravenous theophylline when given frusemide.[3] Serum-theophylline concentrations returned to normal when frusemide and theophylline were given more than 2 hours apart.

The possibility that adverse effects such as hypokalaemia may be potentiated by concomitant administration of theophylline and diuretics should be borne in mind.

1. Conlon PF, *et al.* Effect of intravenous furosemide on serum theophylline concentration. *Am J Hosp Pharm* 1981; **38:** 1345–7.
2. Carpentiere G, *et al.* Furosemide and theophylline. *Ann Intern Med* 1985; **103:** 957.
3. Toback JW, Gilman ME. Theophylline-furosemide inactivation. *Pediatrics* 1983; **71:** 140–1.

Gastro-intestinal drugs. Concomitant oral administration of *antacids* does not appear to affect the total absorption of theophylline from the gut.[1-5] However, some studies have shown a reduction in the rate of absorption from both immediate-[1] and modified-release theophylline preparations[2] following concurrent administration of antacids. Also an increase in peak serum-theophylline concentrations has been noted with certain modified-release formulations.[3]

Cimetidine inhibits the oxidative metabolism of theophylline reducing its clearance by 20 to 35% and prolonging its serum half-life;[6-8] toxic effects have been reported.[6] It has been recommended that the dose of aminophylline should be reduced by about one-third if cimetidine is used concomitantly.[6] This inhibition of theophylline metabolism may be enhanced by liver disease,[9] but there is wide interindividual variation. The reduction in clearance may be greater in smokers.[10] Studies have suggested that *ranitidine* does not significantly inhibit theophylline metabolism,[11-14] even at very high doses.[15] However, there have been occasional reports of theophylline toxicity after concomitant ranitidine therapy.[16-18] *Famotidine*[19] has also been reported to not alter theophylline disposition but one small study found a significant decrease in theophylline clearance in some patients with chronic obstructive pulmonary disease.[20] *Etintidine*[21] has reduced the clearance of theophylline and prolonged its elimination half-life. *Omeprazole*[22] and *lansoprazole*[23] have been reported to produce a modest increase in theophylline clearance.

Loperamide has been reported to decrease the rate but not the extent of theophylline absorption from a modified-release preparation, while in the same study *metoclopramide* was found to have no significant effect on either the rate or extent of absorption.[24]

1. Arnold LA, *et al.* Effect of an antacid on gastrointestinal absorption of theophylline. *Am J Hosp Pharm* 1979; **36:** 1059–62.
2. Shargel L, *et al.* Effect of antacid on bioavailability of theophylline from rapid and timed-release drug products. *J Pharm Sci* 1981; **70:** 599–602.
3. Darzentas LJ, *et al.* Effect of antacid on bioavailability of a sustained-release theophylline preparation. *Drug Intell Clin Pharm* 1983; **17:** 555–7.
4. Myhre KI, Walstad RA. The influence of antacid on the absorption of two different sustained-release formulations of theophylline. *Br J Clin Pharmacol* 1983; **15:** 683–7.
5. Muir JF, *et al.* Lack of effect of magnesium-aluminium hydroxide on the absorption of theophylline given as a pH-dependent sustained-release preparation. *Eur J Clin Pharmacol* 1993; **44:** 85–8.
6. Bauman JH, *et al.* Cimetidine-theophylline interaction: report of four patients. *Ann Allergy* 1982; **48:** 100–2.
7. Vestal RE, *et al.* Cimetidine inhibits theophylline clearance in patients with chronic obstructive pulmonary disease: a study using stable isotope methodology during multiple oral dose administration. *Br J Clin Pharmacol* 1983; **15:** 411–18.
8. Roberts RK, *et al.* Cimetidine-theophylline interaction in patients with chronic obstructive airways disease. *Med J Aust* 1984; **140:** 279–80.
9. Gugler R, *et al.* The inhibition of drug metabolism by cimetidine in patients with liver cirrhosis. *Klin Wochenschr* 1984; **62:** 1126–31.
10. Grygiel JJ, *et al.* Differential effects of cimetidine on theophylline metabolic pathways. *Eur J Clin Pharmacol* 1984; **26:** 335–40.
11. Breen KJ, *et al.* Effects of cimetidine and ranitidine on hepatic drug metabolism. *Clin Pharmacol Ther* 1982; **31:** 297–300.
12. Segger JS, *et al.* No evidence for interaction between ranitidine and theophylline. *Arch Intern Med* 1987; **147:** 179–80.
13. Adebayo GI. Effects of equimolar doses of cimetidine and ranitidine on theophylline elimination. *Biopharm Drug Dispos* 1989; **10:** 77–85.
14. Boehning W. Effect of cimetidine and ranitidine on plasma theophylline in patients with chronic obstructive airways disease treated with theophylline and corticosteroids. *Eur J Clin Pharmacol* 1990; **38:** 43–5.
15. Kelly HW, *et al.* Ranitidine at very large doses does not inhibit theophylline elimination. *Clin Pharmacol Ther* 1986; **39:** 577–81.
16. Fernandes E, Melewicz FM. Ranitidine and theophylline. *Ann Intern Med* 1984; **100:** 459.
17. Gardner ME, Sikorski GW. Ranitidine and theophylline. *Ann Intern Med* 1985; **102:** 559.
18. Hegman GW, Gilbert RP. Ranitidine-theophylline interaction—fact or fiction? *DICP Ann Pharmacother* 1991; **25:** 21–5.
19. Chremos AN, *et al.* Famotidine does not interfere with the disposition of theophylline in man: comparison to cimetidine. *Clin Pharmacol Ther* 1986; **39:** 187.
20. Dal Negro R, *et al.* Famotidine and theophylline pharmacokinetics: an unexpected cimetidine-like interaction in patients with chronic obstructive pulmonary disease. *Clin Pharmacokinet* 1993; **24:** 255–8.
21. Huang S-M, *et al.* Etintidine-theophylline interaction study in humans. *Biopharm Drug Dispos* 1987; **8:** 561–9.
22. Cavuto NJ, *et al.* Effect of omeprazole on theophylline clearance in poor metabolizers of omeprazole. *Clin Pharmacol Ther* 1995; **57:** 215.
23. Kokufu T, *et al.* Effects of lansoprazole on pharmacokinetics and metabolism of theophylline. *Eur J Clin Pharmacol* 1995; **48:** 391–5.
24. Bryson JC, *et al.* Effect of altering small bowel transit time on sustained release theophylline absorption. *J Clin Pharmacol* 1989; **29:** 733–8.

General anaesthetics. There have been several reports, some of which are cited below,[1,2] of increased cardiotoxicity when patients taking theophylline were anaesthetised with *halothane*. There was also an early report of seizures and tachycardia attributed to an interaction between theophylline and *ketamine*.[3]

1. Barton MD. Anesthetic problems with aspirin-intolerant patients. *Anesth Analg* 1975; **54:** 376–80.
2. Richards W, *et al.* Cardiac arrest associated with halothane anesthesia in a patient receiving theophylline. *Ann Allergy* 1988; **61:** 83–4.
3. Hirschman CA, *et al.* Ketamine-aminophylline-induced decrease in seizure threshold. *Anesthesiology* 1982; **56:** 464–7.

Idrocilamide. The muscle relaxant idrocilamide has been reported to increase the half-life and decrease the clearance of theophylline.[1]

1. Lacroix C, *et al.* Influence de l'idrocilamide sur le métabolisme de la théophylline. *Rev Pneumol Clin* 1986; **42:** 164–6.

Neuromuscular blockers. For reference to resistance to neuromuscular block with pancuronium in patients receiving aminophylline, see p.1307.

Oral contraceptives. Oral contraceptives have been reported to decrease the clearance of theophylline by about 30%, and serum concentrations may be increased,[1-3] due to the inhibitory effects of oral contraceptives on hepatic P450 enzymes.

1. Tornatore KM, *et al.* Effect of chronic oral contraceptive steroids on theophylline disposition. *Eur J Clin Pharmacol* 1982; **23:** 129–34.
2. Gardner MJ, *et al.* Effects of tobacco smoking and oral contraceptive use on theophylline disposition. *Br J Clin Pharmacol* 1983; **16:** 271–80.
3. Roberts RK, *et al.* Oral contraceptive steroids impair the elimination of theophylline. *J Lab Clin Med* 1983; **101:** 821–5.

Smoking. Certain components of tobacco smoke, notably aromatic hydrocarbons, induce hepatic drug-metabolising enzymes and cigarette smoking has been reported[1-3] to increase theophylline clearance and shorten its elimination half-life. The inductive effect of smoking may override factors that tend to decrease theophylline clearance, such as old age.[4] The duration of enzyme induction after stopping smoking is uncertain; theophylline clearance decreased by 38% after one week of abstinence from smoking in one study,[5] while others have found changes in clearance persisting for at least 3 months.[1] Tobacco chewing has also been reported to increase theophylline clearance,[6] but nicotine chewing gum appears to have no effect.[5]

1. Hunt SN, *et al.* Effect of smoking on theophylline disposition. *Clin Pharmacol Ther* 1976; **19:** 546–51.
2. Jusko WJ, *et al.* Enhanced biotransformation of theophylline in marihuana and tobacco smokers. *Clin Pharmacol Ther* 1978; **24:** 406–10.
3. Grygiel JJ, Birkett DJ. Cigarette smoking and theophylline clearance and metabolism. *Clin Pharmacol Ther* 1981; **30:** 491–6.
4. Cusack B, *et al.* Theophylline kinetics in relation to age: the importance of smoking. *Br J Clin Pharmacol* 1980; **10:** 109–14.
5. Lee BL, *et al.* Cigarette abstinence, nicotine gum, and theophylline disposition. *Ann Intern Med* 1987; **106:** 553–5.
6. Rockwood R, Henann N. Smokeless tobacco and theophylline clearance. *Drug Intell Clin Pharm* 1986; **20:** 624–5.

Sympathomimetics. The effect of beta-adrenoceptor agonists on the pharmacokinetics of theophylline is unclear. Whereas some studies have found that concomitant administration of *orciprenaline*[1] or *terbutaline*[2] had no effect on theophylline disposition, others have shown an increase in theophylline clearance following the concurrent use of *isoprenaline*[3,4] or *terbutaline*.[5,6]

Concurrent administration of theophylline with beta-adrenoceptor agonists can potentiate adverse effects including hypokalaemia,[7,8] hyperglycaemia,[7] tachycardia,[7,8] hypertension,[7] and tremor.[9] Of 9 patients reported to the UK Committee on Safety of Medicines with hypokalaemia during such combined therapy, 4 had clinical sequelae of cardiorespiratory arrest, intestinal pseudo-obstruction, or confusion. Monitoring of serum-potassium concentrations was recommended in patients with severe asthma receiving concomitant treatment with beta-adrenoceptor agonists and xanthine derivatives.[10]

The possibility of an interaction with *phenylpropanolamine* should also be borne in mind, as it has been shown to reduce the clearance of theophylline significantly.[11]

1. Conrad KA, Woodworth JR. Orciprenaline does not alter theophylline elimination. *Br J Clin Pharmacol* 1981; **12:** 756–7.
2. Snidow J, *et al.* Acute effects of short-term subcutaneous terbutaline on theophylline disposition. *Eur J Clin Pharmacol* 1987; **32:** 191–3.
3. Hemstreet MP, *et al.* Effect of intravenous isoproterenol on theophylline kinetics. *J Allergy Clin Immunol* 1982; **69:** 360–4.
4. Griffith JA, Kozloski GD. Isoproterenol-theophylline interaction: possible potentiation by other drugs. *Clin Pharm* 1990; **9:** 54–7.
5. Danziger Y, *et al.* Reduction of serum theophylline levels by terbutaline in children with asthma. *Clin Pharmacol Ther* 1985; **37:** 469–71.
6. Garty M, *et al.* Increased theophylline clearance in asthmatic patients due to terbutaline. *Eur J Clin Pharmacol* 1989; **36:** 25–8.
7. Smith SR, Kendall MJ. Potentiation of the adverse effects of intravenous terbutaline by oral theophylline. *Br J Clin Pharmacol* 1986; **21:** 451–3.
8. Whyte KF, *et al.* Salbutamol induced hypokalaemia: the effect of theophylline alone and in combination with adrenaline. *Br J Clin Pharmacol* 1988; **25:** 571–8.
9. van der Vet APH, *et al.* Pharmacodynamics (lungfunction tests, tremor measurements and cAMP determinations) of a single dose of 0.5 mg terbutaline subcutaneously during sustained-release theophylline medication in patients with asthmatic bronchitis. *Int J Clin Pharmacol Ther Toxicol* 1986; **24:** 569–73.
10. Committee on Safety of Medicines. β_2 agonists, xanthines and hypokalaemia. *Current Problems 28* 1990.
11. Wilson HA, *et al.* Phenylpropanolamine significantly reduces the clearance of theophylline. *Am Rev Respir Dis* 1991; **143:** A629.

Tacrine. Results of a study in healthy subjects indicated that tacrine reduced theophylline clearance by about 50% and increased plasma-theophylline concentrations. Competitive inhibition by tacrine of theophylline metabolism was proposed.[1]

1. deVries TM, *et al.* Effect of multiple-dose tacrine administration on single-dose pharmacokinetics of digoxin, diazepam, and theophylline. *Pharm Res* 1993; **10** (suppl): S333.

Thiabendazole. Thiabendazole has been reported[1,2] to increase serum-theophylline concentrations and to decrease theophylline clearance. It has been recommended[2] that theophylline dosage should be reduced by 50% when thiabendazole therapy is initiated.

1. Sugar AM, *et al.* Possible thiabendazole-induced theophylline toxicity. *Am Rev Respir Dis* 1980; **122:** 501–3.
2. Lew G, *et al.* Theophylline-thiabendazole drug interaction. *Clin Pharm* 1989; **8:** 225–7.

Ticlopidine. Theophylline elimination half-life was increased and plasma clearance was decreased in 10 healthy subjects after the administration of ticlopidine 500 mg daily by mouth for 10 days.[1]

1. Colli A, *et al.* Ticlopidine-theophylline interaction. *Clin Pharmacol Ther* 1987; **41:** 358–62.

Vaccines. Transient inhibition of the hepatic metabolism of theophylline, possibly secondary to interferon production, resulting in increased theophylline serum half-life and concentration has been reported after BCG vaccination[1] and influenza vaccination.[2,3] Other studies have not been able to confirm the interaction with influenza vaccine.[4-7] The differing findings are probably due to differences in vaccine; modern purified subvirion vaccines which do not induce interferon production do not appear to alter theophylline metabolism.[8,9]

1. Gray JD, *et al.* Depression of theophylline elimination following BCG vaccination. *Br J Clin Pharmacol* 1983; **16:** 735–7.
2. Renton KW, *et al.* Decreased elimination of theophylline after influenza vaccination. *Can Med Assoc J* 1980; **123:** 288–90.
3. Walker S, *et al.* Serum theophylline levels after influenza vaccination. *Can Med Assoc J* 1981; **125:** 243–4.
4. Goldstein RS, *et al.* Decreased elimination of theophylline after influenza vaccination. *Can Med Assoc J* 1982; **126:** 470.
5. Fischer RG, *et al.* Influence of trivalent influenza vaccine on serum theophylline levels. *Can Med Assoc J* 1982; **126:** 1312–13.
6. Britton L, Ruben FL. Serum theophylline levels after influenza vaccination. *Can Med Assoc J* 1982; **126:** 1375.

7. Patriarca PA, *et al.* Influenza vaccination and warfarin or theophylline toxicity in nursing-home residents. *N Engl J Med* 1983; **308:** 1601–2.
8. Stults BM, Hashisaki PA. Influenza vaccination and theophylline pharmacokinetics in patients with chronic obstructive lung disease. *West J Med* 1983; **139:** 651–4.
9. Winstanley PA, *et al.* Lack of effect of highly purified subunit influenza vaccination on theophylline metabolism. *Br J Clin Pharmacol* 1985; **20:** 47–53.

Zileuton. Zileuton prolongs the half-life and reduces the clearance of theophylline when given concomitantly;[1] dosage of theophylline should be reduced to avoid toxicity when both drugs are given together, and plasma theophylline concentrations should be monitored.

1. Granneman GR, *et al.* Effect of zileuton on theophylline pharmacokinetics. *Clin Pharmacokinet* 1995; **29** (suppl 2): 77–83.

Pharmacokinetics

Theophylline is rapidly and completely absorbed from liquid preparations, capsules, and uncoated tablets; the rate, but not the extent of absorption is decreased by food and food may also affect theophylline clearance. Modified-release preparations of theophylline can provide adequate plasma concentrations usually when administered every 12 hours. However, there is a considerable variability in their absorption characteristics and in the effect of food. It is generally recommended that if a patient is transferred from one such preparation to another then the dose should be retitrated. Rectal absorption is rapid from enemas, but may be slow and erratic from suppositories. Absorption following intramuscular injection is slow and incomplete. Peak serum-theophylline concentrations occur 1 to 2 hours after ingestion of liquid preparations, capsules, and uncoated tablets, and generally about 4 hours after ingestion of modified-release preparations.

Theophylline is approximately 40% bound to plasma proteins, but in neonates, or adults with liver disease, binding is reduced. Optimum therapeutic serum concentrations are generally considered to range from 10 to 20 μg per mL (55 to 110 μmol per litre) although some consider a lower range appropriate (see Therapeutic Drug Monitoring, below).

Theophylline is metabolised in the liver to 1,3-dimethyluric acid, 1-methyluric acid, and 3-methylxanthine. These metabolites are excreted in the urine. In adults, about 10% of a dose of theophylline is excreted unchanged in the urine, but in neonates around 50% is excreted unchanged, and a large proportion is excreted as caffeine. Considerable interindividual differences in the rate of hepatic metabolism of theophylline result in large variations in clearance, serum concentrations, and half-lives. Hepatic metabolism is further affected by factors such as age, smoking, disease, diet, and drug interactions. The serum half-life of theophylline in an otherwise healthy, non-smoking asthmatic adult is 6 to 12 hours, in children 1 to 5 hours, in cigarette smokers 4 to 5 hours, and in neonates and premature infants 10 to 45 hours. The serum half-life of theophylline may be increased in the elderly and in patients with heart failure or liver disease.

Theophylline crosses the placenta; it also enters breast milk.

Absorption. DIURNAL VARIATION. Higher serum concentrations may be achieved more quickly when a dose of oral theophylline is given in the morning than when a similar dose is given at night,[1-3] although not every study has found this.[4] When modified-release preparations are given 12-hourly, this diurnal variation can result in higher pre-dose serum-theophylline concentrations in the morning than in the evening,[5,6] which could have important consequences when adjusting doses. The most widely accepted explanation for the circadian variation in theophylline pharmacokinetics is slower absorption at night,[2,3,6,7] since no diurnal variation in metabolic clearance has been observed.[6-8] Resorption of theophylline from the bladder[9] and the effects of supine posture[10,11] have also been suggested as contributory factors, although night-workers still exhibit slower theophylline absorption at night.[12] Changing the times of dosing from 11am and 11pm to 5am and 5pm respectively abolished circadian variation in trough serum-theophylline concentrations.[13,14]

1. Lesko LJ, *et al.* Temporal variations in trough serum theophylline concentrations at steady state. *J Pharm Sci* 1980; **69:** 358–9.
2. Thompson PJ, *et al.* Pharmacokinetics of a single evening dose of slow release theophylline in patients with chronic lung disease. *Br J Clin Pharmacol* 1981; **12:** 443–4.
3. Taylor DR, *et al.* Circadian variation in plasma theophylline concentrations during maintenance therapy with a sustained-release preparation in patients with obstructive airways disease. *Br J Clin Pharmacol* 1984; **18:** 27–30.
4. Trnavská Z, *et al.* Pharmacokinetics of once-daily theophylline dose following the morning versus evening administration. *Arzneimittelforschung* 1989; **39:** 1149–51.
5. Jonkman JHG, van der Boon WJV. Nocturnal theophylline plasma concentrations. *Lancet* 1983; **i:** 1278–9.
6. Coulthard KP, *et al.* Bioavailability and diurnal variation in absorption of sustained release theophylline in asthmatic children. *Eur J Clin Pharmacol* 1983; **25:** 667–72.
7. Taylor DR, *et al.* Investigation of diurnal changes in the disposition of theophylline. *Br J Clin Pharmacol* 1983; **16:** 413–16.
8. St-Pierre MV, *et al.* Temporal variation in the disposition of theophylline and its metabolites. *Clin Pharmacol Ther* 1985; **38:** 89–95.
9. Wood JH, Garrettson LK. An explanation of circadian rhythm for theophylline and other drugs. *Lancet* 1983; **ii:** 570.
10. Warren J. Theophylline concentrations and posture. *Lancet* 1983; **ii:** 850.
11. Warren JB, *et al.* Posture and theophylline kinetics. *Br J Clin Pharmacol* 1985; **19:** 707–9.
12. Decourt S, *et al.* Pharmacokinetics of theophylline in night-workers. *Br J Clin Pharmacol* 1982; **13:** 567–9.
13. Jackson SHD, *et al.* Is circadian variation in theophylline trough serum concentrations determined by time of dosing? *Br J Clin Pharmacol* 1984; **17:** 777–9.
14. Jackson SHD, *et al.* Circadian variation in theophylline absorption during chronic dosing with a slow release theophylline preparation and the effect of clock time of dosing. *Br J Clin Pharmacol* 1988; **26:** 73–7.

FOOD. The effect of food on the absorption of theophylline from modified-release formulations of theophylline and its derivatives has been reviewed.[1] Substantial but variable effects have been reported but it is difficult to predict whether a particular modified-release theophylline formulation will be affected. Some formulations are not affected by the presence of food but for others increases or decreases in the rate and/or extent of absorption have been reported. The composition and fluid content of the food appears to be important and a rapid release of theophylline ('dose-dumping') has occurred with some formulations following a meal, especially one with a high fat content.

A diet high in protein and low in carbohydrate has been reported to increase theophylline clearance, and *vice versa*.[2-6] The consumption of methylxanthines, particularly caffeine, in the diet may decrease theophylline clearance (see under Interactions, above).

1. Jonkman JHG. Food interactions with sustained-release theophylline preparations: a review. *Clin Pharmacokinet* 1989; **16:** 162–79.
2. Kappas A, *et al.* Influence of dietary protein and carbohydrate on antipyrine and theophylline metabolism in man. *Clin Pharmacol Ther* 1976; **20:** 643–53.
3. Feldman CH, *et al.* Effect of dietary protein and carbohydrate on theophylline metabolism in children. *Pediatrics* 1980; **66:** 956–62.
4. Feldman CH, *et al.* Interaction between nutrition and theophylline metabolism in children. *Ther Drug Monit* 1982; **4:** 69–76.
5. Juan D, *et al.* Effects of dietary protein on theophylline pharmacokinetics and caffeine and aminopyrine breath tests. *Clin Pharmacol Ther* 1986; **40:** 187–94.
6. Juan D, *et al.* Impairment of theophylline clearance by a hypocaloric low-protein diet in chronic obstructive pulmonary disease. *Ther Drug Monit* 1990; **12:** 111–14.

PERCUTANEOUS ABSORPTION. Application of theophylline sodium glycinate in hydroxymethylcellulose gel[1] or choline theophyllinate in hydrogel discs[2] under an occlusive dressing to the skin of preterm infants increased or maintained therapeutic theophylline concentrations. Percutaneous administration of theophylline is an attractive alternative route of administration in neonates although with increasing age the skin matures and the amount of drug absorbed is reduced.

1. Evans N, *et al.* In vitro release of theophylline with a view to systemic percutaneous treatment in the preterm neonate. *J Pharm Pharmacol* 1984; **36** (suppl): 10P.
2. Cartwright RG, *et al.* Transdermal delivery of theophylline to premature infants using a hydrogel disc system. *Br J Clin Pharmacol* 1990; **29:** 533–9.

Metabolism and excretion. AGE. From approximately one year of age until adolescence, children have a rapid theophylline clearance.[1] Premature infants and those under one year of age have a slower clearance[2,3] due to immature metabolic pathways.[3-5] In neonates the capacity of hepatic cytochrome P450 enzymes is much reduced compared with older children and adults, and *N*-demethylation and oxidation reactions play a minor role in the metabolism of theophylline.[4-6] Neonates are, however, capable of methylating theophylline at the N7 position to form caffeine which is present at about one-third the concentration of theophylline at steady state.[5,6] The proportion of theophylline excreted unchanged is also increased in premature neonates and decreases with age as hepatic enzyme systems develop.[6] More rapid clearance on the first day of life in premature neonates has been reported.[7] Models of population pharmacokinetics in premature neonates have been used to calculate appropriate dosage of theophylline in premature infants according to postnatal age and body-weight.[8]

Some studies have demonstrated a progressive decline in clearance throughout adult years[9] whereas others have not.[10] Similarly, some studies have noted a decreased clearance in the elderly[11,12] but others have found no significant change.[13,14]

1. Zaske DE, *et al.* Oral aminophylline therapy: increased dosage requirements in children. *JAMA* 1977; **237:** 1453–5.
2. Aranda JV, *et al.* Pharmacokinetic aspects of theophylline in premature newborns. *N Engl J Med* 1976; **295:** 413–16.
3. Kraus DM, *et al.* Alterations in theophylline metabolism during the first year of life. *Clin Pharmacol Ther* 1993; **54:** 351–9.
4. Grygiel JJ, Birkett DJ. Effect of age on patterns of theophylline metabolism. *Clin Pharmacol Ther* 1980; **28:** 456–62.
5. Tserng K-Y, *et al.* Theophylline metabolism in premature infants. *Clin Pharmacol Ther* 1981; **29:** 594–600.
6. Tserng K-Y, *et al.* Developmental aspects of theophylline metabolism in premature infants. *Clin Pharmacol Ther* 1983; **33:** 522–8.
7. Stile IL, *et al.* Pharmacokinetics of theophylline in premature infants on the first day of life. *Clin Ther* 1986; **8:** 336–41.
8. Lee TC, *et al.* Theophylline population pharmacokinetics from routine monitoring data in very premature infants with apnoea. *Br J Clin Pharmacol* 1996; **41:** 191–200.
9. Randolph WC, *et al.* The effect of age on theophylline clearance in normal subjects. *Br J Clin Pharmacol* 1986; **22:** 603–5.
10. Wiffen JK, *et al.* Does theophylline clearance alter within the adult age range? *Br J Clin Pharmacol* 1984; **17:** 219P.
11. Antal EJ, *et al.* Theophylline pharmacokinetics in advanced age. *Br J Clin Pharmacol* 1981; **12:** 637–45.
12. Jackson SHD, *et al.* The relationship between theophylline clearance and age in adult life. *Eur J Clin Pharmacol* 1989; **36:** 29–34.
13. Bauer LA, Blouin RA. Influence of age on theophylline clearance in patients with chronic obstructive pulmonary diseased. *Clin Pharmacokinet* 1981; **6:** 469–74.
14. Fox RW, *et al.* Theophylline kinetics in a geriatric group. *Clin Pharmacol Ther* 1983; **34:** 60–7.

DOSAGE REGIMEN. There is evidence that the elimination of theophylline is dose-dependent and that at high serum concentrations, a small change in dose of a theophylline preparation could cause a disproportionate increase in serum-theophylline concentration, due to a reduction in clearance.[1-3] However, it is not clear that this effect is clinically significant when serum-theophylline concentrations are within the therapeutic range.[4-8] It has also been suggested that repeated oral dosing of theophylline might result in a decrease of clearance compared with pre-treatment values.[9]

1. Weinberger M, Ginchansky E. Dose-dependent kinetics of theophylline disposition in asthmatic children. *J Pediatr* 1977; **91:** 820–4.
2. Tang-Liu DD-S, *et al.* Nonlinear theophylline elimination. *Clin Pharmacol Ther* 1982; **31:** 358–69.
3. Butcher MA, *et al.* Dose-dependent pharmacokinetics with single daily dose slow release theophylline in patients with chronic lung disease. *Br J Clin Pharmacol* 1982; **13:** 241–3.
4. Koëter GH, *et al.* Pharmacokinetics of sustained release theophylline in low and high multidose regimens. *Br J Clin Pharmacol* 1981; **12:** 647–51.
5. Rovei V, *et al.* Pharmacokinetics of theophylline: a dose-range study. *Br J Clin Pharmacol* 1982; **14:** 769–78.
6. Gundert-Remy U, *et al.* Non-linear elimination processes of theophylline. *Eur J Clin Pharmacol* 1983; **24:** 71–8.
7. Brown PJ, *et al.* Lack of dose dependent kinetics of theophylline. *Eur J Clin Pharmacol* 1983; **24:** 525–7.
8. Milavetz G, *et al.* Dose dependency for absorption and elimination rates of theophylline: implications for studies of bioavailability. *Pharmacotherapy* 1984; **4:** 216–20.
9. Efthimiou H, *et al.* Influence of chronic dosing on theophylline clearance. *Br J Clin Pharmacol* 1984; **17:** 525–30.

GENDER. A higher theophylline clearance and shorter elimination half-life has been reported in healthy premenopausal female subjects than in healthy male subjects, probably due to sex-related differences in hepatic metabolism.[1] Changes in the pharmacokinetics of theophylline have also been reported in females according to the stage of the menstrual cycle.[2,3]

1. Nafziger AN, Bertino JS. Sex-related differences in theophylline pharmacokinetics. *Eur J Clin Pharmacol* 1989; **37:** 97–100.
2. Bruguerolle B, *et al.* Influence of the menstrual cycle on theophylline pharmacokinetics in asthmatics. *Eur J Clin Pharmacol* 1990; **39:** 59–61.
3. Nagata K, *et al.* Increased theophylline metabolism in the menstrual phase of healthy women. *J Allergy Clin Immunol* 1997; **100:** 39–43.

Pregnancy and breast feeding. The pharmacokinetics of theophylline may be altered during pregnancy and the post-partum period requiring close monitoring of serum-theophylline concentrations.

In a study of 12 neonates whose mothers received various theophylline preparations throughout their pregnancies[1] maternal, cord, and neonatal heelstick theophylline concentrations were not notably different, and ranged from 2.3 to 19.6 μg per mL. Transient jitteriness was seen in 2 neonates and tachycardia in one, at cord theophylline concentrations of 11.7 to 17 μg per mL. There were no instances of vomiting, seizure, arrhythmias, diarrhoea, or feeding disturbances which had been reported previously.

Neonatal theophylline toxicity should not occur in breast-feeding women taking appropriate doses of theophylline (see under Precautions, above).

1. Labovitz E, Spector S. Placental theophylline transfer in pregnant asthmatics. *JAMA* 1982; **247:** 786–8.

Protein binding. Albumin is the major plasma binding protein for theophylline, binding is pH-dependent, and the percentage of theophylline bound at physiological pH is reported to range from about 35 to 45%.[1,2] Some studies have found the plasma protein binding of theophylline to be concentration dependent,[3] but others have not confirmed this.[1,4] Protein binding has been reported to be slightly but significantly higher in patients with bronchial asthma than in healthy controls.[5] Reduced protein binding occurs in patients with hypoalbuminaemia;[6,7] it has also been found in obese subjects[8] possibly due to elevated concentrations of free fatty acids which can displace theophylline from binding sites.

1. Buss D, *et al.* Determinants of the plasma protein binding of theophylline in health. *Br J Clin Pharmacol* 1983; **15:** 399–405.
2. Brørs O, *et al.* Binding of theophylline in human serum determined by ultrafiltration and equilibrium dialysis. *Br J Clin Pharmacol* 1983; **15:** 393–7.
3. Gundert-Remy U, Hildebrandt R. Binding of theophylline and its metabolites to human plasma proteins. *Br J Clin Pharmacol* 1983; **16:** 573–4.
4. Buss DC, *et al.* Protein binding of theophylline. *Br J Clin Pharmacol* 1985; **19:** 529–31.
5. Trnavská Z. Theophylline protein binding. *Arzneimittelforschung* 1990; **40:** 166–9.
6. Leopold D, *et al.* The ex vivo plasma protein binding of theophylline in renal disease. *Br J Clin Pharmacol* 1985; **19:** 823–5.
7. Connelly TJ, *et al.* Characterization of theophylline binding to serum proteins in pregnant and nonpregnant women. *Clin Pharmacol Ther* 1990; **47:** 68–72.
8. Shum L, Jusko WJ. Effects of obesity and ancillary variables (dialysis time, drug, albumin, and fatty acid concentrations) on theophylline serum protein binding. *Biopharm Drug Dispos* 1989; **10:** 549–62.

Therapeutic drug monitoring. Dosage requirements of theophylline preparations vary widely between subjects and even vary with time in individuals, since serum-theophylline concentrations are influenced by a number of factors including disease states, concurrent medication, diet, smoking, and age. Serious toxicity is related to serum concentration and may not be preceded by minor symptoms. For these reasons it is recommended that serum-theophylline concentrations should be monitored if theophylline is to be used safely. The generally accepted optimal serum concentration is between 10 and 20 μg per mL,[1-3] but this should be regarded as a guide and not a rigid barrier and clinical decisions should never be based solely on the serum concentration.[1] The therapeutic range in the treatment of neonatal apnoea is usually considered to be 5 to 15 μg per mL although some babies may respond at lower concentrations.[4] Some now consider that this is a more appropriate range in asthma (except perhaps acute severe asthma).[5] It has been suggested that pulmonary function tests provide a better guide in long-term therapy with theophylline.[6]

Serum-theophylline concentrations were originally measured by spectrophotometry but this is subject to considerable interference from other drugs. High performance liquid chromatography is now the method of choice when extreme accuracy is important and the enzyme multiplied immunoassay technique (EMIT) has become popular because of its rapidity and adaptability to processing large batches.[2] Devices are also available which provide serum-theophylline measurements within several minutes using monoclonal antibody technology.[2,7]

The use of salivary concentrations for monitoring theophylline dosage requirements has been suggested,[8,9] but poor correlations between salivary- and serum-theophylline concentrations, and errors in serum concentration predictions have been reported.[10-13] Salivary sampling may be useful in children to avoid invasive procedures when adjusting doses or checking compliance.[14,15] Measurement of saliva-theophylline concentrations has also been suggested as a means of assessing compliance in elderly patients.[13]

1. Hampson JP. The theophylline "therapeutic window"—fact or fallacy? *Pharm J* 1988; **241:** 722–4.
2. Bierman CW, Williams PV. Therapeutic monitoring of theophylline: rationale and current status. *Clin Pharmacokinet* 1989; **17:** 377–84.
3. Holford N, *et al.* Theophylline target concentration in severe airways obstruction—10 or 20 mg/L. A randomised concentration-controlled trial. *Clin Pharmacokinet* 1993; **25:** 495–505.
4. Edwards C. Theophylline and caffeine. *Pharm J* 1986; **237:** 128–9.
5. Hardy CC, Smith J. Adverse reactions profile: theophylline and aminophylline. *Prescribers' J* 1997; **37:** 96–101.
6. Ashutosh K, *et al.* Use of serum theophylline level as a guide to optimum therapy in patients with chronic obstructive lung disease. *J Clin Pharmacol* 1990; **30:** 324–9.
7. Clifton GD, *et al.* Accuracy and time requirements for use of three rapid theophylline assay methods. *Clin Pharm* 1988; **7:** 462–6.
8. Plavsic F, *et al.* Theophylline concentration in saliva as a guide for individualization of its therapeutic use. *Br J Clin Pharmacol* 1981; **11:** 533–4.
9. Blanchard J, *et al.* Serum/saliva correlations for theophylline in asthmatics. *J Clin Pharmacol* 1991; **31:** 565–70.
10. Hendeles L, *et al.* Unpredictability of theophylline saliva measurements in chronic obstructive pulmonary disease. *J Allergy Clin Immunol* 1977; **60:** 335–8.
11. Culig J, *et al.* Saliva theophylline concentrations after a single oral dose. *Br J Clin Pharmacol* 1982; **13:** 243–5.
12. Jackson AH, *et al.* Reproducibility of saliva and plasma theophylline levels following single dose administration of two sustained release preparations. *Br J Clin Pharmacol* 1983; **15:** 407–10.
13. Gardiner ME, *et al.* Salivary theophylline levels in the elderly. *Aust J Hosp Pharm* 1986; **16:** 4–6.
14. Goldsworthy SJ, Kemp M. Salivary and urine theophylline levels in the management of childhood asthma. *Br J Clin Pharmacol* 1981; **11:**, 434P.
15. Bidat E, *et al.* Traitement par théophylline à libération prolongée: surveillance par dosage salivaire chez l'enfant. *Presse Med* 1990; **19:** 158–61.

Uses and Administration

Theophylline relaxes bronchial smooth muscle, relieves bronchospasm, and has a stimulant effect on respiration. It stimulates the myocardium and central nervous system, decreases peripheral resistance and venous pressure, and causes diuresis. It is still not clear how theophylline exerts these effects. Inhibition of phosphodiesterase with a resulting increase in intracellular cyclic adenosine monophosphate (cyclic AMP) does occur, but not apparently at concentrations normally used for clinical effect. Other proposed mechanisms of action include adenosine receptor antagonism, prostaglandin antagonism, and effects on intracellular calcium, but these actions also appear to occur only with high doses.

Theophylline is used as a bronchodilator in the management of reversible airways obstruction, such as in asthma. Although selective $beta_2$ adrenoceptor stimulants ($beta_2$ agonists) such as salbutamol are generally the preferred bronchodilators for initial treatment, theophylline is commonly used as an adjunct to $beta_2$ agonist and corticosteroid therapy in patients requiring an additional bronchodilating effect. Some patients with chronic obstructive pulmonary disease can also exhibit a beneficial response to theophylline therapy. Theophylline is also used to relieve apnoea in neonates. It was formerly used in the treatment of heart failure, angina pectoris, and for its diuretic action, but more effective drugs are now available.

Theophylline may be given in the anhydrous form or as the hydrate. Doses of theophylline are usually expressed as anhydrous theophylline.

The pharmacokinetics of theophylline may be altered by a number of factors including age, smoking, disease, diet, and drug interactions (see above under Interactions and Pharmacokinetics). Theophylline doses should therefore be adjusted for each individual patient according to clinical response, adverse effects, and serum-theophylline concentrations. Optimum therapeutic serum concentrations of theophylline are traditionally considered to range from 10 to 20 μg per mL (55 to 110 μmol per litre) and toxic effects are more common above 20 μg per mL. A range of 5 to 15 μg per mL may be effective, and associated with fewer adverse effects. For long-term administration, once a maintenance dose has been established, monitoring of serum-theophylline concentrations at 6- to 12-monthly intervals has been recommended.

In the management of **acute severe bronchospasm**, theophylline may be given *intravenously by slow injection or infusion*, though usually aminophylline is preferred (see p.748). (Anhydrous theophylline 1 mg is approximately equivalent to 1.17 mg anhydrous aminophylline or 1.27 mg aminophylline hydrate.) In patients not currently receiving theophylline, aminophylline, or other xanthine-containing medications, a suggested loading dose of 4 to 5 mg per kg body-weight may be given by intravenous infusion over 20 to 30 minutes followed by a suggested maintenance dose of 0.4 mg per kg per hour. Lower doses should be used in the elderly and those with cor pulmonale, heart failure, or liver disease; smokers may require a higher maintenance dose (see under Precautions, above). In obese patients dosage should be calculated in terms of lean or ideal body-weight. Some authorities do not consider a loading dose is necessary unless the patient's condition is deteriorating.

Suggested doses for children (not taking theophylline or other xanthine medication) are theophylline 4 to 5 mg per kg by intravenous infusion over 20 to 30 minutes, followed by maintenance doses of: in children 1 to 9 years, 0.8 mg per kg per hour; in children over 9 years, 0.6 to 0.7 mg per kg per hour.

Intravenous theophylline therapy is best avoided in patients already taking theophylline, aminophylline, or other xanthine-containing medication but, if considered necessary, serum-theophylline concentrations should be monitored and the initial dose should be calculated on the basis that each 0.5 mg of theophylline per kg of lean body-weight will result in an increase of serum theophylline concentration of 1 μg per mL.

In the treatment of **acute bronchospasm** which has not required intravenous therapy, theophylline has been given *by mouth* in conventional dosage forms; modified-release preparations are not suitable. In the USA, one suggested oral regimen for adults and children not currently taking theophylline or xanthine-containing products is 5 mg per kg, to produce an average peak serum concentration of 10 μg per mL, and followed by appropriate oral maintenance doses. These are given every 6 to 8 hours in adults, and every 4 to 6 hours in children. Doses should again be reduced in the elderly and those with cor pulmonale, heart failure, or liver disease; smokers may require a higher maintenance dose.

In the long-term management of **chronic bronchospasm**, theophylline may be given *by mouth* in doses ranging from 300 to 1000 mg daily in divided doses as conventional tablets, capsules, liquid preparations, or modified-release preparations.

For conventional dosage forms the divided doses are generally given every 6 to 8 hours. However, modified-release preparations are more commonly used as they reduce the need for frequent dosing, especially in patients with a rapid theophylline clearance. A usual dose of modified-release theophylline is 175 to 500 mg every 12 hours, though the bioavailability of different modified-release theophylline preparations may not be comparable and retitration of dosage may be required if the patient is changed from one modified-release preparation to another.

Initially, low doses of theophylline should be given and they should be gradually adjusted according to clinical response and serum-theophylline measurements. In the USA a preferred approach to initial dosage titration, in adults and children weighing over 45 kg, may be to begin with 300 mg daily, in divided doses, for 3 days; if well tolerated to increase the total daily dose to 400 mg for 3 days, and then 600 mg for a further 3 days, before titrating to a final dose based on serum-theophylline concentrations.

The total dose of some modified-release preparations may be given as a single daily dose, for example, in the evening if nocturnal symptoms are a problem.

Elderly patients may require lower doses due to reduced theophylline clearance.

In the UK, suggested oral doses for children weighing 20 to 35 kg (about 6 to 12 years old) are approximately half the adult dose; dosage recommendations for children aged 2 to 6 years are scarce and inconsistent, but one manufacturer recommends approximately quarter the adult dose; administration to children under 2 years is not recommended. In the USA, dosage guidelines recommend the following *maximum* daily doses of theophylline (when serum-theophylline concentrations are *not* being monitored): children aged 1 to 9 years up to 24 mg per kg body-weight, children aged 9 to 12 years up to 20 mg per kg, children aged 12 to 16 years up to 18 mg per kg, patients aged 16 years and above up to 13 mg per kg; a total daily dose of 900 mg should not be exceeded in the absence of monitoring, and some advocate monitoring at all doses above 600 mg daily.

Intramuscular injection and administration by suppository are not recommended due to severe local irritation, although theophylline may be administered rectally by enema.

When given as a respiratory stimulant in **neonatal apnoea**, the suggested dosage of theophylline, usually as a liquid oral dosage form, is as follows in infants not currently receiving theophylline or other xanthines: a loading dose of 5 mg per kg, followed by 1 mg per kg every 12 hours in infants with a postnatal age less than 24 days, or 1.5 mg per kg every 12 hours in those of postnatal age 24 days or more.

There are topical cosmetic preparations containing theophylline derivatives, particularly aminophylline, that are promoted for the local reduction of body fat.

Theophylline monoethanolamine (theophylline olamine), theophylline calcium salicylate, theophylline and sodium acetate (theophylline sodium acetate), theophylline sodium glycinate (theophylline sodium aminoacetate), theophylline calcium glycinate, and theophylline glycinate have all been used similarly to theophylline.

General references.

1. Vasallo R, Lipsky JJ. Theophylline: recent advances in the understanding of its mode of action and uses in clinical practice. *Mayo Clin Proc* 1998; **73:** 346–54.

Administration. Various methods have been proposed for estimating theophylline pharmacokinetic parameters to enable optimisation of initial dosage but none should be substituted for the subsequent determination of serum-theophylline concentrations and clearance at steady state.[1-3]

Asmus and colleagues noted in 1997 that dosage requirements for theophylline had declined relative to those of historical controls, apparently due to a downward shift in theophylline clearance in the US population (perhaps due to environmental changes, such as a decrease in exposure to tobacco smoke).[4] They suggested that earlier dosage guidelines for theophylline needed to be revised in the light of these data, so that the initial dose did not exceed 300 mg daily by mouth—for an approach to initial dosage titration consonant with this view, see Uses and Administration, above.

1. Erdman SM, *et al.* An updated comparison of drug dosing methods part II: theophylline. *Clin Pharmacokinet* 1991; **20:** 280–92.
2. Hogue SL, Phelps SJ. Evaluation of three theophylline dosing equations for use in infants up to one year of age. *J Pediatr* 1993; **123:** 651–6.
3. Lee TC, *et al.* Theophylline population pharmacokinetics from routine monitoring data in very premature infants with apnoea. *Br J Clin Pharmacol* 1996; **41:** 191–200.
4. Asmus MJ, *et al.* Apparent decrease in population clearance of theophylline: implications for dosage. *Clin Pharmacol Ther* 1997; **62:** 483–9.

ADMINISTRATION IN THE ELDERLY. For reference to altered pharmacokinetics of theophylline in the elderly, see under Metabolism and Excretion in Pharmacokinetics, above.

ADMINISTRATION IN INFANTS. Theophylline clearance is reduced in premature neonates and infants under one year of age due to an immature hepatic microsomal enzyme system (see under Metabolism and Excretion in Pharmacokinetics, above).

Theophylline dosage guidelines for infants under one year of age have been suggested by the FDA.[1] Loading dose, when clinically indicated: 1 mg per kg body-weight for each 2 μg per mL desired increase in the serum-theophylline concentration. Initial maintenance doses: preterm infants up to 40 weeks postconception age (gestational age at birth plus postnatal age), 1 mg per kg every 12 hours; term infants (either at birth or 40 weeks postconception) up to 4 weeks postnatal, 1 to 2 mg per kg every 12 hours; infants aged 4 to 8 weeks, 1 to 2 mg per kg every 6 hours; infants aged over 8 weeks, 1 to 3 mg per kg every 6 hours. However, the FDA dosing regimen above has been reported to result in subtherapeutic serum-theophylline concentrations in the majority of newborns[2] and is considered by some to be inadequate.[2,3] The final maintenance dose and dosage interval should be guided by serum-theophylline concentrations obtained after steady-state has been achieved. The FDA recommends that serum concentrations should be kept below 20 μg per mL for infants and 10 μg per mL for neonates.[1]

Others consider a theophylline concentration in serum of 5 to 15 μg per mL to be appropriate for the treatment of neonatal apnoea.[4] A suggested dose regimen for the treatment of apnoea in neonates is a loading dose of theophylline 5.5 to 6 mg per kg followed by maintenance doses of either 1 mg per kg every 8 hours or 2 mg per kg every 12 hours.[4] Postconceptional age may have a slight influence on theophylline clearance but postnatal age was thought to be more significant.[2]

1. Anonymous. Use of theophylline in infants. *FDA Drug Bull* 1985; **15:** 16–17.
2. Gilman JT, Gal P. Inadequacy of FDA dosing guidelines for theophylline use in neonates. *Drug Intell Clin Pharm* 1986; **20:** 481–4.
3. Murphy JE, *et al.* New FDA guidelines for theophylline dosing in infants. *Clin Pharm* 1986; **5:** 16.
4. Kriter KE, Blanchard J. Management of apnea in infants. *Clin Pharm* 1989; **8:** 577–87.

PERCUTANEOUS ADMINISTRATION. For reference to the use of percutaneous administration of theophylline in preterm infants, see under Absorption in Pharmacokinetics, above.

Asthma. Theophylline may be used in the treatment of asthma (p.745) as an adjunct to $beta_2$ agonists and corticosteroid therapy when an additional bronchodilator is indicated. Modified-release preparations can be useful in the control of nocturnal asthma.

Cardiac arrhythmias. While theophylline is no longer used in heart failure, there are reports of it being tried in other cardiac conditions usually when other treatment has failed.[1-3]

1. Viskin S, *et al.* Aminophylline for bradyasystolic cardiac arrest refractory to atropine and epinephrine. *Ann Intern Med* 1993; **118:** 279–81.
2. Sra JS, *et al.* Comparison of cardiac pacing with drug therapy in the treatment of neurocardiogenic (vasovagal) syncope with bradycardia or asystole. *N Engl J Med* 1993; **328:** 1085–90.
3. Bertolet BD, *et al.* Theophylline for the treatment of atrioventricular block after myocardial infarction. *Ann Intern Med* 1995; **123:** 509–11.

Cheyne-Stokes respiration. Oral theophylline considerably reduced Cheyne-Stokes respiration (periodic breathing) and episodes of central apnoea in a study in 15 patients with stable heart failure and left ventricular systolic dysfunction.[1] This was associated with an improvement in arterial oxygen saturation during sleep. There was no significant change in cardiac function, although pulmonary function did improve.

1. Javaheri S, *et al.* Effect of theophylline on sleep-disordered breathing in heart failure. *N Engl J Med* 1996; **335:** 562–7.

Chronic obstructive pulmonary disease. In the treatment of chronic obstructive pulmonary disease (COPD, p.747), the bronchodilators of first choice are usually either an antimuscarinic such as ipratropium bromide, or a $beta_2$ agonist such as salbutamol, given by inhalation. However the addition of theophylline, administered by mouth, may be of value in some patients to maximise respiratory function and for its positive cardiac inotropic effects.

Erythrocytosis. Erythrocytosis (an elevation in red-cell mass with normal plasma volume) can develop in up to 15% of renal-transplant recipients several months after transplantation. Post-transplantation erythrocytosis is usually self-limiting but weekly phlebotomy may be required to avoid thrombo-embolic complications. Theophylline 8 mg per kg body-weight daily by mouth has significantly reduced haematocrit, red-cell mass, and serum-erythropoietin concentrations during 8 weeks of treatment in 8 patients with erythrocytosis after renal transplantation.[1] The need for weekly phlebotomy to lower the haematocrit was eliminated after one week of treatment with theophylline and it may provide an alternative to such phlebotomies in renal transplant patients. Others have also found theophylline to be of benefit.[2] However, there is some evidence that an ACE inhibitor may be more effective than theophylline for this purpose.[3] The adenosine-antagonist action of theophylline may be responsible for this effect as there is *in-vitro* evidence that the production of erythropoietin is modulated by adenosine.

1. Bakris GL, *et al.* Effects of theophylline on erythropoietin production in normal subjects and in patients with erythrocytosis after renal transplantation. *N Engl J Med* 1990; **323:** 86–90.
2. Ilan Y, *et al.* Erythrocytosis after renal transplantation: the response to theophylline treatment. *Transplantation* 1994; **57:** 661–4.
3. Ok E, *et al.* Comparison of the effects of enalapril and theophylline on polycythemia after renal transplantation. *Transplantation* 1995; **59:** 1623–45.

Hyposmia. Theophylline is reported to be effective in the treatment of hyposmia and to act by increasing the receptor level of adenylate cyclase activity to stimulate olfactory receptor growth and sensitivity.[1] Theophylline is particularly effective in type II hyposmia. Patients with type I hyposmia or anosmia commonly require the addition of systemic corticosteroids.

1. Henkin RI. Hyposmia in woman with asthma and allergic rhinitis. *JAMA* 1991; **266:** 583.

Methotrexate neurotoxicity. Aminophylline by intravenous infusion or theophylline by mouth relieved the acute neurotoxicity of methotrexate (p.547) in some children[1] possibly through an anti-adenosine effect.

1. Bernini JC, *et al.* Aminophylline for methotrexate-induced neurotoxicity. *Lancet* 1995; **345:** 544–7.

Neonatal apnoea. Apnoea is a cessation of respiratory airflow due to lack of respiratory effort or airway obstruction.[1,2] Apnoea of infancy has been defined as cessation of breathing either lasting 20 seconds or more or associated with bradycardia, cyanosis, pallor, and marked hypotonia, for which no specific cause can be identified.[1] Premature infants (less than 37 weeks' gestation) can exhibit periodic breathing with pathological apnoea; this may be considered to be apnoea of prematurity and usually resolves as the infant approaches term and the neurological systems controlling ventilation mature.[1,2]

The management of neonatal apnoea for which no underlying disorder can be found may involve supportive measures such as water beds and cardiorespiratory monitoring. Methylxanthines such as caffeine and theophylline are respiratory and CNS stimulants and can be of benefit.[1,2] However, it is important that any underlying seizure disorder is ruled out before methylxanthine therapy is initiated, as caffeine and theophylline can exacerbate seizures.[1]

Administration of either caffeine (as the citrate) or theophylline has been found to reduce the number and severity of apnoeic episodes within 24 to 48 hours,[3-5] although studies have mostly been restricted to use in premature infants. Appropriate serum concentrations are considered to be 5 to 15 μg per mL for theophylline (see also under Administration in Infants, above) and 8 to 20 μg per mL for caffeine.[1] Higher doses of caffeine (to produce a desired serum concentration of 26 to 40 μg per mL) have been used to obtain a faster response (within 8 hours) without apparent side-effects.[5] During the first year of life, the elimination half-life of both caffeine and theophylline decreases significantly as the infant's capacity for hepatic metabolism increases; regular monitoring of serum concentrations and constant dosage adjustments are therefore required.[1] Administration by the oral route is generally preferred.[1] Caffeine appears to have a number of advantages over theophylline including a wider therapeutic index, fewer peripheral adverse effects, and a longer half-life enabling once-daily administration, but the lack of a suitable readily available preformulated preparation limits its use.[1] Also, caffeine has been reported to be effective in some children unresponsive to theophylline.[2]

As the patient gets older or becomes asymptomatic (for at least 4 to 8 weeks), xanthine therapy can be withdrawn on a trial basis to see if apnoea will recur.

In infants with apnoea which does not respond to xanthine therapy, treatment with doxapram, another central respiratory stimulant, may be considered.[1,2] Doxapram is as effective as theophylline, and may also be of benefit as an addition to xanthine therapy[6,7] but must be administered by continuous intravenous infusion and blood pressure must be monitored for signs of hypertension.[2] Adverse effects such as irritability and convulsions may also be a problem.[2]

1. Kriter KE, Blanchard J. Management of apnea in infants. *Clin Pharm* 1989; **8:** 577–87.
2. Ruggins NR. Pathophysiology of apnoea in preterm infants. *Arch Dis Child* 1991; **66:** 70–73.
3. Murat I, *et al.* The efficacy of caffeine in the treatment of recurrent idiopathic apnea in premature infants. *J Pediatr* 1981; **99:** 984–9.
4. Autret E, *et al.* Comparaison de deux doses d'entretien différentes de caféine dans le traitment des apnées du prématuré. *Therapie* 1985; **40:** 235–9.
5. Scanlon JEM, *et al.* Caffeine or theophylline for neonatal apnoea? *Arch Dis Child* 1992; **67:** 425–8.
6. Eyal F, *et al.* Aminophylline versus doxapram in idiopathic apnea of prematurity: a double-blind controlled study. *Pediatrics* 1985; **75:** 709–13.
7. Peliowski A, Finer NN. A blinded, randomized, placebo-controlled trial to compare theophylline and doxapram for the treatment of apnea of prematurity. *J Pediatr* 1990; **116:** 648–53.

Preparations

USP 23: Theophylline and Guaifenesin Capsules; Theophylline and Guaifenesin Oral Solution; Theophylline Capsules; Theophylline Extended-release Capsules; Theophylline in Dextrose Injection; Theophylline Sodium Glycinate Elixir; Theophylline Sodium Glycinate Tablets; Theophylline Tablets; Theophylline, Ephedrine Hydrochloride, and Phenobarbital Tablets.

Proprietary Preparations (details are given in Part 3)

Aust.: Aerodyne; Afonilum†; Euphyllin; Pulmidur; Respicur; Theohexal; Theoplus; Theospirex; Unifyl; ***Austral.:*** Austyn; Elixophyllin†; Nuelin; Slo-Bid†; Theo-Dur; ***Belg.:*** Theo-Dur; Theolair; Theophyllard; Xanthium; ***Canad.:*** Apo-Theo; Pulmophylline; Quibron-T; Slo-Bid; Somophyllin†; Theo-Dur; Theo-SR; Theochron; Theolair; Uniphyl; ***Fr.:*** Armophylline†; Ceetraphylline†; Dilatrane; Euphylline; Theolair; Theostat; Xanthium; ***Ger.:*** Aerobin; Afonilum; Afonilum novo; afpred-THEO; Bilordyl†; Bronchoparat; Bronchoretard; Contiphyllin; Cronasma; Ditenate N†; duraphyllin; Etheophyl; Euphyllin; Euphyllin 200†; Euphylong; Flui-Theophylline; Myocardon N; Parasthman†; Perasthman N; Pulmidur; Pulmo-Timelets; Solosin; Theo; Theolair; Theophyllard; Unilair; Uniphyllin; ***Irl.:*** Lasma; Nuelin; Pro-Vent; Slo-Phyllin; Theo-Dur; Theolan; Uniphyllin Continus; Zepholin; ***Ital.:*** Aminomal; Diffumal; Euphyllina Rilcon; Euphyllina Ritardo; Respicur; Sabidal Retiolt†; Slo-Phyllin†; Somofillina†; Tefamin; Teobid; Teonova; Teoplus†; Teoval/R†; Theo-24; Theo-Dur; Theolair; ***Jpn:*** Theolong; ***Mon.:*** Techniphylline†; ***Neth.:*** Euphylong; Pediaphyllin PL†; Theo₂†; Theolair; Theolin; Unilair; ***Norw.:*** Euphyllin; Nuelin; Theo-Dur; ***S.Afr.:*** Alcophyllin; Biophyllin; Bronchophen; Chronophyllin; Euphyllin; Microphyllin; Nuelin; Pulmophyllin; Somophyllin†; Theo-Dur; Theoplus; Uni-Dur; Uniphyl; Vernthol†; ***Spain:*** Asmo; Chantaline; Godafilin†; Histafilin; Neo Elixifilin; Piridasmin†; Pulmeno; Teodelin; Teogel†; Teolixir; Theo Max; Theo-Dur; Theolair; Theoplus; Unilong; Vent Retard; ***Swed.:*** Euphylong; Theo-Dur; ***Switz.:*** Escophylline; Euphyllin; Euphylong; Sodip-phylline; Theolair; Theon†; Unifyl; Xantivent; ***UK:*** Biophylline†; Lasma; Nuelin; Slo-Phyllin; Theo-Dur; Uniphyllin Continus; ***USA:*** Accurbron; Aerolate; Aquaphyllin; Asmalix; Bronkodyl†; Constant-T†; Duraphyl†; Elixomin; Elixophyllin; Lanophyllin; Quibron-T; Respbid; Slo-Bid; Slo-Phyllin; Sustaire; T-Phyl; Theo-24; Theo-Dur; Theo-Sav†; Theo-X; Theobid Duracaps; Theochron; Theoclear; Theolair; Theospan-SR; Theostat; Theovent; Uni-Dur; Uniphyl.

Multi-ingredient: ***Aust.:*** Ambredin; Asthma 23 D; Asthma-Bisolvon; Bellasthman; Bronchisan; Eudur; Neobiphyllin†; Peripherin; Perphyllon; Theo-Lanicor; Theo-Lanitop; Theocaradrin; Thilocombin; ***Austral.:*** Elixophyllin-KI†; ***Belg.:*** Asperal-B†; Perphyllone†; Pneumogenol†; Theophylline Sedative Bruneau†; ***Canad.:*** Tedral; Theo-Bronc; ***Fr.:*** Asthmasedine†; Hypnasmine; Pneumogeine; Tedralan; Uromil; ***Ger.:*** Adenovasin†; Asthma-Bisolvon†; Broncho-Binotal†; Broncho-Euphyllin; Cordalin-Strophanthin†; Coritrat†; Ditenate†; Eudur; Neobiphyllin; Neobiphyllin-Clys; Par-Isalon†; Peripherin†; Perspiran N†; Priatan-N†; Theo-Lanicor†; Theo-Lanitop†; ***Irl.:*** Franol; Franol Expectorant; ***Ital.:*** Lisomucil Teofillina†; Perventil†; ***S.Afr.:*** Actophlem; Alcophyllex; Diatussin; Framol†; Lipostabil; Metaxol; Solphyllex; Solphyllin; Tedral†; Theophen; Theophen Comp; ***Spain:*** Angiofiline†; Dexabronchisan†; Elixifilin; Muco Teolixir†; Novofilin; Pelsonfilina†; Tedral†; Teolixir Compositum; Winasma†; ***Switz.:*** Dilaphylline†; Eudur†; Neo-Biphyllin; ***UK:*** Anestan†; Do-Do; Franol; Franol Plus; Franolyn Expectorant; Labophylline†; ***USA:*** Asbron G†; Bronkaid†; Bronkolixir†; Bronkotabs†; Elixophyllin-GG; Elixophyllin-KI; Glyceryl-T; Hydrophed; Marax; Mudrane GG†; Primatene; Primatene Dual Action; Quadrinal; Quibron; Slo-Phyllin GG; Synophylate-GG†; Tedral†; Tedrigen; Theo-Organidin†; Theodrine; Theomax DF.

Tiacrilast (1256-d)

Tiacrilast *(USAN, rINN).*

Ro-22-3747/000 (tiacrilast); Ro-22-3747/007 (tiacrilast sodium). (*E*)-6-(Methylthio)-4-oxo-3(4*H*)-quinazolineacrylic acid.

$C_{12}H_{10}N_2O_3S$ = 262.3.

CAS — 78299-53-3 (tiacrilast); 111868-63-4 (tiacrilast sodium).

NOTE. Tiacrilast Sodium is *USAN.*

Tiacrilast is an anti-allergic drug with a stabilising action on mast cells resembling that of sodium cromoglycate (p.762). It has been investigated for the management of asthma and allergic rhinitis.

Tiotropium Bromide (16866-y)

Tiotropium Bromide *(rINN).*

6β,7β-Epoxy-3β-hydroxy-8-methyl-1α*H*,5α*H*-tropanium bromide di-2-thienylglycolate.

$C_{19}H_{22}BrNO_4S_2$ = 472.4.

CAS — 139404-48-1.

Tiotropium bromide is a quaternary ammonium antimuscarinic structurally related to ipratropium (p.754) and with a prolonged bronchodilator action. It is under investigation in the treatment of reversible airways obstruction.

References.

1. Maesen FP, *et al.* Tiotropium bromide, a new long-acting antimuscarinic bronchodilator: a pharmacodynamic study in patients with chronic obstructive pulmonary disease (COPD). *Eur Respir J* 1995; **8:** 1506–13.
2. O'Connor BJ, *et al.* Prolonged effect of tiotropium bromide on methacholine-induced bronchoconstriction in asthma. *Am J Respir Crit Care Med* 1996; **154:** 876–80.

Tranilast (12988-j)

Tranilast *(USAN, rINN).*

MK-341; N-5'. *N*-(3,4-Dimethoxycinnamoyl)anthranilic acid.

$C_{18}H_{17}NO_5$ = 327.3.

CAS — 53902-12-8.

Adverse Effects and Precautions

Adverse effects reported with tranilast have included gastro-intestinal disturbances, headache, drowsiness or insomnia, dizziness, malaise, and skin rashes and generalised pruritus. Surveillance has suggested an incidence of 2.4% of adverse effects most of which were gastro-intestinal. Rarely, liver function disturbance or jaundice, cystitis-like symptoms, anaemia, palpitations, oedema, facial flushing, and stomatitis may occur.

The manufacturers advise against the use of tranilast in pregnancy because of teratogenicity in *animal* studies.

It should not be used for the treatment of acute asthma attacks. The general cautions described under Sodium Cromoglycate (p.762) also apply.

Uses and Administration

Tranilast has a stabilising action on mast cells resembling that of sodium cromoglycate (p.762). It is also stated to inhibit collagen synthesis in fibroblasts. It is given by mouth in the prophylactic management of asthma (p.745) and in allergic rhinitis (p.400) and eczema (p.1073). It is also used in the management of keloids and hypertrophic scarring, and is under investigation for the prevention of restenosis following coronary artery revascularisation procedures. Adults have been given 100 mg three times daily; 5 mg per kg body-weight daily in divided doses has been suggested for children.

For a mention of possible benefit from tranilast in cutaneous sarcoidosis see p.1028.

Preparations

Proprietary Preparations (details are given in Part 3)
Jpn: Rizaben.

Tretoquinol Hydrochloride (2110-y)

Tretoquinol Hydrochloride *(pINNM).*

AQ-110 (tretoquinol); Ro-07-5965; Trimethoquinol Hydrochloride; Trimetoquinol Hydrochloride. (−)-1,2,3,4-Tetrahydro-1-(3,4,5-trimethoxybenzyl)isoquinoline-6,7-diol hydrochloride monohydrate.

$C_{19}H_{23}NO_5,HCl,H_2O$ = 399.9.

CAS — 30418-38-3 (tretoquinol); 18559-59-6 (tretoquinol hydrochloride, anhydrous).

Pharmacopoeias. In *Jpn.*

Tretoquinol is a direct-acting sympathomimetic reported to have a selective action on beta$_2$ receptors (beta$_2$ agonist). It has properties similar to those of salbutamol (see p.758). It is given as the hydrochloride for its bronchodilating properties in the management of reversible airways obstruction, as in asthma (p.745) or in some patients with chronic obstructive pulmonary disease (p.747). A usual dose by mouth is 2 to 4 mg of tretoquinol hydrochloride two to three times daily. It has also been given by injection.

Preparations

Proprietary Preparations (details are given in Part 3)
Jpn: Inolin.

Tulobuterol Hydrochloride (17020-r)

Tulobuterol Hydrochloride *(BANM, rINNM).*

C-78. 2-*tert*-Butylamino-1-*o*-chlorophenylethanol hydrochloride.

$C_{12}H_{18}ClNO,HCl$ = 264.2.

CAS — 41570-61-0 (tulobuterol); 56776-01-3 (tulobuterol hydrochloride).

Pharmacopoeias. In *Jpn.*

Tulobuterol is a direct-acting sympathomimetic with mainly beta-adrenergic activity and a selective action on beta$_2$ receptors (beta$_2$ agonist). It has properties similar to those of salbutamol (see p.758).

Tulobuterol is used as a bronchodilator in the management of reversible airways obstruction, as in asthma (p.745) and in some patients with chronic obstructive pulmonary disease (p.747). It is given by mouth as the hydrochloride. The initial oral dose in adults is 1 or 2 mg of tulobuterol hydrochloride twice daily, increased to 2 mg three times daily if necessary. A suggested dose for children is: 6 to 10 years, 0.5 to 1 mg twice daily; over 10 years, 1 to 2 mg twice daily.

Tulobuterol is also given as the base, by inhalation from a metered dose inhaler: the usual dose is 2 inhalations of 400 μg as required.

A transdermal formulation is under investigation.

References to the transdermal formulation of tulobuterol.

1. Uematsu T, *et al.* The pharmacokinetics of the β$_2$-adrenoceptor agonist, tulobuterol, given transdermally and by inhalation. *Eur J Clin Pharmacol.* 1993; **44:** 361–4.
2. Iikura Y, *et al.* Pharmacokinetics and pharmacodynamics of the tulobuterol patch, HN-078, in childhood asthma. *Ann Allergy* 1995; **74:** 147–51.

Preparations

Proprietary Preparations (details are given in Part 3)
Aust.: Bremax; ***Belg.:*** Respacal; ***Ger.:*** Atenos; Brelomax; ***Jpn:*** Hokunalin; ***UK:*** Brelomax†; Respacal.

Zafirlukast (10561-k)

Zafirlukast *(BAN, USAN, rINN).*

ICI-204219. Cyclopentyl 3-{2-methoxy-4-[(*o*-tolylsulfonyl)-carbamoyl]benzyl}-1-methylindole-5-carbamate.

$C_{31}H_{33}N_3O_6S$ = 575.7.

CAS — 107753-78-6.

Adverse Effects and Precautions

Zafirlukast is generally well tolerated: headache, an increased incidence of respiratory tract infection, and gastro-intestinal disturbances have occasionally been reported. Elevations in liver enzyme values have occurred, but symptomatic hepatitis or hyperbilirubinaemia appear to be rare. Other adverse effects reported in patients receiving zafirlukast include generalised pain, myalgia, fever, and dizziness. There have been a few reports of Churg-Strauss syndrome in patients receiving zafirlukast (see Vasculitic Syndromes, below).

Zafirlukast should not be used for the treatment of acute asthma attacks. The general cautions described under sodium cromoglycate (p.762) also apply. Zafirlukast is contra-indicated in moderate or severe renal impairment, and in those with hepatic impairment or cirrhosis.

Vasculitic syndromes. Wechsler and colleagues reported pulmonary infiltrates and eosinophilia, resembling the Churg-Strauss syndrome, together with dilated cardiomyopathy, following the withdrawal of corticosteroid therapy in 8 patients receiving zafirlukast.[1] Symptoms responded to withdrawal of zafirlukast and treatment with corticosteroids, with or without cyclophosphamide. It has been suggested that the patients' original asthmatic symptoms had been part of an unrecognised vasculitic syndrome that was unmasked by the corticosteroid withdrawal.[2] However, others have reported Churg-Strauss syndrome associated with zafirlukast in a patient who had not been receiving corticosteroids.[3]

1. Wechsler ME, *et al.* Pulmonary infiltrates, eosinophilia, and cardiomyopathy following corticosteroid withdrawal in patients with asthma receiving zafirlukast. *JAMA* 1998; **279:** 455–7.
2. Churg A, Churg J. Steroids and Churg-Strauss syndrome. *Lancet* 1998; **352:** 32–3.
3. Katz RS, Papernik M. Zafirlukast and Churg-Strauss syndrome. *JAMA* 1998; **279:** 1949.

Interactions

Zafirlukast is metabolised by hepatic cytochrome P450, specifically the CYP2C9 and CYP3A4 isoforms. In consequence, interactions may occur with drugs primarily metabolised by these enzyme systems. Patients receiving warfarin may develop prolongation of the prothrombin time and anticoagulant dosage should be adjusted accordingly. Terfenadine and theophylline may both reduce plasma concentrations of zafirlukast; erythromycin appears to reduce zafirlukast bioavailability. In contrast, increased plasma concentrations of zafirlukast have been seen when given concomitantly with high doses of aspirin.

Pharmacokinetics

Zafirlukast is rapidly absorbed from the gastro-intestinal tract following oral administration, with peak plasma concentrations generally within 3 hours of a dose. The absolute bioavailability is uncertain, but administration with food reduces both the rate and extent of absorption, decreasing bioavailability by about 40%. Zafirlukast is about 99% bound to plasma protein. It is extensively metabolised in the liver (see Interactions, above) and excreted principally in faeces, as unchanged drug and metabolites. About 10% of a dose is excreted in urine. The terminal elimination half-life of zafirlukast is about 10 hours. Studies in *animals* suggest that small amounts cross the placenta; it is also distributed in low concentrations into breast milk.

Uses and Administration

Zafirlukast is a selective antagonist of the leukotriene D_4 receptor, stimulation of which by circulating leukotrienes is thought to play a role in the pathogenesis of asthma. It suppresses both early and late bronchoconstrictor responses to inhaled antigens or irritants, but has no bronchodilator properties and is not suitable for the management of acute attacks of asthma.

Zafirlukast is used in the management of chronic asthma. It is given by mouth in doses of 20 mg twice daily, taken at least 1 hour before or 2 hours after meals.

General references.

1. Adkins JC, Brogden RN. Zafirlukast: a review of its pharmacology and therapeutic potential in the management of asthma. *Drugs* 1998; **55:** 121–44.

Asthma. Zafirlukast blocks leukotriene- and antigen-induced bronchoconstriction in asthmatic subjects,[1,2] and produces modest improvement in mild-to-moderate asthma,[3] probably of a similar order to that seen with sodium cromoglycate.[4] However, its benefits are at best modest, and corticosteroids remain the drugs of choice for regular prophylactic therapy of mild to moderate asthma.[5] Revised US guidelines for the management of asthma (p.745) permit the use of zafirlukast as an alternative to cromoglycate, nedocromil, or inhaled corticosteroids in patients with mild persistent asthma, who cannot be managed with inhaled beta$_2$ agonists on an as-needed basis alone.

1. Smith LJ, *et al.* Inhibition of leukotriene D_4-induced bronchoconstriction in subjects with asthma: a concentration-effect study of ICI 204,219. *Clin Pharmacol Ther* 1993; **54:** 430–6.
2. Nathan RA, *et al.* Inhaled ICI 204,219 blocks antigen-induced bronchoconstriction in subjects with bronchial asthma. *Chest* 1994; **105:** 483–8.
3. Suissa S, *et al.* Effectiveness of the leukotriene receptor antagonist zafirlukast for mild-to-moderate asthma: a randomized, double-blind, placebo-controlled trial. *Ann Intern Med* 1997; **126:** 177–83.
4. Nathan RA, *et al.* Effects of 13 weeks of treatment with ICI 204,219 (Accolate) or cromolyn sodium (Intal) in patients with mild to moderate asthma. *J Allergy Clin Immunol* 1995; **95:** 388.
5. Anonymous. Zafirlukast for asthma. *Med Lett Drugs Ther* 1996; **38:** 111–12.

Preparations

Proprietary Preparations (details are given in Part 3)
Irl.: Accolate; ***UK:*** Accolate; ***USA:*** Accolate.

Zileuton (9332-j)

Zileuton *(BAN, USAN, rINN).*

A-64077; Abbott-64077. (±)-1-(1-Benzo[*b*]thien-2-ylethyl)-*N*-hydroxyurea.

$C_{11}H_{12}N_2O_2S$ = 236.3.

CAS — 111406-87-2.

Adverse Effects

Zileuton has been associated with raised liver enzyme values, gastro-intestinal disturbances, urticaria, headache, and leucopenia in a few patients. It should not be used in patients with hepatic impairment or active liver disease.

Zileuton is not suitable for the treatment of acute asthma attacks.

Interactions

Zileuton has been reported to impair the metabolism of some drugs metabolised via hepatic cytochrome P450, including theophylline, and the *R*- but not the *S*-enantiomer of warfarin.

Pharmacokinetics

Zileuton is reported to be well absorbed from the gastro-intestinal tract following oral administration, with peak plasma concentrations occurring about 2 hours after a dose. It is apparently widely distributed and is about 93% bound to plasma protein. It is extensively metabolised in the liver, and excreted in the urine, largely as glucuronide metabolites. The elimination half-life is reported to be about 2 hours.

References.

1. Wong SL, *et al.* The pharmacokinetics of single oral doses of zileuton 200 to 800 mg, its enantiomers, and its metabolites, in normal healthy volunteers. *Clin Pharmacokinet* 1995; **29** (suppl 2): 9–21.
2. Awni WM, *et al.* Pharmacokinetics and pharmacodynamics of zileuton after oral administration of single and multiple dose regimens of zileuton 600 mg in healthy volunteers. *Clin Pharmacokinet* 1995; **29** (suppl 2): 22–33.
3. Braeckman RA, *et al.* The pharmacokinetics of zileuton in healthy young and elderly volunteers. *Clin Pharmacokinet* 1995; **29** (suppl 2): 42–8.
4. Awni WM, *et al.* Population pharmacokinetics of zileuton, a selective 5-lipoxygenase inhibitor, in patients with rheumatoid arthritis. *Eur J Clin Pharmacol* 1995; **48:** 155–60.

Uses and Administration

Zileuton is an orally active 5-lipoxygenase inhibitor. It is used in the management of chronic asthma but has no bronchodilator properties and is not suitable for the management of acute attacks. Zileuton is given by mouth, in doses of 600 mg 4 times daily.

It has also been tried in some other disorders including arthritis, allergic rhinitis, and inflammatory bowel disease.

Asthma. Zileuton has been found to be of some benefit in asthma, including that provoked by external stimuli such as cold air, exercise, and NSAIDs. Revised US guidelines for the management of asthma (p.745) permit its use as an alternative to cromoglycate, nedocromil or inhaled corticosteroids in patients with mild persistent asthma who cannot be managed with inhaled $beta_2$ agonists on an as-needed basis alone.

References.

1. McGill KA, Busse WW. Zileuton. *Lancet* 1996; **348:** 519–24.
2. Israel E, *et al.* The effects of a 5-lipoxygenase inhibitor on asthma induced by cold, dry air. *N Engl J Med* 1990; **323:** 1740–4.
3. Israel E, *et al.* The effect of inhibition of 5-lipoxygenase by zileuton in mild-to-moderate asthma. *Ann Intern Med* 1993; **119:** 1059–66.
4. Israel E, *et al.* Effect of treatment with zileuton, a 5-lipoxygenase inhibitor, in patients with asthma: a randomized controlled trial. *JAMA* 1996; **275:** 931–6.

Inflammatory bowel disease. Despite initial hopes that inhibition of lipoxygenase might prove of benefit in patients with ulcerative colitis,[1] a study in patients with mild or moderately active relapsing ulcerative colitis found that its symptomatic benefits were confined to those not already receiving sulphasalazine.[2] For a discussion of inflammatory bowel disease and its management, see p.1171.

1. Laursen LS, *et al.* Selective 5-lipoxygenase inhibition in ulcerative colitis. *Lancet* 1990; **335:** 683–5.
2. Laursen LS, *et al.* Selective 5-lipoxygenase inhibition by zileuton in the treatment of relapsing ulcerative colitis: a randomized double-blind placebo-controlled multicentre trial. *Eur J Gastroenterol Hepatol* 1994; **6:** 209–15.

Rhinitis. A study in 8 patients with allergic rhinitis (p.400) found that a single dose of zileuton 800 mg reduced the response to a nasal antigen challenge 3 hours later,[1] including reduced sneezing and nasal congestion.

1. Knapp HR. Reduced allergen-induced nasal congestion and leukotriene synthesis with an orally active 5-lipoxygenase inhibitor. *N Engl J Med* 1990; **323:** 1745–8.

Cardiovascular Drugs

This chapter describes drugs used principally in the management of cardiovascular disorders, as well as the choice of treatment for a particular disorder. Lipid regulating drugs, which also have a role in cardiovascular disease, are described elsewhere (p.1265) as are blood products, plasma expanders, and haemostatics (p.701).

Cardiovascular Drug Groups

Although very diverse, cardiovascular drugs can be broadly classified according to their pharmacological action. Basic details of the major groups follow, together with lists of the drugs described in this chapter.

ACE inhibitors

The main uses of ACE (angiotensin-converting enzyme) inhibitors are in the management of heart failure, hypertension, and myocardial infarction. Their actions and uses are discussed in more detail on p.805.

Described in this chapter are

Alacepril	Moexipril
Benazepril	Moveltipril
Captopril	Pentopril
Ceronapril	Perindopril
Cilazapril	Quinapril
Delapril	Ramipril
Enalapril	Spirapril
Enalaprilat	Temocapril
Fosinopril	Teprotide
Imidapril	Trandolapril
Libenzapril	Zofenopril
Lisinopril	

Adrenergic neurone blockers

Adrenergic neurone blockers are used in hypertension although they have largely been superseded by other drugs less likely to cause orthostatic hypotension. They have been also used in open-angle glaucoma.

Adrenergic neurone blockers act by selectively inhibiting transmission in postganglionic adrenergic nerves. They are believed to act mainly by preventing the release of noradrenaline at nerve endings; they cause the depletion of noradrenaline stores in peripheral sympathetic nerve terminals. They do not prevent the secretion of catecholamines by the adrenal medulla.

Described in this chapter are

Bethanidine	Guanadrel
Debrisoquine	Guanethidine
Guabenxan	Guanoxan

Alpha blockers

Alpha blockers are used mainly in the management of hypertension and benign prostatic hyperplasia. Some of them have other uses, for example, phenoxybenzamine, prazosin, and tolazoline are also used in peripheral vascular disease, phenoxybenzamine is used in the management of phaeochromocytoma, and tolazoline may be employed in pulmonary hypertension.

Alpha blockers are also known as alpha-adrenergic antagonists or alpha-adrenergic receptor antagonists. Some of the alpha blockers have particular affinities for one of the two subtypes of the alpha adrenoceptor, namely the alpha$_1$ adrenoceptor (α_1 receptor) or the alpha$_2$ adrenoceptor (α_2 receptor). Drugs such as indoramin or prazosin are much more potent in blocking alpha$_1$ than alpha$_2$ adrenoceptors and are often termed selective alpha$_1$ blockers. Blockade of alpha$_1$ adrenoceptors inhibits the vasoconstriction induced by endogenous catecholamines. Both arteriolar and venous vasodilatation may occur resulting in a fall in blood pressure because of decreased peripheral resistance. Blockade of alpha$_2$ adrenoceptors with a selective drug such as yohimbine (p.1645) can conversely lead to a rise in blood pressure. With phenoxybenzamine and phentolamine, which broadly have similar affinities for both the alpha$_1$ and alpha$_2$ subtypes of receptor, any increase in blood pressure due to alpha$_2$ blockade is prevented by the inhibition of vasoconstriction caused by alpha$_1$ blockade. Alpha blockers also act at alpha adrenoceptors in nonvascular smooth muscle, for example in the bladder where alpha blockade produces decreased resistance to urinary outflow. Most alpha blockers are reversible or 'competitive' inhibitors of alpha adrenoceptors; phenoxybenzamine is an irreversible or 'non-competitive' blocker of alpha adrenoceptors.

Described in this chapter are

Alfuzosin	Prazosin
Bunazosin	Tamsulosin
Doxazosin	Terazosin
Indoramin	Tolazoline
Naftopidil	Trimazosin
Phenoxybenzamine	Urapidil
Phentolamine	

Angiotensin II receptor antagonists

Angiotensin II receptor antagonists are used in the management of hypertension. They act mainly by selective blockade of AT$_1$ receptors thus reducing the pressor effects of angiotensin II.

Described in this chapter are

Candesartan	Tasosartan
Eprosartan	Telmisartan
Irbesartan	Valsartan
Losartan	

Antiarrhythmics

Drugs used in the management of cardiac arrhythmias form a diverse group of drugs. Many of them, such as beta blockers, digoxin, lignocaine (p.1293), magnesium (p.1157), and phenytoin (p.352) have important actions in addition to their antiarrhythmic properties and thus, as well as being employed in the treatment of cardiac arrhythmias, have a wide range of other clinical applications.

Various methods of classifying antiarrhythmics (formerly described as cardiac depressants) may be employed.

The most widely used classification of antiarrhythmics is that proposed by Vaughan Williams and later modified by Harrison. This classification is based largely on *in-vitro* electrophysiological effects of the drugs on myocardial cells. The action potential involved in the contraction of cardiac muscle consists of several phases (Figure 1) controlled by ionic movements across the myocardial cell membrane.

Figure 1. The action potential.

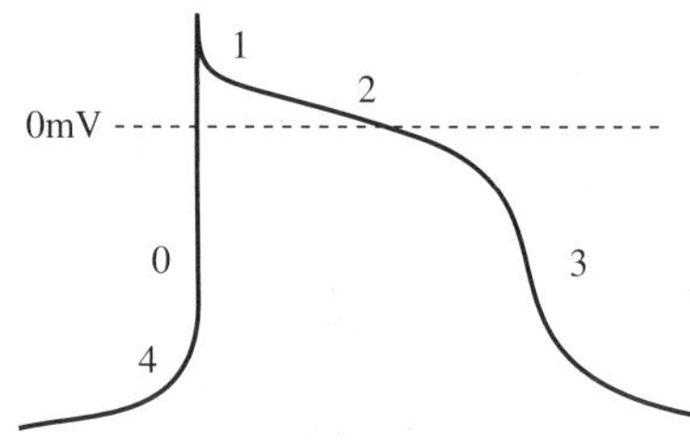

When the cell is excited it becomes depolarised due to an increase in sodium conductance and a consequent fast influx of sodium ions (phase 0) lasting a few milliseconds, followed by a transient outward current probably carried by potassium ions (phase 1). A slow influx of ions, mainly calcium ions, forms phase 2 of the cardiac action potential which is known as the 'plateau' phase. The cell finally repolarises (phase 3) due to an increase in potassium conductance and an efflux of potassium ions which returns it to its initial resting membrane potential (phase 4). In specialised cardiac tissue such as the sino-atrial node and atrioventricular node the resting cell membrane spontaneously depolarises and initiates action potentials, due mainly to decreased potassium conductance. The tissues of the nodes are dependent predominantly on calcium transport for the depolarisation phase of the action potential, whereas the atria and ventricles are mainly sodium-dependent.

A typical normal ECG trace is shown in Figure 2.

Figure 2. A normal ECG trace.

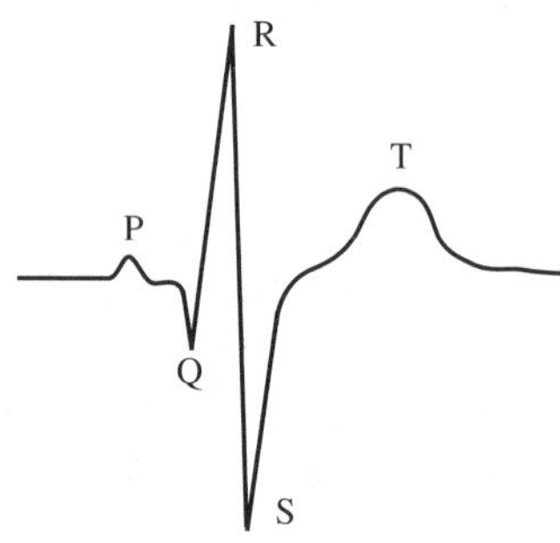

Class I includes drugs which directly interfere with depolarisation of the cell membrane (membrane-stabilising agents) by blocking the fast inward current of sodium into cardiac cells; they also have local anaesthetic properties. They are subdivided into 3 further groups according to their effects on factors such as the duration of the cardiac action potential, the rate of change of the depolarisation phase of the cardiac action potential, the fibrillation threshold, conduction properties, and atrial and ventricular refractoriness.

Class Ia drugs slow the rate of change of the depolarisation phase of the action potential, moderately prolong the repolarisation phase, and prolong the PR, QRS, and QT intervals on ECG recording.

Described in this chapter are

Ajmaline	Pirmenol
Cibenzoline	Procainamide
Disopyramide	Quinidine
Hydroquinidine	Recainam
Lorajmine	

Class Ib drugs have a limited effect on the rate of change of the depolarisation phase of the action potential, shorten the repolarisation phase, shorten the QT interval, and elevate the fibrillation threshold.

Described in this chapter are

Aprindine	Recainam
Mexiletine	Tocainide

Class Ic drugs markedly slow the rate of change of the depolarisation phase of the action potential, have little effect on the repolarisation phase, and markedly prolong the PR and QRS intervals.

Described in this chapter are

Diprafenone	Lorcainide
Encainide	Pilsicainide
Flecainide	Propafenone
Indecainide	Recainam

Class II drugs are characterised by beta-blocking activity.

Described in this chapter are

Beta blockers (but sotalol has predominantly class III activity)	Bretylium

Class III drugs prolong the repolarisation phase of the action potential.

Described in this chapter are

Acecainide	Cibenzoline
Amiodarone	Dofetilide
Azimilide	Ibutilide
Bretylium	Sotalol
Bunaftine	

Class IV drugs block the slow inward calcium current (calcium-channel blockers) although not all drugs that fall into the broad general category of calcium-channel blockers share the same specific properties.

Described in this chapter are

Cibenzoline	Verapamil

Class V drugs reduce the slope of the slow diastolic depolarisation in pacemaking cells of the sino-atrial node.

Described in this chapter are

Alinidine

Many antiarrhythmics have actions typical of more than one class of compound making allocation to one specific class difficult. In some cases this results in multiple classification; an example is bretylium which has class II and III actions. However, in other cases a compound has been allocated to only one class even though it does display additional properties typical of another class; thus propafenone is usually recognised as a class Ic drug although it does possess some beta-blocking activity; beta blockers such as propranolol are traditionally described as class II drugs despite possessing some class I actions; sotalol has some class II actions typical of the beta blockers generally, but has predominantly class III activity and is usually described as a class III drug. Some drugs such as adenosine and digoxin do not fit into the Vaughan Williams classification at all.

The Vaughan Williams classification has been criticised because the electrophysiological action of the antiarrhythmic drugs is not clearly related to their effectiveness in treating a particular arrhythmia in an individual patient. A more clinically useful method might be to categorise the drugs according to the cardiac tissues which each affects. Thus drugs which act on the sino-atrial node include beta blockers, class IV antiarrhythmics, and cardiac glycosides such as digoxin; class I and class III antiarrhythmics act on the ventricles; and drugs acting on atrial arrhythmias include class Ia, Ic, and III antiarrhythmics and beta blockers. Class Ia and III antiarrhythmics act on accessory pathways and drugs acting on the atrioventricular node include class Ic and IV antiarrhythmics, beta blockers, and cardiac glycosides. A simplification of this scheme is to classify drugs into those that act on both ventricular and supraventricular arrhythmias such as amiodarone, beta blockers, disopyramide, procainamide, and quinidine, those that act mainly on ventricular arrhythmias such as lignocaine, mexiletine, and phenytoin, and those that act mainly on supraventricular arrhythmias such as verapamil.

References.

1. Vaughan Williams EM. Classification of antidysrhythmic drugs. *Pharmacol Ther* 1975; **1:** 115–38.
2. Harrison DC. Current classification of antiarrhythmic drugs as a guide to their rational clinical use. *Drugs* 1986; **31:** 93–5.
3. Frumin H, *et al.* Classification of antiarrhythmic drugs. *J Clin Pharmacol* 1989; **29:** 387–94.
4. Nattel S. Antiarrhythmic drug classifications: a critical appraisal of their history, present status, and clinical relevance. *Drugs* 1991; **41:** 672–701.
5. Vaughan Williams EM. Classifying antiarrhythmic actions: by facts or speculation. *J Clin Pharmacol* 1992; **32:** 964–77.

Anticoagulants

Anticoagulants are used in the treatment and prophylaxis of thrombo-embolic disorders. They may be divided into direct anticoagulants such as the heparins, low-molecular-weight heparins, and heparinoids and indirect anticoagulants such as the coumarin and indanedione derivatives.

Direct anticoagulants

Heparin inhibits clotting of blood *in vitro* and *in vivo* by enhancing the action of antithrombin III. Antithrombin III, which is present in plasma, inhibits the activity of activated clotting factors including thrombin (factor IIa) and activated factor X (factor Xa). With normal therapeutic doses heparin has an inhibitory effect on both thrombin and factor Xa. The low doses that are given subcutaneously for the prophylaxis of thrombo-embolism have a selective effect on antithrombin III's inhibition of factor Xa. Very high doses are reported to reduce the activity of antithrombin III. Heparin also has some effect on platelet function, inhibits the formation of a stable fibrin clot, and has an antilipaemic effect.

Low-molecular-weight heparins are salts of fragments of heparin produced by chemical or enzymatic depolymerisation of the heparin molecule. Commercially available low-molecular-weight heparins differ in their method of production, molecular-weight range, and degree of sulphation. Like heparin, these compounds enhance the action of antithrombin III but they are characterised by a higher ratio of anti-factor Xa to anti-factor IIa (antithrombin activity) than heparin. The possibility that such selective factor-Xa inhibition would result in antithrombotic activity without anticoagulant and hence haemorrhagic effects has not been fully confirmed by clinical experience in humans. Low-molecular-weight heparins also have less effect on platelet aggregation than heparin.

Direct thrombin inhibitors such as bivalirudin and hirudins are also used.

Described in this chapter are

Ardeparin	Low-molecular-weight Heparins
Bivalirudin	Nadroparin
Certoparin	Parnaparin
Dalteparin	Reviparin
Enoxaparin	Tinzaparin
Heparin	
Hirudin	

The term *heparinoid* includes heparin derivatives and has also been used more loosely to include naturally occurring and synthetic highly sulphated polysaccharides of similar structure, such as danaparoid and dermatan sulphate. Some compounds have been described in many ways; some of the terms used include sulphated glucosaminoglycans, glycosaminoglycan polysulphate compounds, or sulphated mucopolysaccharides.

Described in this chapter are

Danaparoid	Sodium Apolate
Dermatan Sulphate	Sulodexide
Pentosan Polysulphate Sodium	

Indirect anticoagulants

Indirect anticoagulants act by depressing the hepatic vitamin K-dependent synthesis of coagulation factors II (prothrombin), VII, IX, and X, and of the anticoagulant protein C and its cofactor protein S. Warfarin, a coumarin, is the main drug used, but indanediones such as phenindione are also available. Since they act indirectly, they have no effect on existing clots. Also as the coagulation factors involved have half-lives ranging from 6 to 60 hours, several hours are required before an effect is observed. A therapeutic effect is usually apparent by 24 hours, but the peak effect may not be achieved until 2 or 3 days after a dose; the overall effect may last for 5 days.

Described in this chapter are

Anisindione	Phenindione
Dicoumarol	Phenprocoumon
Ethyl Biscoumacetate	Tioclomarol
Fluindione	Warfarin
Nicoumalone	

Antiplatelet drugs

Platelet aggregation is important in haemostasis (p.704) and is also involved in thrombus formation, particularly in the arterial circulation. Antiplatelet drugs reduce platelet aggregation and are used to prevent further thrombo-embolic events in patients who have suffered myocardial infarction, ischaemic stroke or transient ischaemic attacks, or unstable angina, and for primary prevention of a thrombo-embolic event in patients at risk. Some are also used for the prevention of reocclusion or restenosis following angioplasty and bypass procedures.

Antiplatelet drugs act through a wide range of mechanisms. Aspirin (p.16) is the most widely used and studied; it acts by irreversibly inhibiting platelet cyclo-oxygenase and thus preventing synthesis of thromboxane A_2. Reversible cyclo-oxygenase inhibitors such as indobufen are also available, and thromboxane synthase inhibitors (pirmagrel) and thromboxane receptor antagonists (sulotroban) may also be used.

Drugs that interfere with adenosine metabolism have an antiplatelet effect and those used include some prostaglandins, which act by increasing platelet cyclic adenosine monophosphate levels; ticlopidine, which interferes with adenosine diphosphate mediated platelet activation; and the adenosine reuptake inhibitor dipyridamole.

Thrombin inhibitors such as heparin and the hirudins have antiplatelet and anticoagulant effects; argatroban is used specifically as an antiplatelet drug. Glycoprotein IIb/IIIa receptor antagonists, such as abciximab, eptifibatide, and tirofiban, interfere with the final step in platelet aggregation and are used mainly as adjuncts in reperfusion and revascularisation procedures.

Described in this chapter are

Abciximab	Picotamide
Argatroban	Pirmagrel
Clopidogrel	Sarpogrelate
Cloricromen	Sibrafiban
Dipyridamole	Sulotroban
Ditazole	Ticlopidine
Eptifibatide	Tirofiban
Indobufen	Trapidil
Ketanserin	Triflusal
Lamifiban	Xemilofiban
Orbofiban	

References.

1. Schrör K. Antiplatelet drugs: a comparative review. *Drugs* 1995; **50:** 7–28.

Beta blockers

Beta blockers are competitive antagonists at beta-adrenergic receptor sites and are used in the management of cardiovascular disorders such as hypertension, angina pectoris, cardiac arrhythmias, and myocardial infarction. They are also given to control symptoms of sympathetic overactivity in alcohol withdrawal, anxiety states, hyperthyroidism, and tremor and in the prophylaxis of migraine and of bleeding associated with portal hypertension. Some beta blockers are used as eye drops to reduce raised intra-ocular pressure in glaucoma and ocular hypertension. Their actions and uses are discussed in more detail on p.828.

Described in this chapter are

Acebutolol	Flestolol
Alprenolol	Indenolol
Amosulalol	Labetalol
Arotinolol	Levobunolol
Atenolol	Levomoprolol
Befunolol	Medroxalol
Betaxolol	Mepindolol
Bevantolol	Metipranolol
Bisoprolol	Metoprolol
Bopindolol	Nadolol
Bucindolol	Nebivolol
Bufetolol	Nipradilol
Bufuralol	Oxprenolol
Bunitrolol	Penbutolol
Bupranolol	Pindolol
Carazolol	Practolol
Carteolol	Propranolol
Carvedilol	Sotalol
Celiprolol	Talinolol
Cloranolol	Tertatolol
Dilevalol	Tilisolol
Epanolol	Timolol
Esmolol	

Calcium-channel blockers

The main use of calcium-channel blockers is in the management of angina pectoris and hypertension; some are also employed in cardiac arrhythmias.

Calcium-channel blockers, also known as calcium antagonists, calcium-entry blockers, and slow-channel blockers, inhibit the cellular influx of calcium which is responsible for maintenance of the plateau phase of the action potential. Thus calcium-channel blockers primarily affect tissues in which depolarisation is dependent upon calcium rather than sodium influx, and these include vascular smooth muscle, myocardial cells, and cells within the sino-atrial (SA) and atrioventricular (AV) nodes. The main actions of the calcium-channel blockers include dilatation of coronary and peripheral arteries and arterioles with little or no effect on venous tone, a negative inotropic action, reduction of heart rate, and slowing of AV conduction. However, the effects of individual drugs, and therefore their uses, are modified by their selectivity of action at different tissue sites and by baroreceptor reflexes.

Calcium-channel blockers may be classified according to their chemical structure. There are three major groups that are highly specific blockers of calcium channels.

Dihydropyridine calcium-channel blockers (such as nifedipine) have a greater selectivity for vascular smooth muscle than for myocardium and therefore their main effect is vasodilatation. They have little or no action at the SA or AV nodes and negative inotropic activity is rarely seen at therapeutic doses. They are used for their antihypertensive and anti-anginal properties. Some dihydropyridine derivatives, for example nimodipine, cross the blood-brain barrier and are used in cerebral ischaemia.

Benzothiazepine calcium-channel blockers (such as diltiazem) and **phenylalkylamine** calcium-channel blockers (such as verapamil) have less selective vasodilator activity than dihydropyridine derivatives; they have a direct effect on myocardium causing depression of SA and AV nodal conduction. They are used for their antiarrhythmic, anti-anginal, and antihypertensive properties.

Recently, a new class of calcium-channel blockers has come under investigation. These drugs act principally on fast T-type calcium channels unlike conventional calcium-channel blockers that act on slow L-type channels. Mibefradil is an example of a T-type calcium-channel blocker.

For further discussion of the actions and uses of the three main groups of calcium-channel blockers, see Nifedipine, p.916, Diltiazem, p.854, and Verapamil, p.960, respectively.

Described in this chapter are

Amlodipine	Lidoflazine
Anipamil	Manidipine
Aranidipine	Mibefradil
Barnidipine	Nicardipine
Benidipine	Nifedipine
Bepridil	Nilvadipine
Cilnidipine	Nimodipine
Diltiazem	Nisoldipine
Efonidipine	Nitrendipine
Felodipine	Perhexiline
Isradipine	Tiapamil
Lacidipine	Verapamil
Lercanidipine	

Cardiac inotropes

Positive cardiac inotropes increase the force of contraction of the myocardium and are therefore used in the management of acute and chronic heart failure. Some inotropes also increase or decrease the heart rate (positive or negative chronotropes), provide vasodilatation (inodilators), or improve myocardial relaxation (positive lusitropes), and these additional properties influence the choice of drug in specific situations. Drugs that are used predominantly for their inotropic effects include the cardiac glycosides and phosphodiesterase inhibitors; sympathomimetics are employed as inotropes but also have other important uses.

References.

1. Feldman AM. Classification of positive inotropic agents. *J Am Coll Cardiol* 1993; **22:** 1223–7.
2. Cuthbertson BH, *et al.* Inotropic agents in the critically ill. *Br J Hosp Med* 1996; **56:** 386–91.

Cardiac glycosides, such as digoxin, possess positive inotropic activity which is mediated by inhibition of sodium-potassium adenosine triphosphatase (Na/K-ATPase). They also reduce conductivity in the heart, particularly through the atrioventricular node, and therefore have a negative chronotropic effect. The cardiac glycosides have very similar pharmacological effects but differ considerably in their speed of onset and duration of action. They are used to slow the heart rate in supraventricular arrhythmias, especially atrial fibrillation, and are also given in chronic heart failure.

Described in this chapter are

Acetyldigitoxin	Lanatoside C
Acetyldigoxin	Medigoxin
Cymarin	Meproscillarin
Deslanoside	Ouabain
Digitalis Lanata Leaf	Peruvoside
Digitalis Leaf	Proscillaridin
Digitoxin	Strophanthin-K
Digoxin	

Phosphodiesterase inhibitors are also potent inotropes; they also have vasodilator effects. They are used in the short-term treatment of severe heart failure.

Described in this chapter are

Amrinone	Olprinone
Enoximone	Pimobendan
Milrinone	Vesnarinone

Centrally acting antihypertensives

Centrally acting antihypertensives include alpha$_2$-adrenoceptor agonist such as clonidine and methyldopa. Stimulation of alpha$_2$ adrenoceptors in the CNS results in a reduction in sympathetic tone and a fall in blood pressure. Heart rate is also reduced. They are used in the management of hypertension, although other drugs with fewer adverse effects are generally preferred. Some have a role in the management of glaucoma. Clonidine is also used in migraine prophylaxis and menopausal flushing, and forms part of the treatment of opioid withdrawal.

Described in this chapter are

Apraclonidine	Guanoxabenz
Azepexole	Methyldopa
Brimonidine	Moxonidine
Clonidine	Rilmenidine
Guanabenz	Tiamenidine
Guanfacine	Tolonidine

Diuretics

Diuretics promote the excretion of water and electrolytes by the kidneys. They are used in the treatment of heart failure or in hepatic, renal, or pulmonary disease when salt and water retention has resulted in oedema or ascites. Diuretics are also used, either alone, or in association with other drugs, in the treatment of hypertension.

The principal groups of diuretics are as follows.

Carbonic anhydrase inhibitors are weak diuretics and are used mainly to reduce raised intra-ocular pressure.

Described in this chapter are

Acetazolamide	Dorzolamide
Brinzolamide	Methazolamide
Dichlorphenamide	

'Loop' or **'high-ceiling' diuretics** produce an intense, dose-dependent diuresis of relatively short duration.

Described in this chapter are

Azosemide	Frusemide
Bumetanide	Piretanide
Ethacrynic Acid	Torasemide
Etozolin	

Osmotic diuretics raise the osmolality of plasma and renal tubular fluid. They are used to reduce or prevent cerebral oedema, to reduce raised intra-ocular pressure, and in acute renal failure.

Described in this chapter are

Isosorbide	Mannitol

Potassium-sparing diuretics have a relatively weak diuretic effect and are normally used in conjunction with thiazide or loop diuretics.

Described in this chapter are

Amiloride	Spironolactone
Canrenoate Potassium	Triamterene
Canrenone	

Thiazides (benzothiadiazines), such as bendrofluazide and hydrochlorothiazide, and certain other compounds, such as metolazone, with structural similarities to the thiazides, inhibit sodium and chloride reabsorption in the kidney tubules and produce a corresponding increase in potassium excretion.

Described in this chapter are

Althiazide	Indapamide
Bemetizide	Mebutizide
Bendrofluazide	Mefruside
Benzthiazide	Methyclothiazide
Buthiazide	Meticrane
Chlorothiazide	Metolazone
Chlorthalidone	Polythiazide
Clopamide	Quinethazone
Cyclopenthiazide	Teclothiazide
Cyclothiazide	Trichlormethiazide
Epithiazide	Tripamide
Hydrochlorothiazide	Xipamide
Hydroflumethiazide	

Ganglion blockers

Ganglion blockers are antihypertensives that inhibit the transmission of nerve impulses in both sympathetic and parasympathetic ganglia. The sympathetic blockade produces peripheral vasodilatation. There is also a direct vasodilator effect on peripheral blood vessels. Ganglion blockers are used for inducing controlled hypotension during surgical procedures and for the emergency treatment of hypertensive crises, although sodium nitroprusside is usually preferred.

Described in this chapter are

Mecamylamine	Trimetaphan

Nitrates

Nitrates are peripheral and coronary vasodilators used in the management of angina pectoris, heart failure, and myocardial infarction. Some of them may also be used to control blood pressure during surgery. Nitrates are believed to exert their vasodilator effect through nitric oxide (p.923) stimulating guanylate cyclase in the vascular smooth muscle cells; this results in an increase in cyclic guanosine monophosphate. This nucleotide induces relaxation probably by lowering the free calcium concentration in the cytosol. Nitrates are thus termed nitrovasodilators. In their action on vascular muscle venous dilatation predominates over dilatation of the arterioles. Venous dilatation decreases venous return as a result of venous pooling and lowers left ventricular diastolic volume and pressure (termed a reduction in preload). The smaller or less important dilatation of arterioles reduces both peripheral vascular resistance and left ventricular pressure at systole (termed a reduction in afterload). The consequent effect is a reduction in the primary determinants of myocardial oxygen demand. The effect on preload is not shared by beta blockers or calcium-channel blockers. Nitrates also have a coronary vasodilator effect which improves regional coronary blood flow to ischaemic areas resulting in improved oxygen supply to the myocardium.

Described in this chapter are

Erythrityl Tetranitrate	Pentaerythritol Tetranitrate
Glyceryl Trinitrate	Propatylnitrate
Isosorbide Dinitrate	Sodium Nitroprusside
Isosorbide Mononitrate	Tenitramine
Linsidomine	Trolnitrate
Mannityl Hexanitrate	
Molsidomine	

Potassium-channel openers

Potassium-channel openers (potassium-channel activators) are used in the management of angina pectoris and hypertension. They have a direct relaxant effect on smooth muscle. They act at potassium channels to allow cellular efflux of potassium which hyperpolarises the cell membrane and leads to a reduction in intracellular calcium. The reduction in intracellular calcium produces relaxation of smooth muscle. Activation of potassium channels in blood vessels produces vasodilatation. Potassium-channel openers may also have potential use in other conditions caused by smooth muscle contraction, for example asthma and urinary incontinence.

Described in this chapter are

Cromakalim	Pinacidil
Nicorandil	

Sympathomimetics

Sympathomimetics produce either direct or indirect stimulation of adrenergic receptors and have various actions depending on the specific receptors involved. Stimulation of α_1 receptors produces smooth muscle contraction; in the cardiovascular system this leads to vasoconstriction and increased blood pressure. Stimulation of β_1 receptors has an inotropic effect and also increases heart rate. Stimulation of β_2 receptors leads to smooth muscle relaxation and produces vasodilatation.

Sympathomimetics have a wide range of uses. In cardiovascular disorders, they are mainly used for their $alpha_1$ and $beta_1$ properties to provide haemodynamic support in the management of acute heart failure and shock. The partial $beta_1$-agonist xamoterol has a role in chronic heart failure.

Described in this chapter are

Adrenaline	Mephentermine
Amezinium	Metaraminol
Arbutamine	Methoxamine
Denopamine	Midodrine
Dimetofrine	Noradrenaline
Dobutamine	Norfenefrine
Docarpamine	Octodrine
Dopamine	Octopamine
Dopexamine	Oxedrine
Etilefrine	Oxilofrine
Gepefrine	Pholedrine
Ibopamine	Prenalterol
Isoprenaline	Xamoterol

Thrombolytics

Thrombolytics are used in the treatment of thrombo-embolic disorders such as myocardial infarction, peripheral arterial thrombo-embolism, and venous thrombo-embolism (deep-vein thrombosis and pulmonary embolism). They are also used to clear blocked cannulas and shunts.

Thrombolytics activate plasminogen to form plasmin, a proteolytic enzyme that degrades fibrin and thus produces dissolution of clots. Some thrombolytics, such as alteplase, act only on fibrin-bound plasminogen and have little effect on circulating, unbound plasminogen; these thrombolytics are termed fibrin-specific agents. Thrombolytics, such as streptokinase, that affect circulating, unbound as well as fibrin-bound plasminogen are termed fibrin-nonspecific agents.

Described in this chapter are

Alteplase	Plasmin
Anistreplase	Plasminogen
Defibrotide	Reteplase
Duteplase	Saruplase
Lanoteplase	Staphylokinase
Monteplase	Streptokinase
Nasaruplase	Urokinase

Vasodilators

Vasodilator is a broad term applied to a wide range of drugs that produce dilatation of blood vessels. The main groups of drugs producing vasodilatation are ACE inhibitors (p.805), nitrates (above), and direct-acting vasodilators.

Direct-acting vasodilators act predominantly on the arterioles reducing peripheral resistance and producing a fall in blood pressure. Their main use is in hypertension, although other drugs are generally preferred. Some of them are used in hypertensive crises.

Described in this chapter are

Cadralazine	Hydralazine
Diazoxide	Minoxidil
Dihydralazine	Picodralazine
Endralazine	Todralazine
Flosequinan	Tolazoline

Other vasodilators may be divided into those used for ischaemic heart disease and those used mainly for cerebral and peripheral vascular disorders. Some drugs originally regarded as vasodilators and used for cerebral and peripheral vascular disorders are now thought to improve microcirculatory flow disturbances by altering the rheological properties of blood or tissue metabolism.

Vasodilators used in Ischaemic Heart Disease

Described in this chapter are

Capobenic Acid	Fendiline
Chromonar	Imolamine
Cinepazet	Oxyfedrine
Cloridarol	Trapidil
Dilazep	Trimetazidine
Efloxate	Visnadine
Etafenone	

Vasodilators used in Cerebral and Peripheral Vascular Disorders

Described in this chapter are

Bamethan	Inositol Nicotinate
Bencyclane	Naftidrofuryl
Buflomedil	Niceritrol
Butalamine	Nicofuranose
Calcitonin Gene-related Peptide	Nicotinyl Alcohol
Cetiedil	Oxpentifylline
Cinepazide	Papaveroline
Cyclandelate	Pentifylline
Di-isopropylammonium Dichloroacetate	Pipratecol
Fasudil	Propentofylline
Hepronicate	Raubasine
Ifenprodil	Suloctidil
	Thymoxamine
	Xanthinol Nicotinate

Management of Cardiovascular Disorders

Management of the main cardiovascular disorders is discussed below. These overviews focus on pharmacological therapy, but other options are also mentioned where they form an important part of treatment.

Advanced cardiac life support

Cardiac arrest is the cessation of effective cardiac mechanical activity and is usually a result of ischaemic heart disease in adults and respiratory or circulatory failure in children. It may be associated with four arrhythmias, namely **ventricular fibrillation, pulseless ventricular tachycardia, asystole**, and **electromechanical dissociation**. Ventricular fibrillation is the commonest in adults and asystole in children. In ventricular fibrillation and pulseless ventricular tachycardia there is chaotic electrical and mechanical activity; in asystole a total absence of both activities; and in electromechanical dissociation an absence of mechanical activity, or undetectable activity, in the presence of some electrical activity.

Cardiac arrest is an emergency situation and should be treated by the institution of full life support measures. European guidelines[1] (adopted in the UK) based on a statement issued by the International Liaison Committee on Resuscitation[2] and American[3] guidelines for advanced life support and the immediate period of cardiac arrest have been published and, apart from some differences in detail, are broadly similar. In order to maintain cardiorespiratory function, basic life support (cardiopulmonary resuscitation) consisting of chest compression and ventilation (mouth-to-mouth/mask) should be instituted immediately and continued during the resuscitation attempt. Subsequent procedures will depend to some extent on the type of arrhythmia present. For the commonest, ventricular fibrillation, rapid defibrillation is of paramount importance and should not be delayed by other necessary measures such as the administration of oxygen, intubation, and the provision of intravenous access. Defibrillation is intended to produce momentary asystole and allow the natural pacemakers to resume normal activity. Adrenaline is given principally to increase the efficacy of basic life support rather than as an adjunct to defibrillation although evidence that it improves survival is limited; through its alpha agonist effects it increases myocardial and cerebral blood flow. A dose of 1 mg of adrenaline is regarded as the 'standard' dose. A higher dose of 5 mg has been used in some clinical trials, although there is as yet no evidence that this dose is associated with an improvement in overall survival rate. In the case of asystole, atropine may be given to block excess vagal tone. Other drugs that may be given during resuscitation attempts include antiarrhythmics such as lignocaine, bretylium, or amiodarone, buffering agents such as intravenous sodium bicarbonate for acidosis, and calcium, magnesium, or potassium salts for known deficiencies. Specific guidelines for the different types of arrhythmia are as follows.

Ventricular fibrillation and **pulseless ventricular tachycardia**

These are treated in the same way. The European guidelines for adults[1] emphasise that the first defibrillating shock must be administered as quickly as possible. In cases of witnessed cardiac arrest a precordial thump, which sometimes aborts the arrhythmia if given within 30 seconds of the loss of cardiac output, may be given before attaching the monitor/defibrillator. However, the attachment of the defibrillator must not be delayed; the initial direct current shock (200J) is followed as necessary by a second (200J) and a third (360J) shock if the preceding shock is not successful. If the initial group of three shocks is unsuccessful, chest compression and ventilation should be continued and further shocks given. Adrenaline 1 mg intravenously should be administered before the next set of three shocks (each of 360J). This loop of adrenaline and three shocks (360J) should be repeated as necessary. Endotracheal administration of adrenaline may be employed if intravenous access cannot be obtained, but doses 2 to 3 times greater than those given intravenously are suggested. However, some workers consider that these doses are likely to be ineffective.[4] After a total of three loops other drugs (such as those described above) may be employed as appropriate. Meanwhile, the adrenaline and 3-shock loops continue for as long as defibrillation is indicated. The total number of loops is a matter of judgement but a resuscitation attempt may reasonably last for anything from 10 minutes to 1 hour.

The American guidelines[3] follow a similar pattern to the European ones although they also give instances where higher-dose adrenaline regimens may be employed.

The basic management of **ventricular fibrillation in children** is the same as in adults, but the energies used for defibrillation and the doses of drugs used are different.[3,5] The initial dose of adrenaline recommended in the International[5] and American[3] guidelines is 10 μg per kg body-weight by intravenous or intraosseous injection but all subsequent doses are of 100 μg per kg. Endotracheal administration is an alternative route if an intravenous or intraosseous access cannot be obtained; the suggested endotracheal dose is 100 μg per kg for both initial and subsequent doses.[3,5]

In survivors of ventricular fibrillation and pulseless ventricular tachycardia in whom it is considered there is a high risk of **recurrence**, implantable cardioverter defibrillators may be employed. Drug therapy may also be used prophylactically as outlined under Ventricular Tachycardia in Cardiac Arrhythmias, below.

Asystole and **electromechanical dissociation**

In general, the prognosis of patients with these arrhythmias is much less favourable than those with ventricular fibrillation or pulseless ventricular tachycardia, although there are certain causes such as hypovolaemia, hypoxia, pneumothorax, pulmonary embolism, drug overdose, hypothermia, and electrolyte imbalances that may respond to treatment and these should be considered and the appropriate therapy given promptly once resuscitation has been instituted. As described above, a precordial thump may be appropriate if the cardiac arrest is witnessed. Once ventricular fibrillation or tachycardia is positively excluded, cardiopulmonary resuscitation should be instituted immediately and adrenaline 1 mg should be given intravenously every 3 minutes. In asystole a single dose of atropine 3 mg intravenously is also administered to block vagal activity.[1,2] In the American guidelines[3] atropine is recommended in repeated doses of 1 mg to a total of 0.04 mg per kg body-weight rather than as a single dose of 3 mg. Three further cycles of adrenaline and chest compression and ventilation follow (but no more atropine); then high-dose adrenaline (5 mg) may be considered although its value is said to be unproved.[1,2] Other drugs (such as buffering agents) may be considered. Cardiac pacing is instituted once there is evidence of electrical activity. Resuscitation should generally continue for at least 20 to 30 minutes from the time of collapse; prolonged resuscitation is not usually undertaken as recovery rarely occurs after 15 minutes of asystole if there has been no response.

As ventricular fibrillation is unusual in **children**, a precordial thump and defibrillation are not included as routine in the paediatric guidelines for asystole or electromechanical dissociation. The initial dose of adrenaline recommended is 10 μg per kg body-weight followed by subsequent doses of 100 μg per kg given by intravenous or intraosseous injection.[3,5] Adrenaline may be given by the endotracheal route in doses of 100 μg per kg.[3,5] Atropine has not been shown to be necessary.[3]

1. Advanced Life Support Working Group of the European Resuscitation Council. The 1998 European Resuscitation Council guidelines for adult advanced life support. *Br Med J* 1998; **316:** 1863–9. [Also published in *Resuscitation* 1998; **37:** 81–90.]

2. ALS Working Group of the International Liaison Committee on Resuscitation. The universal algorithm. *Resuscitation* 1997; **34:** 109–11.
3. Emergency Cardiac Care Committee and Subcommittees, American Heart Association. Guidelines for cardiopulmonary resuscitation and emergency cardiac care. *JAMA* 1992; **268:** 2171–2295.
4. McCrirrick A, Monk CR. Comparison of i.v. and intra-tracheal administration of adrenaline. *Br J Anaesth* 1994; **72:** 529–32.
5. Nadkarni V, *et al.* Paediatric life support: an advisory statement by the Paediatric Life Support Working Group of the International Liaison Committee on Resuscitation. *Resuscitation* 1998; **34:** 115–27. [NB. Contains incorrect adrenaline dose in figure 3.]

Angina pectoris

Angina pectoris is a syndrome that arises from an inadequate myocardial oxygen supply (myocardial ischaemia). The prominent symptom is transient precordial distress ranging from discomfort to severe pain. Some patients may also experience dyspnoea, nausea, sweating, and left arm discomfort. Myocardial oxygen supply depends upon coronary blood flow which normally increases to meet increased oxygen demands. Ischaemia occurs when blood flow cannot be increased or is reduced and may be due to a fixed obstruction in the coronary arteries, vasoconstriction, thrombus formation, or platelet aggregation.

Three main types of angina have been described: stable angina; unstable angina; and Prinzmetal's angina. These should not be regarded as discrete groups as more than one type is usually present in the patient with angina.

Stable angina (effort angina) is angina which is usually precipitated by exertion and relieved by rest. It is often called chronic stable angina and as the name implies the frequency, intensity, and duration of the attacks are stable. The predominant underlying disorder is coronary atherosclerosis causing a fixed obstruction in one or more coronary arteries. While the restricted coronary blood flow is still adequate for oxygenation of the unstressed heart, it is not capable of being increased to meet the increase in myocardial oxygen demand that may occur during exercise, cold exposure, emotional stress, or after eating.

Unstable angina (acute coronary insufficiency or intermediate coronary syndrome) represents symptom complexes intermediate between stable angina pectoris and myocardial infarction. Three subgroups are recognised: angina that presents from the beginning as severe and frequent attacks; an increase in the frequency, intensity, and/or duration of previously stable angina, often with diminishing responsiveness to sublingual nitrates (crescendo angina); and recurring or prolonged angina at rest. In unstable angina the decreased coronary artery blood flow is usually caused by disruption of an atherosclerotic plaque which leads to platelet adhesion and aggregation, thrombus formation, and vasoconstriction, thus resulting in partial occlusion of one or more coronary arteries. The coronary blood flow can be so restricted that it does not meet the oxygenation demands of the unstressed heart. Patients with unstable angina are at an increased risk of sudden death and myocardial infarction, and those with rest pain are at the greatest risk.

Prinzmetal's angina (variant angina) is a rare form of angina caused by coronary vasospasm and is usually associated with atherosclerosis. It occurs spontaneously at rest and with greater frequency during the night or early hours of the morning. It carries a considerable risk of progression to myocardial infarction and may be considered as part of the spectrum of unstable angina. Prolonged vasospasm may also lead to ventricular arrhythmias, heart block, or death.

In addition to the types of angina described above periods of **silent myocardial ischaemia** (asymptomatic transient myocardial ischaemia) in which there is no anginal pain have been identified during ECG monitoring. In some patients all such episodes are asymptomatic. However, asymptomatic ischaemic episodes also occur in patients with angina and seem to be more common than symptomatic episodes. It is not clear why some episodes of ischaemia are symptomatic while others are not.

Treatment depends on the type of angina and involves management of acute anginal pain and long-term management to prevent angina attacks. This treatment, which is described in more detail below, includes drug therapy (nitrates, beta blockers, and calcium-channel blockers), coronary artery bypass surgery, and percutaneous transluminal coronary angioplasty. While antianginal treatment can abolish or control attacks of angina, it does not treat the underlying cause of the ischaemia and patients should be assessed for risk factors for ischaemic heart disease and the appropriate lifestyle changes made (see Atherosclerosis, below). Lipid lowering therapy should also be considered. Aspirin is used in the prevention of myocardial infarction (below), stroke (below), and other vascular events in patients with unstable and stable angina.[1-3] Aspirin has also been tried in subjects with no evidence of ischaemic heart disease to prevent the development of angina but the results from one large study are not encouraging,[4] and its use in low risk subjects such as these is not recommended.[1]

Anti-anginal drugs act in a variety of ways. Glyceryl trinitrate and other organic *nitrates* have a vasodilator effect with venodilatation predominating over dilatation of the arterioles. Dilatation of veins decreases venous return as a result of venous pooling and lowers left ventricular diastolic volume and pressure (together termed a reduction in preload). The smaller or less important dilatation of arterioles reduces both peripheral vascular resistance and left ventricular pressure at systole (termed a reduction in afterload). The consequence of these effects is a reduction in myocardial oxygen demand. Also the vasodilator effect improves regional coronary blood flow to ischaemic areas, and alleviates coronary spasm. *Beta blockers* cause a slowing of the heart rate and reduction in contractility and therefore reduce myocardial oxygen demand. *Calcium-channel blockers* reduce the work of the heart by dilating peripheral arteries. They also act on the coronary circulation preventing spasm.

Percutaneous transluminal coronary *angioplasty* is a means of mechanically dilating coronary arteries using a balloon that has been passed down a catheter and inflated at the appropriate sites. Nitrates and calcium-channel blockers may be given to alleviate coronary spasm due to the procedure. Coronary artery *bypass surgery* abolishes or reduces episodes of angina in the majority of patients but if preventative measures are not successful angina reappears after several years. Restenosis and thrombo-embolic complications may follow angioplasty or bypass surgery and a wide variety of drugs have been investigated for prophylaxis; for further details, see Reperfusion and Revascularisation Procedures, below. Alternative surgical methods such as plaque removal and stenting are also being investigated.[5]

Treatment of stable angina. Management of the patient with stable angina includes treatment of contributory conditions such as anaemia, control of risk factors for atherosclerosis (see below) including lipid-lowering therapy, antiplatelet therapy, and therapy to increase blood flow to the ischaemic myocardium as well as to reduce myocardial oxygen demand.[6-8]

Treatment of infrequent angina episodes (less than about 2 attacks per week) usually consists of glyceryl trinitrate given when required, generally sublingually; alternatively, a buccal tablet or spray formulation may be used. Isosorbide dinitrate, in the form of sublingual tablets or spray, may be used, although it has a slower onset of action than glyceryl trinitrate. Glyceryl trinitrate in sublingual or buccal forms may also be used by patients before an activity or circumstance that might precipitate an attack.

When episodes occur more frequently then sublingual glyceryl trinitrate, at least on its own, may no longer be appropriate, and regular symptomatic treatment has to be considered. Such treatment includes other nitrate therapy, beta blockers, or calcium-channel blockers, and these treatments may be used individually or in combination. Choice depends upon patient characteristics and any concurrent medical conditions.

Beta blockers are the mainstay of therapy and some suggest they should be used as first-line treatment if sublingual glyceryl trinitrate is not adequate.[8] The different beta blockers appear to be equally effective in stable angina.

A calcium-channel blocker may be used as an alternative in patients unable to tolerate a beta blocker. There has been concern regarding the safety of short-acting nifedipine preparations in patients with angina but recent studies indicate similar outcomes in patients receiving either long-acting calcium-channel blockers or beta blockers.[9,10] Care is required in selecting an appropriate drug since not all calcium-channel blockers have the same properties. Dihydropyridines should not be used without beta blockers since response is often variable and angina may even be provoked in some patients because of the effect of increasing heart rate.[6,11,12]

Nitrate therapy for these more frequent attacks including modified-release forms of glyceryl trinitrate, for example transdermal patches, and the long-acting nitrates such as isosorbide dinitrate or isosorbide mononitrate is used in patients with left ventricular dysfunction. Diminished effectiveness or tolerance occurs, particularly with nitrate preparations that produce sustained plasma concentrations, and dosage regimens including a nitrate-free period are commonly used (see p.875).

Alternative drugs that may be used as monotherapy in the management of stable angina include the potassium-channel openers such as nicorandil.

Where optimal therapy with a single agent fails to control symptoms, combination therapy may be used. There is additional benefit from concomitant nitrate and beta blocker therapy, since nitrates can moderate the excessive effects that beta blockers may have in increasing left ventricular diastolic volume and pressure and in inducing bradycardia. Calcium-channel blockers may also be used with nitrates; the combination of verapamil or diltiazem with a nitrate may be preferrable to a combination of nifedipine (or other dihydropyridine derivative) with nitrates as both nifedipine and nitrates cause reflex tachycardia, hypotension, and headaches.

Combination therapy with beta blockers and calcium-channel blockers improves exercise tolerance[8] but adverse effects may be a problem. A beta blocker with nifedipine or another dihydropyridine is preferred and is probably least hazardous.[6,13,14] Verapamil is best avoided in such combinations as its use with a beta blocker increases the risk of impaired cardiac conduction (see Verapamil, p.962). Caution with any combination of a calcium-channel blocker with a beta blocker is particularly necessary in patients with pre-existing conduction disorders or moderate to severe left ventricular dysfunction as the use of calcium-channel blockers may actually increase mortality.[13]

Triple therapy using a nitrate, a beta blocker, and a calcium-channel blocker may sometimes be used although it is likely to be associated with more adverse effects.

If medical treatment does not control the angina the patient should be investigated to determine suitability for coronary angioplasty or coronary artery bypass surgery. Angioplasty is ideally suited to patients with single-vessel disease, good left ventricular function, and stable angina, although the technique is also used in patients with more complex disease, impaired left ventricular function, and unstable angina.[15] Coronary artery bypass surgery is generally the preferred technique in patients with multivessel disease, or disease of the major coronary arteries, impaired left ventricular function, and severe symptoms.[16] Age of the patient also influences the choice of technique; angioplasty may be favoured in the elderly as operative risks are higher in this group.[15]

Treatment of unstable angina. Unstable angina is generally regarded as an emergency and those patients with a change in the pattern of previously stable angina or with recurring or prolonged angina at rest should be hospitalised. The aim of treatment is to control the attacks and prevent the condition progressing to myocardial infarction and death. Once the patient has been stabilised the underlying factors can be treated or controlled and long-term prophylaxis set up to guard against any further ischaemic attacks.

Initial treatment[17-20] depends on the severity of the ischaemia. All patients with unstable angina should receive aspirin, and heparin should also be considered. Nitrates and beta blockers are given to control symptoms and to relieve ischaemia. Calcium-channel blockers may also be used if there is vasospasm or if the patient fails to respond to the other drugs.

Aspirin is routinely included in the initial treatment. It inhibits platelet aggregation and reduces the incidence of myocardial infarction and death, although it has not been shown to reduce the number of ischaemic episodes or to relieve pain during the acute phase. Ticlopidine may be an alternative if aspirin is not tolerated.[18,19] Glycoprotein IIb/IIIa inhibitors such as abciximab, eptifibatide,[39] and tirofiban are more potent inhibitors of platelet aggregation and may have a role in addition to aspirin. Beneficial results have been reported in patients receiving tirofiban and aspirin alone[21] or in combination with heparin therapy.[22]

Heparin is given by continuous intravenous infusion to reduce thrombin generation and fibrin formation. Most people recommend that the infusion be continued for 6 or 7 days.[17] It reduces the number of ischaemic episodes and major cardiovascular events during the acute phase,[18] although it has been suggested that heparin must be started early to be effective.[17] Although some reserve heparin for high risk patients a recent meta-analysis[23] suggests that a combination of aspirin and heparin should be used in most patients. Reactivation of unstable angina has been reported in patients discontinuing intravenous heparin;[24] combination with aspirin or gradual discontinuation may prevent this effect.[20] Subcutaneous heparin may be an alternative.[25] Low-molecular-weight heparins in combination with aspirin also appear to be effective[26-28] and may be given for longer periods than standard heparin, but their role in patient therapy is not clearly established.[29] Direct thrombin inhibitors such as the recombinant hirudin, lepirudin, have also been tried.[30]

The initial nitrate treatment is given intravenously to produce a fast response and to provide better dose control than can be achieved with other routes. Glyceryl trinitrate or isosorbide dinitrate are used. Generally the intravenous nitrate is only given during the acute phase, and once the patient is stabilised the infusion is withdrawn, usually within about 48 hours. Sublingual glyceryl trinitrate may be tried initially in patients with less severe symptoms.

Treatment with a beta blocker is started during the acute phase to reduce myocardial oxygen demand. Initially, the intravenous route may be employed and then followed by oral administration.[18,19] Beta blockers with intrinsic sympathomimetic activity do not reduce resting heart rate and are not recommended.[17]

Calcium-channel blockers may be added to therapy although some authorities doubt their value and consider they should be reserved for patients with angina refractory to treatment with the above drugs.[17-20] However, calcium-channel blockers are the drugs of choice if the angina has a vasospastic aetiology, for example in Prinzmetal's angina. The choice of calcium-channel blocker is described under the treatment of stable angina above.

Thrombolytics such as alteplase, streptokinase, and urokinase have been given intravenously in unstable angina. Although small-scale studies reported some benefit the results were variable. Two studies have investigated alteplase (the TIMI-IIIB study[31] with 1473 patients) and anistreplase (the UNASEM study[32] involving 159 patients). Thrombolysis failed to improve outcome and was associated with an excess of bleeding complications. Low-dose regimens are also being investigated and may have benefits.[20] However, thrombolytic therapy is not recommended for routine treatment of unstable angina.[33]

Drug treatment is usually successful in stabilising angina in about 80% of patients and these patients should continue to take aspirin and a beta blocker. Some patients are given a long-acting nitrate for long-term prophylaxis, although nitrates have not been shown to protect against subsequent cardiovascular events.[17-19] Some advocate giving long-term oral anticoagulation but it is not clear that this offers any advantage over aspirin.[17]

Having controlled the acute phase the patient should be assessed to see if angioplasty or coronary artery bypass surgery would be helpful. Measures should also be adopted to control recognised risk factors (see Atherosclerosis, below).

Patients with unstable angina who do not respond to full medical treatment, as above, within 48 hours should undergo emergency angiography in preparation for angioplasty or coronary artery bypass surgery.

Treatment of Prinzmetal's angina. This should be treated like unstable angina with the addition of a calcium-channel blocker; the selection of an appropriate calcium-channel blocker is described above under the treatment of stable angina. Once stabilised, maintenance should include a nitrate, or calcium-channel blocker, or both to protect against further spasm. Surgery may be considered in some patients.

Treatment of silent myocardial ischaemia. Increasing recognition is being given to silent myocardial ischaemia as a potential risk factor for future cardiovascular morbidity and mortality and current research is being undertaken to assess whether suppressing such episodes can improve long-term outcome. Although many of the therapies used in angina reduce the incidence of silent ischaemia it is not yet clear whether complete suppression of ischaemia affects prognosis.[10,34-37] Other studies have suggested that periods of ischaemia may protect the heart during subsequent myocardial infarction[38] and further work is needed to reconcile these findings.

1. Antiplatelet Trialists' Collaboration. Collaborative overview of randomised trials of antiplatelet therapy–I: prevention of death, myocardial infarction, and stroke by prolonged antiplatelet therapy in various categories of patients. *Br Med J* 1994; **308:** 81–106. Correction. *ibid.*; 1540.
2. Hennekens CH, *et al.* Aspirin as a therapeutic agent in cardiovascular disease: a statement for healthcare professionals from the American Heart Association. *Circulation* 1997; **96:** 2751–3.
3. Eccles M, *et al.* North of England evidence based guideline development project: guideline on the use of aspirin as secondary prophylaxis for vascular disease in primary care. *Br Med J* 1998; **316:** 1303–9.
4. Manson JE, *et al.* Aspirin in the primary prevention of angina pectoris in a randomized trial of United States physicians. *Am J Med* 1990; **89:** 772–6.
5. Corr L. New methods of making blocked coronary arteries patent again. *Br Med J* 1994; **309:** 579–83.
6. Shub C. Stable angina pectoris 3: medical treatment. *Mayo Clin Proc* 1990; **65:** 256–73.
7. Chan P, *et al.* The role of nitrates, beta blockers, and calcium antagonists in stable angina pectoris. *Am Heart J* 1988; **116:** 838–48.
8. North of England Stable Angina Guideline Development Group. North of England evidence based guidelines development project: summary version of evidence based guideline for the primary care management of stable angina. *Br Med J* 1996; **312:** 827–32.
9. Rehnqvist N, *et al.* Effects of metoprolol vs verapamil in patients with stable angina pectoris: the Angina Prognosis Study in Stockholm (APSIS). *Eur Heart J* 1996; **17:** 76–81.
10. Dargie HJ, *et al.* Total Ischaemic Bruden European Trial (TIBET): effects of ischaemia and treatment with atenolol, nifedipine SR and their combination on outcome in patients with chronic stable angina. *Eur Heart J* 1996; **17:** 104–12.
11. Kenny J. Calcium channel blocking agents and the heart. *Br Med J* 1985; **291:** 1150–2.
12. Horowitz JD, Powell AC. Calcium antagonist drugs in the management of cardiovascular disease: current status. *Med J Aust* 1989; **150:** 591–5.
13. Packer M. Combined beta-adrenergic and calcium-entry blockade in angina pectoris. *N Engl J Med* 1989; **320:** 709–18.
14. Strauss WE, Parisi AF. Combined use of calcium-channel and beta-adrenergic blockers for the treatment of chronic stable angina: rationale, efficacy, and adverse effects. *Ann Intern Med* 1988; **109:** 570–81.
15. ACC/AHA Task Force. Guidelines for percutaneous transluminal coronary angioplasty: a report of the American College of Cardiology/American Heart Association Task Force on assessment of diagnostic and therapeutic cardiovascular procedures (subcommittee on percutaneous transluminal coronary angioplasty). *J Am Coll Cardiol* 1988; **12:** 529–45.
16. ACC/AHA Task Force. Guidelines and indications for coronary artery bypass graft surgery: a report of the American College of Cardiology/American Heart Association Task Force on assessment of diagnostic and therapeutic cardiovascular procedures (subcommittee on coronary artery bypass graft surgery). *Circulation* 1991; **83:** 1125–73.
17. McMurray J, McLenachan J. Unstable angina. *Prescribers' J* 1990; **30:** 165–73.
18. Kar S, *et al.* The high-risk unstable angina patient: an approach to treatment. *Drugs* 1992; **43:** 837–48.
19. Braunwald E, *et al.* Diagnosing and managing unstable angina. *Circulation* 1994; **90:** 613–22.
20. Brunelli C, *et al.* Recognition and treatment of unstable angina. *Drugs* 1996; **52:** 196–208.
21. The Platelet Receptor Inhibition in Ischemic Syndrome Management (PRISM) study Investigators. A comparison of aspirin plus tirofiban with aspirin plus heparin for unstable angina. *N Engl J Med* 1998; **338:** 1498–1505.
22. The Platelet Receptor Inhibition in Ischemic Syndrome Management in Patients Limited by Unstable Signs and Symptoms (PRISM-PLUS) Study Investigators. Inhibition of the platelet glycoprotein IIb/IIIa receptor with tirofiban in unstable angina and non-Q-wave myocardial infarction. *N Engl J Med* 1998; **338:** 1488–97.
23. Oler A, *et al.* Adding heparin to aspirin reduces the incidence of myocardial infarction and death in patients with unstable angina: a meta-analysis. *JAMA* 1996; **276:** 811–15.
24. Théroux P, *et al.* Reactivation of unstable angina after the discontinuation of heparin. *N Engl J Med* 1992; **327:** 141–5.
25. Serneri GGN, *et al.* Randomised comparison of subcutaneous heparin, intravenous heparin, and aspirin in unstable angina. *Lancet* 1995; **345:** 1201–4. Correction. *ibid.*; **346:** 130.
26. Fragmin During Instability in Coronary Artery Disease (FRISC) Study Group. Low-molecular-weight heparin during instability in coronary artery disease. *Lancet* 1996; **347:** 561–8.
27. Gurfinkel EP, *et al.* Low molecular weight heparin versus regular heparin or aspirin in the treatment of unstable angina and silent ischemia. *J Am Coll Cardiol* 1995; **26:** 313–18.
28. Cohen M, *et al.* A comparison of low-molecular-weight heparin with unfractionated heparin for unstable coronary artery disease. *N Engl J Med* 1997; **337:** 447–52.
29. Spinler SA, Nawarskas JJ. Low-molecular-weight heparins for acute coronary syndromes. *Ann Pharmacother* 1998; **32:** 103–110.
30. Organization to Assess Strategies for Ischemic Syndromes (OASIS) Investigators. Comparison of the effects of two doses of recombinant hirudin compared with heparin in patients with acute myocardial ischemia without ST elevation: a pilot study. *Circulation* 1997; **96:** 769–77.
31. The TIMI IIIB Investigators. Effects of tissue plasminogen activator and a comparison of early invasive and conservative strategies in unstable angina and non-Q-wave myocardial infarction: results of the TIMI IIIB trial. *Circulation* 1994; **89:** 1545–56.
32. Bär FW, *et al.* Thrombolysis in patients with unstable angina improves the angiographic but not the clinical outcome: results of UNASEM, a multicenter, randomized, placebo-controlled, clinical trial with anistreplase. *Circulation* 1992; **86:** 131–7.
33. Anderson HV. Intravenous thrombolysis in refractory unstable angina pectoris. *Lancet* 1995; **346:** 1113–14.
34. Bertolet BD, Pepine CJ. Daily life cardiac ischaemia: should it be treated? *Drugs* 1995; **49:** 176–95.
35. Pepine CJ, *et al.* Effects of treatment on outcome in mildly symptomatic patients with ischaemia during daily life: the Atenolol Silent Ischaemia Study (ASIST). *Circulation* 1994; **90:** 762–8.
36. Knatterud GL, *et al.* Effects of treatment strategies to suppress ischemia in patients with coronary artery disease: 12-week results of the Asymptomatic Cardiac Ischemia Pilot (ACIP) Study. *J Am Coll Cardiol* 1994; **24:** 11–20.
37. Rogers W, *et al.* Asymptomatic Cardiac Ischemia Pilot (ACIP) study: 1 year follow-up. *Circulation* 1994; **90:** I-17.
38. Yellon DM, *et al.* Angina reassessed: pain or protector? *Lancet* 1996; **347:** 1159–62.
39. The PURSUIT Trial Investigators. Inhibition of platelet glycoprotein IIb/IIIa with eptifibatide in patients with acute coronary syndromes. *N Engl J Med* 1998; **339:** 436–43.

Ascites

Ascites is the accumulation of fluid within the peritoneal cavity. Alcoholic hepatic cirrhosis is probably the commonest underlying cause in the western world; others include malignant neoplasms, heart failure, and tuberculosis. The following discussion is restricted mainly to **cirrhotic ascites**.

The mechanism of ascites formation in hepatic cirrhosis has been explained in terms of the underfill and overflow theories, and more recently, the vasodilatation hypothesis. Whatever the mechanism, ascites formation is linked to renal sodium and water retention partly as a result of increased circulating renin and aldosterone concentrations. Portal hypertension and hypoalbuminaemia may be contributory factors. More details may be found in reviews of the pathophysiology of ascites formation.[1-3]

Small amounts of ascitic fluid may go undetected but as it accumulates abdominal distension becomes apparent, and there is a feeling of discomfort. There may be respiratory distress and cardiac dysfunction in severe cases. Peripheral oedema may, or may not, be present. Patients are at risk of primary (spontaneous) bacterial peritonitis (p.136).

Management[1-6] depends on the severity of ascites but the mainstays are dietary sodium restriction and diuretic treatment. In mild to moderate ascites, sodium restriction alone may sometimes be effective but most patients also require diuretics. Bed rest has been advocated but not all workers consider its value proven. Response is monitored by measuring the daily reduction in body weight. The diuretic of choice is the aldosterone antagonist spironolactone, with the addition of a loop diuretic such as frusemide if necessary. Amiloride or another potassium-sparing diuretic may be used as an alternative to spironolactone if adverse effects are a problem. Spironolactone together with frusemide from the outset has also been employed. In tense or refractory ascites, large-volume or total paracentesis (removal of ascitic fluid by drainage) is often used initially; patients may then be maintained on diuretics or repeated paracentesis may be used. Plasma volume replacement with albumin or dextrans after paracentesis is usual, particularly if large volumes are removed. Where ascites remains refractory or repeated paracentesis is not tolerated various shunting procedures have been tried, although their role is not established. In severe cases liver transplantation may be necessary.

In **malignant ascites**, that is ascites due to malignant neoplasms, paracentesis is often necessary but spironolactone may be of benefit in some patients.

1. Roberts LR, Kamath PS. Ascites and hepatorenal syndrome: pathophysiology and management. *Mayo Clin Proc* 1996; **71:** 874–81.
2. Stanley AJ, *et al.* Pathophysiology and management of portal hypertension 2: cirrhotic ascites. *Br J Hosp Med* 1997; **58:** 74–8.
3. Jalan R, Hayes PC. Hepatic encephalopathy and ascites. *Lancet* 1997; **350:** 1309–15.
4. Gerbes AL. Medical treatment of ascites in cirrhosis. *J Hepatol* 1993; **17** (suppl 2): S4–S9.
5. Runyon BA. Care of patients with ascites. *N Engl J Med* 1994; **330:** 337–42.
6. Bataller R, *et al.* Practical recommendations for the treatment of ascites and its complications. Drugs 1997; **54:** 571–80.

Atherosclerosis

Atherosclerosis is the narrowing and hardening of medium and large arteries that results from the development of lipid-rich lesions (atheromas) in their intimal lining. Three main lesions are recognised: fatty streaks, fibrous plaques, and complicated lesions. Fatty streaks develop from infancy and are composed of lipid-filled macrophages (foam cells). Formerly fatty streaks were considered to be precursors of fibrous plaques, although it seems that the origins of the two types of lesions may not be identical. Fibrous plaques consist of lipid-rich smooth muscle cells and macrophages with a connective-tissue matrix that may subsequently undergo calcification, necrosis, thrombosis, and haemorrhage to form complicated lesions. When the atheroma becomes sufficiently large it can block the lumen of the artery although occlusion occurs more commonly when there is thrombosis at the site of a recently ruptured atheromatous plaque. Reduction or total blockage of blood supply results in ischaemia and the clinical events of angina pectoris (above), myocardial infarction (below), peripheral vascular disease (intermittent claudication) (below), and stroke (ischaemic stroke) (below). The term **ischaemic heart disease** (coronary heart or coronary artery disease) encompasses angina pectoris and myocardial infarction and is the most common manifestation of atherosclerosis; in most industrialised countries ischaemic heart disease is a leading cause of death. However, atherosclerosis is essentially a generalised condition and can affect most arteries throughout the body. Thus, the patient with peripheral vascular disease is also likely to develop or to have evidence of ischaemic heart disease and those with ischaemic heart disease may also have atherosclerotic deterioration of other arteries. The term atherosclerotic disease has been used to cover all such manifestations of atherosclerosis.

Epidemiological studies have identified various **risk factors** associated with the development of atherosclerosis. The three major ones are hypercholesterolaemia, hypertension, and smoking. Other characteristics which contribute to the risk include advancing age, male sex, diabetes, obesity, lack of exercise, family history of atherosclerotic disease, abnormal blood clotting factors, in particular raised fibrinogen concentrations, and hyperhomocysteinaemia. The same risk factors apply to all the main forms of atherosclerotic disease although there may be differences in their relative importance. For example the predominant risk factor for stroke is high blood pressure, whereas diabetes and smoking are most strongly linked with peripheral vascular disease. Individuals with a large increase in only one risk factor, such as those with high blood pressure or high blood-cholesterol concentrations are in a minority. Most cases of atherosclerotic disease occur in individuals with mild or moderate increases in *several* risk factors; the presence of more than one risk factor enhances the overall risk for developing atherosclerotic disease, that is, they are not simply additive. The aim is to **prevent** the development of atherosclerotic disease by abolishing or reducing these risk factors. It requires both individual intervention for those at high risk and a population approach to reduce the overall levels of risk factors in the general populace. These approaches have been the subject of guidelines[1,2,15] and reviews.[3-7] Most studies have been in men, but the prevention of atherosclerosis in women has also been reviewed.[8,9]

Individual intervention entails identification of those who are at high risk of developing atherosclerotic disease or who have already suffered a clinical event, and modifying those characteristics that place them at risk by instituting lifestyle changes and specific treatment as appropriate. Intervention is clearly beneficial in those at high risk. For example, treatment of hypercholesterolaemia reduces the incidence of ischaemic heart disease (see Hyperlipidaemias, p.1265) and treatment of hypertension substantially reduces the incidence of stroke, although it does not seem to have such a clear effect on ischaemic heart disease (see Hypertension, below). Intervention in those with only mildly to moderately increased risk levels, which has been mainly in middle-aged men, has been somewhat less successful but is nevertheless recommended. The following lifestyle changes are recommended. Patients should be advised not to smoke, to avoid obesity, to increase exercise, to moderate their alcohol intake, and to adopt a low-fat diet. Women have a lower risk of atherosclerotic disease than men of a comparable age, although the difference narrows with increasing age postmenopausally. Oestrogens, with or without progestogens, given as hormone replacement therapy (HRT) might reduce the incidence of cardiovascular disease in postmenopausal women (see p.1436).

General screening methods fail to identify all individuals at risk of atherosclerotic disease and a **population approach** is also required. This involves general health education and promotion to encourage the lifestyle changes listed above that are associated with lower risk levels. As atheroma development may begin in childhood a healthy diet should be encouraged from an early age. These efforts, though, probably produce only modest changes in risk factors.[10] The incidence of ischaemic heart disease is falling in many populations, although preliminary analysis of the WHO MONICA project results (Monitoring the Trends and Determinants in Cardiovascular Diseases) did not find any correlation with reduction in risk factors. Thus, research continues into the pathogenesis of atherosclerosis and the identification of further risk factors.

Other possible approaches to the management of atherosclerosis include the use of drugs that interfere with atherogenesis (the development of atheromas). *Oxidation* of low-density lipoprotein (LDL) is thought to be a crucial step in atherogenesis[11-13] and dietary antoxidants such as vitamins E and C, betacarotene, and polyphenol compounds found in various foods including red wine have received much attention for their possible role in the prevention of atherosclerosis (see Vitamins, p.1333).

Hyperhomocysteinaemia is an independent risk factor for atherosclerosis, although at present the mechanism by which homocysteine promotes atherosclerosis is unknown,[14] and there is growing interest in assessing the effect of folic acid in the primary or secondary prevention of atherosclerosis (see p.1341).

1. Wood D, *et al.* Joint British recommendations on prevention of coronary heart disease in clinical practice. *Heart* 1998; **80** (suppl 2): S1–S29.
2. Wood D, *et al.* Prevention of coronary heart disease in clinical practice: recommendations of the second joint task force of European and other societies on coronary prevention. *Eur Heart J* 1998; **19:** 1434–1503.
3. Rose G. Epidemiology of atherosclerosis. In: Wolfe JHN, ed. *ABC of vascular diseases.* London: BMJ Publishing Group, 1992: 1–3.
4. Truswell AS. Reducing the risk of coronary heart disease. In: Truswell AS, ed. *ABC of nutrition.* 2nd ed. London: BMJ Publishing Group, 1992; 1–5.
5. Manson JE, *et al.* The primary prevention of myocardial infarction. *N Engl J Med* 1992; **326:** 1406–16.
6. Henderson A. Coronary heart disease: overview. *Lancet* 1996; **348:** s1–s4.
7. 27th Bethesda Conference. Matching the intensity of risk factor management with the hazard for coronary disease events. *J Am Coll Cardiol* 1996; **27:** 957–1047.
8. Wenger NK, *et al.* Cardiovascular health and disease in women. *N Engl J Med* 1993; **329:** 247–56.
9. Rich-Edwards JW, *et al.* The primary prevention of coronary heart disease in women. *N Engl J Med* 1995; **332:** 1758–66.
10. Ebrahim S, Davey Smith G. Systematic review of randomised controlled trials of multiple risk factor interventions for preventing coronary heart disease. *Br Med J* 1997; **314:** 1666–74.
11. Esterbauer H, *et al.* Lipid peroxidation and its role in atherosclerosis. *Br Med Bull* 1993; **49:** 566–76.
12. Witztum JL. The oxidation hypothesis of atherosclerosis. *Lancet* 1994; **344:** 793–5.
13. Diaz MN, *et al.* Antioxidants and atherosclerotic heart disease. *N Engl J Med* 1997; **337:** 408–16.
14. Welch GN, Loscalzo J. Homocysteine and atherothrombosis. *N Engl J Med* 1998; **338:** 1042–50.
15. Grundy SM, *et al.* Primary prevention of coronary heart disease: guidance from Framingham. A statement for healthcare professionals from the AHA task force on risk reduction. *Circulation* 1998; **97:** 1876–87.

Cardiac arrhythmias

The heart acts as a pump and maintains circulation of the blood by alternate contraction and relaxation of cardiac muscle (the myocardium). It generally contracts at a rate of 70 to 75 beats per minute in a healthy 70-kg person at rest. The normal heart rhythm, known as *sinus rhythm*, originates in specialised cardiac cells called *pacemaker cells* in the *sino-atrial (SA)* or *sinus node* and has been defined as a sinus node rate of 60 to 100 per minute. Each heart beat or contraction is initiated by generation of an *action potential* (see Antiarrhythmics, p.776) in the SA node; the electrical impulse spreads over both atria, causing them to contract, and on to the *atrioventricular (AV) node*. From the AV node it spreads through the bundle of His and down the Purkinje fibres to the ventricles, causing them to contract. It is the movement of ions across the cardiac cell membrane that generates the action potential. The electrical changes involved can be recorded on an electrocardiogram (ECG). Other cardiac cells which are located outside the sinus node are also capable of initiating impulses. These cells are termed *ectopic pacemakers* and can be found in the atrioventricular junction and in the His-Purkinje system. The normal rate of impulse initiation by these ectopic pacemakers is less than that of the sinus node and therefore they do not normally initiate the heart beat but may become dominant in certain circumstances such as: if the intrinsic rate of the ectopic pacemaker rises above that of the sinus node; if the sinus node rate falls below that of the ectopic pacemaker; or when a normal sinus node impulse is prevented from conducting through the heart (heart block) leaving the ectopic pacemaker to fire at its own intrinsic rate.

A **cardiac arrhythmia** can be defined in simple terms as any abnormality of rate, regularity, or site of origin of the cardiac impulse or as a disturbance in conduction that causes an abnormal sequence of activation. **Palpitation** is a term used to describe an unacceptable awareness of a beating heart by the patient. This may occur normally in circumstances such as emotion, exercise, or stress or may occur in association with arrhythmias. Clinically, arrhythmias may be classified by presumed site of origin, namely as **supraventricular arrhythmias** (including **atrial arrhythmias** and **atrioventricular junctional arrhythmias**) or as **ventricular arrhythmias**. Classification can also be based on rate as either bradyarrhythmias (slow) or tachyarrhythmias (fast). It is the group of tachyarrhythmias that are discussed in more detail here.

Bradyarrhythmias are caused by sinus node dysfunction that disturbs the conduction of impulses from the sinus node to the atria. **Atrioventricular block** indicates disturbance of conduction of the atrial impulse to the ventricles. In first-degree block the impulse is delayed. It is usually asymptomatic but may progress to second- or third-degree block. In second-degree block the impulse is blocked intermittently and in third-degree block there is a complete block. **Atrioventricular dissociation** indicates a condition in which ventricular activity is faster, and independent of, the atrial activity. Bradyarrhythmias may be treated with either atropine or with isoprenaline, although cardiac pacing is the treatment of choice.

For **tachyarrhythmias** a classification or diagnosis based on the precise mechanism of the arrhythmia would also be desirable but this is not always clear. In many of the clinically relevant arrhythmias, however, the mechanism is one of re-entry. Re-entry occurs when the initial impulse does not die out but continues to propagate and reactivate the heart.

Diagnosis and management. Cardiac arrhythmias can range from little more than asymptomatic ECG abnormalities through to severe or life-threatening events. Treatment can be with antiarrhythmics or with non-pharmacological methods.

The precise identification of an arrhythmia is not always easy, but is important for correct management. The inappropriate use of an antiarrhythmic for a specific arrhythmia can not only be ineffective but, in view of the proarrhythmic potential of most of them, may even be deleterious. Identification and diagnosis should be based on clinical symptoms and on characteristic ECG features as well as on other specialised tests and features relevant to individual arrhythmias. A typical normal ECG trace is shown in Figure 2 under Antiarrhythmics, p.776. An arrhythmia with a narrow QRS complex is always supraventricular in origin whereas a broad QRS complex can indicate either a supraventricular or ventricular origin hence the diagnostic difficulties.

Ectopic beats, extrasystoles, or **premature contractions** can arise in either the atria or the ventricles and, although their precise meaning and definition differs, for practical purposes they can be considered equivalent. Generally, they cause few or no symptoms and usually have no prognostic value although some patients suffer distressing symptoms or palpitations.

Atrial fibrillation is the commonest cardiac arrhythmia and has been the subject of several reviews.[1-15] The mechanism of the arrhythmia in atrial fibrillation is one of re-entry. Atrial fibrillation is often associated with underlying cardiovascular disease, notably ischaemic or hypertensive heart disease, or less frequently today with rheumatic heart disease; hyperthyroidism and acute alcohol intoxication can also be causes. In some patients there is no obvious cause in which case the arrhythmia is described as 'lone' atrial fibrillation. Atrial fibrillation is relatively common following cardiothoracic surgery, but is usually self-limiting. It is characterised by an irregular and very rapid atrial rate (usually more than 300 beats per minute) and as the atrioventricular node is incapable of conducting all the impulses adequately, the increased ventricular response results in a rapid and totally irregular ventricular rate. The atrial fibrillation may be paroxysmal (intermittent) but is more usually chronic (persistent). Although atrial fibrillation can cause distressing symptoms such as severe palpitations and exercise intolerance it is not usually immediately life-threatening, but does result in long-term morbidity and mortality. The condition leads to left atrial dilatation and reduced cardiac output with stasis of blood in the left atrium. This can result in thrombus formation and subsequent systemic embolisation, notably ischaemic stroke. Thrombo-embolic events are relatively rare in lone atrial fibrillation (where no other cardiovascular disease is present) but the risk is very much increased in concomitant cardiovascular disease, especially so in rheumatic heart disease.

Management options for atrial fibrillation include treatment to slow the increased ventricular response, or cardioversion to restore a normal sinus rhythm. Anticoagulation may also be necessary to prevent thrombo-embolic episodes.

Digoxin has traditionally been used to slow an increased ventricular rate but beta blockers or calcium-channel blockers such as diltiazem or verapamil are preferred by some as they are usually considered more effective, especially in controlling the increased rates that may occur during exercise. If necessary, a combination of digoxin with either a beta blocker or a calcium-channel blocker may be employed. All these drugs act by slowing the conduction through the atrioventricular node. They do not, however, have an antifibrillatory action and do not restore sinus rhythm. Catheter ablation of atrioventricular conduction pathways followed by permanent pacing may be necessary in patients intolerant or unresponsive to drug therapy.

Restoration of sinus rhythm provides far better relief of symptoms than merely controlling the increased ventricular rate. If the fibrillation is of recent onset, usually less than 48 hours when there is no risk of precipitating thrombo-embolism, sinus rhythm can be restored either by synchronised direct current cardioversion or by pharmacological cardioversion. Drugs employed, either orally or intravenously, for cardioversion are usually class I antiarrhythmics (see p.776 for an explanation of the classification of antiarrhythmics), including disopyramide, flecainide, procainamide, propafenone, or quinidine. These drugs terminate atrial fibrillation by prolongation of atrial refractoriness, thus reducing the number of re-entry circuits in the atria. Amiodarone, a class III drug, may also be used and has the dual properties of ventricular rate control and antifibrillatory action. Sotalol, a beta blocker with class III antiarrhythmic activity in addition to the class II activity of beta blockers in general, also has this dual action. Direct current cardioversion has the advantage of restoring sinus rhythm more rapidly and effectively than that achieved by drugs but has the disadvantage that it needs to be performed under general anaesthesia.

Once sinus rhythm has been achieved, or in cases of paroxysmal atrial fibrillation, long-term maintenance drug therapy needs to be considered. The drugs used for this are broadly similar to those used for pharmacological cardioversion, namely the class I or class III antiarrhythmics. Surgery or implantable cardioversion devices are also options available for some patients.

The problem of **thrombo-embolic** events, principally ischaemic stroke, resulting from atrial fibrillation has been the subject of several reviews[16-21] as well as being addressed in the general reviews quoted above. If atrial fibrillation has been present for 48 hours or more it is generally recognised that there is a potential risk of causing systemic embolisation once sinus rhythm is restored. It is therefore recommended that oral anticoagulation with warfarin should be given for 2 to 4 weeks before cardioversion is attempted. If immediate cardioversion is necessary, administration of intravenous heparin followed by transoesophageal echocardiography to exclude the presence of thrombi has been suggested.[8,10,13] Control of the ventricular rate as outlined above should also be undertaken during this period. Anticoagulation is usually continued for up to 4 weeks following successful cardioversion.

Anticoagulation may also be undertaken for long-term **prophylaxis of stroke** in selected patients. The risk of stroke is increased about 17-fold in atrial fibrillation associated with rheumatic heart disease and the benefits of long-term prophylaxis with warfarin are well-established. For non-rheumatic heart disease the risk is less, but is still increased by about 5-fold and affects many more patients. The results of recent studies (AFASAK,[22] BAATAF,[23] CAFA,[24] SPAF I,[25] SPINAF/VASP,[26] and SPAF II[27]) have also clearly demonstrated a beneficial effect of warfarin in the primary prevention of stroke in patients with non-rheumatic atrial fibrillation. The design of these studies has, however, been criticised and a meta-analysis of the trials (excluding SPAF II) found that warfarin had no significant effect on fatal stroke incidence and produced only a small reduction in major stroke incidence.[28] Warfarin may also be of benefit in the secondary prevention of stroke in patients with non-rheumatic atrial fibrillation (see, for example, the EAFT study[29]). However, the benefits of anticoagulation need to be balanced against the risk of increased bleeding episodes, notably stroke due to intracranial haemorrhage, induced by warfarin. As the risk of thrombo-embolism is influenced by different factors and variables, oral anticoagulation is recommended for specific groups with high risk factors such as increasing age, ischaemic or hypertensive heart disease, heart failure, hyperthyroidism, or history or evidence of thrombo-embolism. Aspirin[30] and indobufen[31] have also been shown to have some, albeit limited, effect and may be possible alternatives in patients with contra-indications to warfarin. A low-intensity fixed-dose warfarin regimen combined with aspirin has been examined (SPAF III) in patients with high risk factors to try to reduce the risk of warfarin-induced haemorrhage, but the degree of anticoagulation was insufficient for stroke prevention.[32]

Atrial flutter is an arrhythmia somewhat similar in nature to atrial fibrillation and has been discussed in reviews of atrial arrhythmias.[3,5] Like atrial fibrillation it is characterised by a rapid (about 300 beats per minute) atrial rate, although the atrial rhythm is more regular and organised, and by a corresponding increase in the ventricular rate. It is far less common than atrial fibrillation to which it often degenerates if left untreated or it may revert to normal sinus rhythm in some cases. Unlike atrial fibrillation, atrial flutter does not usually carry an increased risk of thrombo-embolic episodes. Management strategies for atrial flutter are broadly similar to those outlined above for atrial fibrillation, namely controlling the increased ventricular response rate and cardioversion. However, in general terms drug therapy for either of these interventions is less successful in flutter than in fibrillation. Cardioversion with drug therapy has a relatively low success rate and cardiac pacing is usually employed which often results in a self-terminating atrial fibrillation. Synchronised direct current cardioversion may be employed to restore sinus rhythm if pacing fails.

Other atrial arrhythmias include **atrial premature beats** and **atrial tachycardia**. Premature beats are usually asymptomatic but if symptoms are severe (the awareness of a pause between normal beats) beta blockers may be employed.[5] Atrial tachycardia may also be treated with beta blockers but if it is due to digoxin toxicity, withdrawal of digoxin may be all that is required.[5]

Paroxysmal supraventricular tachycardia is a re-entry arrhythmia. The term paroxysmal atrial tachycardia was used, but became obsolete when it was realised that many such arrhythmias arise in the atrioventricular junction rather than in atrial muscle.[33] The re-entry circuit can be either due to an accessory atrioventricular pathway between the atria and ventricles or re-entry can occur at the site of the node itself. It is a relatively common arrhythmia occurring in otherwise healthy individuals. It may resolve spontaneously or reflex vagal stimulation, with respiratory manoeuvres, prompt squatting, or pressure over one carotid sinus may restore normal sinus rhythm. If symptoms associated with the rapid heart rate are severe, treatment will be needed. For termination of paroxysmal supraventricular tachycardia adenosine given intravenously is often the drug of choice;[33,34] intravenous verapamil is an alternative. Digoxin or beta blockers, also given intravenously, have been tried but appear to offer no advantage over adenosine or verapamil and are less effective.[33,34] Long-term maintenance therapy to prevent recurrence is required in some patients. Oral drugs are employed and may include beta blockers, digoxin, disopyramide, flecainide, quinidine, or verapamil. As discussed under atrial fibrillation above, beta blockers, digoxin, and calcium-channel blockers such as verapamil act by delaying impulses along the atrioventricular conduction system whereas the class I drugs act on atrial refractoriness. However, for symptomatic patients in whom an accessory atrioventricular pathway is the cause or for atrioventricular nodal re-entry tachycardia, a non-pharmacological method, namely radiofrequency ablation of the affected tissue is said to be the treatment of choice.[33,35]

Patients with the Wolff-Parkinson-White syndrome,[36] a congenital abnormality characterised by an accessory atrioventricular conduction pathway known as a Kent bundle, may be at special risk of developing atrial fibrillation or paroxysmal supraventricular tachycardia. Great care is necessary with the choice of antiarrhythmic in such patients.

Supraventricular tachycardia can occur rarely *in utero* and is associated with hydrops fetalis and perinatal mortality and morbidity. Antiarrhythmic drugs given either to the mother (usually flecainide) or directly to the fetus by intraperitoneal or intravascular administration (usually amiodarone) may be used to terminate these arrhythmias.[37]

Ventricular tachycardia is a re-entry arrhythmia[38-40] often associated with underlying cardiovascular disease such as myocardial infarction or cardiomyopathies or with digoxin toxicity. The heart rate is about 120 to 250 beats per minute and the tachycardia, which arises in the ventricles below the atrioventricular node, can be paroxysmal consisting of short self-terminating episodes or can be sustained (lasting 30 seconds or longer). Although ventricular tachycardia can be asymptomatic (if the episodes are non-sustained) it is potentially a serious condition which may lead to reduced cardiac output, shock, and progression to ventricular fibrillation. It is one of the most common causes of sudden unexplained cardiac death. The ECG trace of ventricular tachycardia has sometimes been confused with that of supraventricular tachycardia but since the treatments differ markedly, every effort should be made to obtain the correct diagnosis.

The initial treatment of ventricular tachycardia depends largely on the haemodynamic status of the patient. If the patient has sustained ventricular tachycardia or has pulseless non-sustained ventricular tachycardia, both of which tend to be associated with instability and a poorer prognosis, defibrillation, as outlined under Advanced Cardiac Life Support (above), should be initiated. In the more stable patient, intravenous drug therapy may be employed for acute termination of the tachycardia. Lignocaine has been the drug of choice; other class I drugs such as disopyramide, flecainide, mexiletine, procainamide, or quinidine are alternatives, as is the class III drug amiodarone. In some patients with non-sustained ventricular tachycardia, beta blockers may be adequate and in one study[41] sotalol appeared to be superior to lignocaine for the acute termination of sustained tachycardia. Non-pharmacological methods of management include ablation either by radiofrequency or surgery, and electrical techniques such as pacing or cardioversion.

Following restoration of normal sinus rhythm maintenance drug therapy needs to be considered to prevent recurrences. Implantation of a cardioverter defibrillator is recommended in patients surviving sustained ventricular tachycardia (see below). Long-term prophylaxis is generally not warranted in low risk patients such as those who have experienced asymptomatic non-sustained ventricular tachycardia. In the past, the choice of drug for maintenance was largely empirical and was often a class I drug or a beta blocker or amiodarone given orally. Electrophysiological testing and electrocardiographic monitoring may be used to determine antiarrhythmic efficacy long term. In the former, drug efficacy is assessed invasively by using programmed ventricular stimulation in an attempt to reproduce the ventricular tachycardia, then giving the antiarrhythmic and repeating the stimulus to determine whether the tachycardia remains inducible. Electrocardiographic monitoring is non-invasive and ambulatory monitoring (Holter monitoring) is frequently employed. No significant difference in the success of drug therapy (imipramine, mexiletine, pirmenol, procainamide, propafenone, quinidine, or sotalol) selected by the two monitoring methods was shown in the ESVEM study.[42] A further analysis by the ESVEM investigators,[43] compared the relative efficacies of the above drugs and found that sotalol was the most effective. However, it has been suggested that ambulatory monitoring and electrophysiological testing should be regarded as complementary rather than alternative means of evaluating drug therapy.[44,45]

Cardiac arrest is the cessation of effective cardiac mechanical activity and may be associated with four arrhythmias, namely **ventricular fibrillation, pulseless ventricular tachycardia, asystole,** and **electromechanical dissociation**. In ventricular fibrillation and pulseless ventricular tachycardia there is chaotic electrical and mechanical activity; in asystole a total absence of both activities; and in electromechanical dissociation an absence of mechanical activity or undetectable activity in the presence of some electrical activity. In adults, ventricular fibrillation is the commonest of these four arrhythmias causing cardiac arrest. All are emergencies and should be treated by the institution of full life support measures as described on p.779. European[46-48] and American[49] guidelines are broadly similar. Antiarrhythmics such as lignocaine, bretylium, or amiodarone may be necessary. Survivors of ventricular fibrillation and pulseless ventricular tachycardia have a high risk of recurrence of arrhythmia and until recently either an implantable cardioverter defibrillator or drug therapy (as outlined above under Ventricular Tachycardia) has been employed in these patients prophylactically. However, a recent study in 1016 patients comparing the two methods found a greater reduction in mortality with implantable cardioverter defibrillators[50] and the American College of Cardiology/American Heart Association now recommend implantable defibrillators as preferred first-line therapy.[51] If drug therapy is used, beta blockers are particularly recommended in patients who survive ventricular fibrillation.[52]

Ventricular arrhythmias may be associated with **heart disease** such as myocardial infarction or heart failure. Ventricular tachycardia and ventricular fibrillation are common early after **acute myocardial infarction**. Lignocaine may be given prophylactically after myocardial infarction to patients at high risk of ventricular fibrillation. Asymptomatic premature ventricular arrhythmias in subjects who have previously suffered a myocardial infarction are also common and are recognised as a risk factor for subsequent sudden cardiac death. Suppressing such arrhythmias might be expected to reduce the incidence of sudden death but results have not been promising. A large multicentre study was set up in the USA (the Cardiac Arrhythmia Suppression Trial known as CAST) and the class I antiarrhythmics encainide, flecainide, and moracizine were selected following a preliminary study[53] (CAPS; the Cardiac Arrhythmia Pilot Study) in which they had been shown to suppress premature ventricular depolarisations in post-infarction patients. After an average of 10 months of daily treatment with one of the active agents or placebo both the class Ic antiarrhythmics encainide and flecainide were withdrawn from the CAST study because patients receiving either of them showed a higher than expected mortality rate.[54,55] Moracizine, which is a class I antiarrhythmic with activities corresponding to a, b, and c subclasses, was not implicated in increasing mortality at the CAST I assessment,[54] so the study continued as CAST II to compare this antiarrhythmic against placebo. In late 1991 an increased mortality with moracizine was also documented and the study was halted.[56]

Following publication of the CAST studies some workers looked at other class I antiarrhythmic drugs. A meta-analysis of trials utilising quinidine was undertaken[57] as it was believed that this agent had gained in popularity after the adverse CAST results. However, this meta-analysis suggested that quinidine was associated with at least as high a proportion of adverse events, such as death and early proarrhythmia, as the class Ic drugs flecainide and propafenone. A study of *d*-sotalol, a class III antiarrhythmic, in patients with left ventricular dysfunction following myocardial infarction was stopped early because of increased mortality in the treatment group.[58]

Until recently, meta-analyses[59,60] of prophylactic antiarrhythmic therapy have concluded that the only class of drugs with proven benefit after myocardial infarction is the beta blockers. Some limited success has been seen with amiodarone in asymptomatic arrhythmias after myocardial infarction (BASIS: the Basel Antiarrhythmic Study of Infarct Survival,[61] CAMIAT: the Canadian Amiodarone Myocardial Infarction Arrhythmia Trial,[62] and EMIAT: the European Myocardial Infarct Amiodarone Trial[63]). Both CAMIAT and EMIAT reported a reduction in risk of arrhythmic death, but neither study showed a reduction in total mortality. However, meta-analysis of studies using amiodarone found a small reduction in total mortality suggesting that amiodarone might be of benefit after myocardial infarction in patients, such as those with heart failure, at high risk of arrhythmic death.[64] Thus, prophylactic antiarrhythmic therapy for asymptomatic arrhythmias with drugs other than beta blockers and possibly amiodarone is not practised routinely.

Attempts have been made to reduce deaths from ventricular arrhythmias in patients with severe **heart failure** (below); results with the antiarrhythmic amiodarone have been conflicting.

Drugs used to treat arrhythmias can have a **proarrhythmic** effect, that is they can exacerbate or induce arrhythmias of all types. **Torsade de pointes** is a potentially lethal ventricular tachycardia with a characteristic ECG pattern and is often associated with drug-induced prolongation of the QT interval.[65,66] Drugs responsible include antiarrhythmics and several non-cardiac drugs[67] including phenothiazines, tricyclic antidepressants, antihistamines such as astemizole and terfenadine, antibacterials such as erythromycin, the antimalarial halofantrine, and the lipid lowering drug probucol. The ventricular tachycardia is often non-sustained, but may persist for long enough to cause syncope or it may even progress to ventricular fibrillation. If torsade de pointes is drug-induced withdrawal and subsequent avoidance of the offending drug is mandatory. Electrolyte disturbances appear to contribute to torsade de pointes and initial therapy is with magnesium given intravenously together with temporary pacing of the atria or ventricles as appropriate. Isoprenaline may be given cautiously to increase the heart rate and shorten the QT interval, until pacing is instituted.

1. Pritchett ELC. Management of atrial fibrillation. *N Engl J Med* 1992; **326:** 1264–71.
2. Clark A, Cotter L. Cardioversion in atrial fibrillation. *Br J Hosp Med* 1993; **49:** 256–61.
3. Geraets DR, Kienzle MG. Atrial fibrillation and atrial flutter. *Clin Pharm* 1993; **12:** 721–35.
4. Murgatroyd FD, Camm AJ. Current concepts in atrial fibrillation. *Br J Hosp Med* 1993; **49:** 546–60.
5. Murgatroyd FD, Camm AJ. Atrial arrhythmias. *Lancet* 1993; **341:** 1317–22.
6. Nattel S, *et al.* The treatment of atrial fibrillation: an evaluation of drug therapy, electrical modalities and therapeutic considerations. *Drugs* 1994; **48:** 345–71.
7. Anonymous. The antiarrhythmic treatment of atrial fibrillation. *Drug Ther Bull* 1996; **34:** 41–5.
8. Blackshear JL, *et al.* Management of atrial fibrillation in adults: prevention of thromboembolism and symptomatic treatment. *Mayo Clin Proc* 1996; **71:** 150–60.
9. Channer KS. Treatment of atrial fibrillation. *Prescribers' J* 1996; **36:** 146–53.
10. Gilligan DM, *et al.* The management of atrial fibrillation. *Am J Med* 1996; **101:** 413–21.
11. Golzari H, *et al.* Atrial fibrillation: restoration and maintenance of sinus rhythm and indications for anticoagulation therapy. *Ann Intern Med* 1996; **125:** 311–23.
12. Lip GYH, ed. *ABC of atrial fibrillation.* London: BMJ Publishing Group, 1996.
13. Prystowsky EN, *et al.* Management of patients with atrial fibrillation: a statement for healthcare professionals from the Subcommittee on Electrocardiography and Electrophysiology, American Heart Association. *Circulation* 1996; **93:** 1262–77.
14. Narayan SM, *et al.* Atrial fibrillation. *Lancet* 1997; **350:** 943–50.
15. Jung F, DiMarco JP. Treatment strategies for atrial fibrillation. *Am J Med* 1998; **104:** 272–86.
16. Lowe GDO. Antithrombotic treatment and atrial fibrillation. *Br Med J* 1992; **305:** 1445–6.
17. Marchant BG, Timmis AD. Benefits and risks of thrombolytic, anticoagulant and antiplatelet therapies in atrial fibrillation. *Br J Hosp Med* 1993; **49:** 186–190.
18. White HD. Aspirin or warfarin for non-rheumatic atrial fibrillation? *Lancet* 1994; **343:** 683–4.
19. Lowe GDO. Use of anticoagulants in atrial fibrillation. *Prescribers' J* 1994; **34:** 91–101.
20. Nelson KM, Talbert RL. Preventing stroke in patients with nonrheumatic atrial fibrillation. *Am J Hosp Pharm* 1994; **51:** 1175–83.
21. Anonymous. Warfarin or aspirin for non-rheumatic atrial fibrillation? *Drug Ther Bull* 1994; **32:** 57–60. Correction. *ibid.*; 80.
22. Petersen P, *et al.* Placebo-controlled, randomised trial of warfarin and aspirin for prevention of thromboembolic complications in chronic atrial fibrillation: the Copenhagen AFASAK Study. *Lancet* 1989; **i:** 175–9.
23. Boston Area Anticoagulation Trial in Atrial Fibrillation Investigators. The effect of low-dose warfarin on the risk of stroke in patients with nonrheumatic atrial fibrillation. *N Engl J Med* 1990; **323:** 1505–11.
24. Connolly SJ, *et al.* Canadian Atrial Fibrillation Anticoagulation (CAFA) Study. *J Am Coll Cardiol* 1991; **18:** 349–55.
25. Stroke Prevention in Atrial Fibrillation Investigators. Stroke Prevention in Atrial Fibrillation Study: final results. *Circulation* 1991; **84:** 527–39.
26. Ezekowitz MD, *et al.* Warfarin in the prevention of stroke associated with nonrheumatic atrial fibrillation. *N Engl J Med* 1992; **327:** 1406–12.
27. Stroke Prevention in Atrial Fibrillation Investigators. Warfarin versus aspirin for prevention of thromboembolism in atrial fibrillation: Stroke Prevention in Atrial Fibrillation II Study. *Lancet* 1994; **343:** 687–91.
28. Green CJ, *et al.* Anticoagulation in chronic nonvalvular atrial fibrillation: a critical appraisal and meta-analysis. *Can J Cardiol* 1997; **13:** 811–15.
29. EAFT (European Atrial Fibrillation Trial) Study Group. Secondary prevention in non-rheumatic atrial fibrillation after transient ischaemic attack or minor stroke. *Lancet* 1993; **342:** 1255–62.
30. The Atrial Fibrillation Investigators. The efficacy of aspirin in patients with atrial fibrillation: analysis of pooled data from 3 randomised trials. *Arch Intern Med* 1997; **157:** 1237–40.
31. Morocutti C, *et al.* Indobufen versus warfarin in the secondary prevention of major vascular events in nonrheumatic atrial fibrillation. *Stroke* 1997; **28:** 1015–21.
32. Stroke Prevention in Atrial Fibrillation Investigators. Adjusted-dose warfarin versus low-intensity, fixed-dose warfarin plus aspirin for high-risk patients with atrial fibrillation: Stroke Prevention in Atrial Fibrillation III randomised clinical trial. *Lancet* 1996; **348:** 633–8.
33. Ganz LI, Friedman PL. Supraventricular tachycardia. *N Engl J Med* 1995; **332:** 162–73.
34. Kugler JD, Danford DA. Management of infants, children, and adolescents with paroxysmal supraventricular tachycardia. *J Pediatr* 1996; **129:** 324–38.
35. Kuck K-H, Schlüter M. Junctional tachycardia and the role of catheter ablation. *Lancet* 1993; **341:** 1386–91.
36. Gaita F, *et al.* Wolff-Parkinson-White syndrome: identification and management. *Drugs* 1992; **43:** 185–200.
37. Owen P, Cameron A. Fetal tachyarrhythmias. *Br J Hosp Med* 1997; **58:** 142–4.
38. Dancy M. Diagnosis and management of ventricular tachycardia. *Postgrad Med J* 1992; **68:** 406–14.
39. Campbell RWF. Ventricular ectopic beats and non-sustained ventricular tachycardia. *Lancet* 1993; **341:** 1454–8.
40. Shenasa M, *et al.* Ventricular tachycardia. *Lancet* 1993; **341:** 1512–19.
41. Ho DSW, *et al.* Double-blind trial of lignocaine versus sotalol for acute termination of spontaneous sustained ventricular tachycardia. *Lancet* 1994; **344:** 18–23.
42. Mason JW. A comparison of electrophysiologic testing with Holter monitoring to predict antiarrhythmic-drug efficacy for ventricular tachyarrhythmias. *N Engl J Med* 1993; **329:** 445–51.
43. Mason JW. A comparison of seven antiarrhythmic drugs in patients with ventricular tachyarrhythmias. *N Engl J Med* 1993; **329:** 452–8.
44. Ward DE, Camm AJ. Dangerous ventricular arrhythmias—can we predict drug efficacy? *N Engl J Med* 1993; **329:** 498–9.
45. Murgatroyd F. Malignant arrhythmias: tribulations post ESVEM. *Lancet* 1993; **342:** 569.
46. Chamberlaine D, *et al.* Guidelines for advanced life support: a statement by the Advanced Life Support Working Party of the European Resuscitation Council, 1992. *Resuscitation* 1992; **24:** 111–121.
47. European Resuscitation Council Working Party. Adult advanced cardiac life support: the European Resuscitation Council guidelines 1992 (abridged). *Br Med J* 1993; **306:** 1589–93.
48. Paediatric Life Support Working Party of the European Resuscitation Council. Guidelines for paediatric life support. *Br Med J* 1994; **308:** 1349–55. Correction. *ibid.*; 1563.
49. Emergency Cardiac Care Committee and Subcommittees, American Heart Association. Guidelines for cardiopulmonary resuscitation and emergency cardiac care. *JAMA* 1992; **268:** 2171–2295.
50. The Antiarrhythmics versus Implantable Defibrillators (AVID) Investigators. A comparison of antiarrhythmic-drug therapy with implantable defibrillators in patients resuscitated from near-fatal ventricular arrhythmias. *N Engl J Med* 1997; **337:** 1576–83.
51. Gregoratos G, *et al.* ACC/AHA guidelines for implantation of cardiac pacemakers and antiarrhythmia devices: a report of the American College of Cardiology/American Heart Association Task Force on Practice Guidelines (Committee on Pacemaker Implantation). *J Am Coll Cardiol* 1998; **31:** 1175–1209.
52. O'Nunain S, Ruskin J. Cardiac arrest. *Lancet* 1993; **341:** 1641–7.
53. The CAPS Investigators. The Cardiac Arrhythmia Pilot Study. *Am J Cardiol* 1986; **57:** 91–5.
54. The Cardiac Arrhythmia Suppression Trial (CAST) Investigators. Preliminary report: effect of encainide and flecainide on mortality in a randomized trial of arrhythmia suppression after myocardial infarction. *N Engl J Med* 1989; **321:** 406–12.
55. Echt DS, *et al.* Mortality and morbidity in patients receiving encainide, flecainide, or placebo: the Cardiac Arrhythmia Suppression Trial. *N Engl J Med* 1991; **324:** 781–8.
56. The Cardiac Arrhythmia Suppression Trial II Investigators. Effect of the antiarrhythmic agent moricizine on survival after myocardial infarction. *N Engl J Med* 1992; **327:** 227–33.
57. Morganroth J, Goin JE. Quinidine-related mortality in the short-to-medium-term treatment of ventricular arrhythmias: a meta-analysis. *Circulation* 1991; **84:** 1977–83.
58. Waldo AL, *et al.* Effect of d-sotalol on mortality in patients with left ventricular dysfunction after recent and remote myocardial infarction. *Lancet* 1996; **348:** 7–12. Correction. *ibid.*; 416.
59. Teo KK, *et al.* Effects of prophylactic antiarrhythmic drug therapy in acute myocardial infarction: an overview of results from randomized controlled trials. *JAMA* 1993; **270:** 1589–95.

60. McAlister FA, Teo KK. Antiarrhythmic therapies for the prevention of sudden cardiac death. *Drugs* 1997; **54:** 235–52.
61. Pfisterer ME, *et al.* Long-term benefit of 1-year amiodarone treatment for persistent complex ventricular arrhythmias after myocardial infarction. *Circulation* 1993; **87:** 309–11.
62. Cairns JA, *et al.* Randomised trial of outcome after myocardial infarction in patients with frequent or repetitive ventricular premature depolarisations: CAMIAT. *Lancet* 1997; **349:** 675–82.
63. Julian DG, *et al.* Randomised trial of effect of amiodarone on mortality in patients with left-ventricular dysfunction after recent myocardial infarction: EMIAT. *Lancet* 1997; **349:** 667–74. Corrections. *ibid.*; 1180 and 1776.
64. Amiodarone Trials Meta-Analysis Investigators. Effect of prophylactic amiodarone on mortality after acute myocardial infarction and in congestive heart failure: meta-analysis of individual data from 6500 patients in randomised trials. *Lancet* 1997; **350:** 1417–24.
65. Ben-David J, Zipes DP. Torsades de pointes and proarrhythmia. *Lancet* 1993; **341:** 1578–82.
66. Thomas SHL. Drugs and the QT interval. *Adverse Drug React Bull* 1997; **182:** 691–4.
67. Doig JC. Drug-induced cardiac arrhythmias: incidence, prevention and management. *Drug Safety* 1997; **17:** 265–75.

Cardiomyopathies

Cardiomyopathy is a term used to describe heart muscle disease. It is usually applied to a condition of unknown cause (idiopathic). Known causes of disorders of heart muscle such as systemic or pulmonary hypertension, ischaemic heart disease, valvular heart disease, congenital abnormalities, metabolic disorders, inflammatory or infectious diseases, and drug-induced conditions are excluded by some authorities when defining cardiomyopathy. Three distinct types of cardiomyopathy are generally recognised, namely dilated cardiomyopathy, hypertrophic cardiomyopathy, and restrictive cardiomyopathy; the dilated and hypertrophic forms are the two major types. The management of the individual forms has been reviewed.[1-7]

In **dilated cardiomyopathy** (previously known as congestive cardiomyopathy) the main finding is one of dilated and poorly contracting ventricles and a low cardiac output; this is systolic dysfunction. The right, left, or both ventricles may be affected. Although there may be some ventricular hypertrophy, because of the dilatation there is no overall increase in the thickness of the ventricle walls. Dilated cardiomyopathy may be asymptomatic for some time but the initial manifestations are commonly those of heart failure; chest pain, systemic and pulmonary embolism, and arrhythmias may also occur. If symptomatic heart failure is present, management should generally follow the conventional strategies for heart failure as outlined on p.785 and includes the use of ACE inhibitors, diuretics, digoxin, and vasodilators (hydralazine and oral nitrates such as isosorbide dinitrate). One particular problem in dilated cardiomyopathy, because of blood stasis due to the poorly contracting ventricle, is the risk of systemic and pulmonary thrombo-embolism. Thus, chronic oral anticoagulation has been suggested for these patients although the current view appears to recommend it only in those with atrial fibrillation, previous systemic embolism, or severe left ventricular dysfunction.[1,8] Arrhythmias should be treated as appropriate (see under Cardiac Arrhythmias, above); amiodarone may be particularly suitable as it has no negative inotropic effect. Low-dose amiodarone may also be used in patients at high risk of sudden death, but its efficacy has not yet been confirmed.[1]

Beta blockers have negative inotropic properties and have not generally been considered to be a part of the usual management of most patients with heart failure, although this view is changing. They may have a role as additional therapy in some patients with idiopathic dilated cardiomyopathy.[9-11] A large number of studies have demonstrated significant improvements in cardiac function,[9] but the effect on mortality has been less clear. The MDC trial (Metoprolol in Dilated Cardiomyopathy)[12,13] and the early results of the CIBIS study (Cardiac Insufficiency Bisoprolol Study)[14] demonstrated an improvement in cardiac function and symptoms, together with prevention of clinical deterioration, but neither study demonstrated a significant effect on overall mortality. However, another trial evaluating carvedilol therapy in patients with heart failure, including patients with dilated cardiomyopathy, was terminated early because mortality was significantly reduced in the carvedilol groups[15] and the extended CIBIS trial (CIBIS II)[22] using bisoprolol was also terminated early because of favourable results. A further long-term study[16] using metoprolol has also reported a significantly higher survival rate in those receiving metoprolol for up to 7 years. Symptomatic improvement has also been reported with the calcium-channel blocker diltiazem.[17]

A number of surgical treatments have been tried but cardiac transplantation remains the principal method of improving survival in these patients. Other therapies that have been tried include growth hormone, thyroxine, oxpentifylline, and immunosuppressants for presumed myocarditis.

In **hypertrophic cardiomyopathy** (previously known as obstructive cardiomyopathy) there is, as the name implies, ventricular hypertrophy but the ventricles are not dilated. This leads to diastolic dysfunction since diastolic filling is impaired by the stiff hypertrophied ventricular walls. It is an inherited condition occurring as an autosomal dominant trait and can occur at any age although presentation during the second decade of life is common. Patients may be asymptomatic or may experience chest pain, syncope, dyspnoea, or arrhythmias. Sudden death associated with emotional stress or exercise is not an uncommon finding and patients should avoid strenuous exercise.

Patients should be investigated for the presence of any arrhythmias and treated appropriately (see Cardiac Arrhythmias, above) although this may not necessarily prevent sudden death. Atrial fibrillation is particularly important and is probably most effectively treated with amiodarone.[3,4] Anticoagulation should be considered in all patients with sustained atrial fibrillation.[3-5]

Beta blockers may be used for control of symptoms. They curtail emotion- or exercise-induced tachycardia. Anginal pain is also reduced and syncopal attacks may be prevented. Calcium-channel blockers (usually verapamil) also improve symptoms and exercise tolerance and may be considered in those who continue to have disabling symptoms or who are unable to tolerate beta blockers.[18] However, in a crossover study[19] exercise capacity was not improved by either verapamil or nadolol, although most patients preferred one or other of the drugs rather than placebo and quality of life did appear to be improved by verapamil. Other drugs that may provide symptomatic relief include disopyramide, which is used for its negative inotropic effect. Diuretics may be needed for congestive symptoms but may also reduce cardiac output. Surgery to reduce outflow obstruction may be of benefit in some patients whose symptoms are resistant to drug therapy.[3-5]

The risk of sudden death is difficult to assess, particularly in asymptomatic patients. Neither beta blockers nor verapamil, as used for possible symptomatic relief, prevent ventricular arrhythmias. Low-dose amiodarone may have a role in high risk patients, but this remains to be confirmed;[20,21] implantable cardioverter-defibrillators are also used in some patients.

In **restrictive cardiomyopathy** the filling of the ventricles is impaired, often due to endomyocardial fibrosis, resulting in predominantly diastolic dysfunction. Diuretics may improve congestive symptoms but should be used cautiously as they may decrease cardiac output. Arrhythmias should be treated if they are symptomatic and anticoagulation is advised, particularly in patients with atrial fibrillation, valvular disorders, or a low cardiac output.[6]

1. Dec GW, Fuster V. Idiopathic dilated cardiomyopathy. *N Engl J Med* 1994; **331:** 1564–75.
2. Burch M, Runciman M. Dilated cardiomyopathy. *Arch Dis Child* 1996; **74:** 479–81.
3. Spirito P, *et al.* The management of hypertrophic cardiomyopathy. *N Engl J Med* 1997; **336:** 775–85.
4. Maron BJ. Hypertrophic cardiomyopathy. *Lancet* 1997; **350:** 127–33.
5. Elliott PM, McKenna WJ. Management of hypertrophic cardiomyopathy. *Br J Hosp Med* 1996; **55:** 419–23.
6. Kushwaha SS, *et al.* Restrictive cardiomyopathy. *N Engl J Med* 1997; **336:** 267–76.
7. Oakley C. Aetiology, diagnosis, investigation, and management of cardiomyopathies. *Br Med J* 1997; **315:** 1520–4.
8. Cheng JWM, Spinler SA. Should all patients with dilated cardiomyopathy receive chronic anticoagulation? *Ann Pharmacother* 1994; **28:** 604–9.
9. Hjalmarson Å, Waagstein F. The role of β-blockers in the treatment of cardiomyopathy and ischaemic heart failure. *Drugs* 1994; **47** (suppl 4): 31–40.
10. Barnett DB. Beta-blockers in heart failure: a therapeutic paradox. *Lancet* 1994; **343:** 557–8.
11. Asseman P, *et al.* Why do beta-blockers help in idiopathic dilated cardiomyopathy—frequency mismatch? *Lancet* 1994; **344:** 803–4.
12. Waagstein F, *et al.* Beneficial effects of metoprolol in idiopathic dilated cardiomyopathy. *Lancet* 1993; **342:** 1441–6.
13. The Metoprolol in Dilated Cardiomyopathy (MDC) Trial Study Group. 3-year follow-up of patients randomised in the metoprolol in dilated cardiomyopathy trial. *Lancet* 1998; **351:** 1180–1.
14. CIBIS Investigators and Committees. A randomized trial of β-blockade in heart failure: the cardiac insufficiency bisoprolol study (CIBIS). *Circulation* 1994; **90:** 1765–73.
15. Packer M, *et al.* The effect of carvedilol on morbidity and mortality in patients with chronic heart failure. *N Engl J Med* 1996; **334:** 1349–55.
16. Di Lenarda A, *et al.* Long term survival effect of metoprolol in dilated cardiomyopathy. *Heart* 1998; **79:** 337–44.
17. Figulla HR, *et al.* Diltiazem improves cardiac function and exercise capacity in patients with idiopathic dilated cardiomyopathy: results of the Diltiazem in Dilated Cardiomyopathy Trial. *Circulation* 1996; **94:** 346–52.
18. Lorell BH. Use of calcium channel blockers in hypertrophic cardiomyopathy. *Am J Med* 1985; **78** (suppl 2B): 43–54.
19. Gilligan DM, *et al.* A double-blind, placebo-controlled crossover trial of nadolol and verapamil in mild and moderately symptomatic hypertrophic cardiomyopathy. *J Am Coll Cardiol* 1993; **21:** 1672–9.
20. Clark AL, Coates AJS. Screening for hypertrophic cardiomyopathy. *Br Med J* 1993; **306:** 409–10.
21. Prasad K, Frenneaux MP. Hypertrophic cardiomyopathy: is there a role for amiodarone? *Heart* 1998; **79:** 317–18.
22. CIBIS-II Investigators and Committees. The Cardiac Insufficiency Bisoprolol Study II (CIBIS-II): a randomised trial. *Lancet* 1999; **353:** 9–13.

Cerebrovascular disease

The term 'cerebrovascular disease' may cover disorders of the cerebral circulation such as ischaemic stroke and subarachnoid haemorrhage (see Stroke, below), but is often used to cover the rather vague concept of cerebrovascular insufficiency.

At one time it was believed that the dementia associated with Alzheimer's disease (p.1386) was due to cerebrovascular insufficiency and many drugs with vasodilator activity have been tried, but overall there is little convincing evidence of benefit. Ergot derivatives such as co-dergocrine mesylate and nicergoline have been the most commonly used; however, any effectiveness is now attributed to their action as metabolic enhancers or nootropic drugs rather than to vasodilatation and their place in therapy has still to be established. Calcium-channel blockers such as nimodipine are under investigation. Other vasodilators used have included buflomedil, cyclandelate, isoxsuprine, naftidrofuryl, oxpentifylline, and propentofylline.

Heart failure

Heart failure is a diagnosis made in a patient with a known or suspected cardiac disorder who presents with dyspnoea, fatigue, and oedema (peripheral and/or pulmonary).[1,2] It may be graded as mild, moderate, or severe depending upon whether symptoms such as dyspnoea and fatigue appear on ordinary physical exertion, on little exertion, or at rest, respectively. Another grading system (that of the New York Heart Association) has four grades (grades I, II, III, IV), again partly classified on appearance of symptoms in relation to exertion (with grade IV representing the most severe form). The discussion that follows focuses on the chronic form of heart failure. The management of acute heart failure resulting in cardiogenic shock is covered under Shock, below.

Heart failure is a common condition and is a consequence of cardiac abnormality, injury, or cardiovascular stress such as hypertension or valve disorders. Myocardial infarction is a leading cause of heart failure. Other cardiovascular disorders that may lead to heart failure include cardiomyopathies and cor pulmonale. Infections causing myocardial damage and cardiotoxicity arising from alcoholism or induced by drugs may also be precipitating factors. The increased demands put on the heart by chronic severe anaemia or hyperthyroidism can also be causes.

Echocardiography is the most useful investigative procedure in patients with heart failure. It enables structural changes to be observed and rapidly identifies patients with potentially correctable abnormalities such as valvular disease. Although dysfunction of either the right or left ventricle (right- or left-sided heart failure) may occur in isolation, dysfunction of both ventricles is likely to be present to some extent; however, in most patients, and especially in those with heart failure following myocardial infarction, the predominant finding is that of a dilated and poorly contracting left ventricle. This represents left ventricular systolic dysfunction in which the ejection fraction and the cardiac output is low. Isolated left ventricular diastolic dysfunction, in which there is impaired ventricular filling but a normal ejection fraction, can also result in heart failure although this is less common; cardiac output may be normal but does not increase in response to exercise. Diastolic dysfunction is more common in the elderly and also occurs in some cardiomyopathies (see p.785); many patients have both diastolic and systolic dysfunction. As mentioned above, the term heart failure is usually employed to represent a symptomatic condition. However, echocardiographic investigation of some patients, especially those in the early postmyocardial infarction period, does reveal that asymptomatic left ventricular dysfunction occurs and many of these patients are treated in an attempt to prevent the development of full symptomatic disease. In theory, left ventricular systolic and diastolic dysfunction should be treated in different ways[3] but in some of the drug therapy trials no complete characterisation of ventricular dynamics has been attempted and in such cases recommendations can only be made on the basis of a clinical diagnosis of heart failure.

Traditionally, heart failure has been defined as a condition in which the heart is unable to provide an adequate blood flow to meet the metabolic demands of the body and has been thought of in purely haemodynamic terms.[4] It is now appreciated that compensatory neurohormonal mechanisms play just as important a role in its development.[3,4]

Myocardial injury or impairment leads to an inability of the ventricles to empty adequately during systole. The resulting ventricular dilatation increases wall tension and initially leads to an increase in contraction while the decrease in cardiac output and blood pressure results in activation of the sympathetic nervous system, leading to an increase in the force and frequency of contraction. An increase in wall stress also occurs in the atria leading to secretion of atrial natriuretic peptide; this inhibits the release of noradrenaline but also has direct vasodilator and natriuretic actions that lower the haemodynamic load on the heart. Thus, in the short term, compensation for myocardial injury can occur and cardiac output may be maintained. In the long term, these compensatory haemodynamic and neurohormonal mechanisms become ineffective. Ventricular dilatation progresses, the sympathetic nervous system and renin-angiotensin system are persistently activated, ventricular hypertrophy occurs, and ventricular function deteriorates progressively.

Management. Heart failure is a progressively disabling condition associated with considerable morbidity and mortality. Management is aimed therefore not only at providing symptomatic relief, but also at improving prognosis. Reviews[1,2,5-10] and guidelines[11,12] have been published concerning management, although it has been suggested that the variable nature of heart failure may limit their use as absolute guidelines for therapy.[13]

Any underlying cause of heart failure should be corrected and certain non-pharmacological interventions may be beneficial. Weight reduction should be attempted in the overweight; moderate salt restriction may be undertaken; and, although in acute heart failure bed rest becomes necessary, in controlled chronic heart failure the patients should be encouraged to take normal exercise. Drug therapy of heart failure is based on the use of ACE inhibitors, diuretics, cardiac glycosides, and vasodilators. Other drugs which may have a role include beta blockers, some calcium-channel blockers, and angiotensin II receptor antagonists.

Diuretics have been the mainstay in the treatment of heart failure.[14] They provide very effective symptomatic control in patients with peripheral or pulmonary oedema and rapidly relieve dyspnoea. If symptoms of fluid retention are only mild, a *thiazide diuretic* such as *bendrofluazide* or *hydrochlorothiazide*, may be adequate. However, in most cases, especially in moderate or severe fluid retention, a *loop diuretic* such as *frusemide* will be necessary. Combination treatment with diuretics that behave synergistically by acting at different sites (the principle of sequential nephron blockade), namely a loop diuretic with a thiazide or potassium-sparing diuretic, may be needed in some patients, especially when there is diuretic resistance.[15-17]

However, diuretics are not a sufficient treatment on their own as clinical stability tends to deteriorate over time. In addition, there have been no long-term trials assessing the effect of diuretics on prognosis, and drugs that have been shown to have a mortality benefit are also required.

ACE inhibitors given orally produce clinical benefit in all stages of chronic heart failure additional to that seen with diuretics. They relieve symptoms such as dyspnoea and improve exercise tolerance. In addition, unlike with diuretics, studies have demonstrated that ACE inhibitors improve survival and reduce the progression of mild or moderate heart failure to more severe stages.[18] ACE inhibitors may also be beneficial in asymptomatic left ventricular dysfunction.[19] The Studies of Left Ventricular Dysfunction (SOLVD)[20] trials indicated that ACE inhibitors, in this case enalapril, might protect against myocardial infarction, unstable angina, and cardiac death in patients with either symptomatic or asymptomatic heart failure. ACE inhibitors are now recommended,[11,12,21] therefore, in all patients with symptomatic heart failure, including those receiving diuretic therapy, and should also be given to all patients with significantly reduced left ventricular ejection fraction, whether or not they have symptoms.

ACE inhibitors have also been given to patients shortly after suffering myocardial infarction but before the development of symptomatic heart failure and appear to be beneficial. However, it is not yet clear which patients should receive such therapy or when the optimum time to start ACE inhibitors is (see under Myocardial Infarction, below).

The precise mode of action of ACE inhibitors in heart failure is not completely understood but appears to be a result of both haemodynamic and neurohormonal mechanisms. They are vasodilators and cause both arteriolar and venous dilatation, mainly through reduction of angiotensin II formation. They also attenuate the ventricular dilatation and prevent the ventricular remodelling that develops after a myocardial injury. It has also been suggested that they may protect against the development of arrhythmias.[22]

Cardiac glycosides such as *digoxin* or *digitoxin* have an extremely long history in the management of heart failure. They are positive inotropes and increase the contractility of the heart thereby increasing cardiac output. Additional effects in heart failure appear to be due to neuroendocrine suppression such as inhibition of the sympathetic nervous system and indirect arterial vasodilatation. Long-term therapy produces symptomatic improvement, increases exercise tolerance, and decreases the risk of clinical deterioration but has no effect on mortality.[23]

The benefit of cardiac glycosides in heart failure accompanied by atrial fibrillation is not disputed although there is still continuing debate over the benefit in patients with sinus rhythm. There is evidence that withdrawal of digoxin from patients receiving diuretics (the PROVED trial)[24] or ACE inhibitors (the RADIANCE study)[25] carries a considerable risk of clinical deterioration if they are stable on such combination therapy. However, the large DIG study[23] found that digoxin, given in addition to diuretics and ACE inhibitors, had no effect on mortality. Digoxin may therefore have a role in patients who remain symptomatic despite ACE inhibitor and diuretic therapy.[11,12,26,27]

ACE inhibitors are but one of a heterogeneous group of drugs that can be described as *vasodilators*, but have different mechanisms of action.[28] The effects of various vasodilators in heart failure have been studied in a series of Vasodilator-Heart Failure Trials (V-HeFT).[29] Oral nitrates, such as *isosorbide dinitrate*, produce a predominantly venous dilatation whereas *hydralazine* produces arterial vasodilatation and they are thus used in combination. They alleviate peripheral vasoconstriction and produce symptomatic control including a benefit on exercise tolerance but are of somewhat limited efficacy in long-term control. A modest improvement in long-term survival has been noted but this effect is less than that observed with the ACE inhibitors. The combination of isosorbide dinitrate with hydralazine has been recommended in patients with left ventricular dysfunction who are unable to tolerate ACE inhibitors; they may also be used as adjuncts in patients who remain symptomatic despite therapy with ACE inhibitors, diuretics, and digoxin.

Angiotensin II receptor antagonists are being investigated as alternatives to ACE inhibitors. The ELITE study,[30] which compared *losartan* with captopril in elderly patients with heart failure, found that both drugs had similar effects on renal function but other adverse effects were fewer with losartan. Losartan might also have a mortality benefit but further studies are needed to confirm this finding.

Beta blockers have negative inotropic properties and have generally been contra-indicated in patients with heart failure. However, persistent activation of the sympathetic nervous system appears to be associated with disease progression and beta blockers might therefore be beneficial in the long-term management of heart failure.[31-34] Recent studies with *carvedilol* have suggested a positive effect on mortality in patients with varying degrees of heart failure.[35,36] A systematic overview,[37] and a meta-analysis,[38] of trials using various beta blockers (including the carvedilol trials) support the finding of a reduction in mortality, but both concluded that further large, long-term studies were required. One such study, the CIBIS II trial,[54] has shown a significant reduction in all-cause mortality in patients receiving *bisoprolol*. The effects of beta blocker therapy on quality of life are also not yet clear.[39] If beta blockers are used they must be introduced cautiously since symptoms may initially worsen.[40,41] Beta blockers do appear to be of value in heart failure due to idiopathic dilated cardiomyopathy (see under Cardiomyopathies, above) and possibly in isolated diastolic dysfunction.

Despite reservations about the use of *calcium-channel blockers* in heart failure[42] (they have often been contra-indicated because of their negative inotropic activity), their use as adjuncts is being investigated. In the PRAISE study,[43] *amlodipine* had no adverse effect on morbidity or mortality in patients with severe heart failure also receiving diuretics, ACE inhibitors, and digoxin. Amlodipine might therefore be a suitable treatment for angina or hypertension in such patients. The potential additive effect of *felodipine* when used with an ACE inhibitor is under investigation in the V-HeFT III study.[29]

Phosphodiesterase inhibitors have a dual action being both positive inotropes and vasodilators. In theory, this is an attractive combination of mechanisms for use in heart failure but in general this group of drugs has not lived up to early expectations. Although short-term haemodynamic variables are improved, long-term oral use has been associated either with an unacceptable incidence of adverse effects (*amrinone*) or with an increased mortality rate (*enoximone*[44] and *milrinone*[45]). Thus, these phosphodiesterase inhibitors have been reserved for intravenous use in the short-term treatment of severe heart failure unresponsive to other treatment.[46-48] More recently introduced phosphodiesterase inhibitors include *vesnarinone* and *pimobendan*; they also have calcium-sensitising properties. Initial studies with vesnarinone[49] indicated a survival benefit but a larger trial has shown an increased mortality in patients receiving vesnarinone. The place of these drugs in the management of heart failure remains unclear.

Although *antiarrhythmics* are not routinely recommended in the management of heart failure, those that do not have a negative inotropic effect may have a role since sudden deaths have been attributed to ventricular arrhythmias in patients with severe heart failure. A meta-analysis[50] of 5 trials involving 1452 patients with symptomatic compensated heart failure indicated that *amiodarone* reduced the rate of arrhythmic or sudden death in high-risk patients and that this resulted in an overall reduction in mortality.

Several *miscellaneous drugs*, such as *flosequinan* (an arterial and venous vasodilator), *epoprostenol* (a prostaglandin), and *xamoterol* (a partial β_1-adrenoceptor agonist) have been tried in heart failure but have proved either disappointing or have been associated with excessive toxicity or an increased mortality rate. Of these drugs only xamoterol is still employed and is indicated only in chronic mild heart failure. Pulsed β-stimulant therapy with *dobutamine* has been investigated but the oral dopamine agonist *ibopamine* appears to increase mortality.[51] Other drugs that are being studied in heart failure include *candoxatril*, which acts by inhibiting the metabolism of atrial natriuretic peptide, and *endothelin antagonists* such as *bosentan*. The role of *antithrombotic* therapy in patients with heart failure remains unclear.[52]

Some patients with refractory heart failure may be suitable for surgical management. Heart transplantation is the optimum surgical therapy but availability is limited and a number of methods for augmenting the heart muscle or reducing ventricular dilatation are being investigated.[53]

1. Dargie HJ, McMurray JJV. Diagnosis and management of heart failure. *Br Med J* 1994; **308:** 321–8.
2. Cohn JN. The management of chronic heart failure. *N Engl J Med* 1996; **335:** 490–8.
3. Gaasch WH. Diagnosis and treatment of heart failure based on left ventricular systolic or diastolic dysfunction. *JAMA* 1994; **271:** 1276–80.
4. Packer M. Pathophysiology of chronic heart failure. *Lancet* 1992; **340:** 88–92.
5. Packer M. Treatment of chronic heart failure. *Lancet* 1992; **340:** 92–5.
6. Baker DW, *et al.* Management of heart failure: 1. pharmacologic treatment. *JAMA* 1994; **272:** 1361–6.
7. Kleber FX, Wensel R. Current guidelines for the treatment of congestive heart failure. *Drugs* 1996; **51:** 89–98.
8. Bonarjee VVS, Dickstein K. Novel drugs and current therapeutic approaches in the treatment of heart failure. *Drugs* 1996; **51:** 347–58.
9. Forker AD. A cardiologist's perspective on evolving concepts in the management of congestive heart failure. *J Clin Pharmacol* 1996; **36:** 973–84.
10. Cleland JGF, *et al.* Successes and failures of current treatment of heart failure. *Lancet* 1998; **352** (suppl): 19–28.
11. ACC/AHA Task Force. Guidelines for the evaluation and management of heart failure: report of the American College of Cardiology/American Heart Association Task Force on Practice Guidelines (Committee on Evaluation and Management of Heart Failure). *Circulation* 1995; **92:** 2764–84.
12. Task Force of the Working Group on Heart Failure of the European Society of Cardiology. The treatment of heart failure. *Eur Heart J* 1997; **18:** 736–53.
13. Parmley WW. Clinical practice guidelines: does the cookbook have enough recipes? *JAMA* 1994; **272:** 1374–5.
14. Anonymous. Diuretics for heart failure. *Drug Ther Bull* 1994; **32:** 83–5.
15. Channer KS, *et al.* Thiazides with loop diuretics for severe congestive heart failure. *Lancet* 1990; **i:** 922–3.
16. Ellison DH. The physiologic basis of diuretic synergism: its role in treating diuretic resistance. *Ann Intern Med* 1991; **114:** 886–94.
17. Knauf H, Mutschler E. Low-dose segmental blockade of the nephron rather than high-dose diuretic monotherapy. *Eur J Clin Pharmacol* 1993; **44** (suppl 1): S63–S68.
18. Garg R, Yusuf S. Overview of randomized trials of angiotensin-converting enzyme inhibitors on mortality and morbidity in patients with heart failure. *JAMA* 1995; **273:** 1450–6.
19. Nelson KM, Yeager BF. What is the role of angiotensin-converting enzyme inhibitors in congestive heart failure and after myocardial infarction? *Ann Pharmacother* 1996; **30:** 986–93.
20. The SOLVD Investigators. Effects of enalapril on mortality and the development of heart failure in asymptomatic patients with reduced left ventricular ejection fractions. *N Engl J Med* 1992; **327:** 685–91.
21. Eccles M, *et al.* North of England evidence based development project; guideline for angiotensin converting enzyme inhibitors in primary care management of adults with symptomatic heart failure. *Br Med J* 1998; **316:** 1369–75.
22. Campbell RWF. ACE inhibitors and arrhythmias. *Heart* 1996; **76** (suppl 3): 79–82.
23. The Digitalis Investigation Group. The effect of digoxin on mortality and morbidity in patients with heart failure. *N Engl J Med* 1997; **336:** 525–33.
24. Uretsky NF, *et al.* Randomized study assessing the effect of digoxin withdrawal in patients with mild to moderate chronic congestive heart failure: results of the PROVED trial. *J Am Coll Cardiol* 1993; **22:** 955–62.
25. Packer M, *et al.* Withdrawal of digoxin from patients with chronic heart failure treated with angiotensin-converting-enzyme inhibitors. *N Engl J Med* 1993; **329:** 1–7.
26. Packer M. End of the oldest controversy in medicine: are we ready to conclude the debate on digitalis? *N Engl J Med* 1997; **336:** 575–6.
27. Riaz K, Forker AD. Digoxin use in congestive heart failure: current status. *Drugs* 1998; **55:** 747–58.
28. Stevenson LW, Fonarow G. Vasodilators: a re-evaluation of their role in heart failure. *Drugs* 1992; **43:** 15–36.
29. Cohn JN. Vasodilators in heart failure: conclusions from V-HeFT II and rationale for V-HeFT III. *Drugs* 1994; **47** (suppl 4): 47–58.
30. Pitt B, *et al.* Randomised trial of losartan versus captopril in patients over 65 with heart failure (Evaluation of Losartan in the Elderly Study, ELITE). *Lancet* 1997; **349:** 747–52.
31. Sackner-Bernstein JD, Mancini DM. Rationale for treatment of patients with chronic heart failure with adrenergic blockade. *JAMA* 1995; **274:** 1462–7.
32. Krum H. β-adrenoceptor blockers in chronic heart failure—a review. *Br J Clin Pharmacol* 1997; **44:** 111–18.
33. Eichhorn EJ. Restoring function in failing hearts: the effects of beta blockers. *Am J Med* 1998; **104:** 163–9.
34. White CM. Catecholamines and their blockade in congestive heart failure. *Am J Health-Syst Pharm* 1998; **55:** 676–82.
35. Packer M, *et al.* The effect of carvedilol on morbidity and mortality in patients with chronic heart failure. *N Engl J Med* 1996; **334:** 1349–55.
36. Australia/New Zealand Heart Failure Research Collaborative Group. Randomised, placebo-controlled trial of carvedilol in patients with congestive heart failure due to ischaemic heart disease. *Lancet* 1997; **349:** 375–80.
37. Doughty RN, *et al.* Effects of beta-blocker therapy on mortality in patients with heart failure; a systematic overview of randomized controlled trials. *Eur Heart J* 1997; **18:** 560–5.
38. Heindenreich PA, *et al.* Effect of beta-blockade on mortality in patients with heart failure: a meta-analysis of randomized clinical trials. *J Am Coll Cardiol* 1997; **30:** 27–34.
39. Hjalmarson Å, *et al.* The role of β-blockers in left ventricular dysfunction and heart failure. *Drugs* 1997; **54:** 501–10.
40. Cleland JGF, Swedberg K. Carvedilol for heart failure, with care. *Lancet* 1996; **347:** 1199–1201.
41. Krum H. β-Blockers in chronic heart failure: paradox proven? *Med J Aust* 1996; **164:** 581–2.
42. Piepho RW. Calcium antagonist use in congestive heart failure: still a bridge too far? *J Clin Pharmacol* 1995; **35:** 443–53.
43. Packer M, *et al.* Effect of amlodipine on morbidity and mortality in severe chronic heart failure. *N Engl J Med* 1996; **335:** 1107–14.
44. Uretsky BF, *et al.* Multicenter trial of oral enoximone in patients with moderate to moderately severe congestive heart failure: lack of benefit compared with placebo. *Circulation* 1990; **82:** 774–80.
45. Packer M, *et al.* Effect of oral milrinone on mortality in severe chronic heart failure. *N Engl J Med* 1991; **325:** 1468–75.
46. Fischer TA, *et al.* Current status of phosphodiesterase inhibitors in the treatment of congestive heart failure. *Drugs* 1992; **44:** 928–45.
47. Packer M. The search for the ideal positive inotropic agent. *N Engl J Med* 1993; **329:** 210–2.
48. Nony P, *et al.* Evaluation of the effect of phosphodiesterase inhibitors on mortality in chronic heart failure patients: a meta-analysis. *Eur J Clin Pharmacol* 1994; **46:** 191–6.
49. Feldman AM, *et al.* Effects of vesnarinone on morbidity and mortality in patients with heart failure. *N Engl J Med* 1993; **329:** 149–55.
50. Amiodarone Trials Meta-Analysis Investigators. Effect of prophylactic amiodarone on mortality after acute myocardial infarction and in congestive heart failure: meta-analysis of individual data from 6500 patients in randomised trials. *Lancet* 1997; **350:** 1417–24.
51. Hampton JR, *et al.* Randomised study of effect of ibopamine on survival in patients with advanced severe heart failure. *Lancet* 1997; **349:** 971–7.
52. Ezekowitz M. Antithrombotics for left-ventricular impairment? *Lancet* 1998; **351:** 1904.
53. Taggart DP, Westaby S. Surgical management of heart failure. *Br Med J* 1997; **314:** 453–4.
54. CIBIS-II Investigators and Committees. The Cardiac Insufficiency Bisoprolol Study II (CIBIS-II): a randomised trial. *Lancet* 1999; **353:** 9–13.

High-altitude disorders

Rapid ascent (ascent without time to acclimatise) to high altitudes may produce a spectrum of illness (altitude illness) ranging from the usually benign acute mountain sickness to life-threatening pulmonary oedema and cerebral oedema. Factors influencing the development of altitude illness include rate of ascent, altitude attained, and length of stay at altitude. Individual susceptibility is also an important factor. Ascent to altitudes of 2000 to 3000 metres (6500 to 9750 feet) produces no ill effects in most people although susceptible individuals may be affected at altitudes as low as 2000 metres.[1] Symptoms of altitude illness occur in about 50% of people ascending rapidly to altitudes of over 4000 metres (13 000 feet)[1] and in about 75% of people at 4500 metres (14 625 feet);[2] they are severe (pulmonary oedema or cerebral oedema) in about 4%.[1]

Symptoms of **acute mountain sickness** include headache, which is worse in the supine position, nausea, vomiting, anorexia, lethargy, insomnia, and dizziness. These may develop during ascent, but characteristically occur 6 to 48 hours after arrival at altitude. They are usually short-lived and resolve after a few days at altitude. In a very few people symptoms persist for longer. Chronic mountain sickness, characterised by persistent severe hypoxia and polycythaemia, may develop during prolonged residence at high altitude. The discussion that follows is limited to management of the acute forms. A small proportion of people with acute mountain sickness suddenly deteriorate and develop pulmonary oedema or cerebral oedema both of which may be life-threatening. Occasionally, pulmonary or cerebral oedema develops without symptoms of acute mountain sickness. Symptoms of **pulmonary oedema** include rapid onset of breathlessness and tachypnoea at rest, and a dry cough which may develop into haemoptysis. Symptoms of **cerebral oedema** include increasing headache, ataxia, mental disturbances, drowsiness and eventually coma. Pulmonary and cerebral oedema frequently occur together.

The **pathogenesis** of altitude illness is not fully understood, and it is not known whether the mechanisms of acute mountain sickness and pulmonary or cerebral oedema differ in nature or merely degree.[3] Hypoxia, a result of the reduced partial pressure of oxygen at high altitudes is considered the primary stimulus in the development of altitude illness.[1-3] When ascent to high altitudes occurs gradually the bicarbonate concentration and the pH of extracellular fluid falls progressively. The falling pH increases the sensitivity of chemoreceptors to hypoxia and so permits greater ventilation, thus allowing acclimatisation. Rapid ascent to high altitudes does not allow time for these changes to occur and although the hypoxia stimulates hyperventilation, it produces a respiratory alkalosis which limits the ventilatory response to hypoxia.[3] The hypoxaemia produced leads to alterations in fluid and electrolyte balance and haemodynamic changes responsible for the symptoms of altitude illness. Symptoms are often worse at night when ventilation is reduced leading to a worsening of the hypoxaemia.[2]

Prophylaxis. Altitude illness may be avoided by ascending to high altitudes slowly and thereby allowing time for acclimatisation. This may be achieved by staying for 2 to 5 days at 2000 to 3000 metres and avoiding strenuous physical activity,[2,4] thus allowing the body to adapt to the reduced oxygen pressure and to ascend above 3000 metres without sickness. Acclimatisation may also be achieved when going above 3000 metres by limiting the rate of ascent to 300 metres a day with an intermediate night or two resting at a particular altitude.[1] Some recommend that after a couple of days this rate of ascent should be further reduced to 150 metres a day.[5]

However, when time for acclimatisation is limited or when abrupt arrival at high altitude (for instance by air) cannot be avoided, drug prophylaxis may be considered. Prophylaxis should also be considered for those individuals who have developed symptoms on ascending to high altitudes on previous occasions.

Acetazolamide is the most frequently used drug. It produces a mild metabolic acidosis which has the effect of stimulating chemoreceptors to produce an increase in the rate of respiration and tidal volume, and it therefore accelerates the process of acclimatisation. Although acetazolamide has diuretic actions it does not prevent fluid retention or prevent or protect against pulmonary or cerebral oedema. A reduction in the frequency of acute mountain sickness of about 30 to 50% has been reported with acetazolamide.[2] It improves sleep hypoxaemia and quality of sleep, reduces proteinuria, improves exercise performance, and reduces loss of muscle mass, probably by improving oxygen supply to the tissues.[3] Acetazolamide should be taken on the day of ascent or 1 or 2 days before ascent to altitudes above 3000 metres, and continued for at least 5 days at the higher altitudes.[2,4] Some have cautioned that the use of acetazolamide to prevent symptoms of acute mountain sickness may encourage too rapid an ascent and perhaps increase the risk of developing pulmonary or cerebral oedema.[3]

Dexamethasone has also been effective in the prevention of acute mountain sickness. The rationale for its use is that mild brain oedema is thought to contribute to the symptoms of acute mountain sickness.[2] However, as the side-effects associated with dexamethasone are more severe than those associated with acetazolamide, it is not considered suitable for prophylaxis in healthy people.[1] If it is used, dexamethasone should be taken on the day of ascent to high altitude (above 3000 metres), continued for 3 days at the higher altitudes, and then tapered over 5 days.[2]

Spironolactone has also shown some benefit, but it has only been investigated in a few people.[1]

Nifedipine has been shown to lower pulmonary artery pressure and to protect against pulmonary oedema in people susceptible to the development of pulmonary symptoms at altitude[6] but is not usually recommended for prophylaxis due to the risk of adverse effects.

Aspirin was reported[7] to reduce the incidence of headache in a small study in people with a history of headache at high altitude.

Treatment. Once symptoms of altitude illness develop the course of action should be determined by the severity and nature of the symptoms.

1. When symptoms are *mild* and are not suggestive of pulmonary or cerebral oedema, rest and mild analgesics for headache are usually all that is required; symptoms resolve within a few days and further ascent is possible.[2] *Acetazolamide* may have some benefit in relieving symptoms although it has only been studied in small numbers of patients.[8] If mild symptoms of pulmonary oedema are present, such as dyspnoea and cough, rest with supplementary oxygen and further oxygen at night may resolve the symptoms and allow further ascent;[4] however signs and symptoms at altitude may be confusing and it is always safest to descend. The use of hypnotics at altitude is not generally advised since there is a risk that respiratory depression may further reduce oxygen saturation. However, a small study[9] using the short-acting benzodiazepine *temazepam* reported that sleep quality was improved without an alteration in mean oxygen saturation.

2. When symptoms are *moderate to severe*, are progressing, or are suggestive of cerebral oedema, immediate descent is necessary. Descending by as little as 300 metres is beneficial.[2] Various drugs and therapies have been given to alleviate symptoms and to facilitate descent and should also be employed when immediate descent is not possible. For example, *dexamethasone* can reduce the symptoms of acute mountain sickness and might be used in emergencies.[10,11] Portable hyperbaric chambers are available[1,12] and provide rapid but short-term improvement. They may be useful in combination with dexamethasone, which has a more sustained effect.[13]

If pulmonary oedema is present, oxygen, which relieves hypoxia and reduces pulmonary hypertension, should be given;[1] *nifedipine*, which suppresses the exaggerated hypoxic pulmonary vasoconstrictor response seen in people with pulmonary oedema, has provided benefit.[14,15] Positive pressure expiration by use of a mask may also be useful;[1] it has the effect of increasing oxygen saturation and partial pressure of carbon dioxide at altitude. Inhalation of nitric oxide has also been reported to improve oxygenation but administration may not be feasible at altitude.[16]

People with cerebral oedema should be given *dexamethasone* and oxygen therapy.

1. Beeley JM, *et al.* Environmental hazards and health. *Br Med Bull* 1993; **49:** 305–25.
2. Johnson TS, Rock PB. Acute mountain sickness. *N Engl J Med* 1988; **319:** 841–5.
3. Dickinson JG. Acetazolamide in acute mountain sickness. *Br Med J* 1987; **295:** 1161–2.
4. Anonymous. High altitude sickness. *Med Lett Drugs Ther* 1992; **34:** 84–6.
5. Pollard AJ. Altitude induced illness. *Br Med J* 1992; **304:** 1324–5.
6. Bärtsch P, *et al.* Prevention of high-altitude pulmonary edema by nifedipine. *N Engl J Med* 1991; **325:** 1284–9.
7. Burtscher M, *et al.* Aspirin for prophylaxis against headache at high altitudes: randomised, double blind, placebo controlled trial. *Br Med J* 1998; **316:** 1057–8.
8. Grissom CK, *et al.* Acetazolamide in the treatment of acute mountain sickness: clinical efficacy and effect on gas exchange. *Ann Intern Med* 1992; **116:** 461–5.
9. Dubowitz G. Effect of temazepam on oxygen saturation and sleep quality at high altitude: randomised placebo controlled crossover trial. *Br Med J* 1998; **316:** 587–9.
10. Ferrazzini G, *et al.* Successful treatment of acute mountain sickness with dexamethasone. *Br Med J* 1987; **294:** 1380–2.
11. Levine BD, *et al.* Dexamethasone in the treatment of acute mountain sickness. *N Engl J Med* 1989; **321:** 1707–13.
12. Bärtsch P, *et al.* Treatment of acute mountain sickness by simulated descent: a randomised controlled trial. *Br Med J* 1993; **306:** 1098–1101.
13. Keller H-R, *et al.* Simulated descent v dexamethasone in treatment of acute mountain sickness: a randomised trial. *Br Med J* 1995; **310:** 1232–5.
14. Oelz O, *et al.* Nifedipine for high altitude pulmonary oedema. *Lancet* 1989; **2:** 1241–4. Correction. *ibid.* 1991; **337:** 556.
15. Jamieson A, Kerr GW. Treatment of high-altitude pulmonary oedema. *Lancet* 1992; **340:** 1468.
16. Scherrer U, *et al.* Inhaled nitric oxide for high-altitude pulmonary edema. *N Engl J Med* 1996; **334:** 624–9.

Hypertension

Hypertension, particularly essential or primary hypertension, is widespread and although usually asymptomatic, is a major risk factor for stroke and to some extent ischaemic heart disease. Series of reviews in *Br Med Bull*[1], a 1994 *Lancet* octet, and a 1996 issue of *JAMA* have addressed various aspects of hypertension including definitions, classifications, origins, risk factors, non-pharmacological and pharmacological treatment interventions, and target-organ disease. National[2-4] and international[5,6] guidelines on management have also been published.

Definitions. The term *blood pressure* generally means arterial blood pressure, that is the pressure of the blood on artery walls. It is usually measured indirectly in the brachial artery just above the elbow using a mercury sphygmomanometer and is expressed in mmHg. Two measurements are made: *systolic* or maximum blood pressure (achieved during ventricular contraction of the heart) and *diastolic* or minimum blood pressure (achieved during ventricular dilatation). *Hypertension* means a higher than 'normal' blood pressure. Many factors influence blood pressure, resulting in a bell-shaped distribution curve in the general population, and in consequence it is difficult to define an absolute norm. An arbitrary definition of *normal* adult blood pressure[3,5] is a systolic pressure below 140 mmHg together with a diastolic pressure below 90 mmHg (i.e. below 140/90 mmHg). US guidelines[3] also cite an *optimal* blood pressure, with respect to cardiovascular risk, of less than 120/80 mmHg. Although there is some evidence that the systolic pressure is an important predictor of risk,[63] hypertension has frequently been defined in terms of diastolic pressure alone.

Hypertension is often classified as mild, moderate, or severe. However, these terms may be misleading since absolute cardiovascular risk also depends on other factors (see below). In the US guidelines[3] a staging system is preferred for classification, as follows:

stage 1: 140–159/90–99 mmHg;

stage 2: 160–179/100–109 mmHg;

stage 3: ≥180/≥110 mmHg.

When systolic and diastolic pressure fall into different categories the higher value is used for classification purposes. Similar values are given in the WHO/ISH (International Society of Hypertension) guidelines.[5] Classification and subsequent treatment decisions should be based on blood pressure measurements taken on several occasions over a period that varies according to the severity of hypertension and should also take into account the absence, presence, or extent of target-organ damage. Ambulatory blood pressure monitoring may be used in some cases.[3,4,7]

In *malignant* or *accelerated hypertension* rapidly progressing severe hypertension is associated with retinopathy and often renal impairment.

Isolated systolic hypertension occurs mainly in the elderly and has been defined as systolic pressure over 160 mmHg[2,4] (or 140 mmHg or more[3,5]) and diastolic pressure under 90 mmHg.

Origins. In the majority of cases of hypertension the cause is unknown, and it is suspected that such *primary* or *essential* hypertension is multifactorial in origin, and that genotype, as well as external factors such as diet and body-weight, may play a role. Hypertension may also be associated with surgery and pregnancy and is prevalent in diabetics. In a limited number of cases hypertension is *secondary* to some other condition, such as renal disease, Cushing's syndrome, phaeochromocytoma, or the adverse effects of drugs such as oestrogens, and such causes may be suspected particularly in resistant or malignant hypertension. Although treatment of the underlying condition will generally be desirable, the resultant hypertension will not necessarily be abolished by this.

Management of hypertension. Most of what follows relates to primary or essential hypertension in adults. Hypertensive crises and hypertension associated with surgery, diabetes, renal disease, or pregnancy are also discussed below under separate headings.

Hypertension may be discovered because of adverse vascular events, especially in the eyes, brain, kidneys, or heart, but is more often asymptomatic and only discovered on routine measurement of blood pressure. As already mentioned, the dividing line between normal and raised blood pressure is fairly arbitrary, but may be defined as the level of blood pressure above which intervention has been shown to reduce the associated cardiovascular risk. It is well-established that hypertension is a risk factor for the development of stroke, heart failure, and renal damage, and to a lesser extent ischaemic heart disease, and a reduction in blood pressure is generally beneficial, although mortality remains higher than in non-hypertensives.[8] However, it is important to assess hypertension in the context of other cardiovascular risk factors such as increasing age, male gender, postmenopausal status, previous cardiovascular events, target-organ disease such as left ventricular hypertrophy or renal disease, smoking, diabetes, dyslipidaemia, obesity, and sedentary life-style. The main clinical problem is whether, or when, to treat so-called mild hypertension. The term 'mild' can be misleading since the risk of cardiovascular disease can range from low to high in patients with only mild hypertension depending on whether, or what, other associated risk factors are present.

In addition to specific antihypertensive treatment other cardiovascular risk factors should be reduced and coexisting disease dealt with. Guidelines on the management of hypertension may differ in detail, but reflect judgement on when intervention, both non-pharmacological and pharmacological, is justified.

Non-pharmacological treatment. In patients with mild hypertension control of blood pressure by non-pharmacological means may be attempted and patients requiring drug therapy to reduce their blood pressure will also benefit from such life-style changes. A number of non-pharmacological options have been recommended as reducing blood pressure[3,4,9,10] and these include: reduction in excess weight; reduction in excess alcohol consumption; reduction in sodium intake; adequate exercise. Tobacco smoking, a major risk factor for cardiovascular disease, should also be stopped. Other interventions tried, but with less evidence of benefit include: increased intake of potassium, magnesium, and calcium; increased polyunsaturated fat intake and reduced saturated fat intake; and relaxation therapies for stress reduction.

These life-style changes may also be promoted in the population as a whole, or in individuals most likely to develop hypertension, in strategies for the *primary prevention* of high blood pressure.

Pharmacological treatment. What needs to be decided before embarking on drug therapy of hypertension is: when to intervene with antihypertensive drugs, what the treatment goal is, and what drug regimen to choose. In patients with mild to moderate hypertension drug treatment should not be initiated until after an adequate period of observation including monitoring of blood pressure; this may extend to 3 to 6 months although the higher the blood pressure the shorter the observation period.

When to intervene with antihypertensive drugs depends on a number of factors. The British Hypertension Society[2,4] recommends that *younger patients* (under 60 years) should definitely be treated if diastolic blood pressure is 100 mmHg or more, and may be treated if diastolic blood pressure is between 90 and 99 mmHg (especially in those with other cardiovascular risk factors, with target-organ damage such as left ventricular hypertrophy, with renal impairment, or with diabetes); younger patients with systolic blood pressure above 160 mmHg should also be treated, irrespective of the diastolic pressure. For *elderly patients* (over 60 years) the benefit of treating hypertension has been established in several trials.[11-13,63] The British Hypertension Society recommends that those with systolic blood pressure of 160 mmHg or more (isolated systolic hypertension), diastolic blood pressure of 90 mmHg or more, or both, should be treated with antihypertensive drugs. For very old people (those over 80 years) the benefit of initiating therapy is less clear, although those already being treated should continue. Some authorities in the UK have noted that benefit is evident up to at least 85 years of age and have considered a strict age limit to drug therapy to probably be inappropriate.

US[3] and WHO[5] guidelines differ in some respects from those of the UK on when to intervene. The US guidelines[3] consider treatment to be indicated when systolic is 140 mmHg or more and diastolic 90 mmHg or more particularly in the presence of other cardiovascular risk factors or target-organ disease. Drug treatment is also indicated in patients with lower pressures if they have target-organ disease or are diabetic. WHO[5] offers detailed guidance for the management of mild hypertension (defined as diastolic pressure between 90 and 105 mmHg and/or systolic pressure between 140 and 180 mmHg) based on the results of repeated blood pressure measurements over at least 3 months.

Treatment goals, according to the British Hypertension Society guidelines,[2,4] are the reduction of diastolic blood pressure to less than 90 mmHg and systolic blood pressure to less than 160 mmHg (although the latter is less well established). Lower blood pressure targets have been suggested by some, for example, less than 125 mmHg systolic and less than 85 mmHg diastolic,[14] and WHO guidelines[5,6] suggest a goal of at least 120–130/80 mmHg in young patients with mild hypertension. US guidelines[3] have cited an optimal blood pressure of less than 120/80 mmHg although their suggested goal is below 140/90 mmHg. However, there has been concern that the over-aggressive reduction of diastolic pressure might increase the risk of ischaemic heart disease and optimal treatment is still being assessed.[15,16] There is some evidence that effective blood-pressure control to maintain the diastolic pressure below 90 mmHg (at about 85 mmHg) reduces the rate of cardiovascular events, but lower pressures (of around 70 mmHg) may not provide any further benefit.[17]

The drug regimen may include drugs from a number of groups that have antihypertensive effects. These groups have differing pharmacological actions although the precise mechanism is not understood in all cases. Thiazide diuretics and beta blockers have been the mainstay of drug therapy for hypertension, but more recently the availability of other drug groups such as calcium-channel blockers, ACE inhibitors, and alpha blockers, as well as concern about the possible metabolic effects of thiazides and beta blockers has led to increasing use of these newer drugs.

Choice of initial therapy has been controversial.[18,19] Studies such as the TOMHS[20] (comparing chlorthalidone, acebutolol, amlodipine, enalapril, and doxazosin), and a similar study[21] (comparing hydrochlorothiazide, atenolol, diltiazem, captopril, prazosin, and clonidine), have shown that the response to, and tolerance of, the 5 main types of antihypertensive drug is similar. Each type will provide control in about 50% of patients, although the response may also depend on individual factors such as age[22] and race.[23] However, the national and international guidelines[2-5] all continue to rank diuretics (particularly thiazides) and beta blockers as the first-line drugs of choice since only they had been adequately tested in long-term mortality/morbidity studies in hypertensive subjects. A systematic review and meta-analysis[24] came to a similar conclusion. ACE inhibitors, calcium-channel blockers, and alpha blockers, as well as angiotensin II receptor antagonists, are generally considered to be alternative first-line drugs, the ultimate choice depending on the presence or absence of contra-indications, on adverse effects, and on co-existing disease. In one of the *Lancet* octet papers, Swales[25] concluded that, in the absence of other data, beta blockers seemed preferable first-line therapy in younger patients and low-dose diuretics in elderly patients, although beta blockers would be first choice in post-myocardial infarction patients with no evidence of heart failure. Beta blockers and ACE inhibitors appear to be less effective in Afro-Caribbean blacks, whereas ACE inhibitors may be preferable in patients with left ventricular dysfunction. Angiotensin II receptor antagonists may be considered as an alternative to ACE inhibitors when persistent cough associated with the latter is unacceptable. The role of calcium-channel blockers is controversial;[26] although they have been widely used, the safety of short-acting calcium-channel blockers has recently been questioned and some recommend that they should be avoided (see under Adverse Effects of Nifedipine, p.916).

Having decided what drug to use, treatment is started at the lowest recommended dose.[27] If this is ineffective or only partially effective the dose may be increased (except in the case of thiazide diuretics where there is generally no additional benefit, but more adverse effects); alternatively another first-line drug may either be substituted (sequential therapy) or added. Two-drug combinations will control blood pressure in a higher proportion of patients although the effects of the two drugs may not be fully additive.[28] Combination therapy also allows lower doses of the individual drugs to be used with a consequent reduction in adverse effects. The most effective combinations involve drugs that act on different physiological systems; appropriate combinations include: a diuretic plus a beta blocker, an ACE inhibitor, or an alpha blocker; a calcium-channel blocker plus an ACE inhibitor, an alpha blocker, or (except with verapamil) a beta blocker; an alpha blocker plus any other class. A 3-drug combination may sometimes be required, especially in severe hypertension. (The formerly widely used 'stepped-care' approach entailed a diuretic or beta blocker as step 1, a diuretic with a beta blocker as step 2, and addition of usually a vasodilator as step 3.) In patients who maintain an elevated diastolic blood pressure despite triple therapy the possibility of secondary hypertension should be considered, although factors such as non-compliance, NSAID use, or alcohol abuse may contribute to resistance.[29,30]

Other classes of antihypertensive drugs that are sometimes used include centrally acting drugs such as clonidine, methyldopa, and the less sedating moxonidine, and direct-acting drugs such as hydralazine and minoxidil. Older drugs like the adrenergic neurone blocker guanethidine and the rauwolfia alkaloid reserpine are rarely recommended now. Renin inhibitors, endopeptidase inhibitors, and endothelin antagonists are under investigation.

Withdrawal of drug treatment. It has been standard teaching that drug treatment for hypertension is continued indefinitely, but there have been some reports of successful withdrawal in selected patients.[31,32] Some guidelines[2,3] suggest that, once hypertension is controlled, a reduction in dosage or even withdrawal of antihypertensive drugs may be possible in patients with mild hypertension provided that blood pressure is consistently controlled, there is no evidence of target-organ damage, and blood pressure continues to be monitored. In these patients, non-pharmacological measures should be continued indefinitely.

Hypertensive crises. Patients with severe hypertension may be divided into those in whom there is evidence of rapid or progressive CNS, cardiovascular, or renal deterioration (hypertensive *emergencies*) and those with no evidence of target-organ damage (urgent hypertensive crises or hypertensive *urgencies*).[33] In the former case the goal is a reduction in mean arterial blood pressure by 25%, or a fall in diastolic blood pressure to 100 to 110 mmHg, over a period of several minutes to several hours depending on the clinical situation; intravenous therapy is often required although oral therapy may be adequate. In the latter case a drastic reduction in blood pressure is inappropriate and oral therapy is preferred, with the aim of a reduction in blood pressure over several hours to days. It should be remembered in both situations that a too rapid reduction of blood pressure may be detrimental and may lead to cerebral infarction and blindness, to deterioration in renal function, and to myocardial ischaemia.

If oral treatment can be given and there is no evidence of ongoing target-organ damage, standard initiation of antihypertensive therapy is appropriate, although the patient should be closely monitored. If there is no evidence of heart failure or asthma then a beta blocker has often been the treatment of choice.[34] A calcium-channel blocker such as nifedipine, given orally, may be used as an alternative. Diuretics are less suitable since patients may initially be fluid depleted but they may be added after two to three days, treatment with other antihypertensive drugs to maintain blood pressure control.[34] Other drugs that have been used for a rapid effect include the centrally acting drug clonidine, the ACE inhibitor captopril, and the alpha blocker prazosin (especially when there are increased circulating catecholamines), but caution is needed since they may all lower blood pressure abruptly and for this reason, they are not generally recommended as initial therapy. Nifedipine and captopril have also been administered sublingually for a faster onset,[35] but again care is needed since their rapid action may be detrimental. There appears to be no clearly defined clinical advantage for sublingual as opposed to oral administration and some consider that nifedipine should not be used.[36]

In the emergency situation, when parenteral therapy is required, choice of therapy depends on concomitant clinical conditions.[37] Sodium nitroprusside has most often been the drug of choice, given by intravenous infusion.[38,39] Alternatives include intravenous labetalol, nicardipine, hydralazine (in eclampsia), glyceryl trinitrate (in patients with coronary ischaemia), phentolamine (in phaeochromocytoma and other states associated with catecholamine excess such as the MAOI-tyramine interaction), trimetaphan (in patients with aortic dissection),[38,39] fenoldopam,[37] and urapidil.[40]

Hypertensive emergencies in children have been managed successfully with intravenous infusions of labetalol and/or sodium nitroprusside.[41]

Hypertension during surgery. Despite earlier concern over the risks of administering antihypertensive drugs to patients about to undergo surgery, substantial subsequent data have confirmed that it is not only safe but probably preferable to continue such medication up to and including the morning of surgery.[42]

Perioperative hypertension may occur as a result of surgery and frequently needs to be controlled with parenteral antihypertensives since oral administration in such patients may not be possible. The parenteral drug of choice is often sodium nitroprusside; others include glyceryl trinitrate (especially after coronary artery bypass), diazoxide, hydralazine, labetalol, and methyldopa.[38]

Hypertension in diabetic patients. Hypertension occurs with twice the frequency in the diabetic compared with the nondiabetic population, and up to 50% of patients with type 2 diabetes mellitus become hypertensive.[43] The reasons proposed for this increased prevalence are controversial, but some have implicated insulin resistance.[44] In addition to being a major risk factor for atherosclerosis in large blood vessels, hypertension in diabetes appears to contribute to small vessel disease and is a risk factor for diabetic nephropathy and possibly for diabetic retinopathy. The UK Prospective Diabetes Study (UKPDS) Group has reported[45] that tight control of blood pressure (with a target of <150/85 mmHg) reduces the risk of diabetes-related death and diabetic complications, including diabetic retinopathy, in type 2 diabetics.

The threshold for intervention with drug treatment may be lower in diabetic than in non-diabetic hypertensive patients. All the first-line antihypertensive drugs can be used in diabetics, but because of the potential adverse effects of diuretics and beta blockers on glucose and lipid metabolism, treatment with an ACE inhibitor or calcium-channel blocker has been preferred; alpha blockers may also be acceptable.[2] ACE inhibitors are reported to reduce insulin resistance. They may be particularly effective in patients with nephropathy, as there is evidence of benefit in preserving renal function; they have been reported to decrease proteinuria and preserve glomerular filtration rate in diabetic patients independently of changes in systemic blood pressure.[46] However, in the UKPDS treatment with an ACE inhibitor (captopril) or a beta blocker (atenolol) was equally effective in reducing the risk of diabetic complications, although the ACE inhibitor was better tolerated.[47]

Hypertension and renal disease. Hypertension is closely linked with the kidney—the kidney may have a role in the pathogenesis of hypertension and it may also be a prime target of damage caused by hypertension. Both renal parenchymal disorders and renovascular disorders may be associated with hypertension. In the former, hypertension is often resistant to treatment and a combination of drugs, including vasodilators, may be required.

Renovascular hypertension has been defined as arterial hypertension resulting from obliteration or compression of one or both renal arteries, the commonest cause being stenosis due to atherosclerosis. Underperfusion of the kidney leads to increased release of renin and a consequent rise in blood pressure. However, the relationship between renovascular hypertension and renal artery stenosis is not clear cut; the two conditions may simply co-exist or hypertension may cause the stenosis rather than the other way round.[48]

Renovascular hypertension may be difficult to distinguish clinically, but carries a worse prognosis than essential hypertension, may be less amenable to treatment, carries a higher risk of progression to accelerated or malignant hypertension, and may result in irreversible ischaemic failure of the affected kidney.

Diagnostic methods used to detect renovascular hypertension include imaging and functional tests. The captopril-renin test is one of the latter (see under ACE inhibitors on p.809 for further details); renal scintigraphy with and without ACE inhibition is also used.

Blood pressure in renovascular hypertension can often be lowered by antihypertensive drugs, particularly ACE inhibitors and calcium-channel blockers.[49] However, medical treatment may not prevent progression of stenosis and there are concerns about possible harmful effects of blood pressure reduction on the function of the affected kidney.[48] Adverse effects on renal function are a particular concern with ACE inhibitors since, in patients with bilateral renal artery stenosis or stenosis to a solitary kidney, renal perfusion may be dependent on angiotensin II. Although some consider renovascular disease to be a contra-indication to the use of ACE inhibitors, they may be needed to control blood pressure in some patients. However, they should be used cautiously and in low doses[50] and renal function needs to be monitored with great care (see under Precautions for ACE inhibitors, p.807). Alternatives to medical treatment are renal angioplasty or surgery.

Hypertension in pregnancy. Hypertension in pregnancy may be life-threatening to both mother and fetus. It may be pre-existing or may develop for the first time during pregnancy when it may range from transient hypertension late in pregnancy through to pre-eclampsia and eclampsia. Definitions vary, but hypertension presenting before 20 weeks' gestation generally continues long-term and is considered chronic hypertension, while pregnancy-induced hypertension (gestational hypertension) usually presents after the 20th week. Pregnancy-induced hypertension has been defined by some as a blood pressure of 140/90 mmHg or more on at least two occasions a minimum of 6 hours apart in a previously normotensive woman, and whose blood pressure has returned to normal limits by the sixth week post partum.[51] Pre-eclampsia entails increased blood pressure together with proteinuria, and, sometimes, abnormal coagulation and liver function, and oedema; it may progress to eclampsia, a convulsive phase.

Recommendations about the level of blood pressure which warrants treatment during pregnancy have been controversial. Mild hypertension carries little immediate risk for the mother or fetus and treatment is unlikely to be beneficial.[52] A US working group has recommended that treatment with antihypertensive drugs should be restricted to pregnant patients with a diastolic blood pressure of 100 mmHg or more,[3] although lower limits have been suggested.[62] However, women with mild hypertension are at an increased risk of developing pre-eclampsia, regardless of whether they receive antihypertensives, and should be closely monitored.

Mothers with *pre-existing* hypertension should continue their antihypertensive treatment although ACE inhibitors and angiotensin II receptor antagonists are contra-indicated in pregnancy. Methyldopa or beta blockers are effective first-line antihypertensives in mild to moderate hypertension and comparative studies have shown little difference between them in the outcome of pregnancy; however, methyldopa has the advantage of reassuring long-term safety results in the infant. Nifedipine may also be used.[53] Diuretics are not generally recommended for controlling hypertension in pregnancy because of the theoretical risk of exacerbating the volume depletion of pre-eclampsia.

In patients with pre-eclampsia the aim of treatment is to prevent maternal complications while allowing fetal maturation; delivery is the definitive treatment. Oral therapy may be appropriate although intravenous antihypertensives are used in acute pre-eclampsia or when delivery is imminent. For oral treatment methyldopa or a beta blocker is considered first-line. If this fails to reduce blood pressure adequately then it is usual to add a vasodilator such as hydralazine or prazosin;[51] a calcium-channel blocker such as nifedipine is also effective.[54] In the emergency control of hypertension in patients with severe pre-eclampsia or eclampsia intravenous hydralazine has been widely used; sodium nitroprusside has also been effective.[51] Other parenteral antihypertensives tried have included diazoxide, labetalol, clonidine,[3] and glyceryl trinitrate.[54]

The management of seizures associated with eclampsia is discussed on p.338.

Prevention of pre-eclampsia. It was hoped that prevention of pre-eclampsia might be possible by reducing the local platelet aggregation thought to be responsible for some of its manifestations. Several small studies suggested that low-dose aspirin reduced the risk of pregnancy-induced hypertension and intra-uterine growth retardation in high-risk patients.[55] However, larger studies in women at lower risk generally failed to confirm this benefit[56,57] and in one[57] the risk of abruptio placentae was higher in those taking aspirin. Findings of the CLASP (Collaborative Low-dose Aspirin Study in Pregnancy) multicentre study[58] involving over 9000 women considered to be at increased risk of pre-eclampsia or intra-uterine growth retardation did not support the routine prophylactic or therapeutic use of antiplatelet therapy in all such women. A further study[59] in high-risk women also failed to show any benefit, although administration of aspirin appeared to be safe for mother and fetus. The CLASP workers suggested that the only women in whom low-dose aspirin may be justified are those at especially high risk of early-onset pre-eclampsia severe enough to warrant very preterm delivery. The role of calcium supplementation in the prevention of pre-eclampsia is controversial. Although small studies and a meta-analysis[60] indicated that calcium supplementation during pregnancy reduced the risk of pre-eclampsia, this was not confirmed in a larger randomised study.[61]

1. Reid J, Swales JD, eds. Hypertension in theory and practice. *Br Med Bull* 1994; **50:** 235–515.
2. Sever P, *et al.* Management guidelines in essential hypertension: report of the second working party of the British Hypertension Society. *Br Med J* 1993; **306:** 983–7.
3. Joint National Committee. The sixth report of the joint national committee on prevention, detection, evaluation, and treatment of high blood pressure (JNC VI). *Arch Intern Med* 1997; **157:** 2413–46. Correction. *ibid.* 1998; **158:** 573.
4. British Hypertension Society. *Management guidelines in essential hypertension: modified recommendations based on the report by the Second Working Party of the British Hypertension Society.* Middlesex: British Hypertension Society, 1997.
5. Guidelines Sub-Committee. 1993 guidelines for the management of mild hypertension: memorandum from a WHO/ISH meeting. *Bull WHO* 1993; **71:** 503–17.
6. WHO. Hypertension control: report of a WHO expert committee. *WHO Tech Rep Ser 862* 1996.
7. Prasad N, Isles C. Ambulatory blood pressure monitoring: a guide for general practitioners. *Br Med J* 1996; **313:** 1535–41.
8. Andersson OK, *et al.* Survival in treated hypertension: follow up study after two decades. *Br Med J* 1998; **317:** 167–71.
9. Ramsay LE, *et al.* Non-pharmacological therapy of hypertension. *Br Med Bull* 1994; **50:** 494–508.
10. Alderman MH. Non-pharmacological treatment of hypertension. *Lancet* 1994; **344:** 307–11.
11. Dahlöf B, *et al.* Morbidity and mortality in the Swedish Trial in Old Patients with Hypertension (STOP-Hypertension). *Lancet* 1991; **338:** 1281–5.
12. SHEP Cooperative Research Group. Prevention of stroke by antihypertensive drug treatment in older persons with isolated systolic hypertension: final results of the Systolic Hypertension in the Elderly Program (SHEP). *JAMA* 1991; **265:** 3255–64.
13. MRC Working Party. Medical Research Council trial of treatment of hypertension in older patients: principal results. *Br Med J* 1992; **304:** 405–12.
14. Fletcher AE, Bulpitt CJ. How far should blood pressure be lowered? *N Engl J Med* 1992; **326:** 251–4.
15. The HOT Study Group. The Hypertension Optimal Treatment Study (The HOT Study). *Blood Pressure* 1993; **2:** 62–8.
16. Staessen JA. Potential adverse effects of blood pressure lowering—J-curve revisited. *Lancet* 1996; **348:** 696–7.
17. Hansson L, *et al.* Effects of intensive blood-pressure lowering and low-dose aspirin in patients with hypertension: principal results of the Hypertension Optimal Treatment (HOT) randomised trial. *Lancet* 1998; **351:** 1755–62.
18. Chalmers J. The treatment of hypertension. *Br J Clin Pharmacol* 1996; **42:** 29–35.
19. Kaplan NM, Gifford RW. Choice of initial therapy for hypertension. *JAMA* 1996; **275:** 1577–80.
20. Neaton JD, *et al.* Treatment of mild hypertension study: final results. *JAMA* 1993; **270:** 713–24.
21. Materson BJ, *et al.* Single-drug therapy for hypertension in men: a comparison of six antihypertensive agents with placebo. *N Engl J Med* 1993; **328:** 914–21. Correction. *ibid.* 1994; **330:** 1689.
22. Bennet NE. Hypertension in the elderly. *Lancet* 1994; **344:** 447–9.
23. Kaplan NM. Ethnic aspects of hypertension. *Lancet* 1994; **344:** 450–2.
24. Psaty BM, *et al.* Health outcomes associated with antihypertensive therapies used as first-line agents: a systematic review and meta-analysis. *JAMA* 1997; **277:** 739–45.
25. Swales JD. Pharmacological treatment of hypertension. *Lancet* 1994; **344:** 380–5.
26. Cutler JA. Calcium-channel blockers for hypertension—uncertainty continues. *N Engl J Med* 1998; **338:** 679–81.
27. Johnston GD. Selecting appropriate antihypertensive drug dosages. *Drugs* 1994; **47:** 567–75.
28. Lyons D, *et al.* Drug treatment: present and future. *Br Med Bull* 1994; **50:** 472–93.
29. McInnes GT, Semple PF. Hypertension: investigation, assessment and diagnosis. *Br Med Bull* 1994; **50:** 443–59.
30. Padfield PL. Resistant hypertension. *Prescribers' J* 1997; **37:** 69–76.
31. van den Bosch WJHM, *et al.* Withdrawal of antihypertensive drugs in selected patients. *Lancet* 1994; **343:** 1157.
32. Aylett MJ, *et al.* Withdrawing antihypertensive drugs. *Lancet* 1994; **343:** 1512.
33. Calhoun DA, Oparil S. Treatment of hypertensive crisis. *N Engl J Med* 1990; **323:** 1177–83.
34. Semple PF. Emergency treatment of hypertension. *Prescribers' J* 1989; **29:** 62–9.
35. Anonymous. Hypertensive emergencies. *Lancet* 1991; **338:** 220–1.
36. Grossman E, *et al.* Should a moratorium be placed on sublingual nifedipine capsules for hypertensive emergencies and pseudoemergencies? *JAMA* 1996; **276:** 1328–31.
37. Grossman E, *et al.* Comparative tolerability profile of hypertensive crisis treatments. *Drug Safety* 1998; **19:** 99–122.
38. Gifford RW. Management of hypertensive crises. *JAMA* 1991; **266:** 829–35.
39. Kaplan NM. Management of hypertensive emergencies. *Lancet* 1994; **344:** 1335–8.
40. Hirschl MM. Guidelines for the drug treatment of hypertensive crises. *Drugs* 1995; **50:** 991–1000.
41. Deal JE, *et al.* Management of hypertensive emergencies. *Arch Dis Child* 1992; **67:** 1089–92.
42. Goldman L. Cardiac risks and complications of noncardiac surgery. *Ann Intern Med* 1983; **98:** 504–13.
43. Barnett AH. Diabetes and hypertension. *Br Med Bull* 1994; **50:** 397–407.
44. Reaven GM, *et al.* Hypertension and associated metabolic abnormalities—the role of insulin resistance and the sympathoadrenal system. *N Engl J Med* 1996; **334:** 374–81.
45. UK Prospective Diabetes Study Group. Tight blood pressure control and risk of macrovascular and microvascular complications in type 2 diabetes: UKPDS 38. *Br Med J* 1998; **317:** 703–13.
46. Kaisiske BL, *et al.* Effect of antihypertensive therapy on the kidney in patients with diabetes: a meta-regression analysis. *Ann Intern Med* 1993; **118:** 129–38.
47. UK Prospective Diabetes Study Group. Efficacy of atenolol and captopril in reducing risk of macrovascular and microvascular complications in type 2 diabetes: UKPDS 39. *Br Med J* 1998; **317:** 713–20.
48. Derkx FHM, Schalekamp MADH. Renal artery stenosis and hypertension. *Lancet* 1994; **344:** 237–9.
49. Rosenthal T. Drug therapy of renovascular hypertension. *Drugs* 1993; **45:** 895–909.
50. Navis G, *et al.* ACE inhibitors and the kidney: a risk-benefit assessment. *Drug Safety* 1996; **15:** 200–211.
51. Broughton Pipkin F, Rubin PC. Pre-eclampsia—the 'disease of theories'. *Br Med Bull* 1994; **50:** 381–96.
52. Teoh TG, Redman CW. Management of pre-existing disorders in pregnancy: hypertension. *Prescribers' J* 1996; **36:** 28–36.
53. Sibai BM. Treatment of hypertension in pregnant women. *N Engl J Med* 1996; **335:** 257–65.
54. Mushambi MC, *et al.* Recent developments in the pathophysiology and management of pre-eclampsia. *Br J Anaesth* 1996; **76:** 133–48.
55. Imperiale TF, Petrulis AS. A meta-analysis of low-dose aspirin for the prevention of pregnancy-induced hypertensive disease. *JAMA* 1991; **266:** 260–4.
56. Italian Study of Aspirin in Pregnancy. Low-dose aspirin in prevention and treatment of intrauterine growth retardation and pregnancy-induced hypertension. *Lancet* 1993; **341:** 396–400.
57. Sibai BM, *et al.* Prevention of preeclampsia with low-dose aspirin in healthy, nulliparous pregnant women. *N Engl J Med* 1993; **329:** 1213–18.
58. CLASP (Collaborative Low-dose Aspirin Study in Pregnancy) Collaborative Group. CLASP: a randomised trial of low-dose aspirin for the prevention and treatment of pre-eclampsia among 9364 pregnant women. *Lancet* 1994; **343:** 619–29.
59. Caritis S, *et al.* Low-dose aspirin to prevent preeclampsia in women at high risk. *N Engl J Med* 1998; **338:** 701–5.
60. Bucher HC, *et al.* Effect of calcium supplementation on pregnancy-induced hypertension and preeclampsia: a meta-analysis of randomized controlled trials. *JAMA* 1996; **275:** 1113–17.
61. Levine RJ, *et al.* Trial of calcium to prevent preeclampsia. *N Engl J Med* 1997; **337:** 69–76.
62. Rey É. Report of the Canadian Hypertension Society Consensus Conference: pharmacologic treatment of hypertensive disorders in pregnancy. *Can Med Assoc J* 1997; **157:** 1245–54.
63. Staessen JA, *et al.* Randomised double-blind comparison of placebo and active treatment for older patients with isolated systolic hypertension. *Lancet* 1997; **350:** 757–64. Correction. *ibid.*; 1636.

Hypotension

As discussed under Hypertension (above) many factors influence blood pressure making it difficult to define an absolute norm. An arbitrary definition of *normal* adult blood pressure[1,2] is a systolic pressure below 140 mmHg together with a diastolic pressure below 90 mmHg (i.e. below 140/90 mmHg). US guidelines[1] also cite an *optimal* blood pressure, with respect to cardiovascular risk, of less than 120/80 mmHg. Unlike hypertension, for which national and international guidelines have been developed, there does not appear to be an accepted definition of either low blood pressure or hypotension.

Despite such shortcomings over definition, the existence of several forms of hypotensive disease is recognised.

Hypotension can occur after haemorrhage or in other forms of shock and the management of this acute and potentially dangerous form of low blood pressure is usually with vasopressor sympathomimetics, notably noradrenaline or dopamine, and is described under Shock (below). Another situation in which acute hypotension can develop is during anaesthesia and surgery; spinal or epidural block is associated with a greater risk than many other forms of anaesthesia. Again, sympathomimetics, and ephedrine particularly, are used as vasopressors,[3] and this topic is discussed further on p.1060.

Chronic forms of hypotension also exist and include orthostatic (postural) hypotension and neurally mediated hypotension. The management of orthostatic hypotension is discussed on p.1040 under fludrocortisone which is usually the first pharmacological treatment to be tried in this condition. Neurally mediated hypotension, which has also been known as neurocardiogenic syncope, neurally mediated syncope, vasodepressor syncope, or vasovagal syncope, is a common cause of recurrent lightheadedness (presyncope) and syncope in persons with structurally normal hearts. It is characterised by a paradoxical neurocardiogenic reflex that ultimately results in vasodilatation, bradycardia, and hypotension. Fludrocortisone, a beta blocker (such as atenolol or metoprolol), and disopyramide are reported to be standard drugs used.[4-6] Antimuscarinics, such as propantheline bromide, have also been tried. Selective serotonin reuptake inhibitors have been suggested for refractory cases.[6] In a few patients cardiac pacing may be required.

One contentious issue is whether general and non-specific symptoms of ill health such as mental and physical fatigue, depression, and anxiety can be attributed to a low blood pressure (for example, a systolic pressure below 110 mmHg or diastolic pressure below 60 mmHg).[7] In the UK and the USA such an association has never been accepted whereas in some European countries (e.g. Germany) a wide range of pharmaceutical preparations usually containing a sympathomimetic has been available for treatment. Some evidence is being presented to support the theory,[8,9] as well as to suggest a possible link between the chronic fatigue syndrome and neurally mediated hypotension,[4,5] although implications for treatment are far from clear.

1. Joint National Committee. The sixth report of the joint national committee on prevention, detection, evaluation, and treatment of high blood pressure (JNC VI). *Arch Intern Med* 1997; **157:** 2413–46. Correction. *ibid.* 1998; **158:** 573.
2. Guidelines Sub-Committee. 1993 guidelines for the management of mild hypertension: memorandum from a WHO/ISH meeting. *Bull WHO* 1993; **71:** 503–17.
3. McCrae AF, Wildsmith JAW. Prevention and treatment of hypotension during central neural block. *Br J Anaesth* 1993; **70:** 672–80.
4. Rowe PC, *et al.* Is neurally mediated hypotension an unrecognised cause of chronic fatigue? *Lancet* 1995; **345:** 623–4.
5. Bou-Holaigah I, *et al.* The relationship between neurally mediated hypotension and the chronic fatigue syndrome. *JAMA* 1995; **274:** 961–7.
6. Lazarus JC, Mauro VF. Syncope: pathophysiology, diagnosis, and pharmacotherapy. *Ann Pharmacother* 1996; **30:** 994–1005.
7. Mann A. Psychiatric symptoms and low blood pressure. *Br Med J* 1992; **304:** 64–5.
8. Rosengren A, *et al.* Low systolic blood pressure and self perceived wellbeing in middle aged men. *Br Med J* 1993; **306:** 243–6.
9. Barrett-Connor E, Palinkas LA. Low blood pressure and depression in older men: a population based study. *Br Med J* 1994; **308:** 446–9.

Kawasaki disease

Cardiac effects including coronary artery abnormalities are the major complications of Kawasaki disease, also known as mucocutaneous lymph node syndrome of childhood. Normal immunoglobulin and aspirin are used in its initial management, and antiplatelet therapy, usually with aspirin, may be continued long term to prevent coronary thrombosis. Further details concerning the overall management of Kawasaki disease are provided under Normal Immunoglobulins, p.1524.

Myocardial infarction

Myocardial infarction is defined as necrosis of heart muscle caused by coronary artery occlusion, usually due to thrombosis at the site of a recently ruptured atheromatous plaque; in a few patients coronary embolism or spasm, arteritis, spontaneous thrombosis, or a sudden severe rise in blood pressure, as in phaeochromocytoma, is responsible. The immediate consequence of coronary occlusion is myocardial ischaemia which leads to impaired contractility, arrhythmias, and eventually myocardial cell death. The lay term 'heart attack' describes both sudden cardiac death and myocardial infarction. Sudden death often occurs before treatment is possible and is usually due to ventricular fibrillation. The majority of patients resuscitated from ventricular fibrillation develop features of myocardial infarction or have coronary artery disease. The initial symptoms of acute myocardial infarction are usually chest pain, breathlessness, and sweating. The chest pain is typically severe and resembles that of angina pectoris, being precordial with radiation to the neck, lower jaw, and left arm. Other symptoms include nausea and vomiting, bradycardia, hypotension, and apprehension. Half of all myocardial infarcts are said to be silent, that is asymptomatic.

The introduction of aspirin and thrombolytics like streptokinase transformed the management of acute myocardial infarction and many more people now survive the initial attack and achieve a better recovery of left ventricular function.[1] Further improvement in survival and morbidity should be possible if more candidates for thrombolysis can be identified and treated early and if the risks of recurrence and haemorrhage can be reduced as a result of the continuing development of thrombolytics and of adjunctive antiplatelet and antithrombin drugs.

Numerous large-scale studies have helped to establish various aspects of treatment and more are planned.

Guidelines for the early management of myocardial infarction[2-4] emphasise the importance of the rapid provision of life support, adequate pain relief, accurate diagnosis, immediate administration of aspirin, and, where appropriate, thrombolytic treatment ideally commencing within 90 minutes of the call for help. The immediate aims are to relieve pain and anxiety and to reopen the occluded artery (reperfusion or revascularisation) as soon as possible thus limiting damage to the heart. After reperfusion long-term management aims to maintain patency and to treat or protect against complications of the post-infarction period such as arrhythmias, left ventricular failure, persistent angina, and venous thrombo-embolism. Cardiac rupture and aneurysms may also occur after myocardial infarction. The ideal is of course to prevent myocardial infarction from occurring in the first place.

The **management** of myocardial infarction is discussed in more detail under the headings Early Management (of the acute phase), Long-term Management (including secondary prevention), and Primary Prevention (in healthy subjects and those with risk factors).

Early management. Those patients with myocardial infarction who develop ventricular fibrillation very quickly, often within the first hour after the onset of symptoms of infarction, die before they reach hospital; this is often referred to as sudden cardiac death. Ventricular fibrillation is treated by defibrillation followed by adrenaline and possibly lignocaine if defibrillation alone is unsuccessful (see under Advanced Cardiac Life Support, above, for further details). Treatment must be instituted quickly and in order to achieve this there are paramedic ambulance teams experienced in defibrillation and programmes aimed at educating the public in the basic techniques of cardiopulmonary resuscitation. Patients with suspected myocardial infarction should be admitted to hospital and where possible managed in a coronary care unit.

As already stated, the immediate priority in patients with myocardial infarction is relief of pain and anxiety. Pain should be relieved with an opioid analgesic, usually diamorphine or morphine given intravenously (see Myocardial Infarction Pain, p.10); an antiemetic such as metoclopramide intravenously may also be necessary. An inhaled mixture of nitrous oxide and oxygen (Entonox) has sometimes been used to provide pain relief before arrival in hospital; sublingual glyceryl trinitrate or an alternative fast-acting nitrate may also be given. A benzodiazepine may be useful for anxiety.

Reperfusion is usually achieved with a thrombolytic such as streptokinase given intravenously and the antiplatelet drug aspirin by mouth;[5] the additive benefit of streptokinase and aspirin was established by, for example, the ISIS-2 study.[6] Aspirin can be given immediately and the thrombolytic as soon as an ECG has been performed to confirm the diagnosis. Some also give heparin at this stage. Alternatively, reperfusion may be achieved with angioplasty.

A *diagnosis* is made mainly from clinical history, particularly typical chest pain lasting more than 30 minutes (although this is absent in many patients), and a characteristic ECG. Rapid diagnosis is important so that, if indicated, thrombolysis can be given as soon as possible. The greatest benefit from thrombolysis appears to be achieved in patients with an ECG demonstrating ST-segment elevation or new left bundle-branch block.[1,2] Other diagnostic techniques include measurement of cardiac enzymes and echocardiography.

Thrombolysis. Thrombolytics are given intravenously to break up the thrombus or clot and restore the patency of the coronary artery thereby limiting infarct size and irreversible damage to the myocardium. Several large studies have established that thrombolytics can preserve left ventricular function and improve short-term and one-year mortality figures;[7,8] benefit has been maintained in 5-year[9] and 10-year[10] follow-up studies, although one study failed to show an improvement in 3- to 8-year survival rate.[11] Reduction of ECG abnormalities and modification of ventricular remodelling may contribute to the benefits seen with thrombolytics. It is generally accepted that, subject to an appropriate ECG and provided there are no contra-indications (see Precautions under Streptokinase, p.950), the sooner thrombolytic treatment is started the better. Trials such as the GISSI-1 study[12] and the ISIS-2 study[6] helped to establish that mortality is reduced if thrombolytics are administered within 6 hours of the onset of symptoms[13] and further studies provided evidence[14,15] that patients presenting within 12 hours should receive a thrombolytic. There is insufficient experience to determine whether the benefits outweigh the risks when thrombolytics are given later than 12 hours.[13] There have been some reports of early excess mortality on days 0 to 1 ('early hazard') attributed to cardiac rupture in patients with other known risk factors for early hazard (over 64 years of age, female sex, raised blood pressure on admission) given late thrombolytic treatment (after 6 hours).[13,16,17] Thus the ideal is to give a thrombolytic as soon as possible. The British Heart Foundation Working Group[2] has recommended administration within 90 minutes of alerting the general practitioner or ambulance service ('call to needle' time); an American group[18] has recommended injection within 70 minutes. Once in hospital, the time between admission and administration of a thrombolytic (the 'door to needle' time) varies widely and could be improved; a median interval of 3 to 4½ hours between onset of pain and the start of treatment has been cited for British hospitals.[19] Prehospital thrombolysis by general practitioners[20-23] or paramedics,[18,22] after ECG diagnosis, is feasible and can reduce the interval between symptom onset and administration of the thrombolytic.

Streptokinase has been the most widely used thrombolytic. Several large studies have compared clinical benefit in terms of improved left ventricular function and mortality and have shown no difference between streptokinase and other thrombolytics, including saruplase,[24] the tissue plasminogen activator alteplase,[25] anistreplase,[26] and reteplase[27] in overall efficacy. In the GUSTO-I study,[28] accelerated or 'front loaded' alteplase (that is, rapid intravenous administration over 1½ hours rather than the conventional 3 hours) was more effective than streptokinase, although the study was criticised for not comparing like with like. On the other hand, alteplase might be associated with a greater risk of stroke than streptokinase.[29] Another study (GUSTO-III)[30] comparing bolus injections of reteplase with accelerated alteplase found no difference in mortality rate. Factors such as cost, method of administration, and contra-indications help to determine the choice of thrombolytic, but ensuring that a thrombolytic is administered as soon as possible is probably more important than which is given.[5,31] If streptokinase or anistreplase, so-called antigenic thrombolytics, have been administered recently, non-antigenic agents such as alteplase or urokinase should be given.

The overall effectiveness of thrombolytics is limited by persistent coronary occlusion, re-occlusion, and infrequent but serious bleeding complications including intracranial haemorrhage. Different thrombolytic administration regimens, such as bolus injections of reteplase and combinations of thrombolytics for example alteplase with streptokinase and alteplase with saruplase, are being investigated in attempts to improve patency rates. A study[32] comparing double-bolus administration of alteplase with accelerated alteplase was terminated early when excess deaths were found in the group receiving bolus injections. If re-occlusion occurs further thrombolytic therapy may be given. Alternatively angioplasty may be performed (see below). Antiplatelet and antithrombin drugs are given as adjuncts to thrombolytics.

Antiplatelet drugs. The value of giving aspirin by mouth, as an antiplatelet drug, was shown by the ISIS-2 study[6] in which aspirin started during the first 24 hours after myocardial infarction reduced mortality and also reduced the incidence of re-infarction and stroke. Combination with streptokinase proved to be more effective than either streptokinase or aspirin alone. Aspirin should therefore be taken as soon as possible when myocardial infarction is suspected and the tablet chewed so that some buccal absorption occurs. Despite the clear benefits of aspirin therapy, it still appears to be underused.[33,34] New antiplatelets, such as abciximab, are under investigation as adjuncts to thrombolytic therapy.

Anticoagulants. Heparin was widely used in acute myocardial infarction before thrombolytics were available, but the necessity for adjuvant therapy with heparin in addition to aspirin is not certain.[35] Many centres administer parenteral heparin with or shortly after the thrombolytic to prevent the re-occlusion of the coronary artery often associated with thrombolysis. Alteplase appears to open occluded arteries more rapidly but to cause re-occlusion more often than streptokinase, and thus heparin has been regarded by some as particularly necessary when alteplase is used. The ISIS-3 study[26] indicated that the addition of subcutaneous heparin (from about 4 hours after randomisation) did have a slight advantage over a thrombolytic and aspirin alone, but the benefit was not large and there was no substantial difference in mortality, whereas the incidence of major bleeds and haemorrhagic stroke was increased. An overview of randomised studies[36] found that in patients receiving aspirin, addition of heparin (either intravenous or subcutaneous) produced a small reduction in mortality but was associated with an excess of major bleeds. The authors concluded that the routine addition of heparin to aspirin could not be justified. Alternatives to heparin such as the thrombin inhibitor hirudin are also under investigation although results so far have been disappointing. Studies (GUSTO-IIa,[37] TIMI-9A,[38] and HIT-III[39]) comparing heparin with a recombinant hirudin had to be stopped because of higher than expected haemorrhagic stroke rates. In GUSTO-IIa and TIMI-9A a higher stroke rate was also seen in the heparin group. Use of higher doses of heparin than in GUSTO-I and inclusion of high-risk patients may explain the stroke incidence. GUSTO-IIa and TIMI-9A restarted as GUSTO-IIb[40] and TIMI-9B,[41] respectively, using lower doses of heparin and the recombinant hirudin desirudin. The results of GUSTO-IIb[40] showed that desirudin was still associated with increased haemorrhage although not with major bleeding and produced only a small benefit over heparin. TIMI-9B[41] reported no difference between heparin and desirudin. The authors suggested that desirudin may have advantages over heparin as it has a more consistent anticoagulant effect that reduces the need to adjust infusion rates and it may be useful in patients who develop heparin-induced thrombocytopenia. Other thrombin inhibitors under investigation include argatroban and bivalirudin. Heparin may also be given prophylactically to myocardial infarction patients at risk of developing left ventricular mural thrombosis with subsequent systemic embolisation. Patients with complications following myocardial infarction who are likely to be immobile for several days should also receive heparin prophylaxis.

Angioplasty. Percutaneous transluminal coronary angioplasty is effective at re-opening occluded coronary arteries and immediate angioplasty (termed primary angioplasty) has been performed as an alternative method of reperfusion to thrombolysis. Studies have compared the two methods. A substudy of GUSTO-IIb suggested that angioplasty may have a small advantage over thrombolysis,[42] although in another study thrombolytic therapy was as effective and cheaper than primary angioplasty.[43] A review of randomised studies comparing primary angioplasty with thrombolysis concluded that primary angioplasty was associated with lower mortality and re-infarction rates at hospital discharge or 30 days post myocardial infarction.[44] However, the numbers of patients included in these studies were small and until larger studies with longer follow-up periods have been conducted no definitive recommendations can be made on the choice of angioplasty or thrombolysis. Where angioplasty is available it may be considered for patients in whom thrombolytics are contra-indicated or in patients at highest risk such as those over 75 years of age, or those with anterior infarction, persistent tachycardia, cardiogenic shock, or sustained hypotension.[45] Since angioplasty is only available in specialised cardiac centres, thrombolysis will remain the method of reperfusion for the majority of patients. Angioplasty may also be considered when thrombolytic therapy has failed to unblock the artery (so-called 'rescue' angioplasty). Angioplasty has been used in attempts to abolish residual stenoses that usually remain after thrombolysis and that may re-occlude, although such use within hours or days of thrombolysis has not been successful.[46] The associated therapy, such as antithrombotic therapy, that is usually necessary in conjunction with angioplasty to prevent restenosis is discussed under Reperfusion and Revascularisation Procedures (below).

Thus, at present, standard early therapy for the majority of patients with myocardial infarction is streptokinase with aspirin, and possibly heparin. Other early treatment options include beta blockers, nitrates, ACE inhibitors, magnesium, and calcium-channel blockers.

Beta blockers. Before thrombolytics were widely used the intravenous administration of beta blockers, such as atenolol and metoprolol, in the early period following myocardial infarction was associated with a reduction in mortality. Contributory mechanisms were considered to be a reduction in size of infarction or number of re-infarctions and an antiarrhythmic effect, although the ISIS-1 study[47] suggested that beta blockers improved early survival by reducing the incidence of cardiac rupture. The role of beta blockers in the thrombolytic era is less certain, but an overview of randomised studies[48] indicated that early use of intravenous beta blockers definitely reduced mortality after myocardial infarction. They appear to be less popular in the UK than in the US.[49]

Nitrates. The use of intravenous nitrates (glyceryl trinitrate or sodium nitroprusside), started within 24 hours of the onset of pain, has been associated with a reduction in mortality in patients with acute myocardial infarction,[50] although this was before the routine use of thrombolytics, and in a more recent study molsidomine and its active metabolite linsidomine (a nitric oxide donor) had no effect on mortality.[51] Nevertheless, the empirical use of intravenous glyceryl trinitrate in the acute phase of myocardial infarction is widespread and appears to be safe, as was demonstrated in the GISSI-3 study;[52] these workers considered that glyceryl trinitrate could be given when clinically indicated in addition to thrombolysis, aspirin, and a beta blocker.

ACE inhibitors. Early treatment with ACE inhibitors as an adjunct to standard thrombolytic therapy is less well established than post-infarction treatment. Favourable results have been reported in the GISSI-3[52] and the ISIS-4[53] studies where lisinopril and captopril, respectively, were given by mouth starting within 24 hours of the onset of chest pain and in the Chinese Cardiac Study[54] (CCS-1) where captopril was given by mouth within 36 hours of the onset of symptoms. In the GISSI-3 study the beneficial effects were maintained at 6 months.[55] However, the CONSENSUS II study was terminated early when it was found that enalapril, given intravenously as enalaprilat and begun within 24 hours of the onset of chest pain, did not improve survival during the 180 days after infarction.[56] A substudy on some of the patients did however suggest that they may have benefited from early treatment since left ventricular dilatation was attenuated.[57] An interaction between aspirin and enalapril was postulated as one of the reasons for the overall lack of benefit seen and further analysis of the CONSENSUS II results found that the beneficial effect of enalapril was reduced in those patients already taking aspirin.[58] A systematic review of the CONSENSUS II, GISSI-3, ISIS-4, and CCS-1 studies found lower 30-day cumulative mortality and incidence of non-fatal heart failure among ACE inhibitor recipients.[59] However, the size of benefit in these studies of largely unselected patients is much smaller than in the studies of patients with left ventricular dysfunction. The authors of ISIS-4[53] recommended that early treatment with an ACE inhibitor should be considered in all patients, except those with cardiogenic shock or persistent severe hypotension, and that treatment should be reviewed after a few weeks and continued in those with left ventricular dysfunction. This view is supported by the guidelines of the American College of Cardiology and American Heart Association.[4] Others[60,61] consider that routine early treatment with an ACE inhibitor in unselected patients is not warranted and such use should be reserved for patients with signs of heart failure (see under Long-term Management, below). The European Society of Cardiology recognises that there are valid arguments for both views and advocates the early use of an ACE inhibitor if symptoms of heart failure appear.[3]

Magnesium. Magnesium has an important physiological role in maintaining the ion balance in muscle including the myocardium. Administration of magnesium might have an antiarrhythmic effect and might protect the myocardium against reperfusion injury and in an overview of studies in patients with suspected myocardial infarction administration of intravenous magnesium, generally within 12 hours of the onset of chest pain, had reduced mortality.[62] The beneficial effect on mortality appeared to be confirmed by the LIMIT-2 study[63] and at follow-up an average of 2.7 years later;[64] there was no evidence of an antiarrhythmic effect. Unfortunately in the large ISIS-4 study[53] magnesium had no effect on mortality. No benefit was seen in any of the subgroups, including those not receiving thrombolytics. The LIMIT-2 workers[64] considered that timing of magnesium administration in relation to thrombolytic therapy or spontaneous reperfusion was likely to be critical. In their study a loading injection of magnesium was given before thrombolysis and a maintenance infusion of magnesium continued over the following 24 hours. In the ISIS-4 study magnesium was given after thrombolysis was started; it was intended that magnesium be started immediately after the early lytic phase, that is, in the first hour or so. At present, the routine use of magnesium cannot be recommended.

Calcium-channel blockers. Studies have not shown a reduction in mortality when calcium-channel blockers are given in the early phase of acute myocardial infarction. However, since myocardial stunning has been linked to intracellular calcium overload[65] there has been speculation that calcium-channel blockers might benefit patients about to undergo reperfusion. This is yet to be confirmed.

Metabolic support. Infusions containing glucose, insulin, and potassium have been used in small numbers of patients with the aim of providing metabolic support in the acute phase of myocardial infarction. A meta-analysis of randomised controlled trials that were performed before the widespread use of thrombolytics found that mortality was reduced in recipients of glucose-insulin-potassium.[66] Reduced mortality has also been reported in diabetic patients with myocardial infarction given insulin-glucose infusions (see Myocardial Infarction under Insulin, p.329). The role of metabolic support in acute myocardial infarction may warrant further investigation.

Long-term management. Patients who survive the immediate post-myocardial infarction period remain at high risk for cardiovascular mortality. The main predictors of poor outcome are the extent of left ventricular dysfunction, residual myocardial ischaemia, and ventricular arrhythmias. Follow-up should include the identification and modification of risk factors for ischaemic heart disease (see under Atherosclerosis, abovelp.782). Exercise testing can be used after myocardial infarction to help identify those at high risk for recurrent ischaemic events and to select patients needing coronary angiography.[67] In patients who develop angina soon after myocardial infarction, exercise testing may be unhelpful and potentially hazardous, although many will need angiography to determine whether angioplasty or bypass surgery is required. Myocardial imaging techniques and pharmacological stress testing may also have a role (see Ischaemic Heart Disease under Dipyridamole, p.857).

Drug therapy is also important in the long-term management of patients following myocardial infarction. *Aspirin*, given during the acute phase and then continued for one to two years, has been shown to reduce mortality and re-infarction rates. Studies[68] and a meta-analysis[69] have confirmed the benefit of prolonged antiplatelet treatment in the secondary prevention of myocardial infarction and patients should probably receive antiplatelet therapy indefinitely.[4] Alternative antiplatelet drugs such as clopidogrel, sulphinpyrazone, or ticlopidine may be considered in the few patients intolerant of aspirin. The routine long-term use of *oral anticoagulation* after the acute phase of myocardial infarction has been difficult to justify. In the ASPECT study,[70] such treatment had only a limited effect on mortality but did reduce the risk of cerebrovascular events and of re-infarction; as expected there was an increased incidence of bleeding complications. Those at high risk of systemic embolism because of atrial fibrillation, heart failure, or mobile mural thrombus will require prophylaxis with oral anticoagulants, but for other patients aspirin will probably be preferred.[71,72] Addition of low-dose warfarin (1 or 3 mg) to low-dose aspirin (80 mg) has not conferred clinical benefit above that achieved with moderate-dose aspirin alone (160 mg).[73] Long-term prophylactic treatment with oral *beta blockers* (usually propranolol, metoprolol, or timolol) has reduced mortality and the rate of re-infarction. In patients with no contra-indications to beta-blocker therapy (see Precautions, p.829) they are usually started before hospital discharge and continued for a minimum of one year. Some only use them in patients with hypertension or angina pectoris following myocardial infarction; their use in low-risk, asymptomatic patients is more controversial. However, a recent survey of 201 752 patients who had suffered a myocardial infarction found that low-risk patients and those with conditions often considered to be contra-indications also benefited from administration of a beta blocker.[92] Beta blockers seem to be underused particularly in elderly patients even though there is clear evidence of benefit in this group.[74] *Calcium-channel blockers* are not routinely used in the long-term management of myocardial infarction although in selected patients without heart failure verapamil or diltiazem may be of some benefit if beta blockers are contra-indicated. *ACE inhibitors* reduce left ventricular remodelling, a process which sometimes follows myocardial infarction and is a recognised precursor of symptomatic heart failure. Myocardial infarction patients with left ventricular dysfunction benefit from long-term oral administration of ACE inhibitors such as captopril (the SAVE study),[75] ramipril (the AIRE and AIRE extension (AIREX) studies),[76-78] or trandolapril (the TRACE study)[79] started about 3 days, or more, after infarction. As noted under Early Management (above), favourable results have been reported with ACE inhibitors started early and continued for at least four to six weeks. An expert panel[80] has recommended that all patients with signs of left ventricular dysfunction at any time after an acute myocardial infarction should receive prompt treatment with an ACE inhibitor (provided there were no contra-indications) and that such treatment should be long term. The ACE inhibitor could be started within 24 hours of onset of the infarction. The panel were unable to agree on whether all infarction patients should receive early treatment with an ACE inhibitor. There is some evidence that ACE inhibitors may reduce re-infarction rates and this is being investigated in large-scale studies.[81] *Statins*, such as simvastatin and pravastatin, have a more marked cholesterol-lowering effect than older lipid regulating drugs and studies have shown them to be effective in the primary and secondary prevention of myocardial infarction in patients with hypercholesterolaemia. More recently, their benefit has also been demonstrated in patients with average, rather than elevated, cholesterol concentrations. Thus, their use has been advocated in all patients who have suffered a myocardial infarction (see Hyperlipidaemias, p.1265). Some patients, for example those with myocardial ischaemia or poor left ventricular function may require the long-term administration of *nitrates*, but recent studies have thrown doubt on the routine use of nitrates or other nitric oxide donors. In the GISSI-3 study[52] there was no significant benefit from the use of transdermal glyceryl trinitrate for 6 weeks post-infarction; in the ISIS-4 study[53] oral isosorbide mononitrate had no effect on 35-day mortality, and in the ESPRIM study[51] molsidomine had no effect on 35-day or longer term mortality. Patients with acute myocardial infarction may have magnesium deficiency and long-term treatment with *oral magnesium* has been tried, but in one study was associated with an increased risk of adverse cardiac events and could not be recommended for secondary prevention.[82]

Post-infarction problems such as heart failure (left ventricular dysfunction), angina pectoris, and arrhythmias are discussed on p.785, p.780, and p.782, respectively.

Primary prevention. Myocardial infarction is one of the principal causes of death in industrialised countries. Risk factors and general preventive measures are discussed under Atherosclerosis, above. The beneficial effects of lowering raised blood pressure and cholesterol concentrations on cardiac mortality rates are discussed under Hypertension, above, and Hyperlipidaemias, p.1265, respectively. See also above for the protective effect of statins.

The benefit of taking *aspirin* as an antiplatelet drug following myocardial infarction is well-established, but its role in primary prevention has been less clear. Two large studies in the UK[83] and in the US[84] in healthy male physicians produced conflicting results. In the UK study there was no reduction in the incidence of fatal and non-fatal myocardial infarction in those who had taken aspirin, while the US study did show a reduction in subjects 50 years of age or older. A large observational study in healthy US nurses[85] indicated that aspirin might reduce the risk of first myocardial infarction in women. The American Heart Association[86,87] states that aspirin may be warranted for middle-aged and older men whose risks of a first myocardial infarction outweigh the possible adverse effects of long-term use. Aspirin may also reduce the risk of first myocardial infarction in patients with stable chronic angina.[88] The Antiplatelet Trialists' Collaboration[69] concluded that aspirin or some other antiplatelet regimen offers worthwhile protection against myocardial infarction in a wide range of patients at high risk of occlusive vascular disease, but that benefit was not established for primary prevention in low risk subjects. The Thrombosis Prevention Trial[89] in males at high risk of developing occlusive vascular disease and the Hypertension Optimal Treatment (HOT) trial[90] have, more recently, confirmed that aspirin reduces the incidence of myocardial infarction in these at-risk groups. The Thrombosis Prevention Trial also investigated the use of low-intensity *warfarin* and found that its use reduced the incidence of ischaemic heart disease (defined as coronary death or myocardial infarction). A greater reduction in ischaemic heart disease incidence was seen with a combination of aspirin and low-intensity warfarin but there was increased incidence of fatal stroke. Low-intensity warfarin may be a possible alternative to aspirin therapy in high-risk males intolerant of aspirin although careful selection of subjects is necessary to minimise risk of bleeding. Studies of Left Ventricular Dysfunction (SOLVD) trials have indicated that *ACE inhibitors*, in this case enalapril,[91] might protect against myocardial infarction, unstable angina, and cardiac death in patients with symptomatic or asymptomatic heart failure.

1. Anderson HV, Willerson JT. Thrombolysis in acute myocardial infarction. *N Engl J Med* 1993; **329:** 703–9.
2. Weston CFM, *et al.* Guidelines for the early management of patients with myocardial infarction. *Br Med J* 1994; **308:** 767–71.
3. The Task Force on the Management of Acute Myocardial Infarction of the European Society of Cardiology. Acute myocardial infarction: pre-hospital and in-hospital management. *Eur Heart J* 1996; **17:** 43–63.
4. Ryan TJ, *et al.* ACC/AHA guidelines for the management of patients with acute myocardial infarction: a report of the American College of Cardiology/American Heart Association Task Force on Practice Guidelines (Committee on Management of Acute Myocardial Infarction). *J Am Coll Cardiol* 1996; **28:** 1328–1428.
5. Collins R, *et al.* Aspirin, heparin, and fibrinolytic therapy in suspected acute myocardial infarction. *N Engl J Med* 1997; **336:** 847–60.
6. Second International Study of Infarct Survival Collaborative Group. Randomised trial of intravenous streptokinase, oral aspirin, both, or neither among 17 187 cases of suspected acute myocardial infarction: ISIS-2. *Lancet* 1988; **ii:** 349–60.
7. Gruppo Italiano per lo Studio della Streptochinasi nell'Infarto Miocardico (GISSI). Long-term effects of intravenous thrombolysis in acute myocardial infarction: final report of the GISSI study. *Lancet* 1987; **ii:** 871–4.
8. Wilcox RG, *et al.* Effects of alteplase in acute myocardial infarction: 6-month results from the ASSET study. *Lancet* 1990; **335:** 1175–8.
9. Simoons ML, *et al.* Long-term benefit of early thrombolytic therapy in patients with acute myocardial infarction: 5 year follow-up of a trial conducted by the Interuniversity Cardiology Institute of the Netherlands. *J Am Coll Cardiol* 1989; **14:** 1609–15.
10. Baigent C, *et al.* ISIS-2: 10 year survival among patients with suspected acute myocardial infarction in randomised comparison of intravenous streptokinase, oral aspirin, both, or neither. *Br Med J* 1998; **316:** 1337–43.
11. Cerqueira MD, *et al.* Long-term survival in 618 patients from the Western Washington streptokinase in myocardial infarction trials. *J Am Coll Cardiol* 1992; **20:** 1452–9.
12. Gruppo Italiano per lo Studio della Streptochinasi nell'Infarto Miocardico (GISSI). Effectiveness of intravenous thrombolytic treatment in acute myocardial infarction. *Lancet* 1986; **i:** 397–402.
13. Fibrinolytic Therapy Trialists' (FTT) Collaborative Group. Indications for fibrinolytic therapy in suspected acute myocardial infarction: collaborative overview of early mortality and major morbidity results from all randomised trials of more than 1000 patients. *Lancet* 1994; **343:** 311–22.
14. LATE Study Group. Late assessment of thrombolytic efficacy (LATE) study with alteplase 6–24 hours after onset of acute myocardial infarction. *Lancet* 1993; **342:** 759–66.
15. EMERAS (Estudio Multicéntrico Estreptoquinasa Repúblicas de América del Sur) Collaborative Group. Randomised trial of late thrombolysis in patients with suspected acute myocardial infarction. *Lancet* 1993; **342:** 767–72.
16. Davis RC. Fibrinolytic therapy in suspected acute myocardial infarction. *Lancet* 1994; **343:** 912.
17. Carlsson J, *et al.* Fibrinolytic therapy in suspected acute myocardial infarction. *Lancet* 1994; **343:** 912–13.
18. Weaver WD, *et al.* Prehospital-initiated vs hospital-initiated thrombolytic therapy: the myocardial infarction triage and intervention trial. *JAMA* 1993; **270:** 1211–16.
19. Cobbe SM. Thrombolysis in myocardial infarction. *Br Med J* 1994; **308:** 216–17.
20. GREAT Group. Feasibility, safety, and efficacy of domiciliary thrombolysis by general practitioners: Grampian region early anistreplase trial. *Br Med J* 1992; **305:** 548–53.
21. The European Myocardial Infarction Project Group. Prehospital thrombolytic therapy in patients with suspected acute myocardial infarction. *N Engl J Med* 1993; **329:** 383–9.
22. Grijseels EWM, *et al.* Pre-hospital thrombolytic therapy with either alteplase or streptokinase: practical applications, complications and long-term results in 529 patients. *Eur Heart J* 1995; **16:** 1833–8.
23. Rawles J. Magnitude of benefit from earlier thrombolytic treatment in acute myocardial infarction: new evidence from Grampian region early anistreplase trial (GREAT). *Br Med J* 1996; **312:** 212–15.
24. PRIMI Trial Study Group. Randomised double-blind trial of recombinant pro-urokinase against streptokinase in acute myocardial infarction. *Lancet* 1989; **i:** 863–8.
25. GISSI-2 and International Study Group. Six-month survival in 20 891 patients with acute myocardial infarction randomized between alteplase and streptokinase with or without heparin. *Eur Heart J* 1992; **13:** 1692–7.
26. Third International Study of Infarct Survival Collaborative Group. ISIS-3: a randomised comparison of streptokinase vs tissue plasminogen activator vs anistreplase and of aspirin plus heparin vs aspirin alone among 41 299 cases of suspected acute myocardial infarction. *Lancet* 1992; **339:** 753–70.
27. International Joint Efficacy Comparison of Thrombolytics. Randomised, double-blind comparison of reteplase double-bolus administration with streptokinase in acute myocardial infarction (INJECT): trial to investigate equivalence. *Lancet* 1995; **346:** 329–36.
28. The GUSTO Investigators. An international randomized trial comparing four thrombolytic strategies for acute myocardial infarction. *N Engl J Med* 1993; **329:** 673–82.
29. Vaitkus PT, *et al.* Stroke complicating acute myocardial infarction: a meta-analysis of risk modification by anticoagulation and thrombolytic therapy. *Arch Intern Med* 1992; **152:** 2020–4.
30. The Global Use of Strategies to Open Occluded Coronary Arteries (GUSTO III) Investigators. A comparison of reteplase with alteplase for acute myocardial infarction. *N Engl J Med* 1997; **337:** 1118–23.
31. Ridker PM, *et al.* Large-scale trials of thrombolytic therapy for acute myocardial infarction: GISSI-2, ISIS-3, and GUSTO-1. *Ann Intern Med* 1993; **119:** 530–2.
32. The Continuous Infusion versus Double-Bolus Administration of Alteplase (COBALT) Investigators. A comparison of continuous infusion of alteplase with double-bolus administration for acute myocardial infarction. *N Engl J Med* 1997; **337:** 1124–30.
33. Moher M, Johnson N. Use of aspirin by general practitioners in suspected acute myocardial infarction. *Br Med J* 1994; **308:** 760.
34. Wyllie HR, Dunn FG. Pre-hospital opiate and aspirin administration in patients with suspected myocardial infarction. *Br Med J* 1994; **308:** 760–1.
35. Ridker PM, *et al.* Are both aspirin and heparin justified as adjuncts to thrombolytic therapy for acute myocardial infarction. *Lancet* 1993; **341:** 1574–7.
36. Collins R, *et al.* Clinical effects of anticoagulant therapy in suspected acute myocardial infarction: systematic overview of randomised trials. *Br Med J* 1996; **313:** 652–9.
37. The Global Use of Strategies to Open Occluded Coronary Arteries (GUSTO) IIa Investigators. Randomized trial of intravenous heparin versus recombinant hirudin for acute coronary syndromes. *Circulation* 1994; **90:** 1631–7.
38. Antman EM, *et al.* Hirudin in acute myocardial infarction: safety report from the Thrombolysis and Thrombin Inhibition in Myocardial Infarction (TIMI) 9A trial. *Circulation* 1994; **90:** 1624–30.
39. Neuhaus K-L, *et al.* Safety observations from the pilot phase of the randomized r-Hirudin for Improvement of Thrombolysis (HIT-III) study: a study of the Arbeitsgemeinschaft Leitender Kardiologischer Krankenhausärzte (ALKK). *Circulation* 1994; **90:** 1638–42.
40. The Global Use of Strategies to Open Occluded Coronary Arteries (GUSTO) IIb Investigators. A comparison of recombinant hirudin with heparin for the treatment of acute coronary syndromes. *N Engl J Med* 1996; **335:** 775–82.
41. Antman EM. Hirudin in acute myocardial infarction: thrombolysis and thrombin inhibition in myocardial infarction (TIMI) 9B trial. *Circulation* 1996; **94:** 911–21.
42. The Global Use of Strategies to Open Occluded Coronary Arteries in Acute Coronary Syndromes (GUSTO IIb) Angioplasty Substudy Investigators. A clinical trial comparing primary coronary angioplasty with tissue plasminogen activator for acute myocardial infarction. *N Engl J Med* 1997; **336:** 1621–8. Correction. *ibid.;* **337:** 287.
43. Every NR, *et al.* A comparison of thrombolytic therapy with primary coronary angioplasty for acute myocardial infarction. *N Engl J Med* 1996; **335:** 1253–60.
44. Weaver WD, *et al.* Comparison of primary coronary angioplasty and intravenous thrombolytic therapy for acute myocardial infarction: a quantitative review. *JAMA* 1997; **278:** 2093–8. Correction. *ibid.* 1998; **279:** 1876.
45. Lange RA, Hillis LD. Immediate angioplasty for acute myocardial infarction. *N Engl J Med* 1993; **328:** 726–8.
46. Landau C, *et al.* Percutaneous transluminal coronary angioplasty. *N Engl J Med* 1994; **330:** 981–93.
47. First International Study of Infarct Survival Collaborative Group. Mechanisms for the early mortality reduction produced by beta-blockade started early in acute myocardial infarction: ISIS-1. *Lancet* 1988; **i:** 921–3.
48. Teo KK, *et al.* Effects of prophylactic antiarrhythmic drug therapy in acute myocardial infarction: an overview of results from randomized controlled trials. *JAMA* 1993; **270:** 1589–95.
49. Owen A. Intravenous β blockade in acute myocardial infarction. *Br Med J* 1998; **317:** 226–7.
50. Yusuf S, *et al.* Effect of intravenous nitrates on mortality in acute myocardial infarction: an overview of the randomised trials. *Lancet* 1988; **i:** 1088–92.
51. European Study of Prevention of Infarct with Molsidomine (ESPRIM) Group. The ESPRIM trial: short-term treatment of acute myocardial infarction with molsidomine. *Lancet* 1994; **344:** 91–7.
52. Gruppo Italiano per lo Studio della Sopravvivenza nell'Infarto Miocardico. GISSI-3: effects of lisinopril and transdermal glyceryl trinitrate singly and together on 6-week mortality and ventricular function after acute myocardial infarction. *Lancet* 1994; **343:** 1115–22.
53. ISIS-4 (Fourth International Study of Infarct Survival) Collaborative Group. ISIS-4: a randomised factorial trial assessing early oral captopril, oral mononitrate, and intravenous magnesium sulphate in 58 050 patients with suspected acute myocardial infarction. *Lancet* 1995; **345:** 669–85.
54. Chinese Cardiac Study collaborative group. Oral captopril versus placebo among 13 634 patients with suspected acute myocardial infarction: interim report from the Chinese Cardiac Study (CCS-1). *Lancet* 1995; **345:** 686–7.
55. Gruppo Italiano per lo Studio della Sopravvivenza nell'Infarto Miocardico. Six-month effects of early treatment with lisinopril and transdermal glyceryl trinitrate singly and together withdrawn six weeks after acute myocardial infarction: the GISSI-3 trial. *J Am Coll Cardiol* 1996; **27:** 337–44.
56. Swedberg K, *et al.* Effects of the early administration of enalapril on mortality in patients with acute myocardial infarction: results of the Cooperative New Scandinavian Enalapril Survival Study II (CONSENSUS II). *N Engl J Med* 1992; **327:** 678–84.
57. Bonarjee VVS, *et al.* Attenuation of left ventricular dilatation after acute myocardial infarction by early initiation of enalapril therapy. *Am J Cardiol* 1993; **72:** 1004–9.

58. Nguyen KN, *et al.* Interaction between enalapril and aspirin on mortality after acute myocardial infarction: subgroup analysis of the Cooperative New Scandinavian Enalapril Survival Study II (CONSENSUS II). *Am J Cardiol* 1997; **79:** 115–19.
59. ACE Inhibitor Myocardial Infarction Collaborative Group. Indications for ACE inhibitors in the early treatment of acute myocardial infarction: systematic overview of individual data from 100 000 patients in randomized trials. *Circulation* 1998; **97:** 2202–12.
60. Ertl G, Jugdutt B. ACE inhibition after myocardial infarction: can megatrials provide answers? *Lancet* 1994; **344:** 1068–9.
61. Hall AS, *et al.* Inhibition of the renin-angiotensin system after acute myocardial infarction—treat first, select later? *Heart* 1996; **76** (suppl 3): 73–8.
62. Teo KK, *et al.* Effects of intravenous magnesium in suspected acute myocardial infarction: overview of randomised trials. *Br Med J* 1991; **303:** 1499–1503.
63. Woods KL, *et al.* Intravenous magnesium sulphate in suspected acute myocardial infarction: results of the second Leicester Intravenous Magnesium Intervention Trial (LIMIT-2). *Lancet* 1992; **339:** 1553–8.
64. Woods KL, Fletcher S. Long-term outcome after intravenous magnesium sulphate in suspected acute myocardial infarction: the second Leicester Intravenous Magnesium Intervention Trial (LIMIT-2). *Lancet* 1994; **343:** 816–19.
65. Anonymous. Myocardial stunning. *Lancet* 1991; **337:** 585–6.
66. Fath-Ordoubadi F, Beatt KJ. Glucose-insulin-potassium therapy for treatment of acute myocardial infarction: an overview of randomized placebo-controlled trials. *Circulation* 1997; **96:** 1152–6.
67. Northridge DB, Hall RJC. Post-myocardial-infarction exercise testing in the thrombolytic era. *Lancet* 1994; **343:** 1175–6.
68. CAPRIE Steering Committee. A randomised, blinded, trial of clopidogrel versus aspirin in patients at risk of ischaemic events (CAPRIE). *Lancet* 1996; **348:** 1329–39.
69. Antiplatelet Trialists' Collaboration. Collaborative overview of randomised trials of antiplatelet therapy—I: prevention of death, myocardial infarction, and stroke by prolonged antiplatelet therapy in various categories of patients. *Br Med J* 1994; **308:** 81–106. Correction. *ibid.*: 1540.
70. Anticoagulants in the Secondary Prevention of Events in Coronary Thrombosis (ASPECT) Research Group. Effects of long-term oral anticoagulant treatment on mortality and cardiovascular morbidity after myocardial infarction. *Lancet* 1994; **343:** 499–503.
71. Cairns JA. Oral anticoagulants or aspirin after myocardial infarction? *Lancet* 1994; **343:** 497–8.
72. Julian DG, *et al.* A comparison of aspirin and anticoagulation following thrombolysis for myocardial infarction (the AFTER Study): a multicentre unblinded randomised clinical trial. *Br Med J* 1996; **313:** 1429–31.
73. Coumadin Aspirin Reinfarction Study (CARS) Investigators. Randomised double-blind trial of fixed low-dose warfarin with aspirin after myocardial infarction. *Lancet* 1997; **350:** 389–96.
74. Soumerai SB, *et al.* Adverse outcomes of underuse of β-blockers in elderly survivors of acute myocardial infarction. *JAMA* 1997; **277:** 115–21.
75. Pfeffer MA, *et al.* Effect of captopril on mortality and morbidity in patients with left ventricular dysfunction after myocardial infarction: results of the Survival and Ventricular Enlargement Trial. *N Engl J Med* 1992; **327:** 669–77.
76. The Acute Infarction Ramipril Efficacy (AIRE) Study Investigators. Effect of ramipril on mortality and morbidity of survivors of acute myocardial infarction with clinical evidence of heart failure. *Lancet* 1993; **342:** 821–8.
77. Hall AS, *et al.* Follow-up study of patients randomly allocated ramipril or placebo for heart failure after acute myocardial infarction: AIRE extension (AIREX) study. *Lancet* 1997; **349:** 1493–7.
78. Cleland JGF, *et al.* Effect of ramipril on morbidity and mode of death among survivors of acute myocardial infarction with clinical evidence of heart failure: a report from the AIRE study investigators. *Eur Heart J* 1997; **18:** 41–51.
79. Køber L, *et al.* A clinical trial of the angiotensin-converting-enzyme inhibitor trandolapril in patients with left ventricular dysfunction after myocardial infarction. *N Engl J Med* 1995; **333:** 1670–6.
80. Latini R, *et al.* ACE inhibitor use in patients with myocardial infarction: summary of evidence from clinical trials. *Circulation* 1995; **92:** 3132–7.
81. Reynolds G, *et al.* What have the ACE-inhibitor trials in post-myocardial patients with left ventricular dysfunction taught us? *Eur J Clin Pharmacol* 1996; **49:** S35–S39.
82. Galløe AM, *et al.* Influence of oral magnesium supplementation on cardiac events among survivors of an acute myocardial infarction. *Br Med J* 1993; **307:** 585–7.
83. Peto R, *et al.* Randomised trial of prophylactic daily aspirin in British male doctors. *Br Med J* 1988; **296:** 313–16.
84. Steering Committee of the Physicians Health Study Research Group. Final report on the aspirin component of the ongoing physicians' health study. *N Engl J Med* 1989; **321:** 129–35.
85. Manson JE, *et al.* A prospective study of aspirin use and primary prevention of cardiovascular disease in women. *JAMA* 1991; **266:** 521–7.
86. Fuster V, *et al.* Aspirin as a therapeutic agent in cardiovascular disease. *Circulation* 1993; **87:** 659–75.
87. Hennekens CH, *et al.* Aspirin as a therapeutic agent in cardiovascular disease: a statement for healthcare professionals from the American Heart Association. *Circulation* 1997; **96:** 2751–3.
88. Juul-Möller S, *et al.* Double-blind trial of aspirin in primary prevention of myocardial infarction in patients with stable chronic angina pectoris. *Lancet* 1992; **340:** 1421–5.
89. The Medical Research Council's General Practice Research Framework. Thrombosis prevention trial: randomised trial of low-intensity oral anticoagulation with warfarin and low-dose aspirin in the primary prevention of ischaemic heart disease in men at increased risk. *Lancet* 1998; **351:** 233–41.
90. Hansson L, *et al.* Effects of intensive blood-pressure lowering and low-dose aspirin in patients with hypertension: principal results of the Hypertension Optimal Treatment (HOT) randomised trial. *Lancet* 1998; **351:** 1755–62.
91. Yusuf S, *et al.* Effect of enalapril on myocardial infarction and unstable angina in patients with low ejection fractions. *Lancet* 1992; **340:** 1173–8.
92. Gottlieb SS, *et al.* Effect of beta-blockade on mortality among high-risk and low-risk patients after myocardial infarction. *N Engl J Med* 1998; **339:** 489–97.

Patent ductus arteriosus

The ductus arteriosus is a vascular channel present in the fetal circulation that connects the pulmonary artery and the descending aorta. In some infants the ductus arteriosus fails to close, a condition known as persistent patent ductus arteriosus. Details of its management are given on p.47.

Peripheral arterial thrombo-embolism

Occlusion of the peripheral arteries may occur due to embolism or thrombosis (see Thrombo-embolic Disorders, below). Sudden or acute occlusion causes reduction of blood flow to the distal portions of the limb and may lead to critical limb ischaemia. Emergency treatment with surgery or thrombolytic drugs is often required to restore blood flow and preserve the limb.

Acute peripheral arterial thrombo-embolism produces pain, pallor, and coldness in the affected limb. Numbness and paraesthesia may occur and if the clot is not removed, gangrene develops. Sudden onset is usually due to occlusion by an embolus. The heart is a frequent source of emboli; atrial fibrillation, cardiomyopathy, myocardial infarction, and valvular heart disease are all associated with peripheral arterial embolism. Peripheral arterial thrombosis often has a more gradual onset due to collateral vessels maintaining some perfusion of the limb. Thrombosis is usually the result of thrombus formation at a site of atheroma in an atherosclerotic artery; thus it may occur in patients with chronic occlusive arterial disease (see Peripheral Vascular Disease, below). Thrombosis is now more common than pure embolism although the two may co-exist.

Sudden arterial occlusion requires emergency treatment to restore circulation and to avoid gangrene and possible amputation of the limb. Where there is imminent danger to the limb surgery is necessary to rapidly restore blood flow. In patients with **embolism** in otherwise healthy arteries surgical removal of the embolus by catheter (embolectomy) is used and usually results in restoration of blood flow. Sudden arterial occlusion due to **thrombosis** where gangrene is imminent requires emergency bypass surgery to restore blood flow; surgical removal of a thrombus (thrombectomy) is not usually successful as most arterial thromboses are superimposed on atheromatous plaques, particularly in elderly patients, and thrombectomy adds to the intimal damage.

Where the risk from ischaemia is less acute, angiography may be performed to confirm the type of occlusion and intra-arterial thrombolysis may be used as initial therapy, particularly if the cause is thrombotic.[1-3] This method is particularly useful for occlusion of smaller vessels, distal occlusions in surgically inaccessible small arteries, or in patients too ill to undergo surgery. However, it is a slower method of restoring blood flow and its use in limb-threatening ischaemia is controversial.[4] The TOPAS study[5] reported no significant difference in outcomes in patients with acute arterial occlusion treated initially with thrombolysis or surgery, although the rate of bleeding complications was higher with thrombolysis. It has therefore been suggested that thrombolysis may be appropriate for initial therapy in acute occlusion, providing this will not lead to an unacceptable delay in reperfusion.[6] However, others[7] consider that thrombolysis should not be used as first-line therapy due to the lack of significant benefit and the increased risk of bleeding.

Thrombolytics may be administered intravenously, but intra-arterial administration of low doses of thrombolytics directly into the clot is often used. Despite the use of low doses the risk of major haemorrhage is still about 10%. Continuous intra-arterial infusion, pulse infusion, and different thrombolytics are used; the optimal technique and choice of thrombolytic are unclear. Alteplase, streptokinase, and urokinase are all used. Local treatment with low-dose streptokinase or urokinase infused into the clot is successful in about 50 to 80% of patients and recanalisation is sustained for a year in 50%. Thrombolytic therapy is more likely to be successful if it is begun soon after thrombosis occurs. If no lysis has occurred within the first 12 to 24 hours the procedure is unlikely to be successful, but where thrombolysis is occurring infusion has been continued for several days. There is rather less experience with alteplase; it is claimed to produce more rapid thrombolysis than streptokinase although studies have been too small to provide evidence of reduced limb loss or mortality.[1] On completion of thrombolytic therapy angiography should be repeated to identify the underlying abnormalities that caused the original occlusion. The lesions can then be treated by balloon angioplasty or surgical repair, and this should be done as soon as possible to avoid rethrombosis, which occurs in about 10 to 30% of patients.

Intra-arterial thrombolysis may also be used in conjunction with surgical techniques, particularly when surgery fails to restore blood flow due to distal occlusions.[8-11]

Adjunctive treatment with antithrombotics, such as heparin and aspirin, is often given to patients with peripheral arterial thrombo-embolism to prevent propagation of the clot and also to prevent post-operative thrombo-embolic complications. However, there is an increased risk of serious bleeding complications if heparin is used with thrombolytic therapy.[5] Where the occlusion has been due to embolism, the patient should be investigated for a possible source of emboli and long-term anticoagulation should be considered to prevent recurrent embolism.

1. Wolfe JH. Critical limb ischaemia. *Prescribers' J* 1994; **34:** 50–8.
2. Beattie DK, Davies AH. Management of the acutely ischaemic limb. *Br J Hosp Med* 1996; **55:** 204–8.
3. Ludlam CA, *et al.* Guidelines for the use of thrombolytic therapy. *Blood Coag Fibrinol* 1995; **6:** 273–85.
4. Hawkins DW, Hirsh J. Antithrombotic drugs for thromboembolic disorders: a lesson in evidence-based medicine. *Am J Health-Syst Pharm* 1997; **54:** 1992–4.
5. Ouriel K, *et al.* A comparison of recombinant urokinase with vascular surgery as initial treatment for acute arterial occlusion of the legs. *N Engl J Med* 1998; **338:** 1105–15.
6. Working Party on Thrombolysis in the Management of Limb Ischemia. Thrombolysis in the management of lower limb peripheral arterial occlusion—a consensus document. *Am J Cardiol* 1998; **81:** 207–18.
7. Porter JM. Thrombolysis for acute arterial occlusion of the legs. *N Engl J Med* 1998; **338:** 1148–50.
8. Earnshaw JJ, Beard JD. Intraoperative use of thrombolytic agents. *Br Med J* 1993; **307:** 638–9.
9. Chester JF, *et al.* Peroperative t-PA thrombolysis. *Lancet* 1991; **337:** 861–2.
10. Verstraete M. Use of thrombolytic drugs in non-coronary disorders. *Drugs* 1989; **38:** 801–21.
11. Anonymous. Non-coronary thrombolysis. *Lancet* 1990; **335:** 691–3.

Peripheral vascular disease

The term peripheral vascular disease may be used to cover venous and arterial diseases of the limbs, but is often confined to arterial disease, as is the discussion that follows.

For details of venous diseases, see under Venous Thrombo-embolism, below.

Peripheral arterial disease can be divided into obstructive or occlusive disease and vasospastic disease and these two types are described in turn.

The commonest form of **occlusive arterial disease** is caused by **atherosclerosis**. It may well be only one manifestation of a generalised atherosclerotic process and sufferers also usually experience, or are at increased risk of, ischaemic heart disease. **Thromboangiitis obliterans** (Buerger's disease) is also an occlusive arterial disease, but, rather than being caused by atherosclerosis, it is a result of inflammatory and proliferative lesions in medium and small arteries and veins of the limbs. The lesions are predominantly thrombotic in nature. It progresses more rapidly than atherosclerotic disease; severe ulceration and gangrene, necessitating amputation, may often occur. Sufferers are typically heavy smokers. **Intermittent claudication** is a major feature of occlusive arterial disease of the lower limbs and is characterised by pain which develops during exercise and which disappears at rest. The pain is due to **ischaemia** (insufficient oxygen supply) resulting from the obstruction or vasoconstriction of peripheral arteries. Pain at rest may occur in severe forms of disease. Ischaemia may also result in trophic changes in the skin. In severe or advanced disease, ulceration of skin and tissues can occur and may even progress to gangrene. The cause of arterial obstruction, and therefore the precursor of ischaemia, is often atherosclerosis; ischaemia is commonly precipitated by thrombosis. Smoking causes vasoconstriction and is frequently a contributory factor.

Management. Patients with occlusive arterial disease should adopt a lifestyle that minimises cardiovascular risk factors, as described under Atherosclerosis, above. They should be advised not to smoke; in the case of thromboangiitis obliterans, cessation of smoking is essential to halt progression of the disease. Supervised exercise programmes may help to improve walking distance in patients with intermittent claudication. In common with other atherosclerotic diseases, such as angina and myocardial infarction, antiplatelet therapy has been investigated in patients with peripheral arterial disease. Early studies indicated that *aspirin*, with or without dipyridamole, may have some effect in delaying the progression of peripheral arterial diseases. An overview of trials[1] of antiplatelet therapies demonstrated that patients with peripheral vascular disease, peripheral grafts, or peripheral angioplasty benefit additionally in terms of fewer subsequent vascular events such as myocardial infarction and stroke. Thus it is suggested that antiplatelet therapy be considered as routine prophylactic treatment in these patients. The dose of aspirin generally used in the trials was 75 to 325 mg daily. Ticlopidine[1] or clopidogrel[2] may be suitable alternatives in patients unable to tolerate aspirin. Since patients with occlusive arterial disease have a high risk of ischaemic heart disease, lipid lowering therapy should also be considered.

Many other drugs have been employed in the treatment of occlusive arterial disease, but studies have often been unsatisfactory and their efficacy and/or overall place in management remains to be firmly established.

Naftidrofuryl and *oxpentifylline* are used in intermittent claudication to increase the time and distance walked before the onset of pain, but evidence of benefit has generally been unconvincing.[3-6] Although often described as *vasodilators*, any purported benefit with this type of drug may be due to actions on blood cells or blood rheology rather than vasodilatation. In any case, drugs with vasodilatory actions do not preferentially dilate affected arteries and those to ischaemic tissue may be fully dilated already. Administration of vasodilators will result in dilatation of arteries supplying non-ischaemic tissues elsewhere in the body and thus blood may actually be diverted away from the affected ischaemic area—the so-called 'steal' phenomenon; this is a known risk with all vasodilators, but especially with powerful arterial vasodilators such as hydralazine and this type of drug is not suitable for use in peripheral arterial disease. Other drugs that have been promoted for the treatment of intermittent claudication include cinnarizine, cyclandelate, and inositol nicotinate.[5,6]

Ketanserin inhibits vasoconstriction and also changes indices of blood rheology, but results in intermittent claudication have been inconsistent.

Certain *prostaglandins* cause vasodilatation and prevent platelet aggregation and some have appeared promising in the presence of advanced disease or complications. A beneficial effect on rest pain has been noted and some ulcers have either regressed or healed; in selected patients this form of therapy has avoided the need for amputation. Prostaglandins employed include *alprostadil* or *epoprostenol*, both intra-arterially or intravenously, *iloprost* intravenously, and *dinoprostone* topically.

If intermittent claudication is severe **non-pharmacological** techniques such as bypass surgery, endarterectomy, or percutaneous transluminal angioplasty should be considered. Following these procedures, treatment to prevent postoperative thrombosis and restenosis may be necessary (see Reperfusion and Revascularisation Procedures, below).

Sudden or **acute arterial occlusion** due to emboli or to thrombosis may occur in 10% of patients with atherosclerotic disease, but is rare in thromboangiitis obliterans. The initial approach has been surgical removal; dissolution of the thrombus using local or systemic thrombolytic therapy may be considered. For further details, see Peripheral Arterial Thrombo-embolism, above.

Vasospastic arterial disease is due to an inappropriate response to temperature, usually cold, when vasoconstriction and/or vasospasm occurs. The most important of these disorders is Raynaud's syndrome. Other vasospastic conditions include acrocyanosis, chilblains, and erythromelalgia.

In **Raynaud's syndrome**, paroxysmal attacks of pallor and cyanosis, usually of the digits, occur in response to cold, or sometimes emotional stress. Erythema replaces the cyanosis as the attacks resolve. The cause of primary Raynaud's syndrome (Raynaud's disease) is unknown. Features identified include intense vasoconstriction or vasospasm, disturbance of sympathetic nerve supply, changes in circulating catecholamines, enhanced platelet aggregation, red cell deformability, and fibrinolysis. It is probable that not all cases are due to the same mechanism. It has been suggested that the underlying defect may not be an overreaction to the initial cold insult but be a defect in the normal ensuing adaptive response. Secondary Raynaud's syndrome (Raynaud's phenomenon) frequently co-exists with arterial occlusive disease such as thromboangiitis obliterans (see above) and connective tissue disorders, in particular scleroderma (systemic sclerosis). Trauma and certain drugs, notably beta blockers and ergotamine, may also be responsible for inducing secondary Raynaud's syndrome.

Management. In mild cases of Raynaud's syndrome, where attacks are infrequent and of limited severity, protective measures to keep warm are the mainstay of treatment; this involves wearing appropriate clothing and the use of appliances such as heated gloves. Patients should also stop smoking because of the vasoconstriction caused. Any underlying or co-existing disease or cause in secondary Raynaud's syndrome should be treated. Drug therapy is indicated in more severe cases. It is directed towards producing vascular smooth muscle relaxation and vasodilatation in order to improve resting blood flow, thereby reducing the extent of tissue ischaemia. Some drugs may also act by modifying platelet aggregation or blood rheology. As with occlusive arterial disease many drugs have been tried in Raynaud's syndrome. This perhaps reflects the large number of differing mechanisms of defect that have been proposed.[7-13]

Calcium-channel blockers have been of benefit in Raynaud's syndrome, but it is not entirely clear which of their pharmacological actions is responsible. The most widely used and studied is *nifedipine*.

Thymoxamine, an alpha blocker with vasodilating activity is also widely employed. Other alpha blockers, for example, phenoxybenzamine and prazosin as well as reserpine have been used although in some cases side-effects have limited their usefulness.

Cinnarizine, *naftidrofuryl*, *oxpentifylline*, and *nicotinic acid derivatives* such as inositol nicotinate have had widespread use in Raynaud's syndrome but, as for occlusive arterial disease, evidence of efficacy is lacking.

In severe Raynaud's syndrome complicated by ulceration and gangrene, as in occlusive disease, *prostaglandins* have been promising. *Alprostadil*, *epoprostenol*, and *iloprost* have been administered by intravenous infusion. In some cases the beneficial effects have persisted for a few months after treatment and two or three infusions given at intervals over the winter months have prevented the severe complications of Raynaud's suffered in previous years. Iloprost orally has also been reported to reduce the severity of attacks. Prostaglandins applied topically in ulcerative cases include *dinoprostone*.

Small studies or anecdotal reports have noted variable effects with many *other drugs* including the ACE inhibitors captopril and enalapril,[14] the serotonin reuptake inhibitors fluoxetine and venlafaxine, topical nitrates such as glyceryl trinitrate, ketanserin, piracetam, and sodium nitroprusside. None of these therapies appears, however, to have come into widespread use. The potent vasodilator calcitonin gene-related peptide has recently shown promise.

Acrocyanosis is characterised by a persistent blue discoloration of the skin. There is an abnormal constriction of arterioles, even at normal environmental conditions and this is potentiated by cold. **Chilblains** are an inflammatory condition (perniosis) affecting the extremities and symptoms include erythema, pruritus, and ulceration; they may be acute or chronic. Chilblains occur more commonly in cold damp conditions. Acrocyanosis and chilblains do not generally require specific treatment; smoking cessation, protection from the cold, or symptomatic antipruritic treatment are often sufficient. However, if severe, the drugs described above under Raynaud's syndrome may be considered. **Erythromelalgia** is a vasospastic condition usually provoked by heat. It is characterised by painful, red extremities together with a burning sensation and increased skin temperature of the affected area. Thrombocythaemia is the most common underlying cause and indeed erythromelalgia may be the presenting feature; in thrombocythaemia arteriolar occlusion may occur as a result of platelet aggregation. Small doses of aspirin have produced considerable relief in some patients, presumably by preventing platelet aggregation. Beta blockers may also be of some help. Attacks should be prevented wherever possible by avoiding exposure to heat.

1. Antiplatelet Trialists' Collaboration. Collaborative overview of randomised trials of antiplatelet treatment—I: prevention of death, myocardial infarction, and stroke by prolonged antiplatelet therapy in various categories of patients. *Br Med J* 1994; **308:** 81–106.
2. CAPRIE Steering Committee. A randomised, blinded, trial of clopidogrel versus aspirin in patients at risk of ischaemic events (CAPRIE). *Lancet* 1996; **348:** 1329–39.
3. Cameron HA, *et al.* Drug treatment of intermittent claudication: a critical analysis of the methods and findings of published clinical trials, 1965–1985. *Br J Clin Pharmacol* 1988; **26:** 569–76.
4. Radack K, Wyderski RJ. Conservative management of intermittent claudication. *Ann Intern Med* 1990; **113:** 135–46.
5. Anonymous. Do drugs help intermittent claudication? *Drug Ther Bull* 1990; **28:** 1–2.
6. Waller D, Chant A. Intermittent claudication. *Prescribers' J* 1995; **35:** 64–70.
7. Belch JJF, Ho M. Pharmacotherapy of Raynaud's phenomenon. *Drugs* 1996; **52:** 682–95.
8. Roath S. Management of Raynaud's phenomenon: focus on newer treatments. *Drugs* 1989; **37:** 700–12.
9. Cooke ED, Nicolaides AN. Raynaud's syndrome. *Br Med J* 1990; **300:** 553–5.
10. Black C. Update on Raynaud's phenomenon. *Br J Hosp Med* 1994; **52:** 555–8.
11. Black CM. Raynaud's phenomenon. *Prescribers' J* 1994; **34:** 125–33.
12. Isenberg DA, Black C. Raynaud's phenomenon, scleroderma, and overlap syndromes. *Br Med J* 1995; **310:** 795–8.
13. Report of a Meeting of Physicians and Scientists. Raynaud's phenomenon. *Lancet* 1995; **346:** 283–90.
14. Challenor VF. Angiotensin converting enzyme inhibitors in Raynaud's phenomenon. *Drugs* 1994; **48:** 864–7.

Phaeochromocytoma

Phaeochromocytoma is a rare catecholamine-secreting tumour of the adrenal medulla and its diagnosis and management have been reviewed.[1,2]

Patients are usually hypertensive and suffer headache, palpitations, and excessive sweating; the hypertension may be either episodic or sustained. However, if the tumour is predominantly adrenaline-secreting, tachyarrhythmias may be associated with a normal or even decreased arterial pressure and if the tumour secretes mainly noradrenaline, vasoconstriction may lead to contraction of the venous pool and hypovolaemia. If the effects of the release of catecholamines are not controlled a life-threatening crisis ultimately ensues and may range from a shock-like syndrome with multiple organ failure to hypertensive crisis, depending on the predominance of the catecholamine secreted.

For a diagnosis of phaeochromocytoma, history and clinical symptoms are important, but a firm diagnosis may require further investigative techniques. Plasma concentrations of adrenaline and noradrenaline and urinary concentrations of these catecholamines and their metabolites are indicators of the presence of a tumour and precise location can be established by procedures such as computerised axial tomography, magnetic resonance imaging, or scintigraphy with ^{131}I-iobenguane (^{131}I-*m*-iodobenzylguanidine). Early tests used agents such as glucagon, histamine, or tyramine as provocation tests in which positive cases would develop hypertensive surges but these tests are now considered obsolete. Alternatively, tests may be employed in which drugs such as clonidine that suppress catecholamine release are given; in patients with phaeochromocytoma catecholamine concentrations are unaffected whereas in normal patients they are decreased after such drug administration.

Although surgery to remove the tumour is the ultimate treatment goal, the initial step in management must be the prevention of the pressor effects of catecholamines. Alpha blockers such as phenoxybenzamine, phentolamine, or prazosin are used. Initial doses should be small and increased gradually until all signs of pressor activity are suppressed. Once, but not until, alpha blockade is successfully established, tachycardia can be controlled by the cautious use of a beta blocker. A $beta_1$-selective blocker is preferred so that peripheral $beta_2$-mediated vasodilatation is unaffected. α-Methyltyrosine, which suppresses catecholamine synthesis, may be tried in selected patients such as those resistant to alpha blockade or those with heart failure in whom the effects of alpha or beta blockade may be undesirable.

Once the pressor effects of catecholamine secretion are controlled, surgery can be contemplated. Agents used for premedication and anaesthesia should be chosen so as to avoid those which may cause pressor responses or tachycardia. Although the opioids, anaesthetic agents, and neuromuscular blocking agents chosen should suppress the adrenergic response to surgical stimuli, such conventional measures will still not be adequate to prevent catecholamine release when the tumour is handled. Thus, potent vasodilators such as sodium nitroprusside or glyceryl trinitrate have been given intravenously to prevent dangerously high arterial pressures; the alpha blocker phentolamine has also been advocated although tachycardia is invariably a problem. Cardioselective beta blockers such as atenolol may be given, often in high dosage, to control tachycardia during surgery.

If it proves impossible to remove all the active tissue of a phaeochromocytoma during surgery, maintenance therapy with alpha and beta blockade needs to be continued or α-methyltyrosine may be used. Alternatively, ^{131}I-iobenguane has been given in high doses sufficient to cause radionecrosis.

1. Hull CJ. Phaeochromocytoma: diagnosis, preoperative preparation and anaesthetic management. *Br J Anaesth* 1986; **58:** 1453–68.
2. Foo M, *et al.* Phaeochromocytoma. *Br J Hosp Med* 1995; **54:** 318–21.

Pulmonary hypertension

Pulmonary hypertension, unless otherwise specified, refers to pulmonary arterial pressure. The criteria depend on altitude, but in a resting individual at sea level a pulmonary arterial pressure greater than 20 mmHg establishes a diagnosis; at higher altitudes, correspondingly higher pressures occur and at about 15 000 feet a value greater than 25 mmHg signifies pulmonary hypertension.

Two subsets of pulmonary hypertension are recognised. Primary pulmonary hypertension is uncommon and patients have no underlying disease known to cause an elevation of the pulmonary arterial pressure. Secondary pulmonary hypertension, in contrast, is far more prevalent and patients have some form of cardiopulmonary disorder that can lead to the development of pulmonary hypertension.

Primary pulmonary hypertension has been reviewed.[1,26,27] It has been recorded in patients of all ages and in both sexes but women in the fourth decade of life are those typically seen. Initial complaints include dyspnoea on exertion, fatigue, and chest discomfort or pain. In advanced disease, cor pulmonale (an enlargement of the right ventricle due to either dilatation, hypertrophy, or both) occurs and may progress to right-sided heart failure. The pulmonary arteries may be affected by thrombo-embolic disease. Primary pulmonary hypertension is a progressive and incurable disease and patients appear to be prone to sudden death.

The aim of treatment is to decrease the pulmonary arterial pressure, preferably in conjunction with an increase in cardiac output. Many drugs with vasodilating effects have been investigated in pulmonary hypertension,[2,3] the rationale usually being based upon their application in systemic hypertension. Unfortunately, the vast majority have been unsatisfactory. Although most vasodilators do reduce pulmonary arterial pressure they are not selective for the pulmonary circulation and therefore also reduce systemic blood pressure producing undesirable, or sometimes intolerable, side-effects. In some cases vasodilators have been ineffective in reducing pulmonary arterial pressure. Of all the vasodilators studied the most promising appear to be calcium-channel blockers and the prostaglandin epoprostenol. Improved survival over a 5-year period has been noted in some patients treated with high-dose *calcium-channel blockers*.[4] However, not all patients respond and because of concerns about previously reported adverse effects in patients with primary pulmonary hypertension given these drugs it has been advised that an acute response test should be performed before embarking on long term treatment.[3,4] Although oral calcium-channel blockers may be used for the test, shorter-acting vasodilators such as intravenous epoprostenol, intravenous adenosine, or inhaled nitric oxide, are generally employed.[1] *Epoprostenol* was originally introduced into the management of primary pulmonary hypertension to sustain patients long enough for them to have heart-lung transplantation. Recently, encouraging results (sustained clinical improvement and probable improved survival) have been reported in some patients given long-term intravenous therapy by portable infusion pumps.[5-8] Continuous infusion of the more stable analogue iloprost may also be effective.[9] Administration by inhalation may avoid some of the complications of long-term intravenous access and beneficial responses have been reported with inhaled epoprostenol[10,11] and with iloprost.[10] Therapy with beraprost sodium, an epoprostenol analogue that can be given orally, has also been tried.[12] Lung or heart-lung transplantation may be required in patients who do not respond to vasodilator therapy.[1] Patients with primary pulmonary hypertension have an increased risk of thrombo-embolism and *oral anticoagulants* are recommended on a long term basis for most patients as they may improve survival.[4] *Diuretics*[4,5] and *digoxin*[4,5] are given as necessary for associated right-sided heart failure.

Secondary pulmonary hypertension, as mentioned above, is a consequence of established cardiopulmonary disorders and clinical manifestations are dominated by those of the underlying condition. Management thus basically constitutes appropriate treatment of the underlying condition, although inhaled nitric oxide may be used in acutely ill patients.[13]

Disorders of left ventricular function, such as may occur after myocardial infarction (above) or in mitral valve disease, can increase pulmonary venous pressure, which in turn increases pulmonary arterial pressure. Chronic obstructive pulmonary disease (p.747) is the commonest respiratory cause of pulmonary hypertension. Diseases of the lung parenchyma which can lead to pulmonary hypertension include alveolar disorders such as the respiratory distress syndromes (p.1017) and inflammatory interstitial diseases such as sarcoidosis (p.1028) and idiopathic fibrosing alveolitis (p.1024). Disorders affecting the pulmonary vessels themselves such as thrombo-embolic disease (below) and systemic lupus erythematosus (p.1029) can also be causes of pulmonary hypertension.

Persistent pulmonary hypertension of the newborn, sometimes also termed persistent fetal circulation, is, as the name implies, a form of pulmonary hypertension specifically affecting neonates. It can be primary in nature (that is, idiopathic, affecting infants with an anatomically normal heart and no pulmonary disease) or secondary, being associated with a number of cardiopulmonary conditions including congenital heart disease, diaphragmatic hernia, meconium aspiration, respiratory distress syndrome, or sepsis. The pulmonary hypertension and altered vasoreactivity lead to a right-to-left shunting of blood across the patent ductus arteriosus or foramen ovale and this often results in critical hypoxaemia.

Management has included high-frequency oscillatory ventilation (to achieve optimal lung inflation) and extracorporeal membrane oxygenation; alkalosis induced by mechanical hyperventilation has decreased pulmonary arterial pressure and improved oxygenation in some patients.[14,15] Vasodilators have also been employed, but, as discussed above, their use is generally restricted because of their non-selectivity for the pulmonary circulation. *Tolazoline* has been the vasodilator most commonly employed. One report[16] has described the use of inhaled *epoprostenol* in two neonates, a method of administration that may overcome the problems of systemic vasodilatation. *Magnesium sulphate* intravenously has also been reported[17-19] to have potential use as a vasodilator, and intravenous *adenosine* has also been tried.[20] Current interest is, however, being focused on the use of inhaled *nitric oxide*[14,15] which is a potent, selective pulmonary vasodilator. Studies[21-23] have shown that it can cause marked improvement in oxygenation and a reduction in the need for extracorporeal membrane oxygenation, but no effect on mortality has been demonstrated. Although there have been concerns that use of inhaled nitric oxide might adversely affect neurodevelopmental outcome more than conventional therapy, this was not confirmed in infants followed up for up to 2 years.[24] Use of inhaled nitric oxide in combination with high-frequency oscillatory ventilation may have additional benefits.[25]

1. Rubin LJ. Primary pulmonary hypertension. *N Engl J Med* 1997; **336:** 111–17.
2. Weir EK, *et al.* The acute administration of vasodilators in primary pulmonary hypertension: experience from the National Institutes of Health Registry on Primary Pulmonary Hypertension. *Am Rev Respir Dis* 1989; **140:** 1623–30.
3. Barnes PJ, Liu SF. Regulation of pulmonary vascular tone. *Pharmacol Rev* 1995; **47:** 87–131.
4. Rich S, *et al.* The effect of high doses of calcium-channel blockers on survival in primary pulmonary hypertension. *N Engl J Med* 1992; **327:** 76–81.
5. Barst RJ, *et al.* Survival in primary pulmonary hypertension with long-term continuous intravenous prostacyclin. *Ann Intern Med* 1994; **121:** 409–15. Correction. *ibid.* 1995; **122:** 238.
6. Barst RJ, *et al.* A comparison of continuous intravenous epoprostenol (prostacyclin) with conventional therapy for primary pulmonary hypertension. *N Engl J Med* 1996; **334:** 296–301.
7. Shapiro SM, *et al.* Primary pulmonary hypertension: improved long-term effects and survival with continuous intravenous epoprostenol infusion. *J Am Coll Cardiol* 1997; **30:** 343–9.
8. McLaughlin VV, *et al.* Reduction in pulmonary vascular resistance with long-term epoprostenol (prostacyclin) therapy in primary pulmonary hypertension. *N Engl J Med* 1998; **338:** 273–7.
9. Higenbottam TW, *et al.* Treatment of pulmonary hypertension with the continuous infusion of a prostacyclin analogue, iloprost. *Heart* 1998; **79:** 175–9.
10. Olschewski H, *et al.* Aerosolized prostacyclin and iloprost in severe pulmonary hypertension. *Ann Intern Med* 1996; **124:** 820–4.
11. Mikhail G, *et al.* An evaluation of nebulized prostacyclin in patients with primary and secondary pulmonary hypertension. *Eur Heart J* 1997; **18:** 1499–1504.
12. Okano Y, *et al.* Orally active prostacyclin analogue in primary pulmonary hypertension. *Lancet* 1997; **349:** 1365. Correction. *ibid.*; **350:** 1406.
13. Cuthbertson BH, *et al.* Use of inhaled nitric oxide in British intensive therapy units. *Br J Anaesth* 1997; **78:** 696–700.
14. Kinsella JP, Abman SH. Recent developments in the pathophysiology and treatment of persistent pulmonary hypertension of the newborn. *J Pediatr* 1995; **126:** 853–64.
15. Mupanemunda RH, Edwards AD. Treatment of newborn infants with inhaled nitric oxide. *Arch Dis Child* 1995; **72:** F131–F134.
16. Bindl L, *et al.* Aerosolised prostacyclin for pulmonary hypertension in neonates. *Arch Dis Child* 1994; **71:** F214–F216.
17. Abu-Osba YK, *et al.* Treatment of severe persistent pulmonary hypertension of the newborn with magnesium sulphate. *Arch Dis Child* 1992; **67:** 31–5.
18. Tolsa J-F, *et al.* Magnesium sulphate as an alternative and safe treatment for severe persistent pulmonary hypertension of the newborn. *Arch Dis Child* 1995; **72:** F184–F187.
19. Wu T-Z, *et al.* Persistent pulmonary hypertension of the newborn treated with magnesium sulfate in premature neonates. *Pediatrics* 1995; **96:** 472–4.
20. Konduri GG, *et al.* Adenosine infusion improves oxygenation in term infants with respiratory failure. *Pediatrics* 1996; **97:** 295–300.
21. The Neonatal Inhaled Nitric Oxide Study Group. Inhaled nitric oxide in full-term and nearly full-term infants with hypoxic respiratory failure. *N Engl J Med* 1997; **336:** 597–604.
22. Roberts JD, *et al.* Inhaled nitric oxide and persistent pulmonary hypertension of the newborn. *N Engl J Med* 1997; **336:** 605–10.
23. Davidson D, *et al.* Inhaled nitric oxide for the early treatment of persistent pulmonary hypertension of the term newborn: a randomized, double-masked, placebo-controlled, dose-response, multicenter study. *Pediatrics* 1998; **101:** 325–34.
24. Rosenberg AA, *et al.* Longitudinal follow-up of a cohort of newborn infants treated with inhaled nitric oxide for persistent pulmonary hypertension. *J Pediatr* 1997; **131:** 70–5.
25. Kinsella JP, *et al.* Randomized, multicenter trial of inhaled nitric oxide and high-frequency oscillatory ventilation in severe, persistent pulmonary hypertension of the newborn. *J Pediatr* 1997; **131:** 55–62.
26. Gaine SP, Rubin LJ. Primary pulmonary hypertension. *Lancet* 1998; **352:** 719–25.
27. Peacock A, Raeside D. Pulmonary hypertension. *Prescribers' J* 1998; **38:** 158–66.

Raised intracranial pressure

The intracranial compartment consists of brain parenchyma, vascular tissue, and cerebrospinal fluid (CSF). Since the skull is a rigid structure a change in the volume of any one of these compartments will raise intracranial pressure. This may be due to the formation of cerebral oedema following head injury or around tumours, mass-lesions such as tumours or haemorrhage, CNS infections, or metabolic disorders. Other mechanisms which can raise intracranial pressure include increased dural sinus venous pressure, increased resistance to CSF outflow, and an increased rate of formation of CSF. In conditions such as benign intracranial hypertension there may be no obvious cause. Raised intracranial pressure (intracranial hypertension) can produce irreversible damage to the CNS and is potentially fatal; herniation of brain tissue can occur and reduced cerebral blood flow can lead to cerebral ischaemia. Symptoms of raised intracranial pressure include headache, which is frequently worse in the morning and may wake the patient from sleep, vomiting, drowsiness, and visual disturbances; most patients have papilloedema on examination.

The management of raised intracranial pressure has been reviewed.[1-4] There are several ways of reducing pressure, the choice of treatment being determined mainly by the underlying cause. Whatever the cause, in acutely raised intracranial pressure the initial aim is to reduce the volume of the intracranial contents as quickly as possible to prevent brain damage. For patients with haematoma or tumours the treatment of choice is frequently surgery but other methods may be used to control intracranial pressure before surgery.

Intracranial pressure monitoring can be helpful in guiding therapy since reducing the intracranial pressure too far is also deleterious. Patients may be sedated to avoid elevations of intracranial pressure due to unnecessary movement but if this is ineffective the use of neuromuscular blocking agents such as pancuronium or atracurium with artificial ventilation should be considered. Hyperventilation reduces the intracranial pressure by constricting the cerebral blood vessels and controlled hyperventilation may be employed. Raising the patient's head to promote venous drainage and restriction of fluid intake may be helpful to reduce intracranial pressure, but care is needed to avoid compromising the circulation. Removal of CSF through a ventricular catheter may also be effective.

The mainstay of pharmacological treatment for acutely raised intracranial pressure is diuretic therapy, usually with an osmotic diuretic. Mannitol is most commonly used but urea, glycerol, and hypertonic glucose solutions have also been employed. Osmotic diuretics act by increasing the osmolality of plasma and drawing water out of the tissues, as well as by promoting an osmotic diuresis. They should not be given to patients with intracranial bleeding after head injury since they can exacerbate the bleeding,[5] and should also be avoided in patients who are already dehydrated. *Mannitol* has been suggested for control of raised intracranial pressure of various origins including severe head injury,[4,6] and cerebral oedema in hepatic failure,[7] and is often used to control intracranial pressure prior to surgery.[4,6,8] Mannitol has also produced beneficial responses in *children* with raised intracranial pressure from birth asphyxia,[9] diabetic ketoacidosis,[10] or Reye's syndrome.[11,12] Beneficial effects with osmotic diuretics such as mannitol or glycerol in patients following stroke have not been demonstrated (see Stroke, below). The use of osmotic diuretics to reduce intracranial pressure in patients with cerebral malaria is not routinely recommended and is controversial in other CNS infections.

In addition to its ability to lower intracranial pressure *glycerol* is reported to be able to increase blood flow to areas of brain ischaemia.[1] It has been used by mouth or intravenously in an attempt to reduce cerebral oedema and raised intracranial pressure in a variety of conditions including Reye's syndrome[13] and meningitis;[14] it has been reported to be ineffective in hepatic coma.[15] Some patients have experienced severe adverse effects including haemolysis, haemoglobinuria, and renal failure. Strongly *hyperosmotic glucose* solutions (25 to 50%) have been used to reduce raised intracranial pressure and cerebral oedema caused by delirium or acute alcohol intoxication.

If control is required for more than a few hours, repeated doses or continuous administration of osmotic diuretics may be required. Fluid and electrolyte balance and plasma osmolality should be closely monitored.

Loop diuretics such as *frusemide* are also effective and may be used as alternatives to osmotic diuretics, particularly where a sustained effect is required. They may increase the effect of osmotic diuretics and may be used as adjuncts, usually given after the osmotic diuretic. Frusemide decreases cerebral water content and possibly also reduces secretion of CSF. It may be preferred to mannitol in patients undergoing neurosurgery.[16]

Corticosteroids have an accepted and important role in the management of raised intracranial pressure associated with tumour-induced cerebral oedema. They may be used intravenously in high doses to control acutely raised intracranial pressure due to a rapidly expanding tumour. Lower doses are given orally for maintenance or where the onset of cerebral oedema is more insidious. Corticosteroids have also been tried in patients with head injury or stroke but their effectiveness is not proven and their adverse effects may outweigh any benefit. Further studies are needed to clarify their role in head injury.[17]

The use of barbiturate-induced coma with intravenous *thiopentone* or *pentobarbitone* for raised intracranial pressure has been controversial but it may be of benefit in patients refractory to conventional therapies. In addition to their effect on intracranial pressure barbiturates may be able to protect the brain from ischaemia. Gamma-hydroxybutyrate has been tried similarly to reduce intracranial pressure and protect against ischaemia.[18,19]

Small studies[20,21] indicated that intravenous *dimethyl sulphoxide* might be of use for raised intracranial pressure refractory to other therapy but there have been problems with fluid overload and difficulties with administration.[20]

Benign intracranial hypertension (pseudotumour cerebri) is a rare disorder of unknown cause in which there is a raised intracranial pressure in the absence of an intracranial mass or obstruction to CSF outflow. Patients are often obese and tend to be young and female. Although the condition is not life-threatening and is often self-limiting, it may be a chronic condition and treatment is required to prevent visual loss and to alleviate symptoms.

Management of mild symptoms usually involves diuretic treatment with frusemide, a thiazide, or acetazolamide. Corticosteroids may be used to control acute symptoms but long-term adverse effects limit their use. Repeated lumbar puncture to remove CSF may relieve symptoms and has been used every 2 to 5 days to induce remission. In patients who cannot be controlled medically surgical methods such as lumboperitoneal shunting may be required. There has been an anecdotal report of beneficial effects with *octreotide* in a small number of patients.[22]

Acetazolamide has also been tried in the treatment of patients with chronically raised intracranial pressure due to cryptococcal meningitis.[23]

1. Woster PS, LeBlanc KL. Management of elevated intracranial pressure. *Clin Pharm* 1990; **9:** 762–72.
2. Lyons MK, Meyer FB. Cerebrospinal fluid physiology and the management of increased intracranial pressure. *Mayo Clin Proc* 1990; **65:** 684–707.
3. Heinemeyer G. Clinical pharmacokinetic considerations in the treatment of increased intracranial pressure. *Clin Pharmacokinet* 1987; **13:** 1–25.
4. Dearden NM. Management of raised intracranial pressure after severe head injury. *Br J Hosp Med* 1986; **36:** 94–103.
5. Williams B. Management of raised ICP after severe head injury. *Br J Hosp Med* 1987; **37:** 85.
6. Bullock R, Teasdale G. Head injuries—II. *Br Med J* 1990; **300:** 1576–9.
7. Canalese J, *et al.* Controlled trial of dexamethasone and mannitol for the cerebral oedema of fulminant hepatic failure. *Gut* 1982; **23:** 625–9.
8. Andrews CJH. Intracranial aneurysms: perioperative management. *Br J Hosp Med* 1989; **41:** 485–8.
9. Levene MI, Evans DH. Medical management of raised intracranial pressure after severe birth asphyxia. *Arch Dis Child* 1985; **60:** 12–16.
10. Bello FA, Sotos JF. Cerebral oedema in diabetic ketoacidosis in children. *Lancet* 1990; **336:** 64.
11. Shaywitz BA, *et al.* Prolonged continuous monitoring of intracranial pressure in severe Reye's syndrome. *Pediatrics* 1977; **59:** 595–605.
12. Newman SL, *et al.* Reye's syndrome: success of supportive care. *N Engl J Med* 1978; **299:** 1079.
13. Nahata MC, *et al.* Variations in glycerol kinetics in Reye's syndrome. *Clin Pharmacol Ther* 1981; **29:** 782–7.
14. Kilpi T, *et al.* Oral glycerol and intravenous dexamethasone in preventing neurologic and audiologic sequelae of childhood bacterial meningitis. *Pediatr Infect Dis J* 1995; **14:** 270–8.
15. Record CO, *et al.* Glycerol therapy for cerebral oedema complicating fulminant hepatic failure. *Br Med J* 1975; **ii:** 540.
16. Cottrell JE, *et al.* Furosemide- and mannitol-induced changes in intracranial pressure and serum osmolality and electrolytes. *Anesthesiology* 1977; **47:** 28–30.
17. Alderson P, Roberts I. Corticosteroids in acute traumatic brain injury: systematic review of randomised controlled trials. *Br Med J* 1997; **314:** 1855–9.
18. Escuret E, *et al.* Gamma hydroxy butyrate as a substitute for barbiturate therapy in comatose patients with head injuries. *Acta Neurol Scand* 1979; **60** (suppl 72): 38–9.
19. Strong AJ, *et al.* Reduction of raised intracranial pressure (ICP) by gamma-hydroxybutyric acid following severe head injury. *Br J Surg* 1983; **70:** 303.
20. Marshall LF, *et al.* Dimethyl sulfoxide for the treatment of intracranial hypertension: a preliminary trial. *Neurosurgery* 1984; **14:** 659–63.
21. Karaca M, *et al.* Dimethyl sulphoxide lowers ICP after closed head trauma. *Eur J Clin Pharmacol* 1991; **40:** 113–14.
22. Antaraki A, *et al.* Octreotide in benign intracranial hypertension. *Lancet* 1993; **342:** 1170.
23. Johnston SRD, *et al.* Raised intracranial pressure and visual complications in AIDS patients with cryptococcal meningitis. *J Infect* 1992; **24:** 185–9.

Reperfusion and revascularisation procedures

Percutaneous transluminal angioplasty and bypass grafting are non-pharmacological procedures employed in the management of atherosclerotic arterial disease associated with angina pectoris (above), myocardial infarction (above), and peripheral vascular disease (above) to aid revascularisation and reperfusion. In coronary disease the use of stents to keep the arteries patent is also gaining acceptance.[1,2] Newer methods of plaque removal are also being tried. Patients undergoing such revascularisation are at risk of further thrombo-embolic events leading to myocardial infarction, ischaemic stroke, or death either shortly after the procedure or in the long term as a consequence of restenosis of the artery.[3] Thus adjunctive drug therapy is given with the aim of preventing perioperative thrombosis and long-term restenosis and the following discussion focuses on this aspect rather than on the choice or merits of any given technique for particular patient groups.

Heparin is given in conjunction with coronary angioplasty[4] or bypass surgery[5] to decrease the risk of perioperative thrombosis but has no role in the long-term prevention of restenosis. In one study there were fewer acute ischaemic events early after angioplasty when recombinant hirudin was given instead of heparin, but no longer term benefit was seen.[6] Oral anticoagulants such as warfarin do not appear to be used routinely either perioperatively or for long-term prophylaxis in the UK[5] or the USA[7] although they are said to be popular in parts of Europe.[5] Nitrates[4] or calcium-channel blockers[4,8] may be employed during coronary angioplasty if vasospasm is likely to be a problem, but again have no routine role in long-term prevention of restenosis.

Antiplatelet drugs have a role in preventing both acute occlusion and restenosis. Aspirin is most commonly used and is usually started around the time of angioplasty or bypass grafting and continued long-term as discussed further below. Abciximab is an antiplatelet drug that acts by blocking glycoprotein IIb/IIIa receptors and its beneficial effect in preventing perioperative occlusion in patients undergoing coronary angioplasty has been demonstrated in three large studies. Two of the studies (EPIC[9] and CAPTURE[10]) included only patients at high risk of abrupt vessel closure, while the third study (EPILOG[11]) included unselected patients. Follow-up at 6 months[12] and 3 years[13] has been reported after the EPIC study and at 6 months after the EPILOG study[11] and in these studies where abciximab was infused intravenously immediately before angioplasty and continued for 12 hours the initial beneficial effects have been maintained at follow-up. In the CAPTURE study where abciximab was given for 18 to 24 hours pre-procedure and for 1 hour post-procedure the initial beneficial effects were lost at 6-month follow-up.[10] Abciximab in these studies was given in addition to aspirin and heparin. Use of abciximab is associated with bleeding complications and other glycoprotein IIb/IIIa-receptor antagonists, such as eptifibatide[14] and tirofiban,[32] that have a shorter duration of action and therefore may be safer to use, are under investigation; however, 6-month results in the tirofiban study[32] have been disappointing with no reduction in the incidence of restenosis being found.

Coronary stents (metallic mesh tubes that are inflated across a stenosis and thus permanently embedded in the vessel wall) were introduced in the early 1990s and were initially used to prevent restenosis occurring after coronary angioplasty. They are now also used increasingly as an alternative to angioplasty and to treat acute or threatened vessel closure complicating angioplasty. Thrombotic occlusion occurring 2 to 14 days following stent implantation (subacute stent thrombosis) led to the use of intensive anticoagulation/antiplatelet regimens consisting of aspirin, dipyridamole, dextran, heparin, and warfarin.[15,16] These regimens were associated with a high incidence of bleeding complications and less intensive antiplatelet therapy has been investigated since thrombosis appears to be associated with platelet activation rather than coagulation.[17] Incomplete stent implantation is also thought to contribute to the risk of subacute stent thrombosis.[3] A regimen of aspirin with ticlopidine, in addition to heparin during the procedure appears to be effective[18-20] and is now used if the stent has been positioned adequately and the risk of thrombosis is considered to be low. The intensive regimen is still recommended if stenting is performed for abrupt closure following angioplasty or in other cases where risk of thrombosis is high.[15] A low-molecular-weight heparin given for 1 month after the procedure is used additionally by some practitioners. Abciximab is also under investigation.[21] Local drug delivery using heparin-coated stents is also being tried.[22]

Several pathological processes are believed to be responsible for the development of restenosis[2,4,23] and include platelet aggregation and thrombus formation, neointimal hyperplasia, elastic recoil, and vascular remodelling. Therefore, a wide variety of drugs has been investigated in an attempt to prevent restenosis.[23] Drugs employed have included antithrombotics (heparin, low-molecular-weight heparins, hirudin, and warfarin), antiplatelets (primarily aspirin but also dipyridamole and ticlopidine and prostaglandins such as epoprostenol and ciprostene), antiproliferatives (ACE inhibitors, colchicine, lanreotide, and trapidil), antoxidants (probucol), calcium-channel blockers, and lipid regulating drugs (fish oils and statins). Radiotherapy is being investigated for prevention of neointimal hyperplasia following coronary stent implantation. Local gene delivery is also under investigation as a possible treatment for restenosis. In general, with the exception of antiplatelet drugs such as aspirin, and possibly lanreotide, probucol, and trapidil, results have been either disappointing or equivocal and further evaluation is needed.

The value of antiplatelet drugs, and aspirin in particular, following coronary or peripheral angioplasty or after bypass procedures has been confirmed by the Antiplatelet Trialists' Collaboration.[24] This overview showed that such treatment reduces not only the risk of occlusion or restenosis but also reduces the incidence of major vascular events such as myocardial infarction or stroke and of death. Aspirin is sometimes started shortly before the procedures and sometimes shortly after. The rationale for delaying the initiation of therapy has been the belief that perioperative bleeding could be reduced but this does not appear to be an important factor[24] and the comment has been made[25] that trials which failed to show a benefit were those in which antiplatelet therapy had been delayed until the second or third postoperative day. The optimum dose and duration of therapy also needs to be established.[24]

Promising results in terms of reduction in restenosis and of adverse vascular events following coronary angioplasty have been reported with lanreotide[26,27] and trapidil.[28,29] Reduction in restenosis following coronary angioplasty has also been reported with probucol.[30] The drugs have been used in addition to standard therapies such as heparin and aspirin. However, experience with them is still very limited compared with the knowledge accumulated with aspirin for long-term prophylaxis. Benefit has been observed when lanreotide was given for about 5 days around the time of angioplasty whereas trapidil was given for up to 6 months postangioplasty. Probucol was given for a month before and 6 months after angioplasty. Both lanreotide and trapidil may act by reducing smooth muscle cell proliferation thus reducing neointimal hyperplasia. Probucol may act by reducing formation of active metabolites at the angioplasty site and thus preventing endothelial dysfunction; other actions have also been proposed.

Atherosclerosis in saphenous-vein coronary bypass grafts is a frequent cause of obstruction in the years following bypass surgery, especially in patients with hyperlipidaemia. Aggressive lowering of LDL-cholesterol using mainly statins may be beneficial in these patients.[31]

1. Corr L. New methods of making blocked coronary arteries patent again. *Br Med J* 1994; **309:** 579–83.
2. Goldberg S, *et al.* Coronary artery stents. *Lancet* 1995; **345:** 1523–4.
3. O'Meara JJ, Dehmer GJ. Care of the patient and management of complications after percutaneous coronary artery interventions. *Ann Intern Med* 1997; **127:** 458–71.
4. Landau C, *et al.* Percutaneous transluminal coronary angioplasty. *N Engl J Med* 1994; **330:** 981–93.
5. Wolfe JH. Critical limb ischaemia. *Prescribers' J* 1994; **34:** 50–8.
6. Serruys PW, *et al.* A comparison of hirudin with heparin in the prevention of restenosis after coronary angioplasty. *N Engl J Med* 1995; **333:** 757–63.
7. Nwasokwa ON. Coronary artery bypass graft disease. *Ann Intern Med* 1995; **123:** 528–45.
8. Vahanian A, Iung B. Role of calcium channel blockers in reducing acute ischaemia and preventing restenosis in PTCA. *Drugs* 1996; **52** (suppl 4): 9–16.
9. The EPIC Investigators. Use of a monoclonal antibody directed against the platelet glycoprotein IIb/IIIa receptor in high-risk coronary angioplasty. *N Engl J Med* 1994; **330:** 956–61.
10. The CAPTURE Investigators. Randomised placebo-controlled trial of abciximab before and during coronary intervention in refractory unstable angina: the CAPTURE study. *Lancet* 1997; **349:** 1429–35. Correction. *ibid.*; **350:** 744.
11. The EPILOG Investigators. Platelet glycoprotein IIb/IIIa receptor blockade and low-dose heparin during percutaneous coronary revascularization. *N Engl J Med* 1997; **336:** 1689–96.
12. Topol EJ, *et al.* Randomised trial of coronary intervention with antibody against platelet IIb/IIIa integrin for reduction of clinical restenosis: results at six months. *Lancet* 1994; **343:** 881–6.
13. Topol EJ, *et al.* Long-term protection from myocardial ischemic events in a randomized trial of brief integrin β_3 blockade with percutaneous coronary intervention. *JAMA* 1997; **278:** 479–84.
14. The IMPACT-II Investigators. Randomised placebo-controlled trial of effect of eptifibatide on complications of percutaneous coronary intervention: IMPACT-II. *Lancet* 1997; **349:** 1422–8.
15. Pepine CJ, *et al.* ACC Expert Consensus document: coronary artery stents. *J Am Coll Cardiol* 1996; **28:** 782–94.
16. Mauro LS, *et al.* Introduction to coronary artery stents and their pharmacotherapeutic management. *Ann Pharmacother* 1997; **31:** 1490–8.
17. Bittl JA. Advances in coronary angioplasty. *N Engl J Med* 1996; **335:** 1290–1302. Correction. *ibid.* 1997; **336:** 670.
18. Schömig A, *et al.* A randomized comparison of antiplatelet and anticoagulant therapy after the placement of coronary-artery stents. *N Engl J Med* 1996; **334:** 1084–9.
19. Hall P, *et al.* A randomized comparison of combined ticlopidine and aspirin therapy versus aspirin therapy alone after successful intravascular ultrasound-guided stent implantation. *Circulation* 1996; **93:** 215–22.
20. Lablanche J-M, *et al.* Combined antiplatelet therapy with ticlopidine and aspirin: a simplified approach to intracoronary stent management. *Eur Heart J* 1996; **17:** 1373–80.
21. The EPISTENT Investigators. Randomised placebo-controlled and balloon-angioplasty-controlled trial to assess safety of coronary stenting with use of platelet glycoprotein-IIb/IIIa blockade. *Lancet* 1998; **352:** 87–92.
22. Serruys PW, *et al.* Randomised comparison of implantation of heparin-coated stents with balloon angioplasty in selected patients with coronary artery disease (Benestent II). *Lancet* 1998; **352:** 673–81. Correction. *ibid.*; 1478.
23. Herrman J-PR, *et al.* Pharmacological approaches to the prevention of restenosis following angioplasty: the search for the holy grail? *Drugs* 1993; **46:** 18–52 and 249–62.
24. Antiplatelet Trialists' Collaboration. Collaborative overview of randomised trials of antiplatelet therapy—maintenance of vascular graft or arterial patency by antiplatelet therapy. *Br Med J* 1994; **308:** 159–68.
25. Underwood MJ, More RS. The aspirin papers. *Br Med J* 1994; **308:** 71–2.
26. Emanuelsson H, *et al.* Long-term effects of angiopeptin treatment in coronary angioplasty: reduction of clinical events but not angiographic restenosis. *Circulation* 1995; **91:** 1689–96.
27. Eriksen UH, *et al.* Randomised double-blind Scandinavian trial of angiopeptin versus placebo for the prevention of clinical events and restenosis after coronary balloon angioplasty. *Am Heart J* 1995; **130:** 1–8.
28. Okamoto S, *et al.* Effects of trapidil (triazolopyrimidine), a platelet-derived growth factor antagonist, in preventing restenosis after percutaneous transluminal coronary angioplasty. *Am Heart J* 1992; **123:** 1439–44.
29. Maresta A, *et al.* Trapidil (triazolopyrimidine), a platelet-derived growth factor antagonist, reduces restenosis after percutaneous transluminal coronary angioplasty: results of the randomized, double-blind STARC study. *Circulation* 1994; **90:** 2710–15.
30. Tardif J-C, *et al.* Probucol and multivitamins in the prevention of restenosis after coronary angioplasty. *N Engl J Med* 1997; **337:** 365–72.
31. The Post Coronary Artery Bypass Graft Trial Investigators. The effect of aggressive lowering of low-density lipoprotein cholesterol levels and low-dose anticoagulation on obstructive changes in saphenous-vein coronary-artery bypass grafts. *N Engl J Med* 1997; **336:** 153–62.
32. Gibson CM, *et al.* Six-month angiographic and clinical follow-up of patients prospectively randomized to receive either tirofiban or placebo during angioplasty in the RESTORE trial. *J Am Coll Cardiol* 1998; **32:** 28–34.

Shock

Shock is a complex clinical syndrome of multiple aetiologies. A traditional approach has been to place the cause of shock into one of several basic groups. Commonly used groupings are hypovolaemic shock, cardiogenic shock, septic shock, and anaphylactic shock. These are the types included below.

The common factor in all types of shock is a failure of the circulatory system to maintain cellular perfusion and function. A patient in decompensated shock classically presents with hypotension, tachycardia, and tachypnoea and has cold, clammy cyanotic skin and dulled mental alertness that may progress to stupor or coma; oliguria or anuria are also frequent. Complications of shock include disseminated intravascular coagulation due to platelet sludging and microvascular insufficiency, acute respiratory distress syndrome (previously termed 'shock lung') (p.1017), and acute renal failure. The terms multiple organ failure syndrome (MOFS) and multiple organ dysfunction syndrome (MODS) are applied to the consequences of shock where several organs or body systems have become hypoperfused and are unable to maintain their normal function.

In *hypovolaemic shock* fluid losses can arise from haemorrhagic or non-haemorrhagic causes. Haemorrhage can be from internal sources such as severe gastro-intestinal bleeding or external such as in traumatic injury. Causes of non-haemorrhagic hypovolaemia include severe vomiting and diarrhoea, polyuria, or burns. Hypovolaemia can also be present in most other forms of shock.

Cardiogenic shock has a number of causes but the underlying feature is usually acute heart failure with an inadequate stroke volume. It is most commonly associated with acute myocardial infarction. Other disorders that may result in cardiogenic shock include valvular heart disease, some cardiomyopathies, and some severe cardiac arrhythmias such as ventricular tachycardia or ventricular fibrillation. Shock due to circulatory disorders is also sometimes classified as cardiogenic shock. Like hypovolaemia, cardiac and circulatory problems may be seen in other forms of shock as well as in cardiogenic shock.

Septic shock may occur as a complication of infectious disease and is described and defined in more detail under Septicaemia, p.141.

Anaphylactic shock (p.816) is commonly a type I hypersensitivity reaction to various allergens such as drugs, foods, and insect venoms. A clinically identical reaction can, however, be provoked by a type II mechanism, as in blood transfusion reactions, or a type III mechanism, as in drug-induced serum sickness reactions.

Management. The management of shock falls into general supportive and symptomatic measures that may be applicable in all forms of shock and primary specific therapies directed against any underlying cause.

General measures include correction of electrolyte disturbances, correction of hypovolaemia and hypotension, and improving cardiac output. Pain and respiratory problems often accompany shock and may necessitate the administration of intravenous opioid analgesics and oxygen therapy.

Electrolyte disturbances (p.1147) should be managed conventionally; this may include the administration of sodium bicarbonate for acidosis. An adequate diuresis should be maintained in order to prevent renal failure.

Correction of hypovolaemia is important in all forms of shock. Various options are available[1-5] and the choice is not always clear. If haemorrhage has resulted in loss of approximately 50% or more of total blood volume then transfusion of whole blood is required, although for initial therapy volume expansion is more important. If haemorrhage is less severe, red cells together with plasma expanders may be adequate. In non-haemorrhagic hypovolaemia, plasma expanders alone are employed. However, debate continues concerning the relative merits of crystalloid or colloid solutions for volume expansion. Crystalloids (such as glucose or sodium chloride solutions) rapidly expand both the intravascular and extravascular compartments and it is argued by some that this is necessary as the interstitial space becomes depleted in hypovolaemia. Colloids (such as albumin, dextrans, gelatins, and hydroxyethyl starches) expand the intravascular space more effectively than crystalloids, and thus smaller volumes are employed leading to less haemodilution, although the exact significance of this has been questioned. A systematic review[6] of trials comparing the effect of volume replacement with colloid or crystalloid solutions in critically ill patients concluded that there was a small increase in mortality associated with the use of colloids. A further review[7] looking specifically at the use of albumin solutions in critically ill patients, including patients with hypovolaemia, reported that data suggested an increased mortality in those receiving the colloid. However, the conclusions of both reviews have been criticised,[8-10] and in practice a mixture of colloids and crystalloids tends to be given. Another potential concern with the use of colloids is that some have the potential to cause hypersensitivity reactions including anaphylaxis.

Successful correction of hypovolaemia may alleviate hypotension in some cases, but cardiac output may remain depressed and signs of impaired organ perfusion may persist, necessitating additional therapy. Further measures are also frequently needed if there is profound hypotension; blood pressure in shock can be extremely low (sometimes a systolic pressure of less than 70 mmHg) despite fluid replacement. In patients with profound **hypotension** or a **low cardiac output** sympathomimetics are usually employed.[11-13] Their precise effects on the vasculature vary and choice depends on individual patient characteristics and the type of shock.[14] In cardiogenic or hypovolaemic shock cardiac output is usually low but peripheral resistance is high and drugs that have predominantly inotropic effects are most suitable. Dopamine or dobutamine are often chosen. Dopamine is widely used in all forms of shock; in low doses it may maintain renal perfusion although higher doses cause vasoconstriction, and it is often used in combination with other inotropes. Dobutamine causes peripheral vasodilatation and is useful where hypotension is not significant. Noradrenaline causes peripheral vasoconstriction and should be reserved for severe hypotension. It is particularly useful in septic shock where the cardiac output is usually high but peripheral resistance is low. It is often given in combination with more potent inotropes such as dobutamine or adrenaline. Adrenaline has also been used alone but renal artery vasoconstriction may limit its use, and it has also been reported to cause lactic acidosis.[15] Phosphodiesterase inhibitors such as amrinone and milrinone, which have positive inotropic activity, can also be considered in low cardiac output states;[12] like dopamine they also produce peripheral vasodilatation. Vasodilators such as intravenous glyceryl trinitrate or sodium nitroprusside can be beneficial for patients in shock with a low cardiac output but a high diastolic pressure (more than 110 mmHg).[11,13] They act by reducing cardiac afterload. Caution must however by observed because of the risk of precipitating hypotension.

In **septic shock** appropriate antibacterial therapy should be given as outlined under Septicaemia on p.141. Methods of inhibiting endogenous mediators released in response to sepsis that are thought to be responsible for the haemodynamic effects are also under investigation but clinical benefits have not yet been demonstrated.[16]

Adrenaline is the cornerstone of management in **anaphylactic shock** (see p.816).

1. Donaldson MDJ, *et al.* Massive blood transfusion. *Br J Anaesth* 1992; **69:** 621–30.
2. Huskisson L. Intravenous volume replacement: which fluid and why? *Arch Dis Child* 1992; **67:** 649–53.
3. Shaw A, *et al.* Pathophysiological basis of burn management. *Br J Hosp Med* 1994; **52:** 583–7.
4. Cone A. The use of colloids in clinical practice. *Br J Hosp Med* 1995; **54:** 155–9.
5. Nolan JP, Parr MJA. Aspects of resuscitation in trauma. *Br J Anaesth* 1997; **79:** 226–40.
6. Schierhout G, Roberts I. Fluid resuscitation with colloid or crystalloid solutions in critically ill patients: a systematic review of randomised trials. *Br Med J* 1998; **316:** 961–4.
7. Cochrane Injuries Group Albumin Reviewers. Human albumin administration in critically ill patients: systematic review of randomised controlled trials. *Br Med J* 1998; **317:** 235–40.
8. Watts J. Fluid resuscitation with colloid or crystalloid solutions. *Br Med J* 1998; **317:** 277.
9. Wyncoll DLA, *et al.* Fluid resuscitation with colloid or crystalloid solutions. *Br Med J* 1998; **317:** 278–9.
10. Beale RJ, *et al.* Human albumin administration in critically ill patients. *Br Med J* 1998; **317:** 884.
11. Emergency Cardiac Care Committee and Subcommittees, American Heart Association. Guidelines for cardiopulmonary resuscitation and emergency cardiac care. *JAMA* 1992; **268:** 2171–2295.
12. Barnard MJ, Linter SPK. Acute circulatory support. *Br Med J* 1993; **307:** 35–41.
13. Califf RM, Bengtson JR. Cardiogenic shock. *N Engl J Med* 1994; **330:** 1724–30.
14. Cuthbertson BH, *et al.* Inotropic agents in the critically ill. *Br J Hosp Med* 1996; **56:** 386–91.
15. Day NPJ, *et al.* The effects of dopamine and adrenaline infusions on acid-base balance and systemic haemodynamics in severe infection. *Lancet* 1996; **348:** 219–23.
16. Glauser MP. The inflammatory cytokines: new developments in the pathophysiology and treatment of septic shock. *Drugs* 1996; **52** (suppl 2): 9–17.

Stroke

Stroke, sometimes called a cerebrovascular accident, is the major consequence of cerebrovascular disease and has been defined as an acute neurological dysfunction of vascular origin with sudden (within seconds) or at least rapid (within hours) occurrence of symptoms and signs corresponding to the involvement of focal areas of the brain.[1] If signs and symptoms persist for more than 24 hours the event is termed a completed stroke whereas if they disappear within a few minutes or hours, or at most within 24 hours, the event is termed a transient ischaemic attack.

Strokes may be ischaemic (infarction-related) or haemorrhagic. **Ischaemic stroke** is by far the commonest type and may result from arterial occlusion caused by local thrombosis in the vessels of the brain at sites of atheroma or, more often, by thrombo-embolism arising from outside the brain and lodging in the cerebral vessels. An example of the latter is cardio-embolic infarction associated with atrial fibrillation or acute myocardial infarction. Such arterial occlusion results in inadequate cerebral perfusion, depriving the brain of glucose and oxygen, and stroke occurs. About 20% of patients with acute ischaemic stroke experience worsening of symptoms within a few days of onset. This is termed progressing stroke, stroke-in-evolution, or unstable stroke, and occurs when the thrombotic process is incomplete. **Transient ischaemic attacks** are acute episodes of focal neurological deficit or monocular visual loss (amaurosis fugax), mainly due to ischaemia associated with atherothrombosis, but unlike stroke last less than 24 hours and often only minutes. They are usually of sudden onset with complete clinical recovery but a tendency to recur. Patients suffering these attacks are at an increased risk of stroke. **Haemorrhagic stroke** is secondary to subarachnoid or to intracerebral haemorrhage. *Subarachnoid haemorrhage* is bleeding into the fluid-filled subarachnoid space between the brain and the skull, and usually occurs after rupture of an aneurysm; other causes include arteriovenous malformations and hypertensive microaneurysms. *Intracerebral haemorrhage* is bleeding into the parenchyma of the brain, and may result from rupture of arteries damaged by chronic hypertension. Haemorrhage produces a focal haematoma causing a local increase in pressure which may lead to further bleeding and enlargement of the haematoma. The increase in pressure in the area of the haematoma may also produce local ischaemia.

Clinical presentation of stroke can vary enormously in severity and combination of signs and symptoms, and depends on the site of infarction or haemorrhage. Neurological deficits may include impairments to speech, balance, vision, touch sensation, and movement. Patients have been classed as major or minor stroke (reversible ischaemic neurological deficit) victims according to their degree of recovery at a given time after the stroke.

It is important to diagnose the type of stroke correctly because management is very different and what might be of benefit in patients with cerebral infarction might be dangerous in those with haemorrhage. Haemorrhagic stroke is typically of sudden onset with severe headaches, vomiting, and rapid deterioration of consciousness – all signs of raised intracranial pressure – but mild to moderate haemorrhage may be difficult to distinguish from infarction on the basis of clinical signs alone. Computed tomography (CT) is a surer way of distinguishing between haemorrhagic and ischaemic stroke. Magnetic resonance imaging may also be useful. Recent guidelines[2,3] have emphasised that, as in myocardial infarction, early recognition of symptoms and prompt evaluation and treatment of stroke are of vital importance; the European Ad Hoc Consensus Group[2] recommend admittance to hospital within one hour of symptom onset. Where possible patients should be managed within a stroke unit.

Diagnosis of transient ischaemic attacks usually rests on the patient's history as these short attacks are seldom witnessed by a physician and there are no objective confirmatory tests.

Management of stroke can be divided into: primary prevention, that is prior to any stroke or transient ischaemic attack in patients at risk or even apparently healthy people; treatment of acute stroke, either ischaemic or haemorrhagic; and secondary prevention, that is after a stroke or transient ischaemic attack has occurred.

Primary prevention

Primary prevention[4,5] is important, especially as treatment for acute stroke remains largely unsatisfactory. Prevention strategies require the identification of risk factors and if possible their modification in individuals at high risk and in the population as a whole. A major risk factor for stroke of any type appears to be hypertension and its treatment has reduced mortality from stroke. Atrial fibrillation, acute myocardial infarction, and valvular diseases may be sources of cardiogenic embolism[6] and are major risk factors for ischaemic stroke. Patients with these disorders may require prophylaxis with anticoagulants or antiplatelet drugs. For further details, see Cardiac Arrhythmias, above and Myocardial Infarction, above, respectively. Smoking is another major risk factor. Other risk factors identified include obesity, high fibrinogen concentrations, diabetes mellitus, oral contraceptive use (but see p.1429), diet, alcohol intake, and a family history of stroke. Many of these are also risk factors for ischaemic heart disease or atherosclerosis and similar preventive measures may apply (see Atherosclerosis, above). The relationship between plasma-cholesterol concentrations and risk of stroke is not clear, but a reduced incidence of stroke has been reported recently in studies of patients receiving statins[7,8] (see Hyperlipidaemias, p.1265).

Endarterectomy for carotid artery stenosis is an established method for the secondary prevention of stroke, but its role in primary prevention is less clear. A recent study[9] carried out in asymptomatic patients with carotid stenosis found that treatment with surgery, aspirin, and risk factor reduction produced a greater reduction in ischaemic stroke than aspirin and risk factor reduction alone. However, since the overall risk of stroke in this group of patients is already low, endarterectomy cannot be recommended for primary prevention of ischaemic stroke until those patients at highest risk of stroke can be identified.[10]

Primary prevention of stroke in healthy people has also been investigated. The US[11] and British[12] physicians' studies of aspirin in the prevention of cardiovascular and cerebrovascular disease both showed a slight non-significant increase in the number of disabling strokes which, in the US study, were attributed to cerebral haemorrhage. However, the American Heart Association[13] has suggested that the use of aspirin may be justified when patients have evidence of atherosclerotic disease or risk factors for stroke, as the high risk of ischaemic stroke that is reduced by aspirin outweighs the increased risk of haemorrhagic stroke. This may not be so in practice; both the Thrombosis Prevention Trial[60] in men at increased risk of ischaemic heart disease and the Hypertension Optimal Treatment (HOT) trial[61] in hypertensive patients reported little or no effect on the overall incidence of stroke.

Treatment

The aim of treatment in **acute ischaemic stroke** is early reversal or limitation of the degree of brain dysfunction by treatment, given as soon as possible after the onset of symptoms, that will re-establish cerebral blood flow, limit ischaemic neuronal injury, and reduce cerebral oedema.[14-17,58] General supportive measures include restoring systemic blood pressure, ensuring adequate oxygenation and fluid and electrolyte balances, avoiding hypercapnia and hyperglycaemia, and abolishing seizures. Many specific measures have been tried, but with the exception of aspirin, which has shown a small benefit, and possibly alteplase in selected patients, there is none that can be recommended routinely.

Antithrombotic therapy with antiplatelet agents, heparin, and thrombolytics would be expected to be of benefit in the treatment of cerebral infarction and the re-establishment of cerebral blood flow. However, the presence of haemorrhage must be excluded and the risk of potentiating spontaneous secondary brain haemorrhage (haemorrhagic transformation) must be borne in mind.

Antiplatelet drugs. The rationale for using aspirin is based on its effectiveness in patients with myocardial infarction where the underlying vascular pathology is similar to that in ischaemic stroke. Aspirin has been evaluated in two large studies—the International Stroke Trial (IST)[18] and the Chinese Acute Stroke Trial (CAST).[19] The combined results of these studies[19] found that aspirin 160 mg[19] or 300 mg[18] daily started within 48 hours of symptom onset produced about 9 fewer deaths or nonfatal strokes per 1000 patients in the first few weeks following ischaemic stroke.

Heparin. Anticoagulation should prevent further thrombus formation and limit the size of the cerebral infarct in acute ischaemic stroke. The International Stroke Trial[18] which evaluated two dosages of heparin (5000 units or 12 500 units subcutaneously twice a day) found no benefit from either regimen and the higher dose particularly was associated with haemorrhagic stroke and bleeding. It has previously been considered that patients with cardio-embolic stroke are likely to benefit from heparin therapy,[20] even though there is a special risk of haemorrhagic transformation in these patients which means that early anticoagulation is often hazardous. However, the International Stroke Trial[18] failed to show any benefit in this group. An initial study of a low-molecular-weight heparin produced favourable results at follow-up after 6 months.[21] No improvement in outcome was reported after 3 months in a study of danaparoid given in acute ischaemic stroke.[22] Ancrod is also under investigation. Early small studies of intravenous heparin in stroke-in-evolution were encouraging but have not been confirmed.[23-25]

Low-dose subcutaneous heparin may be indicated to reduce the risk of venous thrombo-embolism (deep-vein thrombosis and pulmonary embolism) associated with stroke.

Thrombolytics. Stroke is normally considered a contra-indication to the use of thrombolytics, and clearly they would be inappropriate in haemorrhagic stroke. However, when stroke is associated with thrombotic occlusion there is evidence, as with myocardial infarction, that a degree of neuronal recovery is possible if the occlusion is reversed sufficiently quickly. Early small studies suggested a fall in early death,[16] although subsequent randomised trials (three with streptokinase,[26-29] one with alteplase[30]) produced disappointing results with the exception of one with alteplase given within 3 hours of the onset of stroke (NINDS—National Institute of Neurological Disorders and Stroke rt-PA Stroke Trial).[31] The studies using streptokinase—MAST-E (Multicentre Acute Stroke Trial-Europe),[26,32] ASK (Australian Streptokinase Trial),[27] and MAST-I (Multicentre Acute Stroke Trial-Italy)[28,29]—were terminated early because of adverse outcomes (intracranial bleeding and increased mortality) in the treatment groups. The study investigating alteplase given within 6 hours of the onset of symptoms (ECASS I—European Cooperative Acute Stroke Study)[30] reported that, although some patients might benefit, overall alteplase was associated with higher mortality rates and an increase in some intracranial bleeding (parenchymal haemorrhage). The NINDS randomised study[31] of alteplase, given within 3 hours of the onset of ischaemic stroke, appeared to improve clinical outcome despite an increased incidence of symptomatic intracerebral haemorrhage. A second ECASS study (ECASS II)[59] that hoped to confirm the findings of the NINDS study failed to confirm a statistical benefit for alteplase over placebo and treatment differences were similar whether patients received alteplase within 3 hours or between 3 and 6 hours. On the basis of the NINDS study, alteplase given within 3 hours of the onset of ischaemic stroke has been recommended for selected patients in some guidelines on stroke management[2,3] and, despite their own disappointing results, the ECASS II investigators upheld this view. However, these recommendations have been criticised.[33,34] It has been pointed out[35,36] that very few patients will be eligible for treatment with alteplase, since the time of onset of symptoms is often uncertain and in many patients more than 3 hours elapses before a definite diagnosis of ischaemic stroke is made. In addition, the NINDS study[31] excluded patients with severe stroke and those taking anticoagulants. The rationale for exclusion of patients with severe stroke is that haemorrhagic transformation is more likely to occur with large areas of infarction.[35] However, size of infarct is difficult to identify by CT scanning.[35] Anticoagulants or antiplatelets are also contra-indicated in the first 24 hours after administration of alteplase. The poor results obtained in studies using streptokinase have led to recommendations that streptokinase should be avoided in ischaemic stroke,[2,3] although an overview of thrombolytic studies[36] suggested that streptokinase may not be worse than alteplase and that the apparent hazards of streptokinase may be accounted for by differences in trial design (for example concomitant use of anticoagulants) and in patient population. Thus, while alteplase can be considered for those few patients meeting the entry criteria for the NINDS study, further large studies are required to establish more clearly the role of thrombolytics in acute ischaemic stroke.

The intra-arterial administration of thrombolytics is under investigation.

Other attempts to improve cerebral blood flow have included haemodilution with *dextran* or *pentastarch,* but both of these approaches have been disappointing.

Ischaemia leads to a complex series of biochemical changes, the 'ischaemic cascade', resulting eventually in cell necrosis. The process is incompletely understood, but steps include calcium influx and release of neurotransmitters. Drugs acting at different steps in this ischaemic cascade, sometimes termed neuroprotectants, have been tried in acute ischaemic stroke in the hope of limiting the damage caused by ischaemia. Although results of studies so far have been largely disappointing, this is an area of active research and many trials of neuroprotectants are underway. Recent studies are focusing more on starting treatment with these drugs in the first few hours following ischaemic stroke.[37] Drugs that are or have been under investigation include:

calcium-channel blockers such as nimodipine. In addition to increasing cerebral blood flow they may prevent brain cell necrosis by limiting transcellular calcium influx, but results have been conflicting;[38,39]

chlormethiazole, which may act through an agonist effect on GABA receptors;

citicoline, a derivative of choline and cytidine, thought to prevent accumulation of toxic free fatty acids and to contribute to repair of damaged neuronal tissue;

epoprostenol, a prostaglandin thought to inhibit a stage of the ischaemic cascade;

fibroblast growth factors that stimulate blood vessel formation and tissue repair processes;

glycine antagonists, which block neuronal influx of calcium;

GM-1 ganglioside, a monosialoganglioside which reduces excitatory amino acid related neurotoxicity;

lubeluzole, a glutamate antagonist;

magnesium sulphate;

naftidrofuryl, which has a direct effect on cerebral intracellular metabolism and protects cells against the results of ischaemia;

N-methyl-D-aspartate (NMDA)-receptor antagonists such as aptiganel, dextrorphan, dextromethorphan, dizocilpine, ketamine, and selfotel might reduce ischaemic neuronal injury by preventing fatal influx of calcium;

oxpentifylline reduces viscosity of blood and this effect may be beneficial in ischaemic tissue;

tirilazad, a lipid peroxidation inhibitor (also used in subarachnoid haemorrhage).

Hypoxia and hypocapnia have been demonstrated in some patients with ischaemic stroke and are likely to contribute to ischaemic injury both directly and via cerebral vasoconstriction. There are anecdotal reports and some small studies on the use of *hyperbaric oxygen therapy* but its clinical value remains unknown.

Cerebral oedema associated with ischaemic stroke may be a mixture of intracellular oedema associated with cell damage (part of the ischaemic cascade) and interstitial vasogenic oedema. Treatment with *corticosteroids* or hyperosmolar diuretics such as *glycerol* or *mannitol* in an attempt to reduce the cerebral oedema have been disappointing.[40]

Patients who survive the acute event should be investigated to see if there is a cardiac source of emboli (see under Secondary Prevention of Stroke, below) and to determine whether surgery will be beneficial. Blood screening should also be carried out for polycythaemia, thrombocytosis, and abnormal coagulation functions.

Subarachnoid haemorrhage. Subarachnoid haemorrhage is associated with high morbidity and mortality, early deaths being due to damage from initial bleeding, recurrence of bleeding, and infarction. Infarction is often a result of vasospasm which is one of the pathophysiological mechanisms that contributes to stopping the bleeding; clot formation and increasing intracranial pressure are other processes involved. Up to a quarter of patients with subarachnoid haemorrhage develop delayed cerebral ischaemia mainly between days 5 and 14 after the initial bleed, again vasospasm may be a contributory factor. Early medical treatment aims to prevent delayed cerebral ischaemia, to prevent rebleeding, and to stabilise the patient until surgery can be carried out to clip the aneurysm or correct the arteriovenous malformation and thus prevent further haemorrhage.[41,42] Plasma volume should be maintained to prevent delayed cerebral ischaemia; a fluid intake of 3 litres per day has been recommended. Nimodipine is of benefit and should be started as soon as possible after diagnosis of subarachnoid haemorrhage. Antifibrinolytic drug therapy with tranexamic acid or aminocaproic acid has been used to prevent rebleeding, particularly if surgery is to be delayed, although this might result in an increased incidence of ischaemic complications. Paradoxically, rebleeding has been noted in patients given high doses of aminocaproic acid after subarachnoid haemorrhage (see Adverse Effects, Effects on the Blood, under Aminocaproic Acid, p.711). Headache can be managed with analgesics such as paracetamol, dextropropoxyphene, or codeine; aspirin should be avoided. Localised haematomas may be amenable to surgical evacuation. Tirilazad, a lipid peroxidation inhibitor, may be given to male patients with subarachnoid haemorrhage.

Intracerebral haemorrhage. Outcome of intracerebral haemorrhage depends on the location and size of the haematoma (determined by computed tomography), on the level of consciousness, and on the progression of neurological signs, and development of increased intracranial pressure.[43] Any known cause of bleeding such as warfarin anticoagulation, should be reversed. Blood pressure should be lowered when it is very high (>170 mmHg systolic), but hypoperfusion should be avoided. Labetalol has been used to reduce blood pressure. Surgical drainage of the haematoma may sometimes be possible. Raised intracranial pressure may be reduced by medical decompression using intubation with forced hyperventilation, mannitol or glycerol, and corticosteroids.

Secondary prevention

Once patients have suffered a stroke, risk factors should be identified (see Primary Prevention, above) and appropriate changes made in lifestyle. Hypertension requires treatment and surgery may be necessary in patients with aneurysms, arteriovenous malformations, or carotid stenoses. Patients who have suffered ischaemic stroke or transient ischaemic attacks are at risk of further stroke, myocardial infarction, or sudden death.[44-47] Nearly 20% of ischaemic strokes are secondary to cardiogenic emboli[9] and, as mentioned for primary prevention, antithrombotic therapy may be required.

Antiplatelet drugs. Long-term prophylaxis with aspirin reduces the risk of future serious vascular events including stroke in patients who have already suffered an ischaemic stroke or transient ischaemic attack,[45,46,48-50] regardless of age.[51] Medium doses of 75 to 325 mg of aspirin daily have been most widely studied. Dipyridamole given alone has also been shown to be effective for secondary prevention of ischaemic stroke[52] and may be used in patients unable to tolerate aspirin; the combination of aspirin and dipyridamole has produced additive protective effects.[52] Ticlopidine[53-55] or clopidogrel[56] may also be used in patients unable to tolerate aspirin and appear to be at least as effective.

Anticoagulants. The value of oral anticoagulants to prevent recurrent transient ischaemic attacks or stroke in patients with transient ischaemic attacks is unclear. One study was terminated early because of a high rate of major bleeding complications in the patients receiving an oral anticoagulant.[57] They have generally been used only in those who continue to experience transient ischaemic attacks despite treatment with aspirin. Oral anticoagulants may be started in these patients following anticoagulation with heparin. Long-term aspirin therapy may then be substituted.

1. WHO. Stroke—1989: recommendations on stroke prevention, diagnosis, and therapy: report of the WHO task force on stroke and other cerebrovascular disorders. *Stroke* 1989; **20:** 1407–31.
2. The European Ad Hoc Consensus Group. European strategies for early intervention in stroke: a report of an Ad Hoc Consensus Group meeting. *Cerebrovasc Dis* 1996; **6:** 315–24.
3. Adams HP, *et al.* Guidelines for thrombolytic therapy for acute stroke: a supplement to the guidelines for the management of patients with acute ischaemic stroke. *Circulation* 1996; **94:** 1167–74 [also published in *Stroke* 1996; **27:** 1711–18].
4. Marmot MG, Poulter NR. Primary prevention of stroke. *Lancet* 1992; **339:** 344–7.
5. Bronner LL, *et al.* Primary prevention of stroke. *N Engl J Med* 1995; **333:** 1392–1400.
6. Hart RG. Cardiogenic embolism to the brain. *Lancet* 1992; **339:** 589–94.
7. Crouse JR, *et al.* Reductase inhibitor monotherapy and stroke prevention. *Arch Intern Med* 1997; **157:** 1305–10.
8. Bucher HC, *et al.* Effect of HMGcoA reductase inhibitors on stroke: a meta-analysis of randomized, controlled trials. *Ann Intern Med* 1998; **128:** 89–95.
9. Executive Committee for the Asymptomatic Carotid Atherosclerosis Study. Endarterectomy for asymptomatic carotid artery stenosis. *JAMA* 1995; **273:** 1421–8.
10. Warlow C. Endarterectomy for asymptomatic carotid stenosis? *Lancet* 1995; **345:** 1254–5.
11. Steering committee of the Physicians' Health Study Research Group. Final report on the aspirin component of the ongoing physicians' health study. *N Engl J Med* 1989; **321:** 129–35.
12. Peto R, *et al.* Randomised trial of prophylactic daily aspirin in British male doctors. *Br Med J* 1988; **296:** 313–16.
13. Fuster V, *et al.* Aspirin as a therapeutic agent in cardiovascular disease. *Circulation* 1993; **87:** 659–75.
14. Sandercock P, Willems H. Medical treatment of acute ischaemic stroke. *Lancet* 1992; **339:** 537–9.
15. Sila CA. Prophylaxis and treatment of stroke: the state of the art in 1993. *Drugs* 1993; **45:** 329–37.
16. Bath PMW. Treating acute ischaemic stroke. *Br Med J* 1995; **311:** 139–40.
17. Adams HP, *et al.* Guidelines for the management of patients with acute ischemic stroke: a statement for healthcare professionals from a special writing group of the Stroke Council, American Heart Association. *Stroke* 1994; **25:** 1901–14.
18. International Stroke Trial Collaborative Group. The International Stroke Trial (IST): a randomised trial of aspirin, subcutaneous heparin, both, or neither among 19 435 patients with acute ischaemic stroke. *Lancet* 1997; **349:** 1569–81.
19. CAST (Chinese Acute Stroke Trial) Collaborative Group. CAST: randomised placebo-controlled trial of early aspirin use in 20 000 patients with acute ischaemic stroke. *Lancet* 1997; **349:** 1641–9.
20. Sandercock PAG, *et al.* Antithrombotic therapy in acute ischaemic stroke: an overview of the completed randomised trials. *J Neurol Neurosurg Psychiatry* 1993; **56:** 17–25.

21. Kay R, *et al.* Low-molecular-weight heparin for the treatment of acute ischemic stroke. *N Engl J Med* 1995; **333:** 1588–93.
22. The Publications Committee for the Trial of ORG 10172 in Acute Stroke Treatment (TOAST) Investigators. Low molecular weight heparinoid, ORG 10172 (danaparoid), and outcome after acute ischemic stroke: a randomized controlled trial. *JAMA* 1998; **279:** 1265–72.
23. Harper GD, Castleden CM. Drug therapy in patients with recent stroke. *Br Med Bull* 1990; **46:** 181–201.
24. Jonas S. Anticoagulant therapy in cerebrovascular disease: review and meta-analysis. *Stroke* 1988; **19:** 1043–8.
25. Sherman DG, *et al.* Antithrombotic therapy for cerebrovascular disorders. *Chest* 1989; **95** (suppl): 140S-155S.
26. Hommel M, *et al.* Termination of trial of streptokinase in severe acute ischaemic stroke. *Lancet* 1995; **345:** 57.
27. Donnan GA, *et al.* Trials of streptokinase in severe acute ischaemic stroke. *Lancet* 1995; **345:** 578–9.
28. Multicentre Acute Stroke Trial - Italy (MAST-I) Group. Randomised controlled trial of streptokinase, aspirin, and combination of both in treatment of acute ischaemic stroke. *Lancet* 1995; **346:** 1509–14.
29. Tognoni G, Roncaglioni MC. Dissent: an alternative interpretation of MAST-I. *Lancet* 1995; **346:** 1515.
30. Hacke W, *et al.* Intravenous thrombolysis with recombinant tissue plasminogen activator for acute hemispheric stroke: the European Cooperative Acute Stroke Study (ECASS). *JAMA* 1995; **274:** 1017–25.
31. The National Institute of Neurological Disorders and Stroke rt-PA Stroke Study Group. Tissue plasminogen activator for acute ischemic stroke. *N Engl J Med* 1995; **333:** 1581–7.
32. The Multicenter Acute Stroke Trial—Europe Study Group. Thrombolytic therapy with streptokinase in acute ischemic stroke. *N Engl J Med* 1996; **335:** 145–50.
33. Caplan LR. Stroke thrombolysis—growing pains. *Mayo Clin Proc* 1997; **72:** 1090–2.
34. Caplan LR, *et al.* Should thrombolytic therapy be the first-line treatment for acute ischemic stroke? Thrombolysis—not a panacea for ischemic stroke. *N Engl J Med* 1997; **337:** 1309–10.
35. Muir KW. Thrombolysis for stroke: pushed out of the window? *Br J Clin Pharmacol* 1996; **42:** 681–2.
36. Wardlaw JM, *et al.* Systematic review of evidence on thrombolytic therapy for acute ischaemic stroke. *Lancet* 1997; **350:** 607–14.
37. Fisher M, Bogousslavsky J. Further evolution toward effective therapy for acute ischemic stroke. *JAMA* 1998; **279:** 1298–1303.
38. Gelmers HJ, Hennerici M. Effect of nimodipine on acute ischemic stroke: pooled results from five randomized trials. *Stroke* 1990; **21** (suppl IV): IV-81–IV-84.
39. The American Nimodipine Study Group. Clinical trial of nimodipine in acute ischemic stroke. *Stroke* 1992; **23:** 3–8.
40. Anonymous. Treatment for stroke? *Lancet* 1991; **337:** 1129–31.
41. Powell M. Subarachnoid haemorrhage. *Prescribers' J* 1990; **30:** 173–9.
42. van Gijn J. Subarachnoid haemorrhage. *Lancet* 1992; **339:** 653–5.
43. Caplan LR. Intracerebral haemorrhage. *Lancet* 1992; **339:** 656–8.
44. Warlow C. Secondary prevention of stroke. *Lancet* 1992; **339:** 724–7.
45. American College of Physicians. Guidelines for medical treatment for stroke prevention. *Ann Intern Med* 1994; **121:** 54–5.
46. Matchar DB, *et al.* Medical treatment for stroke prevention. *Ann Intern Med* 1994; **121:** 41–53.
47. Warlow CP, Davenport RJ. The management of transient ischaemic attacks. *Prescribers' J* 1996; **36:** 1–8.
48. Antiplatelet Trialists' Collaboration. Collaborative overview of randomised trials of antiplatelet therapy—I: prevention of death, myocardial infarction, and stroke by prolonged antiplatelet therapy in various categories of patients. *Br Med J* 1994; **308:** 81–106. Correction. *ibid.*; 1540.
49. Hennekens CH, *et al.* Aspirin as a therapeutic agent in cardiovascular disease: a statement for healthcare professionals from the American Heart Association. *Circulation* 1997; **96:** 2751–3.
50. Sherman DG, *et al.* Antithrombotic therapy for cerebrovascular disorders: an update. *Chest* 1995; **108** (suppl 4): 444S–456S.
51. Sivenius J, *et al.* Antiplatelet treatment in elderly people with transient ischaemic attacks or ischaemic strokes. *Br Med J* 1995; **310:** 25–6.
52. Diener HC, *et al.* European Stroke Prevention Study 2: dipyridamole and acetylsalicylic acid in the secondary prevention of stroke. *J Neurol Sci* 1996; **143:** 1–13.
53. Hass WK, *et al.* A randomized trial comparing ticlopidine hydrochloride with aspirin for the prevention of stroke in high-risk patients. *N Engl J Med* 1989; **321:** 501–7.
54. Harbison JW. Ticlopidine versus aspirin for the prevention of recurrent stroke: analysis of patients with minor stroke from the ticlopidine aspirin stroke study. *Stroke* 1992; **23:** 1723–7.
55. Bellavance A. Efficacy of ticlopidine and aspirin for prevention of reversible cerebrovascular ischemic events: the ticlopidine aspirin stroke study. *Stroke* 1993; **24:** 1452–7.
56. CAPRIE Steering Committee. A randomised, blinded, trial of clopidogrel versus aspirin in patients at risk of ischaemic events (CAPRIE). *Lancet* 1996; **348:** 1329–39.
57. The Stroke Prevention in Reversible Ischemia Trial (SPIRIT) Study Group. A randomized trial of anticoagulants versus aspirin after cerebral ischemia of presumed arterial origin. *Ann Neurol* 1997; **42:** 857–65.
58. Various. Stroke. *Lancet* 1998; **352** (suppl 3): 1–30.
59. Hacke W, *et al.* Randomised double-blind placebo-controlled trial of thrombolytic therapy with intravenous alteplase in acute ischaemic stroke (ECASS II). *Lancet* 1998; **352:** 1245–51.
60. The Medical Research Council's General Practice Research Framework. Thrombosis prevention trial: randomised trial of low-intensity oral anticoagulation with warfarin and low-dose aspirin in the primary prevention of ischaemic heart disease in men at increased risk. *Lancet* 1998; **351:** 233–41.
61. Hansson L, *et al.* Effects of intensive blood-pressure lowering and low-dose aspirin in patients with hypertension: principal results of the Hypertension Optimal Treatment (HOT) randomised trial. *Lancet* 1998; **351:** 1755–62.

Thrombo-embolic disorders

The term thrombo-embolic disorder has been applied loosely to cardiovascular disorders associated with thrombus and embolus formation in blood vessels. A **thrombus** is a stationary blood clot composed of fibrin and platelets and other cellular elements. **Thrombosis** is occlusion of a vein or artery by a thrombus. An **embolus** is a fragment of blood clot, atheromatous material, or other foreign matter carried along in the blood stream. Occlusion of a blood vessel by an embolus is termed **embolism** or **thrombo-embolism**.

Formation of blood clots in the body is the result of a coagulation cascade (see p.704). Under normal circumstances systemic coagulation is prevented by natural antithrombotic systems that limit blood clots to sites of vascular injury. Thrombo-embolic disorders occur when there is an imbalance between these systems. Three factors are involved, namely damage to the endothelial lining of blood vessels, reduced blood flow, or changes in the coagulation mechanisms of the blood. A further factor that increases the risk of clotting is the presence of an artificial surface in contact with the blood, for example mechanical heart valves, intravascular catheters, or during extracorporeal circulation procedures. Thrombo-embolism can occur in any part of the circulation, including the heart and the capillaries, but the characteristics of the thrombi, the consequences, and the management of thrombo-embolism depend to a large extent upon whether the arterial or venous system is involved.

The mainstay of management for thrombo-embolic disorders is antithrombotic drugs. These act at different sites in the coagulation cascade and include anticoagulants and antiplatelet drugs, which are used to limit the extent of thrombosis or thrombo-embolism and to prevent further thrombo-embolic events occurring, and thrombolytics, which are used to lyse the clot.

Arterial thrombo-embolism is almost always a consequence of damage to the endothelium due to atherosclerosis (above); the atheroma may block the blood vessel or, more commonly, occlusion is a result of thrombus formation at a site of a recently ruptured atheromatous plaque. Arterial thrombi contain more platelets than venous thrombi and tend to remain fixed, but emboli may break off and occlude distal vessels. Arterial emboli may also result from thrombosis within the heart, for example due to arrhythmias or valvular heart disorders.

Thrombosis or thrombo-embolism in the arterial circulation produces ischaemia in the tissues perfused by the artery leading to infarction. It may therefore result in myocardial infarction (above) or unstable angina (above) if it occurs in coronary arteries, stroke (above) if it occurs in cerebral arteries, or critical limb ischaemia if it occurs in peripheral arteries (above).

Venous thrombo-embolism (below) is usually a consequence of stasis of the blood, but other factors such as local trauma or coagulation activation are also required. Reduced venous blood flow occurs in many conditions, including obesity, heart failure, and during prolonged immobilisation. Abnormal clotting may occur in conditions such as malignancy, pregnancy, and the nephrotic syndrome, or during oestrogen therapy; it may also be due to inherited or acquired clotting disorders or thrombophilias (see below). Surgical operations are particularly associated with venous thrombo-embolism; trauma activates clotting factors and reduced blood flow may occur during the procedure and recovery period.

Venous thrombi have a 'red tail' of fibrin and red cells that may occlude the vein but which often separates to form an embolus; this is most likely during the early stages when the thrombus is only loosely attached. Thrombosis or thrombo-embolism in the venous circulation produces oedema or inflammation in the tissue drained by the affected vein. The commonest type of venous thrombosis is deep-vein thrombosis which is associated especially with immobility and the post-operative period. Pulmonary embolism is the most serious complication of deep-vein thrombosis and occurs when part of the thrombus migrates in the circulation and becomes lodged in the pulmonary artery. Hypercoagulable states may result in deep-vein thrombosis or more generalised clotting in microvessels (microvessel thrombosis), such as thrombotic thrombocytopenic purpura or purpura fulminans (see Thrombotic Microangiopathies, p.726).

Thrombophilias are acquired or inherited disorders of the clotting system in which the antithrombotic mechanisms are impaired. Inherited deficiencies of antithrombin III, protein C and protein S all predispose to thrombo-embolism. More recently, resistance to activated protein C has been identified as a major cause of inherited thrombophilia and appears to be due to a mutation in the factor V gene (factor V Leiden). Acquired thrombophilias are more common and may occur secondary to disorders such as malignancy, infection, or collagen-vascular disorders; in many cases antiphospholipid antibodies (such as lupus anticoagulant) are present.

Inherited thrombophilias generally result in venous thrombo-embolism; this is often recurrent and may occur in unusual sites or at a young age. They often present when some further risk factor is present, such as pregnancy, use of combined oral contraceptives, or surgery, but the value of screening asymptomatic patients remains unclear. Acquired thrombophilias may lead to arterial or venous thrombo-embolism.

Patients with thrombophilias who develop thrombo-embolism should be treated conventionally, with anticoagulants or thrombolytics as appropriate. There continues to be debate regarding the duration of therapy, with some authorities recommending life-long anticoagulant therapy following a single episode and others recommending life-long therapy only in those with recurrent thrombosis. If anticoagulation is not continued, thromboprophylaxis should be given during high risk situations. Thromboprophylaxis is probably also necessary during pregnancy, particularly in women with antiphospholipid antibodies who are at risk for recurrent fetal loss, but the risks to the fetus from anticoagulant therapy must also be considered (see Venous Thrombo-embolism, below).

References.

1. Haines ST, Bussey HI. Thrombosis and the pharmacology of antithrombotic agents. *Ann Pharmacother* 1995; **29:** 892–905.
2. Anonymous. Management of patients with thrombophilia. *Drug Ther Bull* 1995; **33:** 6–8.
3. WHO. Inherited thrombophilia: memorandum from a joint WHO/International Society on Thrombosis and Haemostasis meeting. *Bull WHO* 1997; **75:** 177–89.
4. Price DT, Ridker PM. Factor V Leiden mutation and the risks for thromboembolic disease: a clinical perspective. *Ann Intern Med* 1997; **127:** 895–903.

Valvular heart disease

Valvular heart disease affects the normal function of the heart and leads to disorders of the blood circulation. The principal cause of valvular disease world-wide is rheumatic endocarditis. Other causes include congenital abnormalities, cardiovascular disorders such as ischaemic heart disease and hypertension, and degenerative disorders. Any of the heart valves may be affected but disorders of the aortic and mitral valves are most significant; more than one valve may be involved in some patients.

The symptoms of valvular heart disease depend upon the valve that is affected, and whether the problem is stenosis or regurgitation. All valve disorders place a haemodynamic burden on the heart and ultimately lead to heart failure.[1] Other consequences include the development of pulmonary hypertension and arrhythmias. Infective endocarditis and thrombo-embolic disorders, in particular stroke or systemic embolism, are important complications.

The main aims of treatment in patients with valvular heart disease are to reduce symptoms, prevent complications, and reduce mortality. In symptomatic patients, standard treatment for heart failure (see above) may be of benefit, although improvement is not generally sustained. Choice of therapy depends upon the valve affected; vasodilators should not be used in patients with aortic stenosis.[2] Arrhythmias should be treated with standard antiarrhythmics (see above). Surgical treatment is necessary in most patients and generally involves valve replacement, although valve repair may be suitable in some cases, particularly for mitral regurgitation. Valve replacement alleviates symptoms but does not remove the risks of endocarditis or thrombo-embolism. Bioprosthetic (tissue) or mechanical valves may be used; the latter are longer lasting, but pose a greater risk for thrombo-embolism.

In asymptomatic patients and in those who have had valve replacement, the main aim of therapy is to prevent the complications of bacterial endocarditis and of systemic embolism from thrombus formation within the heart.[3] Antibiotic prophylaxis should be given to all patients with valvular heart disease as indicated (see Endocarditis, p.120). Long-term thrombo-embolism prophylaxis is only required in patients with another risk factor for embolisation, such as concurrent atrial fibrillation, a dilated left atrium, or previous systemic embolism,[4] and in those with mechanical replacement valves.

Long-term treatment with an oral anticoagulant such as warfarin is generally regarded as essential for patients with a mechanical prosthetic heart valve.[3,5] The risk of thrombo-embolism depends upon the type and position of the valve and the presence of other risk factors. In the UK, a target INR of 3.5 is recommended,[6] but there is evidence that lower intensities may be effective while reducing the risk of bleeding.[7,8] In the USA, the recommended target INR is 2.5 to 3.5,[4,9] although a lower range of 2.0 to 3.0 may be adequate and is recommended where there is a high risk of bleeding. A higher level of anticoagulation may be considered in patients with caged-ball or caged-disk valves.[9]

For patients with bioprosthetic heart valves anticoagulants are recommended for the first 3 months after replacement.[3,5] Thereafter, long-term oral anticoagulant therapy is generally considered unnecessary for valves placed in the aortic position.[4] For patients with atrial fibrillation, a dilated left atrium, left atrial thrombus, or a history of systemic embolism, continued anticoagulation is usually recommended.[4,5,9] An INR of 2.0 to 3.0 appears adequate for patients with bioprosthetic heart valves.[4,5,9,10]

The value of adding an antiplatelet drug to anticoagulant therapy in patients with artificial heart valves is unclear. There is some evidence of benefit in all patients with mechanical prosthetic valves but the risk of bleeding is increased and they are currently only recommended as adjuncts in patients with other risk factors,[3,5] although they may be considered in other patients.[9] Dipyridamole has been preferred to aspirin because of the lower risk of bleeding complications when used in conjunction with warfarin, but low-dose aspirin may have benefits. Aspirin may also be considered in patients with bioprosthetic valves who are at intermediate risk but who do not require oral anticoagulants.[3,4] It has been suggested[11] that all patients with prosthetic valves should receive low-dose aspirin given its additional benefits in preventing cardiovascular disease.

The use of anticoagulants is controversial in patients with infective endocarditis because of the substantial increase in risk of haemorrhage in these patients. Oral anticoagulants should generally be continued in patients who have prosthetic heart valves, unless complications occur.[5] Anticoagulation may also be considered for patients with endocarditis who have other risk factors for systemic embolism.

Pregnancy is a known risk-factor for thrombo-embolism and patients with valvular heart disease who become pregnant are therefore at increased risk. However, long-term prophylaxis with an oral anticoagulant such as warfarin presents a problem since warfarin is generally contra-indicated in pregnancy (see Adverse Effects under Warfarin, p.964). Women with mechanical prosthetic valves must continue anticoagulation but it is usually recommended that subcutaneous heparin should be substituted for warfarin.[3,4] A dose of 17 500 to 20 000 units subcutaneously every 12 hours, together with aspirin 100 mg daily, has been suggested;[12] intravenous administration is an alternative but low-dose subcutaneous heparin is not suitable since it provides inadequate protection against prosthetic valve thrombosis.[13] Ideally heparin should be started before conception, or as soon after as possible, and should be continued at least until the 12th week to avoid the risk of warfarin embryopathy. If necessary, warfarin may then be reintroduced, although heparin is also recommended at term (to avoid an anticoagulated neonate). Low-dose aspirin may be used as an adjunct to heparin or warfarin.[5] However, a retrospective study[14] reported satisfactory outcomes following use of warfarin during the first trimester of pregnancy and some authorities[2] recommend continued use of oral anticoagulants throughout pregnancy in most patients. Low-molecular-weight heparins or heparinoids may also be an alternative to heparin in pregnant patients, but experience with these drugs is limited and they are not currently recommended.[3,13]

1. Carabello BA, Crawford FA. Valvular heart disease. *N Engl J Med* 1997; **337:** 32–41.
2. Prendergast BD, *et al.* Valvular heart disease: recommendations for investigation and management. *J R Coll Physicians Lond* 1996; **30:** 309–15.
3. Coulshed DS, *et al.* Drug treatment associated with heart valve replacement. *Drugs* 1995; **49:** 897–911.
4. Hirsh J, Fuster V. Guide to anticoagulant therapy part 2: oral anticoagulants. *Circulation* 1994; **89:** 1469–80.
5. Vongpatanasin W, *et al.* Prosthetic heart valves. *N Engl J Med* 1996; **335:** 407–16.
6. British Society for Haematology: British Committee for Standards in Haematology—Haemostasis and Thrombosis Task Force. Guidelines on oral anticoagulation: third edition. *Br J Haematol* 1998; **101:** 374–87.
7. Saour JN, *et al.* Trial of different intensities of anticoagulation in patients with prosthetic heart valves. *N Engl J Med* 1990; **322:** 428–32.
8. Cannegieter SC, *et al.* Optimal oral anticoagulant therapy in patients with mechanical heart valves. *N Engl J Med* 1995; **333:** 11–17.
9. Stein PD, *et al.* Antithrombotic therapy in patients with mechanical and biological prosthetic heart valves. *Chest* 1995; **108** (suppl): 371S–379S.
10. Turpie AGG, *et al.* Randomised comparison of two intensities of oral anticoagulant therapy after tissue heart valve replacement. *Lancet* 1988; **i:** 1242–5.
11. Tiede DJ, *et al.* Modern management of prosthetic valve anticoagulation. *Mayo Clin Proc* 1998; **73:** 665–80.
12. Ginsberg JS, Barron WM. Pregnancy and prosthetic heart valves. *Lancet* 1994; **344:** 1170–2.
13. Maternal and Neonatal Haemostasis Working Party of the Haemostasis and Thrombosis Task. Guidelines on the prevention, investigation and management of thrombosis associated with pregnancy. *J Clin Pathol* 1993; **46:** 489–96.
14. Sbarouni E, Oakley CM. Outcome of pregnancy in women with valve prostheses. *Br Heart J* 1994; **71:** 196–201.

Venous thrombo-embolism

The term venous thrombo-embolism embraces both deep-vein thrombosis and pulmonary embolism; the two often co-exist and should be considered as a single clinical entity. In deep-vein thrombosis a thrombus forms, frequently in the pockets of valves, and blocks the veins of the lower limbs or main pelvic veins. Pulmonary embolism occurs when the thrombus or part of it migrates in the circulation and blocks the pulmonary artery. About 70% of patients with confirmed pulmonary embolism have thrombosis in their deep leg veins and about 40% of patients with confirmed deep-vein thrombosis have silent pulmonary embolism. Proximal deep-vein thrombosis is associated with a higher risk of pulmonary embolism than distal deep-vein thrombosis.

Venous thrombo-embolism is a common but underdiagnosed condition and the cause of considerable morbidity and mortality, especially among hospitalised patients. Various factors underlie the development of thrombosis and there are a number of conditions that predispose patients to venous thrombo-embolism (see Thrombo-embolic Disorders, above).

Symptoms of *deep-vein thrombosis* include a tender and swollen calf; increased temperature, cyanosis, and engorgement of the superficial veins of the affected limb; fever; and tachycardia. However, about half of all cases may be symptomless. In the longer term chronic venous insufficiency and venous ulceration often occur (post-phlebitic or post-thrombotic syndrome). As most clinical signs of deep-vein thrombosis are non-specific, the diagnosis should always be confirmed before committing a patient to long-term anticoagulation treatment. Noninvasive diagnostic techniques such as ultrasound and impedence plethysmography are usually adequate but venography may be required;[1] an iodine-125-labelled fibrinogen uptake test has also been used. *Pulmonary embolism* may present in a number of ways depending on its extent and duration. Acute massive embolism causes serious haemodynamic disturbance with a sudden reduction in cardiac output and circulatory collapse. The most common form of pulmonary embolism seen, however, is acute minor embolism where the patient may present with pleuritic pain, haemoptysis, dyspnoea, tachycardia, and fever. Diagnosis may involve perfusion/ventilation scans or angiography.[2]

Prophylaxis of venous thrombo-embolism. Prophylaxis with anticoagulants aims to prevent deep-vein thrombosis and hence pulmonary embolism in patients at risk. It appears to be underused.[3-5] Ideally all medical and surgical hospital inpatients should be assessed for risk factors and should receive prophylaxis according to their degree of risk at least until discharge or, for those at higher risk, after discharge. A prophylactic regimen should be chosen for a particular patient after balancing the degree of risk against the potential complications of prophylaxis. Guidelines have been published by the British Society for Haematology[6] and the American College of Chest Physicians.[7]

Patients can be categorised as being at low, medium, or high risk of venous thrombo-embolism according to the duration and type of operation in those undergoing surgery, to age, and to the presence of other risk factors.[8] Low-risk patients include young patients undergoing short operative procedures. Older age, operations lasting longer than 30 minutes, and a history of thrombophilia or previous thrombo-embolism indicate medium risk. Orthopaedic surgery is associated with a high risk of venous thrombo-embolism in all patients. Other patients at high risk include those with multiple risk factors. Non-surgical patients are also at risk of thrombo-embolism, particularly if they are immobile, but there is less experience with prophylaxis in this group of patients. Pregnancy is also a risk factor and is discussed in more detail below.

Methods of prophylaxis may be physical or pharmacological. Physical methods, which increase venous velocity, include elevation of the legs, early ambulation, graduated compression stockings, and intermittent pneumatic compression boots. Pharmacological methods generally involve anticoagulation usually with heparin, low-molecular-weight heparins, or an oral anticoagulant. Other therapies that have been used include antiplatelet drugs, dihydroergotamine, dextrans, antithrombin III, and, more recently, heparinoids such as danaparoid. Ancrod has been used in patients who have developed heparin-induced thrombocytopenia or thrombosis.

For low-risk surgical patients general measures such as early ambulation and the use of graduated compression stockings are generally considered adequate. Moderate- and high-risk patients generally require pharmacological methods, although physical methods (particularly intermittent compression devices) may be used in those who are at high risk from bleeding complications. Physical methods are not suitable in patients with significant peripheral vascular disease. In practice, a combination of mechanical methods (particularly graduated compression stockings) and pharmacological methods is often used, and may give better protection than either method alone.[7]

For moderate-risk patients, such as those undergoing general surgical procedures lasting more than 30 minutes, low-dose subcutaneous heparin ('standard heparin prophylaxis') is the most widely used pharmacological method, a typical regimen being 5000 units subcutaneously 2 hours pre-operatively, then every 8 or 12 hours postoperatively for 7 days or until the patient is mobile.[6] Subcutaneous low-molecular-weight heparins may be used as an alternative. High-risk patients usually require higher doses of heparin with laboratory monitoring (adjusted-dose heparin); alternatively subcutaneous low-molecular-weight heparins or oral anticoagulants may be used.

Many studies have examined the use of *low-dose subcutaneous heparin* for surgical thrombo-embolism prophylaxis. In an overview[9] of more than 70 randomised studies in 16 000 patients heparin reduced the risk of subclinical deep-vein thrombosis by 67% in general surgery, 68% in orthopaedic surgery, and 75% in urological surgery. There was also a 40% reduction in non-fatal cases of pulmonary embolism, a 64% reduction in fatal cases, and a 47% reduction of all cases. Surgical thrombo-embolism prophylaxis with heparin also decreased total mortality.

Adjusted-dose heparin may be more effective in higher risk patients but the need for laboratory monitoring and the risk of bleeding complications limit its use. *Low-molecular-weight heparins* have a number of potential advantages, including less frequent administration and no need for monitoring, and they are being used increasingly. It was hoped that they might also reduce the risk of bleeding but this has not been clearly demonstrated. Generally, studies have shown low-molecular-weight heparins to be at least as effective as unfractionated or standard heparin, but a number of meta-analyses have come to differing conclusions regarding superiority. The evidence suggests that low-molecular-weight heparins are superior in orthopaedic surgery,[10-13] particularly with regard to proximal deep-vein thrombosis.[12] In general surgery both types of heparin appear to be of equivalent efficacy, although one analysis[11] reported that low-molecular-weight heparins were superior. A recent large study[14] showed low-molecular-weight heparins to be as effective as heparin for prophylaxis after major abdominal surgery and to be associated with fewer bleeding complications. Two recent meta-analyses of 45 studies[15] and 56 studies[16] respectively evaluated the efficacy of several prophylactic methods (such as aspirin, dextran, oral anticoagulants, heparin, heparin with dihydroergotamine, low-molecular-weight heparins, and intermittent pneumatic compression) against deep-vein thrombosis following major hip surgery and concluded that low-molecular-weight heparins should be the method of choice. Low-molecular-weight heparins may also be more effective than unfractionated heparin in patients with major trauma.[17]

The optimum duration of prophylaxis is unclear. Prophylaxis is usually only continued during hospitalisation but 2 studies[18,19] have shown an increased risk for venographically detected deep-vein thrombosis up to a month after discharge. This risk was reduced by low-molecular-weight heparin but the clinical significance of this finding has been questioned.[20]

Oral anticoagulants have not been so widely used as subcutaneous heparin. Amstutz *et al.*[21] described 'a low-dose' warfarin regimen (initially 10 mg), given on the night of surgery and continued for 3 weeks after, in 3000 total hip replacements. There were 14 cases (0.5%) of pulmonary embolism, none fatal. Bleeding complications occurred in 44 operations (1.5%) although the incidence depended on the type of hip prosthesis used. A fixed minidose warfarin regimen (1 mg daily) starting a mean of 20 days before gynaecological surgery was effective[22] but a similar regimen in patients having hip or knee joint replacements was not.[23,24] In another study[25] warfarin, in a low-dose regimen [dose not stated but not fixed] beginning 10 to 14 days before total hip replacement, was much more effective than external pneumatic compression in preventing proximal vein thrombi, but was less effective in preventing calf vein thrombosis. 'Less intense' warfarin (an international normalised ratio of 2.0 to 3.0 — see Warfarin, p.969 for further details), not to be confused with minidose warfarin, is one of the prophylactic methods recommended by authorities in the USA for selected high risk general surgical patients and for hip surgery.[7] When compared with low-molecular-weight heparins it was slightly less effective in preventing deep-vein thrombosis after hip or knee replacements, but there were fewer bleeding complications with warfarin; adjusted-dose warfarin was started on the evening of the day of surgery in an initial dose of 10 mg.[26]

Antiplatelet drugs such as aspirin have been considered less effective antithrombotics than anticoagulants in the venous circulation and to be of limited value in preventing venous thrombo-embolism. However, a collaborative overview[27] of all relevant randomised trials available by March 1990 indicated that antiplatelet prophylaxis should be reconsidered since all the evidence demonstrated a reduction in the incidence of deep-vein thrombosis and pulmonary embolism in a wide range of surgical patients and possible benefit in high-risk medical patients. Aspirin alone was the most widely used antiplatelet regimen. Others included aspirin with dipyridamole; hydroxychloroquine; and ticlopidine. This advice did attract some criticism[28] but was defended.[29]

Of the other drugs tried for surgical thrombo-embolism prophylaxis, *dihydroergotamine* can reduce venous stasis by vasoconstriction of capacitance vessels and has enhanced postoperative prophylaxis when used in association with low-dose heparin, but there is a risk of peripheral ischaemia[6] and it is no longer widely used. *Dextrans* (dextran 70 or dextran 40) alone, or with dihydroergotamine, have also been used for prophylaxis, but their administration involves the infusion of 500 to 1000 mL of fluid, a procedure which is cumbersome and may interfere with fluid balance. *Antithrombin III* (an endogenous inhibitor of thrombin and the cofactor through which heparin acts) used together with heparin has reduced the risk of venous thrombo-embolism in patients undergoing total knee arthroplasty.[30] The direct thrombin inhibitor desirudin has also been shown to be effective and was reported to be superior to both low-dose subcutaneous heparin[31] and to a low-molecular-weight heparin[32] in patients undergoing hip replacement surgery. Bivalirudin has also been tried.

The role of prophylaxis of thrombo-embolism in the non-surgical setting is much less clear.[33] One study[34] showed that very-low-dose warfarin (average daily dose of 2.6 mg) was safe and effective in patients receiving chemotherapy for metastatic breast cancer, a situation in which the high risk of thrombo-embolic disease is well recognised. Prophylaxis with low-molecular-weight heparin has been shown to be effective in patients with immobilisation of the leg.[35] Standard unfractionated heparin prophylaxis, however, had no effect on mortality in patients admitted to hospital with infection.[36]

Treatment of venous thrombo-embolism. Treatment of *deep-vein thrombosis*[37] aims to prevent the development of pulmonary embolism, to prevent extension of the thrombus, and to reduce the long-term complications of chronic venous insufficiency and venous ulceration. Non-pharmacological therapy may include bed rest with the foot of the bed raised, limb exercise, and graduated compression stockings.[38] These measures may be adequate in patients with small thrombi confined to the calf veins, although this is controversial. Heparin and oral anticoagulants are the mainstay of treatment; they prevent further thrombosis while allowing natural thrombolytic mechanisms to act on the existing clot. Anticoagulants may be used in combination with non-pharmacological methods; graduated compression stockings may reduce the risk of post-phlebitic symptoms in patients receiving anticoagulants.[39] Thrombolytics, or very rarely surgical thrombectomy, may be used for very extensive thrombosis.[40]

Heparin has an immediate effect whereas oral anticoagulants such as warfarin take several days to achieve their full anticoagulant effect. Heparin is therefore used for initial therapy and oral anticoagulants are used for maintenance. Doses of unfractionated heparin and oral anticoagulants must be adjusted according to laboratory monitoring. In the initial treatment of deep-vein thrombosis, current UK recommendations[6] are for an intravenous loading dose of heparin 5000 units followed by 1000 to 2000 units per hour by continuous intravenous infusion or 15 000 units by subcutaneous injection every 12 hours. In the USA,[40] a similar 5000 unit loading dose is given, followed by 1400 units per hour intravenously or 17 500 units every 12 hours subcutaneously. A meta-analysis suggested that heparin twice daily by subcutaneous injection is more effective and at least as safe as continuous intravenous heparin in the initial treatment of deep-vein thrombosis.[41] Low-molecular-weight heparins are also an alternative. A number of meta-analyses have shown them to be at least as effective and safe as unfractionated heparin in the treatment of deep-vein thrombosis;[42,43] similar results were found in a large study involving patients with both deep-vein thrombosis and pulmonary embolism.[44] Two studies[45,46] have also shown low-molecular-weight heparins to be safe and effective for the outpatient treatment of deep-vein thrombosis and it is likely that their use will increase.

Treatment with an oral anticoagulant (usually warfarin) may be started at the same time as heparin, or 3 to 4 days before it is discontinued. A standard loading dose is usually given, and dosage is then adjusted to maintain the international normalised ratio (INR) within recommended limits.[40,47] Heparin should be continued until the INR has been in the therapeutic range for at least 2 days;[40,48] a period of about 5 days is usually adequate if warfarin has been started on day 1.[49] The optimum duration of oral anticoagulation has been debated and probably depends upon the presence of risk factors. Prevention of disease recurrence must be balanced against minimising the risk of haemorrhagic complications. A multicentre study in the UK[50] indicated that, for postoperative deep-vein thrombosis or pulmonary embolism, anticoagulation for 4 weeks may be adequate; patients with idiopathic venous thrombo-embolism, however, may require anticoagulants for 3 months. Another multicentre study in Sweden[51] found that although six months of treatment with warfarin after a first episode of venous thrombo-embolism led to a lower cumulative recurrence rate than 6 weeks of treatment, this difference only occurred between 6 weeks and 6 months and the rates remained nearly parallel thereafter. In the light of evidence from this and other studies, Chesterman[52] concluded that anticoagulant treatment might reasonably be stopped after 4 to 6 weeks in patients with reversible risk factors for venous thrombo-embolism such as surgery, trauma, or temporary immobilisation. Similar recommendations have been made by the American Heart Association.[40] Lifelong treatment may be considered in patients with repeated thrombo-embolic episodes or with a continuing risk factor.

Ancrod or the recombinant hirudin, lepirudin, may be used as an alternative to heparin in patients who have developed heparin-induced thrombocytopenia or thrombosis. A heparinoid such as danaparoid or a low-molecular-weight heparin may also be suitable, although there may be cross-reactivity. In patients who have other contra-indications to anticoagulation or in whom thrombosis recurs despite anticoagulation, insertion of a vena caval filter may be appropriate.[40] The use of filters in conjunction with anticoagulation has also been investigated.[53] Although the incidence of pulmonary embolism was reduced during the first 12 days, no effect on mortality was shown at 2 years.

Therapy with thrombolytics such as streptokinase is controversial[54] but is generally reserved for very extensive thrombosis. Patients with more recent thrombi, incomplete occlusion, and proximal rather than distal thrombus location respond best.[55] Thrombolysis has not been shown to improve mortality in patients with deep-vein thrombosis and the main indication is to reduce the incidence of post-phlebitic syndrome. Since thrombolytic activity fades when infusion stops, heparin followed by oral anticoagulation is given to prevent re-occlusion.

Minor *pulmonary embolism* is treated with heparin and oral anticoagulants as described for deep-vein thrombosis (above). For more severe pulmonary embolism the initial bolus dose of heparin may be doubled[6] and heparin may be continued for 7 to 10 days.[40] Acute massive pulmonary embolism with major haemodynamic disturbance may be treated initially with thrombolytic therapy;[2] surgical methods such as embolectomy or percutaneous catheter fragmentation may be preferred in some patients.[56,57] Streptokinase, urokinase, and alteplase have all been shown to accelerate the lysis of pulmonary emboli and to decrease pulmonary vascular obstruction but no effect on mortality has yet been demonstrated. Comparisons between thrombolytics have been difficult because the doses used in different studies have not always been comparable. Probably more important than the choice of thrombolytic is ensuring that treatment starts quickly.[58] A small study[59] comparing the use of alteplase followed by heparin with heparin alone in pulmonary embolism, suggested that alteplase therapy was associated with more rapid improvement in right-ventricular function and pulmonary perfusion. This result requires confirmation in a larger study.[60]

Venous thrombo-embolism in children. Venous thrombo-embolism is relatively rare in children and has differing epidemiology to that in adults.[61] Although guidelines[62] for its management have been published they generally rely on extrapolation from studies in adults.

Venous thrombo-embolism in pregnancy. Pregnancy is a known risk factor for venous thrombo-embolism and, although the absolute risk is low, pulmonary embolism is the commonest cause of maternal death during pregnancy in the UK. Anticoagulation during pregnancy may be necessary either to prevent or treat venous thrombo-embolism; continued anticoagulation may also be needed in pregnant patients at risk of systemic embolism because of valvular heart disease or prosthetic heart valves (see above).

Oral anticoagulants such as warfarin cross the placenta and may harm the fetus; they are generally contra-indicated during pregnancy. Heparin does not appear to cross the placenta and despite potential maternal complications such as osteoporosis and thrombocytopenia remains the anticoagulant of choice in pregnancy.

The management of venous thrombo-embolism in pregnancy has been reviewed[63,64] and guidelines have been published in the UK.[65] **Prophylactic anticoagulation** is not necessary in all pregnancies, but should be considered in women at special risk of venous thrombo-embolism either because of a history of thrombo-embolism and/or a thrombophilic abnormality such as inherited deficiency of antithrombin III, protein C, or protein S or acquired thrombophilia due to antiphospholipid antibodies in plasma. Patients must be managed individually and current strategies differ. In those women with a history of thrombo-embolism but without thrombophilic abnormalities some authors recommend prophylactic anticoagulation intrapartum and for 6 weeks post partum provided there has been only one episode of thrombo-embolism and there are no additional risk factors; others advocate prophylaxis with subcutaneous heparin throughout pregnancy. Although standard low-dose heparin has been recommended, higher doses may be necessary.[63-65] Those with inherited or acquired thrombophilic abnormalities but no evidence of thrombosis do not necessarily require anticoagulation, but must be assessed carefully.

If acute venous thrombo-embolism occurs during pregnancy it should be **treated** with intravenous heparin as in non-pregnant patients (see above). Antenatal patients need to continue anticoagulation for the rest of their pregnancy, usually by substituting adjusted-dose subcutaneous heparin every 12 hours after 6 to 10 days of intravenous therapy; low-molecular-weight heparins may be an alternative.[40,63] If the patient has already had her baby, treatment can be continued with oral warfarin. Special care must be taken at delivery. Patients receiving full therapeutic doses of heparin should have their dose reduced on the day of delivery; this may not be necessary in those on lower prophylactic doses of heparin. If possible patients receiving warfarin should be changed to heparin 2 or 3 weeks before labour or delivery and not later than 36 weeks' gestation. Anticoagulants should be continued after delivery, but can usually be stopped after 6 weeks; the total duration of treatment should be at least 3 months.[40]

During pregnancy, especially the third trimester, laboratory monitoring of anticoagulation may be less reliable because high procoagulant concentrations particularly of factor VIII and fibrinogen, may result in low activated partial thromboplastin time (APTT) values despite adequate heparin concentrations in plasma.

1. Kearon C, *et al.* Noninvasive diagnosis of deep venous thrombosis. *Ann Intern Med* 1998; **128:** 663–77.
2. British Thoracic Society, Standards of Care Committee. Suspected acute pulmonary embolism: a practical approach. *Thorax* 1997; **52** (suppl 4): S1–S24.
3. Anderson FA, *et al.* Physician practices in the prevention of venous thromboembolism. *Ann Intern Med* 1991; **115:** 591–5.
4. Thomboembolic Risk Factors (THRIFT) Consensus Group. Risk of and prophylaxis for venous thromboembolism in hospital patients. *Br Med J* 1992; **305:** 567–74.
5. The Venous Thromboembolism Study Group of the Spanish Society of Clinical Pharmacology. Multicentre hospital drug utilization study on the prophylaxis of venous thromboembolism. *Br J Clin Pharmacol* 1994; **37:** 255–9.
6. Colvin BT, Barrowcliffe TW. The British Society for Haematology guidelines on the use and monitoring of heparin 1992: second revision. *J Clin Pathol* 1993; **46:** 97–103.
7. Clagett GP, *et al.* Prevention of venous thromboembolism. *Chest* 1995; **108** (suppl): 312S–334S.
8. Verstraete M. Prophylaxis of venous thromboembolism. *Br Med J* 1997; **314:** 123–5.
9. Collins R, *et al.* Reduction in fatal pulmonary embolism and venous thrombosis by perioperative administration of subcutaneous heparin: overview of results of randomized trials in general, orthopedic, and urologic surgery. *N Engl J Med* 1988; **318:** 1162–73.
10. Nurmohamed MT, *et al.* Low-molecular-weight heparin versus standard heparin in general and orthopaedic surgery: a meta-analysis. *Lancet* 1992; **340:** 152–6.
11. Leizorovicz A, *et al.* Low molecular weight heparin in prevention of perioperative thrombosis. *Br Med J* 1992; **305:** 913–20.
12. Anderson DR, *et al.* Efficacy and cost of low-molecular-weight heparin compared with standard heparin for the prevention of deep vein thrombosis after total hip arthroplasty. *Ann Intern Med* 1993; **119:** 1105–12.
13. Koch A, *et al.* Low molecular weight heparin and unfractionated heparin in thrombosis prophylaxis after major surgical intervention: update of previous meta-analyses. *Br J Surg* 1997; **84:** 750–9.
14. Kakkar VV, *et al.* Low molecular weight versus standard heparin for prevention of venous thromboembolism after major abdominal surgery. *Lancet* 1993; **341:** 259–65.
15. Simonneau G, Leizorovicz A. Prophylactic treatment of postoperative thrombosis: a meta-analysis of the results from trials assessing various methods used in patients undergoing major orthopaedic (hip and knee) surgery. *Clin Trials Meta-Analysis* 1993; **28:** 177–91.
16. Imperiale TF, Speroff T. A meta-analysis of methods to prevent venous thromboembolism following total hip replacement. *JAMA* 1994; **271:** 1780–5. Correction. *ibid.* 1995; **273:** 288.
17. Geerts WH, *et al.* A comparison of low-dose heparin with low-molecular-weight heparin as prophylaxis against venous thromboembolism after major trauma. *N Engl J Med* 1996; **335:** 701–7.
18. Planes A, *et al.* Risk of deep-venous thrombosis after hospital discharge in patients having undergone total hip replacement: double-blind randomised comparison of enoxaparin versus placebo. *Lancet* 1996; **348:** 224–8.
19. Bergqvist D, *et al.* Low-molecular-weight heparin (enoxaparin) as prophylaxis against venous thromboembolism after total hip replacement. *N Engl J Med* 1996; **335:** 696–700.
20. Anderson DR, *et al.* Enoxaparin as prophylaxis against thromboembolism after total hip replacement. *N Engl J Med* 1997; **336:** 585.
21. Amstutz HC, *et al.* Warfarin prophylaxis to prevent mortality from pulmonary embolism after total hip replacement. *J Bone Joint Surg (Am)* 1989; **71A:** 321–6.
22. Poller L, *et al.* Fixed minidose warfarin: a new approach to prophylaxis against venous thrombosis after major surgery. *Br Med J* 1987; **295:** 1309–12.
23. Fordyce MJF, *et al.* Efficacy of fixed minidose warfarin prophylaxis in total hip replacement. *Br Med J* 1991; **303:** 219–20.
24. Dale C, *et al.* Prevention of venous thrombosis with minidose warfarin after joint replacement. *Br Med J* 1991; **303:** 224.
25. Francis CW, *et al.* Comparison of warfarin and external pneumatic compression in prevention of venous thrombosis after total hip replacement. *JAMA* 1992; **267:** 2911–15.
26. Hull R, *et al.* A comparison of subcutaneous low-molecular-weight heparin with warfarin sodium for prophylaxis against deep-vein thrombosis after hip or knee implantation. *N Engl J Med* 1993; **329:** 1370–6.
27. Antiplatelet Trialists' Collaboration. Collaborative overview of randomised trials of antiplatelet therapy—III: reduction in venous thrombosis and pulmonary embolism by antiplatelet prophylaxis among surgical and medical patients. *Br Med J* 1994; **308:** 235–46.
28. Cohen AT, *et al.* Antiplatelet treatment for thromboprophylaxis: a step forward or backwards? *Br Med J* 1994; **309:** 1213–15.
29. Collins R, *et al.* Antiplatelet therapy for thromboprophylaxis: the need for careful consideration of the evidence from randomised trials. *Br Med J* 1994; **309:** 1215–17.
30. Francis CW, *et al.* Prevention of venous thrombosis after total knee arthroplasty: comparison of antithrombin III and low-dose heparin with dextran. *J Bone Joint Surg (Am)* 1990; **72-A:** 976–82.
31. Eriksson BI, *et al.* Prevention of deep-vein thrombosis after total hip replacement: direct thrombin inhibition with recombinant hirudin, CGP 39393. *Lancet* 1996; **347:** 635–9.
32. Eriksson BI, *et al.* A comparison of recombinant hirudin with a low-molecular-weight heparin to prevent thromboembolic complications after total hip replacement. *N Engl J Med* 1997; **337:** 1329–35.
33. Lederle FA. Heparin prophylaxis for medical patients? *Ann Intern Med* 1998; **128:** 768–70.
34. Levine M, *et al.* Double-blind randomised trial of very-low-dose warfarin for prevention of thromboembolism in stage IV breast cancer. *Lancet* 1994; **343:** 886–9.
35. Kock H-J, *et al.* Thromboprophylaxis with low-molecular-weight heparin in outpatients with plaster-cast immobilisation of the leg. *Lancet* 1995; **346:** 459–61.
36. Gårdlund B. Randomised, controlled trial of low-dose heparin for prevention of fatal pulmonary embolism in patients with infectious diseases. *Lancet* 1996; **347:** 1357–61.
37. Shetty HG. Management of deep-vein thrombosis. *Prescribers' J* 1997; **37:** 166–72.
38. McCollum C. Avoiding the consequences of deep vein thrombosis. *Br Med J* 1998; **317:** 696.
39. Brandjes DPM, *et al.* Randomised trial of effect of compression stockings in patients with symptomatic proximal-vein thrombosis. *Lancet* 1997; **349:** 759–62.
40. Hirsh J, Hoak J. Management of deep vein thrombosis and pulmonary embolism: a statement for healthcare professionals. *Circulation* 1996; **93:** 2212–45.
41. Hommes DW, *et al.* Subcutaneous heparin compared with continuous intravenous heparin administration in the initial treatment of deep vein thrombosis. *Ann Intern Med* 1992; **116:** 279–84.
42. Siragusa S, *et al.* Low-molecular-weight heparins and unfractionated heparin in the treatment of patients with acute venous thromboembolism: results of a meta-analysis. *Am J Med* 1996; **100:** 269–77.
43. Leizorovicz A. Comparison of the efficacy and safety of low molecular weight heparins and unfractionated heparin in the initial treatment of deep venous thrombosis: an updated meta-analysis. *Drugs* 1996; **52** (suppl 7): 30–7.
44. The Columbus Investigators. Low-molecular-weight heparin in the treatment of patients with venous thromboembolism. *N Engl J Med* 1997; **337:** 657–62.
45. Levine M, *et al.* A comparison of low-molecular-weight heparin administered primarily at home with unfractionated heparin administered in the hospital for proximal deep-vein thrombosis. *N Engl J Med* 1996; **334:** 677–81.
46. Koopman MMW, *et al.* Treatment of venous thrombosis with intravenous unfractionated heparin administered in the hospital as compared with subcutaneous low-molecular-weight heparin administered at home. *N Engl J Med* 1996; **334:** 682–7. Correction. *ibid.* 1997; **337:** 1251.
47. British Society for Haematology: British Committee for Standards in Haematology—Haemostasis and Thrombosis Task Force. Guidelines on oral anticoagulation: third edition. *Br J Haematol* 1998; **101:** 374–87.
48. Ginsberg JS. Management of venous thromboembolism. *N Engl J Med* 1996; **335:** 1816–28.
49. Hull RD, *et al.* Heparin for 5 days as compared with 10 days in the initial treatment of proximal venous thrombosis. *N Engl J Med* 1990; **322:** 1260–4.
50. Research Committee of the British Thoracic Society. Optimum duration of anticoagulation for deep-vein thrombosis and pulmonary embolism. *Lancet* 1992; **340:** 873–6.
51. Schulman S, *et al.* A comparison of six weeks with six months of oral anticoagulant therapy after a first episode of venous thromboembolism. *N Engl J Med* 1995; **332:** 1661–5.
52. Chesterman CN. After a first episode of venous thromboembolism. *Br Med J* 1995; **311:** 700–1.
53. Decousus H, *et al.* A clinical trial of vena caval filters in the prevention of pulmonary embolism in patients with proximal deep-vein thrombosis. *N Engl J Med* 1998; **338:** 409–15.
54. Hawkins DW, Hirsh J. Antithrombotic drugs for thromboembolic disorders: a lesson in evidence-based medicine. *Am J Health-Syst Pharm* 1997; **54:** 1992–4.
55. Rogers LQ, Lutcher CL. Streptokinase therapy for deep vein thrombosis: a comprehensive review of the English literature. *Am J Med* 1990; **88:** 389–95.
56. Gulba DC, *et al.* Medical compared with surgical treatment for massive pulmonary embolism. *Lancet* 1994; **343:** 576–7.
57. Goldhaber SZ. Pulmonary embolism. *N Engl J Med* 1998; **339:** 93–104.
58. Anonymous. Thrombolysis for pulmonary embolism. *Lancet* 1992; **340:** 21–2.
59. Goldhaber SZ, *et al.* Alteplase versus heparin in acute pulmonary embolism: randomised trial assessing right-ventricular function and pulmonary perfusion. *Lancet* 1993; **341:** 507–11.
60. ten Cate JW. Thrombolytic treatment of pulmonary embolism. *Lancet* 1993; **341:** 1315–16.
61. David M, Andrew M. Venous thromboembolic complications in children. *J Pediatr* 1993; **123:** 337–46.
62. Andrew M, *et al.* Guidelines for antithrombotic therapy in pediatric patients. *J Pediatr* 1998; **132:** 575–88.
63. Nelson-Piercy C. Obstetric thromboprophylaxis. *Br J Hosp Med* 1996; **55:** 404–8.
64. Toglia MR, Weg JG. Venous thromboembolism during pregnancy. *N Engl J Med* 1996; **335:** 108–14.
65. Maternal and Neonatal Haemostasis Working Party of the Haemostasis and Thrombosis Task. Guidelines on the prevention, investigation and management of thrombosis associated with pregnant. *J Clin Pathol* 1993; **46:** 489–96.

Abciximab (14557-q)

Abciximab *(BAN, USAN, rINN).*

c7E3. Immunoglobulin G (human-mouse monoclonal c7E3 clone p7E3V_HhC_γ4 Fab fragment anti-human platelet glycoprotein IIb/IIIa complex), disulphide with human-mouse monoclonal c7E3 clone p7E3V_κhC_κ light chain.

$C_{2101}H_{3229}N_{551}O_{673}S_{15}$ = 47455.4.

CAS — 143653-53-6.

Adverse Effects and Precautions

Bleeding during the first 36 hours after administration is the most common adverse effect of abciximab and therefore it should not be given to patients who are actively bleeding or to patients at increased risk of haemorrhage, including those with haemorrhagic disorders, cerebrovascular disorders, uncontrolled hypertension, or who have recently undergone major surgery. Abciximab should be discontinued if serious uncontrolled bleeding occurs or emergency surgery is required. Abciximab should not be given to patients with severe renal or hepatic impairment. Thrombocytopenia may occur and platelet counts should be monitored before and following administration of abciximab. Antibodies may develop 2 to 4 weeks after administration and hypersensitivity reactions could occur on administration of other monoclonal antibodies or following re-treatment with abciximab; thus readministration is not recommended. Hypersensitivity reactions have not been noted after a single administration but the possibility should be considered. Other side-effects include hypotension, nausea and vomiting, back pain, chest pain, headache, haematoma, bradycardia, fever, and vascular disorders.

Pharmacokinetics

Following intravenous administration of abciximab free plasma concentrations fall rapidly due to binding to platelet receptors. Platelet function recovers over about 48 hours although abciximab may remain in the circulation for up to 10 days in a platelet-bound state.

Uses and Administration

Abciximab is the Fab fragment of the chimaeric monoclonal antibody 7E3. It binds to the glycoprotein IIb/IIIa receptor on the surface of platelets. This prevents binding of fibrinogen, von Willebrand factor, and other adhesive molecules to the receptor sites and inhibits platelet aggregation. It is used as an adjunct to heparin and aspirin therapy for the prevention of acute ischaemic complications in patients undergoing percutaneous transluminal coronary procedures including angioplasty, atherectomy, and stenting. It is also used in patients with unstable angina who are candidates for such procedures.

Abciximab is given intravenously as a bolus injection over one minute in a dose of 250 μg per kg body-weight followed immediately by an infusion of 0.125 μg per kg per minute (to a maximum dose of 10 μg per minute). In patients with unstable angina the bolus dose followed by the infusion should be started up to 24 hours before the possible angioplasty and continued for 12 hours after the intervention; for patients undergoing angioplasty the bolus should be given 10 to 60 minutes before the intervention followed by the infusion for 12 hours.

General references.

1. Faulds D, Sorkin EM. Abciximab (c7E3 Fab): a review of its pharmacology and therapeutic potential in ischaemic heart disease. *Drugs* 1994; **48:** 583–98.

Angioplasty. Percutaneous transluminal coronary angioplasty is a non-pharmacological procedure employed in the management of atherosclerotic arterial disease to aid revascularisation and reperfusion (p.797). Heparin is usually given during the procedure to prevent perioperative thrombosis and aspirin is given as an antiplatelet drug to reduce long-term stenosis. Abciximab has a role as an adjunct to heparin and aspirin in various groups of patients undergoing angioplasty. In the EPIC study,[1] which included only patients at high risk for abrupt vessel closure, acute ischaemic events and complications of angioplasty were reduced but there was also a significant increase in bleeding complications. In those given abciximab as a bolus injection immediately before angioplasty followed by intravenous infusion for 12 hours there was also a reduction in restenosis at 6 months[2] and at 3 years.[3] Similar results were obtained in the EPILOG study,[4] which used a lower dose of heparin and included unselected patients. However, in the CAPTURE study,[5] in which abciximab was given for 18 to 24 hours before angioplasty and for 1 hour after, the initial benefit was not maintained at 6 months.

Abciximab is also being investigated as an adjunct to angioplasty in patients with acute myocardial infarction, and as an adjunct to thrombolysis in patients with acute myocardial infarction who are not undergoing angioplasty. It also has a role in patients undergoing coronary stenting procedures.[6]

1. The EPIC Investigators. Use of a monoclonal antibody directed against the platelet glycoprotein IIb/IIIa receptor in high-risk coronary angioplasty. *N Engl J Med* 1994; **330:** 956–61.
2. Topol EJ, *et al.* Randomised trial of coronary intervention with antibody against platelet IIb/IIIa integrin for reduction of clinical restenosis: results at six months. *Lancet* 1994; **343:** 881–6.
3. Topol EJ, *et al.* Long-term protection from myocardial ischemic events in a randomized trial of brief integrin β_3 blockade with percutaneous coronary intervention. *JAMA* 1997; **278:** 479–84.
4. The EPILOG Investigators. Platelet glycoprotein IIb/IIIa receptor blockade and low-dose heparin during percutaneous coronary revascularization. *N Engl J Med* 1997; **336:** 1689–96.
5. The CAPTURE Investigators. Randomised placebo-controlled trial of abciximab before and during coronary intervention in refractory unstable angina: the CAPTURE study. *Lancet* 1997; **349:** 1429–35.
6. The EPISTENT Investigators. Randomised placebo-controlled and balloon-angioplasty-controlled trial to assess safety of coronary stenting with use of platelet glycoprotein-IIb/IIIa blockade. *Lancet* 1998; **352:** 87–92.

Preparations

Proprietary Preparations (details are given in Part 3)

Austral.: ReoPro; ***Fr.:*** ReoPro; ***Ger.:*** ReoPro; ***Irl.:*** ReoPro; ***Ital.:*** ReoPro; ***Neth.:*** ReoPro; ***Norw.:*** ReoPro; ***S.Afr.:*** ReoPro; ***Spain:*** ReoPro; ***Swed.:*** ReoPro; ***Switz.:*** ReoPro; ***UK:*** ReoPro; ***USA:*** ReoPro.

Acadesine (14674-l)

Acadesine *(BAN, USAN, rINN).*

GP-1-110; GP-1-110-0. 5-Amino-1-(β-D-ribofuranosyl)imidazole-4-carboxamide.

$C_9H_{14}N_4O_5$ = 258.2.

CAS — 2627-69-2.

Acadesine is a purine nucleoside analogue reported to have cardioprotective effects. It is being investigated in the management of myocardial ischaemia particularly in patients undergoing coronary artery bypass graft surgery. Acadesine may act by influencing metabolism in ischaemic cells to enhance release of adenosine, which protects against further ischaemia, in preference to inosine following breakdown of adenosine monophosphate.

References.

1. Europe/Canada Perioperative Ischemia Research Group. Multinational study of the effect of acadesine on major cardiovascular outcomes associated with CABG surgery. *J Am Coll Cardiol* 1993; 21 (suppl): 150A.
2. Leung JM, *et al.* An initial multicenter, randomized controlled trial on the safety and efficacy of acadesine in patients undergoing coronary artery bypass graft surgery. *Anesth Analg* 1994; **78:** 420–34.
3. Alkhulaifi AM, Pugsley WB. Role of acadesine in clinical myocardial protection. *Br Heart J* 1995; **73:** 304–5.
4. Mangano DT. Effects of acadesine on myocardial infarction, stroke, and death following surgery: a meta-analysis of the 5 international randomized trials. *JAMA* 1997; **277:** 325–32.

ACE Inhibitors (17463-h)

Angiotensin-converting Enzyme Inhibitors.

There appear to be few significant differences between ACE inhibitors. They may be distinguished from each other by the presence or absence of a sulfhydryl group, whether they are prodrugs or not, their route of elimination, and their affinity for angiotensin-converting enzyme in vascular and other tissue, although whether these characteristics modify pharmacodynamics and therefore clinical efficacy is uncertain. Differences in these characteristics do however influence onset and duration of action of ACE inhibitors.

Adverse Effects and Treatment

ACE inhibitors all appear to have a similar spectrum of adverse effects although at one time some, such as taste disturbances and skin reactions, were attributed to the presence of a sulfhydryl group as in captopril.

They include hypotension, dizziness, fatigue, headache, gastro-intestinal disturbances, taste disturbances, persistent dry cough and other upper respiratory tract symptoms, skin rashes (including erythema multiforme and toxic epidermal necrolysis), angioedema, hypersensitivity reactions, renal impairment, hyperkalaemia, hyponatraemia, and blood disorders.

Pronounced hypotension may occur at the start of therapy with ACE inhibitors, particularly in patients with heart failure and in sodium- or volume-depleted patients (for example, those who have received previous diuretic therapy). In patients with ischaemic heart disease or cerebrovascular disease a severe fall in blood pressure could result in myocardial infarction or cerebrovascular accident.

Deterioration in renal function, including increasing blood concentrations of urea and creatinine, and reversible acute renal failure have been reported. This occurs mainly in patients with existing renal or renovascular dysfunction or heart failure and may be aggravated by hypovolaemia. Proteinuria has also occurred and in some patients has progressed to nephrotic syndrome.

Other adverse effects reported with ACE inhibitors include chest pain, palpitations, tachycardia, stomatitis, abdominal pain, pancreatitis, hepatocellular injury or cholestatic jaundice, alopecia, neutropenia and agranulocytosis (especially in patients with renal failure and in those with collagen vascular disorders such as systemic lupus erythematosus and scleroderma), thrombocytopenia, anaemias, muscle cramps, paraesthesias, mood and sleep disturbances, and impotence.

ACE inhibitors may be toxic to the fetus (see Pregnancy under Precautions, below).

Most of the adverse effects of ACE inhibitors are reversible on withdrawing therapy. Symptomatic hypotension, including that following overdosage, generally responds to volume expansion with an intravenous infusion of sodium chloride 0.9%. Specific therapy with angiotensin amide (p.824) may be considered if conventional therapy is ineffective.

General reviews.

1. Parish RC, Miller LJ. Adverse effects of angiotensin converting enzyme (ACE) inhibitors: an update. *Drug Safety* 1992; **7:** 14–31.
2. Alderman CP. Adverse effects of the angiotensin-converting enzyme inhibitors. *Ann Pharmacother* 1996; **30:** 55–61.

Angioedema. See under Hypersensitivity, below.

Cough. Treatment with ACE inhibitors has been associated with the development of cough in up to 20% of hypertensive patients; cough may be less troublesome in those with heart failure,[1] although the incidence may be higher.[2] The cough is reported to be persistent, paroxysmal, and non-productive; it causes irritation of the throat, may be accompanied by voice changes (hoarseness or huskiness), and is often worse when lying down.[1,3,4] It is more common in women and non-smokers, and may be delayed in onset by weeks or even months.

The majority of reports of this adverse effect concern captopril and enalapril,[3,4] but it has also occurred in patients receiving many of the newer ACE inhibitors,[5] suggesting that the effect is common to all drugs of this class.

The mechanism that produces the reaction is uncertain. The sensitivity of the cough reflex is increased.[6] Prostaglandins released in the respiratory tract have been proposed as mediators,[3] but other mediators such as bradykinin[7] or substance P,[8] both of which are substrates for ACE, have been suggested. However, attempts to demonstrate a link between the effects of ACE inhibitors on cough, and bronchial hyperreactivity of the type found in obstructive airways disease and asthma have produced conflicting evidence: while Bucknall and colleagues found evidence of bronchial hyperreactivity in 6 patients with cough and two with evidence of exacerbated asthma when receiving ACE inhibitors,[9] Boulet and others failed to find evidence of airflow obstruction or bronchial hyperreactivity in 15 patients after treatment with captopril.[10]

Where the patient can tolerate the cough, it may be reasonable to continue treatment; in some cases reducing the dose may help. Spontaneous recovery or improvement in the cough has been reported.[11] Changing to an alternative ACE inhibitor is not advised since it is rarely effective.[6] Drugs that inhibit prostaglandin synthesis including the NSAIDs sulindac[12] and indomethacin,[13] and the calcium-channel blocker nifedipine[13] have been reported to suppress the cough, but NSAIDs and ACE inhibitors may interact adversely (see under Interactions, below). Inhaled bupivacaine,[14] inhaled sodium cromoglycate,[15,16] oral baclofen,[17] and oral picotamide,[18] have also been reported to be of help. However, in many patients there will be no alternative but to withdraw the ACE inhibitor.[4]

1. Anonymous. Cough caused by ACE inhibitors. *Drug Ther Bull.* 1994; **32:** 28 and 55–6.
2. Ravid D, *et al.* Angiotensin-converting enzyme inhibitors and cough: a prospective evaluation in hypertension and congestive heart failure. *J Clin Pharmacol* 1994; **34:** 1116–20.
3. Coulter DM, Edwards IR. Cough associated with captopril and enalapril. *Br Med J* 1987; **294:** 1521–3.
4. Berkin KE, Ball SG. Cough and angiotensin converting enzyme inhibition. *Br Med J* 1988; **296:** 1279–80.
5. Israili ZH, Hall WD. Cough and angioneurotic edema associated with angiotensin-converting enzyme inhibitor therapy. *Ann Intern Med* 1992; **117:** 234–42.
6. Overlack A. ACE inhibitor-induced cough and bronchospasm. *Drug Safety* 1996; **15:** 72–8.
7. Ferner RE, *et al.* Effects of intradermal bradykinin after inhibition of angiotensin converting enzyme. *Br Med J* 1987; **294:** 1119–20.
8. Morice AH, *et al.* Angiotensin-converting enzyme and the cough reflex. *Lancet* 1987; **ii:** 1116–18.
9. Bucknall CE, *et al.* Bronchial hyperreactivity in patients who cough after receiving angiotensin converting enzyme inhibitors. *Br Med J* 1988; **296:** 86–8.
10. Boulet L-P, *et al.* Pulmonary function and airway responsiveness during long-term therapy with captopril. *JAMA* 1989; **261:** 413–16.
11. Reisin L, Schneeweiss A. Spontaneous disappearance of cough induced by angiotensin-converting enzyme inhibitors (captopril or enalapril). *Am J Cardiol* 1992; **70:** 398–9.
12. Nicholls MG, Gilchrist NL. Sulindac and cough induced by converting enzyme inhibitors. *Lancet* 1987; **i:** 872.
13. Fogari R, *et al.* Effects of nifedipine and indomethacin on cough induced by angiotensin-converting enzyme inhibitors: a double-blind, randomized, cross-over study. *J Cardiovasc Pharmacol* 1992; **19:** 670–3.
14. Brown RC, Turton CWG. Cough and angiotensin converting enzyme inhibition. *Br Med J* 1988; **296:** 1741.
15. Keogh A. Sodium cromoglycate prophylaxis for angiotensin-converting enzyme inhibitor cough. *Lancet* 1993; **341:** 560.
16. Hargreaves MR, Benson MK. Inhaled sodium cromoglycate in angiotensin-converting enzyme inhibitor cough. *Lancet* 1995; **345:** 13–16.
17. Dicpinigaitis PV. Use of baclofen to suppress cough induced by angiotensin-converting enzyme inhibitors. *Ann Pharmacother* 1996; **30:** 1242–5.
18. Malini PL, *et al.* Thromboxane antagonism and cough induced by angiotensin-converting-enzyme inhibitor. *Lancet* 1997; **350:** 15–18.

Effects on the blood. A number of blood disorders have occurred in patients receiving ACE inhibitors, although there have been few reports in the literature. A reduction in haemoglobin concentration and haematocrit may occur but is not usually clinically significant. Cases of neutropenia and agranulocytosis (particularly in patients with renal or collagen vascular disorders), and thrombocytopenia have been noted. Aplastic anaemia has also occurred[1,2] and may be fatal.[2]

1. Kim CR, *et al.* Captopril and aplastic anemia. *Ann Intern Med* 1989; **111:** 187–8.
2. Harrison BD, *et al.* Fatal aplastic anaemia associated with lisinopril. *Lancet* 1995; **346:** 247–8.

Effects on the kidneys. The complex, and sometimes apparently contradictory, effects of ACE inhibitors on the kidney have been reviewed in detail.[1,2] In the normal kidney the effects of ACE inhibition depend on the state of activation of the renin-angiotensin-aldosterone system, and therefore on the state of sodium balance. In normal individuals with unrestricted sodium intake the renin-angiotensin-aldosterone system is suppressed; the increase in renal blood flow observed with captopril administration probably involves other mechanisms. Sodium restriction leads to activation of the renin-angiotensin-aldosterone system with a consequent reduction in renal blood flow and glomerular filtration rate due to renal vasoconstriction; this effect is reversed by ACE inhibitors. In patients with essential hypertension ACE inhibition has generally been reported to result in an increase in effective renal blood flow despite the reduction in arterial blood pressure. However, there are only minor changes in glomerular filtration rate, and filtration fraction falls since the pressure within the glomerulus is reduced due to the pronounced renal vasodilatation. The increase in renal blood flow is more pronounced during sodium restriction and in younger patients.

These effects increase or maintain renal blood flow and are generally beneficial. However, in patients with renovascular hypertension they may provoke problems. Severe renal function loss or even anuria have been reported in patients with a single transplanted kidney with renal artery stenosis, or patients with bilateral renal artery disease. The frequency of clinically significant renal function loss during long-term treatment with captopril in patients at risk has been reported to be about 6%. The stenotic kidney maintains its filtering capacity by preferential vasoconstriction of the efferent arterioles, a mechanism mainly mediated by the renin-angiotensin system; under ACE inhibition, vasodilatation of the efferent arterioles combined with the drop in arterial pressure can result in a critical decrease in filtration pressure. Sodium depletion contributes to renal function loss in this setting, and most patients developing renal insufficiency have been using diuretics; sodium repletion can restore renal function despite continuation of ACE inhibition.

Patients with heart failure may also be at risk of a decline in renal function on long-term ACE inhibitor therapy. This is because in chronic heart failure, angiotensin-II mediated systemic and renal vasoconstriction is more important in the maintenance of renal perfusion pressure than in normal or hypertensive persons. The decline may be alleviated by reduction of the dosage of diuretics or liberalisation of dietary salt intake, despite continuation of the ACE inhibitor.

In addition to these pathophysiological effects ACE inhibitors may induce membranous glomerulopathy or interstitial nephritis. The former has been associated with captopril use, particularly at high doses, but is rare, and seems less likely to occur at the lower doses favoured today. The proteinuria usually clears without appreciable renal function loss irrespective of whether or not the drug is continued, although persistent proteinuria and renal function loss have been described. Proven interstitial nephritis has also been reported rarely, and may possibly be due to an allergic mechanism.

1. Gans ROB, *et al.* Renal effects of angiotensin-I converting enzyme inhibitors. *Neth J Med* 1988; **32:** 247–64.
2. Navis G, *et al.* ACE inhibitors and the kidney: a risk-benefit assessment. *Drug Safety* 1996; **15:** 200–11.

Effects on the liver. Reporting on 3 cases of liver disease apparently caused or aggravated by captopril, Bellary *et al.*[1] noted that jaundice due to captopril is usually predominantly cholestatic in nature but acute hepatocellular injury has also been observed. Of 29 cases of liver dysfunction due to captopril and reported to the Committee on Safety of Medicines in the UK, 9 had hepatocellular jaundice, with 2 deaths; 8 were cholestatic jaundice, with 1 fatality; and 3 patients had hepatorenal syndrome, all of whom died. Worldwide, excluding the UK, 164 cases of hepatic adverse reactions had been notified to the WHO by January 1989. The incidence of such reactions is estimated at 0.09 per 1000 patients but this is likely to be an underestimate. As with chlorpromazine-induced cholestasis resolution may take a long time and captopril should be withdrawn immediately at the earliest hint of liver sensitivity. Hepatotoxicity has also been reported with enalapril and lisinopril.[2]

1. Bellary SV, *et al.* Captopril and the liver. *Lancet* 1989; **ii:** 514.
2. Hagley MT, *et al.* Hepatotoxicity associated with angiotensin-converting enzyme inhibitors. *Ann Pharmacother* 1993; **27:** 228–31.

Effects on the mouth. Aphthous and tongue ulcers may occur during treatment with ACE inhibitors. There have been a few reports of a 'scalded mouth syndrome', described as similar to being scalded by hot liquids, associated with captopril,[1] enalapril,[1] and lisinopril[2] therapy.

1. Vlasses PH, *et al.* "Scalded mouth" caused by angiotensin-converting enzyme inhibitors. *Br Med J* 1982; **284:** 1672–3.
2. Savino LB, Haushalter NM. Lisinopril-induced "scalded mouth syndrome." *Ann Pharmacother* 1992; **26:** 1381–2.

Effects on the nervous system. Encephalopathy and focal neurological signs,[1] and peripheral neuropathy,[2,3] including Guillain-Barré neuropathy,[3] have been reported in patients receiving captopril. Some central nervous effects of captopril may be attributable to alterations in cerebral blood flow. In a study in patients with severe heart failure Britton and others noted that while cerebral blood flow in patients aged under 65 was improved by a single dose of captopril 12.5 mg, in patients aged over 70 there was a 13% reduction in cerebral blood flow.[4] Two patients in whom captopril 6.25 mg produced impaired consciousness and paraesthesias, and dizziness, blurred vision, and aphasia, were found to have stenosis of the carotid arteries.[5] Agitation, panic, extreme depression, and insomnia was reported in a patient 4 weeks after starting treatment with enalapril; depressive episodes recurred on rechallenge.[6] There have been reports of mania possibly precipitated by captopril,[7] and visual hallucinations have been reported in association with captopril and enalapril therapy.[8]

1. Rapoport S, Zyman P. Captopril and central nervous system effects. *Ann Intern Med* 1983; **98:** 1023.
2. Samanta A, Burden AC. Peripheral neuropathy due to captopril. *Br Med J* 1985; **291:** 1172.
3. Chakraborty TK, Ruddell WSJ. Guillain-Barré neuropathy during treatment with captopril. *Postgrad Med J* 1987; **63:** 221–2.
4. Britton KE, *et al.* Angiotensin-converting-enzyme inhibitors and treatment of heart failure. *Lancet* 1985; **ii:** 1236.
5. Jensen H, *et al.* Carotid artery stenosis exposed by an adverse effect of captopril. *Br Med J* 1986; **293:** 1073–4.
6. Ahmad S. Enalapril-induced acute psychosis. *DICP Ann Pharmacother* 1991; **25:** 558–9.
7. Peet M, Peters S. Drug-induced mania. *Drug Safety* 1995; **12:** 146–53.
8. Haffner CA, *et al.* Hallucinations as an adverse effect of angiotensin converting enzyme inhibition. *Postgrad Med J* 1993; **69:** 240.

Effects on the pancreas. According to Dabaghi,[1] the manufacturers of captopril, enalapril, and lisinopril all have data on file on drug-associated pancreatitis. In 1994 the UK Committee on Safety of Medicines[2] noted that there had been 23 reports of pancreatitis associated with ACE inhibitors (captopril 11, enalapril 10, fosinopril 1, and quinapril 1) although whether or not this was causal was not certain.

1. Dabaghi S. ACE inhibitors and pancreatitis. *Ann Intern Med* 1991; **115:** 330–1.
2. Committee on Safety of Medicines/Medicines Control Agency. Drug-induced pancreatitis. *Current Problems* 1994; **20:** 2–3.

Effects on the respiratory system. Cough is a recognised adverse effect of ACE inhibitors but evidence for a link with bronchial hyperreactivity or airways obstruction is controversial (see above). In reports of adverse respiratory reactions to ACE inhibitors submitted to the Swedish Adverse Drug Reactions Advisory Committee and to WHO, symptoms of airway obstruction such as dyspnoea, asthma, and bronchospasm occurred rarely, usually within the first few weeks of treatment.[1] However, Inman *et al.*[2] questioned the evidence for a causal link between ACE inhibitors and these symptoms.

Severe nasal obstruction was associated with enalapril treatment in a 45-year-old woman with a history of mild rhinorrhoea and sneezing. Symptoms cleared within 2 days of stopping enalapril and recurred on rechallenge.[3]

There have been case reports of pneumonitis associated with treatment with captopril[4] and perindopril.[5]

1. Lunde H, *et al.* Dyspnoea, asthma, and bronchospasm in relation to treatment with angiotensin converting enzyme inhibitors. *Br Med J* 1994; **308:** 18–21.
2. Inman WHW, *et al.* Angiotensin converting enzyme inhibitors and asthma. *Br Med J* 1994; **308:** 593–4.
3. Fennerty A, *et al.* Enalapril-induced nasal blockage. *Lancet* 1986; **ii:** 1395–6.
4. Kidney JC, *et al.* Captopril and lymphocytic alveolitis. *Br Med J* 1989; **299:** 981.
5. Benard A, *et al.* Perindopril-associated pneumonitis. *Eur Respir J* 1996; **9:** 1314–16.

Effects on skeletal muscle. A report of severe muscle pain and weakness, accompanied by morning stiffness, in a patient taking enalapril. Symptoms resolved within a few days of discontinuing the drug.[1]

1. Leloët X, *et al.* Pseudopolymyalgia rheumatica during treatment with enalapril. *Br Med J* 1989; **298:** 325.

Effects on the skin. Skin rashes may occur during treatment with ACE inhibitors; they have been reported in 1 to 6% of patients receiving captopril. Angioedema is also an adverse effect of ACE inhibitors (see under Hypersensitivity, below). There have been reports of bullous pemphigoid,[1] hyperhidrosis,[2] Kaposi's sarcoma,[3] lichen planus,[4] onycholysis,[5,6] pemphigus,[7,8] and cutaneous hypersensitivity vasculitis[9] associated with administration of captopril. Onycholysis has also occurred with enalapril[10] and pemphigus with enalapril[11,12] and ramipril.[13] Lichen planus pemphigoides has been reported with ramipril.[14] A severe cutaneous reaction, resembling early mycosis fungoides, and possibly allergic in nature, has been reported following administration of captopril or enalapril.[15] Captopril has also been reported to exacerbate psoriasis.[16] Vulvovaginal pruritus with dysuria[17] has been noted in a patient receiving enalapril.

1. Mallet L, *et al.* Bullous pemphigoid associated with captopril. *DICP Ann Pharmacother* 1989; **23:** 63.
2. Morse MH. Hyperhidrosis: a possible side effect of captopril treatment. *Br Med J* 1984; **289:** 1272.
3. Puppin D, *et al.* Kaposi's sarcoma associated with captopril. *Lancet* 1990; **336:** 1251–2.
4. Cox NH, *et al.* Lichen planus associated with captopril: a further disorder demonstrating the 'tin-tack' sign. *Br J Dermatol* 1989; **120:** 319–21.
5. Brueggemeyer CD, Ramirez G. Onycholysis associated with captopril. *Lancet* 1984; **i:** 1352–3.
6. Borders JV. Captopril and onycholysis. *Ann Intern Med* 1986; **105:** 305–6.
7. Parfrey PS, *et al.* Captopril-induced pemphigus. *Br Med J* 1980; **281:** 194.
8. Butt A, Burge SM. Pemphigus vulgaris induced by captopril. *Br J Dermatol* 1995; **132:** 315–16.
9. Miralles R, *et al.* Captopril and vasculitis. *Ann Intern Med* 1988; **109:** 514.
10. Gupta S, *et al.* Nail changes with enalapril. *Br Med J* 1986; **293:** 140.
11. Kuechle MK, *et al.* Angiotensin-converting enzyme inhibitor-induced pemphigus: three case reports and literature review. *Mayo Clin Proc* 1994; **69:** 1166–71.
12. Frangogiannis NG, *et al.* Pemphigus of the larynx and esophagus. *Ann Intern Med* 1995; **122:** 803–4.
13. Vignes S, *et al.* Ramipril-induced superficial pemphigus. *Br J Dermatol* 1996; **135:** 657–8.
14. Ogg GS, *et al.* Ramipril-associated lichen planus pemphigoides. *Br J Dermatol* 1997; **136:** 412–14.
15. Furness PN, *et al.* Severe cutaneous reactions to captopril and enalapril; histological study and comparison with early mycosis fungoides. *J Clin Pathol* 1986; **39:** 902–7.
16. Hamlet NW, *et al.* Does captopril exacerbate psoriasis? *Br Med J* 1987; **295:** 1352.
17. Heckerling PS. Enalapril and vulvovaginal pruritus. *Ann Intern Med* 1990; **112:** 879–80.

Gynaecomastia. Painful unilateral gynaecomastia was reported in a patient with systemic lupus erythematosus and impaired renal function who was given captopril for hypertension.[1] In view of reports of breast enlargement in women given penicillamine it was suggested that the sulfhydryl structure might be responsible; however, gynaecomastia has also been reported in two patients receiving enalapril,[2,3] which does not contain the sulfhydryl grouping.

1. Markusse HM, Meyboom RHB. Gynaecomastia associated with captopril. *Br Med J* 1988; **296:** 1262–3.
2. Nakamura Y, *et al.* Gynaecomastia induced by angiotensin converting enzyme inhibitor. *Br Med J* 1990; **300:** 541.
3. Llop R, *et al.* Gynecomastia associated with enalapril and diazepam. *Ann Pharmacother* 1994; **28:** 671–2.

Hypersensitivity. Some of the adverse effects of ACE inhibitors might be mediated by the immune system, but evidence of specific hypersensitivity reactions seems to be limited. Coleman and colleagues demonstrated the presence of an IgG antibody to captopril in the serum of 2 of 45 patients receiving the drug but did not demonstrate any clinical significance to this.[1] A reaction resembling serum sickness was reported in one patient given captopril, with deposition of immune complexes in the glomerular basement membrane, and symptoms of rash, arthralgia, epidermolysis, fever, and lymphadenopathy.[2] Eosinophilia has also been reported in a number of patients.[3] The formation of antinuclear antibodies and lupus-like reactions have been described.[4,5]

Treatment with ACE inhibitors (enalapril, captopril, or lisinopril) has been associated with the development of **anaphylactoid reactions** in patients undergoing high-flux haemodialysis using polyacrylonitrile membrane (AN69).[6,7] The Committee on Safety of Medicines (CSM) in the UK has advised that the combined use of ACE inhibitors and such membranes should be avoided.[8] Similar anaphylactoid reactions have occurred in patients taking ACE inhibitors while being treated for severe hypercholesterolaemia by extracorporeal removal of low-density lipoproteins (LDL-apheresis) with dextran sulphate columns.[9] These reactions are thought to be bradykinin-mediated. Some have averted them by prolonging the interval between the last dose of ACE inhibitor and dextran sulphate apheresis[10] whereas others found this to be ineffective, but did prevent anaphylactoid reactions in one patient using the bradykinin receptor antagonist icatibant.[11] There have also been rare reports of severe anaphylactoid reactions occurring during desensitisation with Hymenoptera venom (e.g. bee or wasp venom) in patients receiving ACE inhibitors.

Angioedema is a known adverse effect of ACE inhibitors[12-15] and is reported to occur in 0.1 to 0.2% of patients.[14,15] There is no evidence that angioedema results from an immunological mechanism in these patients and it has been suggested that the effect is due to impaired kinin degradation. However, angioedema has been reported with lisinopril in a patient who had previously tolerated captopril.[16] The onset of angioedema has usually been within hours or at most a week of starting treatment with the ACE inhibitor,[14] but can occur after prolonged therapy for several months or years.[17-19] Visceral angioedema presenting as abdominal pain with diarrhoea, nausea, and vomiting, has been reported in a patient receiving enalapril.[20] If angioedema occurs the ACE inhibitor should be withdrawn and if there is swelling affecting the tongue, glottis, or larynx likely to cause airway obstruction, adrenaline should be given (see p.815).

1. Coleman JW, *et al.* Drug-specific antibodies in patients receiving captopril. *Br J Clin Pharmacol* 1986; **22:** 161–5.
2. Hoorntje SJ, *et al.* Serum-sickness-like syndrome with membranous glomerulopathy in patient on captopril. *Lancet* 1979; **ii:** 1297.
3. Kayanakis JG, *et al.* Eosinophilia during captopril treatment. *Lancet* 1980; **ii:** 923.
4. Schwartz D, *et al.* Enalapril-induced antinuclear antibodies. *Lancet* 1990; **336:** 187.
5. Pelayo M, *et al.* Drug-induced lupus-like reaction and captopril. *Ann Pharmacother* 1993; **27:** 1541–2.
6. Verresen L, *et al.* Angiotensin-converting-enzyme inhibitors and anaphylactoid reactions to high-flux membrane dialysis. *Lancet* 1990; **336:** 1360–2.
7. Tielmans C, *et al.* ACE inhibitors and anaphylactoid reactions to high-flux membrane dialysis. *Lancet* 1991; **337:** 370–1.
8. Committee on Safety of Medicines. Anaphylactoid reactions to high-flux polyacrylonitrile membranes in combination with ACE inhibitors. *Current Problems 33* 1992.
9. Olbricht CJ, *et al.* Anaphylactoid reactions, LDL apheresis with dextran sulphate, and ACE inhibitors. *Lancet* 1992; **340:** 908–9.
10. Keller C, *et al.* LDL-apheresis with dextran sulphate and anaphylactoid reactions to ACE inhibitors. *Lancet* 1993; **341:** 60–1.

11. Davidson DC, *et al.* Prevention with icatibant of anaphylactoid reactions to ACE inhibitor during LDL apheresis. *Lancet* 1994; **343:** 1575.
12. Wood SM, *et al.* Angio-oedema and urticaria associated with angiotensin converting enzyme inhibitors. *Br Med J* 1987; **294:** 91–2.
13. Hedner T, *et al.* Angio-oedema in relation to treatment with angiotensin converting enzyme inhibitors. *Br Med J* 1992; **304:** 941–6.
14. Israili ZH, Hall WD. Cough and angioneurotic edema associated with angiotensin-converting enzyme inhibitor therapy: a review of the literature and pathophysiology. *Ann Intern Med* 1992; **117:** 234–42.
15. Vleeming W, *et al.* ACE inhibitor-induced angioedema. *Drug Safety* 1998; **18:** 171–88.
16. McElligott S, *et al.* Angioedema after substituting lisinopril for captopril. *Ann Intern Med* 1992; **116:** 426–7.
17. Chin HL, Buchan DA. Severe angioedema after long-term use of an angiotensin-converting enzyme inhibitor. *Ann Intern Med* 1990; **112:** 312–13.
18. Edwards TB. Adverse effects of ACE inhibitors. *Ann Intern Med* 1993; **118:** 314.
19. Chu TJ, Chow N. Adverse effects of ACE inhibitors. *Ann Intern Med* 1993; **118:** 314.
20. Mullins RJ, *et al.* Visceral angioedema related to treatment with an ACE inhibitor. *Med J Aust* 1996; **165:** 319–21.

Overdosage. There have been reports of overdosage with captopril,[1,2] enalapril,[3-6] and lisinopril.[7,8] The main adverse effect is hypotension which usually responds to supportive treatment and volume expansion. Pressor agents are rarely required. Infusion of angiotensin amide may be considered if hypotension persists.[5,6,8]

1. Augenstein WL, *et al.* Captopril overdose resulting in hypotension. *JAMA* 1988; **259:** 3302–5.
2. Graham SR, *et al.* Captopril overdose. *Med J Aust* 1989; **151:** 111.
3. Waeber B, *et al.* Self poisoning with enalapril. *Br Med J* 1984; **288:** 287–8.
4. Lau CP. Attempted suicide with enalapril. *N Engl J Med* 1986; **315:** 197.
5. Jackson T, *et al.* Enalapril overdose treated with angiotensin infusion. *Lancet* 1993; **341:** 703.
6. Newby DE, *et al.* Enalapril overdose and the corrective effect of intravenous angiotensin II. *Br J Clin Pharmacol* 1995; **40:** 103–4.
7. Dawson AH, *et al.* Lisinopril overdose. *Lancet* 1990; **335:** 487–8.
8. Trilli LE, Johnson KA. Lisinopril overdose and management with intravenous angiotensin II. *Ann Pharmacother* 1994; **28:** 1165–8.

Precautions

ACE inhibitors should not be used in patients with aortic stenosis or outflow tract obstruction. They should not generally be used in patients with renovascular disease or suspected renovascular disease, but are occasionally necessary for severe resistant hypertension in such patients when they should only be given with great caution and under close specialist supervision. It should be noted that the elderly or patients with peripheral vascular diseases or generalised atherosclerosis may be at high risk because they may have clinically silent renovascular disease. Renal function should be assessed in all patients prior to administration of ACE inhibitors. Patients with existing renal disease or taking high doses should be monitored regularly for proteinuria. Regular white blood cell counts may be necessary in patients with collagen vascular disorders, such as systemic lupus erythematosus and scleroderma, or in patients receiving immunosuppressive therapy, especially when they also have impaired renal function.

Patients with heart failure and patients who are likely to be salt or water depleted—for example, those receiving concomitant treatment with diuretics or dialysis—may experience symptomatic hypotension during the initial stages of ACE inhibitor therapy. Treatment should therefore be started under close medical supervision, using a low dose and with the patient in a recumbent position to minimise this effect.

Anaphylactoid reactions have occurred in patients taking ACE inhibitors during haemodialysis using high-flux polyacrylonitrile membranes, during LDL-apheresis with dextran sulphate columns, and during desensitisation with Hymenoptera venom.

ACE inhibitors have been reported to produce harmful effects in *animal* fetuses following large maternal doses and should not be used during pregnancy (see below).

Diarrhoea. Several reports have indicated that life-threatening hypotension and signs of renal failure may develop in patients receiving captopril[1-3] or enalapril[3] following volume depletion due to diarrhoea.

1. McMurray J, Matthews DM. Effect of diarrhoea on a patient taking captopril. *Lancet* 1985; **i:** 581.
2. Benett PR, Cairns SA. Captopril, diarrhoea, and hypotension. *Lancet* 1985; **i:** 1105.
3. McMurray J, Matthews DM. Consequences of fluid loss in patients treated with ACE inhibitors. *Postgrad Med J* 1987; **63:** 385–7.

Hepatic cirrhosis. It has been suggested that in patients with cirrhosis captopril could cause a marked reduction in arterial pressure and severely compromise renal function since maintenance of glomerular filtration rate might be mediated by angiotensin II in these patients.[1] This theory was supported by Wood *et al.* who reported a reduction in glomerular filtration rate in response to a fall in mean arterial pressure in 4 patients with resistant ascites secondary to hepatic cirrhosis.[2] The fall in mean arterial pressure was associated with postural hypotension and increasing encephalopathy. Jørgensen *et al.* reported severe confusion in 2 patients with cirrhosis during treatment with captopril 6.25 to 12.5 mg three times daily.[3]

1. Ring T. Captopril and resistant ascites: a word of caution. *Lancet* 1983; **ii:** 165.
2. Wood LJ, *et al.* Adverse effects of captopril in treatment of resistant ascites, a state of functional bilateral renal artery stenosis. *Lancet* 1985; **ii:** 1008–9.
3. Jørgensen F, *et al.* Captopril and resistant ascites. *Lancet* 1983; **ii:** 405.

Huntington's disease. A report of a woman with Huntington's disease whose condition deteriorated dramatically during treatment with captopril and improved on withdrawal of the drug.[1]

1. Goldblatt J, Bryer A. Huntington's disease: deterioration in clinical state during treatment with angiotensin converting enzyme inhibitor. *Br Med J* 1987; **294:** 1659–60.

Peripheral vascular disease. Patients with peripheral vascular disease may have a high incidence of renal artery stenosis and are therefore at high risk of renal failure with ACE inhibitor therapy (see Effects on the Kidneys, above). Mild renal artery stenosis was found in 64 of 374 patients (17%) with peripheral vascular disease and severe renal artery stenosis in 52 (14%); the stenosis was bilateral in 43 (12%).[1] Renal function should be carefully monitored in any patient with peripheral vascular disease who receives ACE inhibitors.

1. Salmon P, Brown MA. Renal artery stenosis and peripheral vascular disease: implications for ACE inhibitor therapy. *Lancet* 1990; **336:** 321.

Pregnancy. There is evidence from *animal* studies that administration of ACE inhibitors during pregnancy is associated with fetal toxicity and an increase in still-births.[1] Several case reports have described the development of fetal renal failure, with oligohydramnios or neonatal anuria, in the offspring of mothers receiving captopril[2-4] or enalapril;[5,6] there have been fetal[4] and neonatal[3] deaths. Withdrawal of the ACE inhibitor might result in reversal of the renal dysfunction.[6] A review of the subject has concluded that when ACE inhibitors are stopped in the first trimester the baby is likely to be born at or near term and of normal birth-weight whereas continued treatment carries a risk of early delivery and low birth-weight.[7] There are also 2 case reports in which maternal captopril[8] or enalapril[9] therapy, in association with other drugs, was associated with birth defects including defective ossification of the skull. A literature search up to the end of 1989 indicated that the use of ACE inhibitors during pregnancy can cause severe disturbances of fetal and neonatal renal function, pulmonary hypoplasia, and long-lasting neonatal anuria.[10] Analysis of pregnancy outcome in more than 100 000 women in Tennessee found that 19 had been exposed to an ACE inhibitor during pregnancy.[11] Of the 19 infants, 2 were preterm and had serious life-threatening conditions. One had prolonged anuria requiring dialysis; the mother had probably taken enalapril during the second and third trimesters, but had a renal transplant and was also receiving other drugs. The other had microcephaly and a large occipital encephalocele; the mother had probably taken captopril during the first and second trimesters.

The FDA has re-emphasised that ACE inhibitors can cause injury and even death to the developing fetus in the second and third trimester.[12] A review of the available experimental and clinical data concluded that the use of ACE inhibitors should be avoided in all trimesters of pregnancy.[13]

1. Broughton Pipkin F, *et al.* Possible risk with captopril in pregnancy: some animal data. *Lancet* 1980; **i:** 1256.
2. Boutroy M-J, *et al.* Captopril administration in pregnancy impairs fetal angiotensin converting enzyme activity and neonatal adaptation. *Lancet* 1984; **ii:** 935–6.
3. Guignard JP, *et al.* Persistent anuria in a neonate: a side effect of captopril? *Int J Pediatr Nephrol* 1981; **2:** 133.
4. Knott PD, *et al.* Congenital renal dysgenesis possibly due to captopril. *Lancet* 1989; **i:** 451.
5. Schubiger G, *et al.* Enalapril for pregnancy-induced hypertension: acute renal failure in a neonate. *Ann Intern Med* 1988; **108:** 215–16. Correction. *ibid.*: 777.
6. Broughton Pipkin F, *et al.* ACE inhibitors in pregnancy. *Lancet* 1989; **ii:** 96–7.
7. Anonymous. Are ACE inhibitors safe in pregnancy? *Lancet* 1989; **ii:** 482–3.
8. Duminy PC, Burger P du T. Fetal abnormality associated with use of captopril during pregnancy. *S Afr Med J* 1981; **60:** 805.
9. Mehta N, Modi N. ACE inhibitors in pregnancy. *Lancet* 1989; **ii:** 96.
10. Hanssens M, *et al.* Fetal and neonatal effects of treatment with angiotensin-converting enzyme inhibitors in pregnancy. *Obstet Gynecol* 1991; **78:** 128–35.
11. Piper JM, *et al.* Pregnancy outcome following exposure to angiotensin-converting enzyme inhibitors. *Obstet Gynecol* 1992; **80:** 429–32.
12. Nightingale SL. Warnings on use of ACE inhibitors in second and third trimester of pregnancy. *JAMA* 1992; **267:** 2445.
13. Shotan A, *et al.* Risk of angiotensin-converting enzyme inhibition during pregnancy: experimental and clinical evidence, potential mechanisms, and recommendations for use. *Am J Med* 1994; **96:** 451–6.

Interactions

Excessive hypotension may occur when ACE inhibitors are used concurrently with diuretics, other antihypertensives, or other agents, including alcohol, that lower blood pressure. An additive hyperkalaemic effect is possible in patients receiving ACE inhibitors with potassium-sparing diuretics, potassium supplements (including potassium-containing salt substitutes), or other drugs that can cause hyperkalaemia (such as cyclosporin or indomethacin) and serum-potassium concentrations should be monitored. Potassium-sparing diuretics and potassium supplements should be stopped before initiating ACE inhibitors in patients with heart failure. However, ACE inhibitor therapy does not obviate the possible need for potassium supplementation in patients receiving potassium-wasting diuretics and potassium concentrations should also be monitored in these patients. The adverse effects of ACE inhibitors on the kidneys may be potentiated by other drugs, such as NSAIDs, that can affect renal function.

General references.

1. Shionoiri H. Pharmacokinetic drug interactions with ACE inhibitors. *Clin Pharmacokinet* 1993; **25:** 20–58.
2. Mignat C, Unger T. ACE inhibitors: drug interactions of clinical significance. *Drug Safety* 1995; **12:** 334–7.

Allopurinol. For reports of reactions in patients taking captopril and allopurinol, see under Allopurinol, p.391.

Antacids. Administration of captopril with antacids reduced the bioavailability of captopril although this did not significantly alter the effects on blood pressure and heart rate.[1] The bioavailability of fosinopril, and possibly other ACE inhibitors, may also be reduced by concurrent antacid administration.

1. Mäntylä R, *et al.* Impairment of captopril bioavailability by concomitant food and antacid intake. *Int J Clin Pharmacol Ther Toxicol* 1984; **22:** 626–9.

Antidiabetics. Hypoglycaemia was noted by Ferriere and colleagues in 3 type 1 diabetics when captopril was added to their therapeutic regimen; it was also seen in one type 2 diabetic, in whom withdrawal of hypoglycaemic drugs became necessary.[1] Subsequent study suggested that the effect was due to enhanced insulin sensitivity.[1] Similar instances of a reduction in blood sugar in both non-diabetic[2] and diabetic[3] patients given enalapril have occurred. Two case-control studies in diabetic patients receiving insulin or oral hypoglycaemics suggested that patients treated with ACE inhibitors were at increased risk of developing severe hypoglycaemia.[4,5] However, other studies in diabetic patients given captopril or enalapril have failed to find any significant alterations in blood-glucose control,[6,7] and ACE inhibitors have been favoured by some as first-line drugs in the treatment of hypertension in diabetic patients (see p.788).

1. Ferriere M, *et al.* Captopril and insulin sensitivity. *Ann Intern Med* 1985; **102:** 134–5.
2. Helgeland A, *et al.* Enalapril, atenolol, and hydrochlorothiazide in mild to moderate hypertension: a comparative multicentre study in general practice in Norway. *Lancet* 1986; **i:** 872–5.
3. McMurray J, Fraser DM. Captopril, enalapril, and blood glucose. *Lancet* 1986; **i:** 1035.
4. Herings RMC, *et al.* Hypoglycaemia associated with use of inhibitors of angiotensin converting enzyme. *Lancet* 1995; **345:** 1195–8.
5. Morris AD, *et al.* ACE inhibitor use is associated with hospitalization for severe hypoglycemia in patients with diabetes. *Diabetes Care* 1997; **20:** 1363–7.
6. Passa P, *et al.* Enalapril, captopril, and blood glucose. *Lancet* 1986; **i:** 1447.
7. Winocour P, *et al.* Captopril and blood glucose. *Lancet* 1986; **ii:** 461.

Azathioprine. Leucopenia has been reported in a patient given captopril with azathioprine; the effect did not occur when either drug was given alone.[1] In a similar report, neutropenia in a patient receiving a regimen including azathioprine and captopril did not recur when captopril was reintroduced following withdrawal of azathioprine.[2]

1. Kirchertz EJ, *et al.* Successful low dose captopril rechallenge following drug-induced leucopenia. *Lancet* 1981; **i:** 1363.
2. Edwards CRW, *et al.* Successful reintroduction of captopril following neutropenia. *Lancet* 1981; **i:** 723.

Cyclosporin. An additive hyperkalaemic effect with ACE inhibitors and cyclosporin is possible. Also, acute renal failure has been reported in 2 patients receiving cyclosporin after renal transplantation following administration of enalapril.[1] Renal function recovered when the ACE inhibitor was withdrawn.

1. Murray BM, *et al.* Enalapril-associated acute renal failure in renal transplants: possible role of cyclosporine. *Am J Kidney Dis* 1990; **16:** 66–9.

Cytokines. An additive hyperkalaemic effect may occur when ACE inhibitors are administered with *epoetins*. ACE inhibitors have also been reported to antagonise the haematopoietic effects of epoetins.

Marked hypotension occurred in three patients[1] receiving ACE inhibitors who were given *interleukin-3* following chemotherapy; blood pressure returned to normal when the ACE inhibitors were discontinued.

1. Dercksen MW, *et al.* Hypotension induced by interleukin-3 in patients on angiotensin-converting enzyme inhibitors. *Lancet* 1995; **345:** 448.

Digoxin. For reports of an increase in serum-digoxin concentrations during therapy with ACE inhibitors, see p.850.

Diuretics. Excessive hypotension may occur when ACE inhibitors are used concurrently with diuretics. Deterioration in renal function has also been reported (see under Metolazone, p.907).

General anaesthetics. Marked hypotension may occur during general anaesthesia in patients receiving ACE inhibitors. In addition corrected cerebral blood flow was significantly lower in 11 patients who received captopril before general anaesthesia induced with thiopentone and maintained with nitrous oxide and enflurane, than in 9 patients pretreated with metoprolol and 9 untreated controls.[1] The age range was comparable in all groups, being within 20 and 48 years. Although there were no complications of anaesthesia associated with captopril pretreatment, discontinuation of ACE inhibitor therapy before anaesthesia should be considered.

1. Jensen K, *et al.* Cerebral blood flow during anaesthesia: influence of pretreatment with metoprolol or captopril. *Br J Anaesth* 1989; **62:** 321–3.

Gold salts. The nitritoid reaction (flushing, nausea, dizziness, and hypotension associated with the first weeks of gold treatment) occurred soon after commencing treatment with an ACE inhibitor (captopril, lisinopril, or enalapril) in 4 patients who had been receiving sodium aurothiomalate for at least 2 years.[1]

1. Healey LA, Backes MB. Nitritoid reactions and angiotensin-converting-enzyme inhibitors. *N Engl J Med* 1989; **321:** 763.

Interferons. Severe granulocytopenia has been reported[1] in three patients with mixed cryoglobulinaemia treated with interferon alfa-2a who also received ACE inhibitors. The effect was considered to be due to synergistic haematological toxicity. However, in a further report,[2] two patients developed only mild granulocytopenia that was reversible despite continued therapy, while a third patient retained a normal granulocyte count.

1. Casato M, *et al.* Granulocytopenia after combined therapy with interferon and angiotensin-converting enzyme inhibitors: evidence for a synergistic hematologic toxicity. *Am J Med* 1995; **99:** 386–91.
2. Jacquot C, *et al.* Granulocytopenia after combined therapy with interferon and angiotensin-converting enzyme inhibitors: evidence for a synergistic hematologic toxicity. *Am J Med* 1996; **101:** 235–6.

Lithium. For reports of lithium toxicity in patients taking ACE inhibitors, see p.293.

NSAIDs. *Indomethacin* and possibly other NSAIDs, including aspirin, have been reported to reduce or abolish the hypotensive action of ACE inhibitors. Some have proposed that part of the hypotensive effect of ACE inhibitors is prostaglandin-dependent, which might explain this interaction with drugs such as NSAIDs that block prostaglandin synthesis. However, in a double-blind study Gerber *et al.*[1] found that indomethacin did not influence the hypotensive effect of captopril or enalapril in patients with essential hypertension, suggesting that the effects on prostaglandins are not significant.

The possibility of an interaction between low-dose *aspirin* and ACE inhibitors may be of concern, especially in patients with heart failure. Hall *et al.*[2] reported that aspirin appeared to counteract the vasodilator activity of enalapril in patients with severe heart failure although the clinical implications for patients with less severe left ventricular dysfunction are not clear. A review[3] of the evidence for such an interaction concluded that the data were inconclusive and further study was required.

The combination of NSAIDs and ACE inhibitors may also have variable effects on renal function since they act at different parts of the glomerulus.[4] When given to patients whose kidneys are underperfused, for example because of heart failure, liver cirrhosis, or haemorrhage, renal function may deteriorate. However, specific patient groups without reduced renal perfusion may benefit from combining an NSAID with an ACE inhibitor.

Indomethacin, and possibly other NSAIDs, may have an additive hyperkalaemic effect.

1. Gerber JG, *et al.* The hypotensive action of captopril and enalapril is not prostacyclin dependent. *Clin Pharmacol Ther* 1993; **54:** 523–32.
2. Hall D, *et al.* Counteraction of the vasodilator effects of enalapril by aspirin in severe heart failure. *J Am Coll Cardiol* 1992; **20:** 1549–55.
3. Cleland JGF, *et al.* Is aspirin safe for patients with heart failure? *Br Heart J* 1995; **74:** 215–19.
4. Sturrock NDC, Struthers AD. Non-steroidal anti-inflammatory drugs and angiotensin converting enzyme inhibitors: a commonly prescribed combination with variable effects on renal function. *Br J Clin Pharmacol* 1993; **35:** 343–8.

Probenecid. Administration of probenecid to four healthy subjects during intravenous infusion of captopril caused increases in the steady-state plasma-captopril concentration. The interaction was considered to be due to a reduction of tubular secretion of captopril by probenecid.[1]

1. Singhvi SM, *et al.* Renal handling of captopril: effect of probenecid. *Clin Pharmacol Ther* 1982; **32:** 182–9.

Pharmacokinetics

Most ACE inhibitors are given by mouth. Apart from captopril and lisinopril, they are generally prodrugs and following absorption undergo rapid metabolism by ester hydrolysis to the active diacid form; for example, enalapril is converted to enalaprilat. Metabolism occurs mainly in the liver. Excretion as active drug or active metabolite is principally in the urine; some, such as benazeprilat and fosinoprilat are also excreted via the biliary tract. Elimination of the diacid is polyphasic and there is a prolonged terminal elimination phase, which is considered to represent binding to the angiotensin-converting enzyme at a saturable binding site. This bound fraction does not contribute to accumulation of drug following multiple doses. The terminal elimination half-life does not therefore predict the kinetics observed with multiple dosing and the effective half-life for accumulation is the value usually quoted.

Reviews.

1. Burnier M, Biollaz J. Pharmacokinetic optimisation of angiotensin converting enzyme (ACE) inhibitor therapy. *Clin Pharmacokinet* 1992; **22:** 375–84.
2. Hoyer J, *et al.* Clinical pharmacokinetics of angiotensin converting enzyme (ACE) inhibitors in renal failure. *Clin Pharmacokinet* 1993; **24:** 230–54.

Uses and Administration

ACE inhibitors are antihypertensive drugs that act as vasodilators and reduce peripheral resistance. They inhibit angiotensin-converting enzyme (ACE), which is involved in the conversion of angiotensin I to angiotensin II. Angiotensin II stimulates the synthesis and secretion of aldosterone and raises blood pressure via a potent direct vasoconstrictor effect. ACE is identical to bradykininase or kininase II and ACE inhibitors may reduce the degradation of bradykinin. They may also affect enzymes involved in the generation of prostaglandins. The pharmacological actions of ACE inhibitors are thought to be primarily due to the inhibition of the renin-angiotensin-aldosterone system, but since they also effectively reduce blood pressure in patients with low renin concentrations other mechanisms are probably also involved. ACE inhibitors produce a reduction in both preload and afterload in patients with heart failure. They also reduce left ventricular remodelling, a process that sometimes follows myocardial infarction. Normally, renal blood flow is increased without a change in glomerular filtration rate. ACE inhibitors also have the property of reducing proteinuria associated with glomerular kidney disease.

ACE inhibitors are used in the treatment of hypertension and heart failure and are given to improve survival following myocardial infarction. They are also used in the treatment of diabetic nephropathy. Administration is generally by mouth.

In some hypertensive patients there may be a precipitous fall in blood pressure when starting therapy with an ACE inhibitor and the first dose should preferably be given at bedtime; if possible, any diuretic therapy should be stopped a few days beforehand and resumed later if necessary.

In patients with heart failure taking loop diuretics, severe first-dose hypotension is common on introduction of an ACE inhibitor, but temporary withdrawal of the diuretic may cause rebound pulmonary oedema. Thus treatment should be initiated with a low dose under close medical supervision.

Action. Although the main target for ACE inhibitors was initially thought to be the endocrine renin-angiotensin system in the circulation it is now recognised that this mechanism alone cannot readily explain all the actions of ACE inhibitors.[1] It is now clear that endogenous renin-angiotensin systems exist in many tissues and that ACE inhibitors may have localised effects.[2] It is thought that this may underlie some of the long-term effects of ACE inhibition, including increased arterial wall compliance, improved left ventricular function in heart failure, regression of vascular and left ventricular hypertrophy, and delayed progression of diabetic nephropathy. Although ACE inhibitors differ in their degree of binding to tissue ACE and in their tissue distribution, there is at present no evidence that this is clinically significant.[1] However, novel compounds with greater tissue specificity may have new therapeutic implications.

It has been suggested[3] that ACE inhibitors may exercise their antihypertensive effects, at least in part, by inhibiting calcium-mobilisation in vascular tissue. Whether this represents direct calcium-channel blocking properties or is mediated via tissue renin-angiotensin systems warrants further investigation. ACE inhibitors also have effects on the kinin system and there is some evidence that the cardiovascular actions of ACE inhibitors also involve localised accumulation of kinins.[4]

1. Anonymous. ACE inhibitors and tissue binding. *Lancet* 1990; **336:** 718–20.
2. Zarnke KB, Feldman RD. Direct angiotensin converting enzyme inhibitor-mediated venodilation. *Clin Pharmacol Ther* 1996; **59:** 559–68.
3. Jeremy JY, *et al.* ACE inhibitors and tissue binding. *Lancet* 1990; **336:** 1189.
4. Linz W, *et al.* Contribution of kinins to the cardiovascular actions of angiotensin-converting enzyme inhibitors. *Pharmacol Rev* 1995; **47:** 25–49.

Ascites. Conflicting responses have been reported following the use of captopril in ascites resistant to conventional diuretic treatment (p.781). Shepherd *et al.* reported a reduction in pulmonary oedema and ascites in a patient with liver disease with captopril 25 mg three times daily.[1] However, administration of captopril in patients with cirrhosis has been associated with severe adverse effects (see Hepatic Cirrhosis, under Precautions, above). Interestingly, Noto *et al.* reported that doses of captopril 300 mg daily reduced resistant ascites in a study of 10 patients;[2] at these doses the effect appeared to be linked to reduced aldosterone secretion and not to the suppressed haemodynamic vascular effects induced by angiotensin II reported at lower doses.

1. Shepherd AN, *et al.* Captopril and resistant ascites. *Lancet* 1983; **i:** 1391–2.
2. Noto R, *et al.* Captopril and resistant ascites in cirrhotic patients with various stages of portal hypertension. *Curr Ther Res* 1986; **40:** 733–8.

Bartter's syndrome. Captopril has been reported to produce beneficial responses in patients with Bartter's syndrome[1-5] (p.1150), which is characterised by hyperaldosteronism, hypokalaemia, and hyperreninaemia, but with normal or reduced blood pressure.[1-4]

1. Aurell M, Rudin A. Effects of captopril in Bartter's syndrome. *N Engl J Med* 1981; **304:** 1609.
2. Hené RJ, *et al.* Long-term treatment of Bartter's syndrome with captopril. *Br Med J* 1982; **285:** 695.
3. James JM, Davies D. The use of captopril in Bartter's syndrome. *Br Med J* 1984; **289:** 162.
4. Savastano A, *et al.* Treatment of Bartter's disease with captopril: a case report. *Curr Ther Res* 1986; **39:** 408–13.
5. Jest P, *et al.* Angiotensin-converting enzyme inhibition as a therapeutic principle in Bartter's syndrome. *Eur J Clin Pharmacol* 1991; **41:** 303–5.

Diabetic retinopathy. It has been reported[1] that administration of an ACE inhibitor may reduce the progression of retinopathy in non-hypertensive patients with insulin-dependent diabetes mellitus (p.315). However, progression of retinopathy was a secondary end-point of the study and it was suggested that further studies were needed to confirm the beneficial results.

1. Chaturvedi N, *et al.* Effect of lisinopril on progression of retinopathy in normotensive people with type 1 diabetes. *Lancet* 1998; **351:** 28–31.

Erythrocytosis. Erythrocytosis may occur following renal transplantation and is usually treated by phlebotomy, although oral theophylline may be an alternative (see p.773).

Enalapril, in a dose of 10 mg daily by mouth, however, was reported to be more effective than theophylline in one study.[1] A second study[2] reported effective reductions in haematocrit with a dose of enalapril 2.5 mg daily. Beneficial responses have also been reported with captopril[3] and lisinopril.[4]

1. Ok E, *et al.* Comparison of the effects of enalapril and theophylline on polycythemia after renal transplantation. *Transplantation* 1995; **59:** 1623–45.
2. Beckingham IJ, *et al.* A randomized placebo-controlled study of enalapril in the treatment of erythrocytosis after renal transplantation. *Nephrol Dial Transplant* 1995; **10:** 2316–20.
3. Hernández E, *et al.* Usefulness and safety of treatment with captopril in posttransplant erythrocytosis. *Transplant Proc* 1995; **27:** 2239–41.
4. MacGregor MS, *et al.* Treatment of postrenal transplant erythrocytosis. *Nephron* 1996; **74:** 517–21.

Heart failure. ACE inhibitors given orally produce clinical benefit in all stages of chronic heart failure (p.785) additional to that seen with diuretics. They relieve symptoms and improve survival and reduce the progression of mild or moderate heart failure to more severe stages. Thus, many authorities now advocate that most patients, even if asymptomatic with diuretics alone, should be treated with ACE inhibitors. The optimum dose of ACE inhibitors in heart failure and their role in diastolic dysfunction are not yet clear. ACE inhibitors may also be beneficial in patients with heart failure associated with valve disorders.

The mechanism of action in heart failure is not yet clear. A comparison of captopril with glyceryl trinitrate indicated that captopril is both a potent venodilator and an arterial vasodilator, which reduces both preload and afterload (in contrast to glyceryl trinitrate, which predominantly reduces preload), and it was suggested that venodilatation, rather than simply vasodilatation, may be significantly associated with improved survival in patients with cardiac failure.[1] The haemodynamic and neurohormonal consequences of ACE inhibition play a part[2] and there may be indirect prevention of cardiac arrhythmias.[3] ACE inhibitors also appear to reduce left ventricular hypertrophy. It has also been proposed that captopril's free-radical scavenging property may have a role,[4] although another study[5] did not confirm this effect.

Captopril and enalapril have both been used in infants with severe heart failure (see p.837, and p.864, respectively).

1. Capewell S, *et al.* Acute and chronic arterial and venous effects of captopril in congestive cardiac failure. *Br Med J* 1989; **299:** 942–5.
2. Deedwania PC. Angiotensin-converting enzyme inhibitors in congestive heart failure. *Arch Intern Med* 1990; **150:** 1798–1805.
3. Wesseling H, *et al.* Cardiac arrhythmias—a new indication for angiotensin-converting enzyme inhibitors? *J Hum Hypertens* 1989; **3** (suppl 1): 89–95.
4. Chopra M, *et al.* Captopril: a free radical scavenger. *Br J Clin Pharmacol* 1989; **27:** 396–9.
5. Lapenna D, *et al.* Captopril has no significant scavenging antioxidant activity in human plasma in vitro or in vivo. *Br J Clin Pharmacol* 1996; **42:** 451–6.

Hypertension. The role of ACE inhibitors, in the management of hypertension has been reviewed.[1] ACE inhibitors, along with calcium-channel blockers, and alpha blockers, are generally considered to be alternative first-line drugs to diuretics and beta blockers in the treatment of hypertension (see p.788). ACE inhibitors may be particularly useful in diabetic patients due to their beneficial effects on the kidney. Other suggested advantages include their lack of adverse effects on serum lipids, a reduction in left ventricular hypertrophy,[2] and a reduction in plasma fibrinogen levels.[3] However, the clinical significance of these effects is not yet established.

The antihypertensive actions of ACE inhibitors may be potentiated by drugs that activate the renin-angiotensin system. Hence, combination therapy with diuretics or with calcium-channel blockers may be particularly useful.

1. Burris JF. The expanding role of angiotensin converting enzyme inhibitors in the management of hypertension. *J Clin Pharmacol* 1995; **35:** 337–42.
2. Schmieder RE, *et al.* Reversal of left ventricular hypertrophy in essential hypertension: a meta-analysis of randomized double-blind studies. *JAMA* 1996; **275:** 1507–13.
3. Fogari R, *et al.* Effects of different antihypertensive drugs on plasma fibrinogen in hypertensive patients. *Br J Clin Pharmacol* 1995; **39:** 471–6.

DIAGNOSIS OF RENOVASCULAR HYPERTENSION. Captopril has been used to diagnose renovascular hypertension: the increase in plasma renin activity following blockade of the conversion of angiotensin I to angiotensin II being greater in renovascular hypertension than in primary hypertension.[1] A review of methods for detecting renovascular hypertension[2] noted that accuracy of the captopril test may be lower in younger patients, black patients, and those with impaired renal function. However, the test may be a useful diagnostic tool for use in selected patients by specialised centres.[2,3] Captopril has also been given to enhance the sensitivity and specificity of renal scintigraphy.[2]

1. Muller FB, *et al.* The captopril test for identifying renovascular disease in hypertensive patients. *Am J Med* 1986; **80:** 633–44.
2. Mann SJ, Pickering TG. Detection of renovascular hypertension: state of the art 1992. *Ann Intern Med* 1992; **117:** 845–53.
3. McCarthy JE, Weder AB. The captopril test and renovascular hypertension: a cautionary tale. *Arch Intern Med* 1990; **150:** 493–5.

Ischaemic heart disease. In the SAVE[1] and SOLVD[2] studies, administration of ACE inhibitors to patients with heart failure was noted to lead to a reduction in the incidence of myocardial infarction. ACE inhibitors have therefore been investigated in the management of atherosclerosis (p.782) and ischaemic heart disease but with conflicting results. In the TREND study,[3] administration of quinapril for 6 months was reported to improve endothelial dysfunction in patients with ischaemic heart disease. However, apparently no effects on the progression of atherosclerosis or the incidence of cardiac events were found in the QUIET study [not yet published], which used a lower dose of quinapril given for 3 years. A lack of acute anti-ischaemic effect has also been found with short-term administration of captopril and enalapril in patients with stable angina,[4] and with enalapril in Prinzmetal's angina.[5]

1. Pfeffer MA, *et al.* Effect of captopril on mortality and morbidity in patients with left ventricular dysfunction after myocardial infarction: results of the Survival and Ventricular Enlargement Trial. *N Engl J Med* 1992; **327:** 669–77.
2. Yusuf S, *et al.* Effect of enalapril on myocardial infarction and unstable angina in patients with low ejection fractions. *Lancet* 1992; **340:** 1173–8.
3. Mancini GBJ, *et al.* Angiotensin-converting enzyme inhibition with quinapril improves endothelial vasomotor dysfunction in patients with coronary artery disease: the TREND (Trial on Reversing Endothelial Dysfunction) study. *Circulation* 1996; **94:** 258–65.
4. Longobardi G, *et al.* Failure of protective effect of captopril and enalapril on exercise and dipyridamole-induced myocardial ischemia. *Am J Cardiol* 1995; **76:** 255–8.
5. Guazzi M, *et al.* Ineffectiveness of angiotensin converting enzyme inhibition (enalapril) on overt and silent myocardial ischemia in vasospastic angina and comparison with verapamil. *Clin Pharmacol Ther* 1996; **59:** 476–81.

Kidney disorders. Although ACE inhibitors may adversely affect renal function (see under Adverse Effects and Treatment, above), and although pre-existing renal dysfunction is considered a reason for caution in administering these drugs, ACE inhibitors can have beneficial effects in diabetic and nondiabetic renal disease. Hypertension is closely linked with the kidney—the kidney is important in the normal control of blood pressure and may have a role in the pathogenesis of hypertension; it may also be a prime target of damage caused by hypertension.[1] ACE inhibitors tend to improve renal haemodynamics in patients with hypertension and may slow the rate of loss of renal function. However, they also have an antiproteinuric effect that is independent of their antihypertensive action.[2-5] Proteinuria is an important indicator of glomerular kidney disease (p.1021) of various causes and may range from asymptomatic to severe. Diabetic nephropathy (p.315) is often associated with hypertension and may progress from microalbuminuria to the nephrotic syndrome and end-stage renal failure.

Most experience has been gained in patients with overt diabetic nephropathy, in whom the use of ACE inhibitors now appears to be of established benefit whether they are hypertensive or normotensive or whether they have type 1 or type 2 diabetes mellitus. They may also impede progression of microalbuminuria in early diabetic nephropathy,[4-7] and have been recommended, in conjunction with tight glycaemic control, in all diabetic patients with microalbuminuria.[8]

ACE inhibitors may also be of benefit in renal disease unrelated to diabetes, although their role is not yet established. A number of studies[9-12,15] have reported that ACE inhibitors reduce both proteinuria and the rate of decline of renal function in patients with various non-diabetic renal disorders, and a meta-analysis[13] concluded that ACE inhibitors are more effective than other antihypertensives in reducing the incidence of end-stage renal disease.

Patients with systemic sclerosis (see Scleroderma, p.501) are considered to be at high risk of adverse effects from ACE inhibitors; however there is evidence that these drugs are of benefit in the management of scleroderma-associated hypertension and renal crisis.[14]

1. Raine EG. Hypertension and the kidney. *Br Med Bull* 1994; **50:** 322–41.
2. Kasiske BL, *et al.* Effect of antihypertensive therapy on the kidney in patients with diabetes: a meta-regression analysis. *Ann Intern Med* 1993; **118:** 129–38.
3. Lewis EJ, *et al.* The effect of angiotensin-converting-enzyme inhibition on diabetic nephropathy. *N Engl J Med* 1993; **329:** 1456–62.
4. Viberti G, *et al.* Effect of captopril on progression to clinical proteinuria in patients with insulin-dependent diabetes mellitus and microalbuminuria. *JAMA* 1994; **271:** 275–9.
5. Ravid M, *et al.* Long-term stabilizing effect of angiotensin-converting enzyme inhibition on plasma creatinine and on proteinuria in normotensive type II diabetic patients. *Ann Intern Med* 1993; **118:** 577–81.
6. Laffel LMB, *et al.* The beneficial effect of angiotensin-converting enzyme inhibition with captopril on diabetic nephropathy in normotensive IDDM patients with microalbuminuria. *Am J Med* 1995; **99:** 497–504.
7. The EUCLID Study Group. Randomised placebo-controlled trial of lisinopril in normotensive patients with insulin-dependent diabetes and normoalbuminuria or microalbuminuria. *Lancet* 1997; **349:** 1787–92.
8. Mogensen CE, *et al.* Prevention of diabetic renal disease with special reference to microalbuminuria. *Lancet* 1995; **346:** 1080–4.
9. Gansevoort RT, *et al.* Long-term benefits of the antiproteinuric effect of angiotensin-converting enzyme inhibition in nondiabetic renal disease. *Am J Kidney Dis* 1993; **22:** 202–6.
10. Hannedouche T, *et al.* Randomised controlled trial of enalapril and β blockers in non-diabetic chronic renal failure. *Br Med J* 1994; **309:** 833–7.
11. Maschio G, *et al.* Effect of the angiotensin-converting-enzyme inhibitor benazepril on the progression of chronic renal insufficiency. *N Engl J Med* 1996; **334:** 939–45.
12. The GISEN Group (Gruppo Italiano di Studi Epidemiologici in Nefrologia). Randomised placebo-controlled trial of effect of ramipril on decline in glomerular filtration rate and risk of terminal renal failure in proteinuric, non-diabetic nephropathy. *Lancet* 1997; **349:** 1857–63.
13. Giatras I, *et al.* Effect of angiotensin-converting enzyme inhibitors on the progression of nondiabetic renal disease: a meta-analysis of randomized trials. *Ann Intern Med* 1997; **127:** 337–45.
14. Steen VD, *et al.* Outcome of renal crisis in systemic sclerosis: relation to availability of angiotensin converting enzyme (ACE) inhibitors. *Ann Intern Med* 1990; **113:** 352–7.
15. Ruggenenti P, *et al.* Renal function and requirement for dialysis in chronic nephropathy patients on long-term ramipril: REIN follow-up trial. *Lancet* 1998; **352:** 1252–6.

Myocardial infarction. ACE inhibitors may be of benefit in both the prevention and treatment of myocardial infarction (p.791). They have an established role in the management of patients following acute myocardial infarction,[1,2] particularly in patients with left ventricular dysfunction. They may also have a role in the primary or secondary prevention of myocardial infarction in certain at-risk or susceptible patient groups.

1. Borghi C, Ambrosioni E. A risk-benefit assessment of ACE inhibitor therapy post-myocardial infarction. *Drug Safety* 1996; **14:** 277–87.
2. Murdoch DR, McMurray JJV. ACE inhibitors in acute myocardial infarction. *Hosp Med* 1998; **59:** 111–15.

Peripheral vascular disease. ACE inhibitors are among many drugs that have been tried in Raynaud's syndrome, a vasospastic peripheral arterial disease (p.794). Variable effects have been reported. In a patient with Raynaud's syndrome captopril improved blood circulation in the fingers both acutely and during long-term therapy with a dose of 37.5 mg daily; the effect was apparently related to its effects on kinins rather than inhibition of angiotensin II formation.[1] However, a double-blind crossover study in 15 patients with Raynaud's phenomenon given captopril 25 mg or placebo three times daily for 6 weeks found that the drug improved blood flow but not the frequency or severity of attacks,[2] and a similar study in patients given enalapril failed to find any subjective or objective benefits.[3] It should also be borne in mind that patients with peripheral vascular disease have a high incidence of renal artery stenosis, and may be at increased risk of renal failure if given ACE inhibitors,[4] although this need not preclude their use in such patients if monitoring of renal function is adequate.[5]

In one patient, peripheral ischaemia induced by ergotamine was rapidly reversed by captopril.[6]

1. Miyazaki S, *et al.* Relief from digital vasospasm by treatment with captopril and its complete inhibition by serine proteinase inhibitors in Raynaud's phenomenon. *Br Med J* 1982; **284:** 310–11.
2. Rustin MHA, *et al.* The effect of captopril on cutaneous blood flow in patients with primary Raynaud's phenomenon. *Br J Dermatol* 1987; **117:** 751–8.
3. Challenor VF, *et al.* Subjective and objective assessment of enalapril in primary Raynaud's phenomenon. *Br J Clin Pharmacol* 1991; **31:** 477–80.
4. Salmon P, Brown MA. Renal artery stenosis and peripheral vascular disease: implications for ACE inhibitor therapy. *Lancet* 1990; **336:** 321.
5. Walley T, Roberts D. ACE inhibitors and peripheral vascular disease. *Lancet* 1990; **336:** 810.
6. Zimran A, *et al.* Treatment with captopril for peripheral ischaemia induced by ergotamine. *Br Med J* 1984; **288:** 364.

Acebutolol Hydrochloride (6302-q)

Acebutolol Hydrochloride *(BANM, rINNM)*.

Acebutololi Hydrochloridum; IL-17803A; M&B-17803A. (±)-3′-Acetyl-4′-(2-hydroxy-3-isopropylaminopropoxy)butyranilide hydrochloride.

$C_{18}H_{28}N_2O_4,HCl = 372.9.$

CAS — 37517-30-9 (± acebutolol); 34381-68-5 (± acebutolol hydrochloride).

NOTE. Acebutolol is *USAN*.

Pharmacopoeias. In *Eur.* (see p.viii), *Jpn*, and *US*.

A white or almost white crystalline powder. Freely **soluble** in water and in alcohol; very slightly soluble in acetone and in dichloromethane; practically insoluble in ether. A 1% solution in water has a pH of 4.5 to 7.0.

Store in airtight containers. Protect from light.

Adverse Effects, Treatment, and Precautions

As for beta blockers, p.828.

Effects on the circulation. A report of near-fatal shock occurring within 40 minutes of acebutolol 400 mg in an elderly patient with chronic bronchitis and angina pectoris.[1]

1. Tirlapur VG, *et al.* Shock syndrome after acebutolol. *Br J Clin Pract* 1986; **40:** 33–4.

Effects on immune response. An increase in antinuclear antibodies has been observed with acebutolol.[1] One report of a lupus syndrome in an elderly patient receiving acebutolol and clonidine described remission of symptoms when acebutolol was withdrawn, but the high antinuclear antibody titre persisted for more than 9 months.[2]

1. Wilson JD. Antinuclear antibodies and cardiovascular drugs. *Drugs* 1980; **19:** 292–305.
2. Hourdebaigt-Larrusse P, *et al.* Une nouvelle observation de lupus induit par acébutolol. *Ann Cardiol Angeiol (Paris)* 1985; **34:** 421–3.

Effects on the liver. Six cases of liver toxicity associated with acebutolol were reported in the USA to the Food and Drug Administration between 1985 and 1989.[1] The syndrome consisted of markedly elevated transaminase concentrations, moderately elevated alkaline phosphatase concentrations, fever, and other constitutional symptoms. The duration of therapy before onset of symptoms ranged from 10 to 31 days; five patients received a dose of 400 mg per day; the dose was unspecified in the sixth patient. The syndrome resolved when acebutolol was discontinued. Two patients were rechallenged and the syndrome reappeared.

1. Tanner LA, *et al.* Hepatic toxicity after acebutolol therapy. *Ann Intern Med* 1989; **111:** 533–4.

Effects on respiratory function. A report of pleurisy and pulmonary granulomas in a patient receiving acebutolol and a diuretic; acebutolol was considered to be responsible.[1] Hypersensitivity pneumonitis has also been reported in a patient taking acebutolol.[2]

1. Wood GM, *et al.* Pleurisy and pulmonary granulomas after treatment with acebutolol. *Br Med J* 1982; **285:** 936.
2. Akoun GM, *et al.* Acebutolol-induced hypersensitivity pneumonitis. *Br Med J* 1983; **286:** 266–7.

Hypersensitivity. See under Effects on Immune Response, and under Effects on Respiratory Function, above.

Pregnancy. Both acebutolol and its active metabolite diacetolol cross the placenta. In a study[1] in 29 pregnant women who had received acebutolol for at least one month before delivery, there was evidence of bradycardia in 12 of the 31 offspring and tachypnoea in 6.

1. Boutroy MJ, *et al.* Infants born to hypertensive mothers treated by acebutolol. *Dev Pharmacol Ther* 1982; **4** (suppl 1): 109–15.

Interactions

The interactions associated with beta blockers are discussed on p.829.

Pharmacokinetics

Acebutolol is well absorbed from the gastro-intestinal tract, but undergoes extensive first-pass metabolism in the liver. Although the bioavailability of acebutolol is reported to be only about 40%, the major metabolite diacetolol is active. Following oral administration, peak plasma concentrations of acebutolol and diacetolol are reached in approximately 2 and 4 hours, respectively.

Acebutolol and diacetolol are widely distributed in the body, but they have low to moderate lipid solubility and penetration into the CSF is poor. They cross the placenta and higher concentrations are achieved in breast milk than in maternal plasma. Acebutolol is not appreciably bound to plasma proteins; it is about 50% bound to erythrocytes. The plasma elimination half-life for acebutolol and diacetolol is 3 to 4 hours and 8 to 13 hours respectively. Half-life values for acebutolol and diacetolol may be increased in the elderly and the half-life for diacetolol may be prolonged up to 32 hours in patients with severe renal impairment. Acebutolol and diacetolol are excreted in the urine and in the bile and may undergo enterohepatic recycling; acebutolol is also reported to be excreted directly from the intestinal wall. Acebutolol and diacetolol are removed by dialysis.

Uses and Administration

Acebutolol is a cardioselective beta blocker (p.828). It is reported to have some intrinsic sympathomimetic activity and membrane stabilising properties.

Acebutolol is used in the management of hypertension (p.788), angina pectoris (p.780), and cardiac arrhythmias (p.782).

Acebutolol is used as the hydrochloride, but doses are usually expressed in terms of the base. It is generally given by mouth although slow intravenous injection has been employed for the emergency treatment of arrhythmias.

In **hypertension** the usual initial dose is 400 mg once daily by mouth or 200 mg twice daily, increased if necessary after 2 weeks according to the patient's response, to 400 mg twice daily. Doses up to 1.2 g daily in divided doses may be given.

The usual dose for **angina pectoris** is 400 mg once daily by mouth or 200 mg twice daily but up to 300 mg three times daily may be required and total daily doses of 1.2 g have been given.

The usual initial dose for **cardiac arrhythmias** is 200 mg twice daily by mouth but up to 1.2 g daily in divided doses has been required.

Reduced doses may be required in patients with impaired renal function; suggested guidelines are to reduce the dose by 50% when glomerular filtration rate is between 25 and 50 mL per minute and by 75% when glomerular filtration rate is below 25 mL per minute. It has been recommended that doses greater than 800 mg daily should be avoided in elderly patients.

Action. Acebutolol is generally considered to be a cardioselective beta blocker but there has been considerable controversy as to the degree of its selectivity and the selectivity of its primary metabolite, diacetolol.[1-3] In a review of beta blockers, Feely *et al.*[4] have stated that acebutolol is less cardioselective than other drugs such as atenolol or metoprolol, and Feely and Maclean propose[5] that this may be because the metabolite accumulates during chronic dosage to reach concentrations which affect both $beta_1$ and $beta_2$ receptors since cardioselectivity is only a relative phenomenon and is dose-related. This remains uncertain and there is some evidence[6] that at least after single doses, diacetolol is actually more cardioselective than acebutolol itself.

1. Whitsett TL, *et al.* Comparison of the $beta_1$ and $beta_2$ adrenoceptor blocking properties of acebutolol and propranolol. *Chest* 1982; **82:** 668–73.
2. Nair S, *et al.* The effect of acebutolol, a beta adrenergic blocking agent, and placebo on pulmonary functions in asthmatics. *Int J Clin Pharmacol Ther Toxicol* 1981; **19:** 519–26.
3. Leary WP, *et al.* Respiratory effects of acebutolol hydrochloride: a new selective beta-adrenergic blocking agent. *S Afr Med J* 1973; **47:** 1245–8.
4. Feely J, *et al.* Beta-blockers and sympathomimetics. *Br Med J* 1983; **286:** 1043–7.
5. Feely J, Maclean D. New drugs: beta blockers and sympathomimetics. *Br Med J* 1983; **286:** 1972.
6. Thomas MS, Tattersfield AE. Comparison of beta-adrenoceptor selectivity of acebutolol and its metabolite diacetolol with metoprolol and propranolol in normal man. *Eur J Clin Pharmacol* 1986; **29:** 679–83.

Preparations

Proprietary Preparations (details are given in Part 3)

Aust.: Sectral; ***Belg.:*** Sectral; ***Canad.:*** Monitan; Rhotral; Sectral; ***Fr.:*** Sectral; ***Ger.:*** Neptal; Prent; ***Irl.:*** Sectral; ***Ital.:*** Acecor; Alol†; Prent; Sectral; ***Neth.:*** Prent†; Sectral; ***S.Afr.:*** Sectral; ***Spain:*** Sectral; ***Switz.:*** Prent†; Sectral; ***UK:*** Sectral; ***USA:*** Sectral.

Multi-ingredient: ***Belg.:*** Sectrazide; ***Ger.:*** Sali-Prent; Tredalat; ***Irl.:*** Secadrex; ***Neth.:*** Secadrex; ***S.Afr.:*** Secadrex; ***Spain:*** Secadrex; ***UK:*** Secadrex.

Acecainide Hydrochloride (7776-m)

Acecainide Hydrochloride *(USAN, rINNM).*

N-Acetylprocainamide Hydrochloride; ASL-601; NAPA. 4′-[(2-Diethylaminoethyl)carbamoyl]acetanilide hydrochloride.

$C_{15}H_{23}N_3O_2,HCl = 313.8.$

CAS — 32795-44-1 (acecainide); 34118-92-8 (acecainide hydrochloride).

Acecainide is the acetylated form of procainamide (p.934) but has class III antiarrhythmic activity (p.776). It has been tried for the treatment of premature ventricular contractions and ventricular arrhythmias.

References.

1. Harron DWG, Brogden RN. Acecainide (N-acetylprocainamide): a review of its pharmacodynamic and pharmacokinetic properties, and therapeutic potential in cardiac arrhythmias. *Drugs* 1990; **39:** 720–40.

Acetazolamide (2301-x)

Acetazolamide *(BAN, rINN).*

Acetazolam; Acetazolamidum. 5-Acetamido-1,3,4-thiadiazole-2-sulphonamide; *N*-(5-Sulphamoyl-1,3,4-thiadiazol-2-yl)acetamide.

$C_4H_6N_4O_3S_2 = 222.2.$

CAS — 59-66-5.

Pharmacopoeias. In *Chin., Eur.* (see p.viii), *Int., Jpn, Pol.,* and *US.*

A white to yellowish-white, odourless, crystalline powder. Very slightly **soluble** in water; sparingly soluble in practically boiling water; slightly soluble in alcohol; practically insoluble in ether; dissolves in dilute solutions of alkali hydroxides.

Acetazolamide Sodium (2302-r)

Acetazolamide Sodium *(BANM, rINNM).*

Sodium Acetazolamide.

$C_4H_5N_4NaO_3S_2 = 244.2.$

CAS — 1424-27-7.

Acetazolamide sodium 275 mg is approximately equivalent to 250 mg of acetazolamide. A freshly prepared 10% solution in water has a pH of 9.0. to 10.0.

Solutions of acetazolamide sodium in glucose 5% and sodium chloride 0.9% were stable for 5 days at 25° with a loss of potency of less than 7.2%.[1] At 5° the loss of potency in both solutions was less than 6% after 44 days of storage. Small reductions in pH were recorded possibly due to the formation of acetic acid during the decomposition of acetazolamide. At −10° the loss in potency after 44 days of storage was less than 3% in both solutions. Results were similar in samples thawed in tap water and in a microwave oven.

An oral suspension of acetazolamide 25 mg per mL prepared from tablets with the aid of sorbitol solution 70% was stable for at least 79 days at 5°, 22°, and 30°. It was recommended that the formulation be maintained at pH 4 to 5 and stored in amber glass bottles.[2]

1. Parasrampuria J, *et al.* Stability of acetazolamide sodium in 5% dextrose or 0.9% sodium chloride injection. *Am J Hosp Pharm* 1987; **44:** 358–60.
2. Alexander KS, *et al.* Stability of acetazolamide in suspension compounded from tablets. *Am J Hosp Pharm* 1991; **48:** 1241–4.

Adverse Effects

Acetazolamide can commonly cause malaise, fatigue, depression, excitement, headache, weight loss, and gastro-intestinal disturbances. Drowsiness and paraesthesia involving numbness and tingling of the face and extremities are common particularly with high doses. Diuresis can be troublesome, but generally abates after a few days of continuous therapy. Acidosis may develop during treatment and is generally mild but severe metabolic acidosis has occasionally been reported, especially in elderly or diabetic patients or those with impaired renal function.

Blood dyscrasias occur rarely and may include aplastic anaemia, agranulocytosis, leucopenia, thrombocytopenia, and thrombocytopenic purpura. Acetazolamide therapy can give rise to crystalluria, renal calculi, and renal colic; renal lesions, possibly due to a hypersensitivity reaction, have also been reported. Other adverse reactions include allergic skin reactions, fever, thirst, dizziness, ataxia, alterations in taste, transient myopia, and tinnitus and hearing disturbances. Hypokalaemia may occur but is generally transient and rarely clinically significant.

Intramuscular injections are painful owing to the alkalinity of the solution.

A retrospective review[1] of 222 patients with glaucoma indicating that those aged 40 years or less tolerated treatment with carbonic anhydrase inhibitors much better than older patients.

1. Shrader CE, *et al.* Relationship of patient age and tolerance to carbonic anhydrase inhibitors. *Am J Ophthalmol* 1983; **96:** 730–3.

Effects on the blood. Severe, often fatal, blood dyscrasias have been reported in patients taking acetazolamide,[1-4] including thrombocytopenic purpura,[1] pancytopenia,[2] and aplastic anaemia.[4] By 1989, the National Registry of Drug-Induced Ocular Side Effects in the USA[5] had received reports of haematological reactions possibly due to carbonic anhydrase inhibitors in 139 patients of which 50 (36%) were fatal. The majority of deaths were due to aplastic anaemia. Over half the reactions occurred during the first six months of therapy. There has been considerable debate over the value of periodic blood analysis in patients taking carbonic anhydrase inhibitors for prolonged periods;[6-11] the US National Registry has recommended[12] that initial and 6-monthly blood analysis should be undertaken.

1. Corbett JT. Acetazolamide and purpura. *Br Med J* 1958; **1:** 1122–3.
2. Englund GW. Fatal pancytopenia and acetazolamide therapy. *JAMA* 1969; **210:** 2282.
3. Inman WHW. Study of fatal bone marrow depression with special reference to phenylbutazone and oxyphenbutazone. *Br Med J* 1977; **1:** 1500–5.
4. Niven BI, Manoharan A. Acetazolamide-induced anaemia. *Med J Aust* 1985; **142:** 120.
5. Fraunfelder FT, Bagby GC. Possible hematologic reactions associated with carbonic anhydrase inhibitors. *JAMA* 1989; **261:** 2257.
6. Alm A, *et al.* Monitoring acetazolamide treatment. *Acta Ophthalmol (Copenh)* 1982; **60:** 24–34.
7. Johnson T, Kass MA. Hematologic reactions to carbonic anhydrase inhibitors. *Am J Ophthalmol* 1986; **101:** 128–9.
8. Zimran A, Beutler E. Can the risk of acetazolamide-induced aplastic anemia be decreased by periodic monitoring of blood cell counts? *Am J Ophthalmol* 1987; **104:** 654–8.
9. Lichter PR. Carbonic anhydrase inhibitors, blood dyscrasias, and standard-of-care. *Ophthalmology* 1988; **95:** 711–12.
10. Mogk LG, Cyrlin MN. Blood dyscrasias and carbonic anhydrase inhibitors. *Ophthalmology* 1988; **95:** 768–71.
11. Miller RD. Hematologic reactions to carbonic anhydrase inhibitors. *Am J Ophthalmol* 1985; **100:** 745–6.
12. Fraunfelder FT, *et al.* Hematologic reactions to carbonic anhydrase inhibitors. *Am J Ophthalmol* 1985; **100:** 79–81.

Effects on the electrolyte balance. Acetazolamide has been reported to cause symptomatic metabolic acidosis in the elderly, in diabetic patients, and in patients with renal impairment.[1-5] Raised plasma-acetazolamide concentrations have been reported in elderly patients, probably attributable to reduced renal function, and in 6 of 9 glaucoma patients this was associated with hyperchloraemic metabolic acidosis.[6] A single-dose study[7] in 4 elderly patients indicated that acetazolamide clearance was reduced and that this correlated with renal function. Urea and electrolyte concentrations should be measured before and during treatment with acetazolamide in the elderly and in other patients such as diabetics who may have renal impairment. The elderly may require reduced doses.

1. Maisey DN, Brown RD. Acetazolamide and symptomatic metabolic acidosis in mild renal failure. *Br Med J* 1981; **283:** 1527–8.
2. Goodfield M, *et al.* Acetazolamide and symptomatic metabolic acidosis in mild renal failure. *Br Med J* 1982; **284:** 422.
3. Reid W, Harrower ADB. Acetazolamide and symptomatic metabolic acidosis in mild renal failure. *Br Med J* 1982; **284:** 1114.
4. Heller I, *et al.* Significant metabolic acidosis induced by acetazolamide: not a rare complication. *Arch Intern Med* 1985; **145:** 1815–17.
5. Parker WA, Atkinson B. Acetazolamide therapy and acid-base disturbance. *Can J Hosp Pharm* 1987; **40:** 31–4.
6. Chapron DJ, *et al.* Acetazolamide blood concentrations are excessive in the elderly: propensity for acidosis and relationship to renal function. *J Clin Pharmacol* 1989; **29:** 348–53.
7. Chapron DJ, *et al.* Influence of advanced age on the disposition of acetazolamide. *Br J Clin Pharmacol* 1985; **19:** 363–71.

Effects on endocrine function. Hirsutism occurred in a 2½-year-old girl after treatment for 16 months with acetazolamide for congenital glaucoma.[1] There was no evidence of virilisation.

1. Weiss IS. Hirsutism after chronic administration of acetazolamide. *Am J Ophthalmol* 1974; **78:** 327–8.

Effects on the kidneys. Large reductions in glomerular filtration rate were observed during treatment with carbonic anhydrase inhibitors in 3 type 1 diabetics with nephropathy and glaucoma.[1] Kidney function improved when the carbonic anhydrase inhibitor was withdrawn.

1. Skøtt P, *et al.* Effect of carbonic anhydrase inhibitors on glomerular filtration rate in diabetic nephropathy. *Br Med J* 1987; **294:** 549.

Effects on the liver. For a report of liver damage associated with acetazolamide administration, see Hypersensitivity, below.

Effects on the skin. Rashes, including severe skin reactions such as erythema multiforme, Stevens-Johnson syndrome, and toxic epidermal necrolysis, have been reported during acetazolamide administration; the fact that acetazolamide is a sulphonamide-derivative has been suggested as a cause for these reactions. Photosensitivity has also been noted rarely.

A severe exacerbation of rosacea occurred in one patient following the use of acetazolamide for glaucoma; the rosacea improved on withdrawal of acetazolamide and relapsed again on its reintroduction.[1]

1. Shah P, *et al.* Severe exacerbation of rosacea by oral acetazolamide. *Br J Dermatol* 1993; **129:** 647–8.

Extravasation. A report of extravasation in a patient following the administration of acetazolamide intravenously which resulted in severe ulceration necessitating surgical procedures to repair the skin defect.[1] It was recommended that 1 to 2 mL of sodium citrate 3.8% should be injected subcutaneously near the site of extravasation in order to neutralise the alkaline effects of the acetazolamide injection.

1. Callear A, Kirkby G. Extravasation of acetazolamide. *Br J Ophthalmol* 1994; **78:** 731.

Hypersensitivity. A 54-year-old man with glaucoma who was treated with acetazolamide 500 mg daily for 26 days developed a generalised erythematous rash and became delirious, dehydrated, markedly jaundiced, with peripheral circulatory failure, and died from cholestatic jaundice with hepatic coma and anuria.[1] Drug-induced hypersensitivity and hepatitis due to acetazolamide was suspected.

Anaphylaxis has also been reported[2] following a single oral dose in a patient who had not previously received acetazolamide. However, the patient was hypersensitive to sulphonamides and the reaction may have been caused by cross sensitivity.

1. Kristinsson A. Fatal reaction to acetazolamide. *Br J Ophthalmol* 1967; **51:** 348–9.
2. Tzanakis N, *et al.* Anaphylactic shock after a single oral intake of acetazolamide. *Br J Ophthalmol* 1998; **82:** 588.

Precautions

Acetazolamide is contra-indicated in the presence of sodium or potassium depletion, in hyperchloraemic acidosis, in conditions such as Addison's disease and adrenocortical insufficiency, and in marked hepatic or renal impairment. Encephalopathy may be precipitated in patients with hepatic dysfunction. It should not be given in chronic angle-closure glaucoma since it may mask deterioration of the condition. It should be given with care to patients likely to develop acidosis or with diabetes mellitus; severe metabolic acidosis may occur in the elderly and in patients with impaired renal function. Acetazolamide may increase the risk of hyperglycaemia in diabetic patients. Periodic monitoring of plasma electrolytes and blood count is recommended during long-term therapy and patients should be cautioned to report any unusual skin rashes. Acetazolamide is teratogenic in *animals.*

For a brief discussion of metabolic acidosis in patients with diabetes or impaired renal function, see under Adverse Effects, Effects on the Electrolyte Balance, above.

For a report of renal function impairment in patients with diabetic nephropathy associated with carbonic anhydrase inhibitors, see under Adverse Effects, Effects on the Kidneys, above.

Interference with laboratory estimations. Acetazolamide interfered with an HPLC method of assay for theophylline[1] resulting in an unnecessary dose reduction and worsening apnoea in an infant. Kelsey and colleagues[2] pointed out that the interference depended on the solvent used in the extraction, and presented evidence to suggest that acetazolamide may not interfere with other assay methods for theophylline.

1. Mecrow IK, Goldie BP. Acetazolamide interferes with theophylline assay. *Lancet* 1987; **i:** 558.
2. Kelsey HC, *et al.* Interference by acetazolamide in theophylline assay depends on the method. *Lancet* 1987; **ii:** 403.

Old age. A single-dose study[1] of acetazolamide in 4 elderly subjects indicated that the elderly have a reduced capacity to clear acetazolamide from plasma correlating with creatinine clearance; that they have reduced plasma protein binding which offsets the reduced unbound clearance; and that these factors predispose the elderly to enhanced accumulation of acetazolamide in erythrocytes.

Plasma-acetazolamide concentrations exceeded the therapeutic range (5.0 to 10.0 μg per mL) in 9 of 12 elderly patients receiving acetazolamide for glaucoma or metabolic alkalosis.[2] Hyperchloraemic metabolic acidosis was detected in 6 of 9 glaucoma patients. The excessive plasma concentrations were attributed to age-related reductions in renal function. It was suggested that elderly patients may require reduced doses of acetazolamide.

For reports of symptomatic metabolic acidosis associated with use of acetazolamide in the elderly, see under Adverse Effects, Effects on the Electrolyte Balance, above.

1. Chapron DJ, *et al.* Influence of advanced age on the disposition of acetazolamide. *Br J Clin Pharmacol* 1985; **19:** 363–71.
2. Chapron DJ, *et al.* Acetazolamide blood concentrations are excessive in the elderly: propensity for acidosis and relationship to renal function. *J Clin Pharmacol* 1989; **29:** 348–53.

Interactions

By rendering the urine alkaline acetazolamide reduces the urinary excretion and so may enhance the effects of drugs such as amphetamines, ephedrine, and quinidine; urinary alkalinisation also reduces the effects of hexamine and its compounds. Acetazolamide may enhance antiepileptic-induced osteomalacia. Concurrent administration of acetazolamide and aspirin may result in severe acidosis and increase CNS toxicity. Acetazolamide may affect fluid and electrolyte balance leading to interactions similar to those of the thiazide diuretics (see Hydrochlorothiazide, p.887). Unlike thiazides, acetazolamide may increase the excretion of lithium.

Antacids. The use of concurrent sodium bicarbonate therapy enhances the risk of renal calculus formation in patients taking acetazolamide.[1]

1. Rubenstein MA, Bucy JG. Acetazolamide-induced renal calculi. *J Urol (Baltimore)* 1975; **114:** 610–12.

Antiepileptics. For severe osteomalacia in patients taking acetazolamide with phenytoin and other antiepileptics, see p.356.

Benzodiazepines. Ventilatory depression in a mountain climber with acute mountain sickness was considered to be due to the potentiation of triazolam by acetazolamide.[1]

1. Masuyama S, *et al.* 'Ondine's Curse': side effect of acetazolamide? *Am J Med* 1989; **86:** 637.

Local anaesthetics. For the effect of acetazolamide on procaine, see p.1299.

Salicylates. Salicylates have been shown to displace acetazolamide from plasma protein binding sites and reduce its renal clearance,[1] leading to elevated plasma-acetazolamide concentrations. In addition acidosis produced by acetazolamide may increase salicylate toxicity by enhancing salicylate tissue penetration.[2] Severe metabolic acidosis has been reported[3] in patients with normal renal function during treatment with acetazolamide and salicylates.

Concurrent use of salicylates and acetazolamide should be avoided if possible, particularly if renal dysfunction is present. If the combination is used, patients should be carefully monitored for symptoms of central nervous system toxicity such as lethargy, confusion, somnolence, tinnitus, and anorexia.

1. Sweeney KR, *et al.* Toxic interaction between acetazolamide and salicylate: case report and a pharmacokinetic explanation. *Clin Pharmacol Ther* 1986; **40:** 518–24.
2. Anderson CJ, *et al.* Toxicity of combined therapy with carbonic anhydrase inhibitors and aspirin. *Am J Ophthalmol* 1978; **86:** 516–19.
3. Cowan RA, *et al.* Metabolic acidosis induced by carbonic anhydrase inhibitors and salicylates in patients with normal renal function. *Br Med J* 1984; **289:** 347–8.

Pharmacokinetics

Acetazolamide is fairly rapidly absorbed from the gastro-intestinal tract with peak plasma concentrations occurring about 2 hours after administration by mouth. It has been estimated to have a plasma half-life of about 3 to 6 hours. It is tightly bound to carbonic anhydrase and high concentrations are present in tissues containing this enzyme, particularly red blood cells and the renal cortex; it is highly bound to plasma proteins. It is excreted unchanged in the urine and has been detected in breast milk.

References.

1. Lehmann B, *et al.* The pharmacokinetics of acetazolamide in relation to its use in the treatment of glaucoma and to its effects as an inhibitor of carbonic anhydrases. *Adv Biosci* 1969; **5:** 197–217.
2. Söderman P, *et al.* Acetazolamide excretion into human breast milk. *Br J Clin Pharmacol* 1984; **17:** 599–600.

Uses and Administration

Acetazolamide is an inhibitor of carbonic anhydrase with weak diuretic activity and is used mainly in the management of glaucoma. Other indications include epilepsy and high-altitude disorders.

By inhibiting the reaction catalysed by carbonic anhydrase in the renal tubules, acetazolamide increases the excretion of bicarbonate and of cations, chiefly sodium and potassium, and so promotes an alkaline diuresis. When given by mouth, its effect begins within 60 to 90 minutes and lasts for 8 to 12 hours.

Continuous administration of acetazolamide is associated with metabolic acidosis and an accompanying loss of diuretic activity. Therefore, although acetazolamide has been used as a diuretic, its effectiveness diminishes with continuous use and it has largely been superseded by drugs such as the thiazides or frusemide. For **diuresis** the usual dose is 250 to 375 mg by mouth daily or on alternate days; intermittent therapy is required for a continued effect.

By inhibiting carbonic anhydrase in the eye acetazolamide decreases the formation of aqueous humour and so decreases intra-ocular pressure. It is used in the pre-operative management of angle-closure **glaucoma**, or as an adjunct in the treatment of open-angle glaucoma. In the treatment of glaucoma the usual dose is 250 to 1000 mg by mouth daily, in divided doses for amounts over 250 mg daily; modified-release preparations are also available.

Acetazolamide is also used, either alone or in association with other antiepileptics, for the treatment of various forms of **epilepsy** in doses of 250 to 1000 mg daily by mouth. A suggested dose for children with epilepsy is 8 to 30 mg per kg body-weight daily by mouth; the total daily dose should not exceed 750 mg.

When oral administration is impracticable, similar doses of acetazolamide sodium may be given by intramuscular or preferably by intravenous injection.

Acetazolamide is also used to prevent or ameliorate the symptoms of **high-altitude disorders**. Prompt descent will still be necessary if severe symptoms such as cerebral oedema or pulmonary oedema occur. The usual dose is 500 to 1000 mg daily by mouth.

Epilepsy. Acetazolamide may be used in the treatment of epilepsy (p.335) as an alternative to conventional first-line antiepileptics for refractory partial seizures with or without secondary generalisation. It is also effective in a number of other refractory forms of epilepsy including atypical absence, tonic, atonic, myoclonic, and menstruation-related seizures (catamenial epilepsy).[1-4] Beneficial responses have also been reported with acetazolamide in combination with carbamazepine in refractory partial seizures.[5] It is believed to act by inhibition of carbonic anhydrase in glial cells in the CNS.[6] The major drawback to the chronic use of acetazolamide is the rapid development of tolerance,[6,7] but this may be delayed or prevented by using it as adjunctive therapy to other antiepileptics. Acetazolamide has been shown to have greater activity in children than in adults.[1]

1. Millichap JG. Acetazolamide in treatment of epilepsy. *Lancet* 1987; **ii:** 163.
2. Shorvon SD. Medical assessment and treatment of chronic epilepsy. *Br Med J* 1991; **302:** 363–6.
3. Resor SR, Resor LD. Chronic acetazolamide monotherapy in the treatment of juvenile myoclonic epilepsy. *Neurology* 1990; **40:** 1677–81.
4. Reiss WG, Oles KS. Acetazolamide in the treatment of seizures. *Ann Pharmacother* 1996; **30:** 514–19.
5. Oles KS, *et al.* Use of acetazolamide as an adjunct to carbamazepine in refractory partial seizures. *Epilepsia* 1989; **30:** 74–8.
6. Rogawski MA, Porter RJ. Antiepileptic drugs: pharmacological mechanisms and clinical efficacy with consideration of promising developmental stage compounds. *Pharmacol Rev* 1990; **42:** 223–86.
7. Hankey GJ, Stewart-Wynne EG. Management of non-convulsive status epilepticus. *Lancet* 1987; **i:** 1427.

Glaucoma. Acetazolamide may be given orally or parenterally in the acute management of angle-closure glaucoma (p.1387) and to minimise rises in intra-ocular pressure associated with ocular surgery.[1,2] It may also be given orally in the long-term management of primary and secondary open-angle glaucoma but is usually used as a second-line drug and added to topical beta blocker therapy. However, up to 50% of patients are unable to tolerate oral therapy because of adverse effects[3] although topical carbonic anhydrase inhibitors such as dorzolamide (p.862) may be better tolerated. Attempts have been made to reduce the adverse effects of acetazolamide by modifying the dosage schedule. A single-dose study[4] showed that doses of acetazolamide greater than 63 mg produced no greater reductions in intra-ocular pressure in patients with ocular hypertension. Ledger-Scott and Hurst[5] reported that acetazolamide 250-mg tablets twice daily controlled intra-ocular pressure adequately while producing fewer adverse effects than 250 mg four times daily and suggested that there was no advantage in using the modified-release capsule formulation (500 mg twice daily). A study in patients with open-angle glaucoma[6] found that most patients were adequately controlled by a single night-time dose of acetazolamide 500 mg either as tablets or modified-release capsules. The night-time dose also reduced the severity of adverse effects compared with the same dose given in the morning, and could aid compliance.

1. Ladas ID, *et al.* Prophylactic use of acetazolamide to prevent intraocular pressure elevation following Nd-YAG laser posterior capsulotomy. *Br J Ophthalmol* 1993; **77:** 136–8.
2. Edmunds B, Canning CR. The effect of prophylactic acetazolamide in patients undergoing extensive retinal detachment repair. *Eye* 1996; **10:** 328–30.
3. Hurvitz LM, *et al.* New developments in the drug treatment of glaucoma. *Drugs* 1991; **41:** 514–32.
4. Friedland BR, *et al.* Short-term dose response characteristics of acetazolamide in man. *Arch Ophthalmol* 1977; **95:** 1809–12.
5. Ledger-Scott M, Hurst J. Comparison of the bioavailability of two acetazolamide formulations. *Pharm J* 1985; **235:** 451.
6. Joyce PW, Mills KB. Comparison of the effect of acetazolamide tablets and sustets on diurnal intraocular pressure in patients with chronic simple glaucoma. *Br J Ophthalmol* 1990; **74:** 413–16.

High-altitude disorders. Acetazolamide is the most frequently used drug for the prophylaxis of high-altitude disorders (p.787). It accelerates the process of acclimatisation, thus reducing the incidence of acute mountain sickness and associated symptoms such as headache, nausea, vomiting, and lethargy. Acetazolamide may have some benefit in relieving symptoms once they have developed although experience is limited. It does not prevent or protect against pulmonary or cerebral oedema.

Macular oedema. For mention of the use of acetazolamide to treat macular oedema associated with uveitis, see Uveitis, p.1030.

Ménière's disease. In Ménière's disease (p.400) high concentrations of carbonic anhydrase are found in the labyrinth, and acetazolamide, a carbonic anhydrase inhibitor, has been tried for both diagnosis and treatment.[1] Acetazolamide 500 mg by intravenous injection has been suggested for diagnosis of fluctuating Ménière's disease. Treatment with oral acetazolamide has not been particularly effective and has been associated with a high incidence of side-effects.[2]

1. Brookes GB. Ménière's disease: a practical approach to management. *Drugs* 1983; **25:** 77–89.
2. Brookes GB, Booth JB. Oral acetazolamide in Ménière's disease. *J Laryngol Otol* 1984; **98:** 1087–95.

Neuromuscular disorders. Acetazolamide may be of benefit in a number of neuromuscular disorders, including hypokalaemic periodic paralysis (p.1150). Acetazolamide 375 to 500 mg daily was effective in 2 patients with severe paralysis and was well tolerated.[1] Preliminary observations in 5 other patients given acetazolamide showed a striking improvement in 3. In treating a further 12 patients,[2] doses of 125 mg of acetazolamide were given three times daily to children and 250 mg two to six times daily to adults. There was dramatic improvement in 10 of the 12 and this lasted for up to 43 months. Chronic weakness between attacks in 10 patients was improved in 8.

Acetazolamide may reduce the frequency of attacks in patients with hyperkalaemic periodic paralysis (p.1149). It has also been used in episodic ataxia.[3]

1. Resnick JS, *et al.* Acetazolamide prophylaxis in hypokalemic periodic paralysis. *N Engl J Med* 1968; **278:** 582–6.
2. Griggs RC, *et al.* Acetazolamide treatment of hypokalemic periodic paralysis: prevention of attacks and improvement of persistent weakness. *Ann Intern Med* 1970; **73:** 39–48.
3. Melberg A, *et al.* Loss of control after a cup of coffee. *Lancet* 1997; **350:** 1220.

Raised intracranial pressure. Acetazolamide has been used to reduce raised intracranial pressure (p.796). It has a role in the management of benign intracranial hypertension, and has also been tried in the treatment of patients with chronically raised intracranial pressure due to cryptococcal meningitis.[1]

1. Johnston SRD, *et al.* Raised intracranial pressure and visual complications in AIDS patients with cryptococcal meningitis. *J Infect* 1992; **24:** 185–9.

Preparations

BP 1998: Acetazolamide Tablets;
USP 23: Acetazolamide for Injection; Acetazolamide Tablets.

Proprietary Preparations (details are given in Part 3)
Aust.: Diamox; Diureticum†; ***Austral.:*** Diamox; ***Belg.:*** Diamox; ***Canad.:*** Diamox; Novo-Zolamide; ***Fr.:*** Defiltran; Diamox; ***Ger.:*** Diamox; Diuramid; Glaupax; ***Irl.:*** Diamox; Glaupax; ***Ital.:*** Diamox; ***Neth.:*** Diamox; Glaupax; ***Norw.:*** Diamox; Glaupax; ***S.Afr.:*** Diamox; ***Spain:*** Diamox; Edemox; ***Swed.:*** Diamox; Glaupax†; ***Switz.:*** Diamox; Glaupax; ***UK:*** Diamox; ***USA:*** Ak-Zol†; AZM-Tab; Dazamide; Diamox; Storzolamide†.

Acetyldigitoxin (5802-t)

Acetyldigitoxin (*rINN*).

α-Acetyldigitoxin; Digitoxin 3‴-Acetate; α-Digitoxin Monoacetate. 3β-[(O-3-O-Acetyl-2,6-dideoxy-β-D-*ribo*-hexopyranosyl-(1→4)-O-2,6-dideoxy-β-D-*ribo*-hexopyranosyl-(1→4)-2,6-dideoxy-β-D-*ribo*-hexopyranosyl)oxy]-14-hydroxy-5β,14β-card-20(22)-enolide.

$C_{43}H_{66}O_{14}$ = 807.0.

CAS — 1111-39-3.

Acetyldigitoxin is a cardiac glycoside with positive inotropic activity derived from lanatoside A. It has the general properties of digoxin (p.849) and has been used similarly in the management of some cardiac arrhythmias and in heart failure.

Acetyldigoxin (5803-x)

Desglucolanatoside C. 3β-[(O-3-O-Acetyl-2,6-dideoxy-β-D-*ribo*-hexopyranosyl-(1→4)-O-2,6-dideoxy-β-D-*ribo*-hexopyranosyl-(1→4)-2,6-dideoxy-β-D-*ribo*-hexopyranosyl)oxy]-12β,14-dihydroxy-5β,14β-card-20(22)-enolide (α-acetyldigoxin); 3β-[(O-4-O-Acetyl-2,6-dideoxy-β-D-*ribo*-hexopyranosyl-(1→4)-O-2,6-dideoxy-β-D-*ribo*-hexopyranosyl-(1→4)-2,6-dideoxy-β-D-*ribo*-hexopyranosyl)oxy]-12β,14-dihydroxy-5β,14β-card-20(22)-enolide (β-acetyldigoxin).

$C_{43}H_{66}O_{15}$ = 823.0.

CAS — 5511-98-8 (α-acetyldigoxin); 5355-48-6 (β-acetyldigoxin).

Pharmacopoeias. Aust. includes a monograph for α-acetyldigoxin.

Acetyldigoxin is a cardiac glycoside with positive inotropic activity. It has the general properties of digoxin (p.849) and has been used similarly in the management of some cardiac arrhythmias (p.782) and in heart failure (p.785). Both the α- and β-isomers have been used in usual maintenance doses of 200 to 400 μg daily by mouth.

Preparations

Proprietary Preparations (details are given in Part 3)
Aust.: Corotal; Lanatilin; Novodigal; Sandolanid; ***Belg.:*** Novodigal; ***Ger.:*** Digilateral†; Digostada; Digotab; Digox; Digoxin "Dier"; Gladixol N; Kardiamed; Longdigox†; Novodigal; Sandolanid†; Stillacor; ***Ital.:*** Beta-Acigoxin†; Cardioreg; Cedigossina†; ***Spain:*** Agolanid†; ***Switz.:*** Cedigocine†.

Multi-ingredient: ***Aust.:*** Digi-Aldopur; Gladixol; ***Ger.:*** Cormelian-Digotab†; Digo-Sensit†; Esberilan†; Lanadigin-EL†; Nitro-Novodigal†; Novo-Card-Fludilat†; Spirodigal†.

Adenosine (18724-z)

Adenosine (*BAN, USAN*).

SR-96225. 6-Amino-9-β-D-ribofuranosyl-9*H*-purine.

$C_{10}H_{13}N_5O_4$ = 267.2.

CAS — 58-61-7.

Pharmacopoeias. In Ger.

Stability. Adenosine was found to be stable[1] when it was mixed with glucose 5%, lactated Ringer's, sodium chloride 0.9%, or a mixture of glucose 5% and lactated Ringer's and stored in polypropylene syringes or PVC bags.

1. Ketkar VA, *et al.* Stability of undiluted and diluted adenosine at three temperatures in syringes and bags. *Am J Health-Syst Pharm* 1998; **55:** 466–70.

Adverse Effects and Precautions

Adverse effects of adenosine are usually transient, lasting less than a minute, due to its very short plasma half-life. They include nausea, lightheadedness, flushing, headache, angina-like chest pain, and dyspnoea. Bronchospasm has been reported. Like other antiarrhythmics, adenosine may worsen arrhythmias. Bradycardia and heart block have been reported. The larger doses given by intravenous infusion may rarely produce hypotension and tachycardia.

Adenosine is contra-indicated in patients with second- or third-degree atrioventricular block or in those with sick sinus syndrome. It is also contra-indicated in asthmatic subjects and should be used with caution in patients with obstructive pulmonary disease. Intravenous infusion of adenosine should be used with caution in patients who may develop hypotensive complications such as those with autonomic dysfunction, pericarditis, or stenotic valvular heart disease.

Use of Belzer solution [University of Wisconsin (UW) solution] for the hypothermic storage of kidneys prior to transplantation has been associated with bradycardia, prolonged PR intervals, and heart block.[1,2] The solution contains hetastarch, allopurinol, glutathione, and adenosine, and adenosine was considered to be the arrhythmogenic factor. Some centres had used the solution to flush kidneys before implantation,[2] a use for which it was never intended.[3] When used properly the adenosine in solution is catabolised to hypoxanthine and inosine which do not cause cardiac problems, but this takes some time in hypothermic conditions.[3]

1. Prien T, *et al.* Bradyarrhythmia with University of Wisconsin preservation solution. *Lancet* 1989; **i:** 1319–20.
2. Vanrenterghem Y, *et al.* University of Wisconsin preservation solute and bradyarrhythmia. *Lancet* 1989; **ii:** 745.
3. Belzer FO. Correct use of University of Wisconsin preservation solution. *Lancet* 1990; **335:** 362.

Effects on the heart. Adenosine may worsen arrhythmias. A prospective study[1] in 200 patients reported an incidence of atrial fibrillation of 12% following bolus injection of adenosine 12 mg used to terminate paroxysmal supraventricular tachycardia. Haemodynamically unstable proarrhythmia occurred in 2 patients with the Wolff-Parkinson-White syndrome and palpitations[2] after standard intravenous doses of adenosine were given.

1. Strickberger SA, *et al.* Adenosine-induced atrial arrhythmia: a prospective analysis. *Ann Intern Med* 1997; **127:** 417–22.
2. Exner DV, *et al.* Proarrhythmia in patients with the Wolff-Parkinson-White syndrome after standard doses of intravenous adenosine. *Ann Intern Med* 1995; **122:** 351–2.

Effects on the respiratory system. Acute exacerbation of asthma is well known following inhalation of adenosine. Recently there have been reports of bronchospasm occurring in patients with asthma[1,2] or a history of asthma[3] following the intravenous administration of adenosine. Bronchospasm following adenosine given intravenously produced respiratory failure in a patient with obstructive pulmonary disease.[4]

1. DeGroff CG, Silka MJ. Bronchospasm after intravenous administration of adenosine in a patient with asthma. *J Pediatr* 1994; **125:** 822–3.
2. Drake I, *et al.* Bronchospasm induced by intravenous adenosine. *Hum Exp Toxicol* 1994; **13:** 263–5.
3. Hintringer F, *et al.* Supraventricular tachycardia. *N Engl J Med* 1995; **333:** 323.
4. Burkhart KK. Respiratory failure following adenosine administration. *Am J Emerg Med* 1993; **11:** 249–50.

Migraine. A 35-year-old man with a history of migraine developed symptoms identical to those of his usual episodes of migraine immediately following two intravenous bolus doses of adenosine.[1]

1. Brown SGA, Waterer GW. Migraine precipitated by adenosine. *Med J Aust* 1995; **162:** 389–91.

Interactions

Dipyridamole inhibits adenosine uptake and therefore may potentiate the action of adenosine; if concurrent use of the two drugs is essential the dosage of adenosine should be reduced. Theophylline and other xanthines are inhibitors of adenosine.

Pharmacokinetics

Following intravenous administration adenosine is rapidly taken up by an active transport system into erythrocytes and vascular endothelial cells where it is metabolised to inosine and adenosine monophosphate. The plasma half-life is less than 10 seconds.

Uses and Administration

Adenosine is an endogenous nucleoside involved in many biological processes. It acts as an antiarrhythmic by stimulating adenosine (A_1) receptors and slowing conduction through the atrioventricular node. It does not fit into the usual classification of antiarrhythmics (p.776). It also produces peripheral vasodilatation by stimulating adenosine (A_2) receptors.

Adenosine is used to restore sinus rhythm in the treatment of **paroxysmal supraventricular tachycardia** including that associated with the Wolff-Parkinson-White syndrome. It is also used for the differential diagnosis of broad or narrow complex supraventricular tachycardias and diagnostically in myocardial imaging.

In the treatment of paroxysmal supraventricular tachycardia, the usual initial dose of adenosine is 3 mg by rapid intravenous injection. If this dose is ineffective within 1 to 2 minutes, 6 mg may be given and if necessary, 12 mg after a further 1 to 2 minutes. This dosage regimen is also used for differential diagnosis of supraventricular tachycardias. A dose of 0.0375 to 0.25 mg per kg body-weight is reported to be effective in children.

In myocardial imaging adenosine is given by intravenous infusion in a dose of 0.14 mg per kg per minute for 6 minutes. The radionuclide is injected after 3 minutes of the infusion.

Adenosine appears to have been tried with carmustine in the treatment of brain neoplasms.

Adenosine triphosphate (p.1543), in the form of the disodium salt, has been used as an antiarrhythmic.

Cardiac arrhythmias. Adenosine is used for the termination of paroxysmal supraventricular tachycardia[1-4] (p.782), including that associated with the Wolff-Parkinson-White syndrome, and may often be the drug of choice. Following bolus intravenous injection of adenosine, there is a rapid response and the extremely short plasma half-life (less than 10 seconds) allows dosage titration every 1 to 2 minutes so that most episodes can be controlled within 5 minutes without the danger of drug accumulation.

It has been used successfully in pregnant women with paroxysmal supraventricular tachycardia[5-8] and cardioversion of fetal supraventricular tachycardia by direct fetal therapy with adenosine has been reported.[9,10]

Adenosine can be used for the differential **diagnosis** of broad complex tachycardia where the mechanism is not known.[1] If the cause is supraventricular, adenosine will terminate the arrhythmia or produce atrioventricular block to reveal the underlying atrial rhythm. If the cause is ventricular, adenosine will have no effect on the tachycardia, but if verapamil is given to these patients severe hypotension and cardiac arrest can occur.

1. Faulds D, *et al.* Adenosine: an evaluation of its use in cardiac diagnostic procedures, and in the treatment of paroxysmal supraventricular tachycardia. *Drugs* 1991; **41:** 596–624.
2. Garratt CJ, *et al.* Adenosine and cardiac arrhythmias. *Br Med J* 1992; **305:** 3–4.
3. Rankin AC, *et al.* Adenosine and the treatment of supraventricular tachycardia. *Am J Med* 1992; **92:** 655–64.
4. Anonymous. Adenosine for acute cardiac arrhythmias. *Drug Ther Bull* 1993; **31:** 49–50.
5. Mason BA, *et al.* Adenosine in the treatment of maternal paroxysmal supraventricular tachycardia. *Obstet Gynecol* 1992; **80:** 478–80.
6. Afridi I, *et al.* Termination of supraventricular tachycardia with intravenous adenosine in a pregnant woman with Wolff-Parkinson-White syndrome. *Obstet Gynecol* 1992; **80:** 481–3.
7. Hagley MT, Cole PL. Adenosine use in pregnant women with supraventricular tachycardia. *Ann Pharmacother* 1994; **28:** 1241–2.
8. Hagley MT, *et al.* Adenosine use in a pregnant patient with supraventricular tachycardia. *Ann Pharmacother* 1995; **29:** 938.
9. Blanch G, *et al.* Cardioversion of fetal tachyarrhythmia with adenosine. *Lancet* 1994; **344:** 1646.
10. Kohl T, *et al.* Direct fetal administration of adenosine for the termination of incessant supraventricular tachycardia. *Obstet Gynecol* 1995; **85:** 873–4.

Ischaemic heart disease. Adenosine produces coronary vasodilatation and has been used to provide a pharmacological stress in patients undergoing assessment of their ischaemic heart disease when exercise stress is inappropriate. It has been given to such patients being evaluated either by thallium-201 myocardial imaging[1] or by stress echocardiography.[2]

1. Mohiuddin SM, *et al.* Thallium-201 myocardial imaging in patients with coronary artery disease: comparison of intravenous adenosine and oral dipyridamole. *Ann Pharmacother* 1992; **26:** 1352–7.
2. Martin TW, *et al.* Comparison of adenosine, dipyridamole, and dobutamine in stress echocardiography. *Ann Intern Med* 1992; **116:** 190–6.

Pulmonary hypertension. A randomised placebo-controlled study[1] in 18 term infants with persistent pulmonary hypertension of the newborn (p.796) indicated that intravenous infusion of adenosine improved oxygenation without causing hypotension or tachycardia. Larger studies were needed to assess any effect on mortality and/or the need for extracorporeal membrane oxygenation.

1. Konduri GG, *et al.* Adenosine infusion improves oxygenation in term infants with respiratory failure. *Pediatrics* 1996; **97:** 295–300.

Preparations

Proprietary Preparations (details are given in Part 3)
Aust.: Adrekar; ***Austral.:*** Adenocor; Adenoscan; ***Belg.:*** Adenocor; ***Canad.:*** Adenocard; ***Fr.:*** Krenosin; ***Ger.:*** Adrekar; ***Irl.:*** Adenocor; ***Ital.:*** Krenosin; ***Neth.:*** Adenocor; Adenoscan; ***Norw.:*** Adenocor; ***S.Afr.:*** Adenocor; ***Spain:*** Adenocor; ***Swed.:*** Adenocor†; ***Switz.:*** Krenosine; ***UK:*** Adenocor; Adenoscan; ***USA:*** Adenocard; Adenoscan.

Multi-ingredient: ***Aust.:*** Laevadosin; Vitasic; ***Fr.:*** Vitacic; Vitaphakol; ***Ger.:*** Adenopurin†; Adenovasin†; Hepatofalk; Laevadosin†; Ophtovitol†; Ordinal retard†; Pentavenon†; Ton-O_2 (Tonozwei)†; Vitaphakol N†; Vitasic†; Vitreolent Plus; ***Ital.:*** Neo-Epat†; ***Spain:*** Vitaphakol; ***Switz.:*** Vitaphakol.

Adrenaline (2041-c)

Adrenaline *(BAN)*.

Epinephrine *(rINN)*; Epinefrina; Epinephrinum; Epirenamine; Levorenin; Suprarenin. (*R*)-1-(3,4-Dihydroxyphenyl)-2-methylaminoethanol.

$C_9H_{13}NO_3$ = 183.2.

CAS — 51-43-4.

NOTE. ADN and EPN are codes approved by the BP for use on single unit doses of eye drops containing adrenaline where the individual container may be too small to bear all the appropriate labelling information.

Pharmacopoeias. In *Br., Chin., Fr., Int., It., Jpn, Neth., Pol.,* and *US.* *US* also includes the racemic substances Racepinephrine (Racepinefrine *(rINN)*) and Racepinephrine Hydrochloride (Racepinefrine Hydrochloride *(rINNM)*).

Adrenaline is an active principle of the medulla of the adrenal gland. It may be obtained from the adrenal glands of certain mammals or it may be prepared synthetically. Endogenous adrenaline and the monograph substance are the laevo isomer.

A white or creamy-white, odourless, crystalline powder or granules. It darkens in colour on exposure to air and light.

BP **solubilities** are: sparingly soluble in water; practically insoluble in alcohol and in ether. Adrenaline dissolves in solutions of mineral acids and in solutions of sodium or potassium hydroxide, but not in solutions of ammonia or of the alkali carbonates. USP solubilities are: very slightly soluble in water and in alcohol; insoluble in chloroform, in ether, and in fixed and volatile oils.

Solutions in water are alkaline to litmus. It is unstable in neutral or alkaline solution which rapidly becomes red on exposure to air. **Store** in airtight containers, preferably in which the air has been replaced by nitrogen. Protect from light.

Adrenaline Acid Tartrate (2042-k)

Adrenaline Acid Tartrate *(BANM)*.

Epinephrine Bitartrate *(rINNM)*; Adrenaline Bitartrate; Adrenaline Tartrate; Adrenalini Bitartras; Adrenalini Tartras; Adrenalinii Tartras; Adrenalinium Hydrogentartaricum; Epinephrine Hydrogen Tartrate; Epirenamine Bitartrate.

$C_9H_{13}NO_3,C_4H_6O_6$ = 333.3.

CAS — 51-42-3.

Pharmacopoeias. In *Eur.* (see p.viii), *Int.*, and *US*.

A white to greyish-white or light brownish-grey, odourless, crystalline powder. It slowly darkens on exposure to air and light. Adrenaline acid tartrate 1.8 mg is approximately equivalent to 1 mg of adrenaline.

Soluble 1 in 3 of water; slightly soluble in alcohol; practically insoluble in chloroform and ether. A solution in water is acid to litmus, with a pH of about 3.5.

Store in airtight containers, preferably in a vacuum-sealed tube or in an atmosphere of inert gas. Protect from light.

Studies on the stability of adrenaline injections.

1. Taylor JB, *et al.* Effect of sodium metabisulphite and anaerobic processing conditions on the oxidative degradation of adrenaline injection BP [1980]. *Pharm J* 1984; **232:** 646–8.

Adrenaline Hydrochloride (9501-z)

Adrenaline Hydrochloride *(BANM)*.

Epinephrine Hydrochloride *(rINNM)*.

$C_9H_{13}NO_3,HCl$ = 219.7.

CAS — 55-31-2.

Adrenaline hydrochloride 1.2 mg is approximately equivalent to 1 mg of adrenaline.

Adverse Effects

Adrenaline is a potent sympathomimetic and may exhibit the adverse effects typical of both alpha- and beta-adrenoceptor stimulation. It can thus produce a wide range of adverse effects, most of which mimic the results of excessive stimulation of the sympathetic nervous system. Side-effects such as anxiety, dyspnoea, hyperglycaemia, restlessness, palpitations, tachycardia (sometimes with anginal pain), tremors, sweating, hypersalivation, weakness, dizziness, headache, and coldness of extremities may occur even with low doses. Overdosage may cause cardiac arrhythmias and a sharp rise in blood pressure (sometimes leading to cerebral haemorrhage and pulmonary oedema); these effects may occur at normal dosage in susceptible subjects.

Since adrenaline does not readily cross the blood-brain barrier, its central effects, which encompass anxiety, fear, restlessness, insomnia, confusion, irritability, and psychotic states, may be largely a somatic response to its peripheral effects. Anorexia, nausea, and vomiting, may occur similarly.

The peripheral adverse effects of adrenaline are complex and mediated via its action on the various types of adrenergic receptor (see under Uses and Administration, below). Stimulation of alpha-adrenergic (mainly $alpha_1$) receptors produces vasoconstriction leading to hypertension, and this alpha-mediated hypertension may induce reflex bradycardia. On the other hand, stimulation of $beta_1$ adrenergic receptors in the heart produces tachycardia and cardiac arrhythmias. Finally, stimulation of $beta_2$ receptors produces vasodilatation with flushing and hypotension (apparent if the vasoconstricting alpha effects are blocked).

In relation to some of the other adverse effects of adrenaline, difficulty in micturition with urinary retention is a characteristic of $alpha_1$ receptor stimulation whereas muscle tremor and hypokalaemia are characteristics of $beta_2$ receptor stimulation.

The potent alpha-adrenergic effects of adrenaline may lead to gangrene following the vasoconstriction that is induced by infiltration of adrenaline-containing local anaesthetic solutions into digits. Extravasation of parenterally administered adrenaline similarly causes intense vasoconstriction, resulting in tissue necrosis and sloughing.

Topical application of adrenaline to mucosal surfaces also causes vasoconstriction, which may induce hypoxia leading to compensatory rebound congestion of the mucosa.

Inhalations of adrenaline have been associated with epigastric pain (which was caused by swallowing a portion of the inhalation and could be minimised by rinsing the mouth and throat with water after inhaling).

Adrenaline eye drops may produce severe smarting, blurred vision, and photophobia on instillation; they may also leave melanin-like deposits in the cornea and conjunctiva, which have caused obstruction of the naso-lachrymal ducts. Repeated ocular administration of adrenaline may cause oedema, hyperaemia, and inflammation of the eyes.

Other sympathomimetics have adverse effects that resemble those of adrenaline to a greater or lesser extent according to their relative agonist activities on the different receptors. For example, noradrenaline, whose alpha adrenergic effects predominate, may produce severe hypertension, whereas isoprenaline, whose beta adrenergic effects predominate, may produce severe tachycardia.

Systemic side-effects may occasionally follow the local or topical administration of sympathomimetics; this may often be in relation to the use of eye drops for the treatment of glaucoma.[1] Psychiatric side-effects including hallucinations and paranoia have also occurred following both proper and improper use of sympathomimetics in decongestant preparations.[2]

1. Everitt DE, Avorn J. Systemic effects of medications used to treat glaucoma. *Ann Intern Med* 1990; **112:** 120–5.

2. Anonymous. Drugs that cause psychiatric symptoms. *Med Lett Drugs Ther* 1993; **35:** 65–70.

Effects on the eyes. In addition to the possibility of pigment deposition and local pain (see above) adrenaline eye drops have been associated with maculopathy. During 4 years, 15 patients showed reactions to adrenaline eye drops, usually 2% of the hydrochloride or acid tartrate, while some used 1% epinephryl borate.[1] Blurring and distortion of vision were followed by decreased visual acuity, and by the appearance of oedema and sometimes haemorrhage in the macular region. A few patients developed cysts near the fovea. These effects appeared within a few weeks of, or several months after, commencement of therapy and were usually reversible. All except 1 of the patients were aphakic (devoid of lens). In a study of 200 consecutive patients receiving adrenaline therapy, 23 were aphakic in one or both eyes, and 7 experienced these reactions to adrenaline.

1. Kolker AE, Becker B. Epinephrine maculopathy. *Arch Ophthalmol* 1968; **79:** 552–62.

Effects on the heart. A review of the arrhythmogenic effects of vasopressor sympathomimetics[1] concluded that dopamine and adrenaline were associated with the highest risk, mainly of dose-related sinus tachycardia and ventricular arrhythmias. The clinical significance of most arrhythmias occurring with dopamine was considered questionable, however; supraventricular or ventricular arrhythmias occurring with adrenaline were most likely in patients receiving general anaesthesia or with underlying disorders of cardiac conduction. The risk with noradrenaline was uncertain, though there are few clinical reports, while phenylephrine and methoxamine were thought unlikely to cause problems. Overall the frequency of serious problems with this class of drugs did not seem to be high, and benefits outweighed the risks in most patients.

1. Tisdale JE, *et al.* Proarrhythmic effects of intravenous vasopressors. *Ann Pharmacother* 1995; **29:** 269–81.

Overdosage. A report of inadvertent administration to a 13-month-old infant of a solution containing racemic adrenaline (racepinephrine) meant for nebulisation.[1] The infant received the equivalent of approximately 327 μg per kg body-weight of *l*-adrenaline intravenously. Marked pallor, pulselessness, and profound bradycardia ensued, but the child responded to cardiopulmonary resuscitation and was subsequently discharged with no evidence of long-term sequelae.

1. Kurachek SC, Rockoff MA. Inadvertent intravenous administration of racemic epinephrine. *JAMA* 1985; **253:** 1441–2.

Treatment of Adverse Effects

Because of the short duration of the adverse effects of adrenaline, due to inactivation in the body, treatment of severe toxic reactions in hypersensitive patients or after overdose is primarily supportive. Prompt injection of a rapidly acting alpha-adrenoceptor blocker, such as phentolamine, followed by a beta blocker such as propranolol, has been tried to counteract the pressor and arrhythmogenic effects of adrenaline; rapidly-acting vasodilators such as glyceryl trinitrate have also been used.

Precautions

Adrenaline should be used with great caution in patients who may be particularly susceptible to its cardiovascular actions, notably those with pre-existing arrhythmias or tachycardia, Prinzmetal's angina, thrombo-embolic disorders, or a history of ischaemic heart disease. Extreme care is also needed in conditions which predispose a patient to adverse effects on the heart, such as hyperthyroidism; elevated thyroid hormone concentrations may also enhance receptor sensitivity. The use of adrenaline is generally inappropriate where there is pre-existing hypertension and it increases the risk of ischaemia in the extremities of patients with occlusive vascular disease. Special care is also needed in the elderly who may have pre-existing coronary or cerebrovascular disease.

Special care is also needed if adrenaline is given to patients with diabetes mellitus (both because of its vasoconstrictor actions and because of its metabolic effects on blood sugar). It should be avoided in phaeochromocytoma.

Adrenaline eye drops are contra-indicated in angle-closure glaucoma unless an iridectomy has been carried out.

When adrenaline is used for circulatory support, correction of hypovolaemia, metabolic acidosis, and hypoxia or hypercapnia should be carried out beforehand or concomitantly.

Precautions that need to be observed for *other sympathomimetics* resemble those for adrenaline, but vary to a greater or lesser extent according to their relative agonist activities on the different receptors. For example, noradrenaline, whose alpha adrenergic effects predominate, is a particular hazard in hypertension, whereas a beta-adrenergic agonist such as isoprenaline is a particular hazard in tachycardia. It also needs to be borne in mind that since non-catecholamine sympathomimetics have a longer duration of action than catecholamines, side-effects are more likely to be sustained and, in particular, that any rise in blood pressure is liable to be prolonged.

Abuse. A number of sympathomimetics, particularly those available without prescription, have been subject to abuse. The use of sympathomimetics by athletes is prohibited by the International Olympic Committee,[1] although there is little evidence that they increase physical ability or stamina.

1. MacAuley D. Drugs in sport. *Br Med J* 1996; **313:** 211–15.

Contact lenses. Discussion of drug-induced staining of soft-contact lenses.[1] Adrenochrome staining of contact lenses of patients using adrenaline eye drops has been reported. Melanin deposits may also become locked into the lens; such deposits may be broken down by hydrogen peroxide but in practice the lens is usually discarded. Patients prescribed drugs likely to cause this problem should be given appropriate warning. The prodrug, dipivefrine hydrochloride (p.1572) has been used without staining soft lenses.

1. Ingram DV. Spoiled soft contact lenses. *Br Med J* 1986; **292:** 1619.

Infection. A small open study[1] in patients critically ill with severe sepsis or malaria has suggested that the use of adrenaline as an inotrope and vasopressor in patients with severe infection causes the development of lactic acidosis. However, adrenaline is widely used in the treatment of septic shock, and others have pointed out that 20 of the 23 patients involved in the former study had responded to fluids, a situation in which the use of inotropic or vasopressor support was considered questionable.[2]

1. Day NPJ, *et al.* The effects of dopamine and adrenaline infusions on acid-base balance and systemic haemodynamics in severe infection. *Lancet* 1996; **348:** 219–23. Correction. *ibid.*; 902.

2. Barry B, Bodenham A. Effects of dopamine and adrenaline infusions in severe infection. *Lancet* 1996; **348:** 1099–1100.

Interactions

Interactions with adrenaline are complex and often hazardous; they stem primarily from its agonist actions on alpha- and beta-adrenoceptors.

Hazardous arrhythmias are a risk if adrenaline is used in patients anaesthetised with *cyclopropane, halothane,* or other *volatile anaesthetics* which sensitise the myocardium to its beta-adrenergic effects.

The vasoconstrictor and pressor effects of adrenaline, mediated by its alpha-adrenergic action, may be enhanced by the concomitant administration of drugs with similar effects, such as *ergot alkaloids* or *oxytocin*.

Because adrenaline increases blood pressure, special care is advisable in patients receiving *antihypertensive therapy*. Moreover, adrenaline specifically reverses the antihypertensive effects of *adrenergic neurone blockers* such as *guanethidine* with the risk of severe hypertension. Severe hypertension (followed by reflex bradycardia) may also develop if adrenaline is given with a *beta blocker (especially a non-selective beta blocker)* since the beta blocker opposes the beta adrenergic action of adrenaline, leaving its alpha adrenergic effect unopposed; for details see below. Conversely, the bronchoconstrictor effect of a *beta blocker (especially a non-selective beta blocker)* antagonises the $beta_2$ (bronchodilating) effect of adrenaline and constitutes a serious hazard. It should also be noted that in patients on non-cardioselective beta blockers, severe anaphylaxis may not respond to adrenaline (see below). Complex interactions also occur with *alpha-adrenoceptor blockers* such as *phenoxybenzamine* and *phentolamine* which oppose the alpha adrenergic action of adrenaline leaving its beta adrenergic effect unopposed, thus resulting in both antihypertensive and cardiac-accelerating effects; nevertheless, use is made of this blood pressure reduction to reverse hypertension in adrenaline overdosage (see also under Treatment of Adverse Effects, above). For a warning concerning hypotension associated with adrenaline-induced reversal of alpha-blockade in phenothiazine overdosage, see under Chlorpromazine, p.651.

Although caution is still necessary, the action of adrenaline or noradrenaline may be only slightly enhanced by an *MAOI*, since they are direct acting and inactivation by uptake into nerves and tissues is not inhibited. Dangerous hypertensive interactions are, however, a risk if dopamine (which has indirect-acting properties) is given concomitantly with an *MAOI (including an RIMA)*. Hazardous hypertensive interactions are also a major risk if dexamphetamine, dopexamine, ephedrine, isometheptene, mephentermine, metaraminol, methylphenidate, phentermine, phenylephrine, phenylpropanolamine, pseudoephedrine, and many other sympathomimetics are given concomitantly with an *MAOI (including an RIMA)*. For additional warnings see under Phenelzine (p.305) and Moclobemide (p.299).

Administration of adrenaline or noradrenaline with *tricyclic antidepressants* (which inhibit their re-uptake) carries a risk of inducing hypertension and arrhythmias. In the case of local anaesthetic preparations containing adrenaline there is no clinical evidence of dangerous interactions with either *tricyclic antidepressants* or *MAOIs*, but great care needs to be taken to avoid inadvertent intravenous administration of the local anaesthetic preparations. (For a warning to avoid local anaesthetics containing noradrenaline, see under Adverse Effects of Noradrenaline, p.924).

The hypokalaemic effect of adrenaline may be potentiated by other drugs that cause potassium loss, including *corticosteroids*, *potassium-depleting diuretics*, and *aminophylline* or *theophylline*; patients receiving high doses of beta$_2$-adrenergic agonists concomitantly should have their plasma-potassium concentration monitored (see Salbutamol, p.759). Hypokalaemia may also result in increased susceptibility to cardiac arrhythmias caused by *digoxin* and other *cardiac glycosides*.

In addition to their interactions with *MAOIs* (cited above) the interactions of *other sympathomimetics* resemble those of adrenaline to a greater or lesser extent, according to their relevant agonist activities on the different receptors. For some details of specific interactions see under individual monographs.

Beta blockers. Patients given adrenaline (including the low doses used with local anaesthetics) while receiving non-selective beta blockers such as *propranolol* can develop elevated blood pressure due to alpha-mediated vasoconstriction, followed by reflex bradycardia, and occasionally cardiac arrest;[1] the bronchodilator effects of adrenaline are also inhibited. In contrast, cardioselective beta blockers such as *metoprolol*, which act preferentially at beta$_1$ adrenergic receptors, do not prevent adrenaline-induced vasodilatation via beta$_2$ receptors, and in consequence blood pressure and heart rate change only minimally. Low doses of cardioselective beta blockers do not appear to interfere with sympathomimetic (isoprenaline)-induced bronchodilatation,[2] although the effect of larger doses is uncertain.

Propranolol has also been shown to inhibit the favourable pressor and bronchodilator responses to adrenaline when given for anaphylaxis.[3] Thus, patients receiving long-term treatment with some non-cardioselective beta blockers who develop anaphylaxis may be relatively refractory to adrenaline.

1. Jay GT, Chow MSS. Interaction of epinephrine and β-blockers. *JAMA* 1995; **274:** 1830–2.
2. Decalmer PBS, *et al.* Beta blockers and asthma. *Br Heart J* 1978; **40:** 184–9.
3. Newman BR, Schultz LK. Epinephrine-resistant anaphylaxis in a patient taking propranolol hydrochloride. *Ann Allergy* 1981; **47:** 35–7.

General anaesthetics. In a review in 1967[1] the sensitisation of the myocardium to β-adrenergic stimulation caused by some anaesthetics was considered to be of clinical importance when adrenaline was injected into an operation area to reduce bleeding. It had previously been considered that adrenaline could not be given when the patient had been anaesthetised with *cyclopropane, halothane*, or similar volatile anaesthetics but it had become evident that adrenaline could be used so long as the dose was small and other factors likely to increase the irritability of the myocardium, such as carbon-dioxide retention, hypoxia, or the simultaneous use of cocaine were avoided. It appeared[2] that provided the solution of adrenaline was not stronger than 1 in 100 000 and that the rate of injection did not exceed 10 mL per 10 minutes or 30 mL an hour no serious results should ensue under *halothane* or *trichloroethylene* anaesthesia. The technique was considered inappropriate for use with cyclopropane although some disagreed with this view admitting, however, that the risk of arrhythmias was higher with cyclopropane than with halothane or trichloroethylene.[2]

There have, however, been fatalities reported in patients who underwent surgery which involved the use of halothane and adrenaline.[3]

1. Anonymous. Anaesthetics and the heart. *Lancet* 1967; **i:** 484–5.
2. Katz RL, Epstein RA. The interaction of anesthetic agents and adrenergic drugs to produce cardiac arrhythmias. *Anesthesiology* 1968; **29:** 763.
3. Buzik SC. Fatal interaction? Halothane, epinephrine and tooth implant surgery. *Can Pharm J* 1990; **123:** 68–9 and 81.

Local anaesthetics. It is common practice to administer adrenaline with a local anaesthetic to produce vasoconstriction when the lowest effective concentration of adrenaline should be used. However, with *cocaine* there is a risk of cardiac arrhythmias and the use, for example, of cocaine and adrenaline paste in otolaryngology may be hazardous. See p.1291 for references to this interaction.

Pharmacokinetics

As a result of enzymatic degradation in the gut and first-pass metabolism in the liver, adrenaline is almost totally inactive when given by mouth. Systemic absorption can occur following topical application for example of eye drops. Adrenaline acts rapidly following intramuscular and subcutaneous injection; this latter route is, however, sometimes considered to be slower and therefore less reliable and predictable for emergency use. Although absorption is slowed by local vasoconstriction it can be hastened by massaging the injection site.

Most adrenaline that is either injected into the body or released into the circulation from the adrenal medulla, is very rapidly inactivated by processes which include uptake into adrenergic neurones, diffusion, and enzymatic degradation in the liver and body tissues. The half-life of circulating adrenaline is only about 1 minute. One of the enzymes responsible for the chemical inactivation of adrenaline is catechol-*O*-methyltransferase (COMT), the other is monoamine oxidase (MAO). In general, adrenaline is methylated to metanephrine by COMT followed by oxidative deamination by MAO and eventual conversion to 4-hydroxy-3-methoxymandelic acid (formerly termed vanillylmandelic acid; VMA), or oxidatively deaminated by MAO and converted to 3,4-dihydroxymandelic acid which, in turn, is methylated by COMT, once again to 4-hydroxy-3-methoxymandelic acid; the metabolites are excreted in the urine mainly as their glucuronide and ethereal sulphate conjugates.

The ability of catechol-*O*-methyltransferase to effect introduction of a methyl group is an important step in the chemical inactivation of adrenaline and similar catecholamines (in particular, noradrenaline). It means that the termination of the pharmacological response of catecholamines is not simply dependent upon monoamine oxidase. In its role of neurotransmitter intraneuronal catecholamine (mainly noradrenaline) is, however, enzymatically regulated by monoamine oxidase.

Adrenaline crosses the placenta to enter fetal circulation.

Uses and Administration

Adrenaline is an active principle of the adrenal medulla which is used as a direct-acting sympathomimetic; for an outline of the actions of sympathomimetics, see below. It has a somewhat more marked effect on beta-adrenoceptors than on alpha-adrenoceptors, and this property explains many aspects of its pharmacology; in addition, its actions vary considerably according to the dose given, and the consequent reflex compensating responses of the body.

In practice, major effects of adrenaline include increased speed and force of cardiac contraction (with lower doses this causes increased systolic pressure yet reduced diastolic pressure since overall peripheral resistance is lowered, but with higher doses both systolic and diastolic pressure are increased as stimulation of peripheral alpha-receptors increases peripheral resistance); blood flow to skeletal muscle is increased (reduced with higher doses); there is relaxation of bronchial smooth muscle; metabolic effects result in hyperglycaemia as well as markedly increased oxygen consumption; blood flow in the kidneys, mucosa, and skin is reduced; there is little direct effect on cerebral blood flow.

Adrenaline has an important role in the management of acute allergic reactions and can be life saving in patients with anaphylactic shock (below). It is also used in advanced cardiac life support (below). Adrenaline has been given subcutaneously in the treatment of acute asthma but more selective drugs are available, and it has no role in the chronic management of asthma (p.745). It has been given by nebulisation in severe croup (p.1020). Adrenaline is used for a number of other indications including the control of minor bleeding from the skin and mucous membranes, in ophthalmology chiefly for the management of open-angle (simple) glaucoma (p.1387), and also as an adjunct to local anaesthesia (p.1283). Adrenaline was formerly incorporated into creams used in the treatment of rheumatic and muscular disorders, and in rectal preparations used in the treatment of haemorrhoids. Racepinephrine (racemic adrenaline) or racepinephrine hydrochloride has been used for bronchodilatation.

Adrenaline is given by subcutaneous or intramuscular injection. In extreme emergencies, where a more rapid effect is required, adrenaline may be given as a dilute solution (1 in 10 000 or 1 in 100 000) by very slow intravenous injection or by slow intravenous infusion. Intraosseous administration, usually into the marrow of the tibia, is sometimes used as an alternative to the intravenous route. Adrenaline has sometimes been injected directly in the heart; current guidelines for the management of cardiac emergencies do not include that route but recommend administration via a central vein. Endotracheal administration is occasionally employed when intravenous access cannot be obtained. Adrenaline may be applied topically and can be administered by inhalation. Aqueous solutions of adrenaline are usually prepared using the acid tartrate or the hydrochloride but the dosage is generally stated in terms of the equivalent content of adrenaline.

The usual dose of adrenaline in **anaphylactic shock** is 0.5 to 1 mg (0.5 to 1 mL of a 1 in 1000 solution) by intramuscular injection repeated as necessary every 10 minutes. A dose of 0.3 mg (0.3 mL of a 1 in 1000 solution) may be appropriate for emergency self-administration. Children's doses range from 100 to 500 μg depending on age; 50 μg may be used in infants under 1 year of age. If intravenous administration is required the dose is 500 μg for adults and 10 μg per kg body-weight for children, as a more dilute 1 in 10 000 solution at a rate of 1 mL (100 μg) or less per minute.

In **advanced cardiac life support** the initial dose of adrenaline for adults is 1 mg intravenously (10 mL of a 1 in 10 000 solution), preferably into a central vein, and this may be repeated as often as every 2 to 3 minutes in some circumstances for up to an hour. Depending on the arrhythmia the dose may be increased after three injections of 1 mg to 5 mg or 100 μg per kg. Children may be given intravenous doses of 10 μg per kg initially then 100 μg per kg. Intraosseous doses are the same as those used intravenously. Endotracheal doses are 2 to 3 times the intravenous dose for adults; children may be given 100 μg per kg.

Adrenaline relaxes the bronchial musculature and has sometimes been injected subcutaneously or intramuscularly in the management of **acute asthmatic attacks**. However, in general, the use of adrenaline in asthma has been superseded by beta$_2$-selective sympathomimetics, such as salbutamol, which can alleviate bronchospasm with fewer effects on the heart. If adrenaline is to be used, the suggested adult dose is 0.3 to 0.5 mL of a 1 in 1000 aqueous solution (300 to 500 μg); children have received 0.01 mL per kg body-weight (10 μg per kg) to a maximum of 0.5 mL (500 μg). Aqueous solutions with an adrenaline content equivalent to 1 in 100 have occasionally been used by inhalation as a spray to alleviate asthmatic attacks; these solutions must never be confused with the weaker strength used for injection. Pressurised aerosols delivering metered doses equivalent to approximately 160 μg to 275 μg of adrenaline have also been used; adults have received 1 or 2 metered inhalations repeated, if necessary, after 3 hours.

Adrenaline is frequently added to **local anaesthetics** to retard diffusion and limit absorption, to prolong the duration of effect, and to lessen the danger of toxicity. A concentration of 1 in 200 000 (5 μg per mL) is usually used; adrenaline should not be added when procedures involve digits, ears, nose, penis, or scrotum owing to the risk of ischaemic tissue necrosis. A concentration of up to 1 in 80 000 (12.5 μg per mL) may be used in dental preparations where the total dose administered is small.

Adrenaline constricts arterioles and capillaries and causes blanching when applied locally to mucous membranes and exposed tissues. It is used as an aqueous solution in strengths up to a 1 in 1000 dilution to check capillary **bleeding**, epistaxis, and bleeding from superficial wounds and abrasions, but it does not stop internal haemorrhage. It is usually applied as a spray or on pledgets of cotton wool or gauze.

In ophthalmology, adrenaline solutions of 1 in 100 (1%) or 1 in 200 (0.5%) are used to reduce intra-ocular pressure in open-angle (simple) **glaucoma** and ocular hypertension. An adrenaline borate complex is also used in ophthalmology.

Actions of sympathomimetics

Sympathomimetics have actions similar to those that follow stimulation of postganglionic sympathetic (or adrenergic) nerves. The three naturally occurring sympathomimetics are adrenaline, noradrenaline, and dopamine. All three are catecholamines, i.e. their aromatic portion is catechol (which is characterised by hydroxy groups at adjacent positions of a benzene ring) and the aliphatic portion is an amine. Despite widespread use of the term 'adrenergic' for sympathetic nerves, the physiological functions of adrenaline itself are predominantly metabolic. It is noradrenaline that is the endogenous neurotransmitter at postganglionic sympathetic nerves. Dopamine acts peripherally on the renal, mesenteric, and coronary vascular beds. Both noradrenaline and dopamine also have key roles as neurotransmitters within the CNS, but (in common with adrenaline) are highly polar and cannot cross the blood-brain barrier.

These three catecholamines differ markedly in effect according to their specificity for different adrenergic receptors.

Adrenergic receptors are divided into alpha- and beta-adrenoceptors. These are then subdivided into $alpha_1$ (postsynaptic) and $alpha_2$ (mainly presynaptic) types, and into $beta_1$, $beta_2$, and $beta_3$ receptors. A third distinct group of receptors which occur primarily within the CNS are described as dopaminergic and at least 5 subtypes are known (see p.1128); D_1 receptors also occur within renal, mesenteric, and coronary vascular beds.

Stimulation of these different receptors produces the following effects:

- stimulation of $alpha_1$ receptors produces vasoconstriction, particularly in the vessels of the skin and mucosa, abdominal viscera, and kidney; this results in an increase in blood pressure, sometimes with compensatory reflex bradycardia; $alpha_1$ stimulation also results in contraction of other smoother muscle, including the urinary sphincter and the uterus, and induces mydriasis in the eye
- stimulation of $alpha_2$ receptors appears to play a role in feedback inhibition of neurotransmitter release and may be involved in the inhibition of intestinal activity; it also plays a role in the inhibition of insulin secretion
- stimulation of $beta_1$ receptors produces an increase in the rate and force of contraction of the heart, increased conduction velocity, and greater automaticity
- stimulation of $beta_2$ receptors produces vasodilatation, bronchodilatation, uterine relaxation, and a decrease in gastro-intestinal motility; it also results in release of insulin and enhances gluconeogenesis and glycogenolysis
- stimulation of $beta_3$ receptors is thought to have a role in lipolysis and thermogenesis
- stimulation of D_1 receptors produces vasodilatation of renal, mesenteric, and coronary vessels.

The pattern of activity of the three catecholamines is complex and influenced not only by receptor specificity, but also by feedback mechanisms and receptor distribution. In broad terms:

- adrenaline is a potent agonist at both alpha and beta receptors
- noradrenaline is a potent agonist at alpha and $beta_1$ receptors, but has little effect on $beta_2$ receptors
- dopamine in low doses activates D_1 receptors; in higher doses it activates $beta_1$ and then alpha receptors, and also provokes release of noradrenaline from nerve terminals.

Other sympathomimetic drugs are analogues of the catecholamines and according to their structure either act directly on adrenergic receptors (e.g. phenylephrine) or indirectly (e.g. ephedrine, which also has direct actions). Indirect actions are achieved by displacing noradrenaline from storage vesicles within the nerve terminals. In practice many sympathomimetics have both direct and indirect actions.

Catecholamines have a fleeting action and are inactive by mouth whereas their analogues have a prolonged action and are active by mouth; the analogues are also less polar than the catecholamines and can often cross the blood-brain barrier. This ability to cross the blood-brain barrier explains why some sympathomimetics (e.g. dexamphetamine) have marked central stimulant effects. It may also explain the seemingly paradoxical antihypertensive effect of $alpha_2$ adrenergic agonists (e.g. clonidine) since their central effects may outweigh their effects in vascular smooth muscle.

Advanced cardiac life support. Adrenaline has an important role in advanced cardiac life support (p.779) since, through its alpha agonist effects, it increases myocardial and cerebral blood flow and thereby the efficacy of cardiopulmonary resuscitation or basic life support procedures. Depending on the arrhythmia that has led to cardiac arrest treatment starts with cardiopulmonary resuscitation and defibrillation. If these measures fail to restore a conventional rhythm, the next step involves the administration of adrenaline.

For adults, adrenaline is given in a dose of 1 mg ideally intravenously into a central vein. If such venous access is not practicable adrenaline may be given through a peripheral vein followed by a flush of 20 mL or more of sodium chloride injection; however, the response is slower than with central venous injection. This intravenous dose of 1 mg may be given approximately every 3 minutes[1,2] or 3 to 5 minutes[3] in further cycles of cardiopulmonary resuscitation and, if necessary, shocks. If the 1-mg dose of adrenaline fails, a higher dose of 5 mg[1-3] or 100 μg per kg body-weight[3] may sometimes be considered. In ventricular fibrillation or pulseless ventricular tachycardia, a resuscitation attempt may reasonably last for anything from 10 minutes to 1 hour with adrenaline 1 mg intravenously being administered every 3 minutes during this period. Where the arrest is associated with asystole it is unlikely that a response will be achieved after 15 minutes.[1,2]

The initial dose of 1 mg is reported to be based on the dose that was given by intracardiac injection, so it would be expected that a higher dose would be required for intravenous administration. However, studies[4-6,10] have failed to show any survival benefit with the use of doses higher than the 1-mg dose as used above.[3]

The intravenous dose for children is 10 μg per kg as the first dose; second and subsequent doses are 100 μg per kg[3,7] or possibly 200 μg per kg.[3] However, as with adults the use of the higher dose has been questioned and a retrospective study[8] found no improvement in outcome.

The intraosseous route is a practicable alternative to intravenous injection for adults as well as for children, although the guidelines only give doses for children which are identical to those given intravenously. Alternatively, adrenaline can be administered through the endotracheal tube that will have been inserted, but only if the intravenous or intraosseous administration is delayed. Endotracheal doses for adults should be 2 to 3 times those used intravenously; for children doses of 100 μg per kg have been suggested. The adrenaline solution should be diluted and administered deeply using a catheter; several rapid ventilations or inflations should follow. It is recognised that the endotracheal route is imperfect[1-3,7] and some workers consider it to be ineffective.[9]

1. Advanced Life Support Working Group of the European Resuscitation Council. The 1998 European Resuscitation Council guidelines for adult advanced life support. *Br Med J* 1998; **316:** 1863–9. [Also published in *Resuscitation* 1998; **37:** 81–90.]
2. ALS Working Group of the International Liaison Committee on Resuscitation. The universal algorithm. *Resuscitation* 1997; **34:** 109–11.
3. Emergency Cardiac Care Committee and Subcommittees, American Heart Association. Guidelines for cardiopulmonary resuscitation and emergency cardiac care. *JAMA* 1992; **268:** 2171–2295.
4. Stiell IG, *et al.* High-dose epinephrine in adult cardiac arrest. *N Engl J Med* 1992; **327:** 1045–50.
5. Brown CG, *et al.* A comparison of standard-dose and high-dose epinephrine in cardiac arrest outside the hospital. *N Engl J Med* 1992; **327:** 1051–5.
6. Callaham M, *et al.* A randomized clinical trial of high-dose epinephrine and norepinephrine vs standard-dose epinephrine in prehospital cardiac arrest. *JAMA* 1992; **268:** 2667–72.
7. Nadkarni V, *et al.* Paediatric life support: an advisory statement by the Paediatric Life Support Working Group of the International Liaison Committee on Resuscitation. *Resuscitation* 1997; **34:** 115–27. [NB. Contains incorrect adrenaline dose in figure 3.]
8. Carpenter TC, Stenmark KR. High-dose epinephrine is not superior to standard-dose epinephrine in pediatric in-hospital cardiopulmonary arrest. *Pediatrics* 1997; **99:** 403–8.
9. McCrirrick A, Monk CR. Comparison of i.v. and intra-tracheal administration of adrenaline. *Br J Anaesth* 1994; **72:** 529–32.
10. Gueugniaud P-Y, *et al.* A comparison of repeated high doses and repeated standard doses of epinephrine for cardiac arrest outside the hospital. *N Engl J Med* 1998; **339:** 1595–1601.

Anaphylactic shock. Anaphylactic shock is usually a type 1 hypersensitivity reaction (p.399). It is a medical emergency and prompt treatment of laryngeal oedema, bronchospasm, and hypotension is necessary. Adrenaline is the cornerstone of management[1-6] although it may not always be effective.[3]

In early anaphylaxis, vasodilatation is the main pathological change and cardiac output and blood flow to skin and muscle may be increased enabling subcutaneous and intramuscular absorption of adrenaline to be sufficiently rapid and effective.[1] The intramuscular route is generally preferred although the subcutaneous route may be used, especially by patients treating themselves. Prefilled syringes for intramuscular or subcutaneous administration of adrenaline are available for those known to be at high risk of developing anaphylactic shock. Such syringes mean that patients can self-administer their initial emergency treatment; they should still seek medical assistance as additional treatment may be required.[3] In the early stages adrenaline may be administered by inhalation and is sometimes taken with an antihistamine,[7] but this should not be a substitute for the administration of adrenaline by injection in patients with a history of acute attacks. As anaphylaxis progresses the intravascular volume becomes depleted, shock occurs, and at this stage the intravenous route is probably necessary to enable absorption.[1] The general principles used in the management of hypovolaemia and hypotension in shock are outlined on p.798.

The dose of adrenaline for intramuscular injection is usually 0.5 to 1 mg (0.5 to 1 mL of a 1 in 1000 solution) which may be repeated at about 10-minute intervals, according to blood pressure and pulse, until improvement occurs. Some use lower doses of 0.2 to 0.5 mg (0.2 to 0.5 mL of a 1 in 1000 solution) for intramuscular or subcutaneous injection. A more dilute solution of 1 in 10 000 is used for slow intravenous administration when the dose is 500 μg (5 mL) given at a rate of 100 μg (1 mL) per minute, stopping when a response has been obtained.

The intramuscular or subcutaneous dose for children using the 1 in 1000 solution ranges from: 50 μg (0.05 mL) for those under 1 year; 100 μg (0.1 mL) for those aged 1 year; 200 μg (0.2 mL) for a two-year-old; 300 μg (0.3 mL) for those aged 3 to 4 years; 400 μg (0.4 mL) for a five-year-old; and 500 μg (0.5 mL) for children aged 6 to 12 years. These doses may need to be halved in children 2 years and older who are underweight. The intravenous dose for children, employing the 1 in 10 000 solution, is 10 μg (0.1 mL) per kg body-weight.

A slow intravenous injection of an antihistamine, such as chlorpheniramine 10 to 20 mg, may be given immediately after the adrenaline and repeated over the subsequent 24 to 48 hours to prevent relapse. Although antihistamines are particularly effective in the management of angioedema, pruritus, and urticaria, they remain second-line treatment. Intravenous corticosteroids have little place in the immediate management of anaphylaxis, since their beneficial effects are delayed for several hours but in severely ill patients early administration of hydrocortisone 100 to 300 mg as the sodium succinate may help prevent deterioration after the primary treatment has been given. Also some consider that asthmatics who have relatively recently undergone regular corticosteroid treatment may benefit from hydrocortisone.[3] Patients should also receive oxygen as required.

Continuing deterioration with circulatory collapse, bronchospasm, or laryngeal oedema requires further treatment including intravenous fluids, intravenous aminophylline, a nebulised β_2-agonist (such as salbutamol or terbutaline), assisted respiration (if necessary), and possibly, emergency tracheostomy. Noradrenaline may be necessary if the hypotension does not respond to adrenaline and intravenous fluids.[2]

It should be remembered that patients receiving some non-cardioselective beta blockers may be relatively refractory to the effects of adrenaline used for anaphylactic shock (see under Interactions for Adrenaline, above); in such cases the use of a more selective $beta_2$-agonist such as salbutamol by intravenous injection should be considered. Glucagon is another alternative to adrenaline in such patients.[2,8]

Other measures to control anaphylaxis include desensitisation in patients who have reacted to bee or wasp venom.[9] Patients with idiopathic anaphylaxis have benefited from prophylaxis with a corticosteroid and antihistamine, sometimes with a beta agonist.[10]

1. Fisher M. Treating anaphylaxis with sympathomimetic drugs. *Br Med J* 1992; **305:** 1107–8.
2. Anonymous. Adrenaline for anaphylaxis. *Drug Ther Bull* 1994; **32:** 19–21.
3. Patel L, *et al.* Management of anaphylactic reactions to food. *Arch Dis Child* 1994; **71:** 370–5.
4. Fisher M. Treatment of acute anaphylaxis. *Br Med J* 1995; **311:** 731–3. Correction. *ibid.*; 937.
5. Ewan PW. Anaphylaxis. *Br Med J* 1998; **316:** 1442–5. Correction. *ibid.*; 1587.
6. Ewan PW. Treatment of anaphylactic reactions. *Prescribers' J* 1997; **37:** 125–32.
7. Hourihane JO'B, Warner JO. Management of anaphylactic reactions to food. *Arch Dis Child* 1995; **72:** 274.
8. Lang DM. Anaphylactoid and anaphylactic reactions: hazards of β-blockers. *Drug Safety* 1995; **12:** 299–304.
9. Frew AJ, *et al.* Injection immunotherapy. *Br Med J* 1993; **307:** 919–23.
10. Wong S, *et al.* Outcome of prophylactic therapy for idiopathic anaphylaxis. *Ann Intern Med* 1991; **114:** 133–6.

Haemorrhage. Adrenaline has a long history of being applied topically to check minor bleeding. It constricts arterioles and capillaries and causes blanching. It has sometimes been used as an adjunct to other measures in the control of bleeding peptic ulcers (p.1174). Injection of adrenaline under endoscopic control is highly effective in controlling bleeding peptic ulcers, but does not produce permanent thrombosis of the vessels; combination of adrenaline with the use of a contact thermal probe may confer an advantage.[1]

1. Chung SSC, *et al.* Randomised comparison between adrenaline injection alone and adrenaline injection plus heat probe treatment for actively bleeding ulcers. *Br Med J* 1997; **314:** 1307–11.

Priapism. For reference to adrenaline in low dosage and dilute solution being given by intracavernosal injection to reverse priapism, see under Alprostadil, p.1413.

Preparations

BP 1998: Adrenaline Eye Drops *(Neutral Adrenaline Eye Drops)*; Adrenaline Injection; Adrenaline Solution; Bupivacaine and Adrenaline Injection; Dilute Adrenaline Injection 1 in 10,000; Lidocaine and Adrenaline Injection;
USP 23: Bupivacaine Hydrochloride and Epinephrine Injection; Cocaine and Tetracaine Hydrochlorides and Epinephrine Topical Solution; Epinephrine Bitartrate for Ophthalmic Solution; Epinephrine Bitartrate Inhalation Aerosol; Epinephrine Bitartrate Ophthalmic Solution; Epinephrine Inhalation Aerosol; Epinephrine Inhalation Solution; Epinephrine Injectable Oil Suspension; Epinephrine Injection; Epinephrine Nasal Solution; Epinephrine Ophthalmic Solution; Epinephryl Borate Ophthalmic Solution; Lidocaine Hydrochloride and Epinephrine Injection; Prilocaine and Epinephrine Injection; Procaine Hydrochloride and Epinephrine Injection; Racepinephrine Inhalation Solution.

Proprietary Preparations (details are given in Part 3)
Aust.: Eppystabil; Glycirenan; Suprarenin; ***Austral.:*** Epifrin†; Epipen; Eppy/N†; Medihaler-Epi; ***Belg.:*** Epifrin†; Isopto Epinal†; ***Canad.:*** Bronkaid; Epi EZ; Epifrin; Epipen; Medihaler-Epi†; Vaponefrin; ***Fr.:*** Anahelp; Anakit; Dyspne-Inhal; Eppy; Glauposine†; ***Ger.:*** Anaphylaxie-Besteck; Epiglaufrin†; Fastjekt; Suprarenin; ***Irl.:*** Epifrin†; Eppy; Simplene; ***Ital.:*** Eppy; Fastjekt; ***Neth.:*** Eppy†; ***S.Afr.:*** Ana-Guard; Epifrin†; Epipen; Eppy; Medihaler-Epi†; Simplene; ***Spain:*** Isopto Epinal†; ***Swed.:*** Epipen; Eppy; Glaufrin; ***Switz.:*** Epifrin†; Eppy/N†; Gingi-Pak; Medihaler-Epi; Orostat; Surgident; ***UK:*** Epipen; Eppy; Medihaler-Epi†; Simplene; ***USA:*** AsthmaHaler Mist; AsthmaNefrin; Bronitin Mist; Bronkaid Mist Suspension†; Epifrin; Epinal; Epipen; Eppy/N; Glaucon; Medihaler-Epi†; microNefrin; Nephron; Primatene Mist; Primatene Mist Suspension; S-2; Sus-Phrine; Vaponefrin.

Multi-ingredient: ***Austral.:*** Rectinol; ***Belg.:*** Glaucofrin; ***Canad.:*** Ana-Kit; E-Pilo; ***Fr.:*** Glaucadrine; Sirop Boin; ***Ger.:*** Bormelin N-Adrenalin†; Bronchovydrin†; Brox-Aerosol N†; Glaucadrin†; Links-Glaukosan†; Mydrial-Atropin†; Piladren†; Suprexon; ***Irl.:*** Ganda; ***Ital.:*** Asman-Valeas†; Pilodren; Rinantipiol; ***Neth.:*** Glaucofrin; Suprexon; ***S.Afr.:*** Ganda†; ***Spain:*** Antihemorroidal†; Coliriocilina Adren Astr; Epistaxol; Xilorroidal†; ***Switz.:*** Glaucadrine; Haemocortin; Medi-Kord; Suprexon; ***UK:*** Ganda; ***USA:*** Ana-Kit; Bronkaid Mist; E-Pilo; Emergent-Ez; PE.

Used as an adjunct in: ***Aust.:*** Carbostesin; Neo-Xylestesin; Neo-Xylestesin forte; Scandonest; Ubistesin; Ultracain Dental; Xylanaest; Xylocain; ***Austral.:*** Citanest; Marcain; Nurocain; Nurocain with Sympathin†; Xylocaine; ***Belg.:*** Citanest; Marcaine; Xylocaine; ***Canad.:*** Citanest; Marcaine; Sensorcaine; Ultracaine D-S; Xylocaine; ***Fr.:*** Alphacaine; Duranest; Marcaine; Xylocaine; ***Ger.:*** Anaesthol; Carbostesin; Lidocaton; Meaverin; Meaverin "A" mit Adrenalin; Mepivastesin forte†; neo-Novutox†; Scandicain; Ubistesin; Ultracain D-S; Ultracain-Suprarenin; Xylestesin-A; Xylestesin-S; Xylocain; Xylocitin; Xylonest; ***Irl.:*** Marcain; Xylocaine; ***Ital.:*** Bupiforan; Carbocaina; Citocartin; Ecocain; Lident Adrenalina; Lident Andrenor; Marcaina; Mepi-Mynol; Mepicain; Mepident; Mepiforan; Optocain; Septanest; Ultracain D-S; Xilo-Mynol; Xylestesina S†; Xylocaina; Xylonor; ***Neth.:*** Citanest; Marcaine; Scandicaine; Ultracain D-S; Xylocaine; ***Norw.:*** Marcain; Xylocain; ***S.Afr.:*** Lidocaton†; Macaine; Pharmacaine†; Scandonest; Xylotox; ***Spain:*** Anestesia Loc Braun C/A; Anestesia Topi Braun C/A; Meganest; Scandinibsa; Stoma Anestesia Dental; Ultracain; Xilonibsa; Xylonor Especial; ***Swed.:*** Carbocain; Citanest; Duranest†; Marcain; Xylocain; ***Switz.:*** Carbostesin; Lidocaton; Lignospan; Rapidocaine; Rudocaine; Scandicain; Scandonest; Septanest; Ubistesin; Ultracaine D-S; Xylestesin-S "special"; Xylocain; Xylonest; Xylonor; ***UK:*** AccuSite†; Lignostab-A; Marcain; Pensacaine with Adrenaline†; Xylocaine; Xylotox; ***USA:*** Citanest; Duranest; Marcaine; Octocaine; Sensorcaine; Xylocaine.

Ajmaline (7777-b)

Ajmalina; Ajmalinum; Rauwolfine. (17*R*,21*R*)-Ajmalan-17,21-diol.

$C_{20}H_{26}N_2O_2$ = 326.4.
CAS — 4360-12-7.

Pharmacopoeias. In *Aust.*, *It.*, and *Jpn.*
Aust. and *It.* also include Ajmaline Monohydrate and Ajmaline Monoethanolate.

Ajmaline is an alkaloid obtained from the root of *Rauwolfia serpentina* (Apocynaceae).

Adverse Effects

Ajmaline depresses the conductivity of the heart, and at high doses can cause heart block. At very high doses it may produce a negative inotropic effect. High doses may cause cardiac arrhythmias, coma, and death. Arrhythmias have also been reported after usual intravenous doses (see below). Adverse neurological effects have been reported including eye twitching, convulsions, and respiratory depression. Hepatotoxicity and agranulocytosis may occasionally occur.

Effects on the heart. Electrophysiologic study[1] in 1955 patients revealed that ajmaline 1 mg per kg intravenously could induce arrhythmias; 63 developed a supraventricular arrhythmia and 7 an atrioventricular re-entrant tachycardia.

1. Brembilla-Perrot B, Terrier de la Chaise A. Provocation of supraventricular tachycardias by an intravenous class I antiarrhythmic drug. *Int J Cardiol* 1992; **34:** 189–98.

Precautions

As for Quinidine, p.939.

Interactions

Concurrent oral administration of quinidine with ajmaline gave considerably increased plasma concentrations of ajmaline in 4 healthy subjects; the elimination half-life of ajmaline was increased about twofold.[1] The pharmacokinetics of quinidine did not seem to be affected by the presence of ajmaline.

1. Hori R, *et al.* Quinidine-induced rise in ajmaline plasma concentration. *J Pharm Pharmacol* 1984; **36:** 202–4.

Uses and Administration

Ajmaline is a class Ia antiarrhythmic (p.776). It is used in the treatment of supraventricular and ventricular arrhythmias (p.782). The usual dose of ajmaline by mouth is 100 to 300 mg daily. It is also given by intravenous injection in a dose of 1 mg per kg body-weight at a maximum rate of 10 mg per minute, or by intramuscular injection in a dose of 50 to 150 mg daily.

Ajmaline is also used as the hydrochloride, monoethanolate, and as the phenobarbitone salt.

Preparations

Proprietary Preparations (details are given in Part 3)
Aust.: Gilurytmal; ***Belg.:*** Gilurytmal†; ***Ger.:*** Gilurytmal; Tachmalin; ***Ital.:*** Aritmina; Ritmos†; Ritmosedina†; ***Spain:*** Gilurytmal.

Multi-ingredient: ***Ger.:*** Coritrat†; Digi-Pulsnorma†; Diuraupur sine†; Diuraupur†; Pulsnorma†; ***Spain:*** Diu Rauwiplus.

Alacepril (18737-x)

Alacepril *(rINN)*.
DU-1219. *N*-{1-[(*S*)-3-Mercapto-2-methylpropionyl]-L-prolyl}-3-phenyl-L-alanine acetate (ester).

$C_{20}H_{26}N_2O_5S$ = 406.5.
CAS — 74258-86-9.

Alacepril is an ACE inhibitor (p.805) used in the treatment of hypertension. It is converted to captopril and desacetylalacepril (DU-1227) in the body following oral administration.

Preparations

Proprietary Preparations (details are given in Part 3)
Jpn: Cetapril.

Alfuzosin Hydrochloride (12287-p)

Alfuzosin Hydrochloride *(BANM, USAN, rINNM)*.
Alfuzosini Hydrochloridum; SL-77499-10; SL-77499 (alfuzosin). *N*-{3-[4-Amino-6,7-dimethoxyquinazolin-2-yl(methyl)amino]propyl}tetrahydro-2-furamide hydrochloride.

$C_{19}H_{27}N_5O_4,HCl$ = 425.9.
CAS — 81403-80-7 (alfuzosin); 81403-68-1 (alfuzosin hydrochloride).

Pharmacopoeias. In *Eur.* (see p.viii).

A white or almost white, slightly hygroscopic, crystalline powder. Freely **soluble** in water; sparingly soluble in alcohol; practically insoluble in dichloromethane. A 2% solution in water has a pH of 4 to 6. **Store** in airtight containers. Protect from light.

Adverse Effects, Treatment, and Precautions

As for Prazosin Hydrochloride, p.932. Alfuzosin may be more selective for the urinary tract and vasodilatory effects may be less frequent.

References.

1. Lukacs B, *et al.* Safety profile of 3 months' therapy with alfuzosin in 13,389 patients suffering from benign prostatic hypertrophy. *Eur Urol* 1996; **29:** 29–35.

Pharmacokinetics

Alfuzosin hydrochloride is readily absorbed after oral administration and peak plasma concentrations generally occur 0.5 to 3 hours after a dose; bioavailability is about 64%. It is extensively metabolised in the liver to inactive metabolites and excreted primarily in faeces via the bile. Only about 11% of a dose is excreted unchanged in the urine. Alfuzosin has a plasma elimination half-life of 3 to 5 hours. It is 90% bound to plasma proteins.

References.

1. Scott MG, *et al.* Haemodynamic and pharmacokinetic evaluation of alfuzosin in man: a dose ranging study and comparison with prazosin. *Eur J Clin Pharmacol* 1989; **37:** 53–8.

Uses and Administration

Alfuzosin is an alpha$_1$-adrenoceptor blocker (p.776) with actions similar to those of prazosin (p.933). It is used in the symptomatic treatment of urinary obstruction caused by benign prostatic hyperplasia (p.1446) and has been tried in the treatment of hypertension.

Alfuzosin is given by mouth as the hydrochloride. Like other alpha$_1$-adrenoceptor blockers, it may cause collapse in some patients after the first dose, which should therefore be given just before bedtime to reduce the risk. In benign prostatic hyperplasia, the usual dose is 2.5 mg three times daily, increased to 10 mg daily if necessary. Doses may need to be reduced in patients with hepatic impairment. Dose reduction may also be necessary in the elderly and in those with renal impairment; alternatively, modified-release preparations may be preferred.

References.

1. Leto di Priolo S, *et al.* Dose-titration study of alfuzosin, a new alpha$_1$-adrenoceptor blocker, in essential hypertension. *Eur J Clin Pharmacol* 1988; **35:** 25–30.
2. Jardin A, *et al.* Alfuzosin for treatment of benign prostatic hypertrophy. *Lancet* 1991; **337:** 1457–61.
3. Wilde MI, *et al.* Alfuzosin: a review of its pharmacodynamic and pharmacokinetic properties, and therapeutic potential in benign prostatic hyperplasia. *Drugs* 1993; **45:** 410–29.

Preparations

Proprietary Preparations (details are given in Part 3)
Fr.: Urion; Xatral; ***Ger.:*** Urion; UroXatral; ***Irl.:*** Xatral; ***Ital.:*** Benestan; Mittoval; Xatral; ***Neth.:*** Xatral; ***Spain:*** Alfetim; Benestan; Dalfaz; ***Swed.:*** Xatral; ***Switz.:*** Xatral; ***UK:*** Xatral.

Alinidine (7779-g)

Alinidine *(BAN, rINN)*.
ST-567 (alinidine); ST-567-BR (alinidine hydrobromide). *N*-Allyl-2,6-dichloro-*N*-(2-imidazolin-2-yl)aniline.

$C_{12}H_{13}Cl_2N_3$ = 270.2.
CAS — 33178-86-8.

Alinidine resembles clonidine in chemical structure, but has been reported to differ in pharmacological action. It causes bradycardia probably due to a direct effect on the heart. It has been suggested that its properties may represent a fifth class of antiarrhythmic action (p.776).

References.

1. Millar JS, Vaughan Williams EM. Anion antagonism—a fifth class of antiarrhythmic action? *Lancet* 1981; **i:** 1291–3.
2. Nawrath H. A fifth class of antiarrhythmic action? *Lancet* 1981; **ii:** 209–10.
3. Harron DWG, *et al.* Alinidine pharmacokinetics following acute and chronic dosing. *Br J Clin Pharmacol* 1982; **13:** 821–7.

Alprenolol Benzoate (15827-r)

Alprenolol Benzoate *(BANM, rINNM)*.
Alprenololi Benzoas. (±)-1-(2-Allylphenoxy)-3-isopropylaminopropan-2-ol benzoate.

$C_{22}H_{29}NO_4$ = 371.5.
Pharmacopoeias. In *Eur.* (see p.viii).

A white crystalline powder or colourless crystals. Slightly **soluble** in water; soluble in alcohol. **Protect** from light.

Alprenolol Hydrochloride (6303-p)

Alprenolol Hydrochloride *(BANM, USAN, rINNM)*.
Alprenololi Hydrochloridum; H56/28. (±)-1-(2-Allylphenoxy)-3-isopropylaminopropan-2-ol hydrochloride.

$C_{15}H_{23}NO_2,HCl$ = 285.8.
CAS — 13655-52-2 (alprenolol); 13707-88-5 (alprenolol hydrochloride).
Pharmacopoeias. In *Eur.* (see p.viii) and *Jpn.*

A white crystalline powder or colourless crystals. Very **soluble** in water; freely soluble in alcohol and in dichloromethane. **Protect** from light.

Adverse Effects, Treatment, and Precautions

As for beta blockers, p.828.

Hypersensitivity. A report of contact eczema in workers exposed to alprenolol.[1]

1. Ekenvall L, Forsbeck M. Contact eczema produced by a β-adrenergic blocking agent (alprenolol). *Contact Dermatitis* 1978; **4:** 190–4.

Interactions

The interactions associated with beta blockers are discussed on p.829.

Pharmacokinetics

Alprenolol is almost completely absorbed from the gastro-intestinal tract but is subject to considerable first-pass metabolism in the liver. Peak plasma concentrations are achieved about 1 hour after a dose. It has high lipid solubility. Alprenolol is about 85% bound to plasma proteins. It is distributed into breast milk. It is metabolised in the liver, primarily to 4-hydroxyalprenolol, which is active. The plasma half-life of alprenolol is about 3 hours and the plasma half-life of 4-hydroxyalprenolol is about 20 minutes. It is excreted in the urine mainly in the form of its metabolites.

Uses and Administration

Alprenolol is a non-cardioselective beta blocker (p.828). It is reported to have intrinsic sympathomimetic activity and some membrane-stabilising properties.

Alprenolol is used in the management of hypertension (p.788), angina pectoris (p.780), and cardiac arrhythmias (p.782).

It is given by mouth, as the benzoate or hydrochloride; doses have been expressed in terms of the base or of the hydrochloride.

In **hypertension** the usual initial dose is 200 mg daily, in divided doses by mouth, increased weekly according to the response of the patient up to a total of 800 mg daily in divided doses. The usual dose for **angina pectoris**, **cardiac arrhythmias**, and other cardiac disorders is 50 to 100 mg four times daily. It may be necessary to reduce the dose in patients with renal or hepatic impairment.

Preparations

Proprietary Preparations (details are given in Part 3)
Austral.: Aptin†; ***Belg.:*** Aptine; ***Ger.:*** Aptin; ***Ital.:*** Aptin†; ***Neth.:*** Aptine; ***Norw.:*** Aptin; ***Swed.:*** Aptin N.

Alseroxylon (852-l)

CAS — 8001-95-4.

Alseroxylon is a mixture of selected alkaloid hydrochlorides from *Rauwolfia serpentina* and has properties and uses similar to those described under reserpine (see p.942).

Alteplase (16956-z)

Alteplase *(BAN, USAN, rINN).*

G-11035; G-11044; G-11021 (2-chain form); Recombinant Tissue-type Plasminogen Activator; rt-PA.

CAS — 105857-23-6.

Pharmacopoeias. In *Eur.* (see p.viii) and *US.*

A glycosylated protein of 527 residues having the amino acid sequence of human tissue plasminogen activator (t-PA) and produced by recombinant DNA technology.

A study by Lee and others[1] concluded that alteplase should not be mixed in the same container with dobutamine, dopamine, glyceryl trinitrate or heparin, as there was evidence of incompatibility, although a subsequent study found no incompatibility between alteplase and glyceryl trinitrate.[2] Another study, by Frazin,[3] found that dilution of a proprietary preparation of alteplase (Activase) to 0.09 and 0.16 mg per mL with 5% glucose injection resulted in precipitation of the drug. Alteplase is formulated with arginine as a solubilising agent, and dilution with 5% glucose to concentrations below 0.5 mg of alteplase per mL makes precipitation possible. Dilution with 0.9% sodium chloride is possible to concentrations down to 0.2 mg per mL before precipitation becomes a risk.

1. Lee CY, *et al.* Visual and spectrophotometric determination of compatibility of alteplase and streptokinase with other injectable drugs. *Am J Hosp Pharm* 1990; **47:** 606–8.
2. Lam XM, *et al.* Stability and activity of alteplase with injectable drugs commonly used in cardiac therapy. *Am J Health-Syst Pharm* 1995; **52:** 1904–9.
3. Frazin BS. Maximal dilution of Activase. *Am J Hosp Pharm* 1990; **47:** 1016.

Units

The activity of alteplase can be measured in terms of international units using the second International Standard for tissue plasminogen activator established in 1987, although doses are generally expressed by weight. The specific activity of alteplase is 580 000 international units per mg.

Adverse Effects, Treatment, and Precautions

As for Streptokinase, p.948. Allergic reactions are less likely with alteplase and repeated administration is possible.

Infusion of alteplase produces considerable thrombin generation which may result from direct activation of the coagulation system by plasmin or by positive feedback of the coagulation system by clot-bound thrombin. This excessive thrombin generation was considered a possible cause of myocardial infarction in a patient undergoing thrombolytic therapy with alteplase for venous thrombosis.[1] Infusion of streptokinase produced no evidence of excessive thrombin generation.

1. Baglin TP, *et al.* Thrombin generation and myocardial infarction during infusion of tissue-plasminogen activator. *Lancet* 1993; **341:** 504–5.

Hypersensitivity. An anaphylactoid reaction to alteplase occurred in a patient with a history of atopy.[1] For comment on this unexpected reaction, see Hypersensitivity under the Adverse Effects of Streptokinase, p.949.

1. Purvis JA, *et al.* Anaphylactoid reaction after injection of alteplase. *Lancet* 1993; **341:** 966–7.

Interactions

As for Streptokinase, p.950.

Glyceryl trinitrate. Although thrombolytics and nitrates are both frequently used in acute myocardial infarction one report has suggested that this combination may result in impaired thrombolysis. Concurrent intravenous administration of alteplase and glyceryl trinitrate to 36 patients with acute myocardial infarction produced lower plasma-antigen concentrations of tissue-plasminogen activator than alteplase given alone to 11 patients.[1] Reperfusion was sustained in only 44% of patients receiving both drugs compared with 91% of patients receiving alteplase alone. The authors of a subsequent study[2] suggested that these lower plasma concentrations may be due to increased hepatic metabolism of alteplase as a result of glyceryl trinitrate's effect of increasing hepatic blood flow.

1. Nicolini FA, *et al.* Concurrent nitroglycerin therapy impairs tissue-type plasminogen activator-induced thrombolysis in patients with acute myocardial infarction. *Am J Cardiol* 1994; **74:** 662–6.
2. Romeo F, *et al.* Concurrent nitroglycerin administration reduces the efficacy of recombinant tissue-type plasminogen activator in patients with acute anterior wall myocardial infarction. *Am Heart J* 1995; **130:** 692–7.

Pharmacokinetics

Alteplase is cleared rapidly from the plasma, mainly by metabolism in the liver.

References.

1. Krause J. Catabolism of tissue-type plasminogen activator (t-PA), its variants, mutants and hybrids. *Fibrinolysis* 1988; **2:** 133–42.

Uses and Administration

Alteplase is a thrombolytic drug. It is a predominantly single-chain form of the endogenous enzyme tissue plasminogen activator and is produced by recombinant DNA technology. Like endogenous tissue plasminogen activator, alteplase converts fibrin-bound plasminogen to the active form plasmin, resulting in fibrinolysis and dissolution of clots. The mechanisms of fibrinolysis are discussed further under Haemostasis on p.704. Alteplase has relatively little effect on circulating, unbound plasminogen and thus may be termed a fibrin-specific agent. Fibrin specificity was thought to be required for reducing the risk of haemorrhage associated with the use of thrombolytics, although currently available fibrin-specific agents do not produce less bleeding than nonspecific thrombolytics (see Haemorrhage under Adverse Effects of Streptokinase, p.949).

Alteplase is used similarly to streptokinase (p.950) in the treatment of thrombo-embolic disorders, particularly myocardial infarction (p.791) and venous thrombo-embolism (p.802). Alteplase may also be used in patients with acute ischaemic stroke (p.799).

In the treatment of acute **myocardial infarction**, alteplase is given intravenously as soon as possible after the onset of symptoms in a total dose of 100 mg; a total dose of 1.5 mg per kg body-weight is suggested for patients weighing less than 65 kg. The total dose of 100 mg may be given either over 1½ hours (accelerated or 'front-loaded' alteplase) or over 3 hours. The accelerated schedule has been recommended where administration is within 6 hours of myocardial infarction, while the 3-hour schedule has been recommended where administration is more than 6 hours after myocardial infarction. Administration over 1½ hours is as follows: 15 mg as an intravenous bolus, then 0.75 mg per kg body-weight, up to a maximum of 50 mg, by intravenous infusion over 30 minutes, followed by the remainder infused over the subsequent 60 minutes. Administration over 3 hours is as follows: 10 mg as an intravenous bolus, then 50 mg by intravenous infusion over 1 hour, followed by a further 40 mg infused over the subsequent 2 hours.

In the treatment of **pulmonary embolism** 100 mg may be given by intravenous infusion over 2 hours.

In acute **ischaemic stroke**, alteplase is given within 3 hours of the onset of symptoms in a dose of 0.9 mg per kg up to a maximum total dose of 90 mg. The dose is administered intravenously over 60 minutes with 10% being given as a bolus during the first minute.

General references.

1. Gillis JC, *et al.* Alteplase: a reappraisal of its pharmacological properties and therapeutic use in acute myocardial infarction. *Drugs* 1995; **50:** 102–36.
2. Wagstaff AJ, *et al.* Alteplase: a reappraisal of its pharmacology and therapeutic use in vascular disorders other than acute myocardial infarction. *Drugs* 1995; **50:** 289–316.

Catheters and cannulas. Alteplase has been used successfully to clear thrombi in central venous catheters.[1,2] Doses typically employed have been 2 mg injected as a bolus into the blocked catheter. In two children[3] alteplase in doses of 0.01 to 0.05 mg per kg body-weight per hour intravenously has been used for venous thrombosis associated with indwelling intravascular catheters.

1. Paulsen D, *et al.* Use of tissue plasminogen activator for reopening of clotted dialysis catheters. *Nephron* 1993; **64:** 468–9.
2. Haire WD, *et al.* Urokinase versus recombinant tissue plasminogen activator in thrombosed central venous catheters: a double-blinded, randomized trial. *Thromb Haemost* 1994; **72:** 543–7.
3. Doyle E, *et al.* Thrombolysis with low dose tissue plasminogen activator. *Arch Dis Child* 1992; **67:** 1483–4.

Intracardiac thrombosis. Alteplase has been used, in a dose of 100 mg given intravenously over two hours, for thrombosis of prosthetic heart valves.[1]

Alteplase has been used successfully in a neonate to treat intracardiac thrombosis associated with the use of a central venous line.[2] A dose of 0.5 mg per kg body-weight given over 10 minutes was followed by infusion of 0.2 mg per kg per hour for three days.

1. Astengo D, *et al.* Recombinant tissue plasminogen activator for prosthetic mitral-valve thrombosis. *N Engl J Med* 1995; **333:** 259.
2. Van Overmeire B, *et al.* Intracardiac thrombus formation with rapidly progressive heart failure in the neonate: treatment with tissue type plasminogen activator. *Arch Dis Child* 1992; **67:** 443–5.

Microvessel thrombosis. Alteplase has been used in a number of conditions where the underlying pathology is occlusion of small blood vessels by microthrombi.

Purpura and loss of circulation in the hands of a patient recovering from **fulminant meningococcaemia**[1] responded to intra-arterial infusion of alteplase 0.02 to 0.04 mg per kg body-weight per hour for 22 hours in the right hand, and 0.02 mg per kg per hour for 11 hours in the left. Perfusion was successfully restored to both hands, and full function subsequently attained in them. Improvement was also achieved when alteplase was given to 2 infants with septic shock and purpura fulminans caused by meningococcal infection.[2]

Six patients[3] with ulcers caused by **livedoid vasculitis** and refractory to conventional treatment were treated with alteplase 10 mg infused intravenously over 4 hours daily for 14 days. Most ulcers healed rapidly; one patient required retreatment with concomitant anticoagulation.

A 4-year-old girl[4] with **haemolytic uraemic syndrome** (see under Thrombotic Microangiopathies, p.726) responded to treatment with an intravenous infusion of alteplase 0.2 mg per kg per hour for 5 hours, subsequently reduced to 0.05 mg per kg per hour for 14 days.

Alteplase has been tried in a few patients with **veno-occlusive disease of the liver**, a serious complication of bone-marrow transplantation that may be caused by diffuse thrombi in the hepatic venules. However, results have been mixed.[5-7]

1. Keeley SR, *et al.* Tissue plasminogen activator for gangrene in fulminant meningococcaemia. *Lancet* 1991; **337:** 1359.
2. Zenz W, *et al.* Recombinant tissue plasminogen activator treatment in two infants with fulminant meningococcemia. *Pediatrics* 1995; **96:** 144–8.
3. Klein KL, Pittelkow MR. Tissue plasminogen activator for treatment of livedoid vasculitis. *Mayo Clin Proc* 1992; **67:** 923–33.
4. Kruez W, *et al.* Successful treatment of haemolytic uraemic syndrome with recombinant tissue-type plasminogen activator. *Lancet* 1993; **341:** 1665–6.
5. Laporte JP, *et al.* Alteplase for hepatic veno-occlusive disease complicating bone-marrow transplantation. *Lancet* 1992; **339:** 1057.
6. Rosti G, *et al.* Alteplase for hepatic veno-occlusive disease after bone-marrow transplantation. *Lancet* 1992; **339:** 1481–2.
7. Ringdén O, *et al.* Alteplase for hepatic veno-occlusive disease after bone-marrow transplantation. *Lancet* 1992; **340:** 546–7.

Peripheral arterial thrombo-embolism. Thrombolytics, including alteplase, may be used in the management of peripheral arterial thrombo-embolism (p.794). Alteplase has been injected intravenously or intra-arterially directly into the clot as an alternative to surgical treatment of the occlusion. It has also been infused intra-arterially to remove distal clots during a surgical procedure. Alteplase is claimed to produce more rapid thrombolysis than streptokinase although studies have been too small to provide evidence of reduced limb loss or mortality.[1] The most common dose range is 0.5 to 1 mg per hour given intra-arterially.[1-3] An intravenous dose of 0.5 mg per kg body-weight per hour for the first hour followed by 0.25 mg per kg per hour until clot lysis occurred has been used in infants.[4] Where a thrombolytic is used to remove distal clots during a surgical procedure alteplase has been given intra-arterially as three doses of 5 mg at 10-minute intervals.[5]

1. Wolfe JH. Critical limb ischaemia. *Prescribers' J* 1994; **34:** 50–8.
2. Anonymous. Non-coronary thrombolysis. *Lancet* 1990; **335:** 691–3.
3. Ward AS, *et al.* Peripheral thrombolysis with tissue plasminogen activator: results of two treatment regimens. *Arch Surg* 1994; **129:** 861–5.
4. Zenz W, *et al.* Tissue plasminogen activator (alteplase) treatment for femoral artery thrombosis after cardiac catheterisation in infants and children. *Br Heart J* 1993; **70:** 382–5.
5. Chester JF, *et al.* Peroperative t-PA thrombolysis. *Lancet* 1991; **337:** 861–2.

Preparations

USP 23: Alteplase for Injection.

Proprietary Preparations (details are given in Part 3)
Aust.: Actilyse; Besopartin; ***Austral.:*** Actilyse; ***Belg.:*** Actilyse; ***Canad.:*** Activase; Lysatec rt-PA†; ***Fr.:*** Actilyse; ***Ger.:*** Actilyse; ***Irl.:*** Actilyse; ***Ital.:*** Actilyse; Actiplas; ***Neth.:*** Actilyse; ***Norw.:*** Actilyse; ***S.Afr.:*** Actilyse; ***Spain:*** Actilyse; ***Swed.:*** Actilyse; ***Switz.:*** Actilyse; ***UK:*** Actilyse; ***USA:*** Activase.

Althiazide (12345-h)

Althiazide *(USAN).*

Altizide *(rINN)*; P-1779. 3-Allylthiomethyl-6-chloro-3,4-dihydro-2*H*-1,2,4-benzothiadiazine-7-sulphonamide 1,1-dioxide.

$C_{11}H_{14}ClN_3O_4S_3$ = 383.9.

CAS — 5588-16-9.

Althiazide is a thiazide diuretic (see Hydrochlorothiazide, p.885) that is used in the treatment of oedema and hypertension. It is frequently used in combination with spironolactone.

Preparations

Proprietary Preparations (details are given in Part 3)

Multi-ingredient: ***Belg.:*** Aldactazine; ***Fr.:*** Aldactazine; Practazin; Prinactizide; Spiroctazine; ***Spain:*** Aldactacine.

Amezinium Methylsulphate (12353-h)

Amezinium Metilsulfate *(rINN)*. 4-Amino-6-methoxy-1-phenylpyridazinium methylsulphate.

$C_{12}H_{15}N_3O_5S$ = 313.3.

CAS — 30578-37-1.

Amezinium methylsulphate is a sympathomimetic (see Adrenaline, p.813) which is used for its vasopressor effects in the treatment of hypotensive states. It is given by mouth and also by slow intravenous injection.

Preparations

Proprietary Preparations (details are given in Part 3)
Belg.: Regulton; ***Ger.:*** Regulton; Supratonin; ***Jpn:*** Risumic.

Amiloride Hydrochloride (2304-d)

Amiloride Hydrochloride *(BANM, USAN, rINNM).*

Amiloridi Hydrochloridum; Amipramizide; Cloridrato de Amilorida; MK-870. *N*-Amidino-3,5-diamino-6-chloropyrazine-2-carboxamide hydrochloride dihydrate.

$C_6H_8ClN_7O,HCl,2H_2O$ = 302.1.

CAS — 2609-46-3 (amiloride); 2016-88-8 (amiloride hydrochloride, anhydrous); 17440-83-4 (amiloride hydrochloride, dihydrate).

NOTE. Compounded preparations of amiloride hydrochloride and frusemide in the proportions, by weight, 1 part to 8 parts have the British Approved Name Co-amilofruse.

Compounded preparations of amiloride hydrochloride and hydrochlorothiazide in the proportions, by weight, 1 part to 10 parts have the British Approved Name Co-amilozide.

Compounded preparations of amiloride hydrochloride and hydrochlorothiazide in USP 23 may be represented by the name Co-amilozide.

Pharmacopoeias. In *Eur.* (see p.viii), *Int.*, and *US.*

A pale yellow to yellowish-green, odourless or almost odourless powder. Slightly **soluble** in water and in alcohol; practically insoluble in acetone, in chloroform, in ether, and in ethyl acetate; freely soluble in dimethyl sulphoxide; sparingly soluble in methyl alcohol. **Protect** from light.

Adverse Effects

Amiloride can cause hyperkalaemia, particularly in elderly patients, diabetics, and patients with impaired renal function. Hyponatraemia has been reported in patients receiving combination therapy with amiloride and other diuretics. Amiloride may cause nausea, vomiting, abdominal pain, diarrhoea or constipation, paraesthesia, thirst, dizziness, skin rash, pruritus, weakness, muscle cramps, headache, and minor psychiatric or visual changes. Orthostatic hypotension and rises in blood-urea-nitrogen concentrations have been reported.

Effects on the electrolyte balance. Reports of metabolic acidosis associated with amiloride or triamterene[1] and with co-amilozide.[2]

1. Kushner RF, Sitrin MD. Metabolic acidosis: development in two patients receiving a potassium-sparing diuretic and total parenteral nutrition. *Arch Intern Med* 1986; **146:** 343–5.
2. Wan HH, Lye MDW. Moduretic-induced metabolic acidosis and hyperkalaemia. *Postgrad Med J* 1980; **56:** 348–50.

POTASSIUM. Hyperkalaemia is the main adverse effect when amiloride is given alone but may also occur when amiloride is given in combination with a potassium-wasting diuretic. Severe hyperkalaemia has been reported during co-amilozide therapy, particularly in patients with impaired renal function.[1,2] Wan and Lye[3] reported severe hyperkalaemia accompanied by metabolic acidosis in one such patient.

1. Whiting GFM, *et al.* Severe hyperkalaemia with Moduretic. *Med J Aust* 1979; **1:** 409.
2. Jaffey L, Martin A. Malignant hyperkalaemia after amiloride/hydrochlorothiazide treatment. *Lancet* 1981; **i:** 1272.
3. Wan HH, Lye MDW. Moduretic-induced metabolic acidosis and hyperkalaemia. *Postgrad Med J* 1980; **56:** 348–50.

SODIUM. For reports of severe hyponatraemia in patients taking amiloride with potassium-wasting diuretics, see Hydrochlorothiazide, p.886.

Effects on the skin. For a report of photosensitivity reactions in patients taking co-amilozide, see Hydrochlorothiazide, p.886.

Precautions

Amiloride has the same precautions as spironolactone with regard to hyperkalaemia (see p.946). It should be discontinued at least 3 days before glucose-tolerance tests are given to patients with diabetes mellitus because of the risks if patients are hyperkalaemic.

Interactions

There is an increased risk of hyperkalaemia if amiloride is given concomitantly with potassium supplements or with other potassium-sparing diuretics. Hyperkalaemia may also occur in patients receiving ACE inhibitors, NSAIDs, cyclosporin, or trilostane concomitantly. In patients receiving amiloride with NSAIDs or cyclosporin the risk of nephrotoxicity may also be increased. Diuretics may reduce the excretion of lithium and increase the risk of lithium toxicity, but this does not appear to occur with amiloride. Hyponatraemia may occur in patients receiving a combination of potassium-sparing diuretic with a thiazide; this risk may be increased in patients receiving chlorpropamide. Amiloride may reduce the ulcer-healing properties of carbenoxolone. As with other diuretics, amiloride may enhance the effects of other antihypertensive drugs.

Digoxin. For the effects of amiloride on digoxin clearance, see under Digoxin, p.851.

Quinidine. For a report of amiloride producing arrhythmias in patients receiving quinidine, see p.940.

Pharmacokinetics

Amiloride is incompletely absorbed from the gastro-intestinal tract; bioavailability of about 50% is reported and is reduced by food. It is not significantly bound to plasma proteins and has a plasma half-life of 6 to 9 hours; the terminal half-life may be 20 hours or more. It is excreted unchanged by the kidneys.

General references.

1. Weiss P, *et al.* The metabolism of amiloride hydrochloride in man. *Clin Pharmacol Ther* 1969; **10:** 401–6.

Hepatic impairment. In patients with acute hepatitis the terminal half-life of amiloride was 33 hours compared with 21 hours in healthy subjects.[1] The proportion of the dose excreted in the urine was increased from 49 to 80%.

1. Spahn H, *et al.* Pharmacokinetics of amiloride in renal and hepatic disease. *Eur J Clin Pharmacol* 1987; **33:** 493–8.

Renal impairment. Studies of the pharmacokinetics of amiloride[1,2] have reported an increase in terminal elimination half-life from 20 hours in healthy subjects to 100 hours in patients with end-stage renal disease. The natriuretic effect of amiloride was reduced[1] in patients with creatinine clearance below 50 mL per minute. In patients with renal impairment administration of amiloride could aggravate potassium retention due to renal disease. Studies in elderly patients have demonstrated increased half-life[3] and steady-state concentrations[4] associated with reduced renal function.

1. Knauf H, *et al.* Limitation on the use of amiloride in early renal failure. *Eur J Clin Pharmacol* 1985; **28:** 61–6.
2. Spahn H, *et al.* Pharmacokinetics of amiloride in renal and hepatic disease. *Eur J Clin Pharmacol* 1987; **33:** 493–8.
3. Sabanathan K, *et al.* A comparative study of the pharmacokinetics and pharmacodynamics of atenolol, hydrochlorothiazide and amiloride in normal young and elderly subjects and elderly hypertensive patients. *Eur J Clin Pharmacol* 1987; **32:** 53–60.
4. Ismail Z, *et al.* The pharmacokinetics of amiloride-hydrochlorothiazide combination in the young and elderly. *Eur J Clin Pharmacol* 1989; **37:** 167–71.

Uses and Administration

Amiloride is a mild diuretic which appears to act mainly on the distal renal tubules. It is described as potassium-sparing since, like spironolactone, it increases the excretion of sodium and reduces the excretion of potassium. Unlike spironolactone, however, it does not act by specifically antagonising aldosterone. Amiloride does not inhibit carbonic anhydrase. It takes effect about 2 hours after administration by mouth and its diuretic action reaches a peak in 6 to 10 hours and has been reported to persist for about 24 hours.

Amiloride diminishes the kaliuretic effects of other diuretics, and may produce an additional natriuretic effect. It is mainly used as an adjunct to thiazide diuretics such as hydrochlorothiazide and loop diuretics such as frusemide, to conserve potassium in those at risk from hypokalaemia during the long-term treatment of oedema associated with hepatic cirrhosis (including ascites, p.781) and heart failure (p.785). It is also used in combination with other diuretics in the treatment of hypertension (p.788). Diuretic-induced hypokalaemia and its management, including the role of potassium-sparing diuretics such as amiloride, is discussed under Effects on the Electrolyte Balance in the Adverse Effects of Hydrochlorothiazide, p.885.

Amiloride by inhalation has also been investigated in the management of cystic fibrosis patients with lung disease (see below).

In the treatment of **oedema** amiloride is given by mouth as the hydrochloride and doses are expressed in terms of the anhydrous substance. The usual dose is 5 to 10 mg daily which may be increased, if necessary, to a maximum of 20 mg daily. Similar doses are used to reduce potassium loss in patients receiving thiazide or loop diuretics.

Potassium supplements should not be given.

Cystic fibrosis. Pulmonary disease is the major cause of mortality in cystic fibrosis (p.119). Experimental treatment aimed at modifying the pulmonary disease process has included the administration of amiloride by inhalation.[1,2] No evidence of pulmonary or systemic toxicity was seen in 14 patients treated for 25 weeks.[1] The mechanism of action is unclear but could be the sodium-channel blocking effect[1] or anti-inflammatory effects[3] of amiloride. Henkin[4] has expressed concern over possible consequences of the inhibition of endogenous urokinase by amiloride although Knowles *et al.*[5] considered this to be unlikely at the concentrations studied.

1. Knowles MR, *et al.* A pilot study of aerosolized amiloride for the treatment of lung disease in cystic fibrosis. *N Engl J Med* 1990; **322:** 1189–94.
2. App EM, *et al.* Acute and long-term amiloride inhalation in cystic fibrosis lung disease: a rational approach to cystic fibrosis therapy. *Am Rev Respir Dis* 1990; **141:** 605–12.
3. Gallo RL. Aerosolized amiloride for the treatment of lung disease in cystic fibrosis. *N Engl J Med* 1990; **323:** 996–7.
4. Henkin J. Aerosolized amiloride for the treatment of lung disease in cystic fibrosis. *N Engl J Med* 1990; **323:** 997.
5. Knowles MR, *et al.* Aerosolized amiloride for the treatment of lung disease in cystic fibrosis. *N Engl J Med* 1990; **323:** 997–8.

Diabetes insipidus. Thiazide diuretics are commonly used in nephrogenic diabetes insipidus (p.1237) and NSAIDs may also be employed; both result in an overall decrease in urine production. Addition of amiloride to hydrochlorothiazide has been reported to be at least as effective as hydrochlorothiazide plus indomethacin in 5 patients.[1] In addition, amiloride obviated the need for potassium supplements.

1. Knoers N, Monnens LAH. Amiloride-hydrochlorothiazide versus indomethacin-hydrochlorothiazide in the treatment of nephrogenic diabetes insipidus. *J Pediatr* 1990; **117:** 499–502.

Renal calculi. Patients with idiopathic hypercalciuria and a history of renal calculi are usually given a thiazide diuretic such as hydrochlorothiazide to reduce calcium excretion (p.888). In patients with calcium oxalate calculi an inherited cellular defect in oxalate transport may also be involved and this might be corrected by amiloride.[1]

1. Baggio B, *et al.* An inheritable anomaly of red-cell oxalate transport in "primary" calcium nephrolithiasis correctable with diuretics. *N Engl J Med* 1986; **314:** 599–604.

Preparations

BP 1998: Amiloride Tablets; Co-amilofruse Tablets; Co-amilozide Oral Solution; Co-amilozide Tablets;
USP 23: Amiloride Hydrochloride and Hydrochlorothiazide Tablets; Amiloride Hydrochloride Tablets.

Proprietary Preparations (details are given in Part 3)
Aust.: Midamor; ***Austral.:*** Amidal; Kaluril; Midamor; Midoride; ***Canad.:*** Midamor; ***Fr.:*** Modamide; ***Irl.:*** Berkamil; ***Neth.:*** Midamor; ***Norw.:*** Midamor; ***Swed.:*** Amikal†; Midamor; ***Switz.:*** Midamor; ***UK:*** Amilamont; Amilospare; Berkamil; Midamor†; ***USA:*** Midamor.

Multi-ingredient: ***Aust.:*** Aldoretic; Amiloretik; Amilorid comp; Lanuretic; Loradur; Moducrin; Moduretic; ***Austral.:*** Amizide; Hydrozide; Modizide; Moduretic; ***Belg.:*** Belidral; Frusamil; Kalten; Moduretic; ***Canad.:*** Apo-Amilzide; Moduret; Novamilor; Nu-Amilzide; ***Fr.:*** Logirene; Moducren; Moduretic; ***Ger.:*** Amiduret; Amilo-OPT†; Amiloretik; Amilorid comp; Amilothiazid; Amilozid; Aquaretic; Combiprotect†; Diaphal; Dignoretik; Diursan; durarese; Esmalorid; Hydrocomp; Minoremed†; Modu-Puren; Moducrin; Moduretik; Rhefluin; Tensoflux; ***Irl.:*** Amizide†; Buram; Clonuretic; Fru-Co; Frumil; Lasoride; Moducren; Moduret; Moduretic; Navispare; ***Ital.:*** Moduretic; ***Neth.:*** Elkin; Hykaten†; Moducren; Moduretic; ***Norw.:*** Moduretic Mite; Normorix; ***S.Afr.:*** Acumod; Adco-Retic; Aldoretic; Amiloretic; Amizide; Aquadrex†; Arcanaretic†; Betaretic; Cliniretic†; Diutec; Hexaretic; Moducren; Moduretic; Servatrin; Trimolex†; ***Spain:*** Ameride; Diuzine; Donicer; Frusamil†; Kalten; ***Swed.:*** Amiloferm; Moduretic; Normorix; Sparkal; ***Switz.:*** Aldoretic; Amilo-basan; Amilorid comp; Betadiur; Comilorid; Ecodurex; Esmaloride†; Frumil; Grodurex; Hydrolid; Kalten; Modisal†; Moducren; Moduretic; Rhefluin; ***UK:*** Amilco; Amilmaxco; Aridil; Burinex A; Delvas; Fresmoo Co; Fru-Co; Frumil; Frusemek; Hypertane†; Kalten; Lasoride; Moducren; Moduret; Moduretic; Navispare; Synuretic; Vasetic†; Zida-Co; ***USA:*** Moduretic.

Amiodarone Hydrochloride (7780-f)

Amiodarone Hydrochloride *(BANM, rINNM).*

Amiodaroni Hydrochloridum; L-3428 (amiodarone); 51087N (amiodarone hydrochloride); SKF-33134-A (amiodarone). 2-Butylbenzofuran-3-yl 4-(2-diethylaminoethoxy)-3,5-di-iodophenyl ketone hydrochloride.

$C_{25}H_{29}I_2NO_3,HCl = 681.8.$

CAS — 1951-25-3 (amiodarone); 19774-82-4 (amiodarone hydrochloride).

NOTE. Amiodarone is *USAN.*

Pharmacopoeias. In *Chin.* and *Eur.* (see p.viii).

A white or almost white, fine crystalline powder. Very slightly **soluble** in water; sparingly soluble in alcohol; soluble in methyl alcohol; freely soluble in dichloromethane; very slightly soluble in hexane. **Protect** from light.

Adsorption. There was a rapid fall in the concentration of solutions of amiodarone hydrochloride by 10% in 3 hours followed by a steady decrease to 60% of the initial concentration after 5 days' storage in flexible polyvinyl chloride bags at ambient temperature.[1] When amiodarone solutions were perfused through polyvinyl chloride giving sets the concentration had fallen to 82% after 15 minutes. Similar losses were not observed from solutions stored in glass or rigid polyvinyl chloride bottles, and the losses were attributed to the presence of the plasticiser, di-2-ethylhexylphthalate.

1. Weir SJ, *et al.* Sorption of amiodarone to polyvinyl chloride infusion bags and administration sets. *Am J Hosp Pharm* 1985; **42:** 2679–83.

Incompatibility. Amiodarone injection has been reported to be incompatible with aminophylline,[1] flucloxacillin,[2] heparin,[3] and sodium bicarbonate.[4] The manufacturer states that it is incompatible with sodium chloride solutions.

1. Hasegawa GR, Eder JF. Visual compatibility of amiodarone hydrochloride injection with other injectable drugs. *Am J Hosp Pharm* 1984; **41:** 1379–80.
2. Taylor A, Lewis R. Amiodarone and injectable drug incompatibility. *Pharm J* 1992; **248:** 533.
3. Cairns CJ. Incompatibility of amiodarone. *Pharm J* 1986; **236:** 68.
4. Korth-Bradley JM. Incompatibility of amiodarone hydrochloride and sodium bicarbonate injections. *Am J Health-Syst Pharm* 1995; **52:** 2340.

Stability. An oral suspension prepared from tablets and containing amiodarone hydrochloride 5 mg per mL was stable for 3 months at 4° and 6 weeks at 25°.[1]

1. Nahata MC. Stability of amiodarone in an oral suspension stored under refrigeration and at room temperature. *Ann Pharmacother* 1997; **31:** 851–2.

Adverse Effects and Treatment

Adverse effects are common with amiodarone; many are dose-related and reversible with reduction in dose.

Adverse cardiovascular effects associated with amiodarone include severe bradycardia, sinus arrest, and conduction disturbances. Severe hypotension may follow intravenous administration particularly, though not exclusively, at rapid infusion rates. Amiodarone may also give rise to ventricular tachyarrhythmias; torsade de pointes appears to be less of a problem with amiodarone than other antiarrhythmics. Rarely, heart failure may be precipitated or aggravated.

Amiodarone is reported to reduce the peripheral transformation of thyroxine (T_4) to tri-iodothyronine (T_3) and to increase the formation of reverse-T_3. It can affect thyroid function and may induce hypo- or hyperthyroidism.

There have been reports of severe pulmonary toxicity including pulmonary fibrosis and interstitial pneumonitis. These effects are usually reversible on withdrawal of amiodarone but are potentially fatal.

Amiodarone can adversely affect the liver. There may be abnormal liver function tests and cirrhosis or hepatitis; fatalities have been reported.

Prolonged treatment with amiodarone causes the development of benign yellowish-brown corneal microdeposits in the majority of patients, sometimes associated with coloured haloes of light; these are reversible on stopping therapy. Photosensitivity reactions are also common and more rarely blue-grey discoloration of the skin may occur.

Other adverse effects reported include peripheral neuropathy, myopathy, ataxia, tremor, nausea, vomiting, a metallic taste, nightmares, headaches, sleeplessness, and epididymitis.

Thrombophlebitis can occur if amiodarone is injected regularly or infused for prolonged periods into a peripheral vein. Rapid intravenous administration has been associated with anaphylactic shock, hot flushes, sweating, and nausea.

It has been suggested that amiodarone-induced phospholipidosis may explain some of its adverse effects. Amiodarone's iodine content contributes to its thyrotoxicity.

Reviews of the adverse effects of amiodarone.

1. Naccarelli GV, *et al.* Adverse effects of amiodarone: pathogenesis, incidence and management. *Med Toxicol Adverse Drug Exp* 1989; **4:** 246–53.
2. Kerin NZ, *et al.* Long-term efficacy and toxicity of high- and low-dose amiodarone regimens. *J Clin Pharmacol* 1989; **29:** 418–23.
3. Perkins MW, *et al.* Intraoperative complications in patients receiving amiodarone: characteristics and risk factors. *DICP Ann Pharmacother* 1989; **23:** 757–63.
4. Vrobel TR, *et al.* A general overview of amiodarone toxicity: its prevention, detection, and management. *Prog Cardiovasc Dis* 1989; **31:** 393–426.
5. Morgan DJR. Adverse reactions profile: amiodarone. *Prescribers' J* 1991; **31:** 104–11.
6. Committee on Safety of Medicines/Medicines Control Agency. Amiodarone (Cordarone X). *Current Problems* 1996; **22:** 3–4.

Effects on the eyes. Slit-lamp examination showed corneal abnormalities in 103 of 105 patients treated with amiodarone for 3 months to 7 years.[1] The most advanced abnormality comprised whorled patterns with uniform granular opacities. The corneal deposits became denser if amiodarone dosage was increased and regressed if dosage was reduced. Ocular symptoms were reported in only 12 patients. These were photophobia (3 patients), visual haloes (2), blurring of vision (1), and lid irritation (6), but lid irritation was considered a photosensitive skin reaction and blurred vision was probably not due to amiodarone. No patient had any deterioration in visual acuity attributable to amiodarone. In 16 patients amiodarone was withdrawn with complete clearing of corneal abnormalities within 7 months and routine ophthalmological monitoring was considered unnecessary in patients without ocular symptoms. However, optic neuropathy[2] and neuritis with visual impairment have been reported in association with amiodarone and the manufacturers recommend that annual ophthalmological examinations should be performed.

A sicca syndrome with diminished tear and saliva production has been reported[3] during amiodarone treatment.

1. Ingram DV, *et al.* Ocular changes resulting from therapy with amiodarone. *Br J Ophthalmol* 1982; **66:** 676–9.
2. Feiner LA, *et al.* Optic neuropathy and amiodarone therapy. *Mayo Clin Proc* 1987; **62:** 702–17.
3. Dickinson EJ, Wolman RL. Sicca syndrome associated with amiodarone therapy. *Br Med J* 1986; **293:** 510.

Effects on the genital system. Epididymal swelling and scrotal pain have been reported.[1,2] Symptoms occurred 7 to 20 months after the start of treatment with amiodarone and resolved within 10 weeks despite continuation of amiodarone in some patients. In one patient[2] the concentration of desethylamiodarone in semen was five times the concentration in serum.

Brown discoloration of semen and sweat has also been associated with amiodarone therapy.[3]

1. Gasparich JP, *et al.* Non-infectious epididymitis associated with amiodarone therapy. *Lancet* 1984; **ii:** 1211–12.
2. Ward MJ, *et al.* Association of seminal desethylamiodarone concentration and epididymitis with amiodarone treatment. *Br Med J* 1988; **296:** 19–20.
3. Adams PC, *et al.* Amiodarone in testis and semen. *Lancet* 1985; **i:** 341.

Effects on the heart. Amiodarone has the potential to provoke arrhythmias, but a review of the literature[1] indicated that the frequency of proarrhythmic events, including torsade de pointes, was low.

1. Hohnloser SH, *et al.* Amiodarone-associated proarrhythmic effects: a review with special reference to torsade de pointes tachycardia. *Ann Intern Med* 1994; **121:** 529–35.

Effects on lipids. Amiodarone increases phospholipid concentrations in tissues and this may be responsible for some of its adverse effects.[1] Also serum cholesterol concentrations can increase independently of any effect on the thyroid.[2,3] The effect on triglyceride concentrations is not clear.[3]

1. Kodavanti UP, Mehendale HM. Cationic amphiphilic drugs and phospholipid storage disorder. *Pharmacol Rev* 1990; **42:** 327–54.
2. Wiersinga WM, *et al.* An increase in plasma cholesterol independent of thyroid function during long-term amiodarone therapy: a dose-dependent relationship. *Ann Intern Med* 1991; **114:** 128–32.
3. Lakhdar AA, *et al.* Long-term amiodarone therapy raises serum cholesterol. *Eur J Clin Pharmacol* 1991; **40:** 477–80.

Effects on the liver. Amiodarone-induced elevation of liver enzyme concentrations without clinical symptoms of hepatic dysfunction occurs in some patients.[1] However, hepatic injury which may be severe[2] and sometimes fatal[3-7] has been reported. Hepatitis and cirrhosis have occurred and histological changes resemble those in alcoholic liver disease. Severe reversible cholestasis with hyperbilirubinaemia has also been reported.[2] Hepatotoxicity may not occur for several years after starting amiodarone but rapidly progressive fatal hepatic failure has occurred[6] only one month after starting treatment. Liver enzymes may remain elevated and hepatic injury continue to develop for several months after discontinuing amiodarone. Acute hepatitis occurring within 24 hours of intravenous administration of amiodarone has been reported.[8]

1. Simon JB, *et al.* Amiodarone hepatotoxicity simulating alcoholic liver disease. *N Engl J Med* 1984; **311:** 167–72.
2. Morse RM, *et al.* Amiodarone-induced liver toxicity. *Ann Intern Med* 1988; **109:** 838–40.

3. Lim PK, *et al.* Neuropathy and fatal hepatitis in a patient receiving amiodarone. *Br Med J* 1984; **288:** 1638–9.
4. Tordjman K, *et al.* Amiodarone and the liver. *Ann Intern Med* 1985; **102:** 411–12.
5. Rinder HM, *et al.* Amiodarone hepatotoxicity. *N Engl J Med* 1986; **314:** 318–19.
6. Lwakatare JM, *et al.* Fatal fulminating liver failure possibly related to amiodarone treatment. *Br J Hosp Med* 1990; **44:** 60–1.
7. Richer M, Robert S. Fatal hepatotoxicity following oral administration of amiodarone. *Ann Pharmacother* 1995; **29:** 582–6.
8. Pye M, *et al.* Acute hepatitis after parenteral amiodarone administration. *Br Heart J* 1988; **59:** 690–1.

Effects on the lungs. Pulmonary toxicity is one of the most severe adverse effects associated with amiodarone therapy and may occur in up to 10% of patients.[1] Interstitial and alveolar infiltration,[2] fibrosis,[3] and pneumonitis[4] have been reported. Patients often present with increasing dyspnoea, cough, and pleuritic chest pain. Most patients respond to withdrawal of amiodarone and, if necessary, treatment with corticosteroids[2] but fatalities have occurred.[3,5] Two patients with amiodarone pulmonary toxicity died less than 1 hour and 24 hours, respectively after pulmonary angiography.[6] Pulmonary toxicity appears to be dose-related[2] in some patients, but an immunological reaction occurring at low doses[4] appears to be the cause in others.

1. Martin WJ, Rosenow EC. Amiodarone pulmonary toxicity: recognition and pathogenesis. *Chest* 1988; **93:** 1067–75 (part 1) and 1242–8 (part 2).
2. Marchlinski FE, *et al.* Amiodarone pulmonary toxicity. *Ann Intern Med* 1982; **97:** 839–45.
3. Morera J, *et al.* Amiodarone and pulmonary fibrosis. *Eur J Clin Pharmacol* 1983; **24:** 591–3.
4. Venet A, *et al.* Five cases of immune-mediated amiodarone pneumonitis. *Lancet* 1984; **i:** 962–3.
5. Committee on Safety of Medicines. Recurrent ventricular tachycardia: adverse drug reactions. *Br Med J* 1986; **292:** 50.
6. Wood DL, *et al.* Amiodarone pulmonary toxicity: report of two cases associated with rapidly progressive fatal adult respiratory distress syndrome after pulmonary angiography. *Mayo Clin Proc* 1985; **60:** 601–3.

Effects on mental state. Delirium occurred 17 days after starting amiodarone therapy in a 66-year-old man.[1] Mental status returned to normal on withdrawal of amiodarone.

1. Trohman RG, *et al.* Amiodarone-induced delirium. *Ann Intern Med* 1988; **108:** 68–9.

Effects on the nervous system. Of 10 patients treated with amiodarone for more than 2 years, 3 patients had evidence of peripheral neuropathy.[1] Initial results suggested that neuropathy correlated with high doses and high serum concentrations of amiodarone.

1. Fraser AG, McQueen INF. Adverse reactions during treatment with amiodarone hydrochloride. *Br Med J* 1983; **287:** 612.

Effects on the pancreas. Pancreatitis has been reported[1] in one patient 4 days after the initiation of amiodarone therapy. Symptoms resolved following withdrawal of the drug but returned on re-exposure.

1. Bosch X, Bernadich O. Acute pancreatitis during treatment with amiodarone. *Lancet* 1997; **350:** 1300.

Effects on the skin and hair. The most common adverse skin reaction associated with amiodarone therapy is photosensitivity. This is a phototoxic rather than a photoallergic reaction[1-3] and the wavelengths responsible extend from the long-wave ultraviolet (UVA) into the visible light range.[1] Affected patients should be advised to wear protective clothing and avoid exposure to sunlight. Topical sunblock preparations, such as those containing zinc or titanium oxides, may reduce the risk of reaction and a reduction in amiodarone dosage may also be useful.[1] Although pyridoxine has been reported[4] to protect against amiodarone-induced photosensitivity, results from a double-blind placebo-controlled study[5] indicated that it may enhance the photosensitivity. Photosensitivity may continue for several weeks after withdrawal of amiodarone due to its extensive distribution.

Blue-grey[2,3] and golden-brown[3] pigmentation of light-exposed skin have been reported during long-term amiodarone therapy. The pigmentation is usually slowly reversible on withdrawing amiodarone but may not completely disappear. The mean concentrations of amiodarone and its desethyl metabolite in light-exposed pigmented skin have been found to be 10 times the concentrations in non-exposed skin.[2]

Cutaneous vasculitis,[6,7] exfoliative dermatitis,[8] and fatal toxic epidermal necrolysis[9] have been reported during amiodarone therapy. Alopecia[10,11] has been associated with amiodarone therapy but increased hair growth,[3] possibly due to the vasodilatory activity of amiodarone, has also been reported.

1. Ferguson J, *et al.* Prevention of amiodarone-induced photosensitivity. *Lancet* 1984; **ii:** 414.
2. Zachary CB, *et al.* The pathogenesis of amiodarone-induced pigmentation and photosensitivity. *Br J Dermatol* 1984; **110:** 451–6.
3. Ferguson J, *et al.* A study of cutaneous photosensitivity induced by amiodarone. *Br J Dermatol* 1985; **113:** 537–49.
4. Kaufmann G. Pyridoxine against amiodarone-induced photosensitivity. *Lancet* 1984; **i:** 51–2.
5. Mulrow JP, *et al.* Pyridoxine and amiodarone-induced photosensitivity. *Ann Intern Med* 1985; **103:** 68–9.
6. Starke ID, Barbatis C. Cutaneous vasculitis associated with amiodarone therapy. *Br Med J* 1985; **291:** 940.
7. Gutierrez R, *et al.* Vasculitis associated with amiodarone treatment. *Ann Pharmacother* 1994; **28:** 537.
8. Moots RJ, Banerjee A. Exfoliative dermatitis after amiodarone treatment. *Br Med J* 1988; **296:** 1332–3.
9. Bencini PL, *et al.* Toxic epidermal necrolysis and amiodarone treatment. *Arch Dermatol* 1985; **121:** 838.
10. Samanta A, *et al.* Adverse reactions during treatment with amiodarone hydrochloride. *Br Med J* 1983; **287:** 503.
11. Samuel LM, *et al.* Amiodarone and hair loss. *Postgrad Med J* 1992; **68:** 771.

Effects on thyroid function. The majority of euthyroid patients receiving amiodarone therapy remain clinically euthyroid. However, serum concentrations of thyroid hormones may be altered and can complicate the interpretation of thyroid function tests. Administration of amiodarone results in a reduction of the peripheral conversion of thyroxine (T_4) to tri-iodothyronine (T_3) with a resulting increase in T_4, a modest fall in T_3, and an increase in reverse-T_3 concentrations; the basal serum-TSH (thyroid-stimulating hormone; thyrotrophin) concentration rises transiently during the first several months of treatment.[1-4]

Occasionally patients become clinically hypo- or hyperthyroid and the prevalence appears to correlate with dietary iodine intake. The incidence of hyperthyroidism in amiodarone-treated patients in West Tuscany, Italy, an area where iodine intake is low, was 9.6% compared with an incidence of 2% in similar patients in Worcester, USA, an area where iodine intake is normal. The incidence of hypothyroidism in these patients was 5% and 22% respectively.[1] Each amiodarone molecule contains 2 atoms of iodine, representing about 37.5% of the mass of amiodarone hydrochloride; hence each 200-mg tablet contains about 75 mg of iodine.[1,5] This large iodine load probably contributes to the development of hypo- or hyperthyroidism in patients with an underlying subclinical thyroid defect. Auto-immune mechanisms may also contribute and antithyroid antibodies have developed during amiodarone therapy.

Assessment of thyroid function is recommended in patients before starting amiodarone treatment and periodically during treatment. Patients with amiodarone-induced hyperthyroidism may present with tachycardia, tremor, weight loss, nervousness, irritability, reappearance of angina, or a worsening of arrhythmia. An ultrasensitive TSH assay should be used to confirm the diagnosis of hypo- or hyperthyroidism.

Hypothyroidism is usually treated with thyroxine starting with a low dose and gradually increasing until control is achieved; amiodarone may be continued.[1-4]

Hyperthyroidism may be treated with the thiourea drugs carbimazole, methimazole, or propylthiouracil;[1-6] although withdrawal of amiodarone has been advocated it may be continued if necessary. Potassium perchlorate has also been used[5] with a thiourea to reduce the thyroid iodine load. Radio-iodine can be used[1] but may not be effective if the uptake of radio-iodine by the thyroid is low due to the iodine load from amiodarone. Corticosteroids may also be used.[2-4] Thyroidectomy has been successfully used[7] in the treatment of resistant amiodarone-induced hyperthyroidism.

1. Figge HL, Figge J. The effects of amiodarone on thyroid hormone function: a review of the physiology and clinical manifestations. *J Clin Pharmacol* 1990; **30:** 588–95.
2. Harjai KJ, Licata AA. Effects of amiodarone on thyroid function. *Ann Intern Med* 1997; **126:** 63–73.
3. Kumar A, Borsey DQ. Amiodarone-related thyroid dysfunction. *Br J Hosp Med* 1994; **52:** 283–9.
4. Newman CM, *et al.* Amiodarone and the thyroid: a practical guide to the management of thyroid dysfunction induced by amiodarone therapy. *Heart* 1998; **79:** 121–7.
5. Reichert LJM, de Rooy HAM. Treatment of amiodarone induced hyperthyroidism with potassium perchlorate and methimazole during amiodarone treatment. *Br Med J* 1989; **298:** 1547–8.
6. Davies PH, *et al.* Treatment of amiodarone induced thyrotoxicosis with carbimazole alone and continuation of amiodarone. *Br Med J* 1992; **305:** 224–5.
7. Farwell AP, *et al.* Thyroidectomy for amiodarone-induced thyrotoxicosis. *JAMA* 1990; **263:** 1526–8.

Precautions

Amiodarone should not be given to patients with bradycardia, atrioventricular block, severe hypotension, or severe respiratory failure. It may be used with caution in patients with heart failure. Electrolyte disorders should be corrected before starting treatment. The use of amiodarone should be avoided in patients with iodine sensitivity, disorders of the thyroid gland, or with a history of thyroid disorders. Patients taking amiodarone should avoid exposure to sunlight. Amiodarone is contra-indicated in breast-feeding women.

Thyroid function should be monitored regularly in order to detect amiodarone-induced hyper- or hypothyroidism. Thyroxine, tri-iodothyronine, and thyrotrophin (thyroid-stimulating hormone; TSH) concentrations should be measured; clinical assessment alone is unreliable. See also under Effects on Thyroid Function in Adverse Effects and Treatment, above.

Tests of liver and pulmonary function also should be carried out regularly in patients on long-term therapy. Ophthalmological examinations should be performed annually. Although urinary excretion is not a major route for the elimination of amiodarone or its metabolites, some have nevertheless advised caution in patients with moderate or severe renal impairment because of the possibility of iodine accumulation.

Intravenous injections of amiodarone should be given slowly: if prolonged or repeated infusions are envisaged, the use of a central venous catheter should be considered.

Administration. For the problems of controlling the delivery rate of amiodarone by intravenous infusion, see under Uses and Administration, below.

Breast feeding. Amiodarone may be excreted in significant amounts in breast milk[1,2] and is therefore contra-indicated in women who are breast feeding.

1. Pitcher D, *et al.* Amiodarone in pregnancy. *Lancet* 1983; **i:** 597–8.
2. Plomp TA, *et al.* Use of amiodarone during pregnancy. *Eur J Obstet Gynecol Reprod Biol* 1992; **43:** 201–7.

Pregnancy. Each 200-mg tablet of amiodarone contains about 75 mg of iodine. The uncertainty as to the effect of this iodine on the fetus has largely limited the use of amiodarone in pregnancy since iodine freely crosses the placenta and may cause thyroid disorders in the fetus. There are reports[1-3] of the use of amiodarone during pregnancy without any adverse effects appearing in the neonate, although transient biochemical hyperthyroidism or hypothyroidism in two neonates has been reported.[4] Amiodarone and desethylamiodarone both cross the placenta and at delivery their respective concentrations in cord blood are about 10% and 25% of the maternal plasma concentrations.

1. Pitcher D, *et al.* Amiodarone in pregnancy. *Lancet* 1983; **i:** 597–8.
2. Robson DJ, *et al.* Use of amiodarone during pregnancy. *Postgrad Med J* 1985; **61:** 75–7.
3. Rey E, *et al.* Effects of amiodarone during pregnancy. *Can Med Assoc J* 1987; **136:** 959–60.
4. Plomp TA, *et al.* Use of amiodarone during pregnancy. *Eur J Obstet Gynecol Reprod Biol* 1992; **43:** 201–7.

Interactions

Amiodarone should be used with caution with other drugs liable to induce bradycardia, such as beta blockers or calcium-channel blockers, and with other antiarrhythmic drugs. Concomitant administration with arrhythmogenic drugs, for example phenothiazine antipsychotics, tricyclic antidepressants, halofantrine, and terfenadine, should be avoided. The effects of warfarin and other oral anticoagulants and of clonazepam may be enhanced by concomitant administration of amiodarone, and plasma concentrations of cyclosporin, digoxin, flecainide, phenytoin, procainamide, and quinidine may be raised. Further information on these interactions is given under the individual drug monographs. Plasma-amiodarone concentrations may be decreased by phenytoin and increased by cimetidine and other inhibitors of metabolising enzymes including HIV-protease inhibitors.

Reviews.

1. Marcus FI. Drug interactions with amiodarone. *Am Heart J* 1983; **106:** 924–30.
2. Lesko LJ. Pharmacokinetic drug interactions with amiodarone. *Clin Pharmacokinet* 1989; **17:** 130–40.

Cimetidine. Cimetidine inhibits hepatic metabolism and an increase in the serum-amiodarone concentration has been reported[1] in 8 out of 12 patients given amiodarone and cimetidine concurrently.

1. Hogan C, *et al.* Cimetidine-amiodarone interaction. *J Clin Pharmacol* 1988; **28:** 909.

Phenytoin. The interaction between phenytoin and amiodarone resulting in increased plasma-phenytoin concentrations is widely recognised (see p.354). However, phenytoin is a hepatic enzyme inducer and has been reported[1] to decrease serum-amiodarone concentrations by 32 and 49% after 1 and 2 weeks of concurrent administration.

1. Nolan PE, *et al.* Effect of phenytoin on the clinical pharmacokinetics of amiodarone. *J Clin Pharmacol* 1990; **30:** 1112–19.

Pharmacokinetics

Amiodarone is absorbed variably and erratically from the gastro-intestinal tract.

Amiodarone is extensively distributed to body tissues and accumulates notably in muscle and fat; it has been reported to be 96% bound to plasma proteins. The terminal elimination half-life is about 50 days with a range of about 20 to 100 days due to its extensive tissue distribution. On stopping prolonged amiodarone therapy a pharmacological effect is evident for a month or more. One metabolite, desethylamiodarone, has been identified and this also has antiarrhythmic properties. There is very little urinary excretion of amiodarone or its metabolites, the major route of excretion being in faeces via the bile; some enterohepatic recycling may occur. Amiodarone and desethylamiodarone are reported to cross the placenta and to appear in breast milk.

Following intravenous injection the maximum effect is achieved within 1 to 30 minutes and persists for 1 to 3 hours.

Reviews.

1. Latini R, *et al.* Clinical pharmacokinetics of amiodarone. *Clin Pharmacokinet* 1984; **9:** 136–56.

Uses and Administration

Amiodarone is predominantly a class III antiarrhythmic (p.776). It is used in the control of ventricular and supraventricular **arrhythmias**, including arrhythmias associated with Wolff-Parkinson-White syndrome. It has been tried as an antiarrhythmic to prevent arrhythmias in patients with myocardial infarction or heart failure.

Amiodarone is given by mouth as the hydrochloride in initial doses of 200 mg three times daily for a week, then 200 mg twice daily for a week, and then a usual maintenance dosage of 200 mg or less daily, according to the patient's response. Loading doses of up to 1600 mg daily for 1 to 3 weeks, followed by 600 to 800 mg daily for a month, and usual maintenance doses of up to 400 mg daily, are used in the USA. Consideration should be given to potential adverse effects, and patients should be given the minimum effective dose.

Amiodarone hydrochloride may be given intravenously where facilities for close monitoring of cardiac function and resuscitation are available. It is given by intravenous infusion usually in a dose of 5 mg per kg body-weight in 250 mL of glucose 5%, infused over 20 minutes to 2 hours; further doses may be given up to a maximum in 24 hours of 1.2 g in up to 500 mL of glucose 5%. Repeated infusions are preferably made through a central venous catheter. In emergencies it may also be given in doses of 150 to 300 mg in 10 to 20 mL of glucose by slow intravenous injection over a period of not less than 3 minutes; a second injection should not be given until at least 15 minutes after the first. The UK manufacturers state that sodium chloride is not a suitable vehicle for administration of amiodarone hydrochloride injection.

General references.

1. Gill J, *et al.* Amiodarone: an overview of its pharmacological properties, and review of its therapeutic use in cardiac arrhythmias. *Drugs* 1992; **43:** 69–110.
2. Podrid PJ. Amiodarone: reevaluation of an old drug. *Ann Intern Med* 1995; **122:** 689–70.
3. Swanton H. Amiodarone. *Br J Hosp Med* 1997; **58:** 329–32.

Administration. Addition of amiodarone hydrochloride to an intravenous infusion solution reduces the drop size delivered[1,2] and the reduction in size is greater as the concentration of amiodarone is increased. This resulted in a reduction of about 30% in the expected delivery rate when amiodarone hydrochloride 1200 mg was administered in glucose 5% 500 mL.[1] The reduction in drop size has been attributed to a reduction in surface tension caused by inclusion of Tween 80 [polysorbate 80] in the commercial injection.[1] Allowances should be made for the changes in drop size causing a reduction of the delivery rate of infusions of amiodarone hydrochloride.

1. Capps PA, Robertson AL. Influence of amiodarone injection on the delivery rate of intravenous fluids. *Pharm J* 1985; **234:** 14–15.
2. Chouhan UM, Lynch E. Amiodarone intravenous infusion. *Pharm J* 1985; **235:** 466.

Cardiac arrhythmias. Amiodarone is an effective drug for the management of supraventricular and ventricular arrhythmias[1-3,15] (p.782). It is useful for the treatment of supraventricular arrhythmias associated with the Wolff-Parkinson-White syndrome[2,3] and for both the acute conversion and long-term management of atrial fibrillation.[3] It has been used orally and intravenously in infants and children[4,5] and has been given by various routes to terminate fetal arrhythmias.[13] It is also useful for controlling both atrial and ventricular arrhythmias associated with hypertrophic **cardiomyopathy**[2,3] and may reduce the incidence of sudden death in these patients. It is effective in the management of malignant ventricular arrhythmias although there are few comparative studies with other antiarrhythmics.[1-3] Amiodarone's relative lack of negative inotropic activity compared with class I antiarrhythmics makes it particularly useful for ventricular arrhythmias associated with impaired left ventricular function.[2] See under Heart Failure, below, for the use of amiodarone in the treatment of **heart failure**.

Amiodarone has also been investigated in patients with asymptomatic ventricular arrhythmias surviving **myocardial infarction** (BASIS: the Basel Antiarrhythmic Study of Infarct Survival,[6,7] CAMIAT: the Canadian Amiodarone Myocardial Infarction Arrhythmia Trial,[8] and EMIAT: the European Myocardial Infarct Amiodarone Trial[9]). Improved mortality rates were reported in the BASIS study,[6,7] but neither CAMIAT[8] nor EMIAT[9] showed a reduction in total mortality, although both studies reported a reduction in risk of arrhythmic death. However, meta-analysis of studies using amiodarone found a small reduction in total mortality suggesting that amiodarone might be of benefit after myocardial infarction in patients, such as those with heart failure, at high risk of arrhythmic death.[14]

While amiodarone can cause torsade de pointes it appears to do so rarely[10,11] and patients who have experienced this form of ventricular tachycardia as a result of other antiarrhythmic therapy have been given amiodarone subsequently without a recurrence.[12] However, amiodarone has generally been withheld until other appropriate antiarrhythmics have been tried because of its toxicity and the difficulty of instituting and evaluating other therapies after discontinuation of amiodarone.[1,3] The lower doses of amiodarone employed in Europe may be more acceptable than the higher doses that have been used in the US.

1. Mason JW. Amiodarone. *N Engl J Med* 1987; **316:** 455–66. Correction. *ibid.*; 760.
2. Counihan PJ, McKenna WJ. Risk-benefit assessment of amiodarone in the treatment of cardiac arrhythmias. *Drug Safety* 1990; **5:** 286–304.
3. Katritsis D, Camm AJ. Amiodarone in long term prophylaxis. *Drugs* 1991; **41** (suppl 2): 54–66.
4. Shuler CO, *et al.* Efficacy and safety of amiodarone in infants. *Am Heart J* 1993; **125:** 1430–2.
5. Figa FH, *et al.* Clinical efficacy and safety of intravenous amiodarone in infants and children. *Am J Cardiol* 1994; **74:** 573–7.
6. Burkart F, *et al.* Effect of antiarrhythmic therapy on mortality in survivors of myocardial infarction with asymptomatic complex ventricular arrhythmias: Basel Antiarrhythmic Study of Infarct Survival (BASIS). *J Am Coll Cardiol* 1990; **16:** 1711–18.
7. Pfisterer ME, *et al.* Long-term benefit of 1-year amiodarone treatment for persistent complex ventricular arrhythmias after myocardial infarction. *Circulation* 1993; **87:** 309–11.
8. Cairns JA, *et al.* Randomised trial of outcome after myocardial infarction in patients with frequent or repetitive ventricular premature depolarisations: CAMIAT. *Lancet* 1997; **349:** 675–82.
9. Julian DG, *et al.* Randomised trial of effect of amiodarone on mortality in patients with left-ventricular dysfunction after recent myocardial infarction: EMIAT. *Lancet* 1997; **349:** 667–74. Corrections. *ibid.*; 1180 and 1776.
10. Naccarelli GV, *et al.* Adverse effects of amiodarone: pathogenesis, incidence and management. *Med Toxicol Adverse Drug Exp* 1989; **4:** 246–53.
11. Hohnloser SH, *et al.* Amiodarone-associated proarrhythmic effects: a review with special reference to torsade de pointes tachycardia. *Ann Intern Med* 1994; **121:** 529–35.
12. Mattioni TA, *et al.* Amiodarone in patients with previous drug-mediated torsade de pointes: long-term safety and efficacy. *Ann Intern Med* 1989; **111:** 574–80.
13. Flack NJ, *et al.* Amidoarone given by three routes to terminate fetal atrial flutter associated with severe hydrops. *Obstet Gynecol* 1993; **82:** 714–16.
14. Amiodarone Trials Meta-Analysis Investigators. Effect of prophylactic amiodarone on mortality after acute myocardial infarction and in congestive heart failure: meta-analysis of individual data from 6500 patients in randomised trials. *Lancet* 1997; **350:** 1417–24.
15. Desai AD, *et al.* The role of intravenous amiodarone in the management of cardiac arrhythmias. *Ann Intern Med* 1997; **127:** 294–303. Correction. *ibid.* 1998; **128:** 505.

Heart failure. Although antiarrhythmics are not routinely recommended in the management of heart failure (p.785), those such as amiodarone that have no significant negative inotropic effect may have a role in some patients since sudden deaths have been attributed to ventricular arrhythmias in patients with severe heart failure. In the GESICA study (Grupo de Estudio de la Sobrevida en la Insuficiencia Cardiaca en Argentina)[1] amiodarone appeared to reduce mortality in patients with severe chronic heart failure, but without symptomatic ventricular arrhythmias. An improvement in functional capacity was also noted. The decrease in mortality appeared to be greater than could be expected from antiarrhythmic activity alone. However, in the CHF-STAT study (Survival Trial of Antiarrhythmic Therapy in Congestive Heart Failure)[2] involving patients with heart failure and premature ventricular contractions, overall survival did not appear to be improved by amiodarone. A meta-analysis[3] including these and 3 further trials concluded that amiodarone reduced the rate of arrhythmic or sudden death in high-risk patients and that this resulted in an overall reduction in mortality.

1. Doval HC, *et al.* Randomised trial of low-dose amiodarone in severe congestive heart failure. *Lancet* 1994; **344:** 493–8.
2. Singh SN, *et al.* Amiodarone in patients with congestive heart failure and asymptomatic ventricular arrhythmia. *N Engl J Med* 1995; **333:** 77–82.
3. Amiodarone Trials Meta-Analysis Investigators. Effect of prophylactic amiodarone on mortality after acute myocardial infarction and in congestive heart failure: meta-analysis of individual data from 6500 patients in randomised trials. *Lancet* 1997; **350:** 1417–24.

Preparations

BP 1998: Amiodarone Intravenous Infusion; Amiodarone Tablets.

Proprietary Preparations (details are given in Part 3)
Aust.: Sedacoron; ***Austral.:*** Aratac; Cordarone X; ***Belg.:*** Cordarone; ***Canad.:*** Cordarone; ***Fr.:*** Corbionax; Cordarone; ***Ger.:*** Cordarex; Tachydaron; ***Irl.:*** Cordarone X; ***Ital.:*** Amiodar; Cordarone; ***Neth.:*** Cordarone; ***Norw.:*** Cordarone; ***S.Afr.:*** Cordarone X; ***Spain:*** Ortacrone†; Trangorex; ***Swed.:*** Cordarone; ***Switz.:*** Cordarone; ***UK:*** Amidox; Cordarone X; ***USA:*** Cordarone; Pacerone.

Amlodipine Besylate (10499-b)

Amlodipine Besylate *(BANM, USAN).*

Amlodipine Besilate *(rINNM)*; Amlodipine Monobenzenesulphonate; UK-48340-26; UK-48340-11 (amlodipine maleate). 3-Ethyl 5-methyl 2-(2-aminoethoxymethyl)-4-(2-chlorophenyl)-1,4-dihydro-6-methylpyridine-3,5-dicarboxylate monobenzenesulphonate.

$C_{20}H_{25}ClN_2O_5,C_6H_6O_3S$ = 567.1.

CAS — 88150-42-9 (amlodipine); 111470-99-6 (amlodipine besylate); 88150-47-4 (amlodipine maleate).

NOTE. Amlodipine Maleate is *USAN*.

Amlodipine besylate 6.9 mg is approximately equivalent to 5 mg of amlodipine.

Adverse Effects, Treatment, and Precautions

As for dihydropyridine calcium-channel blockers (see Nifedipine, p.916).

Of 1091 patients prescribed amlodipine for hypertension, 128 (11.7%) discontinued the drug because of adverse effects.[1] The commonest side-effects were ankle oedema, flushing, headache, skin rash, and fatigue.

1. Benson E, Webster J. The tolerability of amlodipine in hypertensive patients. *Br J Clin Pharmacol* 1995; **39:** 578P–579P.

Interactions

As for dihydropyridine calcium-channel blockers (see Nifedipine, p.918).

Pharmacokinetics

Amlodipine is well absorbed following oral administration with peak blood concentrations occurring after 6 to 12 hours. The bioavailability is about 60 to 65%. It has a prolonged terminal elimination half-life of 35 to 50 hours and steady-state plasma concentrations are not achieved until after 7 to 8 days of administration. Amlodipine is extensively metabolised in the liver; metabolites are mostly excreted in urine together with less than 10% of a dose as unchanged drug. Amlodipine is reported to be about 97.5% bound to plasma protein.

General reviews.

1. Meredith PA, Elliott HL. Clinical pharmacokinetics of amlodipine. *Clin Pharmacokinet* 1992; **22:** 22–31.

Absorption. Results of studies involving 24 healthy subjects indicated that absorption of amlodipine from a capsule was equivalent to that from a solution, suggesting that the slow transfer of amlodipine into the blood is a property of the drug not of the dosage form; it was also shown that absorption was not affected by food.[1]

1. Faulkner JK, *et al.* Absorption of amlodipine unaffected by food: solid dose equivalent to solution dose. *Arzneimittelforschung* 1989; **39:** 799–801.

Metabolism. Characterisation of the metabolites of amlodipine in *animals* and in human subjects.[1] Metabolism of amlodipine is complex and extensive, and in common with other dihydropyridines oxidation to the pyridine analogue represents a major step. About 5% of a dose was recovered from urine as unchanged amlodipine.

1. Beresford AP, *et al.* Biotransformation of amlodipine. *Arzneimittelforschung* 1989; **39:** 201–9.

Uses and Administration

Amlodipine is a dihydropyridine calcium-channel blocker with actions similar to those of nifedipine (p.919). It is used in the management of hypertension (p.788) and angina pectoris (p.780).

Amlodipine is given by mouth as the besylate, but doses are usually expressed in terms of the base.

In **hypertension** the usual initial dose is 5 mg once daily, increased, if necessary, to 10 mg once daily. Similar doses are given in the treatment of stable **angina** and Prinzmetal's angina.

Reviews.

1. Murdoch D, Heel RC. Amlodipine: a review of its pharmacodynamic and pharmacokinetic properties, and therapeutic use in cardiovascular disease. *Drugs* 1991; **41:** 478–505.
2. Haria M, Wagstaff AJ. Amlodipine: a reappraisal of its pharmacological properties and therapeutic use in cardiovascular disease. *Drugs* 1995; **50:** 560–86.

Preparations

Proprietary Preparations (details are given in Part 3)
Aust.: Norvasc; ***Austral.:*** Norvasc; ***Belg.:*** Amlor; ***Canad.:*** Norvasc; ***Fr.:*** Amlor; ***Ger.:*** Norvasc; ***Irl.:*** Istin; ***Ital.:*** Antacal; Monopina; Norvasc; ***Jpn:*** Amlodin; ***Neth.:*** Norvasc; ***Norw.:*** Norvasc; ***S.Afr.:*** Norvasc; ***Spain:*** Astudal; Norvas; ***Swed.:*** Norvasc; ***Switz.:*** Norvasc; ***UK:*** Istin; ***USA:*** Norvasc.

Multi-ingredient: ***USA:*** Lotrel.

Amosulalol Hydrochloride (18755-f)

Amosulalol Hydrochloride *(rINNM)*.

YM-09538. (±)-5-(1-Hydroxy-2-{[2-(*o*-methoxyphenoxy)ethyl]amino}ethyl)-*o*-toluenesulphonamide hydrochloride.

$C_{18}H_{24}N_2O_5S,HCl = 416.9$.

CAS — 85320-68-9 (amosulalol); 70958-86-0 (amosulalol hydrochloride); 93633-92-2 (amosulalol hydrochloride).

Amosulalol is a beta blocker (p.828). In addition, it has alpha-blocking activity. It is given by mouth as the hydrochloride in the management of hypertension.

Preparations

Proprietary Preparations (details are given in Part 3)
Jpn: Lowgan.

Amrinone (12373-g)

Amrinone *(BAN, USAN, rINN)*.

Win-40680. 5-Amino-3,4′-bipyridyl-6(1*H*)-one.

$C_{10}H_9N_3O = 187.2$.

CAS — 60719-84-8.

Pharmacopoeias. In US.

Protect from light.

Amrinone Lactate (18497-x)

Amrinone Lactate *(BANM, rINNM)*.

$C_{10}H_9N_3O,C_3H_6O_3 = 277.3$.

CAS — 75898-90-7.

Amrinone lactate injection has been reported to be physically **incompatible** with glucose-containing solutions and with frusemide.

Amrinone lactate 1.48 mg is approximately equivalent to 1 mg of amrinone.

Amrinone, as the lactate salt, was reported[1] to be visually and chemically compatible with digoxin, potassium chloride, procainamide hydrochloride, propranolol hydrochloride, and verapamil hydrochloride, at a range of concentrations in sodium chloride 0.45%. Precipitation occurred when amrinone was mixed with sodium bicarbonate injection, probably because of the reduced solubility of amrinone in alkaline solutions.

1. Riley CM, Junkin P. Stability of amrinone and digoxin, procainamide hydrochloride, propranolol hydrochloride, sodium bicarbonate, potassium chloride, or verapamil hydrochloride in intravenous admixtures. *Am J Hosp Pharm* 1991; **48:** 1245–52.

Adverse Effects

Amrinone produces gastro-intestinal disturbances that may necessitate withdrawal of treatment. It produces dose-dependent thrombocytopenia. Hepatotoxicity may occur, particularly during long-term oral treatment. Hypotension and cardiac arrhythmias have been reported. Other adverse effects include headache, fever, chest pain, hypersensitivity reactions including myositis and vasculitis, nail discoloration, and decreased tear production. Local pain and burning may occur at the site of intravenous injection.

The adverse effects associated with oral administration have made this route unacceptable and amrinone is now only employed intravenously for short-term use. Studies with other inotropic phosphodiesterase inhibitors have shown that their prolonged oral administration can increase the mortality rate.

References.

1. Wynne J, *et al.* Oral amrinone in refractory congestive heart failure. *Am J Cardiol* 1980; **45:** 1245–9.
2. Wilmshurst PT, Webb-Peploe MM. Side effects of amrinone therapy. *Br Heart J* 1983; **49:** 447–51.
3. Wilmshurst PT, *et al.* The effects of amrinone on platelet count, survival and function in patients with congestive cardiac failure. *Br J Clin Pharmacol* 1984; **17:** 317–24.
4. Silverman BD, *et al.* Clinical effects and side effects of amrinone: a study of 24 patients with chronic congestive heart failure. *Arch Intern Med* 1985; **145:** 825–9.
5. Webster MWI, Sharpe DN. Adverse effects associated with the newer inotropic agents. *Med Toxicol* 1986; **1:** 335–42.
6. Mattingly PM, *et al.* Pancytopenia secondary to short-term, high-dose intravenous infusion of amrinone. *DICP Ann Pharmacother* 1990; **24:** 1172–4.
7. Ross MP, *et al.* Amrinone-associated thrombocytopenia: pharmacokinetic analysis. *Clin Pharmacol Ther* 1993; **53:** 661–7.

Precautions

Amrinone should be used with caution in severe obstructive aortic or pulmonary valvular disease or in hypertrophic cardiomyopathy. Blood pressure and heart rate should be monitored during parenteral amrinone administration. The fluid and electrolyte balance should be maintained. Platelet counts and liver function should also be monitored.

Pharmacokinetics

Amrinone is rapidly absorbed from the gastro-intestinal tract although it is no longer given orally because of an unacceptable level of adverse effects when administered by this route. The half-life is variable and has been reported to be about 4 hours in healthy subjects and about 6 hours in patients with heart failure after intravenous administration. Binding to plasma proteins is generally low. Amrinone is partially metabolised in the liver and excreted in the urine as the unchanged drug and its metabolites; up to about 40% is excreted as unchanged drug after intravenous administration. About 18% of an orally administered dose has been detected in the faeces over 72 hours.

General references.

1. Rocci ML, Wilson H. The pharmacokinetics and pharmacodynamics of newer inotropic agents. *Clin Pharmacokinet* 1987; **13:** 91–109. Correction. *ibid.* 1988; **14:** (contents page).

Infants. For reference to the pharmacokinetics of amrinone in neonates and infants, see under Uses and Administration, below.

Renal impairment. Studies in a child with multi-organ failure and anuria[1] and in 3 adults with anuria following cardiac surgery[2] have shown that amrinone is effectively removed by haemofiltration but clearance varies widely between patients. Non-renal clearance may also be altered in critically ill patients and monitoring of plasma-amrinone concentrations has been suggested.[2]

1. Lawless S, *et al.* Effect of continuous arteriovenous haemofiltration on pharmacokinetics of amrinone. *Clin Pharmacokinet* 1993; **25:** 80–2.
2. Hellinger A, *et al.* Elimination of amrinone during continuous veno-venous haemofiltration after cardiac surgery. *Eur J Clin Pharmacol* 1995; **48:** 57–9.

Uses and Administration

Amrinone is a phosphodiesterase inhibitor which has vasodilator and positive inotropic properties. It is used in the management of heart failure (p.785). Although amrinone is effective when administered orally this route has been associated with an unacceptable level of adverse effects, and the drug is now only given intravenously for the short-term management of heart failure unresponsive to other forms of therapy.

The mode of action has not been fully determined, but appears to involve an increase in cyclic adenosine monophosphate concentration secondary to inhibition of phosphodiesterase leading to an increased contractile force in cardiac muscle.

Amrinone is administered intravenously as the lactate and doses are expressed in terms of the base. The recommended initial loading dose is 750 µg per kg body-weight by slow intravenous injection over 2 to 3 minutes. This is followed by a maintenance infusion, although the loading dose may be repeated after 30 minutes if necessary. Maintenance doses are 5 to 10 µg per kg per minute by infusion to a usual maximum total dose (including loading doses) of 10 mg per kg in 24 hours. Doses of up to 18 mg per kg per day have been used for short periods in a limited number of patients.

General references.

1. Colucci WS, *et al.* New positive inotropic agents in the treatment of congestive heart failure: mechanisms of action and recent clinical developments. *N Engl J Med* 1986; **314:** 349–58.

Administration in infants. Pharmacokinetic and pharmacodynamic studies[1,2] in infants undergoing cardiac surgery indicated that the dose needed for infants to achieve a plasma-amrinone concentration of 2 to 7 µg per mL was an initial intravenous bolus of 3.0 to 4.5 mg per kg in divided doses followed by a continuous infusion of 10 µg per kg per minute. It was suggested that neonates should receive a similar bolus dose followed by a continuous infusion of 3 to 5 µg per kg per minute. In a further study[3] that also included some older children, amrinone clearance and volume of distribution varied widely between patients but did not appear to be related to age.

1. Lawless S, *et al.* Amrinone in neonates and infants after cardiac surgery. *Crit Care Med* 1989; **17:** 751–4.
2. Lawless ST, *et al.* The acute pharmacokinetics and pharmacodynamics of amrinone in pediatric patients. *J Clin Pharmacol* 1991; **31:** 800–3.
3. Allen-Webb EM, *et al.* Age-related amrinone pharmacokinetics in a pediatric population. *Crit Care Med* 1994; **22:** 1016–24.

Preparations

USP 23: Amrinone Injection.

Proprietary Preparations (details are given in Part 3)
Belg.: Inocor; ***Canad.:*** Inocor; ***Fr.:*** Inocor; ***Ger.:*** Wincoram; ***Ital.:*** Inocor; Vesistol†; ***Jpn:*** Amcoral; ***Spain:*** Wincoram; ***Swed.:*** Inocor; ***Switz.:*** Inocor†; ***USA:*** Inocor.

Ancrod (4804-y)

Ancrod *(BAN, USAN, rINN)*.

CAS — 9046-56-4.

Ancrod is an enzyme obtained from the venom of the Malayan pit-viper (*Calloselasma rhodostoma = Agkistrodon rhodostoma*).

Units

The first International Reference Preparation of ancrod was established in 1976 and contains 55 units in 16.90 mg of purified ancrod (1 unit in about 307 µg).

Adverse Effects and Treatment

Haemorrhage may occur during treatment with ancrod and usually responds to its withdrawal. If severe it may be treated by an antivenom, each mL of which is sufficient to neutralise 70 units of ancrod. An initial dose of 0.2 mL is given subcutaneously, followed in the absence of untoward reaction after 30 minutes by 0.8 mL intramuscularly; in the absence of untoward reaction 1 mL is then given intravenously 30 minutes later. In emergency the intramuscular dose may be omitted in the absence of untoward reaction to the subcutaneous dose. In life-threatening haemorrhage it may be necessary to give the antivenom intravenously without prior test doses but with adrenaline, antihistamines, and corticosteroids available against the possibility of anaphylactic shock. Fibrinogen 5 g or 1 litre of fresh blood or plasma should also be given to restore the fibrinogen concentration. Cryoprecipitate may also be used.

Precautions

As for Heparin, p.880.

Ancrod should not be given to patients with severe infections or disseminated intravascular coagulation. It should be used cautiously in patients with cardiovascular disorders that may be complicated by defibrination. It is very important that when ancrod is given by intravenous infusion it should be administered slowly to prevent the formation of large amounts of unstable fibrin.

High doses of ancrod have caused fetal death in *animals* as a result of placental haemorrhage and ancrod is not, therefore, recommended during pregnancy.

Interactions

Ancrod should not be administered concomitantly with antifibrinolytics such as aminocaproic acid or with plasma volume expanders such as dextrans.

Uses and Administration

Ancrod is an anticoagulant. It reduces the blood concentration of fibrinogen by the cleavage of microparticles of fibrin which are rapidly removed from the circulation by fibrinolysis or phagocytosis. It reduces blood viscosity but has no effect on established thrombi. Haemostatic concentrations of fibrinogen are normally restored in about 12 hours and normal concentrations in 10 to 20 days.

Ancrod may be used in the treatment of thrombo-embolic disorders (p.801), particularly in deep-vein thrombosis and to prevent thrombosis after surgery in patients requiring anticoagulation but who have developed heparin-induced thrombocytopenia or thrombosis (see p.802). It is under investigation in the treatment of ischaemic stroke and has also been given for priapism.

For treatment of thrombo-embolic disorders ancrod is given by intravenous infusion in an initial dose of 1 to 2 units per kg body-weight in 250 to 500 mL of sodium chloride 0.9% or dextrose 5% over at least 12 hours. Maintenance doses of 0.5 to 1 unit per kg in 250 to 500 mL of infusion fluid are given over 24 hours. The blood-fibrinogen concentrations may be used to monitor treatment.

For the prevention of deep-vein thrombosis after surgery for fractured neck of a femur, 4 units per kg have been given by subcutaneous injection postoperatively, followed by 1 unit per kg daily for 4 days. Resistance has developed to ancrod.

References.

1. Cole CW, *et al.* Heparin-associated thrombocytopenia and thrombosis: optimal therapy with ancrod. *Can J Surg* 1990; **33:** 207–10.
2. Demers C, *et al.* Rapid anticoagulation using ancrod for heparin-induced thrombocytopenia. *Blood* 1991; **78:** 2194–7.

Preparations

Proprietary Preparations (details are given in Part 3)
Aust.: Arwin; ***Canad.:*** Arvin; ***Ger.:*** Arwin; ***Spain:*** Arvin; ***UK:*** Arvin†.

Angiotensin Amide (2044-t)

Angiotensin Amide *(BAN, USAN).*

Angiotensinamide *(rINN)*; NSC-107678. Asn-Arg-Val-Tyr-Val-His-Pro-Phe; [1-Asparagine,5-valine]angiotensin II.

$C_{49}H_{70}N_{14}O_{11}$ = 1031.2.

CAS — 11128-99-7 (angiotensin II); 53-73-6 (angiotensin amide).

Adverse Effects and Precautions

Rapid infusion of angiotensin amide may readily cause very severe hypertension. It should be given with caution to patients with cardiovascular disease or heart failure.

Interactions

Angiotensin amide should not be given to patients being treated with an MAOI or within 14 days of stopping such treatment as a hypertensive crisis may be precipitated.

Pharmacokinetics

Angiotensin amide is rapidly inactivated in the tissues and circulation by peptidase enzymes. When given intravenously it has a duration of action of only a few minutes.

Uses and Administration

Angiotensin amide is a vasopressor related to the naturally occurring peptide angiotensin II. It increases the peripheral resistance mainly in cutaneous, splanchnic, and renal blood vessels. The increased blood pressure is accompanied by a reflex reduction in heart rate, and cardiac output may also be reduced.

Angiotensin amide has been used in the treatment of hypotension associated with shock. It has also been given in the management of overdosage of ACE inhibitors, when conventional therapy has been ineffective.

For the management of hypotension, it is given by continuous intravenous infusion; concentrations have ranged from 1 to 10 mg per litre in sodium chloride 0.9%, glucose 5%, or other suitable diluent. Doses are adjusted according to blood pressure response; doses of up to 10 μg per minute may be adequate. Blood pressure must be monitored continuously during the infusion. Once the patient's condition improves the dosage should be reduced gradually before withdrawal.

References to the use of angiotensin amide in ACE inhibitor overdosage.

1. Jackson T, *et al.* Enalapril overdose treated with angiotensin infusion. *Lancet* 1993; **341:** 703.
2. Newby DE, *et al.* Enalapril overdose and the corrective effect of intravenous angiotensin II. *Br J Clin Pharmacol* 1995; **40:** 103–4.

Preparations

Proprietary Preparations (details are given in Part 3)
Ger.: Hypertensin†; ***Switz.:*** Hypertensine†.

Anipamil (3328-c)

Anipamil *(rINN).*

2-{3-[(*m*-Methoxyphenethyl)methylamino]propyl}-2-(*m*-methoxyphenyl)-tetradecanenitrile.

$C_{34}H_{52}N_2O_2$ = 520.8.

CAS — 83200-10-6.

Anipamil is a calcium-channel blocker related to verapamil (see p.960) which has been investigated in the treatment of hypertension and angina pectoris.

References.

1. Dies R, *et al.* Antihypertensive efficacy of anipamil in mild to moderate hypertension. *J Cardiovasc Pharmacol* 1989; **13** (suppl 4): S76–8.
2. Sørum C, *et al.* Efficacy of anipamil, a phenylalkylamine calcium antagonist, in treatment of angina pectoris. *J Cardiovasc Pharmacol* 1994; **24:** 841–5.

Anisindione (4805-j)

Anisindione *(BAN, rINN).*

2-(4-Methoxyphenyl)indan-1,3-dione.

$C_{16}H_{12}O_3$ = 252.3.

CAS — 117-37-3.

Anisindione is an orally administered indanedione anticoagulant with actions similar to those of warfarin sodium (p.964). It is used in the management of thrombo-embolic disorders (p.801) but, as the indanediones are generally more toxic than warfarin (see phenindione, p.928), its use is limited.

The usual initial dose is 300 mg on the first day, 200 mg on the second day, and 100 mg on the third. The maintenance dose may range from 25 to 250 mg daily according to coagulation tests.

During treatment with anisindione the urine may be coloured pink or orange.

Preparations

Proprietary Preparations (details are given in Part 3)
USA: Miradon.

Anistreplase (16996-d)

Anistreplase *(BAN, USAN, rINN).*

Anisoylated Plasminogen Streptokinase Activator Complex; APSAC; BRL-26921. *p*-Anisoylated (human) lys-plasminogen streptokinase activator complex (1:1).

CAS — 81669-57-0.

The manufacturer recommends that anistreplase should be **stored** at 2° to 8°.

Adverse Effects, Treatment, and Precautions

As for Streptokinase, p.948. Like streptokinase, anistreplase appears to be antigenic and may be neutralised by streptokinase antibodies.

Back pain. For references to back pain associated with anistreplase infusion, see under Streptokinase, p.948.

Interactions

As for Streptokinase, p.950.

Pharmacokinetics

Anistreplase is reported to be cleared from plasma at about half the rate of streptokinase and to have a fibrinolytic half-life of about 90 minutes. It is metabolised to the plasminogen-streptokinase complex at a steady rate.

References.

1. Gemmill JD, *et al.* A comparison of the pharmacokinetic properties of streptokinase and anistreplase in acute myocardial infarction. *Br J Clin Pharmacol* 1991; **31:** 143–7.

Uses and Administration

Anistreplase is a thrombolytic drug. It consists of a complex of the lys-form of plasminogen and streptokinase with the addition of a *p*-anisoyl group that prevents the complex activating plasminogen to plasmin. Following intravenous injection the anisoyl group undergoes deacylation at a steady rate to release the active complex which converts plasminogen to plasmin, a proteolytic enzyme which has fibrinolytic effects. The mechanisms of fibrinolysis are dilscussed further under Haemostasis on p.704.

Anistreplase is used similarly to streptokinase (p.950) in the treatment of thrombo-embolic disorders, principally to clear occlusions in coronary vessels in patients with acute myocardial infarction (p.791). It is given as a single intravenous injection in a dose of 30 units over 4 to 5 minutes, as soon as possible after the onset of symptoms.

Preparations

Proprietary Preparations (details are given in Part 3)
Aust.: Eminase; ***Belg.:*** Eminase; ***Fr.:*** Eminase; ***Ger.:*** Eminase; ***Irl.:*** Eminase†; ***Ital.:*** Eminase†; Multilase; ***Neth.:*** Eminase; ***Spain:*** Iminase; ***Switz.:*** Eminase; ***UK:*** Eminase; ***USA:*** Eminase.

Apraclonidine Hydrochloride

(3917-j)

Apraclonidine Hydrochloride *(BANM, USAN, rINNM).*

AL-02145 (apraclonidine); Aplonidine Hydrochloride; NC-14; p-Aminoclonidine. 2-[(4-Amino-2,6-dichlorophenyl)imino]imidazolidine hydrochloride; 2,6-Dichloro-N^1-imidazolidin-2-ylidene-*p*-phenylenediamine hydrochloride.

$C_9H_{10}Cl_2N_4$,HCl = 281.6.

CAS — 66711-21-5 (apraclonidine); 73218-79-8 (apraclonidine hydrochloride).

NOTE. APR is a code approved by the BP for use on single unit doses of eye drops containing apraclonidine hydrochloride where the individual container may be too small to bear all the appropriate labelling information.

Pharmacopoeias. In US.

A white to off-white, odourless or practically odourless powder. **Soluble** 1 in 34 of water, 1 in 74 of alcohol, and 1 in 13 of methyl alcohol; practically insoluble in chloroform, in ethyl acetate, and in hexanes. A 1% solution has a pH between 5.0 and 6.6. **Store** in airtight containers. Protect from light.

Apraclonidine hydrochloride 11.5 mg is approximately equivalent to 10 mg of apraclonidine.

Adverse Effects and Precautions

Adverse effects following perioperative instillation of apraclonidine into the eye include hyperaemia, lid retraction, conjunctival blanching, and mydriasis. Some patients may develop an exaggerated reduction in intra-ocular pressure. Following regular instillation an ocular intolerance reaction may occur, characterised by hyperaemia, ocular pruritus, increased tearing, ocular discomfort, and oedema of the lids and conjunctiva. Other adverse effects reported include dry mouth and nose, conjunctivitis, blurred vision, asthenia, headache, and taste disturbances. Systemic absorption may occur after application to the eye and may result in adverse effects similar to those of clonidine (p.841). Cardiovascular effects have been reported, therefore apraclonidine should be used with caution in patients with severe cardiovascular disease, including hypertension, and in patients with a history of vasovagal attacks. Drowsiness may also occur. Depression has rarely been associated with use of apraclonidine and it should be used with caution in depressed patients. Apraclonidine is contra-indicated in patients taking MAOIs; there is a possible risk of hypertension in patients receiving sympathomimetics or tricyclic antidepressants.

Uses and Administration

Apraclonidine is an alpha$_2$-adrenoceptor agonist derived from clonidine (p.841). It reduces intra-ocular pressure when instilled into the eye and is used in patients undergoing eye surgery and as an adjunct in the management of glaucoma. The reduction in intra-ocular pressure begins within an hour of instillation and is maximal after about three to five hours.

Apraclonidine is used as the hydrochloride, but the strength of an ophthalmic solution is usually expressed in terms of the base.

To control or prevent a postoperative increase in intra-ocular pressure in patients undergoing anterior segment laser surgery, one drop of a 1% solution is instilled into the eye one hour before surgery and a second drop is instilled immediately upon completion of surgery.

For short-term adjunctive therapy in patients with raised intra-ocular pressure not controlled by conventional therapy, one or two drops of a 0.5% solution may be instilled into the affected eye or eyes three times daily.

Glaucoma and ocular hypertension. Apraclonidine administered topically lowers intra-ocular pressure, probably by reducing production of aqueous humour, and is used to control intra-ocular pressure in patients undergoing eye surgery and for short-term treatment in patients with glaucoma (p.1387).

Apraclonidine 1% eye drops applied pre-operatively and/or post-operatively have been reported to minimise increases in intra-ocular pressure following ocular laser surgery[1-3] and surgical removal of cataracts.[4] The combination of apraclonidine 1% and pilocarpine 4% has been reported to produce additional benefit over either drug administered alone.[5] The manufacturers recommend that a concentration of 1% apraclonidine should be used, although satisfactory results have been reported using 0.5% eye drops.[3]

Apraclonidine may be used for short-term therapy to control intra-ocular pressure in patients with glaucoma not adequately controlled by other drugs to delay surgery or laser treatment. Long-term use has also been reported[6] but is limited by a high incidence of ocular adverse effects and the development of tachyphylaxis.

1. Robin AL. Argon laser trabeculoplasty medical therapy to prevent the intraocular pressure rise associated with argon laser trabeculoplasty. *Ophthalmic Surg* 1991; **22:** 31–7.
2. Rao BS, Badrinath SS. Efficacy and safety of apraclonidine in patients undergoing anterior segment laser surgery. *Br J Ophthalmol* 1989; **73:** 884–7.
3. Rosenberg LF, *et al.* Apraclonidine and anterior segment laser surgery: comparison of 0.5% versus 1.0% apraclonidine for prevention of postoperative intraocular pressure rise. *Ophthalmology* 1995; **102:** 1312–18.
4. Wiles SB, *et al.* Control of intraocular pressure with apraclonidine hydrochloride after cataract extraction. *Am J Ophthalmol* 1991; **111:** 184–8.
5. Dapling RB, *et al.* Influence of apraclonidine and pilocarpine alone and in combination on post laser trabeculoplasty pressure rise. *Br J Ophthalmol* 1994; **78:** 30–2.
6. Araujo SV, *et al.* Long term effect of apraclonidine. *Br J Ophthalmol* 1995; **79:** 1098–1101.

Preparations

USP 23: Apraclonidine Ophthalmic Solution.

Proprietary Preparations (details are given in Part 3)
Aust.: Iopidine; ***Austral.:*** Iopidine; ***Belg.:*** Iopidine; ***Canad.:*** Iopidine; ***Fr.:*** Iopidine; ***Ger.:*** Iopidine; ***Irl.:*** Iopidine; ***Ital.:*** Iopidine; ***Norw.:*** Iopidine; ***S.Afr.:*** Iopidine; ***Spain:*** Iopimax; ***Swed.:*** Iopidine; ***UK:*** Iopidine; ***USA:*** Iopidine.

Aprindine Hydrochloride (7781-d)

Aprindine Hydrochloride *(BANM, USAN, rINNM).*

AC-1802; Compound 83846; Compound 99170 (aprindine). *N*-(3-Diethylaminopropyl)-*N*-indan-2-ylaniline hydrochloride; *NN*-Diethyl-*N'*-indan-2-yl-*N'*-phenyltrimethylenediamine hydrochloride.

$C_{22}H_{30}N_2,HCl$ = 358.9.

CAS — 37640-71-4 (aprindine); 33237-74-0 (aprindine hydrochloride).

Adverse Effects and Precautions

Adverse effects of aprindine hydrochloride are usually dose-related and most commonly affect the CNS. They include tremor, vertigo, ataxia, diplopia, memory impairment, hallucinations, and convulsions. Gastro-intestinal effects include nausea, vomiting, and bloating. There have been reports of agranulocytosis which may be fatal. Hepatitis and cholestatic jaundice have occasionally been reported; blood and liver function tests should be performed during treatment.

Aprindine is contra-indicated in patients with advanced heart failure or severe conduction disturbances. Some manufacturers have recommended that aprindine should not be used in patients with parkinsonism or convulsive disorders. It should be used with caution in patients with bradycardia, hypotension, and hepatic or renal function impairment.

Interactions

Steady-state plasma-aprindine concentrations increased in 2 patients after the initiation of amiodarone therapy and coincided with the appearance of adverse effects.[1]

1. Southworth W, *et al.* Possible amiodarone-aprindine interaction. *Am Heart J* 1982; **104:** 323.

Pharmacokinetics

Aprindine is readily absorbed from the gastro-intestinal tract. It has a long plasma half-life, usually between 20 and 27 hours, and is about 85 to 95% bound to plasma proteins. It is excreted in the urine and the bile.

Uses and Administration

Aprindine is a class Ib antiarrhythmic (p.776) used in the management of ventricular and supraventricular arrhythmias (p.782).

Aprindine is given as the hydrochloride in usual doses of 100 mg daily by mouth; doses may range from 50 to 200 mg daily. If necessary initial doses of up to 300 mg daily may be given under strict surveillance for the first 2 to 3 days. Therapy should be monitored by ECG during initial stabilisation of the dose and intermittently thereafter. It has also been given intravenously.

References.

1. Danilo P. Aprindine. *Am Heart J* 1979; **97:** 119–24.

Preparations

Proprietary Preparations (details are given in Part 3)
Aust.: Ritmusin†; ***Belg.:*** Fiboran; ***Fr.:*** Fiboran; ***Ger.:*** Amidonal; ***Spain:*** Fiboran.

Aranidipine (17286-n)

Aranidipine *(rINN).*

(±)-Acetonyl methyl 1,4-dihydro-2,6-dimethyl-4-(*o*-nitrophenyl)-3,5-pyridinedicarboxylate.

$C_{19}H_{20}N_2O_7$ = 388.4.

CAS — 86780-90-7.

Aranidipine is a calcium-channel blocker used in the management of hypertension.

Arbutamine Hydrochloride (14332-y)

Arbutamine Hydrochloride *(BANM, USAN, rINNM).*

GP-2-121-3 (arbutamine or arbutamine hydrochloride). (*R*)-4-(1-Hydroxy-2-[4-(4-hydroxyphenyl)butylamino]ethyl)-pyrocatechol hydrochloride.

$C_{18}H_{23}NO_4,HCl$ = 353.8.

CAS — 128470-16-6 (arbutamine); 125251-66-3 (arbutamine hydrochloride).

Arbutamine hydrochloride has beta agonist properties and like dobutamine (p.860) has been used for cardiac stress testing in patients unable to exercise. For such a purpose an initial dose of 0.1 μg per kg body-weight is given intravenously by a computer-controlled delivery system over 1 minute, and the heart rate response is measured. The device then calculates the difference between the desired and actual heart rate and adjusts the infusion rate accordingly up to a maximum rate of 0.8 μg per kg per minute and a maximum total dose of 10 μg per kg.

References.

1. Anonymous. Arbutamine for stress testing. *Med Lett Drugs Ther* 1998; **40:** 19–20.

Preparations

Proprietary Preparations (details are given in Part 3)
Swed.: Genesa; ***USA:*** Genesa.

Ardeparin Sodium (17068-j)

Ardeparin Sodium *(USAN, rINN).*

WY-90493-RD.

CAS — 9041-08-1.

Ardeparin sodium is prepared by peroxide degradation of heparin obtained from the intestinal mucosa of pigs. The end chain structure appears to be the same as the starting material with no unusual sugar residues present. The molecular weight of 98% of the components is between 2000 and 15 000 and the average molecular weight is about 5500 to 6500. The degree of sulphation is about 2.7 per disaccharide unit.

Ardeparin sodium is a low-molecular-weight heparin (p.899) with anticoagulant activity used for the prevention of postoperative venous thrombo-embolism (p.802). It is given by subcutaneous injection in a dose of 50 units per kg body-weight every 12 hours, beginning on the evening of the day of surgery or the following morning and continuing for up to 14 days or until the patient is fully ambulant.

Preparations

Proprietary Preparations (details are given in Part 3)
USA: Normiflo.

Argatroban (19453-c)

Argatroban *(USAN, rINN).*

DK-7419; GN-1600; MCI-9038; MD-805. (2*R*,4*R*)-4-Methyl-1-[(*S*)-N^2-{[(*RS*)-1,2,3,4-tetrahydro-3-methyl-8-quinolyl]sulfonyl}arginyl]pipecolic acid.

$C_{23}H_{36}N_6O_5S$ = 508.6.

CAS — 74863-84-6 (anhydrous argatroban); 141396-28-3 (argatroban monohydrate).

Argatroban is a synthetic thrombin inhibitor with antiplatelet activity being investigated in thrombo-embolic disorders, including in patients with heparin-induced thrombocytopenia.

Preparations

Proprietary Preparations (details are given in Part 3)
Jpn: Novastan.

Arotinolol Hydrochloride (18779-q)

Arotinolol Hydrochloride *(rINNM).*

S-596. (±)-5-[2-{[3-(*tert*-Butylamino)-2-hydroxypropyl]thio}-4-thiazolyl]-2-thiophenecarboxamide hydrochloride.

$C_{15}H_{21}N_3O_2S_3,HCl$ = 408.0.

CAS — 68377-92-4 (arotinolol).

Pharmacopoeias. In *Jpn.*

Arotinolol is a non-cardioselective beta blocker (p.828). In addition, it has alpha$_1$-blocking activity. It is given by mouth as the hydrochloride in the management of hypertension, cardiac disorders, and essential tremor.

Preparations

Proprietary Preparations (details are given in Part 3)
Jpn: Almarl.

Atenolol (6304-s)

Atenolol *(BAN, USAN, rINN).*

Atenololum; ICI-66082. 4-(2-Hydroxy-3-isopropylaminopropoxy)phenylacetamide; 2-{*p*-[2-Hydroxy-3-(isopropylamino)propoxy]phenyl}acetamide.

$C_{14}H_{22}N_2O_3$ = 266.3.

CAS — 29122-68-7; 60966-51-0 (±).

NOTE. Compounded preparations of atenolol and chlorthalidone in the proportions, by weight, 4 parts to 1 part have the British Approved Name Co-tenidone.

Compounded preparations of atenolol and chlorthalidone in USP 23 may be represented by the name Co-tenidone.

Pharmacopoeias. In *Chin., Eur.* (see p.viii), and *US.*

A white or almost white powder. Sparingly **soluble** in water; soluble in dehydrated alcohol; slightly soluble in dichloromethane; practically insoluble in ether.

Stability. There was no appreciable loss of atenolol from an extemporaneously prepared liquid preparation containing atenolol 2 mg per mL for up to 40 days when stored at 5° or 25°.[1] The liquid was prepared by triturating crushed tablets with a diluent containing alcohol 1%, saccharin 0.05%, and macrogol '8000' 33%. Sediment formed in each container, but was considered to be due to insoluble tablet excipients rather than precipitation of atenolol.

1. Garner SS, *et al.* Stability of atenolol in an extemporaneously compounded oral liquid. *Am J Hosp Pharm* 1994; **51:** 508–11.

Adverse Effects, Treatment, and Precautions

As for beta blockers, p.828.

Breast feeding. For a report of bradycardia in a neonate following ingestion of atenolol in breast milk, see under Pharmacokinetics, below.

Effects on the gastro-intestinal tract. Reports of sclerosing peritonitis[1] and retroperitoneal fibrosis[2] in patients taking atenolol.

1. Nielsen BV, Pedersen KG. Sclerosing peritonitis associated with atenolol. *Br Med J* 1985; **290:** 518.
2. Johnson JN, McFarland J. Retroperitoneal fibrosis associated with atenolol. *Br Med J* 1980; **280:** 864.

Effects on the heart. Atenolol 2.5 mg by intravenous injection induced atrial fibrillation in 6 of 12 predisposed patients.[1]

1. Rassmussen K, *et al.* Atrial fibrillation induced by atenolol. *Eur Heart J* 1982; **3:** 276–81.

Effects on lipid metabolism. For a report of acute pancreatitis in a patient taking atenolol and metoprolol, see p.829.

Effects on the liver. A report of reversible cholestatic hepatitis in a patient receiving atenolol[1] and hepatic dysfunction in another.[2]

1. Schwartz MS, *et al.* Atenolol-associated cholestasis. *Am J Gastroenterol* 1989; **84:** 1084–6.
2. Yusuf SW, Mishra RM. Hepatic dysfunction associated with atenolol. *Lancet* 1995; **346:** 192.

Effects on vision. Visual symptoms without headache were associated with atenolol for migraine prophylaxis in a patient who had experienced a similar reaction with nadolol.[1]

1. Kumar KL, Cooney TG. Visual symptoms after atenolol therapy for migraine. *Ann Intern Med* 1990; **112:** 712–13. Correction. *ibid.*; **113:** 257.

Hypotension. Precipitous falls in blood pressure in patients with malignant hypertension may cause ischaemic damage to vital organs. Initiating treatment with 1 or 2 oral drugs is considered appropriate but not without risk. Two cases of hypotension following a single oral dose of atenolol 100 mg (27-year-old woman) and following 2 oral doses of atenolol 50 mg (51-year-old woman) have been reported.[1] The women had presented with severe hypertension, hyponatraemia, hypokalaemia, and high renin activity. There was a transient elevation of serum creatinine in both patients indicating kidney ischaemia. Renal artery thrombosis believed to be due to the hypotensive effect of atenolol was reported in a 70-year-old man with a history of circulatory and cardiac disorders.[2] He had received atenolol 100 mg for treatment of moderate hypertension.

1. Kholeif M, Isles C. Profound hypotension after atenolol in severe hypertension. *Br Med J* 1989; **298:** 161–2.
2. Shaw AB, Gopalka SK. Renal artery thrombosis caused by antihypertensive treatment. *Br Med J* 1982; **285:** 1617.

Overdosage. Ventricular asystole occurred in a man who had taken a massive overdose of atenolol.[1]

1. Stinson J, *et al.* Ventricular asystole and overdose with atenolol. *Br Med J* 1992; **305:** 693.

Interactions

The interactions associated with beta blockers are discussed on p.829.

Pharmacokinetics

Atenolol is incompletely absorbed from the gastrointestinal tract; following oral administration about 50% is absorbed. Peak plasma concentrations are reached in 2 to 4 hours. Atenolol has low lipid solubility. It crosses the placenta and is distributed into breast milk where concentrations higher than those in maternal plasma have been achieved. Only small amounts are reported to cross the blood-brain barrier, and plasma-protein binding is minimal. The plasma half-life is about 6 to 7 hours. Atenolol undergoes little or no hepatic metabolism and is excreted mainly in the urine.

Breast feeding. Atenolol diffuses into breast milk and is present in milk in concentrations similar[1] to or higher[2] than those in maternal blood. Bradycardia associated with ingestion of atenolol in breast milk has been reported in a 5-day-old term infant. The baby improved when breast feeding was discontinued.[3]

1. Thorley KJ, McAinsh J. Levels of the beta-blockers atenolol and propranolol in the breast milk of women treated for hypertension in pregnancy. *Biopharm Drug Dispos* 1983; **4:** 299–301.
2. White WB, *et al.* Atenolol in human plasma and breast milk. *Obstet Gynecol* 1984; **63:** 42S–44S.
3. Schimmel MS, *et al.* Toxic effects of atenolol consumed during breast feeding. *J Pediatr* 1989; **114:** 476–8.

Pregnancy. In 6 women who had taken atenolol for at least 6 days up to the time of delivery concentrations of atenolol in maternal and umbilical serum were approximately equal. In a further woman who had discontinued treatment one day before delivery atenolol was not found in maternal or umbilical serum.[1] The half-life of atenolol in neonates born to mothers who had been receiving atenolol ranged from 10.5 to 34.6 hours (mean 16.1 hours) in a study of 35 term infants.[2] Atenolol concentrations were determined in cord blood and in neonatal blood 24 hours after delivery. The range of elimination rate was 4 times slower than in adults, a difference expected based on renal excretion of atenolol.

1. Melander A, *et al.* Transplacental passage of atenolol in man. *Eur J Clin Pharmacol* 1978; **14:** 93–4.
2. Rubin PC, *et al.* Atenolol elimination in the neonate. *Br J Clin Pharmacol* 1983; **16:** 659–62.

Uses and Administration

Atenolol is a cardioselective beta blocker (p.828). It is reported to lack intrinsic sympathomimetic activity and membrane-stabilising properties.

Atenolol is used in the management of hypertension (p.788), angina pectoris (p.780), cardiac arrhythmias (p.782), and myocardial infarction (p.791). It may also be used in the prophylactic treatment of migraine (p.443).

In **hypertension** atenolol is given by mouth in a dose of 50 to 100 mg daily, as a single dose, although 50 mg daily is generally adequate. The full effect is usually evident within 1 to 2 weeks.

The usual dose for **angina pectoris** is 50 to 100 mg daily by mouth, given as single or divided doses. Although up to 200 mg daily has been given for angina pectoris additional benefit is not usually obtained from higher doses of atenolol.

For the emergency treatment of **cardiac arrhythmias** atenolol may be given by intravenous injection in a dose of 2.5 mg injected at a rate of 1 mg per minute, repeated if necessary every 5 minutes to a maximum total dosage of 10 mg. Alternatively atenolol may be given by intravenous infusion, a dose of 150 μg per kg body-weight being administered over 20 minutes. The injection or infusion procedure may be repeated every 12 hours if necessary. When control is achieved maintenance doses of 50 to 100 mg daily may be given by mouth.

Atenolol is also used in the early management of acute **myocardial infarction**. Treatment should be given within 12 hours of the onset of chest pain; atenolol 5 to 10 mg should be given by slow intravenous injection at a rate of 1 mg per minute and followed after 15 minutes with 50 mg by mouth, provided no adverse effects result. A further 50 mg may be given by mouth after 12 hours, and subsequent dosage maintained, after a further 12 hours, with 100 mg daily.

In the prophylaxis of **migraine** a dose of 50 to 100 mg daily by mouth has been used.

Reduced doses may be required in patients with impaired renal function, as follows. When creatinine clearance is 15 to 35 mL per minute suggested doses are 50 mg daily by mouth or 10 mg once every two days intravenously. When creatinine clearance is less than 15 mL per minute suggested doses are 25 mg daily or 50 mg on alternate days by mouth or 10 mg once every four days intravenously.

Preparations

BP 1998: Atenolol Injection; Atenolol Oral Solution; Atenolol Tablets; Co-tenidone Tablets;
USP 23: Atenolol and Chlorthalidone Tablets; Atenolol Injection; Atenolol Tablets.

Proprietary Preparations (details are given in Part 3)
Aust.: Arcablock; Atenobene; Atenolan; Betasyn; Tenormin; *Austral.:* Anselol; Atehexal; Noten; Tenlol; Tenormin; Tensig; *Belg.:* Tenormin; *Canad.:* Novo-Atenol; Nu-Atenol; Tenolin; Tenormin; *Fr.:* Betatop; Tenormine; *Ger.:* Atebeta; Atehexal; Atendol; Ateno; Atenomerck; Atereal; Blocotenol; Cuxanorm; Dignobeta; duratenol; Evitocor; Falitonsin; Jenatenol; Juvental; Taraskon†; Teno; teno-basan†; Tenormin; Tonoprotect; Unibloc†; *Irl.:* Amolin; Antipressan; Atecor; Ateni; Atenogen; Atenomel; Tenormin; Trantalol; *Ital.:* Atenol; Seles Beta; Tenormin; *Neth.:* Tenormin; Unibloc; *Norw.:* Alinor; Coratol; Tenormin; Uniloc; *S.Afr.:* Atenoblok; Aterol; B-Vasc; Clinaten†; Hexa-Blok; Ten-Bloka; Tenormin; Venapulse†; *Spain:* Blokium; Neatenol; Tenormin; *Swed.:* Alinor†; Selinol; Tenormin; Uniloc; *Switz.:* Atenil; ateno-basan mite; Atesifar; Cardaxen; Selobloc†; Servitenol; Tenat; Tenormin; *UK:* Antipressan; Atenix; Tenormin; Totamol; Vasaten†; *USA:* Tenormin.

Multi-ingredient: *Aust.:* Arcablock comp; Atenolan comp; Atenolol comp; Beta-Adalat; Nif-Ten; Polinorm; Tenoretic; *Belg.:* Beta-Adalat; Kalten; Tenif; Tenoretic; *Canad.:* Tenoretic; *Fr.:* Beta-Adalate; Tenordate; *Ger.:* Atehexal comp; Ateno comp; Atenolol AL comp; Atenolol comp; Atenomerck comp; Blocotenol comp; Bresben; Diu-Atenolol; duratenol comp; Evitocor plus; Nif-Ten; Sigabloc; Teneretic; TRI-Normin; *Irl.:* Atenetic; Beta-Adalat; Cotenomel; Nif-Ten; Tenchlor; Tenoret; Tenoretic; *Ital.:* Ataclor; Atenigron; Atinorm; Carmian; Clortanol; Diube; Eupres; Igroseles; Mixer; Nif-Ten; Nor-Pa; Normopress; Target; Tenolone; Tenoretic; *Neth.:* Beta-Adalat†; Hykaten†; Nif-Ten; Tenoretic; *S.Afr.:* Adco-Loten; Ateren; Tenchlor; Tenoret†; Tenoretic; Venachlor†; *Spain:* Betasit Plus; Blokium Diu; Kalten; Neatenol Diu; Neatenol Diuvas; Normopresil; Tenoretic; *Switz.:* ateno-basan comp.; Beta-Adalat; Cardaxen plus; Cotenolol; Kalten; Nif-Atenil; Nif-Ten; Tenoretic; *UK:* AtenixCo; Beta-Adalat; Kalten; Tenben; Tenchlor; Tenif; Tenoret; Tenoretic; Totaretic; *USA:* Tenoretic.

Atrial Natriuretic Peptide (3930-e)

Atrial natriuretic peptide (ANP) is an endogenous substance secreted by the heart that possesses diuretic and natriuretic properties. It has also been called atrial natriuretic factor (ANF), atriopeptin, auriculin, or cardionatrin, and is the 28-membered carboxy terminus of a precursor containing 126 amino acid residues and stored in the heart. Atrial peptides have also been synthesised. The name anaritide has been applied to an atrial natriuretic peptide with the structure *N*-L-arginyl-[8-L-methionine-21a-L-phenylalanine-21b-L-arginine-21c-L-tyrosine]-atriopeptin-21. Carperitide is the name applied to recombinant human atrial natriuretic peptide.

Natriuretic peptides related structurally to atrial natriuretic peptide have been discovered and include brain natriuretic peptide (BNP; B-type natriuretic peptide), originally isolated from porcine brain, although it is now recognised that the cardiac ventricle is the main source, and ularitide (urodilatin), present in human urine.

Atrial natriuretic peptide and brain natriuretic peptide are closely involved in fluid and electrolyte homoeostasis and in the regulation of blood pressure, together with other complex systems such as the renin-angiotensin-aldosterone cascade. Their physiological and pathological role and potential clinical applications are under investigation. Plasma concentrations of atrial natriuretic peptide and brain natriuretic peptide have been used as indicators of cardiac function. Anaritide and ularitide are being studied for possible use in acute renal failure and brain natriuretic peptide for use in acute heart failure. Carperitide has recently been introduced for use in acute heart failure.

Human atrial natriuretic peptide and available synthetic analogues have a short half-life and have to be given parenterally. Long-acting analogues, particularly if stable when given by mouth, would greatly increase the therapeutic potential. The half-life of atrial natriuretic peptide may be prolonged by atriopeptidase inhibitors (neutral endopeptidase inhibitors; neutral metalloendopeptidase inhibitors), and several compounds with this property are also under investigation, including candoxatril the prodrug of candoxatrilat (p.836), Sch-42495, and ecadotril (sinorphan). Compounds that inhibit both neutral endopeptidase and angiotensin-converting enzyme are also being studied.

References.

1. Tan ACITL, *et al.* Atrial natriuretic peptide: an overview of clinical pharmacology and pharmacokinetics. *Clin Pharmacokinet* 1993; **24:** 28–45.
2. Deutsch A, *et al.* Atrial natriuretic peptide and its potential role in pharmacotherapy. *J Clin Pharmacol* 1994; **34:** 1133–47.
3. Struthers AD. Ten years of natriuretic peptide research: a new dawn for their diagnostic and therapeutic use? *Br Med J* 1994; **308:** 1615–19.
4. Richards AM. The renin-angiotensin-aldosterone system and the cardiac natriuretic peptides. *Heart* 1996; **76** (suppl 3): 36–44.
5. Wilkins MR, *et al.* The natriuretic-peptide family. *Lancet* 1997; **349:** 1307–10.
6. Allgren RL, *et al.* Anaritide in acute tubular necrosis. *N Engl J Med* 1997; **336:** 828–34.
7. Levin ER, *et al.* Natriuretic peptides. *N Engl J Med* 1998; **339:** 321–8.

Azepexole (18795-q)

Azepexole *(BAN, rINN)*.

BHT-933 (azepexole dihydrochloride). 6-Ethyl-5,6,7,8-tetrahydro-4*H*-[1,3]oxazolo[4,5-*d*]azepin-2-ylamine.

$C_9H_{15}N_3O = 181.2$.

CAS — 36067-73-9.

Azepexole is reported to have selective alpha$_2$-adrenoceptor agonist properties similar to those of clonidine (p.841). It is also reported to have antitussive properties.

Azimilide (17812-q)

Azimilide *(BAN, rINN)*.

NE-10064 (azimilide hydrochloride). 1-{[5-(*p*-Chlorophenyl)furfurylidene]amino}-3-[4-(4-methyl-1-piperazinyl)butyl]hydantoin.

$C_{23}H_{28}ClN_5O_3 = 458.0$.

CAS — 149908-53-2 (azimilide); 149888-94-8 (azimilide hydrochloride).

NOTE. Azimilide Dihydrochloride is *USAN*.

Azimilide is a class III antiarrhythmic (p.776) under investigation.

Azosemide (12415-d)

Azosemide *(USAN, rINN)*.

BM-02001; Ple-1053. 2-Chloro-5-(1*H*-tetrazol-5-yl)-4-(2-thenylamino)benzenesulphonamide.

$C_{12}H_{11}ClN_6O_2S_2 = 370.8$.

CAS — 27589-33-9.

Azosemide is a diuretic with actions similar to those of frusemide (p.871).

Preparations

Proprietary Preparations (details are given in Part 3)
Ger.: Luret.

Bamethan Sulphate (9207-s)

Bamethan Sulphate *(BANM, rINNM)*.

Bamethan Sulfate *(USAN)*. 2-Butylamino-1-(4-hydroxyphenyl)ethanol sulphate.

$(C_{12}H_{19}NO_2)_2,H_2SO_4$ = 516.6.

CAS — 3703-79-5 (bamethan); 5716-20-1 (bamethan sulphate).

Pharmacopoeias. In *Jpn* and *Pol.*

Bamethan sulphate is a vasodilator used in the management of peripheral vascular disorders.

Bamethan nicotinate has been used similarly.

Preparations

Proprietary Preparations (details are given in Part 3)
Aust.: Provascul; Vasculat; ***Ger.:*** Emasex A; Vasculat†; ***Ital.:*** Angiolast†; Vasculat†; ***Spain:*** Vasculat; ***Switz.:*** Vasculat†.

Multi-ingredient: ***Fr.:*** Escinogel; ***Ger.:*** Emasex-N; Heweven P 7†; Medigel; Theo-Hexanicit†; Veno-Tablinen†; ***Spain:*** Lotanal†.

Barnidipine Hydrochloride (15254-d)

Barnidipine Hydrochloride *(rINNM)*.

LY-198561; Mepirodipine Hydrochloride; YM-730; YM-09730-5. (+)-(3′*S*,4*S*)-1-Benzyl-3-pyrrolidinyl methyl 1,4-dihydro-2,6-dimethyl-4-(*m*-nitrophenyl)-3,5-pyridinedicarboxylate hydrochloride.

$C_{27}H_{29}N_3O_6$,HCl = 528.0.

CAS — 104713-75-9 (barnidipine); 104757-53-1 (barnidipine hydrochloride).

Barnidipine is a dihydropyridine calcium-channel blocker with general properties similar to those of nifedipine (p.916). It is given by mouth as the hydrochloride in the management of hypertension.

Preparations

Proprietary Preparations (details are given in Part 3)
Jpn: Hypoca.

Befunolol Hydrochloride (16528-a)

Befunolol Hydrochloride *(rINNM)*.

BFE-60. 7-[2-Hydroxy-3-(isopropylamino)propoxy]-2-benzofuranyl methyl ketone hydrochloride.

$C_{16}H_{21}NO_4$,HCl = 327.8.

CAS — 39552-01-7 (befunolol); 39543-79-8 (befunolol hydrochloride).

Befunolol is a beta blocker (p.828). It is used as the hydrochloride in the management of ocular hypertension and open-angle glaucoma (p.1387). Eye drops containing befunolol hydrochloride 0.25%, 0.5%, or 1% are instilled twice daily.

Preparations

Proprietary Preparations (details are given in Part 3)
Aust.: Glauconex; ***Belg.:*** Glauconex; ***Fr.:*** Bentos; ***Ger.:*** Glauconex; ***Ital.:*** Betaclar; ***Jpn:*** Bentos; ***Neth.:*** Glauconex†.

Bemetizide (12423-d)

Bemetizide *(BAN, rINN)*.

Diu-60. 6-Chloro-3,4-dihydro-3-(α-methylbenzyl)-2*H*-1,2,4-benzothiadiazine-7-sulphonamide 1,1-dioxide.

$C_{15}H_{16}ClN_3O_4S_2$ = 401.9.

CAS — 1824-52-8.

Bemetizide is a thiazide diuretic (see Hydrochlorothiazide, p.885) that is used, often in combination with triamterene, in the treatment of oedema and hypertension.

Preparations

Proprietary Preparations (details are given in Part 3)

Multi-ingredient: ***Aust.:*** Dehydrosin; Diucomb; ***Belg.:*** Diucomb; ***Fr.:*** Tensigradyl; ***Ger.:*** cardiotensin†; dehydro sanol tri; dehydro sanol†; dehydro tri mite; Diucomb; pertenso†; ***Switz.:*** Diucomb.

Benazepril Hydrochloride (18951-m)

Benazepril Hydrochloride *(BANM, USAN, rINNM)*.

CGS-14824A (benazepril or benazepril hydrochloride). {(3*S*)-3-[(1*S*)-1-Ethoxycarbonyl-3-phenylpropylamino]-2,3,4,5-tetrahydro-2-oxo-1*H*-1-benzazepin-1-yl}acetic acid hydrochloride; 1-Carboxymethyl-3-[1-ethoxycarbonyl-3-phenyl-(1*S*)-propylamino]-2,3,4,5-tetrahydro-1*H*-1(3*S*)-benzazepin-2-one hydrochloride.

$C_{24}H_{28}N_2O_5$,HCl = 461.0.

CAS — 86541-75-5 (benazepril); 86541-74-4 (benazepril hydrochloride).

Adverse Effects, Treatment, and Precautions

As for ACE inhibitors, p.805.

Interactions

As for ACE inhibitors, p.807.

Pharmacokinetics

Benazepril acts as a prodrug of the diacid benazeprilat, its active metabolite. Following oral administration at least 37% of a dose of benazepril is absorbed. Benazepril is almost completely metabolised in the liver to benazeprilat. Peak plasma concentrations of benazeprilat following an oral dose of benazepril have been achieved after 1 to 2 hours in the fasting state or after 2 to 4 hours in the nonfasting state. Both benazepril and benazeprilat are about 95% bound to plasma proteins. Benazeprilat is excreted mainly in the urine; about 11 to 12% is excreted in the bile. The effective half-life for accumulation of benazeprilat is 10 to 11 hours following multiple doses of benazepril. The elimination of benazeprilat is slowed in renal impairment. Small amounts of benazepril and benazeprilat are distributed into breast milk.

References.

1. Kaiser G, *et al.* Pharmacokinetics of the angiotensin converting enzyme inhibitor benazepril HCl (CGS 14 824A) in healthy volunteers after single and repeated administration. *Biopharm Drug Dispos* 1989; **10:** 365–76.
2. Kaiser G, *et al.* Pharmacokinetics of a new angiotensin-converting enzyme inhibitor, benazepril hydrochloride, in special populations. *Am Heart J* 1989; **117:** 746–51.
3. Kaiser G, *et al.* Pharmacokinetics and pharmacodynamics of the ace inhibitor benazepril hydrochloride in the elderly. *Eur J Clin Pharmacol* 1990; **38:** 379–85.
4. Macdonald N-J, *et al.* A comparison in young and elderly subjects of the pharmacokinetics and pharmacodynamics of single and multiple doses of benazepril. *Br J Clin Pharmacol* 1993; **36:** 201–4.

Uses and Administration

Benazepril is an ACE inhibitor (p.805). It is used in the treatment of hypertension (p.788) and heart failure (p.785).

Benazepril owes its activity to benazeprilat to which it is converted after oral administration. The haemodynamic effects are seen within 1 hour of a single oral dose and the maximum effect occurs after about 2 to 4 hours, although the full effect may not develop for 1 to 2 weeks during chronic dosing. The haemodynamic action lasts for about 24 hours, allowing once-daily dosing. Benazepril is given by mouth as the hydrochloride, but doses are usually expressed in terms of the base.

In the treatment of **hypertension**, the usual initial dose is 10 mg once daily. An initial dose of 5 mg once daily is suggested for patients with renal impairment or who are receiving a diuretic; if possible the diuretic should be withdrawn 2 or 3 days before benazepril is started and resumed later if necessary. The usual maintenance dose is 20 to 40 mg daily, which may be given in 2 divided doses if control is inadequate with a single dose.

In the treatment of **heart failure** the usual initial dose is 2.5 mg once daily, adjusted according to response to a maximum dose of 20 mg daily.

Preparations

Proprietary Preparations (details are given in Part 3)

Aust.: Cibacen; ***Belg.:*** Cibacen; ***Canad.:*** Lotensin; ***Fr.:*** Briem; Cibacene; ***Ger.:*** Cibacen; ***Irl.:*** Cibacen; ***Ital.:*** Cibacen; Tensanil; Zinadril; ***Neth.:*** Cibacen; ***S.Afr.:*** Cibace; ***Spain:*** Cibacen; Labopal; ***Switz.:*** Cibacen; ***USA:*** Lotensin.

Multi-ingredient: ***Aust.:*** Cibadrex; ***Fr.:*** Briazide; Cibadrex; ***Ger.:*** Cibadrex; ***Ital.:*** Cibadrex; Tensadiur; Zinadiur; ***Neth.:*** Cibadrex; ***S.Afr.:*** Cibadrex; ***Swed.:*** Cibadrex†; ***Switz.:*** Cibadrex; ***USA:*** Lotensin HCT; Lotrel.

Bencyclane Fumarate (9208-w)

Bencyclane Fumarate *(rINNM)*.

Bencyclane Hydrogen Fumarate. 3-(1-Benzylcycloheptyloxy)-*NN*-dimethylpropylamine hydrogen fumarate.

$C_{19}H_{31}NO,C_4H_4O_4$ = 405.5.

CAS — 2179-37-5 (bencyclane); 14286-84-1 (bencyclane fumarate).

Pharmacopoeias. In *Jpn*.

Bencyclane fumarate is a vasodilator used in the management of peripheral (p.794) and cerebral vascular disorders (p.785) in usual doses of 100 to 200 mg three times a day by mouth. It has also been given intravenously.

Bencyclane acephyllinate is also used.

Preparations

Proprietary Preparations (details are given in Part 3)
Aust.: Ludilat; ***Ger.:*** Fludilat; ***Ital.:*** Angiociclan†; ***Switz.:*** Fludilat.

Multi-ingredient: ***Ger.:*** Card-Fludilat†; Novo-Card-Fludilat†; ***Ital.:*** Tensilene†; ***Spain:*** Dilangio Compositum; Dilapres.

Bendrofluazide (2306-h)

Bendrofluazide *(BAN)*.

Bendroflumethiazide *(rINN)*; Bendrofluaz.; Bendroflumethiazidum; Benzydroflumethiazide; FT-81. 3-Benzyl-3,4-dihydro-6-trifluoromethyl-2*H*-1,2,4-benzothiadiazine-7-sulphonamide 1,1-dioxide.

$C_{15}H_{14}F_3N_3O_4S_2$ = 421.4.

CAS — 73-48-3.

Pharmacopoeias. In *Chin., Eur.* (see p.viii), and *US*.

A white or cream-coloured, odourless or almost odourless, crystalline powder.

Practically **insoluble** in water; soluble in alcohol; freely soluble in acetone. **Store** in airtight containers.

Adverse Effects, Treatment, and Precautions

As for Hydrochlorothiazide, p.885.

Overdosage. Tonic-clonic convulsions occurred in a previously healthy 14-year-old girl following ingestion of bendrofluazide 150 to 200 mg.[1] The convulsions were not associated with any measurable disturbance of serum electrolytes.

1. Hine KR, *et al.* Bendrofluazide convulsions. *Lancet* 1982; **i:** 564.

Interactions

As for Hydrochlorothiazide, p.887.

Pharmacokinetics

Bendrofluazide has been reported to be completely absorbed from the gastro-intestinal tract and to have a plasma half-life of about 3 or 4 hours. It is highly bound to plasma protein. There are indications that bendrofluazide is fairly extensively metabolised; about 30% is excreted unchanged in the urine.

References.

1. Beermann B, *et al.* Pharmacokinetics of bendroflumethiazide. *Clin Pharmacol Ther* 1977; **22:** 385–8.
2. Beermann B, *et al.* Pharmacokinetics of bendroflumethiazide in hypertensive patients. *Eur J Clin Pharmacol* 1978; **13:** 119–24.

Uses and Administration

Bendrofluazide is a thiazide diuretic with actions and uses similar to those of hydrochlorothiazide (p.887). It is used for oedema, including that associated with heart failure (p.785), and for hypertension (p.788). Other indications have included the suppression of lactation.

Diuresis is initiated in about 2 hours and lasts for 12 to 18 hours or longer.

In the treatment of **oedema** the usual initial dose is 5 to 10 mg by mouth daily or on alternate days; in some cases initial doses of up to 20 mg may be necessary. Maintenance dosage schedules have varied from 2.5 to 10 mg once to three times weekly in the UK to 2.5 to 5 mg daily or intermittently in the USA.

In the treatment of **hypertension** bendrofluazide 2.5 mg daily, either alone or in conjunction with other antihypertensive drugs, is usually adequate although doses of up to 20 mg daily have sometimes been suggested.

A suggested initial dose for children is up to 400 μg per kg body-weight daily, reduced to 50 to 100 μg per kg for maintenance.

In susceptible patients potassium supplements or a potassium-sparing diuretic may be necessary, but see hydrochlorothiazide.

A suggested dose of bendrofluazide to suppress lactation is 5 mg twice daily for about 5 days.

Preparations

BP 1998: Bendroflumethiazide Tablets;
USP 23: Bendroflumethiazide Tablets; Nadolol and Bendroflumethiazide Tablets.

Proprietary Preparations (details are given in Part 3)
Aust.: Sinesalin†; *Austral.:* Aprinox; Benzide†; *Canad.:* Naturetin; *Fr.:* Naturine; *Ger.:* Esbericid†; Sinesalin†; *Irl.:* Centyl; *Neth.:* Pluryl†; *Norw.:* Centyl; *Swed.:* Salures; *Switz.:* Sinesalin; *UK:* Aprinox; Berkozide; Centyl†; Neo-NaClex; *USA:* Naturetin.

Multi-ingredient: *Aust.:* Inderetic; Pressimedin; Sali-Aldopur; Solgeretik; *Belg.:* Inderetic; *Canad.:* Corzide; *Fr.:* Precyclan; Tensionorme; *Ger.:* Docidrazin; Docirectic; Pertenso N; Sali-Aldopur; Solgeretik†; Sotaziden N; Spirostada comp; Tensoflux; *Irl.:* Centyl K; Corgaretic; Inderetic; Prestim; *Ital.:* Notens†; *Neth.:* Inderetic; Prestim; *Norw.:* Centyl med Kaliumklorid; *S.Afr.:* Corgaretic; Inderetic; Mendrome†; *Spain:* Betadipresan Diu; Neatenol Diu; Neatenol Diuvas; Spirometon; *Swed.:* Salures-K; *Switz.:* Corgaretic; Inderetic; Pressimed; Saluretin; *UK:* Centyl K†; Corgaretic; Inderetic; Inderex; Neo-NaClex-K; Prestim; Tenben; *USA:* Corzide; Rauzide.

Benidipine Hydrochloride (4595-x)

Benidipine Hydrochloride *(rINNM).*

KW-3049; Nakadipine Hydrochloride. (±)-(R^*)-3-[(R^*)-1-Benzyl-3-piperidyl]methyl 1,4-dihydro-2,6-dimethyl-4-(*m*-nitrophenyl)-3,5-pyridinedicarboxylate hydrochloride.

$C_{28}H_{31}N_3O_6,HCl$ = 542.0.

CAS — 105979-17-7 (benidipine); 91599-74-5 (benidipine hydrochloride).

Benidipine is a dihydropyridine calcium-channel blocker with general properties similar to those of nifedipine (p.916). It is given by mouth as the hydrochloride in the treatment of hypertension.

Preparations

Proprietary Preparations (details are given in Part 3)
Jpn: Coniel.

Benzthiazide (2307-m)

Benzthiazide *(BAN, rINN).*

P-1393. 3-Benzylthiomethyl-6-chloro-2*H*-1,2,4-benzothiadiazine-7-sulphonamide 1,1-dioxide.

$C_{15}H_{14}ClN_3O_4S_3$ = 431.9.

CAS — 91-33-8.

Pharmacopoeias. In US.

A white crystalline powder with a characteristic odour. Practically **insoluble** in water and chloroform; slightly soluble in acetone; soluble 1 in 480 of alcohol; freely soluble in dimethylformamide and in solutions of fixed alkali hydroxides; soluble 1 in 2900 of ether. **Store** in airtight containers.

Benzthiazide is a thiazide diuretic with properties similar to those of hydrochlorothiazide (p.885). It is used for oedema, including that associated with heart failure (p.785), and for hypertension (p.788).

Diuresis is initiated in about 2 hours and lasts for 12 to 18 hours.

The initial dose in the treatment of oedema is 50 to 200 mg by mouth daily, followed by a maintenance dose of 25 to 150 mg daily or intermittently. In the treatment of hypertension, an initial dose of 12.5 to 25 mg daily, either alone or in conjunction with other antihypertensive drugs, may be adequate although the US manufacturers have recommended 50 to 100 mg daily. The maintenance dose should be adjusted to the lowest effective dose for the patient, but some have required up to 200 mg daily. Benzthiazide may be given in single or divided doses. A suggested initial dose in children is 1 to 4 mg per kg body-weight daily in divided doses.

In susceptible patients potassium supplements or a potassium-sparing diuretic may be necessary, but see hydrochlorothiazide.

Preparations

USP 23: Benzthiazide Tablets.

Proprietary Preparations (details are given in Part 3)
S.Afr.: Diurin†; *USA:* Exna.

Multi-ingredient: *Ger.:* Sali-Raufuncton†; *Irl.:* Dytide†; *Switz.:* Dyrenium compositum; *UK:* Dytide.

Bepridil Hydrochloride (12435-b)

Bepridil Hydrochloride *(BANM, USAN, rINNM).*

CERM-1978; Org-5730. *N*-Benzyl-*N*-(3-isobutoxy-2-pyrrolidin-1-ylpropyl)aniline hydrochloride monohydrate.

$C_{24}H_{34}N_2O,HCl,H_2O$ = 421.0.

CAS — 64706-54-3 (bepridil); 49571-04-2 (bepridil); 64616-81-5 (anhydrous bepridil hydrochloride); 74764-40-2 (bepridil hydrochloride monohydrate).

Bepridil is a calcium-channel blocker (p.778) with properties similar to nifedipine (p.916). It also has antiarrhythmic activity. It is not related chemically to other calcium-channel blockers such as diltiazem, nifedipine, or verapamil.

Bepridil is used as the hydrochloride in angina pectoris (p.780) in doses of 200 to 400 mg daily by mouth. Elderly patients may require reduced doses. Ventricular arrhythmias, including torsade de pointes, and agranulocytosis have been associated with bepridil and, as a result, it is usually reserved for patients who have not responded adequately to other antianginal drugs.

References.

1. Hollingshead LM, *et al.* Bepridil: a review of its pharmacological properties and therapeutic use in stable angina pectoris. *Drugs* 1992; **44:** 835–57.
2. Awni WM, *et al.* Pharmacokinetics of bepridil and two of its metabolites in patients with end-stage renal disease. *J Clin Pharmacol* 1995; **35:** 379–83.

Preparations

Proprietary Preparations (details are given in Part 3)
Belg.: Cordium; *Fr.:* Cordium; *USA:* Vascor.

Beta Blockers (6300-v)

Beta blockers (beta-adrenoceptor blocking drugs or antagonists) can be characterised by their affinity for $beta_1$ or $beta_2$ receptor subtypes, intrinsic sympathomimetic activity, membrane-stabilising activity, blockade of alpha-adrenergic receptors, and pharmacokinetic properties including differences in lipid solubility (see Table 1, p.831, under Uses and Administration for some of these characteristics).

Beta blockers have different affinities for $beta_1$ or $beta_2$ receptors. $Beta_1$ receptors are found mainly in the heart while $beta_2$ receptors are in noncardiac tissue, including bronchial tissue, peripheral blood vessels, uterus, and pancreas. While propranolol affects both $beta_1$ and $beta_2$ receptors, other drugs such as atenolol and metoprolol, have greater affinity for $beta_1$ receptors and are described as cardioselective. However, selectivity is relative and, as doses are increased, activity at $beta_2$ receptors becomes clinically important.

Some beta blockers, such as acebutolol, celiprolol, oxprenolol, and pindolol, also possess intrinsic (partial) sympathomimetic activity in that they activate beta receptors in the absence of catecholamines and are therefore partial agonists. Beta blockers with intrinsic sympathomimetic activity produce less resting bradycardia than beta blockers without.

At high blood concentrations, propranolol and some other beta blockers also possess a membrane-stabilising effect. This effect may not be evident at therapeutic doses but may be important in overdose. Some beta blockers, such as carvedilol and labetalol, may also block $alpha_1$ receptors. Blockade of $alpha_1$ receptors produces vasodilatation. Other beta blockers, such as bevantolol and celiprolol also have vasodilator properties. Various mechanisms, including $alpha_1$ blockade, $beta_2$ stimulation, and direct vasodilator activity may contribute to the vasodilator effect.

Sotalol is a beta blocker that also has class III antiarrhythmic activity.

Adverse Effects and Treatment

The most frequent and serious adverse effects of these drugs are related to their beta adrenergic blocking activity. Among the most serious adverse effects are heart failure, heart block, and bronchospasm. Troublesome subjective side-effects include fatigue and coldness of the extremities. Reactions may be more severe following intravenous than oral administration; ocular use has also been associated with systemic adverse effects. When beta blockers are used for long-term treatment of asymptomatic diseases such as hypertension, subjective side-effects may be an important determinant of patient compliance.

Cardiovascular effects include bradycardia and hypotension; heart failure or heart block may be precipitated in patients with underlying cardiac disorders. Abrupt withdrawal of beta blockers may exacerbate angina and may lead to sudden death. For further details on withdrawal of beta blockers, see below. Reduced peripheral circulation can produce coldness of the extremities and may exacerbate peripheral vascular disease such as Raynaud's syndrome.

Bronchospasm may be precipitated in susceptible patients due to blockade of $beta_2$ receptors in bronchial smooth muscle. Drugs with selectivity for $beta_1$ receptors or with intrinsic sympathomimetic activity at $beta_2$ receptors may be less likely to induce bronchospasm (but see under Precautions, below). Pneumonitis, pulmonary fibrosis, and pleurisy have also been reported.

Central nervous system effects include depression, dizziness, hallucinations, confusion, and sleep disturbances including nightmares. Coma and convulsions have been reported following beta-blocker overdosage. Beta blockers which are lipid soluble are more likely to enter the brain and would be expected to be associated with a higher incidence of CNS adverse effects, although this is not proven.

Fatigue is a common side-effect experienced with beta blockers. Paraesthesia, peripheral neuropathy, and myopathies, including muscle cramps, have been reported.

Adverse gastro-intestinal effects include nausea and vomiting, diarrhoea, constipation, and abdominal cramping.

Beta blockers interfere with carbohydrate and lipid metabolism and can produce hypoglycaemia, hyperglycaemia, and changes in blood concentrations of triglycerides and cholesterol (see below for further details).

Skin rash, pruritus, and reversible alopecia have occurred with use of beta blockers.

Decreased tear production, blurred vision, and soreness are among the ocular symptoms which have been reported. Adverse effects specific to ocular use are also discussed below.

Haematological reactions include nonthrombocytopenic purpura, thrombocytopenia, and rarely agranulocytosis. Transient eosinophilia can occur.

Other adverse effects reported with some beta blockers include a lupus-like syndrome, male impotence, sclerosing peritonitis, and retroperitoneal fibrosis.

For reference to the treatment of adverse effects, see under Overdosage, below.

Carcinogenicity. An apparent excess of deaths from cancer was noted in elderly men, but not women, given atenolol during a trial of antihypertensive treatment.[1] However, two subsequent studies found no evidence of a link between atenolol and cancer.[2,3]

1. MRC Working Party. Medical Research Council trial of treatment of hypertension in older adults: principal results. *Br Med J* 1992; **304:** 405–12.
2. Fletcher AE, *et al.* Cancer mortality and atenolol treatment. *Br Med J* 1993; **306:** 622–3.
3. Hole DJ, *et al.* Incidence of and mortality from cancer in hypertensive patients. *Br Med J* 1993; **306:** 609–11.

Effects on carbohydrate metabolism. The sympathetic nervous system is involved in the control of carbohydrate metabolism and blockade of adrenergic receptors by beta blockers can interfere with carbohydrate and insulin regulation; both hypoglycaemia and hyperglycaemia have been reported. Propranolol-induced hypoglycaemia was first noted in adult type 1 diabetic patients in the late 1960s. In a review of drug-induced hypoglycaemia, Seltzer[1] considered 49 cases of severe hypoglycaemia associated with non-selective beta blockers. These events occurred in the following circumstances:

nondiabetic patients taking propranolol and undergoing regular haemodialysis; neonates of mothers who took propranolol until a few hours before delivery; infants who received propranolol; and both diabetic and nondiabetic patients on long-term propranolol who were nutritionally compromised or had liver disease. In type 1 diabetes mellitus beta blockers mask the adrenaline-mediated symptoms of hypoglycaemia such as tachycardia and tremor, and may delay the recovery from hypoglycaemia in glucose-treated patients. Numerous studies have been undertaken to determine the role of beta blockers' cardioselectivity and lipid solubility in blood sugar control. The optimal beta blocker for use in patients with diabetes mellitus appears to be a $beta_1$ cardioselective drug with little or no lipophilicity.[2]

The use of beta blockers has also been associated with hyperglycaemia[3,4] and diabetes mellitus.[5,6]

1. Seltzer HS. Drug-induced hypoglycemia. *Endocrinol Metab Clin North Am* 1989; **18:** 163–83.
2. O'Byrne S, Feely J. Effects of drugs on glucose tolerance in non-insulin-dependent diabetics (part 1). *Drugs* 1990; **40:** 6–18.
3. Veterans Administration Cooperative Study Group on Antihypertensive Agents. Propranolol or hydrochlorothiazide alone for the initial treatment of hypertension IV: effect on plasma glucose and glucose tolerance. *Hypertension* 1985; **7:** 1008–16.
4. Pollare T, *et al.* Sensitivity to insulin during treatment with atenolol and metoprolol: a randomised, double blind study of effects on carbohydrate and lipoprotein metabolism in hypertensive patients. *Br Med J* 1989; **298:** 1152–7.
5. Skarfors ET, *et al.* Do antihypertensive drugs precipitate diabetes in predisposed men? *Br Med J* 1989; **298:** 1147–52.
6. Samuelsson O, *et al.* Diabetes mellitus in treated hypertension: incidence, predictive factors and the impact of non-selective beta-blockers and thiazide diuretics during 15 years treatment of middle-aged hypertensive men in the Primary Prevention Trial in Göteborg, Sweden. *J Hum Hypertens* 1994; **8:** 257–63.

Effects on lipid metabolism. The adrenergic system is involved in the control of lipid metabolism. Thus, beta blockers may have some effect on plasma-lipid concentrations. Plasma concentrations of very low density lipoprotein and triglyceride may be raised in patients taking beta blockers and concentrations of high density lipoprotein reduced. Plasma concentrations of low density lipoprotein are usually unchanged. These effects may be less pronounced with $beta_1$ cardioselective drugs, beta blockers with intrinsic sympathomimetic activity,[1] and beta blockers that also block alpha-adrenergic receptors. For example, pindolol,[2,3] a beta blocker with intrinsic sympathomimetic activity and arotinolol[4] and carvedilol[5] that possess alpha-adrenergic blocking properties are reported to have no adverse effects on plasma-lipid concentrations. However, a patient taking atenolol and metoprolol, both $beta_1$ cardioselective drugs, developed acute pancreatitis as a result of severe hypertriglyceridaemia.[6]

Exercise has been suggested to have a favourable impact on lipid profiles and 2 studies[7,8] have investigated the role of exercise in attenuating the effects of beta blockers on lipids. Neither study showed that exercise improved the lipid profile in patients given beta blockers. However, the anticipated deterioration in lipid profile may have been attenuated.[7]

1. Krone W, Nägele H. Effects of antihypertensives on plasma lipids and lipoprotein metabolism. *Am Heart J* 1988; **116:** 1729–34.
2. Hunter Hypertension Research Group. Effects of pindolol, or a pindolol/clopamide combination preparation, on plasma lipid levels in essential hypertension. *Med J Aust* 1989; **150:** 646–52.
3. Terént A, *et al.* Long-term effect of pindolol on lipids and lipoproteins in men with newly diagnosed hypertension. *Eur J Clin Pharmacol* 1989; **36:** 347–50.
4. Sasaki J, *et al.* Effects of arotinolol on serum lipid and apolipoprotein levels in patients with mild essential hypertension. *Clin Ther* 1989; **11:** 580–3.
5. Hauf-Zachariou U, *et al.* A double-blind comparison of the effects of carvedilol and captopril on serum lipid concentrations in patients with mild to moderate essential hypertension and dyslipidaemia. *Eur J Clin Pharmacol* 1993; **45:** 95–100.
6. Durrington PN, Cairns SA. Acute pancreatitis: a complication of beta-blockade. *Br Med J* 1982; **284:** 1016.
7. Morton AR, *et al.* Alterations in plasma lipids consequent to endurance training and beta-blockade. *Med Sci Sports Exerc* 1989; **21:** 288–92.
8. Arvan S, Rueda BG. Nonselective beta-receptor blocker effect on high density lipoprotein cholesterol after chronic exercise. *J Am Coll Cardiol* 1988; **12:** 662–8.

Effects following ophthalmic use. Ophthalmic administration of beta blockers may produce the following localised effects: ocular irritation (including hypersensitivity), blepharitis, keratitis, decreased corneal sensitivity, visual disturbances, diplopia, and ptosis. Uveitis has been reported with metipranolol eye drops.[1]

Topical beta blockers may produce corneal anaesthesia. Older patients using these eye drops may be at greater risk of decreased corneal sensitivity or corneal anaesthesia with the consequent risk of keratitis.[2]

Systemic absorption may occur following the use of beta blockers in eye drops. Excess drug can drain into the lachrymal ducts to be absorbed through the nasal mucosa. Absorption also occurs via the ophthalmic and facial veins. Following such absorption the beta blocker reaches the systemic circulation without undergoing first-pass hepatic metabolism. The main systemic effects associated with topical ocular administration of beta blockers are on the pulmonary, cardiovascular, and central nervous systems.[3]

Fifty-six cases of alopecia associated with ocular use of beta blockers have been reported to the National Registry of Drug-induced Ocular Side Effects in the US.[4]

Beta blockers given orally can adversely affect serum-lipoprotein concentrations; however, a study of the effect of timolol 0.5% administered topically twice daily to both eyes of 19 patients showed no effect on lipoprotein concentrations at 5 and 15 weeks.[5]

1. Akingbehin T, Villada JR. Metipranolol-associated granulomatous anterior uveitis. *Br J Ophthalmol* 1991; **75:** 519–23.
2. Weissman SS, Asbell PA. Effects of topical timolol (0.5%) and betaxolol (0.5%) on corneal sensitivity. *Br J Ophthalmol* 1990; **74:** 409–12.
3. Everitt DE, Avorn J. Systemic effects of medications used to treat glaucoma. *Ann Intern Med* 1990; **112:** 120–5.
4. Fraunfelder FT, *et al.* Alopecia possibly secondary to topical ophthalmic β-blockers. *JAMA* 1990; **263:** 1493–4.
5. West J, Longstaff S. Topical timolol and serum lipoproteins. *Br J Ophthalmol* 1990; **74:** 663–4.

Hypersensitivity. For the suggestion that beta blockers may exacerbate anaphylactic reactions, see under Precautions, below.

Overdosage. Many cases of beta-blocker overdosage are uneventful, but some patients develop severe and occasionally fatal cardiovascular depression. Effects can include bradycardia, cardiac conduction block, hypotension, heart failure, and cardiogenic shock. Convulsions, coma, respiratory depression, and bronchoconstriction can also occur, although infrequently. Most reports of serious toxic reactions following overdosage concern beta blockers with significant membrane-stabilising activity, such as propranolol or oxprenolol.[1] Overdosage of beta blockers with intrinsic sympathomimetic activity may present with tachycardia and hypertension.[2] Overdosage of sotalol, a beta blocker with class II and III antiarrhythmic properties, usually presents as ventricular tachyarrhythmia.[1,2] **Treatment** involves gastric lavage and activated charcoal for patients presenting with a history of recent acute ingestion.[1-3] When indicated, additional measures are instituted to counter hypotension.[2,3] Mild hypotension may respond to fluid administration; if hypotension continues, glucagon or sympathomimetics may be used, either alone[1-3] or in combination.[2,3] Very large doses of sympathomimetics may be required; infusion rates of up to 333 μg per minute of isoprenaline have been used.[3] Bradycardia may be treated with atropine, sympathomimetics, or a pacemaker.

A patient who failed to respond to the usual management for beta-blocker overdosage responded to treatment with enoximone.[4]

1. Critchley JAJH, Ungar A. The management of acute poisoning due to β-adrenoceptor antagonists. *Med Toxicol* 1989; **4:** 32–45.
2. Pentel PR, Salerno DM. Cardiac drug toxicity: digitalis glycosides and calcium-channel and β-blocking agents. *Med J Aust* 1990; **152:** 88–94.
3. Taboulet P, *et al.* Pathophysiology and management of self-poisoning with beta-blockers. *Clin Toxicol* 1993; **31:** 531–51.
4. Hoeper MM, Boeker KHW. Overdose of metoprolol treated with enoximone. *N Engl J Med* 1996; **335:** 1538.

Precautions

Beta blockers should not be given to patients with bronchospasm or asthma or to those with a history of obstructive airways disease. This contra-indication applies even to those beta blockers considered to be cardioselective. However, some authorities consider that a cardioselective beta blocker might be used with extreme caution when there is no alternative treatment. Other contra-indications include metabolic acidosis, sinus bradycardia, or partial heart block. Although a few beta blockers may be used as part of the management of heart failure, in general, beta blockers should not be given to patients with heart failure unless the heart failure is controlled and even then great care is still necessary. Patients with phaeochromocytoma should not receive beta blockers without concomitant alpha-adrenoceptor blocking therapy.

Beta blockers may mask the symptoms of hyperthyroidism and of hypoglycaemia. They may unmask myasthenia gravis. Psoriasis may be aggravated. Patients with a history of anaphylaxis to an antigen may be more reactive to repeated challenge with the antigen while taking beta blockers (see Hypersensitivity, below).

The dose may need to be reduced in patients with renal or hepatic dysfunction.

Abrupt withdrawal of beta blockers has sometimes resulted in angina, myocardial infarction, ventricular arrhythmias, and death. Patients on long-term treatment with a beta blocker should have their medication discontinued gradually over a period of 1 to 2 weeks. Some authorities have advocated their gradual and temporary withdrawal prior to anaesthesia in order to provide better control of the circulatory system. If beta blockers are not discontinued prior to anaesthesia, an agent such as atropine may be given to counter increases in vagal tone. Anaesthetics causing myocardial depression, such as ether, cyclopropane, and trichloroethylene, are best avoided. Awareness by the anaesthetist that beta blockers are being taken is of the greatest importance.

Administration of beta blockers to pregnant women shortly before delivery has occasionally resulted in bradycardia and other adverse effects such as hypoglycaemia and hypotension in the neonate. Many beta blockers are distributed into breast milk.

Similar precautions should be observed when beta blockers are applied topically as eye drops since systemic absorption can occur.

Effects on the eyes. Beta blockers may reduce tear flow, leading to irritation of the eye in wearers of contact lenses and potentially to the dehydration of soft lenses.[1] Older patients using beta blocker eye drops may be at greater risk of corneal anaesthesia. See also Effects Following Ophthalmic Use under Adverse Effects, above.

1. McGuire T. Drugs interfering with contact lenses. *Aust J Hosp Pharm* 1987; **17:** 55–6.

Hypersensitivity. There have been reports of several patients whose anaphylactic reactions to stings or other antigens were potentiated by their concomitant beta-blocker therapy.[1-3]

For the effect of adrenaline in the management of anaphylaxis in patients on beta-blocker therapy, see Interactions under Adrenaline, p.815.

1. Hannaway PJ, Hopper GDK. Severe anaphylaxis and drug-induced beta-blockade. *N Engl J Med* 1983; **308:** 1536.
2. Pedersen DL. Hymenoptera stings and beta-blockers. *Lancet* 1989; **ii:** 619.
3. Lang DM. Anaphylactoid and anaphylactic reactions: hazards of β-blockers. *Drug Safety* 1995; **12:** 299–304.

Pregnancy. The use of a beta blocker from early in pregnancy has been associated with growth retardation of the fetus.[1] However, beta blockers are still considered one of the first-line drugs in mild to moderate hypertension in pregnancy. Many beta blockers cross the placenta and administration of beta blockers to pregnant women shortly before delivery has occasionally resulted in bradycardia and other adverse effects such as hypoglycaemia and hypotension in the neonate.

1. Butters L, *et al.* Atenolol in essential hypertension during pregnancy. *Br Med J* 1990; **301:** 587–9.

Withdrawal. The abrupt withdrawal of beta blockers may lead to rebound hypertension or overshoot hypertension where the patient's blood pressure is higher than before treatment. Angina can be exacerbated, myocardial infarction induced, and fatalities have occurred.[1,2]

1. Houston MC, Hodge R. Beta-adrenergic blocker withdrawal syndromes in hypertension and other cardiovascular diseases. *Am Heart J* 1988; **116:** 515–23.
2. Psaty BM, *et al.* The relative risk of incident coronary heart disease associated with recently stopping the use of β-blockers. *JAMA* 1990; **263:** 1653–7.

Interactions

Both pharmacodynamic and pharmacokinetic interactions have been reported with beta blockers. **Pharmacodynamic** interactions may occur with drugs whose actions enhance or antagonise the various effects of beta blockers at $beta_1$ and $beta_2$ receptors. Thus, interactions may occur with drugs that interfere with the antihypertensive effect, cardiodepressant effect, effect on carbohydrate metabolism, or effect on bronchial $beta_2$ receptors of beta blockers. The characteristics of the individual beta blocker must therefore be borne in mind when considering likely interactions. For more details on the characteristics of different beta blockers, see above. Drugs that enhance the antihypertensive effects of beta blockers, such as ACE inhibitors, calcium-channel blockers, and clonidine may be useful in controlling hypertension. Drugs that cause hypotension such as aldesleukin and general anaesthetics also enhance the antihypertensive effects of beta blockers while other drugs, for example NSAIDs, antagonise the antihypertensive effects. Concomitant use of beta blockers with other cardiac depressants such as amiodarone, diltiazem, and verapamil can precipitate bradycardia and heart block. Sotalol is particularly prone to interactions with other drugs affecting cardiac conduction (see p.945). Beta blockers may potentiate bradycardia due to digoxin. In diabetic patients beta blockers can reduce the response to insulin and oral hypoglycaemics through their effects on pancreatic beta receptors. Blockade of peripheral beta receptors interferes with the effects of sympathomimetics; patients on beta blockers, especially non-selective beta blockers, may develop elevated blood pressure if they are given adrenaline and the bronchodilator effects of adrenaline are also inhibited. The response to adrenaline given for anaphylaxis may be reduced in patients on long-term treatment with beta blockers (see Adrenaline, p.815).

Pharmacokinetic interactions occur with drugs that alter the absorption or metabolism of beta blockers. Although these interactions may alter the beta blocker plasma concentration, they are not usually clinically significant since there is no association between plasma concentrations and therapeutic effect or toxicity and there are wide interindividual differences in steady-state plasma concentrations of beta blockers. Drugs that reduce absorption include aluminium salts (but see also below) and bile-acid binding resins such as cholestyramine. Metabolism of beta blockers can be increased by concomitant treatment with drugs such as barbiturates and rifampicin and decreased with drugs such as cimetidine, erythromycin, fluvoxamine, and hydralazine. Drugs that alter hepatic blood flow also affect metabolism of beta blockers. For example, cimetidine and hydralazine decrease hepatic blood flow and this contributes to the decreased hepatic clearance seen with these drugs. Drugs that influence hepatic metabolism affect beta blockers, such as labetalol, propranolol, and timolol, that are extensively metabolised while beta blockers that are excreted largely unchanged, for example atenolol and nadolol, are unaffected.

Since systemic absorption can occur following ocular use of beta blockers the possibility of interactions with concomitant drugs should be considered.

See below for further details of interactions of beta blockers.

General references.

1. McDevitt DG. Interactions that matter: 12. β-adrenoceptor antagonists. *Prescribers' J* 1988; **28:** 25–30.
2. Blaufarb I, *et al.* β-Blockers: drug interactions of clinical significance. *Drug Safety* 1995; **13:** 359–70.

Anaesthetics. Anaesthetics that cause myocardial depression, such as *ether, cyclopropane,* and *trichloroethylene* should preferably be avoided in patients on beta blockers (see under Precautions, above).

Antacids. Bioavailability of metoprolol was increased when given concurrently with an antacid containing aluminium and magnesium salts but the bioavailability of atenolol was reduced by concurrent administration of this antacid. Variable results on bioavailability of propranolol have been reported when aluminium hydroxide was given with propranolol.[1]

1. Gugler R, Allgayer H. Effects of antacids on the clinical pharmacokinetics of drugs: an update. *Clin Pharmacokinet* 1990; **18:** 210–19.

Antiarrhythmics. Concomitant use of beta blockers with antiarrhythmic drugs and other drugs affecting cardiac conduction can precipitate bradycardia and heart block.

Bradycardia, cardiac arrest, and ventricular fibrillation have been reported shortly after initiation of beta blocker treatment in patients receiving *amiodarone.*[1] Concurrent administration of *flecainide* and propranolol produced additive negative inotropic effects on the heart and increased serum concentrations of both drugs.[2] In a pharmacokinetic study in 12 healthy males, concomitant administration of *propafenone* and propranolol resulted in increases in serum-propranolol concentrations but only modest enhancement of beta-blocking activity.[3] An increase in serum-metoprolol concentration has been reported following concurrent administration of propafenone and metoprolol.[4] The metabolism of metoprolol may be decreased by *quinidine.*[5] Both quinidine and beta blockers have a negative inotropic action on the heart; bradycardia[6] and hypotension[7] have occurred in patients receiving quinidine and beta blockers.

For a report of reduced clearance of *disopyramide* by concomitant administration of atenolol, see p.859.

The interactions of sotalol are discussed on p.945.

1. Lesko LJ. Pharmacokinetic drug interactions with amiodarone. *Clin Pharmacokinet* 1989; **17:** 130–40.
2. Holtzman JL, *et al.* The pharmacodynamic and pharmacokinetic interaction of flecainide acetate with propranolol: effects on cardiac function and drug clearance. *Eur J Clin Pharmacol* 1987; **33:** 97–9.
3. Kowey PR, *et al.* Interaction between propranolol and propafenone in healthy volunteers. *J Clin Pharmacol* 1989; **29:** 512–17.
4. Wagner F, *et al.* Drug interaction between propafenone and metoprolol. *Br J Clin Pharmacol* 1987; **24:** 213–20.
5. Leemann T, *et al.* Single-dose quinidine treatment inhibits metoprolol oxidation in extensive metabolizers. *Eur J Clin Pharmacol* 1986; **29:** 739–41.
6. Dinai Y, *et al.* Bradycardia induced by interaction between quinidine and ophthalmic timolol. *Ann Intern Med* 1985; **103:** 890–1.
7. Loon NR, *et al.* Orthostatic hypotension due to quinidine and propranolol. *Am J Med* 1986; **81:** 1101–4.

Antibacterials. Serum-atenolol concentrations were reduced by concurrent administration of *ampicillin* given in doses of 1 g by mouth in 6 healthy subjects.[1] Plasma concentrations of propranolol,[2] metoprolol,[3] and bisoprolol[4] may be reduced by concomitant *rifampicin* administration.

1. Schäfer-Korting M, *et al.* Atenolol interaction with aspirin, allopurinol, and ampicillin. *Clin Pharmacol Ther* 1983; **33:** 283–8.
2. Shaheen O, *et al.* Influence of debrisoquin phenotype on the inducibility of propranolol metabolism. *Clin Pharmacol Ther* 1989; **45:** 439–43.
3. Bennett PN, *et al.* Effect of rifampicin on metoprolol and antipyrine kinetics. *Br J Clin Pharmacol* 1982; **13:** 387–91.
4. Kirch W, *et al.* Interaction of bisoprolol with cimetidine and rifampicin. *Eur J Clin Pharmacol* 1986; **31:** 59–62.

Anticoagulants. For the effect of beta blockers on the pharmacokinetics of some oral anticoagulants, see p.968.

Antidepressants. Bradycardia and heart block, occurring shortly after the introduction of treatment with *fluoxetine*, have been reported in patients receiving metoprolol[1] and propranolol.[2] Possible mechanisms include impaired conduction through the atrioventricular node and inhibition by fluoxetine of the oxidative metabolism of beta blockers.

Fluvoxamine inhibits oxidative metabolism, and increased plasma concentrations of propranolol have been noted in patients receiving fluvoxamine.

1. Walley T, *et al.* Interaction of metoprolol and fluoxetine. *Lancet* 1993; **341:** 967–8.
2. Drake WM, Gordon GD. Heart block in a patient on propranolol and fluoxetine. *Lancet* 1994; **343:** 425–6.

Antihypertensives. An enhanced antihypertensive effect is seen when other antihypertensives are given concomitantly. However, some combinations should be avoided (see Calcium-channel Blockers, below). Beta blockers can potentiate the severe postural hypotension that may follow the initial dose of prazosin (see p.933) and can exacerbate rebound hypertension following withdrawal of clonidine treatment (see p.841).

Antimalarials. Some antimalarials, for example *halofantrine, mefloquine*, and *quinine* can cause cardiac conduction defects. Cardiopulmonary arrest has occurred after a single dose of mefloquine in a patient taking propranolol[1] (see p.433).

1. Anonymous. Mefloquine for malaria. *Med Lett Drugs Ther* 1990; **32:** 13–14.

Anxiolytics and antipsychotics. Plasma concentrations of some beta blockers may be reduced by *barbiturates.*[1-3] Increased plasma-propranolol concentrations and bioavailability and reduced metabolism have been reported in healthy subjects also given *chlorpromazine.*[4]

See p.664 for the effect of beta blockers on the pharmacokinetics of some *benzodiazepines.*

1. Sotaniemi EA, *et al.* Plasma clearance of propranolol and sotalol and hepatic drug-metabolizing enzyme activity. *Clin Pharmacol Ther* 1979; **26:** 153–61.
2. Haglund K, *et al.* Influence of pentobarbital on metoprolol plasma levels. *Clin Pharmacol Ther* 1979; **26:** 326–9.
3. Seideman P, *et al.* Decreased plasma concentrations and clinical effects of alprenolol during combined treatment with pentobarbitone in hypertension. *Br J Clin Pharmacol* 1987; **23:** 267–71.
4. Vestal RE, *et al.* Inhibition of propranolol metabolism by chlorpromazine. *Clin Pharmacol Ther* 1979; **25:** 19–24.

Calcium-channel blockers. Concurrent administration of calcium-channel blockers and beta blockers has resulted in hypotension, bradycardia, conduction defects, and cardiac failure.[1]

Beta blockers should be avoided in combination with cardiodepressant calcium-channel blockers such as *verapamil* (see p.962) and *diltiazem.*[2] Although they are reportedly safe in combination with the dihydropyridines such as *nifedipine,*[3] heart failure and severe hypotension have been reported (see under Nifedipine, p.918). Reported pharmacokinetic interactions include increased plasma concentrations of propranolol and of metoprolol with concurrent administration of diltiazem[4] or verapamil,[1] and increased plasma concentrations of propranolol with *nicardipine.*[5]

1. Lam YWF, Shepherd AMM. Drug interactions in hypertensive patients: pharmacokinetic, pharmacodynamic and genetic considerations. *Clin Pharmacokinet* 1990; **18:** 295–317.
2. Beevers DG, Wilkins MR. Drug treatment I: first choice agents. In: *ABC of Hypertension.* 2nd ed. London: British Medical Association, 1987: 25–7.
3. Reid JL. First-line and combination treatment for hypertension. *Am J Med* 1989; **86** (suppl 4A): 2–5.
4. Tateishi T, *et al.* Effect of diltiazem on the pharmacokinetics of propranolol, metoprolol and atenolol. *Eur J Clin Pharmacol* 1989; **36:** 67–70.
5. Schoors DF, *et al.* Influence of nicardipine on the pharmacokinetics and pharmacodynamics of propranolol in healthy volunteers. *Br J Clin Pharmacol* 1990; **29:** 497–501.

Ergot derivatives. *Nicergoline* enhanced the cardiac depressant action of propranolol in healthy subjects.[1]

For reports of enhanced vasoconstrictor action in patients taking *ergot alkaloids* and beta blockers, see p.446.

1. Boismare F, *et al.* Potentiation by an alpha-adrenolytic agent, nicergoline, of the cardiac effects of propranolol. *Methods Find Exp Clin Pharmacol* 1983; **5:** 83–8.

Histamine H_2-receptor antagonists. Plasma concentrations of propranolol and metoprolol may be increased by *cimetidine*;[1] pharmacokinetic studies indicate that cimetidine exerts its effect by reducing hepatic blood flow and impairing beta blocker metabolism. Cimetidine has been reported to increase the bioavailability of labetalol.[1]

1. Smith SR, Kendall MJ. Ranitidine versus cimetidine: a comparison of their potential to cause clinically important drug interactions. *Clin Pharmacokinet* 1988; **15:** 44–56.

Local anaesthetics. For details of the effect of beta blockers in reducing the clearance of *bupivacaine*, see p.1287, and of *lignocaine*, see p.1294.

NSAIDs. The antihypertensive effect of beta blockers may be impaired by concurrent administration of some NSAIDs, possibly due to their inhibition of renal synthesis of vasodilatory prostaglandins. This interaction probably occurs with all beta blockers but may not occur with all NSAIDs. For example, *sulindac* appears to affect blood pressure control less than *indomethacin.*[1]

1. Lam YWF, Shepherd AMM. Drug interactions in hypertensive patients: pharmacokinetic, pharmacodynamic and genetic considerations. *Clin Pharmacokinet* 1990; **18:** 295–317.

Opioid analgesics. Bioavailability of propranolol and metoprolol was increased in subjects given *dextropropoxyphene.*[1] Intravenous administration of *morphine* may increase serum concentrations of esmolol.[2]

1. Lundborg P, *et al.* The effect of propoxyphene pretreatment on the disposition of metoprolol and propranolol. *Clin Pharmacol Ther* 1981; **29:** 263–4.
2. Lowenthal DT, *et al.* Clinical pharmacology, pharmacodynamics and interactions with esmolol. *Am J Cardiol* 1985; **56:** 14F–17F.

Oral contraceptives. Plasma-metoprolol concentrations were increased in some women taking oral contraceptives.[1]

1. Kendall MJ, *et al.* Metoprolol pharmacokinetics and the oral contraceptive pill. *Br J Clin Pharmacol* 1982; **14:** 120–2.

Parasympathomimetics. For the effect of beta blockers on the response to *anticholinesterases*, see p.1394.

Skeletal muscle relaxants. For the effects of beta blockers on skeletal muscle relaxants, see under Atracurium, p.1306.

Thyroid drugs. For a discussion of thyroid status and its effect on plasma-propranolol concentrations and the effects of propranolol on *thyroid hormone* metabolism, see p.1498.

Xanthines. For details of reduced *theophylline* clearance in patients receiving beta blockers, see p.769.

Pharmacokinetics

Beta blockers differ widely in their pharmacokinetic properties. Differences in lipid solubility contribute to these varying pharmacokinetic properties. Beta blockers with low lipid solubility (hydrophilic beta blockers) include atenolol and nadolol. Beta blockers with high lipid solubility (lipophilic beta blockers) include alprenolol and propranolol. Generally, those with low lipid solubility tend to be less readily absorbed from the gastro-intestinal tract, to be less extensively metabolised, to have low plasma-protein binding, to have relatively long plasma half-lives, and to cross the blood-brain barrier less readily than beta blockers with high lipid solubility. Beta blockers cross the placenta and most are known to distribute into breast milk.

There is no clear correlation between plasma concentrations of beta blockers and therapeutic activity, especially when the beta blocker undergoes metabolism to active metabolites.

Uses and Administration

Beta blockers are competitive antagonists of the effects of catecholamines at beta-adrenergic receptor sites and are used in a variety of disorders, especially those affecting the cardiovascular system.

Two subtypes of beta-adrenergic receptors are recognised; $beta_1$ and $beta_2$. Blockade of $beta_1$ receptors reduces heart rate, myocardial contractility, and the rate of conduction of impulses through the conducting system. These effects are termed class II antiarrhythmic actions (p.776). Other effects of blockade of $beta_1$ receptors include suppression of adrenergic-induced renin release and lipolysis. Effects produced by blockade of $beta_2$ receptors include increased bronchial resistance and inhibition of catecholamine-induced glucose metabolism. $Beta_1$ receptors are found mainly in the heart while $beta_2$ receptors are found in noncardiac tissue, including bronchial tissue and peripheral blood vessels, although it is now recognised that in some organs, including the heart, both receptor subtypes are present. $Beta_2$ receptors may have a role in regulation of heart rate.

Individual beta blockers differ according to their pharmacological properties. See Table 1, below, for some of these characteristics and above. Beta blockers also differ widely in their pharmacokinetic properties (see above).

Beta blockers are used in the treatment of hypertension (p.788), angina pectoris (p.780), cardiac arrhythmias (p.782), and myocardial infarction (p.791). They are also used to control symptoms of sympathetic overactivity in the management of alcohol withdrawal (p.1099), in anxiety disorders (below), in hyperthyroidism (p.1489), and in tremor (below). Beta blockers are used in the prophylaxis of migraine (below) and of variceal bleeding associated with portal hypertension (p.1576). They are also used, in conjunction with an alpha-blocker, in the initial management of phaeochromocytoma (below). Some beta blockers are instilled as eye drops in the management of ocular hypertension and glaucoma (below).

The selection of a specific beta blocker for an individual patient depends on the condition being treated and patient characteristics such as liver and kidney function or existing disease such as diabetes. Patient tolerability also varies for different beta blockers. The characteristics of the beta blocker, for example, $beta_1$ selectivity and intrinsic sympathomimetic activity may also influence selection. However, the clinical significance of these properties is debated. $Beta_1$ selectivity may be clinically significant in patients with insulin-dependent diabetes mellitus.

Many of the newer beta blockers, such as carvedilol and celiprolol, have additional pharmacological properties such as vasodilator activity. These newer beta blockers have not yet been tested in large clinical trials and some practitioners advise that until they have, the older beta blockers, for example acebutolol, atenolol, metoprolol, pindolol, propranolol, and timolol should be preferred.

1. Hampton JR. Choosing the right β-blocker: a guide to selection. *Drugs* 1994; **48:** 549–68.
2. Brown MJ. To β block or better block? *Br Med J* 1995; **311:** 701–2.
3. Anonymous. Too many beta-blockers. *Drug Ther Bull* 1996; **34:** 49–52.

Anxiety disorders. Beta blockers have been used in patients with various anxiety disorders (p.635), including generalised anxiety disorders, panic disorders, and performance anxiety.[1] However, the role of beta blockers in anxiety disorders remains to be established.[2,3] Their benefits do not appear to be particularly great and they are probably most useful in reducing symptoms mediated through beta stimulation such as tremor or palpitations. Improvement usually occurs within 1 to 2 hours with relatively low doses of beta blockers (propranolol 40 mg, oxprenolol 40 to 80 mg, nadolol 40 mg). Some patients require higher doses and longer periods of treatment for a beneficial effect. A beta blocker may also be useful[4] in the management of pronounced somatic anxiety symptoms during withdrawal from opioids (p.67) or benzodiazepines (p.661).

1. Tyrer P. Current status of β-blocking drugs in the treatment of anxiety disorders. *Drugs* 1988; **36:** 773–83.
2. Manchanda R. Propranolol—the wonder drug for psychiatric disorders? *Br J Hosp Med* 1988; **39:** 267–71.
3. Manchanda R. Propranolol in anxiety. *Br J Hosp Med* 1988; **40:** 323.
4. DoH. *Drug misuse and dependence: guidelines on clinical management.* London: HMSO, 1991.

Cardiomyopathy. See under Heart Failure, below.

Extrapyramidal disorders. Beta blockers (in low doses) have been suggested for the management of antipsychotic-induced akathisia (see under Chlorpromazine, p.650).

Glaucoma and ocular hypertension. Topical beta blockers are often the drugs of first choice[1] for the initial treatment and maintenance of open-angle glaucoma and other chronic glaucomas (p.1387). They are believed to inhibit beta receptors in the ciliary epithelium and reduce the secretion of aqueous humour. Clinical studies have established that timolol, betaxolol, levobunolol, metipranolol, and carteolol are effective, generally reducing intra-ocular pressure to a similar extent.[2-6] Details on doses of these drugs are provided under the individual monographs. The possibility of systemic effects following topical use needs to be borne in mind (see above), especially in the elderly.[7]

Beta blockers are frequently combined with other ocular hypotensive drugs with different modes of action for optimum pressure control. However, Allen and Epstein[8] reported that the addition of adrenaline eye drops to treatment with timolol (a non-cardioselective beta blocker) did not result in an additive effect. On the other hand the addition of adrenaline to treatment with betaxolol (a cardioselective beta blocker) did result in additional benefit.[8]

Beta blockers have also been used for prophylaxis of postoperative ocular hypertension.[9,10]

1. Frishman WH, *et al.* Topical ophthalmic β-adrenergic blockade for the treatment of glaucoma and ocular hypertension. *J Clin Pharmacol* 1994; **34:** 795–803.
2. LeBlanc RP, *et al.* Timolol: long-term Canadian Multicentre Study. *Can J Ophthalmol* 1985; **20:** 128–30.
3. Stewart RH, *et al.* Betaxolol vs timolol: a six-month double-blind comparison. *Arch Ophthalmol* 1986; **104:** 46–8.
4. Geyer O, *et al.* Levobunolol compared with timolol: a four-year study. *Br J Ophthalmol* 1988; **72:** 892–6.
5. Krieglstein GK, *et al.* Levobunolol and metipranolol: comparative ocular hypotensive efficacy, safety, and comfort. *Br J Ophthalmol* 1987; **71:** 250–3.
6. Scoville B, *et al.* A double-masked comparison of carteolol and timolol in ocular hypertension. *Am J Ophthalmol* 1988; **105:** 150–4.
7. O'Donoghue E. β Blockers and the elderly with glaucoma: are we adding insult to injury? *Br J Ophthalmol* 1995; **79:** 794–6.
8. Allen RC, Epstein DL. Additive effect of betaxolol and epinephrine in primary open angle glaucoma. *Arch Ophthalmol* 1986; **104:** 1178–84.
9. West DR, *et al.* Comparative efficacy of the β-blockers for the prevention of increased intraocular pressure after cataract extraction. *Am J Ophthalmol* 1988; **106:** 168–73.
10. Odberg T. Primary argon laser trabeculoplasty after pretreatment with timolol. *Acta Ophthalmol (Copenh)* 1990; **68:** 317–19.

Heart failure. Beta blockers have negative inotropic properties and have generally been contra-indicated in patients with heart failure. However, they may be of value in some patients with heart failure due to idiopathic dilated cardiomyopathy (p.785). The beta blocker most commonly used is metoprolol although alprenolol, bisoprolol, bucindolol, carvedilol, labetalol, and practolol have also been studied. Beta blockers may also be of value in hypertrophic cardiomyopathy. They are employed to curtail tachycardia, reduce anginal pain, and prevent syncope. Beta blockers are also under investigation in heart failure (p.785) where persistent activation of the sympathetic nervous system appears to be associated with disease progression. Beta blockers might therefore be beneficial in the long-term management of heart failure and a systematic review[1] and a meta-analysis[2] of trials using various beta blockers have suggested that they may improve mortality. However, both concluded that further large, long-term studies were required and several studies are underway to clarify the role of beta blockers. Carvedilol has been the most commonly used beta blocker.

1. Doughty RN, *et al.* Effects of beta-blocker therapy on mortality in patients with heart failure; a systematic overview of randomized controlled trials. *Eur Heart J* 1997; **18:** 560–5.
2. Heidenreich PA, *et al.* Effect of beta-blockade on mortality in patients with heart failure: a meta-analysis of randomized clinical trials. *J Am Coll Cardiol* 1997; **30:** 27–34.

Hypotension. A beta blocker (such as atenolol or metoprolol) is reported to be one of the standard drugs used in the management of neurally mediated hypotension (p.790).

Migraine. Beta blockers (usually propranolol) are considered by many to be the drugs of choice in patients requiring prophylactic treatment for migraine (p.443). Their mechanism of action in this disorder is not fully understood. Other beta blockers reported to be effective are those that, like propranolol, possess no intrinsic sympathomimetic activity and include atenolol, metoprolol, nadolol, and timolol.

Beta blockers may sometimes also be of benefit in patients with chronic tension-type headache (p.444).

Peripheral vascular disease. Beta blockers may cause coldness of the extremities and have been reported to induce secondary Raynaud's syndrome. However, they may be of some help in the management of erythromelalgia (see under Peripheral Vascular Disease on p.794).

Phaeochromocytoma. Beta blockers are used, in conjunction with an alpha blocker, in the initial management of phaeochromocytoma (p.795). Beta blockers reduce the responses to the beta-adrenoceptor stimulating effects of adrenaline. Treatment must be started with the alpha blocker and only when alpha blockade is successfully established can tachycardia be controlled by the cautious use of a beta blocker. A $beta_1$-selective blocker is preferred so that peripheral $beta_2$-mediated vasodilatation is unaffected. In most cases modest doses are sufficient although higher doses may be required for a tumour that is predominantly adrenaline-secreting.

Tension-type headache. See under Migraine, above.

Tremor. Tremor is a rhythmical oscillation of part of the body caused by involuntary contraction of opposing muscles. It may occur during action, maintenance of posture, or at rest and varies in frequency and amplitude. Resting tremor is associated mainly with parkinsonism, the treatment of which is discussed on p.1128, whereas action tremor, which includes postural tremor and kinetic tremor, occurs in a wide variety of disorders and treatment of the underlying disorder may remove the tremor. Drugs such as bronchodilators, tricyclic

Table 1. Characteristics of beta blockers.

Beta blocker	$Beta_1$ selectivity	Intrinsic sympathomimetic activity	Membrane-stabilising activity
Acebutolol	+	+	+
Alprenolol	0	+	0
Atenolol	+	0	0
Betaxolol	+	0	0
Bisoprolol	+	0	0
Carteolol	0	+	–
Celiprolol	+	+	–
Esmolol	+	0	0
Labetalol	0	0	0
Levobunolol	0	0	0
Metipranolol	0	0	0
Metoprolol	+	0	0
Nadolol	0	0	0
Oxprenolol	0	+	+
Penbutolol	0	0	0
Pindolol	0	++	0
Propranolol	0	0	++
Sotalol	0	0	0
Timolol	0	0	0

0 = absent or low; + = moderate; ++ = high; – = no information

antidepressants, lithium, and caffeine may induce tremor; withdrawal of the causative drug usually alleviates the tremor. However, tremor often has no known underlying cause. Such tremor is referred to as essential tremor or benign essential tremor; it is usually postural and tends to affect the hands, head, voice, and sometimes the legs and trunk. It is exacerbated by emotional stress and anxiety. Essential tremor may appear at any age and is a lifelong condition that may progress with increasing age. In many cases there is a family history of the disorder (familial essential tremor).

Mild cases of essential tremor may require no regular treatment with drugs. Single doses of a beta blocker or a benzodiazepine may be useful in acute circumstances to control exacerbations provoked by stress. A single dose of propranolol usually produces a maximum effect after 1 to 2 hours and the effect may persist for several hours. Small amounts of alcohol may also provide effective temporary relief of essential tremor, although its regular use is obviously discouraged.

For more severe cases of essential tremor long-term drug treatment may be required (and may also be tried in other forms of tremor).[1-3] A beta blocker (usually propranolol) is often the first drug used. Up to 70% of people have been reported to respond, although the average tremor reduction is only about 50 to 60%. The beneficial effect appears to be predominantly due to blockade of peripheral beta$_2$ receptors on extrafusal muscle fibres and muscle spindles, although there may also be a CNS effect. Adverse effects may be troublesome on long-term use. Primidone may also be tried[4] although there may be a high incidence of acute adverse reactions following initial doses. Concern has been expressed that patients may become tolerant to these drugs given long-term. However, three small studies found a reduced response in only a few patients.[5-7] Local injection of botulinum A toxin has been tried in refractory essential tremor. In very severe disabling cases, surgery (thalamotomy) may have to be considered.

1. Hallett M. Classification and treatment of tremor. *JAMA* 1991; **266:** 1115–17.
2. Wills AJ. Essential tremor and related disorders. *Br J Hosp Med* 1995; **54:** 21–6.
3. Findley LJ. Essential tremor. *Br J Hosp Med* 1986; **35:** 388–92.
4. Koller WC, Royse VL. Efficacy of primidone in essential tremor. *Neurology* 1986; **36:** 121–4.
5. Koller WC, Vetere-Overfield B. Acute and chronic effects of propranolol and primidone in essential tremor. *Neurology* 1989; **39:** 1587–8.
6. Calzetti S, *et al.* Clinical and computer-based assessment of long-term therapeutic efficacy of propranolol in essential tremor. *Acta Neurol Scand* 1990; **81:** 392–6.
7. Sasso E, *et al.* Primidone in the long-term treatment of essential tremor: a prospective study with computerized quantitative analysis. *Clin Neuropharmacol* 1990; **13:** 67–76.

Betaxolol Hydrochloride (12439-p)

Betaxolol Hydrochloride *(BANM, USAN, rINNM)*.

ALO-1401-02; Betaxololi Hydrochloridum; SL-75212-10. 1-{4-[2-(Cyclopropylmethoxy)ethyl]phenoxy}-3-isopropylaminopropan-2-ol hydrochloride.

$C_{18}H_{29}NO_3,HCl = 343.9$.

CAS — 63659-18-7 (betaxolol); 63659-19-8 (betaxolol hydrochloride).

Pharmacopoeias. In *Eur.* (see p.viii) and *US.*

A white or almost white crystalline powder. Very **soluble** to freely soluble in water; freely soluble in alcohol, in chloroform, and in methyl alcohol; soluble in dichloromethane; practically insoluble in ether. A 2% solution in water has a pH of 4.5 to 6.5. **Store** in airtight containers. Protect from light.

Adverse Effects, Treatment, and Precautions

As for beta blockers, p.828.

Systemic side-effects have occasionally followed topical use of the eye drops; local irritation and photophobia have been reported.

Myocardial infarction occurred in an 81-year-old man shortly after administration of a single eye drop of betaxolol 0.5% solution.[1] He was also taking atenolol and indapamide for hypertension.

1. Chamberlain TJ. Myocardial infarction after ophthalmic betaxolol. *N Engl J Med* 1989; **321:** 1342.

Interactions

The interactions associated with beta blockers are discussed on p.829.

Since systemic absorption can follow ophthalmic use of beta blockers the possibility of interactions occurring with betaxolol eye drops should also be considered.

Pharmacokinetics

Betaxolol is completely absorbed from the gastro-intestinal tract and undergoes only minimal first-pass metabolism, resulting in a high oral bioavailability of 80 to 90%. It has high lipid solubility. Betaxolol is about 50% bound to plasma proteins. It crosses the placenta and is distributed into breast milk where higher concentrations have been achieved than in maternal blood. The plasma elimination half-life of betaxolol ranges from 16 to 20 hours. The primary route of elimination is via hepatic metabolism and urinary excretion; only about 15% is excreted in the urine as unchanged drug.

Pregnancy. The pharmacokinetics of betaxolol were investigated in the perinatal period in 28 pregnant hypertensive patients receiving doses of 10 to 40 mg daily.[1] Pharmacokinetic values were similar to those observed in non-pregnant patients. Umbilical-cord concentrations were similar to maternal blood concentrations and showed a negative correlation between concentration in cord blood and timing of the last dose of betaxolol. Thus the betaxolol concentration in the newborn can be considerably reduced by discontinuing drug administration to the mother 16 to 18 hours before birth. The blood-betaxolol half-life in the neonates ranged from 14.8 to 38.5 hours. The mean apparent half-life in infants with gestational age less than 36 weeks was about 32% higher than in full-term neonates. Betaxolol concentrations in milk and/or colostrum were determined in 3 mothers. In all samples the milk-to-blood ratio was greater than 2.

1. Morselli PL, *et al.* Placental transfer and perinatal pharmacokinetics of betaxolol. *Eur J Clin Pharmacol* 1990; **38:** 477–83.

Uses and Administration

Betaxolol is a cardioselective beta blocker (p.828). It is reported to lack intrinsic sympathomimetic activity. Betaxolol has some membrane-stabilising activity.

Betaxolol is used as the hydrochloride in the management of hypertension (p.788) and glaucoma (p.1387).

In **hypertension** betaxolol hydrochloride is given in initial doses of 10 to 20 mg as a single daily dose by mouth; doses may be increased if necessary after 1 to 2 weeks according to the patient's response, to 40 mg daily. Initial doses of 5 to 10 mg daily are suggested for elderly patients. Reduced dosages should also be used in patients with severe renal impairment.

Eye drops containing the equivalent of 0.25 or 0.5% betaxolol as the hydrochloride are instilled twice daily to reduce raised intra-ocular pressure in ocular hypertension and open-angle **glaucoma**.

General references.

1. Buckley MM-T, *et al.* Ocular betaxolol: a review of its pharmacological properties, and therapeutic efficacy in glaucoma and ocular hypertension. *Drugs* 1990; **40:** 75–90.

Speech disorders. A 50-year-old man who had stuttered since childhood obtained striking improvement in his stuttering (p.674) when he was given betaxolol 20 mg daily for essential hypertension.[1]

1. Burris JF, *et al.* Betaxolol and stuttering. *Lancet* 1990; **335:** 223.

Preparations

USP 23: Betaxolol Ophthalmic Solution; Betaxolol Tablets.

Proprietary Preparations (details are given in Part 3)
Aust.: Betoptic; ***Austral.:*** Betoptic; Betoquin; ***Belg.:*** Betoptic; Kerlone; ***Canad.:*** Betoptic; Kerlone; ***Fr.:*** Betoptic; Kerlone; ***Ger.:*** Betoptima; Kerlone; ***Irl.:*** Betoptic; ***Ital.:*** Betoptic; Kerlon; ***Neth.:*** Betoptic†; Kerlon; ***Norw.:*** Betoptic; ***S.Afr.:*** Betoptic; ***Spain:*** Betoptic; Kerlone†; Oxodal; ***Swed.:*** Betoptic; Kerlon; ***Switz.:*** Betoptic; Kerlon; ***UK:*** Betoptic; Kerlone; ***USA:*** Betoptic; Kerlone.

Multi-ingredient: ***USA:*** Kerledex.

Bethanidine Sulphate (854-j)

Bethanidine Sulphate *(BANM)*.

Betanidine Sulphate *(pINNM)*; Betanidini Sulfas; Bethanidine Sulfate *(USAN)*; BW-467-C-60; NSC-106563. 2-Benzyl-1,3-dimethylguanidine sulphate.

$(C_{10}H_{15}N_3)_2,H_2SO_4 = 452.6$.

CAS — 55-73-2 (bethanidine); 114-85-2 (bethanidine sulphate).

Pharmacopoeias. In *Eur.* (see p.viii) and *Jpn.*

A white powder. Freely **soluble** in water; sparingly soluble in alcohol; practically insoluble in ether.

Adverse Effects, Treatment, and Precautions

As for Guanethidine Monosulphate, p.878. Postural hypotension with transient sweating and headache may occur.

Interactions

As for Guanethidine Monosulphate, p.878.

Pharmacokinetics

Bethanidine is rapidly but incompletely absorbed from the gastro-intestinal tract. It is excreted unchanged in the urine and may accumulate to some extent in patients with impaired renal function.

References.

1. Shen D, *et al.* Pharmacokinetics of bethanidine in hypertensive patients. *Clin Pharmacol Ther* 1975; **17:** 363–73.

Uses and Administration

Bethanidine is an antihypertensive with actions and uses similar to those of guanethidine monosulphate (p.878), but it causes less depletion of noradrenaline stores. It also has a more rapid onset, together with a shorter duration of action, than guanethidine.

Bethanidine is used in the management of hypertension (p.788), although it has largely been superseded by other drugs less likely to cause orthostatic hypotension. It appears to have been tried in ventricular fibrillation.

Bethanidine is given by mouth as the sulphate.

The usual initial dose is 5 to 10 mg three times daily. The dosage may then be increased by 5 to 10 mg three times daily at brief intervals according to the response of the patient. The maintenance dose is normally in the range 100 to 200 mg daily.

For rapid blood pressure control, an initial dose of 20 mg of bethanidine sulphate may be given and increased by 10 to 20 mg every 4 to 6 hours.

Preparations

Proprietary Preparations (details are given in Part 3)
Irl.: Esbatal†; ***UK:*** Bendogen†.

Bevantolol Hydrochloride (12440-n)

Bevantolol Hydrochloride *(BANM, USAN, rINNM)*.

CI-775; NC-1400. 1-(3,4-Dimethoxyphenethylamino)-3-*m*-tolyloxypropan-2-ol hydrochloride.

$C_{20}H_{27}NO_4,HCl = 381.9$.

CAS — 59170-23-9 (bevantolol); 42864-78-8 (bevantolol hydrochloride).

Bevantolol is a cardioselective beta blocker (p.828). It is reported to be lacking in significant intrinsic sympathomimetic activity. It has weak membrane-stabilising properties and also has vasodilator activity.

Bevantolol is moderately lipid-soluble. It is reported to be virtually completely absorbed from the gastro-intestinal tract and to undergo moderate first-pass metabolism, resulting in a bioavailability of about 60%. It is extensively metabolised and excreted largely in urine as metabolites and small amounts of unchanged drug; the elimination half-life has been reported as 1.5 hours.

Bevantolol has been given by mouth as the hydrochloride in the management of hypertension and angina pectoris.

References.

1. Frishman WH, *et al.* Bevantolol: a preliminary review of its pharmacodynamic and pharmacokinetic properties, and therapeutic efficacy in hypertension and angina pectoris. *Drugs* 1988; **35:** 1–21.

Preparations

Proprietary Preparations (details are given in Part 3)
Neth.: Ranestol†.

Multi-ingredient: ***Neth.:*** Ranezide†.

Bietaserpine (12443-b)

Bietaserpine *(pINN)*.

1-(2-Diethylaminoethyl)reserpine; DL-152; S-1210. Methyl 1-(2-diethylaminoethyl)-18-*O*-(3,4,5-trimethoxybenzoyl)reserpate.

$C_{39}H_{53}N_3O_9 = 707.9$.

CAS — 53-18-9.

Bietaserpine is an antihypertensive with properties and uses similar to reserpine (p.942). It has been given as the tartrate.

Preparations

Proprietary Preparations (details are given in Part 3)

Multi-ingredient: ***Spain:*** Bietapres Complex†; Bietapres†.

Bisoprolol Fumarate (18615-w)

Bisoprolol Fumarate *(BANM, USAN, rINNM).*

CL-297939; EMD-33512 (bisoprolol or bisoprolol fumarate). 1-[4-(2-Isopropoxyethoxymethyl)phenoxy]-3-isopropylaminopropan-2-ol fumarate.

$(C_{18}H_{31}NO_4)_2,C_4H_4O_4$ = 767.0.

CAS — 66722-44-9 (bisoprolol); 66722-45-0 (bisoprolol fumarate); 104344-23-2 (bisoprolol fumarate).

Adverse Effects, Treatment, and Precautions

As for beta blockers, p.828.

Interactions

The interactions associated with beta blockers are discussed on p.829.

Pharmacokinetics

Bisoprolol is almost completely absorbed from the gastro-intestinal tract and undergoes only minimal first-pass metabolism resulting in an oral bioavailability of about 90%. Peak plasma concentrations are reached 2 to 4 hours after oral administration. Bisoprolol is about 30% bound to plasma proteins. It has a plasma elimination half-life of 10 to 12 hours. Bisoprolol is moderately lipid-soluble. Approximately 50% of a dose is metabolised in the liver and it is excreted in urine as unchanged drug and metabolites.

Uses and Administration

Bisoprolol is a cardioselective beta blocker (p.828). It is reported to be devoid of intrinsic sympathomimetic and membrane-stabilising properties.

Bisoprolol is given as the fumarate in the management of **hypertension** (p.788) and **angina pectoris** (p.780). It is under investigation in **heart failure** (p.785).

The usual dose of bisoprolol fumarate is 5 to 10 mg by mouth as a single daily dose; the maximum recommended dose is 20 mg daily. It is suggested that in patients with severe renal impairment (creatinine clearance less than 20 mL per minute) or severe hepatic dysfunction the dose should not exceed 10 mg daily.

References.

1. Lancaster SG, Sorkin EM. Bisoprolol: a preliminary review of its pharmacodynamic and pharmacokinetic properties, and therapeutic efficacy in hypertension and angina pectoris. *Drugs* 1988; **36:** 256–85.
2. Johns TE, Lopez LM. Bisoprolol: is this just another beta-blocker for hypertension or angina? *Ann Pharmacother* 1995; **29:** 403–14.

Preparations

Proprietary Preparations (details are given in Part 3)
Aust.: Concor; ***Belg.:*** Emconcor; Isoten; ***Fr.:*** Detensiel; Soprol; ***Ger.:*** Bisobloc; Bisomerck; Concor; Cordalin; Fondril; ***Irl.:*** Emcor; ***Ital.:*** Concor; ***Neth.:*** Bisobloc; Emcor; ***S.Afr.:*** Concor; ***Spain:*** Emconcor; Euradal; Godal; ***Swed.:*** Emconcor; ***Switz.:*** Concor; ***UK:*** Emcor; Monocor; ***USA:*** Zebeta.

Multi-ingredient: ***Aust.:*** Concor Plus; ***Belg.:*** Emcoretic; Maxsoten; ***Ger.:*** Concor Plus; Fondril-5 HCT; ***Neth.:*** Emcoretic; ***Spain:*** Emcoretic; ***Switz.:*** Concor Plus; ***UK:*** Monozide; ***USA:*** Ziac.

Bivalirudin (17816-e)

Bivalirudin *(BAN, USAN, rINN).*

BG-8967; Hirulog.

$C_{98}H_{138}N_{24}O_{33}$ = 2180.3.

CAS — 128270-60-0.

Bivalirudin, an analogue of the peptide hirudin (p.883), is a direct thrombin inhibitor under investigation as an anticoagulant in arterial thrombo-embolic disorders such as unstable angina and myocardial infarction. It is also under investigation as an adjunct in angioplasty procedures.

References.

1. Lidón R-M, *et al.* A pilot, early angiographic patency study using a direct thrombin inhibitor as adjunctive therapy to streptokinase in acute myocardial infarction. *Circulation* 1994; **89:** 1567–72.
2. Fuchs J, *et al.* Hirulog in the treatment of unstable angina: results of the Thrombin Inhibition in Myocardial Ischemia (TIMI) 7 trial. *Circulation* 1995; **92:** 727–33.
3. Bittl JA, *et al.* Treatment with bivalirudin (Hirulog) as compared with heparin during coronary angioplasty for unstable or postinfarction angina. *N Engl J Med* 1995; **333:** 764–9.
4. White HD, *et al.* Randomized, double-blind comparison of hirulog versus heparin in patients receiving streptokinase and aspirin for acute myocardial infarction (HERO). *Circulation* 1997; **96:** 2155–61.

Bopindolol Malonate (16544-a)

Bopindolol Malonate *(rINNM).*

Bopindolol Hydrogen Malonate; LT-31-200. (±)-1-(*tert*-Butylamino)-3-[(2-methylindol-4-yl)oxy]propan-2-ol benzoate malonate.

$C_{23}H_{28}N_2O_3,C_3H_4O_4$ = 484.5.

CAS — 62658-63-3 (bopindolol); 82857-38-3 (bopindolol malonate).

Bopindolol is a non-cardioselective beta blocker (p.828). It is reported to possess some intrinsic sympathomimetic activity.

It is used as the malonate in the management of hypertension (p.788) and angina pectoris (p.780) in daily doses equivalent to 0.5 to 2 mg of bopindolol by mouth.

References.

1. Harron DWG, *et al.* Bopindolol: review of its pharmacodynamic and pharmacokinetic properties and therapeutic efficacy. *Drugs* 1991; **41:** 130–49.

Preparations

Proprietary Preparations (details are given in Part 3)
Aust.: Sandonorm; ***Ger.:*** Wandonorm; ***Switz.:*** Sandonorm.

Multi-ingredient: ***Switz.:*** Sandoretic.

Bosentan (17405-z)

Bosentan *(USAN, rINN).*

Ro-47-0203/029. *p-tert*-Butyl-*N*-[6-(2-hydroxyethoxy)-5-(*o*-methoxyphenoxy)-2-(2-pyrimidinyl)-4-pyrimidinyl]benzenesulfonamide.

$C_{27}H_{29}N_5O_6S$ = 551.6.

CAS — 147536-97-8 (anhydrous bosentan); 157212-55-0 (bosentan monohydrate).

Bosentan is an endothelin receptor antagonist under investigation in the management of hypertension and heart failure.

References.

1. Krum H, *et al.* The effect of an endothelin-receptor antagonist, bosentan, on blood pressure in patients with essential hypertension. *N Engl J Med* 1998; **338:** 784–90.

Bretylium Tosylate (855-z)

Bretylium Tosylate *(BAN, USAN).*

Bretylium Tosilate *(rINN)*; ASL-603. (2-Bromobenzyl)ethyldimethylammonium toluene-4-sulphonate.

$C_{11}H_{17}BrN,C_7H_7O_3S$ = 414.4.

CAS — 59-41-6 (bretylium); 61-75-6 (bretylium tosylate).

Pharmacopoeias. In Br. and US.

A white, crystalline, hygroscopic powder. Freely **soluble** in water, in alcohol, and in methyl alcohol; practically insoluble in ether, in ethyl acetate, and in petroleum spirit. A 5% solution in water has a pH of 5.0 to 6.5.

Store in airtight containers. Protect from light.

Adverse Effects, Treatment, and Precautions

The most common adverse effect following administration of bretylium is hypotension which may be severe. Bretylium may also cause a transient initial increase in blood pressure and heart rate, and a worsening of cardiac arrhythmias due to a release of noradrenaline. Nausea and vomiting may occur particularly during rapid intravenous infusion. Intramuscular injection of bretylium can lead to local tissue necrosis and muscle atrophy, which can be avoided by limiting the volume and varying the site of the injection (see Uses and Administration, below). Care should be taken when administering bretylium to patients with impaired renal function and doses should be reduced. Caution is also required in patients with severe aortic stenosis or pulmonary hypertension who may be unable to increase cardiac output in response to the fall in peripheral resistance produced by bretylium.

Effects on body temperature. Bretylium tosylate administered by intravenous infusion was considered to be the cause of hyperthermia in a 59-year-old-man.[1] Six similar cases had been reported to the manufacturer in the USA.

1. Thibault J. Hyperthermia associated with bretylium tosylate injection. *Clin Pharm* 1989; **8:** 145–6.

Effects on the cardiovascular system. Seven patients with recent myocardial infarction, 3 with and 4 without left ventricular failure, received bretylium tosylate 5 to 10 mg per kg body-weight intravenously.[1] Initial transient tachycardia and hypertension, and late sustained bradycardia, hypotension with decreased vascular resistance, and increased calf blood flow and venous capacitance occurred in all 7 patients. Bretylium should be used cautiously in patients with hypotension as it might cause a significant reduction in arterial pressure.

1. Chatterjee K, *et al.* Cardiovascular effects of bretylium tosylate in acute myocardial infarction. *JAMA* 1973; **223:** 757–60.

Interactions

Bretylium may exacerbate arrhythmias caused by digitalis toxicity. If sympathomimetics are required to reverse bretylium-induced hypotension, great care should be exercised since their effects may be enhanced.

Pharmacokinetics

Bretylium tosylate is incompletely absorbed from the gastro-intestinal tract. It is well absorbed following intramuscular administration. It is not metabolised in the body and is largely excreted unchanged in the urine. The half-life is reported to be between 4 and 17 hours in patients with normal renal function and is prolonged in patients with impaired renal function. Bretylium is dialysable.

Reviews.

1. Rapeport WG. Clinical pharmacokinetics of bretylium. *Clin Pharmacokinet* 1985; **10:** 248–56.

Uses and Administration

Bretylium is a quaternary ammonium agent with class II and class III antiarrhythmic activity (p.776); it causes an initial release of noradrenaline and then blocks adrenergic transmission by preventing noradrenaline release from adrenergic nerve endings. It suppresses ventricular fibrillation and other ventricular arrhythmias, but the exact mode of action has yet to be determined.

It is given parenterally as the tosylate for the treatment of immediately life-threatening ventricular arrhythmias and for the short-term control of ventricular arrhythmias resistant to standard treatment (see p.782). If a positive response is to be seen in patients with ventricular fibrillation it usually occurs within minutes. However, a delay of up to several hours may occur before peak antiarrhythmic activity is achieved and therefore it should only be used in other ventricular arrhythmias if the arrhythmia is resistant to more rapidly acting drugs.

In immediately life-threatening ventricular arrhythmias such as **ventricular fibrillation** a suggested dose is 5 mg per kg body-weight as an undiluted 5% (50 mg per mL) solution by rapid intravenous injection, in association with other resuscitative measures and cardioversion, increased to 10 mg per kg if the ventricular fibrillation persists, and repeated as necessary up to a total dose of 30 mg per kg.

For the control of **ventricular arrhythmias** that are not immediately life-threatening bretylium may be given under ECG monitoring by intramuscular or slow intravenous injection. The patient should be supine or closely observed for postural hypotension. A dose of 5 to 10 mg per kg by either route may be repeated initially every 1 to 2 hours until the arrhythmia is controlled and subsequently every 6 hours intravenously or 6 to 8 hours intramuscularly for maintenance therapy. The patient should be changed to an oral antiarrhythmic as soon as possible. For intramuscular administration an undiluted 5% (50 mg per mL) solution is used; the site of intramuscular injections should be varied on repeated injection and not more than 5 mL should be given into any one site. Nausea and vomiting during intravenous administration can be avoided by administering the injection over not less than 8 minutes although a period of 15 to 30 minutes is preferred: the injection is diluted to 10 mg per mL with glucose 5% or sodium chloride 0.9%. Alternatively an intravenous infusion of 1 to 2 mg per minute has been recommended.

Doses should be reduced in patients with renal impairment.

Bretylium tosylate was originally used in the treatment of hypertension but because of poor gastric absorption and the development of tolerance during long-term therapy it has been superseded by other drugs.

Preparations

BP 1998: Bretylium Injection;
USP 23: Bretylium Tosylate in Dextrose Injection; Bretylium Tosylate Injection.

Proprietary Preparations (details are given in Part 3)
Austral.: Bretylate†; Critifib†; ***Belg.:*** Bretylate; ***Canad.:*** Bretylate; ***Fr.:*** Bretylate†; ***Irl.:*** Bretylate; ***Neth.:*** Bretylate†; ***S.Afr.:*** Bretylol†; ***UK:*** Bretylate; ***USA:*** Bretylol†.

Brimonidine Tartrate (1925-r)

Brimonidine Tartrate *(BANM, USAN, rINNM).*

AGN-190342-LF; UK-14304-18. 5-Bromo-6-(2-imidazolin-2-ylamino)quinoxaline D-tartrate.

$C_{11}H_{10}BrN_5,C_4H_6O_6$ = 442.2.

CAS — 59803-98-4 (brimonidine); 79570-19-7 (brimonidine tartrate).

Adverse Effects and Precautions

As for Apraclonidine Hydrochloride, p.824.

Uses and Administration

Brimonidine is an alpha$_2$-adrenoceptor agonist with actions and uses similar to those of apraclonidine (p.824). It is used to lower intra-ocular pressure in patients with open-angle glaucoma or ocular hypertension (p.1387), as an alternative to or as an adjunct to topical beta blocker therapy. The reduction in intra-ocular pressure is maximal about two hours after topical application.

Brimonidine is used as the tartrate. In the management of glaucoma or ocular hypertension one drop of a 0.2% solution is instilled into the affected eye or eyes two or three times daily.

References.

1. Anonymous. Brimonidine—an alpha$_2$-agonist for glaucoma. *Med Lett Drugs Ther* 1997; **39:** 54–5.

Preparations

Proprietary Preparations (details are given in Part 3)
Austral.: Alphagan; ***Swed.:*** Alphagan; ***UK:*** Alphagan; ***USA:*** Alphagan.

Brinzolamide (9711-h)

Brinzolamide *(USAN, rINN).*

AL-4862. (*R*)-4-(Ethylamino)-3,4-dihydro-2-(3-methoxypropyl)-2*H*-thieno[3,2-e]-1,2-thiazine-6-sulfonamide 1,1-dioxide.

$C_{12}H_{21}N_3O_5S_3$ = 383.5.

CAS — 138890-62-7.

Brinzolamide is a carbonic anhydrase inhibitor with general properties similar to those of dorzolamide (p.862). It is used topically to reduce intra-ocular pressure in the management of glaucoma and ocular hypertension.

Preparations

Proprietary Preparations (details are given in Part 3)
USA: Azopt.

Bucindolol Hydrochloride (12462-q)

Bucindolol Hydrochloride *(BANM, USAN, rINNM).*

MJ-13105-1. 2-[2-Hydroxy-3-(2-indol-3-yl-1,1-dimethylethylamino)propoxy]benzonitrile hydrochloride.

$C_{22}H_{25}N_3O_2,HCl$ = 399.9.

CAS — 71119-11-4 (bucindolol); 70369-47-0 (bucindolol hydrochloride).

Bucindolol is a non-cardioselective beta blocker (p.828). It is reported to possess intrinsic sympathomimetic activity as well as weak alpha$_1$-blocking activity, and also has direct vasodilating activity. Bucindolol, as the hydrochloride, has been investigated in the management of hypertension and cardiac disorders.

Bufetolol Hydrochloride (6305-w)

Bufetolol Hydrochloride *(rINNM).*

Y-6124. 1-*tert*-Butylamino-3-(2-tetrahydrofurfuryloxyphenoxy)propan-2-ol hydrochloride.

$C_{18}H_{29}NO_4,HCl$ = 359.9.

CAS — 53684-49-4 (bufetolol); 35108-88-4 (bufetolol hydrochloride).

Pharmacopoeias. In *Jpn.*

Bufetolol is a beta blocker (p.828). It has been given as the hydrochloride by mouth in the management of various cardiovascular disorders.

Preparations

Proprietary Preparations (details are given in Part 3)
Ital.: Adobiol†.

Buflomedil Hydrochloride (12465-w)

Buflomedil Hydrochloride *(BANM, rINNM).*

LL-1656. 2′,4′,6′-Trimethoxy-4-(pyrrolidin-1-yl)butyrophenone hydrochloride.

$C_{17}H_{25}NO_4,HCl$ = 343.8.

CAS — 55837-25-7 (buflomedil); 35543-24-9 (buflomedil hydrochloride).

Adverse Effects

Buflomedil has been reported to cause gastro-intestinal disturbances, headache, vertigo, syncope, rash, pruritus, and paraesthesia. Overdosage may produce severe hypotension, tachycardia, and convulsions.

References.

1. Bachand RT, Dubourg AY. A review of long-term safety data with buflomedil. *J Int Med Res* 1990; **18:** 245–52.

Pharmacokinetics

Buflomedil hydrochloride is absorbed from the gastro-intestinal tract and peak plasma concentrations are reached 1.5 to 4 hours following oral administration. Buflomedil is subject to first-pass metabolism; bioavailability is reported to be between 50 and 80%.

Buflomedil is widely distributed. Binding to plasma proteins is dose-dependent and varies between 60 and 80% at therapeutic concentrations. Buflomedil is metabolised in the liver and is mainly excreted in the urine both as unchanged drug and metabolites. The elimination half-life is about 2 to 3 hours. Elimination may be impaired in patients with renal or hepatic impairment.

Uses and Administration

Buflomedil hydrochloride is a vasodilator used in the treatment of cerebrovascular (p.785) and peripheral vascular disease (p.794). Usual doses by mouth are 300 to 600 mg daily, by intramuscular injection up to 100 mg daily, by slow intravenous injection up to 200 mg daily, and by intravenous infusion up to 400 mg daily.

References.

1. Clissold SP, *et al.* Buflomedil: a review of its pharmacodynamic and pharmacokinetic properties, and therapeutic efficacy in peripheral and cerebral vascular diseases. *Drugs* 1987; **33:** 430–60.

Preparations

Proprietary Preparations (details are given in Part 3)
Aust.: Loftyl; ***Belg.:*** Loftyl; ***Fr.:*** Fonzylane; Loftyl; ***Ger.:*** Bufedil; Buflo-Puren; Buflo-Reu; Bufloхeal; Defluina; ***Ital.:*** Bufene; Buflan; Buflocit; Buflofar; Bufoxin; Emoflux; Flomed; Flupress; Irrodan; Loftyl; Medil; Perfudan; Pirxane; ***Neth.:*** Loftyl; ***S.Afr.:*** Loftyl; ***Spain:*** Lofton; Sinoxis; ***Switz.:*** Loftyl.

Bufuralol Hydrochloride (6306-e)

Bufuralol Hydrochloride *(BANM, rINNM).*

Ro-03-4787. 2-*tert*-Butylamino-1-(7-ethylbenzofuran-2-yl)ethanol hydrochloride.

$C_{16}H_{23}NO_2,HCl$ = 297.8.

CAS — 54340-62-4 (bufuralol); 60398-91-6 (bufuralol hydrochloride).

Bufuralol is a non-cardioselective beta blocker (p.828). It has high intrinsic sympathomimetic activity.

Bumetanide (2310-r)

Bumetanide *(BAN, USAN, rINN).*

Bumetanidum; Ro-10-6338. 3-Butylamino-4-phenoxy-5-sulphamoylbenzoic acid.

$C_{17}H_{20}N_2O_5S$ = 364.4.

CAS — 28395-03-1.

Pharmacopoeias. In *Chin., Eur.* (see p.viii), *Jpn*, and *US.*

A white crystalline powder. Practically **insoluble** to slightly soluble in water; soluble in acetone and in alcohol; slightly soluble in dichloromethane and in ether; soluble in alkaline solutions. **Store** in airtight containers. Protect from light.

Adverse Effects

As for Frusemide, p.871. Bumetanide may cause muscle pain, particularly at high doses.

Effects on the ears. Early reports suggested that bumetanide might be less ototoxic than frusemide.[1] However, both drugs can cause deafness, especially when given in large doses to patients with renal impairment.

1. Ward A, Heel RC. Bumetanide: a review of its pharmacodynamic and pharmacokinetic properties and therapeutic use. *Drugs* 1984; **28:** 426–64.

Effects on the muscles. Bumetanide, particularly in high doses in patients with chronic renal impairment, may cause severe musculoskeletal pain. A curious muscle stiffness distinct from cramp, with tenderness to compression and pain on movement, was noted in association with bumetanide therapy in 4 patients with end-stage renal failure.[1] The calf muscles were the first to be affected; shoulder girdle and thigh muscle tenderness also occurred in 2 patients, and one patient also had neck stiffness. The side-effect appeared to be dose-related for the individual patients.

1. Barclay JE, Lee HA. Clinical and pharmacokinetic studies on bumetanide in chronic renal failure. *Postgrad Med J* 1975; **51** (suppl 6): 43–6.

Effects on the skin. Bullous pemphigoid developed in one patient approximately 6 weeks after starting therapy with bumetanide.[1] Healing occurred after withdrawal of the drug without the need for corticosteroid treatment.

1. Boulinguez S, *et al.* Bullous pemphigoid induced by bumetanide. *Br J Dermatol* 1998; **138:** 548–9.

Precautions

Bumetanide's precautions and contra-indications are generally dependent on its effects on fluid and electrolyte balance and are similar to those of the thiazide diuretics (see Hydrochlorothiazide, p.887).

Interactions

As for Frusemide, p.872.

Pharmacokinetics

Bumetanide is almost completely and fairly rapidly absorbed from the gastro-intestinal tract; the bioavailability is reported to be about 80 to 95%. It has a plasma elimination half-life of about 1 to 2 hours. It is about 95% bound to plasma proteins. About 80% of the dose is excreted in the urine, approximately 50% as unchanged drug, and 10 to 20% in the faeces.

References to the pharmacokinetics of bumetanide in healthy subjects.

1. Halladay SC, *et al.* Diuretic effect and metabolism of bumetanide in man. *Clin Pharmacol Ther* 1977; **22:** 179–87.
2. Pentikäinen PJ, *et al.* Fate of [^{14}C]-bumetanide in man. *Br J Clin Pharmacol* 1977; **4:** 39–44.
3. Holazo AA, *et al.* Pharmacokinetics of bumetanide following intravenous, intramuscular, and oral administrations to normal subjects. *J Pharm Sci* 1984; **73:** 1108–13.
4. McCrindle JL, *et al.* Effect of food on the absorption of frusemide and bumetanide in man. *Br J Clin Pharmacol* 1996; **42:** 743–6.

Hepatic impairment. In a study of 8 patients with chronic hepatic disease,[1] the diuretic response to bumetanide 1 mg was impaired but bumetanide excretion rates were normal.

1. Marcantonio LA, *et al.* The pharmacokinetics and pharmacodynamics of the diuretic bumetanide in hepatic and renal disease. *Br J Clin Pharmacol* 1983; **15:** 245–52.

Renal impairment. Renal excretion of bumetanide has been shown to be reduced in patients with chronic renal impairment with a subsequent attenuation of diuretic effect.[1-3] Lau and colleagues[2] reported that the cumulative pharmacodynamic effects of oral and intravenous doses were essentially similar in patients with renal impairment and that transition from intravenous to oral maintenance regimens should pose no special problems.

1. Marcantonio LA, *et al.* The pharmacokinetics and pharmacodynamics of the diuretic bumetanide in hepatic and renal disease. *Br J Clin Pharmacol* 1983; **15:** 245–52.

2. Lau HSH, *et al.* Kinetics, dynamics, and bioavailability of bumetanide in healthy subjects and patients with chronic renal failure. *Clin Pharmacol Ther* 1986; **39:** 635–45.
3. Howlett MR, *et al.* Metabolism of the diuretic bumetanide in healthy subjects and patients with renal impairment. *Eur J Clin Pharmacol* 1990; **38:** 583–6.

Uses and Administration

Although chemically unrelated, bumetanide is a loop diuretic with actions and uses similar to those of frusemide (p.872). Bumetanide is used in the treatment of oedema associated with heart failure (p.785) and with renal and hepatic disorders. It is given in high doses in the management of oliguria due to renal failure or insufficiency. Bumetanide has also been used in hypertension (p.788).

Diuresis is initiated within about 30 minutes to an hour after a dose by mouth, reaches a maximum at 1 to 2 hours, and lasts for about 4 hours but may be prolonged to 6 hours after high doses; after intravenous injection its effects are evident within a few minutes and last for about 2 hours. As a general guide bumetanide 1 mg produces a diuretic effect similar to frusemide 40 mg although this should not be used for direct substitution at higher doses.

In the treatment of **oedema** the usual dose is 1 mg by mouth in the morning or early evening; a second dose may be given 6 to 8 hours later if necessary. A dose of 0.5 mg daily may be adequate in some elderly patients.

In refractory oedema higher doses may be necessary, usually starting at a dose of 5 mg daily. Dose increments of 5 mg every 12 to 24 hours as required have been advocated although other sources have suggested a maximum total dose of 10 mg daily. Twice daily dosing may be preferred at higher doses. For maintenance therapy doses may be given daily or intermittently. In an emergency or when oral therapy cannot be given 0.5 to 1 mg may be administered by intramuscular or slow intravenous injection, subsequently adjusted according to the patient's response. A recommended dose for pulmonary oedema is 1 to 2 mg by intravenous injection, repeated 20 minutes later if necessary. Alternatively, 2 to 5 mg may be given over 30 to 60 minutes in 500 mL of a suitable infusion fluid.

In the treatment of **hypertension** bumetanide has been given in doses of 0.5 to 2 mg daily by mouth.

In susceptible patients potassium supplements or potassium-sparing diuretics may be necessary, but see under hydrochlorothiazide (Uses and Administration, p.887). When very high doses of bumetanide are used careful laboratory control is essential as described under the uses for frusemide (p.872; high-dose therapy).

General references.

1. Ward A, Heel RC. Bumetanide: a review of its pharmacodynamic and pharmacokinetic properties and therapeutic use. *Drugs* 1984; **28:** 426–64.

Preparations

BP 1998: Bumetanide and Slow Potassium Tablets; Bumetanide Injection; Bumetanide Oral Solution; Bumetanide Tablets;
USP 23: Bumetanide Injection; Bumetanide Tablets.

Proprietary Preparations (details are given in Part 3)
Aust.: Burinex; ***Austral.:*** Burinex; ***Belg.:*** Burinex; ***Canad.:*** Burinex; ***Fr.:*** Burinex; ***Ger.:*** Burinex; Fordiuran†; ***Irl.:*** Burinex; ***Ital.:*** Burinex†; Fontego; ***Neth.:*** Burinex; ***Norw.:*** Burinex; ***S.Afr.:*** Burinex; ***Spain:*** Butinat†; Farmadiuril; Fordiuran; ***Swed.:*** Burinex; ***Switz.:*** Burinex; ***UK:*** Betinex; Burinex; ***USA:*** Bumex.

Multi-ingredient: ***Irl.:*** Buram; Burinex K; ***Norw.:*** Burinex K; ***S.Afr.:*** Burinex K†; ***UK:*** Burinex A; Burinex K.

Bunaftine Citrate (7782-n)

Bunaftine Citrate *(rINNM)*.

Bunaphtine Citrate. *N*-Butyl-*N*-(2-diethylaminoethyl)-1-naphthamide dihydrogen citrate.

$C_{21}H_{30}N_2O,C_6H_8O_7$ = 518.6.

CAS — 32421-46-8 (bunaftine).

Bunaftine is reported to have class III antiarrhythmic activity (p.776) and has been given by mouth as the citrate and by intramuscular injection as the hydrochloride for the treatment of cardiac arrhythmias.

Preparations

Proprietary Preparations (details are given in Part 3)
Ital.: Meregon†.

Bunazosin Hydrochloride (18560-e)

Bunazosin Hydrochloride *(rINNM)*.

E-643. 1-(4-Amino-6,7-dimethoxy-2-quinazolinyl)-4-butyrylhexahydro-1*H*-1,4-diazepine monohydrochloride.

$C_{19}H_{27}N_5O_3,HCl$ = 409.9.

CAS — 80755-51-7 (bunazosin); 52712-76-2 (bunazosin hydrochloride).

Pharmacopoeias. In *Jpn.*

Bunazosin is an alpha$_1$-adrenoceptor blocker (p.776) with general properties similar to those of prazosin (p.932). It is given by mouth as the hydrochloride in the management of hypertension.

Preparations

Proprietary Preparations (details are given in Part 3)
Ger.: Andante; ***Jpn:*** Detantol.

Bunitrolol Hydrochloride (6307-l)

Bunitrolol Hydrochloride *(rINNM)*.

Ko-1366 (bunitrolol). 2-(3-*tert*-Butylamino-2-hydroxypropoxy)benzonitrile hydrochloride.

$C_{14}H_{20}N_2O_2,HCl$ = 284.8.

CAS — 34915-68-9 (bunitrolol); 23093-74-5 (bunitrolol hydrochloride).

Bunitrolol is a beta blocker (p.828). It is given as the hydrochloride by mouth in the management of cardiovascular disorders.

Preparations

Proprietary Preparations (details are given in Part 3)
Aust.: Stresson; ***Ger.:*** Stresson†.

Bupranolol Hydrochloride (6309-j)

Bupranolol Hydrochloride *(rINNM)*.

B-1312; KL-255. 1-*tert*-Butylamino-3-(6-chloro-*m*-tolyloxy)propan-2-ol hydrochloride.

$C_{14}H_{22}ClNO_2,HCl$ = 308.2.

CAS — 14556-46-8 (bupranolol); 15148-80-8 (bupranolol hydrochloride).

Pharmacopoeias. In *Jpn.*

Bupranolol is a beta blocker (p.828). It is given as the hydrochloride in usual doses of 100 to 400 mg daily by mouth in the management of cardiovascular disorders.

Bupranolol eye drops in concentrations of 0.05 to 0.5% have been used in the management of glaucoma (p.1387).

Preparations

Proprietary Preparations (details are given in Part 3)
Aust.: Adomed; ***Ger.:*** Betadrenol; Ophtorenin†; ***Ital.:*** Betadrenol†.

Multi-ingredient: ***Aust.:*** Beta-Isoket†; Betamed; ***Ger.:*** Beta-Isoket†; cardiotensin†; Oxycardin†; pertenso†.

Butalamine Hydrochloride (9215-s)

Butalamine Hydrochloride *(BANM, rINNM)*.

LA-1221. *NN*-Dibutyl-*N'*-(3-phenyl-1,2,4-oxadiazol-5-yl)ethylenediamine hydrochloride.

$C_{18}H_{28}N_4O,HCl$ = 352.9.

CAS — 22131-35-7 (butalamine); 56974-46-0 (butalamine hydrochloride).

Butalamine hydrochloride is a vasodilator given in the management of peripheral (p.794) and cerebral vascular disorders (p.785) in a usual dose of 80 to 240 mg daily by mouth.

Preparations

Proprietary Preparations (details are given in Part 3)
Ger.: Adrevil; ***Ital.:*** Surheme†; ***Spain:*** Surem.

Multi-ingredient: ***Fr.:*** Oxadilene.

Buthiazide (2311-f)

Buthiazide *(USAN)*.

Butizide *(rINN)*; Isobutylhydrochlorothiazide; Thiabutazide. 6-Chloro-3,4-dihydro-3-isobutyl-2*H*-1,2,4-benzothiadiazine-7-sulphonamide 1,1-dioxide.

$C_{11}H_{16}ClN_3O_4S_2$ = 353.8.

CAS — 2043-38-1.

Buthiazide is a thiazide diuretic with properties similar to those of hydrochlorothiazide (p.885). It is used for oedema, including that associated with heart failure (p.785), and for hypertension (p.788).

Buthiazide is given by mouth in doses of 5 to 15 mg daily or on 2 or 3 days weekly for the treatment of oedema. It is also given in doses of 2.5 to 10 mg daily for hypertension, either alone or in conjunction with other antihypertensive drugs.

Preparations

Proprietary Preparations (details are given in Part 3)
Aust.: Saltucin; ***Ger.:*** Saltucin.

Multi-ingredient: ***Aust.:*** Aldactone Saltucin; Modenol; Suprenoat; Torrat; ***Ger.:*** Aldactone Saltucin; Modenol; Sembrina-Saltucin†; Torrat; Tri-Torrat; ***Ital.:*** Kadiur; Saludopin; ***S.Afr.:*** Aldazide; Saltucin Co†; ***Switz.:*** Aldozone; Modenol†; Sali-Spiroctan; Torrat†.

Cadralazine (16559-h)

Cadralazine *(BAN, rINN)*.

CGP-18684/E; ISF-2469. Ethyl 3-{6-[ethyl(2-hydroxypropyl)amino]pyridazin-3-yl}carbazate.

$C_{12}H_{21}N_5O_3$ = 283.3.

CAS — 64241-34-5.

Cadralazine is a vasodilator with actions and uses similar to those of hydralazine (p.883). In the treatment of hypertension (p.788) it is given in doses of 10 to 15 mg daily, as a single dose by mouth.

Reviews.

1. McTavish D, *et al.* Cadralazine: a review of its pharmacodynamic and pharmacokinetic properties, and therapeutic potential in the treatment of hypertension. *Drugs* 1990; **40:** 543–60.

Cadralazine is reported not to produce the lupus-like syndrome seen in some patients receiving hydralazine.[1,2]

1. Andersson OK. Cadralazine did not produce the SLE-syndrome when hydralazine did. *Eur J Clin Pharmacol* 1987; **31:** 741.
2. Mulder H. Conversion of drug-induced SLE-syndrome by the vasodilating agent cadralazine. *Eur J Clin Pharmacol* 1990; **38:** 303.

Preparations

Proprietary Preparations (details are given in Part 3)
Ital.: Cadraten; Cadrilan.

Cafedrine Hydrochloride (12500-x)

Cafedrine Hydrochloride *(BANM, pINNM)*.

H-8351; Kafedrin Hydrochloride. 7-[2-(β-Hydroxy-α-methylphenethylamino)ethyl]theophylline hydrochloride.

$C_{18}H_{23}N_5O_3,HCl$ = 393.9.

CAS — 58166-83-9 (cafedrine).

Cafedrine hydrochloride is a derivative of theophylline (p.765), used in the treatment of hypotensive states in a usual dose of 100 to 400 mg daily by mouth.

Preparations

Proprietary Preparations (details are given in Part 3)
Ital.: Akrinor†.

Multi-ingredient: ***Aust.:*** Akrinor; ***Fr.:*** Praxinor; ***Ger.:*** Akrinor; ***S.Afr.:*** Akrinor; ***Spain:*** Bifort; ***Switz.:*** Akrinor.

Calcitonin Gene-related Peptide (18900-z)

CGRP.

Calcitonin gene-related peptide is an endogenous peptide derived from the calcitonin gene. It has vasodilating activity and is under investigation in the management of peripheral vascular disease (Raynaud's syndrome), heart failure, and for ischaemia following neurosurgery for subarachnoid haemorrhage.

For details of the endogenous substance and its pharmacological effects, see under Calcitonins, p.735.

References.

1. Shawket S, *et al.* Selective suprasensitivity to calcitonin-gene-related peptide in the hands in Raynaud's phenomenon. *Lancet* 1989; **ii:** 1354–7.
2. Bunker CB, *et al.* Calcitonin gene-related peptide and Raynaud's phenomenon. *Lancet* 1990; **335:** 239.
3. Johnston FG, *et al.* Effect of calcitonin-gene-related peptide on postoperative neurological deficits after subarachnoid haemorrhage. *Lancet* 1990; **335:** 869–72.
4. Shawkett S, *et al.* Prolonged effect of CGRP in Raynaud's patients: a double-blind randomised comparison with prostacyclin. *Br J Clin Pharmacol* 1991; **32:** 209–13.
5. Shekhar YC, *et al.* Effects of prolonged infusion of human alpha calcitonin gene-related peptide on haemodynamics, renal blood flow and hormone levels in congestive heart failure. *Am J Cardiol* 1991; **67:** 732–6.
6. European CGRP in Subarachnoid Haemorrhage Study Group. Effect of calcitonin-gene-related peptide in patients with delayed postoperative cerebral ischaemia after aneurysmal subarachnoid haemorrhage. *Lancet* 1992; **339:** 831–4.
7. Bunker CB, *et al.* Calcitonin gene-related peptide in treatment of severe peripheral vascular insufficiency in Raynaud's phenomenon. *Lancet* 1993; **342:** 80–2.

Candesartan Cilexetil (17153-e)

Candesartan Cilexetil (*BANM, USAN, rINNM*).

CV-11974 (candesartan); TCV-116. (±)-1-Hydroxyethyl 2-ethoxy-1-[*p*-(*o*-1*H*-tetrazol-5-ylphenyl)benzyl]-7-benzimidazolecarboxylate, cyclohexyl carbonate ester.

$C_{33}H_{34}N_6O_6$ = 610.7.

CAS — 139481-59-7 (candesartan); 145040-37-5 (candesartan cilexetil).

Adverse Effects and Precautions

As for Losartan Potassium, p.899.

Pharmacokinetics

Candesartan cilexetil is an ester prodrug that is hydrolysed in the body to the active form candesartan. It is absorbed from the gastro-intestinal tract with an absolute bioavailability for candesartan of about 40% following administration of candesartan cilexetil as a solution and about 14% following administration as tablets. Peak plasma concentrations of candesartan occur about 3 to 4 hours after oral administration. Candesartan is more than 99% bound to plasma proteins. It is excreted in urine and bile mainly as unchanged drug and a small amount of inactive metabolites. The terminal elimination half-life is approximately 9 hours.

Uses and Administration

Candesartan is an angiotensin II receptor antagonist with actions similar to those of losartan (p.899). It is used in the management of hypertension (p.788).

Candesartan is administered by mouth as the ester prodrug candesartan cilexetil. The onset of antihypertensive effect occurs about 2 hours after administration and the maximum effect is achieved within about 4 weeks after initiating therapy.

In the management of hypertension candesartan cilexetil is given in an initial dose of 4 mg once daily. A lower initial dose of 2 mg once daily is suggested for patients with renal or hepatic impairment. The dose should be adjusted according to response. The usual maintenance dose is 8 mg once daily with a maximum dose of 16 mg once daily.

Preparations

Proprietary Preparations (details are given in Part 3)
Swed.: Atacand; ***UK:*** Amias; ***USA:*** Atacand.

Candoxatril (12037-y)

Candoxatril (*BAN, USAN, rINN*).

UK-79300. *cis*-4-{1-[(*S*)-2-(Indan-5-yloxycarbonyl)-3-(2-methoxyethoxy)propyl]cyclopentylcarbonylamino}cyclohexanecarboxylic acid.

$C_{29}H_{41}NO_7$ = 515.6.

CAS — 118785-03-8; 123122-55-4.

Candoxatril is an ester prodrug which is hydrolysed in the body following oral administration to its active form candoxatrilat. Candoxatrilat is a neutral endopeptidase (neutral metalloendopeptidase) inhibitor. It is a potent inhibitor of the endopeptidase responsible for the metabolism of atrial natriuretic peptide (ANP) (p.826); inhibition of this enzyme results in raised ANP concentrations with consequent natriuresis and suppression of the renin-angiotensin-aldosterone system. Candoxatril is under investigation in the management of hypertension and heart failure.

The active (+)-enantiomer of the competitive atriopeptidase inhibitor candoxatrilat (UK-69578) has been shown by Barclay and others to be twice as potent as the racemic form in inhibiting degradation of atrial natriuretic peptide (ANP) *in vitro*;[1] Northridge and colleagues, using the racemic form, have shown it to be a potent and selective inhibitor of endopeptidase 24.11 and intravenous infusions in doses of up to 10 mg per kg body-weight over 20 minutes in 16 healthy subjects were well tolerated, and increased endogenous circulating ANP concentrations with associated diuresis and natriuresis; similar results were obtained in 6 men with chronic heart failure.[2] Richards and co-workers found similar results on administration of the orally active prodrug candoxatril 25 or 50 mg to 6 subjects; both doses produced an increase in plasma ANP, peak enhancement occurring 2 to 3 hours after administration.[3] Plasma renin activity and plasma aldosterone concentrations were reduced by candoxatril treatment and natriuresis increased, but blood pressure and heart rate were not affected.[3] Candoxatril has also been shown to reduce the elimination of exogenous ANP in patients with chronic heart failure.[4] However, the endopeptidase enzyme is not specific for ANP and candoxatril has also been reported to increase plasma concentrations of endothelin and calcitonin gene-related peptide.[5]

1. Barclay PL, *et al.* Inhibitory potencies of UK-69578 and thiorphan. *Lancet* 1990; **336:** 754–5.
2. Northridge DB, *et al.* Effects of UK 69578: a novel atriopeptidase inhibitor. *Lancet* 1989; **ii:** 591–3.
3. Richards M, *et al.* Inhibition of endopeptidase EC24 11 in humans: renal and endocrine effects. *Hypertension* 1990; **16:** 269–76.
4. Motwani JG, *et al.* Dose-ranging effects of candoxatril on elimination of exogenous atrial natriuretic peptide in chronic heart failure. *Clin Pharmacol Ther* 1993; **54:** 661–9.
5. McDowell G, *et al.* The effect of the neutral endopeptidase inhibitor drug, candoxatril, on circulating levels of two of the most potent vasoactive peptides. *Br J Clin Pharmacol* 1997; **43:** 329–32.

Canrenoate Potassium (2313-n)

Canrenoate Potassium (*BANM, USAN*).

Potassium Canrenoate (*rINN*); Aldadiene Potassium; MF-465a; SC-14266. Potassium 17-hydroxy-3-oxo-17α-pregna-4,6-diene-21-carboxylate.

$C_{22}H_{29}KO_4$ = 396.6.

CAS — 4138-96-9 (canrenoic acid); 2181-04-6 (canrenoate potassium).

Pharmacopoeias. In *Jpn.*

Adverse Effects and Precautions

As for Spironolactone, p.946. Irritation or pain may occur at the site of injection.

Effects on endocrine function. A lower incidence of gynaecomastia has been reported in patients with hepatic cirrhosis and ascites during treatment with canrenoate potassium compared with equivalent doses of spironolactone[1] and spironolactone-induced gynaecomastia disappeared when spironolactone was replaced by canrenoate potassium in a patient with hyperaldosteronism.[2] This suggests that metabolites other than canrenone (a common metabolite of both canrenoate and spironolactone thought to be responsible for their activity) or possibly spironolactone itself may be responsible for the anti-androgenic effects of spironolactone.[3,4]

1. Bellati G, Idéo G. Gynaecomastia after spironolactone and potassium canrenoate. *Lancet* 1986; **i:** 626.
2. Dupont A. Disappearance of spironolactone-induced gynaecomastia during treatment with potassium canrenoate. *Lancet* 1985; **ii:** 731.
3. Gardiner P. Spironolactone and potassium canrenoate metabolism. *Lancet* 1985; **ii:** 1432.
4. Overdiek JWPM, Merkus FWHM. Spironolactone metabolism and gynaecomastia. *Lancet* 1986; **i:** 1103.

Interactions

As for Spironolactone, p.947.

Uses and Administration

Canrenoate potassium is a potassium-sparing diuretic with actions and uses similar to those of spironolactone (p.947). Canrenone is a metabolite common to both drugs, but its contribution to the pharmacological action is unclear. Canrenoate potassium is used in the treatment of refractory oedema associated with heart failure (p.785) or hepatic disease when an injectable aldosterone antagonist is required. It may be given in doses of 200 to 400 mg daily, increasing to 800 mg daily in exceptional cases, by slow intravenous injection over a period of 2 to 3 minutes per 200 mg or by intravenous infusion in glucose 5% or sodium chloride 0.9%.

Preparations

Proprietary Preparations (details are given in Part 3)
Aust.: Aldactone; Osiren; ***Belg.:*** Canrenol; Soldactone; ***Fr.:*** Soludactone; ***Ger.:*** Aldactone; Kalium-Can; Osyrol; ***Ital.:*** Kanrenol; Luvion; Venactone; ***Neth.:*** Soldactone; Spiroctan†; ***Norw.:*** Soldactone; ***S.Afr.:*** Soldactone†; ***Swed.:*** Soldactone; ***Switz.:*** Soldactone; Spiroctan; ***UK:*** Spiroctan-M.

Multi-ingredient: ***Ital.:*** Kadiur.

Canrenone (2312-d)

Canrenone (*USAN, pINN*).

SC-9376. 17-Hydroxy-3-oxo-17α-pregna-4,6-diene-21-carboxylic acid γ-lactone.

$C_{22}H_{28}O_3$ = 340.5.

CAS — 976-71-6.

Canrenone is a potassium-sparing diuretic with properties similar to those of spironolactone (p.946) and is used in the treatment of refractory oedema associated with heart failure (p.785) or hepatic disease, and in hypertension (p.788). It is a metabolite of both spironolactone and canrenoate potassium (above). It is given in usual doses of 50 to 200 mg daily by mouth. Doses of up to 300 mg daily may be required in some patients.

Preparations

Proprietary Preparations (details are given in Part 3)
Belg.: Contaren; ***Ital.:*** Luvion.

Capobenic Acid (12520-n)

Capobenic Acid (*USAN, rINN*).

C-3 (capobenic acid and sodium salt). 6-(3,4,5-Trimethoxybenzamido)hexanoic acid.

$C_{16}H_{23}NO_6$ = 325.4.

CAS — 21434-91-3 (capobenic acid); 27276-25-1 (capobenate sodium).

Capobenic acid is a coronary vasodilator that has been used in ischaemic heart disease and the management of heart failure.

Preparations

Proprietary Preparations (details are given in Part 3)
Spain: Pectoris†.

Captopril (856-c)

Captopril (*BAN, USAN, rINN*).

Captoprilum; SQ-14225. 1-[(2*S*)-3-Mercapto-2-methylpropionyl]-L-proline.

$C_9H_{15}NO_3S$ = 217.3.

CAS — 62571-86-2.

NOTE. Compounded preparations of captopril and hydrochlorothiazide in the proportions, by weight, 2 parts to 1 part have the British Approved Name Co-zidocapt.

Pharmacopoeias. In *Chin., Eur.* (see p.viii), and *US.*

A white or off-white crystalline powder which may have a characteristic sulphide-like odour. Freely **soluble** in water, in alcohol, in chloroform, in dichloromethane, and in methyl alcohol. It dissolves in dilute solutions of alkali hydroxides. A 2% solution in water has a pH of 2.0 to 2.6. **Store** in airtight containers.

Stability. Although captopril itself is relatively stable at temperatures up to 50°,[1] and extemporaneously prepared powders (made by triturating the tablets with lactose) have been reported to be stable for at least 12 weeks at room temperature,[2] aqueous solutions are subject to oxidative degradation, mainly to captopril disulphide,[1] which increases with increase in pH above 4.[3] The manufacturers report that a liquid form prepared from pulverised tablets in distilled water containing 1 mg of captopril per mL retained 96.6% of the original concentration of drug after storage at room temperature for 5 days, but they advise that since it contains no preservative it should be used within 2 days of preparation.[4] Others have reported wide variations in stability depending upon the formulation. The shelf-life of a solution of captopril 1 mg per mL prepared from crushed tablets and tap water[5] was estimated to be 27 days when stored at 5°. In another study[6] captopril disappeared at a much faster rate in tap water than in sterile water for irrigation; in the sterile water captopril was stable for at least 3 days when stored at 5°. Increased stability has been reported following the addition of sodium ascorbate to the solution,[7] and with captopril powder rather than crushed tablets.[8] A 1 mg per mL preparation made with crushed tablets and undiluted syrup has also been reported to be stable for 30 days at 5° and may be more palatable than aqueous formulations.[9]

1. Lund W, Cowe HJ. Stability of dry powder formulations. *Pharm J* 1986; **237:** 179–80.
2. Taketomo CK, *et al.* Stability of captopril in powder papers under three storage conditions. *Am J Hosp Pharm* 1990; **47:** 1799–1801.
3. Timmins P, *et al.* Factors affecting captopril stability in aqueous solution. *Int J Pharmaceutics* 1982; **11:** 329–36.
4. Andrews CD, Essex A. Captopril suspension. *Pharm J* 1986; **237:** 734–5.
5. Pereira CM, Tam YK. Stability of captopril in tap water. *Am J Hosp Pharm* 1992; **49:** 612–15.
6. Anaizi NH, Swenson C. Instability of aqueous captopril solutions. *Am J Hosp Pharm* 1993; **50:** 486–8.
7. Nahata MC, *et al.* Stability of captopril in three liquid dosage forms. *Am J Hosp Pharm* 1994; **51:** 95–6.
8. Chan DS, *et al.* Degradation of captopril in solutions compounded from tablets and standard powder. *Am J Hosp Pharm* 1994; **51:** 1205–7.
9. Lye MYF, *et al.* Effects of ingredients on stability of captopril in extemporaneously prepared oral liquids. *Am J Health-Syst Pharm* 1997; **54:** 2483–7.

Adverse Effects, Treatment, and Precautions

As for ACE inhibitors, p.805.

Captopril has been reported to cause false positive results in tests for acetone in urine.

Results of postmarketing surveillance in 30 515 hypertensive patients receiving captopril showed that 4.9% had their therapy discontinued because of adverse effects thought to be due to the drug. The mean initial daily dose was 46 mg; at final evaluation the mean daily dose was 58 mg. The adverse effect most commonly reported was headache (in 1.8%); others included dizziness (1.6%), rashes (1.1%), nausea (1.0%), taste disturbances (0.9%), and cough (0.8%).[1] This study excluded patients with impaired renal function but an earlier survey in 6737 patients who received captopril alone or in combination found that rash and dysgeusia were more frequent in patients with impaired renal function (occurring in 6.2% and 3.2% respectively of those receiving 150 mg daily or less of captopril) than in those with normal serum creatinine (4.3% and 2.2%). The frequency of both symptoms was somewhat higher in those given higher doses. Symptoms of hypotension occurred in about 5% of patients and were not influenced by dose or renal function.[2] The cumulative frequency of withdrawal due to adverse reactions was estimated at 5.8% in this study, which is similar to that in the larger survey. In another postmarketing surveillance study involving more than 60 000 patients, captopril was withdrawn in 8.9% because of adverse effects.[3]

For further reference to some of these adverse effects, see under ACE Inhibitors, p.805.

1. Schoenberger JA, *et al.* Efficacy, safety, and quality-of-life assessment of captopril antihypertensive therapy in clinical practice. *Arch Intern Med* 1990; **150:** 301–6.
2. Jenkins AC, *et al.* Captopril in hypertension: seven years later. *J Cardiovasc Pharmacol* 1985; **7** (suppl 1): S96–S101.
3. Chalmers D, *et al.* Postmarketing surveillance of captopril for hypertension. *Br J Clin Pharmacol* 1992; **34:** 215–23.

Interactions

As for ACE inhibitors, p.807.

Pharmacokinetics

About 60 to 75% of a dose of captopril is absorbed from the gastro-intestinal tract and peak plasma concentrations are achieved within about an hour. Absorption has been reported to be reduced in the presence of food, but see under Absorption, below. Captopril is about 30% bound to plasma proteins. It crosses the placenta and is found in breast milk at about 1% of maternal blood concentrations. It is largely excreted in the urine, 40 to 50% as unchanged drug, the rest as disulphide and other metabolites. The elimination half-life has been reported to be 2 to 3 hours but this is increased in renal failure. Captopril is removed by haemodialysis.

Reviews.

1. Duchin KL, *et al.* Pharmacokinetics of captopril in healthy subjects and in patients with cardiovascular diseases. *Clin Pharmacokinet* 1988; **14:** 241–59.

Absorption. The bioavailability and peak plasma concentrations of captopril have been shown to be reduced by 25 to 55% on administration with food in single dose studies[1-4] and with chronic dosing.[5] However, Izumi *et al.* found insignificant differences in these parameters between the fasting and nonfasting states,[6] and their study, as well as those of Müller *et al.*[3] and Mäntylä *et al.*,[4] indicated that food intake had no effect on the antihypertensive activity of captopril.

1. Williams GM, Sugerman AA. The effect of a meal, at various times relative to drug administration, on the bioavailability of captopril. *J Clin Pharmacol* 1982; **22:** 18A.
2. Singhvi SM, *et al.* Effect of food on the bioavailability of captopril in healthy subjects. *J Clin Pharmacol* 1982; **22:** 135–40.
3. Müller HM, *et al.* The influence of food intake on pharmacodynamics and plasma concentration of captopril. *J Hypertens* 1985; **3** (suppl 2): S135–6.
4. Mäntylä R. *et al.* Impairment of captopril bioavailability by concomitant food and antacid intake. *Int J Clin Pharmacol Ther Toxicol* 1984; **22:** 626–9.
5. Öhman KP, *et al.* Pharmacokinetics of captopril and its effects on blood pressure during acute and chronic administration and in relation to food intake. *J Cardiovasc Pharmacol* 1985; **7** (suppl 1): S20–4.
6. Izumi Y, *et al.* Influence of food on the clinical effect of angiotensin I converting enzyme inhibitor (SQ 14225). *Tohoku J Exp Med* 1983; **139:** 279–86.

Renal impairment. A study of 9 patients with chronic renal failure undergoing dialysis found that peak plasma concentrations of captopril were 2.5 times higher and peak concentrations of the disulphide metabolites were 4 times higher than in patients with normal renal function following a single dose of captopril.[1] Peak concentrations occurred later in uraemic patients and the apparent half-life of total captopril was 46 hours in uraemic patients compared with 2.95 hours in patients with normal renal function.

1. Drummer OH, *et al.* The pharmacokinetics of captopril and captopril disulfide conjugates in uraemic patients on maintenance dialysis: comparison with patients with normal renal function. *Eur J Clin Pharmacol* 1987; **32:** 267–71.

Uses and Administration

Captopril is a sulfhydryl-containing ACE inhibitor (p.805). It is used in the management of hypertension (p.788), in heart failure (p.785), following myocardial infarction (p.791), and in diabetic nephropathy (p.809).

Following oral administration captopril produces a maximum effect within 1 to 2 hours, although the full effect may not develop for several weeks during chronic dosing. The duration of action is dose-dependent and may persist for 6 to 12 hours.

In the treatment of **hypertension** the initial dose is 12.5 mg twice daily by mouth, increased gradually at intervals of 2 to 4 weeks according to the response. The usual maintenance dose is 25 to 50 mg twice daily and should not normally exceed 50 mg three times daily. If hypertension is not satisfactorily controlled at this dosage, addition of a second drug or substitution of an alternative drug should be considered. In the USA higher doses of up to 150 mg three times daily have been suggested for patients with hypertension uncontrolled by lower doses of captopril in conjunction with diuretic therapy. Since there may be a precipitous fall in blood pressure in some patients when starting therapy with an ACE inhibitor, the first dose should preferably be given at bedtime and if diuretics are already being taken they should be stopped, if possible, for a few days before introducing captopril. An initial dose of 6.25 mg twice daily is recommended if captopril is given in addition to a diuretic or to elderly patients.

In the treatment of **heart failure** severe first-dose hypotension on introduction of an ACE inhibitor is common in patients on loop diuretics, but their temporary withdrawal may cause rebound pulmonary oedema. Thus an initial dose of 6.25 to 12.5 mg of captopril is given by mouth under close medical supervision; the usual maintenance dose is 25 mg two or three times daily, and doses should not normally exceed 50 mg three times daily. Again, in the USA higher doses of up to 150 mg three times daily have been suggested.

Following **myocardial infarction**, captopril is used prophylactically in clinically stable patients with symptomatic or asymptomatic left ventricular dysfunction to improve survival, delay the onset of symptomatic heart failure, and reduce recurrent infarction. It may be started 3 days after myocardial infarction in an initial dose of 6.25 mg by mouth, increased over several weeks to 150 mg daily in divided doses if tolerated.

In **diabetic nephropathy** (microalbuminuria greater than 30 mg per day) in type 1 diabetics, 75 to 100 mg of captopril may be given daily, in divided doses, by mouth. Other antihypertensives may be used with captopril if a further reduction in blood pressure is required. In patients with severe renal impairment (creatinine clearance less than 30 mL per minute) the initial dose of captopril should be 12.5 mg twice daily and if a diuretic also needs to be given a loop diuretic should be chosen rather than a thiazide.

Administration. Captopril is generally given orally. Sublingual[1] and intravenous[2,3] administration has also been tried, but these routes are not established.

1. Angeli P, *et al.* Comparison of sublingual captopril and nifedipine in immediate treatment of hypertensive emergencies: a randomized, single-blind clinical trial. *Arch Intern Med* 1991; **151:** 678–82.
2. Savi L, *et al.* A new therapy for hypertensive emergencies: intravenous captopril. *Curr Ther Res* 1990; **47:** 1073–81.
3. Langes K, *et al.* Efficacy and safety of intravenous captopril in congestive heart failure. *Curr Ther Res* 1993; **53:** 167–76.

Administration in children. Experience with captopril in children is limited. The UK manufacturers have suggested an initial dose of 0.3 mg per kg body-weight increased as necessary to a maximum of 6 mg per kg daily given in two or three divided doses. They do not recommend captopril for the treatment of mild to moderate hypertension in children.

Captopril, given in an initial dose of 0.25 mg per kg body-weight daily, increased to up to 2.5 or 3.5 mg per kg daily in 3 divided doses has also been reported to produce benefit in infants with severe heart failure secondary to congenital defects (predominantly manifesting as left-to-right shunt).[1,2]

1. Scammell AM, *et al.* Captopril in treatment of infant heart failure: a preliminary report. *Int J Cardiol* 1987; **16:** 295–301.
2. Shaw NJ, *et al.* Captopril in heart failure secondary to a left to right shunt. *Arch Dis Child* 1988; **63:** 360–3.

Nitrate tolerance. For reference to the use of captopril as a sulfhydryl donor in the management of nitrate tolerance, see under Precautions of Glyceryl Trinitrate, p.875.

Preparations

BP 1998: Captopril Tablets;
USP 23: Captopril and Hydrochlorothiazide Tablets; Captopril Tablets.

Proprietary Preparations (details are given in Part 3)
Aust.: Debax; Lopirin; ***Austral.:*** Acenorm; Capace; Capoten; Captohexal; Enzace; ***Belg.:*** Capoten; ***Canad.:*** Capoten; Nu-Capto; ***Fr.:*** Captolane; Lopril; ***Ger.:*** ACE-Hemmer; Acenorm; Adocor; Capto; Capto-dura Cor; Capto-ISIS; Capto-Puren Cor; Captobeta; Captoflux; Captogamma; Captohexal; Captomerck; Captopress; Captoreal; cor tensobon; Coronorm; Epicordin; Esparil; Lopirin Cor; Mundil; Sansanal; Sigacap Cor; Tensiomin-Cor; Tensobon; Tensostad; ***Irl.:*** Aceomel; Capoten; Captor; Geroten; ***Ital.:*** Acepress; Capoten; ***Neth.:*** Capoten; ***Norw.:*** Capoten; ***S.Afr.:*** Capace; Capoten; ***Spain:*** Alopresin; Capoten; Cesplon; Dardex; Dilabar; Garanil; Tensoprel; ***Swed.:*** Capoten; ***Switz.:*** Lopirin; Tensobon; ***UK:*** Acepril; Capoten; ***USA:*** Capoten.

Multi-ingredient: ***Aust.:*** Capozide; Captocomp; Captopril Compositum; Veracapt; ***Fr.:*** Captea; Ecazide; ***Ger.:*** Capozide; Tensobon comp; ***Irl.:*** Capozide; ***Ital.:*** Acediur; Aceplus; ***Neth.:*** Aceplus; Capozide; ***S.Afr.:*** Capozide; ***Spain:*** Alopresin Diu; Cesplon Plus; Decresco; Dilabar Diu; Ecadiu; Ecazide; Eutiman†; ***Swed.:*** Capozid; ***Switz.:*** Capozide; Tensobon comp; ***UK:*** Acezide; Capozide; ***USA:*** Capozide.

Carazolol (12521-h)

Carazolol *(BAN, rINN)*.

BM-51052. 1-(Carbazol-4-yloxy)-3-isopropylaminopropan-2-ol.

$C_{18}H_{22}N_2O_2$ = 298.4.

CAS — 57775-29-8.

Carazolol is a beta blocker (p.828). It is given in doses of 5 to 30 mg daily by mouth in the management of various cardiovascular disorders.

Preparations

Proprietary Preparations (details are given in Part 3)
Aust.: Conducton; ***Ger.:*** Conducton.

Carteolol Hydrochloride (12533-g)

Carteolol Hydrochloride *(BANM, USAN, rINNM)*.

Abbott-43326; OPC-1085. 5-(3-*tert*-Butylamino-2-hydroxypropoxy)-3,4-dihydroquinolin-2(1*H*)-one hydrochloride.

$C_{16}H_{24}N_2O_3,HCl$ = 328.8.

CAS — 51781-06-7 (carteolol); 51781-21-6 (carteolol hydrochloride).

Pharmacopoeias. In *Br.*, *Jpn*, and *US*.

White crystals or a white crystalline powder. **Soluble** in water; very slightly soluble in alcohol and in glacial acetic acid; sparingly soluble in methyl alcohol; practically insoluble in ether. A 1% solution in water has a pH of 5.0 to 6.0.

Store in airtight containers.

Adverse Effects, Treatment, and Precautions

As for beta blockers, p.828.

Systemic side-effects may follow topical use of the eye drops; local irritation, blurred vision, and photophobia have also been reported.

Interactions

The interactions associated with beta blockers are discussed on p.829.

Since systemic absorption can follow ophthalmic use of beta blockers, the possibility of interactions occurring with carteolol eye drops should also be considered.

Pharmacokinetics

Carteolol, given as the hydrochloride, is well absorbed from the gastro-intestinal tract with a peak plasma concentration being reached within 1 to 3 hours of oral administration. It has low lipid solubility. Approximately 20 to 30% is protein bound. The plasma half-life is reported to be 5 to 6 hours. The major route of elimination is renal with 50 to 70% of carteolol being excreted unchanged in the urine. Major metabolites are 8-hydroxycarteolol and glucuronic acid conjugates of carteolol and 8-hydroxycarteolol. The 8-hydroxycarteolol metabolite is active; its half-life is reported to be 8 to 12 hours. Because the main route of elimination is renal carteolol accumulates in patients with renal disease.

Uses and Administration

Carteolol is a non-cardioselective beta blocker (see p.828). It is reported to possess intrinsic sympathomimetic activity.

Carteolol is used as the hydrochloride in the management of glaucoma (p.1387), hypertension (p.788), and some cardiac disorders such as angina pectoris (p.780) and cardiac arrhythmias (p.782).

Eye drops containing carteolol hydrochloride 1% or 2% are instilled twice daily to reduce raised intra-ocular pressure in open-angle **glaucoma** and ocular hypertension.

In **hypertension** carteolol hydrochloride is given in initial doses of 2.5 mg once daily by mouth, increased, if necessary according to the patient's response, to 10 mg once daily. In cardiac disorders such as **angina pectoris** and **arrhythmias** carteolol hydrochloride has been employed in doses of 10 to 30 mg daily.

The oral dose of carteolol hydrochloride should be reduced in patients with renal impairment. It is suggested that the dosage interval should be increased from 24 hours to 48 hours in patients with a creatinine clearance of 20 to 60 mL per minute and to 72 hours in patients with a creatinine clearance of less than 20 mL per minute.

Preparations

BP 1998: Carteolol Eye Drops;
USP 23: Carteolol Hydrochloride Ophthalmic Solution; Carteolol Hydrochloride Tablets.

Proprietary Preparations (details are given in Part 3)
Aust.: Endak; ***Belg.:*** Carteol; ***Fr.:*** Carteol; Mikelan; ***Ger.:*** Arteoptic; Endak; ***Irl.:*** Teoptic; ***Ital.:*** Carteol; ***Jpn:*** Mikelan; ***Neth.:*** Teoptic; ***S.Afr.:*** Mikelan; ***Spain:*** Arteolol; Arteoptic†; Elebloc; Mikelan; ***Swed.:*** Arteoptic; ***Switz.:*** Arteoptic; ***UK:*** Cartrol†; Teoptic; ***USA:*** Cartrol; Ocupress.

Multi-ingredient: ***Fr.:*** Carpilo.

Carvedilol (18917-n)

Carvedilol *(BAN, USAN, rINN).*

BM-14190. 1-Carbazol-4-yloxy-3-[2-(2-methoxyphenoxy)ethylamino]propan-2-ol.

$C_{24}H_{26}N_2O_4$ = 406.5.

CAS — 72956-09-3.

Adverse Effects, Treatment, and Precautions

As for beta blockers, p.828.

Liver function abnormalities, reversible on stopping treatment with carvedilol, have been reported rarely. Carvedilol is not recommended in patients with hepatic dysfunction. Acute renal failure and renal abnormalities have been reported in patients with heart failure who also suffered from diffuse vascular disease and/or renal impairment.

Effects on lipid metabolism. Beta blockers may affect plasma-lipid concentrations (p.829), although these effects may be less pronounced with beta blockers that also block alpha-adrenergic receptors. Carvedilol has been reported to have no adverse effects on plasma-lipid concentrations.[1]

1. Hauf-Zachariou U, *et al.* A double-blind comparison of the effects of carvedilol and captopril on serum lipid concentrations in patients with mild to moderate essential hypertension and dyslipidaemia. *Eur J Clin Pharmacol* 1993; **45:** 95–100.

Interactions

The interactions associated with beta blockers are discussed on p.829.

Pharmacokinetics

Carvedilol is well absorbed from the gastro-intestinal tract but is subject to considerable first-pass metabolism in the liver; the absolute bioavailability is about 25%. Peak plasma concentrations occur 1 to 2 hours after administration. It has high lipid solubility. Carvedilol is more than 98% bound to plasma proteins. It is extensively metabolised in the liver, the metabolites being excreted mainly in the bile. The elimination half-life is about 6 to 10 hours. Carvedilol has been shown to accumulate in breast milk in *animals*.

References.

1. Neugebauer G, *et al.* Stereoselective disposition of carvedilol in man after intravenous and oral administration of the racemic compound. *Eur J Clin Pharmacol* 1990; **38:** S108–S111.
2. McTavish D, *et al.* Carvedilol: a review of its pharmacodynamic and pharmacokinetic properties, and therapeutic efficacy. *Drugs* 1993; **45:** 232–58.
3. Morgan T. Clinical pharmacokinetics and pharmacodynamics of carvedilol. *Clin Pharmacokinet* 1994; **26:** 335–46.

Uses and Administration

Carvedilol is a non-cardioselective beta blocker (p.828). It also has vasodilating properties that are attributed mainly to its blocking activity at $alpha_1$ receptors; at higher doses calcium-channel blocking activity may contribute.

Carvedilol is used in the management of hypertension (p.788), angina pectoris (p.780), and heart failure (p.785).

In **hypertension** carvedilol is given in an initial dose of 12.5 mg once daily by mouth, increased after two days to 25 mg once daily. Alternatively, an initial dose of 6.25 mg is given twice daily, increased after one to two weeks to 12.5 mg twice daily. The dose may be increased further, if necessary, at intervals of at least two weeks, to 50 mg once daily or in divided doses. A dose of 12.5 mg once daily may be adequate for elderly patients.

In **angina pectoris** an initial dose of 12.5 mg is given twice daily by mouth, increased after two days to 25 mg twice daily.

In **heart failure** 3.125 mg is given by mouth twice daily for two weeks. The dose may then be increased, if tolerated, to 6.25 mg twice daily. The dosage should be increased as tolerated at intervals of at least two weeks to a maximum recommended dose of 25 mg twice daily for patients weighing less than 85 kg or 50 mg twice daily for patients weighing more than 85 kg.

References.

1. Ruffolo RR, *et al.* The pharmacology of carvedilol. *Eur J Clin Pharmacol* 1990; **38:** S82–8.
2. McTavish D, *et al.* Carvedilol: a review of its pharmacodynamic and pharmacokinetic properties, and therapeutic efficacy. *Drugs* 1993: **45:** 232–58.
3. Morgan T. Clinical pharmacokinetics and pharmacodynamics of carvedilol. *Clin Pharmacokinet* 1994; **26:** 335–46.
4. Louis WJ, *et al.* A risk-benefit assessment of carvedilol in the treatment of cardiovascular disorders. *Drug Safety* 1994; **11:** 86–93.
5. Krum H, *et al.* Double-blind, placebo-controlled study of the long-term efficacy of carvedilol in patients with severe chronic heart failure. *Circulation* 1995; **92:** 1499–1506.
6. Packer M, *et al.* The effect of carvedilol on morbidity and mortality in patients with chronic heart failure. *N Engl J Med* 1996; **334:** 1349–55.
7. Australia/New Zealand Heart Failure Research Collaborative Group. Randomised, placebo-controlled trial of carvedilol in patients with congestive heart failure due to ischaemic heart disease. *Lancet* 1997; **349:** 375–80.
8. Dunn CJ, *et al.* Carvedilol: a reappraisal of its pharmacological properties and therapeutic use in cardiovascular disorders. *Drugs* 1997; **54:** 161–85.
9. Frishman WH. Carvedilol. *N Engl J Med* 1998; **339:** 1759–65.

Administration in the elderly. The manufacturer of carvedilol recommends an initial dose of 12.5 mg once daily in hypertension. A study in 16 elderly patients (mean age 70 years) given single doses of 12.5 mg and 25 mg found a high incidence of postural hypotension[1] and the authors suggested that a starting dose lower than 12.5 mg may be necessary in elderly patients.

1. Krum H, *et al.* Postural hypotension in elderly patients given carvedilol. *Br Med J* 1994; **309:** 775–6.

Preparations

Proprietary Preparations (details are given in Part 3)
Aust.: Dilatrend; ***Belg.:*** Dimitone; Kredex; ***Ger.:*** Dilatrend; Querto; ***Ital.:*** Carvipress; Dilatrend; Kredex; ***Neth.:*** Eucardic; ***Norw.:*** Dilatrend; Kredex; ***S.Afr.:*** Dilatrend; ***Spain:*** Coropres; Kredex; ***Swed.:*** Eucardic; Kredex; ***Switz.:*** Dilatrend; ***UK:*** Eucardic; ***USA:*** Coreg.

Celiprolol Hydrochloride (16573-d)

Celiprolol Hydrochloride *(BANM, USAN, rINNM).*

3-{3-Acetyl-4-[3-(*tert*-butylamino)-2-hydroxypropoxy]phenyl}-1,1-diethylurea hydrochloride.

$C_{20}H_{33}N_3O_4,HCl$ = 416.0.

CAS — 56980-93-9 (celiprolol); 57470-78-7 (celiprolol hydrochloride).

Adverse Effects, Treatment, and Precautions

As for beta blockers, p.828.

Tremor and palpitations associated with intrinsic sympathomimetic activity at $beta_2$ receptors have been reported.

Interactions

The interactions associated with beta blockers are discussed on p.829.

Pharmacokinetics

Celiprolol is absorbed from the gastro-intestinal tract in a non-linear fashion; the percentage of the dose absorbed increases with increasing dose. The plasma elimination half-life is about 5 to 6 hours. Celiprolol crosses the placenta. It has low lipid solubility. Metabolism is minimal and celiprolol is mainly excreted unchanged in the urine and faeces.

Uses and Administration

Celiprolol is a cardioselective beta blocker (p.828). It is reported to possess intrinsic sympathomimetic activity and direct vasodilator activity. Celiprolol is used as the hydrochloride in the management of **hypertension** (p.788) and **angina pectoris** (p.780). The usual dose of celiprolol hydrochloride is 200 to 400 mg once daily by mouth. Reduced doses may be required in patients with impaired renal function; suggested guidelines are to reduce the dose by 50% when creatinine clearance is between 15 and 40 mL per minute, but not to use at all when it is below 15 mL per minute.

References.

1. Riddell JG, *et al.* Celiprolol: a preliminary review of its pharmacodynamic and pharmacokinetic properties and its therapeutic use in hypertension and angina pectoris. *Drugs* 1987; **34:** 438–58.
2. Milne RJ, Buckley MM-T. Celiprolol: an updated review of its pharmacodynamic and pharmacokinetic properties, and therapeutic efficacy in cardiovascular disease. *Drugs* 1991; **41:** 941–69.
3. Anonymous. Celiprolol: theory and practice. *Lancet* 1991; **338:** 1426–7.
4. Anonymous. Celiprolol—a better beta blocker? *Drug Ther Bull* 1992; **30:** 35–6.
5. Kendall MJ, Rajman I. A risk-benefit assessment of celiprolol in the treatment of cardiovascular disease. *Drug Safety* 1994; **10:** 220–32.
6. Riddell J. Drugs in focus 18: celiprolol. *Prescribers' J* 1996; **36:** 165–8.

Preparations

Proprietary Preparations (details are given in Part 3)
Aust.: Selectol; ***Belg.:*** Selectol; ***Fr.:*** Celectol; ***Ger.:*** Celipro; Corliprol†; Selectol; ***Irl.:*** Selectol; ***Neth.:*** Dilanorm; ***Spain:*** Cardem; Jofurol†; Moderator; ***Switz.:*** Corliprol†; Selectol; ***UK:*** Celectol.

Multi-ingredient: ***Aust.:*** Selecturon.

Ceronapril (5772-g)

Ceronapril *(USAN, rINN).*

Ceranapril; SQ-29852. 1-[(2S)-6-Amino-2-hydroxyhexanoyl]-L-proline hydrogen (4-phenyl-butyl)phosphonate.

$C_{21}H_{33}N_2O_6P$ = 440.5.

CAS — 111223-26-8.

Ceronapril is an ACE inhibitor (p.805) under investigation.

Ceronapril is a phosphoryl-containing ACE inhibitor that is active in its own right rather than being a prodrug. It is well absorbed by mouth with a 66% bioavailability and undergoes negligible biotransformation. Peak serum concentrations are reported to occur 4 hours after a dose and the plasma half-life is about 15 hours, giving it a prolonged duration of effect.[1]

1. Salvetti A. Newer ACE inhibitors: a look at the future. *Drugs* 1990; **40:** 800–28.

Certoparin Sodium (17408-a)

Certoparin Sodium (rINN).

NOTE. Certoparin is *BAN*, although this appears to be the sodium salt.

Certoparin sodium is prepared by amyl nitrite degradation of heparin obtained from the intestinal mucosa of pigs. The majority of the components have a 2-*O*-sulpho-α-L-idopyranosuronic acid structure at the non-reducing end and a 6-*O*-sulpho-2,5-anhydro-D-mannose structure at the reducing end of their chain. The molecular weight of 70% of the components is less than 10 000 and the average molecular weight is about 6000. The degree of sulphation is about 2 to 2.5 per disaccharide unit.

Units

As for Low-molecular-weight Heparins, p.899.

Adverse Effects and Treatment

As for Low-molecular-weight Heparins, p.899.

Precautions and Interactions

As for Low-molecular-weight Heparins, p.900.

Pharmacokinetics

Certoparin sodium is rapidly and completely absorbed following subcutaneous injection. Peak plasma activity is reached within 2 to 4 hours. The half-life of anti-factor Xa activity is about 4 hours.

Uses and Administration

Certoparin sodium is a low-molecular-weight heparin (p.899) with anticoagulant activity used for the prevention of postoperative venous thromboembolism (p.802). It is given by subcutaneous injection in a dose of 3000 units 1 to 2 hours before the procedure, followed by 3000 units daily for 7 to 10 days or until the patient is fully ambulant.

References.

1. Kock H-J, *et al.* Thromboprophylaxis with low-molecular-weight heparin in outpatients with plaster-cast immobilisation of the leg. *Lancet* 1995; **346:** 459–61.

Preparations

Proprietary Preparations (details are given in Part 3)
Aust.: Sandoparin; Troparin; ***Ger.:*** Mono-Embolex NM; ***Switz.:*** Sandoparine; ***UK:*** Alphaparin.

Multi-ingredient: ***Aust.:*** Embolex; Troparin compositum; ***Ger.:*** Embolex NM; ***Switz.:*** Embolex LM†.

Cetiedil Citrate (9217-e)

Cetiedil Citrate (USAN, rINNM).

2-(Perhydroazepin-1-yl)ethyl α-cyclohexyl-α-(3-thienyl)acetate dihydrogen citrate monohydrate.

$C_{20}H_{31}NO_2S,C_6H_8O_7,H_2O$ = 559.7.

CAS — 14176-10-4 (cetiedil); 16286-69-4 (anhydrous cetiedil citrate).

Cetiedil citrate is a vasodilator with antimuscarinic activity used in the management of peripheral vascular disorders (p.794) in doses of 400 to 600 mg daily by mouth.

Sickle-cell disease. Cetiedil is reported to have an antisickling effect and has been tried in sickle-cell crises (p.703).[1,2]

1. Cabannes R, *et al.* Acute painful sickle-cell crises in children: a double-blind, placebo-controlled evaluation of efficacy and safety of cetiedil. *Clin Trials J* 1983; **20:** 207–18.
2. Benjamin LJ, *et al.* A collaborative, double-blind randomized study of cetiedil citrate in sickle cell crisis. *Blood* 1986; **67:** 1442–7.

Preparations

Proprietary Preparations (details are given in Part 3)
Fr.: Stratene; Vasocet; ***Ital.:*** Stratene†; ***Spain:*** Huberdilat.

Chlorothiazide (2316-b)

Chlorothiazide (BAN, rINN).

Chlorothiazidum; Clorotiazida. 6-Chloro-2*H*-1,2,4-benzothiadiazine-7-sulphonamide 1,1-dioxide.

$C_7H_6ClN_3O_4S_2$ = 295.7.

CAS — 58-94-6.

Pharmacopoeias. In *Eur.* (see p.viii) and *US.*

A white or almost white, odourless, crystalline powder. Very slightly **soluble** in water; slightly soluble in alcohol, in methyl alcohol, and in pyridine; sparingly soluble in acetone; freely soluble in dimethylformamide and dimethyl sulphoxide; practically insoluble in ether and chloroform. It dissolves in dilute solutions of alkali hydroxides. Alkaline solutions undergo decomposition due to hydrolysis upon standing or heating.

Chlorothiazide Sodium (2317-v)

Chlorothiazide Sodium (BANM, USAN, rINNM).

Sodium Chlorothiazide.

$C_7H_5ClN_3NaO_4S_2$ = 317.7.

CAS — 7085-44-1.

Chlorothiazide sodium 537 mg is approximately equivalent to 500 mg of chlorothiazide. The alkaline nature of chlorothiazide in injectable form suggests that **incompatibilities** with acidic drugs could be expected; the US manufacturer states that the injection may be diluted with glucose or sodium chloride solutions.

Adverse Effects, Treatment, and Precautions

As for Hydrochlorothiazide, p.885. Chlorothiazide sodium injection is alkaline: when administering chlorothiazide by intravenous infusion, care should be taken to ensure that extravasation does not occur.

Interactions

As for Hydrochlorothiazide, p.887.

Pharmacokinetics

Chlorothiazide is incompletely and variably absorbed from the gastro-intestinal tract. It has been estimated to have a plasma half-life of 45 to 120 minutes although the clinical effects last for up to about 12 hours. It is excreted unchanged in the urine. Chlorothiazide crosses the placental barrier and small amounts are reported to be distributed into breast milk.

Uses and Administration

Chlorothiazide is a thiazide diuretic with actions and uses similar to those of hydrochlorothiazide (p.887). It is used for oedema, including that associated with heart failure (p.785), and for hypertension (p.788).

Following oral administration of chlorothiazide diuresis usually occurs in about 2 hours, reaches a maximum at about 4 hours, and is maintained for 6 to 12 hours.

In the treatment of **oedema** the usual dose of chlorothiazide is 0.25 to 1 g by mouth once or twice daily; therapy on alternate days or on 3 to 5 days weekly may be adequate. The dose should not normally exceed 2 g daily.

In the treatment of **hypertension** the usual initial dose is 250 to 500 mg daily by mouth, given as a single or divided dose. A dose of 125 mg may be adequate in some patients. Patients may rarely require up to 1 g daily.

In susceptible patients potassium supplements or potassium-sparing diuretics may be necessary, but see hydrochlorothiazide.

A suggested dose of chlorothiazide in children is up to 25 mg per kg body-weight by mouth daily in two divided doses. Infants up to the age of 6 months may require up to 35 mg per kg daily in two divided doses.

Chlorothiazide has also been given intravenously as the sodium salt, in doses similar to those given by mouth. It is not suitable for subcutaneous or intramuscular injection and extravasation should be avoided. The diuretic effect lasts for up to 2 hours following intravenous injection.

Preparations

BP 1998: Chlorothiazide Tablets;
USP 23: Chlorothiazide Oral Suspension; Chlorothiazide Sodium for Injection; Chlorothiazide Tablets; Methyldopa and Chlorothiazide Tablets; Reserpine and Chlorothiazide Tablets.

Proprietary Preparations (details are given in Part 3)
Austral.: Chlotride; ***Irl.:*** Saluric; ***Neth.:*** Chlotride; ***UK:*** Saluric; ***USA:*** Diachlor; Diurigen; Diuril.

Multi-ingredient: ***Canad.:*** Supres; ***Ital.:*** Ipogen; ***USA:*** Aldoclor; Chloroserpine†; Diupres†.

Chlorthalidone (2318-g)

Chlorthalidone (BAN, USAN).

Chlortalidone (rINN); Chlortalidonum; Clorotalidona; G-33182; NSC-69200. 2-Chloro-5-(1-hydroxy-3-oxoisoindolin-1-yl)benzenesulphonamide.

$C_{14}H_{11}ClN_2O_4S$ = 338.8.

CAS — 77-36-1.

NOTE. Compounded preparations of chlorthalidone and atenolol in the proportions, by weight, 1 part to 4 parts have the British Approved Name Co-tenidone.

Pharmacopoeias. In *Eur.* (see p.viii), *Int.*, and *US.*

A white or yellowish-white crystalline powder.

Practically **insoluble** in water, in chloroform, in dichloromethane, and in ether; slightly soluble in alcohol; soluble in methyl alcohol and in acetone; dissolves in dilute solutions of alkali hydroxides.

Adverse Effects, Treatment, and Precautions

As for Hydrochlorothiazide, p.885.

Interactions

As for Hydrochlorothiazide, p.887.

Anticoagulants. For references to the interaction between *warfarin* and chlorthalidone, see p.968.

Pharmacokinetics

Chlorthalidone is erratically absorbed from the gastro-intestinal tract. It has a prolonged elimination half-life from plasma and blood of 40 to 60 hours and is highly bound to red blood cells; the receptor to which it is bound has been identified as carbonic anhydrase. Chlorthalidone is much less strongly bound to plasma proteins. Chlorthalidone is mainly excreted unchanged in the urine. It crosses the placental barrier and is distributed into breast milk.

References.

1. Riess W, *et al.* Pharmacokinetic studies with chlorthalidone (Hygroton®) in man. *Eur J Clin Pharmacol* 1977; **12:** 375–82.
2. Mulley BA, *et al.* Placental transfer of chlorthalidone and its elimination in maternal milk. *Eur J Clin Pharmacol* 1978; **13:** 129–31.
3. Fleuren HLJ, *et al.* Absolute bioavailability of chlorthalidone in man: a cross-over study after intravenous and oral administration. *Eur J Clin Pharmacol* 1979; **15:** 35–50.
4. Fleuren HLJ, *et al.* Dose-dependent urinary excretion of chlorthalidone. *Clin Pharmacol Ther* 1979; **25:** 806–12.
5. Mulley BA, *et al.* Pharmacokinetics of chlorthalidone: dependence of biological half life on blood carbonic anhydrase levels. *Eur J Clin Pharmacol* 1980; **17:** 203–7.

Uses and Administration

Chlorthalidone is a diuretic with actions and uses similar to those of the thiazide diuretics (see Hydrochlorothiazide, p.887) even though it does not contain a thiazide ring system. It is used for oedema, including that associated with heart failure (p.785), and for hypertension (p.788). Other indications include diabetes insipidus (p.1237).

Diuresis is initiated in about 2 hours and lasts for 48 to 72 hours.

In the treatment of **oedema** the usual initial dose is 25 to 50 mg daily by mouth. In severe cases a daily dose of 100 to 200 mg may be given. If possible lower doses should be used for maintenance; 25 to 50 mg daily or on alternate days may be adequate.

The usual dose in the treatment of **hypertension** is 25 mg daily, either alone or in conjunction with other antihypertensives, increasing to 50 mg daily if necessary.

A suggested dose for children is up to 2 mg per kg body-weight daily on alternate days.

In **diabetes insipidus** an initial dose of 100 mg twice daily has been recommended reduced to a maintenance dose of 50 mg daily.

In the US, a preparation is available with improved bioavailability; suggested doses range from 30 to 120 mg daily for oedema and 15 to 50 mg daily for hypertension.

In susceptible patients potassium supplements or a potassium-sparing diuretic may be necessary, but see hydrochlorothiazide.

Preparations

BP 1998: Chlortalidone Tablets; Co-tenidone Tablets;
USP 23: Atenolol and Chlorthalidone Tablets; Chlorthalidone Tablets; Clonidine Hydrochloride and Chlorthalidone Tablets.

Proprietary Preparations (details are given in Part 3)
Aust.: Hygroton; ***Austral.:*** Hygroton; ***Belg.:*** Hygroton; ***Canad.:*** Hygroton; Novo-Thalidone; ***Fr.:*** Hygroton; Hygroton-Quart†; ***Ger.:*** Hydro-long; Hygroton; Odemo-Genat†; ***Irl.:*** Hygroton†; ***Ital.:*** Igroton; Urolin†; Zambesil; ***Neth.:*** Hygroton; ***Norw.:*** Hygroton; ***S.Afr.:*** Axamin†; Hygroton; Renidone†; ***Spain:*** Higrotona; ***Swed.:*** Hygroton†; ***Switz.:*** Hygroton; ***UK:*** Hygroton; ***USA:*** Hygroton; Hylidone; Thalitone.

Multi-ingredient: ***Aust.:*** Arcablock comp; Atenolan comp; Atenolol comp; Combipresan; Darebon; Logroton; Polinorm; Selecturon; Tenoretic; Trasitensin; Trepress; ***Belg.:*** Logroton; Tenoretic; ***Canad.:*** Combipres; Hygroton-Reserpine†; Tenoretic; ***Fr.:*** Logroton; Trasitensine; ***Ger.:*** Atehexal comp; Ateno comp; Atenolol AL comp; Atenolol comp; Atenomerck comp; Blocotenol comp; Combipresan; Darebon; Diu-Atenolol; duratenol comp; Evitocor plus; Impresso; Prelis comp; Sigabloc; Teneretic; Trasitensin; Trepress; TRI-Normin; ***Irl.:*** Atenetic; Cotenomel; Hygroton-K†; Lopresoretic†; Tenchlor; Tenoret; Tenoretic; ***Ital.:*** Ataclor; Atenigron; Biotens; Carmian; Clortanol; Combipresan†; Diube; Diurolab†; Eupres; Igroseles; Igroton-Lopresor; Igroton-Reserpina; Pressalolo Diuretico; Target; Tenolone; Tenoretic; Trandiur; Trasitensin; ***Neth.:*** Logroton; Tenoretic; ***S.Afr.:*** Adco-Loten; Ateren; Hygroton-Reserpine; Logroton†; Tenchlor; Tenoret†; Tenoretic; Venachlor†; ***Spain:*** Aldoleo; Betasit Plus; Blokium Diu; Higrotona Reserpina; Normopresil; Resnedal; Tenoretic; Trasitensin; ***Swed.:*** Hygroton-K†; ***Switz.:*** ateno-basan comp.; Cardaxen plus; Cotenolol; Hygroton-K†; Hygroton-Reserpine; Logroton; Sandoretic; Slow-Trasitensine; Tenoretic; Trasitensine; Trepress; ***UK:*** AtenixCo; Hygroton-K†; Kalspare; Lopresoretic†; Tenchlor; Tenoret; Tenoretic; Totaretic; ***USA:*** Combipres; Demi-Regroton; Kerledex; Regroton; Tenoretic.

Chromonar Hydrochloride (9218-l)

Chromonar Hydrochloride *(USAN)*.

Carbocromen Hydrochloride *(rINNM)*; A-27053; AG-3; Cassella-4489; NSC-110430. Ethyl 3-(2-diethylaminoethyl)-4-methylcoumarin-7-yloxyacetate hydrochloride.

$C_{20}H_{27}NO_5,HCl = 397.9.$

CAS — 804-10-4 (chromonar); 655-35-6 (chromonar hydrochloride).

Chromonar hydrochloride is a vasodilator used in ischaemic heart disease in usual doses of 150 to 900 mg daily by mouth.

Ischaemic heart disease is discussed under Atherosclerosis (p.782) and the treatment of its clinical manifestations is described under Angina Pectoris (p.780) and Myocardial Infarction (p.791).

Preparations

Proprietary Preparations (details are given in Part 3)
Belg.: Intensain†; ***Ger.:*** Intensain; ***Ital.:*** Cardiocap; Cromene†; ***Spain:*** Intensain†.

Multi-ingredient: ***Aust.:*** Coro-Lanitop; ***Ger.:*** Intensain-Lanicor†; Intensain-Lanitop†.

Cibenzoline (15315-x)

Cibenzoline *(BAN, rINN)*.

Cifenline *(USAN)*; Ro-22-7796; Ro-22-7796/001 (cibenzoline succinate); UP-339-01. (±)-2-(2,2-Diphenylcyclopropyl)-2-imidazoline.

$C_{18}H_{18}N_2 = 262.3.$

CAS — 53267-01-9 (cibenzoline); 100678-32-8 (cibenzoline succinate).

Adverse Effects and Precautions

Cibenzoline may cause neurological and gastro-intestinal side-effects including vertigo, tremor, nausea, vomiting, and diarrhoea. Other adverse effects include fatigue, visual disturbances, and hypoglycaemia. Like other antiarrhythmics it can cause arrhythmias and may reduce blood pressure.

Cibenzoline is contra-indicated in patients with heart block and severe heart failure. It should be used with caution in renal impairment when doses should be reduced.

Effects on the neuromuscular system. A myasthenia-form syndrome with acute respiratory failure has been described[1] in one patient with impaired renal function who ingested a cibenzoline overdose.

1. Similowski T, *et al.* Neuromuscular blockade with acute respiratory failure in a patient receiving cibenzoline. *Thorax* 1997; **52:** 582–4.

Hypoglycaemia. Cibenzoline therapy was associated with severe hypoglycaemia in a 67-year-old patient.[1] The plasma-cibenzoline concentration on admission to hospital was 1800 ng per mL which would probably be considered toxic since the accepted therapeutic trough range is 200 to 600 ng per mL.

1. Hilleman DE, *et al.* Cibenzoline-induced hypoglycemia. *Drug Intell Clin Pharm* 1987; **21:** 38–40.

Interactions

Increased blood concentrations and prolonged half-lives of cibenzoline occurred in healthy subjects given cimetidine.[1] The interaction did not occur with ranitidine. The probable reason was that cimetidine, but not ranitidine, inhibited the metabolism of cibenzoline although the clinical importance was not known.

1. Massarella JW. The effects of cimetidine and ranitidine on the pharmacokinetics of cibenzoline. *Br J Clin Pharmacol* 1991; **31:** 481–3.

Pharmacokinetics

Cibenzoline is well absorbed from the gastro-intestinal tract following oral administration, with a bioavailability of about 90%. It is about 50 to 60% bound to plasma proteins. About 60% of a dose is excreted unchanged in the urine and the elimination half-life is reported to be about 7 hours.

References.

1. Brazzell RK, *et al.* Pharmacokinetics and pharmacodynamics of intravenous cibenzoline in normal volunteers. *J Clin Pharmacol* 1985; **25:** 418–23.
2. Massarella JW, *et al.* Pharmacokinetics of cibenzoline after single and repetitive dosing in healthy volunteers. *J Clin Pharmacol* 1986; **26:** 125–30.

Uses and Administration

Cibenzoline is an antiarrhythmic drug. It possesses class Ia activity but also has some class III and class IV properties (p.776). It is used in the management of ventricular and supraventricular arrhythmias (p.782).

Cibenzoline succinate is given by mouth in a dose equivalent to cibenzoline base 260 to 390 mg daily. A dosage of 130 mg daily in two divided doses is recommended in elderly patients. Cibenzoline may also be given parenterally; the usual initial dose is the equivalent of 1 mg per kg body-weight cibenzoline base over 2 minutes followed by either 8 mg per kg over 24 hours by infusion or by oral therapy. Dosage should be reduced in renal impairment.

Administration in the elderly. The renal and non-renal clearance of cibenzoline was found to decrease with increasing age in healthy subjects.[1] The mean elimination half-life was 7 hours in the 20- to 30-year age group and 10.5 hours in the 70- to 80-year age group. The reduction in renal clearance was considered to be related to the decrease in creatinine clearance with increasing age. The results suggested that older patients may need lower doses than younger patients to maintain therapeutic plasma-cibenzoline concentrations.

1. Brazzell RK, *et al.* Age and cibenzoline disposition. *Clin Pharmacol Ther* 1984; **36:** 613–19.

Administration in renal impairment. A study in patients with normal or impaired renal function has suggested that in renal impairment initial loading doses of cibenzoline may be equivalent to those used in normal renal function although maintenance doses should be reduced to about two-thirds of normal.[1]

1. Aronoff G, *et al.* Bioavailability and kinetics of cibenzoline in patients with normal and impaired renal function. *J Clin Pharmacol* 1991; **31:** 38–44.

Preparations

Proprietary Preparations (details are given in Part 3)
Belg.: Cipralan; ***Fr.:*** Cipralan; Exacor.

Cicletanine Hydrochloride (13232-n)

Cicletanine Hydrochloride *(BANM, rINNM)*.

(±)-BN-1270 (cicletanine); (±)-Cycletanide Hydrochloride; Win-90000 (cicletanine). (±)-3-(*p*-Chlorophenyl)-1,3-dihydro-6-methylfuro[3,4-*c*]pyridin-7-ol hydrochloride.

$C_{14}H_{12}ClNO_2,HCl = 298.2.$

CAS — 89943-82-8 (cicletanine); 82747-56-6 (cicletanine hydrochloride).

NOTE. Cicletanine is *USAN*.

Cicletanine hydrochloride is a diuretic with properties similar to those of the thiazide diuretics (see Hydrochlorothiazide, p.885). It is used in the treatment of hypertension (p.788) in a usual dose of 50 to 100 mg daily by mouth.

References.

1. Ferry N, *et al.* Influence of renal insufficiency on the pharmacokinetics of cicletanine and its effects on urinary excretion of electrolytes and prostanoids. *Br J Clin Pharmacol* 1988; **25:** 359–66
2. Guinot P, *et al.* Determination of the optimal dose of the antihypertensive drug cicletanine hydrochloride in man. *Arzneimittelforschung* 1989; **39:** 86–9.
3. Singer DRJ, *et al.* A comparison of the acute effects of cicletanine and bendrofluazide on urinary electrolytes and plasma potassium in essential hypertension. *Eur J Clin Pharmacol* 1990; **39:** 227–32.

Preparations

Proprietary Preparations (details are given in Part 3)
Fr.: Tenstaten; ***Ger.:*** Justar.

Cilazapril (18620-q)

Cilazapril *(BAN, USAN, rINN)*.

Ro-31-2848 (anhydrous cilazapril); Ro-31-2848/006 (cilazapril monohydrate). (1*S*,9*S*)-9-[(*S*)-1-Ethoxycarbonyl-3-phenylpropylamino]-10-oxoperhydropyridazino[1,2-*a*][1,2]diazepine-1-carboxylic acid monohydrate.

$C_{22}H_{31}N_3O_5,H_2O = 435.5.$

CAS — 88768-40-5 (anhydrous cilazapril); 92077-78-6 (cilazapril monohydrate).

Cilazapril 1.04 mg as the monohydrate is approximately equivalent to 1 mg of anhydrous cilazapril.

Adverse Effects, Treatment, and Precautions

As for ACE inhibitors, p.805.

Interactions

As for ACE inhibitors, p.807.

Pharmacokinetics

Cilazapril acts as a prodrug of the diacid cilazaprilat, its active metabolite. Following oral administration and absorption of cilazapril it is rapidly metabolised in the liver to cilazaprilat, the bioavailability of which is about 60%. Peak plasma concentrations of cilazaprilat occur within 2 hours of an oral dose of cilazapril. Cilazaprilat is eliminated unchanged in the urine. The effective half-life of cilazaprilat is reported to be 9 hours following once-daily dosing. The elimination of cilazaprilat is reduced in renal impairment. Both cilazapril and cilazaprilat are removed to a limited extent by haemodialysis.

Reviews.

1. Kelly JG, O'Malley K. Clinical pharmacokinetics of the newer ACE inhibitors: a review. *Clin Pharmacokinet* 1990; **19:** 177–96.
2. Kloke HJ, *et al.* Pharmacokinetics and haemodynamic effects of the angiotensin converting enzyme inhibitor cilazapril in hypertensive patients with normal and impaired renal function. *Br J Clin Pharmacol* 1996; **42:** 615–20.

Uses and Administration

Cilazapril is an ACE inhibitor (p.805). It is used in the treatment of hypertension (p.788) and heart failure (p.785).

Cilazapril owes its activity to cilazaprilat to which it is converted after oral administration. The haemodynamic effects are seen within 1 hour of a single oral dose and the maximum effect occurs after about 3 to 7 hours. The haemodynamic action persists for about 24 hours, allowing once-daily dosing. Cilazapril is given by mouth as the monohydrate, but doses are expressed in terms of the anhydrous substance.

In the treatment of **hypertension** the initial dose is 1 to 1.25 mg once daily. Since there may be a precipitous fall in blood pressure in some patients when starting therapy with an ACE inhibitor, the first dose should preferably be given at bedtime. In the elderly or those taking diuretics, a usual initial dose is 0.5 mg daily. If possible the diuretic should be withdrawn 2 to 3 days before cilazapril is started and resumed later if necessary. In patients with mild to moderate renal impairment a usual initial dose is 0.5 mg daily and in those with severe renal impairment 0.25 to 0.5 mg once or twice weekly. Particular caution is required in patients with renovascular hypertension (see Precautions under ACE Inhibitors, p.807) or in liver impairment. An initial dose of 0.25 mg daily may be appropriate in these patients. Maintenance doses range from 2.5 to 5 mg daily.

In the treatment of **heart failure** severe first-dose hypotension on introduction of an ACE inhibitor is common in patients on loop diuretics, but their temporary withdrawal may cause rebound pulmonary oedema. Thus therapy should be initiated with a low dose under close medical supervision. Cilazapril is given in an initial dose of 0.5 mg once daily, increased if tolerated to a usual maintenance dose of 1 to 2.5 mg once daily. The usual maximum dose is 5 mg daily.

References.

1. Deget F, Brogden RN. Cilazapril: a review of its pharmacodynamic and pharmacokinetic properties, and therapeutic potential in cardiovascular disease. *Drugs* 1991; **41:** 799–820.

Preparations

Proprietary Preparations (details are given in Part 3)
Aust.: Inhibace; ***Austral.:*** Inhibace; ***Belg.:*** Inhibace; ***Canad.:*** Inhibace; ***Fr.:*** Justor; ***Ger.:*** Dynorm; ***Irl.:*** Vascace; ***Ital.:*** Inibace; Initiss; ***Neth.:*** Vascase; ***S.Afr.:*** Inhibace; ***Spain:*** Inhibace; Inocar; ***Swed.:*** Inhibace; ***Switz.:*** Inhibace; ***UK:*** Vascace.

Multi-ingredient: ***Aust.:*** Inhibace Plus; ***Belg.:*** Co-Inhibace; ***Ger.:*** Dynorm Plus; ***Ital.:*** Inibace Plus; Initiss Plus; ***Neth.:*** Vascase Plus; ***S.Afr.:*** Inhibace Plus; ***Spain:*** Inhibace Plus; Inocar Plus; ***Swed.:*** Inhibace comp; ***Switz.:*** Inhibace Plus.

Cilnidipine (15885-p)

Cilnidipine *(rINN).*

FRC-8653. (±)-(*E*)-Cinnamyl 2-methoxyethyl 1,4-dihydro-2,6-dimethyl-4-(*m*-nitrophenyl)-3,5-pyridinedicarboxylate.

$C_{27}H_{28}N_2O_7$ = 492.5.

CAS — 132203-70-4.

Cilnidipine is a calcium-channel blocker (p.778) given by mouth in the management of hypertension.

Cilostazol (1981-g)

Cilostazol *(USAN, pINN).*

OPC-21; OPC-13013. 6-[4-(1-Cyclohexyl-1*H*-tetrazol-5-yl)butoxy]-3,4-dihydrocarbostyril.

$C_{20}H_{27}N_5O_2$ = 369.5.

CAS — 73963-72-1.

Cilostazol is reported to be an inhibitor of platelet aggregation and a vasodilator. It is used in the management of peripheral vascular disorders.

References.

1. Vehara S, Hirayama A. Effects of cilostazol on platelet function. *Arzneimittelforschung* 1989; **39:** 1531–4.
2. Ochiai M, *et al.* Uses of cilostazol, a novel antiplatelet agent, in post-Palmaz-Schatz stenting regimen. *Am J Cardiol* 1997; **79:** 1471–4.

Preparations

Proprietary Preparations (details are given in Part 3)
Jpn: Pletaal.

Cinepazet Maleate (9219-y)

Cinepazet Maleate *(BANM, USAN, pINNM).*

Cinepazic Acid Ethyl Ester Maleate. Ethyl 4-(3,4,5-trimethoxycinnamoyl)piperazin-1-ylacetate hydrogen maleate.

$C_{20}H_{28}N_2O_6,C_4H_4O_4$ = 508.5.

CAS — 23887-41-4 (cinepazet); 50679-07-7 (cinepazet maleate).

Cinepazet maleate is a vasodilator that has been used in angina pectoris.

Preparations

Proprietary Preparations (details are given in Part 3)
Ital.: Vascoril†.

Cinepazide Maleate (9220-g)

Cinepazide Maleate *(BANM, rINNM).*

MD-67350. 1-(Pyrrolidin-1-ylcarbonylmethyl)-4-(3,4,5-trimethoxycinnamoyl)piperazine hydrogen maleate.

$C_{22}H_{31}N_3O_5,C_4H_4O_4$ = 533.6.

CAS — 23887-46-9 (cinepazide); 26328-04-1 (cinepazide maleate).

Cinepazide maleate is a vasodilator which has been used in peripheral vascular disorders, but has been withdrawn from the market in some countries following reports of agranulocytosis.

Preparations

Proprietary Preparations (details are given in Part 3)
Ital.: Vasodistal†.

Clonidine Hydrochloride (857-k)

Clonidine Hydrochloride *(BANM, USAN, rINNM).*

Clonidini Hydrochloridum; ST-155; ST-155-BS (clonidine). 2-(2,6-Dichloroanilino)-2-imidazoline hydrochloride; 2,6-Dichloro-*N*-(imidazolidin-2-ylidene)aniline hydrochloride.

$C_9H_9Cl_2N_3,HCl$ = 266.6.

CAS — 4205-90-7 (clonidine); 4205-91-8 (clonidine hydrochloride).

Pharmacopoeias. In *Chin., Eur.* (see p.viii), *Jpn, Pol.,* and *US.*

A white or almost white, crystalline powder. **Soluble** in water and in dehydrated alcohol. The Ph. Eur. states that a 5% solution in water has a pH of 4.0 to 5.0; the USP specifies 3.5 to 5.5. **Store** in airtight containers.

Adverse Effects and Treatment

Drowsiness, dry mouth, dizziness, and headache commonly occur during the initial stages of therapy with clonidine. Constipation is also common, and other adverse effects which have been reported include depression, anxiety, fatigue, nausea, anorexia, parotid pain, sleep disturbances, vivid dreams, impotence and loss of libido, urinary retention or incontinence, slight orthostatic hypotension, and dry, itching, or burning sensations in the eye. Fluid retention may occur and is usually transient, but may be responsible for a reduction in the hypotensive effect during continued treatment. Clonidine may cause rashes and pruritus, and these are more common with the use of transdermal delivery systems. Less frequently, bradycardia, including sinus bradycardia with atrioventricular block, other ECG disturbances, heart failure, hallucinations, cramp, Raynaud's syndrome, gynaecomastia, and transient abnormalities in liver function tests have been reported. Large doses have been associated with initial increases in blood pressure and transient hyperglycaemia, although these do not persist during continued therapy.

Symptoms of overdosage include transient hypertension or profound hypotension, bradycardia, sedation, miosis, respiratory depression, convulsions, and coma. Treatment consists of general supportive measures. An alpha-adrenoceptor blocker may be given if necessary.

Sudden withdrawal of clonidine may produce rebound hypertension—see under Precautions, below.

A transdermal clonidine "patch" dislodged during sleep was accidentally transferred to the skin of the patient's 9-month-old child who was sharing the bed.[1] The child subsequently showed signs of somnolence, irritability, and increased fluid intake, presumably due to a dry mouth.

1. Reed MT, Hamburg EL. Person-to-person transfer of transdermal drug-delivery systems: a case report. *N Engl J Med* 1986; **314:** 1120–1.

Abuse. Despite its central effects and ability to cause a form of physical dependence there was no evidence of recreational use of clonidine and the likelihood of abuse was rated as very low.[1] However, clonidine may potentiate the psychoactive effects of morphine and abuse has been reported.[2]

1. WHO. WHO expert committee on drug dependence: twenty-fifth report. *WHO Tech Rep Ser 775* 1989.
2. Sullivan JT, *et al.* Does clonidine alter the abuse potential of morphine? *Clin Pharmacol Ther* 1995; **57:** 163.

Effects on the gastro-intestinal tract. Constipation is a relatively common adverse effect of clonidine, the US manufacturer reporting an incidence of about 10%. Several cases of ileus or pseudo-obstruction of the bowel in patients receiving clonidine have been reported;[1-3] withdrawal of clonidine was associated with a return of bowel function to normal. Abdominal pain mimicking acute appendicitis occurred in another patient prescribed clonidine; symptoms recurred on restarting the drug and subsided when it was withdrawn.[4]

1. Davidov M, *et al.* The antihypertensive effects of an imidazoline compound. *Clin Pharmacol Ther* 1967; **8:** 810–16.
2. Bear R, Steer K. Pseudo-obstruction due to clonidine. *Br Med J* 1976; **1:** 197.
3. Bauer GE, Hellestrand KJ. Pseudo-obstruction due to clonidine. *Br Med J* 1976; **1:** 769.
4. Mjörndal T, Mellbring G. Abdominal pain associated with clonidine. *Br Med J* 1986; **292:** 174.

Effects on the heart. Clonidine has been associated with impaired atrioventricular conduction in a few patients,[1,2] although some of these may have had underlying conduction defects and had previously received digitalis, which may have contributed to their condition. Other electrocardiographic abnormalities may occur, and sudden death has been reported in 3 children receiving clonidine and methylphenidate,[3] although the significance of these reports has been questioned.[4]

1. Kibler LE, Gazes PC. Effect of clonidine on atrioventricular conduction. *JAMA* 1977; **238:** 1930–2.
2. Abiuso P, Abelow G. Atrioventricular dissociation in a patient receiving clonidine. *JAMA* 1978; **240:** 108–9.
3. Maloney MJ, Schwam, JS. Clonidine and sudden death. *Pediatrics* 1995; **96:** 1176–7.
4. Blackman JA, *et al.* Clonidine and electrocardiograms. *Pediatrics* 1996; **98:** 1223–4.

Effects on mental function. There have been occasional reports of disturbed mental state in patients given clonidine.[1-3]

1. Lavin P, Alexander CP. Dementia associated with clonidine therapy. *Br Med J* 1975; **1:** 628.
2. Enoch MD, Hammad GEM. Acute hallucinosis due to clonidine. *Curr Med Res Opin* 1977; **4:** 670–1.
3. Brown MJ, *et al.* Clonidine hallucinations. *Ann Intern Med* 1980; **93:** 456–7.

Effects on the skin. Skin reactions have been reported in up to 50% of patients receiving clonidine by a transdermal delivery system.[1] Localised erythema and irritation during early treatment are usually mild, but allergic contact dermatitis may develop.[2-4] In a brief review, Dick *et al.* suggested that skin reactions became commoner when treatment was continued for several months, and reported that although only mild skin reactions had been observed in their trial of transdermal clonidine during 8 to 14 weeks of treatment in 15 patients, severe skin reactions occurred after an average of 20 weeks in 4 of 5 patients who continued treatment.[5] Despite a claim that skin reactions were due to a component in the delivery system and not to clonidine itself,[6] Boekhorst and Groth obtained positive patch tests to clonidine in several of their patients.[2,4] Subsequent reaction to oral clonidine in patients who develop skin reactions to the transdermal delivery system is reported to be rare.[7,8]

1. Carmichael AJ. Skin sensitivity and transdermal drug delivery: a review of the problem. *Drug Safety* 1994; **10:** 151–9.
2. Groth H, *et al.* Allergic skin reactions to transdermal clonidine. *Lancet* 1983; **ii:** 850–1.
3. McMahon FG, Weber MA. Allergic skin reactions to transdermal clonidine. *Lancet* 1983; **ii:** 851.
4. Boekhorst JC. Allergic contact dermatitis with transdermal clonidine. *Lancet* 1983; **ii:** 1031–2.
5. Dick JBC, *et al.* Skin reactions to long-term transdermal clonidine. *Lancet* 1987; **i:** 516.
6. Anonymous. Transdermal clonidine sensitiser identified? *Pharm J* 1984; **233:** 16.
7. Bigby M. Transdermal clonidine dermatitis. *JAMA* 1987; **258:** 1819.
8. Burris JF. Transdermal clonidine dermatitis. *JAMA* 1987; **258:** 1819–20.

PEMPHIGOID. Report of anogenital cicatricial pemphigoid associated with long-term therapy with clonidine.[1]

1. van Joost T, *et al.* Drug-induced anogenital cicatricial pemphigoid. *Br J Dermatol* 1980; **102:** 715–18.

Hypersensitivity. See Effects on the Skin, above.

Overdosage. Analysis by the National Poisons Information Service[1] of poisoning by clonidine in 133 children and 37 adults reported that there were no deaths but clinical features were often severe. Supportive measures were usually adequate but atropine was often needed for severe and persistent bradycardia. Forced diuresis was not advised because hypotension could be enhanced and there was no evidence that excretion of clonidine was increased.

Although naloxone has been suggested as an antidote for clonidine overdose a study by Rogers and Cubeddu failed to note any reversal of the hypotensive effects of clonidine 300 μg in 6 hypertensive subjects receiving naloxone by intravenous infusion.[2] In a retrospective analysis of 47 children with clonidine poisoning Wiley and colleagues studied 19 who had received naloxone, and of these only 3 showed definite improvement;[3] it was concluded that naloxone is at best an inconsistent antidote for clonidine poisoning.

Severe symptoms of overdosage have also been reported following the ingestion of clonidine transdermal patches.[4]

1. Stein B, Volans GN. Dixarit overdose: the problem of attractive tablets. *Br Med J* 1978; **2:** 667–8.
2. Rogers JF, Cubeddu LX. Naloxone does not antagonise the antihypertensive effect of clonidine in essential hypertension. *Clin Pharmacol Ther* 1983; **34:** 68–73.
3. Wiley JF, *et al.* Clonidine poisoning in young children. *J Pediatr* 1990; **116:** 654–8.
4. Raber JH, *et al.* Clonidine patch ingestion in an adult. *Ann Pharmacother* 1993; **27:** 719–22. Correction. *ibid.*; 1143.

Precautions

Clonidine should be used with caution in patients with cerebrovascular disease, ischaemic heart disease including myocardial infarction, renal impairment, occlusive peripheral vascular disorders such as Raynaud's disease, or those with a history of depression.

Clonidine causes drowsiness and patients should not drive or operate machinery where loss of attention could be dangerous. The effects of other CNS depressants may be enhanced.

Withdrawal of clonidine therapy should be gradual as sudden discontinuation may cause rebound hypertension, sometimes severe. Symptoms of increased catecholamine release such as agitation, sweating, tachycardia, headache, and nausea may also occur. Beta blockers can exacerbate the rebound hypertension and if clonidine is being given concurrently with a beta-blocking drug, clonidine should not be discontinued until several days after the withdrawal of the beta blocker. It has been suggested that patients should be warned of the risk of missing a dose or stopping the drug without consulting their doctor and should carry a reserve supply of tablets.

Although hypotension may occur during anaesthesia in clonidine-treated patients clonidine should not be withdrawn, indeed if necessary it should be given intravenously during the operation to avoid the risk of rebound hypertension. Intravenous injections of clonidine should be given slowly to avoid a possible transient pressor effect especially in patients already receiving other antihypertensives such as guanethidine or reserpine.

Diabetes mellitus. The effects of clonidine on carbohydrate metabolism appear to be variable. There are studies which suggest that administration of clonidine does not affect carbohydrate metabolism in diabetics[1] or non-diabetic hypertensive patients.[2] However, Okada and colleagues reported a diabetic patient in whom clonidine administration was associated with elevated fasting blood-glucose values,[3] and increased insulin requirements were noted in a diabetic child treated with clonidine for tics.[4] Guthrie and others studied 10 diabetic hypertensive patients and found that clonidine impaired response to an acute glucose load but did not significantly affect diabetic control over a 10-week period.[5] Problems may arise when clonidine is given to patients with autonomic neuropathy: both severe postural hypotension[6] and paradoxical hypertension[7] have been reported following administration of clonidine to diabetics with autonomic denervation.

For discussion of the use of clonidine in diabetic diarrhoea see below.

1. Nilsson-Ehle P, *et al.* Lipoproteins and metabolic control in hypertensive type II diabetics treated with clonidine. *Acta Med Scand* 1988; **224:** 131–4.
2. Molitch ME, *et al.* Effects of antihypertensive medications on carbohydrate metabolism. *Curr Ther Res* 1986; **39:** 398–407.
3. Okada S, *et al.* Effect of clonidine on insulin secretion: a case report. *J Int Med Res* 1986; **14:** 299–302.
4. Mimouni-Bloch A, Mimouni M. Clonidine-induced hyperglycemia in a young diabetic girl. *Ann Pharmacother* 1993; **27:** 980.
5. Guthrie GP, *et al.* Clonidine in patients with diabetes and mild hypertension. *Clin Pharmacol Ther* 1983; **34:** 713–17.
6. Moffat B. Postural hypotension induced by clonidine in insulin dependent diabetes. *Br Med J* 1985; **290:** 822.
7. Young E, *et al.* Paradoxical hypertension from clonidine. *Ann Intern Med* 1984; **101:** 282–3.

ECT. Maximal ECT stimuli were unsuccessful in producing seizures in 4 of 7 treatment attempts in a 66-year-old patient receiving concomitant clonidine therapy.[1] It was suggested that clonidine may elevate the seizure threshold.

1. Elliott RL. Case report of a potential interaction between clonidine and electroconvulsive therapy. *Am J Psychiatry* 1983; **140:** 1237–8.

Porphyria. Clonidine hydrochloride has been associated with clinical exacerbations of porphyria and is considered unsafe in porphyric patients.[1]

1. Moore MR, McColl KEL. *Porphyria: drug lists.* Glasgow: Porphyria Research Unit, University of Glasgow, 1991.

Interactions

The hypotensive effect of clonidine may be enhanced by diuretics, other antihypertensives, and drugs that cause hypotension. However, beta blockers may exacerbate rebound hypertension following clonidine withdrawal (see Precautions, above), and tricyclic antidepressants may antagonise the hypotensive effect. The sedative effect of clonidine may be enhanced by CNS depressants.

Antidepressants. Although tricyclic antidepressants commonly cause orthostatic hypotension, they may antagonise the hypotensive effects of clonidine. Briant and colleagues, in a study in 5 hypertensive patients receiving clonidine and a diuretic found that *desipramine* 75 mg daily resulted in a loss of blood pressure control in 4.[1] Increase in blood pressure generally occurred in the second week of treatment, but one patient had a dramatic rise in blood pressure within 24 hours of starting treatment. The mechanism is thought to be due to a central interaction between clonidine and the tricyclic antidepressant, although a peripheral effect cannot be completely excluded.[2] Loss of blood pressure control also occurred in a patient receiving guanfacine, another alpha$_2$-adrenoceptor agonist, when *amitriptyline* was given concomitantly.[3] The reaction recurred with *imipramine*. However, in another study clonidine was given to 11 patients receiving *amitriptyline* or *imipramine*, and 10 achieved good blood pressure control, although 4 developed an acute rise in blood pressure when methyldopa or guanethidine was added to the regimen.[4] *Maprotiline*[5] or *mianserin*[6] do not appear to interact with clonidine.

1. Briant RH, *et al.* Interaction between clonidine and desipramine in man. *Br Med J* 1973; **1:** 522–3.
2. van Spanning HW, van Zwieten PA. The interference of tricyclic antidepressants with the central hypotensive effect of clonidine. *Eur J Pharmacol* 1973; **24:** 402–4.
3. Buckley M, Feely J. Antagonism of antihypertensive effect of guanfacine by tricyclic antidepressants. *Lancet* 1991; **337:** 1173–4.
4. Raftos J, *et al.* Clonidine in the treatment of severe hypertension. *Med J Aust* 1973; **1:** 786–93.
5. Gundert-Remy U, *et al.* Lack of interaction between the tetracyclic antidepressant maprotiline and the centrally acting antihypertensive drug clonidine. *Eur J Clin Pharmacol* 1983; **25:** 595–9.
6. Elliott HL, *et al.* Absence of an effect of mianserin on the actions of clonidine or methyldopa in hypertensive patients. *Eur J Clin Pharmacol* 1983; **24:** 15–19.

Antipsychotics. Acute, severe hypotension occurred in 2 agitated hypertensive patients following administration of clonidine and either *chlorpromazine* or *haloperidol*. Both patients had mitral insufficiency.[1]

1. Fruncillo RJ, *et al.* Severe hypotension associated with concurrent clonidine and antipsychotic medication. *Am J Psychiatry* 1985; **142:** 274.

Dopaminergic antiparkinsonian drugs. For a report of the inhibition of the therapeutic effect of *levodopa* by clonidine, see p.1139.

Immunosuppressants. For a report of clonidine increasing whole blood-*cyclosporin* concentrations, see p.522.

Pharmacokinetics

Following oral administration clonidine is well absorbed from the gastro-intestinal tract, with peak plasma concentrations observed after about 3 to 5 hours. About 50% of an administered dose is metabolised in the liver. It is excreted in the urine as unchanged drug and metabolites, 40 to 60% of an oral dose being excreted in 24 hours as unchanged drug; about 20% of a dose is excreted in the faeces, probably via enterohepatic circulation. The elimination half-life has been variously reported to range between 6 and 24 hours, extended to up to 41 hours in patients with impaired renal function.

Clonidine is absorbed through the skin; absorption is reported to be better when applied to the chest or arm than when applied to the thigh. Therapeutic plasma concentrations are achieved 2 or 3 days after application of a transdermal delivery system and are roughly equivalent to trough concentrations achieved after oral dosage. Therapeutic plasma concentrations are maintained for about 8 hours after removal of the delivery system and then decline slowly over several days.

Reviews.

1. Lowenthal DT, *et al.* Clinical pharmacokinetics of clonidine. *Clin Pharmacokinet* 1988; **14:** 287–310.

Pregnancy. A study in 5 pregnant women treated with clonidine for pre-eclampsia[1] reported an average ratio of cord- to plasma-concentrations of 0.87, indicating placental transfer of clonidine.

1. Boutroy MJ, *et al.* Clonidine placental transfer and neonatal adaption. *Early Hum Dev* 1988; **17:** 275–86.

Uses and Administration

Clonidine is an imidazoline antihypertensive that appears to act centrally to reduce sympathetic tone, resulting in a fall in diastolic and systolic blood pressure and a reduction in heart rate. The exact mechanism is unclear; clonidine stimulates alpha$_2$-adrenoceptors and central imidazoline receptors, but it is not known which receptors mediate which effects. It also acts peripherally, and this peripheral activity may be responsible for the transient increase in blood pressure seen during rapid intravenous administration as well as contributing to the hypotensive effect during chronic administration. Peripheral resistance is reduced during continuous treatment. Cardiovascular reflexes remain intact so postural hypotension occurs infrequently.

Clonidine is used in the management of hypertension (p.788), including hypertensive crises, although other drugs with fewer adverse effects are now generally preferred. It may be given in conjunction with a thiazide diuretic, but combination with a beta blocker should be avoided where possible. Clonidine has also been used in the prophylactic treatment of migraine or recurrent vascular headaches and in the treatment of menopausal flushing. It is also used in conjunction with opioids in the management of cancer pain (p.8) and has been tried for various other forms of pain (below). Other uses of clonidine have included the symptomatic treatment of opioid withdrawal (below), the diagnosis of phaeochromocytoma (below), and administration as eye drops in the management of glaucoma (p.1387). It has also been tried in Tourette's syndrome (below) and numerous other disorders.

Clonidine is used as the hydrochloride. When given by mouth, its haemodynamic effects appear in about 30 to 60 minutes, reaching a maximum after 2 to 4 hours and lasting up to 8 hours. Tolerance to clonidine has been reported. Withdrawal of clonidine should be gradual because of the risk of rebound hypertension.

In **hypertension**, the usual initial dose of clonidine hydrochloride is 50 to 100 μg three times daily by mouth (or in the US, 100 μg twice daily), increased every second or third day according to the response of the patient; the usual maintenance dose is 300 to 1200 μg daily but doses of 1800 μg or more daily may sometimes be required. Clonidine may also be given in a modified-release formulation which enables once or twice daily dosage, or by transdermal delivery systems applied once a week, which each deliver 100 to 300 μg of clonidine base daily at a constant rate.

Clonidine hydrochloride may be given by slow intravenous injection over 10 to 15 minutes in hypertensive crises, usually in doses of 150 to 300 μg. The effect usually appears within 10 minutes, but transient hypertension may precede hypotension if the injection is administered too rapidly. The hypotensive effect reaches a maximum about 30 to 60 minutes after administration and the duration is about 3 to 7 hours; up to 750 μg may be given intravenously over 24 hours. Although oral administration does not produce a sufficiently rapid hypotensive effect for use in an emergency situation, a dose of 100 to 200 μg initially followed by 50 to 100 μg every hour until control of blood pressure is achieved or a maximum of 500 to 800 μg is reached, has been recommended for the control of severe hypertension.

In the prophylaxis of **migraine** or recurrent vascular headaches and in the treatment of **menopausal flushing**, a dose of 50 μg twice daily by mouth has been employed, increased, if there is no remission after 2 weeks, to 75 μg twice daily.

In the management of severe **cancer pain**, clonidine hydrochloride may be given by continuous epidural infusion in combination with an opioid, in an initial dose of 30 μg per hour, adjusted according to response.

Anxiety disorders. Clonidine has been tried in various anxiety disorders (p.635) but evidence of efficacy is limited. A review[1] of the use of clonidine in panic disorder considered that it might be useful as a last-line anxiolytic in patients unresponsive to standard treatment as occasional success had been obtained in a few patients. There have also been isolated reports of small numbers of patients with post-traumatic stress disorder who have benefited from treatment with clonidine.[2]

1. Puzantian T, Hart LL. Clonidine in panic disorder. *Ann Pharmacother* 1993; **27:** 1351–3.
2. Harmon RJ, Riggs PD. Clonidine for posttraumatic stress disorder in preschool children. *J Am Acad Child Adolesc Psychiatry* 1996; **35:** 1247–9.

Cardiac arrhythmias. Atrial fibrillation (p.782) is managed by treatment to slow the increased ventricular responses or by cardioversion. Control of ventricular rate is usually achieved with digoxin, beta blockers, or calcium-channel blockers but clonidine, which reduces sympathetic tone and thus reduces heart rate, has also been tried. In preliminary studies, clonidine 75 μg given by mouth as a single dose (repeated after 2 hours, if necessary)[1] or as a twice daily dose,[2] either alone[1] or in addition to digoxin,[2] controlled rapid atrial fibrillation in clinically and haemodynamically stable patients.

1. Roth A, *et al.* Clonidine for patients with rapid atrial fibrillation. *Ann Intern Med* 1992; **116:** 388–90.
2. Scardi S, *et al.* Oral clonidine for heart rate control in chronic atrial fibrillation. *Lancet* 1993; **341:** 1211–12.

Diarrhoea. Some studies have shown that clonidine possesses antidiarrhoeal properties. Clonidine may stimulate alpha$_2$-adrenoceptors on enterocytes thus promoting fluid and electrolyte absorption and inhibiting anion secretion. It may also modify intestinal motility or rectal sphincter tone.

Most experience with clonidine is in diabetic diarrhoea (p.315). Diabetic diarrhoea is chronic diarrhoea of unknown cause which occurs in 10 to 22% of patients with diabetes mellitus and is often associated with automatic neuropathy. It often responds poorly to treatment with conventional antidiarrhoeal drugs. The pathophysiology is poorly understood, but loss of adrenergic innervation to intestinal mucosa may be a contributory mechanism. Clonidine 100 to 600 μg by mouth every 12 hours reduced diabetic diarrhoea in 3 patients with type 1 diabetes[1] and good results have also been reported in such patients when transdermal clonidine was used.[2,3] Benefit has also been reported in patients with symptoms of diabetic gastroparesis in addition to diarrhoea.[3,4] However, oral (but perhaps not transdermal) clonidine may worsen orthostatic hypotension in patients with diabetic diarrhoea which may limit its usefulness.[5]

1. Fedorak RN, *et al.* Treatment of diabetic diarrhea with clonidine. *Ann Intern Med* 1985; **102:** 197–9.
2. Sacerdote, A. Topical clonidine for diabetic diarrhea. *Ann Intern Med* 1986; **105:** 139.
3. Sacerdote AS. Topical clonidine and diabetic gastroparesis. *Ann Intern Med* 1990; **112:** 796.
4. Migliore A, *et al.* Diabetic diarrhea and clonidine. *Ann Intern Med* 1988; **109:** 170–1.
5. Ogbonnaya KI, Arem R. Diabetic diarrhea: pathophysiology, diagnosis, and management. *Arch Intern Med* 1990; **150:** 262–7.

Extrapyramidal disorders. There is limited evidence[1] from studies of small numbers of patients that clonidine might reduce symptoms of antipsychotic-induced akathisia and tardive dyskinesia (p.650). However, adverse effects such as sedation and hypotension may limit use.

1. Ahmed I, Takeshita J. Clonidine: a critical review of its role in the treatment of psychiatric disorders. *CNS Drugs* 1996; **6:** 53–70.

Growth retardation. Clonidine has been reported to be a stimulant of growth hormone release, presumably as a result of central alpha-adrenergic stimulation, and has been tried in the diagnosis and management of growth retardation (p.1237). It may be given orally as a provocative test for growth hormone deficiency,[1,2] particularly in children,[3] although some consider measurement of circulating somatomedins to be more useful than provocative tests. It has also been tried in growth retardation, both in children with growth hormone deficiency and in short children without proven deficiency, but results have been contradictory and largely unsatisfactory.[4-9]

1. Gil-Ad I, *et al.* Oral clonidine as a growth hormone stimulation test. *Lancet* 1979; **ii:** 278–80.
2. Hoffman WH, *et al.* Relationship of plasma clonidine to growth hormone concentrations in children and adolescents. *J Clin Pharmacol* 1989; **29:** 538–42.
3. Hindmarsh PC, Swift PGF. An assessment of growth hormone provocation tests. *Arch Dis Child* 1995; **72:** 362–8.
4. Pintor C, *et al.* Clonidine treatment for short stature. *Lancet*; 1987; **i:** 1226–30.
5. Pescovitz OH, Tan E. Lack of benefit of clonidine treatment for short stature in a double-blind, placebo-controlled trial. *Lancet* 1988; **ii:** 874–7.
6. Anonymous. Alternatives to growth hormone. *Lancet* 1989; **i:** 820–2.
7. Suri D, *et al.* Clonidine for short stature. *Lancet* 1989; **i:** 508.
8. Müller EE, *et al.* Clonidine for short stature. *Lancet* 1989; **i:** 1395.
9. Allen DB. Effects of nightly clonidine administration on growth velocity in short children without growth hormone deficiency: a double-blind, placebo-controlled study. *J Pediatr* 1993; **122:** 32–6.

Hyperactivity. Drug treatment of attention deficit hyperactivity disorder (p.1476) is usually initiated with a central stimulant. Improvement was reported with clonidine 4 to 5 μg per kg body-weight daily for 8 weeks in 10 children;[1] in another study clonidine either orally or transdermally was as effective as methylphenidate.[2] These small studies have suggested that clonidine may have a favourable effect, although there have probably not been controlled trials in adequate numbers of children and adverse effects may also be a problem.[3]

1. Hunt RD, *et al.* Clonidine benefits children with attention deficit disorder and hyperactivity: report of a double-blind placebo-crossover therapeutic trial. *J Am Acad Child Psychiatry* 1985; **24:** 617–29.
2. Hunt RD. Treatment effects of oral and transdermal clonidine in relation to methylphenidate: an open pilot study in ADD-H. *Psychopharmacol Bull* 1987; **23:** 111–14.
3. Anonymous. Clonidine for treatment of attention-deficit/hyperactivity disorder. *Med Lett Drugs Ther* 1996; **38:** 109–110.

Menopausal disorders. Although hormone replacement therapy is the mainstay of treatment for menopausal disorders (p.1437) clonidine has been of some use in countering vasomotor symptoms in patients who cannot receive hormone replacement therapy;[1,2] however, some studies have failed to demonstrate a reduction in hot flushes. The adverse effects reported in normotensive women, including orthostatic hypotension, may mean that it is best reserved for women who are also hypertensive.

1. Young RL, *et al.* Management of menopause when estrogen cannot be used. *Drugs* 1990; **40:** 220–30.
2. Lucero MA, McCloskey WW. Alternatives to estrogen for the treatment of hot flashes. *Ann Pharmacother* 1997; **31:** 915–17.

Migraine. Propranolol and pizotifen are probably the most well-established drugs for prophylaxis of migraine (p.443). Many other drugs have been used, including clonidine, but a review of clinical trials[1] indicated that it was a poor first choice and seemed unlikely to work even as a last resort. It has been used in patients whose attacks may be precipitated by tyramine-containing foods.

1. Anonymous. Clonidine in migraine prophylaxis—now obsolete. *Drug Ther Bull* 1990; **28:** 79–80.

Organ and tissue transplantation. A preliminary study indicating that clonidine 100 to 200 μg daily from a transdermal patch reduced the frequency of cyclosporin-associated nephrotoxicity in bone-marrow transplant patients.[1] However, such concomitant therapy is not yet generally accepted in the prevention of toxicity, and clonidine administration may increase cyclosporin blood concentrations (see p.522).

1. Luke J, *et al.* Prevention of cyclosporine-induced nephrotoxicity with transdermal clonidine. *Clin Pharm* 1990; **9:** 49–53.

Orthostatic hypotension. Clonidine has produced beneficial effects in a few patients with orthostatic hypotension (p.1040), including orthostatic hypotension due to autonomic neuropathy.[1] Its use in this condition is somewhat paradoxical as orthostatic hypotension may occur as an adverse effect of clonidine therapy.

1. Acott PD, *et al.* Effectiveness of clonidine in congenital orthostatic hypotension. *J Pediatr* 1990; **116:** 666–7.

Pain. Administration of opioids and local anaesthetics by the epidural or intrathecal routes can produce effective analgesia but adverse effects are common. Many other drugs, including clonidine, have been tried by these routes, alone or as adjuncts. Clonidine is thought to produce analgesia by a direct action on alpha$_2$-adrenoceptors in the spinal cord. Some studies of clonidine given *epidurally* alone in a dose of 2 μg per kg body-weight[1] or 150 μg[2] have produced satisfactory pain relief, although duration of action was short. Higher doses have also been used.[3] Hypotension and sedation have been reported as frequent side-effects and an editorial on epidural clonidine[4] considered it unlikely that clonidine would be useful as a sole analgesic drug although it may have a role in combination with opioids and/or local anaesthetics. Clonidine has been given epidurally in combination with various opioids and has produced satisfactory analgesia in postoperative pain,[5] neurogenic pain,[6] and labour pain;[7] the combination is also used in chronic pain due to cancer. Clonidine has also been given epidurally with local anaesthetics and enhanced analgesia has been reported in postoperative pain[8] and labour pain.[9] Epidural clonidine combined with both an opioid and a local anaesthetic may increase the duration of analgesia during labour, but adverse effects on the fetal heartbeat may limit this use.[10] The combination of clonidine and bupivacaine has also produced enhanced analgesia in a study in children undergoing lower limb orthopaedic surgery;[11] clonidine was given epidurally in a dose of 2 μg per kg body-weight. Clonidine and bupivacaine have been given intrathecally[12] and may produce less urinary retention than the combination of morphine with bupivacaine.[13] Long-term intrathecal administration of clonidine in combination with midazolam has also been reported[14] and may be effective in refractory neurogenic or musculoskeletal pain.

Analgesia has also been reported following administration of clonidine by other routes. A study comparing intravenous and epidural clonidine 150 μg in 10 patients with back pain reported that *intravenous* clonidine produced better analgesia, although pain relief was poor following administration by either route.[15] However, a study[3] in postoperative patients using an initial dose of clonidine 8 μg per kg body-weight followed by bolus doses of 30 μg as required found that the epidural and intravenous routes were both effective but the epidural route produced less sedation. In another study,[16] *intramuscular* injection of clonidine 2 μg per kg was as effective as the same dose given epidurally for relief of postoperative pain. Clonidine has some effect when given *orally*[17-20] but the effect is much less marked than following parenteral administration. Premedication with oral clonidine has also been reported to provide effective postoperative analgesia in children.[21] *Transdermal* clonidine has also been tried for postoperative analgesia.[22]

The role of clonidine in the management of pain remains to be established. For further discussion of the management of various types of pain, see p.4.

1. Bonnet F, *et al.* Postoperative analgesia with extradural clonidine. *Br J Anaesth* 1989; **63:** 465–9.
2. Lund C, *et al.* Comparison of the effects of extradural clonidine with those of morphine on postoperative pain, stress responses, cardiopulmonary function and motor and sensory block. *Br J Anaesth* 1989; **63:** 516–19.
3. Bernard J-M, *et al.* Comparison of intravenous and epidural clonidine for postoperative patient-controlled analgesia. *Anesth Analg* 1995; **81:** 706–12.
4. Macdonald R. Extradural clonidine—the need for well designed controlled trials. *Br J Anaesth* 1994; **72:** 255–7.
5. Carabine UA, *et al.* Extradural clonidine infusions for analgesia after total hip replacement. *Br J Anaesth* 1992; **68:** 338–43.
6. Tamsen A, Gordh T. Epidural clonidine produces analgesia. *Lancet* 1984; **ii:** 231–2.
7. Buggy DJ, MacDowell C. Extradural analgesia with clonidine and fentanyl compared with 0.25% bupivacaine in the first stage of labour. *Br J Anaesth* 1996; **76:** 319–21.
8. Carabine UA, *et al.* Extradural clonidine and bupivacaine for postoperative analgesia. *Br J Anaesth* 1992; **68:** 132–5.
9. O'Meara ME, Gin T. Comparison of 0.125% bupivacaine with 0.125% bupivacaine and clonidine as extradural analgesia in the first stage of labour. *Br J Anaesth* 1993; **71:** 651–6.
10. Chassard D, *et al.* Extradural clonidine combined with sufentanil and 0.0625% bupivacaine for analgesia in labour. *Br J Anaesth* 1996; **77:** 458–62.
11. Lee JJ, Rubin AP. Comparison of a bupivacaine-clonidine mixture with plain bupivacaine for caudal analgesia in children. *Br J Anaesth* 1994; **72:** 258–62.
12. Bonnet F, *et al.* Prevention of tourniquet pain by spinal isobaric bupivacaine with clonidine. *Br J Anaesth* 1989; **63:** 93–6.
13. Gentili M, Bonnet F. Spinal clonidine produces less urinary retention than spinal morphine. *Br J Anaesth* 1996; **76:** 872–3.
14. Borg PAJ, Krijnen HJ. Long-term intrathecal administration of midazolam and clonidine. *Clin J Pain* 1996; **12:** 63–8.
15. Carroll D, *et al.* Single-dose, randomized, double-blind, double-dummy cross-over comparison of extradural and I.V. clonidine in chronic pain. *Br J Anaesth* 1993; **71:** 665–9.
16. Bonnet F, *et al.* Clonidine-induced analgesia in postoperative patients: epidural versus intramuscular administration. *Anesthesiology* 1990; **72:** 423–7.
17. Glynn CF, *et al.* Role of spinal noradrenergic system in transmission of pain in the patients with spinal cord injury. *Lancet* 1986; **ii:** 1249–50.
18. Petros AJ, Wright RMB. Epidural and oral clonidine in domiciliary control of deafferentation pain. *Lancet* 1987; **i:** 1034.
19. Tan Y-M, Croese J. Clonidine and diabetic patients with leg pains. *Ann Intern Med* 1986; **105:** 633–4.
20. Benhamon D, *et al.* Addition of oral clonidine to postoperative patient-controlled analgesia with i.v. morphine. *Br J Anaesth* 1994; **72:** 537–40.
21. Mikawa K, *et al.* Oral clonidine premedication reduces postoperative pain in children. *Anesth Analg* 1996; **82:** 225–30.
22. Segal IS, *et al.* Clinical efficacy of oral transdermal clonidine combinations during the perioperative period. *Anesthesiology* 1991; **74:** 220–5.

Phaeochromocytoma. Clonidine acts centrally to suppress catecholamine release and may be used in the diagnosis of phaeochromocytoma (p.795). Experience gained with the clonidine suppression test (as described by Bravo *et al.*[1]) and a review of published studies indicated that it is of value in selected patients with moderately elevated plasma and/or urinary catecholamine concentrations.[2]

1. Bravo EL, *et al.* Clonidine-suppression test: a useful aid in the diagnosis of pheochromocytoma. *N Engl J Med* 1981; **305:** 623–6.
2. Sjoberg RJ, *et al.* The clonidine suppression test for pheochromocytoma. *Arch Intern Med* 1992; **152:** 1193–7.

Premedication. Clonidine has been administered pre-operatively for its sedative, anxiolytic and analgesic effects and to provide haemodynamic stability and reduce anaesthetic requirements. Clonidine may attenuate the perioperative stress response and has been shown to reduce perioperative oxygen consumption, which is a marker of sympathetic activation.[1]

1. Taittonen MT, *et al.* Effect of clonidine and dexmedetomidine premedication on perioperative oxygen consumption and haemodynamic state. *Br J Anaesth* 1997; **78:** 400–406.

Restless legs syndrome. Numerous drugs have been tried for the treatment of restless legs syndrome (see Parasomnias, p.639). Symptomatic improvement has been reported with clonidine in a number of case studies[1,2] and small controlled trials,[3] but side-effects may limit its use.

1. Handwerker JV, Palmer RF. Clonidine in the treatment of "restless leg" syndrome. *N Engl J Med* 1985; **313:** 1228–9.
2. Zoe A, *et al.* High-dose clonidine in a case of restless legs syndrome. *Ann Pharmacother* 1994; **28:** 878–81.
3. Wagner ML, *et al.* Randomized, double-blind, placebo-controlled study of clonidine in restless legs syndrome. *Sleep* 1996; **19:** 52–8.

Shivering. Numerous drugs, including clonidine, have been tried for the treatment of postoperative shivering (p.1219).

Clonidine's central and peripheral effects could both account for its antishivering activity, but some have suggested that it acts by resetting the central threshold for shivering. In preliminary studies a small intravenous dose of clonidine 75 μg or 30 μg stopped shivering after general anaesthesia[1] or epidural anaesthesia,[2] respectively. Administration of clonidine intra-operatively has also been reported to reduce the incidence of postoperative shivering.[3,4]

1. Joris J, *et al.* Clonidine and ketanserin both are effective treatment for postanesthetic shivering. *Anesthesiology* 1993; **79:** 532–9.
2. Capogna G, Celleno D. IV clonidine for post-extradural shivering in parturients: a preliminary study. *Br J Anaesth* 1993; **71:** 294–5.
3. Steinfath M, *et al.* Clonidine administered intraoperatively prevents postoperative shivering. *Br J Clin Pharmacol* 1995; **39:** 580P–581P.
4. Vanderstappen I, *et al.* The effect of prophylactic clonidine on postoperative shivering: a large prospective double-blind study. *Anaesthesia* 1996; **51:** 351–5.

Spasticity. Clonidine, given alone or as an adjunct to baclofen, has been tried in patients with various forms of spasticity (p.1303) including those refractory to baclofen.[1-4]

1. Nance PW, *et al.* Clonidine in spinal cord injury. *Can Med Assoc J* 1985; **133:** 41–2.
2. Donovan WH, *et al.* Clonidine effect on spasticity: a clinical trial. *Arch Phys Med Rehabil* 1988; **69:** 193–4.
3. Sandford PR, *et al.* Clonidine in the treatment of brainstem spasticity: case report. *Am J Phys Med Rehabil* 1992; **71:** 301–303.
4. Middleton JW, *et al.* Intrathecal clonidine and baclofen in the management of spasticity and neuropathic pain following spinal cord injury: a case study. *Arch Phys Med Rehabil* 1996; **77:** 824–6.

Tourette's syndrome. Clonidine is one of many drugs that have been tried in the management of Tourette's syndrome (see Tics under Extrapyramidal Disorders, p.636).

Disturbance of monoamine metabolism (including dopamine, noradrenaline, and serotonin) has been implicated in Tourette's syndrome. Clonidine is thought to reduce central noradrenergic activity and may also affect other neurochemical systems and these properties may account for its beneficial effects in this disorder. Studies of clonidine in Tourette's syndrome have produced mixed results,[1-5] although this may reflect the difficulty in study design for a disease that can vary considerably in severity and presence of comorbid conditions and whose symptoms wax and wane. Nevertheless, clonidine has been used as an alternative to the commonly used dopamine antagonist antipsychotics, such as haloperidol and pimozide, when side-effects of antipsychotics limit their use. Although it appears to be less effective than these drugs,[2] clonidine has been reported to successfully control symptoms in some children with Tourette's syndrome unresponsive to haloperidol.[1]

1. Cohen DJ, *et al.* Clonidine in Tourette's syndrome. *Lancet* 1979; **ii:** 551–3.
2. Shapiro AK, *et al.* Treatment of Gilles de la Tourette's syndrome with clonidine and neuroleptics. *Arch Gen Psychiatry* 1983; **40:** 1235–40.
3. Leckman JF, *et al.* Short- and long-term treatment of Tourette's syndrome with clonidine: a clinical perspective. *Neurology* 1985; **35:** 343–51.
4. Goetz CG, *et al.* Clonidine and Gilles de la Tourette's syndrome: double-blind study using objective rating methods. *Ann Neurol* 1987; **21:** 307–10.
5. Leckman JF, *et al.* Clonidine treatment of Gilles de la Tourette's syndrome. *Arch Gen Psychiatry* 1991; **48:** 324–8.

Withdrawal syndromes. ALCOHOL. Although drug treatment of alcohol withdrawal (p.1099) is usually with a benzodiazepine, clonidine has sometimes been used to good effect,[1,2] although it does not have any effect on convulsions or delirium tremens[3] and should not be used as sole therapy.

1. Guthrie SK. The treatment of alcohol withdrawal. *Pharmacotherapy* 1989; **9:** 131–43.
2. Ip Yam PC, *et al.* Clonidine in the treatment of alcohol withdrawal in the intensive care unit. *Br J Anaesth* 1992; **68:** 106–8.
3. Anonymous. Alcohol problems in the general hospital. *Drug Ther Bull* 1991; **29:** 69–71.

OPIOIDS ANALGESICS. Clonidine has been reported to be useful in controlling withdrawal symptoms following abrupt discontinuation of opioids (p.67). Treatment is required for about 10 days following methadone withdrawal and less for withdrawal from diamorphine.[1] Most studies have reported favourable results, although studies by Preston *et al.*[2] and Jasinski *et al.*[3] suggest that subjective response may be less favourable. However, the maximum dose of clonidine used by Preston *et al.* was 300 μg twice daily: Camí *et al.* used initial doses of up to 1.35 mg daily[4] and Washton *et al.*[5] found that a dose of 100 to 200 μg every 4 to 6 hours was necessary: doses of up to 17 μg per kg body-weight daily have been used.[6] The major drawback of clonidine therapy is the tendency to cause hypotension, and this may limit its usefulness in some patients.

Charney *et al.* reported the use of clonidine in combination with naltrexone to shorten the withdrawal syndrome and achieved withdrawal within 6 days.[7] Subsequent modification to the regimen allowed 38 of 40 patients addicted to methadone to withdraw completely in 4 to 5 days.[8] Patients required a mean of 2.3 mg of clonidine on the first day which reduced but did not abolish symptoms. A further modification was reported by Brewer and colleagues to allow opioid withdrawal with minimal drop-out over 2 to 3 days.[9]

Clonidine has also been used in the management of neonatal opioid dependence (p.67) in infants born to opioid-addicted mothers maintained on methadone.[10,11] Hoder and colleagues reported benefit in 6 of 7 such infants given an initial clonidine dose of 0.5 to 1.0 μg per kg body-weight by mouth, increased over 1 to 2 days to 3 to 5 μg per kg daily in divided doses. Total length of treatment ranged from 6 to 17 days. The infant who failed to respond was born to a mother also receiving haloperidol, desipramine, and theophylline.[11]

1. Cook C, *et al.* Opiate withdrawal: inpatient versus outpatient programmes. *Br Med J* 1986; **293:** 506.
2. Preston KL, *et al.* Self-administration of clonidine, oxazepam, and hydromorphone by patients undergoing methadone detoxification. *Clin Pharmacol Ther* 1985; **38:** 219–27.
3. Jasinski DR, *et al.* Clonidine in morphine withdrawal: differential effects on signs and symptoms. *Arch Gen Psychiatry* 1985; **42:** 1063–6.
4. Camí J, *et al.* Efficacy of clonidine and of methadone in the rapid detoxification of patients dependent on heroin. *Clin Pharmacol Ther* 1985; **38:** 336–41.
5. Washton AM, *et al.* Clonidine for outpatient opiate detoxification. *Lancet* 1980; **i:** 1078–9.
6. Gold MS, *et al.* Clonidine and opiate withdrawal. *Lancet* 1980; **ii:** 1078–9.
7. Charney DS, *et al.* Clonidine and naltrexone: a safe, effective, and rapid treatment of abrupt withdrawal from methadone therapy. *Arch Gen Psychiatry* 1982; **39:** 1327–32.
8. Charney DS, *et al.* The combined use of clonidine and naltrexone as a rapid, safe, and effective treatment of abrupt withdrawal from methadone. *Am J Psychiatry* 1986; **143:** 831–7.
9. Brewer C, *et al.* Opioid withdrawal and naltrexone induction in 48-72 hours with minimal drop-out, using a modification of the naltrexone-clonidine technique. *Br J Psychiatry* 1988; **153:** 340–3.
10. Hoder EL, *et al.* Clonidine in neonatal narcotic-abstinence syndrome. *N Engl J Med* 1981; **305:** 1284.
11. Hoder EL, *et al.* Clonidine treatment of neonatal narcotic abstinence syndrome. *Psychiatry Res* 1984; **13:** 243–51.

SMOKING. Nicotine dependence may be managed using behavioural or psychological counselling. In addition, nicotine replacement therapy (p.1608) can help alleviate withdrawal symptoms. A number of other drugs, including clonidine, have also been investigated. Clonidine has been studied in doses of 100 to 400 μg daily by mouth[1-4] and 100 or 200 μg daily by the transdermal route.[5-7] However, conflicting results have been reported and adverse effects are reported to be common. It might be of use in selected patients who experience severe agitation and anxiety on cessation of smoking.[8] In some studies any benefit has been largely confined to women.[1,3,7]

1. Glassman AH, *et al.* Heavy smokers, smoking cessation and clonidine: results of a double-blind, randomized trial. *JAMA* 1988; **259:** 2863–6.
2. Franks P, *et al.* Randomized, controlled trial of clonidine for smoking cessation in a primary care setting. *JAMA* 1989; **262:** 3011–13.
3. Glassman AH, *et al.* Smoking cessation, clonidine, and vulnerability to nicotine among dependent smokers. *Clin Pharmacol Ther* 1993; **54:** 670–9.
4. Gourlay S, *et al.* A placebo-controlled study of three clonidine doses for smoking cessation. *Clin Pharmacol Ther* 1994; **55:** 64–9.
5. Ornish SA, *et al.* Effects of transdermal clonidine treatment on withdrawal symptoms associated with smoking cessation: a randomized, controlled trial. *Arch Intern Med* 1988; **148:** 2027–31.
6. Prochazka AV, *et al.* Transdermal clonidine reduced some withdrawal symptoms but did not increase smoking cessation. *Arch Intern Med* 1992; **152:** 2065–9.
7. Hilleman DE, *et al.* Randomized, controlled trial of transdermal clonidine for smoking cessation. *Ann Pharmacother* 1993; **27:** 1025–8.
8. Gourlay SG, Benowitz NL. Is clonidine an effective smoking cessation therapy? *Drugs* 1995; **50:** 197–207.

Preparations

BP 1998: Clonidine Injection; Clonidine Tablets;
USP 23: Clonidine Hydrochloride and Chlorthalidone Tablets; Clonidine Hydrochloride Tablets.

Proprietary Preparations (details are given in Part 3)
Aust.: Cantanidin†; Catanidin; Catapresan; Isoglaucon; ***Austral.:*** Catapres; Dixarit†; ***Belg.:*** Catapressan; Dixarit; Paracefan†; ***Canad.:*** Catapres; Dixarit; ***Fr.:*** Barclyd†; Catapressan; ***Ger.:*** Aruclonin; Catapresan; Clonistada; Dispaclonidin; Dixarit; Haemiton; Haemiton-Augentropfen†; Isoglaucon; Mirfat; Paracefan; Tenso-Timelets†; ***Irl.:*** Catapres; Dixarit; ***Ital.:*** Adesipress-TTS; Catapresan; Ipotensium†; Isoglaucon; ***Neth.:*** Catapresan; Dixarit; ***Norw.:*** Catapresan; ***S.Afr.:*** Catapres; Dixarit; ***Spain:*** Catapresan; Isoglaucon; ***Swed.:*** Catapresan; ***Switz.:*** Catapresan; ***UK:*** Catapres; Dixarit; ***USA:*** Catapres.

Multi-ingredient: ***Aust.:*** Combipresan; ***Canad.:*** Combipres; ***Ger.:*** Combipresan; Haemiton compositum; ***Ital.:*** Combipresan†; ***Spain:*** Dilapres; Sali Catapresan†; ***USA:*** Combipres.

Clopamide (2320-d)

Clopamide *(BAN, USAN, rINN).*

DT-327. 4-Chloro-*N*-(2,6-dimethylpiperidino)-3-sulphamoylbenzamide; *cis*-3-(Aminosulphonyl)-4-chloro-*N*-(2,6-dimethyl-1-piperidinyl)benzamide.

$C_{14}H_{20}ClN_3O_3S = 345.8.$

CAS — 636-54-4.

Clopamide is a diuretic with properties similar to those of the thiazide diuretics (see Hydrochlorothiazide, p.885) even though it does not contain a thiazide ring system. It is used for oedema, including that associated with heart failure (p.785), and for hypertension (p.788).

Diuresis is initiated in 1 to 2 hours, reaches a maximum in about 3 to 6 hours, and lasts for up to 24 hours.

In the treatment of oedema the usual dose is 10 to 40 mg daily by mouth; frequency may be reduced for maintenance. The usual dose in the treatment of hypertension is 5 to 10 mg daily, either alone, or in conjunction with other antihypertensives.

In susceptible patients potassium supplements or a potassium-sparing diuretic may be necessary, but see hydrochlorothiazide.

Preparations

Proprietary Preparations (details are given in Part 3)
Fr.: Brinaldix†; ***Ger.:*** Brinaldix; ***Ital.:*** Brinaldix†; ***Neth.:*** Brinaldix†; ***Swed.:*** Brinaldix†.

Multi-ingredient: ***Aust.:*** Brinerdin; Viskaldix; ***Belg.:*** Viskaldix; ***Fr.:*** Viskaldix; ***Ger.:*** Briserin N; Viskaldix; ***Irl.:*** Viskaldix; ***Ital.:*** Brinerdina; ***Neth.:*** Brinerdin†; Viskaldix; ***S.Afr.:*** Brinerdin; Viskaldix†; ***Spain:*** Brinerdina; ***Switz.:*** Brinerdine; Viskaldix; ***UK:*** Viskaldix.

Clopidogrel Bisulphate (3672-s)

Clopidogrel Bisulphate *(BANM, rINNM).*

Clopidogrel Bisulfate *(USAN)*; Clopidogrel Hydrogen Sulphate; SR-25990C. Methyl (*S*)-2-chlorophenyl(4,5,6,7-tetrahydrothieno[3,2-c]pyridin-5-yl)acetate bisulphate; Methyl (+)-(*S*)-α-(*o*-chlorophenyl)-6,7-dihydrothieno[3,2-c]pyridine-5(4*H*)-acetate sulphate.

$C_{16}H_{16}ClNO_2S,H_2SO_4 = 419.9.$

CAS — 113665-84-2 (clopidogrel); 94188-84-8 (clopidogrel); 120202-66-6 (clopidogrel bisulphate).

Adverse Effects and Precautions

As for Ticlopidine, p.953. The incidence of blood dyscrasias may be lower with clopidogrel.

Interactions

As for Ticlopidine, p.953.

Pharmacokinetics

Clopidogrel is rapidly but incompletely absorbed following oral administration; absorption appears to be about 50%. It is a prodrug and is extensively metabolised in the liver following absorption, mainly to the inactive carboxylic acid derivative. The active metabolite appears to be a thiol derivative but has not been identified in plasma. Clopidogrel and the carboxylic acid derivative are highly protein bound. Clopidogrel and its metabolites are excreted about equally in urine and in faeces.

Uses and Administration

Clopidogrel bisulphate is an analogue of ticlopidine (p.953) with similar actions and uses. It is given prophylactically as an alternative to aspirin in patients at risk of thrombo-embolic disorders such as myocardial infarction (p.791), peripheral arterial disease (p.794), and stroke (p.799). The usual dose is 75 mg once daily by mouth.

References.

1. CAPRIE Steering Committee. A randomised, blinded, trial of clopidogrel versus aspirin in patients at risk of ischaemic events (CAPRIE). *Lancet* 1996; **348:** 1329–39.
2. Anonymous. Clopidogrel for reduction of atherosclerotic events. *Med Lett Drugs Ther* 1998; **40:** 59–60.
3. Hankey GJ. Clopidogrel: a new safe and effective antiplatelet agent. But unanswered questions remain. *Med J Aust* 1997; **167:** 120–1.
4. Sharis PJ, *et al.* The antiplatelet effects of ticlopidine and clopidogrel. *Ann Intern Med* 1998; **129:** 394–405.

Preparations

Proprietary Preparations (details are given in Part 3)
UK: Plavix; ***USA:*** Plavix.

Cloranolol Hydrochloride (12591-c)

Cloranolol Hydrochloride *(rINNM).*

GYKI-41099. 1-(*tert*-Butylamino)-3-(2,5-dichlorophenoxy)propan-2-ol hydrochloride.

$C_{13}H_{19}Cl_2NO_2,HCl = 328.7.$

CAS — 39563-28-5 (cloranolol).

Cloranolol is a beta blocker (p.828). It is given by mouth as the hydrochloride in the management of various cardiovascular disorders.

Preparations

Proprietary Preparations (details are given in Part 3)
Multi-ingredient: ***Hung.:*** Tobanum.

Cloricromen (14754-l)

Cloricromen *(rINN)*.

Ethyl ({8-chloro-3-[2-(diethylamino)ethyl]-4-methyl-2-oxo-2*H*-1-benzopyran-7-yl}oxy)acetate.

$C_{20}H_{26}ClNO_5$ = 395.9.

CAS — 68206-94-0.

Cloricromen is an antiplatelet drug with vasodilating activity and is used in thrombo-embolic disorders (p.801). It is given as the hydrochloride in arterial vascular disorders where there is a risk of thrombosis. It may be given by mouth in a dose of 100 mg two or three times daily or intravenously in a dose of 30 mg daily.

Preparations

Proprietary Preparations (details are given in Part 3)
Ital.: Assogen; Proendotel.

Cloridarol (9221-q)

Cloridarol *(rINN)*.

Clobenfurol. α-(Benzofuran-2-yl)-α-(4-chlorophenyl)methanol.

$C_{15}H_{11}ClO_2$ = 258.7.

CAS — 3611-72-1.

Cloridarol is a vasodilator used in ischaemic heart disease in usual doses of 250 to 500 mg daily by mouth.

Ischaemic heart disease is discussed under Atherosclerosis (p.782) and the treatment of its clinical manifestations is described under Angina Pectoris (p.780) and Myocardial Infarction (p.791).

Preparations

Proprietary Preparations (details are given in Part 3)
Ital.: Menacor†; ***Spain:*** Menoxicor.

Cromakalim (3034-h)

Cromakalim *(BAN, rINN)*.

BRL-34915. (±)-*trans*-3,4-Dihydro-3-hydroxy-2,2-dimethyl-4-(2-oxopyrrolidin-1-yl)-2*H*-chromene-6-carbonitrile.

$C_{16}H_{18}N_2O_3$ = 286.3.

CAS — 94470-67-4 (cromakalim); 94535-50-9 (levcromakalim).

Cromakalim is a potassium-channel opening vasodilator (p.778). Cromakalim and its (−)-enantiomer, levcromakalim (lemakalim), have been investigated in the management of hypertension and have also been tried in patients with asthma.

Action. The potassium-channel opening activity of cromakalim leads to hyperpolarisation of smooth muscle cells and consequently vasodilatation. Webb and co-workers found that infusion of cromakalim at rates of up to 10 μg per minute into the brachial artery for 15 minutes produced dose-dependent arterioselective vasodilatation,[1] and similar observations were made by Fox and colleagues in subjects given oral cromakalim.[2] How well such actions translate into antihypertensive effects remains to be decided. Donnelly and others found that addition of cromakalim 1 mg daily to treatment with atenolol in 10 poorly-controlled hypertensive subjects produced only modest additional reductions in blood pressure, lasting about 3 hours from administration.[3] Levcromakalim may be more effective and was reported to control blood pressure over 24 hours following oral administration in 14 hypertensive patients.[4]

Cromakalim has also been found to stimulate renin release.[5,6]

1. Webb DJ, *et al.* The potassium channel opening drug cromakalim produces arterioselective vasodilation in the upper limbs of healthy volunteers. *Br J Clin Pharmacol* 1989; **27:** 757–61.
2. Fox JS, *et al.* Cardiovascular effects of cromakalim (BRL34915) in healthy volunteers. *Br J Clin Pharmacol* 1991; **32:** 45–9.
3. Donnelly R, *et al.* Clinical studies with cromakalim in normotensive and hypertensive subjects. *Br J Clin Pharmacol* 1990; **30:** 314P-15P.
4. Suzuki S, *et al.* Antihypertensive effect of levcromakalim in patients with essential hypertension: study by 24-h ambulatory blood pressure monitoring. *Arzneimittelforschung* 1995; **45:** 859–64.
5. Ferrier CP, *et al.* Stimulation of renin secretion by potassium-channel activation with cromakalim. *Eur J Clin Pharmacol* 1989; **36:** 443–7.
6. Lijnen P, *et al.* Humoral and cellular effects of the K^+-channel activator cromakalim in man. *Eur J Clin Pharmacol* 1989; **37:** 609–11.

Asthma. In a study involving 23 patients a single dose of cromakalim 0.25 or 0.5 mg was more effective than placebo in reducing the early-morning fall in FEV_1 associated with nocturnal asthma.[1] However, cromakalim 1.5 mg did not have a significant effect, perhaps because a high incidence of associated headache impaired testing. In a second study in a further 8 patients with nocturnal asthma given cromakalim 0.25 or 0.5 mg or placebo at night for 5 days the mean early morning fall in FEV_1 was 28.7% after placebo but only 19% after cromakalim 0.25 mg, and 14.9% after cromakalim 0.5 mg. Cromakalim at these doses had no effect on blood pressure or heart rate in these normotensive subjects.

The usual drugs used in the treatment of asthma are discussed on p.745.

1. Williams AJ, *et al.* Attenuation of nocturnal asthma by cromakalim. *Lancet* 1990; **336:** 334–6.

Cyclandelate (9222-p)

Cyclandelate *(BAN, rINN)*.

BS-572. 3,3,5-Trimethylcyclohexyl mandelate.

$C_{17}H_{24}O_3$ = 276.4.

CAS — 456-59-7.

Pharmacopoeias. In *Jpn.*

Adverse Effects

Nausea, gastro-intestinal distress, or flushing may follow high doses of cyclandelate.

Other adverse effects reported include tingling, tachycardia, sweating, dizziness, and headache.

Precautions

Cyclandelate is contra-indicated in the acute phase of a cerebrovascular accident. It should be used with caution in patients with severe obliterative coronary artery disease or cerebrovascular disease.

Uses and Administration

Cyclandelate is a vasodilator used in the management of cerebrovascular (p.785) and peripheral vascular disorders (p.794). It is given by mouth in a dosage of up to 1.6 g daily in divided doses although a daily dose of 400 to 800 mg may be adequate.

Preparations

Proprietary Preparations (details are given in Part 3)
Aust.: Cyclospasmol†; ***Belg.:*** Cyclospasmol; ***Canad.:*** Cyclospasmol; ***Fr.:*** Cyclergine; Cyclospasmol; Novodil; Vascunormyl; ***Ger.:*** Natil; Spasmocyclon; ***Ital.:*** Ciclospasmol; ***Neth.:*** Cyclospasmol†; ***Swed.:*** Cyclomandol; ***UK:*** Cyclobral†; ***USA:*** Cyclan†; Cyclospasmol†.

Multi-ingredient: ***Ger.:*** Eucebral-N.

Cyclopenthiazide (2323-m)

Cyclopenthiazide *(BAN, USAN, rINN)*.

Cyclopenthiaz.; NSC-107679; Su-8341. 6-Chloro-3-cyclopentylmethyl-3,4-dihydro-2*H*-1,2,4-benzothiadiazine-7-sulphonamide 1,1-dioxide.

$C_{13}H_{18}ClN_3O_4S_2$ = 379.9.

CAS — 742-20-1.

NOTE. Compounded preparations of cyclopenthiazide and oxprenolol hydrochloride in the proportions, by weight, 1 part to 640 parts have the British Approved Name Co-prenozide.

Pharmacopoeias. In *Br.*

A white, odourless or almost odourless powder. Practically **insoluble** in water; soluble in alcohol and in acetone; very slightly soluble in ether; practically insoluble in chloroform.

Cyclopenthiazide is a thiazide diuretic with properties similar to those of hydrochlorothiazide (p.885). It is used for oedema, including that associated with heart failure (p.785), and for hypertension (p.788).

Diuresis is induced in 1 to 3 hours, reaches a maximum in 4 to 8 hours, and lasts up to about 12 hours.

In the treatment of oedema the usual initial dose is 0.25 to 0.5 mg daily by mouth; up to 1 mg daily may be given in heart failure. The dose should be reduced to the lowest effective dose for maintenance; 0.5 mg on alternate days may be adequate. In the treatment of hypertension the usual dose is 0.25 to 0.5 mg daily either alone, or in conjunction with other antihypertensives. The maximum effective daily dose of cyclopenthiazide has been reported to be 1.5 mg, and to be rarely required.

In susceptible patients potassium supplements or a potassium-sparing diuretic may be necessary, but see hydrochlorothiazide.

Preparations

BP 1998: Cyclopenthiazide Tablets.

Proprietary Preparations (details are given in Part 3)
Austral.: Navidrex†; ***Irl.:*** Navidrex†; ***Neth.:*** Navidrex†; ***Switz.:*** Navidrex†; ***UK:*** Navidrex.

Multi-ingredient: ***Irl.:*** Navidrex-K†; Navispare; Trasidrex; ***S.Afr.:*** Lenurex-K†; Navidrex-K†; Serpasil-Navidrex-K†; Trasidrex; ***UK:*** Navispare; Trasidrex.

Cyclothiazide (2324-b)

Cyclothiazide *(BAN, USAN, rINN)*.

Compound 35483; MDi-193. 6-Chloro-3,4-dihydro-3-(norborn-5-en-2-yl)-2*H*-1,2,4-benzothiadiazine-7-sulphonamide 1,1-dioxide.

$C_{14}H_{16}ClN_3O_4S_2$ = 389.9.

CAS — 2259-96-3.

Cyclothiazide is a thiazide diuretic (see Hydrochlorothiazide, p.885) that is used, usually in combination preparations, in the management of oedema and hypertension.

Preparations

Proprietary Preparations (details are given in Part 3)
Multi-ingredient: ***Fr.:*** Cycloteriam; ***Spain:*** Sali Catapresan†.

Cymarin (5808-h)

K-Strophanthin-α. 3β-[(2,6-Dideoxy-3-*O*-methyl-β-D-*ribo*-hexopyranosyl)oxy]-5,14-dihydroxy-19-oxo-5β,14β-card-20(22)-enolide.

$C_{30}H_{44}O_9$ = 548.7.

CAS — 508-77-0.

NOTE. Do not confuse with Strophanthin-K (p.951).

A glycoside extracted from the roots of *Apocynum cannabinum.*

Cymarin is a cardiac glycoside with positive inotropic activity. Its actions are similar to those of digoxin (p.849) and it has been used in the management of heart failure.

Preparations

Proprietary Preparations (details are given in Part 3)
Ger.: Alvonal MR†.

Dalteparin Sodium (14676-j)

Dalteparin Sodium *(BAN, USAN, rINN)*.

Dalteparinum Natricum; Kabi-2165.

CAS — 9041-08-1.

NOTE. The name tedelparin sodium has been applied to this substance.

Pharmacopoeias. In *Eur.* (see p.viii).

Dalteparin sodium is prepared by nitrous acid degradation of heparin obtained from the intestinal mucosa of pigs. The majority of the components have a 2-*O*-sulpho-α-L-idopyranosuronic acid structure at the non-reducing end and a 6-*O*-sulpho-2,5-anhydro-D-mannitol structure at the reducing end of their chain. The molecular weight of 90% of the components is between 2000 and 9000 and the mass-average molecular mass ranges between 5600 and 6400, with a characteristic value of about 6000. The degree of sulphation is 2 to 2.5 per disaccharide unit.

The Ph. Eur. specifies that potency is not less than 110 units and not more than 210 units of anti-factor Xa activity per mg with reference to the dried substance and that the ratio of anti-factor Xa activity to anti-factor IIa (antithrombin) activity is between 1.9 and 3.2.

Units

As for Low-molecular-weight Heparins, p.899.

Adverse Effects and Treatment

As for Low-molecular-weight Heparins, p.899.

Precautions and Interactions

As for Low-molecular-weight Heparins, p.900.

Pharmacokinetics

Dalteparin is almost completely absorbed following subcutaneous administration, with a bioavailability of about 87%. Peak plasma activity is reached in about 4 hours. The terminal half-life is about 2 hours following intravenous injection and 3 to 5 hours following subcutaneous injection. Dalteparin is excreted via the kidneys and the half-life is prolonged in patients with renal impairment.

Uses and Administration

Dalteparin sodium is a low-molecular-weight heparin (p.899) with anticoagulant properties. It is used in the treatment and prophylaxis of venous thrombo-embolism (p.802) and to prevent clotting during extracorporeal circulation. It is also used in the management of unstable angina (p.780).

Dalteparin is administered by subcutaneous or intravenous injection. Doses are expressed in terms of units of anti-factor Xa activity.

For prophylaxis of venous thrombo-embolism during surgical procedures, 2500 units of dalteparin sodium are given by subcutaneous injection 1 to 2 hours before the procedure. For patients at moderate risk of thrombosis this is followed by 2500 units once daily for 5 to 7 days or until the patient is fully ambulant. For patients at high risk, 2500 units are given 1 to 2 hours before and 8 to 12 hours after the procedure followed by 5000 units daily. Alternatively, 5000 units may be given the evening before surgery followed by 5000 units each subsequent evening. This dosage may be continued for up to 5 weeks following hip replacement surgery.

In the treatment of established deep-vein thrombosis dalteparin sodium is given subcutaneously in a dose of 200 units per kg body-weight daily. This may be given as a single dose or, in patients at higher risk of bleeding, in two divided doses. The maximum recommended dose is 18 000 units daily.

For prevention of clotting in the extracorporeal circulation during haemodialysis or haemofiltration in adults with chronic renal insufficiency an intravenous injection of dalteparin sodium 30 to 40 units per kg is followed by an intravenous infusion of 10 to 15 units per kg per hour. A single injection of 5000 units may be given for a haemodialysis or haemofiltration session lasting less than 4 hours. The dose of dalteparin sodium should be reduced in patients at high risk of bleeding complications or who are in acute renal failure; in such patients an intravenous injection of 5 to 10 units per kg is followed by an infusion of 4 to 5 units per kg per hour.

In the management of unstable angina, dalteparin sodium is given subcutaneously in a dose of 120 units per kg every 12 hours; the maximum recommended dose is 10 000 units every 12 hours. Treatment is continued for 5 to 8 days and low-dose aspirin should be given concomitantly.

Reversal of effects. Severe bleeding with dalteparin may be reduced by the slow intravenous injection of protamine sulphate; 1 mg of protamine sulphate is stated to inhibit the effects of 100 units of dalteparin sodium.

References.

1. Dunn CJ, Sorkin EM. Dalteparin sodium: a review of its pharmacology and clinical use in the prevention and treatment of thromboembolic disorders. *Drugs* 1996; **52:** 276–305.
2. Howard PA. Dalteparin: a low-molecular-weight heparin. *Ann Pharmacother* 1997; **31:** 192–203.

Preparations

Proprietary Preparations (details are given in Part 3)
Aust.: Fragmin; ***Austral.:*** Fragmin; ***Belg.:*** Fragmin; ***Canad.:*** Fragmin; ***Fr.:*** Fragmine; ***Ger.:*** Fragmin; ***Ital.:*** Fragmin; ***Neth.:*** Fragmin; ***Norw.:*** Fragmin; ***S.Afr.:*** Fragmin; ***Spain:*** Boxol; Fragmin; ***Swed.:*** Fragmin; ***Switz.:*** Fragmin; Low Liquemine; ***UK:*** Fragmin; ***USA:*** Fragmin.

Danaparoid Sodium (3155-e)

Danaparoid Sodium *(BAN, USAN, rINN).*

Org-10172.

CAS — 83513-48-8.

Danaparoid sodium is a low-molecular-weight heparinoid derived from porcine intestinal mucosa. It contains a mixture of the sodium salts of heparan sulphate, dermatan sulphate, and chondroitin sulphate in an approximate ratio of 21:3:1. The average molecular weight is about 5500 to 6000.

Adverse Effects and Treatment

Haemorrhage may occur after administration of danaparoid sodium, although there is a possible decreased risk of bleeding complications compared with heparin. Liver enzymes may be transiently elevated. Other adverse effects include hypersensitivity reactions, thrombocytopenia, and pain at the site of injection.

Protamine sulphate only partially neutralises the anticoagulant effect of danaparoid sodium and cannot be relied on to reverse bleeding associated with overdosage.

Precautions

As for Heparin, p.880.

Danaparoid sodium should not be administered to patients who have developed thrombocytopenia with heparin if they demonstrate cross-reactivity in an *in-vitro* test.

Pharmacokinetics

Following subcutaneous administration of danaparoid sodium, peak anti-factor Xa activity is reached in approximately 4 to 5 hours. The elimination half-lives of anti-factor Xa and anti-factor IIa (antithrombin) activities are approximately 25 and 7 hours, respectively. Danaparoid sodium is excreted in the urine.

Uses and Administration

Danaparoid sodium is a low-molecular-weight heparinoid. It is an anticoagulant and, like heparin (p.881), enhances the action of antithrombin III. Similarly to low-molecular-weight heparins (p.899) it is characterised by a higher ratio of anti-factor Xa to anti-factor IIa (antithrombin) activity than heparin, but is reported to be a much more selective inhibitor of factor Xa than the low-molecular-weight heparins. It was therefore hoped that danaparoid might be associated with a low incidence of bleeding complications, although this is yet to be established.

Danaparoid sodium is used in the prophylaxis of venous thrombo-embolism (p.802) in patients undergoing surgery. It may be used in patients with heparin-associated thrombocytopenia providing there is no cross-reactivity.

Doses of danaparoid sodium are expressed in terms of units of anti-factor Xa activity. It is given by subcutaneous injection in a dose of 750 units twice daily for 7 to 10 days. The first dose should be given 1 to 4 hours before surgery.

References to the use of danaparoid sodium.

1. Henny CP, *et al.* Use of a new heparinoid as anticoagulant during acute haemodialysis of patients with bleeding complications. *Lancet* 1983; **i:** 890–3.
2. Turpie AGG, *et al.* Double-blind randomised trial of Org 10172 low-molecular-weight heparinoid in prevention of deep-vein thrombosis in thrombotic stroke. *Lancet* 1987; **i:** 523–6.
3. Massey EW, *et al.* Large-dose infusions of heparinoid ORG 10172 in ischemic stroke. *Stroke* 1990; **21:** 1289–92.
4. Turpie AGG, *et al.* A low-molecular-weight heparinoid compared with unfractionated heparin in the prevention of deep vein thrombosis in patients with acute ischemic stroke: a randomized, double-blind study. *Ann Intern Med* 1992; **117:** 353–7.
5. Boon DMS, *et al.* Heparin-induced thrombocytopenia and antithrombotic therapy. *Lancet* 1994; **344:** 1296.
6. de Valk HW, *et al.* Comparing subcutaneous danaparoid with intravenous unfractionated heparin for the treatment of venous thromboembolism: a randomized controlled trial. *Ann Intern Med* 1995; **123:** 1–9.
7. Skoutakis VA. Danaparoid in the prevention of thromboembolic complications. *Ann Pharmacother* 1997; **31:** 876–87.
8. Wilde MI, Markham A. Danaparoid: a review of its pharmacology and clinical use in the management of heparin-induced thrombocytopenia. *Drugs* 1997; **54:** 903–24.

Preparations

Proprietary Preparations (details are given in Part 3)
Austral.: Orgaran; ***Canad.:*** Orgaran; ***Neth.:*** Orgaran; ***Swed.:*** Orgaran; ***UK:*** Orgaran; ***USA:*** Orgaran.

Debrisoquine Sulphate (860-l)

Debrisoquine Sulphate *(BANM, rINNM).*

Debrisoquin Sulfate *(USAN)*; Isocaramidine Sulphate; Ro-5-3307/1. 1,2,3,4-Tetrahydroisoquinoline-2-carboxamidine sulphate.

$(C_{10}H_{13}N_3)_2,H_2SO_4$ = 448.5.

CAS — 1131-64-2 (debrisoquine); 581-88-4 (debrisoquine sulphate).

Pharmacopoeias. In Br.

A white odourless or almost odourless crystalline powder. Sparingly **soluble** in water; very slightly soluble in alcohol; practically insoluble in chloroform and ether. A 3% solution in water has a pH of 5.3 to 6.8. **Protect** from light.

Debrisoquine sulphate 12.8 mg is approximately equivalent to 10 mg of debrisoquine.

Adverse Effects, Treatment, and Precautions

As for Guanethidine Monosulphate, p.878.

Diarrhoea is rare with debrisoquine sulphate. Abrupt cessation of treatment should be avoided as this may lead to rebound hypertension.

The metabolism of debrisoquine is subject to genetic polymorphism and non-metabolisers may show a marked response to doses that have little or no effect in metabolisers.

Interactions

As for Guanethidine Monosulphate, p.878.

Pharmacokinetics

Debrisoquine is rapidly absorbed from the gastro-intestinal tract. The major metabolite is 4-hydroxydebrisoquine; metabolism is subject to genetic polymorphism.

Pre-systemic metabolism of debrisoquine to its metabolite 4-hydroxydebrisoquine occurred in 15 patients with hypertension and 4 healthy subjects.[1] Results indicated that debrisoquine or its metabolite could inhibit this metabolism and therefore increases in the dose of debrisoquine could produce disproportionate decreases in blood pressure. The estimated half-life of elimination for debrisoquine and 4-hydroxydebrisoquine ranged from 11.5 to 26 hours and from 5.8 to 14.5 hours respectively. A further study of one healthy subject indicated that debrisoquine was actively taken up by platelets and that this was responsible for its long half-life.

1. Silas JH, *et al.* The disposition of debrisoquine in hypertensive patients. *Br J Clin Pharmacol* 1978; **5:** 27–34.

Genetic polymorphism. A review of polymorphic drug metabolism.[1] Debrisoquine, along with sparteine and a number of other drugs is a substrate for a polymorphic cytochrome P450 enzyme, coded by a gene mapped to chromosome 22. Patients homozygous for the mutant allele are termed poor metabolisers and express little or none of the enzyme. The prevalence of the poor-metaboliser phenotype is about 5% in most Caucasian populations, while studies in other genetic groups have indicated a range of about 2 to 10% although in some groups, such as the Japanese, poor metabolisers have yet to be identified. Poor metabolisers of debrisoquine are unable to 4-hydroxylate the drug adequately to its inactive metabolite and are thus prone to excessive hypotension. A number of other drugs are metabolised by the same enzyme, including antidepressants such as amitriptyline, imipramine, and nortriptyline, other antihypertensives such as indoramin, antiarrhythmics like encainide, flecainide, and propafenone, analgesics like phenacetin, beta blockers such as metoprolol, propranolol, and timolol, hypoglycaemics like phenformin, and opioids such as codeine and dextromethorphan. However, the clinical consequences of polymorphism in patients receiving these drugs depend on the relative activity and toxicity of parent drug and metabolite, and the availability and relative importance of other routes of metabolism. Determination of phenotype is generally performed by administration of a test drug and assay of parent drug and metabolite in urine collected over a defined period of time. Although debrisoquine or sparteine may be used for this purpose, dextromethorphan (which yields phenotype assignments in agreement with those obtained after debrisoquine, is widely available, and has not been reported to cause toxicity after single doses even in poor metabolisers) is recommended as ideal.

1. Relling MV. Polymorphic drug metabolism. *Clin Pharm* 1989; **8:** 852–63.

Uses and Administration

Debrisoquine is an antihypertensive with actions and uses similar to those of guanethidine monosulphate (p.878), but it causes less depletion of noradrenaline stores. When administered by mouth, debrisoquine is reported to act within about 4 to 10 hours and to have effects lasting for 9 to 24 hours. It is used in the management of hypertension (p.788), although it has largely been superseded by other drugs.

Debrisoquine is given by mouth as the sulphate, but doses are usually expressed in terms of the base.

The usual initial dose is 10 to 20 mg once or twice daily. The daily dose is then increased by 10 to 20 mg, according to the severity of the condition, every 3 or 4 days. The usual maintenance dose is 20 to 120 mg daily, but 300 mg or more daily may be given.

For reference to the use of debrisoquine in identifying metabolic phenotypes, see under Genetic Polymorphism, above.

Preparations

BP 1998: Debrisoquine Tablets.

Proprietary Preparations (details are given in Part 3)
Irl.: Declinax†; ***UK:*** Declinax.

Defibrotide (18626-y)

Defibrotide *(BAN, rINN).*

Polydeoxyribonucleotides from bovine lung with molecular weight between 45 000 and 55 000.

Defibrotide is a deoxyribonucleic acid derivative that has antithrombotic and fibrinolytic properties. Defibrotide's mechanism of action is uncertain; it appears to increase levels of prostaglandin E_2 and prostacyclin, to alter platelet activity, and to increase tissue plasminogen activator function at the same time as decreasing activity of tissue plasminogen activator inhibitor. It is used in the management of thrombo-embolic disorders and is under investigation for the treatment of thrombotic thrombocytopenic purpura. Oral and parenteral formulations have been used in doses of up to 800 mg daily.

References.

1. Palmer KJ, Goa KL. Defibrotide: a review of its pharmacodynamic and pharmacokinetic properties, and therapeutic use in vascular disorders. *Drugs* 1993; **45:** 259–94.

Preparations

Proprietary Preparations (details are given in Part 3)
Ital.: Dasovas†; Noravid; Prociclide.

Delapril Hydrochloride (2850-m)

Delapril Hydrochloride *(USAN, rINNM).*

Alindapril Hydrochloride; CV-3317; Indalapril Hydrochloride; REV-6000A. Ethyl (S)-2-{[(S)-1-(carboxymethyl-2-indanylcarbamoyl)ethyl]amino}-4-phenylbutyrate hydrochloride.

$C_{26}H_{32}N_2O_5,HCl = 489.0.$

CAS — 83435-66-9 (delapril); 83435-67-0 (delapril hydrochloride).

Delapril is an ACE inhibitor (p.805). It is converted in the body to two metabolites to which it owes its activity. It is given by mouth as the hydrochloride in the treatment of hypertension (p.788), in usual maintenance doses of 30 to 60 mg daily in two divided doses.

References.

1. Shionoin H, *et al.* Antihypertensive effect of delapril during long-term treatment in hypertensive patients. *Curr Ther Res* 1989; **45:** 813–20.
2. Kelly JG, O'Malley K. Clinical pharmacokinetics of the newer ACE inhibitors: a review. *Clin Pharmacokinet* 1990; **19:** 177–96.
3. Salvetti A. Newer ACE inhibitors: a look at the future. *Drugs* 1990; **40:** 800–28.

Preparations

Proprietary Preparations (details are given in Part 3)
Ital.: Delaket; ***Jpn:*** Adecut.
Multi-ingredient: ***Ital.:*** Delapride; Dinapres.

Denopamine (19049-b)

Denopamine *(rINN).*

TA-064. (−)-(R)-α-{[(3,4-Dimethoxyphenethyl)amino]methyl}-p-hydroxybenzyl alcohol.

$C_{18}H_{23}NO_4 = 317.4.$

CAS — 71771-90-9.

Denopamine is an oral sympathomimetic (see Adrenaline, p.813) with predominantly beta-adrenergic activity selective to $beta_1$ receptors ($beta_1$ agonist). It acts as a partial agonist (see Xamoterol, p.971) and is under investigation for the treatment of heart failure.

References.

1. Satoh Y, *et al.* Short-term effects of denopamine on anaerobic threshold and related parameters in patients with chronic heart failure: a double-blind crossover study. *Clin Pharmacol Ther* 1993; **53:** 562–9.

Preparations

Proprietary Preparations (details are given in Part 3)
Jpn: Kalgut.

Dermatan Sulphate (10810-a)

LMW-DS (depolymerised dermatan sulphate); MF-701; OP-370 (depolymerised dermatan sulphate).

CAS — 54328-33-5 (dermatan sulphate, sodium salt).

Dermatan sulphate is a naturally occurring glycosaminoglycan under investigation as an anticoagulant and antithrombotic. The sodium salt is a component of the heparinoid, danaparoid sodium (p.846). Low-molecular-weight (depolymerised) dermatan sulphate is also being investigated.

References.

1. Dawes J, *et al.* The pharmacokinetics of dermatan sulphate MF701 in healthy human volunteers. *Br J Clin Pharmacol* 1991; **32:** 361–6.
2. Lane DA, *et al.* Dermatan sulphate in haemodialysis. *Lancet* 1992; **339:** 334–5.
3. Cofrancesco E, *et al.* Dermatan sulphate in acute leukaemia. *Lancet* 1992; **339:** 1177–8.
4. Agnelli G, *et al.* Randomised, double-blind, placebo-controlled trial of dermatan sulphate for prevention of deep vein thrombosis in hip fracture. *Thromb Haemost* 1992; **67:** 203–8.
5. Gianese F, *et al.* The pharmacokinetics and pharmacodynamics of dermatan sulphate MF701 during haemodialysis for chronic renal failure. *Br J Clin Pharmacol* 1993; **35:** 335–9.
6. Agnelli G, *et al.* Dermatan sulphate in heparin-induced thrombocytopenia. *Lancet* 1994; **344:** 1295–6.
7. Legnani C, *et al.* Acute and chronic effects of a new low molecular weight dermatan sulphate (Desmin 370) on blood coagulation and fibrinolysis in healthy subjects. *Eur J Clin Pharmacol* 1994; **47:** 247–52.

Deserpidine (861-y)

Deserpidine *(BAN, rINN).*

Canescine; 11-Desmethoxyreserpine; Raunormine; Recanescine. Methyl 11-demethoxy-O-(3,4,5-trimethoxybenzoyl)reserpate.

$C_{32}H_{38}N_2O_8 = 578.7.$

CAS — 131-01-1.

An ester alkaloid isolated from the root of *Rauwolfia canescens.*

Deserpidine has properties similar to those described under reserpine (p.942) and has been used in the treatment of hypertension and psychoses.

Preparations

Proprietary Preparations (details are given in Part 3)
Multi-ingredient: ***Canad.:*** Dureticyl†; ***Ital.:*** Enduronil; ***USA:*** Enduronyl; Oreticyl†.

Deslanoside (5809-m)

Deslanoside *(BAN, rINN).*

Deacetyl-lanatoside C; Desacetyl-lanatoside C; Deslanosídeo; Deslanosidum. 3-[(O-β-D-Glucopyranosyl-(1→4)-O-2,6-dideoxy-β-D-*ribo*-hexopyranosyl-(1→4)-O-2,6-dideoxy-β-D-*ribo*-hexopyranosyl-(1→4)-O-2,6-dideoxy-β-D-*ribo*-hexopyranosyl)oxy]-12,14-dihydroxy-3β,5β,12β-card-20(22)-enolide.

$C_{47}H_{74}O_{19} = 943.1.$

CAS — 17598-65-1.

Pharmacopoeias. In *Chin., Eur.* (see p.viii), *Jpn,* and *US.*

A white, crystalline or finely crystalline hygroscopic powder. Practically **insoluble** in water and in ether; very slightly soluble in alcohol. **Store** in airtight, glass containers at a temperature not exceeding 10°. Protect from light.

Deslanoside, a cardiac glycoside with positive inotropic activity, is a derivative of lanatoside C. It has the general properties of digoxin (p.849) and has been used similarly in the management of some cardiac arrhythmias (p.782) and in heart failure (p.785).

Deslanoside is usually reserved for the treatment of emergencies although digoxin is generally preferred. Its effects occur about 5 to 10 minutes after intravenous administration and the full action on the heart is exerted after about 2 hours. It has a half-life of about 33 hours and its effects persist for 2 to 5 days.

A suggested rapid digitalising dose of deslanoside is up to 1.6 mg given by intravenous injection as a single dose or in two divided doses. Maintenance treatment with a cardiac glycoside given by mouth may be started within 12 hours of parenteral digitalisation with deslanoside.

Preparations

USP 23: Deslanoside Injection.

Proprietary Preparations (details are given in Part 3)
Aust.: Cedilanid; ***Fr.:*** Cedilanide; ***Ital.:*** Desaci†.
Multi-ingredient: ***Ger.:*** Conjunctisan-A.

Diazoxide (862-j)

Diazoxide *(BAN, USAN, rINN).*

Diazoxidum; NSC-64198; Sch-6783; SRG-95213. 7-Chloro-3-methyl-2H-1,2,4-benzothiadiazine 1,1-dioxide.

$C_8H_7ClN_2O_2S = 230.7.$

CAS — 364-98-7.

Pharmacopoeias. In *Eur.* (see p.viii), *Int.,* and *US.*

A white or almost white fine or crystalline powder. Practically **insoluble** to sparingly soluble in water; slightly soluble in alcohol; very soluble in strong alkaline solutions and in dilute solutions of alkali hydroxides; freely soluble in dimethylformamide; practically insoluble in ether. Liquid preparations should be **stored** protected from light.

Adverse Effects

In addition to inappropriate hypotension and hyperglycaemia (which includes ketoacidosis and hyperosmolar nonketotic coma), side-effects during prolonged therapy frequently include oedema due to salt and water retention, which may result in precipitation of heart failure. Other adverse effects include dysgeusia, nausea, anorexia, and other gastro-intestinal disturbances; mild hyperuricaemia; extrapyramidal symptoms; eosinophilia and thrombocytopenia; dyspnoea; hypertrichosis; and headache, dizziness, tinnitus, and blurred vision. Hypersensitivity has occurred, manifesting as rashes, leucopenia, and fever.

Alopecia has been reported in infants born to mothers taking diazoxide.

During intravenous therapy, particularly following large intravenous boluses, adverse effects may be associated with an inappropriately rapid reduction in the blood pressure: coronary ischaemia leading to angina, cardiac arrhythmias, marked ECG changes, tachycardia, palpitations, and bradycardia; cerebral ischaemia leading to confusion, convulsions, loss of consciousness, and neurological deficit; impaired renal function; symptoms of vasodilatation.

Diazoxide may cause a burning sensation in the vein used for injection; extravasation of the alkaline solution is painful.

Effects on the blood. A 26-year-old man with hypertension developed reversible haemolytic anaemia when treated with diazoxide by mouth on 3 separate occasions.[1]

1. Best RA, Clink HM. Haemolysis associated with diazoxide, used for the control of hypertension. *Postgrad Med J* 1975; **51:** 402–4.

Effects on the hair. *Hirsutism* and *hypertrichosis* are different types of excessive hair growth, but the terms have often been used interchangeably. Hirsutism is androgen-related whereas hypertrichosis is thought to be independent from hormone stimulation. Hypertrichosis is acknowledged to be a frequent adverse effect of diazoxide in children receiving long-term treatment for idiopathic hypoglycaemia.[1] Two such children had unusually deep (low-pitched) voices as well as marked hypertrichosis.[2] A woman on continuous diazoxide therapy who developed so-called hirsutism without signs of virilisation had raised serum concentrations of androgens.[3]

Alopecia has been reported in infants born to mothers who had been on long-term treatment with diazoxide during pregnancy.

1. Burton JL, *et al.* Hypertrichosis due to diazoxide. *Br J Dermatol* 1975; **93:** 707–11.
2. West RJ. Side effects of diazoxide. *Br Med J* 1978; **2:** 506.
3. Hallengren B, Hökfelt B. Increase of serum androgens during diazoxide treatment. *Lancet* 1984; **ii:** 1044–5.

Extrapyramidal effects. In a study of 100 hypertensive patients receiving diazoxide, the incidence of extrapyramidal symptoms was 15%.[1]

1. Pohl JEF. Development and management of extrapyramidal symptoms in hypertensive patients treated with diazoxide. *Am Heart J* 1975; **89:** 401–2.

Pancreatitis. Ten patients with severe hypertension and renal failure were treated with diazoxide in a last attempt to avert nephrectomy; 1 patient developed acute pancreatitis and another diabetic ketoacidosis.[1] Both patients recovered from these effects when diazoxide was withdrawn.

1. De Broe M, *et al.* Oral diazoxide for malignant hypertension. *Lancet* 1972; **i:** 1397.

Pregnancy. Transplacental transfer of diazoxide was considered to be responsible for an inappropriately low plasma-insulin concentration in an infant whose mother had received diazoxide 150 mg daily for 47 days prior to delivery.[1]

1. Smith MJ, *et al.* Neonatal hyperglycaemia after prolonged maternal treatment with diazoxide. *Br Med J* 1982; **284:** 1234.

Voice changes. In addition to marked hypertrichosis, 2 children who had received diazoxide for several years were noted to have unusually deep (low-pitched) voices.[1]

1. West RJ. Side effects of diazoxide. *Br Med J* 1978; **2:** 506.

Treatment of Adverse Effects

Treatment is largely symptomatic. Severe hyperglycaemia may be corrected by giving insulin: less severe hyperglycaemia is reported to respond to tolbutamide. Hypotension may be managed with intravenous fluids. Severe hypotension may require sympathomimetic drugs. Antiparkinsonian drugs, such as procyclidine, have been given to control extrapyramidal effects while a loop diuretic may be required for salt and water retention. Diazoxide can be removed from the body by dialysis but recovery is relatively low owing to extensive protein binding.

Precautions

Diazoxide should be used with care in patients with impaired cardiac or cerebral circulation and in patients with aortic coarctation, arteriovenous shunt, or other cardiac disorders in which an increase in cardiac output could be detrimental. During prolonged therapy blood-glucose concentrations and blood pressure should be monitored and the blood should be examined regularly for signs of leucopenia and thrombocytopenia; in children, bone and psychological maturation and growth should be regularly assessed. Caution is necessary in patients with renal impairment.

If given during parturition, diazoxide may delay delivery unless oxytocin is given concomitantly.

Pregnancy. For reports of sedation, hypotonia, hypoventilation, or apnoea among infants born to mothers given both diazoxide and chlormethiazole edisylate for the treatment of toxaemia of pregnancy, see Chlormethiazole Edisylate, p.647.

Interactions

The hyperglycaemic, hyperuricaemic, and hypotensive actions of diazoxide may be enhanced by diuretics. Administration of diazoxide with other antihypertensives or vasodilators may lead to increased risk of hypotension.

Chlorpromazine. A report of *chlorpromazine* enhancing the hyperglycaemic effect of diazoxide in a 2-year-old child.[1]

1. Aynsley-Green A, Illig R. Enhancement by chlorpromazine of hyperglycaemic action of diazoxide. *Lancet* 1975; **ii:** 658–9.

Phenytoin. For the effect of diazoxide on serum-phenytoin concentrations, see p.355.

Pharmacokinetics

Diazoxide is readily absorbed from the gastro-intestinal tract and more than 90% bound to plasma proteins, although protein binding is decreased in uraemic patients. Its plasma half-life has been estimated to range from about 20 to 45 hours but values of up to 60 hours have been reported. The half-life is reported to be prolonged in renal impairment and shorter for children. The plasma half-life greatly exceeds the duration of vascular activity. Diazoxide is partly metabolised in the liver and is excreted in the urine both unchanged and in the form of metabolites; only small amounts are recovered from the faeces. It crosses the placenta and the blood-brain barrier.

Children. A pharmacokinetic study of diazoxide in 4 children with hypoglycaemia revealed a plasma half-life of 9.5 to 24 hours, which is considerably shorter than that in adults.[1]

1. Pruitt AW, *et al.* Disposition of diazoxide in children. *Clin Pharmacol Ther* 1973; **14:** 73–82.

Uses and Administration

Diazoxide increases the concentration of glucose in the plasma; it inhibits the secretion of insulin by the beta cells of the pancreas, and may increase the hepatic output of glucose. When administered intravenously, it produces a fall in blood pressure by a vasodilator effect on the arterioles and a reduction in peripheral resistance. Diazoxide is closely related structurally to the thiazide diuretics, but has an antidiuretic action and thus produces fluid and electrolyte retention; a loop diuretic may be given concomitantly to reduce fluid retention.

Diazoxide is used by mouth in the management of intractable hypoglycaemia and intravenously in the management of hypertensive crises (p.788), particularly when first-line agents such as sodium nitroprusside are ineffective or unsuitable. Diazoxide is not given by mouth in the chronic treatment of hypertension because of the severity of the adverse effects produced.

In **hypoglycaemia**, diazoxide is given in an initial dose of 3 to 5 mg per kg body-weight daily in 2 or 3 divided doses by mouth, then the dosage is adjusted according to the needs of the patient. Usual maintenance doses are from 3 to 8 mg per kg daily but total doses of up to 1 g daily have been given to adults with islet cell tumours. In neonates and infants, an initial dose of 10 mg per kg daily in 3 divided doses has been suggested; usual maintenance doses have ranged from 8 to 15 mg per kg daily, in 2 or 3 divided doses, although up to 20 mg per kg daily has been suggested in children with leucine-sensitive hypoglycaemia. The hyperglycaemic effect normally begins within 1 hour of administration and lasts for up to 8 hours.

In **hypertensive crises**, a single bolus intravenous injection of 300 mg will produce a rapid fall in blood pressure, but such a rapid fall may be hazardous and injection of 1 to 3 mg per kg body-weight within 30 seconds, up to a maximum dose of 150 mg, and repeated after 5 to 15 minutes if required, is now preferred.

Reduced doses may be necessary in patients with impaired renal function.

Preparations

BP 1998: Diazoxide Injection; Diazoxide Tablets;
USP 23: Diazoxide Capsules; Diazoxide Injection; Diazoxide Oral Suspension.

Proprietary Preparations (details are given in Part 3)
Austral.: Hyperstat†; ***Belg.:*** Hyperstat; ***Canad.:*** Hyperstat; Proglycem; ***Fr.:*** Hyperstat; Proglicem; ***Ger.:*** Hypertonalum; Proglicem; ***Irl.:*** Eudemine†; ***Ital.:*** Hyperstat; Proglicem; ***Neth.:*** Hyperstat; Proglicem; ***S.Afr.:*** Hyperstat; ***Spain:*** Hyperstat; ***Swed.:*** Hyperstat; ***Switz.:*** Hyperstat; Proglicem; ***UK:*** Eudemine; ***USA:*** Hyperstat; Proglycem.

Dichlorphenamide (2325-v)

Dichlorphenamide *(BAN)*.
Diclofenamide *(rINN)*; Diclofenamidum. 4,5-Dichlorobenzene-1,3-disulphonamide.
$C_6H_6Cl_2N_2O_4S_2$ = 305.2.
CAS — 120-97-8.
Pharmacopoeias. In *Chin., Jpn*, and *US.*

Dichlorphenamide is an inhibitor of carbonic anhydrase with properties similar to those of acetazolamide (p.810). When given by mouth, its effect begins within 1 hour and lasts for 6 to 12 hours.

Dichlorphenamide is used to reduce intra-ocular pressure in glaucoma (p.1387). The usual initial adult dose is 100 to 200 mg by mouth, then 100 mg every 12 hours until the desired response is obtained, followed by a maintenance dose of 25 to 50 mg one to three times daily. Dichlorphenamide sodium has been given by injection.

Preparations

USP 23: Dichlorphenamide Tablets.

Proprietary Preparations (details are given in Part 3)
Aust.: Glaucol; ***Austral.:*** Daranide; ***Belg.:*** Oratrol; ***Irl.:*** Daranide; ***Ital.:*** Antidrasi; Fenamide; Glaumid; ***Spain:*** Glauconide; Oratrol; Tensodilen†; ***Swed.:*** Oralcon; ***Switz.:*** Oratrol; ***UK:*** Daranide†; ***USA:*** Daranide.

Dicoumarol (4811-l)

Dicoumarol *(rINN)*.
Bishydroxycoumarin; Dicoumarin; Dicumarol *(USAN)*; Melitoxin. 3,3′-Methylenebis(4-hydroxycoumarin).
$C_{19}H_{12}O_6$ = 336.3.
CAS — 66-76-2.
Pharmacopoeias. In *Int.*

Adverse Effects, Treatment, and Precautions

As for Warfarin Sodium, p.964, although gastro-intestinal side-effects are reported to occur more frequently. The absorption of dicoumarol is affected by food.

Interactions

The interactions associated with oral anticoagulants are discussed in detail under warfarin (p.965). Specific references to interactions involving dicoumarol can be found under the headings for the following drug groups: analgesics; antiarrhythmics; antibacterials; antidepressants; antidiabetics; antiepileptics; antigout drugs; anxiolytic sedatives; gastro-intestinal drugs; lipid regulating drugs; sex hormones; and vitamins.

Pharmacokinetics

Dicoumarol is slowly and erratically absorbed from the gastro-intestinal tract and is extensively bound to plasma protein. It is metabolised in the liver and is excreted in the urine, mainly as metabolites.

Uses and Administration

Dicoumarol is an orally administered coumarin anticoagulant with actions similar to those of warfarin sodium (p.969). It is used in the management of thrombo-embolic disorders (p.801). The initial dose of dicoumarol is usually 200 to 300 mg with a daily maintenance dose according to coagulation tests of 25 to 200 mg.

Because of its unpredictability of response and high incidence of gastro-intestinal effects, dicoumarol has been largely replaced by warfarin sodium.

Preparations

Proprietary Preparations (details are given in Part 3)
Swed.: Apekumarol.

Digitalis Leaf (5812-r)

Digit. Fol.; Digit. Leaf; Digitale Pourprée; Digitalis; Digitalis Folium; Digitalis Purpureae Folium; Feuille de Digitale; Fingerhutblatt; Folha de Dedaleira; Foxglove Leaf; Hoja de Digital.

NOTE. The term 'digitalis' is often used to describe the entire class of cardiac glycosides.

Pharmacopoeias. In *Chin., Eur.* (see p.viii), *Jpn*, and *US.*

The dried leaves of *Digitalis purpurea* (Scrophulariaceae). Digitalis leaf contains a number of glycosides, including digitoxin, gitoxin, and gitaloxin. The Ph. Eur. specifies the potency as not less than 0.3% of cardenolic glycosides calculated as digitoxin. The USP specifies a potency of 1 USP unit in 100 mg.

Store in airtight containers. Protect from light.

Digitalis contains cardiac glycosides with positive inotropic activity and has the general properties described under digoxin (p.849). It has been used similarly in the management of heart failure. However, when treatment with a cardiac glycoside is required a single glycoside is preferred to digitalis, and digoxin or digitoxin are most commonly used.

Digitalis is used in herbal and homoeopathic medicine.

Preparations

USP 23: Digitalis Capsules; Digitalis Tablets.

Proprietary Preparations (details are given in Part 3)
Ger.: Digitalysat†; Digophton.

Multi-ingredient: ***Aust.:*** Augentropfen Stulln; ***Ger.:*** Augentropfen Stulln Mono; Robusanon†; Strophanthus-Strath†; Unguentum Lymphaticum; Valeriana-Digitalysat (Valdig)†; ***Switz.:*** Augentonicum; Collypan.

Digitalis Lanata Leaf (5814-d)

Austrian Digitalis; Austrian Foxglove; Digitalis Lanatae Folium; Woolly Foxglove Leaf.
CAS — 17575-20-1 (lanatoside A).
Pharmacopoeias. In *Aust.*

The dried leaves of the woolly foxglove, *Digitalis lanata* (Scrophulariaceae), containing about 1 to 1.4% of a mixture of cardioactive glycosides, including digoxin, digitoxin, acetyldigoxin, acetyldigitoxin, lanatoside A, and deslanoside.

Digitalis lanata leaf is used as a source for the manufacture of digoxin and other glycosides.

Digitoxin (5815-n)

Digitoxin *(BAN, rINN)*.
Digitaline Cristallisée; Digitoxinum; Digitoxoside. 3β-[(*O*-2,6-Dideoxy-β-D-*ribo*-hexopyranosyl-(1→4)-*O*-2,6-dideoxy-β-D-*ribo*-hexopyranosyl-(1→4)-2,6-dideoxy-β-D-*ribo*-hexopyranosyl)oxy]-14β-hydroxy-5β-card-20(22)-enolide.
$C_{41}H_{64}O_{13}$ = 764.9.
CAS — 71-63-6.
Pharmacopoeias. In *Chin., Eur.* (see p.viii), *Int., Jpn*, and *US.*

A crystalline glycoside obtained from suitable species of *Digitalis.*

It is a white or pale buff-coloured, odourless, microcrystalline powder. Practically **insoluble** in water; soluble 1 in 150 of alcohol and 1 in 40 of chloroform; slightly soluble in methyl alcohol; very slightly soluble in ether; freely soluble in a mixture of equal volumes of chloroform and methyl alcohol. **Store** in airtight containers. Protect from light.

Binding to an inline intravenous filter containing a cellulose ester membrane accounted for a reduction in digitoxin concentration of up to 25% from solutions of digitoxin 200 μg in 50 mL of glucose 5% or sodium chloride 0.9%.[1] Pretreatment of the filter with a polymer coating reduced adsorbance by about half.[2]

Digitoxin was found to be adsorbed onto glass and plastic in substantial amounts from simple aqueous solutions but not from solutions in 30% alcohol, or in plasma, or urine.[3]

1. Butler LD, *et al.* Effect of inline filtration on the potency of low-dose drugs. *Am J Hosp Pharm* 1980; **37:** 935–41.
2. Kanke M, *et al.* Binding of selected drugs to a "treated" inline filter. *Am J Hosp Pharm* 1983; **40:** 1323–8.
3. Molin L, *et al.* Solubility, partition, and adsorption of digitalis glycosides. *Acta Pharm Suec* 1983; **20:** 129–44.

Adverse Effects, Treatment, and Precautions

As for Digoxin, below. Toxicity may be more prolonged after withdrawal of digitoxin because of the longer half-life.

References.

1. Lely AH, van Enter CHJ. Large-scale digitoxin intoxication. *Br Med J* 1970; **3:** 737–40.
2. Gilfrich H-J, *et al.* Treatment of massive digitoxin overdose by charcoal haemoperfusion and cholestyramine. *Lancet* 1978; **i:** 505.
3. Pond S, *et al.* Treatment of digitoxin overdose with oral activated charcoal. *Lancet* 1981; **ii:** 1177–8.

Interactions

As for Digoxin, below. Since digitoxin is significantly metabolised in the liver it may be affected by drugs that induce microsomal enzymes, such as some antiepileptics.

Antibacterials. Acute heart failure has been reported in a patient taking digitoxin when treatment with *rifampicin* and isoniazid was started with plasma-digitoxin concentrations falling from a pretreatment steady-state value of 27 ng per mL to 10 ng per mL. The reduction in the digitoxin concentration was attributed to induction of digitoxin metabolism by rifampicin.[1]

Digitoxin toxicity has been described in 2 patients following addition of *azithromycin* to their therapy.[2]

1. Boman G, *et al.* Acute cardiac failure during treatment with digitoxin—an interaction with rifampicin. *Br J Clin Pharmacol* 1980; **10:** 89–90.
2. Thalhammer F, *et al.* Azithromycin-related toxic effects of digitoxin. *Br J Clin Pharmacol* 1998; **45:** 91–2.

Antineoplastics and immunosuppressants. A mean overall increase of 109% was seen in digitoxin clearance in 5 patients during concomitant treatment with *aminoglutethimide*. The interaction was attributed to the induction of hepatic enzymes by aminoglutethimide.[1]

1. Lønning PE, *et al.* Effect of aminoglutethimide on antipyrine, theophylline, and digitoxin disposition in breast cancer. *Clin Pharmacol Ther* 1984; **36:** 796–802.

Calcium-channel blockers. Steady-state concentrations of digitoxin in the plasma increased by an average of 35% over 2 to 3 weeks in 8 of 10 patients when *verapamil* 240 mg daily was added to their therapy. Total body clearance and extrarenal clearance of digitoxin were reduced by 27% and 29% respectively although renal excretion was unchanged. Plasma-digitoxin concentrations increased by a mean of 21% in 5 of 10 patients treated with *diltiazem* but were not increased by concomitant treatment with *nifedipine*.[1]

1. Kuhlman J. Effects of verapamil, diltiazem, and nifedipine on plasma levels and renal excretion of digitoxin. *Clin Pharmacol Ther* 1985; **38:** 667–73.

Diuretics. *Spironolactone* has been reported to decrease the half-life and the urinary elimination of unchanged digitoxin when given for at least 10 days to 8 patients on oral maintenance digitoxin therapy.[1] However, increased digitoxin half-life has been reported[2] in 3 healthy subjects when spironolactone was added to digitoxin therapy. The interaction was judged to be of minor clinical importance.

1. Wirth KE, *et al.* Metabolism of digitoxin in man and its modification by spironolactone. *Eur J Clin Pharmacol* 1976; **9:** 345–54.
2. Carruthers SG, Dujovne CA. Cholestyramine and spironolactone and their combination in digitoxin elimination. *Clin Pharmacol Ther* 1980; **27:** 184–7.

Pharmacokinetics

Digitoxin is readily and completely absorbed from the gastro-intestinal tract. Therapeutic plasma concentrations may range from 10 to 35 ng per mL but there is considerable interindividual variation. Digitoxin is extensively (more than 90%) bound to plasma protein. It is very slowly eliminated from the body and is metabolised in the liver. Most metabolites are inactive; the major active metabolite is digoxin. Enterohepatic recycling occurs and digitoxin is excreted in the urine, mainly as metabolites. It is also excreted in the faeces and this route becomes significant in renal impairment. Digitoxin has an elimination half-life of up to 7 days or more. The half-life is generally unchanged in renal impairment.

The pharmacokinetics of digitoxin may be affected by age and by concurrent diseases (see under Uses and Administration, below).

Uses and Administration

Digitoxin is a cardiac glycoside with positive inotropic activity. It has actions similar to those of digoxin (below) and is used in the management of some cardiac arrhythmias (p.782) and in heart failure (p.785).

Digitoxin is completely and readily absorbed when given by mouth. It is the most potent of the digitalis glycosides and is the most cumulative in action. The onset of its action is slower than that of the other cardiac glycosides; following oral administration its effects may be evident in about 2 hours and its full effects in about 12 hours. Its effects persist for about 3 weeks.

As described under digoxin, dosage should be carefully adjusted to the needs of the individual patient. Steady-state therapeutic plasma concentrations of digitoxin may range from 10 to 35 ng per mL; higher values may be associated with toxicity. Digoxin may be more suitable for rapid digitalisation. In adults an initial dose of 600 µg of digitoxin by mouth may be given for rapid digitalisation, followed by 400 µg after 4 to 6 hours, then 200 µg every 4 to 6 hours as necessary; the maximum total dose is usually 1.6 mg. For slow digitalisation 200 µg may be given twice daily for 4 days. The maintenance dose varies from 50 to 300 µg once daily, the usual dose being 150 µg daily. Digitoxin may also be given in similar doses by slow intravenous injection when vomiting or other conditions prevent administration by mouth. It has also been given intramuscularly but injections may be irritant.

Suggested doses of digitoxin for rapid digitalisation in children, to be given in 3 or more divided doses daily by mouth or by injection, are: premature and full-term infants, 22 µg per kg body-weight; 2 weeks to 1 year, 45 µg per kg; 1 to 2 years, 40 µg per kg; and over 2 years, 30 µg per kg. For maintenance one-tenth of the total digitalising dose may be given daily.

Administration in children. Children were found to have a greater volume of distribution of digitoxin than adults and a shorter mean half-life, although individual variation was considerable. The increase in total clearance in children compared with adults was attributed to greater metabolic clearance. Digitalisation doses of 20 µg per kg body-weight were well tolerated.[1]

1. Larsen A, Storstein L. Digitoxin kinetics and renal excretion in children. *Clin Pharmacol Ther* 1983; **33:** 717–26.

Administration in the elderly. Digitoxin half-life, apparent volume of distribution, and clearance were not found to differ in elderly subjects compared with young adults following intravenous injection in a single-dose study. The long half-life may make once weekly dosing possible in poorly compliant patients.[1]

1. Donovan MA, *et al.* The effect of age on digitoxin pharmacokinetics. *Br J Clin Pharmacol* 1981; **11:** 401–2.

Administration in renal disease. The pharmacokinetics of digitoxin were changed significantly in 5 patients with the nephrotic syndrome. The apparent volume of distribution of digitoxin was increased and protein binding decreased. Such patients should be maintained at lower serum-digitoxin concentrations than other patients but will need larger doses because of the shortened serum half-life and the increased renal excretion of digitoxin and its cardioactive metabolites.[1]

1. Storstein L. Studies on digitalis VII: influence of nephrotic syndrome on protein binding, pharmacokinetics, and renal excretion of digitoxin and cardioactive metabolites. *Clin Pharmacol Ther* 1976; **20:** 158–66.

Preparations

BP 1998: Digitoxin Tablets;
USP 23: Digitoxin Injection; Digitoxin Tablets.

Proprietary Preparations (details are given in Part 3)

Aust.: Digimerck; Ditaven; ***Belg.:*** Digitaline; Digitasid†; ***Canad.:*** Digitaline; ***Fr.:*** Digitaline; ***Ger.:*** Coramedan; Digicor†; Digimed; Digimerck; Digipural†; Ditaven; mono-glycocard†; Tardigal†; ***Norw.:*** Digitrin; ***Spain:*** Digitaline†; ***Swed.:*** Digitrin; ***Switz.:*** Digitaline†; ***USA:*** Crystodigin.

Multi-ingredient: ***Aust.:*** Ditaven comp; ***Fr.:*** Ditavene; ***Switz.:*** Augentonicum; Optazine.

Digoxin (5801-a)

Digoxin *(BAN, rINN)*.

Digoxinum; Digoxosidum. 3β-[(*O*-2,6-Dideoxy-β-D-*ribo*-hexopyranosyl-(1→4)-*O*-2,6-dideoxy-β-D-*ribo*-hexopyranosyl-(1→4)-2,6-dideoxy-β-D-*ribo*-hexopyranosyl)oxy]-12β,14β-dihydroxy-5β-card-20(22)-enolide.

$C_{41}H_{64}O_{14}$ = 780.9.

CAS — 20830-75-5.

Pharmacopoeias. In *Chin., Eur.* (see p.viii), *Int., Jpn, Pol.,* and *US.*

A cardiac glycoside obtained from the leaves of *Digitalis lanata*. It occurs as odourless, colourless or white crystals or a white or almost white powder.

Practically **insoluble** in water and in ether; slightly soluble in chloroform and in alcohol; freely soluble in pyridine and in a mixture of equal volumes of dichloromethane and methyl alcohol. **Store** in airtight containers. Protect from light.

Adverse Effects

Digoxin and the other cardiac glycosides commonly produce side-effects because the margin between the therapeutic and toxic doses is small; plasma concentrations of digoxin in excess of 2 ng per mL are considered to be an indication that the patient is at special risk although there is considerable interindividual variation. There have been many fatalities, particularly due to cardiac toxicity.

Nausea, vomiting, and anorexia may be among the earliest symptoms of digoxin toxicity or overdosage; diarrhoea and abdominal pain may occur. Certain neurological effects are also common symptoms of digoxin overdosage and include headache, facial pain, fatigue, weakness, dizziness, drowsiness, disorientation, mental confusion, bad dreams and more rarely delirium, acute psychoses, and hallucinations. Convulsions have been reported. Visual disturbances including blurred vision may occur; colour vision may be affected with objects appearing yellow or less frequently green, red, brown, blue, or white. Hypersensitivity reactions are rare; thrombocytopenia has been reported. The cardiac glycosides may have some oestrogenic activity and occasionally cause gynaecomastia at therapeutic doses.

Rapid intravenous injection of digoxin may cause vasoconstriction and transient hypertension. Intramuscular or subcutaneous injection can cause local irritation.

The most serious adverse effects are those on the heart. Toxic doses may cause or aggravate heart failure. Supraventricular or ventricular arrhythmias and defects of conduction are common and may be an early indication of excessive dosage. In general the incidence and severity of arrhythmias is related to the severity of the underlying heart disease. Almost any arrhythmia may ensue, but particular note should be made of supraventricular tachycardia, especially atrioventricular (AV) junctional tachycardia and atrial tachycardia with block. Ventricular arrhythmias including extrasystoles, sinoatrial block, sinus bradycardia, and AV block may also occur.

Hypokalaemia predisposes to digoxin toxicity; adverse reactions to digoxin may be precipitated if there is potassium depletion such as may be caused by the prolonged administration of diuretics. Hyperkalaemia occurs in acute overdosage.

As digoxin has a shorter half-life than digitalis or digitoxin any toxic effects will tend to resolve more rapidly.

General references to digitalis toxicity.

1. Beller GA, *et al.* Digitalis intoxication: a prospective clinical study with serum level concentrations. *N Engl J Med* 1971; **284:** 989–97.
2. Bullock RE, Hall RJC. Digitalis toxicity and poisoning. *Adverse Drug React Acute Poisoning Rev* 1982; **1:** 201–22.
3. Aronson JK. Digitalis intoxication. *Clin Sci* 1983; **64:** 253–8.
4. George CF. Digitalis intoxication: a new approach to an old problem. *Br Med J* 1983; **286:** 1533–4.
5. Pentel PR, Salerno DM. Cardiac drug toxicity: digitalis glycosides and calcium-channel and β-blocking agents. *Med J Aust* 1990; **152:** 88–94.
6. Wells TG, *et al.* Age-related differences in digoxin toxicity and its treatment. *Drug Safety* 1992; **7:** 135–51.

7. Johnston GD. Adverse reaction profile: digoxin. *Prescribers' J* 1993; **33:** 29–35.
8. Kernan WN, *et al.* Incidence of hospitalization for digitalis toxicity among elderly Americans. *Am J Med* 1994; **96:** 426–31.
9. Li-Saw-Hee FL, Lip GYH. How safe it digoxin? *Adverse Drug React Bull* 1998; (Feb): 715–18.

Adverse effects reported in elderly patients with toxic plasma-digoxin concentrations have included chorea,[1] profuse watery diarrhoea,[2] and dysphagia with dysphonia.[3]

1. Mulder LJMM, *et al.* Generalised chorea due to digoxin toxicity. *Br Med J* 1988; **296:** 1262.
2. Andrews PA, Wilkinson PR. Diarrhoea as a side effect of digoxin. *Br Med J* 1990; **301:** 1398.
3. Cordeiro MF, Arnold KG. Digoxin toxicity presenting as dysphagia and dysphonia. *Br Med J* 1991; **302:** 1025.

Effects on the blood. An association between several cardiovascular drugs, including digitalis glycosides (digoxin and acetyldigoxin), and agranulocytosis was found in an international study[1] although the incidence was low.

1. Kelly JP, *et al.* Risks of agranulocytosis and aplastic anemia in relation to the use of cardiovascular drugs: the international agranulocytosis and aplastic anemia study. *Clin Pharmacol Ther* 1991; **49:** 330–41.

Hypersensitivity. Hypersensitivity reactions to cardiac glycosides are rare but skin reactions have been reported. An 86-year-old man developed a generalised, pruritic, erythematous rash following administration of digoxin intravenously.[1] The rash recurred following rechallenge with digoxin tablets.

1. Martin SJ, Shah D. Cutaneous hypersensitivity reaction to digoxin. *JAMA* 1994; **271:** 1905.

Treatment of Adverse Effects

In the early stages of *acute poisoning* the stomach should be emptied by emesis or lavage. Activated charcoal may be given to reduce the absorption and enterohepatic recycling of cardiac glycosides; cholestyramine and colestipol have also been tried. Attempts to remove cardiac glycosides by haemodialysis or peritoneal dialysis have generally been ineffective and the value of haemoperfusion is controversial. Forced diuresis with frusemide is generally ineffective and may be dangerous; serious electrolyte imbalance may result from the use of such potent diuretics.

Cardiac toxicity in acute or chronic poisoning should be treated under ECG control and serum electrolytes should be monitored. Antiarrhythmic treatment may be necessary and should be determined by the specific arrhythmia present (see p.782). Atropine is given intravenously to correct bradycardia and in patients with heart block. Pacing may be necessary if atropine is not effective. Potassium chloride may be given in hypokalaemic patients provided that renal function is normal and heart block is not present. Potassium has also been given to normokalaemic patients but caution is needed since hyperkalaemia can occur rapidly. Other electrolyte imbalance should be corrected.

In *massive overdosage* progressive hyperkalaemia occurs and is fatal unless reversed. Glucose infusions and injections of soluble insulin have been given and, if the hyperkalaemia is refractory, dialysis may be tried. Massive life-threatening overdosage has been treated successfully with digoxin-specific antibody fragments (p.979).

For the treatment of *chronic poisoning* temporary withdrawal of digoxin or other cardiac glycosides may be all that is necessary, with subsequent doses adjusted according to the needs of the patient. Serum electrolytes should be measured and the ECG monitored. Potassium supplements should be given to correct hypokalaemia.

Reviews on the management of digitalis poisoning.

1. Allen NM, Dunham GD. Treatment of digitalis intoxication with emphasis on the clinical use of digoxin immune Fab. *DICP Ann Pharmacother* 1990; **24:** 991–8.
2. Dick M, *et al.* Digitalis intoxication recognition and management. *J Clin Pharmacol* 1991; **31:** 444–7.

Precautions

Digoxin is generally contra-indicated in patients with hypertrophic obstructive cardiomyopathy unless there is severe cardiac failure, since the outflow obstruction may be worsened. It is also contra-indicated in patients with the Wolff-Parkinson-White syndrome or other evidence of an accessory pathway, especially if it is accompanied by atrial fibrillation, since ventricular tachycardia or fibrillation may be precipitated. Digoxin is not an appropriate form of therapy for any ventricular arrhythmia.

Digoxin toxicity is common and may result from raised plasma concentrations or an increase in sensitivity to digoxin. Almost any deterioration in the condition of the heart or circulation may increase the sensitivity to digoxin and it should be used with caution in all patients with cardiovascular disease. Early signs of digoxin toxicity should be watched for and the heart rate should generally be maintained above 60 beats per minute. Toxicity may result from administering loading doses too rapidly and from accumulation of maintenance doses as well as from acute poisoning.

Digoxin should be used with caution in partial heart block since complete heart block may be induced; it should also be used with care in sinus node disorders. Caution is also required in acute myocarditis (such as rheumatic carditis), in acute myocardial infarction, in advanced heart failure, and in severe pulmonary disease, due to the increased myocardial sensitivity. Digoxin may also enhance the occurrence of arrhythmias in patients undergoing cardioversion and should be withdrawn 1 to 2 days before such procedures if possible. If cardioversion is essential and digoxin has already been given, low energy shocks must be used.

Electrolyte imbalances may affect the sensitivity to digoxin, as may thyroid dysfunction. The effects of digoxin are enhanced by hypokalaemia, hypomagnesaemia, hypercalcaemia, hypoxia, and hypothyroidism and doses may need to be reduced until these conditions are corrected. Resistance to the effects of digoxin may occur in hyperthyroidism. Digoxin should be given with care to patients who may have already received cardiac glycosides and it has been suggested that the initial dose should be reduced if the patient has received them in the preceding 2 weeks.

Digoxin doses should generally be reduced and plasma-digoxin concentrations monitored in patients with impaired renal function, in the elderly, and in premature infants (see under Uses and Administration, below).

Gastro-intestinal disorders. Absorption from tablet formulations of digoxin may be decreased in patients with malabsorption syndromes or small bowel resections due to inadequate dissolution and it has been recommended that liquid dosage forms of digoxin should be used in patients with small bowel resections.[1] However, only 40 to 60% of a digoxin dose administered as elixir was absorbed in one patient with a small bowel resection[2] compared with about 80% in patients with normal gastro-intestinal function, suggesting a need for slightly increased oral maintenance doses of digoxin in patients with small bowel resections. In a further patient with a similar resection[3] a therapeutic plasma-digoxin concentration was not achieved with any oral formulation.

1. Kumer KP, *et al.* Perspectives on digoxin absorption from small bowel resections. *Drug Intell Clin Pharm* 1983; **17:** 121–3.
2. Vetticaden SJ, *et al.* Digoxin absorption in a patient with short-bowel syndrome. *Clin Pharm* 1986; **5:** 62–4.
3. Ehrenpreis ED, *et al.* Malabsorption of digoxin tablets, gel caps, and elixir in a patient with an end jejunostomy. *Ann Pharmacother* 1994; **28:** 1239–40.

Heart surgery. Patients undergoing cardiac surgery appear to have increased sensitivity to digoxin toxicity and thus an increased risk of arrhythmias.[1] Digoxin has been found[2] to be no better than placebo in preventing postoperative arrhythmias in patients following coronary artery bypass surgery and actually induced supraventricular arrhythmias in 2 patients. Arrhythmias compatible with digoxin intoxication have occurred postoperatively[1] although serum-digoxin concentrations ranged from 0 to 2.8 ng per mL and it may be that the surgical procedures or increased sensitivity to digoxin caused them.

1. Rose MR, *et al.* Arrhythmias following cardiac surgery: relation to serum digoxin levels. *Am Heart J* 1975; **89:** 288–94.
2. Weiner B, *et al.* Digoxin prophylaxis following coronary artery bypass surgery. *Clin Pharm* 1986; **5:** 55–8.

Interference with digoxin assays. The presence of endogenous digoxin-like substances in neonates, and in patients with liver or kidney dysfunction may be responsible for elevated values or false-positive results in some plasma-digoxin assays.[1] Some patients may have antibodies that react with the assay system and produce falsely elevated values.[2] Prednisolone[1] and spironolactone[1,3] might each interfere with plasma-digoxin assays; spironolactone may also produce actual changes in digoxin concentrations (see below).

1. Yosselson-Superstine S. Drug interferences with plasma assays in therapeutic drug monitoring. *Clin Pharmacokinet* 1984; **9:** 67–89.
2. Liendo C, *et al.* A new interference in some digoxin assays: anti-murine heterophilic antibodies. *Clin Pharmacol Ther* 1996; **60:** 593–8.
3. Foukaridis GN. Influence of spironolactone and its metabolite canrenone on serum digoxin assays. *Ther Drug Monit* 1990; **12:** 82–4.

Pregnancy. There is considerable evidence that digoxin crosses the placenta freely with serum-digoxin concentrations at term similar in the newborn and mother. No significant adverse effects attributed to digoxin have been noted in the fetus or neonate although adverse fetal effects, including fetal death, have been reported in mothers with digitalis toxicity. Some concern has been expressed that maternal digitalis therapy may occasionally cause low birth-weights in infants of mothers with heart disease, but the underlying disease might also be important.[1] The presence of endogenous digoxin-like immunoreactive substances in the serum of pregnant women and neonates could make the interpretation of digoxin assays difficult. In one study,[2] high concentrations of endogenous digoxin-like immunoreactivity in cord blood suggested that it might be synthesised during delivery, in which case the placental transfer of digoxin might be overestimated.

1. Rotmensch HH, *et al.* Management of cardiac arrhythmias during pregnancy: current concepts. *Drugs* 1987; **33:** 623–33.
2. Lupoglazoff JM, *et al.* Endogenous digoxin-like immunoreactivity during pregnancy and at birth. *Br J Clin Pharmacol* 1993; **35:** 251–4.

Interactions

There may be interactions between digoxin and drugs which alter its absorption, interfere with its excretion, or have additive effects on the myocardium. Drugs which cause electrolyte disturbances increase the risk of toxicity from cardiac glycosides. Thiazides and loop *diuretics* cause hypokalaemia and also hypomagnesaemia which may lead to cardiac arrhythmias. Other causes of hypokalaemia include treatment with *corticosteroids, beta$_2$ agonists* (such as salbutamol), *amphotericin, sodium polystyrene sulphonate, carbenoxolone*, and dialysis. Hypercalcaemia may also increase toxicity and intravenous administration of *calcium salts* is best avoided in patients taking cardiac glycosides. Serum-digoxin concentrations may be significantly increased by *quinidine*, *amiodarone*, and *propafenone* and reduction of digoxin dosage may be required. Other antiarrhythmic drugs may have additive effects on the myocardium increasing the likelihood of adverse effects; *beta blockers* may potentiate bradycardia due to digoxin. *Calcium-channel blockers* may increase digoxin concentrations.

Reviews of drug interactions occurring with digoxin.

1. Rodin SM, Johnson BF. Pharmacokinetic interactions with digoxin. *Clin Pharmacokinet* 1988; **15:** 227–44.
2. Magnani B, Malini PL. Cardiac glycosides: drug interactions of clinical significance. *Drug Safety* 1995; **12:** 97–109.

ACE inhibitors. Although increased serum-digoxin concentrations have been reported in patients with severe chronic heart failure given the ACE inhibitor *captopril*,[1] other studies have failed to confirm this effect.[2,3] Studies with various other ACE inhibitors have also failed to show any significant effect on serum-digoxin concentrations. However, ACE inhibitors may cause a deterioration in renal function and this could lead to an increase in serum-digoxin concentration due to impaired digoxin excretion.[4]

1. Cleland JGF, *et al.* Interaction of digoxin and captopril. *Br J Clin Pharmacol* 1984; **17:** 214P.
2. Magelli C, *et al.* Lack of effect of captopril on serum digoxin in congestive heart failure. *Eur J Clin Pharmacol* 1989; **36:** 99–100.
3. Rossi GP, *et al.* Effect of acute captopril administration on digoxin pharmacokinetics in normal subjects. *Curr Ther Res* 1989; **46:** 439–44.
4. Mignat C, Unger T. ACE inhibitors: drug interactions of clinical significance. *Drug Safety* 1995; **12:** 334–47.

Alpha blockers. *Prazosin*[1] has been reported to increase the mean plasma-digoxin concentration in patients receiving a maintenance dose of digoxin.

1. Çopur S, *et al.* Effects of oral prazosin on total plasma digoxin levels. *Fundam Clin Pharmacol* 1988; **2:** 13–17.

Antiarrhythmics. An interaction between digoxin and *amiodarone* resulting in increases in plasma concentrations of digoxin has been reported[1-5] on several occasions and plasma-digoxin concentration may be doubled.[5] An increase in serum-digoxin concentrations of 68 to 800% has been reported[2] during amiodarone therapy in children. The interaction does not appear to be due to a reduction in urinary excretion alone[3,4] and seems to be dose-related. It has been recommended[1,6] that the initial dose of digoxin should be halved when amiodarone is given concurrently.

1. Moysey JO, *et al.* Amiodarone increases plasma digoxin concentrations. *Br Med J* 1981; **282:** 272.
2. Koren G, *et al.* Digoxin toxicity associated with amiodarone therapy in children. *J Pediatr* 1984; **104:** 467–70.
3. Douste-Blazy P, *et al.* Influence of amiodarone on plasma and urine digoxin concentrations. *Lancet* 1984; **i:** 905.
4. Mingardi G. Amiodarone and plasma digoxin levels. *Lancet* 1984; **i:** 1238.
5. Johnston A, *et al.* The digoxin-amiodarone interaction. *Br J Clin Pharmacol* 1987; **24:** 253P.
6. Naccarelli GV, *et al.* Adverse effects of amiodarone: pathogenesis, incidence and management. *Med Toxicol Adverse Drug Exp* 1989; **4:** 246–53.

Disopyramide appears to have no clinically significant effect on the pharmacokinetics of digoxin in healthy subjects[1,2] but has been reported to modify the cardiovascular effects of digoxin.[1]

1. Elliott HL, *et al.* Pharmacodynamic and pharmacokinetic evaluation of the interaction between digoxin and disopyramide. *Br J Clin Pharmacol* 1982; **14:** 141P.
2. Risler T, *et al.* On the interaction between digoxin and disopyramide. *Clin Pharmacol Ther* 1983; **34:** 176–80.

Administration of *flecainide* 200 mg twice daily to 15 healthy subjects taking digoxin caused a mean increase of 24% in predose digoxin concentrations and of 13% in digoxin concentrations 6 hours after the digoxin dose.[1] It was considered that in most cases these increases in plasma-digoxin concentrations would not present a clinical problem, but that patients with higher plasma-digoxin concentrations or atrioventricular nodal dysfunction should be monitored.

1. Weeks CE, *et al.* The effect of flecainide acetate, a new antiarrhythmic, on plasma digoxin levels. *J Clin Pharmacol* 1986; **26:** 27–31.

Increased serum-digoxin concentrations have been reported when *propafenone* is given concurrently.[1-4] There is considerable interindividual variation in the extent of the interaction; increases in serum-digoxin concentrations of up to 254% have been reported. If digoxin and propafenone are given concurrently, the dose of digoxin should be reduced and serum-digoxin concentration should be monitored.

1. Nolan PE, *et al.* Effects of coadministration of propafenone on the pharmacokinetics of digoxin in healthy volunteer subjects. *J Clin Pharmacol* 1989; **29:** 46–52.
2. Calvo MV, *et al.* Interaction between digoxin and propafenone. *Ther Drug Monit* 1989; **11:** 10–15.
3. Zalzstein E, *et al.* Interaction between digoxin and propafenone in children. *J Pediatr* 1990; **116:** 310–12.
4. Bigot M-C, *et al.* Serum digoxin levels related to plasma propafenone levels during concomitant treatment. *J Clin Pharmacol* 1991; **31:** 521–6.

Quinidine causes an increase in serum-digoxin concentration in almost all patients given the two drugs concurrently.[1-3] The serum-digoxin concentration may increase by up to 500% but is usually approximately doubled.[1] Signs and symptoms of digoxin toxicity may occur although some workers[4] have suggested that these may be accounted for by an additive effect of the 2 drugs rather than by the effect on serum-digoxin concentration. The exact mechanism of interaction is not clear but a substantial decrease in the renal and nonrenal clearance of digoxin has been demonstrated.[5] The distribution volume of digoxin may also be reduced[2] reflecting impaired tissue binding, and there is increased systemic availability.[1] It is generally recommended that the dose of digoxin is halved in digitalised patients who are to be given quinidine.[2] Subsequently serum-digoxin concentrations should be monitored, especially during the first 1 to 2 weeks after which the new steady-state digoxin concentration should be achieved.[2]

1. Bigger JT, Leahey EB. Quinidine and digoxin: an important interaction. *Drugs* 1982; **24:** 229–39.
2. Pedersen KE. Digoxin interactions: the influence of quinidine and verapamil on the pharmacokinetics and receptor binding of digitalis glycosides. *Acta Med Scand* 1985; **697** (suppl): 1–40.
3. Mordel A, *et al.* Quinidine enhances digitalis toxicity at therapeutic serum digoxin levels. *Clin Pharmacol Ther* 1993; **53:** 457–62.
4. Walker AM, *et al.* Drug toxicity in patients receiving digoxin and quinidine. *Am Heart J* 1983; **105:** 1025–8.
5. Hedman A, *et al.* Interactions in the renal and biliary elimination of digoxin: stereoselective difference between quinine and quinidine. *Clin Pharmacol Ther* 1990; **47:** 20–6.

For a discussion on the interaction between digoxin and *verapamil*, see under Calcium-channel Blockers, below.

Antibacterials. Approximately 10% of patients receiving digoxin may metabolise 40% or more of the drug to cardioinactive metabolites.[1] Gut flora contribute greatly to this process, and the administration of antibacterials such as *erythromycin* or *tetracycline* to these patients appears to reduce this metabolic process resulting in higher serum concentrations.[2] Digoxin toxicity has been reported in digitalised patients given erythromycin,[3,4] clarithromycin,[5-7] and roxithromycin.[8] Oral *neomycin* may reduce serum-digoxin concentrations by reducing digoxin absorption.

Rifampicin may reduce serum-digitoxin concentrations by inducing its metabolism (see p.849). Digoxin is mainly excreted unchanged in the urine but rifampicin has been reported[9] to increase digoxin dose requirements substantially in 2 patients dependent on dialysis. When rifampicin was discontinued digoxin requirements fell by about 50%.

1. Doherty JE. A digoxin-antibiotic drug interaction. *N Engl J Med* 1981; **305:** 827–8.
2. Lindenbaum J, *et al.* Inactivation of digoxin by the gut flora: reversal by antibiotic therapy. *N Engl J Med* 1981; **305:** 789–94.
3. Maxwell DL, *et al.* Digoxin toxicity due to interaction of digoxin with erythromycin. *Br Med J* 1989; **298:** 572.
4. Morton MR, Cooper JW. Erythromycin-induced digoxin toxicity. *DICP Ann Pharmacother* 1989; **23:** 668–70.
5. Midoneck SR, Etingin OR. Clarithromycin-related toxic effects of digoxin. *N Engl J Med* 1995; **333:** 1505.
6. Nawarskas JJ, *et al.* Digoxin toxicity secondary to clarithromycin therapy. *Ann Pharmacother* 1997; **31:** 864–6.
7. Laberge P, Martineau P. Clarithromycin-induced digoxin intoxication. *Ann Pharmacother* 1997; **31:** 999–1002.
8. Corallo CE, Rogers IR. Roxithromycin-induced digoxin toxicity. *Med J Aust* 1996; **165:** 433–4.
9. Gault H, *et al.* Digoxin-rifampin interaction. *Clin Pharmacol Ther* 1984; **35:** 750–4.

Antidiabetics. Subtherapeutic plasma-digoxin concentrations were noted in a diabetic woman receiving *acarbose* and digoxin concurrently.[1] The plasma concentration of digoxin increased to a therapeutic level when acarbose was discontinued.

1. Serrano JS, *et al.* A possible interaction of potential clinical interest between digoxin and acarbose. *Clin Pharmacol Ther* 1996; **60:** 589–92.

Antiepileptics. *Phenytoin* caused a marked decrease in steady-state serum-digoxin concentrations when administered with digoxin and acetyldigoxin to 6 healthy subjects for 7 days.[1] Total digoxin clearance was increased by an average of 27% and elimination half-life was reduced by an average of 30%. This interaction may be more likely with digitoxin, since digitoxin is more dependent on the liver for elimination.

A brief report of an open study[2] in 12 subjects indicated a slight but significant decrease in digoxin bioavailability when *topiramate* was given concomitantly, although half-life and renal clearance of digoxin did not appear to be affected.

1. Rameis H. On the interaction between phenytoin and digoxin. *Eur J Clin Pharmacol* 1985; **29:** 49–53.
2. Liao S, Palmer M. Digoxin and topiramate drug interaction study in male volunteers. *Pharm Res* 1993; **10** (suppl): S405.

Antifungals. Two men given *itraconazole* while receiving digoxin developed signs and symptoms of digoxin toxicity and elevated serum-digoxin concentrations.[1,2]

Additive adverse effects due to hypokalaemia may occur when digoxin is given with *amphotericin*.

1. Rex J. Itraconazole–digoxin interaction. *Ann Intern Med* 1992; **116:** 525.
2. Alderman CP, Jersmann HPA. Digoxin–itraconazole interaction. *Med J Aust* 1993; **159:** 838–9.

Antimalarials. In 6 subjects given *quinine sulphate,* total body clearance of digoxin after an intravenous dose was decreased by 26%, primarily through a reduction in nonrenal clearance.[1] Increased urinary excretion of digoxin was consistent with alterations in the nonrenal clearance of digoxin and might be due to changes in the metabolism or biliary secretion of digoxin. Quinine increased the mean elimination half-life of digoxin from 34.2 to 51.8 hours but did not consistently change the volume of distribution.

An increase in the plasma-digoxin concentration, but without symptoms of toxicity, was noted in two women given *hydroxychloroquine* (for rheumatoid arthritis) in addition to long-term digoxin therapy.[2]

1. Wandell M, *et al.* Effect of quinine on digoxin kinetics. *Clin Pharmacol Ther* 1980; **28:** 425–30.
2. Leden I. Digoxin–hydroxychloroquine interaction? *Acta Med Scand* 1982; **211:** 411–12.

Antineoplastics and immunosuppressants. The absorption of digoxin from tablets was reduced by an average of 45.6% in patients undergoing antineoplastic therapy.[1] Also the steady-state concentration of digoxin after administration of β-acetyldigoxin has been reduced in patients undergoing antineoplastic therapy.[2] The interaction was considered to be due to reduced absorption of digitalis glycosides when the gastro-intestinal mucosa is damaged and might be minimised by administering digoxin in the form of liquid-filled capsules[1] or by giving digitoxin.[2]

Increased serum-digoxin concentrations with symptoms of toxicity have been reported in patients when *cyclosporin* was added to their digoxin therapy.[3,4]

1. Bjornsson TD, *et al.* Effects of high-dose cancer chemotherapy on the absorption of digoxin in two different formulations. *Clin Pharmacol Ther* 1986; **39:** 25–8.
2. Kuhlmann J. Inhibition of digoxin absorption but not of digitoxin during cytostatic drug therapy. *Arzneimittelforschung* 1982; **32:** 698–704.
3. Dorian P, *et al.* Digoxin-cyclosporine interaction: severe digitalis toxicity after cyclosporine treatment. *Clin Invest Med* 1988; **ii:** 108–12.
4. Robieux I, *et al.* The effects of cardiac transplantation and cyclosporine therapy on digoxin pharmacokinetics. *J Clin Pharmacol* 1992; **32:** 338–43.

Antithyroid drugs. Reduced peak serum-digoxin concentrations were noted in 9 of 10 healthy subjects following administration of a single oral dose of *carbimazole* although conversely in the tenth subject digoxin concentrations rose.[1] Caution is also needed since changes in thyroid function may affect sensitivity to digoxin independently of serum concentrations (see Precautions, above).

1. Rao BR, *et al.* Influence of carbimazole on serum levels and haemodynamic effects of digoxin. *Clin Drug Invest* 1997; **13:** 350–4.

Benzodiazepines. Raised serum-digoxin concentrations have been reported in patients also taking *diazepam*[1] or *alprazolam*.[2,3] The clearance of digoxin was reduced by these benzodiazepines.

1. Castillo-Ferrando JR, *et al.* Digoxin levels and diazepam. *Lancet* 1980; **ii:** 368.
2. Tollefson G, *et al.* Alprazolam-related digoxin toxicity. *Am J Psychiatry* 1984; **141:** 1612–14.
3. Guven H, *et al.* Age-related digoxin-alprazolam interaction. *Clin Pharmacol Ther* 1993; **54:** 42–4.

Calcium-channel blockers. Studies on interactions between digoxin and calcium-channel blockers appear to show that *verapamil* increases plasma-digoxin concentrations[1-3] by up to 70%. The effect of *nifedipine* is not as clear. Although it has been reported[1] to produce a 45% increase in plasma-digoxin concentrations, other studies[4,5] have reported little or no increase and the interaction is unlikely to be of clinical significance for most patients. Studies on the interaction between digoxin and *diltiazem* have also produced conflicting results. Increases in plasma-digoxin concentrations of 20% and up to 59% have been reported[6,7] and an increase in medigoxin concentrations[7] of up to 51%. However, other studies[8,9] have shown no diltiazem-induced change in digoxin pharmacokinetics or plasma concentration. *Bepridil,*[10] *gallopamil,*[1] *mibefradil,*[11] *nisoldipine,*[12] and *nitrendipine*[13] have all been reported to increase plasma-digoxin concentrations. Bepridil increased the concentration by 34% and it was recommended that patients given this combination be monitored carefully. *Felodipine*[14,15] and *isradipine*[3] have both been reported to increase peak serum-digoxin concentrations, but steady-state digoxin concentrations were not affected and the interactions were unlikely to be of clinical relevance.

The mechanism of interaction between calcium-channel blockers and digoxin is not completely understood but appears to be related to decreased renal and nonrenal clearance of digoxin. The pharmacodynamic effects of digoxin and calcium-channel blockers may also be additive.

1. Belz GG, *et al.* Interaction between digoxin and calcium antagonists and antiarrhythmic drugs. *Clin Pharmacol Ther* 1983; **33:** 410–17.
2. Pedersen KE, *et al.* Influence of verapamil on the inotropism and pharmacokinetics of digoxin. *Eur J Clin Pharmacol* 1983; **25:** 199–206.
3. Rodin SM, *et al.* Comparative effects of verapamil and isradipine on steady-state digoxin kinetics. *Clin Pharmacol Ther* 1988; **43:** 668–72.
4. Schwartz JB, Migliore PJ. Effect of nifedipine on serum digoxin concentration and renal digoxin clearance. *Clin Pharmacol Ther* 1984; **36:** 19–24.
5. Kleinbloesem CH, *et al.* Interactions between digoxin and nifedipine at steady state in patients with atrial fibrillation. *Ther Drug Monit* 1985; **7:** 372–6.
6. Rameis H, *et al.* The diltiazem-digoxin interaction. *Clin Pharmacol Ther* 1984; **36:** 183–9.
7. Oyama Y, *et al.* Digoxin-diltiazem interaction. *Am J Cardiol* 1984; **53:** 1480–1.
8. Beltrami TR, *et al.* Lack of effects of diltiazem on digoxin pharmacokinetics. *J Clin Pharmacol* 1985; **25:** 390–2.
9. Elkayam U, *et al.* Effect of diltiazem on renal clearance and serum concentration of digoxin in patients with cardiac disease. *Am J Cardiol* 1985; **55:** 1393–5.
10. Belz GG, *et al.* Digoxin and bepridil: pharmacokinetic and pharmacodynamic interactions. *Clin Pharmacol Ther* 1986; **39:** 65–71.
11. Siepmann M, *et al.* The interaction of the calcium antagonist RO 40-5967 with digoxin. *Br J Clin Pharmacol* 1995; **39:** 491–6.
12. Kirch W, *et al.* Influence of nisoldipine on haemodynamic effects and plasma levels of digoxin. *Br J Clin Pharmacol* 1986; **22:** 155–9.
13. Kirch W, *et al.* Nitrendipine increases digoxin plasma levels dose dependently. *J Clin Pharmacol* 1986; **26:** 553.
14. Rehnqvist N, *et al.* Pharmacokinetics of felodipine and effect on digoxin plasma levels in patients with heart failure. *Drugs* 1987; **34** (suppl 3): 33–42.
15. Dunselman PHJM, *et al.* Digoxin-felodipine interaction in patients with congestive heart failure. *Eur J Clin Pharmacol* 1988; **35:** 461–5.

Diuretics. *Amiloride* administration increased renal clearance of digoxin and reduced the extrarenal digoxin clearance in 6 healthy subjects after a single intravenous dose of digoxin.[1] Amiloride also inhibited the digoxin-induced positive inotropic effect, but the clinical implications in cardiac patients are unknown. A further study[2] failed to confirm this effect.

Spironolactone and its metabolites have been reported to interfere with serum-digoxin determinations by radio-immunoassay or fluorescence-polarisation immunoassay resulting in falsely elevated measurements.[3,4] The interference with digoxin assays is neither consistent nor predictable and serum-digoxin concentrations should be interpreted with caution when the 2 drugs are given concomitantly, especially since spironolactone has also been reported to decrease digoxin clearance by a median of 26% resulting in a true increase in the serum-digoxin concentration.[5]

Diuretic therapy with *triamterene* in association with a thiazide or loop diuretic increased the mean serum-digoxin concentration; this interaction was considered unlikely to be of clinical importance, except perhaps in patients with renal impairment.[6]

1. Waldorff S, *et al.* Amiloride-induced changes in digoxin dynamics and kinetics: abolition of digoxin-induced inotropism with amiloride. *Clin Pharmacol Ther* 1981; **30:** 172–6.
2. Richter JP, *et al.* The acute effects of amiloride and potassium canrenoate on digoxin-induced positive inotropium in healthy volunteers. *Eur J Clin Pharmacol* 1993; **45:** 195–6.
3. Paladino JA, *et al.* Influence of spironolactone on serum digoxin concentration. *JAMA* 1984; **251:** 470–1.
4. Foukaridis GN. Influence of spironolactone and its metabolite canrenone on serum digoxin assays. *Ther Drug Monit* 1990; **12:** 82–4.
5. Waldorff S, *et al.* Spironolactone-induced changes in digoxin kinetics. *Clin Pharmacol Ther* 1978; **24:** 162–7.
6. Impivaara O, Iisalo E. Serum digoxin concentrations in a representative digoxin-consuming adult population. *Eur J Clin Pharmacol* 1985; **27:** 627–32.

Gastro-intestinal drugs. A number of gastro-intestinal drugs can affect the absorption of digoxin by binding to the digoxin or by changing gastro-intestinal motility. The problem has often been related to the bioavailability of the digoxin formulation and appears to be less important with currently used preparations. Some *antacids*,[1,2] particularly liquid formulations, and *adsorbents*[1] such as kaolin-pectin, can reduce the absorption of digoxin from the gastro-intestinal tract and administration should probably be separated by at least 2 hours. *Activated charcoal*, and *ion-exchange resins* such as cholestyramine and colestipol, also reduce digoxin absorption. *Sucralfate*[3] may also reduce the absorption of digoxin. *Omeprazole* and possibly other gastric acid inhibitors may reduce the gastro-intestinal metabolism and enhance the absorption of unchanged digoxin,[4] although the clinical relevance of this is uncertain.[5]

Drugs such as *metoclopramide* which increase gastro-intestinal motility can reduce the absorption of digoxin, especially if digoxin is given as a slowly dissolving formulation. Reduced absorption of digoxin has occurred when digoxin and metoclopramide have been given concurrently.[6] Conversely, *anticholinergics* reduce motility, and propantheline has increased digoxin absorption.

Sulphasalazine has been found to impair the absorption of digoxin and to reduce the serum-digoxin concentration,[7] but the mechanism is unclear.

1. Rodin SM, Johnson BF. Pharmacokinetic interactions with digoxin. *Clin Pharmacokinet* 1988; **15:** 227–44.
2. Gugler R, Allgayer H. Effects of antacids on the clinical pharmacokinetics of drugs: an update. *Clin Pharmacokinet* 1990; **18:** 210–19.
3. Rey AM, Gums JG. Altered absorption of digoxin, sustained-release quinidine, and warfarin with sucralfate administration. *DICP Ann Pharmacother* 1991; **25:** 745–6.
4. Cohen AF, *et al.* Influence of gastric acidity on the bioavailability of digoxin. *Ann Intern Med* 1991; **115:** 540–5.
5. Oosterhuis B, *et al.* Minor effect of multiple dose omeprazole on the pharmacokinetics of digoxin after a single oral dose. *Br J Clin Pharmacol* 1991; **32:** 569–72.
6. Johnson BF, *et al.* Effect of metoclopramide on digoxin absorption from tablets and capsules. *Clin Pharmacol Ther* 1984; **36:** 724–30.
7. Juhl RP, *et al.* Effect of sulfasalazine on digoxin bioavailability. *Clin Pharmacol Ther* 1976; **20:** 387–94.

Ginseng. Raised serum-digoxin concentrations (but without signs of digoxin toxicity) have been noted in an elderly male patient following the use of Siberian ginseng (*Eleutherococcus senticosus*).[1] However, concentrations remained high even when digoxin was discontinued and returned to within the therapeutic range only after the ginseng was stopped. Siberian ginseng contains eleutherosides, which are chemically related to cardiac glycosides such as digoxin, and the assay may have measured these compounds, or their derivatives, as well as digoxin.

1. McRae S. Elevated serum digoxin levels in a patient taking digoxin and Siberian ginseng. *Can Med Assoc J* 1996; **155:** 293–5.

NSAIDs. An increase in serum-digoxin concentration has been reported with *aspirin, ibuprofen, indomethacin, fenbufen*, and *diclofenac*.[1] Potentially toxic serum-digoxin concentrations occurred in preterm infants[2] with patent ductus arteriosus on digoxin therapy when given indomethacin by mouth in a mean total dose of 0.32 mg per kg body-weight and it was recommended that the dose of digoxin should be halved initially if indomethacin is also given. Lack of increase in serum-digoxin concentrations has also been reported with concomitant aspirin or indomethacin, as well as with *ketoprofen*, and *tiaprofenic acid*[1] but some of these studies were in healthy subjects and it is advised that digoxin therapy be monitored carefully whenever any NSAID is initiated or discontinued in digitalised patients.

1. Verbeeck RK. Pharmacokinetic drug interactions with nonsteroidal anti-inflammatory drugs. *Clin Pharmacokinet* 1990; **19:** 44–66.
2. Koren G, *et al.* Effects of indomethacin on digoxin pharmacokinetics in preterm infants. *Pediatr Pharmacol* 1984; **4:** 25–30.

Skeletal muscle relaxants. *Pancuronium* or *suxamethonium* may interact with digitalis glycosides resulting in an increased incidence of arrhythmias; the interaction is more likely with pancuronium.[1]

1. Bartolone RS, Rao TLK. Dysrhythmias following muscle relaxant administration in patients receiving digitalis. *Anesthesiology* 1983; **58:** 567–9.

Sympathomimetics. A single intravenous[1,2] or oral[3] dose of *salbutamol* has been reported to decrease steady-state serum-digoxin concentrations by up to 16% and 22% respectively in healthy subjects. Although salbutamol had no significant effect on the concentration of digoxin in skeletal muscle, it was considered that increased binding to skeletal muscle could explain the interaction. Beta$_2$ agonists such as salbutamol can also cause hypokalaemia which may increase susceptibility to digoxin-induced arrhythmias.

1. Edner M, Jogestrand T. Effect of salbutamol on digoxin concentration in serum and skeletal muscle. *Eur J Clin Pharmacol* 1989; **36:** 235–8.
2. Edner M, *et al.* Effect of salbutamol on digoxin pharmacokinetics. *Eur J Clin Pharmacol* 1992; **42:** 197–201.
3. Edner M, Jogestrand T. Oral salbutamol decreases serum digoxin concentration. *Eur J Clin Pharmacol* 1990; **38:** 195–7.

Pharmacokinetics

The absorption of digoxin from the gastro-intestinal tract is variable depending upon the formulation used. About 70% of the administered dose is absorbed from tablets which comply with BP or USP specifications, 80% is absorbed from an elixir, and over 90% is absorbed from liquid-filled soft gelatin capsules. The generally accepted therapeutic plasma concentration range is from 0.5 to 2.0 ng per mL but there is considerable interindividual variation. Digoxin has a large volume of distribution and is widely distributed in tissues, including the heart, brain, erythrocytes, and skeletal muscle. The concentration of digoxin in the myocardium is considerably higher than in plasma. From 20 to 30% is bound to plasma protein. Digoxin has been detected in cerebrospinal fluid and breast milk; it also crosses the placenta. It has an elimination half-life of 1.5 to 2 days.

Digoxin is mainly excreted unchanged in the urine by glomerular filtration and tubular secretion; reabsorption also occurs. Extensive metabolism has been reported in a minority of patients (see under Metabolism and Excretion, below). Excretion of digoxin is proportional to the glomerular filtration rate. After intravenous injection 50 to 70% of the dose is excreted unchanged. Digoxin is not removed from the body by dialysis, and only small amounts are removed by exchange transfusion and during cardiopulmonary bypass.

Reviews of the clinical pharmacokinetics of digoxin.

1. Iisalo E. Clinical pharmacokinetics of digoxin. *Clin Pharmacokinet* 1977; **2:** 1–16.
2. Aronson JK. Clinical pharmacokinetics of digoxin 1980. *Clin Pharmacokinet* 1980; **5:** 137–49.
3. Mooradian AD. Digitalis: an update of clinical pharmacokinetics, therapeutic monitoring techniques and treatment recommendations. *Clin Pharmacokinet* 1988; **15:** 165–79.

Absorption. Studies in 6 healthy subjects demonstrated that ingestion of food decreased the rate but not the extent of absorption of concurrently administered digoxin.[1]

1. Johnson BF, *et al.* Effect of a standard breakfast on digoxin absorption in normal subjects. *Clin Pharmacol Ther* 1978; **23:** 315–19.

Bioavailability. Large variations in the content, disintegration, and dissolution of solid dosage forms of digoxin preparations have led to large variations in plasma concentrations from different proprietary preparations. Other factors involved in varying bioavailability include the pharmaceutical formulation and presentation (capsules, solution, or tablets), particle size, and biological factors. Serious problems occurred in the UK[1] in 1972 and in Israel[2] in 1975 following changes in the manufacturing procedure for Lanoxin leading to a twofold increase in bioavailability.

1. Anonymous. Therapeutic non-equivalence. *Br Med J* 1972; **3:** 599–600.
2. Danon A, *et al.* An outbreak of digoxin intoxication. *Clin Pharmacol Ther* 1977; **21:** 643–6.

Distribution and protein binding. Digoxin has been reported to be 5 to 60% bound to plasma proteins,[1] depending partly on the method of measurement, but the figure is usually around 20%. Protein binding is reduced in patients undergoing haemodialysis; mean reductions of about 8 and 10% have been reported.[1,2] Injection of heparin has produced a similar reduction.[2]

Digoxin is widely distributed to tissues and serum-digoxin concentrations have been reported to be increased during immobilisation[3] and decreased during exercise[4,5] due to changes in binding to tissues such as skeletal muscle.

1. Storstein L. Studies on digitalis V: the influence of impaired renal function, hemodialysis, and drug interaction on serum protein binding of digitoxin and digoxin. *Clin Pharmacol Ther* 1976; **20:** 6–14.
2. Storstein L, Janssen H. Studies on digitalis VI: the effect of heparin on serum protein binding of digitoxin and digoxin. *Clin Pharmacol Ther* 1976; **20:** 15–23.
3. Pedersen KE, *et al.* Effects of physical activity and immobilization on plasma digoxin concentration and renal digoxin clearance. *Clin Pharmacol Ther* 1983; **34:** 303–8.
4. Joreteg T, Jogestrand T. Physical exercise and digoxin binding to skeletal muscle: relation to exercise intensity. *Eur J Clin Pharmacol* 1983; **25:** 585–8.
5. Joreteg T, Jogestrand T. Physical exercise and binding of digoxin to skeletal muscle—effect of muscle activation frequency. *Eur J Clin Pharmacol* 1984; **27:** 567–70.

Infants and neonates. Digoxin has been widely used in the treatment of cardiac disorders in neonates and infants and its pharmacokinetics in this age group have been reviewed.[1,2] In full-term neonates or infants, 80 to 90% of a dose of digoxin administered by mouth in liquid form is absorbed, with peak plasma concentrations occurring within 30 to 120 minutes. The rate of absorption may be slower in preterm and low birth-weight infants, with peak concentrations achieved at 90 to 180 minutes, and may be significantly reduced in severe heart failure and in malabsorption syndromes. After the intravenous administration of digoxin there is a rapid distribution phase with an apparent half-life of 20 to 40 minutes followed by a slower exponential decay of plasma concentrations. In full-term neonates, digoxin has an apparent volume of distribution of 6 to 10 litres per kg body-weight. Low birth-weight infants have a volume of distribution of 4.3 to 5.7 litres per kg while in older infants the volume may range from 10 to 22 litres per kg which is 1.5 to 2 times reported adult values. This large volume of distribution in full-term neonates and infants is thought to be due to increased tissue binding, a larger extracellular fluid volume, and slightly lower plasma protein binding.

The apparent plasma half-life in healthy and sick neonates is generally very long and may range from 20 to 70 hours in full-term neonates or from 40 to 180 hours in preterm neonates. Digoxin is eliminated at a considerably faster rate in infants than in neonates and, in parallel with maturation of kidney function, a marked increase in clearance rate is usually observed between the second and third month of life. The large apparent volume of distribution, higher clearance values, and greater concentrations of digoxin in the myocardial tissue and red cells of infants might justify the traditional assumption that infants tolerate digoxin better than adults and that higher doses are consequently needed in infants. However, studies have shown that in infants, as in adults, toxic signs become evident at plasma-digoxin concentrations above 3 ng per mL and that the therapeutic range may be 1.5 to 2 ng per mL.

1. Morselli PL, *et al.* Clinical pharmacokinetics in newborns and infants: age-related differences and therapeutic implications. *Clin Pharmacokinet* 1980; **5:** 485–527.
2. Besunder JB, *et al.* Principles of drug biodisposition in the neonate: a critical evaluation of the pharmacokinetic-pharmacodynamic interface. *Clin Pharmacokinet* 1988; **14:** 189-216 (part I) and 261–86 (part II).

Metabolism and excretion. Although digoxin is reported to be excreted mainly unchanged in the urine there is evidence to suggest that metabolism may sometimes be extensive. Metabolites that have been detected in the urine include digoxigenin, dihydrodigoxigenin, the mono- and bisdigitoxosides of digoxigenin, and dihydrodigoxin. Digoxigenin mono- and bisdigitoxosides are known to be cardioactive whereas dihydrodigoxin is probably much less active than digoxin.[1]

In about 10% of patients there is considerable reduction to cardio-inactive metabolites, chiefly dihydrodigoxin, and 40% or more of a dose may be excreted in the urine as dihydrodigoxin.[2-4] Bacterial flora in the gastro-intestinal tract appear to be responsible for this metabolism and antibacterial agents can arrest the process. Oral digoxin formulations with a high bioavailability are mostly absorbed in the stomach and upper small intestine and little digoxin is available in the lower intestine for bacterial degradation to dihydrodigoxin.[4]

1. Iisalo E. Clinical pharmacokinetics of digoxin. *Clin Pharmacokinet* 1977; **2:** 1–16.
2. Doherty JE. A digoxin-antibiotic drug interaction. *N Engl J Med* 1981; **305:** 827–8.
3. Rund DG, *et al.* Decreased digoxin cardioinactive-reduced metabolites after administration of an encapsulated liquid concentrate. *Clin Pharmacol Ther* 1983; **34:** 738–43.
4. Lofts F, *et al.* Digoxin metabolism to reduced products: clinical significance. *Br J Clin Pharmacol* 1986; **21:** 600P.

Old age. For references to alterations in the pharmacokinetics of digoxin in the elderly, see under Uses and Administration, below.

Renal impairment. For references to alterations in the pharmacokinetics of digoxin in patients with renal impairment, see under Uses and Administration, below.

Uses and Administration

Digoxin is a cardiac glycoside used in the management of supraventricular arrhythmias, particularly atrial fibrillation (p.782), and in heart failure (p.785).

The principal actions of digoxin are an increase in the force of myocardial contraction (positive inotropic activity) and a reduction in the conductivity of the heart, particularly in conduction through the atrioventricular (AV) node. Digoxin also has a direct action on vascular smooth muscle and indirect effects mediated primarily by the autonomic nervous system, and particularly by an increase in vagal activity. There are also reflex alterations in autonomic activity due to the effects on the circulation. Overall, these actions result in positive inotropic effects, negative chronotropic effects, and decreased AV nodal activity.

Cardiac arrhythmias. In atrial arrhythmias direct and indirect actions cause a decrease in the conduction velocity through the AV node and an increase in the effective refractory period thus reducing ventricular rate. In addition there is a decrease in the refractory period of the cardiac muscle and depression of the sinus node partly in response to the increase in vagal activity.

Digoxin is thus given to slow the increased ventricular rate that occurs in response to atrial fibrillation, although other drugs may be preferred; treatment is usually long term. In atrial flutter, the ventricular rate is normally more difficult to control with digoxin. Direct current cardioversion is the preferred method of treatment, but treatment with digoxin may restore sinus rhythm, or it may convert the flutter to fibrillation and sinus rhythm may then be induced by subsequent withdrawal of digoxin. In patients with the Wolff-Parkinson-White syndrome together with atrial fibrillation, digoxin can cause rapid ventricular rates, and possibly ventricular fibrillation, and should be avoided. It may be given to relieve an attack of paroxysmal supraventricular tachycardia and has also been given to prevent further attacks.

Heart failure. Digoxin and other cardiac glycosides directly inhibit the activity of the enzyme sodium-potassium adenosine triphosphatase (Na/K-ATPase) which is required for the active transport of sodium from myocardial cells. The result is a gradual increase in the intracellular sodium concentration and a decrease in the intracellular potassium concentration. The increased concentration of sodium inside the cells leads to an increase in the intracellular calcium concentration with enhancement of mechanical contractile activity and an increased inotropic effect.

When used in heart failure the increased force of myocardial contraction results in increased cardiac output, decreased end-systolic volume, decreased heart size, and decreased end-diastolic pressure and volume. Increased blood flow through the kidneys results in diuresis with a reduction in oedema and blood volume. The decrease in pulmonary venous pressure relieves dyspnoea and orthopnoea. Digoxin may thus provide symptomatic improvement in patients with heart failure and is mainly used for adjunctive therapy.

Dosage. When given by mouth, digoxin may take effect within about 2 hours and the maximum effect may be reached in about 6 hours. Initially a loading dose may be given to digitalise the patient, although this may not be necessary in, for example, mild heart failure.

Dosage should be carefully adjusted to the needs of the individual patient. Factors which may be considered include the patient's age, lean body-mass, renal status, thyroid status, electrolyte balance, degree of tissue oxygenation, and the nature of the underlying cardiac or pulmonary disease. Bearing in mind the above factors, steady-state plasma-digoxin concentrations (in a specimen taken at least 6 hours after a dose) of 0.5 to 2 ng per mL are generally considered acceptable. For reference to therapeutic drug monitoring, see below.

If rapid digitalisation is required then a loading dose is given to allow for the large volume of distribution. A total loading dose of 750 to 1500 μg of digoxin may be given by mouth during the initial 24-hour period; a dose towards the upper end of this range should be given in divided doses. If there is less urgency digitalisation may be achieved more slowly with doses of 250 μg once or twice daily. Steady-state plasma concentrations are achieved in about 7 days in patients with normal renal function. The usual maintenance dose of digoxin is 125 to 250 μg by mouth daily, but may range from 62.5 to 500 μg daily. In elderly patients therapy should generally be initiated gradually and with smaller doses (but see under Administration in the Elderly, below).

In urgent cases, provided that the patient has not been treated with cardiac glycosides during the previous 2 weeks, digoxin may be given intravenously initially. The intravenous dose ranges from 0.5 to 1 mg and produces a definite effect on the heart rate in about 10 minutes, reaching a maximum within about 2 hours. It is administered by intravenous infusion, either as a single dose given over 2 or more hours, or in divided doses each over 10 to 20 minutes. Maintenance treatment is then usually given by mouth. Digoxin has also been given intramuscularly but this route is not generally recommended since such injections may be painful and tissue damage has been reported. Digoxin should not be given subcutaneously as it may give rise to intense local irritation.

Children's doses are complex. They are based on body-weight and the developmental stage of the child as well as on response. Premature infants are especially sensitive to digoxin but, along with all other neonates, infants, and children up to about 10 years of age, still require doses that are higher per kg body-weight than those used for adults. Preterm infants receive lower doses than full-term infants, while children aged 2 to 10 years require lower doses than children up to 2 years of age. As an indication of the doses employed, oral loading doses recommended by manufacturers in the UK range from 25 to 45 μg per kg body-weight over 24 hours and in the USA the range is 20 to 60 μg per kg; the range for intravenous loading doses given over 24 hours is 20 to 35 μg per kg in the UK and 15 to 50 μg per kg in the USA.

Doses should be reduced in patients with renal impairment.

General reviews on the actions and uses of digoxin and the other cardiac glycosides.

1. Opie LH. Digitalis and sympathomimetic stimulants. *Lancet* 1980; **i:** 912–18.
2. Taggart AJ, McDevitt DG. Digitalis: its place in modern therapy. *Drugs* 1980; **20:** 398–404.
3. Chamberlain DA. Digitalis: where are we now? *Br Heart J* 1985; **54:** 227–33.
4. Doherty JE. Clinical use of digitalis glycosides: an update. *Cardiology* 1985; **72:** 225–54.
5. Smith TW. Digitalis: mechanisms of action and clinical use. *N Engl J Med* 1988; **318:** 358–65.
6. Riaz K, Forker AD. Digoxin use in congestive heart failure: current status. *Drugs* 1998; **55:** 747–58.

Administration in the elderly. The volume of distribution of digoxin and the elimination half-life increase with age.[1] Therefore there are problems in giving digoxin to elderly patients since steady-state plasma concentrations may not be reached for up to 2 weeks. Fears of toxicity have led some practitioners to use a fixed 'geriatric' dose of 62.5 μg daily. However, such a dose can produce subtherapeutic concentrations.[2] The routine use of very low doses of digoxin in the elderly is inappropriate and dosage should be individualised.

1. McMurray J, McDevitt DG. Treatment of heart failure in the elderly. *Br Med Bull* 1990; **46:** 202–29.
2. Nolan L, *et al.* The need for reassessment of digoxin prescribing for the elderly. *Br J Clin Pharmacol* 1989; **27:** 367–70.

Administration in renal impairment. A review of the pharmacokinetics of cardiac glycosides in patients with renal impairment.[1] The rate but not the extent of digoxin absorption is reduced in renal impairment but this is unlikely to be clinically important. Plasma-protein binding may also be reduced but since digoxin is poorly bound to these proteins and has a large apparent volume of distribution this also is unlikely to be important. The apparent volume of distribution is reduced by one-third to one-half and the loading dose of digoxin should therefore be reduced; an oral loading dose of 10 μg per kg body-weight is suggested. Non-renal clearance of digoxin is unaffected or only slightly reduced but renal clearance is reduced, the extent being closely related to creatinine clearance. The elimination half-life of digoxin is prolonged and it therefore takes longer to reach steady state and longer for toxicity to resolve. Because of the reduction in renal clearance of digoxin, maintenance doses must be reduced in line with renal function. Serum-digoxin concentration should be monitored although the presence of digoxin-like immunoreactive substances may make interpretation difficult. In addition, the presence of hyperkalaemia in patients with renal impairment may reduce sensitivity to the effects of digoxin.[2]

Since digoxin has such a large distribution volume, procedures such as peritoneal dialysis and haemodialysis remove only very small amounts of drug from the body and no dosage supplement is needed.

1. Aronson JK. Clinical pharmacokinetics of cardiac glycosides in patients with renal dysfunction. *Clin Pharmacokinet* 1983; **8:** 155–78.
2. Matzke GR, Frye RF. Drug administration in patients with renal insufficiency: minimising renal and extrarenal toxicity. *Drug Safety* 1997; **16:** 205–31.

Therapeutic drug monitoring. Digoxin has a narrow therapeutic index. It is generally considered that plasma-digoxin concentrations required for a therapeutic effect are usually between 0.5 and 2.0 ng per mL.[1-3] The factor for converting ng per mL to nmol per litre is 1.28.[1]

Digoxin dosage can be calculated in uncomplicated cases by considering the patient's weight, renal function, and clinical status. Therapeutic drug monitoring is *not* considered to be necessary in patients with a satisfactory clinical response to conventional doses in the absence of signs or symptoms of toxicity.[1,2] Measurement of plasma-digoxin concentrations is useful if poor compliance is suspected, if response is poor or there is a deterioration in response without apparent reason, if renal function is fluctuating, when it is unknown if a cardiac glycoside has been previously taken, during drug interactions, and to confirm clinical toxicity.[1,3,4] A plasma concentration should never be considered in isolation and should be used with other patient data as an important component in clinical decision making. This is particularly important in the diagnosis of digoxin toxicity since signs and symptoms of toxicity may be difficult to distinguish from the underlying disease and can occur within the usual therapeutic range.

A number of factors may influence the response to digoxin and thus the interpretation of digoxin assays. These include renal impairment, extremes of age, thyroid disease, patient compliance, drug interactions, and electrolyte disturbances.[1-4] Variations in the bioavailability of different digoxin preparations have also caused problems. Renal impairment and hypokalaemia are two of the most important factors affecting dosage of digoxin and whenever plasma-digoxin concentrations are assayed renal function and plasma potassium should also be measured. The interpretation of digoxin assays is further confounded by the presence of digoxin-like immunoreactive substances in patients with renal or hepatic impairment, in pregnant women, and in neonates. Blood samples for digoxin assay should be taken at least 6 hours after a dose to allow for distribution.[1,3,4]

The usefulness of plasma-digoxin concentrations in the diagnosis of toxicity in children is unclear. For children older than 12 months the adult guidelines can probably be followed and for younger children the trend for increased risk of toxicity at increased plasma-digoxin concentrations appears to hold but the threshold for toxicity may be higher especially in children less than 3 months old.[1] It has been suggested that determination of electrolyte concentrations in erythrocytes (a measure of sodium-potassium ATPase inhibition) may be a more accurate means of diagnosing digoxin toxicity in adults[5] and children.[6]

1. Aronson JK. Indications for the measurement of plasma digoxin concentrations. *Drugs* 1983; **26:** 230–42.
2. Lee TH, Smith TW. Serum digoxin concentration and diagnosis of digitalis toxicity: current concepts. *Clin Pharmacokinet* 1983; **8:** 279–85.
3. Aronson JK, Hardman M. Digoxin. *Br Med J* 1992; **305:** 1149–52.
4. Brodie MJ, Feely J. Practical clinical pharmacology: therapeutic drug monitoring and clinical trials. *Br Med J* 1988; **296:** 1110–14.
5. van Boxtel CJ, *et al.* Red blood cell electrolytes for monitoring digoxin therapy in adults. *Ther Drug Monit* 1985; **7:** 191–6.
6. Loes MW, *et al.* Relation between plasma and red-cell electrolyte concentrations and digoxin levels in children. *N Engl J Med* 1978; **299:** 501–4.

Preparations

BP 1998: Digoxin Injection; Digoxin Tablets; Paediatric Digoxin Injection; Paediatric Digoxin Oral Solution;
USP 23: Digoxin Elixir; Digoxin Injection; Digoxin Tablets.

Proprietary Preparations (details are given in Part 3)
Aust.: Lanicor; Novodigal; ***Austral.:*** Lanoxin; ***Belg.:*** Lanoxin; ***Canad.:*** Lanoxin; ***Ger.:*** Digacin; Dilanacin; Lanacard†; Lanicor; Lenoxin; Novodigal; ***Irl.:*** Lanoxin; ***Ital.:*** Cardioreg†; Digomal; Eudigox; Lanicor†; Lanoxin; ***Neth.:*** Lanoxin; ***Norw.:*** Lanoxin; ***S.Afr.:*** Lanoxin; Purgoxin; ***Spain:*** Lanacordin; ***Swed.:*** Lanacrist; Lanoxin; ***Switz.:*** Lanoxin; ***UK:*** Lanoxin; ***USA:*** Lanoxicaps; Lanoxin.

Multi-ingredient: ***Aust.:*** Card-Lamuran†; Gradulon; Theo-Lanicor; ***Ger.:*** Card-Dusodril†; Card-Fludilat†; Card-Instenon†; Card-Lamuran†; Coroverlan-Digoxin†; Crataelanat; Digi-Nitronal†; Digi-Pulsnorma†; Digi-Tromcardin†; Gradulon s. T.†; Intensain-Lanicor†; Stutgeron-Digoxin†; Theo-Lanicor†.

Dihydralazine Sulphate (864-c)

Dihydralazine Sulphate *(BANM, rINNM).*

Dihydralazini Sulfas Hydricus; Dihydralazinum Sulfuricum; Dihydrallazine Sulphate. Phthalazine-1,4-diyldihydrazine sulphate.

$C_8H_{10}N_6,H_2SO_4,2\frac{1}{2}H_2O = 333.3.$

CAS — 484-23-1 (dihydralazine); 7327-87-9 (dihydralazine sulphate).

Pharmacopoeias. In *Eur.* (see p.viii) and *Pol.*
Swiss includes Dihydralazine Mesylate.

White or slightly yellow crystalline powder. Slightly **soluble** in water; practically insoluble in alcohol; dissolves in dilute mineral acids.

Dihydralazine is a vasodilator with actions and uses similar to those of hydralazine (p.883). It is given by mouth as the sulphate, but doses are usually expressed in terms of the base. In hypertension (p.788) the usual initial dose is 12.5 mg by mouth twice daily. Up to 200 mg daily has been given; in some countries higher doses have been recommended in the management of heart failure (p.785).

Other salts of dihydralazine used in oral preparations include the hydrochloride and the tartrate. The mesylate is given by injection.

Preparations

Proprietary Preparations (details are given in Part 3)
Aust.: Nepresol; ***Belg.:*** Nepresol; ***Fr.:*** Nepressol; ***Ger.:*** Depressan; Dihyzin; Nepresol; ***Ital.:*** Nepresol†; ***Neth.:*** Nepresol; ***Norw.:*** Nepresol; ***S.Afr.:*** Nepresol; ***Swed.:*** Nepresol; ***Switz.:*** Nepresol.

Multi-ingredient: ***Aust.:*** Adelphan-Esidrex; Adelphan-Esidrex-K†; Elfanex; ***Fr.:*** Trasipressol; ***Ger.:*** Adelphan-Esidrix; Adelphan†; Elfanex†; Obsilazin N; pertenso†; Tri-Torrat; Triniton; ***Ital.:*** Adelfan-Esidrex†; Adelfan†; Axiten Tre†; Ipogen; Vallizina†; ***S.Afr.:*** Adelphane-Esidrex†; ***Spain:*** Adelfan-Esidrex; Adelfan†; Bietapres Complex†; ***Switz.:*** Adelphan-Esidrex; Adelphan-Esidrex-K†; Adelphan†.

Di-isopropylammonium Dichloroacetate

(9223-s)

Di-isopropylamine Dichloroacetate; Di-isopropylamine Dichloroethanoate; DIPA-DCA.

$C_8H_{17}Cl_2NO_2 = 230.1.$

CAS — 660-27-5.

Di-isopropylammonium dichloroacetate is a vasodilator which has been given in peripheral and cerebral vascular disorders. Preparations containing it have sometimes been described as 'pangamic acid' (p.1614).

Preparations

Proprietary Preparations (details are given in Part 3)
Ger.: B 15 APS†; Disotat; Oxypangam; ***Ital.:*** Kalodil†.

Multi-ingredient: ***Austral.:*** Pamica†; ***Ger.:*** Jasivita†; Sklerocedin N†; ***Ital.:*** Binevrilplus†; Liedasi†; ***Spain:*** Menalgil B6; Vitaber A E.

Dilazep Hydrochloride (9224-w)

Dilazep Hydrochloride *(rINNM).*

Asta C-4898. Perhydro-1,4-diazepin-1,4-diylbis(trimethylene 3,4,5-trimethoxybenzoate) dihydrochloride.

$C_{31}H_{44}N_2O_{10},2HCl = 677.6.$

CAS — 35898-87-4 (dilazep); 20153-98-4 (dilazep hydrochloride).

Pharmacopoeias. In *Jpn.*

Dilazep hydrochloride is a vasodilator used in ischaemic heart disease in doses of 150 to 300 mg daily by mouth.

Ischaemic heart disease is discussed under Atherosclerosis (p.782) and the treatment of its clinical manifestations is described under Angina Pectoris (p.780) and Myocardial Infarction (p.791).

Preparations

Proprietary Preparations (details are given in Part 3)
Ger.: Cormelian†; ***Ital.:*** Cormelian; ***Spain:*** Coratoline†.

Multi-ingredient: ***Ger.:*** Cormelian-Digotab†.

Dilevalol (18629-c)

Dilevalol *(BAN, pINN).*

R,R-Labetalol; Sch-19927 (dilevalol hydrochloride). 5-{(*R*)-1-Hydroxy-2-[(*R*)-1-methyl-3-phenylpropylamino]ethyl}salicylamide.

$C_{19}H_{24}N_2O_3 = 328.4.$

CAS — 75659-07-3 (dilevalol); 75659-08-4 (dilevalol hydrochloride).

NOTE. Dilevalol Hydrochloride is *USAN.*

Dilevalol is a beta blocker (p.828). It also has vasodilating activity. Dilevalol was formerly used as the hydrochloride in the treatment of hypertension. It was withdrawn from the world market in 1990 due to reports of hepatotoxicity.

Diltiazem Hydrochloride (9225-e)

Diltiazem Hydrochloride *(BANM, USAN, rINNM).*

CRD-401; Diltiazemi Hydrochloridum; Latiazem Hydrochloride; MK-793 (diltiazem malate). (+)-*cis*-3-Acetoxy-5-(2-dimethylaminoethyl)-2,3-dihydro-2-(4-methoxyphenyl)-1,5-benzothiazepin-4(5*H*)-one hydrochloride; (2*S*,3*S*)-5-(2-Dimethylaminoethyl)-2,3,4,5- tetrahydro-2-(4-methoxyphenyl)-4-oxo-1,5-benzothiazepin-3-yl acetate hydrochloride.

$C_{22}H_{26}N_2O_4S,HCl = 451.0.$

CAS — 42399-41-7 (diltiazem); 33286-22-5 (diltiazem hydrochloride); 144604-00-2 (diltiazem malate).

NOTE. Diltiazem Malate is *USAN.*

Pharmacopoeias. In *Chin., Eur.* (see p.viii), *Jpn,* and *US.*

A white odourless crystalline powder or small crystals. Freely **soluble** in water, chloroform, dichloromethane, formic acid, and methyl alcohol; sparingly soluble in dehydrated alcohol; practically insoluble in ether.

The pH of a 1% solution in water is 4.3 to 5.3. **Store** in airtight containers. Protect from light.

Stability. A stability study of diltiazem hydrochloride and two of its metabolites[1] indicated that the degradation of diltiazem *in vitro* was enhanced at acid pH and elevated temperature; about 25% of a sample in plasma was lost after 24 hours at 37°, whereas there was no appreciable loss at 25°. In 1*N* hydrochloric acid at 25°, 59.5% of the sample was degraded in 24 hours. The main degradation product was desacetyldiltiazem, which is not a major metabolite *in vivo.*[1]

1. Caillé G, *et al.* Stability study of diltiazem and two of its metabolites using a high performance liquid chromatographic method. *Biopharm Drug Dispos* 1989; **10:** 107–14.

Adverse Effects

Treatment with diltiazem is generally well tolerated. Headache, ankle oedema, hypotension, dizziness, flushing, fatigue, and nausea and other gastro-intestinal disturbances (including anorexia, vomiting, constipation or diarrhoea, taste disturbances, and weight gain) may occur. Gingival hyperplasia has been reported. Rashes, possibly due to hypersensitivity, are normally mild and transient, but in a few cases erythema multiforme or exfoliative dermatitis has developed. Transient elevations in liver enzyme values, and occasionally hepatitis, have been reported.

Diltiazem may depress cardiac conduction and has occasionally led to atrioventricular block, bradycardia, and rarely asystole or sinus arrest.

Overdosage with diltiazem may be associated with bradycardia, with or without atrioventricular conduction defects, and hypotension.

Diltiazem has been shown to cause teratogenicity in *animal* studies.

For discussion of the possibility that calcium-channel blockers might be associated with increased cardiovascular mortality, see under Adverse Effects of Nifedipine, p.916.

Abuse. Abuse of diltiazem by body builders and rugby players has been alleged. Such abuse is possibly because of evidence that diltiazem increases maximum oxygen consumption after training. A body builder who admitted to taking diltiazem in high doses suffered severe abdominal cramps.[1]

1. Richards H, *et al.* Use of diltiazem in sport. *Br Med J* 1993; **307:** 940.

Angioedema. Periorbital angioedema, accompanied by pruritus or burning and erythema developed in 2 patients given diltiazem.[1]

1. Sadick NS, *et al.* Angioedema from calcium channel blockers. *J Am Acad Dermatol* 1989; **21:** 132–3.

Effects on the blood. A report of thrombocytopenia in association with diltiazem.[1]

1. Lehav M, Arav R. Diltiazem and thrombocytopenia. *Ann Intern Med* 1989; **110:** 327.

Effects on carbohydrate metabolism. Although raised blood-glucose concentrations and insulin requirements have been reported in a patient with insulin-dependent diabetes mellitus during diltiazem therapy, particularly at high doses,[1] a study in 11 obese black women, who were nondiabetic but had a family history of non-insulin-dependent diabetes, failed to find any effect of diltiazem 240 mg daily on plasma-glucose and C-peptide concentrations, nor any clinical signs of glucose intolerance.[2]

1. Pershadsingh HA, *et al.* Association of diltiazem therapy with increased insulin resistance in a patient with type I diabetes mellitus. *JAMA* 1987; **257:** 930–1.
2. Jones BJ, *et al.* Effects of diltiazem hydrochloride on glucose tolerance in persons at risk for diabetes mellitus. *Clin Pharm* 1988; **7:** 235–8.

Effects on the ears. There have been isolated reports[1] of tinnitus associated with several calcium-channel blockers including nifedipine, nicardipine, nitrendipine, diltiazem, verapamil, and cinnarizine.

1. Narváez M, *et al.* Tinnitus with calcium-channel blockers. *Lancet* 1994; **343:** 1229–30.

Effects on the heart. ATRIOVENTRICULAR BLOCK. Atrioventricular block appears to be uncommon in patients receiving diltiazem, but is potentially serious when it occurs. Prescription-event monitoring of a cohort of 10 119 patients for 1 year revealed 22 reports of atrioventricular block during diltiazem treatment. At least 8 patients had third-degree heart block, and 12 required a pacemaker; 3 died within 72 hours of the onset of heart block.[1] A high proportion of these patients were also receiving beta blockers,[1] which is in line with other reports.[2,3] (See also Beta Blockers under Interactions, below.) There is some evidence that the incidence of this effect may depend on the serum concentration of diltiazem. In a study in patients receiving diltiazem after myocardial infarction, patients with serum-diltiazem concentrations greater than 150 ng per mL were more likely to experience atrioventricular block than patients with concentrations of diltiazem below this value.[4]

1. Waller PC, Inman WHW. Diltiazem and heart block. *Lancet* 1989; **i:** 617.
2. Hossack KF. Conduction abnormalities due to diltiazem. *N Engl J Med* 1982; **307:** 953–4.
3. Ishikawa T, *et al.* Atrioventricular dissociation and sinus arrest induced by oral diltiazem. *N Engl J Med* 1983; **309:** 1124–5.
4. Nattel S, *et al.* Determinants and significance of diltiazem plasma concentrations after acute myocardial infarction. *Am J Cardiol* 1990; **66:** 1422–8.

MYOCARDIAL INFARCTION. Results from at least one large multicentre study (the Multicenter Diltiazem Postinfarction Trial) suggest that diltiazem, although apparently of benefit after myocardial infarction in patients with normal left ventricular function (as indicated by absence of pulmonary congestion), was associated with an increased risk of cardiac death or nonfatal re-infarction in patients with impaired left ventricular function.[1] Long-term follow-up[2] indicated that diltiazem also increased the risk of late-onset heart failure in postinfarction patients with left ventricular dysfunction.

1. The Multicenter Diltiazem Postinfarction Trial Research Group. The effect of diltiazem on mortality and reinfarction after myocardial infarction. *N Engl J Med* 1988; **319:** 385–92.
2. Goldstein RE, *et al.* Diltiazem increases late-onset congestive heart failure in postinfarction patients with early reduction in ejection fraction. *Circulation* 1991; **83:** 52–60.

WITHDRAWAL. Life-threatening coronary vasospasm, that was fatal in one patient, occurred in 4 patients following coronary revascularisation for unstable angina.[1] Treatment with a calcium-channel blocker (diltiazem or nifedipine) had been discontinued between 8 and 18 hours before the procedure and this abrupt withdrawal was thought to be responsible for the rebound vasospasm. The coronary vasospasm was managed with glyceryl trinitrate and nifedipine.

Withdrawal of diltiazem over a 4-day period from a patient with stable angina pectoris was followed by recurrence of anginal attacks.[2] Ambulatory ECG monitoring confirmed worsening myocardial ischaemia that responded to re-introduction of diltiazem. Two further patients experienced a similar withdrawal effect.

1. Engelman RM, *et al.* Rebound vasospasm after coronary revascularization in association with calcium antagonist withdrawal. *Ann Thorac Surg* 1984; **37:** 469–72.
2. Subramanian VB, *et al.* Calcium antagonist withdrawal syndrome: objective demonstration with frequency-modulated ambulatory ST-segment monitoring. *Br Med J* 1983; **286:** 520–1.

Effects on the kidneys. Diltiazem may be of benefit in various kidney disorders (see under Uses, below). However, there are a few reports of acute renal failure associated with diltiazem administration.[1,2] Acute interstitial nephritis has been proposed as a mechanism.[2,3]

1. ter Wee PM, *et al.* Acute renal failure due to diltiazem. *Lancet* 1984; **ii:** 1337–8.
2. Abadín JA, *et al.* Probable diltiazem-induced acute interstitial nephritis. *Ann Pharmacother* 1998; **32:** 656–8.
3. Achenbach V, *et al.* Acute renal failure due to diltiazem. *Lancet* 1985; **i:** 176.

Effects on mental function. By September 1989, eight cases of mental depression (severe in two) associated with diltiazem therapy had been gathered by the WHO collaborative programme for international drug monitoring.[1] Time of onset of symptoms varied from a few hours to a few months after starting treatment with diltiazem. There was some evidence that the problem might be dose-related as 5 of the 8 cases were receiving doses of 180 mg daily or more.

Psychoses have been reported rarely in association with diltiazem. One patient[2] who developed hallucinations (both auditory and visual) and paranoid delusions after 2 days of diltiazem therapy was subsequently treated with nifedipine without abnormal effects. A patient[3] with bipolar affective disorder that had been well-controlled by lithium carbonate for some years developed acute psychosis with extrapyramidal symptoms of cogwheel rigidity and ataxia, which was thought to represent an interaction between diltiazem and lithium.

1. Biriell C, *et al.* Depression associated with diltiazem. *Br Med J* 1989; **299:** 796.
2. Bushe CJ. Organic psychosis caused by diltiazem. *J R Soc Med* 1988; **81:** 296–7.
3. Binder EF. Diltiazem-induced psychosis and a possible diltiazem-lithium interaction. *Arch Intern Med* 1991; **151:** 373–4.

Effects on the mouth. A study involving 115 patients who had received nifedipine, diltiazem, or verapamil for at least 3 months indicated that gingival hyperplasia is an important side-effect that may occur with calcium-channel blockers in general.[1]

1. Steele RM, *et al.* Calcium antagonist-induced gingival hyperplasia. *Ann Intern Med* 1994; **120:** 663–4.

Effects on the nervous system. Akathisia has been reported in a 62-year-old patient one day after starting treatment with diltiazem. Symptoms disappeared when treatment was withdrawn and recurred on rechallenge after the third dose of diltiazem.[1] Similar symptoms in association with mania have also been reported in a 56-year-old patient given diltiazem.[2]

1. Jacobs MB. Diltiazem and akathisia. *Ann Intern Med* 1983; **99:** 794–5.
2. Brink DD. Diltiazem and hyperactivity. *Ann Intern Med* 1984; **100:** 459–60.

PARKINSONISM. Parkinsonism developed in an elderly patient with heart disease and hypertension when diltiazem was added to existing drug therapy.[1] Symptoms worsened over 3 months but improved significantly when diltiazem was slowly discontinued. On rechallenge severe tremor, impaired gait, and cogwheel rigidity recurred, but resolved when the drug was again discontinued except for slight residual cogwheel rigidity.

See also under Effects on Mental Function, above.

1. Dick RS, Barold SS. Diltiazem-induced parkinsonism. *Am J Med* 1989; **87:** 95–6.

Effects on the skin. A variety of skin disorders have been associated with diltiazem therapy, including acute pustular dermatitis,[1,2] cutaneous vasculitis,[3,4] erythema multiforme,[5,6] pruritic macular rashes,[7] severe toxic erythema,[8] and subacute lupus erythematosus-like eruptions.[9] Analysis of cutaneous adverse reactions to diltiazem indicated that acne, rash, and urticaria were among the commonest; there were a few reports of exfoliative dermatitis, erythema multiforme and Stevens Johnson syndrome, and one report of toxic epidermal necrolysis.[10]

For a report of periorbital skin rash associated with diltiazem, see under Angioedema, above.

Cross-sensitivity, manifest as a pruritic maculopapular rash, has been reported between diltiazem and amlodipine.[11]

1. Lambert DG, *et al.* Acute generalized exanthematous pustular dermatitis induced by diltiazem. *Br J Dermatol* 1988; **118:** 308–9.
2. Vicente-Calleja JM, *et al.* Acute generalized exanthematous pustulosis due to diltiazem: confirmation by patch testing. *Br J Dermatol* 1997; **137:** 837–9.
3. Carmichael AJ, Paul CJ. Vasculitic leg ulcers associated with diltiazem. *Br Med J* 1988; **297:** 562.
4. Sheehan-Dare RA, Goodfield MJ. Severe cutaneous vasculitis induced by diltiazem. *Br J Dermatol* 1988; **119:** 134.
5. Berbis P, *et al.* Diltiazem associated erythema multiforme. *Dermatologica* 1989; **179:** 90.
6. Sanders CJG, Neumann HAM. Erythema multiforme, Stevens-Johnson syndrome, and diltiazem. *Lancet* 1993; **341:** 967.
7. Wirebaugh SR, Geraets DR. Reports of erythematous macular skin eruptions associated with diltiazem therapy. *DICP Ann Pharmacother* 1990; **24:** 1046–9.
8. Wakeel RA, *et al.* Severe toxic erythema caused by diltiazem. *Br Med J* 1988; **296:** 1071.
9. Crowson AN, Magro CM. Diltiazem and subacute cutaneous lupus erythematosus-like lesions. *N Engl J Med* 1995; **333:** 1429.
10. Stern R, Khalsa JH. Cutaneous adverse reactions associated with calcium channel blockers. *Arch Intern Med* 1989; **149:** 829–32.
11. Baker BA, Cacchione JG. Dermatologic cross-sensitivity between diltiazem and amlodipine. *Ann Pharmacother* 1994; **28:** 118–19.

Overdosage. See under Treatment of Adverse Effects, below.

Treatment of Adverse Effects

In overdosage with diltiazem by mouth the stomach should be emptied by lavage; activated charcoal may be administered. Hypotension may require plasma expanders, intravenous calcium gluconate or calcium chloride, and a sympathomimetic such as dopamine or isoprenaline. Bradycardia may be treated with atropine, isoprenaline, or cardiac pacing.

Overdosage. The consequences and treatment of diltiazem overdosage are similar to those described under nifedipine (p.918), although death and life-threatening complications might be more common with diltiazem.[1] According to Roper[2] 6 cases of fatal overdose with diltiazem had been reported. He advocated the measurement of diltiazem concentrations to assist in diagnosis and management of overdosage, but Lip and Ferner[3] disputed its value.

The following are individual reports of overdosage with diltiazem.

A 58-year-old patient who took approximately 10.8 g of diltiazem developed hypotension and complete heart block. Dopamine, isoprenaline, and calcium chloride were required to maintain the blood pressure. The ECG reverted to sinus rhythm after 31 hours. The plasma-diltiazem concentration was 1670 ng per mL 43 hours after ingestion and fell to 12.1 ng per mL over a further 55.5 hours with an elimination half-life of 7.9 hours.[4]

In a further case a 50-year-old patient took 5.88 g of diltiazem with alcohol, and developed severe junctional bradycardia, hypotension, and reduced cardiac function that did not respond to intravenous calcium gluconate. The maximum plasma-diltiazem concentration of 6090 ng per mL occurred 7 hours after presentation. Approximately half the dose was vomited after treatment with activated charcoal. The patient was treated with cardiac pacing and a dopamine infusion; he reverted to sinus rhythm within 24 hours, and a subsequent episode of atrial fibrillation was treated successfully with digoxin.[5]

Charcoal haemoperfusion had a limited effect in improving the clearance of diltiazem in an 18-year-old patient who had taken 14.94 g of diltiazem.[6] The patient developed severe hypotension, complete heart block, and acute renal failure. Supportive care included cardiac pacing and numerous vasopressors including intravenous glucagon and infusions of dopamine, adrenaline, and noradrenaline.

1. Buckley NA, *et al.* Overdose with calcium channel blockers. *Br Med J* 1994; **308:** 1639.
2. Roper TA. Overdose of diltiazem. *Br Med J* 1994; **308:** 1571.
3. Lip GYH, Ferner RE. Overdose of diltiazem. *Br Med J* 1994; **309:** 193.
4. Malcolm N, *et al.* Massive diltiazem overdosage: clinical and pharmacokinetic observations. *Drug Intell Clin Pharm* 1986; **20:** 888.
5. Ferner RE, *et al.* Pharmacokinetics and toxic effects of diltiazem in massive overdose. *Hum Toxicol* 1989; **8:** 497–9.
6. Williamson KM, Dunham GD. Plasma concentrations of diltiazem and desacetyldiltiazem in an overdose situation. *Ann Pharmacother* 1996; **30:** 608–11.

Precautions

Diltiazem is contra-indicated in patients with the sick sinus syndrome, pre-existing second- or third-degree atrioventricular block, or marked bradycardia, and should be used with care in patients with lesser degrees of atrioventricular block or bradycardia. Diltiazem has been associated with the development of heart failure and great care is required in patients with impaired left ventricular function. Sudden withdrawal of diltiazem might be associated with an exacerbation of angina.

Treatment with diltiazem should commence with reduced doses in elderly patients and in patients with impaired liver or kidney function.

Breast feeding. Concentrations of diltiazem were almost the same in serum and breast milk from a woman receiving diltiazem 60 mg four times daily by mouth.[1] The results show that diltiazem is freely diffusible in human milk, and it should not be given to nursing women until more information becomes available concerning its safety in infants.

1. Okada M, *et al.* Excretion of diltiazem in human milk. *N Engl J Med* 1985; **312:** 992–3.

Porphyria. Diltiazem was considered to be unsafe in patients with acute porphyria because it has been shown to be porphyrinogenic in *animals* or *in-vitro* systems.[1]

1. Moore MR, McColl KEL. *Porphyria: drug lists.* Glasgow: Porphyria Research Unit. University of Glasgow, 1991.

Renal impairment. A 44-year-old man with end-stage renal failure requiring haemodialysis developed hypotension, bradycardia, metabolic acidosis, hyperkalaemia, and acute congestive heart failure about 60 hours after his last haemodialysis.[1] The patient had been taking diltiazem 60 mg three times a day. The symptoms were attributed to diltiazem toxicity due to accumulation of diltiazem and its metabolites which are poorly dialysed and normally excreted partially in the urine.

1. Patel R, *et al.* Toxic effects of diltiazem in a patient with chronic renal failure. *J Clin Pharmacol* 1994; **34:** 273–4.

Interactions

Increased depression of cardiac conduction with risk of bradycardia and atrioventricular block may occur when diltiazem is given with other cardiac depressants such as amiodarone, beta blockers, digoxin, and mefloquine. Enhanced antihypertensive effect may occur with concomitant use of other antihypertensive drugs or drugs that cause hypotension such as aldesleukin and antipsychotics. Diltiazem is extensively metabolised in the liver by the cytochrome P450 enzyme system; interactions may be expected with enzyme inducers, such as carbamazepine, phenobarbitone, phenytoin, and rifampicin, and enzyme inhibitors, such as cimetidine.

Antidepressants. For a report of diltiazem increasing the bioavailability of imipramine and nortriptyline, see p.277.

Antiepileptics. For a report of diltiazem administration precipitating carbamazepine and phenytoin toxicity, see p.342 and p.356, respectively.

Anxiolytics. For the effect of diltiazem on plasma-buspirone concentrations, see p.644.

Benzodiazepines. For a potential interaction between diltiazem and midazolam or triazolam, see Calcium-channel Blockers under Interactions of Diazepam, p.664.

Beta blockers. Profound bradycardia has been reported in a number of patients when diltiazem was prescribed with a beta blocker.[1,2] Tateishi and colleagues have shown that diltiazem decreases the clearance of a single dose of propranolol or metoprolol, though not atenolol, and suggest that elevated concentrations of beta blocker may be responsible for the bradycardic effects.[3] This is unlikely to be the full story, however, since atenolol, which was unaffected in this study, has been implicated in producing bradycardia when diltiazem was added in a patient with myocardial ischaemia.[2]

1. Hassell AB, Creamer JE. Profound bradycardia after the addition of diltiazem to a β blocker. *Br Med J* 1989; **298:** 675.
2. Nagle RE, *et al.* Diltiazem and heart block. *Lancet* 1989; **i:** 907.
3. Tateishi T, *et al.* Effect of diltiazem on the pharmacokinetics of propranolol, metoprolol and atenolol. *Eur J Clin Pharmacol* 1989; **36:** 67–70.

Calcium-channel blockers. For the effect of diltiazem and nifedipine on each others plasma concentrations, see p.918.

Cyclosporin. For reports of a potentially beneficial interaction between diltiazem and cyclosporin, see Transplantation under Uses and Administration, below.

Digoxin. For a discussion of interactions between digoxin and calcium-channel blockers including diltiazem, see p.851.

General anaesthetics. Two patients on diltiazem therapy developed impaired myocardial conduction during anaesthesia with enflurane;[1] one of the patients had severe sinus bradycardia that progressed to asystole. Additive cardiodepressant effects of diltiazem and enflurane were considered responsible.

1. Hantler CB, *et al.* Impaired myocardial conduction in patients receiving diltiazem therapy during enflurane anesthesia. *Anesthesiology* 1987; **67:** 94–6.

Histamine H_2-receptor antagonists. Cimetidine administration caused increases in plasma-diltiazem concentrations and in plasma-deacetyldiltiazem concentrations in 6 subjects given a single dose of diltiazem 60 mg by mouth. Ranitidine produced a similar, though less marked effect.[1]

1. Winship LC, *et al.* The effect of ranitidine and cimetidine on single-dose diltiazem pharmacokinetics. *Pharmacotherapy* 1985; **5:** 16–19.

Lithium. Neurotoxicity has been reported in patients receiving lithium and diltiazem.[1,2] See also under Effects on Mental Function, above.

1. Valdiserri EV. A possible interaction between lithium and diltiazem: case report. *J Clin Psychiatry* 1985; **46:** 540–1.
2. Binder EF, *et al.* Diltiazem-induced psychosis and a possible diltiazem–lithium interaction. *Arch Intern Med* 1991; **151:** 373–4.

Theophylline. For the effect of diltiazem on plasma-theophylline concentrations, see p.769.

Pharmacokinetics

Diltiazem is rapidly and almost completely absorbed from the gastro-intestinal tract following oral administration, but undergoes extensive first-pass hepatic metabolism. The bioavailability has been reported to be about 40%, although there is considerable interindividual variation in plasma concentrations. Diltiazem is about 80% bound to plasma proteins. It is distributed into breast milk. It is extensively metabolised in the liver; one of the metabolites, desacetyldiltiazem has been reported to have 25 to 50% of the activity of the parent compound. The half-life of diltiazem is reported to be about 3 to 5 hours. Approximately 2 to 4% of a dose is excreted in urine as unchanged diltiazem with the remainder excreted as metabolites in bile and urine. Diltiazem is poorly dialysable.

General reviews.

1. Kelly JG, O'Malley K. Clinical pharmacokinetics of calcium antagonists: an update. *Clin Pharmacokinet* 1992; **22:** 416–33.

Studies of the pharmacokinetics of diltiazem in healthy subjects after single and multiple doses,[1-3] indicating that bioavailability was increased after multiple doses, probably because of decreased presystemic elimination.[3]

1. Höglund P, Nilsson L-G. Pharmacokinetics of diltiazem and its metabolites after repeated multiple-dose treatments in healthy volunteers. *Ther Drug Monit* 1989; **11:** 543–50.
2. Höglund P, Nilsson L-G. Pharmacokinetics of diltiazem and its metabolites after repeated single dosing in healthy volunteers. *Ther Drug Monit* 1989; **11:** 551–7.
3. Höglund P, Nilsson L-G. Pharmacokinetics of diltiazem and its metabolites after single and multiple dosing in healthy volunteers. *Ther Drug Monit* 1989; **11:** 558–66.

Renal impairment. The pharmacokinetics of diltiazem and its major metabolite desacetyldiltiazem in patients with severely impaired renal function were similar to those in patients with normal renal function.[1] Nevertheless, reduced doses may be necessary in patients with renal impairment. See also under Precautions, above.

1. Pozet N, *et al.* Pharmacokinetics of diltiazem in severe renal failure. *Eur J Clin Pharmacol* 1983; **24:** 635–8.

Uses and Administration

Diltiazem hydrochloride is a benzothiazepine calcium-channel blocker (p.778). It is a peripheral and coronary vasodilator with limited negative inotropic activity but its vasodilator properties are less marked than those of the dihydropyridine calcium-channel blocker nifedipine (p.916). Unlike nifedipine, diltiazem inhibits cardiac conduction, particularly at the sino-atrial and atrioventricular nodes. Diltiazem is used in the management of angina pectoris (p.780) and hypertension (p.788). In some countries it is available for intravenous administration in the treatment of various cardiac arrhythmias (atrial fibrillation or flutter and paroxysmal supraventricular tachycardia) (p.782).

Diltiazem hydrochloride is given by mouth in the treatment of angina pectoris and hypertension and is available in a number of formulations for administration once, twice, or three times daily. The variety of formulations means that dosage is dependent on the preparation used.

In **angina pectoris** an initial dose is 60 mg by mouth three times daily (or 30 mg four times daily in the USA), increased if necessary to 360 mg daily; up to 480 mg daily has sometimes been given. Formulations suitable for once- or twice-daily administration may be used in doses of 180 to 360 mg daily.

In **hypertension** diltiazem hydrochloride may be given as modified-release capsules or tablets. Depending on the formulation, an initial dose is 60 to 120 mg twice daily, increased as required to a maximum of 360 mg daily. Formulations suitable for once-daily administration may be given in similar daily doses.

Reduced doses may be required in the elderly or those with impaired renal or hepatic function; the dose should not be increased if the heart rate drops below 50 beats per minute.

In **cardiac arrhythmias** an initial dose of 0.25 mg per kg body-weight by bolus intravenous injection over 2 minutes has been suggested; a further dose of 0.35 mg per kg may be administered after 15 minutes if the response is inadequate. Subsequent doses should be individualised for each patient. For those with atrial fibrillation or flutter, a continued reduction in heart rate may be achieved with an intravenous infusion of diltiazem hydrochloride after the bolus injection. An initial infusion rate of 5 to 10 mg per hour, may be increased as necessary in increments of 5 mg per hour up to a rate of 15 mg per hour. The infusion may be continued for up to 24 hours.

General reviews.

1. Buckley MM-T, *et al.* Diltiazem: a reappraisal of its pharmacological properties and therapeutic use. *Drugs* 1990; **39:** 757–806.
2. Anonymous. Calcium antagonists for cardiovascular disease. *Drug Ther Bull* 1993; **31:** 81–4.
3. Fisher M, Grotta J. New uses for calcium channel blockers: therapeutic implications. *Drugs* 1993; **46:** 961–75.
4. Weir MR. Diltiazem: ten years of clinical experience in the treatment of hypertension. *J Clin Pharmacol* 1995; **35:** 220–32.

Action. The haemodynamic and electrophysiological effects of diltiazem appear to resemble those of verapamil more than those of nifedipine.[1] It inhibits sino-atrial and atrioventricular nodal function in clinically employed doses. The effects on sino-atrial function are more pronounced than those observed after verapamil. Diltiazem causes a decrease in the rate-pressure product indicating that decreased oxygen demand is a likely mechanism of action in relieving angina pectoris. Like verapamil, but unlike nifedipine, diltiazem does not appear to cause significant increases in coronary blood flow. The negative inotropic effect of diltiazem is presumably counteracted by afterload reduction.

1. Soward AL, *et al.* The haemodynamic effects of nifedipine, verapamil and diltiazem in patients with coronary artery disease: a review. *Drugs* 1986; **32:** 66–101.

Asthma. Studies have indicated that inhaled diltiazem has no clinically important effect on exercise-induced bronchospasm in asthmatics although oral diltiazem was found to have a modest protective effect. Oral diltiazem had little or no effect against histamine- or methacholine-induced bronchospasm.[1]

For a brief discussion of the role of calcium-channel blockers in asthma (p.745), see under Nifedipine, p.920.

1. Massey KL, Hendeles L. Calcium antagonists in the management of asthma: breakthrough or ballyhoo? *Drug Intell Clin Pharm* 1987; **21:** 505–9.

Cardiomyopathies. Symptomatic improvement has been reported in patients with dilated cardiomyopathy (p.785) given diltiazem.[1]

1. Figulla HR, *et al.* Diltiazem improves cardiac function and exercise capacity in patients with idiopathic dilated cardiomyopathy: results of the Diltiazem in Dilated Cardiomyopathy Trial. *Circulation* 1996; **94:** 346–52.

Kidney disorders. Calcium-channel blockers may be of benefit in various forms of kidney disorder (see Nifedipine, p.921). Diltiazem has been reported to reduce urinary protein excretion without exacerbating pre-existing renal dysfunction in diabetic patients.[1,2] A small study[3] in 15 hypertensive patients with non-insulin-dependent diabetes mellitus, albuminuria, and renal impairment found that diltiazem only reduced urinary albumin excretion when patients received a restricted dietary sodium intake of 50 mEq per day.

Diltiazem may also reduce the nephrotoxicity associated with certain drugs. Reduced nephrotoxicity has been reported when diltiazem is given to healthy subjects receiving the aminoglycoside antibiotic netilmicin,[4] but diltiazem does not appear to modify the acute renal failure associated with tubular damage which may be caused by methotrexate.[5] Diltiazem may reduce cyclosporin-induced nephrotoxicity (see Transplantation, below).

1. Bakris GL. Effects of diltiazem or lisinopril on massive proteinuria associated with diabetes mellitus. *Ann Intern Med* 1990; **112:** 707–8.
2. Demarie BK, Bakris GL. Effects of different calcium antagonists on proteinuria associated with diabetes mellitus. *Ann Intern Med* 1990; **113:** 987–8.
3. Bakris GL, Smith A. Effects of sodium intake on albumin excretion in patients with diabetic nephropathy treated with long-acting calcium antagonists. *Ann Intern Med* 1996; **125:** 201–4.
4. Lortholary O, *et al.* Calcium antagonists and aminoglycoside nephrotoxicity. *Am J Med* 1990; **88:** 445.
5. Deray G, *et al.* The effects of diltiazem on methotrexate-induced nephrotoxicity. *Eur J Clin Pharmacol* 1989; **37:** 337–40.

Migraine. For reference to the use of calcium-channel blockers, including diltiazem, in the management of migraine, see under Nifedipine, p.921.

Myocardial infarction. Studies have not shown a reduction in mortality when calcium-channel blockers are given in the **early** phase of acute myocardial infarction (p.791). However, since myocardial stunning has been linked to intracellular calcium overload[1] there has been speculation that calcium-channel blockers might benefit patients about to undergo reperfusion. This is yet to be confirmed. Diltiazem started within 24 to 72 hours after the onset of infarction and continued for up to 14 days has been reported to protect against re-infarction and refractory angina in patients recovering from acute non-Q-wave infarction.[2] Calcium-channel blockers are not routinely used in the **long-term** management of myocardial infarction although in selected patients without heart failure verapamil or diltiazem may be of some benefit. In a study by the Multicenter Diltiazem Postinfarction Trial (MDPIT) research group,[3] diltiazem in a standard dose of 240 mg daily reduced 1-year mortality and re-infarction rates in patients without left ventricular dysfunction, but increased such adverse events in those with left ventricular dysfunction. Re-analysis of the Multicenter Diltiazem Postinfarction Trial provided further evidence that diltiazem should be avoided in postinfarction patients with left ventricular dysfunction.[4]

1. Anonymous. Myocardial stunning. *Lancet* 1991; **337:** 585–6.
2. Gibson RS, *et al.* Diltiazem and reinfarction in patients with non-Q-wave myocardial infarction: results of a double-blind, randomized, multicenter trial. *N Engl J Med* 1986; **315:** 423–9.
3. The Multicenter Diltiazem Postinfarction Trial Research Group. The effect of diltiazem on mortality and reinfarction after myocardial infarction. *N Engl J Med* 1988; **319:** 385–92.
4. Goldstein RE, *et al.* Diltiazem increases late-onset congestive heart failure in post-infarction patients with early reduction in ejection fraction. *Circulation* 1991; **83:** 52–60.

Oesophageal motility disorders. Calcium-channel blockers have been tried in patients with oesophageal motility disorders (p.1174) because of their ability to relax smooth muscle. Diltiazem in doses of 150 mg by mouth has been reported to decrease the amplitude and duration of peristaltic contractions in patients with the nutcracker oesophagus, but the results of preliminary studies of diltiazem in patients with oesophageal disorders have conflicted, and it appears that decreases in oesophageal pressure may not correlate with alleviation of pain.[1]

1. Richter JE, *et al.* Esophageal chest pain: current controversies in pathogenesis, diagnosis, and therapy. *Ann Intern Med* 1989; **110:** 66–78.

Peripheral vascular disease. Vasospastic arterial disease (p.794) is due to an inappropriate response to temperature, usually cold, when vasoconstriction and/or vasospasm occurs. The most important of these disorders is Raynaud's syndrome. Calcium-channel blockers have been of benefit, but it is not entirely clear which of their pharmacological actions is responsible. The most widely used and studied is nifedipine (see p.921).

Although some studies have reported that diltiazem 120 or 180 mg daily in divided doses produces significant subjective improvement in the majority of patients with Raynaud's syndrome not all investigators have found similar improvement in objective parameters, and there is no evidence to date on the long-term efficacy of diltiazem or its effect on sequelae of the disease such as digital gangrene.[1]

1. Buckley MM-T, *et al.* Diltiazem: a reappraisal of its pharmacological properties and therapeutic use. *Drugs* 1990; **39:** 757–806.

Proctalgia fugax. Beneficial response to diltiazem was reported by Boquet *et al.* in a patient with proctalgia fugax.[1] A similar case was seen by Jonard and Essamri who found that diltiazem 60 mg decreased the resting pressure of the internal anal sphincter by a mean of 20.6% in all but 1 of 13 patients, and concluded that smooth muscle relaxation may explain the effect of diltiazem in proctalgia fugax.[2]

1. Boquet J, *et al.* Diltiazem for proctalgia fugax. *Lancet* 1986; **i:** 1493.
2. Jonard P, Essamri B. Diltiazem and internal anal sphincter. *Lancet* 1987; **i:** 754.

Transplantation. Diltiazem increases blood-cyclosporin concentrations when given by mouth in doses of 60 to 180 mg daily to transplant patients receiving cyclosporin therapy.[1-3] In consequence, cyclosporin doses can be reduced by about one-third, at a considerable saving in cost.[2,3] In addition to this effect, which is apparently due to non-competitive inhibition of cyclosporin metabolism by diltiazem,[4] there is evidence of improved renal graft-function in patients given the combined therapy, suggesting that diltiazem may reduce cyclosporin-induced nephrotoxicity.[1,2]

1. Wagner K, Neumayer H-H. Prevention of delayed graft function in cadaver kidney transplants by diltiazem. *Lancet* 1985; **ii:** 1355–6.
2. Neumayer H-H, Wagner K. Diltiazem and economic use of cyclosporin. *Lancet* 1986; **ii:** 523.
3. Bourge RC, *et al.* Diltiazem-cyclosporine interaction in cardiac transplant recipients: impact on cyclosporine dose and medication costs. *Am J Med* 1991; **90:** 402–4.
4. Brockmöller J, *et al.* Pharmacokinetic interaction between cyclosporin and diltiazem. *Eur J Clin Pharmacol* 1990; **38:** 237–42.

Preparations

USP 23: Diltiazem Hydrochloride Extended-release Capsules; Diltiazem Hydrochloride Tablets.

Proprietary Preparations (details are given in Part 3)
Aust.: Cardiacton; Corazem; Dilatame; Dilzem; Gewazem; ***Austral.:*** Auscard; Cardcal; Cardizem; Coras; Diltahexal; Diltiamax;

Dilzem; Vasocardol†; *Belg.:* Tildiem; *Canad.:* Cardizem; Novo-Diltazem; Nu-Diltiaz; *Fr.:* Bi-Tildiem; Deltazen; Diacor; Dilrene; Mono-Tildiem; Tildiem; *Ger.:* Corazet; Dil-Sanorania; Diltahexal; Diltaretard; Dilti; Dilti-Essex†; Diltiamerck; Diltiuc; Dilzem; Dilzereal; Dilzicardin; *Irl.:* Adizem; Diltam; Dilzem; Entrydil; Metazem; Tildiem; *Ital.:* Altiazem; Angidil; Angipress; Angizem; Carzem; Citizem; Diladel; Dilem; Diliter; Dilzene; Etyzem; Longazem; Tiakem; Tiazen; Tildiem; Zilden; *Jpn:* Herbesser; *Neth.:* Diloc; Surazem; Tildiem; *Norw.:* Cardizem; Kardil; *S.Afr.:* Anzem; Dilatam; Tilazem; Zildem; *Spain:* Angiodrox; Cardiser; Carreldon; Clobendian; Convectal; Corolater; Cronodine; Dilaclan; Diltiwas; Dinisor; Doclis; Lacerol; Masdil; Tilker; Uni Masdil; *Swed.:* Cardizem; Coramil; *Switz.:* Coridil; Dilzem; Ubicor†; *UK:* Adizem; Angiozem; Angitil; Britiazim†; Calazem; Calcicard; Dilcardia; Dilzem; Slozem; Tildiem; Viazem XL; Zemtard; *USA:* Cardizem; Dilacor XR; Tiazac.

Multi-ingredient: *UK:* Adizem-XL Plus†.

Dimetofrine Hydrochloride (2051-a)

Dimetofrine Hydrochloride *(rINNM)*.

Dimetophrine Hydrochloride. 4-Hydroxy-3,5-dimethoxy-α-[(methylamino)methyl]benzyl alcohol hydrochloride.

$C_{11}H_{17}NO_4,HCl = 263.7$.

CAS — 22950-29-4 (dimetofrine); 22775-12-8 (dimetofrine hydrochloride).

Dimetofrine hydrochloride is a sympathomimetic (see Adrenaline, p.813) used for its vasopressor effects in usual doses of 300 to 400 mg daily by mouth in the treatment of hypotensive states; it is also given by intramuscular injection or intravenous infusion.

Preparations

Proprietary Preparations (details are given in Part 3)
Ital.: Pressamina; *Spain:* Dovida†.

Diprafenone Hydrochloride (3923-l)

Diprafenone Hydrochloride *(rINNM)*.

(±)-2′-[2-Hydroxy-3-(*tert*-pentylamino)propoxy]-3-phenylpropiophenone hydrochloride.

$C_{23}H_{31}NO_3,HCl = 406.0$.

CAS — 81447-80-5 (diprafenone); 86342-43-0 (diprafenone hydrochloride).

Diprafenone hydrochloride is a class Ic antiarrhythmic (p.776) structurally related to propafenone. It has some beta-adrenoceptor blocking activity.

References.

1. Trenk D, *et al.* Pharmacokinetic characterization of the antiarrhythmic drug diprafenone in man. *Eur J Clin Pharmacol* 1989; **37:** 313–16.
2. Wagner F, *et al.* Evaluation of the beta-adrenoceptor blocking activity of the class Ic antiarrhythmic drug diprafenone in man. *Eur J Clin Pharmacol* 1989; **36:** 579–82.
3. Koytchev R, *et al.* Influence of food on the bioavailability and some pharmacokinetic parameters of diprafenone—a novel antiarrhythmic agent. *Eur J Clin Pharmacol* 1996; **50:** 315–19.

Dipyridamole (9226-l)

Dipyridamole *(BAN, USAN, rINN)*.

Dipyridamolum; NSC-515776; RA-8. 2,2′,2″,2‴-[(4,8-Dipiperidinopyrimido[5,4-*d*]pyrimidine-2,6-diyl)dinitrilo]tetraethanol.

$C_{24}H_{40}N_8O_4 = 504.6$.

CAS — 58-32-2.

Pharmacopoeias. In *Chin., Eur.* (see p.viii), *Jpn, Pol.,* and *US.*

An intensely yellow, crystalline powder or needles. Ph. Eur. **solubilities** are: practically insoluble in water and in ether; soluble in alcohol; freely soluble in acetone; it dissolves in dilute solutions of mineral acids. USP solubilities are: slightly soluble in water; very soluble in chloroform, in alcohol, and in methyl alcohol; very slightly soluble in acetone and in ethyl acetate. **Store** in airtight containers. Protect from light.

Adverse Effects, Treatment, and Precautions

Gastric disturbances, including nausea, vomiting, and diarrhoea, headache, dizziness, faintness, facial flushing, and skin rash may occur after administration of dipyridamole. Dipyridamole can also induce chest pain or lead to a worsening of the symptoms of angina. Cardiac arrhythmias have been reported in patients given dipyridamole during thallium-201 imaging. Aminophylline may reverse some of the adverse effects.

When dipyridamole is given by mouth care is required in patients with hypotension, unstable angina, aortic stenosis, recent myocardial infarction, heart failure, or coagulation disorders. Many of these conditions may become contra-indications when dipyridamole is used intravenously and details are given under Myocardial Imaging, below.

Effects on the biliary tract. Gallstones containing unconjugated dipyridamole were removed from two patients who had been taking dipyridamole for 15 and 10 years, respectively.[1]

1. Moesch C, *et al.* Biliary drug lithiasis: dipyridamole gallstones. *Lancet* 1992; **340:** 1352–3.

Effects on the heart. Transient myocardial ischaemia occurred in 4 patients with unstable angina and multivessel coronary artery disease during oral treatment with dipyridamole.[1] See under Myocardial Imaging, below, for additional reports.

1. Keltz TN, *et al.* Dipyridamole-induced myocardial ischemia. *JAMA* 1987; **257:** 1515–16.

Effects on the muscles. Symptoms resembling acute pseudopolymyalgia rheumatica developed in a patient taking dipyridamole.[1]

1. Chassagne P, *et al.* Pseudopolymyalgia rheumatica with dipyridamole. *Br Med J* 1990; **301:** 875.

Effects on taste. A report of a disagreeable taste associated with other gastro-intestinal symptoms occurring in one patient taking dipyridamole.[1] Two similar cases had been reported to the CSM.

1. Willoughby JMT. Drug-induced abnormalities of taste sensation. *Adverse Drug React Bull* 1983; **100:** 368–71.

Myocardial imaging. Dipyridamole may be used in association with thallium-201 in myocardial stress imaging. Safety data from over 3900 patients has been summarised.[1] Adverse effects which occurred within 24 hours after intravenous administration of dipyridamole (mean dose 0.56 mg per kg body-weight) were recorded. Ten patients had major adverse effects and 1820 patients experienced minor adverse effects. Myocardial infarction occurred in 4 patients, 3 of whom had unstable angina before thallium-201 myocardial scanning. Six patients developed acute bronchospasm, 4 of whom had a history of asthma or had wheezing before administration of dipyridamole. Adverse effects considered to be minor included chest pain in 19.7% of patients, ST-T-segment depression in 7.5%, ventricular extrasystoles in 5.2%, headache in 12.2%, dizziness in 11.8%, nausea in 4.6%, and hypotension in 4.6%. Aminophylline was effective in relieving symptoms of adverse effects in 97% of 454 patients.

An anaphylaxis-like reaction has been reported in one patient.[2]

In a review of pharmacological stress testing, Beller[3] suggested that with appropriate patient selection and adequate monitoring, the incidence of life-threatening adverse reactions is negligible. Beller also considered that dipyridamole-thallium-201 imaging could be safely performed in the early post-myocardial infarction period. Caution should be exercised in patients with acute unstable angina or a history of bronchospasm. However, the manufacturers contra-indicate the injection of dipyridamole in subvalvular aortic stenosis, aortic disease, hypotension associated with recent myocardial infarction, significant valvular disease, uncompensated heart failure, conduction defects, or arrhythmias.

1. Ranhosky A, *et al.* The safety of intravenous dipyridamole thallium myocardial perfusion imaging. *Circulation* 1990; **81:** 1205–9.
2. Weinmann P, *et al.* Anaphylaxis-like reaction induced by dipyridamole during myocardial scintigraphy. *Am J Med* 1994; **97:** 488.
3. Beller GA. Pharmacologic stress imaging. *JAMA* 1991; **265:** 633–8.

Interactions

Dipyridamole may enhance the actions of oral anticoagulants due to its antiplatelet effect. It inhibits the reuptake of adenosine and may enhance its effects; the dose of adenosine must be reduced if the two drugs are given concomitantly. Dipyridamole may also inhibit the uptake of fludarabine and may reduce its efficacy.

The absorption of dipyridamole may be reduced by drugs such as antacids that increase gastric pH.

Anticoagulants. Dipyridamole may induce bleeding in patients receiving oral anticoagulants without altering prothrombin times, see under Warfarin, p.968.

Xanthines. Xanthines may antagonise some of the effects of dipyridamole due to their action as adenosine antagonists. Aminophylline may be used to reverse some of the adverse effects of dipyridamole. Administration of caffeine intravenously has been reported[1] to attenuate the haemodynamic response to dipyridamole and it has been suggested that caffeine should be avoided for at least 24 hours before the test in patients receiving dipyridamole for myocardial imaging.

1. Smits P, *et al.* Dose-dependent inhibition of the hemodynamic response to dipyridamole by caffeine. *Clin Pharmacol Ther* 1991; **50:** 529–37.

Pharmacokinetics

Dipyridamole is incompletely absorbed from the gastro-intestinal tract with peak plasma concentrations occurring about 75 minutes after oral administration. Dipyridamole is highly bound to plasma proteins. A terminal half-life of 10 to 12 hours has been reported. Dipyridamole is metabolised in the liver and is mainly excreted as glucuronides in the bile. Excretion may be delayed by enterohepatic recirculation. A small amount is excreted in the urine.

References.

1. Mahony C, *et al.* Dipyridamole kinetics. *Clin Pharmacol Ther* 1982; **31:** 330–8.
2. Mahony C, *et al.* Plasma dipyridamole concentrations after two different dosage regimens in patients. *J Clin Pharmacol* 1983; **23:** 123–6.

Uses and Administration

Dipyridamole is an adenosine reuptake inhibitor and phosphodiesterase inhibitor with antiplatelet and vasodilating activity and is used in thrombo-embolic disorders (p.801). Oral dipyridamole is used in association with an oral anticoagulant for the prophylaxis of thrombo-embolism following cardiac valve replacement (p.801). The usual adult dose is 300 to 600 mg daily by mouth in divided doses before meals. Children may be given 5 mg per kg body-weight by mouth daily in divided doses.

It has been given either alone or with aspirin in the management of myocardial infarction (p.791) and stroke (p.799). For the secondary prevention of stroke or transient ischaemic attack it may be given as a modified-release preparation in a dose of 200 mg twice daily.

Dipyridamole administered intravenously results in marked coronary vasodilatation and is used in stress testing in patients with ischaemic heart disease (see below).

General references.

1. Rivey MP, *et al.* Dipyridamole: a critical evaluation. *Drug Intell Clin Pharm* 1984; **18:** 869–80.
2. FitzGerald GA. Dipyridamole. *N Engl J Med* 1987; **316:** 1247–57.
3. Gibbs CR, Lip GYH. Do we still need dipyridamole? *Br J Clin Pharmacol* 1998; **45:** 323–8.

Ischaemic heart disease. Scintigraphy with thallium-201 is used to assess coronary artery disease. Perfusion abnormalities due to coronary artery disease are usually absent at rest but are present during stress. The stress is usually supplied by exercise, but when exercise is inappropriate a pharmacological stress can be supplied by dipyridamole which is usually given intravenously in a dose of 560 μg per kg body-weight over 4 minutes. Thallium-201 is given immediately after completion of the infusion of dipyridamole. Initial images are obtained 5 minutes after drug administration and delayed images are obtained 2.5 to 4 hours later. Dipyridamole (300 to 400 mg) has also been given as an oral suspension; thallium-201 is given about 45 minutes later to coincide with peak dipyridamole-serum concentrations.

Dipyridamole has also been used in echocardiography.[1,2] The intravenous dipyridamole dose used to obtain maximum sensitivity is often higher (750 to 840 μg per kg) than the dose used in scintigraphy.[1] Dobutamine echocardiography might prove to be more sensitive and better tolerated.[3]

1. Beller GA. Pharmacologic stress imaging. *JAMA* 1991; **265:** 633–8.
2. Buchalter MB, *et al.* Dipyridamole echocardiography: the bedside stress test for coronary artery disease. *Postgrad Med J* 1990; **66:** 531–5.
3. Martin TW, *et al.* Comparison of adenosine, dipyridamole, and dobutamine in stress echocardiography. *Ann Intern Med* 1992; **116:** 190–6.

Preparations

BP 1998: Dipyridamole Tablets;
USP 23: Dipyridamole Tablets.

Proprietary Preparations (details are given in Part 3)
Aust.: Persantin; *Austral.:* Persantin; *Belg.:* Agredamol†; Didamol; Dipyridan; Persantine; *Canad.:* Novo-Dipiradol; Persantine; *Fr.:* Cleridium; Coronarine; Diphar†; Perkod†; Persantine; Prandiol†; Protangix†; *Ger.:* Curantyl; Persantin; *Irl.:* Perclodin†; Persantin; Pyridamel†; *Ital.:* Coribon†; Corosan; Coroxin†; Novodil; Persantin; Platelet†; Stenocor†; Stimolcardio†; Trancocard†; Viscor†; *Neth.:* Persantin; *Norw.:* Persantin; *S.Afr.:* Dipyrol; Persantin; Plato; *Spain:* Miosen; Persantin; *Swed.:* Persantin; *Switz.:* Natyl; Persantine; *UK:* Cerebrovase; Modaplate; Persantin; Vasyrol†; *USA:* Persantine.

Multi-ingredient: *Aust.:* Anxiocard†; Duplinal; Persumbran†; Thrombosantin; *Canad.:* Asasantine; *Ger.:* Asasantin; Oxygenabund†; Persumbran†; *Ital.:* Persumbrax; *Spain:* Asasantin; *Switz.:* Asasantine†; *UK:* Asasantin.

Disopyramide (7783-h)

Disopyramide (BAN, USAN, rINN).

Disopyramidum; SC-7031. 4-Di-isopropylamino-2-phenyl-2-(2-pyridyl)butyramide.

$C_{21}H_{29}N_3O$ = 339.5.

CAS — 3737-09-5.

Pharmacopoeias. In *Eur.* (see p.viii) and *Jpn.*

A white or almost white powder. Slightly **soluble** in water; soluble in alcohol; freely soluble in dichloromethane. **Protect** from light.

Disopyramide Phosphate (7784-m)

Disopyramide Phosphate (BANM, USAN, rINNM).

Disopyramidi Phosphas; SC-13957.

$C_{21}H_{29}N_3O,H_3PO_4$ = 437.5.

CAS — 22059-60-5.

Pharmacopoeias. In *Eur.* (see p.viii) and *US.*

A white or practically white odourless or almost odourless powder. Disopyramide phosphate 1.3 g is approximately equivalent to 1 g of disopyramide. **Soluble** to freely soluble in water; slightly to sparingly soluble in alcohol; practically insoluble in chloroform, in dichloromethane, and in ether. A 5% solution in water has a pH of 4.0 to 5.0. **Store** in airtight containers. Protect from light.

Adverse Effects and Treatment

The adverse effects most commonly associated with disopyramide therapy relate to its antimuscarinic properties and are dose-related. They include dry mouth, blurred vision, urinary hesitancy, impotence, and constipation; the most serious effect is urinary retention. Gastro-intestinal effects which are less common include nausea, bloating, and abdominal pain. Other adverse effects reported include skin rashes, hypoglycaemia, dizziness, fatigue, muscle weakness, headache, and urinary frequency. Insomnia and depression have also been associated with disopyramide administration. There have been rare reports of psychosis, cholestatic jaundice, elevated liver enzymes, thrombocytopenia, and agranulocytosis. Disopyramide has cardiac depressant properties, and may induce cardiac arrhythmias particularly ventricular tachycardia and fibrillation, heart block and conduction disturbances, heart failure, and hypotension.

Over-rapid intravenous injection of disopyramide may cause profuse sweating and severe cardiovascular depression.

In overdose cardiovascular and antimuscarinic effects are pronounced, and there may be apnoea, loss of consciousness, loss of spontaneous respiration, and asystole. Treatment of overdosage is symptomatic and supportive.

A review of the adverse effects associated with the class Ia antiarrhythmic drugs disopyramide, procainamide, and quinidine, and their clinical management.[1]

1. Kim SY, Benowitz NL. Poisoning due to class IA antiarrhythmic drugs quinidine, procainamide and disopyramide. *Drug Safety* 1990; **5:** 393–420.

During long-term therapy with disopyramide 400 to 1600 mg daily in 40 patients, 28 (70%) had one or more adverse effects.[1] Dry mouth occurred in 15 (38%), constipation in 12 (30%), blurred vision in 11 (28%), urinary hesitancy in 9 (23%), nausea in 9 (23%), impotence in 2 (5%), and dyspareunia in one patient (3%). In addition 3 of the 9 patients had worsening of heart failure due to disopyramide. Adverse effects were sufficiently severe for disopyramide to be discontinued in 7 patients, and for dosage reductions in another 7.

1. Bauman JL, *et al.* Long-term therapy with disopyramide phosphate: side effects and effectiveness. *Am Heart J* 1986; **111:** 654–60.

Effects on the blood. Granulocytopenia was associated on 2 occasions with the use of disopyramide phosphate in a 61-year-old man.[1]

1. Conrad ME, *et al.* Agranulocytosis associated with disopyramide therapy. *JAMA* 1978; **240:** 1857–8.

Effects on the eyes. The antimuscarinic activity of disopyramide may cause adverse effects on the eyes such as dilated pupils,[1] severe blurring of vision,[1] and acute glaucoma.[2,3] Disopyramide should be avoided in patients with glaucoma and used with caution if there is a family history of glaucoma.

1. Frucht J, *et al.* Ocular side effects of disopyramide. *Br J Ophthalmol* 1984; **68:** 890–1.
2. Trope GE, Hind VMD. Closed-angle glaucoma in patient on disopyramide. *Lancet* 1978, **i:** 329.
3. Ahmad S. Disopyramide: pulmonary complications and glaucoma. *Mayo Clin Proc* 1990; **65:** 1030–1.

Effects on the heart. Disopyramide has a strong negative inotropic effect and reversible heart failure has been reported[1] following administration of disopyramide. As many as 50% of patients with a previous history of heart failure may have a recurrence of the disease with an incidence of less than 5% in other patients.

As disopyramide can prolong the QT interval seen on the ECG it can induce ventricular tachyarrhythmias. A case of fatal torsade de pointes has been reported.[2]

1. Podrid PJ, *et al.* Congestive heart failure caused by oral disopyramide. *N Engl J Med* 1980; **302:** 614–17.
2. Schattner A, *et al.* Fatal torsade de pointes following jaundice in a patient treated with disopyramide. *Postgrad Med J* 1989; **65:** 333–4.

Effects on the liver. Cholestatic jaundice with raised liver enzyme values has been associated with disopyramide treatment.[1-3] Laboratory and clinical abnormalities disappear on withdrawal of disopyramide although liver enzyme values may remain elevated for several months.

Severe hepatocellular damage with disseminated intravascular coagulation[4] has also been reported.

1. Craxi A, *et al.* Disopyramide and cholestasis. *Ann Intern Med* 1980; **93:** 150–1.
2. Edmonds ME, Hayler AM. *Eur J Clin Pharmacol* 1980; **18:** 285–6.
3. Bakris GL, *et al.* Disopyramide-associated liver dysfunction. *Mayo Clin Proc* 1983; **58:** 265–7.
4. Doody PT. Disopyramide hepatotoxicity and disseminated intravascular coagulation. *South Med J* 1982; **75:** 496–8.

Effects on mental state. Agitation and distress leading to paranoia and auditory and visual hallucinations have been reported[1,2] in patients shortly after starting disopyramide therapy. Complete recovery occurred on withdrawal of disopyramide.

1. Falk RH, *et al.* Mental distress in patient on disopyramide. *Lancet* 1977; **i:** 858–9.
2. Padfield PL, *et al.* Disopyramide and acute psychosis. *Lancet* 1977; **i:** 1152.

Effects on the nervous system. Peripheral neuropathy affecting the feet and severe enough to prevent walking was associated with disopyramide in a 72-year-old patient.[1] There was gradual improvement on withdrawal of disopyramide with the patient being symptom-free after 4 months.

A 75-year-old woman with atrial fibrillation suffered a tonic-clonic seizure followed by respiratory arrest after receiving disopyramide 150 mg intravenously over a period of 10 minutes.[2] On recovery she complained of a dry mouth and blurred vision and it was considered that the seizure was caused by the antimuscarinic action of disopyramide, although it may have been due to a direct stimulant action.

1. Dawkins KD, Gibson J. Peripheral neuropathy with disopyramide. *Lancet* 1978; **i:** 329.
2. Johnson NM, *et al.* Epileptiform convulsion with intravenous disopyramide. *Lancet* 1978; **ii:** 848.

Effects on sexual function. A report of impotence in a patient taking disopyramide which was abolished when the plasma concentration was reduced from 14 to 3 μg per mL.[1] This effect was probably due to the antimuscarinic activity of disopyramide although the patient did not report any other antimuscarinic symptoms such as dry mouth.

1. McHaffie DJ, *et al.* Impotence in patient on disopyramide. *Lancet* 1977; **i:** 859.

Effects on the urinary tract. A report of 9 cases of urinary retention associated with disopyramide therapy and a review of the literature.[1] It was observed that urinary retention secondary to disopyramide therapy was most likely to develop in male patients over the age of 65 in whom there was some pre-existing renal dysfunction: there was an increased risk in patients with evidence of prostatic hyperplasia.

1. Danziger LH, Horn JR. Disopyramide-induced urinary retention. *Arch Intern Med* 1983; **143:** 1683–6.

Hypersensitivity. Worsening of ventricular arrhythmia and an anaphylactoid reaction occurred in a 58-year-old man after a single dose of disopyramide 300 mg by mouth.[1] Two hours after the dose he complained of a swollen tongue and difficulty in breathing. He became cyanotic and was given diphenhydramine 25 mg intravenously, which resulted in improvement of his respiratory status.

1. Porterfield JG, *et al.* Respiratory difficulty after use of disopyramide. *N Engl J Med* 1980; **303:** 584.

Hypoglycaemia. Following reports to the manufacturer of hypoglycaemia associated with administration of disopyramide, 2 controlled studies were conducted in healthy subjects.[1] Disopyramide produced a small decrease in blood-glucose concentration but there were no symptoms of hypoglycaemia. It was considered that the glucose-lowering effect may be clinically significant in patients with renal or hepatic impairment.

1. Strathman I, *et al.* Hypoglycemia in patients receiving disopyramide phosphate. *Drug Intell Clin Pharm* 1983; **17:** 635–8.

Overdosage. A 2-year-old boy suffered hypotension, cardiac arrhythmias, and convulsions and died 28 hours after ingestion of 600 mg of disopyramide.[1] In a report[2] of 5 cases of fatal overdosage with disopyramide the most common clinical finding appeared to be an early loss of consciousness following an episode of respiratory arrest. Four of the patients initially responded to resuscitation but subsequently deteriorated rapidly, with cardiac arrhythmias and loss of spontaneous respiration; in 4 of the cases post-mortem examination demonstrated pulmonary congestion secondary to left ventricular failure.

1. Hutchison A, Kilham H. Fatal overdosage of disopyramide in a child. *Med J Aust* 1978; **2:** 335–6.
2. Hayler AM, *et al.* Fatal overdosage with disopyramide. *Lancet* 1978; **i:** 968–9.

Precautions

Disopyramide is contra-indicated in patients with complete heart block or cardiogenic shock. It should be used with extreme caution in patients with conductive tissue disease or uncompensated heart failure. If disopyramide is used to treat atrial tachycardia it may be necessary to pre-treat with digoxin; see Quinidine, p.939. Hypokalaemia should be corrected before treatment with disopyramide is initiated since the effectiveness of disopyramide may be diminished. Care should be taken in patients susceptible to hypoglycaemia, including those with heart failure, renal or hepatic impairment, and patients taking beta blockers or alcohol.

Intravenous injections of disopyramide should be given slowly to avoid hypotension and it is recommended that facilities for cardiac monitoring and defibrillation should be available when the injection is used.

Dosage reduction may be necessary in patients with renal or hepatic impairment and in patients with heart failure.

Owing to its antimuscarinic properties, disopyramide should be avoided in patients with glaucoma or a tendency to urinary retention, as in benign prostatic hyperplasia, and also in patients with myasthenia gravis due to the risk of precipitating a myasthenic crisis. It should be used with caution in patients with a family history of glaucoma.

For dosage adjustments in the elderly and in patients with abnormal hepatic or renal function, see under Uses and Administration, below.

Breast feeding. Disopyramide is excreted in breast milk and milk to plasma ratios of 0.4, about 0.5, and 0.9 have been reported.[1-3] Disopyramide has been detected in the plasma of breast-fed infants, but was not associated with adverse effects. Disopyramide treatment should not be considered a contra-indication to breast feeding although the infant should be monitored for adverse effects, especially antimuscarinic effects.

1. MacKintosh D, Buchanan N. Excretion of disopyramide in human breast milk. *Br J Clin Pharmacol* 1985; **19:** 856–7.
2. Hoppu K, *et al.* Disopyramide and breast feeding. *Br J Clin Pharmacol* 1986; **21:** 553.
3. Barnett DB, *et al.* Disopyramide and its N-monodesalkyl metabolite in breast milk. *Br J Clin Pharmacol* 1982; **14:** 310–12.

Pregnancy. One patient received disopyramide 200 mg every 8 hours from 26 weeks' gestation until delivery without any adverse effects,[1] but doses of 100 to 300 mg were associated with initiation of uterine contractions in a second patient in week 32 of pregnancy.[2] A double-blind, placebo-controlled study[3] involving 20 women hospitalised for induction of labour confirmed that disopyramide induces uterine contractions. All 10 women given disopyramide 150 mg every 6 hours for 48 hours had initiation of contractions and in 8 delivery was induced. It was considered that disopyramide should not be used as an antiarrhythmic during pregnancy.

1. Shaxted EJ, Milton PJ. Disopyramide in pregnancy: a case report. *Curr Med Res Opin* 1979; **6:** 70–2.
2. Leonard RF, *et al.* Initiation of uterine contractions by disopyramide during pregnancy. *N Engl J Med* 1978; **299:** 84–5.
3. Tadmor OP, *et al.* The effect of disopyramide on uterine contractions during pregnancy. *Am J Obstet Gynecol* 1990; **162:** 482–6.

Interactions

Disopyramide should be used with caution in association with other cardiac depressants including beta blockers and other class I antiarrhythmics. Concomitant use of disopyramide and other antimuscarinic drugs produces enhanced antimuscarinic effects.

Anti-anginals. For reference to disopyramide reducing the effectiveness of sublingual isosorbide dinitrate, see p.893.

Antiarrhythmics. The cardiac depressant effects of disopyramide are additive to those of other class I antiarrhythmic drugs.[1] Brief mention has been made of the prolongation of the QT interval, a factor associated with torsade de pointes, when *amiodarone* and disopyramide were given together.[2] Also the serum concentration of disopyramide has been increased by concurrent administration of *quinidine*;[3] there was a reciprocal decrease in the serum-quinidine concentration but this was less important clinically.

1. Ellrodt G, Singh BN. Adverse effects of disopyramide (Norpace): toxic interactions with other antiarrhythmic agents. *Heart Lung* 1980; **9:** 469–74.
2. Tartini R, *et al.* Dangerous interaction between amiodarone and quinidine. *Lancet* 1982; **i:** 1327–9.
3. Baker BJ, *et al.* Concurrent use of quinidine and disopyramide: evaluation of serum concentrations and electrocardiographic effects. *Am Heart J* 1983; **105:** 12–15.

Antibacterials. The metabolism of disopyramide may be increased by enzyme inducers such as *rifampicin*;[1,2] the increased clearance of disopyramide may lead to subtherapeutic plasma concentrations. Elevation of serum-disopyramide concentrations with ventricular tachycardia occurred[3] in 2 patients when *erythromycin* was added to disopyramide therapy. Ventricular fibrillation developed in a 74-year-old woman 6 days after *clarithromycin* was added to disopyramide therapy.[4] The elimination half-life of disopyramide was found to be markedly prolonged.

1. Aitio M-L, *et al.* The effect of enzyme induction on the metabolism of disopyramide in man. *Br J Clin Pharmacol* 1981; **11:** 279–85.
2. Staum JM. Enzyme induction: rifampin-disopyramide interaction. *DICP Ann Pharmacother* 1990; **24:** 701–3.
3. Ragosta M, *et al.* Potentially fatal interaction between erythromycin and disopyramide. *Am J Med* 1989; **86:** 465–6.
4. Paar D, *et al.* Life-threatening interaction between clarithromycin and disopyramide. *Lancet* 1997; **349:** 326–7.

Antiepileptics. The enzyme inducers *phenytoin*[1] and *phenobarbitone* may increase the clearance of disopyramide.

1. Aitio M-L, *et al.* The effect of enzyme induction on the metabolism of disopyramide in man. *Br J Clin Pharmacol* 1981; **11:** 279–85.

Beta blockers. Bradycardia,[1,2] severe hypotension,[1] and asystole,[1] with one fatality,[1] have been reported following the intravenous injection of disopyramide 20 minutes after intravenous *practolol*. Both drugs have negative inotropic effects which are additive when they are administered in close succession, but separation of the drugs by 2 hours prevented the development of these adverse effects.[2] A pharmacokinetic interaction may also occur with beta blockers since the clearance of disopyramide has been reported[3] to be reduced by approximately 16% during concomitant treatment with *atenolol*.

1. Cumming AD, Robertson C. Interaction between disopyramide and practolol. *Br Med J* 1979; **2:** 1264.
2. Gelipter D, Hazell M. Interaction between disopyramide and practolol. *Br Med J* 1980; **280:** 52.
3. Bonde J, *et al.* Atenolol inhibits the elimination of disopyramide. *Eur J Clin Pharmacol* 1985; **28:** 41–3.

Pharmacokinetics

Disopyramide is readily and almost completely absorbed from the gastro-intestinal tract, peak plasma concentrations being attained about 0.5 to 3 hours after oral administration.

Disopyramide is partially metabolised in the liver; the major metabolite is mono-*N*-dealkylated disopyramide which retains some antiarrhythmic and antimuscarinic activity. The major route of excretion is through the kidney, approximately 50% as the unchanged drug, 20% as the *N*-dealkylated metabolite, and 10% as other metabolites. About 10% is excreted in the faeces. The clearance of disopyramide does not appear to be influenced by urinary pH.

The therapeutic plasma concentration range is generally accepted as 2 to 6 μg per mL. Within this range, protein binding is reported to be 50 to 65%, but the degree of binding varies with the plasma concentration and this limits the usefulness of plasma concentration monitoring as a guide to therapy. Estimations of the plasma half-life of disopyramide range from about 4 to 10 hours. The half-life is increased in renal and hepatic impairment, and in cardiac failure.

Disopyramide crosses the placental barrier and is distributed into breast milk.

Reviews.

1. Siddoway LA, Woosley RL. Clinical pharmacokinetics of disopyramide. *Clin Pharmacokinet* 1986; **11:** 214–22.

Metabolism. Mono-*N*-dealkylated disopyramide, the major metabolite of disopyramide, produced no substantial cardiac effects after a single dose in healthy subjects, but produced greater antimuscarinic effects than disopyramide.[1]

1. Chiang W-T, *et al.* Kinetics and dynamics of disopyramide and its dealkylated metabolite in healthy subjects. *Clin Pharmacol Ther* 1985; **38:** 37–44.

Protein binding. The binding of disopyramide to plasma proteins shows considerable interindividual variation[1,2] and is concentration-dependent[2,3] with the unbound fraction increasing with rising plasma-disopyramide concentrations. Disopyramide is bound mostly to alpha-1-acid glycoprotein, for which it has a high affinity, but there is also a second low-affinity binding site which may be on albumin.[1,2] Increased plasma concentrations of alpha-1-acid glycoprotein are associated with increased binding of disopyramide;[3] significantly reduced protein binding of disopyramide is observed in Chinese subjects[4] compared with Caucasians and this is consistent with a lower concentration of alpha-1-acid glycoprotein in Chinese people. Age also affects the protein binding of disopyramide[3] with reduced binding in neonates and increased binding in geriatric patients compared with healthy adults. Decreased protein binding during the third trimester of pregnancy with increased binding one month postpartum has been reported[5] and correlates with the changes in the plasma concentration of alpha-1-acid glycoprotein during pregnancy.

1. David BM, *et al.* Plasma binding of disopyramide. *Br J Clin Pharmacol* 1980; **9:** 614–18.
2. Giacomini KM, Blaschke TF. Effect of concentration-dependent binding to plasma proteins on the pharmacokinetics and pharmacodynamics of disopyramide. *Clin Pharmacokinet* 1984; **9** (suppl 1): 42–8.
3. Holt DW, *et al.* Effect of age and plasma concentrations of albumin and α_1-acid glycoprotein on protein binding of disopyramide. *Br J Clin Pharmacol* 1983; **16:** 344–5.
4. Zhou H-H, *et al.* Differences in plasma binding of drugs between caucasians and Chinese subjects. *Clin Pharmacol Ther* 1990; **48:** 10–17.
5. Echizen H, *et al.* Plasma protein binding of disopyramide in pregnant and postpartum women, and in neonates and their mothers. *Br J Clin Pharmacol* 1990; **29:** 423–30.

Uses and Administration

Disopyramide is a class Ia antiarrhythmic (p.776) with a depressant action on the heart similar to that of quinidine (p.940). It also has antimuscarinic and negative inotropic properties.

Disopyramide is used in the management of supraventricular and ventricular **arrhythmias** (p.782).

It may be given by mouth as either the base or the phosphate or intravenously as the phosphate; doses are expressed in terms of the base. The usual oral dose is 300 to 800 mg daily in divided doses adjusted according to the patient's response. A modified-release preparation can be used, enabling 12-hourly dosage intervals. A maximum daily dose of 800 mg should not usually be exceeded. An initial loading dose of 200 to 300 mg may be given.

Disopyramide may be given by slow intravenous injection in a dose of 2 mg per kg body-weight to a maximum of 150 mg, at a rate not exceeding 30 mg per minute, followed by 200 mg by mouth immediately on completion of the injection and every 8 hours for 24 hours with subsequent maintenance doses usually in the range of 500 to 750 mg daily; if the arrhythmia recurs on completion of the intravenous injection it may be repeated, but a total intravenous dose of 4 mg per kg (maximum, 300 mg) should not be exceeded in the first hour, nor should the total by both intravenous and oral routes exceed 800 mg in 24 hours. Alternatively, the initial intravenous injection may be followed by intravenous infusion of 0.4 mg per kg per hour (or 20 to 30 mg per hour) to a maximum of 800 mg daily. Patients receiving disopyramide intravenously or in high oral doses should be monitored by ECG.

Dosage reduction may be necessary in patients with hepatic or renal impairment. Doses should also be adjusted in patients with heart failure to compensate for the prolonged half-life.

An optimum dosage regimen for children has not been fully established, but the following oral doses have been used: under 1 year, 10 to 30 mg per kg body-weight per day; age 1 to 4 years, 10 to 20 mg per kg per day; age 4 to 12 years, 10 to 15 mg per kg per day; age 12 to 18 years, 6 to 15 mg per kg per day.

Reviews.

1. Brogden RN, Todd PA. Disopyramide: a reappraisal of its pharmacodynamic and pharmacokinetic properties, and therapeutic use in cardiac arrhythmias. *Drugs* 1987; **34:** 151–87.

Action. A study in 6 patients with atrial flutter suggesting that the antiarrhythmic activity of racemic disopyramide resides in the S(+)-enantiomer.[1]

1. Lima JJ, *et al.* Antiarrhythmic activity and unbound concentrations of disopyramide enantiomers in patients. *Ther Drug Monit* 1990; **12:** 23–8.

Administration in the elderly. The clearance of disopyramide was reduced in elderly non-smoking patients compared with young subjects, but the reduction was less marked in elderly patients who smoked more than 20 cigarettes daily.[1] It was recommended that the dose of disopyramide should be reduced by approximately 30% in elderly non-smokers.

See also under Protein Binding in Pharmacokinetics, above.

1. Bonde J, *et al.* The influence of age and smoking on the elimination of disopyramide. *Br J Clin Pharmacol* 1985; **20:** 453–8.

Administration in hepatic impairment. Dosage reduction should be considered for patients with liver impairment who demonstrate prolonged disopyramide plasma half-lives. Also the plasma concentration of alpha-1-acid glycoprotein is significantly reduced in patients with liver cirrhosis[1,2] and its binding capacity for disopyramide is reduced.[1] This is associated with an increase in the free fraction of disopyramide such that measurement of total disopyramide in plasma may not be a safe indicator for dosing, and a therapeutic range 50% lower than in patients with normal hepatic function should be considered.[2]

1. Bonde J, *et al.* Kinetics of disopyramide in decreased hepatic function. *Eur J Clin Pharmacol* 1986; **31:** 73–7.
2. Echizen H, *et al.* Protein binding of disopyramide in liver cirrhosis and in nephrotic syndrome. *Clin Pharmacol Ther* 1986; **40:** 274–80.

Administration in renal impairment. Disopyramide is excreted mainly in the urine and alterations in its pharmacokinetics might be expected in renal impairment. A significant reduction in disopyramide clearance with an increase in elimination half-life has been observed[1] in patients with chronic renal failure and dosage reductions are generally recommended if creatinine clearance is less than 40 to 60 mL per minute. Patients with a creatinine clearance less than 40 mL per minute should not be given modified-release preparations of disopyramide.

At therapeutic concentrations disopyramide is not significantly removed by haemodialysis;[2] the half-life is similar both on and off dialysis (16.8 versus 16.1 hours). An increased free fraction of disopyramide has been observed[3] during haemodialysis associated with an elevation in free fatty acids in plasma and in such cases free plasma-disopyramide concentrations should be monitored.

1. Francois B, *et al.* Pharmacokinetics of disopyramide in patients with chronic renal failure. *Eur J Drug Metab Pharmacokinet* 1983; **8:** 85–92.
2. Sevka MJ, *et al.* Disopyramide hemodialysis and kinetics in patients requiring long-term hemodialysis. *Clin Pharmacol Ther* 1981; **29:** 322–6.
3. Horiuchi T, *et al.* Inhibitory effect of free fatty acids on plasma protein binding of disopyramide in haemodialysis patients. *Eur J Clin Pharmacol* 1989; **36:** 175–80.

Hypotension. Disopyramide is reported to be one of the standard drugs used in the management of neurally mediated hypotension (p.790).

Preparations

BP 1998: Disopyramide Capsules; Disopyramide Phosphate Capsules;
USP 23: Disopyramide Phosphate Capsules; Disopyramide Phosphate Extended-release Capsules.

Proprietary Preparations (details are given in Part 3)
Aust.: Rythmodan; ***Austral.:*** Norpace; Rythmodan; ***Belg.:*** Dirytmin; Rythmodan; ***Canad.:*** Norpace; Rythmodan; ***Fr.:*** Isorythm; Rythmodan; ***Ger.:*** Diso-Duriles; Disonorm; Norpace; Rythmodul; ***Irl.:*** Dirythmin†; Rythmodan; ***Ital.:*** Ritmodan; ***Neth.:*** Dirytmin; Ritmoforine; Rythmodan; ***Norw.:*** Dirytmin†; Durbis; ***S.Afr.:*** Norpace; Rythmodan; ***Spain:*** Dicorynan; ***Swed.:*** Dirytmin; Durbis; ***Switz.:*** Norpace; ***UK:*** Dirythmin; Isomide; Rythmodan; ***USA:*** Norpace.

Ditazole (2639-d)

Ditazole *(rINN)*.

Diethamphenazole; S-222. 2,2′-[(4,5-Diphenyloxazol-2-yl)imino]diethanol.

$C_{19}H_{20}N_2O_3$ = 324.4.

CAS — 18471-20-0.

Ditazole is an inhibitor of platelet aggregation used in the management of thrombo-embolic disorders (p.801) in doses of 400 mg two or three times daily by mouth.

Preparations

Proprietary Preparations (details are given in Part 3)
Ital.: Ageroplas†; ***Spain:*** Ageroplas.

Dobutamine Hydrochloride (2052-t)

Dobutamine Hydrochloride *(BANM, USAN, rINNM)*.

46236; Compound 81929 (dobutamine); Dobutamini Hydrochloridum; LY-174008 (dobutamine tartrate). (±)-4-{2-[3-(4-Hydroxyphenyl)-1-methylpropylamino]ethyl}pyrocatechol hydrochloride; (±)-4-{2-[3-(4-Hydroxyphenyl)-1-methylpropylamino]ethyl}benzene-1,2-diol hydrochloride.

$C_{18}H_{23}NO_3,HCl$ = 337.8.

CAS — 34368-04-2 (dobutamine); 49745-95-1 (dobutamine hydrochloride); 101626-66-8 (dobutamine tartrate).

Pharmacopoeias. In *Chin., Eur.* (see p.viii), *Jpn*, and *US.*

A white to practically white, crystalline powder. Sparingly **soluble** in water; the Ph. Eur. states that it is sparingly soluble in alcohol and soluble in methyl alcohol, the USP states the reverse. **Store** at 15° to 30° in airtight containers. Protect from light.

Incompatibility. Dobutamine is incompatible with alkaline solutions such as sodium bicarbonate 5% and alkaline drugs such as aminophylline, frusemide, and thiopentone sodium; the manufacturers also suggest that it is physically incompatible with bumetanide, calcium gluconate, insulin, diazepam, and phenytoin, and incompatibility with heparin has also been reported.

References to the stability and compatibility of dobutamine infusions.[1-3]

1. Lee CY, *et al.* Visual and spectrophotometric determination of compatibility of alteplase and streptokinase with other injectable drugs. *Am J Hosp Pharm* 1990; **47:** 606–8.
2. Yamashita SK, *et al.* Compatibility of selected critical care drugs during simulated Y-site administration. *Am J Health-Syst Pharm* 1996; **53:** 1048–51.
3. Chiu MF, Schwartz ML. Visual compatibility of injectable drugs used in the intensive care unit. *Am J Health-Syst Pharm* 1997; **54:** 64–5.

Adverse Effects

The principal adverse effects of dobutamine are dose-related increases in heart rate and blood pressure, ectopic beats, angina or chest pain, and palpitations; dosage should be reduced or temporarily stopped if they occur. Ventricular tachycardia may occur rarely. Other adverse effects that have occurred occasionally include hypotension, dyspnoea, paraesthesias, headache, nausea and vomiting, and leg cramps.

For the adverse effects of sympathomimetics in general, see Adrenaline, p.813.

For reference to fatalities occurring in patients given dobutamine, see Heart Failure in Uses and Administration, below.

Effects on body temperature. A 71-year-old woman with heart failure developed a fever on 2 separate occasions 8 to 12 hours after starting an infusion of dobutamine.[1]

1. Robison-Strane SR, Bubik JS. Dobutamine-induced fever. *Ann Pharmacother* 1992; **26:** 1523–4.

Effects on the heart. For reference to severe cardiovascular complications of dobutamine stress echocardiography, see Diagnosis and Testing, below.

Effects on the skin. A report of troublesome pruritus of the scalp associated with dobutamine infusion.[1]

1. McCauley CS, Blumenthal MS. Dobutamine and pruritus of the scalp. *Ann Intern Med* 1986; **105:** 966.

Hypersensitivity. There has been a report[1] of redness, swelling, itching and a sensation of warmth around the site of infusion of dobutamine in one patient. These symptoms recurred when the infusion was given again one week later.

1. Cernek PK. Dermal cellulitis—a hypersensitivity reaction from dobutamine hydrochloride. *Ann Pharmacother* 1994; **28:** 964.

Overdosage. A report has been published describing an accidental overdose of dobutamine.[1] The patient received a dobutamine intravenous infusion at a rate of more than 130 μg per kg body-weight per minute for 30 minutes, this being three times the recommended maximum. Characteristic side-effects of dobutamine such as emesis, palpitations, chest pain, dyspnoea, and paraesthesia did develop together with urinary incontinence, an effect not previously associated with dobutamine.

1. Paulman PM, *et al.* Dobutamine overdose. *JAMA* 1990; **264:** 2386–7.

Precautions

For precautions to be observed with sympathomimetics in general, see Adrenaline, p.814.

Dobutamine hydrochloride should be avoided or used only with great caution in patients with marked obstruction of cardiac ejection, such as idiopathic hypertrophic subaortic stenosis. It should also be used with caution in patients with acute myocardial infarction, and in cardiogenic shock complicated by severe hypotension. Hypovolaemia should be corrected before treatment.

Interference with diagnostic tests. Contamination of blood samples with dobutamine has been reported to produce falsely decreased creatinine values in an enzymatic test.[1] Colorimetric measurements of creatinine were not affected.

1. Daly TM, *et al.* "Bouncing" creatinine levels. *N Engl J Med* 1996; **334:** 1749–50.

Interactions

Although it is less likely than adrenaline to produce ventricular arrhythmias, dobutamine should be used with extreme caution during anaesthesia with cyclopropane, halothane, and other volatile anaesthetics. The inotropic effects of dobutamine on the heart are reversed by beta blockade, and there may then be vasoconstriction and an increase in blood pressure due to dopamine's alpha agonist effects.

For the interactions of sympathomimetics in general, see Adrenaline, p.814.

Pharmacokinetics

Like adrenaline (p.815), dobutamine is inactive when given by mouth, and it is rapidly inactivated in the body by similar processes. It has a half-life of about 2 minutes. Conjugates of dobutamine and its major metabolite 3-*O*-methyldobutamine are excreted primarily in urine, with small amounts eliminated in the faeces.

The primary mechanism of clearance of dobutamine appears to be distribution to other tissues, and not metabolism or elimination. It has a half-life of about 2 minutes and plasma concentrations of dobutamine reach steady-state about 10 to 12 minutes after the start of an infusion. Dobutamine is used mainly for the short-term treatment of heart failure and any pharmacokinetic changes in this condition have no clinical implications in dosage titration.[1]

Steinberg and Notterman reviewed the pharmacokinetics of dobutamine and other cardiovascular drugs in children[2] and considered that further study was required to explain the different findings that had been reported.

1. Shammas FV, Dickstein K. Clinical pharmacokinetics in heart failure: an updated review. *Clin Pharmacokinet* 1988; **15:** 94–113.
2. Steinberg C, Notterman DA. Pharmacokinetics of cardiovascular drugs in children: inotropes and vasopressors. *Clin Pharmacokinet* 1994; **27:** 345–67.

Uses and Administration

Dobutamine is a sympathomimetic (see Adrenaline, p.815) with direct effects on $beta_1$-adrenergic receptors, which confer upon it a prominent inotropic action on the heart. It also has some alpha and $beta_2$-agonist properties. Dobutamine differs from dopamine in not having the specific dopaminergic properties of dopamine which induce renal mesenteric vasodilatation. However, like dopamine, the inotropic action of dobutamine on the heart is associated with less cardiac-accelerating effect than that of isoprenaline.

Dobutamine is used to increase the contractility of the heart in acute heart failure, as occurs in cardiogenic shock (p.798) and myocardial infarction (p.791); it is also used in septic shock. Other circumstances in which its inotropic activity may be useful are during cardiac surgery and positive end-expiratory pressure ventilation (PEEP).

Dobutamine is given as the hydrochloride but doses are expressed in terms of the base. It is administered by intravenous infusion as a dilute solution (0.25 to 5 mg per mL), in glucose 5% or sodium chloride 0.9%; other fluids may also be suitable and the manufacturers' guidelines should be consulted.

In the management of **acute heart failure**, dobutamine is given at a usual rate of 2.5 to 10 μg per kg body-weight per minute, according to the patient's heart rate, blood pressure, cardiac output, and urine output. A range of 0.5 up to 40 μg per kg per minute has occasionally been required. It has been recommended that treatment with dobutamine should be discontinued gradually.

Dobutamine is also employed as an alternative to exercise in **cardiac stress testing**. A solution containing 1 mg per mL is employed for this purpose, administered via an infusion pump. A dose of 5 μg per kg per minute is infused for 8 minutes; the dose is then increased by increments of 5 μg per kg per minute up to a maximum of 20 μg per kg per minute, with each dose being infused for 8 minutes before the next incremental increase. The ECG should be monitored continuously and the infusion terminated if arrhythmias, marked ST segment depression, or other adverse effects occur.

General references.

1. Majerus TC, *et al.* Dobutamine: ten years later. *Pharmacotherapy* 1989; **9:** 245–59.

Action. *Animal* studies show that the ability of dobutamine to stimulate $alpha_1$- and $beta_2$-adrenergic receptors appears to be as great as its $beta_1$-stimulant properties, and it has been proposed that the inotropic action results from a combination of alpha-stimulant activity on myocardial $alpha_1$ receptors, a property residing mainly in the (−)-enantiomer, with $beta_1$ stimulation by the (+)-enantiomer; peripherally, alpha-mediated vasoconstriction would be opposed by the $beta_2$-agonist properties of the (+)-enantiomer, resulting in the net inotropic action with relatively little effect on blood pressure seen with the racemic mixture used clinically.[1]

Dobutamine has a thermogenic effect,[2] but using it to increase oxygen delivery and consumption and the cardiac index in critically ill patients did not improve patient outcome and in some cases might have been harmful.[3]

1. Ruffolo RR. The mechanism of action of dobutamine. *Ann Intern Med* 1984; **100:** 313–14.
2. Bhatt SB, *et al.* Effect of dobutamine on oxygen supply and uptake in healthy volunteers. *Br J Anaesth* 1992; **69:** 298–303.
3. Hayes MA, *et al.* Elevation of systemic oxygen delivery in the treatment of critically ill patients. *N Engl J Med* 1994; **330:** 1717–22.

Cardiac surgery. Dobutamine and dopamine are each used for inotropic support in patients undergoing cardiac surgery. A comparison in children[1] suggests that dobutamine may be preferred to dopamine since the latter could cause pulmonary vasoconstriction.

1. Booker PD, *et al.* Comparison of the haemodynamic effects of dopamine and dobutamine in young children undergoing cardiac surgery. *Br J Anaesth* 1995; **74:** 419–23.

Diagnosis and testing. Dynamic exercise is the established mode of stress for the assessment of cardiac function. In patients who are unable to exercise, a dobutamine infusion is the best alternative way of producing a stress.[1] Dobutamine stress echocardiography, which can often involve the additional administration of atropine, has been reported to be more sensitive and better tolerated than adenosine or dipyridamole stress echocardiography.[2] It might also have a useful prognostic role.[3-5] However there have been instances of severe cardiovascular complications attributable to dobutamine.[6-8]

1. Nihoyannopoulos P. Stress echocardiography. *Br J Hosp Med* 1997; **57:** 31–5.
2. Martin TW, *et al.* Comparison of adenosine, dipyridamole, and dobutamine in stress echocardiography. *Ann Intern Med* 1992; **116:** 190–6.
3. Poldermans D, *et al.* Dobutamine-atropine stress echocardiography and clinical data for predicting late cardiac events in patients with suspected coronary artery disease. *Am J Med* 1994; **97:** 119–25.
4. Cigarroa CG, *et al.* Dobutamine stress echocardiography identifies hibernating myocardium and predicts recovery of left ventricular function after coronary revascularization. *Circulation* 1993; **88:** 430–6.
5. Elhendy A, *et al.* Relation between ST segment elevation during dobutamine stress test and myocardial viability after a recent myocardial infarction. *Heart* 1997; **77:** 115–21.
6. Picano E, *et al.* Safety and tolerability of dobutamine-atropine stress echocardiography: a prospective, multicentre study. *Lancet* 1994; **344:** 1190–2.
7. Mathew J, *et al.* Transmural myocardial ischaemia during dobutamine stress echocardiography. *Lancet* 1995; **346:** 383–4.
8. Reisenhofer B, *et al.* Cardiac rupture during dobutamine stress test. *Ann Intern Med* 1998; **128:** 605.

Heart failure. Dobutamine may be used in the management of acute heart failure, as discussed under Shock, p.798. It may also have a role as a bridge to transplantation in patients with severe chronic heart failure (p.785). In less severe cases, conflicting results have been reported. Adamopoulos *et al.*,[1] for example, reported that pulsed therapy with dobutamine (30 minutes daily for 4 days each week for 3 weeks) could produce similar improvements to those achieved with exercise. However, sudden death occurred in patients receiving dobutamine as infusions for 48 hours per week, and one study[2] was halted for this reason.

1. Adamopoulos S, *et al.* Effects of pulsed β-stimulant therapy on β-adrenoceptors and chronotropic responsiveness in chronic heart failure. *Lancet* 1995; **345:** 344–9.
2. Dies F, *et al.* Intermittent dobutamine in ambulatory outpatients with chronic cardiac failure. *Circulation* 1986; **74:** (suppl II): 38.

Preparations

USP 23: Dobutamine for Injection; Dobutamine Injection.

Proprietary Preparations (details are given in Part 3)
Aust.: Dobutrex; ***Austral.:*** Dobutrex; ***Belg.:*** Dobutrex; ***Canad.:*** Dobutrex; ***Fr.:*** Dobutrex; ***Ger.:*** Dobutrex; ***Irl.:*** Dobutrex; Posiject; ***Ital.:*** Dobutrex; ***Neth.:*** Dobutrex; ***Norw.:*** Dobutrex; ***S.Afr.:*** Dobutrex; ***Spain:*** Dobutrex; ***Swed.:*** Dobuject; Dobutrex; ***Switz.:*** Dobutrex; ***UK:*** Dobutrex; Posiject; ***USA:*** Dobutrex.

Docarpamine (6470-d)

Docarpamine *(rINN)*.

TA-870. (−)-(*S*)-2-Acetamido-*N*-(3,4-dihydroxyphenethyl)-4-(methylthio)butyramide bis(ethyl carbonate) ester.

$C_{21}H_{30}N_2O_8S$ = 470.5.

CAS — 74639-40-0.

Docarpamine is an orally active prodrug of dopamine (p.861) that is used in the treatment of acute heart failure. The usual dose is 2.25 g of docarpamine daily by mouth, in 3 divided doses.

References.

1. Nishizaki S, *et al.* Acute effects of an orally active dopamine prodrug (TA-870) on systemic haemodynamics and renal functions. *Drug Invest* 1991; **3:** 118–25.

Preparations

Proprietary Preparations (details are given in Part 3)
Jpn: Tanadopa.

Dofetilide (10888-k)

Dofetilide *(BAN, USAN, rINN)*.

UK-68798. β-[(*p*-Methanesulfonamidophenethyl)methyl-amino]methanesulfono-*p*-phenetidide.

$C_{19}H_{27}N_3O_5S_2$ = 441.6.

CAS — 115256-11-6.

Dofetilide is a class III antiarrhythmic (p.776) under investigation.

References.

1. Tham TCK, *et al.* Pharmacodynamics and pharmacokinetics of the novel class III antiarrhythmic drug UK-68,798 in man. *Br J Clin Pharmacol* 1991; **31:** 243P–244P.
2. Crijns HJGM, *et al.* Atrial flutter can be terminated by a class III antiarrhythmic drug but not by a class 1C drug. *Eur Heart J* 1994; **15:** 1403–8.
3. Bashir Y, *et al.* Electrophysiologic profile and efficacy of intravenous dofetilide (UK-68,798), a new class III antiarrhythmic drug, in patients with sustained monomorphic ventricular tachycardia. *Am J Cardiol* 1995; **76:** 1040–44.

Dopamine Hydrochloride (2053-x)

Dopamine Hydrochloride *(BANM, USAN, pINNM)*.

ASL-279; Dopamini Hydrochloridum; 3-Hydroxytyramine Hydrochloride. 4-(2-Aminoethyl)pyrocatechol hydrochloride; 4-(2-Aminoethyl)benzene-1,2-diol hydrochloride.

$C_8H_{11}NO_2$,HCl = 189.6.

CAS — 51-61-6 (dopamine); 62-31-7 (dopamine hydrochloride).

Pharmacopoeias. In *Chin., Eur.* (see p.viii), *Int., Jpn,* and *US.*

A white or almost white crystalline powder. Freely **soluble** in water and in solutions of alkali hydroxides; soluble in alcohol and in methyl alcohol; sparingly soluble in acetone and in dichloromethane; practically insoluble in ether and in chloroform. A 4% solution has a pH of between 3.0 and 5.5. **Store** in airtight containers. Protect from light.

Incompatibility. Dopamine is inactivated in alkaline solutions such as sodium bicarbonate 5% and is incompatible with alkaline drugs such as frusemide and thiopentone sodium; incompatibility with insulin has also been reported, and the manufacturers state that it is incompatible with ampicillin and with amphotericin, and that mixtures with gentamicin sulphate, cephalothin sodium, or oxacillin sodium should be avoided.

References to the stability and incompatibility of dopamine infusions.[1-3]

1. Lee CY, *et al.* Visual and spectrophotometric determination of compatibility of alteplase and streptokinase with other injectable drugs. *Am J Hosp Pharm* 1990; **47:** 606–8.
2. Yamashita SK, *et al.* Compatibility of selected critical care drugs during simulated Y-site administration. *Am J Health-Syst Pharm* 1996; **53:** 1048–51.
3. Chiu MF, Schwartz ML. Visual compatibility of injectable drugs used in the intensive care unit. *Am J Health-Syst Pharm* 1997; **54:** 64–5.

Adverse Effects

The most common adverse effects of dopamine infusion are ectopic beats, tachycardia, anginal pain, palpitations, hypotension, vasoconstriction, nausea and vomiting, headache, and dyspnoea. More rarely, bradycardia and cardiac conduction abnormalities, piloerection, and raised BUN have been reported; hypertension has occurred, particularly in overdosage. Extravasation may lead to tissue necrosis and sloughing.

For the adverse effects of sympathomimetics in general, see Adrenaline, p.813.

Effects on the endocrine system. Dopamine infusion, even at low doses (2.5 µg per kg body-weight per minute) was found to decrease serum concentrations of prolactin in critically ill patients.[1] This was considered undesirable because of the immunomodulatory role of prolactin in the endocrine response to stress.

1. Bailey AR, Burchett KR. Effect of low-dose dopamine on serum concentrations of prolactin in critically ill patients. *Br J Anaesth* 1997; **78:** 97–9.

Effects on the heart. For mention of the arrhythmogenic effects of dopamine on the heart, see p.814.

Ischaemia and gangrene. Ischaemia and gangrene has been reported on several occasions following dopamine infusions.[1-4] Dopamine is converted to noradrenaline which is a known powerful vasoconstrictor and is also noted to be associated with vascular problems if extravasation occurs.

1. Alexander CS, *et al.* Pedal gangrene associated with the use of dopamine. *N Engl J Med* 1975; **293:** 591.
2. Julka NK, Nora JR. Gangrene aggravation after use of dopamine. *JAMA* 1976; **253:** 2812–13.
3. Boltax RS, *et al.* Gangrene resulting from infiltrated dopamine solution. *N Engl J Med* 1977; **296:** 823.
4. Maggi JC, *et al.* Gangrene in a neonate following dopamine therapy. *J Pediatr* 1982; **100:** 323–5.

Treatment of Adverse Effects

Since the half-life of dopamine is only about 2 minutes most adverse effects can be corrected by discontinuing or reducing the rate of infusion. If these measures fail excessive vasoconstriction and hypertension may be treated with an alpha-adrenoceptor blocking agent such as phentolamine mesylate intravenously.

Relief from tissue necrosis and pain due to extravasation may be produced by immediate infiltration with phentolamine as described under Noradrenaline, p.924.

Topical glyceryl trinitrate ointment has been used successfully to improve capillary blood flow in patients with dopamine-induced ischaemia of the digits.[1,2]

1. Gibbs NM, Oh TE. Nitroglycerine ointment for dopamine induced peripheral digital ischaemia. *Lancet* 1983; **ii:** 290.
2. Coakley J. Nitroglycerin ointment for dopamine-induced peripheral ischaemia. *Lancet* 1983; **ii:** 633.

Precautions

Dopamine should not be used in patients with phaeochromocytoma or hyperthyroidism, nor in the presence of uncorrected tachyarrhythmias or ventricular fibrillation. Care is required and low doses should be used in patients with shock secondary to myocardial infarction. Patients with a history of peripheral vascular disease are at increased risk of ischaemia of the extremities. Hypovolaemia should be corrected before beginning dopamine infusion.

For precautions to be observed with sympathomimetics in general, see Adrenaline, p.814.

Dependence. There may be difficulty in weaning patients off dopamine. For example, there has been a report of a patient with intra-abdominal sepsis who received dopamine in an intensive care unit.[1] When attempts were made to withdraw dopamine, hypotension resulted. Withdrawal of dopamine was made possible by substitution with ibopamine, a dopamine agonist.

1. Milner AR, *et al.* Ibopamine substitution in a dopamine-dependent patient. *Lancet* 1993; **342:** 1555.

Interactions

Although it is less likely than adrenaline to produce ventricular arrhythmias, dopamine should be used with extreme caution during anaesthesia with cyclopropane, halothane, and other volatile anaesthetics. In patients treated with MAOIs, the dose of dopamine should be reduced substantially; a suggested starting dose is one tenth of the usual dose.

For the interactions of sympathomimetics in general, see Adrenaline, p.814.

Antiepileptics. Following a report in 1976 to the FDA by Rapp of hypotension in patients given *phenytoin* in addition to dopamine infusion, Smith and Lomas[1] studied the potential interaction, and found that dopamine given by intravenous infusion concomitantly with phenytoin infusion to *dogs*, did not alter the CNS effects of phenytoin nor result in hypotension and cardiovascular collapse. Large doses of phenytoin alone had a reproducible hypotensive effect which was reduced by dopamine, suggesting a possible supportive role in phenytoin-induced hypotension.

1. Smith RD, Lomas TE. Modification of cardiovascular responses to intravenous phenytoin by dopamine in dogs: evidence against an adverse interaction. *Toxicol Appl Pharmacol* 1978; **45:** 665–73.

Vasodilators. Fatal hypotension occurred in a man given *tolazoline* in addition to dopamine.[1]

1. Carlon GC. Fatal association of tolazoline and dopamine. *Chest* 1979; **76:** 336.

Pharmacokinetics

The vasoconstrictor properties of dopamine preclude its administration by subcutaneous or intramuscular administration. Like adrenaline (p.815) it is inactive when given by mouth, and it is rapidly inactivated in the body by similar processes, with a half-life of about 2 minutes. Dopamine is a metabolic precursor of noradrenaline and a proportion is excreted as the metabolic products of noradrenaline. Nevertheless, the majority appears to be directly metabolised into dopamine-related metabolic products.

References.

1. Banner W, *et al.* Nonlinear dopamine pharmacokinetics in pediatric patients. *J Pharmacol Exp Ther* 1989; **249:** 131–3.
2. Padbury JF, *et al.* Pharmacokinetics of dopamine in critically ill newborn infants. *J Pediatr* 1990; **117:** 472–6.
3. Notterman DA, *et al.* Dopamine clearance in critically ill infants and children: effect of age and organ system dysfunction. *Clin Pharmacol Ther* 1990; **48:** 138–47.
4. Bhatt-Mehta V, *et al.* Dopamine pharmacokinetics in critically ill newborn infants. *Eur J Clin Pharmacol* 1991; **40:** 593–7.
5. Steinberg C, Notterman DA. Pharmacokinetics of cardiovascular drugs in children: inotropes and vasopressors. *Clin Pharmacokinet* 1994; **27:** 345–67.

Uses and Administration

The catecholamine, dopamine, is a sympathomimetic (see Adrenaline, p.815) with both direct and indirect effects. It is formed in the body by the decarboxylation of levodopa, and is both a neurotransmitter in its own right (notably in the brain) and a precursor of noradrenaline. Dopamine differs from adrenaline and noradrenaline in dilating renal and mesenteric blood vessels and increasing urine output, apparently by a specific dopaminergic mechanism. This effect is predominant at low infusion rates (about 2 µg per kg body-weight per minute); at slightly higher infusion rates (around 2 to 10 µg per kg per minute) it also stimulates $beta_1$-adrenergic receptors in the myocardium, and at 10 to 20 µg per kg per minute the effects of alpha adrenergic stimulation predominate, such as vasoconstriction. The inotropic action of dopamine on the heart is associated with less cardiac-accelerating effect, and a lower incidence of arrhythmias, than that of isoprenaline.

Dopamine also inhibits release of prolactin from the anterior pituitary.

Dopamine is used in acute heart failure, as occurs in cardiogenic shock (p.798) and myocardial infarction (p.791); it is also employed in renal failure, in cardiac surgery, and in septic shock.

Dopamine is administered as the hydrochloride by intravenous infusion as a dilute solution (usually 1.6 or 3.2 mg per mL, although more dilute solutions may be used where fluid expansion is not a problem), in glucose 5%, sodium chloride 0.9%, or other suitable diluents; many fluids are suitable and the manufacturers' data sheets or literature should be consulted. The initial rate is 2 to 5 µg per kg body-weight per minute, gradually increased by 5 to 10 µg per kg per minute according to the patient's blood pressure, cardiac output, and urine output. Up to 20 to 50 µg per kg per minute may be required in seriously ill patients; higher doses have been given. A reduction in urine flow, without hypotension, may indicate a need to reduce the dose. To avoid tissue necrosis dopamine is best administered into a large vein high up in a limb, preferably the arm. It has been recommended that on gradual discontinuation of dopamine care should be taken to avoid undue hypotension associated with very low dosage levels where vasodilatation could predominate.

Concentrations of dopamine are reduced in the brains of patients with parkinsonism; increased brain-dopamine concentrations are accordingly beneficial in this condition. In practice, as dopamine is not active by mouth and does not readily cross the blood-brain barrier, its precursor, levodopa is given for treatment. For the use of dopaminergics in parkinsonism, see p.1128.

Surgery and intensive care. As well as being used for its inotropic effect in cardiac surgery dopamine has been given in low doses for renal protection in patients at risk, such as those undergoing major surgery or in intensive care. It has recently been pointed out[1] that there is little evidence of the value of this use of dopamine as a renal protectant. This view was prompted by a small study[2] that found no renal benefit in patients given dopamine after major vascular surgery but the possibility of an increased incidence of myocardial infarction. There is also uncertainty about the benefits of dopamine infusion as a treatment for acute renal failure:[3] subgroup analysis of data from a study of the effects of atrial natriuretic peptide in acute tubular necrosis was unable to demonstrate convincing evidence for improved survival or a reduced need for dialysis associated with dopamine therapy.[4] It seems to be generally agreed that controlled studies of the role of dopamine are overdue.[3,5,6]

1. Thompson BT, Cockrill BA. Renal-dose dopamine: a siren song? *Lancet* 1994; **344:** 7–8.
2. Baldwin L, *et al.* Effect of postoperative low-dose dopamine on renal function after elective major vascular surgery. *Ann Intern Med* 1994; **120:** 744–7.
3. Cuthbertson BH, Noble DW. Dopamine in oliguria. *Br Med J* 1997; **314:** 690–1.
4. Chertow GM, *et al.* Is the administration of dopamine associated with adverse or favourable outcomes in acute renal failure? *Am J Med* 1996; **101:** 49–53.
5. Lindner A, Sherrard DJ. Acute renal failure. *N Engl J Med* 1996; **335:** 1320–1.
6. McCrory C, Cunningham AJ. Low-dose dopamine: will there ever be a scientific rationale? *Br J Anaesth* 1997; **78:** 350–1.

Preparations

BP 1998: Dopamine Intravenous Infusion;
USP 23: Dopamine Hydrochloride and Dextrose Injection; Dopamine Hydrochloride Injection.

Proprietary Preparations (details are given in Part 3)
Austral.: Intropin†; ***Belg.:*** Dynatra; ***Canad.:*** Intropin; Revimine†; ***Ger.:*** Cardiosteril†; ***Irl.:*** Intropin; ***Ital.:*** Revivan; ***Jpn:*** Inovan; Predopa; ***Neth.:*** Dynatra; Intropin†; ***S.Afr.:*** Dopamed†; Dynos; Intropin; ***Swed.:*** Abbodop; Giludop; Intropin; ***UK:*** Intropin†; ***USA:*** Intropin.

Multi-ingredient: ***Fr.:*** Tensophoril†.

Dopexamine Hydrochloride (18632-e)

Dopexamine Hydrochloride *(BANM, USAN, rINNM).*

FPL-60278 (dopexamine); FPL-60278AR. 4-{2-[6-(Phenethylamino)hexylamino]ethyl}pyrocatechol dihydrochloride.

$C_{22}H_{32}N_2O_2,2HCl = 429.4.$

CAS — 86197-47-9 (dopexamine); 86484-91-5 (dopexamine dihydrochloride).

Dopexamine is inactivated in alkaline solutions such as sodium bicarbonate 5%.

Adverse Effects and Precautions

The most common adverse effect of dopexamine administration is tachycardia; transient hypotension may also occur. Other adverse effects include arrhythmias and ECG changes, exacerbation of heart failure, nausea and vomiting, tremor, headache, sweating, and dyspnoea.

Dopexamine should not be used in patients with left ventricular outlet obstruction such as aortic stenosis or in phaeochromocytoma or thrombocytopenic patients. It should be used with caution in patients with ischaemic heart disease or following myocardial infarction. Care is also required in the presence of hypokalaemia or hyperglycaemia. Pre-existing hypotension and reduced vascular resistance should be corrected before beginning dopexamine administration.

For the adverse effects of sympathomimetics in general, and precautions to be observed, see Adrenaline, p.813.

Interactions

Dopexamine may potentiate the effects of noradrenaline and some other sympathomimetics by inhibiting neuronal uptake of noradrenaline.

For the interactions of sympathomimetics in general, see Adrenaline, p.814.

Pharmacokinetics

Dopexamine has a short half-life in blood of about 6 or 7 minutes. It is subject to biliary and renal excretion.

Uses and Administration

Dopexamine is a sympathomimetic (see Adrenaline, p.815) with direct and indirect effects. It stimulates beta$_2$ adrenoceptors and peripheral dopamine receptors and also inhibits the neuronal reuptake of noradrenaline. These actions result in an increased cardiac output, peripheral vasodilatation, and an increase in renal and mesenteric blood flow.

Dopexamine hydrochloride is used to provide short-term haemodynamic support that may be required after cardiac surgery or in exacerbations of chronic heart failure. It is given as an intravenous infusion of either 400 or 800 μg per mL in glucose 5% or sodium chloride 0.9% through a central or large peripheral vein; more concentrated solutions may be given via a central vein but concentrations should not exceed 4 mg per mL. The initial dose is generally 0.5 μg per kg body-weight per minute and is then increased to 1 μg per kg per minute; further increases, in increments of 0.5 to 1 μg per kg per minute at intervals of not less than 15 minutes, may be made up to a total of 6 μg per kg per minute if necessary. Heart rate, blood pressure, urine output, and cardiac output should be monitored. On withdrawal, the dose of dopexamine hydrochloride should be reduced gradually.

The pharmacological properties and therapeutic uses of dopexamine have been reviewed.[1,2] Fitton and Benfield concluded that although dopexamine hydrochloride may prove to be a useful alternative to dopamine and dobutamine in the treatment of acute heart failure (cardiogenic shock, p.798) and the postoperative management of low cardiac output conditions, controlled studies are required to establish its efficacy and tolerability with respect to that of established therapies.[2] Much the same view was expressed in a later commentary;[3] the lack of comparative studies on the outcome of such treatment meant that it was difficult to identify advantages to employing dopexamine. An unblinded study in patients undergoing surgery who were thought to be at high risk of postsurgical complications did suggest that perioperative dopexamine reduced mortality and complications.[4]

Dopexamine has also been used in acutely deteriorating chronic heart failure when it appears that systemic vasodilatation is more pronounced than with dopamine or dobutamine.[3]

1. Smith GW, Filcek SAL. Dopexamine hydrochloride: a novel dopamine receptor agonist for the acute treatment of low cardiac output states. *Cardiovasc Drug Rev* 1989; **7:** 141–59.
2. Fitton A, Benfield P. Dopexamine hydrochloride. *Drugs* 1990; **39:** 308–30.
3. Anonymous. Dopexamine after cardiac surgery. *Drug Ther Bull* 1995; **33:** 30–2.
4. Boyd O, *et al.* A randomized clinical trial of the effect of deliberate perioperative increase of oxygen delivery on mortality in high-risk surgical patients. *JAMA* 1993; **270:** 2699–2707.

Preparations

Proprietary Preparations (details are given in Part 3)

Fr.: Dopacard; ***Irl.:*** Dopacard; ***Neth.:*** Dopacard†; ***Swed.:*** Dopacard; ***Switz.:*** Dopacard; ***UK:*** Dopacard.

Dorzolamide Hydrochloride (17057-e)

Dorzolamide Hydrochloride *(BANM, USAN, rINNM).*

L-671152 (dorzolamide); MK-507; MK-0507. (4S,6S)-4-(Ethylamino)-5,6-dihydro-6-methyl-4H-thieno[2,3-b]thiopyran-2-sulphonamide 7,7-dioxide hydrochloride.

$C_{10}H_{16}N_2O_4S_3,HCl = 360.9.$

CAS — 120279-96-1 (dorzolamide); 130693-82-2 (dorzolamide hydrochloride).

Adverse Effects and Precautions

Local ocular adverse effects may occur following the use of dorzolamide eye drops and include conjunctivitis, keratitis, burning or stinging, eyelid inflammation or irritation, and blurred vision. It may be absorbed systemically, resulting in adverse effects, precautions, and interactions similar to those of acetazolamide (see p.810). Other side-effects reported are headache, bitter taste, fatigue, and nausea.

Uses and Administration

Dorzolamide is a carbonic anhydrase inhibitor with actions similar to those of acetazolamide (p.811). It is used topically in the management of open-angle **glaucoma** and ocular hypertension (p.1387), either alone or as adjunctive therapy with a topical beta blocker.

Dorzolamide is administered as eye drops containing dorzolamide hydrochloride equivalent to 2% of the base. When used as monotherapy the usual dose is one drop three times daily; a twice daily regimen is recommended when used in conjunction with a beta blocker.

Preparations

Proprietary Preparations (details are given in Part 3)
Aust.: Trusopt; ***Austral.:*** Trusopt; ***Belg.:*** Trusopt; ***Canad.:*** Trusopt; ***Fr.:*** Trusopt; ***Ger.:*** Trusopt; ***Irl.:*** Trusopt; ***Ital.:*** Trusopt; ***Neth.:*** Trusopt; ***Norw.:*** Trusopt; ***S.Afr.:*** Trusopt; ***Spain:*** Trusopt; ***Swed.:*** Trusopt; ***Switz.:*** Trusopt; ***UK:*** Trusopt; ***USA:*** Trusopt.

Multi-ingredient: ***UK:*** Cosopt; ***USA:*** Cosopt.

Doxazosin Mesylate (16611-y)

Doxazosin Mesylate *(BANM, USAN).*

Doxazosin Mesilate *(rINNM)*; Doxazosin Methanesulphonate; UK-33274-27. 2-[4-(2,3-Dihydro-1,4-benzodioxin-2-ylcarbonyl)piperazin-1-yl]-6,7-dimethoxyquinazolin-4-ylamine methanesulphonate; 1-(4-Amino-6,7-dimethoxyquinazolin-2-yl)-4-(1,4-benzodioxan-2-ylcarbonyl)piperazine methanesulphonate.

$C_{23}H_{25}N_5O_5,CH_3SO_3H = 547.6.$

CAS — 74191-85-8 (doxazosin); 77883-43-3 (doxazosin mesylate).

Doxazosin mesylate 1.2 mg is approximately equivalent to 1 mg of doxazosin.

Adverse Effects, Treatment, and Precautions

As for Prazosin Hydrochloride, p.932.

Effects on mental function. For a report of acute psychosis associated with doxazosin administration, see under Adverse Effects of Prazosin Hydrochloride, p.932.

Hypotension. Six of 18 hypertensive patients exhibited first-dose postural hypotension after receiving doxazosin 1 mg; three others had substantial but asymptomatic reductions in supine systolic blood pressure following the first dose.[1] The effect might have been exacerbated since all these patients were receiving concomitant beta blocker or diuretic therapy, or both. A further patient, who was also taking methyldopa, withdrew from the study with persistent postural hypotension.

1. Oliver RM, *et al.* The pharmacokinetics of doxazosin in patients with hypertension and renal impairment. *Br J Clin Pharmacol* 1990; **29:** 417–22.

Urinary incontinence. For reference to urinary incontinence associated with doxazosin, see under Adverse Effects of Prazosin Hydrochloride, p.932.

Pharmacokinetics

Doxazosin is well absorbed after oral administration, peak blood concentrations occurring 2 hours after a dose. Oral bioavailability is about 65%. It is extensively metabolised in the liver, and excreted in faeces as metabolites and a small amount of unchanged drug. Elimination from plasma is biphasic, with a mean terminal half-life of about 22 hours. The pharmacokinetics are not altered in patients with impaired renal function. Doxazosin is extensively bound to plasma proteins and is not removed by dialysis.

Reviews.

1. Elliott HL, *et al.* Pharmacokinetic overview of doxazosin. *Am J Cardiol* 1987; **59:** 78G–81G.

Uses and Administration

Doxazosin is an $alpha_1$-adrenoceptor blocker (p.776) with actions and uses similar to those of prazosin (p.933), but a longer duration of action. It is used in the management of hypertension (p.788) and in benign prostatic hyperplasia (p.1446) to relieve urinary obstruction.

Doxazosin is given by mouth as the mesylate, but doses are usually expressed in terms of the base. Following an oral dose maximum reduction in blood pressure is reported to occur after 2 to 6 hours and the effects are maintained for 24 hours, permitting once daily dosage.

To avoid the risk of collapse which may occur in some patients after the first dose, the initial dose is 1 mg, preferably at bedtime. Dosage may be increased after 1 or 2 weeks according to response. Usual maintenance doses for hypertension are up to 4 mg once daily; doses of 16 mg daily should not be exceeded. For benign prostatic hyperplasia the usual maintenance dose is 2 to 4 mg daily; doses of 8 mg daily should not be exceeded.

Reviews.

1. Fulton B, *et al.* Doxazosin: an update of its clinical pharmacology and therapeutic applications in hypertension and benign prostatic hyperplasia. *Drugs* 1995; **49:** 295–320.

Preparations

Proprietary Preparations (details are given in Part 3)
Aust.: Prostadilat; Supressin; ***Austral.:*** Carduran; ***Canad.:*** Cardura; ***Ger.:*** Cardular; Diblocin; ***Irl.:*** Cardura; ***Ital.:*** Benur; Cardura; Dedralen; Normothen; ***Neth.:*** Cardura; ***Norw.:*** Carduran; ***S.Afr.:*** Cardura; ***Spain:*** Carduran; Progandol; ***Swed.:*** Alfadil; ***UK:*** Cardura; ***USA:*** Cardura.

Duteplase (13784-w)

Duteplase *(rINN).*

245-L-Methionine Plasminogen Activator; SM-9527.

$C_{2736}H_{4174}N_{914}O_{824}S_{46}$ = 64529.1.

CAS — 120608-46-0.

Duteplase is a thrombolytic drug. It is a biosynthetic derivative of endogenous tissue plasminogen activator and has been used similarly to alteplase (p.818) in the treatment of thrombo-embolic disorders, particularly myocardial infarction.

References.

1. Hayashi H, *et al.* Effects of intravenous SM-9527 (double-chain tissue plasminogen activator) on left ventricular function in the chronic stage of acute myocardial infarction. *Clin Cardiol* 1993; **16:** 409–14.

Preparations

Proprietary Preparations (details are given in Part 3)
Jpn: Solclot.

Efloxate (9227-y)

Efloxate *(rINN).*

7-(Carbethoxymethoxy)flavone; Efloxatum; Ethyl Flavone-7-oxyacetate; 7-Ethyloxyacetate Flavone; Flavone-7-ethyloxyacetate; Rec 1/0185. Ethyl 4-oxo-2-phenyl-4*H*-chromen-7-yloxyacetate.

$C_{19}H_{16}O_5$ = 324.3.

CAS — 119-41-5.

Efloxate is a vasodilator that has been used in ischaemic heart disease.

Preparations

Proprietary Preparations (details are given in Part 3)
Fr.: Recordil†; ***Ital.:*** Dilatan Kore†; Recordil†.

Efonidipine (15889-l)

Efonidipine *(rINN).*

Cyclic 2,2-dimethyltrimethylene ester of 2-(*N*-benzylanilino)ethyl (±)-1,4-dihydro-2,6-dimethyl-4-(*m*-nitrophenyl)-5-phosphononicontinate.

$C_{34}H_{38}N_3O_7P$ = 631.7.

CAS — 111011-63-3.

Efonidipine is a dihydropyridine calcium-channel blocker with general properties similar to those of nifedipine (p.916) and is used in the treatment of hypertension.

Enalapril (17599-a)

Enalapril *(BAN, rINN).*

N-{*N*-[(*S*)-1-Ethoxycarbonyl-3-phenylpropyl]-L-alanyl}-L-proline.

$C_{20}H_{28}N_2O_5$ = 376.4.

CAS — 75847-73-3.

Enalapril Maleate (12969-e)

Enalapril Maleate *(BANM, USAN, rINNM).*

MK-421. *N*-{*N*-[(*S*)-1-Ethoxycarbonyl-3-phenylpropyl]-L-alanyl}-L-proline hydrogen maleate.

$C_{20}H_{28}N_2O_5,C_4H_4O_4$ = 492.5.

CAS — 76095-16-4.

Pharmacopoeias. In US.

An off-white crystalline powder. Sparingly **soluble** in water; soluble in alcohol; freely soluble in methyl alcohol and in dimethylformamide; slightly soluble in semipolar organic solvents; practically insoluble in nonpolar organic solvents.

Enalaprilat (16618-x)

Enalaprilat *(BAN, USAN, rINN).*

Enalaprilic acid; MK-422. *N*-{*N*-[(*S*)-1-Carboxy-3-phenylpropyl]-L-alanyl}-L-proline dihydrate.

$C_{18}H_{24}N_2O_5,2H_2O$ = 384.4.

CAS — 76420-72-9 (anhydrous enalaprilat); 84680-54-6 (enalaprilat dihydrate).

Pharmacopoeias. In US.

A white or nearly white, hygroscopic, crystalline powder. **Soluble** 1 in 200 of water, 1 in 68 of methyl alcohol, and 1 in 40 of dimethylformamide; slightly soluble in isopropyl alcohol; very slightly soluble in acetone, in alcohol, and in hexane; practically insoluble in chloroform.

Enalaprilat 1.38 mg as the dihydrate is approximately equivalent to 1.25 mg of anhydrous enalaprilat.

Enalaprilat was visually incompatible with phenytoin sodium in sodium chloride 0.9%, producing a crystalline precipitate; there was also some visual evidence of incompatibility when mixed with amphotericin in glucose 5%.[1]

1. Thompson DF, *et al.* Visual compatibility of enalaprilat with selected intravenous medications during simulated Y-site injection. *Am J Hosp Pharm* 1990; **47:** 2530–1.

Adverse Effects, Treatment, and Precautions

As for ACE inhibitors, p.805.

Postmarketing surveillance for enalapril was carried out by prescription-event monitoring of 12 543 patients.[1] There were 374 skin events including facial oedema or angioedema in 29 (leading to withdrawal of treatment in 10), 15 cases of photosensitivity, and urticaria in 32 (leading to withdrawal in 5). Syncope and dizziness occurred in 155 and 483 patients respectively, sometimes in association with hypotension. Hypotension occurred in 218 patients, 71 in the first month. Treatment was stopped in 121 patients with hypotension, and dosage reduced in 36. Other adverse effects reported included headache (in 310 patients), paraesthesias (126), taste disturbances (25), conjunctivitis (67), tachycardia (194), cough (360), renal failure (82), muscle cramp (96), diarrhoea (236), and nausea and vomiting (326). Of 1098 deaths only 10, due to renal failure, were thought possibly related to enalapril therapy. Dysgeusia and skin reactions appeared to be less common than has been reported for captopril, but precise comparisons were difficult; the range of adverse effects was similar.[2]

Deafness was a possible side-effect of enalapril noted earlier;[2] it was reported in 19 of the 12 543 patients monitored, but only while they were taking enalapril, there being no record of deafness after treatment stopped.

For further reference to some of these adverse effects, see under ACE Inhibitors, p.805.

1. Inman WHW, *et al.* Postmarketing surveillance of enalapril I: results of prescription-event monitoring. *Br Med J* 1988; **297:** 826–9.
2. Inman WHW, Rawson NSB. Deafness with enalapril and prescription event monitoring. *Lancet* 1987; **i:** 872.

Breast feeding. Following administration of a single dose of enalapril 20 mg to 5 lactating women enalaprilat was detected in breast milk in concentrations of 1 to 2.3 ng per mL (mean peak 1.72 ng per mL); enalapril was also present (mean peak 1.74 ng per mL). This compared with peak serum values of 39 to 112 ng per mL for enalaprilat and 92 to 151 ng per mL for enalapril. Although enalapril and its metabolite are thus present in small amounts in breast milk it was calculated that the average total daily dose to the neonate would only be about 2 μg of enalaprilat.[1]

1. Redman CWG, *et al.* The excretion of enalapril and enalaprilat in human breast milk. *Eur J Clin Pharmacol* 1990; **38:** 99.

Porphyria. Enalapril has been associated with clinical exacerbations of porphyria and is considered unsafe in porphyric patients.[1]

1. Moore MR, McColl KEL. *Porphyria: drug lists.* Glasgow: Porphyria Research Unit, University of Glasgow, 1991.

Interactions

As for ACE inhibitors, p.807.

Pharmacokinetics

Enalapril acts as a prodrug of the diacid enalaprilat, its active form, which is poorly absorbed by mouth. Following oral administration about 60% of a dose of enalapril is absorbed from the gastro-intestinal tract and peak plasma concentrations are achieved within about 1 hour. Enalapril is extensively hydrolysed in the liver to enalaprilat; peak plasma concentrations of enalaprilat are achieved 3 to 4 hours after an oral dose of enalapril. About 60% of an oral dose is excreted in urine, as enalaprilat and unchanged drug, the rest in the faeces. Enalaprilat is 50 to 60% bound to plasma proteins; its elimination is multiphasic but its effective half-life for accumulation following multiple doses of enalapril is reported to be about 11 hours in patients with normal renal function. Enalaprilat is removed by haemodialysis and by peritoneal dialysis.

References.

1. MacFadyen RJ, *et al.* Enalapril clinical pharmacokinetics and pharmacokinetic-pharmacodynamic relationships: an overview. *Clin Pharmacokinet* 1993; **25:** 274–82.
2. Ulm EH, *et al.* Enalapril maleate and a lysine analogue (MK-521): disposition in man. *Br J Clin Pharmacol* 1982; **14:** 357–62.
3. Till AE, *et al.* Pharmacokinetics of repeated single oral doses of enalapril maleate (MK-421) in normal volunteers. *Biopharm Drug Dispos* 1984; **5:** 273–80.

Renal impairment. Comparison of the pharmacokinetics of enalapril in 6 diabetics with persistent proteinuria and glomerular filtration rates (GFR) of 44.1 to 58.4 mL per minute with those in 8 age-matched controls showed that in the diabetic group the peak serum concentration of enalaprilat was higher, the time to peak concentration longer, renal clearance lower, and the areas under the concentration/time curve greater than in controls.[1] Renal clearance of enalaprilat in the diabetics ranged from 56 to 66 mL per minute compared with 105 to 133 mL per minute in controls; clearance correlated with GFR.

1. Baba T, *et al.* Enalapril pharmacokinetics in diabetic patients. *Lancet* 1989; **i:** 226–7.

Uses and Administration

Enalapril is an ACE inhibitor (p.805) used in the treatment of hypertension (p.788) and heart failure (p.785). It may also be given prophylactically to patients with asymptomatic left ventricular dysfunction to delay the onset of symptomatic heart failure and to those with left ventricular dysfunction to reduce the incidence of coronary ischaemic events, including myocardial infarction (p.791).

Enalapril owes its activity to enalaprilat to which it is converted after oral administration. The haemodynamic effects are seen within 1 hour of a single oral dose and the maximum effect occurs after about 4 to 6 hours, although the full effect may not develop for several weeks during chronic dosing. The haemodynamic action lasts for about 24 hours, allowing once-daily dosing. Enalapril is given by mouth as the maleate.

Enalaprilat is not absorbed by mouth but is given by intravenous injection; its haemodynamic effects develop within 15 minutes of injection and reach a peak in 1 to 4 hours. The action lasts for about 6 hours at recommended doses. Enalaprilat is given as the dihydrate, but doses are expressed in terms of the anhydrous substance.

In the treatment of **hypertension**, an initial dose of 5 mg of enalapril maleate daily may be given by mouth. Since there may be a precipitous fall in blood pressure in some patients when starting therapy with an ACE inhibitor, the first dose should preferably be given at bedtime. An initial dose of 2.5 mg daily should be given to patients with renal impairment or to those who are receiving a diuretic; if possible, the diuretic should be withdrawn 2 or 3 days before enalapril is started and resumed later if necessary. An initial dose of 2.5 mg is also recommended in elderly patients. The usual maintenance dose is 10 to 20 mg given once daily, although doses of up to 40 mg daily may be required in severe hypertension. It may be given in 2 divided doses if control is inadequate with a single dose.

When oral therapy of hypertension is impractical enalaprilat may be given in a dose of 1.25 mg by slow intravenous injection over 5 minutes, repeated every 6 hours if necessary; the initial dose should be halved in patients with renal impairment (creatinine clearance less than 30 mL per minute) or those who are receiving a diuretic.

In the management of **heart failure**, severe first-dose hypotension on introduction of an ACE inhibitor is common in patients on loop diuretics, but their temporary withdrawal may cause rebound pulmonary oedema. Thus treatment should be initiated with a low dose under close medical supervision. In patients with heart failure or asymptomatic left ventricular dysfunction enalapril maleate is given by mouth in an initial dose of 2.5 mg daily. The usual maintenance dose is 20 mg daily as a single dose or in 2 divided doses.

Administration in children. Enalapril has been given to infants with severe heart failure in doses of 0.1 to 0.5 mg per kg body-weight daily as an oral suspension produced by suspending a crushed tablet in water.[1] In this study one infant, with severe myocarditis, developed hypotension and the drug had to be withdrawn; the remaining 7 showed clinical improvement on a mean enalapril dose of 0.26 mg per kg daily and were able markedly to reduce the dose of concomitant diuretic required. Another study in 10 infants found that enalapril was less bioavailable and probably had a shorter duration of action in infants than in adults, and that doses of 0.08 mg per kg daily were inadequate in the treatment of infant heart failure.[2] A larger study in 63 infants and children (median age 5.4 months) with heart failure found enalapril 0.36 mg per kg daily to be of benefit, whereas there was no improvement with a lower dose of 0.24 mg per kg daily.[3]

1. Frenneaux M, *et al.* Enalapril for severe heart failure in infancy. *Arch Dis Child* 1989; **64:** 219–23.
2. Lloyd TR, *et al.* Orally administered enalapril for infants with congestive heart failure: a dose-finding study. *J Pediatr* 1989; **114:** 650–4.
3. Leversha AM, *et al.* Efficacy and dosage of enalapril in congenital and acquired heart disease. *Arch Dis Child* 1994; **70:** 35–9.

Preparations

USP 23: Enalapril Maleate and Hydrochlorothiazide Tablets; Enalapril Maleate Tablets.

Proprietary Preparations (details are given in Part 3)

Aust.: Mepril; Regomed; Renitec; ***Austral.:*** Amprace; Renitec; ***Belg.:*** Renitec; ***Canad.:*** Vasotec; ***Fr.:*** Renitec; ***Ger.:*** Pres; Pres iv; Xanef; ***Irl.:*** Innovace; ***Ital.:*** Converten; Enapren; Naprilene; ***Neth.:*** Renitec; ***Norw.:*** Renitec; ***S.Afr.:*** Renitec; ***Spain:*** Acetensil; Baripril; Bitensil; Clipto; Controlvas; Corprilor; Crinoren; Dabonal; Ditensor; Herten; Hipoartel; Iecatec; Insup; Nacor; Naprilene; Neotensin; Pressitan; Reca; Renitec; Ristalen; ***Swed.:*** Renitec; ***Switz.:*** Reniten; ***UK:*** Innovace; ***USA:*** Vasotec.

Multi-ingredient: ***Aust.:*** Co-Renitec; ***Belg.:*** Co-Renitec; ***Canad.:*** Vaseretic; ***Fr.:*** Co-Renitec; ***Ger.:*** Pres plus; Renacor; ***Irl.:*** Innozide; ***Ital.:*** Acesistem; Condiuren; Vasoretic; ***Neth.:*** Co-Renitec; Renitec Plus; ***Norw.:*** Renitec Comp; ***S.Afr.:*** Co-Renitec; ***Spain:*** Acediur; Acetensil Plus; Baripril Diu; Bitensil Diu; Co-Renitec; Crinoretic; Dabonal Plus; Ditenside; Hipoartel Plus; Neotensin Diu; Pressitan Plus; ***Swed.:*** Synerpril; ***Switz.:*** Co-Reniten; ***UK:*** Innozide; ***USA:*** Lexxel; Teczem; Vaseretic.

Enalkiren (10781-g)

Enalkiren *(USAN, rINN).*

Abbott-64662. (αS)-α-[(αS)-α-(3-Amino-3-methylbutyramido)-*p*-methoxyhydrocinnamamido]-*N*-[(1S,2R,3S)-1-(cyclohexylmethyl)-2,3-dihydroxy-5-methylhexyl]imidazole-4-propionamide.

$C_{35}H_{56}N_6O_6$ = 656.9.

CAS — 113082-98-7.

Enalkiren inhibits the actions of renin and thus prevents the conversion of angiotensinogen into angiotensin I. Enalkiren is given intravenously. It is under investigation in the management of hypertension and heart failure.

A number of renin antagonists are under investigation as specific inhibitors of the renin-angiotensin system.[1,2] Enalkiren is a dipeptide that has no oral activity but that has been shown to reduce blood pressure when given intravenously. Enalkiren 0.03, 0.1, 0.3, and 1.0 mg per kg body-weight was given as intravenous boli at 45-minute intervals to 17 patients with mild-to-moderate hypertension who were receiving hydrochlorothiazide and a controlled-sodium diet. Systolic and diastolic blood pressure fell after all doses of enalkiren; subsequent comparison in the same patients suggested that enalkiren 0.03 mg per kg produced an equivalent fall in blood pressure to that obtained after a single dose of enalaprilat 0.625 mg intravenously.[3]

1. Frishman WH, *et al.* Renin inhibition: a new approach to cardiovascular therapy. *J Clin Pharmacol* 1994; **34:** 873–80.
2. Rongen GA, *et al.* Clinical pharmacokinetics and efficacy of renin inhibitors. *Clin Pharmacokinet* 1995; **29:** 6–14.
3. Griffiths AN, *et al.* The hypotensive effect of increasing doses of enalkiren, a dipeptide renin inhibitor, compared with enalaprilat in hypertensive patients. *Br J Clin Pharmacol* 1990; **29:** 614P–15P.

Encainide Hydrochloride (7785-b)

Encainide Hydrochloride *(BANM, USAN, rINNM).*

MJ-9067-1 (encainide). (±)-2′-[2-(1-Methyl-2-piperidyl)ethyl]-*p*-anisanilide hydrochloride.

$C_{22}H_{28}N_2O_2,HCl$ = 388.9.

CAS — 37612-13-8 (encainide); 66778-36-7 (encainide); 66794-74-9 (encainide hydrochloride).

Encainide is a class Ic antiarrhythmic (p.776) and was used for the treatment of severe or life-threatening ventricular arrhythmias. As a result of encainide causing an increase in mortality rates in post-infarction patients in the Cardiac Arrhythmia Suppression Trial (CAST) (p.782) encainide was withdrawn from the market. Doses which were built up gradually did not generally exceed 200 mg daily by mouth.

Endralazine Mesylate (12688-h)

Endralazine Mesylate *(BANM, USAN).*

Endralazine Mesilate *(rINNM)*; BQ-22-708; Compound 22-708. 6-Benzoyl-5,6,7,8-tetrahydropyrido[4,3-c]pyridazin-3-yl-hydrazone monomethanesulfonate.

$C_{14}H_{15}N_5O,CH_4O_3S$ = 365.4.

CAS — 39715-02-1 (endralazine); 65322-72-7 (endralazine mesylate).

Endralazine is a vasodilator with properties similar to those of hydralazine (p.883). It has been used as the mesylate in the treatment of hypertension.

Enoxaparin Sodium (13424-s)

Enoxaparin Sodium *(BAN, USAN, rINN).*

Enoxaparinum Natricum; PK-10169; RP-54563.

CAS — 9041-08-1.

Pharmacopoeias. In Eur. (see p.viii).

Enoxaparin sodium is prepared by alkaline depolymerisation of heparin benzyl ester obtained from the intestinal mucosa of pigs. The majority of the components have a 2-*O*-sulpho-4-desoxy-4-α-L-*threo*-hex-4-enopyranosuronic acid structure at the non-reducing end of their chain. The mass-average molecular mass ranges between 3500 and 5500 and the average value is about 4500. The degree of sulphation is about 2 per disaccharide unit.

The Ph. Eur. specifies that potency is not less than 90 units and not more than 125 units of anti-factor Xa activity per mg with reference to the dried substance and that the ratio of anti-factor Xa activity to anti-factor IIa (antithrombin) activity is between 3.3 and 5.3.

Units

As for Low-molecular-weight Heparins, p.899.

Adverse Effects and Treatment

As for Low-molecular-weight Heparins, p.899.

Precautions and Interactions

As for Low-molecular-weight Heparins, p.900.

Pharmacokinetics

Enoxaparin is rapidly absorbed following subcutaneous injection with a bioavailability of about 92%. Peak plasma activity is reached within 1 to 5 hours. The elimination half-life is about 4 to 5 hours but anti-factor Xa activity persists for up to 24 hours following a 40-mg dose. Enoxaparin is metabolised in the liver and excreted in the urine, as unchanged drug and metabolites.

Uses and Administration

Enoxaparin sodium is a low-molecular-weight heparin (p.899) with anticoagulant properties. It is used in the treatment and prophylaxis of venous thrombo-embolism (p.802) and to prevent clotting during extracorporeal circulation. It is also used in the management of unstable angina (p.780).

In the prophylaxis of venous thrombo-embolism during surgical procedures, patients at low to moderate risk are given 20 mg (2000 units) of enoxaparin sodium by subcutaneous injection once daily for 7 to 10 days or until the patient is ambulant; the first dose is given approximately 2 hours pre-operatively. In patients at high risk the dose should be increased to 40 mg (4000 units) once daily with the initial dose given approximately 12 hours before the procedure. Alternatively, a dose of 30 mg (3000 units) may be given subcutaneously twice daily, starting within 12 to 24 hours after the operation.

For the treatment of deep-vein thrombosis enoxaparin sodium is given subcutaneously in a dose of 1 mg (100 units) per kg body-weight every 12 hours for 5 days or until oral anticoagulation is established.

For prevention of clotting in the extracorporeal circulation during haemodialysis, enoxaparin sodium 1 mg (100 units) per kg is introduced into the arterial line of the circuit at the beginning of the dialysis session. A further dose of 0.5 to 1 mg (50 to 100 units) per kg may be given if required. The dose should be reduced in patients at high risk of haemorrhage.

In the management of unstable angina, enoxaparin sodium is given subcutaneously in a dose of 1 mg (100 units) per kg every 12 hours. Treatment is usually continued for 2 to 8 days and low-dose aspirin should be given concomitantly.

Reversal of effects. Severe bleeding with enoxaparin may be reduced by the slow intravenous injection of protamine sulphate; 1 mg of protamine sulphate is stated to inhibit the effects of 1 mg (100 units) of enoxaparin sodium.

References.

1. Noble S, *et al.* Enoxaparin: a reappraisal of its pharmacology and clinical applications in the prevention and treatment of thromboembolic disease. *Drugs* 1995; **49:** 388–410.
2. Noble S, Spencer CM. Enoxaparin: a review of its clinical potential in the management of coronary artery disease. *Drugs* 1998; **56:** 259–72.

Preparations

Proprietary Preparations (details are given in Part 3)

Aust.: Lovenox; ***Austral.:*** Clexane; ***Belg.:*** Clexane; ***Canad.:*** Lovenox; ***Fr.:*** Lovenox; ***Ger.:*** Clexane; ***Irl.:*** Clexane; ***Ital.:*** Clexane; Trombenox; ***Neth.:*** Clexane; ***Norw.:*** Klexane; ***S.Afr.:*** Clexane; ***Spain:*** Clexane; Decipar; Plaucina†; ***Swed.:*** Klexane; ***Switz.:*** Clexane; ***UK:*** Clexane; ***USA:*** Lovenox.

Enoximone (16805-d)

Enoximone *(BAN, USAN, rINN)*.

Fenoximone; MDL-17043; MDL-19438; RMI-17043; YMDL-17043. 4-Methyl-5-[4-(methylthio)benzoyl]-4-imidazolin-2-one.

$C_{12}H_{12}N_2O_2S$ = 248.3.

CAS — 77671-31-9.

Crystal formation has been observed when enoximone injection was mixed in glass containers or syringes; the manufacturer recommends that only plastic containers or syringes are used for dilutions. The manufacturer also recommends that only sodium chloride 0.9% or water be used as diluents. Glucose solutions should not be used as a diluent since crystal formation may occur.

Adverse Effects

Long-term oral treatment with enoximone has been reported to increase the mortality rate and enoximone is now only employed intravenously for short-term use.

The commonest adverse effects of enoximone affect the gastro-intestinal tract and include diarrhoea, nausea, and vomiting. Other adverse effects include headache, insomnia, chills, oliguria, fever, urinary retention, and limb pain. There have been reports of thrombocytopenia and abnormal liver enzyme values.

Enoximone may cause ventricular and supraventricular tachyarrhythmias, ectopic beats, and hypotension.

A report of tonic-clonic convulsions in a patient given enoximone 6 μg per kg body-weight per minute by intravenous infusion. The convulsions subsided when enoximone was discontinued.[1]

1. Appadurai I, *et al.* Convulsions induced by enoximone administered as a continuous intravenous infusion. *Br Med J* 1990; **300:** 613–14.

Hyperosmolality occurred in an infant during intravenous infusion of enoximone 20 μg per kg body-weight per minute. The probable cause was propylene glycol in the enoximone injection providing a dose of 2.4 mg per kg per minute.[1]

1. Huggon I, *et al.* Hyperosmolality related to propylene glycol in an infant treated with enoximone infusion. *Br Med J* 1990; **301:** 19–20.

Precautions

Enoximone should be used with caution in patients with hypertrophic cardiomyopathy or severe obstructive aortic or pulmonary valvular disease.

Blood pressure, heart rate, ECG, and fluid and electrolyte status should be monitored during therapy. Platelet count and liver enzyme values should also be monitored.

Extravasation should be avoided during administration.

The injection has a high pH (approximately 12) and must be diluted before use (but see above).

Hepatic and renal impairment. The elimination half-life of enoximone was 2.16 hours in a patient with hepatic impairment and 1.33 hours in a patient with renal impairment both given enoximone intravenously. The mean elimination half-life in patients with normal hepatic and renal function was 1.26 hours. It was suggested that patients with renal impairment should be monitored and have plasma concentrations measured during continuous infusions and that in hepatic disease the dosage may need to be modified.[1]

1. Desager JP, *et al.* Plasma enoximone concentrations in cardiac patients. *Curr Ther Res* 1990; **47:** 743–52.

Pharmacokinetics

Enoximone is absorbed from the gastro-intestinal tract but it is no longer administered orally due to an increased mortality rate in some long-term studies. The plasma elimination half-life varies widely; it may be about 1 to 4 hours in healthy volunteers and about 3 to 8 hours in patients with heart failure, but longer values have been reported. Enoximone is about 85% bound to plasma proteins. It is metabolised in the liver and is excreted in the urine, mainly as metabolites. Following intravenous administration about 70% of a dose is excreted in the urine as metabolites and less than 1% as unchanged drug.

General references.

1. Rocci ML, Wilson H. The pharmacokinetics and pharmacodynamics of newer inotropic agents. *Clin Pharmacokinet* 1987; **13:** 91–109. Correction. *ibid.* 1988; **14:** (contents page).

Uses and Administration

Enoximone is a phosphodiesterase inhibitor similar to amrinone (p.823) with positive inotropic and vasodilator activity. It is given intravenously in the short-term management of heart failure. In some long-term studies it was given by mouth, but an increased mortality rate was reported.

The usual initial dose of enoximone by intravenous injection is 0.5 to 1.0 mg per kg body-weight given at a rate not greater than 12.5 mg per minute. This may be followed by doses of 0.5 mg per kg every 30 minutes until a satisfactory response is obtained or a total dose of 3 mg per kg has been given. Alternatively, the initial dose may be given as a continuous intravenous infusion in a dose of 90 μg per kg per minute over 10 to 30 minutes until the desired response is achieved.

For maintenance therapy the initial dose (up to a total of 3 mg per kg) may be repeated as required every 3 to 6 hours or a continuous or intermittent infusion may be given in a dose of 5 to 20 μg per kg per minute.

The total dose over 24 hours should not exceed 24 mg per kg.

Dosage may need to be reduced in patients with renal impairment.

General references.

1. Vernon MW, *et al.* Enoximone: a review of its pharmacological properties and therapeutic potential. *Drugs* 1991; **42:** 997–1017.

Beta blocker overdosage. Enoximone, given intravenously as a bolus dose of 0.5 mg per kg body-weight followed by an infusion of 15 μg per kg per minute, successfully increased the cardiac output and stroke volume in a woman who had ingested 10 g of metoprolol.[1] It was suggested that enoximone may be useful in such patients since its action does not involve the beta-adrenergic system.

1. Hoeper MM, Boeker KHW. Overdose of metoprolol treated with enoximone. *N Engl J Med* 1996; **335:** 1538.

Heart failure. Enoximone is one of several drugs that may be used in heart failure (p.785), but because of an increased mortality rate reported following long-term oral administration it is only given intravenously for short-term management of heart failure unresponsive to other forms of therapy. In a comparison of oral enoximone and placebo in patients with moderate to moderately severe heart failure,[1] enoximone was no better than placebo in improving exercise duration over the 16-week study period. The overall incidence of adverse effects was similar in the two groups, although mortality was higher in the enoximone group; 5 patients on active treatment died but no deaths occurred in the placebo group.

1. Uretsky BF, *et al.* Multicenter trial of oral enoximone in patients with moderate to moderately severe congestive heart failure: lack of benefit compared with placebo. *Circulation* 1990; **82:** 774–80.

Preparations

Proprietary Preparations (details are given in Part 3)
Belg.: Perfan; ***Fr.:*** Perfane; ***Ger.:*** Perfan; ***Irl.:*** Perfan; ***Ital.:*** Perfan; ***Neth.:*** Perfan; ***UK:*** Perfan.

Epanolol (18637-c)

Epanolol *(BAN, rINN)*.

ICI-141292. (*RS*)-*N*-[2-(3-*o*-Cyanophenoxy-2-hydroxypropylamino)ethyl]-2-(4-hydroxyphenyl)acetamide.

$C_{20}H_{23}N_3O_4$ = 369.4.

CAS — 86880-51-5.

Epanolol is reported to be a cardioselective beta blocker (p.828). It has some intrinsic sympathomimetic activity.

References.

1. Frishshman WH, Lydén L, eds. Symposium on patient preference in antianginal therapy. *Drugs* 1989; **38** (suppl 2): 1–91.

Epithiazide (2327-q)

Epithiazide *(BAN, USAN)*.

Epitizide *(rINN)*; NSC-108164; P-2105. 6-Chloro-3,4-dihydro-3-(2,2,2-trifluoroethylthiomethyl)-2*H*-1,2,4-benzothiadiazine-7-sulphonamide 1,1-dioxide.

$C_{10}H_{11}ClF_3N_3O_4S_3$ = 425.9.

CAS — 1764-85-8.

Epithiazide is a thiazide diuretic (see Hydrochlorothiazide, p.885) used in the treatment of oedema and hypertension, often in combination with triamterene.

Preparations

Proprietary Preparations (details are given in Part 3)
Multi-ingredient: ***Belg.:*** Dyta-Urese; ***Neth.:*** Dyta-Urese.

Eprosartan (17512-a)

Eprosartan *(BAN, USAN, rINN)*.

SKF-108566. (*E*)-2-Butyl-1-(*p*-carboxybenzyl)-α-2-thienylimidazole-5-acrylic acid; (*E*)-α-{2-Butyl-5-[2-carboxy-3-(2-thienyl)prop-1-enyl]-1*H*-imidazol-1-yl}-*p*-toluic acid.

$C_{23}H_{24}N_2O_4S$ = 424.5.

CAS — 133040-01-4 (eprosartan); 144143-96-4 (eprosartan mesylate).

Eprosartan is an angiotensin II receptor antagonist with general properties similar to those of losartan (p.899). It is used as the mesylate in the management of hypertension.

Reviews.

1. McClellan KJ, Balfour JA. Eprosartan. *Drugs* 1998; **55:** 713–18.

Preparations

Proprietary Preparations (details are given in Part 3)
Irl.: Teveten; ***Swed.:*** Teveten.

Eproxindine (16633-t)

Eproxindine *(rINN)*.

(±)-*N*-[3-(Diethylamino)-2-hydroxypropyl]-3-methoxy-1-phenylindole-2-carboxamide.

$C_{23}H_{29}N_3O_3$ = 395.5.

CAS — 83200-08-2.

Eproxindine has been studied for its antiarrhythmic activity.

A report of sudden cardiorespiratory arrest and death[1] in an apparently healthy subject shortly after receiving eproxindine 400 mg by intravenous infusion during the course of a clinical study. He was subsequently found to have received a depot injection of flupenthixol the previous day. Displacement of flupenthixol from its plasma binding sites by eproxindine may have been responsible for the fatal cardiotoxicity although an idiosyncratic reaction to eproxindine could also have been a possible explanation.[2]

1. Darragh A, *et al.* Sudden death of a volunteer. *Lancet* 1985; **i:** 93–4.
2. Simister JM, Jorgensen A. Sudden death of a volunteer. *Lancet* 1985; **i:** 343.

Eptifibatide (15030-q)

Eptifibatide *(rINN)*.

Integrelin. N^6-Amidino-N^2-(3-mercaptopropionyl)-L-lysylglycyl-L-α-aspartyl-L-tryptophyl-L-prolyl-L-cysteinamide, cyclic (1→6)-disulfide.

$C_{35}H_{49}N_{11}O_9S_2$ = 832.0.

Eptifibatide is an antiplatelet drug that inhibits glycoprotein IIb/IIIa. It is used, usually in combination with aspirin and heparin, in the management of unstable angina and in patients undergoing coronary angioplasty procedures.

In the management of **unstable angina**, eptifibatide is given in an initial dose of 180 μg per kg body-weight by intravenous injection, followed by 2 μg per kg per minute by intravenous infusion, for up to 72 hours.

In patients undergoing **angioplasty**, eptifibatide is given in an initial dose of 135 μg per kg by intravenous injection immediately before the procedure, followed by 0.5 μg per kg per minute by intravenous infusion, for 20 to 24 hours.

References.

1. Tcheng JE, *et al.* Multicenter, randomized, double-blind, placebo-controlled trial of the platelet integrin glycoprotein IIb/IIIa blocker integrelin in elective coronary intervention. *Circulation* 1995; **91:** 2151–7.
2. The IMPACT-II Investigators. Randomised placebo-controlled trial of effect of eptifibatide on complications of percutaneous coronary intervention: IMPACT-II. *Lancet* 1997; **349:** 1422–8.
3. The PURSUIT Trial Investigators. Inhibition of platelet glycoprotein IIb/IIIa with eptifibatide in patients with acute coronary syndromes. *N Engl J Med* 1998; **339:** 436–43.

Preparations

Proprietary Preparations (details are given in Part 3)
USA: Integrilin.

Erythrityl Tetranitrate (9229-z)

Erythrityl Tetranitrate *(USAN)*.

Eritrityl Tetranitrate; Erythritol Tetranitrate; Erythrol Nitrate or Tetranitrate; Nitroerythrite; Nitroerythrol; NSC-106566; Tetranitrol. Butane-1,2,3,4-tetrol tetranitrate.

$C_4H_6(O.NO_2)_4$ = 302.1.

CAS — 7297-25-8.

Pharmacopoeias. Diluted erythrityl tetranitrate is included in *Aust.* (25% in lactose) and *US* (in lactose or other suitable inert excipient; the strength is not specified).

Diluted erythrityl tetranitrate is a mixture of erythrityl tetranitrate and lactose or other suitable inert excipients, the excipients being added to minimise the risk of explosion.

It is a white powder with a slight odour of nitric oxides. **Store** at a temperature not exceeding 40° in airtight containers.

CAUTION. *Undiluted erythrityl tetranitrate can be exploded by percussion or excessive heat.*

Erythrityl tetranitrate is a vasodilator with general properties similar to those of glyceryl trinitrate (p.875). When administered sublingually its effects are evident within 5 minutes and when swallowed within 30 minutes.

Erythrityl tetranitrate is used in angina pectoris (p.780). It is used before an activity or stress which might provoke an attack or for long-term management; it is not suitable for the treatment of acute anginal pain. The usual dose is 5 to 10 mg sublingually or by mouth three or four times daily, increased as necessary up to 100 mg daily.

Preparations

USP 23: Erythrityl Tetranitrate Tablets.

Proprietary Preparations (details are given in Part 3)
Ital.: Cardilate; *USA:* Cardilate†.

Esmolol Hydrochloride (16636-f)

Esmolol Hydrochloride *(BANM, USAN, rINNM)*.

ASL-8052. Methyl 3-[4-(2-hydroxy-3-isopropylaminopropoxy)phenyl]propionate hydrochloride.

$C_{16}H_{25}NO_4,HCl$ = 331.8.

CAS — 84057-94-3 (esmolol); 103598-03-4 (± esmolol); 81161-17-3 (esmolol hydrochloride).

Incompatibility. The manufacturers advise against admixture with sodium bicarbonate because of incompatibility. Esmolol hydrochloride could be given in glucose injection (5%) or sodium chloride injection (0.9%). Esmolol hydrochloride (600 mg) was visually compatible and chemically stable for at least 24 hours when mixed with aminophylline (100 mg), heparin sodium (5000 units), bretylium tosylate (100 mg), or procainamide hydrochloride (400 mg) in polyvinyl chloride bags containing glucose 5% (100 mL).[1] Esmolol hydrochloride was considered visually and chemically compatible with sodium nitroprusside when studied in concentrations intended to maximise potential interactions (sodium nitroprusside 200 µg per mL and esmolol hydrochloride 10 mg per mL) in glucose 5% (250 mL, protected from light).[2]

1. Schaaf LJ, *et al.* Stability of esmolol hydrochloride in the presence of aminophylline, bretylium tosylate, heparin sodium, and procainamide hydrochloride. *Am J Hosp Pharm* 1990; **47:** 1567–71.
2. Karnatz NN, *et al.* Stability of esmolol hydrochloride and sodium nitroprusside in intravenous admixtures. *Am J Hosp Pharm* 1989; **46:** 101–4.

Adverse Effects, Treatment, and Precautions

As for beta blockers, p.828.

Hypotension is the most frequently reported adverse effect associated with the infusion of esmolol hydrochloride; it generally resolves within 30 minutes once the dosage is reduced or the infusion is discontinued. Local irritation at the site of infusion, inflammation, induration, and thrombophlebitis have occurred and necrosis is a hazard of extravasation. These local effects have occurred with concentrations of 20 mg per mL and it is recommended that they should not exceed 10 mg per mL and that the infusion should not be made into a small vein.

Effects on the CNS. Generalised tonic-clonic seizures in an elderly patient given esmolol hydrochloride.[1]

1. Das G, Ferris JC. Generalized convulsions in a patient receiving ultra short-acting beta-blocker infusion. *Drug Intell Clin Pharm* 1988; **22:** 484–5.

Interactions

The interactions associated with beta blockers are discussed on p.829.

For references to interactions with morphine and suxamethonium, see under Opioid Analgesics, p.830 and Skeletal Muscle Relaxants, p.830, respectively.

Pharmacokinetics

Following intravenous administration of esmolol hydrochloride the drug is rapidly hydrolysed by esterases in the red blood cells. Steady-state blood concentrations are reached within 30 minutes with doses of 50 to 300 µg per kg body-weight per minute. The time to steady-state may be reduced to 5 minutes by the administration of an appropriate loading dose. Blood concentrations are reported to decline in a biphasic manner with a distribution half-life of about 2 minutes and an elimination half-life of approximately 9 minutes. Esmolol has low lipid solubility. It is excreted in urine, primarily as the de-esterified metabolite.

Uses and Administration

Esmolol is a cardioselective short-acting beta blocker (p.828). It is reported to be lacking in intrinsic sympathomimetic and membrane-stabilising properties.

Esmolol is used as the hydrochloride in the management of supraventricular arrhythmias (p.782). It is also used for the control of hypertension (p.788) and tachycardia during the perioperative period.

Esmolol hydrochloride is administered intravenously at a concentration not exceeding 10 mg per mL.

For the rapid temporary control of ventricular rate in patients with **supraventricular arrhythmias**, a loading dose of 500 µg per kg body-weight over 1 minute is followed by an initial maintenance infusion of 50 µg per kg per minute for 4 minutes. If the response is satisfactory this maintenance infusion should be continued at 50 µg per kg per minute. If a suitable response is not obtained within the initial 5 minutes a further loading dose of 500 µg per kg over 1 minute may be given and the maintenance infusion may be increased to 100 µg per kg per minute for 4 minutes. This procedure may be repeated until a satisfactory response is obtained, increasing the maintenance infusion each time by 50 µg per kg per minute to a maximum of 200 µg per kg per minute. Little additional benefit is obtained from further increases in maintenance dosage. Once a satisfactory response is obtained infusion may be continued, if necessary, for up to 48 hours.

When transferring a patient to another antiarrhythmic drug, the infusion rate of esmolol hydrochloride is reduced by 50% thirty minutes after administration of the alternative drug, and may be discontinued one hour after the second dose of that drug.

In the control of perioperative **hypertension** and tachycardia, esmolol hydrochloride may be given intravenously as follows:

during anaesthesia, a loading dose of 80 mg over 15 to 30 seconds followed by an infusion of 150 µg per kg per minute, increased as necessary up to 300 µg per kg per minute; on waking from anaesthesia, an infusion of 500 µg per kg per minute for 4 minutes, followed by an infusion of 300 µg per kg per minute as required; postoperatively, a stepped dosage schedule, as described under control of supraventricular arrhythmias above, although maintenance infusions may be increased up to 300 µg per kg per minute as necessary.

References.

1. Benfield P, Sorkin EM. Esmolol: a preliminary review of its pharmacodynamic and pharmacokinetic properties, and therapeutic efficacy. *Drugs* 1987; **33:** 392–412.
2. Wiest D. Esmolol: a review of its therapeutic efficacy and pharmacokinetic characteristics. *Clin Pharmacokinet* 1995; **28:** 190–202.

Tetanus. For reference to the use of esmolol in controlling autonomic hyperactivity associated with tetanus, see under Labetalol, p.896.

Preparations

Proprietary Preparations (details are given in Part 3)
Aust.: Brevibloc; *Austral.:* Brevibloc; *Canad.:* Brevibloc; *Fr.:* Brevibloc; *Irl.:* Brevibloc; *S.Afr.:* Brevibloc; *Switz.:* Brevibloc; *UK:* Brevibloc; *USA:* Brevibloc.

Etafenone Hydrochloride (9230-p)

Etafenone Hydrochloride *(rINNM)*.

LG-11457. 2′-(2-Diethylaminoethoxy)-3-phenylpropiophenone hydrochloride.

$C_{21}H_{27}NO_2,HCl$ = 361.9.

CAS — 90-54-0 (etafenone); 2192-21-4 (etafenone hydrochloride).

Etafenone hydrochloride is a vasodilator that has been given by mouth or by intravenous or intramuscular injection in ischaemic heart disease.

Preparations

Proprietary Preparations (details are given in Part 3)
Aust.: Baxacor†; *Ger.:* Baxacor†; *Ital.:* Baxacor†; Dialicor†.

Multi-ingredient: *Aust.:* Baxanitrat†; Seda-baxacor†; *Ger.:* Seda Baxacor†.

Ethacrynic Acid (2363-e)

Ethacrynic Acid *(BAN, USAN)*.

Etacrynic Acid *(rINN)*; Acidum Etacrynicum; Etacrynsäure; MK-595; NSC-85791. [2,3-Dichloro-4-(2-ethylacryloyl)phenoxy]acetic acid; [2,3-Dichloro-4-(2-methylene-1-oxobutyl)phenoxy]acetic acid.

$C_{13}H_{12}Cl_2O_4$ = 303.1.

CAS — 58-54-8.

Pharmacopoeias. In *Chin., Eur.* (see p.viii), *Jpn, Pol.*, and *US*.

A white or almost white, odourless or almost odourless, crystalline powder. Very slightly **soluble** in water; soluble 1 in 1.6 of alcohol, 1 in 6 of chloroform, and 1 in 3.5 of ether; dissolves in ammonia and in dilute aqueous solutions of alkali hydroxides and carbonates.

CAUTION. *Ethacrynic acid, especially in the form of dust, is irritating to the skin, eyes, and mucous membranes.*

Sodium Ethacrynate (2328-p)

Sodium Ethacrynate *(BANM)*.

Sodium Etacrynate *(rINNM)*; Etacrynate Sodium; Ethacrynate Sodium *(USAN)*.

$C_{13}H_{11}Cl_2NaO_4$ = 325.1.

CAS — 6500-81-8.

Pharmacopoeias. In *Chin.*

Solutions of sodium ethacrynate containing the equivalent of ethacrynic acid 0.1% have a pH of 6.3 to 7.7. Solutions are relatively stable at about pH 7 at room temperatures for short periods and less stable at higher pH values and temperatures. They are **incompatible** with solutions with a pH below 5. The injection should be **protected** from light.

Adverse Effects

As for Frusemide, p.871. Gastro-intestinal disturbances may be more common and severe with ethacrynic acid; profuse watery diarrhoea is an indication for stopping therapy. Gastro-intestinal bleeding has been associated with ethacrynic acid and tinnitus and deafness, particularly following high dose parenteral administration may be more common. Other adverse effects include confusion, fatigue, nervousness, and apprehensiveness. Haematuria has been reported rarely.

Local irritation and pain may follow intravenous injection.

Effects on carbohydrate metabolism. Although ethacrynic acid is generally considered to have less pronounced effects on carbohydrate metabolism than frusemide or the thiazide diuretics, adverse effects have been reported. Russell[1] observed reductions in glucose tolerance following ethacrynic acid 200 mg daily for 6 weeks similar to those produced by hydrochlorothiazide 200 mg daily. The effect was most pronounced in diabetic patients. Hyperosmolar hyperglycaemic coma[2] and symptomatic hypoglycaemia with convulsions[3] have been reported in patients receiving high doses of ethacrynic acid.

1. Russell RP, *et al.* Metabolic and hypotensive effects of ethacrynic acid: comparative study with hydrochlorothiazide. *JAMA* 1968; **205:** 11–16.
2. Cowley AJ, Elkeles RS. Diabetes and therapy with potent diuretics. *Lancet* 1978; **i:** 154.
3. Maher JF, Schreiner GE. Studies on ethacrynic acid in patients with refractory edema. *Ann Intern Med* 1965; **62:** 15–29.

Effects on the ears. Drug-induced deafness occurred in 2 of 184 patients given ethacrynic acid intravenously.[1,2] Deafness accompanied by nystagmus was reported in a patient[3] following an intravenous infusion of ethacrynic acid. Symptoms resolved within 1 hour. He had previously been taking frusemide and ethacrynic acid orally.

1. Boston Collaborative Drug Surveillance Program. Drug-induced deafness: a cooperative study. *JAMA* 1973; **224:** 515–16.
2. Porter J, Jick H. Drug-induced anaphylaxis, convulsions, deafness, and extrapyramidal symptoms. *Lancet* 1977; **i:** 587–8.
3. Gomolin IH, Garshick E. Ethacrynic acid-induced deafness accompanied by nystagmus. *N Engl J Med* 1980; **303:** 702.

Precautions

Ethacrynic acid's precautions and contra-indications are generally dependent on its effects on fluid and electrolyte balance and are similar to those of the thiazide diuretics (see Hydrochlorothiazide, p.887).

Interactions

As for Frusemide, p.872. The risks of gastro-intestinal bleeding may be enhanced by concurrent administration of ethacrynic acid with other gastric irritants or with anticoagulants.

For reference to the interaction between warfarin and ethacrynic acid, see p.968.

Pharmacokinetics

Ethacrynic acid is fairly rapidly absorbed from the gastro-intestinal tract. The plasma half-life is 30 to 60 minutes. It is excreted both in the bile and the urine, partly unchanged and partly in the form of metabolites. It is extensively bound to plasma proteins.

Uses and Administration

Although chemically unrelated, ethacrynic acid is a loop diuretic with actions and uses similar to those of frusemide (p.872). Ethacrynic acid is used in the treatment of oedema associated with heart failure (p.785) and with renal and hepatic disorders.

Diuresis is initiated within about 30 minutes after a dose by mouth, and lasts for about 6 to 8 hours; after intravenous injection of its sodium salt, the effects are evident within a few minutes and last for about 2 hours.

In the treatment of **oedema**, the usual initial dose is 50 mg by mouth in the morning, taken with or immediately after food. The dose may be increased, if necessary, by 25- to 50-mg increments daily to the minimum effective dose. Severe cases have required gradual titration of the ethacrynic acid dosage up to a maximum of 400 mg daily, but the effective dose range is usually between 50 and 150 mg daily. Dosage of more than 50 mg daily should be given in divided doses, and it is preferable for all doses to be taken with food. Maintenance doses may be taken daily or intermittently.

In emergencies, such as acute pulmonary oedema, or when oral therapy cannot be given, ethacrynic acid may be given intravenously. It is administered as its salt, sodium ethacrynate, but doses are expressed in terms of the base. The usual dose is 50 mg, or 0.5 to 1 mg per kg body-weight as a 1 mg per mL solution in glucose 5% (provided the pH is above 5) or sodium chloride 0.9%, given by slow intravenous injection either directly or into the tubing of a running infusion. Should a subsequent injection be required the site should be changed to avoid thrombophlebitis. Single doses of 100 mg have been given intravenously in critical situations. It is not suitable for subcutaneous or intramuscular injection.

For children over 2 years of age a suggested initial dose of ethacrynic acid is 25 mg daily by mouth, cautiously increased as necessary by 25 mg daily.

In susceptible patients potassium supplements or potassium-sparing diuretics may be necessary, but see under hydrochlorothiazide (Uses and Administration, p.887). If very high doses of ethacrynic acid are used careful laboratory control is essential as described under frusemide (p.872; high-dose therapy).

Preparations

BP 1998: Etacrynic Acid Tablets; Sodium Etacrynate Injection; ***USP 23:*** Ethacrynate Sodium for Injection; Ethacrynic Acid Tablets.

Proprietary Preparations (details are given in Part 3)
Aust.: Edecrin; ***Austral.:*** Edecril; ***Canad.:*** Edecrin; ***Ger.:*** Hydromedin; Uregyt; ***Irl.:*** Edecrin; ***Ital.:*** Edecrin; Reomax; ***Neth.:*** Edecrin; ***Norw.:*** Edecrin†; ***Swed.:*** Edecrina; ***UK:*** Edecrin; ***USA:*** Edecrin; Sodium Edecrin.

Ethyl Biscoumacetate (4813-j)

Ethyl Biscoumacetate *(BAN, rINN).*

Aethylis Biscoumacetas; Ethyldicoumarol; Ethylis Biscoumacetas; Neodicumarinum. Ethyl bis(4-hydroxycoumarin-3-yl)acetate.

$C_{22}H_{16}O_8$ = 408.4.
CAS — 548-00-5.
Pharmacopoeias. In *Fr.* and *It.*

Adverse Effects, Treatment, and Precautions

As for Warfarin Sodium, p.964.

Interactions

The interactions associated with oral anticoagulants are discussed in detail under warfarin (p.965). Specific references to interactions involving ethyl biscoumacetate can be found under the headings for the following drug groups: analgesics; antifungals; antigout drugs; central stimulants; corticosteroids and corticotrophin; and diuretics.

Pharmacokinetics

Ethyl biscoumacetate is readily absorbed from the gastro-intestinal tract and is extensively bound to plasma proteins. It is metabolised in the liver; the inactive metabolites are excreted in the urine. Reported plasma half-life ranges from 2 to 3.5 hours.

Ethyl biscoumacetate crosses the placenta and has been reported to appear in only small amounts in breast milk.

Uses and Administration

Ethyl biscoumacetate is an orally administered coumarin anticoagulant with actions similar to those of warfarin sodium (p.969). It has been used in the management of thrombo-embolic disorders (p.801).

It has been given in a dose of 600 to 1200 mg on the first day, 300 to 600 mg on the second day, with subsequent doses generally in the range of 300 to 450 mg daily according to coagulation tests, administered in 3 to 4 divided doses.

Preparations

Proprietary Preparations (details are given in Part 3)
Fr.: Tromexane†.

Etilefrine Hydrochloride (2061-x)

Etilefrine Hydrochloride *(rINNM).*

Ethyladrianol Hydrochloride; Ethylnorphenylephrine Hydrochloride; Etilefrini Hydrochloridum; M-I-36. 2-Ethylamino-1-(3-hydroxyphenyl)ethanol hydrochloride.

$C_{10}H_{15}NO_2$,HCl = 217.7.
CAS — 709-55-7 (etilefrine); 943-17-9 (etilefrine hydrochloride).
Pharmacopoeias. In *Eur.* (see p.viii) and *Jpn.*

White crystalline powder or colourless crystals. Freely **soluble** in water; soluble in alcohol; practically insoluble in dichloromethane. **Store** in airtight containers. Protect from light.

Etilefrine is a direct-acting sympathomimetic (see Adrenaline, p.813) with $beta_1$ agonist properties, and some alpha and $beta_2$ agonist actions. It is used for the treatment of hypotensive states. It is given as the hydrochloride by mouth in usual doses of 5 or 10 mg three times daily; controlled-release dosage forms are also employed in doses of 25 mg once or twice daily. Etilefrine hydrochloride can also be given parenterally.

Etilefrine in the form of etilefrine polistirex is used in the management of rhinitis.

Preparations

Proprietary Preparations (details are given in Part 3)
Aust.: Amphodyn mono; Circupon; Effortil; ***Belg.:*** Effortil; ***Fr.:*** Effortil; ***Ger.:*** Adrenam; Bioflutin-N; Cardanat; Cardialgine; Circupon RR; Circuvit E; Confidol; Effortil; Eti-Puren; Etil; Kreislauf Katovit; Logomed Kreislauf-Tabletten; Thomasin; Tonus-forte-Tablinen; ***Ital.:*** Effortil; ***Norw.:*** Effortil; ***S.Afr.:*** Effortil; ***Spain:*** Efortil; ***Swed.:*** Effortil; ***Switz.:*** Circupon; Effortil.

Multi-ingredient: ***Aust.:*** Agilan; Amphodyn; Effortil comp; Hypodyn; Influbene; ***Ger.:*** Agit plus; Amphodyn; Dihydergot plus; Effortil plus; Ergolefrin; Ergomimet plus; Poikiloton†; ***Switz.:*** Addergit†; Amphodyn special†; Dihydergot plus; Effortil plus; Influbene†.

Etozolin (12722-e)

Etozolin *(USAN, rINN).*

Gö-687; W-2900A. Ethyl (3-methyl-4-oxo-5-piperidinothiazolidin-2-ylidene)acetate.

$C_{13}H_{20}N_2O_3S$ = 284.4.
CAS — 73-09-6.

Etozolin is a loop diuretic with properties similar to those of frusemide (p.871), but with a longer duration of action. It is used in the treatment of oedema and hypertension. Etozolin is reported to be rapidly metabolised to ozolinone which also has diuretic activity.

References.

1. Knauf H, *et al.* Pharmacodynamics and kinetics of etozolin/ozolinone in hypertensive patients with normal and impaired kidney function. *Eur J Clin Pharmacol* 1984; **26:** 687–93.
2. Beermann B, Grind M. Clinical pharmacokinetics of some newer diuretics. *Clin Pharmacokinet* 1987; **13:** 254–66.

Preparations

Proprietary Preparations (details are given in Part 3)
Aust.: Elkapin; ***Ger.:*** Elkapin; ***Ital.:*** Elkapin; ***Spain:*** Diuzolin†; Elkapin.

Fasudil Hydrochloride (15275-v)

Fasudil Hydrochloride *(rINNM).*

AT-877; HA-1077. Hexahydro-1-(5-isoquinolylsulfonyl)-1*H*-1,4-diazepine hydrochloride.

$C_{14}H_{17}N_3O_2S$,HCl = 327.8.
CAS — 103745-39-7 (fasudil); 105628-07-7 (fasudil hydrochloride).

Fasudil is a vasodilator used as the hydrochloride in the management of cerebrovascular disorders.

Felodipine (16801-t)

Felodipine *(BAN, USAN, rINN).*

Felodipinum; H-154/82. Ethyl methyl 4-(2,3-dichlorophenyl)-1,4-dihydro-2,6-dimethylpyridine-3,5-dicarboxylate.

$C_{18}H_{19}Cl_2NO_4$ = 384.3.
CAS — 72509-76-3; 86189-69-7.
Pharmacopoeias. In *Eur.* (see p.viii).

A white or light yellow crystalline powder. Practically **insoluble** in water; freely soluble in acetone, in absolute alcohol, in methyl alcohol, and in dichloromethane.
Protect from light.

Adverse Effects, Treatment, and Precautions

As for dihydropyridine calcium-channel blockers (see Nifedipine, p.916).

Interactions

As for dihydropyridine calcium-channel blockers (see Nifedipine, p.918).

Pharmacokinetics

Felodipine is almost completely absorbed from the gastro-intestinal tract after oral administration but undergoes extensive first-pass metabolism, with a bioavailability of about 15% (range 10 to 25%). It is extensively metabolised in the gut and the liver and is excreted almost entirely as metabolites, about 70% of a dose being excreted in urine and the remainder in faeces. The terminal elimination half-life is reported to be about 11 to 16 hours following oral administration of an immediate-release preparation, but longer with a modified-release formulation. Felodipine is about 99% bound to plasma protein (mainly albumin).

General reviews.

1. Dunselman PHJM, Edgar B. Felodipine clinical pharmacokinetics. *Clin Pharmacokinet* 1991; **21:** 418–30.

Hepatic impairment. In 9 patients with liver cirrhosis given felodipine 0.75 mg by intravenous infusion over 20 minutes and 10 mg by mouth as single doses on separate occasions the mean oral bioavailability was 17.1% which was not significantly different from published values in healthy subjects, but the maximum plasma concentrations were almost twice as high as normal, apparently due to reduced systemic clearance and volume of distribution.[1] The fact that bioavailability was not increased suggests that much pre-systemic metabolism takes place in the gut rather than the liver. Although increased adverse effects were not associated with the raised felodipine concentrations in this study it is recommended that therapy in cirrhotic patients be initiated at lower doses than in patients with normal liver function.

1. Regårdh CG, *et al.* Pharmacokinetics of felodipine in patients with liver disease. *Eur J Clin Pharmacol* 1989; **36:** 473–9.

Uses and Administration

Felodipine is a dihydropyridine calcium-channel blocker with actions similar to those of nifedipine (p.919). It is used in the treatment of hypertension (p.788) and angina pectoris (p.780).

Felodipine is given by mouth, generally in a modified-release formulation for administration once daily in the morning. In **hypertension** the usual initial dose is 5 mg daily by mouth, adjusted as required; the usual maintenance dose is 2.5 to 10 mg daily and doses above 20 mg daily are not usually needed. In **angina** the usual initial dose is 5 mg daily increased if necessary to 10 mg daily.

Lower doses may be required in the elderly and in patients with impaired liver function.

Reviews.

1. Saltiel E, *et al.* Felodipine: a review of its pharmacodynamic and pharmacokinetic properties, and therapeutic use in hypertension. *Drugs* 1988; **36:** 387–428.
2. Todd PA, Faulds D. Felodipine: a review of the pharmacology and therapeutic use of the extended release formulation in cardiovascular disorders. *Drugs* 1992; **44:** 251–77.
3. Walton T, Symes LR. Felodipine and isradipine: new calcium-channel-blocking agents for the treatment of hypertension. *Clin Pharm* 1993; **12:** 261–75.

Preparations

Proprietary Preparations (details are given in Part 3)
Aust.: Munobal; Plendil; ***Austral.:*** Agon; Felodur; Plendil; ***Belg.:*** Plendil; Renedil; ***Canad.:*** Plendil; Renedil; ***Fr.:*** Flodil; ***Ger.:*** Modip; Munobal; ***Irl.:*** Plendil; ***Ital.:*** Feloday; Plendil; Prevex; ***Neth.:*** Plendil; Renedil; ***Norw.:*** Plendil; ***S.Afr.:*** Plendil; ***Spain:*** Fensel; Perfudal; Plendil; Preslow; ***Swed.:*** Hydac; Plendil; ***Switz.:*** Munobal; Plendil; ***UK:*** Plendil; ***USA:*** Plendil.

Multi-ingredient: ***Aust.:*** Logimax; ***Belg.:*** Logimat; ***Fr.:*** Logimax; ***Norw.:*** Logimax; ***Spain:*** Logimax; ***Swed.:*** Logimax; ***Switz.:*** Logimax; ***USA:*** Lexxel.

Fendiline Hydrochloride (9233-e)

Fendiline Hydrochloride *(pINNM).*

N-(2-Benzhydrylethyl)-α-methylbenzylamine hydrochloride.

$C_{23}H_{25}N,HCl$ = 351.9.

CAS — 13042-18-7 (fendiline); 13636-18-5 (fendiline hydrochloride).

Fendiline hydrochloride is a calcium-channel blocker used as a vasodilator in ischaemic heart disease in usual doses of 150 mg daily, in divided doses, by mouth.

Ischaemic heart disease is discussed under Atherosclerosis (p.782) and the treatment of its clinical manifestations is described under Angina Pectoris (p.780) and Myocardial Infarction (p.791).

Preparations

Proprietary Preparations (details are given in Part 3)
Aust.: Sensit; ***Ger.:*** Sensit; ***Ital.:*** Cordan†; Difmecor; Fendilar†; Olbiacor; Sensit-F; ***Switz.:*** Sensit.

Multi-ingredient: ***Ger.:*** Digo-Sensit†.

Fenoldopam Mesylate (17955-f)

Fenoldopam Mesylate *(BANM, USAN).*

Fenoldopam Mesilate *(rINNM)*; SKF-82526-j. 6-Chloro-2,3,4,5-tetrahydro-1-(*p*-hydroxyphenyl)-1*H*-3-benzazepine-7,8-diol methanesulfonate.

$C_{17}H_{20}ClNO_6S$ = 401.9.

CAS — 67227-56-9 (fenoldopam); 67227-57-0 (fenoldopam mesylate).

Adverse Effects and Precautions

The adverse effects of fenoldopam are mainly due to vasodilatation and include hypotension, flushing, dizziness, headache, and reflex tachycardia. Nausea and vomiting, and ECG abnormalities have also been reported. Hypokalaemia has occurred and serum-electrolyte concentrations should be monitored during therapy. Fenoldopam may increase intra-ocular pressure and it should be used with caution in patients with glaucoma. Caution is also required in patients in whom hypotension could be deleterious, such as those with acute cerebral infarction or haemorrhage. Blood pressure and heart rate should be monitored.

Interactions

The hypotensive effects of fenoldopam may be enhanced by other drugs with hypotensive actions. Beta blockers may block the reflex tachycardia that occurs with fenoldopam and concomitant use is not recommended.

Pharmacokinetics

Steady-state plasma concentrations of fenoldopam are reached about 20 minutes after commencing continuous intravenous infusion. Fenoldopam is extensively metabolised with only about 4% of a dose being excreted unchanged. It is metabolised by conjugation (mainly glucuronidation, methylation, and sulphation). Fenoldopam and its metabolites are excreted predominantly in the urine, the remainder being excreted in the faeces. The elimination half-life of fenoldopam is about five minutes.

Uses and Administration

Fenoldopam is a dopamine agonist which is reported to have a selective action at dopamine D_1-receptors, leading to vasodilatation. It is given intravenously as the mesylate in the short-term management of severe hypertension (p.788). It has also been tried in heart failure.

In the management of hypertensive crises, fenoldopam mesylate is given by continuous intravenous infusion as a solution containing 40 μg per mL. The dose should be adjusted according to response, in usual increments of 0.05 to 0.1 μg per kg bodyweight per minute at 15-minute intervals. The usual dose range is from 0.1 to 1.6 μg per kg per minute.

Reviews.

1. Brogden RN, Markham A. Fenoldopam: a review of its pharmacodynamic and pharmacokinetic properties and intravenous clinical potential in the management of hypertensive urgencies and emergencies. *Drugs* 1997; **54:** 634–50.
2. Post JB, Frishman WH. Fenoldopam: a new dopamine agonist for the treatment of hypertensive urgencies and emergencies. *J Clin Pharmacol* 1998; **38:** 2–13.

Heart failure. Diuretics, ACE inhibitors, cardiac glycosides, and vasodilators are the main drugs used in the management of heart failure (p.785).

Fenoldopam given orally has been investigated in small studies of patients with heart failure. In a study in 20 patients with moderately severe heart failure (New York Heart Association grades II to III) fenoldopam 50 mg three times daily by mouth, increased where tolerated to 100 mg three times daily, was given to 10 while the remainder received placebo.[1] One patient in the fenoldopam group died, and 2 were withdrawn due to worsening heart failure, as was 1 patient in the placebo group, and a further patient receiving fenoldopam withdrew for unknown reasons. Among the remaining patients there was no difference between groups in exercise tolerance, symptoms, or ejection fraction. There was no evidence from this preliminary study of any benefit in heart failure from oral fenoldopam.[1] In contrast to these results, King and others[2] have reported improvements in exercise tolerance and symptoms in similarly classified patients given fenoldopam 100 mg two or three times daily for 8 weeks, compared with placebo. These apparently contradictory results might be due to differences in the statistical power of the studies, but it should also be noted that both studies used oral fenoldopam, which is poorly bioavailable. Resolution of the role of fenoldopam in heart failure awaits the results of larger studies.

1. MacDonald TM, *et al.* A preliminary study of the dopamine DA_1 agonist fenoldopam in the treatment of chronic left ventricular failure due to ischaemic heart disease. *Eur J Clin Pharmacol* 1990; **38:** 199–201.
2. King BD, *et al.* Efficacy of fenoldopam (SKF 82526) in chronic congestive heart failure. *Circulation* 1987; **76** (suppl IV): 71.

Hypertension. Fenoldopam has a short duration of action and poor oral bioavailability necessitating frequent large oral doses, and better results have been obtained with intravenous infusions.[1] The rapid onset of its hypotensive action and its short elimination half-life suggest a role in patients requiring rapid blood pressure reduction.[2] Comparative studies with sodium nitroprusside in patients with severe hypertension requiring urgent therapy have shown fenoldopam to be effective in rapidly lowering blood pressure and, in contrast to nitroprusside, urine output, creatinine clearance, and sodium excretion were increased by fenoldopam.[1,3] In view of the beneficial renal haemodynamic effects, and the fact that it is well tolerated, fenoldopam may offer advantages over current therapy in the acute treatment of severe hypertension in patients with impaired renal function.[3]

For a discussion of the treatment of hypertension, including hypertensive crises, see p.788.

1. Horn PT, Murphy MB. Therapeutic applications of drugs acting on peripheral dopamine receptors. *J Clin Pharmacol* 1990; **30:** 674–9.
2. Weber RR, *et al.* Pharmacokinetic and pharmacodynamic properties of intravenous fenoldopam, a dopamine$_1$-receptor agonist, in hypertensive patients. *Br J Clin Pharmacol* 1988; **25:** 17–21.
3. Shusterman NH, *et al.* Fenoldopam, but not nitroprusside, improves renal function in severely hypertensive patients with impaired renal function. *Am J Med* 1993; **95:** 161–8.

Preparations

Proprietary Preparations (details are given in Part 3)
USA: Corlopam.

Fenquizone Potassium (12745-a)

Fenquizone Potassium *(rINNM).*

MG-13054 (fenquizone). 7-Chloro-1,2,3,4-tetrahydro-4-oxo-2-phenylquinazoline-6-sulphonamide, monopotassium salt.

$C_{14}H_{12}ClN_3O_3S,K$ = 376.9.

CAS — 20287-37-0 (fenquizone); 52246-40-9 (fenquizone potassium).

NOTE. Fenquizone is *USAN.*

Fenquizone potassium is a diuretic that is used in the treatment of oedema and hypertension (p.788) in doses equivalent to 10 to 20 mg of fenquizone daily by mouth.

References.

1. Beermann B, Grind M. Clinical pharmacokinetics of some newer diuretics. *Clin Pharmacokinet* 1987; **13:** 254–66.
2. Costa FV, *et al.* Hemodynamic and humoral effects of chronic antihypertensive treatment with fenquizone: importance of aldosterone response. *J Clin Pharmacol* 1990; **30:** 254–61.

Preparations

Proprietary Preparations (details are given in Part 3)
Ital.: Idrolone.

Flecainide Acetate (12753-a)

Flecainide Acetate *(BANM, USAN, rINNM).*

R-818. *N*-(2-Piperidylmethyl)-2,5-bis(2,2,2-trifluoroethoxy)benzamide acetate.

$C_{17}H_{20}F_6N_2O_3,C_2H_4O_2$ = 474.4.

CAS — 54143-55-4 (flecainide); 54143-56-5 (flecainide acetate).

Pharmacopoeias. In *Eur.* (see p.viii) and *US.*

A white to slightly off-white very hygroscopic crystalline powder. **Soluble** in water; soluble to freely soluble in alcohol; very soluble in dilute acetic acid; practically insoluble in dilute hydrochloric acid. A 2.5% solution in water has a pH of 6.7 to 7.1. **Protect** from light.

Stability. Storage of an extemporaneously prepared flecainide syrup in a refrigerator led to crystallisation of the drug and the administration of a toxic dose.[1] Oral liquid formulations of flecainide should be freshly reconstituted from a powder before each dose.

1. Stuart AG, *et al.* Is there a genetic factor in flecainide toxicity? *Br Med J* 1989; **298:** 117–18.

Adverse Effects

The most common adverse effects caused by flecainide affect the central nervous system and include dizziness, visual disturbances, and lightheadedness. Nausea, vomiting, headache, tremor, peripheral neuropathy, ataxia, and paraesthesia may also occur. These effects are generally transient and respond to dosage reduction. There have been isolated cases of photosensitivity. Disturbances of liver function have been reported rarely. Corneal deposits, pulmonary fibrosis, and pneumonitis have occurred during long-term therapy. Cardiovascular effects are less common, but can be serious and sometimes fatal. Ventricular tachyarrhythmias have been reported, particularly in patients with a history of ventricular tachyarrhythmias and taking high doses of flecainide. Flecainide produced an increased mortality rate when it was assessed for the control of asymptomatic ventricular arrhythmias in patients who had previously suffered a myocardial infarction (see Cardiac Arrhythmias under Uses and Administration, below).

Report of the non-cardiac adverse effects of flecainide from one short-term and 3 longer term studies.[1] The most common adverse effects during both short- and long-term studies were dizziness and visual disturbances which occurred in about 30% of patients. Headache and nausea both occurred in about 10% of patients. Other adverse effects reported include dyspnoea, chest pain, asthenia, fatigue, and tremor. Therapy was discontinued due to non-cardiac adverse effects in 10% of patients in the short-term trial, and in 6% of those in the chronic studies. A review of 60 studies using flecainide[2] reported that non-cardiac side-effects (mainly gastro-intestinal and CNS adverse effects) occurred in 12% of patients. In the UK, the Committee on Safety of Medicines (CSM) had received reports of neurological (4 patients with sensory neuropathy, 2 with ataxia), corneal (2 with corneal deposits), and pulmonary (3 with pulmonary fibrosis and pneumonitis) reactions associated with the long-term use of flecainide.[3]

1. Gentzkow GD, Sullivan JY. Extracardiac adverse effects of flecainide. *Am J Cardiol* 1984; **53:** 101B–105B.
2. Hohnloser SH, Zabel M. Short- and long-term efficacy and safety of flecainide acetate for supraventricular arrhythmias. *Am J Cardiol* 1992; **70:** 3A–10A.
3. Committee on Safety of Medicines. Multi-system adverse reactions following long-term flecainide therapy. *Current Problems 31* 1991.

Effects on the blood. Severe granulocytopenia believed to be related to flecainide acetate occurred in a 66-year-old man 3 months after starting therapy with the drug.[1] Haematological findings suggested an immune-mediated reaction in which flecainide binds to normal neutrophils with subsequent recognition by specific antibodies resulting in enhanced destruction of mature granulocytes in peripheral blood and bone marrow.

1. Samlowski WE, *et al.* Flecainide-induced immune neutropenia: documentation of a hapten-mediated mechanism of cell destruction. *Arch Intern Med* 1987; **147:** 383–4.

Effects on the eyes. In addition to visual disturbance, corneal deposits have been reported in association with flecainide therapy.[1]

1. Ulrik H, *et al.* Corneal deposits associated with flecainide. *Br Med J* 1991; **302:** 506–7.

Effects on the heart. Like many antiarrhythmics, flecainide can have proarrhythmic effects.[1,2] Further information is also given in Cardiac Arrhythmias under Uses and Administration, below.

1. Falk RH. Flecainide-induced ventricular tachycardia and fibrillation in patients treated for atrial fibrillation. *Ann Intern Med* 1989; **111:** 107–11.
2. Herre JM, *et al.* Inefficacy and proarrhythmic effects of flecainide and encainide for sustained ventricular tachycardia and ventricular fibrillation. *Ann Intern Med* 1990; **113:** 671–6.

Effects on the liver. Elevated liver enzymes and jaundice, reversible on stopping treatment, have been reported rarely in association with flecainide therapy.

Conjugated hyperbilirubinaemia with jaundice developed in a newborn infant following maternal treatment with flecainide for fetal supraventricular tachycardia.[1]

1. Vanderhal AL, *et al.* Conjugated hyperbilirubinemia in a newborn infant after maternal (transplacental) treatment with flecainide acetate for fetal tachycardia and fetal hydrops. *J Pediatr* 1995; **126:** 988–90.

Effects on the lungs. Reports[1,2] of interstitial pneumonitis associated with flecainide therapy.

1. Akoun GM, *et al.* Flecainide-associated pneumonitis. *Lancet* 1991; **337:** 49.
2. Hanston P, *et al.* Flecainide-associated interstitial pneumonitis. *Lancet* 1991; **337:** 371–2.

Effects on mental state. Dysarthria and visual hallucinations were associated with elevated plasma concentration of flecainide (2500 ng per mL) in 1 patient.[1] A serial rise and fall in plasma-bilirubin concentration during flecainide therapy also suggested possible direct hepatotoxicity.

1. Ramhamadany E, *et al.* Dysarthria and visual hallucinations due to flecainide toxicity. *Postgrad Med J* 1986; **62:** 61–2.

Effects on the nervous system. Peripheral neuropathy in one patient taking flecainide long term has been described; symptoms regressed after drug withdrawal.[1] In the UK the Committee on Safety of Medicines had received four other reports possibly associated with flecainide and three reports of aggravation of pre-existing neuropathy.[1]

1. Palace J, *et al.* Flecainide induced peripheral neuropathy. *Br Med J* 1992; **305:** 810.

Lupus erythematosus. A brief report of a patient who developed painful eye movement during treatment with flecainide.[1] The pain resolved when treatment was withdrawn, but recurred when flecainide was restarted, and was accompanied by lateral rectus spasm, a facial rash, and positive antinuclear factor, suggestive of lupus erythematosus.

1. Skander M, Isaacs PET. Flecainide, ocular myopathy, and antinuclear factor. *Br Med J* 1985; **291:** 450.

Treatment of Adverse Effects

In overdosage by mouth the stomach should be emptied by lavage. Treatment is largely symptomatic and supportive and may need to be continued for extended periods of time because of the long half-life and the possibility of non-linear elimination at very high doses. Haemodialysis or haemoperfusion are unlikely to enhance elimination.

Life-threatening ventricular tachycardia occurred in a young woman following ingestion of flecainide acetate 3.8 g, diazepam 50 mg, loperamide 20 mg, and alcohol 100 g.[1] The serum-flecainide concentration on admission, 2 hours after the overdose, was 3700 ng per mL. Treatment included mechanical ventilation, intravenous dopamine and an intravenous sodium load for cardiogenic shock, and intravenous physostigmine salicylate to protect against cardiotoxicity. The stomach was emptied by lavage followed by activated charcoal and forced diarrhoea with mannitol. Forced diuresis was performed but probably had a negligible effect owing to the extensive distribution of flecainide into the tissues. The serum-flecainide concentration 9 hours after the overdose was 1680 ng per mL; it continued to decline thereafter at a slower rate.

1. Winkelmann BR, Leinberger H. Life-threatening flecainide toxicity: a pharmacodynamic approach. *Ann Intern Med* 1987; **106:** 807–14.

Failure of haemoperfusion to reduce flecainide intoxication in a patient with terminal renal failure and undergoing haemodialysis.[1]

1. Braun J, *et al.* Failure of haemoperfusion to reduce flecainide intoxication: a case study. *Med Toxicol* 1987; **2:** 463–7.

Precautions

Flecainide treatment should be instituted in hospitalised patients and pacing rescue should be available when it is used in patients with conduction defects. Its use is limited to serious or life-threatening arrhythmias and it should not be given to control asymptomatic arrhythmias especially in patients with a history of myocardial infarction (see Cardiac Arrhythmias under Uses and Administration, below). Flecainide has some negative inotropic activity and may precipitate or aggravate heart failure in patients with compromised left ventricular function and some authorities, such as those in the UK, recommend that flecainide should not be used in patients with heart failure. Flecainide has been shown to increase the endocardial pacing threshold and should be used with caution in patients with pacemakers. Electrolyte imbalances should be corrected before initiating flecainide therapy. Reduction of dosage may be necessary in patients with impaired renal function; extreme caution is needed in patients with pronounced hepatic impairment.

Pregnancy. Flecainide crosses the placenta and is distributed into breast milk, further details of which are given under Pharmacokinetics, below.

For a report of hyperbilirubinaemia in an infant following maternal treatment with flecainide, see under Effects on the Liver, above.

Interactions

Concomitant administration of flecainide with other antiarrhythmics or arrhythmogenic drugs may increase the incidence of cardiac arrhythmias. Concomitant use with a beta blocker produces additive negative inotropic effects. Flecainide undergoes metabolism in the liver and its activity may be influenced by other drugs affecting the enzymes responsible for its metabolism.

Antiarrhythmics. *Amiodarone* increases the plasma-flecainide concentration when the two drugs are given concomitantly.[1] It has been recommended that to maintain plasma-flecainide concentrations similar to those obtained during flecainide monotherapy, the dose of flecainide should be reduced by about half, but because the effect of amiodarone differs widely between patients, the plasma-flecainide concentration should be monitored. The clearance of flecainide may be decreased by *quinidine* in patients who are extensive metabolisers, since quinidine inhibits the enzyme responsible for the metabolism of flecainide.[2] Cardiogenic shock and asystole has been described in two patients receiving flecainide when *verapamil* was added to their therapy.[3]

1. Shea P, *et al.* Flecainide and amiodarone interaction. *J Am Coll Cardiol* 1986; **7:** 1127–30.
2. Birgersdotter UM, *et al.* Stereoselective genetically-determined interaction between chronic flecainide and quinidine in patients with arrhythmias. *Br J Clin Pharmacol* 1992; **33:** 275–80.
3. Buss J, *et al.* Asystole and cardiogenic shock due to combined treatment with verapamil and flecainide. *Lancet* 1992; **340:** 546.

Antimalarials. *Quinine* has been reported to inhibit metabolism of flecainide in healthy subjects without altering its renal elimination, resulting in a reduction of total clearance and prolongation of the elimination half-life.[1]

1. Munafo A, *et al.* Altered flecainide disposition in healthy volunteers taking quinine. *Eur J Clin Pharmacol* 1990; **38:** 269–73.

Beta blockers. Concurrent administration of flecainide and *propranolol* in healthy subjects increases the plasma concentration of both drugs. The negative inotropic effects of the two drugs on cardiac function are at most only additive, but treatment with this combination should be initiated with caution in patients with impaired left ventricular function.[1] Addition of *sotalol* to flecainide therapy has produced profound bradycardia and atrioventricular block followed by cardiac arrest and death in a man with ventricular tachycardia.[2]

1. Holtzman JL, *et al.* The pharmacodynamic and pharmacokinetic interaction of flecainide acetate with propranolol: effects on cardiac function and drug clearance. *Eur J Clin Pharmacol* 1987; **33:** 97–9.
2. Warren R, *et al.* Serious interactions of sotalol with amiodarone and flecainide. *Med J Aust* 1990; **152:** 277.

Food. Milk feeds reduced the absorption of flecainide in an infant who required a dose of 40 mg per kg body-weight daily to control supraventricular tachycardias. When milk feeds were replaced by glucose, the serum-flecainide concentration increased from 990 to 1824 ng per mL. Milk-fed infants on high doses of flecainide should have the dose reduced if milk is stopped or reduced.[1]

1. Russell GAB, Martin RP. Flecainide toxicity. *Arch Dis Child* 1989; **64:** 860–2.

Histamine H_2-antagonists. *Cimetidine* has been reported to increase the bioavailability of flecainide in healthy subjects, probably due to a decrease in the biotransformation of flecainide. Elimination half-life and renal clearance were unchanged.[1]

1. Tjandra-Maga TB, *et al.* Altered pharmacokinetics of oral flecainide by cimetidine. *Br J Clin Pharmacol* 1986; **22:** 108–10.

Pharmacokinetics

Flecainide is almost completely absorbed after oral administration and does not undergo extensive first-pass hepatic metabolism. Flecainide is metabolised to 2 major metabolites, *m-O*-dealkylated flecainide and *m-O*-dealkylated lactam of flecainide, both of which may have some activity. Its metabolism is subject to genetic polymorphism (see below). Flecainide is excreted mainly in the urine, approximately 30% as unchanged drug and the remainder as metabolites. About 5% is excreted in the faeces. Excretion of flecainide is decreased in renal impairment, heart failure, and in alkaline urine. Haemodialysis removes only about 1% of an oral dose as unchanged flecainide.

The therapeutic plasma concentration range is generally accepted as 200 to 1000 ng per mL. The elimination half-life of flecainide is about 20 hours and it is about 40% bound to plasma proteins.

Flecainide crosses the placenta and is distributed into breast milk.

Breast feeding. Flecainide 100 mg every 12 hours by mouth was given to 11 healthy women beginning 1 day after delivery and continuing for 5½ days.[1] The mean milk to plasma ratios on study days 2 to 5 were 3.7, 3.2, 3.5, and 2.6 respectively but it was considered that the risk to breast-fed infants of ingesting toxic amounts of flecainide in breast milk was very low. The mean elimination half-life of flecainide from milk was 14.7 hours, very similar to the plasma elimination half-life.

1. McQuinn RL, *et al.* Flecainide excretion in human breast milk. *Clin Pharmacol Ther* 1990; **48:** 262–7.

Metabolism. Oxidative metabolism is an important route of flecainide elimination.[1] A number of other drugs, such as sparteine and debrisoquine, which also undergo oxidative metabolism display a genetic polymorphism and extensive metabolisers and poor metabolisers can be identified. A similar type of genetic polymorphism has been demonstrated for flecainide and the 5 to 10% of the population who are poor metabolisers for sparteine and debrisoquine will also have a restricted capacity to metabolise flecainide. The mean elimination half-life of flecainide in poor metabolisers was found to be 11.8 hours compared with 6.8 hours in extensive metabolisers and the amounts of a dose excreted as unchanged drug in the urine were 51% and 31% respectively. These differences in pharmacokinetics will not be of clinical importance as long as renal function is not impaired since the reduced metabolic clearance in poor metabolisers can be compensated by increased renal elimination. However, if patients with impaired renal function are to be given flecainide their metabolic phenotype should be identified and special care taken with dosage adjustments in poor metabolisers.

1. Mikus G, *et al.* The influence of the sparteine-debrisoquin phenotype on the disposition of flecainide. *Clin Pharmacol Ther* 1989; **45:** 562–7.

Pregnancy. A study of the pharmacokinetics of flecainide, given to a mother during the third trimester of pregnancy for the treatment of fetal supraventricular tachycardia,[1] indicated that close to term flecainide crosses the placenta easily without accumulating in fetal blood, but with a high concentration in the amniotic fluid.

See also under Effects on the Liver, above.

1. Bourget P, *et al.* Flecainide distribution, transplacental passage and accumulation in the amniotic fluid during the third trimester of pregnancy. *Ann Pharmacother* 1994; **28:** 1031–4.

Uses and Administration

Flecainide is a class Ic antiarrhythmic (p.776) used for the treatment of severe symptomatic ventricular arrhythmias (sustained ventricular tachycardia or premature ventricular contractions or non-sustained ventricular tachycardia resistant to other therapy) and severe symptomatic supraventricular arrhythmias (atrioventricular nodal reciprocating tachycardia, arrhythmias associated with the Wolff-Parkinson-White syndrome, and paroxysmal atrial fibrillation).

Flecainide is administered orally or intravenously as the acetate. Treatment should be started in hospital. A suggested therapeutic plasma concentration range is 200 to 1000 ng per mL. Doses may need to be reduced in patients with renal impairment.

In ventricular **arrhythmias** the usual initial dose of flecainide acetate by mouth is 100 mg twice daily; the usual maximum total dose is 400 mg daily. The dose should be adjusted after 3 to 5 days and reduced once control has been achieved. In supraventricular arrhythmias the usual initial dose is 50 mg twice daily by mouth with a maximum total dose of 300 mg daily.

For rapid control of arrhythmias flecainide acetate 2 mg per kg body-weight may be administered intravenously over 10 to 30 minutes, to a maximum dose of 150 mg; the ECG should be monitored. If longer term parenteral therapy is necessary therapy is initiated by intravenous injection of 2 mg per kg over 30 minutes, as above, then continued by intravenous infusion of 1.5 mg per kg over the first hour, and 0.1 to 0.25 mg per kg per hour thereafter. The maximum cumulative dose in the first 24 hours should not exceed 600 mg. Infusion should not generally continue for more than 24 hours and oral administration should be substituted as soon as possible.

Flecainide has also been tried in the treatment of refractory neurogenic pain.

Administration. Flecainide is usually given by mouth or intravenously, but was reported to be rapidly and reliably absorbed after rectal administration as a solution in healthy subjects.[1] The mean time to achieve peak serum concentration was 0.67 hours and the mean bioavailability was 98% compared with 1 hour and 78% for an oral solution and 4 hours and 81% for a tablet. The absorption of rectally administered flecainide in 2 critically ill patients was good in one but poor in the other[2] and it was recommended that rectal administration be reserved for patients unresponsive to maximal parenteral therapy and in whom oral or nasogastric administration cannot be used.

1. Lie-A-Huen L, *et al.* Absorption kinetics of oral and rectal flecainide in healthy subjects. *Eur J Clin Pharmacol* 1990; **38:** 595–8.
2. Quattrocchi FP, Karim A. Flecainide acetate administration by enema. *DICP Ann Pharmacother* 1990; **24:** 1233–4.

Cardiac arrhythmias. Asymptomatic premature ventricular arrhythmias in subjects who have previously suffered a myocardial infarction are recognised as a risk factor for subsequent sudden cardiac death.[1] Suppressing such arrhythmias in this group might be expected to reduce the incidence of sudden death and it was to test this hypothesis that a large multi-centre study was set up in the USA (the Cardiac Arrhythmia Suppression Trial known as CAST).[2,3] Encainide, flecainide, and moracizine were the antiarrhythmics studied, but unfortunately all three were associated with increased mortality and it is now accepted that these drugs should not be used prophylactically in post-infarction patients with asymptomatic arrhythmias.

Licensed indications for flecainide cover severe symptomatic ventricular and supraventricular arrhythmias including sustained ventricular tachycardia, premature ventricular contractions resistant to other therapy, atrioventricular nodal reciprocating tachycardias, arrhythmias associated with the Wolff-Parkinson-White syndrome, and paroxysmal atrial fibrillation. Flecainide has been found to be effective in such arrhythmias,[4-7] and groups of patients successfully treated have included children.[8-10] Maternal administration of flecainide has been successful in treating fetal arrhythmias.[11-13]

For further discussion on the management of cardiac arrhythmias, with mention of flecainide, see p.782.

1. Task Force of the Working Group on Arrhythmias of the European Society of Cardiology. CAST and beyond: implications of the cardiac arrhythmias suppression trial. *Circulation* 1990; **81:** 1123–7. [Simultaneous publication occurred in *Eur Heart J* 1990; **11:** 194–9].
2. The Cardiac Arrhythmia Suppression Trial (CAST) Investigators. Preliminary report: effect of encainide and flecainide on mortality in a randomized trial of arrhythmia suppression after myocardial infarction. *N Engl J Med* 1989; **321:** 406–12.
3. Echt DS, *et al.* Mortality and morbidity in patients receiving encainide, flecainide, or placebo: The Cardiac Arrhythmia Suppression Trial. *N Engl J Med* 1991; **324:** 781–8.
4. Hohnloser SH, Zabel M. Short- and long-term efficacy and safety of flecainide acetate for supraventricular arrhythmias. *Am J Cardiol* 1992; **70:** 3A–10A.
5. Anderson J, *et al.* Flecainide acetate for paroxysmal supraventricular tachyarrhythmias. *Am J Cardiol* 1994; **74:** 578–84.
6. Dorian P, *et al.* A randomized comparison of flecainide versus verapamil in paroxysmal supraventricular tachycardia. *Am J Cardiol* 1996; **77:** 89A–95A.
7. Aliot E, *et al.* Comparison of the safety and efficacy of flecainide versus propafenone in hospital out-patients with symptomatic paroxysmal atrial fibrillation/flutter. *Am J Cardiol* 1996; **77:** 66A–71A.
8. Till JA, *et al.* Treatment of refractory supraventricular arrhythmias with flecainide acetate. *Arch Dis Child* 1987; **62:** 247–52.
9. Till JA, *et al.* Use of flecainide in children. *Lancet* 1989; **ii:** 326.
10. O'Sullivan JJ, *et al.* Digoxin or flecainide for prophylaxis of supraventricular tachycardia in infants? *J Am Coll Cardiol* 1995; **26:** 991–4.
11. Wren C, Hunter S. Maternal administration of flecainide to terminate and suppress fetal tachycardia. *Br Med J* 1988; **296:** 249.
12. Perry JC, *et al.* Fetal supraventricular tachycardia treated with flecainide acetate. *J Pediatr* 1991; **118:** 303–5.
13. Smoleniec JS, *et al.* Intermittent fetal tachycardia and fetal hydrops. *Arch Dis Child* 1991; **66:** 1160–1.

Pain. Neurogenic pain (p.10) is often insensitive to opioid analgesics, and various drugs, including flecainide, have been tried. Beneficial results were achieved with flecainide 100 mg twice daily by mouth in the control of severe pain associated with malignant infiltration of nerves.[1,2] Unfortunately, a controlled trial had to be abandoned[3] when flecainide was withdrawn following its association with increased mortality in post-infarction patients. Nevertheless, flecainide may be of value in refractory neurogenic pain, usually as a second- or third-line drug in patients with advanced cancer, but with neither a history of, nor suspected, ischaemic heart disease.[4]

1. Dunlop R, *et al.* Analgesic effects of oral flecainide. *Lancet* 1988; **i:** 420–1.
2. Sinnott C, *et al.* Flecainide in cancer nerve pain. *Lancet* 1991; **337:** 1347.
3. Dunlop RJ, *et al.* Flecainide in cancer nerve pain. *Lancet* 1991; **337:** 1347.
4. Davis CL, Hardy JR. Palliative care. *Br Med J* 1994; **308:** 1359–62.

Preparations

USP 23: Flecainide Acetate Tablets.

Proprietary Preparations (details are given in Part 3)
Aust.: Aristocor; ***Austral.:*** Tambocor; ***Belg.:*** Tambocor; ***Canad.:*** Tambocor; ***Fr.:*** Flecaine; ***Ger.:*** Tambocor; ***Irl.:*** Tambocor; ***Ital.:*** Almarytm; ***Neth.:*** Tambocor; ***Norw.:*** Tambocor; ***S.Afr.:*** Tambocor; ***Spain:*** Apocard; Corflene†; ***Swed.:*** Tambocor; ***Switz.:*** Tambocor; ***UK:*** Tambocor; ***USA:*** Tambocor.

Flestolol (18708-z)

Flestolol *(rINN)*.

ACC-9089 (flestolol sulphate). (±)-{2-[(2,3-Dihydroxypropyl)amino]-2-methylpropyl}urea 3-o-fluorobenzoate.

$C_{15}H_{22}FN_3O_4$ = 327.4.

CAS — 87721-62-8 (flestolol); 88844-73-9 (flestolol sulphate).

NOTE. Flestolol Sulfate is *USAN*.

Flestolol is a short-acting beta blocker (p.828). It has been given intravenously as the sulphate.

References.

1. Barton SD, *et al.* Flestolol: an ultra-short-acting beta-adrenergic blocking agent. *J Clin Pharmacol* 1986; **26** (suppl A): A36–9.

Flosequinan (18878-w)

Flosequinan *(BAN, USAN, rINN)*.

BTS-49465. 7-Fluoro-1-methyl-3-methylsulphinyl-4-quinolone.

$C_{11}H_{10}FNO_2S$ = 239.3.

CAS — 76568-02-0.

Flosequinan is a direct-acting arteriovenous vasodilator that was used as an adjunct to the conventional treatment of heart failure, but has been withdrawn from the market following findings of excess mortality.

References.

1. Barnett DB. Flosequinan. *Lancet* 1993; **341:** 733–6.
2. Anonymous. Flosequinan for heart failure. *Med Lett Drugs Ther* 1993; **35:** 23–4.
3. Anonymous. Flosequinan for chronic heart failure? *Drug Ther Bull* 1993; **31:** 47–8.
4. Anonymous. Flosequinan withdrawn. *Lancet* 1993; **342:** 235.
5. Kamali F, Edwards C. Possible role of metabolite in flosequinan-related mortality. *Clin Pharmacokinet* 1995; **29:** 396–403.

Preparations

Proprietary Preparations (details are given in Part 3)
UK: Manoplax†; ***USA:*** Manoplax†.

Fluindione (4815-c)

Fluindione *(rINN)*.

Fluorindione; LM-123. 2-(4-Fluorophenyl)indan-1,3-dione.

$C_{15}H_9FO_2$ = 240.2.

CAS — 957-56-2.

Fluindione is an orally administered indanedione anticoagulant with actions similar to those of warfarin sodium (p.964). It is used in the management of thrombo-embolic disorders (p.801) but, as the indanediones are generally more toxic than warfarin (see Phenindione, p.928), its use is limited.

The usual initial dose is 20 mg daily; the dose is then adjusted according to coagulation tests.

Preparations

Proprietary Preparations (details are given in Part 3)
Fr.: Previscan.

Fosinopril Sodium (965-r)

Fosinopril Sodium *(BANM, USAN, rINNM)*.

SQ-28555. (4*S*)-4-Cyclohexyl-1-{[(*RS*)-2-methyl-1-(propionyloxy)propoxy](4-phenylbutyl)phosphinoylacetyl}-L-proline, sodium salt.

$C_{30}H_{45}NNaO_7P$ = 585.6.

CAS — 97825-24-6 (fosinopril); 98048-97-6 (fosinopril); 88889-14-9 (fosinopril sodium).

Adverse Effects, Treatment, and Precautions

As for ACE inhibitors, p.805.

Interactions

As for ACE inhibitors, p.807.

Pharmacokinetics

Fosinopril acts as a prodrug of the diacid fosinoprilat, its active metabolite. Following oral administration about 36% of a dose of fosinopril is absorbed. Fosinopril is rapidly and completely hydrolysed to fosinoprilat in both gastro-intestinal mucosa and liver. Peak plasma concentrations of fosinoprilat are achieved about 3 hours after an oral dose of fosinopril. Fosinoprilat is excreted both in urine and in the faeces via the bile; it has been detected in breast milk. Fosinoprilat is more than 95% bound to plasma protein. The effective half-life for accumulation of fosinoprilat following multiple doses of fosinopril is about 11.5 hours in patients with hypertension and about 14 hours in patients with heart failure.

References.

1. Singhvi SM, *et al.* Disposition of fosinopril sodium in healthy subjects. *Br J Clin Pharmacol* 1988; **25:** 9–15.
2. Kostis JB, *et al.* Fosinopril: pharmacokinetics and pharmacodynamics in congestive heart failure. *Clin Pharmacol Ther* 1995; **58:** 660–5.

Renal impairment. Total body clearance of fosinoprilat, the active metabolite of fosinopril, is slower in patients with impaired renal function. However, pharmacokinetic studies in patients with varying degrees of renal dysfunction,[1-4] including those requiring dialysis, indicate that decreases in renal clearance may be compensated for, at least in part, by increases in hepatic clearance.

1. Hui KK, *et al.* Pharmacokinetics of fosinopril in patients with various degrees of renal function. *Clin Pharmacol Ther* 1991; **49:** 457–67.
2. Gehr TWB, *et al.* Fosinopril pharmacokinetics and pharmacodynamics in chronic ambulatory peritoneal dialysis patients. *Eur J Clin Pharmacol* 1991; **41:** 165–9.
3. Sica DA, *et al.* Comparison of the steady-state pharmacokinetics of fosinopril, lisinopril and enalapril in patients with chronic renal insufficiency. *Clin Pharmacokinet* 1991; **20:** 420–7.
4. Gehr TWB, *et al.* The pharmacokinetics and pharmacodynamics of fosinopril in haemodialysis patients. *Eur J Clin Pharmacol* 1993; **45:** 431–6.

Uses and Administration

Fosinopril is an ACE inhibitor (p.805). It is used in the treatment of hypertension (p.788) and heart failure (p.785).

Fosinopril owes its activity to fosinoprilat to which it is converted after oral administration. The haemodynamic effects are seen within 1 hour of a single oral dose and the maximum effect occurs after 2 to 6 hours, although the full effect may not develop for several weeks during chronic dosing. The haemodynamic action lasts for about 24 hours, allowing once-daily dosing. Fosinopril is given by mouth as the sodium salt.

In the treatment of **hypertension** the initial dose is 10 mg once daily. Since there may be a precipitous fall in blood pressure in some patients when starting therapy with an ACE inhibitor, the first dose should preferably be given at bedtime. Usual maintenance doses range from 10 to 40 mg once daily. In patients already receiving diuretic therapy the diuretic should be withdrawn if possible several days before commencing fosinopril, and resumed later if necessary.

In the management of **heart failure**, severe first-dose hypotension on introduction of an ACE inhibitor is common in patients on loop diuretics, but their temporary withdrawal may cause rebound pulmonary oedema. Thus treatment should be initiated with a low dose under close medical supervision. Fosinopril is given in an initial dose of 10 mg once daily and, if well tolerated, increased to up to 40 mg once daily.

Reviews.

1. Murdoch D, McTavish D. Fosinopril: a review of its pharmacodynamic and pharmacokinetic properties, and therapeutic potential in essential hypertension. *Drugs* 1992; **43:** 123–40.
2. Wagstaff AJ, *et al.* Fosinopril: a reappraisal of its pharmacology and therapeutic efficacy in essential hypertension. *Drugs* 1996; **51:** 777–91.
3. Davis R, *et al.* Fosinopril: a review of its pharmacology and clinical efficacy in the management of heart failure. *Drugs* 1997; **54:** 103–16.

Preparations

Proprietary Preparations (details are given in Part 3)
Aust.: Fositens; ***Austral.:*** Monopril; ***Belg.:*** Fosinil; ***Canad.:*** Monopril; ***Fr.:*** Fozitec; ***Ger.:*** Dynacil; Fosinorm; ***Ital.:*** Eliten; Fosipres; Tensogard; ***Neth.:*** NewAce; ***S.Afr.:*** Monopril; ***Spain:*** Fositens; Hiperlex; Tenso Stop; ***Swed.:*** Monopril; ***Switz.:*** Fositen; ***UK:*** Staril; ***USA:*** Monopril.

Multi-ingredient: ***Ital.:*** Elidiur; Fosicombi; Tensozide; ***Swed.:*** Monopril comp; ***Switz.:*** Fosicomp.

Frusemide (2331-m)

Frusemide *(BAN)*.

Furosemide *(USAN, rINN)*; Furosemidum; LB-502. 4-Chloro-*N*-furfuryl-5-sulphamoylanthranilic acid.

$C_{12}H_{11}ClN_2O_5S$ = 330.7.

CAS — 54-31-9.

NOTE. Compounded preparations of frusemide and amiloride hydrochloride in the proportions, by weight, 8 parts to 1 part have the British Approved Name Co-amilofruse.

Pharmacopoeias. In *Chin., Eur.* (see p.viii), *Int., Jpn, Pol.,* and *US.*

A white or slightly yellow, odourless, crystalline powder. Practically **insoluble** in water and in dichloromethane; very slightly soluble in chloroform; sparingly soluble in alcohol; slightly soluble in ether; soluble or freely soluble in acetone and in dimethylformamide; soluble in methyl alcohol; dissolves in dilute aqueous solutions of alkali hydroxides. **Protect** from light.

Solutions for injection are prepared with the aid of sodium hydroxide, giving solutions with a pH of 8.0 to 9.3. Such solutions should not be mixed or diluted with glucose injection or other acidic solutions.

Incompatibilities. Frusemide injection has been reported[1] to be visually incompatible with injections of diltiazem hydrochloride, dobutamine hydrochloride, dopamine hydrochloride, labetalol hydrochloride, midazolam hydrochloride, milrinone lactate, nicardipine hydrochloride, and vecuronium bromide. Incompatibility has also been noted with parenteral nutrient solutions[2] and with cisatracurium besylate.[3]

1. Chiu MF, Schwartz ML. Visual compatibility of injectable drugs used in the intensive care unit. *Am J Health-Syst Pharm* 1997; **54:** 64–5.
2. Trissel LA, *et al.* Compatibility of parenteral nutrient solutions with selected drugs during simulated Y-site administration. *Am J Health-Syst Pharm* 1997; **54:** 1295–1300.
3. Trissel LA, *et al.* Compatibility of cisatracurium besylate with selected drugs during simulated Y-site administration. *Am J Health-Syst Pharm* 1997; **54:** 1735–41.

Adverse Effects

The most common side-effect associated with frusemide therapy is fluid and electrolyte imbalance including hyponatraemia, hypokalaemia, and hypochloraemic alkalosis, particularly after large doses or prolonged administration. Because of their shorter duration of action, the risk of hypokalaemia may be less with loop diuretics such as frusemide than with thiazide diuretics. Unlike the thiazide diuretics, frusemide increases the urinary excretion of calcium. Nephrocalcinosis has been reported when frusemide has been used to treat preterm infants.

Frusemide may provoke hyperglycaemia and glycosuria, but probably to a lesser extent than the thiazide diuretics. It may cause hyperuricaemia and precipitate attacks of gout in some patients.

Signs of electrolyte imbalance include headache, hypotension, muscle cramps, dry mouth, thirst, weakness, lethargy, drowsiness, restlessness, oliguria, cardiac arrhythmias, and gastro-intestinal disturbances.

Other side-effects are relatively uncommon, and include blurred vision, yellow vision, dizziness, headache, and orthostatic hypotension. Skin rashes and photosensitivity reactions, although rare, may be severe and hypersensitivity reactions including interstitial nephritis, vasculitis, and fever occur rarely. Pancreatitis is more common at high doses and cholestatic jaundice has been reported. Bone marrow depression may occur rarely: agranulocytosis, thrombocytopenia, and leucopenia have been reported. Tinnitus and deafness may rarely occur in particular during rapid high-dose parenteral frusemide therapy. Rarely, deafness may be permanent particularly if frusemide has been given to patients taking other ototoxic drugs.

The most commonly encountered adverse effects attributable to frusemide are fluid depletion and electrolyte disturbances arising from frusemide's diuretic action. These effects are dose-dependent[1,2] and serious disturbances can result from over enthusiastic use of loop diuretics in oedematous patients.[3] In a survey of 553 hospital inpatients[1] receiving frusemide 220 patients (40%) experienced 480 adverse reactions. Electrolyte disturbances occurred in 130 (23.5%) patients and extracellular volume depletion in 50 (9%). Adverse reactions were more common in patients with liver disease, and hepatic coma occurred in 20 patients with hepatic cirrhosis. A similar survey in 585 hospital inpatients[2] revealed 177 adverse effects in 123 patients (21%). These included volume depletion in 85 patients (14.5%), hypokalaemia in 21 (3.6%), and hyponatraemia in 6 (1%). Hypokalaemia was considered to be life-threatening in 2 patients. Hyperuricaemia occurred in 54 patients (9.2%), of whom 40 also had volume depletion, and clinical gout developed in 2.

Decreases in blood pressure and increases in haematocrit values following the introduction of frusemide treatment were considered to have contributed to the pathogenesis of stroke in 3 elderly patients.[4] It was suggested that the use of powerful high-ceiling diuretics such as frusemide could cause cerebral ischaemia and should be avoided in the treatment of hypertension in the elderly. Over enthusiastic use of frusemide or co-amilofruse was also considered responsible for leg ischaemia or superficial gangrene in 5 elderly patients.[5]

1. Naranjo CA, *et al.* Frusemide-induced adverse reactions during hospitalization. *Am J Hosp Pharm* 1978; **35:** 794–8.
2. Lowe J, *et al.* Adverse reactions to frusemide in hospital inpatients. *Br Med J* 1979; **2:** 360–2.
3. Plumb VJ, James TN. Clinical hazards of powerful diuretics: furosemide and ethacrynic acid. *Mod Concepts Cardiovasc Dis* 1978; **47:** 91–4.
4. Jansen PAF, *et al.* Contribution of inappropriate treatment for hypertension to pathogenesis of stroke in the elderly. *Br Med J* 1986; **293:** 914–17.
5. O'Rourke DA, Hede JE. Reversible leg ischaemia due to diuretics. *Br Med J* 1978; **1:** 1114.

Effects on the ears. Ototoxicity and deafness during frusemide therapy is most frequently associated with elevated blood concentrations resulting from rapid intravenous infusion[1] or delayed excretion in patients with impaired renal function.[2] In a report[3] of 29 cases of frusemide-induced deafness reported to the Food and Drug Administration in the USA, most patients had concomitant renal disease or had received frusemide intravenously. Eight patients had also received another ototoxic drug. However, deafness occurred in 11 patients following oral administration, and in 4 of these hearing loss occurred in the absence of renal disease or other ototoxic drugs. Hearing loss was generally transient, lasting from one half to 24 hours, but permanent hearing loss occurred in 3 patients, one of whom had taken frusemide orally. Deafness was not always associated with high doses; six patients had received a total of 200 mg or less of frusemide.

See also under Precautions, below.

1. Heidland A, Wigand ME. Einfluss hoher furosemiddosen auf die gehörfunktion bei urämie. *Klin Wochenschr* 1970; **48:** 1052–6.
2. Schwartz GH, *et al.* Ototoxicity induced by furosemide. *N Engl J Med* 1970; **282:** 1413–14.
3. Gallagher KL, Jones JK. Furosemide-induced ototoxicity. *Ann Intern Med* 1979; **91:** 744–5.

Effects on the electrolyte balance. CALCIUM. Frusemide increases renal calcium excretion. There is a danger of hypocalcaemic tetany during frusemide administration in hypoparathyroid patients[1] and it has also been reported[2] in a patient with latent hypoparathyroidism following thyroidectomy.

The decrease in serum-calcium concentrations could also induce hyperparathyroidism. In a study involving 36 patients with heart failure frusemide administration was associated with elevations in both parathyroid hormone and alkaline phosphatase concentrations, possibly indicating accelerated bone remodelling such as that found in primary hyperparathyroidism.[3]

For reports of hypercalciuria, rickets, renal calculi, and hyperparathyroidism in neonates treated with frusemide, see under Effects in Infants and Neonates, below.

1. Gabow PA, *et al.* Furosemide-induced reduction in ionized calcium in hypoparathyroid patients. *Ann Intern Med* 1977; **86:** 579–81.
2. Bashey A, MacNee W. Tetany induced by frusemide in latent hypoparathyroidism. *Br Med J* 1987; **295:** 960–1.
3. Elmgreen J, *et al.* Elevated serum parathyroid hormone concentration during treatment with high ceiling diuretics. *Eur J Clin Pharmacol* 1980; **18:** 363–4.

MAGNESIUM, POTASSIUM, AND SODIUM. For discussions of the effects of diuretics on these electrolytes see under the Adverse Effects of Hydrochlorothiazide, p.885.

Effects in infants and neonates. Frusemide is commonly used in the treatment of cardiac and pulmonary disorders in premature infants and neonates. This age group appears to be particularly susceptible to adverse effects arising from the increase in urinary calcium excretion which occurs during long-term frusemide therapy. Increases in parathyroid hormone concentration[1,2] and evidence of bone resorption[1,3] support the suggestion that the increased calcium loss causes secondary hyperparathyroidism. There have been reports of decreased mineral content of bone,[1,3] rickets,[4] fractures,[3] and renal calcification.[1,5-7] Hufnagle's observation[5] that renal calcification could be reversed by the addition of a thiazide diuretic was supported by Noe.[6] There is evidence[8] that frusemide-related renal calcifications in very low birth-weight infants might be associated with long-term impairment of kidney function. Renal calcification has also been reported following frusemide administration in older infants.[9] Salmon[10] has suggested that a sodium deficit in infants treated with frusemide for heart failure may contribute to a failure to thrive.

Concern has been expressed over the finding[11] that frusemide use in premature infants with respiratory distress syndrome increases the incidence of patent ductus arteriosus. The mechanism is thought to be connected with stimulation of renal prostaglandin E_2. However, the increased incidence of patent ductus arteriosus did not adversely affect the mortality in infants treated with frusemide, and a subsequent study[12] failed to find any increase in the incidence of patent ductus arteriosus in infants treated with frusemide compared with a control group. Paradoxically frusemide has been used in the management of delayed closure of ductus (see Patent Ductus Arteriosus under Uses and Administration, below). There is a possibility that frusemide may not be effective in infants receiving indomethacin[13] but frusemide can prevent the decline in urine output which occurs during indomethacin administration.[14,15]

1. Venkataraman PS, *et al.* Secondary hyperparathyroidism and bone disease in infants receiving long-term furosemide therapy. *Am J Dis Child* 1983; **187:** 1157–61.
2. Vileisis RA. Furosemide effect on mineral status of parenterally nourished premature neonates with chronic lung disease. *Pediatrics* 1990; **85:** 316–22.
3. Morgan MEI, Evans SE. Osteopenia in very low birthweight infants. *Lancet* 1986; **ii:** 1399–1400.
4. Chudley AE, *et al.* Nutritional rickets in 2 very low birthweight infants with chronic lung disease. *Arch Dis Child* 1980; **55:** 687–90.
5. Hufnagle KG, *et al.* Renal calcifications: a complication of long-term furosemide therapy in preterm infants. *Pediatrics* 1982; **70:** 360–3.
6. Noe HN, *et al.* Urolithiasis in pre-term neonates associated with furosemide therapy. *J Urol (Baltimore)* 1984; **132:** 93–4.
7. Pearse DM, *et al.* Sonographic diagnosis of furosemide-induced nephrocalcinosis in newborn infants. *J Ultrasound Med* 1984; **3:** 553–6.
8. Downing GJ, *et al.* Kidney function in very low birth weight infants with furosemide-related renal calcifications at ages 1 to 2 years. *J Pediatr* 1992; **120:** 599–604.
9. Alon US, *et al.* Nephrocalcinosis and nephrolithiasis in infants with congestive heart failure treated with furosemide. *J Pediatr* 1994; **125:** 149–51.
10. Salmon AP, *et al.* Sodium balance in infants with severe congestive heart failure. *Lancet* 1989; **ii:** 875.
11. Green TP, *et al.* Furosemide promotes patent ductus arteriosus in premature infants with respiratory-distress syndrome. *N Engl J Med* 1983; **308:** 743–8.
12. Yeh TF, *et al.* Early furosemide therapy in premature infants (≤ 2000 gm) with respiratory distress syndrome: a randomized controlled trial. *J Pediatr* 1984; **105:** 603–9.
13. Friedman Z, *et al.* Urinary excretion of prostaglandin E following the administration of furosemide and indomethacin to sick low-birth-weight infants. *J Pediatr* 1978; **93:** 512–15.
14. Yeh TF, *et al.* Furosemide prevents the renal side effects of indomethacin therapy in premature infants with patent ductus arteriosus. *J Pediatr* 1982; **101:** 433–7.
15. Nahata MC, *et al.* Furosemide can prevent decline in urine output in infants receiving indomethacin for patent ductus closure: a multidose study. *Infusion* 1988; **12:** 11–12 and 15.

Effects on lipid metabolism. Most studies into the effects of diuretics on blood-lipid concentrations have used thiazides (see Hydrochlorothiazide, p.886). The few studies into the effects of frusemide suggest that, like thiazides, it may adversely influence blood-lipid concentrations during short-term administration.[1]

1. Ames RP. The effects of antihypertensive drugs on serum lipids and lipoproteins I: diuretics. *Drugs* 1986; **32:** 260–78.

Precautions

Frusemide's precautions and contra-indications which are dependent on its effects on fluid and electrolyte balance are similar to those of the thiazide diuretics (see Hydrochlorothiazide, p.887). Although frusemide is used in high doses for oliguria due to chronic or acute renal insufficiency it should not be given in anuria or in renal failure due to nephrotoxic or hepatotoxic drugs nor in renal failure associated with hepatic coma. Frusemide should not be given in pre-comatose states associated with hepatic cirrhosis. It should be used with care in patients with prostatic hyperplasia or impairment of micturition since it can precipitate acute urinary retention.

To reduce the risk of ototoxicity, frusemide should not be injected intravenously at a rate exceeding 4 mg per minute.

Frusemide should be used with caution in pregnancy and in breast-feeding mothers since it crosses the placenta and also appears in breast milk. Frusemide may compromise placental perfusion by reducing maternal blood volume; it may also inhibit lactation.

Hepatic impairment. In patients with chronic cardiac failure and moderate liver congestion, high-dose frusemide therapy could produce increases in liver enzymes suggestive of hepatitis.[1] Special care should be taken with the dosage and mode of administration of frusemide in such patients to avoid severe ischaemic liver damage caused by a drop in systemic blood pressure.

As with the thiazides, frusemide should be avoided in patients with severe liver impairment.

1. Lang I, *et al.* Furosemide and increases in liver enzymes. *Ann Intern Med* 1988; **109:** 845.

Hypoparathyroidism. For comments on the possibility of hypocalcaemic tetany in hypoparathyroid patients taking frusemide, see under Adverse Effects, above.

Infants and neonates. Several studies[1-3] have shown frusemide to be a potent displacer of bilirubin from albumin binding sites and it should be used with caution in jaundiced infants. Wennberg[2] found that on a molar basis chlorothiazide, frusemide, and ethacrynic acid were at least as potent as sulphafurazole in displacing bilirubin from albumin. Doses of frusemide 1 mg per kg body-weight probably do not produce a significant increase in free bilirubin in most jaundiced infants,[2,3] although doses greater than 1.5 mg per kg or repeated dosing could potentially do so.[3] Chlorothiazide 15 to 20 mg per kg would not be an appropriate alternative to frusemide[2] since it could produce higher plasma bilirubin concentrations in jaundiced infants.

In addition, there is some evidence from an *in vitro* study[4] that bilirubin may displace frusemide from binding sites to a greater extent in neonates than in adults. The clearance of frusemide is much slower in neonates than in adults, with an eightfold prolongation in plasma half-life, and this should be taken into account during repeat dosing.[3]

1. Shankaran S, Poland RL. The displacement of bilirubin from albumin by furosemide. *J Pediatr* 1977; **90:** 642–6.
2. Wennberg RP, *et al.* Displacement of bilirubin from human albumin by three diuretics. *J Pediatr* 1977; **90:** 647–50.
3. Aranda JV, *et al.* Pharmacokinetic disposition and protein binding of furosemide in newborn infants. *J Pediatr* 1978; **93:** 507–11.
4. Viani A, Pacifici GM. Bilirubin displaces furosemide from serum protein: the effect is greater in newborn infants than adult subjects. *Dev Pharmacol Ther* 1990; **14:** 90–5.

Porphyria. Frusemide has been associated with clinical exacerbations of porphyria and is considered unsafe in porphyric patients.[1]

1. Moore MR, McColl KEL. *Porphyria: drug lists.* Glasgow: Porphyria Research Unit, University of Glasgow, 1991.

Interactions

The interactions of frusemide that are due to its effects on fluid and electrolyte balance are similar to those of hydrochlorothiazide (see p.887).

Frusemide may enhance the nephrotoxicity of cephalosporin antibacterials such as cephalothin and can enhance the ototoxicity of aminoglycoside antibacterials and other ototoxic drugs.

Anticoagulants. For reference to the lack of interaction between warfarin and frusemide, see p.968.

Antiepileptics. The diuretic effect of frusemide has been shown to be substantially reduced by concomitant antiepileptic therapy.[1,2] The mean diuretic effect of frusemide 20 mg or 40 mg by mouth in patients on antiepileptic therapy was 68% and 51% that of healthy controls respectively.[1]

For the effect of frusemide on phenobarbitone, see p.351.

Symptomatic hyponatraemia has been associated with the concomitant use of frusemide or hydrochlorothiazide with carbamazepine.[3]

1. Ahmad S. Renal insensitivity to frusemide caused by chronic anticonvulsant therapy. *Br Med J* 1974; **3:** 657–9.
2. Fine A, *et al.* Malabsorption of frusemide caused by phenytoin. *Br Med J* 1977; **2:** 1061–2.
3. Yassa R, *et al.* Carbamazepine, diuretics, and hyponatremia: a possible interaction. *J Clin Psychiatry* 1987; **48:** 281–3.

Diuretics. Severe electrolyte disturbances may occur in patients given metolazone concurrently with frusemide.

Hypnotics. A syndrome of flushing, tachycardia, elevated blood pressure, and severe diaphoresis was reported following intravenous administration of frusemide to 6 patients who had received chloral hydrate orally during the preceding 24 hours.[1] The reaction recurred in 1 patient on a subsequent occasion when given both drugs but not when frusemide was administered without chloral hydrate. A subsequent retrospective study[2] among 43 patients who had received both chloral hydrate and frusemide showed that 1 patient had suffered a similar reaction; of 2 further patients who had possibly been affected, 1 had subsequently taken both drugs without adverse effects. A similar interaction has been reported in an 8-year-old child.[3]

1. Malach M, Berman N. Furosemide and chloral hydrate: adverse drug interaction. *JAMA* 1975; **232:** 638–9.
2. Pevonka MP, *et al.* Interaction of chloral hydrate and furosemide: a controlled retrospective study. *Drug Intell Clin Pharm* 1977; **11:** 332–5.
3. Dean RP, *et al.* Interaction of chloral hydrate and intravenous furosemide in a child. *Clin Pharm* 1991; **10:** 385–7.

Lithium. For reports of a possible increase in plasma-lithium concentrations in patients receiving loop diuretics, see p.294.

NSAIDs. NSAIDs may antagonise the diuretic effect of frusemide and other diuretics.[1] Concomitant administration of NSAIDs with diuretics may increase the risk of nephrotoxicity, although it has also been suggested that frusemide may protect against the renal effects of indomethacin in infants (see Effects in Infants and Neonates, above).

1. Webster J. Interactions of NSAIDs with diuretics and β-blockers: mechanisms and clinical implications. *Drugs* 1985; **30:** 32–41.

Probenecid. Probenecid has been shown[1-4] to reduce the renal clearance of frusemide and reduce the diuretic effect.[2,3]

1. Honari J, *et al.* Effects of probenecid on furosemide kinetics and natriuresis in man. *Clin Pharmacol Ther* 1977; **22:** 395–401.
2. Odlind B, Beermann B. Renal tubular secretion and effects of furosemide. *Clin Pharmacol Ther* 1980; **27:** 784–90.
3. Smith DE, *et al.* Preliminary evaluation of furosemide-probenecid interaction in humans. *J Pharm Sci* 1980; **69:** 571–5.
4. Vree TB, *et al.* Probenecid inhibits the renal clearance of frusemide and its acyl glucuronide. *Br J Clin Pharmacol* 1995; **39:** 692–5.

Smoking. Miller has reviewed[1,2] the effects of tobacco smoking on the pharmacokinetics of frusemide. Nicotine inhibits diuresis and diminishes the diuretic effect of frusemide. However, this effect is attenuated in habitual smokers.

1. Miller LG. Recent developments in the study of the effects of cigarette smoking on clinical pharmacokinetics and clinical pharmacodynamics. *Clin Pharmacokinet* 1989; **17:** 90–108.
2. Miller LG. Cigarettes and drug therapy: pharmacokinetic and pharmacodynamic considerations. *Clin Pharm* 1990; **9:** 125–35.

Xanthines. For the effect of frusemide on theophylline, see p.770.

Pharmacokinetics

Frusemide is fairly rapidly absorbed from the gastro-intestinal tract; bioavailability has been reported to be about 60 to 70% but absorption is variable and erratic. The half-life of frusemide is up to about 2 hours although it is prolonged in neonates and in patients with renal and hepatic insufficiency. It is up to 99% bound to plasma albumin, and is mainly excreted in the urine, largely unchanged. There is also some excretion via the bile and non-renal elimination is considerably increased in renal impairment. Frusemide crosses the placental barrier and is distributed into breast milk. The clearance of frusemide is not increased by haemodialysis.

The pharmacokinetics of frusemide have been extensively reviewed.[1-6] The development of an analytical method using HPLC with fluorescence has produced greater sensitivity and more consistent results. Absorption following oral dosing is erratic and is subject to large inter- and intra-individual variation. It is influenced by the dosage form, underlying disease processes, and by the presence of food. Frusemide absorption in patients with heart failure has been reported to be even more erratic than in healthy subjects. The bioavailability of frusemide from oral dosage forms is also highly variable with reported values ranging from 20 to 100%. It is influenced by factors affecting absorption but the poor solubility of frusemide does not appear to have a major influence on bioavailability and *in vitro* dissolution data may not reflect *in vivo* bioavailability. Bioavailability tends to be decreased by about 10% in patients with renal disease, and slightly increased in liver disease. Values are erratic in patients with heart disease.

Frusemide is highly bound to plasma proteins, almost exclusively to albumin. The proportion of free (unbound) frusemide is higher in patients with heart disease, renal impairment, and cirrhosis of the liver. Patients with liver disease also have an increased apparent volume of distribution which is proportionally greater than the observed decrease in protein binding. Patients with nephrotic syndrome have significant proteinuria and secondary hypoalbuminaemia. This results in reduced protein binding in the blood, particularly at higher blood concentrations, and binding to proteins present in the urine, which may account for the resistance to frusemide therapy reported in these patients.

A glucuronide metabolite of frusemide is produced in varying amounts. The site of metabolism is unknown at present. There is debate over another potential metabolite, 4-chloro-5-sulfamoyl anthranilic acid (CSA). Hammarlund-Udenaes and Benet[3] have argued that it is an artefact produced during the extraction procedures although there is some evidence to refute this.[4]

A half-life for frusemide in healthy subjects has generally been reported in the range of 30 to 120 minutes. In patients with end-stage renal disease the average half-life is 9.7 hours. The half-life may be slightly longer in patients with hepatic dysfunction and a range of 50 to 327 minutes has been reported in patients with heart failure. In severe multi-organ failure the half-life may range from 20 to 24 hours.

Frusemide clearance is influenced by age, underlying disease state, and drug interactions. Clearance reduces with increasing age, probably due to declining renal function. Impaired renal function in renal or cardiac disease reduces renal clearance, although this may be compensated by increases in non-renal clearance. Hepatic impairment has little impact on clearance. Renal and non-renal clearance may be reduced by probenecid and indomethacin.

The effectiveness of frusemide as a diuretic depends upon it reaching its site of action, the renal tubules, unchanged. Approximately one-half to two-thirds of an intravenous dose or one-quarter to one-third of an oral dose are excreted unchanged, the difference being largely due to the poor bioavailability from the oral route. The effect of frusemide is more closely related to its urinary excretion than to the plasma concentration. Urinary excretion may be reduced in renal impairment due to reduced renal blood flow and reduced tubular secretion.

1. Cutler RE, Blair AD. Clinical pharmacokinetics of frusemide. *Clin Pharmacokinet* 1979; **4:** 279–96.
2. Benet LZ. Pharmacokinetics/pharmacodynamics of furosemide in man: a review. *J Pharmacokinet Biopharm* 1979; **7:** 1–27.
3. Hammarlund-Udenaes M, Benet LZ. Furosemide pharmacokinetics and pharmacodynamics in health and disease—an update. *J Pharmacokinet Biopharm* 1989; **17:** 1–46.
4. Ponto LLB, Schoenwald RD. Furosemide (frusemide): a pharmacokinetic/pharmacodynamic review (part I). *Clin Pharmacokinet* 1990; **18:** 381–408.
5. Ponto LLB, Schoenwald RD. Furosemide (frusemide): a pharmacokinetic/pharmacodynamic review (part II). *Clin Pharmacokinet* 1990; **18:** 460–71.
6. Vrhovac B, *et al.* Pharmacokinetic changes in patients with oedema. *Clin Pharmacokinet* 1995; **28:** 405–18.

Infants and neonates. The half-life of frusemide in term and preterm neonates is markedly prolonged compared with that in adults.[1,2] Half-lives of 4.5 to 46 hours have been reported and it has been suggested that the prolongation may be greater in preterm than in term neonates. This effect is due primarily to immature renal function and if repeated doses are necessary over a short period accumulation may occur.[1]

1. Besunder JB, *et al.* Principles of drug biodisposition in the neonate: a critical evaluation of the pharmacokinetic-pharmacodynamic interface (part II). *Clin Pharmacokinet* 1988; **14:** 261–86.
2. Aranda JV, *et al.* Pharmacokinetic disposition and protein binding of furosemide in newborn infants. *J Pediatr* 1978; **93:** 507–11.

Uses and Administration

Frusemide is a potent diuretic with a rapid action. Like the other loop or high-ceiling diuretics it is used in the treatment of oedema associated with heart failure (below), including pulmonary oedema, and with renal and hepatic disorders (but see under Precautions, above) and may be effective in patients unresponsive to thiazide diuretics. It is also used in high doses in the management of oliguria due to renal failure or insufficiency. Frusemide is also used in the treatment of hypertension (p.788), either alone or together with other antihypertensives.

Frusemide inhibits the reabsorption of electrolytes primarily in the thick ascending limb of the loop of Henle and also in the distal renal tubules. It may also have a direct effect in the proximal tubules. Excretion of sodium, potassium, calcium, and chloride ions is increased and water excretion enhanced. It has no clinically significant effect on carbonic anhydrase. See below for further reference to its mechanism of action.

Administration and dosage. Frusemide's effects are evident within 30 minutes to 1 hour after a dose by mouth, peak at 1 to 2 hours, and last for about 4 to 6 hours; after intravenous injection its effects are evident in about 5 minutes and last for about 2 hours. It is given by mouth, usually in the morning. Alternatively it may be administered intramuscularly or intravenously as the sodium salt; doses are expressed in terms of frusemide base. Whether by direct intravenous injection or by infusion the rate of intravenous administration should not exceed 4 mg per minute.

Unlike the thiazide diuretics where, owing to their flat dose-response curve, very little is gained by increasing the dose, frusemide has a steep dose-response curve, which gives it a wide therapeutic range.

In the treatment of **oedema**, the usual initial dose is 40 mg once daily by mouth, adjusted as necessary according to response. Mild cases may respond to 20 mg daily or 40 mg on alternate days. Some patients may require doses of 80 mg or more daily given as one or two doses daily, or intermittently. Severe cases may require gradual titration of the frusemide dosage up to 600 mg daily. In an emergency or when oral therapy cannot be given, 20 to 50 mg of frusemide may be administered by intramuscular or slow intravenous injection; if necessary further doses may be given, increasing by 20-mg increments and not given more often than every 2 hours. If doses greater than 50 mg are required it is recommended that they be given by slow intravenous infusion. For pulmonary oedema, sources in the USA have recommended that if an initial slow intravenous injection of 40 mg does not produce a satisfactory response within one hour, the dose may be increased to 80 mg given slowly intravenously.

For children, the usual dose by mouth is 1 to 3 mg per kg body-weight daily up to a maximum of 40 mg daily; suggested doses by injection are 0.5 to 1.5 mg per kg daily up to a maximum of 20 mg daily.

In the treatment of **hypertension**, frusemide is given in doses of 40 to 80 mg daily by mouth, either alone, or in conjunction with other antihypertensives.

In susceptible patients potassium supplements or potassium-sparing diuretics such as amiloride (p.819) may be necessary, but see under Hydrochlorothiazide (Uses and Administration, p.887).

High-dose therapy. In the management of **oliguria** in acute or chronic renal failure where the glomerular filtration rate is less than 20 mL per minute frusemide 250 mg diluted to 250 mL in a suitable diluent is infused over one hour. If urine output is insufficient within the next hour, this dose may be followed by 500 mg added to an appropriate infusion fluid, the total volume of which must be governed by the patient's state of hydration, and infused over approximately 2 hours. If a satisfactory urine output has still not been achieved within one hour of the end of the second infusion then a third dose of 1 g may be infused over approximately 4 hours. The rate of infusion should never exceed 4 mg per minute. In oliguric patients with significant fluid overload, the injection may be given without dilution directly into the vein, using a constant rate infusion pump with a micrometer screw-gauge adjustment; the rate of administration should still never exceed 4 mg per minute. Patients who do not respond to a dose of 1 g probably require dialysis. If the response to either method of administration is satisfactory, the effective dose (of up to 1 g) may then be repeated every 24 hours. Dosage adjustments should subsequently be made according to the patient's response. Alternatively, treatment may be maintained by mouth; 500 mg should be given by mouth for each 250 mg required by injection.

When used in chronic renal insufficiency, an initial dose of 250 mg may be given by mouth, increased, if necessary in steps of 250 mg every 4 to 6 hours to a maximum of 1.5 g in 24 hours; in exceptional cases up to 2.0 g in 24 hours may be given. Dosage adjustments should subsequently be made according to the patient's response.

During treatment with these high-dose forms of frusemide therapy, careful laboratory control is essential. Fluid balance and electrolytes should be carefully controlled and, in particular, in patients with shock, measures should be taken to correct the blood pressure and circulating blood volume, before commencing this type of treatment. High-dose frusemide therapy is contra-indicated in renal failure caused by nephrotoxic or hepatotoxic drugs, and in renal failure associated with hepatic coma.

Action. The mechanism of action of frusemide is not fully understood.[1] It appears to act primarily by inhibiting active reabsorption of chloride ions in the ascending limb of the loop of Henle. Urinary excretion of sodium, chloride, potassium, hydrogen, calcium, magnesium, ammonium, bicarbonate, and possibly phosphate is increased; the chloride excretion exceeds that of sodium and there is an enhanced exchange of sodium for potassium leading to greater excretion of potassium. The resulting low osmolality of the medulla inhibits the reabsorption of water by the kidney. There is a possibility that frusemide may also act at a more proximal site.

In addition to its diuretic actions, frusemide has been shown to increase peripheral venous capacitance and reduce forearm blood flow. It also reduces renal vascular resistance with a resultant increase in renal blood flow the degree of which is proportional to the initial resistance.

Frusemide administration has been shown to increase plasma-renin activity, plasma-noradrenaline concentrations, and plasma-arginine-vasopressin concentrations. Alterations in the renin-angiotensin-aldosterone system may play a part in the development of acute tolerance. Frusemide increases renal-prostaglandin concentrations but it is not known whether this is due to increased synthesis or inhibition of degradation or both. Prostaglandins appear to mediate the diuretic/natriuretic action. The primary effects appear to be alterations in renal haemodynamics with subsequent increases in electrolyte and fluid excretion.

The diuretic response to frusemide is related to the concentration in the urine not in the plasma. Frusemide is delivered to the renal tubules by a nonspecific organic acid pump in the proximal tubules.[1]

In some cases sodium intake may be sufficient to overcome the diuretic effect, and limiting sodium intake could restore responsiveness.[2]

1. Ponto LLB, Schaenwald RD. Furosemide (frusemide): a pharmacokinetic/pharmacodynamic review (part I). *Clin Pharmacokinet* 1990; **18:** 381–408.
2. Brater DC. Resistance to loop diuretics: why it happens and what to do about it. *Drugs* 1985; **30:** 427–43.

Administration. Continuous intravenous infusion of loop diuretics may be more effective than intermittent intravenous bolus injection and may provide a more consistent urine flow with fewer alterations in urine balance.[1] Bumetanide was more effective by continuous infusion than by bolus administration in 8 patients with severe chronic renal insufficiency.[2] In 20 patients with chronic heart failure requiring high-dose frusemide therapy, administration of frusemide by continuous infusion was more effective than the same dose by bolus injection.[3] The lower plasma concentrations associated with continuous infusion may also reduce the risk of toxicity.

1. Yelton SL, *et al.* The role of continuous infusion loop diuretics. *Ann Pharmacother* 1995; **29:** 1010–14.
2. Rudy DW, *et al.* Loop diuretics for chronic renal insufficiency: a continuous infusion is more efficacious than bolus therapy. *Ann Intern Med* 1991; **115:** 360–6.
3. Dormans TPJ, *et al.* Diuretic efficacy of high dose furosemide in severe heart failure: bolus injection versus continuous infusion. *J Am Coll Cardiol* 1996; **28:** 376–82.

Ascites. Dietary sodium restriction and diuretics are mainstays of the management of cirrhotic ascites (p.781). Spironolactone is usually the diuretic of first choice, but frusemide may be added to therapy as necessary.

Asthma. Inhaled frusemide solutions have been shown to prevent exercise-induced bronchoconstriction in asthmatic patients[1] and to inhibit both early and late reactions induced by specific allergen challenge in allergic asthmatics.[2] Inhaled frusemide is considered to produce a response profile similar to that of sodium cromoglycate.[2] The potential for clinical applications remains unclear and frusemide is not a part of the accepted schedules for the treatment of asthma (p.745). However, research into the mode of action of frusemide on the bronchial mucosa may shed light on the pathophysiology of asthma.[2,3]

A number of mechanisms have been suggested. These include changes in the local osmotic and ionic environment leading to reduced responsiveness of epithelial receptors to inflammatory stimuli,[1,2] release of bronchodilatory prostaglandins,[3] inhibition of inflammatory mediators,[4] resolution of mucosal oedema,[5] or inhibition of epithelial nerves.[2,6] Fujimura *et al.*[7] demonstrated a protective effect during methacholine challenge and suggested a direct effect on bronchial responsiveness, although Bianco *et al.*[8] considered that this would only play a minor role.

1. Bianco S, *et al.* Prevention of exercise-induced bronchoconstriction by inhaled frusemide. *Lancet* 1988; **ii:** 252–5.
2. Bianco S, *et al.* Protective effect of inhaled furosemide on allergen-induced early and late asthmatic reactions. *N Engl J Med* 1989; **321:** 1069–73.
3. Anonymous. Inhaled frusemide and asthma. *Lancet* 1990; **335:** 944–6.
4. Anderson SD, *et al.* Inhibition by furosemide of inflammatory mediators from lung fragments. *N Engl J Med* 1991; **324:** 131.
5. Lloyd EL. Frusemide and prevention of bronchoconstriction. *Lancet* 1988; **ii:** 564.
6. Chung KF, Barnes PJ. Inhaled frusemide and asthma. *Lancet* 1990; **335:** 1539.
7. Fujimura M, *et al.* Effect of inhaled furosemide on bronchial responsiveness to methacholine. *N Engl J Med* 1990; **322:** 935–6.
8. Bianco S, *et al.* Effect of inhaled furosemide on bronchial responsiveness to methacholine. *N Engl J Med* 1990; **322:** 936.

Bronchopulmonary dysplasia. Bronchopulmonary dysplasia is a major cause of chronic lung disease in infants. Treatment often involves the use of corticosteroids (see p.1018). Additional supportive therapy may include the use of diuretics such as frusemide.

Rush and colleagues[1] reported that alternate-day therapy with frusemide 4 mg per kg by mouth produced modest benefits in pulmonary status in the absence of a diuretic effect, and few adverse effects. Stefano and Bhutani[2] also reported improved pulmonary function in infants given frusemide 1 mg per kg parenterally following packed red blood cell transfusions, given to improve oxygen-carrying capacity. One report[3] has described the successful use of nebulised frusemide in a dose of 1 mg per kg body-weight; again pulmonary status was improved without production of diuresis or renal side-effects. However, a single inhaled dose of 1 mg per kg failed to improve pulmonary mechanics in another study involving infants with more severe disease.[4]

Caution must be exercised in administering frusemide to infants, particularly for extended periods. The immaturity of the renal system can result in unexpectedly high blood concentrations and extended half lives. Fluid and electrolyte balances should therefore be monitored carefully. Neonates appear to be particularly susceptible to increases in urinary calcium concentrations following long-term frusemide administration. There have also been reports[5] of an increased incidence of patent ductus arteriosus in infants given frusemide, although this did not adversely affect the mortality.

1. Rush MG, *et al.* Double-blind, placebo-controlled trial of alternate-day furosemide therapy in infants with chronic bronchopulmonary dysplasia. *J Pediatr* 1990; **117:** 112–18.
2. Stefano JL, Bhutani VK. Role of furosemide therapy after booster-packed erythrocyte transfusions in infants with bronchopulmonary dysplasia. *J Pediatr* 1990; **117:** 965–8.
3. Rastogi A, *et al.* Nebulized furosemide in infants with bronchopulmonary dysplasia. *J Pediatr* 1994; **125:** 976–9.
4. Kugelman A, *et al.* Pulmonary effect of inhaled furosemide in ventilated infants with severe bronchopulmonary dysplasia. *Pediatrics* 1997; **99:** 71–5.
5. Green TP, *et al.* Furosemide promotes patent ductus arteriosus in premature infants with the respiratory-distress syndrome. *N Engl J Med* 1983; **308:** 743–8.

Haemolytic uraemic syndrome. Renal failure is a possible consequence of the haemolytic-uraemic syndrome (see under Thrombotic Microangiopathies, p.726). Correction of any hypovolaemic state with adequate fluids and of oliguria by inducing diuresis with frusemide may be used to prevent this.

Of 54 children with haemolytic-uraemic syndrome given intravenous frusemide 2.5 to 4 mg per kg body-weight every 3 to 4 hours immediately after diagnosis 24% eventually required dialysis.[1] In contrast, a retrospective analysis of 39 patients treated conservatively showed that 82% had required dialysis. The results therefore suggested that high-dose frusemide could prevent the progression of oliguria to anuria in these patients by increasing urate clearance.

1. Rousseau E, *et al.* Decreased necessity for dialysis with loop diuretic therapy in hemolytic uremic syndrome. *Clin Nephrol* 1990; **34:** 22–5.

Heart failure. Diuretics have been the mainstay in the treatment of heart failure (p.785) but drugs such as ACE inhibitors that have been shown to improve mortality are now generally recommended for first line therapy along with diuretics. Diuretics provide very effective symptomatic control in patients with peripheral or pulmonary oedema and rapidly relieve dyspnoea. If symptoms of fluid retention are only mild, a thiazide diuretic such as bendrofluazide or hydrochlorothiazide, may be adequate. However, in most cases, especially in moderate or severe fluid retention, a loop diuretic such as frusemide will be necessary. Combination treatment with diuretics that behave synergistically by acting at different sites (the principle of sequential nephron blockade), namely a loop diuretic with a thiazide or potassium-sparing diuretic, may be needed in some patients, especially when there is diuretic resistance.

Patients have been successfully treated using continuous intravenous infusions[1] or high doses (up to 8 g daily) of frusemide given by intravenous infusion[2,3] or by mouth.[3] Hattersley and colleagues[4] reported a patient who was successfully maintained on intravenous frusemide at home. Combination of frusemide with thiazide diuretics[5] or metolazone[6,7] has been reported. There is a danger of overdiuresis with both of these strategies, and careful monitoring of electrolytes and renal function is essential.[8] Delivery of frusemide to the renal tubules may be enhanced by combined therapy with hydralazine[9] or captopril.[10] The use of captopril and frusemide may also correct hyponatraemia without fluid restriction.[11] In elderly patients not responding adequately to low-dose frusemide together with optimum doses of ACE inhibitors, increasing the dose of frusemide (to an average of 297 mg daily by mouth) has been reported[12] to be of benefit. However, caution is necessary when administering frusemide with antihypertensives and especially ACE inhibitors since these combinations can result in sudden and profound hypotension and renal toxicity. Low-dose dopamine infusion has been suggested as an alternative to high-dose frusemide infusion and may cause less toxicity. In a study[13] in patients with severe refractory heart failure receiving optimal therapy with ACE inhibitors, oral diuretics, nitrates, and digoxin, additional therapy with low-dose intravenous dopamine (4 μg per kg body-weight per minute) and low-dose oral frusemide (80 mg daily) was as effective as intravenous high-dose frusemide (10 mg per kg daily) but caused less hypokalaemia and renal impairment.

1. Lawson DH, *et al.* Continuous infusion of frusemide in refractory oedema. *Br Med J* 1978; **2;** 476.
2. O'Rourke MF, *et al.* High-dose furosemide in cardiac failure. *Arch Intern Med* 1984; **144:** 2429.
3. Gerlag PGG, van Meijel JJM. High-dose furosemide in the treatment of refractory congestive heart failure. *Arch Intern Med* 1988; **148:** 286–91.
4. Hattersley AT, *et al.* Home intravenous diuretic therapy for patient with refractory heart failure. *Lancet* 1989; **i:** 446.
5. Channer KS, *et al.* Thiazides with loop diuretics for severe congestive heart failure. *Lancet* 1990; **335:** 922–3.
6. Aravot DJ, *et al.* Oral metolazone plus frusemide for home therapy in patients with refractory heart failure. *Lancet* 1989; **i:** 727.
7. Friedland JS, Ledingham JGG. Oral metolazone plus frusemide for home therapy in patients with refractory heart failure. *Lancet* 1989; **i:** 727–8.
8. Oster JR, *et al.* Combined therapy with thiazide-type and loop diuretic agents for resistant-sodium retention. *Ann Intern Med* 1983; **99:** 405–6.
9. Nomura A, *et al.* Effect of furosemide in congestive heart failure. *Clin Pharmacol Ther* 1981; **30:** 177–82.
10. Dzau VJ, Hollenberg NK. Renal response to captopril in severe heart failure: role of furosemide in natriuresis and reversal of hyponatremia. *Ann Intern Med* 1984; **100:** 777–82.
11. Hamilton RW, Buckalew VM. Sodium, water, and congestive heart failure. *Ann Intern Med* 1984; **100:** 902–4.
12. Waterer G, Donaldson M. High-dose frusemide for cardiac failure. *Lancet* 1995; **346:** 254.
13. Cotter G, *et al.* Increased toxicity of high-dose furosemide versus low-dose dopamine in the treatment of refractory congestive heart failure. *Clin Pharmacol Ther* 1997; **62:** 187–93.

Hypercalcaemia. Hypercalcaemia (p.1148) usually results from an underlying disease and long-term management involves treating the cause. However, if significant symptoms are present, treatment is necessary to reduce plasma-calcium concentrations. This primarily involves rehydration, but loop diuretics such as frusemide have been used following rehydration to promote urinary calcium excretion.

Patent ductus arteriosus. The usual initial treatment for a haemodynamically significant ductus is reduction of fluid intake, correction of anaemia, support of respiration, and the administration of a diuretic. If that fails to control symptoms then indomethacin is generally given to promote closure of the ductus (see p.47).

Frusemide is often chosen as the diuretic. It is effective and widely used but there has been concern that it may promote delayed ductus closure (see Effects in Infants and Neonates under Adverse Effects, above). However, the concurrent use of frusemide does not seem to inhibit duct closure during treatment with indomethacin and may reduce adverse renal effects of indomethacin.

Raised intracranial pressure. Osmotic diuretics such as mannitol are first-line drugs for the management of raised intracranial pressure (p.796) but loop diuretics such as frusemide may be employed as adjuncts.

Tinnitus. Treatment of tinnitus (p.1297) is difficult and a wide variety of therapeutic drugs has been tried, including frusemide which has been reported to be effective in some patients, but is rarely used because of problems with adverse effects.

Preparations

BP 1998: Co-amilofruse Tablets; Furosemide Injection; Furosemide Tablets;
USP 23: Furosemide Injection; Furosemide Tablets.

Proprietary Preparations (details are given in Part 3)
Aust.: Furon; Lasix; ***Austral.:*** Lasix; Uremide; Urex; ***Belg.:*** Lasix; ***Canad.:*** Lasix; Novo-Semide; Uritol†; ***Fr.:*** Furosemix†; Lasilix; ***Ger.:*** Diurapid; durafurid; Fumarenid†; Furanthril; Furo; Furo-Puren; Furobeta; Furomed; Furorese; Fusid; Hydro-rapid; Lasix; Odemase; Sigasalur; ***Irl.:*** Dryptal; Lasix; ***Ital.:*** Lasix; ***Neth.:*** Fusid†; Lasiletten; Lasix; Vesix†; ***Norw.:*** Diural; Furix; Lasix; ***S.Afr.:*** Aquarid; Arcanamide†; Hydrex; Lasix; Puresis; Uremide; ***Spain:*** Diurolasa†; Seguril; ***Swed.:*** Diural†; Furix; Furoscand; Impugan; Lasix; ***Switz.:*** Diuresal†; Diurix; furo-basan; Furodrix; Furosifar; Fursol; Hydro-Rapid-Tablinen†; Impugan; Lasix; Oedemex; ***UK:*** Dryptal†; Froop; Frumax; Frusid; Frusol; Lasix; Rusyde; Tenkafruse; ***USA:*** Lasix.

Multi-ingredient: ***Aust.:*** Furo-Aldopur; Furolacton; Hydrotrix; Lasilacton; Lasitace; Normotensin; Spirono comp; Terbolan; ***Belg.:*** Frusamil; ***Fr.:*** Aldalix; Logirene; ***Ger.:*** Betasemid; Diaphal; duraspiron-comp.; Furesis comp; Furo-Aldopur; Furorese Comp; Hydrotrix; Nortensin†; Osyrol Lasix; Spiro comp; Spiro-D; Spiro-D-Tablinen†; Spironolacton Plus; ***Irl.:*** Diumide-K Continus; Fru-Co; Frumil; Frusene; Lasikal; Lasix + K†; Lasoride; ***Ital.:*** Betasemid†; Fluss 40; Lasitone; Lasix-Reserpin†; Spirofur; ***Neth.:*** Elkin; ***Spain:*** Frusamil†; Salidur; ***Switz.:*** Diumid+K†; Frumil; Furosemid comp; Furospir; Hydrotrix; Lasilactone; ***UK:*** Aridil; Diumide-K Continus; Froop Co; Fru-Co; Frumil; Frusemek; Frusene; Lasikal; Lasilactone; Lasipressin†; Lasix + K†; Lasoride.

Gallopamil Hydrochloride (16819-g)

Gallopamil Hydrochloride *(BANM, rINNM).*

D-600 (gallopamil); Methoxyverapamil Hydrochloride. 5-[*N*-(3,4-Dimethoxyphenethyl)-*N*-methylamino]-2-(3,4,5-trimethoxyphenyl)-2-isopropylvaleronitrile hydrochloride.

$C_{28}H_{40}N_2O_5,HCl = 521.1.$

CAS — 16662-47-8 (gallopamil).

Gallopamil is a calcium-channel blocker (see p.778) with antiarrhythmic activity and is chemically related to verapamil. It is used in chronic cardiac insufficiency, angina pectoris, and cardiac arrhythmias. Gallopamil hydrochloride is given by mouth in doses of 25 to 50 mg every 6 to 12 hours up to a maximum total dose of 200 mg daily.

Angina pectoris. Calcium-channel blockers are widely used in angina pectoris, the overall management of which is discussed on p.780.

Gallopamil has been reported[1] to improve subjective and objective symptoms of angina pectoris without causing severe adverse effects. The most frequently used dosage was gallopamil 50 mg two or three times daily, and full effectiveness was usually reached 4 weeks after the start of therapy. Therapeutic success was defined as good in 73% of cases. The most frequent adverse effects were gastric discomfort, bradycardia, and atrioventricular prolongation: therapy was discontinued in 4 patients due to cardiac adverse reactions.

Gallopamil has also been reported[2] to increase the antiischaemic effect of isosorbide mononitrate in patients with angina.

1. Sućić M, Schiemann J. Multizentrische gallopamil-langzeitstudie bei patienten mit koronarer herzkrankheit. *Arzneimittelforschung* 1984; **34:** 1587–94.
2. Stauch M, *et al.* Lack of tolerance after chronic administration of controlled-release isosorbide-5-mononitrate: interaction of nitrate and gallopamil. *Eur J Clin Pharmacol* 1990; **38** (suppl 1): S31–4.

Pharmacokinetics. A single-dose study of intravenous and oral gallopamil hydrochloride in healthy subjects indicated that the drug was almost completely metabolised, only a very small amount being excreted as unchanged drug.[1] Approximately equal amounts were excreted in urine and faeces, mainly as conjugated metabolites.

1. Weymann J, *et al.* Metabolism of the calcium antagonist gallopamil in man. *Arzneimittelforschung* 1989; **39:** 605–7.

Preparations

Proprietary Preparations (details are given in Part 3)
Aust.: Procorum; ***Ger.:*** Procorum; ***Ital.:*** Algocor; Procorum.

Gepefrine Tartrate (11602-a)

Gepefrine Tartrate *(rINNM).*

(+)-(*S*)-*m*-(2-Aminopropyl)phenol tartrate.

$C_9H_{13}NO,C_4H_6O_6 = 301.3.$

CAS — 18840-47-6 (gepefrine).

Gepefrine is a sympathomimetic (see Adrenaline, p.813) used as the tartrate in doses of up to 30 mg three times daily in the treatment of hypotensive states.

Preparations

Proprietary Preparations (details are given in Part 3)
Ger.: Pressionorm†; Wintonin.

Glyceryl Trinitrate (9237-z)

Glonoin; GTN; Nitroglycerin; Nitroglycerol; NTG; Trinitrin; Trinitroglycerin. Propane-1,2,3-triol trinitrate.

$C_3H_5(O.NO_2)_3 = 227.1.$

CAS — 55-63-0.

Pharmacopoeias. Chin., Eur. (see p.viii), and *US* include glyceryl trinitrate as diluted solutions.

Undiluted glyceryl trinitrate is a white to pale yellow, thick, flammable, explosive liquid. Slightly **soluble** in water; soluble in acetone, in alcohol, in carbon disulphide, in chloroform, in dichloromethane, in ether, in ethyl acetate, in glacial acetic acid, and in methyl alcohol.

Glyceryl Trinitrate Solution (Ph. Eur.) is a solution of glyceryl trinitrate in alcohol (96%). It is a clear, colourless, to slightly yellow solution. **Miscible** with acetone and dehydrated alcohol.

Diluted Nitroglycerin (USP 23) is a mixture of glyceryl trinitrate with lactose, glucose, alcohol, propylene glycol, or other suitable inert excipient. When diluted in either alcohol or propylene glycol it is a clear, colourless, or pale yellow liquid. When diluted with lactose, it is a white odourless powder.

Dilution of 1% alcoholic solutions with an equal volume of water produces a clear solution; dilution with twice its volume of water produces a turbid mixture from which glyceryl trinitrate deposits on standing; careless handling can then lead to explosion. Glyceryl trinitrate is saponified by strong alkalis.

Store in airtight containers protected from light. Diluted solutions (1%) should be stored at 2° to 15°; more concentrated solutions may be stored at 15° to 20°.

CAUTION. *Undiluted glyceryl trinitrate can be exploded by percussion or excessive heat and only exceedingly small amounts should be isolated.*

Incompatibility. Studies have found glyceryl trinitrate to be incompatible with phenytoin[1] and alteplase.[2]

1. Klamerus KJ, *et al.* Stability of nitroglycerin in intravenous admixtures. *Am J Hosp Pharm* 1984; **41:** 303–5.
2. Lee CY, *et al.* Visual and spectrophotometric determination of compatibility of alteplase and streptokinase with other injectable drugs. *Am J Hosp Pharm* 1990; **47:** 606–8.

Stability. INTRAVENOUS SOLUTIONS. The loss of glyceryl trinitrate from solution by adsorption or absorption into some plastics of intravenous administration equipment has been recognised for some years,[1,2] although adsorption does not appear to occur to any great extent with polyolefin[3] or polyethylene.[4-6] It is not only infusion containers and plastic tubing that may be involved; some inline filters can adsorb glyceryl trinitrate.[7,8]

1. Crouthamel WG, *et al.* Loss of nitroglycerin from plastic intravenous bags. *N Engl J Med* 1978; **299:** 262.
2. Roberts MS, *et al.* The availability of nitroglycerin from parenteral solutions. *J Pharm Pharmacol* 1980; **32:** 237–44.
3. Wagenknecht DM, *et al.* Stability of nitroglycerin solutions in polyolefin and glass containers. *Am J Hosp Pharm* 1984; **41:** 1807–11.
4. Martens HJ, *et al.* Sorption of various drugs in polyvinyl chloride, glass, and polyethylene-lined infusion containers. *Am J Hosp Pharm* 1990; **47:** 369–73.
5. Schaber DE, *et al.* Nitroglycerin adsorption to a combination polyvinyl chloride, polyethylene intravenous administration set. *Drug Intell Clin Pharm* 1985; **19:** 572–5.
6. Tracy TS, *et al.* Nitroglycerin delivery through a polyethylene-lined intravenous administration set. *Am J Hosp Pharm* 1989; **46:** 2031–5.
7. Baaske DM, *et al.* Nitroglycerin compatibility with intravenous fluid filters, containers, and administration sets. *Am J Hosp Pharm* 1980; **37:** 201–5.
8. Kanke M, *et al.* Binding of selected drugs to a "treated" inline filter. *Am J Hosp Pharm* 1983; **40:** 1323–8.

TABLETS. Many studies have demonstrated that glyceryl trinitrate tablets are unstable and subject to considerable loss of potency in contact with packaging components such as adhesive labels, cotton and rayon fillers, and plastic bottles and caps. Both the Council of the Royal Pharmaceutical Society of Great Britain and the Food and Drug Administration in the USA have issued packaging and dispensing guidelines. Glyceryl trinitrate tablets should be dispensed only in glass containers sealed with a foil lined cap and containing no cotton wool wadding. In addition, the Council of the Royal Pharmaceutical Society of Great Britain recommends that no more than 100 tablets should be supplied and that the container should be labelled with an indication that any tablets should be discarded after eight weeks in use.

Adverse Effects

Glyceryl trinitrate may cause flushing of the face, dizziness, tachycardia, and throbbing headache. Large doses cause vomiting, restlessness, blurred vision, hypotension (which can be severe), syncope, and rarely cyanosis, and methaemoglobinaemia; impairment of respiration and bradycardia may ensue. Contact dermatitis has been reported in patients using topical glyceryl trinitrate preparations; local irritation and erythema may also occur. Preparations applied to the oral mucosa frequently produce a localised burning sensation.

Chronic poisoning may occur in industry but tolerance develops when glyceryl trinitrate is regularly handled and nitrate dependence can lead to severe withdrawal symptoms in subjects abruptly removed from chronic exposure. Loss of such tolerance is rapid and may cause poisoning on re-exposure. Tolerance may occur during clinical use and is usually associated with preparations that produce sustained plasma concentrations.

Effects on the heart. Tachycardia, hypotension, and bradycardia are recognised adverse cardiac effects of glyceryl trinitrate. Rarely reported adverse effects include asystole[1] and complete heart block.[2]

1. Ong EA, *et al.* Nitroglycerin-induced asystole. *Arch Intern Med* 1985; **145:** 954.
2. Lancaster L, Fenster PE. Complete heart block after sublingual nitroglycerin. *Chest* 1983; **84:** 111–12.

Effects on taste. A 61-year-old man experienced loss of bitter and salty taste sensations 2 weeks after addition of glyceryl trinitrate patches to his post-myocardial infarction drug regimen.[1] The patient experienced complete loss of taste after 6 weeks; his taste sensation returned to normal within one week of discontinuing glyceryl trinitrate patches. Taste sensation was again altered on rechallenge.

1. Ewing RC, *et al.* Ageusia associated with transdermal nitroglycerin. *Clin Pharm* 1989; **8:** 146–7.

Hypersensitivity. Contact dermatitis has been reported in patients using glyceryl trinitrate ointment and patches.[1] Both glyceryl trinitrate and formulation components may be involved in these reactions.

1. Carmichael AJ. Skin sensitivity and transdermal drug delivery: a review of the problem. *Drug Safety* 1994; **10:** 151–9.

Intravenous administration. Some commercial formulations of glyceryl trinitrate for intravenous use may contain substantial quantities of alcohol in the solvent. There have been several reports of alcohol intoxication occurring in patients during high-dose intravenous glyceryl trinitrate infusion.[1-3] In one patient[3] who required glyceryl trinitrate 2 mg per minute, a blood-alcohol concentration of 2.67 mg per mL was reported. Polyvinyl chloride tubing had been used for the infusion and the authors suggested that adsorption of glyceryl trinitrate onto the tubing may have increased the dose requirement and thus the amount of alcohol given.

Propylene glycol is also used as a solvent in some commercial formulations of glyceryl trinitrate. Infusion of solutions with propylene glycol can lead to hyperosmolarity: see Fluid and Electrolyte Homoeostasis under Propylene Glycol, p.1622, for details.

1. Shook TL, *et al.* Ethanol intoxication complicating intravenous nitroglycerin therapy. *Ann Intern Med* 1984; **101:** 498–9.
2. Daly TJ, *et al.* "Cocktail"-coronary care. *N Engl J Med* 1984; **310:** 1123.
3. Korn SH, Comer JB. Intravenous nitroglycerin and ethanol intoxication. *Ann Intern Med* 1985; **102:** 274.

Treatment of Adverse Effects

Syncope and hypotension should be treated by keeping the patient in a recumbent position with the head lowered. The administration of oxygen, with assisted respiration, may be necessary in severe poisoning and infusion of plasma expanders or suitable electrolyte solutions may be required to maintain the circulation. If methaemoglobinaemia occurs methylene blue may be given intravenously. In the case of severe poisoning with tablets the stomach should be emptied by lavage.

Precautions

Glyceryl trinitrate should not be used in patients with severe hypotension, hypovolaemia, marked anaemia, heart failure due to obstruction (including constrictive pericarditis), or raised intracranial pressure due to head trauma or cerebral haemorrhage. Glyceryl trinitrate may increase intra-ocular pressure in patients with angle-closure glaucoma and it is recommended by some that it should be avoided in such patients.

It should be used with caution in patients with severely impaired renal or hepatic function, hypothyroidism, malnutrition, or hypothermia. Metal-containing transdermal systems should be removed before cardioversion or diathermy.

Nitrate tolerance. Organic nitrates can lose their anti-anginal and anti-ischaemic effects in some patients.[1] Tolerance tends to develop in the majority of patients on continuous therapy and higher nitrate doses appear to induce attenuation in response to a greater degree than lower doses.[2]

The mechanisms of nitrate tolerance are incompletely understood. Organic nitrates are believed to exert their vasodilator effect by stimulating guanylate cyclase and thus increasing the formation of cyclic guanosine monophosphate. To stimulate guanylate cyclase, organic nitrates must be converted to the active form which requires the presence of cysteine or another thiol. Repeated doses of a nitrate exhaust tissue stores of sulfhydryl groups and this is one mechanism that may account for the development of tolerance.[3] The activation of neurohumoral systems, which counteract the effects of organic nitrates, has also been proposed as a mechanism.[4]

One method proposed to avoid the development of tolerance is to provide a nitrate-free interval. With transdermal glyceryl trinitrate systems, the patch can be removed at night. For oral, buccal, and ointment preparations, the dose given at the end of the day can be omitted. Whether a nitrate-free interval is necessary for all patients has not been determined as many patients receiving continuous nitrates do not experience clinical tolerance.[2] A transdermal patch has been developed that has a higher release rate during the first than during the second part of a 24-hour period, and it was hoped that this would prevent the development of tolerance, although results so far have not been promising.[5] Another method under investigation includes the administration of a sulfhydryl donor such as acetylcysteine (see also p.1054), methionine, or captopril.[6] Other drugs studied include hydralazine, which may act by reducing neurohumoral activation.[7]

1. Parker JO. Nitrate tolerance: a problem during continuous nitrate administration. *Eur J Clin Pharmacol* 1990; **38** (suppl 1): S21–S25.
2. Flaherty JT. Nitrate tolerance: a review of the evidence. *Drugs* 1989; **37:** 523–50.
3. Kukovetz WR, Holzmann S. Mechanisms of nitrate-induced vasodilatation and tolerance. *Eur J Clin Pharmacol* 1990; **38** (suppl 1): S9–S14.
4. Maxwell SRJ, Kendall MJ. An update on nitrate tolerance: can it be avoided? *Postgrad Med J* 1992; **68:** 857–66.
5. Wiegand A, *et al.* Pharmacodynamic and pharmacokinetic evaluation of a new transdermal delivery system with a time-dependent release of glyceryl trinitrate. *J Clin Pharmacol* 1992; **32:** 77–84.
6. Elkayam U. Tolerance to organic nitrates: evidence, mechanisms, clinical relevance, and strategies for prevention. *Ann Intern Med* 1991; **114:** 667–77.
7. Gogia H, *et al.* Prevention of tolerance to hemodynamic effects of nitrates with concomitant use of hydralazine in patients with chronic heart failure. *J Am Coll Cardiol* 1995; **26:** 1575–80.

Transdermal patches. An explosion occurred during defibrillation in a patient with a glyceryl trinitrate transdermal patch on the left side of the chest.[1] There was no visible injury to the patient. Subsequent studies suggested that this was caused by an electrical arc between the defibrillator paddle and the aluminium backing of the patch rather than explosion of the glyceryl trinitrate.

Although some recommend removal of transdermal patches prior to diathermy, a maximum rise in patch temperature of only 2.2° was reported when patches were exposed to a maximum power density of 800 watts per m^2. It was considered that exposure of transdermal patches to microwave diathermy, for example as part of physiotherapy treatment, was unlikely to cause direct thermal injury to the wearer.[2]

1. Babka JC. Does nitroglycerin explode? *N Engl J Med* 1983; **309:** 379.
2. Moseley H, *et al.* The influence of microwave radiation on transdermal delivery systems. *Br J Dermatol* 1990; **122:** 361–3.

Interactions

The hypotensive effects of glyceryl trinitrate may be enhanced by alcohol, and by vasodilators and other drugs with hypotensive actions. The effectiveness of sublingual and buccal tablet preparations may be reduced by drugs that cause dry mouth since dissolution may be delayed.

For the effects of glyceryl trinitrate on alteplase, see p.818, on dihydroergotamine mesylate, see p.446, and on heparin, see p.881.

Antimuscarinics. Delayed dissolution of glyceryl trinitrate tablets due to dry mouth has been reported in a patient taking imipramine[1] and in a patient treated with atropine;[2] this effect should be considered whenever glyceryl trinitrate sublingual tablets are given to patients taking other drugs that can cause dry mouth. Use of the lingual spray[2] rather than a sublingual tablet or addition of 1 mL of saline under the tongue[3] may be used to overcome the problem.

1. Robbins LJ. Dry mouth and delayed dissolution of sublingual nitro-glycerin. *N Engl J Med* 1983; **309:** 985.
2. Kimchi A. Dry mouth and delayed dissolution of nitroglycerin. *N Engl J Med* 1984; **310:** 1122.
3. Rasler FE. Ineffectiveness of sublingual nitroglycerin in patients with dry mucous membranes. *N Engl J Med* 1986; **314:** 181.

Pharmacokinetics

Glyceryl trinitrate is rapidly absorbed from the oral mucosa. It is also well absorbed from the gastro-intestinal tract and through the skin. Bioavailability is less than 100% following administration by any of these routes due to pre-systemic clearance; bioavailability is further reduced following oral administration owing to extensive first-pass metabolism in the liver.

Therapeutic effect is apparent within 1 to 3 minutes of administration of sublingual tablets, sublingual spray, or buccal tablets; within 30 to 60 minutes of administration of an ointment or transdermal patch; and within 1 to 2 minutes following intravenous administration.

Duration of action is about 30 to 60 minutes with sublingual tablets or spray and 3 to 5 hours with modified-release buccal tablets. Transdermal patches are designed to release a stated amount of drug over 24 hours, while therapeutic effects following application of glyceryl trinitrate ointment 2% persist for up to 8 hours. Duration of action following intravenous administration is about 3 to 5 minutes.

Glyceryl trinitrate is widely distributed with a large apparent volume of distribution. It is taken up by smooth muscle cells of blood vessels and the nitrate group is cleaved to inorganic nitrite and then to nitric oxide. This reaction requires the presence of cysteine or another thiol, see Nitrate Tolerance under Precautions, above. Glyceryl trinitrate also undergoes hydrolysis in plasma and is rapidly metabolised in the liver by glutathione-organic nitrate reductase to dinitrates and mononitrates. The dinitrates are less potent vasodilators than glyceryl trinitrate; the mononitrates may have some vasodilator activity.

References.

1. Bogaert MG. Clinical pharmacokinetics of glyceryl trinitrate following the use of systemic and topical preparations. *Clin Pharmacokinet* 1987; **12:** 1–11.
2. Thadani U, Whitsett T. Relationship of pharmacokinetic and pharmacodynamic properties of the organic nitrates. *Clin Pharmacokinet* 1988; **15:** 32–43.
3. Ridout G, *et al.* Pharmacokinetic considerations in the use of newer transdermal formulations. *Clin Pharmacokinet* 1988; **15:** 114–31.

Uses and Administration

Glyceryl trinitrate is a nitrovasodilator used in the management of angina pectoris (p.780), heart failure (p.785), and myocardial infarction (below). Other indications include inducing hypotension and controlling hypertension during surgery.

Glyceryl trinitrate is believed to exert its vasodilator effect through nitric oxide stimulating guanylate cyclase in the vascular smooth muscle cells; this results in an increase in cyclic guanosine monophosphate. This nucleotide induces relaxation probably by lowering the free calcium concentration in the cytosol. In its action on vascular muscle venous dilatation predominates over dilatation of the arterioles. Venous dilatation decreases venous return as a result of venous pooling and lowers left ventricular diastolic volume and pressure (termed a reduction in preload). The smaller or less important dilatation of arterioles reduces both peripheral vascular resistance and left ventricular pressure at systole (termed a reduction in afterload). The consequent effect is a reduction in the primary determinants of myocardial oxygen demand. The effect on preload is not shared by beta blockers or calcium-channel blockers. Glyceryl trinitrate also has a coronary vasodilator effect which improves regional coronary blood flow to ischaemic areas resulting in improved oxygen supply to the myocardium.

Glyceryl trinitrate may be administered by the sublingual, buccal, oral, transdermal, or intravenous route. The dose and choice of formulation depend upon the clinical situation.

In the management of **acute angina** glyceryl trinitrate is given as sublingual tablets, a sublingual aerosol spray, or buccal tablets, which all produce a rapid onset of therapeutic effect and provide rapid relief of anginal pain. These dosage forms may also be used before an activity or stress which might provoke an attack. One sublingual tablet (usual strength 300 to 600 μg) is placed under the tongue. The dose may be repeated as required but patients should be advised to seek medical care if pain persists after a total of 3 doses within 15 minutes. If an aerosol spray is used one or two sprays of 400 μg each are directed onto or under the tongue, then the mouth is closed; three sprays may be used if necessary. Buccal tablets of glyceryl trinitrate are placed between the upper lip and gum (see below for precautions to be observed during use). A dose of 1 or 2 mg is usually sufficient, although 3 mg may be needed in some cases.

In the long-term management of **stable angina** glyceryl trinitrate is given as modified-release tablets or capsules, transdermal formulations, or buccal tablets, which all provide a long duration of action. Dosage varies according to the specific formulation. In the UK, for example, modified-release oral tablets are available that allow doses of up to 12.8 mg to be given up to three times daily. The transdermal formulations available are ointments and patches. With the ointment a measured amount (½ to 2 inches of glyceryl trinitrate ointment 2%) is applied 3 or 4 times daily, or every 3 to 4 hours if necessary, to the chest, arm, thigh, or back. Transdermal patches applied to the chest, upper arm, or shoulder are more convenient. Patches are generally designed to release glyceryl trinitrate at a constant rate; they are available in a range of sizes, releasing an average of 2.5 to 20 mg of glyceryl trinitrate over 24 hours (0.1 to 0.8 mg per hour). A maximum daily dose of 20 mg has been suggested. Glyceryl trinitrate ointment and patches should be applied to a fresh area of skin and several days should elapse before re-application to formerly used sites. Buccal tablets are used in doses of 1 to 5 mg three times daily. The tablets are retained in the buccal cavity; the rate of dissolution of the tablet can be increased by touching the tablet with the tongue or drinking hot liquids. It is common practice to remove the tablets at bedtime because of the risk of aspiration. Also patients using buccal tablets should be advised to alternate placement sites and pay close attention to oral hygiene. The tablets are not intended to be chewed; if the buccal tablet is inadvertently swallowed, another may be placed in the buccal cavity.

Tolerance tends to develop in the majority of patients on continuous nitrate therapy and nitrate-free intervals are often employed to avoid this problem (see above under Precautions, Nitrate Tolerance for further details).

In the management of **unstable angina** glyceryl trinitrate may be given by intravenous infusion. Manufacturers' guidelines for dilution of glyceryl trinitrate injection specify glucose 5% or sodium chloride 0.9% as the diluent. During intravenous administration of glyceryl trinitrate there should be haemodynamic monitoring of the patient with the dose being adjusted gradually to produce the desired response. The plastic used in the infusion equipment may adsorb glyceryl trinitrate (see above) and allowance may have to be made for this. The usual initial dose for unstable angina is 5 to 10 μg per minute. Most patients respond to doses between 10 and 200 μg per minute, although higher doses may be required in some cases. The sublingual and buccal routes may also be used; doses of up to 5 mg as buccal tablets may be required to relieve pain in patients with unstable angina.

In the management of acute **heart failure** glyceryl trinitrate is given intravenously in an initial dose of 5 to 25 μg per minute. Buccal tablets have been used in doses of 5 mg repeated as needed until symptoms are controlled. In chronic heart failure buccal tablets may be given in doses of 5 to 10 mg three times daily.

Glyceryl trinitrate is also used intravenously in acute **myocardial infarction**, and to induce hypotension or control hypertension during **surgery**. The initial dose is 5 to 25 μg per minute, adjusted according to response. The usual range is 10 to 200 μg per minute but some surgical patients may require up to 400 μg per minute.

Glyceryl trinitrate has also been used as transdermal patches in the prophylactic treatment of **phlebitis and extravasation** secondary to venous cannulation. One 5-mg patch is applied distal to the intravenous site; after 3 to 4 days the patch should be replaced at a different skin site. This treatment should continue only as long as the intravenous infusion is maintained.

Anal fissure. Nitrates such as glyceryl trinitrate are being studied in the treatment of chronic anal fissure (p.1311) because of their ability to relax the anal sphincter. Topical application of glyceryl trinitrate ointment in concentrations of 0.2 to 0.8% has relieved pain and aided healing of anal fissures both in uncontrolled[1-3] and controlled studies.[4] Follow-up[6] of some of the patients indicated that after 24 to 38 months most had not experienced further problems or had had occasional recurrences which in the majority of cases had responded to further topical treatment. Encouraging results have also been obtained in an uncontrolled study using a 1% ointment of isosorbide dinitrate.[5]

1. Gorfine SR. Topical nitroglycerin therapy for anal fissures and ulcers. *N Engl J Med* 1995; **333:** 1156–7.
2. Lund JN *et al.* Use of glyceryl trinitrate ointment in the treatment of anal fissure. *Br J Surg* 1996; **83:** 776–7.
3. Watson SJ, *et al.* Topical glyceryl trinitrate in the treatment of chronic anal fissure. *Br J Surg* 1996; **83:** 771–5.
4. Lund JN, Scholefield JH. A randomised, prospective, double-blind, placebo-controlled trial of glyceryl trinitrate ointment in treatment of anal fissure. *Lancet* 1997; **349:** 11–14. Correction. *ibid.*; 656.
5. Schouten WR, *et al.* Pathophysiological aspects and clinical outcome of intra-anal application of isosorbide dinitrate in patients with chronic anal fissure. *Gut* 1996; **39:** 465–9.
6. Lund JN, Scholefield JH. Follow-up of patients with chronic anal fissure treated with topical glyceryl trinitrate. *Lancet* 1998; **352:** 1681.

Erectile dysfunction. Erectile dysfunction (p.1614) has been managed by the penile injection of drugs such as papaverine or alprostadil although oral treatment with sildenafil is now available. Penile injections are not always acceptable to the patient and a number of studies have investigated topical therapies, mostly glyceryl trinitrate applied either as ointment or as a transdermal delivery system to the penis.[1-4] Such treatment can produce erections in some subjects, although response rates vary. However, patients must wear a condom to protect their partner from the effects. The mechanism of action of glyceryl trinitrate is believed to be due to smooth muscle relaxation and vasodilatation which are necessary prerequisites for penile erection.

Isosorbide dinitrate as a cream also containing aminophylline and co-dergocrine mesylate has produced some benefit[5] although a further study[6] failed to confirm these results.

1. Heaton JPW, *et al.* Topical glyceryl trinitrate causes measurable penile arterial dilation in impotent men. *J Urol (Baltimore)* 1990; **143:** 729–31.
2. Meyhoff HH, *et al.* Non-invasive management of impotence with transcutaneous nitroglycerin. *Br J Urol* 1992; **69:** 88–90.
3. Nunez BD, Anderson DC. Nitroglycerin ointment in the treatment of impotence. *J Urol (Baltimore)* 1993; **150:** 1241–3.
4. Anderson DC, Seifert CF. Topical nitrate treatment of impotence. *Ann Pharmacother* 1993; **27:** 1203–5.
5. Gomaa A, *et al.* Topical treatment of erectile dysfunction: randomised double blind placebo controlled trial of cream containing aminophylline, isosorbide dinitrate, and co-dergocrine mesylate. *Br Med J* 1996; **312:** 1512–15.
6. Naude JH, Le Roux PJ. Topical treatment of erectile dysfunction did not show results. *Br Med J* 1998; **316:** 1318.

Gallstones. Endoscopic removal of gallstones (p.1642) in a small series of 15 patients was facilitated by glyceryl trinitrate 1.2 to 3.6 mg applied as a spray to the tongue. Glyceryl trinitrate 1.2 mg was shown to relax the sphincter of Oddi to approximately 30% of its normal pressure.[1] The ability of glyceryl trinitrate to relax smooth muscle has also been employed to relieve biliary colic (p.8) in 3 patients with gallstones;[2] in one of these patients standard managements for the pain such as oral opioids had been only moderately effective.

1. Staritz M, *et al.* Nitroglycerine dilatation of sphincter of Oddi for endoscopic removal of bileduct stones. *Lancet* 1984; **i:** 956.
2. Hassel B. Treatment of biliary colic with nitroglycerin. *Lancet* 1993; **342:** 1305.

Myocardial infarction. The management of myocardial infarction (p.791) can involve numerous drug therapies including nitrates.

Nitrovasodilatation with intravenous glyceryl trinitrate or sodium nitroprusside, started within 24 hours of the onset of pain, has been associated with a reduction in mortality.[1] Its role is not certain but the empirical use of intravenous glyceryl trinitrate (in addition to standard treatment with a thrombolytic, oral aspirin, and an intravenous beta blocker) in the acute phase of myocardial infarction is widespread and appears to be safe, as was demonstrated in the GISSI-3 study.[2] In this study glyceryl trinitrate was administered by intravenous infusion during the first 24 hours, starting at 5 μg per minute and increasing by 5 to 20 μg per minute every 5 minutes for the first half hour until systolic blood pressure fell by at least 10% provided it remained above 90 mmHg; after 24 hours it was replaced by a transdermal patch providing 10 mg daily.

Some patients, for example those with myocardial ischaemia or poor left ventricular function, may require the long-term administration of nitrates, but recent studies have thrown doubt on their routine use. In the GISSI-3 study there was no significant benefit when assessed 6 weeks[2] and 6 months[3] post-infarction from the use of transdermal glyceryl trinitrate and in the ISIS-4 study[4] oral isosorbide mononitrate apparently had no effect on 35-day mortality.

1. Yusuf S, *et al.* Effect of intravenous nitrates on mortality in acute myocardial infarction: an overview of the randomised trials. *Lancet* 1988; **i:** 1088–92.
2. Gruppo Italiano per lo Studio della Sopravvivenza nell'Infarto Miocardico. GISSI-3: effects of lisinopril and transdermal glyceryl trinitrate singly and together on 6-week mortality and ventricular function after acute myocardial infarction. *Lancet* 1994; **343:** 1115–22.
3. Gruppo Italiano per lo Studio della Sopravvivenza nell'Infarto Miocardico. Six-month effects of early treatment with lisinopril and transdermal glyceryl trinitrate singly and together withdrawn six weeks after myocardial infarction: the GISSI-3 trial. *J Am Coll Cardiol* 1996; **27:** 337–44.
4. ISIS-4 (Fourth International Study of Infarct Survival) Collaborative Group. ISIS-4: a randomised factorial trial assessing early oral captopril, oral mononitrate, and intravenous magnesium sulphate in 58 050 patients with suspected acute myocardial infarction. *Lancet* 1995; **345:** 669–85.

Obstetrics and gynaecology. The smooth muscle relaxant properties of glyceryl trinitrate have been employed in various obstetric or gynaecological situations although the reports are basically only anecdotal or include small numbers of patients. The intravenous injection of glyceryl trinitrate 50 to 100 μg repeated to a total dose of 200 μg if necessary has produced sufficient uterine relaxation in postpartum women for the manual extraction of retained placentas.[1,2] Administration by sublingual spray has also been used successfully to facilitate breech extraction in one set of twins.[3]

Glyceryl trinitrate has been given as a sublingual spray to relax the cervix prior to IUD insertion. In a series of over 100 patients one or two doses of 400 μg sublingually were usually adequate.[4]

Beneficial preliminary results have been reported in 13 women with possible premature labour (p.760) following application of glyceryl trinitrate patches to the abdomen.[5] Uterine relaxation allowed prolongation of pregnancy of between 1 and 87 days although the difficulty in proving efficacy is well recognised as early contractions may not always progress to premature labour.

Transdermal glyceryl trinitrate has been tried for controlling pain in severe and moderate-to-severe dysmenorrhoea[6,7] (p.9).

Glyceryl trinitrate has been given intravenously in the management of pre-eclampsia (see under Hypertension, p.788) and is reported to reduce blood pressure without compromising uterine blood flow.[8]

Isosorbide mononitrate administered vaginally has been found to produce cervical ripening[9] and may be an alternative to prostaglandins for this purpose before first trimester termination of pregnancy (p.1412).

1. DeSimone CA, *et al.* Intravenous nitro-glycerin aids manual extraction of a retained placenta. *Anesthesiology* 1990; **73:** 787.
2. Lowenwirt IP, *et al.* Safety of intravenous glyceryl trinitrate in management of retained placenta. *Aust N Z J Obstet Gynaecol* 1997; **37:** 20–4.
3. Greenspoon JS, Kovacic A. Breech extraction facilitated by glyceryl trinitrate sublingual spray. *Lancet* 1991; **338:** 124–5.

4. Yadava RP. Sublingual glyceryl trinitrate spray facilitates IUD insertion. *Br J Sex Med* 1990; **17:** 217.
5. Lees C, *et al.* Arrest of preterm labour and prolongation of gestation with glyceryl trinitrate, a nitric oxide donor. *Lancet* 1994; **343:** 1325–6.
6. Pittrof R, *et al.* Crossover study of glyceryl trinitrate patches for controlling pain in women with severe dysmenorrhoea. *Br Med J* 1996; **312:** 884.
7. The Transdermal Nitroglycerine/Dysmenorrhoea Study Group. Transdermal nitroglycerine in the management of pain associated with primary dysmenorrhoea: a multinational pilot study. *J Int Med Res* 1997; **25:** 41–4.
8. Grunewald C, *et al.* Effects of nitroglycerin on the uterine and umbilical circulation in severe preeclampsia. *Obstet Gynecol* 1995; **86:** 600–4.
9. Thomson AJ, *et al.* Randomised trial of nitric oxide donor versus prostaglandin for cervical ripening before first-trimester termination of pregnancy. *Lancet* 1998; **352:** 1093–6.

Oesophageal motility disorders. A variety of oesophageal disorders may produce non-cardiac chest pain, similar to that of angina pectoris, from which they must be differentiated. Achalasia is obstruction caused by failure of the lower oesophageal sphincter to relax and permit passage of food into the stomach. Nitrates such as isosorbide dinitrate have been reported to produce effective relaxation[1] although the treatment of choice is mechanical dilatation of the sphincter, or if necessary surgery. Nitrates have also been tried in an attempt to relax the smooth muscle in oesophageal spasm, but results are often disappointing.[2] For a discussion of the overall management of such oesophageal motility disorders, including mention of the use of nitrates, see p.1174.

Nitrates may also be employed in oesophageal disorders such as variceal haemorrhage (see below).

1. Gelfond M, *et al.* Isosorbide dinitrate and nifedipine treatment of achalasia: a clinical, manometric and radionuclide evaluation. *Gastroenterology* 1982; **83:** 963–9.
2. Richter JE, *et al.* Esophageal chest pain: current controversies in pathogenesis, diagnosis, and therapy. *Ann Intern Med* 1989; **110:** 66–78.

Peripheral vascular disease. In peripheral vascular disease (p.794) nitrates have been tried as vasodilators and smooth muscle relaxants in order to improve resting blood flow. Glyceryl trinitrate has been applied topically in patients with Raynaud's syndrome[1,2] and in distal limb ischaemia[3] resulting in some benefit but this form of therapy is not widely used in these disorders.

1. Franks AG. Topical glyceryl trinitrate as adjunctive treatment in Raynaud's disease. *Lancet* 1982; **i:** 76–7.
2. Coppock JS, *et al.* Objective relief of vasospasm by glyceryl trinitrate in secondary Raynaud's phenomenon. *Postgrad Med J* 1986; **62:** 15–18.
3. Fletcher S, *et al.* Locally applied transdermal nitrate patches for the treatment of ischaemic rest pain. *Int J Clin Pract* 1997; **51:** 324–5.

Pulmonary hypertension. Administration of glyceryl trinitrate to patients with primary pulmonary hypertension (p.796) results in a fall in total pulmonary resistance in most patients.[1,2] However, pulmonary vasoconstriction may not be a pathogenic factor in this condition and in the absence of any controlled clinical trials, the use of vasodilators in the treatment of primary pulmonary hypertension must remain controversial.[3]

1. Pearl RG, *et al.* Acute hemodynamic effects of nitroglycerin in pulmonary hypertension. *Ann Intern Med* 1983; **99:** 9–13.
2. Weir EK, *et al.* The acute administration of vasodilators in primary pulmonary hypertension. *Am Rev Respir Dis* 1989; **140:** 1623–30.
3. Packer M. Is it ethical to administer vasodilator drugs to patients with primary pulmonary hypertension? *Chest* 1989; **95:** 1173–5.

Quinine oculotoxicity. Intravenous nitrate administration has been advised for the management of quinine oculotoxicity (p.440) and its benefit may be due to an increase in retinal vascular bed flow.[1]

1. Moore D, *et al.* Research into quinine ocular toxicity. *Br J Ophthalmol* 1992; **76:** 703.

Variceal haemorrhage. The usual treatment in variceal haemorrhage (p.1576) is injection sclerotherapy which may be performed during the emergency endoscopy procedure. Where endoscopy is unavailable drug therapy may be used and it may also have a role when sclerotherapy fails. Vasoconstrictors that are used include vasopressin and its analogue terlipressin given together with glyceryl trinitrate which counteracts the adverse cardiac effects of vasopressin, while potentiating its beneficial effects on portal pressure.

Prophylaxis of a first bleed in patients with portal hypertension is controversial since about 70% of patients who have varices will never bleed. It is postulated that a reduction in portal pressure to below 12 mmHg is necessary to reduce the incidence of variceal bleeding and that treatment with beta blockers alone does not achieve this. More effective drugs are being sought and isosorbide mononitrate (as adjunctive therapy with a beta blocker) is under investigation, both for prophylaxis of a first bleed[1,2] and in the prevention of rebleeding.[3] Early emergency treatment (before endoscopy) with terlipressin given intravenously and glyceryl trinitrate transdermally controlled bleeding and lowered mortality rates in patients with gastro-intestinal bleeding and a history or clinical signs of cirrhosis.[4]

1. Angelico M, *et al.* Isosorbide-5-mononitrate versus propranolol in the prevention of first bleeding in cirrhosis. *Gastroenterology* 1993; **104:** 1460–5.
2. Merkel C, *et al.* Randomised trial of nadolol alone or with isosorbide mononitrate for primary prophylaxis of variceal bleeding in cirrhosis. *Lancet* 1996; **348:** 1677–81.
3. Villanueva C, *et al.* Nadolol plus isosorbide mononitrate compared with sclerotherapy for the prevention of variceal rebleeding. *N Engl J Med* 1996; **334:** 1624–9.
4. Levacher S, *et al.* Early administration of terlipressin plus glyceryl trinitrate to control active upper gastrointestinal bleeding in cirrhotic patients. *Lancet* 1995; **346:** 865–8.

Venepuncture. Local topical application of glyceryl trinitrate patches to skin adjacent to intravenous infusion sites is used in the prophylactic treatment of phlebitis and extravasation.

Local application of glyceryl trinitrate 1 to 2 mg as ointment was found to be a useful aid to venepuncture in a study of 50 patients undergoing surgery,[1] but conflicting results have been reported in children and neonates.[2,3]

1. Hecker JF, *et al.* Nitroglycerine ointment as an aid to venepuncture. *Lancet* 1983; **i:** 332–3.
2. Vaksmann G, *et al.* Nitroglycerine ointment as aid to venous cannulation in children. *J Pediatr* 1987; **111:** 89–91.
3. Maynard EC, Oh W. Topical nitroglycerin ointment as an aid to insertion of peripheral venous catheters in neonates. *J Pediatr* 1989; **114:** 474–6.

Preparations

BP 1998: Glyceryl Trinitrate Tablets;
USP 23: Nitroglycerin Injection; Nitroglycerin Ointment; Nitroglycerin Tablets.

Proprietary Preparations (details are given in Part 3)
Aust.: Deponit; Minitran; Nitro Mack; Nitro-Dur; Nitroderm; Nitrolingual; Nitronal; Nitrong; Nitrozell; Perlinganit; ***Austral.:*** Anginine; Minitran; Nitradisc; Nitro-Bid; Nitro-Dur; Nitrolate†; Nitrolingual; Transderm-Nitro; Tridil†; ***Belg.:*** Deponit; Diafusor; Minitran; Nitro-Dyl; Nitrobaat†; Nitroderm; Nitrolingual; Nitrong; Nysconitrine; Willlong; ***Canad.:*** Minitran; Nitro-Bid†; Nitro-Dur; Nitrogard†; Nitroject†; Nitrol; Nitrolingual; Nitrong; Nitrostat; Transderm-Nitro; Tridil; ***Fr.:*** Cordipatch; Corditrine; Diafusor; Discotrine; Lenitral; Natirose†; Natispray; Nitriderm TTS; Optizor; Trinipatch; Trinitran†; ***Ger.:*** Aquo-Trinitrosan; Corangin Nitrokapseln; Coro-Nitro; Deponit; Gilustenon; Herwicard 0,8†; Maycor†; MinitranS; neos nitro OPT; Nitradisc; Nitrangin; Nitrangin forte; Nitro Mack; Nitro Pohl†; Nitro Rorer†; Nitro-Gesanit†; Nitro-Pflaster-ratiopharm; Nitroderm TTS; Nitroglin†; Nitrokapseln-ratiopharm; Nitrolingual; Nitronal; nitroperlinit†; Nitrorectal†; Nitrozell†; Perlinganit; Trinitrosan; Turicard; ***Irl.:*** Angised; Deponit; Glytrin; Nitro-Dur; Nitrocine; Nitrocontin Continus†; Nitrolingual; Nitronal; Percutol†; Suscard; Sustac; Transiderm-Nitro; Tridil; ***Ital.:*** Adesitrin; Angiospray†; Deponit; Minitran; Natispray; Nitro-Dur; Nitro-Retard†; Nitrocor†; Nitroderm TTS; Nitrong†; Nitrosylon; Perganit; Suscard†; Top-Nitro; Triniplas; Trinitrina; Venitrin; ***Jpn:*** Millisrol; Vasolator; ***Neth.:*** Angonit†; Deponit; Minitran; Nitro Pohl; Nitro-Dur; Nitrobaat; Nitrolingual; Nitrostat; Nitrozell†; Probucard†; Transiderm-Nitro; Trinipatch; ***Norw.:*** Minitran; Nitradisc; Nitro-Dur; Nitrolingual; Nitromex; Nitrong†; Nitroretard†; Nitroven; Suscard; Transiderm-Nitro; ***S.Afr.:*** Angised; Nitradisc; Nitrocine; Nitroderm TTS; Nitrolingual; Nitronal†; Nitrong†; Tridil; ***Spain:*** Cardiodisco; Colenitral; Cordiplast; Diafusor; Minitran; Nitradisc; Nitro Dur; Nitroderm TTS; Nitropacin; Nitroplast; Nitrotard; Solinitrina; Vernies; ***Swed.:*** Angiplex†; Minitran; Nitroglyn†; Nitrolingual; Nitromex; Nitrong; Nitroretard†; Perlinganit; Suscard; Transiderm-Nitro; ***Switz.:*** Aquo-Trinitrosan†; Deponit; Minitran; Natispray; Niong retard; Nitro Mack; Nitro-Dur; Nitroderm TTS; Nitrolingual; Nitromint; Nitronal; Perlinganit; Trinitrine; ***UK:*** Coro-Nitro; Deponit; Glytrin†; Minitran; Nitro-Dur; Nitrocine; Nitrocontin Continus†; Nitrolingual; Nitromin; Nitronal; Percutol; Suscard; Sustac; Transiderm-Nitro; Tridil†; ***USA:*** Deponit; Minitran; Nitrek; Nitro-Bid; Nitro-Derm; Nitro-Dur; Nitro-Time; Nitrodisc; Nitrogard; Nitroglyn; Nitrol; Nitrolingual; Nitrong; Nitrospan†; Nitrostat; NTS; Transderm-Nitro; Transdermal-NTG; Tridil.

Multi-ingredient: ***Aust.:*** Myocardon; Spasmocor; ***Ger.:*** Adenovasin†; Angiocardyl N; Baldronit cum Nitro†; Digi-Nitronal†; Eukliman†; Gallolingual†; Govil†; Myocardetten†; Nitrangin compositum; Nitro-Praecordin N; Nitrodurat†; Seda Nitro Mack†; Steno-Valocordin†; ***Ital.:*** Nitromaxitate†; ***Spain:*** Cafinitrina; ***USA:*** Emergent-Ez.

Guabenxan (12800-s)

Guabenxan *(rINN)*.

(1,4-Benzodioxan-6-ylmethyl)guanidine.

$C_{10}H_{13}N_3O_2$ = 207.2.

CAS — 19889-45-3.

Guabenxan is an antihypertensive with properties similar to guanethidine (below). It has been given by mouth as the sulphate.

Preparations

Proprietary Preparations (details are given in Part 3)

Multi-ingredient: ***Fr.:*** Tensigradyl.

Guanabenz Acetate (865-k)

Guanabenz Acetate *(USAN, rINNM)*.

NSC-68982 (guanabenz); Wy-8678 (guanabenz). (2,6-Dichlorobenzylideneamino)guanidine acetate.

$C_8H_8Cl_2N_4,C_2H_4O_2$ = 291.1.

CAS — 5051-62-7 (guanabenz); 23256-50-0 (guanabenz acetate).

Pharmacopoeias. In *Jpn* and *US*.

A white or almost white powder with not more than a slight odour. Sparingly **soluble** in water and in dilute hydrochloric acid; soluble in alcohol and in propylene glycol. A 0.7% solution in water has a pH of 5.5 to 7.0. **Store** in airtight containers. Protect from light.

Guanabenz acetate 5 mg is approximately equivalent to 4 mg of guanabenz.

Adverse Effects and Precautions

As for Clonidine Hydrochloride, p.841.

Overdosage. Report of 2 cases of overdosage with guanabenz.[1] The main symptoms were lethargy, drowsiness, bradycardia, and hypotension. A 45-year-old woman who had taken 200 to 240 mg of guanabenz with alcohol recovered following gastric lavage and intravenous fluids: a 3-year-old child who had taken 12 mg of guanabenz responded to atropine and dopamine. Naloxone had little effect in either patient.

1. Hall AH, *et al.* Guanabenz overdose. *Ann Intern Med* 1985; **102:** 787–8.

Pharmacokinetics

Following oral administration guanabenz is well absorbed and undergoes extensive first-pass metabolism. Peak plasma concentrations occur about 2 to 5 hours after a dose. It is about 90% bound to plasma protein. Guanabenz is mainly excreted in urine, almost entirely as metabolites; about 10 to 30% is excreted in faeces. The average elimination half-life is reported to range from 4 to 14 hours.

Uses and Administration

Guanabenz is an alpha$_2$-adrenoceptor agonist with actions and uses similar to those of clonidine (p.842). It is used in the management of hypertension (p.788), either alone or in conjunction with other antihypertensives, particularly thiazide diuretics.

Guanabenz is given by mouth as the acetate, but doses are usually expressed in terms of the base.

In hypertension, it is given in a usual dose of 4 mg twice a day initially increasing by increments of 4 to 8 mg per day every 1 to 2 weeks according to the patient's response. Doses of up to 32 mg twice daily have been used.

Preparations

USP 23: Guanabenz Acetate Tablets.

Proprietary Preparations (details are given in Part 3)
Aust.: Rexitene; Wytensin; ***Ger.:*** Wytensin†; ***Ital.:*** Rexitene†; ***Switz.:*** Tenelid†; ***USA:*** Wytensin.

Multi-ingredient: ***Ital.:*** Rexitene Plus†.

Guanadrel Sulphate (867-t)

Guanadrel Sulphate *(rINNM)*.

CL-1388R; Guanadrel Sulfate *(USAN)*; U-28288D. 1-(Cyclohexanespiro-2′-[1′,3′]dioxolan-4′-ylmethyl)guanidine sulphate; 1-(1,4-Dioxaspiro[4.5]dec-2-ylmethyl)guanidine sulphate.

$(C_{10}H_{19}N_3O_2)_2,H_2SO_4$ = 524.6.

CAS — 40580-59-4 (guanadrel); 22195-34-2 (guanadrel sulphate).

Pharmacopoeias. In *US*.

A white to off-white crystalline powder. **Soluble** in water; sparingly soluble in methyl alcohol; slightly soluble in alcohol and in acetone.

Adverse Effects, Treatment, and Precautions

As for Guanethidine Monosulphate, below. Guanadrel has been reported to cause less diarrhoea and orthostatic hypotension on rising in the morning than guanethidine, but more than methyldopa. However, orthostatic symptoms seem to occur with a similar frequency to guanethidine during the day. Guanadrel may cause fewer CNS effects than methyldopa.

Interactions

As for Guanethidine Monosulphate, below.

Pharmacokinetics

Guanadrel is rapidly and almost completely absorbed from the gastro-intestinal tract, with a reported bioavailability of about 85%. It is widely distributed throughout the body and about 20% is bound to plasma proteins. It is reported not to cross the blood-brain barrier. Plasma concentrations decline in a biphasic manner: the half-life varies widely between individuals, in the initial phase from 1 to 4 hours, and in the terminal phase from 5 to 45 hours, with a mean of about 10 hours. Guanadrel is metabolised in the liver and approximately 85% is excreted in the urine over 24 hours as the unchanged drug and its metabolites. About 40 to 50% of the drug is excreted unchanged.

Uses and Administration

Guanadrel is an antihypertensive with actions and uses similar to those of guanethidine monosulphate (below). Following oral administration, guanadrel acts within 2 hours with the maximum effect after 4 to 6 hours. The hypotensive effect is reported to last for 4 to 14 hours following a single dose. It is used in the management of hypertension (p.788), although it has largely been superseded by other drugs less likely to cause orthostatic hypotension.

Guanadrel is given by mouth as the sulphate. The usual initial dose is 5 mg twice daily adjusted at weekly or monthly intervals according to the patient's response. The maintenance dose is normally in the range of 20 to 75 mg daily in two or more divided doses.

Administration in renal impairment. Renal and non-renal clearance of guanadrel were decreased in 16 patients with impaired renal function compared with 6 healthy subjects, and this was reflected in a prolongation of the terminal elimination half-life from a mean of 3.69 hours to 6.8, 12.6, and 19.2 hours in patients with mild, moderate, and severe renal insufficiency, respectively.[1] Dosage adjustment would be preferable in patients with impaired kidney function given guanadrel, perhaps by giving the daily dose every 2 to 3 days in mild to moderate insufficiency and 5 days in severe insufficiency.

1. Halstenson CE, *et al.* Disposition of guanadrel in subjects with normal and impaired renal function. *J Clin Pharmacol* 1989; **29:** 128–32.

Preparations

USP 23: Guanadrel Sulfate Tablets.

Proprietary Preparations (details are given in Part 3)
USA: Hylorel.

Guanethidine Monosulphate (869-r)

Guanethidine Monosulphate *(BANM, rINNM)*.

Guanethidine Monosulfate *(USAN)*; Guanethidini Monosulfas; NSC-29863 (guanethidine hemisulphate); Su-5864 (guanethidine hemisulphate). 1-[2-(Perhydroazocin-1-yl)ethyl]guanidine monosulphate.

$C_{10}H_{22}N_4,H_2SO_4$ = 296.4.

CAS — 55-65-2 (guanethidine); 60-02-6 (guanethidine hemisulphate); 645-43-2 (guanethidine monosulphate).

Pharmacopoeias. In *Eur.* (see p.viii), *Jpn*, and *US*.
Chin. includes the hemisulphate, $(C_{10}H_{22}N_4)_2,H_2SO_4$.

A colourless crystalline powder. Freely **soluble** in water; practically insoluble in alcohol and in ether. A 2% solution in water has a pH of 4.7 to 5.7. **Protect** from light.

Adverse Effects

The commonest side-effects with guanethidine are severe postural and exertional hypotension and diarrhoea which may be particularly troublesome during the initial stages of therapy and during the dose adjustment. Dizziness, syncope, muscle weakness, and lassitude are liable to occur, especially on rising from sitting or lying. Postural hypotension may be severe enough to provoke angina, signs of renal insufficiency, and transient cerebral ischaemia. Other frequent side-effects are bradycardia, failure of ejaculation, fatigue, headache, salt and water retention and oedema, which may be accompanied by breathlessness and may occasionally precipitate overt heart failure.

Nausea, vomiting, dry mouth, nasal congestion, parotid tenderness, blurring of vision, depression, myalgia, muscle tremor, paraesthesias, hair loss, dermatitis, disturbed micturition, priapism, aggravation or precipitation of asthma, and exacerbation of peptic ulcer have also been reported. It has been reported that guanethidine may possibly cause anaemia, leucopenia, and thrombocytopenia.

When guanethidine is used as eye drops, common side-effects are conjunctival hyperaemia and miosis. Burning sensations and ptosis have also occurred. Superficial punctate keratitis has been reported particularly following prolonged administration of concentrated solutions.

Treatment of Adverse Effects

Withdrawal of guanethidine or reduction in dosage reverses many side-effects. If overdosage occurs the stomach should be emptied by lavage and activated charcoal may be given. Diarrhoea may be controlled by reducing dosage or giving codeine phosphate, or antimuscarinics. Hypotension may respond to placing the patient in the supine position with the feet raised. If hypotension is severe it may be necessary to give intravenous fluid replacement and small doses of vasopressors may be given cautiously. The patient must be observed for several days.

Precautions

Guanethidine should not be given to patients with phaeochromocytoma, as it may cause a hypertensive crisis, or to patients with heart failure not caused by hypertension.

It should be used with caution in patients with renal impairment, cerebrovascular disorders, or ischaemic heart disease, or with a history of peptic ulceration or asthma. Exercise and heat may increase the hypotensive effect of guanethidine, and dosage requirements may be reduced in patients who develop fever.

There may be an increased risk of cardiovascular collapse or cardiac arrest in patients undergoing surgery while taking guanethidine, but authorities differ as to whether the drug should be discontinued before elective surgery. Some authorities recommend discontinuation up to 2 or 3 weeks beforehand. In patients undergoing emergency procedures or where treatment has not been interrupted large doses of atropine should be given before induction of anaesthesia.

Patients undergoing treatment with eye drops containing guanethidine should be examined regularly for signs of conjunctival damage.

Interactions

Patients taking guanethidine may show increased sensitivity to the action of adrenaline, amphetamine, and other sympathomimetics resulting in exaggerated pressor effects. The hypotensive effects may also be antagonised by tricyclic antidepressants, MAOIs, and phenothiazine derivatives and related antipsychotics (although phenothiazines may also exacerbate postural hypotension—see below). In the UK the manufacturers suggest that treatment with MAOIs should be stopped at least 14 days before beginning guanethidine, although in the USA a minimum of a week has been recommended as adequate. It has been reported that oral contraceptives may reduce the hypotensive action of guanethidine. Concurrent administration of digitalis with guanethidine may cause excessive bradycardia.

The hypotensive effects of guanethidine may be enhanced by thiazide diuretics, other antihypertensives, and levodopa. Alcohol may cause orthostatic hypotension in patients taking guanethidine.

Phenothiazines. The reported antagonism between guanethidine and chlorpromazine was not considered of clinical relevance under most conditions. However, both phenothiazines and adrenergic neurone blockers could produce postural hypotension.[1]

1. Prasad A. Interaction. *Pharm J* 1990; **245:** 320.

Pharmacokinetics

Guanethidine is variably and incompletely absorbed from the gastro-intestinal tract with less than 50% of the dose reaching the systemic circulation. It is actively taken up into adrenergic neurones by the mechanism responsible for noradrenaline reuptake. A plasma concentration of 8 ng per mL is reported to be necessary for adrenergic blockade, but the dose required to achieve this varies between individuals due to differences in absorption and metabolism. It is partially metabolised in the liver, and is excreted in the urine as metabolites and unchanged guanethidine. It has a terminal half-life of about 5 days. Guanethidine does not penetrate the blood-brain barrier significantly.

Uses and Administration

Guanethidine is an antihypertensive which acts by selectively inhibiting transmission in postganglionic adrenergic nerves. It is believed to act mainly by preventing the release of noradrenaline at nerve endings; it causes the depletion of noradrenaline stores in peripheral sympathetic nerve terminals. It does not prevent the secretion of catecholamines by the adrenal medulla.

When administered by mouth its maximal effects may take 1 to 2 weeks to appear on continued dosing and persist for 7 to 10 days after treatment has been stopped. It causes an initial reduction in cardiac output but its main hypotensive effect is to cause peripheral vasodilatation; it reduces the vasoconstriction which normally results from standing up and which is the result of reflex sympathetic nervous activity. In the majority of patients it reduces the standing blood pressure but has a less marked effect on the supine blood pressure. When applied topically to the eye guanethidine reduces the production of aqueous humour.

Guanethidine is used in the management of hypertension (p.788) and in the topical treatment of open-angle glaucoma (p.1387). Eye drops of guanethidine have also been used for lid retraction associated with hyperthyroidism. Guanethidine may also be used in the management of neurological pain syndromes (see below).

Guanethidine is used in the treatment of hypertension when other drugs have proved inadequate, although it has largely been superseded by other drugs less likely to cause orthostatic hypotension. It is often given in conjunction with a diuretic or sometimes with another antihypertensive. Tolerance to guanethidine has occurred in some patients; this may be countered by intensive diuretic therapy.

In **hypertension**, the usual initial dose of guanethidine monosulphate is 10 mg daily by mouth. This is increased by increments of 10 mg every 7 days according to the response of the patient although some authorities recommend intervals of 2 to 3 weeks between increments to avoid accumulation. The usual maintenance dose varies from 25 to 50 mg daily as a single dose but up to 300 mg daily may be given. Children have been given 200 µg per kg bodyweight daily with increments of 200 µg per kg every 1 to 3 weeks until a satisfactory response is achieved; a dose of about 1.5 mg per kg daily may be required.

Smaller doses of guanethidine are needed when it is given concomitantly with other antihypertensives or diuretics.

Guanethidine monosulphate has been given intramuscularly in the treatment of hypertensive crises, including severe pre-eclampsia, but more suitable drugs are available. An intramuscular dose of 10 to 20 mg is reported to produce a fall in blood pressure within 30 minutes, reaching a maximum in 1 to 2 hours and lasting for 4 to 6 hours. When given by intravenous injection guanethidine may produce an initial hypertensive effect and hence when given intravenously should be given by slow intravenous infusion.

Eye drops containing guanethidine monosulphate 1 or 3% together with adrenaline 0.2 or 0.5%, respectively, are used in the treatment of open-angle **glaucoma**. Guanethidine monosulphate 5% eye drops, without adrenaline, have also been used for open-angle glaucoma and for the lid retraction which may accompany hyperthyroidism.

Pain syndromes. Sympathetic nerve blocks may be used in the management of acute or chronic pain associated with a well-defined anatomical site. Guanethidine has been used for intravenous regional sympathetic block in the management of neurogenic pain including central pain syndromes (p.8), to reduce pain and to maintain blood flow. Open studies[1,2] have shown benefit from guanethidine, and the effects of serial blocks appear to be cumulative.[3] Guanethidine has been suggested as a suitable treatment for reflex sympathetic dystrophy.[4] However, Jadad *et al.*[5] conducted a review of the literature and a double-blind trial in patients with reflex sympathetic dystrophy and failed to find any benefit from guanethidine. The trial had to be terminated early due to unacceptable adverse effects. Interestingly a small double-blind study in patients with rheumatoid arthritis found that regional sympathetic blockade with guanethidine 15 mg in 13 produced a significant improvement in pain intensity and pinch strength compared with placebo in 11. Grip strength, tenderness, and morning stiffness were not improved.[6]

Intravenous regional sympathetic blockade using guanethidine has also been reported in the management of frostbite[7] (see also p.895).

For a discussion of sympathetic pain syndromes, see p.11.

1. Hannington-Kiff JG. Relief of causalgia in limbs by regional intravenous guanethidine. *Br Med J* 1979; **2:** 367–8.
2. Loh L, *et al.* Pain due to lesions of central nervous system removed by sympathetic block. *Br Med J* 1981; **282:** 1026–8.
3. Parry CBW, Withrington RH. Painful disorders of peripheral nerves. *Postgrad Med J* 1984; **60:** 869–75.
4. Yasuda JM, Schroeder DJ. Guanethidine for reflex sympathetic dystrophy. *Ann Pharmacother* 1994; **28:** 338–41.
5. Jadad AR, *et al.* Intravenous regional sympathetic blockade for pain relief in reflex sympathetic dystrophy: a systematic review and a randomized, double-blind crossover study. *J Pain Symptom Manage* 1995; **10:** 13–20.
6. Levine JD, *et al.* Clinical response to regional intravenous guanethidine in patients with rheumatoid arthritis. *J Rheumatol* 1986; **13:** 1040–3.
7. Kaplan R, *et al.* Treatment of frostbite with guanethidine. *Lancet* 1981; **ii:** 940–1.

Preparations

BP 1998: Guanethidine Tablets;
USP 23: Guanethidine Monosulfate Tablets.

Proprietary Preparations (details are given in Part 3)
Aust.: Ismelin; ***Austral.:*** Ismelin; ***Canad.:*** Ismelin†; ***Fr.:*** Ismeline; ***Irl.:*** Ismelin†; ***Ital.:*** Visutensil; ***Neth.:*** Ismelin†; ***S.Afr.:*** Ismelin†; ***Switz.:*** Ismelin; Ismeline†; ***UK:*** Ismelin; ***USA:*** Ismelin.

Multi-ingredient: ***Aust.:*** Thilodigon; ***Canad.:*** Ismelin Esidrix†; ***Fr.:*** Esimil†; ***Ger.:*** Esimil; Suprexon; Thilodigon; ***Irl.:*** Ganda; ***Neth.:*** Suprexon; ***S.Afr.:*** Ganda†; ***Switz.:*** Suprexon; ***UK:*** Ganda; ***USA:*** Esimil.

Guanfacine Hydrochloride (12806-z)

Guanfacine Hydrochloride *(BANM, USAN, rINNM).*

BS-100-141; LON-798. *N*-Amidino-2-(2,6-dichlorophenyl)acetamide hydrochloride.

$C_9H_9Cl_2N_3O,HCl = 282.6.$

CAS — 29110-47-2 (guanfacine); 29110-48-3 (guanfacine hydrochloride).

Pharmacopoeias. In *US.*

Store in airtight containers. Protect from light.

Guanfacine hydrochloride 1.15 mg is approximately equivalent to 1 mg of guanfacine.

Adverse Effects and Precautions

As for Clonidine Hydrochloride, p.841. Rebound hypertension may occur but is delayed due to the longer half-life.

Reviews.

1. Jerie P. Clinical experience with guanfacine in long-term treatment of hypertension, part II: adverse reactions to guanfacine. *Br J Clin Pharmacol* 1980; **10** (suppl 1): 157S–164S.
2. Board AW, *et al.* A postmarketing evaluation of guanfacine hydrochloride in mild to moderate hypertension. *Clin Ther* 1988; **10:** 761–75.

Withdrawal. Rapid reduction of the guanfacine dosage resulted in rebound hypertension leading to generalised seizures and coma in a 47-year-old patient with renal failure who was receiving haemodialysis.[1] There was evidence to suggest that concomitant administration of phenobarbitone enhanced metabolism of guanfacine and was considered to have contributed to the development of the withdrawal effect.

1. Kiechel JR, *et al.* Pharmacokinetic aspects of guanfacine withdrawal syndrome in a hypertensive patient with chronic renal failure. *Eur J Clin Pharmacol* 1983; **25:** 463–6.

Interactions

As for Clonidine Hydrochloride, p.842.

Pharmacokinetics

Following oral administration guanfacine is rapidly absorbed, peak plasma concentrations occurring 1 to 4 hours after ingestion. The oral bioavailability is reported to be about 80%. It is about 70% bound to plasma proteins. It is excreted in urine as unchanged drug and metabolites; about 50% of a dose is reported to be eliminated unchanged. The normal elimination half-life ranges from 10 to 30 hours, tending to be longer in older patients than in young ones.

Results in patients with normal and impaired renal function suggested that non-renal elimination of guanfacine plays an important role in patients with renal impairment since clearance and serum concentrations were not significantly altered in such patients.[1]

1. Kirch W, *et al.* Elimination of guanfacine in patients with normal and impaired renal function. *Br J Clin Pharmacol* 1980; **10** (suppl 1): 33S–35S.

Uses and Administration

Guanfacine is a centrally acting $alpha_2$-adrenoceptor agonist with actions and uses similar to those of clonidine (p.842). It is used in the management of hypertension, either alone or in conjunction with other antihypertensives, particularly thiazide diuretics. However, other antihypertensives are usually preferred (p.788).

Guanfacine is given by mouth as the hydrochloride, but doses are usually expressed in terms of the base.

In hypertension it is given in usual initial doses of 1 mg daily increasing after 3 to 4 weeks to 2 mg daily if necessary.

Reviews.

1. Cornish LA. Guanfacine hydrochloride: a centrally acting antihypertensive agent. *Clin Pharm* 1988; **7:** 187–97.

Preparations

USP 23: Guanfacine Tablets.

Proprietary Preparations (details are given in Part 3)
Belg.: Estulic; ***Fr.:*** Estulic; ***Ger.:*** Estulic; ***Irl.:*** Akfen; ***Jpn:*** Estulic†; ***Neth.:*** Estulic; ***Spain:*** Estulic†; ***Switz.:*** Estulic†; ***USA:*** Tenex.

Guanoxabenz Hydrochloride (12808-k)

Guanoxabenz Hydrochloride *(rINNM).*

43-663 (guanoxabenz). 1-(2,6-Dichlorobenzylideneamino)-3-hydroxyguanidine hydrochloride.

$C_8H_8Cl_2N_4O,HCl = 283.5.$

CAS — 24047-25-4 (guanoxabenz); 7473-70-3 (guanoxabenz).

NOTE. Guanoxabenz is *USAN.*

Guanoxabenz hydrochloride is a centrally acting antihypertensive.

Guanoxan Sulphate (871-z)

Guanoxan Sulphate *(BANM, rINNM).*

3-01003; Guanoxan Sulfate *(USAN).* 1-(1,4-Benzodioxan-2-ylmethyl)guanidine sulphate; 1-(2,3-Dihydro-1,4-benzodioxin-2-ylmethyl)guanidine sulphate.

$(C_{10}H_{13}N_3O_2)_2,H_2SO_4 = 512.5.$

CAS — 2165-19-7 (guanoxan); 5714-04-5 (guanoxan sulphate).

Guanoxan is an antihypertensive with properties similar to those of guanethidine (p.878). It was formerly used in the management of hypertension. Liver damage has followed treatment with guanoxan.

Adverse effects. Of 96 patients treated with guanoxan, 26 had some derangement of liver function tests, severe in 10; four of these developed jaundice and 1 of the 4 patients died with chronic hepatic necrosis.[1]

1. Cotton SG, Montuschi E. Guanoxan. *Br Med J* 1967; **3:** 174.

Botulism. The treatment of botulism usually involves administration of antitoxin and supportive therapy (see p.1506). Drug treatment has been used to reverse neuromuscular blockade. Guanoxan in an initial dose of 5 mg, increased to 15 mg twice daily improved respiratory difficulties and ability to swallow in an elderly patient with botulism.[1]

1. Neal KR, Dunbar EM. Improvement in bulbar weakness with guanoxan in type B botulism. *Lancet* 1990; **335:** 1286–7.

Heparan Sulphate (19289-x)

Heparan Sulfate; Heparitin Sulfate; Suleparoid.

CAS — 9050-30-0 (heparan sulphate); 57459-72-0 (heparan sulphate, sodium salt).

NOTE. Suleparoid Sodium is *rINN.*

Heparan sulphate is a naturally occurring glycosaminoglycan given orally in the management of thrombo-embolic disorders. The sodium salt (suleparoid sodium) is a component of the heparinoid, danaparoid sodium (p.846).

Preparations

Proprietary Preparations (details are given in Part 3)
Ital.: Aremin; Arteven; Clarema; Hemovasal; Iparen; Tavidan; Tromir; Tronan; Vas; Vasorema; Vepar.

Heparin (11401-s)

Heparin *(BAN).*

Heparinum.

CAS — 9005-49-6.

NOTE. Heparin is often described in the literature as standard heparin or unfractionated heparin to distinguish it from low-molecular-weight heparins.

Heparin is an anionic polysaccharide of mammalian origin with irregular sequence. It consists principally of alternating iduronate and glucosamine residues most of which are sulphated. It may be described as a sulphated glucosaminoglycan. Heparin has the characteristic property of delaying the clotting of freshly shed blood. It may be prepared from the lungs of oxen or the intestinal mucosa of oxen, pigs, or sheep.

Heparin Calcium (4801-w)

Heparin Calcium *(BANM).*

Calcium Heparin; Heparinum Calcicum.

CAS — 37270-89-6.

Pharmacopoeias. In *Eur.* (see p.viii) and *US.*

The calcium salt of heparin. The Ph. Eur. specifies that heparin calcium intended for use in the manufacture of a parenteral dosage form contains not less than 150 international units per mg and heparin calcium not intended for use in the manufacture of a parenteral dosage form contains not less than 120 international units per mg, both calculated with reference to the dried substance. The USP specifies a potency, calculated on the dried basis, of not less than 140 USP units in each mg. The USP states that USP heparin units are *not* equivalent to international units. The USP requires that the source of the material be stated on the label.

A white or almost white moderately hygroscopic powder. Freely **soluble** in water. A 1% solution in water has a pH of 5 to 8. **Store** in airtight containers.

Incompatibility. See Heparin Sodium below.

Heparin Sodium (4802-e)

Heparin Sodium *(BANM, rINN).*

Heparinum Natricum; Sodium Heparin; Soluble Heparin.

CAS — 9041-08-1.

Pharmacopoeias. In *Chin., Eur.* (see p.viii), *Jpn,* and *US.*

The sodium salt of heparin. The Ph. Eur. specifies that heparin sodium intended for use in the manufacture of a parenteral dosage form contains not less than 150 international units per mg and heparin sodium not intended for use in the manufacture of a parenteral dosage form contains not less than 120 international units per mg, both calculated with reference to the dried substance. The USP specifies a potency, calculated on the dried basis, of not less than 140 USP units in each mg. The USP states that USP heparin units are *not* equivalent to international units. The USP requires that the source of the material be stated on the label.

A white or almost white, odourless or almost odourless, moderately hygroscopic powder. Ph. Eur. solubilities are: freely **soluble** in water and a 1% solution has a pH of 5.5 to 8.0. The USP solubilities are: soluble 1 in 20 of water and a 1% solution has a pH of 5.0 to 7.5. **Store** in airtight containers. The USP recommends storage below 40°, preferably between 15 and 30°, unless otherwise specified by the manufacturer.

Incompatibility. Incompatibility has been reported between heparin calcium or sodium and alteplase, amikacin sulphate, amiodarone hydrochloride, ampicillin sodium, aprotinin, benzylpenicillin potassium or sodium, cephalothin sodium, ciprofloxacin lactate, cytarabine, dacarbazine, daunorubicin hydrochloride, diazepam, dobutamine hydrochloride, doxorubicin hydrochloride, droperidol, erythromycin lactobionate, gentamicin sulphate, haloperidol lactate, hyaluronidase, hydrocortisone sodium succinate, kanamycin sulphate, methicillin sodium, netilmicin sulphate, some opioid analgesics, oxytetracycline hydrochloride, some phenothiazines, polymyxin B sulphate, streptomycin sulphate, tetracycline hydrochloride, tobramycin sulphate, vancomycin hydrochloride, and vinblastine sulphate. Heparin sodium has also been reported to be incompatible with cisatracurium besylate,[1] labetalol hydrochloride,[2] and nicardipine hydrochloride.[3] Although visually compatible,[4] cefmetazole sodium is reported to inactivate heparin sodium.

Glucose can have variable effects,[5,6] but glucose-containing solutions are generally considered suitable diluents for heparin. Incompatibility has also been reported between heparin and fat emulsion.

1. Trissel LA, *et al.* Compatibility of cisatracurium besylate with selected drugs during simulated Y-site administration. *Am J Health-Syst Pharm* 1997; **54:** 1735–41.
2. Yamashita SK, *et al.* Compatibility of selected critical care drugs during simulated Y-site administration. *Am J Health-Syst Pharm* 1996; **53:** 1048–51.
3. Chiu MF, Schwartz ML. Visual compatibility of injectable drugs used in the intensive care unit. *Am J Health-Syst Pharm* 1997; **54:** 64–5.

4. Hutching SR, *et al.* Compatibility of cefmetazole sodium with commonly used drugs during Y-site delivery. *Am J Health-Syst Pharm* 1996; **53:** 2185–8.
5. Anderson W, Harthill JE. The anticoagulant activity of heparins in dextrose solutions. *J Pharm Pharmacol* 1982; **34:** 90–6.
6. Wright A, Hecker J. Long term stability of heparin in dextrose-saline intravenous fluids. *Int J Pharm Pract* 1995; **3:** 253–5.

Units

The fourth International Standard for porcine heparin was established in 1983. The USP states that USP and international units are not equivalent, although doses expressed in either appear to be essentially the same.

Adverse Effects

Heparin can give rise to haemorrhage as a consequence of its action. It can also cause thrombocytopenia, either through a direct effect or through an immune effect producing a platelet-aggregating antibody. Consequent platelet aggregation and thrombosis may therefore exacerbate the condition being treated. The incidence of thrombocytopenia is reported to be greater with bovine than porcine heparin.

Hypersensitivity reactions may occur, as may local irritant effects, and skin necrosis. Alopecia and osteoporosis resulting in spontaneous fractures have occurred after prolonged use of heparin.

Effects on the adrenal glands. Aull and colleagues[1] have reported two cases of heparin-induced hypoaldosteronism resulting in persistent hyperkalaemia. In reviewing previous reports they concluded that, although all patients treated with heparin may have reduced aldosterone concentrations, most are able to compensate through increased renin production. Patients on prolonged heparin therapy or those unable to compensate, such as patients with diabetes mellitus or renal insufficiency[1] or those on concomitant therapy with ACE inhibitors[2] may present with symptoms. It has been suggested[3] that serum-potassium concentration should be monitored in all patients receiving heparin for 3 or more days, particularly if there are other risk factors.

Adrenal insufficiency secondary to adrenal haemorrhage has also been associated with heparin administration; heparin-induced thrombocytopenia may be implicated.[4]

1. Aull L, *et al.* Heparin-induced hyperkalemia. *DICP Ann Pharmacother* 1990; **24:** 244–6.
2. Durand D, *et al.* Inducing hyperkalemia by converting enzyme inhibitors and heparin. *Kidney Int* 1988; **34** (suppl 25): S196–7.
3. Oster JR, *et al.* Heparin-induced aldosterone suppression and hyperkalemia. *Am J Med* 1995; **98:** 575–86.
4. Dahlberg PJ, *et al.* Adrenal insufficiency secondary to adrenal hemorrhage: two case reports and a review of cases confirmed by computed tomography. *Arch Intern Med* 1990; **150:** 905–9.

Effects on the blood. *Haemorrhage* is a recognised risk with heparin.[1] The risk may be lower with continuous intravenous infusion than with intermittent intravenous injection, although results from 6 studies were contradictory.[2]

Heparin has been associated with the development of *thrombocytopenia*. The reported incidence has varied greatly; up to 6% appears to be a reasonable estimate[3,4] although up to 10% has also been quoted.[5] Thrombocytopenia induced by heparin may be of two types. The first is an acute, but usually mild, fall in platelet count occurring within 1 to 4 days of initiation of therapy and which often resolves without cessation of treatment. A direct effect of heparin on platelet aggregation appears to be responsible. The second type of thrombocytopenia, which has an immunological basis, is more serious. It usually occurs after 7 to 11 days of heparin although its onset may be more rapid in patients previously exposed to heparin. It is often associated with thrombo-embolic complications due to platelet-rich thrombi (the 'white clot syndrome') or, more rarely, bleeding. Of 34 cases of heparin-associated thrombocytopenia reported to the Committee on Safety of Medicines (CSM) in the UK from 1964 to 1989, bleeding or thrombo-embolic complications occurred in 11 patients, seven of whom died.[3] This type of thrombocytopenia appears to occur more frequently with bovine heparin than with heparin from other species[6] and it has been proposed that in susceptible patients antibody reacts with heparin bound to platelets and endothelial cells.[7] Patients with lupus anticoagulant may also be more susceptible.[8] The reaction is independent of dose or route of administration; there are reports of thrombocytopenia after use of heparin flushes[9] or heparin-coated catheters.[10] The CSM recommend monitoring of platelet counts in patients given heparin for more than 5 days.[3] Patients previously exposed to heparin may be sensitised to it and after re-exposure should have a platelet count before the 5 days are up.[11]

Treatment should be stopped immediately in those who develop thrombocytopenia. It should be noted, however, that thrombosis has occurred in patients whose reduction in platelet count was relatively mild and who may not be considered to be thrombocytopenic.[12-15] On withdrawal of heparin, a low-molecular-weight heparin or a heparinoid such as danaparoid[16,17] may be tried, provided that an *in-vitro* platelet aggregation test is negative, i.e. there is no cross-reactivity with heparin. Low-molecular-weight heparins are not without risk, but in one study the incidence of induced thrombocytopenia was less than with unfractionated heparin.[18] Alternatively, oral anticoagulation may be initiated, although an increased risk of venous limb gangrene has been reported[19] with warfarin. Ancrod,[20] dermatan sulphate,[21] hirudins,[22] and argatroban[22] have also been used. Thrombocytopenia has been managed with aspirin and dipyridamole or with normal immunoglobulin.[23] A fibrinolytic such as urokinase has been used in a few cases of occlusive thrombosis.[24,25]

There may be a relationship between heparin-induced thrombocytopenia and skin necrosis (see below).

1. Walker AM, Jick H. Predictors of bleeding during heparin therapy. *JAMA* 1980; **244:** 1209–12.
2. Morabia A. Heparin doses and major bleedings. *Lancet* 1986; **i:** 1278–9.
3. Committee on Safety of Medicines. Heparin-induced thrombocytopenia. *Current Problems 28* 1990.
4. Derlon A, *et al.* Thrombopénies induites par l'héparine: symptomatologie, détection, fréquence. *Therapie* 1988; **43:** 199–203.
5. Aster RH. Heparin-induced thrombocytopenia and thrombosis. *N Engl J Med* 1995; **332:** 1374–6
6. Bell WR, Royall RM. Heparin-associated thrombocytopenia: a comparison of three heparin preparations. *N Engl J Med* 1980; **303:** 902–7.
7. Cines DB, *et al.* Immune endothelial-cell injury in heparin-associated thrombocytopenia. *N Engl J Med* 1987; **316:** 581–9.
8. Auger WR, *et al.* Lupus anticoagulant, heparin use, and thrombocytopenia in patients with chronic thromboembolic pulmonary hypertension: a preliminary report. *Am J Med* 1995; **99:** 392–6.
9. Heeger PS, Backstrom JT. Heparin flushes and thrombocytopenia. *Ann Intern Med* 1986; **105:** 143.
10. Laster JL, *et al.* Thrombocytopenia associated with heparin-coated catheters in patients with heparin-associated antiplatelet antibodies. *Arch Intern Med* 1989; **149:** 2285–7.
11. Hunter JB, *et al.* Heparin induced thrombosis: an important complication of heparin prophylaxis for thromboembolic disease in surgery. *Br Med J* 1993; **307:** 53–5.
12. Phelan BK. Heparin-associated thrombosis without thrombocytopenia. *Ann Intern Med* 1983; **99:** 637–8.
13. Trono DP, *et al.* Thrombocytopenia and heparin-associated thrombosis. *Ann Intern Med* 1984; **100:** 464–5.
14. Ramirez-Lassepas M, Cipolle RJ. Heparin and thrombocytopenia. *Ann Intern Med* 1984; **100:** 613.
15. Hach-Wunderle V, *et al.* Heparin-associated thrombosis despite normal platelet counts. *Lancet* 1994; **344:** 469–70.
16. Magnani HN. Management of heparin induced thrombocytopenia. *Br Med J* 1993; **307:** 203–4.
17. Boon DMS, *et al.* Heparin-induced thrombocytopenia and antithrombotic therapy. *Lancet* 1994; **344:** 1296.
18. Warkentin TE, *et al.* Heparin-induced thrombocytopenia in patients treated with low-molecular- weight heparin or unfractionated heparin. *N Engl J Med* 1995; **332:** 1330–5.
19. Warkentin TE, *et al.* The pathogenesis of venous limb gangrene associated with heparin-induced thrombocytopenia. *Ann Intern Med* 1997; **127:** 804–12.
20. Soutar RL, Ginsberg JS. Ancrod for heparin induced thrombocytopenia. *Br Med J* 1993; **306:** 1410.
21. Agnelli G, *et al.* Dermatan sulphate in heparin-induced thrombocytopenia. *Lancet* 1994; **344:** 1295–6.
22. Warkentin TE. Heparin-induced thrombocytopenia: pathogenesis, frequency, avoidance and management. *Drug Safety* 1997; **17:** 325–41.
23. Frame JN, *et al.* Correction of severe heparin-associated thrombocytopenia with intravenous immunoglobulin. *Ann Intern Med* 1989; **111:** 946–7.
24. Krueger SK, *et al.* Thrombolysis in heparin-induced thrombocytopenia with thrombosis. *Ann Intern Med* 1985; **103:** 159.
25. Clifton GD, Smith MD. Thrombolytic therapy in heparin-associated thrombocytopenia with thrombosis. *Clin Pharm* 1986; **5:** 597–601.

Effects on the bones. Osteoporosis is a rare complication of long term heparin treatment.[1] Available evidence suggests that bone demineralisation is dose- and duration-dependent but conclusive evidence about the risk of developing clinically important disease is difficult to obtain. Women receiving 20 000 units of heparin daily for more than 5 months may be at increased risk but the possibility that only a subgroup is susceptible must also be considered. It was originally believed that bone changes were irreversible but recent evidence suggests that they may, in fact, be reversible.

1. Maternal and Neonatal Haemostasis Working Party of the Haemostasis and Thrombosis Task. Guidelines on the prevention, investigation and management of thrombosis associated with pregnancy. *J Clin Pathol* 1993; **46:** 489–96.

Effects on the liver. Reports of increases in transaminase values in patients given therapeutic[1-3] or prophylactic[3] doses of heparin. The abnormality usually resolved on discontinuation of heparin.

1. Sonnenblick M, *et al.* Hyper-transaminasemia with heparin therapy. *Br Med J* 1975; **3:** 77.
2. Dukes GE, *et al.* Transaminase elevations in patients receiving bovine or porcine heparin. *Ann Intern Med* 1984; **100:** 646–50.
3. Monreal M, *et al.* Adverse effects of three different forms of heparin therapy: thrombocytopenia, increased transaminases, and hyperkalaemia. *Eur J Clin Pharmacol* 1989; **37:** 415–18.

Effects on serum lipids. Administration of heparin leads to the release of lipoprotein lipase into the plasma. Postprandial lipidaemia is reduced due to increased hydrolysis of triglycerides into free fatty acids and glycerol. Raised concentrations of free fatty acids have been reported following heparin administration, but the magnitude of this effect may have been overestimated.[1] Rebound hyperlipidaemia may occur when heparin is withdrawn. With long-term administration reserves of lipoprotein lipase may be depleted; severe hypertriglyceridaemia reported in a pregnant woman was attributed to long-term heparin prophylaxis that was thought to have resulted in lipoprotein lipase deficiency.[2]

1. Riemersma RA, *et al.* Heparin-induced lipolysis, an exaggerated risk. *Lancet* 1981; **ii:** 471.
2. Watts GF, *et al.* Lipoprotein lipase deficiency due to long-term heparinization presenting as severe hypertriglyceridaemia in pregnancy. *Postgrad Med J* 1991; **67:** 1062–4.

Effects on sexual function. There have been several reports of priapism associated with the administration of heparin. The prognosis is poor, impotence following more often than in priapism of other aetiologies. The mechanism of heparin-induced priapism is unclear.[1]

1. Baños JE, *et al.* Drug-induced priapism: its aetiology, incidence and treatment. *Med Toxicol* 1989; **4:** 46–58.

Effects on the skin. Skin necrosis is a rare complication of heparin administration.[1,2] It may be a localised reaction at the site of subcutaneous injection or possibly be related to heparin-induced thrombocytopenia (see above). An immune mechanism may be responsible.

Eczematous plaque reactions have developed several days after initiation of subcutaneous heparin. A type IV hypersensitivity reaction has been implicated.[3] Low-molecular-weight heparins may be an alternative but cross-reactivity can occur.[4]

1. Ulrick PJ, Manoharan A. Heparin-induced skin reaction. *Med J Aust* 1984; **140:** 287–9.
2. Fowlie J, *et al.* Heparin-associated skin necrosis. *Postgrad Med J* 1990; **66:** 573–5.
3. Bircher AJ, *et al.* Eczematous infiltrated plaques to subcutaneous heparin: a type IV allergic reaction. *Br J Dermatol* 1990; **123:** 507–14.
4. O'Donnell BF, Tan CY. Delayed hypersensitivity reactions to heparin. *Br J Dermatol* 1993; **129:** 634–6.

Treatment of Adverse Effects

Slight haemorrhage due to overdosage can usually be treated by withdrawing heparin. Severe bleeding may be reduced by the slow intravenous administration of protamine sulphate (p.993). The dose is dependent on the amount of heparin to be neutralised and ideally should be titrated against assessments of the coagulability of the patient's blood. As heparin is being continuously excreted the dose should be reduced if more than 15 minutes have elapsed since heparin administration; for example, if protamine sulphate is given 30 minutes after heparin the dose may be reduced to about one-half. Not more than 50 mg of protamine sulphate should be injected for any one dose; patients should be carefully monitored as further doses may be required. The Ph. Eur. specifies that 1 mg of protamine sulphate precipitates not less than 100 international units of heparin sodium, but adds that this potency is based on a specific reference batch of heparin sodium. The UK manufacturer has stated that each mg of protamine sulphate will usually neutralise the anticoagulant effect of at least 80 international units of heparin (lung) or at least 100 international units of heparin (mucous). The US manufacturer has stated that each mg of protamine sulphate neutralises approximately 90 USP units of heparin (lung) or about 115 USP units of heparin (mucous).

For reference to the treatment of heparin-induced thrombocytopenia and associated thrombo-embolic complications, see Effects on the Blood under Adverse Effects, above.

Precautions

Heparin should not be given to patients who are haemorrhaging. In general it should not be given to patients at serious risk of haemorrhage, although it has been used with very careful control; patients at risk include those with haemorrhagic blood disorders, thrombocytopenia, peptic ulcers, cerebrovascular disorders, bacterial endocarditis, severe hypertension, oesophageal varices, or patients who have recently undergone surgery at sites where haemorrhage would be an especial risk. Severe kidney and liver impairment are considered by some to be contra-indications. Heparin should not be given by intramuscular injection. Since heparin has caused thrombocytopenia with severe thrombo-embolic complications, platelet counts should be monitored in patients receiving heparin for more than a few days. Heparin should be discontinued if thrombocytopenia develops. A test dose has been recommended for patients with a history of allergy.

Dosage of heparin may need to be reduced in old people; elderly women appear to be especially susceptible to haemorrhage after heparin administration.

The preservatives used in heparin preparations have been implicated in unwanted effects. Benzyl alcohol has been suspected of contributing to heparin's toxicity in neonates (see p.1103). Chlorbutol present in another heparin preparation caused a sharp fall in blood pressure.[1]

1. Bowler GMR, *et al.* Sharp fall in blood pressure after injection of heparin containing chlorbutol. *Lancet* 1986; **i:** 848–9.

Catheters and cannulas. Serum concentrations of sodium and potassium could be falsely elevated in samples obtained through heparin-bonded umbilical catheters due to release of benzalkonium chloride used in the manufacturing process of some catheters.[1] It was unknown if the amount of benzalkonium chloride released would be toxic to small premature neonates.

1. Gaylord MS, *et al.* Release of benzalkonium chloride from a heparin-bonded umbilical catheter with resultant factitious hypernatremia and hyperkalemia. *Pediatrics* 1991; **87:** 631–5.

Local anaesthesia. Some authorities recommend that spinal or epidural anaesthesia be avoided in patients receiving heparin because of the risk of haematoma formation and compression of the spinal cord. The necessity for this contra-indication in patients receiving low-dose heparin is controversial.[1]

1. Stow PJ, Burrows FA. Anticoagulants in anaesthesia. *Can J Anaesth* 1987; **34:** 632–49.

Pregnancy. Heparin does not cross the placenta, and therefore adverse effects on the fetus would not be expected.[1,2] In reviewing the literature, however, Hall *et al.*[1] reported 2 spontaneous abortions and 17 still-births in 135 pregnancies exposed to heparin; 29 infants were premature, 10 of whom died. Ginsberg and Hirsh[2] carried out an independent literature review and found a drop of adverse outcomes in heparin-treated patients from 21.7 to 10.4% when pregnancies with co-morbid conditions were excluded. A further drop to 3.6% was observed when cases of prematurity with normal outcome were also excluded. The death rate of 2.5% and prematurity rate of 6.8% in heparin-treated patients was similar to that found in the normal population. They concluded that heparin appears safer for the fetus than warfarin when used during pregnancy.

1. Hall JG, *et al.* Maternal and fetal sequelae of anticoagulation during pregnancy. *Am J Med* 1980; **68:** 122–40.
2. Ginsberg JS, Hirsh J. Optimum use of anticoagulants in pregnancy. *Drugs* 1988; **36:** 505–12.

Interactions

Heparin should be used with care in conjunction with oral anticoagulants or drugs, such as aspirin and dipyridamole, which affect platelet function. Concomitant use of NSAIDs may also increase the risk of haemorrhage. Other drugs which affect the coagulation process and which may therefore increase the risk of haemorrhage include dextran injections, thrombolytic enzymes such as streptokinase, high doses of penicillins and some cephalosporins, some contrast media, asparaginase, and epoprostenol. Estimations of oral anticoagulant control may be modified by heparin's action on prothrombin.

ACE inhibitors. For reference to hyperkalaemia in patients on heparin and ACE inhibitors, see Effects on the Adrenal Glands under Adverse Effects, above.

Alcohol. Heavy drinkers were at greater risk of major heparin-associated bleeding than moderate drinkers or non-drinkers.[1]

1. Walker AM, Jick H. Predictors of bleeding during heparin therapy. *JAMA* 1980; **244:** 1209–12.

Aprotinin. For comment on the use of heparin with aprotinin, see under Surgery in Aprotinin, p.712.

Glyceryl trinitrate. Glyceryl trinitrate has been reported to reduce the activity of heparin when both drugs are administered simultaneously by the intravenous route.[1] This effect has been seen even at low doses of glyceryl trinitrate.[2] Propylene glycol present in the glyceryl trinitrate formulation may contribute to the effect,[3] or it may not.[1] No interaction was reported when glyceryl trinitrate was administered immediately after heparin.[4]

1. Habbab MA, Haft JI. Heparin resistance induced by intravenous nitroglycerin. *Arch Intern Med* 1987; **147:** 857–60.
2. Brack MJ, *et al.* The effect of low dose nitroglycerine on plasma heparin concentrations and activated partial thromboplastin times. *Blood Coag Fibrinol* 1993; **4:** 183–6.
3. Col J, *et al.* Propylene glycol-induced heparin resistance during nitroglycerin infusion. *Am Heart J* 1985; **110:** 171–3.
4. Bode V, *et al.* Absence of drug interaction between heparin and nitroglycerin. *Arch Intern Med* 1990; **150:** 2117–19.

Tobacco smoking. Reduced half-life and increased elimination of heparin have been reported in smokers compared with non-smokers.[1]

1. Cipolle RJ, *et al.* Heparin kinetics: variables related to disposition and dosage. *Clin Pharmacol Ther* 1981; **29:** 387–93.

Pharmacokinetics

Heparin is not absorbed from the gastro-intestinal tract. Following intravenous or subcutaneous injection heparin is extensively bound to plasma proteins. It does not cross the placenta and it is not distributed into breast milk. The half-life of heparin depends on the dose and route of administration as well as the method of calculation and is subject to wide inter- and intra-individual variation; a range of 1 to 6 hours with an average of 1.5 hours has been cited. It may be slightly prolonged in renal impairment, decreased in patients with pulmonary embolism, and either increased or decreased in patients with liver disorders. Heparin is taken up by the reticuloendothelial system. It is excreted in the urine, mainly as metabolites, although, following administration of large doses, up to 50% may be excreted unchanged.

References.

1. Estes JW. Clinical pharmacokinetics of heparin. *Clin Pharmacokinet* 1980; **5:** 204–20.
2. Kandrotas RJ. Heparin pharmacokinetics and pharmacodynamics. *Clin Pharmacokinet* 1992; **22:** 359–74.

Uses and Administration

Heparin is an anticoagulant used principally in the treatment and prophylaxis of thrombo-embolic disorders (p.801). It is often described as standard heparin or unfractionated heparin to distinguish it from low-molecular-weight heparins (p.899).

It inhibits clotting of blood *in vitro* and *in vivo* through its action on antithrombin III. Antithrombin III, which is present in plasma, inhibits the activity of activated clotting factors including thrombin (factor IIa) and activated factor X (factor Xa); heparin increases the rate of this inhibition, but in a manner that is dependent on its dose. With normal therapeutic doses heparin has an inhibitory effect on both thrombin and factor Xa. Thus the conversion of fibrinogen to fibrin is blocked through the thrombin inhibition, while the conversion of prothrombin to thrombin is blocked by the inhibition of factor Xa. The low doses that are given subcutaneously for the prophylaxis of thrombo-embolism have a selective effect on antithrombin III's inhibition of factor Xa. Very high doses are reported to reduce the activity of antithrombin III. Heparin also has some effect on platelet function, inhibits the formation of a stable fibrin clot, and has an antilipaemic effect. For an explanation of the coagulation cascade, see p.704.

Heparin is used in the treatment and prophylaxis of venous thrombo-embolism (deep-vein thrombosis and pulmonary embolism, p.802), especially prophylaxis in surgical patients and in those pregnant women at particular risk. It is also used in the management of arterial thrombo-embolism including that associated with unstable angina pectoris (p.780), myocardial infarction (p.791), acute peripheral arterial occlusion (p.794), and stroke (p.799). It is often used as a precursor to oral anticoagulation and is withdrawn once the oral anticoagulant is exerting its full effect.

Heparin has been tried in the treatment of disseminated intravascular coagulation. It is also used to prevent coagulation during haemodialysis and other extracorporeal circulatory procedures such as cardiopulmonary bypass. Other uses include the anticoagulation of blood for transfusion or blood samples and the flushing of catheters and cannulas to maintain patency.

Heparin and its salts are constituents of many topical preparations for the treatment of various inflammatory disorders.

Administration and dosage. Heparin is administered intravenously, preferably by continuous infusion, or by subcutaneous injection. It may be given as the calcium or sodium salt and it is generally accepted that there is little difference in their effects. Oral formulations of heparin are under investigation.

Doses of heparin for treatment (sometimes termed 'full-dose' heparin), and in some cases prophylaxis, of thrombo-embolism should be monitored and determined as discussed below under Control of Heparin Therapy. The subcutaneous doses of heparin commonly used for prophylaxis and often termed 'low-dose' subcutaneous heparin do not require routine monitoring. A test dose has been recommended for patients with a history of allergy. Although international and USP units are not strictly equivalent, doses expressed in either appear to be essentially the same. The following doses of heparin are broadly in the line with British Society for Haematology guidelines.

For **treatment of venous thrombo-embolism**, an intravenous loading dose of 5000 to 10 000 units is followed by continuous intravenous infusion of 1000 to 2000 units per hour or subcutaneous injection of 15 000 units every 12 hours. Alternatively, intermittent intravenous injection of 5000 to 10 000 units every 4 to 6 hours is suggested on some data sheets. Children and small adults are given a lower intravenous loading dose followed by maintenance with continuous intravenous infusion of 15 to 25 units per kg body-weight per hour or subcutaneous injection of 250 units per kg every 12 hours.

For **prophylaxis** of **postoperative venous thrombo-embolism**, subcutaneous doses used are 5000 units 2 hours before surgery then every 8 to 12 hours for 7 days or until the patient is ambulant. Similar doses are used to prevent thrombo-embolism during pregnancy in mothers with a history of deep-vein thrombosis or pulmonary embolism; the dosage may need to be increased to 10 000 units every 12 hours during the third trimester.

In the management of **unstable angina** or acute **peripheral arterial embolism,** heparin may be given by continuous intravenous infusion in the same doses as those recommended for the treatment of venous thrombo-embolism. Suggested doses for the prevention of re-occlusion of the coronary arteries following thrombolytic therapy in **myocardial infarction** include either 2000 units of heparin intravenously followed by 12 500 units subcutaneously every 12 hours after streptokinase, or 5000 units intravenously followed by 1000 units per hour intravenously after alteplase; a dose of 12 500 units subcutaneously every 12 hours for at least 10 days may be used to prevent mural thrombosis.

Control of Heparin Therapy. Treatment with full-dose heparin must be monitored to ensure that the dose is providing the required effect on antithrombin III. The most commonly used test to monitor the action of heparin is the activated partial thromboplastin time (APTT). The APTT of patients on full-dose heparin should generally be maintained at 1.5 to 2.5 times the control value although the optimum therapeutic range varies between individual laboratories depending on the APTT reagent in use. Regular monitoring is essential preferably on a daily basis. Prophylaxis with low-dose subcutaneous heparin is not routinely monitored; the APTT is not significantly prolonged in these patients. A dose-adjusted regimen to maintain minimal prolongation of the APTT may be required in patients with malignancy or undergoing orthopaedic surgery to ensure adequate protection against thrombo-embolism. Other tests used include the activated clotting time (ACT). The value of measurements of heparin concentration in the blood remains to be established.

General references to anticoagulation with heparin.

1. Hirsh J. Heparin. *N Engl J Med* 1991; **324:** 1565–74.
2. Cruickshank MK, *et al.* A standard heparin nomogram for the management of heparin therapy. *Arch Intern Med* 1991; **151:** 333–7
3. Freedman MD. Pharmacodynamics, clinical indications, and adverse effects of heparin. *J Clin Pharmacol* 1992; **32:** 584–96.
4. Hyers TM. Heparin therapy: regimens and treatment considerations. *Drugs* 1992; **44:** 738–49.
5. Colvin BT, Barrowcliffe TW. The British Society for Haematology guidelines on the use and monitoring of heparin 1992: second revision. *J Clin Pathol* 1993; **46:** 97–103.
6. Brill-Edwards P, *et al.* Establishing a therapeutic range for heparin therapy. *Ann Intern Med* 1993; **119:** 104–9.
7. Raschke RA, *et al.* The weight-based heparin dosing nomogram compared with a "standard care" nomogram: a randomized controlled trial. *Ann Intern Med* 1993; **119:** 874–81.
8. Hirsh J, Fuster V. Guide to anticoagulant therapy part 1: heparin. *Circulation* 1994; **89:** 1449–68.

Action. Heparin is well established as an anticoagulant and antithrombotic and acts primarily by binding to and enhancing the activity of antithrombin III. However, the physiological role of endogenous heparin has not been clearly defined, despite its presence in mast cells, its ability to interact with numerous proteins, and its close structural similarity to heparan sulphate the ubiquitous cell-surface glycosaminoglycan.[1,2] Endogenous heparin activity may have a role in protecting against atherosclerosis.[3] Non-anticoagulant properties of heparin have been reported to include anti-inflammatory activity, with a possible application in, for example, asthma.[4] A major obstacle to the use of heparin itself for non-anticoagulant purposes would be the risk of bleeding.

1. Lane DA, Adams L. Non-anticoagulant uses of heparin. *N Engl J Med* 1993; **329:** 129–30.
2. Page CP. Proteoglycans: the "Teflon" of the airways? *Thorax* 1997; **52:** 924–5.
3. Engelberg H. Actions of heparin in the atherosclerotic process. *Pharmacol Rev* 1996; **48:** 327–52.
4. Martineau P, Vaughan LM. Heparin inhalation for asthma. *Ann Pharmacother* 1995; **29:** 71–2.

Catheters and cannulas. Solutions of heparin sodium 10 or 100 units per mL in sodium chloride 0.9% are used for the flushing of intravenous catheters, cannulas, and other indwelling intravenous infusion devices used for intermittent administration (heparin locks). Several studies[1-6] and a meta-analysis[7] have, however, been unable to demonstrate any major advantage of either strength of heparin sodium solution over sodium chloride 0.9% alone in terms of maintenance of cannula patency or reduction in incidence of thrombophlebitis, and sodium chloride 0.9% is therefore recommended for cannulas intended to be in place for 48 hours or less. Reduced use of heparin flush solutions could minimise the risk of adverse effects to heparin such as thrombocytopenia and reduce the risk of incompatibilities with intravenously administered drugs.

Use of heparin-coated catheters or the addition of heparin to intravenous fluids such as total parenteral nutrition solutions has also been tried in an attempt to maintain indwelling intravenous infusion devices (but see under Precautions, above). Continuous infusion of heparin-containing fluids may prolong the patency of peripheral arterial catheters.[7]

Very low doses of warfarin (1 mg daily) may protect against thrombosis in patients with central venous catheters.[8]

1. Epperson EL. Efficacy of 0.9% sodium chloride injection with and without heparin for maintaining indwelling intermittent injection sites. *Clin Pharm* 1984; **3:** 626–9.
2. Hamilton RA, *et al.* Heparin sodium versus 0.9% sodium chloride injection for maintaining patency of indwelling intermittent infusion devices. *Clin Pharm* 1988; **7:** 439–43.
3. Lombardi TP, *et al.* Efficacy of 0.9% sodium chloride injection with or without heparin sodium for maintaining patency of intravenous catheters in children. *Clin Pharm* 1988; **7:** 832–6.
4. Shaw P, Baker D. Flushing solutions for indwelling intravenous catheters. *Pharm J* 1988; **241:** 122–3.
5. Garrelts JC, *et al.* Comparison of heparin and 0.9% sodium chloride injection in the maintenance of indwelling intermittent iv devices. *Clin Pharm* 1989; **8:** 34–9.
6. Nelson TJ, Graves SM. 0.9% Sodium chloride injection with and without heparin for maintaining peripheral indwelling intermittent-infusion devices in infants. *Am J Health-Syst Pharm* 1998; **55:** 570–3.
7. Randolph AG, *et al.* Benefit of heparin in peripheral venous and arterial catheters: systematic review and meta-analysis of randomised controlled trials. *Br Med J* 1998; **316:** 969–75.
8. Bern MM, *et al.* Very low doses of warfarin can prevent thrombosis in central venous catheters: a randomized prospective trial. *Ann Intern Med* 1990; **112:** 423–8.

Disseminated intravascular coagulation. Heparin has been used with some success in disseminated intravascular coagulation (p.706) associated with a variety of conditions. However, this use is considered by some to be controversial and should be reserved for specific situations where the risk of bleeding is relatively minor in comparison with the possible beneficial effect on formation of microthromboses. The maximum dose given intravenously is usually 1000 units per hour because of the risk of bleeding.[1]

1. Colvin BT, Barrowcliffe TW. The British Society for Haematology guidelines on the use and monitoring of heparin 1992: second revision. *J Clin Pathol* 1993; **46:** 97–103.

Extracorporeal circulation. Anticoagulation with heparin is necessary during procedures such as cardiopulmonary bypass and haemodialysis and haemofiltration.[1] In the case of bypass, heparin is added to the crystalloid solution and any stored blood used for priming the bypass machine and is given intravenously before cannulation of the heart and major blood vessels. Activated clotting time (ACT) is monitored throughout. After bypass is discontinued, anticoagulation can be reversed with protamine but caution is advised because of potential toxicity on the cardiopulmonary circulation.

At the start of haemodialysis sessions patients generally receive a loading dose of heparin followed by continuous infusion into the exit line of the extracorporeal circuit until about one hour before the end of dialysis. The dose of heparin varies widely depending on body-weight, volume of the extracorporeal circulation, dialysis membrane biocompatibility, and pump speed.

1. Colvin BT, Barrowcliffe TW. The British Society for Haematology guidelines on the use and monitoring of heparin 1992; second revision. *J Clin Pathol* 1993; **46:** 97–103.

Fat embolism syndrome. Fat embolism syndrome results from the presence of fat droplets in the lung or peripheral microvasculature and may lead to respiratory failure or neurological symptoms. It most commonly follows traumatic fracture of the pelvis or long bones, in which case the fat emboli are probably derived from bone marrow. Treatment of fat embolism syndrome is mainly supportive although specific treatments have been tried.[1] Heparin has been used because of its effects on lipoprotein lipase (see under Effects on Serum Lipids, above) but both improved survival and increased mortality have been reported and the available evidence does not support its use. Corticosteroids have also been tried; they do not appear to have a clear benefit in established fat embolism syndrome but may prevent its development in patients with fractures.

1. Van Besouw J-P, Hinds CJ. Fat embolism syndrome. *Br J Hosp Med* 1989; **42:** 304–11.

Idiopathic thrombocytopenic purpura. Subcutaneous administration of a low dose of heparin improved platelet counts in a small number of patients with idiopathic thrombocytopenic purpura (p.1023) that was resistant to standard corticosteroid therapy.[1] However, heparin may itself cause thrombocytopenia, even at very low doses (see under Adverse Effects, above).

1. Shen ZX, *et al.* Thrombocytopoietic effect of heparin given in chronic immune thrombocytopenic purpura. *Lancet* 1995; **346:** 220–1.

Pregnancy. Heparin is the anticoagulant of choice for use in pregnancy although it is not without risk for the fetus, (see above), and for the mother.

Guidelines on thrombosis associated with pregnancy have been published in the UK.[1] Pregnant women may require anticoagulation for the treatment or prophylaxis of venous thrombo-embolism (p.802), or for the prevention of systemic thrombo-embolism associated with prosthetic heart valves (p.801). Patients with a history of thrombo-embolism or a thrombophilic abnormality such as inherited deficiencies of antithrombin III, protein C, or protein S or acquired antiphospholipid antibodies may be at particular risk. Administration of heparin to women with antiphospholipid antibodies may also decrease the risk of fetal loss that has been associated with this disorder.[2,3]

1. Maternal and Neonatal Haemostatis Working Party of the Haemostasis and Thrombosis Task. Guidelines on the prevention, investigation and management of thrombosis associated with pregnancy. *J Clin Pathol* 1993; **46:** 489–96.
2. Rosove MH, *et al.* Heparin therapy for pregnant women with lupus anticoagulant or anticardiolipin antibodies. *Obstet Gynecol* 1990; **75:** 630–4.
3. Rai R, *et al.* Randomised controlled trial of aspirin and aspirin plus heparin in pregnant women with recurrent miscarriage associated with phospholipid antibodies (or antiphospholipid antibodies). *Br Med J* 1997; **314:** 253–7.

Reperfusion and revascularisation procedures. Heparin is widely used in patients undergoing angioplasty or bypass surgery (p.797) to prevent perioperative thrombosis of the operated artery. It is frequently used in conjunction with aspirin or other antiplatelet drugs. However, it appears to have no role in the long-term prevention of restenosis, although heparin-coated stents may have potential benefits.

Preparations

BP 1998: Heparin Injection;
USP 23: Anticoagulant Heparin Solution; Heparin Calcium Injection; Heparin Lock Flush Solution; Heparin Sodium Injection.

Proprietary Preparations (details are given in Part 3)
Aust.: Calciparin; Liquemin; Thrombophob; Thrombophob-S; ***Austral.:*** Calcihep; Calciparine; Caprin†; Uniparin; ***Belg.:*** Calparine; Liquemine; ***Canad.:*** Calcilean; Hepalean; Hepalean-Lok; ***Fr.:*** Calciparine; Liquemine†; Percase†; ***Ger.:*** Ariven; Calciparin; Depot-Thrombophob-N; Enelbin-Venen Salbe; Essaven 60 000; Hemeran; Hepa-Gel; Hepa-Salbe; Hepaplus; Hepathromb; Hepathrombin; Juwoment Sport; Liquemin N; Logomed Sport-Gel; Logomed Venen-Salbe; Perivar; Praecivenin†; Sportino; Thrombareduct; Thrombo-Vetren†; Thrombophob; Traumalitan; Trirutin; Venalitan; Venalitan N; Venelbin N; Venoflexil†; Venoruton Heparin; Vetren; Zuk Hepagel†; ***Irl.:*** Calciparine; Hep-Rinse; Heplok; Hepsal; Minihep; Monoparin; Multiparin; Pump-Hep†; Unihep; Uniparin; ***Ital.:*** Ateroclar; Calciparina; Chemyparin; Clarisco; Croneparina; Disebrin; Ecabil; Ecafast; Ecasolv; Emoklar; Eparical; Eparinlider; Eparinovis; Epsoclar; Isoclar; Lioton; Liquemin; Normoparin; Reoflus; ***Neth.:*** Calparine; Liquemin†; Minihep; Tromboliquine†; ***S.Afr.:*** Calciparine; Pularin†; Thrombophob; ***Spain:*** Calciparina; Menaven; ***Swed.:*** Noparin†; ***Switz.:*** Calciparine; Gelparine; HepaGel; Liquemine; Ruscovarin; Thrombophob†; ***UK:*** Calciparine; Canusal; Hep-Flush; Heplok; Hepsal; Minihep; Monoparin; Multiparin; Pump-Hep; Unihep; Uniparin; ***USA:*** Calciparine†; Hep-Lock; Hep-Pak†.

Multi-ingredient: ***Aust.:*** Ambenat; Contractubex; Derivon; Ditaven comp; Dolo-Menthoneurin; Etrat; Ichthalgan forte; Pasta Cool; Pertrombon; Thrombion; Thrombophob; Venobene; Venosin; Venostasin†; Vetren; ***Belg.:*** Thrombophob†; ***Canad.:*** Lipactin; ***Fr.:*** Cirkan a la Prednacinolone; Ditavene; Esberiven; Neoparyl-B_{12}†; Peridil-Heparine†; ***Ger.:*** Arnica Kneipp Salbe; Arnika plus; Arthro-Menthoneurin†; Contractubex; Cycloarthrin†; Dolo-Menthoneurin; Dolo-Rubriment; Dolobene; Enelbin-Salbe forte†; Enelbin-Salbe N; Essaven; Essaven 50 000†; Essaven Tri-Complex; Etrat Sportgel; Etrat Sportsalbe†; Fibraflex†; Hamoagil†; Haven†; Heparin 30 000-ratiopharm/ Heparin 50 000-ratiopharm†; Heparin Comp; Hepathrombin-Procto†; Ichthalgan; Jossathromb†; Kelofibrase; Lipactin; Neo-Gallonorm†; NeyGeront "N" (Revitorgan-Dilutionen "N" Nr. 64); Ostochont; Pan†; Pe-Ce Ven N; Pentavenon†; Phlogase†; Robusanon†; Sensicutan; Sportofit†; Sportupac N; Thrombimed†; Thrombo-Enelbin N†; Thrombocutan†; Trauma-Puren; Turgostad†; varico sanol Beincreme†; Venalot†; Venoplant; Venostasin; Venothromb†; Vetren†; ***Ital.:*** Epartisone†; Essaven; Facocinerin†; Flebogamma†; Flebs; Idracemi Eparina; Luxazone Eparina; Proctosoll; Recto Menaderm†; Reparil; Rubidiosin Composto; Venotrauma; Via Mal Trauma Gel; Vit Eparin; Xantervit Eparina; ***S.Afr.:*** Essaven; Thrombophob; ***Spain:*** Essavenon; Recto Menaderm; Sol Dial Perit†; Venacol; Venoplant; ***Swed.:*** Orstanorm med heparin†; ***Switz.:*** Assan; Assan-Thermo; Bonactin; Butaparin; Contractubex; Contugel†; Demovarin; Dolo-Arthrosenex; Dolo-Menthoneurin†; Dolobene; Gorgonium; Hepabuzone; Heparinol†; Hepathrombine; Keli-med; Keppur; Lipactin; Lyman; Ralur; Rollbene; Sportusal; Venalot; Venoplant N; Venostasin comp†.

Heparinoids (3872-k)

The term heparinoid includes heparin derivatives and has also been used more loosely to include naturally occurring and synthetic highly-sulphated polysaccharides of similar structure. Such compounds have been described in many ways; some of the terms used include sulphated glucosaminoglycans; glycosaminoglycan polysulphate compounds; or sulphated mucopolysaccharides.

The following anticoagulants may be described as heparinoids: danaparoid sodium (p.846), pentosan polysulphate sodium (p.928), sodium apolate (p.943), and sulodexide (p.951).

Heparinoid preparations are available with uses ranging from anticoagulation to the alleviation of inflammation (applied topically); some are claimed to have hypolipidaemic properties.

The proprietary names listed below refer to preparations containing undefined or less readily defined heparinoids that are used in a range of conditions including musculoskeletal and joint disorders, haemorrhoids, lipid disorders, and thrombo-embolic disorders.

Preparations

Proprietary Preparations (details are given in Part 3)

Aust.: Hemeran; Hirudoid; ***Austral.:*** Hirudoid; ***Belg.:*** Hemeran; Hirudoid; ***Ger.:*** Arteparon†; Etrat Sportsalbe MPS; Hirudoid; ***Ital.:*** Angioflux; Ateran; Ateroid; Ateroxide; Condral; Erevan; Flebeparoid†; Glicamin; Gluparin; Hirudoid; Lasoven; Liparoid†; Lipostat; Lipostop; Matrix; Provenal; Ravenol; Suloves; Treparin; ***Neth.:*** Hirudoid; ***Norw.:*** Hirudoid; ***S.Afr.:*** Arteparon†; ***Spain:*** Arteparon†; Dinoven; Heparilene†; Hirudoid; ***Swed.:*** Hirudoid; ***Switz.:*** Hemeran; Hirudoid; ***UK:*** Hirudoid.

Multi-ingredient: ***Aust.:*** Bayolin; Lasonil; Lemuval; Mobilat; Mobilisin; Mobilisin plus; Moviflex; ***Austral.:*** Lasonil; Movelat; ***Belg.:*** Bayoline†; Lasonil; Mobilat; Mobilisin; ***Fr.:*** Bayoline†; Lasonil; ***Ger.:*** Bayolin†; Dignowell; Dolo Mobilat; Lasonil; Mobilat; Mobilisin; opino heparinoid†; Sanaven; Thermo Mobilisin; ***Irl.:*** Bayolin†; ***Ital.:*** Artrocur; Flebs; Flogogin; Geriavit†; Herbavit; Lasonil; Lasonil H; Lasoproct; Lasoreuma; Lisiflen†; Mobilat; Mobilisin; Sinteroid†; Traumal; ***Neth.:*** Lasonil; Mobilat; ***S.Afr.:*** Flexilat†; Mobilat; ***Spain:*** Duvaline Compositum†; Lasonil; Movilat; Movilisin; ***Switz.:*** Dolo-Veniten; Lasonil†; Mobilat; Mobilisin; Moviflex; Prelloran; ***UK:*** Anacal; Bayolin†; Lasonil; Movelat.

Hepronicate (9238-c)

Hepronicate (*rINN*).

Heptylidynetris(methylene nicotinate).

$C_{28}H_{31}N_3O_6$ = 505.6.

CAS — 7237-81-2.

Hepronicate is a vasodilator that has been used in the treatment of peripheral vascular disorders.

Preparations

Proprietary Preparations (details are given in Part 3)
Jpn: Megrin†.

Hexobendine Hydrochloride (9239-k)

Hexobendine Hydrochloride (*BANM, rINNM*).

ST-7090. *NN'*-Ethylenebis(3-methylaminopropyl 3,4,5-trimethoxybenzoate) dihydrochloride.

$C_{30}H_{44}N_2O_{10}$,2HCl = 665.6.

CAS — 54-03-5 (hexobendine); 50-62-4 (hexobendine hydrochloride).

NOTE. Hexobendine is *USAN*.

Hexobendine hydrochloride is a vasodilator used in ischaemic heart disease in usual doses of 180 to 270 mg daily, in divided doses, by mouth. It may also be given by intravenous or intramuscular injection.

Ischaemic heart disease is discussed under Atherosclerosis (p.782) and the treatment of its clinical manifestations is described under Angina Pectoris (p.780) and Myocardial Infarction (p.791).

Preparations

Proprietary Preparations (details are given in Part 3)
Aust.: Ustimon; ***Spain:*** Ustimon.

Multi-ingredient: ***Aust.:*** Instenon; ***Ger.:*** Card-Instenon†; Instenon†; ***Spain:*** Vasperdil.

Hirudin (5344-s)

Hirudine.

Desirudin (17413-z)

Desirudin (*BAN, USAN, rINN*).

CGP-39393. 63-Desulfohirudin (*Hirudo medicinalis* isoform HV1).

$C_{287}H_{440}N_{80}O_{110}S_6$ = 6963.4.

CAS — 120993-53-5.

Lepirudin (19770-g)

Lepirudin (*BAN, pINN*).

HBW-023. 1-L-Leucine-2-L-threonine-63-desulfohirudin (*Hirudo medicinalis* isoform HV1).

$C_{287}H_{440}N_{80}O_{111}S_6$ = 6979.4.

CAS — 138068-37-8.

Hirudin is a 65-amino-acid protein that is a direct inhibitor of thrombin. It has been extracted from leeches (p.897) and this form is used in various topical preparations. Recombinant hirudins that have been produced include desirudin and lepirudin (HBW-023). Lepirudin is used as an anticoagulant in patients with heparin-associated thrombocytopenia and recombinant hirudins are being investigated in arterial thrombo-embolic disorders such as myocardial infarction and unstable angina, as adjuncts in angioplasty procedures, and in the prevention of postoperative venous thrombo-embolism. Analogues of hirudin, such as bivalirudin (p.833) are also under investigation.

In the management of thrombo-embolism in patients with heparin-induced thrombocytopenia lepirudin is given in an initial dose of 0.4 mg per kg body-weight (to a maximum dose of 44 mg) by slow intravenous injection. This is followed by a maintenance dose of 0.15 mg per kg per hour (to a maximum dose per hour of 16.5 mg) by continuous intravenous infusion, adjusted according to response, usually for 2 to 10 days. Doses should be reduced in patients with renal impairment.

Recombinant hirudins are under investigation as alternatives to heparin in the early management of myocardial infarction (p.791). Initial studies comparing heparin with desirudin[1,2] or lepirudin[3] had to be stopped because of higher than expected haemorrhagic stroke rates,[4,5] and subsequent studies using lower doses of desirudin[6,7] failed to show a clear benefit over heparin. The role of hirudins therefore remains to be confirmed.

Recombinant hirudins are also being investigated in unstable angina[8,9] (p.780), in patients undergoing percutaneous transluminal angioplasty[10] (p.797), and in the prevention of postoperative venous thrombo-embolism[11,12] (p.802).

1. The Global Use of Strategies to Open Occluded Coronary Arteries (GUSTO) IIa Investigators. Randomized trial of intravenous heparin versus recombinant hirudin for acute coronary syndromes. *Circulation* 1994; **90:** 1631–7.
2. Antman EM, *et al.* Hirudin in acute myocardial infarction: safety report from the Thrombolysis and Thrombin Inhibition in Myocardial Infarction (TIMI) 9A trial. *Circulation* 1994; **90:** 1624–30.
3. Neuhaus K-L, *et al.* Safety observations from the pilot phase of the randomized r-Hirudin for Improvement of Thrombolysis (HIT-III) study: a study of the Arbeitsgemeinschaft Leitender Kardiologischer Krankenhausärzte (ALKK). *Circulation* 1994; **90:** 1638–42.
4. Zeymer U, Neuhaus K-L. Hirudin and excess bleeding: implications for future use. *Drug Safety* 1995; **12:** 234–9.
5. Conrad KA. Clinical pharmacology and drug safety: lessons from hirudin. *Clin Pharmacol Ther* 1995; **58:** 123–6.
6. The Global Use of Strategies to Open Occluded Coronary Arteries (GUSTO) IIb Investigators. A comparison of recombinant hirudin with heparin for the treatment of acute coronary syndromes. *N Engl J Med* 1996; **335:** 775–82.
7. Antman EM. Hirudin in acute myocardial infarction: thrombolysis and thrombin inhibition in myocardial infarction (TIMI) 9B trial. *Circulation* 1996; **94:** 911–21.
8. Topol EJ, *et al.* Recombinant hirudin for unstable angina pectoris: a multicenter, randomized angiographic trial. *Circulation* 1994; **89:** 1557–66.
9. Organization to Assess Strategies for Ischemic Syndromes (OASIS) Investigators. Comparison of the effects of two doses of recombinant hirudin compared with heparin in patients with acute myocardial ischemia without ST elevation: a pilot study. *Circulation* 1997; **96:** 769–77.
10. Serruys PW, *et al.* A comparison of hirudin with heparin in the prevention of restenosis after coronary angioplasty. *N Engl J Med* 1995; **333:** 757–63.
11. Eriksson BI, *et al.* Prevention of deep-vein thrombosis after total hip replacement: direct thrombin inhibition with recombinant hirudin, CGP 39393. *Lancet* 1996; **347:** 635–9.
12. Eriksson BI, *et al.* A comparison of recombinant hirudin with a low-molecular-weight heparin to prevent thromboembolic complications after total hip replacement. *N Engl J Med* 1997; **337:** 1329–35.

Preparations

Proprietary Preparations (details are given in Part 3)
Aust.: Irudil; ***Fr.:*** Hirucreme; ***Neth.:*** Refludan; ***Swed.:*** Refludan; ***UK:*** Refludan; Revasc; ***USA:*** Refludan.

Multi-ingredient: ***Ger.:*** Dolo-Exhirud†.

Hydralazine Hydrochloride (878-f)

Hydralazine Hydrochloride (*BANM, rINNM*).

Apressinum; Hydralazini Hydrochloridum; Hydrallazine Hydrochloride; Idralazina. 1-Hydrazinophthalazine hydrochloride.

$C_8H_8N_4$,HCl = 196.6.

CAS — 86-54-4 (hydralazine); 304-20-1 (hydralazine hydrochloride).

NOTE. Hydralazine Polistirex (hydralazine and sulphonated diethenylbenzene-ethenylbenzene copolymer complex) is *USAN*.

Pharmacopoeias. In *Eur.* (see p.viii), *Int., Jpn,* and *US.*

A white to off-white odourless or almost odourless crystalline powder. **Soluble** 1 in 25 of water and 1 in 500 of alcohol; very slightly soluble in dichloromethane and in ether. A 2% solution in water has a pH of 3.5 to 4.2. **Store** in airtight containers. Protect from light.

Incompatible with glucose solutions.

Discoloration of hydralazine injection was observed on several occasions after storage in a syringe for up to 12 hours.[1] Hydralazine reacts with metals and therefore the injection should be prepared using a non-metal filter and should be used as quickly as possible after being drawn through a needle into a syringe.

A study of the rate of degradation of hydralazine hydrochloride, 1 mg per mL in sweetened, aqueous oral liquids showed that glucose, fructose, lactose, and maltose reduced the stability of the drug.[2] In solutions containing mannitol or sorbitol, there was less than 10% degradation of hydralazine after 3 weeks.

1. Enderlin G. Discoloration of hydralazine injection. *Am J Hosp Pharm* 1984; **41:** 634.
2. Das Gupta V, *et al.* Stability of hydralazine hydrochloride in aqueous vehicles. *J Clin Hosp Pharm* 1986; **11:** 215–23.

Adverse Effects

Toxic effects occur frequently with hydralazine, particularly tachycardia, palpitations, angina pectoris, severe headache, and gastro-intestinal disturbances such as anorexia, nausea, vomiting, and diarrhoea. These adverse effects, together with flushing, dizziness, and nasal congestion, which occur less often, may be seen at the start of treatment, especially if the dose is increased quickly. They generally subside with continued treatment. Other less common side-effects include postural hypotension, fluid retention with oedema and weight gain, conjunctivitis, lachrymation, tremor, and muscle cramps.

Hydralazine may deplete pyridoxine in the body, and can produce peripheral neuropathy with numbness and tingling of the extremities. Occasionally, hepatotoxicity, blood dyscrasias, difficulty in urinating, glomerulonephritis, constipation, paralytic ileus, depression, and anxiety occur.

Hypersensitivity reactions may occur. Fever, chills, pruritus, and rashes have been reported. Haemolytic anaemia and eosinophilia may occur.

Following the prolonged use of large doses antinuclear antibodies may develop and a condition resembling systemic lupus erythematosus may occur. The incidence is greater in slow acetylators, patients with renal impairment, women, and patients taking more than 100 mg of hydralazine daily. The symptoms usually disappear when the drug is withdrawn; some patients may require treatment with corticosteroids.

Following acute overdosage, hypotension, tachycardia, myocardial ischaemia, dysrhythmias, shock, and coma may occur.

Paradoxical severe hypertension followed administration of hydralazine by mouth or intramuscularly on 3 occasions in a patient with renal artery stenosis.[1]

1. Webb DB, White JP. Hypertension after taking hydrallazine. *Br Med J* 1980; **280:** 1582.

Carcinogenicity. There was no evidence from a survey of 1978 patients with lung or colorectal cancer and 6807 controls that use of hydralazine was associated with an increased risk of these neoplasms.[1]

1. Kaufman DW, *et al.* Hydralazine use in relation to cancers of the lung, colon, and rectum. *Eur J Clin Pharmacol* 1989; **36:** 259–64.

Effects on the blood. PREGNANCY. Report of 3 cases of thrombocytopenia in neonates whose mothers had been treated with hydralazine for some months before delivery.[1] The thrombocytopenia and bleeding was transient with full recovery occurring within a few weeks. No adverse effects were noticed in the mothers.

1. Widerlöv E, *et al.* Hydralazine-induced neonatal thrombocytopenia. *N Engl J Med* 1980; **303:** 1235.

Effects on the kidneys. Rapidly progressive glomerulonephritis with focal and segmental lesions, usually accompanied by necrosis and crescent formation, have been reported in patients receiving hydralazine.[1-3] The condition is reported to be associated with the presence of antinuclear antibodies,[3] and Kincaid-Smith and Whitworth reported that of 4 female patients who developed the syndrome all were slow acetylators,[2] factors associated with the development of hydralazine-induced lupus erythematosus.[4] However, renal involvement is much less common in drug-induced lupus,[4] and Björck and colleagues report that in their experience of 15 such cases men and women and fast and slow acetylators were equally affected;[3] in addition these authors note that criteria for systemic lupus erythematosus were not usually fulfilled in these patients and suggest that the condition should be distinguished from lupus nephritis. Immediate withdrawal of hydralazine generally results in some improvement in renal function but complete recovery is uncommon; severe cases may require immunosuppressive therapy.[3]

1. Björck S, *et al.* Rapidly progressive glomerulonephritis after hydralazine. *Lancet* 1983; **ii:** 42.
2. Kincaid-Smith P, Whitworth JA. Hydralazine-associated glomerulonephritis. *Lancet* 1983; **ii:** 348.
3. Björck S, *et al.* Hydralazine-induced glomerulonephritis. *Lancet* 1985; **i:** 392.
4. Hughes GRV. Recent developments in drug-associated systemic lupus erythematosus. *Adverse Drug React Bull* 1987; (Apr.): 460–3.

Effects on the skin. Pruritus and skin rashes have been reported with hydralazine use.

A 59-year-old woman who had been taking hydralazine 25 mg three times a day for 6 months developed symptoms of Sweet's syndrome (erythematous plaques and nodules and haemorrhagic blisters) initially diagnosed as a vasculitis.[1] Symptoms began to subside on withdrawal of hydralazine but recurred when hydralazine was reintroduced. The condition resolved on discontinuation of hydralazine and treatment with prednisolone.

1. Gilmour E, *et al.* Drug-induced Sweet's syndrome (acute febrile neutrophilic dermatosis) associated with hydralazine. *Br J Dermatol* 1995; **133:** 490–1.

Lupus erythematosus. Drug-associated lupus erythematosus is a well-documented adverse effect of hydralazine therapy. Onset is typically delayed from 1 month to 5 years from the start of treatment, and the most common symptoms are arthralgia or arthritis, usually non-deforming, in up to 95% of patients, fever and myalgia in about 50%, and pleuropulmonary involvement, manifesting as pleurisy, pleural effusions, or pulmonary infiltrates in up to 30%.[1-3] Renal involvement is reported to be less common than in idiopathic systemic lupus erythematosus and there is some uncertainty as to whether the glomerulonephritis sometimes seen in patients receiving hydralazine should be considered lupus nephritis—see under Effects on the Kidneys, above. Nonetheless a 20% incidence of renal involvement has been reported.[1] Other complications and symptoms that have been associated with lupus erythematosus in patients taking hydralazine include cutaneous vasculitis,[4-6] orogenital and cutaneous ulceration,[7] bilateral retinal vasculitis,[8] reactive hypoglycaemia (although the attribution is uncertain),[9] life-threatening cardiac tamponade,[10] and hoarseness and stridor secondary to vocal cord palsy, which progressed to respiratory arrest.[11] Skin rashes are reported to be less prominent than with the idiopathic form of the disease.[1] Fatalities have occurred,[12] but appear to be rare. Estimates of the overall incidence of hydralazine-associated lupus erythematosus vary from about 1.2 to 5% or more.[13-16] The syndrome appears to occur only in patients who develop antinuclear antibodies while receiving hydralazine, but the incidence of positive antinuclear antibody tests is much higher than that of lupus, at up to 60%, so the presence of antinuclear antibodies alone is not diagnostic.[15] There is a strong relationship with drug dose,[14,16] acetylator status,[13,15,16] and patient gender,[16] the syndrome being more common in slow acetylators and women, and in patients receiving 100 mg daily or more.

Although it has been reported that hydralazine-associated lupus was more frequent in patients with the HLA-DR4 antigen[17] this was not confirmed by others[18] and subsequent work has suggested that the association is rather with the non-expressing or null forms of the adjacent complement C4 gene.[19] Hydralazine can inactivate complement C4 *in vitro*[20] and might exacerbate complement deficiency (which is known to be associated with idiopathic systemic lupus erythematosus) in patients with an already low level of C4 due to a null allele.[19]

1. Hughes GRV. Recent developments in drug-associated systemic lupus erythematosus. *Adverse Drug React Bull* 1987; (Apr.): 460–3.
2. Cohen MG, Prowse MV. Drug-induced rheumatic syndromes: diagnosis, clinical features and management. *Med Toxicol Adverse Drug Exp* 1989; **4:** 199–218.
3. Price EJ, Venables PJW. Drug-induced lupus. *Drug Safety* 1995; **12:** 283–90.
4. Bernstein RM, *et al.* Hydrallazine-induced cutaneous vasculitis. *Br Med J* 1980; **280:** 156–7.
5. Peacock A, Weatherall D. Hydralazine-induced necrotising vasculitis. *Br Med J* 1981; **282:** 1121–2.
6. Finlay AY, *et al.* Hydrallazine-induced necrotising vasculitis. *Br Med J* 1981; **282:** 1703–4.
7. Neville E, *et al.* Orogenital ulcers, SLE and hydrallazine. *Postgrad Med J* 1981; **57:** 378–9.
8. Doherty M, *et al.* Hydralazine induced lupus syndrome with eye disease. *Br Med J* 1985; **290:** 675.
9. Blackshear PJ, *et al.* Reactive hypoglycaemia and insulin autoantibodies in drug-induced lupus erythematosus. *Ann Intern Med* 1983; **99:** 182–4.
10. Anandadas JA, Simpson P. Cardiac tamponade, associated with hydralazine therapy, in a patient with rapid acetylator status. *Br J Clin Pract* 1986; **40:** 305–6.
11. Chong WK, *et al.* Acute laryngeal stridor with respiratory arrest in drug induced systemic lupus erythematosus. *Br Med J* 1988; **297:** 660–1.
12. Sturman SG, *et al.* Fatal hydralazine-induced systemic lupus erythematosus. *Lancet* 1988; **ii:** 1304.
13. Bing RF, *et al.* Hydrallazine in hypertension: is there a safe dose? *Br Med J* 1980; **281:** 353–4.
14. Freestone S, *et al.* Incidence of hydrallazine-associated autoimmune disease. *Br J Clin Pharmacol* 1982; **13:** 291P–292P.
15. Mansilla-Tinoco R, *et al.* Hydralazine, antinuclear antibodies, and the lupus syndrome. *Br Med J* 1982; **284:** 936–9.
16. Cameron HA, Ramsay LE. The lupus syndrome induced by hydralazine: a common complication with low dose treatment. *Br Med J* 1984; **289:** 410–12.
17. Batchelor JR, *et al.* Hydralazine-induced systemic lupus erythematosus: influence of HLA-DR and sex on susceptibility. *Lancet* 1980; **i:** 1107–9.
18. Brand C, *et al.* Hydralazine-induced lupus: no association with HLA-DR4. *Lancet* 1984; **i:** 462.
19. Speirs C, *et al.* Complement system protein C4 and susceptibility to hydralazine-induced systemic lupus erythematosus. *Lancet* 1989; **i:** 922–4.
20. Sim E, *et al.* Drugs that induce systemic lupus erythematosus inhibit complement component C4. *Lancet* 1984; **ii:** 422–4.

Treatment of Adverse Effects

Withdrawal of hydralazine or reduction of the dosage causes the reversal of many side-effects. Peripheral neuropathy has been reported to be alleviated by pyridoxine.

If overdosage occurs the stomach should be emptied by gastric lavage. Activated charcoal may be administered. Symptomatic and supportive treatment, including plasma expanders for shock and a beta blocker for tachycardia, should be given as necessary. Severe hypotension may respond to placing the patient in the supine position with the feet raised. If possible, pressor drugs should be avoided. If a pressor is necessary, one should be chosen that will not cause tachycardia or exacerbate arrhythmias; adrenaline should not be used.

Precautions

Hydralazine is contra-indicated in patients with severe tachycardia, dissecting aortic aneurysm, heart failure with high cardiac output, cor pulmonale, or myocardial insufficiency due to mechanical obstruction, for example aortic or mitral stenosis or constrictive pericarditis. Hydralazine is also contra-indicated in patients with idiopathic systemic lupus erythematosus and related disorders.

Hydralazine-induced vasodilatation produces myocardial stimulation. It should therefore be used with caution in patients with ischaemic heart disease since it can increase angina and it should not be given to patients following myocardial infarction until their condition has stabilised. Patients with suspected or confirmed ischaemic heart disease should be given hydralazine under cover of a beta blocker, which should be started a few days before hydralazine, in order to prevent myocardial stimulation. If given to patients with heart failure they should be monitored for postural hypotension and tachycardia during the initial stages of therapy, preferably in hospital. If treatment with hydralazine is to be stopped in patients with heart failure it should generally be withdrawn gradually. Hydralazine should be used with caution in patients with cerebrovascular disorders.

The dose of hydralazine should be reduced or the dosage interval prolonged in patients with impaired renal or hepatic function. Complete blood counts and antinuclear antibody determinations should be carried out periodically during long-term therapy. Urine analysis (for microhaematuria and proteinuria) is also recommended.

Hydralazine is teratogenic in some species of *animals* and should therefore be avoided during the first two trimesters of pregnancy.

Patients may experience impaired reactions, especially at the start of therapy, and should not drive or operate machinery if affected.

Porphyria. Hydralazine has been associated with clinical exacerbations of porphyria and is considered unsafe in porphyric patients.[1]

1. Moore MR, McColl KEL. *Porphyria: drug lists*. Glasgow: Porphyria Research Unit, University of Glasgow, 1991.

Pregnancy and breast feeding. Hydralazine should be avoided during the first two trimesters of pregnancy.

Hydralazine concentrations were found to be similar in maternal and umbilical-cord blood in a study of 6 women being treated with hydralazine for pronounced hypertension during pregnancy.[1] Hydralazine was determined in the breast milk of 1 mother, but amounts detected were unlikely to produce clinically relevant concentrations in the infant.

For a report of thrombocytopenia occurring in neonates following maternal treatment with hydralazine during pregnancy, see Effects on the Blood under Adverse Effects, above.

1. Liedholm H, *et al.* Transplacental passage and breast milk concentrations of hydralazine. *Eur J Clin Pharmacol* 1982; **21:** 417–19.

Interactions

The hypotensive effect of hydralazine may be enhanced by other agents with a hypotensive action. Severe hypotension may occur if hydralazine and diazoxide are given concurrently. However, some interactions with antihypertensives may be beneficial: thiazide diuretics also counteract the fluid retention caused by hydralazine, and beta blockers diminish the cardiac-accelerating effects.

Indomethacin. Indomethacin 100 mg daily did not attenuate the hypotensive effect of hydralazine in a study in 9 healthy subjects,[1] but another study[2] showed that indomethacin 200 mg daily did attenuate the hypotensive effect of hydralazine but not the effects on heart rate, renal or limb blood flow, or plasma-catecholamine concentration.

1. Jackson SHD, Pickles H. Indomethacin does not attenuate the effects of hydralazine in normal subjects. *Eur J Clin Pharmacol* 1983; **25:** 303–5.
2. Cinquegrani MP, Liang C. Indomethacin attenuates the hypotensive action of hydralazine. *Clin Pharmacol Ther* 1986; **39:** 564–70.

Pharmacokinetics

Hydralazine is rapidly absorbed from the gastro-intestinal tract but undergoes considerable first-pass metabolism by acetylation in the gastro-intestinal mucosa and liver. The rate of metabolism is genetically determined and depends upon the acetylator status of the individual. The bioavailability of hydralazine has been reported to be about 35% in slow acetylators and less in fast acetylators; thus plasma concentrations after a given dose are higher in slow acetylators.

Peak concentrations have been reported to occur in the plasma after about one hour. Hydralazine is chiefly present in plasma as a hydrazone conjugate with pyruvic acid. Plasma protein binding is about 90%. The drug is widely distributed, notably into arterial walls.

Systemic metabolism in the liver is by hydroxylation of the ring system and conjugation with glucuronic acid; most sources suggest that N-acetylation is not of major importance in systemic clearance and that therefore acetylator status does not affect elimination. Hydralazine is excreted mainly in urine as metabolites.

The apparent average half-life for hydralazine has been reported to vary from about 45 minutes to about 8 hours, with a number of sources giving the average as about 2 to 4 hours. Some of the variation may be due to problems with the analytical procedures—see below. The half-life is prolonged in renal impairment and may be up to 16 hours in patients with a creatinine clearance of less than 20 mL per minute.

Hydralazine crosses the placenta and is distributed into breast milk.

Attempts to describe the pharmacokinetics of hydralazine have been plagued by the instability of the drug itself in plasma and in alkaline solutions, and the instability of its circulating metabolites during analysis, and has meant that many techniques for the measurement of hydralazine have proved non-selective and yield overestimates of unchanged drug.[1] Studies using less selective methods have yielded an apparent bioavailability for oral hydralazine of 38 to 69% in slow acetylators and 22 to 32% in fast acetylators; in contrast, more selective assays have yielded values of 31 to 35% and 10 to 16% for slow and rapid acetylators respectively. Similarly, hydralazine plasma clearance is lower and the half-life longer when based upon the results of non-selective assay procedures; mean elimination half-life has ranged from 2.2 to 3.6 hours based upon these methods compared with 0.67 to 0.96 hours using a more selective assay. Improved pharmacokinetic data has indicated that while the first-pass effect is dependent upon acetylator phenotype, systemic clearance is only minimally dependent upon acetylation. The formation of the pyruvic acid hydrazone, which is without significant vasodilator activity, contributes to extrahepatic phenotype-independent clearance.

Although some workers have correlated the hypotensive effect of hydralazine with the serum concentrations,[2] others have been unable to do so.[3] Moreover, the duration of hypotensive effect has been shown to exceed considerably that predicted from the rate of elimination.[4,5] Possible explanations are the accumulation of hydralazine at its sites of action in the arterial walls[6] or the existence of active metabolites.[7-9]

Concurrent intake of food has been found by Melander *et al.* to enhance considerably the bioavailability of hydralazine[10] but Shepherd *et al.* demonstrated food-related reductions in plasma-hydralazine concentrations with reduced vasodilator effect.[11] The discrepancy was thought to be due to the greater specificity of the assay used in the latter study and to differences in the timing of food and hydralazine administration in the two studies.[12,13]

1. Ludden TM, *et al.* Clinical pharmacokinetics of hydralazine. *Clin Pharmacokinet* 1982; **7:** 185–205.
2. Zacest R, Koch-Weser J. Relation of hydralazine plasma concentration to dosage and hypotensive action. *Clin Pharmacol Ther* 1972; **13:** 420–5.
3. Talseth T, *et al.* Hydralazine slow-release: observations on serum profile and clinical efficacy in man. *Curr Ther Res* 1977; **21:** 157–68.

4. O'Malley K, *et al.* Duration of hydralazine action in hypertension. *Clin Pharmacol Ther* 1975; **18:** 581–6.
5. Shepherd AMM, *et al.* Hydralazine kinetics after single and repeated oral doses. *Clin Pharmacol Ther* 1980; **28:** 804–11.
6. Moore-Jones D, Perry HM. Radioautographic localization of hydralazine-1-C_{14} in arterial walls. *Proc Soc Exp Biol Med* 1966; **122:** 576–9.
7. Barron K, *et al.* Comparative evaluation of the in vitro effects of hydralazine and hydralazine acetonide on arterial smooth muscle. *Br J Pharmacol* 1977; **61:** 345–9.
8. Haegele KD, *et al.* Identification of hydrallazine and hydrallazine hydrazone metabolites in human body fluids and quantitative in vitro comparisons of their smooth muscle relaxant activity. *Br J Clin Pharmacol* 1978; **5:** 489–94.
9. Reece PA, *et al.* Interference in assays for hydralazine in humans by a major plasma metabolite, hydralazine pyruvic acid hydrazone. *J Pharm Sci* 1978; **67:** 1150–3.
10. Melander A, *et al.* Enhancement of hydralazine bioavailability by food. *Clin Pharmacol Ther* 1977; **22:** 104–7.
11. Shepherd AMM, *et al.* Effect of food on blood hydralazine levels and response in hypertension. *Clin Pharmacol Ther* 1984; **36:** 14–18.
12. Shepherd AMM, *et al.* Concomitant food intake does enhance the bioavailability and effect of hydralazine. *Clin Pharmacol Ther* 1985; **38:** 475–6.
13. Melander A, *et al.* Concomitant food intake does enhance the bioavailability and effect of hydralazine. *Clin Pharmacol Ther* 1985; **38:** 475.

Uses and Administration

Hydralazine is a direct-acting vasodilator which acts predominantly on the arterioles. It reduces blood pressure and peripheral resistance but produces fluid retention. Tachycardia and an increase in cardiac output occur mainly as a reflex response to the reduction in peripheral resistance. Hydralazine tends to improve renal and cerebral blood flow and its effect on diastolic pressure is more marked than on systolic pressure.

Hydralazine hydrochloride is given by mouth for the treatment of hypertension (p.788), usually in conjunction with a beta blocker and a thiazide diuretic. In addition to an additive antihypertensive effect, this combination reduces the reflex tachycardia and fluid retention caused by hydralazine. It may be given intravenously in hypertensive crises. Hydralazine has also been used together with a nitrate vasodilator in the management of heart failure (but see Precautions, above). For further discussion of this use of hydralazine, see below.

The dose of hydralazine should be reduced or the dosage interval prolonged in patients with impaired renal or hepatic function.

In **hypertension**, the usual initial dose of hydralazine hydrochloride is 40 to 50 mg daily by mouth in divided doses, increased according to the patient's response. In the UK it is suggested that a dose of 100 mg daily, in divided doses, should rarely be exceeded, although the recommended maximum dose is 200 mg daily; doses above 100 mg daily are associated with an increased incidence of lupus erythematosus, particularly in women and in slow acetylators.

In hypertensive crises, hydralazine hydrochloride may be given by slow intravenous injection or by intravenous infusion. A recommended dose is 5 to 10 mg intravenously over 20 minutes, repeated if necessary after 20 to 30 minutes. Alternatively infusion of 200 to 300 µg per minute intravenously is suggested; the usual maintenance dose range is 50 to 150 µg per minute. Hydralazine hydrochloride has also been given by intramuscular injection.

Heart failure. The value of hydralazine when given alone in heart failure (p.785) is equivocal. A review by Packer points out that although it increases cardiac output and decreases systemic resistance in patients with heart failure the doses required to produce benefit are unpredictable and may be as high as 3 g daily.[1] Patients with marked left ventricular dilatation and secondary mitral regurgitation appear to respond best, but in others the drug may compromise peripheral perfusion without an improvement in cardiac performance. Adverse reactions require discontinuation of therapy in up to 25% of patients, while nearly 30% on long-term treatment develop haemodynamic and clinical tolerance.[1] Meta-analysis of a number of studies[2] of vasodilator therapy for heart failure has failed to show a benefit in terms of improved functional status or reduced mortality in patients given hydralazine alone. However, there is evidence from the Veterans Administration Cooperative Study[3] of reduced mortality from the use of hydralazine with nitrates and this has been confirmed in a second study (V-HeFTII),[4] although hydralazine with isosorbide dinitrate was less effective than enalapril. In these two studies,[3,4] the dose of hydralazine was increased gradually to 300 mg daily and that of isosorbide dinitrate to 160 mg daily, provided that they were tolerated by the patient. Both drugs were given by mouth in divided doses.

See above for precautions necessary in patients with heart failure.

1. Packer M. The role of vasodilator therapy in the treatment of severe chronic heart failure. *Drugs* 1986; **32** (suppl 5): 13–26.
2. Mulrow CD, *et al.* Relative efficacy of vasodilator therapy in chronic congestive heart failure: implications of randomized trials. *JAMA* 1988; **259:** 3422–6.
3. Cohn JN, *et al.* Effect of vasodilator therapy on mortality in chronic congestive heart failure: results of a Veterans Administration cooperative study. *N Engl J Med* 1986; **314:** 1547–52.
4. Cohn JN, *et al.* A comparison of enalapril with hydralazine-isosorbide dinitrate in the treatment of chronic congestive heart failure. *N Engl J Med* 1991; **325:** 303–10.

IN CHILDREN. Although somewhat limited, there is some experience with hydralazine in infants and children with heart failure. Single intravenous injections of 500 µg per kg bodyweight have produced increases in stroke volume index and cardiac index in 13 infants aged between 2 and 13 months with heart failure and dilated cardiomyopathy.[1] Oral hydralazine therapy was given to 10 of these infants in addition to treatment with digitalis and a diuretic. At a follow-up of 3 to 38 months, 8 patients were asymptomatic. One child showed no apparent improvement after 3 months of therapy, and one child died. A similar study in 10 infants and children aged between 3 and 36 months with primary myocardial disease reported benefit from treatment with oral hydralazine in doses up to 4 mg per kg daily, in addition to digoxin and diuretics.[2] Follow-up for up to 42 months indicated marked improvement in cardiac size in 5 patients and improvement or normalisation of the ECG in 6.

1. Artman M, *et al.* Hemodynamic effects of hydralazine in infants with idiopathic dilated cardiomyopathy and congestive heart failure. *Am Heart J* 1987; **113:** 144–50.
2. Rao PS, Andaya WG. Chronic afterload reduction in infants and children with primary myocardial disease. *J Pediatr* 1986; **108:** 530–4.

Preparations

BP 1998: Hydralazine Injection; Hydralazine Tablets;
USP 23: Hydralazine Hydrochloride Injection; Hydralazine Hydrochloride Oral Solution; Hydralazine Hydrochloride Tablets; Reserpine, Hydralazine Hydrochloride, and Hydrochlorothiazide Tablets.

Proprietary Preparations (details are given in Part 3)
Austral.: Alphapress; Apresoline; ***Canad.:*** Apresoline; Novo-Hylazin; Nu-Hydral; ***Irl.:*** Apresoline; ***Ital.:*** Apresolin†; Ipolina†; ***Neth.:*** Apresoline; ***Norw.:*** Apresolin; ***S.Afr.:*** Apresoline; Hyperex†; Hyperphen; Rolazine; ***Spain:*** Hydrapres; ***Swed.:*** Apresolin; ***Switz.:*** Slow-Apresoline†; ***UK:*** Apresoline; ***USA:*** Apresoline.

Multi-ingredient: ***Aust.:*** Polinorm; Trepress; Triloc; ***Canad.:*** Ser-Ap-Es; ***Ger.:*** Docidrazin; Impresso; Pertenso N; Treloc; Trepress; TRI-Normin; ***Spain:*** Betadipresan; Betadipresan Diu; Neatenol Diuvas; Tensiocomplet; ***Switz.:*** Trepress; ***USA:*** Apresazide; Aprozide†; Cam-ap-es†; HHR†; Hydra-zide; Hydrap-ES; Marpres; Ser-Ap-Es; Tri-Hydroserpine; Unipres†.

Hydrochlorothiazide (2333-v)

Hydrochlorothiazide *(BAN, rINN).*

Hidroclorotiazida; Hydrochlorothiazidum. 6-Chloro-3,4-dihydro-2*H*-1,2,4-benzothiadiazine-7-sulphonamide 1,1-dioxide.

$C_7H_8ClN_3O_4S_2$ = 297.7.

CAS — 58-93-5.

NOTE. Compounded preparations of hydrochlorothiazide and amiloride hydrochloride in the proportions, by weight, 10 parts to 1 part have the British Approved Name Co-amilozide.
Compounded preparations of hydrochlorothiazide and captopril in the proportions, by weight, 1 part to 2 parts have the British Approved Name Co-zidocapt.
Compounded preparations of triamterene and hydrochlorothiazide in the proportions, by weight, 2 parts to 1 part have the British Approved Name Co-triamterzide.
Compounded preparations containing hydrochlorothiazide in USP 23 may be represented by the following names:
Co-amilozide for amiloride hydrochloride and hydrochlorothiazide;
Co-spironozide for spironolactone and hydrochlorothiazide; and
Co-triamterzide for triamterene and hydrochlorothiazide.

Pharmacopoeias. In *Chin., Eur.* (see p.viii), *Int., Jpn, Pol.,* and *US.*

A white or almost white, almost odourless crystalline powder. Slightly or very slightly **soluble** in water; sparingly soluble in alcohol and in methyl alcohol; soluble in acetone; freely soluble in dimethylformamide, in *n*-butylamine, and in solutions of alkali hydroxides; practically insoluble in ether, in chloroform, and in dilute mineral acids.

Adverse Effects

Hydrochlorothiazide and other thiazide diuretics may cause a number of metabolic disturbances especially at high doses. They may provoke hyperglycaemia and glycosuria in diabetic and other susceptible patients. They may cause hyperuricaemia and precipitate attacks of gout in some patients. Administration of thiazide diuretics may be associated with electrolyte imbalances including hypochloraemic alkalosis, hyponatraemia, and hypokalaemia. Hypokalaemia intensifies the effect of digitalis on cardiac muscle and administration of digitalis or its glycosides may have to be temporarily suspended. Patients with cirrhosis of the liver are particularly at risk from hypokalaemia. Hyponatraemia may occur in patients with severe heart failure who are very oedematous, particularly with large doses in conjunction with restricted salt in the diet. The urinary excretion of calcium is reduced. Hypomagnesaemia has also occurred. Adverse changes in plasma lipids have also been noted but their clinical significance is unclear.

Signs of electrolyte imbalance include dry mouth, thirst, weakness, lethargy, drowsiness, restlessness, muscle pain and cramps, seizures, oliguria, hypotension, and gastro-intestinal disturbances.

Other side-effects include anorexia, gastric irritation, nausea, vomiting, constipation, diarrhoea, headache, dizziness, photosensitivity reactions, postural hypotension, paraesthesia, impotence, and yellow vision. Hypersensitivity reactions include skin rashes, fever, pulmonary oedema, and pneumonitis. Cholestatic jaundice, pancreatitis, and blood dyscrasias including thrombocytopenia and, more rarely, granulocytopenia, leucopenia, and aplastic and haemolytic anaemia have been reported.

Intestinal ulceration has occurred following the administration of tablets containing thiazides with an enteric-coated core of potassium chloride (see also under Potassium, p.1161).

Effects on the blood. Individual case reports of intravascular immune haemolysis in patients taking hydrochlorothiazide and methyldopa.[1-3] In each of these 3 cases the hydrochlorothiazide was identified as the probable cause of haemolysis on serological data, although methyldopa could have been a contributory factor. One of these patients died[3] during the haemolytic episode although post-mortem examination failed to reveal a cause of death.

1. Vila JM, *et al.* Thiazide-induced immune hemolytic anemia. *JAMA* 1976; **236:** 1723–4.
2. Garratty G, *et al.* Acute immune intravascular hemolysis due to hydrochlorothiazide. *Am J Clin Pathol* 1981; **76:** 73–8.
3. Beck ML, *et al.* Fatal intravascular immune hemolysis induced by hydrochlorothiazide. *Am J Clin Pathol* 1984; **81:** 791–4.

Effects on the electrolyte balance. MAGNESIUM AND POTASSIUM. The clinical consequences of diuretic-induced hypokalaemia have been controversial.[1-3] Of major concern has been the possibility that diuretic-induced hypokalaemia could predispose to cardiac arrhythmias and sudden cardiac death in some patients, and it has been suggested that this could explain the lower than expected reduction in deaths due to ischaemic heart disease found in some hypertension trials. Indeed, some case-control studies[4,5] have suggested an association between an increased risk of sudden cardiac death and the use of thiazides or other non-potassium-sparing diuretics; the addition of a potassium supplement had little effect on this risk, whereas addition of a potassium-sparing diuretic to the thiazide lowered the risk.[4] However, Papademetriou and colleagues observed no reduction in cardiac arrhythmias following the correction of hypokalaemia[6] nor any evidence of increased arrhythmias associated with diuretic-induced hypokalaemia.[7] Several reviews[8,9] have argued that there is no proof of a causal relationship between hypokalaemia and serious dysrhythmias and this was endorsed by a more recent randomised study.[10]

It is generally agreed that routine potassium supplementation in patients taking diuretics is unnecessary unless the serum-potassium concentration falls below 3.0 mmol per litre. Potassium replacement or conservation is likely to be necessary in patients at risk from the cardiac effects of hypokalaemia[11] such as those with severe heart disease, those taking digitalis preparations or high doses of diuretics, and in patients with severe liver disease.

The amount of potassium in fixed combination diuretic and potassium preparations has long been considered insufficient to correct hypokalaemia and the effectiveness of oral potassium supplements in increasing body stores of potassium has been questioned.[12-14] Hypokalaemia may be overcome by adding a potassium-sparing diuretic such as amiloride or triamterene[15] to the regimen, but there is a danger of hyperkalaemia if they are used indiscriminately. The *routine* use of fixed-dose combination preparations of a thiazide or loop diuretic with a potassium-sparing diuretic is considered unnecessary.[16] Potassium-sparing diuretics will not correct the potassium deficit unrelated to diuretic therapy in patients with severe heart failure.[17] Administration of a thiazide in combination with a beta blocker may ameliorate diuretic-induced hypokalaemia, but will not necessarily correct it completely. Hypokalaemia has been reported[18-20] in patients taking fixed-dose combinations of thiazides and beta blockers.

Potassium supplementation alone may not be sufficient to correct hypokalaemia in patients who are also deficient in magnesium,[21] although Papademetriou[22] considered this unlikely to be of clinical significance. Magnesium depletion has also been implicated as a risk factor for arrhythmias.[9,23]

1. Materson BJ. Diuretic-associated hypokalemia. *Arch Intern Med* 1985; **145:** 1966–7.
2. Kaplan NM, *et al.* Potassium supplementation in hypertensive patients with diuretic-induced hypokalemia. *N Engl J Med* 1985; **312:** 746–9.
3. Kassirer JP, Harrington JT. Fending off the potassium pushers. *N Engl J Med* 1985; **312:** 785–7.
4. Siscovick DS, *et al.* Diuretic therapy for hypertension and the risk of primary cardiac arrest. *N Engl J Med* 1994; **330:** 1852–7.
5. Hoes AW, *et al.* Diuretics, β-blockers, and the risk for sudden cardiac death in hypertensive patients. *Ann Intern Med* 1995; **123:** 481–7.
6. Papademetriou V, *et al.* Diuretic-induced hypokalemia in uncomplicated systemic hypertension: effect of plasma potassium correction on cardiac arrhythmias. *Am J Cardiol* 1983; **52:** 1017–22.
7. Papademetriou V, *et al.* Thiazide therapy is not a cause of arrhythmia in patients with systemic hypertension. *Arch Intern Med* 1988; **148:** 1272–6.
8. Harrington JT, *et al.* Our national obsession with potassium. *Am J Med* 1982; **73:** 155–9.
9. Freis ED. Critique of the clinical importance of diuretic-induced hypokalemia and elevated cholesterol level. *Arch Intern Med* 1989; **149**: 2640–8.
10. Siegel D, *et al.* Diuretics, serum and intracellular electrolyte levels, and ventricular arrhythmias in hypertensive men. *JAMA* 1992; **267:** 1083–9.
11. Anonymous. Potassium-sparing diuretics—when are they really needed? *Drug Ther Bull* 1985; **23:** 17–20.
12. Jackson PR, *et al.* Relative potency of spironolactone, triamterene and potassium chloride in thiazide-induced hypokalaemia. *Br J Clin Pharmacol* 1982; **14:** 257–63.
13. Shenfield GM. Fixed combination drug therapy. *Drugs* 1982; **23:** 462–80.
14. Papademetriou V, *et al.* Effectiveness of potassium chloride or triamterene in thiazide hypokalemia. *Arch Intern Med* 1985; **145:** 1986–90.
15. Kohvakka A. Maintenance of potassium balance during long-term diuretic therapy in chronic heart failure patients with thiazide-induced hypokalemia: comparison of potassium supplementation with potassium chloride and potassium-sparing agents, amiloride and triamterene. *Int J Clin Pharmacol Ther Toxicol* 1988; **26:** 273–7.
16. Anonymous. Routine use of potassium-sparing diuretics. *Drug Ther Bull* 1991; **29:** 85–7.
17. Davidson C, *et al.* The effects of potassium supplements, spironolactone or amiloride on the potassium status of patients with heart failure. *Postgrad Med J* 1978; **54:** 405–9.
18. Skehan JD, *et al.* Hypokalaemia induced by a combination of a beta-blocker and a thiazide. *Br Med J* 1982; **284:** 83.
19. Odugbesan O, *et al.* Hazards of combined beta-blocker/diuretic tablets. *Lancet* 1985; **i:** 1221–2.
20. Jacobs L. Hypokalaemia with beta-blocker/thiazide combinations. *J R Coll Gen Pract* 1986; **36:** 39.
21. Dyckner T. Relation of cardiovascular disease to potassium and magnesium deficiencies. *Am J Cardiol* 1990; **65:** 44–6.
22. Papademetriou V. Magnesium depletion and thiazide hypokalemia. *Arch Intern Med* 1986; **146:** 1026.
23. Ryan MP. Diuretics and potassium/magnesium depletion: directions for treatment. *Am J Med* 1987; **82** (suppl 3A): 38–47.

SODIUM. Diuretic therapy is a common cause of hyponatraemia.[1-3] Dilutional hyponatraemia may occur in patients with heart failure, but hyponatraemia may also result from sodium depletion[1] or inappropriate antidiuretic hormone secretion.[4] Other suggested mechanisms include decreased renal clearance of free water, hypomagnesaemia, and intracellular potassium depletion.[3,5] There have been a number of reports suggesting that hyponatraemia may be a particular problem with combinations of hydrochlorothiazide and potassium-sparing diuretics,[6-8] especially in elderly patients. The effect may be exacerbated by the relatively high doses of thiazide present in some fixed-dose preparations.[9] The symptoms of hyponatraemia may be non-specific and include nausea, lethargy, weakness, mental confusion, and anorexia,[1,2] but it may be an important cause of morbidity.[2,5] Severe sequelae of hyponatraemia include tonic-clonic seizures[10] and clinical features resembling subarachnoid haemorrhage.[11,12] Some patients, especially the elderly, may be particularly susceptible to the hyponatraemic effects of thiazide diuretics, possibly as a result of inappropriate secretion of antidiuretic hormone.[4] Plasma electrolyte concentrations should be monitored in patients receiving long-term diuretic therapy.[3,10] Friedman[5] has demonstrated that measurement of serum-sodium concentration and body-weight following a single dose of thiazide could be useful in identifying patients at increased risk of developing hyponatraemia.

1. Roberts CJC, *et al.* Hyponatraemia: adverse effect of diuretic treatment. *Br Med J* 1977; **1:** 210.
2. Kennedy PGE, *et al.* Severe hyponatraemia in hospital inpatients. *Br Med J* 1978; **2:** 1251–3.
3. Walters EG, *et al.* Hyponatraemia associated with diuretics. *Br J Clin Pract* 1987; **41:** 841–4.
4. Sonnenblick M, *et al.* Thiazide-induced hyponatremia and vasopressin release. *Ann Intern Med* 1989; **110:** 751.
5. Friedman E, *et al.* Thiazide-induced hyponatremia: reproducibility by single dose rechallenge and an analysis of pathogenesis. *Ann Intern Med* 1989; **110:** 24–30.
6. Strykers PH, *et al.* Hyponatremia induced by a combination of amiloride and hydrochlorothiazide. *JAMA* 1984; **252:** 389.
7. Roberts CJC, *et al.* Hyponatraemia induced by a combination of hydrochlorothiazide and triamterene. *Br Med J* 1984; **288:** 1962.
8. Millson D, *et al.* Hyponatraemia and Moduretic (amiloride plus hydrochlorothiazide). *Br Med J* 1984; **289:** 1308–9.
9. Bayer AJ, *et al.* Plasma electrolytes in elderly patients taking fixed combination diuretics. *Postgrad Med J* 1986; **62:** 159–62.
10. Johnston C, *et al.* Hyponatraemia and Moduretic-grand mal seizures: a review. *J R Soc Med* 1989; **82:** 479–83.
11. Benfield GFA, *et al.* Dilutional hyponatraemia masquerading as subarachnoid haemorrhage in patient on hydrochlorothiazide/amiloride/timolol combined drug. *Lancet* 1986; **ii:** 341.
12. Bain PG, *et al.* Thiazide-induced dilutional hyponatraemia masquerading as subarachnoid haemorrhage. *Lancet* 1986; **ii:** 634.

Effects on the gallbladder. There is an increased risk of patients taking thiazide diuretics developing cholecystitis, with some indication that risk increases with the duration of treatment.[1,2] van der Linden and colleagues[2] also concluded that this increased risk was confined to patients with pre-existing gallstones. In a study in 10 healthy subjects,[3] hydrochlorothiazide was found to induce modest changes in biliary lipid concentrations although it was not associated with supersaturation of the bile. It was concluded that these changes could not wholly explain any increase in gallbladder disease in patients taking thiazides. However, evidence is conflicting. Porter[4] and Kakar[5] both found no association between thiazide use and cholecystitis, except possibly in women who are not overweight.[5]

1. Rosenberg L, *et al.* Thiazides and acute cholecystitis. *N Engl J Med* 1980; **303:** 546–8.
2. van der Linden W, *et al.* Acute cholecystitis and thiazides. *Br Med J* 1984; **289:** 654–5.
3. Angelin B. Effect of thiazide treatment on biliary lipid composition in healthy volunteers. *Eur J Clin Pharmacol* 1989; **37:** 95–6.
4. Porter JB, *et al.* Acute cholecystitis and thiazides. *N Engl J Med* 1981; **304:** 954–5.
5. Kakar F, *et al.* Thiazide use and the risk of cholecystectomy in women. *Am J Epidemiol* 1986; **124:** 428–33.

Effects on glucose metabolism. The adverse effects of thiazide diuretics on glucose metabolism, such as insulin resistance, impaired glucose tolerance, precipitation of overt diabetes, and worsening of diabetic control, are well established but appear to be dose-related and may not be significant at lower doses (for example, hydrochlorothiazide 6.25 or 12.5 mg).[1] However, higher doses, for example bendrofluazide 5 mg twice daily, as used in the Medical Research Council Study on Mild to Moderate Hypertension[2] resulted in an incidence of glucose intolerance that led to withdrawal from the study of 9.38 per 1000 patient-years in men and 6.01 per 1000 patient-years in women compared with 2.51 and 0.82 per 1000 patient-years respectively in patients taking placebo.

In a study[3] in 16 non-diabetic hypertensive patients, bendrofluazide, in a dose of 1.25 mg daily, had no effect on insulin sensitivity whereas a daily dose of 5 mg produced hepatic insulin resistance.

1. Neutel JM. Metabolic manifestations of low-dose diuretics. *Am J Med* 1996; **101** (suppl 3A): 71S–82S.
2. Greenburg G. Adverse reactions to bendrofluazide and propranolol for the treatment of mild hypertension: report of Medical Research Council Working Party on Mild to Moderate Hypertension. *Lancet* 1981; **ii:** 539–43.
3. Harper R, *et al.* Effects of low dose versus conventional dose thiazide diuretic on insulin action in essential hypertension. *Br Med J* 1994; **309:** 226–30.

Effects on the kidneys. Thiazide diuretics can produce acute renal failure either from over-enthusiastic use producing saline depletion and hypovolaemia or, occasionally, as a result of a hypersensitivity reaction.[1] Acute interstitial nephritis has been reported.[2,3] They can occasionally cause the formation of non-opaque urate calculi.[4]

1. Curtis JR. Diseases of the urinary system: drug-induced renal disorders: I. *Br Med J* 1977; **2:** 242–4.
2. Linton AL, *et al.* Acute interstitial nephritis due to drugs: review of the literature with a report of nine cases. *Ann Intern Med* 1980; **93:** 735–41.
3. Anonymous. Case records of the Massachusetts General Hospital: case 42-1983. *N Engl J Med* 1983; **309:** 970–8.
4. Curtis JR. Diseases of the urinary system: drug-induced renal disorders: II. *Br Med J* 1977; **2:** 375–7.

Effects on lipids. Thiazide diuretics have been reported to adversely affect the plasma-lipid profile in the short term by increasing concentrations of low-density and very low-density lipoprotein cholesterol, as well as of triglycerides, but not of high-density lipoprotein cholesterol.[1] These effects are probably dose-related[2] and it has been argued that changes in plasma lipids are likely to be slight at the relatively low doses of thiazide diuretics now used in the treatment of hypertension. The available evidence has also suggested that these lipid changes may not persist long-term,[3] but this is by no means established. In the Treatment of Mild Hypertension Study (TOMHS),[4] plasma total cholesterol concentrations were increased after 12 months in patients receiving chlorthalidone but this effect was no longer present after 24 months. However, overall there is still concern in some quarters that any hyperlipidaemic effect might offset the benefits of treating hypertension in patients at risk of ischaemic heart disease.

1. Ames R. Effects of diuretic drugs on the lipid profile. *Drugs* 1988; **36** (suppl 2): 33–40.
2. Carlsen JE, *et al.* Relation between dose of bendrofluazide, antihypertensive effect, and adverse biochemical effects. *Br Med J* 1990; **300:** 975–8.
3. Freis ED. Critique of the clinical importance of diuretic-induced hypokalemia and elevated cholesterol level. *Arch Intern Med* 1989; **149:** 2640–8.
4. Grimm RH, *et al.* Long-term effects on plasma lipids of diet and drugs to treat hypertension. *JAMA* 1996; **275:** 1549–56.

Effects on respiratory function. Acute interstitial pneumonitis and acute pulmonary oedema are rare but potentially dangerous complications of thiazide therapy and may be due to a hypersensitivity reaction. A number of cases have been reported,[1-6] frequently following a single dose of hydrochlorothiazide or chlorothiazide. The presenting symptoms could be mistakenly attributed to myocardial infarction.

1. Steinberg AD. Pulmonary edema following ingestion of hydrochlorothiazide. *JAMA* 1968; **204:** 167–9.
2. Beaudry C, Laplante L. Severe allergic pneumonitis from hydrochlorothiazide. *Ann Intern Med* 1973; **78:** 251–3.
3. Parfrey NA, Herlong HF. Pulmonary oedema after hydrochlorothiazide. *Br Med J* 1984; **288:** 1880.
4. Watrigant Y, *et al.* Pneumopathie à l'hydrochlorothiazide d'évolution subaiguë: etude cytologique du lavage broncho-alvéolaire. *Rev Mal Respir* 1986; **4:** 227–9.
5. Klein MD. Noncardiogenic pulmonary edema following hydrochlorothiazide ingestion. *Ann Emerg Med* 1987; **16:** 901–3.
6. Bowden FJ. Non-cardiogenic pulmonary oedema after ingestion of chlorothiazide. *Br Med J* 1989; **298:** 605.

Effects on sexual function. Adverse effects on sexual function have been reported in hypertensive patients receiving thiazide diuretics and other antihypertensives but it is not clear how much this is due to the underlying disease and how much is due to the drugs. In the Medical Research Council Study on Mild to Moderate Hypertension[1] the incidence of impotence in men receiving bendrofluazide or placebo was 19.58 and 0.89 per 1000 patient-years, respectively. In the Treatment of Mild Hypertension Study (TOMHS),[2] which randomised patients to treatment with one of five groups of antihypertensives, the incidence of erectile dysfunction in men was relatively low but was highest in the diuretic group (chlorthalidone treatment). The incidence was significantly higher in chlorthalidone recipients than in placebo recipients at 24 months (17.1 and 8.1% respectively), but the difference was no longer significant at 48 months (18.3 and 16.7% respectively).

1. Greenburg G. Adverse reactions to bendrofluazide and propranolol for the treatment of mild hypertension: report of Medical Research Council Working Party on Mild to Moderate Hypertension. *Lancet* 1981; **ii:** 539–43.
2. Grimm RH, *et al.* Long-term effects on sexual function of five antihypertensive drugs and nutritional hygienic treatment in hypertensive men and women: Treatment of Mild Hypertension Study (TOMHS). *Hypertension* 1997; **29:** 8–14.

Effects on the skin. A variety of rashes and skin reactions has been reported in patients taking hydrochlorothiazide and other thiazide diuretics. *Photosensitivity* reactions are among the most frequently reported skin reactions. In Australia[1] co-amilozide was the preparation most commonly implicated in photosensitivity reactions in reports to the Australian Drug Reactions Advisory Committee, although this may reflect the high usage of this preparation. The most likely mechanism is thought to be phototoxicity[1,2] involving mainly UVA radiation although UVB may be involved in some cases.[2] Chronic photosensitivity does not usually occur following withdrawal of the drug[2] although photosensitivity may persist for longer in some patients than in others.[2,3] Eruptions resembling *lichen planus*[4] and *subacute cutaneous lupus erythematosus*[5-7] may be due to photosensitivity reactions.

Other reported skin reactions include *vasculitis*,[8,9] *erythema multiforme*,[9] and *pseudoporphyria*.[10]

1. Stone K. Photosensitivity reactions to drugs. *Aust J Pharm* 1985; **66:** 415–18.
2. Addo HA, *et al.* Thiazide-induced photosensitivity: a study of 33 subjects. *Br J Dermatol* 1987; **116:** 749–60.
3. Robinson HN, *et al.* Thiazide diuretic therapy and chronic photosensitivity. *Arch Dermatol* 1985; **121:** 522–4.
4. Graham-Brown R. Lichen planus and lichen-planus-like reactions. *Br J Hosp Med* 1986; **36:** 281–4.
5. Jones SK, *et al.* Thiazide diuretic-induced subacute cutaneous lupus-like syndrome. *Br J Dermatol* 1985; **113** (suppl 29): 25.
6. Reed BR, *et al.* Subacute cutaneous lupus erythematosus associated with hydrochlorothiazide therapy. *Ann Intern Med* 1985; **103:** 49–51.
7. Darken M, McBurney EI. Subacute cutaneous lupus erythematosus-like drug eruption due to combination diuretic hydrochlorothiazide and triamterene. *J Am Acad Dermatol* 1988; **18:** 38–42.
8. Björnberg A, Gisslén H. Thiazides: a cause of necrotising vasculitis? *Lancet* 1965; **ii:** 982–3.
9. Hardwick N, Saxe N. Patterns of dermatology referrals in a general hospital. *Br J Dermatol* 1986; **115:** 167–76.
10. Motley RS. Pseudoporphyria due to Dyazide in a patient with vitiligo. *Br Med J* 1990; **300:** 1468.

Gout. Thiazide diuretics have been associated with hyperuricaemia and gout in some patients. In the Medical Research Council Study on Mild to Moderate Hypertension,[1] men receiving bendrofluazide had higher incidences of gout than those receiving placebo (12.23 and 1.03 per 1000 patient-years, respectively). The risk appears to be dose-related; in a retrospective study[2] in patients aged 65 or older receiving antihypertensive therapy, there was a significantly increased risk of starting anti-gout therapy in patients receiving the equivalent of 25 mg hydrochlorothiazide or more daily, but not in those receiving lower doses.

1. Greenburg G. Adverse reactions to bendrofluazide and propranolol for the treatment of mild hypertension: report of Medical Research Council Working Party on Mild to Moderate Hypertension. *Lancet* 1981; **ii:** 539–43.
2. Gurwitz JH, *et al.* Thiazide diuretics and the initiation of anti-gout therapy. *J Clin Epidemiol* 1997; **50:** 953–9.

Withdrawal. For a report of oedema following withdrawal of thiazide diuretics, see under Precautions, below.

Treatment of Adverse Effects

Hypokalaemia in patients treated with thiazide diuretics may be avoided or treated by concurrent administration of potassium or a potassium-sparing diuretic (but see the discussion on potassium supplements, under Effects on Electrolyte Balance in Adverse Effects, above). Potassium loss can also be reduced by moderate sodium restriction. With the exception of patients with conditions such as liver failure or kidney disease, chloride deficiency is usually mild and does not require specific treatment. Apart from the rare occasions when it is life-threatening, dilutional hyponatraemia is best treated with water restriction rather than salt therapy; in true hyponatraemia, appropriate replacement is the treatment of choice (see p.1150).

In massive overdosage, treatment should be symptomatic and directed at fluid and electrolyte replacement. In the case of recent ingestion gastric lavage should be carried out.

Precautions

All diuretics produce changes in fluid and electrolyte balance (see under Adverse Effects, above). They should be used with caution in patients with existing fluid and electrolyte disturbances or who are at risk from changes in fluid and electrolyte balance, such as the elderly. They should be avoided in patients with severe hepatic impairment, in whom encephalopathy may be precipitated. Patients with hepatic cirrhosis are also more likely to develop hypokalaemia. Hyponatraemia may occur in patients with severe heart failure who are very oedematous, particularly with large doses of thiazides in conjunction with restricted salt in the diet. All patients should be carefully observed for signs of fluid and electrolyte imbalance, especially in the presence of vomiting or during parenteral fluid therapy. Thiazide diuretics should not be given to patients with Addison's disease.

Diuretics should also be given with caution in renal impairment since they can further reduce renal function. Most thiazide diuretics are not effective in patients with a creatinine clearance of less than 30 mL per minute. They should not be used in patients with severe renal impairment or anuria.

Thiazides may precipitate attacks of gout in susceptible patients. They may cause hyperglycaemia and aggravate or unmask diabetes mellitus. Blood-glucose concentrations should be monitored in patients taking antidiabetics, since requirements may change. Thiazides can reduce urinary excretion of calcium, sometimes resulting in mild hypercalcaemia; thiazides should not be given to patients with pre-existing hypercalcaemia. There is a possibility that thiazide diuretics may exacerbate or activate systemic lupus erythematosus in susceptible patients. For a suggestion that thiazide diuretics may increase the risk of developing gallstones, see under Effects on the Gallbladder, above.

Thiazides cross the placenta and there have been reports of neonatal jaundice, thrombocytopenia, and electrolyte imbalances following maternal treatment. Reductions in maternal blood volume could also adversely affect placental perfusion. Thiazide diuretics are distributed into breast milk. Treatment with large doses of thiazide diuretics can inhibit lactation.

Hyperparathyroidism. Hypertension is a complication of primary hyperparathyroidism but thiazides have often been withheld for fear of exacerbating hypercalcaemia. However, no differences in plasma-calcium concentrations were found in 13 patients who received thiazides intermittently for up to 18 months. It was therefore concluded that thiazide diuretics are not contra-indicated in such patients.[1] They should, however, be stopped before parathyroid function is tested.

1. Farquhar CW, *et al.* Failure of thiazide diuretics to increase plasma calcium in mild primary hyperparathyroidism. *Postgrad Med J* 1990; **66:** 714–16.

Withdrawal. In patients with mild hypertension whose blood pressure is consistently controlled, reduction in dosage on withdrawal of antihypertensive drugs may be possible. Serious oedema occurred in 8 patients with controlled hypertension within 2 weeks of abrupt withdrawal of thiazide diuretics.[1] Thiazides were resumed and gradually tapered without recurrence of oedema.

1. Brandspigel K. Diuretic-withdrawal edema. *N Engl J Med* 1986; **314:** 515.

Interactions

Many of the interactions of hydrochlorothiazide and other thiazide diuretics are due to their effects on fluid and electrolyte balance. Diuretic-induced hypokalaemia may enhance the toxicity of digitalis glycosides and may also increase the risk of arrhythmias with drugs that prolong the QT interval, such as astemizole, terfenadine, halofantrine, pimozide, and sotalol. Thiazides may enhance the neuromuscular blocking action of competitive muscle relaxants, such as tubocurarine, probably by their hypokalaemic effect. The potassium-depleting effect of diuretics may be enhanced by corticosteroids, corticotrophin, beta$_2$ agonists such as salbutamol, carbenoxolone, or amphotericin.

Diuretics may enhance the effect of other antihypertensives, particularly the first-dose hypotension that occurs with alpha blockers or ACE inhibitors. Postural hypotension associated with diuretic therapy may be enhanced by concomitant ingestion of alcohol, barbiturates, or opioids. The antihypertensive effects of diuretics may be antagonised by drugs that cause fluid retention, such as corticosteroids, NSAIDs, or carbenoxolone. Thiazides have been reported to diminish the response to pressor amines, such as noradrenaline, but the clinical significance of this effect is uncertain.

Thiazide diuretics should not usually be administered concomitantly with lithium since the association may lead to toxic blood concentrations of lithium (see p.294). Other drugs for which increased toxicity has been reported when given concomitantly with thiazides include allopurinol and tetracyclines. Thiazides may alter the requirements for hypoglycaemic drugs in diabetic patients.

Antibacterials. Severe hyponatraemia has been reported in patients taking trimethoprim with co-amilozide[1] and hydrochlorothiazide.[2]

1. Eastell R, Edmonds CJ. Hyponatraemia associated with trimethoprim and a diuretic. *Br Med J* 1984; **289:** 1658–9.
2. Hart TL, *et al.* Hyponatremia secondary to thiazide-trimethoprim interaction. *Can J Hosp Pharm* 1989; **42:** 243–6.

Anticoagulants. For reference to a lack of interaction between warfarin and thiazide diuretics, see p.968.

Antiepileptics. Report of symptomatic hyponatraemia associated with concomitant use of hydrochlorothiazide or frusemide and carbamazepine.[1]

1. Yassa R, *et al.* Carbamazepine, diuretics, and hyponatremia: a possible interaction. *J Clin Psychiatry* 1987; **48:** 281–3.

Bile-acid binding resins. Gastro-intestinal absorption of both chlorothiazide and hydrochlorothiazide has been reported to be reduced by colestipol and cholestyramine.[1-3] In a study in healthy subjects[2] cholestyramine had the greatest effect on hydrochlorothiazide, decreasing absorption by 85% compared with a decrease of 43% with colestipol. Even when cholestyramine was administered 4 hours after hydrochlorothiazide[3] reductions of absorption of at least 30 to 35% could be expected.

1. Kauffman RE, Azarnoff DL. Effect of colestipol on gastrointestinal absorption of chlorothiazide in man. *Clin Pharmacol Ther* 1973; **14:** 886–90.
2. Hunninghake DB, *et al.* The effect of cholestyramine and colestipol on the absorption of hydrochlorothiazide. *Int J Clin Pharmacol Ther Toxicol* 1982; **20:** 151–4.
3. Hunninghake DB, Hibbard DM. Influence of time intervals for cholestyramine dosing on the absorption of hydrochlorothiazide. *Clin Pharmacol Ther* 1986; **39:** 329–34.

Calcium salts. The milk-alkali syndrome, characterised by hypercalcaemia, metabolic alkalosis, and renal failure, developed in a patient taking chlorothiazide and moderately large doses of calcium carbonate.[1] Patients taking thiazide diuretics may be at increased risk of developing the milk-alkali syndrome because of their reduced ability to excrete excess calcium. Hypercalcaemia may also occur in patients taking thiazides with drugs that increase calcium levels, such as vitamin D.

1. Gora ML, *et al.* Milk-alkali syndrome associated with use of chlorothiazide and calcium carbonate. *Clin Pharm* 1989; **8:** 227–9.

Dopaminergics. For a report of increased amantadine toxicity associated with hydrochlorothiazide and triamterene, see p.1130.

NSAIDs. Discussion of antagonism of the diuretic actions of thiazides by NSAIDs.[1]

1. Webster J. Interactions of NSAIDs with diuretics and β-blockers: mechanisms and clinical implications. *Drugs* 1985; **30:** 32–41.

Pharmacokinetics

Hydrochlorothiazide is fairly rapidly absorbed from the gastro-intestinal tract. It is reported to have a bioavailability of about 65 to 70%. It has been estimated to have a plasma half-life of between about 5 and 15 hours and appears to be preferentially bound to red blood cells. It is excreted mainly unchanged in the urine. Hydrochlorothiazide crosses the placental barrier and is distributed into breast milk.

References.

1. Beermann B, *et al.* Absorption, metabolism, and excretion of hydrochlorothiazide. *Clin Pharmacol Ther* 1976: **19:** 531–7.
2. Beermann B, Groschinsky-Grind M. Pharmacokinetics of hydrochlorothiazide in man. *Eur J Clin Pharmacol* 1977; **12:** 297–303.
3. Beermann B, Groschinsky-Grind M. Pharmacokinetics of hydrochlorothiazide in patients with congestive heart failure. *Br J Clin Pharmacol* 1979: **7:** 579–83.

Uses and Administration

Hydrochlorothiazide and the other thiazide diuretics are used in the treatment of oedema associated with heart failure (p.785) and with renal and hepatic disorders. They are also used in hypertension (p.788), either alone or together with other antihypertensives such as ACE inhibitors (p.805) and beta blockers (p.828). Other indications have included the treatment of oedema accompanying the premenstrual syndrome, the prevention of water retention associated with corticosteroids and oestrogens, the treatment of diabetes insipidus (below), and the prevention of renal calculus formation in patients with hypercalciuria (below).

Thiazides are moderately potent diuretics and exert their diuretic effect by reducing the reabsorption of electrolytes from the renal tubules, thereby increasing the excretion of sodium and chloride ions, and consequently of water. They act mainly at the beginning of the distal tubules. The excretion of other electrolytes, notably potassium and magnesium, is also increased. The excretion of calcium is reduced. They also reduce carbonic-anhydrase activity so that bicarbonate excretion is increased, but this effect is generally small compared with the effect on chloride excretion and does not appreciably alter the pH of the urine. They may also reduce the glomerular filtration rate.

Their hypotensive effect is probably partly due to a reduction in peripheral resistance; they also enhance the effects of other antihypertensives. Paradoxically, thiazides have an antidiuretic effect in patients with diabetes insipidus.

Administration and dosage. Thiazides are usually given in the morning so that sleep is not interrupted by diuresis. Diuresis is initiated in about 2 hours following the oral administration of hydrochlorothiazide, reaches a maximum in about 4 hours, and lasts for 6 to 12 hours.

The dosage of thiazides should be adjusted to the minimum effective dose, especially in the elderly, and in recent years there has been a definite trend towards lower doses. In general lower doses are required for the treatment of hypertension than for oedema, although the maximum therapeutic effect may not be seen for several weeks.

They may be given to patients with mild renal impairment, but thiazides are generally not effective at a creatinine clearance of less than 30 mL per minute. Some have recommended that the dose of hydrochlorothiazide should be halved when there is moderate renal impairment (a creatinine clearance of 30 to 70 mL per minute).

Hydrochlorothiazide is given by mouth.

In the treatment of **oedema** the usual dose is 25 to 100 mg daily, reduced to a dose of 25 to 50 mg daily or intermittently; in severe cases initial doses of up to 200 mg daily have been recommended, but the more powerful loop diuretics (see Frusemide, p.871) are preferred in such patients.

In the treatment of **hypertension** the usual dose of hydrochlorothiazide is 25 to 50 mg daily, either alone, or in conjunction with other antihypertensives. In some patients an initial dose of 12.5 mg may be sufficient. Doses of up to 100 mg have been recommended but are rarely necessary.

In the treatment of nephrogenic **diabetes insipidus** an initial dose of up to 100 mg daily has been suggested.

A suggested initial dose for children has been 1 to 2 mg per kg body-weight daily in 2 divided doses. Infants under 6 months may need doses of up to 3 mg per kg daily.

The routine use of potassium supplements is no longer recommended in patients taking thiazide diuretics. Clinically significant hypokalaemia is unlikely to occur with the low doses used in hypertension. However, the concomitant administration of a potassium-sparing diuretic such as amiloride (p.819) or, less usually, a potassium supplement may be necessary in patients at risk from hypokalaemia such as those taking digitalis preparations, those with cirrhosis of the liver, those receiving high doses of diuretics long-term, and those taking other potassium-depleting drugs concurrently.

Bronchopulmonary dysplasia. Bronchopulmonary dysplasia (p.1018) is a major cause of chronic lung disease in infants. Treatment often involves the use of corticosteroids. Additional supportive therapy has included the use of diuretics such as frusemide (p.873); results with hydrochlorothiazide or spironolactone have been more ambiguous. No beneficial effects on lung function or oxygenation were found in a study of 12 infants after 1 week of treatment with hydrochlorothiazide and spironolactone.[1] However, hydrochlorothiazide and spironolactone therapy was found to improve total respiratory system compliance with decreased lung damage and increased survival rate in 34 premature infants with bronchopulmonary dysplasia after 8 weeks of therapy.[2] In the latter study frusemide was also administered if clinically indicated.

1. Engelhardt B, *et al.* Effect of spironolactone-hydrochlorothiazide on lung function in infants with chronic bronchopulmonary dysplasia. *J Pediatr* 1989; **114:** 619–24.
2. Albersheim SG, *et al.* Randomized, double-blind, controlled trial of long-term diuretic therapy for bronchopulmonary dysplasia. *J Pediatr* 1989; **115:** 615–20.

Diabetes insipidus. Thiazide diuretics are used in nephrogenic diabetes insipidus (p.1237), sometimes combined with potassium-sparing diuretics. For instance, hydrochlorothiazide with amiloride was effective in controlling nephrogenic diabetes insipidus in 5 boys and compared favourably with treatment with hydrochlorothiazide in combination with indomethacin.[1] Treatment was well tolerated in 4 patients. Abdominal pain and anorexia necessitated withdrawal of amiloride in the fifth patient after six months of treatment. The use of hydrochlorothiazide with amiloride also obviated the need for potassium supplements, which were required with hydrochlorothiazide and indomethacin.

1. Knoers N, Monnens LAH. Amiloride-hydrochlorothiazide versus indomethacin-hydrochlorothiazide in the treatment of nephrogenic diabetes insipidus. *J Pediatr* 1990; **117:** 499–502.

Hypoparathyroidism. In hypoparathyroidism (p.733), treatment is usually with oral vitamin D compounds to correct the hypocalcaemia. Thiazide diuretics may be useful in some patients. Beneficial effects on serum-calcium concentrations in patients with hypoparathyroidism have been reported following treatment with chlorthalidone plus dietary salt restriction[1] and with bendrofluazide.[2] However, chlorthalidone has not been found to be effective in all patients,[3] and the reduction in urinary calcium excretion by thiazides has been shown to be diminished in patients with hypoparathyroidism[4] suggesting that this effect may be dependent on the presence of active parathyroid hormone. Care should be taken when administering diuretics to hypoparathyroid patients with co-existing adrenal insufficiency[3] or metabolic alkalosis.[5]

1. Porter RH, *et al.* Treatment of hypoparathyroid patients with chlorthalidone. *N Engl J Med* 1978; **298:** 577–81.
2. Newman GH, *et al.* Effect of bendrofluazide on calcium reabsorption in hypoparathyroidism. *Eur J Clin Pharmacol* 1984; **27:** 41–6.
3. Gertner JM, Genel M. Chlorthalidone for hypoparathyroidism. *N Engl J Med* 1978; **298:** 1478.
4. Middler S, *et al.* Thiazide diuretics and calcium metabolism. *Metabolism* 1973; **22:** 139–45.
5. Barzel US. Chlorthalidone for hypoparathyroidism. *N Engl J Med* 1978; **289:** 1478.

Ménière's disease. In Ménière's disease (p.400) there is an excess of endolymph fluid in the ear and diuretics such as hydrochlorothiazide have been used in attempts to relieve symptoms by reducing the amount of fluid.

Osteoporosis. Although some studies have indicated beneficial effects of thiazide diuretics on bone (reduced rates of bone loss[1] and a reduced risk of hip fracture[2-4]) a comprehensive analysis involving 9704 women over the age of 65 years[5] showed only a small effect on bone mass, no effect on the risk for falls, and no overall protective effect against fractures. Thus, thiazides have no established role in the prevention or treatment of osteoporosis (p.731). They might, however, be useful to reduce hypercalciuria in patients taking glucocorticoids[6] but serum-potassium concentrations should be monitored closely.

1. Wasnich R, *et al.* Effect of thiazide on rates of bone mineral loss: a longitudinal study. *Br Med J* 1990; **301:** 1303–5. Correction. *ibid.* 1991; **302:** 218.
2. LaCroix AZ, *et al.* Thiazide diuretic agents and the incidence of hip fracture. *N Engl J Med* 1990; **322:** 286–90.
3. Ray WA, *et al.* Long-term use of thiazide diuretics and risk of hip fracture. *Lancet* 1989; **i:** 687–90.
4. Felson DT, *et al.* Thiazide diuretics and the risk of hip fracture: results from the Framingham Study. *JAMA* 1991; **265:** 370–3.
5. Cauley JA, *et al.* Effects of thiazide diuretic therapy on bone mass, fractures, and falls. *Ann Intern Med* 1993; **118:** 666–73.
6. Lukert BP, Raisz LG. Glucocorticoid-induced osteoporosis: pathogenesis and management. *Ann Intern Med* 1990; **112:** 352–64.

Renal calculi. Normal urine contains calcium, oxalate, and phosphate in amounts greater than their normal aqueous solubility; this supersaturation is maintained by a variety of inhibitors of crystallisation, both organic and inorganic. However, increases in the concentrations of crystalline substances in the urine, or decreases in the relative proportions of crystallisation inhibitors, may render individuals susceptible to the formation of renal calculi (kidney stones).

Renal calculi consist of crystalline components arranged around an organic matrix. They are typically formed in the calices or renal pelvis, and may become lodged in the ureter. About 1 to 5% of the population are affected, and although some patients only ever develop a single stone, between 50 and 80% of patients experience subsequent recurrences. Calcium-containing stones (usually calcium oxalate and calcium phosphate in variable proportions) account for the vast majority of occurrences although stones of other compositions including cystine, uric acid, or magnesium ammonium phosphate, are occasionally seen.

Patients with renal calculi may be asymptomatic or may pass small stones with relatively little discomfort. However, passage of a larger stone down the ureter may be accompanied by excruciating pain (renal or ureteral colic), obstruction, and trauma; there may also be associated infection.

Treatment. Treatment of existing stones, if any, is essentially surgical, while medical treatment is aimed at prevention of recurrence. In the acute episode analgesics may be required for the pain (see Colic Pain, p.8) but if there is no obstruction, infection, or other complication conservative treatment is favoured, with the patient being monitored radiographically over several weeks to see if the stone will pass of its own accord. Where intervention is considered necessary, it may be by open or endoscopic surgery, or shock wave lithotripsy, in which focussed shock waves are used to shatter the stone. Antibacterials may be needed for infection (see p.149 for urinary-tract infections).

In the prevention of recurrence it is important to identify, and where possible correct, any underlying disease process or biochemical or anatomical abnormality. Certain general measures are also appropriate. Patients should drink a minimum of 3 litres of fluid daily in order to maintain an adequate volume of urine. In hot climates or working environments a higher volume of fluid should be taken.

Dietary restrictions may be appropriate in some cases. Traditionally, dairy products and other foods rich in calcium, as well as calcium-containing antacids and vitamin D supplements, have been avoided in patients with calcium-containing stones. However, recent studies have found an inverse relationship between dietary calcium intake and the risk of stone formation in men[1] and in women,[2] and restriction of dietary calcium is probably not necessary.[3] Conversely, calcium supplements do appear to increase the risk of stone formation and should be avoided, although the reason for this difference is not clear.[2] Limitation of the intake of animal protein and oxalate-rich foods, including tea, is also probably appropriate in such patients,[4] and sodium restriction may also be beneficial.

In patients with idiopathic hypercalciuria (i.e. when excessive calcium excretion cannot be linked to hyperparathyroidism, sarcoidosis, malignancy, or some other underlying condition) and a history of renal calculi a **thiazide diuretic** is usually given. Such therapy has generally[5,6] though not universally[7] been found effective, although the benefit may decline with time. A potassium supplement, or combination with the potassium-sparing diuretic amiloride, may be necessary to avoid hypokalaemia. Hydrochlorothiazide or amiloride have also been reported to be of benefit in patients with a history of calcium oxalate stones due to a defect in oxalate transport,[8] while thiazide treatment or oral phosphates have been found effective in decreasing urinary calcium excretion in patients with absorptive hypercalciuria.[9] Where thiazide treatment is ineffective treatment with sodium cellulose phosphate may be considered, together with a magnesium supplement. Sodium cellulose phosphate is of value in patients with excessive intestinal calcium absorption.[10] Phosphate salts[10] or magnesium salts[11,12] which act as nonspecific inhibitors of urinary crystallisation may also be used.

In patients with reduced citrate excretion treatment with potassium citrate may be useful in preventing stone recurrence;[13] by increasing urinary pH, it may also be helpful in patients with uric acid stones. Allopurinol has also been suggested, both for uric acid and for calcium oxalate stone prevention, although the latter has been a matter of debate.[14,15]

In patients with struvite (magnesium ammonium phosphate) stones, which are associated with bacterial infection and result from the action of bacterial urease, control may be difficult to achieve using antibacterials alone; acetohydroxamic acid, an inhibitor of bacterial urease, has been given as an adjunct.[16,17] Penicillamine may be of benefit in preventing cystine stones in patients with cystinuria (p.991).

1. Curhan GC, *et al.* A prospective study of dietary calcium and other nutrients and the risk of symptomatic kidney stones. *N Engl J Med* 1993; **328:** 833–8.
2. Curhan GC, *et al.* Comparison of dietary calcium with supplemental calcium and other nutrients as factors affecting the risk for kidney stones in women. *Ann Intern Med* 1997; **126:** 497–504.
3. Coe FL, *et al.* Diet and calcium: the end of an era? *Ann Intern Med* 1997; **126:** 553–5.
4. Lemann J. Composition of the diet and calcium kidney stones. *N Engl J Med* 1993; **328:** 880–2.
5. Yendt ER, *et al.* The use of thiazides in the prevention of renal calculi. *Can Med Assoc J* 1970; **102:** 614–20.
6. Laerum E, Larsen S. Thiazide prophylaxis of urolithiasis: a double-blind study in general practice. *Acta Med Scand* 1984; **215:** 383–9.
7. Scholz D, *et al.* Double-blind study with thiazide in recurrent calcium lithiasis. *J Urol (Baltimore)* 1982; **128:** 903–7.
8. Baggio B, *et al.* An inheritable anomaly of red-cell oxalate transport in "primary" calcium nephrolithiasis correctable with diuretics. *N Engl J Med* 1986; **314:** 599–604.
9. Insogna KL, *et al.* Trichlormethiazide and oral phosphate therapy in patients with absorptive hypercalciuria. *J Urol (Baltimore)* 1989; **141:** 269–74.
10. Pak CYC. Formation of renal stones may be prevented by restoring normal urinary composition. *Proc Eur Dial Transplant Assoc* 1983; **20:** 371–85.
11. Melnick I, *et al.* Magnesium therapy for recurring calcium oxalate urinary calculi. *J Urol (Baltimore)* 1971; **105:** 119–22.
12. Johansson G, *et al.* Biochemical and clinical effects of the prophylactic treatment of renal calcium stones with magnesium hydroxide. *J Urol (Baltimore)* 1980; **124:** 770–4.
13. Pak CYC, Fuller C. Idiopathic hypocitraturic calcium-oxalate nephrolithiasis successfully treated with potassium citrate. *Ann Intern Med* 1986; **104:** 33–7.
14. Ettinger B, *et al.* Randomized trial of allopurinol in the prevention of calcium oxalate calculi. *N Engl J Med* 1986; **315:** 1386–9.
15. Tiselius H-G, *et al.* Clinical results of allopurinol treatment in prevention of calcium oxalate stone formation. *J Urol (Baltimore)* 1986; **136:** 50–3.
16. Martelli A, *et al.* Acetohydroxamic acid therapy in infected renal stones. *Urology* 1981; **17:** 320–2.
17. Williams JJ, *et al.* A randomized double-blind study of acetohydroxamic acid in struvite nephrolithiasis. *N Engl J Med* 1984; **311:** 760–4.

Preparations

BP 1998: Co-amilozide Oral Solution; Co-amilozide Tablets; Co-triamterzide Tablets; Hydrochlorothiazide Tablets;
USP 23: Amiloride Hydrochloride and Hydrochlorothiazide Tablets; Captopril and Hydrochlorothiazide Tablets; Enalapril Maleate and Hydrochlorothiazide Tablets; Hydrochlorothiazide Tablets; Methyldopa and Hydrochlorothiazide Tablets; Metoprolol Tartrate and Hydrochlorothiazide Tablets; Propranolol Hydrochloride and Hydrochlorothiazide Extended-release Capsules; Propranolol Hydrochloride and Hydrochlorothiazide Tablets; Reserpine and Hydrochlorothiazide Tablets; Reserpine, Hydralazine Hydrochloride, and Hydrochlorothiazide Tablets; Spironolactone and Hydrochlorothiazide Tablets; Timolol Maleate and Hydrochlorothiazide Tablets; Triamterene and Hydrochlorothiazide Capsules; Triamterene and Hydrochlorothiazide Tablets.

Proprietary Preparations (details are given in Part 3)
Aust.: Dithiazid†; Esidrex; ***Austral.:*** Dichlotride; ***Belg.:*** Dichlotride; Esidrex; ***Canad.:*** Apo-Hydro; HydroDiuril; Novo-Hydrazide; ***Fr.:*** Esidrex; ***Ger.:*** Disalunil; diu-melusin; Esidrix; Thiazid-Wolff†; ***Irl.:*** HydroSaluric; ***Ital.:*** Esidrex; Idrodiuvis†; ***Neth.:*** Dichlotride; Esidrex; ***Norw.:*** Dichlotride; Esidrex; ***S.Afr.:*** Dichlotride; ***Spain:*** Acuretic; Esidrex; Hidrosaluretil; ***Swed.:*** Dichlotride; Esidrex; ***Switz.:*** Esidrex; ***UK:*** Esidrex†; HydroSaluric; ***USA:*** Diaqua; Esidrix; Hydro-Chlor; Hydro-Z; HydroDiuril; Hydromal; Hydrozide; Microzide; Mictrin; Oretic; Thiuretic.

Multi-ingredient: ***Aust.:*** Accuzide; Acecomb; Adelphan-Esidrex; Adelphan-Esidrex-K†; Aldoretic; Amiloretik; Amilorid comp; Beloc comp; Capozide; Captopril Compositum; Cibadrex; Co-Renitec; Concor Plus; Confit; Corindocomb; Deverol mit Thiazid; Diurid; Dytide H; Elfanex; Hypren plus; Inderal comp; Inhibace Plus; Lanuretic; Loradur; Metolol compositum; Moducrin; Moduretic; Prinzide; Resaltex; Salodiur; Seloken retard Plus; Supergan; Supracid; Tardurol; Triamteren comp; Triloc; Tritazide; Zestoretic; ***Austral.:*** Amizide; Dyazide; Hydrene; Hydrozide; Modizide; Moduretic; ***Belg.:*** Accuretic; Belidral; Co-Inhibace; Co-Renitec; Dytenzide; Emcoretic; Esidrex-K†; Kalten; Maxsoten; Maxzide; Moduretic; Novazyd; Sectrazide; Selozide; Uractazide; Zestoretic; Zok-Zid; ***Canad.:*** Aldactazide; Aldoril; Apo-Amilzide; Apo-Methazide; Apo-Triazide; Dyazide; Hydropres; Inderide; Ismelin Esidrix†; Moduret; Novamilor; Novo-Doparil; Novo-Spirozine; Novo-Triamzide; Nu-Amilzide; Nu-Triazide; Prinzide; Ser-Ap-Es; Serpasil-Esidrix†; Timolide; Vaseretic; Viskazide; Zestoretic; ***Fr.:*** Acuilix; Briazide; Captea; Cibadrex; Co-Renitec; Ecazide; Esimil†; Hyzaar; Koretic; Moducren; Moduretic; Prestole; Prinzide; Zestoretic; ***Ger.:*** Accuzide; Acercomp; Adelphan-Esidrix; Amiduret; Amilo-OPT†; Amiloretik; Amilorid comp; Amilothiazid; Amilozid; Aquaretic; Barotonal; Beloc comp; Beloc-Zok comp; Beta-Nephral; Beta-Turfa; Betathiazid; Betathiazid A; Calmoserpin†; Capozide; Cibadrex; Combiprotect†; Concor Plus; Coric plus; Corindocomb; Delix plus; Dignoretik; Disalpin; Diu Venostasin; Diu-Tonolytril†; Diuretikum Verla; Diursan; Diutensat; Diutensat comp; Dociteren; Dociton Dytide H†; duradiuret; durarese; Dynorm Plus; Dytide H; Elfanex†; Esimil; Esiteren; Fondril-5 HCT; Haemiton compositum; Hydrocomp; Hypertorr; Jenateren comp; Manimon; Metocomp; Meto-thiazid; Metodura comp; Metohexal Comp; Metostad Comp; Minoremed†; Modu-Puren; Moducrin; Moduretik; Nephral; Pres plus; Propra comp; Renacor; Resaltex; Rhefluin; Risicordin; Sali-Puren; Slimin†; Sotaziden†; Spironothiazid; Tensobon comp; Thiazid-comp.; Trasicor Esidrix†; Treloc; Tri-Thiazid; Tri-Thiazid Reserpin; Triampur; Triamteren comp; Triamteren-H; Triarese; Triazid; Triniton; Turfa; Veratide; Vesdil plus; ***Irl.:*** Accuretic; Amizide†; Capozide; Carace Plus; Clonuretic; Co-Betaloc; Dyazide; Hydromet; Innozide; Moducren; Moduret; Moduretic; Secadrex; Sotazide†; Zestoretic; ***Ital.:*** Accuretic; Acediur; Aceplus; Acequide; Acesistem; Adelfan-Esidrex†; Aldactazide; Aldotride†; Cibadrex; Condiuren; Diertina Ipotensiva†; Elidiur; Fosicombi; Hizaar; Idroquark; Inibace Plus; Initiss Plus; Losazid; Medozide; Moduretic; Neo-Lotan Plus; Prinzide; Quinazide; Raufluin†; Raunova Plus†; Selozide; Sermidrina†; Sfigmoreg†; Spiridazide; Tensadiur; Tensozide; Triamteril Complex†; Triatec HCT; Vallizina†; Vasoretic; Zestoretic; Zinadiur; ***Neth.:*** Aceplus; Acuzide; Capozide; Cibadrex; Co-Renitec; Dytenzide; Emcoretic; Hydromet†; Hykaten†; Hyzaar; Moducren; Moduretic; Novazyd; Ranezide†; Renitec Plus; Secadrex; Selokomb; Tritazide; Vascase Plus; Zestoretic; ***Norw.:*** Cozaar Comp; Moduretic Mite; Normorix; Renitec Comp; Vivatec Comp; Zestoretic; ***S.Afr.:*** Accuretic; Acumod; Adco-Retic; Adelphane-Esidrex†; Aldoretic; Amiloretic; Amizide; Aquadrex†; Arcanaretic†; Betaretic; Capozide; Cibadrex; Cliniretic†; Co-Renitec; Cozaar Comp; Diutec; Dyazide; Hexaretic; Hydromet†; Inhibace Plus; Loretic; Moducren; Moduretic; Renezide; Secadrex; Servatrin; Sotazide†; Trimolex†; Urirex-K†; Urizide; Zestoretic; ***Spain:*** Acediur; Acetensil Plus; Adelfan-Esidrex; Alopresin Diu; Ameride; Baripril Diu; Bicetil; Bietapres Complex†; Bietapres†; Bitensil Diu; Cesplon Plus; Co-Renitec; Crinoretic; Dabonal Plus; Decresco; Dilabar Diu; Dilapres; Ditenside; Diu Rauwiplus; Diuzine; Doneka Plus; Donicer; Ecadiu; Ecazide; Emcoretic; Eutiman†; Flebo Stop; Hipoartel Plus; Hydromet†; Inhibace Plus; Inocar Plus; Kalten; Lidaltrin Diu; Miscidon; Neotensin Diu; Picten†; Pressitan Plus; Prinivil Plus; Prosanon†; Rulun; Secadrex; Secubar Diu; Selopresin; Tensiocomplet; Urocaudal Tiazida; Zestoretic; ***Swed.:*** Accupro Comp; Amiloferm; Capozid; Cibadrex†; Esidrex-K†; Hydromet; Inhibace comp; Moduretic; Monopril comp; Normorix; Sparkal; Synerpril; Triatec comp; Zestoretic; ***Switz.:*** Accuretic; Adelphan-Esidrex; Adelphan-Esidrex-K†; Aldoretic; Amilo-basan; Amilorid comp; Betadiur; Capozide; Cibadrex; Co-Reniten; Comilorid; Concor Plus; Dyazide; Ecodurex; Esidrex-K†; Fosicomp; Grodurex; Hydrolid; Inhibace Plus; Kalten; Modisal†; Moducren; Moduretic; Prinzide; Rhefluin; Spironothiazid; Synureticum; t/h-basan; Tensobon comp; Triatec comp; Zestoretic; ***UK:*** Accuretic; Acezide; Adizem-XL Plus†; Amilco; Amilmaxco; Capozide; Carace Plus; Co-Betaloc; Cozaar Comp; Delvas; Dyazide; Hydromet†; Hypertane†; Innozide; Kalten; Moducren; Moduret; Moduretic; Monozide; Secadrex; Sotazide†; Synuretic; Tolerzide†; Triamaxco; Triamco; Vasetic†; Zestoretic; Zida-Co; ***USA:*** Aldactazide; Aldoril; Apresazide; Aprozide†; Cam-ap-es†; Capozide; Dyazide; Esimil; HHR†; Hydra-zide; Hydrap-ES; Hydro-Serp; Hydropres; Hydroserpine; Hydrosine†; Hyzaar; Inderide; Lopressor HCT; Lotensin HCT; Marpres; Maxzide; Moduretic; Normozide†; Oreticyl†; Prinzide; Ser-Ap-Es; Timolide; Tri-Hydroserpine; Unipres†; Uniretic; Vaseretic; Zestoretic; Ziac.

Hydroflumethiazide (2334-g)

Hydroflumethiazide (*BAN, rINN*).

Hydroflumethiazidum; Trifluoromethylhydrothiazide. 3,4-Dihydro-6-trifluoromethyl-2*H*-1,2,4-benzothiadiazine-7-sulphonamide 1,1-dioxide.

$C_8H_8F_3N_3O_4S_2$ = 331.3.

CAS — 135-09-1.

NOTE. Compounded preparations of equal parts by weight of hydroflumethiazide and spironolactone have the British Approved Name Co-flumactone.

Pharmacopoeias. In Br. and US.

White or cream-coloured, odourless or almost odourless, glistening crystals or crystalline powder. Practically **insoluble** to very slightly soluble in water; soluble in alcohol; freely soluble in acetone; practically insoluble in chloroform and in ether. **Store** in airtight containers.

Adverse Effects, Treatment, and Precautions

As for Hydrochlorothiazide, p.885.

Interactions

As for Hydrochlorothiazide, p.887.

Pharmacokinetics

Hydroflumethiazide is incompletely but fairly rapidly absorbed from the gastro-intestinal tract. It is reported to have a beta-phase biological half-life of about 17 hours and a metabolite with a longer half-life which is extensively bound to red blood cells. Hydroflumethiazide is excreted in the urine; its metabolite has also been detected in the urine.

References.

1. Yakatan GJ, *et al.* Pharmacokinetics of orally administered hydroflumethiazide in man. *J Clin Pharmacol* 1977; **17:** 37–47.
2. McNamara PJ, *et al.* Absorption kinetics of hydroflumethiazide. *J Clin Pharmacol* 1978; **18:** 190–3.
3. Brørs O, *et al.* Pharmacokinetics of a single dose of hydroflumethiazide in health and in cardiac failure. *Eur J Clin Pharmacol* 1978; **14:** 29–37.
4. Brørs O, *et al.* Excretion of hydroflumethiazide in bile and urine of man. *Eur J Clin Pharmacol* 1979; **15:** 287–9.
5. Brørs O, Jacobsen S. Distribution and elimination of hydroflumethiazide in man. *Eur J Clin Pharmacol* 1979; **16:** 125–31.

Uses and Administration

Hydroflumethiazide is a thiazide diuretic with actions and uses similar to those of hydrochlorothiazide (p.887). It is used for oedema, including that associated with heart failure (p.785), and for hypertension (p.788).

Diuresis is initiated in about 2 hours and has been reported to last for up to 24 hours.

In the treatment of **oedema** the usual initial dose by mouth is 50 to 100 mg daily, in one or two divided doses, reduced to a dose of 25 to 50 mg on alternate days or intermittently. Doses of up to 200 mg daily may be required by some patients. In the treatment of **hypertension** the usual dose is 25 to 50 mg daily either alone, or in conjunction with other antihypertensives. An initial dose of 12.5 mg has been suggested.

A suggested initial dose for children is 1 mg per kg body-weight daily, reduced for maintenance.

In susceptible patients potassium supplements or a potassium-sparing diuretic may be necessary, but see hydrochlorothiazide.

Preparations

BP 1998: Hydroflumethiazide Tablets;
USP 23: Hydroflumethiazide Tablets.

Proprietary Preparations (details are given in Part 3)
Ital.: Rivosil†; ***UK:*** Hydrenox†; ***USA:*** Diucardin; Saluron.

Multi-ingredient: ***Irl.:*** Aldactide; Rautrax†; ***Ital.:*** Diuritens†; ***S.Afr.:*** Protensin-M; Rautrax†; ***UK:*** Aldactide; Spiro-Co; ***USA:*** Salutensin.

Hydroquinidine Hydrochloride (7786-v)

Dihydrochinidin Hydrochloride; Dihydroquinidine Hydrochloride; Hydroconchinine Hydrochloride. (8*R*,9*S*)-10,11-Dihydro-6′-methoxycinchonan-9-ol hydrochloride.

$C_{20}H_{26}N_2O_2,HCl$ = 362.9.

CAS — 1435-55-8 (hydroquinidine); 1476-98-8 (hydroquinidine hydrochloride).

Pharmacopoeias. In Fr.

Hydroquinidine is an antiarrhythmic with actions and uses similar to those of quinidine (p.938). It is given as the hydrochloride in a usual maintenance dose of 600 mg daily by mouth in divided doses.

Hydroquinidine alginate has also been employed as an antiarrhythmic.

Preparations

Proprietary Preparations (details are given in Part 3)
Fr.: Serecor; ***Spain:*** Algiquin†; Lentoquine.

Ibopamine Hydrochloride (12838-d)

Ibopamine Hydrochloride (*BANM, rINNM*).

SB-7505 (ibopamine); SKF-100168 (ibopamine). 4-(2-Methylaminoethyl)-*o*-phenylene di-isobutyrate hydrochloride.

$C_{17}H_{25}NO_4,HCl$ = 343.8.

CAS — 66195-31-1 (ibopamine); 75011-65-3 (ibopamine hydrochloride).

NOTE. Ibopamine is *USAN*.

Adverse Effects and Precautions

Ibopamine should not be used in patients with severe heart failure in whom, similarly to xamoterol (p.970), it has been reported to increase the risk of death.

For the adverse effects of sympathomimetics in general, and precautions to be observed, see Adrenaline, p.813.

A multicentre study (PRIME II) of the use of ibopamine in patients with severe (NYHA class III or IV) heart failure found that the drug was associated with an increased risk of death:[1] the study was stopped early. Subgroup analysis found that use of an antiarrhythmic drug was independently predictive of an adverse effect in ibopamine-treated patients. In a commentary, Niebauer and Coats[2] point out that excess mortality in heart failure has also been reported with dobutamine and xamoterol, and with flosequinan and the phosphodiesterase inhibitors amrinone, enoximone, milrinone, and vesnarinone, all of which produce positive inotropic effects through catecholamine-receptor stimulation or post-receptor pathway stimulation. The association with antiarrhythmic therapy in the ibopamine study might reflect an interaction with amiodarone, the most commonly used antiarrhythmic in this study, or might simply be a marker for patients at risk of ibopamine-induced tachyarrhythmias.

1. Hampton JR, *et al.* Randomised study of effect of ibopamine on survival in patients with advanced severe heart failure. *Lancet* 1997; **349:** 971–7.
2. Niebauer J, Coats AJS. Treating chronic heart failure: time to take stock. *Lancet* 1997; **349:** 966–7.

Interactions

It has been recommended that ibopamine should not be given to patients receiving amiodarone in the light of the increased mortality seen in the PRIME II study in patients receiving both drugs (see above), although it is not clear that this represents a genuine interaction.

For the interactions of sympathomimetics in general, see Adrenaline, p.814.

Uses and Administration

Ibopamine is rapidly converted after oral administration to its active metabolite, epinine, which is a peripheral dopamine agonist with vasodilating properties and a weak positive inotropic effect; at high concentrations it has a stimulant action on alpha- and beta-adrenoceptors.

Ibopamine has been used in the management of heart failure (p.785). It is given as the hydrochloride but doses are often expressed in terms of the base. Doses of 100 to 200 mg by mouth two or three times daily have been used, in combination with a diuretic.

References.

1. Henwood JM, Todd PA. Ibopamine: a preliminary review of its pharmacodynamic and pharmacokinetic properties and therapeutic efficacy. *Drugs* 1988; **36:** 11–31.
2. Spencer C, *et al.* Ibopamine: a review of its pharmacodynamic and pharmacokinetic properties, and therapeutic use in congestive heart failure. *Drugs Aging* 1993; **3:** 556–84.
3. Rousseau MF, *et al.* Progression of left ventricular dysfunction secondary to coronary artery disease, sustained neurohormonal activation and effects of ibopamine therapy during long-term therapy with angiotensin-converting enzyme inhibitor. *Am J Cardiol* 1994; **73:** 488–93.
4. Dohmen HJM, *et al.* Comparison of captopril and ibopamine in mild to moderate heart failure. *Heart* 1997; **78:** 285–90.

Preparations

Proprietary Preparations (details are given in Part 3)
Aust.: Escandine; ***Belg.:*** Idopamil; Scandine; ***Ital.:*** Inopamil; Scandine; ***Neth.:*** Inopamil; ***Spain:*** Erfolgan; Escandine.

Ibutilide Fumarate (13799-k)

Ibutilide Fumarate *(BANM, USAN, rINNM).*

U-70226E. (±)-4′-[4-(Ethylheptylamino)-1-hydroxybutyl]methanesulfonanilide fumarate (2:1).

$(C_{20}H_{36}N_2O_3S)_2,C_4H_4O_4$ = 885.2.

CAS — 122647-31-8 (ibutilide); 122647-32-9 (ibutilide fumarate).

Adverse Effects

Adverse cardiovascular effects associated with ibutilide include heart block, hypotension, hypertension, and bradycardia. Like other antiarrhythmic drugs it can cause arrhythmias, including torsade de pointes. Other adverse effects include nausea and vomiting.

Interactions

Concomitant administration of ibutilide with other antiarrhythmics or drugs that prolong the QT interval, for example tricyclic antidepressants and phenothiazines, should be avoided.

Pharmacokinetics

Ibutilide is widely distributed in the body following intravenous administration. It has low plasma protein binding (about 40%) and undergoes extensive metabolism in the liver to form several metabolites. Ibutilide is excreted mainly in the urine as metabolites with about 19% being excreted in the faeces. The elimination half-life is reported to range from 2 to 12 hours.

Uses and Administration

Ibutilide is a class III antiarrhythmic (p.776) used in the management of **atrial fibrillation** or **flutter** (p.782).

Ibutilide is given intravenously as the fumarate. The ECG should be monitored continuously during infusion and for at least 4 hours after administration. The recommended dose for patients weighing 60 kg or more is 1 mg of ibutilide fumarate given intravenously over 10 minutes. This dose may be repeated, if necessary, 10 minutes after completion of the first dose. The infusion should be stopped as soon as the arrhythmia is terminated. A dose of 0.01 mg per kg body-weight is recommended for patients weighing less than 60 kg.

References.

1. Foster RH, *et al.* Ibutilide: a review of its pharmacological properties and clinical potential in the acute management of atrial flutter and fibrillation. *Drugs* 1997; **54:** 312–30.
2. Granberry MC. Ibutilide: a new class III antiarrhythmic agent. *Am J Health-Syst Pharm* 1998; **55:** 255–60.

Preparations

Proprietary Preparations (details are given in Part 3)
Neth.: Corvert; ***Swed.:*** Corvert; ***USA:*** Corvert.

Ifenprodil Tartrate (9241-e)

Ifenprodil Tartrate *(rINNM).*

RC-61-91. (±)-2-(4-Benzylpiperidino)-1-(4-hydroxyphenyl)propan-1-ol tartrate.

$(C_{21}H_{27}NO_2)_2,C_4H_6O_6$ = 801.0.

CAS — 23210-56-2 (ifenprodil); 23210-58-4 (ifenprodil tartrate).

Pharmacopoeias. In *Jpn.*

Ifenprodil tartrate is a vasodilator, with alpha-adrenoceptor blocking properties, used in peripheral vascular disorders (p.794). It is given in usual doses of 40 to 60 mg daily by mouth or up to 15 mg daily by deep intramuscular injection, slow intravenous injection, or intravenous infusion.

Preparations

Proprietary Preparations (details are given in Part 3)
Fr.: Vadilex.

Imidapril (5366-z)

Imidapril *(BAN, rINN).*

TA-6366 (imidapril hydrochloride). (S)-3-{N-[(S)-1-Ethoxycarbonyl-3-phenylpropyl]-L-alanyl}-1-methyl-2-oxoimidazoline-4-carboxylic acid.

$C_{20}H_{27}N_3O_6$ = 405.4.

CAS — 89371-37-9 (imidapril); 89396-94-1 (imidapril hydrochloride).

Imidapril is an ACE inhibitor (p.805). It is converted in the body into its active metabolite imidaprilat and is given by mouth as the hydrochloride for the treatment of hypertension (p.788), in a usual dose of 5 to 10 mg once daily.

References.

1. Vandenburg MJ, *et al.* Dose-finding studies with imidapril—a new ACE inhibitor. *Br J Clin Pharmacol* 1994; **37:** 265–72.
2. Harder S, *et al.* Single dose and steady state pharmacokinetics and pharmacodynamics of the ACE-inhibitor imidapril in hypertensive patients. *Br J Clin Pharmacol* 1998; **45:** 377–80.

Preparations

Proprietary Preparations (details are given in Part 3)
Jpn: Novarok; Tanatril.

Imolamine Hydrochloride (9242-l)

Imolamine Hydrochloride *(BANM, rINNM).*

LA-1211. 2-(5-Imino-3-phenyl-1,2,4-oxadiazolin-4-yl)triethylamine hydrochloride.

$C_{14}H_{20}N_4O,HCl$ = 296.8.

CAS — 318-23-0 (imolamine); 15823-89-9 (imolamine hydrochloride).

Imolamine hydrochloride is a vasodilator used in angina pectoris (p.780) in doses of up to 90 mg daily by mouth.

Preparations

Proprietary Preparations (details are given in Part 3)
Aust.: Irri-Cor†; ***Spain:*** Coremax†.

Indapamide (2335-q)

Indapamide *(BAN, USAN, rINN).*

Indapamidum; SE-1520. 4-Chloro-N-(2-methylindolin-1-yl)-3-sulphamoylbenzamide.

$C_{16}H_{16}ClN_3O_3S$ = 365.8.

CAS — 26807-65-8 (anhydrous).

Pharmacopoeias. In *Eur.* (see p.viii) and *US.*

White to off-white crystalline powder. Practically **insoluble** in water; soluble in alcohol, in methyl alcohol, in acetonitrile, in glacial acetic acid, and in ethyl acetate; slightly to very slightly soluble in ether; very slightly soluble in chloroform. **Protect** from light.

Adverse Effects, Treatment, and Precautions

As for Hydrochlorothiazide, p.885.

Indapamide has been claimed to produce few adverse biochemical effects at the usual dose of 2.5 mg daily. However, adverse biochemical effects have been reported in individual patients, including severe hypokalaemia[1] and hyponatraemia,[2,3] and with the trend towards using lower doses of thiazide diuretics in hypertension, it may be that indapamide has no clinical advantage over low-dose thiazide diuretics.

Several studies have reported no changes in blood-glucose concentrations during indapamide treatment,[4-6] although elevated blood-glucose concentrations have been reported in individual patients.[7,8] There have been reports of increases in total cholesterol[4] and of no change.[5]

1. Rodat O, Hamelin J-P. Hypokaliémie au cours d'un traitement par l'indapamide. *Nouv Presse Med* 1978; **7:** 3054.
2. Read SJ, *et al.* Hyponatraemia and raised creatine kinase level associated with indapamide. *Med J Aust* 1994; **161:** 607–8.
3. Chan TYK. Indapamide-induced severe hyponatremia and hypokalemia. *Ann Pharmacother* 1995; **29:** 1124–8.
4. Prisant LM, *et al.* Biochemical, endocrine, and mineral effects of indapamide in black women. *J Clin Pharmacol* 1990; **30:** 121–6.
5. Leonetti G, *et al.* Long-term effects of indapamide: final results of a two-year Italian multicenter study in systemic hypertension. *Am J Cardiol* 1990; **65:** 674–714.
6. Velussi M, *et al.* Treatment of mild-to-moderate hypertension with indapamide in type II diabetics: midterm (six months) evaluation. *Curr Ther Res* 1988; **44:** 1076–86.
7. Slotkoff L. Clinical efficacy and safety of indapamide in the treatment of edema. *Am Heart J* 1983; **106:** 233–7.
8. Beling S, *et al.* Long term experience with indapamide. *Am Heart J* 1983; **106:** 258–62.

Effects on the kidneys. Acute interstitial nephritis was associated with indapamide treatment in a 74-year-old patient.[1]

1. Newstead CG, *et al.* Interstitial nephritis associated with indapamide. *Br Med J* 1990; **300:** 1344.

Effects on the skin. Sixteen cases of skin rash attributed to indapamide had been reported to the Netherlands Centre for Monitoring of Adverse Reactions to Drugs.[1] All patients had taken indapamide 2.5 mg daily for hypertension. The skin rash was accompanied by fever in 5 cases. In all cases the rash subsided within 14 days of indapamide being stopped, and 11 patients subsequently took thiazides, frusemide, or clopamide without recurrence. Among 188 cases of skin rash attributed to indapamide reported to the WHO Collaborating Centre for International Drug Monitoring were 4 cases of erythema multiforme and 2 of epidermal necrolysis. A further case of toxic epidermal necrolysis was reported by Black and colleagues.[2]

1. Stricker BHC, Biriell C. Skin reactions and fever with indapamide. *Br Med J* 1987; **295:** 1313–14.
2. Black RJ, *et al.* Toxic epidermal necrolysis associated with indapamide. *Br Med J* 1990; **301:** 1280–1.

Interactions

As for Hydrochlorothiazide, p.887.

Pharmacokinetics

Indapamide is rapidly and completely absorbed from the gastro-intestinal tract. Elimination is biphasic with a half-life in whole blood of about 14 hours. Indapamide is strongly bound to red blood cells. It is extensively metabolised. About 60 to 70% of the dose has been reported to be excreted in the urine; only about 5 to 7% is excreted unchanged. About 16 to 23% of the administered dose is excreted in the faeces. Indapamide is not removed by haemodialysis but does not accumulate in patients with impaired renal function.

References.

1. Beermann B, Grind M. Clinical pharmacokinetics of some newer diuretics. *Clin Pharmacokinet* 1987; **13:** 254–66.

Uses and Administration

Indapamide is a diuretic with actions and uses similar to those of the thiazide diuretics (see Hydrochlorothiazide, p.887) even though it does not contain a thiazide ring system. It is used for hypertension (p.788), and also for oedema, including that associated with heart failure (p.785).

In some countries indapamide is described as the hemihydrate. In the treatment of **hypertension** the usual dose by mouth is 1.25 to 2.5 mg once daily, either alone, or in conjunction with other antihypertensives; at higher doses the diuretic effect may become apparent without appreciable additional antihypertensive effect although the US manufacturers have suggested that the dose may be increased to 5 mg after 4 weeks. In the treatment of **oedema** the usual dose is 2.5 mg once daily increasing to 5 mg daily after 1 week if necessary.

In susceptible patients potassium supplements or a potassium-sparing diuretic may be necessary, but see hydrochlorothiazide.

Reviews.

1. Chaffman M, *et al.* Indapamide: a review of its pharmacodynamic properties and therapeutic efficacy in hypertension. *Drugs* 1984; **28:** 189–235.

Preparations

USP 23: Indapamide Tablets.

Proprietary Preparations (details are given in Part 3)
Aust.: Fludex; ***Austral.:*** Dapa-tabs; Insig; Napamide; Naride; Natrilix; ***Belg.:*** Fludex; ***Canad.:*** Lozide; ***Fr.:*** Fludex; ***Ger.:*** Natrilix; Sicco; ***Irl.:*** Agelan; Clonilix; Inamide; Natrilix; ***Ital.:*** Damide; Indaflex; Indamol; Indolin; Ipamix; Millibar; Natrilix; Pressural; Veroxil; ***Neth.:*** Fludex; ***S.Afr.:*** Dapamax; Daptril; Hydro-Less; Natrilix; ***Spain:*** Extur; Tertensif; ***Switz.:*** Fludex; ***UK:*** Natramid; Natrilix; Opumide; ***USA:*** Lozol.

Multi-ingredient: ***Ital.:*** Atinorm; Delapride; Dinapres; Nor-Pa; Normopress.

Indecainide Hydrochloride (19340-q)

Indecainide Hydrochloride *(USAN, rINNM).*

LY-135837; Ricainide. 9-[3-(Isopropylamino)propyl]fluorene-9-carboxamide hydrochloride.

$C_{20}H_{24}N_2O,HCl$ = 344.9.

CAS — 74517-78-5 (indecainide); 73681-12-6 (indecainide hydrochloride).

Indecainide is a class Ic antiarrhythmic drug (p.776).

References.

1. Morganroth J, *et al.* Efficacy safety and pharmacokinetics of indecainide—a new IC antiarrhythmic agent. *J Clin Pharmacol* 1984; **24:** 414.
2. Giardina E-GV, *et al.* Effect of indecainide in patients with left ventricular dysfunction. *Clin Pharmacol Ther* 1990; **48:** 582–9.

Indenolol Hydrochloride (12849-m)

Indenolol Hydrochloride *(BANM, rINNM)*.

Sch-28316Z (indenolol); YB-2.

$C_{15}H_{21}NO_2,HCl = 283.8.$

CAS — 60607-68-3 (indenolol); 68906-88-7 (indenolol hydrochloride).

Pharmacopoeias. In *Jpn.*

A 2:1 tautomeric mixture of 1-(inden-7-yloxy)-3-isopropylaminopropan-2-ol hydrochloride and 1-(inden-4-yloxy)-3-isopropylaminopropan-2-ol hydrochloride.

Indenolol is a non-cardioselective beta blocker (p.828). It is reported to possess potent membrane-stabilising properties and intrinsic sympathomimetic activity.

Indenolol is used as the hydrochloride in the management of various cardiovascular disorders in doses of 30 to 180 mg daily by mouth.

Preparations

Proprietary Preparations (details are given in Part 3)
Belg.: Vasocor†; ***Ital.:*** Securpres; ***Jpn:*** Pulsan.

Indobufen (12850-t)

Indobufen *(rINN)*.

K-3920. (±)-2-[4-(1-Oxo-isoindolin-2-yl)phenyl]butyric acid.

$C_{18}H_{17}NO_3 = 295.3.$

CAS — 63610-08-2.

Indobufen is an inhibitor of platelet aggregation used in various thrombo-embolic disorders (p.801) in doses of 200 to 400 mg daily by mouth given in 2 divided doses. It is also given parenterally as the sodium salt in similar doses. For patients with renal impairment or those over the age of 65, it has been recommended that the dose is reduced to 100 to 200 mg daily.

References.

1. Wiseman LR, *et al.* Indobufen: a review of its pharmacodynamic and pharmacokinetic properties, and therapeutic efficacy in cerebral, peripheral and coronary vascular disease. *Drugs* 1992; **44:** 445–64.

Preparations

Proprietary Preparations (details are given in Part 3)
Aust.: Ibustrin; ***Ital.:*** Ibustrin.

Indoramin Hydrochloride (879-d)

Indoramin Hydrochloride *(BANM, USAN, rINNM)*.

Wy-21901 (indoramin). *N*-[1-(2-Indol-3-ylethyl)-4-piperidyl]benzamide hydrochloride.

$C_{22}H_{25}N_3O,HCl = 383.9.$

CAS — 26844-12-2 (indoramin); 33124-53-7 (indoramin hydrochloride); 38821-52-2 (indoramin hydrochloride).

Pharmacopoeias. In *Br.*

A white or almost white powder. It exhibits polymorphism. Slightly **soluble** in water; sparingly soluble in alcohol; very slightly soluble in ether; soluble in methyl alcohol. A 2% suspension in water has a pH of 4.0 to 5.5. **Protect** from light.

Indoramin hydrochloride 11.0 mg is approximately equivalent to 10 mg of indoramin.

Adverse Effects, Treatment, and Precautions

The most common adverse effects in patients receiving indoramin are sedation and dizziness; dry mouth, nasal congestion, headache, fatigue, depression, weight gain (almost certainly due to fluid retention), and failure of ejaculation may also occur. Tachycardia does not seem to be a problem with therapeutic doses. Extrapyramidal disturbances have been reported.

Following overdosage, coma, convulsions, and hypotension may occur; hypothermia has been reported in *animals*. In acute poisoning the stomach should be emptied by lavage and appropriate symptomatic and supportive care given.

Indoramin should be avoided in patients with heart failure; it has been recommended that incipient heart failure should be controlled before giving indoramin. Caution should be observed in patients with hepatic or renal insufficiency, a history of depression, epilepsy, or Parkinson's disease. Elderly patients may respond to lower doses.

Because indoramin can cause drowsiness care should be taken in patients who drive or operate machinery.

Effects on mental function. Sleep disturbances and vivid dreams were reported during a study in hypertensive patients when indoramin was added to therapy with a thiazide diuretic and a beta blocker.[1]

1. Marshall AJ, *et al.* Evaluation of indoramin added to oxprenolol and bendrofluazide as a third agent in severe hypertension. *Br J Clin Pharmacol* 1980; **10:** 217–21.

Overdosage. A 43-year-old woman with a long history of heavy alcohol intake died after taking 100 tablets of indoramin 25 mg.[1] The main clinical features were deep sedation, respiratory depression, hypotension and convulsions. Although the hypotension was satisfactorily controlled the effects on the central nervous system were resistant to treatment and proved fatal. Other clinical features included areflexia, metabolic acidosis, tachycardia, and later bradyarrhythmias.

1. Hunter R. Death due to overdose of indoramin. *Br Med J* 1982; **285:** 1011.

Interactions

The hypotensive effects of indoramin may be enhanced by the concomitant administration of diuretics and other antihypertensives. It has been reported that the concomitant ingestion of alcohol can increase the rate and extent of absorption and the sedative effects of indoramin (see below) and that indoramin should not be given to patients already receiving MAOIs.

Alcohol. In a study in 9 healthy subjects alcohol 0.5 g per kg body-weight significantly enhanced plasma concentrations of indoramin following ingestion of indoramin 50 mg compared with placebo.[1] The effect was most marked in the early period, corresponding to the absorptive phase. The mean maximum plasma concentration of indoramin was increased from 15.0 to 23.7 ng per mL by concomitant alcohol administration; the area under the concentration/time curve was increased by 25%. Alcohol did not affect the pharmacokinetics of intravenous indoramin. The results suggest that alcohol increases indoramin bioavailability either by enhancing absorption or reducing first-pass metabolism. Since the combination was more sedative than either drug alone patients taking indoramin should be advised not to drink alcohol if they intend to drive or operate machinery.

1. Abrams SML, *et al.* Pharmacokinetic interaction between indoramin and ethanol. *Hum Toxicol* 1989; **8:** 237–41.

Pharmacokinetics

Indoramin is readily absorbed from the gastro-intestinal tract and undergoes extensive first-pass metabolism. It is reported to be about 90% bound to plasma proteins. It has a half-life of about 5 hours which is reported to be prolonged in elderly patients. It is extensively metabolised and is excreted mainly as metabolites in the urine and faeces. There is evidence to suggest that some metabolites may retain some alpha-adrenoceptor blocking activity.

The plasma half-life of indoramin in 5 healthy elderly subjects following a single oral dose ranged from 6.6 to 32.8 hours with a mean of 14.7 hours.[1] The increased half-life may have been caused by reduced clearance in elderly patients.

1. Norbury HM, *et al.* Pharmacokinetics of oral indoramin in elderly and middle-aged female volunteers. *Eur J Clin Pharmacol* 1984; **27:** 247–9.

Uses and Administration

Indoramin is a selective and competitive $alpha_1$-adrenoceptor antagonist (p.776) with actions similar to those of prazosin (p.933); it is also reported to have membrane-stabilising properties and to be a competitive antagonist at histamine H_1 and 5-hydroxytryptamine receptors. Indoramin is used in the management of hypertension (p.788) and in benign prostatic hyperplasia (p.1446) to relieve urinary obstruction. It has also been used in the prophylactic treatment of migraine.

Indoramin is given by mouth as the hydrochloride, but doses are usually expressed in terms of the base.

In hypertension, the initial dose is 25 mg twice daily, increased in steps of 25 or 50 mg at intervals of 2 weeks to a maximum of 200 mg daily in 2 or 3 divided doses.

In benign prostatic hyperplasia, the initial dose is 20 mg twice daily, increased if necessary by 20 mg at 2-week intervals, to a maximum of 100 mg daily in divided doses.

Lower doses may be required in the elderly.

Reviews.

1. Holmes B, Sorkin EM. Indoramin: a review of its pharmacodynamic and pharmacokinetic properties, and therapeutic efficacy in hypertension and related vascular, cardiovascular and airway diseases. *Drugs* 1986; **31:** 467–99.

Migraine. Propranolol and pizotifen are probably the most well-established drugs for prophylaxis of migraine (p.443). Many other drugs have been used including indoramin. In one double-blind study,[1] indoramin in a dose of 25 mg twice daily was reported to be as effective as dihydroergotamine mesylate in reducing the frequency of migraine attacks.

1. Pradalier A, *et al.* Etude comparative indoramine versus dihydroergotamine dans le traitement préventif de la migraine. *Therapie* 1988; **43:** 293–7.

Preparations

BP 1998: Indoramin Tablets.

Proprietary Preparations (details are given in Part 3)
Aust.: Wypresin; ***Fr.:*** Vidora; ***Ger.:*** Wydora; ***Irl.:*** Baratol; Doralese; ***Ital.:*** Indorene†; Vidora†; ***S.Afr.:*** Baratol; ***Spain:*** Orfidora; ***UK:*** Baratol; Doralese.

Inositol Nicotinate (9243-y)

Inositol Nicotinate *(BAN, rINN)*.

Inositol Niacinate *(USAN)*; NSC-49506; Win-9154. *meso*-Inositol hexanicotinate; *myo*-Inositol hexanicotinate.

$C_{42}H_{30}N_6O_{12} = 810.7.$

CAS — 6556-11-2.

Pharmacopoeias. In *Br.*

A white or almost white odourless or almost odourless powder. Practically **insoluble** in water, in alcohol, in acetone, and in ether; sparingly soluble in chloroform. It dissolves in dilute mineral acids.

Inositol nicotinate is a vasodilator and is believed to be slowly hydrolysed to nicotinic acid. It is given by mouth in the management of peripheral vascular disorders (p.794). The usual dose is 3 g daily given in divided doses. The dose may be increased to 4 g daily if necessary.

Inositol nicotinate has been used in hyperlipidaemias.

Preparations

BP 1998: Inositol Nicotinate Tablets.

Proprietary Preparations (details are given in Part 3)
Ger.: Hamovannad; Hexanicit; Nicolip; ***Irl.:*** Hexogen; Hexopal; ***Jpn:*** Hexanicit†; ***Neth.:*** Palohex†; ***Swed.:*** Hexanicit; ***UK:*** Hexopal.

Multi-ingredient: ***Aust.:*** Bendigon†; Prospervital; ***Canad.:*** Formula CI; ***Ger.:*** Anti-Lipide-ratiopharm†; durasklerai†; Jasivita†; Lioftal s. T.†; Migranex spezial N†; Nico-Padutin†; Pentavenon†; Theo-Hexanicit†; Veno-Hexanicit; Venosan†; Vit-O_2 (Vitozwei)†; Zellaforte N Plus; ***Ital.:*** Vasonicit Composto†; Vasonicit†; ***S.Afr.:*** Geratar; ***Spain:*** Venosan; Vertigum; ***Switz.:*** Hexafene; Venosan.

Irbesartan (17634-v)

Irbesartan *(BAN, USAN, rINN)*.

BMS-186295; SR-47436. 2-Butyl-3-[*p*-(*o*-1*H*-tetrazol-5-ylphenyl)benzyl]-1,3-diazaspiro[4.4]non-1-en-4-one.

$C_{25}H_{28}N_6O = 428.5.$

CAS — 138402-11-6.

Adverse Effects and Precautions

As for Losartan Potassium, p.899.

Pharmacokinetics

Irbesartan is rapidly absorbed from the gastro-intestinal tract with an oral bioavailability of 60 to 80%. It undergoes some metabolism in the liver to inactive metabolites. Peak plasma concentrations of irbesartan occur 1.5 to 2 hours after an oral dose. Irbesartan is about 90% bound to plasma proteins. It is excreted as unchanged drug and metabolites in the bile and in urine; after oral or intravenous administration approximately 20% of the dose is excreted in the urine, with less than 2% as unchanged drug. The terminal elimination half-life is about 11 to 15 hours.

References.

1. Sica DA, *et al.* The pharmacokinetics of irbesartan in renal failure and maintenance hemodialysis. *Clin Pharmacol Ther* 1997; **62:** 610–18.
2. Marino MR, *et al.* Pharmacokinetics and pharmacodynamics of irbesartan in healthy subjects. *J Clin Pharmacol* 1998; **38:** 246–55.
3. Marino MR, *et al.* Pharmacokinetics and pharmacodynamics of irbesartan in patients with hepatic cirrhosis. *J Clin Pharmacol* 1998; **38:** 347–56.

Uses and Administration

Irbesartan is an angiotensin II receptor antagonist with actions similar to those of losartan (p.899). It is used in the management of hypertension (p.788) and is under investigation in other cardiovascular disorders.

Irbesartan is administered by mouth. Following an oral dose the hypotensive effect peaks within 3 to 6 hours and persists for at least 24 hours. The maximum hypotensive effect is achieved within 4 to 6 weeks after initiating therapy.

In hypertension, irbesartan is given in a dose of 150 mg once daily increased, if necessary, to 300 mg once daily. A lower initial dose of 75 mg once daily may be considered in elderly patients over 75 years, for patients with intravascular volume depletion, and for those receiving haemodialysis.

Reviews.

1. Gillis JC, Markham A. Irbesartan: a review of its pharmacodynamic and pharmacokinetic properties and therapeutic use in the management of hypertension. *Drugs* 1997; **54:** 885–902.
2. Anonymous. Irbesartan for hypertension. *Med Lett Drugs Ther* 1998; **40:** 18–19.

Preparations

Proprietary Preparations (details are given in Part 3)
Irl.: Aprovel; ***Neth.:*** Aprovel; ***Swed.:*** Aprovel; ***UK:*** Aprovel; ***USA:*** Avapro.

Isoprenaline (14807-s)

Isoprenaline *(BAN, rINN)*.

Isopropylarterenol; Isopropylnoradrenaline; Isoproterenol. 1-(3,4-Dihydroxyphenyl)-2-isopropylaminoethanol.

$C_{11}H_{17}NO_3$ = 211.3.

CAS — 7683-59-2.

Isoprenaline Hydrochloride (2074-h)

Isoprenaline Hydrochloride *(BANM, rINNM)*.

Isopropylarterenol Hydrochloride; Isopropylnoradrenaline Hydrochloride; Isoproterenol Hydrochloride.

$C_{11}H_{17}NO_3,HCl$ = 247.7.

CAS — 51-30-9.

Pharmacopoeias. In *Chin., Eur.* (see p.viii), *Int., Jpn,* and *US.*

A white or almost white, odourless or almost odourless, crystalline powder. It gradually darkens on exposure to air and light. **Soluble** 1 in 3 of water and 1 in 50 of alcohol; less soluble in dehydrated alcohol; practically insoluble in chloroform, in dichloromethane, and in ether. A 1% solution in water has a pH of about 5 and a 5% solution has a pH of 4.3 to 5.5. Solutions become pink to brownish-pink on standing exposed to air and almost immediately so when made alkaline. **Store** in airtight containers. Protect from light.

Isoprenaline Sulphate (2075-m)

Isoprenaline Sulphate *(BANM, rINNM)*.

Isoprenalini Sulfas; Isopropylarterenol Sulphate; Isopropylnoradrenaline Sulphate; Isoproterenol Sulfate.

$(C_{11}H_{17}NO_3)_2,H_2SO_4,2H_2O$ = 556.6.

CAS — 299-95-6 (anhydrous isoprenaline sulphate); 6700-39-6 (isoprenaline sulphate dihydrate).

Pharmacopoeias. In *Eur.* (see p.viii), *Int., Pol.,* and *US.*

A white or almost white, odourless crystalline powder. It gradually darkens on exposure to light and air. Isoprenaline sulphate 1.32 mg is approximately equivalent to 1 mg of isoprenaline or to 1.17 mg of the hydrochloride. **Soluble** 1 in 4 of water; very slightly soluble in alcohol, chloroform, and ether. A 1% solution in water has a pH of about 5. Solutions become pink to brownish-pink on standing exposed to air, and almost immediately so when made alkaline. **Store** in airtight containers. Protect from light.

Adverse Effects and Precautions

The adverse effects of isoprenaline may include tachycardia and cardiac arrhythmias, palpitations, hypotension, tremor, headache, sweating, and facial flushing. Prolonged use of isoprenaline has been associated with swelling of the parotid glands. Special caution is needed in the presence of ischaemic heart disease, diabetes mellitus, and hyperthyroidism.

Prolonged use of isoprenaline tablets sublingually has been reported to cause severe damage to the teeth due to the acidic nature of the drug. Sublingual use or inhalation may colour the saliva or sputum red.

For the adverse effects of sympathomimetics in general, and precautions for their use, see Adrenaline, p.813.

Increased mortality. For a discussion of the increased mortality and morbidity that has sometimes been observed in asthmatic patients and reference to an early epidemic associated with isoprenaline inhalers, see p.753.

Interactions

Isoprenaline should not be given concomitantly with other potent $beta_1$ agonists such as adrenaline.

For the interactions of sympathomimetics in general, see Adrenaline, p.814.

Theophylline. For reports of increased theophylline clearance following concomitant use of isoprenaline, see p.770.

Pharmacokinetics

As a result of sulphate conjugation in the gut, isoprenaline is considerably less active following administration by mouth than following parenteral administration. It is absorbed through the oral mucosa and has accordingly been given sublingually, but absorption by this route remains very erratic. Isoprenaline in the body is resistant to metabolism by monoamine oxidase, but is metabolised by catechol-*O*-methyltransferase in the liver, lungs, and other tissues, this metabolite being subsequently conjugated before excretion in the urine. Whereas the sulphate conjugate of isoprenaline is inactive the methylated metabolite exhibits weak activity.

Following intravenous injection isoprenaline has a plasma half-life of about one to several minutes according to whether the rate of injection is rapid or slow; it is almost entirely excreted in the urine as unchanged drug and metabolites within 24 hours. A much slower onset of action and a more extended initial half-life has been demonstrated following oral administration. Isoprenaline is reported to have a duration of action of up to about 2 hours after inhalation; it has been demonstrated that a large proportion of an inhaled dose is swallowed.

References.

1. Blackwell EW, *et al.* The fate of isoprenaline administered by pressurized aerosols. *Br J Pharmacol* 1970; **39:** 194P–195P.
2. Conolly ME, *et al.* Metabolism of isoprenaline in dog and man. *Br J Pharmacol* 1972; **46:** 458–72.
3. Blackwell EW, *et al.* Metabolism of isoprenaline after aerosol and direct intrabronchial administration in man and dog. *Br J Pharmacol* 1974; **50:** 587–91.
4. Reyes G, *et al.* The pharmacokinetics of isoproterenol in critically ill pediatric patients. *J Clin Pharmacol* 1993; **33:** 29–34.

Uses and Administration

Isoprenaline is a sympathomimetic (see Adrenaline, p.815) that acts almost exclusively on beta-adrenergic receptors. It stimulates the CNS. It has a powerful stimulating action on the heart and increases cardiac output, excitability, and rate; it also causes peripheral vasodilatation and produces a fall in diastolic blood pressure and usually maintains or slightly increases systolic blood pressure. In addition, isoprenaline has bronchodilating properties.

Isoprenaline has been used in a variety of cardiac disorders. It may be used for the temporary prevention or control of Stokes-Adams attacks although for long-term management the use of a pacemaker is preferable. Isoprenaline may be useful in severe bradycardia unresponsive to atropine, although again cardiac pacing is preferred. It has also been advocated as an adjunct for other cardiac disorders including shock (p.798) and torsade de pointes (see p.782). It has been used in the diagnosis of congenital heart defects.

In the management of **cardiac disorders**, isoprenaline is usually given as the hydrochloride by slow intravenous infusion under ECG control. Infusion rates may range from 0.5 to 10 μg per minute depending on the clinical condition of the patient; 1 to 4 μg per minute may be adequate to correct bradycardia but higher rates of 4 to 8 μg per minute may be required for acute Stokes-Adams attacks. Isoprenaline hydrochloride can be given by intracardiac injection in extreme cases. It has also been given subcutaneously or intramuscularly in initial doses of 200 μg (as 1 mL of a 0.02% solution) and by slow intravenous injection in initial doses of 20 to 60 μg (as 1 to 3 mL of a 0.002% solution); doses are subsequently adjusted according to ventricular rate. Tablets of isoprenaline hydrochloride have been administered by mouth or sublingually.

Isoprenaline has been used as a bronchodilator in the management of **reversible airways obstruction** but sympathomimetics with a selective action on $beta_2$ receptors, such as salbutamol, are now preferred (see Asthma, p.745). It is given as the sulphate or hydrochloride usually by inhalation; sublingual tablets and intravenous injections have also been used. The adult dosage has generally been 1 to 3 inhalations of isoprenaline sulphate 80 μg by metered dose inhaler, repeated if necessary after not less than 30 minutes up to a maximum of 8 treatments in 24 hours. An aerosol inhaler which delivers metered doses of 400 μg has also been employed. Solutions containing about 0.1% isoprenaline hydrochloride may be administered by nebulisation; solutions up to 1% have been used in a hand-bulb nebuliser. Isoprenaline hydrochloride has also been given by sublingual administration in the management of bronchospasm in usual doses of 10 to 15 mg three or four times daily.

Preparations

BP 1998: Isoprenaline Injection;
USP 23: Acetylcysteine and Isoproterenol Hydrochloride Inhalation Solution; Isoproterenol Hydrochloride and Phenylephrine Bitartrate Inhalation Aerosol; Isoproterenol Hydrochloride Inhalation Aerosol; Isoproterenol Hydrochloride Injection; Isoproterenol Hydrochloride Tablets; Isoproterenol Inhalation Solution; Isoproterenol Sulfate Inhalation Aerosol; Isoproterenol Sulfate Inhalation Solution.

Proprietary Preparations (details are given in Part 3)
Aust.: Ingelan; Medihaler-Iso; ***Austral.:*** Isuprel; Medihaler-Iso†; ***Belg.:*** Isuprel; Medihaler-Iso; ***Canad.:*** Isuprel; ***Fr.:*** Isuprel; ***Ger.:*** Bellasthman†; Ingelan; Kattwilon N; ***Irl.:*** Saventrine; ***Neth.:*** Medihaler-Iso; ***S.Afr.:*** Imuprel; Lenoprel†; Medihaler-Iso†; Saventrine†; ***Spain:*** Aleudrina; ***Switz.:*** Isuprel†; ***UK:*** Medihaler-Iso†; Saventrine; ***USA:*** Isuprel; Medihaler-Iso; Norisodrine Aerotrol†.

Multi-ingredient: ***Ger.:*** afdosa-duo†; Duo-Medihaler†; Ingelan; Intal compositum†; Older†; ***Ital.:*** Frenal Compositum†; ***Neth.:*** Lomudal Compositum†; ***S.Afr.:*** Lomudal Comp†; ***Spain:*** Aldo Asma; Frenal Compositum; ***Switz.:*** Mucobronchyl; ***UK:*** Intal Compound†; Medihaler-duo†; ***USA:*** Duo-Medihaler†; Norisodrine with Calcium Iodide.

Isosorbide (2336-p)

Isosorbide *(BAN, USAN, rINN)*.

AT-101; NSC-40725. 1,4:3,6-Dianhydro-D-glucitol.

$C_6H_{10}O_4$ = 146.1.

CAS — 652-67-5.

Pharmacopoeias. In *Jpn.*
US includes Isosorbide Concentrate.

Isosorbide Concentrate (USP 23) is an aqueous solution containing 70.0 to 80.0% w/w of isosorbide. A colourless to slightly yellow liquid. **Soluble** in water and in alcohol. **Store** in airtight containers. Protect from light.

Isosorbide is an osmotic diuretic with properties similar to those of mannitol (p.900). It is reported to cause less nausea and vomiting than other oral osmotic diuretics.

Isosorbide is used for short-term reduction of intra-ocular pressure in acute glaucoma or prior to surgery (p.1387). The usual dose is 1 to 3 g per kg body-weight by mouth 2 to 4 times daily. The onset of action is usually within 30 minutes and lasts for up to 5 or 6 hours.

Preparations

USP 23: Isosorbide Concentrate; Isosorbide Oral Solution.

Proprietary Preparations (details are given in Part 3)
USA: Ismotic.

Isosorbide Dinitrate (9245-z)

Isosorbide Dinitrate *(BAN, USAN, rINN)*.

ISDN; Isosorbidi Dinitras; Sorbide Nitrate. 1,4:3,6-Dianhydro-D-glucitol 2,5-dinitrate.

$C_6H_8N_2O_8$ = 236.1.

CAS — 87-33-2.

Pharmacopoeias. In *Chin., Jpn*, and *Pol.*

Eur. (see p.viii) and *US* include diluted isosorbide dinitrate.

Undiluted isosorbide dinitrate is a white crystalline powder. Very slightly **soluble** in water; sparingly soluble in alcohol; very soluble in acetone; freely soluble in chloroform.

Diluted isosorbide dinitrate is a mixture of isosorbide dinitrate (usually about 25%) with lactose, mannitol, or other suitable inert excipients, the latter being added to minimise the risk of explosion. It may contain up to 1% of a suitable stabiliser such as ammonium phosphate. The solubility of the diluted product depends on the diluent and its concentration. **Store** in airtight containers. Protect from light.

CAUTION. *Undiluted isosorbide dinitrate may explode if subjected to percussion or excessive heat.*

Stability. The loss of isosorbide dinitrate from solution during infusion was found to be 30% with polyvinyl chloride plastic intravenous infusion sets but negligible when polyolefin or glass delivery systems were used.[1] Another study reported a 23% decrease in isosorbide dinitrate concentration after 24 hours of storage at 21° in polyvinyl chloride containers; most of the loss occurred in the first 6 hours. Loss of potency was not noted when isosorbide dinitrate was stored under similar conditions in glass bottles or polyethylene, nylon, and polypropylene laminated bags.[2]

1. Kowaluk EA, *et al.* Drug loss in polyolefin infusion systems. *Am J Hosp Pharm* 1983; **40:** 118–19.
2. Martens HJ, *et al.* Sorption of various drugs in polyvinyl chloride, glass, and polyethylene-lined infusion containers. *Am J Hosp Pharm* 1990; **47:** 369–73.

Adverse Effects, Treatment, and Precautions

As for Glyceryl Trinitrate, p.875.

Effects on the blood. Haemolysis occurred in 2 patients with glucose-6-phosphate dehydrogenase deficiency during treatment with isosorbide dinitrate.[1]

1. Aderka D, *et al.* Isosorbide dinitrate-induced hemolysis in G6PD-deficient subjects. *Acta Haematol (Basel)* 1983; **69:** 63–4.

Headache. The most common adverse effect of nitrate therapy is headache which usually decreases after a few days. There has been a report[1] of a severe continuous unilateral headache with an oculosympathetic paresis on the same side associated with isosorbide dinitrate therapy.

1. Mueller RA, Meienberg O. Hemicrania with oculosympathetic paresis from isosorbide dinitrate. *N Engl J Med* 1983; **308:** 458–9.

Hypersensitivity. Laryngeal oedema developed on two occasions in a woman following the administration of isosorbide dinitrate spray;[1] nifedipine was also given sublingually which on the second occasion caused a noticeable increase in the laryngeal swelling induced by the nitrate.

1. Silfvast T, *et al.* Laryngeal oedema after isosorbide dinitrate spray and sublingual nifedipine. *Br Med J* 1995; **311:** 232.

Oedema. Reports of ankle oedema associated with isosorbide dinitrate therapy in 3 patients with cardiac failure.[1]

1. Rodger JC. Peripheral oedema in patients treated with isosorbide dinitrate. *Br Med J* 1981; **283:** 1365–6.

Tolerance. Continuous administration of organic nitrates is associated with tolerance to their haemodynamic effects; for an overview of nitrate tolerance see under Precautions for Glyceryl Trinitrate, p.875.

A study in 12 patients with chronic stable angina[1] showed that following treatment for one week with isosorbide dinitrate 30 mg two or three times daily, treadmill-walking time was longer throughout a 5-hour testing period compared with placebo. In contrast, after treatment for one week with isosorbide dinitrate 30 mg four times daily, treadmill-walking time was prolonged at one hour but not at 3 or 5 hours. These results support the concept that clinical efficacy of isosorbide dinitrate is maintained if administered in a dose schedule which provides a nitrate-free or a low-nitrate period.

The effect of sublingual isosorbide dinitrate in patients receiving chronic therapy with isosorbide dinitrate was evaluated in 24 patients with angina.[2] Sublingual administration produced less reduction of aortic systolic pressure and left ventricular end-diastolic pressure and less dilatation of coronary artery diameter in patients who received chronic isosorbide dinitrate therapy compared with patients not receiving chronic therapy.

1. Parker JO, *et al.* Effect of intervals between doses on the development of tolerance to isosorbide dinitrate. *N Engl J Med* 1987; **316:** 1440–4.
2. Naito H, *et al.* Effects of sublingual nitrate in patients receiving sustained therapy of isosorbide dinitrate for coronary artery disease. *Am J Cardiol* 1989; **64:** 565–68.

Interactions

As for Glyceryl Trinitrate, p.875.

Disopyramide. The effectiveness of sublingual isosorbide dinitrate was reduced in a patient taking disopyramide.[1] The interaction was considered to be due to diminished salivary secretions caused by the antimuscarinic action of disopyramide which inhibited the dissolution of the sublingual isosorbide dinitrate tablet.

1. Barletta MA, Eisen H. Isosorbide dinitrate-disopyramide phosphate interaction. *Drug Intell Clin Pharm* 1985; **19:** 764.

Pharmacokinetics

Like glyceryl trinitrate, isosorbide dinitrate is readily absorbed from the oral mucosa. Isosorbide dinitrate is also readily absorbed following administration by mouth but owing to extensive first-pass metabolism in the liver and pre-systemic clearance its bioavailability is reduced. Isosorbide dinitrate is also absorbed through the skin from an ointment basis.

Following sublingual administration, anti-anginal effect is apparent within 2 to 5 minutes and persists for about 2 hours. Following oral administration of conventional tablets, anti-anginal activity is present in less than one hour and lasts for 4 to 6 hours.

Isosorbide dinitrate is widely distributed with a large apparent volume of distribution. It is taken up by smooth muscle cells of blood vessels and the nitrate group is cleaved to inorganic nitrite and then to nitric oxide. It is also rapidly metabolised in the liver to the major active metabolites isosorbide 2-mononitrate and isosorbide 5-mononitrate (see Isosorbide Mononitrate, below).

After sublingual administration, isosorbide dinitrate has a plasma half-life of 45 to 60 minutes. Plasma half-lives of 20 minutes and 4 hours have been reported following intravenous and oral administration, respectively. During prolonged administration, the half-life is increased due to accumulation of the isosorbide 5-mononitrate metabolite which reduces hepatic isosorbide dinitrate extraction. Both primary metabolites have longer half-lives than the parent compound.

References.

1. Abshagen U, *et al.* Pharmacokinetics and metabolism of isosorbide-dinitrate after intravenous and oral administration. *Eur J Clin Pharmacol* 1985; **27:** 637–44.
2. Straehl P, Galeazzi RL. Isosorbide dinitrate bioavailability, kinetics, and metabolism. *Clin Pharmacol Ther* 1985; **38:** 140–9.
3. Thadani U, Whitsett T. Relationship of pharmacokinetic and pharmacodynamic properties of the organic nitrates. *Clin Pharmacokinet* 1988; **15:** 32–43.
4. Schneider W, *et al.* Concentrations of isosorbide dinitrate, isosorbide-2-mononitrate and isosorbide-5-mononitrate in human vascular and muscle tissue under steady-state conditions. *Eur J Clin Pharmacol* 1990; **38:** 145–7.
5. Vogt D, *et al.* Pharmacokinetics and haemodynamic effects of ISDN following different dosage forms and routes of administration. *Eur J Clin Pharmacol* 1994; **46:** 319–24.
6. Bergami A, *et al.* Pharmacokinetics of isosorbide dinitrate in healthy volunteers after 24-hour intravenous infusion. *J Clin Pharmacol* 1997; **37:** 828–33.

Uses and Administration

Isosorbide dinitrate is a vasodilator with general properties similar to those of glyceryl trinitrate (p.875). It is used in the management of angina pectoris (p.780) and of heart failure (p.785). It has also been investigated in myocardial infarction (p.791).

Isosorbide dinitrate may be administered by the sublingual, oral, transdermal, or intravenous route.

In **angina** isosorbide dinitrate may be given as sublingual tablets or spray for the relief of an acute attack, although glyceryl trinitrate may be preferred because it has a faster onset of action. Isosorbide dinitrate may also be used before an activity or stress which might provoke an attack. The usual dose in acute angina is 2.5 to 10 mg sublingually. As an alternative, one to three sprays (1.25 mg per spray) may be directed under the tongue.

Isosorbide dinitrate is also used in the long-term management of angina in oral doses of 30 to 120 mg daily in divided doses according to the patient's needs. Increases in dosage should be gradual to avoid side-effects. Up to 240 mg daily in divided doses may be necessary. Modified-release formulations may be used in equivalent doses. Transdermal preparations such as topical sprays or ointments may also be used.

Isosorbide dinitrate is given by intravenous infusion for unstable angina. The dose is titrated according to patient response; doses in the range of 2 to 12 mg per hour are usually suitable but up to 20 mg per hour may be necessary in some patients. The plastic used in the infusion equipment may adsorb isosorbide dinitrate (see above) and allowance may have to be made for this.

During percutaneous transluminal coronary angioplasty isosorbide dinitrate can be given by the intracoronary route. Only injections of isosorbide dinitrate which are approved for intracoronary administration should be given by this route as preparations intended for normal intravenous administration may contain additives that are harmful if injected into diseased coronary vessels. The usual dose is 1 mg as a bolus before balloon inflation. The maximum recommended dose is 5 mg within a 30-minute time period.

Isosorbide dinitrate is also used in the management of **heart failure**. It is given in doses of 5 to 15 mg sublingually every 2 to 3 hours, or in oral doses of 30 to 160 mg daily in divided doses. Oral doses of up to 240 mg daily may be required. The intravenous route may also be employed using the intravenous doses given above for angina.

As well as being used in cardiovascular disorders, nitrates such as isosorbide dinitrate have been tried in a number of other conditions including anal fissure, erectile dysfunction, and oesophageal motility disorders such as achalasia and spasm. Further details of these uses are given under Glyceryl Trinitrate (p.876).

Preparations

BP 1998: Isosorbide Dinitrate Tablets;

USP 23: Isosorbide Dinitrate Chewable Tablets; Isosorbide Dinitrate Extended-release Capsules; Isosorbide Dinitrate Extended-release Tablets; Isosorbide Dinitrate Sublingual Tablets; Isosorbide Dinitrate Tablets.

Proprietary Preparations (details are given in Part 3)

Aust.: Cedocard; Hexanitrat; Isoket; Isomack; Maydil; Sorbidilat; Vasorbate; ***Austral.:*** Isogen†; Isordil; Isotrate†; Nitro-Spray†; Sorbidin; ***Belg.:*** Cedocard; Isocard; Isordil; Sorbitrate; ***Canad.:*** Apo-ISDN; Cedocard; Coradur; Coronex†; Isordil; Novo-Sorbide; ***Fr.:*** Disorlon; Isocard; Langoran; Risordan; Sorbitrate†; ***Ger.:*** Corovliss; Dignonitrat; duranitrat; EureCor†; Isdin†; Iso Mack; Iso-Puren; Isodinit; isoforce†; Isoket; Isostenase; Jenacard; Maycor; Nitro-Tablinen; Nitrosorbon; Rifloc†; Sorbidilat†; TD Spray Iso Mack; Vermicet†; ***Irl.:*** Cedocard; Imtack; Isoket; Isordil; Soni-Slo; Vascardin†; ***Ital.:*** Carvasin; Diniket; Nitrosorbide; ***Jpn:*** Nitorol; ***Neth.:*** Cedocard; Isordil; Prodicard; ***Norw.:*** Sorbangil; ***S.Afr.:*** Angi-Spray; Dilanid; Iso Mack†; Isoket; Isordil; ***Spain:*** Edistol†; Iso; Isordil†; Maycor; ***Swed.:*** Cardopax†; Sorbangil; ***Switz.:*** Acordin; Cedocard†; Iso Mack; Isoday; Isoket; Sorbidilat; ***UK:*** Cedocard; Imtack†; Isocard; Isoket; Isordil; Jeridin; Soni-Slo; Sorbichew; Sorbid; Sorbitrate; Vascardin†; ***USA:*** Dilatrate; Iso-Bid†; Isordil; Isotrate; Sorbitrate.

Multi-ingredient: ***Aust.:*** Acordin; Baxanitrat†; Beta-Isoket†; Viskenit; ***Ger.:*** Beta-Isoket†; Nitrisken†; Nitroduratt†; Oxycardin†; Stenoptin; ***Ital.:*** Stenodilate†; ***Switz.:*** Viskenit†.

Isosorbide Mononitrate (15336-h)

Isosorbide Mononitrate *(BAN, USAN, rINN)*.

AHR-4698; BM-22145; IS-5-MN; Isosorbide-5-mononitrate; Isosorbidi Mononitras. 1,4:3,6-Dianhydro-D-glucitol 5-nitrate.

$C_6H_9NO_6$ = 191.1.

CAS — 16051-77-7.

Pharmacopoeias. Eur. (see p.viii) includes diluted isosorbide mononitrate.

Undiluted isosorbide mononitrate is a white, crystalline powder. Freely **soluble** in water, in acetone, in alcohol, and in dichloromethane.

Diluted isosorbide mononitrate is a mixture of isosorbide mononitrate with lactose or mannitol. The solubility of the diluted product depends on the diluent and its concentration. **Protect** from light.

Adverse Effects, Treatment, and Precautions

As for Glyceryl Trinitrate, p.875.

Interactions

As for Glyceryl Trinitrate, p.875.

Pharmacokinetics

Isosorbide mononitrate is readily absorbed from the gastro-intestinal tract. Following oral administration of conventional tablets, peak plasma levels are reached in about 1 hour; onset of action occurs within 20 minutes and lasts for about 8 to 10 hours. Unlike isosorbide dinitrate, isosorbide mononitrate does not undergo first-pass hepatic metabolism and bioavailability is nearly 100%. Isosorbide mononitrate is widely distributed with a large apparent volume of distribution. It is taken up by smooth muscle cells of blood vessels and the nitrate group is cleaved to inorganic nitrite and then to nitric oxide. Isosorbide mononitrate is metabolised to inactive metabolites, including isosorbide and isosorbide glucuronide. Only about 2% of isosorbide mononitrate is excreted unchanged in the urine. An elimination half-life of about 4 to 5 hours has been reported.

References.

1. Taylor T, *et al.* Isosorbide 5-mononitrate pharmacokinetics in humans. *Biopharm Drug Dispos* 1981; **2:** 255–63.
2. Thadani U, Whitsett T. Relationship of pharmacokinetic and pharmacodynamic properties of the organic nitrates. *Clin Pharmacokinet* 1988; **15:** 32–43.
3. McClennen W, *et al.* The plasma concentrations of isosorbide 5-mononitrate (5-ISMN) administered in an extended-release form to patients with acute myocardial infarction. *Br J Clin Pharmacol* 1995; **39:** 704–8.
4. Hutt V, *et al.* Evaluation of the pharmacokinetics and absolute bioavailability of three isosorbide-5-mononitrate preparations in healthy volunteers. *Arzneimittelforschung* 1995; **45:** 142–5.
5. Baxter T, Eadie CJ. Twenty-four hour plasma profile of sustained-release isosorbide mononitrate in healthy volunteers and in patients with chronic stable angina: two open label trials. *Br J Clin Pharmacol* 1997; **43:** 333–5.

Uses and Administration

Isosorbide mononitrate is an active metabolite of the vasodilator isosorbide dinitrate and is used in the long-term management of angina pectoris (p.780) and heart failure (p.785). It has also been investigated in myocardial infarction (below).

The usual oral dose is 20 mg two or three times daily, although doses ranging from 20 to 120 mg daily have been given. Modified-release oral preparations have been developed for use in angina.

Myocardial infarction. Long-term management of myocardial infarction (p.791) can involve numerous drug therapies and some patients, for example those with myocardial ischaemia or poor left ventricular function, may require the long-term administration of nitrates, although recent studies have thrown doubt on their routine use. In the GISSI-3 study[1] there was no significant benefit when assessed 6 weeks post-infarction from the use of transdermal glyceryl trinitrate and in the ISIS-4 study[2] oral isosorbide mononitrate apparently had no effect on 35-day mortality.

1. Gruppo Italiano per lo Studio della Sopravvivenza nell'Infarto Miocardico. GISSI-3: effects of lisinopril and transdermal glyceryl trinitrate singly and together on 6-week mortality and ventricular function after acute myocardial infarction. *Lancet* 1994; **343:** 1115–22.
2. ISIS-4 (Fourth International Study of Infarct Survival) Collaborative Group. ISIS-4: a randomised factorial trial assessing early oral captopril, oral mononitrate, and intravenous magnesium sulphate in 58 050 patients with suspected acute myocardial infarction. *Lancet* 1995; **345:** 669–85.

Termination of pregnancy. For mention of the use of isosorbide mononitrate to ripen the cervix before termination of pregnancy, see under Glyceryl Trinitrate, p.876.

Variceal haemorrhage. For reference to the use of isosorbide mononitrate (as adjunctive therapy with a beta blocker) in the prevention of variceal haemorrhage, see under Glyceryl Trinitrate, p.877.

Preparations

Proprietary Preparations (details are given in Part 3)
Aust.: Corangin; Elantan; Epicordin; Imdur; Isomonat; Mono Mack; Monoket; Myocardon mono; Olicardin; Sorbimon; ***Austral.:*** Duride; Imdur; Imtrate; Monodur; ***Belg.:*** Pentacard; Promocard; ***Canad.:*** Imdur; Ismo; ***Fr.:*** Monicor; Oxycardin†; ***Ger.:*** Coleb; Conpin; Corangin; Corvasal†; duramonitat; Elantan; IS 5 Mono; Ismo; Isomonit; Isomonoreal; Moni; Monit-Puren; Mono Mack; Mono Maycor; Mono-Wolff; Monobeta; Monoclair; Monolong; Monopur; Monostenase; Olicard; Orasorbil; Sigacora; Turimonit; ***Irl.:*** Elantan; Imdur; Isomel; Isotrate; ***Ital.:*** Duronitrin; Elan; Ismo; Kiton; Leicester Retard; Monocinque; Monoket; Nitrex; Orasorbil; Vasdilat; ***Neth.:*** Ismo; Mono Mack†; Mono-Cedocard; Promocard; ***Norw.:*** Imdur; Ismo; Monoket; ***S.Afr.:*** Angitrate; Elantan; Imdur; Ismo; Mono Mack†; ***Spain:*** Cardiovas; Coronur; Dolak; Imdur†; Ismo†; Isonitril; Olicard; Pancardiol; Percorina; Pertil; Titrane; Uniket; ***Swed.:*** Fem-Mono; Imdur; Ismo; Monoket; ***Switz.:*** Corangine; Elantan; Etimonis; Imdur; Ismo; Olicard†; ***UK:*** Angeze; Dynamin; Elantan; Imdur; Isib; Ismo; Isotard; Isotrate†; MCR-50; Modisal; Monit; Mono-Cedocard; Monomax; Monosorb; ***USA:*** Imdur; Ismo; Monoket.

Isradipine (19367-a)

Isradipine *(BAN, USAN, rINN).*

PN-200-110. Isopropyl methyl 4-(2,1,3-benzoxadiazol-4-yl)-1,4-dihydro-2,6-dimethylpyridine-3,5-dicarboxylate.

$C_{19}H_{21}N_3O_5$ = 371.4.

CAS — 75695-93-1.

Pharmacopoeias. In *US.*

A yellow fine crystalline powder. **Protect** from light.

Stability. An oral preparation of isradipine 1 mg per mL, prepared using the powder from capsules of isradipine suspended in syrup[1] and stored at 4°, was stable when tested at 7, 16, 22, 28, and 35 days after preparation.

1. MacDonald JL, *et al.* Stability of isradipine in an extemporaneously compounded oral liquid. *Am J Hosp Pharm* 1994; **51:** 2409–11.

Adverse Effects, Treatment, and Precautions

As for dihydropyridine calcium-channel blockers (see Nifedipine, p.916).

In a multicentre study involving 74 patients allocated to antihypertensive therapy with isradipine 2.5 to 10 mg twice daily, and 72 allocated to treatment with hydrochlorothiazide, adverse effects were reported in 44 of the isradipine group but only 29 of the thiazide group.[1] Flushing, palpitation, and oedema were more common in patients receiving isradipine, while headache, dizziness, and dyspnoea were reported in both groups with similar frequency. In another study,[2] spontaneously reported adverse effects occurred less frequently in patients taking isradipine (18.4% of 103 patients) than in those taking amlodipine (33.3% of 102 patients). In particular, ankle oedema was more frequent, severe, and prolonged than the oedema reported in patients taking isradipine. A multicentre study comparing isradipine and enalapril antihypertensive therapy[3] reported adverse effects in 51% of 71 patients taking isradipine and 45% of 64 patients taking enalapril. The commonest side-effects with isradipine were dizziness (14%), oedema (10%), fatigue (9%), headache (9%), and pruritus (7%).

1. Carlsen JE, Køber L. Blood pressure lowering effect and adverse events during treatment of arterial hypertension with isradipine and hydrochlorothiazide. *Drug Invest* 1990; **2:** 10–16.
2. Hermans L, *et al.* At equipotent doses, isradipine is better tolerated than amlodipine in patients with mild-to-moderate hypertension: a double-blind, randomized, parallel-group study. *Br J Clin Pharmacol* 1994; **38:** 335–40.
3. Johnson BF, *et al.* A multicenter comparison of adverse reaction profiles of isradipine and enalapril at equipotent doses in patients with essential hypertension. *J Clin Pharmacol* 1995; **35:** 484–92.

Interactions

As for dihydropyridine calcium-channel blockers (see Nifedipine, p.918).

Pharmacokinetics

Isradipine is almost completely absorbed from the gastro-intestinal tract following a dose by mouth but undergoes extensive first-pass metabolism; the bioavailability is reported to be 15 to 24%. Peak plasma concentrations occur about 2 hours after oral administration. Isradipine is extensively metabolised in the liver. About 70% of an oral dose is reported to be excreted in urine, the remainder in faeces as metabolites. The terminal elimination half-life is often stated to be about 8 hours although a value of less than 4 hours has also been reported. Isradipine is about 95% bound to plasma protein.

In single-dose and steady-state studies of the pharmacokinetics of isradipine in 9 hypertensive subjects using a specific high performance liquid chromatographic assay, isradipine was found to be rapidly absorbed with peak concentrations occurring 1.2 (steady state) to 1.5 (single dose) hours after administration.[1] The mean terminal elimination half-life at steady state was 3.8 hours, suggesting that duration of action is likely to be short and that isradipine would need to be administered at least twice daily. There was considerable inter-individual variation in the pharmacokinetics. In an earlier study[2] in healthy subjects the effective half-life of isradipine was calculated to be 8.8 hours, but radiolabelled isradipine was used and the assay method might have been less specific for unchanged drug.

1. Shenfield GM, *et al.* The pharmacokinetics of isradipine in hypertensive subjects. *Eur J Clin Pharmacol* 1990; **38:** 209–11.
2. Tse FLS, Jaffe JM. Pharmacokinetics of PN 200-110 (isradipine), a new calcium antagonist, after oral administration in man. *Eur J Clin Pharmacol* 1987; **32:** 361–5.

Hepatic impairment. Systemic availability following a radiolabelled dose of isradipine 5 mg by mouth was no different at 15.6% in 7 patients with non-cirrhotic chronic liver disease from the value of 16.5% in 8 healthy subjects.[1] However, in 8 patients with cirrhosis of the liver availability was markedly increased to a mean of 36.9%; this was associated with decreased clearance (1.6 L per minute, compared with 9.9 in controls). Terminal half-life, as measured after intravenous administration, was greater at 11.9 hours in cirrhotic patients than the 5.1 hours seen in controls.

1. Cotting J, *et al.* Pharmacokinetics of isradipine in patients with chronic liver disease. *Eur J Clin Pharmacol* 1990; **38:** 599–603.

Uses and Administration

Isradipine is a dihydropyridine calcium-channel blocker with actions similar to those of nifedipine (p.919). It is used in the treatment of **hypertension** (p.788).

The usual initial dose of isradipine is 2.5 mg by mouth twice daily increased if necessary after 3 to 4 weeks to 5 mg twice daily. Some patients may require 10 mg twice daily. In elderly patients and those with impaired hepatic or renal function an initial dose of 1.25 mg twice daily may be preferable; a maintenance dose of 2.5 or 5 mg once daily may sometimes be sufficient.

A modified-release preparation allowing once-daily dosing is available in some countries.

Reviews.

1. Fitton A, Benfield P. Isradipine: a review of its pharmacodynamic and pharmacokinetic properties, and therapeutic use in cardiovascular disease. *Drugs* 1990; **40:** 31–74.
2. Walton T, Symes LR. Felodipine and isradipine: new calcium-channel blocking agents for the treatment of hypertension. *Clin Pharm* 1993; **12:** 261–75.
3. Brogden RN, Sorkin EM. Isradipine: an update of its pharmacodynamic and pharmacokinetic properties and therapeutic efficacy in the treatment of mild to moderate hypertension. *Drugs* 1995; **49:** 618–49.

Preparations

Proprietary Preparations (details are given in Part 3)
Aust.: Lomir; ***Belg.:*** Lomir; ***Canad.:*** Dynacirc†; ***Fr.:*** Icaz; ***Ger.:*** Lomir; Vascal; ***Irl.:*** Prescal; ***Ital.:*** Clivoten; Esradin; Lomir; ***Neth.:*** Lomir; ***Norw.:*** Lomir; ***S.Afr.:*** Dynacirc; ***Spain:*** Lomir; Vaslan; ***Swed.:*** Lomir; ***Switz.:*** Lomir; ***UK:*** Prescal; ***USA:*** Dynacirc.

Ketanserin Tartrate (12881-m)

Ketanserin Tartrate *(BANM, rINNM).*

R-49945; R-41468 (ketanserin). 3-{2-[4-(4-Fluorobenzoyl)piperidino]ethyl}quinazoline-2,4(1*H*,3*H*)-dione tartrate.

$C_{22}H_{22}FN_3O_3,C_4H_6O_6$ = 545.5.

CAS — 74050-98-9 (ketanserin).

NOTE. Ketanserin is *USAN.*

Ketanserin tartrate 27.6 mg is approximately equivalent to 20 mg of ketanserin.

Adverse Effects and Precautions

Ketanserin has been reported to cause sedation, fatigue, light-headedness, dizziness, headache, dry mouth, and gastro-intestinal disturbances. Oedema has been reported rarely. In patients with predisposing factors chronic administration of ketanserin has been associated with the development of ventricular arrhythmias; ketanserin should be used with caution in patients taking antiarrhythmics or those with second- or third-degree atrioventricular block. Care should be taken to avoid the development of hypokalaemia in patients taking ketanserin, for example if diuretics are given concomitantly.

Because ketanserin may cause drowsiness care should be taken in patients who drive or operate machinery.

Ketanserin is reported to be better tolerated in elderly than in younger patients.

Profound hypotension occurred in 2 patients one hour after taking ketanserin 40 mg by mouth.[1] Both patients were also taking a beta blocker which may have exacerbated the reaction.

1. Waller PC, *et al.* Profound hypotension after the first dose of ketanserin. *Postgrad Med J* 1987; **63:** 305–7.

Interactions

The hypotensive effects of ketanserin may be enhanced by diuretics and other antihypertensive drugs. Ketanserin should be used with caution in patients taking antiarrhythmics or drugs that cause hypokalaemia since the risk of arrhythmias is increased.

Pharmacokinetics

Ketanserin is rapidly absorbed from the gastro-intestinal tract but has a bioavailability of about 50% due to first-pass hepatic metabolism. Peak plasma concentrations occur between half and 2 hours after a dose by mouth. Ketanserin is about 95% bound to plasma proteins. The terminal half-life is stated to be between 13 and 18 hours but some studies report that following multiple doses the half-life is 19 to 29 hours. The metabolite ketanserinol has a terminal half-life of 31 to 35 hours following multiple doses, and it has been suggested that reconversion of ketanserinol to ketanserin may be responsible for the prolonged half-life of the parent compound during chronic administration.

Following oral administration about 68% of a dose is excreted in urine, and 24% in faeces, mainly as metabolites. Studies in *animals* suggest that ketanserin may cross the placenta and that some is present, together with metabolites, in breast milk.

References.

1. Kurowski M. Bioavailability and pharmacokinetics of ketanserin in elderly subjects. *Eur J Clin Pharmacol* 1985; **28:** 411–17.
2. Persson B, *et al.* Pharmacokinetics of ketanserin in patients with essential hypertension. *Eur J Clin Pharmacol* 1987; **32:** 259–65.
3. Persson B, *et al.* Clinical pharmacokinetics of ketanserin. *Clin Pharmacokinet* 1991; **20:** 263–79.

Uses and Administration

Ketanserin is a serotonin antagonist with a high affinity for peripheral serotonin-2 (5-HT_2) receptors and thus inhibits serotonin-induced vasoconstriction, bronchoconstriction, and platelet aggregation. It also has some $alpha_1$-antagonist and histamine H_1 antagonist properties, but the clinical significance of these is controversial.

Ketanserin is used in the management of hypertension (p.788) and has also been tried in a variety of other conditions (see below).

Ketanserin is given as the tartrate, but doses are usually expressed in terms of the base.

Ketanserin produces a gradual hypotensive effect when administered by mouth, and 2 or 3 months of therapy may be required to produce the maximum reduction in blood pressure. Following intravenous injection a fall in blood pressure is generally produced in one or two minutes and lasts for 30 to 60 minutes.

In **hypertension** the usual initial dose is 20 mg twice daily by mouth, increasing, if necessary, after 1 month, to 40 mg twice daily. It has also been given by intravenous or intramuscular injection in doses of 5 to 30 mg.

Action. Ketanserin has antagonist activity at both 5-HT_2 and α_1-adrenergic receptors, and the relative contribution of these and other mechanisms, including depression of the renin-angiotensin-aldosterone system, sympathetic inhibition, depletion of monoamine stores, and central nervous effects to the antihypertensive effect is still being investigated.[1] Experiments with ritanserin suggest that 5-HT_2 antagonism alone, either at central or peripheral sites, does not lower arterial pressure. Evidence for a role of α_1-adrenoceptor antagonism is conflicting, but there is some evidence that these two mechanisms of action act to potentiate antihypertensive effects. There is no clear unconflicting evidence for any central effect or for action on the renin-angiotensin system; an apparent partial depletion of catecholamine and indoleamine stores has been noted, as well as evidence for a direct effect on transmembrane sodium transport systems, but the contribution, if any, of these actions to the drug's antihypertensive effects remains to be determined.

1. Brogden RN, Sorkin EM. Ketanserin: a review of its pharmacodynamic and pharmacokinetic properties, and therapeutic potential in hypertension and peripheral vascular disease. *Drugs* 1990; **40:** 903–49.

Administration in hepatic impairment. The half-life and volume of distribution of ketanserin were decreased in patients with cirrhosis but the area under the concentration-time curve was markedly increased. The rate of metabolism was reduced. The results suggested that the dosage should be reduced or the dosage interval increased when ketanserin is given to patients with cirrhosis.[1]

1. Lebrec D, *et al.* Pharmacokinetics of ketanserin in patients with cirrhosis. *Clin Pharmacokinet* 1990; **19:** 160–6.

Administration in renal impairment. Results from a study in 12 patients with chronic renal impairment, of whom 6 required haemodialysis, suggested that no adjustment of the standard dose of ketanserin 20 mg twice daily was required in patients with renal impairment.[1]

1. Barendregt JNM, *et al.* Ketanserin pharmacokinetics in patients with renal failure. *Br J Clin Pharmacol* 1990; **29:** 715–23.

Carcinoid syndrome. The management of carcinoid syndrome (p.477) is mainly symptomatic and serotonin antagonists including ketanserin are among the drugs that have been used.

Frostbite. Frostbite is tissue damage resulting from freezing of the tissues and cold-induced vasoconstriction. The initial treatment is rapid rewarming and administration of analgesics. Spontaneous healing of necrotic tissue may occur slowly, although surgical amputation may be required. Sympathetic blockade, including regional guanethidine (p.878), has been suggested in the early stages. There has also been a report of rapid healing in a patient with severe bilateral frostbite following treatment with ketanserin.[1]

1. Vayssairat M, *et al.* Does ketanserin relieve frostbite? *Practitioner* 1986; **230:** 406–7.

Glaucoma and ocular hypertension. Ketanserin 0.5% eye drops can reduce intra-ocular pressure in normal and glaucomatous eyes;[1] their value if any in the treatment of glaucoma and ocular hypertension (p.1387) remains to be determined.

1. Costagliola C, *et al.* Effect of topical ketanserin administration on intraocular pressure. *Br J Ophthalmol* 1993; **77:** 344–8.

Peripheral vascular disease. Ketanserin is one of many drugs tried in the management of peripheral vascular disease (p.794) but results have been conflicting. Details of studies of ketanserin in intermittent claudication and Raynaud's syndrome are given below; see also Frostbite, above, and Wounds and Ulcers, below.

INTERMITTENT CLAUDICATION. Evidence of benefit from ketanserin in patients with intermittent claudication is equivocal. De Cree and others reported that ketanserin 20 to 40 mg three times daily in 11 patients improved the distance these patients could travel before forced to stop by claudication pain (claudication distance), when compared with placebo in 9 others.[1] There was evidence of improvement in the collateral circulation. However, Bounameaux and colleagues found that treatment with ketanserin had no effect on,[2] or actually worsened[3,4] claudication distance (depending on the statistical analysis),[4] in 18 patients, whereas 19 given placebo showed some improvement. The improvement in blood flow reported by De Cree has also been questioned. Beckers and co-workers examined macrocirculatory and microcirculatory blood flow in 6 patients who had received ketanserin in maintenance doses of 40 mg three times daily for a year and found no effect compared with placebo in 5 further patients.[5] The multicentre Prevention of Atherosclerotic Complications with Ketanserin Trial (PACK),[6] involving 3899 patients with intermittent claudication, suggested that ketanserin might be of benefit in preventing limb amputation in some patients, although this was the result of subgroup analysis.

1. De Cree J, *et al.* Placebo-controlled double-blind trial of ketanserin in treatment of intermittent claudication. *Lancet* 1984; **ii:** 775–9.
2. Bounameaux H, *et al.* Placebo-controlled, double-blind, two-centre trial of ketanserin in intermittent claudication. *Lancet* 1985; **ii:** 1268–71.
3. Ramsay LE. Ketanserin in intermittent claudication. *Lancet* 1986; **i:** 619.
4. Verhaeghe R. Ketanserin in intermittent claudication. *Lancet* 1986; **i:** 619.
5. Beckers RCY, *et al.* Effect of ketanserin on macrocirculatory and microcirculatory blood flow in patients with intermittent claudication: a prospective randomized study. *Eur J Clin Pharmacol* 1989; **37:** 295–6.
6. Prevention of Atherosclerotic Complications with Ketanserin Trial Group. Prevention of atherosclerotic complications: controlled trial of ketanserin. *Br Med J* 1989; **298:** 424–30. Correction. *ibid.*: 644.

RAYNAUD'S SYNDROME. There is some evidence of benefit from the use of ketanserin in Raynaud's syndrome. Stranden and colleagues reported that ketanserin 10 mg by intravenous injection into the hand produced an increase in finger blood-flow and skin temperature in 8 of 9 patients with primary or secondary Raynaud's syndrome.[1] Despite this, however, clinical results have been somewhat contradictory. Roald and Seem reported clinical improvement in 8 of 10 patients given ketanserin in a relatively-high dose of 40 mg three times daily for Raynaud's syndrome secondary to connective-tissue disorders,[2] but a similar study by Engelhart in 9 patients with Raynaud's syndrome secondary to scleroderma failed to note any benefit from this dose of ketanserin and found intolerable adverse effects to be common.[3] Comparisons with other drugs have also produced conflicting results. Kirch and co-workers found neither ketanserin 40 mg twice daily nor nifedipine 20 mg twice daily to be effective in relieving secondary Raynaud's syndrome in 10 patients with connective tissue disorders,[4] but a study by Codella and colleagues in 28 patients found some evidence for limited benefit of ketanserin 40 mg twice daily, which was considered to give a good response by 69.2% of patients compared with only 30% when given nifedipine 10 mg three times daily.[5] Probably the largest controlled trial, involving 112 patients with primary and 110 patients with secondary Raynaud's syndrome, found that treatment with ketanserin 40 mg three times daily produced a 34% decrease in frequency of attacks, compared with only 18% with placebo.[6] There was no difference in the duration or severity of attacks, nor was there any difference in the response of patients with primary or secondary disease.

1. Stranden E, *et al.* Treatment of Raynaud's phenomenon with the 5-HT_2-receptor antagonist ketanserin. *Br Med J* 1982; **285:** 1069–71.
2. Roald OK, Seem E. Treatment of Raynaud's phenomenon with ketanserin in patients with connective tissue disorders. *Br Med J* 1984; **289:** 577–9.
3. Engelhart M. Ketanserin in the treatment of Raynaud's phenomenon associated with generalized scleroderma. *Br J Dermatol* 1988; **119:** 751–4.
4. Kirch W, *et al.* Ketanserin versus nifedipine in secondary Raynaud's phenomenon. *Vasa* 1987; **16:** 77–80.
5. Codella O, *et al.* Controlled comparison of ketanserin and nifedipine in Raynaud's phenomenon. *Angiology* 1989; **40:** 114–21.
6. Coffman JD, *et al.* International study of ketanserin in Raynaud's phenomenon. *Am J Med* 1989; **87:** 264–8.

Shivering. Numerous drugs, including ketanserin, have been tried for the treatment of postoperative shivering (p.1219).

In a preliminary study ketanserin 10 mg intravenously stopped shivering after general anaesthesia.[1]

1. Joris J, *et al.* Clonidine and ketanserin both are effective treatment for postanesthetic shivering. *Anesthesiology* 1993; **79:** 532–9.

Wounds and ulcers. Systemic administration of ketanserin has been reported to improve healing in various ulcers associated with impaired blood flow,[1,2] although others have found little benefit.[3] Several placebo-controlled studies[4-6] have reported improved healing of decubitus, venous, and ischaemic ulcers following the application of ketanserin as a 2% ointment. However, when ketanserin was applied topically as a 2% gel to surgical wounds no improvement in healing rate was found and it was suggested that ketanserin is only of benefit where the blood supply is compromised.[7]

The management of wounds and ulcers in general is described on p.1076.

1. Roald OK, Seem E. Treatment of Raynaud's phenomenon with ketanserin in patients with connective tissue disorders. *Br Med J* 1984; **289:** 577–8.
2. Rustin MHA, *et al.* Chronic leg ulceration with livedoid vasculitis, and response to oral ketanserin. *Br J Dermatol* 1989; **120:** 101–5.
3. Cox NH, Dufton PA. Treatment of Raynaud's phenomenon with ketanserin. *Br Med J* 1984; **289:** 1078–9.
4. Tytgat H, van Asch H. Topical ketanserin in the treatment of decubitus ulcers: a double-blind study with 2% ketanserin ointment against placebo. *Adv Therapy* 1988; **5:** 143–52.
5. Roelens P. Double-blind placebo-controlled study with topical 2% ketanserin ointment in the treatment of venous ulcers. *Dermatologica* 1989; **178:** 98–102.
6. Janssen PAJ, *et al.* Use of topical ketanserin in the treatment of skin ulcers: a double-blind study. *J Am Acad Dermatol* 1989; **21:** 85–90.
7. Lawrence CM, *et al.* The effect of ketanserin on healing of fresh surgical wounds. *Br J Dermatol* 1995; **132:** 580–6.

Preparations

Proprietary Preparations (details are given in Part 3)

Belg.: Sufrexal; ***Ital.:*** Ket†; Perketan; Serepress; Sufrexal; ***Neth.:*** Ketensin; ***Switz.:*** Sufrexal†.

Labetalol Hydrochloride (6311-p)

Labetalol Hydrochloride *(BANM, USAN, rINNM)*.

AH-5158A; Ibidomide Hydrochloride; Labetaloli Hydrochloridum; Sch-15719W. 5-[1-Hydroxy-2-(1-methyl-3-phenylpropylamino)ethyl]salicylamide hydrochloride; 2-Hydroxy-5-[1-hydroxy-2-(1-methyl-3-phenylpropylamino)ethyl]benzamide hydrochloride.

$C_{19}H_{24}N_2O_3,HCl = 364.9.$

CAS — 36894-69-6 (labetalol); 32780-64-6 (labetalol hydrochloride).

Pharmacopoeias. In *Eur.* (see p.viii) and *US.*

A white or almost white powder. **Soluble** to sparingly soluble in water and in alcohol; practically insoluble in chloroform, in dichloromethane, and in ether. A 1% solution in water has a pH of 4 to 5. **Store** in airtight containers. Protect from light.

Incompatibility. Labetalol hydrochloride is considered compatible with standard intravenous solutions such as glucose 5% and sodium chloride 0.9%. However, precipitation has been reported when labetalol hydrochloride is added to sodium bicarbonate injection 5%.[1] The precipitate is probably labetalol base.[2]

A study investigating the compatibility and stability of labetalol with various drugs used in intensive care settings[3] found that labetalol hydrochloride 1 mg per mL (in glucose 5%) was stable for up to 4 hours at 20 to 25° in combination with dobutamine 2.5 mg per mL, dopamine hydrochloride 1.6 mg per mL, glyceryl trinitrate 0.2 mg per mL, morphine sulphate 0.5 mg per mL, or ranitidine 0.6 mg per mL. The drugs were mixed together in Y-site administration sets. Incompatibilities have been reported with frusemide 10 mg per mL,[4] heparin 100 units per mL,[5] insulin 1 unit per mL,[5] and thiopentone[4] [no concentration specified]. In all cases a white precipitate formed immediately on mixing with labetalol hydrochloride 5 mg per mL (in glucose 5%).

1. Yuen P-HC, *et al.* Compatibility and stability of labetalol hydrochloride in commonly used intravenous solutions. *Am J Hosp Pharm* 1983; **40:** 1007–9.
2. Alam AS. Identification of labetalol precipitate. *Am J Hosp Pharm* 1984; **41:** 74.
3. Hassan E, *et al.* Stability of labetalol hydrochloride with selected critical care drugs during simulated Y-site injection. *Am J Hosp Pharm* 1994; **51:** 2143–5.
4. Chiu MF, Schwartz ML. Visual compatibility of injectable drugs used in the intensive care unit. *Am J Health-Syst Pharm* 1997; **54:** 64–5.
5. Yamashita SK, *et al.* Compatibility of selected critical care drugs during simulated Y-site administration. *Am J Health-Syst Pharm* 1996; **53:** 1048–51.

Adverse Effects

The adverse effects following beta blockade are described on p.828. Labetalol's alpha-blocking activity also contributes to its adverse effects. Postural hypotension may be a problem with high doses or at the start of treatment. Other effects include scalp tingling, nasal congestion, muscle weakness, dyspnoea, tremor, urinary retention, hepatitis, and jaundice. Male sexual function may be impaired to a greater extent than with beta blockade alone.

In a summary of clinical experience with labetalol, Goa *et al.*[1] reported that the most frequent adverse effects during oral therapy are dizziness, fatigue, headache, scalp tingling, nasal congestion, and gastro-intestinal symptoms. Dizziness was the most troublesome adverse effect and was reported in 3 to 12% of patients. Hypotension occurs and may be asymptomatic. Dizziness, scalp tingling, and nasal congestion are associated with alpha-adrenoceptor blockade. Adverse effects attributed specifically to beta blockade include exacerbation of asthma, Raynaud's phenomenon, CNS depression, nightmares, and heart failure; these adverse effects tend to occur at a lower incidence than those attributed to alpha blockade.

1. Goa KL, *et al.* Labetalol: a reappraisal of its pharmacology, pharmacokinetics and therapeutic use in hypertension and ischaemic heart disease. *Drugs* 1989; **37:** 583–627.

Effects on the liver. By 1990, the US Food and Drug Administration had received 11 reports of hepatocellular damage associated with labetalol therapy.[1] Three patients died. Liver function should be monitored and labetalol discontinued in patients who develop liver function abnormalities. The *R,R*-isomer of labetalol, dilevalol, was withdrawn from the market because of hepatotoxicity.[2]

1. Clark JA, *et al.* Labetalol hepatotoxicity. *Ann Intern Med* 1990; **113:** 210–13.
2. Harvengt C. Labetalol hepatotoxicity. *Ann Intern Med* 1991; **114:** 341.

Hypersensitivity. Hypersensitivity reactions may manifest as fever.[1] Anaphylactoid reaction to labetalol has also been reported.[2]

1. D'Arcy PF. Drug reactions and interactions: drug fever with labetalol. *Int Pharm J* 1987; **1:** 43–4.
2. Ferree CE. Apparent anaphylaxis from labetalol. *Ann Intern Med* 1986; **104:** 729–30.

Overdosage. Acute oliguric renal failure developed after a short period of moderate hypotension in a patient who ingested labetalol 16 g. Renal function subsequently recovered.[1] Renal failure has also been reported following ingestion of labetalol 6 g.[2] The patient recovered following treatment with glucagon, isoprenaline, and dialysis.

1. Smit AJ, *et al.* Acute renal failure after overdose of labetalol. *Br Med J* 1986; **293:** 1142–3.
2. Korzets A, *et al.* Acute renal failure associated with a labetalol overdose. *Postgrad Med J* 1990; **66:** 66–7.

Precautions

As for beta blockers, p.829.

Because labetalol causes postural hypotension it is recommended that injections are administered to patients when they are lying down and that patients should remain lying down for the following 3 hours.

Labetalol should be withdrawn from patients who develop signs of liver impairment.

Interactions

The interactions associated with beta blockers are discussed on p.829.

Labetalol may enhance the effect of halothane on blood pressure.

Pharmacokinetics

Labetalol is readily absorbed from the gastro-intestinal tract, but is subject to considerable first-pass metabolism. Bioavailability varies widely between patients and may be increased in the presence of food. Peak plasma concentrations occur about 1 to 2 hours after an oral dose. Labetalol has low lipid solubility and only very small amounts appear to cross the blood-brain barrier in *animals*. It is about 50% protein bound. Labetalol crosses the placenta and is distributed into breast milk. Labetalol is metabolised predominantly in the liver, the metabolites being excreted in the urine together with only small amounts of unchanged labetalol; its major metabolite has not been found to have significant alpha- or beta-adrenoceptor blocking effects. Excretion also occurs in the faeces via the bile. The elimination half-life at steady state is reported to be 8 hours. Following intravenous infusion, the elimination half-life is about 5.5 hours. Labetalol is not removed by dialysis.

Old age. Data from 4 single-dose studies and 3 multidose studies were analysed to determine the effect of age on the pharmacokinetics of labetalol hydrochloride given by mouth.[1] Age did not appear to be a significant factor in oral clearance in elderly patients receiving labetalol for long-term management of hypertension.

1. Rocci ML, *et al.* Effects of age on the elimination of labetalol. *Clin Pharmacokinet* 1989; **17:** 452–7.

Pregnancy and breast feeding. The concentration of labetalol hydrochloride is lower in amniotic fluid and fetal plasma than in maternal plasma. A ratio of infant to maternal drug concentration of 0.2 to 0.8 has been reported based on concentration in infant cord blood at delivery.[1]

In 2 of 3 studies, the concentration of labetalol in breast milk was substantially less than in maternal plasma. In the third study, the concentration of drug in milk exceeded maternal plasma concentration in 2 of 3 mothers. In one infant, the plasma-labetalol concentration was similar to that of the mother.[1] The half-life of labetalol was reported as 24 hours in a neonate of 37 weeks' gestation whose mother had received labetalol 600 mg daily for 11 weeks prior to delivery.[2]

1. Goa KL, *et al.* Labetalol: a reappraisal of its pharmacology, pharmacokinetics and therapeutic use in hypertension and ischaemic heart disease. *Drugs* 1989; **37:** 583–627.
2. Haraldsson A, Geven W. Half-life of maternal labetalol in a premature infant. *Pharm Weekbl (Sci)* 1989; **11:** 229–31.

Uses and Administration

Labetalol is a non-cardioselective beta blocker (p.828). It is reported to possess some intrinsic sympathomimetic and membrane-stabilising activity. In addition, it has selective $alpha_1$-blocking properties which decrease peripheral vascular resistance. The ratio of alpha- to beta-blocking activity has been estimated to be about 1:3 following oral administration and 1:7 following intravenous administration.

Labetalol is used as the hydrochloride in the management of hypertension (p.788). It is also used to induce hypotension during surgery. Labetalol decreases blood pressure more rapidly than other beta blockers; the full antihypertensive effect may be seen within 1 to 3 hours of an oral dose.

In **hypertension** labetalol hydrochloride is usually given in an initial dose of 100 mg twice daily by mouth with food, gradually increased if necessary according to the response of the patient and standing blood pressure, to 200 to 400 mg twice daily; total daily doses of 2.4 g have occasionally been required. An initial dose of 50 mg twice daily has been recommended for elderly patients.

For the emergency treatment of hypertension labetalol hydrochloride may be given by slow intravenous injection. In the UK a dose of 50 mg, over a period of at least 1 minute, is recommended; if necessary this dose may be repeated at intervals of 5 minutes until a total of 200 mg has been given. In the USA an initial dose of 20 mg is recommended, given over 2 minutes; subsequent doses of 40 to 80 mg may be given every 10 minutes if necessary up to a maximum of 300 mg. Blood pressure should be monitored, and the patient should remain supine during intravenous administration and for 3 hours afterwards, to avoid excessive postural hypotension. Following bolus intravenous injection a maximum effect is usually obtained within 5 minutes and usually lasts up to 6 hours, although it may extend as long as 18 hours.

Labetalol hydrochloride has also been given by intravenous infusion in usual doses of 2 mg per minute. Suggested concentrations for intravenous infusions are 1 mg per mL or 2 mg per 3 mL of suitable diluent. In hypertension in pregnancy, labetalol infusion may be started at the rate of 20 mg per hour, then doubled every 30 minutes until a satisfactory response is obtained or a dose of 160 mg per hour is reached. In hypertension following myocardial infarction, labetalol infusion may be started at the rate of 15 mg per hour and gradually increased until a satisfactory response is obtained or a dose of 120 mg per hour is reached.

A recommended initial dose in **hypotensive anaesthesia** is 10 to 20 mg intravenously, with increments of 5 to 10 mg if satisfactory hypotension is not achieved after 5 minutes. A higher initial dose may be required if halothane anaesthesia is not used (see under Interactions of Beta Blockers, p.829).

Action. Labetalol hydrochloride has 2 optical centres; it is used as the racemic mixture of the 4 stereoisomers. The *R,R*-isomer is responsible for the beta-blocking activity and has limited alpha-blocking activity; it also has beta-adrenergic mediated peripheral vasodilating activity. The *S,R*-isomer has the most potent alpha-blocking activity. The *S,S*-isomer has some alpha-blocking activity and the *R,S*-isomer does not appear to have either alpha- or beta-adrenergic blocking effect.[1] The *R,R*-isomer, dilevalol (p.854), appears to be hepatotoxic.

1. Gold EH, *et al.* Synthesis and comparison of some cardiovascular properties of the stereoisomers of labetalol. *J Med Chem* 1982; **25:** 1363–70.

Tetanus. Autonomic overactivity, usually due to excessive catecholamine release, may occur as a complication of tetanus. Intravenous labetalol has been used successfully to control the cardiovascular effects.[1] Labetalol has both alpha- and beta-blocking properties. Unopposed beta blockade may produce severe hypertension and is thus not usually recommended, although esmolol, a short-acting beta blocker has been used.[2]

Management of the neuromuscular manifestations of tetanus is discussed on p.1304.

1. Domenighetti GM, *et al.* Hyperadrenergic syndrome in severe tetanus: extreme rise in catecholamines responsive to labetalol. *Br Med J* 1984; **288:** 1483–4.
2. King WW, Cave DR. Use of esmolol to control autonomic instability of tetanus. *Am J Med* 1991; **91:** 425–8.

Preparations

BP 1998: Labetalol Injection; Labetalol Tablets;
USP 23: Labetalol Hydrochloride Injection; Labetalol Hydrochloride Tablets.

Proprietary Preparations (details are given in Part 3)
Aust.: Trandate; ***Austral.:*** Presolol; Trandate; ***Belg.:*** Trandate; ***Canad.:*** Trandate; ***Fr.:*** Trandate; ***Ger.:*** Trandate†; ***Irl.:*** Trandate; ***Ital.:*** Abetol; Alfabetal; Amipress; Ipolab; Lolum†; Mitalolo†;

Pressalolo; Trandate; *Neth.:* Trandate; *Norw.:* Trandate; *S.Afr.:* Trandate; *Spain:* Trandate; *Swed.:* Trandate; *Switz.:* Trandate; *UK:* Labrocol; Trandate; *USA:* Normodyne; Trandate.

Multi-ingredient: *Ital.:* Biotens; Diurolab†; Pressalolo Diuretico; Trandiur; *USA:* Normozide†.

Lacidipine (2495-d)

Lacidipine *(BAN, USAN, rINN).*

GR-43659X; GX-1048. Diethyl 4-{2-[(*tert*-butoxycarbonyl)vinyl]phenyl}-1,4-dihydro-2,6-dimethylpyridine-3,5-dicarboxylate.

$C_{26}H_{33}NO_6$ = 455.5.

CAS — 103890-78-4.

Adverse Effects, Treatment, and Precautions

As for dihydropyridine calcium-channel blockers (see Nifedipine, p.916).

Interactions

As for dihydropyridine calcium-channel blockers (see Nifedipine, p.918).

Pharmacokinetics

Lacidipine is rapidly but poorly absorbed from the gastro-intestinal tract following oral administration and undergoes extensive first-pass metabolism; the bioavailability has been reported to be 2 to 9%, or 18.5% (range 4 to 52%) using a more sensitive assay method. Lacidipine is eliminated by metabolism in the liver and metabolites are excreted mainly by the biliary route. About 70% of an oral dose is eliminated in the faeces, the remainder in the urine. The average steady-state terminal elimination half-life of lacidipine is 13 to 19 hours. It is more than 95% bound to plasma proteins.

Uses and Administration

Lacidipine is a dihydropyridine calcium-channel blocker with actions similar to those of nifedipine (p.919). It is used in the treatment of **hypertension** (p.788).

The usual initial dose of lacidipine is 2 mg once daily by mouth increased if necessary after 3 to 4 weeks or more to 4 mg daily; a further increase in dose to 6 mg daily may be necessary in some patients.

Reviews.

1. Lee CR, Bryson HM. Lacidipine: a review of its pharmacodynamic and pharmacokinetic properties and therapeutic potential in the treatment of hypertension. *Drugs* 1994; **48:** 274–96.
2. Anonymous. Lacidipine—a once-daily calcium antagonist for hypertension. *Drug Ther Bull* 1994; **32:** 60–1. Correction. *ibid.*; 96.

Preparations

Proprietary Preparations (details are given in Part 3)
Belg.: Motens; *Fr.:* Caldine; *Ital.:* Aponil; Lacipil; Lacirex; Viapres; *Neth.:* Motens; *S.Afr.:* Zascal†; *Spain:* Lacimen; Lacipil; Motens; *Swed.:* Midotens; *Switz.:* Motens; *UK:* Motens.

Lamifiban (17727-w)

Lamifiban *(USAN, rINN).*

Ro-44-9883; Ro-44-9883/000. ({1-[*N*-(*p*-Amidinobenzoyl)-L-tyrosyl]-4-piperidyl}oxy)acetic acid.

$C_{24}H_{28}N_4O_6$ = 468.5.

CAS — 144412-49-7.

Lamifiban is an antiplatelet drug that acts by blocking glycoprotein IIb/IIIa receptors. It is under investigation for the management of thrombo-embolic disorders, such as unstable angina.

References.

1. Théroux P, *et al.* Platelet membrane receptor glycoprotein IIb/IIIa antagonism in unstable angina: the Canadian Lamifiban Study. *Circulation* 1996; **94:** 899–905.
2. The PARAGON Investigators. International, randomized, controlled trial of lamifiban (a platelet glycoprotein IIb/IIIa inhibitor), heparin, or both in unstable angina. *Circulation* 1998; **97:** 2386–95.

Lanatoside C (5819-v)

Lanatoside C *(BAN, rINN).*

Celanide; Celanidum; Lanatosidum C. 3-[(*O*-β-D-Glucopyranosyl-(1→4)-*O*-3-acetyl-2,6-dideoxy-β-D-*ribo*-hexopyranosyl-(1→4)-*O*-2,6-dideoxy-β-D-*ribo*-hexopyranosyl-(1→4)-*O*-2,6-dideoxy-β-D-*ribo*-hexopyranosyl)oxy]-12,14-dihydroxy-3β,5β,12β-card-20(22)-enolide.

$C_{49}H_{76}O_{20}$ = 985.1.

CAS — 17575-22-3.

Pharmacopoeias. In *Eur.* (see p.viii), *Jpn,* and *Pol.*

A glycoside obtained from digitalis lanata leaf. It occurs as white or yellowish, hygroscopic crystals or crystalline powder.

Practically **insoluble** in water and in ether; soluble in methyl alcohol. **Store** in airtight, well-filled, glass containers at a temperature not exceeding 10°. Protect from light.

Lanatoside C is a cardiac glycoside with positive inotropic activity. It has general properties similar to those of digoxin (p.849) and has been used in the treatment of some cardiac arrhythmias and in heart failure.

Mixtures of lanatosides A, B, and C have also been used.

Preparations

Proprietary Preparations (details are given in Part 3)
Aust.: Cedilanid; *Ger.:* Cedilanid†; Celadigal†; *Irl.:* Cedilanid†; *Ital.:* Cedilanid†; *S.Afr.:* Cedilanid†; *Switz.:* Celanate†.

Multi-ingredient: *Ger.:* Pandigal†.

Lanoteplase (9235-y)

Lanoteplase *(rINN).*

$C_{2184}H_{3323}N_{633}O_{666}S_{29}$ = 50032.5.

CAS — 171870-23-8.

Lanoteplase is a thrombolytic under investigation in acute myocardial infarction.

Leech (4816-k)

Blutegel; Hirudo; Sangsue; Sanguessugas; Sanguisuga.

Pharmacopoeias. In *Chin.*

Hirudo medicinalis is the leech commonly used in medicine and is a fresh-water annelid.

Leeches are used for withdrawing blood from congested areas and have been found to be of value in plastic surgery. The buccal secretion of the leech contains the anticoagulant hirudin (p.883). The part to be bitten may be moistened with sugar solution before applying the leech. Once used a leech should not be applied to another patient.

There have been reports of wound infection from *Aeromonas hydrophila* transmitted by leeches. Prolonged bleeding may occur from the site of attachment once the leech has been removed.

References.

1. Braidwood PS. The medicinal leech. *Pharm J* 1987; **239:** 766–7.
2. Abrutyn E. Hospital-associated infection from leeches. *Ann Intern Med* 1988; **109:** 356–8.
3. Adams SL. The medicinal leech; a page from the annelids of internal medicine. *Ann Intern Med* 1988; **109:** 399–405.
4. Menage MJ, Wright G. Use of leeches in a case of severe periorbital haematoma. *Br J Ophthalmol* 1991; **75:** 755–6.
5. Anonymous. Hirudins: return of the leech? *Lancet* 1992; **340:** 579–80.

Precautions. Dickson *et al.*[1] reported a case of wound infection due to *Aeromonas hydrophila* acquired from leeches used for decongestion in plastic surgery. Subsequently Mercer *et al.*[2] reported 6 cases of similar infection occurring over a period of 3 years when they would have used leeches on about 30 patients—an infection rate of 20%. All but one of the strains were resistant to penicillin and ampicillin; successful treatment was with amoxycillin, with or without clavulanic acid, or with cefuroxime.

1. Dickson WA, *et al.* An unusual source of hospital wound infection. *Br Med J* 1984; **289:** 1727–8.
2. Mercer NSG, *et al.* Medical leeches as sources of wound infection. *Br Med J* 1987; **294:** 937.

Preparations

Proprietary Preparations (details are given in Part 3)
Aust.: Exhirud; *Ger.:* Exhirud.

Multi-ingredient: *Ger.:* HAEMO-Exhirud; *Ital.:* Hirudex.

Lercanidipine Hydrochloride (17047-s)

Lercanidipine Hydrochloride *(BANM, rINNM).*

Masnidipine Hydrochloride; R-75; Rec-15-2375. (±)-2-[(3,3-Diphenylpropyl)methylamino]-1,1-dimethylethyl methyl 1,4-dihydro-2,6-dimethyl-4-(*m*-nitrophenyl)-3,5-pyridinedicarboxylate hydrochloride.

$C_{36}H_{41}N_3O_6$,HCl = 648.2.

CAS — 100427-26-7 (lercanidipine); 132866-11-6 (lercanidipine hydrochloride).

Adverse Effects, Treatment, and Precautions

As for dihydropyridine calcium-channel blockers (see Nifedipine, p.916).

Interactions

As for dihydropyridine calcium-channel blockers (see Nifedipine, p.918).

Pharmacokinetics

Lercanidipine is completely absorbed from the gastro-intestinal tract following oral administration but undergoes extensive saturable first-pass metabolism. Peak plasma concentrations occur about 1.5 to 3 hours after oral administration. Lercanidipine is rapidly and widely distributed. It is more than 98% bound to plasma proteins. Lercanidipine is extensively metabolised mainly to inactive metabolites and about 50% of an oral dose is excreted in the urine. The terminal elimination half-life is about 2 to 5 hours.

Uses and Administration

Lercanidipine is a dihydropyridine calcium-channel blocker with actions similar to those of nifedipine (p.919). It is used in the treatment of **hypertension** (p.788).

Lercanidipine is given by mouth as the hydrochloride in a usual initial dose of 10 mg daily before food increased if necessary after at least 2 weeks to 20 mg daily.

Preparations

Proprietary Preparations (details are given in Part 3)
Neth.: Lerdip; *UK:* Zanidip.

Levobunolol Hydrochloride (6312-s)

Levobunolol Hydrochloride *(BANM, USAN, rINNM).*

(−)-Bunolol Hydrochloride; *l*-Bunolol Hydrochloride; W-7000A. (−)-5-(3-*tert*-Butylamino-2-hydroxypropoxy)-3,4-dihydronaphthalen-1(2*H*)-one hydrochloride; (−)-5-(3-*tert*-Butylamino-2-hydroxypropoxy)-1,2,3,4-tetrahydronaphthalen-1-one hydrochloride.

$C_{17}H_{25}NO_3$,HCl = 327.8.

CAS — 47141-42-4 (levobunolol); 27912-14-7 (levobunolol hydrochloride).

Pharmacopoeias. In *Br.* and *US.*

A white or pinkish white odourless crystalline powder. **Soluble** to freely soluble in water; slightly to sparingly soluble in alcohol; soluble in methyl alcohol; slightly soluble in chloroform. A 5% solution in water has a pH between 4.5 and 6.5. **Protect** from light.

Adverse Effects, Treatment, and Precautions

As for beta blockers, p.828.

Systemic effects have followed topical use of the eye drops; local irritation and blurred vision have also occurred.

Effects on respiratory function. A 42-year-old female developed a wheeze, which lasted about 20 minutes, approximately 8 hours after starting treatment with one drop in each eye of levobunolol 0.25%.[1] A second dose was instilled 12 hours after the first dose and after about 2½ hours the patient developed severe respiratory distress requiring hospitalisation.

1. Stubbs GM. Betagan drops. *Med J Aust* 1994; **161:** 576.

Interactions

The interactions associated with beta blockers are discussed on p.829.

Pharmacokinetics

Some systemic absorption is reported to occur following topical application to the eye. Following oral administration levobunolol is rapidly and almost completely absorbed from the gastro-intestinal tract. It is extensively metabolised in the liver; the principal metabolite, dihydrolevobunolol, is reported to possess beta blocking activity. The metabolites and a certain amount of unchanged drug are excreted in the urine.

Uses and Administration

Levobunolol is a non-cardioselective beta blocker (p.828). It is reported to lack intrinsic sympathomimetic activity and membrane-stabilising properties.

Levobunolol is used as the hydrochloride to reduce raised intra-ocular pressure in open-angle glaucoma and ocular hypertension (p.1387). The usual dosage is one drop of a 0.5% solution instilled once or twice daily. Other regimens include 1 to 2 drops of a 0.25% solution instilled twice daily.

Preparations

BP 1998: Levobunolol Eye Drops;
USP 23: Levobunolol Hydrochloride Ophthalmic Solution.

Proprietary Preparations (details are given in Part 3)
Aust.: Vistagan; ***Austral.:*** Betagan; ***Belg.:*** Betagan; ***Canad.:*** Betagan; Ophtho-Bunolol; ***Fr.:*** Betagan; ***Ger.:*** Vistagan; ***Irl.:*** Betagan; ***Ital.:*** Vistagan; ***Neth.:*** Betagan†; ***S.Afr.:*** Betagan; ***Spain:*** Betagan; ***Swed.:*** Betagan; ***Switz.:*** Vistagan; ***UK:*** Betagan; ***USA:*** Ak-Beta; Betagan.

Multi-ingredient: ***Canad.:*** Probeta.

Levomoprolol Hydrochloride (19406-s)

Levomoprolol Hydrochloride (*rINNM*).
(−)-(*S*)-Moprolol Hydrochloride. (−)-(*S*)-1-(Isopropylamino)-3-(*o*-methoxyphenoxy)-2-propanol hydrochloride.
$C_{13}H_{21}NO_3,HCl = 275.8.$
CAS — 77164-20-6 (levomoprolol).

Levomoprolol is a beta blocker (p.828). It is the (−)-enantiomer of moprolol and is responsible for moprolol's beta-blocking activity.

Both moprolol hydrochloride and levomoprolol hydrochloride have been given in the management of hypertension.

Preparations

Proprietary Preparations (details are given in Part 3)
Ital.: Levotensin†.

Multi-ingredient: ***Ital.:*** Betalevo†; Minusten†.

Libenzapril (5467-x)

Libenzapril (*USAN, rINN*).
CGS-16617. *N*-[(3*S*)-1-(Carboxymethyl)-2,3,4,5-tetrahydro-2-oxo-1*H*-1-benzazepin-3-yl]-L-lysine.
$C_{18}H_{25}N_3O_5 = 363.4.$
CAS — 97878-35-8; 109214-55-3.

Libenzapril is an ACE inhibitor (p.805) that is under investigation in the management of hypertension.

References.

1. Waeber G, *et al.* Effects of prolonged administration of the angiotensin converting enzyme inhibitor CGS 16617 in normotensive volunteers. *Eur J Clin Pharmacol* 1989; **36:** 587–91.
2. Morgan JM, *et al.* Inhibition of angiotensin-converting enzyme with libenzapril in normotensive males. *J Clin Pharmacol* 1994; **34:** 1177–82.

Lidoflazine (9250-l)

Lidoflazine (*BAN, USAN, rINN*).
McN-JR-7904; Ordiflazine; R-7904. 4-[3-(4,4′-Difluorobenzhydryl)propyl]piperazin-1-ylaceto-2′,6′-xylidide.
$C_{30}H_{35}F_2N_3O = 491.6.$
CAS — 3416-26-0.
Pharmacopoeias. In *Belg.*

Adverse Effects

Side-effects associated with lidoflazine include gastro-intestinal upset, transient dizziness, tinnitus and headache. Central effects such as hallucinations have occurred. Lidoflazine may also cause or aggravate sinus bradycardia, atrioventricular block, and ventricular arrhythmias.

Uses and Administration

Lidoflazine is a calcium-channel blocker (p.778) that reduces atrioventricular conduction. It has been used in angina pectoris (p.780). A recommended oral dosage schedule was 60 mg daily initially for the first week, increased at weekly intervals to 60 mg three times daily. Higher doses, up to 120 mg three times daily, have been given.

Preparations

Proprietary Preparations (details are given in Part 3)
Ger.: Clinium†.

Linsidomine Hydrochloride (5469-f)

Linsidomine Hydrochloride (*rINNM*).
3-Morpholinosydnonimine hydrochloride.
$C_6H_{10}N_4O_2,HCl = 206.6.$
CAS — 33876-97-0 (linsidomine); 16142-27-1 (linsidomine hydrochloride).

Linsidomine is a nitrovasodilator and a metabolite of molsidomine (p.912). It is given as the hydrochloride via the intracoronary route in doses of 0.6 to 1 mg in the management of coronary artery spasm and to facilitate vasodilatation during coronary angiography. Additional doses may be required; the maximum total dose is 2 mg. It is also given by intravenous infusion in the management of unstable angina (p.780), in an initial dose of 1 mg per hour, adjusted according to response.

References.

1. Delonca J, *et al.* Comparative efficacy of the intravenous administration of linsidomine, a direct nitric oxide donor, and isosorbide dinitrate in severe unstable angina: a French multicentre study. *Eur Heart J* 1997; **18:** 1300–6.

Preparations

Proprietary Preparations (details are given in Part 3)
Fr.: Corvasal.

Lisinopril (16878-k)

Lisinopril (*BAN, USAN, rINN*).
Lisinoprilum; MK-521. *N*-{*N*-[(*S*)-1-Carboxy-3-phenylpropyl]-L-lysyl}-L-proline dihydrate.
$C_{21}H_{31}N_3O_5,2H_2O = 441.5.$
CAS — 76547-98-3 (anhydrous lisinopril); 83915-83-7 (lisinopril dihydrate).
Pharmacopoeias. In *Eur.* (see p.viii) and *US.*

A white crystalline powder. **Soluble** 1 in 10 of water and 1 in 70 of methyl alcohol; practically insoluble in alcohol, in acetone, in chloroform, and in ether.

Lisinopril 2.72 mg as the dihydrate is approximately equivalent to 2.5 mg of anhydrous lisinopril.

Adverse Effects, Treatment, and Precautions

As for ACE inhibitors, p.805.

Interactions

As for ACE inhibitors, p.807.

Pharmacokinetics

Lisinopril is slowly and incompletely absorbed following oral administration. About 25% of a given dose is absorbed on average, but the absorption varies considerably between individuals, ranging from about 6 to 60%. It is already an active diacid and does not need to be metabolised *in vivo*. Peak concentrations in plasma are reported to occur after about 7 hours. Lisinopril is reported not to be significantly bound to plasma proteins. It is excreted unchanged in the urine. The effective half-life for accumulation following multiple doses is 12 hours in patients with normal renal function. Lisinopril is removed by haemodialysis.

References.

1. Till AE, *et al.* The pharmacokinetics of lisinopril in hospitalized patients with congestive heart failure. *Br J Clin Pharmacol* 1989; **27:** 199–204.
2. Neubeck M, *et al.* Pharmacokinetics and pharmacodynamics of lisinopril in advanced renal failure: consequence of dose adjustment. *Eur J Clin Pharmacol* 1994; **46:** 537–43.

Uses and Administration

Lisinopril is an ACE inhibitor (p.805). It is used in the treatment of hypertension (p.788) and heart failure (p.785), prophylactically after myocardial infarction (p.791), and in diabetic nephropathy (p.809).

The haemodynamic effects of lisinopril are seen within 1 to 2 hours of a single oral dose and the maximum effect occurs after about 6 hours, although the full effect may not develop for several weeks during chronic dosing. The haemodynamic action lasts for about 24 hours following once-daily dosing. Lisinopril is given by mouth as the dihydrate, but doses are expressed in terms of the anhydrous substance.

In the treatment of **hypertension** the initial dose is 2.5 mg daily; if possible, diuretic therapy should be withdrawn 2 or 3 days before lisinopril is started and resumed later if required. Since there may be a precipitous fall in blood pressure in some patients when starting therapy with an ACE inhibitor, the first dose should preferably be given at bedtime. Higher initial doses have been used and in the USA 10 mg of lisinopril daily is suggested for patients with uncomplicated hypertension, not on diuretic therapy, and without substantial renal impairment. The usual maintenance dose is 10 to 20 mg given once daily, though up to 40 mg daily may be given if necessary.

In the management of **heart failure**, severe first-dose hypotension on introduction of an ACE inhibitor is common in patients on loop diuretics, but their temporary withdrawal may cause rebound pulmonary oedema. Thus treatment should be initiated with a low dose under close medical supervision. Lisinopril is given by mouth in an initial dose of 2.5 mg daily. In the USA an initial dose of 5 mg daily is suggested. Usual maintenance doses range from 5 to 20 mg daily.

Following **myocardial infarction**, treatment with lisinopril may be started within 24 hours of the onset of symptoms in an initial dose of 5 mg once daily for two days, then increased to 10 mg once daily. An initial dose of 2.5 mg once daily is recommended for patients with a low systolic blood pressure.

In **diabetic nephropathy**, the initial dose is 2.5 mg once daily. In normotensive insulin-dependent diabetics the maintenance dose is 10 mg daily, increased to 20 mg daily if necessary to achieve a sitting diastolic blood pressure below 75 mmHg. In hypertensive non-insulin-dependent diabetics, the dose should be adjusted to achieve a sitting diastolic blood pressure below 90 mmHg.

Reviews.

1. Noble TA, Murray KM. Lisinopril: a nonsulfhydryl angiotensin-converting enzyme inhibitor. *Clin Pharm* 1988; **7:** 659–69.
2. Armayor GM, Lopez LM. Lisinopril: a new angiotensin-converting enzyme inhibitor. *Drug Intell Clin Pharm* 1988; **22:** 365–72.
3. Lancaster SG, Todd PA. Lisinopril: a preliminary review of its pharmacodynamic and pharmacokinetic properties, and therapeutic use in hypertension and congestive heart failure. *Drugs* 1988; **35:** 646–69.
4. Goa KL, *et al.* Lisinopril: a review of its pharmacology and clinical efficacy in the early management of acute myocardial infarction. *Drugs* 1996; **52:** 564–88.
5. Goa KL, *et al.* Lisinopril: a review of its pharmacology and use in the management of the complications of diabetes mellitus. *Drugs* 1997; **53:** 1081–1105.

Preparations

USP 23: Lisinopril Tablets.

Proprietary Preparations (details are given in Part 3)
Aust.: Acemin; Prinivil; ***Austral.:*** Prinivil; Zestril; ***Belg.:*** Novatec; Zestril; ***Canad.:*** Prinivil; Zestril; ***Fr.:*** Prinivil; Zestril; ***Ger.:*** Acerbon; Coric; ***Irl.:*** Carace; Zestril; ***Ital.:*** Alapril; Prinivil; Zestril; ***Neth.:*** Novatec; Zestril; ***Norw.:*** Vivatec; Zestril; ***S.Afr.:*** Prinivil; Zestril; ***Spain:*** Doneka; Prinivil; Secubar; Zestril; ***Swed.:*** Vivatec; Zestril; ***Switz.:*** Prinil; Zestril; ***UK:*** Carace; Zestril; ***USA:*** Prinivil; Zestril.

Multi-ingredient: ***Aust.:*** Acecomb; Prinzide; Zestoretic; ***Belg.:*** Novazyd; Zestoretic; ***Canad.:*** Prinzide; Zestoretic; ***Fr.:*** Prinzide; Zestoretic; ***Ger.:*** Acercomp; Coric plus; ***Irl.:*** Carace Plus; Zestoretic; ***Ital.:*** Prinzide; Zestoretic; ***Neth.:*** Novazyd; Zestoretic; ***Norw.:*** Vivatec Comp; Zestoretic; ***S.Afr.:*** Zestoretic; ***Spain:*** Doneka Plus; Prinivil Plus; Secubar Diu; Zestoretic; ***Swed.:*** Zestoretic; ***Switz.:*** Prinzide; Zestoretic; ***UK:*** Carace Plus; Zestoretic; ***USA:*** Prinzide; Zestoretic.

Lorajmine Hydrochloride (7787-g)

Lorajmine Hydrochloride (*USAN, rINNM*).
Chloroacetylajmaline Hydrochloride; Win-11831. Ajmaline 17-chloroacetate hydrochloride.
$C_{22}H_{27}ClN_2O_3,HCl = 439.4.$
CAS — 47562-08-3 (lorajmine); 40819-93-0 (lorajmine hydrochloride).
Pharmacopoeias. In *It.*

Lorajmine is a class Ia antiarrhythmic (p.776) related to ajmaline (p.817). It has been given as the hydrochloride by mouth and by intravenous or intramuscular injection in the management of cardiac arrhythmias.

Preparations

Proprietary Preparations (details are given in Part 3)
Ital.: Ritmos Elle†.

Lorcainide Hydrochloride (7788-q)

Lorcainide Hydrochloride *(BANM, USAN, rINNM).*

Isocainide Hydrochloride; R-15889; Socainide Hydrochloride.

4'-Chloro-*N*-(1-isopropyl-4-piperidyl)-2-phenylacetanilide hydrochloride.

$C_{22}H_{27}ClN_2O,HCl = 407.4.$

CAS — 59729-31-6 (lorcainide); 58934-46-6 (lorcainide hydrochloride).

Lorcainide is a class Ic antiarrhythmic (p.776) that has been used for the management of ventricular and supraventricular arrhythmias. It has been given by mouth and by intravenous infusion as the hydrochloride.

Preparations

Proprietary Preparations (details are given in Part 3)
Ger.: Remivox†.

Losartan Potassium (11145-s)

Losartan Potassium *(BANM, USAN, rINNM).*

DuP-753; E-3340; MK-0954. 2-Butyl-4-chloro-1-[*p*-(*o*-1*H*-tetrazol-5-ylphenyl)benzyl]imidazole-5-methanol potassium.

$C_{22}H_{22}ClKN_6O = 461.0.$

CAS — 114798-26-4 (losartan); 124750-99-8 (losartan potassium).

Adverse Effects

Adverse effects of losartan have been reported to be usually mild and transient, and include dizziness and dose-related orthostatic hypotension. Hypotension may occur particularly in patients with volume depletion (for example those who have received high-dose diuretics). Impaired renal function and, rarely, rash, angioedema, and raised alanine aminotransferase may occur. Hyperkalaemia and myalgia have been reported. Losartan appears less likely than ACE inhibitors to cause cough.

Angioedema. Angioedema is a recognised adverse effect of ACE inhibitors and is thought to be due to accumulation of bradykinins. However, there have been case reports[1] of angioedema in patients receiving losartan, which does not affect bradykinin levels.

1. Acker CG, Greenberg A. Angioedema induced by the angiotensin II blocker losartan. *N Engl J Med* 1995; **333:** 1572.

Effects on the liver. Raised liver enzyme values have occurred rarely in patients receiving losartan. Severe, acute hepatotoxicity developed in a patient one month after losartan was substituted for enalapril because of ACE inhibitor-induced cough.[1] The patient recovered when losartan was withdrawn but symptoms and raised liver enzyme concentrations recurred following rechallenge.

1. Bosch X. Losartan-induced hepatotoxicity. *JAMA* 1997; **278:** 1572.

Effects on the skin. Atypical cutaneous lymphoid infiltrates developed in two patients while they were receiving losartan for hypertension.[1] In both cases the lesions disappeared within a few weeks of stopping the drug.

1. Viraben R, *et al.* Losartan-associated atypical cutaneous lymphoid hyperplasia. *Lancet* 1997; **350:** 1366.

Effects on taste. Taste disturbance progressing to complete taste loss occurred[1] in a patient receiving losartan for hypertension. Taste returned to normal several weeks after discontinuing losartan therapy.

1. Schlienger RG, *et al.* Reversible ageusia associated with losartan. *Lancet* 1996; **347:** 471–2.

Migraine. Severe migraine has been reported[1] in a patient following administration of losartan. The patient had no history of migraine and symptoms recurred on rechallenge.

1. Ahmad S. Losartan and severe migraine. *JAMA* 1995; **274:** 1266–7.

Pancreatitis. Acute pancreatitis has been reported[1,2] in two patients receiving losartan. However, one of the patients subsequently developed pancreatitis unrelated to losartan.[3] The other patient[2] had also developed acute pancreatitis during enalapril therapy.

1. Bosch X. Losartan-induced acute pancreatitis. *Ann Intern Med* 1997; **127:** 1043–4.
2. Birck R, *et al.* Pancreatitis after losartan. *Lancet* 1998; **351:** 1178.
3. Bosch X. Correction: losartan, pancreatitis, and microlithiasis. *Ann Intern Med* 1998; **129:** 755.

Precautions

Losartan is contra-indicated in pregnancy and breast feeding. It should be used with caution in patients with renal artery stenosis. Reduced doses may be required in patients with renal impairment and should be considered in patients with hepatic impairment. Patients with volume depletion (for example those who have received high-dose diuretic therapy) may experience hypotension, which may be minimised by initiating treatment with a low dose of losartan. Since hyperkalaemia may occur, serum-potassium concentrations should be monitored, especially in the elderly and patients with renal impairment, and the concomitant use of potassium-sparing diuretics should be avoided.

Pharmacokinetics

Losartan is readily absorbed from the gastro-intestinal tract following oral administration, with an oral bioavailability of about 33%. It undergoes first-pass metabolism to form an active carboxylic acid metabolite E-3174 (EXP-3174), which has greater pharmacological activity than losartan, and some inactive metabolites. Peak plasma concentrations of losartan and E-3174 occur about 1 hour and 3 to 4 hours, respectively, after an oral dose. Both losartan and E-3174 are more than 98% bound to plasma proteins. Losartan is excreted in the urine, and in the faeces via bile, as unchanged drug and metabolites. Following oral dosing about 35% of the dose is excreted in the urine and about 60% in the faeces. The terminal elimination half-lives of losartan and E-3174 are about 1.5 to 2.5 hours and 3 to 9 hours, respectively.

References.

1. Lo M-W, *et al.* Pharmacokinetics of losartan, an angiotensin II receptor antagonist, and its active metabolite EXP3174 in humans. *Clin Pharmacol Ther* 1995; **58:** 641–9.
2. Ohtawa M, *et al.* Pharmacokinetics and biochemical efficacy after single and multiple oral administration of losartan, an orally active nonpeptide angiotensin II receptor antagonist, in humans. *Br J Clin Pharmacol* 1993; **35:** 290–7.
3. Csajka C, *et al.* Pharmacokinetic-pharmacodynamic profile of angiotensin II receptor antagonists. *Clin Pharmacokinet* 1997; **32:** 1–29.

Uses and Administration

Losartan is an angiotensin II receptor antagonist with antihypertensive activity due mainly to selective blockade of AT_1 receptors and the consequent reduced pressor effect of angiotensin II. It is used in the management of hypertension (p.788) and may have a role in patients who are unable to tolerate ACE inhibitors. It has also been tried in heart failure (p.785) and in myocardial infarction (p.791).

Losartan is given by mouth as the potassium salt.

In hypertension the usual dose is 50 mg once daily. The maximum effect is achieved in about 3 to 6 weeks after initiating treatment. The dose may be increased, if necessary, to 100 mg daily in one or two divided doses. An initial dose of 25 mg once daily is suggested for the elderly over 75 years-of-age, and for patients with moderate to severe renal impairment (creatinine clearance less than 20 mL per minute), or intravascular fluid depletion. A reduced dose should also be considered for patients with hepatic impairment.

References.

1. Anonymous. Losartan—a new antihypertensive. *Drug Ther Bull* 1995; **33:** 73–4.
2. Johnston CI. Angiotensin receptor antagonists: focus on losartan. *Lancet* 1995; **346:** 1403–7.
3. Carr AA, Prisant LM. Losartan: first of a new class of angiotensin antagonists for the management of hypertension. *J Clin Pharmacol* 1996; **36:** 3–12.
4. Goa KL, Wagstaff AJ. Losartan potassium: a review of its pharmacology, clinical efficacy and tolerability in the management of hypertension. *Drugs* 1996; **51:** 820–45.
5. Schaefer KL, Porter JA. Angiotensin II receptor antagonists: the prototype losartan. *Ann Pharmacother* 1996; **30:** 625–36.
6. Burrell LM. A risk-benefit assessment of losartan potassium in the treatment of hypertension. *Drug Safety* 1997; **16:** 56–65.

Uricosuric action. In a study[1] in healthy volunteers losartan was found to reduce serum uric acid concentration and increase urinary uric acid excretion in a dose-dependent manner.

1. Nakashima M, *et al.* Pilot study of the uricosuric effect of DuP-753, a new angiotensin II receptor antagonist, in healthy subjects. *Eur J Clin Pharmacol* 1992; **42:** 333–5.

Preparations

Proprietary Preparations (details are given in Part 3)
Aust.: Cosaar; ***Austral.:*** Cozaar; ***Belg.:*** Cozaar; ***Canad.:*** Cozaar; ***Fr.:*** Cozaar; ***Ger.:*** Lorzaar; ***Irl.:*** Cozaar; ***Ital.:*** Lortaan; Losaprex; Neo-Lotan; ***Neth.:*** Cozaar; ***Norw.:*** Cozaar; ***S.Afr.:*** Cozaar; ***Spain:*** Cozaar; ***Swed.:*** Cozaar; ***Switz.:*** Cosaar; ***UK:*** Cozaar; ***USA:*** Cozaar.

Multi-ingredient: ***Fr.:*** Hyzaar; ***Ital.:*** Hizaar; Losazid; Neo-Lotan Plus; ***Neth.:*** Hyzaar; ***Norw.:*** Cozaar Comp; ***S.Afr.:*** Cozaar Comp; ***UK:*** Cozaar Comp; ***USA:*** Hyzaar.

Low-molecular-weight Heparins

(18636-z)

Depolymerised Heparins; Heparina Massae Molecularis Minoris; LMW Heparins; Low-molecular-mass Heparins.

Pharmacopoeias. In *Eur.* (see p.viii).

Low-molecular-weight heparins are salts of sulphated glucosaminoglycans and have a mass-average molecular mass of less than 8000. They are obtained by fractionation or depolymerisation of heparin of natural origin and, depending on the method of production, display different chemical structures at the reducing and non-reducing end of the polysaccharide chains.

The Ph. Eur. specifies that potency is not less than 70 units of anti-factor Xa activity per mg with reference to the dried substance and that the ratio of anti-factor Xa activity to anti-factor IIa (antithrombin) activity is not less than 1.5.

A white or almost white hygroscopic powder. Freely **soluble** in water. A 1% solution in water has a pH of 5.5 to 8.0. **Store** in airtight containers.

Units

The first International Standard for low-molecular-weight heparin was established in 1986 and is used to calibrate products for both anti-factor Xa and anti-factor IIa activities. Potency is expressed in terms of units of anti-factor Xa activity per mg and the ratio of anti-factor Xa to anti-factor IIa activity. This ratio differs for individual low-molecular-weight heparins and neither they nor unfractionated heparin can be used interchangeably unit for unit.

Adverse Effects

As for Heparin, p.880; a possible decreased risk of bleeding complications compared with heparin has not been established (see below).

Effects on the adrenal glands. Hyperkalaemia related to hypoaldosteronism has been reported in a patient treated with a low-molecular-weight heparin. In a study of 12 patients given enoxaparin and 15 given nadroparin the mean plasma-aldosterone concentration decreased after 4 days of treatment. This was accompanied by an increase in the mean serum-potassium concentration. Both values returned towards normal after withdrawal of therapy.[1]

1. Levesque H, *et al.* Low molecular weight heparins and hypoaldosteronism. *Br Med J* 1990; **300:** 1437–8.

Effects on the blood. It was hoped that, because of their higher ratio of anti-factor Xa to anti-thrombin activity compared with heparin, low-molecular-weight heparins might cause less bleeding while maintaining their antithrombotic activity. Although *animal* studies found a lower incidence of bleeding for an equivalent antithrombotic effect this is yet to be established in clinical studies in humans.[1-3] Some large studies have suggested less bleeding with low-molecular-weight heparins than with unfractionated heparin.[4,5] Despite this it is thought that the risk may well be similar.[6,7]

Thrombocytopenia has also been reported with low-molecular-weight heparins[8-10] although in one study the incidence was less than with unfractionated heparin.[11]

There has also been a report of thrombocytosis in one patient receiving enoxaparin.[12]

1. Hirsh J. From unfractionated heparins to low molecular weight heparins. *Acta Chir Scand* 1990; (suppl 556): 42–50.
2. Verstraete M. Pharmacotherapeutic aspects of unfractionated and low molecular weight heparins. *Drugs* 1990; **40:** 498–530.
3. Borris LC, Lassen MR. A comparative review of the adverse effect profiles of heparins and heparinoids. *Drug Safety* 1995; **12:** 26–31.
4. Levine MN, *et al.* Prevention of deep vein thrombosis after elective hip surgery: a randomized trial comparing low molecular weight heparin with standard unfractionated heparin. *Ann Intern Med* 1991; **114:** 545–51.

5. Hull RD, *et al.* Subcutaneous low-molecular-weight heparin compared with continuous intravenous heparin in the treatment of proximal-vein thrombosis. *N Engl J Med* 1992; **326:** 975–82. Correction. *ibid.* **327:** 140.
6. Thomas DP. Bleeding after low-molecular-weight heparin. *Lancet* 1992; **339:** 1119.
7. Lensing AWA, *et al.* Bleeding after low-molecular-weight heparin. *Lancet* 1992; **339:** 1119–20.
8. Eichinger S, *et al.* Thrombocytopenia associated with low-molecular-weight heparin. *Lancet* 1991; **337:** 1425–6.
9. Lecompte T, *et al.* Thrombocytopenia associated with low-molecular-weight heparin. *Lancet* 1991; **338:** 1217.
10. Tardy B, *et al.* Thrombocytopenia associated with low-molecular-weight heparin. *Lancet* 1991; **338:** 1217.
11. Warkentin TE, *et al.* Heparin-induced thrombocytopenia in patients treated with low-molecular-weight heparin or unfractionated heparin. *N Engl J Med* 1995; **332:** 1330–5.
12. Rizzieri DA, *et al.* Thrombocytosis associated with low-molecular-weight heparin. *Ann Intern Med* 1996; **125:** 157.

Effects on the skin. Skin necrosis at the site of enoxaparin injection has been reported in 2 patients.[1] A third patient developed necrosis at enoxaparin injection sites when enoxaparin was substituted for heparin;[2] an association with heparin-induced thrombocytopenia was suggested.

A delayed eczematous reaction developed at the site of previous injections in a woman who had been receiving certoparin for 5 months.[3] There was no reaction when therapy was changed to an alternative low-molecular-weight heparin.

1. Fried M, *et al.* Enoxaparin-induced skin necrosis. *Ann Intern Med* 1996; **125:** 521–2.
2. Tonn ME, *et al.* Enoxaparin-associated dermal necrosis: a consequence of cross-reactivity with heparin-mediated antibodies. *Ann Pharmacother* 1997; **31:** 323–6.
3. Bircher AJ, *et al.* Delayed hypersensitivity to one low-molecular-weight heparin with tolerance of other low-molecular-weight heparins. *Br J Dermatol* 1995; **132:** 461–3.

Hypersensitivity. Reports of hypersensitivity reactions associated with low-molecular-weight heparins are rare. However, a patient being treated with enoxaparin 20 mg subcutaneously daily developed a widespread pruritic urticaria and swelling of lips and tongue after three days of treatment.[1] Antihistamines and prednisone given with enoxaparin failed to control the reaction and enoxaparin treatment was stopped after a further three days. Urticaria and angioedema rapidly resolved on withdrawal of enoxaparin.

1. Odeh M, Oliven A. Urticaria and angioedema induced by low-molecular-weight heparin. *Lancet* 1992; **340:** 972–3.

Treatment of Adverse Effects

Severe bleeding with low-molecular-weight heparins, usually caused by accidental overdosage, may be reduced by the slow intravenous administration of protamine sulphate (p.993). The recommended doses of protamine sulphate are given in the individual monographs and should completely neutralise the anti-thrombin effect of the low-molecular-weight heparin but will only partially neutralise the anti-factor-Xa effect. Not more than 50 mg of protamine sulphate should be injected for any one dose.

Precautions

As for Heparin, p.880.

Low-molecular-weight heparins should not be administered to patients who have developed thrombocytopenia with heparin and who have a positive *in-vitro* platelet aggregation test (that is, cross-reactivity) with the particular low-molecular-weight heparin to be used.

Local anaesthesia. Spinal and epidural haematomas, sometimes leading to paralysis, have occurred in patients receiving low-molecular-weight heparin in association with spinal or epidural anaesthesia or analgesia.[1] The risk of haematoma appeared to be higher in patients who had indwelling catheters or who were receiving concomitant therapy with other drugs that affect haemostasis.

1. Wysowski DK, *et al.* Spinal and epidural hematoma and low-molecular-weight heparin. *N Engl J Med* 1998; **338:** 1774.

Interactions

As for Heparin, p.881.

Pharmacokinetics

Although the precise pharmacokinetic parameters of different low-molecular-weight heparins vary (see individual monographs), they generally have a greater bioavailability after subcutaneous injection and a longer half-life than heparin.

References.

1. Kandrotas RJ. Heparin pharmacokinetics and pharmacodynamics. *Clin Pharmacokinet* 1992; **22:** 359–74.

Uses and Administration

Low-molecular-weight heparins are salts of fragments of heparin produced by chemical or enzymatic depolymerisation of the heparin molecule. Commercially available low-molecular-weight heparins differ in their method of production, molecular-weight range, and degree of sulphation. Like heparin (p.881), these compounds enhance the action of antithrombin III but they are characterised by a higher ratio of anti-factor Xa to anti-factor IIa (antithrombin) activity than heparin. The possibility that such selective factor-Xa inhibition would result in antithrombotic activity without anticoagulant and hence haemorrhagic effects has not been fully confirmed by clinical experience in humans. Low-molecular-weight heparins also have less effect on platelet aggregation than heparin. They have no significant effect on blood coagulation tests such as activated partial thromboplastin time (APTT). Therapy may be monitored by measurement of plasma-anti-factor-Xa activity.

Low-molecular-weight heparins are used in the management of venous thrombo-embolism (deep-vein thrombosis and pulmonary embolism, p.802). They are used for prophylaxis, particularly during surgery, and for treatment of established thrombo-embolism. They are administered by subcutaneous injection once or twice daily; laboratory monitoring is not generally necessary. They are also given intravenously to prevent coagulation during haemodialysis and other extracorporeal circulatory procedures, and subcutaneously in the management of unstable angina (p.780).

Doses are expressed either in terms of the weight of low-molecular-weight heparin or in terms of units of anti-factor Xa activity. Since low-molecular-weight heparins differ in their relative inhibition of factor Xa and thrombin, doses, even when expressed in terms of anti-factor-Xa activity, cannot be equated. Different preparations of the same low-molecular-weight heparin may also have different doses depending on the reference preparation used.

References.

1. Verstraete M. Pharmacotherapeutic aspects of unfractionated and low molecular weight heparins. *Drugs* 1990; **40:** 498–530.
2. Hirsh J. From unfractionated heparins to low molecular weight heparins. *Acta Chir Scand* 1990; (suppl 556): 42–50.
3. Freedman MD. Low molecular weight heparins: an emerging new class of glycosaminoglycan antithrombotics. *J Clin Pharmacol* 1991; **31:** 298–306.
4. Colvin BT, Barrowcliffe TW. The British Society for Haematology guidelines on the use and monitoring of heparin 1992: second revision. *J Clin Pathol* 1993; **46:** 97–103.
5. Green D, *et al.* Low molecular weight heparin: a critical analysis of clinical trials. *Pharmacol Rev* 1994; **46:** 89–109.
6. Nurmohamed MT, *et al.* Low molecular weight heparin(oid)s: clinical investigations and practical recommendations. *Drugs* 1997; **53:** 736–51.
7. Weitz JI. Low-molecular-weight heparins. *N Engl J Med* 1997; **337:** 688–98. Correction. *ibid.*: 1567.

Lubeluzole (17435-r)

Lubeluzole *(BAN, rINN).*

R-87926. (S)-1-{4-[1,3-Benzothiazol-2-yl(methyl)amino]piperidino}-3-(3,4-difluorophenoxy)propan-2-ol.

$C_{22}H_{25}F_2N_3O_2S$ = 433.5.

CAS — 144665-07-6.

Lubeluzole is a neuroprotectant under investigation for ischaemic stroke.

Manidipine Dihydrochloride (6487-s)

Manidipine Dihydrochloride *(rINNM).*

CV-4093; Franidipine Dihydrochloride. 2-[4-(Diphenylmethyl)-1-piperazinyl]ethyl methyl (±)-1,4-dihydro-2,6-dimethyl-4-(*m*-nitrophenyl)-3,5-pyridinedicarboxylate dihydrochloride.

$C_{35}H_{38}N_4O_6,2HCl$ = 683.6.

CAS — 120092-68-4 (manidipine); 89226-75-5 (manidipine dihydrochloride); 126229-12-7 (manidipine dihydrochloride).

Manidipine is a dihydropyridine calcium-channel blocker (see Nifedipine, p.916). It is given by mouth as the dihydrochloride in the management of hypertension.

References.

1. Takabatake, T, *et al.* Renal effects of manidipine hydrochloride: a new calcium antagonist in hypertensive patients. *Eur J Clin Pharmacol* 1993; **45:** 321–5.

Preparations

Proprietary Preparations (details are given in Part 3)
Ital.: Iperten; Vascoman; ***Jpn:*** Calslot.

Mannitol (2338-w)

Cordycepic Acid; E421; Manita; Manitol; Manna Sugar; Mannite; Mannitolum. D-Mannitol.

$C_6H_{14}O_6$ = 182.2.

CAS — 69-65-8.

Pharmacopoeias. In *Chin., Eur.* (see p.viii), *Int., Jpn, Pol.,* and *US.*

A hexahydric alcohol related to mannose ($C_6H_{12}O_6$ = 180.2). It is isomeric with sorbitol. A white odourless crystalline powder or granules with a sweet taste.

Freely **soluble** in water; very slightly soluble in alcohol; slightly soluble in pyridine; practically insoluble in ether; soluble in alkaline solutions. Supersaturated aqueous solutions are prepared with the aid of heat. Any crystals which form during storage of the injection should be dissolved by warming before use; this may be a particular problem with the 20 and 25% injections which are supersaturated. A 5.07% solution in water is iso-osmotic with serum.

Mannitol should never be added to whole blood for transfusion or given through the same set by which blood is being infused. For details of the adverse effects of mannitol on red blood cells, see Effects on the Blood under Adverse Effects, below.

Adverse Effects

The most common side-effect associated with mannitol therapy is fluid and electrolyte imbalance including circulatory overload and acidosis at high doses. The expansion of extracellular volume can precipitate pulmonary oedema and patients with diminished cardiac reserve are at special risk. The shift of fluid from the intracellular to extracellular compartment can cause tissue dehydration; dehydration of the brain, particularly in patients with renal failure, may give rise to CNS symptoms.

When given by mouth, mannitol causes diarrhoea. Intravenous infusion of mannitol has been associated with nausea, vomiting, thirst, headache, dizziness, chills, fever, tachycardia, chest pain, hyponatraemia, dehydration, blurred vision, urticaria, and hypotension or hypertension. Large doses have been associated rarely with acute renal failure. Hypersensitivity reactions have occurred.

Extravasation of the solution may cause oedema and skin necrosis; thrombophlebitis may occur.

Severe mannitol intoxication was reported in 8 patients with renal failure who had received large, and sometimes enormous, amounts of mannitol intravenously over 1 to 3 days.[1] These patients had CNS involvement out of proportion to uraemia, severe hyponatraemia, a large osmolality gap, and fluid overload. Six patients were treated with haemodialysis and this was considered to be more effective than peritoneal dialysis, which was used in 1 patient.

1. Borges HF, *et al.* Mannitol intoxication in patients with renal failure. *Arch Intern Med* 1982; **142:** 63–6.

Effects on the blood. Agglutination and irreversible crenation of erythrocytes occurred when blood was mixed with varying proportions of a 10% mannitol solution.[1] It was suggested that intravenous infusions should be carefully controlled and administered at a slow rate. This observation could have particular relevance to patients with sickle-cell disease.[2,3] Samson[4] commented that, although agglutination and crenation had been observed *in vitro*, dilutional effects would make *in-vivo* interaction with blood cells less likely.

1. Roberts BE, Smith PH. Hazards of mannitol infusions. *Lancet* 1966; **ii:** 421–2.
2. Konotey-Ahulu FID. Hazards of mannitol infusions. *Lancet* 1966; **ii:** 591.
3. Roberts BE, Smith PH. Hazards of mannitol infusions. *Lancet* 1966; **ii:** 591.
4. Samson JH. Hazards of mannitol infusions. *Lancet* 1966; **ii:** 1191.

Effects on the gastro-intestinal tract. Potentially explosive intracolonic concentrations of hydrogen gas were detected in 6 out of 10 patients given mannitol prior to colonoscopy.[1] However, Trotman and Walt[2] and Avgerinos and colleagues[3] considered the risk of explosion to be small when air insufflation and suction were used during the colonoscopy procedure.

1. La Brooy SJ, *et al.* Potentially explosive colonic concentrations of hydrogen after bowel preparation with mannitol. *Lancet* 1981; **i:** 634–6.
2. Trotman I, Walt R. Mannitol and explosions. *Lancet* 1981; **i:** 848.
3. Avgerinos A, *et al.* Bowel preparation and the risk of explosion during colonoscopic polypectomy. *Gut* 1984; **25:** 361–4.

Effects on the kidneys. Focal osmotic nephrosis occurred in a patient after the administration of mannitol 20% intravenously.[1]

Acute oliguric renal failure has been associated with the administration of large doses of mannitol to patients with previously normal renal function.[2-4]

1. Goodwin WE, Latta H. Focal osmotic nephrosis due to the therapeutic use of mannitol: a case of perirenal hematoma after renal biopsy. *J Urol (Baltimore)* 1970; **103:** 11–14.
2. Whelan TV, *et al.* Acute renal failure associated with mannitol intoxication. *Arch Intern Med* 1984; **144:** 2053–5.
3. Goldwasser P, Fotino S. Acute renal failure following massive mannitol infusion: appropriate response of tubuloglomerular feedback? *Arch Intern Med* 1984; **144:** 2214–16.
4. Rabetoy GM, *et al.* Where the kidney is concerned, how much mannitol is too much? *Ann Pharmacother* 1993; **27:** 25–8.

Precautions

Mannitol is contra-indicated in patients with pulmonary congestion or pulmonary oedema, intracranial bleeding (except during craniotomy), heart failure (in patients with diminished cardiac reserve, expansion of the extracellular fluid may lead to fulminating heart failure), metabolic oedema with abnormal capillary fragility, and in patients with renal failure unless a test dose has produced a diuretic response (if urine flow is inadequate, expansion of the extracellular fluid may lead to acute water intoxication).

Mannitol should not be administered with whole blood.

All patients given mannitol should be carefully observed for signs of fluid and electrolyte imbalance and renal function should be monitored.

Pharmacokinetics

Only small amounts of mannitol are absorbed from the gastro-intestinal tract. Following intravenous injection mannitol is excreted rapidly by the kidneys before any very significant metabolism can take place in the liver. Mannitol does not cross the blood-brain barrier or penetrate the eye. An elimination half-life of about 100 minutes has been reported.

Uses and Administration

Mannitol is an osmotic agent. Although an isomer of sorbitol, it has little energy value, since it is largely eliminated from the body before any metabolism can take place.

Mannitol is mainly used, with adequate rehydration, to increase urine flow in patients with acute renal failure and to reduce raised intracranial pressure (p.796) and treat cerebral oedema. It is also used in the short-term management of glaucoma (p.1387), especially to reduce intra-ocular pressure prior to ophthalmic surgery, and to promote the excretion of toxic substances by forced diuresis.

Other indications include bladder irrigation during transurethral resection of the prostate in order to reduce haemolysis and oral administration as an osmotic laxative for bowel preparation. Mannitol is used as a diluent and excipient in pharmaceutical preparations and as a bulk sweetener.

When administered parenterally, mannitol raises the osmotic pressure of the plasma thus drawing water out of body tissues and produces an osmotic diuresis. Reduction of cerebrospinal and intra-ocular fluid pressure occurs within 15 minutes of the start of a mannitol infusion and lasts for 3 to 8 hours after the infusion is discontinued; diuresis occurs after 1 to 3 hours.

When used as an osmotic diuretic, mannitol is administered by intravenous infusion. Careful monitoring of fluid balance, electrolytes, renal function, and vital signs is necessary during infusion to prevent fluid and electrolyte imbalance, including circulatory overload and tissue dehydration. Solutions containing more than 15% of mannitol may crystallise during storage, particularly at low temperatures; crystals may be redissolved by warming before use; the administration set should include a filter.

Mannitol may be used to treat patients with **renal failure** (oliguria) or those suspected of inadequate renal function after correction of plasma volume, provided a test dose of about 200 mg per kg body-weight given by rapid intravenous infusion of a 15 to 25% solution over 3 to 5 minutes produces a diuresis of at least 30 to 50 mL per hour during the next 2 to 3 hours; a second test dose is permitted if the response to the first is inadequate. The usual adult dose of mannitol ranges from 50 to 100 g by intravenous infusion of a 5 to 25% solution. The rate of administration is usually adjusted to maintain a urine flow of at least 30 to 50 mL per hour.

For children, a dose of 0.25 to 2 g per kg body-weight has been suggested.

The total dosage, the concentration, and the rate of administration depend on the fluid requirement, the urinary output, and the nature and severity of the condition being treated. Mannitol infusion has also been used to prevent acute renal failure during cardiovascular and other types of surgery, or following trauma.

To reduce **raised intracranial** or **intra-ocular pressure** mannitol may be given by intravenous infusion as a 15 to 25% solution in a dose of 0.25 to 2 g per kg body-weight over 30 to 60 minutes. Rebound increases in intracranial or intra-ocular pressure may occur but are less frequent than with urea.

During **transurethral prostatic resection** a 2.5 to 5% solution of mannitol has been used for irrigating the bladder.

Ciguatera poisoning. Ciguatera poisoning occurs as a result of the consumption of certain fish contaminated with ciguatoxin found throughout the Caribbean and Indopacific. Symptoms can be severe, including a bizarre reversal of hot and cold sensation, and may last several weeks.[1] Treatment is usually symptomatic since there is no specific antidote. Dramatic reversal of neuromuscular symptoms with slower resolution of gastro-intestinal upset has been reported following administration of mannitol 1 g per kg body-weight by intravenous infusion over 30 to 45 minutes in the acute phase of the illness.[2-4] Treatment with mannitol may also be beneficial up to a week after poisoning.[5] Amitriptyline (p.273) has been found on several occasions[6-8] to relieve neurological symptoms (dysaesthesias and paraesthesias) and pruritus.

1. Bignall J. Ciguatera poisoning in Hong Kong. *Lancet* 1994; **344:** 1698.
2. Palafox NA, *et al.* Successful treatment of ciguatera fish poisoning with intravenous mannitol. *JAMA* 1988; **259:** 2740–2.
3. Pearn JH, *et al.* Ciguatera and mannitol: experience with a new treatment regimen. *Med J Aust* 1989; **151:** 77–80.
4. Williamson J. Ciguatera and mannitol: a successful treatment. *Med J Aust* 1990; **153:** 306–7.
5. Fenner PJ, *et al.* A Queensland family with ciguatera after eating coral trout. *Med J Aust* 1997; **166:** 473–5.
6. Bowman PB. Amitriptyline and ciguatera. *Med J Aust* 1984; **140:** 802.
7. Davis RT, Villar LA. Symptomatic improvement with amitriptyline in ciguatera fish poisoning. *N Engl J Med* 1986; **315:** 65.
8. Calvert GM, *et al.* Treatment of ciguatera fish poisoning with amitriptyline and nifedipine. *J Toxicol Clin Toxicol* 1987; **25:** 423–8.

Gastro-intestinal disorders. BOWEL PREPARATION. Mannitol, 1000 mL of a 10% solution or 500 mL of 10 or 20% solution by mouth, has been reported to be effective in preparing the bowel for surgical and diagnostic procedures.[1,2] The potential for formation of explosive gas in the bowel should be borne in mind (see under Adverse Effects, above).

1. Palmer KR, Khan AN. Oral mannitol: a simple and effective bowel preparation for barium enema. *Br Med J* 1979; **2:** 1038.
2. Newstead GL, Morgan BP. Bowel preparation with mannitol. *Med J Aust* 1979; **2:** 582–3.

DIAGNOSIS AND TESTING. Mannitol has been used in combination with lactulose[1,2] and with cellobiose[3,4] in the detection of abnormal small bowel permeability, particularly that occurring in coeliac disease. For further information on the use of differential sugar absorption tests, see Lactulose, p.1196.

1. Pearson ADJ, *et al.* The gluten challenge—biopsy v permeability. *Arch Dis Child* 1983; **58:** 653.
2. Cooper BT. Intestinal permeability in coeliac disease. *Lancet* 1983; **i:** 658–9.
3. Juby LD, *et al.* Cellobiose/mannitol sugar test—a sensitive tubeless test for coeliac disease: results on 1010 unselected patients. *Gut* 1989; **30:** 476–80.
4. Hodges S, *et al.* Cellobiose: mannitol differential permeability in small bowel disease. *Arch Dis Child* 1989; **64:** 853–5.

Preparations

BP 1998: Mannitol Intravenous Infusion;
USP 23: Mannitol in Sodium Chloride Injection; Mannitol Injection.

Proprietary Preparations (details are given in Part 3)
Aust.: Osmofundin 20%; ***Austral.:*** Mede-Prep; Osmitrol; ***Canad.:*** Osmitrol; ***Fr.:*** Manicol; ***Ger.:*** Eufusol M 20†; Mannit-Losung; Osmofundin 15%; Osmosteril 20%; Thomaemannit; ***Ital.:*** Isotol; Mannistol; ***Switz.:*** Mannite; ***USA:*** Osmitrol; Resectisol.

Multi-ingredient: ***Aust.:*** Osmofundin 10%; Resectal; ***Belg.:*** Alcon Eye Gel; ***Fr.:*** Lycaon†; Lyptocodine; Rectolax†; ***Ger.:*** Osmofundin 10%; Osmofundin 20%†; Osmosteril 10%; ***Ital.:*** Malto Mannite Magnesiaca†; ***Spain:*** Jorkil; Salcedogen; Salcemetic; Salmagne; ***Swed.:*** Somanol; ***Switz.:*** Bigasan; Cital; Purisole.

Mannityl Hexanitrate (9251-y)

Mannitol Hexanitrate *(rINN)*; Nitromannite; Nitromannitol.

$C_6H_8(O.NO_2)_6$ = 452.2.

CAS — 15825-70-4.

Mannityl hexanitrate has general properties similar to those of glyceryl trinitrate (p.875) and has been used in angina pectoris.

Preparations

Proprietary Preparations (details are given in Part 3)
Multi-ingredient: ***Ital.:*** Nitromaxitate†.

Mebutamate (7063-c)

Mebutamate *(BAN, USAN, rINN).*

W-583. 2-sec-Butyl-2-methyltrimethylene dicarbamate.

$C_{10}H_{20}N_2O_4$ = 232.3.

CAS — 64-55-1.

Mebutamate is a carbamate with general properties similar to those of meprobamate (p.678). It has been given by mouth in some countries as an adjunct in the treatment of hypertension in doses of 300 mg up to four times daily.

Preparations

Proprietary Preparations (details are given in Part 3)
Ital.: Axiten†; Butatensin†; Mebutina†; Sigmafon; Vallene†.

Multi-ingredient: ***Ital.:*** Axiten Tre†; Vallizina†; ***Spain:*** Vallene Complex†.

Mebutizide (2339-e)

Mebutizide *(rINN).*

6-Chloro-3-(1,2-dimethylbutyl)-3,4-dihydro-2*H*-1,2,4-benzothiadiazine-7-sulphonamide 1,1-dioxide.

$C_{13}H_{20}ClN_3O_4S_2$ = 381.9.

CAS — 3568-00-1.

Mebutizide is a thiazide diuretic (see Hydrochlorothiazide, p.885) which is used in the treatment of oedema and hypertension.

Preparations

Proprietary Preparations (details are given in Part 3)
Belg.: Neoniagar.

Multi-ingredient: ***Ital.:*** Betalevo†; Minusten†; ***Spain:*** Triniagar; Vallene Complex†.

Mecamylamine Hydrochloride (880-c)

Mecamylamine Hydrochloride *(BANM, rINNM).*

Mecamine Hydrochloride. *N*-Methyl-2,3,3-trimethylbicyclo[2.2.1]hept-2-ylamine hydrochloride.

$C_{11}H_{21}N,HCl$ = 203.8.

CAS — 60-40-2 (mecamylamine); 826-39-1 (mecamylamine hydrochloride).

Pharmacopoeias. In US.

Store in airtight containers.

Adverse Effects, Treatment, and Precautions

As for Trimetaphan Camsylate, p.958. The administration of mecamylamine may cause tremor, convulsions, choreiform movements, insomnia, sedation, dysarthria, and mental aberrations.

Pharmacokinetics

Mecamylamine hydrochloride is almost completely absorbed from the gastro-intestinal tract. It diffuses across the placenta and crosses the blood-brain barrier. About 50% of the dose is excreted unchanged in the urine over 24 hours, but the rate is diminished in alkaline urine.

Uses and Administration

Mecamylamine hydrochloride is a ganglion blocker with actions similar to those of trimetaphan (p.959). It is used in the management of hypertension (p.788), although other antihypertensives with fewer adverse effects are preferred.

The usual initial dosage is 2.5 mg twice daily, gradually increased or decreased, usually by increments of 2.5 mg at intervals of not less than 2 days, until a satisfactory response is obtained. Tolerance may develop.

Smoking cessation. Mecamylamine is a centrally acting nicotine antagonist that might be of some benefit in assisting withdrawal from smoking.[1] In one study, addition of oral mecamylamine therapy appeared to enhance the effectiveness of nicotine skin patches.[2] Smoking cessation is discussed under Nicotine, p.1608.

1. Nunn-Thompson CL, Simon PA. Pharmacotherapy for smoking cessation. *Clin Pharm* 1989; **8:** 710–20.
2. Rose JE, *et al.* Mecamylamine combined with nicotine skin patch facilitates smoking cessation beyond nicotine patch treatment alone. *Clin Pharmacol Ther* 1994; **56:** 86–99.

Preparations

USP 23: Mecamylamine Hydrochloride Tablets.

Proprietary Preparations (details are given in Part 3)
USA: Inversine.

Medigoxin (5820-r)

Medigoxin *(BAN).*

Metildigoxin *(rINN)*; β-Methyl Digoxin; β-Methyldigoxin. 3β-[(*O*-2,6-Dideoxy-4-*O*-methyl-D-*ribo*-hexopyranosyl-(1→4)-*O*-2,6-dideoxy-D-*ribo*-hexopyranosyl-(1→4)-2,6-dideoxy-D-*ribo*-hexopyranosyl)oxy]-12β,14-dihydroxy-5β,14β-card-20(22)-enolide.

$C_{42}H_{66}O_{14}$ = 795.0.

CAS — 30685-43-9.

Pharmacopoeias. In *Jpn.* as $C_{42}H_{66}O_{14}$,½C_3H_6O.

Adverse Effects, Treatment, and Precautions

As for Digoxin, p.849.

Interactions

As for Digoxin, p.850.

For a report of an interaction between medigoxin and diltiazem, see Calcium-channel Blockers, under Interactions of Digoxin, p.851.

Pharmacokinetics

Medigoxin is rapidly and almost completely absorbed from the gastro-intestinal tract and at steady state a half-life of 54 to 60 hours has been reported. Demethylation to digoxin occurs. About 60% of an oral or intravenous dose is excreted in the urine as unchanged drug and metabolites over 7 days.

Hepatic impairment. Hepatic demethylation of medigoxin was reduced in 12 patients with cirrhosis of the liver compared with 12 healthy subjects. This resulted in a reduction in medigoxin clearance, a smaller volume of distribution, and a significantly higher serum concentration.[1]

1. Rameis H, *et al.* Changes in metildigoxin pharmacokinetics in cirrhosis of the liver: a comparison with β-acetyldigoxin. *Int J Clin Pharmacol Ther Toxicol* 1984; **22:** 145–51.

Renal impairment. For reference to the pharmacokinetics of medigoxin in patients with renal impairment, see under Uses and Administration, below.

Uses and Administration

Medigoxin is a cardiac glycoside with positive inotropic activity. It has actions similar to those of digoxin (p.853) and may be used in the treatment of some cardiac arrhythmias (p.782) and in heart failure (p.785).

The onset of action of medigoxin is more rapid than that of digoxin. When medigoxin is given by mouth an effect may appear within 5 to 20 minutes and a maximum effect on the myocardium may be seen in 15 to 30 minutes. The duration of action is similar to or a little longer than that of digoxin; therapeutic plasma concentrations are also similar. In stabilised patients a dose of 300 μg of medigoxin is as effective as 500 μg of digoxin.

Medigoxin may be given by mouth or intravenously. Initial doses of 150 to 600 μg daily by mouth may be given depending upon whether rapid or slow digitalisation is desired; digitalisation is usually performed over 2 to 4 days and the larger doses are given in divided daily doses. A daily dose of 400 μg intravenously for 3 days may also be employed. Maintenance therapy is continued with 50 to 300 μg daily by mouth in divided doses.

Dosage should be reduced in patients with renal impairment.

Administration in renal impairment. Fairly good nonlinear correlation was found between creatinine clearance and medigoxin half-life in a study of 15 patients with chronic renal impairment, including 8 undergoing haemodialysis, and 4 patients with heart failure and unimpaired renal function. The mean elimination half-life was 5.62 days in patients undergoing dialysis (clearance essentially 0 mL per minute) and 3.41 days in the other patients with chronic renal impairment (clearance 15 to 50 mL per minute) compared with 1.49 days in patients with normal renal function (clearance 62 to 96 mL per minute). It was recommended that patients undergoing dialysis should be given 30 to 50% of the usual dose initially.[1] Other studies have suggested that dose reduction may be necessary in renal impairment when creatinine clearance is below 50 mL per minute per 1.48 m² body-surface.[2]

1. Trovato GM, *et al.* Relationship between β-methyl-digoxin pharmacokinetic and degree of renal impairment. *Curr Ther Res* 1983; **33:** 158–64.
2. Tsutsumi K, *et al.* Pharmacokinetics of beta-methyldigoxin in subjects with normal and impaired renal function. *J Clin Pharmacol* 1993; **33:** 154–60.

Preparations

Proprietary Preparations (details are given in Part 3)
Aust.: Lanitop; ***Belg.:*** Lanitop; ***Ger.:*** Lanitop; ***Ital.:*** Cardiolan; Lanitop; Miopat; ***Jpn:*** Lanirapid; ***Spain:*** Lanirapid; ***Switz.:*** Lanitop.

Multi-ingredient: ***Aust.:*** Coro-Lanitop; Theo-Lanitop; ***Ger.:*** Intensain-Lanitop†; Theo-Lanitop†.

Medroxalol Hydrochloride (12921-a)

Medroxalol Hydrochloride *(BANM, USAN, rINNM).*

MDL-81968A; RMI-81968A. 5-{1-Hydroxy-2-[1-methyl-3-(3,4-methylenedioxyphenyl)propylamino]ethyl}salicylamide hydrochloride; 5-{2-[3-(1,3-Benzodioxol-5-yl)-1-methylpropylamino]-1-hydroxyethyl}salicylamide hydrochloride.

$C_{20}H_{24}N_2O_5$,HCl = 408.9.

CAS — 56290-94-9 (medroxalol); 70161-10-3 (medroxalol hydrochloride).

Medroxalol hydrochloride is reported to have alpha- and beta-blocking activity and has been investigated in the treatment of hypertension.

Mefruside (2340-b)

Mefruside *(BAN, USAN, rINN).*

Bay-1500; FBA-1500. 4-Chloro-*N*¹-methyl-*N*¹-(tetrahydro-2-methylfurfuryl)benzene-1,3-disulphonamide.

$C_{13}H_{19}ClN_2O_5S_2$ = 382.9.

CAS — 7195-27-9.

Pharmacopoeias. In *Jpn.*

Mefruside is a diuretic with properties similar to those of the thiazide diuretics (see Hydrochlorothiazide, p.885) even though it does not contain a thiazide ring system. It is used for oedema, including that associated with heart failure (p.785), and for hypertension (p.788).

Diuresis is initiated in about 2 to 4 hours and reaches a maximum between 6 and 12 hours.

In the treatment of oedema the usual dose is 25 to 50 mg daily by mouth, increasing if necessary to 75 to 100 mg. For long-term therapy a dose of 25 to 50 mg every second or third day is preferable.

In the treatment of hypertension the usual dose is 25 mg daily, either alone, or in conjunction with other antihypertensives; initial doses of 25 to 50 mg daily have been recommended; alternate-day maintenance dosage may be used.

In susceptible patients potassium supplements or a potassium-sparing diuretic may be necessary, but see hydrochlorothiazide.

Preparations

Proprietary Preparations (details are given in Part 3)
Ger.: Baycaron; ***Irl.:*** Baycaron; ***Neth.:*** Baycaron; ***Norw.:*** Baycaron; ***Swed.:*** Baycaron†; ***UK:*** Baycaron.

Multi-ingredient: ***Aust.:*** Bendigon†; ***Ger.:*** Bendigon N; Caprinol†; duranifin Sali; Nifehexal Sali; Sali-Adalat; Sali-Prent; Sali-Presinol; ***Ital.:*** Rexitene Plus†.

Mephentermine Sulphate (2078-g)

Mephentermine Sulphate *(BANM, rINNM).*

Mephentermine Sulfate; Mephentermini Sulfas; Mephetedrine Sulphate; Sulfato de Mefentermina. *N*,α,α-Trimethylphenethylamine sulphate dihydrate.

$(C_{11}H_{17}N)_2$,H_2SO_4,$2H_2O$ = 460.6.

CAS — 100-92-5 (mephentermine); 1212-72-2 (anhydrous mephentermine sulphate); 6190-60-9 (mephentermine sulphate dihydrate).

Pharmacopoeias. In *Chin.*

US has anhydrous or dihydrate.

White odourless crystals or crystalline powder. Mephentermine base 15 mg is approximately equivalent to 21 mg of mephentermine sulphate. **Soluble** 1 in 18 of water and 1 in 220 of alcohol; practically insoluble in chloroform. Solutions in water have a pH of about 6. **Protect** from light.

Adverse Effects, Treatment, and Precautions

Mephentermine may produce CNS stimulation, especially in overdosage; anxiety, drowsiness, incoherence, hallucinations, and convulsions have been reported.

Although the central stimulant effects of mephentermine are much less than those of amphetamine its use may lead to dependence of the amphetamine type.

The hypertensive effects of mephentermine may be treated with an alpha-adrenergic blocker such as phentolamine mesylate.

For the adverse effects of sympathomimetics in general, and precautions to be observed, see Adrenaline, p.813.

Interactions

For the interactions of sympathomimetics in general, see Adrenaline, p.814.

Pharmacokinetics

Mephentermine acts in about 5 to 15 minutes following intramuscular injection and has a duration of action of up to about 4 hours; it acts almost immediately following intravenous injection with a duration of action of up to about 30 minutes. It is rapidly metabolised in the body by demethylation; hydroxylation may follow. It is excreted as unchanged drug and metabolites in the urine; excretion is more rapid in acidic urine.

Uses and Administration

Mephentermine is a sympathomimetic (see Adrenaline, p.815) with mainly indirect effects on adrenergic receptors. It has alpha- and beta-adrenergic activity, and a slight stimulating effect on the central nervous system. It has an inotropic effect on the heart.

Mephentermine sulphate has been used to maintain blood pressure in hypotensive states, for example following spinal anaesthesia. Typical doses are the equivalent of up to 45 mg of mephentermine base by slow intravenous injection, or 15 to 30 mg intramuscularly.

Preparations

USP 23: Mephentermine Sulfate Injection.

Proprietary Preparations (details are given in Part 3)
USA: Wyamine.

Multi-ingredient: *USA:* Emergent-Ez.

Mepindolol Sulphate (12928-h)

Mepindolol Sulphate *(BANM, rINNM).*

LF-17895 (mepindolol); SHE-222. 1-Isopropylamino-3-(2-methylindol-4-yloxy)propan-2-ol sulphate.

$(C_{15}H_{22}N_2O_2)_2$,H_2SO_4 = 622.8.

CAS — 23694-81-7 (mepindolol); 56396-94-2 (mepindolol sulphate).

Mepindolol, the methyl analogue of pindolol, is a non-cardioselective beta blocker (p.828). It is reported to possess intrinsic sympathomimetic activity.

Mepindolol is used by mouth as the sulphate in the management of cardiovascular disorders including hypertension.

Preparations

Proprietary Preparations (details are given in Part 3)
Aust.: Corindolan; ***Ger.:*** Corindolan; ***Ital.:*** Betagon; Mepicor†.

Multi-ingredient: ***Aust.:*** Corindocomb; ***Ger.:*** Corindocomb.

Meproscillarin (5821-f)

Meproscillarin *(BAN, rINN).*

Knoll 570; Ky-18; 4′-*O*-Methylproscillaridin; Rambufaside. 14-Hydroxy-3β-[(4-*O*-methyl-α-L-rhamnopyranosyl)oxy]-14β-bufa-4,20,22-trienolide.

$C_{31}H_{44}O_8$ = 544.7.

CAS — 33396-37-1.

Meproscillarin, the methyl ether of the cardiac glycoside proscillaridin, is a positive inotrope with general properties similar to those of digoxin (p.849). It has been given by mouth in heart failure (p.785) in usual maintenance doses of 500 to 750 μg daily in divided doses.

Dose reduction of meproscillarin was not considered to be necessary for patients with chronic renal failure.[1]

1. Twittenhoff WD, *et al.* Zur frage der kumulation von meproscillarin bei niereninsuffizienz. *Arzneimittelforschung* 1978; **28:** 562–5.

Preparations

Proprietary Preparations (details are given in Part 3)
Ger.: Clift†.

Mersalyl Acid (2345-s)

Acidum Mersalylicum; Mersal. Acid; Mersalylum Acidum. A mixture of {3-[2-(carboxymethoxy)benzamido]-2-methoxypropyl}hydroxymercury and its anhydrides.

$C_{13}H_{17}HgNO_6$ = 483.9.

CAS — 486-67-9 ($C_{13}H_{17}HgNO_6$).

Mersalyl Sodium (2346-w)

Mersalyl *(pINN).* The sodium salt of mersalyl acid.

$C_{13}H_{16}HgNNaO_6$ = 505.8.

CAS — 492-18-2.

Mersalyl acid, in the form of its salts, is a powerful diuretic that acts on the renal tubules, increasing the excretion of sodium and chloride, in approximately equal amounts, and of water. Organic mercurial diuretics were widely used prior to the introduction of thiazide and other diuretics but have now been almost completely superseded by these orally active drugs which are both potent and less toxic. For details of the adverse effects of mersalyl sodium, see *Martindale*. 29th ed. p.997.

Mersalyl acid was usually given by injection as the sodium salt in conjunction with theophylline as this lessened the local irritant reaction and increased absorption. It was given by deep intramuscular injection after a test dose for hypersensitivity. Other organic mercurial diuretics include chlormerodrin, meralluride, mercaptomerin sodium, mercurophylline sodium, and merethoxylline procaine. They were mainly administered by intramuscular injection or, for those which were less irritant, subcutaneous injection.

Metaraminol Tartrate (2079-q)

Metaraminol Tartrate (*BANM, rINNM*).

Hydroxynorephedrine Bitartrate; Metaradrine Bitartrate; Metaraminol Acid Tartrate; Metaraminol Bitartrate. (−)-2-Amino-1-(3-hydroxyphenyl)propan-1-ol hydrogen tartrate.

$C_9H_{13}NO_2,C_4H_6O_6$ = 317.3.

CAS — 54-49-9 (metaraminol); 33402-03-8 (metaraminol tartrate).

Pharmacopoeias. In Br., Chin., and US.

An odourless or almost odourless, white, crystalline powder. Metaraminol tartrate 9.5 mg is approximately equivalent to 5 mg of metaraminol. Freely **soluble** in water; sparingly soluble in alcohol; practically insoluble in chloroform and ether. A 5% solution in water has a pH of 3.2 to 3.5.

Adverse Effects, Treatment, and Precautions

Metaraminol has a longer duration of action than adrenaline or noradrenaline and therefore an excessive vasopressor response may cause a prolonged rise in blood pressure. Tachycardia or other arrhythmias may also occur. Metaraminol may reduce placental perfusion and should be avoided during pregnancy.

The hypertensive effects of metaraminol may be treated with an alpha-adrenoceptor blocker such as phentolamine.

Tissue necrosis can occur as a result of accidental extravasation during intravenous injection. Infiltration with phentolamine may be beneficial if extravasation occurs.

For the adverse effects of sympathomimetics in general, and precautions to be observed, see Adrenaline, p.813.

Interactions

For the interactions of sympathomimetics in general, see Adrenaline, p.814.

Pharmacokinetics

Metaraminol acts about 10 minutes after intramuscular injection with a duration of action of up to about 1 hour. Effects are seen 1 to 2 minutes after intravenous injection with a duration of action of about 20 minutes.

Uses and Administration

Metaraminol is a sympathomimetic (see Adrenaline, p.815) with direct and indirect effects on adrenergic receptors. It has alpha- and beta-adrenergic activity, the former being predominant. Metaraminol has an inotropic effect and acts as a peripheral vasoconstrictor, thus increasing cardiac output, peripheral resistance, and blood pressure. Coronary blood flow is increased and the heart rate slowed.

Metaraminol tartrate is used for its pressor action in **hypotensive states** such as those that may occur following spinal anaesthesia. Doses are expressed in terms of the base. An intravenous infusion of 15 to 100 mg per 500 mL of glucose 5% or sodium chloride 0.9% may be used for maintaining the blood pressure, the rate of administration being adjusted according to blood pressure response. Higher concentrations have been given. As the maximum effects are not immediately apparent, at least 10 minutes should elapse before increasing the dose and the possibility of a cumulative effect should be borne in mind. In an emergency an initial dose of 0.5 to 5 mg may be given by direct intravenous injection followed by an intravenous infusion as above.

Metaraminol tartrate has also been given by intramuscular or subcutaneous injection for the prevention of hypotension in doses equivalent to 2 to 10 mg of metaraminol. Subcutaneous injection increases the risk of local tissue necrosis and sloughing.

Diagnosis and testing. The use of metaraminol as a provocative test in the diagnosis of familial Mediterranean fever has been described.[1] Intravenous infusion of metaraminol 10 mg in 500 mL of sodium chloride 0.9% provoked typical symptoms of the disease in 21 patients but this did not occur in 21 control subjects. However, the use of metaraminol for such a purpose has been questioned in terms of safety and possible adverse effects that may be produced.[2,3] Additionally, the specificity, and therefore the reliability, of the test has been doubted.[4]

1. Barakat MH, *et al.* Metaraminol provocative test: a specific diagnostic test for familial Mediterranean fever. *Lancet* 1984; **i:** 656–7.
2. Cattan D, *et al.* Metaraminol provocation test for familial Mediterranean fever. *Lancet* 1984; **i:** 1130–1.
3. Buades J, *et al.* The metaraminol test and adverse cardiac effects. *Ann Intern Med* 1989; **111:** 259–60.
4. Ben-Chetrit E, *et al.* Dopamine-β-hydroxylase activity in familial Mediterranean fever. *Lancet* 1990; **335:** 176.

Priapism. Metaraminol in low dosage and dilute solution, by intracavernosal injection, has been used successfully to treat priapism associated with a variety of conditions; these have included drug-induced priapism,[1] as a complication of chronic myeloid leukaemia,[2] associated with haemodialysis,[3] and during spinal block[4] or fentanyl-induced general anaesthesia.[4] It may be used to reverse the effects of alprostadil or papaverine given for the management of some types of erectile dysfunction. However, this use of metaraminol by intracavernosal injection has been associated with fatal hypertensive crisis (see also Alprostadil, p.1413).

Alternatives include the use of corporal aspiration followed by intracavernosal phenylephrine in low dosage and dilute solution in patients with low-flow priapism (due to decreased penile venous outflow);[5] in high-flow priapism (due to increased arterial inflow), which is less of an emergency, embolisation of the source of abnormal inflow is used. Surgery is usually favoured in low-flow priapism unresponsive to drug therapy. Phenylpropanolamine[5] and pseudoephedrine[6] have both been given by mouth as an alternative to phenylephrine or metaraminol injection.

1. Brindley GS. New treatment for priapism. *Lancet* 1984; **ii:** 220–1.
2. Stanners A, Colin-Jones D. Metaraminol for priapism. *Lancet* 1984; **ii:** 978.
3. Branger B, *et al.* Metaraminol for haemodialysis-associated priapism. *Lancet* 1985; **i:** 641.
4. Tsai SK, Hong CY. Intracavernosal metaraminol for treatment of intraoperative penile erection. *Postgrad Med J* 1990; **66:** 831–3.
5. Harmon WJ, Nehra A. Priapism: diagnosis and management. *Mayo Clin Proc* 1997; **72:** 350–5.
6. Millard RJ, *et al.* Risks of self-injection therapy for impotence. *Med J Aust* 1996; **165:** 117–18.

Preparations

BP 1998: Metaraminol Injection;
USP 23: Metaraminol Bitartrate Injection.

Proprietary Preparations (details are given in Part 3)
Austral.: Aramine; ***Belg.:*** Aramine; ***Ital.:*** Levicor; ***Neth.:*** Aramine†; ***Norw.:*** Aramine; ***UK:*** Aramine; ***USA:*** Aramine.

Methazolamide (2347-e)

Methazolamide (*BAN, rINN*).

N-(4-Methyl-2-sulphamoyl-Δ^2-1,3,4-thiadiazolin-5-ylidene)acetamide.

$C_5H_8N_4O_3S_2$ = 236.3.

CAS — 554-57-4.

Pharmacopoeias. In US.

A white or faintly yellow crystalline powder with a slight odour. Very slightly **soluble** in water and in alcohol; slightly soluble in acetone; soluble in dimethylformamide. **Protect** from light.

Adverse Effects and Precautions

As for Acetazolamide, p.810.

Cholestatic hepatitis with jaundice, rash, and subsequent pure red cell aplasia was associated with methazolamide in 1 patient.[1] Drug-induced hypersensitivity was suspected as the cause of the reaction.

1. Krivoy N, *et al.* Methazolamide-induced hepatitis and pure RBC aplasia. *Arch Intern Med* 1981; **141:** 1229–30.

Pharmacokinetics

Methazolamide is absorbed from the gastro-intestinal tract more slowly than acetazolamide. It has been reported not to be extensively bound to plasma protein, and to have a half-life of about 14 hours. About 15 to 30% of the dose is excreted in the urine; the fate of the remainder is unknown.

Uses and Administration

Methazolamide is an inhibitor of carbonic anhydrase with actions similar to those of acetazolamide (p.811). It is used in the management of glaucoma (p.1387) in doses of 50 to 100 mg two or three times daily by mouth. Its action is less prompt but of longer duration than that of acetazolamide, lasting for 10 to 18 hours.

The diuretic activity of methazolamide is less pronounced than that of acetazolamide.

Preparations

USP 23: Methazolamide Tablets.

Proprietary Preparations (details are given in Part 3)
Austral.: Neptazane; ***Canad.:*** Neptazane; ***USA:*** GlaucTabs; Neptazane.

Methoserpidine (881-k)

Methoserpidine (*BAN, rINN*).

10-Methoxydeserpidine. Methyl 11-demethoxy-10-methoxy-*O*-(3,4,5-trimethoxybenzoyl)reserpate.

$C_{33}H_{40}N_2O_9$ = 608.7.

CAS — 865-04-3.

Methoserpidine has properties similar to those described under reserpine (p.942) and has been used in the treatment of hypertension.

Methoxamine Hydrochloride

(2080-d)

Methoxamine Hydrochloride (*BANM, rINNM*).

Methoxamedrine Hydrochloride. 2-Amino-1-(2,5-dimethoxyphenyl)propan-1-ol hydrochloride.

$C_{11}H_{17}NO_3,HCl$ = 247.7.

CAS — 390-28-3 (methoxamine); 61-16-5 (methoxamine hydrochloride).

Pharmacopoeias. In Br., Chin., and US.

Colourless or white plate-like crystals or white crystalline powder; odourless or almost odourless.

Soluble 1 in 2.5 of water and 1 in 12 of alcohol; very slightly soluble or practically insoluble in chloroform and ether. A 2% solution in water has a pH of 4.0 to 6.0. **Protect** from light.

Adverse Effects, Treatment, and Precautions

Methoxamine may induce a desire to micturate and a pilomotor reaction (goose flesh). The hypertensive effects of methoxamine may be treated with an alpha-adrenoceptor blocker such as phentolamine. Atropine may be given if reflex bradycardia is significant.

For the adverse effects of sympathomimetics in general, and precautions to be observed, see Adrenaline, p.813.

Interactions

For the interactions of sympathomimetics in general, see Adrenaline, p.814.

Pharmacokinetics

Methoxamine acts within about 2 minutes of intravenous injection and within about 15 to 20 minutes of intramuscular injection; the duration of action of these two routes is about 10 to 15 minutes and about 1.5 hours respectively.

Uses and Administration

Methoxamine is a sympathomimetic (see Adrenaline, p.815) with mainly direct effects on adrenergic receptors. It has alpha-adrenergic activity entirely; beta-adrenergic activity is not demonstrable and beta-adrenoceptor blockade has been postulated. Methoxamine causes prolonged peripheral vasoconstriction and consequently a rise in arterial blood pressure. It has little effect on the heart, though reflex bradycardia may occasionally occur. It has a marked pilomotor effect but does not stimulate the central nervous system or cause bronchodilatation. It markedly reduces blood flow to the kidney.

Methoxamine hydrochloride is used for its pressor action in **hypotensive states** (p.790), notably in general or spinal anaesthesia; it may be used in patients who have received cyclopropane or halothane anaesthesia. It is given intramuscularly in usual doses of 10 to 15 mg (range 5 to 20 mg). As the maximum effects are not immediately apparent, about 15 minutes should elapse before repeating a dose. In an emergency 3 to 5 mg may be given by slow intravenous injection (at a rate of 1 mg per minute); doses of up to 10 mg have been employed. In children, doses of 70 to 280 μg per kg body-weight intramuscularly or 40 to 70 μg per kg by slow intravenous injection have been suggested.

Methoxamine hydrochloride may be given for **paroxysmal supraventricular tachycardia** unresponsive to other therapies (p.782) in doses of 10 mg by slow intravenous injection over 3 to 5 minutes.

Methoxamine hydrochloride is also used for its vasoconstrictor effect in the management of **nasal congestion** (p.1052). It has been administered by nasal drops or a spray as a 0.25% solution.

Preparations

BP 1998: Methoxamine Injection.

Proprietary Preparations (details are given in Part 3)

Aust.: Vasoxine; ***Austral.:*** Vasylox Junior†; ***Canad.:*** Vasoxyl; ***Irl.:*** Vasoxine; ***Spain:*** Idasal†; ***UK:*** Vasoxine; ***USA:*** Vasoxyl.

Multi-ingredient: ***Spain:*** Idasal Antibiotico†.

Methyclothiazide (2348-l)

Methyclothiazide *(BAN, USAN, rINN)*.

NSC-110431. 6-Chloro-3-chloromethyl-3,4-dihydro-2-methyl-2*H*-1,2,4-benzothiadiazine-7-sulphonamide 1,1-dioxide.

$C_9H_{11}Cl_2N_3O_4S_2$ = 360.2.

CAS — 135-07-9.

Pharmacopoeias. In *US.*

A white or almost white, odourless or almost odourless, crystalline powder. Very slightly **soluble** in water and chloroform; soluble 1 in 92.5 of alcohol and 1 in 2700 of ether; sparingly soluble in methyl alcohol; freely soluble in acetone and in pyridine.

Methyclothiazide is a thiazide diuretic with properties similar to those of hydrochlorothiazide (see p.885). It is used for oedema, including that associated with heart failure (p.785), and for hypertension (p.788).

Diuresis is initiated in about 2 hours, reaches a peak at about 6 hours, and lasts for 24 hours or more.

In the treatment of oedema the usual initial dose is 2.5 to 5 mg by mouth daily, increasing to a maximum dose of 10 mg daily if necessary. In the treatment of hypertension the usual dose is 2.5 to 5 mg daily, either alone, or in conjunction with other antihypertensives. Doses of up to 10 mg daily have been suggested, but this may not result in an increased hypotensive effect.

Children have been given a dose of 50 to 200 μg per kg body-weight daily.

In susceptible patients potassium supplements or a potassium-sparing diuretic may be necessary, but see hydrochlorothiazide.

Preparations

USP 23: Methyclothiazide Tablets.

Proprietary Preparations (details are given in Part 3)

Austral.: Enduron; ***Canad.:*** Duretic†; ***Swed.:*** Enduronа†; ***UK:*** Enduron†; ***USA:*** Aquatensen; Enduron.

Multi-ingredient: ***Canad.:*** Dureticyl†; ***Fr.:*** Isobar; ***Ital.:*** Enduronil; ***USA:*** Diutensen-R; Enduronyl.

Methyldopa (882-a)

Methyldopa *(BAN, USAN, rINN)*.

Alpha-methyldopa; Methyldopum; Methyldopum Hydratum; Metildopa; MK-351. (−)-3-(3,4-Dihydroxyphenyl)-2-methyl-L-alanine sesquihydrate; (−)-2-Amino-2-(3,4-dihydroxybenzyl)propionic acid sesquihydrate.

$C_{10}H_{13}NO_4,1\frac{1}{2}H_2O$ = 238.2.

CAS — 555-30-6 (anhydrous methyldopa); 41372-08-1 (methyldopa sesquihydrate).

Pharmacopoeias. In *Eur.* (see p.viii), *Int., Jpn,* and *US.*

Colourless or almost colourless crystals or a white to yellowish-white odourless fine powder which may contain friable lumps. Methyldopa 1.13 g is approximately equivalent to 1 g of anhydrous methyldopa.

Ph. Eur. **solubilities** are: slightly soluble in water; very slightly soluble in alcohol; practically insoluble in ether; freely soluble in dilute mineral acids. USP solubilities are: sparingly soluble in water; slightly soluble in alcohol; practically insoluble in ether; very soluble in 3N hydrochloric acid. **Protect** from light.

Methyldopate Hydrochloride (883-t)

Methyldopate Hydrochloride *(BANM, USAN)*.

Cloridrato de Metildopato. The hydrochloride of the ethyl ester of anhydrous methyldopa; Ethyl (−)-2-amino-2-(3,4-dihydroxybenzyl)propionate hydrochloride.

$C_{12}H_{17}NO_4,HCl$ = 275.7.

CAS — 2544-09-4 (methyldopate); 2508-79-4 (methyldopate hydrochloride).

Pharmacopoeias. In *Br.* and *US.*

A white or almost white, odourless or almost odourless, crystalline powder. Freely **soluble** in water, in alcohol, and in methyl alcohol; slightly soluble in chloroform; practically insoluble in ether. A 1% solution in water has a pH of 3 to 5. **Protect** from light.

Incompatibility. A haze developed over 3 hours when methyldopate hydrochloride 1 g per litre was mixed with amphotericin 200 mg per litre in glucose injection; crystals were produced with methohexitone sodium 200 mg per litre in sodium chloride injection, but a haze developed when they were mixed in glucose injection. A crystalline precipitate occurred with tetracycline hydrochloride 1 g per litre in glucose injection, and with sulphadiazine sodium 4 g per litre in glucose injection or sodium chloride injection.[1]

1. Riley BB. Incompatibilities in intravenous solutions. *J Hosp Pharm* 1970; **28:** 228–40.

Adverse Effects

The adverse effects of methyldopa are mostly consequences of its pharmacological action. The incidence of adverse effects overall may be as high as 60% but most are transient or reversible. Drowsiness is common, especially initially and following an increase in dosage. Dizziness and lightheadedness may be associated with postural hypotension, and nausea, headache, weakness and fatigue, and decreased libido and impotence have also been reported quite frequently.

The mental and neurological effects of methyldopa have included impaired concentration and memory, mild psychoses, depression, disturbed sleep and nightmares, paraesthesias, Bell's palsy, involuntary choreoathetotic movements, and parkinsonism.

In addition to postural hypotension, methyldopa is frequently associated with fluid retention and oedema, which responds to diuretics, but may rarely progress to heart failure. Angina pectoris may be aggravated. Bradycardia, syncope, and prolonged carotid sinus hypersensitivity have been reported. Intravenous administration of methyldopate has been associated with a paradoxical rise in blood pressure.

Methyldopa may produce gastro-intestinal disturbances including nausea and vomiting, diarrhoea, constipation, and rarely pancreatitis and colitis. A black or sore tongue, and inflammation of the salivary glands, have occurred, and dry mouth is quite common.

A positive Coombs' test may occur in 10 to 20% of all patients on prolonged therapy but only a small proportion develop haemolytic anaemia. Thrombocytopenia and leucopenia, notably granulocytopenia, have occurred and warrant prompt discontinuation. Other hypersensitivity effects have included myocarditis, fever, eosinophilia, and disturbances of liver function. Hepatitis may develop, particularly in the first 2 or 3 months of therapy, and is generally reversible on discontinuation, but fatal hepatic necrosis has occurred. Antinuclear antibodies may develop and cases of a lupus-like syndrome have been reported.

Other adverse effects that have been reported in patients receiving methyldopa include rashes, lichenoid and granulomatous eruptions, toxic epidermal necrolysis, a flu-like syndrome (of fever, myalgia, and mild arthralgia), nocturia, uraemia, nasal stuffiness, and retroperitoneal fibrosis. Hyperprolactinaemia may occur, with breast enlargement or gynaecomastia, galactorrhoea, and amenorrhoea.

Methyldopa may occasionally cause urine to darken on exposure to the air because of the breakdown of the drug or its metabolites.

Reviews.

1. Furhoff A-K. Adverse reactions with methyldopa—a decade's reports. *Acta Med Scand* 1978; **203:** 425–8.
2. Lawson DH, *et al.* Adverse reactions to methyldopa with particular reference to hypotension. *Am Heart J* 1978; **96:** 572–9.

Effects on the blood. HAEMOLYTIC ANAEMIA. An analysis of drug-induced blood dyscrasias reported to the Swedish Adverse Drug Reaction Committee for the 10-year period 1966-75 showed that haemolytic anaemia attributable to methyldopa had been reported on 69 occasions and had caused 3 deaths. This represented the vast majority of all the reports of drug-induced haemolytic anaemia.[1] However, the actual incidence of haemolytic anaemia in patients receiving methyldopa is quite low; data from the Boston Collaborative Drug Surveillance Program indicated that only 2 of 1067 patients receiving methyldopa developed haemolytic anaemia,[2] an incidence of about 0.2%. The proportion of patients with a positive Coombs' test is much higher, being variously reported at 10 to 20%.[3-5] It has been suggested that the high incidence of autoantibody formation may be due to inhibition of suppressor T-cells by methyldopa[4] while the relatively low incidence of resultant haemolysis may be due to drug-associated impairment of the reticuloendothelial system which would normally clear the antibody-sensitised cells from the circulation.[5]

1. Böttiger LE, *et al.* Drug-induced blood dyscrasias. *Acta Med Scand* 1979; **205:** 457–61.
2. Lawson DH, *et al.* Adverse reactions to methyldopa with particular reference to hypotension. *Am Heart J* 1978; **96:** 572–9.
3. Carstairs K, *et al.* Methyldopa and haemolytic anaemia. *Lancet* 1966; **i:** 201.
4. Kirtland HH, *et al.* Methyldopa inhibition of suppressor-lymphocyte function: a proposed cause of autoimmune hemolytic anemia. *N Engl J Med* 1980; **302:** 825–32.
5. Kelton JG. Impaired reticuloendothelial function in patients treated with methyldopa. *N Engl J Med* 1985; **313:** 596–600.

Effects on the gastro-intestinal tract. COLITIS. Report of 6 cases of colitis associated with methyldopa.[1] An auto-immune mechanism was proposed.

1. Graham CF, *et al.* Acute colitis with methyldopa. *N Engl J Med* 1981; **304:** 1044–5.

DIARRHOEA. Severe chronic diarrhoea was associated with methyldopa therapy for 2 years in a 62-year-old woman. Diarrhoea stopped immediately after discontinuation of methyldopa.[1] In another case severe diarrhoea in an elderly senile patient, that had persisted for 7 years and worsened with age, stopped when methyldopa was withdrawn and recurred, after a delay, when the drug was given again in a lower dose. Discontinuation of methyldopa resulted in complete freedom from diarrhoea and faecal incontinence within 7 days.[2]

1. Quart BD, Guglielmo BJ. Prolonged diarrhea secondary to methyldopa therapy. *Drug Intell Clin Pharm* 1983; **17:** 462.
2. Gloth FM, Busby MJ. Methyldopa-induced diarrhea: a case of iatrogenic diarrhea leading to request for nursing home placement. *Am J Med* 1989; **87:** 480–1.

PANCREATITIS. Increases in serum- and urinary-amylase activity accompanied by fever and suggestive of pancreatitis were associated with methyldopa in 2 patients.[1] One patient also had symptoms of severe pancreatitis. Symptoms reappeared on rechallenge in both patients. A further report of acute pancreatitis in a patient who had recently begun methyldopa therapy (with a diuretic) also confirmed a recurrence of symptoms on rechallenge.[2] In contrast to the acute form, chronic pancreatitis is not generally attributable to drug ingestion.[3] However Ramsay and colleagues reported a case of florid chronic pancreatitis, with exocrine and endocrine insufficiency and heavy calcification over 30 months, associated with 2 periods of methyldopa treatment.[4] Symptoms in this patient who was also receiving a thiazide, included severe diabetic ketoacidosis.

1. van der Heide H, *et al.* Pancreatitis caused by methyldopa. *Br Med J* 1981; **282:** 1930–1.
2. Anderson JR, *et al.* Drug-associated recurrent pancreatitis. *Dig Surg* 1985; **2:** 24–6.
3. Banergee AK, *et al.* Drug-induced acute pancreatitis. *Med Toxicol Adverse Drug Exp* 1989; **4:** 186–98.
4. Ramsay LE, *et al.* Methyldopa-induced chronic pancreatitis. *Practitioner* 1982; **226:** 1166–9.

Effects on the heart. MYOCARDITIS. Sudden death in a number of patients receiving methyldopa has been associated with the presence of myocarditis, often in association with hepatitis and pneumonitis.[1,2] The effect is thought to be due to hypersensitivity. Hypersensitivity myocarditis is generally marked by ECG changes, a slight rise in cardiac enzymes, cardiomegaly, and persistent sinus tachycardia, along with peripheral blood eosinophilia, and most patients will recover within days if the drug is withdrawn in time.[3]

1. Mullick FG, McAllister HA. Myocarditis associated with methyldopa therapy. *JAMA* 1977; **237:** 1699–1701. Correction. *ibid.*; **238:** 399.
2. Seeverens H, *et al.* Myocarditis and methyldopa. *Acta Med Scand* 1982; **211:** 233–5.
3. Anonymous. Myocarditis related to drug hypersensitivity. *Lancet* 1985; **ii:** 1165–6.

Effects on the liver. Rodman and colleagues have reported on 6 cases of hepatitis in patients taking methyldopa and reviewed 77 cases from the literature.[1] Most patients presented with symptoms including malaise, fatigue, anorexia, weight loss, nausea, and vomiting, and histopathological changes resembling those of viral hepatitis. Fever occurred in 28 of the 83 patients; rashes and eosinophilia occurred rarely. Symptoms usually began 1 to 4 weeks after the first dose of methyldopa. Clinically apparent jaundice occurred as early as 1 week and as late as 3 years after the initiation of therapy, although only 6 or 7 patients presented with jaundice later than 3 months. Liver damage was not dose-related and had features suggestive of an immunologically-mediated hypersensitivity reaction. The histological changes included chronic active hepatitis, massive fatal necrosis, and cirrhosis.

In an analysis by Sotaniemi and others of 36 patients with liver damage due to methyldopa, hepatic injury tended to occur in 2 phases—acute and chronic.[2] Acute liver damage developed within a few months of starting treatment with methyldopa, and was considered to be an allergic reaction to methyldopa metabolites. The chronic form usually occurred at least a year after starting methyldopa, and was characterised by an accumulation of fat in the liver. Recovery after withdrawal of methyldopa was directly related to duration of exposure and degree of liver damage. There was also a suggestion of genetic predisposition, as acute methyldopa-induced liver damage occurred in 4 members of a family. Neuberger and co-workers have suggested that idiosyncratic metabolism of methyldopa in susceptible patients is responsible for expression of an antigen on the surface of liver cells with which circulating antibodies react.[3]

See also under Fever, below.

1. Rodman JS, *et al.* Methyldopa hepatitis: a report of six cases and review of the literature. *Am J Med* 1976; **60:** 941–8.
2. Sotaniemi EA, *et al.* Hepatic injury and drug metabolism in patients with alpha-methyldopa-induced liver damage. *Eur J Clin Pharmacol* 1977; **12:** 429–35.
3. Neuberger J, *et al.* Antibody mediated hepatocyte injury in methyldopa induced hepatotoxicity. *Gut* 1985; **26:** 1233–9.

Effects on mental function. Anecdotal reports have implicated methyldopa in producing disturbances of mental acuity including inability to concentrate, an impaired calculating ability, and forgetfulness.[1-3] These have been confirmed to some extent by psychometric studies. Solomon and others reported impaired verbal memory but not visual memory in 10 patients receiving methyldopa with a diuretic.[4] A crossover study by Johnson and colleagues in 16 patients also indicated impairment of cognitive function by methyldopa.[5]

1. Adler S. Methyldopa-induced decrease in mental activity. *JAMA* 1974; **230:** 1428–9.
2. Ghosh SK. Methyldopa and forgetfulness. *Lancet* 1976; **i:** 202–3.
3. Fernandez PG. Alpha methyldopa and forgetfulness. *Ann Intern Med* 1976; **85:** 128.
4. Solomon S, *et al.* Impairment of memory function by antihypertensive medication. *Arch Gen Psychiatry* 1983; **40:** 1109–12.
5. Johnson B, *et al.* Effects of methyldopa on psychometric performance. *J Clin Pharmacol* 1990; **30:** 1102–5.

DEPRESSION. Depression has been associated with methyldopa therapy, although the exact relationship is unclear.[1] One review[2] reported the incidence to be 3.6% and suggested that depression was more common in patients with a previous history.

1. Patten SB, Love EJ. Drug-induced depression. *Drug Safety* 1994; **10:** 203–19.
2. Paykel ES, *et al.* Psychiatric side effects of antihypertensive drugs other than reserpine. *J Clin Psychopharmacol* 1982; **2:** 14–39.

Effects on the nervous system. Involuntary choreoathetotic movements resembling those of Huntington's chorea began in a 59-year-old man with cerebrovascular disease following increase of his methyldopa dose from 1 to 1.5 g daily. He recovered when methyldopa therapy was withdrawn.[1] In another report methyldopa was associated with the development of bilateral choreiform movements in a patient without cerebrovascular disease but with chronic renal failure.[2]

1. Yamadori A, Albert ML. Involuntary movement disorder caused by methyldopa. *N Engl J Med* 1972; **286:** 610.
2. Neil EM, Waters AK. Generalized choreiform movements as a complication of methyldopa therapy in chronic renal failure. *Postgrad Med J* 1981; **57:** 732–3.

Effects on sexual function. Methyldopa has been associated with numerous cases of sexual dysfunction. In males failure to maintain erection, decreased libido, impaired ejaculation, and gynaecomastia have occurred, while in females decreased libido, painful breast enlargement, and delayed or absent orgasm have been reported.[1] The reported incidence varies and there is some evidence that sexual dysfunction may be underreported: Alexander and Evans found that while only 2 of 30 men receiving methyldopa spontaneously reported erection failure the actual incidence on questioning was 16 of 30.[2]

1. Stevenson JG, Umstead GS. Sexual dysfunction due to antihypertensive agents. *Drug Intell Clin Pharm* 1984; **18:** 113–21.
2. Alexander WD, Evans JI. Side effects of methyldopa. *Br Med J* 1975; **2:** 501.

Fever. Report of 78 cases of methyldopa-induced fever.[1] Fever occurred 5 to 35 days after the first exposure to methyldopa in 77 patients and one day after recommencing methyldopa in the remaining patient. Rigors, headache, and myalgia were common accompanying symptoms, but eosinophilia and skin rashes were not seen. The majority of patients did not appear seriously ill, but 4 patients presented the picture of septic shock. Biochemical evidence of liver damage was found in 61% of patients but jaundice was uncommon. In the majority of patients, symptoms were relieved within 48 hours of the withdrawal of the drug.

1. Stanley P, Mijch A. Methyldopa: an often overlooked cause of fever and transient hepatocellular dysfunction. *Med J Aust* 1986; **144:** 603–5.

Lupus erythematosus. The incidence of antinuclear antibodies was 13% in 269 hypertensive patients taking methyldopa (irrespective of other medication), compared with 3.8% in 448 hypertensive patients not taking methyldopa.[1] Apart from the occasional case of methyldopa-induced lupus, however, patients did not appear to be at risk.

1. Wilson JD, *et al.* Antinuclear antibodies in patients receiving non-practolol beta-blockers. *Br Med J* 1978; **1:** 14–16.

Overdosage. Ingestion of methyldopa 2.5 g produced coma, hypothermia, hypotension, bradycardia, and dry mouth in a 19-year-old man.[1] The serum-methyldopa concentration 10 hours after ingestion was 19.2 μg per mL compared with serum concentrations of approximately 2 μg per mL in patients receiving therapeutic doses of methyldopa. The patient recovered following treatment with intravenous fluids.

1. Shnaps Y, *et al.* Methyldopa poisoning. *J Toxicol Clin Toxicol* 1982; **19:** 501–3.

Retroperitoneal fibrosis. A 60-year-old patient developed retroperitoneal fibrosis and a positive direct Coombs' test associated with methyldopa given in a daily dose of 750 mg with bendrofluazide 2.5 mg for about 5 years.[1]

1. Iversen BM, *et al.* Retroperitoneal fibrosis during treatment with methyldopa. *Lancet* 1975; **ii:** 302–4.

Treatment of Adverse Effects

Withdrawal of methyldopa or reduction in dosage causes the reversal of many side-effects. If overdosage occurs the stomach may be emptied by lavage. Treatment is largely symptomatic, but if necessary, intravenous fluid infusions may be given to promote urinary excretion, and vasopressors given cautiously. Severe hypotension may respond to placing the patient in the supine position with the feet raised.

Methyldopa is dialysable.

Precautions

Methyldopa should be used with caution in patients with impaired kidney or liver function or with a history of haemolytic anaemia, liver disease, or depression. Care is also advisable in patients with parkinsonism. It should not be given to patients with active liver disease or depression and it is not recommended for phaeochromocytoma. Methyldopa has been reported to aggravate porphyria.

It is advisable to make periodic blood counts and to perform liver-function tests at intervals during the first 6 to 12 weeks of treatment or if the patient develops an unexplained fever. Patients taking methyldopa may produce a positive response to a direct Coombs' test; if blood transfusion is required, prior knowledge of a positive direct Coombs' test reaction will aid cross matching.

Methyldopa may cause sedation; if affected patients should not drive or operate machinery.

Porphyria. Methyldopa has been associated with acute attacks of porphyria and is considered unsafe in patients with acute porphyria.[1]

1. Moore MR, McColl KEL. *Porphyria: drug lists.* Glasgow: Porphyria Research Unit, University of Glasgow, 1991.

Pregnancy and breast feeding. Methyldopa is commonly used in the management of hypertension occurring during pregnancy (p.788). There is little evidence of adverse effects on fetal development. However, methyldopa crosses the placenta[1] and reduced blood pressure has been reported in the infants of mothers given methyldopa.[2] There has also been a report of tremor in 7 infants associated with maternal methyldopa therapy during pregnancy.[3] Depressed cerebrospinal fluid noradrenaline concentrations were noted in the 3 infants examined leading to successful treatment of the other 4 infants with atropine: tremor was abolished in 2 and substantially reduced in the other 2 infants.

A small amount of methyldopa may be distributed into breast milk.[1]

1. Jones HMR, Cummings AJ. A study of the transfer of α-methyldopa to the human foetus and newborn infants. *Br J Clin Pharmacol* 1978; **6:** 432–4.
2. Whitelaw A. Maternal methyldopa treatment and neonatal blood pressure. *Br Med J* 1981; **283:** 471.
3. Bódis J, *et al.* Methyldopa in pregnancy hypertension and the newborn. *Lancet* 1982; **ii:** 498–9.

Interactions

The hypotensive effects of methyldopa are potentiated by diuretics, other antihypertensives, and drugs with hypotensive effects. However, there have been reports of paradoxical antagonism of the hypotensive effects by tricyclic antidepressants, antipsychotics, and beta blockers. Sympathomimetics may also antagonise the hypotensive effects.

There may be an interaction between methyldopa and MAOIs and care is required if they are given concomitantly.

Patients receiving methyldopa may require lower doses of general anaesthetics.

Alpha blockers. Urinary incontinence occurred on concomitant administration of methyldopa and *phenoxybenzamine* in a patient who had undergone bilateral lumbar sympathectomy.[1]

1. Fernandez PG, *et al.* Urinary incontinence due to interaction of phenoxybenzamine and α-methyldopa. *Can Med Assoc J* 1981; **124:** 174–5.

Antipsychotics. Antipsychotics may enhance the hypotensive effects of methyldopa but a paradoxical increase in blood pressure has also been reported. A woman with systemic lupus erythematosus taking *trifluoperazine* up to 15 mg daily and prednisone up to 120 mg daily was given methyldopa up to 2 g and triamterene for high blood pressure. Her blood pressure rose further to 200/140 mmHg. After discontinuation of trifluoperazine blood pressure returned to 160/100 mmHg.[1]

In another report, 2 patients with essential hypertension who had been receiving methyldopa for 3 years and 18 months respectively developed symptoms of dementia within days of concurrent administration of *haloperidol* for anxiety.[2] In both patients the symptoms resolved rapidly on discontinuation of haloperidol.

1. Westervelt FB, Atuk NO. Methyldopa-induced hypertension. *JAMA* 1974; **227:** 557.
2. Thornton WE. Dementia induced by methyldopa with haloperidol. *N Engl J Med* 1976; **294:** 1222.

Cephalosporins. A report of a pustular pruritic eruption following administration of *cephazolin sodium* to a patient receiving methyldopa.[1] A previous similar case has been reported in a patient receiving *cephradine* and methyldopa.

1. Stough D, *et al.* Pustular eruptions following administration of cefazolin: a possible interaction with methyldopa. *J Am Acad Dermatol* 1987; **16:** 1051–2.

Digoxin. Syncope associated with carotid sinus hypersensitivity has been reported to be possibly enhanced by methyldopa in a patient taking digoxin and chlorthalidone.[1] In another report,[2] sinus bradycardia developed in 2 patients taking methyldopa and digoxin concomitantly.

1. Bauernfeind R, *et al.* Carotid sinus hypersensitivity with alpha methyldopa. *Ann Intern Med* 1978; **88:** 214–15.
2. Davis JC, *et al.* Sinus node dysfunction caused by methyldopa and digoxin. *JAMA* 1981; **245:** 1241–3.

Iron. Following results in healthy subjects which indicated that the absorption of methyldopa was reduced by 73% and 61% respectively when taken with a dose of ferrous sulphate or ferrous gluconate, 5 hypertensive patients receiving methyldopa were also given ferrous sulphate 325 mg three times daily for 2 weeks.[1] All patients experienced a rise in systolic pressure, and 4 had a rise in diastolic pressure, associated with ferrous sulphate administration, amounting to more than 15/10 mmHg in some patients after 2 weeks. Blood pressure fell again when the iron therapy was discontinued.

1. Campbell N, *et al.* Alteration of methyldopa absorption, metabolism, and blood pressure control caused by ferrous sulfate and ferrous gluconate. *Clin Pharmacol Ther* 1988; **43:** 381–6.

Levodopa. For reference to a mutual interaction between methyldopa and levodopa, see p.1139.

Lithium. For reference to the development of lithium toxicity on concurrent administration of methyldopa, see p.294.

Sympathomimetics. A 31-year-old man whose hypertension was well controlled with methyldopa and oxprenolol suffered a severe hypertensive episode when he took a preparation for a cold containing *phenylpropanolamine.*[1]

1. McLaren EH. Severe hypertension produced by interaction of phenylpropanolamine with methyldopa and oxprenolol. *Br Med J* 1976; **2:** 283–4.

Pharmacokinetics

Following oral administration methyldopa is variably and incompletely absorbed, apparently by an amino-acid active transport system. The mean bioavailability has been reported to be about 50%. It is extensively metabolised and is excreted in urine mainly as unchanged drug and the O-sulphate conjugate. It crosses the blood-brain barrier and is decarboxylated in the central nervous system to active alphamethylnoradrenaline.

The elimination is biphasic with a half-life of about 1.7 hours in the initial phase; the second phase is more prolonged. Clearance is decreased and half-life prolonged in renal insufficiency. Plasma protein binding is reported to be minimal. Methyldopa crosses the placenta; small amounts are distributed into breast milk.

Uses and Administration

Methyldopa is an antihypertensive that is thought to have a predominantly central action. It is decarboxylated in the CNS to alpha-methylnoradrenaline which is thought to stimulate alpha$_2$-adrenoceptors resulting in a reduction in sympathetic tone and a fall in blood pressure. It may also act as a false neurotransmitter, and have some inhibitory actions on plasma renin activity. Methyldopa reduces the tissue concentrations of dopamine, noradrenaline, adrenaline, and serotonin.

Methyldopa is used in the management of hypertension (p.788), although other drugs with fewer adverse effects are generally preferred. Methyldopa may, however, be the treatment of choice for hypertension in pregnancy. Oedema and tolerance sometimes associated with methyldopa therapy may be reduced when it is given with a thiazide diuretic.

Methyldopa is given by mouth as the sesquihydrate, but doses are usually expressed in terms of anhydrous methyldopa. For hypertensive crises, methyldopa has been given intravenously as methyldopate hydrochloride.

When methyldopa is administered by mouth its effects reach a maximum in 4 to 6 hours following a single dose, although the maximum hypotensive effect may not occur until the second or third day of continuous treatment; some effect is usually apparent for 48 hours after withdrawal of methyldopa. When administered intravenously the hypotensive effect may be obtained within 4 to 6 hours and last for 10 to 16 hours. It lowers the standing, and to a lesser extent the supine, blood pressure.

In **hypertension**, the usual initial dose by mouth is 250 mg of methyldopa two or three times daily for 2 days; this is then adjusted by small increments or decrements not more frequently than every 2 days according to the response of the patient. Although higher doses have been given it is generally considered that no advantage can be gained by giving doses larger than 3 g daily. The usual maintenance dosage is 0.5 to 2 g of methyldopa daily. In the elderly an initial dose of 125 mg twice daily has been recommended; this dose may be increased gradually if necessary, but should not exceed 2 g daily.

A suggested initial dose for children has been 10 mg per kg body-weight daily in 2 to 4 divided doses, increased as necessary to a maximum of 65 mg per kg or 3 g daily whichever is less.

The usual dose by intravenous injection is 250 to 500 mg of methyldopate hydrochloride in 100 mL of 5% glucose injection administered over 30 to 60 minutes every 6 hours. It is suggested that the dose should not exceed 1 g every 6 hours. A suggested dose for children is 5 to 10 mg per kg body-weight every 6 hours. The maximum recommended daily dose for children is 65 mg per kg or 3 g, whichever is less.

Preparations

BP 1998: Methyldopa Tablets; Methyldopate Injection;
USP 23: Methyldopa and Chlorothiazide Tablets; Methyldopa and Hydrochlorothiazide Tablets; Methyldopa Oral Suspension; Methyldopa Tablets; Methyldopate Hydrochloride Injection.

Proprietary Preparations (details are given in Part 3)
Aust.: Aldometil; Presinol; ***Austral.:*** Aldomet; Aldopren; Hydopa; Nudopa; ***Belg.:*** Aldomet; Presinol†; ***Canad.:*** Aldomet; Novo-Medopa; Nu-Medopa; ***Fr.:*** Aldomet; Equibar†; ***Ger.:*** Dopegyt; Presinol; Sembrina; ***Irl.:*** Aldomet; Dopagen†; Dopamet; Elanpres†; Meldopa; ***Ital.:*** Aldomet; Elanpress†; Medopren; Presinol†; ***Neth.:*** Aldomet; Sembrina; ***Norw.:*** Aldomet; Dopamet; Medopal†; ***S.Afr.:*** Aldomet; Alphamex†; Arcanadopa†; Hy-Po-Tone; Normopress; Pharmet†; Sinepress; ***Spain:*** Aldomet; ***Swed.:*** Aldomet; Dopamet†; ***Switz.:*** Aldomet; Dopamet; ***UK:*** Aldomet; Dopamet†; Medomet; Metalpha; ***USA:*** Aldomet.

Multi-ingredient: ***Aust.:*** Aldoretic; ***Canad.:*** Aldoril; Apo-Methazide; Novo-Doparil; Supres; ***Ger.:*** Caprinol†; Sali-Presinol; Sembrina-Saltucin†; ***Irl.:*** Hydromet; ***Ital.:*** Aldotride†; Medozide; Saludopin; ***Neth.:*** Hydromet†; ***S.Afr.:*** Aldoretic; Hydromet†; ***Spain:*** Hydromet†; Picten†; ***Swed.:*** Hydromet; ***Switz.:*** Aldoretic; ***UK:*** Hydromet†; ***USA:*** Aldoclor; Aldoril.

Meticrane (12953-m)

Meticrane *(rINN).*

SD-17102. 6-Methylthiochroman-7-sulphonamide 1,1-dioxide.

$C_{10}H_{13}NO_4S_2$ = 275.3.

CAS — 1084-65-7.

Meticrane is a thiazide diuretic (see Hydrochlorothiazide, p.885) that has been used in the treatment of hypertension.

Metipranolol (6313-w)

Metipranolol *(BAN, USAN, rINN).*

BMOI-004; Methypranolol; VUAB-6453 (SPOFA); VUFB-6453. 1-(4-Acetoxy-2,3,5-trimethylphenoxy)-3-isopropylaminopropan-2-ol; 4-(2-Hydroxy-3-isopropylaminopropoxy)-2,3,6-trimethylphenyl acetate.

$C_{17}H_{27}NO_4$ = 309.4.

CAS — 22664-55-7.

NOTE. MPR is a code approved by the BP for use on single unit doses of eye drops containing metipranolol where the individual container may be too small to bear all the appropriate labelling information.

Adverse Effects, Treatment, and Precautions

As for beta blockers, p.828.

Conjunctivitis, conjunctival leukoplakia, transient stinging, as well as other ocular adverse effects have been reported with metipranolol eye drops. Granulomatous anterior uveitis has been reported mainly in the UK and it has been suggested that this effect may be associated with changes induced by radiation sterilisation of metipranolol eye drops in their final container.

Systemic adverse effects may occur following ocular administration.

Effects on the lungs. Acute pulmonary oedema, secondary to the negative inotropic and chronotropic effects of beta blockade, developed in a 72-year-old woman who had been applying one drop daily of metipranolol 0.3% eye drops to each eye for about six weeks.[1] Symptoms cleared over about 10 hours, but reappeared following accidental rechallenge. It was suggested that drug had accumulated over the six-week period, possibly due to deficient metabolism.

1. Johns MD, Ponte CD. Acute pulmonary edema associated with ocular metipranolol use. *Ann Pharmacother* 1995; **29:** 370–3.

Interactions

The interactions associated with beta blockers are discussed on p.829.

Since systemic absorption can follow ophthalmic use of beta blockers, the possibility of interactions occurring with metipranolol eye drops should also be considered.

Uses and Administration

Metipranolol is a non-cardioselective beta blocker (p.828). It is reported to be largely lacking in intrinsic sympathomimetic activity and membrane-stabilising properties.

Metipranolol is used in the management of open-angle glaucoma. (p.1387). It has also been used in the management of cardiovascular disorders.

To reduce raised intra-ocular pressure in open-angle **glaucoma** and ocular hypertension, metipranolol is instilled in the affected eye in usual doses of one drop of a 0.1 or 0.3% solution twice daily.

In **cardiovascular disorders** it has been given in doses of 5 to 20 mg by mouth two or three times daily.

References.

1. Battershill PE, Sorkin EM. Ocular metipranolol: a preliminary review of its pharmacodynamic and pharmacokinetic properties, and therapeutic efficacy in glaucoma and ocular hypertension. *Drugs* 1988; **36:** 601–15.

Preparations

Proprietary Preparations (details are given in Part 3)
Aust.: Beta-Ophtiole; ***Belg.:*** Beta-Ophtiole; ***Fr.:*** Betanol†; ***Ger.:*** Betamann; Disorat†; ***Ital.:*** Turoptin; ***Neth.:*** Beta-Ophtiole; ***S.Afr.:*** Beta-Ophtiole; ***Switz.:*** Turoptin; ***USA:*** OptiPranolol.

Multi-ingredient: ***Aust.:*** Betacarpin; Torrat; ***Belg.:*** Normoglaucon; ***Ger.:*** Normoglaucon; Torrat; Tri-Torrat; ***Ital.:*** Ripix; ***Neth.:*** Normoglaucon; ***Switz.:*** Ripix; Torrat†.

Metirosine (15325-f)

Metirosine *(BAN, rINN).*

L-588357-0; Metyrosine *(USAN)*; MK-781. (−)-α-Methyl-L-tyrosine; 4-Hydroxy-α-methylphenylalanine.

$C_{10}H_{13}NO_3$ = 195.2.

CAS — 672-87-7 (metirosine); 620-30-4 (racemetirosine).

NOTE. The term α-methyltyrosine (α-MPT; α-MT; α-methyl-*p*-tyrosine) is used below since although metirosine, the (−)-isomer, is the active form the manufacturers state that some racemate (racemetirosine; (±)-α-methyl-DL-tyrosine) is produced during synthesis but that the material supplied contains mainly (−)-isomer with a small amount of (+)-isomer.
The code name MK-781, applied to earlier investigational material, may have described a racemate or a preparation containing a smaller proportion of (−)-isomer than the product now available commercially.
Potency of the proprietary preparation (Demser) is expressed in terms of metirosine.

Pharmacopoeias. In US.

Adverse Effects

Sedation occurs in almost all patients receiving α-methyltyrosine. Extrapyramidal symptoms including trismus and frank parkinsonism; anxiety, depression, and psychic disturbances including hallucinations, disorientation, and confusion; and diarrhoea have also been reported. Crystalluria, transient dysuria, and haematuria have been seen in a few patients. Other adverse effects reported occasionally include slight swelling of the breast, galactorrhoea, nasal stuffiness, decreased salivation, gastro-intestinal disturbances, headache, impotence or failure of ejaculation, and hypersensitivity reactions. Eosinophilia, raised serum aspartate aminotransferase, and peripheral oedema have been reported rarely.

Neuroleptic malignant syndrome occurred after the use of the dopamine-depleting drugs tetrabenazine and α-methyltyrosine in a patient with Huntington's chorea.[1]

1. Burke RE, *et al.* Neuroleptic malignant syndrome caused by dopamine-depleting drugs in a patient with Huntington disease. *Neurology* 1981; **31:** 1022–6.

Precautions

To minimise the risk of crystalluria, patients receiving α-methyltyrosine should have a fluid intake sufficient to maintain a urine volume of at least 2 litres daily and their urine should be examined regularly for the presence of crystals.

α-Methyltyrosine has sedative effects and patients should be warned of the hazards of driving a motor vehicle or operating machinery while receiving the drug. Symptoms of psychic stimulation and insomnia may occur when α-methyltyrosine is withdrawn.

When α-methyltyrosine is used pre-operatively in patients with phaeochromocytoma, blood pressure and the ECG should be monitored continuously during surgery as the danger of hypertensive crises and arrhythmias is not obviated. Concomitant alpha-adrenoceptor blockade (e.g. with phentolamine) may be required; a beta blocker or lignocaine, may be needed for the management of arrhythmias. Blood volume must be maintained during and after surgery, particularly if an alpha-adrenoceptor blocker is used concurrently, in order to avoid hypotension.

Interactions

The sedative effects of α-methyltyrosine may be potentiated by alcohol and other CNS depressants. Concomitant administration with phenothiazines or haloperidol may exacerbate extrapyramidal effects.

Pharmacokinetics

α-Methyltyrosine is well absorbed from the gastro-intestinal tract and is excreted mainly unchanged by the kidneys. A plasma half-life of 3.4 to 7.2 hours has been reported. Less than 1% of a dose may be excreted as the metabolites α-methyldopa, α-methyldopamine, α-methylnoradrenaline, and α-methyltyramine.

Uses and Administration

α-Methyltyrosine is an inhibitor of the enzyme tyrosine hydroxylase, and consequently of the synthesis of catecholamines. It is used to control the symptoms of excessive sympathetic stimulation in patients with phaeochromocytoma (p.795) and decreases the frequency and severity of hypertensive attacks and related symptoms in most patients. It may be given for pre-operative preparation, to those patients for whom surgery is contra-indicated, or for long-term management in those with malignant phaeochromocytoma.

α-Methyltyrosine is given by mouth in a dose of 250 mg four times daily, increased daily by 250 mg or 500 mg to a maximum of 4 g daily in divided doses. The optimum dose, achieved by monitoring clinical symptoms and catecholamine excretion, is usually in the range of 2 to 3 g daily and when used pre-operatively it should be given for at least 5 to 7 days before surgery.

The concomitant use of alpha-adrenoceptor blockers may be necessary.

α-Methyltyrosine is not effective in controlling essential hypertension.

α-Methyltyrosine has also been tried in patients with schizophrenia.

Preparations

USP 23: Metyrosine Capsules.

Proprietary Preparations (details are given in Part 3)
Neth.: Demser†; ***UK:*** Demser; ***USA:*** Demser.

Metolazone (2349-y)

Metolazone *(BAN, USAN, rINN).*

SR-720-22. 7-Chloro-1,2,3,4-tetrahydro-2-methyl-4-oxo-3-o-tolylquinazoline-6-sulphonamide.

$C_{16}H_{16}ClN_3O_3S$ = 365.8.

CAS — 17560-51-9.

Pharmacopoeias. In US.

Store in airtight containers. Protect from light.

Adverse Effects and Treatment

As for Hydrochlorothiazide, p.885. Metolazone has also been reported to cause palpitations, chest pain, and chills.

Effects on the blood. Profound neutropenia was observed in a 58-year-old woman within 10 days of starting treatment with metolazone.[1] Neutropenia persisted for a further 10 days after metolazone was withdrawn. No other haematological abnormalities were observed.

1. Donovan KL. Neutropenia and metolazone. *Br Med J* 1989; **299:** 981.

Effects on the nervous system. Two patients experienced acute muscle cramps with impairment of consciousness and epileptiform movements after taking metolazone 5 mg (single dose) or 2.5 mg daily for 3 days.[1]

1. Fitzgerald MX, Brennan NJ. Muscle cramps, collapse, and seizures in two patients taking metolazone. *Br Med J* 1976; **1:** 1381–2.

Precautions

As for Hydrochlorothiazide, p.887. Severe electrolyte disturbances may occur when metolazone and frusemide are used concurrently.

Interactions

As for Hydrochlorothiazide, p.887.

ACE inhibitors. Deterioration in renal function occurred in a 65-year-old woman when metolazone 5 mg [daily] was added to treatment with *captopril*, frusemide, spironolactone, and digoxin for heart failure.[1] An interaction between captopril and metolazone was suspected and both drugs were discontinued with a subsequent return to normal renal function. It was suggested that natriuresis and a fall in blood pressure caused by the diuretic may have compromised an already low renal perfusion pressure when autoregulatory mechanisms were blocked by captopril.

1. Hogg KJ, Hillis WS. Captopril/metolazone induced renal failure. *Lancet* 1986; **i:** 501–2.

Antidiabetics. Hypoglycaemia occurred in a patient with type 2 diabetes mellitus controlled with *glibenclamide* 40 hours after initiation of therapy with metolazone 5 mg daily.[1] Studies of protein binding *in vitro* did not reveal any evidence of displacement of glibenclamide from binding sites.

1. George S, *et al.* Possible protein binding displacement interaction between glibenclamide and metolazone. *Eur J Clin Pharmacol* 1990; **38:** 93–5.

Cyclosporin. An increase in serum-creatinine concentration in a renal transplant patient was attributed to a toxic drug interaction between metolazone and cyclosporin.[1] Serum-creatinine concentrations returned to pretreatment values when metolazone was discontinued.

1. Christensen P, Leski M. Nephrotoxic drug interaction between metolazone and cyclosporin. *Br Med J* 1987; **294:** 578.

Pharmacokinetics

Metolazone is slowly and incompletely absorbed from the gastro-intestinal tract. An average of about 65% of the administered dose has been reported to be absorbed following an oral dose in healthy subjects, and an average of about 40% in patients with cardiac disease. In some countries a formulation with enhanced bioavailability is available. About 95% of the drug is bound in the circulation; about 50 to 70% to the red blood cells and between 15 and 33% to plasma proteins. The half-life has been reported to be 8 to 10 hours in whole blood, and 4 to 5 hours in plasma, but the diuretic effect persists for up to 24 hours or more. About 70 to 80% of the amount of metolazone absorbed is excreted in the urine, of which 80 to 95% is excreted unchanged. The remainder is excreted in the bile and some enterohepatic circulation has been reported. Metolazone crosses the placental barrier and is distributed into breast milk.

References.

1. Tilstone WJ, *et al.* Pharmacokinetics of metolazone in normal subjects and in patients with cardiac or renal failure. *Clin Pharmacol Ther* 1974; **16:** 322–9.

Uses and Administration

Metolazone is a diuretic with actions and uses similar to those of the thiazide diuretics (see Hydrochlorothiazide, p.887) even though it does not contain a thiazide ring system. It is used for oedema, including that associated with heart failure (p.785), and for hypertension (p.788).

Unlike thiazides in general, metolazone is reported to be effective in patients with a glomerular filtration rate of less than 20 mL per minute. Diuresis is initiated in about 1 hour, reaches a peak in about 2 hours, and the effect lasts for 12 to 24 hours depending on the dose.

In some countries a preparation is available with enhanced bioavailability which is effective in lower doses than conventional formulations. Doses given in *Martindale* refer to the conventional tablet formulation unless otherwise stated.

In the treatment of **oedema** the usual dose is 5 to 10 mg by mouth daily; in some cases doses of 20 mg or more may be required. It has been recommended that not more than 80 mg should be given in any 24-hour period. In refractory cases, metolazone has been used in combination with frusemide or other loop diuretics, but the electrolyte balance should be monitored closely.

In the treatment of **hypertension** the usual dose is 2.5 to 5 mg daily either alone, or in conjunction with other antihypertensives. An initial dose of 1.25 mg has also been suggested. The dosage may be adjusted after 3 to 4 weeks according to response. A maintenance dose of 5 mg on alternate days has been suggested.

Formulations with enhanced bioavailability are given in doses of 0.5 to 1 mg daily in the treatment of hypertension. They are not bioequivalent to the conventional tablet formulation and should not be used interchangeably.

In susceptible patients potassium supplements or a potassium-sparing diuretic may be necessary, but see hydrochlorothiazide.

Preparations

USP 23: Metolazone Tablets.

Proprietary Preparations (details are given in Part 3)
Aust.: Birobin; ***Austral.:*** Diulo†; ***Canad.:*** Zaroxolyn; ***Ger.:*** Zaroxolyn; ***Irl.:*** Zaroxolyn; ***Ital.:*** Zaroxolyn; ***S.Afr.:*** Zaroxolyn; ***Spain:*** Diondel†; ***Swed.:*** Zaroxolyn; ***Switz.:*** Zaroxolyne; ***UK:*** Metenix 5; Xuret†; ***USA:*** Diulo; Mykrox; Zaroxolyn.

Metoprolol Tartrate (6314-e)

Metoprolol Tartrate *(BANM, USAN, rINNM).*

CGP-2175E; H-93/26; Metoprololi Tartras. (±)-1-Isopropylamino-3-[4-(2-methoxyethyl)phenoxy]propan-2-ol tartrate.

$(C_{15}H_{25}NO_3)_2,C_4H_6O_6$ = 684.8.

CAS — 54163-88-1 (metoprolol); 37350-58-6 (± metoprolol); 56392-17-7 (± metoprolol tartrate).

Pharmacopoeias. In *Chin.*, *Eur.* (see p.viii) and *US.*
US also includes Metoprolol Fumarate.

A white crystalline powder or colourless crystals. Very **soluble** in water; freely soluble in alcohol, in chloroform, and in dichloromethane; slightly soluble in acetone; practically insoluble in ether. A 10% solution in water has a pH of between 6 and 7. **Store** in airtight containers. Protect from light.

Stability. Metoprolol tartrate 0.4 mg per mL in glucose 5% or sodium chloride 0.9% was stable for 36 hours when stored at 24° in polyvinyl chloride bags.[1]

1. Belliveau PP, *et al.* Stability of metoprolol tartrate in 5% dextrose injection or 0.9% sodium chloride injection. *Am J Hosp Pharm* 1993; **50:** 950–2.

Adverse Effects, Treatment, and Precautions

As for beta blockers, p.828.

Effects on bones and joints. Five cases of arthralgia associated with the use of metoprolol had been reported to the FDA; 6 reports of similar symptoms associated with propranolol, and one with atenolol, had been reported.[1] A polymyalgia rheumatic-like syndrome has also been reported in one patient.[2]

1. Sills JM, Bosco L. Arthralgia associated with β-adrenergic blockade. *JAMA* 1986; **255:** 198–9.
2. Snyder S. Metoprolol-induced polymyalgia-like syndrome. *Ann Intern Med* 1991; **114:** 96–7.

Effects on the gastro-intestinal tract. Reports of retroperitoneal fibrosis in a patient who had been taking metoprolol and nifedipine[1] and of sclerosing peritonitis in a patient receiving metoprolol.[2]

1. Thompson J, Julian DG. Retroperitoneal fibrosis associated with metoprolol. *Br Med J* 1982; **284:** 83–4.
2. Clark CV, Terris R. Sclerosing peritonitis associated with metoprolol. *Lancet* 1983; **i:** 937.

Effects on hearing. Loss of hearing in a patient receiving metoprolol appeared to be dose-related;[1] hearing gradually improved over several months once the drug was withdrawn.

1. Fäldt R, *et al.* β Blockers and loss of hearing. *Br Med J* 1984; **289:** 1490–2.

Effects on lipid metabolism. Beta blockers may increase serum-triglyceride concentrations. For a report of acute pancreatitis provoked by severe hypertriglyceridaemia in a patient taking atenolol and metoprolol, see p.829.

Effects on the liver. Acute hepatitis associated with metoprolol has been reported in a 56-year-old woman.[1] The hepatotoxicity could not be explained by deficient oxidation of metoprolol; drug oxidation phenotyping showed she was an extensive metaboliser of debrisoquine and hence metoprolol.

For debate as to whether the polymorphic oxidation of metoprolol contributes to the incidence of adverse effects, see under Pharmacokinetics, below.

1. Larrey D, *et al.* Metoprolol-induced hepatitis: rechallenge and drug oxidation phenotyping. *Ann Intern Med* 1988; **108:** 67–8.

Interactions

The interactions associated with beta blockers are discussed on p.829.

Pharmacokinetics

Metoprolol is readily and completely absorbed from the gastro-intestinal tract but is subject to considerable first-pass metabolism. Peak plasma concentrations vary widely and occur about 1.5 to 2 hours after a single oral dose. It is moderately lipid-soluble.

Metoprolol is widely distributed, it crosses the blood-brain barrier, the placenta, and is distributed into breast milk. It is slightly bound to plasma protein. It is extensively metabolised in the liver by oxidative deamination, *O*-dealkylation followed by oxidation, and aliphatic hydroxylation. The metabolites are excreted in the urine together with only small amounts of unchanged metoprolol. The rate of hydroxylation to α-hydroxymetoprolol is reported to be determined by genetic polymorphism; the half-life of metoprolol in fast hydroxylators is stated to be 3 to 4 hours, whereas in poor hydroxylators it is about 7 hours.

Metabolism. It has been reported[1-3] that metoprolol exhibits a debrisoquine-type genetic polymorphism with poor metabolisers of metoprolol also being poor metabolisers of debrisoquine. However, some workers have disputed these findings.[4] In addition, the clinical relevance of the polymorphism, if it exists, has been questioned, since there has been no correlation shown between poor metaboliser status and increased incidence of adverse effects.[5,6]

The subject may be further confused by variations in the phenotype between ethnic groups. Although the incidence of the poor metaboliser phenotype in whites of European origin is reported to be about 9%, a study in 138 Nigerians[7] failed to identify evidence of polymorphic metabolism, and the authors caution against extrapolation of data between different racial groups.

1. Lennard MS, *et al.* Defective metabolism of metoprolol in poor hydroxylators of debrisoquine. *Br J Clin Pharmacol* 1982; **14:** 301–3.
2. Lennard MS, *et al.* Oxidation phenotype—a major determinant of metoprolol metabolism and response. *N Engl J Med* 1982; **307:** 1558–60.
3. McGourty JC, *et al.* Metoprolol metabolism and debrisoquine oxidation polymorphism—population and family studies. *Br J Clin Pharmacol* 1985; **20:** 555–66.
4. Jack DB, *et al.* Lack of evidence for polymorphism in metoprolol metabolism. *Br J Clin Pharmacol* 1983; **16:** 188–90.
5. Regårdh CG, Johnsson G. Interindividual variations in metoprolol metabolism—some clinical and other observations. *Br J Clin Pharmacol* 1984; **17:** 495–6.
6. Clark DWJ, *et al.* Adverse effects from metoprolol are not generally associated with oxidation status. *Br J Clin Pharmacol* 1984; **18:** 965–6.
7. Iyun AO, *et al.* Metoprolol and debrisoquin metabolism in Nigerians: lack of evidence for polymorphic oxidation. *Clin Pharmacol Ther* 1986; **40:** 387–94.

Old age. Several studies[1-3] indicate that age-related physiological changes have negligible effects on the pharmacokinetics of metoprolol.

1. Quarterman CP, *et al.* The effect of age on the pharmacokinetics of metoprolol and its metabolites. *Br J Clin Pharmacol* 1981; **11:** 287–94.
2. Regårdh CG, *et al.* Pharmacokinetics of metoprolol and its metabolite α-OH-metoprolol in healthy, non-smoking, elderly individuals. *Eur J Clin Pharmacol* 1983; **24:** 221–6.
3. Larsson M, *et al.* Pharmacokinetics of metoprolol in healthy, elderly, non-smoking individuals after a single dose and two weeks of treatment. *Eur J Clin Pharmacol* 1984; **27:** 217–22.

Pregnancy and breast feeding. The clearance of metoprolol was increased fourfold in 5 pregnant women during the last trimester, compared with that some months after delivery; this was probably due to enhanced hepatic metabolism in the pregnant state.[1]

The disposition of metoprolol was investigated in newborn infants of mothers treated with metoprolol 50 to 100 mg twice daily.[2] In 15 of the 17 neonates plasma-metoprolol concentrations increased in the first 2 to 5 hours of the post-natal period, then declined over the next 15 hours; 5 of these infants had no detectable metoprolol concentrations in the umbilical plasma. No infant demonstrated signs of beta blockade.

Only a small amount appears to be distributed into breast milk.

1. Högstedt S, *et al.* Increased oral clearance of metoprolol in pregnancy. *Eur J Clin Pharmacol* 1983; **24:** 217–20.
2. Lundborg P, *et al.* Disposition of metoprolol in the newborn. *Br J Clin Pharmacol* 1981; **12:** 598–600.

Renal impairment. A study of the pharmacokinetics of metoprolol and its renally excreted metabolite α-hydroxymetoprolol in normal subjects and subjects with renal impairment.[1] Following a single dose of a sustained-release tablet of metoprolol, similar plasma-metoprolol concentrations and values for the area under the concentration/time curve were reported in both groups. Mean plasma concentrations of α-hydroxymetoprolol were increased two to threefold in subjects with renal impairment compared with normal subjects but such a rise was not considered likely to contribute to beta blockade.

1. Lloyd P, *et al.* The effect of impaired renal function on the pharmacokinetics of metoprolol after single administration of a 14/190 metoprolol OROS system. *Am Heart J* 1990; **120:** 478–82.

Uses and Administration

Metoprolol is a cardioselective beta blocker (p.828). It is reported to lack intrinsic sympathomimetic activity and to have little or no membrane-stabilising activity.

It is used in the management of hypertension (p.788), angina pectoris (p.780), cardiac arrhythmias (p.782), and myocardial infarction (p.791). It is also used in the management of hyperthyroidism (p.1489) and migraine (p.443). Metoprolol is under investigation in dilated cardiomyopathy (p.785).

Metoprolol is given as the tartrate. The fumarate and succinate salts are used in some modified-release tablets.

Reduced doses are given to patients with hepatic dysfunction.

In **hypertension** metoprolol tartrate is usually given in an initial dose of 100 mg daily by mouth, increased weekly according to the response of the patient to 400 mg daily; it may be taken as a single daily dose or twice daily. A usual maintenance dose is 100 to 200 mg daily. Some manufacturers recommend that the dose should be taken with or immediately following a meal.

The usual dose for **angina pectoris** is 50 to 100 mg two or three times daily by mouth.

In the treatment of **cardiac arrhythmias** the usual dose is 50 mg two or three times daily by mouth, increased if necessary up to 300 mg daily in divided doses.

For the emergency treatment of cardiac arrhythmias metoprolol tartrate may be given intravenously in an initial dose of up to 5 mg administered at a rate of 1 to 2 mg per minute; this may be repeated, if necessary, at intervals of 5 minutes to a total dose of 10 to 15 mg. When acute arrhythmias have been controlled, maintenance therapy may be started with doses not exceeding 50 mg three times daily by mouth 4 to 6 hours after intravenous therapy.

Arrhythmias may be prevented on induction of anaesthesia or controlled during anaesthesia, by the slow intravenous injection of 2 to 4 mg; further injections of 2 mg may be repeated as necessary to a maximum total dose of 10 mg.

Metoprolol is also used as an adjunct in the early management of acute **myocardial infarction.** Treatment should be given within 12 hours of the onset of chest pain; metoprolol tartrate 5 mg should be given intravenously at 2-minute intervals to a total of 15 mg, where tolerated. This should be followed, after 15 minutes, by the commencement of oral treatment, in patients who have received the full intravenous dose, with 50 mg every 6 hours for 2 days. In patients who have failed to tolerate the full intravenous dose a reduced oral dose should be given as and when their condition permits. Subsequent maintenance dosage is 100 mg given twice daily by mouth. In patients who did not receive metoprolol by intravenous injection as part of the early management of myocardial infarction, metoprolol 100 mg twice daily by mouth may be started once the clinical condition of the patient stabilises.

As an adjunct in the treatment of **hyperthyroidism** metoprolol tartrate may be given in doses of 50 mg four times daily by mouth. Doses of 100 to 200 mg are given daily in divided doses for **migraine** prophylaxis.

General references.

1. Plosker GL, Clissold SP. Controlled release metoprolol formulations: a review of their pharmacodynamic and pharmacokinetic properties, and therapeutic use in hypertension and ischaemic heart disease. *Drugs* 1992; **43:** 382–414.

Preparations

BP 1998: Metoprolol Injection; Metoprolol Tartrate Tablets;
USP 23: Metoprolol Tartrate and Hydrochlorothiazide Tablets; Metoprolol Tartrate Injection; Metoprolol Tartrate Tablets.

Proprietary Preparations (details are given in Part 3)
Aust.: Beloc; Lanoc; Lopresor; Metohexal; Metolol; Metoros; Seloken; ***Austral.:*** Betaloc; Lopresor; Metohexal; Minax; ***Belg.:*** Lopresor; Seloken; Selozok; ***Canad.:*** Betaloc; Lopresor; Novo-Metoprol; Nu-Metop; ***Fr.:*** Lopressor; Seloken; ***Ger.:*** Azumetop; Beloc; Beloc-Zok; Dignometoprol; Jeprolol; Lopresor; Meprolol; Meto; Meto-Tablinen; Metobeta; Metodura; Metohexal; Metomerck; Prelis; Sigaprolol; ***Irl.:*** Betaloc; Betazok; Lopresor; Metocor; Metop; Topromel; ***Ital.:*** Beprolo†; Lopresor; Seloken; ***Neth.:*** Lopresor; Selokeen; ***Norw.:*** Selo-Zok; Seloken; ***S.Afr.:*** Lopresor; Lopresor Oros†; ***Spain:*** Lopresor; Seloken; ***Swed.:*** Metoprofermt†; Seloken; Seloken ZOC; ***Switz.:*** Beloc-Zok; Lopresor; ***UK:*** Arbralene; Betaloc; Lopresor; Mepranix; ***USA:*** Lopressor; Toprol XL.

Multi-ingredient: ***Aust.:*** Beloc comp; Logimax; Logroton; Metolol compositum; Seloken retard Plus; Triloc; ***Belg.:*** Logimat; Logroton; Selozide; Zok-Zid; ***Fr.:*** Logimax; Logroton; ***Ger.:*** Belnif; Beloc comp; Beloc-Zok comp; Meto-comp; Meto-thiazid; Metodura comp; Metohexal Comp; Metostad Comp; Prelis comp; Treloc; ***Irl.:*** Co-Betaloc; Lopresoretic†; ***Ital.:*** Igroton-Lopresor; Selozide; ***Neth.:*** Logroton; Selokomb; ***Norw.:*** Logimax; ***S.Afr.:*** Logroton†; ***Spain:*** Logimax; Selopresin; ***Swed.:*** Logimax; ***Switz.:*** Logimax; Logroton; ***UK:*** Co-Betaloc; Lopresoretic†; ***USA:*** Lopressor HCT.

Mexiletine Hydrochloride (7789-p)

Mexiletine Hydrochloride *(BANM, USAN, rINNM)*.

Kö-1173; Mexiletini Hydrochloridum. 1-Methyl-2-(2,6-xylyloxy)ethylamine hydrochloride.

$C_{11}H_{17}NO,HCl$ = 215.7.

CAS — 31828-71-4 (mexiletine); 5370-01-4 (mexiletine hydrochloride).

Pharmacopoeias. In *Chin., Eur.* (see p.viii), *Jpn,* and *US.*

A white or almost white, crystalline powder. Freely **soluble** in water and in methyl alcohol; slightly soluble in acetonitrile; sparingly soluble in dichloromethane; practically insoluble in ether. A 10% solution in water has a pH of 3.5 to 5.5. **Store** in airtight containers.

Adverse Effects and Treatment

Mexiletine has a narrow therapeutic ratio: many adverse effects of mexiletine are dose-related and will respond to dosage reduction but may be severe enough to necessitate discontinuation of mexiletine and the institution of symptomatic and supportive therapy. Toxicity is commonly seen with oral or parenteral loading doses when plasma concentrations are high.

The most common adverse effects affect the gastro-intestinal tract and CNS. Effects on the gastro-intestinal tract include nausea, vomiting, constipation, and diarrhoea. Effects on the nervous system include tremor, confusion, lightheadedness, dizziness, blurred vision and other visual disturbances, sleep disturbances, and speech difficulties. The most frequent cardiovascular effects are hypotension, sinus bradycardia, atrioventricular dissociation, and atrial fibrillation. As with other antiarrhythmics mexiletine may exacerbate arrhythmias. Other adverse effects which have been reported include skin rashes, abnormal liver function tests, thrombocytopenia, positive antinuclear factor titres, and convulsions. The Stevens-Johnson syndrome has been reported rarely.

In a study involving 100 patients with ventricular arrhythmias given mexiletine, the drug had to be discontinued in 49 patients due to intolerable adverse effects.[1] The most common intolerable effects affected the gastro-intestinal system (27%) and included nausea (10%), vomiting (6%), heartburn (6%), and oesophageal spasm (3%). Intolerable adverse effects affecting the CNS occurred in 10% of patients and these were most commonly tremor (4%), ataxia (2%), dyskinesia (1%), and tinnitus (1%). When mexiletine was used in combination with another antiarrhythmic, the incidence of intolerable adverse effects was 56%.

Tolerable adverse effects with mexiletine alone were transient and dose-dependent and occurred in 18% of patients. They most commonly affected the gastro-intestinal tract. No irreversible adverse effects were reported and no proarrhythmic effects were seen.

1. Kerin NZ, *et al.* Mexiletine: long-term efficacy and side effects in patients with chronic drug-resistant potentially lethal ventricular arrhythmias. *Arch Intern Med* 1990; **150:** 381–4.

Effects on the lungs. Pulmonary fibrosis has been reported in one elderly patient receiving mexiletine; the manufacturer was aware of three other cases.[1]

1. Bero CJ, Rihn TL. Possible association of pulmonary fibrosis with mexiletine. *DICP Ann Pharmacother* 1991; **25:** 1329–31.

Precautions

Mexiletine should be used with special caution in patients with sinus node dysfunction, conduction defect, bradycardia, hypotension, cardiogenic shock, heart failure, or hepatic impairment. ECG and blood pressure monitoring should be carried out during treatment.

Absorption of mexiletine may be delayed after myocardial infarction.

Pregnancy. A normal infant was born to a woman given mexiletine with propranolol for the control of ventricular tachycardia during the third trimester of pregnancy.[1] During the first 6 hours after delivery the infant had a heart rate of only 90 beats per minute, probably due to the propranolol; it was normal thereafter. At delivery the concentration of mexiletine in the serum of the mother and the infant was the same.

1. Timmis AD, *et al.* Mexiletine for control of ventricular dysrhythmias in pregnancy. *Lancet* 1980; **ii:** 647–8.

Interactions

Mexiletine undergoes extensive metabolism in the liver and plasma concentrations of mexiletine may be reduced by the concurrent administration of drugs which induce hepatic enzymes such as phenytoin and rifampicin.

Absorption of mexilitine may be delayed by concurrent administration of drugs that slow gastric emptying such as opioid analgesics and atropine. The rate of absorption may be increased by metoclopramide; the extent of absorption is unaffected.

Drugs that acidify or alkalinise the urine enhance or reduce the rate of elimination of mexiletine, respectively.

Mexiletine has been reported to increase theophylline concentrations (p.768) and to precipitate lignocaine toxicity (p.1294).

References.

1. Wing LMH, *et al.* The effect of administered mexiletine. *Br J Clin Pharmacol* 1980; **9:** 505–9.
2. Begg EJ, *et al.* Enhanced metabolism of mexiletine after phenytoin administration. *Br J Clin Pharmacol* 1982; **14:** 219–23.
3. Pentikäinen PJ, *et al.* Effect of rifampicin treatment on the kinetics of mexiletine. *Eur J Clin Pharmacol* 1982; **23:** 261–6.

Pharmacokinetics

Mexiletine is readily and almost completely absorbed from the gastro-intestinal tract although absorption may be delayed after myocardial infarction.

Mexiletine is metabolised in the liver to a number of metabolites. It is excreted in the urine, mainly in the form of its metabolites with about 10% excreted as unchanged mexiletine; the clearance of mexiletine is increased in acid urine.

Mexiletine is widely distributed throughout the body and is about 50 to 70% bound to plasma proteins. Mexiletine crosses the placenta and is distributed into breast milk. It has an elimination half-life of about 10 hours in healthy subjects but this may be prolonged in patients with heart disease, hepatic impairment, or severe renal impairment. Its therapeutic effect has been correlated with plasma concentrations of 0.5 to 2 μg per mL, but the margin between therapeutic and toxic concentrations is narrow, and severe toxicity may occur within this range.

References.

1. Campbell NPS, *et al.* The clinical pharmacology of mexiletine. *Br J Clin Pharmacol* 1978; **6:** 103–8.
2. Johnston A, *et al.* The effect of spontaneous changes in urinary pH on mexiletine plasma concentrations and excretion during chronic administration to healthy volunteers. *Br J Clin Pharmacol* 1979; **8:** 349–52.
3. Lewis AM, *et al.* Mexiletine in human blood and breast milk. *Postgrad Med J* 1981; **57:** 546–7.
4. Mitchell BG, *et al.* Mexiletine disposition: individual variation in response to urine acidification and alkalinisation. *Br J Clin Pharmacol* 1983; **16:** 281–4.
5. Pentikäinen PJ, *et al.* Pharmacokinetics of oral mexiletine in patients with acute myocardial infarction. *Eur J Clin Pharmacol* 1983; **25:** 773–7.
6. Lledó P, *et al.* Influence of debrisoquine hydroxylation phenotype on the pharmacokinetics of mexiletine. *Eur J Clin Pharmacol* 1993; **44:** 63–7.

Uses and Administration

Mexiletine is a class Ib antiarrhythmic (p.776) with actions similar to those of lignocaine (p.1295), to which it is structurally related. Unlike lignocaine it undergoes little hepatic first-pass metabolism and is suitable for oral administration.

Mexiletine is used for the treatment of ventricular **arrhythmias**.

It is given by mouth as the hydrochloride in an initial loading dose of 400 mg followed by 200 to 250 mg three or four times daily, starting 2 hours after the loading dose. Higher loading doses (for example, of 600 mg) may be necessary in patients after myocardial infarction to overcome delayed absorption, especially if they have received an opioid analgesic. The usual maintenance dosage of mexiletine is 600 to 900 mg daily in divided doses; doses up to 1200 mg daily may be given. Use of a modified-release preparation allows administration every 12 hours.

Mexiletine may be given by slow intravenous injection of the hydrochloride in doses of 100 to 250 mg at a rate of 25 mg per minute, followed by an infusion at a rate of 250 mg over 1 hour, 250 mg over the next 2 hours, and then at about 0.5 mg per minute for maintenance, according to the patient's response; when appropriate the patient may be transferred to oral therapy with doses of 200 to 250 mg of the hydrochloride three or four times daily. Alternatively, an initial intravenous dose of 200 mg at a rate of 25 mg per minute, may be followed by an oral dose of 400 mg on completion of the injection, with subsequent oral therapy as before.

Mexiletine has also been tried in the treatment of refractory neurogenic **pain**.

Reviews of mexiletine.

1. Campbell RWF. Mexiletine. *N Engl J Med* 1987; **316:** 29–34.
2. Monk JP, Brogden RN. Mexiletine: a review of its pharmacodynamic and pharmacokinetic properties, and therapeutic use in the treatment of arrhythmias. *Drugs* 1990; **40:** 374–411. Correction. *ibid.* 1991; **41:** 377.

Administration in children. The dose of mexiletine in children should be titrated according to the concentration in plasma.[1] In a 2-week-old girl and a 20-month-old boy high oral doses of 25 and 15 mg per kg body-weight respectively were needed to produce therapeutic concentrations in plasma and control of tachycardia.

1. Holt DW, *et al.* Paediatric use of mexiletine and disopyramide. *Br Med J* 1979; **2:** 1476–7.

Administration in the elderly. The rate of absorption of mexiletine was slower in a group of 7 elderly subjects compared with 8 young subjects given mexiletine 100 mg by mouth, but the extent of absorption was probably not affected.[1] Elimination of mexiletine was not significantly different between the 2 groups and there was no pharmacokinetic basis for dosage modification of mexiletine in the elderly.

1. Grech-Bélanger O, *et al.* Pharmacokinetics of mexiletine in the elderly. *J Clin Pharmacol* 1989; **29:** 311–15.

Administration in renal impairment. The pharmacokinetics of mexiletine were not significantly modified in patients with chronic renal failure when the creatinine clearance was above 10 mL per minute and these patients could be given usual doses of mexiletine.[1] However, in patients with a creatinine clearance below 10 mL per minute the steady-state plasma concentration and half-life were increased and in these patients mexiletine dosage should be adjusted according to plasma-mexiletine concentrations.

Continuous ambulatory peritoneal dialysis did not influence the clearance of mexiletine in a patient with chronic renal failure.[2]

1. El Allaf D, *et al.* Pharmacokinetics of mexiletine in renal insufficiency. *Br J Clin Pharmacol* 1982; **14:** 431–5.
2. Guay DRP, *et al.* Mexiletine clearance during peritoneal dialysis. *Br J Clin Pharmacol* 1985; **19:** 857–8.

Cardiac arrhythmias. Several studies[1-4] showed that mexiletine could reduce the incidence of ventricular arrhythmias (p.782) after acute myocardial infarction but no significant reduction in mortality was demonstrated.

The long-term efficacy of mexiletine in the treatment of ventricular arrhythmias refractory to other drug therapy has also been the subject of several studies,[5-8] but, although it may be effective in the treatment of some such patients, adverse effects may limit the usefulness of mexiletine in long-term therapy.

1. Chamberlain DA, *et al.* Oral mexiletine in high-risk patients after myocardial infarction. *Lancet* 1980; **ii** 1324–7.
2. Bell JA, *et al.* A trial of prophylactic mexiletine in home coronary care. *Br Heart J* 1982; **48:** 285–90.
3. Halinen MO, *et al.* Antiarrhythmic efficacy of combined intravenous and oral mexiletine in acute myocardial infarction: a double blind placebo-controlled study. *Eur Heart J* 1984; **5:** 675–83.
4. IMPACT Research Group. International mexiletine and placebo antiarrhythmic coronary trial: I: report on arrhythmia and other findings. *J Am Coll Cardiol* 1984; **4:** 1148–63.
5. Stein J, *et al.* Long-term mexiletine for ventricular arrhythmia. *Am Heart J* 1984; **107:** 1091–8.
6. Rutledge JC, *et al.* Clinical evaluation of oral mexiletine therapy in the treatment of ventricular arrhythmias. *J Am Coll Cardiol* 1985; **6:** 780–4.
7. Nademanee K, *et al.* Mexiletine: double-blind comparison with procainamide in PVC suppression and open-label sequential comparison with amiodarone in life-threatening ventricular arrhythmias. *Am Heart J* 1985; **110:** 923–31.
8. Poole JE, *et al.* Intolerance and ineffectiveness of mexiletine in patients with serious ventricular arrhythmias. *Am Heart J* 1986; **112:** 322–6.

Pain. Neurogenic pain (p.10) is often insensitive to opioid analgesics and various drugs, including mexiletine, have been tried. Mexiletine has been tried in painful diabetic neuropathy (p.9) although results have been conflicting.[1-3,7] Two of the studies that reported no difference between treatment and placebo groups found that a subset of patients (those with stabbing or burning pain, heat sensations, and formication) appeared to benefit.[2,3]

Other painful states in which mexiletine has been reported to be of benefit include: Dercum's disease (a condition involving painful fatty deposits),[4] central pain (thalamic pain syndrome) (p.8),[5] and severe scrotal and inguinal pain after radiation for prostate cancer.[6]

1. Dejgård A, *et al.* Mexiletine for treatment of chronic painful diabetic neuropathy. *Lancet* 1988; **i:** 9–11.
2. Stracke H, *et al.* Mexiletine in the treatment of diabetic neuropathy. *Diabetes Care* 1992; **15:** 1550–5.
3. Wright JM, *et al.* Mexiletine in the symptomatic treatment of diabetic peripheral neuropathy. *Ann Pharmacother* 1997; **31:** 29–34.
4. Petersen P, *et al.* Treating the pain of Dercum's disease. *Br Med J* 1984; **288:** 1880.
5. Awerbuch GI, Sandyk R. Mexiletine for thalamic pain syndrome. *Int J Neurosci* 1990; **55:** 129–33.
6. Colclough G, *et al.* Mexiletine for chronic pain. *Lancet* 1993; **342:** 1484–5.
7. Oskarsson P, *et al.* Efficacy and safety of mexiletine in the treatment of painful diabetic neuropathy. *Diabetes Care* 1997; **20:** 1594–7.

Preparations

BP 1998: Mexiletine Capsules; Mexiletine Injection;
USP 23: Mexiletine Hydrochloride Capsules.

Proprietary Preparations (details are given in Part 3)
Aust.: Mexitil; ***Austral.:*** Mexitil; ***Belg.:*** Mexitil; ***Canad.:*** Mexitil; ***Fr.:*** Mexitil; ***Ger.:*** Mexitil; ***Irl.:*** Mexitil; ***Ital.:*** Mexitil; ***Neth.:*** Mexitil; ***Norw.:*** Mexitil; ***S.Afr.:*** Mexitil; ***Spain:*** Mexitil; ***Swed.:*** Mexitil; ***Switz.:*** Mexitil; ***UK:*** Mexitil; ***USA:*** Mexitil.

Mibefradil Dihydrochloride (19405-p)

Mibefradil Dihydrochloride *(USAN, rINNM).*

Mibefradil Hydrochloride *(BANM)*; Ro-40-5967 (mibefradil); Ro-40-5967/001 (mibefradil dihydrochloride). (1*S*,2*S*)-(2-{[3-(2-Benzimidazolyl)propyl]methylamino}ethyl)-6-fluoro-1,2,3,4-tetrahydro-1-isopropyl-2-naphthyl methoxyacetate dihydrochloride.

$C_{29}H_{38}FN_3O_3,2HCl = 568.6.$

CAS — 116644-53-2 (mibefradil); 116666-63-8 (mibefradil dihydrochloride).

Mibefradil is a calcium-channel blocker that acts principally on fast T-type calcium channels unlike conventional calcium-channel blockers that act on slow L-type channels (see p.778). Mibefradil was introduced for the management of hypertension and angina pectoris but was withdrawn worldwide several months later due to increasing reports of serious interactions with a wide range of drugs.

Preparations

Proprietary Preparations (details are given in Part 3)
Austral.: Posicor†; ***Irl.:*** Posicor†; ***Neth.:*** Posicor†; ***UK:*** Posicor†; ***USA:*** Posicor†.

Midodrine Hydrochloride (12959-s)

Midodrine Hydrochloride *(BANM, USAN, rINNM).*

A-4020 Linz; ST-1085 (midodrine or midodrine hydrochloride); St. Peter-224. 2-Amino-*N*-(β-hydroxy-2,5-dimethoxyphenethyl)acetamide hydrochloride; (*RS*)-N^1-(β-Hydroxy-2,5-dimethoxyphenethyl)glycinamide hydrochloride.

$C_{12}H_{18}N_2O_4,HCl = 290.7.$

CAS — 42794-76-3 (midodrine); 3092-17-9 (midodrine hydrochloride).

Adverse Effects, Treatment, and Precautions

The most serious adverse effect of midodrine is supine hypertension. Paraesthesias, dysuria, pilomotor reaction (goose flesh), pruritus and rashes have been reported. The hypertensive effects of midodrine may be treated with an alpha-adrenoceptor blocker such as phentolamine.

For the adverse effects of sympathomimetics in general, and precautions to be observed, see Adrenaline, p.813.

Interactions

For the interactions of sympathomimetics in general, see Adrenaline, p.814.

Pharmacokinetics

Midodrine is well absorbed from the gastro-intestinal tract and undergoes enzymatic hydrolysis in the systemic circulation to its active metabolite, de-glymidodrine (desglymidodrine, ST-1059). Midodrine itself reaches its peak plasma concentrations about half an hour after a dose by mouth, and has a plasma half-life of about 25 minutes. The active metabolite reaches its peak plasma concentration about an hour after oral administration and has a terminal elimination half-life of about 3 hours. De-glymidodrine undergoes some further metabolism in the liver. Midodrine is primarily excreted in the urine as metabolites and a small amount of unchanged drug.

Uses and Administration

Midodrine is a direct-acting sympathomimetic (see Adrenaline, p.815) with selective alpha agonist activity; the main active moiety has been stated to be its major metabolite, deglymidodrine. It acts as a peripheral vasoconstrictor but has no direct cardiac stimulatory effects.

Midodrine hydrochloride is used in the treatment of hypotensive states (p.790) and in particular of orthostatic hypotension (p.1040). Alpha agonist drugs such as midodrine have also been used as an adjunct in the management of urinary incontinence (p.454).

In **hypotensive states**, a usual initial dose of midodrine hydrochloride is 2.5 mg twice daily by mouth adjusted gradually according to the patient's response; up to 10 mg three times daily may be required.

A suggested dose for **urinary incontinence** is 2.5 to 5 mg by mouth two to three times daily.

Midodrine hydrochloride can also be given in similar doses by slow intravenous injection. It has also been used in the treatment of retrograde ejaculation in a dose of 10 to 40 mg intravenously.

References.

1. McTavish D, Goa KL. Midodrine: a review of its pharmacological properties and therapeutic use in orthostatic hypotension and secondary hypotensive disorders. *Drugs* 1989; **38:** 757–77.
2. Jankovic J, *et al.* Neurogenic orthostatic hypotension: a double-blind, placebo-controlled study with midodrine. *Am J Med* 1993; **95:** 38–48.
3. Fouad-Tarazi FM, *et al.* Alpha sympathomimetic treatment of autonomic insufficiency with orthostatic hypotension. *Am J Med* 1995; **99:** 604–10.
4. Low PA, *et al.* Efficacy of midodrine vs placebo in neurogenic orthostatic hypotension: a randomized, double-blind multicenter study. *JAMA* 1997; **277:** 1046–51. Correction. *ibid.*; **278:** 388.

Preparations

Proprietary Preparations (details are given in Part 3)
Aust.: Gutron; ***Canad.:*** Amatine; ***Fr.:*** Gutron; ***Ger.:*** Gutron; ***Irl.:*** Midon; ***Ital.:*** Gutron; ***Switz.:*** Gutron; ***USA:*** ProAmatine.

Milrinone (16896-t)

Milrinone *(BAN, USAN, rINN).*

Win-47203-2. 1,6-Dihydro-2-methyl-6-oxo[3,4′-bipyridine]-5-carbonitrile.

$C_{12}H_9N_3O = 211.2.$

CAS — 78415-72-2.

Milrinone Lactate (13500-v)

Milrinone Lactate *(BANM, rINNM).*

$C_{12}H_9N_3O,C_3H_6O_3 = 301.3.$

Milrinone lactate injection is reported to be **incompatible** with frusemide and bumetanide, and it should not be diluted with sodium bicarbonate injection. Milrinone lactate 1.43 mg is approximately equivalent to 1 mg of milrinone.

Adverse Effects and Precautions

Prolonged oral treatment with milrinone has increased the mortality rate and milrinone is now only employed intravenously for short-term use.

Supraventricular and ventricular arrhythmias, hypotension, angina-like chest pain, and headache have been reported. Hypokalaemia, tremor, and thrombocytopenia may occur.

Milrinone should be used with caution in patients with severe obstructive aortic or pulmonary valvular disease or with hypertrophic cardiomyopathy. Since milrinone may facilitate conduction through the atrioventricular node it can increase the ventricular response rate in patients with atrial flutter or fibrillation. Digitalisation should be considered in these patients before milrinone therapy is started.

Blood pressure, heart rate, ECG, and fluid and electrolyte balance should be monitored during milrinone therapy.

Pharmacokinetics

Milrinone is rapidly and almost completely absorbed from the gastro-intestinal tract, but is only given intravenously because of an increased mortality rate associated with prolonged administration via the oral route. It is about 70% bound to plasma proteins. Elimination occurs mainly via the urine; about 83% of a dose is excreted as unchanged drug. The elimination half-life is about 2.3 hours.

General references.

1. Rocci ML, Wilson H. The pharmacokinetics and pharmacodynamics of newer inotropic agents. *Clin Pharmacokinet* 1987; **13:** 91–109. Correction. *ibid.* 1988; **14:** (contents page).

Uses and Administration

Milrinone is a phosphodiesterase inhibitor similar to amrinone (p.823) with positive inotropic and vasodilator activity. It is, however, reported to have greater positive inotropic activity than amrinone. It is given intravenously, as the lactate, in the short-term management of severe heart failure unresponsive to other forms of therapy and in acute heart failure following cardiac surgery. In some longer-term studies milrinone was given by mouth, but an increased mortality rate was reported.

Doses of milrinone lactate are expressed in terms of the base. The recommended initial loading dose is 50 µg of milrinone per kg body-weight given over 10 minutes followed by a continuous maintenance infusion. The maintenance infusion may be titrated between 0.375 and 0.75 µg per kg per minute but a total daily dose of 1.13 mg per kg should not be exceeded.

Dosage should be reduced in patients with renal impairment.

Administration in children. Pharmacokinetic studies[1,2] have suggested that steady-state plasma concentrations of milrinone are lower in children than in adults given similar doses, and that milrinone clearance is faster in children. It has been suggested[1] that in children an initial loading dose of 75 µg per kg body-weight should be administered, followed by maintenance infusions of 0.75 µg per kg per minute, increased to 1.0 µg per kg per minute if required. An additional bolus dose of 25 µg per kg was recommended before each increase of 0.25 µg per kg per minute in infusion rate.

1. Lindsay CA, *et al.* Pharmacokinetics and pharmacodynamics of milrinone lactate in pediatric patients with septic shock. *J Pediatr* 1998; **132:** 329–34.
2. Ramamoorthy C, *et al.* Pharmacokinetics and side effects of milrinone in infants and children after open heart surgery. *Anesth Analg* 1998; **86:** 283–9.

Heart failure. Milrinone is one of several drugs that may be used in heart failure (p.785), but because of an increased mortality rate reported following long-term oral administration it is usually only given intravenously for short-term management of heart failure unresponsive to other forms of therapy. However, more recently longer-term continuous intravenous administration for up to 8 weeks has been studied in patients awaiting heart transplantation and appeared to be well tolerated.[1] Intermittent administration on several days a week has also been tried.[2] When compared with digoxin, milrinone by mouth was found to be less effective and when used in conjunction with digoxin milrinone provided no additional benefit.[3] The PROMISE study (Prospective Randomized Milrinone Survival Evaluation)[4] showed that oral milrinone increased morbidity and mortality in patients with severe chronic heart failure.

1. Mehra MR, *et al.* Safety and clinical utility of long-term intravenous milrinone in advanced heart failure. *Am J Cardiol* 1997; **80:** 61–4.
2. Cesario D, *et al.* Beneficial effects of intermittent home administration of the inotrope/vasodilator milrinone in patients with end-stage congestive heart failure: a preliminary study. *Am Heart J* 1998; **135:** 121–9.
3. DiBianco R, *et al.* A comparison of oral milrinone, digoxin, and their combination in the treatment of patients with chronic heart failure. *N Engl J Med* 1989; **320:** 677–83.
4. Packer M, *et al.* Effect of oral milrinone on mortality in severe chronic heart failure. *N Engl J Med* 1991; **325:** 1468–75.

Preparations

Proprietary Preparations (details are given in Part 3)
Aust.: Corotrop; ***Austral.:*** Primacor; ***Belg.:*** Corotrope; ***Canad.:*** Primacor; ***Fr.:*** Corotrope; ***Ger.:*** Corotrop; ***Neth.:*** Corotrope; ***Spain:*** Corotrope; ***Swed.:*** Corotrop; ***Switz.:*** Corotrop; ***UK:*** Primacor; ***USA:*** Primacor.

Minoxidil (884-x)

Minoxidil *(BAN, USAN, rINN).*

Minoxidilum; U-10858. 2,6-Diamino-4-piperidinopyrimidine 1-oxide.

$C_9H_{15}N_5O = 209.2.$

CAS — 38304-91-5.

Pharmacopoeias. In *Eur.* (see p.viii) and *US.*

A white or off-white crystalline powder. Slightly **soluble** in water; soluble in alcohol and in propylene glycol; soluble or sparingly soluble in methyl alcohol; very slightly soluble in ether; practically insoluble in acetone, in chloroform, in ethyl acetate, and in petroleum spirit. **Protect** from light.

Adverse Effects and Treatment

Adverse effects commonly caused by minoxidil include reflex tachycardia, fluid retention accompanied by weight gain, oedema, and sometimes deterioration of existing heart failure and changes in the ECG. Hypertrichosis develops in up to 80% of patients within 3 to 6 weeks of the start of minoxidil therapy but is slowly reversible on discontinuation. Pericardial effusion, sometimes with associated tamponade, has been reported in about 3% of patients. Pericarditis may also occur. Administration of minoxidil may aggravate or uncover angina pectoris. Other less frequent adverse effects include headache, nausea, gynaecomastia and breast tenderness, polymenorrhoea, allergic skin rashes, Stevens-Johnson syndrome, and thrombocytopenia.

Reflex tachycardia can be overcome by the concomitant administration of a beta blocker or methyldopa, and a diuretic (usually a loop diuretic) is used to reduce fluid retention. If excessive hypotension occurs, an intravenous infusion of normal saline can be given to maintain the blood pressure. If a pressor agent is necessary, drugs such as adrenaline which can aggravate tachycardia should be avoided; phenylephrine, angiotensin amide, vasopressin, or dopamine may be given if there is evidence of inadequate perfusion of a vital organ.

Topical application of minoxidil may be associated with contact dermatitis, pruritus, local burning, and flushing; sufficient may be absorbed to produce systemic adverse effects.

Two haemorrhagic lesions with Kaposi's features appeared on the forehead, an unusual location for HIV-associated Kaposi's sarcoma, in an HIV-positive patient who had applied topical minoxidil there for 3 months.[1] In another, healthy, patient an angioma of the scalp developed after 2 months of topical minoxidil therapy. The patient had had a similar lesion as a baby. Minoxidil may induce angiogenesis or may stimulate endothelial cells, fibroblasts, and muscle cells to proliferate. Care should be taken when minoxidil is applied to the skin of people who are predisposed to neo-angiogenesis, or who are HIV-positive.

For other effects of minoxidil on the skin following topical application, see below.

1. Pavlovitch JH, *et al.* Angiogenesis and minoxidil. *Lancet* 1990; **336:** 889.

Effects on the cardiovascular system. Application of topical minoxidil 2% solution twice daily (giving a dose of 40 mg) in 20 subjects produced an increase in left-ventricular mass and end-diastolic volume, and in cardiac output, when compared with placebo in a further 15.[1] It is uncertain what effects this might have in otherwise healthy subjects long-term, or whether the increase in left-ventricular mass would continue and give further reason for concern. In patients with coronary artery disease, however, the increased cardiac work might aggravate ischaemic symptoms.

1. Leenen FHH, *et al.* Topical minoxidil: cardiac effects in bald man. *Br J Clin Pharmacol* 1988; **26:** 481–5.

Effects on the eyes. Bilateral optic neuritis and retinitis occurred in a patient during treatment with minoxidil for hypertension following a renal transplant.[1] The patient was also taking prednisolone and azathioprine.

1. Gombos GM. Bilateral optic neuritis following minoxidil administration. *Ann Ophthalmol* 1983; **15:** 259–61.

Effects on the hair. The hypertrichosis associated with minoxidil taken orally makes it unsuitable generally for use in women. As well as frequent hypertrichosis, there have been reports of changes in hair colour in patients receiving minoxidil.[1] In addition one case has been reported of increased hair loss, followed by subsequent regrowth of differently-coloured hair.[2] Substantial hair loss occurred in a woman patient following withdrawal of minoxidil and she had to wear a wig.[3]

Severe hypertrichosis has also been reported in 5 of 56 women applying minoxidil 5% solution topically for androgenetic alopecia.[4] Facial, arm, and leg hypertrichosis were reported 2 to 3 months after starting treatment. Hypertrichosis had disappeared 5 months after discontinuation of minoxidil.

1. Traub YM, *et al.* Treatment of severe hypertension with minoxidil. *Isr J Med Sci* 1975; **11:** 991–8.
2. Ingles RM, Kahn T. Unusual hair changes with minoxidil therapy. *Int J Dermatol* 1983; **22:** 120–2.
3. Kidwai BJ, George M. Hair loss with minoxidil withdrawal. *Lancet* 1992; **340:** 609–10.
4. Peluso AM, *et al.* Diffuse hypertrichosis during treatment with 5% topical minoxidil. *Br J Dermatol* 1997; **136:** 118–20.

Effects on skeletal muscle. A polymyalgia syndrome, manifesting as fatigue, anorexia, weight loss, and severe pain in the shoulders and pelvic girdle was seen in 4 men using topical minoxidil.[1] All symptoms improved within 2 to 4 weeks of withdrawing the drug. In 2 of the patients rechallenge produced a relapse of the symptoms.

1. Colamarino R, *et al.* Polymyalgia and minoxidil. *Ann Intern Med* 1990; **113:** 256–7.

Effects on the skin. Although skin reactions to systemic minoxidil do not appear to be common, a case of classic Stevens-Johnson syndrome has been reported in a patient receiving minoxidil.[1] The syndrome responded to withdrawal and steroid therapy; subsequent rechallenge provoked a recurrence. In another patient extensive erythematous weeping rash, with lesions consistent with actinic keratosis also appeared to be due to minoxidil; bullous lesions recurred on re-exposure.[2] Following topical application itching, scaling, flushing, and dermatitis have been the most common adverse effects; allergic contact dermatitis has been reported in rare instances.[3]

For other lesions associated with Kaposi's sarcoma and angioma and for effects on the hair, see above.

1. DiSantis DJ, Flanagan J. Minoxidil-induced Stevens-Johnson syndrome. *Arch Intern Med* 1981; **141:** 1515.
2. Ackerman BH, *et al.* Pruritic rash with actinic keratosis and impending exfoliation in a patient with hypertension managed with minoxidil. *Drug Intell Clin Pharm* 1988; **22:** 702–3.
3. Clissold SP, Heel RC. Topical minoxidil: a preliminary review of its pharmacodynamic properties and therapeutic efficacy in alopecia areata and alopecia androgenetica. *Drugs* 1987; **33:** 107–22.

Precautions

Minoxidil is contra-indicated in phaeochromocytoma. It should be used with caution after a recent myocardial infarction, and in patients with pulmonary hypertension, angina pectoris, chronic heart failure, and significant renal impairment.

Topical application of minoxidil should be restricted to the scalp; it should not be applied to inflamed scalp skin or areas affected by psoriasis, severe sunburn, or severe excoriations, due to the risk of increased absorption. Patients being treated for hypertension should be monitored if topical minoxidil is used concurrently.

AIDS. For recommendations that topical minoxidil should be used with caution in HIV-positive patients, see under Adverse Effects, above.

Pregnancy and breast feeding. A patient who took minoxidil, propranolol, and frusemide throughout pregnancy delivered a normal infant at 37 weeks. Pregnancy was uneventful.[1] Subsequent studies showed that minoxidil was rapidly distributed into breast milk achieving similar concentrations to those in the plasma. No adverse effects were seen in the infant after 2 months but it was considered that prolonged exposure during breast feeding could be deleterious to the infant.

1. Valdivieso A, *et al.* Minoxidil in breast milk. *Ann Intern Med* 1985; **102:** 135.

Interactions

The antihypertensive effect of minoxidil may be enhanced by concomitant use of other hypotensive drugs. Severe orthostatic hypotension may occur if minoxidil and sympathetic blocking drugs such as guanethidine or bethanidine are given concurrently.

Topical minoxidil should not be used with other topical agents known to enhance absorption, such as corticosteroids, retinoids, or occlusive ointment bases.

Pharmacokinetics

About 90% of an oral dose of minoxidil has been reported to be absorbed from the gastro-intestinal tract. The plasma half-life is about 4.2 hours although the haemodynamic effect may persist for up to 75 hours, presumably due to accumulation at its site of action. Minoxidil is not bound to plasma proteins. It is distributed into breast milk. Minoxidil is extensively metabolised by the liver. It requires sulphation to become active, but the major metabolite is a glucuronide conjugate. Minoxidil is excreted predominantly in the urine mainly in the form of metabolites. Minoxidil and its metabolites are dialysable.

Following topical application between 0.3 and 4.5% of the total applied dose of minoxidil is absorbed from intact scalp.

References.

1. Pacifici GM, *et al.* Minoxidil sulphation in human liver and platelets: a study of interindividual variability. *Eur J Clin Pharmacol* 1993; **45:** 337–41.

Uses and Administration

Minoxidil is an antihypertensive that acts predominantly by causing direct peripheral vasodilatation of the arterioles. It produces effects on the cardiovascular system similar to those of hydralazine (p.885). Minoxidil is administered by mouth for the treatment of severe hypertension unresponsive to standard therapy (p.788). When applied topically to the scalp minoxidil may stimulate hair growth to a limited extent and is used in the treatment of alopecia.

In the treatment of **hypertension** minoxidil is given with a beta blocker or methyldopa to diminish the cardiac-accelerating effects, and with a diuretic, usually a loop diuretic, to control oedema. Following a single dose by mouth, the maximum hypotensive effect usually occurs after 2 to 3 hours, although the full effects may not occur until after 3 to 7 days of continuous treatment. The action may persist for up to 75 hours. An initial dose of 5 mg of minoxidil daily (or 2.5 mg daily in the elderly) is gradually increased at intervals of not less than 3 days to 40 or 50 mg daily according to the patient's response; in exceptional circumstances up to 100 mg daily has been given. If more rapid control of blood pressure is required, dosage adjustments may be made every 6 hours with careful monitoring. The daily dose may be given as a single dose or in 2 divided doses. For children 12 years of age or under, the recommended initial dose is 200 μg per kg body-weight daily, increased in steps of 100 to 200 μg per kg at intervals of not less than 3 days, until control of blood pressure has been achieved or a maximum of 1 mg per kg or 50 mg daily has been reached.

Reduced doses may be required in patients with impaired renal function.

In the treatment of **male-pattern baldness** (alopecia androgenetica) 1 mL of a 2% or 5% solution of minoxidil is applied twice daily to the scalp.

Administration in renal impairment. A study of the pharmacokinetics of minoxidil in patients with varying degrees of renal function impairment found that the non-renal clearance was also impaired as renal function worsened.[1] Substantial accumulation of minoxidil might occur in these patients during multiple-dose therapy. It was advised that minoxidil therapy be initiated with smaller doses or a longer dose interval in patients with renal insufficiency.

1. Halstenson CE, *et al.* Disposition of minoxidil in patients with various degrees of renal function. *J Clin Pharmacol* 1989; **29:** 798–802.

Alopecia. Although topical minoxidil clearly has some effect on hair growth in alopecia (p.1073), increases in pigmented non-vellus hair may be due to thickening and pigmentation of existing vellus rather than new growth.[1] As a result cosmetically acceptable hair growth may occur in less than 10% of patients with male-pattern baldness (alopecia androgenetica),[2-4] and fewer still among those with alopecia areata,[4] despite the fact that higher-strength 5% solutions have been tried in the latter condition.[4] One study indicated that combination of topical minoxidil with 0.5% dithranol cream was more effective than either treatment alone in patients with alopecia areata.[5] The hair is lost again when treatment is stopped,[2-4] and even with continued use there is a waning of effect.[2,4] Minoxidil may be more effective in retarding the progression of male-pattern baldness than in reversing it,[1] and users are advised to abandon treatment if there is insufficient benefit after a year.[3]

A review of recent controlled trials, that were conducted mostly in men,[6] concluded that topical minoxidil 2% had only a minimal to modest effect on promoting hair regrowth in alopecia androgenetica and needed to be used indefinitely; some workers believed it to be more effective in females than in males, although another review of controlled studies in women[7] concluded that the effectiveness of minoxidil in female alopecia androgenetica was yet to be demonstrated and that larger trials were required. Minoxidil appeared to have no beneficial effect on alopecia areata.[6]

1. Katz HI. Topical minoxidil: review of efficacy and safety. *Cutis* 1989; **43:** 94–8.
2. de Groot AC, *et al.* Minoxidil: hope for the bald? *Lancet* 1987; **i:** 1019–22.
3. Shrank AB. Treating young men with hair loss. *Br Med J* 1989; **298:** 847–8.
4. Anonymous. Topical minoxidil does little for baldness. *Drug Ther Bull* 1989; **27:** 74–5.
5. Fiedler VC, *et al.* Treatment-resistant alopecia areata. *Arch Dermatol* 1990; **126:** 756–9.
6. Anonymous. Topical minoxidil for baldness: a reappraisal. *Med Lett Drugs Ther* 1994; **36:** 9–10.
7. Wong WM, Seifert L. Minoxidil used in female alopecia. *Ann Pharmacother* 1994; **28:** 290–1.

CHEMOTHERAPY-INDUCED ALOPECIA. Minoxidil 2% solution was applied daily to the scalp of a boy with acute lymphoblastic leukaemia whose hair had failed to regrow satisfactorily following intensive chemotherapy.[1] Almost normal hair growth was achieved over a period of nine months that was attributed to the application of minoxidil.

A small study[2] in women undergoing chemotherapy found that topical minoxidil applied throughout the duration of antineoplastic therapy and for up to 4 months afterwards reduced the duration of alopecia by an average of 50 days.

Other methods for reducing chemotherapy-induced alopecia are described under the Treatment of Adverse Effects of Antineoplastics, p.474.

1. Vickers MA, Barton CJ. Minoxidil induced hair growth after leukaemia treatment? *Arch Dis Child* 1995; **73:** 184.
2. Duvic M, *et al.* A randomized trial of minoxidil in chemotherapy-induced alopecia. *J Am Acad Dermatol* 1996; **35:** 74–8.

Preparations

USP 23: Minoxidil Tablets; Minoxidil Topical Solution.

Proprietary Preparations (details are given in Part 3)
Aust.: Loniten; Moxiral; Regaine; ***Austral.:*** Loniten; Ralogaine; Regaine; ***Belg.:*** Lonnoten; Neoxidil; Regaine; ***Canad.:*** Apo-Gain; Loniten; Minoxigaine; Rogaine; ***Fr.:*** Alopexy; Alostil; Lonoten; Neoxidil; Regaine; ***Ger.:*** Lonolox; ***Irl.:*** Loniten; Regaine; ***Ital.:*** Aloxidil; Loniten; Minotricon†; Minovital; Minoximen; Normoxidil; Pierminox†; Prexidil†; Regaine; Tricoxidil; ***Neth.:*** Lonnoten; Regaine; ***Norw.:*** Regaine; ***S.Afr.:*** Loniten; Regaine; ***Spain:*** Crecisan†; Kapodin; Kresse; Lacovin; Loniten; Pilovital; Regaine; Riteban; Trico†; ***Swed.:*** Regaine; ***Switz.:*** Alopexy; Loniten; Neocapil; Regaine; ***UK:*** Loniten; Regaine; ***USA:*** Loniten; Minodyl†; Rogaine.

Mivazerol (14644-g)

Mivazerol *(rINN)*.

UCB-22073.

CAS — 125472-02-8.

Mivazerol is an alpha$_2$-adrenoceptor agonist under investigation for the prevention of perioperative complications resulting from myocardial ischaemia in patients with ischaemic heart disease undergoing non-cardiac surgery.

Moexipril Hydrochloride (17803-g)

Moexipril Hydrochloride *(BANM, USAN, rINNM)*.

CI-925; RS-10085-197; SPM-925. (3*S*-{2[*R**(*R**)],3*R**})-2-(2-{[1-(Ethoxycarbonyl)-3-phenylpropyl]amino}-1-oxopropyl)-1,2,3,4-tetrahydro-6,7-dimethoxy-3-isoquinoline-carboxylic acid hydrochloride.

$C_{27}H_{34}N_2O_7,HCl = 535.0.$

CAS — 103775-10-6 (moexipril); 82586-52-5 (moexipril hydrochloride).

Adverse Effects, Treatment, and Precautions

As for ACE inhibitors, p.805.

Interactions

As for ACE inhibitors, p.807.

Pharmacokinetics

Moexipril acts as a prodrug of the diacid moexiprilat, its active metabolite. Following oral administration moexipril is rapidly but incompletely absorbed and is metabolised to moexiprilat in the gastro-intestinal mucosa and liver. Absorption is reduced in the presence of food. The bioavailability of moexiprilat is about 13% following oral moexipril administration, and peak plasma concentrations of moexiprilat are reached in about 1.5 hours. Both moexipril and moexiprilat are moderately bound to plasma proteins. Moexipril is excreted predominantly in the urine as moexiprilat, unchanged drug, and other metabolites; some moexiprilat may also be excreted in the faeces. The functional elimination half-life of moexiprilat is about 12 hours.

Uses and Administration

Moexipril is an ACE inhibitor (p.805). It is used in the treatment of hypertension (p.788).

Moexipril owes its activity to moexiprilat, to which it is converted after oral administration. The haemodynamic effects are seen about 1 hour after an oral dose and the maximum effect occurs after about 3 to 6 hours, although the full effect may not develop for 2 to 4 weeks during chronic dosing. Moexipril is given by mouth as the hydrochloride.

In the treatment of **hypertension**, the usual initial dose of moexipril hydrochloride is 7.5 mg once daily. An initial dose of 3.75 mg once daily, given under close medical supervision, is suggested for patients who are receiving a diuretic; if possible the diuretic should be withdrawn 2 or 3 days before moexipril is started and resumed later if necessary. An initial dose of 3.75 mg once daily is also recommended for patients with renal or liver impairment, the elderly, and those also receiving nifedipine. The usual maintenance dose is 7.5 to 30 mg daily, which may be given in 2 divided doses if control is inadequate with a single dose.

Reviews.

1. Brogden RN, Wiseman LR. Moexipril: a review of its use in the management of essential hypertension. *Drugs* 1998; **55:** 845–60.

Preparations

Proprietary Preparations (details are given in Part 3)
Ital.: Femipres; Primoxil; ***UK:*** Perdix; ***USA:*** Univasc.

Multi-ingredient: ***USA:*** Uniretic.

Molsidomine (12971-v)

Molsidomine *(BAN, USAN, rINN)*.

CAS-276; Morsydomine; SIN-10. *N*-Ethoxycarbonyl-3-morpholinosydnonimine.

$C_9H_{14}N_4O_4 = 242.2.$

CAS — 25717-80-0.

Molsidomine is a nitrovasodilator used in angina pectoris (p.780). It may also be used in heart failure (p.785) and following myocardial infarction (p.791).

It is given by mouth in usual doses of 1 to 4 mg two to four times daily. It is also given by injection in single doses of 2 to 4 mg and doses of 2 mg may be repeated at intervals of at least 2 hours if necessary; total doses of up to 40 mg daily have been given. Infusions may be employed at a rate of up to 3 mg per hour.

Molsidomine is metabolised to linsidomine (p.898), an active metabolite.

The pharmacokinetics of molsidomine have been reviewed.[1] Molsidomine is metabolised in the liver to linsidomine and other morpholine derivatives. Prolonged elimination half-lives of molsidomine and linsidomine due to reduced plasma clearance have been reported in patients with liver cirrhosis.[2]

Molsidomine tends to degrade into morpholine (even when protected from the light), a compound considered potentially carcinogenic. This finding and evidence that molsidomine is carcinogenic in *animals* have led to the suspension of marketing of molsidomine on two occasions,[3] although in the second instance only certain formulations were affected by the suspension.

1. Rosenkranz B, *et al.* Clinical pharmacokinetics of molsidomine. *Clin Pharmacokinet* 1996; **30:** 372–84.
2. Spreux-Varoquaux O, *et al.* Pharmacokinetics of molsidomine and its active metabolite, linsidomine, in patients with liver cirrhosis. *Br J Clin Pharmacol* 1991; **32:** 399–401.
3. Anonymous. Corvaton Tropfen. *Dtsch Apotheker Ztg* 1989; **129** (49): VI.

Myocardial infarction. Although intravenous nitrates (glyceryl trinitrate or sodium nitroprusside) may be used in the management of acute myocardial infarction (p.791), molsidomine and its active metabolite linsidomine (a nitric oxide donor) had no effect on mortality.[1]

1. European Study of Prevention of Infarct with Molsidomine (ESPRIM) Group. The ESPRIM trial: short-term treatment of acute myocardial infarction with molsidomine. *Lancet* 1994; **344:** 91–7.

Preparations

Proprietary Preparations (details are given in Part 3)
Aust.: Molsidolat†; ***Belg.:*** Corvaton; ***Fr.:*** Corvasal; ***Ger.:*** Corvaton; duracoron; Molsicor; Molsihexal; ***Ital.:*** Molsidolat†; Molsiton†; ***Spain:*** Corangor†; Corpea; Molsidain; ***Switz.:*** Corvaton.

Monteplase (17638-s)

Monteplase *(rINN)*.

E-6010.

$C_{2569}H_{3896}N_{746}O_{783}S_{39} = 59009.6.$

CAS — 156616-23-8.

Monteplase is a thrombolytic drug related to alteplase (p.818) used in the treatment of myocardial infarction.

References.

1. Kawai C, *et al.* Randomized, double-blind multicenter trial of a novel modified t-PA, E6010 by i.v. bolus injection in treatment of acute myocardial infarction (AMI): comparison with native t-PA. *J Am Coll Cardiol* 1995; **25** (Special issue): 5A.

Moracizine Hydrochloride (12978-l)

Moracizine Hydrochloride *(BANM, rINNM)*.

EN-313 (moracizine). Ethyl [10-(3-morpholinopropionyl)phenothiazin-2-yl]carbamate hydrochloride.

$C_{22}H_{25}N_3O_4S,HCl = 464.0.$

CAS — 31883-05-3 (moracizine); 29560-58-5 (moracizine hydrochloride).

NOTE. Moricizine is *USAN*.

Pharmacopoeias. In US.

A white to off-white crystalline powder. **Soluble** in water and in alcohol. **Store** in airtight containers.

Adverse Effects

The most common adverse effects associated with moracizine therapy affect the central nervous system and the gastro-intestinal tract and include dizziness, headache, fatigue, nausea, and abdominal pain. Other adverse effects include dyspnoea, dry mouth, blurred vision, impotence, and urinary-tract disorders. There have been occasional reports of fever, thrombocytopenia, hepatic dysfunction, hypothermia, and skin rash.

Like other antiarrhythmics moracizine can provoke or worsen arrhythmias. This may range from an increase in the frequency of premature ventricular contractions to induction or worsening of ventricular tachycardia.

An increased mortality rate occurred when moracizine was tested in the control of asymptomatic ventricular arrhythmias in post-infarction patients (see Cardiac Arrhythmias under Uses and Administration, below).

Fever with elevated creatine phosphokinase and hepatic transaminase concentrations was associated with moracizine administration in 2 patients.[1] The fever abated within 48 hours of withdrawing moracizine and recurred within 24 hours of rechallenge in both patients. Results suggested a similarity to the neuroleptic malignant syndrome which has been attributed to other phenothiazine derivatives.

1. Miura DS, *et al.* Ethmozine toxicity: fever of unknown origin. *J Clin Pharmacol* 1986; **26:** 153–5.

Precautions

As for Flecainide Acetate, p.869.

Pharmacokinetics

Moracizine is readily and almost completely absorbed from the gastro-intestinal tract. It undergoes significant first-pass hepatic metabolism so that the bioavailability following oral administration is about 38%. Moracizine is extensively metabolised and some of the numerous metabolites may be active. It induces its own metabolism; the plasma elimination half-life is about 2 hours following multiple doses. Although plasma concentrations are reduced with multiple dosing, clinical response is not affected. It is about 95% bound to plasma proteins. Moracizine is distributed into breast milk. Approximately 56% of a dose is excreted in the faeces and approximately 39% in the urine.

References.

1. Benedek IH, *et al.* Enzyme induction by moricizine: time course and extent in healthy subjects. *J Clin Pharmacol* 1994; **34:** 167–75.

Uses and Administration

Moracizine is a phenothiazine compound with class I antiarrhythmic activity (p.776) but which does not readily fall into the subclasses a, b, or c. It is used as the hydrochloride in the treatment of serious symptomatic ventricular **arrhythmias**. Moracizine hydrochloride is given in a usual dose of 600 to 900 mg daily by mouth in 2 or 3 divided doses. Doses, which should be given initially in hospital, should be adjusted at intervals of not less than 3 days. If rapid control of life-threatening arrhythmias is essential a suggested initial dose is 400 to 500 mg followed by 200 mg every 8 hours.

Patients with hepatic or renal impairment should be started on a dosage of 600 mg or less daily and monitored closely.

General reviews of moracizine published before[1-3] and after[4] the results of the Cardiac Arrhythmia Suppression Trial (CAST II), in which moracizine was associated with increased mortality (see Cardiac Arrhythmias, below).

1. Fitton A, Buckley MM-T. Moricizine: a review of its pharmacological properties, and therapeutic efficacy in cardiac arrhythmias. *Drugs* 1990; **40:** 138–67.
2. Carnes CA, Coyle JD. Moricizine: a novel antiarrhythmic agent. *DICP Ann Pharmacother* 1990; **24:** 745–53.
3. Mann HJ. Moricizine: a new class I antiarrhythmic. *Clin Pharm* 1990; **9:** 842–52.
4. Clyne CA, *et al.* Moricizine. *N Engl J Med* 1992; **327:** 255–60.

Cardiac arrhythmias. Asymptomatic premature ventricular arrhythmias in subjects who have previously suffered a myocardial infarction are recognised as a risk factor for subsequent sudden cardiac death.[1] Suppressing such arrhythmias in this group might be expected to reduce the incidence of sudden death and it was to test this hypothesis that a large multicentre study was set up in the USA (the Cardiac Arrhythmia Suppression Trial known as CAST).[2,3] Encainide, flecainide, and moracizine were the antiarrhythmics studied, but encainide and flecainide, and later moracizine,[4] were all associated with increased mortality. It is now accepted that these drugs should not be used prophylactically in post-infarction patients with asymptomatic arrhythmias.

Licensed indications for moracizine cover severe symptomatic ventricular arrhythmias (p.782).

1. Task Force of the Working Group on Arrhythmias of the European Society of Cardiology. CAST and beyond: implications of the cardiac arrhythmias suppression trial. *Circulation* 1990; **81:** 1123–7. [Simultaneous publication occurred in *Eur Heart J* 1990; **11:** 194–9.]
2. The Cardiac Arrhythmia Suppression Trial (CAST) Investigators. Preliminary report: effect of encainide and flecainide on mortality in a randomized trial of arrhythmia suppression after myocardial infarction. *N Engl J Med* 1989; **321:** 406–12.
3. Echt DS, *et al.* Mortality and morbidity in patients receiving encainide, flecainide, or placebo: the Cardiac Arrhythmia Suppression Trial. *N Engl J Med* 1991; **324:** 781–8.
4. The Cardiac Arrhythmia Suppression Trial II Investigators. Effect of the antiarrhythmic agent moricizine on survival after myocardial infarction. *N Engl J Med* 1992; **327:** 227–33.

Preparations

USP 23: Moricizine Hydrochloride Tablets.

Proprietary Preparations (details are given in Part 3)
Irl.: Ethmozine; *UK:* Ethmozine; *USA:* Ethmozine.

Moveltipril (5508-y)

Moveltipril *(rINN)*.

Altiopril; MC-838 (moveltipril calcium). [*R*-(*R**,*S**)]-1-[3-{[2-[(Cyclohexylcarbonyl)amino]-1-oxopropyl]thio}-2-methyl-1-oxopropyl]-L-proline.

$C_{19}H_{30}N_2O_5S$ = 398.5.

CAS — 85856-54-8 (moveltipril); 85921-53-5 (moveltipril calcium).

Moveltipril is an ACE inhibitor (p.805). It is under investigation as the calcium salt in the management of hypertension.

Moveltipril contains a captopril moiety in its structure but it is unclear whether it is converted *in vivo* to captopril or is metabolised to other active metabolites containing the sulfhydryl group.[1] Studies in *animals* have demonstrated a hypotensive effect equivalent to that of captopril but with a slower onset and more prolonged duration of action.

1. Salvetti A. Newer ACE inhibitors: a look at the future. *Drugs* 1990; **40:** 800–28.

Moxonidine (19534-k)

Moxonidine *(BAN, rINN)*.

BDF-5895; BE-5895. 4-Chloro-5-(2-imidazolin-2-ylamino)-6-methoxy-2-methylpyrimidine.

$C_9H_{12}ClN_5O$ = 241.7.

CAS — 75438-57-2.

Adverse Effects and Treatment

Moxonidine has similar adverse effects to clonidine (p.841) but causes less sedation. The incidence of dry mouth may also be lower.

Precautions

Moxonidine should not be used in patients with conduction disorders, bradycardia, severe arrhythmias, severe heart failure, severe ischaemic heart disease, severe liver or renal impairment, or a history of angioedema. The manufacturer suggests that It should also be avoided in patients with intermittent claudication or Raynaud's disease, Parkinson's disease, epilepsy, glaucoma, and depression.

Although rebound hypertension has not been reported following moxonidine withdrawal it should not be stopped abruptly but should be withdrawn gradually over 2 weeks. In patients who are receiving a beta blocker concomitantly, the beta blocker should be stopped several days before moxonidine is withdrawn.

Interactions

The hypotensive effect of moxonidine may be enhanced by other antihypertensives and drugs that cause hypotension. The effect of sedatives and hypnotics, including benzodiazepines, may be enhanced by moxonidine.

Pharmacokinetics

Moxonidine is well absorbed following oral administration and has a bioavailability of about 88%. Peak plasma concentrations occur 0.5 to 3 hours after an oral dose. It is excreted almost entirely in the urine as unchanged drug and metabolites; about 50 to 75% of an oral dose is excreted as unchanged drug. The mean plasma elimination half-life is 2 to 3 hours and is prolonged in renal impairment. Moxonidine is about 7% bound to plasma proteins.

Uses and Administration

Moxonidine is a centrally acting antihypertensive structurally related to clonidine (p.841). It appears to act through stimulation of central imidazoline receptors to reduce sympathetic tone, and also has alpha$_2$-adrenoceptor agonist activity. It is used in the treatment of hypertension (p.788).

In the treatment of hypertension, moxonidine is given by mouth in a usual initial dose of 200 μg once daily. The dose may be increased if necessary, after 3 weeks, to 400 μg daily in one or two divided doses, and after a further 3 weeks, to a maximum dose of 600 μg daily in two divided doses. The dose should be reduced in patients with renal impairment.

References.

1. Kirch W, *et al.* Pharmacodynamic action and pharmacokinetics of moxonidine after single oral administration in hypertensive patients. *J Clin Pharmacol* 1990; **30:** 1088–95.
2. MacPhee GJA, *et al.* A comparison of the haemodynamic and behavioural effects of moxonidine and clonidine in normotensive subjects. *Br J Clin Pharmacol* 1992; **33:** 261–7.
3. Chrisp P, Faulds D. Moxonidine: a review of its pharmacology, and therapeutic use in essential hypertension. *Drugs* 1992; **44:** 993–1012.
4. Schachter M, *et al.* Safety and tolerability of moxonidine in the treatment of hypertension. *Drug Safety* 1998; **19:** 191–203.

Preparations

Proprietary Preparations (details are given in Part 3)
Aust.: Normoxin; *Fr.:* Physiotens; *Ger.:* Cynt; Physiotens; *Neth.:* Normatens; *Switz.:* Physiotens; *UK:* Physiotens.

Nadolol (6315-l)

Nadolol *(BAN, USAN, rINN)*.

SQ-11725. (2*R*,3*S*)-5-(3-*tert*-Butylamino-2-hydroxypropoxy)-1,2,3,4-tetrahydronaphthalene-2,3-diol.

$C_{17}H_{27}NO_4$ = 309.4.

CAS — 42200-33-9.

Pharmacopoeias. In *US.*

White or off-white, practically odourless, crystalline powder. **Soluble** in water at pH 2; freely soluble in alcohol and in methyl alcohol; slightly soluble in chloroform, in dichloromethane, in isopropyl alcohol, and in water at pH 7 to 10; practically insoluble in acetone, in ether, in hexane, and in trichloroethane.

Adverse Effects, Treatment, and Precautions

As for beta blockers, p.828.

Hypersensitivity. Hypersensitivity pneumonitis was associated with nadolol in a patient prescribed the drug for migraine.[1] Symptoms improved when nadolol was withdrawn.

1. Levy MB, *et al.* Nadolol and hypersensitivity pneumonitis. *Ann Intern Med* 1986; **105:** 806–7.

Interactions

The interactions associated with beta blockers are discussed on p.829.

Pharmacokinetics

Nadolol is incompletely absorbed from the gastro-intestinal tract to give peak plasma concentrations about 3 or 4 hours after a dose. It has low lipid solubility. Nadolol is widely distributed and appears in breast milk where higher concentrations have been achieved than in maternal serum. It is only about 30% bound to plasma proteins. It does not appear to be metabolised and is excreted mainly in the urine. The plasma half-life has been reported as ranging from about 12 to 24 hours. Nadolol is reported to be dialysable.

In 4 patients with mild hypertension given nadolol 2 mg by mouth or intravenously, the elimination half-life from plasma was an average of 10 to 12 hours (a range of 5.9 to 12.2 hours following intravenous administration, and a range of 9.6 to 14.2 hours following oral administration). Calculations based on urinary excretion and plasma concentration data suggested that about 33% was absorbed after oral administration. There was evidence of biliary as well as urinary excretion since after intravenous administration about 73% was excreted in urine and 23% in faeces. Nadolol did not appear to be metabolised.[1] In a similar study of therapeutic oral doses, terminal half-lives ranging from 14 to 17 hours were reported for nadolol 80 mg given as a single dose and the same dose daily in a multiple dosage regimen.[2]

1. Dreyfuss J, *et al.* Metabolic studies in patients with nadolol: oral and intravenous administration. *J Clin Pharmacol* 1977; **17:** 300–7.
2. Dreyfuss J, *et al.* Pharmacokinetics of nadolol, a beta-receptor antagonist: administration of therapeutic single- and multiple-dosage regimens to hypertensive patients. *J Clin Pharmacol* 1979; **19:** 712–20.

Breast feeding. Concentrations of nadolol in breast milk following administration of nadolol 80 mg daily by mouth for 5 days were determined in 12 lactating normotensive women.[1] The mean nadolol concentration in milk for the 24 hours after the last dose was 357 ng per mL; the mean serum-nadolol concentration was only 77 ng per mL during the same time period.

1. Devlin RG, Fleiss PM. Nadolol excretion in human milk. *Clin Pharmacol Ther* 1981; **29:** 240.

Children. The pharmacokinetics of nadolol given intravenously and orally were studied in six children aged 3 months to 14 years.[1] The elimination half-lives for the two oldest children aged 10 and 14 years were 7.3 and 15.7 hours, respectively. These values are similar to those reported for adults whereas in the children 22 months-of-age or younger, shorter half-lives of 3.2 to 4.3 hours were found. The authors considered that the shorter half-lives were probably a result of a reduction in the total apparent volume of distribution of nadolol in the youngest children. Elimination rates were similar after either intravenous or oral administration.

1. Mehta AV, *et al.* Pharmacokinetics of nadolol in children with supraventricular tachycardia. *J Clin Pharmacol* 1992; **32:** 1023–7.

Uses and Administration

Nadolol is a non-cardioselective beta blocker (p.828). It is reported to lack intrinsic sympathomimetic and membrane-stabilising activity. Nadolol is used in the management of hypertension (p.788), angina pectoris (p.780), and cardiac arrhythmias (p.782).

It is also used in the management of hyperthyroidism (p.1489) and migraine (p.443).

In the treatment of **hypertension**, nadolol is usually given in an initial dose of 40 to 80 mg daily by mouth, increased weekly according to the response of the patient to 240 mg or more daily.

In **angina pectoris**, the usual initial dose is 40 mg daily, increased weekly according to the response of the patient to usual doses of up to 160 mg daily; some patients may require up to 240 mg daily. Doses of 40 to 160 mg daily have also been given for **cardiac arrhythmias**.

Similar doses of 40 to 160 mg daily are used in **migraine** prophylaxis.

In the management of **hyperthyroidism**, doses of 80 to 160 mg daily have been given; most patients are reported to require the higher dose.

Patients with renal impairment may require a lower dose or less frequent administration. One method of dose adjustment is to increase the dosage interval according to the patient's creatinine clearance. For patients with a creatinine clearance between 31 and 50 mL per minute, nadolol is given every 24 to 36 hours; for patients with a clearance between 10 and 30 mL per minute, administration is every 24 to 48 hours; for those with a clearance of less than 10 mL per minute, the dosage interval is 40 to 60 hours.

Preparations

USP 23: Nadolol and Bendroflumethiazide Tablets; Nadolol Tablets.

Proprietary Preparations (details are given in Part 3)
Aust.: Solgol; ***Belg.:*** Corgard; ***Canad.:*** Corgard; ***Fr.:*** Corgard; ***Ger.:*** Solgol; ***Irl.:*** Corgard; ***Ital.:*** Corgard; ***S.Afr.:*** Corgard; ***Spain:*** Corgard; Solgol; ***Switz.:*** Corgard; ***UK:*** Corgard; ***USA:*** Corgard.

Multi-ingredient: ***Aust.:*** Solgeretik; ***Canad.:*** Corzide; ***Ger.:*** Solgeretik†; Sotaziden N; ***Irl.:*** Corgaretic; ***S.Afr.:*** Corgaretic; ***Switz.:*** Corgaretic; ***UK:*** Corgaretic; ***USA:*** Corzide.

Nadoxolol Hydrochloride (12992-w)

Nadoxolol Hydrochloride *(rINNM)*.

LL-1530. 3-Hydroxy-4-(1-naphthyloxy)butyramide oxime hydrochloride.

$C_{14}H_{16}N_2O_3,HCl = 296.7.$

CAS — 54063-51-3 (nadoxolol); 35991-93-6 (nadoxolol hydrochloride).

Nadoxolol hydrochloride is an antiarrhythmic used in doses of 0.75 to 1.5 g daily by mouth.

Preparations

Proprietary Preparations (details are given in Part 3)
Fr.: Bradyl.

Nadroparin Calcium (4871-n)

Nadroparin Calcium *(BAN, rINN)*.

CY-216; Nadroparinum Calcicum.

Pharmacopoeias. In *Eur.* (see p.viii).

Nadroparin calcium is prepared by nitrous acid depolymerisation of heparin obtained from the intestinal mucosa of pigs. The majority of the components have a 2-*O*-sulpho-α-L-idopyranosuronic acid structure at the non-reducing end and a 6-*O*-sulpho-2,5-anhydro-D-mannitol structure at the reducing end of their chain. The mass-average molecular mass ranges between 3600 and 5000, with a characteristic value of 4300. The mass percentage of chains lower than 2000 is not more than 15%. The degree of sulphation is about 2.1 per disaccharide unit.

The Ph. Eur. specifies that potency is not less than 95 units and not more than 130 units of anti-factor Xa activity per mg with reference to the dried substance and that the ratio of anti-factor Xa activity to anti-factor IIa (antithrombin) activity is between 2.5 and 4.0.

Nadroparin calcium is a low-molecular-weight heparin (p.899) with anticoagulant properties. It is used in the treatment and prophylaxis of venous thrombo-embolism (p.802) and to prevent clotting during extracorporeal circulation.

Doses are expressed in terms of anti-factor Xa activity (anti-Xa units) although different values may be encountered in the literature depending upon the reference preparation used. For prophylaxis of venous thrombo-embolism during surgery, patients at moderate risk of thrombosis are given 2850 anti-Xa units (Ph. Eur.) or 3075 anti-Xa units (WHO standard) of nadroparin calcium by subcutaneous injection daily for at least 7 days or until the patient is ambulant; the first dose is given 2 to 4 hours before the procedure. For patients at high risk of thrombosis the dose is adjusted according to bodyweight. Usual doses are 38 anti-Xa units (Ph. Eur.) or 41 anti-Xa units (WHO standard) per kg 12 hours before surgery, 12 hours postoperatively and then daily until 3 days after the procedure; the dose is then increased by 50% to 57 anti-Xa units (Ph. Eur.) or 61 anti-Xa units (WHO standard) per kg daily. The total duration of treatment should be at least 10 days.

For the treatment of thrombo-embolism, nadroparin calcium is given in a dose of 85 anti-Xa units (Ph. Eur.) or 92 anti-Xa units (WHO standard) per kg by subcutaneous injection every 12 hours for 10 days.

For prevention of clotting in the extracorporeal circulation during haemodialysis sessions lasting less than 4 hours, nadroparin calcium is administered into the arterial line of the circuit at the beginning of the dialysis session. The usual dose is 70 anti-Xa units (WHO standard) per kg; doses expressed in anti-Xa units (Ph. Eur.) are 2850 units for patients weighing less than 50 kg, 3800 units for patients weighing 50 to 69 kg, and 5700 units for patients weighing 70 kg or more. Doses should be reduced in patients at high risk of haemorrhage.

References.

1. Barradell LB, Buckley MM. Nadroparin calcium: a review of its pharmacology and clinical applications in the prevention and treatment of thromboembolic disorders. *Drugs* 1992; **44:** 858–88.

Preparations

Proprietary Preparations (details are given in Part 3)
Austral.: Fraxiparine; ***Belg.:*** Fraxiparine; ***Fr.:*** Fraxiparine; ***Ger.:*** Fraxiparin; ***Ital.:*** Fraxiparina; Seleparina; ***Neth.:*** Fraxiparine; ***Spain:*** Fraxiparina; ***Swed.:*** Fraxiparine; ***Switz.:*** Fraxiparine.

Naftidrofuryl Oxalate (9256-a)

Naftidrofuryl Oxalate *(BANM, rINNM)*.

EU-1806; LS-121; Nafronyl Oxalate *(USAN)*. 2-Diethylaminoethyl 3-(1-naphthyl)-2-tetrahydrofurfurylpropionate hydrogen oxalate.

$C_{24}H_{33}NO_3,C_2H_2O_4 = 473.6.$

CAS — 31329-57-4 (naftidrofuryl); 3200-06-4 (naftidrofuryl oxalate).

Pharmacopoeias. In *Br.* and *Fr.*

A fine white powder with a characteristic odour. Freely **soluble** in water and in alcohol; sparingly soluble in acetone; practically insoluble in ether. **Store** in airtight containers.

Adverse Effects

Naftidrofuryl oxalate given orally may cause nausea and epigastric pain. Rash has been reported occasionally. Hepatitis or hepatic failure has occurred rarely. Convulsions may occur at high doses. Depression of cardiac conduction may occur following overdosage. Following intravenous administration cardiac arrhythmias, hypotension, and convulsions have been reported and intravenous preparations have been withdrawn from the market (see below).

In early 1995 the Committee on Safety of Medicines in the UK published details of adverse reactions to naftidrofuryl.[1] Following parenteral administration of naftidrofuryl 47 reports of 79 reactions had been received, the most serious consequences being cardiac arrhythmias (9), convulsions (3), and hypotension (2). It was also noted that two fatal cases of cardiac arrest had occurred in Germany following bolus intravenous doses and it was stressed that the drug must not be given as a bolus but as a slow intravenous infusion. Additionally, 16 reports, including one fatality, of hepatitis or hepatic failure associated with oral naftidrofuryl had been received although this appeared to be a rare reaction.

Later in 1995, following a review conducted in the UK and Europe, it was announced by the CSM that intravenous naftidrofuryl was to be withdrawn.[2] It was considered that the risks of cardiac and neurological toxicity outweighed the benefits of intravenous administration in peripheral vascular disease. The oral form of naftidrofuryl would remain available.

1. Committee on Safety of Medicines/Medicines Control Agency. Adverse reactions with naftidrofuryl (Praxilene). *Current Problems* 1995; **21:** 2.
2. Committee on Safety of Medicines/Medicines Control Agency. Withdrawal of naftidrofuryl infusion (Praxilene Forte). *Current Problems* 1995; **21:** 7.

Effects on the kidneys. Calcium oxalate crystals in the renal tubules of 2 patients with acute renal failure[1] were associated with the high amounts of oxalate they had received when naftidrofuryl oxalate was administered intravenously.

1. Moesch C, *et al.* Renal intratubular crystallisation of calcium oxalate and naftidrofuryl oxalate. *Lancet* 1991; **338:** 1219–20.

Effects on the liver. Severe hepatitis was associated with naftidrofuryl therapy in a 60-year-old patient.[1] Liver function tests had returned to normal one year after naftidrofuryl was discontinued.

1. de Caestecker JS, Heading RC. Naftidrofuryl-induced acute hepatic necrosis. *Postgrad Med J* 1986; **62:** 309–10.

Uses and Administration

Naftidrofuryl oxalate is used as a vasodilator in the treatment of peripheral (p.794) and cerebral vascular disorders (p.785). It is also claimed to enhance cellular oxidative capacity thereby protecting cells against the results of ischaemia.

Naftidrofuryl oxalate is given by mouth in usual doses of 100 to 200 mg three times daily for peripheral vascular disorders and 100 mg three times daily for cerebrovascular disorders.

Naftidrofuryl oxalate has also been administered parenterally. However, intravenous administration has been associated with serious adverse effects (see above) and intravenous preparations have been withdrawn.

Cramp. Quinine is traditionally the standard treatment for nocturnal cramp (see under Muscle Spasm, p.1303) but because of concern about efficacy and potential for adverse effects, several other drugs have been investigated for this condition. One small study[1] involving 14 patients found a modified-release preparation containing the equivalent of naftidrofuryl oxalate 300 mg twice daily reduced cramp frequency and increased cramp-free days. The precise mode of action by which naftidrofuryl exerted its beneficial effect was not known.

1. Young JB, Connolly MJ. Naftidrofuryl treatment for rest cramp. *Postgrad Med J* 1993; **69:** 624–6.

Stroke. Naftidrofuryl is one of many drugs (sometimes referred to as neuroprotectants) that have been tried in acute ischaemic stroke (p.799). It is believed to act on cerebral intracellular metabolism protecting the cells against the results of ischaemia. Results of a double-blind placebo-controlled study of naftidrofuryl in 91 patients with acute stroke indicated that the extent of recovery was greater following 12 weeks of treatment with oral naftidrofuryl and patients were able to leave hospital on average 25 days sooner than patients taking placebo.[1] A placebo-controlled study[2] in 100 patients with acute stroke given naftidrofuryl initially by intravenous infusion [preparation no longer available] for 10 days followed by 9 months of oral treatment, showed no effect on death rate but an improvement was seen in neurological recovery.

1. Admani AK. New approach to treatment of recent stroke. *Br Med J* 1978; **2:** 1678–9.
2. Steiner TJ, Rose FC. Towards a model stroke trial: the single-centre naftidrofuryl study. *Neuroepidemiology* 1986; **5:** 121–47.

Preparations

BP 1998: Naftidrofuryl Capsules.

Proprietary Preparations (details are given in Part 3)
Aust.: Dusodril; Naftodril; ***Belg.:*** Praxilene; ***Fr.:*** Di-Actane; Gevatran; Naftilux; Praxilene; ***Ger.:*** Artocoron; Azunaftil; Dusodril; Luctor; Nafti; Nafti-ratiopharm; Naftilong; ***Irl.:*** Praxilene; Vasolate†; ***Ital.:*** Esedril; Praxilene; ***Spain:*** Praxilene; ***Switz.:*** Praxilene; Sodipryl retard; ***UK:*** Praxilene; Stimlor.

Multi-ingredient: ***Ger.:*** Card-Dusodril†.

Naftopidil (2756-v)

Naftopidil *(rINN)*.

BM-15275; KT-611. (±)-4-(o-Methoxyphenyl)-α-[(1-naphthyloxy)methyl]-1-piperazineethanol.

$C_{24}H_{28}N_2O_3 = 392.5.$

CAS — 57149-07-2.

Naftopidil is a peripheral $alpha_1$-adrenoceptor antagonist which is structurally related to urapidil (p.959) and has similar general properties. It is under investigation in the management of hypertension.

Nasaruplase (17099-r)

Nasaruplase *(rINN)*.

Prourokinase (enzyme-activating) (human clone pA3/pD2/pF1 protein moiety), glycosylated.

CAS — 99821-44-0.

Nasaruplase is a thrombolytic.

Nebivolol Hydrochloride (2966-z)

Nebivolol Hydrochloride *(BANM, rINNM)*.

R-67555; R-65824 (nebivolol). (1*RS*,1′*RS*)-1,1′-[(2*RS*,2′*SR*)-Bis(6-fluorochroman-2-yl)]-2,2′-iminodiethanol hydrochloride.

$C_{22}H_{25}F_2NO_4,HCl = 441.9.$

CAS — 99200-09-6 (nebivolol).

NOTE. Nebivolol is *USAN*.

Nebivolol is a cardioselective beta blocker (p.828). It is also reported to have vasodilating activity but to lack intrinsic sympathomimetic activity. Nebivolol is used in the management of hypertension (p.788). It is given by mouth as the hydrochloride although doses are expressed in terms of the base. The usual dose is 5 mg daily.

References.

1. Fitzgerald JD, ed. First international nebivolol investigators' meeting. *Drug Invest* 1991; **3** (suppl 1): 1–203.
2. Lacourcière Y, *et al.* Comparative effects of a new cardioselective beta-blocker nebivolol and nifedipine sustained-release on 24-hour ambulatory blood pressure and plasma lipoproteins. *J Clin Pharmacol* 1992; **32:** 660–6.
3. Goldstein M, *et al.* Administration of nebivolol after coronary artery bypass in patients with altered left ventricular function. *J Cardiovasc Pharmacol* 1993; **22:** 253–8.

Preparations

Proprietary Preparations (details are given in Part 3)
Aust.: Nebilet; ***Ger.:*** Nebilet; ***Neth.:*** Nebilet.

Nicardipine Hydrochloride (13008-c)

Nicardipine Hydrochloride *(BANM, USAN, rINNM).*

RS-69216; RS-69216-XX-07-0; YC-93. 2-[Benzyl(methyl)amino]ethyl methyl 1,4-dihydro-2,6-dimethyl-4-(3-nitrophenyl)pyridine-3,5-dicarboxylate hydrochloride.

$C_{26}H_{29}N_3O_6,HCl = 516.0.$

CAS — 55985-32-5 (nicardipine); 54527-84-3 (nicardipine hydrochloride).

Pharmacopoeias. In *Jpn.*

Incompatibilities. The manufacturers recommend that a solution containing nicardipine hydrochloride 0.1 mg per mL is used for intravenous infusion. Suitable diluents are solutions of glucose or sodium chloride; sodium bicarbonate and lactated Ringer's are incompatible with nicardipine infusion.

Adverse Effects, Treatment, and Precautions

As for dihydropyridine calcium-channel blockers (see Nifedipine, p.916).

Interactions

As for dihydropyridine calcium-channel blockers (see Nifedipine, p.918).

Pharmacokinetics

Nicardipine is rapidly absorbed from the gastro-intestinal tract but is subject to saturable first-pass hepatic metabolism. Bioavailability of about 35% has been reported following a 30-mg dose at steady state. The pharmacokinetics of nicardipine are non-linear due to the saturable first-pass hepatic metabolism and an increase in dose may produce a disproportionate increase in plasma concentration. There is also considerable interindividual variation in plasma-nicardipine concentrations. Nicardipine is highly bound to plasma proteins (more than 95%). Nicardipine is extensively metabolised in the liver and is excreted in the urine and faeces, mainly as inactive metabolites. The terminal plasma half-life is about 8.6 hours, thus steady-state plasma concentrations are achieved after 2 to 3 days of dosing three times a day.

References.

1. Graham DJM, *et al.* Pharmacokinetics of nicardipine following oral and intravenous administration in man. *Postgrad Med J* 1984; **60** (suppl 4): 7–10.
2. Graham DJM, *et al.* The metabolism and pharmacokinetics of nicardipine hydrochloride in man. *Br J Clin Pharmacol* 1985; **20:** 23S–8S.
3. Porchet HC, Dayer P. Serum concentrations and effects of (±)-nicardipine compared with nifedipine in a population of healthy subjects. *Clin Pharmacol Ther* 1990; **48:** 155–60.

Uses and Administration

Nicardipine hydrochloride is a dihydropyridine calcium-channel blocker with actions and uses similar to nifedipine (p.919). It is used in the management of hypertension (p.788) and angina pectoris (p.780).

Nicardipine hydrochloride is generally given by mouth although the intravenous route has been employed for the short-term treatment of hypertension.

Oral doses of nicardipine hydrochloride are similar for both **hypertension** and **angina**. An initial dose of 20 mg by mouth three times a day is recommended. The dose may be increased at intervals of 3 days until the required effect is achieved. The effective dose range is between 60 and 120 mg per day, the usual dose being 30 mg three times a day; in hypertensive patients a maintenance dose of 30 or 40 mg twice daily may be possible. Modified-release preparations of nicardipine hydrochloride for administration twice daily are also available.

Nicardipine hydrochloride may be administered by slow intravenous infusion as a 0.1 mg per mL solution in the short-term treatment of hypertension. An initial infusion rate of 5 mg per hour is recommended, increased, as necessary, up to a maximum of 15 mg per hour and subsequently reduced to 3 mg per hour.

Reduced doses of nicardipine hydrochloride and longer dosing intervals may be necessary in patients with impaired liver function.

General reviews.

1. Sorkin EM, Clissold SP. Nicardipine: a review of its pharmacodynamic and pharmacokinetic properties, and therapeutic efficacy, in the treatment of angina pectoris, hypertension and related cardiovascular disorders. *Drugs* 1987; **33:** 296–345.
2. Frishman WH. New therapeutic modalities in hypertension: focus on a new calcium antagonist—nicardipine. *J Clin Pharmacol* 1989; **29:** 481–7.
3. Anonymous. Nicardipine: another calcium antagonist. *Drug Ther Bull* 1989; **27:** 89–90.

Administration in neonates. Intravenous infusion of nicardipine was used successfully in 8 preterm infants (gestational age 28 to 36 weeks) for the management of hypertension.[1] Infusions were continued for periods of 3 to 36 days. No hypotension, oedema, or tachycardia were observed.

1. Gouyon JB, *et al.* Intravenous nicardipine in hypertensive preterm infants. *Arch Dis Child* 1997; **76:** F126–F127.

Cerebrovascular disorders. Nicardipine has been reported to increase cerebral blood flow[1] and has been investigated for possible benefit in haemorrhagic and ischaemic stroke[2,3] (p.799), although nimodipine (p.922) is the dihydropyridine calcium-channel blocker usually used. Nicardipine has also been tried[4] in patients with cerebrovascular insufficiency. However, studies have produced inconclusive results.

1. Savage I, James I. The effect of nicardipine hydrochloride on cerebral blood flow in normotensive volunteers. *Br J Clin Pharmacol* 1986; **21:** 591P–2P.
2. Rosenbaum D, *et al.* Early treatment of ischemic stroke with a calcium antagonist. *Stroke* 1991; **22:** 437–41.
3. Yao L, Ding D. Effect of nicardipine on somatosensory evoked potentials in patients with acute cerebral infarction. *J Neurol Neurosurg Psychiatry* 1990; **53:** 844–6.
4. Silva APE, Diament CK. Nicardipine versus cinnarizine in cerebrovascular insufficiency. *Curr Ther Res* 1988; **43:** 888–99.

Renal transplantation. Like other calcium-channel blockers nicardipine increases blood-cyclosporin concentrations when the 2 drugs are given concurrently.[1,2] However, in contrast to reports of benefit from the concurrent use of nifedipine and cyclosporin (p.922), Kessler and colleagues did not note any improvement in renal function when nicardipine and cyclosporin were given together in renal transplant patients.[2]

1. Todd P, *et al.* Nicardipine interacts with cyclosporin. *Br J Dermatol* 1989; **121:** 820.
2. Kessler M, *et al.* Influence of nicardipine on renal function and plasma cyclosporin in renal transplant patients. *Eur J Clin Pharmacol* 1989; **36:** 637–8.

Preparations

Proprietary Preparations (details are given in Part 3)
Aust.: Karden; ***Belg.:*** Rydene; ***Canad.:*** Cardene; ***Fr.:*** Loxen; ***Ger.:*** Antagonil; ***Irl.:*** Cardene; ***Ital.:*** Bionicard; Cardioten; Cardip; Cordipina; Farnic†; Lisanirc; Neucor; Nicant; Nicapress; Nicardal; Nicardium; Nicarpin; Nimicor; Niven; Perdipina; Ranvil; Vasodin; ***Jpn:*** Perdipine; ***Neth.:*** Cardene; ***Spain:*** Dagan; Flusemide; Lecibral; Lincil; Lucenfal; Nerdipina; Vasonase; Vatrasin; ***UK:*** Cardene; ***USA:*** Cardene.

Niceritrol (9258-x)

Niceritrol *(BAN, rINN).*

PETN. Pentaerythritol tetranicotinate; 2,2-Bis(hydroxymethyl)propane-1,3-diol tetranicotinate.

$C_{29}H_{24}N_4O_8 = 556.5.$

CAS — 5868-05-3.

NOTE. The synonym PETN has been applied to both niceritrol and pentaerythritol tetranitrate.

Pharmacopoeias. In *Jpn.*

Niceritrol, an ester of pentaerythritol and nicotinic acid, has general properties similar to those of nicotinic acid (p.1351), to which it is slowly hydrolysed. Niceritrol is used as a lipid regulating drug in hyperlipidaemias (p.1265) in initial doses of 250 mg three times daily by mouth, gradually increased to 1 g three times daily.

It has also been used as a vasodilator in the treatment of peripheral vascular disorders (p.794).

References.

1. Curtis LD, *et al.* Clinical and laboratory responses to niceritrol in the treatment of hypercholesterolaemia. *Postgrad Med J* 1988; **64:** 672–5.
2. Seo H, *et al.* Effect of niceritrol on the glucose metabolism in type II diabetes mellitus associated with hyperlipidemia. *Curr Ther Res* 1988; **44:** 189–99.

Preparations

Proprietary Preparations (details are given in Part 3)
Spain: Perycit†; ***Swed.:*** Perycit.

Nicofuranose (9259-r)

Nicofuranose *(BAN, rINN).*

ES-304; Tetranicotinoylfructofuranose; Tetranicotinoylfructose. β-D-Fructofuranose 1,3,4,6-tetranicotinate.

$C_{30}H_{24}N_4O_{10} = 600.5.$

CAS — 15351-13-0.

Nicofuranose is a vasodilator and lipid regulating drug with general properties similar to those of nicotinic acid (p.1351), to which it is slowly hydrolysed. It has been given in the management of peripheral vascular disorders and hyperlipidaemias.

Preparations

Proprietary Preparations (details are given in Part 3)
Irl.: Bradilan†; ***UK:*** Bradilan†.

Nicorandil (16912-m)

Nicorandil *(BAN, USAN, rINN).*

SG-75. *N*-[2-(Nitroxy)ethyl]-3-pyridinecarboxamide.

$C_8H_9N_3O_4 = 211.2.$

CAS — 65141-46-0.

Adverse Effects and Precautions

Adverse effects reported with nicorandil are headache which is usually transitory and occurring at the start of therapy, cutaneous vasodilatation and flushing, nausea, vomiting, dizziness, and weakness. A reduction in blood pressure and/or an increase in heart rate may occur with high doses.

Nicorandil is contra-indicated in patients with cardiogenic shock, left ventricular failure with low filling pressures, and hypotension. It should be avoided, or used only with caution, in patients with hypovolaemia, low systolic blood pressure, or acute pulmonary oedema.

Oral ulceration. Painful, large aphthous ulcers on the tongue and oral mucosa have been reported[1,2] in patients receiving nicorandil for angina. The ulcers were resistant to treatment but healed when nicorandil was withdrawn.

1. Cribier B, *et al.* Chronic buccal ulceration induced by nicorandil. *Br J Dermatol* 1998; **138:** 372–3.
2. Desruelles F, *et al.* Giant oral aphthous ulcers induced by nicorandil. *Br J Dermatol* 1998; **138:** 712–13.

Pharmacokinetics

Nicorandil is absorbed from the gastro-intestinal tract and maximum plasma concentrations are achieved 30 to 60 minutes after administration by mouth. Metabolism is mainly by denitration and approximately 20% of an administered dose is excreted in the urine mainly as metabolites. The elimination half-life is about one hour. Nicorandil is only slightly bound to plasma proteins.

Uses and Administration

Nicorandil is a nitrate derivative of nicotinamide (p.1351) and acts as a vasodilator. It is a potassium-channel opener (p.778) providing vasodilatation of arterioles and large coronary arteries and its nitrate component produces venous vasodilatation through stimulation of guanylate cyclase. It is used in angina pectoris (p.780). The usual initial dose by mouth is 10 mg twice daily (or 5 mg twice daily in patients susceptible to headache), increased as necessary to a maximum of 30 mg twice daily; the usual therapeutic dose is in the range of 10 to 20 mg twice daily.

References.

1. Frampton J, *et al.* Nicorandil: a review of its pharmacology and therapeutic efficacy in angina pectoris. *Drugs* 1992; **44:** 625–55.
2. Anonymous. Nicorandil for angina. *Drug Ther Bull* 1995; **33:** 89–92.
3. Goldschmidt M, *et al.* Nicorandil: a potassium channel opening drug for treatment of ischemic heart disease. *J Clin Pharmacol* 1996; **36:** 559–72.

Preparations

Proprietary Preparations (details are given in Part 3)
Aust.: Dancor; ***Fr.:*** Adancor; Ikorel; ***Jpn:*** Sigmart; ***Neth.:*** Dancor†; Ikorel; ***Switz.:*** Dancor; ***UK:*** Ikorel.

Nicotinyl Alcohol (9261-z)

Nicotinyl Alcohol *(BAN, USAN).*

3-Hydroxymethylpyridine; Nicotinic Alcohol; NSC-526046; NU-2121; 3-Pyridinemethanol; β-Pyridylcarbinol; Ro-1-5155. 3-Pyridylmethanol.

$C_6H_7NO = 109.1.$

CAS — 100-55-0.

Nicotinyl Alcohol Tartrate (9262-c)

Nicotinyl Alcohol Tartrate *(BANM).*

Nicotinyl Tartrate. 3-Pyridylmethanol hydrogen tartrate; 3-Pyridylmethanol hydrogen (2*R*,3*R*)-tartrate.

$C_6H_7NO,C_4H_6O_6 = 259.2.$

CAS — 6164-87-0.

Pharmacopoeias. In *Br.*

A white or almost white odourless or almost odourless crystalline powder. Nicotinyl alcohol tartrate 2.4 g is approximately equivalent to 1 g of nicotinyl alcohol. Freely **soluble** in water; slightly soluble in alcohol; practically insoluble in chloroform and in ether. A 5% solution in water has a pH of 2.8 to 3.7.

Adverse Effects and Precautions

Nicotinyl alcohol may cause flushing of the skin of the face and neck, dizziness, faintness, nausea and vomiting, and hypotension. Skin rashes and urticaria have been reported. Glucose tolerance may be impaired particularly at higher doses, and abnormal liver function tests indicating hepatotoxicity have been reported when high doses are used for long periods.

It should be used with care in diabetic or pre-diabetic patients.

Effects on the liver. A report of hepatic lesions in 2 patients following long-term administration of nicotinyl alcohol (1.35 to 1.5 g per day).[1]

1. Keller C, *et al.* Unusual but reversible hepatic lesions following long-term treatment with pyridylcarbinol for familial hypercholesterolemia. *Klin Wochenschr* 1988; **66:** 647–50.

Uses and Administration

Nicotinyl alcohol is a vasodilator and lipid regulating drug with general properties similar to those of nicotinic acid (p.1352), to which it is partly hydrolysed.

Nicotinyl alcohol tartrate is given by mouth in the management of peripheral vascular disorders (p.794) in usual doses equivalent to 25 to 50 mg of nicotinyl alcohol 4 times daily or as a modified-release preparation in doses equivalent to 150 to 300 mg of nicotinyl alcohol twice daily.

Nicotinyl alcohol tartrate is also used in Ménière's disease and in hyperlipidaemias.

Preparations

BP 1998: Nicotinyl Alcohol Tablets.

Proprietary Preparations (details are given in Part 3)

Canad.: Roniacol Supraspan†; ***Ger.:*** Radecol; Ronicol†; ***Irl.:*** Ronicol†; ***Ital.:*** Ronicol†; Selcarbinol†; ***Neth.:*** Ronicol†; ***Swed.:*** Ronicol†; ***Switz.:*** Ronicol†; ***UK:*** Ronicol.

Multi-ingredient: ***Aust.:*** Thilocombin; ***Ger.:*** Lipofacton†; LP-Truw†; ***S.Afr.:*** Lipaten; ***Switz.:*** Liaptene†.

Nicoumalone (4817-a)

Nicoumalone *(BAN)*.

Acenocoumarol *(rINN)*; Acenocumarin; G-23350. 4-Hydroxy-3-[1-(4-nitrophenyl)-3-oxobutyl]coumarin.

$C_{19}H_{15}NO_6$ = 353.3.

CAS — 152-72-7.

Pharmacopoeias. In Br.

An almost white to buff-coloured odourless or almost odourless powder. Practically **insoluble** in water and in ether; slightly soluble in alcohol and in chloroform; dissolves in aqueous solutions of alkali hydroxides.

Adverse Effects, Treatment, and Precautions

As for Warfarin Sodium, p.964.

Interactions

The interactions associated with oral anticoagulants are discussed in detail under warfarin (p.965). Specific references to interactions involving nicoumalone can be found there under the headings for the following drug groups: analgesics; antiarrhythmics; antibacterials; antifungals; antigout drugs; antihistamines; antineoplastics; antiplatelets; diuretics; gastro-intestinal drugs; lipid regulating drugs; prostaglandins; sex hormones; and vaccines.

Pharmacokinetics

Nicoumalone is readily absorbed from the gastro-intestinal tract and is excreted chiefly in the urine mainly as metabolites. Nicoumalone is extensively bound to plasma proteins. Figures reported for elimination half-life vary; 8 to 11 hours appears a reasonable range. Nicoumalone crosses the placenta; only small quantities have been detected in breast milk. Nicoumalone is administered as a racemic mixture; the *R*-isomer is reported to be more potent. The stereo-isomers have different pharmacokinetics.

Uses and Administration

Nicoumalone is an orally administered coumarin anticoagulant with actions similar to those of warfarin sodium (p.969). It is used in the management of thrombo-embolic disorders (p.801). The usual dose on the first day is 8 to 12 mg, on the second day 4 to 8 mg; subsequent maintenance doses range from 1 to 8 mg depending on the response. Nicoumalone is given in a single dose at the same time every day.

Preparations

BP 1998: Acenocoumarol Tablets.

Proprietary Preparations (details are given in Part 3)

Aust.: Sintrom; ***Belg.:*** Sintrom; ***Canad.:*** Sintrom; ***Fr.:*** Mini-sintrom; Sintrom; ***Ger.:*** Sintrom†; ***Irl.:*** Sinthrome†; ***Ital.:*** Sintrom; ***Neth.:*** Sintrom Mitis; ***Spain:*** Sintrom; ***Switz.:*** Sintrom; ***UK:*** Sinthrome.

Nifedipine (9263-k)

Nifedipine *(BAN, USAN, rINN)*.

Bay-a-1040; Nifedipina; Nifedipinum. Dimethyl 1,4-dihydro-2,6-dimethyl-4-(2-nitrophenyl)pyridine-3,5-dicarboxylate.

$C_{17}H_{18}N_2O_6$ = 346.3.

CAS — 21829-25-4.

Pharmacopoeias. In *Chin., Eur.* (see p.viii), *Jpn,* and *US.*

A yellow crystalline powder. Practically **insoluble** in water; soluble 1 in 10 of acetone; sparingly soluble in absolute alcohol. When exposed to daylight or to certain wavelengths of artificial light it is converted to a nitrosophenylpyridine derivative, while exposure to ultraviolet light leads to formation of a nitrophenylpyridine derivative. Solutions should be prepared in the dark or under light of wavelength greater than 420 nm, immediately before use.

Store in airtight containers. Protect from light.

Mention of the use of yellow food colourings such as curcumin to slow photodegradation of nifedipine solutions.[1]

1. Thoma K, Klimek R. Photostabilization of drugs in dosage forms without protection from packaging materials. *Int J Pharmaceutics* 1991; **67:** 169–75.

Adverse Effects

The most common adverse effects of nifedipine are associated with its vasodilatory action and often diminish on continued therapy. They include dizziness, flushing, headache, hypotension, peripheral oedema, tachycardia, and palpitations. Nausea and other gastro-intestinal disturbances, increased micturition frequency, lethargy, eye pain, and mental depression have also occurred. A paradoxical increase in ischaemic chest pain may occur at the start of treatment and in a few patients excessive fall in blood pressure has led to cerebral or myocardial ischaemia or transient blindness.

There have been reports of rashes (including erythema multiforme), fever, and abnormalities in liver function due to hypersensitivity reactions. Gingival hyperplasia has been reported.

Overdosage may be associated with bradycardia and hypotension.

Nifedipine has been reported to be teratogenic in *animals.*

Since 1995 there have been reports and reviews that have implicated calcium-channel blockers (particularly short-acting nifedipine and high doses) in increasing cardiovascular[1] and overall mortality[2] and risks of cancer and haemorrhage. Other safety concerns include links with depression and suicide. In response, the US National Heart, Lung, and Blood Institute issued a statement warning that short-acting nifedipine should be used with great caution (if at all), especially at higher doses, in the treatment of hypertension, angina, and myocardial infarction,[3] and in some countries short-acting nifedipine preparations have been withdrawn. However, there has been much debate and controversy over the reports that questioned the safety of calcium-channel blockers.[4-6]

A review by the WHO/ISH pointed out that much of the evidence for adverse effects comes from observational studies or small randomised studies and concluded that, as there was insufficient evidence to confirm either benefit or harm, current recommendations on the management of angina, hypertension, and myocardial infarction should remain unchanged.[7] In addition, many of the studies that have led to the negative reports employed the older short-acting calcium-channel blockers. The calcium-channel blockers used now are largely modified-release formulations of short half-life blockers or are calcium-channel blockers with long half-lives.

Since the WHO/ISH review was published, a placebo-controlled study investigating the effects of calcium-channel blockers on cardiovascular events (SYST-EUR) has been reported.[8] A reduction in incidence of stroke and cardiovascular events was found in 4695 elderly patients treated with nitrendipine (and enalapril and hydrochlorothiazide in addition if necessary) for isolated systolic hypertension. Two further large long-term randomised studies in hypertension are underway—the Antihypertensive and Lipid Lowering treatment to prevent Heart Attack Trial (ALLHAT) and the Anglo-Scandinavian Coronary Outcomes Trial (ASCOT)—that should clarify the effects of calcium-channel blockers on morbidity and mortality.

1. Psaty BM, *et al.* The risk of myocardial infarction associated with antihypertensive drug therapies. *JAMA* 1995; **274:** 620–5.
2. Furberg CD, *et al.* Nifedipine: dose-related increase in mortality in patients with coronary heart disease. *Circulation* 1995; **92:** 1326–31.
3. McCarthy M. US NIH issues warning on nifedipine. *Lancet* 1995; **346:** 689–90.
4. Opie LH, Messerli FH. Nifedipine and mortality: grave defects in the dossier. *Circulation* 1995; **92:** 1068–72.
5. Grossman E, Messerli FH. Calcium antagonists in cardiovascular disease: a necessary controversy but an unnecessary panic. *Am J Med* 1997; **102:** 147–9.
6. Stanton AV. Calcium channel blockers. *Br Med J* 1998; **316:** 1471–3.
7. Ad Hoc Subcommittee of the Liaison Committee of the World Health Organisation and the International Society of Hypertension. Effects of calcium antagonists on the risks of coronary heart disease, cancer and bleeding. *J Hypertens* 1997; **15:** 105–15.
8. Staessen JA, *et al.* Randomised double-blind comparison of placebo and active treatment for older patients with isolated systolic hypertension. *Lancet* 1997; **350:** 757–64. Correction. *ibid.*; 1636.

Cancer occurrence. An observational study carried out between 1988 and 1992 suggested that calcium-channel blockers are associated with an increased risk of cancer.[1] Subsequent studies have produced conflicting results.[2-4] A review by the WHO/ISH concluded that there is no good evidence that calcium-channel blockers increase cancer risk.[5] Long-term morbidity and mortality studies are currently underway that should yield further information.[6]

1. Pahor M, *et al.* Calcium-channel blockade and incidence of cancer in aged populations. *Lancet* 1996; **348:** 493–7.
2. Jick H, *et al.* Calcium-channel blockers and risk of cancer. *Lancet* 1997; **349:** 525–8.
3. Rosenberg L, *et al.* Calcium channel blockers and the risk of cancer. *JAMA* 1998; **279:** 1000–4.
4. Braun S, *et al.* Calcium channel blocking agents and risk of cancer in patients with coronary heart disease. *J Am Coll Cardiol* 1998; **31:** 804–8.
5. *Ad Hoc* Subcommittee of the Liaison Committee of the World Health Organisation and the International Society of Hypertension. Effects of calcium antagonists on the risks of coronary heart disease, cancer and bleeding. *J Hypertens* 1997; **15:** 105–15.
6. Howes LG, Edwards CT. Calcium antagonists and cancer: is there really a link? *Drug Safety* 1998; **18:** 1–7.

Effects on the blood. Treatment with nifedipine significantly reduces the ability of platelets to aggregate *in vitro*[1] and results indicating inhibition of platelet function in healthy subjects receiving oral (but not intravenous) nifedipine have been reported.[2,3] Thus, concern has been expressed[4] that calcium-channel blockers may have the potential to produce haemorrhagic complications in surgical patients (specifically, those undergoing coronary bypass surgery). Major surgical bleeding was associated with nimodipine in patients undergoing cardiac valve replacement,[5] although it has been used in other situations apparently without an increased risk of bleeding.[6] A prospective cohort study in 1636 elderly hypertensive patients[7] reported that calcium-channel blockers were associated with an increased risk of gastro-intestinal haemorrhage compared with beta blockers. However, a review instigated by the WHO/ISH[8] (International Society of Hypertension) concluded that although it is not possible to rule out modest effects on bleeding calcium-channel blockers do not seem to be associated with large haemorrhagic risk.

1. Ośmiałwska Z, *et al.* Effect of nifedipine monotherapy on platelet aggregation in patients with untreated essential hypertension. *Eur J Clin Pharmacol* 1990; **39:** 403–4.
2. Winther K, *et al.* Dose-dependent effects of verapamil and nifedipine on in vivo platelet function in normal volunteers. *Eur J Clin Pharmacol* 1990; **39:** 291–3.
3. Walley TJ, *et al.* The effects of intravenous and oral nifedipine on ex vivo platelet function. *Eur J Clin Pharmacol* 1989; **37:** 449–52.
4. Becker RC, Alpert JS. The impact of medical therapy on hemorrhagic complications following coronary artery bypass grafting. *Arch Intern Med* 1990; **150:** 2016–21.
5. Wagenknecht LE, *et al.* Surgical bleeding: unexpected effect of a calcium antagonist. *Br Med J* 1995; **310:** 776–7.
6. Öhman J and others. Surgical bleeding and calcium antagonists. *Br Med J* 1995; **311:** 388–9. (Several letters.)
7. Pahor M, *et al.* Risk of gastrointestinal haemorrhage with calcium antagonists in hypertensive persons over 67 years old. *Lancet* 1996; **347:** 1061–5.
8. Ad Hoc Subcommittee of the Liaison Committee of the World Health Organisation and the International Society of Hypertension. Effects of calcium antagonists on the risks of coronary heart disease, cancer and bleeding. *J Hypertens* 1997; **15:** 105–15.

Effects on the brain. Cerebral ischaemia[1,2] has been reported in small numbers of patients given nifedipine.

1. Nobile-Orazio E, Sterzi R. Cerebral ischaemia after nifedipine treatment. *Br Med J* 1981; **283:** 948.
2. Schwartz M, *et al.* Oral nifedipine in the treatment of hypertensive urgency: cerebrovascular accident following a single dose. *Arch Intern Med* 1990; **150:** 686–7.

Effects on carbohydrate metabolism. There are reports of deterioration of diabetes,[1] reduction in glucose tolerance,[2] and development of diabetes[1,3] in patients receiving treatment with nifedipine. Nifedipine has also been reported to increase plasma-glucose concentrations.[3,4] However, other reports and studies have found no change in glucose tolerance in either diabetic or non-diabetic patients taking nifedipine.[5-10]

See also Diabetes Mellitus under Precautions, below.

1. Bhatnagar SK, *et al.* Diabetogenic effects of nifedipine. *Br Med J* 1984; **289:** 19.
2. Giugliano D, *et al.* Impairment of insulin secretion in man by nifedipine. *Eur J Clin Pharmacol* 1980; **18:** 395–8.
3. Zezulka AV, *et al.* Diabetogenic effects of nifedipine. *Br Med J* 1984; **289:** 437–8.
4. Charles S, *et al.* Hyperglycaemic effect of nifedipine. *Br Med J* 1981; **283:** 19–20.

5. Harrower ADB, Donnelly T. Hyperglycaemic effect of nifedipine. *Br Med J* 1981; **283:** 796.
6. Greenwood RH. Hyperglycaemic effect of nifedipine. *Br Med J* 1982; **284:** 50.
7. Abadie E, Passa P. Diabetogenic effects of nifedipine. *Br Med J* 1984; **289:** 438.
8. Antonelli D. Nifedipine and fasting glycemia. *Ann Intern Med* 1985; **104:** 125–6.
9. Whitcroft I, *et al.* Calcium antagonists do not impair long-term glucose control in hypertensive non-insulin dependent diabetics (NIDDS). *Br J Clin Pharmacol* 1986; **22:** 208P.
10. Tentorio A, *et al.* Insulin secretion and glucose tolerance in non-insulin dependent diabetic patients after chronic nifedipine treatment. *Eur J Clin Pharmacol* 1989; **36:** 311–13.

Effects on the ears. There have been isolated reports[1] of tinnitus associated with several calcium-channel blockers including nifedipine, nicardipine, nitrendipine, diltiazem, verapamil, and cinnarizine.

1. Narváez M, *et al.* Tinnitus with calcium-channel blockers. *Lancet* 1994; **343:** 1229–30.

Effects on the eyes. Individual reports have implicated nifedipine in the development of transient retinal ischaemia and blindness,[1] and of periorbital oedema.[2] In a postmarketing survey painful or stinging eyes were more common in patients receiving nifedipine (178 of 757 evaluable) than in those given captopril (45 of 289), although the cause was uncertain.[3] Nifedipine has also been suggested as a risk factor in the development of cataract,[4,5] but the numbers involved in this analysis are small[6] and it is possible that the risk, if it exists,[7] relates to hypertension rather than nifedipine treatment.[6]

1. Pitlik S, *et al.* Transient retinal ischaemia induced by nifedipine. *Br Med J* 1983; **287:** 1845–6.
2. Silverstone PH. Periorbital oedema caused by nifedipine. *Br Med J* 1984; **288:** 1654.
3. Coulter DM. Eye pain with nifedipine and disturbance of taste with captopril: a mutually controlled study showing a method of postmarketing surveillance. *Br Med J* 1988; **296:** 1086–8.
4. van Heyningen R, Harding JJ. Do aspirin-like analgesics protect against cataract? *Lancet* 1986; **i:** 1111–13.
5. Harding JJ, van Heyningen R. Drugs, including alcohol, that act as risk factors for cataract, and possible protection against cataract by aspirin-like analgesics and cyclopenthiazide. *Br J Ophthalmol* 1988; **72:** 809–14.
6. van Heyningen R, Harding JJ. Aspirin-like analgesics and cataract. *Lancet* 1986; **ii:** 283.
7. Kewitz H, *et al.* Aspirin and cataract. *Lancet* 1986; **ii:** 689.

Effects on the heart. The use of nifedipine has been associated with the development of various heart disorders in some patients. Complete heart block has been reported in an elderly patient who had previously developed heart block with verapamil,[1] and sudden circulatory collapse has been reported in 4 patients receiving nifedipine who underwent routine coronary bypass surgery.[2] One patient died despite all attempts at resuscitation.[2] However, probably the majority of reports have concerned the development or aggravation of cardiac ischaemia, up to and including frank myocardial infarction following administration of short-acting nifedipine.[3-6] Such cases appear to be chiefly associated with a too-rapid fall in blood pressure following the use of sublingual nifedipine for hypertensive urgencies or emergencies,[5,6] or occur in patients with a history of ischaemic heart disease.[3,4]

For discussion of the effects of calcium-channel blockers on cardiovascular mortality, see above.

1. Chopra DA, Maxwell RT. Complete heart block with low dose nifedipine. *Br Med J* 1984; **288:** 760.
2. Goiti JJ. Calcium channel blocking agents and the heart. *Br Med J* 1985; **291:** 1505.
3. Sia STB, *et al.* Aggravation of myocardial ischaemia by nifedipine. *Med J Aust* 1985; **142:** 48–50.
4. Boden WE, *et al.* Nifedipine-induced hypotension and myocardial ischemia in refractory angina pectoris. *JAMA* 1985; **253:** 1131–5.
5. O'Mailia JJ, *et al.* Nifedipine-associated myocardial ischemia or infarction in the treatment of hypertensive urgencies. *Ann Intern Med* 1987; **107:** 185–6.
6. Leavitt AD, Zweifler AJ. Nifedipine, hypotension, and myocardial injury. *Ann Intern Med* 1988; **108:** 305–6.

WITHDRAWAL. Exacerbation of coronary ischaemia and thrombosis of arteriovenous graft could have resulted from withdrawal of nifedipine in 1 patient.[1] Abrupt withdrawal of nisoldipine from 15 patients with stable angina pectoris after 6 weeks of therapy resulted in severe unstable angina in 2 patients and acute myocardial infarction in 1 patient.[2] It was postulated that the withdrawal effect could be due to an increase in sensitivity of vascular α_2 adrenoceptors to circulating adrenaline.

1. Mysliwiec M, *et al.* Calcium antagonist withdrawal syndrome. *Br Med J* 1983; **286:** 1898.
2. Mehta J, Lopez LM. Calcium-blocker withdrawal phenomenon: increase in affinity of alpha$_2$ adrenoceptors for agonist as a potential mechanism. *Am J Cardiol* 1986; **58:** 242–6.

Effects on the kidneys. Calcium-channel blockers may be of benefit in various forms of kidney disorder (see under Uses and Administration, below). However, reversible deterioration in renal function without any appreciable accompanying decline in systemic arterial blood pressure has been reported in 4 patients with underlying renal insufficiency receiving nifedipine[1] and nifedipine has increased urinary protein excretion and exacerbated renal impairment in fourteen type 2 diabetic patients.[2]

Excessive diuresis has occurred in a patient given nifedipine for angina pectoris[3] and nocturia in 9 patients referred for prostatic surgery was also attributed to nifedipine.[4]

1. Diamond JR, *et al.* Nifedipine-induced renal dysfunction: alterations in renal hemodynamics. *Am J Med* 1984; **77:** 905–9.
2. Demarie BK, Bakris GL. Effects of different calcium antagonists on proteinuria associated with diabetes mellitus. *Ann Intern Med* 1990; **113:** 987–8.
3. Antonelli D, *et al.* Excessive nifedipine diuretic effect. *Br Med J* 1984; **288:** 760.
4. Williams G, Donaldson RM. Nifedipine and nocturia. *Lancet* 1986; **i:** 738.

Effects on the liver. A number of cases of hepatitis, apparently due to a hypersensitivity reaction, and frequently accompanied by fever, sweating, chills, rigor, and arthritic symptoms, have been reported in patients receiving nifedipine.[1-4]

1. Rotmensch HH, *et al.* Lymphocyte sensitisation in nifedipine-induced hepatitis. *Br Med J* 1980; **281:** 976–7.
2. Davidson AR. Lymphocyte sensitisation in nifedipine-induced hepatitis. *Br Med J* 1980; **281:** 1354.
3. Abramson M, Littlejohn GO. Hepatic reactions to nifedipine. *Med J Aust* 1985; **142:** 47–8.
4. Shaw DR, *et al.* Nifedipine hepatitis. *Aust N Z J Med* 1987; **17:** 447–8.

Effects on the menstrual cycle. Menorrhagia in 2 women[1] and menstrual irregularity with heavy bleeding in another[2] have been reported in association with nifedipine treatment.

1. Rodger JC, Torrance TC. Can nifedipine provoke menorrhagia? *Lancet* 1983; **ii:** 460.
2. Singh G, *et al.* Can nifedipine provoke menorrhagia? *Lancet* 1983; **ii:** 1022.

Effects on mental function. Insomnia, hyperexcitability, pacing, agitation, and depression were reported[1] in a patient in association with nifedipine therapy. The symptoms disappeared within 2 days of withdrawal of nifedipine. Four further cases of major depression, that developed within a week of commencing nifedipine and resolved within a week of discontinuing the drug have been reported.[2]

Recently, 2 epidemiological studies suggested that calcium-channel blockers may promote suicide.[3]

1. Ahmad S. Nifedipine-induced acute psychosis. *J Am Geriatr Soc* 1984; **32:** 408.
2. Hullett FJ, *et al.* Depression associated with nifedipine-induced calcium channel blockade. *Am J Psychiatry* 1988; **145:** 1277–9.
3. Lindberg G, *et al.* Use of calcium channel blockers and risk of suicide: ecological findings confirmed in population based cohort study. *Br Med J* 1998; **316:** 741–5.

Effects on the mouth. GINGIVAL HYPERPLASIA. A number of reports have implicated nifedipine in the development of gingival hyperplasia.[1-4] In most cases it has occurred about 1 to 6 months after starting therapy and has resolved following withdrawal of nifedipine. A patient who had taken nifedipine for 12 years developed gingival hyperplasia shortly after the dosage of nifedipine was increased.[5] Amlodipine has also induced gingival overgrowth.[6] A study involving 115 patients who had received nifedipine, diltiazem, or verapamil for at least 3 months indicated that gingival hyperplasia is an important side-effect that may occur with calcium-channel blockers in general.[7]

1. Ramon Y, *et al.* Gingival hyperplasia caused by nifedipine—a preliminary report. *Int J Cardiol* 1984; **5:** 195–204.
2. van der Wall EE, *et al.* Gingival hyperplasia induced by nifedipine, an arterial vasodilating drug. *Oral Surg* 1985; **60:** 38–40.
3. Shaftic AA, *et al.* Nifedipine-induced gingival hyperplasia. *Drug Intell Clin Pharm* 1986; **20:** 602–5.
4. Jones CM. Gingival hyperplasia associated with nifedipine. *Br Dent J* 1986; **160:** 416–17.
5. Johnson RB. Nifedipine-induced gingival overgrowth. *Ann Pharmacother* 1997; **31:** 935.
6. Ellis JS, *et al.* Gingival sequestration of amlodipine and amlodipine-induced gingival overgrowth. *Lancet* 1993; **341:** 1102–3.
7. Steele RM, *et al.* Calcium antagonist-induced gingival hyperplasia. *Ann Intern Med* 1994; **120:** 663–4.

PAROTITIS. Acute swelling of the parotid glands occurred in a patient after sublingual administration of nifedipine.[1]

1. Bosch X, *et al.* Nifedipine-induced parotitis. *Lancet* 1986; **ii:** 467.

Effects on the neuromuscular system. Severe muscle cramps have been reported in a few patients taking nifedipine;[1,2] In one patient[2] the cramps were associated with widespread paraesthesia. Reversible myoclonic dystonia associated with nifedipine has been reported in one patient.[3] Severe rhabdomyolysis developed in a patient with a transplanted kidney who was receiving an intravenous infusion of nifedipine.[4] The patient recovered rapidly once the infusion was stopped.

1. Keidar S, *et al.* Muscle cramps during treatment with nifedipine. *Br Med J* 1982; **285:** 1241–2.
2. Macdonald JB. Muscle cramps during treatment with nifedipine. *Br Med J* 1982; **285:** 1744.
3. de Medina A, *et al.* Nifedipine and myoclonic dystonia. *Ann Intern Med* 1985; **104:** 125.
4. Horn S, *et al.* Severe rhabdomyolysis in a kidney-transplant recipient receiving intravenous nifedipine. *Lancet* 1995; **346:** 848–9.

Effects on the peripheral circulation. An erythromelalgia-like eruption occurred in a 44-year-old patient 8 weeks after starting therapy with nifedipine. Symptoms included severe burning pain and swelling in the feet and lower legs, which were fiery red, tender, and warm to the touch. Symptoms resolved in 2 days when nifedipine was discontinued.[1] Similar effects have been reported in other patients on nifedipine.[2-4] Erythromelalgia has also been reported with nicardipine.[5] This type of erythromelalgia may be termed secondary erythermalgia.[6]

1. Fisher JR, *et al.* Nifedipine and erythromelalgia. *Ann Intern Med* 1983; **98:** 671–2.
2. Grunwald Z. Painful edema, erythematous rash, and burning sensation due to nifedipine. *Drug Intell Clin Pharm* 1982; **16:** 492.
3. Brodmerkel GJ. Nifedipine and erythromelalgia. *Ann Intern Med* 1983; **99:** 415.
4. Sunahara JF, *et al.* Possible erythromelalgia-like syndrome associated with nifedipine in a patient with Raynaud's phenomenon. *Ann Pharmacother* 1996; **30:** 484–6.
5. Levesque H, *et al.* Erythromelalgia induced by nicardipine (inverse Raynaud's phenomenon?) *Br Med J* 1989; **298:** 1252–3.
6. Drenth JPH, Michiels JJ. Three types of erythromelalgia. *Br Med J* 1990; **301:** 454–5.

Effects on the respiratory system. There have been some reports of pulmonary oedema being precipitated by nifedipine therapy in patients with aortic stenosis.[1,2] Nifedipine has also been reported to exacerbate impaired tissue oxygenation in patients with cor pulmonale secondary to obstructive airways disease.[3]

For a report of exacerbation of laryngeal oedema, see under Hypersensitivity, below.

1. Gillmar DJ, Kark P. Pulmonary oedema precipitated by nifedipine. *Br Med J* 1980; **280:** 1420–1.
2. Aderka D, Pinkhas J. Pulmonary oedema precipitated by nifedipine. *Br Med J* 1984; **289:** 1272.
3. Kalra L, Bone MF. Nifedipine and impaired oxygenation in patients with chronic bronchitis and cor pulmonale. *Lancet* 1989; **i:** 1135–6.

Effects on the skin. The commonest skin reactions to nifedipine have been rash, pruritus, urticaria, alopecia, and exfoliative dermatitis;[1] there have been a few reports of erythema multiforme and the Stevens-Johnson syndrome.[1] Erythema multiforme occurred in one patient following substitution of amlodipine for nifedipine[2] and cross-sensitivity, manifest as a pruritic maculopapular rash, has been reported between amlodipine and diltiazem.[3] Generalised pruritus has been reported with amlodipine.[4] Severe photosensitivity reactions,[5] nonthrombocytopenic purpuric rashes,[6] and telangiectasias,[7] including photodistributed facial telangiectasias with amlodipine[8] and with nifedipine[9] (that recurred 3 years later with amlodipine), have also been reported.

For reference to erythromelalgia, see under Effects on the Peripheral Circulation, above.

1. Stern R, Khalsa JH. Cutaneous adverse reactions associated with calcium channel blockers. *Arch Intern Med* 1989; **149:** 829–32.
2. Bewley AP, *et al.* Erythema multiforme following substitution of amlodipine for nifedipine. *Br Med J* 1993; **307:** 241.
3. Baker BA, Cacchione JG. Dermatologic cross-sensitivity between diltiazem and amlodipine. *Ann Pharmacother* 1994; **28:** 118–19.
4. Orme S, *et al.* Generalised pruritus associated with amlodipine. *Br Med J* 1997; **315:** 463.
5. Thomas SE, Wood ML. Photosensitivity reactions associated with nifedipine. *Br Med J* 1986; **292:** 992.
6. Oren R, *et al.* Nifedipine-induced nonthrombocytopenic purpura. *DICP Ann Pharmacother* 1989; **23:** 88.
7. Tsele E, Chu AC. Nifedipine and telangiectasias. *Lancet* 1992; **339:** 365–6.
8. Basarab T, *et al.* Calcium antagonist-induced photo-exposed telangiectasia. *Br J Dermatol* 1997; **136:** 974–5.
9. Collins P, Ferguson J. Photodistributed nifedipine-induced facial telangiectasia. *Br J Dermatol* 1993; **129:** 630–3.

Effects on taste. Although distortion of taste and smell has been reported in 2 patients taking nifedipine,[1] a large survey involving 922 patients receiving nifedipine and 343 taking captopril did not show any association of taste disturbances with nifedipine.[2]

1. Levenson JL, Kennedy K. Dysomia, dysgeusia, and nifedipine. *Ann Intern Med* 1985; **102:** 135–6.
2. Coulter DM. Eye pain with nifedipine and disturbance of taste with captopril: a mutually controlled study showing a method of postmarketing surveillance. *Br Med J* 1988; **296:** 1086–8.

Gynaecomastia. Unilateral gynaecomastia developed in 3 men 4, 6, and 26 weeks after starting nifedipine therapy.[1]

1. Clyne CAC. Unilateral gynaecomastia and nifedipine. *Br Med J* 1986; **292:** 380.

Haemorrhage. See under Effects on the Blood, above.

Hypersensitivity. Nifedipine is associated with various hypersensitivity reactions including skin rashes and effects on the liver (see above).

Nifedipine, given sublingually, exacerbated laryngeal swelling that developed in a woman following the use of isosorbide dinitrate spray.[1]

1. Silfvast T, *et al.* Laryngeal oedema after isosorbide dinitrate spray and sublingual nifedipine. *Br Med J* 1995; **311:** 232.

Oedema. Peripheral oedema of the feet and ankles is a common side-effect of nifedipine and other dihydropyridine calcium-channel blockers. It occurs typically 2 or more weeks after starting treatment and is caused by pre-capillary arteriolar dilatation rather than fluid retention.[1] Evidence from a study in 10 diabetic subjects beginning nifedipine therapy, 5 of whom developed ankle oedema, suggested that nifedipine abolished the reflex vasoconstriction produced when the feet are below the level of the heart which is believed to prevent excessive fluid filtration into the tissues.[2]

The oedema usually lessens with time and may respond to simple measures such as elevation of the feet or to a reduction in dosage. If oedema persists the calcium-channel blocker should be withdrawn.[1]

1. Maclean D, MacConnachie AM. Selective side-effects: peripheral oedema with dihydropyridine calcium antagonists. *Prescribers' J* 1991; **31:** 4–6.
2. Williams SA, *et al.* Dependent oedema and attenuation of postural vasoconstriction associated with nifedipine therapy for hypertension in diabetic patients. *Eur J Clin Pharmacol* 1989; **37:** 333–5.

Overdosage. See under Treatment of Adverse Effects, below.

Treatment of Adverse Effects

In overdosage with nifedipine by mouth the stomach should be emptied by lavage; activated charcoal may be administered. Supportive and symptomatic care should be given. Hypotension may respond to placing the patient in the supine position with the feet raised and the administration of plasma expanders, although cardiac overload should be avoided. If hypotension is not corrected, calcium gluconate or calcium chloride should be given intravenously. Glucagon may also be used. If hypotension persists, intravenous administration of a sympathomimetic such as isoprenaline, dopamine, or noradrenaline may also be necessary. Bradycardia may be treated with atropine, isoprenaline, or cardiac pacing. Dialysis is not useful as nifedipine is highly protein bound. Plasmapheresis may be beneficial.

In a discussion of overdosage with calcium-channel blockers, Kenny[1] considered the consequences and treatment to be similar for verapamil and nifedipine. However, Buckley and others,[2] writing from Australia, considered death and life-threatening complications to be much more common with verapamil than with diltiazem and more common with diltiazem than nifedipine (and presumably other dihydropyridine calcium-channel blockers). They suggested that, whereas most nifedipine poisonings would respond to supportive treatment with intravenous fluids, verapamil frequently caused profound bradycardia and hypotension requiring aggressive and intensive therapy including thorough gastro-intestinal decontamination and high doses of calcium intravenously. Reports of overdosage have so far related mainly to verapamil, as illustrated by a review of cases in Australia[3] from the same group of workers.

The following are two of the few published reports of nifedipine overdosage. In one, hypotension, tachycardia, and flushing, followed by hypokalaemia, were seen in a patient who took nifedipine 600 mg as modified-release tablets together with an overdose of paracetamol, but there was no evidence of heart block.[4] After initial administration of ipecacuanha syrup the patient was given calcium gluconate intravenously, and subsequently activated charcoal and lactulose. Absorption of nifedipine was essentially complete 10 hours after ingestion. Potassium chloride was given by mouth to treat hypokalaemia and acetylcysteine was used to manage the paracetamol poisoning.

Third degree atrioventricular block, progressing to asystole, developed in a 14-month-old child who ingested approximately 800 mg of nifedipine.[5] During cardiopulmonary resuscitation a total of 700 mg of calcium chloride was given, together with atropine, adrenaline, and sodium bicarbonate. The stomach was subsequently emptied by gastric lavage and activated charcoal given. The patient remained tachycardic and hypotensive, with evidence of pulmonary oedema and hyperglycaemia, and was treated with intravenous electrolytes and dopamine infusions and assisted ventilation, together with phenobarbitone to control subsequent tonic-clonic seizures. She eventually made an apparently complete recovery apart from a moderate speech delay.

1. Kenny J. Treating overdose with calcium channel blockers. *Br Med J* 1994; **308:** 992–3.
2. Buckley NA, *et al.* Overdose with calcium channel blockers. *Br Med J* 1994; **308:** 1639.
3. Howarth DM, *et al.* Calcium channel blocking drug overdose: an Australian series. *Hum Exp Toxicol* 1994; **13:** 161–6.
4. Ferner RE, *et al.* Pharmacokinetics and toxic effects of nifedipine in massive overdose. *Hum Exp Toxicol* 1990; **9:** 309–11.
5. Wells TG, *et al.* Nifedipine poisoning in a child. *Pediatrics* 1990; **86:** 91–4.

Precautions

Nifedipine should be used with caution in patients with hypotension, in patients whose cardiac reserve is poor, and in those with heart failure since deterioration of heart failure has been noted. Nifedipine should not be used in cardiogenic shock, in patients who have recently suffered a myocardial infarction, or in acute unstable angina. Nifedipine should not be used to treat an anginal attack in chronic stable angina. In patients with severe aortic stenosis nifedipine may increase the risk of developing heart failure. Sudden withdrawal of nifedipine might be associated with an exacerbation of angina. The dose may need to be reduced in patients with hepatic impairment.

Nifedipine should be discontinued in patients who experience ischaemic pain following its administration.

Nifedipine is reported to be teratogenic in *animals* and may inhibit labour, but it has been used in hypertension in pregnancy (see below).

Diabetes mellitus. Nifedipine may modify insulin and glucose responses (see Effects on Carbohydrate Metabolism under Adverse Effects, above) calling for adjustments in antidiabetic therapy. Also some studies have suggested that nifedipine may worsen proteinuria and renal dysfunction in diabetic patients with some degree of renal insufficiency,[1,2] but other studies, (see Kidney Disorders under Uses and Administration, below), have suggested that nifedipine treatment may prevent or retard the progression of albuminuria.

Some studies have suggested that patients with diabetes mellitus[3,4] or impaired glucose metabolism[5] may be more susceptible to adverse cardiovascular effects of calcium-channel blockers (see above). The calcium-channel blockers used in these studies were nisoldipine, amlodipine, and isradipine (long-acting or intermediate-acting calcium-channel blockers). However, two of the studies[3,4] compared the calcium-channel blocker with an ACE inhibitor and it has been suggested that ACE inhibitors may have a protective effect in patients with diabetes that is additional to their antihypertensive action. Thus, ACE inhibitors may be particularly beneficial in these patients rather than calcium-channel blockers being particularly harmful.[6] Large randomised studies are underway that should provide further information.

1. Mimran A, *et al.* Contrasting effects of captopril and nifedipine in normotensive patients with incipient diabetic nephropathy. *J Hypertens* 1988; **6:** 919–23.
2. Demarie BK, Bakris GL. Effects of different calcium antagonists on proteinuria associated with diabetes mellitus. *Ann Intern Med* 1990; **113:** 987–8.
3. Estacio RO, *et al.* The effect of nisoldipine as compared with enalapril on cardiovascular outcomes in patients with non-insulin-dependent diabetes and hypertension. *N Engl J Med* 1998; **338:** 645–52. Correction. *ibid.*; **339:** 1339.
4. Tatti P, *et al.* Outcome results of the fosinopril versus amlodipine cardiovascular events randomized trial (FACET) in patients with hypertension and NIDDM. *Diabetes Care* 1998; **21:** 597–603.
5. Byington RP, *et al.* Isradipine, raised glycosylated haemoglobin, and risk of cardiovascular events. *Lancet* 1997; **350:** 1075–6.
6. Poulter NR. Calcium channel blockers and cardiovascular risk in diabetes. *Lancet* 1998; **351:** 1809–10.

Interference with laboratory estimations. Nifedipine may give falsely elevated spectrophotometric values of urinary vanillylmandelic acid; HPLC estimations are unaffected.

Porphyria. Nifedipine is considered to be unsafe in patients with acute porphyria because it has been associated with acute attacks.[1]

1. Moore MR, McColl KEL. *Porphyria: drug lists.* Glasgow: Porphyria Research Unit, University of Glasgow, 1991.

Withdrawal. Sudden withdrawal of nifedipine might be associated with an exacerbation of angina.

For a report of life-threatening coronary vasospasm occurring following withdrawal of nifedipine before a revascularisation procedure, see under Diltiazem, p.854.

Interactions

Nifedipine may enhance the antihypertensive effects of other antihypertensive drugs such as beta blockers although the combination is generally well tolerated. Enhanced antihypertensive effects may also be seen with concomitant use of drugs such as aldesleukin and antipsychotics that cause hypotension. Nifedipine may modify insulin and glucose responses (see Effects on Carbohydrate Metabolism, above) and therefore diabetic patients may need to adjust their antidiabetic treatment when receiving nifedipine. Nifedipine is extensively metabolised in the liver by the cytochrome P450 enzyme system, and interactions may occur with other drugs, such as quinidine, sharing the same metabolic pathway, and with enzyme inducers, such as carbamazepine, phenytoin, and rifampicin, and enzyme inhibitors, such as cimetidine and erythromycin.

Alcohol. A study involving 10 healthy subjects showed that the area under the concentration-time profile for nifedipine 20 mg by mouth was increased by 54% when taken with alcohol, and maximum pulse rate was achieved more rapidly, which was in line with *animal* and *in-vitro* studies suggesting that the metabolism of nifedipine is inhibited by alcohol.[1]

1. Qureshi S, *et al.* Nifedipine-alcohol interaction. *JAMA* 1990; **264:** 1660–1.

Antiarrhythmics. Nifedipine and *quinidine* probably have a common metabolic pathway in the liver and might be expected to interact if given concurrently. In one study,[1] quinidine appeared to inhibit nifedipine metabolism resulting in increased serum concentrations of nifedipine; quinidine concentrations were unchanged.

For the effect of nifedipine on serum-quinidine concentrations, see p.940.

1. Bowles SK, *et al.* Evaluation of the pharmacokinetic and pharmacodynamic interaction between quinidine and nifedipine. *J Clin Pharmacol* 1993; **33:** 727–31.

Antidiabetics. See Diabetes Mellitus under Precautions and Effects on Carbohydrate Metabolism under Adverse Effects, above.

Antiepileptics. The effects of dihydropyridine calcium-channel blockers may be reduced by enzyme-inducing antiepileptics such as *carbamazepine, phenobarbitone*, and *phenytoin*.[1-3] In contrast, *sodium valproate* has been reported to increase plasma-nimodipine concentrations.[3]

For reports of an interaction between nifedipine and *phenytoin* resulting in raised serum-phenytoin concentration, see p.356.

1. Capewell S, *et al.* Reduced felodipine bioavailability in patients taking anticonvulsants. *Lancet* 1988; **ii:** 480–2.
2. Schellens JHM, *et al.* Influence of enzyme induction and inhibition on the oxidation of nifedipine, sparteine, mephenytoin and antipyrine in humans as assessed by a "cocktail" study design. *J Pharmacol Exp Ther* 1989; **249:** 638–45.
3. Tartara A, *et al.* Differential effects of valproic acid and enzyme-inducing anticonvulsants on nimodipine pharmacokinetics in epileptic patients. *Br J Clin Pharmacol* 1991; **32:** 335–40.

Antifungals. Azole antifungals inhibit the cytochrome P450 enzyme system and may therefore interfere with metabolism of calcium-channel blockers. Two women who had been taking felodipine for about a year developed peripheral oedema a few days after starting treatment with *itraconazole*.[1] Plasma-felodipine concentrations that were measured in one of the women before and during a subsequent course of itraconazole increased considerably when the two drugs were taken concomitantly. A similar interaction has been reported when itraconazole therapy was started in a patient already taking nifedipine.[2]

1. Neuvonen PJ, Suhonen R. Itraconazole interacts with felodipine. *J Am Acad Dermatol* 1995; **33:** 134–5.
2. Tailor SAN, *et al.* Peripheral edema due to nifedipine-itraconazole interaction: a case report. *Arch Dermatol* 1996; **132:** 350–2.

Antihistamines. Severe angina developed in a patient stabilised on nifedipine who took *terfenadine* 60 mg for seasonal allergy. The pain resolved within an hour or two.[1]

1. Falkenberg HM. Possible interaction report. *Can Pharm J* 1988; **121:** 294.

Antineoplastics. For a report of increased *vincristine* toxicity in children also receiving itraconazole and nifedipine concomitantly, see p.570.

Beta blockers. Although nifedipine is often used in combination with beta blockers without untoward effects, heart failure has been reported in a few patients with angina who were given nifedipine in addition to treatment with a beta blocker.[1,2] Severe hypotension has been reported in 1 of 15 angina patients given nifedipine and atenolol;[3] withdrawal of the beta blocker precipitated severe unstable angina in this patient. Severe hypotension in a patient was attributed to the use of nifedipine in conjunction with propranolol, and was thought to have contributed to fatal myocardial infarction.[4]

1. Anastassiades CJ. Nifedipine and beta-blocker drugs. *Br Med J* 1980; **281:** 1251–2.
2. Robson RH, Vishwanath MC. Nifedipine and beta-blockade as a cause of cardiac failure. *Br Med J* 1982; **284:** 104.
3. Opie LH, White DA. Adverse interaction between nifedipine and β-blockade. *Br Med J* 1980; **281:** 1462.
4. Staffurth JS, Emery P. Adverse interaction between nifedipine and beta-blockade. *Br Med J* 1981; **282:** 225.

Calcium-channel blockers. Plasma concentrations of nifedipine were increased in a study in 6 healthy subjects when pretreated with *diltiazem*; the elimination half-life of nifedipine was prolonged from 2.54 hours to 3.40 hours after pretreatment with diltiazem 30 mg daily and to 3.47 hours after 90 mg daily. The effect was probably due to reduced hepatic metabolism of nifedipine.[1] Nifedipine and diltiazem are reported to be metabolised by the same hepatic enzyme and, conversely, pretreatment with nifedipine has resulted in increased concentrations of diltiazem.[2]

1. Tateishi T, *et al.* Dose dependent effect of diltiazem on the pharmacokinetics of nifedipine. *J Clin Pharmacol* 1989; **29:** 994–7.
2. Tateishi T, *et al.* The effect of nifedipine on the pharmacokinetics and dynamics of diltiazem: the preliminary study in normal volunteers. *J Clin Pharmacol* 1993; **33:** 738–40.

Digoxin. For the effect of nifedipine and other dihydropyridine calcium-channel blockers on digoxin, see p.851.

Food. Grapefruit juice inhibits the cytochrome P450 enzyme system, particularly in the intestinal wall, and concomitant oral administration with calcium-channel blockers has been shown to increase markedly bioavailability of the calcium-channel blocker;[1-3] calcium-channel blockers administered intravenously appear to be unaffected.[4] Most calcium-channel blockers should not therefore be taken orally at the same time as grapefruit juice.[5]

See also Absorption under Pharmacokinetics, below.

1. Bailey DG, *et al.* Interaction of citrus juices with felodipine and nifedipine. *Lancet* 1991; **337:** 268–9.
2. Bailey DG, *et al.* Effect of grapefruit juice and naringin on nisoldipine pharmacokinetics. *Clin Pharmacol Ther* 1993; **54:** 589–94.
3. Lundahl J, *et al.* Relationship between time of intake of grapefruit juice and its effect on pharmacokinetics and pharmacodynamics of felodipine in healthy subjects. *Eur J Clin Pharmacol* 1995; **49:** 61–7.
4. Rashid TJ, *et al.* Factors affecting the absolute bioavailability of nifedipine. *Br J Clin Pharmacol* 1995; **40:** 51–8.
5. Committee on Safety of Medicines/Medicines Control Agency. Drug interactions with grapefruit juice. *Current Problems* 1997; **23:** 2.

Histamine H_2-receptor antagonists. Pharmacokinetic studies have indicated that concurrent administration of nifedipine and *cimetidine* can increase the bioavailability of nifedipine;[1-4] Renwick *et al.* and Smith *et al.* showed an increase in the area under the plasma concentration-time curve of between 77 and 92%.[2,3] Kirch *et al.* also showed a potentiation of the hypotensive effect of nifedipine by cimetidine in 7 hypertensive patients.[1] The mechanism of the interaction was thought to be due to inhibition of the cytochrome P450 system by cimetidine and thus inhibition of the metabolism of nifedipine.

Ranitidine was found to have little effect on the pharmacokinetics of nifedipine, although Kirch *et al.* were able to show an increase in the bioavailability of nifedipine during ranitidine administration.[5] *Famotidine* has been reported not to interact with nifedipine.[6]

1. Kirch W, *et al.* Einflußvon cimetidin und ranitidin auf pharmakokinetik und antihypertensiven effekt von nifedipin. *Dtsch Med Wochenschr* 1983; **108:** 1757–61.
2. Renwick AG, *et al.* Factors affecting the pharmacokinetics of nifedipine. *Eur J Clin Pharmacol* 1987; **32:** 351–5.
3. Smith SR, *et al.* Ranitidine and cimetidine: drug interactions with single dose and steady-state nifedipine administration. *Br J Clin Pharmacol* 1987; **23:** 311–15.
4. Schwartz JB, *et al.* Effect of cimetidine or ranitidine administration on nifedipine pharmacokinetics and pharmacodynamics. *Clin Pharmacol Ther* 1988; **43:** 673–80.
5. Kirch W, *et al.* Ranitidine increases bioavailability of nifedipine. *Clin Pharmacol Ther* 1985; **37:** 204.
6. Kirch W, *et al.* Negative effects of famotidine on cardiac performance assessed by noninvasive hemodynamic measurements. *Gastroenterology* 1989; **96:** 1388–92.

Immunosuppressants. Flushing, paraesthesias, and rashes were reported in 2 patients given nifedipine 40 mg daily while taking *cyclosporin* for psoriasis.[1] A study in 8 psoriatic patients indicated that administration of nifedipine with cyclosporin resulted in reduced recovery of the principal metabolite of nifedipine, presumably because cyclosporin reduced nifedipine metabolism through competition for the cytochrome P450 metabolising enzymes.

For reference to the effects of calcium-channel blockers on cyclosporin concentrations in blood, see p.522. For the possible protective effect of nifedipine against cyclosporin-induced nephrotoxicity, see Transplantation under Uses and Administration, below.

For the effect of nifedipine on *tacrolimus*, see p.563.

1. McFadden JP, *et al.* Cyclosporin decreases nifedipine metabolism. *Br Med J* 1989; **299:** 1224.

Magnesium salts. Profound hypotension has been reported in 2 women in whom a single dose of nifedipine 10 mg by mouth was added to treatment with magnesium sulphate infusion for pre-eclampsia; both women were also receiving methyldopa.[1] Neuromuscular blockade has been reported in 2 women following concomitant use of nifedipine and intravenous magnesium sulphate. In one woman receiving nifedipine as a tocolytic, symptoms of neuromuscular blockade occurred immediately on injection of magnesium sulphate and resolved within 25 minutes of stopping the injection.[2] In another woman who was receiving a magnesium sulphate infusion for pre-eclampsia, symptoms developed 30 minutes after the second of 2 doses of nifedipine had been administered and improved following administration of calcium gluconate injection.[3]

1. Waisman GD, *et al.* Magnesium plus nifedipine: potentiation of hypotensive effect in pre-eclampsia? *Am J Obstet Gynecol* 1988; **159:** 308–9.
2. Snyder SW, Cardwell MS. Neuromuscular blockade with magnesium sulfate and nifedipine. *Am J Obstet Gynecol* 1989; **161:** 35–6.
3. Ben-Ami M, *et al.* The combination of magnesium sulphate and nifedipine: a cause of neuromuscular blockade. *Br J Obstet Gynaecol* 1994; **101:** 262–3.

Tobacco smoking. In a study of the effects of cigarette smoking and the treatment of angina with nifedipine, propranolol, or atenolol, smoking was shown to have direct and adverse effects on the heart and to interfere with the efficacy of all 3 anti-anginal drugs, with nifedipine being the most affected.[1]

1. Deanfield J, *et al.* Cigarette smoking and the treatment of angina with propranolol, atenolol, and nifedipine. *N Engl J Med* 1984; **310:** 951–4.

Xanthines. For the effect of nifedipine on *theophylline*, see p.769.

Pharmacokinetics

Nifedipine is rapidly and almost completely absorbed from the gastro-intestinal tract, but undergoes extensive hepatic first-pass metabolism. Bioavailability after oral administration of liquid-filled capsules is between 45 and 75%, but is lower for longer-acting formulations. Following administration by mouth peak blood concentrations are reported to occur after 30 minutes with liquid-filled capsules.

Nifedipine is about 92 to 98% bound to plasma proteins. It is distributed into breast milk. It is extensively metabolised in the liver and 70 to 80% of a dose is excreted in the urine almost entirely as inactive metabolites. The half-life is about 2 hours following intravenous administration or administration of liquid-filled capsules.

General reviews.

1. Kelly JG, O'Malley K. Clinical pharmacokinetics of calcium antagonists: an update. *Clin Pharmacokinet* 1992; **22:** 416–33.

A review of the pharmacokinetics of nifedipine.[1] Studies of the pharmacokinetics of nifedipine have been complicated by the difficulty in preparing a stable intravenous formulation and the problems in developing a sufficiently sensitive and specific method of analysis. Nearly 100% of an oral dose of nifedipine is absorbed in the small intestine although the bioavailability from capsules is 45 to 68%. The rate of absorption from both oral and sublingual capsules varies widely among individuals: there has been a report that high plasma-nifedipine concentrations are achieved more rapidly if the capsule is bitten and swallowed than from standard oral and sublingual administration. The absorption of nifedipine from tablets is slower than from capsules, with maximum plasma concentrations occurring at 1.6 to 4.2 hours compared with 0.5 to 2.17 hours, and absorption may still be occurring at 24 to 32 hours after administration.

Nifedipine undergoes almost complete hepatic oxidation to 3 pharmacologically inactive metabolites which are excreted in the urine. It has been reported that following oral administration 30 to 40% of the amount absorbed is metabolised during the first pass through the liver. The elimination half-life of nifedipine is apparently dependent upon the dosage form in which it is administered, with half-lives of 6 to 11 hours, 2 to 3.4 hours, and 1.3 to 1.8 hours measured after oral tablet, oral capsule, and intravenous administration respectively. The total systemic clearance of nifedipine from plasma ranges from 27 to about 66 litres per hour. Renal impairment does not substantially alter nifedipine pharmacokinetics.

1. Sorkin EM, *et al.* Nifedipine: a review of its pharmacodynamic and pharmacokinetic properties, and therapeutic efficacy, in ischaemic heart disease, hypertension and related cardiovascular disorders. *Drugs* 1985; **30:** 182–274.

Absorption. Although studies have indicated that the absorption of nifedipine may be affected by administration with food the results appear to vary depending upon the nifedipine preparation used. Hirasawa and colleagues[1] reported a reduction in peak plasma-nifedipine concentrations, and a delay in achieving them, when nifedipine *capsules* were given after a meal compared with 30 minutes before. In contrast, Ueno and others reported that bioavailability of nifedipine and maximum serum concentrations were markedly increased when a *modified-release tablet* (Adalat L) was given after a meal rather than fasting.[2] The same group has reported that a *modified-release capsule* containing uncoated and enteric-coated granules (Sepamit R) had essentially the same bioavailability when taken before or after a meal.[3]

See also under Interactions, Food, above.

1. Hirasawa K, *et al.* Effect of food ingestion on nifedipine absorption and haemodynamic response. *Eur J Clin Pharmacol* 1985; **28:** 105–7.
2. Ueno K, *et al.* Effect of food on nifedipine sustained-release preparation. *DICP Ann Pharmacother* 1989; **23:** 662–5.
3. Ueno K, *et al.* Effect of a light breakfast on the bioavailability of sustained-release nifedipine. *DICP Ann Pharmacother* 1991; **25:** 317–19.

Hepatic impairment. The pharmacokinetics of nifedipine were found to be considerably altered in 7 patients with liver cirrhosis.[1] Systemic plasma clearance was substantially reduced and the elimination half-life was considerably longer than in healthy subjects. In addition, systemic availability of oral nifedipine was much higher in patients with cirrhosis and was complete in 3 patients with surgical portacaval shunt. Patients with liver cirrhosis seemed to be more sensitive to the effects of nifedipine on diastolic blood pressure and heart rate, and this could be explained by the higher free drug concentrations observed. It was concluded that lower doses of nifedipine may be required in patients with liver cirrhosis, and the patient's response should be closely monitored.

1. Kleinbloesem CH, *et al.* Nifedipine: kinetics and hemodynamic effects in patients with liver cirrhosis after intravenous and oral administration. *Clin Pharmacol Ther* 1986; **40:** 21–8.

Interindividual variation. A study in 53 Dutch subjects found a bimodal distribution of plasma concentrations of nifedipine following a single oral dose; it was proposed that the higher plasma concentrations in 17% of subjects represented a slow metaboliser phenotype, with the majority of the population being fast metabolisers.[1] Although further studies[2,3] in European populations have not confirmed these results, a study in 12 Mexican subjects supported the concept of polymorphic metabolism, with 5 fast and 7 slow metabolisers, a much higher proportion of slow metabolisers than in the European studies.[4] Studies have also reported a markedly increased area under the concentration-time curve (AUC) in South Asian,[5,6] Mexican,[7] and Nigerian[8] subjects compared with Caucasians. The difference did not appear to be due to diet.[5,6] The initial dose of nifedipine might need to be lower in these ethnic groups. CYP3A4 is believed to be the isoenzyme involved in metabolism of dihydropyridine calcium-channel blockers.

1. Kleinbloesem CH, *et al.* Variability in nifedipine pharmacokinetics and dynamics: a new oxidation polymorphism in man. *Biochem Pharmacol* 1984; **33:** 3721–4.
2. Renwick AG, *et al.* The pharmacokinetics of oral nifedipine—a population study. *Br J Clin Pharmacol* 1988; **25:** 701–8.
3. Lobo J, *et al.* The intra- and inter-subject variability of nifedipine pharmacokinetics in young volunteers. *Eur J Clin Pharmacol* 1986; **30:** 57–60.
4. Hoyo-Vadillo C, *et al.* Pharmacokinetics of nifedipine slow release tablet in Mexican subjects: further evidence for an oxidation polymorphism. *J Clin Pharmacol* 1989; **29:** 816–20.
5. Ahsan CH, *et al.* Ethnic differences in the pharmacokinetics of oral nifedipine. *Br J Clin Pharmacol* 1991; **31:** 399–403.
6. Ahsan CH, *et al.* The influences of dose and ethnic origins on the pharmacokinetics of nifedipine. *Clin Pharmacol Ther* 1993; **54:** 329–38.
7. Castañeda-Hernández G, *et al.* Interethnic variability in nifedipine disposition: reduced systemic plasma clearance in Mexican subjects. *Br J Clin Pharmacol* 1996; **41:** 433–4.
8. Sowunmi A, *et al.* Ethnic differences in nifedipine kinetics: comparisons between Nigerians, Caucasians and South Asians. *Br J Clin Pharmacol* 1995; **40:** 489–93.

Uses and Administration

Nifedipine is a dihydropyridine calcium-channel blocker (p.778). It is a peripheral and coronary vasodilator, but, unlike the calcium-channel blockers verapamil or diltiazem, has little or no effect on cardiac conduction and negative inotropic activity is rarely seen at therapeutic doses. Administration of nifedipine results primarily in vasodilatation, with reduced peripheral resistance, blood pressure, and afterload, increased coronary blood flow, and a reflex increase in heart rate. This in turn results in an increase in myocardial oxygen supply and cardiac output. Nifedipine has no antiarrhythmic activity. Nicardipine and newer dihydropyridines such as amlodipine, felodipine, isradipine, and lacidipine may be even more selective than nifedipine for vascular smooth muscle. Nimodipine acts particularly on cerebral blood vessels. Most of the dihydropyridine calcium-channel blockers (nifedipine and lacidipine are exceptions) are chiral compounds used as racemic mixtures.

Nifedipine is used in the management of hypertension; in the prophylaxis of angina pectoris (p.780), particularly when a vasospastic element is present, as in Prinzmetal's angina; and in the treatment of

Raynaud's syndrome. Nifedipine has also been tried in numerous non-vascular disorders.

Nifedipine is usually given by mouth. It is available in a number of formulations. Liquid-filled capsules with a relatively rapid onset but short duration of action are administered three times daily. This short-acting preparation is not recommended for the management of hypertension (see below). There are also tablets and capsules with a slower onset and longer duration of action, enabling twice-daily administration; although these are often referred to by nomenclature implying extended or sustained release they should be distinguished from the true extended-release preparations available in some countries that allow administration once daily. Nifedipine is normally given with or after food.

Doses of nifedipine are dependent upon the formulation used; they may need to be reduced in the elderly or those with impaired liver function.

In the management of **hypertension** a long-acting preparation of nifedipine may be given in doses of 10 to 40 mg twice daily, 30 to 90 mg once daily, or 20 to 100 mg once daily, depending on the preparation used.

In the management of **angina pectoris**, nifedipine may be given as a long-acting preparation in a dose of 10 to 40 mg twice daily or 30 to 90 mg once daily, depending on the preparation. Alternatively, the liquid-filled capsules may be given in an initial dose of 5 to 10 mg three times daily; the usual range is 5 to 20 mg three times daily.

Nifedipine has been administered by injection via a coronary catheter for the treatment of coronary spasm during coronary angiography and balloon angioplasty. Blood pressure and heart rate should be monitored carefully.

In the management of **Raynaud's syndrome**, nifedipine may be given as liquid-filled capsules in a dose of 5 to 20 mg three times daily.

General reviews.

1. Sorkin EM, *et al.* Nifedipine. *Drugs* 1985; **30:** 182–274.
2. Anonymous. Nifedipine in myocardial ischaemia, systemic hypertension, and other cardiovascular disorders. *Ann Intern Med* 1986; **105:** 714–29.
3. Anonymous. Calcium antagonists for cardiovascular disease. *Drug Ther Bull* 1993; **31:** 81–4.
4. Fisher M, Grotta J. New uses for calcium channel blockers: therapeutic implications. *Drugs* 1993; **46:** 961–75.

Administration. Reviews of the various modified-release nifedipine formulations.

1. Murdoch D, Brogden RN. Sustained release nifedipine formulations: an appraisal of their current uses and prospective roles in the treatment of hypertension, ischaemic heart disease and peripheral vascular disorders. *Drugs* 1991; **41:** 737–79.
2. Anonymous. Nifedipine: a new life with GITS? *Lancet* 1992; **340:** 1507–8.
3. Devane JG, *et al.* New developments in sustained-release antihypertensive therapy: formulation and pharmacokinetic considerations. *Am J Cardiol* 1992; **69:** 23E–27E.

Administration in children. Nifedipine has been administered sublingually to children aged 6 to 15 years with acute severe hypertension in a mean dose of 0.24 mg per kg bodyweight (range 0.18 to 0.32 mg per kg).[1] Sublingual administration is difficult in younger children, but nifedipine has successfully been administered rectally, as a pierced capsule with sufficient of the contents withdrawn to give a dose in the range 0.2 to 0.5 mg per kg body-weight;[2] it has also been given intranasally in a dose of 0.4 mg per kg.[3]

1. Evans JHC, *et al.* Sublingual nifedipine in acute severe hypertension. *Arch Dis Child* 1988; **63:** 975–7.
2. Uchiyama M, Ogawa I. Rectal nifedipine in acute severe hypertension in young children. *Arch Dis Child* 1989; **64:** 632–3.
3. Lopez-Herce J, *et al.* Treatment of hypertensive crisis with intranasal nifedipine. *Crit Care Med* 1988; **9:** 914.

Amaurosis fugax. Relief of vasospasm might explain the efficacy of the calcium-channel blockers nifedipine and verapamil in a few patients with amaurosis fugax (see under Stroke, p.799) unresponsive to anticoagulants or antiplatelet agents.[1]

1. Winterkorn JMS, *et al.* Brief report: treatment of vasospastic amaurosis fugax with calcium-channel blockers. *N Engl J Med* 1993; **329:** 396–8.

Asthma. Since calcium is important in airway smooth muscle contraction, degranulation of mast cells, and secretion of mucus,[1] there has been some interest in the potential role of calcium-channel blockers in the treatment of asthma (p.745). However, the results of clinical studies have shown little benefit and it has been suggested that the chief roles of calcium-channel blockers may be in the treatment of angina and hypertension in asthmatic patients (in whom drugs such as the beta blockers would be unsuitable)[1-3] and as a pharmacological tool in investigating the role of calcium in airway physiology.[1,2]

1. Löfdahl C-G, Barnes PJ. Calcium channel blockade and asthma—the current position. *Eur J Respir Dis* 1985; **67:** 233–7.
2. Fanta CH. Calcium-channel blockers in prophylaxis and treatment of asthma. *Am J Cardiol* 1985; **55:** 202B–9B.
3. Massey KL, Hendeles L. Calcium antagonists in the management of asthma: breakthrough or ballyhoo? *Drug Intell Clin Pharm* 1987; **21:** 505–9.

Atherosclerosis. The use of drugs that interfere with atherogenesis (the development of atheromas) has been suggested as a means of reducing diseases associated with atherosclerosis (p.782). Calcium is thought to be necessary for several steps in atherogenesis and studies in *animals* have shown that calcium-channel blockers slow the development and progression of atherosclerotic lesions. However, studies in humans have been less convincing.[1]

1. Borcherding SM, *et al.* Calcium-channel antagonists for prevention of atherosclerosis. *Ann Pharmacother* 1993; **27:** 61–7.

Cardiomyopathies. Calcium-channel blockers may have a role in some forms of cardiomyopathy (p.785). In *hypertrophic cardiomyopathy* verapamil is probably the calcium-channel blocker of choice (see p.963). Nifedipine does not appear to reduce left ventricular outflow tract obstruction, and conflicting results have been demonstrated with respect to improvement in the diastolic function abnormality with this drug.[1] The use of calcium-channel blockers in *dilated cardiomyopathy* is not usually advisable.

1. Richardson PJ. Calcium antagonists in cardiomyopathy. *Br J Clin Pract* 1988; **42** (suppl 60): 33–7.

Cough. Nifedipine has been reported to reduce the severity of cough induced by captopril,[1] possibly by inhibiting prostaglandin synthesis. For further details on cough associated with ACE inhibitors, see p.805.

1. Fogari R, *et al.* Effects of nifedipine and indomethacin on cough induced by angiotensin-converting enzyme inhibitors: a double-blind, randomized, cross-over study. *J Cardiovasc Pharmacol* 1992; **19:** 670–3.

Epilepsy. Calcium-channel blockers have been tried in various forms of epilepsy but are not the usual form of therapy (see p.335). There were preliminary reports of beneficial results with nifedipine in patients with refractory epilepsy.[1,2] Wen pointed out that although theory supports a potential role for calcium-channel blockers in treating epilepsy, nifedipine, which is largely protein bound and unlikely to cross the blood-brain barrier in large amounts, is less likely to be a suitable choice than a drug with greater CNS penetration such as nimodipine.[3] However, neither nifedipine[4] nor nimodipine[5] were of benefit when given as adjunctive therapy in controlled studies of patients with refractory epilepsy.

1. Larkin JG, *et al.* Nifedipine for epilepsy: a pilot study. *Br Med J* 1988; **296:** 530–1.
2. Sander JWAS, Shorvon SD. Nifedipine for epilepsy? *Br Med J* 1988; **296:** 1070.
3. Wen P. Nifedipine for epilepsy? *Br Med J* 1988; **296:** 1069.
4. Brodie MJ, *et al.* A double-blind, crossover, placebo-controlled trial of adjuvant nifedipine in refractory epilepsy. *Br J Clin Pharmacol* 1990; **29:** 592P-593P.
5. Meyer FB, *et al.* Nimodipine as an add-on therapy for intractable epilepsy. *Mayo Clin Proc* 1995; **70:** 623–7.

Gastro-intestinal spasm. Nifedipine 20 mg by mouth produced complete pain relief within 2 hours in 11 of 14 patients with acute intestinal colic (p.1170) due to bacillary or amoebic dysentery.[1] This compared with pain relief in only 2 of 14 control patients given placebo. The results suggest a spasmolytic activity of nifedipine on intestinal muscles.

1. Al-Waili NSD. Nifedipine in intestinal colic. *JAMA* 1990; **263:** 3258.

Hiccup. Hiccups (p.655) result from involuntary spasmodic contraction of the diaphragm. Intractable hiccups resolved completely with nifedipine 20 mg every 8 hours in 1 patient.[1] In a further 7 such patients,[2] nifedipine in doses of 20 to 80 mg daily stopped hiccups in 4 and improved them in a 5th.

1. Mukhopadhyay P, *et al.* Nifedipine for intractable hiccups. *N Engl J Med* 1986; **314:** 1256.
2. Lipps DC, *et al.* Nifedipine for intractable hiccups. *Neurology* 1990; **40:** 531–2.

High-altitude disorders. Nifedipine lowers pulmonary artery pressure and is one of several drugs that are used in high-altitude disorders (p.787), success being reported for both the treatment[1,2] and prevention[2,3] of symptoms of pulmonary oedema. In a study conducted at 4559 m above sea-level[1] nifedipine 10 mg sublingually, then 20 mg as a controlled-release dosage form was given to 6 subjects with symptoms of high-altitude pulmonary oedema. The sublingual dose was repeated if tolerated after 15 minutes and the subjects subsequently received controlled-release nifedipine 20 mg every 6 hours whilst they remained at high altitude. Symptoms of high-altitude pulmonary oedema were relieved within 1 hour of beginning nifedipine and radiographic signs of oedema regressed during treatment despite remaining at high altitude for 36 hours and participating in mountaineering activities. Raised pulmonary arterial pressure was also reduced to control values by nifedipine. Successful treatment of pulmonary oedema in a climber at 6550 m has been described with doses of 20 mg every 8 hours for 36 hours and such doses also prevented the development of symptoms in 2 climbers who had taken nifedipine from the start of the climb.[2] Doses of 20 mg every 8 hours have been reported to allow rapid ascent to 4559 m without development of pulmonary oedema in 9 of 10 subjects who received nifedipine compared with 4 of 11 who received only placebo.[3] However, the point has been made that although it is reasonable that many climbers carry nifedipine in case of an attack, prophylactic nifedipine should not be considered an alternative to slow ascent and acclimatisation.[4]

1. Oelz O, *et al.* Nifedipine for high altitude pulmonary oedema. *Lancet* 1989; **ii:** 1241–4. Correction. *ibid.* 1991; **337:** 556.
2. Jamieson A, Kerr GW. Treatment of high-altitude pulmonary oedema. *Lancet* 1992; **340:** 1468.
3. Bärtsch P, *et al.* Prevention of high-altitude pulmonary oedema by nifedipine. *N Engl J Med* 1991; **325:** 1284–9.
4. A'Court CHD, *et al.* Doctor on a mountaineering expedition. *Br Med J* 1995; **310:** 1248–52.

Hypertension. Calcium-channel blockers are generally considered to be alternative first-line drugs to diuretics and beta blockers in the treatment of hypertension (p.788), although the safety of short-acting calcium-channel blockers has recently been questioned (see under Adverse Effects, above). Two-drug combinations, for example, a dihydropyridine calcium-channel blocker plus a beta blocker or an ACE inhibitor may be necessary.

In **hypertensive crises**, if oral treatment can be given, a calcium-channel blocker such as nifedipine has been widely used. Nifedipine has been administered sublingually, or by biting the capsule and swallowing the contents,[1] for a faster onset of action,[2] but such use may cause dangerous hypotension and the US Joint National Committee on hypertension[3] and others[4] have concluded that such use is unacceptable. Some calcium-channel blockers, for example nicardipine, are available for intravenous administration and may be given when a parenteral antihypertensive drug is considered necessary. One study concluded that intravenous nicardipine was as effective as sodium nitroprusside in the treatment of postoperative hypertension.[5]

For reference to the rectal, intranasal, and sublingual administration of nifedipine to children with acute severe hypertension, see under Administration in Children, above.

A calcium-channel blocker has been suggested for **hypertension in pregnancy** if first-line treatment with methyldopa or a beta blocker fails to reduce blood pressure adequately. Nifedipine is reported to be teratogenic in *animals* and may inhibit labour, but it has been tried in a limited number of patients with pre-eclampsia. Although Constantine and colleagues reported a high rate of caesarean deliveries, premature births and small-for-date infants in patients given nifedipine as a second-line drug[6] assessment of the role of nifedipine is difficult because outcome is often poor in such severely compromised pregnancies.[7] Hanretty and others found that nifedipine 20 mg as tablets lowered blood pressure in 9 women in the third trimester with normal haemodynamics without compromising blood flow in the fetus,[7] which is in line with similar results reported by Pirhonen and colleagues,[8] despite fetal nifedipine concentrations that may be 75% of maternal values 2 to 3 hours after sublingual administration.[9] In a randomised controlled study carried out by Fenakel and co-workers[10] nifedipine 10 to 30 mg sublingually followed by 10 mg as capsules by mouth every 6 hours increasing to 20 mg every 4 hours if necessary, was compared with hydralazine 12.5 mg intravenously as required followed by 20 to 30 mg by mouth every 6 hours, with added methyldopa if necessary. Both groups also received intravenous magnesium sulphate. Effective control of blood pressure was achieved in 23 of 24 patients given nifedipine compared with only 17 of 25 given hydralazine and 9 nifedipine patients achieved term delivery compared with only 2 of those receiving hydralazine. The average gestational age was greater in infants in the nifedipine group; hence these neonates weighed more and had fewer neonatal complications when compared with neonates from the hydralazine treated group.[10]

1. Gifford RW. Management of hypertensive crises. *JAMA* 1991; **266:** 829–35.
2. Angeli P, *et al.* Comparison of sublingual captopril and nifedipine in immediate treatment of hypertensive emergencies. *Arch Intern Med* 1991; **151:** 678–82.
3. Joint National Committee. The sixth report of the joint national committee on prevention, detection, evaluation, and treatment of high blood pressure (JNC VI). *Arch Intern Med* 1997; **157:** 2413–46. Correction. *ibid.* 1998; **158:** 573.
4. Grossman E, *et al.* Should a moratorium be placed on sublingual nifedipine capsules given for hypertensive emergencies and pseudoemergencies? *JAMA* 1996; **276:** 1328–31.
5. Halpern NA, *et al.* Postoperative hypertension: a multicenter, prospective, randomized comparison between intravenous nicardipine and sodium nitroprusside. *Crit Care Med* 1992; **20:** 1637–43.
6. Constantine G, *et al.* Nifedipine as a second line antihypertensive drug in pregnancy. *Br J Obstet Gynaecol* 1987; **94:** 1136–42.
7. Hanretty KP, *et al.* Effect of nifedipine on Doppler flow velocity waveforms in severe pre-eclampsia. *Br Med J* 1989; **299:** 1205–6.

8. Pirhonen JP, *et al.* Uterine and fetal flow velocity wave forms in hypertensive pregnancy: the effect of a single dose of nifedipine. *Obstet Gynecol* 1990; **76:** 37–41.
9. Pirhonen JP, *et al.* Single dose of nifedipine in normotensive pregnancy: nifedipine concentrations, hemodynamic responses, and uterine and fetal flow velocity waveforms. *Obstet Gynecol* 1990; **76:** 807–11.
10. Fenakel K, *et al.* Nifedipine in the treatment of severe preeclampsia. *Obstet Gynecol* 1991; **77:** 331–7.

Irritable bowel syndrome. In irritable bowel syndrome (p.1172), pain or discomfort may be associated with spasm of the smooth muscle of the gut. Calcium-channel blockers might alleviate symptoms by reducing colonic motility, but the results of small trials have not been encouraging.

Kidney disorders. Although nifedipine may adversely affect renal function (see under Adverse Effects, above) there is evidence that calcium-channel blockers, like ACE inhibitors (p.809), may be of benefit in various forms of kidney disorder. Hypertension is closely linked with the kidney—the kidney is important in the normal control of blood pressure and may have a role in the pathogenesis of hypertension; it may also be a prime target of damage caused by hypertension.[1] Proteinuria is an important indicator of glomerular kidney disease (p.1021) of various causes and the effects of calcium-channel blockers on proteinuria and renal dysfunction have been studied in a variety of patients. Results have been mixed,[2-6] although reviews of the available evidence[7-9] suggest that calcium-channel blockers do have a protective effect on renal function over and above that due to the control of hypertension.

Nifedipine has also been reported to protect against cyclosporin-induced nephrotoxicity in renal transplant patients (see Transplantation, below).

1. Raine EG. Hypertension and the kidney. *Br Med Bull* 1994; **50:** 322–41.
2. Demarie BK, Bakris GL. Effects of different calcium antagonists on proteinuria associated with diabetes mellitus. *Ann Intern Med* 1990; **113:** 987–8.
3. Melbourne Diabetic Nephropathy Study Group. Comparison between perindopril and nifedipine in hypertensive and normotensive diabetic patients with microalbuminuria. *Br Med J* 1991; **302:** 210–16.
4. Reams G, *et al.* The effect of nifedipine GITS on renal function in hypertensive patients with renal insufficiency. *J Clin Pharmacol* 1991; **31:** 468–72.
5. Abbott K, *et al.* Effects of dihydropyridine calcium antagonists on albuminuria in patients with diabetes. *J Clin Pharmacol* 1996; **36:** 274–9.
6. Bouhanick B, *et al.* Equivalent effects of nicardipine and captopril on urinary albumin excretion of type 2, non-insulin-dependent diabetic subjects with mild to moderate hypertension. *Therapie* 1996; **51:** 41–7.
7. Valentino VA, *et al.* A perspective on converting enzyme inhibitors and calcium channel antagonists in diabetic renal disease. *Arch Intern Med* 1991; **151:** 2367–72.
8. Epstein M. Calcium antagonists and renal protection: current status and future perspectives. *Arch Intern Med* 1992; **152:** 1573–84.
9. Reams GP. Calcium channel blockers: do they offer renal protection? *J Hum Hypertens* 1993; **7:** 211–19.

Migraine and cluster headache. Drugs with calcium-channel blocking activity have been given in the management of headaches considered to have a vascular component such as migraine (p.443) and cluster headache (p.443).

In migraine prophylaxis, of those drugs with calcium-channel blocking activity studied, flunarizine (p.411) has the best documented efficacy, and verapamil may be useful. Other calcium-channel blockers such as diltiazem, nifedipine, and nimodipine have been tried, but results have been conflicting.

Beneficial effects have been reported[1,2] with calcium-channel blockers in the prevention of cluster headache during cluster periods. Verapamil appears to have been the most widely used calcium-channel blocker for cluster headache prophylaxis. In one double-blind study verapamil was found to be of similar efficacy to lithium[3] and appeared to produce fewer adverse effects.

1. Jónsdóttir M, *et al.* Efficacy, side effects and tolerance compared during headache treatment with three different calcium blockers. *Headache* 1987; **27:** 364–9.
2. Gabai IJ, Spierings ELH. Prophylactic treatment of cluster headache with verapamil. *Headache* 1989; **29:** 167–8.
3. Bussone G, *et al.* Double blind comparison of lithium and verapamil in cluster headache prophylaxis. *Headache* 1990; **30:** 411–17.

Oesophageal motility disorders. Calcium-channel blockers have been tried in disorders of oesophageal motility (p.1174) because of their ability to relax smooth muscle.

Results from a number of studies have indicated that nifedipine, usually in doses of 10 to 20 mg sublingually may be of benefit in patients with achalasia, reducing lower oesophageal sphincter pressure and producing symptomatic improvement.[1-5] Although dilatation or cardiomyotomy is the treatment of choice, Coccia and colleagues found that results in 14 patients given nifedipine 10 to 20 mg sublingually 30 minutes before meals were as good as those in 16 further patients treated with dilatation on follow-up for a mean of 21 months.[5] This was in contrast to the study of Robertson and others which found nifedipine to be ineffective in the treatment of achalasia, in comparison with dilatation which was effective.[6] The reasons for the apparent lack of effect of nifedipine in this latter study may be the use of a lower dose, and insufficient time allowed for the effects of nifedipine to develop.[5] However, there is evidence from the study of Gelfond and co-workers that nifedipine may not be as effective as isosorbide dinitrate in the drug therapy of achalasia.[2]

Nifedipine has also been reported to be of benefit in 'nutcracker oesophagus',[3] and diffuse oesophageal spasm,[7] but recent studies in these conditions have produced disappointing results and suggest that decreases in oesophageal pressure may not correlate with an alleviation of pain.[8]

1. Bortolotti M, Labò G. Clinical and manometric effects of nifedipine in patients with esophageal achalasia. *Gastroenterology* 1981; **80:** 39–44.
2. Gelfond M, *et al.* Isosorbide dinitrate and nifedipine treatment of achalasia: a clinical, manometric and radionuclide evaluation. *Gastroenterology* 1982; **83:** 963–9.
3. Traube M, *et al.* Effects of nifedipine in achalasia and in patients with high-amplitude peristaltic esophageal contractions. *JAMA* 1984; **252:** 1733–6.
4. Román FJ, *et al.* Effects of nifedipine in achalasia and patients with high-amplitude peristaltic esophageal contractions. *JAMA* 1985; **253:** 2046.
5. Coccia G, *et al.* Prospective clinical and manometric study comparing pneumatic dilatation and sublingual nifedipine in the treatment of oesophageal achalasia. *Gut* 1991; **32:** 604–6.
6. Robertson CS, *et al.* Quantitative assessment of the response to therapy in achalasia of the cardia. *Gut* 1989; **30:** 768–73.
7. Nasrallah SM. Nifedipine in the treatment of diffuse oesophageal spasm. *Lancet* 1982; **ii:** 1285.
8. Richter JE, *et al.* Esophageal chest pain: current controversies in pathogenesis, diagnosis, and therapy. *Ann Intern Med* 1989; **110:** 66–78.

Peripheral vascular disease. Vasospastic arterial disease (p.794) is due to an inappropriate response to temperature, usually cold, when vasoconstriction and/or vasospasm occurs. The most important of these disorders is Raynaud's syndrome. Calcium-channel blockers have been of benefit in Raynaud's syndrome, but it is not entirely clear which of their pharmacological actions is responsible. The most widely used and studied is nifedipine. Evidence of subjective benefit has been seen both in primary idiopathic disease[1-4] and in Raynaud's phenomenon secondary to systemic sclerosis,[2,3,5,6] systemic lupus erythematosus,[2,3] rheumatoid arthritis,[3] and cancer chemotherapy.[7] Objective improvement as demonstrated by evidence of improved digital blood flow has been demonstrated in some[4,5,8,9] but not all[6] studies. Doses have varied; 10 mg of nifedipine twice daily initially, increased after a week to a maximum of 20 mg twice daily has been suggested,[10] but in many studies doses of up to 60 mg daily have been used, although side-effects have proved intolerable in some patients given such doses.[6]

Other vasospastic conditions include acrocyanosis, chilblains, and erythromelalgia. Nifedipine in doses of 20 to 60 mg daily has been reported to be of benefit in the treatment of established chilblains and in the prevention of relapse.[11]

1. Roath S. Management of Raynaud's phenomenon: focus on newer treatments. *Drugs* 1989; **37:** 700–12.
2. Smith CD, McKendry RJR. Controlled trial of nifedipine in the treatment of Raynaud's phenomenon. *Lancet* 1982; **ii:** 1299–1301.
3. Kahan A, *et al.* Nifedipine for Raynaud's phenomenon. *Lancet* 1983; **i:** 131.
4. Gasser P. Reaction of capillary blood cell velocity in nailfold capillaries to nifedipine and ketanserin in patients with vasospastic disease. *J Int Med Res* 1991; **19:** 24–31.
5. Thomas RHM, *et al.* Nifedipine in the treatment of Raynaud's phenomenon in patients with systemic sclerosis. *Br J Dermatol* 1987; **117:** 237–41.
6. Rademaker M, *et al.* Comparison of intravenous infusions of iloprost and oral nifedipine in treatment of Raynaud's phenomenon in patients with systemic sclerosis: a double blind randomised study. *Br Med J* 1989; **298:** 561–4.
7. Hantel A, *et al.* Nifedipine and oncologic Raynaud phenomenon. *Ann Intern Med* 1988; **108:** 767.
8. Nilsson H, *et al.* Treatment of digital vasospastic disease with the calcium-entry blocker nifedipine. *Acta Med Scand* 1984; **215:** 135–9.
9. Finch MB, *et al.* The peripheral vascular effects of nifedipine in Raynaud's disease. *Br J Clin Pharmacol* 1986; **21:** 100P–101P.
10. Grigg MH, Wolfe JHN. Raynaud's syndrome and similar conditions. *Br Med J* 1991; **303:** 913–16.
11. Rustin MHA, *et al.* The treatment of chilblains with nifedipine: the results of a pilot study, a double-blind placebo-controlled randomized study and a long-term open trial. *Br J Dermatol* 1989; **120:** 267–75.

Phaeochromocytoma. Pharmacological management of phaeochromocytoma (p.795) is principally achieved by alpha-adrenergic blockade and tachycardia may subsequently be controlled by cautious addition of a beta blocker. There is also some limited experience of the use of nifedipine. A patient with a noradrenaline-secreting phaeochromocytoma experienced great improvement in cardiovascular symptoms during treatment with nifedipine.[1] Symptomatic relief was associated with a pronounced decline in elevated urinary noradrenaline concentrations and it was suggested that nifedipine could interfere with the release of noradrenaline from phaeochromocytoma tissue. However, very high plasma concentrations of noradrenaline persisted in a patient with phaeochromocytoma despite abolition of the associated increase in blood pressure by nifedipine.[2] It was suggested that nifedipine was interfering with the action of noradrenaline by acting directly on the vascular smooth muscle. A similar result was obtained by Favre and Vallotton.[3] In a review of 10 cases of childhood phaeochromocytoma Deal and colleagues reported that 4 were treated with nifedipine but adequate preoperative control of blood pressure was achieved with nifedipine alone only in 2. Nonetheless, although phenoxybenzamine and propranolol remained the drug of first choice for catecholamine blockade, results with nifedipine were considered encouraging.[4]

1. Serfas D, *et al.* Phaeochromocytoma and hypertrophic cardiomyopathy: apparent suppression of symptoms and noradrenaline secretion by calcium-channel blockade. *Lancet* 1983; **ii:** 711–13.
2. Lenders JWM, *et al.* Treatment of a phaeochromocytoma of the urinary bladder with nifedipine. *Br Med J* 1985; **290:** 1624–5.
3. Favre L, Vallotton MB. Nifedipine in pheochromocytoma. *Ann Intern Med* 1986; **104:** 125.
4. Deal JE, *et al.* Phaeochromocytoma—investigation and management of 10 cases. *Arch Dis Child* 1990; **65:** 269–74.

Premature labour. Although beta-adrenoceptor agonists are the drugs most commonly used as tocolytic agents for the prevention of premature labour (p.760), some success has been achieved with calcium-channel blockers such as nifedipine, either given alone or added to beta agonists. Labour was successfully postponed in a patient treated with nifedipine 20 mg three times a day and terbutaline 5 mg 4-hourly by mouth.[1] Terbutaline 0.25 mg up to 4 times a day by subcutaneous injection was also occasionally necessary. Nifedipine was administered from the 26th week of pregnancy for 55 days. A normal, healthy infant was delivered in the 36th week of pregnancy. Read and Wellby found that nifedipine 30 mg initially, then 20 mg every 8 hours by mouth, in 20 patients, was more effective in suppressing premature labour than ritodrine given intravenously or no treatment.[2] Similar results were reported in a more recent study in 185 women using nifedipine in an initial dose of up to 40 mg followed by 60 to 160 mg daily.[3] Nifedipine was also associated with fewer maternal side-effects than ritodrine. However, a similar study in 33 patients by Ferguson and others found nifedipine to be no more effective than ritodrine infusion, although associated with a lower incidence of adverse effects.[4] Similar results have been reported with nicardipine.[5]

1. Kaul AF, *et al.* The management of preterm labor with the calcium channel-blocking agent nifedipine combined with the β-mimetic terbutaline. *Drug Intell Clin Pharm* 1985; **19:** 369–71.
2. Read MD, Wellby DE. The use of a calcium antagonist (nifedipine) to suppress preterm labour. *Br J Obstet Gynaecol* 1986; **93:** 933–7.
3. Papatsonis DNM, *et al.* Nifedipine and ritodrine in the management of preterm labor: a randomized multicenter trial. *Obstet Gynecol* 1997; **90:** 230–4.
4. Ferguson JE, *et al.* A comparison of tocolysis with nifedipine or ritodrine: analysis of efficacy and maternal, fetal, and neonatal outcome. *Am J Obstet Gynecol* 1990; **163:** 105–11.
5. Jannet D, *et al.* Nicardipine versus salbutamol in the treatment of premature labor: a prospective randomized study. *Eur J Obstet Gynecol Reprod Biol* 1997; **73:** 11–16.

Pulmonary hypertension. Vasodilators have been tried in primary pulmonary hypertension (p.796) on the premise that pulmonary vasoconstriction is an important component of the condition. Calcium-channel blockers are the most widely-used vasodilators in primary pulmonary hypertension. Six patients treated with oral nifedipine 40 to 120 mg daily reported symptomatic improvement in dyspnoea and absence of syncope on follow-up for between 4 and 14 months.[1] Five of the patients showed haemodynamic improvement.[1] A review[2] of the drug treatment of primary pulmonary hypertension reported a further 4 cases of clear benefit from oral nifedipine following both acute and chronic administration in primary pulmonary hypertension. However, treatment failures have occurred with nifedipine, and at least one death has been reported shortly after starting therapy.[2] Other reports have also stressed the potentially deleterious effects of nifedipine (or other vasodilator) therapy in pulmonary hypertension. Increased dyspnoea and a fall in arterial PO_2 have been reported in a patient with primary pulmonary hypertension given nifedipine, probably due to preferential vasodilatation of underventilated hypoxic tissues resulting in an increased physiological shunt.[3] Invasive investigations, notably blood-gas monitoring, is therefore recommended when giving nifedipine to these patients[2,3] and it has been advised that an acute response test should be performed before embarking on long-term treatment.[4] Improved survival over a 5-year period has been noted in a study in patients treated with high doses of calcium-channel blockers (nifedipine or diltiazem).[4]

1. Rubin LJ, *et al.* Treatment of primary pulmonary hypertension with nifedipine: a hemodynamic and scintigraphic evaluation. *Ann Intern Med* 1983; **99:** 433–8.
2. McLeod AA, Jewitt DE. Drug treatment of primary pulmonary hypertension. *Drugs* 1986; **31:** 177–84.
3. Krol RC, *et al.* Primary pulmonary hypotension, nifedipine, and hypoxemia. *Ann Intern Med* 1984; **100:** 163.
4. Rich S, *et al.* The effect of high doses of calcium-channel blockers on survival in primary pulmonary hypertension. *N Engl J Med* 1992; **327:** 76–81.

Tardive dyskinesia. Calcium-channel blockers have been tried in the treatment of tardive dyskinesia[1] (see under Extrapyramidal Disorders, p.650). However, results have been mixed and there is concern that, if their action is mediated through an antidopaminergic effect, they may only temporarily mask symptoms or exacerbate them in the long term.[1]

1. Cates M, *et al.* Are calcium-channel blockers effective in the treatment of tardive dyskinesia? *Ann Pharmacother* 1993; **27:** 191–6.

Transplantation. Retrospective analysis of 106 cyclosporin-treated renal transplant patients found that patients receiving nifedipine for hypertension had better graft function, despite shorter graft duration requiring higher dosage of cyclosporin, than equivalent hypertensive patients receiving other drug treatment. Nifedipine appears to be of potential value as a protective agent against cyclosporin-induced nephrotoxicity.[1] Subsequent studies have similarly reported improved graft function[2] in patients receiving nifedipine and suggest that graft survival is also improved.[3]

See also Kidney Disorders, above.

For a report of adverse effects attributed to reduced metabolism of nifedipine in patients taking cyclosporin, see under Interactions, above.

1. Feehally J, *et al.* Does nifedipine ameliorate cyclosporin A nephrotoxicity? *Br Med J* 1987; **295:** 310.
2. Shin GT, *et al.* Effect of nifedipine on renal allograft function and survival beyond one year. *Clin Nephrol* 1997; **47:** 33–6.
3. Weinrauch LA, *et al.* Role of calcium channel blockers in diabetic renal transplant patients: preliminary observations on protection from sepsis. *Clin Nephrol* 1995; **44:** 185–92.

Urticaria. Oral antihistamines are the main drugs used in the management of urticaria (p.1076). Addition of a calcium-channel blocker, such as nifedipine, has been suggested for patients unresponsive to treatment with oral antihistamines alone, but results have been mixed.[1,2]

1. Lawlor F, *et al.* Calcium antagonist in the treatment of symptomatic dermographism: low-dose and high-dose studies with nifedipine. *Dermatologica* 1988; **177:** 287–91.
2. Bressler RB, *et al.* Therapy of chronic idiopathic urticaria with nifedipine: demonstration of beneficial effect in a double-blinded, placebo-controlled, crossover trial. *J Allergy Clin Immunol* 1989; **83:** 756–63.

Preparations

BP 1998: Nifedipine Capsules;
USP 23: Nifedipine Capsules.

Proprietary Preparations (details are given in Part 3)
Aust.: Adalat; Buconif†; Einalat; Fedip; Gewadilat; Majolat; Nifebene; Nifecard; Ospocard; Unidipin; ***Austral.:*** Adalat; Adapine; Anpine†; Nifecard; Nyefax; ***Belg.:*** Adalat; ***Canad.:*** Adalat; Apo-Nifed; Novo-Nifedin; Nu-Nifed; ***Fr.:*** Adalate; Chronadalate; Nifelate†; ***Ger.:*** Adalat; Aprical; Cisday; Cordicant; Corinfar; Corotrend; Dignokonstant; duranifin; Jedipin; Nife; Nife-Puren; Nife-Wolff; Nifeclair; Nifecor; Nifedipat; Nifehexal; Nifelat; Nifical; Nifreal; Pidilat; ***Irl.:*** Adalat; Nifed; Nifensar; Pinifed; Systepin; Vasofed; ***Ital.:*** Adalat; Anifed; Citilat; Coral; Nifedicor; Nifedin; ***Neth.:*** Adalat; ***Norw.:*** Adalat; ***S.Afr.:*** Adalat; Anginor; Cardifen; Clinolat†; Nifedalat; Nifidine; Vasofed; ***Spain:*** Adalat; Cordilan; Dari; Dilcor; Pertensal; ***Swed.:*** Adalat; ***Switz.:*** Adalat; Adapress†; Aldipine; Antamex†; Corotrend; Ecodipine; Fedip; nife-basan; Nifedicor; Servidipine†; Unidipine†; ***UK:*** Adalat; Adipine; Angiopine; Calanif; Calcilat; Cardilate MR; Coracten; Coroday; Fortipine; Hypolar Retard; Nifedipress; Nifedotard; Nifensar XL†; Nimodrel; Nivaten; Slofedipine; Tensipine; Unipine XL; Vasad†; ***USA:*** Adalat; Procardia.

Multi-ingredient: ***Aust.:*** Beta-Adalat; Nif-Ten; Pontuc; ***Belg.:*** Beta-Adalat; Tenif; ***Fr.:*** Beta-Adalate; Tenordate; ***Ger.:*** Belnif; Bresben; duranifin Sali; Nif-Ten; Nifehexal Sali; Pontuc; Sali-Adalat; Tredalat; ***Irl.:*** Beta-Adalat; Nif-Ten; ***Ital.:*** Mixer; Nif-Ten; ***Neth.:*** Beta-Adalat†; Nif-Ten; ***Switz.:*** Beta-Adalat; Nif-Atenil; Nif-Ten; ***UK:*** Beta-Adalat; Nifelease; Tenif.

Nilvadipine (2192-p)

Nilvadipine (*BAN, USAN, rINN*).

CL-287389; FK-235; Nivadipine; SKF-102362. 5-Isopropyl 3-methyl 2-cyano-1,4-dihydro-6-methyl-4-(*m*-nitrophenyl)-3,5-pyridinedicarboxylate.

$C_{19}H_{19}N_3O_6$ = 385.4.

CAS — 75530-68-6.

Nilvadipine is a dihydropyridine calcium-channel blocker with general properties similar to those of nifedipine (p.916). It is used in the management of hypertension (p.788). Nilvadipine is given by mouth as a modified-release preparation in a usual dose of up to 16 mg daily.

References.

1. Takata Y, *et al.* Elevated plasma nilvadipine concentration after single and chronic oral administration to patients with chronic liver disease. *Eur J Clin Pharmacol* 1992; **42:** 475–9.

Preparations

Proprietary Preparations (details are given in Part 3)
Aust.: Arcadipin; Tensan; ***Ger.:*** Escor; Nivadil; ***Irl.:*** Nivadil; ***Jpn:*** Nivadil.

Nimodipine (16914-v)

Nimodipine (*BAN, USAN, rINN*).

Bay-e-9736; Nimodipinum. Isopropyl 2-methoxyethyl 1,4-dihydro-2,6-dimethyl-4-(3-nitrophenyl)pyridine-3,5-dicarboxylate.

$C_{21}H_{26}N_2O_7$ = 418.4.

CAS — 66085-59-4.

Pharmacopoeias. In *Eur.* (see p.viii).

A light yellow or yellow crystalline powder. Practically **insoluble** in water; sparingly soluble in absolute alcohol; freely soluble in ethyl acetate. It exhibits polymorphism. Exposure to ultraviolet light leads to formation of a nitrophenylpyridine derivative. Solutions should be prepared in the dark or under light of wavelength greater than 420 nm, immediately before use.

Protect from light.

The manufacturer states that solutions of nimodipine are **incompatible** with some plastics, including polyvinyl chloride.

Adverse Effects, Treatment, and Precautions

As for dihydropyridine calcium-channel blockers (see Nifedipine, p.916).

Nimodipine should be administered with caution to patients with cerebral oedema or severely raised intracranial pressure.

Marked bradycardia developed in a patient with acute ischaemic stroke during treatment with nimodipine and was suspected to be related to the drug therapy.[1]

1. Fagan SC, Nacci N. Nimodipine and bradycardia in acute stroke—drug or disease? *DICP Ann Pharmacother* 1991; **25:** 247–9.

Interactions

As for dihydropyridine calcium-channel blockers (see Nifedipine, p.918).

Pharmacokinetics

Nimodipine is rapidly absorbed from the gastro-intestinal tract following oral administration but undergoes extensive first-pass metabolism in the liver. The oral bioavailability is reported to be about 13%. It readily crosses the blood-brain barrier. Nimodipine is extensively metabolised in the liver. It is excreted in faeces via the bile, and in urine, almost entirely as metabolites. The terminal elimination half-life is reported to be about 9 hours but the initial decline in plasma concentrations is very much more rapid, equivalent to a half-life of 1 to 2 hours. Nimodipine is about 95% bound to plasma protein.

Uses and Administration

Nimodipine is a dihydropyridine calcium-channel blocker that has the general properties of nifedipine (p.919), but acts particularly on cerebral blood vessels. It is used in cerebrovascular disorders (see below), particularly in the prevention and treatment of ischaemic neurological deficits caused by arterial vasospasm following subarachnoid haemorrhage.

For the prophylaxis of neurological deficit nimodipine is given by mouth in a dose of 60 mg every 4 hours. Treatment should begin within 4 days of **subarachnoid haemorrhage** and should continue for 21 days. In patients with impaired hepatic function the initial dose should be halved to 30 mg every 4 hours.

Once cerebral ischaemia occurs, neurological deficit may be treated by intravenous infusion of nimodipine. It should be given via a bypass into a running intravenous infusion into a central vein. The initial dose should be nimodipine 1 mg per hour for 2 hours, increased (providing no severe decrease in blood pressure is observed) to 2 mg per hour. The starting dose should be reduced to 0.5 mg or less per hour in patients weighing less than 70 kg, in those with unstable blood pressure, or in those with impaired hepatic function. Infusion should be continued for at least 5 and no more than 14 days.

General reviews.

1. Langley MS, Sorkin EM. Nimodipine: a review of its pharmacodynamic and pharmacokinetic properties, and therapeutic potential in cerebrovascular disease. *Drugs* 1989; **37:** 669–99.

Cerebrovascular disorders. As described under Uses and Administration, above, nimodipine is used orally and intravenously in the prevention and treatment of ischaemic neurological deficits caused by arterial vasospasm following subarachnoid haemorrhage (see Stroke, p.799). In addition to dilating cerebral blood vessels and improving cerebral blood flow, nimodipine may also prevent or reverse ischaemic damage to the brain by limiting transcellular calcium influx.

These effects have led to the investigation of nimodipine in other conditions associated with cerebral ischaemia. Studies of nimodipine given orally following ischaemic stroke have produced conflicting results.[1,2] However, a meta-analysis[3] of controlled studies suggested that nimodipine is beneficial if given within 12 hours of stroke onset and a further study is underway to confirm these findings. In a controlled study of 155 patients suffering a cardiac arrest, nimodipine was given by intravenous infusion for 24 hours.[4] Nimodipine had no effect on overall survival, although it did improve survival of patients in whom advanced life support was delayed for more than 10 minutes after arrest. Nimodipine has also been tried in dementia (p.1386). Two multicentre studies involving a total of 755 patients with dementia of vascular or degenerative origin given nimodipine for up to 6 months reported improvements in cognitive function and disability.[5]

1. Gelmers HJ, *et al.* A controlled trial of nimodipine in acute ischemic stroke. *N Engl J Med* 1988; **318:** 203–7.
2. Trust Study Group. Randomised, double-blind, placebo-controlled trial of nimodipine in acute stroke. *Lancet* 1990; **336:** 1205–9.
3. Mohr JP, *et al.* Meta-analysis of oral nimodipine trials in acute ischemic stroke. *Cerebrovasc Dis* 1994; **4:** 197–203.
4. Roine RO, *et al.* Nimodipine after resuscitation from out-of-hospital ventricular fibrillation: a placebo-controlled, double-blind, randomized trial. *JAMA* 1990; **264:** 3171–7.
5. Parnetti L, *et al.* Nimodipine Study Group. Mental deterioration in old age: results of two multicenter, clinical trials with nimodipine. *Clin Ther* 1993; **15:** 394–406.

Migraine. For reference to the use of calcium-channel blockers, including nimodipine, in the management of migraine, see under Nifedipine, p.921.

Pain. Results in two patients indicated that intravenous nimodipine enhanced the effect of epidural morphine in the treatment of cancer pain.[1] Epidural nimodipine alone produced intense but short-lasting analgesia.

1. Filos KS, *et al.* Analgesia with epidural nimodipine. *Lancet* 1993; **342:** 1047.

Preparations

Proprietary Preparations (details are given in Part 3)
Aust.: Nimotop; ***Austral.:*** Nimotop; ***Belg.:*** Nimotop; ***Canad.:*** Nimotop; ***Fr.:*** Nimotop; ***Ger.:*** Nimotop; ***Irl.:*** Nimotop; ***Ital.:*** Nimotop; Periplum; ***Neth.:*** Nimotop; ***Norw.:*** Nimotop; ***S.Afr.:*** Nimotop; ***Spain:*** Admon; Brainal; Calnit; Kenesil; Modus; Nimotop; Remontal; ***Swed.:*** Nimotop; ***Switz.:*** Nimotop; ***UK:*** Nimotop; ***USA:*** Nimotop.

Nipradilol (19579-q)

Nipradilol (*rINN*).

K-351; Nipradolol. 8-[2-Hydroxy-3-(isopropylamino)propoxy]-3-chromanol,3-nitrate.

$C_{15}H_{22}N_2O_6$ = 326.3.

CAS — 81486-22-8.

Nipradilol is a beta blocker (p.828). It is also reported to have direct vasodilating activity. It is used in the management of hypertension and angina pectoris.

References.

1. Okumura H, *et al.* Effect of long-term therapy with nipradilol on esophageal varices in patients with compensated cirrhosis: results of a multicenter open study. *Arzneimittelforschung* 1994; **44:** 1250–4.

Preparations

Proprietary Preparations (details are given in Part 3)
Jpn: Hypadil†.

Nisoldipine (13022-j)

Nisoldipine (*BAN, USAN, rINN*).

Bay-k-5552. Isobutyl methyl 1,4-dihydro-2,6-dimethyl-4-(2-nitrophenyl)pyridine-3,5-dicarboxylate.

$C_{20}H_{24}N_2O_6$ = 388.4.

CAS — 63675-72-9.

Adverse Effects, Treatment, and Precautions

As for dihydropyridine calcium-channel blockers (see Nifedipine, p.916).

Interactions

As for dihydropyridine calcium-channel blockers (see Nifedipine, p.918).

Pharmacokinetics

Nisoldipine is well absorbed from the gastro-intestinal tract after oral administration, but undergoes rapid and extensive first-pass metabolism in the gut wall and liver and bioavailability has been reported to be only about 4 to 8%. About 60 to 80% of an oral dose is excreted in the urine and the remainder in the faeces, mainly as metabolites. The terminal elimination half-life is about 7 to 12 hours. Nisoldipine is highly bound to plasma proteins (99%).

The results of a study[1] in 11 patients receiving nisoldipine 10 mg once or twice daily by mouth indicated that the pharmacokinetics of nisoldipine could best be described by an open 2-compartment model. Peak plasma concentrations occurred one hour after a single oral dose, and varied greatly between the patients. The mean plasma elimination half-life was 11.4 hours after a single dose and 14.0 hours after repeated dosing, which was longer than had been previously reported, perhaps reflecting the greater sensitivity of the assay.

In another study oral but not intravenous administration of nisoldipine increased liver blood flow in 10 healthy subjects and thus affected its own systemic availability.[2] Variations in liver blood flow may account for the interindividual variation in the pharmacokinetics of nisoldipine.

1. Ottosson A-M, *et al.* Analysis and pharmacokinetics of nisoldipine in hypertensive patients. *Curr Ther Res* 1989; **45:** 347–58.
2. van Harten J, *et al.* Variability in the pharmacokinetics of nisoldipine as caused by differences in liver blood flow response. *J Clin Pharmacol* 1989; **29:** 714–21.

Uses and Administration

Nisoldipine is a dihydropyridine calcium-channel blocker with actions and uses similar to those of nifedipine (p.919). It is used in the management of hypertension (p.788) and angina pectoris (p.780).

Nisoldipine is given by mouth usually as a modified-release preparation. Doses are similar for both **hypertension** and **angina**. An initial dose of 10 mg once daily has been recommended. The usual maintenance dose is 20 to 40 mg once daily.

Reviews.

1. Mitchell J, *et al.* Nisoldipine: a new dihydropyridine calcium-channel blocker. *J Clin Pharmacol* 1993; **33:** 46–52.
2. Plosker GL, Faulds D. Nisoldipine coat-core: a review of its pharmacology and therapeutic efficacy in hypertension. *Drugs* 1996; **52:** 232–53.
3. Langtry HD, Spencer CM. Nisoldipine coat-core; a review of its pharmacodynamic and pharmacokinetic properties and clinical efficacy in the management of ischaemic heart disease. *Drugs* 1997; **53:** 867–84.

Preparations

Proprietary Preparations (details are given in Part 3)
Aust.: Syscor; ***Belg.:*** Syscor; ***Ger.:*** Baymycard; ***Ital.:*** Syscor; Zadipina; ***Neth.:*** Sular; Syscor; ***Spain:*** Cornel; Syscor; ***Swed.:*** Syscor; ***Switz.:*** Syscor; ***UK:*** Syscor; ***USA:*** Sular.

Nitrendipine (16915-g)

Nitrendipine *(BAN, USAN, rINN)*.

Bay-e-5009; Nitrendipinum. Ethyl methyl 1,4-dihydro-2,6-dimethyl-4-(3-nitrophenyl)pyridine-3,5-dicarboxylate.

$C_{18}H_{20}N_2O_6$ = 360.4.

CAS — 39562-70-4.

Pharmacopoeias. In *Eur.* (see p.viii).

A yellow crystalline powder. Practically **insoluble** in water; sparingly soluble in absolute alcohol and in methyl alcohol; freely soluble in ethyl acetate. It exhibits polymorphism. Exposure to ultraviolet light leads to formation of a nitrophenylpyridine derivative. Solutions should be prepared in the dark or under light of wavelength greater than 420 nm, immediately before use.

Protect from light.

Adverse Effects, Treatment, and Precautions

As for dihydropyridine calcium-channel blockers (see Nifedipine, p.916).

Interactions

As for dihydropyridine calcium-channel blockers (see Nifedipine, p.918).

Pharmacokinetics

Nitrendipine is reported to be well absorbed following oral administration but undergoes extensive first-pass metabolism; the absolute oral bioavailability is reported to range from about 10 to 20%, depending in part on the dosage form.

Nitrendipine is extensively metabolised in the liver and is excreted as metabolites, mainly in urine, with small amounts in the faeces. Although early studies reported a terminal elimination half-life of about 2 to 4 hours, later studies, using more sensitive assay procedures, have recorded values between about 10 and 22 hours. Nitrendipine is about 98% bound to plasma proteins.

References.

1. Soons PA, Breimer DD. Stereoselective pharmacokinetics of oral and intravenous nitrendipine in healthy male subjects. *Br J Clin Pharmacol* 1991; **32:** 11–16.

Uses and Administration

Nitrendipine is a dihydropyridine calcium-channel blocker with actions similar to those of nifedipine (p.919). It is used in the treatment of **hypertension** (p.788).

The usual dose is 20 mg daily as a single dose by mouth or as 2 divided doses. The dose may be increased to 20 mg twice daily if necessary for the control of resistant hypertension. In the elderly, and in patients with liver disease, an initial dose of 10 mg daily has been recommended.

Reviews.

1. Goa KL, Sorkin EM. Nitrendipine: a review of its pharmacodynamic and pharmacokinetic properties, and therapeutic efficacy in the treatment of hypertension. *Drugs* 1987; **33:** 123–55.
2. Santiago TM, Lopez LM. Nitrendipine: a new dihydropyridine calcium-channel antagonist for the treatment of hypertension. *DICP Ann Pharmacother* 1990; **24:** 167–75.

Preparations

Proprietary Preparations (details are given in Part 3)
Aust.: Baypress; ***Belg.:*** Baypress; ***Fr.:*** Baypress; Nidrel; ***Ger.:*** Bayotensin; Nitrendepat; Nitrepress; ***Ital.:*** Baypress; Deiten; ***Neth.:*** Baypress; ***Spain:*** Baypresol; Gericin; Monopress; Niprina; Sub Tensin; Tensogradal; Trendinol; Vastensium; ***Switz.:*** Baypress.

Nitric Oxide (15530-b)

Mononitrogen Monoxide; Nitrogen Monoxide.

NO = 30.01.

Nitric oxide is an endogenous chemical messenger whose predominant effect is as a vasodilator. Nitric oxide is also involved in platelet aggregation, neurotransmission, and the immune system, and possesses antimicrobial, antitumour, and antiviral activity.

Nitric oxide is synthesised from L-arginine and is now recognised to be the same substance as endothelium-derived relaxing factor (EDRF). Synthesis from L-arginine is by the enzyme, nitric oxide synthase. Three isoforms of this enzyme have been identified. Constitutive isoforms occur in endothelial cells (such as in vascular endothelium, platelets, and the heart) and neuronal cells (in some central and peripheral neurones). Small amounts of nitric oxide are regularly produced by these systems. In contrast, an inducible nitric oxide synthase isoform is expressed only after activation by external stimuli such as in infection or inflammation and larger amounts of nitric oxide are produced. This inducible nitric oxide synthase may be expressed in a wide range of cells, including macrophages and cells in vascular smooth muscle, the heart, gastro-intestinal tract, and liver. Once released, nitric oxide acts by stimulating guanylate cyclase in vascular smooth muscle cells, but is rapidly inactivated by oxidation to nitrite and nitrate and reaction with haemoglobin to form methaemoglobin. Nitric oxide has a half-life of only a few seconds.

Inhaled nitric oxide is a highly selective pulmonary vasodilator and is being studied in a variety of bronchopulmonary disorders including pulmonary hypertension and respiratory distress syndromes.

Organic nitrates such as glyceryl trinitrate (p.874) and other nitrovasodilators such as sodium nitroprusside (p.943) are now believed to exert their vasodilator action through nitric oxide. Such molecules are referred to as nitric oxide donors.

Excess or insufficient production of endogenous nitric oxide is thought to occur in many diseases and this has led to trials of nitric oxide donors or nitric oxide synthase inhibitors in various conditions. For example, enhanced synthesis of endogenous nitric oxide by the inducible isoform of nitric oxide synthase is thought to be involved in the severe hypotension of septic shock and this has led to the investigation of nitric oxide synthase inhibitors, such as targinine (p.1634).

General reviews.

1. Änggård E. Nitric oxide: mediator, murderer, and medicine. *Lancet* 1994; **343:** 1199–1206.
2. Holden K. Nitric oxide—from exhaust fumes to medical revolution. *Pharm J* 1994; **252:** 402–7.
3. Lowenstein CJ, *et al.* Nitric oxide: a physiologic messenger. *Ann Intern Med* 1994; **120:** 227–37.
4. Vallance P, Collier J. Biology and clinical relevance of nitric oxide. *Br Med J* 1994; **309:** 453–7.
5. Edwards AD. The pharmacology of inhaled nitric oxide. *Arch Dis Child* 1995; **72:** F127–F130.
6. Lunn RJ. Inhaled nitric oxide therapy. *Mayo Clin Proc* 1995; **70:** 247–55.
7. Quinn AC, *et al.* Nitric oxide: an endogenous gas. *Br J Anaesth* 1995; **74:** 443–51.
8. Zoritch B. Nitric oxide and asthma. *Arch Dis Child* 1995; **72:** 259–62.
9. Loscalzo J. Nitric oxide and vascular disease. *N Engl J Med* 1995; **333:** 251–3.
10. Brett SJ, Evans TW. Nitric oxide: physiological roles and therapeutic implications in the lung. *Br J Hosp Med* 1996; **55:** 487–90.
11. Finer N. Inhaled nitric oxide in neonates. *Arch Dis Child* 1997; **77:** F81–F84.

Inhaled nitric oxide is a potent and highly selective pulmonary vasodilator and thus offers potential advantages over other vasodilators that may cause unwanted systemic effects. It is being widely investigated in persistent pulmonary hypertension of the newborn and other conditions leading to hypoxic respiratory failure in neonates and in the acute respiratory distress syndrome (see below).

Nitric oxide has also been tried in the neonatal respiratory distress syndrome,[1,2] in primary pulmonary hypertension,[3,4] and in pulmonary hypertension associated with a wide range of conditions including heart failure,[5] post-cardiac surgery,[6] and high-altitude disorders.[7]

1. Peliowski A, *et al.* Inhaled nitric oxide for premature infants after prolonged rupture of the membranes. *J Pediatr* 1995; **126:** 450–3.
2. Skimming JW, *et al.* Nitric oxide inhalation in infants with respiratory distress syndrome. *J Pediatr* 1997; **130:** 225–30.
3. Kinsella JP, *et al.* Selective and sustained pulmonary vasodilation with inhalational nitric oxide therapy in a child with idiopathic pulmonary hypertension. *J Pediatr* 1993; **122:** 803–6.
4. Goldman AP, *et al.* Is it time to consider domiciliary nitric oxide? *Lancet* 1995; **345:** 199–200.
5. Matsumoto A, *et al.* Inhaled nitric oxide and exercise capacity in congestive heart failure. *Lancet* 1997; **349:** 999–1000. Correction. *ibid.*; **350:** 818.
6. Haydar A, *et al.* Inhaled nitric oxide for postoperative pulmonary hypertension in patients with congenital heart defects. *Lancet* 1992; **340:** 1545.
7. Scherrer U, *et al.* Inhaled nitric oxide for high-altitude pulmonary edema. *N Engl J Med* 1996; **334:** 624–9.

Adverse effects and precautions. Inhaled nitric oxide appears to be relatively free of toxicity although some side-effects have occurred. A potential complication is methaemoglobinaemia but this is probably related to the dose and the risk does not appear to be increased during low-dose (20 ppm) therapy.[1] Another possible adverse event is an increased risk of bleeding due to inhibition of platelet aggregation by nitric oxide.[2-5] Motor neuron disease in a patient with alcoholism has been partly attributed[6] to the use of nitric oxide for pulmonary hypertension. Rebound pulmonary hypertension has been recorded[7] in some children following withdrawal of nitric oxide therapy. Increasing the inhaled concentration of oxygen while inhaled nitric oxide is being withdrawn has been suggested[8] for preventing the sudden deterioration in oxygenation that occurs in some infants on withdrawal of nitric oxide. Inhaled nitric oxide is a selective pulmonary vasodilator. However, severe systemic hypotension has been reported[9] following initiation of inhaled nitric oxide therapy in a neonate with severe left ventricular dysfunction.

Some of the toxicity of inhaled nitric oxide may be due to nitrogen dioxide that is formed from nitric oxide in the presence of high oxygen concentrations. Some practitioners recommend monitoring concentrations of inspired nitric oxide and nitrogen dioxide.[10]

Nitric oxide is a potential carcinogen and consideration must be given to limiting exposure of healthcare personnel to nitric oxide and nitrogen dioxide.[11]

1. Kinsella JP, Abman SH. Methaemoglobin during nitric oxide therapy with high-frequency ventilation. *Lancet* 1993; **342:** 615.
2. Högman M, *et al.* Bleeding time prolongation and NO inhalation. *Lancet* 1993; **341:** 1664–5.
3. Joannidis M, *et al.* Inhaled nitric oxide. *Lancet* 1996; **348:** 1448–9.
4. Cheung P-Y, *et al.* Inhaled nitric oxide and inhibition of platelet aggregation in critically ill neonates. *Lancet* 1998; **351:** 1181–2.
5. George TN, *et al.* The effect of inhaled nitric oxide therapy on bleeding time and platelet aggregation in neonates. *J Pediatr* 1998; **132:** 731–4.
6. Tsai GE, Gastfriend DR. Nitric oxide-induced motor neuron disease in a patient with alcoholism. *N Engl J Med* 1995; **332:** 1036.
7. Miller OI, *et al.* Rebound pulmonary hypertension on withdrawal from inhaled nitric oxide. *Lancet* 1995; **346:** 51–2.

8. Aly H, *et al.* Weaning strategy with inhaled nitric oxide treatment in persistent pulmonary hypertension of the newborn. *Arch Dis Child* 1997; **76:** F118–F122.
9. Henrichsen T, *et al.* Inhaled nitric oxide can cause severe systemic hypotension. *J Pediatr* 1996; **129:** 183.
10. Cuthbertson BH, *et al.* Use of inhaled nitric oxide in British intensive therapy units. *Br J Anaesth* 1997; **78:** 696–700.
11. Committee on Safety of Medicines/Medicines Control Agency. Inhaled nitric oxide. *Current Problems* 1996; **22:** 8.

Acute respiratory distress syndrome. Although inhalation of nitric oxide has been reported[1,2] to improve oxygenation in patients with acute respiratory distress syndrome (p.1017), a small randomised trial[3] and a multicentre study[2] have reported no effect on mortality; other studies have shown that response to nitric oxide therapy is very variable. Further studies are underway to confirm the benefits of nitric oxide in patients with the acute respiratory distress syndrome.[4] Simultaneous intravenous administration of almitrine, a pulmonary vasoconstrictor, has been reported to increase arterial oxygenation more than nitric oxide alone.[5]

1. Rossaint R, *et al.* Inhaled nitric oxide for the adult respiratory distress syndrome. *N Engl J Med* 1993; **328:** 399–405.
2. Dellinger RP, *et al.* Effects of inhaled nitric oxide in patients with acute respiratory distress syndrome: results of a randomized phase II trial. *Crit Care Med* 1998; **26:** 15–23.
3. Troncy E, *et al.* Should we treat acute respiratory distress syndrome with inhaled nitric oxide? *Lancet* 1997; **350:** 111–12.
4. Young JD. The use of inhaled nitric oxide in the acute respiratory distress syndrome. *Br J Hosp Med* 1997; **57:** 126–7.
5. Wysocki M, *et al.* Additive effect on gas exchange of inhaled nitric oxide and intravenous almitrine bismesylate in the adult respiratory distress syndrome. *Intensive Care Med* 1994; **20:** 254–9.

Persistent pulmonary hypertension in newborns. Inhaled nitric oxide is being widely investigated in persistent pulmonary hypertension of the newborn[1,2] (p.796). Studies have shown marked improvement in oxygenation[3] although one study suggested this may not be sustained.[4] Two multicentre controlled studies[5,6] have found that inhaled nitric oxide reduces the use of extracorporeal membrane oxygenation but neither study showed any effect on mortality. Some neonates may not respond to nitric oxide therapy; one study found that neonates with pulmonary hypoplasia and dysplasia may have decreased sensitivity to nitric oxide.[4] Another study reported that some neonates who failed to respond to nitric oxide were successfully treated with a combination of nitric oxide and high-frequency oscillatory ventilation.[7] There have been concerns that use of inhaled nitric oxide might adversely affect neurodevelopmental outcome more than conventional therapy, but this was not confirmed in infants followed up for up to 2 years.[8]

1. Kinsella JP, Abman SH. Recent developments in the pathophysiology and treatment of persistent pulmonary hypertension of the newborn. *J Pediatr* 1995; **126:** 853–64.
2. Mupanemunda RH, Edwards AD. Treatment of newborn infants with inhaled nitric oxide. *Arch Dis Child* 1995; **72:** F131–F134.
3. Davidson D, *et al.* Inhaled nitric oxide for the early treatment of persistent pulmonary hypertension of the term newborn: a randomized, double-masked, placebo-controlled, dose-response, multicenter study. *Pediatrics* 1998; **101:** 325–34.
4. Goldman AP, *et al.* Four patterns of response to inhaled nitric oxide for persistent pulmonary hypertension of the newborn. *Pediatrics* 1996; **98:** 706–13.
5. The Neonatal Inhaled Nitric Oxide Study Group. Inhaled nitric oxide in full-term and nearly full-term infants with hypoxic respiratory failure. *N Engl J Med* 1997; **336:** 597–604. Correction. *ibid.*; **337:** 434.
6. Roberts JD, *et al.* Inhaled nitric oxide and persistent pulmonary hypertension of the newborn. *N Engl J Med* 1997; **336:** 605–10.
7. Kinsella JP, *et al.* Randomized, multicenter trial of inhaled nitric oxide and high-frequency oscillatory ventilation in severe, persistent pulmonary hypertension of the newborn. *J Pediatr* 1997; **131:** 55–62.
8. Rosenberg AA, *et al.* Longitudinal follow-up of a cohort of newborn infants treated with inhaled nitric oxide for persistent pulmonary hypertension. *J Pediatr* 1997; **131:** 70–5.

Noradrenaline (9506-x)

Noradrenaline (*BAN*).

Norepinephrine (*rINN*); Norepirenamine. (*R*)-2-Amino-1-(3,4-dihydroxyphenyl)ethanol.

$C_8H_{11}NO_3$ = 169.2.

CAS — 51-41-2.

Pharmacopoeias. Jpn includes the racemic form.

Noradrenaline Acid Tartrate (2087-q)

Noradrenaline Acid Tartrate (*BANM*).

Norepinephrine Bitartrate (*USAN, rINNM*); Arterenol Acid Tartrate; *l*-Arterenol Bitartrate; Levarterenol Acid Tartrate; Levarterenol Bitartrate; Levarterenoli Bitartras; Noradrenaline Bitartrate; Noradrenaline Tartrate; Noradrenalini Tartras; *l*-Norepinephrine Bitartrate.

$C_8H_{11}NO_3,C_4H_6O_6,H_2O$ = 337.3.

CAS — 51-40-1 (noradrenaline acid tartrate, anhydrous); 69815-49-2 (noradrenaline acid tartrate, monohydrate).

Pharmacopoeias. In Chin., Eur. (see p.viii), Pol., and US.

A white or faintly grey, odourless, crystalline powder. It darkens on exposure to air and light. Noradrenaline acid tartrate 2 micrograms is approximately equivalent to 1 microgram of noradrenaline. **Soluble** 1 in 2.5 of water and 1 in 300 of alcohol; practically insoluble in chloroform and ether. Solutions in water have a pH of about 3.5. **Store** in airtight containers, or preferably, in a sealed tube under vacuum or an inert gas. Protect from light.

Incompatibility. Noradrenaline acid tartrate is strongly acidic in solution, and would be expected to be incompatible with drugs having an alkaline pH. The manufacturers in the UK state that solutions are reportedly incompatible with alkalis and oxidising agents, barbiturates, chlorpheniramine, chlorothiazide, nitrofurantoin, novobiocin, phenytoin, sodium bicarbonate, sodium iodide, and streptomycin. Incompatibility with insulin has also been reported.[1]

1. Yamashita SK, *et al.* Compatibility of selected critical care drugs during simulated Y-site administration. *Am J Health-Syst Pharm* 1996; **53:** 1048–51.

Noradrenaline Hydrochloride (9505-t)

Noradrenaline Hydrochloride (*BANM*).

Norepinephrine Hydrochloride (*rINNM*); Noradrenalini Hydrochloridum.

$C_8H_{11}NO_3,HCl$ = 205.6.

CAS — 329-56-6.

Pharmacopoeias. In *Eur.* (see p.viii).

A white or brownish white, crystalline powder. It becomes coloured on exposure to air and light. Noradrenaline hydrochloride 1.2 micrograms is approximately equivalent to 1 microgram of noradrenaline. Very **soluble** in water; slightly soluble in alcohol. A 2% solution in water has a pH of 3.5 to 4.5. **Store** in airtight containers, or preferably, in a sealed tube under vacuum or an inert gas. Protect from light.

Adverse Effects

Noradrenaline is an extremely potent peripheral vasoconstrictor and hypertension (possibly associated with reflex bradycardia), headache, and peripheral ischaemia, which may be severe enough to result in gangrene of the extremities, are among the potential adverse effects.

Noradrenaline is a severe tissue irritant and only very dilute solutions should be injected. The needle must be inserted well into the vein to avoid extravasation, otherwise severe phlebitis and sloughing may occur.

For the adverse effects of sympathomimetics in general, see Adrenaline, p.813.

Severe headache, once with fatal cerebral haemorrhage, had been reported in dental patients who had received injections of lignocaine 2% with noradrenaline 1 in 25 000. It was suggested that a concentration of noradrenaline 1 in 25 000 was too high and could not be justified and that a concentration of 1 in 80 000 was to be preferred.[1] However, authorities in the UK now consider that noradrenaline should not be used as a vasoconstrictor in local anaesthetic solutions since it presents no advantages over adrenaline and carries additional hazard.

1. Boakes AJ, *et al.* Adverse reactions to local anaesthetic/vasoconstrictor preparations: a study of the cardiovascular responses to Xylestesin and Hostacain-with-Noradrenaline. *Br Dent J* 1972; **133:** 137–40.

Treatment of Adverse Effects

The hypertensive effects of noradrenaline may be treated with an alpha-adrenoceptor blocker such as phentolamine. If extravasation occurs, infiltration with phentolamine (see p.930) as soon as possible, and certainly within 12 hours, may relieve pain and prevent tissue necrosis.

Precautions

Noradrenaline must be avoided in the presence of hypertension and blood pressure and infusion rate must be monitored frequently. Noradrenaline-induced cardiac arrhythmias are more likely in patients with hypoxia or hypercapnia. Hypovolaemia should be corrected before starting noradrenaline infusion.

Noradrenaline may reduce placental perfusion throughout pregnancy and some consider that it and similar vasoconstrictor sympathomimetics are best avoided; also in late pregnancy noradrenaline provokes uterine contractions which can result in fetal asphyxia.

For the precautions to be observed with sympathomimetics in general, see Adrenaline, p.814.

Interactions

For the interactions of the sympathomimetics in general, see Adrenaline, p.814.

Pharmacokinetics

Like adrenaline (p.815), noradrenaline is inactive when given by mouth, and it is rapidly inactivated in the body by similar processes. When given intravenously it is extensively metabolised and only small amounts are excreted unchanged in the urine of healthy subjects.

Uses and Administration

The catecholamine, noradrenaline, is a direct-acting sympathomimetic (see Adrenaline, p.815) with pronounced effects on alpha-adrenergic receptors and less marked effects on beta-adrenergic receptors. It is a neurotransmitter, stored in granules in nerve axons, which is released at the terminations of post ganglionic adrenergic nerve fibres when they are stimulated; some is also present in the adrenal medulla from which it is liberated together with adrenaline. A major effect of noradrenaline is to raise systolic and diastolic blood pressure (which is accompanied by reflex slowing of the heart rate). This is a result of its alpha-stimulant effects which cause vasoconstriction, with reduced blood flow in the kidneys, liver, skin, and usually skeletal muscle. The pregnant uterus also contracts; high doses liberate glucose from the liver and have other hormonal effects similar to those of adrenaline. There is little stimulation of the central nervous system. Beta-stimulant effects of noradrenaline have a positive inotropic action on the heart, but there is little bronchodilator effect.

Noradrenaline is used for the emergency restoration of blood pressure in acute hypotensive states (p.790). It has been used in local anaesthesia to diminish the absorption and localise the effect of the local anaesthetic (p.1283) but adrenaline is now preferred (see also under Adverse Effects, above). Locally applied solutions have been used to control bleeding in upper gastro-intestinal haemorrhage and similar disorders.

In **acute hypotensive states**, noradrenaline is administered as the acid tartrate by intravenous infusion of a solution containing the equivalent of 4 µg of the base per mL in glucose 5%, or sodium chloride 0.9% and glucose 5%. To avoid tissue necrosis the infusion should be administered through a central venous catheter or into a large vein high up in a limb, preferably the arm. Some sources have suggested that addition of phentolamine 5 to 10 mg per litre to the infusion may prevent sloughing, should extravasation occur, without affecting the vasopressor action. The infusion is usually given initially at a rate of 2 to 3 mL per minute (8 to 12 µg per minute) and adjusted according to the blood pressure response. Blood pressure is initially recorded every 2 minutes and the rate of infusion continuously monitored. The infusion must not be stopped suddenly but should be gradually withdrawn to avoid disastrous falls in blood pressure. The average maintenance dose is 0.5 to 1 mL per minute (2 to 4 µg per minute), but there is a wide variation and higher doses may be required. The concentration of the infusion may be altered according to clinical needs. Alternatively a solution containing the equivalent of 40 µg of the base per mL may be given at an initial rate of 0.16 to 0.33 mL per minute via a central venous catheter, using a syringe pump or drip counter. Noradrenaline may also be given parenterally as the hydrochloride in the management of hypotensive states.

Similar doses may be given to restore blood pressure following **cardiac arrest**. In patients with cardiac standstill, a more concentrated solution of the acid tartrate equivalent to 100 µg of the base per mL can be given by rapid intravenous or intracardiac injection; a dose of 0.5 to 0.75 mL (50 to 75 µg of noradrenaline) has been suggested which may be repeated if necessary.

Preparations

BP 1998: Noradrenaline Injection;
USP 23: Norepinephrine Bitartrate Injection; Propoxycaine and Procaine Hydrochlorides and Norepinephrine Bitartrate Injection.

Proprietary Preparations (details are given in Part 3)
Austral.: Levophed; ***Belg.:*** Levophed; ***Canad.:*** Levophed; ***Ger.:*** Arterenol; ***Irl.:*** Levophed; ***Ital.:*** Noradrec†; ***Spain:*** Adrenor; ***UK:*** Levophed; ***USA:*** Levophed.

Used as an adjunct in: ***Aust.:*** Neo-Xylestesin forte; Scandonest; ***Austral.:*** Nurocain with Sympathin†; ***Ger.:*** Anaesthol; Meaverin "N" mit Noradrenaline; Neo-Lidocaton; Nor-Anaesthol; Scandicain "N3"†; Xylestesin; Xylestesin-S; ***Ital.:*** Lident Andrenor; Neo-Lidocaton†; Xylestesina S†; Xylestesina†; Xylonor; ***S.Afr.:*** Scandonest; Xylotox; ***Spain:*** Anestecidan Noradrenalin†; Cidancaina†; Llorentecaina Noradrenal; Stoma Anestesia Dental; Xylonor Especial; ***Switz.:*** Neo-Lidocaton†; Scandonest; Xylestesin-F; Xylestesin-S "special"; Xylonor; ***UK:*** Lignostab-N†; ***USA:*** Ravocaine and Novocain.

Norfenefrine Hydrochloride (2089-s)

Norfenefrine Hydrochloride *(rINNM)*.

Norphenylephrine Hydrochloride; *m*-Norsynephrine Hydrochloride; WV-569. 2-Amino-1-(3-hydroxyphenyl)ethanol hydrochloride.

$C_8H_{11}NO_2,HCl = 189.6$.

CAS — 536-21-0 (norfenefrine); 15308-34-6 (norfenefrine hydrochloride).

NOTE. *m*-Octopamine has been used as a synonym for norfenefrine. Care should be taken to avoid confusion between the 2 compounds.

Norfenefrine is a sympathomimetic (see Adrenaline, p.813) with predominantly alpha-adrenergic activity. It is used as the hydrochloride for its vasopressor effect in the treatment of hypotensive states (p.790). The usual dose is 15 mg three times daily by mouth, as a controlled-release preparation, but doses of up to 45 mg three times daily have been given. Norfenefrine hydrochloride has also been given by injection.

Preparations

Proprietary Preparations (details are given in Part 3)
Aust.: Novadral; ***Ger.:*** Energona; Esbuphon†; Hypolind†; Novadral; Stagural†; ***Swed.:*** Nevadral Retard†; ***Switz.:*** Novadral.

Multi-ingredient: ***Ger.:*** Adyston; Normotin-P†; Normotin-R; Ordinal Forte; Ordinal retard†; Tonovit†; ***Switz.:*** Ortho-Maren retard.

Octodrine (6344-k)

Octodrine *(USAN, rINN)*.

SKF-51. 1,5-Dimethylhexylamine.

$C_8H_{19}N = 129.2$.

CAS — 543-82-8.

Octodrine is a sympathomimetic (see Adrenaline, p.813) with predominantly alpha-adrenergic activity. It is given by mouth as the camsylate, in combination with norfenefrine (p.925), in the treatment of hypotensive states. Octodrine phosphate has been used as an ingredient of preparations for obstructive airways disease.

Preparations

Proprietary Preparations (details are given in Part 3)

Multi-ingredient: ***Aust.:*** Ambredin; ***Ger.:*** Ordinal Forte; Ordinal retard†.

Octopamine (2090-h)

Octopamine *(rINN)*.

β,4-Dihydroxyphenethylamine; *p*-Hydroxymandelamine; ND-50; Noroxedrine; *p*-Norsynephrine. 2-Amino-1-(4-hydroxyphenyl)ethanol.

$C_8H_{11}NO_2 = 153.2$.

CAS — 104-14-3.

NOTE. *m*-Octopamine has been used as a synonym for norfenefrine. Care should be taken to avoid confusion between the 2 compounds.

Octopamine is a sympathomimetic (see Adrenaline, p.813) with predominantly alpha-adrenergic activity. It has been given by mouth as the hydrochloride or the tartrate in the treatment of hypotensive states.

Preparations

Proprietary Preparations (details are given in Part 3)
Aust.: Norphen†; ***Ger.:*** Norphen†; ***Ital.:*** Norden†.

Multi-ingredient: ***Ger.:*** Norphenovit N†.

Olprinone (17438-n)

Olprinone *(rINN)*.

1,2-Dihydro-5-imidazo[1,2-*a*]pyridin-6-yl-6-methyl-2-oxonicotinonitrile.

$C_{14}H_{10}N_4O = 250.3$.

CAS — 106730-54-5.

Olprinone is a phosphodiesterase inhibitor used as a cardiac inotrope in acute heart failure.

Orbofiban Acetate (5599-s)

Orbofiban Acetate *(USAN, rINNM)*.

SC-57099-B. *N*-{[(3*S*)-1-(*p*-Amidinophenyl)-2-oxo-3-pyrrolidinyl]carbamoyl}-β-alanine ethyl ester monoacetate quadrantihydrate.

$C_{17}H_{23}N_5O_4,C_2H_4O_2,\frac{1}{4}H_2O = 426.0$.

CAS — 163250-90-6 (orbofiban); 165800-05-5 (orbofiban acetate).

Orbofiban is a glycoprotein IIb/IIIa-receptor antagonist under investigation as an antiplatelet drug in unstable angina and myocardial infarction.

Ouabain (5823-n)

Acocantherin; G-Strophanthin; Ouabainum; Strophanthin-G; Strophanthinum; Strophanthoside-G; Uabaina; Ubaína. 3β-(α-L-Rhamnopyranosyloxy)-1β,5,11α,14,19-pentahydroxy-5β,14β-card-20(22)-enolide octahydrate.

$C_{29}H_{44}O_{12},8H_2O = 728.8$.

CAS — 630-60-4 (anhydrous ouabain); 11018-89-6 (ouabain octahydrate).

Pharmacopoeias. In *Eur.* (see p.viii), *Jpn*, and *Pol.*

A glycoside obtained from the seeds of *Strophanthus gratus* or from the wood of *Acokanthera schimperi* or *A. ouabaio* (Apocynaceae).

Colourless crystals or white crystalline powder. Sparingly **soluble** in water and alcohol; practically insoluble in ether and in ethyl acetate. **Protect** from light.

Ouabain is a cardiac glycoside with positive inotropic activity. It has general properties similar to those of digoxin (p.849) and may be used in the treatment of heart failure (p.785).

Ouabain takes effect in 3 to 10 minutes following intravenous injection and exerts its full action on the heart within 30 minutes to 2 hours; the effect persists for 1 to 3 days.

In heart failure ouabain has been given by slow intravenous injection in a dose of up to 250 µg. Ouabain may also be given by mouth for maintenance treatment in a dose of up to 24 mg daily.

An endogenous digitalis-like factor, known to be present in plasma, was identified as a steroid produced by the adrenal cortex and identical to ouabain.[1] As a sodium pump inhibitor it had the potential to affect sodium homoeostasis and blood pressure regulation, but whether authentic ouabain circulates in human plasma and is of adrenocortical origin, and also what function it might have, is still debated.[2] A study involving human placenta extracts suggested the substance may be a structurally related bufenolide but could not confirm its endogenous origin.[3]

1. Anonymous. Welcome to ouabain—a new steroid hormone. *Lancet* 1991; **338:** 543–4.
2. Nicholls MG, *et al.* Ouabain: a new steroid hormone? *Lancet* 1995; **346:** 1381–2.
3. Hilton PJ, *et al.* An inhibitor of the sodium pump obtained from human placenta. *Lancet* 1996; **348:** 303–5.

Preparations

Proprietary Preparations (details are given in Part 3)
Aust.: Strodival†; ***Ger.:*** Melostrophan†; Purostrophan†; Strodival; Strophocor N.

Multi-ingredient: ***Ger.:*** Cor-Neo-Nervacit-S†; Crataegutt-Strophanthin†; Purostrophyll†; Strophanon†.

Oxedrine (9510-c)

Oxedrine *(BAN)*.

Sympaethaminum; Synephrine. (*RS*)-1-(4-Hydroxyphenyl)-2-(methylamino)ethanol.

$C_9H_{13}NO_2 = 167.2$.

CAS — 94-07-5.

NOTE. *m*-Synephrine has been used as a synonym for phenylephrine. Care should be taken to avoid confusion between the two compounds.

Oxedrine Hydrochloride (11485-g)

Oxedrine Hydrochloride *(BANM)*.

$C_9H_{13}NO_2,HCl = 203.7$.

Oxedrine Tartrate (2092-b)

Oxedrine Tartrate *(BANM)*.

Aetaphen. Tartrat.; Aethaphenum Tartaricum; Oxedrini Tartras; Oxyphenylmethylaminoethanol Tartrate; Sinefrina Tartrato; Synephrine Tartrate.

$(C_9H_{13}NO_2)_2,C_4H_6O_6 = 484.5$.

CAS — 16589-24-5 (oxedrine tartrate); 67-04-9 (oxedrine tartrate, ±).

Pharmacopoeias. In *It.*

Oxedrine is a sympathomimetic (see Adrenaline, p.813) given as the tartrate in the treatment of hypotensive states in doses of about 100 to 150 mg three times daily by mouth; it has also been given by subcutaneous, intramuscular, or intravenous injection.

The hydrochloride and tartrate are used in eye drops as an ocular decongestant.

Preparations

Proprietary Preparations (details are given in Part 3)
Aust.: Sympatol; ***Ger.:*** Fraxipos N†; Sympatol; ***Ital.:*** Sympatol; ***Switz.:*** Sympalept; Sympatol†.

Multi-ingredient: ***Aust.:*** Dacrin; Pasuma-Dragees; ***Fr.:*** Antalyre; Chibro-Boraline†; Dacrine†; Dacryne; Dacryoboraline; Dulcidrine†; Polyfra; Posine; Sedacollyre; Uvicol; ***Ger.:*** Dacrin; hypo-loges†; Ophtalmin; Pasgensin; Solupen-D; Solupen†; Sympatocard†; Sympatovit†; ***Ital.:*** Broncobeta†; Torfanolo†; ***Switz.:*** Chibro-Boraline; Dacrine; Demo-Rhinil†.

Oxilofrine Hydrochloride (11409-k)

Oxilofrine Hydrochloride *(rINNM)*.

p-Hydroxyephedrine Hydrochloride; Methylsynephrine Hydrochloride; Oxyephedrine Hydrochloride. *erythro*-*p*-Hydroxy-α-[1-(methylamino)ethyl]benzyl alcohol hydrochloride.

$C_{10}H_{15}NO_2,HCl = 217.7$.

CAS — 942-51-8.

Oxilofrine is a sympathomimetic related to ephedrine (p.1059). It is used as the hydrochloride in the treatment of hypotensive states in usual doses of 16 mg three times daily by mouth, although higher doses have been given. Its salts have been used in antitussive preparations.

Preparations

Proprietary Preparations (details are given in Part 3)
Aust.: Carnigen; ***Ger.:*** Carnigen.

Multi-ingredient: ***Canad.:*** Cophylac; ***Ger.:*** Diben-amid†.

Oxpentifylline (9267-r)

Oxpentifylline *(BAN)*.

Pentoxifylline *(USAN, rINN)*; BL-191; Pentoxifyllinum. 3,7-Dimethyl-1-(5-oxohexyl)xanthine.

$C_{13}H_{18}N_4O_3 = 278.3$.

CAS — 6493-05-6.

Pharmacopoeias. In *Eur.* (see p.viii) and *Jpn.*

A white or almost white crystalline powder. **Soluble** in water; sparingly soluble in alcohol; very slightly soluble in ether; freely soluble in dichloromethane. **Protect** from light.

Adverse Effects

Oxpentifylline can cause nausea, gastro-intestinal disturbances, dizziness, and headache. Flushing, angina, palpitations, cardiac arrhythmias, and hypersensitivity reactions may also occur. Bleeding events have been reported rarely, usually in association with bleeding risk factors.

Overdosage with oxpentifylline may be associated with fever, faintness, flushing, hypotension, drowsiness, agitation, and seizures.

Haemorrhage. Three major bleeding episodes including 2 fatal cerebral haemorrhages were reported in a group of patients receiving oxpentifylline 400 mg three times daily together with nicoumalone for intermittent claudication.[1] Gastro-intestinal bleeding occurred in a 67-year-old patient with a history of duodenal ulcer following a single dose of oxpentifylline for optic neuropathy.[2]

1. APIC Study Group. Acenocoumarol and pentoxifylline in intermittent claudication: a controlled clinical study. *Angiology* 1989; **40:** 237–48.
2. Oren R, *et al.* Pentoxifylline-induced gastrointestinal bleeding. *DICP Ann Pharmacother* 1991; **25:** 315–16.

Overdosage. A 22-year-old woman who took oxpentifylline 4 to 6 g with suicidal intent experienced severe bradycardia and first- and second-degree atrioventricular block; other side-effects included nausea, vomiting, abdominal cramps, hypokalaemia, excitation, and insomnia.[1] She recovered after intensive supportive and symptomatic treatment.

1. Sznajder IJ, *et al.* First and second degree atrioventricular block in oxpentifylline overdose. *Br Med J* 1984; **288:** 26.

Precautions

Oxpentifylline should be avoided in cerebral haemorrhage, extensive retinal haemorrhage, and acute myocardial infarction. It should be used with caution in patients with ischaemic heart disease or hypotension. The dose of oxpentifylline may need to be adjusted in patients with impaired renal function or severe liver impairment.

Hepatic impairment. The elimination half-life of oxpentifylline and the 5-hydroxyhexyl metabolite is prolonged in patients with cirrhosis.[1]

1. Rames A, *et al.* Pharmacokinetics of intravenous and oral pentoxifylline in healthy volunteers and in cirrhotic patients. *Clin Pharmacol Ther* 1990; **47:** 354–9.

Interactions

Oxpentifylline may potentiate the effect of antihypertensives. High parenteral doses of oxpentifylline may enhance the hypoglycaemic action of insulin in diabetic patients. Oxpentifylline should not be given concomitantly with ketorolac as there is reported to be an increased risk of bleeding and/or prolongation of the prothrombin time. There may also be an increased risk of bleeding during concomitant use with meloxicam.

Pharmacokinetics

Oxpentifylline is readily absorbed from the gastro-intestinal tract but undergoes first-pass hepatic metabolism. Some metabolites are active. The apparent plasma half-life of oxpentifylline is reported to be 0.4 to 0.8 hours; that of the metabolites varies from 1.0 to 1.6 hours. In 24 hours most of a dose is excreted in the urine mainly as metabolites and less than 4% is recovered in the faeces. Elimination of oxpentifylline is decreased in elderly patients and patients with hepatic disease. Oxpentifylline and its metabolites are distributed into breast milk.

References.

1. Beermann B, *et al.* Kinetics of intravenous and oral pentoxifylline in healthy subjects. *Clin Pharmacol Ther* 1985; **37:** 25–8.
2. Smith RV, *et al.* Pharmacokinetics of orally administered pentoxifylline in humans. *J Pharm Sci* 1986; **75:** 47–52.
3. Witter FR, Smith RV. The excretion of pentoxifylline and its metabolites into human breast milk. *Am J Obstet Gynecol* 1985; **151:** 1094–7.
4. Paap CM, *et al.* Multiple-dose pharmacokinetics of pentoxifylline and its metabolites during renal insufficiency. *Ann Pharmacother* 1996; **30:** 724–9.

Uses and Administration

Oxpentifylline is a xanthine derivative used as a vasodilator in the treatment of peripheral (p.794) and cerebral vascular disorders (p.785). It also reduces blood viscosity probably by effects on erythrocyte deformability, platelet adhesion, and platelet aggregation. Oxpentifylline is reported to increase blood flow to ischaemic tissues and improve tissue oxygenation in patients with peripheral vascular disease and to increase oxygen tension in the cerebral cortex and in the cerebrospinal fluid. Oxpentifylline inhibits production of the cytokine, tumour necrosis factor alpha (TNFα) and this property is under investigation in a number of diseases (see below).

In the treatment of peripheral vascular disease the usual dose of oxpentifylline is 400 mg three times daily by mouth in a modified-release formulation, reducing to 400 mg twice daily if adverse effects are troublesome. Doses should be taken with meals to reduce gastro-intestinal disturbances. Beneficial effects may not be evident until after 2 to 6 weeks of treatment. Oxpentifylline may also be administered by intravenous infusion.

General references.

1. Ward A, Clissold SP. Pentoxifylline: a review of its pharmacodynamic and pharmacokinetic properties, and its therapeutic efficacy. *Drugs* 1987; **34:** 50–97.
2. Samlaska CP, Winfield EA. Pentoxifylline. *J Am Acad Dermatol* 1994; **30:** 603–21.

Oxpentifylline inhibits production of tumour necrosis factor alpha (TNFα), a cytokine that is implicated in the pathogenesis of many diseases and investigative work with oxpentifylline is being, or has been, carried out in many such disorders. Studies have been performed in patients with AIDS,[1,2] acute respiratory distress syndrome,[3] cerebral malaria,[4] diabetes mellitus,[5-10] inflammatory bowel disease,[11] Kawasaki disease,[12] infertility (males),[13-15] severe sepsis or septic shock,[16] recurrent aphthous stomatitis,[17] toxic epidermal necrolysis,[18] and various vasculitic syndromes.[19,20] Oxpentifylline has also been tried for reducing the toxicity of procedures and treatments associated with bone-marrow transplantation[21-23] including graft-versus-host disease.[24] Although promising results have been reported in some of these studies, the place of oxpentifylline in the overall management of these disorders remains to be established.

1. Luke DR, *et al.* Phase I/II study of pentoxifylline with zidovudine on HIV-1 growth in AIDS patients. *Int J Clin Pharmacol Ther Toxicol* 1993; **31:** 343–50.
2. Reeves GEM, *et al.* Pentoxifylline to treat Mycobacterium avium complex exacerbation in late-stage HIV infection. *Med J Aust* 1996; **166:** 446.
3. Wenstone R, Wilkes RG. Clinical management of ARDS. *Br J Anaesth* 1994; **72:** 617–19.
4. Di Perri, *et al.* Pentoxifylline as a supportive agent in the treatment of cerebral malaria in children. *J Infect Dis* 1995; **171:** 1317–22.
5. MacDonald MJ, *et al.* Pentoxifylline in the treatment of children with new-onset type I diabetes mellitus. *JAMA* 1994; **271:** 27–8.
6. Campbell RK. Clinical update on pentoxifylline therapy for diabetes-induced peripheral vascular disease. *Ann Pharmacother* 1993; **27:** 1099–1105.
7. Sulerte SB, Ferrari E. Diabetic retinal vascular complications and erythrocyte filtrability: results of a 2-year follow-up study with pentoxifylline. *Pharmatherapeutica* 1985; **4:** 341–50.
8. White JR, *et al.* Effects of pentoxifylline on proteinuria in normotensive patients with diabetes mellitus. *DICP Ann Pharmacother* 1990; **24:** 1043–5.
9. Guerrero-Romero F, *et al.* Pentoxifylline reduces proteinuria in insulin-dependent and non-insulin dependent diabetic patients. *Clin Nephrol* 1995; **43:** 116–21.
10. Sebag J, *et al.* Effects of pentoxifylline on choroidal blood flow in nonproliferative diabetic retinopathy. *Angiology* 1994; **45:** 429–33.
11. Bauditz J, *et al.* Treatment with tumour necrosis factor inhibitor oxpentifylline does not improve corticosteroid dependent chronic active Crohn's disease. *Gut* 1997; **40:** 470–4.
12. Matsubara T, *et al.* Treatment of Kawasaki disease with pentoxifylline, an inhibitor of TNF-α transcription. *Clin Res* 1994; **42:** 1A.
13. Wang C, *et al.* Comparison of the effectiveness of placebo, clomiphene citrate, mesterolone, pentoxifylline, and testosterone rebound therapy for the treatment of idiopathic oligospermia. *Fertil Steril* 1983; **40:** 358–65.
14. Marrama P, *et al.* Further studies on the effects of pentoxifylline on sperm count and sperm motility in patients with idiopathic oligo-asthenozoospermia. *Andrologia* 1985; **17:** 612–16.
15. Craft I, Shrivastav P. Treatment of male infertility. *Lancet* 1994; **344:** 191–2.
16. Staubach K-H, *et al.* Effect of pentoxifylline in severe sepsis: results of a randomized, double-blind, placebo-controlled study. *Arch Surg* 1998; **133:** 94–100.
17. Pizarro A, *et al.* Treatment of recurrent aphthous stomatitis with pentoxifylline. *Br J Dermatol* 1995; **133:** 659–60.
18. Redondo P, *et al.* Toxic epidermal necrolysis: treatment with pentoxifylline. *Br J Dermatol* 1994; **130:** 688–9.
19. Calderón MJ, *et al.* Successful treatment of cutaneous PAN with pentoxifylline. *Br J Dermatol* 1993; **128:** 706–7.
20. Nürnberg W, *et al.* Synergistic effects of pentoxifylline and dapsone in leucocytoclastic vasculitis. *Lancet* 1994; **343:** 491.
21. Bianco J, *et al.* Pentoxifylline diminishes regimen related toxicity in patients undergoing bone marrow transplantation. *Blood* 1990; **76** (suppl 1): 528A.
22. Beelen DW, *et al.* Constant intravenous pentoxifylline infusions in allogeneic marrow transplant recipients: results of a dose escalation study. *Bone Marrow Transplant* 1993; **12:** 363–70.
23. Clift RA, *et al.* A randomized controlled trial of pentoxifylline for the prevention of regimen-related toxicities in patients undergoing allogeneic marrow transplantation. *Blood* 1993; **82:** 2025–30.
24. Vogelsang GB, Morris LE. Prevention and management of graft-versus-host disease: practical recommendations. *Drugs* 1993; **45:** 668–76.

Preparations

Proprietary Preparations (details are given in Part 3)

Aust.: Haemodyn; Pentomer; Pentoxi; Trental; Vasonit; ***Austral.:*** Trental; ***Belg.:*** Torental; ***Canad.:*** Trental; ***Fr.:*** Pentoflux; Torental; ***Ger.:*** Agapurin; Azupentat; Claudicat; durapental; Pento-Puren; Pentohexal; Pentox; Ralofekt; Rentylin; Trental; ***Irl.:*** Trental; ***Ital.:*** Trental; ***Neth.:*** Trental; ***Norw.:*** Trental; ***S.Afr.:*** Trental; ***Spain:*** Elorgan; Hemovas; Retimax; ***Switz.:*** Dinostral; Pentoxi; Trental; ***UK:*** Trental; ***USA:*** Trental.

Oxprenolol Hydrochloride (6317-j)

Oxprenolol Hydrochloride (*BANM, USAN, rINNM*).

Ba-39089; Oxprenololi Hydrochloridum; Oxyprenolol Hydrochloride. 1-(o-Allyloxyphenoxy)-3-isopropylaminopropan-2-ol hydrochloride.

$C_{15}H_{23}NO_3,HCl = 301.8$.

CAS — 6452-71-7 (oxprenolol); 6452-73-9 (oxprenolol hydrochloride).

NOTE. Compounded preparations of oxprenolol hydrochloride and cyclopenthiazide in the proportions, by weight, 640 parts to 1 part have the British Approved Name Co-prenozide.

Pharmacopoeias. In *Eur.* (see p.viii), *Jpn, Pol.,* and *US.*

A white or almost white crystalline powder. Very to freely **soluble** in water; freely soluble in alcohol and chloroform; sparingly soluble in acetone; practically insoluble in ether. A 10% solution in water has a pH of 4 to 6. **Protect** from light.

Adverse Effects, Treatment, and Precautions

As for beta blockers, p.828.

Effects on the gastro-intestinal tract. Retroperitoneal fibrosis in one patient associated with the use of oxprenolol.[1]

1. McCluskey DR, *et al.* Oxprenolol and retroperitoneal fibrosis. *Br Med J* 1980; **281:** 1459–60.

Hypersensitivity. A report of oxprenolol-induced drug fever in a patient which was confirmed by a challenge test.[1]

1. Hasegawa K, *et al.* Drug fever due to oxprenolol. *Br Med J* 1980; **281:** 27–8.

Overdosage. A report of rhabdomyolysis and myoglobinuria complicating severe overdosage with oxprenolol.[1]

1. Schofield PM, *et al.* Recovery after severe oxprenolol overdose complicated by rhabdomyolysis. *Hum Toxicol* 1985; **4:** 57–60.

Interactions

The interactions associated with beta blockers are discussed on p.829.

Pharmacokinetics

Oxprenolol is well absorbed from the gastro-intestinal tract, but is subject to first-pass metabolism resulting in variable bioavailability (20 to 70%). Peak plasma concentrations have been reported to occur about 1 or 2 hours after a dose. Oxprenolol is 80% bound to plasma proteins. Oxprenolol is metabolised in the liver and almost entirely excreted in the urine. Oxprenolol diffuses across the placenta and is present in breast milk. It is moderately lipid-soluble and crosses the blood-brain barrier. An elimination half-life of 1 to 2 hours has been reported.

Pregnancy and breast feeding. A study of the placental transfer of oxprenolol and its passage into breast milk in 32 pregnant women receiving oxprenolol in association with dihydralazine (Trasipressol).[1] At delivery the mean maternal plasma concentration was 0.386 nmol per mL compared with 0.071 and 0.081 nmol per mL in plasma from the umbilical artery and vein respectively. Oxprenolol plasma concentrations in the newborn ranged from 0 to 0.186 nmol per mL during the first 24 hours of life. The concentrations of oxprenolol in breast milk 3 to 6 days after delivery ranged from 0 to 1.342 nmol per mL, and the milk to plasma concentration ratio was 0.45:1. Based on the highest milk concentration observed it was calculated that a breast-fed infant could receive, at a maximum, a daily dose at least sixty times less than an average daily dose (240 mg daily) taken by a hypertensive adult.

1. Sioufi A, *et al.* Oxprenolol placental transfer, plasma concentrations in newborns and passage into breast milk. *Br J Clin Pharmacol* 1984; **18:** 453–6.

Uses and Administration

Oxprenolol is a non-cardioselective beta blocker (p.828). It is reported to possess intrinsic sympathomimetic and membrane-stabilising activity.

Oxprenolol is used as the hydrochloride in the management of hypertension (p.788), angina pectoris (p.780), and cardiac arrhythmias (p.782). It is also used in anxiety disorders (p.635).

In **hypertension** oxprenolol hydrochloride is given by mouth in a usual dose of 80 to 160 mg daily in two or three divided doses. The dose may be increased at weekly or fortnightly intervals until a satisfactory response is achieved. The usual maximum dose is 320 mg daily although up to 480 mg daily has been allowed. Modified-release tablets may be given once daily in a dose of up to 320 mg.

The usual dose for **angina pectoris** is 80 to 160 mg daily in two or three divided doses with a usual maximum of 320 mg daily. For **cardiac arrhythmias** a dose of 40 mg daily to not more than 240 mg daily in two or three divided doses may be used.

For the emergency treatment of cardiac arrhythmias oxprenolol hydrochloride has been given by slow intravenous injection or by the intramuscular route.

Oxprenolol hydrochloride is given by mouth in usual doses of 40 to 80 mg daily, either as a single dose or in two divided doses, to relieve **anxiety** in stressful situations.

Preparations

BP 1998: Oxprenolol Tablets;
USP 23: Oxprenolol Hydrochloride Extended-release Tablets; Oxprenolol Hydrochloride Tablets.

Proprietary Preparations (details are given in Part 3)

Aust.: Trasicor; ***Austral.:*** Corbeton; Trasicor†; ***Belg.:*** Trasicor; ***Canad.:*** Slow-Trasicor; Trasicor; ***Fr.:*** Trasicor; ***Ger.:*** Trasicor; ***Irl.:*** Slow-Trasicor; Trasicor; ***Ital.:*** Trasicor†; ***Neth.:*** Trasicor; ***Norw.:*** Trasicor; ***S.Afr.:*** Lo-Tone†; Ornel†; Slow-Trasicor†; Trasicor; ***Spain:*** Trasicor; ***Swed.:*** Trasicor†; ***Switz.:*** Slow-Trasicor; Trasicor; ***UK:*** Apsolox†; Oxyprenix; Slow-Pren†; Slow-Trasicor; Trasicor.

Multi-ingredient: ***Aust.:*** Trasitensin; Trepress; ***Fr.:*** Trasipressol; Trasitensine; ***Ger.:*** Impresso; Trasicor Esidrix†; Trasitensin; Trepress; ***Irl.:*** Trasidrex; ***Ital.:*** Tensilene†; Trasitensin; ***S.Afr.:*** Trasidrex; ***Spain:*** Trasitensin; ***Switz.:*** Slow-Trasitensine; Trasitensine; Trepress; ***UK:*** Trasidrex.

Oxyfedrine Hydrochloride (9268-f)

Oxyfedrine Hydrochloride *(BANM, rINNM).*

D-563; Oxifedrini Chloridum. L-3-(β-Hydroxy-α-methylphenethylamino)-3′-methoxypropiophenone hydrochloride.

$C_{19}H_{23}NO_3,HCl$ = 349.9.

CAS — 15687-41-9 (oxyfedrine); 16777-42-7 (oxyfedrine hydrochloride).

Oxyfedrine hydrochloride has vasodilator properties and is used in angina pectoris (p.780), and myocardial infarction (p.791).

It is given in doses of 8 to 24 mg three times daily by mouth. It may also be given by slow intravenous injection or intravenous infusion. Oxyfedrine is metabolised to phenylpropanolamine (p.1067).

Preparations

Proprietary Preparations (details are given in Part 3)
Aust.: Ildamen; ***Ger.:*** Ildamen; Myofedrin; ***Ital.:*** Ildamen†; ***Spain:*** Ildamen†; ***Switz.:*** Ildamen†.

Multi-ingredient: ***Ger.:*** Seda-ildamen†.

Pamabrom (13073-h)

Pamabrom *(USAN).*

2-Amino-2-methylpropan-1-ol 8-bromotheophyllinate.

$C_4H_{11}NO,C_7H_7BrN_4O_2$ = 348.2.

CAS — 606-04-2.

Pharmacopoeias. In *US.*

Pamabrom is a mild diuretic that has been used, in combination with analgesics and antihistamines, for symptomatic relief of the premenstrual syndrome.

Preparations

Proprietary Preparations (details are given in Part 3)
USA: Fluidex with Pamabrom; Maximum Strength Aqua-Ban.

Multi-ingredient: ***Canad.:*** Midol Extra Strength†; Midol PMS Extra Strength; Pamprin; Trendar PMS; ***USA:*** Bayer Select Maximum Strength Menstrual; Fem-1; Fem-Etts†; Lurline PMS; Maximum Strength Midol PMS†; Midol PMS; Pamprin; Premsyn PMS; Teen Midol.

Papaveroline (13077-g)

Papaveroline *(BAN, rINN).*

1-(3,4-Dihydroxybenzyl)isoquinoline-6,7-diol.

$C_{16}H_{13}NO_4$ = 283.3.

CAS — 574-77-6.

Papaveroline is a vasodilator which has been used in the treatment of vascular disorders.

Preparations

Proprietary Preparations (details are given in Part 3)
Ital.: Modus†.

Pargyline Hydrochloride (886-f)

Pargyline Hydrochloride *(BANM, USAN, rINNM).*

A-19120; MO-911; NSC-43798. *N*-Methyl-*N*-2-propynylbenzylamine hydrochloride; Benzylmethylprop-2-ynylamine hydrochloride.

$C_{11}H_{13}N,HCl$ = 195.7.

CAS — 555-57-7 (pargyline); 306-07-0 (pargyline hydrochloride).

Adverse Effects, Treatment, and Precautions

The adverse effects and precautions of pargyline are similar to those of phenelzine and other MAOIs (p.302). Muscle twitching and extrapyramidal disorders have been reported. There have been reports of heart failure in patients with reduced cardiac reserve. Hypoglycaemia has occurred in some patients. As with other MAOIs severe toxic reactions may occur if pargyline is taken simultaneously with certain other drugs or foods (see p.303).

Uses and Administration

Pargyline hydrochloride is an MAOI that has been used in the treatment of moderate to severe hypertension although less toxic drugs are preferred.

Parnaparin Sodium (10349-y)

Parnaparin Sodium *(BAN, rINN).*

OP-21-23; Parnaparinum Natricum.

Pharmacopoeias. In *Eur.* (see p.viii).

Parnaparin sodium is prepared by hydrogen peroxide and copper(II) acetate depolymerisation of heparin obtained from the intestinal mucosa of pigs and cattle. The majority of the components have a 2-*O*-sulpho-α-L-idopyranosuronic acid structure at the non-reducing end and a 2-*N*,6-*O*-disulpho-D-glucosamine structure at the reducing end of their chain. The mass-average molecular mass ranges between 4000 and 6000, with a characteristic value of about 5000. The mass percentage of chains lower than 3000 is not more than 30%. The degree of sulphation is 2.0 to 2.6 per disaccharide unit. The Ph. Eur. specifies that potency is not less than 75 units and not more than 110 units of anti-factor Xa activity per mg with reference to the dried substance and that the ratio of anti-factor Xa activity to anti-factor IIa (antithrombin) activity is between 1.5 and 3.0.

Parnaparin sodium is a low-molecular-weight heparin (p.899) with anticoagulant activity used in the prevention of postoperative venous thrombo-embolism (p.802). For general surgical procedures it is given by subcutaneous injection in a dose of 3200 units 2 hours before the procedure, followed by 3200 units once daily for 7 days or until the patient is fully ambulant. For higher risk or orthopaedic patients a dose of 4250 units is given 12 hours before the procedure, followed by 4250 units 12 hours postoperatively and then once daily for 10 days.

References.

1. Frampton JE, Faulds D. Parnaparin: a review of its pharmacology, and clinical application in the prevention and treatment of thromboembolic and other vascular disorders. *Drugs* 1994; **47:** 652–76.

Preparations

Proprietary Preparations (details are given in Part 3)
Ital.: Fluxum; Minidalton.

Penbutolol Sulphate (6318-z)

Penbutolol Sulphate *(BANM, rINNM).*

Hoe-39-893d; Hoe-893d; Penbutolol Hemisulphate; Penbutolol Sulfate *(USAN).* (*S*)-1-*tert*-Butylamino-3-(2-cyclopentylphenoxy)propan-2-ol hemisulphate.

$(C_{18}H_{29}NO_2)_2,H_2SO_4$ = 680.9.

CAS — 38363-40-5 (penbutolol); 38363-32-5 (penbutolol sulphate).

Pharmacopoeias. In *Jpn* and *US.*

A white to off-white crystalline powder. **Soluble** in water and methyl alcohol. **Store** in airtight containers. Protect from light.

Adverse Effects, Treatment, and Precautions

As for beta blockers, p.828.

Interactions

The interactions associated with beta blockers are discussed on p.829.

Pharmacokinetics

Penbutolol is readily absorbed from the gastro-intestinal tract and peak plasma concentrations occur about 1 or 3 hours after a dose. Penbutolol is 80 to 98% bound to plasma proteins. It has a high lipid solubility. It is extensively metabolised in the liver by hydroxylation and glucuronidation, the metabolites being excreted in the urine together with only small amounts of unchanged penbutolol. A plasma elimination half-life of about 20 hours has been reported.

Glucuronidation was considered more prominent than hydroxylation in the metabolism of penbutolol and its activity was not altered in patients with renal insufficiency.[1]

1. Bernard N, *et al.* Pharmacokinetics of penbutolol and its metabolites in renal insufficiency. *Eur J Clin Pharmacol* 1985; **29:** 215–19.

Uses and Administration

Penbutolol is a non-cardioselective beta blocker (p.828). It is reported to possess some intrinsic sympathomimetic activity but lacks membrane-stabilising properties.

Penbutolol is used as the sulphate in the management of hypertension (p.788). It may also be used in cardiac disorders such as angina pectoris (p.780).

In **hypertension** penbutolol sulphate is given in initial doses of 20 mg daily by mouth; the dose may be increased if necessary to 40 to 80 mg daily. Maximum antihypertensive efficacy is reported to occur within 2 weeks in patients given a dose of 20 mg daily but about 4 weeks may be required for maximum effect in patients given 10 mg daily.

Penbutolol sulphate has also been used in similar doses in cardiac disorders such as **angina**.

References.

1. Frishman WH, Covey S. Penbutolol and carteolol: two new beta-adrenergic blockers with partial agonism. *J Clin Pharmacol* 1990; **30:** 412–21.
2. Schlanz KD, Thomas RL. Penbutolol: a new beta-adrenergic blocking agent. *DICP Ann Pharmacother* 1990; **24:** 403–8.

Preparations

USP 23: Penbutolol Sulfate Tablets.

Proprietary Preparations (details are given in Part 3)
Aust.: Betapressin; ***Fr.:*** Betapressine; ***Ger.:*** Betapressin; ***Ital.:*** Betapressin†; Ipobar†; ***Spain:*** Blocotin†; ***Switz.:*** Betapressine†; ***USA:*** Levatol.

Multi-ingredient: ***Aust.:*** Normotensin; ***Ger.:*** Betarelix; Betasemid; ***Ital.:*** Betasemid†; ***UK:*** Lasipressin†.

Pentaerythritol Tetranitrate (9270-c)

Pentaerythritol Tetranitrate *(BAN).*

Pentaerithrityl Tetranitrate *(rINN)*; Erynite; Nitropentaerythrol; Nitropenthrite; Pentaerythritolum Tetranitricum; Pentanitrol; PETN. 2,2-Bis(hydroxymethyl)propane-1,3-diol tetranitrate.

$C_5H_8N_4O_{12}$ = 316.1.

CAS — 78-11-5.

NOTE. The synonym PETN has been applied to both niceritrol and pentaerythritol tetranitrate.

Pharmacopoeias. In *Pol.*

Eur. (see p.viii) and *US* include as diluted pentaerythritol tetranitrate.

Undiluted pentaerythritol tetranitrate is practically **insoluble** in water; slightly soluble in alcohol and in ether; soluble in acetone.

Diluted pentaerythritol tetranitrate is a mixture of pentaerythritol tetranitrate with lactose, mannitol, or other suitable inert excipients, the latter being added to minimise the risk of explosion. **Store** in airtight containers at a temperature not exceeding 40°. Protect from light.

CAUTION. *Undiluted pentaerythritol tetranitrate can be exploded by percussion or excessive heat.*

Pentaerythritol tetranitrate is a vasodilator with general properties similar to those of glyceryl trinitrate (p.875) but its duration of action is more prolonged.

It is used in angina pectoris (p.780) in oral doses of 30 to 240 mg daily, in divided doses, before a meal. It is also given as modified-release preparations.

Pentaerythritol trinitrate, an active metabolite of pentaerythritol tetranitrate, has also been used clinically under the name pentrinitrol.

Preparations

BP 1998: Pentaerythrityl Tetranitrate Tablets;
USP 23: Pentaerythritol Tetranitrate Tablets.

Proprietary Preparations (details are given in Part 3)
Aust.: Dilcoran; ***Canad.:*** Peritrate; ***Fr.:*** Nitrodex; Peritrate†; ***Ger.:*** Dilcoran; Nirason N; Pentalong; ***Irl.:*** Mycardol; ***Ital.:*** Niscodil†; Peritrate; ***S.Afr.:*** Peritrate†; ***Spain:*** Peritrate†; ***Switz.:*** Nitrodex; ***UK:*** Mycardol; ***USA:*** Duotrate†; Pentylan; Peritrate†.

Multi-ingredient: ***Aust.:*** Lenticor†; Spasmocor; ***Ger.:*** Adenopurin†; Govil†; Nitro-Crataegutt; Nitro-Novodigal†; Nitro-Obsidan; Pentaneural†; VisanoCor N; ***Ital.:*** Stenodilate†.

Pentifylline (639-q)

Pentifylline *(BAN, rINN).*

1-Hexyltheobromine; SK7. 1-Hexyl-3,7-dimethylxanthine.

$C_{13}H_{20}N_4O_2$ = 264.3.

CAS — 1028-33-7.

Pentifylline is a xanthine derivative used as a vasodilator in the management of peripheral or cerebral vascular disorders.

Preparations

Proprietary Preparations (details are given in Part 3)
Ger.: Cosaldon.

Multi-ingredient: ***Aust.:*** Cosaldon; ***Fr.:*** Cosadon†; ***Ger.:*** Cosaldon A; ***S.Afr.:*** Cosaldon.

Pentopril (18950-h)

Pentopril *(USAN, rINN).*

CGS-13945. Ethyl (α*R*,γ*R*,2*S*)-2-carboxy-α,γ-dimethyl-δ-oxo-1-indolinevalerate.

$C_{18}H_{23}NO_5$ = 333.4.

CAS — 82924-03-6.

Pentopril is an ACE inhibitor (p.805). It is converted in the body into its active diacid metabolite CGS-13934. It has been investigated in the treatment of hypertension.

Pentosan Polysulphate Sodium (4821-j)

Pentosan Polysulphate Sodium *(BAN)*.

Pentosan Polysulfate Sodium *(USAN, rINN)*; PZ-68; Sodium Pentosan Polysulphate; Sodium Xylanpolysulphate; SP-54.

CAS — 37319-17-8; 116001-96-8.

A mixture of linear polymers of β-1→4-linked xylose, usually sulphated at the 2- and 3-positions and occasionally (approximately 1 in every 4 residues) substituted at the 2-position with 4-*O*-methyl-α-D-glucuronic acid 2,3-*O*-sulphate. The average molecular weight lies between 4000 and 6000 with a total molecular weight range of 1000 to 40 000.

Adverse Effects and Precautions

As for Heparin, p.880. Gastro-intestinal disturbances may also occur.

Uses and Administration

Pentosan polysulphate sodium is a heparinoid with anticoagulant and fibrinolytic properties; it may also have hypolipidaemic and anti-inflammatory effects. It is used in thrombo-embolic disorders, although its anticoagulant effect is less than that of heparin. It is also used in the management of interstitial cystitis (see below) and has been tried in a number of other conditions. Pentosan polysulphate sodium has been administered orally, parenterally, and by topical application.

In the management of interstitial cystitis, pentosan polysulphate sodium is given orally in a dose of 100 mg three times a day.

Cystitis. Pentosan polysulphate sodium has been used in inflammatory conditions of the bladder, including interstitial cystitis (p.1377), and is postulated to act by enhancing the protective effect of mucins at the bladder surface. However, double-blind placebo-controlled studies have differed concerning its efficacy in the treatment of interstitial cystitis.[1] Any benefit is usually apparent within 12 to 16 weeks of commencing treatment and only occurs in a minority of patients.[2]

Administration of pentosan polysulphate sodium by mouth controlled haemorrhage in 5 patients with radiation cystitis.[3]

1. Ryan PG, Wallace DMA. Are we making progress in the drug treatment of disorders of the bladder, prostate, and penis? *J Clin Pharm Ther* 1990; **15:** 1–12.
2. Anonymous. Pentosan for interstitial cystitis. *Med Lett Drugs Ther* 1997; **39:** 56.
3. Parsons CL. Successful management of radiation cystitis with sodium pentosanpolysulfate. *J Urol (Baltimore)* 1986; **136:** 813–14.

Preparations

Proprietary Preparations (details are given in Part 3)

Aust.: Polyanion; ***Canad.:*** Elmiron; ***Fr.:*** Hemoclar; Lelong Contusions†; ***Ger.:*** Fibrezym; ***Ital.:*** Fibrase; ***S.Afr.:*** Tavan-SP 54; ***Spain:*** Fibrocid.

Multi-ingredient: ***Aust.:*** Flexurat; Thrombocid; ***Fr.:*** Collyrex; Keratosane; ***Ger.:*** Flexurat; Phlebex†; Probaphen†; Thrombocid; ***Spain:*** Anso; Plasmaclar; Rulun; Thrombocid; ***Switz.:*** Thrombocid.

Perhexiline Maleate (9272-a)

Perhexiline Maleate *(BANM, USAN, rINNM)*.

WSM-3978G. 2-(2,2-Dicyclohexylethyl)piperidine hydrogen maleate.

$C_{19}H_{35}N,C_4H_4O_4$ = 393.6.

CAS — 6621-47-2 (perhexiline); 6724-53-4 (perhexiline maleate).

Perhexiline maleate may be used in the long-term management of severe angina pectoris (p.780) in patients who have not responded to other anti-anginal drugs. Its mode of action is complex but may be partly due to calcium antagonism.

The usual dose is 100 to 200 mg daily by mouth in 2 divided doses; it is generally recommended not to administer more than 300 mg daily although doses of 400 mg daily have been necessary in some patients.

Perhexiline occasionally produces severe adverse effects including peripheral neuropathy affecting all four limbs with associated papilloedema, severe and occasionally fatal hepatic toxicity, and metabolic abnormalities with marked weight loss, hypertriglyceridaemia, and profound hypoglycaemia. It is contra-indicated in patients with impaired hepatic or renal function. Perhexiline should be administered with caution to diabetic patients.

Preparations

Proprietary Preparations (details are given in Part 3)

Austral.: Pexid; ***Belg.:*** Pexid; ***Fr.:*** Pexid†; ***Ger.:*** Pexid†.

Perindopril (729-s)

Perindopril *(BAN, USAN, rINN)*.

McN-A-2833; S-9490. (2S,3aS,7aS)-1-{*N*-[(*S*)-1-Ethoxycarbonylbutyl]-L-alanyl}perhydroindole-2-carboxylic acid.

$C_{19}H_{32}N_2O_5$ = 368.5.

CAS — 82834-16-0.

Perindopril Erbumine (13519-c)

Perindopril Erbumine *(BANM, USAN, rINNM)*.

McN-A-2833-109; Perindopril *tert*-Butylamine; S-9490-3.

$C_{19}H_{32}N_2O_5,C_4H_{11}N$ = 441.6.

CAS — 107133-36-8.

Adverse Effects, Treatment, and Precautions

As for ACE inhibitors, p.805.

Although a study[1] of perindopril administration to patients with stable chronic heart failure reported no significant first-dose hypotension, there has been a case report[2] of ischaemic stroke possibly associated with hypotension in a patient with post-infarction heart failure following a single dose of perindopril. Standard precautions as for other ACE inhibitors (p.807) should be followed when initiating perindopril therapy.

1. MacFadyen RJ, *et al.* Differences in first dose response to angiotensin converting enzyme inhibition in congestive heart failure: a placebo controlled study. *Br Heart J* 1991; **66:** 206–11.
2. Bagger JP. Adverse event with first-dose perindopril in congestive heart failure. *Lancet* 1997; **349:** 1671–2.

Interactions

As for ACE inhibitors, p.807.

Pharmacokinetics

Perindopril acts as a prodrug of the diacid perindoprilat, its active form. Following oral administration perindopril is rapidly absorbed and extensively metabolised, mainly in the liver, to perindoprilat and inactive metabolites including glucuronides. The presence of food is reported to reduce the conversion of perindopril to perindoprilat. Peak plasma concentrations of perindoprilat are achieved 3 to 4 hours after an oral dose of perindopril. About 75% of an oral dose is excreted in the urine as unchanged drug, as perindoprilat, and as other metabolites; the remainder is excreted in the faeces. Perindoprilat is about 10 to 20% bound to plasma proteins; its elimination is biphasic with a distribution half-life of about 5 hours and an elimination half-life of 25 to 30 hours, the latter half-life probably representing strong binding to angiotensin-converting enzyme. The excretion of perindoprilat is decreased when there is renal impairment. Both perindopril and perindoprilat are removed by dialysis.

References.

1. Lecocq B, *et al.* Influence of food on the pharmacokinetics of perindopril and the time course of angiotensin-converting enzyme inhibition in serum. *Clin Pharmacol Ther* 1990; **47:** 397–402.
2. Verpooten GA, *et al.* Single dose pharmacokinetics of perindopril and its metabolites in hypertensive patients with various degrees of renal insufficiency. *Br J Clin Pharmacol* 1991; **32:** 187–92.
3. Sennesael J, *et al.* The pharmacokinetics of perindopril and its effects on serum angiotensin converting enzyme activity in hypertensive patients with chronic renal failure. *Br J Clin Pharmacol* 1992; **33:** 93–9.
4. Thiollet M, *et al.* The pharmacokinetics of perindopril in patients with liver cirrhosis. *Br J Clin Pharmacol* 1992; **33:** 326–8.
5. Guérin A, *et al.* The effect of haemodialysis on the pharmacokinetics of perindoprilat after long-term perindopril. *Eur J Clin Pharmacol* 1993; **44:** 183–7.

Uses and Administration

Perindopril is an ACE inhibitor (p.805). It is used in the treatment of hypertension (p.788) and heart failure (p.785)

Perindopril is converted in the body into its active metabolite perindoprilat. ACE inhibition is reported to occur within 1 hour of a dose, to be at a maximum at about 4 to 8 hours, and to be maintained for 24 hours. Perindopril is given by mouth as the erbumine salt.

In the treatment of **hypertension** perindopril erbumine is given in an initial dose of 2 mg once daily. Since there may be a precipitous fall in blood pressure in some patients when starting therapy with an ACE inhibitor, the first dose should preferably be given at bedtime. The dose may be increased according to response to a maximum of 8 mg daily. The usual maintenance dose is 4 mg daily. Higher doses are suggested in the USA, with a maximum dose of 16 mg daily in uncomplicated hypertensive patients. Patients receiving diuretics should have the diuretic discontinued 2 or 3 days before starting perindopril if possible, and resumed later if necessary.

In the management of **heart failure**, severe first-dose hypotension on introduction of an ACE inhibitor is common in patients on loop diuretics, but their temporary withdrawal may cause rebound pulmonary oedema. Thus treatment should be initiated with a low dose under close medical supervision. Perindopril is given in an initial dose of 2 mg in the morning. The usual maintenance dose is 4 mg daily.

A reduction in dosage may be necessary in patients with impaired renal function.

References.

1. Todd PA, Fitton A. Perindopril: a review of its pharmacological properties and therapeutic use in cardiovascular disorders. *Drugs* 1991; **42:** 90–114.
2. Doyle AE, ed. Angiotensin-converting enzyme (ACE) inhibition: benefits beyond blood pressure control. *Am J Med* 1992; **92** (suppl 4B): 1S–107S.

Preparations

Proprietary Preparations (details are given in Part 3)

Aust.: Coversum; ***Austral.:*** Coversyl; ***Belg.:*** Coversyl; ***Canad.:*** Coversyl; ***Fr.:*** Coversyl; ***Ger.:*** Coversum; ***Irl.:*** Coversyl; ***Ital.:*** Coversyl; Procaptan; ***Neth.:*** Coversyl; ***S.Afr.:*** Coversyl; ***Spain:*** Coversyl; ***Switz.:*** Coversum; ***UK:*** Coversyl; ***USA:*** Aceon.

Peruvoside (13098-e)

(3β,5β)-3-[(6-Deoxy-3-*O*-methyl-α-L-glucopyranosyl)oxy]-14-hydroxy-19-oxocard-20(22)-enolide.

$C_{30}H_{44}O_9$ = 548.7.

CAS — 1182-87-2.

A cardiac glycoside obtained from the seeds of *Thevetia neriifolia* (Apocynaceae), related to thevetin A.

Peruvoside has been used orally in the management of heart failure.

Preparations

Proprietary Preparations (details are given in Part 3)

Ital.: Nerial†.

Phenindione (4818-t)

Phenindione *(BAN, rINN)*.

Fenindione; Phenylindanedione; Phenylinium. 2-Phenylindan-1,3-dione.

$C_{15}H_{10}O_2$ = 222.2.

CAS — 83-12-5.

Pharmacopoeias. In Br. and Fr.

Soft, odourless or almost odourless, white or creamy-white crystals. Very slightly **soluble** in water; slightly soluble in alcohol and in ether; freely soluble in chloroform. Solutions are yellow to red.

Adverse Effects and Treatment

As for Warfarin Sodium, p.964. However, phenindione and the other indanediones are generally more toxic than warfarin sodium with hypersensitivity reactions involving many organs and sometimes resulting in death. Some of the reactions include skin rashes and exfoliative dermatitis, pyrexia, diarrhoea, vomiting, sore throat, liver and kidney damage, myocarditis, agranulocytosis, leucopenia, eosinophilia, and a leukaemoid syndrome.

Phenindione may discolour the urine pink or orange and this is independent of any haematuria. Taste disturbances have been reported.

Effects on the gastro-intestinal tract. There have been cases of paralytic ileus, one fatal, associated with phenindione.[1,2]

1. Menon IS. Phenindione and paralytic ileus. *Lancet* 1966; **i:** 1421–2.
2. Nash AG. Phenindione and paralytic ileus. *Lancet* 1966; **ii:** 51–2.

Precautions

As for Warfarin Sodium, p.965.

Phenindione is not recommended in pregnancy. Unlike warfarin significant quantities have been detected in breast milk so it should not be given to breast-feeding women.

Interactions

The interactions associated with oral anticoagulants are described in detail under warfarin (p.965). Specific references to interactions involving phenindione can be found there under the headings for the following drug groups: analgesics; antibacterials; antifungals; antiplatelets; anxiolytic sedatives; gastro-intestinal drugs; lipid regulating drugs; and sex hormones.

Pharmacokinetics

Phenindione is absorbed from the gastro-intestinal tract. It diffuses across the placenta and is distributed into breast milk. Metabolites of phenindione excreted in the urine are responsible for any discoloration.

Uses and Administration

Phenindione is an orally administered indanedione anticoagulant with actions similar to those of warfarin sodium (p.969). It is used in the management of thrombo-embolic disorders (p.801), but because of its higher incidence of severe adverse effects it is now rarely employed.

The usual initial dose of phenindione is 200 mg on the first day, 100 mg on the second day, and then maintenance doses of 50 to 150 mg daily according to coagulation tests.

Preparations

BP 1998: Phenindione Tablets.

Proprietary Preparations (details are given in Part 3)
Austral.: Dindevan; ***Fr.:*** Pindione; ***UK:*** Dindevan.

Phenoxybenzamine Hydrochloride

(892-x)

Phenoxybenzamine Hydrochloride *(BANM, rINNM).*

SKF-688A. Benzyl(2-chloroethyl)(1-methyl-2-phenoxyethyl)amine hydrochloride.

$C_{18}H_{22}ClNO,HCl = 340.3.$

CAS — 59-96-1 (phenoxybenzamine); 63-92-3 (phenoxybenzamine hydrochloride).

Pharmacopoeias. In *Br., Chin.,* and *US.*

A white or almost white, odourless or almost odourless, crystalline powder. Sparingly **soluble** in water; freely soluble in alcohol and in chloroform.

Adverse Effects and Treatment

The adverse effects of phenoxybenzamine are primarily due to its alpha-adrenoceptor blocking activity. They include postural hypotension and dizziness, reflex tachycardia, nasal congestion, and miosis. Inhibition of ejaculation may occur. These effects may be minimised by using a low initial dose of phenoxybenzamine, and may diminish with continued administration, but the hypotensive effect can be exaggerated by exercise, heat, a large meal, or alcohol ingestion. Other side-effects include dryness of the mouth, drowsiness, fatigue, and confusion. Gastro-intestinal effects are usually slight. When phenoxybenzamine is administered intravenously, idiosyncratic profound hypotension can occur within a few minutes of starting the infusion. Convulsions have been reported after rapid intravenous infusion of phenoxybenzamine.

Severe hypotension may occur in overdose and treatment includes support of the circulation by postural measures and parenteral fluid volume replacement. Sympathomimetics are considered to be of little value, and adrenaline is contra-indicated since it also stimulates beta-receptors causing increased hypotension and tachycardia. Sources differ as to the value of noradrenaline in overcoming alpha-receptor blockade.

Phenoxybenzamine has been shown to be mutagenic in *in vitro* tests and carcinogenic in *rodents.*

Precautions

Phenoxybenzamine should be given with care to patients with heart failure, ischaemic heart disease, cerebrovascular disease, or renal impairment, and should be avoided if a fall in blood pressure would be dangerous. Phenoxybenzamine may aggravate the symptoms of respiratory infections.

When given intravenously, phenoxybenzamine hydrochloride should always be diluted and given by infusion. Intravenous fluids must always be given beforehand to ensure an adequate circulating blood volume and to prevent a precipitous fall in blood pressure. Care should be taken to avoid extravasation.

Interactions

Since phenoxybenzamine only blocks alpha-receptors, leaving the beta-receptors unopposed, concomitant administration of drugs, such as adrenaline, which also stimulate beta-receptors, may enhance the cardiac-accelerating and hypotensive action of phenoxybenzamine.

Pharmacokinetics

Phenoxybenzamine is incompletely and variably absorbed from the gastro-intestinal tract. The maximum effect is attained in about 1 hour after an intravenous dose. Following oral administration the onset of action is gradual over several hours and persists for 3 or 4 days following a single dose. The plasma half-life is about 24 hours. Phenoxybenzamine is metabolised in the liver and excreted in the urine and bile, but small amounts remain in the body for several days. The duration of action is thought to depend on the rate of synthesis of new alpha receptors following irreversible covalent bonding to existing alpha receptors by a reactive intermediate of phenoxybenzamine.

Uses and Administration

Phenoxybenzamine is a powerful alpha-adrenoceptor blocker (p.776) with a prolonged duration of action; it binds covalently to alpha-receptors in smooth muscle to produce an irreversible ('non-competitive') blockade. A single large dose of phenoxybenzamine can cause alpha-adrenoceptor blockade for 3 days or longer.

Phenoxybenzamine is used in the management of phaeochromocytoma. It has also been employed in severe shock (p.798) and in the treatment of urinary retention (p.454).

Phenoxybenzamine is used as the hydrochloride. It is given by mouth or by intravenous infusion as a dilute solution.

In phaeochromocytoma it is used to control the hypertension associated with excessive catecholamine release during the pre-operative period and in patients whose tumours are inoperable. A beta blocker may also be given to control tachycardia, but not before alpha blockade has completely suppressed the pressor effects of the phaeochromocytoma. The usual initial dose of phenoxybenzamine hydrochloride is 10 mg once or twice daily by mouth, increased gradually, according to the patient's response, to a usual dose of 1 to 2 mg per kg body-weight daily in 2 divided doses. It may be given intravenously for operative cover in patients with phaeochromocytoma. A suggested daily dose is 1 mg per kg intravenously in 200 mL of sodium chloride 0.9% infused over at least 2 hours. A similar intravenous dose in 200 to 500 mL of sodium chloride 0.9% has been given in the management of severe shock.

For urinary retention due to neurogenic bladder a dose of 10 mg twice daily by mouth has been given.

Erectile dysfunction. Intracavernous injection of phenoxybenzamine hydrochloride in a dose of 5 to 6 mg has been tried in erectile dysfunction[1,2] (p.1614). However, phenoxybenzamine injection is painful, and its effects are slow in onset,[3] and other treatments are generally preferred.

1. Brindley GS. Cavernosal alpha-blockade: a new technique for investigating and treating erectile impotence. *Br J Psychiatry* 1983; **143:** 332–7.
2. Keogh EJ. Treatment of impotence by intrapenile injections of papaverine and phenoxybenzamine: a double blind, controlled trial. *Aust N Z J Med* 1989; **19:** 108–12.
3. Anonymous. Vasoactive intracavernous pharmacotherapy for impotence: papaverine and phentolamine. *JAMA* 1990; **264:** 752–4.

Phaeochromocytoma. Phenoxybenzamine is widely used in the initial suppression of the pressor effects produced by catecholamines secreted by phaeochromocytoma[1] (p.795). The non-competitive adrenergic blockade produced means that surges of catecholamine release cannot override the inhibition as may occur with a competitive blocker. However, since phenoxybenzamine blocks alpha$_2$-receptors as well as alpha$_1$-receptors it should be used with great caution in patients with marginal coronary perfusion with or without angina. Phenoxybenzamine may be preferred to prazosin for the initial control of hypertension when the patient is intensely vasoconstricted and the plasma volume reduced since prazosin can cause severe initial hypotension. The treatment should be started at a low dose and increased gradually until the response is achieved. If additional beta blockade is required, it should never be given until alpha blockade has completely suppressed the pressor effects of the tumour.

1. Hull CJ. Phaeochromocytoma: diagnosis, preoperative preparation and anaesthetic management. *Br J Anaesth* 1986; **58:** 1453–68.

Preparations

BP 1998: Phenoxybenzamine Capsules;
USP 23: Phenoxybenzamine Hydrochloride Capsules.

Proprietary Preparations (details are given in Part 3)
Aust.: Dibenzyran; ***Austral.:*** Dibenyline; ***Belg.:*** Dibenyline; ***Ger.:*** Dibenzyran; ***Irl.:*** Dibenyline†; ***Neth.:*** Dibenyline; ***S.Afr.:*** Dibenyline†; ***UK:*** Dibenyline; ***USA:*** Dibenzyline.

Phenprocoumon (4819-x)

Phenprocoumon *(BAN, USAN, rINN).*

Phenylpropylhydroxycoumarin. 4-Hydroxy-3-(1-phenylpropyl)coumarin.

$C_{18}H_{16}O_3 = 280.3.$

CAS — 435-97-2.

Adverse Effects and Treatment

As for Warfarin Sodium, p.964.

Effects on the liver. A woman who had twice previously developed jaundice while taking phenprocoumon developed jaundice and parenchymal liver damage when, after some years, phenprocoumon was again given.[1] Two other cases of phenprocoumon-associated hepatitis have been reported.[2]

1. den Boer W, Loeliger EA. Phenprocoumon-induced jaundice. *Lancet* 1976; **i:** 912.
2. Slagboom G, Loeliger EA. Coumarin-associated hepatitis: report of two cases. *Arch Intern Med* 1980; **140:** 1028–9.

Precautions

As for Warfarin Sodium, p.965.

Interactions

The interactions associated with oral anticoagulants are discussed in detail under warfarin (p.965). Specific references to interactions involving phenprocoumon can be found there under the headings for the following drug groups: analgesics; antiarrhythmics; antidepressants; antidiabetics; antigout drugs; gastro-intestinal drugs; lipid regulating drugs; prostaglandins; and sex hormones.

Pharmacokinetics

Phenprocoumon is readily absorbed from the gastro-intestinal tract and is extensively bound to plasma proteins. A half-life of 5 to 6 days has been reported. It is excreted in the urine and faeces as conjugated hydroxy metabolites and parent compound. Phenprocoumon is administered as a racemic mixture; the *S*-isomer is reported to be more potent. The stereo-isomers have different pharmacokinetics.

References.

1. Husted S, Andreasen F. Individual variation in the response to phenprocoumon. *Eur J Clin Pharmacol* 1977; **11:** 351–8.
2. Toon S, *et al.* Metabolic fate of phenprocoumon in humans. *J Pharm Sci* 1985; **74:** 1037–40.

Uses and Administration

Phenprocoumon is an orally administered coumarin anticoagulant with actions similar to those of warfarin sodium (p.969). It is used in the management of thrombo-embolic disorders (p.801). Initial doses of up to 15 mg on the first day followed by up to 9 mg on the second day are used. Maintenance doses are usually from 1.5 to 6 mg daily, depending on the response.

Preparations

Proprietary Preparations (details are given in Part 3)
Aust.: Marcoumar; ***Belg.:*** Marcoumar; ***Ger.:*** Falithrom; Marcumar; Phenpro; ***Neth.:*** Marcoumar; ***Spain:*** Marcumar†; ***Switz.:*** Marcoumar.

Phentolamine Mesylate (894-f)

Phentolamine Mesylate *(BANM)*.

Phentolamine Mesilate *(rINNM)*; Phentolamine Methanesulphonate; Phentolamini Mesilas. 3-[*N*-(2-Imidazolin-2-ylmethyl)-*p*-toluidino]phenol methanesulphonate.

$C_{17}H_{19}N_3O,CH_4SO_3 = 377.5$.

CAS — 50-60-2 (phentolamine); 73-05-2 (phentolamine hydrochloride); 65-28-1 (phentolamine mesylate).

Pharmacopoeias. In *Chin., Eur.* (see p.viii), and *US.*

A white or off-white slightly hygroscopic, odourless crystalline powder.

Soluble 1 in 1 of water, 1 in 4 of alcohol, and 1 in 700 of chloroform; practically insoluble in dichloromethane. Solutions slowly deteriorate on storage.

Store in airtight containers. Protect from light.

Adverse Effects and Treatment

The adverse effects of phentolamine are primarily due to its alpha-adrenoceptor blocking activity and include orthostatic hypotension and tachycardia. Myocardial infarction and cerebrovascular spasm or occlusion have been reported occasionally, usually in association with marked hypotension; flushing, sweating, and feelings of apprehension may accompany hypotensive episodes. Anginal pain and arrhythmias have been reported rarely. Nausea, vomiting, and diarrhoea may also occur. Other side-effects include weakness, dizziness, flushing, and nasal stuffiness. Hypoglycaemia has been reported following overdosage.

Severe hypotension may occur in overdosage although phentolamine has a short duration of action. Treatment may include keeping the patient's legs raised and the administration of a plasma expander. Noradrenaline may be administered cautiously to overcome alpha-adrenoceptor blockade. Adrenaline is contra-indicated since it also stimulates beta receptors causing increased hypotension and tachycardia.

When injected into the corpus cavernosum of the penis phentolamine has been associated with local pain; induration and fibrosis may occur with repeated use. Priapism has occurred.

Precautions

Phentolamine should not generally be given to patients with angina pectoris or other evidence of ischaemic heart disease. Care should be taken in patients with peptic ulcer disease, which may be exacerbated.

Interactions

Since phentolamine only blocks alpha-receptors, concomitant use of drugs such as adrenaline may lead to severe hypotension and tachycardia due to unopposed beta-adrenoceptor stimulation.

Pharmacokinetics

Following intravenous administration, the half-life of phentolamine has been reported to be 19 minutes. It is extensively metabolised and about 13% of an intravenous dose is excreted unchanged in the urine.

Uses and Administration

Phentolamine is an alpha-adrenoceptor blocker (p.776) which also has a direct action on vascular smooth muscle. It produces vasodilatation, an increase in cardiac output, and has a positive inotropic effect, but is reported to have little effect on the blood pressure of patients with essential hypertension. The alpha-receptor blocking action is reported to be transient and incomplete; it is reversible ('competitive').

Phentolamine is given in the management of hypertensive crises associated with surgery for phaeochromocytoma (p.795) and due to excessive catecholamine release. It has been employed for the differential diagnosis of phaeochromocytoma, but has largely been superseded by estimations of catecholamines in blood and urine.

Phentolamine is also used to prevent or treat dermal necrosis and sloughing associated with the intravenous infusion or extravasation of noradrenaline. It has been tried in the treatment of erectile dysfunction (p.1614).

Phentolamine is given by injection as the mesylate. In patients undergoing surgery for phaeochromocytoma, the UK dose is 2 to 5 mg of phentolamine mesylate given intravenously and repeated if necessary; blood pressure should be monitored. In the USA the usual dose is 5 mg given intravenously or intramuscularly. A dose of 1 mg intravenously has been suggested for children.

For prevention of dermal necrosis during intravenous infusion of noradrenaline, 10 mg of phentolamine mesylate is added to each litre of solution containing noradrenaline. For treatment following extravasation of noradrenaline, 5 to 10 mg of phentolamine mesylate in 10 mL of saline is injected into the affected area.

Injections of phentolamine mesylate, usually in association with papaverine, into the corpora cavernosa of the penis, have been used in the treatment of impotence due to erectile failure. The oral route is also being investigated.

Pancreatic pain. Pain due to pancreatitis is usually treated with opioid analgesics (see p.10). Long-term relief of pain has been reported in a patient with chronic pancreatitis following an intravenous infusion of phentolamine.[1]

1. McCleane GJ. Phentolamine abolishes the pain of chronic pancreatitis. *Br J Hosp Med* 1996; **55:** 521.

Preparations

BP 1998: Phentolamine Injection;
USP 23: Phentolamine Mesylate for Injection.

Proprietary Preparations (details are given in Part 3)
Austral.: Regitine; ***Belg.:*** Regitine; ***Canad.:*** Rogitine; ***Ger.:*** Regitin†; ***Irl.:*** Rogitine†; ***Neth.:*** Regitine; ***S.Afr.:*** Regitine†; ***Switz.:*** Regitine; ***UK:*** Rogitine; ***USA:*** Regitine.

Multi-ingredient: ***Aust.:*** Androskat; ***Neth.:*** Androskat.

Pholedrine Sulphate (2096-p)

Pholedrine Sulphate *(BANM, rINNM)*.

Isodrine Sulphate; Sympropaminum (pholedrine). 4-(2-Methylaminopropyl)phenol sulphate.

$(C_{10}H_{15}NO)_2,H_2SO_4 = 428.5$.

CAS — 370-14-9 (pholedrine); 6114-26-7 (pholedrine sulphate).

Pholedrine is a sympathomimetic (see Adrenaline, p.813) given by mouth as the sulphate in combination with other drugs in the treatment of hypotensive states. It is also an ingredient of preparations promoted for vascular disorders.

Preparations

Proprietary Preparations (details are given in Part 3)

Multi-ingredient: ***Ger.:*** Adyston; Jatamansin†; Kontagripp-RR†; Pentavenon†; Venosan†; Zellaforte N Plus; ***Spain:*** Venosan; ***Switz.:*** Ortho-Maren retard; Venosan.

Picodralazine (13114-a)

Picodralazine *(rINN)*.

Picodralazinum. 1-Hydrazino-4-(4-pyridylmethyl)phthalazine.

$C_{14}H_{13}N_5 = 251.3$.

CAS — 17692-43-2.

Picodralazine is a peripheral vasodilator structurally related to hydralazine (p.883) that has been used in the treatment of hypertension.

Preparations

Proprietary Preparations (details are given in Part 3)

Multi-ingredient: ***Spain:*** Vallene Complex†.

Picotamide (3939-x)

G-137; Picotamidum Monohydricum. 4-Methoxy-*N,N'*-bis(3-pyridinylmethyl)-1,3-benzenedicarboxamide monohydrate.

$C_{21}H_{20}N_4O_3,H_2O = 394.4$.

CAS — 32828-81-2 (anhydrous picotamide); 80530-63-8 (picotamide monohydrate); 86247-87-2 (picotamide tartrate).

Pharmacopoeias. In *Eur.* (see p.viii).

A white or almost white, polymorphic, crystalline powder. Slightly **soluble** in water; soluble in dehydrated alcohol and in dichloromethane; dissolves in dilute mineral acids.

Picotamide is a thromboxane synthase inhibitor and thromboxane receptor antagonist with antiplatelet activity. It is given by mouth in thrombo-embolic disorders (p.801) in initial doses of 900 to 1200 mg daily in divided doses, reducing to a maintenance dose of 300 to 600 mg daily.

References.

1. Berrettini M, *et al.* "In vitro" and "ex vivo" effects of picotamide, a combined thromboxane A_2-synthase inhibitor and -receptor antagonist, on human platelets. *Eur J Clin Pharmacol* 1990; **39:** 495–500.
2. Modesti PA, *et al.* Acute reduction of TxA_2 platelet binding sites after in vivo administration of a TxA_2 receptor inhibitor. *Br J Clin Pharmacol* 1991; **31:** 439–43.
3. Balsano F, *et al.* Effect of picotamide on the clinical progression of peripheral vascular disease: a double-blind placebo-controlled study. *Circulation* 1993; **87:** 1563–9.

ACE inhibitor-induced cough. Cough is a recognised adverse effect of ACE inhibitor administration and has been treated with a number of drugs (see p.805). Administration of picotamide led to the disappearance of cough in 8 of 9 patients receiving enalapril for hypertension,[1] suggesting that thromboxanes may be involved in the aetiology of ACE inhibitor-induced cough.

1. Malini PL, *et al.* Thromboxane antagonism and cough induced by angiotensin-converting-enzyme inhibitor. *Lancet* 1997; **350:** 15–18.

Preparations

Proprietary Preparations (details are given in Part 3)
Ital.: Plactidil.

Pilsicainide Hydrochloride (991-d)

Pilsicainide Hydrochloride *(rINNM)*.

SUN-1165. Tetrahydro-1*H*-pyrrolizine-7a(5*H*)-aceto-2′,6′-xylidide hydrochloride.

$C_{17}H_{24}N_2O,HCl = 308.8$.

CAS — 88069-67-4 (pilsicainide).

Pilsicainide hydrochloride is an antiarrhythmic with class Ic activity (p.776).

References.

1. Takabatake T, *et al.* Pharmacokinetics of SUN 1165, a new antiarrhythmic agent, in renal dysfunction. *Eur J Clin Pharmacol* 1991; **40:** 411–14.

Pimobendan (19663-m)

Pimobendan *(USAN, rINN)*.

UDCG-115. 4,5-Dihydro-6-[2-(*p*-methyoxyphenyl)-5-benzimidazolyl]-5-methyl-3(2*H*)-pyridazinone.

$C_{19}H_{18}N_4O_2 = 334.4$.

CAS — 74150-27-9; 118428-36-7.

Pimobendan is a phosphodiesterase inhibitor with calcium-sensitising properties. It has positive inotropic and vasodilator activity and has been tried in the management of heart failure. Studies with other inotropic phosphodiesterase inhibitors have shown that their prolonged oral administration can increase the mortality rate.

References.

1. Przechera M, *et al.* Pharmacokinetic profile and tolerability of pimobendan in patients with terminal renal insufficiency. *Eur J Clin Pharmacol* 1991; **40:** 107–11.
2. The Pimobendan in Congestive Heart Failure (PICO) Investigators. Effect of pimobendan on exercise capacity in patients with heart failure: main results from the Pimobendan in Congestive Heart Failure (PICO) trial. *Heart* 1996; **76:** 223–31.

Pinacidil (16954-y)

Pinacidil *(USAN, rINN)*.

P-1134. (±)-2-Cyano-1-(4-pyridyl)-3-(1,2,2-trimethylpropyl)guanidine; (±)-*N″*-Cyano-*N*-4-pyridinyl-*N′*-(1,2,2-trimethylpropyl)guanidine.

$C_{13}H_{19}N_5 = 245.3$.

CAS — 60560-33-0 (anhydrous pinacidil); 85371-64-8 (pinacidil monohydrate).

Adverse Effects and Precautions

The most common adverse effects in patients receiving pinacidil are reported to be headache, oedema and fluid retention, dizziness, palpitations, and tachycardia. ECG changes, hypertrichosis, flushing, tiredness, postural hypotension, nasal congestion, and gastro-intestinal disturbances have also been reported. Many adverse effects are dose-related.

Oedema may be reduced by concomitant administration of a thiazide diuretic.

Pinacidil should be used with caution in patients with symptomatic ischaemic heart disease, cerebrovascular insufficiency, renal or hepatic dysfunction, or pre-existing tachyarrhythmias.

Pharmacokinetics

Pinacidil is reported to be rapidly absorbed from the gastro-intestinal tract. It is metabolised in the liver, principally to pinacidil-*N*-oxide, and excreted in urine as metabolites and a small amount of unchanged drug. The elimination half-life has been reported to range from 1.6 to 2.9 hours after administration of standard tablets. Pinacidil is about 65% bound to plasma protein.

In a study of the clinical pharmacokinetics of pinacidil in 406 patients receiving 12.5 to 75 mg twice daily as a modified-release capsule, clearance of pinacidil and pinacidil-*N*-oxide was reduced in patients with impaired renal function, and in older as compared with younger patients.[1] Clearance was also lower in white than in non-white patients. Dosage titration should be cautious in the elderly and in patients with renal dysfunction. A study of the variable metabolism of pinacidil found that it was independent of other metabolic polymorphisms of oxidation, and was probably due to variations in the isozymes of cytochrome P450.[2]

1. Goldberg MR, *et al.* Clinical pharmacokinetics of pinacidil, a potassium channel opener, in hypertension. *J Clin Pharmacol* 1989; **29:** 33–40.
2. Ayesh R, *et al.* Variable metabolism of pinacidil: lack of correlation with the debrisoquine and trimethylamine C- and N-oxidative polymorphisms. *Br J Clin Pharmacol* 1989; **27:** 423–8.

Uses and Administration

Pinacidil is a potassium-channel opener (p.778) that produces direct peripheral vasodilatation of the arterioles. It reduces blood pressure and peripheral resistance and produces fluid retention. Tachycardia and an increase in cardiac output occur mainly as a reflex response to the reduction in peripheral resistance.

Pinacidil is used in the management of hypertension (p.788).

In hypertension, the usual initial dose is 12.5 mg given twice daily by mouth as a modified-release preparation, increased if necessary at intervals of 1 to 2 weeks to a maximum of 100 to 150 mg daily in divided doses. Usual maintenance doses are 25 mg twice daily.

Reviews.

1. Friedel HA, Brogden RN. Pinacidil: a review of its pharmacodynamic and pharmacokinetic properties, and therapeutic potential in the treatment of hypertension. *Drugs* 1990; **39:** 929–67.

Preparations

Proprietary Preparations (details are given in Part 3)
Irl.: Pindac.

Pindolol (6319-c)

Pindolol *(BAN, USAN, rINN).*

LB-46; Pindololum; Prindolol; Prinodolol. 1-(Indol-4-yloxy)-3-isopropylaminopropan-2-ol.

$C_{14}H_{20}N_2O_2$ = 248.3.

CAS — 13523-86-9.

Pharmacopoeias. In *Eur.* (see p.viii), *Jpn*, and *US*.

A white or almost white crystalline powder. Practically **insoluble** in water; slightly soluble in methyl alcohol; very slightly soluble in chloroform; dissolves in dilute mineral acids. **Protect** from light.

Adverse Effects, Treatment, and Precautions

As for beta blockers, p.828.

Effects on lipid metabolism. Beta blockers can affect plasma-lipid concentrations, although these effects may be less pronounced with beta blockers possessing intrinsic sympathomimetic activity (p.829). Administration of pindolol in patients with hypertension is not associated with any increases in total plasma-cholesterol concentrations or falls in high density lipoprotein fraction.[1,2]

1. Hunter Hypertension Research Group. Effects of pindolol, or a pindolol/clopamide combination preparation, on plasma lipid levels in essential hypertension. *Med J Aust* 1989; **150:** 646–52.
2. Terént A, *et al.* Long-term effect of pindolol on lipids and lipoproteins in men with newly diagnosed hypertension. *Eur J Clin Pharmacol* 1989; **36:** 347–50.

Tremor. Fine tremor in the extremities of 5 patients during pindolol therapy was considered to have been due to its partial agonist activity.[1]

1. Hod H, *et al.* Pindolol-induced tremor. *Postgrad Med J* 1980; **56:** 346–7.

Interactions

The interactions associated with beta blockers are discussed on p.829.

Pharmacokinetics

Pindolol is almost completely absorbed from the gastro-intestinal tract and peak plasma concentrations are obtained about 1 to 2 hours after a dose. About 40 to 60% is reported to be bound to plasma proteins. It is moderately lipid-soluble. Pindolol is distributed into breast milk. It is only partially metabolised in the liver and is excreted in the urine both unchanged and in the form of metabolites. A plasma elimination half-life of 3 to 4 hours has been reported in healthy adults. The half-life may be prolonged in elderly hypertensive patients, and in patients with renal or hepatic failure.

Uses and Administration

Pindolol is a non-cardioselective beta blocker (p.828). It is reported to have intrinsic sympathomimetic actions but little membrane-stabilising activity.

Pindolol is used in the management of hypertension (p.788), angina pectoris (p.780), and other cardiovascular disorders. It is also used in glaucoma (p.1387).

In **hypertension** pindolol is usually given initially in a dosage of 5 mg two or three times daily by mouth, subsequently increased according to the patient's response; additional benefit is rarely obtained from doses higher than 45 mg daily, although doses up to 60 mg daily have been given. A once-daily dosage regimen has been reported to be adequate for some patients.

The usual dose for **angina pectoris** is 2.5 to 5 mg up to three times daily; however, doses of up to 10 mg three times daily have been suggested.

Pindolol eye drops in concentrations of 0.5 to 1% are used in the management of **glaucoma**.

Orthostatic hypotension. Many drugs have been tried in the management of orthostatic hypotension (p.1040) although none is entirely satisfactory. The successful treatment of 4 patients, with severe orthostatic hypotension because of chronic autonomic failure, with pindolol has been reported.[1] However, pindolol was of no benefit in 5 patients with postural hypotension due to autonomic failure associated with multiple system atrophy.[2] Others[3] have also reported lack of effect.

1. Man in't Veld AJ, *et al.* Effects of β-adrenoceptor agonists and antagonists in patients with peripheral autonomic neuropathy. *Br J Clin Pharmacol* 1982; **13:** 367S–74S.
2. Davies B, *et al.* Pindolol in postural hypotension: the case for caution. *Lancet* 1981; **ii:** 982–3.
3. Goldstraw P, Waller DG. Pindolol in orthostatic hypotension. *Br Med J* 1981; **283:** 310.

Preparations

BP 1998: Pindolol Tablets;
USP 23: Pindolol Tablets.

Proprietary Preparations (details are given in Part 3)
Aust.: Visken; ***Austral.:*** Barbloc; Visken; ***Belg.:*** Visken; ***Canad.:*** Novo-Pindol; Nu-Pindol; Visken; ***Fr.:*** Visken; ***Ger.:*** durapindol; Glauco-Stulln; Pectobloc†; Pinbetol†; Pindoptan; Pindoreal; Visken; ***Irl.:*** Visken; ***Ital.:*** Visken; ***Neth.:*** Visken; ***Norw.:*** Decreten†; Hexapindol; Visken; ***S.Afr.:*** Visken; ***Swed.:*** Hexapindol; Visken; ***Switz.:*** Bedrenal†; Betapindol; Viskene; ***UK:*** Visken; ***USA:*** Visken.

Multi-ingredient: ***Aust.:*** Viskaldix; Viskenit; ***Belg.:*** Viskaldix; ***Canad.:*** Viskazide; ***Fr.:*** Viskaldix; ***Ger.:*** Nitrisken†; Viskaldix; ***Irl.:*** Viskaldix; ***Neth.:*** Viskaldix; ***S.Afr.:*** Viskaldix†; ***Switz.:*** Viskaldix; Viskenit†; ***UK:*** Viskaldix.

Pipratecol (9274-x)

Pipratecol *(rINN).*

711-SE. 1-(3,4-Dihydroxyphenyl)-2-[4-(2-methoxyphenyl)piperazin-1-yl]ethanol.

$C_{19}H_{24}N_2O_4$ = 344.4.

CAS — 15534-05-1.

Pipratecol is a vasodilator given in conjunction with raubasine (p.941) in the treatment of cerebrovascular disorders.

Preparations

Proprietary Preparations (details are given in Part 3)
Multi-ingredient: ***Ital.:*** Isosarpan†.

Piretanide (13130-a)

Piretanide *(BAN, USAN, rINN).*

Hoe-118; S73-4118. 4-Phenoxy-3-(pyrrolidin-1-yl)-5-sulphamoylbenzoic acid.

$C_{17}H_{18}N_2O_5S$ = 362.4.

CAS — 55837-27-9.

Adverse Effects

As for Frusemide, p.871. Muscle cramps have been reported following high doses of piretanide.

Precautions

Piretanide's precautions and contra-indications which are dependent on its effects on fluid and electrolyte balance are similar to those of the thiazide diuretics (see Hydrochlorothiazide, p.887). Patients with impaired micturition or prostatic hyperplasia may develop retention of urine with piretanide.

Interactions

As for Frusemide, p.872.

Pharmacokinetics

Piretanide has been reported to be almost completely absorbed following oral administration. It is extensively bound to plasma proteins, and is reported to have a half-life of about 1 hour.

References.

1. Beermann B, Grind M. Clinical pharmacokinetics of some newer diuretics. *Clin Pharmacokinet* 1987; **13:** 254–66.

Uses and Administration

Piretanide is a loop diuretic with actions and uses similar to those of frusemide (p.872). In the treatment of hypertension (p.788) it is given in a usual dose of 6 to 12 mg daily by mouth. The sodium salt is given by injection.

References.

1. Clissold SP, Brogden RN. Piretanide: a preliminary review of its pharmacodynamic and pharmacokinetic properties, and therapeutic efficacy. *Drugs* 1985; **29:** 489–530.

Preparations

Proprietary Preparations (details are given in Part 3)
Aust.: Arelix; ***Fr.:*** Eurelix; ***Ger.:*** Arelix; ***Irl.:*** Arelix; ***Ital.:*** Tauliz; ***Neth.:*** Arelix†; ***S.Afr.:*** Arelix; ***Spain:*** Midaten; Perbilen; ***Switz.:*** Arelix; Pirenex; ***UK:*** Arelix†.

Multi-ingredient: ***Aust.:*** Trialix; ***Ger.:*** Arelix ACE; Betarelix; ***Irl.:*** Trialix; ***Switz.:*** Trialix.

Pirmagrel (18947-q)

Pirmagrel *(USAN, rINN).*

CGS-13080. Imidazo[1,5-*a*]pyridine-5-hexanoic acid.

$C_{13}H_{16}N_2O_2$ = 232.3.

CAS — 85691-74-3.

Pirmagrel is a thromboxane synthase inhibitor with antiplatelet activity under investigation in thrombo-embolic disorders.

References.

1. Mickelson JK, *et al.* Thromboxane synthase inhibition with CGS 13080 improves coronary blood flow after streptokinase-induced thrombolysis. *Am Heart J* 1987; **113:** 1345–52.
2. Kim YD, *et al.* Effects of CGS-13080, a thromboxane inhibitor, on pulmonary vascular resistance in patients after mitral valve replacement surgery. *Circulation* 1988; **78** (suppl 1): I44–I50.
3. Chouinard ML, *et al.* Pharmacokinetics and biochemical efficacy of pirmagrel, a thromboxane synthase inhibitor, in renal allograft recipients. *Clin Pharmacol Ther* 1992; **52:** 597–604.

Pirmenol Hydrochloride (16955-j)

Pirmenol Hydrochloride *(USAN, rINNM).*

CI-845. (±)-*cis*-2,6-Dimethyl-α-phenyl-α-2-pyridyl-1-piperidinebutanol hydrochloride.

$C_{22}H_{30}N_2O,HCl$ = 374.9.

CAS — 68252-19-7 (pirmenol); 61477-94-9 (pirmenol hydrochloride).

Pirmenol hydrochloride is an antiarrhythmic with class Ia activity (p.776).

References.

1. Hampton EM, *et al.* Initial and long-term outpatient experience with pirmenol for control of ventricular arrhythmias. *Eur J Clin Pharmacol* 1986; **31:** 15–22.
2. Stringer KA, *et al.* Enhanced pirmenol elimination by rifampin. *J Clin Pharmacol* 1988; **28:** 1094–7.
3. Janiczek N, *et al.* Pharmacokinetics of pirmenol enantiomers and pharmacodynamics of pirmenol racemate in patients with premature ventricular contractions. *J Clin Pharmacol* 1997; **37:** 502–13.

Plasmin (3739-l)

Plasmin *(BAN).*

Fibrinolysin (Human) *(rINN)*; Fibrinase; Plasmin (Human).

CAS — 9001-90-5 (plasmin); 9004-09-5 (human plasmin).

Plasmin is a proteolytic enzyme derived from the activation of human plasminogen. Plasmin derived from cattle (bovine plasmin) and other animals is also available. Plasmin converts fibrin into soluble products and also hydrolyses some other proteins. Its role in haemostasis is described further on p.704.

Plasmin is used (generally as bovine plasmin) in conjunction with deoxyribonuclease for the debridement of wounds. It was formerly given parenterally for the treatment of thrombotic disorders.

Preparations

Proprietary Preparations (details are given in Part 3)

Multi-ingredient: ***Aust.:*** Fibrolan; ***Austral.:*** Elase; ***Canad.:*** Elase; Elase-Chloromycetin; ***Fr.:*** Elase; ***Ger.:*** Fibrolan; Fibrolan mit Chloromycetin†; ***Ital.:*** Elase; ***Neth.:*** Elase; ***Spain:*** Parkelase; Parkelase Chloromycetin; ***Switz.:*** Fibrolan; ***USA:*** Elase; Elase-Chloromycetin.

Plasminogen (13140-x)

Plasminogen *(BAN).*

CAS — 9001-91-6.

Plasminogen is the specific substance derived from plasma which, when activated to plasmin, has the property of lysing fibrinogen, fibrin, and some other proteins. Its role in haemostasis is described further on p.704. Plasminogen has been investigated as a thrombolytic and has been used in combination with other blood products in wound-sealant preparations.

Preparations

Proprietary Preparations (details are given in Part 3)

Multi-ingredient: ***Aust.:*** Tissucol; Tissucol Duo Quick; ***Canad.:*** Tisseel†; ***Ger.:*** Tissucol Duo S; Tissucol Fibrinkleber tiefgefroren; Tissucol-Kit; ***Spain:*** Tissucol; ***Swed.:*** Tisseel Duo Quick; ***Switz.:*** Tissucol; ***UK:*** Tisseel.

Polythiazide (2352-p)

Polythiazide *(BAN, USAN, rINN).*

NSC-108161; P-2525. 6-Chloro-3,4-dihydro-2-methyl-3-(2,2,2-trifluoroethylthiomethyl)-2*H*-1,2,4-benzothiadiazine-7-sulphonamide 1,1-dioxide.

$C_{11}H_{13}ClF_3N_3O_4S_3$ = 439.9.

CAS — 346-18-9.

Pharmacopoeias. In Br. and US.

A white or almost white crystalline powder with an alliaceous odour. Practically **insoluble** in water and in chloroform; slightly to sparingly soluble in alcohol; soluble in methyl alcohol and acetone. **Store** in airtight containers. Protect from light.

Adverse Effects, Treatment, and Precautions

As for Hydrochlorothiazide, p.885.

Interactions

As for Hydrochlorothiazide, p.887.

Pharmacokinetics

Polythiazide is fairly readily absorbed from the gastro-intestinal tract. It has been estimated to have a plasma elimination half-life of about 26 hours. More than 80% may be bound to plasma proteins. It is excreted mainly in the urine as unchanged polythiazide and metabolites.

References.

1. Hobbs DC, Twomey TM. Kinetics of polythiazide. *Clin Pharmacol Ther* 1978; **23:** 241–6.

Uses and Administration

Polythiazide is a thiazide diuretic with actions and uses similar to those of hydrochlorothiazide (p.887). It is used for oedema, including that associated with heart failure (p.785), and for hypertension (p.788).

Diuresis is initiated within about 2 hours after administration, and lasts for 24 to 48 hours.

In the treatment of **oedema** the usual dose is 1 to 4 mg by mouth daily. In the treatment of **hypertension** the usual dose is stated to be 2 to 4 mg daily, either alone or in conjunction with other antihypertensives although doses of only 0.5 mg to 1.0 mg may be adequate.

In susceptible patients potassium supplements or a potassium-sparing diuretic may be necessary, but see hydrochlorothiazide.

Preparations

BP 1998: Polythiazide Tablets;
USP 23: Polythiazide Tablets.

Proprietary Preparations (details are given in Part 3)

Belg.: Renese; ***Ger.:*** Drenusil†; ***Irl.:*** Nephril; ***Norw.:*** Renese†; ***Swed.:*** Renese†; ***UK:*** Nephril; ***USA:*** Renese.

Multi-ingredient: ***Ger.:*** Drenusil-R†; Polypress; ***USA:*** Minizide; Renese R.

Practolol (6320-s)

Practolol *(BAN, USAN, pINN).*

AY-21011; ICI-50172. 4′-(2-Hydroxy-3-isopropylaminopropoxy)acetanilide.

$C_{14}H_{22}N_2O_3$ = 266.3.

CAS — 6673-35-4.

Practolol is a cardioselective beta blocker (p.828). It is reported to possess intrinsic sympathomimetic activity. Its use was restricted by its serious adverse effects. In particular, the 'oculomucocutaneous syndrome' of serious adverse effects on the skin, eyes, and mucous membranes, deafness, systemic lupus erythematosus, and sclerosing peritonitis, which may be fatal, was associated with practolol.

Prajmalium Bitartrate (7790-n)

Prajmalium Bitartrate *(BAN, rINN).*

GT-1012; NPAB. *N*-Propylajmalinium hydrogen tartrate.

$C_{23}H_{33}N_2O_2,C_4H_5O_6$ = 518.6.

CAS — 35080-11-6 (prajmalium); 2589-47-1 (prajmalium bitartrate).

Adverse Effects and Precautions

As for Ajmaline, p.817.

Effects on the liver. Cholestatic jaundice associated with pruritus, chills, and eosinophilia[1] was attributed to an allergic reaction to prajmalium bitartrate in a patient 20 days after the start of treatment.

1. Rotmensch HH, *et al.* Cholestatic jaundice: an immune response to prajmalium bitartrate. *Postgrad Med J* 1980; **56:** 738–41.

Effects on mental state. Confusion and disorientation in time and place[1] occurred on 2 occasions in a 67-year-old man given prajmalium bitartrate 100 mg daily for the control of tachycardia; the confusion rapidly disappeared when prajmalium was withdrawn.

1. Lessing JB, Copperman IJ. Severe cerebral confusion produced by prajmalium bitartrate. *Br Med J* 1977; **2:** 675.

Uses and Administration

Prajmalium is a class I antiarrhythmic (p.776) which is the *N*-propyl derivative of ajmaline (p.817). It is given by mouth as the bitartrate in the management of cardiac arrhythmias (p.782) in initial doses of 60 to 80 mg daily. Maintenance doses of 20 to 40 mg daily in divided doses are used.

Preparations

Proprietary Preparations (details are given in Part 3)

Aust.: Neo-Gilurytmal; ***Ger.:*** Neo-Gilurytmal; ***Ital.:*** Neo Aritmina; ***Spain:*** Neo Gilurytmal; ***Switz.:*** Neo-Gilurytmal†.

Multi-ingredient: ***Spain:*** Cresophene.

Prazosin Hydrochloride (896-n)

Prazosin Hydrochloride *(BANM, USAN, rINNM).*

CP-12299-1; Furazosin Hydrochloride; Prazosini Hydrochloridum. 2-[4-(2-Furoyl)piperazin-1-yl]-6,7-dimethoxyquinazolin-4-ylamine hydrochloride.

$C_{19}H_{21}N_5O_4,HCl$ = 419.9.

CAS — 19216-56-9 (prazosin); 19237-84-4 (prazosin hydrochloride).

Pharmacopoeias. In *Chin., Eur.* (see p.viii), and *US.*

A white to tan-coloured powder. Very slightly to slightly **soluble** in water and in alcohol; slightly soluble in methyl alcohol and in dimethylformamide; practically insoluble in chloroform and in acetone. **Store** in airtight containers. Protect from light.

Prazosin hydrochloride 1.1 mg is approximately equivalent to 1 mg of prazosin.

Adverse Effects

Prazosin hydrochloride can cause postural hypotension and it may be severe and produce syncope following the initial dose; it may be preceded by tachycardia. This reaction can be avoided by starting treatment with a low dose, preferably at night (see Uses and Administration, below).

The more common side-effects include dizziness, drowsiness, headache, lack of energy, nausea, and palpitations, and may diminish with continued prazosin therapy or with a reduction in dosage. Other adverse effects include oedema, chest pain, dyspnoea, constipation, diarrhoea, vomiting, depression and nervousness, sleep disturbances, vertigo, hallucinations, paraesthesia, nasal congestion, epistaxis, dryness of mouth, urinary frequency and incontinence, reddened sclera, blurred vision, tinnitus, abnormal liver enzyme values, pancreatitis, arthralgia, skin rashes, pruritus, and diaphoresis. Impotence and priapism have also been reported.

General reviews.

1. Carruthers SG. Adverse effects of α_1-adrenergic blocking drugs. *Drug Safety* 1994; **11:** 12–20.

Effects on the cardiovascular system. Postural hypotension, preceded by tachycardia and sometimes producing syncope, is an established side-effect of prazosin following the initial dose. Sinus bradycardia was associated with prazosin in a patient who experienced light headedness following each daily dose.[1]

1. Ball J. Symptomatic sinus bradycardia due to prazosin. *Lancet* 1994; **343:** 121.

Effects on the gastro-intestinal tract. Faecal incontinence in a 52-year-old man receiving prazosin was exacerbated by haemorrhoidectomy and appeared to be due to diminished resting anal tone, presumably because of smooth muscle relaxation secondary to alpha-adrenoceptor blockade.[1] Symptoms ceased almost immediately on discontinuing the drug.

1. Holmes SAV, *et al.* Faecal incontinence resulting from α_1-adrenoceptor blockade. *Lancet* 1990; **336:** 685–6.

Effects on mental function. Psychiatric symptoms including confusion, paranoia, and hallucinations developed in 3 patients associated with prazosin treatment.[1] Two of the patients had chronic renal failure and the renal function of the third was mildly impaired. Acute psychosis has also been reported with doxazosin.[2]

1. Chin DKF, *et al.* Neuropsychiatric complications related to use of prazosin in patients with renal failure. *Br Med J* 1986; **293:** 1347.
2. Evans M, *et al.* Drug induced psychosis with doxazosin. *Br Med J* 1997; **314:** 1869.

Hypersensitivity. Urticaria and angioedema were attributed to prazosin in a 70-year-old woman.[1]

1. Ruzicka T, Ring J. Hypersensitivity to prazosin. *Lancet* 1983; **i:** 473–4.

Lupus erythematosus. One study has reported the formation of antinuclear antibodies in patients receiving prazosin,[1] but this is not in agreement with other reports,[2,3] and commentators consider the association unproven.[4] There is no evidence of the development of lupus erythematosus.[1]

1. Marshall AJ, *et al.* Positive antinuclear factor tests with prazosin. *Br Med J* 1979; **1:** 165–6.
2. Wilson JD, *et al.* Antinuclear factor in patients on prazosin. *Br Med J* 1979; **1:** 553–4.
3. Melkild A, Gaarder PI. Does prazosin induce formation of antinuclear factor? *Br Med J* 1979; **1:** 620–1.
4. Kristensen BØ. Does prazosin induce formation of antinuclear factor? *Br Med J* 1979; **1:** 621.

Urinary incontinence. There have been reports of urinary incontinence developing in patients receiving prazosin. Analysis by Mathew and colleagues[1] of 56 cases reported to the

Australian Adverse Drug Reactions Advisory Committee indicated that typically symptoms appeared within a day or two of the commencement of prazosin and persisted until the drug was withdrawn or the dose reduced. Both stress and urge incontinence were experienced, sometimes in the same patient. Of the 56 patients, 51 were women and most were elderly. In a study[2] in women attending a hypertension clinic urinary incontinence was reported in 40.8% of 49 women receiving alpha blockers (prazosin, terazosin, or doxazosin) and in 16.3% of controls. Incontinence might be due to a reduction in urethral pressure induced by alpha-adrenoceptor blockade.

Interestingly, faecal incontinence has also been reported with prazosin—see Effects on the Gastro-intestinal Tract, above.

1. Mathew TH, *et al.* Urinary incontinence secondary to prazosin. *Med J Aust* 1988; **148:** 305–6.
2. Marshall HJ, Beevers DG. α-Adrenoceptor blocking drugs and female urinary incontinence: prevalence and reversibility. *Br J Clin Pharmacol* 1996; **42:** 507–9.

Treatment of Adverse Effects

If overdosage occurs the stomach should be emptied by lavage. Severe hypotension may respond to placing the patient in the supine position with the feet raised. The effects of gross overdosage may be treated by infusions of volume expanders, and if necessary cautious intravenous infusion of a vasopressor. Prazosin is not removed by dialysis.

Precautions

Treatment with prazosin should be introduced cautiously because of the risk of sudden collapse following the initial dose. Especial caution is necessary in patients with renal or hepatic impairment and in the elderly.

Prazosin is not recommended for the treatment of heart failure caused by mechanical obstruction, for example aortic or mitral valve stenosis, pulmonary embolism, and restrictive pericardial disease. It should be used with caution in patients with angina pectoris. Prazosin may cause drowsiness or dizziness; patients so affected should not drive or operate machinery.

Cerebral haemorrhage. Hypotension with disturbance of consciousness occurred in 3 patients with recent cerebral haemorrhage following an initial dose of prazosin 0.5 mg.[1]

1. Lin M-S, Hsieh W-J. Prazosin-induced first-dose phenomenon possibly associated with hemorrhagic stroke: a report of three cases. *Drug Intell Clin Pharm* 1987; **21:** 723–6.

Tolerance. Packer and colleagues have reported that despite initially favourable responses to prazosin in a study of 27 patients with severe chronic heart failure, the effects became rapidly attenuated after 48 hours despite continued treatment: complete loss of haemodynamic efficacy was noted in 58% of 24 patients who completed the study.[1] Long-term tolerance was not accompanied by changes in plasma renin activity or in body-weight and could not be prevented by concomitant treatment with spironolactone. Only 30 to 40% of patients with heart failure treated with prazosin showed notable long-term haemodynamic benefits. Although disagreeing about the mechanism, this confirms the earlier report of Bayliss and others, who noted beneficial haemodynamic effects when a single dose of prazosin was given to 19 patients with chronic heart failure, but no benefit from long-term therapy in 16.[2] In this study there was evidence of activation of the sympathetic and renin-angiotensin-aldosterone systems associated with fluid retention, which persisted despite high doses of frusemide in some patients.

1. Packer M, *et al.* Role of the renin-angiotensin system in the development of hemodynamic and clinical tolerance to long-term prazosin therapy in patients with severe chronic heart failure. *J Am Coll Cardiol* 1986; **7:** 671–80.
2. Bayliss J, *et al.* Clinical importance of the renin-angiotensin system in chronic heart failure: double blind comparison of captopril and prazosin. *Br Med J* 1985; **290:** 1861–5.

Interactions

The hypotensive effects of prazosin may be enhanced by the concomitant administration of diuretics and other antihypertensives, and by alcohol and other drugs that cause hypotension. The risk of first-dose hypotension may be particularly increased in patients receiving beta blockers or calcium-channel blockers.

Analgesics. Indomethacin reduced prazosin-induced hypotension in 4 of 9 subjects.[1]

1. Rubin P, *et al.* Studies on the clinical pharmacology of prazosin II: the influence of indomethacin and of propranolol on the action and disposition of prazosin. *Br J Clin Pharmacol* 1980; **10:** 33–9.

Antidepressants and antipsychotics. A patient who was taking chlorpromazine and amitriptyline developed acute agitation on receiving prazosin.[1] The symptoms settled rapidly when prazosin was discontinued. Antidepressants and antipsychotics may enchance the hypotensive effect of prazosin and other alpha blockers.

1. Bolli P, Simpson FO. New vasodilator drugs for hypertension. *Br Med J* 1974; **1:** 637.

Calcium-channel blockers. An enhanced hypotensive effect has been reported in normotensive subjects given prazosin and *verapamil* concurrently; the effect may be due in part to enhanced bioavailability of prazosin.[1] Markedly increased hypotensive responses have also been reported with combined use of prazosin and *nifedipine*,[2,3] although the validity of such reports has been questioned.[4]

1. Pasanisi F, *et al.* Combined alpha adrenoceptor antagonism and calcium channel blockade in normal subjects. *Clin Pharmacol Ther* 1984; **36:** 716–23.
2. Jee LD, Opie LH. Acute hypotensive response to nifedipine added to prazosin in treatment of hypertension. *Br Med J* 1983; **287:** 1514.
3. Jee LD, Opie LH. Acute hypotensive response to nifedipine added to prazosin. *Br Med J* 1984; **288:** 238–9.
4. Elliott HL, *et al.* Acute hypotensive response to nifedipine added to prazosin. *Br Med J* 1984; **288:** 238.

Digoxin. For reference to the effect of prazosin on serum-digoxin concentrations, see under Digoxin, p.850.

Pharmacokinetics

Prazosin is readily absorbed from the gastro-intestinal tract with peak plasma concentrations occurring 1 to 3 hours after an oral dose. The bioavailability is variable and a range of 43 to 85% has been reported. Prazosin is highly bound to plasma protein. It is extensively metabolised in the liver and some of the metabolites are reported to have hypotensive activity. It is excreted as the metabolites and 5 to 11% as unchanged prazosin mainly in the faeces via the bile. Less than 10% is excreted in the urine. Small amounts are distributed into breast milk. Its duration of action is longer than would be predicted from its relatively short plasma half-life of about 2 to 4 hours. Half-life is reported to be increased to about 7 hours in patients with heart failure.

Old age. The bioavailability of prazosin was significantly reduced in the elderly, about 40% less unchanged drug reaching the systemic circulation compared with the young.[1] This was attributed to a reduction in the absorption from the gastro-intestinal tract. The half-life was also prolonged in the elderly and this was associated with an increase in the volume of distribution at steady state. However, it was considered unlikely that these effects would have major clinical significance.

1. Rubin PC, *et al.* Prazosin disposition in young and elderly subjects. *Br J Clin Pharmacol* 1981; **12:** 401–4.

Protein binding. Although Brunner and Müller have reported that prazosin was about 80 to 85% bound to serum albumin and only about 10 to 30% bound to α_1-acid glycoprotein *in vitro*,[1] this study does not take account of potential interactions between the binding proteins *in vivo*, and binding to α_1-acid glycoprotein might be more significant in clinical practice. A subsequent study by Sager and others has indicated that variations in prazosin protein binding pre- and post-operatively were related to variations in concentration of the glycoprotein.[2]

1. Brunner F, Müller WE. Prazosin binding to human α_1-acid glycoprotein (orosomucoid), human serum albumin, and human serum: further characterisation of the 'single drug binding site' of orosomucoid. *J Pharm Pharmacol* 1985; **37:** 305–9.
2. Sager G, *et al.* Binding of prazosin and propranolol at variable α_1-acid glycoprotein and albumin concentrations. *Br J Clin Pharmacol* 1989; **27:** 229–34.

Uses and Administration

Prazosin is an alpha blocker (p.776) that acts by selective blockade of alpha$_1$-adrenoceptors. It is used in the management of hypertension (p.788), Raynaud's syndrome (below), and benign prostatic hyperplasia (p.1446). It has also been used in heart failure (p.785).

Prazosin produces peripheral dilatation of both arterioles and veins and reduction of peripheral resistance, usually without reflex tachycardia. It reduces both standing and supine blood pressure with a greater effect on the diastolic pressure. It is reported to have no effect on renal blood flow or glomerular filtration rate, and has little effect on cardiac output in hypertensive patients. In patients with heart failure, prazosin reduces both preload and afterload and produces an improvement in cardiac output. Tolerance may develop during the treatment of heart failure. In benign prostatic hyperplasia, prazosin may relieve the symptoms of urinary obstruction by reducing smooth muscle tone in the prostate and bladder neck.

Prazosin is given by mouth as the hydrochloride, but doses are usually expressed in terms of the base. Following oral administration the hypotensive effect is seen within 2 to 4 hours and persists for several hours.

A low starting dose is given in the evening to lessen the risk of collapse which may occur in some patients after the first dose (see Adverse Effects, above). Doses may need to be reduced in the elderly and in patients with renal or hepatic impairment.

In **hypertension**, the usual initial dose in the UK is 500 μg two or three times daily for 3 to 7 days; if tolerated the dose may then be increased to 1 mg two or three times daily for a further 3 to 7 days, and thereafter gradually increased, according to the patient's response, to a usual maximum of 20 mg daily in divided doses. In the US the recommended starting dose is 1 mg two or three times daily. Although sources in the UK recommend 20 mg as a maximum daily dose, sources in the USA report that a few patients may obtain benefit from up to 40 mg daily in divided doses. However, the usual maintenance dose is between 6 and 15 mg daily. Smaller doses may be required in patients concurrently taking other antihypertensive drugs. Modified-release preparations may allow once daily dosing.

In **Raynaud's syndrome** and in **benign prostatic hyperplasia** an initial dose of 500 μg twice a day may be given increasing to a maintenance dose not exceeding 2 mg twice a day.

In **heart failure**, treatment has been started with 500 μg two to four times daily and increased gradually according to response; the usual maintenance dose has been 4 to 20 mg daily.

Muscle cramp. Skeletal muscle cramp may occur during haemodialysis, possibly due to activation of the sympathetic nervous system. Prazosin was reported[1] to reduce the incidence of cramp in 4 of 5 patients with frequent haemodialysis-associated muscle cramp. However, the incidence of hypotension was also increased and might limit the use of prazosin for this indication.

1. Sidhom OA, *et al.* Low-dose prazosin in patients with muscle cramps during hemodialysis. *Clin Pharmacol Ther* 1994; **56:** 445–51.

Peripheral vascular disease. Alpha blockers, including prazosin, may be used in the management of Raynaud's syndrome (p.794). Studies of the benefits of prazosin have produced varying results. Nielsen and colleagues reported a short-term reduction in number and duration of attacks in 5 of 7 patients given prazosin 2 mg daily but only 1 patient had complete relief from attacks and few could tolerate doses higher than 6 mg daily.[1] Improvements were not maintained during continued treatment for 2 months. Wollersheim and others and Allegra and others have both reported benefit from prazosin 1 mg two or three times daily, in the majority of patients, but the latter study suggested greater benefit in Raynaud's disease (the primary, idiopathic form) than in secondary Raynaud's syndrome,[2] whereas no such difference was found by Wollersheim's study.[3] In a subsequent study Wollersheim and Thien found higher doses of prazosin (2 mg or 4 mg three times daily) to be no more effective than 1 mg three times daily, and associated with a significantly greater incidence of adverse effects.[4]

1. Nielsen SL, *et al.* Prazosin treatment of primary Raynaud's phenomenon. *Eur J Clin Pharmacol* 1983; **24:** 421–3.
2. Allegra C, *et al.* Pharmacological treatment of Raynaud's phenomenon: a new therapeutic approach. *Curr Ther Res* 1986; **40:** 303–11.
3. Wollersheim H, *et al.* Double-blind, placebo-controlled study of prazosin in Raynaud's phenomenon. *Clin Pharmacol Ther* 1986, **40:** 219–25.
4. Wollersheim H, Thien T. Dose-response study of prazosin in Raynaud's phenomenon: clinical effectiveness versus side effects. *J Clin Pharmacol* 1988; **28:** 1089–93.

Phaeochromocytoma. Prazosin has been used successfully to overcome the pressor effects of catecholamines released by phaeochromocytoma[1] (p.795). Since it selectively blocks alpha$_1$-adrenoceptors, tachycardia following prazosin treatment is much less marked than following phentolamine or phenoxybenzamine and it may be of particular value in managing phaeochromocytoma crisis. Prazosin is also preferable if the tumour is predominantly adrenaline-secreting. However, the marked hypotensive effect is more pronounced than with other vasodilators such as phenoxybenzamine. Prazosin has also been advocated for control of hypertension during surgical treatment, but its use is limited to the pre-operative phase of management because no parenteral preparation is available.

1. Hull CJ. Phaeochromocytoma: diagnosis, preoperative preparation and anaesthetic management. *Br J Anaesth* 1986; **58:** 1453–68.

Scorpion stings. Stings from the Indian Red Scorpion (*Mesobuthus tamulus*) are potentially fatal. The scorpion venom is a potent sympathetic stimulator resulting in high circulating catecholamines, hypertension, arrhythmias, pulmonary oedema, and circulatory failure. Antivenom is generally ineffective and treatment for cardiotoxicity is supportive (see p.1533). Prazosin, given orally, appears to be beneficial and has been suggested[1] as first-line treatment, except in cases of severe pulmonary oedema.

1. Bawaskar HS, Bawaskar PH. Scorpion envenoming and the cardiovascular system. *Trop Doct* 1997; **27:** 6–9.

Preparations

BP 1998: Prazosin Tablets;
USP 23: Prazosin Hydrochloride Capsules.

Proprietary Preparations (details are given in Part 3)
Aust.: Minipress; ***Austral.:*** Minipress; Prasig; Pressin; ***Belg.:*** Minipress; ***Canad.:*** Apo-Prazo; Minipress; Novo-Prazin; Nu-Prazo; ***Fr.:*** Alpress; Minipress; ***Ger.:*** Adversuten; duramipress; Eurex; Minipress; ***Irl.:*** Hypovase; ***Ital.:*** Minipress†; ***Neth.:*** Minipress; ***Norw.:*** Peripress†; ***S.Afr.:*** Minipress; Pratsiol; ***Spain:*** Minipres; ***Swed.:*** Peripress†; ***Switz.:*** Minipress; ***UK:*** Alphavase; Hypovase; ***USA:*** Minipress.

Multi-ingredient: ***Ger.:*** Polypress; ***USA:*** Minizide.

Prenalterol Hydrochloride (13164-v)

Prenalterol Hydrochloride *(BANM, USAN, rINNM)*.

C-50005/A-Ba (racemate); CGP-7760B; H133/22; H-80/62 (racemate). (*S*)-1-(4-Hydroxyphenoxy)-3-isopropylaminopropan-2-ol hydrochloride.

$C_{12}H_{19}NO_3$,HCl = 261.7.

CAS — 57526-81-5 (prenalterol); 61260-05-7 (prenalterol hydrochloride).

Prenalterol is a sympathomimetic (see Adrenaline, p.813) with stimulant effects on $beta_1$-adrenoceptors. It has an inotropic action on the heart with relatively little chronotropic effect. Prenalterol hydrochloride has been administered parenterally in the treatment of heart failure and shock. It has also been promoted for the reversal of beta blockade.

Preparations

Proprietary Preparations (details are given in Part 3)
Norw.: Hyprenan; ***Swed.:*** Hyprenan.

Procainamide Hydrochloride (7791-h)

Procainamide Hydrochloride *(BANM, rINNM)*.

Novocainamidum; Procainamidi Chloridum; Procainamidi Hydrochloridum. 4-Amino-*N*-(2-diethylaminoethyl)benzamide hydrochloride.

$C_{13}H_{21}N_3O$,HCl = 271.8.

CAS — 51-06-9 (procainamide); 614-39-1 (procainamide hydrochloride).

Pharmacopoeias. In *Chin., Eur.* (see p.viii), *Int., Jpn, Pol.,* and *US.*

A white to tan-coloured, odourless, hygroscopic, crystalline powder. Very **soluble** in water; soluble to freely soluble in alcohol; slightly soluble in acetone and in chloroform; very slightly soluble to practically insoluble in ether. A 10% solution in water has a pH of 5.0 to 6.5. **Store** in airtight containers. Protect from light.

Stability. Procainamide is more stable in neutral solutions, such as sodium chloride, than in acidic solutions, such as glucose, but patients requiring intravenous procainamide often have heart failure and cannot tolerate the sodium load associated with sodium chloride injections. The stability of procainamide in glucose 5% injection is improved by neutralising the glucose injection using sodium bicarbonate, or storing the admixture at 5°. The concentration of procainamide remained above 90% of the initial concentration for 24 hours if the glucose injection was first neutralised and this was considered more practical than refrigeration if extended stability was required.[1]

The compound formed by mixing procainamide hydrochloride with glucose 5% infusion was shown to be a mixture of α- and β-glucosylamines[2] and about 10 to 15% of the procainamide was lost in this way after 10 hours at room temperature.

An oral liquid[3] prepared from procainamide capsules containing 5, 50, or 100 mg per mL of the hydrochloride was stable for at least 6 months when stored at 4 to 6°.

1. Raymond GG, *et al.* Stability of procainamide hydrochloride in neutralized 5% dextrose injection. *Am J Hosp Pharm* 1988; **45:** 2513–17.
2. Sianipar A, *et al.* Chemical incompatibility between procainamide hydrochloride and glucose following intravenous admixture. *J Pharm Pharmacol* 1994; **46:** 951–5.
3. Metras JI, *et al.* Stability of procainamide hydrochloride in an extemporaneously compounded oral liquid. *Am J Hosp Pharm* 1992; **49:** 1720–4.

Adverse Effects

Cardiac effects occur particularly during intravenous administration of procainamide and in overdose. Rapid intravenous administration may result in severe hypotension, ventricular fibrillation, and asystole. High plasma concentrations are also associated with impaired cardiac conduction.

Hypersensitivity reactions to procainamide are common. Procainamide is a frequent cause of drug-induced systemic lupus erythematosus (SLE) and the incidence has been reported to be as high as 30% of patients taking procainamide over prolonged periods. Antinuclear antibodies may be detected in a high proportion of patients, but they do not necessarily develop the symptoms of SLE that include arthralgia, arthritis, myalgia, pleural effusion, pericarditis, and fever. Agranulocytosis, eosinophilia, neutropenia, thrombocytopenia, and haemolytic anaemia have been reported. Other symptoms of hypersensitivity not necessarily related to SLE may also occur including hepatomegaly, angioedema, skin rashes, pruritus, urticaria, flushing, and hypergammaglobulinaemia.

Anorexia, nausea, vomiting, a bitter taste, and diarrhoea are more common with higher oral doses. Effects on the central nervous system such as mental depression, dizziness, and psychosis with hallucinations, have been reported.

Out of 488 hospitalised patients in the Boston Collaborative Drug Surveillance Program who had received procainamide, 45 experienced acute adverse effects attributed to the drug.[1] Life-threatening reactions included heart block in 3, tachyarrhythmias in 2, and bradycardia and/or hypotension in 2. Other reactions included gastro-intestinal upsets in 19, pyrexia in 8, bradycardia and hypotension in 5, tachyarrhythmias in 3, heart block in 1, eosinophilia in 1, and urticaria in 1 patient.

1. Lawson DH, Jick H. Adverse reactions to procainamide. *Br J Clin Pharmacol* 1977; **4:** 507–11.

Effects on the blood. Adverse haematological effects reported during procainamide therapy include neutropenia,[1-3] agranulocytosis,[2-6] thrombocytopenia,[5] haemolytic anaemia,[7] and pancytopenia.[8] These disorders are usually reversible on withdrawing procainamide although some fatalities have been reported.[3,4] It has been suggested[2,6] that agranulocytosis or severe neutropenia is more likely in patients taking modified-release preparations, but others have found no difference in the incidence between modified-release and conventional-release preparations.[3] An increased risk of agranulocytosis with procainamide has been documented in one large study.[9] Although the precise estimate of excess risk could not be calculated, the order of magnitude was about 3 per million exposed for up to one week. This excess risk was low and of little relevance in the initial choice of therapy.

1. Riker J, *et al.* Bone marrow granulomas and neutropenia associated with procainamide. *Arch Intern Med* 1978; **138:** 1731–2.
2. Ellrodt AG, *et al.* Severe neutropenia associated with sustained-release procainamide. *Ann Intern Med* 1984; **100:** 197–201.
3. Meyers DG, *et al.* Severe neutropenia associated with procainamide: comparison of sustained release and conventional preparations. *Am Heart J* 1985; **109:** 1393–5.
4. Fleet S. Agranulocytosis, procainamide, and phenytoin. *Ann Intern Med* 1984; **100:** 616–17.
5. Christensen DJ, *et al.* Agranulocytosis, thrombocytopenia, and procainamide. *Ann Intern Med* 1984; **100:** 918.
6. Thompson JF, *et al.* Procainamide agranulocytosis: a case report and review of the literature. *Curr Ther Res* 1988; **44:** 872–81.
7. Kleinman S, *et al.* Positive direct antiglobulin tests and immune hemolytic anemia in patients receiving procainamide. *N Engl J Med* 1984; **311:** 809–12.
8. Bluming AZ, *et al.* Severe transient pancytopenia associated with procainamide ingestion. *JAMA* 1976; **236:** 2520–1.
9. Kelly JP, *et al.* Risks of agranulocytosis and aplastic anemia in relation to the use of cardiovascular drugs: The International Agranulocytosis and Aplastic Anemia Study. *Clin Pharmacol Ther* 1991; **49:** 330–41.

Effects on the gastro-intestinal tract. Pseudo-obstruction of the bowel occurred in a diabetic patient when given procainamide both orally and intravenously. It was believed that the anticholinergic properties of procainamide, together with the diabetic state, contributed to the severe hypomotility of the gastro-intestinal tract.[1]

1. Peterson AM, *et al.* Procainamide-induced pseudo-obstruction in a diabetic patient. *DICP Ann Pharmacother* 1991; **25:** 1334–5.

Effects on the heart. Procainamide has been associated with the development of torsade de pointes.[1,2] Elevated plasma concentrations of the major metabolite *N*-acetylprocainamide were present in 1 patient[1] and haemodialysis was used to reduce the plasma concentration and control the arrhythmia.

1. Nguyen KPV, *et al.* N-Acetylprocainamide, torsades de pointes, and hemodialysis. *Ann Intern Med* 1986; **104:** 283–4.
2. Habbab MA, El-Sherif N. Drug-induced torsades de pointes: role of early afterdepolarizations and dispersion of repolarization. *Am J Med* 1990; **89:** 241–6.

Effects on the liver. Reports of granulomatous hepatitis[1] and intrahepatic cholestasis[2,3] due to hypersensitivity reactions in patients taking procainamide. Fever and elevation of liver enzyme values also occurred. The reactions were reversible on withdrawing procainamide.

1. Rotmensch HH, *et al.* Granulomatous hepatitis: a hypersensitivity response to procainamide. *Ann Intern Med* 1978; **89:** 646–7.
2. Ahn C-S, Tow DE. Intrahepatic cholestasis due to hypersensitivity reaction to procainamide. *Arch Intern Med* 1990; **150:** 2589–90.
3. Chuang LC, *et al.* Possible case of procainamide-induced intrahepatic cholestatic jaundice. *Ann Pharmacother* 1993; **27:** 434–7.

Effects on the muscles. Reports of 3 patients in whom procainamide caused severe generalised skeletal muscle weakness[1-3] with respiratory failure[1,2] within a few days of starting therapy. Concentrations of procainamide and its *N*-acetyl metabolite exceeded the normal therapeutic ranges and rapid recycling peritoneal dialysis was used to remove the drug in 1 patient.[2] Adverse muscle symptoms are a feature of procainamide-induced lupus erythematosus (see below), but in such instances symptoms usually develop on long-term treatment.

1. Lewis CA, *et al.* Myopathy after short term administration of procainamide. *Br Med J* 1986; **292:** 593–4.
2. Javaheri S, *et al.* Diaphragmatic paralysis. *Am J Med* 1989; **86:** 623–4.
3. Sayler DJ, DeJong DJ. Possible procainamide-induced myopathy. *DICP Ann Pharmacother* 1991; **25:** 436.

Lupus erythematosus. Procainamide is one of the most common causes of drug-induced lupus erythematosus.[1-3] Antinuclear antibodies are present in the majority of patients on long-term therapy but the clinical syndrome develops in only up to 30%. The development of antinuclear antibodies is more likely in slow acetylators than in rapid acetylators; also the antibodies appear earlier in treatment in slow acetylators.[4] The clinical syndrome may include fever, polyarthritis, arthralgia, myalgia, and pleuropulmonary and pericardial features, and is usually spontaneously reversible on withdrawal of procainamide.

1. Hughes GRV. Recent developments in drug-associated systemic lupus erythematosus. *Adverse Drug React Bull* 1987; (Apr.): 460–3.
2. Mitchell JA, *et al.* Immunotoxic side-effects of drug therapy. *Drug Safety* 1990; **5:** 168–78.
3. Price EJ, Venables PJW. Drug-induced lupus. *Drug Safety* 1995; **12:** 283–90.
4. Woosley RL, *et al.* Effect of acetylator phenotype on the rate at which procainamide induces antinuclear antibodies and the lupus syndrome. *N Engl J Med* 1978; **298:** 1157–9.

Treatment of Adverse Effects

In overdosage treatment is largely symptomatic and supportive. The ECG, blood pressure, and renal function should be monitored. Supportive measures include correction of hypotension, assisted respiration, and electrical pacing. Haemodialysis or haemoperfusion increase the elimination of procainamide and *N*-acetylprocainamide.

Systemic lupus erythematosus will normally respond to withdrawal of procainamide but corticosteroids may be required.

Dialysis. There are reports of haemodialysis and haemoperfusion being effective in reducing concentrations of procainamide and *N*-acetylprocainamide.[1-3]

1. Atkinson AJ, *et al.* Hemodialysis for severe procainamide toxicity: clinical and pharmacokinetic observations. *Clin Pharmacol Ther* 1976; **20:** 585–92.
2. Braden GL, *et al.* Hemoperfusion for treatment of N-acetylprocainamide intoxication. *Ann Intern Med* 1986; **105:** 64–5.
3. Domoto DT, *et al.* Removal of toxic levels of N-acetylprocainamide with continuous arteriovenous hemofiltration or continuous arteriovenous hemodiafiltration. *Ann Intern Med* 1987; **106:** 550–2.

Precautions

Procainamide is contra-indicated in patients with heart block or systemic lupus erythematosus, and should be used with caution in those with myocardial damage or severe organic heart disease. Some authorities consider that it should not be used in heart failure or hypotension. Patients with torsade de pointes may deteriorate if given procainamide. If procainamide is used to treat atrial tachycardia it may be necessary to pre-treat with digoxin. Procainamide should preferably not be used in patients with myasthenia gravis or digoxin toxicity. There may be cross-sensitivity between procaine and procainamide.

Accumulation of procainamide may occur in patients with heart failure, renal insufficiency, or impaired hepatic function and dosage reduction may be necessary.

Regular blood tests should be carried out in patients receiving procainamide, and screening for lupus erythematosus and serum antinuclear factor should be carried out before and regularly during therapy.

Grave hypotension may follow intravenous administration of procainamide; it should be injected slowly under ECG control.

Breast feeding. There was evidence of accumulation of procainamide and *N*-acetylprocainamide in the breast milk of a woman taking procainamide 500 mg four times a day.[1] However, it was considered that the amount ingested by an infant would not be expected to yield clinically significant plasma concentrations.

1. Pittard WB, Glazier H. Procainamide excretion in human milk. *J Pediatr* 1983; **102:** 631–3.

Interactions

Procainamide may enhance the effects of antihypertensives, other antiarrhythmics, antimuscarinics, and neuromuscular blocking drugs, and diminish those of parasympathomimetics, such as neostigmine. Procainamide is actively secreted by kidney tubules and interactions are possible with other drugs secreted by the same pathway, such as cimetidine and trimethoprim.

Alcohol. The total body clearance of procainamide is increased by alcohol[1] and the elimination half-life reduced. The acetylation rate of procainamide is also increased resulting in a greater proportion of drug present as the active metabolite *N*-acetylprocainamide.

1. Olsen H, Mørland J. Ethanol-induced increase in procainamide acetylation in man. *Br J Clin Pharmacol* 1982; **13:** 203–8.

Antiarrhythmics. Amiodarone given orally alters the pharmacokinetic properties of an intravenous dose of procainamide,[1] decreasing clearance and prolonging the plasma elimination half-life. The dosage of intravenous procainamide should be reduced by 20 to 30% during concurrent drug administration.

1. Windle J, *et al.* Pharmacokinetic and electrophysiologic interactions of amiodarone and procainamide. *Clin Pharmacol Ther* 1987; **41:** 603–10.

Antibacterials. The renal clearance of procainamide and *N*-acetylprocainamide is reduced by trimethoprim[1] through competition for renal tubular secretion. Serum concentrations may be increased with a resulting increase in pharmacodynamic response.

1. Vlasses PH, *et al.* Trimethoprim decreases the renal clearance of procainamide and N-acetylprocainamide. *Clin Pharmacol Ther* 1986; **39:** 233.

Gastro-intestinal drugs. Adsorption of procainamide by antacids[1] can reduce the bioavailability of procainamide and it is recommended that they are not administered concomitantly. Histamine H_2-antagonists compete with other basic drugs for renal tubular secretion. Cimetidine reduces the renal clearance of procainamide and *N*-acetylprocainamide[2,3] and a dosage reduction may be necessary. Increases[4,5] and decreases[5] in renal and metabolic clearances of procainamide have been reported when ranitidine is administered concomitantly.

1. Al-Shora HI, *et al.* Interactions of procainamide, verapamil, guanethidine and hydralazine with adsorbent antacids and antidiarrhoeal mixtures. *Int J Pharmaceutics* 1988; **47:** 209–13.
2. Christian CD, *et al.* Cimetidine inhibits renal procainamide clearance. *Clin Pharmacol Ther* 1984; **36:** 221–7.
3. Somogyi A, *et al.* Cimetidine-procainamide pharmacokinetic interaction in man: evidence of competition for tubular secretion of basic drugs. *Eur J Clin Pharmacol* 1983; **25:** 339–45.
4. Somogyi A, Bochner F. Dose and concentration dependent effect of ranitidine on procainamide disposition and renal clearance in man. *Br J Clin Pharmacol* 1984; **18:** 175–81.
5. Rocci ML, *et al.* Ranitidine-induced changes in the renal and hepatic clearances of procainamide are correlated. *J Pharmacol Exp Ther* 1989; **248:** 923–8.

Pharmacokinetics

Procainamide is readily and almost completely absorbed from the gastro-intestinal tract.

Procainamide is widely distributed throughout the body and is only about 15 to 20% bound to plasma proteins. The therapeutic effect of procainamide has been correlated with plasma concentrations of about 3 to 10 μg per mL in most patients, progressively severe toxicity being noted at concentrations above 12 μg per mL.

Some procainamide undergoes acetylation in the liver to *N*-acetylprocainamide. This metabolite is also called acecainide (p.810) and has antiarrhythmic properties. The rate of acetylation of procainamide is genetically determined, there being slow and fast acetylators. Procainamide also undergoes hydrolysis in plasma to para-aminobenzoic acid.

Procainamide is excreted in the urine following active renal secretion, 30 to 70% as unchanged procainamide, with the remainder as *N*-acetylprocainamide and other metabolites. The elimination half-life of procainamide is 2.5 to 5 hours and that of its acetyl metabolite 6 to 7 hours. *N*-Acetylprocainamide may represent a significant fraction of the total drug in the circulation.

Procainamide crosses the placental barrier and is distributed into breast milk.

References.

1. Grasela TH, Sheiner LB. Population pharmacokinetics of procainamide from routine clinical data. *Clin Pharmacokinet* 1984; **9:** 545–54.

Bioavailability. Modified-release procainamide preparations have been shown[1] to produce similar steady-state serum concentrations of procainamide and *N*-acetylprocainamide when compared with equivalent total doses of immediate-release capsules. However, tablet matrices of a modified-release preparation have been recovered from the stools of a patient with diarrhoea[2] and 3.5 g of procainamide was recovered in these matrices over an 18-hour collection period; the patient had correspondingly low plasma-procainamide concentrations.

1. Vlasses PH, *et al.* Immediate-release and sustained-release procainamide: bioavailability at steady state in cardiac patients. *Ann Intern Med* 1983; **98:** 613–14.
2. Woosley RL, *et al.* Antiarrhythmic therapy: clinical pharmacology update. *J Clin Pharmacol* 1984; **24:** 295–305.

Uses and Administration

Procainamide hydrochloride is a class Ia antiarrhythmic (p.776); it has properties similar to those of quinidine (p.940).

Procainamide hydrochloride tends to be used for the short-term management of severe or symptomatic **arrhythmias** (p.782). It is used for the treatment of ventricular arrhythmias particularly those resistant to lignocaine and those following myocardial infarction. It may also be used to maintain sinus rhythm after cardioversion of atrial fibrillation.

Therapeutic effect is generally associated with plasma concentrations of 3 to 10 μg per mL. The dose of procainamide hydrochloride required will depend on the age, renal and hepatic function, and underlying cardiac condition of the patient: an adult with normal renal function generally requires up to 50 mg per kg body-weight daily by mouth in divided doses every 3 to 6 hours. Higher doses may be necessary for atrial arrhythmias. Modified-release preparations are available. A dose of 40 to 60 mg per kg body-weight daily by mouth in 4 to 6 divided doses has been suggested for children.

In an emergency and under continuous ECG and blood pressure monitoring, procainamide hydrochloride may be given intravenously. The injection should be diluted in a 5% solution of glucose to permit better control of the speed of injection, and should be given in doses of 100 mg every 5 minutes at a rate not exceeding 50 mg per minute until the arrhythmia has been suppressed or a maximum dose of 1 g has been reached. A response may be obtained after 100 to 200 mg has been given and more than 500 or 600 mg is not generally required. Alternatively, procainamide hydrochloride may be administered by continuous infusion of 500 to 600 mg over 25 to 30 minutes. Therapeutic plasma concentrations may then be maintained by giving an infusion in a 5% solution of glucose, at a rate of 2 to 6 mg per minute. When transferring to oral therapy, a period of about 3 to 4 hours should elapse between the last intravenous dose and the first oral dose.

Procainamide hydrochloride has also been given intramuscularly.

Administration in children. In a study in 5 children treated with procainamide for various cardiac arrhythmias the mean elimination half-life was found to be 1.7 hours, and the plasma clearance was higher than that reported in adults.[1] In contrast the total serum clearance of procainamide in 3 neonates with supraventricular tachycardia was found to be similar to that in adults and the mean elimination half-life was 5.3 hours.[2] A loading dose of 10 to 12 mg per kg body-weight intravenously was given followed by a continuous infusion of 20 to 75 μg per kg per minute.

1. Singh S, *et al.* Procainamide elimination kinetics in pediatric patients. *Clin Pharmacol Ther* 1982; **32:** 607–11.
2. Bryson SM, *et al.* Therapeutic monitoring and pharmacokinetic evaluation of procainamide in neonates. *DICP Ann Pharmacother* 1991; **25:** 68–71.

Administration in the elderly. Reduced renal clearance of procainamide in the elderly.[1]

1. Reidenberg MM, *et al.* Aging and renal clearance of procainamide and acetylprocainamide. *Clin Pharmacol Ther* 1980; **28:** 732–5.

Administration in hepatic impairment. In 20 healthy subjects and 20 patients with chronic liver disease given a single dose of procainamide hydrochloride 500 mg by mouth about 64 and 33% respectively of the administered dose was excreted in the urine within 6 hours.[1] Decreased procainamide acetylation in the patients compared with the control group was not correlated with the severity of liver disease whereas decreased procainamide hydrolysis and increased procainamide-derived aminobenzoic acid acetylation appeared to be related to the degree of hepatic impairment. It was suggested that the decrease in excretion of procainamide and its metabolites in the urine of the patients with liver disease could be due to an impairment in oral absorption since renal function was within the normal range but the variations in acetylation and hydrolysis were related to hepatic function.

1. du Souich P, Erill S. Metabolism of procainamide and p-aminobenzoic acid in patients with chronic liver disease. *Clin Pharmacol Ther* 1977; **22:** 588–95.

Administration in renal impairment. Procainamide is excreted in the urine, largely as unchanged drug, and accumulation, especially of the active acetyl metabolite,[1] may occur in renal insufficiency. Haemodialysis and haemoperfusion increase the clearance of procainamide and *N*-acetylprocainamide (see Treatment of Adverse Effects, above).

1. Vlasses PH, *et al.* Lethal accumulation of procainamide metabolite in renal insufficiency. *Drug Intell Clin Pharm* 1984; **18:** 493–4.

Preparations

BP 1998: Procainamide Injection; Procainamide Tablets;
USP 23: Procainamide Hydrochloride Capsules; Procainamide Hydrochloride Extended-release Tablets; Procainamide Hydrochloride Injection; Procainamide Hydrochloride Tablets.

Proprietary Preparations (details are given in Part 3)
Austral.: Pronestyl; ***Belg.:*** Pronestyl†; ***Canad.:*** Procan; Pronestyl; ***Irl.:*** Pronestyl; ***Ital.:*** Procamide; ***Neth.:*** Pronestyl; ***S.Afr.:*** Pronestyl; ***Spain:*** Biocoryl; ***Switz.:*** Pronestyl; ***UK:*** Pronestyl; ***USA:*** Procanbid; Pronestyl.

Multi-ingredient: ***Ger.:*** Coritrat†; Rhythmochin I†; Rhythmochin II (cum sedativo)†.

Propafenone Hydrochloride (13177-w)

Propafenone Hydrochloride *(BANM, USAN, rINNM)*.

Fenopraine Hydrochloride; SA-79; WZ-884642; WZ-884643. 2′-(2-Hydroxy-3-propylaminopropoxy)-3-phenylpropiophenone hydrochloride.

$C_{21}H_{27}NO_3,HCl = 377.9$.

CAS — 54063-53-5 (propafenone); 34183-22-7 (propafenone hydrochloride).

Pharmacopoeias. In *Chin.* and *US.*

A white powder. **Soluble** in hot water and in methyl alcohol; slightly soluble in alcohol and in chloroform; very slightly soluble in acetone; practically insoluble in ether and in toluene. A 0.5% solution has a pH of 5.0 to 6.2. **Store** in airtight containers. Protect from light.

Adverse Effects

Propafenone can cause disturbances in cardiac conduction which can result in bradycardia, heart block, and sinus arrest. It may aggravate heart failure and may cause hypotension. In common with other antiarrhythmics, propafenone may induce or worsen arrhythmias in some patients.

Among the most common adverse effects are gastro-intestinal intolerance, dry mouth, a bitter or metallic taste, dizziness, blurred vision, headache, and fatigue. Convulsions, blood dyscrasias, liver disorders, lupus erythematosus, skin rashes, and impotence have also been reported. Increased breathlessness and worsening of asthma have been reported.

Effects on the heart. Fatal exacerbation of ventricular tachycardia was associated with propafenone therapy in a 63-year-old man.[1]

1. Nathan AW, *et al.* Fatal ventricular tachycardia in association with propafenone, a new class IC antiarrhythmic agent. *Postgrad Med J* 1984; **60:** 155–6.

Effects on the liver. A review of liver injury secondary to propafenone therapy has concluded it is a rare occurrence and appears to be due to hepatocellular injury, cholestasis, or a combination.[1]

1. Spinler SA, *et al.* Propafenone-induced liver injury. *Ann Pharmacother* 1992; **26:** 926–8.

Effects on mental state. Delusions, hallucinations, and paranoia have been reported in an elderly patient following two doses of propafenone. The manufacturer had received reports of mania and psychosis.[1] Amnesia developed in a 61-year-old man six days after starting treatment with propafenone.[2] Symptoms resolved 6 to 7 hours after discontinuing the drug.

1. Robinson AJ. Paranoia after propafenone. *Pharm J* 1991; **247:** 556.
2. Jones RJ, *et al.* Probable propafenone-induced transient global amnesia. *Ann Pharmacother* 1995; **29:** 586–90.

Effects on the nervous system. Myoclonus has been reported in one patient receiving propafenone.[1] Peripheral neuropathy developed in a patient 10 months after starting treatment with propafenone.[2] Symptoms had resolved 6 months after stopping the drug.

1. Chua TP, *et al.* Myoclonus associated with propafenone. *Br Med J* 1994; **308:** 113.
2. Galasso PJ, *et al.* Propafenone-induced peripheral neuropathy. *Mayo Clin Proc* 1995; **70:** 469–72.

Lupus erythematosus. Symptoms of lupus erythematosus and raised antinuclear antibody titres were associated with propafenone therapy on 2 occasions in a 63-year-old woman.[1]

1. Guindo J, *et al.* Propafenone and a syndrome of the lupus erythematosus type. *Ann Intern Med* 1986; **104:** 589.

Precautions

Propafenone is contra-indicated in patients with uncontrolled heart failure, conduction disturbances including heart block unless controlled by artificial pacing, cardiogenic shock not arrhythmia-induced, severe bradycardia, or pronounced hypotension. It may alter the endocardial pacing threshold and adjustment may be necessary in patients with pacemakers.

Propafenone's beta-blocking activity can exacerbate obstructive airways disease; it should be used with great caution in patients with this disease and if the disease is severe then propafenone is contra-indicated. Propafenone may aggravate myasthenia gravis and should be avoided in patients with this condition. Electrolyte disturbances should be corrected before initiating propafenone treatment. Propafenone should be used with caution in patients with hepatic or renal impairment.

Pregnancy and breast feeding. Experience in one patient given propafenone throughout the last trimester of pregnancy indicated that despite transplacental diffusion propafenone could safely be used at this time without harm to the fetus. Propafenone and its metabolite were excreted in breast milk although it was considered that the amount would have represented a markedly subtherapeutic dose to the infant who in any case was not breast fed.[1]

1. Libardoni M, *et al.* Transfer of propafenone and 5-OH-propafenone to foetal plasma and maternal milk. *Br J Clin Pharmacol* 1991; **32:** 527–8.

Interactions

Propafenone is extensively metabolised by the hepatic mixed function oxidase system and plasma-propafenone concentrations may be reduced by inducers of this system such as rifampicin; enzyme inhibitors, such as cimetidine and quinidine, may increase plasma-propafenone concentrations (see below). Propafenone itself may alter the plasma concentrations of other drugs given concomitantly, possibly by interfering with their metabolism. Drugs affected include beta blockers, cyclosporin, desipramine, digoxin, theophylline, and warfarin. Details are given under the individual drug monographs.

Rifampicin has lowered steady-state plasma concentrations of propafenone with the reappearance of arrhythmia.[1] *Quinidine* inhibits the hepatic metabolism of propafenone and has raised plasma-propafenone concentrations in extensive metabolisers;[2] the plasma concentration of the active 5-hydroxy metabolite was reduced and that of the *N*-depropyl metabolite increased but there was no change in the clinical response. *Cimetidine* has also been reported[3] to raise plasma-propafenone concentrations. The mean steady-state concentration increased by 22% but the wide interindividual variability meant this change was not significant.

1. Castel JM, *et al.* Rifampicin lowers plasma concentrations of propafenone and its antiarrhythmic effect. *Br J Clin Pharmacol* 1990; **30:** 155–6.
2. Funck-Brentano C, *et al.* Genetically-determined interaction between propafenone and low dose quinidine: role of active metabolites in modulating net drug effect. *Br J Clin Pharmacol* 1989; **27:** 435–44.
3. Pritchett ELC, *et al.* Pharmacokinetic and pharmacodynamic interactions of propafenone and cimetidine. *J Clin Pharmacol* 1988; **28:** 619–24.

Pharmacokinetics

Propafenone is readily and almost completely absorbed from the gastro-intestinal tract. It is metabolised in the liver and the extent of metabolism is genetically determined. In subjects with the extensive metaboliser phenotype there is extensive first-pass metabolism to two active metabolites, 5-hydroxypropafenone and *N*-depropylpropafenone, and to other minor inactive metabolites. In the small proportion of subjects with the slow metaboliser phenotype little or no 5-hydroxypropafenone is formed. The bioavailability of propafenone is dependent upon metaboliser phenotype but more importantly on dosage as the first-pass metabolism is saturable. In practice doses are high enough to compensate for differences in phenotype. Propafenone and its metabolites also undergo glucuronidation.

Propafenone is extensively (more than 95%) protein bound.

Propafenone is excreted in the urine and faeces mainly in the form of conjugated metabolites. The elimination half-life is reported to be 2 to 10 hours in extensive metabolisers and 10 to 32 hours in slow metabolisers.

Propafenone crosses the placenta and is distributed into breast milk.

General references.

1. Hii JTY, *et al.* Clinical pharmacokinetics of propafenone. *Clin Pharmacokinet* 1991; **21:** 1–10.

Uses and Administration

Propafenone hydrochloride is a class Ic antiarrhythmic (p.776) with some negative inotropic and beta-adrenoceptor blocking activity. It is used in the management of supraventricular and ventricular **arrhythmias**.

The usual initial dose by mouth is 150 mg three times daily and this may be increased, if necessary, at intervals of 3 to 4 days up to a maximum of 300 mg three times daily. Patients of less than 70 kg body-weight should be given reduced doses; the elderly may also respond to reduced doses. Doses may need to be reduced if hepatic function is impaired.

Propafenone hydrochloride has also been given by slow intravenous injection or by infusion.

General references.

1. Bryson HM, *et al.* Propafenone: a reappraisal of its pharmacology, pharmacokinetics and therapeutic use in cardiac arrhythmias. *Drugs* 1993; **45:** 85–130.

Administration in renal impairment. Propafenone is extensively metabolised and the metabolites formed are excreted in the urine and faeces. A study of the effect of renal function on disposition of propafenone found that renal impairment did not alter the pharmacokinetics of propafenone or 5-hydroxypropafenone.[1] Nevertheless, the manufacturers advise that caution is necessary if propafenone is administered to patients with impaired renal function.

1. Fromm MF, *et al.* Influence of renal function on the steady-state pharmacokinetics of the antiarrhythmic propafenone and its phase I and phase II metabolites. *Eur J Clin Pharmacol* 1995; **48:** 279–83.

Cardiac arrhythmias. Early reviews[1-4] showed propafenone, a class Ic antiarrhythmic, to be effective in a large variety of cardiac arrhythmias (p.782) including ventricular arrhythmias and supraventricular arrhythmias such as atrial flutter and atrial fibrillation. It has been used successfully to treat arrhythmias in children.[5,8] However, the results of the Cardiac Arrhythmia Suppression Trial (known as CAST), demonstrating that other class I antiarrhythmics (encainide, flecainide, and moracizine) were associated with an increased mortality rate when used for asymptomatic ventricular arrhythmias in post-infarction patients, led to many drugs of this class being restricted to severe or life-threatening ventricular arrhythmias; this restriction has also applied to propafenone in many countries although, in some, use in supraventricular arrhythmias is permitted. As well as having antiarrhythmic actions propafenone also has some beta-adrenoceptor blocking activity and this theoretically may be beneficial in post-infarction patients, but in the absence of data showing safety and efficacy of propafenone in this situation such use is not considered warranted.[4] A more recent review[6] acknowledges a general trend against the use of class Ic antiarrhythmics, including propafenone, in patients with nonsustained ventricular arrhythmias. Another[7] supports it use in supraventricular arrhythmias.

1. Siddoway LA, Woosley RL. Propafenone: a promising new antiarrhythmic agent. *Cardiovasc Rev Rep* 1986; **7:** 153–5 and 158–9.
2. Harron DWG, Brogden RN. Propafenone: a review of its pharmacodynamic and pharmacokinetic properties, and therapeutic use in the treatment of arrhythmias. *Drugs* 1987; **34:** 617–47.
3. Chow MSS, *et al.* Propafenone: a new antiarrhythmic agent. *Clin Pharm* 1988; **7:** 869–77.
4. Funck-Brentano C, *et al.* Propafenone. *N Engl J Med* 1990; **322:** 518–25.
5. Heusch A, *et al.* Clinical experience with propafenone for cardiac arrhythmias in the young. *Eur Heart J* 1994; **15:** 1050–6.
6. Capucci A, Boriani G. Propafenone in the treatment of cardiac arrhythmias: a risk-benefit appraisal. *Drug Safety* 1995; **12:** 55–72.
7. Kishore AGR, Camm AJ. Guidelines for the use of propafenone in treating supraventricular arrhythmias. *Drugs* 1995; **50:** 250–62.
8. Janoušek J, Paul T. Safety of oral propafenone in the treatment of arrhythmias in infants and children (European Retrospective Multicenter Study). *Am J Cardiol* 1998; **81:** 1121–4.

Preparations

Proprietary Preparations (details are given in Part 3)

Aust.: Asonacor; Metronom; Rhythmocor; Rytmonorma; ***Belg.:*** Rytmonorm; ***Canad.:*** Rythmol; ***Fr.:*** Rythmol; ***Ger.:*** Propa-Oramon†; Propafen; Propamerck; Propastad; Prorynorm; Rytmogenat; Rytmonorm; Tachyfenon; ***Irl.:*** Arythmol; ***Ital.:*** Rytmonorm; ***Neth.:*** Rytmonorm; ***S.Afr.:*** Rythmol; ***Spain:*** Rytmonorm; ***Swed.:*** Rytmonorm; ***Switz.:*** Rytmonorm; ***UK:*** Arythmol; ***USA:*** Rythmol.

Propatylnitrate (9276-f)

Propatylnitrate *(BAN, rINN)*.

ETTN; Ettriol Trinitrate; Propatyl Nitrate *(USAN)*; Trinettriol; Win-9317. 2-Ethyl-2-hydroxymethylpropane-1,3-diol trinitrate.

$C_6H_{11}N_3O_9$ = 269.2.

CAS — 2921-92-8.

Propatylnitrate is a vasodilator with general properties similar to those of glyceryl trinitrate (p.875) and is used in angina pectoris (p.780). It is given in doses of 10 mg sublingually for acute attacks or 5 mg three times daily for long-term management.

Preparations

Proprietary Preparations (details are given in Part 3)

Spain: Etrynit†.

Propentofylline (239-j)

Propentofylline *(BAN, rINN)*.

HWA-285. 3-Methyl-1-(5-oxohexyl)-7-propylxanthine.

$C_{15}H_{22}N_4O_3$ = 306.4.

CAS — 55242-55-2.

Propentofylline is a xanthine derivative that is being investigated in cerebrovascular disorders. It has been reported to slow progression of dementia in Alzheimer's disease (p.1386).

Propranolol Hydrochloride (6301-g)

Propranolol Hydrochloride *(BANM, USAN, rINNM).*

AY-64043; ICI-45520; NSC-91523; Propranololi Hydrochloridum. (±)-1-Isopropylamino-3-(1-naphthyloxy)propan-2-ol hydrochloride.

$C_{16}H_{21}NO_2$,HCl = 295.8.

CAS — 525-66-6 (propranolol); 13013-17-7 (±-propranolol); 318-98-9 (propranolol hydrochloride); 3506-09-0 (±-propranolol hydrochloride).

Pharmacopoeias. In *Chin., Eur.* (see p.viii), *Int., Jpn, Pol.,* and *US.*

A white or off-white, odourless crystalline powder.

Soluble in water and alcohol; slightly soluble in chloroform; practically insoluble in ether.

In aqueous solutions propranolol decomposes with oxidation of the isopropylamine side-chain, accompanied by a reduction in pH and discoloration of the solution. Solutions are most stable at pH 3 and decompose rapidly when alkaline.

Adverse Effects, Treatment, and Precautions

As for beta blockers, p.828.

Effects on the gastro-intestinal tract. A report of retroperitoneal fibrosis associated with propranolol in one patient.[1]

1. Pierce JR, *et al.* Propranolol and retroperitoneal fibrosis. *Ann Intern Med* 1981; **95:** 244.

Overdosage. A case of severe propranolol overdosage with the patient in electromechanical dissociation responded dramatically to treatment with calcium chloride.[1]

For general information on the management of overdosage with beta blockers, see p.829.

1. Brimacombe JR, *et al.* Propranolol overdose—a dramatic response to calcium chloride. *Med J Aust* 1991; **155:** 267–8.

Interactions

The interactions associated with beta blockers are discussed on p.829.

Pharmacokinetics

Propranolol is almost completely absorbed from the gastro-intestinal tract, but is subject to considerable hepatic tissue binding and first-pass metabolism. Peak plasma concentrations occur about 1 to 2 hours after an oral dose. Plasma concentrations vary greatly between individuals. It has high lipid solubility. Propranolol crosses the blood-brain barrier and the placenta. The drug is distributed into breast milk. Propranolol is more than 90% bound to plasma proteins. It is metabolised in the liver, the metabolites being excreted in the urine together with only small amounts of unchanged propranolol; at least one of its metabolites (4-hydroxypropranolol) is considered to be biologically active but the contribution of metabolites to its overall activity is uncertain. The plasma half-life of propranolol is about 3 to 6 hours. Propranolol is reported not to be significantly dialysable.

Breast feeding. Propranolol diffuses into breast milk. A milk/plasma ratio range of 0.33 to 1.65 was reported in a study of 3 lactating women.[1] It was calculated that the maximum dose likely to be ingested by a breast-fed infant would be less than 0.1% of the maternal dose.

1. Smith MT, *et al.* Propranolol, propranolol glucuronide, and naphthoxylactic acid in breast milk and plasma. *Ther Drug Monit* 1983; **5:** 87–93.

Pregnancy. A study in 6 pregnant patients (32 to 36 weeks' gestation) showed that the disposition of propranolol 120 mg by mouth and 10 mg intravenously was not altered in pregnancy compared with the post-natal period.[1] Another study[2] in 13 pregnant patients given propranolol to control hypertension demonstrated that the pharmacokinetics of propranolol and most of its major metabolites were not altered during pregnancy. Samples at term[3] in 10 of the women showed that propranolol and all of its known metabolites were present in maternal plasma, cord plasma, and neonatal plasma. At delivery plasma protein binding of propranolol was reported as 87.5% in maternal plasma and 67.2% in cord plasma. Similar results for maternal and cord plasma protein binding have been reported by others.[4]

1. O'Hare MFO, *et al.* Pharmacokinetics of propranolol during pregnancy. *Eur J Clin Pharmacol* 1984; **27:** 583–7.
2. Smith MT, *et al.* Chronic propranolol administration during pregnancy: maternal pharmacokinetics. *Eur J Clin Pharmacol* 1983; **25:** 481–90.
3. Smith MT, *et al.* Metabolism of propranolol in the human maternal-placental-foetal unit. *Eur J Clin Pharmacol* 1983; **24:** 727–32.
4. Wood M, Wood AJJ. Changes in plasma drug binding and α_1-acid glycoprotein in mother and newborn infant. *Clin Pharmacol Ther* 1981; **29:** 522–6.

Uses and Administration

Propranolol is a non-cardioselective beta blocker (p.828). It is reported to have membrane-stabilising properties, but does not possess intrinsic sympathomimetic activity.

Propranolol is used as the hydrochloride in the management of hypertension (p.788), phaeochromocytoma (p.795), angina pectoris (p.780), myocardial infarction (p.791), and cardiac arrhythmias (p.782). It is also used in hypertrophic subaortic stenosis. It is used to control symptoms of sympathetic overactivity in the management of hyperthyroidism (p.1489), anxiety disorders (p.635), and tremor (p.831). Other indications include the prophylaxis of migraine (p.443) and of upper gastro-intestinal bleeding in patients with portal hypertension (see Variceal Haemorrhage under Ethanolamine Oleate, p.1576).

Propranolol hydrochloride is usually given by mouth. In **hypertension** propranolol hydrochloride is given in initial doses of 40 to 80 mg twice daily increased as required to a usual range of 160 to 320 mg daily; some patients may require up to 640 mg daily. Propranolol is *not* suitable for the emergency treatment of hypertension; it should not be given intravenously in hypertension.

In **phaeochromocytoma**, 60 mg daily may be given on 3 pre-operative days always in association with alpha blockade. If the tumour is inoperable prolonged treatment may be given with a daily dose of 30 mg.

In **angina,** initial doses of propranolol hydrochloride 40 mg given 2 or 3 times daily are increased as required to a usual range of 120 to 240 mg daily. Some patients may require up to 320 mg daily.

Propranolol hydrochloride is administered within 5 to 21 days of **myocardial infarction** in doses of 40 mg given four times daily for 2 or 3 days followed by 80 mg twice daily. Another regimen is to give 180 to 240 mg daily in divided doses.

Propranolol may be given in doses of 30 to 160 mg daily in divided doses in the long-term management of **cardiac arrhythmias**. For the emergency treatment of cardiac arrhythmias, propranolol hydrochloride may be given by slow intravenous injection in a dose of 1 mg injected over a period of 1 minute, repeated if necessary every 2 minutes until a maximum total of 10 mg has been given in conscious patients and 5 mg in patients under anaesthesia. Patients receiving propranolol intravenously should be carefully monitored.

In **hypertrophic subaortic stenosis,** the usual dose of propranolol hydrochloride is 10 to 40 mg given three to four times daily.

In **hyperthyroidism** propranolol hydrochloride is given in doses of 10 to 40 mg three or four times daily. Intravenous administration may be necessary; the dose is 1 mg injected over 1 minute, repeated at 2-minute intervals until a response is observed or to a maximum dose of 10 mg in conscious patients or 5 mg in patients under anaesthesia.

A suggested dose for **anxiety** is 40 mg daily; this may be increased to 40 mg two or three times daily.

Essential tremor may be treated with 40 mg given two to three times daily; the dose can be increased at weekly intervals to 160 mg daily although doses up to 320 mg daily may be necessary.

An initial dose of 40 mg two or three times daily is used in **migraine** prophylaxis; the dose can be increased at weekly intervals up to 160 mg daily. Some patients have been given 240 mg daily.

In **portal hypertension,** propranolol hydrochloride should be given in initial doses of 40 mg twice daily; the dose may be increased as required up to 160 mg twice daily.

Children. Propranolol hydrochloride has been used in the treatment of hypertension in children in initial doses of 1 mg per kg body-weight daily in divided doses by mouth, increased as required to a usual range of 2 to 4 mg per kg daily in divided doses. For arrhythmias, phaeochromocytoma, and hyperthyroidism, the suggested dose is 250 to 500 µg per kg three or four times daily by mouth. Children requiring intravenous administration may be given 25 to 50 µg per kg injected slowly with appropriate monitoring; this dose may be repeated three or four times daily. Children under 12 years of age may be given 20 mg two or three times daily for the prophylactic management of migraine.

Administration in hepatic impairment. A study of the effects of cirrhosis on the disposition of propranolol during steady-state oral administration in 9 normal subjects and 7 with cirrhosis demonstrated a mean threefold increase in unbound propranolol concentrations in the blood in patients with cirrhosis when compared with the controls. Mean half-lives for the 2 groups were 11.2 and 4 hours respectively.[1] Another study of the pharmacokinetics of propranolol given as a single dose of a 20-mg tablet and as a 160-mg controlled-release preparation daily for 7 days in 10 patients with cirrhosis and portal hypertension demonstrated higher plasma concentrations in patients with severe liver disease compared with those reported in normal controls.[2] Similar pharmacokinetic findings have been reported by others.[3]

In patients with severe liver disease, it has been suggested that propranolol therapy be started at a low dose such as 20 mg three times daily, or 80 mg of a controlled-release preparation given once daily,[2] or 160 mg of a controlled-release preparation given every other day.[3] Monitoring of beta blockade is essential; checking the heart rate[2] or exercise testing[3] have been suggested as suitable methods to assess the extent of beta blockade in patients with cirrhosis.

1. Wood AJJ, *et al.* The influence of cirrhosis on steady-state blood concentrations of unbound propranolol after oral administration. *Clin Pharmacokinet* 1978; **3:** 478–87.
2. Arthur MJP, *et al.* Pharmacology of propranolol in patients with cirrhosis and portal hypertension. *Gut* 1985; **26:** 14–19.
3. Calès P, *et al.* Pharmacodynamic and pharmacokinetic study of propranolol in patients with cirrhosis and portal hypertension. *Br J Clin Pharmacol* 1989; **27:** 763–70.

Administration in renal impairment. A study of the pharmacokinetics of propranolol in 11 patients with chronic renal insufficiency showed no impairment in the elimination kinetics of propranolol compared with 8 subjects with normal renal function.[1] Peak concentrations of propranolol reported in patients with chronic renal failure have been 2 to 3 times higher than those reported in patients receiving dialysis or normal subjects.[1,2] Additional studies indicate that there is no pharmacokinetic reason to amend the dosage of propranolol in patients with renal impairment.[3]

Findings from a study in 8 patients on haemodialysis include a slight elevation of propranolol-plasma concentrations, no elevation of plasma concentration of 4-hydroxypropranolol, but extremely high plasma concentrations of other propranolol metabolites.[4]

1. Lowenthal DT, *et al.* Pharmacokinetics of oral propranolol in chronic renal disease. *Clin Pharmacol Ther* 1974; **16:** 761–9.
2. Bianchetti G, *et al.* Pharmacokinetics and effects of propranolol in terminal uraemic patients and in patients undergoing regular dialysis treatment. *Clin Pharmacokinet* 1976; **1:** 373–84.
3. Wood AJJ, *et al.* Propranolol disposition in renal failure. *Br J Clin Pharmacol* 1980; **10:** 561–6.
4. Stone WJ, Walle T. Massive propranolol metabolite retention during maintenance hemodialysis. *Clin Pharmacol Ther* 1980; **28:** 449–55.

Preparations

BP 1998: Propranolol Injection; Propranolol Tablets;
USP 23: Propranolol Hydrochloride and Hydrochlorothiazide Extended-release Capsules; Propranolol Hydrochloride and Hydrochlorothiazide Tablets; Propranolol Hydrochloride Extended-release Capsules; Propranolol Hydrochloride Injection; Propranolol Hydrochloride Tablets.

Proprietary Preparations (details are given in Part 3)
Aust.: Inderal; Proprahexal; ***Austral.:*** Deralin; Inderal; ***Belg.:*** Inderal; ***Canad.:*** Inderal; Novo-Pranol; ***Fr.:*** Avlocardyl; Hemipralon; ***Ger.:*** Beta-Tablinen; Beta-Timelets†; Dociton; Efektolol; Elbrol; Indobloc; Intermigran†; Obsidan; Propabloc; Prophylux; Propra; Propra-ratiopharm; Propranur; ***Irl.:*** Antarol†; Berkolol; Creanol†; Duranol†; Half Inderal; Inderal; Tiperal; ***Ital.:*** Inderal; ***Neth.:*** Inderal; ***Norw.:*** Inderal; Pranolol; Pronovan; ***S.Afr.:*** Cardiblok; Cardimax; Cardispare; Dynablok†; Hipranol†; Inderal; Indoblok†; Nolol; Norpro†; Pressanol†; Prodorol; Pur-Bloka; Rexigen†; ***Spain:*** Sumial; ***Swed.:*** Inderal; ***Switz.:*** Bedranol†; Betaprol; Inderal; Servanolol†; ***UK:*** Angilol; Apsolol; Bedranol SR; Berkolol; Beta-Prograne; Betadur CR; Cardinol; Half Beta-Pro-

grane; Half Betadur CR; Half Inderal; Inderal; Lopranol LA; Probeta LA; Propanix; Sloprolol†; *USA:* Betachron; Inderal.

Multi-ingredient: ***Aust.:*** Inderal comp; Inderetic; Tardurol; ***Belg.:*** Inderetic; ***Canad.:*** Inderide; ***Ger.:*** Beta-Nephral; Beta-Turfa; Betathiazid; Betathiazid A; Diutensat comp; Docidrazin; Dociretic; Dociteren; Dociton Dytide H†; Euchon†; Manimon; Nitro-Obsidan; Obsilazin N; Pertenso N; Propra comp; ***Irl.:*** Inderetic; Spiroprop†; ***Neth.:*** Inderetic; ***S.Afr.:*** Inderetic; ***Spain:*** Betadipresan; Betadipresan Diu; ***Switz.:*** Inderetic; ***UK:*** Inderetic; Inderex; ***USA:*** Inderide.

Proscillaridin (5826-b)

Proscillaridin *(BAN, USAN, rINN).*

2936; A-32686; Proscillaridin A; PSC-801. 14-Hydroxy-3β-(α-L-rhamnopyranosyloxy)-14β-bufa-4,20,22-trienolide.

$C_{30}H_{42}O_8$ = 530.6.

CAS — 466-06-8.

A glycoside obtained from *Drimia maritima* (Liliaceae).

Proscillaridin is a cardiac glycoside and positive inotrope with general properties similar to those of digoxin (p.849). It is reported to have a rapid onset and a short duration of action.

Proscillaridin is used in the treatment of heart failure (p.785). It is given by mouth in usual initial and usual maintenance doses of 1 to 1.5 mg daily; maintenance doses may range from 0.5 to 2.5 mg daily as required.

Preparations

Proprietary Preparations (details are given in Part 3)
Aust.: Caradrin; ***Austral.:*** Talusin; ***Ger.:*** Talusin; ***Irl.:*** Talusin†; ***Ital.:*** Caradrin†; Stellarid†; Talusin†; ***S.Afr.:*** Talusin†; ***Swed.:*** Talusin†; ***Switz.:*** Talusin.

Multi-ingredient: ***Aust.:*** Taluvian†; Theocaradrin; ***Ger.:*** Taluvian†; Theo-Talusin†; Tromscillan†; ***Ital.:*** Neo Gratusminal†; Teostellarid†; ***Switz.:*** Theo-Talusin.

Quinalbital (13197-j)

Chinalbitale; Chinalbitalum.

$C_{20}H_{26}N_2O_2,C_{11}H_{18}N_2O_3$ = 552.7.

Quinalbital is the hydroquinidine salt (see p.889) of amylobarbitone and has been used in the treatment of cardiac arrhythmias.

Preparations

Proprietary Preparations (details are given in Part 3)
Ital.: Amosedil†.

Quinapril Hydrochloride (491-m)

Quinapril Hydrochloride *(BANM, USAN, rINNM).*

CI-906 (quinapril). (3S)-2-{N-[(S)-1-Ethoxycarbonyl-3-phenylpropyl]-L-alanyl}-1,2,3,4-tetrahydro-isoquinoline-3-carboxylic acid hydrochloride.

$C_{25}H_{30}N_2O_5$,HCl = 475.0.

CAS — 85441-61-8 (quinapril); 82586-55-8 (quinapril hydrochloride).

Quinapril hydrochloride 10.8 mg is approximately equivalent to 10.0 mg of quinapril.

Adverse Effects, Treatment, and Precautions

As for ACE inhibitors, p.805.

Interactions

As for ACE inhibitors, p.807.

Antibacterials. Quinapril has been reported to reduce the absorption of tetracyclines due to the presence of magnesium carbonate in the tablet formulation.

Pharmacokinetics

Quinapril acts as a prodrug of the diacid quinaprilat, its active metabolite. Following oral administration about 60% of a dose is absorbed. Quinapril is metabolised mainly in the liver to quinaprilat and inactive metabolites. Peak plasma concentrations of quinaprilat are achieved within 2 hours of an oral dose of quinapril. Up to 60% of an oral dose of quinapril is excreted in the urine as quinaprilat, other metabolites, and unchanged drug, with the rest being excreted in the faeces. Quinaprilat is about 97% bound to plasma proteins. The effective half-life for accumulation of quinaprilat is approximately 3 hours following multiple doses of quinapril; a long terminal phase half-life of 25 hours may represent strong binding of quinaprilat to angiotensin-converting enzyme.

The pharmacokinetics of both quinapril and quinaprilat are affected by renal and hepatic impairment.

References.

1. Begg EJ, *et al.* The pharmacokinetics and pharmacodynamics of quinapril and quinaprilat in renal impairment. *Br J Clin Pharmacol* 1990; **30:** 213–20.
2. Halstenson CE, *et al.* The pharmacokinetics of quinapril and its active metabolite, quinaprilat, in patients with various degrees of renal function. *J Clin Pharmacol* 1992; **32:** 344–50.
3. Wolter K, Fritschka E. Pharmacokinetics and pharmacodynamics of quinaprilat after low dose quinapril in patients with terminal renal failure. *Eur J Clin Pharmacol* 1993; **44** (suppl 1): S53–6.
4. Begg EJ, *et al.* The pharmacokinetics of quinapril and quinaprilat in patients with congestive heart failure. *Br J Clin Pharmacol* 1994; **37:** 302–4.
5. Squire IB, *et al.* Haemodynamic response and pharmacokinetics after the first dose of quinapril in patients with congestive heart failure. *Br J Clin Pharmacol* 1994; **38:** 117–23.
6. Breslin E, *et al.* A pharmacodynamic and pharmacokinetic comparison of intravenous quinaprilat and oral quinapril. *J Clin Pharmacol* 1996; **36:** 414–21.

Uses and Administration

Quinapril is an ACE inhibitor (p.805). It is used in the treatment of hypertension (p.788) and heart failure (p.785).

Quinapril is converted in the body to its active metabolite quinaprilat. The haemodynamic effects are seen within 1 hour of a single dose by mouth and the maximum effect occurs after about 2 to 4 hours, although the full effect may not develop for 1 to 2 weeks during chronic administration. The haemodynamic action persists for about 24 hours, allowing once-daily dosing. Quinapril is given by mouth as the hydrochloride, but doses are expressed in terms of quinapril.

In the treatment of **hypertension** the initial dose is 10 mg once daily. Since there may be a precipitous fall in blood pressure in some patients when starting therapy with an ACE inhibitor, the first dose should preferable be given at bedtime. An initial dose of 2.5 mg daily is recommended in the elderly, in patients with renal impairment, or in those receiving a diuretic; if possible, the diuretic should be withdrawn 2 or 3 days before quinapril is started and resumed later if necessary. The usual maintenance dose is 20 to 40 mg daily, as a single dose or divided into 2 doses, although up to 80 mg daily has been given.

In the management of **heart failure**, severe first-dose hypotension on introduction of an ACE inhibitor is common in patients on loop diuretics, but their temporary withdrawal may cause rebound pulmonary oedema. Thus treatment should be initiated with a low dose under close medical supervision. Quinapril is given in an initial dose of 2.5 mg daily. Usual maintenance doses range from 10 to 20 mg daily, usually in 2 divided doses; up to 40 mg daily has been given.

Quinaprilat is given intravenously.

Reviews.

1. Wadworth AN, Brogden RN. Quinapril: a review of its pharmacological properties, and therapeutic efficacy in cardiovascular disorders. *Drugs* 1991; **41:** 378–99.
2. Plosker GL, Sorkin EM. Quinapril: a reappraisal of its pharmacology and therapeutic efficacy in cardiovascular disorders. *Drugs* 1994; **48:** 227–52.

Preparations

Proprietary Preparations (details are given in Part 3)
Aust.: Accupro; Continucor; ***Austral.:*** Accupril; Asig; ***Belg.:*** Accupril; ***Canad.:*** Accupril; ***Fr.:*** Acuitel; Korec; ***Ger.:*** Accupro; ***Irl.:*** Accupro; ***Ital.:*** Accuprin; Acequin; Quinazil; ***Neth.:*** Acupril; ***S.Afr.:*** Accupril; ***Spain:*** Acuprel; Acuretic; Ectren; Lidaltrin; ***Swed.:*** Accupro; ***Switz.:*** Accupro; ***UK:*** Accupro; ***USA:*** Accupril.

Multi-ingredient: ***Aust.:*** Accuzide; ***Belg.:*** Accuretic; ***Fr.:*** Acuilix; Koretic; ***Ger.:*** Accuzide; ***Irl.:*** Accuretic; ***Ital.:*** Accuretic; Acequide; Quinazide; ***Neth.:*** Acuzide; ***S.Afr.:*** Accuretic; ***Spain:*** Bicetil; Lidaltrin Diu; ***Swed.:*** Accupro Comp; ***Switz.:*** Accuretic; ***UK:*** Accuretic.

Quinethazone (2354-w)

Quinethazone *(BAN, rINN).*

Chinethazonum. 7-Chloro-2-ethyl-1,2,3,4-tetrahydro-4-oxoquinazoline-6-sulphonamide.

$C_{10}H_{12}ClN_3O_3S$ = 289.7.

CAS — 73-49-4.

Quinethazone is a diuretic which is related chemically to metolazone and has properties similar to those of the thiazide diuretics (see Hydrochlorothiazide, p.885). It is used for oedema, including that associated with heart failure (p.785), and for hypertension (p.788).

Diuresis is initiated within about 2 hours after administration, reaches a peak after 6 hours, and lasts for 18 to 24 hours.

In the treatment of oedema the usual dose is 50 to 100 mg by mouth daily; in some cases doses of 200 mg daily may be necessary.

In the treatment of hypertension the usual dose is 50 to 100 mg daily, either alone, or in conjunction with other antihypertensives. An initial dose of 25 mg daily has also been suggested.

In susceptible patients potassium supplements or a potassium-sparing diuretic may be necessary, but see hydrochlorothiazide.

Preparations

Proprietary Preparations (details are given in Part 3)
Austral.: Aquamox†; ***Ital.:*** Aquamox†; ***Neth.:*** Aquamox†; ***USA:*** Hydromox.

Multi-ingredient: ***Ital.:*** Ipotex†.

Quinidine (7771-r)

Quinidine *(BAN).*

Chinidinum; Quinidina. (8R,9S)-6′-Methoxycinchonan-9-ol; (+)-(αS)-α-(6-Methoxy-4-quinolyl)-α-[(2R,4S,5R)-(5-vinylquinuclidin-2-yl)]methanol.

$C_{20}H_{24}N_2O_2$ = 324.4.

CAS — 56-54-2 (anhydrous quinidine); 63717-04-4 (quinidine dihydrate); 72402-50-7 (± quinidine).

An isomer of quinine, obtained from the bark of species of *Cinchona* and their hybrids. The USP (under Quinidine Gluconate) also allows quinidine obtained from *Remijia pedunculata*, or prepared from quinine. It contains up to 20% of hydroquinidine, a closely allied base with similar chemical, physical, and physiological properties.

Quinidine Bisulphate (7772-f)

Quinidine Bisulphate *(BANM).*

$C_{20}H_{24}N_2O_2,H_2SO_4$ = 422.5.

CAS — 747-45-5 (anhydrous quinidine bisulphate); 6151-39-9 (quinidine bisulphate tetrahydrate).

Pharmacopoeias. In Br.

Colourless, odourless or almost odourless crystals. The BP specifies not more than 15% of hydroquinidine bisulphate (dihydroquinidine bisulphate). Quinidine bisulphate (anhydrous) 260 mg is approximately equivalent to 200 mg of quinidine (anhydrous). Freely **soluble** in water and in alcohol; practically insoluble in ether. A 1% solution in water has a pH of 2.6 to 3.6. **Protect** from light.

Quinidine Gluconate (7773-d)

Quinidine Gluconate *(BANM).*

Quinidinium Gluconate.

$C_{20}H_{24}N_2O_2,C_6H_{12}O_7$ = 520.6.

CAS — 7054-25-3.

Pharmacopoeias. In US.

A white odourless powder. The USP specifies not more than 20% of hydroquinidine gluconate (dihydroquinidine gluconate). Quinidine gluconate (anhydrous) 321 mg is approximately equivalent to 200 mg of quinidine (anhydrous). Freely **soluble** in water; slightly soluble in alcohol. **Protect** from light.

More than 40% of a dose of quinidine gluconate was lost when the drug was administered by intravenous infusion using a PVC infusion bag and tubing.[1]

1. Darbar D, *et al.* Loss of quinidine gluconate injection in a polyvinyl chloride infusion system. *Am J Health-Syst Pharm* 1996; **53:** 655–8.

Quinidine Polygalacturonate (7774-n)

Quinidine poly(D-galacturonate) hydrate.

$C_{20}H_{24}N_2O_2,(C_6H_{10}O_7)_x,xH_2O$.

CAS — 27555-34-6 (anhydrous quinidine polygalacturonate); 65484-56-2 (quinidine polygalacturonate hydrate).

Quinidine Sulphate (7775-h)

Quinidine Sulphate *(BANM)*.

Chinidini Sulfas; Chinidinsulfate; Chinidinum Sulfuricum; Quinidine Sulfate; Quinidini Sulfas.

$(C_{20}H_{24}N_2O_2)_2,H_2SO_4,2H_2O$ = 782.9.

CAS — 50-54-4 (anhydrous quinidine sulphate); 6591-63-5 (quinidine sulphate dihydrate).

Pharmacopoeias. In *Eur.* (see p.viii), *Int., Jpn, Pol.,* and *US.*

White, or almost white, odourless, fine crystalline powder, or fine, silky, needle-like white or colourless crystals, darkening on exposure to light. The Ph. Eur. specifies not more than 15% of hydroquinidine sulphate (dihydroquinidine sulphate); the USP specifies not more than 20%. Quinidine sulphate (dihydrate) 241 mg and quinidine sulphate (anhydrous) 230 mg are each approximately equivalent to 200 mg of quinidine (anhydrous).

Soluble 1 in 100 of water, 1 in 10 of alcohol, and 1 in 15 of chloroform; soluble in boiling water; practically insoluble in acetone and in ether. A 1% solution in water has a pH of 6.0 to 6.8. **Protect** from light.

Adverse Effects and Treatment

Quinidine and its salts cause both cardiac and extracardiac adverse effects. They commonly cause gastro-intestinal irritation with nausea, vomiting, and diarrhoea.

Hypersensitivity similar to that occurring with quinine may also occur and a test dose should be given to each patient (see Uses and Administration, below). Reactions include respiratory difficulties, urticaria, pruritus, skin rashes, purpura, thrombocytopenia and other blood dyscrasias, and, rarely, fever and anaphylaxis. Granulomatous hepatitis and a lupus-like syndrome have been reported.

Quinidine may give rise to cinchonism (see Quinine, p.439) with tinnitus, impaired hearing, visual disturbances, headache, confusion, vertigo, vomiting, and abdominal pain; it is usually associated with large doses, but may occur in idiosyncratic subjects given small doses.

Quinidine may induce hypotension; this is a special risk with intravenous administration. It may precipitate ventricular arrhythmias.

In quinidine overdosage, the cardiac symptoms of intoxication predominate. Quinidine is cumulative in action and inappropriately high plasma concentrations may induce ECG changes, heart block, asystole, ventricular tachycardia, ventricular fibrillation, syncope, seizures, coma, and sometimes death. Treatment of adverse effects and overdosage is symptomatic and supportive.

A review of adverse effects associated with the class Ia antiarrhythmic drugs quinidine, disopyramide, and procainamide, and their clinical management.[1]

1. Kim SY, Benowitz NL. Poisoning due to class IA antiarrhythmic drugs quinidine, procainamide and disopyramide. *Drug Safety* 1990; **5:** 393–420.

Effects on the blood. Quinidine-induced thrombocytopenia is not uncommon and it is one of the best documented drugs known to cause drug-dependent thrombocytopenia. The reaction is considered to be a hypersensitivity reaction probably due to the binding of quinidine to the platelet surface causing production of auto-antibodies and subsequent platelet lysis.[1] The antigenic constituent of the platelet membrane may be glycoprotein Ib although other surface glycoproteins have also been implicated.[2] Highly specific quinidine-dependent platelet antibodies have been found in the serum of patients with quinidine-induced thrombocytopenia;[3] the antibodies reacted with quinidine and the isomerically similar desmethoxy derivative cinchonine, but not with quinine. Once formed such antibodies may remain detectable for over 2 years.

A second mechanism has been proposed in which quinidine-autoantibody complexes are formed and then deposited on the platelet causing lysis.[2]

See also under Effects on the Skin, below.

1. Mitchell JA, *et al.* Immunotoxic side-effects of drug therapy. *Drug Safety* 1990; **5:** 168–78.
2. Stricker RB, Shuman MA. Quinidine purpura: evidence that glycoprotein V is a target platelet antigen. *Blood* 1986; **67:** 1377–81.
3. Reid DM, Shulman NR. Drug purpura due to surreptitious quinidine intake. *Ann Intern Med* 1988; **108:** 206–8.

Effects on the eyes. Corneal deposits resembling those found in keratopathy developed in a patient who had been taking quinidine for 2 years.[1] Symptoms had improved and both corneas had cleared completely within 2 months of stopping the drug.

A small number of patients have also been identified[2] who developed uveitis during quinidine treatment.

1. Zaidman GW. Quinidine keratopathy. *Am J Ophthalmol* 1984; **97:** 247–9.
2. Fraunfelder FW, Rosenbaum JT. Drug-induced uveitis: incidence, prevention and treatment. *Drug Safety* 1997; **17:** 197–207.

Effects on the joints. Quinidine has been associated with the development of reversible, symmetrical polyarthritis in several patients.[1-3] No biochemical or immunological abnormalities were found and the reaction was considered to be distinct from quinidine-induced lupus erythematosus (see below). Symptoms resolved within 1 week of withdrawing quinidine.

1. Kertes P, Hunt D. Polyarthritis complicating quinidine treatment. *Br Med J* 1982; **284:** 1373–4.
2. Cohen MG, *et al.* Two distinct quinidine-induced rheumatic syndromes. *Ann Intern Med* 1988; **108:** 369–71.
3. Naschitz JE, Yeshurun D. Quinidine and rheumatic syndromes. *Ann Intern Med* 1988; **109:** 248–9.

Effects on the liver. Hypersensitivity reactions involving the liver have been reported in about 2% of patients receiving quinidine.[1,2] The main clinical symptom is fever[1-3] but skin rash,[1-3] purpura,[2] and hepatomegaly[1] may also occur. Liver enzyme values are raised[1-4] and the platelet count may be reduced.[3] The reaction is reversible on withdrawing quinidine with fever resolving in about 48 hours and liver enzymes values returning to normal within about 2 weeks. Liver biopsy often shows granulomatous hepatitis,[1-3] but other inflammatory changes[2] and cholestatic jaundice[4] have been found.

1. Geltner D, *et al.* Quinidine hypersensitivity and liver involvement: a survey of 32 patients. *Gastroenterology* 1976; **70:** 650–2.
2. Knobler H, *et al.* Quinidine-induced hepatitis. *Arch Intern Med* 1986; **146:** 526–8.
3. Bramlet DA, *et al.* Granulomatous hepatitis as a manifestation of quinidine hypersensitivity. *Arch Intern Med* 1980; **140:** 395–7.
4. Hogan DB, *et al.* Unusual hepatotoxic reaction to quinidine. *Can Med Assoc J* 1984; **130:** 973.

Effects on mental state. Gradually progressive cerebral dysfunction characterised by intermittent confusion, agitation, restlessness, personality change, and paranoid features occurred in a 62-year-old man who had taken quinidine for about 15 years.[1] Within 24 hours of discontinuing quinidine there was a marked improvement and after 5 days he had returned to normal with no cognitive deficits. It was considered that quinidine precipitated or exacerbated the functional psychosis in this patient.

1. Johnson AG, *et al.* A functional psychosis precipitated by quinidine. *Med J Aust* 1990; **153:** 47–9.

Effects on the skin. Skin reactions reported with quinidine include exacerbation of psoriasis,[1] blue-grey pigmentation,[2] and photosensitivity.[3] Purpuric bruising has occurred in one person who was subjected to inhalation of quinidine dust in the workplace.[4]

1. Harwell WB. Quinidine-induced psoriasis. *J Am Acad Dermatol* 1983; **9:** 278.
2. Mahler R, *et al.* Pigmentation induced by quinidine therapy. *Arch Dermatol* 1986; **122:** 1062–4.
3. Marx JL, *et al.* Quinidine photosensitivity. *Arch Dermatol* 1983; **119:** 39–43.
4. Salom IL. Purpura due to inhaled quinidine. *JAMA* 1991; **266:** 1220.

Hypoglycaemia. Mean plasma-insulin concentrations increased and mean plasma-glucose concentrations decreased in 8 healthy subjects and 10 patients with malaria given quinidine intravenously.[1] Profound hypoglycaemia occurred in one patient with cerebral malaria and acute renal failure. These effects were considered to be associated with stimulation of β-cell secretion of insulin by quinidine and it was concluded that hypoglycaemia may occur in any severely ill fasting patient given parenteral quinidine.

1. Phillips RE, *et al.* Hypoglycaemia and antimalarial drugs: quinidine and release of insulin. *Br Med J* 1986; **292:** 1319–21.

Lupus erythematosus. There are several well-documented reports of quinidine-induced lupus erythematosus.[1-4] The syndrome involves polyarthritis with a positive antinuclear antibody test. Symptoms do not usually occur until several months after starting quinidine and resolve slowly on withdrawing the drug. A recurrence of lupus-like symptoms has occurred in patients with a previous reaction to procainamide.[2]

1. West SG, *et al.* Quinidine-induced lupus erythematosus. *Ann Intern Med* 1984; **100:** 840–2.
2. Amadio P, *et al.* Procainamide, quinidine, and lupus erythematosus. *Ann Intern Med* 1985; **102:** 419.
3. Lavie CJ, *et al.* Systemic lupus erythematosus (SLE) induced by quinidine. *Arch Intern Med* 1985; **145:** 446–8.
4. Cohen MG, *et al.* Two distinct quinidine-induced rheumatic syndromes. *Ann Intern Med* 1988; **108:** 369–71.

Oesophageal stricture. Oesophageal stricture occurred in 3 patients taking quinidine and was associated with ulceration in 2.[1] A literature review showed that quinidine and potassium chloride were the drugs most commonly implicated in stricture formation. Stricture also occurred more commonly following ingestion of modified-release formulations.

1. McCord GS, Clouse RE. Pill-induced esophageal strictures: clinical features and risk factors for development. *Am J Med* 1990; **88:** 512–18.

Precautions

Quinidine sulphate is contra-indicated in patients with complete heart block. An initial test dose of quinidine should always be given to detect hypersensitivity; positive responders should not be given quinidine nor should patients who have previously experienced quinidine hypersensitivity. It should be used with extreme caution in patients with incomplete heart block, and uncompensated heart failure. Care is also required in patients with myasthenia gravis as it can exacerbate the symptoms and may reduce the effectiveness of parasympathomimetic drugs. Antiarrhythmic therapy with quinidine should be initiated with extreme caution, if at all, during acute infections or fever as hypersensitivity reactions may be masked.

When quinidine is used to treat atrial flutter or fibrillation, the reduction in atrioventricular block may result in a very rapid ventricular rate. This can be avoided by prior digitalisation. However, quinidine is contra-indicated in digitalis overdosage as concomitant administration of quinidine with digoxin results in markedly increased plasma concentrations of digoxin.

Reduced dosage should be considered for the elderly, for patients with hepatic or renal impairment, and on the occasions when it is used in cardiac failure.

Pregnancy and breast feeding. A report on the administration of quinidine sulphate to one woman throughout pregnancy.[1] Concentrations in the infant's serum at delivery were similar to the mother's although amniotic fluid concentrations were raised. Quinidine diffused freely into the mother's milk and, although the infant would have received a dose far below the therapeutic dose, she was advised not to breast feed because of potential quinidine accumulation in the immature newborn liver.

1. Hill LM, Malkasian GD. The use of quinidine sulfate throughout pregnancy. *Obstet Gynecol* 1979; **54:** 366–8.

Interactions

Quinidine is used in combination with other antiarrhythmic drugs but caution is required with such combinations (see below). Concomitant use with other arrhythmogenic drugs should be avoided.

Quinidine is metabolised in the liver and interactions may occur through inhibition or enhancement of hepatic metabolism. Rifampicin, phenobarbitone, and phenytoin increase hepatic metabolism of quinidine and increased doses of quinidine may be needed if one of these drugs is added to quinidine therapy.

Urinary excretion of quinidine is dependent on urinary pH; drugs which increase urinary pH such as sodium bicarbonate, some antacids, and carbonic anhydrase inhibitors tend to increase the plasma concentration of quinidine since the proportion of nonionised drug in the urine is increased allowing greater renal tubular reabsorption.

As well as being affected by a range of drugs quinidine can in its turn affect other compounds which include oral anticoagulants, antihypertensives, muscle relaxants, antimuscarinics, and beta blockers. These interactions are discussed under the monographs for those drugs.

Antiarrhythmics. *Amiodarone* may increase the plasma concentration of quinidine, increasing the risk of toxicity; prolongation of the QT interval with torsade de pointes has been reported.[1] This interaction is probably due to amiodarone inhibiting hepatic or renal clearance of quinidine or displacing quinidine from binding sites. If the two drugs are used together the dose of quinidine may need to be reduced and the patient should be closely monitored. *Verapamil* given intravenously has been reported[2] to cause severe hypotension in patients also receiving quinidine by mouth. Studies *in vitro* suggest this is due to the additive blockade of α-adrenergic receptors by both drugs and the simultaneous blockade of calcium channels by verapamil. Quinidine may increase the plasma concentration of other antiarrhythmics when administered concomitantly (see Ajmaline, p.817, Digoxin, p.851, Disopyramide, p.859, Flecainide Acetate, p.869, and Propafenone Hydrochloride, p.936).

1. Lesko LJ. Pharmacokinetic drug interactions with amiodarone. *Clin Pharmacokinet* 1989; **17:** 130–40.
2. Maisel AS, *et al.* Hypotension after quinidine plus verapamil. *N Engl J Med* 1985; **312:** 167–70.

Antibacterials. *Erythromycin* might inhibit the hepatic metabolism of quinidine.[1]

1. Spinler SA, *et al.* Possible inhibition of hepatic metabolism of quinidine by erythromycin. *Clin Pharmacol Ther* 1995; **57:** 89–94.

Antifungals. *Ketoconazole* temporarily increased the plasma-quinidine concentration in one patient through reduced hepatic elimination.[1] Another antifungal that inhibits hepatic metabolism, *itraconazole*, has also been reported[2] to increase plasma-quinidine concentrations.

1. McNulty RM, *et al.* Transient increase in plasma quinidine concentrations during ketoconazole-quinidine therapy. *Clin Pharm* 1989; **8:** 222–5.
2. Kaukonen K-M, *et al.* Itraconazole increases plasma concentrations of quinidine. *Clin Pharmacol Ther* 1997; **62:** 510–17.

Beta blockers. Sinus bradycardia in a patient prescribed quinidine by mouth and *timolol* eye drops,[1] and orthostatic hypotension with quinidine and *atenolol*[2] have occurred. Administration of quinidine or the beta blocker alone was well tolerated in each case with no adverse effects.

1. Dinai Y, *et al.* Bradycardia induced by interaction between quinidine and ophthalmic timolol. *Ann Intern Med* 1985; **103:** 890–1.
2. Manolis AS, Estes NAM. Orthostatic hypotension due to quinidine and atenolol. *Am J Med* 1987; **82:** 1083–4.

Calcium-channel blockers. *Nifedipine* has been reported[1] to reduce plasma-quinidine concentrations and up to 20 mg of quinidine per kg body-weight failed to increase the plasma concentration. Withdrawal of nifedipine resulted in a doubling of the quinidine concentration. A pharmacokinetic and pharmacodynamic study in healthy subjects, however, failed to show that modified-release *felodipine* or nifedipine had any effect on quinidine disposition.[2] Another study in healthy subjects suggested that quinidine may inhibit nifedipine metabolism.[3]

1. Green JA, *et al.* Nifedipine-quinidine interaction. *Clin Pharm* 1983; **2:** 461–5.
2. Bailey DG, *et al.* Quinidine interaction with nifedipine and felodipine: pharmacokinetic and pharmacodynamic evaluation. *Clin Pharmacol Ther* 1993; **53:** 354–9.
3. Bowles SK, *et al.* Evaluation of the pharmacokinetic and pharmacodynamic interaction between quinidine and nifedipine. *J Clin Pharmacol* 1993; **33:** 727–31.

Diuretics. *Carbonic anhydrase inhibitors* tend to increase plasma-quinidine concentrations due to increased renal tubular reabsorption of quinidine.

Administration of *amiloride* to 10 patients receiving quinidine therapy produced arrhythmias in 4 of the patients.[1] It was suggested that additive sodium-channel blockade may be responsible.

1. Wang L, *et al.* Amiloride-quinidine interaction: adverse outcomes. *Clin Pharmacol Ther* 1994; **56:** 659–67.

Histamine H_2-receptor antagonists. *Cimetidine* inhibits the hepatic metabolism of quinidine and increases in plasma concentration and half-life with a reduction in clearance have been reported.[1-3]

1. Hardy BG, *et al.* Effect of cimetidine on the pharmacokinetics and pharmacodynamics of quinidine. *Am J Cardiol* 1983; **52:** 172–5.
2. Kolb KW, *et al.* Effect of cimetidine on quinidine clearance. *Ther Drug Monit* 1984; **6:** 306–12.
3. MacKichan JJ, *et al.* Effect of cimetidine on quinidine bioavailability. *Biopharm Drug Dispos* 1989; **10:** 121–5.

Pharmacokinetics

Quinidine is rapidly absorbed from the gastro-intestinal tract, peak plasma concentrations being achieved about 1.5 hours after oral administration of quinidine sulphate and about 4 hours after quinidine gluconate; its bioavailability is variable, owing to first-pass metabolism in the liver.

Quinidine is metabolised in the liver to a number of metabolites, at least some of which are pharmacologically active. It is excreted in the urine, mainly in the form of its metabolites. The proportion excreted unchanged is dependent on urinary pH; in acidic urine about 20% is excreted as unchanged quinidine but in alkaline urine this is reduced to about 5% due to increased renal tubular reabsorption.

Quinidine is widely distributed throughout the body and is 80 to 90% bound to plasma proteins including α_1-acid glycoprotein. It has a plasma half-life of about 6 to 8 hours but this may show wide variation. Its therapeutic effect has been correlated with plasma concentrations within about 2 to 7 μg per mL. However, plasma concentrations can be misleading as, depending on the assay method, quinidine may not be differentiated from its metabolites. It has been suggested that with specific assays quinidine concentrations of 1 μg or less per mL may be all that are required.

Quinidine crosses the placental barrier and is distributed into breast milk. Small amounts are removed by haemodialysis.

Considerable intersubject and intrasubject variability in the pharmacokinetics of quinidine have been noted[1] with the half-life ranging from about 1 to 16 hours regardless of whether the drug was administered as a tablet, capsule, oral solution, or intramuscular injection. There may also be considerable variations in absorption pharmacokinetic parameters depending upon the formulation and the salt used.[2,3] The effect of food on absorption is not clear.[4,5] The heart condition being treated or associated with the arrhythmia may alter quinidine's pharmacokinetics[6,7] as may the age of the patient.[8-10] Hepatic impairment may affect protein binding and prolong quinidine's half-life.[11] Protein binding increases in patients with renal impairment, although it returns to normal during dialysis procedures.[12] Accumulation of quinidine metabolites may occur in patients with renal dysfunction.[13-15]

1. Mason WD, *et al.* Comparative plasma concentrations of quinidine following administration of one intramuscular and three oral formulations to 13 human subjects. *J Pharm Sci* 1976; **65:** 1325–9.
2. Frigo GM, *et al.* Comparison of quinidine plasma concentration curves following oral administration of some short- and long-acting formulations. *Br J Clin Pharmacol* 1977; **4:** 449–54.
3. Mahon WA, *et al.* Comparative bioavailability study of three sustained release quinidine formulations. *Clin Pharmacokinet* 1987; **13:** 118–24.
4. Woo E, Greenblatt DJ. Effect of food on enteral absorption of quinidine. *Clin Pharmacol Ther* 1980; **27:** 188–93.
5. Martinez MN, *et al.* Effect of dietary fat content on the bioavailability of a sustained release quinidine gluconate tablet. *Biopharm Drug Dispos* 1990; **11:** 17–29.
6. Ueda CT, Dzindzio BS. Quinidine kinetics in congestive heart failure. *Clin Pharmacol Ther* 1978; **23:** 158–64.
7. Ueda CT, Dzindzio BS. Bioavailability of quinidine in congestive heart failure. *Br J Clin Pharmacol* 1981; **11:** 571–7.
8. Drayer DE, *et al.* Prevalence of high (3S)-3-hydroxyquinidine/quinidine ratios in serum, and clearance of quinidine in cardiac patients with age. *Clin Pharmacol Ther* 1980; **27:** 72–5.
9. Szefler SJ, *et al.* Rapid elimination of quinidine in pediatric patients. *Pediatrics* 1982; **70:** 370–5.
10. Pickoff AS, *et al.* Age-related differences in the protein binding of quinidine. *Dev Pharmacol Ther* 1981; **3:** 108–15.
11. Kessler KM, *et al.* Quinidine pharmacokinetics in patients with cirrhosis or receiving propranolol. *Am Heart J* 1978; **96:** 627–35.
12. Kessler KM, Perez GO. Decreased quinidine plasma protein binding during haemodialysis. *Clin Pharmacol Ther* 1981; **30:** 121–6.
13. Kessler KM, *et al.* Quinidine elimination in patients with congestive heart failure or poor renal function. *N Engl J Med* 1974; **290:** 706–9.
14. Drayer DE, *et al.* Steady-state serum levels of quinidine and active metabolites in cardiac patients with varying degrees of renal function. *Clin Pharmacol Ther* 1978; **24:** 31–9.
15. Hall K, *et al.* Clearance of quinidine during peritoneal dialysis. *Am Heart J* 1982; **104:** 646–7.

Uses and Administration

Quinidine is a class Ia antiarrhythmic (p.776). It also has antimuscarinic and alpha-adrenoceptor blocking properties. Quinidine is used to maintain sinus rhythm after cardioversion of atrial fibrillation, and for the suppression of supraventricular and ventricular **arrhythmias**.

Quinidine is an isomer of quinine and may be used as an alternative to quinine in the treatment of **malaria** when quinine is not immediately available.

Strengths of preparations and doses of quinidine salts used have been expressed in a variety of ways; as well as expressing in terms of the salt actually being employed equivalences in terms of anhydrous quinidine base or quinidine sulphate dihydrate have commonly been used.

For the management of cardiac arrhythmias, quinidine sulphate is given by mouth in usual doses of 200 to 400 mg three or four times daily. Doses of up to 600 mg every 2 to 4 hours have been given for the treatment of supraventricular tachycardias to a maximum of 4 g a day; these higher doses should only be given with frequent monitoring of the electrocardiogram and plasma concentration. An initial test dose of 200 mg should always be given to detect hypersensitivity.

Quinidine is also given by mouth as a range of salts including the bisulphate, the gluconate, and the polygalacturonate.

Modified-release formulations are generally preferred as the plasma concentration profile is smoother and doses can be given at 8- to 12-hourly intervals.

Quinidine has been given intramuscularly or by slow intravenous injection, but absorption from the intramuscular route can be erratic and incomplete, and the intravenous route is associated with a risk of severe hypotension. Suggested parenteral doses of quinidine gluconate are: intramuscularly, 600 mg initially then up to 400 mg repeated every 2 hours if necessary; by intravenous infusion 800 mg diluted to a volume of 50 mL with 5% glucose and given at a rate of 1 mL per minute with electrocardiogram and blood-pressure monitoring.

General references.

1. Grace AA, Camm AJ. Quinidine. *N Engl J Med* 1998; **338:** 35–45.

Cardiac arrhythmias. Quinidine is a class Ia antiarrhythmic and has been used in the management of supraventricular and ventricular arrhythmias (p.782), but like other antiarrhythmics it may precipitate arrhythmias. The CAST (Cardiac Arrhythmia Suppression Trial) studies demonstrated that other class I antiarrhythmics (encainide, flecainide, and moracizine) were associated with an increased mortality rate when used for asymptomatic ventricular arrhythmias in post-infarction patients and led to many drugs of this class being restricted to severe or life-threatening arrhythmias. A meta-analysis of trials utilising quinidine was undertaken as it was believed this drug had gained in popularity after the adverse CAST results. This meta-analysis[1] suggested that quinidine was associated with at least as high a proportion of adverse events, such as death and early proarrhythmia, as the class Ic drugs flecainide and propafenone. It was, however, emphasised that these results do not necessarily apply to the use of quinidine for the treatment of life-threatening or sustained ventricular arrhythmias.

1. Morganroth J, Goin JE. Quinidine-related mortality in the short-to-medium-term treatment of ventricular arrhythmias: a meta-analysis. *Circulation* 1991; **84:** 1977–83.

Cramps. Although quinidine would be expected to have similar efficacy to quinine in preventing nocturnal cramps, quinine is preferred due to its lower potential for cardiotoxicity.[1] For a discussion of the usual treatment of nocturnal cramp, see under Muscle Spasm, p.1303.

1. Beeley L. *Br Med J* 1991; **302:** 33.

Hiccup. Quinidine is one of several drugs that have been tried in intractable hiccups and for details of a protocol for the control of hiccups which eventually leads to oral administration of quinidine, see Chlorpromazine Hydrochloride, p.655.

Malaria. Although quinidine might theoretically be superior to quinine as an antimalarial it is more likely to cause cardiac toxicity and hypersensitivity and WHO[1,2] has recommended that oral or parenteral formulations of quinidine should only be used when quinine is not immediately available. In this situation intravenous infusions of quinidine could be used to initiate treatment for severe chloroquine-resistant malaria under close control, preferably with continuous ECG monitoring and frequent measurements of blood pressure. Patients should be transferred to oral therapy with quinine, or, if not available, quinidine as soon as possible.

In the USA, the Centers for Disease Control[3] have recommended parenteral quinidine gluconate as the drug of choice for the treatment of complicated falciparum malaria, but only because parenteral quinine was not available there.

Quinidine is given intravenously as the gluconate and doses have been expressed in terms of the base or salt. Phillips *et al.*[4] have used a regimen where the equivalent of 15 mg of the base per kg body-weight was infused over 4 hours as a loading dose followed by the equivalent of 7.5 mg of the base per kg every 8 hours for 7 days given either as infusions over 4 hours or by mouth when the patient was able to tolerate oral therapy. An alternative regimen used by Miller *et al.*[5] consisted of a loading dose of 10 mg of quinidine gluconate per kg given by intravenous infusion over a period of 1 to 2 hours followed by a constant intravenous infusion of 0.02 mg per kg per minute for a maximum of 72 hours or until oral therapy with quinine can be instituted to complete a total 3-day course of treatment. It is generally recommended that loading doses should not be used if the patient has received quinine or quinidine within the previous 24 hours or mefloquine within the preceding 7 days.[2]

The overall management of malaria is discussed in the chapter on Antimalarials, p.422.

1. WHO. Practical chemotherapy of malaria: report of a WHO scientific group. *WHO Tech Rep Ser 805* 1990.
2. Gilles HM. *Management of severe and complicated malaria.* Geneva: WHO, 1991.
3. Centers for Disease Control. Treatment with quinidine gluconate of persons with severe Plasmodium falciparum infection: discontinuation of parenteral quinine from CDC drug service. *MMWR* 1991; **40** (RR-4): 21–3.
4. Phillips RE, *et al.* Intravenous quinidine for the treatment of severe falciparum malaria: clinical pharmacokinetic studies. *N Engl J Med* 1985; **312:** 1273–8.
5. Miller KD, *et al.* Treatment of severe malaria in the United States with a continuous infusion of quinidine gluconate and exchange transfusion. *N Engl J Med* 1989; **321:** 65–70.

Preparations

BP 1998: Quinidine Sulphate Tablets;
USP 23: Quinidine Gluconate Extended-release Tablets; Quinidine Gluconate Injection; Quinidine Sulfate Capsules; Quinidine Sulfate Extended-release Tablets; Quinidine Sulfate Tablets.

Proprietary Preparations (details are given in Part 3)
Aust.: Galactoquin; ***Austral.:*** Kinidin; Quinidex†; ***Belg.:*** Cardioquine†; Kinidine Durettes; Longacor†; ***Canad.:*** Biquin; Cardioquin; Natisedine; Quinaglute†; Quinate; Quinidex; Quinobarb; ***Fr.:*** Cardioquine; Longacor; Quinidurule; ***Ger.:*** Galactoquin†; Natisedine†; Optochinidin retard; ***Irl.:*** Kinidin; ***Ital.:*** Chinteina; Longachin; Naticardina; Natisedina; Neochinidin†; Quinaglute†; Ritmocor; Solfachinid†; ***Neth.:*** Cardioquin; Kiditard†; Kinidine; Natisedine†; ***Norw.:*** Kinidin; Systodin; ***S.Afr.:*** Quinaglute; ***Spain:*** Cardioquine; Longacor; Natisedina†; Quinicardina; ***Swed.:*** Kinidin; ***Switz.:*** Kinidin; Longacor; ***UK:*** Kiditard†; Kinidin; ***USA:*** Cardioquin; Duraquin†; Quinaglute; Quinalan; Quinidex; Quinora.

Multi-ingredient: ***Ger.:*** Circovegetalin compositum†; Circovegetalin†; Cordichin; Coritrat†; Eucard†; Rhythmochin I†; Rhythmochin II (cum sedativo)†.

Ramipril (16975-a)

Ramipril *(BAN, USAN, rINN).*

HOE-498; Ramiprilum. (2*S*,3a*S*,6a*S*)-1-{*N*-[(*S*)-1-Ethoxycarbonyl-3-phenylpropyl]L-alanyl}perhydrocyclopenta[*b*]pyrrole-2-carboxylic acid.

$C_{23}H_{32}N_2O_5$ = 416.5.

CAS — 87333-19-5.

Pharmacopoeias. in *Eur.* (see p.viii).

A white or almost white, crystalline powder. Sparingly **soluble** in water; freely soluble in methyl alcohol. **Protect** from light.

Adverse Effects, Treatment, and Precautions

As for ACE inhibitors, p.805.

Interactions

As for ACE inhibitors, p.807.

Pharmacokinetics

Ramipril acts as a prodrug of the diacid ramiprilat, its active metabolite. Following oral administration at least 50 to 60% is absorbed. Ramipril is metabolised in the liver to ramiprilat; other metabolites are inactive. Peak plasma concentrations of ramiprilat are achieved 2 to 4 hours after an oral dose of ramipril. About 60% of an oral dose is excreted in the urine, the rest in the faeces. Ramiprilat is about 56% bound to plasma proteins. The effective half-life for accumulation of ramiprilat is 13 to 17 hours following multiple doses of ramipril 5 to 10 mg, but is much longer for doses of 1.25 to 2.5 mg daily. The clearance of ramiprilat is reduced in renal impairment.

Reviews.

1. Meisel S, *et al.* Clinical pharmacokinetics of ramipril. *Clin Pharmacokinet* 1994; **26:** 7–15.
2. van Griensven JMT, *et al.* Pharmacokinetics, pharmacodynamics and bioavailability of the ACE inhibitor ramipril. *Eur J Clin Pharmacol* 1995; **47:** 513–8.

Uses and Administration

Ramipril is an ACE inhibitor (p.805). It is used in the treatment of hypertension (p.788), heart failure (p.785), and following myocardial infarction (p.791) to improve survival in patients with clinical evidence of heart failure.

Ramipril owes its activity to ramiprilat to which it is converted after oral administration. The haemodynamic effects are seen within 1 to 2 hours of a single oral dose and the maximum effect occurs after about 3 to 6 hours, although the full effect may not develop for several weeks during chronic dosing. The haemodynamic effect is maintained for at least 24 hours, allowing once-daily dosing.

In the treatment of **hypertension** an initial dose of 1.25 mg once daily is given by mouth. Since there may be a precipitous fall in blood pressure when starting therapy with an ACE inhibitor, the first dose should preferably be given at bedtime. Patients receiving diuretics should, if possible, have the diuretic discontinued 2 to 3 days before starting ramipril, and resumed later if necessary. The usual maintenance dose is 2.5 to 5 mg daily as a single dose, although up to 10 mg daily may be required. In the USA an initial dose of 2.5 mg once daily in hypertensive patients not receiving a diuretic and a maintenance dose of 2.5 to 20 mg daily have been suggested.

In the management of **heart failure**, severe first-dose hypotension on introduction of an ACE inhibitor is common in patients on loop diuretics, but their temporary withdrawal may cause rebound pulmonary oedema. Thus treatment should be initiated with a low dose under close medical supervision; high doses of diuretics should be reduced before starting ramipril. Ramipril is given in an initial dose of 1.25 mg once daily. The usual maximum dose is 10 mg daily; doses of 2.5 mg or more daily may be taken in 1 or 2 divided doses.

Following **myocardial infarction**, treatment with ramipril may be started in hospital 3 to 10 days after the infarction at a usual initial dose of 2.5 mg twice daily, increased after two days to 5 mg twice daily. The usual maintenance dose is 2.5 to 5 mg twice daily.

A reduction in dosage of ramipril may be necessary in patients with impaired renal function.

References.

1. Todd PA, Benfield P. Ramipril: a review of its pharmacological properties and therapeutic efficacy in cardiovascular disorders. *Drugs* 1990; **39:** 110–35.
2. Frampton JE, Peters DH. Ramipril: an updated review of its therapeutic use in essential hypertension and heart failure. *Drugs* 1995; **49:** 440–66.
3. The Acute Infarction Ramipril Efficacy (AIRE) Study Investigators. Effect of ramipril on mortality and morbidity of survivors of acute myocardial infarction with clinical evidence of heart failure. *Lancet* 1993; **342:** 821–8.

Preparations

Proprietary Preparations (details are given in Part 3)
Aust.: Hypren; Tritace; ***Austral.:*** Ramace; Tritace; ***Belg.:*** Ramace; Tritace; ***Canad.:*** Altace; ***Fr.:*** Triatec; ***Ger.:*** Delix; Vesdil; ***Irl.:*** Pramace†; Tritace; ***Ital.:*** Quark; Triatec; Unipril; ***Neth.:*** Tritace; ***Norw.:*** Triatec; ***S.Afr.:*** Ramace; Tritace; ***Spain:*** Acovil; Carasel; ***Swed.:*** Pramace; Triatec; ***Switz.:*** Triatec; Vesdil; ***UK:*** Tritace; ***USA:*** Altace.

Multi-ingredient: ***Aust.:*** Hypren plus; Lasitace; Trialix; Tritazide; ***Ger.:*** Arelix ACE; Delix plus; Vesdil plus; ***Irl.:*** Trialix; ***Ital.:*** Idroquark; Triatec HCT; ***Neth.:*** Tritazide; ***Swed.:*** Triatec comp; ***Switz.:*** Trialix; Triatec comp.

Ranolazine Hydrochloride (3760-s)

Ranolazine Hydrochloride *(USAN, rINNM).*

RS-43285. (±)-4-[2-Hydroxy-3-(*o*-methoxyphenoxy)propyl]-1-piperazineaceto-2′,6′-xylidide dihydrochloride.

$C_{24}H_{33}N_3O_4,2HCl$ = 500.5.

CAS — 95635-55-5 (ranolazine); 95635-56-6 (ranolazine hydrochloride).

Ranolazine hydrochloride is under investigation for use in angina pectoris.

Raubasine (9277-d)

Ajmalicine; Alkaloid F; δ-Yohimbine. Methyl 16,17-didehydro-19α-methyl-18-oxayohimban-16-carboxylate.

$C_{21}H_{24}N_2O_3$ = 352.4.

CAS — 483-04-5.

Raubasine is an alkaloid obtained from *Rauwolfia serpentina* (Apocynaceae).

Raubasine is a vasodilator related chemically to reserpine (below). It has been given by mouth and by injection in peripheral and cerebral vascular disorders.

Preparations

Proprietary Preparations (details are given in Part 3)
Aust.: Lamuran; ***Canad.:*** Hydrosarpan†; ***Ger.:*** Lamuran†; ***Ital.:*** Circolene†; Lamuran; Sarpan†; ***S.Afr.:*** Melanex.

Multi-ingredient: ***Aust.:*** Card-Lamuran†; Defluina; Modenol; ***Fr.:*** Cristanyl†; Duxil; Iskedyl; ***Ger.:*** Card-Lamuran†; ***Ital.:*** Isosarpan†; ***S.Afr.:*** Saltucin Co†; ***Spain:*** Duxor; Iskedyl; Isquebral; Salvalion; ***Switz.:*** Modenol†.

Rauwolfia Serpentina (898-m)

Chotachand; Rauvolfia; Rauwolfia; Rauwolfiae Radix; Rauwolfiawurzel.

CAS — 8063-17-0 (rauwolfia).

Pharmacopoeias. In *Ger.* (not less than 1% of total alkaloids) and *US.*

The dried roots of *Rauwolfia serpentina* (Apocynaceae). It contains not less than 0.15% of reserpine-rescinnamine group alkaloids calculated as reserpine.

Rauwolfia serpentina contains numerous alkaloids, the most active as hypotensive agents being the ester alkaloids, reserpine and rescinnamine. Other alkaloids present have structures related to reserpic acid, but are not esterified, and include ajmaline (rauwolfine), ajmalinine, ajmalicine, isoajmaline (isorauwolfine), serpentine, rauwolfinine, and sarpagine. **Store** at 15° to 30° in a dry place.

The actions of rauwolfia serpentina are those of its alkaloids and it has been used for the same purposes as reserpine, below. It has been administered by mouth as the powdered whole root.

Rauwolfia vomitoria has also been used.

The crude drug has been used in India for centuries as preparations such as Sarpagandha, in the treatment of insomnia and certain forms of mental illness.

Preparations

USP 23: Powdered Rauwolfia Serpentina; Rauwolfia Serpentina Tablets.

Proprietary Preparations (details are given in Part 3)
Belg.: Raudosal†; ***Ger.:*** Arte Rautin forte S; Rivadescin†; ***USA:*** Rauverid†.

Multi-ingredient: ***Ger.:*** Diuraupur sine†; Diuraupur†; Hyperforat-forte; Mistelan†; Nerviguttum†; Raufuncton N; Rauwoplant; ***Irl.:*** Rautrax†; ***S.Afr.:*** Rautrax†; ***Spain:*** Diu Rauwiplus; Rulun; ***UK:*** Hypercal-B†; ***USA:*** Rauzide.

Recainam (1515-m)

Recainam *(BAN, rINN).*

Wy-42362. 1-[3-(Isopropylamino)propyl]-3-(2,6-xylyl)urea.

$C_{15}H_{25}N_3O$ = 263.4.

CAS — 74738-24-2 (recainam); 74752-07-1 (recainam hydrochloride); 74752-08-2 (recainam tosylate).

NOTE. Recainam Hydrochloride and Recainam Tosylate are *USAN.*

Recainam is an antiarrhythmic with class Ia, class Ib, and class Ic activity (p.776).

Remikiren (15920-a)

Remikiren *(rINN).*

Ro-42-5892. (α*S*)-α-[(α*S*)-α-[(*tert*-Butylsulfonyl)methyl]hydrocinnamamido]-*N*-[(1*S*,2*R*,3*S*)-1-(cyclohexylmethyl)-3-cyclopropyl-2,3-dihydroxypropyl]imidazole-4-propionamide.

$C_{33}H_{50}N_4O_6S$ = 630.8.

CAS — 126222-34-2.

Remikiren inhibits the actions of renin and thus prevents the conversion of angiotensinogen into angiotensin I. It is active by mouth and is under investigation in the management of hypertension and heart failure.

A number of renin antagonists are under investigation as specific inhibitors of the renin-angiotensin system.[1,2] Remikiren is a nonpeptide that is active intravenously and orally, but it is reported to have a very low oral bioavailability.

1. Frishman WH, *et al.* Renin inhibition: a new approach to cardiovascular therapy. *J Clin Pharmacol* 1994; **34:** 873–80.
2. Rongen GA, *et al.* Clinical pharmacokinetics and efficacy of renin inhibitors. *Clin Pharmacokinet* 1995; **29:** 6–14.

Rescinnamine (900-b)

Rescinnamine *(BAN, rINN).*

Methyl-O-(3,4,5-trimethoxycinnamoyl)reserpate.

$C_{35}H_{42}N_2O_9$ = 634.7.

CAS — 24815-24-5.

An ester alkaloid isolated from the root of *Rauwolfia serpentina* or *R. vomitoria.*

Rescinnamine has properties similar to those described under reserpine (below) and has been used in the treatment of hypertension.

Preparations

Proprietary Preparations (details are given in Part 3)
USA: Moderil†.

Multi-ingredient: ***Aust.:*** Modenol; ***Ger.:*** Diuraupur sine†; Diuraupur†; ***S.Afr.:*** Saltucin Co†; ***Spain:*** Diu Rauwiplus; ***Switz.:*** Modenol†.

Reserpine (901-v)

Reserpine *(BAN, rINN).*

Reserpinum. Methyl 11,17α-dimethoxy-18β-(3,4,5-trimethoxybenzoyloxy)-3β,20α-yohimbane-16β-carboxylate; Methyl O-(3,4,5-trimethoxybenzoyl)reserpate.

$C_{33}H_{40}N_2O_9$ = 608.7.

CAS — 50-55-5.

Pharmacopoeias. In *Chin., Eur.* (see p.viii), *Int., Jpn, Pol.,* and *US.*

An alkaloid obtained from the roots of certain species of *Rauwolfia* (Apocynaceae), mainly *Rauwolfia serpentina* and *R. vomitoria,* or by synthesis. The material obtained from natural sources may contain closely related alkaloids.

It occurs as odourless, small white or pale buff to slightly yellow-coloured crystals or crystalline powder. It darkens slowly on exposure to light but more rapidly when in solution.

Ph. Eur. **solubilities** are: practically insoluble in water and ether; very slightly soluble in alcohol. USP solubilities are: insoluble in water; very slightly soluble in ether; soluble 1 in 1800 of alcohol and 1 in 6 of chloroform; freely soluble in acetic acid. Reserpine is **unstable** in the presence of alkalis, particularly when the drug is in solution. **Store** in airtight containers. Protect from light.

Adverse Effects

Side-effects commonly include nasal congestion, headache and CNS symptoms including depression, drowsiness, dizziness, lethargy, nightmares, and symptoms of increased gastro-intestinal tract motility including diarrhoea, abdominal cramps, and, at higher doses, increased gastric acid secretion. Respiratory distress, cyanosis, anorexia, and lethargy may occur in infants whose mothers have received reserpine prior to delivery.

Higher doses may cause flushing, bradycardia, severe depression which may lead to suicide, and extrapyramidal effects. Hypotension, coma, convulsions, respiratory depression and hypothermia also occur in overdosage. Hypotension is also more common in patients following a cerebrovascular accident.

Breast engorgement and galactorrhoea, gynaecomastia, increased prolactin concentrations, decreased libido, impotence, sodium retention, oedema, decreased or increased appetite, weight gain, miosis, dry mouth, sialorrhoea, dysuria, rashes, pruritus, and thrombocytopenic purpura have also been reported.

Reserpine has been shown to be tumorigenic in *rodents* following administration of large doses. Several reports have suggested an association between the ingestion of reserpine and the development of neoplasms of the breast (see below) but other surveys have failed to confirm the association.

Neoplasms of the breast. Epidemiological studies by the Boston Collaborative Drug Surveillance Program,[1] Armstrong *et al.*[2] and Heinonen *et al.*[3] found that the incidence of breast cancer was up to 3 to 4 times greater in hypertensive women treated with rauwolfia preparations than in control groups, and the findings were subsequently supported to some degree by a further study by Armstrong *et al.*[4] The studies were criticised especially for the selections of control series[5-7] although the validity of the criticisms was itself questioned.[8-10] Subsequent studies, however, have failed to find an association between reserpine and breast cancer[11-17] although the difficulties in proving no association were discussed by Jick.[10]

1. Boston Collaborative Drug Surveillance Program. Reserpine and breast cancer. *Lancet* 1974; **ii:** 669–71.
2. Armstrong B, *et al.* Retrospective study of the association between use of rauwolfia derivatives and breast cancer in English women. *Lancet* 1974; **ii:** 672–5.
3. Heinonen OP, *et al.* Reserpine use in relation to breast cancer. *Lancet* 1974; **ii:** 675–7.
4. Armstrong B, *et al.* Rauwolfia derivatives and breast cancer in hypertensive women. *Lancet* 1976; **ii:** 8–12.
5. Immich H. Rauwolfia derivatives and cancer. *Lancet* 1974; **ii:** 774–5.
6. Mann RD, *et al.* Rauwolfia derivatives and breast cancer. *Lancet* 1974; **ii:** 966.
7. Siegel C, Laska E. Rauwolfia derivatives and breast cancer. *Lancet* 1974; **ii:** 966–7.
8. Boston Collaborative Drug Surveillance Program Research Group. Rauwolfia derivatives and breast cancer. *Lancet* 1974; **ii:** 1315–16.
9. Heinonen OP, Shapiro S. Rauwolfia derivatives and breast cancer. *Lancet* 1974; **ii:** 1316.
10. Jick H. Reserpine and breast cancer: a perspective. *JAMA* 1975; **233:** 896–7.
11. Mack TM, *et al.* Reserpine and breast cancer in a retirement community. *N Engl J Med* 1975; **292:** 1366–71.
12. O'Fallon WM, *et al.* Rauwolfia derivatives and breast cancer. *Lancet* 1975; **ii:** 292–6.
13. Laska EM, *et al.* Matched-pairs study of reserpine use and breast cancer. *Lancet* 1975; **ii:** 296–300.
14. Christopher LJ, *et al.* A multicentre study of rauwolfia derivatives and breast cancer. *Eur J Clin Pharmacol* 1977; **11:** 409–17.
15. Labarthe DR, O'Fallon WM. Reserpine and breast cancer: a community-based longitudinal study of 2000 hypertensive women. *JAMA* 1980; **243:** 2304–10.
16. Curb JD, *et al.* Reserpine and breast cancer in the Hypertension Detection and Follow-up Program. *Hypertension* 1982; **4:** 307–11.
17. Friedman GD. Rauwolfia and breast cancer: no relation found in long term users age fifty and over. *J Chron Dis* 1983; **36:** 367–70.

Treatment of Adverse Effects

Withdrawal of reserpine or reduction of the dosage causes the reversal of many side-effects although mental disorders may persist for months and hypotensive effects may persist for weeks after the cessation of treatment. If overdosage occurs the stomach should be emptied by lavage even if several hours have elapsed after ingestion. Treatment is generally supportive and symptomatic. Severe hypotension may respond to placing the patient in the supine position with the feet raised. Direct-acting sympathomimetics may be effective for treatment of severe hypotension, but should be given with caution. The patient must be observed for at least 72 hours.

Precautions

Reserpine should not be used in patients with depression or a history of depression, with active peptic ulcer, or ulcerative colitis, and in patients with Parkinson's disease. It should also be avoided in phaeochromocytoma.

It should be used with caution in debilitated or elderly patients, and in the presence of cardiac arrhythmias, myocardial infarction, renal insufficiency, gallstones, epilepsy, or allergic conditions such as bronchial asthma.

If used in patients requiring electroconvulsive therapy an interval of at least 7 to 14 days should be allowed to elapse between the last dose of reserpine and the commencement of the shock treatment.

It is probably not necessary to discontinue treatment with reserpine during anaesthesia, although the effects of CNS depressants may be enhanced by reserpine.

Interactions

Patients taking reserpine may be hypersensitive to adrenaline and other direct-acting sympathomimetics which should not be given except to antagonise reserpine. The effects of indirect-acting sympathomimetics such as ephedrine may be decreased by reserpine. The hypotensive effects of reserpine are enhanced by thiazide diuretics and other antihypertensives. Reserpine may cause excitation and hypertension in patients receiving MAOIs. Concurrent administration of digitalis or quinidine may cause cardiac arrhythmias. Reserpine may enhance the effects of CNS depressants.

Pharmacokinetics

Reserpine is absorbed from the gastro-intestinal tract with a reported bioavailability of 50%. It is extensively metabolised and is excreted slowly in the urine and faeces. About 8% has been reported to be excreted in the urine in the first 4 days, mainly as metabolites; about 60% has been reported to be excreted in the faeces in the first 4 days, mainly unchanged. Reserpine crosses the placenta and the blood-brain barrier and also appears in breast milk.

Uses and Administration

Reserpine is an antihypertensive drug that causes depletion of noradrenaline stores in peripheral sympathetic nerve terminals and depletion of catecholamine and serotonin stores in the brain, heart, and many other organs resulting in a reduction in blood pressure, bradycardia, and CNS depression. The hypotensive effect is mainly due to a reduction in cardiac output and a reduction in peripheral resistance. Cardiovascular reflexes are partially inhibited, but postural hypotension is rarely a problem at the doses used in hypertension. When given by mouth the full effect is only reached after several weeks of continued treatment and persists for up to 6 weeks after treatment is discontinued.

Reserpine has been used in the management of hypertension (p.788) and in chronic psychoses (p.636) such as schizophrenia. It has also been tried in the treatment of Raynaud's syndrome (p.794).

In hypertension, reserpine is given by mouth in an initial dose of up to 500 μg daily for about 2 weeks, subsequently reduced to the lowest dose necessary to maintain the response; some sources have recommended an initial dose of 100 μg. A maintenance dose of about 250 μg daily is usually adequate and 500 μg should not normally be exceeded. To reduce side-effects and tolerance smaller doses of reserpine may be given in conjunction with a thiazide diuretic.

Reserpine has been used in chronic psychoses in daily doses of up to 1 mg.

Preparations

USP 23: Reserpine and Chlorothiazide Tablets; Reserpine and Hydrochlorothiazide Tablets; Reserpine Elixir; Reserpine Injection; Reserpine Tablets; Reserpine, Hydralazine Hydrochloride, and Hydrochlorothiazide Tablets.

Proprietary Preparations (details are given in Part 3)
Canad.: Serpasil; ***Ital.:*** Serpasil†; ***Spain:*** Serpasol†; ***USA:*** Sandril†; Serpalan.

Multi-ingredient: ***Aust.:*** Adelphan-Esidrex; Adelphan-Esidrex-K†; Bendigon†; Brinerdin; Darebon; Elfanex; Modenol; Pressimedin; Resaltex; Supergan; Suprenoat; Terbolan; ***Canad.:*** Hydropres; Hygroton-Reserpine†; Ser-Ap-Es; Serpasil-Esidrix†; ***Fr.:*** Tensionorme; ***Ger.:*** Adelphan-Esidrix; Adelphan†; Barotonal; Bendigon N; Briserin N; Calmoserpin†; Caprinol†; Darebon; Disalpin; Diuraupur†; Drenusil-R†; Durotan; Elfanex†; Modenol; Nortensin†; Rau-D-Tablinen†; Resaltex; Tonamyl†; Tri-Thiazid Reserpin; Triniton; ***Ital.:*** Adelfan-Esidrex†; Adelfan†; Axiten Tre†; Brinerdina; Diertina Ipotensiva†; Diuritens†; Igroton-Reserpina; Ipotex†; Lasix-Reserpin†; Raufluin†; Sermidrina†; Sfigmoreg†; ***Neth.:*** Brinerdin†; ***S.Afr.:*** Adelphane-Esidrex†; Brinerdin; Hygroton-Reserpine; Protensin-M; Saltucin Co†; Serpasil-Navidrex-K†; ***Spain:*** Adelfan-Esidrex; Adelfan†; Brinerdina; Diu Rauwiplus; Endofren†; Higrotona Reserpina; Neo Endofren†; Picten†; Resnedal; Tensiocomplet; ***Switz.:*** Adelphan-Esidrex; Adelphan-Esidrex-K†; Adelphan†; Brinerdine; Hygroton-Reserpine; Modenol†; Pressimed; ***USA:*** Cam-ap-es†; Chloroserpine†; Demi-Regroton; Diupres†; Diutensen-R; HHR†; Hydrap-ES; Hydro-Serp; Hydropres; Hydroserpine; Hydrosine†; Marpres; Metatensin; Regroton; Renese R; Salutensin; Ser-Ap-Es; Tri-Hydroserpine; Unipres†.

Reteplase (17311-s)

Reteplase *(BAN, USAN, rINN).*

BM-06.022; rPA. 173-L-Serine-174-L-tyrosine-175-L-glutamine-173–527-plasminogen activator (human tissue-type).

$C_{1736}H_{2653}N_{499}O_{522}S_{22}$ = 39571.1.

CAS — 133652-38-7.

A nonglycosylated protein produced by recombinant DNA technology that consists of selected domains of human tissue plasminogen activator.

Adverse Effects, Treatment, and Precautions

As for Streptokinase, p.948.

Interactions

As for Streptokinase, p.950.

Pharmacokinetics

Reteplase is reported to have a fibrinolytic half-life of about 1.6 hours in patients with myocardial infarction.

Uses and Administration

Reteplase is a thrombolytic drug. It converts plasminogen to plasmin, a proteolytic enzyme which has fibrinolytic effects. The mechanisms of fibrinolysis are discussed further under Haemostasis on p.704.

Reteplase is used similarly to streptokinase (p.950) in the management of coronary occlusion in myocardial infarction (p.791). It is given intravenously as soon as possible after the onset of symptoms. The dose is 10 units given by slow intravenous injection (but over not more than 2 minutes) and this dose of 10 units is repeated once 30 minutes after the start of the first injection.

General references.

1. Noble S, McTavish D. Reteplase: a review of its pharmacological properties and clinical efficacy in the management of acute myocardial infarction. *Drugs* 1996; **52:** 589–605.

Preparations

Proprietary Preparations (details are given in Part 3)
Fr.: Rapilysin; ***Ger.:*** Rapilysin; ***Swed.:*** Rapilysin; ***UK:*** Rapilysin; ***USA:*** Retavase.

Reviparin Sodium (15402-t)

Reviparin Sodium *(BAN, rINN)*.

Reviparin sodium is prepared by nitrous acid depolymerisation of heparin obtained from the intestinal mucosa of pigs. The majority of the components have a 2-*O*-sulpho-α-L-idopyranosuronic acid structure at the non-reducing end and a 6-*O*-sulpho-2,5-anhydro-D-mannitol structure at the reducing end of their chain. The mass-average molecular mass ranges between 3150 and 5150 with a characteristic value of about 4150. The degree of sulphation is about 2.1 per disaccharide unit.

Reviparin sodium is a low-molecular-weight heparin (p.899) with anticoagulant activity used in the prevention of postoperative venous thrombo-embolism.

References.

1. The Columbus Investigators. Low-molecular-weight heparin in the treatment of patients with venous thromboembolism. *N Engl J Med* 1997; **337:** 657–62.

Preparations

Proprietary Preparations (details are given in Part 3)
Fr.: Clivarine; ***Ger.:*** Clivarin; ***Swed.:*** Clivarin.

Rilmenidine Phosphate (14744-w)

Rilmenidine Phosphate *(rINNM)*.

Oxaminozoline Phosphate; Rilmenidine Acid Phosphate; Rilmenidine Hydrogen Phosphate; S-3341-3. 2-[(Dicyclopropylmethyl)amino]-2-oxazoline phosphate.

$C_{10}H_{16}N_2O,H_3PO_4$ = 278.2.

CAS — 54187-04-1 (rilmenidine); 85409-38-7 (rilmenidine phosphate).

Rilmenidine is a centrally acting antihypertensive that appears to act through stimulation of central imidazoline receptors and also has alpha$_2$-adrenoceptor agonist activity. It has general properties similar to those of clonidine (p.841), but is reported to cause less sedation and central adverse effects. In the management of hypertension (p.788) it has been given as the phosphate, in doses equivalent to 1 mg of base daily, as a single dose by mouth; this may be increased if necessary, after 1 month, to 2 mg daily in divided doses.

References.

1. Fillastre JP, Vanhoutte PM, eds. Second international symposium on rilmenidine. *Am J Med* 1989; **87** (suppl 3C): 1S–74S.

Preparations

Proprietary Preparations (details are given in Part 3)
Fr.: Hyperium.

Saralasin Acetate (902-g)

Saralasin Acetate *(BANM, USAN, rINNM)*.

P-113; The acetate of 1-Sar-8-Ala-angiotensin II. The hydrated acetate of Sar-Arg-Val-Tyr-Val-His-Pro-Ala; [1-(*N*-Methylglycine)-5-L-valine-8-L-alanine]-angiotensin II acetate hydrate.

$C_{42}H_{65}N_{13}O_{10}$, xCH_3COOH, xH_2O = 912.0 (saralasin).

CAS — 34273-10-4 (saralasin); 54194-01-3 (anhydrous saralasin); 39698-78-7 (saralasin acetate, hydrate).

Saralasin acetate is a competitive antagonist of angiotensin II and thus blocks its pressor action. It is also a partial agonist and causes a transient initial rise in blood pressure. Saralasin has a short half-life and has been used in the differential diagnosis of renovascular hypertension: following intravenous administration, saralasin commonly causes a fall in blood pressure in patients with renovascular hypertension, whereas patients with low-renin essential hypertension may have a sustained pressor response. The reaction is affected by sodium balance and patients are normally mildly depleted of sodium before the test. False positive and false negative results are numerous, and the use of saralasin has largely been superseded by the ACE inhibitors.

Preparations

Proprietary Preparations (details are given in Part 3)
Ger.: Sarenin NT†.

Sarpogrelate Hydrochloride (14655-s)

Sarpogrelate Hydrochloride *(rINNM)*.

(±)-2-(Dimethylamino)-1-{[*o*-(*m*-methoxyphenethyl)phenoxy]methyl}ethyl hydrogen succinate hydrochloride.

$C_{24}H_{31}NO_6$,HCl = 466.0.

CAS — 125926-17-2 (sarpogrelate).

Sarpogrelate is an inhibitor of platelet aggregation used in thrombo-embolic disorders. It has been given by mouth as the hydrochloride.

Preparations

Proprietary Preparations (details are given in Part 3)
Jpn: Anplag.

Saruplase (248-z)

Saruplase *(BAN, rINN)*.

Prourokinase (enzyme-activating) (human clone pUK4/pUK18), non-glycosylated; Recombinant Human Single-Chain Urokinase-type Plasminogen Activator; scuPA.

$C_{2031}H_{3121}N_{585}O_{601}S_{31}$ = 46343.1.

CAS — 99149-95-8.

Saruplase is a thrombolytic drug. It is a urokinase-type plasminogen activator with a single chain structure prepared via recombinant DNA technology and is converted to urokinase (p.959) in the body by plasmin. It also has some intrinsic plasminogen-activating properties and is reported to have greater selectivity for fibrin-bound plasminogen than for plasma plasminogen. Saruplase is under investigation in the thrombolytic therapy of acute myocardial infarction and ischaemic stroke.

References.

1. Koster RW, *et al.* Pharmacokinetics and pharmacodynamics of saruplase, an unglycosylated single-chain urokinase-type plasminogen activator, in patients with acute myocardial infarction. *Thromb Haemost* 1994; **72:** 740–4.

Sibrafiban (10240-d)

Sibrafiban *(rINN)*.

Ethyl (*Z*)-[(1-{*N*-[(*p*-hydroxyamidino)benzoyl]-L-alanyl}-4-piperidyl)oxy] acetate.

$C_{20}H_{28}N_4O_6$ = 420.5.

Sibrafiban is a glycoprotein IIb/IIIa-receptor antagonist under investigation as an antiplatelet drug in unstable angina and myocardial infarction.

References.

1. Cannon CP, *et al.* Randomized trial of an oral platelet glycoprotein IIb/IIIa antagonist, sibrafiban, in patients after an acute coronary syndrome: results of the TIMI 12 trial. *Circulation* 1998; **97:** 340–9.

Sodium Apolate (13240-n)

Sodium Apolate *(BAN, rINN)*.

Lyapolate Sodium *(USAN)*; Sodium Lyapolate. Poly(sodium ethylenesulphonate).

$(C_2H_3NaO_3S)_n$.

CAS — 25053-27-4.

Sodium apolate is a synthetic heparinoid anticoagulant. It has been employed in the topical treatment of haematomas and superficial thromboses and for the relief of sprains and contusions.

Preparations

Proprietary Preparations (details are given in Part 3)
Ger.: Pergagel†.

Multi-ingredient: ***Austral.:*** Pergalen†; ***Fr.:*** Pergalen†; ***Ger.:*** Pergalen†.

Sodium Nitroprusside (903-q)

Disodium (*OC*-6-22)-Pentakis(cyano-*C*)nitrosylferrate Dihydrate; Natrii Nitroprussias; Sodium Nitroferricyanide Dihydrate; Sodium Nitroprussiate. Sodium nitrosylpentacyanoferrate(III) dihydrate.

$Na_2Fe(CN)_5NO,2H_2O$ = 297.9.

CAS — 14402-89-2 (anhydrous sodium nitroprusside); 13755-38-9 (sodium nitroprusside dihydrate).

Pharmacopoeias. In *Chin.*, *Eur.* (see p.viii), *Int.*, and *US.*

Reddish-brown almost odourless crystals or powder. Freely **soluble** in water; slightly soluble in alcohol; very slightly soluble in chloroform.

Store in airtight containers. Protect from light.

CAUTION. *Solutions of sodium nitroprusside decompose when exposed to light and must be protected during infusion by wrapping the container with aluminium foil or some other light-proof material. Nitroprusside will react with minute quantities of organic and inorganic substances forming highly coloured products. If this occurs the solution should be discarded. Solutions should not be used more than 24 hours after preparation.*

Stability in solution. The instability of sodium nitroprusside solutions has been the subject of considerable investigation. Schumacher has stated that it was more stable in acid than in alkaline solution,[1] but a later study by Hargrave found that whereas the initial light-induced darkening of a 1% solution was independent of pH, further degradation leading to the development of a blue precipitate required an acid pH.[2] If protected from light by wrapping in aluminium foil sodium nitroprusside 50 or 100 μg per mL was found to be stable in 5% glucose, lactated Ringer's, and normal saline solutions for 48 hours.[3] In clinical practice the infusion container should be opaque or protected with foil, but an amber giving set may be used in conjunction, which allows visual monitoring of the infusion.[4,5]

Various substances have been reported to increase the stability of nitroprusside solutions, including dimethyl sulphoxide,[6] glycerol,[1] sodium citrate,[1] and other salts with anionic chelating potential such as sodium acetate or phosphate.[1] In contrast sodium bisulphite and the hydroxybenzoates are reported to reduce stability.[1]

1. Schumacher GE. Sodium nitroprusside injection. *Am J Hosp Pharm* 1966; **23:** 532.
2. Hargrave RE. Degradation of solutions of sodium nitroprusside. *J Hosp Pharm* 1974; **32:** 188–91.
3. Mahony C, *et al.* In vitro stability of sodium nitroprusside solutions for intravenous administration. *J Pharm Sci* 1984; **73:** 838–9.
4. Davidson SW, Lyall D. Sodium nitroprusside stability in light-protective administration sets. *Pharm J* 1987; **239:** 599–601.
5. Lyall D. Sodium nitroprusside stability. *Pharm J* 1988; **240:** 5.
6. Asker AF, Gragg R. Dimethyl sulfoxide as a photoprotective agent for sodium nitroprusside solutions. *Drug Dev Ind Pharm* 1983; **9:** 837–48.

Adverse Effects

Sodium nitroprusside rapidly reduces blood pressure and is converted in the body to cyanide and then thiocyanate. Its adverse effects can be attributed mainly to excessive hypotension and excessive cyanide accumulation; thiocyanate toxicity may also occur, especially in patients with renal impairment. Intravenous infusion of sodium nitroprusside may produce nausea and vomiting, apprehension, headache, dizziness, restlessness, perspiration, palpitations, retrosternal discomfort, abdominal pain, and muscle twitching, but these effects may be reduced by slowing the rate of infusion.

An excessive amount of cyanide in plasma (more than 0.08 μg per mL), because of overdosage or depletion of endogenous thiosulphate (which converts cyanide to thiocyanate *in vivo*), may result in tachycardia, sweating, hyperventilation, arrhythmias, and profound metabolic acidosis. Metabolic acidosis may be the first sign of cyanide toxicity. Methaemoglobinaemia may also occur.

Adverse effects attributed to thiocyanate include tinnitus, miosis, and hyperreflexia; confusion, hallucinations, and convulsions have also been reported.

Other adverse effects include thrombocytopenia and phlebitis.

Effects on the blood. THROMBOCYTOPENIA. Platelet counts decreased in 7 of 8 patients with heart failure 1 to 6 hours after intravenous infusion of nitroprusside was started.[1] The counts began to return to normal 24 hours after the infusion was stopped.

1. Mehta P, *et al.* Nitroprusside lowers platelet count. *N Engl J Med* 1978; **299:** 1134.

Effects on the gastro-intestinal tract. Five out of 38 patients who were given sodium nitroprusside intravenously for controlled hypotension during surgery developed symptoms of adynamic ileus postoperatively.[1] The authors suggested that the symptoms could be secondary to intestinal ischaemia due to diminished mesenteric arterial blood flow. However, other explanations have been proposed including sympathetic stimulation[2,3] or the concomitant use of opioid analgesics.[4]

1. Chen JW, *et al.* Adynamic ileus following induced hypotension. *JAMA* 1985; **253:** 633.
2. Gelman S. Adynamic ileus following induced hypotension. *JAMA* 1985; **254:** 1721.
3. Lampert BA. Adynamic ileus following induced hypotension. *JAMA* 1985; **254:** 1721.
4. Lemmo J, Karnes J. Adynamic ileus following induced hypotension. *JAMA* 1985; **254:** 1721.

Effects on intracranial pressure. Turner and colleagues have reported that intracranial pressure rose significantly while the mean blood pressure was 90 or 80% of initial values in 14 normocapnic patients given an infusion of sodium nitroprusside to produce controlled hypotension prior to neurosurgery; values reverted towards normal at mean blood pressures of 70% of controls.[1] A similar but insignificant trend occurred in 5 hypocapnic patients. In another report Griswold and others have noted a rise in intracranial pressure following the use of nitroprusside in a patient with Reye's syndrome.[2]

1. Turner JM, *et al.* Intracranial pressure changes in neurosurgical patients during hypotension induced with sodium nitroprusside or trimetaphan. *Br J Anaesth* 1977; **49:** 419–24.
2. Griswold WR, *et al.* Nitroprusside-induced intracranial hypertension. *JAMA* 1981; **246:** 2679–80.

Phlebitis. Acute transient phlebitis has occurred following sodium nitroprusside administration.[1]

1. Miller R, Stark DCC. Acute phlebitis from nitroprusside. *Anesthesiology* 1978; **49:** 372.

Treatment of Adverse Effects

Side-effects due to excessive hypotension may be treated by slowing or discontinuing the infusion.

For details of the treatment of cyanide poisoning see Hydrocyanic Acid, p.1407. Thiocyanate can be removed by dialysis. Hydroxocobalamin can be given to reduce cyanide concentrations, but is of little value in acute poisoning because of the large quantities required.

A review of the literature[1] concluded that hydroxocobalamin was safe and effective in the prevention and treatment of cyanide toxicity due to nitroprusside although, as the manufacturers have pointed out, hydroxocobalamin is probably impractical in acute treatment of cyanide poisoning because of the large amount required. In a study involving 14 patients requiring nitroprusside hypotensive anaesthesia,[2] blood-cyanide concentrations of those who concomitantly received an intravenous infusion of hydroxocobalamin 100 mg in 100 mL of glucose injection at a rate of 12.5 mg per 30 minutes throughout the duration of nitroprusside administration, were decreased compared with those who received nitroprusside alone. They received a total of 87.5 to 100 mg of hydroxocobalamin.

1. Zerbe NF, Wagner BKJ. Use of vitamin B_{12} in the treatment and prevention of nitroprusside-induced cyanide toxicity. *Crit Care Med* 1993; **21:** 465–7.

2. Cottrell JE, *et al.* Prevention of nitroprusside-induced cyanide toxicity with hydroxocobalamin. *N Engl J Med* 1978; **298:** 809–11.

Precautions

Sodium nitroprusside should not be used in the presence of compensatory hypertension (for example, in arteriovenous shunts or coarctation of the aorta). It should be used with caution in patients with impaired hepatic function, in patients with low plasma-cobalamin concentrations or Leber's optic atrophy. Some authorities consider that it is contra-indicated in such patients if the impairment is severe. It should also be used with caution in patients with impaired renal or pulmonary function and with particular caution in patients with impaired cerebrovascular circulation. The use of hydroxocobalamin before and during administration of sodium nitroprusside, has been advocated. Thiocyanate, a metabolite of sodium nitroprusside, inhibits iodine binding and uptake and sodium nitroprusside should be used with caution in patients with hypothyroidism. The plasma-thiocyanate concentration should be monitored if treatment continues for more than 3 days and should not exceed 100 μg per mL although toxicity may be apparent at lower thiocyanate concentrations. Thiocyanate concentrations do not reflect cyanide toxicity and cyanide concentrations should also be monitored; the blood concentration of cyanide should not exceed 1 μg per mL and the plasma concentration should not exceed 0.08 μg per mL. The acid-base balance should also be monitored. Care should be taken to ensure that extravasation does not occur.

Tachyphylaxis. Tachyphylaxis to sodium nitroprusside was associated with high plasma concentrations of cyanide without metabolic acidosis in 3 patients undergoing hypotensive anaesthesia.[1]

1. Cottrell JE, *et al.* Nitroprusside tachyphylaxis without acidosis. *Anesthesiology* 1978; **49:** 141–2.

Withdrawal. Rebound haemodynamic changes, including hypertension and increased heart rate, occurred 10 to 30 minutes after discontinuation of intravenous sodium nitroprusside infusion in a study in 20 patients with heart failure.[1] The changes generally resolved spontaneously within 1 to 3 hours after drug withdrawal and produced only minimal exacerbation of symptoms in most patients, although 3 patients developed pulmonary oedema 20 to 30 minutes after stopping the nitroprusside infusion that required reinstitution of nitroprusside in 2 of them. A study investigating a possible mechanism for this effect[2] found that plasma-renin concentrations were increased during infusion of nitroprusside and remained elevated for 30 minutes after the infusion was stopped. It was suggested that this persistence of elevated plasma-renin concentrations after clearance of short-lived nitroprusside may be responsible for the rebound effects.

1. Packer M, *et al.* Rebound hemodynamic events after the abrupt withdrawal of nitroprusside in patients with severe chronic heart failure. *N Engl J Med* 1979; **301:** 1193–7.
2. Cottrell JE, *et al.* Rebound hypertension after sodium nitroprusside-induced hypotension. *Clin Pharmacol Ther* 1980; **27:** 32–6.

Interactions

Enhanced hypotension should be expected if sodium nitroprusside is used concomitantly with other antihypertensive drugs or drugs that produce hypotension.

Alteplase. Sodium nitroprusside infusion prolonged the fibrinolytic activity of alteplase when given concomitantly to *animals*; use of nitrovasodilators with alteplase may be responsible for the enhanced bleeding tendency seen in some patients on thrombolytic therapy.[1]

1. Korbut R, *et al.* Prolongation of fibrinolytic activity of tissue plasminogen activator by nitrovasodilators. *Lancet* 1990; **335:** 669.

Pharmacokinetics

Sodium nitroprusside is converted in the erythrocytes to cyanide. Nitric oxide is also released *in vivo*. Cyanide is metabolised in the liver to thiocyanate by the enzyme rhodanase in the presence of thiosulphate and slowly excreted in the urine. The plasma half-life of thiocyanate is reported to be about 3 days, but may be much longer in patients with renal impairment.

Reviews.

1. Schulz V. Clinical pharmacokinetics of nitroprusside, cyanide, thiosulphate and thiocyanate. *Clin Pharmacokinet* 1984; **9:** 239–51.

Metabolism. Although Bisset and colleagues questioned the liberation of cyanide from nitroprusside *in vivo*, suggesting that reported values were due to photodecomposition prior to infusion of nitroprusside, or flaws in the assay technique, or both,[1,2] Vesey and co-workers have shown that incubation of nitroprusside with blood (but not with assay reagents) produced significant amounts of cyanide *in vitro*,[3] and have provided further evidence for breakdown of nitroprusside to cyanide *in vivo*.[4]

1. Bisset WIK, *et al.* Sodium nitroprusside and cyanide release: reasons for re-appraisal. *Br J Anaesth* 1981; **53:** 1015–18.
2. Butler AR, *et al.* Sodium nitroprusside and cyanide release. *Br J Anaesth* 1982; **54:** 792–3.
3. Vesey CJ, *et al.* Decay of nitroprusside I: in vitro. *Br J Anaesth* 1990; **64:** 696–703.
4. Vesey CJ, *et al.* Decay of nitroprusside II: in vivo. *Br J Anaesth* 1990; **64:** 704–9.

Uses and Administration

Sodium nitroprusside is a short-acting hypotensive drug with a duration of action of 1 to 10 minutes. It produces peripheral vasodilatation and reduces peripheral resistance by a direct action on both veins and arterioles. It has been termed a nitrovasodilator because it releases nitric oxide *in vivo*. Its effects appear within a few seconds of intravenous infusion. Sodium nitroprusside is used in the treatment of hypertensive crises (p.788) and to produce controlled hypotension during general anaesthesia. It has also been used to reduce preload and afterload in severe heart failure (p.785) including that associated with myocardial infarction (p.791).

It is given by continuous intravenous infusion of a solution containing 50 to 200 μg per mL. A controlled infusion device must be used. The solution should be prepared immediately before use by dissolving sodium nitroprusside in 5% glucose injection and then diluting with 5% glucose; the solution must be protected from light during administration. Blood pressure should be monitored closely during administration and care should be taken to prevent extravasation. In general, treatment should not continue for more than 72 hours. If required for several days blood and plasma concentrations of cyanide should be monitored and should not exceed 1 μg per mL and 0.08 μg per mL respectively; thiocyanate concentrations in serum should also be measured if infusion continues for more than 72 hours and should not exceed 100 μg per mL. Since rebound hypertension has been reported when sodium nitroprusside is withdrawn, the infusion should be tailed off gradually over 10 to 30 minutes.

For **hypertensive crises** in patients not receiving antihypertensive drugs, a suggested initial dose is 0.3 μg per kg body-weight per minute increasing gradually under close supervision until the desired reduction in blood pressure is achieved. The average dose required to maintain the blood pressure 30 to 40% below the pretreatment diastolic blood pressure is 3 μg per kg per minute and the usual dose range is 0.5 to 6 μg per kg per minute. Lower doses should be used in patients already receiving other antihypertensives. The maximum recommended rate is about 8 μg per kg per minute in the UK, and 10 μg per kg per minute in the USA; infusions at these rates should be used for no longer than 10 minutes and should be stopped after 10 minutes if there is no response. If there is a response, sodium nitroprusside should ideally be given for only a few hours to avoid the risk of cyanide toxicity. An alternative antihypertensive that can be given by mouth should be introduced as soon as possible.

For the **induction of hypotension** during anaesthesia a maximum dose of 1.5 μg per kg body-weight per minute is recommended.

In **heart failure** an initial dose of 10 to 15 μg per minute has been recommended increasing by increments of 10 to 15 μg per minute every 5 to 10 minutes until the initial response is seen. The usual dosage range is 10 to 200 μg per minute and the dose should not exceed 280 μg per minute or 4 μg per kg body-weight per minute.

Sodium nitroprusside is also used as a reagent for detecting ketones in urine.

Administration in children. Although experience is more limited than with adults sodium nitroprusside has been successfully used in infants and children. Luderer and colleagues reported continuous infusion of nitroprusside at a rate of 2 to 4 μg per kg body-weight per minute for 28 days in an 11-year-old child with refractory hypertension, without any signs of thiocyanate toxicity.[1] Benitz and others reported on the use of sodium nitroprusside in 58 neonates with cardiovascular disorders or respiratory distress syndrome.[2] A usual initial dose of 0.25 to 0.5 μg per kg per minute was given, and the rate then repeatedly doubled at intervals of 15 to 20 minutes until the desired effect was achieved, or adverse effects supervened or it was judged ineffective. The maximum rate did not exceed 6.0 μg per kg per minute. Reviewing their experience over 10 years, Deal and others had used infusion of sodium nitroprusside in doses of 0.5 to 8 μg per kg per minute to produce controlled reduction of blood pressure in 28 children with hypertensive crises; 16 had also received labetalol.[3]

1. Luderer JR, *et al.* Long-term administration of sodium nitroprusside in childhood. *J Pediatr* 1977; **91:** 490–1.
2. Benitz WE, *et al.* Use of sodium nitroprusside in neonates: efficacy and safety. *J Pediatr* 1985; **106:** 102–10.
3. Deal JE, *et al.* Management of hypertensive emergencies. *Arch Dis Child* 1992; **67:** 1089–92.

Ergotamine poisoning. For the use of sodium nitroprusside in the treatment of cyanosis of the extremities due to ergotamine overdosage, see Ergotamine Tartrate, p.446.

Peripheral vascular disease. Many drugs have been tried in Raynaud's syndrome, a vasospastic peripheral arterial disease (p.794). There was reference to clinical improvement with sodium nitroprusside infusion in the management of 2 children with severe Raynaud's disease[1] and it was suggested that sodium nitroprusside might be useful in the management of acute attacks of Raynaud's syndrome, but it does not appear to have come into widespread use.

1. Burns EC, *et al.* Raynaud's disease. *Arch Dis Child* 1985; **60:** 537–41.

Preparations

BP 1998: Sodium Nitroprusside Intravenous Infusion;
USP 23: Sodium Nitroprusside for Injection.

Proprietary Preparations (details are given in Part 3)

Belg.: Nipride†; ***Canad.:*** Nipride; ***Fr.:*** Nipride†; Nitriate; ***Ger.:*** nipruss; ***Irl.:*** Nipride; ***Neth.:*** Nipride†; ***S.Afr.:*** Hypoten; ***Spain:*** Nitroprussiat; ***Swed.:*** Nipride†; ***Switz.:*** Nipride†; ***UK:*** Nipride†; ***USA:*** Nitropress.

Sotalol Hydrochloride (6322-e)

Sotalol Hydrochloride *(BANM, USAN, rINNM)*.

MJ-1999; *d,l*-Sotalol Hydrochloride. 4′-(1-Hydroxy-2-isopropylaminoethyl)methanesulphonanilide hydrochloride.

$C_{12}H_{20}N_2O_3S,HCl = 308.8$.

CAS — 3930-20-9 (sotalol); 959-24-0 (sotalol hydrochloride).

Pharmacopoeias. In *Br.*

A white or almost white powder. Freely **soluble** in water; slightly soluble in alcohol; practically insoluble in chloroform.

Adverse Effects, Treatment, and Precautions

As for beta blockers, p.828.

Torsade de pointes has been reported in patients given sotalol, usually due to prolongation of the QT interval. The QT interval should be monitored; extreme caution is required if the QT interval exceeds 0.50 seconds and sotalol should be discontinued or the dose reduced if the QT interval exceeds 0.55 seconds. As hypokalaemia or hypomagnesaemia may predispose patients to arrhythmias, serum-electrolyte concentrations should be monitored before and during treatment with sotalol.

Sotalol is contra-indicated in patients with renal impairment whose creatinine clearance is less than 10 mL per minute.

Effects on the gastro-intestinal tract. A report of retroperitoneal fibrosis associated with the use of sotalol.[1]

1. Laakso M, *et al.* Retroperitoneal fibrosis associated with sotalol. *Br Med J* 1982; **285:** 1085–6.

Effects on the heart. Atypical ventricular tachycardia ('torsade de pointes') has been reported in patients receiving sotalol and may be associated with prolongation of the QT interval.[1,2] Hypokalaemia may contribute to sotalol's proarrhythmic effect and was considered relevant in 8 of 12 patients who developed ventricular tachycardia when given sotalol in association with hydrochlorothiazide; 4 patients were also receiving other drugs known to prolong the QT interval.[3] A meta-analysis[4] of 22 clinical trials involving 3135 patients who had taken sotalol orally found women to be at increased risk of developing torsade de pointes. Torsade de pointes developed in 44 (1.9%) of 2336 men and in 33 (4.1%) of 799 women.

In one patient torsade de pointes was treated successfully with magnesium sulphate by intravenous infusion and withdrawal of sotalol.[5]

1. Kontopoulos A, *et al.* Sotalol-induced torsade de pointes. *Postgrad Med J* 1981; **57:** 321–3.
2. Krapf R, Gertsch M. Torsade de pointes induced by sotalol despite therapeutic plasma sotalol concentrations. *Br Med J* 1985; **290:** 1784–5.
3. McKibbin JK, *et al.* Sotalol, hypokalaemia, syncope, and torsade de pointes. *Br Heart J* 1984; **541:** 157–62.
4. Lehmann MH, *et al.* Sex difference in risk of torsade de pointes with d,l-sotalol. *Circulation* 1996; **94:** 2534–41.
5. Arstall MA, *et al.* Sotalol-induced torsade de pointes: management with magnesium infusion. *Postgrad Med J* 1992; **68:** 289–90.

Interactions

Sotalol should not be given concurrently with other drugs that prolong the QT interval due to the increased risk of precipitating ventricular arrhythmias. Thus sotalol should not be given with antiarrhythmics such as amiodarone, disopyramide, procainamide, or quinidine, phenothiazine antipsychotics, tricyclic antidepressants, the antihistamines astemizole and terfenadine, erythromycin, halofantrine, pentamidine, sultopride, or vincamine. Also, sotalol should not be given with drugs that cause electrolyte disturbances such as diuretics.

Other interactions associated with beta blockers are discussed on p.829.

Pharmacokinetics

Sotalol is virtually completely absorbed from the gastro-intestinal tract and peak plasma concentrations are obtained about 2 to 4 hours after a dose. The plasma elimination half-life is about 10 to 20 hours. Sotalol has low lipid solubility. Very little is metabolised and it is excreted unchanged in the urine. Binding to plasma proteins is reported to be low. It crosses the placenta and is distributed into breast milk where higher concentrations have been achieved than in maternal serum. Only small amounts are reported to cross the blood-brain barrier and enter the CSF. Sotalol is removed by dialysis.

General references.

1. Singh BN, *et al.* Sotalol: a review of its pharmacodynamic and pharmacokinetic properties, and therapeutic use. *Drugs* 1987; **34:** 311–49.
2. Fitton A, Sorkin EM. Sotalol: an updated review of its pharmacological properties and therapeutic use in cardiac arrhythmias. *Drugs* 1993; **46:** 678–719.

Breast feeding. Sotalol is distributed into breast milk. Milk to serum ratios have been reported to range from 2.43 to 5.64.[1] It was calculated that a breast-fed infant may receive 20 to 23% of a maternal dose.

1. Hackett LP, *et al.* Excretion of sotalol in breast milk. *Br J Clin Pharmacol* 1990; **29:** 277–8.

Pregnancy. The pharmacokinetics of sotalol in 6 healthy pregnant subjects. The systemic clearance of sotalol following an intravenous dose was significantly higher during pregnancy than in the postnatal period, and the mean elimination half-life shorter (6.6 versus 9.3 hours) although the latter difference was not significant. Clearance following an oral dose was also higher during pregnancy than afterwards, but half-lives (10.9 versus 10.3 hours) and mean bioavailability were similar. The changes were probably due to alterations in renal function in the antenatal period.[1]

1. O'Hare MF, *et al.* Pharmacokinetics of sotalol during pregnancy. *Eur J Clin Pharmacol* 1983; **24:** 521–4.

Stereo-isomers. A pharmacokinetic study in 6 subjects given *d*-sotalol in doses of 0.25 to 2 mg per kg body-weight by intravenous infusion and a single dose of 100 mg by mouth.[1] Results suggest that *d*-sotalol has a linear pharmacokinetic profile over the doses studied. The oral absorption of *d*-sotalol was almost complete; peak concentrations were reached between 3 and 4 hours after oral administration. Unchanged *d*-sotalol was mainly excreted in the urine; an average of 75% of an intravenous dose was excreted in the urine within 48 hours. The elimination half-life averaged 7.2 and 7.5 hours following intravenous and oral administration respectively.

See under Action in Uses and Administration, below for further information on the stereo-isomers of sotalol.

1. Poirier JM, *et al.* The pharmacokinetics of d-sotalol and d,l-sotalol in healthy volunteers. *Eur J Clin Pharmacol* 1990; **38:** 579–82.

Uses and Administration

Sotalol is a non-cardioselective beta blocker (p.828). It is reported to lack both intrinsic sympathomimetic and membrane-stabilising properties. In addition to the class II antiarrhythmic activity of beta blockers, sotalol lengthens the duration of the action potential resulting in class III antiarrhythmic activity. For a classification and explanation of antiarrhythmic activity, see p.776.

Sotalol is used in the management of ventricular and supraventricular **arrhythmias** (p.782). It was also formerly used in the management of angina pectoris, hypertension, and myocardial infarction but, because of its proarrhythmic effect, it is no longer recommended for these indications. Its use in arrhythmias is restricted to severe disturbances. It should not be used in patients with asymptomatic ventricular arrhythmias.

Sotalol is usually given orally as the hydrochloride. Initiation of treatment should be in hospital with suitable monitoring facilities. The QT interval is monitored before the start of treatment and whenever the dosage is adjusted (see Precautions above). Plasma-electrolyte concentrations and renal function should also be monitored. The dosage is individualised according to the response of the patient. Doses are increased gradually allowing two or three days between dosing increments. A suggested initial dose of sotalol hydrochloride is 80 mg daily by mouth given as a single dose or in two divided doses. Most patients respond to doses of 160 to 320 mg daily (usually given in two divided doses). Some patients may require doses as high as 640 mg daily.

Sotalol may be given intravenously as the hydrochloride to control acute arrhythmias, to substitute for oral therapy, and for programmed electrical stimulation. To control acute arrhythmias, a dose of 20 to 120 mg (0.5 to 1.5 mg per kg body-weight) is given intravenously over 10 minutes. This dose may be repeated every six hours if necessary. To substitute for oral therapy an intravenous infusion of 0.2 to 0.5 mg per kg per hour may be used. The total daily dose should not exceed 640 mg. For programmed electrical stimulation (to test antiarrhythmic efficacy) an initial dose of 1.5 mg per kg of sotalol hydrochloride is given over 10 to 20 minutes, followed by an intravenous infusion of 0.2 to 0.5 mg per kg per hour.

The dose should be reduced in patients with renal impairment. The following dosage reductions have been recommended for both the oral and intravenous routes: half the dose in patients whose creatinine clearance is between 30 and 60 mL per minute, and quarter the dose in patients whose creatinine clearance is between 10 and 30 mL per minute. When sotalol is given orally the dosage interval may also be increased. At least five or six doses should be given before incremental dosage adjustments are made.

The use of sotalol as described above is as the racemic mixture; *d*-sotalol is under investigation as an antiarrhythmic (see under Action, below).

General references.

1. Fitton A, Sorkin EM. Sotalol: an updated review of its pharmacological properties and therapeutic use in cardiac arrhythmias. *Drugs* 1993; **46:** 678–719.
2. Nappi JM, McCollam PL. Sotalol: a breakthrough antiarrhythmic? *Ann Pharmacother* 1993; **27:** 1359–68.
3. Zanetti LAF. Sotalol: a new class III antiarrhythmic agent. *Clin Pharm* 1993; **12:** 883–91.
4. Hohnloser SH, Woosley RL. Sotalol. *N Engl J Med* 1994; **331:** 31–8.

Action. Sotalol is used as the racemic mixture of the two stereoisomers, *d*-sotalol ((+)-sotalol) and *l*-sotalol ((−)-sotalol). A comparison of the effects of *d*-sotalol and racemic sotalol in 6 healthy subjects[1] demonstrated that the beta-blocking activity resided almost entirely in the *l*-isomer, while the effects on the QT interval, which are consistent with type III antiarrhythmic activity, appear to be due to both isomers. A study in 8 healthy subjects also demonstrated a lack of beta blockade by *d*-sotalol.[2] This would suggest that the electrophysiological effects of sotalol are unrelated to its beta-blocking properties. *d*-Sotalol has been investigated as an antiarrhythmic.[3] However, a preliminary placebo-controlled study in patients with myocardial infarction at high risk of arrhythmia due to impaired left ventricular function was terminated early when increased mortality was seen in the treatment group.[4,5]

1. Johnston GD, *et al.* A comparison of the cardiovascular effects of (+)-sotalol and (±)-sotalol following intravenous administration in normal volunteers. *Br J Clin Pharmacol* 1985; **20:** 507–10.
2. Yasuda SU, *et al.* d-Sotalol reduces heart rate in vivo through a β-adrenergic receptor-independent mechanism. *Clin Pharmacol Ther* 1993; **53:** 436–42.
3. Advani SV, Singh BN. Pharmacodynamic, pharmacokinetic and antiarrhythmic properties of d-sotalol, the dextro-isomer of sotalol. *Drugs* 1995; **49:** 664–79.
4. Choo V. SWORD slashed. *Lancet* 1994; **344:** 1358.
5. Waldo AL, *et al.* Effect of d-sotalol on mortality in patients with left ventricular dysfunction after recent and remote myocardial infarction. *Lancet* 1996; **348:** 7–12. Correction. *ibid.*; 416.

Administration in renal impairment. Sotalol is excreted mainly by the renal route and elimination is therefore slower in patients with reduced renal function. Reduced doses and/or increased dosage intervals should be used (see above). In a study of 10 hypertensive patients with varying degrees of renal impairment, Berglund and colleagues[1] reported that the apparent first-order elimination rate constant and plasma clearance of sotalol correlated with glomerular filtration rate. Another study[2] compared kinetics in patients with normal renal function, renal insufficiency and renal failure. Elimination half-lives of 8.1 and 24.2 hours were reported in patients with creatinine clearance values above 39 mL per minute and clearance values between 8 and 38 mL per minute, respectively. It was suggested that an increase in the dosage interval to 48 or 72 hours may be necessary to compensate for longer half-lives. Caution is required when sotalol is administered to patients on dialysis; a half-life of 33.9 hours was reported in patients with renal failure but this fell to 5.8 hours during dialysis which removed approximately 43% of sotalol.

1. Berglund G, *et al.* Pharmacokinetics of sotalol after chronic administration to patients with renal insufficiency. *Eur J Clin Pharmacol* 1980; **18:** 321–6.
2. Blair AD, *et al.* Sotalol kinetics in renal insufficiency. *Clin Pharmacol Ther* 1981; **29:** 457–63.

Preparations

BP 1998: Sotalol Injection; Sotalol Tablets.

Proprietary Preparations (details are given in Part 3)
Aust.: Sotacor; ***Austral.:*** Cardol; Sotacor; ***Belg.:*** Sotalex; ***Canad.:*** Sotacor; ***Fr.:*** Sotalex; ***Ger.:*** CorSotalol; Darob; Gilucor; Rentibloc; Sota-saar; Sotabeta; Sotahexal; Sotalex; Sotaryt; Sotastad; Tachytalol; ***Irl.:*** Sotacor; ***Ital.:*** Betades; Sotalex; ***Neth.:*** Sotacor; ***Norw.:*** Sotacor; ***S.Afr.:*** Sotacor; ***Spain:*** Sotapor; ***Swed.:*** Darob; Sotacor; ***Switz.:*** Sotalex; ***UK:*** Beta-Cardone; Sotacor; ***USA:*** Betapace.

Multi-ingredient: ***Ger.:*** Sotazident†; ***Irl.:*** Sotazide†; ***S.Afr.:*** Sotazide†; ***Swed.:*** Sotacor/ASA†; ***UK:*** Sotazide†; Tolerzide†.

Spirapril Hydrochloride (2542-j)

Spirapril Hydrochloride *(BANM, USAN, rINNM).*

Sch-33844. (*S*)-7-{*N*-[(*S*)-1-Ethoxycarbonyl-3-phenylpropyl]-L-alanyl}-1,4-dithia-7-azaspiro[4.4]nonane-8-carboxylic acid hydrochloride.

$C_{22}H_{30}N_2O_5S_2$,HCl = 503.1.

CAS — 83647-97-6 (spirapril); 94841-17-5 (spirapril hydrochloride).

Spirapril is an ACE inhibitor (p.805) that is used in the management of hypertension. It owes its activity to the diacid spiraprilat, to which it is converted after oral administration.

References.

1. Noble S, Sorkin EM. Spirapril: a preliminary review of its pharmacology and therapeutic efficacy in the treatment of hypotension. *Drugs* 1995; **49:** 750–66.
2. Widimský J, *et al.* Czech and Slovak spirapril intervention study (CASSIS): a randomized, placebo and active-controlled, double-blind multicentre trial in patients with congestive heart failure. *Eur J Clin Pharmacol* 1995; **49:** 95–102.

Preparations

Proprietary Preparations (details are given in Part 3)
Aust.: Sandopril; ***Ital.:*** Setrilan; ***Switz.:*** Cardiopril; ***USA:*** Renormax.

Spironolactone (2355-e)

Spironolactone *(BAN, rINN).*

Espironolactona; SC-9420; Spirolactone; Spironolactonum. 7α-Acetylthio-3-oxo-17α-pregn-4-ene-21,17β-carbolactone; (7α,17α)-7-(Acetylthio)-17-hydroxy-3-oxo-pregn-4-ene-21-carboxylic acid γ-lactone.

$C_{24}H_{32}O_4S$ = 416.6.

CAS — 52-01-7.

NOTE. Compounded preparations of equal parts by weight of spironolactone and hydroflumethiazide have the British Approved Name Co-flumactone.

Compounded preparations of spironolactone and hydrochlorothiazide in USP 23 may be represented by the name Co-spironozide.

Pharmacopoeias. In *Chin., Eur.* (see p.viii), *Int., Jpn, Pol.,* and *US.*

A white or yellowish-white crystalline powder; it has a slight characteristic odour. Practically **insoluble** in water; soluble in alcohol and in ethyl acetate; freely soluble in chloroform; slightly soluble in ether, in methyl alcohol, and in fixed oils. **Protect** from light.

Stability. There was no appreciable loss of spironolactone from extemporaneously prepared suspensions of spironolactone, 2.5, 5.0, and 10.0 mg per mL, in a cherry syrup after storage for 2 weeks at 5° or 30° or at ambient room temperature under intense fluorescent light.[1] Degradation was less than 5% for samples stored for 4 weeks, but was more noticeable in suspensions with a higher initial concentration. There were no changes in colour or odour. Bacterial and fungal counts were well within acceptable limits after 4 weeks at 30°.

1. Mathur LK, Wickman A. Stability of extemporaneously compounded spironolactone suspensions. *Am J Hosp Pharm* 1989; **46:** 2040–2.

Adverse Effects

Spironolactone may give rise to headache and drowsiness, and gastro-intestinal disturbances, including cramp and diarrhoea. Ataxia, mental confusion, and skin rashes have been reported as side-effects. Gynaecomastia is not uncommon and in rare cases breast enlargement may persist. Other endocrine disorders include hirsutism, deepening of the voice, menstrual irregularities, and impotence. Transient increases in blood-urea-nitrogen concentrations may occur and mild acidosis has been reported. Spironolactone has been demonstrated to cause tumours in *rats.*

Spironolactone may cause hyponatraemia and hyperkalaemia.

A survey indicated that of 788 patients who received spironolactone 164 developed side-effects.[1] These included hyperkalaemia in 8.6%, dehydration in 3.4%, hyponatraemia in 2.4%, gastro-intestinal disorders in 2.3%, neurological disorders in 2%, rash, and gynaecomastia. Hyperkalaemia was associated with renal insufficiency and the administration of potassium supplements: only 2.8% of nonazotaemic patients not receiving potassium chloride developed hyperkalaemia, while 42.1% of those with marked azotaemia and treated with potassium chloride became hyperkalaemic.

In a study of 54 patients (53 female, 1 male) taking spironolactone 200 mg daily for hirsutism or acne adverse effects were reported in 91%.[2] Menstrual disturbances occurred in 72% of patients, breast tenderness in 39%, dry skin in 39%, and breast enlargement in 24%. Other adverse effects included nausea and vomiting, dizziness, headache, drowsiness, and skin rashes. Two patients developed a chloasma-like pigmentation of the face. The gynaecological effects were reduced in patients taking oral contraceptives.

1. Greenblatt DG, Koch-Weser J. Adverse reactions to spironolactone: a report from the Boston Collaborative Drug Surveillance Program. *JAMA* 1973; **225:** 40–3.
2. Hughes BR, Cunliffe WJ. Tolerance of spironolactone. *Br J Dermatol* 1988; **118:** 687–91.

Carcinogenicity. Breast cancer was reported in 5 patients taking spironolactone and hydrochlorothiazide for prolonged periods[1] although Jick and Armstrong[2] suggested that the association with spironolactone therapy was unlikely to be causal.

Although the *rat* may not be an appropriate model for determining long-term safety in man,[3,4] evidence of carcinogenicity in this species prompted the Committee on Safety of Medicines to limit the product licences of spironolactone-containing products to exclude use in essential hypertension or idiopathic oedema in the UK.[5]

1. Loube SD, Quirk RA. Breast cancer associated with administration of spironolactone. *Lancet* 1975; **i:** 1428–9.
2. Jick H, Armstrong B. Breast cancer and spironolactone. *Lancet* 1975; **ii:** 368–9.
3. Lumb G, *et al.* Effects in animals of chronic administration of spironolactone—a review. *J Environ Pathol Toxicol* 1978; **i:** 641–60.
4. Wagner BM. Long-term toxicology studies of spironolactone in animals and comparison with potassium canrenoate. *J Drug Dev* 1987; **1** (suppl 2): 7–11.
5. Committee on Safety of Medicines. Spironolactone. *Current Problems* 1988; 21.

Effects on the blood. Agranulocytosis has been reported[1,2] in association with the administration of spironolactone.

1. Stricker BHC, Oei TT. Agranulocytosis caused by spironolactone. *Br Med J* 1984; **289:** 731.
2. Whitling AM, *et al.* Spironolactone-induced agranulocytosis. *Ann Pharmacother* 1997; **31:** 582–5.

Effects on the electrolyte balance. CALCIUM. A report[1] suggested that spironolactone may have a calcium-sparing effect, in addition to its well known potassium-sparing properties.

1. Puig JG, *et al.* Hydrochlorothiazide versus spironolactone: long-term metabolic modifications in patients with essential hypertension. *J Clin Pharmacol* 1991; **31:** 455–61.

POTASSIUM. There have been a number of reports[1-3] of severe hyperkalaemia in patients taking spironolactone, including those with impaired renal function and those with a high potassium intake from either dietary sources or as potassium supplements. In the Boston Collaborative Drug Surveillance Program[4] hyperkalaemia was reported in 42.1% of patients with uraemia taking spironolactone and receiving potassium supplements compared with 2.8% of those without uraemia and not receiving potassium supplements. Two deaths were attributed to hyperkalaemia in patients taking spironolactone and potassium chloride. Potassium supplements should be avoided in patients receiving spironolactone, and plasma-potassium concentrations should be carefully monitored in those with impaired renal function.

1. Pongpaew C, *et al.* Hyperkalemic cardiac arrhythmia secondary to spironolactone. *Chest* 1973; **63:** 1023–5.
2. Udezue EO, Harrold BP. Hyperkalaemic paralysis due to spironolactone. *Postgrad Med J* 1980; **56:** 254–5.
3. O'Reilly PH, *et al.* Life-threatening hyperkalaemia after bladder decompression for high pressure chronic retention. *Lancet* 1987; **ii:** 859.
4. Greenblatt DJ, Koch-Weser J. Adverse reactions to spironolactone: a report from the Boston Collaborative Drug Surveillance Program. *JAMA* 1973; **225:** 40–3.

Effects on endocrine function. Spironolactone has been associated with a number of disturbances of endocrine function. The most prominent in men is gynaecomastia which appears to be related to both dose and duration of treatment. Incidences of 62%[1] and 100%[2] have been reported. Gynaecomastia has also been accompanied by impotence.[3,4] The effects are generally reversible on discontinuing treatment. Reversal of male-pattern baldness has also been reported.[5]

In women symptoms include breast enlargement and tenderness.[6] The incidence of menstrual abnormalities may be high: unspecified disturbances have been reported in 33 of 53 women,[6] secondary amenorrhoea in 6 of 9,[7] and secondary and primary amenorrhoea in 1 and 2 patients, respectively.[8] Hughes and Cunliffe[6] found the incidence of gynaecological disturbances to be lower in women taking oral contraceptives than in those using other methods of contraception.

The mechanism of the effects of spironolactone on the endocrine system is unclear. Loriaux and colleagues[9] suggested that although spironolactone affects testosterone synthesis, the more likely explanation was its anti-androgenic action, and reduction in 17-hydroxylase activity. Rose and colleagues[10] demonstrated an alteration in the testosterone/oestrogen ratio due to an increase in testosterone clearance and increased peripheral conversion to oestradiol. In addition, spironolactone is reported to inhibit binding of dihydrotestosterone to receptors.

1. Huffman DH, *et al.* Gynecomastia induced in normal males by spironolactone. *Clin Pharmacol Ther* 1978; **24:** 465–73.
2. Bellati G, Idéo G. Gynaecomastia after spironolactone and potassium canrenoate. *Lancet* 1986; **i:** 626.
3. Greenblatt DJ, Koch-Weser J. Gynecomastia and impotence complications of spironolactone therapy. *JAMA* 1973; **223:** 82.
4. Greenlaw C. Spironolactone induced gynecomastia: a case report. *Drug Intell Clin Pharm* 1977; **11:** 70–3.
5. Thomas PS. Hair: wanted and unwanted. *Br Med J* 1986; **293:** 698.
6. Hughes BR, Cunliffe WJ. Tolerance of spironolactone. *Br J Dermatol* 1988; **118:** 687–91.
7. Levitt JI. Spironolactone therapy and amenorrhea. *JAMA* 1970; **211:** 2014–15.
8. Potter C, *et al.* Primary and secondary amenorrhea associated with spironolactone therapy in chronic liver disease. *J Pediatr* 1992; **121:** 141–3.
9. Loriaux DL, *et al.* Spironolactone and endocrine dysfunction. *Ann Intern Med* 1976; **85:** 630–6.
10. Rose LI, *et al.* Pathophysiology of spironolactone-induced gynecomastia. *Ann Intern Med* 1977; **87:** 398–403.

Effects on lipid metabolism. Unlike thiazide diuretics, spironolactone appeared not to increase serum-cholesterol concentrations in a study of 23 patients.[1]

1. Ames RP, Peacock PB. Serum cholesterol during treatment of hypertension with diuretic drugs. *Arch Intern Med* 1984; **144:** 710–14.

Effects on the liver. Hepatic toxicity characterised by cholestatic lesions has been reported in a patient receiving spironolactone.[1] Only one previously published case of spironolactone-associated hepatic toxicity was known to the authors.

1. Renkes P, *et al.* Spironolactone and hepatic toxicity. *JAMA* 1995; **273:** 376–7.

Effects on the skin. A report of lichen-planus-like skin eruptions which developed in a 62-year-old woman who was taking digoxin, propranolol, diazepam, spironolactone, and iron tablets.[1] Flares of the lichen-planus-like eruption seemed to be associated with administration of spironolactone and there was evidence of resolution when spironolactone was withdrawn. Cutaneous vasculitis was associated with spironolactone treatment on 3 occasions in an 80-year-old man.[2] A chloasma-like pigmentation of the face was reported in 2 patients receiving spironolactone for hirsutism or acne.[3]

1. Downham TF. Spironolactone-induced lichen planus. *JAMA* 1978; **240:** 1138.
2. Phillips GWL, Williams AJ. Spironolactone induced vasculitis. *Br Med J* 1984; **288:** 368.
3. Hughes BR, Cunliffe WJ. Tolerance of spironolactone. *Br J Dermatol* 1988; **118:** 687–91.

Hypersensitivity. Eosinophilia and a rash developed in 2 patients with alcoholic cirrhosis while taking spironolactone.[1]

1. Wathen CG, *et al.* Eosinophilia associated with spironolactone. *Lancet* 1986; **i:** 919–20.

Precautions

Spironolactone should not be used in patients with hyperkalaemia or severe renal impairment. It should be used with care in patients who are at increased risk of developing hyperkalaemia; such patients include the elderly, those with diabetes mellitus, and those with some degree of renal or hepatic impairment. It should also be given with care to patients likely to develop acidosis. Serum electrolytes and blood-urea-nitrogen should be measured periodically. Spironolactone is not suitable for breast-feeding mothers.

Diabetes mellitus. Severe hyperkalaemia in a type 1 diabetic woman with hyporeninaemic hypoaldosteronism given spironolactone.[1]

1. Large DM, *et al.* Hyperkalaemia in diabetes mellitus—potential hazards of coexisting hyporeninaemic hypoaldosteronism. *Postgrad Med J* 1984; **60:** 370–3.

Interference with laboratory estimations. Spironolactone can interfere with some assays for plasma-digoxin concentrations.[1,2] However, spironolactone may also produce actual changes in digoxin concentrations (see p.851) and results of assays should be interpreted with caution.

1. Yosselson-Superstine S. Drug interferences with plasma assays in therapeutic drug monitoring. *Clin Pharmacokinet* 1984; **9:** 67–87.
2. Foukaridis GN. Influence of spironolactone and its metabolite canrenone on serum digoxin assays. *Ther Drug Monit* 1990; **12:** 82–4.

Interactions

There is an increased risk of hyperkalaemia if spironolactone is given concomitantly with potassium supplements or with other potassium-sparing diuretics. Hyperkalaemia may also occur in patients receiving ACE inhibitors, NSAIDs, cyclosporin, or trilostane concomitantly. In patients receiving spironolactone with NSAIDs or cyclosporin the risk of nephrotoxicity may also be increased. Diuretics may reduce the excretion of lithium and increase the risk of lithium toxicity. Hyponatraemia may occur in patients receiving a combination of potassium-sparing diuretic with a thiazide; this risk may be increased in patients receiving chlorpropamide. Spironolactone may reduce the ulcer-healing properties of carbenoxolone. As with other diuretics, spironolactone may enhance the effects of other antihypertensive drugs and may diminish vascular reponses to noradrenaline.

ACE Inhibitors. Hyperkalaemia causing complete heart block was associated with concomitant administration of spironolactone and captopril[1] in a 72-year-old woman. Lakhani[2] reported a similar fatal reaction in a patient taking spironolactone and enalapril. Hyperkalaemia in a 55-year-old patient taking spironolactone and enalapril[3] persisted for over 48 hours despite discontinuation of the drugs and treatment with ion-exchange resin and intravenous glucose and insulin.

1. Lo TCN, Cryer RJ. Complete heart block induced by hyperkalaemia associated with treatment with a combination of captopril and spironolactone. *Br Med J* 1986; **292:** 1672.
2. Lakhani M. Complete heart block induced by hyperkalaemia associated with treatment with a combination of captopril and spironolactone. *Br Med J* 1986; **293:** 271.
3. Morton AR, Crook SA. Hyperkalaemia and spironolactone. *Lancet* 1987; **ii:** 1525.

Aspirin. Administration of aspirin to healthy subjects taking spironolactone has been shown to produce substantial reductions in sodium excretion[1] and to reduce the excretion of spironolactone's active metabolite, canrenone.[2] However, administration of aspirin in therapeutic amounts to hypertensive patients[3] did not alter the effect of spironolactone on blood pressure, serum electrolytes, blood urea nitrogen, or plasma-renin activity.

1. Tweeddale MG, Ogilvie RI. Antagonism of spironolactone-induced natriuresis by aspirin in man. *N Engl J Med* 1973; **289:** 198–200.
2. Ramsay LE, *et al.* Influence of acetylsalicylic acid on the renal handling of a spironolactone metabolite in healthy subjects. *Eur J Clin Pharmacol* 1976; **10:** 43–8.
3. Hollifield JW. Failure of aspirin to antagonize the antihypertensive effect of spironolactone in low-renin hypertension. *South Med J* 1976; **69:** 1034–6.

Cardiac glycosides. For discussions of the effects of spironolactone on digoxin and digitoxin, see p.851 and p.849, respectively. See also Interference with Laboratory Estimations, under Precautions, above.

Mitotane. For a report of the inhibition of the action of mitotane by concomitant administration of spironolactone, see p.553.

Warfarin. For reference to the interaction between warfarin and spironolactone, see p.968.

Pharmacokinetics

Spironolactone is fairly rapidly absorbed from the gastro-intestinal tract, the extent of absorption depending on particle size and formulation. Modern formulations are reported to provide a bioavailability of about 90%. It is about 90% bound to plasma proteins.

Spironolactone is metabolised extensively to a number of metabolites including canrenone and the sulphur-containing 7α-thiomethylspirolactone, both of which are pharmacologically active. The major metabolite may be 7α-thiomethylspirolactone, although it is uncertain to what extent the actions of spironolactone are dependent on the parent compound or its metabolites.

Spironolactone is excreted mainly in the urine and also in the faeces, in the form of metabolites. Spironolactone or its metabolites may cross the placental barrier, and canrenone is distributed into breast milk.

References.

1. Karim A. Spironolactone: disposition, metabolism, pharmacodynamics, and bioavailability. *Drug Metab Rev* 1978; **8:** 151–88.
2. Ho PC, *et al.* Comparison of plasma levels of canrenone and metabolites after base hydrolysis in young and elderly subjects following single and multiple doses of spironolactone. *Eur J Clin Pharmacol* 1984; **27:** 435–9.
3. Ho PC, *et al.* Pharmacokinetics of canrenone and metabolites after base hydrolysis following single and multiple dose oral administration of spironolactone. *Eur J Clin Pharmacol* 1984; **27:** 441–6.
4. Overdiek HWPM, *et al.* New insights into the pharmacokinetics of spironolactone. *Clin Pharmacol Ther* 1985; **38:** 469–74.
5. Gardiner P, *et al.* Spironolactone metabolism: steady-state serum levels of the sulfur-containing metabolites. *J Clin Pharmacol* 1989; **29:** 342–7.

Uses and Administration

Spironolactone, a steroid with a structure resembling that of the natural adrenocortical hormone, aldosterone, acts on the distal portion of the renal tubule as a competitive antagonist of aldosterone. It acts as a potassium-sparing diuretic, increasing sodium and water excretion and reducing potassium excretion.

Spironolactone is reported to have a relatively slow onset of action, requiring 2 or 3 days for maximum effect, and a similarly slow diminishment of action over 2 or 3 days on discontinuation.

Spironolactone is used in the treatment of refractory oedema associated with heart failure (p.785), cirrhosis of the liver (with or without ascites, p.781), or the nephrotic syndrome, and in ascites associated with malignancy. It is frequently given with the thiazides, frusemide, or similar diuretics, where it adds to their natriuretic but diminishes their kaliuretic effects, hence conserving potassium in those at risk from hypokalaemia. Diuretic-induced hypokalaemia and its management, including the role of potassium-sparing diuretics, is discussed under Effects on the Electrolyte Balance in the Adverse Effects of Hydrochlorothiazide, p.885. It has been used in the treatment of essential hypertension (in lower doses than for oedema), but in the UK spironolactone is no longer recommended for use in either essential hypertension or idiopathic oedema; doubts have been expressed over its safety during long-term administration.

Spironolactone is also used in the diagnosis and treatment of primary hyperaldosteronism (below).

Other conditions in which spironolactone has been tried on the basis of its anti-androgenic properties include hirsutism, particularly in the polycystic ovary syndrome.

In the treatment of **oedema**, spironolactone is usually given in an initial dose of 100 mg daily by mouth, subsequently adjusted as necessary; some patients may require doses of up to 400 mg daily. In hepatic cirrhosis with ascites and oedema patients with a urinary sodium/potassium ratio greater than 1 may be given an initial dose of spironolactone 100 mg daily while patients with a ratio of less than 1 may be given initial doses of 200 to 400 mg daily. It is given in doses of 400 mg daily in the presumptive diagnosis of primary **hyperaldosteronism**; in doses of 100 to 400 mg daily for the pre-operative management of hyperaldosteronism; and in the lowest effective dosage for long-term maintenance therapy in the absence of surgery.

A suggested initial dose of spironolactone for children is 1.5 to 3 mg per kg body-weight daily, in divided doses.

Potassium supplements should not be given with spironolactone.

Reviews.

1. Ochs HR, *et al.* Spironolactone. *Am Heart J* 1978; **96:** 389–400.
2. Skluth HA, Gums JG. Spironolactone: a re-examination. *DICP Ann Pharmacother* 1990; **24:** 52–9.

Acne. Spironolactone has been used for its anti-androgenic properties in some cases of acne (p.1072) where standard therapy is unsuccessful. Beneficial responses to oral therapy have been reported in patients with acne from both open[1] and placebo-controlled[2,3] studies. Topical application has been tried[4,5] but response has been variable. It is possible that the vehicle may affect the response. In women, spironolactone may be useful when treatment with an oestrogen is contra-indicated.

1. Burke BM, Cunliffe WJ. Oral spironolactone therapy for female patients with acne, hirsutism or androgenic alopecia. *Br J Dermatol* 1985; **112:** 124–5.
2. Goodfellow A, *et al.* Oral spironolactone improves acne vulgaris and reduces sebum excretion. *Br J Dermatol* 1984; **111:** 209–14.
3. Muhlemann MF, *et al.* Oral spironolactone: an effective treatment for acne vulgaris in women. *Br J Dermatol* 1986; **115:** 227–32.
4. Messina M, *et al.* A new therapeutic approach to acne: an antiandrogen percutaneous treatment with spironolactone. *Curr Ther Res* 1983; **34:** 319–24.
5. Walton S, *et al.* Lack of effect of topical spironolactone on sebum excretion. *Br J Dermatol* 1986; **114:** 261–4.

Bartter's syndrome. Spironolactone may be used to reduce potassium wasting in patients with Bartter's syndrome (p.1150).

Bronchopulmonary dysplasia. Bronchopulmonary dysplasia (p.1018) is a major cause of chronic lung disease in infants. Treatment often involves the use of corticosteroids. Additional supportive therapy has included the use of diuretics such as frusemide (p.873); results with hydrochlorothiazide or spironolactone have been more ambiguous (p.888).

High-altitude disorders. Acetazolamide is generally the drug of choice for prophylaxis of high-altitude disorders (p.787). Anecdotal reports[1-4] and a small-scale double-blind study[5] suggested that spironolactone could be useful in preventing acute mountain sickness, although Meyers[6] reported a deterioration in pulmonary function despite spironolactone prophylaxis in 1 patient.

1. Currie TT, *et al.* Spironolactone and acute mountain sickness. *Med J Aust* 1976; **2:** 168–70.
2. Snell JA, Cordner EP. Spironolactone and acute mountain sickness. *Med J Aust* 1977; **1:** 828.
3. Turnbull G. Spironolactone prophylaxis in mountain sickness. *Br Med J* 1980; **280:** 1453.
4. Rutter LD. Spironolactone prophylaxis in mountain sickness. *Br Med J* 1980; **281:** 618.
5. Brown GV, *et al.* Spironolactone in acute mountain sickness. *Lancet* 1977; **i:** 855.
6. Meyers DH. Spironolactone prophylaxis of mountain sickness. *Br Med J* 1980; **281:** 1569.

Hirsutism. Hirsutism (p.1441) is frequently treated with anti-androgenic drug therapy, usually cyproterone or spironolactone. Spironolactone in doses of 50 to 200 mg daily has produced both subjective and objective improvement in hirsutism in patients with idiopathic hirsutism or polycystic ovary syndrome.[1-4] It is preferably used in combination with oral contraceptives,[5,6] to improve efficacy and menstrual irregularity and to avoid the risk of feminisation to a male fetus. A double-blind placebo-controlled study[7] failed to demonstrate any benefit with spironolactone 100 mg daily in idiopathic hirsutism, whereas another randomised study (not placebo-controlled) found spironolactone 100 mg daily and cyproterone 100 mg daily to be equally effective.[9] Most studies have involved premenopausal women and it has been suggested[4,8] that spironolactone would be useful in women in whom cyproterone is contra-indicated or not tolerated.

1. Cumming DC, *et al.* Treatment of hirsutism with spironolactone. *JAMA* 1982; **247:** 1295–8.
2. Burke BM, Cunliffe WJ. Oral spironolactone therapy for female patients with acne, hirsutism or androgenic alopecia. *Br J Dermatol* 1985; **112:** 124–5.
3. Evans DJ, Burke CW. Spironolactone in the treatment of idiopathic hirsutism and the polycystic ovary syndrome. *J R Soc Med* 1986; **79:** 451–3.
4. Barth JH, *et al.* Spironolactone therapy for hirsute women. *Br J Dermatol* 1988; **119** (suppl 33): 17.
5. Chapman MG, *et al.* Spironolactone in combination with an oral contraceptive: an alternative treatment for hirsutism. *Br J Obstet Gynaecol* 1985; **92:** 983–5.
6. Rittmaster RS. Hirsutism. *Lancet* 1997; **349:** 191–5.
7. McLellan AR, *et al.* Lack of effect of spironolactone on hair shaft diameter in hirsute females. *Postgrad Med J* 1989; **65:** 459–62.
8. West TET. Does spironolactone have a place in treating facial hirsutism in women? *Br Med J* 1988; **296:** 1456.
9. O'Brien RC, *et al.* Comparison of sequential cyproterone acetate/estrogen versus spironolactone/oral contraceptive in the treatment of hirsutism. *J Clin Endocrinol Metab* 1991; **72:** 1008–13.

Hyperaldosteronism. Hyperaldosteronism (aldosteronism) is a disorder characterised by mineralocorticoid excess due to high circulating levels of aldosterone. Mineralocorticoid excess due to other mineralocorticoids is rare. Primary hyperaldosteronism is usually caused by an aldosterone producing adenoma (Conn's syndrome) or primary adrenal hyperplasia. Other causes include aldosterone producing adrenal carcinoma and glucocorticoid-suppressible hyperaldosteronism.

Secondary hyperaldosteronism is more common and results from conditions in which there is activation of the renin-angiotensin-aldosterone system, including diuretic therapy, and oedematous conditions such as heart failure, hepatic cirrhosis, and nephrotic syndrome. Bartter's syndrome (p.1150) also results in hyperaldosteronism.

Most patients with primary hyperaldosteronism are asymptomatic, although they may present with signs or symptoms of mineralocorticoid excess (p.1010). Diagnosis often follows the incidental discovery of hypokalaemia. Symptomatic hypokalaemia (p.1150) may develop in some patients, particularly those receiving diuretic therapy.

Diagnosis is confirmed by the presence of raised plasma and urinary aldosterone concentrations. However, the concentrations may be affected by serum-potassium concentration, posture, and time of day, and interpretation may be difficult. The plasma aldosterone:renin ratio may also be measured. In primary hyperaldosteronism the aldosterone concentration is raised but renin is suppressed whereas in secondary hyperaldosteronism both are raised.

Hyperaldosteronism due to an aldosterone-producing adenoma is usually treated surgically. The aldosterone antagonist spironolactone may be given pre-operatively to lower the blood pressure and normalise the serum potassium. In patients who are not suitable for surgery, long-term medical management involves spironolactone, initially in high doses but reduced to the lowest dose for maintenance. If spironolactone is not tolerated, amiloride may be used as an alternative, but high doses are required. Trilostane, an adrenal suppressant, has also been used to inhibit aldosterone synthesis.

In primary adrenal hyperplasia surgery is not usually effective and medical management with spironolactone or amiloride is required. Additional antihypertensive therapy with ACE inhibitors or calcium-channel blockers may also be needed. Glucocorticoid-suppressible hyperaldosteronism is a rare form and may be treated with dexamethasone. However, this may not control the blood pressure and spironolactone or amiloride may be required in addition.

In secondary hyperaldosteronism the underlying condition should be treated, but spironolactone may be of benefit as part of the therapy.

Precocious puberty. Spironolactone (as an anti-androgen) and testolactone were given to boys with familial precocious puberty (p.1241) for periods of up to 18 months. Rates of growth and bone maturation were restored to normal during combination therapy but not with either drug given alone.[1] However, after further treatment for 2.0 to 4.2 years there was a diminishing response manifested by the recurrence of clinical features of puberty and an increase in the bone maturation rate.[2] Addition of deslorelin appeared to restore the control.

1. Laue L, *et al.* Treatment of familial male precocious puberty with spironolactone and testolactone. *N Engl J Med* 1989; **320:** 496–502.
2. Laue L, *et al.* Treatment of familial male precocious puberty with spironolactone, testolactone, and deslorelin. *J Clin Endocrinol Metab* 1993; **76:** 151–5.

Premenstrual syndrome. Spironolactone has been used for its diuretic and anti-androgenic properties in premenstrual syndrome (p.1456).

Preparations

BP 1998: Spironolactone Tablets;
USP 23: Spironolactone and Hydrochlorothiazide Tablets; Spironolactone Tablets.

Proprietary Preparations (details are given in Part 3)

Aust.: Aldactone; Aldopur; Deverol; Osiren; Spirobene; Spirohexal; ***Austral.:*** Aldactone; Spiractin; Spirotone†; ***Belg.:*** Aldactone; Sincomen†; Uractone; ***Canad.:*** Aldactone; Novo-Spiroton; ***Fr.:*** Aldactone; Flumach; Practon; Spiroctan; Spironone; Spirophar†; ***Ger.:*** Aldace†; Aldactone; Aldopur; Aquareduct; duraspiron; Jenaspiron; Osyrol; Spiro; Spiro-Tablinen; Spirono; Verospiron; ***Irl.:*** Aldactone; Melactone; ***Ital.:*** Aldactone; Idrolattone; Sincomen†; Spiroderm; Spirolang; Uractone; ***Neth.:*** Aldactone; Spiroctan†; ***Norw.:*** Aldactone; Spirix; Spiropal; ***S.Afr.:*** Aldactone; Spiractin; Tensin; ***Spain:*** Aldactone; ***Swed.:*** Aldactone; Spirix; Spiroscand; ***Switz.:*** Aldactone; Osiren†; Spiroctan; Xenalon; ***UK:*** Aldactone; Laractone; Spiretic; Spiroctan; Spirolone; Spirospare; ***USA:*** Alatone; Aldactone.

Multi-ingredient: ***Aust.:*** Aldactone Saltucin; Deverol mit Thiazid; Digi-Aldopur; Furo-Aldopur; Furolacton; Lasilacton; Sali-Aldopur; Spirono comp; Supracid; Suprenoat; ***Belg.:*** Aldactazine; Uractazide; ***Canad.:*** Aldactazide; Novo-Spirozine; ***Fr.:*** Aldactazine; Aldalix; Practazin; Prinactizide; Spiroctazine; ***Ger.:*** Aldactone Saltucin; duraspiron-comp.; Furo-Aldopur; Furorese Comp; Osyrol Lasix; Risicordin; Sali-Aldopur; Spiro comp; Spiro-D; Spiro-D-Tablinen†; Spirodigal†; Spironolacton Plus; Spironothiazid; Spirostada comp; ***Irl.:*** Aldactide; Spiroprop†; ***Ital.:*** Aldactazide; Lasitone; Spiridazide; Spirofur; ***S.Afr.:*** Aldazide; ***Spain:*** Aldactacine; Aldoleo; Miscidon; Resnedal; Spirometon; ***Switz.:*** Aldozone; Furosemid comp; Furospir; Lasilactone; Sali-Spiroctan; Saluretin; Spironothiazid; Synureticum; ***UK:*** Aldactide; Lasilactone; Spiro-Co; ***USA:*** Aldactazide.

Staphylokinase (17142-p)

Staphylokinase is a thrombolytic under investigation for the treatment of thrombo-embolic occlusions, including myocardial infarction.

References.

1. Vanderschueren S, *et al.* A randomized trial of recombinant staphylokinase versus alteplase for coronary artery patency in acute myocardial infarction. *Circulation* 1995; **92:** 2044–9.
2. Vanderschueren S, *et al.* Thrombolytic therapy of peripheral arterial occlusion with recombinant staphylokinase. *Circulation* 1995; **92:** 2050–57.

Streptokinase (3746-e)

Streptokinase *(BAN, rINN).*

Estreptoquinasa; Plasminokinase; Streptokinasum.

CAS — 9002-01-1.

Pharmacopoeias. In *Eur.* (see p.viii).

A protein obtained from culture filtrates of certain strains of *Streptococcus haemolyticus* group C. It has the property of combining with human plasminogen to form plasminogen activator and has been purified to contain not less than 600 international units of streptokinase activity per microgram of nitrogen. After purification it is usually mixed with a buffer and may be stabilised by the addition of suitable substances such as albumin.

A hygroscopic white powder or friable solid. Freely **soluble** in water. A solution in water containing 5000 units per mL has a pH of 6.8 to 7.5. **Store** in sealed containers and protect from light.

Stability. The incorporation of albumin in commercial preparations of streptokinase has reduced the incidence of flocculation with streptokinase solutions. However, flocculation has occurred with small volumes prepared with sodium chloride injection (0.9%) in sterilised glass containers apparently because of residual acid buffers that remain in empty evacuated containers following sterilisation.[1]

1. Thibault L. Streptokinase flocculation in evacuated glass bottles. *Am J Hosp Pharm* 1985; **42:** 278.

Units

The potency of streptokinase is expressed in international units and preparations are assayed using the second International Standard (1989).

The Christensen unit is the quantity of streptokinase that will lyse a standard blood clot completely in 10 minutes and is equivalent to the international unit.

Adverse Effects

In common with other thrombolytics streptokinase may cause haemorrhage, particularly from puncture sites; severe internal bleeding has occurred sometimes and may be difficult to control. Streptokinase is antigenic, and allergic reactions ranging from rashes to rarer, but more serious, anaphylactoid and serum-sickness-like symptoms have occurred. Fever, sometimes high, and associated symptoms such as chills and back or abdominal pain are quite frequent. Nausea and vomiting may occur. There have been a few reports of Guillain-Barré syndrome.

Streptokinase infusion may be associated with hypotension, both direct or as a result of reperfusion; bradycardia and arrhythmias may also occur due to reperfusion. The break-up of existing clots may occasionally produce emboli elsewhere; pulmonary embolism and acute renal failure due to cholesterol embolisation have been reported.

Petch has discussed the risks and benefits of thrombolysis.[1] The benefits of thrombolytic treatment in patients with acute myocardial infarction have to be set against the risk of bleeding. Despite early fears about arrhythmias associated with reperfusion these have not been seen to any extent in clinical practice, but bleeding has presented problems. Major bleeding requiring transfusion was reported in 0.5% of streptokinase-treated patients in the large ISIS 2 study; intracranial haemorrhage has also been seen, although it is rare. Severe embolic complications may follow disintegration of an existing clot. Spectacular bruising around arterial and venous punctures is a familiar sight. In addition, sensitivity reactions to streptokinase are fairly common, although usually mild; proteinuria may be another manifestation of hypersensitivity. Nonetheless, results from the large studies indicate that about 3 in every 100 patients with acute myocardial infarction may have their lives saved by thrombolytic therapy, whereas maybe 1 will suffer a major complication.

An earlier and more detailed review has been provided by Nazari and colleagues.[2]

1. Petch MC. Dangers of thrombolysis. *Br Med J* 1990; **300:** 483–4.
2. Nazari J, *et al.* Adverse reactions to thrombolytic agents: implications for coronary reperfusion following myocardial infarction. *Med Toxicol* 1987; **2:** 274–86.

Back pain. Streptokinase infusion has been associated with the development of very severe low back pain, which resolves within a few minutes of stopping the infusion, and may be severe enough to warrant opioid analgesia.[1-3] The back pain may represent a hypersensitivity reaction. Providing that the pain is controlled and that dissecting aortic aneurysm is not suspected, it may still be possible to complete the streptokinase infusion.[4] Alternatively, immediate substitution with a different thrombolytic has been suggested.[5]

There have also been a few reports of low back pain associated with anistreplase infusion.[6,7]

1. Shah M, Taylor RT. Low back pain associated with streptokinase. *Br Med J* 1990; **301:** 1219.
2. Dickinson RJ, Rosser A. Low back pain associated with streptokinase. *Br Med J* 1991; **302:** 111–12.
3. Porter NJ, Nikoletatos K. Low back pain associated with streptokinase. *Br Med J* 1991; **302:** 112.
4. Lear J, *et al.* Low back pain associated with streptokinase. *Lancet* 1992; **340:** 851.
5. Fishwick D, *et al.* Thrombolysis and low back pain. *Br Med J* 1995; **310:** 504.
6. Hannaford P, Kay CR. Back pain and thrombolysis. *Br Med J* 1992; **304:** 915.
7. Lear J, Rajapakse R. Low back pain associated with anistreplase. *Br Med J* 1993; **306:** 896.

Effects on the blood. Although falls in the haemoglobin value of patients receiving thrombolytics are most likely to be due to blood loss from haemorrhage, Mathiesen and Grunnet have reported a patient who had signs of haemolytic anaemia following intravenous infusion of streptokinase.[1] In a subsequent test *in vitro* the patient's serum caused strong agglutination of streptokinase-treated red blood cells, supporting the view that streptokinase was responsible for the haemolysis.

1. Mathiesen O, Grunnet N. Haemolysis after intravenous streptokinase. *Lancet* 1989; **i:** 1016–17.

Effects on the eyes. Acute uveitis[1,2] and iritis,[3,4] associated with transient renal impairment in one patient,[3] have followed treatment of myocardial infarction with intravenous streptokinase. In one case uveitis was associated with serum sickness[2] and in all of them hypersensitivity to streptokinase was suspected.

1. Kinshuck D. Bilateral hypopyon and streptokinase. *Br Med J* 1992; **305:** 1332.
2. Proctor BD, Joondeph BC. Bilateral anterior uveitis: a feature of streptokinase-induced serum sickness. *N Engl J Med* 1994; **330:** 576–7.
3. Birnbaum Y, *et al.* Acute iritis and transient renal impairment following thrombolytic therapy for acute myocardial infarction. *Ann Pharmacother* 1993; **27:** 1539–40.
4. Gray MY, Lazarus JH. Iritis after treatment with streptokinase. *Br Med J* 1994; **309:** 97.

Effects on the kidneys. Transient proteinuria has been reported following the administration of streptokinase. In some patients proteinuria and impaired renal function have developed about seven days after thrombolytic therapy and have been associated with a syndrome resembling serum sickness,[1,2] suggesting a delayed hypersensitivity reaction; a similar case in a patient receiving anistreplase was associated with Henoch-Schönlein-like vasculitis.[3] These delayed reactions should be distinguished from the transient and apparently self-limiting proteinuria that has been reported in some patients in the first 24 to 72 hours after beginning streptokinase.[4,5] Proteinuria within the first 24 hours has been attributed to deposition of an immune complex in the glomeruli,[6] although haemodynamic and neurohumoral changes associated with acute myocardial infarction may be responsible since proteinuria has occurred in patients not receiving thrombolytic therapy.[7,8]

Streptokinase infusion has also been associated with acute oliguric renal failure due to acute tubular necrosis, apparently as a result of hypotension during the infusion, in a patient with existing renovascular narrowing.[9] Interestingly, it has been pointed out that a variant streptokinase may be the pathogenic agent in glomerulonephritis occurring after *Streptococcus pyogenes* infection.[10]

Renal failure has developed as a consequence of a streptokinase-induced cholesterol embolism, see under Embolism, below.

1. Payne ST, *et al.* Transient impairment of renal function after streptokinase therapy. *Lancet* 1989; **ii:** 1398.
2. Callan MFC, *et al.* Proteinuria and thrombolytic agents. *Lancet* 1990; **335:** 106.
3. Ali A, *et al.* Proteinuria and thrombolytic agents. *Lancet* 1990; **335:** 106–7.
4. Argent N, Adams PC. Proteinuria and thrombolytic agents. *Lancet* 1990; **335:** 106.
5. More RS, Peacock F. Haematuria and proteinuria after thrombolytic therapy. *Lancet* 1990; **336:** 1454.
6. Lynch M, *et al.* Proteinuria with streptokinase. *Lancet* 1993; **341:** 1024.
7. Pickett TM, Hilton PJ. Proteinuria and streptokinase. *Lancet* 1993; **341:** 1538.
8. von Eyben FE, *et al.* Albuminuria with or without streptokinase. *Lancet* 1993; **342:** 365–6.

9. Kalra PA, *et al.* Acute tubular necrosis induced by coronary thrombolytic therapy. *Postgrad Med J* 1991; **67:** 212.
10. Barnham M. Hypersensitivity and streptokinase. *Lancet* 1990; **335:** 535.

Effects on the liver. Raised serum-alanine aminotransferase values, and in some cases raised aspartate aminotransferase activity, were seen more frequently in 95 patients who received streptokinase than in 94 given placebo as part of a study in patients with myocardial infarction.[1] The mechanism for the raised aminotransferase activity was not clear; a concomitant rise in γ-glutamyltransferase activity and bilirubin concentration suggested a hepatic source.

For references to rupture of the liver occurring during treatment with streptokinase, see under Haemorrhage, below.

1. Maclennan AC, *et al.* Activities of aminotransferases after treatment with streptokinase for acute myocardial infarction. *Br Med J* 1990; **301:** 321–2.

Effects on the nervous system. There have been a few reports of Guillain-Barré syndrome following treatment with streptokinase.[1-4] Whether streptokinase was the cause is not certain although its antigenic properties do suggest that induction of an immunological reaction might be responsible.[3]

For discussion of cerebrovascular effects of streptokinase, see under Haemorrhage, below.

1. Eden KV. Possible association of Guillain-Barré syndrome with thrombolytic therapy. *JAMA* 1983; **249:** 2020–1.
2. Leaf DA, *et al.* Streptokinase and the Guillain-Barré syndrome. *Ann Intern Med* 1984; **100:** 617.
3. Barnes D, Hughes RAC. Guillain-Barré syndrome after treatment with streptokinase. *Br Med J* 1992; **304:** 1225.
4. Taylor BV, *et al.* Guillain-Barré syndrome complicating treatment with streptokinase. *Med J Aust* 1995; **162:** 214–15.

Effects on the respiratory system. Fatal acute respiratory distress syndrome occurred in one patient given streptokinase for pulmonary embolism.[1] It was suggested that streptokinase may have caused the pulmonary injury by altering vascular permeability due to generation of fibrinolytic products or via reperfusion oedema.

1. Martin TR, *et al.* Adult respiratory distress syndrome following thrombolytic therapy for pulmonary embolism. *Chest* 1983; **83:** 151–3.

Effects on the skin. Rashes may occur as an allergic reaction to streptokinase. For a report of skin necrosis possibly associated with cholesterol embolisation, see Embolism, below.

Embolism. Thrombolytic therapy has occasionally and paradoxically been associated with further embolism in the patients receiving it. Such embolism may be due to clots that break away from the thrombus being treated, or to cholesterol crystals released following removal of fibrin from atheromatous plaques by thrombolysis.

Hill has described fatal pulmonary embolism apparently due to breakaway from a deep-vein thrombus under treatment,[1] although there is no evidence of a higher rate of such complications with streptokinase than with heparin, and when they do occur a good clinical response is usually seen to continued streptokinase.[2] Stafford and colleagues reported complications due to multiple microemboli in 7 of 475 consecutive patients treated with streptokinase or anistreplase for acute myocardial infarction. The sites of embolism were the legs (in 4) and brain (in 3); one patient apparently had systemic effects with skin infarction and impaired renal function. Five of the 7 patients died.[3]

Cholesterol embolisation can have many clinical manifestations depending on the location of the emboli. A classic presentation is livedo reticularis, gangrenous lower extremities, and acute renal failure.[4,5] Symptoms may appear within a few hours of starting thrombolytic treatment,[6] although in some cases they may not become evident for several days.[7-10]

1. Hill LN. Streptokinase therapy and breakaway pulmonary emboli. *Am J Med* 1991; **90:** 411–12.
2. Rogers LQ, Lutcher CL. Streptokinase therapy and breakaway pulmonary emboli. *Am J Med* 1991; **90:** 412–13.
3. Stafford PJ, *et al.* Multiple microemboli after disintegration of clot during thrombolysis for acute myocardial infarction. *Br Med J* 1989; **299:** 1310–12.
4. Blankenship JC. Cholesterol embolisation after thrombolytic therapy. *Drug Safety* 1996; **14:** 78–84.
5. Wong FKM, *et al.* Acute renal failure after streptokinase therapy in a patient with acute myocardial infarction. *Am J Kidney Dis* 1995; **26:** 508–10.
6. Pochmalicki G, *et al.* Cholesterol embolisation syndrome after thrombolytic therapy for myocardial infarction. *Lancet* 1992; **339:** 58–9.
7. Ridker PM, Michel T. Streptokinase therapy and cholesterol embolization. *Am J Med* 1989; **87:** 357–8.
8. Pirson Y, *et al.* Cholesterol embolism in a renal graft after treatment with streptokinase. *Br Med J* 1988; **296:** 394–5.
9. Dass H, Fescharek R. Skin necrosis induced by streptokinase. *Br Med J* 1994; **309:** 1513–14.
10. Penswick J, Wright AL. Skin necrosis induced by streptokinase. *Br Med J* 1994; **309:** 378.

Haemorrhage. Haemorrhage is a common adverse effect of thrombolytic therapy, particularly where there is existing or concomitant trauma: bleeding or severe bruising has been associated with various therapeutic manipulations including vascular puncture (e.g. injection, phlebotomy, or catheterisation),[1] intramuscular injection of analgesics,[2] the use of an automatic blood-pressure measuring machine,[3] a pre-existing prosthetic abdominal aortic graft,[4] and recent dental extraction.[5] In addition, other disease states may contribute: haemospermia has been reported following thrombolysis in a patient with mild prostatic symptoms,[6] haemorrhagic bullae have been reported in a patient with lichen sclerosus et atrophicus,[7] and diabetic patients are at risk of retinal haemorrhage if they have diabetic retinopathy,[8] although any increase in risk seems to be small.[9]

The problem and its management have been reviewed by Sane and others.[1] Thrombolytics can produce a 'lytic state' due to depletion of the natural plasmin inhibitor α_2-antiplasmin by excess plasmin production, although this correlates only weakly, if at all, with bleeding. Currently available 'fibrin-specific' agents such as alteplase do not produce less bleeding than non-specific thrombolytics such as streptokinase. More than 70% of bleeding episodes occur at vascular puncture sites, so invasive procedures should be avoided if possible; if catheterisation is considered essential meticulous care of the vascular puncture site is necessary. A review of the GUSTO-I Study[10] (40 903 patients) confirmed that invasive procedures are a risk factor for bleeding. Older age, low body-weight, female sex, and African ancestry were other factors that increased the risk of haemorrhage.

Of particular concern is the possibility of intracranial haemorrhage leading to cerebrovascular events.

There has been contradictory evidence of the relative risk with streptokinase and other thrombolytics. A recent assessment of individual patient data collected from a national registry and various large-scale studies confirmed that thrombolytic therapy does cause intracranial haemorrhage in a small number of patients. Risk factors were: advanced age, hypertension on admission, low body-weight, and thrombolysis with current alteplase regimens.[11-13] The benefits and risks must be assessed for each patient and thrombolytic therapy should still be given to the elderly and to those with hypertension if the expected benefits are great.

Rupture of the spleen[14,15] and liver[16] has been reported in patients receiving thrombolytic therapy, and rupture of a follicle has been reported in a menstruating woman.[17] Rupture of the heart with fatal consequences has been reported.[18] However, a review of randomised studies[19] did not suggest an association of cardiac rupture with thrombolytic therapy.

1. Sane DC, *et al.* Bleeding during thrombolytic therapy for acute myocardial infarction: mechanisms and management. *Ann Intern Med* 1989; **111:** 1010–22.
2. Morris GC, Sterry MJG. [case report]. *Br Med J* 1991; **302:** 246.
3. Gibson P. [case report]. *Br Med J* 1991; **302:** 1412.
4. London NJM, *et al.* Systemic thrombolysis causing haemorrhage around a prosthetic abdominal aortic graft. *Br Med J* 1993; **306:** 1530–1.
5. Lustig JP, *et al.* Thrombolytic therapy for acute myocardial infarction after oral surgery. *Oral Surg Oral Med Oral Pathol* 1993; **75:** 547–8.
6. Keeling PJ, Lawson CS. Haemospermia: a complication of thrombolytic therapy. *Br J Hosp Med* 1990; **44:** 244.
7. Dunn HM, Fulton RA. Haemorrhagic bullae in a patient with lichen sclerosus et atrophicus treated with streptokinase. *Heart* 1996; **76:** 448.
8. Caramelli B, *et al.* Retinal haemorrhage after thrombolytic therapy. *Lancet* 1991; **337:** 1356–7.
9. Ward H, Yudkin JS. Thrombolysis in patients with diabetes. *Br Med J* 1995; **310:** 3–4.
10. Berkowitz SD, *et al.* Incidence and predictors of bleeding after contemporary thrombolytic therapy for myocardial infarction. *Circulation* 1997; **95:** 2508–16.
11. Simoons ML, *et al.* Individual risk assessment for intracranial haemorrhage during thrombolytic therapy. *Lancet* 1993; **342:** 1523–8.
12. Aylward PE, *et al.* Relation of increased arterial blood pressure to mortality and stroke in the context of contemporary thrombolytic therapy for acute myocardial infarction: a randomized trial. *Ann Intern Med* 1996; **125:** 891–900.
13. Bovill EG, *et al.* Hemorrhagic events during therapy with recombinant tissue plasminogen activator, heparin, and aspirin for unstable angina (Thrombolysis in Myocardial Ischemia, Phase IIIB trial). *Am J Cardiol* 1997; **79:** 391–6.
14. Wiener RS, Ong LS. Streptokinase and splenic rupture. *Am J Med* 1989; **86:** 249.
15. Blankenship JC, Indeck M. Spontaneous splenic rupture complicating anticoagulant or thrombolytic therapy. *Am J Med* 1993; **94:** 433–7.
16. Eklöf B, *et al.* Spontaneous rupture of liver and spleen with severe intra-abdominal bleeding during streptokinase treatment of deep venous thrombosis. *Vasa* 1977; **6:** 369–71.
17. Müller C-H, *et al.* Near-fatal intra-abdominal bleeding from a ruptured follicle during thrombolytic therapy. *Lancet* 1996; **347:** 1697.
18. Rogers TK, *et al.* Cardiac rupture and fibrinolytic therapy. *Lancet* 1990; **336:** 259–60.
19. Massel DR. How sound is the evidence that thrombolysis increases the risk of cardiac rupture? *Br Heart J* 1993; **69:** 284–7.

Hypersensitivity. Streptokinase is a bacterial protein and has antigenic activity. The formation of streptokinase-neutralising antibodies may reduce the efficacy of subsequent doses and increase the risk of hypersensitivity reactions.

In a series of 25 patients given intravenous streptokinase for myocardial infarction, Jalihal and Morris found that titres of streptokinase-neutralising antibodies rose from a mean neutralisation capacity of 0.16 million units before treatment to a mean of 25.54 million units 2 weeks after treatment, the highest individual titre being 93 million units. After 12 weeks the neutralisation capacity was still sufficient in 24 patients to have neutralised a standard 1.5-million unit dose of streptokinase. After 17 to 34 weeks titres were still high enough in 18 of 20 patients examined to neutralise at least half a standard dose.[1] As these results indicate, administration of standard doses of streptokinase within up to a year of a previous course may lead to reduced effect and up to 12 months is usually stated as the period in which streptokinase should not be repeated (see Precautions, below). However, high titres of neutralising antibodies persisting for up to 4½ years after administration of streptokinase have been reported.[2,3] Since readministration also increases the risk of hypersensitivity reactions, it has been suggested[2,4] that repeat courses should not be given within 4 or more years, and that if a repeat course is needed a non-antigenic thrombolytic such as alteplase or urokinase should be used until it is known whether or not high *in-vitro* titres affect efficacy. Increased titres of streptokinase-neutralising antibodies have also been measured in patients receiving topical streptokinase for wounds.[5]

Anistreplase also appears susceptible to neutralisation by streptokinase antibodies.[6]

Plasmacytosis,[7,8] serum-sickness,[7,9,10] rhabdomyolysis,[11] impaired renal function (see under Effects on the Kidneys, above), uveitis (see under Effects on the Eyes, above), arthritis,[12] and anaphylaxis[13-16] have been reported in patients receiving streptokinase and are thought to represent hypersensitivity reactions, in some cases perhaps due to previous exposure to streptococcal antigens during infection. Back pain (see above) may also represent a hypersensitivity reaction. In some patients there may be a delay of between 1 and 10 days before appearance of the reaction.[17] The incidence of severe hypersensitivity reactions is probably fairly low, however; in the GISSI study anaphylaxis was reported in only 7 of 5860 patients although other hypersensitivity reactions leading to withdrawal of streptokinase were reported in 99 patients, with a further 42 such reactions after completion of the infusion.[14] Some episodes of apparent anaphylaxis seen with streptokinase administration may be plasmin-mediated rather than antibody-antigen reactions. Administration of alteplase, which is considered non-antigenic, produced an anaphylactoid reaction in a patient who had a history of atopy.[18] Plasmin, which activates complement cascade and the kinin system, is formed in quantity after the administration of a thrombolytic. In most patients these effects are clinically insignificant, but in those who are strongly atopic there is the possibility of precipitating an anaphylactoid reaction.

1. Jalihal S, Morris GK. Antistreptokinase titres after intravenous streptokinase. *Lancet* 1990; **335:** 184–5.
2. Elliott JM, *et al.* Neutralizing antibodies to streptokinase four years after intravenous thrombolytic therapy. *Am J Cardiol* 1993; **71:** 640–5.
3. Lee HS, *et al.* Raised levels of antistreptokinase antibody and neutralization titres from 4 days to 54 months after administration of streptokinase or anistreplase. *Eur Heart J* 1993; **14:** 84–9.
4. Jennings K. Antibodies to streptokinase. *Br Med J* 1996; **312:** 393–4.
5. Green C. Antistreptokinase titres after topical streptokinase. *Lancet* 1993; **341:** 1602–3.
6. Binette MJ, Agnone FA. Failure of APSAC thrombolysis. *Ann Intern Med* 1993; **119:** 637.
7. Straub PW, *et al.* Plasmozytose nach thrombolytischer Therapie mit Streptokinase. *Schweiz Med Wochenschr* 1974; **104:** 1891–2.
8. Chan NS, *et al.* Plasmacytosis and renal failure after readministration of streptokinase for threatened myocardial reinfarction. *Br Med J* 1988; **297:** 717–18.
9. Payne ST, *et al.* Transient impairment of renal function after streptokinase therapy. *Lancet* 1989; **ii:** 1398.
10. Callan MFC, *et al.* Proteinuria and thrombolytic agents. *Lancet* 1990; **335:** 106.
11. Montgomery HE, *et al.* Rhabdomyolysis and multiple system organ failure with streptokinase. *Br Med J* 1995; **311:** 1472.
12. Kelly MP, Bielawska C. Recurrence of a reactive arthritis following streptokinase therapy. *Postgrad Med J* 1991; **67:** 402.
13. McGrath KG, Patterson R. Anaphylactic reactivity to streptokinase. *JAMA* 1984; **252:** 1314–17.
14. Gruppo Italiano per lo Studio della Streptochinasi nell'Infarto Miocardico. Effectiveness of intravenous thrombolytic treatment in acute myocardial infarction. *Lancet* 1986; **i:** 397–401.
15. Bednarczyk EM, *et al.* Anaphylactic reaction to streptokinase with first exposure: case report and review of the literature. *DICP Ann Pharmacother* 1989; **23:** 869–72.
16. Tisdale JE, *et al.* Streptokinase-induced anaphylaxis. *DICP Ann Pharmacother* 1989; **23:** 984–7.
17. Seibert WJ, *et al.* Streptokinase morbidity—more common than previously recognised. *Aust N Z J Med* 1992; **22:** 129–33.
18. Purvis JA, *et al.* Anaphylactoid reaction after injection of alteplase. *Lancet* 1993; **341:** 966–7.

Treatment of Adverse Effects

Allergic reactions may require treatment with antihistamines and corticosteroids, which have sometimes been given with streptokinase to reduce the risk of such reactions. Anaphylaxis requires the administration of adrenaline (for further details, see Anaphylactic Shock, p.816).

Severe haemorrhage not controlled by local pressure requires discontinuation of the streptokinase infusion. Tranexamic acid, aminocaproic acid, or aprotinin may be of benefit. Packed red blood cells may be preferable to whole blood for replacement therapy; factor VIII preparations may also be given. Volume expansion may be necessary, but the use of dextrans should be avoided because of their platelet-inhibiting properties.

Precautions

Streptokinase should be used with great care, if at all, in patients at increased risk of bleeding, or those in whom haemorrhage is likely to prove particularly dangerous. It should thus be avoided in patients with active internal bleeding or a recent history of peptic ulcer disease, oesophageal varices, ulcerative colitis or other bleeding gastro-intestinal lesions, in patients with pancreatitis, in patients with coagulation defects including those due to liver or kidney disease, or after recent surgery, parturition, or trauma. It should not be given to patients at increased risk of cerebral bleeding including those with severe hypertension, haemorrhage or recent stroke, or to patients with cerebral neoplasm. It should not be given in pregnancy, particularly in the first 18 weeks because of the risk of placental separation and it has been suggested that it should not be used during heavy vaginal bleeding.

Invasive procedures, including intramuscular injections, should be avoided during, and immediately before and after, streptokinase therapy as they may increase the risk of bleeding. It should be used with care in elderly patients and in patients with diabetic retinopathy. Patients with mitral stenosis associated with atrial fibrillation are more likely to have left heart thrombus which may lead to cerebral embolism following thrombolytic therapy.

The use of streptokinase is contra-indicated in patients with subacute bacterial endocarditis and in streptococcal infection, which may result in the formation of anti-streptokinase antibodies leading to resistance or hypersensitivity. For similar reasons treatment with streptokinase should not be repeated within 12 months of a previous course (even longer periods have been suggested, see Hypersensitivity, under Adverse Effects, above); if thrombolytic therapy is required in this period an alternative non-antigenic drug should be used.

Administration. Overinfusion of streptokinase may occur if a drop-counting infusion pump is employed.[1] This arises as a result of flocculation of the streptokinase solution producing translucent fibres that affect the drop-forming mechanism so increasing the drop size.

For a comment on the incidence of flocculation in streptokinase solutions, see under Stability, above.

1. Schad RF, Jennings RH. Overinfusions of streptokinase. *Am J Hosp Pharm* 1982; **39:** 1850.

Aortic dissection. A report of 4 cases of the inappropriate use of streptokinase in patients with aortic dissection misdiagnosed as myocardial infarction.[1] Thrombolytics are likely to extend aortic dissection and adversely affect the outcome. Of the 2 patients who died, one, who would have been suitable for early operation, died through the delay caused by impaired clotting. Although early intervention with thrombolytics may be of major benefit in acute myocardial infarction it is important that accurate differential diagnosis takes place to exclude conditions such as aortic dissection and prevent avoidable deaths.

1. Butler J, *et al.* Streptokinase in acute aortic dissection. *Br Med J* 1990; **300:** 517–19.

Haemorrhage. Streptokinase should be used with great care, if at all, in patients at increased risk of bleeding, or those in whom haemorrhage is likely to prove particularly dangerous. Thrombolytics are not recommended after prolonged or traumatic cardiopulmonary resuscitation because of the risk of haemorrhage. However, no clinically significant bleeding complications were found in a study in 39 patients with acute myocardial infarction who had a cardiac arrest before or shortly after receiving thrombolysis.[1]

1. Cross SJ, *et al.* Safety of thrombolysis in association with cardiopulmonary resuscitation. *Br Med J* 1991; **303:** 1242.

Pregnancy. Thrombolytics are contra-indicated in pregnancy, although there are a few reports of their use which have been briefly reviewed.[1] In most cases, thrombolytics were given at 28 weeks of pregnancy or later to patients with deep-vein thrombosis, pulmonary embolism, or prosthetic valve thrombosis. There were some reports of favourable maternal and fetal outcomes although therapy was associated with maternal haemorrhage, including spontaneous abortion and minor vaginal bleeding, especially when given near the time of delivery. There was one report of abruptio placentae with fetal death.

1. Roth A, Elkayam U. Acute myocardial infarction associated with pregnancy. *Ann Intern Med* 1996; **125:** 751–62.

Interactions

Oral anticoagulants, heparin, and antiplatelet drugs such as aspirin are often used in conjunction with streptokinase, but may increase the risk of haemorrhage. Other drugs which affect platelet function may do likewise, including allopurinol, dextrans, quinidine, sex hormones, sulphonamides, tetracyclines, valproic acid, and some essential oils.

Pharmacokinetics

Streptokinase is rapidly cleared from the circulation following intravenous administration. Clearance is biphasic with the initial and more rapid phase being due to specific antibodies. A half-life of 23 minutes has been reported for the streptokinase-activator complex.

References.

1. Grierson DS, Bjornsson TD. Pharmacokinetics of streptokinase in patients based on amidolytic activator complex activity. *Clin Pharmacol Ther* 1987; **41:** 304–13.
2. Gemmill JD, *et al.* A comparison of the pharmacokinetic properties of streptokinase and anistreplase in acute myocardial infarction. *Br J Clin Pharmacol* 1991; **31:** 143–7.

Uses and Administration

Streptokinase is a thrombolytic drug derived from various streptococci. It rapidly activates endogenous plasminogen, indirectly by means of a streptokinase-plasminogen complex, to plasmin (p.932), which has fibrinolytic effects and can dissolve intravascular blood clots. The mechanisms of fibrinolysis are discussed further under Haemostasis on p.704. Streptokinase affects circulating, unbound plasminogen as well as fibrin-bound plasminogen and thus may be termed a fibrin-nonspecific thrombolytic agent. This action was thought to contribute to the risk of haemorrhage, although currently available fibrin-specific agents, such as alteplase, do not produce less bleeding than nonspecific thrombolytics (see Haemorrhage under Adverse Effects, above).

Streptokinase is given by intravenous or sometimes intra-arterial infusion in the treatment of thrombo-embolic disorders such as myocardial infarction (p.791), peripheral arterial thrombo-embolism (below), and venous thrombo-embolism (deep-vein thrombosis and pulmonary embolism) (p.802). It has also been tried in unstable angina (p.780) and in ischaemic stroke (p.799), but these uses are less well-established. Streptokinase may be used to clear cannulas and shunts and is used topically in conjunction with streptodornase to clear clots and purulent matter.

In the treatment of **myocardial infarction** a single dose of 1.5 million units of streptokinase is infused intravenously over 1 hour as soon as possible after the onset of symptoms. Coronary catheterisation with the aid of angiography is required for appropriate intracoronary infusion in myocardial infarction, thus restricting administration to suitably equipped centres. An initial intracoronary dose of 10 000 to 25 000 units has been given as a bolus injection followed by an infusion of 2000 to 4000 units per minute. Infusion has been continued until reperfusion has been achieved (usually within about 30 minutes) and for 30 to 60 minutes thereafter, or for 60 to 75 minutes if reperfusion has not been achieved.

In the treatment of **pulmonary embolism** and other **arteriovenous occlusions** an initial loading dose of streptokinase, normally 250 000 units infused intravenously over 30 minutes is given to overcome any resistance due to circulating antibodies. This is followed by infusion of a maintenance dose of 100 000 units per hour for 24 to 72 hours, depending on the condition to be treated. Treatment should be controlled by monitoring the thrombin clotting time, which should be maintained at 2 to 4 times normal values. Since thrombolytic activity rapidly fades when the infusion stops, streptokinase treatment is generally followed by intravenous heparin infusion, and then oral anticoagulation, to prevent re-occlusion. In children, the initial dose should be estimated according to the streptokinase resistance; maintenance doses of 1300 to 1400 units per kg body-weight per hour or 20 units per mL of blood volume per hour have been suggested.

Streptokinase, as a solution containing 1000 units per mL, is used to clear shunts of occluding thrombi; 250 000 units in 2 mL is used to clear occluded cannulas.

General references.

1. Fears R. Biochemical pharmacology and therapeutic aspects of thrombolytic agents. *Pharmacol Rev* 1990; **42:** 201–21.
2. Stringer KA. Beyond thrombolysis: other effects of thrombolytic drugs. *Ann Pharmacother* 1994; **28:** 752–6.
3. Ludlam CA, *et al.* Guidelines for the use of thrombolytic therapy. *Blood Coag Fibrinol* 1995; **6:** 273–85.

Empyema. Thoracic empyema is treated with antibacterials and pleural drainage. Efficient removal of fluid may be impaired by fibrinous clots within the pleural cavity. Intrapleural instillation of streptokinase (100 000 to 750 000 units in up to 100 mL of sodium chloride 0.9%)[1] or urokinase (100 000 to 250 000 units in 100 mL of sodium chloride 0.9%)[1] has been reported to be effective in small series of patients.[1-4]

Intrapericardial instillation of thrombolytics has been tried in a few patients with pericardial empyema to prevent the development of constrictive pericarditis.[5]

1. Temes RT, *et al.* Intrapleural fibrinolytics in management of empyema thoracis. *Chest* 1996; **110:** 102–6.
2. Bouros D, *et al.* Role of streptokinase in the treatment of acute loculated parapneumonic pleural effusions and empyema. *Thorax* 1994; **49:** 852–5.
3. Davies RJO, *et al.* Randomised controlled trial of intrapleural streptokinase in community acquired pleural infection. *Thorax* 1997; **52:** 416–21.
4. Bouros D, *et al.* Intrapleural streptokinase versus urokinase in the treatment of complicated parapneumonic effusions: a prospective, double-blind study. *Am J Respir Crit Care Med* 1997; **155:** 291–5.
5. Winkler W-B, *et al.* Treatment of exudative fibrinous pericarditis with intrapericardial urokinase. *Lancet* 1994; **344:** 1541–2.

Intracardiac thrombosis. Thrombosis of prosthetic heart valves is usually managed surgically. Thrombolysis has been tried and may be useful, especially in critically ill patients. Streptokinase or urokinase are the thrombolytics usually employed, although alteplase has also been used.[1,2]

1. Vasan RS, *et al.* Thrombolytic therapy for prosthetic valve thrombosis: a study based on serial Doppler echocardiographic evaluation. *Am Heart J* 1992; **123:** 1575–80.
2. Silber H, *et al.* The St Jude valve: thrombolysis as the first line of therapy for cardiac valve thrombosis. *Circulation* 1993; **87:** 30–7.

Peripheral arterial thrombo-embolism. Thrombolytics including streptokinase may be used in the management of peripheral arterial thrombo-embolism (p.794). Streptokinase has been injected intravenously or intra-arterially directly into the clot as an alternative to surgical treatment of the occlusion. It has also been infused intra-arterially to remove distal clots during a surgical procedure. The intravenous dose generally used is 250 000 units over 30 minutes followed by 100 000 units per hour. A lower dose of 5000 units per hour has been used intra-arterially directly into the clot[1] and for removal of distal clots during a surgical procedure streptokinase has been given intra-arterially in a dose of 100 000 units over 30 minutes or as five bolus doses of 20 000 units at 5-minute intervals.[2]

1. Anonymous. Non-coronary thrombolysis. *Lancet* 1990; **335:** 691–3.
2. Earnshaw JJ, Beard JD. Intraoperative use of thrombolytic agents. *Br Med J* 1993; **307:** 638–9.

Preparations

BP 1998: Streptokinase Injection.

Proprietary Preparations (details are given in Part 3)
Aust.: Kabikinase; Streptase; ***Austral.:*** Kabikinase; Streptase; ***Belg.:*** Kabikinase; Streptase; ***Canad.:*** Kabikinase; Streptase; ***Fr.:*** Kabikinase; Streptase; ***Ger.:*** Kabikinase; Streptase; ***Irl.:*** Kabikinase; Streptase; ***Ital.:*** Kabikinase†; Streptase; ***Neth.:*** Kabikinase; Streptase; ***Norw.:*** Kabikinase; Streptase; ***S.Afr.:*** Kabikinase; Streptase; ***Spain:*** Kabikinase; Streptase; ***Swed.:*** Kabikinase; Streptase; ***Switz.:*** Kabikinase; Streptase; ***UK:*** Kabikinase; Streptase; ***USA:*** Kabikinase; Streptase.

Multi-ingredient: ***Aust.:*** Varidase; ***Austral.:*** Varidase; ***Belg.:*** Varidase; ***Ger.:*** Varidase; ***Irl.:*** Varidase; ***Ital.:*** Varibiotic†; Varidase; ***Neth.:*** Varidase; ***Norw.:*** Varidase; ***S.Afr.:*** Varidase; ***Spain:*** Ernodasa; Varibiotic; Varidasa; ***Swed.:*** Varidase; ***UK:*** Varidase.

Strophanthin-K (5827-v)

Estrofantina; Kombé Strophanthin; Strophanthin; Strophanthoside-K.

CAS — 11005-63-3.

NOTE. Do not confuse with K-strophanthin-α which is Cymarin (p.845).

Pharmacopoeias. In *Aust.* and *It.*

A mixture of cardiac glycosides from strophanthus, the seeds of *Strophanthus kombe* (Apocynaceae) or other spp., adjusted by admixture with a suitable diluent such as lactose so as generally to possess 40% of the activity of anhydrous ouabain.

Strophanthin-K is a positive inotrope with general properties similar to those of digoxin (p.849). It has been used in the treatment of heart failure p.785. It is poorly absorbed from the gastro-intestinal tract. Strophanthin-K may be given intravenously in doses of 125 to 500 μg daily.

Preparations

Proprietary Preparations (details are given in Part 3)
Aust.: Laevostrophan; ***Ger.:*** Kombetin; ***Ital.:*** Kombetin; Strofopan Vena†.

Multi-ingredient: ***Aust.:*** Laevostrophan compositum; ***Fr.:*** Biocarde; Canteine Bouteille†; Sedibaine; ***Ger.:*** Cordalin-Strophanthin†; Myonasan†; Strophanthus-Strath†; Theokombetin†.

Suloctidil (9278-n)

Suloctidil *(BAN, USAN, rINN).*

CP-556S; MJF-12637. 1-(4-Isopropylthiophenyl)-2-octylaminopropan-1-ol.

$C_{20}H_{35}NOS = 337.6.$

CAS — 54063-56-8.

Suloctidil is a vasodilator that was formerly used in the management of peripheral and cerebral vascular disorders. It is hepatotoxic and fatalities have occurred.

Sulodexide (13285-j)

Sulodexide *(rINN).*

Glucurono-2-amino-2-deoxyglucoglucan sulphate.

CAS — 57821-29-1.

Sulodexide is a heparinoid consisting of a mixture of low-molecular-weight heparin and dermatan sulphate. It is used as a hypolipidaemic and antithrombotic and has been administered by mouth and parenterally.

General references.

1. Ofosu FA. Pharmacological actions of sulodexide. *Semin Thromb Hemost* 1998; **24:** 127–38.

Preparations

Proprietary Preparations (details are given in Part 3)
Ital.: Clarens; Suldex†; Vessel Due F; ***Spain:*** Aterina; Luzone.

Multi-ingredient: ***Ital.:*** Dermoangiopan; Vessiflex; ***Spain:*** Venoflavan†.

Sulotroban (18855-m)

Sulotroban *(BAN, USAN, rINN).*

BM-13177; SKF-95587. [*p*-(2-Benzenesulfonamidoethyl)phenoxy]acetic acid.

$C_{16}H_{17}NO_5S = 335.4.$

CAS — 72131-33-0.

Sulotroban is a thromboxane A_2 antagonist under investigation as an antiplatelet drug.

References.

1. Piper C, *et al.* Pharmacokinetics of the thromboxane A_2 receptor antagonist sulotroban (BM 13177) in renal failure. *Br J Clin Pharmacol* 1989; **28:** 281–8.
2. Pierucci A, *et al.* Improvement of renal function with selective thromboxane antagonism in lupus nephritis. *N Engl J Med* 1989; **320:** 421–5.
3. Savage MP, *et al.* Multi-hospital Eastern Atlantic Restenosis trial II: a placebo-controlled trial of thromboxane blockage in the prevention of restenosis following coronary angioplasty. *Am Heart J* 1991; **122:** 1239–44.
4. Savage MP, *et al.* Effect of thromboxane A_2 blockade on clinical outcome and restenosis after successful coronary angioplasty: Multi-Hospital Eastern Atlantic Restenosis Trial (M-HEART II). *Circulation* 1995; **92:** 3194–3200.

Sympathomimetics (2040-z)

Adverse Effects

The adverse effects of sympathomimetics in general are covered under Adrenaline, p.813. For specific details see under the individual monographs.

Precautions

The precautions for sympathomimetics in general are discussed under Adrenaline, p.814. For specific details see under the individual monographs.

Interactions

The interactions of sympathomimetics with other drugs can be found in Adrenaline, p.814. For specific details see under the individual monographs.

Uses and Administration

Sympathomimetics possess a wide variety of uses and these, together with their pharmacological actions, are discussed further under Adrenaline, p.815.

Syrosingopine (905-s)

Syrosingopine *(BAN, rINN).*

Methyl Carbethoxysyringoyl Reserpate; Su-3118. Methyl *O*-(4-ethoxycarbonyloxy-3,5-dimethoxybenzoyl)reserpate.

$C_{35}H_{42}N_2O_{11} = 666.7.$

CAS — 84-36-6.

Syrosingopine is a derivative of reserpine (p.942) that has been used in the treatment of hypertension.

Preparations

Proprietary Preparations (details are given in Part 3)
Ital.: Neoreserpan†.

Multi-ingredient: ***Ital.:*** Notens†; Raunova Plus†.

Talinolol (1015-g)

Talinolol *(rINN).*

(±)-1-{*p*-[3-(*tert*-Butylamino)-2-hydroxypropoxy]phenyl}-3-cyclohexylurea.

$C_{20}H_{33}N_3O_3 = 363.5.$

CAS — 57460-41-0.

Talinolol is a cardioselective beta blocker (p.828). It is given by mouth in the management of hypertension and other cardiovascular disorders. It may also be given intravenously.

Preparations

Proprietary Preparations (details are given in Part 3)
Ger.: Cordanum.

Tamsulosin Hydrochloride (1543-q)

Tamsulosin Hydrochloride *(BANM, USAN, rINNM).*

LY-253351; R-(−)-YM-12617; YM-617; YM-12617-1. (−)-(*R*)-5-(2-{[2-(*o*-Ethoxyphenoxy)ethyl]amino}-propyl)-2-methoxybenzenesulfonamide hydrochloride.

$C_{20}H_{28}N_2O_5S,HCl = 445.0.$

CAS — 106133-20-4 (tamsulosin); 106463-17-6 (tamsulosin hydrochloride).

Adverse Effects, Treatment, and Precautions

As for Prazosin Hydrochloride, p.932. Tamsulosin should be avoided in severe liver impairment.

Pharmacokinetics

Tamsulosin hydrochloride is absorbed from the gastro-intestinal tract and is almost completely bioavailable. The extent and rate of absorption are reduced in the presence of food. Following oral administration, peak plasma concentrations occur about 1 hour after a dose. Tamsulosin is metabolised slowly in the liver and is excreted mainly in the urine as metabolites and some unchanged drug. The plasma elimination half-life has been reported to be between 4 and 5.5 hours. Tamsulosin is about 99% bound to plasma proteins.

Renal impairment. Plasma-tamsulosin concentrations were reported to be increased in patients with renal impairment when compared with volunteers.[1] However, plasma concentrations of unbound, pharmacologically active drug were similar in both groups and it was suggested that the raised total plasma concentrations were due to an increase in plasma protein binding.

1. Koiso K, *et al.* Pharmacokinetics of tamsulosin hydrochloride in patients with renal impairment: effects of α_1-acid glycoprotein. *J Clin Pharmacol* 1996; **36:** 1029–38.

Uses and Administration

Tamsulosin is an alpha$_1$-adrenoceptor blocker (p.776) with actions similar to those of prazosin (p.933); it is reported to be more selective for the alpha$_{1A}$-adrenoceptor subtype. It is used in the symptomatic treatment of urinary obstruction caused by benign prostatic hyperplasia (p.1446).

Tamsulosin is given by mouth as the hydrochloride. In benign prostatic hyperplasia it is administered in a modified-release formulation, in a dose of 400 μg once daily, after breakfast. The dose may be increased after 2 to 4 weeks, if necessary, to 800 μg once daily.

Reviews.

1. Wilde MI, McTavish D. Tamsulosin: a review of its pharmacological properties and therapeutic potential in the management of symptomatic benign prostatic hyperplasia. *Drugs* 1996; **52:** 883–98.

Preparations

Proprietary Preparations (details are given in Part 3)
Fr.: Omix; ***Ger.:*** Alna; Omnic; ***Irl.:*** Omnic; ***Ital.:*** Omnic; Pradif; ***Jpn:*** Harnal; ***Neth.:*** Omnic; ***UK:*** Flomax; ***USA:*** Flomax.

Tasosartan (17859-f)

Tasosartan *(BAN, USAN, rINN).*

WAY-ANA-756. 5,8-Dihydro-2,4-dimethyl-8-[*p*-(*o*-1*H*-tetrazol-5-ylphenyl)-benzyl]pyrido[2,3*d*]pyrimidin-7(6*H*)-one.

$C_{23}H_{21}N_7O = 411.5.$

CAS — 145733-36-4.

Tasosartan is an angiotensin II receptor antagonist under investigation for the management of hypertension.

References.

1. Oparil S, *et al.* Tolerability profile of tasosartan, a long-acting angiotensin II AT_1 receptor blocker, in the treatment of patients with essential hypertension. *Curr Ther Res* 1997; **58:** 930–43.

Teclothiazide Potassium (2356-l)

Teclothiazide Potassium *(BANM, rINNM).*

Tetrachlormethiazide. 6-Chloro-3,4-dihydro-3-trichloromethyl-2*H*-1,2,4-benzothiadiazine-7-sulphonamide 1,1-dioxide, potassium salt.

$C_8H_7Cl_4N_3O_4S_2,K = 454.2.$

CAS — 4267-05-4 (teclothiazide); 5306-80-9 (teclothiazide potassium).

Teclothiazide potassium is a thiazide diuretic (see Hydrochlorothiazide, p.885) used in the treatment of oedema.

Preparations

Proprietary Preparations (details are given in Part 3)
Multi-ingredient: ***Spain:*** Quimodril.

Telmisartan (17450-x)

Telmisartan *(USAN, rINN).*

BIBR-277-SE. 4′-{[4-Methyl-6-(1-methyl-2-benzimidazolyl)-2-propyl-1-benzimidazolyl]methyl}-2-biphenylcarboxylic acid.

$C_{33}H_{30}N_4O_2 = 514.6.$

CAS — 144701-48-4.

Telmisartan is an angiotensin II receptor antagonist under investigation for the management of hypertension.

Temocapril Hydrochloride (10960-s)

Temocapril Hydrochloride *(BANM, USAN, rINNM).*

CS-622. (+)-(2*S*,6*R*)-6-{[(1*S*)-1-Carboxy-3-phenyl-propyl]amino}tetrahydro-5-oxo-2-(2-thienyl)-1,4-thiazepine-4(5*H*)-acetic acid, 6-ethyl ester, hydrochloride.

$C_{23}H_{28}N_2O_5S_2,HCl = 513.1.$

CAS — 111902-57-9 (temocapril); 110221-44-8 (temocapril hydrochloride).

Temocapril is an ACE inhibitor (p.805). It is used as the hydrochloride in the treatment of hypertension. It owes its activity to the diacid temocaprilat to which it is converted after oral administration.

References.

1. Nakashima M, *et al.* Pharmacokinetics of temocapril hydrochloride, a novel angiotensin converting enzyme inhibitor, in renal insufficiency. *Eur J Clin Pharmacol* 1992; **43:** 657–9.

2. Oguchi H, *et al.* Pharmacokinetics of temocapril and enalapril in patients with various degrees of renal insufficiency. *Clin Pharmacokinet* 1993; **24:** 421–7.
3. Furuta S, *et al.* Pharmacokinetics of temocapril, an ACE inhibitor with preferential biliary excretion, in patients with impaired liver function. *Eur J Clin Pharmacol* 1993; **44:** 383–5.

Preparations

Proprietary Preparations (details are given in Part 3)
Jpn: Acecol.

Tenitramine (13304-n)

NNN'N'-Tetrakis(2-hydroxyethyl)ethylenediamine tetranitrate.

$C_{10}H_{20}N_6O_{12}$ = 416.3.
CAS — 21946-79-2.

Tenitramine is a vasodilator with general properties similar to those of glyceryl trinitrate (p.875) and is used in angina pectoris (p.780). It is given in a usual dose of 10 mg by mouth for acute attacks and 10 mg every six hours for long-term management.

Preparations

Proprietary Preparations (details are given in Part 3)
Ital.: Tenitran.

Teprotide (906-w)

Teprotide *(BAN, USAN, rINN).*

BPF_{9a}; L-Pyroglutamyl-L-tryptophyl-L-prolyl-L-arginyl-L-prolyl-L-glutaminyl-L-isoleucyl-L-prolyl-L-proline; SQ-20881; 2-L-Tryptophan-3-de-L-leucine-4-de-L-proline-8-L-glutamine-bradykinin potentiator B. 5-oxo-Pro-Trp-Pro-Arg-Pro-Gln-Ile-Pro-Pro.

$C_{53}H_{76}N_{14}O_{12}$ = 1101.3.
CAS — 35115-60-7.

Teprotide is a nonapeptide originally found in the venom of *Bothrops jararaca*, a South American pit-viper. It is an ACE inhibitor that was given parenterally and preceded the orally active inhibitors such as captopril. It has a short duration of action and has been used as an investigational tool in hypertension.

Terazosin Hydrochloride (13306-m)

Terazosin Hydrochloride *(BANM, USAN, rINNM).*

Abbott-45975. 1-(4-Amino-6,7-dimethoxyquinazolin-2-yl)-4-(tetrahydro-2-furoyl)piperazine hydrochloride dihydrate; 6,7-Dimethoxy-2-[4-(tetrahydrofuran-2-carbonyl)piperazin-1-yl]quinazolin-4-ylamine hydrochloride dihydrate.

$C_{19}H_{25}N_5O_4,HCl,2H_2O$ = 459.9.
CAS — 63590-64-7 (terazosin); 63074-08-8 (terazosin hydrochloride, anhydrous); 70024-40-7 (terazosin hydrochloride, dihydrate).

Terazosin hydrochloride 1.2 mg is approximately equivalent to 1 mg of terazosin.

Adverse Effects, Treatment, and Precautions

As for Prazosin Hydrochloride, p.932.

Urinary incontinence. For reference to urinary incontinence associated with terazosin, see under Adverse Effects of Prazosin Hydrochloride, p.932.

Interactions

As for Prazosin Hydrochloride, p.933.

Pharmacokinetics

Terazosin is rapidly and almost completely absorbed from the gastro-intestinal tract after oral administration; the bioavailability is reported to be about 90%. Peak plasma concentrations are achieved in about one hour. It is metabolised in the liver; one of the metabolites is reported to possess antihypertensive activity. The half-life in plasma is approximately 12 hours. It is excreted in faeces via the bile, and in the urine, as unchanged drug and metabolites. Terazosin is 90 to 94% protein bound.

Uses and Administration

Terazosin is an alpha$_1$-adrenoceptor blocker (p.776) with actions similar to those of prazosin (p.933), but a longer duration of action.

It is used in the management of hypertension (p.788) and in benign prostatic hyperplasia (p.1446) to relieve urinary obstruction.

Terazosin is given by mouth as the hydrochloride, but doses are usually expressed in terms of the base. Following oral administration its hypotensive effects are seen within 15 minutes and may last for up to 24 hours, permitting once daily dosage.

To avoid the risk of collapse which may occur in some patients after the first dose the initial dose for both hypertension and benign prostatic hyperplasia is 1 mg of terazosin at bedtime, increasing gradually at intervals of 7 days according to the patient's response. For hypertension the usual maintenance dose is 2 to 10 mg once daily and the usual maximum dose is 20 mg daily. In the US, administration of the daily dose in two divided doses has been suggested if 24-hour control of blood pressure proves inadequate. For benign prostatic hyperplasia the usual maintenance dose is 5 to 10 mg once daily.

Reviews.

1. Titmarsh S, Monk JP. Terazosin: a review of its pharmacodynamic and pharmacokinetic properties, and therapeutic efficacy in essential hypertension. *Drugs* 1987; **33:** 461–77.
2. Achari R, Laddu A. Terazosin: a new alpha adrenoceptor blocking drug. *J Clin Pharmacol* 1992; **32:** 520–3.
3. Anonymous. Terazosin for benign prostatic hyperplasia. *Med Lett Drugs Ther* 1994; **36:** 15–16.

Preparations

Proprietary Preparations (details are given in Part 3)
Aust.: Uroflo; Vicard†; ***Austral.:*** Hytrin; ***Belg.:*** Hytrin; ***Canad.:*** Hytrin; ***Ger.:*** Flotrin; Heitrin; ***Irl.:*** Hytrin; ***Ital.:*** Itrin; Teraprost; Urodie; ***Neth.:*** Hytrin; ***S.Afr.:*** Hytrin; ***Spain:*** Deflox; Magnurol; ***Swed.:*** Hytrinex; Sinalfa; ***Switz.:*** Hytrin BPH; Vicard†; ***UK:*** Hytrin; Hytrin BPH; ***USA:*** Hytrin.

Tertatolol Hydrochloride (1143-j)

Tertatolol Hydrochloride *(BANM, rINNM).*

S-2395 (tertatolol or tertatolol hydrochloride); SE-2395 (tertatolol or tertatolol hydrochloride). (±)-1-(*tert*-Butylamino)-3-(thiochroman-8-yloxy)propan-2-ol hydrochloride.

$C_{16}H_{25}NO_2S,HCl$ = 331.9.
CAS — 34784-64-0 (tertatolol); 33580-30-2 (tertatolol hydrochloride).

Tertatolol is a non-cardioselective beta blocker (p.828). It is reported to lack intrinsic sympathomimetic activity.

Tertatolol is given by mouth as the hydrochloride in the management of hypertension (p.788) in single doses of 5 mg daily.

Preparations

Proprietary Preparations (details are given in Part 3)
Belg.: Artex; ***Fr.:*** Artex; ***Ger.:*** Prenalex; ***Irl.:*** Artexal; ***Neth.:*** Artex.

Thymoxamine Hydrochloride (9280-a)

Thymoxamine Hydrochloride *(BANM).*

Moxisylyte Hydrochloride *(rINNM)*; Moxisilita Clorhidrato. 4-(2-Dimethylaminoethoxy)-5-isopropyl-2-methylphenyl acetate hydrochloride.

$C_{16}H_{25}NO_3,HCl$ = 315.8.
CAS — 54-32-0 (thymoxamine); 964-52-3 (thymoxamine hydrochloride).

NOTE. THY is a code approved by the BP for use on single unit doses of eye drops containing thymoxamine hydrochloride where the individual container may be too small to bear all the appropriate labelling information.

Pharmacopoeias. In *Br.* and *Jpn.*

A white odourless or almost odourless crystalline powder. Thymoxamine hydrochloride 45.2 mg is approximately equivalent to 40 mg of thymoxamine. Freely **soluble** in water; soluble in alcohol; freely soluble in chloroform; practically insoluble in ether and petroleum spirit. A 5% solution in water has a pH of 4.5 to 5.5. **Protect** from light.

Adverse Effects

Thymoxamine hydrochloride may cause nausea, diarrhoea, headache, vertigo, flushing of the skin, dry mouth, and nasal congestion. Hepatotoxicity has been reported. Overdosage may cause hypotension.

Transient ptosis has occurred occasionally following ophthalmic application. Prolonged erections or priapism have occurred rarely following intracavernosal injection.

Effects on the liver. Hepatic adverse reactions have been noted with thymoxamine. These first appeared in France following its use in benign prostatic hyperplasia, a condition in which relatively high doses were employed (up to 480 mg daily compared with up to 320 mg daily for peripheral vascular disease). Since then the Committee on Safety of Medicines in the UK has received reports associated with lower doses.[1] Thirteen hepatic reactions, accounting for 17% of all reports of suspected adverse reactions to thymoxamine, had been received and comprised hepatic function abnormalities (3), jaundice (3), cholestatic jaundice (4), hepatitis (2), and hepatitis with jaundice (1). In most cases the reaction occurred within 5 weeks of the start of treatment and resolved on drug withdrawal. In 9 cases the dosage of thymoxamine was known and varied from 80 to 320 mg daily with 7 patients receiving 160 mg or less daily.

1. Committee on Safety of Medicines/Medicines Control Agency. Hepatic reactions with thymoxamine (Opilon). *Current Problems* 1993; **19:** 11–12.

Precautions

Thymoxamine hydrochloride should not be given to patients with active liver disease and should be given with care to patients with diabetes mellitus. Monitoring of liver function is recommended, especially if therapy is prolonged or if high doses are being employed. Intracavernosal injection of thymoxamine is contra-indicated in patients with conditions that predispose to priapism.

Interactions

Thymoxamine may enhance the effects of antihypertensives and the hypotensive effect of thymoxamine may be enhanced by tricyclic antidepressants.

Uses and Administration

Thymoxamine hydrochloride is an alpha-adrenoceptor blocker with vasodilating activity that is used in the treatment of peripheral vascular disease (p.794). The usual dose is the equivalent of 40 mg of thymoxamine four times daily by mouth increased if necessary to 80 mg four times daily. It should be withdrawn if there is no response in 2 weeks.

Intracavernosal injection of thymoxamine hydrochloride by self administration may be employed to treat erectile dysfunction (p.1614). The initial dose is 10 mg; if this is unsuccessful a dose of 20 mg may be used. Thymoxamine should not be injected intracavernosally more than three times a week and there should be at least 48 hours between injections.

Thymoxamine has been used locally in the eye to reverse the mydriasis caused by phenylephrine and other sympathomimetics. It has also been used orally in benign prostatic hyperplasia, although such use has been associated with reports of hepatotoxicity; the doses used in prostatic hyperplasia were generally higher than those in peripheral vascular disease.

Ophthalmic use. References.

1. Relf SJ, *et al.* Thymoxamine reverses phenylephrine-induced mydriasis. *Am J Ophthalmol* 1988; **106:** 251–5.
2. Sharma A, Votruba M. Thymoxamine in the treatment of traumatic mydriasis. *Br J Ophthalmol* 1993; **77:** 681.

Preparations

BP 1998: Moxisylyte Tablets.

Proprietary Preparations (details are given in Part 3)
Fr.: Carlytene; Icavex; Uroalpha†; ***Irl.:*** Opilon; ***Ital.:*** Arlitene; ***Spain:*** Apifor†; ***UK:*** Erecnos; Opilon.

Tiamenidine Hydrochloride (13336-s)

Tiamenidine Hydrochloride *(BANM, USAN, rINNM).*

HOE-42-440; HOE-440 (tiamenidine). (2-Chloro-4-methyl-3-thienyl)-2-imidazolin-2-ylamine hydrochloride.

$C_8H_{10}ClN_3S,HCl$ = 252.2.
CAS — 31428-61-2 (tiamenidine); 51274-83-0 (tiamenidine hydrochloride); 31428-62-3 (tiamenidine hydrochloride).

Tiamenidine hydrochloride is an alpha$_2$-adrenoceptor agonist with general properties similar to those of clonidine (p.841). It has been used in the treatment of hypertension.

Tiapamil (13338-e)

Tiapamil *(BAN, rINN).*

Ditian Tetraoxide; Ro-11-1781; Ro-11-1781/023 (tiapamil hydrochloride); Verocainine. 3,4-Dimethoxyphenethyl{3-[2-(3,4-dimethoxyphenyl)-1,3-dithian-2-yl]propyl}methylamine S,S,S',S'-tetraoxide.

$C_{26}H_{37}NO_8S_2$ = 555.7.
CAS — 57010-31-8 (tiapamil); 87434-83-1 (tiapamil hydrochloride).

NOTE. Tiapamil Hydrochloride is *USAN.*

Tiapamil is an analogue of verapamil (see p.960) with calcium-channel blocking properties that has been tried in the management of angina pectoris and other cardiac disorders and also in the management of hypertension.

References.

1. Eckert M, *et al.* Pharmacokinetics and hemodynamic effects of tiapamil: exercise performance, thallium stress scintigraphy, and radionuclide ventriculography. *J Clin Pharmacol* 1984; **24:** 165–73.
2. Maltz MB, *et al.* Duration of action of tiapamil in stable exercise induced angina. *Eur J Clin Pharmacol* 1987; **32:** 339–42.
3. Balansard P, *et al.* Effect of a new calcium antagonist, tiapamil, in hypertension of the elderly. *Br J Clin Pharmacol* 1984; **18:** 823–9.

Ticlopidine Hydrochloride (13343-p)

Ticlopidine Hydrochloride *(BANM, USAN, rINNM)*.

4-C-32; 53-32C; Ticlopidini Hydrochloridum. 5-(2-Chlorobenzyl)-4,5,6,7-tetrahydrothieno[3,2-*c*]pyridine hydrochloride.

$C_{14}H_{14}ClNS,HCl = 300.2$.

CAS — 55142-85-3 (ticlopidine); 53885-35-1 (ticlopidine hydrochloride).

Pharmacopoeias. In *Eur.* (see p.viii) and *Jpn.*

A white or almost white crystalline powder. Sparingly **soluble** in water and in alcohol; very slightly soluble in ethyl acetate; practically insoluble in ether. A 2.5% solution in water has a pH of 3.5 to 4.0.

Adverse Effects and Precautions

Gastro-intestinal disturbances and skin rashes are the most commonly reported side-effects associated with ticlopidine therapy. Blood dyscrasias, including neutropenia and thrombotic thrombocytopenic purpura, and haemorrhagic disorders have also occurred. There have been reports of hepatitis and cholestatic jaundice. Blood-lipid concentrations may increase during long-term therapy.

Ticlopidine should not be administered to patients with haematopoietic disorders such as neutropenia or thrombocytopenia, haemorrhagic diathesis or other haemorrhagic disorders associated with a prolonged bleeding time, or conditions with an increased risk of bleeding such as gastro-intestinal ulcers, acute cerebral haemorrhage, or severe liver dysfunction. Patients should be monitored every 2 weeks for haematological toxicity during the first 3 months of therapy.

Effects on the blood. Severe neutropenia or agranulocytosis may occur in about 1% of patients given ticlopidine[1,2] and fatal infection has been reported.[3] Neutropenia usually develops within the first three months of therapy and is reversible on discontinuation of ticlopidine, but there has been a report[4] of a delayed reaction that occurred 18 days after ticlopidine was discontinued. Thrombocytopenia and thrombotic thrombocytopenic purpura, sometimes fatal, have also been reported in patients receiving ticlopidine,[5-9,15] although good results have been achieved with ticlopidine as a treatment for thrombotic thrombocytopenic purpura.[10] Aplastic anaemia has occurred.[11,12] The Food and Drug Administration in the US,[13] and the Committee on Safety of Medicines in the UK,[14] recommend complete blood counts every two weeks during the first three months of therapy with ticlopidine.

1. Anonymous. Ticlopidine for prevention of stroke. *Med Lett Drugs Ther* 1992; **34:** 65–6.
2. Love BB, *et al.* Adverse haematological effects of ticlopidine: prevention, recognition and management. *Drug Safety* 1998; **19:** 89–98.
3. Carlson JA, Maesner JE. Fatal neutropenia and thrombocytopenia associated with ticlopidine. *Ann Pharmacother* 1994; **28:** 1236–8.
4. Farver DK, Hansen LA. Delayed neutropenia with ticlopidine. *Ann Pharmacother* 1994; **28:** 1344–6.
5. Takishita S, *et al.* Ticlopidine and thrombocytopenia. *N Engl J Med* 1990; **323:** 1487.
6. Page Y, *et al.* Thrombotic thrombocytopenic purpura related to ticlopidine. *Lancet* 1991; **337:** 774–6.
7. Kovacs MJ, *et al.* Thrombotic thrombocytopenic purpura associated with ticlopidine. *Ann Pharmacother* 1993; **27:** 1060–1.
8. Kupfer Y, Tessler S. Ticlopidine and thrombotic thrombocytopenic purpura. *N Engl J Med* 1997; **337:** 1245.
9. Bennett CL, *et al.* Thrombotic thrombocytopenic purpura associated with ticlopidine: a review of 60 cases. *Ann Intern Med* 1998; **128:** 541–4.
10. Vianelli N, *et al.* Thrombotic thrombocytopenic purpura and ticlopidine. *Lancet* 1991; **337:** 1219.
11. Mataix R, *et al.* Ticlopidine and severe aplastic anaemia. *Br J Haematol* 1992; **80:** 125–6.
12. Mallet L, Mallet J. Ticlopidine and fatal aplastic anemia in an elderly woman. *Ann Pharmacother* 1994; **28:** 1169–71.
13. Wysowksi DK, Bacsanyi J. Blood dyscrasias and hematologic reactions in ticlopidine users. *JAMA* 1996; **276:** 952.
14. Committee on Safety of Medicines/Medicines Control Agency. Ticlopidine and white blood cell disorders. *Current Problems* 1997; **23:** 2.
15. Bennett CL, *et al.* Thrombotic thrombocytopenic purpura after stenting and ticlopidine. *Lancet* 1998; **352:** 1036–7.

Effects on the gastro-intestinal tract. Diarrhoea is a common side-effect of ticlopidine therapy; it usually occurs during the first few months of therapy and resolves within 1 to 2 weeks without stopping therapy. However, there has been a report[1] of chronic diarrhoea and weight loss occurring 2 years after ticlopidine was started; diarrhoea resolved when ticlopidine was withdrawn.

1. Mansoor GA, Aziz K. Delayed chronic diarrhea and weight loss possibly due to ticlopidine therapy. *Ann Pharmacother* 1997; **31:** 870–2.

Effects on the kidneys. A reversible deterioration in renal function has been reported in patients receiving ticlopidine following coronary stent implantation.[1,2]

1. Elsman P, Zijlstra F. Ticlopidine and renal function. *Lancet* 1996; **348:** 273–4.
2. Virdee M, *et al.* Ticlopidine and renal function. *Lancet* 1996; **348:** 1031–2.

Effects on the liver. Cholestatic hepatitis has been reported in patients receiving ticlopidine and is usually reversible when ticlopidine is stopped.[1,2] However, there has been one report of persistent cholestasis following ticlopidine withdrawal.[3] A case of granulomatous hepatitis has also been reported.[4]

1. Cassidy LJ, *et al.* Probable ticlopidine-induced cholestatic hepatitis. *Ann Pharmacother* 1995; **29:** 30–2.
2. Yoder JD, *et al.* More ticlopidine-induced cholestatic jaundice. *Am J Hosp Pharm* 1994; **51:** 1821–2.
3. Colivicchi F, *et al.* Ticlopidine-induced chronic cholestatic hepatitis: a case report. *Curr Ther Res* 1994; **55:** 929–31.
4. Ruiz-Valverde P, *et al.* Ticlopidine-induced granulomatous hepatitis. *Ann Pharmacother* 1995; **29:** 633–4.

Effects on the lungs. Bronchiolitis obliterans-organising pneumonia developed in a 76-year-old woman receiving ticlopidine and prednisone for temporal arteritis.[1] The condition resolved over several months when ticlopidine was withdrawn.

1. Alonso-Martinez JL, *et al.* Bronchiolitis obliterans-organizing pneumonia caused by ticlopidine. *Ann Intern Med* 1998; **129:** 71–2.

Interactions

Ticlopidine should be used with caution in patients receiving other drugs, such as anticoagulants and antiplatelets, that increase the risk of bleeding. Ticlopidine may inhibit the metabolism of other drugs that are metabolised in the liver. The clearance of ticlopidine may be reduced by concomitant cimetidine therapy. Corticosteroids may antagonise the effect of ticlopidine on bleeding time.

Anticoagulants. Concomitant administration of ticlopidine with anticoagulants may increase the risk of bleeding. However, ticlopidine has been reported to antagonise the effect of nicoumalone (see Interactions under Warfarin, p.968).

Phenytoin. For a report of acute phenytoin toxicity in a well-stabilised patient following addition of ticlopidine, see p.356.

Theophylline. For reference to the effect of ticlopidine on theophylline half-life, see p.770.

Pharmacokinetics

Ticlopidine hydrochloride is rapidly and almost completely absorbed from the gastro-intestinal tract. It is extensively bound to plasma proteins. The terminal half-life during chronic dosing is reported to be about 30 to 50 hours. Ticlopidine is extensively metabolised in the liver. Approximately 60% of the administered dose is excreted in the urine as metabolites and 25% in the faeces.

References.

1. Desager J-P. Clinical pharmacokinetics of ticlopidine. *Clin Pharmacokinet* 1994; **26:** 347–55.
2. Buur T, *et al.* Pharmacokinetics and effect of ticlopidine on platelet aggregation in subjects with normal and impaired renal function. *J Clin Pharmacol* 1997; **37:** 108–15.

Uses and Administration

Ticlopidine hydrochloride is an antiplatelet drug used in thrombo-embolic disorders (p.801). It appears to act by inhibiting adenosine diphosphate-mediated platelet aggregation. It is given prophylactically as an alternative to aspirin in patients at risk of thrombotic stroke (p.799) and may also be used in the management of intermittent claudication and ischaemic heart disease and to prevent platelet loss during extracorporeal circulatory procedures.

In the prevention of thrombotic stroke, ticlopidine hydrochloride is given in a dose of 250 mg twice daily by mouth, with meals. Because neutropenia can occur, regular haematological monitoring is recommended for at least the first 12 weeks of treatment.

References.

1. Saltiel E, Ward A. Ticlopidine: a review of its pharmacodynamic and pharmacokinetic properties, and therapeutic efficacy in platelet-dependent disease states. *Drugs* 1987; **34:** 222–62.
2. McTavish D, *et al.* Ticlopidine: an updated review of its pharmacology and therapeutic use in platelet-dependent disorders *Drugs* 1990; **40:** 238–59.
3. Anonymous. Ticlopidine. *Lancet* 1991; **337:** 459–60.
4. Flores-Runk P, Raasch RH. Ticlopidine and antiplatelet therapy. *Ann Pharmacother* 1993; **27:** 1090–8.
5. Schrör K. Antiplatelet drugs: a comparative review. *Drugs* 1995; **50:** 7–28.
6. Sharis PJ, *et al.* The antiplatelet effects of ticlopidine and clopidogrel. *Ann Intern Med* 1998; **129:** 394–405.

Reperfusion and revascularisation procedures. Coronary stents are being used increasingly to treat and prevent restenosis following angioplasty procedures (see p.797). Thrombotic occlusion commonly complicates their use and patients have been aggressively treated with a combination of antiplatelet drugs and anticoagulants. Recent studies, however, suggest that antiplatelet treatment alone may be adequate if the stent has been positioned correctly and the risk of thrombosis is considered to be low. A combination of aspirin with ticlopidine appears to be effective in most patients.[1] In a study[2] comparing a combination of aspirin with either ticlopidine or phenprocoumon fewer cardiac events and fewer haemorrhagic complications occurred in the antiplatelet group. However, another study[3] suggested that aspirin alone may be as effective as ticlopidine with short-term aspirin, and the benefit of adding ticlopidine remains to be confirmed.

Ticlopidine has also been reported[4] to improve the long-term patency of saphenous vein bypass grafts used to treat peripheral vascular disease in the legs.

1. Lablanche J-M, *et al.* Combined antiplatelet therapy with ticlopidine and aspirin: a simplified approach to intracoronary stent management. *Eur Heart J* 1996; **17:** 1373–80.
2. Schömig A, *et al.* A randomized comparison of antiplatelet and anticoagulant therapy after the placement of coronary-artery stents. *N Engl J Med* 1996; **334:** 1084–9.
3. Hall P, *et al.* A randomized comparison of combined ticlopidine and aspirin therapy versus aspirin therapy alone after successful intravascular ultrasound-guided stent implantation. *Circulation* 1996; **93:** 215–22.
4. Becquemin J-P. Effect of ticlopidine on the long-term patency of saphenous-vein bypass grafts in the legs. *N Engl J Med* 1997; **337:** 1726–31.

Preparations

Proprietary Preparations (details are given in Part 3)
Aust.: Ticlodone; Tiklid; ***Austral.:*** Ticlid; ***Belg.:*** Ticlid; ***Canad.:*** Ticlid; ***Fr.:*** Ticlid; ***Ger.:*** Tiklyd; ***Ital.:*** Anagregal; Antigreg; Aplaket; Clox; Fluilast; Klodin; Opteron; Parsilid; Ticlodone; Ticloproge; Ticlosan†; Tiklid; ***Norw.:*** Ticlid; ***Spain:*** Ticlodone; Tiklid; ***Swed.:*** Ticlid; ***Switz.:*** Ticlid; ***UK:*** Ticlid; ***USA:*** Ticlid.

Tienilic Acid (2357-y)

Tienilic Acid *(BAN, rINN)*.

SKF-62698; Ticrynafen *(USAN)*. [2,3-Dichloro-4-(2-thenoyl)phenoxy]acetic acid.

$C_{13}H_8Cl_2O_4S = 331.2$.

CAS — 40180-04-9.

Tienilic acid is a diuretic and was formerly used in the treatment of oedema and hypertension. It has been withdrawn from the market because of reports of severe, sometimes fatal, liver damage.

Tilisolol (3768-k)

Tilisolol *(rINN)*.

N-696 (tilisolol hydrochloride). (±)-4-[3-(*tert*-Butylamino)-2-hydroxypropoxy]-2-methylisocarbostyril.

$C_{17}H_{24}N_2O_3 = 304.4$.

CAS — 85136-71-6.

Tilisolol is a non-cardioselective beta blocker (p.828). It is reported to lack intrinsic sympathomimetic activity. It also has direct vasodilator activity.

Tilisolol is used as the hydrochloride in the management of hypertension.

Timolol Maleate (6323-l)

Timolol Maleate *(BANM, USAN, rINNM)*.

MK-950; Timololi Maleas. (*S*)-1-*tert*-Butylamino-3-(4-morpholino-1,2,5-thiadiazol-3-yloxy)propan-2-ol maleate.

$C_{13}H_{24}N_4O_3S,C_4H_4O_4 = 432.5$.

CAS — 26839-75-8 (timolol); 91524-16-2 (timolol hemihydrate); 26921-17-5 (timolol maleate).

NOTE. TIM is a code approved by the BP for use on single unit doses of eye drops containing timolol maleate where the individual container may be too small to bear all the appropriate labelling information.

Pharmacopoeias. In *Chin., Eur.* (see p.viii), *Int.,* and *US.*

A white or almost white, odourless or almost odourless crystalline powder or colourless crystals. **Soluble** in water; soluble in alcohol and in methyl alcohol; sparingly soluble in chloroform and in propylene glycol; practically insoluble in ether. A 2% solution in water has a pH of 3.8 to 4.3. **Protect** from light.

Adverse Effects, Treatment, and Precautions

As for beta blockers, p.828.

Systemic side-effects have followed topical use of the eye drops; mild local irritation and blurred vision have also been reported.

Effects on the gastro-intestinal tract. Sclerosing peritonitis[1] and retroperitoneal fibrosis[2] have been reported in patients receiving timolol.

1. Baxter-Smith DC, *et al.* Sclerosing peritonitis in patient on timolol. *Lancet* 1978; **ii:** 149.
2. Rimmer E, *et al.* Retroperitoneal fibrosis associated with timolol. *Lancet* 1983; **i:** 300.

Effects following ophthalmic use. Treatment with timolol eye drops for glaucoma was associated with depression and bradycardia in a 74-year-old woman.[1] Rapid withdrawal of the eye drops was followed by a rise in blood pressure and neurological signs of stroke. Severe nausea and vomiting which occurred in a woman being treated with timolol eye drops resolved within a few days of withdrawing treatment.[2] Symptoms recurred on rechallenge.

1. Rao MR, *et al.* Systemic hazards of ocular timolol. *Br J Hosp Med* 1993; **50:** 553.
2. Wolfhagen FHJ, *et al.* Severe nausea and vomiting with timolol eye drops. *Lancet* 1998; **352:** 373.

Interactions

The interactions associated with beta blockers are discussed on p.829.

Since systemic absorption can follow ophthalmic use of beta blockers, the possibility of interactions occurring with timolol eye drops should also be considered.

Pharmacokinetics

Timolol is almost completely absorbed from the gastro-intestinal tract but is subject to moderate first-pass metabolism. Peak plasma concentrations occur about 1 to 2 hours after a dose. It has low to moderate lipid solubility. Protein binding is reported to be low. A plasma half-life of 4 hours has been reported. It is extensively metabolised in the liver, the metabolites being excreted in the urine together with some unchanged timolol. It crosses the placenta and appears in breast milk.

References to the metabolism of timolol being influenced by genetic polymorphism.[1-3]

1. McGourty JC, *et al.* Pharmacokinetics and beta-blocking effects of timolol in poor and extensive metabolizers of debrisoquin. *Clin Pharmacol Ther* 1985; **38:** 409–13.
2. Lewis RV, *et al.* Timolol and atenolol: relationships between oxidation phenotype, pharmacokinetics and pharmacodynamics. *Br J Clin Pharmacol* 1985; **19:** 329–33.
3. Lennard MS, *et al.* Timolol metabolism and debrisoquine oxidation polymorphism: a population study. *Br J Clin Pharmacol* 1989; **27:** 429–34.

Breast feeding. Concentrations of timolol in breast milk were approximately six times greater than those in serum, the values being 5.6 and 0.93 ng per mL respectively, following instillation of timolol 0.5% eye drops twice daily in a lactating woman.[1]

1. Lustgarten JS, Podos SM. Topical timolol and the nursing mother. *Arch Ophthalmol* 1983; **101:** 1381–2.

Uses and Administration

Timolol is a non-cardioselective beta blocker (p.828). It is reported to lack intrinsic sympathomimetic and membrane-stabilising activity.

Timolol is used as the maleate in the management of glaucoma (p.1387), hypertension (p.788), angina pectoris (p.780), and myocardial infarction (p.791). It is also used in the management of migraine (p.443).

Eye drops containing timolol maleate equivalent to 0.25 and 0.5% of timolol are instilled twice daily to reduce **raised intra-ocular pressure** in open-angle **glaucoma** and ocular hypertension. Once-daily instillation may suffice when the intra-ocular pressure has been controlled. Gel-forming eye drops are also available that are instilled once daily.

In **hypertension** timolol maleate is usually given in initial doses of 10 mg daily by mouth, increased according to response at intervals of 7 or more days; usual maintenance doses are 10 to 40 mg daily in single or divided doses, but doses up to 60 mg daily may be required in some patients.

In **angina pectoris** an initial dose of 5 mg two or three times daily has been recommended, increased at intervals of 3 or more days by no more than 10 mg daily initially and 15 mg daily subsequently, in divided doses. Most patients respond to 35 to 45 mg daily in divided doses, but some patients may require up to 60 mg daily.

In patients who have had a **myocardial infarction** timolol maleate is given in initial doses of 5 mg twice daily for 2 days, starting 7 to 28 days after infarction, and increased subsequently in the absence of any contra-indicating adverse effects, to 10 mg twice daily.

Doses of 10 to 20 mg daily of timolol maleate are used in the prophylaxis of **migraine**.

Reduced doses may be required in renal or hepatic impairment.

Preparations

BP 1998: Timolol Eye Drops; Timolol Tablets;
USP 23: Timolol Maleate and Hydrochlorothiazide Tablets; Timolol Maleate Ophthalmic Solution; Timolol Maleate Tablets.

Proprietary Preparations (details are given in Part 3)
Aust.: Blocadren; Timoptic; ***Austral.:*** Blocadren; Optimol; Tenopt; Timoptol; Timoptol-XE; ***Belg.:*** Blocadren; Timoptol; ***Canad.:*** Apo-Timol; Apo-Timop; Beta-Tim; Blocadren; Novo-Timol; Tim-Ak; Timoptic; ***Fr.:*** Digaol; Nyolol; Ophtim; Timacor; Timoptol; ***Ger.:*** Arutimol; Chibro-Timoptol; Dispatim; duratimol; Temserin†; Tim-Ophtal; Timo-Comod; Timoedo; Timohexal; Timomann; Timopos COMOD†; Timosine; Uniget†; ***Irl.:*** Betim†; Blocadren; Timoptol; ***Ital.:*** Blocadren; Droptimol; Oftimolo; Timoptol; ***Mon.:*** Gaoptal; ***Neth.:*** Blocadren; Loptomit; Timoptol; ***Norw.:*** Aquanil; Betim; Blocadren; Oftan; ***S.Afr.:*** Blocadren; Glaucosan; Timoptol; ***Spain:*** Blocadren†; Cusimolol; Nyolol; Timoftol; ***Swed.:*** Aquanil; Blocadren; Optimol; ***Switz.:*** Blocadren; Oftan; Timoptic; ***UK:*** Betim; Blocadren; Glau-opt; Glaucol; Timoptol; ***USA:*** Betimol; Blocadren; Timoptic.

Multi-ingredient: ***Aust.:*** Moducrin; Timpilo; ***Austral.:*** Timpilo; ***Belg.:*** Timpilo†; ***Canad.:*** Timolide; Timpilo; ***Fr.:*** Moducren; Timpilo; ***Ger.:*** Moducrin; Timpilo; ***Irl.:*** Moducren; Prestim; ***Ital.:*** Equiton; Timicon; ***Neth.:*** Moducren; Prestim; Timpilo-2; ***Norw.:*** Fotil; Timpilo; ***S.Afr.:*** Moducren; Servatrin; ***Swed.:*** Fotil; Timpilo; ***Switz.:*** Moducren; Timpilo; ***UK:*** Cosopt; Moducren; Prestim; ***USA:*** Cosopt; Timolide.

Tinzaparin Sodium (14909-z)

Tinzaparin Sodium *(BAN, USAN, rINN).*

Tinzaparinum Natricum.

CAS — 9041-08-1.

Pharmacopoeias. In *Eur.* (see p.viii).

Tinzaparin sodium is prepared by enzymatic depolymerisation, using heparinase from *Flavobacterium heparinum*, of heparin obtained from the intestinal mucosa of pigs. The majority of the components have a 2-*O*-sulpho-4-desoxy-4-α-L-*threo*-hex-4-enopyranosuronic acid structure at the non-reducing end and a 2-*N*,6-*O*-disulpho-D-glucosamine structure at the reducing end of their chain. The mass-average molecular mass ranges between 5500 and 7500, with a characteristic value of about 6500. The mass percentage of chains lower than 2000 is not more than 10%. The degree of sulphation is 1.8 to 2.5 per disaccharide unit.

The Ph. Eur. specifies that potency is not less than 70 units and not more than 120 units of anti-factor Xa activity per mg with reference to the dried substance and that the ratio of anti-factor Xa activity to anti-factor IIa (antithrombin) activity is between 1.5 and 2.5.

Units

As for Low-molecular-weight Heparins, p.899.

Adverse Effects and Treatment

As for Low-molecular-weight Heparins, p.899.

Precautions and Interactions

As for Low-molecular-weight Heparins, p.900.

Pharmacokinetics

Tinzaparin sodium is absorbed following subcutaneous injection with a bioavailability of about 90%. Peak plasma activity is reached within 4 to 6 hours. The elimination half-life is about 90 minutes but detectable anti-factor Xa activity persists for up to 24 hours.

Uses and Administration

Tinzaparin sodium is a low-molecular-weight heparin (p.899) with anticoagulant properties. It is used in the treatment and prophylaxis of venous thrombo-embolism (p.802) and to prevent clotting during extracorporeal circulation.

For prophylaxis of venous thrombo-embolism during general surgical procedures 3500 units of tinzaparin sodium are given by subcutaneous injection 2 hours before the procedure, followed by 3500 units once daily for 7 to 10 days. In patients undergoing orthopaedic surgery a dose of 50 units per kg body-weight has been recommended; alternatively, a dose of 4500 units may be given 12 hours before surgery, followed by 4500 units once daily. For the treatment of venous thrombo-embolism tinzaparin sodium is given in a dose of 175 units per kg by subcutaneous injection once daily for at least 6 days.

For prevention of clotting in the extracorporeal circulation during haemodialysis, tinzaparin sodium may be administered into the arterial side of the dialyser or intravenously. The dialyser may be primed with 5000 units tinzaparin sodium in 500 to 1000 mL sodium chloride 0.9%. For dialysis sessions lasting less than 4 hours a single dose of 2000 to 2500 units tinzaparin sodium is given; for longer sessions an initial dose of 2500 units is followed by an infusion of 750 units per hour.

Reversal of effects. Severe bleeding with tinzaparin sodium may be reduced by the slow intravenous injection of protamine sulphate; 1 mg of protamine sulphate is stated to inhibit the effects of 100 units of tinzaparin sodium.

References.

1. Friedel HA, Balfour JA. Tinzaparin: a review of its pharmacology and clinical potential in the prevention and treatment of thrombo-embolic disorders. *Drugs* 1994; **48:** 638–60.
2. Fegan CD. Tinzaparin as an antithrombotic: an overview. *Hosp Med* 1998; **59:** 145–8.

Preparations

Proprietary Preparations (details are given in Part 3)
Aust.: Logiparin; ***Austral.:*** Logiparin†; ***Belg.:*** Innohep; ***Canad.:*** Innohep; ***Fr.:*** Innohep; ***Ger.:*** Innohep; ***Irl.:*** Innohep; ***Ital.:*** Innohep; Logiparin†; ***Neth.:*** Innohep; ***S.Afr.:*** Logiparin†; ***Swed.:*** Innohep; Logiparin†; ***UK:*** Innohep; Logiparin†.

Tioclomarol (13347-l)

Tioclomarol *(rINN).*

LM-550. 3-[5-Chloro-α-(4-chloro-β-hydroxyphenethyl)-2-thenyl]-4-hydroxycoumarin.

$C_{22}H_{16}Cl_2O_4S$ = 447.3.

CAS — 22619-35-8.

Tioclomarol is an orally administered coumarin anticoagulant with actions similar to those of warfarin sodium (p.964) and is used in the management of thrombo-embolic disorders (p.801). It is given in usual doses of 4 mg daily.

Preparations

Proprietary Preparations (details are given in Part 3)
Fr.: Apegmone.

Tirilazad Mesylate (5845-q)

Tirilazad Mesylate *(BANM, USAN).*

Tirilazad Mesilate *(rINNM)*; U-74006F (tirilazad or tirilazad mesylate). 21-[4-(2,6-Di-1-pyrrolidinyl-4-pyrimidinyl)-1-piperazinyl]-16α-methylpregna-1,4,9(11)-triene-3,20-dione monomethanesulfonate hydrate.

$C_{38}H_{52}N_6O_2,CH_4O_3S,xH_2O$ = 721.0 (anhydrous).

CAS — 110101-66-1 (tirilazad); 111793-42-1 (tirilazad mesylate); 149042-61-5 (tirilazad mesylate).

Tirilazad, a lazaroid, is an inhibitor of lipid peroxidation thought to have a cytoprotective effect against radicals produced in response to tissue trauma. It may be used in the prevention of secondary tissue damage in subarachnoid haemorrhage (see Stroke, p.799). It is under investigation in spinal cord injuries (p.1029). It has also been investigated in head injuries and ischaemic stroke.

In subarachnoid haemorrhage the recommended dose is 1.5 mg per kg body-weight of tirilazad mesylate by intravenous infusion every 6 hours for 8 to 10 days, starting within 48 hours of the onset of haemorrhage. Each dose should be infused over 10 to 30 minutes. This dosage regimen is only recommended for males; tirilazad clearance is higher in females than males and this dosage is ineffective in females.

References.

1. Fleishaker JC, *et al.* Evaluation of the pharmacokinetics and tolerability of tirilazad mesylate, a 21-aminosteroid free radical scavenger: multiple-dose administration. *J Clin Pharmacol* 1993; **33:** 182–90.
2. Hulst LK, *et al.* Effect of age and gender on tirilazad pharmacokinetics in humans. *Clin Pharmacol Ther* 1994; **55:** 378–84.
3. The STIPAS Investigators. Safety study of tirilazad mesylate in patients with acute ischemic stroke (STIPAS). *Stroke* 1994; **25:** 418–23.
4. Haley EC, *et al.* Phase II trial of tirilazad in aneurysmal subarachnoid haemorrhage: a report of the Cooperative Aneurysm Study. *J Neurosurg* 1995; **82:** 786–90.
5. Clark WM, *et al.* Lazaroid: CNS pharmacology and current research. *Drugs* 1995; **50:** 971–83.

Preparations

Proprietary Preparations (details are given in Part 3)
Aust.: Freedox; ***Austral.:*** Freedox; ***Norw.:*** Freedox; ***S.Afr.:*** Freedox; ***Swed.:*** Freedox; ***Switz.:*** Freedox.

Tirofiban Hydrochloride (19429-c)

Tirofiban Hydrochloride *(BANM, USAN, rINNM).*

L-700462; MK-383; MK-0383. *N*-(Butylsulfonyl)-4-[4-(4-piperidyl)butoxy]-L-phenylalanine hydrochloride monohydrate.

$C_{22}H_{36}N_2O_5S,HCl,H_2O$ = 495.1.

CAS — 144494-65-5 (tirofiban); 142373-60-2 (anhydrous tirofiban hydrochloride); 150915-40-5 (tirofiban hydrochloride monohydrate);.

Tirofiban hydrochloride is an antiplatelet drug that acts by blocking glycoprotein IIb/IIIa receptors. It is given intravenously in combination with heparin for the management of unstable angina. It is also under investigation in patients undergoing coronary angioplasty.

References.

1. Barrett JS, *et al.* Pharmacokinetics and pharmacodynamics of MK-383, a selective non-peptide platelet glycoprotein-IIb/IIIa receptor antagonist, in healthy men. *Clin Pharmacol Ther* 1994; **56:** 377–88.
2. The Platelet Receptor Inhibition in Ischemic Syndrome Management (PRISM) Study Investigators. A comparison of aspirin plus tirofiban with aspirin plus heparin for unstable angina. *N Engl J Med* 1998; **338:** 1498–1505.
3. The Platelet Receptor Inhibition in Ischemic Syndrome Management in Patients Limited by Unstable Signs and Symptoms (PRISM-PLUS) Study Investigators. Inhibition of the platelet glycoprotein IIb/IIIa receptor with tirofiban in unstable angina and non-Q-wave myocardial infarction. *N Engl J Med* 1998; **338:** 1488–97.

Preparations

Proprietary Preparations (details are given in Part 3)
USA: Aggrastat.

Tocainide Hydrochloride (7793-b)

Tocainide Hydrochloride *(BANM, rINNM).*

W-36095 (tocainide). 2-Aminopropiono-2′,6′-xylidide hydrochloride.

$C_{11}H_{16}N_2O,HCl$ = 228.7.

CAS — 41708-72-9 (tocainide); 35891-93-1 (tocainide hydrochloride).

NOTE. Tocainide is *USAN.*

Pharmacopoeias. In *Chin.* and *US.*

A fine, white, odourless powder. Freely **soluble** in water and in alcohol; practically insoluble in chloroform and in ether.

Adverse Effects

Tocainide causes severe haematological toxicity leading to neutropenia, agranulocytosis, thrombocytopenia, and aplastic anaemia; fatalities have occurred. Pulmonary toxicity has also proved fatal; patients have developed interstitial pneumonitis, pulmonary fibrosis, and other respiratory disorders.

The most common side-effects are dose-related CNS and gastro-intestinal effects including tremor, dizziness, paraesthesia, lightheadedness, blurred vision, and nausea. These may occur particularly in the initial stages of therapy and may be transient. Other less frequent gastro-intestinal side-effects include vomiting, anorexia, constipation, and diarrhoea. Various mental changes and ataxia have been reported.

Other adverse effects reported include skin rash, lupus erythematosus, sweating, tinnitus, taste disturbances, and liver disorders.

As with other antiarrhythmics, tocainide can cause various cardiac arrhythmias and disturbances of conduction. Bradycardia and hypotension may occur particularly after intravenous administration.

A review of the adverse effects associated with the class Ib antiarrhythmics tocainide, lignocaine, and mexiletine, with guidelines for the clinical management of toxicity.[1]

1. Denaro CP, Benowitz NL. Poisoning due to class 1B antiarrhythmic drugs: lignocaine, mexiletine and tocainide. *Med Toxicol Adverse Drug Exp* 1989; **4:** 412–28.

Effects on the blood. Adverse haematological effects associated with tocainide are serious and have caused fatalities.[1-3] They include agranulocytosis, aplastic anaemia, thrombocytopenia, and neutropenia. The US manufacturer has declared that haematological reactions occur in up to 0.18% of patients and that the mortality rate of patients who develop agranulocytosis is 25%.

These haematological reactions usually occur in the first 12 weeks of treatment and it is therefore recommended that full blood counts are performed weekly during this time and monthly thereafter. Patients should be advised to report promptly any unusual bleeding or bruising, or signs of infection such as fever, sore throat, or chills. The seriousness of these adverse effects limits the use of tocainide.

1. Holmes GI, *et al.* Drug therapy: flecainide and tocainide. *N Engl J Med* 1987; **316:** 344.
2. Volosin K, *et al.* Tocainide associated agranulocytosis. *Am Heart J* 1985; **109:** 1392–3.
3. Morrill GB. Tocainide-induced aplastic anemia. *DICP Ann Pharmacother* 1989; **23:** 90–1.

Effects on the liver. Acute hepatocellular damage in one patient[1] and granulomatous hepatitis in another[2] have been associated with tocainide therapy.

1. Farquhar DL, Davidson NM. Possible hepatotoxicity of tocainide. *Scott Med J* 1984; **29:** 238.
2. Tucker LE. Tocainide-induced granulomatous hepatitis. *JAMA* 1986; **255:** 3362.

Effects on the lungs. Interstitial pneumonitis[1-3] and pulmonary fibrosis[4,5] have been reported in small numbers of patients receiving tocainide.

1. Perlow GM, *et al.* Tocainide-associated interstitial pneumonitis. *Ann Intern Med* 1981; **94:** 489.
2. Van Natta B, *et al.* Irreversible interstitial pneumonitis associated with tocainide therapy. *West J Med* 1988; **149:** 91–2.
3. Ahmad S. Tocainide: interstitial pneumonitis. *J Am Coll Cardiol* 1990; **15:** 1458.
4. Subauste CS, *et al.* Tocainide-induced pulmonary toxicity. *Illinois Med J* 1988; **174:** 287–9.
5. Feinberg L, *et al.* Pulmonary fibrosis associated with tocainide: report of a case with literature review. *Am Rev Respir Dis* 1990; **141:** 505–8.

Effects on mental state. Confusion, paranoia, and hallucinations have been reported[1-3] in a few patients receiving tocainide at recommended doses; all symptoms resolved on discontinuing tocainide. In one patient the reaction was confirmed by rechallenge with tocainide.

1. Currie P, Ramsdale DR. Paranoid psychosis induced by tocainide. *Br Med J* 1984; **288:** 606–7.
2. Harrison DJ, Wathen CG. Paranoid psychosis induced by tocainide. *Br Med J* 1984; **288:** 1010–11.
3. Clarke CWF, El-Mahdi EO. Confusion and paranoia associated with oral tocainide. *Postgrad Med J* 1985; **61:** 79–81.

Effects on the skin. The US Food and Drug Administration received 21 reports of severe dermatologic reactions associated with tocainide therapy during 1985 and 1986.[1] These included erythema multiforme, Stevens-Johnson syndrome, and exfoliative dermatitis. The reaction occurred within 3 weeks of starting tocainide in 67% of patients for whom the duration of treatment was given. Seventeen patients recovered on withdrawal of tocainide, 2 patients died, and the outcome was not available for 2 patients.

1. Arrowsmith JB, *et al.* Severe dermatologic reactions reported after treatment with tocainide. *Ann Intern Med* 1987; **107:** 693–6.

Overdosage. In overdosage with tocainide there may be convulsions, complete heart block, and asystole. Treatment is symptomatic and supportive. Haemodialysis and possibly charcoal haemoperfusion may be helpful. Treatment may need to be continued for a prolonged period due to tocainide's long half-life.

Fatal overdose occurred in a 70-year-old man after taking tocainide 16 g by mouth.[1] Postmortem tocainide concentrations were 384.8 μmol per mL in the blood and 2860 μmol per mL in the urine. Toxic effects included convulsions, complete heart block, multiple ventricular ectopic beats, profound hypotension, evidence of ischaemic cardiac changes, and multiple episodes of asystole which was eventually unresponsive to cardiac pacing.

1. Clarke CWF, El-Mahdi EO. Fatal oral tocainide overdosage. *Br Med J* 1984; **288:** 760.

Precautions

Tocainide should not be used in patients with second or third degree atrioventricular block, in the absence of a pacemaker, or in patients with hypersensitivity to amide-type drugs. It should be used with caution in patients with uncompensated heart failure and in patients receiving other antiarrhythmics. Blood counts should be monitored weekly during the first 12 weeks of therapy and monthly thereafter. Tocainide should be given with caution to patients with impaired renal or hepatic function. Hypokalaemia should be corrected before initiating tocainide therapy.

Interactions

Tocainide is structurally related to lignocaine and concomitant use with lignocaine may produce additive CNS side-effects. Tocainide is metabolised in the liver and enzyme-inducing drugs may reduce the elimination half-life of tocainide.

Tocainide may have a modest inhibitory effect on theophylline metabolism (p.768).

Rifampicin increased the total clearance and reduced the elimination half-life of tocainide in 8 healthy subjects,[1] probably due to an increase in hepatic metabolism of tocainide. A similar interaction should be considered if tocainide is administered concomitantly with other enzyme-inducing drugs such as *phenytoin* or *phenobarbitone.*

Cimetidine has been reported[2] to decrease the bioavailability of tocainide without affecting the renal clearance or half-life. The exact mechanism of the interaction could not be determined but may have been due to reduced absorption of tocainide secondary to a cimetidine-induced increase in gastro-intestinal pH; however, no interaction was observed with *ranitidine.*

1. Rice TL, *et al.* Influence of rifampin on tocainide pharmacokinetics in humans. *Clin Pharm* 1989; **8:** 200–5.
2. North DS, *et al.* The effect of histamine-2 receptor antagonists on tocainide pharmacokinetics. *J Clin Pharmacol* 1988; **28:** 640–3.

Pharmacokinetics

Tocainide is readily and almost completely absorbed from the gastro-intestinal tract.

Tocainide is metabolised to a number of apparently inactive metabolites. It is excreted mainly in the urine, 30 to 50% as unchanged drug.

Tocainide is widely distributed throughout the body and is reported to be about 10% bound to plasma proteins. It has an elimination half-life of about 10 to 20 hours; renal clearance is reduced in alkaline urine but acidification has no effect on excretion. Its therapeutic effect has been correlated with plasma concentrations of about 3 to 10 μg per mL.

Tocainide exists as 2 optically active enantiomers although a 1:1 racemic mixture is used clinically. The pharmacokinetics of the enantiomers are different;[1-3] the R(−)-enantiomer has a faster clearance and shorter elimination half-life than the S(+)-enantiomer. Stereoselective metabolism by liver enzymes has been suggested to explain this difference. The slower clearance of the S(+)-enantiomer means that the S:R plasma concentration ratio will increase with continued administration of tocainide[2] but the clinical significance, if any, has not been established.

In anephric patients[3] both enantiomers are cleared more slowly than in healthy subjects, but the clearance of the S(+)-enantiomer shows a greater relative reduction. Haemodialysis effectively removes both enantiomers.[3]

1. Edgar B, *et al.* The pharmacokinetics of R- and S-tocainide in healthy subjects. *Br J Clin Pharmacol* 1984; **17:** 216P.
2. Thomson AH, *et al.* Pharmacokinetics of R- and S-tocainide in patients with acute ventricular arrhythmias. *Br J Clin Pharmacol* 1986; **21:** 149–54.
3. McErlane KM, *et al.* Stereoselective pharmacokinetics of tocainide in human uraemic patients and in healthy subjects. *Eur J Clin Pharmacol* 1990; **39:** 373–6.

Uses and Administration

Tocainide is a class Ib antiarrhythmic (p.776) with actions similar to those of lignocaine (p.1295) to which it is structurally related. Unlike lignocaine, it undergoes negligible first-pass metabolism and can be given by mouth. Because of its toxicity (see under Adverse Effects, above) tocainide is generally restricted to the treatment of life-threatening ventricular **arrhythmias** (p.782) that cannot be treated by other means.

For treatment of chronic arrhythmias tocainide hydrochloride 1.2 g is given by mouth daily, divided in 2 or 3 doses, the dose being adjusted according to the patient's tolerance and response. Doses above 2.4 g daily are not normally required. Treatment should be initiated in hospital under ECG monitoring. Doses may need to be reduced in patients with renal or hepatic insufficiency. Tocainide hydrochloride was also formerly given intravenously for rapid control of acute arrhythmias.

General references.

1. Holmes B, *et al.* Tocainide: a review of its pharmacological properties and therapeutic efficacy. *Drugs* 1983; **26:** 93–123.
2. Kutalek SP, *et al.* Tocainide: a new oral antiarrhythmic agent. *Ann Intern Med* 1985; **103:** 387–91.
3. Roden DM, Woosley RL. Tocainide. *N Engl J Med* 1986; **315:** 41–5.

Administration in renal impairment. Tocainide is mainly excreted in the urine, and in patients with renal insufficiency the elimination of tocainide is impaired and the half-life prolonged.[1,2] Alterations of urine pH can cause clinically significant alterations in tocainide excretion in patients with mild to moderate renal insufficiency.[2] It has been recommended[1] that the dose of tocainide should be reduced by 50% in patients with severe renal impairment; smaller reductions may be necessary in patients with less severe renal impairment.

Haemodialysis has been reported[1] to remove 25% of tocainide present in the body and a half-life of 8.5 hours was reported; patients may need a supplemental dose of tocainide following haemodialysis.

1. Wiegers U, *et al.* Pharmacokinetics of tocainide in patients with renal dysfunction and during haemodialysis. *Eur J Clin Pharmacol* 1983; **24:** 503–7.
2. Braun J, *et al.* Pharmacokinetics of tocainide in patients with severe renal failure. *Eur J Clin Pharmacol* 1985; **28:** 665–70.

Preparations

USP 23: Tocainide Hydrochloride Tablets.

Proprietary Preparations (details are given in Part 3)
Belg.: Tonocard†; ***Canad.:*** Tonocard; ***Ger.:*** Xylotocan; ***Irl.:*** Tonocard; ***Neth.:*** Tonocard; ***Swed.:*** Tonocard; ***UK:*** Tonocard†; ***USA:*** Tonocard.

Todralazine Hydrochloride (13358-z)

Todralazine Hydrochloride *(BANM, pINNM).*

BT-621; CEPH; Ecarazine Hydrochloride. Ethyl 3-(phthalazin-1-yl)carbazate hydrochloride monohydrate.

$C_{11}H_{12}N_4O_2,HCl,H_2O$ = 286.7.

CAS — 14679-73-3 (todralazine); 3778-76-5 (todralazine hydrochloride, anhydrous).

Pharmacopoeias. In *Jpn* and *Pol.*

Todralazine hydrochloride is an antihypertensive structurally related to hydralazine (p.883) and with similar properties.

Tolazoline Hydrochloride (9281-t)

Tolazoline Hydrochloride *(BANM, rINNM).*

Benzazoline Hydrochloride; Tolazol. Hydrochlor.; Tolazolinium Chloratum. 2-Benzyl-2-imidazoline hydrochloride.

$C_{10}H_{12}N_2,HCl$ = 196.7.

CAS — 59-98-3 (tolazoline); 59-97-2 (tolazoline hydrochloride).

Pharmacopoeias. In *Aust., It., Pol.,* and *US.*

A white to off-white crystalline powder.

Soluble 1 in less than 1 of water, 1 in 2 of alcohol, and 1 in 3 of chloroform; practically insoluble in ether.

Adverse Effects

Side-effects of tolazoline hydrochloride include piloerection, headache, flushing, tachycardia, cardiac arrhythmias, tingling, chilliness, shivering, sweating, nausea, vomiting, diarrhoea, and epigastric pain. Orthostatic hypotension or marked hypertension may occur, especially with large doses. Tolazoline stimulates gastric acid and may exacerbate ulcers. Oliguria, haematuria, myocardial infarction, gastro-intestinal haemorrhage, thrombocytopenia and other blood dyscrasias have been reported.

Intra-arterial injection may be followed by a burning sensation in the limb.

Effects in the neonate. Hypochloraemic metabolic alkalosis,[1] acute renal failure,[2] and duodenal perforation[3] have been reported in neonates given tolazoline.

1. Adams JM, *et al.* Hypochloremic metabolic alkalosis following tolazoline-induced gastric hypersecretion. *Pediatrics* 1980; **65:** 298–300.
2. Trompeter RS, *et al.* Tolazoline and acute renal failure in the newborn. *Lancet* 1981; **i:** 1219.
3. Wilson RG, *et al.* Duodenal perforation associated with tolazoline. *Arch Dis Child* 1985; **60:** 878–9.

Treatment of Adverse Effects

In the event of overdosage hypotension is best treated by keeping the patient recumbent with the head lowered. If necessary the circulation may be maintained by infusion of suitable electrolyte solutions. Hypotension may be treated with ephedrine. Adrenaline is not suitable for the reversal of hypotension induced by alpha-adrenoceptor blockers since it may exacerbate the hypotension by stimulating beta-receptors.

Precautions

Tolazoline hydrochloride should not be given to patients with ischaemic heart disease, hypotension, or after cerebrovascular accident. Since tolazoline hydrochloride stimulates gastric secretion of hydrochloric acid, it should not be used in the presence of peptic ulceration. Pretreatment of infants with antacids may prevent gastro-intestinal bleeding. Tolazoline should be used with caution in patients with mitral stenosis.

Interactions

Tolazoline should not be administered concomitantly with drugs such as adrenaline since the hypotensive effect may be potentiated due to unopposed beta-adrenoceptor stimulation. Tolazoline may cause a disulfiram-like reaction if given with alcohol.

Dopamine. For the effect of tolazoline on dopamine, see p.861.

Ranitidine. Intravenous administration of ranitidine reversed the falls in pulmonary and systemic vascular resistances in 12 children who had been given tolazoline as a pulmonary vasodilator.[1]

1. Bush A, *et al.* Cardiovascular effects of tolazoline and ranitidine. *Arch Dis Child* 1987; **62:** 241–6.

Pharmacokinetics

Tolazoline hydrochloride is absorbed from the gastro-intestinal tract. It is more rapidly absorbed after intramuscular injection. A plasma half-life in neonates of 3 to 10 hours has been reported, although it may be as high as about 40 hours and is inversely related to urine output. Tolazoline hydrochloride is rapidly excreted in the urine, largely unchanged.

Uses and Administration

Tolazoline hydrochloride is a vasodilator that has a direct dilator action on the peripheral blood vessels. It has some alpha-adrenoceptor blocking activity and also stimulates smooth muscle in the gastro-intestinal tract, increases gastro-intestinal secretion, can cause mydriasis, and has a stimulant effect on the heart.

Tolazoline hydrochloride is used to reduce pulmonary artery pressure in persistent pulmonary hypertension in newborn infants with persistent fetal circulation. It has also been used in the treatment of peripheral vascular disease (p.794) and in some ophthalmic conditions.

In pulmonary hypertension in neonates, the usual dose is 1 to 2 mg per kg body-weight over 10 minutes by intravenous infusion followed by 1 to 2 mg per kg per hour thereafter. Infants with reduced urine output may require lower maintenance doses. For additional details on administration in infants, see below.

In peripheral vascular disease doses of 25 to 50 mg have been given four times daily by mouth. Doses of up to 50 mg have been given by subcutaneous, intramuscular, intravenous, or slow intra-arterial injection.

Pulmonary hypertension. Tolazoline and other vasodilators have been tried in persistent pulmonary hypertension in the newborn (p.796) in an attempt to induce selective pulmonary vasodilatation and improve gas exchange. The response is variable and often unsuccessful due to concomitant systemic hypotension, a failure to achieve or sustain pulmonary vasodilatation, and adverse effects. The high incidence of adverse effects seen in neonates given tolazoline has led to several studies investigating the administration of lower doses. One group suggested that a loading dose of 0.5 mg per kg body-weight given intravenously followed by a continuous infusion of 0.5 mg per kg per hour was more appropriate and safer than standard doses.[1] Another study indicated that constant plasma concentrations of tolazoline can be maintained by a dose of 0.16 mg per kg per hour for each 1-mg per kg loading dose.[2]

1. Monin P, *et al.* Treatment of persistent fetal circulation syndrome of the newborn: comparison of different doses of tolazoline. *Eur J Clin Pharmacol* 1987; **31:** 569–73.
2. Ward RM, *et al.* Oliguria and tolazoline pharmacokinetics in the newborn. *Pediatrics* 1986; **77:** 307–15.

Preparations

USP 23: Tolazoline Hydrochloride Injection.

Proprietary Preparations (details are given in Part 3)
Aust.: Vaso-Dilatan; ***Austral.:*** Priscoline; ***Canad.:*** Priscoline†; ***Ger.:*** Priscol; ***Switz.:*** Priscol†; ***USA:*** Priscoline.

Multi-ingredient: ***Switz.:*** Lunadon.

Tolonidine Nitrate (909-y)

Tolonidine Nitrate *(rINNM).*

CERM-10137; ST-375 (tolonidine). 2-(2-Chloro-*p*-toluidino)-2-imidazoline nitrate.

$C_{10}H_{12}ClN_3,HNO_3$ = 272.7.

CAS — 4201-22-3 (tolonidine); 57524-15-9 (tolonidine nitrate).

Tolonidine nitrate is an antihypertensive drug structurally related to clonidine (p.841) and with similar actions. It has been used in the management of hypertension.

Preparations

Proprietary Preparations (details are given in Part 3)
Fr.: Euctan†.

Torasemide (1272-d)

Torasemide *(BAN, rINN).*

AC-4464; BM-02015; Torsemide *(USAN).* 1-Isopropyl-3-(4-*m*-toluidinopyridine-3-sulphonyl)urea.

$C_{16}H_{20}N_4O_3S$ = 348.4.

CAS — 56211-40-6 (torasemide); 72810-59-4 (torasemide sodium).

Adverse Effects, and Precautions

As for Frusemide, p.871.

Interactions

As for Frusemide, p.872.

Pharmacokinetics

Torasemide is well absorbed from the gastro-intestinal tract. Peak serum concentrations are achieved within one hour of administration by mouth. Torasemide is metabolised in the liver and inactive metabolites are excreted in the urine. The elimination half-life of torasemide is approximately 3.5 hours. Torasemide is extensively bound to plasma proteins. In patients with heart failure both hepatic and renal clearance are reduced. In patients with renal impairment, the renal clearance is reduced but total plasma clearance is not significantly altered.

References.

1. Knauf H, Mutschler E. Clinical pharmacokinetics and pharmacodynamics of torasemide. *Clin Pharmacokinet* 1998; **34:** 1–24.

Uses and Administration

Torasemide is a loop diuretic with actions similar to those of frusemide (p.872).

Torasemide is used for oedema associated with heart failure (p.785), including pulmonary oedema, and with renal and hepatic disorders. It is also used in the treatment of hypertension (p.788), either alone or together with other antihypertensives.

Diuresis following oral administration is initiated within 1 hour, reaches a maximum in about 1 to 2 hours, and lasts for up to 8 hours; after intravenous injection its effects are evident within 10 minutes but like oral administration can last up to 8 hours.

In the treatment of **oedema** the usual dose is 5 mg once daily by mouth increased according to response to 20 mg once daily; doses of up to 40 mg daily have been required in some patients. Torasemide may also be given intravenously in usual doses of 10 to 20 mg daily, and not exceeding 40 mg daily. Higher intravenous doses may sometimes be necessary, especially in oedema of renal origin when an initial dose of 20 mg daily may be increased stepwise as necessary to a maximum of 200 mg daily.

In the treatment of **hypertension** torasemide is given in doses of 2.5 to 5 mg daily by mouth; sources in the USA have suggested that doses of up to 10 mg daily may be employed although in the UK doses above 5 mg are considered unlikely to produce additional benefit.

Reviews.

1. Blose JS, *et al.* Torsemide: a pyridine-sulfonylurea loop diuretic. *Ann Pharmacother* 1995; **29:** 396–402.
2. Dunn CJ, *et al.* Torasemide: an update of its pharmacological properties and therapeutic efficacy. *Drugs* 1995; **49:** 121–42.
3. Brater DC. Benefits and risks of torasemide in congestive heart failure and essential hypertension. *Drug Safety* 1996; **14:** 104–120.

Preparations

Proprietary Preparations (details are given in Part 3)
Belg.: Torrem; ***Canad.:*** Demadex; ***Ger.:*** Torem; Unat; ***Ital.:*** Diuremid; Toradiur; ***Neth.:*** Torem†; ***S.Afr.:*** Unat; ***Spain:*** Dilutol; Isodiur; Sutril; ***Swed.:*** Torem; ***Switz.:*** Torem; ***UK:*** Torem; ***USA:*** Demadex.

Trandolapril (2831-d)

Trandolapril *(BAN, rINN).*

RU-44570. Ethyl (2*S*,3a*R*,7a*S*)-1-{(*S*)-*N*-[(*S*)-1-carboxy-3-phenylpropyl]alanyl}hexahydro-2-indolinecarboxylate; (2*S*,3a*R*,7a*S*)-1-{*N*-[(*S*)-1-Ethoxycarbonyl-3-phenylpropyl]-L-alanyl}perhydroindole-2-carboxylic acid.

$C_{24}H_{34}N_2O_5$ = 430.5.

CAS — 87679-37-6.

Adverse Effects, Treatment, and Precautions

As for ACE inhibitors, p.805.

Interactions

As for ACE inhibitors, p.807.

Pharmacokinetics

Trandolapril acts as a prodrug of the diacid trandolaprilat, its active metabolite. Following oral administration of trandolapril the bioavailability of trandolaprilat is 40 to 60%. Trandolapril is metabolised in the liver to trandolaprilat and to some inactive metabolites. Peak plasma concentrations of trandolaprilat are achieved 4 to 6 hours after an oral dose of trandolapril. About 33% of an oral dose is excreted in the urine, mainly as trandolaprilat, the rest is excreted in the faeces. Trandolaprilat is more than 80% bound to plasma proteins. The effective half-life for accumulation of trandolaprilat is 16 to 24 hours following multiple doses of trandolapril.

Impaired renal function decreases the excretion of trandolaprilat.

References.

1. Bevan EG, *et al.* Effect of renal function on the pharmacokinetics and pharmacodynamics of trandolapril. *Br J Clin Pharmacol* 1993; **35:** 128–35.

Uses and Administration

Trandolapril is an ACE inhibitor (p.805). It is used in the treatment of hypertension (p.788) and in left ventricular dysfunction following myocardial infarction (p.791).

Trandolapril owes its activity to trandolaprilat to which it is converted after oral administration. The haemodynamic effects are seen about 1 hour after an oral dose and the maximum effect occurs after 8 to 12 hours. The haemodynamic action lasts for at least 24 hours, allowing once-daily dosing.

In the treatment of **hypertension** the initial dose is 0.5 mg once daily by mouth. Since there may be a precipitous fall in blood pressure in some patients when starting therapy with an ACE inhibitor, the first dose should preferably be given at bedtime. In patients already receiving diuretic therapy, the diuretic should be discontinued, if possible, 2 to 3 days before starting trandolapril and resumed later if necessary. In patients with co-existing heart failure treatment with trandolapril should begin under close medical supervision. The usual maintenance dose for hypertension is 1 to 2 mg once daily, although up to 4 mg once daily may be given.

Following **myocardial infarction**, treatment with trandolapril may be started 3 days after the infarction in an initial dose of 0.5 mg once daily, gradually increased to a maximum of 4 mg once daily. A reduction in dosage may be necessary in patients with renal impairment.

References.

1. Zannad F. Trandolapril: How does it differ from other angiotensin converting enzyme inhibitors? *Drugs* 1993; **46** (suppl 2): 172–82.
2. Wiseman LR, McTavish D. Trandolapril: a review of its pharmacodynamic and pharmacokinetic properties, and therapeutic use in essential hypertension. *Drugs* 1994; **48:** 71–90.
3. Køber L, *et al.* A clinical trial of the angiotensin-converting-enzyme inhibitor trandolapril in patients with left ventricular dysfunction after myocardial infarction. *N Engl J Med* 1995; **333:** 1670–6.

Preparations

Proprietary Preparations (details are given in Part 3)
Austral.: Gopten; Odrik; ***Fr.:*** Gopten; Odrik; ***Ger.:*** Gopten; Udrik; ***Irl.:*** Gopten; Odrik; ***Ital.:*** Gopten; Zeddan; ***Neth.:*** Gopten; ***S.Afr.:*** Gopten; ***Spain:*** Gopten; Odrik; ***Swed.:*** Gopten; ***Switz.:*** Gopten; ***UK:*** Gopten; Odrik; ***USA:*** Mavik.

Multi-ingredient: ***Ger.:*** Tarka; ***Neth.:*** Tarka; ***UK:*** Tarka; ***USA:*** Tarka.

Trapidil (13366-z)

Trapidil *(rINN).*

AR-12008. 7-Diethylamino-5-methyl-1,2,4-triazolo[1,5-*a*]pyrimidine.

$C_{10}H_{15}N_5$ = 205.3.

CAS — 15421-84-8.

Pharmacopoeias. In *Jpn.*

Trapidil is a vasodilator and an inhibitor of platelet aggregation. It is also an antagonist of platelet-derived growth factor. It is used in the management of ischaemic heart disease in doses of 300 to 600 mg daily, in divided doses, by mouth. It may also be given by intravenous injection. Ischaemic heart disease is discussed under Atherosclerosis (p.782) and the treatment of its clinical manifestations is described under Angina Pectoris (p.780) and Myocardial Infarction (p.791). Trapidil may also be used to prevent restenosis following angioplasty (p.797).

References.

1. Okamoto S, *et al.* Effects of trapidil (triazolopyrimidine), a platelet-derived growth factor antagonist, in preventing restenosis after percutaneous transluminal coronary angioplasty. *Am Heart J* 1992; **123:** 1439–44.
2. Maresta A, *et al.* Trapidil (triazolopyrimidine), a platelet-derived growth factor antagonist, reduces restenosis after percutaneous transluminal coronary angioplasty: results of the randomized, double-blind STARC study. *Circulation* 1994; **90:** 2710–15.
3. Harder S, *et al.* Pharmacokinetics of trapidil, an antagonist of platelet derived growth factor, in healthy subjects and in patients with liver cirrhosis. *Br J Clin Pharmacol* 1996; **42:** 443–9.

Preparations

Proprietary Preparations (details are given in Part 3)
Ger.: Rocornal; ***Ital.:*** Avantrin; Travisco; ***Jpn:*** Rocornal†.

Triamterene (2358-j)

Triamterene *(BAN, USAN, rINN).*

NSC-77625; SKF-8542; Triamterenum; Triantereno. 6-Phenylpteridine-2,4,7-triamine; 2,4,7-Triamino-6-phenylpteridine.

$C_{12}H_{11}N_7$ = 253.3.

CAS — 396-01-0.

NOTE. Compounded preparations of triamterene and hydrochlorothiazide in the proportions, by weight, 2 parts to 1 part have the British Approved Name Co-triamterzide.

Compounded preparations of triamterene and hydrochlorothiazide in USP 23 may be represented by the name Co-triamterzide.

Pharmacopoeias. In *Chin., Eur.* (see p.viii), *Jpn,* and *US.*

A yellow odourless crystalline powder. Very slightly **soluble** to practically insoluble in water; very slightly soluble in acetic acid, in alcohol, and in dilute mineral acids; practically insoluble in chloroform, in ether, and in dilute alkali hydroxides; soluble 1 in 30 of formic acid and 1 in 85 of 2-methoxyethanol. Acidified solutions give a blue fluorescence. **Store** in airtight containers. Protect from light.

Adverse Effects

As for Amiloride Hydrochloride, p.819. Triamterene has also been reported to cause photosensitivity reactions, increases in uric acid concentrations, and blood dyscrasias. Renal calculi may occur in susceptible patients, and megaloblastic anaemia has been reported in patients with depleted folic acid stores such as those with hepatic cirrhosis. Reversible renal failure, due either to acute interstitial nephritis or to an interaction with NSAIDs (see under Interactions, below) has occurred.

In a postmarketing surveillance study of 70 898 patients[1] taking a combination of triamterene and hydrochlorothiazide the most common adverse effects were fatigue, dizziness, and nausea. Adverse effects necessitated withdrawal in 8.1% of patients. A subgroup analysis of 21 731 patients[2] indicated that hyperkalaemia was more common in elderly patients and in those with diabetes mellitus.

1. Hollenberg NK, Mickiewicz CW. Postmarketing surveillance in 70,898 patients treated with a triamterene/hydrochlorothiazide combination (Maxzide). *Am J Cardiol* 1989; **63:** 37B–41B.
2. Hollenberg NK, Mickiewicz CW. Hyperkalemia in diabetes mellitus: effect of a triamterene-hydrochlorothiazide combination. *Arch Intern Med* 1989; **149:** 1327–30.

Effects on the blood. Case reports of pancytopenia associated with triamterene therapy.[1,2] Some patients had hepatic cirrhosis and the antifolate activity of triamterene was considered responsible.[2]

1. Castellano G, *et al.* Pancitopenia aguda y megaloblastosis medular durante el tratemiento con triamterene de la ascitis causada por cirrosis hepática: aportación de dos casos. *Gastroenterol Hepatol* 1983; **6:** 540–4.
2. Remacha A, *et al.* Triamterene-induced megaloblastosis: report of two new cases, and review of the literature. *Biol Clin Hematol* 1983; **5:** 127–34.

Effects on the kidneys. There have been a number of reports[1-4] of renal calculi containing triamterene or its metabolites, generally in patients taking triamterene with hydrochlorothiazide. An abnormal urinary sediment was described by Fairley and colleagues[5] in patients taking triamterene which was thought to represent precipitated triamterene. These observations were expanded in a crossover study by Spence and colleagues.[6] Abnormal urinary sediment was seen in 14 of 26 patients while taking triamterene but in none while taking amiloride. Triamterene and its metabolites had been identified by Ettinger and colleagues[7] in 181 of 50 000 renal calculi. Triamterene either formed the nucleus of the stone or was deposited with calcium oxalate or uric acid. One-third of the 181 stones were entirely or predominantly composed of triamterene and its metabolites. Crystal deposition causing intrarenal obstruction and a direct nephrotoxic effect were considered responsible for acute oliguric renal failure following overdosage with triamterene and hydrochlorothiazide.[8] It has been suggested that deposition of triamterene in the urine could also play a part in the development of interstitial nephritis.[6,9]

No evidence of abnormal excretion or metabolism of triamterene has been detected in patients with renal stones,[10,11] but the concentration of the sulphate metabolite has exceeded the apparent maximum solubility.[10-12] White and Nancollas[12] suggest that supersaturation of the urine with triamterene and its metabolites could provide suitable nuclei for the crystallisation of calcium oxalate. Werness and colleagues[13] were unable to demonstrate this and suggested that triamterene and its metabolites could become incorporated into the protein matrix of existing stones. In addition, an epidemiological study reported by Jick and colleagues[14] found no evidence that triamterene use was associated with an increased incidence of renal stones. In assessing the available evidence on renal calculi and triamterene, Woolfson and Mansell[15] considered that contra-indicating the drug in patients with a history of recurrent renal calculi was not yet warranted.

Triamterene has also been associated with transient decline in renal function and the development of renal failure.[16,17] Several mechanisms may be responsible including interstitial nephritis, intrarenal obstruction by crystalline deposits, and an interaction with NSAIDs (see under Interactions, below).[17] Elderly patients may be particularly at risk.[16]

1. Ettinger B, *et al.* Triamterene-induced nephrolithiasis. *Ann Intern Med* 1979; **91:** 745–6.
2. Socolow EL. Triamterene-induced nephrolithiasis. *Ann Intern Med* 1980; **92:** 437.
3. Gault MH, *et al.* Triamterene urolithiasis. *Can Med Assoc J* 1981; **124:** 1556–7.
4. Grunberg RW, Silberg SJ. Triamterene-induced nephrolithiasis. *JAMA* 1981; **245:** 2494–5.
5. Fairley KF, *et al.* Abnormal urinary sediment in patients on triamterene. *Lancet* 1983; **i:** 421–2.
6. Spence JD, *et al.* Effects of triamterene and amiloride on urinary sediment in hypertensive patients taking hydrochlorothiazide. *Lancet* 1985; **ii:** 73–5.
7. Ettinger B, *et al.* Triamterene nephrolithiasis. *JAMA* 1980; **244:** 2443–5.
8. Farge D, *et al.* Dyazide-induced reversible acute renal failure associated with intracellular crystal deposition. *Am J Kidney Dis* 1986; **8:** 445–9.
9. Anonymous. Triamterene and the kidney. *Lancet* 1986; **i:** 424.
10. Ettinger B. Excretion of triamterene and its metabolite in triamterene stone patients. *J Clin Pharmacol* 1985; **25:** 365–8.
11. Sörgel F, *et al.* Metabolic fate and solubility of triamterene—not an explanation for triamterene nephrolithiasis. *J Pharm Sci* 1986; **75:** 129–32.
12. White DJ, Nancollas GH. Triamterene and renal stone formation. *J Urol (Baltimore)* 1982; **127:** 593–7.
13. Werness PG, *et al.* Triamterene urolithiasis: solubility, pK, effect on crystal formation, and matrix binding of triamterene and its metabolites. *J Lab Clin Med* 1982; **99:** 254–62.
14. Jick H, *et al.* Triamterene and renal stones. *J Urol (Baltimore)* 1982; **127:** 224–5.
15. Woolfson RG, Mansell MA. Does triamterene cause renal calculi? *Br Med J* 1991; **303:** 1217–18.
16. Lynn KL, *et al.* Renal failure with potassium-sparing diuretics. *N Z Med J* 1985; **98:** 629–33.
17. Sica DA, Gehr TWB. Triamterene and the kidney. *Nephron* 1989; **51:** 454–61.

Effects on the skin. Photodermatitis has been reported in a patient receiving triamterene.[1] Pseudoporphyria, possibly associated with exposure to sunlight, occurred in a patient with vitiligo during treatment with triamterene and hydrochlorothiazide.[2]

1. Fernández de Corres L, *et al.* Photodermatitis from triamterene. *Contact Dermatitis* 1987; **17:** 114–15.
2. Motley RJ. Pseudoporphyria due to Dyazide in a patient with vitiligo. *Br Med J* 1990; **300:** 1468.

Precautions

As for Amiloride Hydrochloride, p.819. Triamterene should also be given with caution to patients with hyperuricaemia or gout, or a history of renal calculi. Patients with depleted folic acid stores such as those with hepatic cirrhosis may be at increased risk of megaloblastic anaemia.

Triamterene may interfere with the fluorescent measurement of quinidine. It may slightly colour the urine blue.

Interactions

As for Amiloride Hydrochloride, p.819.

For reports of the effects of triamterene on *digoxin*, see p.851, and on *amantadine*, see p.1130.

NSAIDs. There have been several reports of renal failure in patients taking triamterene and NSAIDs.[1,2] Both types of drug are nephrotoxic and in combination the effect appears to be additive.[3-5] It has been suggested that the suppression of urinary prostaglandins by NSAIDs could potentiate the nephrotoxic effects of triamterene.[1]

NSAIDs may also antagonise the diuretic action of triamterene.[6]

1. Favre L, *et al.* Reversible acute renal failure from combined triamterene and indomethacin: a study in healthy subjects. *Ann Intern Med* 1982; **96:** 317–20.
2. Härkönen M, Ekblom-Kullberg S. Reversible deterioration of renal function after diclofenac in patient receiving triamterene. *Br Med J* 1986; **293:** 698–9.
3. Bailey RR. Adverse renal reactions to non-steroidal anti-inflammatory drugs and potassium-sparing diuretics. *Adverse Drug React Bull* 1988; (Aug.): 492–5.
4. Lynn KL, *et al.* Renal failure with potassium-sparing diuretics. *N Z Med J* 1985; **98:** 629–33.
5. Sica DA, Gehr TWB. Triamterene and the kidney. *Nephron* 1989; **51:** 454–61.
6. Webster J. Interactions of NSAIDs with diuretics and β-blockers: mechanisms and clinical implications. *Drugs* 1985; **30:** 32–41.

Pharmacokinetics

Triamterene is variably but fairly rapidly absorbed from the gastro-intestinal tract. The bioavailability has been reported to be about 50%. The plasma half-life has been reported to be about 2 hours. It is estimated to be about 60% bound to plasma proteins. It is extensively metabolised and is mainly excreted in the urine in the form of metabolites with some unchanged triamterene. Triamterene crosses the placental barrier and may be distributed into breast milk.

References.

1. Pruitt AW, *et al.* Variations in the fate of triamterene. *Clin Pharmacol Ther* 1977; **21:** 610–19.
2. Gundert-Remy U, *et al.* Plasma and urinary levels of triamterene and certain metabolites after oral administration to man. *Eur J Clin Pharmacol* 1979; **16:** 39–44.
3. Gilfrich HJ, *et al.* Pharmacokinetics of triamterene after iv administration to man: determination of bioavailability. *Eur J Clin Pharmacol* 1983; **25:** 237–41.
4. Sörgel F, *et al.* Oral triamterene disposition. *Clin Pharmacol Ther* 1985; **38:** 306–12.

Hepatic impairment. Triamterene clearance was markedly decreased in 7 patients with alcoholic cirrhosis and ascites.[1] The diuretic effect lasted for up to 48 hours in cirrhotic patients compared with 8 hours in healthy controls.

1. Villeneuve JP, *et al.* Triamterene kinetics and dynamics in cirrhosis. *Clin Pharmacol Ther* 1984; **35:** 831–7.

Renal impairment. Urinary excretion of triamterene and its metabolite, hydroxytriamterene sulphate, was significantly reduced in patients with renal impairment[1] and in the elderly whose renal function was reduced.[2] Accumulation of the active metabolite was possible in patients with impaired renal function.[1]

1. Knauf H, *et al.* Delayed elimination of triamterene and its active metabolite in chronic renal failure. *Eur J Clin Pharmacol* 1983; **24:** 453–6.
2. Williams RL, *et al.* Absorption and disposition of two combination formulations of hydrochlorothiazide and triamterene: influence of age and renal function. *Clin Pharmacol Ther* 1986; **40:** 226–32.

Uses and Administration

Triamterene is a mild diuretic with potassium-sparing properties which has actions and uses similar to those of amiloride (p.819). It produces a diuresis in about 2 to 4 hours, with a duration of 7 to 9 hours. The full therapeutic effect may be delayed until after several days of treatment.

Triamterene adds to the natriuretic but diminishes the kaliuretic effects of other diuretics. It is mainly used, as an adjunct to thiazide diuretics such as hydrochlorothiazide and loop diuretics such as frusemide, to conserve potassium in those at risk from hypokalaemia during the treatment of refractory oedema associated with hepatic cirrhosis, heart failure (p.785), and the nephrotic syndrome. It is also used in combination with other diuretics in the treatment of hypertension (p.788).

When triamterene is given alone in the treatment of **oedema**, the suggested range of dosage is 150 to 250 mg daily by mouth; 100 mg twice daily, after breakfast and lunch, is considered to be the optimum dose, preferably on alternate days for maintenance therapy. More than 300 mg daily should not be given.

Smaller doses are suggested initially when other diuretics are also being given. When used with hydrochlorothiazide, for example, in the treatment of **hypertension**, an initial dose of 50 mg of triamterene daily has been suggested.

Potassium supplements should not be given.

Preparations

BP 1998: Co-triamterzide Tablets; Triamterene Capsules;
USP 23: Triamterene and Hydrochlorothiazide Capsules; Triamterene and Hydrochlorothiazide Tablets; Triamterene Capsules.

Proprietary Preparations (details are given in Part 3)
Austral.: Dytac†; ***Belg.:*** Dytac†; ***Canad.:*** Dyrenium; ***Ger.:*** Jatropur; ***Irl.:*** Dytac†; ***Neth.:*** Dytac; ***Spain:*** Urocaudal; ***Switz.:*** Dyrenium; ***UK:*** Dytac; ***USA:*** Dyrenium.

Multi-ingredient: ***Aust.:*** Confit; Dehydrosin; Diucomb; Diurid; Dytide H; Hydrotrix; Inderal comp; Resaltex; Salodiur; Tardurol; Triamteren comp; ***Austral.:*** Dyazide; Hydrene; ***Belg.:*** Diucomb; Dyta-Urese; Dytenzide; Maxzide; ***Canad.:*** Apo-Triazide; Dyazide; Novo-Triamzide; Nu-Triazide; ***Fr.:*** Cycloteriam; Isobar; Prestole; ***Ger.:*** Beta-Nephral; Beta-Turfa; Betathiazid; Calmoserpin†; cardiotensin†; dehydro sanol tri; dehydro tri mite; Diu Venostasin; Diu-Tonolytril†; Diucomb; Diuretikum Verla; Diutensat; Diutensat comp; Dociteren; Dociton Dytide H†; duradiuret; Dytide H; Esiteren; Furesis comp; Haemiton compositum; Hydrotrix; Hypertorr; Jenateren comp; Manimon; Neotri; Nephral; pertenso†; Propra comp; Resaltex; Sali-Puren; Slimin†; Thiazid-comp.; Tri-Thiazid; Tri-Thiazid Reserpin; Triampur; Triamteren comp; Triamteren-H; Triarese; Triazid; Turfa; Veratide; ***Irl.:*** Dyazide; Dytide†; Frusene; ***Ital.:*** Fluss 40; Triamteril Complex†; ***Neth.:*** Dyta-Urese; Dytenzide; ***S.Afr.:*** Dyazide; Loretic; Renezide; Urizide; ***Spain:*** Picten†; Salidur; Triniagar; Urocaudal Tiazida; ***Switz.:*** Diucomb; Dyazide; Dyrenium compositum; Hydrotrix; t/h-basan; ***UK:*** Dyazide; Dytide; Frusene; Kalspare; Triamaxco; Triamco; ***USA:*** Dyazide; Maxzide.

Trichlormethiazide (2359-z)

Trichlormethiazide *(rINN)*.

Trichlormethiazidum. 6-Chloro-3-dichloromethyl-3,4-dihydro-2*H*-1,2,4-benzothiadiazine-7-sulphonamide 1,1-dioxide.

$C_8H_8Cl_3N_3O_4S_2$ = 380.7.

CAS — 133-67-5.

Pharmacopoeias. In *Jpn* and *US.*

A white or practically white, odourless or almost odourless, crystalline powder.

Soluble 1 in 1100 of water, 1 in 5000 of chloroform, 1 in 1400 of ether, 1 in 48 of alcohol, 1 in about 9 of dioxan, and 1 in about 4 of dimethylformamide; freely soluble in acetone; soluble in methyl alcohol.

Trichlormethiazide is a thiazide diuretic with properties similar to those of hydrochlorothiazide (p.885). It is used for oedema, including that associated with heart failure (p.785), and for hypertension (p.788).

Diuresis is initiated in about 2 hours, and lasts about 24 hours.

In the treatment of oedema the usual dose by mouth is 1 to 4 mg daily or intermittently. In the treatment of hypertension the usual dose is 2 to 4 mg daily, either alone, or in conjunction with other antihypertensives. In some patients 1 mg daily may be adequate. In children a dose of 70 μg per kg bodyweight daily in one or two doses has been suggested.

In susceptible patients potassium supplements or a potassium-sparing diuretic may be necessary, but see hydrochlorothiazide.

Preparations

USP 23: Trichlormethiazide Tablets.

Proprietary Preparations (details are given in Part 3)
Ger.: Esmarin†; ***Ital.:*** Fluitran†; ***Norw.:*** Fluitran†; ***USA:*** Diurese; Metahydrin; Naqua.

Multi-ingredient: ***Ger.:*** Esmalorid; ***Spain:*** Rulun; ***Switz.:*** Esmaloride†; ***USA:*** Metatensin.

Triflusal (13379-x)

Triflusal *(rINN)*.

Triflusalum; UR-1501. 2-Acetoxy-4-trifluoromethylbenzoic acid.

$C_{10}H_7F_3O_4$ = 248.2.

CAS — 322-79-2.

Pharmacopoeias. In *Eur.* (see p.viii).

A white or almost white powder. Practically **insoluble** in water; very soluble in dehydrated alcohol; freely soluble in dichloromethane. **Store** in airtight containers at a temperature not exceeding 25°.

Triflusal is an inhibitor of platelet aggregation used for the prophylaxis of thrombo-embolic disorders (p.801) in doses of 300 mg daily by mouth and in maintenance therapy in usual doses of 300 to 900 mg daily.

References.

1. McNeely W, Goa KL. Triflusal. *Drugs* 1998; **55:** 823–33.

Preparations

Proprietary Preparations (details are given in Part 3)
Ital.: Disgren; ***Spain:*** Disgren.

Trimazosin Hydrochloride (910-g)

Trimazosin Hydrochloride *(BANM, USAN, rINNM)*.

CP-19106-1. 2-Hydroxy-2-methylpropyl 4-(4-amino-6,7,8-trimethoxyquinazolin-2-yl)piperazine-1-carboxylate hydrochloride monohydrate.

$C_{20}H_{29}N_5O_6,HCl,H_2O$ = 490.0.

CAS — 35795-16-5 (trimazosin); 35795-17-6 (trimazosin hydrochloride, anhydrous); 53746-46-6 (trimazosin hydrochloride, monohydrate).

Trimazosin is an alpha$_1$-adrenoceptor blocker (p.776) that has been used as the hydrochloride in the treatment of hypertension and heart failure.

Preparations

Proprietary Preparations (details are given in Part 3)
Ger.: Cardovar BD†.

Trimetaphan Camsylate (911-q)

Trimetaphan Camsylate *(BAN)*.

Trimetaphan Camsilate *(rINN)*; Méthioplégium; Trimetaphan Camphorsulphonate; Trimetaphani Camsylas; Trimethaphan Camsylate. (+)-1,3-Dibenzylperhydro-2-oxothieno[1',2':1,2]thieno[3,4-*d*]-imidazol-5-ium 2-oxobornane-10-sulphonate; 4,6-Dibenzyl-4,6-diaza-1-thioniatricyclo[6.3.0.0^{3,7}]undecan-5-one 2-oxobornane-10-sulphonate.

$C_{22}H_{25}N_2OS,C_{10}H_{15}O_4S$ = 596.8.

CAS — 7187-66-8 (trimetaphan); 68-91-7 (trimetaphan camsylate).

Pharmacopoeias. In *It., Jpn,* and *US.*

White crystals or white crystalline powder, odourless or with a slight odour. Freely **soluble** in water, in alcohol and in chloroform; practically insoluble in ether. **Store** at a temperature not exceeding 8° in airtight containers.

Incompatible with thiopentone sodium, gallamine triethiodide, iodides, bromides, and strongly alkaline solutions.

Stability. Although the USP recommends storage of trimetaphan camsylate injection between 2° and 8°, Vogenberg and Souney, quoting the manufacturer (*Roche, USA*) have reported that the stability of the commercial injection of trimetaphan camsylate may be maintained for up to 2 weeks at room temperature,[1] while Longland and Rowbotham report (using data from *Roche, UK*) that the shelf-life at room temperature is 1 year,[2] compared with 3 years when stored at 6°.

1. Vogenberg FR, Souney PF. Stability guidelines for routinely refrigerated drug products. *Am J Hosp Pharm* 1983; **40:** 101–2.
2. Longland PW, Rowbotham PC. Stability at room temperature of medicines normally recommended for cold storage. *Pharm J* 1987; **238:** 147–51.

Adverse Effects and Treatment

The adverse effects of trimetaphan are mainly due to ganglionic blockade. A reduction in gastro-intestinal motility may result in constipation and, on prolonged administration, paralytic ileus. Urinary retention, cycloplegia, mydriasis, tachycardia, precipitation of angina, and gastro-intestinal disturbances may occur. Orthostatic hypotension may be severe. Rapid intravenous infusion at rates greater than 5 mg per minute can result in respiratory arrest. Other adverse effects include raised intra-ocular pressure, dry mouth, hypoglycaemia, hypokalaemia, fluid retention, weakness, urticaria, and itching. Trimetaphan crosses the placenta and can cause paralytic or meconium ileus in the neonate.

If severe hypotension occurs, administration of trimetaphan should be stopped and the patient positioned with the head lower than the feet. A vasopressor may be given cautiously if necessary.

Although trimetaphan may increase intra-ocular pressure, a sudden and dramatic reduction of intra-ocular pressure to very low levels was noted in 5 patients undergoing surgery when the systolic blood pressure was reduced to 60 mmHg with trimetaphan infusion.[1]

1. Dias PLR, *et al.* Effect on the intraocular pressure of hypotensive anaesthesia with intravenous trimetaphan. *Br J Ophthalmol* 1982; **66:** 721–4.

Precautions

Trimetaphan should be avoided in patients with asphyxia or respiratory insufficiency, uncorrected anaemia, shock or hypovolaemia, severe arteriosclerosis, severe ischaemic heart disease, or pyloric stenosis and should only be used with extreme caution in those with impaired hepatic or renal function, degenerative disease of the CNS, Addison's disease, prostatic hyperplasia, glaucoma, cerebral or coronary vascular insufficiency, and diabetes. It should be used with care in elderly or debilitated patients and should be avoided in pregnancy. Owing to a histamine-liberating effect it should be used with caution in allergic subjects. Trimetaphan should also be used with caution in patients being treated with other antihypertensives, drugs which depress cardiac function, muscle relaxants, and in those taking corticosteroids. The hypotensive effect is enhanced by general and spinal anaesthetics.

Interactions

For a reference to possible potentiation of neuromuscular blockade by trimetaphan, see Atracurium, p.1307.

Uses and Administration

Trimetaphan is a ganglion blocker which inhibits the transmission of nerve impulses in both sympathetic and parasympathetic ganglia. The sympathetic blockade produces peripheral vasodilatation. Trimetaphan also has a direct vasodilator effect on peripheral blood vessels. It is used for inducing controlled hypotension during surgical procedures although sodium nitroprusside is usually preferred. It acts rapidly to produce a hypotensive response which persists for about 10 to 15 minutes.

Trimetaphan camsylate is administered by slow intravenous infusion of a solution usually containing 1 mg per mL. The infusion is started at the rate of 3 to 4 mg per minute and then adjusted according to the response of the patient. Blood pressure should be closely monitored and should be allowed to rise before wound closure.

Adrenaline should not be infiltrated locally at the site of incision when trimetaphan is being given since this may antagonise the effect of trimetaphan.

Trimetaphan has also been used for the emergency treatment of hypertensive crises (p.788), especially in association with pulmonary oedema or acute dissecting aortic aneurysms, but sodium nitroprusside is often preferred.

Preparations

USP 23: Trimethaphan Camsylate Injection.

Proprietary Preparations (details are given in Part 3)
Canad.: Arfonad†; ***Irl.:*** Arfonad†; ***Ital.:*** Arfonad†; ***UK:*** Arfonad; ***USA:*** Arfonad†.

Trimetazidine Hydrochloride (9282-x)

Trimetazidine Hydrochloride *(BANM, rINNM).*

Trimetazine Hydrochloride. 1-(2,3,4-Trimethoxybenzyl)piperazine dihydrochloride.

$C_{14}H_{22}N_2O_3,2HCl = 339.3.$

CAS — 5011-34-7 (trimetazidine); 13171-25-0 (trimetazidine hydrochloride).

Pharmacopoeias. In *Jpn.*

Trimetazidine hydrochloride is used in angina pectoris (p.780) and in ischaemia of neurosensorial tissues as in Ménière's disease (p.400); 40 to 60 mg is given daily by mouth in divided doses.

References.

1. Harpey C, *et al.* Trimetazidine, a cellular anti-ischemic agent. *Cardiovasc Drug Rev* 1989; **6:** 292–312.

Preparations

Proprietary Preparations (details are given in Part 3)
Fr.: Vastarel; ***Irl.:*** Vastarel; ***Ital.:*** Vastarel; ***Spain:*** Idaptan.

Tripamide (1293-v)

Tripamide *(USAN, rINN).*

ADR-033; E-614. 4-Chloro-*N*-(*endo*-hexahydro-4,7-methanoisoindolin-2-yl)-3-sulphamoylbenzamide.

$C_{16}H_{20}ClN_3O_3S = 369.9.$

CAS — 73803-48-2.

Tripamide is a diuretic structurally related to indapamide. It is used in the treatment of hypertension (p.788) in doses of 15 to 30 mg daily by mouth.

Preparations

Proprietary Preparations (details are given in Part 3)
Jpn: Normonal.

Trolnitrate Phosphate (9283-r)

Trolnitrate Phosphate *(BAN, rINN).*

Aminotrate Phosphate; Nitranolum; Triethanolamine Trinitrate Diphosphate. Nitrilotrisethylene trinitrate diphosphate.

$C_6H_{12}N_4O_9,2H_3PO_4 = 480.2.$

CAS — 7077-34-1 (trolnitrate); 588-42-1 (trolnitrate phosphate).

Trolnitrate phosphate is a vasodilator with general properties similar to those of glyceryl trinitrate (p.875). It has been used in angina pectoris.

Urapidil (11586-e)

Urapidil *(BAN, rINN).*

B-66256M. 6-[3-(4-*o*-Methoxyphenylpiperazin-1-yl)propylamino]-1,3-dimethyluracil.

$C_{20}H_{29}N_5O_3 = 387.5.$

CAS — 34661-75-1.

Urapidil Hydrochloride (14001-k)

Urapidil Hydrochloride *(BANM, rINNM).*

$C_{20}H_{29}N_5O_3,HCl = 423.9.$

CAS — 64887-14-5.

Adverse Effects and Precautions

Urapidil is reported to be well-tolerated, with adverse effects generally transient and most frequent at the beginning of therapy. Dizziness, nausea, headache, fatigue, orthostatic hypotension, palpitations, nervousness, pruritus, and allergic skin reactions have been reported.

It should be used with care in elderly patients and those with severe hepatic insufficiency. Intravenous urapidil should not be used in patients with aortic stenosis.

A report of enuresis associated with the use of urapidil in 2 elderly patients.[1]

1. Jonville A-P, *et al.* Urapidil and enuresis. *Lancet* 1992; **339:** 688.

Pharmacokinetics

Following oral administration urapidil is rapidly absorbed with a reported bioavailability of 70 to 80%. It is extensively metabolised in the liver, principally by hydroxylation, and excreted mostly in urine, as metabolites and 10 to 20% of unchanged drug. Urapidil is reported to be about 80% bound to plasma protein. The elimination half-life is reported to be about 4.7 hours following oral administration as capsules and about 2.7 hours following intravenous administration.

Reviews.

1. Kirsten R, *et al.* Clinical pharmacokinetics of urapidil. *Clin Pharmacokinet* 1988; **14:** 129–40.

Uses and Administration

Urapidil is an antihypertensive drug that is reported to block peripheral alpha$_1$-adrenoceptors (p.776) and to have central actions. It produces a reduction in peripheral resistance and a fall in systolic and diastolic blood pressure, usually without reflex tachycardia.

Urapidil is used in the management of hypertension (p.788), including hypertensive crises.

Urapidil is given by mouth as the base and intravenously as the hydrochloride, but doses are usually expressed in terms of the base. Urapidil fumarate has also been given by mouth.

In hypertension doses of 30 to 90 mg are given twice daily by mouth. In hypertensive crises an initial dose of 25 mg is given by slow intravenous injection over 20 seconds, followed by infusion of 9 to 30 mg per hour.

Reviews.

1. Langtry HD, *et al.* Urapidil: a review of its therapeutic potential in the treatment of hypertension. *Drugs* 1989; **38:** 900–40.

Preparations

Proprietary Preparations (details are given in Part 3)
Aust.: Ebrantil; ***Belg.:*** Ebrantil; ***Fr.:*** Eupressyl; Mediatensyl; ***Ger.:*** Alpha-Depressan; Ebrantil; ***Ital.:*** Ebrantil; Uraprene†; ***Neth.:*** Ebrantil; ***Spain:*** Elgadil; ***Switz.:*** Ebrantil.

Urokinase (3752-s)

Urokinase *(BAN, USAN, rINN).*

Urokinasum.

CAS — 9039-53-6.

Pharmacopoeias. In *Eur.* (see p.viii) and *Jpn.*

An enzyme isolated from human urine or from tissue cultures of human kidney cells that activates plasminogen. The Ph. Eur. specifies urokinase obtained from human urine that consists of a mixture of low (33 000) and high (54 000) molecular weight forms, the high molecular weight form being predominant, and containing not less than 70 000 international units of urokinase activity per mg of protein.

A white or almost white amorphous powder. **Soluble** in water. **Store** in airtight containers at a temperature not exceeding 8°. Protect from light.

Stability. Despite a slight fall in thrombolytic activity after 7 days a mixture of heparin with urokinase suitable for maintaining vascular access devices free of thrombi was stable on incubation at 37° for 21 days.[1]

Urokinase is diluted before administration with glucose 5% or sodium chloride 0.9% injection. A study[2] of the effects of diluent, container, giving set, and drug concentration on adsorption of urokinase found a loss of 15 to 20% of urokinase activity in solutions of glucose 5% containing 1500 units of urokinase per mL stored in polyvinyl chloride (PVC) containers. No loss of activity was measured in solutions of urokinase in sodium chloride 0.9% or in solutions of glucose 5% containing 5000 units of urokinase per mL.

1. Morgan GJ, *et al.* Stability of a heparin urokinase mixture. *Intensive Therapy Clin Monit* 1987; **8:** 89.
2. Patel JP, *et al.* Activity of urokinase diluted in 0.9% sodium chloride injection or 5% dextrose injection and stored in glass or plastic syringes. *Am J Hosp Pharm* 1991; **48:** 1511–14.

Units

The potency of urokinase is expressed in international units. Preparations are assayed using the first International Reference Preparation (1968), a mixture of low molecular weight and high molecular weight urokinases. The first International Standard for high molecular weight urokinase was established in 1989 for use with preparations of this type of urokinase.

Potency used to be expressed in Ploug or Plough units or in CTA units, but these now appear to be obsolete.

Adverse Effects, Treatment, and Precautions

As for Streptokinase, p.948. Serious allergic reactions may be less likely to occur with urokinase than with streptokinase.

Hypersensitivity. Allergic reactions are considered to be less frequent with urokinase than with streptokinase. However, in a series of six patients who had previously been treated with streptokinase,[1] thrombolytic therapy with urokinase for recurrent myocardial infarction was associated with rigors in four patients, two of whom also developed bronchospasm. None of the patients had any history of atopy.

1. Matsis P, Mann S. Rigors and bronchospasm with urokinase after streptokinase. *Lancet* 1992; **340:** 1552.

Interactions

As for Streptokinase, p.950.

Pharmacokinetics

Following intravenous infusion urokinase is cleared rapidly from the circulation by the liver. A plasma half-life of up to 20 minutes has been reported.

Uses and Administration

Urokinase is a thrombolytic drug. It directly converts plasminogen to plasmin, a proteolytic enzyme which has fibrinolytic effects. The mechanisms of fibrinolysis are discussed further under Haemostasis on p.704. Urokinase affects circulating, unbound plasminogen as well as fibrin-bound plasminogen and thus may be termed a fibrin-nonspecific thrombolytic agent. This action was thought to contribute to the risk of haemorrhage, although currently available fibrin-specific agents, such as alteplase, do not produce less bleeding than nonspecific thrombolytics (see Haemorrhage under Adverse Effects of Streptokinase, p.949).

Urokinase is used similarly to streptokinase (p.950) in the management of thrombo-embolic disorders including venous thrombo-embolism (deep-vein thrombosis and pulmonary embolism) (p.802) and coronary occlusion in myocardial infarction (p.791). It is also used in peripheral arterial thrombo-embolism (p.794) and has a specific use in clearing clots following haemorrhage within the eye. Like streptokinase it is used to clear cannulas and shunts of occluding thrombi.

In the treatment of **pulmonary embolism** urokinase is given by intravenous infusion in initial doses of 4400 units per kg body-weight over 10 minutes, followed by 4400 units per kg per hour for 12 hours. Similar doses are used in **deep-vein thrombosis**. Alternatively, 15 000 units per kg may be given as a bolus injection into the pulmonary artery, repeated if necessary at 24-hour intervals for up to three doses; subsequent doses may be adjusted if necessary.

In the management of acute **myocardial infarction** infusion into the coronary arteries of urokinase in a dose of 6000 units per minute, for up to 2 hours, has been recommended; coronary infusion should be preceded by intravenous heparin. Alternatively, urokinase has been given intravenously in usual doses of 2 to 3 million units over 45 to 90 minutes.

In the treatment of **peripheral arterial thrombo-embolism** urokinase is infused into the clot via a catheter at a rate of 4000 units per minute as a solution containing 2500 units per mL; the catheter is advanced into the remaining occlusion every 2 hours until flow resumes, and is then partially withdrawn and an infusion of 1000 units per minute given until the remaining clot has lysed.

To break down clots within the anterior chamber of the eye following internal haemorrhage (hyphaema), solutions of urokinase have been instilled through an incision and the clot fragments removed by aspiration. A dose of 5000 units dissolved in 2 mL of sodium chloride 0.9% injection has been suggested for irrigation of clots in the anterior chamber.

For the clearance of occluded cannulas and shunts up to 25 000 units in 2 to 3 mL of sodium chloride 0.9% injection may be instilled into the affected device and clamped off for 2 to 4 hours; the lysate is then aspirated.

Catheters and cannulas. In a study[1] in 227 paediatric patients with a total of 254 right atrial catheters, catheter occlusion occurred in 58 catheters over 1 year. Clot lysis was achieved in 44 by bolus instillation of 5000 units (1 mL) of urokinase, followed if necessary after 4 hours by a second bolus of 10 000 units in 2 mL. The remaining catheters which did not respond, were infused directly with a solution of urokinase supplying 200 units per kg body-weight per lumen per hour for 24 to 48 hours (or in one patient considered at high risk of intracranial haemorrhage, 100 units per kg per hour) and of the 12 catheters actually studied, 11 responded to this low-dose infusion, with a mean infusion time of 28.7 hours. Blood coagulation profiles were not significantly affected by the urokinase infusion.

Of 434 neonates[2] with central venous catheters, thrombosis developed in 26. Urokinase, given as a bolus of 4400 units per kg over 10 minutes followed by continuous infusion of 4400 units per kg per hour, achieved thrombolysis in 16 of the neonates.

1. Bagnall HA, *et al.* Continuous infusion of low-dose urokinase in the treatment of central venous catheter thrombosis in infants and children. *Pediatrics* 1989; **83:** 963–6.
2. Wever MLG, *et al.* Urokinase therapy in neonates with catheter related central venous thrombosis. *Thromb Haemost* 1995; **73:** 180–5.

Empyema. For the use of urokinase in the management of pericardial and thoracic empyema, see under Streptokinase, p.950.

Intracardiac thrombosis. For the use of urokinase in the management of thrombosis associated with prosthetic heart valves, see under Streptokinase, p.950.

Peritonitis. Antibacterial therapy, given intraperitoneally, is the usual treatment for peritonitis in patients on continuous ambulatory peritoneal dialysis (CAPD) (for further details, see p.136), but some patients relapse. Successful treatment in 3 consecutive patients with recurrent peritonitis on CAPD has been reported[1] using urokinase (5000 units intraperitoneally) without Tenckhoff catheter removal. Oral and intraperitoneal antibacterials were continued throughout the procedure and for a total of 7 days. In a double-blind study,[2] urokinase 5000 units given intraperitoneally followed by antibacterial therapy for 14 days was effective in 8 of 12 patients on CAPD with resistant peritonitis. The mode of action of urokinase in these cases is uncertain, although the rationale for using it has been that lysis of fibrin within the peritoneum and/or catheter might release bacteria trapped in it thus allowing antibacterials to act.

1. Pickering SJ, *et al.* Urokinase for recurrent CAPD peritonitis. *Lancet* 1987; **i:** 1258–9.
2. Innes A, *et al.* Treatment of resistant peritonitis in continuous ambulatory peritoneal dialysis with intraperitoneal urokinase: a double-blind clinical trial. *Nephrol Dial Transplant* 1994; **9:** 797–9.

Preparations

Proprietary Preparations (details are given in Part 3)
Aust.: Abbokinase; Actosolv; Ukidan; ***Austral.:*** Ukidan; ***Belg.:*** Actosolv; ***Canad.:*** Abbokinase; ***Fr.:*** Actosolv; ***Ger.:*** Abbokinase†; Actosolv; Alphakinase; Corase; rheotromb; Ukidan†; ***Ital.:*** Actosolv; Alfakinasi; Kisolv; Persolv Richter; Purochin; Ukidan; ***Jpn:*** Uronase†; ***S.Afr.:*** Ukidan; ***Spain:*** Abbokinase; Uroquidan; ***Swed.:*** Abbokinase; Ukidan; ***Switz.:*** Ukidan; ***UK:*** Ukidan; ***USA:*** Abbokinase.

Valsartan (17122-b)

Valsartan *(BAN, USAN, rINN).*

CGP-48933. *N*-[*p*-(*o*-1*H*-Tetrazol-5-ylphenyl)benzyl]-*N*-valeryl-L-valine; *N*-Pentanoyl-*N*-[2′-(1*H*-tetrazol-5-yl)biphenyl-4-ylmethyl]-L-valine.

$C_{24}H_{29}N_5O_3$ = 435.5.

CAS — 137862-53-4.

Adverse Effects and Precautions

As for Losartan Potassium, p.899. Valsartan is contra-indicated in patients with severe hepatic impairment, cirrhosis, or biliary obstruction.

Pharmacokinetics

Valsartan is rapidly absorbed following oral administration, with a bioavailability of about 23%. It is between 94 and 97% bound to plasma proteins. Valsartan is not significantly metabolised and is excreted mainly via the bile as unchanged drug. The terminal elimination half-life is about 5 to 9 hours. Following an oral dose about 83% is excreted in the faeces and 13% in urine.

Uses and Administration

Valsartan is an angiotensin II receptor antagonist with actions similar to those of losartan potassium (p.899). It is used in the management of hypertension (p.788).

Valsartan is administered by mouth. Following an oral dose the hypotensive effect occurs within 2 hours, is maximal within 4 to 6 hours, and persists for over 24 hours. The maximum hypotensive effect is achieved within 2 to 4 weeks.

In hypertension, valsartan is given in an initial dose of 80 mg once daily. This may be increased, if necessary, to 160 mg once daily, although doses of up to 320 mg once daily have been used. A lower initial dose of 40 mg once daily is suggested for elderly patients over 75 years, and for those with moderate to severe renal impairment (creatinine clearance less than 20 mL per minute), intravascular volume depletion, or hepatic impairment.

References.

1. Müller P, *et al.* Angiotensin II receptor blockade with single doses of valsartan in healthy, normotensive subjects. *Eur J Clin Pharmacol* 1994; **47:** 231–45.
2. Corea L, *et al.* Valsartan, a new angiotensin II antagonist for the treatment of essential hypertension: a comparative study of the efficacy and safety against amlodipine. *Clin Pharmacol Ther* 1996; **60:** 341–6.
3. Benz J, *et al.* Valsartan, a new angiotensin II receptor antagonist: a double-blind study comparing the incidence of cough with lisinopril and hydrochlorothiazide. *J Clin Pharmacol* 1997; **37:** 101–107.
4. Markham A, Goa KL. Valsartan: a review of its pharmacology and therapeutic use in essential hypertension. *Drugs* 1997; **54:** 299–311.

Preparations

Proprietary Preparations (details are given in Part 3)
Ger.: Diovan; ***Irl.:*** Diovan; ***Ital.:*** Tareg; ***Neth.:*** Diovan; ***S.Afr.:*** Diovan; ***Swed.:*** Diovan; ***Switz.:*** Diovan; ***UK:*** Diovan; ***USA:*** Diovan.

Verapamil Hydrochloride (7794-v)

Verapamil Hydrochloride *(BANM, USAN, rINNM).*

CP-16533-1 (verapamil); D-365 (verapamil); Iproveratril Hydrochloride; Verapamili Hydrochloridum. 5-[*N*-(3,4-Dimethoxyphenethyl)-*N*-methylamino]-2-(3,4-dimethoxyphenyl)-2-isopropylvaleronitrile hydrochloride.

$C_{27}H_{38}N_2O_4$,HCl = 491.1.

CAS — 52-53-9 (verapamil); 152-11-4 (verapamil hydrochloride).

Pharmacopoeias. In *Chin., Eur.* (see p.viii), *Int., Jpn,* and *US.*

A white or practically white, practically odourless, crystalline powder. **Soluble** in water; sparingly soluble in alcohol; freely soluble in chloroform; practically insoluble in ether. A 5% solution in water has a pH of 4.5 to 6.5. **Store** in airtight containers. Protect from light.

Incompatibility. Verapamil hydrochloride will precipitate in alkaline solutions. There have been reports of incompatibility with solutions of aminophylline,[1] nafcillin sodium,[2] and sodium bicarbonate.[3]

1. Johnson CE, *et al.* Compatibility of aminophylline and verapamil in intravenous admixtures. *Am J Hosp Pharm* 1989; **46:** 97–100.
2. Tucker R, Gentile JF. Precipitation of verapamil in an intravenous line. *Ann Intern Med* 1984; **101:** 880.
3. Cutie MR. Verapamil precipitation. *Ann Intern Med* 1983; **98:** 672.

Adverse Effects

Treatment with verapamil is generally well tolerated, but adverse effects connected with verapamil's pharmacological effects on cardiac conduction can arise and may be particularly severe in patients with hypertrophic cardiomyopathies. Adverse effects on the heart include bradycardia, atrioventricular block, worsening heart failure, and transient asystole. These effects are more common with parenteral than with oral therapy.

The most troublesome non-cardiac adverse effect is constipation. Nausea may occur but is less frequently reported. Other adverse effects include hypotension, dizziness, flushing, headaches, fatigue, dyspnoea, and peripheral oedema. There have been reports of skin reactions and some cases of abnormal liver function and hepatotoxicity. Gingival hyperplasia has occurred. Gynaecomastia has been reported rarely.

In overdosage there may be severe cardiotoxicity and profound hypotension.

For discussion of the possibility that calcium-channel blockers might be associated with increased cardiovascular mortality, see under Adverse Effects of Nifedipine, p.916.

Cancer occurrence. See under Adverse Effects of Nifedipine, p.916.

Effects on the cardiovascular system. Verapamil has vasodilating properties and negative inotropic activity and may cause adverse cardiovascular effects with worsening of arrhythmias. As discussed below under Precautions certain cardiac disorders put the patient at risk of severe toxicity.

Some references.

1. Radford D. Side effects of verapamil in infants. *Arch Dis Child* 1983; **58:** 465–6.
2. Perrot B, *et al.* Verapamil: a cause of sudden death in a patient with hypertrophic cardiomyopathy. *Br Heart J* 1984; **51:** 352–4.
3. Kirk CR, *et al.* Cardiovascular collapse after verapamil in supraventricular tachycardia. *Arch Dis Child* 1987; **62:** 1265–6.
4. Mohindra SK, Udeani GO. Long-acting verapamil and heart failure. *JAMA* 1989; **261:** 994.
5. Garratt C, *et al.* Degeneration of junctional tachycardia to pre-excited atrial fibrillation after intravenous verapamil. *Lancet* 1989; **ii:** 219.

Effects on the ears. There have been isolated reports[1] of tinnitus associated with several calcium-channel blockers including nifedipine, nicardipine, nitrendipine, diltiazem, verapamil, and cinnarizine.

1. Narváez M, *et al.* Tinnitus with calcium-channel blockers. *Lancet* 1994; **343:** 1229–30.

Effects on the endocrine system. There have been reports of a few patients developing elevated serum-prolactin concentrations during verapamil therapy;[1,2] one of these patients experienced galactorrhoea.[2]

Hyperglycaemia, metabolic acidosis, hyperkalaemia, and bradycardia have occurred[3] following a single dose of modified-release verapamil in a non-diabetic patient who had previously tolerated regular verapamil.

Verapamil has been reported not to affect the release of calcitonin,[4] thyroxine, tri-iodothyronine, thyrotrophin (TSH), follicle-stimulating hormone (FSH), luteinising hormone (LH), or testosterone when given by mouth;[1] however, intravenous administration has been reported to have an inhibitory effect on the release of FSH, LH, and TSH.[5]

1. Semple CG, *et al.* Calcium antagonists and endocrine status: lack of effect of oral verapamil on pituitary-testicular and pituitary-thyroid function. *Br J Clin Pharmacol* 1984; **17:** 179–82.
2. Gluskin LE, *et al.* Verapamil-induced hyperprolactinemia and galactorrhea. *Ann Intern Med* 1981; **95:** 66–7.
3. Roth A, *et al.* Slow-release verapamil and hyperglycemic metabolic acidosis. *Ann Intern Med* 1989; **110:** 171–2.
4. Amado JA, *et al.* No effect of verapamil on calcium stimulated calcitonin release. *Postgrad Med J* 1987; **63:** 23–4.
5. Barbarino A, De Marinis L. Calcium antagonists and hormone release II: effects of verapamil on basal, gonadotrophin-releasing hormone- and thyrotrophin-releasing hormone-induced pituitary hormone release in normal subjects. *J Clin Endocrinol Metab* 1980; **51:** 749–53.

Effects on the liver. Elevated serum concentrations of liver enzymes and bilirubin have been reported during verapamil therapy.[1-4] Clinical symptoms of hepatotoxicity such as abdominal pain, fever, darkened urine, and malaise may occur.[2-4] These reactions might have been due to a hypersensitivity reaction and were reversible on discontinuing verapamil.

1. Brodsky SJ, *et al.* Hepatotoxicity due to treatment with verapamil. *Ann Intern Med* 1981; **94:** 490–1.
2. Stern EH, *et al.* Possible hepatitis from verapamil. *N Engl J Med* 1982; **306:** 612–13.
3. Nash DT, Feer TD. Hepatic injury possibly induced by verapamil. *JAMA* 1983; **249:** 395–6.
4. Guarascio P, *et al.* Liver damage from verapamil. *Br Med J* 1984; **288:** 362–3.

Effects on the mouth. Gingival hyperplasia[1] and oral mucosal injury[2] have been associated with verapamil therapy. A study involving 115 patients who had received nifedipine, diltiazem, or verapamil for at least 3 months indicated that gingival hyperplasia is an important side-effect that may occur with calcium-channel blockers in general.[3]

1. Pernu HE, *et al.* Verapamil-induced gingival overgrowth: a clinical, histologic, and biochemic approach. *J Oral Pathol Med* 1989; **18:** 422–5.
2. Guttenberg SA. Chemical injury of the oral mucosa from verapamil. *N Engl J Med* 1990; **323:** 615.
3. Steele RM, *et al.* Calcium antagonist-induced gingival hyperplasia. *Ann Intern Med* 1994; **120:** 663–4.

Effects on the nervous system. A report of 3 patients who complained of unusual perceptual symptoms, described as painful coldness and numbness or bursting feelings, especially in the legs, in association with oral verapamil therapy.[1]

1. Kumana CR, Mahon WA. Bizarre perceptual disorder of extremities in patients taking verapamil. *Lancet* 1981; **i:** 1324–5.

Effects on the neuromuscular system. A myoclonic, dystonic movement disorder was apparently induced by verapamil in a 70-year-old man.[1]

1. Hicks CB, Abraham K. Verapamil and myoclonic dystonia. *Ann Intern Med* 1985; **103:** 154.

Effects on the peripheral circulation. Persistent disabling burning pain and severe erythema and swelling of the feet occurred in a patient receiving verapamil;[1] it resolved when the drug was discontinued. The condition was diagnosed as secondary erythermalgia, a type of erythromelalgia secondary to a variety of diseases and to vasoactive drugs,[2] including the calcium-channel blocker nifedipine.[1]

1. Drenth JPH, *et al.* Verapamil-induced secondary erythermalgia. *Br J Dermatol* 1992; **127:** 292–4.
2. Drenth JPH, Michiels JJ. Three types of erythromelalgia. *Br Med J* 1990; **301:** 454–5.

Effects on the respiratory tract. A patient with a history of bronchial asthma developed symptoms of acute asthma following administration of a modified-release verapamil preparation;[1] it was possible that excipients, notably alginate, may have been responsible for the reaction.

1. Ben-Noun L. Acute asthma associated with sustained-release verapamil. *Ann Pharmacother* 1997; **31:** 593–5.

Effects on sexual function. Impotence was associated with verapamil therapy in 3 out of 14 men. In one patient normal sexual function returned when verapamil was discontinued and a recurrence of impotence was reported when verapamil therapy was re-instituted.[1]

1. King BD, *et al.* Impotence during therapy with verapamil. *Arch Intern Med* 1983; **143:** 1248–9.

Effects on the skin and hair. The commonest skin reactions to verapamil have been rash, pruritus, alopecia, and urticaria;[1] there have been a few reports of erythema multiforme, the Stevens-Johnson syndrome, and exfoliative dermatitis.[1] Hypertrichosis, over many parts of the body, has been reported in one male patient within about one month of starting verapamil therapy.[2] In one female patient who had been prematurely grey for about 40 years administration of verapamil caused portions of the hair to regrow in its original natural black colour.[3]

1. Stern R, Khalsa JH. Cutaneous adverse reactions associated with calcium channel blockers. *Arch Intern Med* 1989; **149:** 829–32.
2. Sever PS. Hypertrichosis and verapamil. *Lancet* 1991; **338:** 1215–16.
3. Read GM. Verapamil and hair colour change. *Lancet* 1991; **338:** 1520.

Extrapyramidal disorders. Tremor (postural and at rest) diagnosed as parkinsonism developed in a 70-year-old patient 4 months after starting treatment with verapamil. A 79-year-old patient developed symptoms including parkinsonism, rigidity, and bradykinesia 2 years after beginning verapamil therapy. Symptoms disappeared or improved considerably when verapamil was discontinued.[1] Calcium-channel blockers have been tried in the treatment of tardive dyskinesia (see under Nifedipine, Uses, p.921).

1. Padrell MD, *et al.* Verapamil-induced parkinsonism. *Am J Med* 1995; **99:** 436.

Haemorrhage. See Effects on the Blood under Adverse Effects of Nifedipine, p.916.

Overdosage. Acute overdosage with verapamil generally produces cardiovascular symptoms[1-3] such as severe bradycardia, heart block, profound hypotension, and diminished peripheral perfusion with loss of peripheral pulses, cyanosis, and cold hands and feet. Overdosage may be fatal.[3] Haematemesis and gastric ulcers have been reported[4] following ingestion of verapamil 3.2 g.

Long-term treatment with verapamil 240 mg daily[5] in a patient with cirrhosis of the liver led to loss of consciousness, cardiogenic shock, cyanosis, hypotension, severe acidosis, hyperkalaemia, hypothermia, and renal failure. The patient recovered following treatment with high doses of dopamine, noradrenaline, sodium bicarbonate, and sodium chloride.

See also under Treatment of Adverse Effects, below.

1. Perkins CM. Serious verapamil poisoning: treatment with intravenous calcium gluconate. *Br Med J* 1978; **2:** 1127.
2. Crump BJ, *et al.* Lack of response to intravenous calcium in severe verapamil poisoning. *Lancet* 1982; **ii:** 939–40.
3. Orr GM, *et al.* Fatal verapamil overdose. *Lancet* 1982; **ii:** 1218–19.
4. Miller ARO, Ingamells CJ. Gastrointestinal haemorrhage associated with an overdose of verapamil. *Br Med J* 1984; **288:** 1346.
5. Stehle G, *et al.* Cardiogenic shock associated with verapamil in a patient with liver cirrhosis. *Lancet* 1990; **336:** 1079.

Treatment of Adverse Effects

In overdosage with verapamil by mouth the stomach should be emptied by lavage; activated charcoal may be administered. Verapamil is not removed by dialysis. Treatment of cardiovascular effects is supportive and symptomatic. Intravenous infusion of calcium salts is recommended as a specific antagonist to verapamil and may reverse the haemodynamic and electrophysiological effects. A slow intravenous injection or an infusion of calcium gluconate in a dose of 10 to 20 mL of a 10% solution or calcium chloride 1 g has been suggested. If hypotension persists, intravenous administration of a sympathomimetic such as isoprenaline, dopamine, or noradrenaline may also be necessary. Bradycardia may be treated with atropine, isoprenaline, or cardiac pacing.

In a discussion of overdosage with calcium-channel blockers, Kenny[1] considered the consequences and treatment to be similar for verapamil and nifedipine. However, Buckley and others,[2,3] writing from Australia, considered death and life-threatening complications to be much more common with verapamil than with diltiazem and more common with diltiazem than nifedipine, reflecting their relative effects on cardiac conduction. They suggested that, whereas most nifedipine poisonings would respond to supportive treatment with intravenous fluids, verapamil frequently caused profound bradycardia and hypotension requiring aggressive and intensive therapy including thorough gastro-intestinal decontamination and high doses of calcium intravenously. The importance of these measures was noted in a review of intoxication specifically with verapamil.[4] Other treatment of possible benefit in verapamil overdosage includes the specific antidote fampridine.[5]

Overdosage with modified-release preparations of verapamil may result in prolonged toxicity of delayed onset.[6] Conventional-release preparations may also produce prolonged toxicity; elimination half-life was reported to be prolonged to 15 hours and peak plasma concentrations delayed to 6 to 7 hours in a 59-year-old man following ingestion of 2.4 g of verapamil.[7] Rate-limiting absorption at high doses was considered to be the cause.

1. Kenny J. Treating overdose with calcium channel blockers. *Br Med J* 1994; **308:** 992–3.
2. Buckley NA, *et al.* Overdose with calcium channel blockers. *Br Med J* 1994; **308:** 1639.
3. Howarth DM, *et al.* Calcium channel blocking drug overdose: an Australian series. *Hum Exp Toxicol* 1994; **13:** 161–6.
4. Hofer CA, *et al.* Verapamil intoxication: a literature review of overdoses and discussions of therapeutic options. *Am J Med* 1993; **95:** 431–8.
5. Stevens JJWM, Ghosh S. Overdose of calcium channel blockers. *Br Med J* 1994; **309:** 193.
6. Barrow PM, *et al.* Overdose of sustained-release verapamil. *Br J Anaesth* 1994; **72:** 361–5.
7. Buckley CD, Aronson JK. Prolonged half-life of verapamil in a case of overdose: implications for therapy. *Br J Clin Pharmacol* 1995; **39:** 680–3.

Precautions

Verapamil is contra-indicated in hypotension, in cardiogenic shock, in marked bradycardia, in second- or third-degree atrioventricular block, and in uncompensated heart failure. It is also contra-indicated in the sick-sinus syndrome unless a pacemaker is fitted. There is an increased incidence of adverse cardiac effects in patients with hypertrophic cardiomyopathy. In patients with atrial flutter or fibrillation and an accessory pathway with anterograde conduction, for example Wolff-Parkinson-White syndrome, verapamil may induce severe ventricular tachycardia and some authorities contra-indicate its use in such patients.

Special care is required in using verapamil as an antiarrhythmic in infants as they may be more susceptible to verapamil-induced arrhythmias.

Doses of verapamil should be reduced in patients with impaired liver function.

Sudden withdrawal of verapamil might be associated with an exacerbation of angina.

Muscular disorders. Sudden respiratory failure was believed to have been precipitated by intravenous verapamil therapy in a patient with Duchenne's muscular dystrophy.[1]

1. Zalman F, *et al.* Acute respiratory failure following intravenous verapamil in Duchenne's muscular dystrophy. *Am Heart J* 1983; **105:** 510–11.

Interactions

Verapamil should be used with caution in combination with other drugs that have antiarrhythmic or beta-blocking effects. The combination of intravenous verapamil with a beta blocker is especially hazardous (see below). Verapamil is extensively metabolised in the liver and interactions may occur with drugs that inhibit or enhance liver metabolism. Verapamil can itself inhibit the metabolism of other drugs that are subject to hepatic oxidation; increased plasma concentrations of many drugs including *carbamazepine* (p.342), *cyclosporin* (p.522), *midazolam* (see under Diazepam, p.664), and *theophylline* (p.769) may occur. The plasma concentrations of *alcohol* and *digoxin* may also be increased (p.1100 and p.851, respectively).

Analgesics. For a possible interaction of verapamil with *aspirin*, see under Antiplatelets, below.

Antiarrhythmics. Cardiogenic shock and asystole has been described in two patients receiving *flecainide* when verapamil was added to their therapy.[1] Verapamil given intravenously has been reported to cause severe hypotension in patients also receiving *quinidine* by mouth.[2]

1. Buss J, *et al.* Asystole and cardiogenic shock due to combined treatment with verapamil and flecainide. *Lancet* 1992; **340:** 546.
2. Maisel AS, *et al.* Hypotension after quinidine plus verapamil. *N Engl J Med* 1985; **312:** 167–70.

Antibacterials. Acute verapamil toxicity manifested by complete heart block has been reported in one patient following the administration of *ceftriaxone* and *clindamycin*.[1] Displacement of verapamil from binding sites was postulated as the probable mechanism of action. *Rifampicin* is an enzyme-inducing drug and has been reported[2,3] to reduce plasma-verapamil concentrations. A verapamil dose of 1920 mg was required to control supraventricular tachycardia in a patient also taking rifampicin[3] and when rifampicin was withdrawn the plasma-verapamil concentration 9 days later was almost four times higher. A patient taking propranolol and verapamil developed symptomatic bradycardia a few days after starting treatment with *clarithromycin* and on another occasion after starting treatment with *erythromycin*.[4] Inhibition of verapamil metabolism by the antibacterials was proposed as the mechanism for the interaction.

1. Kishore K, *et al.* Acute verapamil toxicity in a patient with chronic toxicity: possible interaction with ceftriaxone and clindamycin. *Ann Pharmacother* 1993; **27:** 877–80.
2. Rahn KH, *et al.* Reduction of bioavailability of verapamil by rifampin. *N Engl J Med* 1985; **312:** 920–1.
3. Barbarash RA. Verapamil-rifampin interaction. *Drug Intell Clin Pharm* 1985; **19:** 559–60.
4. Steenbergen JA, Stauffer VL. Potential macrolide interaction with verapamil. *Ann Pharmacother* 1998; **32:** 387–8.

Antiepileptics. *Phenobarbitone* is a hepatic enzyme-inducing drug and has been reported[1] to increase the clearance of oral and intravenous verapamil and to reduce oral bioavailability in healthy subjects. Plasma protein binding of verapamil was also reduced. Dosage adjustment of verapamil may be needed in patients also taking phenobarbitone. Marked reduction in verapamil concentrations has occurred with *phenytoin*.[2]

1. Rutledge DR, *et al.* Effects of chronic phenobarbital on verapamil disposition in humans. *J Pharmacol Exp Ther* 1988; **246:** 7–13.
2. Woodcock BG, *et al.* A reduction in verapamil concentrations with phenytoin. *N Engl J Med* 1991; **325:** 1179.

Antiplatelets. Calcium-channel blockers can inhibit platelet function (see Effects on the Blood under Adverse Effects of Nifedipine, p.916). Concurrent use of verapamil and *aspirin* in an 85-year-old man was considered to be the cause of ecchymoses and retroperitoneal bleeding that developed about 3 weeks after starting treatment with the combination.[1]

1. Verzino E, *et al.* Verapamil-aspirin interaction. *Ann Pharmacother* 1994; **28:** 536–7.

Anxiolytics. For the effect of verapamil on plasma-buspirone concentrations, see p.644.

Beta blockers. Oral verapamil and beta blockers have been used together in the treatment of angina and hypertension but both drugs have cardiodepressant activity and the combination, if used at all, must be used with extreme caution; bradycardia, heart block, and left ventricular failure have been reported.[1-4] Bradycardia has also been reported[5] in a patient treated with *timolol* eye drops and oral verapamil. Patients with myocardial insufficiency are particularly at risk.[6] The risks are increased when verapamil is given intravenously and the interaction is especially hazardous when both verapamil and the beta blocker are given by this route. Treatment with beta blockers should be discontinued for at least 24 hours before administration of intravenous verapamil.[6]

1. Eisenberg JNH, Oakley GDG. Probable adverse interaction between oral metoprolol and verapamil. *Postgrad Med J* 1984; **60:** 705–6.
2. Hutchison SJ, *et al.* β blockers and verapamil: a cautionary tale. *Br Med J* 1984; **289:** 659–60.
3. Findlay IN, *et al.* β blockers and verapamil: a cautionary tale. *Br Med J* 1984; **289:** 1074.
4. McGourty JC, Silas JH. β blockers and verapamil: a cautionary tale. *Br Med J* 1984; **289:** 1624.
5. Pringle SD, MacEwen CJ. Severe bradycardia due to interaction of timolol eye drops and verapamil. *Br Med J* 1987; **294:** 155–6.
6. McInnes GT. Interactions that matter: calcium blockers. *Prescribers' J* 1988; **28:** 60–4.

Calcium salts. Calcium salts antagonise the pharmacological response to verapamil and are given intravenously to treat adverse effects of verapamil (see under Treatment of Adverse Effects, above). Recurrence of atrial fibrillation has occurred[1] during maintenance verapamil treatment when calcium adipinate and calciferol were given by mouth.

1. Bar-Or D, Yoel G. Calcium and calciferol antagonise effect of verapamil in atrial fibrillation. *Br Med J* 1981; **282:** 1585–6.

Histamine H_2-receptor antagonists. Verapamil is extensively metabolised in the liver and undergoes considerable first-pass metabolism. *Cimetidine* inhibits hepatic oxidative metabolism and may therefore be expected to interact with verapamil. Studies in healthy subjects using single doses of verapamil following pretreatment with cimetidine for up to 8 days have produced conflicting results. The pharmacokinetics of intravenous verapamil were unaltered by cimetidine in some studies,[1,2] but a 21% reduction in clearance and a 50% increase in the elimination half-life were also reported.[3] The pharmacokinetics of oral verapamil were unchanged in one study[2] but two others[1,4] reported a significant increase in bioavailability. Although one of these studies[1] found the interaction had no clinical effects, the other[4] reported an increased clinical effect in 5 of 6 subjects. The interaction with cimetidine appears to be stereoselective since the oral bioavailability of the *S*-enantiomer increased by 35% and that of the *R*-enantiomer by 15%.[4] The clinical significance of this interaction in patients and during long-term verapamil treatment is unknown, but cimetidine should be used with caution in patients receiving verapamil.

1. Smith MS, *et al.* Influence of cimetidine on verapamil kinetics and dynamics. *Clin Pharmacol Ther* 1984; **36:** 551–4.
2. Abernethy DR, *et al.* Lack of interaction between verapamil and cimetidine. *Clin Pharmacol Ther* 1985; **38:** 342–9.
3. Loi C-M, *et al.* Effect of cimetidine on verapamil disposition. *Clin Pharmacol Ther* 1985; **37:** 654–7.
4. Mikus G, *et al.* Interaction of verapamil and cimetidine: stereochemical aspects of drug metabolism, drug disposition and drug action. *J Pharmacol Exp Ther* 1990; **253:** 1042–8.

Lithium. Neurotoxicity has been reported in one patient receiving lithium following the addition of verapamil.[1] Serum-lithium concentrations were still inside the accepted therapeutic range and it was considered that the similar actions of lithium and verapamil on neurosecretory processes may have been responsible. Verapamil has also been reported to decrease serum-lithium concentrations.[2]

1. Price WA, Giannini AJ. Neurotoxicity caused by lithium-verapamil synergism. *J Clin Pharmacol* 1986; **26:** 717–19.
2. Weinrauch LA, *et al.* Decreased serum lithium during verapamil therapy. *Am Heart J* 1984; **108:** 1378–80.

Pharmacokinetics

Verapamil is approximately 90% absorbed from the gastro-intestinal tract, but is subject to very considerable first-pass metabolism in the liver and the bioavailability is only about 20%.

Verapamil exhibits bi- or tri-phasic elimination kinetics and is reported to have a terminal plasma half-life of 2 to 8 hours following a single oral dose or after intravenous administration. After repeated oral doses this increases to 4.5 to 12.0 hours. Verapamil acts within 5 minutes of intravenous administration and in 1 to 2 hours after oral administration with a peak plasma concentration after 1 to 2 hours. There is considerable interindividual variation in plasma concentrations.

Verapamil is about 90% bound to plasma proteins. It is extensively metabolised in the liver to at least 12 metabolites of which norverapamil has been shown to have some activity. About 70% of a dose is excreted by the kidneys in the form of its metabolites but about 16% is also excreted in the bile into the faeces. Less than 4% is excreted unchanged. Verapamil crosses the placenta and is distributed into breast milk.

Reviews.

1. Hamann SR, *et al.* Clinical pharmacokinetics of verapamil. *Clin Pharmacokinet* 1984; **9:** 26–41.
2. Kelly JG, O'Malley K. Clinical pharmacokinetics of calcium antagonists: an update. *Clin Pharmacokinet* 1992; **22:** 416–33.

Breast feeding. Verapamil concentrations in breast milk similar to those found in plasma have been reported[1] in a woman taking verapamil 80 mg four times a day. The maximum concentration measured in breast milk was 300 ng per mL. However, the average concentration in milk in another woman[2] taking 80 mg three times daily was 23% of that in serum. The serum concentration of verapamil in the child was 2.1 ng per mL during treatment and undetectable 38 hours after the last maternal dose. In another patient[3] taking the same dose, the average steady-state concentrations of verapamil and norverapamil in milk were, respectively, 60% and 16% of the concentration in plasma. The ratio between milk and plasma varied during a dosage interval and it is therefore important to know when a sample was obtained if valid conclusions about excretion in breast milk are to be made. No verapamil or norverapamil could be detected in the plasma of the infant.

1. Inove H, *et al.* Level of verapamil in human milk. *Eur J Clin Pharmacol* 1984; **26:** 657–8.
2. Andersen HJ. Excretion of verapamil in human milk. *Eur J Clin Pharmacol* 1983; **25:** 279–80.
3. Anderson P, *et al.* Verapamil and norverapamil in plasma and breast milk during breast feeding. *Eur J Clin Pharmacol* 1987; **31:** 625–7.

Old age. Total verapamil clearance was found to be decreased in elderly (61 years of age or older) hypertensive patients compared with that in young patients, and the elimination half-life was prolonged.[1]

1. Abernethy DR, *et al.* Verapamil pharmacodynamics and disposition in young and elderly hypertensive patients: altered electrocardiographic and hypotensive responses. *Ann Intern Med* 1986; **105:** 329–36.

Stereospecificity. Verapamil is used as a racemic mixture. A series of studies have been carried out to determine whether differences in the pharmacokinetics of the *R*- and *S*-isomers of verapamil could account for observed differences in the plasma concentration-response curve following oral and intravenous administration. After intravenous administration, there were pronounced differences in the pharmacokinetics and protein binding of the 2 isomers;[1] the volume of distribution and total systemic clearance of *S*-verapamil were much higher than those of the *R*-isomer although the terminal half-life was similar. After oral administration of a mixture of *R*- and *S*-verapamil, plasma concentrations of the *R*-isomer were found to be substantially higher than those of the *S*-isomer[2] suggesting stereospecific first-pass hepatic metabolism. Following oral dosing total verapamil concentrations thus consist of a smaller proportion of the more potent *S*-isomer accounting for the apparent lower potency of verapamil when given orally. The proportion of *S*-isomer also depends on the oral formulation; modified-release formulations produce lower proportions of *S*-isomer in plasma than conventional formulations.[3] It has been shown[4] that *S*-verapamil is 3.3 times more potent than the racemic mixture and 11 times more potent than *R*-verapamil. Thus the authors concluded that the cardiac effects of verapamil are related not to the total plasma-verapamil concentration but to the concentration of the *S*-isomer, and conventional plasma concentration monitoring will be of little value in establishing therapeutic plasma concentrations during multiple oral dosing.

1. Eichelbaum M, *et al.* Pharmacokinetics of (+)-, (−)- and (±)-verapamil after intravenous administration. *Br J Clin Pharmacol* 1984; **17:** 453–8.
2. Vogelgesang B, *et al.* Stereoselective first-pass metabolism of highly cleared drugs: studies of the bioavailability of L- and D-verapamil examined with a stable isotope technique. *Br J Clin Pharmacol* 1984; **18:** 733–40.
3. Karim A, Piergies A. Verapamil stereoisomerism: enantiomeric ratios in plasma dependent on peak concentrations, oral input rate, or both. *Clin Pharmacol Ther* 1995; **58:** 174–84.
4. Echizen H, *et al.* Effects of d,l-verapamil on atrioventricular conduction in relation to its stereoselective first-pass metabolism. *Clin Pharmacol Ther* 1985; **38:** 71–6.

Uses and Administration

Verapamil is a calcium-channel blocker (p.778) and a class IV antiarrhythmic (p.776). Verapamil slows conduction through the atrioventricular node, and thus slows the increased ventricular response rate that occurs in atrial fibrillation and flutter. A decrease in both coronary and peripheral vascular resistance together with a sparing effect on myocardial intracellular oxygen consumption appear to be the modes of action in angina. The decrease in peripheral vascular resistance may explain the antihypertensive effect of verapamil. It is used in the control of supraventricular arrhythmias, in the management of angina pectoris, and in the treatment of hypertension. It may also be used in the management of myocardial infarction.

Verapamil may be given intravenously or by mouth as the hydrochloride for the control of supraventricular **arrhythmias**. Intravenous injections should be given under continuous ECG monitoring. When given intravenously a dose of 5 to 10 mg is injected over a period of 2 to 3 minutes; if necessary, a further 5 mg may be injected 5 to 10 minutes after the first. In the USA a second dose of 10 mg given after 30 minutes if required is suggested. Children should be treated with great care; suggested intravenous doses given over at least 2 minutes are: up to 1 year of age, 0.1 to 0.2 mg per kg body-weight; children aged 1 to 15 years, 0.1 to 0.3 mg per kg (to a maximum dose of 5 mg). Smaller doses may be adequate and the injection should be stopped when a response has been obtained.

Oral doses for the treatment of supraventricular arrhythmias are 120 to 480 mg daily in 3 or 4 divided doses, according to the severity of the condition and the patient's response. Suggested oral doses for children are: up to 2 years of age, 20 mg two or three times daily; 2 years and over, 40 to 120 mg two or three times daily according to age and response; great care is still required.

In the management of **angina pectoris,** verapamil hydrochloride is given by mouth in doses of 120 mg three times daily; some patients with angina of effort may respond to 80 mg three times daily, but this lower dose is not likely to be effective in angina at rest or Prinzmetal's variant angina.

In the treatment of **hypertension** the dose of verapamil hydrochloride is generally 160 mg twice daily by mouth with a range of 240 mg to 480 mg daily. A dose of up to 10 mg per kg body-weight daily in divided doses has been suggested for children.

In the management of **myocardial infarction**, verapamil, in a modified-release oral preparation, may be started at least one week after acute infarction (in patients without heart failure). A suggested dose is 360 mg daily in divided doses.

Modified-release oral preparations are also available for use in the treatment of angina and hypertension.

Doses of verapamil should be reduced in patients with impaired liver function.

General reviews.

1. McTavish D, Sorkin EM. Verapamil: an updated review of its pharmacodynamic and pharmacokinetic properties, and therapeutic use in hypertension. *Drugs* 1989; **38:** 19–76.
2. Anonymous. Calcium antagonists for cardiovascular disease. *Drug Ther Bull* 1993; **31:** 81–4.
3. Fisher M, Grotta J. New uses for calcium channel blockers: therapeutic implications. *Drugs* 1993; **46:** 961–75.
4. Brogden RN, Benfield P. Verapamil: a review of its pharmacological properties and therapeutic use in coronary artery disease. *Drugs* 1996; **51:** 792–819.

Administration in the elderly. For a report that the pharmacokinetics of verapamil are altered in the elderly, see Pharmacokinetics, above.

Administration in hepatic impairment. In patients with liver cirrhosis steady-state plasma concentrations of verapamil were double those seen in patients with normal liver function following intravenous administration and 5 times the normal concentration when given by mouth and verapamil dosage must be drastically reduced in these patients, especially when given orally.[1] The elimination half-life was prolonged about fourfold following oral or intravenous administration and thus steady-state plasma concentration will not be reached in patients with liver cirrhosis until about 56 hours after therapy has started.

1. Somogyi A, *et al.* Pharmacokinetics, bioavailability and ECG response of verapamil in patients with liver cirrhosis. *Br J Clin Pharmacol* 1981; **12:** 51–60.

Administration in renal impairment. The pharmacokinetics and pharmacodynamic effects of verapamil are not significantly altered by renal impairment[1] and dosage adjustment is not considered to be necessary. The elimination of verapamil is not altered by haemodialysis,[1,2] haemofiltration,[2] or peritoneal dialysis[2] and no dosage supplement is required in patients undergoing these procedures.

1. Mooy J, *et al.* Pharmacokinetics of verapamil in patients with renal failure. *Eur J Clin Pharmacol* 1985; **28:** 405–10.
2. Beyerlein C, *et al.* Verapamil in antihypertensive treatment of patients on renal replacement therapy—clinical implications and pharmacokinetics. *Eur J Clin Pharmacol* 1990; **39** (suppl 1): S35–S37.

Amaurosis fugax. Relief of vasospasm might explain the efficacy of the calcium-channel blockers nifedipine and verapamil in a few patients with amaurosis fugax (see under Stroke, p.799) unresponsive to anticoagulants or antiplatelets.[1]

1. Winterkorn JMS, *et al.* Brief report: treatment of vasospastic amaurosis fugax with calcium-channel blockers. *N Engl J Med* 1993; **329:** 396–8.

Angina pectoris. Treatment of angina pectoris (p.780) depends on the type of angina and may include the use of nitrates, beta blockers, and calcium-channel blockers such as verapamil either alone or in combination. However, combination of verapamil with a beta blocker has produced adverse effects and this is discussed under Interactions, above.

Bites and stings. Stings by the box-jellyfish (*Chironex fleckeri*) can be fatal due to the effects of the venom on the cardiovascular and respiratory systems and on the kidneys. Studies in *rodents* have reported a beneficial effect of intravenous verapamil in the treatment of box-jellyfish envenomation. It is suggested that intravenous verapamil be used in the acute management of patients with serious box-jellyfish stings since it may reverse the cardiotoxic effects of the venom and allow more time for additional supportive care and for the antivenom to exert its action.[1]

1. Burnett JW. The use of verapamil to treat box-jellyfish stings. *Med J Aust* 1990; **153:** 363.

Cardiac arrhythmias. Verapamil may be used to control supraventricular arrhythmias such as atrial fibrillation and flutter and paroxysmal supraventricular tachycardia (p.782).

It reduces ventricular rate during atrial fibrillation, but should not be used when fibrillation or flutter is associated with an accessory pathway as in the Wolff-Parkinson-White syndrome. Intravenous verapamil has a more rapid onset than digitalis and has a direct depressant effect on the atrioventricular node which persists to a greater extent than that of digitalis during stress and exercise. A bolus dose of 10 mg of verapamil has commonly been recommended for the treatment of acute atrial fibrillation, but Klein and Kaplinsky[1] preferred to give 1 mg by slow injection, repeated at 1-minute intervals. Ventricular fibrillation and severe hypotension have been reported[2] following the administration of intravenous verapamil 5 to 10 mg to patients with the Wolff-Parkinson-White syndrome.

Verapamil may also be given to terminate paroxysmal supraventricular tachycardia, although adenosine may be preferred.

Verapamil has been given to the mother in combination with digoxin in the management of fetal atrial flutter or supraventricular tachycardia.[3] Caution is necessary when verapamil is given to infants to treat their arrhythmias, see Precautions, above.

1. Klein HO, Kaplinsky E. Digitalis and verapamil in atrial fibrillation and flutter: is verapamil now the preferred agent? *Drugs* 1986; **31:** 185–97.
2. McGovern B, *et al.* Precipitation of cardiac arrest by verapamil in patients with Wolff-Parkinson-White syndrome. *Ann Intern Med* 1986; **104:** 791–4.
3. Maxwell DJ, *et al.* Obstetric importance, diagnosis, and management of fetal tachycardias. *Br Med J* 1988; **297:** 107–10.

Cardiomyopathies. Clinical trials have suggested that long-term administration of verapamil improves symptoms and exercise tolerance in many patients with *hypertrophic cardiomyopathy* and it may be considered for the treatment of those patients who continue to have disabling symptoms or who are unable to tolerate beta blockers.[1] The incidence of serious ventricular or supraventricular arrhythmias does not appear to be reduced by verapamil. However, in a crossover study exercise capacity was not improved by verapamil or nadolol although most patients preferred one or other of the drugs rather than placebo and quality of life did appear to be improved by verapamil.[2]

However, patients with hypertrophic cardiomyopathy are especially susceptible to conduction disturbances associated with verapamil since loss of the synchronised contribution of atrial contraction may cause diminished filling of the stiff left ventricle and result in hypotension.[1]

The use of calcium-channel blockers is not standard therapy in *dilated cardiomyopathy* and has resulted in clinical and haemodynamic deterioration.[3] However, symptomatic improvement has been reported with diltiazem over a 24-month period.

For a discussion of the management of cardiomyopathies in general, see p.785.

1. Lorell BH. Use of calcium channel blockers in hypertrophic cardiomyopathy. *Am J Med* 1985; **78** (suppl 2B): 43–54.
2. Gilligan DM, *et al.* A double-blind, placebo-controlled crossover trial of nadolol and verapamil in mild and moderately symptomatic hypertrophic cardiomyopathy. *J Am Coll Cardiol* 1993; **21:** 1672–9.
3. Richardson PJ. Calcium antagonists in cardiomyopathy. *Br J Clin Pract* 1988; **42** (suppl 60): 33–7.

Hypertension. Verapamil may be used for the initial treatment of mild to moderate hypertension (p.788), but is not usually the drug of first choice.[1,2] It may be used as a modified-release or conventional-release formulation. Verapamil may be more effective in elderly patients than in younger patients. Verapamil has been used in pregnant women with severe gestational proteinuric hypertension.[3]

It may also be used in multiple drug regimens to control severe or refractory hypertension[1,2] and will usually have at least an additive effect with other antihypertensives. Extreme caution is needed if verapamil is used in combination with a beta blocker (see under Interactions, above).

1. McTavish D, Sorkin EM. Verapamil: an updated review of its pharmacodynamic and pharmacokinetic properties, and therapeutic use in hypertension. *Drugs* 1989; **38:** 19–76.
2. Kaplan NM. Calcium entry blockers in the treatment of hypertension: current status and future prospects. *JAMA* 1989; **262:** 817–23.
3. Belfort MA, *et al.* Hemodynamic changes associated with intravenous infusion of the calcium antagonists verapamil in the treatment of severe gestational proteinuric hypertension. *Obstet Gynecol* 1990; **75:** 970–4.

Kidney disorders. Calcium-channel blockers may be of benefit in various forms of kidney disorder (see Nifedipine, p.921). Verapamil may also reduce the nephrotoxicity associated with certain drugs. For example, verapamil can prevent cyclosporin-induced deterioration in renal function (see under Transplantation, below) and may possibly reduce nephrotoxicity associated with the aminoglycoside gentamicin.[1]

1. Kazierad DJ, *et al.* The effect of verapamil on the nephrotoxic potential of gentamicin as measured by urinary enzyme excretion in healthy volunteers. *J Clin Pharmacol* 1995; **35:** 196–201.

Malaria. Although studies *in vitro* have shown that verapamil[1] and several other drugs could reverse resistance of *Plasmodium falciparum* to chloroquine, studies in patients with malaria (p.422) have been disappointing as an effect could not be achieved at clinically tolerable doses.

1. Martin SK, *et al.* Reversal of chloroquine resistance in Plasmodium falciparum by verapamil. *Science* 1987; **235:** 899–901.

Malignant neoplasms. Verapamil has been shown to reverse multidrug resistance to antineoplastics in cultured cells and in *animal* studies,[1] but studies in which verapamil was added to therapy for small cell lung cancer[2] or multiple myeloma[3] failed to demonstrate any benefit.

1. Ford JM, Hait WN. Pharmacology of drugs that alter multidrug resistance in cancer. *Pharmacol Rev* 1990; **42:** 155–99.
2. Milroy R, *et al.* A randomised clinical study of verapamil in addition to combination chemotherapy in small cell lung cancer. *Br J Cancer* 1993; **68:** 813–18.
3. Dalton WS, *et al.* A phase III randomized study of oral verapamil as a chemosensitizer to reverse drug resistance in patients with refractory myeloma: a Southwest Oncology Group Study. *Cancer* 1995; **75:** 815–20.

Mania. Although lithium is the mainstay of therapy in mania (p.273) it cannot be used in some patients because of undue toxicity, and is ineffective in others. Verapamil is one of several drugs that have been studied as an alternative.[1] Beneficial responses to verapamil 80 to 120 mg two to four times daily have been reported.[2-5]

1. Höschl C. Do calcium antagonists have a place in the treatment of mood disorders? *Drugs* 1991; **42:** 721–29.
2. Dubovsky SL, *et al.* Effectiveness of verapamil in the treatment of a manic patient. *Am J Psychiatry* 1982; **139:** 502–4.
3. Giannini AJ, *et al.* Antimanic effects of verapamil. *Am J Psychiatry* 1984; **141:** 1602–3.
4. Dubovsky SL, *et al.* Calcium antagonists in mania: a double-blind study of verapamil. *Psychiatry Res* 1986; **18:** 309–20.
5. Giannini AJ, *et al.* Verapamil and lithium in maintenance therapy of manic patients. *J Clin Pharmacol* 1987; **27:** 980–2.

Migraine. For reference to the use of calcium-channel blockers, including verapamil, in the management of migraine and cluster headache, see under Nifedipine, p.921.

Myocardial infarction. Studies have not shown a reduction in mortality when calcium-channel blockers are given in the early phase of acute myocardial infarction (p.791). Results of the Danish Verapamil Infarction Trial (DAVIT I) suggested that early intervention (on admission to hospital) with verapamil might be harmful.[1] However, since myocardial stunning has been linked to intracellular calcium overload[2] there has been speculation that calcium-channel blockers might benefit patients about to undergo reperfusion. This is yet to be confirmed. Calcium-channel blockers are not routinely used in the long-term management of myocardial infarction although in selected patients without heart failure verapamil or diltiazem may be of some benefit. In the DAVIT II study[3] late intervention with verapamil (started in the second week after admission) reduced overall mortality, cardiac events, and reinfarction in such patients although another study[4] found only a benefit in re-infarction rate and not in overall mortality.

1. The Danish Study Group on Verapamil in Myocardial Infarction. The Danish studies on verapamil in acute myocardial infarction. *Br J Clin Pharmacol* 1986; **21:** 197S–204S.
2. Anonymous. Myocardial stunning. *Lancet* 1991; **337:** 585–6.
3. The Danish Study Group on Verapamil in Myocardial Infarction. Effect of verapamil on mortality and major events after acute myocardial infarction (the Danish Verapamil Infarction Trial II–DAVIT II). *Am J Cardiol* 1990; **66:** 779–85.
4. Rengo F, *et al.* A controlled trial of verapamil in patients after acute myocardial infarction: results of the calcium antagonist reinfarction Italian study (CRIS). *Am J Cardiol* 1996; **77:** 365–9.

Transplantation. Cyclosporin is widely used in transplantation to prevent rejection but its use is limited by its nephrotoxicity. A series of studies in renal[1] and heart or lung[2] transplant recipients suggested that verapamil can prevent cyclosporin-induced deterioration in renal function. Although the concentration of cyclosporin in blood was increased by verapamil, kidney function was improved. The incidence of transplant rejection was also reduced by verapamil. The beneficial effect of verapamil therapy on transplant outcome may be related to its ability to protect cells from ischaemia, selective vasodilatation of the afferent renal arterioles, elevation of plasma-cyclosporin concentrations, and inherent immunosuppressive properties. Concomitant use of verapamil also allows lower doses of cyclosporin to be employed.[2]

1. Dawidson I, Rooth P. Improvement of cadaver renal transplantation outcomes with verapamil: a review. *Am J Med* 1991; **90** (suppl 5A): 37S–41S.
2. Chan C, *et al.* A randomized controlled trial of verapamil on cyclosporine nephrotoxicity in heart and lung transplant recipients. *Transplantation* 1997; **63:** 1435–40.

Preparations

BP 1998: Verapamil Injection; Verapamil Tablets;
USP 23: Verapamil Hydrochloride Extended-release Tablets; Verapamil Hydrochloride Injection; Verapamil Hydrochloride Tablets.

Proprietary Preparations (details are given in Part 3)
Aust.: Isoptin; Verapabene; Verexamil; ***Austral.:*** Anpec; Cordilox; Isoptin; Veracaps; ***Belg.:*** Fibrocard†; Isoptine; Lodixal; ***Canad.:*** Apo-Verap; Isoptin; Novo-Veramil; Nu-Verap; Verelan; ***Fr.:*** Arpamyl LP†; Isoptine; Novapamyl; ***Ger.:*** Azupamil; Cardiagutt†; cardibeltin†; Cardioprotect; Dignover; durasoptin; Falicard; Isoptin; Jenapamil; Praecicor; Vera; Verabeta; Veradurat†; Verahexal; Veramex; Veranorm; Veroptinstada; ***Irl.:*** Berkatens; Isoptin; Veramil; Verelan; Verisop; ***Ital.:*** Isoptin; Quasar; ***Jpn:*** Vasolan; ***Neth.:*** Geangin†; Isoptin; ***Norw.:*** Geangin; Isoptin; Verakard; ***S.Afr.:*** Bonceur; Calcicard; Iso-Card; Isoptin; Ravamil; Vasomil; Verahexal; Verpamil†; ***Spain:*** Manidon; Redupres; Univer†; Veratensin; ***Swed.:*** Isoptin; Veraloc; ***Switz.:*** Corpamil; Flamon; Isoptin; Veracim; Veraptin†; Verasifar; ***UK:*** Berkatens; Cordilox; Ethimil; Geangin†; Half Securon; Securon; Univer; Verapress; ***USA:*** Calan; Covera; Isoptin; Verelan.

Multi-ingredient: ***Aust.:*** Captocomp; Confit; Gradulon; Taluvian†; Veracapt; ***Ger.:*** Cordichin; Elthon†; Gradulon s. T.†; Stenoptin; Taluvian†; Tarka; Veratide; ***Neth.:*** Tarka; ***UK:*** Tarka; ***USA:*** Tarka.

Veratrum and Veratrum Alkaloids (14448-h)

Green veratrum consists of the dried rhizome and roots of *Veratrum viride* (Liliaceae) from which are derived the alkaloidal mixtures alkavervir and cryptenamine.

White veratrum consists of the dried rhizome and roots of *Veratrum album* (Liliaceae) from which are derived the alkaloids protoveratrine A and B.

Green Veratrum (913-s)

American Hellebore; American Veratrum; Green Hellebore; Green Hellebore Rhizome; Veratro Verde; Veratrum Viride.
CAS — 8002-39-9.

White Veratrum (914-w)

European Hellebore; Veratrum Album; White Hellebore; White Hellebore Rhizome.

Protoveratrine A (916-l)

Protoverine 6,7-diacetate 3(*S*)-(2-hydroxy-2-methylbutanoate) 15(*R*)-(2-methylbutanoate).
$C_{41}H_{63}NO_{14}$ = 793.9.
CAS — 143-57-7.

Protoveratrine B (917-y)

Neoprotoveratrine; Veratetrine. Protoverine 6,7-diacetate 3(*S*)-(2,3-dihydroxy-2-methylbutanoate) 15(*R*)-(2-methylbutanoate).
$C_{41}H_{63}NO_{15}$ = 809.9.
CAS — 124-97-0 (protoveratrine B); 8053-18-7 (protoveratrines A and B).

Adverse Effects

Veratrum alkaloids may cause nausea and vomiting at conventional therapeutic doses. Other adverse effects include epigastric and substernal burning, sweating, mental confusion, cardiac arrhythmias, dizziness, and hiccup. Profound hypotension and respiratory depression can occur at high doses.

Report of various symptoms of intoxication in 7 patients due to the use of a sneezing powder containing white veratrum alkaloids.[1]

1. Fogh A, *et al.* Veratrum alkaloids in sneezing-powder: a potential danger. *J Toxicol Clin Toxicol* 1983; **20:** 175–9.

Treatment of Adverse Effects

Following oral ingestion of veratrum alkaloids the stomach should be emptied by aspiration and lavage. Excessive hypotension with bradycardia or cardiac arrhythmias can be treated with atropine by intramuscular injection. The patient should be placed in a supine position with the feet raised.

Uses and Administration

White and green veratrum contain a number of pharmacologically active alkaloids that produce centrally mediated peripheral vasodilatation and bradycardia. They have been used in the treatment of hypertension but are generally considered to produce an unacceptably high incidence of adverse effects and have largely been replaced by less toxic antihypertensives.

Both green and white veratrum have also been used as insecticides.

White veratrum has been used, as Veratrum Album, in homoeopathy.

Vesnarinone (3772-y)

Vesnarinone *(USAN, rINN).*
OPC-8212. 1-(1,2,3,4-Tetrahydro-2-oxo-6-quinolyl)-4-veratroylpiperazine.
$C_{22}H_{25}N_3O_4$ = 395.5.
CAS — 81840-15-5.

Vesnarinone is a phosphodiesterase inhibitor with calcium-sensitising properties. It has positive inotropic activity and is given by mouth in the management of heart failure.

Studies with other inotropic phosphodiesterase inhibitors have shown that their prolonged oral administration can increase the mortality rate. In a multicentre study of vesnarinone,[1] doses of 120 mg daily resulted in increased mortality whereas 60 mg daily for 6 months was associated with lower morbidity and mortality. Reversible neutropenia occurred in 2.5% of the patients given 60 mg daily. However, in the larger VEST study, increased mortality was also reported with doses of 30 and 60 mg daily, and the future of this drug appears uncertain.

1. Feldman AM, *et al.* Effects of vesnarinone on morbidity and mortality in patients with heart failure. *N Engl J Med* 1993; **329:** 149–55.

Preparations

Proprietary Preparations (details are given in Part 3)
Multi-ingredient: ***Jpn:*** Arkin-Z.

Visnadine (9284-f)

Visnadine *(BAN, rINN).*
10-Acetoxy-9,10-dihydro-8,8-dimethyl-2-oxo-2*H*,8*H*-pyrano[2,3-*f*]chromen-9-yl 2-methylbutyrate.
$C_{21}H_{24}O_7$ = 388.4.
CAS — 477-32-7.

Visnadine is a vasodilator obtained from *Ammi visnaga* fruit or by synthesis that has been used in coronary, cerebral, and peripheral vascular disorders.
Ammi visnaga fruit is used in herbal preparations.

Preparations

Proprietary Preparations (details are given in Part 3)
Ger.: Carduben; Khellangan N; steno-loges N; ***Spain:*** Vibeline†.
Multi-ingredient: ***Aust.:*** Urelium Neu; ***Ger.:*** Aesrutal S; Cardaminol†; Cardisetten†; Cefedrin N; Hepatofalk Neu; Hevertopect; Oxacant-Khella N; Salusan; Seda-Stenocrat-N†; Silphoscalin†; Stenocrat; Urol†.

Warfarin Sodium (14736-w)

Warfarin Sodium *(BANM, rINNM).*
Sodium Warfarin; Warfarinum Natricum. The sodium salt of 4-hydroxy-3-(3-oxo-1-phenylbutyl)coumarin.
$C_{19}H_{15}NaO_4$ = 330.3.
CAS — 81-81-2 (warfarin); 2610-86-8 (warfarin potassium); 129-06-6 (warfarin sodium).
Pharmacopoeias. In *Chin., Eur.* (see p.viii), *Int.*, and *US.*
Chin., Int., and *US* permit either warfarin sodium or warfarin sodium clathrate. *Eur.* has a separate monograph for warfarin sodium clathrate (see below).
Jpn includes Warfarin Potassium.

The Ph. Eur. describes a white hygroscopic powder. Very **soluble** in water and in alcohol; soluble in acetone; very slightly soluble in dichloromethane and in ether. A 1% solution in water has a pH of 7.6 to 8.6. **Store** in airtight containers. **Protect** from light.
The USP describes a white odourless amorphous powder or crystalline clathrate which is discoloured by light. Very **soluble** in water; freely soluble in alcohol; very slightly soluble in chloroform and in ether. A 1% solution in water has a pH of 7.2 to 8.3. **Protect** from light.
NOTE. Commercial warfarin sodium is racemic.

Adsorption. Studies carried out for periods of 24 hours to 3 months have demonstrated some adsorption of warfarin sodium by polyvinyl chloride when dissolved in 0.9% sodium chloride solution[1,2] or in 5% glucose solution.[3] In one of these studies,[1] adsorption was decreased by buffering the solution from its initial pH of 6.7 to a pH of 7.4. Martens *et al.*[2] could demonstrate no adsorption onto polyethylene-lined or glass infusion containers.

1. Kowaluk EA, *et al.* Interactions between drugs and polyvinyl chloride infusion bags. *Am J Hosp Pharm* 1981; **38:** 1308–14.
2. Martens HJ, *et al.* Sorption of various drugs in polyvinyl chloride, glass, and polyethylene-lined infusion containers. *Am J Hosp Pharm* 1990; **47:** 369–73.
3. Moorhatch P, Chiou WL. Interactions between drugs and plastic intravenous fluid bags: part i: sorption studies on 17 drugs. *Am J Hosp Pharm* 1974; **31:** 72–8.

Incompatibilities. Solutions of warfarin sodium have been reported to be incompatible with adrenaline hydrochloride, amikacin sulphate, metaraminol tartrate, oxytocin, promazine hydrochloride, and tetracycline hydrochloride. Visual incompatibility has been reported[1] with solutions of warfarin sodium mixed with solutions of aminophylline, bretylium tosylate, ceftazidime, cimetidine hydrochloride, ciprofloxacin lactate, dobutamine hydrochloride, esmolol hydrochloride, gentamicin sulphate, labetalol hydrochloride, metronidazole hydrochloride, or vancomycin hydrochloride. Haze was also reported after 24 hours with sodium chloride 0.9%.

1. Bahal SM, *et al.* Visual compatibility of warfarin sodium injection with selected medications and solutions. *Am J Health-Syst Pharm* 1997; **54:** 2599–2600.

Warfarin Sodium Clathrate (4823-c)

Warfarin Sodium Clathrate *(BANM).*

Warfarinum Natricum Clathratum. The clathrate of warfarin sodium with isopropyl alcohol in the molecular proportions 2 to 1 respectively.

Pharmacopoeias. In *Eur.* (see p.viii).
Chin., Int., and *US* permit either warfarin sodium or warfarin sodium clathrate.

A white powder. Very **soluble** in water; freely soluble in alcohol; soluble in acetone; very slightly soluble in dichloromethane and in ether. A 1% solution in water has a pH of 7.6 to 8.6. **Store** in airtight containers. **Protect** from light.

Warfarin sodium clathrate contains approximately 92% of warfarin sodium.

NOTE. Until 1991 the BP, like the USP, allowed the use of either warfarin sodium or warfarin sodium clathrate in the definition of warfarin sodium. The use of the term warfarin sodium in *Martindale* should generally be taken to include the sodium clathrate.

Adverse Effects

The major risk from warfarin therapy is of haemorrhage from almost any organ of the body with the consequent effects of haematomas as well as anaemia. Although good control of warfarin anticoagulation is essential in preventing haemorrhage, bleeding has occurred at therapeutic international normalised ratio (INR) values. In such cases the possibility of an underlying cause such as renal or alimentary tract disease should be investigated. No consistent correlation has been observed between the duration of warfarin anticoagulation and risk of haemorrhage. Skin necrosis (see below) and purple discoloration of the toes (due to cholesterol embolisation) have occasionally occurred. Hypersensitivity reactions are extremely rare. Other effects not necessarily associated with haemorrhage include alopecia, fever, nausea, vomiting, diarrhoea, skin reactions, jaundice, hepatic dysfunction, and pancreatitis.

Warfarin is a recognised teratogen. Given in the first trimester of pregnancy it can cause a fetal warfarin syndrome or warfarin embryopathy characterised by bone stippling (chondrodysplasia punctata) and nasal hypoplasia. CNS abnormalities may develop following administration in any trimester but appear most likely after administration in the second or third trimester. Administration of warfarin during pregnancy has been associated with an increased rate of abortion and still-birth, although this may, in part, be the consequence of an underlying maternal condition. Administration in the late stages of pregnancy is associated with fetal haemorrhage. Reported incidences of the above complications have varied; one estimate is that if a coumarin anticoagulant is taken during pregnancy, one-sixth of pregnancies will result in an abnormal liveborn infant, and one-sixth will result in abortion or still-birth.

Effects on the blood. The incidence and risk of haemorrhage during long-term oral anticoagulation has been studied in patients in clinical trials[1] and in population-based studies.[2-4] The risk of bleeding was generally higher with more intense anticoagulation and in the presence of other risk factors but there was no clear relationship with age.

Withdrawal of warfarin therapy may lead to rebound hypercoagulability and it has been suggested[5] that warfarin should be withdrawn gradually, although there is no clinical evidence to support this.

For the risk of corpus luteum haemorrhage or haematoma associated with ovulation in patients on oral anticoagulants, see under Precautions, below.

1. Levine MN, *et al.* Hemorrhagic complications of long-term anticoagulant therapy. *Chest* 1989; **95** (suppl): 26S–36S.
2. Gitter MJ, *et al.* Bleeding and thromboembolism during anticoagulant therapy: a population-based study in Rochester, Minnesota. *Mayo Clin Proc* 1995; **70:** 725–33.
3. Fihn SD, *et al.* The risk for and severity of bleeding complications in elderly patients treated with warfarin. *Ann Intern Med* 1996; **124:** 970–9.
4. Palareti G, *et al.* Bleeding complications of oral anticoagulant treatment: an inception-cohort, prospective collaborative study (ISCOAT). *Lancet* 1996; **348:** 423–8.
5. Palareti G, Legnani C. Warfarin withdrawal: pharmacokinetic-pharmacodynamic considerations. *Clin Pharmacokinet* 1996; **30:** 300–13.

Effects on the fetus. Reviews of reported fetal complications following exposure to coumarin anticoagulants during pregnancy.

1. Hall JG, *et al.* Maternal and fetal sequelae of anticoagulation during pregnancy. *Am J Med* 1980; **68:** 122–40.
2. Ginsberg JS, Hirsh J. Optimum use of anticoagulants in pregnancy. *Drugs* 1988; **36:** 505–12.

Effects on the liver. There have been a few isolated reports of cholestatic liver damage in patients taking warfarin sodium.[1-3] In these cases hepatic injury resolved on withdrawal of the drug.

1. Rehnqvist N. Intrahepatic jaundice due to warfarin therapy. *Acta Med Scand* 1978; **204:** 335–6.
2. Jones DB, *et al.* Jaundice following warfarin therapy. *Postgrad Med J* 1980; **56:** 671.
3. Adler E, *et al.* Cholestatic hepatic injury related to warfarin exposure. *Arch Intern Med* 1986; **146:** 1837–9.

Effects on sexual function. There are some early reports of priapism in patients taking oral anticoagulants such as warfarin.[1] This adverse effect of warfarin sodium is not described by the UK manufacturers; the US manufacturers consider that no causal relationship has been established.

1. Baños JE, *et al.* Drug-induced priapism: its aetiology, incidence and treatment. *Med Toxicol* 1989; **4:** 46–58.

Effects on the skin and hair. Necrosis of skin and soft tissue associated with coumarin anticoagulant therapy has been reviewed.[1,2] Coumarin-induced necrosis occurs rarely and is characterised by a localised, painful skin lesion, initially erythematous or haemorrhagic in appearance, that becomes bullous and eventually culminates in gangrenous necrosis. Fatalities have occurred. Areas of increased subcutaneous fat such as breast, thigh, and buttocks have most often been involved. The aetiology appears to be thrombotic but the exact pathophysiology is not known. Patients with protein C deficiency appear to be at highest risk. Treatment with coumarin anticoagulants should be discontinued on appearance of skin lesions and vitamin K should be given to reverse their effect. Heparin should be administered to provide anticoagulation. Fresh frozen plasma or protein C concentrates may also have a role in reversing the condition. Surgical intervention is usually required if necrosis does develop.

Other skin reactions have also been reported with coumarins. Vasculitis affecting both legs developed in a 74-year-old woman a few weeks after starting treatment with nicoumalone for deep-vein thrombosis and pulmonary embolism.[3] Nicoumalone treatment was stopped and the skin lesions steadily improved over 15 days. However, the skin lesions reappeared a few hours after re-exposure to a single dose of nicoumalone. The patient had also been taking amiodarone which may have contributed to the reaction.

Increased shedding of telogen hair has been stated to occur in patients given coumarin anticoagulants.[4]

1. Cole MS, *et al.* Coumarin necrosis—a review of the literature. *Surgery* 1988; **103:** 271–7.
2. Comp PC. Coumarin-induced skin necrosis: incidence, mechanisms, management and avoidance. *Drug Safety* 1993; **8:** 128–35.
3. Susano R, *et al.* Hypersensitivity vasculitis related to nicoumalone. *Br Med J* 1993; **306:** 973.
4. Smith AG. Drug-induced disorders of hair and nails. *Adverse Drug React Bull* 1995 (173): 655–8.

Treatment of Adverse Effects

The measures used in the management of bleeding and/or excessive anticoagulation during warfarin therapy, or following warfarin overdosage, depend upon the degree of bleeding, the value of the international normalised ratio (INR), and the degree of thrombo-embolic risk.

If the INR is greater than 5.0 but there is no bleeding or only minor bleeding, warfarin should be temporarily withheld until the INR falls to below 5.0. In some cases where the INR is between 5.0 and 6.0 a reduction in warfarin dose, rather than withdrawal, may be sufficient. For an INR greater than 8.0 administration of phytomenadione (vitamin K_1) should also be considered if there are other risk factors for bleeding; typical doses of phytomenadione are 0.5 mg intravenously or up to 5 mg orally.

If there is any major bleeding warfarin should be stopped and phytomenadione 5 mg by slow intravenous injection given together with a concentrate of factors II, VII, IX, and X. The dose of concentrate should be calculated based on 50 units of factor IX per kg body-weight. If no concentrate is available fresh frozen plasma should be infused (about one litre for an adult), but may not be as effective. It should be remembered that phytomenadione takes several hours to act and large doses may reduce the response to resumed therapy with anticoagulants for a week or more.

If bleeding occurs unexpectedly at therapeutic INR values, the possibility of an underlying cause such as renal or alimentary tract disease should be investigated.

See under Effects on the Skin and Hair, above, for the management of skin and soft tissue necrosis.

Cholestyramine was considered to have increased the elimination of warfarin in a patient being treated for deliberate warfarin overdose.[1] It may be a useful adjunct to vitamin K therapy.

1. Renowden S, *et al.* Oral cholestyramine increases elimination of warfarin after overdose. *Br Med J* 1985; **291:** 513–14.

Precautions

Warfarin should not be given to patients who are haemorrhaging. In general it should not be given to patients at serious risk of haemorrhage, although it has been used with very careful control; patients at risk include those with haemorrhagic blood disorders, peptic ulcers, severe wounds (including surgical wounds), cerebrovascular disorders, and bacterial endocarditis. Severe kidney and liver impairment as well as severe hypertension are considered by some to be contra-indications. Pregnancy is also generally considered to be a contra-indication, especially in the first trimester and during the last few weeks of pregnancy (see Adverse Effects, above).

Many factors may affect anticoagulant control with warfarin. These include vitamin K status, thyroid status, renal impairment, bioavailability differences between warfarin preparations, factors affecting absorption of warfarin, and drug interactions. Such factors may be responsible for apparent resistance to warfarin and a few patients have displayed hereditary resistance. Dosage alterations should be guided by regular monitoring of oral anticoagulant therapy and clinical status. Patients should carry anticoagulant treatment booklets.

A discussion of factors affecting the anticoagulant effect of warfarin sodium.[1]

1. Shetty HGM, *et al.* Clinical pharmacokinetic considerations in the control of oral anticoagulant therapy. *Clin Pharmacokinet* 1989; **16:** 238–53.

Corpus luteum haematoma or haemorrhage was associated with ovulation in 3 women being treated with coumarin anticoagulants.[1] It was suggested that suppression of ovulation be considered for women on anticoagulants during their fertile years, even if sterilisation had been performed.

See Sex Hormones under Interactions, below, for the effect of oral contraceptives on the activity of oral anticoagulants.

1. Bogers J-W, *et al.* Complications of anticoagulant therapy in ovulatory women. *Lancet* 1991; **337:** 618–19.

Interactions

Many compounds interact with warfarin and other oral anticoagulants. Details of these interactions are given below for all oral anticoagulants with different groups of drugs; if the anticoagulant is other than warfarin, then its identity is specified. The major interactions are summarised below.

Drugs generally recognised as diminishing the effects of oral anticoagulants are included in the following list. Further information on the interactions with these drugs and others where the interaction is not so well recognised is provided in the referenced section below.	
acetomenaphthone	ethchlorvynol
alcohol (chronic ingestion without liver impairment)	glutethimide
aminoglutethimide	griseofulvin
barbiturates	nafcillin
carbamazepine	phytomenadione
dichloralphenazone	rifampicin

Drugs recognised or generally reported as enhancing oral anticoagulants are included in the following list. Further information on the interactions with these drugs and others where the interaction is not so well recognised is provided in the referenced section below.	
alcohol (acute ingestion or chronic ingestion with liver impairment)	ethacrynic acid
	ethyloestrenol
	fluconazole
allopurinol	glucagon
amiodarone	itraconazole
aspirin	ketoconazole
cephamandole	metronidazole
chloral hydrate	miconazole
chloramphenicol	norethandrolone
cimetidine	NSAIDs
clofibrate	oymetholone
co-trimoxazole	quinidine
danazol	stanozolol
dextropropoxyphene	sulphinpyrazone
dextrothyroxine	tamoxifen
dipyridamole	thyroid agents
disulfiram	tienilic acid
erythromycin	triclofos sodium

Readers should be aware that while interactions of a pharmacodynamic nature occurring with one anticoagulant may well apply to another, this is not necessarily the case with interactions of a pharmacokinetic nature.

An interaction may be due to increased or decreased anticoagulant metabolism; with warfarin some interacting drugs such as cimetidine, co-trimoxazole, or phenylbutazone have a selective effect on its stereo-isomers. Altered absorption may sometimes play a part, as with cholestyramine. Displacement of oral anticoagulants from plasma protein binding sites has been reported with many drugs, including some analgesics. Not all reports that have recorded an alteration in the pharmacokinetics of the anticoagulant have, however, shown a corresponding change in clinical response.

Interference with the coagulation process may be responsible for the increased risk of haemorrhage when aspirin, clofibrate, or thyroid hormones are used concomitantly with anticoagulants. Many other compounds, such as asparaginase, some contrast media, epoprostenol, streptokinase, and urokinase also carry this risk; while interactions between these compounds and anticoagulants are not discussed further below, the possibility of an increased risk of haemorrhage should be considered when they are used together.

Where there is a risk of serious haemorrhage from an interaction, then use of the 2 drugs is best avoided. In other instances the anticoagulant activity should be carefully monitored so as to increase or decrease the anticoagulant dose as required. Critical periods are when patients stabilised on an anticoagulant commence treatment with an interacting drug, or when patients stabilised on a regimen of an interacting drug and anticoagulant have the interacting drug withdrawn. Depending on the mechanism of the interaction, the clinical response to the interaction may be rapid or may take some days. Interactions involving displacement from plasma protein binding sites are often transient. Readers should also be aware that some interacting drugs do not produce predictable effects; there have for instance been reports of increased as well as decreased anticoagulant activity with disopyramide, phenytoin, quinidine, and oral contraceptives. Another problem occurs with dipyridamole; it can cause bleeding when given to patients taking anticoagulants but without any changes in the measures used for anticoagulant control.

Reviews.

1. Harder S, Thürmann P. Clinically important drug interactions with anticoagulants: an update. *Clin Pharmacokinet* 1996; **30:** 416–44.

Alcohol. Alcohol has a variable effect on warfarin. Heavy regular drinkers may experience a diminished effect, perhaps through enzyme induction, although the effect of warfarin may be increased in the presence of liver impairment; acute ingestion has enhanced the effect of warfarin. A moderate alcohol intake is generally not considered to cause problems.

Alcoholics taking disulfiram will experience an enhanced effect with warfarin (see below).

Analgesics and NSAIDs. All NSAIDs should be used with caution or not at all in patients on warfarin. Many NSAIDs inhibit platelet function to some extent and have an irritant effect on the gastro-intestinal tract, so increasing the risk of haemorrhage. Furthermore, some NSAIDs increase the hypoprothrombinaemic effect of warfarin, possibly by an intrinsic effect on coagulation or by displacement of warfarin from plasma protein-binding sites. Many studies have compared the relative displacing action of a range of NSAIDs *in vitro*, but such studies cannot easily be extrapolated to the clinical situation. Changes in plasma concentration of unbound warfarin resulting from displacement from plasma protein-binding sites are usually transient and are most likely to occur in the first few weeks after an NSAID is added to or withdrawn from warfarin therapy; monitoring of anticoagulant therapy is, therefore, most critical during this period.

In high doses *aspirin* and some other *salicylates* enhance the hypoprothrombinaemic effect of warfarin and should generally be avoided in patients on oral anticoagulant therapy. Low-dose aspirin and warfarin may have a role given concomitantly in some patients but the risk of gastro-intestinal bleeding is increased. The possibility of an interaction with topical salicylate preparations should also be considered.[1,2]

Concurrent administration of *phenylbutazone* and warfarin has led to serious haemorrhage and should be avoided. Phenylbutazone affects the metabolism of the *R*- and *S*- isomers of warfarin in complex and different ways with the net effect of enhancing its anticoagulant activity.[3] Related drugs such as *oxyphenbutazone*, *azapropazone*,[4-6] and *feprazone*[7] behave similarly and should also be avoided.

For the following NSAIDs there are a few studies or isolated reports suggesting that they may enhance the hypoprothrombinaemic effect of warfarin or other specified oral anticoagulant: *diflunisal* (with nicoumalone[8] or warfarin[9]), *flurbiprofen* (with nicoumalone),[10] *indomethacin*,[11,12] *ketoprofen*,[13] *meclofenamate sodium*,[14] *mefenamic acid*,[15] *piroxicam*, (with warfarin[16] or nicoumalone[17]), *sulindac*,[18,19] *tiaprofenic acid* (with nicoumalone),[20] and *tolmetin sodium*.[21] In many cases the result of concomitant therapy was an increased prothrombin time which may or may not be clinically significant; in other cases haemorrhage occurred. It should also be noted that for many of the above NSAIDs, perhaps particularly indomethacin, there are studies (not cited) in which no enhancement of warfarin activity could be demonstrated. NSAIDs with an apparently minimal effect on warfarin activity include *etodolac, ibuprofen, naproxen*, and *tenidap*.

In view of the above considerations, *paracetamol* is recommended as the general analgesic and antipyretic of choice in patients on oral anticoagulant therapy. Caution should, however, be observed since, although it has no effect on the gastric mucosa or on platelet function, some studies (with warfarin, anisindione, dicoumarol, or phenprocoumon)[22,23] and isolated reports[24] have demonstrated an increased risk of bleeding in patients taking regular doses of paracetamol while on an oral anticoagulant.

Opioid analgesics do not generally cause problems, although there have been reports of enhanced anticoagulant activity in patients receiving *tramadol* with warfarin[25] or phenprocoumon.[26] *Dextropropoxyphene*, when used in combination with paracetamol [*co-proxamol*], has increased the effect of warfarin.[27-29] A combination of paracetamol and *codeine* [*co-codamol*] has also enhanced warfarin activity.[30]

Amongst other analgesics, *cinchophen* (with dicoumarol, ethyl biscoumacetate, or phenindione)[31] and *phenyramidol* (with warfarin, dicoumarol, or phenindione)[32] have been reported to enhance the activity of oral anticoagulants and there is the possibility of such an effect with *glafenine* (with phenprocoumon).[33] *Phenazone*, an inducer of enzyme metabolism, reduces plasma concentrations of warfarin and, in contrast with most other analgesics, may necessitate an increase in warfarin dosage.[34]

1. Chow WH, *et al.* Potentiation of warfarin anticoagulation by topical methylsalicylate ointment. *J R Soc Med* 1989; **82:** 501–2.
2. Littleton F. Warfarin and topical salicylates. *JAMA* 1990; **263:** 2888.
3. Banfield C, *et al.* Phenylbutazone-warfarin interaction in man: further stereochemical and metabolic considerations. *Br J Clin Pharmacol* 1983; **16:** 669–75.
4. Powell-Jackson PR. Interaction between azapropazone and warfarin. *Br Med J* 1977; **1:** 1193–4.
5. Green AE, *et al.* Potentiation of warfarin by azapropazone. *Br Med J* 1977; **1:** 1532.
6. Win N, Mitchell DC. Azapropazone and warfarin. *Br Med J* 1991; **302:** 969–70.
7. Chierichetti S, *et al.* Comparison of feprazone and phenylbutazone interaction with warfarin in man. *Curr Ther Res* 1975; **18:** 568–72.
8. Tempero KF, *et al.* Diflunisal: a review of pharmacokinetic and pharmacodynamic properties, drug interactions, and special tolerability studies in humans. *Br J Clin Pharmacol* 1977; **4:** 31S–36S.
9. Serlin MJ, *et al.* The effect of diflunisal on the steady state pharmacodynamics and pharmacokinetics of warfarin. *Br J Clin Pharmacol* 1980; **9:** 287P–8P.
10. Stricker BHC, Delhez JL. Interaction between flurbiprofen and coumarins. *Br Med J* 1982; **285:** 812–13.
11. Koch-Weser J. Hemorrhagic reactions and drug interactions in 500 warfarin-treated patients. *Clin Pharmacol Ther* 1973; **14:** 139.
12. Self TH, *et al.* Drug enhancement of warfarin activity. *Lancet* 1975; **ii:** 557–8.
13. Flessner MF. Prolongation of prothrombin time and severe gastrointestinal bleeding associated with combined use of warfarin and ketoprofen. *JAMA* 1988; **259:** 353.
14. Baragar FD, Smith TC. Drug interaction studies with sodium meclofenamate (Meclomen®). *Curr Ther Res* 1978; **23** (suppl 4): S51–S59.
15. Holmes EL. Pharmacology of the fenamates: IV toleration by normal human subjects. *Ann Phys Med* 1966; **9** (suppl): 36–49.
16. Rhodes RS, *et al.* A warfarin-piroxicam drug interaction. *Drug Intell Clin Pharm* 1985; **19:** 556–8.
17. Bonnabry P, *et al.* Stereoselective interaction between piroxicam and acenocoumarol. *Br J Clin Pharmacol* 1996; **41:** 525–30.
18. Carter SA. Potential effect of sulindac on response of prothrombin-time to oral anticoagulants. *Lancet* 1979; **ii:** 698–9.
19. Ross JRY, Beeley L. Sulindac, prothrombin time, and anticoagulants. *Lancet* 1979; **ii:** 1075.
20. Whittaker SJ, *et al.* A severe, potentially fatal, interaction between tiaprofenic acid and nicoumalone. *Br J Clin Pract* 1986; **40:** 440.
21. Koren JF, *et al.* Tolmetin-warfarin interaction. *Am J Med* 1987; **82:** 1278–9.
22. Antlitz AM, *et al.* Potentiation of oral anticoagulant therapy by acetaminophen. *Curr Ther Res* 1968; **10:** 501–7.
23. Hylek EM, *et al.* Acetaminophen and other risk factors for excessive warfarin anticoagulation. *JAMA* 1998; **279:** 657–62.
24. Boeijinga JJ, *et al.* Interaction between paracetamol and coumarin anticoagulants. *Lancet* 1982; **i:** 506.
25. Scher ML, *et al.* Potential interaction between tramadol and warfarin. *Ann Pharmacother* 1997; **31:** 646–7.
26. Madsen H, *et al.* Interaction between tramadol and phenprocoumon. *Lancet* 1997; **350:** 637.
27. Orme M, *et al.* Warfarin and Distalgesic interaction. *Br Med J* 1976; **1:** 200.
28. Jones RV. Warfarin and Distalgesic interaction. *Br Med J* 1976; **1:** 460.
29. Smith R, *et al.* Propoxyphene and warfarin interaction. *Drug Intell Clin Pharm* 1984; **18:** 822.
30. Bartle WR, Blakely JA. Potentiation of warfarin anticoagulation by acetaminophen. *JAMA* 1991; **265:** 1260.
31. Jarnum S. Cinchophen and acetylsalicylic acid in anticoagulant treatment. *Scand J Clin Lab Invest* 1954; **6:** 91–3.
32. Carter SA. Potentiation of the effect of orally administered anticoagulants by phenyramidol hydrochloride. *N Engl J Med* 1965; **273:** 423–6.
33. Boeijinga JK, van der Vijgh WJF. Double blind study of the effect of glafenine (Glifanan®) on oral anticoagulant therapy with phenprocoumon (Marcumar®). *J Clin Pharmacol* 1977; **12:** 291–6.
34. Whitfield JB, *et al.* Changes in plasma γ-glutamyl transpeptidase activity associated with alterations in drug metabolism in man. *Br Med J* 1973; **1:** 316–18.

Antiarrhythmics. *Amiodarone* has been shown in several studies to increase the activity of warfarin[1-5] and nicoumalone,[6,7] probably through inhibition of metabolism. The potentiating effect of amiodarone has been reported to persist for up to 4 months after its withdrawal.[1] There is an early report of phenprocoumon not being affected by amiodarone.[8] Isolated reports with *disopyramide*[9] and *quinidine*[10] have suggested that these drugs can enhance the anticoagulant effect of warfarin. In 7 patients on warfarin or dicoumarol treated with disopyramide or quinidine, however, all but one needed a small increase in the weekly anticoagulant dose suggesting that the antiarrhythmic had reduced the anticoagulant effect.[11] Since the effect was observed after conversion of atrial fibrillation to sinus rhythm an involvement of haemodynamic factors was postulated. Several studies (not cited) have failed to show an effect of quinidine on warfarin. There are also reports indicating that *propafenone*[12] and *moracizine*[13] can enhance warfarin.

1. Martinowitz U, *et al.* Interaction between warfarin sodium and amiodarone. *N Engl J Med* 1981; **304:** 671–2.
2. Almog S, *et al.* Mechanism of warfarin potentiation by amiodarone: dose—and concentration—dependent inhibition of warfarin elimination. *Eur J Clin Pharmacol* 1985; **28:** 257–61.
3. Watt AH, *et al.* Amiodarone reduces plasma warfarin clearance in man. *Br J Clin Pharmacol* 1985; **20:** 707–9.
4. O'Reilly RA, *et al.* Interaction of amiodarone with racemic warfarin and its separated enantiomorphs in humans. *Clin Pharmacol Ther* 1987; **42:** 290–4.
5. Kerin NZ, *et al.* The incidence, magnitude, and time course of the amiodarone-warfarin interaction. *Arch Intern Med* 1988; **148:** 1779–81.
6. Arboix M, *et al.* The potentiation of acenocoumarol anticoagulant effect by amiodarone. *Br J Clin Pharmacol* 1984; **18:** 355–60.
7. Richard C, *et al.* Prospective study of the potentiation of acenocoumarol by amiodarone. *Eur J Clin Pharmacol* 1985; **28:** 625–9.
8. Verstraete M, *et al.* Dissimilar effect of two anti-anginal drugs belonging to the benzofuran group on the action of coumarin derivatives. *Arch Int Pharmacodyn Ther* 1968; **176:** 33–41.
9. Haworth E, Burroughs AK. Disopyramide and warfarin interaction. *Br Med J* 1977; **2:** 866–7.
10. Gazzaniga AB, Stewart DR. Possible quinidine-induced hemorrhage in a patient on warfarin sodium. *N Engl J Med* 1969; **280:** 711–12.
11. Sylvén C, Anderson P. Evidence that disopyramide does not interact with warfarin. *Br Med J* 1983; **286:** 1181.
12. Kates RE, *et al.* Interaction between warfarin and propafenone in healthy volunteer subjects. *Clin Pharmacol Ther* 1987; **42:** 305–11.
13. Serpa MD, *et al.* Moricizine—warfarin: a possible drug interaction. *Ann Pharmacother* 1992; **26:** 127.

Antibacterials. Several antibacterials have been involved in interactions with warfarin. Only a few reports are of serious effects and it is unlikely that any of the drugs need to be contra-indicated with warfarin; careful control should suffice.

Most of the drugs enhance the effects of warfarin. Apart from possible effects on the metabolism or plasma-protein binding of warfarin, some antibacterials may interfere with platelet function or with the bacterial synthesis of vitamin K in the gastro-intestinal tract and thus have an anticoagulant effect of their own. This is generally considered unlikely to be of clinical significance except, perhaps, in patients with an inadequate vitamin K intake. Fever itself may increase the catabolism of clotting factors and exaggerate a potential antibacterial-warfarin interaction.

There are several reports of an enhanced warfarin response with *co-trimoxazole*; stereospecific inhibition of warfarin metabolism is probably responsible.[1] The interaction is generally attributed to the *sulphamethoxazole* moiety and there are isolated reports suggesting that the activity of warfarin (or other specified oral anticoagulant) may be enhanced by other sulphonamides including *sulphafurazole*,[2] *sulphamethizole*,[3] and *sulphaphenazole* (with phenindione).[4]

There are several reports of potentiation of the effects of warfarin by *erythromycin* or its salts, probably by inhibition of warfarin metabolism. Although no clinically-significant increase in prothrombin time could be demonstrated in 8 non-infected patients, the potential for an interaction was recognised.[5] An enhanced response to warfarin has also been reported with *azithromycin*[6,7] and with *roxithromycin*,[8] including reports of spontaneous bleeding with the latter. *Clarithromycin* may potentiate the effect of nicoumalone[9] and of warfarin,[10] although other factors may also have been involved in this case.

Cephamandole has been reported to enhance the hypoprothrombinaemic response to warfarin.[11,12] Interference with vitamin K synthesis in the gastro-intestinal tract and/or liver has been implicated. Related cephalosporins with an *N*-methylthiotetrazole side chain such as *cefmetazole*, *cefmenoxime*, *cefoperazone*, and *latamoxef* may be expected to behave similarly although there appear to be no reports of an interaction. *Cephazolin*, which has a similar side chain, may also enhance the effect of warfarin to some extent.[12]

There have been a few reports of increased activity of warfarin (or other specified oral anticoagulant) by quinolone antibacterials including *nalidixic acid* (with warfarin[13,14] or nicoumalone[15]), *ciprofloxacin*,[16,17] *norfloxacin*,[18] and *ofloxacin*,[19,20] although for some of these there are also studies indicating no effect (not cited). *Enoxacin* has been reported to decrease the clearance of *R*-warfarin but not *S*-warfarin; no prolongation of prothrombin time occurred.[21]

There are isolated reports suggesting an enhanced effect of warfarin (or other specified oral anticoagulant) with *aminosalicylic acid*,[22] *benzylpenicillin*,[23] *chloramphenicol* (with dicoumarol),[24] *doxycycline*,[25] *isoniazid*,[26] and *neomycin*.[27] Prothrombin times might be prolonged by broad-spectrum antibiotics such as *ampicillin*, but published reports are lacking. Manufacturers' warnings of potentiation of warfarin by *aztreonam*, *trimethoprim*, and *tetracyclines* other than doxycycline appear to have only a theoretical basis. *Metronidazole* is discussed under Antiprotozoals, below.

Rifampicin diminishes the effect of warfarin by induction of metabolising enzymes in the liver. There are several reports of a similar effect with *nafcillin*[28-30] and with *dicloxacillin sodium*.[31,32]

1. O'Reilly RA. Stereo selective interaction of trimethoprim-sulfamethoxazole with the separated enantiomorphs of racemic warfarin in man. *N Engl J Med* 1980; **302** 33–5.
2. Sioris LJ, *et al.* Potentiation of warfarin anticoagulation by sulfisoxazole. *Arch Intern Med* 1980; **140:** 546–7.
3. Lumholtz B, *et al.* Sulfamethizole-induced inhibition of diphenylhydantoin, tolbutamide, and warfarin metabolism. *Clin Pharmacol Ther* 1975; **17:** 731–4.
4. Varma DR, *et al.* Prothrombin response to phenindione during hypoalbuminaemia. *Br J Clin Pharmacol* 1975; **2:** 467–8.
5. Weibert RT, *et al.* Effect of erythromycin in patients receiving long-term warfarin therapy. *Clin Pharm* 1989; **8:** 210–14.
6. Lane G. Increased hypoprothrombinemic effect of warfarin possibly induced by azithromycin. *Ann Pharmacother* 1996; **30:** 884–5.
7. Woldtvedt BR, *et al.* Possible increased anticoagulation effect of warfarin induced by azithromycin. *Ann Pharmacother* 1998; **32:** 269–70.
8. Anonymous. Interaction of warfarin with macrolide antibiotics. *Aust Adverse Drug React Bull* 1995; **14:** 11.
9. Grau E, *et al.* Interaction between clarithromycin and oral anticoagulants. *Ann Pharmacother* 1996; **30:** 1495–6.
10. Recker MW, Kier KL. Potential interaction between clarithromycin and warfarin. *Ann Pharmacother* 1997; **31:** 996–8.
11. Angaran DM, *et al.* The influence of prophylactic antibiotics on the warfarin anticoagulation response in the postoperative prosthetic cardiac valve patient. *Ann Surg* 1984; **199:** 107–11.
12. Angaran DM, *et al.* The comparative influence of prophylactic antibiotics on the prothrombin response to warfarin in the postoperative prosthetic cardiac valve patient: cefamandole, cefazoline, vancomycin. *Ann Surg* 1987; **206:** 155–61.
13. Hoffbrand BI. Interaction of nalidixic acid and warfarin. *Br Med J* 1974; **2:** 666.
14. Leor J, *et al.* Interaction between nalidixic acid and warfarin. *Ann Intern Med* 1987; **107:** 601.
15. Potasman I, Bassan H. Nicoumalone and nalidixic acid interaction. *Ann Intern Med* 1980; **92:** 571.
16. Mott FE, *et al.* Ciprofloxacin and warfarin. *Ann Intern Med* 1989; **111:** 542–3.
17. Kamada AK. Possible interaction between ciprofloxacin and warfarin. *DICP Ann Pharmacother* 1990; **24:** 27–8.
18. Linville T, Matanin D. Norfloxacin and warfarin. *Ann Intern Med* 1989; **110:** 751–2.
19. Leor J, Matetzki S. Ofloxacin and warfarin. *Ann Intern Med* 1988; **109:** 761.
20. Baciewicz AM, *et al.* Interaction of ofloxacin and warfarin. *Ann Intern Med* 1993; **119:** 1223.
21. Toon S, *et al.* Enoxacin-warfarin interaction: pharmacokinetic and stereochemical aspects. *Clin Pharmacol Ther* 1987; **42:** 33–41.
22. Self TH. Interaction of warfarin and aminosalicylic acid. *JAMA* 1973; **223:** 1285.
23. Brown MA, *et al.* Interaction of penicillin-G and warfarin? *Can J Hosp Pharm* 1979; **32:** 18–19.
24. Christensen LK, Skovsted L. Inhibition of drug metabolism by chloramphenicol. *Lancet* 1969; **ii:** 1397–9.
25. Westfall LK, *et al.* Potentiation of warfarin by tetracycline. *Am J Hosp Pharm* 1980; **37:** 1620 and 1625.
26. Rosenthal AR, *et al.* Interaction of isoniazid and warfarin. *JAMA* 1977; **238:** 2177.
27. Udall JA. Drug interference with warfarin therapy. *Clin Med* 1970; **77** (Aug.): 20–5.
28. Qureshi GD, *et al.* Warfarin resistance with nafcillin therapy. *Ann Intern Med* 1984; **100:** 527–9.
29. Fraser GL, *et al.* Warfarin resistance associated with nafcillin therapy. *Am J Med* 1989; **87:** 237–8.
30. Davis RL, *et al.* Warfarin-nafcillin interaction. *J Pediatr* 1991; **118:** 300–3.
31. Krstenansky PM, *et al.* Effect of dicloxacillin sodium on the hypoprothrombinemic response to warfarin sodium. *Clin Pharm* 1987; **6:** 804–6.
32. Mailloux A, *et al.* Potential interaction between warfarin and dicloxacillin. *Ann Pharmacother* 1996; **30:** 1402–7.

Antidepressants. *Amitriptyline* and *nortriptyline* have been reported to prolong the half-life of dicoumarol in healthy subjects.[1,2] The few reports of investigations into the effect of tricyclic antidepressants on warfarin have not been conclusive of an interaction. *Mianserin* and phenprocoumon have been reported not to interact.[3]

Some authorities consider that there is a theoretical risk of increased warfarin activity with *MAOIs* and with *fluvoxamine* and other selective serotonin reuptake inhibitors. Increased warfarin activity has been reported in a few patients taking *fluoxetine*.[4]

One patient required an increase in the dose of warfarin when taking *trazodone*.[5]

1. Vesell ES, *et al.* Impairment of drug metabolism in man by allopurinol and nortriptyline. *N Engl J Med* 1970; **283:** 1484–8.
2. Pond SM, *et al.* Effects of tricyclic antidepressants on drug metabolism. *Clin Pharmacol Ther* 1975; **18:** 191–9.
3. Kopera H, *et al.* Phenprocoumon requirement, whole blood coagulation time, bleeding time and plasma γ-GT in patients receiving mianserin. *Eur J Clin Pharmacol* 1978; **13:** 351–6.
4. Woolfrey S, *et al.* Fluoxetine-warfarin interaction. *Br Med J* 1993; **307:** 241.
5. Hardy J-L, Sirois A. Reduction of prothrombin and partial thromboplastin times with trazodone. *Can Med Assoc J* 1986; **135:** 1372.

Antidiabetics. There have been a few early instances of *tolbutamide* enhancing the activity of dicoumarol.[1] However, this effect has not been observed in later studies involving dicoumarol,[1-3] warfarin,[2] and phenprocoumon,[4] although one study did demonstrate altered dicoumarol pharmacokinetics.[3] An absence of effect has been documented for phenprocoumon and *insulin*, *glibenclamide*, or *glibornuride*,[4] but there is a recent report of glibenclamide enhancing the effect of warfarin.[5]

There has been one early isolated report of bleeding in a patient taking *phenformin* and warfarin.[6] *Metformin* has been reported to diminish phenprocoumon activity.[7]

An enhanced response to warfarin has been reported with *troglitazone*[8] in one patient.

Coumarin anticoagulants may increase the hypoglycaemic effect of *sulphonylureas* (see p.333).

1. Chaplin H, Cassell M. Studies on the possible relationship of tolbutamide to dicumarol in anticoagulant therapy. *Am J Med Sci* 1958; **235:** 706–16.
2. Poucher RL, Vecchio TJ. Absence of tolbutamide effect on anticoagulant therapy. *JAMA* 1966; **197:** 1069–70.
3. Jähnchen E, *et al.* Pharmacokinetic analysis of the interaction between dicoumarol and tolbutamide in man. *Eur J Clin Pharmacol* 1976; **10:** 349–56.
4. Heine P, *et al.* The influence of hypoglycaemic sulphonylureas on elimination and efficacy of phenprocoumon following a single oral dose in diabetic patients. *Eur J Clin Pharmacol* 1976; **10:** 31–6.
5. Jassal SV. *Br Med J* 1991; **303:** 789.
6. Hamblin TJ. Interaction between warfarin and phenformin. *Lancet* 1971; **ii:** 1323.
7. Ohnhaus EE, *et al.* The influence of dimethylbiguanide on phenprocoumon elimination and its mode of action: a drug interaction study. *Klin Wochenschr* 1983; **61:** 851–8.
8. Plowman BK, Morreale AP. Possible troglitazone—warfarin interaction. *Am J Health-Syst Pharm* 1998; **55:** 1071.

Antiepileptics. Barbiturates such as *phenobarbitone* and *primidone* diminish the activity of warfarin and other coumarins through increased metabolism. *Carbamazepine* is reported to have a similar effect.[1,2] Reports of the effect of *phenytoin* on anticoagulants do not provide a clear picture. There are reports of phenytoin enhancing the effects of warfarin[3,4] and a report of initial enhancement followed by decreased anticoagulant action.[5] Phenytoin has been reported to diminish the effect of dicoumarol.[6] Addition of *felbamate* to the therapy of one patient has been reported[7] to necessitate a reduction in warfarin dosage in order to maintain a target INR. In another patient there was a transient increase in response to warfarin when *valproic acid* was commenced.[8] Valproate also inhibits platelet function and caution is required when it is given concomitantly with warfarin.

For the effect of oral anticoagulants on phenytoin, see p.355.

1. Hansen JM, *et al.* Carbamazepine-induced acceleration of diphenylhydantoin and warfarin metabolism in man. *Clin Pharmacol Ther* 1971; **12:** 539–43.
2. Ross JRY, Beeley L. Interaction between carbamazepine and warfarin. *Br Med J* 1980; **280:** 1415–16.
3. Nappi JM. Warfarin and phenytoin interaction. *Ann Intern Med* 1979; **90:** 852.
4. Panegyres PK, Rischbieth RH. Fatal phenytoin warfarin interaction. *Postgrad Med J* 1991; **67:** 98.
5. Levine M, Sheppard I. Biphasic interaction of phenytoin with warfarin. *Clin Pharm* 1984; **3:** 200–3.
6. Hansen JM, *et al.* Effect of diphenylhydantoin on the metabolism of dicoumarol in man. *Acta Med Scand* 1971; **189:** 15–19.
7. Tisdel KA, *et al.* Warfarin—felbamate interaction: first report. *Ann Pharmacother* 1994; **28:** 805.
8. Guthrie SK, *et al.* Hypothesized interaction between valproic acid and warfarin. *J Clin Psychopharmacol* 1995; **15:** 138–9.

Antifungals. *Griseofulvin* has been reported to diminish the activity of warfarin.[1-3] There are several reports indicating that *miconazole*, given either systemically or topically as the oral gel, may enhance the activity of oral anticoagulants (warfarin, ethyl biscoumacetate, nicoumalone, phenindione, and tioclomarol).[4-10] A study in 13 healthy subjects given a single warfarin dose[11] supports case reports[12-14] suggesting that *fluconazole* may increase the anticoagulant activity of warfarin. There are isolated reports of the potentiation of warfarin by *itraconazole*[15] and *ketoconazole*.[16] There has been a single case report of a reduction in the effect of warfarin by *terbinafine*,[17] although others[18] considered that no interaction usually occurs.

1. Cullen SI, Catalano PM. Griseofulvin-warfarin antagonism. *JAMA* 1967; **199:** 582–3.
2. Udall JA. Drug interference with warfarin therapy. *Clin Med* 1970; **77** (Aug.): 20–5.
3. Okino K, Weibert RT. Warfarin-griseofulvin interaction. *Drug Intell Clin Pharm* 1986; **20:** 291–3.
4. Loupi E, *et al.* Interactions médicamenteuses et miconazole: a propos de 10 observations. *Therapie* 1982; **37:** 437–41.
5. Watson PG, *et al.* Drug interaction with coumarin derivative anticoagulants. *Br Med J* 1982; **285:** 1045–6.
6. Colquhoun MC, *et al.* Interaction between warfarin and miconazole oral gel. *Lancet* 1987; **i:** 695–6.
7. Bailey GM, *et al.* Miconazole and warfarin interaction. *Pharm J* 1989; **242:** 183.
8. Ariyaratnam S, *et al.* Potentiation of warfarin anticoagulant activity by miconazole oral gel. *Br Med J* 1997; **314:** 349.
9. Evans J, *et al.* Treating oral candidiasis: potentially fatal. *Br Dent J* 1997; **182:** 452.
10. Pemberton MN, *et al.* Derangement of warfarin anticoagulation by miconazole oral gel. *Br Dent J* 1998; **184:** 68–9.
11. Lazar JD, Wilner KD. Drug interactions with fluconazole. *Rev Infect Dis* 1990; **12** (suppl 3): S327–S333.
12. Seaton TL, *et al.* Possible potentiation of warfarin by fluconazole. *DICP Ann Pharmacother* 1990; **24:** 1177–8.
13. Gericke KR. Possible interaction between warfarin and fluconazole. *Pharmacotherapy* 1993; **13:** 508–9.
14. Baciewicz AM, *et al.* Fluconazole—warfarin interaction. *Ann Pharmacother* 1994; **28:** 1111.
15. Yeh J, *et al.* Potentiation of action of warfarin by itraconazole. *Br Med J* 1990; **301:** 669.
16. Smith AG. Potentiation of oral anticoagulants by ketoconazole. *Br Med J* 1984; **288:** 188–9. Correction. *ibid.*; 608.
17. Warwick JA, Corrall RJ. Serious interaction between warfarin and oral terbinafine. *Br Med J* 1998; **316:** 440.
18. Stockley IH. Terbinafine and warfarin mystery. *Pharm J* 1998; **260:** 408.

Antigout drugs. The two drugs in this group that have mostly been implicated in interactions with anticoagulants are allopurinol and sulphinpyrazone.

With *allopurinol* there are conflicting reports of patients experiencing no interaction or an enhanced anticoagulant effect with dicoumarol,[1] phenprocoumon,[2] or warfarin.[3,4]

Interactions with *sulphinpyrazone* have usually involved warfarin and, apart from one case of a mixed response,[5] have involved increased anticoagulant activity, sometimes with haemorrhage, so calling for careful control. It is still not clear how sulphinpyrazone exerts its effect, but studies point to a stereoselective effect on warfarin metabolism where the *S*-isomer's metabolic clearance is inhibited.[6] It should also be remembered that sulphinpyrazone affects platelets. Sulphinpyrazone has also enhanced the anticoagulant activity of nicoumalone.[7] A significant interaction with phenprocoumon appears unlikely.[8]

Administration of *probenecid* has accelerated the elimination of a single dose of phenprocoumon without effect on the prothrombin time.[9]

Benziodarone has been reported to enhance the effects of warfarin, diphenadione, ethyl biscoumacetate, and nicoumalone, but not of clorindione, dicoumarol, phenindione, or phenprocoumon.[10] A further study[11] confirmed that benziodarone could increase the half-life of ethyl biscoumacetate, but also found that the effect of phenprocoumon was enhanced.

1. Vesell ES, *et al.* Impairment of drug metabolism in man by allopurinol and nortriptyline. *N Engl J Med* 1970; **283:** 1484–8.
2. Jähnchen E, *et al.* Interaction of allopurinol with phenprocoumon in man. *Klin Wochenschr* 1977; **55:** 759–61.
3. Rawlins MD, Smith SE. Influence of allopurinol on drug metabolism in man. *Br J Pharmacol* 1973; **48:** 693–8.
4. Pond SM, *et al.* The effects of allopurinol and clofibrate on the elimination of coumarin anticoagulants in man. *Aust N Z J Med* 1975; **5:** 324–8.
5. Nenci GG, *et al.* Biphasic sulphinpyrazone-warfarin interaction. *Br Med J* 1981; **282:** 1361–2.
6. Toon S, *et al.* The warfarin-sulfinpyrazone interaction: stereochemical considerations. *Clin Pharmacol Ther* 1986; **39:** 15–24.
7. Michot F, *et al.* Über die beeinflussung der gerinnungshemmenden wirkung von acenocoumarol durch sulfinpyrazon. *Schweiz Med Wochenschr* 1981; **111:** 255–60.
8. Heimark LD, *et al.* The effect of sulfinpyrazone on the disposition of pseudoracemic phenprocoumon in humans. *Clin Pharmacol Ther* 1987; **42:** 312–19.
9. Mönig H, *et al.* The effects of frusemide and probenecid on the pharmacokinetics of phenprocoumon. *Eur J Clin Pharmacol* 1990; **39:** 261–5.
10. Pyörälä K, *et al.* Benziodarone (Amplivix®) and anticoagulant therapy. *Acta Med Scand* 1963; **173:** 385–9.
11. Verstraete M, *et al.* Dissimilar effect of two anti-anginal drugs belonging to the benzofuran group on the action of coumarin derivatives. *Arch Int Pharmacodyn Ther* 1968; **176:** 33–41.

Antihistamines. There has been one report[1] of a raised INR and severe epistaxis in a patient receiving long-term nicoumalone following the addition of *cetirizine* to his therapy.

1. Berod T, Mathiot I. Probable interaction between cetirizine and acenocoumarol. *Ann Pharmacother* 1997; **31:** 122.

Antimalarials. The ingestion of large amounts of tonic water by 2 patients necessitated a reduction in their warfarin dosage. The enhanced effect was attributed to the *quinine* content of the tonic water.[1] A woman stabilised on warfarin developed haematuria and a high prothrombin ratio after taking *proguanil* for malaria prophylaxis.[2]

1. Clark DJ. Clinical curio: warfarin and tonic water. *Br Med J* 1983; **286:** 1258.
2. Armstrong G, *et al.* Warfarin potentiated by proguanil. *Br Med J* 1991; **303:** 789.

Antineoplastics. There have been several reports of interactions between warfarin and antineoplastics. No clear picture emerges from these reports which is not surprising considering that antineoplastics are often given in combination and that they can exert their own haematological effects. *Cyclophosphamide* for instance has been associated with an increase in warfarin's activity when given with *methotrexate* and *fluorouracil*,[1] but with a decrease when given with non-antineoplastic drugs.[2] Fluorouracil has also been reported to increase the effect of warfarin when given with levamisole (see below). In one patient, concurrent therapy with warfarin and *cyclosporin* was associated with reduced effect of both drugs;[3] the patient was, however, also receiving phenobarbitone. Increased effects of both drugs were observed in another patient receiving cyclosporin and nicoumalone.[4] *Etoposide* with *vindesine*[5] or with *carboplatin*,[6] *ifosfamide* with *mesna*,[7] and *tamoxifen*[8-10] have all produced an increased anticoagulant effect. *Aminoglutethimide* has led to decreased activity of warfarin or nicoumalone,[11,12] probably due to increased warfarin metabolism. The manufacturers of the anti-androgen *flutamide* state that increases in prothrombin time have been reported after initiation of flutamide therapy in patients on long-term warfarin. *Mercaptopurine*[13] and *mitotane*[14] have also decreased warfarin activity and severe bleeding occurred in a patient on long-term warfarin treatment after discontinuing *azathioprine*.[15]

1. Seifter EJ, *et al.* Possible interactions between warfarin and antineoplastic drugs. *Cancer Treat Rep* 1985; **69:** 244–5.
2. Tashima CK. Cyclophosphamide effect on coumarin anticoagulation. *South Med J* 1979; **72:** 633–4.
3. Snyder DS. Interaction between cyclosporine and warfarin. *Ann Intern Med* 1988; **108:** 311.
4. Campistol JM, *et al.* Interaction between ciclosporin A and Sintrom. *Nephron* 1989; **53:** 291–2.
5. Ward K, Bitran JD. Warfarin, etoposide, and vindesine interactions. *Cancer Treat Rep* 1984; **68:** 817–18.
6. Le AT, *et al.* Enhancement of warfarin response in a patient receiving etoposide and carboplatin chemotherapy. *Ann Pharmacother* 1997; **31:** 1006–8.
7. Hall G, *et al.* Intravenous infusions of ifosfamide/mesna and perturbation of warfarin anticoagulant control. *Postgrad Med J* 1990; **66:** 860–1.
8. Lodwick R, *et al.* Life threatening interaction between tamoxifen and warfarin. *Br Med J* 1987; **295:** 1141.
9. Tenni P, *et al.* Life threatening interaction between tamoxifen and warfarin. *Br Med J* 1989; **298:** 93.
10. Ritchie LD, Grant SMT. Tamoxifen-warfarin interaction: the Aberdeen hospitals drug file. *Br Med J* 1989; **298:** 1253.
11. Lønning PE, *et al.* The influence of a graded dose schedule of aminoglutethimide on the disposition of the optical enantiomers of warfarin in patients with breast cancer. *Cancer Chemother Pharmacol* 1986; **17:** 177–81.
12. Bruning PF, Bonfrèr JGM. Aminoglutethimide and oral anticoagulant therapy. *Lancet* 1983; **ii:** 582.
13. Spiers ASD, Mibashan RS. Increased warfarin requirement during mercaptopurine therapy: a new drug interaction. *Lancet* 1974; **ii:** 221–2.
14. Cuddy PG, *et al.* Influence of mitotane on the hypoprothrombinemic effect of warfarin. *South Med J* 1986; **79:** 387–8.
15. Singleton JD, Conyers L. Warfarin and azathioprine: an important drug interaction. *Am J Med* 1992; **92:** 217.

Antiplatelets. The interaction between anticoagulants and *dipyridamole* is an oddity in that bleeding can occur without any alteration in prothrombin times; special care is therefore required as the usual method of monitoring the anticoagulant effect is of no value. This interaction has involved a small number of patients taking dipyridamole and warfarin or phenindione;[1] inhibition of platelet function by dipyridamole has been implicated. However, in general it does not appear to increase the risk of bleeding.[2]

Interestingly, in a group of patients receiving nicoumalone for thromboprophylaxis, addition of *ticlopidine* was found to significantly increase nicoumalone requirements.[3]

See also under Analgesics and NSAIDs (above).

1. Kalowski S, Kincaid-Smith P. Interaction of dipyridamole with anticoagulants in the treatment of glomerulonephritis. *Med J Aust* 1973; **2:** 164–6.
2. Levine MN, *et al.* Hemorrhagic complications of long-term anticoagulant therapy. *Chest* 1989; **95** (suppl): 26S–36S.
3. Salar A, *et al.* Ticlopidine antagonizes acenocoumarol treatment. *Thromb Haemost* 1997; **77:** 223–4.

Antiprotozoals. *Metronidazole* enhances the activity of warfarin[1,2] through selective inhibition of the metabolism of its *S*-isomer.[3]

1. Kazmier FJ. A significant interaction between metronidazole and warfarin. *Mayo Clin Proc* 1976; **51:** 782–4.
2. Dean RP, Talbert RL. Bleeding associated with concurrent warfarin and metronidazole therapy. *Drug Intell Clin Pharm* 1980; **14:** 864–6.
3. O'Reilly RA. The stereoselective interaction of warfarin and metronidazole in man. *N Engl J Med* 1976; **295:** 354–7.

Antithyroid drugs. See under Thyroid and Antithyroid Drugs, below.

Antivirals. Increased anticoagulation and serum-warfarin concentration necessitating a reduction in warfarin dosage has been noted[1] in a patient given *interferon alfa* for chronic hepatitis C. It was suggested the interaction may have been due to decreased metabolism of warfarin. A similar need for a reduced warfarin dose had also been noted by the authors in patients taking *interferon beta*.

An enhanced response to warfarin has been reported[2] in a patient taking *saquinavir* concomitantly. The mechanism may involve competitive inhibition of warfarin metabolism and might also occur with other HIV-protease inhibitors.

1. Adachi Y, *et al.* Potentiation of warfarin by interferon. *Br Med J* 1995; **311:** 292.
2. Darlington MR. Hypoprothrombinemia during concomitant therapy with warfarin and saquinavir. *Ann Pharmacother* 1997; **31:** 647.

Anxiolytic sedatives, hypnotics, and antipsychotics. *Barbiturates*, by inducing liver metabolism, can reduce the activity of anticoagulants; *glutethimide* has a similar action. The *benzodiazepines* on the other hand do not generally have any effect although there is the rare report of increased or decreased activity.

Although there is an early report suggesting that *chloral hydrate* may decrease the effect of dicoumarol by enzyme induction,[1] later studies and experience indicate an increase in the anticoagulant activity of warfarin.[2-4] However, the increase is only transient and is probably the result of displacement of warfarin from plasma protein binding sites by the metabolite trichloroacetic acid.[2] *Triclofos sodium* appears to increase the activity of warfarin in a similar way.[5]

Reduced anticoagulant activity has been reported with *dichloralphenazone*,[6,7] *ethchlorvynol* (with dicoumarol),[8] and *haloperidol* (with phenindione).[9] Compounds such as *meprobamate* and *methaqualone* appear to have no effect on anticoagulants.

1. Cucinell SA, *et al.* The effect of chloral hydrate on bishydroxycoumarin metabolism: a fatal outcome. *JAMA* 1966; **197:** 366–8.
2. Sellers EM, Koch-Weser J. Kinetics and clinical importance of displacement of warfarin from albumin by acidic drugs. *Ann N Y Acad Sci* 1971; **179:** 213–25.
3. Boston Collaborative Drug Surveillance Program. Interaction between chloral hydrate and warfarin. *N Engl J Med* 1972; **286:** 53–5.
4. Udall JA. Warfarin-chloral hydrate interaction: pharmacological activity and clinical significance. *Ann Intern Med* 1974; **81:** 341–4.
5. Sellers EM, *et al.* Enhancement of warfarin-induced hypoprothrombinemia by triclofos. *Clin Pharmacol Ther* 1972; **13:** 911–15.
6. Breckenridge A, Orme M. Clinical implications of enzyme induction. *Ann N Y Acad Sci* 1971; **179:** 421–3.
7. Whitfield JB, *et al.* Changes in plasma α-glutamyl transpeptidase activity associated with alterations in drug metabolism in man. *Br Med J* 1973; **1:** 316–18.
8. Johansson S-A. Apparent resistance to oral anticoagulant therapy and influence of hypnotics on some coagulation factors. *Acta Med Scand* 1968; **184:** 297–300.
9. Oakley DP, Lautch H. Haloperidol and anticoagulant treatment. *Lancet* 1963; **ii:** 1231.

Beta blockers. There is one report of possible potentiation of the effect of warfarin by *propranolol*.[1] Beta blockers, particularly those with a high lipid solubility such as propranolol, may inhibit the metabolism of warfarin.[2] However, although a number of studies have shown pharmacokinetic interactions between some beta blockers and oral anticoagulants, no effect on anticoagulant activity has been found.

1. Bax NDS, *et al.* Inhibition of drug metabolism by β-adrenoceptor antagonists. *Drugs* 1983; **25** (suppl 2): 121–6.
2. Mantero F, *et al.* Effect of atenolol and metoprolol on the anticoagulant activity of acenocoumarin. *Br J Clin Pharmacol* 1984; **17:** 94S–96S.

Central stimulants. While *methylphenidate hydrochloride* has been reported to increase the half-life of ethyl biscoumacetate,[1] it has also been reported to have no effect on the half-life or on the anticoagulant activity of ethyl biscoumacetate.[2] *Prolintane hydrochloride* also had no effect on ethyl biscoumacetate.[2]

1. Garrettson LK, *et al.* Methylphenidate interaction with both anticonvulsants and ethyl biscoumacetate: a new action of methylphenidate. *JAMA* 1969; **207:** 2053.
2. Hague DE, *et al.* The effect of methylphenidate and prolintane on the metabolism of ethyl biscoumacetate. *Clin Pharmacol Ther* 1971; **12:** 259–62.

Corticosteroids and corticotrophin. There are several early reports of corticosteroids or corticotrophin either enhancing[1] or diminishing[2] the effects of anticoagulants. Matters are further confused by corticosteroids being associated with an increase in the coagulability of the blood.

1. Van Cauwenberge H, Jaques LB. Haemorrhagic effect of ACTH with anticoagulants. *Can Med Assoc J* 1958; **79:** 536–40.
2. Chatterjea JB, Salomon L. Antagonistic effect of ACTH and cortisone on the anticoagulant activity of ethyl biscoumacetate. *Br Med J* 1954; **2:** 790–2.

Dermatological drugs. A patient's warfarin dose had to be increased when he started treatment with *etretinate*.[1]

1. Ostlere LS, *et al.* Reduced therapeutic effect of warfarin caused by etretinate. *Br J Dermatol* 1991; **124:** 505–10.

Disulfiram. Two isolated reports suggesting that disulfiram enhances the activity of warfarin[1,2] were confirmed by a study in 8 healthy subjects.[3] Although inhibition of liver enzymes by disulfiram was considered responsible,[3] a later study[4] suggested that disulfiram acts directly on the liver to increase hypoprothrombinaemia. This interaction is complicated by the variable effects of alcohol on warfarin (see above). Special care is therefore called for when these drugs are used together.

1. Rothstein E. Warfarin effect enhanced by disulfiram. *JAMA* 1968; **206:** 1574–5.
2. Rothstein E. Warfarin effect enhanced by disulfiram (Antabuse). *JAMA* 1972; **221:** 1052–3.
3. O'Reilly RA. Interaction of sodium warfarin and disulfiram (Antabuse®) in man. *Ann Intern Med* 1973; **78:** 73–6.
4. O'Reilly RA. Dynamic interaction between disulfiram and separated enantiomorphs of racemic warfarin. *Clin Pharmacol Ther* 1981; **29:** 332–6.

Diuretics. There have been a number of studies on the effects of diuretics on anticoagulants. *Tienilic acid* produces the most serious interaction enhancing the activity of ethyl biscoumacetate,[1] nicoumalone,[2] and warfarin[3] and has led to haemorrhage; considerable care is obviously required if tienilic acid is used with an anticoagulant. *Ethacrynic acid* has also been reported to enhance the activity of warfarin,[4] but reports do not show as severe an effect as with tienilic acid.

Chlorthalidone[5] and *spironolactone*[6] have both been associated with a reduction in warfarin's activity in healthy subjects and it has been suggested that this might be a consequence of the diuresis concentrating the circulating clotting factors. However, *bumetanide, frusemide*, and the *thiazides* appear to have no effect on warfarin.

1. Detilleux M, *et al.* Potentialisation de l'effet des anticoagulants coumariniques par un nouveau diurétique, l'acide tiénilique. *Nouv Presse Med* 1976; **5:** 2395.
2. Grand A, *et al.* Potentialisation de l'action anticoagulante des anti-vitamines K par l'acide tiénilique. *Nouv Presse Med* 1977; **6:** 2691.
3. McLain DA, *et al.* Adverse reactions associated with ticrynafen use. *JAMA* 1980; **243:** 763–4.
4. Petrick RJ, *et al.* Interaction between warfarin and ethacrynic acid. *JAMA* 1975; **231:** 843–4.
5. O'Reilly RA, *et al.* Impact of aspirin and chlorthalidone on the pharmacodynamics of oral anticoagulant drugs in man. *Ann N Y Acad Sci* 1971; **179:** 173–86.
6. O'Reilly RA. Spironolactone and warfarin interaction. *Clin Pharmacol Ther* 1980; **27:** 198–201.

Gastro-intestinal drugs. Antacids may or may not interact with warfarin. *Bismuth carbonate* and *magnesium trisilicate* for example have been reported to reduce warfarin's absorption,[1] but *aluminium hydroxide* has been observed to have no effect on warfarin or dicoumarol.[2] *Psyllium*[3] and *magnesium hydroxide*[2] have also been reported to have no effect on warfarin, but the latter has increased the plasma concentrations of dicoumarol.[2]

There have been occasional reports of *sucralfate* diminishing the effect of warfarin.[4-6]

Histamine H_2-antagonists have been much studied. There are several reports indicating that *cimetidine* can enhance the anticoagulant effect of warfarin and haemorrhage has occurred. A number of studies show that cimetidine can increase the plasma concentration and half-life of warfarin and that there is a selective inhibitory effect on the metabolism of its *R*-isomer.[7-10] Not all these studies have, however, demonstrated an increase in prothrombin time. The effect of cimetidine on warfarin appears to be dose-dependent[7] and to be subject to interindividual variation;[9,10] the need for careful monitoring of patients receiving both drugs is, therefore, evident. Limited evidence suggests that cimetidine has a similar effect on the metabolism of nicoumalone[11,12] and phenindione[11] but not of phenprocoumon.[13] Studies with *ranitidine* have generally been unable to demonstrate an effect on the metabolism of warfarin,[10,14] although in one study warfarin clearance was reduced.[7] There is one case report suggesting that potentiation of warfarin by ranitidine may occasionally occur.[15]

One study has suggested that *omeprazole* could inhibit the metabolism of *R*-warfarin although a clinically significant effect on the activity of warfarin was unlikely.[16] Similarly, *pantoprazole* appears to have no effect on the pharmacokinetics or pharmacodynamics of warfarin.[17]

A marked increase in the effect of warfarin has been reported in one patient when *cisapride* was added to his therapy.[18]

A reduction in the response to warfarin with development of venous thrombosis has been reported in a patient receiving *mesalazine*.[19]

1. McElnay JC, *et al.* Interaction of warfarin with antacid constituents. *Br Med J* 1978; **2:** 1166.
2. Ambre JJ, Fischer LJ. Effect of coadministration of aluminum and magnesium hydroxides on absorption of anticoagulants in man. *Clin Pharmacol Ther* 1973; **14:** 231–7.
3. Robinson DS, *et al.* Interaction of warfarin and nonsystemic gastrointestinal drugs. *Clin Pharmacol Ther* 1971; **12:** 491–5.
4. Mungall D, *et al.* Sucralfate and warfarin. *Ann Intern Med* 1983; **98:** 557.
5. Rey AM, Gums JG. Altered absorption of digoxin, sustained-release quinidine, and warfarin with sucralfate administration. *DICP Ann Pharmacother* 1991; **25:** 745–6.
6. Parrish RH, *et al.* Sucralfate-warfarin interaction. *Ann Pharmacother* 1992; **26:** 1015–16.
7. Desmond PV, *et al.* Decreased oral warfarin clearance after ranitidine and cimetidine. *Clin Pharmacol Ther* 1984; **35:** 338–41.
8. Choonara IA, *et al.* Stereoselective interaction between the R enantiomer of warfarin and cimetidine. *Br J Clin Pharmacol* 1986; **21:** 271–7.
9. Sax MJ, *et al.* Effect of two cimetidine regimens on prothrombin time and warfarin pharmacokinetics during long-term warfarin therapy. *Clin Pharm* 1987; **6:** 492–5.
10. Toon S, *et al.* Comparative effects of ranitidine and cimetidine on the pharmacokinetics and pharmacodynamics of warfarin in man. *Eur J Clin Pharmacol* 1987; **32:** 165–72.
11. Serlin MJ, *et al.* Cimetidine: interaction with oral anticoagulants in man. *Lancet* 1979; **ii:** 317–19.
12. Gill TS, *et al.* Cimetidine-nicoumalone interaction in man: stereochemical considerations. *Br J Clin Pharmacol* 1989; **27:** 469–74.
13. Harenberg J, *et al.* Cimetidine does not increase the anticoagulant effect of phenprocoumon. *Br J Clin Pharmacol* 1982; **14:** 292–3.
14. Serlin MJ, *et al.* Lack of effect of ranitidine on warfarin action. *Br J Clin Pharmacol* 1981; **12:** 791–4.
15. Baciewicz AM, Morgan PJ. Ranitidine-warfarin interaction. *Ann Intern Med* 1990; **112:** 76–7.
16. Sutfin T, *et al.* Stereoselective interaction of omeprazole with warfarin in healthy men. *Ther Drug Monit* 1989; **11:** 176–84.
17. Duursema L, *et al.* Lack of effect of pantoprazole on the pharmacodynamics and pharmacokinetics of warfarin. *Br J Clin Pharmacol* 1995; **39:** 700–3.
18. Darlington MR. Hypoprothrombinemia induced by warfarin sodium and cisapride. *Am J Health-Syst Pharm* 1997; **54:** 320–1.
19. Marinella MA. Mesalamine and warfarin therapy resulting in decreased warfarin effect. *Ann Pharmacother* 1998; **32:** 841–2.

Ginseng. Reduction in the response to warfarin was reported in a patient after he started taking a ginseng preparation.[1]

1. Janetzky K, Morreale AP. Probable interaction between warfarin and ginseng. *Am J Health-Syst Pharm* 1997; **54:** 692–3.

Glucagon. A dose-dependent enhancement of warfarin's anticoagulant activity has been reported with glucagon.[1]

1. Koch-Weser J. Potentiation by glucagon of the hypoprothrombinemic action of warfarin. *Ann Intern Med* 1970; **72:** 331–5.

Levamisole. An increased INR has been reported[1] in one patient receiving chronic warfarin therapy after addition of *levamisole* and fluorouracil. Inhibition of warfarin metabolism was postulated as the mechanism responsible for the interaction. In a second patient, a similar reaction was reported[2] following administration of levamisole and fluorouracil and an episode of bleeding subsequently occurred after administration of levamisole alone.

1. Scarfe MA, Israel MK. Possible drug interaction between warfarin and combination of levamisole and fluorouracil. *Ann Pharmacother* 1994; **28:** 464–7.
2. Wehbe TW, Warth JA. A case of bleeding requiring hospitalization that was likely caused by an interaction between warfarin and levamisole. *Clin Pharmacol Ther* 1996; **59:** 360–2.

Lipid regulating drugs. *Clofibrate* can enhance the activity of warfarin, sometimes to the point of haemorrhage. The mechanism of this interaction is not clear, but it does not appear to be connected with any pharmacokinetic effect. Similar enhancement of activity has been reported when clofibrate is given to patients taking dicoumarol or phenindione. *Bezafibrate* has been reported to enhance the effect of phenprocoumon,[1] and *fenofibrate*[2] and *gemfibrozil*[3] have been reported to enhance the effect of warfarin.

Hypoprothrombinaemia and bleeding has been reported in 2 patients on warfarin given *lovastatin*.[4] An increased response to warfarin has also been reported[5,6] in a number of patients receiving *fluvastatin* concomitantly. The manufacturers of *simvastatin* state that it has slightly enhanced the effect of warfarin in healthy subjects. Simvastatin has been reported[7] to potentiate the effect of nicoumalone in one patient. However, the INR in a patient on long-term warfarin remained stable on the addition of treatment with simvastatin.[8] The manufacturers of *pravastatin* have not observed any change in warfarin activity in patients given both drugs. However, there has been a report[9] of bleeding in a patient receiving fluindione when pravastatin was added.

Dextrothyroxine increases the anticoagulant effect of warfarin sodium[10,11] and dicoumarol.[12]

An opposite effect may occur with *cholestyramine* which has reduced warfarin's serum concentration[13] and half-life[14] as well as its activity.[13,14] The mechanisms of this interaction include binding of warfarin to cholestyramine and reduced absorption;[13] the enterohepatic recycling of warfarin may also be interrupted.[14] Phenprocoumon's activity has also been reduced by cholestyramine.[15] It should be remembered, however, that cholestyramine can also reduce vitamin K absorption, which may result in hypoprothrombinaemia and bleeding.

Benfluorex[16] and *colestipol*[17] have been reported not to interact with phenprocoumon.

1. Zimmermann R, *et al.* The effect of bezafibrate on the fibrinolytic enzyme system and the drug interaction with racemic phenprocoumon. *Atherosclerosis* 1978; **29:** 477–85.
2. Ascah KJ, *et al.* Interaction between fenofibrate and warfarin. *Ann Pharmacother* 1998; **32:** 765–8.
3. Ahmad S. Gemfibrozil interaction with warfarin sodium (Coumadin). *Chest* 1990; **98:** 1041–2.
4. Ahmad S. Lovastatin: warfarin interaction. *Arch Intern Med* 1990; **150:** 2407.
5. Trilli LE, *et al.* Potential interaction between warfarin and fluvastatin. *Ann Pharmacother* 1996; **30:** 1399–1402.
6. Kline SS, Harrell CC. Potential warfarin-fluvastatin interaction. *Ann Pharmacother* 1997; **31:** 790–1.
7. Grau E, *et al.* Simvastatin-oral anticoagulant interaction. *Lancet* 1996; **347:** 405–6.
8. Gaw A, Wosornu D. Simvastatin during warfarin therapy in hyperlipoproteinaemia. *Lancet* 1992; **340:** 979–80.
9. Trenque T, *et al.* Pravastatin: interaction with oral anticoagulant? *Br Med J* 1996; **312:** 886.
10. Owens JC, *et al.* Effect of sodium dextrothyroxine in patients receiving anticoagulants. *N Engl J Med* 1962; **266:** 76–9.
11. Solomon HM, Schrogie JJ. Change in receptor site affinity: a proposed explanation for the potentiating effect of D-thyroxine on the anticoagulant response to warfarin. *Clin Pharmacol Ther* 1967; **8:** 797–9.
12. Schrogie JJ, Solomon HM. The anticoagulant response to bishydroxycoumarin: II The effect of D-thyroxine, clofibrate, and norethandrolone. *Clin Pharmacol Ther* 1967; **8:** 70–7.
13. Robinson DS, *et al.* Interaction of warfarin and nonsystemic gastrointestinal drugs. *Clin Pharmacol Ther* 1971; **12:** 491–5.
14. Jähnchen E, *et al.* Enhanced elimination of warfarin during treatment with cholestyramine. *Br J Clin Pharmacol* 1978; **5:** 437–40.
15. Meinertz T, *et al.* Interruption of the enterohepatic circulation of phenprocoumon by cholestyramine. *Clin Pharmacol Ther* 1977; **21:** 731–5.
16. De Witte P, Brems HM. Co-administration of benfluorex with oral anticoagulant therapy. *Curr Med Res Opin* 1980; **6:** 478–80.
17. Harvengt C, Desager JP. Effect of colestipol, a new bile acid sequestrant, on the absorption of phenprocoumon in man. *Eur J Clin Pharmacol* 1973; **6:** 19–21.

Pesticides. Chlorinated insecticides have been reported to diminish the activity of warfarin in one patient.[1]

1. Jeffery WH, *et al.* Loss of warfarin effect after occupational insecticide exposure. *JAMA* 1976; **236:** 2881–2.

Piracetam. Piracetam caused an increase in prothrombin time in one patient who had been stabilised on warfarin.[1]

1. Pan HYM, Ng RP. The effect of Nootropil in a patient on warfarin. *Eur J Clin Pharmacol* 1983; **24:** 711.

Prostaglandins. A study in 13 healthy subjects has suggested that *rioprostil* may decrease the anticoagulant activity of nicoumalone and phenprocoumon.[1] The interaction did not appear to have a pharmacokinetic mechanism.

1. Thijssen HHW, Hamulyàk K. The interaction of the prostaglandin E derivative rioprostil with oral anticoagulant agents. *Clin Pharmacol Ther* 1989; **46:** 110–16.

Sex hormones. There have been a number of reports of steroids with anabolic or androgenic properties enhancing the activity of anticoagulants to the point of haemorrhage. Reports have covered *oxymetholone* enhancing warfarin[1-3] and nicoumalone;[4] *stanozolol* enhancing warfarin[5,6] and dicoumarol;[7] *ethyloestrenol* enhancing phenindione;[8] *norethandrolone* enhancing dicoumarol;[9] *methyltestosterone* enhancing phenprocoumon;[10] and *danazol* enhancing warfarin.[11-13] The mechanism of this interaction is not clear although it is considered that it is not due to altered pharmacokinetics. Steroids with a 17-α-alkyl substituent appear to be most involved, but there has been a report of topically applied testosterone, which does not have such a substituent, enhancing warfarin.[14]

Oral contraceptives have also been implicated in interactions. However, while the effects of dicoumarol were diminished by an oestrogen progestogen mixture,[15] those of nicoumalone were enhanced by other oestrogen and progestogen preparations.[16] Oestrogen progestogen contraceptives have increased the clearance of phenprocoumon without altering the anticoagulant effect.[17]

1. Robinson BHB, *et al.* Decreased anticoagulant tolerance with oxymetholone. *Lancet* 1971; **i:** 1356.
2. Longridge RGM, *et al.* Decreased anticoagulant tolerance with oxymetholone. *Lancet* 1971; **ii:** 90.
3. Edwards MS, Curtis JR. Decreased anticoagulant tolerance with oxymetholone. *Lancet* 1971; **ii:** 221.
4. de Oya JC, *et al.* Decreased anticoagulant tolerance with oxymetholone in paroxysmal nocturnal haemoglobinuria. *Lancet* 1971; **ii:** 259.
5. Acomb C, Shaw PW. A significant interaction between warfarin and stanozolol. *Pharm J* 1985; **234:** 73–4.
6. Shaw PW, Smith AM. Possible interaction of warfarin and stanozolol. *Clin Pharm* 1987; **6:** 500–2.
7. Howard W, *et al.* Anabolic steroids and anticoagulants. *Br Med J* 1977; **1:** 1659–60.
8. Vere DW, Fearnley GR. Suspected interaction between phenindione and ethyloestrenol. *Lancet* 1968; **ii:** 281.
9. Schrogie JJ, Solomon HM. The anticoagulant response to bishydroxycoumarin: II The effect of D-thyroxine, clofibrate, and norethandrolone. *Clin Pharmacol Ther* 1967; **8:** 70–7.
10. Husted S, *et al.* Increased sensitivity to phenprocoumon during methyltestosterone therapy. *Eur J Clin Pharmacol* 1976; **10:** 209–16.
11. Goulbourne IA, Macleod DAD. An interaction between danazol and warfarin: case report. *Br J Obstet Gynaecol* 1981; **88:** 950–1.
12. Meeks ML, *et al.* Danazol increases the anticoagulant effect of warfarin. *Ann Pharmacother* 1992; **26:** 641–2.
13. Booth CD. A drug interaction between danazol and warfarin. *Pharm J* 1993; **250:** 439–40.
14. Lorentz SMcQ, Weibert RT. Potentiation of warfarin anticoagulation by topical testosterone ointment. *Clin Pharm* 1985; **4:** 332–4.
15. Schrogie JJ, *et al.* Effect of oral contraceptives on vitamin K-dependent clotting activity. *Clin Pharmacol Ther* 1967; **8:** 670–5.
16. de Teresa E, *et al.* Interaction between anticoagulants and contraceptives: an unsuspected finding. *Br Med J* 1979; **2:** 1260–1.
17. Mönig H, *et al.* Effect of oral contraceptive steroids on the pharmacokinetics of phenprocoumon. *Br J Clin Pharmacol* 1990; **30:** 115–18.

Thyroid and antithyroid drugs. Since response to oral anticoagulants is dependent on thyroid status an interaction between oral anticoagulants and thyroid or antithyroid drugs might be expected. Thyroid compounds do enhance the activity of oral anticoagulants possibly by increased metabolism of clotting factors. Dextrothyroxine is discussed under Lipid Regulating Drugs, above. Antithyroid compounds have not, however, been reported to diminish the effect of anticoagulants and paradoxically *propylthiouracil* has been reported to have caused hypoprothrombinaemia (see p.1491).

Tobacco smoking. Although tobacco smoking may increase warfarin clearance,[1] an appreciable effect on anticoagulant activity appears unlikely.[1,2]

1. Bachmann K, *et al.* Smoking and warfarin disposition. *Clin Pharmacol Ther* 1979; **25:** 309–15.
2. Weiner B, *et al.* Warfarin dosage following prosthetic valve replacement: effect of smoking history. *Drug Intell Clin Pharm* 1984; **18:** 904–6.

Ubidecarenone. Decreased INR values and reduced effect of warfarin has been reported[1] in 3 patients after the addition of ubidecarenone to their therapy.

1. Spigset O. Reduced effect of warfarin caused by ubidecarenone. *Lancet* 1994; **344:** 1372–3.

Vaccines. There have been a few reports of increased prothrombin time and bleeding in warfarin-stabilised patients following *influenza vaccination*. Studies investigating this possible interaction have found only a small or inconsistent increase in warfarin activity[1,2] or no effect.[3-5] One study suggested that influenza vaccine decreases rather than increases the prothrombin time.[6] In a group of patients on long-term nicoumalone therapy, influenza vaccination had no effect on nicoumalone activity.[7]

1. Kramer P, *et al.* Effect of influenza vaccine on warfarin anticoagulation. *Clin Pharmacol Ther* 1984; **35:** 416–18.
2. Weibert RT, *et al.* Effect on influenza vaccine in patients receiving long-term warfarin therapy. *Clin Pharm* 1986; **5:** 499–503.
3. Lipsky BA, *et al.* Influenza vaccination and warfarin anticoagulation. *Ann Intern Med* 1984; **100:** 835–7.
4. Scott AK, *et al.* Lack of effect of influenza vaccination on warfarin in healthy volunteers. *Br J Clin Pharmacol* 1985; **19:** 144P–145P.
5. Gomolin IH. Lack of effect of influenza vaccine on warfarin anticoagulation in the elderly. *Can Med Assoc J* 1986; **135:** 39–41.
6. Bussey HI, Saklad JJ. Effect of influenza vaccine on chronic warfarin therapy. *Drug Intell Clin Pharm* 1988; **22:** 198–201.
7. Souto JC, *et al.* Lack of effect of influenza vaccine on anticoagulation by acenocoumarol. *Ann Pharmacother* 1993; **27:** 365–8.

Vitamins. Since vitamin K reverses the effects of oral anticoagulants, it is not surprising that there have been reports of *acetomenaphthone* and *phytomenadione* reducing anticoagulant activity, or of foods or nutritional preparations containing vitamin K compounds doing the same.

Occasional reports of *ascorbic acid* reducing the activity of warfarin[1,2] have not been confirmed in subsequent studies.[3,4] There have also been isolated reports suggesting that *vitamin E* may enhance the activity of warfarin[5] or dicoumarol.[6]

1. Rosenthal G. Interaction of ascorbic acid and warfarin. *JAMA* 1971; **215:** 1671.
2. Smith EC, *et al.* Interaction of ascorbic acid and warfarin. *JAMA* 1972; **221:** 1166.
3. Hume R, *et al.* Interaction of ascorbic acid and warfarin. *JAMA* 1972; **219:** 1479.
4. Feetam CL, *et al.* Lack of clinically important interaction between warfarin and ascorbic acid. *Toxicol Appl Pharmacol* 1975; **31:** 544–7.
5. Corrigan JJ, Marcus FI. Coagulopathy associated with vitamin E ingestion. *JAMA* 1974; **230:** 1300–1.
6. Schrogie JJ. Coagulopathy and fat-soluble vitamins. *JAMA* 1975; **232:** 19.

Pharmacokinetics

Warfarin sodium is readily absorbed from the gastro-intestinal tract; it can also be absorbed through the skin. It is extensively bound to plasma proteins and its plasma half-life is about 37 hours. It crosses the placenta but does not occur in significant quantities in breast milk. Warfarin is administered as a racemic mixture; the *S*-isomer is reported to be more potent. The *R*- and *S*-isomers are both metabolised in the liver, the *S*-isomer more rapidly than the *R*-isomer; the stereo-isomers may also be affected differently by other drugs (see Interactions, above). Metabolites, with negligible or no anticoagulant activity, are excreted in the urine following reabsorption from the bile.

References.

1. Mungall DR, *et al.* Population pharmacokinetics of racemic warfarin in adult patients. *J Pharmacokinet Biopharm* 1985; **13:** 213–27.
2. Holford NHG. Clinical pharmacokinetics and pharmacodynamics of warfarin: understanding the dose-effect relationship. *Clin Pharmacokinet* 1986; **11:** 483–504.

Uses and Administration

Warfarin is a coumarin anticoagulant used in the treatment and prophylaxis of thrombo-embolic disorders (p.801). It acts by depressing the hepatic vitamin K-dependent synthesis of coagulation factors II (prothrombin), VII, IX, and X, and of the anticoagulant protein C and its cofactor protein S. For an explanation of the coagulation cascade, see p.704. Since warfarin acts indirectly, it has no effect on existing clots. Also as the coagulation factors involved have half-lives ranging from 6 to 60 hours, several hours are required before an effect is observed. A therapeutic effect is usually apparent by 24 hours, but the peak effect may not be achieved until 2 or 3 days after a dose; the overall effect may last for 5 days.

Warfarin is used in the prevention and treatment of venous thrombo-embolism (deep-vein thrombosis and pulmonary embolism, p.802). If an immediate effect on blood coagulation is required, heparin should be given intravenously or subcutaneously to cover the first 2 to 3 days. Warfarin therapy may be initiated concomitantly with or shortly after the initial heparin treatment. Warfarin is also used for the prevention of systemic thrombo-embolism and ischaemic stroke in some patients with atrial fibrillation (p.782), prosthetic heart valves (p.801), or who have suffered a myocardial infarction (p.791). It may also have a role in the prevention of recurrent myocardial infarction and in the management of stroke or transient ischaemic attacks (p.799). Antiplatelet drugs may be given concomitantly.

Some patients may show a hereditary resistance to warfarin. Warfarin is a potent rodenticide although resistance has been reported in *rats*.

Administration and dosage. Warfarin is equally effective either orally or intravenously, but is usually given by mouth. Dosage must be determined individually as discussed below under Control of Anticoagulant Therapy. A usual initial dose of warfarin sodium is 10 mg daily by mouth for 2 days, but may be lower for patients at particular risk of haemorrhage (see Precautions, above). Subsequent maintenance doses usually range from 3 to 9 mg daily. If necessary the same dose may be given by slow intravenous injection. Doses of warfarin sodium should be given at the same time each day. Theoretically sudden discontinuation of warfarin may result in rebound hypercoagulability with risk of thrombosis. Therefore some clinicians tail off long-term treatment over several weeks but the need for this is unclear. Anticoagulant treatment booklets should be carried by patients.

Warfarin has also been given as the potassium salt; warfarin-deanol has been tried.

Control of Oral Anticoagulant Therapy. Treatment with oral anticoagulants must be monitored to ensure that the dose is providing the required effect on the vitamin-K-dependent clotting factors; too small a dose provides inadequate anticoagulation, too large a dose puts the patient at risk of haemorrhage. This monitoring is commonly carried out by checking the clotting property of the patient's plasma using a suitable preparation of thromboplastin and a source of calcium. The time taken for the clot to form due to the effect of the thromboplastin preparation on prothrombin is known as the prothrombin time (PT). The prothrombin time ratio (PTR) is the prothrombin time of the patient's plasma divided by that for a standard plasma sample.

So that there is some consistency in prothrombin time ratios measured at different times or at different laboratories, it is now common practice for the manufacturer or control laboratory to calibrate their batches of thromboplastin against the international reference preparation. This calibration produces an international sensitivity index (ISI) appropriate to that thromboplastin. The laboratory measuring the clotting capacity of a sample of plasma is thus able to convert the prothrombin time ratio to an international normalised ratio (INR) using the sensitivity index through the formula

$$INR = PTR^{(ISI)}$$

Thus a prothrombin time ratio of 2.0 obtained with a thromboplastin with a declared international sensitivity index of 1.5 would be converted to an international normalised ratio of 2.8. An international normalised ratio is therefore equivalent to a prothrombin time ratio carried out using the primary international reference preparation of thromboplastin.

This method of standardisation has taken over from methods involving use of a standard reagent such as the British or Manchester comparative thromboplastin. Also preparations of thromboplastin derived from *rabbit* brain have superseded or are superseding those from human brain because of the dangers of viral transmission.

Recommended target values or ranges of international normalised ratio for patients receiving anticoagulant treatment or cover for various conditions or procedures are given by the British Society for Haematology in the UK and the American College of Chest Physicians and the National Heart, Lung and Blood Institute in the USA. These are given in Table 2, below. An INR within 0.5 units of the target value is generally considered satisfactory. An INR less than 2.0 represents inadequate anticoagulation and an INR greater than 4.5 represents risk of haemorrhage.

Measurements should be carried out before treatment and then daily or on alternate days in the early stages of treatment. Once the dose has been established and the patient well stabilised the measurement can be made at greater but regular intervals, for example every 8 weeks; allowances should be made for any events that might influence the activity of the anticoagulant.

General references to anticoagulation with warfarin sodium.

1. Fennerty A, *et al.* Flexible induction dose regimen for warfarin and prediction of maintenance dose. *Br Med J* 1984; **288:** 1268–70.
2. Scott AK. Warfarin usage: can safety be improved? *Pharmacol Ther* 1989; **42:** 429–57.
3. John RM, Swanton RH. Anticoagulants in cardiovascular diseases. *Br J Hosp Med* 1990; **43:** 207–14.
4. Harrington R, Ansell J. Risk-benefit assessment of anticoagulant therapy. *Drug Safety* 1991; **6:** 54–69.
5. Le DT, *et al.* The international normalized ratio (INR) for monitoring warfarin therapy: reliability and relation to other monitoring methods. *Ann Intern Med* 1994; **120:** 552–8.
6. Fihn SD. Aiming for safe anticoagulation. *N Engl J Med* 1995; **333:** 54–5.
7. Hirsh J, Fuster V. Guide to anticoagulants therapy part 2: oral anticoagulants. *Circulation* 1994; **89:** 1469–80.
8. Hirsh J, *et al.* Oral anticoagulants: mechanism of action, clinical effectiveness, and optimal therapeutic range. *Chest* 1995; **108** (suppl): 231S–246S.
9. Routledge PA. Practical prescribing: warfarin. *Prescribers' J* 1997; **37:** 173–9.
10. British Society for Haematology: British Committee for Standards in Haematology—Haemostasis and Thrombosis Task Force. Guidelines on oral anticoagulation: third edition. *Br J Haematol* 1998; **101:** 374–87.

Table 2. Recommended International Normalised Ratios (INR).

	INR	Condition or procedure
UK	2.5	Pulmonary embolism; deep-vein thrombosis; recurrence of venous thrombo-embolism when no longer on warfarin; symptomatic inherited thrombophilia; atrial fibrillation; cardioversion; mural thrombus; cardiomyopathy.
	3.5	Recurrence of venous thrombo-embolism when on warfarin; antiphospholipid syndrome; mechanical prosthetic heart valves.
US	2.0 to 3.0	Prophylaxis of venous thrombo-embolism in high-risk surgical patients; treatment of venous thrombosis and pulmonary embolism; prophylaxis of systemic embolism in patients with atrial fibrillation, valvular heart disease, bioprosthetic heart valves, or acute myocardial infarction.
	2.5 to 3.5	Prophylaxis in patients with mechanical prosthetic heart valves; prevention of recurrent myocardial infarction.

Action. In a review of warfarin Wessler and Gitel[1] concisely discuss its actions. Before their release into the circulation, factors II, VII, IX, and X are altered by conversion of glutamic acid residues to γ-carboxyglutamic acid residues so that they can bind to phospholipids for activation. Warfarin by inhibiting vitamin K blocks the carboxylation system, so decreasing this binding to phospholipids. Warfarin can also influence the release of proteins deficient in γ-carboxyglutamic acid, although it is not clear how this affects its antithrombotic activity.

Wessler and Gitel comment that warfarin can increase the rate at which plasma inhibits clotting proteases as measured by the rate of factor Xa inhibition. One of the main plasma protease inhibitors is antithrombin III. However, while Winter and Douglas[2] cite studies showing an increase in antithrombin III, they cite other references that show no such increase.

Warfarin also affects protein C and protein S, two other vitamin-K-dependent proteins in the coagulation sequence.[1] Protein C inhibits coagulation factors V and VIII and is augmented by protein S. Warfarin is thus blocking an anticoagulant process and could initially produce a potentially thrombotic state. Depression of protein C has been linked to warfarin-induced skin necrosis (see Effects on the Skin under Adverse Effects, above).

1. Wessler S, Gitel SN. Warfarin: from bedside to bench. *N Engl J Med* 1984; **311:** 645–52.
2. Winter JH, Douglas AS. Familial venous thrombosis. *Postgrad Med J* 1983; **59:** 677–89.

Catheters and cannulas. For mention of the use of oral anticoagulants to prevent thrombosis in patients with indwelling infusion devices, see Heparin Sodium, p.882.

Connective tissue and muscular disorders. For mention of the possible use of low-dose warfarin to treat subcutaneous calcium deposition (calcinosis cutis) in patients with dermatomyositis, see Polymyositis and Dermatomyositis, p.1027.

Preparations

BP 1998: Warfarin Tablets;
USP 23: Warfarin Sodium for Injection; Warfarin Sodium Tablets.

Proprietary Preparations (details are given in Part 3)
Austral.: Coumadin; Marevan; ***Belg.:*** Marevan; ***Canad.:*** Coumadin; Warfilone; ***Fr.:*** Coumadine; ***Ger.:*** Coumadin; ***Ital.:*** Coumadin; ***Norw.:*** Marevan; ***S.Afr.:*** Coumadin†; ***Spain:*** Aldocumar; ***Swed.:*** Waran; ***UK:*** Marevan; ***USA:*** Coumadin; Panwarfin†.

Xamoterol Fumarate (17133-q)

Xamoterol Fumarate *(BANM, USAN, rINNM).*

ICI-118587. N-{2-[2-Hydroxy-3-(4-hydroxyphenoxy)propylamino]ethyl}morpholine-4-carboxamide fumarate.

$(C_{16}H_{25}N_3O_5)_2.C_4H_4O_4 = 794.8.$

CAS — 81801-12-9 (xamoterol); 90730-93-1 (xamoterol fumarate).

Xamoterol fumarate 1.17 mg is approximately equivalent to 1 mg of xamoterol.

Adverse Effects

Xamoterol has been associated with gastro-intestinal side-effects, headache, dizziness, chest pain, palpitations, rash, and muscle cramp.

Bronchospasm, worsening of obstructive airways disease, and hypotension have occurred and may be related to the partial activity of xamoterol as a beta blocker.

Xamoterol has been studied in patients with varying degrees of heart failure but following deterioration and an excess of deaths in those with severe heart failure[1] the licensed indication has been restricted to the treatment of chronic mild heart failure (see under Precautions and under Uses and Administration, below).

1. The Xamoterol in Severe Heart Failure Study Group. Xamoterol in severe heart failure. *Lancet* 1990; **336:** 1–6.

Precautions

Xamoterol is contra-indicated in moderate or severe heart failure because of deterioration during xamoterol therapy. It is also contra-indicated in patients with the following signs or symptoms: shortness of breath or fatigue at rest or on minimal exercise; resting tachycardia or hypotension; acute pulmonary oedema or a history of this condition; peripheral oedema, raised jugular venous pressure, enlarged liver, or third heart sound; need for diuretic therapy equivalent to more than frusemide 40 mg daily; and need for therapy with an ACE inhibitor. If a patient with mild heart failure deteriorates while receiving xamoterol therapy, the drug should be withdrawn.

As with other $beta_1$ agonist sympathomimetics used to increase the force of myocardial contraction xamoterol may exacerbate outflow obstruction in hypertrophic subaortic stenosis. Caution is also required in patients with pre-existing cardiac arrhythmias. Xamoterol is subject to renal excretion and dosage adjustment may be necessary in renal impairment (see Uses and Administration, below).

Xamoterol should be used with caution in patients with obstructive airways disease such as asthma because of its partial effect as a beta blocker.

Interactions

For the interactions of sympathomimetics in general see p.951.

Pharmacokinetics

Xamoterol is poorly absorbed from the gastro-intestinal tract with a bioavailability of only about 5%. It undergoes some metabolism to inactive sulphate conjugates and is excreted mainly in the urine as unchanged drug and metabolites. The half-life has been reported to be around 16 hours.

References.

1. Nicholls DP, *et al.* The pharmacokinetics of xamoterol in liver disease. *Br J Clin Pharmacol* 1989; **28:** 718–21.

2. Marlow HF, *et al.* Relationship between positive inotropic responses and plasma concentrations of xamoterol in middle-aged and elderly patients. *Br J Clin Pharmacol* 1990; **29:** 511–18.

Uses and Administration

Xamoterol is a beta-adrenoceptor partial agonist with a selective action on $beta_1$ receptors (see Actions of Sympathomimetics under Adrenaline, p.815). As a partial agonist it exerts predominantly agonist activity at rest and under conditions of low sympathetic drive which results in improved ventricular function and increased cardiac output; during exercise and during conditions of increased sympathetic drive, such as that occurring in severe heart failure, xamoterol exerts beta-blocking activity.

Xamoterol is used in chronic mild heart failure (p.785) in patients who are not breathless at rest but are limited by symptoms on exertion; it is not suitable for use in patients with moderate to severe heart failure. Xamoterol has been used in orthostatic hypotension secondary to autonomic failure (p.1040).

Xamoterol is used as the fumarate although doses are expressed in terms of the equivalent amount of xamoterol. The recommended initial dose for adults is 200 mg of xamoterol daily by mouth for the first week, increased to 200 mg twice daily depending on response. A dose of 200 mg daily may be sufficient in renal impairment.

References.

1. Anonymous. Xamoterol—more trouble than it's worth? *Drug Ther Bull* 1990; **28:** 53–4.

2. Anonymous. New evidence on xamoterol. *Lancet* 1990; **336:** 24.

Preparations

Proprietary Preparations (details are given in Part 3)

Aust.: Corwil; ***Belg.:*** Corwin; ***UK:*** Corwin.

Xanthinol Nicotinate (9285-d)

Xanthinol Nicotinate *(BAN).*

Xantinol Nicotinate *(rINN)*; SK-331A; Xanthinol Niacinate *(USAN)*. 7-{2-Hydroxy-3-[(2-hydroxyethyl)methylamino]propyl}theophylline nicotinate.

$C_{13}H_{21}N_5O_4,C_6H_5NO_2$ = 434.4.

CAS — 437-74-1.

Pharmacopoeias. In *Pol.*

Xanthinol nicotinate is a vasodilator with general properties similar to those of nicotinic acid (p.1351), to which it is slowly hydrolysed. It is used in the management of peripheral (p.794) and cerebral vascular disorders (p.785) and in hyperlipidaemias (p.1265). Doses of up to 3 g daily may be given by mouth. It has also been given by intramuscular or slow intravenous injection.

Preparations

Proprietary Preparations (details are given in Part 3)

Aust.: Complamin; Frigol; ***Belg.:*** Complamin; ***Canad.:*** Complamin; ***Ger.:*** Complamin; Complamin spezial; ***Ital.:*** Complamin; Vedrin; ***Neth.:*** Complamin; ***Swed.:*** Complamin; ***Switz.:*** Complamin.

Multi-ingredient: ***Spain:*** Duvaline Compositum†; Plasmaclar; Rulun.

Xemilofiban Hydrochloride (18566-k)

Xemilofiban Hydrochloride *(USAN, rINNM).*

SC-54684A. Ethyl (3*S*)-3-{3-[(*p*-amidinophenyl)carbamoyl]propionamido}-4-pentynoate monohydrochloride.

$C_{18}H_{22}N_4O_4,HCl$ = 394.9.

CAS — 149820-74-6 (xemilofiban); 156586-91-3 (xemilofiban hydrochloride).

Xemilofiban is an antiplatelet drug that acts by blocking glycoprotein IIb/IIIa receptors. It is under investigation for the management of thrombo-embolic disorders, such as unstable angina.

Xipamide (2362-w)

Xipamide *(BAN, USAN, rINN).*

Be-1293; MJF-10938. 4-Chloro-5-sulphamoylsalicylo-2′,6′-xylidide; 5-(Aminosulphonyl)-4-chloro-*N*-(2,6-dimethylphenyl)-2-hydroxy-benzamide.

$C_{15}H_{15}ClN_2O_4S$ = 354.8.

CAS — 14293-44-8.

Adverse Effects, Treatment, and Precautions

As for Hydrochlorothiazide, p.885.

Effects on the electrolyte balance. Although reductions in plasma-potassium concentrations with xipamide have been shown to be on average comparable with those produced by thiazide and loop diuretics at equipotent doses,[1] there have been several reports of marked hypokalaemia in individual patients. Asymptomatic hypokalaemia was reported in 4 of 5 patients (serum-potassium concentrations of less than 3.4 mmol per litre) by Weissberg and Kendall[2] and in 3 of 13 patients (serum-potassium concentrations of less than 3.0 mmol per litre) by Raftery.[3] Severe hypokalaemia resulting in ventricular arrhythmias has been reported following xipamide alone[4] or in combination with indapamide.[5] Profound electrolyte disturbances with altered consciousness and ventricular extrasystoles occurred in a patient taking digoxin following the addition of xipamide for 10 days.[6] Boulton and Hardisty have also reported[7] a case of hypokalaemic periodic paralysis associated with xipamide administration.

1. Prichard BNC, Brogden RN. Xipamide: a review of its pharmacodynamic and pharmacokinetic properties and therapeutic efficacy. *Drugs* 1985; **30:** 313–32.

2. Weissberg P, Kendall MJ. Hypokalaemia and xipamide. *Br Med J* 1982; **284:** 975.

3. Raftery EB, *et al.* A study of the antihypertensive action of xipamide using ambulatory intra-arterial monitoring. *Br J Clin Pharmacol* 1981; **12:** 381–5.

4. Altmann P, Hamblin JJ. Ventricular fibrillation induced by xipamide. *Br Med J* 1982; **284:** 494.

5. Boulton AJM, Hardisty CA. Ventricular arrhythmias precipitated by treatment with non-thiazide diuretics. *Practitioner* 1982; **226:** 125–8.

6. Bentley J. Hypokalaemia and xipamide. *Br Med J* 1982; **284:** 975.

7. Boulton AJM, Hardisty CA. Hypokalaemic periodic paralysis precipitated by diuretic therapy and minor surgery. *Postgrad Med J* 1982; **58:** 106–7.

Hepatic impairment. For a recommendation that xipamide should be given with caution to patients with liver disease, see under Pharmacokinetics, below.

Interactions

As for Hydrochlorothiazide, p.887.

Pharmacokinetics

Xipamide has been reported to be well absorbed from the gastro-intestinal tract. Absorption is fairly rapid with peak plasma concentrations occurring within 1 or 2 hours of oral administration. It is 99% bound to plasma proteins, and is excreted in the urine, partly unchanged and partly in the form of the glucuronide metabolite. It is reported to have a plasma half-life of about 5 to 8 hours. In patients with renal impairment excretion in the bile becomes more prominent.

References.

1. Beermann B, Grind M. Clinical pharmacokinetics of some newer diuretics. *Clin Pharmacokinet* 1987; **13:** 254–66.

Hepatic impairment. Xipamide was present in the plasma and in ascitic fluid in patients with liver cirrhosis in proportion to the protein content of the respective compartments.[1] The amount of drug excreted into the urine was much greater in patients with liver disease than in healthy control subjects. This was attributed to a diminution in hepatic elimination, which could result in significant effects on the clinical response to xipamide. Thus patients with cholestasis could have an enhanced response to xipamide. On the other hand cirrhotic patients with the hepatorenal syndrome may be resistant to diuretics. Xipamide should be administered with caution to patients with liver disease.

1. Knauf H, *et al.* Xipamide disposition in liver cirrhosis. *Clin Pharmacol Ther* 1990; **48:** 628–32.

Renal impairment. Following single oral and intravenous doses of xipamide 20 mg the drug appeared to be completely absorbed from the gastro-intestinal tract.[1] The mean elimination half-life in healthy subjects was 7 hours and two-thirds of the clearance was by extrarenal routes. There was some accumulation in patients with chronic renal failure, with a calculated elimination half-life of 9 hours in end-stage renal disease.

1. Knauf H, Mutschler E. Pharmacodynamics and pharmacokinetics of xipamide in patients with normal and impaired kidney function. *Eur J Clin Pharmacol* 1984; **26:** 513–20.

Uses and Administration

Xipamide is a diuretic, structurally related to indapamide, with actions and uses similar to those of the thiazide diuretics (see Hydrochlorothiazide, p.887). It is used for oedema, including that associated with heart failure (p.785), and for hypertension (p.788).

Diuresis is initiated in about 1 or 2 hours, reaches a peak at 4 to 6 hours, and lasts for about 12 hours.

In the treatment of **oedema** the usual initial dose is 40 mg by mouth daily, subsequently reduced to 20 mg daily, according to the patient's response; in resistant cases doses of 80 mg daily may be required. In the treatment of **hypertension** the usual dose is 20 mg daily, as a single morning dose, either alone, or in conjunction with other antihypertensives. In some patients a dose of 10 mg daily may be adequate.

In susceptible patients potassium supplements or a potassium-sparing diuretic may be necessary, but see hydrochlorothiazide.

References.

1. Prichard BNC, Brogden RN. Xipamide: a review of its pharmacodynamic and pharmacokinetic properties and therapeutic efficacy. *Drugs* 1985; **30:** 313–32.

Preparations

Proprietary Preparations (details are given in Part 3)

Aust.: Aquaphoril; ***Belg.:*** Diurexan; ***Fr.:*** Chronexan; Lumitens; ***Ger.:*** Aquaphor; ***Irl.:*** Diurexan; ***Ital.:*** Aquafor; ***S.Afr.:*** Diurexan; ***Spain:*** Demiax; Diurex; ***UK:*** Diurexan.

Multi-ingredient: ***Ger.:*** Durotan; Neotri.

Zofenopril Calcium (3660-v)

Zofenopril Calcium *(BANM, USAN, rINNM).*

SQ-26991. Calcium salt of (4*S*)-1-[(2*S*)-3-(Benzylthio)-2-methylpropionyl]-4-(phenylthio)-L-proline.

$C_{44}H_{44}CaN_2O_8S_4$ = 897.2.

CAS — 81872-10-8 (zofenopril); 81938-43-4 (zofenopril calcium).

Zofenopril is an ACE inhibitor (p.805) that is under investigation as the calcium salt in the management of hypertension and myocardial infarction. It owes its activity to the active metabolite SQ-26333 to which it is converted after oral administration.

References.

1. Lacourcière Y, Provencher P. Comparative effects of zofenopril and hydrochlorothiazide on office and ambulatory blood pressures in mild to moderate essential hypertension. *Br J Clin Pharmacol* 1989; **27:** 371–6.

2. Salvetti A. Newer ACE inhibitors: a look at the future. *Drugs* 1990; **40:** 800–28.

3. Ambrosioni E, *et al.* The effect of the angiotensin-converting-enzyme inhibitor zofenopril on mortality and morbidity after anterior myocardial infarction. *N Engl J Med* 1995; **332:** 80–5.

Chelators Antidotes and Antagonists

The drugs included in this chapter act in a variety of ways to counter the toxic effects of exogenous and endogenous substances in the body. They therefore have applications in the management of poisoning and overdosage, in protecting against the toxic side-effects of drugs such as antineoplastics, and in the management of metabolic disorders such as Wilson's disease where toxic substances accumulate. Some are antagonists, such as the opioid antagonist naloxone, that compete with the poison for receptor sites. There are compounds that inhibit the toxin by reacting with it to form less active or inactive complexes or by interfering with its metabolism; chelators are typical examples of the first group and methionine is an example of the second. Other compounds with a role in the treatment of specific types of poisoning include those such as atropine (p.455) that block essential receptors mediating the toxic effects, or those that reduce the rate of conversion of the poison to a more toxic compound, such as alcohol (p.1099) in methyl alcohol poisoning, or those that bypass the effect of the drug as happens with calcium folinate (p.1342) in methotrexate overdosage. Other specific antagonists include acetylcysteine (p.1052) used in paracetamol poisoning.

Acute poisoning

In the management of suspected acute poisoning it is often impossible to determine the identity of the poison or the size of the dose received. Moreover, specific antidotes and methods of elimination are available for relatively few poisons and the mainstay of treatment for patients with suspected acute poisoning is therefore supportive and symptomatic therapy; in many cases nothing further is required. Symptoms of acute poisoning are frequently non-specific, particularly in the early stages. Maintenance of the airway and ventilation is the most important initial measure; other treatment, for example for cardiovascular or neurological symptoms, may be added as appropriate. Patients who present with loss of consciousness may be given naloxone if opioid overdosage is suspected. Some centres also recommend the routine administration of glucose to all unconscious patients since hypoglycaemia is a common cause of unconsciousness; thiamine is given in addition since glucose administration may precipitate Wernicke's encephalopathy.

Specific antidotes are available for a number of poisons and are the primary treatment where there is severe poisoning with a known toxin. They may be life-saving in such cases but their use is not without hazard and in many situations they are not necessary; their use does not preclude relevant supportive treatment.

Measures to reduce or prevent the absorption of the poison are widely advocated. For inhalational poisoning the victim is removed from the source of poisoning. Some toxins, in particular pesticides, may be absorbed through the skin and clothing is removed and the skin thoroughly washed to avoid continued absorption. Caustic substances are removed from the skin or eyes with copious irrigation. Orally ingested poisons may be actively removed from the stomach by emesis or by gastric lavage, although these measures are of limited value. Activated charcoal may be administered to absorb the toxin.

Induction of emesis has been used in the home situation although its value is questioned; the preferred emetic agent is syrup of ipecacuanha. It should only be used in fully conscious patients and should not be used if the poison is corrosive or petroleum based. Gastric lavage may be indicated for ingestion of non-caustic poisons if less than one to two hours have elapsed since ingestion and is followed by activated charcoal. Whole-bowel irrigation using a non-absorbable osmotic agent such as a macrogol may be useful following ingestion of substances that pass beyond the stomach before being absorbed, such as iron preparations or enteric-coated or modified-release formulations. A single oral dose of activated charcoal is effective for a wide range of toxins, particularly if it is administered within one to two hours of ingestion, although delayed administration may still be useful; it is generally well tolerated although vomiting is common and there is a risk of aspiration if the airway is not adequately protected.

Techniques intended to promote the elimination of poisons from the body such as forced diuresis, haemodialysis, or haemoperfusion are only of value for a limited number of poisons in a few severely poisoned patients. Repeated oral doses of activated charcoal may often be as effective as these more invasive methods.

Poisons Information Centres exist in many countries and should be consulted for more detailed information in specific situations.

Acetylcholinesterase (11228-l)

Acetylcholinesterase is an endogenous enzyme which hydrolyses acetylcholine (p.1389) and thus plays an essential role in cholinergic transmission. It is chiefly found at cholinergic synapses and in the neurones. Unlike the more widely distributed plasma cholinesterase (pseudocholinesterase; butyrylcholinesterase), which can hydrolyse other esters, its actions are relatively selective for choline esters. It has been given by intravenous injection to counteract the effect of overdosage or poisoning with suxamethonium or organophosphorus pesticides.

Preparations

Proprietary Preparations (details are given in Part 3)
Ger.: Serum-Cholinesterase.

Activated Charcoal (686-j)

Carbo Activatus; Decolorising Charcoal.
CAS — 16291-96-6 (charcoal).

Pharmacopoeias. In *Chin., Eur.* (see p.viii), *Int., Jpn,* and *US.*
Fr. and *It.* also include Vegetable Charcoal (Carbo ligni).

A fine, light, odourless, tasteless, black powder, free from grittiness. The Ph. Eur. describes material prepared from vegetable matter by carbonisation processes intended to confer a high adsorbing power. The USP describes the residue from the destructive distillation of various organic materials, treated to increase its adsorptive power.

The Ph. Eur. specifies that it adsorbs not less than 40% of its own weight of phenazone, calculated with reference to the dried substance. The USP has tests for adsorptive power in respect of alkaloids and dyes. Practically **insoluble** in all usual solvents. **Store** in airtight containers.

Adverse Effects and Precautions

Activated charcoal is relatively non-toxic when given by mouth but gastro-intestinal disturbances such as vomiting, constipation, or diarrhoea have been reported. It may colour the faeces black.

Haemoperfusion with activated charcoal has produced various adverse effects including platelet aggregation, charcoal embolism, thrombocytopenia, haemorrhage, hypoglycaemia, hypocalcaemia, hypothermia, and hypotension.

Activated charcoal is contra-indicated when specific oral antidotes such as methionine are used (see Interactions, below).

Effects on the gastro-intestinal tract. Intestinal obstruction[1-4] or faecal impaction, in one case resulting in rectal ulceration,[5] has been reported following multiple oral doses of activated charcoal. Special care should be taken when treating overdoses of drugs with antimuscarinic activity, such as tricyclic antidepressants and phenothiazines.[2] Two cases of pseudo-obstruction, one of which was fatal, have also been reported[6] following the use of activated charcoal and sorbitol with opioid sedation for theophylline poisoning. Care should also be taken to prevent pulmonary aspiration (see below).

1. Watson WA, *et al.* Gastrointestinal obstruction associated with multiple-dose activated charcoal. *J Emerg Med* 1986; **4:** 401–7.
2. Anderson IM, Ware C. Syrup of ipecacuanha. *Br Med J* 1987; **294:** 578.
3. Ray MJ, *et al.* Charcoal bezoar: small-bowel obstruction secondary to amitriptyline overdose therapy. *Dig Dis Sci* 1988; **33:** 106–7.
4. Atkinson SW, *et al.* Treatment with activated charcoal complicated by gastrointestinal obstruction requiring surgery. *Br Med J* 1992; **305:** 563.
5. Mizutani T, *et al.* Rectal ulcer with massive haemorrhage due to activated charcoal treatment in oral organophosphate poisoning. *Hum Exp Toxicol* 1991; **10:** 385–6.
6. Longdon P, Henderson A. Intestinal pseudo-obstruction following the use of enteral charcoal and sorbitol and mechanical ventilation with papaveretum sedation for theophylline poisoning. *Drug Safety* 1992; **7:** 74–7.

Effects on the lungs. Pulmonary aspiration of activated charcoal, sometimes with fatal results, has been reported following oral administration for the treatment of acute poisoning.[1-4] Vomiting has been reported to be fairly common by some,[1,5] but not all,[6] correspondents following activated charcoal administration; the water load resulting from repeated administration of charcoal slurry could contribute to the nausea and vomiting encountered[5] and the use of sorbitol-containing preparations has also been said to contribute to the vomiting.[7] The use of a cuffed endotracheal tube has been recommended for any patient with impaired laryngeal reflexes to prevent aspiration.[4,8]

1. Hoffman JR. Charcoal for gastrointestinal clearance of drugs. *N Engl J Med* 1983; **308:** 157.
2. Harsch HH. Aspiration of activated charcoal. *N Engl J Med* 1986; **314:** 318.
3. Menzies DG, *et al.* Fatal pulmonary aspiration of oral activated charcoal. *Br Med J* 1988; **297:** 459–60.
4. Rau NR, *et al.* Fatal pulmonary aspiration of oral activated charcoal. *Br Med J* 1988; **297:** 918–19.
5. Danel V. Fatal pulmonary aspiration of oral activated charcoal. *Br Med J* 1988; **297:** 684.
6. Levy G. Charcoal for gastrointestinal clearance of drugs. *N Engl J Med* 1983; **308:** 157.
7. McFarland AK, Chyka PA. Selection of activated charcoal products for the treatment of poisonings. *Ann Pharmacother* 1993; **27:** 358–61.
8. Power KJ. Fatal pulmonary aspiration of oral activated charcoal. *Br Med J* 1988; **297:** 919.

Interactions

Activated charcoal diminishes the action of ipecacuanha and other emetics when given concomitantly by mouth; if indicated, emesis should be induced before activated charcoal is administered. Activated charcoal has the potential to reduce the absorption of many drugs from the gastro-intestinal tract and simultaneous oral therapy should therefore be avoided. In the management of acute poisoning, concurrent medication should be administered parenterally. Activated charcoal should not be administered when a specific oral antidote such as methionine is used since adsorption of the antidote may decrease its effectiveness.

Uses and Administration

Activated charcoal can adsorb a wide range of plant and inorganic poisons and many drugs including salicylates, paracetamol, barbiturates, and tricyclic antidepressants; thus when administered by mouth it reduces their systemic absorption from the gastro-intestinal tract and is used in the treatment of acute oral poisoning. It is of no value in the treatment of poisoning by strong acids, alkalis, or other corrosive substances and its adsorptive capacity is too low to be of use in poisoning with iron salts, cyanides, lithium, malathion, dicophane, and some organic solvents such as methyl alcohol or ethylene glycol. Adsorption characteristics can be influenced by charcoal's particle size, thus different responses may be obtained with different preparations.

Activated charcoal is given by mouth usually as a slurry in water. The usual dose is 50 g, but higher doses have been used. For maximum efficacy, activated charcoal should be administered as soon as possible after ingestion of the toxic compound. However, it may be effective several hours after poisoning with certain drugs that slow gastric emptying. In the case of drugs that undergo enterohepatic or enteroenteric recycling (e.g. phenobarbitone and theophylline) *repeated doses* of activated charcoal are of value in enhancing faecal elimination. Doses for repeated administration have varied but typically 50 g may be given every 4 hours or 25 g every 2 hours. Administration may also be via a nasogastric tube.

Mixtures such as 'universal antidote' that contained activated charcoal, magnesium oxide, and tannic acid should not be used; activated charcoal alone is more effective and tannic acid may cause hepatotoxicity.

In the charcoal haemoperfusion treatment of poisoning, activated charcoal may be used to remove drugs from the blood stream. It may be of value in acute severe poisoning by drugs such as the barbiturates, glutethimide, or theophylline when other intensive measures fail to improve the condition of the patient.

Activated charcoal is used in dressings for ulcers and suppurating wounds (p.1076) to reduce malodour and may improve the rate of healing.

Activated charcoal has been used as a marker of intestinal transit and has also been tried in the treatment of flatulence. Both activated charcoal and vegetable charcoal (wood charcoal) are included in preparations for various gastro-intestinal disorders.

Technical grades of activated charcoal have been used as purifying and decolorising agents, for the removal of residual gases in low-pressure apparatus, and in respirators as a protection against toxic gases.

Administration. Activated charcoal is most commonly administered as a slurry in water but this is often found to be unpalatable because of the colour, gritty taste, lack of flavour, and difficulty in swallowing.[1] Efforts have therefore been made to improve its palatability but studies *in vitro* or in healthy subjects have indicated that some foods such as ice cream, milk, and cocoa might inhibit the adsorptive capacity of activated charcoal whereas starches and jams appeared to have no effect.[2,3] Carmellose has been demonstrated to improve palatability though it might also reduce the adsorptive power of activated charcoal.[4-6] Scholtz *et al.*[1] found that activated charcoal formulations containing sorbitol, carmellose sodium, or starch were more palatable and essentially equivalent to the aqueous slurry formulation in efficacy. When chocolate syrup was used as a sweet flavouring agent it had to be added just before administration as the sweetness and flavour disappeared after a few minutes contact with the activated charcoal. Results of a study by Cooney[7] also suggested that saccharin sodium, sucrose, or sorbitol might be suitable flavouring agents for activated charcoal formulations. A survey by McFarland and Chyka[8] of commercially available ready-to-use charcoal preparations in the USA indicated that although differences did exist between the formulations, the clinical significance of such variations was unknown. They highlighted the problems associated with sorbitol-containing products (see also under Poisoning, below) and cautioned against their use, especially for repeated-dose therapy.

1. Scholtz EC, *et al.* Evaluation of five activated charcoal formulations for inhibition of aspirin absorption and palatability in man. *Am J Hosp Pharm* 1978; **35:** 1355–9.
2. Levy G, *et al.* Inhibition by ice cream of the antidotal efficacy of activated charcoal. *Am J Hosp Pharm* 1975; **32:** 289–91.
3. De Neve R. Antidotal efficacy of activated charcoal in presence of jam, starch and milk. *Am J Hosp Pharm* 1976; **33:** 965–6.
4. Mathur LK, *et al.* Activated charcoal–carboxymethylcellulose gel formulation as an antidotal agent for orally ingested aspirin. *Am J Hosp Pharm* 1976; **33:** 717–19.
5. Manes M. Effect of carboxymethylcellulose on the adsorptive capacity of charcoal. *Am J Hosp Pharm* 1976; **33:** 1120, 1122.
6. Mathur LK, *et al.* Effect of carboxymethylcellulose on the adsorptive capacity of charcoal. *Am J Hosp Pharm* 1976; **33:** 1122.
7. Cooney DO. Palatability of sucrose-, sorbitol-, and saccharin-sweetened activated charcoal formulations. *Am J Hosp Pharm* 1980; **37:** 237–9.
8. McFarland AK, Chyka PA. Selection of activated charcoal products for the treatment of poisonings. *Ann Pharmacother* 1993; **27:** 358–61.

Poisoning. The management of acute poisoning is discussed on p.972. The administration of a *single oral dose* of activated charcoal has become a widespread method of preventing the absorption of ingested compounds and may be superior to gastric emptying.[1,2] In addition, *multiple oral doses* of activated charcoal have been found to enhance the elimination of some drugs and toxic substances even after systemic absorption.[3-12] Mechanisms by which activated charcoal may increase drug elimination from the body include interruption of the enterohepatic circulation of drugs excreted into the bile, reduction of the reabsorption of drugs which diffuse or are actively secreted into the intestines, and increased elimination of the drug via the gastro-intestinal tract when co-administered with a laxative to decrease gastro-intestinal transit time,[5] although the practice of giving charcoal with a laxative has been questioned.[8,13] Repeated oral doses of activated charcoal may therefore be considered for compounds that undergo enterohepatic or enteroenteric circulation, have a small volume of distribution, are not extensively bound to plasma proteins, and have a low endogenous clearance. Anecdotal reports and studies in acutely poisoned patients indicate that a technique of giving multiple doses of charcoal may offer an alternative to charcoal haemoperfusion or haemodialysis. However, while activated charcoal is generally well tolerated, major complications do occasionally occur, including pulmonary aspiration and bowel obstruction. Also, use of multiple doses of charcoal preparations containing sorbitol or sodium bicarbonate can result in increased vomiting[14] or in electrolyte disturbances.[8-10] Thus, some have questioned the role of multiple dose therapy.[14,15]

1. Pond SM, *et al.* Gastric emptying in acute overdose: a prospective randomised controlled trial. *Med J Aust* 1995; **163:** 345–9.
2. Albertson TE, *et al.* Superiority of activated charcoal alone compared with ipecac and activated charcoal in the treatment of acute toxic ingestions. *Ann Emerg Med* 1989; **18:** 56–9.
3. Levy G. Gastrointestinal clearance of drugs with activated charcoal. *N Engl J Med* 1982; **307:** 676–8.
4. Park GD, *et al.* Expanded role of charcoal therapy in the poisoned and overdosed patient. *Arch Intern Med* 1986; **146:** 969–73.
5. Pond SM. Role of repeated oral doses of activated charcoal in clinical toxicology. *Med Toxicol* 1986; **1:** 3–11.
6. Anonymous. Repeated oral activated charcoal in acute poisoning. *Lancet* 1987; **i:** 1013–15.
7. Katona BG, *et al.* The new black magic: activated charcoal and new therapeutic uses. *J Emerg Med* 1987; **5:** 9–18.
8. Neuvonen PJ, Olkkola KT. Oral activated charcoal in the treatment of intoxications: role of single and repeated doses. *Med Toxicol* 1988; **3:** 33–58.
9. McLuckie A, *et al.* Role of repeated doses of oral activated charcoal in the treatment of acute intoxications. *Anaesth Intensive Care* 1990; **18:** 375–84.
10. Tenenbein M. Multiple doses of activated charcoal: time for reappraisal? *Ann Emerg Med* 1991; **20:** 529–31.
11. Vale JA, Proudfoot AT. How useful is activated charcoal? *Br Med J* 1993; **306:** 78–9.
12. Bayly GR, Ferner RE. Activated charcoal for drug overdose. *Prescribers' J* 1995; **35:** 12–17.
13. Neuvonen PJ, Olkkola KT. Effect of purgatives on antidotal efficacy of oral activated charcoal. *Hum Toxicol* 1986; **5:** 255–63.
14. McFarland AK, Chyka PA. Selection of activated charcoal products for the treatment of poisonings. *Ann Pharmacother* 1993; **27:** 358–61.
15. Palatnick W, Tenenbein M. Activated charcoal in the treatment of drug overdose: an update. *Drug Safety* 1992; **7:** 3–7.

HAEMOPERFUSION. Haemoperfusion involves the passage of blood through an adsorbent material such as activated charcoal or synthetic hydrophobic polystyrene resins which can retain certain drugs and toxic agents. Early problems with charcoal haemoperfusion such as charcoal embolism, marked thrombocytopenia, fibrinogen loss, and pyrogen reactions have been largely overcome by purification procedures and by coating the carbon with biocompatible polymers. However, transient falls in platelet count, leucocyte count, and circulatory concentrations of clotting factors, calcium, glucose, urea, creatinine, and urate have been reported during haemoperfusion. While there is no substitute for supportive measures, haemoperfusion can significantly reduce the body burden of certain compounds with a low volume of distribution within 4 to 6 hours in some severely poisoned patients; haemoperfusion is not effective for drugs or poisons with very large volumes of distribution.

References.

1. Widdop B, Vale JA. The clinical application and risk-benefit of haemoperfusion. *Hum Toxicol* 1985; **4:** 345.
2. Webb D. Charcoal haemoperfusion in drug intoxication. *Br J Hosp Med* 1993; **49:** 493–6.

Porphyria. Activated charcoal may be used as part of the management of erythropoietic protoporphyria, one of the non-acute porphyrias (p.983). It acts as a sorbent in the gut lumen, interrupting the enterohepatic recycling of protoporphyrin. It has also been tried in a patient with photomutilation diagnosed as having congenital erythropoietic porphyria, a very rare porphyria.[1] Activated charcoal 30 g given by mouth every 3 hours for 36 hours reduced the plasma-porphyrin concentration to normal values by 20 hours and was more effective than cholestyramine or transfusional therapy. After discontinuation of activated charcoal, plasma-porphyrin concentrations rose rapidly to near pretreatment levels within 10 days. Long-term treatment with oral charcoal over a 9-month period effected a clinical remission with low concentrations of plasma and skin porphyrin and an absence of photocutaneous activity. The optimal dose was determined to be 60 g three times a day. However, exacerbation following an initial period of remission has been reported in another patient[2] and total lack of efficacy in a third.[3]

1. Pimstone NR, *et al.* Therapeutic efficacy of oral charcoal in congenital erythropoietic porphyria. *N Engl J Med* 1987; **316:** 390–3.
2. Hift RJ, *et al.* The effect of oral activated charcoal on the course of congenital erythropoietic porphyria. *Br J Dermatol* 1993; **129:** 14–17.
3. Minder EI, *et al.* Lack of effect of oral charcoal in congenital erythropoietic porphyria. *N Engl J Med* 1994; **330:** 1092–4.

Pruritus. Pruritus (p.1075) is usually treated symptomatically. Activated charcoal has been tried in pruritus associated with renal failure. In a double-blind crossover study, administration of activated charcoal 6 g daily by mouth for 8 weeks was more effective than placebo in relieving generalised pruritus in 11 patients undergoing maintenance haemodialysis.[1]

1. Pederson JA, *et al.* Relief of idiopathic generalized pruritus in dialysis patients treated with activated oral charcoal. *Ann Intern Med* 1980; **93:** 446–8.

Preparations

Proprietary Preparations (details are given in Part 3)

Aust.: Kolemed; ***Austral.:*** Ad-Sorb; Carbosorb; CharcoCaps; Charcotabs; Karbons; Prodiarrhoea; ***Belg.:*** Norit; Norit-Carbomix; ***Canad.:*** Charac†; Charcodote Aqueous; ***Fr.:*** Actisorb; Carbomix; Carbonet; Charbon de Belloc; Formocarbine; Mandocarbine†; Splenocarbine; ***Ger.:*** Dregan†; Kohle-Compretten; Kohle-Hevert; Kohle-Pulvis; Kohle-Tabletten; ***Irl.:*** Carbomix; Carbonet; ***Ital.:*** Actisorb†; Carbonet†; Neo Carbone Belloc; ***Neth.:*** Norit; ***Spain:*** Ultra Adsorb; ***Swed.:*** Carbomix; Kolsuspension; Leokol†; Medikol; ***UK:*** Bragg's; Carbomix; Carbonet; Carbosorb†; Clinisorb; Liqui-Char; Lyofoam C; Medicoal; ***USA:*** Actidose-Aqua; Charcoaid; CharcoCaps; Liqui-Char.

Multi-ingredient: ***Aust.:*** Carboguan†; Eucarbon; Intestinol; Sabatif†; ***Austral.:*** Carbosorb S; Kaltocarb; No Gas; ***Belg.:*** Carbobel; Carbolactanose†; Eucarbon; ***Canad.:*** Charcodote; ***Fr.:*** Acticarbine; Actisorb Plus; Carbolevure; Carbonaphtine Pectinee†; Carbophagix; Carbophos; Carbosylane; Digestobiase†; Gastropax; Intesticarbine†; Quinocarbine; ***Ger.:*** Adsorgan†; Aruto-Magenpulver†; Carbomucil†; Dynamol†; Dystomin E†; Kontabletten†; Noventerol†; Pascopankreat†; ***Irl.:*** Actisorb Plus; ***Ital.:*** Actisorb Plus; Carbonesia; Carbosylane Bi-Attivo†; Carbotiol; Carboyoghurt; Cura; Eucarbon; No-Gas; ***Spain:*** Vacuosa Ultra Adsorb†; ***Switz.:*** Carbolevure; Carboticon; Eucarbon; ***UK:*** Acidosis; Actisorb Plus; Carbellon; Kaltocarb; Papaya Plus; ***USA:*** Actidose with Sorbitol; Charcoal Plus; Flatulex; Poison Antidote Kit; Res-Q†.

Amifostine (17040-h)

Amifostine *(BAN, USAN, rINN)*.

Ethiofos; Gammaphos; NSC-296961; WR-2721. S-[2-(3-Aminopropylamino)ethyl] dihydrogen phosphorothioate.

$C_5H_{15}N_2O_3PS$ = 214.2.

CAS — 20537-88-6 (amifostine); 63717-27-1 (amifostine monohydrate).

Incompatibilities. Amifostine has been reported[1] to be physically incompatible with aciclovir sodium, amphotericin, cefoperazone sodium, chlorpromazine hydrochloride, cisplatin, ganciclovir sodium, hydroxyzine hydrochloride, miconazole, minocycline hydrochloride, and prochlorperazine edisylate during simulated Y-site administration.

1. Trissel LA, Martinez JF. Compatibility of amifostine with selected drugs during simulated Y-site administration. *Am J Health-Syst Pharm* 1995; **52:** 2208–12.

Adverse Effects, Treatment, and Precautions

Amifostine may cause a transient reduction, usually in systolic, or, less frequently, in diastolic blood pressure. However, more pronounced reductions in blood pressure may occur and transient loss of consciousness has been reported very rarely. To minimise hypotension, patients should be adequately hydrated before treatment with amifostine begins and should be in a supine position. Amifostine is contra-indicated in patients who are hypotensive or dehydrated. Patients taking antihypertensive drugs should discontinue treatment 24 hours before administration of amifostine. Arterial blood pressure must be monitored during the amifostine infusion and if systolic blood pressure decreases significantly, infusion must stop. It may be continued if blood pressure returns to normal within 5 minutes.

Nausea and vomiting are frequently reported and concurrent antiemetic therapy is recommended.

Amifostine reduces serum-calcium concentrations, although clinical hypocalcaemia has occurred only very rarely in patients who received multiple doses of amifostine within 24 hours. Serum-calcium concentrations should be monitored in patients at risk of hypocalcaemia.

Other side-effects include flushing, chills, somnolence, hiccups, sneezing, and mild skin rashes.

Administration of amifostine over a longer period than the recommended 15 minutes is associated with a higher incidence of side-effects.

The UK manufacturer has contra-indicated amifostine in hepatic or renal impairment, in the very young, and in the elderly owing to a lack of experience with amifostine in such patients.

Uses and Administration

Amifostine, an aminothiol compound, is a cytoprotective agent. It is converted in the body to its active metabolite WR-1065 that protects noncancerous cells against the toxic effects of antineoplastics and ionising radiation. It is used in patients with advanced ovarian cancer to reduce neutropenia-related infection associated with cyclophosphamide and cisplatin therapy and, in patients with advanced solid tumours of non-germ cell origin, to reduce the cumulative renal toxicity associated with repeated cisplatin administration. It is also under investigation in ameliorating the adverse effects of other antineoplastics and of radiation therapy (including dry mouth).

Amifostine is given by intravenous infusion over 15 minutes starting within 30 minutes before administration of antineoplastic therapy. The recommended dose in adults is 910 mg per m^2 body-surface area once daily. The dose should be reduced to 740 mg per m^2 in patients unable to tolerate the full dose. A dose of 740 mg per m^2 is also recommended in patients receiving amifostine to reduce the renal toxicity of cisplatin where the dose of cisplatin is less than 100 mg per m^2.

Adjunct in antineoplastic therapy. Amifostine is rapidly cleared from the plasma following intravenous administration and is dephosphorylated to WR-1065, a free thiol compound, by alkaline phosphatase. WR-1065 readily enters non-malignant cells where it deactivates cytotoxics such as alkylating and platinum-containing antineoplastics and protects against the effects of ionising radiation. The cytoprotective effects of amifostine are reported to be selective for normal cells and not to interfere with the cytotoxic effects of antineoplastics and radiation on malignant cells. Several factors contribute to this selectivity; malignant tumours contain less alkaline phosphatase than normal tissue and WR-1065 is less readily transported into malignant cells. Thus, amifostine has been investigated for reducing adverse effects such as bone-marrow depression and associated suppression of immunity and specific toxicity such as nephrotoxicity with cisplatin.

References.

1. Grdina DJ, Sigdestad CP. Radiation protectors: the unexpected benefits. *Drug Metab Rev* 1989; **20:** 13–42.
2. Lewis C. A review of the use of chemoprotectants in cancer chemotherapy. *Drug Safety* 1994; **11:** 153–62.
3. Glick J, *et al.* A randomized trial of cyclophosphamide and cisplatin ± amifostine in the treatment of advanced epithelial ovarian cancer. *Proc Am Soc Clin Oncol* 1994; **13:** 432.
4. Spencer CM, Goa KL. Amifostine: a review of its pharmacodynamic and pharmacokinetic properties, and therapeutic potential as a radioprotector and cytotoxic chemoprotector. *Drugs* 1995; **50:** 1001–31.
5. Foster-Nora JA, Siden R. Amifostine for protection from antineoplastic drug toxicity. *Am J Health-Syst Pharm* 1997; **54:** 787–800.

Preparations

Proprietary Preparations (details are given in Part 3)

Austral.: Ethyol; ***Canad.:*** Ethyol; ***Fr.:*** Ethyol; ***Ger.:*** Ethyol; ***Neth.:*** Ethyol; ***S.Afr.:*** Ethyol; ***Spain:*** Ethyol; ***UK:*** Ethyol; ***USA:*** Ethyol.

Ammonium Tetrathiomolybdate (10500-b)

Ammonium tetrathiomolybdate is a chelator that aids the elimination of copper from the body. It is under investigation in the treatment of Wilson's disease.

Wilson's disease. Ammonium tetrathiomolybdate forms a complex with protein and copper. When it is taken with food it blocks the intestinal absorption of copper, and when given between meals it combines with albumin- and caeruloplasmin-bound copper. Ammonium tetrathiomolybdate is under investigation for the initial reduction of copper levels in patients with Wilson's disease (p.992); it may be particularly suitable for patients with neurological symptoms.[1,2] Reversible bone marrow depression has been reported in two patients treated with ammonium tetrathiomolybdate.[3]

1. Brewer GJ, *et al.* Treatment of Wilson's disease with ammonium tetrathiomolybdate I: initial therapy in 17 neurologically affected patients. *Arch Neurol* 1994; **51:** 545–54.
2. Brewer GJ, *et al.* Treatment of Wilson disease with ammonium tetrathiomolybdate II: initial therapy in 33 neurologically affected patients and follow-up with zinc therapy. *Arch Neurol* 1996; **53:** 1017–25.
3. Harper PL, Walshe JM. Reversible pancytopenia secondary to treatment with tetrathiomolybdate. *Br J Haematol* 1986; **64:** 851–3.

Amyl Nitrite (9205-q)

Amylis Nitris; Amylium Nitrosum; Azotito de Amilo; Isoamyl Nitrite; Isopentyl Nitrite; Nitrito de Amilo; Pentanolis Nitris.

$C_5H_{11}NO_2$ = 117.1.

Pharmacopoeias. In *Aust., It., Jpn,* and *US.*

A clear, yellow, volatile, flammable liquid with a fragrant odour. B.p. 96°. It consists of the nitrite esters of 3-methylbutan-1-ol and 2-methylbutan-1-ol.

Practically **insoluble** in water; miscible with alcohol, and ether. It is volatile even at low temperatures and is liable to decompose with evolution of nitrogen, particularly if it has become acid in reaction. **Store** in a cool place in airtight containers. Protect from light.

CAUTION. *Amyl nitrite is very flammable and must not be used where it may be ignited.*

Adverse Effects, Treatment, and Precautions

Amyl nitrite inhalation commonly causes flushing, headache, and dizziness; nausea and vomiting, hypotension, restlessness, and tachycardia may also occur. Overdosage may result in cyanosis, syncope, dyspnoea, and muscular weakness, due to vasodilatation and methaemoglobinaemia. Methylene blue administration may be required for severe methaemoglobinaemia but should not be used if cyanide poisoning is suspected since cyanide may be displaced.

Amyl nitrite may increase intra-ocular and intracranial pressure and should be used with caution in patients with glaucoma, recent head trauma, or cerebral haemorrhage.

Abuse. Volatile nitrites (commonly known as 'poppers') have been abused, in the belief that they expand creativity, stimulate music appreciation, promote a sense of abandon in dancing, and intensify sexual experience.[1,2]

Inhalation of amyl, butyl, or isobutyl nitrite has caused headache, tachycardia, syncope, acute psychosis, increased intra-ocular pressure, transient hemiparesis, methaemoglobinaemia, coma, and, rarely, sudden death.[3]

Haemolytic anaemia has been reported in subjects after abuse of volatile nitrites;[4,5] in some subjects, Heinz body formation has been detected.[4] Methaemoglobinaemia has been reported following ingestion of volatile nitrites.[6-9] Symptoms are similar to those of hypoxia[8] and may be reversed by administration of methylene blue.[6-9]

Exposure to amyl nitrite inhalation has led to severe and extensive contact dermatitis around the face with secondary spread elsewhere on the body.[10]

1. Sigell LT, *et al.* Popping and snorting volatile nitrites: a current fad for getting high. *Am J Psychiatry* 1978; **135:** 1216–18.
2. Lockwood B. Poppers: volatile nitrite inhalants. *Pharm J* 1996; **257:** 154–5.
3. Anonymous. Treatment of acute drug abuse reactions. *Med Lett Drugs Ther* 1987; **29:** 83–6.
4. Romeril KR, Concannon AJ. Heinz body haemolytic anaemia after sniffing volatile nitrites. *Med J Aust* 1981; **1:** 302–3.
5. Brandes JC, *et al.* Amyl nitrite-induced, hemolytic anemia. *Am J Med* 1989; **86:** 252–4.
6. Laaban JP, *et al.* Amyl nitrite poppers and methemoglobulinemia. *Ann Intern Med* 1985; **103:** 804–5.
7. Osterloh J, Olson K. Toxicities of alkyl nitrites. *Ann Intern Med* 1986; **104:** 727.
8. Pierce JMT, Nielsen MS. Acute acquired methaemoglobinaemia after amyl nitrite poisoning. *Br Med J* 1989; **298:** 1566.
9. Forsyth RJ, Moulden A. Methaemoglobinaemia after ingestion of amyl nitrite. *Arch Dis Child* 1991; **66:** 152.
10. Bos JD, *et al.* Allergic contact dermatitis to amyl nitrite ('poppers'). *Contact Dermatitis* 1985; **12:** 109.

Uses and Administration

Amyl nitrite is rapidly absorbed on inhalation and may be employed in the immediate treatment of patients with definite cyanide poisoning (p.1407) to induce the formation of methaemoglobin, which combines with the cyanide to form non-toxic cyanmethaemoglobin. The value of such treatment has been questioned since only low levels of methaemoglobin are formed, but other mechanisms may also be important. A suggested procedure is to administer amyl nitrite by inhalation for up to 30 seconds every minute until other measures can be instituted. It has also been suggested for use in the management of hydrogen sulphide poisoning (p.1165).

Amyl nitrite has an action similar to that of glyceryl trinitrate (p.875) and used to be given by inhalation for the relief of acute attacks of angina pectoris but is seldom used now.

Amyl nitrite is used in homoeopathic medicine.

Preparations

USP 23: Amyl Nitrite Inhalant.

Proprietary Preparations (details are given in Part 3)

Multi-ingredient: ***S.Afr.:*** Tripac-Cyano; ***USA:*** Cyanide Antidote Package; Emergent-Ez.

Asoxime Chloride (19298-r)

HI-6.

Asoxime chloride is a cholinesterase reactivator which has been tried in the treatment of poisoning by organophosphorus pesticides and related compounds.

References.

1. Jovanović D, *et al.* A case of unusual suicidal poisoning by the organophosphorus insecticide dimethoate. *Hum Exp Toxicol* 1990; **9:** 49–51.
2. Kušić R, *et al.* HI-6 in man: efficacy of the oxime in poisoning by organophosphorus insecticides. *Hum Exp Toxicol* 1991; **10:** 113–18.

Atipamezole Hydrochloride (5005-y)

Atipamezole Hydrochloride *(BANM, rINNM).*

MPV-1248 (atipamezole). 4-(2-Ethyl-2-indanyl)imidazole hydrochloride.

$C_{14}H_{16}N_2$,HCl = 248.8.

CAS — 104054-27-5 (atipamezole); 104075-48-1 (atipamezole hydrochloride).

NOTE. Atipamezole is *USAN.*

Atipamezole hydrochloride is a selective alpha$_2$-adrenergic receptor antagonist that is used in veterinary medicine to reverse the sedative effects of medetomidine.

Calcium Polystyrene Sulphonate

(5004-l)

Calcium Polystyrene Sulfonate.

CAS — 37286-92-3.

Pharmacopoeias. In *Br.* and *Jpn.*

The calcium salt of sulphonated styrene polymer. A cream to light brown, fine powder, containing not more than 8% of water. The calcium content is not less than 6.5% and not more than 9.5%, calculated with reference to the dried substance. Each g exchanges not less than 1.3 mmol and not more than 2.0 mmol of potassium, calculated with reference to the dried substance. Practically **insoluble** in water and in alcohol. **Store** in airtight containers.

Adverse Effects and Precautions

As for Sodium Polystyrene Sulphonate, p.995. Sorbitol should not be used with calcium polystyrene sulphonate due to the risk of colonic necrosis. Sodium overloading is not a problem with calcium polystyrene sulphonate, but calcium overloading and hypercalcaemia may occur. Patients should be monitored for electrolyte disturbances, especially hypokalaemia and hypercalcaemia. Calcium polystyrene sulphonate should not be used in patients presenting with renal failure together with hypercalcaemia.

Effects on the lungs. An elderly man who died from cardiac arrest was found at necropsy to have bronchopneumonia associated with inhalation of calcium polystyrene sulphonate;[1] the resin had been given by mouth to treat hyperkalaemia.

1. Chaplin AJ, Millard PR. Calcium polystyrene sulphonate: an unusual cause of inhalation pneumonia. *Br Med J* 1975; **3:** 77–8.

Interactions

As for Sodium Polystyrene Sulphonate, p.996. Calcium ions are released from the resin in the gastro-intestinal tract and this may reduce the absorption of tetracycline given by mouth.

Uses and Administration

Calcium polystyrene sulphonate is a cation-exchange resin which exchanges calcium ions for potassium ions and other cations in the gastro-intestinal tract. It is used similarly to sodium polystyrene sulphonate (p.996) to enhance potassium excretion in the treatment of hyperkalaemia (p.1149) and may be preferred to the sodium resin in patients who cannot tolerate an increase in their sodium load.

It is estimated that 1 g of calcium polystyrene sulphonate could bind 1.3 to 2 mmol of potassium but it is unlikely that such figures could be achieved in practice.

It is administered by mouth, in a dose of 15 g up to four times daily, as a suspension in water or syrup or as a sweetened paste. It should not be given in fruit juices that have a high potassium content. A suggested dose for children is up to 1 g per kg body-weight daily in divided doses for acute hyperkalaemia, reduced to a maintenance dose of 500 mg per kg daily in divided doses; the oral route is not recommended for neonates.

When oral administration is difficult, calcium polystyrene sulphonate may be administered rectally as an enema. The usual daily dose is 30 g given as a suspension in 100 mL of 2% methylcellulose '450' and 100 mL of water and retained, if possible, for at least 9 hours. Initial therapy may constitute administration by both oral and rectal routes. Following retention of the enema the colon should be irrigated to remove the resin. Children and neonates may be given rectal doses similar to those suggested for children by mouth.

Preparations

Proprietary Preparations (details are given in Part 3)
Aust.: Sorbisterit; ***Austral.:*** Calcium Resonium; ***Belg.:*** Kayexalate Calcium; ***Canad.:*** Resonium Calcium; ***Fr.:*** Calcium-Sorbisterit; ***Ger.:*** Anti-Kalium; Calcium Resonium; CPS Pulver; Elutit-Calcium; Sorbisterit; ***Irl.:*** Calcium Resonium; ***Jpn:*** Kalimate; ***Neth.:*** Calcium Resonium†; ***Norw.:*** Resonium Calcium; ***Spain:*** Resincalcio; ***Swed.:*** Resonium Calcium; ***Switz.:*** Resonium Calcium†; Sorbisterit; ***UK:*** Calcium Resonium.

Calcium Trisodium Pentetate (1032-q)

Calcium Trisodium Pentetate *(BAN, rINN)*.

Calcium Trisodium DTPA; NSC-34249; Pentetate Calcium Trisodium *(USAN)*; Trisodium Calcium Diethylenetriaminepentaacetate. Calcium trisodium nitrilodiethylenedinitrilopenta-acetate.

$C_{14}H_{18}CaN_3Na_3O_{10}$ = 497.4.

CAS — 12111-24-9 (calcium trisodium pentetate); 67-43-6 (pentetic acid).

NOTE. Pentetic acid is *BAN, USAN,* and *rINN.*

Pharmacopoeias. US includes Pentetic Acid.

Pentetic acid and its salts are chelators with the general properties of the edetates (see Sodium Calciumedetate, p.994). Calcium trisodium pentetate is used in the treatment of poisoning by heavy metals and radioactive metals such as plutonium. Doses of 1 g daily have been administered by slow intravenous infusion for 3 to 5 days. Further treatment may be given after an interval of 3 days.

Calcium pentetate has also been used.

Pentetates, labelled with metallic radionuclides, are used in nuclear medicine (see Indium-111, p.1423, and Technetium-99m, p.1425).

Thalassaemia. Desferrioxamine is used to slow the accumulation of iron in patients with thalassaemia (p.704) who are receiving regular blood transfusions. Calcium pentetate, 0.5 to 1 g by subcutaneous infusion on alternate days or for 5 days each week, was given to 5 patients with thalassaemia who developed auditory neurotoxicity while receiving desferrioxamine and in whom desferrioxamine had to be withdrawn because of high-tone deafness.[1] Calcium pentetate was as effective as desferrioxamine at increasing iron excretion. Hearing improved during treatment. Oral zinc supplements were necessary during treatment with calcium pentetate to maintain adequate plasma-zinc concentrations.

1. Wonke B, *et al.* Reversal of desferrioxamine induced auditory neurotoxicity during treatment with Ca-DTPA. *Arch Dis Child* 1989; **64:** 77–82.

Preparations

Proprietary Preparations (details are given in Part 3)
Ger.: Ditripentat-Heyl.

Deferiprone (3851-l)

Deferiprone *(BAN, rINN)*.

Dimethylhydroxypyridone; L1. 1,2-Dimethyl-3-hydroxypyrid-4-one; 3-Hydroxy-1,2-dimethyl-4-pyridone.

$C_7H_9NO_2$ = 139.2.

CAS — 30652-11-0.

Deferiprone is an orally active iron chelator under investigation in iron overload disorders.

Although desferrioxamine is effective in the treatment of iron overload such as that associated with thalassaemia (p.704), compliance is limited by the need for regular injections. Deferiprone is an orally effective iron chelator that was developed with the aim of overcoming this problem.

Concern has been expressed over the potential toxicity of deferiprone. Preclinical testing in *animals* revealed embryotoxicity, teratogenicity, organ atrophy, and haematological toxicity,[1] and reversible neutropenia or agranulocytosis has been reported in patients.[2-5] In addition, a case of fatal systemic lupus erythematosus has been reported[6] although this could have been related to the patient's thalassaemia rather than to the drug.[7,8] Other reported adverse effects include musculoskeletal and joint pain,[2-5,9] gastro-intestinal intolerance,[2-5] transit liver enzyme abnormalities,[5] and zinc deficiency.[5] One company (Ciba-Geigy) took the decision that the therapeutic safety margin was too narrow to warrant further development.[1] Nevertheless, beneficial responses have been reported,[4,5,10-13] although a recent small study[14] indicated that deferiprone did not adequately control body iron burden long term in patients with thalassaemia and might worsen hepatic fibrosis.

1. Berdoukas V, *et al.* Toxicity of oral iron chelator L1. *Lancet* 1993; **341:** 1088.
2. Hershko C. Development of oral iron chelator L1. *Lancet* 1993; **341:** 1088–9.
3. Kontoghiorghes GJ, *et al.* Future of oral iron chelator deferiprone (L1). *Lancet* 1993; **341:** 1479–80.
4. Olivieri NF, *et al.* Iron-chelator therapy with oral deferiprone in patients with thalassemia major. *N Engl J Med* 1995; **332:** 918–22.
5. Al-Refaie FN, *et al.* Results of long-term deferiprone (L1) therapy: a report by the International Study Group on Oral Iron Chelators. *Br J Haematol* 1995; **91;** 224–9.
6. Mehta J, *et al.* Fatal systemic lupus erythematosus in patient taking oral iron chelator L1. *Lancet* 1991; **337:** 298
7. Berdoukas V. Antinuclear antibodies in patients taking L1. *Lancet* 1991; **337:** 672.
8. Olivieri NF, *et al.* Rarity of systemic lupus erythematosus after oral iron chelator. *Lancet* 1991; **337:** 924.
9. Berkovitch M, *et al.* Arthropathy in thalassaemia patients receiving deferiprone. *Lancet* 1994; **343:** 1471–2.
10. Kontoghiorghes GJ, *et al.* 1,2-dimethyl-3-hydroxypyrid-4-one, an orally active chelator for treatment of iron overload. *Lancet* 1987; **i:** 1294–5.
11. Kontoghiorghes GJ, Hoffbrand AV. Clinical trials with oral iron chelator L1. *Lancet* 1989; **ii:** 1516–17.
12. Agarwal MB, *et al.* Oral iron chelation with L1. *Lancet* 1990; **335:** 601.
13. Olivieri NF, *et al.* Comparison of oral iron chelator L1 and desferrioxamine in iron-loaded patients. *Lancet* 1990; **336:** 1275–9.
14. Olivieri NF, *et al.* Long-term safety and effectiveness of iron-chelation therapy with deferiprone for thalassemia major. *N Engl J Med* 1998; **339:** 417–23.

Desferrioxamine Mesylate (1034-s)

Desferrioxamine Mesylate *(BANM)*.

Deferoxamine Mesilate *(pINNM)*; Ba-33112; Ba-29837 (desferrioxamine hydrochloride); Deferoxamine Mesylate *(USAN)*; Deferoxamini Mesilas; Desferrioxamine Methanesulphonate; NSC-527604 (desferrioxamine). 30-Amino-3,14,25-trihydroxy-3,9,14,20,25-penta-azatriacontane-2,10,13,21,24-pentaone methanesulphonate; *N'*-{5-[(4-{[5-(Acetylhydroxyamino)pentyl]amino}-1,4-dioxobutyl)hydroxyamino]pentyl}-*N*-(5-aminopentyl)-*N*-hydroxy-butanediamide monomethanesulphonate.

$C_{25}H_{48}N_6O_8,CH_3SO_3H$ = 656.8.

CAS — 70-51-9 (desferrioxamine); 138-14-7 (desferrioxamine mesylate); 1950-39-6 (desferrioxamine hydrochloride).

Pharmacopoeias. In Eur. (see p.viii), Int., Jpn, and US.

A white to off-white, odourless or almost odourless, powder. Freely **soluble** in water; very slightly soluble in alcohol; practically insoluble in ether; slightly soluble in methyl alcohol. A 10% solution in water has a pH of 3.7 to 5.5 and a 1% solution in water has a pH of 4.0 to 6.0. **Store** at 2° to 8° in airtight containers. Protect from light.

The manufacturers report that desferrioxamine solutions are **incompatible** with heparin.

Adverse Effects and Treatment

Rapid intravenous injection of desferrioxamine may cause flushing, urticaria, hypotension, and shock. Local pain may occur with subcutaneous or intramuscular injections and pruritus, erythema, and swelling have occurred after prolonged subcutaneous administration. Gastro-intestinal disorders, dysuria, fever, allergic skin rashes, tachycardia, cardiac arrhythmias, convulsions, and leg cramps have been reported. Visual disturbances, including retinal changes, and hearing loss may occur and may be reversible if desferrioxamine is withdrawn. Cataract formation has also been reported. Desferrioxamine therapy may retard growth in very young children.

Reviews of the adverse effects of desferrioxamine.

1. Bentur Y, *et al.* Deferoxamine (desferrioxamine): new toxicities for an old drug. *Drug Safety* 1991; **6:** 37–46.

Effects on the blood. A patient with end-stage renal disease developed reversible thrombocytopenia on 3 separate occasions after intravenous infusions of desferrioxamine for dialysis osteomalacia.[1] Acute fatal aplastic anaemia occurred in a 16-year-old girl with thalassaemia following intravenous administration of high doses of desferrioxamine (80 mg per kg body-weight daily) for 20 days.[2]

1. Walker JA, *et al.* Thrombocytopenia associated with intravenous desferrioxamine. *Am J Kidney Dis* 1985; **6:** 254–6.
2. Sofroniadou K, *et al.* Acute bone marrow aplasia associated with intravenous administration of deferoxamine (desferrioxamine). *Drug Safety* 1990; **5:** 152–4.

Effects on the ear and eye. Lens opacities, retinal pigmentary changes and other retinal abnormalities, and ocular disturbances including loss of colour vision, night blindness, decreased visual acuity, and field defects have been reported in patients receiving long-term or high-dose treatment with desferrioxamine.[1-4] In assessments of patients on long-term therapy with desferrioxamine the incidence of symptomatic and asymptomatic ocular changes has varied from 4% of 52 patients[5] to 66% of 15 patients.[6]

Sensorineural hearing impairment has also been reported.[5,7-12] Tinnitus has been reported in a few patients.[12,13]

Both ophthalmic and auditory abnormalities can improve when desferrioxamine is withdrawn,[1,3,5-10] although sometimes the effects may be irreversible[14] or recovery may only be partial.[8,9]

Several mechanisms for desferrioxamine neurotoxicity have been suggested.[6,8,12,15-18]

1. Davies SC, *et al.* Ocular toxicity of high-dose intravenous desferrioxamine. *Lancet* 1983; **ii:** 181–4.
2. Simon P, *et al.* Desferrioxamine, ocular toxicity, and trace metals. *Lancet* 1983; **ii:** 512–13.
3. Borgna-Pignatti C, *et al.* Visual loss in patient on high-dose subcutaneous desferrioxamine. *Lancet* 1984; **i:** 681.
4. Rubinstein M, *et al.* Ocular toxicity of desferrioxamine. *Lancet* 1985; **i:** 817–18.
5. Cohen A, *et al.* Vision and hearing during deferoxamine therapy. *J Pediatr* 1990; **117:** 326–30.
6. De Virgiliis S, *et al.* Depletion of trace elements and acute ocular toxicity induced by desferrioxamine in patients with thalassaemia. *Arch Dis Child* 1988; **63:** 250–5.
7. Guerin A, *et al.* Acute deafness and desferrioxamine. *Lancet* 1985; **ii:** 39.
8. Olivieri NF, *et al.* Visual and auditory neurotoxicity in patients receiving subcutaneous deferoxamine infusions. *N Engl J Med* 1986; **314:** 869–73.
9. Barratt PS, Toogood IRG. Hearing loss attributed to desferrioxamine in patients with beta-thalassaemia major. *Med J Aust* 1987; **147:** 177–9.
10. Wonke B, *et al.* Reversal of desferrioxamine induced auditory neurotoxicity during treatment with Ca-DTPA. *Arch Dis Child* 1989; **64:** 77–82.
11. Argiolu F, *et al.* Hearing impairment during deferoxamine therapy for thalassemia major. *J Pediatr* 1991; **118:** 826.
12. Porter JB, *et al.* Desferrioxamine ototoxicity: evaluation of risk factors in thalassaemic patients and guidelines for safe dosage. *Br J Haematol* 1989; **73:** 403–9.
13. Marsh MN, *et al.* Tinnitus in a patient with beta-thalassaemia intermedia on long-term treatment with desferrioxamine. *Postgrad Med J* 1981; **57:** 582–4.
14. Bene C, *et al.* Irreversible ocular toxicity from single "challenge" dose of deferoxamine. *Clin Nephrol* 1989; **31:** 45–8.
15. Bentur Y, *et al.* Comparison of deferoxamine pharmacokinetics between asymptomatic thalassemic children and those exhibiting severe neurotoxicity. *Clin Pharmacol Ther* 1990; **47:** 478–82.
16. Rahi AHS, *et al.* Ocular toxicity of desferrioxamine: light microscopic histochemical and ultrastructural findings. *Br J Ophthalmol* 1986; **70:** 373–81.
17. Pall H, *et al.* Ocular toxicity of desferrioxamine – an example of copper promoted auto-oxidative damage? *Br J Ophthalmol* 1989; **73:** 42–7.
18. Arden GB, *et al.* Ocular changes in patients undergoing long-term desferrioxamine treatment. *Br J Ophthalmol* 1984; **68:** 873–7.

Effects on growth rate. Growth retardation has been noted in thalassaemic children undergoing desferrioxamine therapy.[1,2] Growth retardation was related to dose[1,2] and inversely related to iron stores.[1] Also retardation was greater in those who started receiving desferrioxamine at the start of transfusion therapy at approximately 9 months old than in those who started desferrioxamine once iron accumulation was established, after about 3 years. A sharp increase in growth velocity was reported in 15 patients with low ferritin levels following a 50% reduction in desferrioxamine dose.[1]

1. Piga A, *et al.* High-dose desferrioxamine as a cause of growth failure in thalassaemic patients. *Eur J Haematol* 1988; **40:** 380–1.
2. De Virgiliis S, *et al.* Deferoxamine-induced growth retardation in patients with thalassemia major. *J Pediatr* 1988; **113:** 661–9.

Effects on the kidneys. A 14-year-old boy with thalassaemia major and haemosiderosis developed acute renal insufficiency during intravenous infusion of desferrioxamine.[1] Acute decreases in renal function were reported in 3 patients following infusions of desferrioxamine.[2] Two of these patients had received 180 mg per kg body-weight daily and it was suggested[3] that the nephrotoxicity could be related to these high doses, although others reported also having seen reductions in glomerular filtration rates following regular doses.[4]

1. Batey R, *et al.* Acute renal insufficiency occurring during intravenous desferrioxamine therapy. *Scand J Haematol* 1979; **22:** 277–9.
2. Koren G, *et al.* Acute changes in renal function associated with deferoxamine therapy. *Am J Dis Child* 1989; **143:** 1077–80.

3. Li Volti S, *et al.* Acute changes in renal function associated with deferoxamine therapy. *Am J Dis Child* 1990; **144:** 1069–70.
4. Koren G, Bentur Y. Acute changes in renal function associated with deferoxamine. *Am J Dis Child* 1990; **144:** 1070.

Effects on the lungs. A pulmonary syndrome with tachypnoea, hypoxaemia, reduced pulmonary function, and radiographic evidence of diffuse interstitial pneumonia has been reported in patients receiving high-dose intravenous therapy with desferrioxamine.[1,2] It has been suggested that a hypersensitivity reaction was involved.[1,2]

Fatal acute respiratory distress syndrome has occurred in 4 patients; in these cases desferrioxamine infusions had been given for 65 to 92 hours. Pulmonary complications had not been noted in patients given desferrioxamine for less than 24 hours.[3] This report did, however, generate subsequent correspondence disagreeing with the view that prolonged use of desferrioxamine was the cause of the toxicity. Alternative explanations for the pulmonary injury included the administration of above maximum daily doses of desferrioxamine[4] as well as inadequate desferrioxamine therapy.[5]

1. Freedman MH, *et al.* Pulmonary syndrome in patients with thalassemia major receiving intravenous deferoxamine infusions. *Am J Dis Child* 1990; **144:** 565–9.
2. Scanderbeg AC, *et al.* Pulmonary syndrome and intravenous high-dose desferrioxamine. *Lancet* 1990; **336:** 1511.
3. Tenenbein M, *et al.* Pulmonary toxic effects of continuous desferrioxamine administration in acute iron poisoning. *Lancet* 1992; **339:** 699–701.
4. Macarol V, Yawalkar SJ. Desferrioxamine in acute iron poisoning. *Lancet* 1992; **339:** 1601.
5. Shannon M. Desferrioxamine in acute iron poisoning. *Lancet* 1992; **339:** 1601.

Effects on the skin. Desferrioxamine may be used in the management of porphyria cutanea tarda (see p.983). However, lesions resembling porphyria cutanea tarda developed in 3 patients during long-term treatment with desferrioxamine for aluminium toxicity.[1] The lesions worsened on exposure to sun and resolved when desferrioxamine treatment was completed. It was also possible that the lesions were associated with aluminium accumulation. Alopecia was noted in one patient but an association with desferrioxamine therapy could not be established.

1. McCarthy JT, *et al.* Clinical experience with desferrioxamine in dialysis patients with aluminium toxicity. *Q J Med* 1990; **74:** 257–76.

Hypersensitivity. Individual cases of anaphylactoid reactions to desferrioxamine have been reported.[1,2] Rapid intravenous desensitisation was successful in two patients.[1,2] Effects on the lungs have also been attributed to hypersensitivity (see above).

1. Miller KB, *et al.* Rapid desensitisation for desferrioxamine anaphylactic reaction. *Lancet* 1981; **i:** 1059.
2. Bousquet J, *et al.* Rapid desensitisation for desferrioxamine anaphylactoid reactions. *Lancet* 1983; **ii:** 859–60.

Treatment of adverse effects. The adverse effects of desferrioxamine generally respond to dosage reduction. In acute overdosage desferrioxamine may be removed by haemodialysis.

Isoniazid, 50 or 100 mg with pyridoxine, suppressed intolerable adverse effects of desferrioxamine in a patient with Alzheimer's disease.[1] The adverse effects, anorexia and weight loss, were attributed to a toxic metabolite of desferrioxamine generated by the plasma monoamine oxidase enzyme system and isoniazid reduced the formation of this suspect metabolite.

1. Kruck TPA, *et al.* Suppression of deferoxamine mesylate treatment-induced side effects by coadministration of isoniazid in a patient with Alzheimer's disease subject to aluminum removal by ionspecific chelation. *Clin Pharmacol Ther* 1990; **48:** 439–46.

Precautions

Desferrioxamine should be used with caution in patients with impaired renal function since the metal complexes are excreted by the kidneys (in those with severe renal impairment dialysis increases elimination). Skeletal fetal anomalies have occurred in *animals*. The desferrioxamine-iron complex excreted by the kidneys may colour the urine reddish-brown. Desferrioxamine may exacerbate aluminium-related encephalopathy and precipitate seizures. Prophylactic treatment with antiepileptics such as clonazepam has been suggested for patients judged to be at risk. An increased susceptibility to infection, particularly with *Yersinia* species, has been reported in patients with iron overload treated with desferrioxamine. Severe fungal infections have also been reported, predominantly in patients undergoing dialysis. If infection is suspected, treatment with desferrioxamine should be stopped and appropriate antimicrobial treatment given.

The urinary excretion of iron should be regularly monitored during treatment and periodic ophthalmological and audiological examinations are recommended for patients on long-term therapy. Monitoring of cardiac function is also recommended for patients receiving combined treatment with ascorbic acid (see also under Interactions, below).

Inappropriately high dosage in children with low ferritin levels may retard growth, therefore regular checks on height and weight are recommended for children.

Aluminium encephalopathy. The precipitation of dialysis dementia with some fatal outcomes[1-3] has been associated with desferrioxamine treatment for aluminium overload in dialysis patients. McCauley and Sorkin suggested that the effect could be dose related,[2] but Lillevang and Pedersen[3] reported exacerbation of aluminium encephalopathy following the low dose of 0.5 g twice weekly. Sherrard and colleagues[1] suggested that the onset of symptoms could be associated with high concentrations of aluminium observed after desferrioxamine administration. They recommended the use of low doses (for example 10 mg per kg body-weight) given immediately before dialysis in affected patients in conjunction with charcoal haemoperfusion to avoid high serum-aluminium concentrations.

1. Sherrard DJ, *et al.* Precipitation of dialysis dementia by deferoxamine treatment of aluminum related bone disease. *Am J Kidney Dis* 1988; **12:** 126–30.
2. McCauley J, Sorkin I. Exacerbation of aluminium encephalopathy after treatment with desferrioxamine. *Nephrol Dial Transplant* 1989; **4:** 110–14.
3. Lillevang ST, Pedersen FB. Exacerbation of aluminium encephalopathy after treatment with desferrioxamine. *Nephrol Dial Transplant* 1989; **4:** 676.

Infection susceptibility. *Yersinia enterocolitica* is one of the most iron-dependent of all microbes, but unlike most other aerobic bacteria, it produces no detectable iron-binding compounds, or siderophores.[1] Exogenous siderophores, such as desferrioxamine, may enable *Y. enterocolitica* to overcome this handicap[2] and the apparent increased susceptibility to yersiniosis in patients with severe iron overload may therefore be attributable at least in part to desferrioxamine therapy rather than just the increased availability of iron. Infections due to *Y. enterocolitica* have been reported in patients receiving desferrioxamine for acute iron overdosage[3] or for chronic iron overload.[2,4-7] Severe infection with *Y. pseudotuberculosis* has also been reported in a thalassaemic patient on long-term desferrioxamine therapy.[8]

Treatment with desferrioxamine may also increase susceptibility to mucormycosis (p.369). Infections have occurred both in patients with iron overload disorders[9,10] and in those who do not have excessive iron stores.[11-13] Of 26 cases of mucormycosis in patients undergoing treatment with desferrioxamine reviewed by Daly and colleagues[10] 23 patients died; in 19 cases the diagnosis was only made at necropsy and only 9 patients received potentially effective treatment (surgery and/or amphotericin). The organisms responsible were *Rhizopus* species in 13 cases and *Cunninghamella bertholletiae* in 3. In another review of 24 cases of mucormycosis in patients on dialysis,[14] at least 21 were receiving desferrioxamine; infection was fatal in 21 of the 24 patients.

In view of the serious nature of these infections it is important that they should be recognised and treated promptly. It has been suggested that a short course of a suitable antibacterial could be given as prophylaxis to young children from areas with a high incidence of yersiniosis (see Yersinia Enteritis, p.125) who require treatment with desferrioxamine.[15]

1. Anonymous. Yersiniosis today. *Lancet* 1984; **i:** 84–5.
2. Robins-Browne RM, Prpic JK. Desferrioxamine and systemic yersiniosis. *Lancet* 1983; **ii:** 1372.
3. Melby K, *et al.* Septicaemia due to Yersinia enterocolitica after oral overdoses of iron. *Br Med J* 1982; **285:** 467–8.
4. Scharnetzky M, *et al.* Prophylaxis of systemic yersinosis in thalassaemia major. *Lancet* 1984; **i:** 791.
5. Chiu HY, *et al.* Infection with Yersinia enterocolitica in patients with iron overload. *Br Med J* 1986; **292:** 97.
6. Kelly D, *et al.* Yersinia and iron overload. *Br Med J* 1986; **292:** 413.
7. Gallant T, *et al.* Yersinia sepsis in patients with iron overload treated with deferoxamine. *N Engl J Med* 1986; **314:** 1643.
8. Gordts B, *et al.* Yersinia pseudotuberculosis septicaemia in thalassaemia major. *Lancet* 1984; **i:** 41–2.
9. Sane A, *et al.* Deferoxamine treatment as a risk factor for zygomycete infection. *J Infect Dis* 1989; **159:** 151–2.
10. Daly AL, *et al.* Mucormycosis: association with deferoxamine therapy. *Am J Med* 1989; **87:** 468–71.
11. Goodill JJ, Abuelo JG. Mucormycosis–a new risk of deferoxamine therapy in dialysis patients with aluminum or iron overload? *N Engl J Med* 1987; **316:** 54.
12. Windus DW, *et al.* Fatal rhizopus infections in hemodialysis patients receiving deferoxamine. *Ann Intern Med* 1987; **107:** 678–80.
13. Boelaert JR, *et al.* Mucormycosis infections in dialysis patients. *Ann Intern Med* 1987; **107:** 782–3.
14. Boelaert JR, *et al.* Mucormycosis among patients on dialysis. *N Engl J Med* 1989; **321:** 190–1.
15. Hadjiminas JM. Yersiniosis in acutely iron-loaded children treated with desferrioxamine. *J Antimicrob Chemother* 1988; **21:** 680–1.

Pregnancy. Abnormalities in *animals* have been noted following the administration of desferrioxamine in pregnancy. Thus the outcome following iron overdose during pregnancy was studied in 66 patients reported to the Teratology Information Service in London of whom 35 received desferrioxamine.[1] Seven infants of the 66 pregnancies had malformations (severe in only one) and all were associated with maternal overdoses after the first trimester and therefore could not be directly related to either iron or desferrioxamine. It was concluded that treatment of iron overdose with desferrioxamine should not be withheld solely on the grounds of pregnancy.

1. McElhatton PR, *et al.* Outcome of pregnancy following deliberate iron overdose by the mother. *Hum Exp Toxicol* 1993; **12:** 579.

Interactions

Desferrioxamine is usually administered parenterally and thus drug interactions due to chelation with oral metal ions are not a problem.

Ascorbic acid. Ascorbic acid is often given in addition to desferrioxamine to patients with iron overload to achieve better iron excretion. However, early on in treatment when there is excess tissue iron there is some evidence that ascorbic acid may worsen the iron toxicity, particularly to the heart. Thus, ascorbic acid should not be given for the first month after starting desferrioxamine treatment.

Diagnostic tests. Desferrioxamine could interfere with estimations of total iron-binding capacity.[1] It may also interfere with colorimetric iron assays.

Desferrioxamine may distort the results of gallium-67 imaging studies.

1. Bentur Y, *et al.* Misinterpretation of iron-binding capacity in the presence of deferoxamine. *J Pediatr* 1991; **118:** 139–42.

Phenothiazines. Neurological symptoms including loss of consciousness, occurred in 2 patients who received prochlorperazine during desferrioxamine administration.[1] Concomitant use should be avoided.

1. Blake DR, *et al.* Cerebral and ocular toxicity induced by desferrioxamine. *Q J Med* 1985; **56:** 345–55.

Pharmacokinetics

Desferrioxamine mesylate is poorly absorbed from the gastro-intestinal tract. Following parenteral administration, desferrioxamine forms chelates with metal ions and is also metabolised, primarily in the plasma. The iron-desferrioxamine chelate is excreted in the urine and bile. Desferrioxamine is absorbed during peritoneal dialysis if added to the dialysis fluid.

References.

1. Summers MR, *et al.* Studies in desferrioxamine and ferrioxamine metabolism in normal and iron-loaded subjects. *Br J Haematol* 1979; **42:** 547–55.
2. Allain P, *et al.* Pharmacokinetics and renal elimination of desferrioxamine and ferrioxamine in healthy subjects and patients with haemochromatosis. *Br J Clin Pharmacol* 1987; **24:** 207–12.

Uses and Administration

Desferrioxamine is a chelator which has a high affinity for ferric iron. When given by injection it forms a stable water-soluble iron-complex (ferrioxamine) which is readily excreted in the urine and in bile. Desferrioxamine appears to remove both free iron and bound iron from haemosiderin and ferritin but not from haemoglobin, transferrin, or cytochromes. It is estimated that 100 mg of desferrioxamine mesylate could bind about 8.5 mg of iron but it is unlikely that such a figure could be achieved in practice. Desferrioxamine also has an affinity for other trivalent metal ions including aluminium and theoretically 100 mg of the mesylate could bind 4.1 mg of aluminium.

Desferrioxamine increases the excretion of iron from the body and is used in conditions associated with chronic iron overload (such as the iron storage disorders haemochromatosis and haemosiderosis and following repeated transfusions as in thalassaemia) and in acute iron poisoning. It has been used as eye drops in the management of ocular siderosis and corneal rust stains. It is also used to reduce aluminium overload in patients with end-stage renal failure on maintenance dialysis.

Desferrioxamine is administered as the mesylate and may be given by subcutaneous or intravenous infusion, by intramuscular injection, orally, or intraperitoneally.

In the treatment of **chronic iron overload** the dosage and route of administration should be determined for each patient by monitoring urinary iron excretion, with the aim of normalising serum-ferritin concentrations. Continuous subcutaneous infusions, preferably with the aid of a small portable infusion pump, are particularly convenient for ambulant patients and are more effective than intramuscular injections. Continuous intravenous infusion has been recommended for patients incapable of continuing subcutaneous infusions or for those with cardiac problems secondary to iron overload. An initial daily dose of desferrioxamine mesylate 500 mg may be given by subcutaneous infusion or intravenous infusion, increasing until a plateau of iron excretion is reached. The usual effective dose range is 20 to 60 mg per kg body-weight daily. Subcutaneous infusions are administered 4 to 7 times a week depending on the degree of iron overload and are given over 8 to 12 hours, or over 24 hours in some patients. When given by intramuscular injection the initial dose has been 0.5 to 1 g daily as 1 or 2 injections, but again the maintenance dose is determined by response. It has been suggested that in addition to intramuscular treatment, up to 2 g of desferrioxamine mesylate should be given by intravenous infusion for each unit of blood transfused, at a rate not more than 15 mg per kg body-weight per hour at the time of each blood transfusion. Desferrioxamine should be administered separately from the blood. The co-administration of ascorbic acid supplements can enhance the excretion of iron, but should not be started until 1 month after starting desferrioxamine treatment (to reduce the risk of toxicity, see under Interactions, above). Ascorbic acid is given in doses of 200 mg daily for adults or 100 mg daily for infants; it should be administered separately from food since it also enhances iron absorption.

Desferrioxamine has been used as a *diagnostic test* for iron storage disease in patients with normal renal function by injecting 0.5 g of the mesylate intramuscularly and estimating the excretion of iron in the urine collected over the next 6 hours; an excretion of more than 1 mg of iron by the patient under test is suggestive of iron storage disease and more than 1.5 mg can be regarded as pathological.

In the treatment of **acute iron poisoning** the following doses and routes are suggested. In the UK, desferrioxamine mesylate 5 to 10 g in 50 to 100 mL of water may be given by mouth, or by stomach tube, to chelate any iron left in the stomach and prevent further absorption following gastric lavage. To eliminate iron already absorbed, desferrioxamine mesylate should be given intramuscularly or, if the patient is hypotensive or in shock, intravenously by slow infusion. The dose and route of parenteral administration should be adjusted according to the severity of the poisoning, preferably as indicated by the serum-iron concentration and total iron binding capacity, if available, although chelation therapy should be started in patients with significant symptoms without waiting for the results of blood concentrations. In the UK the usual dose of desferrioxamine mesylate is 2 g in adults or 1 g in children by intramuscular injection. Alternatively it may be given by slow intravenous infusion of up to 15 mg per kg body-weight per hour, reducing after 4 to 6 hours to provide a total dose not exceeding 80 mg per kg in 24 hours, although larger doses may be tolerated. In the USA, a recommended procedure is to give desferrioxamine mesylate 1 g initially by intramuscular injection followed by 0.5 g every 4 hours for 2 doses. Subsequent doses of 0.5 g may be administered every 4 to 12 hours to a maximum of 6 g in 24 hours. Alternatively, the same doses may be given by slow intravenous infusion at a rate of not more than 15 mg per kg per hour, but this route of administration is only recommended for patients in a state of cardiovascular collapse.

In the treatment of **aluminium overload** in patients with end-stage renal failure, those undergoing maintenance haemodialysis or haemofiltration may be given desferrioxamine mesylate 5 mg per kg once a week by slow intravenous infusion during the last hour of a dialysis. In patients on peritoneal dialysis (CAPD or CCPD) desferrioxamine mesylate 5 mg per kg may be given once a week, by slow intravenous infusion, subcutaneously, intramuscularly, or intraperitoneally (the recommended route) before the final exchange of the day. For the *diagnosis* of aluminium overload desferrioxamine mesylate 5 mg per kg is administered by slow intravenous infusion during the last hour of haemodialysis. An increase in serum-aluminium concentration, above base-line of more than 150 ng per mL (measured at the start of the next dialysis session) suggests aluminium overload.

Eye drops containing desferrioxamine mesylate 10% have been administered for the treatment of ocular siderosis and corneal rust stains.

Administration. In the absence of a suitable alternative to desferrioxamine as a chelator in chronic iron overload syndromes several attempts have been made to overcome compliance problems encountered with standard parenteral administration by developing oral,[1-3] rectal,[4] or intranasal[5] regimens. Although most regimens produced an increase in urinary iron excretion above base-line, the amount excreted was generally considered to be insufficient to be clinically useful, particularly in young children with low iron stores.[3] However, these alternate routes of administration could be useful as an adjunct in selected patients.[1,5]

Greater success has been reported[6,7] with daily intravenous infusion of desferrioxamine 6 to 12 g over 12 hours[6] or intermittent intravenous infusions in addition to subcutaneous administration[7] in patients poorly compliant with conventional subcutaneous therapy. No major disturbances in vision or hearing were encountered in 8 patients undergoing intensive intravenous treatment for up to 24 months,[6] and established iron-induced heart disease in 2 of these patients improved during therapy. Administration by twice-daily subcutaneous bolus injection has also been reported.[8]

Intraperitoneal administration of desferrioxamine may be used to reduce aluminium levels in patients receiving peritoneal dialysis for chronic renal failure. Good results have also been reported[9] in a patient with haemochromatosis complicated by cirrhosis and cardiomyopathy, in whom a chronic peritoneal dialysis catheter was used to control ascites and to administer desferrioxamine.

1. Callender ST, Weatherall DJ. Iron chelation with oral desferrioxamine. *Lancet* 1980; **ii:** 689.
2. Jacobs A, Chang Ting W. Iron chelation with oral desferrioxamine. *Lancet* 1980; **ii:** 794.
3. Kattamis C, *et al.* Oral desferrioxamine in young patients with thalassaemia. *Lancet* 1981; **i:** 51.
4. Kontoghiorghes G, *et al.* Desferrioxamine suppositories. *Lancet* 1983; **ii:** 454.
5. Gordon GS, *et al.* Intranasal administration of deferoxamine to iron overloaded patients. *Am J Med Sci* 1989; **297:** 280–4.
6. Cohen AR, *et al.* Rapid removal of excessive iron with daily, high-dose intravenous chelation therapy. *J Pediatr* 1989; **115:** 151–5.
7. Sabatino D. Rapid removal of excessive iron in thalassemia by high-dose intravenous chelation therapy. *J Pediatr* 1990; **116:** 157–8.
8. Borgna-Pignatti C, Cohen A. Evaluation of a new method of administration of the iron chelating agent deferoxamine. *J Pediatr* 1997; **130:** 86–8.
9. Swartz RD, Legault DJ. Long-term intraperitoneal deferoxamine for hemochromatosis. *Am J Med* 1996; **100:** 308–12.

Aluminium overload. Aluminium has been implicated in a number of disorders[1] including renal osteodystrophy, dialysis dementia, and Alzheimer's disease (p.1386). Patients with chronic renal failure may be exposed to aluminium from the use of aluminium-containing phosphate binders and from the high concentrations of aluminium sometimes found in tap water used to prepare dialysis fluids. Sources of aluminium in other patients include aluminium-containing antacids, preparations for total parenteral nutrition, contaminated albumin solutions, and environmental and industrial sources.[1] Further references to aluminium toxicity are included under Aluminium (see p.1547).

In patients with chronic renal failure the major sources of aluminium can be substantially reduced by the use of alternative phosphate binders (see Renal Osteodystrophy, p.732) and by reduction in the aluminium concentration of dialysis fluids by reverse osmosis and deionisation.[1] Desferrioxamine may also be used (but see under Precautions, above, for a discussion of aluminium toxicity being exacerbated by desferrioxamine).

Chang and Barre[2] have demonstrated that desferrioxamine greatly increased the removal of aluminium by adsorbent haemoperfusion or haemodialysis. In the treatment of dialysis encephalopathy, desferrioxamine has been reported to have beneficial effects by the mobilisation and removal of aluminium when administered in doses of up to 6 g once a week via the arterial line during the first 2 hours of haemodialysis.[3,4] Of 11 patients with dialysis encephalopathy studied by Milne *et al.*[5] 5 were treated with deionised or reverse-osmosis water alone and all died. The other 6 were treated similarly but were also given desferrioxamine 6 to 10 g intravenously each week at dialysis; 4 of these patients improved but 2 died of progressive dementia.

Although the total amount of aluminium removed with desferrioxamine treatment during peritoneal dialysis may be small compared with the amounts removed during haemodialysis, substantial improvement in early aluminium encephalopathy has been achieved in a patient on continuous ambulatory peritoneal dialysis by using intraperitoneal desferrioxamine.[6] In a study of 27 patients undergoing haemodialysis but without clinical encephalopathy Altmann and colleagues[7] demonstrated impaired cerebral function associated with only mildly elevated plasma-aluminium concentrations. Administration of desferrioxamine to 15 of these patients for 3 months improved psychomotor performance.

Desferrioxamine has produced rapid clinical improvement in patients with dialysis-related bone disease.[8-10] Reduction in the aluminium content of bone was reported in a study of 7 patients by Malluche and colleagues,[8] and in 9 patients by McCarthy and colleagues,[9] but not by Brown and colleagues in a report of 2 patients.[10] Measurement of plasma-aluminium concentrations 24 and 44 hours after administration of desferrioxamine 40 mg per kg body-weight has been used to diagnose aluminium-related osteodystrophy[9,11] but Malluche *et al.*,[8] using a lower dose of desferrioxamine (28.5 mg per kg) and measuring plasma aluminium 5 hours later, found similar increases in patients both with and without bone-aluminium accumulation.

Desferrioxamine therapy has also produced beneficial results in dialysis patients with anaemia[12-14] and has also been found to reverse aluminium-induced resistance to erythropoietin.[15,16]

Prurigo nodularis in chronic aluminium overload has responded to desferrioxamine with resolution of itch and skin lesions.[17]

McLachlan and colleagues[18] found that sustained low doses of desferrioxamine could slow the progression of the dementia of Alzheimer's disease in a study of 48 patients although their results have been questioned.[19,20]

1. Monteagudo FSE, *et al.* Recent developments in aluminium toxicology. *Med Toxicol* 1989; **4:** 1–16.
2. Chang TMS, Barre P. Effect of desferrioxamine on removal of aluminium and iron by coated charcoal haemoperfusion and haemodialysis. *Lancet* 1983; **ii:** 1051–3.
3. Ackrill P, *et al.* Successful removal of aluminium from patient with dialysis encephalopathy. *Lancet* 1980; **ii:** 692–3.
4. Arze RS, *et al.* Reversal of aluminium dialysis encephalopathy after desferrioxamine treatment. *Lancet* 1981; **ii:** 1116.
5. Milne FJ, *et al.* Low aluminium water, desferrioxamine, and dialysis encephalopathy. *Lancet* 1982; **ii:** 502.
6. Payton CD, *et al.* Successful treatment of aluminium encephalopathy by intraperitoneal desferrioxamine. *Lancet* 1984; **i:** 1132–3.
7. Altmann P, *et al.* Disturbance of cerebral function by aluminium in haemodialysis patients without overt aluminium toxicity. *Lancet* 1989; **ii:** 7–12.
8. Malluche HH, *et al.* The use of deferoxamine in the management of aluminum accumulation in bone in patients with renal failure. *N Engl J Med* 1984; **311:** 140–4.
9. McCarthy JT, *et al.* Clinical experience with desferrioxamine in dialysis patients with aluminium toxicity. *Q J Med* 1990; **74:** 257–76.
10. Brown DJ, *et al.* Treatment of dialysis osteomalacia with desferrioxamine. *Lancet* 1982; **ii:** 343–5.
11. Milliner DS, *et al.* Use of deferoxamine infusion test in the diagnosis of aluminium-related osteodystrophy. *Ann Intern Med* 1984; **101:** 775–80.
12. de la Serna F-J, *et al.* Improvement in the erythropoiesis of chronic haemodialysis patients with desferrioxamine. *Lancet* 1988; **i:** 1009–11.
13. Altmann P, *et al.* Aluminium chelation therapy in dialysis patients: evidence for inhibition of haemoglobin synthesis by low levels of aluminium. *Lancet* 1988; **i:** 1012–15.
14. Padovese P, *et al.* Desferrioxamine versus erythropoietin for treatment of dialysis anaemia. *Lancet* 1990; **335:** 1465.
15. Rosenlöf K, *et al.* Erythropoietin, aluminium, and anaemia in patients on haemodialysis. *Lancet* 1990; **335:** 247–9.
16. Zachée P, *et al.* Erythropoietin, aluminium, and anaemia in patients on haemodialysis. *Lancet* 1990; **335:** 1038–9.
17. Brown MA, *et al.* Prurigo nodularis and aluminium overload in maintenance haemodialysis. *Lancet* 1992; **340:** 48.
18. McLachlan DRC, *et al.* Intramuscular desferrioxamine in patients with Alzheimer's disease. *Lancet* 1991; **337:** 1304–8. Correction. *ibid.*: 1618.
19. Davies P. Desferrioxamine for Alzheimer's disease. *Lancet* 1991; **338:** 325.
20. Holleman DR, Goldstone JR. Desferrioxamine for Alzheimer's disease. *Lancet* 1991; **338:** 325.

Iron overload diseases. Chronic iron overload can be caused by inappropriately increased gastro-intestinal absorption, by grossly excessive oral intake over long periods, or by parenteral administration of iron, for example from transfused blood.[1] Excess iron is stored in the form of ferritin and haemosiderin. The term *haemosiderosis* is applied to the accumulation of haemosiderin in body tissues without associated tissue damage; *haemochromatosis* refers to a chronic disease state in which iron overload leads to tissue damage, predominantly in the heart, liver, and pancreas.[1-3] Primary or hereditary haemochromatosis is caused by a genetic defect in iron metabolism which results in excessive gastro-intestinal absorption of iron. The treatment of choice for primary haemochromatosis is phlebotomy,[1-3] but chelation therapy may be needed in patients with anaemia, hypoproteinaemia, or severe cardiac disease.[1,3] Secondary or acquired haemochromatosis is commonly associated with chronic anaemias, in particular thalassaemia, in which excessive iron uptake due to disordered erythropoiesis and excess iron from repeated blood transfusions contribute to iron overload. In these patients the usual therapy is iron chelation with desferrioxamine (see below).

1. Halliday JW, Basset ML. Treatment of iron storage disorders. *Drugs* 1980; **20:** 2077–15.
2. Crawford DHG, Halliday JW. Current concepts in rational therapy for haemochromatosis. *Drugs* 1991; **41:** 875–82.
3. Kirking MH. Treatment of chronic iron overload. *Clin Pharm* 1991; **10:** 775–83.

THALASSAEMIA. Patients homozygous for β-thalassaemia (p.704) have severe anaemia requiring regular blood transfusions. As a consequence of this treatment iron overload develops and the excessive deposition of iron in the myocardium usually results in these patients dying in their second or third decade from arrhythmias or cardiac failure. Desferrioxamine is used to retard the accumulation of iron, the greatest increase in iron excretion being seen in patients given the drug by continuous subcutaneous infusion rather than intramuscular bolus. Better iron excretion may be achieved if patients are given ascorbic acid 100 to 200 mg daily in addition to desferrioxamine (but see Interactions, above).

Desferrioxamine has been shown to improve survival in thalassaemic children given regular systemic therapy,[1-3] and there has also been preliminary evidence that impaired organ function might improve with intensive desferrioxamine therapy. A reduction in liver-iron concentrations and an improvement in liver function was reported in some patients with transfusional iron overload treated with desferrioxamine 2 to 4 g by slow subcutaneous infusion over 12 hours on 6 nights a week,[4] although Maurer and colleagues[5] observed improvement in the degree of hepatic fibrosis in only 2 of 7 patients given desferrioxamine up to 85 mg per kg body-weight daily by subcutaneous injection after 3 to 5 years, despite reductions in iron concentrations. Bronspiegel-Weintrob and colleagues[6] showed that beginning chelation therapy before puberty could help to ensure normal sexual development in patients with thalassaemia major. Studies indicating that desferrioxamine treatment might preserve or possibly improve cardiac function impaired by iron overload in thalassaemic patients[7-9] have been supported by a decrease in mortality from cardiac disease since the introduction of desferrioxamine in Italy,[1] although this continues to be the main cause of death in patients with thalassaemia.[1,2] A recent study[3] in patients with β-thalassaemia demonstrated a markedly improved prognosis for survival without cardiac disease in patients who began chelation therapy with desferrioxamine before iron loading was severe and in whom reduced serum-ferritin concentrations were maintained over a long period. Failure to prevent the accumulation of excess iron or to remove large stores of iron was associated with a poor prognosis at any age. Thus, it is considered advisable to begin chelation therapy as early as possible (in practice usually at 2 to 3 years of age when iron overload becomes significant) to try to prevent organ damage developing.

1. Zurlo MG, *et al.* Survival and causes of death in thalassaemia major. *Lancet* 1989; **ii:** 27–30.
2. Ehlers KH, *et al.* Prolonged survival in patients with beta-thalassemia major treated with deferoxamine. *J Pediatr* 1991; **118:** 540–5.
3. Olivieri NF, *et al.* Survival in medically treated patients with homozygous β-thalassemia. *N Engl J Med* 1994; **331:** 574–8.
4. Hoffbrand AV, *et al.* Improvement in status and liver function in patients with transfusional iron overload with long-term subcutaneous desferrioxamine. *Lancet* 1979; **i:** 947–9.
5. Maurer HS, *et al.* A prospective evaluation of iron chelation therapy in children with severe β-thalassemia: a six-year study. *Am J Dis Child* 1988; **142:** 287–92.
6. Bronspiegel-Weintrob N, *et al.* Effect of age at the start of iron chelation therapy on gonadal function in β-thalassemia major. *N Engl J Med* 1990; **323:** 713–19.
7. Freeman AP, *et al.* Early left ventricular dysfunction and chelation therapy in thalassemia major. *Ann Intern Med* 1983; **99:** 450–4.
8. Marcus RE, *et al.* Desferrioxamine to improve cardiac function in iron-overloaded patients with thalassaemia major. *Lancet* 1984; **i:** 392–3.
9. Wolfe L, *et al.* Prevention of cardiac disease by subcutaneous deferoxamine in patients with thalassemia major. *N Engl J Med* 1985; **312:** 1600–3.

Iron poisoning. Despite the frequency of acute poisoning with iron preparations, no universally accepted treatment protocol exists. It is often difficult to determine the amount of iron ingested, and assessment of clinical symptoms can be misleading since patients may exhibit mild symptoms despite having ingested potentially toxic quantities of iron. Measurement of the serum-iron concentration and the total iron-binding capacity (TIBC) is useful in assessing the severity of poisoning but may not be immediately available and may be misleading. The desferrioxamine challenge test entails giving desferrioxamine 50 mg per kg body-weight (to a maximum dose of 1 g) intramuscularly; if free iron is present, ferrioxamine will be excreted in the urine imparting a classic "vin rosé" colour. However, the results can be difficult to interpret and a negative result does not rule out iron toxicity.

The initial stage of treatment entails removal of unabsorbed iron from the gastro-intestinal tract by induction of emesis and/or gastric lavage, with whole-bowel irrigation as a treatment option in patients suspected of ingesting modified-release preparations or those with radiographic evidence of unabsorbed tablets remaining after gastric lavage. The addition of desferrioxamine to the lavage fluid is controversial since there is little evidence of its efficacy and concern over possible toxic effects of ferrioxamine. However, in the UK it is common practice to leave 5 to 10 g of desferrioxamine in the stomach after gastric lavage. Supportive care should be given as appropriate and may be all that is required in mild poisoning. Activated charcoal is not effective in iron poisoning.

Chelation therapy with desferrioxamine given intramuscularly or intravenously is indicated in patients with impaired consciousness, shock or hypotension; in those with other symptoms of severe poisoning, for example leucocytosis; in those in whom the serum-iron concentration exceeds the TIBC; in those with a positive desferrioxamine challenge test; and those with a serum-iron concentration above 350 μg per 100 mL if TIBC estimations are unavailable. In severe toxicity intravenous desferrioxamine is given immediately without waiting for the results of serum-iron measurements. There is no general agreement on the duration of chelation therapy; among the suggested end-points are the disappearance of the vin rosé coloration of the urine, 24 hours after the disappearance of coloration, and reduction of serum-iron concentrations to less than 100 μg per 100 mL.

General references.

1. Proudfoot AT, *et al.* Management of acute iron poisoning. *Med Toxicol* 1986; **1:** 83–100.
2. Engle JP, *et al.* Acute iron intoxication: treatment controversies. *Drug Intell Clin Pharm* 1987; **21:** 153–9.
3. Mann KV, *et al.* Management of acute iron overdose. *Clin Pharm* 1989; **8:** 428–40.

Malaria. Following the suggestion that iron-deficiency anaemia may offer some protection against infections (see Infections in the Precautions for Iron, p.1346), desferrioxamine was tried in a few patients with malaria.[1,2] Any antimalarial effect of desferrioxamine was thought to be as a result of chelation of parasite-associated iron rather than reduction in body-iron concentrations in the patient. Desferrioxamine given intravenously was reported[3] to shorten the time to regain consciousness in children with cerebral malaria receiving standard therapy with intravenous quinine and oral pyrimethamine-sulfadoxine. However, in a more recent study[4] there was no evidence of a beneficial effect on mortality when desferrioxamine was added to an antimalarial treatment regimen that included a loading dose of quinine.

For a discussion of malaria and its management, see p.422.

1. Gordeuk VR, *et al.* Iron chelation as a chemotherapeutic strategy for falciparum malaria. *Am J Trop Med Hyg* 1993; **48:** 193–7.
2. Thompson DF. Deferoxamine treatment of malaria. *Ann Pharmacother* 1994; **28:** 602–3.
3. Gordeuk V, *et al.* Effect of iron chelation therapy on recovery from deep coma, in children with cerebral malaria. *N Engl J Med* 1992; **327:** 1473–7.
4. Thuma PE, *et al.* Effect of iron chelation therapy on mortality in Zambian children with cerebral malaria. *Trans R Soc Trop Med Hyg* 1998; **92:** 214–18.

Porphyria. The management of various forms of porphyria is discussed on p.983. Desferrioxamine may be used to reduce serum-iron concentrations in porphyria cutanea tarda if phlebotomy is contra-indicated. In a study of 25 patients with porphyria cutanea tarda,[1] subcutaneous infusion of desferrioxamine was found to be as effective as repeated phlebotomies in normalising porphyrin excretion and iron storage. Desferrioxamine was also used successfully to treat haemodialysis-related porphyria cutanea tarda in a 22-year-old man in whom venesection therapy was contra-indicated because of severe anaemia requiring multiple blood transfusion.[2] Each course of intravenous desferrioxamine therapy after the end of 3 haemodialysis sessions was accompanied by a marked decrease in plasma porphyrins, a sharp increase in haematocrit values, and a simultaneous improvement in skin lesions.

1. Rocchi E, *et al.* Iron removal therapy in porphyria cutanea tarda: phlebotomy versus slow subcutaneous desferrioxamine infusion. *Br J Dermatol* 1986; **114:** 621–9.
2. Praga M, *et al.* Treatment of hemodialysis-related porphyria cutanea tarda with deferoxamine. *N Engl J Med* 1987; **316:** 547–8.

Preparations

BP 1998: Desferrioxamine Injection;
USP 23: Deferoxamine Mesylate for Injection.

Proprietary Preparations (details are given in Part 3)
Aust.: Desferal; ***Austral.:*** Desferal; ***Belg.:*** Desferal; ***Canad.:*** Desferal; ***Fr.:*** Desferal; ***Ger.:*** Desferal; ***Irl.:*** Desferal; ***Ital.:*** Desferal; ***Neth.:*** Desferal; ***Norw.:*** Desferal; ***S.Afr.:*** Desferal; ***Spain:*** Desferin; ***Swed.:*** Desferal; ***Switz.:*** Desferal; ***UK:*** Desferal; ***USA:*** Desferal.

Dexrazoxane (19333-p)

Dexrazoxane (*BAN, USAN, rINN*).

ADR-529; ICRF-187; NSC-169780. (+)-(*S*)-4,4′-Propylenebis(piperazine-2,6-dione).

$C_{11}H_{16}N_4O_4$ = 268.3.

CAS — 24584-09-6.

Adverse Effects and Precautions

Dexrazoxane may add to the bone-marrow depression caused by antineoplastics given concurrently and frequent complete blood counts are recommended during therapy. Although dexrazoxane protects against the cardiotoxic effects of anthracyclines cardiac function should continue to be monitored when dexrazoxane is used. Pain on injection has been reported.

It has been recommended that dexrazoxane should only be given to patients who have received a cumulative dose of doxorubicin of 300 mg per m² body-surface and who require continued administration, since there is some evidence that dexrazoxane may reduce the efficacy of the antineoplastic regimen.

Pharmacokinetics

Dexrazoxane is mainly excreted in the urine as unchanged drug and metabolites. The elimination half-life is reported to be about 2 hours.

Uses and Administration

Dexrazoxane is the (+)-enantiomorph of the antineoplastic drug razoxane (p.560) and is a cytoprotective agent that is used to reduce the cardiotoxicity of doxorubicin and other anthracyclines (see Effects on the Heart, p.529). It is hydrolysed to an active metabolite that is similar to edetic acid. This chelates iron within the cells and appears to prevent the formation of the anthracycline-iron complex that is thought to be responsible for cardiotoxicity.

Dexrazoxane is used to reduce the incidence and severity of cardiomyopathy associated with doxorubicin in women with metastatic breast cancer who have received cumulative doses of doxorubicin of 300 mg per m² body-surface and who require continued administration. It is administered as the hydrochloride, by slow intravenous injection or rapid intravenous infusion, starting within 30 minutes before doxorubicin administration. The dose is expressed as the base, calculated on a 10:1 ratio with doxorubicin; typically, 500 mg of dexrazoxane per m² is given for every 50 mg of doxorubicin per m².

Dexrazoxane is also being investigated for use with doxorubicin in various other malignancies.

References.

1. Lewis C. A review of the use of chemoprotectants in cancer chemotherapy. *Drug Safety* 1994; **11:** 153–62.
2. Seifert CF, *et al.* Dexrazoxane in the prevention of doxorubicin-induced cardiotoxicity. *Ann Pharmacother* 1994; **28:** 1063–72.
3. Wexler LH, *et al.* Randomized trial of the cardioprotective agent ICRF-187 in pediatric sarcoma patients treated with doxorubicin. *J Clin Oncol* 1996; **14:** 362–72.
4. Wiseman LR, Spencer CM. Dexrazoxane: a review of its use as a cardioprotective agent in patients receiving anthracycline-based chemotherapy. *Drugs* 1998; **56:** 385–403.

Preparations

Proprietary Preparations (details are given in Part 3)
Canad.: Zinecard; ***Fr.:*** Cardioxane; ***Ital.:*** Cardioxane; Eucardion; ***USA:*** Zinecard.

Dicobalt Edetate (1033-p)

Dicobalt Edetate (*BAN, rINN*).

Cobalt Edetate; Cobalt EDTA; Cobalt Tetracemate. Cobalt [ethylenediaminetetra-acetato(4—)-*N,N′,O,O′*]cobalt(II).

$C_{10}H_{12}Co_2N_2O_8$ = 406.1.

CAS — 36499-65-7.

Adverse Effects and Precautions

Dicobalt edetate may cause hypotension, tachycardia, and vomiting. Anaphylactic reactions have occurred; oedema of the face and neck, sweating, chest pain, cardiac irregularities, and skin rashes have been reported.

The adverse effects of dicobalt edetate are more severe in the absence of cyanide. For this reason dicobalt edetate should not be administered unless cyanide poisoning is definitely confirmed and poisoning is moderate or severe, that is, when consciousness is impaired.

A patient with cyanide toxicity developed severe facial and pulmonary oedema after treatment with dicobalt edetate.[1] When dicobalt edetate is used, facilities for intubation and resuscitation should be immediately available.

1. Dodds C, McKnight C. Cyanide toxicity after immersion and the hazards of dicobalt edetate. *Br Med J* 1985; **291:** 785–6.

Uses and Administration

Dicobalt edetate is a chelator used in the treatment of severe cyanide poisoning (p.1407). Its use arises from the property of cobalt salts to form a relatively non-toxic stable ion-complex with cyanide. Owing to its toxicity, dicobalt edetate should be used only in confirmed cyanide poisoning and never as a precautionary measure. Cyanide poisoning must be treated as quickly as possible. A suggested dose is 300 mg administered by intravenous injection, over about 1 minute, repeated if the response is inadequate; a further dose of 300 mg of dicobalt edetate may be given 5 minutes later if required. For less severe poisoning the injection should be given over 5 minutes. Each injection of dicobalt edetate may be followed immediately by 50 mL of glucose 50% intravenously to reduce toxicity, though the value of giving glucose has been questioned.

Preparations

Proprietary Preparations (details are given in Part 3)
Austral.: Kelocyanor†; ***Fr.:*** Kelocyanor; ***Irl.:*** Kelocyanor; ***S.Afr.:*** Kelocyanor†; ***UK:*** Kelocyanor.

Digoxin-specific Antibody Fragments (19076-q)

Digoxin Immune Fab (Ovine); F(ab).

Store at 2° to 8°. Protect from light.

Adverse Effects and Precautions

Allergic reactions to digoxin-specific antibody fragments have been reported rarely. Patients known to be allergic to sheep protein and patients who have previously received digoxin-specific antibody fragments are likely to be at greater risk of developing an allergic reaction. Blood pressure, ECG, and potassium concentrations should be monitored closely during and after administration.

Uses and Administration

Digoxin-specific antibody fragments are derived from antibodies produced in sheep immunised to digoxin. Digoxin has greater affinity for the antibodies than for tissue-binding sites, and the digoxin-antibody complex is then rapidly excreted in the urine. Digoxin-specific antibody fragments are generally restricted to the treatment of life-threatening digoxin or digitoxin intoxication in which conventional treatment is ineffective. Successful treatment of lanatoside C poisoning has also been reported.

It is estimated that 38 mg of antibody fragments could bind about 0.5 mg of digoxin or digitoxin and the dose calculation is based on this estimate and the body-load of digoxin (based on the amount ingested or ideally from the steady-state plasma concentration). Administration is by intravenous infusion over a 30-minute period. If cardiac arrest is imminent the dose may be given as a bolus. In the case of incomplete reversal or recurrence of toxicity a further dose can be given. In patients considered to be at high risk of an allergic response an intradermal or skin scratch test may be performed.

Clinical studies and reviews of the use of digoxin-specific antibody fragments have confirmed their effectiveness in the treatment of severe digitalis toxicity in the majority of patients.[1-4] An initial response is usually seen within 30 minutes of the end of the infusion with a maximum response after 3 to 4 hours.[3] The main causes of treatment failure or partial response are incorrect diagnosis of digitalis intoxication, inadequate dosage of antibody fragments, and administration to patients already moribund.[3,4] Few adverse reactions have been attributed to the administration of digoxin-specific antibody fragments; a few cases of minor allergic reactions have been reported including erythema, facial swelling, urticaria, and rashes,[2,3] but no anaphylactic reactions have been reported.[1-4] Haemodynamic status normally improves, but withdrawal of the inotropic support provided by digoxin may produce a decline in cardiac function in some patients. There may be dramatic reductions in plasma potassium concentrations.

Treatment has been successful in patients with varying degrees of renal dysfunction.[2,3,5] Elimination of the antibody fragment-digoxin complex may be markedly delayed in severe renal impairment and prolonged monitoring may be required in such patients.[6] Measurement of free serum-digoxin concentrations may be useful.[7] Clifton and colleagues[8] have reported experience with digoxin-specific antibody fragments in a patient with chronic renal failure receiving haemodialysis. The patient had a good clinical response but haemodialysis did not remove the antibody fragment-digoxin complex.

In patients with adequate renal function the half-life of the antibody fragment-digoxin complex has been reported to be about 16 to 20 hours[2] although longer half-lives have been reported.[9] Schaumann and colleagues[10] suggested that the administration of digoxin-specific antibody fragments by infusion over 7 hours following an initial loading dose could be useful in ensuring adequate antibody concentrations are maintained to bind digoxin as it is released from tissue stores over a prolonged period.

Use of the antibody fragments has also been effective in children with severe digitalis intoxication.[11]

1. Smith TW, *et al.* Treatment of life-threatening digitalis intoxication with digoxin-specific Fab antibody fragments: experience in 26 cases. *N Engl J Med* 1982; **307:** 1357–62.
2. Wenger TL, *et al.* Treatment of 63 severely digitalis-toxic patients with digoxin-specific antibody fragments. *J Am Coll Cardiol* 1985; **5:** 118A–123A.
3. Stolshek BS, *et al.* The role of digoxin-specific antibodies in the treatment of digitalis poisoning. *Med Toxicol* 1988; **3:** 167–71.
4. Antman EM, *et al.* Treatment of 150 cases of life-threatening digitalis intoxication with digoxin-specific Fab antibody fragments: final report of a multicenter study. *Circulation* 1990; **81:** 1744–52.
5. Allen NM, *et al.* Clinical and pharmacokinetic profiles of digoxin immune Fab in four patients with renal impairment. *DICP Ann Pharmacother* 1991; **25:** 1315–20.
6. Ujhelyi MR, *et al.* Disposition of digoxin immune Fab in patients with kidney failure. *Clin Pharmacol Ther* 1993; **54:** 388–94.
7. Ujhelyi MR, Robert S. Pharmacokinetic aspects of digoxin-specific Fab therapy in the management of digitalis toxicity. *Clin Pharmacokinet* 1995; **28:** 483–93.
8. Clifton GD, *et al.* Free and total serum digoxin concentrations in a renal failure patient after treatment with digoxin immune Fab. *Clin Pharm* 1989; **8:** 441–5.
9. Gibb I, Parnham A. A star treatment for digoxin overdose? *Br Med J* 1986; **293:** 1171–2.
10. Schaumann W, *et al.* Kinetics of the Fab fragments of digoxin antibodies and of bound digoxin in patients with severe digoxin intoxication. *Eur J Clin Pharmacol* 1986; **30:** 527–33.
11. Woolf AD, *et al.* The use of digoxin-specific Fab fragments for severe digitalis intoxication in children. *N Engl J Med* 1992; **326:** 1739–44.

Preparations

Proprietary Preparations (details are given in Part 3)
Aust.: Digitalis Antidot; ***Austral.:*** Digibind; ***Belg.:*** Digitalis Antidot; ***Canad.:*** Digibind; ***Ger.:*** Digitalis Antidot; ***Swed.:*** Digitalis Antidot; ***Switz.:*** Antidote Anti-Digitale; ***UK:*** Digibind; ***USA:*** Digibind.

Dimercaprol (1036-e)

Dimercaprol *(BAN, rINN).*

BAL; British Anti-Lewisite; Dimercaprolum. 2,3-Dimercaptopropan-1-ol.

$C_3H_8OS_2$ = 124.2.

CAS — 59-52-9.

Pharmacopoeias. In *Chin., Eur.* (see p.viii), *Int., Jpn,* and *US.*

A clear colourless or slightly yellow liquid with an alliaceous odour. **Soluble** in water and in arachis oil; miscible with alcohol, benzyl benzoate, and methyl alcohol. **Store** at 2° to 8° in well-filled airtight containers. Protect from light.

Adverse Effects and Treatment

The most consistent side-effects produced by dimercaprol are hypertension and tachycardia. Other side-effects include nausea, vomiting, headache, burning sensation of the lips, mouth, throat, and eyes, lachrymation and salivation, tingling of the extremities, a sensation of constriction in the throat and chest, muscle pains and muscle spasm, rhinorrhoea, conjunctivitis, sweating, restlessness, and abdominal pain. Transient reductions in the leucocyte count have also been reported. Pain may occur at the injection site and sterile abscesses occasionally develop. In children, fever commonly occurs and persists during therapy. Side-effects are dose-related, relatively frequent, and usually reversible. It has been suggested that oral administration of ephedrine sulphate 30 to 60 mg half an hour before each injection of dimercaprol may reduce side-effects; antihistamines may alleviate some of the symptoms.

Precautions

Dimercaprol should be used with care in patients with hypertension or impaired renal function. It should be discontinued or continued with extreme caution if acute renal insufficiency develops during therapy. Alkalinisation of the urine may protect the kidney during therapy by stabilising the dimercaprol-metal complex. Dimercaprol should not be used in patients with impaired hepatic function unless due to arsenic poisoning. It should not be used in the treatment of poisoning due to cadmium, iron, or selenium as the dimercaprol-metal complexes formed are more toxic than the metals themselves.

Glucose-6-phosphate dehydrogenase deficiency. A report[1] of haemolysis during chelation therapy with dimercaprol and sodium calciumedetate for high blood-lead concentrations in 2 children with a deficiency of glucose-6-phosphate dehydrogenase.

1. Janakiraman N, *et al.* Hemolysis during BAL chelation therapy for high blood lead levels in two G6PD deficient children. *Clin Pediatr (Phila)* 1978; **17:** 485–7.

Pharmacokinetics

After intramuscular injection, maximum blood concentrations of dimercaprol may be attained within 30 to 60 minutes. Dimercaprol is rapidly metabolised and the metabolites and dimercaprol-metal chelates are excreted in the urine and bile. Elimination is essentially complete within 4 hours of a single dose.

Uses and Administration

Dimercaprol is a chelator used in the treatment of acute poisoning by arsenic (p.1551), gold (p.84), and mercury (p.1602); its role in the treatment of poisoning by antimony, bismuth, and thallium is less well established. It is also used, in conjunction with sodium calciumedetate, in acute lead poisoning (p.1595).

The sulfhydryl groups on dimercaprol compete with endogenous sulfhydryl groups on proteins such as enzymes to combine with these metals; chelation by dimercaprol therefore prevents or reverses any inhibition of the sulfhydryl enzymes by the metal and the dimercaprol-metal complex formed is readily excreted by the kidney. Since the complex may dissociate, particularly at acid pH, or be oxidised, the aim of treatment is to provide an excess of dimercaprol in body fluids until the excretion of the metal is complete.

Dimercaprol should be administered by deep intramuscular injection and the injections should be given at different sites. Various dosage schedules are in use.

In the UK a recommended schedule for adults is to give doses of 400 to 800 mg on the first day of treatment, 200 to 400 mg on the second and third days, and 100 to 200 mg on the fourth and subsequent days, all administered in divided doses. Within these dose ranges, the individual dose is determined by body-weight, severity of symptoms, and the causative agent. Single doses should not generally exceed 3 mg per kg body-weight but single doses of up to 5 mg per kg may be required initially in patients with severe acute poisoning. The dose for children is based on body-weight using a similar dose per kg as for adults. A minimum interval of 4 hours between doses appears to reduce side-effects.

In the USA a recommended schedule for severe arsenical or gold poisoning is 3 mg per kg body-weight given at 4-hourly intervals throughout the first 2 days, 4 doses are given on the third day, and 2 doses on each of the next 10 days. In milder cases

2.5 mg per kg is given 4 times daily on each of the first 2 days, twice daily on the third day, and once daily on subsequent days for 10 days. For acute mercurial poisoning an initial injection of 5 mg per kg is followed by 2.5 mg per kg once or twice daily for 10 days.

Some authorities have suggested that doses of up to 5 mg per kg every 4 hours may be required during the first 1 or 2 days of treatment in severe poisoning with gold, mercury, or arsenic.

Dimercaprol is also used in conjunction with sodium calciumedetate (p.994) in the treatment of lead poisoning. It can be of particular value in the treatment of acute lead encephalopathy and a suggested procedure is to administer an initial dose of dimercaprol 4 mg per kg alone followed at 4-hourly intervals by dimercaprol 3 to 4 mg per kg with concomitant doses of sodium calciumedetate administered at a separate site; treatment may be maintained for 2 to 7 days depending on the clinical response.

Preparations

BP 1998: Dimercaprol Injection;
USP 23: Dimercaprol Injection.

Proprietary Preparations (details are given in Part 3)
Ger.: Sulfactin Homburg†.

Multi-ingredient: ***Ital.:*** Sebohermal†.

4-Dimethylaminophenol Hydrochloride

(12658-t)

Dimetamfenol Hydrochloride; 4-DMAP.

$C_8H_{11}NO,HCl$ = 173.6.

CAS — 619-60-3 (4-dimethylaminophenol); 5882-48-4 (4-dimethylaminophenol hydrochloride).

4-Dimethylaminophenol hydrochloride is reported to oxidise haemoglobin to methaemoglobin and has been used in conjunction with sodium thiosulphate as an alternative to sodium nitrite (p.995) in the treatment of cyanide poisoning. Doses of 3 to 4 mg per kg body-weight have been given intravenously.

References.

1. Weger NP. Treatment of cyanide poisoning with 4-dimethylaminophenol (DMAP)–experimental and clinical overview. *Fundam Appl Toxicol* 1983; **3:** 387–96.

Preparations

Proprietary Preparations (details are given in Part 3)
Ger.: 4-DMAP; ***Neth.:*** 4-DMAP.

Diprenorphine Hydrochloride (7302-z)

Diprenorphine Hydrochloride *(BANM, rINNM).*

M5050. (6*R*,7*R*,14*S*)-17-Cyclopropylmethyl-7,8-dihydro-7-(1-hydroxy-1-methylethyl)-6-*O*-methyl-6,14-ethano-17-normorphine hydrochloride; 2-[(−)-(5*R*,6*R*,7*R*,14*S*)-9a-Cyclopropylmethyl-4,5-epoxy-3-hydroxy-6-methoxy-6,14-ethanomorphinan-7-yl]propan-2-ol hydrochloride.

$C_{26}H_{35}NO_4,HCl$ = 462.0.

CAS — 14357-78-9 (diprenorphine); 16808-86-9 (diprenorphine hydrochloride).

Pharmacopoeias. In *BP(Vet).*

A white or almost white crystalline powder. Sparingly **soluble** in water; slightly soluble in alcohol; very slightly soluble in chloroform; practically insoluble in ether. A 2% solution in water has a pH of 4.5 to 6.0. **Protect** from light.

Diprenorphine hydrochloride is an opioid antagonist used in veterinary medicine to reverse the effects of etorphine hydrochloride.

Disodium Edetate (1038-y)

Disodium Edetate *(BAN).*

Disodium Edathamil; Disodium EDTA; Disodium Tetracemate; Edetate Disodium; Natrii Edetas; Sodium Versenate. Disodium dihydrogen ethylenediaminetetra-acetate dihydrate.

$C_{10}H_{14}N_2Na_2O_8,2H_2O$ = 372.2.

CAS — 139-33-3 (anhydrous disodium edetate); 6381-92-6 (disodium edetate dihydrate).

Pharmacopoeias. In *Eur.* (see p.viii), *Int.*, *Jpn*, *Pol.*, and *US.*

A white odourless crystalline powder. **Soluble** in water; sparingly soluble in alcohol; practically insoluble in ether. A 5% solution in water has a pH of 4.0 to 6.0.

Trisodium Edetate (16285-z)

Edetate Trisodium *(USAN).* Trisodium hydrogen ethylenediaminetetra-acetate.

$C_{10}H_{13}N_2Na_3O_8$ = 358.2.

CAS — 150-38-9.

Adverse Effects and Precautions

Disodium and trisodium edetate have similar adverse effects and precautions to sodium calciumedetate (p.994).

Hypocalcaemia can occur if disodium or trisodium edetate is administered by intravenous infusion too rapidly or in too concentrated a solution and tetany, convulsions, respiratory arrest, and cardiac arrhythmias may result.

In addition, they should be used with caution in patients with tuberculosis, impaired cardiac function, or a history of seizures, and are contra-indicated in renal insufficiency. Plasma-electrolyte concentrations, particularly of ionised calcium, should be monitored.

Interactions

Edetates chelate bivalent and trivalent metal ions and may affect the activity of agents such as zinc insulin that contain such ions.

For reference to the inactivation of phenylmercuric salts by disodium edetate, see Phenylmercuric Nitrate, p.1122. For reports of edetates reducing the antimicrobial efficacy of thiomersal, see p.1126.

Uses and Administration

Disodium and trisodium edetate are chelators with a high affinity for calcium, with which they form a stable, soluble complex that is readily excreted by the kidneys. They have been administered intravenously in the emergency treatment of hypercalcaemia (p.1148) and have been used to control digitalis-induced cardiac arrhythmias (p.850) although less toxic agents are generally preferred. They are also used to treat calcium deposits in the eye.

Disodium and trisodium edetate also chelate other polyvalent metals but, unlike sodium calciumedetate, which is saturated with calcium, are not used for the treatment of heavy metal poisoning since hypocalcaemia rapidly develops.

In the treatment of hypercalcaemia, injections containing varying amounts of disodium and trisodium edetate are used. In the UK, the trisodium salt is generally used. A dose of up to 70 mg per kg body-weight daily has been suggested for adults; children may be given up to 60 mg per kg daily. It should be given by slow intravenous infusion over 2 to 3 hours and each gram of trisodium edetate should be diluted with 100 mL of glucose 5% or sodium chloride 0.9%. In the USA, disodium edetate is administered as a mixture of the disodium and trisodium salts. A dose of 50 mg per kg body-weight of disodium edetate in 24 hours by slow intravenous infusion has been suggested for adults with a maximum daily dose of 3 g. Children may be given 40 to 70 mg per kg in 24 hours. The injection should be diluted with sodium chloride 0.9% or glucose 5% to 500 mL for adults or a concentration not greater than 3% for children, and infused over 3 hours or more, preferably 4 to 6 hours. The dosage may be repeated for a further 4 days followed by a two-day interval before subsequent courses of treatment. If necessary, up to fifteen doses may be given in total.

Disodium and trisodium edetate are used in the treatment of calcium deposits from calcium oxide or calcium hydroxide burns of the eye and in the treatment of calcified corneal opacities, either by topical application after removing the appropriate area of corneal epithelium or by iontophoresis. Irrigation has also been suggested for zinc chloride injury to the eye, but treatment may be ineffective unless started within 2 minutes. In the UK a 0.4% solution of the trisodium salt is used for topical application to the eye; in the USA a 0.35 to 1.85% solution of a mixture of the disodium and trisodium salts has been suggested.

Disodium and trisodium edetate are also used in cleaners for contact lenses and as antoxidant synergists in cosmetic and pharmaceutical preparations.

Atherosclerosis. Calcium is thought to be necessary for several steps in atherogenesis and removal of calcium from atherosclerotic plaques using a chelator such as disodium edetate has been proposed.[1,2] However, there is little objective evidence of efficacy and reports of beneficial clinical responses are largely anecdotal or from small scale, short term, or uncontrolled clinical studies,[2,3] and in view of the potential toxicity of such treatment it cannot be recommended;[1-6] there is a report of fatal renal failure in one patient who has undergone such therapy.[4]

For a discussion of atherosclerosis and its prevention, see p.782.

1. Scott J. Chelation therapy—evolution or devolution of a nostrum? *N Z Med J* 1988; **101:** 109–10.
2. Grier MT, Meyers DG. So much writing, so little science: a review of 37 years of literature on edetate sodium chelation therapy. *Ann Pharmacother* 1993; **27:** 1504–9.
3. Rathmann KL, Golightly LK. Chelation therapy of atherosclerosis. *Drug Intell Clin Pharm* 1984; **18:** 1000–3.
4. Magee R. Chelation treatment of atherosclerosis. *Med J Aust* 1985; **142:** 514–15.
5. Wirebaugh SR, Geraets DR. Apparent failure of edetic acid chelation therapy for the treatment of coronary atherosclerosis. *DICP Ann Pharmacother* 1990; **24:** 22–5.
6. Anonymous. EDTA chelation therapy for atherosclerotic cardiovascular disease. *Med Lett Drugs Ther* 1994; **36:** 48.

Preparations

BP 1998: Trisodium Edetate Intravenous Infusion;
USP 23: Edetate Disodium Injection.

Proprietary Preparations (details are given in Part 3)
Fr.: Chelatran; Tracemate; ***Irl.:*** Limclair; ***UK:*** Limclair; ***USA:*** Disotate; Endrate.

Multi-ingredient: ***Canad.:*** Murine Supplemental Tears; ***Fr.:*** Vitaclair†; ***Ger.:*** Complete; Duracare; Oxysept; ***UK:*** Uriflex G; Uriflex R; ***USA:*** Vagisec†.

Edetic Acid (1039-j)

Edetic Acid *(BAN, rINN).*

Edathamil; EDTA; Tetracemic Acid. Ethylenediaminetetra-acetic acid.

$C_{10}H_{16}N_2O_8$ = 292.2.

CAS — 60-00-4.

Pharmacopoeias. In *Br.* and *Ger.* Also in *USNF.*

A white crystalline powder or colourless crystals. Very slightly **soluble** to practically insoluble in water; practically insoluble in alcohol and in chloroform; dissolves in dilute solutions of alkali hydroxides.

Adverse Effects and Precautions

Edetic acid, used as a pharmaceutical excipient, is generally well tolerated. Adverse effects have been reported following inhalation of solutions containing edetic acid.

Inhalation of ipratropium nebuliser solution, containing edetic acid as a preservative, caused bronchoconstriction in 6 of 22 patients with asthma.[1] Inhalation of edetic acid alone produced dose-related bronchoconstriction which persisted for longer than 60 minutes. Preservative-free nebuliser solutions for bronchodilatation are available.

1. Beasley CRW, *et al.* Bronchoconstrictor properties of preservatives in ipratropium bromide (Atrovent) nebuliser solution. *Br Med J* 1987; **294:** 1197–8.

Blood testing. Edetic acid may induce platelet clumping in some specimens collected for blood-cell counting leading to diagnostic errors. The recognition of pseudothrombocytopenia resulting from the use of edetic acid as the anticoagulant in blood samples and the use of alternative anticoagulants have been discussed.[1,2]

1. Lombarts AJPF, de Kieviet W. Recognition and prevention of pseudothrombocytopenia and concomitant pseudoleukocytosis. *Am J Clin Pathol* 1988; **89:** 634–9.
2. Lippi U, *et al.* EDTA-induced platelet aggregation can be avoided by a new anticoagulant also suitable for automated complete blood count. *Haematologica* 1990; **75:** 38–41.

Interactions

Edetic acid and its salts chelate polyvalent metal ions and may affect the activity of agents that contain such ions.

Edetic acid has been reported to enhance the antimicrobial efficacy of some disinfectants such as chloroxylenol (p.1111). However, for a report of edetates reducing the antimicrobial efficacy of thiomersal, see p.1126.

Uses

Edetic acid and its salts are chelators used in pharmaceutical manufacturing and as anticoagulants for blood taken for haematological investigations. Edetates have many industrial applications as chelators; for their use in medicine see Disodium Edetate, p.980, and Sodium Calciumedetate, p.994.

Gallstones. Edetic acid has been suggested as a possible solvent for non-cholesterol gallstones (p.1642).

Preparations

Proprietary Preparations (details are given in Part 3)

Multi-ingredient: *Ital.:* Conta-Lens Wetting; *USA:* Summer's Eve Post-Menstrual; Triv; Vagisec Plus†; Zonite.

Flumazenil (13215-d)

Flumazenil *(BAN, USAN, rINN).*

Flumazenilum; Flumazepil; Ro-15-1788; Ro-15-1788/000.

Ethyl 8-fluoro-5,6-dihydro-5-methyl-6-oxo-4*H*-imidazo[1,5-*a*][1,4]benzodiazepine-3-carboxylate.

$C_{15}H_{14}FN_3O_3$ = 303.3.

CAS — 78755-81-4.

Pharmacopoeias. In *Eur.* (see p.viii).

A white or almost white crystalline powder. Very slightly **soluble** in water; freely soluble in dichloromethane; sparingly soluble in methyl alcohol.

Adverse Effects and Precautions

The adverse effects of flumazenil are generally due to the reversal of benzodiazepine effects and resemble benzodiazepine withdrawal symptoms (see p.661). Nausea, vomiting, dizziness, blurred vision, headache, and flushing may occur. Anxiety, fear, and agitation have been reported following too rapid reversal of sedation. There have been reports of seizures, especially in epileptics. Transient increases in blood pressure and heart rate have been observed. Patients who have received benzodiazepines for prolonged periods are particularly at risk of experiencing withdrawal symptoms.

Because of its short duration of action, patients given flumazenil to reverse benzodiazepine-induced sedation should be kept under close observation; further doses of flumazenil may be necessary. Flumazenil should not be given to epileptic patients who have been receiving benzodiazepines for a prolonged period to control seizures.

In cases of mixed overdose, administration of flumazenil may unmask adverse effects of other psychotropic drugs. In particular, flumazenil should not be used in the presence of severe intoxication with tricyclic and related antidepressants.

Flumazenil should not be given in anaesthesia reversal until the effects of neuromuscular blockade have worn off. Dosage should be adjusted individually. In high-risk or anxious patients, and after major surgery, it may be preferable to maintain some sedation during the early postoperative period. The risk of raising intracranial pressure in patients with head injuries needs to be borne in mind.

Careful titration of dosage is recommended in hepatic impairment.

Cardiac arrhythmias,[1] sometimes preceded by tonic-clonic (grand mal) seizures[2,3] and occasionally fatal,[2] have been reported in several patients following the administration of flumazenil for mixed overdoses with benzodiazepines and other psychotropics. Heart block has also been reported[4] following flumazenil administration in a patient who had taken benzodiazepines, paracetamol, nifedipine, and atenolol. Death from refractory tonic-clonic seizures has been reported in a patient[5] following the use of flumazenil for a mixed overdose with a benzodiazepine and a tricyclic antidepressant.

Death from respiratory failure occurred in an 83-year-old woman following sedation with midazolam[6] despite flumazenil administration, although Birch and Miller[7] considered that this did not represent a failure by flumazenil to reverse the depressive effects on respiration of midazolam. Ventricular fibrillation followed by asystole and death has been reported in one patient given flumazenil during weaning from assisted ventilation (a period during which diazepam had been administered).[8]

1. Short TG, *et al.* Ventricular arrhythmia precipitated by flumazenil. *Br Med J* 1988; **296:** 1070–1.
2. Burr W, *et al.* Death after flumazenil. *Br Med J* 1989; **298:** 1713.
3. Marchant B, *et al.* Flumazenil causing convulsions and ventricular tachycardia. *Br Med J* 1989; **299:** 860.
4. Herd B, Clarke F. Complete heart block after flumazenil. *Hum Exp Toxicol* 1991; **10:** 289.
5. Haverkos GP, *et al.* Fatal seizures after flumazenil administration in a patient with mixed overdose. *Ann Pharmacother* 1994; **28:** 1347–9.
6. Lim AG. Death after flumazenil. *Br Med J* 1989; **299:** 858–9. Correction. *ibid.*: 1531.
7. Birch BRP, Miller RA. Death after flumazenil? *Br Med J* 1990; **300:** 467–8.
8. Katz Y, *et al.* Cardiac arrest associated with flumazenil. *Br Med J* 1992; **304:** 1415.

Effects on mental function. A severe acute psychotic disorder, which developed during treatment with flumazenil in a patient with hepatic encephalopathy, resolved when flumazenil was discontinued.[1]

1. Seebach J, Jost R. Flumazenil-induced psychotic disorder in hepatic encephalopathy. *Lancet* 1992; **339:** 488–9.

Pharmacokinetics

Flumazenil is well absorbed from the gastro-intestinal tract but undergoes extensive first-pass hepatic metabolism and has a systemic bioavailability of about 20%. It is moderately bound to plasma proteins. Following intravenous administration it is extensively metabolised in the liver to the inactive carboxylic acid form, which is excreted predominantly in the urine. The elimination half-life is reported to be about 50 minutes. In patients with impaired hepatic function the clearance of flumazenil is decreased with a resultant prolongation of half-life.

References.

1. Klotz U, *et al.* Pharmacokinetics of the selective benzodiazepine antagonist Ro 15-1788 in man. *Eur J Clin Pharmacol* 1984; **27:** 115–17.
2. Roncari G, *et al.* Pharmacokinetics of the new benzodiazepine antagonist Ro 15-1788 in man following intravenous and oral administration. *Br J Clin Pharmacol* 1986; **22:** 421–8.
3. Breimer LTM, *et al.* Pharmacokinetics and EEG effects of flumazenil in volunteers. *Clin Pharmacokinet* 1991; **20:** 491–6.
4. Jones RDM, *et al.* Pharmacokinetics of flumazenil and midazolam. *Br J Anaesth* 1993; **70:** 286–92.
5. Roncari G, *et al.* Flumazenil kinetics in the elderly. *Eur J Clin Pharmacol* 1993; **45:** 585–7.

Uses and Administration

Flumazenil is a benzodiazepine antagonist which acts competitively at CNS benzodiazepine receptors. It is used in anaesthesia and intensive care to reverse benzodiazepine-induced sedation; it may also be used to treat benzodiazepine overdosage (but see warnings in Precautions, above, and under Benzodiazepine Antagonism: Overdosage, below).

Flumazenil should be administered by slow intravenous injection or infusion.

The usual initial dose for the reversal of benzodiazepine-induced sedation is 200 μg given over 15 seconds, followed at intervals of 60 seconds by further doses of 100 to 200 μg if required, to a maximum total dose of 1 mg or occasionally 2 mg (usual range, 0.3 to 1.0 mg). If drowsiness recurs an intravenous infusion may be used, at a rate of 100 to 400 μg per hour, adjusted according to response. Alternatively, further doses of up to 1 mg, administered in boluses of 200 μg as above, may be given at 20-minute intervals to a maximum of 3 mg in one hour. Patients at risk from the effects of benzodiazepine reversal, such as those dependent on benzodiazepines, should receive smaller bolus injections of 100 μg.

The usual initial dose for the management of benzodiazepine overdose is 200 μg given intravenously over 30 seconds. A further dose of 300 μg can be given after another 30 seconds and can be followed by doses of 500 μg at one-minute intervals if required, to a total dose of 3 mg or occasionally 5 mg. The manufacturers consider that if a dose of up to 5 mg produces no response then further doses are unlikely to be effective. If symptoms of intoxication recur one or two doses of 500 μg may be given as above, with a one-minute interval between doses. This procedure may be repeated at 20-minute intervals. As before a slower rate of administration may be used for 'at risk' patients.

If signs of overstimulation occur during the use of flumazenil, diazepam or midazolam may be given by slow intravenous injection.

General references.

1. Brogden RN, Goa KL. Flumazenil: a reappraisal of its pharmacological properties and therapeutic efficacy as a benzodiazepine antagonist. *Drugs* 1991; **42:** 1061–89.
2. Hoffman EJ, Warren EW. Flumazenil: a benzodiazepine antagonist. *Clin Pharm* 1993; **12:** 641–56.
3. Krenzelok EP. Judicious use of flumazenil. *Clin Pharm* 1993; **12:** 691–2.

Benzodiazepine antagonism. Flumazenil is a specific benzodiazepine antagonist which binds competitively with benzodiazepine receptors. Flumazenil reverses the centrally mediated effects of benzodiazepines. Its effects are evident within a few minutes of intravenous administration, even after substantial doses of benzodiazepines, and last for up to 3 hours depending on the dose and on the characteristics of the benzodiazepine intoxication. In patients who have received benzodiazepines for prolonged periods, flumazenil may precipitate withdrawal syndromes.

POSTOPERATIVE. Flumazenil reduces postoperative sedation and amnesia following induction or maintenance of general anaesthesia with benzodiazepines; however, some patients have increased analgesic requirements, and some patients have experienced anxiety. Reversal of benzodiazepine sedation and amnesia may also be useful in some patients following minor surgery or diagnostic procedures. Sanders *et al.*[1] considered that, although flumazenil may antagonise the obvious effects of sedation, higher cognitive functions may still be impaired and the patient unfit to be discharged safely unaccompanied. There is a risk that sedation may recur if long-acting benzodiazepines have been used.[2-4] Patients who might benefit from sedation reversal include those at increased risk of postoperative complications, those in whom postoperative neurological evaluation would be beneficial, and those who are particularly sensitive to the effects of benzodiazepines.[2,3] In an intensive care unit, flumazenil may assist in weaning sedated patients from mechanical ventilation and in extubation,[3-6] but multiple doses or an infusion may be required due to the short duration of action.[5]

OVERDOSAGE. In benzodiazepine intoxication or mixed overdose, flumazenil may be useful as a diagnostic aid; it may do away with the need for respiratory support, and it may unmask the effects of other intoxicants.[2-7] However, benzodiazepine overdose is rarely lethal but may protect against the toxicity of other drugs, and flumazenil should be used with great caution in mixed overdose, particularly involving tricyclic antidepressants.[8] Repeated doses of flumazenil may be required to maintain consciousness depending on the benzodiazepine responsible and the magnitude of the overdose.

1. Sanders LD, *et al.* Reversal of benzodiazepine sedation with the antagonist flumazenil. *Br J Anaesth* 1991; **66:** 445–53.
2. Anonymous. Flumazenil. *Lancet* 1988; **ii:** 828–30.
3. Klotz U, Kanto J. Pharmacokinetics and clinical use of flumazenil (Ro 15-1788). *Clin Pharmacokinet* 1988; **14:** 1–12.
4. Karavokiros KAT, Tsipis GB. Flumazenil: a benzodiazepine antagonist. *DICP Ann Pharmacother* 1990; **24:** 976–81.
5. Amrein R, *et al.* Flumazenil in benzodiazepine antagonism: actions and clinical use in intoxications and anaesthesiology. *Med Toxicol* 1987; **2:** 411–29.
6. Anonymous. Flumazenil—the first benzodiazepine antagonist. *Drug Ther Bull* 1989; **27:** 39–40.
7. Weinbroum AA, *et al.* A risk-benefit assessment of flumazenil in the management of benzodiazepine overdose. *Drug Safety* 1997; **17:** 181–96.
8. Hoffman RS, Goldfrank LR. The poisoned patient with altered consciousness: controversies in the use of a 'coma cocktail'. *JAMA* 1995; **274:** 562–9.

Benzodiazepine tolerance. Preliminary studies in *animals*[1] and in patients[2] have suggested that flumazenil may reverse tolerance to the anticonvulsant effects of benzodiazepines which occurs during long-term therapy.

1. Gonsalves SF, Gallager DW. Persistent reversal of tolerance to anticonvulsant effects and GABAergic subsensitivity by a single exposure to benzodiazepine antagonist during chronic benzodiazepine administration. *J Pharmacol Exp Ther* 1988; **244:** 79–83.
2. Savic I, *et al.* Feasibility of reversing benzodiazepine tolerance with flumazenil. *Lancet* 1991; **337:** 133–7.

Hepatic encephalopathy. Flumazenil has been tried in hepatic encephalopathy (p.1170). Treatment is based on the suspected role of benzodiazepine-like agonists in the pathogenesis of the disorder. Beneficial responses,[1,2] as well as a lack of response, have been observed in some patients, possibly associated with advanced stages of encephalopathy or cerebral oedema.[2-4]

1. Grimm G, *et al.* Improvement of hepatic encephalopathy treated with flumazenil. *Lancet* 1988; **ii:** 1392–4.
2. Basile AS, *et al.* The pathogenesis and treatment of hepatic encephalopathy: evidence for the involvement of benzodiazepine receptor ligands. *Pharmacol Rev* 1991; **43:** 27–71.
3. Sutherland LR, Minuk GY. Ro 15-1788 and hepatic failure. *Ann Intern Med* 1988; **108:** 158.
4. Klotz U, Walker S. Flumazenil and hepatic encephalopathy. *Lancet* 1989; **i:** 155–6.

Non-benzodiazepine antagonism. Flumazenil blocks the effects of non-benzodiazepines, such as zopiclone and zolpidem, that act via the benzodiazepine receptor. In a double-blind study[1] in healthy volunteers, flumazenil rapidly antagonised clinical sedation induced by zolpidem.

1. Patat A, *et al.* Flumazenil antagonizes the central effects of zolpidem, an imidazopyridine hypnotic. *Clin Pharmacol Ther* 1994; **56:** 430–6.

Preparations

Proprietary Preparations (details are given in Part 3)
Aust.: Anexate; ***Austral.:*** Anexate; ***Belg.:*** Anexate; ***Canad.:*** Anexate; ***Fr.:*** Anexate; ***Ger.:*** Anexate; ***Irl.:*** Anexate; ***Ital.:*** Anexate; ***Neth.:*** Anexate; ***Norw.:*** Anexate; ***S.Afr.:*** Anexate; ***Spain:*** Anexate; ***Swed.:*** Lanexat; ***Switz.:*** Anexate; ***UK:*** Anexate; ***USA:*** Romazicon.

Fomepizole (2184-p)

Fomepizole *(USAN, rINN).*

4-Methylpyrazole; 4-MP. 4-Methyl-1*H*-pyrazole.

$C_4H_6N_2$ = 82.10.

CAS — 7554-65-6.

Fomepizole is an inhibitor of alcohol dehydrogenase. It is used for the treatment of poisoning by ethylene glycol (p.1577), which is converted to toxic metabolites by alcohol dehydrogenase. Fomepizole is given in a dose of 10 or 15 mg per kg body-weight every 12 hours by intravenous infusion over 30 minutes.

Fomepizole has also been investigated for methyl alcohol poisoning.

References.

1. Weintraub M, Standish R. 4-Methylpyrazole: an antidote for ethylene glycol and methanol intoxication. *Hosp Formul* 1988; **23:** 960–9.
2. Baud FJ, *et al.* Treatment of ethylene glycol poisoning with intravenous 4-methylpyrazole. *N Engl J Med* 1988; **319:** 97–100.
3. McMartin KE, Heath A. Treatment of ethylene glycol poisoning with intravenous 4-methylpyrazole. *N Engl J Med* 1989; **320:** 125.
4. Jacobsen D, *et al.* Non-linear kinetics of 4-methylpyrazole in healthy human subjects. *Eur J Clin Pharmacol* 1989; **37:** 599–604.
5. Harry P, *et al.* Efficacy of 4-methylpyrazole in ethylene glycol poisoning: clinical and toxicokinetic aspects. *Hum Exp Toxicol* 1994; **13:** 61–4.

Preparations

Proprietary Preparations (details are given in Part 3)
UK: Antizol; ***USA:*** Antizol.

Fuller's Earth (1610-h)

Terra Fullonica.

CAS — 8031-18-3.

Consists largely of montmorillonite, a native hydrated aluminium silicate, with which very finely divided calcite (calcium carbonate) may be associated.

Fuller's earth is an adsorbent which is used in dusting-powders, toilet powders, and lotions. Fuller's earth of high adsorptive capacity is used in industry as a clarifying and filtering medium.

It has been used in the treatment of paraquat poisoning (p.1409). A dose of 200 to 500 mL of a 30% suspension was administered orally every 2 hours for 3 doses, in association with magnesium sulphate or mannitol to promote diarrhoea and empty the gut.

Glucagon (7711-s)

Glucagon *(BAN, rINN).*

Glucagonum; HGF. His-Ser-Gln-Gly-Thr-Phe-Thr-Ser-Asp-Tyr-Ser-Lys-Tyr-Leu-Asp-Ser-Arg-Arg-Ala-Gln-Asp-Phe-Val-Gln-Trp-Leu-Met-Asn-Thr.

$C_{153}H_{225}N_{43}O_{49}S$ = 3482.8.

CAS — 16941-32-5.

Pharmacopoeias. In *Eur.* (see p.viii) and *US.*

A polypeptide hormone derived from beef or pork pancreas. A white or faintly coloured, almost odourless, fine crystalline powder. Practically **insoluble** in water; soluble in dilute alkalis and acids; practically insoluble in most organic solvents. **Store** at a temperature below 8° in airtight containers. The Ph. Eur. recommends storage preferably at −20°. The USP recommends storage under nitrogen.

A recombinant glucagon is available in some countries.

Adverse Effects

Nausea and vomiting may occur following administration of glucagon. Hypersensitivity reactions and hypokalaemia have also been reported.

Precautions

Glucagon should generally not be given to patients with phaeochromocytoma since it can cause a release of catecholamines producing marked hypertension. Glucagon should be administered with caution to patients with insulinoma as it may induce hypoglycaemia due to its insulin-releasing effect. Glucagon was formerly used to diagnose phaeochromocytoma and insulinoma but this use has been largely abandoned. Caution is also required when it is being employed as a diagnostic aid in diabetic patients.

Glucagon is not effective in patients with marked depletion of liver glycogen stores, as in starvation, adrenal insufficiency, or chronic hypoglycaemia.

Interactions

For a report of glucagon enhancing the anticoagulant effect of warfarin, see p.969.

Pharmacokinetics

Glucagon has a plasma half-life of about 3 to 6 minutes. It is inactivated in the liver, kidneys, and plasma.

Bioavailability. A study in healthy subjects and diabetic patients indicated that the bioavailability following intranasal administration of glucagon was about 30% that following intramuscular administration.[1] However the apparent half-life following intramuscular injection was 28.6 and 31.4 minutes respectively in the two groups, three to four times longer than that observed following either intravenous or intranasal administration, possibly due to slow release of glucagon from the injection site. It was also recognised that the onset of activity was quicker with the intranasal route which was of value in an emergency.

1. Pontiroli AE, *et al.* Pharmacokinetics of intranasal, intramuscular and intravenous glucagon in healthy subjects and diabetic patients. *Eur J Clin Pharmacol* 1993; **45:** 555–8.

Distribution. A study in 19 fasting patients undergoing myelography demonstrated that glucagon was present in CSF at an average of 28% of the concentration in serum.[1] The expected ratio would be 10% if glucagon reached the CSF only through simple diffusion, and it is possible that glucagon, like insulin, is actively transported from blood into CSF.

1. Graner JL, Abraira C. Glucagon in the cerebrospinal fluid. *N Engl J Med* 1985; **312:** 994–5.

Uses and Administration

Glucagon is a polypeptide hormone which is produced by the alpha cells of the pancreatic islets of Langerhans. It is a hyperglycaemic which mobilises glucose by activating hepatic glycogenolysis. It can to a lesser extent stimulate the secretion of pancreatic insulin. Glucagon is administered as glucagon hydrochloride; doses are usually expressed as glucagon (note that 1 unit is equivalent to 1 mg of glucagon). Glucagon is used in the treatment of severe hypoglycaemic reactions induced by insulin, when the patient cannot take glucose by mouth and intravenous glucose is not feasible. It is given by subcutaneous, intramuscular, or intravenous injection in a dose of 1 mg (or 0.5 mg in patients under about 20 kg body-weight). The dose may be repeated after 15 to 20 minutes, but intravenous glucose is to be preferred, and must be given if there is no response. Once the patient has responded sufficiently to take carbohydrate by mouth this should be given to restore liver glycogen stores and prevent secondary hypoglycaemia.

As glucagon reduces the motility of the gastro-intestinal tract it is used as a diagnostic aid in gastro-intestinal radiological examinations. The route of administration is dependent upon the diagnostic procedure. A dose of 1 to 2 mg administered intramuscularly has an onset of action of 4 to 10 minutes and a duration of effect of 10 to 30 minutes; 0.25 to 2 mg given intravenously produces an effect within one minute that lasts for 9 to 25 minutes.

Glucagon possesses positive cardiac inotropic activity but is not generally considered suitable for heart failure. However, as it can bypass blocked beta receptors, it is used in the treatment of beta-blocker overdosage, see Cardiovascular Effects, below.

Intranasal preparations are being developed.

Administration. References to intranasal administration of glucagon in healthy subjects and diabetics.

1. Freychet L, *et al.* Effect of intranasal glucagon on blood glucose levels in healthy subjects and hypoglycaemic patients with insulin-dependent diabetes. *Lancet* 1988; **i:** 1364–6.
2. Pontiroli AE, *et al.* Intranasal glucagon is a remedy for hypoglycemia: studies in healthy subjects and type I diabetic patients. *Diabetes Care* 1989; **12:** 604–8.
3. Pontiroli AE, *et al.* Nasal administration of glucagon and human calcitonin to healthy subjects: a comparison of powders and spray solutions and of different enhancing agents. *Eur J Clin Pharmacol* 1989; **37:** 427–30.
4. Hvidberg A, *et al.* Glucose recovery after intranasal glucagon during hypoglycaemia in man. *Eur J Clin Pharmacol* 1994; **46:** 15–17.

Cardiovascular effects. Glucagon has direct inotropic effects due to its ability to raise cyclic AMP concentrations independently of a response to catecholamines. It is used in the management of beta-blocker overdosage (see p.829); doses of 50 to 150 μg per kg body-weight (or 5 to 10 mg) by intravenous injection, followed by an infusion of 1 to 5 mg per hour if required, have been suggested.

Glucagon may be effective in the management of anaphylactic reactions to contrast media in patients receiving beta blockers.[1,2] A dramatic improvement in refractory hypotension during an anaphylactic reaction to contrast media was described in a 75-year-old man receiving beta blockers following intravenous administration of glucagon.[3]

While it is not regarded as standard treatment for overdosage with calcium-channel blockers, intravenous administration of glucagon 10 mg has been reported to be beneficial.[4]

1. Lieber JJ. Risk for anaphylactoid reaction from contrast media. *Ann Intern Med* 1991; **115:** 985.
2. Lang DM, *et al.* Risk for anaphylactoid reaction from contrast media. *Ann Intern Med* 1991; **115:** 985.
3. Zaloga GP, *et al.* Glucagon reversal of hypotension in a case of anaphylactic shock. *Ann Intern Med* 1986; **105:** 65–6.
4. Walter FG, *et al.* Amelioration of nifedipine poisoning associated with glucagon therapy. *Ann Emerg Med* 1993; **22:** 1234–7.

Diagnosis and testing. PITUITARY FUNCTION. Glucagon stimulates secretion of growth hormone and cortisol (hydrocortisone) and has been used both alone[1,2] and in combination with a beta blocker[3,4] as a test of pituitary function. The test is contra-indicated in patients with heart block, asthma, heart failure, and diabetes mellitus,[4] and severe secondary hypoglycaemia and death has been reported in a 2-year-old child following a glucagon test for growth hormone secretion.[5] In a review of growth hormone provocation tests, Hindmarsh and Swift[6] regarded the glucagon test and the insulin tolerance test as being less useful than the clonidine test.

1. Milner RDG, Burns EC. Investigation of suspected growth hormone deficiency. *Arch Dis Child* 1982; **57:** 944–7.
2. Anonymous. Testing anterior pituitary function. *Lancet* 1986; **i:** 839–41.
3. Colle M, *et al.* Betaxolol and propranolol in glucagon stimulation of growth hormone. *Arch Dis Child* 1984; **59:** 670–2.
4. Abboud CF. Laboratory diagnosis of hypopituitarism. *Mayo Clin Proc* 1986; **61:** 35–48.
5. Shah A, *et al.* Hazards of pharmacologic tests of growth hormone secretion in childhood. *Br Med J* 1992; **304:** 173–4.
6. Hindmarsh PC, Swift PGF. An assessment of growth hormone provocation tests. *Arch Dis Child* 1995; **72:** 362–8.

Gastro-intestinal disorders. The relaxant effect of glucagon on smooth muscle has been used to stop hiccups resulting from distension of the gallbladder[1] and to facilitate passage of swallowed foreign bodies and impacted food boluses which have become lodged in the lower oesophagus.[2,3] Glucagon has also been tried in the management of biliary colic[4] (p.8).

1. Gardner AMN. Glucagon stops hiccups. *Br Med J* 1985; **290:** 822.
2. Cooke MW, Glucksman EE. Swallowed coins. *Br Med J* 1991; **302:** 1607.
3. Farrugia M, *et al.* Radiological treatment of acute oesophageal food impaction. *Br J Hosp Med* 1995; **54:** 410–11.
4. Grossi E, *et al.* Different pharmacological approaches to the treatment of acute biliary colic. *Curr Ther Res* 1986; **40:** 876–82.

Hypoglycaemia. Glucagon is generally used as an alternative to parenteral glucose in hypoglycaemic patients whose consciousness is impaired and who cannot therefore take glucose by mouth. Parenteral glucose corrects the problem at source, and is the preferred treatment (see p.323), but its use is not always possible in the immediate circumstances of an attack, in which case it may be more convenient to use glucagon. Some have advocated its use as a first-line treatment[1] but this does not seem to be the general view; its action relies upon the patient having adequate hepatic glycogen stores which may not always be the case. It has been suggested for the management of hypoglycaemia in infants small for gestational age[2,3] although some authorities consider that it should not be used in premature or small infants.

Continuous infusion of glucagon was reported to be effective in the management of hypoglycaemia in a patient with an extrapancreatic tumour.[4]

1. Gibbins RL. Treating hypoglycaemia in general practice. *Br Med J* 1993; **306:** 600–1.
2. Carter PE, *et al.* Glucagon for hypoglycaemia in infants small for gestational age. *Arch Dis Child* 1988; **63:** 1264.
3. Mehta A. Hyperinsulinaemic hypoglycaemia in small for dates babies. *Arch Dis Child* 1991; **66:** 749.
4. Samaan NA, *et al.* Successful treatment of hypoglycemia using glucagon in a patient with an extrapancreatic tumor. *Ann Intern Med* 1990; **113:** 404–6.

Liver disorders. For references to the use of glucagon with insulin in the treatment of liver disorders, see under Insulin, p.329.

Preparations

BP 1998: Glucagon Injection;
USP 23: Glucagon for Injection.

Proprietary Preparations (details are given in Part 3)
Austral.: GlucaGen; ***Belg.:*** GlucaGen; ***Ger.:*** GlucaGen; ***Irl.:*** GlucaGen; ***Ital.:*** GlucaGen; ***S.Afr.:*** GlucaGen; ***Switz.:*** GlucaGen; ***UK:*** GlucaGen; Glucagon.

Glutathione (588-l)

GSH. *N*-(*N*-L-γ-Glutamyl-L-cysteinyl)glycine.
$C_{10}H_{17}N_3O_6S = 307.3$.
CAS — 70-18-8.

Glutathione is an endogenous peptide with antoxidant and other metabolic functions. It has been used in the treatment of poisoning with a number of compounds including heavy metals. Glutathione sodium has been used similarly. Glutathione has also been tried in idiopathic pulmonary fibrosis and has been used in a number of other conditions including liver disorders, corneal disorders, eczema, and for mitigation of the adverse effects of antineoplastic therapy including the neurotoxicity of cisplatin.

Reviews.

1. Lomaestro BM, Malone M. Glutathione in health and disease: pharmacotherapeutic issues. *Ann Pharmacother* 1995; **29:** 1263–73.

Lung disorders. Glutathione is an important extracellular antoxidant in the lung and high concentrations are found in lung epithelial lining fluid. A deficiency of glutathione may contribute to the epithelial damage that occurs in cryptogenic fibrosing alveolitis (idiopathic pulmonary fibrosis) (p.1024) and to the increased susceptibility to lung infections that occurs in patients with HIV infection (p.599). Preliminary studies have demonstrated beneficial biochemical results with glutathione delivered by aerosol in 10 patients with idiopathic pulmonary fibrosis,[1] and in 14 HIV-seropositive patients,[2] but no clinical effects have been reported.

1. Borok Z, *et al.* Effect of glutathione aerosol on oxidant-antioxidant imbalance in idiopathic pulmonary fibrosis. *Lancet* 1991; **338:** 215–16.
2. Holroyd KJ, *et al.* Correction of glutathione deficiency in the lower respiratory tract of HIV seropositive individuals by glutathione aerosol treatment. *Thorax* 1993; **48:** 985–9.

Preparations

Proprietary Preparations (details are given in Part 3)
Ital.: Gluko; Glutamed; Glutanil; Glutasan; Glutatox†; Gluthion; Glutoxil; Ipatox; Maglut; Novatox; Ridutox; Rition; Scavenger; TAD; Tationil; Thioxene; ***Jpn:*** Atomolan; Glutathin†; Tathion; ***Spain:*** Tition; ***USA:*** Cachexon.

Multi-ingredient: ***Belg.:*** Vitathion; ***Canad.:*** Vitathion-ATP; ***Fr.:*** Vita-Iodurol; Vita-Iodurol ATP; ***Ital.:*** Detoxicon†; Lebersana†; Toxepasi Complex†; ***Spain:*** Higado Potenciado Medic; Toxepasi Complex Forte†.

Haem Derivatives (2164-b)

Heme Derivatives.

Haem is the iron protoporphyrin constituent of haemoglobin and is responsible for its colour and oxygen-carrying capacity. It is used in the management of porphyrias (below). Haem is administered intravenously as its derivatives, although there is some confusion over their terminology. The names haematin and haemin have been used interchangeably although chemically haematin is the hydroxy derivative, formed by the reaction of haemin and sodium carbonate in solution. The arginine salt (haem arginate; haemin arginate) is reported to be more stable.

Haem arginate is used alone or with tin-protoporphyrin (p.1638) in the treatment of acute intermittent porphyria. It is administered by slow intravenous infusion in a dose of 3 to 4 mg per kg body-weight daily, infused over 30 to 45 minutes.

Haematin is used intravenously for the amelioration of acute intermittent porphyria associated with the menstrual cycle in patients unresponsive to other therapy. It is given in a dose of 1 to 4 mg per kg daily for 3 to 14 days as an intravenous infusion over 10 to 15 minutes.

Phlebitis may occur after injection of haematin into small arm veins.

Porphyrias. The porphyrias are a group of inherited and acquired disorders of haem biosynthesis. Deficiencies occur in specific enzymes leading to the accumulation of different porphyrins and porphyrin precursors. They are generally classified as acute or non-acute, reflecting their clinical presentation, or as hepatic or erythropoietic, depending on the site of the enzyme defect. The three most common forms are acute intermittent porphyria, porphyria cutanea tarda, and erythropoietic protoporphyria.

ACUTE PORPHYRIAS. These are inherited disorders characterised by the accumulation of porphyrin precursors, leading to acute attacks of neurovisceral symptoms. The most common form is *acute intermittent porphyria* (acute hepatic porphyria); *variegate porphyria* and *hereditary coproporphyria* are generally less common forms in which there is accumulation of both porphyrin precursors and porphyrins, leading to acute attacks in conjunction with cutaneous symptoms similar to those seen in non-acute porphyrias (see below).

In acute porphyrias the enzyme defect is not complete and only becomes apparent when demand for hepatic haem is increased by drugs, hormones, or nutritional factors. Attacks are rare before puberty and the disorder may remain latent in many patients. The presenting symptom is most commonly severe abdominal pain; other gastro-intestinal symptoms such as nausea and vomiting also occur, along with autonomic effects including hypertension, tachycardia, sweating, pallor, and pyrexia. Neuropathy leads to weakness and paralysis and may progress rapidly to respiratory distress. Psychiatric symptoms are also common, particularly agitation, anxiety, and behavioural disturbances. Attacks are usually precipitated by drugs, alcohol, steroid hormones, reduced caloric intake, or infection. They typically last for several days and are followed by complete recovery, although in some patients chronic abdominal pain may persist without other symptoms.

The primary management of an attack is to remove precipitants and to provide intensive support. *Symptomatic treatment* is complicated by the wide range of drugs that may precipitate porphyria. High doses of parenteral opioids may be required for pain and there is a danger of addiction occurring, particularly if attacks are frequent or if pain persists between attacks. Phenothiazines such as chlorpromazine are useful to control nausea and agitation and their sedative effect may also be beneficial. High doses of propranolol may be required for cardiovascular symptoms. Assisted ventilation may be necessary. *Specific therapy* is aimed at suppressing the haem biosynthetic pathway. A high carbohydrate intake should be ensured in all patients to suppress precursor production; this is given orally to prevent fluid overload but intravenous glucose may be required in patients who are vomiting. Haem administration is also effective; it is given as haematin or as haem arginate and tin-protoporphyrin may be used in conjunction. Prevention of attacks involves avoiding drugs which precipitate porphyria and maintaining an adequate carbohydrate intake. Gonadorelin analogues, such as buserelin, may have a role in preventing attacks related to the menstrual cycle.

NON-ACUTE PORPHYRIAS. These are characterised by the accumulation of porphyrins and usually present with cutaneous symptoms although porphyrins also accumulate in the liver and liver damage commonly occurs. *Porphyria cutanea tarda* (cutaneous hepatic porphyria) is the most common form of porphyria. It is usually an acquired disorder and in most cases there is a history of moderate or heavy alcohol intake. There is usually a raised serum-iron concentration and oestrogen administration has also been implicated. The main clinical symptom is cutaneous photosensitivity leading to bullous dermatosis, pruritus, and skin fragility, in areas exposed to sunlight. *Management* involves protecting the skin from sunlight and trauma and avoiding causative agents such as alcohol and iron. Sunscreen preparations must be based on zinc oxide or titanium dioxide to be effective. Reduction of serum-iron concentrations by phlebotomy is effective in most patients and should be carried out at weekly intervals until remission occurs; desferrioxamine is an alternative method to aid iron excretion but is less effective. Chloroquine and hydroxychloroquine have also been used and may be effective where phlebotomy is contra-indicated; they appear to act by complexing with porphyrins and increasing their excretion but low doses are necessary to avoid exacerbating the condition.

Erythropoietic protoporphyria is a less common non-acute porphyria and is an inherited disorder leading to accumulation of protoporphyrin. Symptoms are cutaneous and there is an acute reaction to sunlight leading to urticaria, pruritus, swelling, redness, and a severe burning sensation; liver damage may also occur. *Management* involves protection of the skin, as for porphyria cutanea tarda. Betacarotene produces benefit in most patients with photosensitivity and canthaxanthin may also be used. Haem administration, as haematin or haem arginate, may be beneficial in suppressing protoporphyrin production. Cholestyramine and activated charcoal reduce protoporphyrin levels by interrupting entero-hepatic recycling; they also bind other porphyrins and may have a role in rare forms of porphyria such as *congenital erythropoietic porphyria*.

References.

1. Moore MR, McColl KEL. *Porphyria: drug lists.* Glasgow: Porphyria Research Unit, University of Glasgow, 1991.
2. Todd DJ. Erythropoietic protoporphyria. *Br J Dermatol* 1994; **131:** 751–66.
3. Elder GH, *et al.* The acute porphyrias. *Lancet* 1997; **349:** 1613–17.
4. Gorchein A. Drug treatment in acute porphyria. *Br J Clin Pharmacol* 1997; **44:** 427–34.

References to haem derivatives in the management of porphyrias.

1. Anonymous. Hemin infusions in acute intermittent porphyria. *Med Lett Drugs Ther* 1984; **26:** 42.
2. Mustajoki P, *et al.* Haem arginate in the treatment of acute hepatic porphyrias. *Br Med J* 1986; **293:** 538–9.
3. Kordač V, Martásek P. Haem arginate in acute hepatic porphyrias. *Br Med J* 1986; **293**: 1098.
4. Tokola O, *et al.* Haem arginate improves hepatic oxidative metabolism in variegate porphyria. *Br J Clin Pharmacol* 1988; **26:** 753–7.
5. Volin L, *et al.* Heme arginate: effects on hemostasis. *Blood* 1988; **71:** 625–8.
6. Herrick AL, *et al.* Controlled trial of haem arginate in acute hepatic porphyria. *Lancet* 1989; **i:** 1295–7.
7. Dover SB, *et al.* Haem-arginate plus tin-protoporphyrin for acute hepatic porphyria. *Lancet* 1991; **338**: 263.
8. Mustajoki P, Nordmann Y. Early administration of heme arginate for acute porphyric attacks. *Arch Intern Med* 1993; **153:** 2004–8.

Preparations

Proprietary Preparations (details are given in Part 3)
Austral.: Panhematin; ***Fr.:*** Normosang; ***USA:*** Panhematin.

Levallorphan Tartrate (7303-c)

Levallorphan Tartrate *(BANM, rINNM).*
(−)-9a-Allylmorphinan-3-ol hydrogen tartrate.
$C_{19}H_{25}NO,C_4H_6O_6 = 433.5$.
CAS — 152-02-3 (levallorphan); 71-82-9 (levallorphan tartrate).
Pharmacopoeias. In *Jpn.*

Levallorphan is an opioid antagonist with properties similar to those of naloxone (p.986); in addition it also possesses some agonist properties. Levallorphan reverses severe opioid-induced respiratory depression but may exacerbate respiratory depression such as that induced by alcohol or other non-opioid central depressants.

It has been used in the treatment of opioid overdosage, to reverse opioid central depression resulting from the use of opioids during surgery, and to reverse neonatal respiratory depression following administration of opioid analgesics to the mother during labour.

Mesna (3726-q)

Mesna *(BAN, USAN, rINN).*
D-7093; Mesnum; UCB-3983. Sodium 2-mercaptoethanesulphonate.
$C_2H_5NaO_3S_2 = 164.2$.
CAS — 19767-45-4.

Solutions of mesna should be **stored** below 30° and protected from light.

Stability. There was no evidence of degradation of mesna when stored in solution with ifosfamide in polyethylene infusion bags at room temperature for 7 hours[1] or in polypropylene syringes at room temperature or at 4° for 4 weeks.[2] However, in the latter study ifosfamide concentrations fell by about 3% after 7 days and 12% after 4 weeks at both temperatures.

1. Shaw IC, Rose JWP. Infusion of ifosphamide plus mesna. *Lancet* 1984; **i:** 1353–4.
2. Rowland CG, *et al.* Infusion of ifosfamide plus mesna. *Lancet* 1984; **ii:** 468.

Adverse Effects and Precautions

Adverse effects which may occur after administration of mesna include gastro-intestinal effects, headache, fatigue, limb pains, depression, hypotension (but see below), and skin rash. Bronchospasm has been reported after administration by nebuliser.

Mesna may produce a false positive result in diagnostic tests for urinary ketones and may produce a false positive or false negative result in diagnostic tests for urinary erythrocytes.

Effects on the blood pressure. Severe hypertension occurred following administration of mesna both in combination with ifosfamide and alone.[1]

1. Gilleece MH, Davies JM. Mesna therapy and hypertension. *DICP Ann Pharmacother* 1991; **25:** 867.

Effects on the nervous system. For reports of severe encephalopathy in patients receiving mesna and ifosfamide, see Ifosfamide, p.540.

Hypersensitivity. Hypersensitivity reactions including rash, fever, nausea, facial and periorbital oedema, ulceration of mucous membranes, and tachycardia have been attributed to mesna.[1-4]

1. Lang E, Goos M. Hypersensitivity to mesna. *Lancet* 1985; **ii:** 329.
2. Seidel A, *et al.* Allergic reactions to mesna. *Lancet* 1991; **338:** 381.
3. Gross WL, *et al.* Allergic reactions to mesna. *Lancet* 1991; **338:** 381–2.
4. D'Cruz D, *et al.* Allergic reactions to mesna. *Lancet* 1991; **338:** 705–6.

Pharmacokinetics

Mesna is rapidly excreted in the urine after oral or intravenous administration as the unchanged drug and as the metabolite mesna disulphide (dimesna). The half-lives of mesna and dimesna are reported to be about 20 minutes and 70 minutes respectively.

References.

1. Burkert H, *et al.* Bioavailability of orally administered mesna. *Arzneimittelforschung* 1984; **34:** 1597–1600.
2. James CA, *et al.* Pharmacokinetics of intravenous and oral sodium 2-mercaptoethane sulphonate (mesna) in normal subjects. *Br J Clin Pharmacol* 1987; **23:** 561–8.
3. El-Yazigi A, *et al.* Pharmacokinetics of mesna and dimesna after simultaneous intravenous bolus and infusion administration in patients undergoing bone marrow transplantation. *J Clin Pharmacol* 1997; **37:** 618–24.

Uses and Administration

Mesna is used for the prophylaxis of urothelial toxicity in patients being treated with the antineoplastics ifosfamide or cyclophosphamide. In the kidney, mesna disulphide, the inactive metabolite of mesna, is reduced to free mesna which has thiol groups that react with the metabolites of ifosfamide and cyclophosphamide, including acrolein, considered to be responsible for the toxic effects on the bladder.

The duration of mesna treatment should equal that of the antineoplastic treatment plus the time taken for the concentration of antineoplastic metabolites in the urine to fall to non-toxic levels. Urinary output should be maintained and the urine monitored for haematuria and proteinuria throughout the treatment period. However, frequent emptying of the bladder should be avoided.

Mesna may be given intravenously or orally for the prophylaxis of urothelial toxicity. Following oral administration, availability of mesna in urine is approximately 50% of that following intravenous administration and excretion in urine is delayed up to 2 hours and is more prolonged. The intravenous preparation may be given orally when it should be added to a flavoured drink; this mixture may be stored in a sealed container in a refrigerator for up to 24 hours. Alternatively, tablets are available.

If ifosfamide or cyclophosphamide is given as an **intravenous bolus**, the *intravenous dose of mesna* is 20% of the dose of the antineoplastic on a weight for weight basis given on 3 occasions over 15 to 30 minutes at intervals of 4 hours beginning at the same time as the antineoplastic injection; thus a total dose of mesna equivalent to 60% of the antineoplastic is given. This regimen is repeated each time the antineoplastic is used. The individual dose of mesna may be increased to 40% of the dose of the antineoplastic and given 4 times at intervals of 3 hours for children and patients at high risk of urotoxicity; in such cases the total dose of mesna is equivalent to 160% of the antineoplastic given. The *oral dose of mesna* is 40% of the dose of the antineoplastic given on 3 occasions at intervals of 4 hours beginning two hours before the antineoplastic injection; thus a total dose of mesna equivalent to 120% of the antineoplastic is given. Alternatively, the initial dose of mesna (20% of the dose of the antineoplastic) may be given *intravenously* followed by two *oral doses* (each 40% of the dose of the antineoplastic) given 2 and 6 hours after the intravenous dose. Any of these regimens may be used if cyclophosphamide is given orally.

If the antineoplastic is given as an **intravenous infusion** over 24 hours, mesna as 20% of the total antineoplastic dose is given by *intravenous injection*, followed by 100% of the total dose by *intravenous infusion* over 24 hours, then followed by 60% by *intravenous infusion* over a further 12 hours. The final 12-hour infusion may be replaced by 3 *intravenous injections* each of 20% of the antineoplastic dose at intervals of 4 hours, the first injection being given 4 hours after the infusion has been stopped; alternatively it may be given *by mouth* in 3 doses each of 40% of the antineoplastic dose, the first dose being given when the 24-hour infusion is stopped, and the second and third doses being given 2 and 6 hours later.

Mesna is also administered by inhalation as a mucolytic in the management of some respiratory-tract disorders. The usual daily dose is 0.6 to 1.2 g administered by a nebuliser; it may also be given by direct endotracheal instillation.

General references.

1. Schoenike SE, Dana WJ. Ifosfamide and mesna. *Clin Pharm* 1990; **9:** 179–91.

Preparations

Proprietary Preparations (details are given in Part 3)
Aust.: Mistabron; Uromitexan; ***Austral.:*** Uromitexan; ***Belg.:*** Mistabron; Mucofluid†; Uromitexan; ***Canad.:*** Uromitexan; ***Fr.:*** Mucofluid; Uromitexan; ***Ger.:*** Mistabronco; Mucofluid†; Uromitexan; ***Irl.:*** Uromitexan; ***Ital.:*** Ausobronc; Mucofluid; Mucolene; Uromitexan; ***Neth.:*** Mistabron; Uromitexan; ***Norw.:*** Uromitexan; ***S.Afr.:*** Mistabron; Uromitexan; ***Spain:*** Mucofluid; Uromitexan; ***Swed.:*** Uromitexan; ***Switz.:*** Mistabron; Uromitexan; ***UK:*** Uromitexan; ***USA:*** Mesnex.

Methionine (605-x)

Methionine *(USAN, rINN).*

M; S-Methionine; L-Methionine; Methioninum. L-2-Amino-4-(methylthio)butyric acid.

$C_5H_{11}NO_2S$ = 149.2.

CAS — 63-68-3.

Pharmacopoeias. In *Eur.* (see p.viii), *Jpn, Pol.,* and *US.*

A white, almost white, or colourless crystalline powder or crystals with a characteristic odour and taste. **Soluble** in water, in warm dilute alcohol, and in dilute mineral acids; practically insoluble in acetone, in dehydrated alcohol, and in ether. A 1% solution in water has a pH of 5.6 to 6.1. **Protect** from light.

DL-Methionine (606-r)

DL-Methioninum; Racemethionine *(USAN).* DL-2-Amino-4-(methylthio)butyric acid.

$C_5H_{11}NO_2S$ = 149.2.

CAS — 59-51-8.

NOTE. The name methionine is often applied to DL-methionine. Co-methiamol is the British Approved Name for compounded preparations of DL-methionine and paracetamol, the proportions being expressed in the form *x/y* where *x* and *y* are the strength in milligrams of DL-methionine and paracetamol respectively.

Pharmacopoeias. In *Eur.* (see p.viii).

An almost white crystalline powder or small flakes. Sparingly **soluble** in water; very slightly soluble in alcohol; practically insoluble in ether; dissolves in dilute acids and in dilute solutions of alkali hydroxides. A 2% solution in water has a pH of 5.4 to 6.1. **Protect** from light.

Adverse Effects and Precautions

Methionine may cause nausea, vomiting, drowsiness, and irritability. Methionine should not be used in patients with acidosis. Methionine may aggravate hepatic encephalopathy in patients with established liver damage; it should be used with caution in patients with severe liver disease.

Interactions

Orally administered methionine may be adsorbed by activated charcoal leading to a diminished effect of methionine if they are given concurrently.

For the antagonism of the antiparkinsonian effect of levodopa by methionine, see p.1139.

Uses and Administration

L-Methionine is an amino acid which is an essential constituent of the diet and is incorporated into amino-acid solutions for parenteral nutrition (p.1331).

Methionine also enhances the synthesis of glutathione and is used as an alternative to acetylcysteine in the treatment of paracetamol poisoning to prevent hepatic damage (see p.72). The literature relating to the use of methionine in paracetamol poisoning is, in general, imprecise as to the form of methionine used. In the UK the usual dose of DL-methionine is 2.5 g by mouth every 4 hours for 4 doses starting less than 10 to 12 hours after ingestion of the paracetamol. Methionine has also been given intravenously. Preparations containing both methionine and paracetamol have been formulated for use in situations where overdosage may occur. However, the issue of whether methionine should be routinely added to paracetamol preparations is contentious for medical and ethical reasons.

Methionine has also been given by mouth to lower urinary pH and as an adjunct in the treatment of liver disorders.

Preparations

Proprietary Preparations (details are given in Part 3)
Aust.: Acimethin; ***Austral.:*** Methnine; ***Ger.:*** Acimethin; ***Switz.:*** Acimethin; ***USA:*** M-Caps; Pedameth; Uracid.

Multi-ingredient: ***Austral.:*** Berberis Complex; Liv-Detox; ***Belg.:*** Verrulyse-Methionine; ***Canad.:*** Amino-Cerv; ***Fr.:*** Cysti-Z; Forcapil; Lobamine-Cysteine; Totephan; Verrulyse-Methionine; ***Ger.:*** Dimaestad†; Hepalipon N; Hepar-Pasc N; Hepsan†; Sulfolitruw†; ***Ital.:*** Agedin Plus; Detoxicon†; Itahepar†; Litrison; Lozione Same AS; Meziv; ***S.Afr.:*** Hepavite; ***Spain:*** Dertrase; Laxante Richelet†; ***Switz.:*** Lobamine-Cysteine; Mechovit; ***UK:*** Fat-Solv; Lipotropic Factors; Pameton; Paradote; ***USA:*** Akoline†; Amino-Cerv.

Methylene Blue (1042-s)

Methylthioninium Chloride *(rINN)*; Azul de Metileno; Blu di Metilene; CI Basic Blue 9; Colour Index No. 52015; Methylenii Caeruleum; Methylthioninii Chloridum; Schultz No. 1038; Tetramethylthionine Chloride Trihydrate. 3,7-Bis(dimethylamino)phenazathionium chloride trihydrate.

$C_{16}H_{18}ClN_3S,3H_2O$ = 373.9.

CAS — 61-73-4 (anhydrous methylene blue); 7220-79-3 (methylene blue trihydrate).

Pharmacopoeias. In *Chin., Fr., It.,* and *US*; in *Aust.* (xH_2O); in *Int.* (anhydrous or $3H_2O$).

Eur. (see p.viii) includes Methylene Blue for External Use.

Dark green, odourless or almost odourless, crystals or crystalline powder with a bronze-like lustre, or a dark blue crystalline powder with a copper-coloured sheen. Solutions in water or alcohol are deep blue in colour. Ph. Eur. **solubilities** are: soluble in water; slightly soluble in alcohol; practically insoluble in ether. USP solubilities are: soluble 1 in 25 of water, 1 in 65 of alcohol; soluble in chloroform. **Protect** from light.

NOTE. Commercial methylene blue may consist of the double chloride of tetramethylthionine and zinc, and is not suitable for medicinal use.

Adverse Effects and Precautions

After intravenous administration of high doses methylene blue may cause nausea, vomiting, abdominal and chest pain, headache, dizziness, mental confusion, profuse sweating, dyspnoea, and hypertension; methaemoglobinaemia and haemolysis may occur. Haemolytic anaemia and hyperbilirubinaemia have been reported in newborn infants following intra-amniotic injection. Oral administration may cause gastro-intestinal disturbances and dysuria.

Methylene blue should not be injected subcutaneously as it has been associated with isolated cases of necrotic abscesses. It should not be given by intrathecal injection as neural damage has occurred.

Pregnancy and the neonate. A study in 30 mothers given a single intravenous dose of naloxone during the second stage of labour, indicated that naloxone rapidly crossed the placental barrier so that some therapeutic effect might be anticipated in most babies.[1] Placental transfer in 7 further mothers given naloxone intramuscularly was considered to be too variable for therapeutic purposes.

In 12 newborn infants given naloxone hydrochloride 35 or 70 μg intravenously via the umbilical vein, the mean plasma half-life of naloxone was 3.53 and 2.65 hours respectively.[2] These half-lives were 2 to 3 times longer than those reported for adults, possibly due to a diminished ability of the newborn to metabolise drugs by conjugation with glucuronic acid. Mean peak plasma concentrations of 8.2 ng per mL in those given 35 μg, and 13.7 ng per mL in those given 70 μg, were reached within 40 minutes of administration but this time was very variable, and in 5 infants peak plasma concentrations were reached within 5 minutes. When naloxone hydrochloride 200 μg was administered intramuscularly to 17 further newborn infants, peak concentrations of 7.4 to 34.6 ng per mL occurred at 0.5 to 2 hours.

1. Hibbard BM, *et al.* Placental transfer of naloxone. *Br J Anaesth* 1986; **58:** 45–8.
2. Moreland TA, *et al.* Naloxone pharmacokinetics in the newborn. *Br J Clin Pharmacol* 1980; **9:** 609–12.

Uses and Administration

Naloxone is a specific opioid antagonist that acts competitively at opioid receptors. It is an effective antagonist of opioids with agonist or mixed agonist-antagonist activity though larger doses may be needed for compounds with the latter activity and for codeine, dextropropoxyphene, and methadone. It is used to reverse opioid central depression, including respiratory depression, induced by natural or synthetic opioids in the following situations: in the treatment of known or suspected opioid overdosage; postoperatively following the use of opioids during surgery; in neonates following the administration of opioid analgesics to the mother during labour.

Naloxone hydrochloride is usually given intravenously for a rapid onset of action which occurs within 2 minutes. The onset of action is only slightly less rapid when it is administered intramuscularly or subcutaneously; sublingual and endotracheal administration have also been suggested. The duration of action of naloxone is dependent on the dose and route of administration; it may be 1 to 4 hours but may also be much shorter.

In the treatment of known or suspected **opioid overdosage**, the initial dose of naloxone hydrochloride is 0.4 to 2 mg given intravenously and repeated if necessary at intervals of 2 to 3 minutes. If no response has been observed after a total dose of 10 mg then the diagnosis of overdosage with drugs other than opioids should be considered. If the patient is suspected of being physically dependent on opioids the dose may be reduced to 0.1 to 0.2 mg to avoid precipitating withdrawal symptoms. In children, the usual initial dose is 10 μg per kg body-weight intravenously followed, if necessary, by a larger dose of 100 μg per kg (for an alternative children's dose suggested in the USA to treat opioid intoxication, see under Administration, below). In both adults and children, if the intravenous route is not feasible the intramuscular or subcutaneous route can be used.

Naloxone hydrochloride may also be used **postoperatively** to reverse central depression resulting from the use of opioids during surgery. A dose of 100 to 200 μg (1.5 to 3 μg per kg) may be given intravenously at intervals of at least 2 minutes, titrated for each patient in order to obtain an optimum respiratory response while maintaining adequate analgesia.

All patients receiving naloxone should be closely observed as the duration of action of some opioids exceeds that of naloxone and repeated doses by intravenous, intramuscular, or subcutaneous injection may be required. Alternatively, to sustain opioid antagonism, an intravenous infusion of naloxone hydrochloride has been suggested. Naloxone hydrochloride 4 μg per mL in sodium chloride 0.9% or glucose 5% may be infused at a rate titrated in accordance with the patient's response, both to the infusion and previous bolus injections; a rate of 0.4 to 0.8 mg per hour has been suggested.

Opioid-induced depression in **neonates** resulting from the administration of opioid analgesics to the mother during labour may be reversed by administering naloxone hydrochloride 10 μg per kg body-weight to the infant by intravenous, intramuscular, or subcutaneous injection, repeated at intervals of 2 to 3 minutes if necessary. Alternatively, a single intramuscular dose of about 60 μg per kg may be given at birth for a more prolonged action. Naloxone should be given with caution to the infants of opioid dependent mothers since withdrawal symptoms can result.

Some opioid analgesics have been formulated in combination with naloxone hydrochloride to reduce their potential for parenteral abuse. Naloxone hydrochloride has also been used cautiously in small doses to diagnose opioid dependence by precipitating the withdrawal syndrome (see below and under Naltrexone Hydrochloride, p.988).

Administration. INFANTS AND CHILDREN. The Committee on Drugs of the American Academy of Pediatrics[1,2] has recommended a dose of 100 μg per kg body-weight by intravenous injection or intratracheal administration for neonates, including premature infants, to the age of 5 years or 20 kg body-weight for treatment of *opioid intoxication*. Children over 5 years or 20 kg body-weight should be given a minimum of 2 mg. These doses may be repeated as necessary to maintain opioid reversal. The use of injections containing 0.02 mg per mL of naloxone hydrochloride are no longer recommended because of the fluid load involved at these doses, especially in small neonates.

1. American Academy of Pediatrics. Emergency drug doses for infants and children and naloxone use in newborns: classification. *Pediatrics* 1989; **83:** 803.
2. American Academy of Pediatrics. Naloxone dosage and route of administration for infants and children: addendum to emergency drug doses for infants and children. *Pediatrics* 1990; **86:** 484–5.

Eating disorders. Endogenous opioids may have a role in the pathophysiology of eating disorders,[1] thus opioid antagonists such as naloxone and naltrexone have been tried in their management. However, their role appears to be limited and opioid antagonists do not form part of the usual management of these conditions.

1. de Zwaan M, Mitchell JE. Opiate antagonists and eating behavior in humans: a review. *J Clin Pharmacol* 1992; **32**; 1060–72.

Non-opioid overdosage. In addition to reversing the effects of exogenous opioids, naloxone also antagonises the action of endogenous opioids. This may explain the varying responses reported to naloxone used in the treatment of overdosage with non-opioids, some of which may modulate endogenous opioids.

Naloxone was successfully used to reverse intoxication with *camylofin* in 2 infants.[1]

Severe central nervous system depression in a 4-year-old boy following *chlorpromazine* ingestion was successfully treated with naloxone.[2]

The response of patients with *clonidine* intoxication to naloxone has been inconsistent. There have been reports of benefit in some patients,[3-8] while other studies have been unable to demonstrate any beneficial effects.[9,10] Hypertension has been reported in some patients following naloxone administration.[5,7,8]

Results suggesting that naloxone may reverse sedation and respiratory depression produced by *benzodiazepines*[11] have not been supported.[12,13]

1. Schvartsman S, *et al.* Camylofin intoxication reversed by naloxone. *Lancet* 1988; **ii:** 1246.
2. Chandavasu O, Chatkupt S. Central nervous system depression from chlorpromazine poisoning: successful treatment with naloxone. *J Pediatr* 1985; **106:** 515–16.
3. Kulig K, *et al.* Naloxone for treatment of clonidine overdose. *JAMA* 1982; **247:** 1697.
4. Niemann JT, *et al.* Reversal of clonidine toxicity by naloxone. *Ann Emerg Med* 1986; **15:** 1229–31.
5. Gremse DA, *et al.* Hypertension associated with naloxone treatment for clonidine poisoning. *J Pediatr* 1986; **108:** 776–8.
6. Wedin GP, Edwards JL. Clonidine poisoning treated with naloxone. *Am J Emerg Med* 1989; **7:** 343–4.
7. Fiser DH, *et al.* Critical care for clonidine poisoning in toddlers. *Crit Care Med* 1990; **18:** 1124–8.
8. Wiley JF, *et al.* Clonidine poisoning in young children. *J Pediatr* 1990; **116:** 654–8.
9. Rogers JF, Cubeddu LX. Naloxone does not antagonize the antihypertensive effect of clonidine in essential hypertension. *Clin Pharmacol Ther* 1983; **34:** 68–73.
10. Banner W, *et al.* Failure of naloxone to reverse clonidine toxic effect. *Am J Dis Child* 1983; **137:** 1170–1.
11. Jordan C, *et al.* Effect of naloxone on respiratory changes after diazepam. *Br J Anaesth* 1979; **51:** 570P.
12. Christensen KN, Hüttel M. Naloxone does not antagonize diazepam-induced sedation. *Anesthesiology* 1979; **51:** 187.
13. Forster A, *et al.* Respiratory depressant effects of different doses of midazolam and lack of reversal with naloxone—a double-blind randomized study. *Anesth Analg* 1983; **62:** 920–4.

Postoperative use. Naloxone is used postoperatively to reverse central depression resulting from the use of opioids during surgery. However, it may antagonise the analgesic effects of the opioids in the control of postoperative pain, and the increasing use of short-acting intravenous opioid analgesics should reduce the need for its use.

Pruritus. For reference to the use of opioid antagonists, including naloxone, in the management of pruritus, see under Nalmefene Hydrochloride, p.986

Reversal of opioid effects. Naloxone has been reported to alleviate some of the adverse effects of opioids without loss of therapeutic efficacy. Naloxone reversed respiratory depression in a patient given intrathecal morphine,[1] and urinary retention in 3 patients after epidural morphine,[2] without reversing analgesia. Naloxone given intravenously has been shown to reverse the delay in gastric emptying induced by opioid analgesics in healthy subjects[3] and in women during labour.[4] In patients receiving long-term opioids, oral naloxone in a daily dose equivalent to 20 to 40% of the daily opioid dose relieved opioid-induced constipation without compromising analgesic control.[5,6] Doses equivalent to 10% or less of the opioid dose were ineffective.[7]

Other opioid antagonists that are under investigation for similar indications include methylnaltrexone.[8]

See also Postoperative Use, above.

1. Jones RDM, Jones JG. Intrathecal morphine: naloxone reverses respiratory depression but not analgesia. *Br Med J* 1980; **281:** 645–6.
2. Rawal N, *et al.* Naloxone reversal of urinary retention after epidural morphine. *Lancet* 1981; **ii:** 1411.
3. Nimmo WS, *et al.* Reversal of narcotic-induced delay in gastric emptying and paracetamol absorption by naloxone. *Br Med J* 1979; **2:** 1189.
4. Frame WT, *et al.* Effect of naloxone on gastric emptying during labour. *Br J Anaesth* 1984; **56:** 263–5.
5. Sykes NP. Oral naloxone in opioid-associated constipation. *Lancet* 1991; **337:** 1475.
6. Sykes NP. Oral naloxone in opioid-associated constipation. *Lancet* 1991; **338:** 582.
7. Robinson BA, *et al.* Oral naloxone in opioid-associated constipation. *Lancet* 1991; **338:** 581–2.
8. Yuan C-S, *et al.* The safety and efficacy of oral methylnaltrexone in preventing morphine-induced delay in oral-cecal transit time. *Clin Pharmacol Ther* 1997; **61:** 467–75.

DIAGNOSTIC USE. Naloxone is used to reverse opioid effects in the diagnosis of opioid overdose, although Hoffman *et al.* have recommended that administration should be restricted to those patients with clinical signs of opioid overdose.[1]

Naloxone has been given intravenously, to precipitate withdrawal symptoms in the diagnosis of opioid dependence and methods that do not induce acute withdrawal have also been investigated. Creighton and Ghodse[2] reported that pupillary dilatation in response to naloxone hydrochloride solution 1 mg per mL applied conjunctivally could distinguish patients with a physical dependence from non-dependent patients who had received opioids on a single occasion as preoperative medication, but this response was not confirmed by Loimer *et al.*[3] using naloxone 0.4 mg per mL solution. Furthermore Sanchez-Ramos and Senay[4] reported withdrawal syndrome and pupillary dilatation occurring in 4 opioid dependent subjects following instillation of naloxone solution 40 mg per mL.

1. Hoffman JR, *et al.* The empiric use of naloxone in patients with altered mental status: a reappraisal. *Ann Emerg Med* 1991; **20:** 246–52.
2. Creighton FJ, Ghodse AH. Naloxone applied to conjunctiva as a test for physical opiate dependence. *Lancet* 1989; **i:** 748–50.
3. Loimer N, *et al.* Conjunctival naloxone is no decision aid in opioid addiction. *Lancet* 1990; **335:** 1107–8.
4. Sanchez-Ramos JR, Senay EC. Ophthalmic naloxone elicits abstinence in opioid-dependent subjects. *Br J Addict* 1987; **82:** 313–15.

Preparations

BP 1998: Naloxone Injection; Neonatal Naloxone Injection;
USP 23: Naloxone Hydrochloride Injection; Pentazocine and Naloxone Hydrochlorides Tablets.

Proprietary Preparations (details are given in Part 3)

Aust.: Narcanti; *Austral.:* Narcan; *Belg.:* Narcan; *Canad.:* Narcan; *Fr.:* Nalone; Narcan; *Ger.:* Narcanti; *Irl.:* Narcan; *Ital.:* Narcan; *Norw.:* Narcanti; *S.Afr.:* Narcan; Zynox; *Swed.:* Narcanti; *Switz.:* Narcan; *UK:* Narcan; *USA:* Narcan.

Used as an adjunct in: Belg.: Valtran; *Ger.:* Tilidalor; Valoron N; *USA:* Talwin NX.

Naltrexone Hydrochloride (7307-x)

Naltrexone Hydrochloride *(BANM, rINNM)*.

EN-1639A. (5*R*)-9a-Cyclopropylmethyl-3,14-dihydroxy-4,5-epoxymorphinan-6-one hydrochloride; 17-(Cyclopropylmethyl)-4,5α-epoxy-3,14-dihydroxymorphinan-6-one hydrochloride.

$C_{20}H_{23}NO_4,HCl$ = 377.9.

CAS — 16590-41-3 (naltrexone); 16676-29-2 (naltrexone hydrochloride).

NOTE. Naltrexone is *USAN*.

Pharmacopoeias. In *US.*

Adverse Effects

Difficulty in sleeping, loss of energy, anxiety, dysphoria, abdominal pain, nausea, vomiting, reduction in appetite, joint and muscle pain, and headache may occur with naltrexone. Other side-effects including dizziness, constipation, diarrhoea, skin rashes, and reduced potency and ejaculatory difficulties have also been reported. Some adverse effects may be associated with opioid withdrawal. Thrombocytopenic purpura has occurred rarely. High doses may cause hepatocellular injury.

Effects on the liver. Increased liver enzyme values were reported in 6 of 40 obese patients receiving naltrexone 50 or 100 mg daily for eight weeks.[1] Five of the six patients had minimally abnormal liver function before naltrexone was administered and liver function tests returned to base-line values or better on discontinuing naltrexone.

Raised transaminase levels were noted in 5 of 26 obese patients after 3 weeks' treatment with naltrexone 300 mg daily; transaminase activity returned to normal when treatment was stopped.[2]

1. Atkinson RL, *et al.* Effects of long-term therapy with naltrexone on body weight in obesity. *Clin Pharmacol Ther* 1985; **38:** 419–22.
2. Mitchell JE. Naltrexone and hepatotoxicity. *Lancet* 1986; **i:** 1215.

Precautions

Naltrexone should be avoided in patients taking opioids for medication or abuse as an acute withdrawal syndrome may be precipitated (see Dependence under Opioid Analgesics, p.67). Withdrawal symptoms may develop within 5 minutes and last up to 48 hours. Naltrexone should be discontinued at least 48 hours before elective surgery involving opioid analgesia. For further precautions when administering naltrexone as an adjunct in the treatment of opioid dependence, see under Uses and Administration, below.

When analgesia is required, larger doses than usual of opioids will be needed and there is an increased risk of respiratory depression and other adverse effects.

Naltrexone should be used with caution in patients with hepatic dysfunction and is contra-indicated in patients with acute hepatitis or liver failure. Regular monitoring of hepatic function has been recommended. Naltrexone should be given with caution to patients with impaired renal function.

Pharmacokinetics

Naltrexone is well absorbed from the gastro-intestinal tract but is subject to considerable first-pass metabolism and may undergo enterohepatic recycling. It is extensively metabolised in the liver and the major metabolite, 6-β-naltrexol may also possess weak opioid antagonist activity. Maximum plasma concentrations of naltrexone and 6-β-naltrexol are achieved in about 1 hour and naltrexone is about 20% bound to plasma proteins at therapeutic doses. The elimination half-life of naltrexone is approximately 4 hours and that of 6-β-naltrexol about 13 hours. Naltrexone and its metabolites are excreted mainly in the urine. Less than 1% of an oral dose of naltrexone is excreted unchanged.

References.

1. Verebey K, *et al.* Naltrexone: disposition, metabolism, and effects after acute and chronic dosing. *Clin Pharmacol Ther* 1976; **20:** 315–28.
2. Wall ME, *et al.* Metabolism and disposition of naltrexone in man after oral and intravenous administration. *Drug Metab Dispos* 1981; **9:** 369–75.
3. Wall ME, *et al.* Naltrexone disposition in man after subcutaneous administration. *Drug Metab Dispos* 1984; **12:** 677–82.
4. Meyer MC, *et al.* Bioequivalence, dose-proportionality, and pharmacokinetics of naltrexone after oral administration. *J Clin Psychiatry* 1984; **45:** 15–19.
5. Chiang CN, *et al.* Kinetics of a naltrexone sustained-release preparation. *Clin Pharmacol Ther* 1984; **36:** 704–8.

Uses and Administration

Naltrexone is a specific opioid antagonist with actions similar to those of naloxone (p.987); however, it is more potent than naloxone and has a longer duration of action.

It is used in the treatment of **opioid dependence** as an aid to maintaining abstinence following opioid withdrawal. Naltrexone treatment should not be started until the patient has been detoxified and abstinent from opioids for at least 7 to 10 days because of the risk of acute withdrawal; abstinence should be verified by analysis of the patient's urine. A *naloxone challenge test* should then be administered to confirm the absence of opioid dependence, as follows: naloxone hydrochloride 200 μg is administered intravenously and the patient observed for 30 seconds for evidence of withdrawal symptoms; if none occur a further dose of 600 μg is given and the patient observed for 30 minutes. A confirmatory rechallenge with naloxone hydrochloride 1.6 mg intravenously may be considered if results are ambiguous. Sources in the USA suggest a naloxone challenge test with a single dose of 800 μg given subcutaneously as an alternative to the intravenous route.

Once a negative naloxone challenge test has been obtained, naltrexone hydrochloride is given by mouth to *treat* opioid dependence. Treatment may be initiated with a dose of 25 mg. If no signs of opioid withdrawal occur subsequent doses may be increased to 50 mg daily. The usual maintenance dose of naltrexone hydrochloride is 350 mg weekly administered as 50 mg daily, but the dosing interval may be lengthened to improve compliance; for example, doses of 100 mg on Monday and Wednesday and 150 mg on Friday may be effective and various other intermittent dosage regimens have been used. Patients should be carefully counselled and warned that attempts to overcome the opioid blockade with large doses of opioids could result in fatal opioid intoxication. Naltrexone hydrochloride is also used as an adjunct in the management of **alcohol dependence** and the recommended dose is 50 mg daily.

Alcohol dependence. Naltrexone may be of use as an adjunct to psychotherapy in maintaining abstinence after alcohol withdrawal in patients with alcohol dependence (p.1099). Short-term studies[1,2] of 12 weeks' duration indicate that it is of benefit for reducing alcohol craving and the severity and number of relapses. Data on long-term efficacy are limited but some benefit may persist after withdrawal of treatment.[3] Reports[4] from patients who continued to drink during therapy suggest that naltrexone may reduce the pleasure associated with drinking, possibly by blocking the effect of endorphins released as a result of alcohol consumption.[5] It is recommended[6] that naltrexone should be given for a minimum of 6 months because of the high relapse rates usually seen during the first 3 to 6 months following alcohol withdrawal. Although naltrexone dose not appear to be hepatotoxic at the dosage of 50 mg daily used for alcohol dependence caution is recommended in patients with liver disease.[6] Concurrent use with disulfiram, which is potentially hepatotoxic, is not usually recommended.[5]

1. Volpicelli JR, *et al.* Naltrexone in the treatment of alcohol dependence. *Arch Gen Psychiatry* 1992; **49:** 876–80.
2. O'Malley SS, *et al.* Naltrexone and coping skills therapy for alcohol dependence: a controlled study. *Arch Gen Psychiatry* 1992; **49:** 881–7.
3. O'Malley SS, *et al.* Six-month follow-up of naltrexone and psychotherapy for alcohol dependence. *Arch Gen Psychiatry* 1996; **53:** 217–24.
4. Volpicelli JR, *et al.* Effect of naltrexone on alcohol "high" in alcoholics. *Am J Psychiatry* 1995; **152:** 613–15.
5. Anonymous. Naltrexone for alcohol dependence. *Med Lett Drugs Ther* 1995; **37:** 64–6.
6. Berg BJ, *et al.* A risk-benefit assessment of naltrexone in the treatment of alcohol dependence. *Drug Safety* 1996; **15:** 274–82.

Opioid dependence. MAINTENANCE. Naltrexone is a long-acting, non-addictive oral opioid antagonist. Although it can be effective in maintaining abstinence in opioid addicts following detoxification, compliance with therapy is difficult to maintain because although it blocks the euphoriant effects of opioids it does not block the craving for narcotics. It is thus most effective in highly motivated addicts with good socio-logical and psychological support to discourage impulsive use of opioids.

For a discussion of the management of opioid dependence, see p.67.

References.

1. Crabtree BL. Review of naltrexone, a long-acting opiate antagonist. *Clin Pharm* 1984; **3:** 273–80.
2. Anonymous. Naltrexone for opioid addiction. *Med Lett Drugs Ther* 1985; **27:** 11–12.
3. Ginzburg HM, MacDonald MG. The role of naltrexone in the management of drug abuse. *Med Toxicol* 1987; **2:** 83–92.
4. Gonzalez JP, Brogden RN. Naltrexone: a review of its pharmacodynamic and pharmacokinetic properties and therapeutic efficacy in the management of opioid dependence. *Drugs* 1988; **35:** 192–213.

RAPID DETOXIFICATION. Combined treatment with clonidine and naltrexone enabled 38 of 40 opioid addicts to withdraw completely from long-term methadone therapy within 4 or 5 days.[1] Modification of the regimen allowed opioid withdrawal over 2 to 3 days.[2] The experimental technique of rapid detoxification with naltrexone while the patient is anaesthetised is controversial.

1. Charney DS, *et al.* The combined use of clonidine and naltrexone as a rapid, safe and effective treatment of abrupt withdrawal from methadone. *Am J Psychiatry* 1986; **143:** 831–7.
2. Brewer C, *et al.* Opioid withdrawal and naltrexone induction in 48–72 hours with minimal drop-out, using a modification of the naltrexone-clonidine technique. *Br J Psychiatry* 1988; **153:** 340–3.

Pruritus. For reference to the use of opioid antagonists, including naltrexone, in pruritus, see under Nalmefene Hydrochloride, p.986.

Preparations

USP 23: Naltrexone Hydrochloride Tablets.

Proprietary Preparations (details are given in Part 3)
Aust.: Nemexin; Revia; ***Canad.:*** Revia; ***Fr.:*** Nalorex; Revia; ***Ger.:*** Nemexin; ***Irl.:*** Nalorex; ***Ital.:*** Antaxone; Nalorex; Narcoral; ***Spain:*** Antaxone; Celupan; ***Switz.:*** Nemexin; ***UK:*** Nalorex; ***USA:*** Depade; Trexan.

Obidoxime Chloride (1043-w)

Obidoxime Chloride *(USAN, rINN)*.

LüH6. 1,1′-[Oxybis(methylene)]bis[4-(hydroxyimino)methyl]pyridinium dichloride.

$C_{14}H_{16}Cl_2N_4O_3$ = 359.2.

CAS — 7683-36-5 (obidoxime); 114-90-9 (obidoxime chloride).

Obidoxime chloride is a cholinesterase reactivator with similar actions and uses to pralidoxime (p.992). It is given in conjunction with atropine in the treatment of organophosphorus poisoning in usual adult doses of 250 mg by slow intravenous injection; it has also been given by intramuscular injection.

References.

1. Thiermann H, *et al.* Cholinesterase status, pharmacokinetics and laboratory findings during obidoxime therapy in organophosphate poisoned patients. *Hum Exp Toxicol* 1997; **16:** 473–80.

Preparations

Proprietary Preparations (details are given in Part 3)
Aust.: Toxogonin; ***Ger.:*** Toxogonin; ***Neth.:*** Toxogonin; ***S.Afr.:*** Toxogonin; ***Swed.:*** Toxogonin; ***Switz.:*** Toxogonine.

Penicillamine (1045-l)

Penicillamine *(BAN, USAN, rINN)*.

D-Penicillamine; Penicillaminum. D-3,3-Dimethylcysteine; D-3-Mercaptovaline.

$C_5H_{11}NO_2S$ = 149.2.

CAS — 52-67-5 (penicillamine); 2219-30-9 (penicillamine hydrochloride).

Pharmacopoeias. In *Eur.* (see p.viii), *Int., Pol.,* and *US.*

A white or almost white, finely crystalline powder with a slight characteristic odour. Freely **soluble** in water; slightly soluble in alcohol; practically insoluble in chloroform and in ether. A 1% solution in water has a pH of 4.5 to 5.5. **Store** in airtight containers.

Adverse Effects and Treatment

Side-effects of penicillamine are frequent. Gastro-intestinal disturbances including anorexia, nausea, and vomiting may occur; oral ulceration and stomatitis have been reported and impaired taste sensitivity is common.

Skin rashes occurring early in treatment are commonly allergic and may be associated with pruritus, urticaria, and fever; they are usually transient but temporary drug withdrawal and treatment with corticosteroids or antihistamines may be required. Lupus erythematosus and pemphigus have been reported. A Stevens-Johnson-like syndrome has been observed during penicillamine treatment. Prolonged use of high doses may affect skin collagen and elastin, resulting in increased skin friability, eruptions resembling elastosis perforans serpiginosa, and a late rash or acquired epidermolysis bullosa (penicillamine dermatopathy) that may necessitate dosage reduction or discontinuation.

Haematological side-effects have included thrombocytopenia and less frequently leucopenia; these are usually reversible but agranulocytosis and aplastic anaemia have occurred and fatalities have been reported. Haemolytic anaemia has also occurred.

Proteinuria occurs frequently and in some patients may progress to glomerulonephritis or nephrotic syndrome. Penicillamine-induced haematuria is rare but normally requires immediate discontinuation.

Other side-effects associated with penicillamine include Goodpasture's syndrome, bronchiolitis and pneumonitis, myasthenia gravis, polymyositis (rarely with cardiac involvement), intrahepatic cholestasis, and pancreatitis.

References describing the range and incidence of adverse effects associated with of D-penicillamine.[1,2] The L or DL forms are much more toxic.[3]

1. Kean WF, *et al.* Efficacy and toxicity of D-penicillamine for rheumatoid disease in the elderly. *J Am Geriatr Soc* 1982; **30:** 94–100.
2. Steen VD, *et al.* The toxicity of D-penicillamine in systemic sclerosis. *Ann Intern Med* 1986; **104:** 699–705.
3. Kean WF, *et al.* Chirality in antirheumatic drugs. *Lancet* 1991; **338:** 1565–8.

Effects on the blood. Of the 18 deaths ascribed to penicillamine reported to the UK Committee on Safety of Medicines between January 1964 and December 1977, fourteen were apparently due to blood disorders, at least 7 of them being marrow aplasias. The myelotoxicity of penicillamine was reviewed in 10 patients with confirmed or suspected marrow depression during penicillamine treatment for rheumatoid arthritis or scleroderma; 6 of these 10 patients died.[1]

Thomas *et al.*[2] reported an incidence of 12 to 27% of penicillamine-induced thrombocytopenia in patients with rheumatoid arthritis. Thrombocytopenia appeared to be due to bone-marrow suppression and a reduced platelet-production rate.

There have been isolated reports[3-5] of thrombotic thrombocytopenic purpura attributed to the use of penicillamine with some fatalaties.

For a brief discussion of the genetic factors influencing myelotoxicity, see under Genetic Factors, below.

1. Kay AGL. Myelotoxicity of D-penicillamine. *Ann Rheum Dis* 1979; **38:** 232–6.
2. Thomas D, *et al.* Thrombokinetics in patients with rheumatoid arthritis treated with D-penicillamine. *Ann Rheum Dis* 1984; **43:** 402–6.
3. Ahmed F, *et al.* Thrombohemolytic thrombocytopenic purpura during penicillamine therapy. *Arch Intern Med* 1978; **138:** 1292–3.
4. Speth PAJ, *et al.* Thrombotic thrombocytopenic purpura associated with D-penicillamine treatment in rheumatoid arthritis. *J Rheumatol* 1982; **9:** 812–13.
5. Trice JM, *et al.* Thrombotic thrombocytopenic purpura during penicillamine therapy in rheumatoid arthritis. *Arch Intern Med* 1983; **143:** 1487–8.

Effects on the breast. Breast enlargement has been reported both in women[1-4] and in men[5] taking penicillamine and may be a rare complication of penicillamine therapy. In some patients breast enlargement was prolonged with poor resolution and others required surgery. Danazol has been used successfully to treat penicillamine-induced breast gigantism.[2-4]

1. Thew DCN, Stewart IM. D penicillamine and breast enlargement. *Ann Rheum Dis* 1980; **39:** 200.
2. Taylor PJ, *et al.* Successful treatment of D-penicillamine-induced breast gigantism with danazol. *Br Med J* 1981; **282:** 362–3.
3. Rooney PJ, Cleland J. Successful treatment of D-penicillamine-induced breast gigantism with danazol. *Br Med J* 1981; **282:** 1627–8.
4. Craig HR. Penicillamine induced mammary hyperplasia: report of a case and review of the literature. *J Rheumatol* 1988; **15:** 1294–7.
5. Reid DM, *et al.* Reversible gynaecomastia associated with D-penicillamine in a man with rheumatoid arthritis. *Br Med J* 1982; **285:** 1083–4.

Effects on the gastro-intestinal tract. There have been isolated reports of acute colitis in patients taking penicillamine.[1,2] Ileal ulceration and stenosis in a patient with Wilson's disease was considered to be related to elastosis probably resulting from long-term penicillamine therapy.[3]

1. Hickling P, Fuller J. Penicillamine causing acute colitis. *Br Med J* 1979; **2:** 367.
2. Grant GB. Penicillamine causing acute colitis. *Br Med J* 1979; **2:** 555.
3. Wassef M, *et al.* Unusual digestive lesions in a patient with Wilson's disease treated with long-term penicillamine. *N Engl J Med* 1985; **313:** 49.

Effects on the heart. For reports of heart block, Stokes-Adams syndrome, and fatal myocarditis in patients taking penicillamine, see under Effects on the Muscles and the Neuromuscular System, Polymyositis, below.

Effects on the kidneys. Proteinuria associated with penicillamine has usually occurred within 4 to 18 months of starting therapy though onset can be later. A greater incidence has been found in patients with rheumatoid arthritis and cystinuria than in those with Wilson's disease. The severity of proteinuria varies; proteinuria of nephrotic proportions usually develops rapidly but resolves on drug cessation. Minimal change, mesangioproliferative, and membranous nephropathy have all been associated with penicillamine treatment and progressive glomerulonephritis has been observed in a few patients who had developed features of Goodpasture's syndrome.[1]

Although there is some evidence of a relationship between nephropathy and penicillamine dose and its rate of increase,[1] Hall and colleagues,[2] in a study of 33 rheumatoid arthritis patients with penicillamine-induced nephropathy, found no correlation with the dose or duration of treatment. Appreciable proteinuria could still be detected 12 months after stopping penicillamine in 40% of their patients, but subsequently resolved in those whose proteinuria was solely related to penicillamine.

Penicillamine was successfully reintroduced and administered for at least 13 months in 5 patients with rheumatoid arthritis who had developed proteinuria during the first course of therapy. Proteinuria did not recur.[3]

Corticosteroids have been used in patients developing rapidly progressive glomerulonephritis[4] but may be unnecessary and potentially hazardous in patients who develop the nephrotic syndrome.[2]

For reports of Goodpasture's syndrome in patients taking penicillamine, see also under Effects on the Respiratory System, below.

For a brief discussion of the genetic factors influencing renal toxicity, see under Genetic Factors, below.

1. Anonymous. Penicillamine nephropathy. *Br Med J* 1981; **282:** 761–2.
2. Hall CL, *et al.* Natural course of penicillamine nephropathy: a long term study of 33 patients. *Br Med J* 1988; **296:** 1083–6.
3. Hill H, *et al.* Resumption of treatment with penicillamine after proteinuria. *Ann Rheum Dis* 1979; **38:** 229–31.
4. Ntoso KA, *et al.* Penicillamine-induced rapidly progressive glomerulonephritis in patients with progressive systemic sclerosis: successful treatment of two patients and a review of the literature. *Am J Kidney Dis* 1986; **8:** 159–63.

Effects on the liver. Seibold *et al.* reported a patient with penicillamine-associated hepatotoxicity and reviewed other reports.[1] Of the 9 patients considered all had liver function profiles consistent with intrahepatic cholestasis; one patient died of acute renal failure but the others improved rapidly after drug withdrawal.[1] In a later report,[2] a 72-year-old man with rheumatoid arthritis developed jaundice approximately 4 weeks after starting penicillamine therapy. Liver biopsy indicated a slight degree of cholangitis with eosinophils in the portal tracts and severe predominantly intrahepatocellular cholestasis. Jaundice cleared within 3 weeks of stopping penicillamine and liver enzyme values approached normal after 6 weeks. Monitoring of liver function and eosinophil counts in the early weeks of penicillamine therapy was recommended.[1]

1. Seibold JR, *et al.* Cholestasis associated with D-penicillamine therapy: case report and review of the literature. *Arthritis Rheum* 1981; **24:** 554–6.
2. Devogelaer JP, *et al.* A case of cholestatic hepatitis associated with D-penicillamine therapy for rheumatoid arthritis. *Int J Clin Pharmacol Res* 1985; **5:**35–8.

Effects on the muscles and the neuromuscular system. Neuromyotonia[1] and profound sensory and motor neuropathy have been reported in patients taking penicillamine. Symptoms improved rapidly after the initiation of pyridoxine supplementation.[2] Low back pain in conjunction with fever and rash developed in a patient during penicillamine treatment.[3] Fever and back pain recurred on rechallenge with penicillamine. It was suggested that an allergic mechanism was involved.

1. Reeback J, *et al.* Penicillamine-induced neuromyotonia. *Br Med J* 1979; **1:** 1464–5.
2. Pool KD, *et al.* Penicillamine-induced neuropathy in rheumatoid arthritis. *Ann Intern Med* 1981; **95:** 457–8.
3. Bannwarth B, *et al.* Low back pain associated with penicillamine. *Br Med J* 1991; **303:** 525.

MYASTHENIA. Myasthenia gravis is a well recognised, though uncommon, complication of long-term penicillamine therapy.[1] Symptoms are similar to those seen with spontaneous myasthenia gravis and include ptosis and diplopia, and generalised weakness, occasionally affecting the respiratory muscles.[1-3] The onset of symptoms usually occurs within 6 to 7 months but may be delayed for a number of years.[3] Myasthenic symptoms usually resolve spontaneously once penicillamine is withdrawn, but some patients require anticholinesterase therapy.[1-3] Acetylcholine receptor antibodies are found in about 75% of affected patients.[2,3] Patients with HLA antigens DRl and Bw35 may have a genetic predisposition to developing myasthenia.[4] Patients with auto-immune diseases may well display an increased susceptibility to drug-induced myasthenia.[3]

1. Delamere JP, *et al.* Penicillamine-induced myasthenia in rheumatoid arthritis: its clinical and genetic features. *Ann Rheum Dis* 1983; **42:** 500–4.
2. Carter H, *et al.* La myasthénie au cours du traitement de la polyarthrite rhumatoïde par la D-pénicillamine. *Therapie* 1984; **39:** 689–95.
3. Katz LJ, *et al.* Ocular myasthenia gravis after D-penicillamine administration. *Br J Ophthalmol* 1989; **73:** 1015–18.
4. Garlepp MJ, *et al.* HLA antigens and acetylcholine receptor antibodies in penicillamine induced myasthenia gravis. *Br Med J* 1983; **286:** 338–40.

POLYMYOSITIS. Penicillamine therapy has been associated rarely with polymyositis and dermatomyositis,[1-6] usually reversible but in some cases fatal.[2] At least two deaths have resulted from myocarditis,[2] and Christensen and Sørensen[4] reported complete heart block and severe Stokes-Adams attacks in patients with polymyositis. It is possible that some patients may have a genetically determined susceptibility to this complication.[5]

1. Wojnarowska F. Dermatomyositis induced by penicillamine. *J R Soc Med* 1980; **73:** 885–6.
2. Doyle DR, *et al.* Fatal polymyositis in D-penicillamine-treated rheumatoid arthritis. *Ann Intern Med* 1983; **98:** 327–30.
3. Renier JC, *et al.* Polymyosite induite par la D-pénicillamine. *Therapie* 1984; **39:** 697–703.
4. Christensen PD, Sørensen KE. Penicillamine-induced polymyositis with complete heart block. *Eur Heart J* 1989; **10:** 1041–4.
5. Carroll GJ, *et al.* Penicillamine induced polymyositis and dermatomyositis. *J Rheumatol* 1987; **14:** 995–1001.
6. Aydintug AO, *et al.* Polymyositis complicating D-penicillamine treatment. *Postgrad Med J* 1991; **67:** 1018–20.

Effects on the respiratory system. Reports of pulmonary haemorrhage associated with progressive renal failure in individual patients treated with penicillamine have commonly been classified as Goodpasture's syndrome,[1,2] although an immune complex syndrome has been suggested.[3] There have been rare reports of obliterative bronchiolitis in patients with rheumatoid arthritis treated with penicillamine.[4-6]

1. Sternlieb I, *et al.* D-Penicillamine induced Goodpasture's syndrome in Wilson's disease. *Ann Intern Med* 1975; **82:** 673–6.
2. Gibson T, *et al.* Goodpasture syndrome and D-penicillamine. *Ann Intern Med* 1976; **84:** 100.
3. Turner-Warwick M. Adverse reactions affecting the lung: possible association with D-penicillamine. *J Rheumatol* 1981; **8** (suppl 7): 166–8.
4. Lyle WH. D-Penicillamine and fatal obliterative bronchiolitis. *Br Med J* 1977; **1:** 105.
5. Epler GR, *et al.* Bronchiolitis and bronchitis in connective tissue disease: a possible relationship to the use of penicillamine. *JAMA* 1979; **242:** 528–32.
6. Murphy KC, *et al.* Obliterative bronchiolitis in two rheumatoid arthritis patients treated with penicillamine. *Arthritis Rheum* 1981; **24:** 557–60.

RHINITIS. Nasal blockage due to grossly oedematous nasal linings and severe disabling watery nasal discharge associated with penicillamine administration was reported in a 76-year-old patient.[1] The patient also had pemphigus foliaceus. The rhinitis resolved promptly when penicillamine was discontinued, as did concurrent bilateral blepharitis.

1. Presley AP. Penicillamine induced rhinitis. *Br Med J* 1988; **296:** 1332.

Effects on the skin. Penicillamine-induced skin lesions have been reviewed.[1] The cutaneous manifestations observed during penicillamine therapy include those resulting from interference with collagen and elastin such as penicillamine dermatopathy, elastosis perforans serpiginosa, and cutis laxa; those associated with auto-immune mechanisms such as pemphigus, pemphigoid, lupus erythematosus, and dermatomyositis; and those classified as acute sensitivity reactions including macular or papular eruptions and urticaria. The effects on collagen and elastin (see below) tend to occur only after prolonged treatment with high doses of penicillamine, as in patients with Wilson's disease or cystinuria, whereas patients with diseases characterised by altered immune systems, such as rheumatoid arthritis, are more prone to develop the antibody-related adverse skin reactions. Acute hypersensitivity reactions tend to occur early in penicillamine treatment, usually within the first 7 to 10 days, and appear not to be dose-related. Lichenoid reactions, stomatitis, nail changes, and adverse effects on hair have also been reported.

1. Levy RS, *et al.* Penicillamine: review and cutaneous manifestations. *J Am Acad Dermatol* 1983; **8:** 548–58.

EPIDERMAL NECROLYSIS. A 56-year-old woman developed agranulocytosis and toxic epidermal necrolysis 7 weeks after starting therapy with penicillamine 250 mg daily for primary biliary cirrhosis.[1]

1. Ward K, Weir DG. Life threatening agranulocytosis and toxic epidermal necrolysis during low dose penicillamine therapy. *Ir J Med Sci* 1981; **150:** 252–3.

INTERFERENCE WITH COLLAGEN AND ELASTIN. Long-term, high-dose treatment with penicillamine can interfere with elastin and collagen production giving rise to increased skin friability, haemorrhagic lesions, miliary papules, and excessive wrinkling and laxity of the skin.[1] Penicillamine dermatopathy, characterised by wrinkling and purpura over bony prominences, was first reported by Sternlieb and Scheinberg.[2] In addition, lesions resembling pseudoxanthoma elasticum have been reported.[3,4] Abnormal elastic tissue has also been reported in patients taking low doses of penicillamine (less than 1 g daily), not only in the skin but also in joint capsules,[5] and elastosis perforans serpiginosa has been reported[6] in a child receiving a low cumulative dose over a short period. In all these cases, histological findings generally show damage to elastic fibres giving them a typical appearance described as "lumpy-bumpy" or "bramble-bush".

For reports of cutis laxa in neonates, see under Pregnancy in Precautions, below.

1. Levy RS, *et al.* Penicillamine: review and cutaneous manifestations. *J Am Acad Dermatol* 1983; **8:** 548–58.
2. Sternlieb I, Scheinberg IH. Penicillamine therapy for hepatolenticular degeneration. *JAMA* 1964; **189:** 748–54.
3. Thomas RHM, *et al.* Pseudoxanthoma elasticum-like skin changes induced by penicillamine. *J R Soc Med* 1984; **77:** 794–8.
4. Bentley-Phillips B. Pseudoxanthoma elasticum-like skin changes induced by penicillamine. *J R Soc Med* 1985; **78:** 787.
5. Dalziel KL, *et al.* Elastic fibre damage induced by low-dose D-penicillamine. *Br J Dermatol* 1990; **123:** 305–12.
6. Sahn EE, *et al.* D-Penicillamine-induced elastosis perforans serpiginosa in a child with juvenile rheumatoid arthritis. *J Am Acad Dermatol* 1989; **20:** 979–88.

LICHEN PLANUS. Observations in some patients reported in the 1980s led to the suggestion that penicillamine might exacerbate or unmask lichen planus.[1,2] However, there do not appear to have been subsequent reports.

1. Powell FC, Rogers RS. Primary biliary cirrhosis, penicillamine, and lichen planus. *Lancet* 1981; **ii:** 525.
2. Powell FC, *et al.* Lichen planus, primary biliary cirrhosis and penicillamine. *Br J Dermatol* 1982; **107:** 616.

PEMPHIGUS. Pemphigus vulgaris[1] and a number of variants including pemphigus foliaceus,[1] herpetiform pemphigus,[2] pemphigus erythematosus,[3] benign mucous membrane pemphigoid,[4] cicatricial pemphigoid,[5] and combined pemphigus and pemphigoid features[6] have been reported with penicillamine therapy.

1. Zone J, *et al.* Penicillamine-induced pemphigus. *JAMA* 1982; **247:** 2705–7.
2. Marsden RA, *et al.* Herpetiform pemphigus induced by penicillamine. *Br J Dermatol* 1977; **97:** 451–2.
3. de Jong MCJM, *et al.* Immunohistochemical findings in a patient with penicillamine pemphigus. *Br J Dermatol* 1980; **102;** 333–7.
4. Lever LR, Wojnarowska F. Benign mucous membrane pemphigoid and penicillamine. *Br J Dermatol* 1985; **113** (suppl 29): 88–9.
5. Shuttleworth D, Graham-Brown RAC. Cicatricial pemphigoid in a D-penicillamine treated patient with rheumatoid arthritis. *Br J Dermatol* 1985; **113** (suppl 29); 89–90.
6. Velthuis PJ, *et al.* Combined features of pemphigus and pemphigoid induced by penicillamine. *Br J Dermatol* 1985; **112:** 615–19.

PSORIASIFORM ERUPTIONS. Two patients with rheumatoid arthritis developed psoriasiform eruptions during penicillamine treatment.[1] In one patient the eruption resolved when penicillamine was stopped but worsened when treatment was restarted.

1. Forgie JC, Highet AS. Psoriasiform eruptions associated with penicillamine. *Br Med J* 1987; **294:** 1101.

SYSTEMIC SCLEROSIS. Penicillamine has been used in the treatment of scleroderma and systemic sclerosis (see under Uses, below). However, systemic sclerosis-like lesions developed in a 14-year-old boy with Wilson's disease who had been treated with penicillamine for 11 years[1] and the suitability of penicillamine for this indication has therefore been questioned.

1. Miyagawa S, *et al.* Systemic sclerosis-like lesions during long-term penicillamine therapy for Wilson's disease. *Br J Dermatol* 1987; **116:** 95–100.

Genetic factors. There is increasing evidence that some patients may have a genetically determined increased susceptibility to the adverse effects of penicillamine. Several studies have suggested that rheumatoid arthritis patients with a poor capacity for producing sulphoxides may be more susceptible to the toxic effects of penicillamine.[1,2] The poor sulphoxidation capacity found in patients with primary biliary cirrhosis could partly explain their high incidence of adverse reactions to penicillamine,[3] although Mitchison and colleagues[4] found no association between penicillamine toxicity and sulphoxidation status in a study of 20 such patients.

In addition to poor sulphoxidation, Emery and colleagues[5] reported increased toxicity in patients possessing the histocompatibility antigen HLA-DR3. Other studies have shown associations between proteinuria and HLA antigens B8 and DR3,[6,7] myasthenia gravis and Bw35 and DR1,[8] thrombocytopenia and HLA antigens DR4,[6,7] A1,[6] and C4BQO,[6] and polymyositis or dermatomyositis and HLA antigens B18, B35, and DR4.[9] However, such associations are insufficiently strong and testing procedures too expensive to make testing sulphoxidation status or HLA-typing useful for identifying high-risk patients.[7,10]

1. Panayi GS, *et al.* Deficient sulphoxidation status and d-penicillamine toxicity. *Lancet* 1983; **i:** 414.
2. Emery P, *et al.* Sulphoxidation status of rheumatoid patients manifesting untoward reactions to chronic D-penicillamine therapy. *Br J Clin Pharmacol* 1984; **18:** 286P.
3. Olomu A, *et al.* Poor sulphoxidation in primary biliary cirrhosis. *Lancet* 1985; **i:** 1504.
4. Mitchison HC, *et al.* D-penicillamine-induced toxicity in primary biliary cirrhosis (PBC): the role of sulphoxidation status. *Gut* 1986; **27:** A622.
5. Emery P, *et al.* D-Penicillamine induced toxicity in rheumatoid arthritis: the role of sulphoxidation status and HLA-DR3. *J Rheumatol* 1984; **11:** 626–32.
6. Stockman A, *et al.* Genetic markers in rheumatoid arthritis: relationship to toxicity from D-penicillamine. *J Rheumatol* 1986; **13:** 269–73.
7. Moens HJB, *et al.* Longterm followup of treatment with D-penicillamine for rheumatoid arthritis: effectivity and toxicity in relation to HLA antigens. *J Rheumatol* 1987; **14:** 1115–19.
8. Garlepp MJ, *et al.* HLA antigens and acetylcholine receptor antibodies in penicillamine induced myasthenia gravis. *Br Med J* 1983; **286:** 338–40.
9. Carroll GJ, *et al.* Penicillamine induced polymyositis and dermatomyositis. *J Rheumatol* 1987; **14:** 995–1001.
10. Hall CL. Penicillamine nephropathy. *Br Med J* 1988; **297:** 137.

Systemic lupus erythematosus. A syndrome resembling lupus erythematosus developed in 6 women with long-standing severe rheumatoid arthritis while being treated with penicillamine;[1] these patients represented an approximate frequency of penicillamine-induced lupus erythematosus of 2%. All 6 had developed previous cutaneous reactions to gold therapy. A case of bullous systemic lupus erythematosus associated with penicillamine administration has also been reported.[2]

1. Chalmers A, *et al.* Systemic lupus erythematosus during penicillamine therapy for rheumatoid arthritis. *Ann Intern Med* 1982; **97:** 659–63.
2. Condon C, *et al.* Penicillamine-induced type II bullous systemic lupus erythematosus. *Br J Dermatol* 1997; **136:** 474–5.

Precautions

Penicillamine is contra-indicated in patients with lupus erythematosus or a history of penicillamine-induced agranulocytosis, aplastic anaemia, or severe thrombocytopenia. It should be used with care, if at all, in patients with renal impairment.

Penicillamine should not be given with other drugs capable of causing similar serious haematological or renal adverse effects, for example gold salts, chloroquine or hydroxychloroquine, or immunosuppressive drugs. Patients who are allergic to penicillin may react similarly to penicillamine but cross-sensitivity appears to be rare (see below).

Patients need to be carefully supervised and observed for side-effects. In particular full blood counts and urinalysis should be carried out; one recommendation is to perform such checks weekly for the first 2 months of treatment and after any change in dosage, and monthly thereafter. Treatment should be withdrawn if there is a fall in white cell or platelet count, or if progressive or serious proteinuria or haematuria occur. Liver function tests have also been recommended at 6-monthly intervals and renal function should be monitored.

Pyridoxine 25 mg daily may be given to patients on long-term therapy, especially if they are on a restricted diet, since penicillamine increases the requirement for this vitamin.

Because of the effect of penicillamine on collagen and elastin and a possible delay in wound healing, it has been suggested that the dose should be reduced to 250 mg daily for 6 weeks prior to surgery and during the postoperative period until healing has taken place.

Anaesthesia. Penicillamine-induced myasthenia in a 57-year-old woman led to prolonged postoperative apnoea necessitating artificial ventilation.[1] The significance of this report in planning anaesthesia for patients with rheumatoid arthritis treated with penicillamine was discussed.

1. Fried MJ, Protheroe DT. D-Penicillamine induced myasthenia gravis: its relevance for the anaesthetist. *Br J Anaesth* 1986; **58:** 1191–3.

Penicillin allergy. Penicillamine is a degradation product of penicillin and patients with penicillin allergy may theoretically have a cross-sensitivity to penicillamine. Reactions due to contamination of penicillamine with trace amounts of penicillin have been eliminated by the use of synthetic penicillamine. Results of a study in 40 patients with penicillin allergy[1] suggested that while cutaneous cross-reactivity with penicillamine had been documented, the risk of a severe allergic reaction to penicillamine in penicillin-allergic patients was probably quite low.

1. Bell CL, Graziano FM. The safety of administration of penicillamine to penicillin-sensitive individuals. *Arthritis Rheum* 1983; **26:** 801–3.

Pregnancy. Penicillamine teratogenicity has been reviewed.[1] Evidence of the embryotoxicity of maternal penicillamine exposure in *animal* studies has been confirmed in man by 5 reports of cutis laxa in neonates of mothers who had taken penicillamine during pregnancy; 3 further reports of intra-uterine brain injury were less characteristic. Nevertheless most pregnancy outcomes were normal. No birth defects have been reported when penicillamine was discontinued in early pregnancy. Unless a safer therapy could be confirmed, penicillamine management of women with Wilson's disease should be continued throughout pregnancy since the benefits outweighed the risks. However, for conditions for which there were safer alternatives it would be prudent to discontinue penicillamine during pregnancy.

1. Rosa FW. Teratogen update: penicillamine. *Teratology* 1986; **33:** 127–31.

Interactions

Penicillamine forms chelates with metal ions and oral absorption of penicillamine may be reduced by concomitant administration of iron and other metals, antacids, and food. Penicillamine should be taken on an empty stomach and it has been recommended that there should be an interval of at least 2 hours between the administration of penicillamine and iron supplements.

Antacids. In a single-dose study in 6 healthy subjects, administration of penicillamine by mouth immediately after food, an oral dose of ferrous sulphate, or a dose of an antacid mixture of aluminium hydroxide, magnesium hydroxide, and simethicone, reduced the plasma concentrations of penicillamine to 52%, 35%, and 66% respectively of those obtained after administration in a fasting state. Results suggested that the reduction in plasma-penicillamine concentrations was associated with decreased penicillamine absorption.[1] Ifan and Welling[2] showed that the reduction of penicillamine plasma concentrations by aluminium- and magnesium-containing antacids was not similarly produced by sodium bicarbonate, and thus the interaction was probably a result of chelation rather than a pH effect.

1. Osman MA, *et al.* Reduction in oral penicillamine absorption by food, antacid, and ferrous sulphate. *Clin Pharmacol Ther* 1983; **33:** 465–70.
2. Ifan A, Welling PG. Pharmacokinetics of oral 500 mg penicillamine: effect of antacids on absorption. *Biopharm Drug Dispos* 1986; **7:** 401–5.

Diazepam. For a report of exacerbation of intravenous diazepam-induced phlebitis by oral penicillamine, see under Diazepam, p.665.

Gold. There have been conflicting reports on the effect of previous gold therapy on the subsequent development of penicillamine toxicity in patients with rheumatoid arthritis.

A multicentre trial group[1] found no evidence of any interaction between gold and penicillamine but Webley and Coomes[2] found that although the overall incidence of side-effects with penicillamine appeared unaffected by prior gold therapy, bone-marrow depression and rashes were more common in those patients previously treated with gold. Hill[3] reported that patients who had to stop gold therapy because of adverse effects were more prone to develop major adverse effects to penicillamine and a study by Dodd *et al.*[4] indicated that patients who reacted adversely to gold were more likely to develop side-effects to penicillamine. Dodd *et al.*[4] also found that the mean interval between finishing gold and beginning penicillamine in patients who developed identical adverse reactions to both drugs was significantly shorter than in those who developed different side-effects or no side-effects; this supported the theory that some adverse reactions to penicillamine might result from the mobilisation of gold previously stored in the tissues during gold therapy. An interval of at least 6 months between gold and penicillamine therapy in patients who had adverse reactions to gold was recommended. In contrast, Smith *et al.*[5] found no evidence that the interval between gold and penicillamine therapy had any influence on the subsequent development of penicillamine toxicity. A genetic susceptibility in certain patients to react adversely to either drug was suggested. However, in a prospective study by Steven *et al.*,[6] prior gold, penicillamine, or levamisole treatment had no influence on the subsequent efficacy or toxicity of any one of these alternative drugs.

There has been a report of gold therapy causing a recurrence of myasthenia that had previously occurred with penicillamine.[7]

1. Multi-centre Trial Group. Absence of toxic or therapeutic interaction between penicillamine and previously administered gold in a trial of penicillamine in rheumatoid disease. *Postgrad Med J* 1974; **50** (suppl 2): 77–8.
2. Webley M, Coomes EN. Is penicillamine therapy in rheumatoid arthritis influenced by previous treatment with gold? *Br Med J* 1978; **2:** 91.
3. Hill H. Penicillamine and previous treatment with gold. *Br Med J* 1978; **2:** 961.
4. Dodd MJ, *et al.* Adverse reactions to D-penicillamine after gold toxicity. *Br Med J* 1980; **280:** 1498–1500.
5. Smith PJ, *et al.* Influence of previous gold toxicity on subsequent development of penicillamine toxicity. *Br Med J* 1982; **285:** 595–6.
6. Steven MM, *et al.* Does the order of second-line treatment in rheumatoid arthritis matter? *Br Med J* 1982; **284:** 79–81.
7. Moore AP, *et al.* Penicillamine induced myasthenia reactivated by gold. *Br Med J* 1984; **288:** 192–3.

Insulin. Unexplained hypoglycaemia in two type 1 diabetics occurred 6 to 8 weeks after penicillamine treatment for rheumatoid arthritis was started.[1] Both patients required a reduction in their insulin dose. It was possible that the reaction was the result of the induction of insulin antibodies.[2]

1. Elling P, Elling H. Penicillamine, captopril, and hypoglycemia. *Ann Intern Med* 1985; **103:** 644–5.
2. Becker RC, Martin RG. Penicillamine-induced insulin antibodies. *Ann Intern Med* 1986; **104:** 127–8.

Iron. Penicillamine plasma concentrations were reduced by 52% when penicillamine was administered after a dose of ferrous sulphate in healthy subjects.[1] Patients stabilised on penicillamine while on oral iron therapy were considered unlikely to respond fully to penicillamine and would be exposed to a large increase in penicillamine absorption with possible adverse reactions if the iron was stopped.[2]

1. Osman MA, *et al.* Reduction in oral penicillamine absorption by food, antacid, and ferrous sulfate. *Clin Pharmacol Ther* 1983; **33:** 465–70.
2. Harkness JAL, Blake DR. Penicillamine nephropathy and iron. *Lancet* 1982; **ii:** 1368–9.

Probenecid. Probenecid reduced the beneficial effects of penicillamine in cystinuria; co-administration in hyperuricaemic cystinuric patients was contra-indicated.[1]

1. Yu T-F, *et al.* Studies on the metabolism of D-penicillamine and its interaction with probenecid in cystinuria and rheumatoid arthritis. *J Rheumatol* 1984; **11:** 467–70.

Pharmacokinetics

Penicillamine is readily absorbed from the gastro-intestinal tract and reaches peak concentrations in the blood within 1 to 3 hours. It is reported to be more than 80% bound to plasma proteins. It is metabolised in the liver and excreted in the urine and faeces mainly as metabolites. Elimination is biphasic with an initial elimination half-life of about 1 to 3 hours followed by a slower phase, suggesting gradual release from tissues.

Reviews.

1. Netter P, *et al.* Clinical pharmacokinetics of D-penicillamine. *Clin Pharmacokinet* 1987; **13:** 317–33.

Uses and Administration

Penicillamine is a chelator which aids the elimination from the body of certain heavy-metal ions, including copper, lead, and mercury, by forming stable soluble complexes with them that are readily excreted by the kidney. It is used in the treatment of Wilson's disease (to promote the excretion of copper), in heavy-metal poisoning such as lead poisoning, in cystinuria (to reduce urinary concentrations of cystine), in severe active rheumatoid arthritis, and in chronic active hepatitis.

Penicillamine is administered by mouth and should be taken on an empty stomach. A low initial dose increased gradually to the minimum optimal maintenance dosage may reduce the incidence of side-effects as well as provide closer control of the condition being treated.

In the treatment of **Wilson's disease**, a dose of 1.5 to 2 g daily in divided doses may be given initially. The optimal dosage to achieve a negative copper balance should be determined initially by regular analysis of 24-hour urinary copper excretion and subsequently by monitoring free copper in the serum. A maintenance dose of 0.75 to 1 g daily may be adequate once remission is achieved and should be continued indefinitely; the UK manufacturers recommend that a maintenance dose of 2 g daily should not be continued for more than a year. In children, a suggested dose is up to 20 mg per kg body-weight daily (minimum 500 mg daily) in divided doses. A dose of up to 20 mg per kg daily is also suggested for the elderly.

In the management of **lead poisoning**, penicillamine may be given in doses of 1 to 2 g daily in divided doses until the urinary lead concentration is stabilised at less than 0.5 mg per day. A recommended dose for children is 20 to 25 mg per kg daily in divided doses. A dose of 20 mg per kg daily is suggested for the elderly.

In **cystinuria**, doses of penicillamine are adjusted according to cystine concentrations in the urine. For the *treatment* of cystinuria and cystine calculi, the dose is usually in the range of 1 to 4 g daily in divided doses; a suggested dose for children is up to 30 mg per kg daily in divided doses. For the *prevention* of cystine calculi, lower doses of 0.25 to 1 g at bedtime may be given. An adequate fluid intake is essential to maintain urine flow during penicillamine administration for cystinuria.

In the treatment of **severe active rheumatoid arthritis** an initial dose of penicillamine 125 to 250 mg daily is increased gradually by the same amount at intervals of 4 to 12 weeks. Remission is usually achieved with maintenance doses of 500 to 750 mg daily in divided doses, but up to 1.5 g daily may be required (one UK manufacturer has reported that up to 2 g daily may be required by a few patients). Improvement may not occur for several months; the USA manufacturers suggest that penicillamine should be discontinued if there is no response after treatment for 3 to 4 months with 1 to 1.5 g daily; in the UK a trial for 12 months is suggested. After remission has been sustained for 6 months an attempt may be made gradually to reduce the dose by 125 to 250 mg daily every 2 to 3 months but relapse may occur. Lower doses may be required in the elderly who may be more susceptible to developing adverse effects. Initial doses of 50 to 125 mg daily have been recommended gradually increased to a maximum of 1 g daily if necessary. In children the maintenance dose is 15 to 20 mg per kg daily; a suggested initial dose is 2.5 to 5 mg per kg or 50 mg daily for one month increased gradually at 4-weekly intervals.

In the management of **chronic active hepatitis**, an initial dose of penicillamine 500 mg daily in divided doses may be given after liver function tests have indicated that the disease has been controlled by corticosteroids; the dose is gradually increased over 3 months to 1.25 g daily with a concurrent reduction in the corticosteroid dose.

Acetylpenicillamine has been used in mercury poisoning.

Chronic active hepatitis. Penicillamine has been tried in chronic active hepatitis (p.1019) as an alternative to prolonged corticosteroid maintenance therapy once control of the disease is achieved. The dose of penicillamine is increased over several months to a suitable maintenance dose with a concurrent reduction in the corticosteroid dose.

Cystinuria. Cystinuria is an inherited disorder of renal amino acid excretion in which there is excessive excretion of cystine (cysteine disulphide), along with ornithine, lysine, and arginine. The low solubility of cystine leads to the formation of cystine stones in the kidney, resulting in pain, haematuria, renal obstruction, and infection. Treatment is primarily aimed at reducing the urinary concentration of cystine to below its solubility limit of 300 to 400 mg per litre at neutral pH. Patients with cystinuria excrete from 400 to 1200 mg cystine daily and should be advised to drink at least 3 litres of water daily, including at night, to maintain a dilute urine. Cystine is more soluble in alkaline urine and urinary alkalinisers such as sodium bicarbonate, sodium citrate, or potassium citrate may be used; however, high doses are required and calcium stone formation may be promoted. In patients where these measures are ineffective or not tolerated penicillamine may be used; it complexes with cysteine to form a more soluble mixed disulphide, therefore reducing cystine excretion, preventing cystine stone formation, and promoting the gradual dissolution of existing stones. Adverse effects are common and tiopronin, which has a similar action, may be used as an alternative. Surgical removal may be necessary for established stones but lithotripsy is not very effective.

Lead poisoning. Penicillamine may be used to treat asymptomatic lead intoxication and to achieve desirable lead-tissue levels in patients with symptomatic lead poisoning once they have received treatment with sodium calciumedetate and dimercaprol (see p.1595).

Primary biliary cirrhosis. Copper accumulation in the liver has been noted in patients with long-lasting cholestatic liver disorders such as primary biliary cirrhosis (p.497) and initial studies[1,2] indicated that penicillamine might be of benefit by increasing the urinary excretion of copper and reducing liver-copper concentrations. It was also suggested that the immunological action of penicillamine might influence the course of the disease.[3] However, preliminary results indicating that penicillamine improved survival in patients with primary biliary cirrhosis[4] were not supported by further studies[5-7] in which penicillamine did not significantly affect the overall survival or prevent progression of the disease. A review by James[8] concluded that the value of penicillamine in the treatment of primary biliary cirrhosis was not proven; there was possibly a marginal decrease in mortality in an intermediate symptomatic group of patients but the incidence of side-effects was probably too high to justify further long and elaborate clinical studies.

1. Deering TB, *et al.* Effect of D-penicillamine on copper retention in patients with primary biliary cirrhosis. *Gastroenterology* 1977; **72:** 1208–12.
2. Jain S, *et al.* A controlled trial of D-penicillamine therapy in primary biliary cirrhosis. *Lancet* 1977; **i:** 831–4.
3. Epstein O, *et al.* Reduction of immune complexes and immunoglobulins induced by D-penicillamine in primary biliary cirrhosis. *N Engl J Med* 1979; **300:** 274–8.
4. Epstein O, *et al.* D-Penicillamine treatment improves survival in primary biliary cirrhosis. *Lancet* 1981; **i:** 1275–7.
5. Matloff DS, *et al.* A prospective trial of D-penicillamine in primary biliary cirrhosis. *N Engl J Med* 1982; **306:** 319–26.
6. Dickson ER, *et al.* Trial of penicillamine in advanced primary biliary cirrhosis. *N Engl J Med* 1985; **312:** 1011–15.
7. Neuberger J, *et al.* Double blind controlled trial of D-penicillamine in patients with primary biliary cirrhosis. *Gut* 1985; **26:** 114–19.
8. James OFW. D-Penicillamine for primary biliary cirrhosis. *Gut* 1985; **26:** 109–13.

Rheumatoid arthritis. *Rheumatoid arthritis* (p.2) and *juvenile chronic arthritis* (p.2) are generally treated using the same methods. Initial drug therapy is usually with an NSAID, which provides symptomatic relief. Penicillamine is one of a diverse group of disease modifying antirheumatic drugs used in an attempt to suppress the rate of cartilage erosion or alter the course of the disease. However, early enthusiasm for penicillamine has been somewhat curtailed by a high incidence of adverse effects.[1] During long-term therapy as many as 50% of patients taking penicillamine have been reported to withdraw from treatment as a consequence of adverse effects.[2] Low doses of penicillamine to reduce the incidence of side-effects have been tried and while doses as low as 125 mg daily have been claimed to be effective in some patients with *rheumatoid arthritis*, a 36-week multicentre double-blind study[3] involving 225 patients concluded that a dose of penicillamine 500 mg daily was only slightly more effective than placebo. A dose of 125 mg daily was not significantly different from either the 500 mg dose or placebo. In patients with *juvenile rheumatoid arthritis* it has been suggested that gold therapy may be preferred to penicillamine since there is greater experience with gold and its efficacy is better established.[4]

1. Taylor HG, Samanta A. Penicillamine in rheumatoid arthritis: a problem of toxicity. *Drug Safety* 1992; **7:** 46–53.
2. Moens HJB, *et al.* Longterm followup of treatment with D-penicillamine for rheumatoid arthritis: effectivity and toxicity in relation to HLA antigens. *J Rheumatol* 1987; **14:** 1115–19.
3. Williams HJ, *et al.* Low-dose D-penicillamine therapy in rheumatoid arthritis: a controlled, double-blind clinical trial. *Arthritis Rheum* 1983; **26:** 581–92.
4. Rosenberg AM. Advanced drug therapy for juvenile rheumatoid arthritis. *J Pediatr* 1989; **114:** 171–8.

Scleroderma. Despite the lack of conclusive evidence in its favour penicillamine, which affects the cross-linking of collagen,[1] has been widely thought to be of benefit in scleroderma (p.501), and perhaps in some visceral manifestations of systemic sclerosis.[2,3] If used, treatment should probably be begun early and continued for several years; therapy for 6 to 12 months is required before any benefit can be observed. A dose of 250 to 500 mg of penicillamine daily has been used.[2]

For a report of sclerodermatous lesions in a patient taking penicillamine for Wilson's disease, see under Adverse Effects, Effects on the Skin, above.

1. Herbert CM, *et al.* Biosynthesis and maturation of skin collagen in scleroderma, and effect of D-penicillamine. *Lancet* 1974; **i:** 187–92.
2. Oliver GF, Winkelmann RK. The current treatment of scleroderma. *Drugs* 1989; **37:** 87–96.
3. Steen VD, *et al.* D-Penicillamine therapy in progressive systemic sclerosis (scleroderma): a retrospective analysis. *Ann Intern Med* 1982; **97:** 652–9.

Wilson's disease. Wilson's disease, or hepatolenticular degeneration, is a rare autosomal disorder of copper accumulation. Excretion of excess copper, which normally occurs via the bile, is impaired in Wilson's disease and total body copper progressively increases. The excess copper accumulates in the liver, brain, and other organs including the kidneys and corneas, and eventually causes tissue damage.

Effective treatment of Wilson's disease depends upon establishing a negative copper balance thereby preventing deposition of more copper and mobilising for excretion excess copper already deposited and this is achieved with copper-reducing drugs. Once negative copper balance has been achieved, maintenance treatment must be continued lifelong. Dietary restriction of copper is not generally considered to be an important part of the treatment of Wilson's disease; patients may be advised to avoid copper-rich foods, such as liver and shellfish, during the first year of treatment and to restrict their consumption thereafter. Symptomatic recovery from copper overload occurs slowly, but is usually complete if treatment is started early enough, and a normal life expectancy can be achieved. However, once irreversible organ damage such as liver cirrhosis has occurred, treatment can only prevent further deterioration; those presenting with end-stage liver disease do not benefit from copper-reducing therapy, and liver transplantation is necessary (although successful medical treatment has been reported in children). The drugs used in the treatment of Wilson's disease are penicillamine, trientine, and zinc. Ammonium tetrathiomolybdate is under investigation.

Penicillamine reduces copper concentrations mainly by chelating copper which is then excreted in the urine. Two molecules of penicillamine combine with one atom of copper. Penicillamine also reduces the affinity of copper for proteins and polypeptides thus allowing removal of copper from tissues and induces synthesis of metallothionein in the liver, a protein that combines with copper to form a non-toxic product. *Trientine* is a less potent copper chelator than penicillamine that competes for copper bound to serum albumin. *Zinc* induces synthesis of metallothionein in the intestine, a protein that has a higher affinity for copper than for zinc, so that absorption of copper from the gastro-intestinal tract is blocked. It is usually given as the acetate as this form is less irritating to the stomach than the sulphate. *Ammonium tetrathiomolybdate* forms a complex with protein and copper. When it is given with food it blocks the intestinal absorption of copper, and when taken between meals it combines with albumin- and caeruloplasmin-bound copper.

CHOICE OF DRUG. Penicillamine is generally regarded as the drug of choice for the initial management of Wilson's disease as it produces a rapid reduction in copper levels. However, in patients with neurological symptoms there may be a worsening of symptoms on initiation of penicillamine (possibly due to transiently increased brain and blood copper concentrations). Some practitioners therefore suggest zinc initially; zinc is not suitable in those requiring rapid reduction of copper levels as it has a slow onset of action. Trientine, which may also exacerbate neurological symptoms, is used in patients intolerant of penicillamine. Ammonium tetrathiomolybdate is under investigation for the initial reduction of copper levels; it may be particularly suitable for patients with neurological symptoms.

Once a negative copper balance is achieved, maintenance therapy must be continued for life. Penicillamine, trientine, and zinc are all used for maintenance treatment. Patients taking penicillamine are also given pyridoxine to prevent deficiency (see under Precautions, above). The adverse effects of penicillamine may be a problem during long-term use and zinc, which has low toxicity, is often preferred. Zinc is also used in patients in the asymptomatic stage of the disease.

References.

1. Tankanow RM. Pathophysiology and treatment of Wilson's disease. *Clin Pharm* 1991; **10:** 839–49.
2. Stremmel W, *et al.* Wilson disease: clinical presentation, treatment, and survival. *Ann Intern Med* 1991; **115:** 720–6.
3. Brewer GJ. Practical recommendations and new therapies for Wilson's disease. *Drugs* 1995; **50:** 240–9.
4. Santos Silva EE, *et al.* Successful medical treatment of severely decompensated Wilson disease. *J Pediatr* 1996; **128:** 285–7.

Preparations

BP 1998: Penicillamine Tablets;
USP 23: Penicillamine Capsules; Penicillamine Tablets.

Proprietary Preparations (details are given in Part 3)

Aust.: Artamin; Distamine; ***Austral.:*** D-Penamine; ***Belg.:*** Kelatin; ***Canad.:*** Cuprimine; Depen; ***Fr.:*** Trolovol; ***Ger.:*** Metalcaptase; Trisorcin; Trolovol; ***Irl.:*** Distamine; ***Ital.:*** Pemine; Sufortan†; ***Neth.:*** Cuprimine; Distamine; Gerodyl†; Kelatin; ***Norw.:*** Cuprimine; ***S.Afr.:*** Metalcaptase; ***Spain:*** Cupripen; Sufortanon; ***Swed.:*** Cuprimine; ***Switz.:*** Mercaptyl; ***UK:*** Distamine; Pendramine; ***USA:*** Cuprimine; Depen.

Multi-ingredient: ***Ger.:*** Trisorcin B_6 N†.

Potassium Polystyrene Sulphonate (13157-g)

Potassium Polystyrene Sulfonate.
CAS — 9011-99-8.

The potassium salt of sulphonated styrene polymer.

Potassium polystyrene sulphonate is a cation-exchange resin that exchanges potassium ions for calcium ions and other cations and is used in the management of hypercalciuria and renal calculi.

Preparations

Proprietary Preparations (details are given in Part 3)
Ger.: Campanyl.

Multi-ingredient: ***Ger.:*** Ujostabil.

Pralidoxime (13533-j)

Pralidoxime *(BAN).*
2-Hydroxyiminomethyl-1-methylpyridinium.
$C_7H_9N_2O$ = 137.2.
CAS — 6735-59-7; 495-94-3.

Pralidoxime Chloride (1050-s)

Pralidoxime Chloride *(BANM, USAN).*
2-Formyl-1-methylpyridinium Chloride Oxime; 2-PAM; 2-PAM Chloride; 2-PAMCl; 2-Pyridine Aldoxime Methochloride.
$C_7H_9ClN_2O$ = 172.6.
CAS — 51-15-0.
Pharmacopoeias. In US.

A white or pale yellow odourless crystalline powder. Freely **soluble** in water.

Pralidoxime Iodide (1048-z)

Pralidoxime Iodide *(BANM, USAN, rINN).*
NSC-7760; 2-PAM Iodide; 2-PAMI.
$C_7H_9IN_2O$ = 264.1.
CAS — 94-63-3.
Pharmacopoeias. In Chin.

Pralidoxime Mesylate (1049-c)

Pralidoxime Mesylate *(BANM, USAN).*
2-PAMM; Pralidoxime Methanesulphonate; P2S.
$C_7H_9N_2O,CH_3O_3S$ = 232.3.
CAS — 154-97-2.

Pralidoxime Methylsulphate (1047-j)

Pralidoxime Methylsulphate *(BANM).*
$C_7H_9N_2O,CH_3SO_4$ = 248.3.
CAS — 1200-55-1.
Pharmacopoeias. In It.

Adverse Effects

The administration of pralidoxime may be associated with drowsiness, dizziness, disturbances of vision, nausea, tachycardia, headache, hyperventilation, and muscular weakness. Tachycardia, laryngospasm, and muscle rigidity have been attributed to administering pralidoxime intravenously at too rapid a rate. Large doses of pralidoxime may cause transient neuromuscular blockade.

Precautions

Pralidoxime should be used cautiously in patients with impaired renal function; a reduction in dosage may be necessary. Caution is also required in administering pralidoxime to patients with myasthenia gravis as it may precipitate a myasthenic crisis. Pralidoxime should not be used to treat poisoning by carbamate pesticides.

When atropine and pralidoxime are given together, the signs of atropinisation may occur earlier than might be expected when atropine is used alone.

Pharmacokinetics

Pralidoxime is not bound to plasma proteins, does not readily pass into the CNS, and is rapidly excreted in the urine partly unchanged and partly as a metabolite. The elimination half-life is approximately 1 to 3 hours.

References.

1. Sidell FR, Groff WA. Intramuscular and intravenous administration of small doses of 2-pyridinium aldoxime methochloride to man. *J Pharm Sci* 1971; **60:** 1224–8.
2. Siddell FR, *et al.* Pralidoxime methansulfonate: plasma levels and pharmacokinetics after oral administration to man. *J Pharm Sci* 1972; **61:** 1136–40.
3. Swartz RD, *et al.* Effects of heat and exercise on the elimination of pralidoxime in man. *Clin Pharmacol Ther* 1973; **14:** 83–9.

Uses and Administration

Pralidoxime is a cholinesterase reactivator. It is used as an adjunct to but *not* as a substitute for atropine in the treatment of poisoning by certain cholinesterase inhibitors. Its main indication is in poisoning due to organophosphorus insecticides or related compounds (see p.1408) when it acts principally by reactivating the enzyme cholinesterase after this enzyme has been inhibited by phosphorylation. It thus restores the enzymatic destruction of acetylcholine at the neuromuscular junction and relieves muscle paralysis; however, concomitant administration of atropine is required to counteract directly the adverse effects of acetylcholine accumulation, particularly at the respiratory centre. Pralidoxime is not equally antagonistic to all organophosphorus anticholinesterases as reactivation is dependent on the nature of the phosphoryl group and the rate at which inhibition becomes irreversible. It is not effective in the treatment of poisoning due to phosphorus, inorganic phosphates, or organophosphates without anticholinesterase activity. It is relatively ineffective in the treatment of poisoning by carbamate insecticides and it should not be used in carbaryl poisoning as it may increase toxicity. The use of pralidoxime has been suggested for the treatment of overdosage by anticholinesterase drugs, including those used to treat myasthenia gravis such as neostigmine; however, it is only slightly effective and its use is not generally recommended.

Pralidoxime is usually given as the chloride or mesylate but the iodide and methylsulphate salts have also been used. Doses are expressed in terms of the salts.

Pralidoxime may be administered by slow intravenous injection over 5 to 10 minutes, by intravenous infusion over 15 to 30 minutes, or by subcutaneous or intramuscular injection; it has also been given orally.

In the treatment of **organophosphorus poisoning** pralidoxime should be given within 24 hours of poisoning to be fully effective as cholinesterase inactivation usually becomes irreversible after this time; however patients with severe poisoning may occasionally respond up to 36 hours or longer after exposure. Injections of *atropine* should be given intravenously or intramuscularly and repeated as necessary until the patient shows signs of atropine toxicity; atropinisation should then be maintained for 48 hours or more. Large amounts of atropine may be required. See under Atropine Sulphate, p.456, for details of dosages. Concomitantly, 1 to 2 g of *pralidoxime*, as the chloride, iodide, or mesylate, should be administered intramuscularly or intravenously and repeated if necessary according to the patient's condition (alternatively, a dose of pralidoxime mesylate of 30 mg per kg body-weight by slow intravenous injection has been suggested by an authoritative UK source). Additional doses may be required every 3 to 8 hours in cases of ingestion (alternatively, in severe poisoning, a continuous infusion of 200 to 500 mg per hour may be administered, titrated against response). A maximum dose of 12 g in 24 hours has been suggested. In children, pralidoxime chloride 20 to 40 mg per kg body-weight or pralidoxime mesylate 20 to 60 mg per kg may be given depending on the severity of poisoning and response to treatment. The dose of pralidoxime may need to be reduced in patients with impaired renal function.

Treatment should preferably be monitored by the determination of blood-cholinesterase concentrations and clinical symptoms. Patients should be closely observed for at least 24 hours following resolution of symptoms.

Other oximes with cholinesterase reactivating properties that have been used similarly include obidoxime chloride (p.988), diacetyl monoxime, and trimedoxime bromide (TMB-4).

Administration. Pralidoxime was administered by continuous intravenous infusion in a dose of 9 to 19 mg per kg bodyweight per hour immediately after a loading dose of 15 to 50 mg per kg to 7 children with symptomatic organophosphorus intoxication.[1] Continuous infusion for 18 to 60 hours was effective and well tolerated. In adults, rates of up to 500 mg per hour have been used for prolonged nicotinic symptoms.[2]

1. Farrar HC, *et al.* Use of continuous infusion of pralidoxime for treatment of organophosphate poisoning in children. *J Pediatr* 1990; **116:** 658–61.
2. Tush GM, Anstead MI. Pralidoxime continuous infusion in the treatment of organophosphate poisoning. *Ann Pharmacother* 1997; **31:** 441–4.

Preparations

USP 23: Pralidoxime Chloride for Injection; Pralidoxime Chloride Tablets.

Proprietary Preparations (details are given in Part 3)
Canad.: Protopam; ***Fr.:*** Contrathion; ***Ital.:*** Contrathion; ***USA:*** Protopam.

Protamine (4999-k)

CAS — 9012-00-4.

Protamine Hydrochloride (11518-f)

Protamine Hydrochloride *(BANM).*

Cloridrato de Protamina; Protamini Hydrochloridum.

Pharmacopoeias. In *Eur.* (see p.viii).

A mixture of the hydrochlorides of basic peptides prepared from the sperm or roe of suitable species of fish, usually from the families Clupeidae or Salmonidae. A white or almost white hygroscopic powder. **Soluble** in water; practically insoluble in alcohol and in ether. **Store** in airtight containers.

Protamine Sulphate (1051-w)

Protamine Sulphate *(BAN).*

Protamine Sulfate *(rINN)*; Protamini Sulfas; Sulfato de Protamina.

CAS — 9009-65-8.

Pharmacopoeias. In *Chin., Eur.* (see p.viii), *Jpn,* and *US.*

A mixture of the sulphates of basic peptides prepared from the sperm, testes, or roe of suitable species of fish, usually from the families Clupeidae or Salmonidae. A white or almost white hygroscopic powder. Sparingly **soluble** in water; practically insoluble in alcohol and in ether. **Store** at 2° to 8° in airtight containers.

Adverse Effects and Precautions

Intravenous injections of protamine sulphate, particularly if given rapidly, may cause hypotension, bradycardia, and dyspnoea. A sensation of warmth, transitory flushing, nausea and vomiting, and lassitude may also occur.

Hypersensitivity reactions can occur; patients at risk include diabetics who have received protamine-insulin preparations, those who have previously undergone procedures such as coronary angioplasty or cardiopulmonary bypass surgery, those allergic to fish, and men who are infertile or who have had a vasectomy. Anaphylactoid reactions have been reported.

Protamine has an anticoagulant effect when administered in the absence of heparin.

When repeated doses of protamine are used to neutralise large doses of heparin a rebound bleeding effect may occur which responds to further doses of protamine. Clotting parameters should be closely monitored in patients undergoing such prolonged procedures.

In a report on 4 patients who received protamine sulphate after cardiac surgery to neutralise the effect of heparin severe adverse reactions including marked hypotension, vascular collapse, and pulmonary oedema were described.[1] Previous reports of similar reactions to protamine were reviewed. A total of 17 patients had immediate anaphylactic reactions; in 1 patient a complement-dependent IgG antibody-mediated reaction had been demonstrated and 3 patients tested for allergy to protamine had positive skin tests. In 15 of these 17 patients there was evidence of previous exposure to protamine; those with a high risk of sensitisation included leucopheresis donors who had received the drug, diabetics using insulin containing protamine, and patients with fish allergy. Suspected reactions to protamine occurred in a further 10 patients after cardiac surgery. However, these reactions were characterised by severe vascular damage manifested as noncardiogenic pulmonary oedema or persistent hypotension and onset was delayed for 30 minutes to several hours. Evidence suggested that these reactions were not antibody mediated; only 2 of 7 evaluable patients had previous exposure. All patients required aggressive therapy.

In a review of the toxicity of protamine[2] adverse cardiovascular responses were considered to be of 3 types, transient hypotension related to rapid drug administration, occasional anaphylactoid responses, and rarely, catastrophic pulmonary vasoconstriction.

1. Holland CL, *et al.* Adverse reactions to protamine sulfate following cardiac surgery. *Clin Cardiol* 1984; **7:** 157–62.
2. Horrow JC. Protamine: a review of its toxicity. *Anesth Analg* 1985; **64:** 348–61.

Uses and Administration

Protamine is a basic protein which combines with heparin to form a stable inactive complex. Protamine is used to neutralise the anticoagulant action of heparin in the treatment of haemorrhage resulting from severe heparin or low-molecular-weight heparin overdosage. It is also used to neutralise the effect of heparin given before surgery and during extracorporeal circulation as in dialysis or cardiac surgery. Protamine is used in some insulin preparations to prolong the effects of insulin. Protamine is usually given as the sulphate, although the hydrochloride may also be used.

Protamine sulphate is administered by slow intravenous injection over a period of about 10 minutes. The dose is dependent on the amount of heparin to be neutralised and ideally should be titrated against assessments of the coagulability of the patient's blood. Protamine sulphate has weak anticoagulating properties and if given in gross excess its anticoagulant action could be significant. As heparin is being continuously excreted the dose should be reduced if more than 15 minutes have elapsed since heparin administration; for example, if protamine sulphate is given 30 minutes after heparin the dose may be reduced to about one-half. Not more than 50 mg of protamine sulphate should be injected for any one dose; patients should be carefully monitored as further doses may be required. The Ph. Eur. specifies that 1 mg of protamine sulphate precipitates not less than 100 units of heparin sodium, but adds that this potency is based on a specific reference batch of heparin sodium. One UK manufacturer has stated that each mg of protamine sulphate will usually neutralise the anticoagulant effect of at least 80 international units of heparin (lung) or at least 100 international units of heparin (mucous). The USA manufacturer has stated that each mg of protamine sulphate neutralises approximately 90 USP units of heparin (lung) or about 115 USP units of heparin (mucous).

Protamine neutralises the anti-thrombin activity of low-molecular-weight heparins but only partially neutralises the anti-factor-Xa effect; 1 mg of protamine sulphate is stated to inhibit the effects of 100 units of dalteparin sodium or 1 mg (100 units) of enoxaparin sodium.

Protamine hydrochloride may be used similarly.

Haemorrhagic disorders. Endogenous production of heparin-like substances may, rarely, be responsible for some bleeding disorders. Protamine could be useful as a diagnostic aid *in vitro* and could be administered intravenously to transiently control bleeding in such patients.[1,2]

1. Tefferi A, *et al.* Circulating heparin-like anticoagulants: report of five consecutive cases and a review. *Am J Med* 1990; **88:** 184–8.
2. Bayly PJM, Thick M. Reversal of post-reperfusion coagulopathy by protamine sulphate in orthotopic liver transplantation. *Br J Anaesth* 1994; **73:** 840–2.

Preparations

BP 1998: Protamine Sulphate Injection;
USP 23: Protamine Sulfate for Injection; Protamine Sulfate Injection.

Proprietary Preparations (details are given in Part 3)
UK: Prosulf.

Prussian Blue (13186-e)

Berlin Blue; CI Pigment Blue 27; Colour Index No. 77510; Ferric Ferrocyanide; Ferric Hexacyanoferrate (II).

$Fe_4[Fe(CN)_6]_3$ = 859.2.

CAS — 14038-43-8; 12240-15-2.

NOTE. The name Prussian Blue (CI Pigment Blue 27) is applied to both ferric hexacyanoferrate (II) and to potassium ferric hexacyanoferrate (II), $KFe[Fe(CN)_6]$ = 306.9 (Colour Index No. 77520).

Prussian blue is used in the treatment of thallium poisoning. When administered by mouth it forms a non-absorbable complex with thallium in the gastro-intestinal tract which is excreted in the faeces. A suggested dose of Prussian blue is 10 g, or 125 mg per kg body-weight, twice daily by mouth or duodenal tube until the urinary excretion of thallium falls to 0.5 mg or less per 24 hours. It has been used similarly for the removal of radiocaesium from the body.

The following treatment of acute thallium poisoning has been suggested:[1] gastric lavage; intravenous fluid challenge with forced diuresis until the 24-hour urinary thallium excretion is below 1 mg; prussian blue 10 g in 100 mL of 15% mannitol twice daily via a duodenal tube until 24-hour urinary thallium excretion is below 0.5 mg; intermittent haemoperfusion or haemodialysis, if possible, especially within 48 hours of ingestion.

1. de Groot G, *et al.* No evidence for general thallium poisoning in Guyana. *Lancet* 1987; **i:** 1084.

Preparations

Proprietary Preparations (details are given in Part 3)
Ger.: Antidotum Thallii Heyl; Radiogardase-Cs.

Sevelamer Hydrochloride (9348-f)

Sevelamer Hydrochloride *(USAN, rINNM).*

GT16-026A. Allylamine polymer with 1-chloro-2,3-epoxypropane hydrochloride.

CAS — 182683-00-7.

Sevelamer hydrochloride is a phosphate binder used for hyperphosphataemia in patients with chronic renal failure.

Silymarin (13236-v)

A mixture of the isomers silibinin, silicristin, and silidianin.

CAS — 65666-07-1.

Pharmacopoeias. Ger. includes Milk Thistle Fruit, the ripe liberated fruit of *Silybum marianum* containing not less than 1.5% of silymarin calculated as silibinin.

The active principle from the fruit of *Silybum marianum* (=*Carduus marianus*) (Compositae). The principal components are the flavonolignans silibinin, silicristin, and silidianin of which silibinin is the major component.

Silibinin (929-k)

Silibinin *(rINN).*

Silybin; Silybum Substance E_6. 3,5,7-Trihydroxy-2-[3-(4-hydroxy-3-methoxyphenyl)-2-(hydroxymethyl)-1,4-benzodioxan-6-yl]-4-chromanone.

$C_{25}H_{22}O_{10}$ = 482.4.

CAS — 22888-70-6.

NOTE. The name silymarin has also been used to denote silibinin.

Silicristin (15705-e)

Silicristin *(rINN).*

Silychristin. 2-[2,3-Dihydro-7-hydroxy-2-(4-hydroxy-3-methoxyphenyl)-3-(hydroxymethyl)-5-benzofuranyl]-3,5,7-trihydroxy-4-chromanone.

$C_{25}H_{22}O_{10}$ = 482.4.

CAS — 33889-69-9.

Silidianin (15706-l)

Silidianin *(rINN).*

Silydianin. (+)-2,3α,3aα,7a-Tetrahydro-7aα-hydroxy-8(*R**)-(4-hydroxy-3-methoxyphenyl)-4-(3α,5,7-trihydroxy-4-oxo-2β-chromanyl)-3,6-methanobenzofuran-7(6α*H*)-one.

$C_{25}H_{22}O_{10}$ = 482.4.

CAS — 29782-68-1.

Silymarin is claimed to be a free radical scavenger and has been used for the treatment of hepatic disorders. Silibinin, one of the active constituents of silymarin, has been used as the disodium dihemisuccinate salt in *Amanita phalloides* poisoning (p.1605). Silymarin is poorly water-soluble and has been given by mouth; disodium silibinin dihemisuccinate is water-soluble and has been given by intravenous injection. Silymarin in doses of up to 140 mg (equivalent to silibinin 60 mg) two or three times daily by mouth has been suggested for hepatic disorders. A dose of silibinin 20 mg per kg body-weight daily by intravenous infusion in 4 divided doses as the disodium dihemisuccinate has been suggested in *Amanita phalloides* poisoning.

Amanita poisoning. Silymarin and silibinin have been found to be effective in preventing hepatic damage following amanita poisoning.[1-3]

1. Vogel G. The anti-amanita effect of silymarin. In: Faulstich H, *et al.*, eds. *Amanita toxins and poisoning*. Baden-Baden: Verlag Gerhad Witzstrock, 1980: 180–7.
2. Lorenz D. Über die anwending von silibinin bei der knollenblätterpilzvergiftung. *Dtsch Arzt* 1982; **79:** 43–5.
3. Hruby K, *et al.* Chemotherapy of Amanita phalloides poisoning with intravenous silibinin. *Hum Toxicol* 1983; **2:** 183–90.

Hepatic disorders. Beneficial responses to silymarin have been reported in patients with liver disorders.[1-3]

1. Cavalieri S. Valutazione clinica controllata del legalon. *Gazz Med Ital* 1974; **133:** 628–35.
2. Salmi HA, Sarna S. Effect of silymarin on chemical, functional, and morphological alterations of the liver: a double-blind controlled study. *Scand J Gastroenterol* 1982; **17:** 517–21.
3. Ferenci P, *et al.* Randomized controlled trial of silymarin treatment in patients with cirrhosis of the liver. *J Hepatol* 1989; **9:** 105–13.

Preparations

Proprietary Preparations (details are given in Part 3)
Aust.: Apihepar; Biogelat Leberschutz; Hepar Pasc Mono; Legalon; Silyhexal; ***Austral.:*** Herbal Liver Formula; Liver Tonic Capsules; Prol; ***Belg.:*** Legalon SIL; ***Fr.:*** Legalon; ***Ger.:*** Alepa; Ardeyhepan N; Carduus-monoplant; Cefasliymarin; Divinal-Hepa; durasilymarin; Hegrimarin; Heliplant; Hepa-loges N; Hepa-Merz Sil; Hepar-Pasc; Heparano N; Heparsyx N; Hepatorell; Hepatos; Heplant; Legalon; Legalon SIL; Logomed Leber-Kapseln; Mariendistel Curarina; Phytohepar; Poikicholan; Probiophyt V; Silibene; Silicur; Silimarit; Silmar; Sulfolitruw H†; Vit-o-Mar; ***Ital.:*** Eparsil; Legalon; Locasil; Marsil; Silepar; Silimarin; Silirex; Silliver; Silmar†; Trissil; ***S.Afr.:*** Legalon; ***Spain:*** Legalon; Silarine; Silimazu; ***Switz.:*** Legalon; Legalon SIL.

Multi-ingredient: ***Aust.:*** Aristochol; Bakanasan Leber-Galle; Hepabene; Pascopankreat; Sanhelios Leber-Galle; Sidroga Leber-Galle-Tee; ***Austral.:*** Herbal Cleanse; Lifesystem Herbal Formula 7 Liver Tonic; Liver Tonic Herbal Formula 6; Silybum Complex; St Mary's Thistle Plus; Super B Plus Liver Tonic; T & T Antioxidant; ***Ger.:*** Asgocholan†; Bilgast†; Bilisan C3; Bilisan forte†; Cefachol N; Cheiranthol; Choanol†; Cholaflux N†; Cholaflux†; Cholhepan N; Cholongal plus†; Cholongal†; Cholosom-Tee; Doppelherz Magenstarkung; Dr. Maurers Magen-Apotheke†; Duoform†; Enzym-Hepaduran†; Esberigal N; Galleb†; Gallexier; Gallitophen†; Galloselect M; Hepaduran†; Hepafungin†; Hepalixier†; Hepar-Pasc N; Heparaxal†; Heparchofid S†; Hepaticum-Medice H; Hepatimed N; Hepatofalk Planta; Hepaton†; Heumann Leber- und Gallentee Solu-Hepar NT; Hevert-Gall S; Iberogast; Jatamansin†; JuCholan S; Legapas comp; LP-Truw†; Marianon; Medichol†; Neo-Gallonorm†; Noricaven†; Pankreaplex N†; Pankreaplex Neu; Pascohepan novo; Pascopankreat†; Pascopnakreat novo; Pascovenol S†; Presselin Hepaticum P; Schwohepan S; Solu-Hepar N†; Spasmo-Bilicura†; Sulfolitruw†; Vasesana-Vasoregulans; Vegomed†; Venacton; ventri-loges; Worishofener Leber- und Gallensteinmittel Dr. Kleinschrod†; ***Ital.:*** Castindia; Venoplant†; Venoplus; ***Neth.:*** Venoplant†; ***Spain:*** Venoplant; ***Switz.:*** Boldocynara N; Demonatur Gouttes pour le foie et la bile; Iberogast; Lapidar 14; Phytomed Hepato; Simepar; Tisane hepatique et biliaire.

Sodium Calciumedetate (1052-e)

Sodium Calciumedetate *(BAN)*.

Sodium Calcium Edetate *(rINN)*; 385; Calcium Disodium Edathamil; Calcium Disodium Edetate; Calcium Disodium Ethylenediaminetetra-acetate; Calcium Disodium Versenate; Calcium EDTA; Disodium Calcium Tetracemate; Edetate Calcium Disodium *(USAN)*; Natrii Calcii Edetas. The calcium chelate of disodium ethylenediaminetetra-acetate; Disodium[(ethylenedinitrilo)tetraacetato]calciate(2−) hydrate.

$C_{10}H_{12}CaN_2Na_2O_8,xH_2O$ = 374.3 (anhydrous).

CAS — 23411-34-9 (sodium calciumedetate, hydrate); 62-33-9 (anhydrous sodium calciumedetate).

Pharmacopoeias. In Eur. (see p.viii), Pol., and US.

US specifies a mixture of the dihydrate and trihydrate but predominantly the dihydrate. *Int.* specifies the dihydrate.

A white or almost white, slightly hygroscopic, odourless, crystalline powder or granules. Freely **soluble** in water; practically insoluble in alcohol and in ether. A 20% solution in water has a pH of 6.5 to 8.0. **Store** in airtight containers.

Adverse Effects

Sodium calciumedetate is nephrotoxic and may cause renal tubular necrosis. Nausea and cramp may also occur. Thrombophlebitis has followed intravenous infusion and may be related to the concentration of the injection. Pain at the intramuscular injection site has been reported. Other side-effects that have been reported include fever, malaise, headache, myalgia, histamine-like responses such as sneezing, nasal congestion, and lachrymation, skin eruptions, transient hypotension, and ECG abnormalities.

Sodium calciumedetate chelates zinc within the body and zinc deficiency has been reported. Displacement of calcium from sodium calciumedetate may lead to hypercalcaemia.

Effects on the kidneys. Of 130 children with lead poisoning who received combined chelation therapy of sodium calciumedetate (25 mg per kg body-weight intramuscularly every 12 hours) and dimercaprol (3 mg per kg intramuscularly every 4 hours) for a total of 5 days, 21 developed clinical evidence of nephrotoxicity and in 4 severe oliguric acute renal failure began 1 or 2 days after chelation therapy was discontinued.[1] Nephrotoxicity was probably attributable to the use of sodium calciumedetate.

1. Moel DI, Kumar K. Reversible nephrotic reactions to a combined 2,3-dimercapto-l-propanol and calcium disodium ethylenediaminetetraacetic acid regimen in asymptomatic children with elevated blood lead levels. *Pediatrics* 1982; **70:** 259–62.

Precautions

Sodium calciumedetate should be used with caution, if at all, in patients with impaired renal function. Daily urinalysis to monitor proteinuria and haematuria and regular monitoring of renal function has been recommended.

Sodium calciumedetate can chelate with several endogenous metals, including zinc, and may increase their excretion; therapy should be intermittent to prevent severe deficiency developing and monitoring of zinc levels may be required (see below).

Sodium calciumedetate should not be given by mouth in the treatment of lead poisoning as it has been suggested that absorption of lead may be increased as a result.

Sodium calciumedetate 500 mg per m^2 body-surface was administered by deep intramuscular injection every 12 hours for 5 days to 10 children with asymptomatic lead poisoning.[1] Lead concentrations in blood decreased to about 58% of the pretreatment values after 5 days of treatment and were essentially unchanged for up to 60 hours after the last dose. Sodium calciumedetate also produced a marked fall in the mean plasma concentration of zinc but this rebounded rapidly after cessation of treatment. Mean urinary-lead excretion increased about 21-fold during the first 24 hours of therapy and urinary-zinc excretion increased about 17-fold. Sodium calciumedetate had little effect on the plasma concentrations or urinary excretion of copper. The results suggested that careful monitoring of zinc was required during treatment with sodium calciumedetate.

1. Thomas DJ, Chisolm JJ. Lead, zinc and copper decorporation during calcium disodium ethylenediamine tetraacetate treatment of lead-poisoned children. *J Pharmacol Exp Ther* 1986; **239:** 829–35.

Pharmacokinetics

Sodium calciumedetate is poorly absorbed from the gastro-intestinal tract. It distributes primarily to the extracellular fluid and does not penetrate cells. It is not significantly metabolised; after intravenous injection about 50% of a dose is excreted in the urine in 1 hour and over 95% in 24 hours.

Uses and Administration

Sodium calciumedetate is the calcium chelate of disodium edetate and is a chelator used in the treatment of lead poisoning (see Lead, Treatment of Adverse Effects, p.1595). It mobilises lead from bone and tissues and aids elimination from the body by forming a stable, water-soluble, lead complex which is readily excreted by the kidneys. It may be used as a diagnostic test for lead poisoning but measurement of blood-lead concentrations is generally preferred.

Sodium calciumedetate is also a chelator of other heavy-metal polyvalent ions, including chromium. A cream containing sodium calciumedetate 10% has been used in the treatment of chrome ulcers and skin sensitivity reactions due to contact with heavy metals.

Edetates have been labelled with metallic radionuclides and used in nuclear medicine. Sodium calciumedetate is also used as a pharmaceutical excipient and as a food additive.

In the treatment of *lead poisoning*, sodium calciumedetate may be administered by intramuscular injection or by intravenous infusion. The intramuscular route may be preferred in patients with lead encephalopathy and increased intracranial pressure in whom excess fluids must be avoided, and also in children, who have an increased risk of incipient encephalopathy. Sodium calciumedetate may initially aggravate the symptoms of lead toxicity due to mobilisation of stored lead and it is commonly given with dimercaprol (p.979) in patients who are symptomatic; the first dose of dimercaprol should preferably be given at least 4 hours before the sodium calciumedetate.

For administration by intravenous infusion, 1 g of sodium calciumedetate should be diluted with 250 to 500 mL of glucose 5% or sodium chloride 0.9%; a concentration of 3% should not be exceeded. The infusion should be administered over a period of at least one hour and infusion times of 8 to 12 hours or longer have been recommended. In the UK, the usual dose is 60 to 80 mg per kg body-weight daily given in two divided doses. In the USA, a dose of 1000 mg per m^2 body-surface daily is suggested for asymptomatic adults and children; a daily dose of 1500 mg per m^2 may be used in patients with symptomatic poisoning. Treatment is given for up to 5 days, repeated if necessary after an interval of at least 2 days. Any further treatment with sodium calciumedetate should then not be recommenced for at least 7 days.

Alternatively, the same daily dose of sodium calciumedetate may be given intramuscularly in 2 to 4 divided doses as a 20% solution. Intramuscular injection of sodium calciumedetate is painful and it is recommended that preservative-free procaine hydrochloride should be added to a concentration of 0.5 to 1.5% to minimise pain; alternatively, lignocaine may be added to a concentration of 0.5%.

As excretion is predominantly renal, an adequate urinary flow must be established and maintained during treatment. In patients with impaired renal function, smaller and less frequent doses have been recommended.

Preparations

BP 1998: Sodium Calcium Edetate Intravenous Infusion;
USP 23: Edetate Calcium Disodium Injection.

Proprietary Preparations (details are given in Part 3)
Ger.: Calciumedetat-Heyl†; ***Irl.:*** Ledclair; ***Ital.:*** Chelante†; ***Switz.:*** Chelintox†; ***UK:*** Ledclair; ***USA:*** Calcium Disodium Versenate.

Sodium Cellulose Phosphate (1053-l)

Cellulose Sodium Phosphate *(USAN)*.

CAS — 9038-41-9; 68444-58-6.

Pharmacopoeias. In US.

The sodium salt of the phosphate ester of cellulose. A free-flowing cream-coloured, odourless powder. The inorganic bound phosphate content is not less than 31.0% and not more than 36.0%; the free phosphate content is not more than 3.5%; and the sodium content is not less than 9.5% and not more than 13.0%, all calculated on the anhydrous basis. Each g exchanges not less than 1.8 mmol of calcium, calculated on the anhydrous basis. Practically **insoluble** in water, in dilute acids, and in most organic solvents.

Adverse Effects and Precautions

Diarrhoea and other gastro-intestinal disturbances have been reported.

Sodium cellulose phosphate should not be administered to patients with primary or secondary hyperparathyroidism, hypomagnesaemia, hypocalcaemia, bone disease, or enteric hyperoxaluria. It should be administered cautiously to pregnant women and children, who have high calcium requirements.

Patients should be monitored for electrolyte disturbances. Uptake of sodium and phosphate may increase and sodium cellulose phosphate should not be given to patients with renal failure or conditions requiring a restricted sodium intake such as heart failure. Theoretically, long-term treatment could result in calcium deficiency; regular monitoring of calcium and parathyroid hormone has therefore been recommended. Sodium cellulose phosphate is not a totally selective exchange resin and the intestinal absorption of other dietary cations may be reduced; magnesium deficiency has been reported but may be corrected by dosage reduction or oral magnesium supplements. Urinary excretion of oxalate may increase and dietary restriction of oxalate intake may be necessary.

Potential complications of long-term sodium cellulose phosphate therapy include secondary hyperparathyroidism and bone disease; deficiency of magnesium, copper, zinc, and iron; and hyperoxaluria. A study in 18 patients[1] with absorptive hypercalciuria and recurrent renal stones indicated that these complications could largely be avoided if patient selection was confined to those with absorptive hypercalciuria (hypercalciuria, intestinal hyperabsorption of calcium, and normal or suppressed parathyroid function); if the dose was adjusted so as not to reduce intestinal calcium absorption or urinary calcium subnormally (the optimal maintenance dose in most patients was 10 g daily); if oral magnesium supplements were provided; and if a moderate dietary restriction of calcium and oxalate was imposed. There was no evidence of zinc, copper, or iron deficiency.

1. Pak CYC. Clinical pharmacology of sodium cellulose phosphate. *J Clin Pharmacol* 1979; **19:** 451–7.

Interactions

Sodium cellulose phosphate binds with calcium and other cations. Administration with calcium or magnesium salts, including cation-donating antacids or laxatives, may reduce the effectiveness of sodium cellulose phosphate. Magnesium supplements are often required in patients receiving sodium cellulose phosphate but should be administered at least one hour before or after any dose of the resin since the absorption of the magnesium may otherwise be impaired.

Uses and Administration

Sodium cellulose phosphate is a cation-exchange resin that exchanges sodium ions for calcium and other divalent cations. When administered by mouth, it binds calcium ions within the stomach and intestine to form a non-absorbable complex which is excreted in the faeces. Theoretically a 5 g dose will bind approximately 350 mg calcium. It is used in the treatment of absorptive hypercalciuria and recurrent formation of calcium-containing renal calculi (p.888), usually in conjunction with a low calcium diet. Sodium cellulose phosphate is also used in the treatment of hypercalcaemia associated with osteopetrosis, sarcoidosis, and vitamin D intoxication, and in idiopathic hypercalcaemia of infancy, although other more effective agents are usually used (see p.1148).

The usual initial dose is 15 g daily by mouth in 3 divided doses with meals reducing to 10 g daily for maintenance. A suggested dose for children is 10 g daily (but see under Adverse Effects and Precautions, above). The powder may be taken dispersed in water or sprinkled onto food. Oral magnesium supplements equivalent to about 60 or 90 mg (about 2.4 or 3.6 mmol) of elemental magnesium twice daily have been recommended for patients taking daily doses of sodium cellulose phosphate 10 or 15 g respectively. The magnesium supplements should not be administered simultaneously with sodium cellulose phosphate.

Sodium cellulose phosphate may also be used for the investigation of calcium absorption.

Preparations

Proprietary Preparations (details are given in Part 3)
Austral.: Calcisorb; ***Belg.:*** Calcisorb; ***Ger.:*** Calcisorb†; ***Neth.:*** Calcisorb; ***S.Afr.:*** Calcisorb†; ***Spain:*** Anacalcit; ***UK:*** Calcisorb; ***USA:*** Calcibind.

Sodium Nitrite (1055-j)

E250; Natrii Nitris; Natrium Nitrosum.
$NaNO_2$ = 69.00.
CAS — 7632-00-0.
Pharmacopoeias. In *Aust., Chin., Int., Swiss,* and *US.*

White or slightly yellow granular powder or white or almost white opaque fused masses or sticks; deliquescent. **Soluble** 1 in 1.5 of water; sparingly soluble in alcohol. Solutions in water are alkaline to litmus. **Store** in airtight containers.

Adverse Effects

Sodium nitrite may cause nausea and vomiting, abdominal pain, dizziness, headache, flushing, cyanosis, tachypnoea, and dyspnoea; vasodilatation resulting in syncope, hypotension, and tachycardia may occur. Overdosage may result in cardiovascular collapse, coma, convulsions, and death. Ionised nitrites readily oxidise haemoglobin to methaemoglobin, causing methaemoglobinaemia.

Sodium nitrite is a precursor for the formation of nitrosamines many of which are carcinogenic in *animals*, but a relationship with human cancer has not been established.

Methaemoglobinaemia has been reported following the consumption of nitrite-contaminated meat.[1,2]

1. Walley T, Flanagan M. Nitrite-induced methaemoglobinaemia. *Postgrad Med J* 1987; **63:** 643–44.
2. Kennedy N, *et al.* Faulty sausage production causing methaemoglobinaemia. *Arch Dis Child* 1997; **76:** 367–8.

Treatment of Adverse Effects

When toxicity results from the ingestion of nitrites, treatment is supportive and symptomatic; oxygen and methylene blue may be required for methaemoglobinaemia although methylene blue should not be administered if cyanide poisoning is suspected since cyanide may be displaced. Exchange transfusion may be considered when methaemoglobinaemia is severe.

Uses and Administration

Sodium nitrite is used in conjunction with sodium thiosulphate in the treatment of cyanide poisoning (p.1407). The sodium nitrite produces methaemoglobinaemia; it is postulated that the cyanide ions combine with the methaemoglobin to produce cyanmethaemoglobin, thus protecting cytochrome oxidase from the cyanide ions, although other mechanisms may have a significant role. As the cyanmethaemoglobin slowly dissociates, the cyanide is converted to relatively non-toxic thiocyanate and is excreted in the urine. Sodium thiosulphate provides an additional source of sulphur for this reaction and this accelerates the process.

The usual dosage regimen in adults is 300 mg of *sodium nitrite* (10 mL of a 3% solution) administered by intravenous injection over 3 to 5 minutes followed by 12.5 g of *sodium thiosulphate* (50 mL of a 25% solution or 25 mL of a 50% solution) administered intravenously over a period of about 10 minutes. A suggested dosage regimen in children is 0.15 to 0.33 mL per kg body-weight, or 6 to 8 mL per m^2 body-surface, of a 3% solution of *sodium nitrite* (approximately 4.5 to 10.0 mg per kg) to a maximum of 10 mL, followed by 1.65 mL per kg, or 28 mL per m^2, of a 25% solution of *sodium thiosulphate* (412.5 mg per kg) to a maximum of 50 mL. The methaemoglobin concentration should not be allowed to exceed 30 to 40%. If symptoms of cyanide toxicity recur, it has been suggested that the injections of nitrite and thiosulphate may be repeated after 30 minutes at half the initial doses.

Sodium nitrite has also been suggested in the treatment of hydrogen sulphide poisoning (see p.1165).

Sodium nitrite has been used as a rust inhibitor. It is also used as a preservative in foods such as cured meats but should not be used in food for infants under the age of 3 months due to the risk of methaemoglobinaemia. Potassium nitrite is also used as a food preservative.

Preparations

USP 23: Sodium Nitrite Injection.

Proprietary Preparations (details are given in Part 3)
Austral.: O A R.

Multi-ingredient: ***Ital.:*** Benzogen Ferri; Citrosil Alcolico Azzuro; Esoform Ferri; Esoform Ferri Alcolico; ***S.Afr.:*** Tripac-Cyano; ***USA:*** Cyanide Antidote Package.

Sodium Phytate (1056-z)

Sodium Fytate *(rINNM)*; Phytate Sodium *(USAN)*; SQ-9343.
The nonasodium salt of *myo*-inositol hexakis(dihydrogen phosphate); Sodium cyclohexanehexyl(hexaphosphate).
$C_6H_9Na_9O_{24}P_6$ = 857.9.
CAS — 83-86-3 (phytic acid); 7205-52-9 (sodium phytate).

Sodium phytate reacts with calcium in the gastro-intestinal tract to form non-absorbable calcium phytate which is excreted in the faeces. Sodium phytate is used in a similar manner to sodium cellulose phosphate (p.995) to reduce the absorption of calcium from the gut in the treatment of hypercalciuria.

Preparations

Proprietary Preparations (details are given in Part 3)
Fr.: Phytat; ***Ger.:*** Alkalovert†.

Multi-ingredient: ***Ger.:*** B 12 Nervinfant†; Nervinfant†; Tussinfantum†.

Sodium Polystyrene Sulphonate

(5009-k)

Sodium Polystyrene Sulfonate.
CAS — 9003-59-2; 9080-79-9; 25704-18-1.
Pharmacopoeias. In *Br., Jpn,* and *US.*

The sodium salt of sulphonated styrene copolymer with divinylbenzene. An odourless, cream to light brown, fine powder containing not more than 7% of water. The sodium content is not less than 9.4% and not more than 11.0%, calculated on the anhydrous basis. Each g exchanges not less than 110 mg (2.81 mmol) and not more than 135 mg (3.45 mmol) of potassium, calculated on the anhydrous basis. Practically **insoluble** in water and in alcohol. **Store** in airtight containers.

Adverse Effects

Anorexia, nausea, vomiting, constipation, and occasionally diarrhoea may develop during treatment with sodium polystyrene sulphonate. Constipation may be severe; large doses in elderly patients and in children may result in faecal impaction and gastro-intestinal concretions have occurred following oral administration to neonates. If necessary a mild laxative may be used to prevent or treat constipation; magnesium-containing laxatives should not be used (see Interactions, below).

Serious potassium deficiency can occur with sodium polystyrene sulphonate and signs of severe hypokalaemia may include irritability, confusion, ECG abnormalities, cardiac arrhythmias, and severe muscle weakness. Like other cation-exchange resins, sodium polystyrene sulphonate is not totally selective and its use may result in other electrolyte disturbances such as hypocalcaemia. Significant sodium retention may also occur, especially in patients with impaired renal function, and may lead to heart failure.

Effects on the gastro-intestinal tract. Colonic necrosis has been reported[1,2] in 6 patients following administration of sodium polystyrene sulphonate in sorbitol as enemas. The inclusion of sorbitol was considered to contribute to this effect,[1,2] although it was subsequently pointed out that colonic irrigation, as recommended by the manufacturer, had not been carried out to remove the residual resin.[3,4]

1. Lillemoe KD, *et al.* Intestinal necrosis due to sodium polystyrene (Kayexalate) in sorbitol enemas: clinical and experimental support for the hypothesis. *Surgery* 1987; **101:** 267–72.
2. Wootton FT, *et al.* Colonic necrosis with Kayexalate-sorbitol enemas after renal transplantation. *Ann Intern Med* 1989; **111:** 947–9.
3. Burnett RJ. Sodium polystyrene-sorbitol enemas. *Ann Intern Med* 1990; **112:** 311–12.
4. Shepard KV. Cleansing enemas after sodium polystyrene sulfonate enemas. *Ann Intern Med* 1990; **112:** 711.

Effects on the lungs. Particles of sodium polystyrene sulphonate were found at autopsy in the lungs of 3 patients who had taken the resin by mouth and were associated with acute bronchitis and bronchopneumonia in 2 and with early bronchitis in the third.[1] It was suggested that rectal administration of sodium polystyrene sulphonate may be preferable, but if administration by mouth is necessary the patient should be positioned carefully to facilitate ingestion of the resin and avoid aspiration.

1. Haupt HM, Hutchins GM. Sodium polystyrene sulfonate pneumonitis. *Arch Intern Med* 1982; **142:** 379–81.

Precautions

Sodium polystyrene sulphonate should not be administered orally to neonates, and is contra-indicated by any route in neonates with reduced gut motility or in any patient with obstructive bowel disease. Care is also needed with rectal administration to neonates and children in order to avoid impaction of the resin. Treatment should be discontinued if clinically significant constipation develops. Sorbitol has been recommended for the prophylaxis and treatment of constipation (but see Effects on the Gastro-intestinal Tract, above); magnesium-containing laxatives should not be used (see Interactions, below).

Patients receiving sodium polystyrene sulphonate should be monitored for electrolyte disturbances, especially hypokalaemia. Since serum concentrations may not always reflect intracellular potassium deficiency, symptoms of hypokalaemia should also be watched for and the decision to stop treatment assessed individually.

Administration of sodium polystyrene sulphonate can result in sodium overloading and it should be used cautiously in patients with renal failure and with conditions requiring a restricted sodium intake, such as heart failure and severe hypertension; calcium polystyrene sulphonate (p.974) may be preferred in these patients.

The possible effects of sodium polystyrene sulphonate on serum electrolytes should be considered when diagnostic measurements are contemplated in patients receiving such treatment.

Following the administration of sodium polystyrene sulphonate retention enemas, the colon should be irrigated to ensure removal of the resin.

Interactions

Sodium polystyrene sulphonate is not totally selective for potassium and may also bind other cations. Metabolic alkalosis has been reported in patients, particularly those with renal impairment, after the concomitant oral administration of sodium polystyrene sulphonate and cation-donating antacids and laxatives such as magnesium hydroxide, aluminium hydroxide, or calcium carbonate; binding of the cation by the resin prevents neutralisation of bicarbonate ions in the small intestine. The potassium-lowering effect of the resin will also be diminished.

Ion-exchange resins may also bind other drugs given concomitantly, reducing their absorption. For reference to such an effect with thyroxine, see p.1498.

Hypokalaemia may exacerbate the adverse effects of digoxin and sodium polystyrene sulphonate should be used with caution in patients receiving cardiac glycosides.

Uses and Administration

Sodium polystyrene sulphonate is a cation-exchange resin which exchanges sodium ions for potassium ions and other cations in the gastro-intestinal tract following oral or rectal administration. The exchanged resin is then excreted in the faeces. Each gram of resin exchanges about 3 mmol of potassium *in vitro*, and about 1 mmol *in vivo*.

Sodium polystyrene sulphonate is used to enhance potassium excretion in the treatment of hyperkalaemia, including that associated with anuria or severe oliguria (caution is demanded due to the sodium content). An effect may not be evident for several hours or longer, and in severe hyperkalaemia, where a rapid effect is required, other measures must also be considered (see p.1149).

Serum-electrolyte concentrations should be monitored throughout treatment and doses given according to the patient's response.

The usual oral dose is 15 g up to four times daily as a suspension in water or syrup or as a sweetened paste. It should not be given in fruit juices that have a high potassium content. A suggested dose for children is up to 1 g per kg body-weight daily by mouth in divided doses for acute hyperkalaemia, reduced to a maintenance dose of 500 mg per kg daily; the oral route is not recommended for neonates.

When oral administration is difficult, sodium polystyrene sulphonate may be administered rectally as an enema. The usual daily dose is 30 g given as a suspension in 100 mL of 2% methylcellulose '450' and 100 mL of water and retained, if possible, for at least 9 hours; higher doses, shorter retention times, and alternative vehicles have also been used. Following retention of the enema the colon should be irrigated to remove the resin. Initial therapy may constitute administration by both oral and rectal routes. Children and neonates may be given rectal doses similar to those suggested for children by mouth; particular care is needed with rectal administration in children as excessive dosage or inadequate dilution could result in impaction of resin.

Other polystyrene sulphonate resins include calcium polystyrene sulphonate (p.974), which is used similarly to the sodium resin; potassium polystyrene sulphonate (p.992), which is used in the treatment of hypercalciuria; aluminium polystyrene sulphonate, which was formerly used in the treatment of hyperkalaemia; and ammonium polystyrene sulphonate, which was formerly used to reduce the absorption of sodium ions.

Preparations

USP 23: Sodium Polystyrene Sulfonate Suspension.

Proprietary Preparations (details are given in Part 3)
Aust.: Resonium A; ***Austral.:*** Resonium A; ***Belg.:*** Kayexalate Sodium; ***Canad.:*** K-Exit†; Kayexalate; ***Fr.:*** Kayexalate; ***Ger.:*** Elutit-Natrium; Resonium A; ***Irl.:*** Resonium A; ***Ital.:*** Kayexalate; ***Neth.:*** Resonium A; ***S.Afr.:*** Kexelate; ***Spain:*** Resinsodio; ***Swed.:*** Resonium; ***Switz.:*** Resonium A; ***UK:*** Resonium A; ***USA:*** Kayexalate; SPS.

Multi-ingredient: *Ger.:* Ujostabil.

Sodium Thiosulphate (1057-c)

Natrii Thiosulfas; Natrium Thiosulfuricum; Sodium Hyposulphite; Sodium Thiosulfate.

$Na_2S_2O_3,5H_2O$ = 248.2.

CAS — 7772-98-7 (anhydrous); 10102-17-7 (pentahydrate).

Pharmacopoeias. In *Chin., Eur.* (see p.viii), *Int., Jpn, Pol.,* and *US.*

Colourless transparent crystals or a coarse crystalline powder; efflorescent in dry air; deliquescent in moist air. It dissolves in its own water of crystallisation at about 49°. **Soluble** 1 in 0.5 of water; practically insoluble in alcohol. A 10% solution in water has a pH of 6.0 to 8.4. **Store** in airtight containers.

Stability. Solutions of sodium thiosulphate 50% stored in air developed cloudiness or a deposit after autoclaving.[1] Addition of sodium phosphate 0.5% or 1.2% improved stability but solutions became cloudy or developed a deposit after 12 and 6 weeks respectively at 25°. Solutions containing sodium bicarbonate 0.5% became cloudy or developed a deposit after 12 weeks at 25°. No significant improvement in stability was obtained when the concentration of sodium thiosulphate was reduced to 30% or 15%, or when the injection was sealed under nitrogen.

1. Anonymous. Sodium thiosulphate injection–effect of additives on stability. *PSGB Lab Rep* P/75/3 1975.

Adverse Effects

Apart from osmotic disturbances sodium thiosulphate is relatively non-toxic. Large doses by mouth have a cathartic action.

Interactions

For reference to the inactivation of phenylmercuric salts by sodium thiosulphate, see Phenylmercuric Nitrate, p.1122.

Pharmacokinetics

Sodium thiosulphate is poorly absorbed from the gastro-intestinal tract. After intravenous injection it is distributed throughout the extracellular fluid and rapidly excreted in the urine.

An intravenous infusion of sodium thiosulphate 12 g per m² body-surface was administered over 6 hours to 8 patients receiving intraperitoneal antineoplastic therapy;[1] in 6 of the patients it was given in conjunction with cisplatin to protect against the adverse effects of cisplatin. The thiosulphate was rapidly eliminated, 95% being excreted within 4 hours of stopping the infusion; on average only 28.5% of the dose was recovered unchanged in the urine. The mean plasma elimination half-life was 80 minutes.

1. Shea M, *et al.* Kinetics of sodium thiosulfate, a cisplatin neutralizer. *Clin Pharmacol Ther* 1984; **35:** 419–25.

Uses and Administration

Sodium thiosulphate is used in the treatment of cyanide poisoning (p.1407). Sodium thiosulphate may be effective alone in less severe cases of cyanide poisoning, but it is often used after administration of sodium nitrite (p.995).

Sodium thiosulphate acts as a sulphur-donating substrate for the enzyme rhodanese, which catalyses the conversion of cyanide to relatively non-toxic thiocyanate, and thus accelerates the detoxification of cyanide.

The usual dosage regimen in adults is 300 mg of *sodium nitrite* (10 mL of a 3% solution) administered by intravenous injection over 3 to 5 minutes followed by 12.5 g of *sodium thiosulphate* (50 mL of a 25% solution or 25 mL of a 50% solution) administered intravenously over a period of about 10 minutes. A suggested dosage regimen in children is 0.15 to 0.33 mL per kg body-weight, or 6 to 8 mL per m² body-surface, of a 3% solution of *sodium nitrite* (approximately 4.5 to 10.0 mg per kg) to a maximum of 10 mL, followed by 1.65 mL per kg, or 28 mL per m², of a 25% solution of *sodium thiosulphate* (412.5 mg per kg) to a maximum of 50 mL. The methaemoglobin concentration should not be allowed to exceed 30 to 40%. If symptoms of cyanide toxicity recur, it has been suggested that the injections of nitrite and thiosulphate may be repeated after 30 minutes at half the initial doses.

Sodium thiosulphate is used as an isotonic 4% solution in the management of extravasation of mustine and has been tried in the management of extravasation of some other antineoplastics (although this is a contentious area, see p.474).

Sodium thiosulphate has been used for its antifungal properties. Sodium thiosulphate and magnesium thiosulphate are included in mixed preparations for a variety of disorders.

Antineoplastic toxicity. Sodium thiosulphate may be used in the management of extravasation of mustine and some other antineoplastics (see p.474).

For a report of sodium thiosulphate given by intravenous infusion reducing the incidence of nephrotoxicity associated with intraperitoneal cisplatin, see under Adverse Effects in Cisplatin, p.514.

Bromate poisoning. Sodium thiosulphate has been administered in the treatment of bromate poisoning[1,2] although its clinical efficacy is unclear.[3] Sodium thiosulphate is thought to act by reducing bromate to the less toxic bromide ion, but experimental evidence is lacking.[3] However, the high morbidity and mortality associated with bromate poisoning may justify the use of this relatively innocuous compound in some clinical circumstances.[4]

1. Lue JN, *et al.* Bromate poisoning from ingestion of professional hair-care neutralizer. *Clin Pharm* 1988; **7:** 66–70.
2. Lichtenberg R, *et al.* Bromate poisoning. *J Pediatr* 1989; **114:** 891–4.
3. McElwee NE, Kearney TE. Sodium thiosulfate unproven as bromate antidote. *Clin Pharm* 1988; **7:** 570, 572.
4. Johnson CE. Sodium thiosulfate unproven as bromate antidote. *Clin Pharm* 1988; **7:** 572.

Preparations

BP 1998: Sodium Thiosulphate Injection;
USP 23: Sodium Thiosulfate Injection.

Proprietary Preparations (details are given in Part 3)
Fr.: Hyposulfene†; ***Ger.:*** S-hydril†.

Multi-ingredient: ***Aust.:*** Schwefelbad Dr Klopfer; ***Belg.:*** ITC; ***Canad.:*** Adasept; ***Fr.:*** Desintex; Desintex Infantile; Desintex-Choline; Intesticarbine†; Rhino-Sulfuryl; Sulfo-Thiorine Pantothenique†; Vagostabyl; ***Ger.:*** Corti Jaikal; Jaikal; Pherajod†; Schwefelbad Dr Klopfer; ***Ital.:*** Istaglobina†; Salicilato Attivato Ana†; Zeta-Bat†; ***S.Afr.:*** Tripac-Cyano; ***Spain:*** Yodo Tio Calci; ***Switz.:*** Sebo Lotion†; Sulfo-Balmiral†; Thiorubrol; ***USA:*** Cyanide Antidote Package; Tinver; Versiclear.

Succimer (1058-k)

Succimer *(BAN, USAN, rINN).*

DIM-SA; DMSA. *meso*-2,3-Dimercaptosuccinic acid; (R^*,S^*)-2,3-Dimercapto-butanedioic acid.

$C_4H_6O_4S_2$ = 182.2.

CAS — 304-55-2.

Adverse Effects and Precautions

Succimer may cause gastro-intestinal disorders, skin rashes, increases in serum transaminase, flu-like symptoms, drowsiness, and dizziness. Mild to moderate neutropenia has been reported in some patients and regular full blood counts are recommended during therapy. Succimer should be used with caution in patients with impaired renal function or a history of hepatic disease.

Pharmacokinetics

Following oral administration succimer is rapidly but incompletely absorbed. It undergoes rapid and extensive metabolism and is excreted mainly in the urine with small amounts excreted in the bile and via the lungs.

References.

1. Dart RC, *et al.* Pharmacokinetics of meso-2,3-dimercaptosuccinic acid in patients with lead poisoning and in healthy adults. *J Pediatr* 1994; **125:** 309–16.

Uses and Administration

Succimer is a chelator structurally related to dimercaprol (p.979). It forms water-soluble chelates with heavy metals and is used in the treatment of lead poisoning. It has also been used in the treatment of poisoning with arsenic or mercury.

Succimer, labelled with a radionuclide, is used in nuclear medicine.

In the treatment of lead poisoning, succimer is given by mouth in a suggested dose of 10 mg per kg body-weight or 350 mg per m^2 body-surface every 8 hours for 5 days then every 12 hours for an additional 14 days. The course of treatment may be repeated if necessary, usually after an interval of not less than 2 weeks.

Lead poisoning. The use of succimer in lead poisoning has been reviewed.[1,2] Although succimer is generally only indicated in children with blood-lead concentrations greater than 45 μg per 100 mL, promising results have also been reported in children with lower blood-lead concentrations.[3] For the management of lead poisoning, see Lead, Treatment of Adverse Effects, p.1595.

1. Anonymous. Succimer—an oral drug for lead poisoning. *Med Lett Drugs Ther* 1991; **33:** 78.
2. Mann KV, Travers JD. Succimer, an oral lead chelator. *Clin Pharm* 1991; **10:** 914–22.
3. Besunder JB, *et al.* Short-term efficacy of oral dimercaptosuccinic acid in children with low to moderate lead intoxication. *Pediatrics* 1995; **96:** 683–7.

Mercury poisoning. Extracorporeal infusion of succimer into the arterial blood line during haemodialysis, a procedure known as extracorporeal regional complexing haemodialysis, produced a substantial clearance of mercury in an anuric patient following intoxication with inorganic mercury.[1] Clearance was approximately ten times greater than that achieved with haemodialysis following intramuscular administration of dimercaprol. For the management of mercury poisoning, see Mercury, Treatment of Adverse Effects, p.1602.

1. Kostyniak PJ, *et al.* Extracorporeal regional complexing haemodialysis treatment of acute inorganic mercury intoxication. *Hum Toxicol* 1990; **9:** 137–41.

Preparations

Proprietary Preparations (details are given in Part 3)
Aust.: Chemet; ***USA:*** Chemet.

Tiopronin (13349-j)

Tiopronin *(rINN).*

Thiopronine. *N*-(2-Mercaptopropionyl)glycine.

$C_5H_9NO_3S$ = 163.2.

CAS — 1953-02-2.

Adverse Effects and Precautions

Tiopronin has similar adverse effects and precautions to those of penicillamine (p.988).

In a study of 140 patients[1] with rheumatoid arthritis receiving long-term treatment with tiopronin, adverse effects necessitated withdrawal of treatment in 56 patients (40%). The majority of adverse effects occurred within the first 6 months of treatment. The most common were those affecting the skin and mucous membranes (46 patients) including stomatitis, pruritus, erythema, and 1 case of pemphigus. Proteinuria developed in 5 patients and nephrotic syndrome in 3. Haematological disorders developed in 13 patients. Gastro-intestinal disorders and ageusia were also reported.

In another study of 74 patients[2] with rheumatoid arthritis adverse effects were reported in 32 patients (43%) and necessitated withdrawal in 24%. The most common adverse effects were ageusia (21%), mucocutaneous lesions (16%), and gastro-intestinal disturbances (14%). Haematological disorders occurred in 5 patients and proteinuria in 3 patients.

In a comparative study in 200 patients,[3] treatment was withdrawn due to toxicity in 27% of patients taking tiopronin and 21% of patients treated with gold.

1. Sany J, *et al.* Etude de la tolérance à long terme de la thiopronine (Acadione) dans le traitement de la polyarthrite rhumatoïde: a propos de 140 cas personnels. *Rev Rhum* 1990; **57:** 105–11.
2. Ehrhart A, *et al.* Effets secondaires dus au traitement par la tiopronine de 74 polyarthrites rhumatoïdes. *Rev Rhum* 1991; **58:** 193–7.
3. Ferraccioli GF, *et al.* Long-term outcome with gold thiosulphate and tiopronin in 200 rheumatoid patients. *Clin Exp Rheumatol* 1989; **7:** 577–81.

Effects on the blood. Leucopenia or thrombocytopenia has been reported in 13 of 140 patients[1] and 5 of 74 patients[2] during long-term studies of tiopronin.

Isolated cases of agranulocytosis[3] and bone marrow aplasia[4] have been reported.

1. Sany J, *et al.* Etude de la tolérance à long terme de la thiopronine (Acadione) dans le traitement de la polyarthrite rhumatoïde: a propos de 140 cas personnels. *Rev Rhum* 1990; **57:** 105–11.
2. Ehrhart A, *et al.* Effets secondaires dus au traitement par la tiopronine de 74 polyarthrites rhumatoïdes. *Rev Rhum* 1991; **58:** 193–7.
3. Corda C, *et al.* Thiopronin-induced agranulocytosis. *Therapie* 1990; **45:** 161.
4. Taillan B, *et al.* Aplasie médullaire au cours d'une polyarthrite rhumatoïde traitée par tiopronine. *Rev Rhum* 1990; **57:** 443–4.

Effects on the kidneys. Proteinuria developed in 3 patients 4 to 14 months after starting treatment with tiopronin for cystinuria.[1] None of the patients had clinical symptoms of nephrotic syndrome. Renal biopsies in 2 patients demonstrated membranous glomerulonephritis. Proteinuria disappeared in all 3 patients 4 to 5 months after tiopronin was discontinued. However, there was histological evidence of irreversible changes and signs of progressive glomerular lesions in one patient.

Proteinuria was reported in 5 patients and nephrotic syndrome in 3 of 140 patients receiving tiopronin long term.[2]

1. Lindell A, *et al.* Membranous glomerulonephritis induced by 2-mercaptopropionylglycine (2-MPG). *Clin Nephrol* 1990; **34:** 108–15.
2. Sany J, *et al.* Etude de la tolérance à long terme de la thiopronine (Acadione) dans le traitement de la polyarthrite rhumatoïde: a propos de 140 cas personnels. *Rev Rhum* 1990; **57:** 105–11.

Effects on the liver. It has been reported[1] that acute liver damage often leading to jaundice has developed in patients given tiopronin; this has led to the Japanese authorities contra-indicating it in patients with a history of hypersensitivity and recommending that serial liver function tests be carried out during treatment.

1. Anonymous. Tiopronin and liver damage. *WHO Drug Inf* 1989; **3:** 139.

Effects on the skin. Mucocutaneous lesions are among the most common adverse effects of tiopronin (see above). Lichenoid eruptions in one patient developed after 2 years of treatment with tiopronin and resolved when tiopronin was withdrawn.[1] Skin patch testing gave a positive response not only to tiopronin but also to penicillamine and captopril, neither of which the patient had taken. It was suggested that the lichenoid reaction was immunologically mediated and that the sulfhydryl group, which is common to all three compounds, could have been responsible.

Skin lesions resembling pemphigus have been reported in a few patients receiving tiopronin.[2,3] The lesions may improve when tiopronin is discontinued;[2] the remaining patients require treatment with a corticosteroid or other immunosuppressant drug, or both.[3]

1. Kurumaji Y, Miyazaki K. Tiopronin-induced lichenoid eruption in a patient with liver disease and positive patch test reaction to drugs with sulfhydryl group. *J Dermatol* 1990; **17:** 176–81.
2. Trotta F, *et al.* Thiopronine-induced pemphigus vulgaris in rheumatoid arthritis. *Scand J Rheumatol* 1984; **13:** 93–5.
3. Verdier-Sevrain S, *et al.* Thiopronine-induced herpetiform pemphigus: report of a case studied by immunoelectron microscopy and immunoblot analysis. *Br J Dermatol* 1994; **130:** 238–40.

Pharmacokinetics

Tiopronin is absorbed from the gastro-intestinal tract. Up to 48% of the dose is reported to be excreted in the urine during the first 4 hours and up to 78% by 72 hours.

References.

1. Carlsson SM, *et al.* Pharmacokinetics of intravenous 2-mercaptopropionylglycine in man. *Eur J Clin Pharmacol* 1990; **38:** 499–503.
2. Carlsson MS, *et al.* Pharmacokinetics of oral tiopronin. *Eur J Clin Pharmacol* 1993; **45:** 79–84.

Uses and Administration

Tiopronin is a sulfhydryl compound and chelator with properties similar to those of penicillamine (p.991). It is given by mouth in the management of cystinuria, in conjunction with adequate hydration and alkalinisation of the urine, in usual doses of 800 mg to 1 g daily in divided doses, rising to 2 g if necessary. Tiopronin should be given on an empty stomach. Tiopronin is administered in similar doses in rheumatoid arthritis. It has been tried in hepatic disorders, heavy-metal poisoning, and as a mucolytic in respiratory disorders, when it may be given by inhalation. It may also be given rectally or by intravenous or intramuscular injection.

The sodium salt has also been used.

Chronic hepatitis. In a 12-week study involving 165 patients with chronic hepatitis (p.1019), the administration of tiopronin 600 mg daily by mouth in divided doses was associated with an improvement in liver function tests regardless of the histological stage of the disease or HBsAg status.[1]

For a comment on liver damage being associated with tiopronin see Adverse Effects, above.

1. Ichida F, *et al.* Therapeutic effects of tiopronin on chronic hepatitis: a double-blind clinical study. *J Int Med Res* 1982; **10:** 325–32.

Cystinuria. Tiopronin may be used as an alternative to penicillamine in the management of cystinuria (p.991). In a multicentre study,[1] 66 patients with cystine nephrolithiasis were treated with tiopronin in doses of up to 2 g daily (mean 1.193 g); ongoing alkali therapy was continued and the same dietary and fluid regimens were maintained. Tiopronin significantly reduced urinary-cystine concentrations and the new stone formation rate. The adverse effects of tiopronin and penicillamine were compared in 49 patients who had been treated with penicillamine before starting the study. Both drugs had similar side-effects; 41 patients had side-effects to penicillamine of which 34 required cessation of drug therapy and 37 patients had side-effects to tiopronin of which 15 required drug withdrawal. However of the 34 patients who had to stop penicillamine therapy because of adverse effects, 22 were able to continue treatment with tiopronin. Of the 17 patients without a history of penicillamine therapy, 11 had adverse effects to tiopronin and 1 discontinued treatment because of proteinuria.

1. Pak CYC, *et al.* Management of cystine nephrolithiasis with alpha-mercaptopropionylglycine. *J Urol (Baltimore)* 1986; **136:** 1003–8.

Lead poisoning. Parenteral administration of tiopronin (30 g over a period of 10 days) to 27 men with symptoms of chronic lead poisoning had a beneficial effect on the biochemical indices of lead poisoning.[1] The mechanism of action was not clear since urinary lead excretion did not change. The usual treatment of lead poisoning is discussed on p.1595.

1. Candura F, *et al.* Sulphydryl compounds in lead poisoning. *Lancet* 1979; **i:** 330.

Mucolytic activity. Studies on the mucolytic activity of tiopronin.

1. Costantini D, *et al.* Evaluation of the therapeutic effectiveness of thiopronine in children with cystic fibrosis. *Curr Ther Res* 1982; **31:** 714–17.
2. Carratù L, *et al.* Clinico-functional and rheological research on mucolytic activity of thiopronine in chronic broncho-pneumopathies. *Curr Ther Res* 1982; **32:** 529–43.

Rheumatoid arthritis. Tiopronin has been reported to have activity comparable to that of gold salts[1] and penicillamine[2] in patients with rheumatoid disease, and could be tried cautiously to treat rheumatoid arthritis (p.2) in patients intolerant of penicillamine.

1. Ferraccioli GF, *et al.* Long-term outcome with gold thiosulphate and tiopronin in 200 rheumatoid patients. *Clin Exp Rheumatol* 1989; **7:** 577–81.
2. Sany J, *et al.* Etude de la tolérance à long terme de la thiopronine (Acadione) dans le traitement de la polyarthrite rhumatoïde: a propos de 140 cas personnels. *Rev Rhum* 1990; **57:** 105–11.

Preparations

Proprietary Preparations (details are given in Part 3)
Fr.: Acadione; ***Ger.:*** Captimer; ***Ital.:*** Epatiol†; Mucolysin; Mucosyt; Thiola; Thiosol; Tioglis†; ***Spain:*** Sutilan†; ***Switz.:*** Mucolysin; ***USA:*** Thiola.

Multi-ingredient: ***Ital.:*** Mucolysin Antibiotico†; ***Spain:*** Hepadigest.

Trientine Dihydrochloride (13377-a)

Trientine Dihydrochloride *(BAN, rINNM).*

MK-0681; Trien Hydrochloride; Trientine Hydrochloride *(USAN)*; Triethylenetetramine Dihydrochloride. 2,2′-Ethylenediiminobis(ethylamine) dihydrochloride; *N,N′*-bis(2-Aminoethyl)-1,2-ethanediamine dihydrochloride.

$C_6H_{18}N_4,2HCl = 219.2.$

CAS — 112-24-3 (trientine); 38260-01-4 (trientine dihydrochloride).

Pharmacopoeias. In US.

A white to pale yellow crystalline powder. Freely **soluble** in water; soluble in methyl alcohol; slightly soluble in alcohol; practically insoluble in chloroform and in ether. A 1% solution in water has a pH of 7.0 to 8.5. **Store** under an inert gas in airtight containers at 2° to 8°. Protect from light.

Adverse Effects and Precautions

Trientine dihydrochloride may cause nausea. Iron deficiency may occur; if iron supplements are given an interval of at least 2 hours between the administration of a dose of trientine and iron has been recommended. Recurrence of symptoms of systemic lupus erythematosus has been reported in a patient who had previously reacted to penicillamine.

Interactions

Chelation of trientine with metal ions in the diet or in mineral supplements may impair the absorption of both. Trientine should not be taken with mineral supplements and should be taken at least one hour apart from food, other drugs, or milk, to reduce the likelihood of absorption being affected. Iron supplements should be taken at least 2 hours before or after trientine.

Uses and Administration

Trientine dihydrochloride is a copper chelator used in a similar way to penicillamine in the treatment of Wilson's disease (p.992). It tends to be used in patients intolerant of penicillamine.

Trientine dihydrochloride is administered by mouth, preferably on an empty stomach. In the USA the usual initial dose in adults is 750 mg to 1250 mg daily in 2 to 4 divided doses increasing to a maximum of 2 g daily if required; daily doses of 1.2 to 2.4 g have been recommended in the UK. In children, the usual initial dose is 500 to 750 mg daily increasing to a maximum of 1.5 g daily if required.

Preparations

USP 23: Trientine Hydrochloride Capsules.

Proprietary Preparations (details are given in Part 3)
USA: Syprine.

Unithiol (1059-a)

DMPS; Unitiol. Sodium 2,3-dimercaptopropanesulphonate.

$C_3H_7NaO_3S_3 = 210.3.$

CAS — 4076-02-2.

Unithiol is a chelator structurally related to dimercaprol (p.979). It is water soluble and reported to be less toxic than dimercaprol. Unithiol is used in the treatment of poisoning by heavy metals including arsenic, lead, inorganic and organic mercury compounds, and chromium. It may be less effective in cadmium poisoning.

Unithiol is given by mouth in doses of 100 mg three or four times daily in chronic poisoning. A dose of 1.2 to 2.4 g has been suggested in acute poisoning. It has also been administered parenterally.

Reviews.

1. Aposhian HV. DMSA and DMPS—water soluble antidotes for heavy metal poisoning. *Ann Rev Pharmacol Toxicol* 1983; **23:** 193–215.
2. Hruby K, Donner A. 2,3-Dimercapto-1-propanesulphonate in heavy metal poisoning. *Med Toxicol* 1987; **2:** 317–23.

Lead poisoning. Unithiol has been tried in chronic lead poisoning. In a study of twelve children[1] it reduced lead concentrations in blood but did not affect the concentrations of copper or zinc in plasma, although the urinary excretion of lead, copper, and zinc was increased during treatment.

The usual chelators used in the management of lead poisoning are discussed under Lead, Treatment of Adverse Effects, on p.1595.

1. Chisolm JJ, Thomas DJ. Use of 2,3-dimercaptopropane-1-sulfonate in treatment of lead poisoning in children. *J Pharmacol Exp Ther* 1985; **235:** 665–9.

Mercury poisoning. Administration of unithiol 100 mg twice daily by mouth for a maximum of 15 days enhanced urinary elimination of mercury in 7 patients with mercury poisoning.[1] The urinary elimination of copper and zinc was also increased in most patients and two developed skin rashes. Unithiol, 50 mg per 10 kg body-weight by intramuscular injection three times a day reducing to 50 mg per 10 kg once a day by the third day of treatment, effectively reduced the half-life of mercury in the blood following poisoning with methylmercury.[2]

There has been a more recent report of 4 weeks of intravenous treatment followed by 3 weeks of oral treatment with unithiol in the successful management of a patient with severe poisoning with mercuric chloride.[3]

For the management of mercury poisoning, see Mercury, Treatment of Adverse Effects, p.1602.

1. Mant TGK. Clinical studies with dimercaptopropane sulphonate in mercury poisoning. *Hum Toxicol* 1985; **4:** 346.
2. Clarkson TW, *et al.* Tests of efficacy of antidotes for removal of methylmercury in human poisoning during the Iraq outbreak. *J Pharmacol Exp Ther* 1981; **218:** 74–83.
3. Toet AE, *et al.* Mercury kinetics in a case of severe mercuric chloride poisoning treated with dimercapto-1-propane sulphonate (DMPS). *Hum Exp Toxicol* 1994; **13:** 11–16.

Wilson's disease. Unithiol 200 mg twice daily[1] was used successfully to maintain cupriuresis in a 13-year-old boy with Wilson's disease after he developed systemic lupus during treatment with penicillamine and with trientine dihydrochloride, which are two of the usual drugs used in Wilson's disease (see p.992). Unithiol was started in two similar patients[1] but both withdrew from treatment, one because of fever and a fall in leucocyte count following a test dose and the other because of intense nausea and taste impairment.

1. Walshe JM. Unithiol in Wilson's disease. *Br Med J* 1985; **290:** 673–4.

Preparations

Proprietary Preparations (details are given in Part 3)
Ger.: Dimaval; Mercuval.

Colouring Agents

Colouring agents have long been used in foods and cosmetics in an attempt to improve the appearance of the product or subject. They are also used in medicinal preparations with the aim of improving their acceptability to patients and this chapter describes the colouring agents used in medicines as well as those used in foods and cosmetics. Such uses are now widely controlled and this has resulted in restrictions on the extent to which colouring agents may be used. Matters of concern that have received considerable publicity include sensitivity reactions (see Tartrazine, p.1001) and hyperactive behaviour (see below).

Colouring agents can be broadly categorised into synthetic dyes and into natural agents (such as canthaxanthin, caramel, carmine, chlorophyll, cochineal, saffron, and turmeric, all of which are described in this chapter). Other compounds which may be used as cosmetic colours or food colours (and which are themselves the natural pigments of the foodstuffs) are anthocyanins (E163) and carotenoids. In this latter group are included bixin (E160b) and norbixin (E160b) which are obtained from annatto (E160b), capsanthin (E160c) which is an extract of paprika, carotenes (E160a) (see Betacarotene, p.1335), lycopene (E160d), beta-apo-8′-carotenal (E160e), and the ethyl ester of beta-apo-8′-carotenoic acid (E160f); lutein (E161b), like canthaxanthin, can be classified either as a carotenoid or as a xanthophyll.

Other agents described in *Martindale* that may be used as food colours include aluminium (p.1547), gold (p.1586), indigo carmine (p.1590), patent blue V (p.1616), riboflavine (p.1362), silver (p.1629), and titanium dioxide (p.1093).

Hyperactivity. Food additives have been implicated in hyperactive behaviour (p.1476) although the role of foods and food additives is not clear. In one double-blind placebo-controlled study,[1] children whose poor behaviour was attributed, by their parents, to the intake of food additives, were given oral challenges with food colours (amaranth, carmoisine, sunset yellow, and tartrazine) in doses far in excess of estimated normal daily intakes. Although the study investigators could measure a worsening of behavioural scores after the food colours, the parents did not note the difference between challenge and placebo periods. Another study[2] of similar design detected a dose-dependent association between tartrazine intake and behavioural changes (irritability, restlessness, and sleep disturbances).

1. Pollock I, Warner JO. Effect of artificial food colours on childhood behaviour. *Arch Dis Child* 1990; **65:** 74–7.
2. Rowe KS, Rowe KJ. Synthetic food coloring and behavior: a dose response effect in a double-blind, placebo-controlled, repeated-measures study. *J Pediatr* 1994; **125:** 691–8.

Allura Red AC (2372-l)

Cl Food Red 17; Colour Index No. 16035; E129; F D & C Red No. 40. Disodium 6-hydroxy-5-(6-methoxy-4-sulphonato-*m*-tolylazo)naphthalene-2-sulphonate.

$C_{18}H_{14}N_2Na_2O_8S_2$ = 496.4.
CAS — 25956-17-6.

Allura red AC is used as a colouring agent in cosmetics and foodstuffs.

Amaranth (2373-y)

Bordeaux S; Cl Acid Red 27; Cl Food Red 9; Colour Index No. 16185; E123; formerly F D & C Red No. 2. It consists mainly of trisodium 3-hydroxy-4-(4-sulphonato-1-naphthylazo)naphthalene-2,7-disulphonate.

$C_{20}H_{11}N_2Na_3O_{10}S_3$ = 604.5.
CAS — 915-67-3.
Pharmacopoeias. In *Fr.*

Amaranth is used as a colouring agent in medicines, foodstuffs, and cosmetics.

Although some evidence of carcinogenicity was found in early *animal* studies, subsequent work failed to confirm these findings and in the UK amaranth is considered suitable for use as a food colour.[1]

1. MAFF. Food advisory committee: final report on the review of the colouring matter in food regulations 1973. *FdAC/REP/4.* London: HMSO, 1987.

Beetroot Red (10150-r)

Beet Red; E162.

Beetroot red is obtained from the roots of red beets, *Beta vulgaris* var. *rubra* (Chenopodiaceae). The main colouring principle consists of betacyanins of which betanine is the main constituent.

Beetroot red is used as a colouring agent for foodstuffs and cosmetics.

Black PN (2375-z)

Brilliant Black BN; Brilliant Black PN; Cl Food Black 1; Colour Index No. 28440; E151; Noir Brillant BN. It consists mainly of tetrasodium 4-acetamido-5-hydroxy-6-[7-sulphonato-4-(4-sulphonatophenylazo)-1-naphthylazo]naphthalene-1,7-disulphonate.

$C_{28}H_{17}N_5Na_4O_{14}S_4$ = 867.7.
CAS — 2519-30-4.
Pharmacopoeias. In *Fr.*

Black PN is used as a colouring agent in medicines, cosmetics, and foods.

Bordeaux B (2376-c)

Azorubrum; Cl Acid Red 17; Colour Index No. 16180. Consists mainly of disodium 3-hydroxy-4-(1-naphthylazo)naphthalene-2,7-disulphonate.

$C_{20}H_{12}N_2Na_2O_7S_2$ = 502.4.
CAS — 5858-33-3.

Bordeaux B was formerly used as a colouring agent for medicines and foods but has been replaced by other colours.

Brilliant Blue FCF (2377-k)

Blue EGS; Cl Acid Blue 9; Cl Food Blue 2; Colour Index No. 42090; E133; F D & C Blue No. 1; Patent Blue AC. Disodium 4′,4″-bis(*N*-ethyl-3-sulphonatobenzylamino)triphenylmethylium-2-sulphonate.

$C_{37}H_{34}N_2Na_2O_9S_3$ = 792.9.
CAS — 3844-45-9.

Brilliant blue FCF is used as a colouring agent in medicines, cosmetics, and foodstuffs.

Brown FK (2378-a)

Chocolate Brown FK; Cl Food Brown 1; E154. A mixture of 6 azo dyes: sodium 2′,4′-diaminoazobenzene-4-sulphonate; sodium 2′,4′-diamino-5′-methylazobenzene-4-sulphonate; disodium 4,4′-(4,6-diamino-1,3-phenylenebisazo) dibenzenesulphonate; disodium 4,4′-(2,4-diamino-1,3-phenylenebisazo) dibenzenesulphonate; disodium 4,4′-(2,4-diamino-5-methyl-1,3-phenylenebisazo) dibenzenesulphonate; trisodium 4,4′,4″-(2,4-diaminobenzene-1,3,5-triazo)tribenzenesulphonate.

CAS — 8062-14-4.

Brown FK is used as a colouring agent for foodstuffs.

Brown HT (2386-a)

Chocolate Brown HT; Cl Food Brown 3; Colour Index No. 20285; E155. Disodium 4,4′-(2,4-dihydroxy-5-hydroxymethyl-1,3-phenylenebisazo)di(naphthalene-1-sulphonate).

$C_{27}H_{18}N_4Na_2O_9S_2$ = 652.6.
CAS — 4553-89-3.

Brown HT is used as a colouring agent for foodstuffs.

Canthaxanthin (2380-l)

Cl Food Orange 8; Colour Index No. 40850; E161(g). β,β-Carotene-4,4′-dione.

$C_{40}H_{52}O_2$ = 564.8.
CAS — 514-78-3.

Canthaxanthin is a carotenoid but unlike betacarotene or β-apo-8′-carotenal it possesses no vitamin A activity. It is given to salmon or trout to colour their flesh. It is also used in cosmetics.

Canthaxanthin has also been given by mouth to produce an artificial suntan, and as an adjunct to betacarotene in the management of erythropoietic protoporphyria (p.983). Such use has led to retinal deposits and in some cases to impairment of vision.

In the UK canthaxanthin has been considered to be suitable for use as a food colour; it was, however, believed that it should be restricted to use as a feed additive for farmed salmon and trout in order to produce a coloration of the fish flesh.[1] This restriction was based partly on reports of retinal changes in humans who had taken canthaxanthin orally, either for the production of an artificial tan by means of pigment deposition in the skin or for the medical treatment of erythropoietic protoporphyria. The retinal changes were an accumulation of bright yellow particles around the macula ('gold speck' maculopathy) and have been associated with altered function of the eye and visual deterioration.[1,2] Although a temporary acceptable daily intake for canthaxanthin was established by the FAO/WHO in 1987 this was not extended in 1990.[2] Long-term toxicity studies in *animals* had indicated a potential for hepatotoxicity although it was acknowledged that the primary problem associated with canthaxanthin was the possible retinal damage.[2] However, subsequent studies failed to confirm hepatotoxicity in humans and an acceptable daily intake was established by the FAO/WHO in 1995.[3]

There has also been a report of fatal aplastic anaemia in one patient who took canthaxanthin in order to produce an artificial tan.[4]

1. MAFF. Food advisory committee: final report on the review of the colouring matter in food regulations 1973. *FdAC/REP/4.* London: HMSO, 1987.
2. FAO/WHO. Evaluation of certain food additives and contaminants: thirty-fifth report of the joint FAO/WHO expert committee on food additives. *WHO Tech Rep Ser 789* 1990.
3. FAO/WHO. Evaluation of certain food additives and contaminants: forty-fourth report of the joint FAO/WHO expert committee on food additives. *WHO Tech Rep Ser 859* 1995.
4. Bluhm R, *et al.* Aplastic anemia associated with canthaxanthin ingested for 'tanning' purposes. *JAMA* 1990; **264:** 1141–2.

Preparations

Proprietary Preparations (details are given in Part 3)

Multi-ingredient: ***Fr.:*** Phenoro; ***Switz.:*** Apotrin; Phenoro†.

Caramel (2381-y)

Burnt Sugar; E150; Sacch. Ust.; Saccharum Ustum.
CAS — 8028-89-5.
Pharmacopoeias. In *USNF.*

Caramel (USNF) is a thick, dark brown liquid, with a characteristic odour and a pleasant bitter taste. **Miscible** with water; immiscible with ether, with chloroform, with acetone, and with petroleum spirit; soluble in alcohol up to 55%. **Store** in airtight containers.

Caramels used as food colours are complex mixtures of compounds prepared by heating carbohydrates (food-grade sweeteners consisting of glucose, fructose, or polymers of these) either alone or in the presence of acids or alkalis (food-grade citric or sulphuric acids or calcium, potassium, or sodium hydroxides, or mixtures of these). The caramels can be classified according to the reactants used in the manufacturing process:

Class I (E150a, plain caramel, spirit caramel, or caustic caramel); no ammonium or sulphite compounds are employed.

Class II (E150b or caustic sulphite caramel); sulphate compounds employed but not ammonium compounds.

Class III (E150c, ammonia caramel, or beer caramel); ammonium compounds employed but not sulphite compounds

Class IV (E150d, sulphite ammonia caramel, or soft-drink caramel); both ammonium and sulphite compounds employed.

Caramel is used as a colouring agent to produce pale yellow to dark brown colours; it is used as a food colour. It has no calorific value.

Some caramels also have flavouring properties.

Carmine (2382-j)

CI Natural Red 4; Colour Index No. 75470; E120.

CAS — 1390-65-4.

Pharmacopoeias. In *Swiss* which specifies the aluminium-calcium lake.

An aluminium lake of the colouring matter of cochineal. It contains carminic acid, an anthraquinone glycoside. Unless precautions are taken during manufacture and transport to prevent contamination, carmine may be infected with salmonella micro-organisms.

Carmine and some of its salts are used as colouring agents in medicines, foodstuffs, and cosmetics.

Carmine passes through the gastro-intestinal tract unchanged and has been used as a faecal 'marker' in a dose of 200 to 500 mg.

Extrinsic allergic alveolitis has been described in one person due to occupational exposure to carmine used as a food additive.[1] Additionally, severe anaphylactic reactions have occurred following the ingestion of food[2,3] (2 patients) and drink[4] (1 patient) containing carmine as a colour.

1. Dietemann-Molard A, *et al.* Extrinsic allergic alveolitis secondary to carmine. *Lancet* 1991; **338:** 460.
2. Beaudouin E, *et al.* Food anaphylaxis following ingestion of carmine. *Ann Allergy Asthma Immunol* 1995; **74:** 427–30.
3. Baldwin JL, *et al.* Popsicle-induced anaphylaxis due to carmine dye allergy. *Ann Allergy Asthma Immunol* 1997; **79:** 415–19.
4. Kägi MK, *et al.* Campari-orange anaphylaxis due to carmine allergy. *Lancet* 1994; **344:** 60–1.

Carmoisine (2384-c)

Azorubine; CI Food Red 3; Colour Index No. 14720; E122. It consists mainly of disodium 4-hydroxy-3-(4-sulphonato-1-naphthylazo)naphthalene-1-sulphonate.

$C_{20}H_{12}N_2Na_2O_7S_2$ = 502.4.

CAS — 3567-69-9.

Pharmacopoeias. In *Fr.*

Carmoisine is used as a colouring agent in foods, medicines, and cosmetics.

Chlorophyll (2385-k)

CI Natural Green 3; Colour Index No. 75810; E140.

CAS — 479-61-8 (chlorophyll a); 519-62-0 (chlorophyll b).

Pharmacopoeias. *US* includes Chlorophyllin Copper Complex Sodium.

Chlorophyll is a green colouring matter of plants. It contains 2 closely related substances, chlorophyll a ($C_{55}H_{72}MgN_4O_5$ = 893.5) and chlorophyll b ($C_{55}H_{70}MgN_4O_6$ = 907.5). The only difference between the 2 chlorophylls is that a methyl side-chain in chlorophyll a is replaced by a formyl group in chlorophyll b.

Oil-soluble chlorophyll derivatives. Replacement of the magnesium atom in the chlorophylls by 2 hydrogen atoms using dilute mineral acids produces olive-green water-insoluble phaeophytins. Copper phaeophytins (sometimes called copper chlorophyll complex;E141) can be formed; these are more stable to acids and to light than the chlorophylls.

Water-soluble chlorophyll derivatives. When the chlorophylls are hydrolysed with alkali, phytyl alcohol and methyl alcohol are split off and green water-soluble chlorophyllins are formed as the potassium or sodium salts. Similar water-soluble compounds can be prepared in which the magnesium is replaced by copper to give copper chlorophyllin complex (E141).

Chlorophylls and chlorophyllins, as well as the copper complexes of these compounds, are employed principally as colouring agents, in foods, medicines, and cosmetics.

Chlorophyll is used as an external application in the treatment of wounds and ulcers. There is no clear evidence that it accelerates healing but it is considered to have a deodorant action. Chlorophyllin and copper chlorophyllin complex are used similarly.

Preparations

Proprietary Preparations (details are given in Part 3)
Austral.: No Odor†; ***Canad.:*** Pals†; ***Ger.:*** Exodor grun†; ***Ital.:*** Derifil†; ***USA:*** Chloresium; Derifil; Innerfresh Pro; Nullo†; Pals.

Multi-ingredient: ***Belg.:*** Ex'ail; ***Fr.:*** Ex'ail; Phytemag; ***Ger.:*** Adebilan†; Anastil†; Bagnisan med Heilbad; Bagnisan S med Rheumabad†; Chlorophyllin Salbe "Schuh"; Dynamol†; Ginseng-Complex "Schuh"; Grune Nervensalbe†; Neuro-Presselin†; Rosmarinsalbe†; Stomasal Med; Stomasal†; Tectivit†; Vulnotox†; ***Ital.:*** Dentovax; ***S.Afr.:*** Dynexan†; ***Spain:*** Balneogel; Balsamo BOI†; Vitavox Pastillas; ***UK:*** Chlorophyll; ***USA:*** Panafil; Prophyllin.

Cochineal (2387-t)

CI Natural Red 4; Coccionella; Coccus; Coccus Cacti; Colour Index No. 75470; E120.

CAS — 1343-78-8.

Pharmacopoeias. In *Br.*

The dried female insect, *Dactylopius coccus* (=*Coccus cacti*) (Coccidae), containing eggs and larvae. It complies with a test for contamination with *Escherichia coli* and salmonellae.

Cochineal, which is a source of carmine, is used as a red colouring agent in food, medicines, and cosmetics.

Cochineal is also used in homoeopathic medicine.

Curcumin (10200-z)

Colour Index No. 75300; E100. 1,7-Bis(4-hydroxy-3-methoxyphenyl)hepta-1,6-diene-3,5-dione.

$C_{21}H_{20}O_6$ = 368.4.

Curcumin is the main colouring component of turmeric (see p.1001).

Curcumin is used as a colouring agent for foodstuffs and cosmetics.

Eosin (2391-z)

CI Acid Red 87; Colour Index No. 45380; D & C Red No. 22; Eosin Y; Éosine Disodique. The disodium salt of 2′,4′,5′,7′-tetrabromofluorescein.

$C_{20}H_6Br_4Na_2O_5$ = 691.9.

CAS — 548-26-5; 17372-87-1.

Pharmacopoeias. In *Fr.*

Eosin has been incorporated in solution-tablets to give a distinctive colour to solutions prepared from them. It is also used in cosmetics.

Erythrosine (2392-c)

CI Food Red 14; Colour Index No. 45430; E127; Erythrosine BS; Erythrosine Sodium; F D & C Red No. 3. The monohydrate of the disodium salt of 2′,4′,5′,7′-tetraiodofluorescein.

$C_{20}H_6I_4Na_2O_5,H_2O$ = 897.9.

CAS — 568-63-8 (anhydrous erythrosine sodium); 16423-68-0 (anhydrous erythrosine sodium); 49746-10-3 (erythrosine sodium monohydrate).

Pharmacopoeias. *Fr.* permits disodium or dipotassium salts.

Red or brownish-red odourless hygroscopic powder. **Soluble** in water forming a bluish-red solution that shows no fluorescence in ordinary light; sparingly soluble in alcohol; soluble in glycerol and propylene glycol; practically insoluble in fats and oils. **Store** in airtight containers.

Erythrosine is used as a colouring agent for medicines and foods. It is also used in cosmetics and as a disclosing agent for plaque on teeth.

Although early *animal* studies had indicated that erythrosine might have an adverse effect on the thyroid gland some authorities,[1] on re-assessing the evidence together with later studies, consider that erythrosine is not genotoxic or mutagenic and that it is suitable for use as a food colour.

1. MAFF. Food advisory committee: final report on the review of the colouring matter in food regulations 1973. *FdAC/REP/4.* London: HMSO, 1987.

Preparations

Proprietary Preparations (details are given in Part 3)
Austral.: Disclo-Gel; Disclo-Tabs; ***Ger.:*** Plaquefarbetabletten†; ***UK:*** Ceplac.

Ferric Oxide (5038-f)

E172 (iron oxides or hydroxides).

CAS — 51274-00-1; 1309-37-1.

Pharmacopoeias. *Fr.* includes monographs for black, brown, red, and yellow forms of ferric oxide. *It.* includes both red and yellow ferric oxide. *USNF* allows the basic colours of red or yellow ferric oxide or mixtures of these.

Ferric Oxide (USNF) is a powder exhibiting two basic colours (red and yellow), or other shades may be produced depending on the blending of the basic colours. **Insoluble** in water and in organic solvents; dissolves in hydrochloric acid upon warming, a small amount of insoluble residue usually remaining.

Ferric oxide is used for tinting pharmaceutical preparations and foodstuffs.

Green S (2394-a)

Acid Brilliant Green BS; Acid Green S; CI Food Green 4; Colour Index No. 44090; E142; Lissamine Green; Wool Green B. Sodium 1-[4-dimethylamino-α-(4-dimethyliminiocyclohexa-2,5-dienylidene)benzyl]-2-hydroxynaphthalene-3,6-disulphonate.

$C_{27}H_{25}N_2NaO_7S_2$ = 576.6.

CAS — 3087-16-9.

Green S is used as a colouring agent in medicines, cosmetics, and foodstuffs.

Studies in *animals* indicated that there is some absorption of green S and caecal enlargement but it was considered that there is a very large margin of safety between the highest estimated intake of green S of 130 μg per person daily and the level at which changes were seen in *animal* studies (500 mg per kg body-weight daily). It was recommended that the use of green S in food is acceptable.[1]

1. MAFF. Food advisory committee: final report on the review of the colouring matter in food regulations 1973. *FdAC/REP/4.* London: HMSO, 1987.

Preparations

BP 1980: Green S and Tartrazine Solution.

Pigment Rubine (10167-q)

E180; Lithol Rubine BK.

Pigment rubine is used as a colouring agent for foodstuffs.

Ponceau 4R (2397-r)

Brilliant Ponceau 4RC; Brilliant Scarlet; CI Food Red 7; Coccine Nouvelle; Cochineal Red A; Colour Index No. 16255; E124; Rouge Cochenille A. Trisodium 7-hydroxy-8-(4-sulphonato-1-naphthylazo)naphthalene-1,3-disulphonate.

$C_{20}H_{11}N_2Na_3O_{10}S_3$ = 604.5.

CAS — 2611-82-7.

Pharmacopoeias. In *Fr.*

Ponceau 4R is used as a colouring agent in medicines, cosmetics, and foods. Sensitivity reactions have been reported.

Quinoline Yellow (2398-f)

Canary Yellow; CI Acid Yellow 3; CI Food Yellow 13; Colour Index No. 47005; Jaune De Quinoléine. The sodium salts of a mixture of the mono- and disulphonic acids of quinophthalone or 2-(2-quinolyl)indanedione.

CAS — 8004-92-0.

NOTE. D & C yellow No.10 and E104 are both used as synonyms or codes for quinoline yellow, but D & C yellow No.10 describes a mixture mainly of the monosulphonic acid of quinophthalone while E104 describes a mixture mainly of the disulphonic acid.

Pharmacopoeias. In *Fr.*

Quinoline yellow is used as a colouring agent in medicines, cosmetics, and foodstuffs.

A severe urticarial reaction in one patient has been attributed to quinoline yellow (E104).[1]

1. Bell T. Colourants and drug reactions. *Lancet* 1991; **338:** 55–6.

Raspberry (2399-d)

Framboise; Fructus Rubi Idaei; Himbeer; Rubus Idaeus.

CAS — 8027-46-1.

The fresh ripe fruit of *Rubus idaeus* (Rosaceae).

Raspberry is used as a colouring and flavouring agent in medicines and foodstuffs.

Red 2G (2400-d)

Acid Red 1; CI Food Red 10; Colour Index No. 18050; E128; Ext. D & C Red No. 11; Geranine 2G. Disodium 5-acetamido-4-hydroxy-3-phenylazonaphthalene-2,7-disulphonate.

$C_{18}H_{13}N_3Na_2O_8S_2$ = 509.4.

CAS — 3734-67-6.

Red 2G is used as a colouring agent in medicines, cosmetics, and foods.

There has been concern that red 2G might produce haemolysis in subjects deficient in glucose-6-phosphate dehydrogenase, but investigations have not confirmed such a risk. However, red 2G might hydrolyse in acid solution to red 10B about which there is inadequate data. Therefore, in the UK it is considered undesirable to use red 2G in foods of high acidity that are subjected to a high temperature during processing and is recommended that the use of red 2G is confined to certain meat products.[1]

1. MAFF. Food advisory committee: final report on the review of the colouring matter in food regulations 1973. FdAC/REP/4. London: HMSO, 1987.

Red Cherry (2401-n)

Acerola; Cerasus; Cerise Rouge; Ginja; Griottier.

Pharmacopoeias. In Fr.

The fresh ripe fruit of varieties of the red or sour cherry, *Prunus cerasus* (Rosaceae).

Red cherry is used as a colouring and flavouring agent. It has also been used in herbal preparations.

Preparations

Proprietary Preparations (details are given in Part 3)

Multi-ingredient: ***Austral.:*** Bio-C Complex; ***Ital.:*** Aprolis†; ***Switz.:*** A Vogel Capsules polyvitaminees; ***UK:*** Vitamin C; ***USA:*** Bio-Acerola C Complex; Citrus-flav C; Ester-C Plus; Ester-C Plus Multi-Mineral; Super Complex C.

Red-Poppy Petal (2402-h)

Coquelicot; Klatschrose; Petalos de Amapola; Rhoead. Pet.; Rhoeados Petalum.

The dried petals of *Papaver rhoeas* (Papaveraceae).

Red-poppy petal has been used as a colouring agent. It is also included in several herbal preparations.

Preparations

Proprietary Preparations (details are given in Part 3)

Multi-ingredient: ***Fr.:*** Actisane Nervosite; Astressane; Nocvalene; ***Ger.:*** Presselin Stoffwechseltee†; ***Ital.:*** Bramserene†; Normalax; Relaten; ***Switz.:*** Baume†; Melissa Tonic; Tisane antitussive et pectorale "H"†; Tisane pectorale et antitussive.

Red-Rose Petal (2403-m)

Fleur de Rose; Flos Rosae; Red Rose Petals; Ros. Pet.; Rosae Gallicae Petala; Rosae Petalum; Rosenblüte.

The petals of the red or Provins rose, *Rosa gallica* (Rosaceae).

Red-rose petal has been employed, as a colouring agent and for its mild astringent properties.

Preparations

Proprietary Preparations (details are given in Part 3)

Multi-ingredient: ***Fr.:*** Ophtalmine; ***Ger.:*** Melrosum Hustensirup N; ***Ital.:*** Gocce D'Erbe†; ***Switz.:*** Tisane diuretique "H"†.

Saffron (2407-q)

Açafrão; Azafrán; CI Natural Yellow 6; Colour Index No. 75100; Croci Stigma; Crocus; Estigmas de Azafrán; Safran.

Pharmacopoeias. In *Aust., Chin.,* and *Jpn.*

The dried stigmas and tops of the styles of *Crocus sativus* (Iridaceae), containing crocines, crocetins, and picrocrocine.

Saffron is used as a food and cosmetic dye and flavouring agent. In some circles it is considered to be a food. It was once widely used for colouring medicines. Saffron has been included in preparations for teething pain. There have been early reports of poisoning with saffron.

Saffron is also used in homoeopathic medicine.

Preparations

Proprietary Preparations (details are given in Part 3)

Multi-ingredient: ***Aust.:*** Zeller-Augenwasser†; ***Belg.:*** Calmant Martou; ***Fr.:*** Delabarre; Laccoderme Dalibour†; ***Ger.:*** Infi-tract N; Schwedentrunk; Schwedentrunk mit Ginseng; ***Ital.:*** Fluxoten; ***Spain:*** Dentomicin; Nani Pre Dental.

Sunset Yellow FCF (2410-h)

CI Food Yellow 3; Colour Index No. 15985; E110; FD & C Yellow No. 6; Jaune Orangé S; Jaune Soleil; Orange Yellow S. Disodium 6-hydroxy-5-(4-sulphonatophenylazo)naphthalene-2-sulphonate.

$C_{16}H_{10}N_2Na_2O_7S_2$ = 452.4.

CAS — 2783-94-0.

Pharmacopoeias. In Fr.

Sunset yellow FCF is used as a colouring agent in foods, medicines, and cosmetics. Sensitivity reactions have been reported.

Although some evidence of carcinogenicity was found in early *animal* studies subsequent work failed to confirm these findings and in the UK sunset yellow FCF is considered suitable for use as a food colour.[1]

1. MAFF. Food advisory committee: final report on the review of the colouring matter in food regulations 1973. *FdAC/REP/4.* London. HMSO, 1987.

Hypersensitivity reactions including severe abdominal cramps[1] and Quincke's oedema[2] have been recorded in single patients receiving medication that was coloured with sunset yellow FCF.

1. Gross PA, *et al.* Additive allergy: allergic gastroenteritis due to yellow dye #6. *Ann Intern Med* 1989; **111:** 87–8.
2. Lévesque H, *et al.* Reporting adverse drug reactions by proprietary name. *Lancet* 1991; **338:** 393.

Preparations

BP 1980: Compound Tartrazine Solution.

Tartrazine (2411-m)

CI Food Yellow 4; Colour Index No. 19140; E102; F D & C Yellow No. 5; Jaune Tartrique; Tartrazin.; Tartrazol Yellow. It consists mainly of trisodium 5-hydroxy-1-(4-sulphonatophenyl)-4-(4-sulphonatophenylazo)pyrazole-3-carboxylate.

$C_{16}H_9N_4Na_3O_9S_2$ = 534.4.

CAS — 1934-21-0.

Pharmacopoeias. In Fr.

Tartrazine is used as a colouring agent in foods, cosmetics, and medicines. Some patients may experience sensitivity reactions.

There have been numerous reports of reactions to tartrazine and these cover angioedema, asthma, urticaria, and anaphylactic shock. Some of the reports have dealt with cross-sensitivity, especially with aspirin, although the connection with aspirin has been questioned.[1] A suggested incidence of tartrazine sensitivity is 1 in 10 000.[2] The mechanism of the reactions may not necessarily be immunological.[3]

In considering the reports of tartrazine sensitivity or intolerance the Food Advisory Committee in the UK[1] reported that similar evidence of intolerance might well be obtained for a variety of natural food ingredients if as many studies were conducted on them as on tartrazine. The Committee considered that tartrazine posed no more problems than other colours or food ingredients and recommended that the continued use of tartrazine in food is acceptable. However, use of tartrazine in medicines appears to be diminishing.

1. MAFF. Food advisory committee: final report on the review of the colouring matter in food regulations 1973. *FdAC/REP/4.* London: HMSO, 1987.
2. Anonymous. Tartrazine: a yellow hazard. *Drug Ther Bull* 1980; **18:** 53–5.
3. Murdoch RD, *et al.* Tartrazine induced histamine release in vivo in normal subjects. *J R Coll Physicians Lond* 1987; **21:** 257–61.

Preparations

BP 1980: Compound Tartrazine Solution; Green S and Tartrazine Solution.

Turmeric (2415-q)

CI Natural Yellow 3; Curcuma; Indian Saffron.

CAS — 458-37-7.

Pharmacopoeias. In *Chin.*

The dried rhizome of *Curcuma longa* (Zingiberaceae).

Turmeric is used principally as a constituent of curry powders and other condiments. Turmeric and its main ingredient curcumin (see p.1000) are used as yellow colouring agents in foods. Turmeric has also been used as an ingredient of preparations indicated for biliary and gastro-intestinal disorders.

There has been some concern about the safety of turmeric oleoresin, an extract of turmeric, following reports of adverse thyroid changes in *pigs.*[1,2]

1. FAO/WHO. Evaluation of certain food additives and contaminants: thirty-fifth report of the joint FAO/WHO expert committee on food additives. *WHO Tech Rep Ser 789* 1990.
2. MAFF. Food advisory committee: final report on the review of the colouring matter in food regulations 1973. *FdAC/REP/4.* London: HMSO, 1987.

Preparations

Proprietary Preparations (details are given in Part 3)

Ger.: Aristochol CC; Choldestal; Logomed Verdauungs-Kapseln†; Meteophyt N; Sergast.

Multi-ingredient: ***Aust.:*** Aktiv Leber- und Gallentee; Bakanasan Leber-Galle; Choleodoron; Claim; Gallo Merz; Kneipp Galle- und Leber-Tee; Krautertee Nr 17; Sanhelios Leber-Galle; Sanvita Leber-Galle; Spasmo Claim; ***Austral.:*** Herbal Digestive Formula; ***Fr.:*** Hepatoum; Solution Buvable Hepatoum†; ***Ger.:*** "Mletzko" Tropfen†; Aristochol†; Basofer†; Bilgast†; Bilisan forte†; Choanol†; Cholaflux N†; Cholaflux†; Cholagogum F; Cholagogum N; Choleodoron; Cholosolm Phyto; Cholosom†; Gallo Merz N; Gastrol S; Heparaxal†; Hepaticum "Mletzko"†; Hepaticum-Medice H; Hepaton†; Hevert-Gall S; Horvilan N; Kneipp Galle- und Leber-Tee N; Medichol†; Meteophyt†; Neo-Gallonorm†; Opobylphyto; Pankreaticum; Paverysat forte; Spasmo Gallo Sanol; Spasmo-CC†; Steigal; Ventracid N; Worishofener Leber- und Gallensteinmittel Dr. Kleinschrod†; Zettagall V†; ***Switz.:*** Demodon†; Digestofluid†; Digestozym†; Globase†; Gouttes bile†; Stago†; Tisane hepatique et biliaire "H"†; ***UK:*** Choleodoron.

Vegetable Carbon (10105-c)

Carbon Black; E153; Vegetable Black.

NOTE. The name Carbon Black has also been used as a synonym for Channel Black, a colouring agent not used in food; care should be taken to avoid confusion between the two compounds.

Vegetable carbon, which consists essentially of finely divided carbon, is produced by the carbonisation of vegetable material such as peat. It is used as a colouring agent for foodstuffs and cosmetics.

Yellow 2G (2419-e)

107; Acid Light Yellow 2G; Acid Yellow 17; CI Food Yellow 5; Colour Index No. 18965. Disodium 2,5-dichloro-4-[5-hydroxy-3-methyl-4-(4-sulphonatophenylazo)pyrazol-1-yl]benzenesulphonate.

$C_{16}H_{10}Cl_2N_4Na_2O_7S_2$ = 551.3.

CAS — 6359-98-4.

Yellow 2G is used as a colouring agent in cosmetics.

Contrast Media

Contrast media are agents that enhance the images obtained from visualisation techniques such as radiography (X-ray imaging, including computed tomography), magnetic resonance imaging, or ultrasound imaging.

In **radiography**, contrast media may be used to increase the absorption of X-rays as they pass through the body, and this is described as *positive contrast*. A gas (air, oxygen, or carbon dioxide) may also be used for visualisation and this is referred to as *negative contrast*. When both gas and contrast medium are used concomitantly the procedure is called *double contrast*. Radiographic contrast media are described further below. Radiographic contrast media may also be used to enhance **computed tomography** images. Tomography is the procedure whereby a selected plane of the subject is visualised using X-rays.

Magnetic resonance imaging also provides sectional images. Contrast agents in magnetic resonance imaging (see below) enhance the images obtained from the absorption of radio waves by atomic nuclei.

In **ultrasound**, contrast agents enhance the images obtained from the reflection of sound waves by different tissues by providing air-liquid interfaces (see below).

Radiographic Contrast Media

Radiographic contrast media contain elements with high atomic numbers that absorb X-rays. The agents most commonly used are *iodinated organic compounds*, whose degree of opacity or radiodensity is directly proportional to their iodine content. *Barium sulphate* is a metal salt with a long established use as a contrast medium. Other heavy atoms have been investigated, but many, such as thorium dioxide and tantalum, were unsuitable due to acute or chronic toxicity.

The iodinated contrast media may be classified as either ionic or nonionic, and additionally as monomeric or dimeric.

The *ionic monomeric* media, such as the diatrizoates, iodamide, and iopanoic acid, generally have very high osmolality when given in concentrations suitable for radiographic visualisation and the resulting hypertonic solutions are associated with a relatively high incidence of adverse effects. Since radiodensity depends solely upon the iodine concentration, and osmolality solely upon the number of particles present in a given weight of solvent, the osmolality of contrast medium solutions can be reduced for a given radiodensity by using an *ionic dimeric* medium, such as iodipamide or ioxaglic acid, that contains twice the number of iodine atoms in each molecule, or by using a *nonionic* medium that does not dissociate into cation and anion. Nonionic media may be *monomeric*, such as iohexol, iopamidol, iopromide, and ioversol, or *dimeric*, for example iotrolan. Thus the best ratio of radiodensity to osmolality is achieved with the nonionic dimeric media.

Choice of radiographic contrast medium. Radiographic techniques to visualise particular structures within the body depend upon the physical and chemical properties of the contrast medium used and upon the way in which it is administered. Some radiographic procedures and the specific contrast media used in them are described below. The likelihood of adverse effects is greater with the older ionic iodinated contrast media, especially in high risk patients (see below), and this also influences the choice of contrast medium.

For **urography** (visualisation of the kidneys and urinary tract) the molecule must be small and highly water-soluble, with low protein-binding, so that glomerular filtration is encouraged with subsequent passage through the urinary tract. For good visualisation high concentrations must be achieved in the urinary tract from the start, and this in turn means high plasma concentrations: contrast media for urography are thus invariably given by the intravenous route. Examples of ionic urographic media include the diatrizoates, iothalamates, and metrizoates. These monomeric ionic media have a relatively high incidence of adverse effects, due in part to their high osmolality and better tolerance may be achieved with compounds of lower osmolality, such as ionic dimeric media (ioxaglic acid) and nonionic media (iohexol, iopamidol, and iopromide).

The requirements for **angiography** (visualisation of the circulatory system) are similar to those for urography in that a water-soluble molecule is required that can be readily distributed through the blood vessels. In addition, the solution should be of low viscosity to facilitate rapid injection and of high radiodensity to counteract the diluting effects of the blood. There are no particular differences between requirements for visualisation of veins (**phlebography** or **venography**) and those for arteries (**arteriography**); however, for **angiocardiography** (visualisation of the heart and heart vessels), or **digital subtraction angiography** where movement of a bolus of contrast medium through the circulation is studied over a period of time, the heart may be exposed to higher-than-usual concentrations of contrast medium and low cardiotoxicity is particularly important. There has been a general trend towards the use of low osmolality media for all types of angiography, since greatly improved tolerance, and in particular less pain on injection, means that procedures can be carried out without general anaesthesia and with less risk of serious adverse effects. Examples of angiographic media include iodixanol, iohexol, iopamidol, iopromide, and ioversol.

For **gastro-intestinal radiography** the principal requirements are that the contrast medium should not be absorbed but should form an even, homogeneous coat on the gastro-intestinal mucosa, without interacting with gut secretions or producing misleading radiographic artifacts. The chief contrast medium for this purpose is barium sulphate, and much effort has been devoted to the production of suitable formulations to improve its coating properties and reduce the formation of bubbles, cracks, and other radiographic artifacts.

The requirements for **cholecystography** and **cholangiography** (visualisation of the gallbladder and biliary tract) depend to some degree on the intended route of administration. In order that the molecule should be preferentially excreted in the bile it should be sufficiently large for biliary excretion and must possess a free carboxy or other acidic group, since the biliary active transport mechanism is an anion transfer process. In addition, the molecule should be protected by virtue of its size or by protein binding from the more rapid renal excretion processes. However, the oral cholecystographic agents need to be absorbed from the gastro-intestinal tract before they become effective, and this imposes a second, and to some extent conflicting, set of requirements. For optimal enteral absorption, molecules should be of relatively small size, sufficiently soluble in gastro-intestinal fluids, and sufficiently lipophilic to pass the cell membranes of the mucosa. Examples of *oral* cholecystographic media include the iopodates, iocetamic acid, iopanoic acid, and sodium tyropanoate. These are relatively small, monomeric molecules and therefore they require conjugation with glucuronic acid within the body to achieve sufficient molecular weight for biliary excretion. They are often given after a fatty meal to enhance absorption and reduce the incidence of inadequate visualisation. The *intravenous* cholecystographic agents do not have to meet the above requirements for enteral absorption and are mostly larger, dimeric molecules that do not require conjugation. They are generally more effective than the oral media. Examples of intravenous cholecystographic media include salts of iodipamide and iotroxic acid.

For **myelography** (visualisation of the structures of the spinal cord) no special requirements other than good tolerance are necessary. Although visualisation was at one time achieved with oily media such as iophendylate these have now mostly been replaced with nonionic water-soluble media. These offer improved tolerance, better visualisation since they are miscible with cerebrospinal fluid, and, unlike the oil-based media, are removed from the subarachnoid space by normal pharmacokinetic mechanisms. Examples include iohexol and iopamidol.

Arthrography (visualisation of the joint capsule) may be performed with many different contrast media provided they are well-diluted before use.

Bronchography (examination of the bronchial tree) is performed with oily or aqueous media, such as iopydol or iopydone.

For **hysterosalpingography** (visualisation of the uterus and fallopian tubes) a water-soluble contrast medium is required. Examples include iotrolan, ioxaglic acid, and metrizoic acid.

Very high radiodensity is required to obtain good visualisation of the lymphatic structures in radiography of the lymphatic system (**lymphography** or **lymphangiography**). In addition, water-soluble media rapidly leave the system and only particulate or water-insoluble media or very large molecules persist within the lymphatic vessels for any length of time. The medium that has been most frequently used is iodised oil. It gives good visualisation of that part of the lymphatic system between the point at which it is infused and the point at which it enters the general circulation, but it is not distributed throughout the whole lymphatic space and has the potential for a number of severe side-effects.

Adverse effects. The adverse effects of iodinated contrast media are described under Diatrizoic Acid, p.1003. Since many of the adverse effects[1,2] of the older ionic iodinated contrast media are associated with their high osmolality, it was hoped that the development of media with reduced osmolality would offer a potential route for the reduction of adverse effects. There is evidence from studies in Australia[3] and Japan[4] which suggests that 'low-risk' patients given conventional high-osmolal media are at greater risk of adverse effects than patients considered 'at-risk' who are given nonionic media. However, although studies comparing high-osmolal versus low-osmolal media[5,6] have found a definite reduction in minor to moderate adverse effects with the latter, they did not demonstrate a reduction in major adverse effects.

Cost considerations mean that low-osmolal media tend to be reserved for patients considered to be at high risk of adverse effects (see Precautions under Diatrizoic Acid, p.1003).

1. Westhoff-Bleck M, *et al.* The adverse effects of angiographic radiocontrast media. *Drug Safety* 1991; **6:** 28–36.
2. Ansell G. Adverse reactions profile: intravascular iodinated radiocontrast media. *Prescribers' J* 1993; **33:** 82–8.
3. Palmer FJ. The RACR Survey of intravenous contrast media reactions: final report. *Australas Radiol* 1988; **32:** 426–8.
4. Katayama H, *et al.* Adverse reactions to ionic and nonionic contrast media: a report from the Japanese Committee on the Safety of Contrast Media. *Radiology* 1990; **175:** 621–8.
5. Kinnison ML, *et al.* Results of randomized controlled trials of low- versus high-osmolality contrast media. *Radiology* 1989; **170:** 381–9.
6. Steinberg EP, *et al.* Safety and cost effectiveness of high-osmolality as compared with low-osmolality contrast material in patients undergoing cardiac angiography. *N Engl J Med* 1992; **326:** 425–30.

HYPERSENSITIVITY. Anaphylactoid reactions to iodinated contrast media are more common with the ionic agents than the nonionic media of lower osmolality. Patients at increased risk are those with a history of asthma or allergy, drug hypersensitivity, adrenal suppression, heart disease, previous reaction to a contrast medium, and those receiving beta blockers or interleukin-2 therapy. In such patients, nonionic media are preferred and beta blockers should be discontinued if possible.

Pretreatment with corticosteroids may be considered for preventing anaphylactoid reactions in high-risk patients and an antihistamine may be given. However, the value is uncertain.

References.

1. Lang DM, *et al.* Increased risk for anaphylactoid reaction from contrast media in patients on β-adrenergic blockers or with asthma. *Ann Intern Med* 1991: **115:** 270–6.
2. Ansell G. Adverse reactions profile: intravascular iodinated radiocontrast media. *Prescribers' J* 1993; **33:** 82–8.
3. Wittbrodt ET, Spinler SA. Prevention of anaphylactoid reactions in high-risk patients receiving radiographic contrast media. *Ann Pharmacother* 1994; **28:** 236–41.
4. Sidhu PS, Dawson P. Corticosteroid prophylaxis in contrast examinations. *Br J Hosp Med* 1997; **58:** 304–6.

THROMBO-EMBOLISM. Angiography is associated with a risk of thrombo-embolism. It has been suggested[1-3] that nonionic contrast media that are the preferred agents in angiography (see above) may contribute to this risk since they have less anticoagulant activity than the ionic contrast media. It is recommended that great care should be taken to prevent mixing of blood and contrast media before injection in angiography.

1. Robertson HJ. Thrombogenic potential of nonionic contrast media. *Mayo Clin Proc* 1990; **65**: 603–4.
2. King BF. Thrombogenic potential of nonionic contrast media. *Mayo Clin Proc* 1990; **65**: 604.
3. Anonymous. Thromboembolism during angiography. *Lancet* 1992; **339**: 1576–8.

Magnetic Resonance Contrast Media

Magnetic resonance contrast media are paramagnetic or superparamagnetic agents that enhance the magnetic resonance image by interfering with the relaxation times of adjacent nuclei. Paramagnetic contrast media include the gadolinium complexes, gadodiamide, gadopentetic acid, and gadoteridol, and the manganese complex mangafodipir trisodium. Superparamagnetic contrast media include the iron compounds ferristene, ferumoxides, and ferumoxsil.

References.

1. Armstrong P, Keevil SF. Magnetic resonance imaging—1: basic principles of image production. *Br Med J* 1991; **303:** 35–40.
2. Armstrong P, Keevil SF. Magnetic resonance imaging—2: clinical uses. *Br Med J* 1991; **303:** 105–9.
3. Edelman RR, Warach S. Magnetic resonance imaging (first of two parts). *N Engl J Med* 1993; **328:** 708–15.
4. Edelman RR, Warach S. Magnetic resonance imaging (second of two parts). *N Engl J Med* 1993; **328:** 785–91.

Ultrasound Contrast Media

Contrast agents for use in ultrasound imaging, termed echocontrast agents or echo-enhancers, have recently been introduced. Microbubbles of gas encapsulated in albumin (p.710), galactose, or fluorocarbons such as perflenapent and perflisopent are examples.

References.

1. Blomley H, Cosgrove D. Contrast agents in ultrasound. *Br J Hosp Med* 1996; **55:** 6–7.

Barium Sulphate (1552-p)

Barii Sulfas; Barii Sulphas; Barium Sulfate; Barium Sulfuricum; Baryum (Sulfate de).

$BaSO_4$ = 233.4.

CAS — 7727-43-7.

Pharmacopoeias. In *Chin., Eur.* (see p.viii), *Int., Jpn, Pol.,* and *US.*

A fine, heavy, white, odourless, powder, free from grittiness.

Practically **insoluble** in water and in organic solvents; very slightly soluble to practically insoluble in acids and alkali hydroxides.

Adverse Effects

Because barium sulphate is almost insoluble it lacks the severe toxicity characteristic of the barium ion; deaths have occurred following the administration of the more soluble barium sulphide in error for the sulphate.

Constipation may occur after oral or rectal barium sulphate administration; impaction, obstruction, and appendicitis have occurred. Surgical removal of faecaliths has sometimes been necessary. Cramping or diarrhoea have also been reported. Venous intravasation has led to the formation of emboli; deaths have occurred. Perforation of the bowel has led to peritonitis, adhesions, granulomas, and a high mortality rate.

ECG abnormalities have occurred during the use of barium sulphate enemas.

Accidental aspiration into the lungs has led to pneumonitis or granuloma formation.

Hypersensitivity. A survey of hypersensitivity reactions to barium preparations found that although barium is inert many of the additives used in formulation have the potential to cause allergic reactions.[1] Of 106 reactions reported or found in the literature, 61% involved the skin and only 8% the respiratory tract; unconsciousness was reported in 8% of cases. In view of the frequency of use of barium preparations, such adverse reactions must be very rare, but radiologists should be aware that they may be somewhat more common than is usually appreciated. A number of severe reactions associated with the use of barium enemas supplied with an inflatable latex cuff may have been due to leaching of components from the latex.[2]

1. Janower ML. Hypersensitivity reactions after barium studies of the upper and lower gastrointestinal tract. *Radiology* 1986; **161:** 139–40.
2. Nightingale SL. Severe adverse reactions to barium enema procedures. *JAMA* 1990; **264:** 2863.

Precautions

Barium sulphate should not be given to patients with intestinal obstruction and care is needed in those with conditions such as pyloric stenosis or lesions which may predispose to obstruction. Adequate hydration should be ensured after the procedure to prevent severe constipation.

It is contra-indicated in patients with gastro-intestinal perforation, and should be avoided, particularly when given rectally, in those at risk of perforation as in acute ulcerative colitis or diverticulitis and following rectal or colonic biopsy, sigmoidoscopy, or radiotherapy.

Uses and Administration

Barium sulphate is used as a contrast medium for X-ray examination of the gastro-intestinal tract involving single- or double-contrast techniques or computed tomography (p.1002).

The dose of barium sulphate is dependent upon the type of examination and technique employed. For examination of the oesophagus, up to 150 mL of a 50 to 200% w/v suspension may be given by mouth. For examination of the stomach and duodenum, up to 300 mL of a 30 to 200% w/v suspension may be given by mouth. For examination of the small intestine, up to 300 mL of a 30 to 150% w/v suspension may be given by mouth. For examination of the colon, up to 2 litres of a 20 to 130% w/v suspension may be administered as an enema.

For double-contrast examination, gas can be introduced into the gastro-intestinal tract by using suspensions of barium sulphate containing carbon dioxide; separate gas-producing preparations based on sodium bicarbonate are also available. Air administered via a tube may be used as an alternative to carbon dioxide.

Reviews.

1. Bentley A, Piper K. Barium sulphate preparations. *Pharm J* 1987; **238:** 138–9.
2. Nolan DJ. Barium examination of the small intestine. *Br J Hosp Med* 1994; **52:** 136–41.

Intussusception. Barium enemas have been recommended in the investigation of children with suspected acute intussusception, a condition where part of the intestine prolapses into the lumen of an adjacent part causing an obstruction. In some cases, the hydrostatic pressure exerted by the enema may reduce the intussusception thus avoiding the need for surgery.[1,2]

1. Anonymous. Acute intussusception in childhood. *Lancet* 1985; **ii:** 250–1.
2. Collins DL, *et al.* Hydrostatic reduction of ileocolic intussusception: a second attempt in the operating room with general anesthesia. *J Pediatr* 1989; **115:** 204–7.

Preparations

BP 1998: Barium Sulphate Oral Suspension;
USP 23: Barium Sulfate for Suspension; Barium Sulfate Suspension.

Proprietary Preparations (details are given in Part 3)
Aust.: Micropaque; Microtrast; Prontobario; Scannotrast; Unibaryt; ***Austral.:*** Medebar; Medescan; Tixobar; ***Belg.:*** EZ Paque-HD†; Micropaque; Polibar†; ***Canad.:*** A C B†; E-Z-Cat; E-Z-HD†; E-Z-Jug†; E-Z-Paque†; Esobar†; Esopho-Cat†; Polibar Liquid†; Polibar Plus†; Polibar Rapid†; Readi-Cat†; Ultra-R; Unibar; ***Fr.:*** Micropaque; Microtrast; Radiopaque†; Telebar†; ***Ger.:*** Falibaryt; Micropaque; Microtrast; Unibaryt; ***Ital.:*** Barytgen†; Mixobar; Prontobario; TAC Esofago; ***Neth.:*** E-Z-HD†; Microbar†; Micropaque; Polibar†; ***Norw.:*** Mixobar; ***Spain:*** Barigraf; Barigraf Tac; Bario Cidan†; Bario Dif; Bario Faes; Bario Faes Ultra; Bario Llorente; Bariopacin; Disperbarium; Justebarin; Micropaque; ***Swed.:*** Barytgen; Mixobar; ***Switz.:*** CAT-Barium (E-Z-CAT); Microbar-Colon; Microbar-HD (E-Z-HD); Micropaque; Polibar-ACB; ***UK:*** Baritop; E-Z-Cat; E-Z-HD; E-Z-Paque; Micropaque; Microtrast†; Polibar; Polibar Rapid; Polibar Viscous; ***USA:*** Anatrast; Baricon; Baro-cat; Barobag†; Baroflave; Barosperse; Enecat; Entrobar; Epi-C; Flo-Coat; HD 200 Plus; HD 85; Liquipake; Prepcat; Tomocat; Tonopaque.

Multi-ingredient: ***Switz.:*** Calcipulpe; Endomethasone.

Diatrizoic Acid (1554-w)

Diatrizoic Acid *(BAN, USAN).*

Acidum Amidotrizoicum; Amidotrizoic Acid; NSC-262168. 3,5-Diacetamido-2,4,6-tri-iodobenzoic acid.

$C_{11}H_9I_3N_2O_4,2H_2O$ = 649.9.

CAS — 117-96-4 (anhydrous diatrizoic acid); 50978-11-5 (diatrizoic acid dihydrate).

Pharmacopoeias. In *Eur.* (see p.viii), *Int., Jpn,* and *US.*

A white or almost white, odourless, crystalline powder, containing approximately 62% of I, calculated on the anhydrous substance.

Very slightly **soluble** in water and in alcohol; soluble in dimethylformamide and in solutions of alkali hydroxides; practically insoluble in ether. **Protect** from light.

Meglumine Diatrizoate (1555-e)

Meglumine Diatrizoate *(BANM).*

Diatrizoate Meglumine; Meglumine Amidotrizoate; Methylglucamine Diatrizoate. *N*-Methylglucamine 3,5-diacetamido-2,4,6-tri-iodobenzoate.

$C_{11}H_9I_3N_2O_4,C_7H_{17}NO_5$ = 809.1.

CAS — 131-49-7.

Pharmacopoeias. In *US.*

An odourless white powder containing approximately 47.1% of I. Freely **soluble** in water. **Incompatibilities** with some antihistamines have been reported.

Sodium Diatrizoate (1556-l)

Sodium Diatrizoate *(BANM).*

Sodium Amidotrizoate *(rINN)*; Diatrizoate Sodium; Natrii Amidotrizoas; NSC-61815. Sodium 3,5-diacetamido-2,4,6-tri-iodobenzoate.

$C_{11}H_8I_3N_2NaO_4$ = 635.9.

CAS — 737-31-5.

Pharmacopoeias. In *Eur.* (see p.viii), *Int., Pol.,* and *US.*

An odourless white or almost white powder. It contains approximately 59.9% of I calculated on the anhydrous substance.

Freely **soluble** in water; slightly soluble in alcohol; practically insoluble in acetone and in ether. **Protect** from light.

Incompatibilities with some antihistamines have been reported.

Adverse Effects and Treatment

Many of the effects of iodinated ionic monomeric contrast media can be attributed to the high osmolality which is a feature of these agents; reducing the osmolality through altering the ionic or molecular profile produces a reduced incidence of adverse effects (see p.1002). The route and speed of administration, and the volume, concentration, and viscosity of the solution also affect the incidence of adverse effects. Most reactions occur within 5 to 10 minutes of injection, but they may be delayed.

Hyperthyroidism has been reported following administration of iodinated contrast media, presumably due to small amounts of iodine present as a contaminant or released by any breakdown of the medium in the body. For the effects of iodine on the thyroid gland, see p.1493.

When given by injection the diatrizoates may cause nausea, a metallic taste, vomiting, flushing and sensations of heat, weakness, dizziness, headache, coughing, rhinitis, sweating, sneezing, lachrymation, visual disturbances, pruritus, salivary gland enlargement, pallor, tachycardia, bradycardia, transient ECG abnormalities, haemodynamic disturbances, and hypotension. Rarely, more severe adverse effects, including convulsions, paralysis, coma, rigors, ventricular fibrillation, pulmonary oedema, circulatory failure, and cardiac arrest have occurred. Occasionally anaphylactoid or hypersensitivity reactions occur; dyspnoea, bronchospasm, angioedema, and severe urticaria have been reported, and reactions have sometimes been fatal. Injections of diatrizoates into the CNS produces severe neurotoxicity.

Deaths have also been recorded due to acute renal failure, which may follow intravenous administration, particularly in dehydrated patients and patients with other predisposing factors (see also under Effects on the Kidneys, and Precautions, below).

Pain may occur at the injection site; extravasation may be followed by tissue damage, thrombophlebitis, thrombosis, venospasm, and embolism (see p.1002).

Fibrinolysis and a possible depressant effect on blood coagulation factors has been reported. Disseminated intravascular coagulation has occurred. Meglumine salts are reportedly better tolerated and produce less pain on injection than sodium salts, but the sodium salts may be associated with a lower incidence of arrhythmias. As a result, the sodium and meglumine salts are often given in combination to minimise adverse effects.

Mild diarrhoea may follow the oral or rectal administration of sodium and meglumine diatrizoates for gastro-intestinal examinations. The accidental aspiration of solutions of these salts has caused fatal pulmonary oedema.

Adverse effects are treated symptomatically and adequate resuscitative facilities should be available when radiographic procedures are to be employed.

Effects on the blood. Reports of diatrizoates adversely affecting the blood.

1. Catterall JR, *et al.* Intravascular haemolysis with acute renal failure after angiocardiography. *Br Med J* 1981; **282:** 779–80.
2. Shojania AM. Immune-mediated thrombocytopenia due to an iodinated contrast medium (diatrizoate). *Can Med Assoc J* 1985; **133:** 123.
3. Fairley S, Ihle BU. Thrombotic microangiopathy and acute renal failure associated with arteriography. *Br Med J* 1986; **293:** 922–3.

Effects on the kidneys. Administration of contrast media may be associated with renal toxicity.[1-3] Estimates of the incidence of nephrotoxicity vary widely, but the figure is probably less than 1% of all patients receiving contrast media and does not appear to differ significantly with ionic or nonionic media. In the majority of patients who develop contrast-medium-induced renal impairment the condition develops within about 24 hours of the procedure, is asymptomatic, and resolves completely within about 10 days. However occasionally the condition may be severe producing oliguria and renal failure that requires dialysis; fatalities have occurred.

The mechanism of nephrotoxicity is not well understood and it seems probable that more than one type of lesion may contribute to the overall incidence of toxicity. Possible mechanisms are tubular necrosis (including that due to anaphylaxis or cardiovascular collapse), traumatic occlusion of the renal arteries, cholesterol embolism, and obstruction of the tubules by protein casts (as in patients with multiple myeloma).

Risk factors include pre-existing renal impairment, especially in patients with diabetes mellitus, and conditions where there is reduced renal blood flow, such as heart failure and dehydration. Old age, repeated administration (over a short period of time), multiple myeloma, and pre-existing hepatic impairment have also been proposed as risk factors.

1. Brezis M, Epstein FH. A closer look at radiocontrast-induced nephropathy. *N Engl J Med* 1989; **320:** 179–81.
2. Parfrey PS, *et al.* Contrast material-induced renal failure in patients with diabetes mellitus, renal insufficiency, or both. *N Engl J Med* 1989; **320:** 143–9.
3. Schwab SJ, *et al.* Contrast nephrotoxicity: a randomized controlled trial of a nonionic and an ionic radiographic contrast agent. *N Engl J Med* 1989; **320:** 149–53.

Precautions

The diatrizoates and similar contrast media should be administered with great caution to patients with asthma or a history of allergy and should be avoided in patients with known hypersensitivity to contrast media or to iodine. An intravenous injection of 0.5 to 1 mL of contrast medium has been given as a test for sensitivity before administration of the main dose but it does not predict hypersensitivity with certainty and severe reactions and fatalities have followed the test dose. Pretreatment with corticosteroids may be considered in patients considered 'at risk' but its value is uncertain (see p.1002). An antihistamine may be given with the corticosteroid.

Caution is needed in patients with severe hepatic or renal impairment or others who may be at increased risk of renal failure; dehydrated patients should have their fluid and electrolyte balance corrected before contrast medium administration. Patients with multiple myeloma may be at particular risk if dehydrated, since precipitation of protein in the renal tubules may lead to anuria and fatal renal failure.

An increased risk of adverse effects has also been reported in patients with severe hypertension, advanced cardiac disease, phaeochromocytoma, sickle-cell disease, or hyperthyroidism. Debilitated, severely ill, very old, or very young patients are also at risk.

Certain problems may be associated with particular radiographic techniques. Administration of diatrizoates or similar hypertonic media into the CNS, e.g. for myelography, should be avoided, and use for cerebral angiography or computed tomography of the brain is contra-indicated in patients with subarachnoid haemorrhage. All intravascular administration requires caution in patients with occlusive vascular disorders. These media should not be given for hysterosalpingography in the presence of infection or inflammation of the pelvic cavity, nor during menstruation or in pregnancy (but all abdominal radiography should be avoided in any case during pregnancy because of the risks of radiation to the fetus).

The administration of iodine-containing contrast media may interfere with thyroid function tests. There may also be interference with blood coagulation tests and certain urine tests.

Neonates. The use of meglumine diatrizoate might have contributed to the death, with bowel necrosis, perforation, and peritonitis, of 2 infants with meconium ileus.[1]

1. Leonidas JC, *et al.* Possible adverse effects of methylglucamine diatrizoate compounds on the bowel of newborn infants with meconium ileus. *Radiology* 1976; **121:** 693–6.

Pharmacokinetics

Diatrizoates are very poorly absorbed from the gastro-intestinal tract. Diatrizoates in the circulation are not significantly bound to plasma proteins. If renal function is not impaired, unchanged diatrizoate is rapidly excreted by glomerular filtration; over 95% of an intravascular dose is reported to be excreted in urine within 24 hours, and about 1 to 2% of a dose may be excreted in faeces. Trace amounts may be detected in other body fluids including tears and saliva. Faecal excretion may increase to 10 to 50% in severe renal impairment. The half-life of diatrizoates has been reported to be 30 to 60 minutes, which can increase to 20 to 140 hours in severe renal impairment. They are removed by haemodialysis and peritoneal dialysis.

The diatrizoates cross the placenta and have been reported to be present in breast milk.

Uses and Administration

The diatrizoates are iodinated ionic monomeric contrast media (p.1002). Both the sodium and the meglumine salt have been widely used in diagnostic radiography including computed tomography (p.1002), but a mixture of both is often preferred to minimise side-effects.

The diatrizoates are used in an extensive range of procedures. The route of administration and the dose employed depend on the type of procedure and the degree and extent of contrast required. They may be given by many routes including the oral, intravenous, intramuscular, subcutaneous, intra-arterial, intra-articular, and intra-osseous. For some procedures, they may be injected into the gallbladder, biliary ducts, or spleen.

Solutions of diatrizoates have also been given as an enema in the treatment of uncomplicated meconium ileus.

Calcium diatrizoate and lysine diatrizoate have also been used as contrast media.

Intussusception. Contrast medium enemas, usually diatrizoate or barium sulphate (p.1003) have been administered as an initial treatment of ileocolic intussusception in children.[1] Surgery is performed if the hydrostatic pressure produced by the enema fails to reduce the intussusception.

1. Collins DL, *et al.* Hydrostatic reduction of ileocolic intussusception: a second attempt in the operating room with general anesthesia. *J Pediatr* 1989; **115**: 204–7.

Preparations

BP 1998: Meglumine Amidotrizoate Injection; Sodium Amidotrizoate Injection;
USP 23: Diatrizoate Meglumine and Diatrizoate Sodium Injection; Diatrizoate Meglumine and Diatrizoate Sodium Solution; Diatrizoate Meglumine Injection; Diatrizoate Sodium Injection; Diatrizoate Sodium Solution.

Proprietary Preparations (details are given in Part 3)
Aust.: Angiografin; Gastrografin; Urografin; Urovison; ***Austral.:*** MD-60; MD-76; MD-Gastroview; ***Canad.:*** Gastrografin; Hypaque; Hypaque-M 76%; MD-76; Reno-M; Renografin; ***Fr.:*** Angiografine; Gastrografine; Radioselectan; ***Ger.:*** Angiografin; Ethibloc Okklusions-Emulsion; Gastrografin; Gastrolux; Peritrast; Peritrast comp; Peritrast-Infusio; Peritrast-Oral CT; Peritrast-Oral-G I; Peritrast-RE; Urografin; Urovison; Urovist†; ***Irl.:*** Hypaque; ***Ital.:*** Angiografin†; Gastrografin; Pielografin†; Selectografin; Urografin†; Urovison†; ***Neth.:*** Angiografin; Gastrografin; Urografin; Urovison; ***Norw.:*** Gastrografin; ***S.Afr.:*** Angiografin; Gastrografin; Urografin; ***Spain:*** Gastrografin; Pielograf; Plenigraf; Radialar 280; Trazograf; Uro Angiografin; Urografin; ***Swed.:*** Gastrografin; Urografin; ***Switz.:*** Ethibloc; Gastrografin; Urografin; ***UK:*** Gastrografin; Hypaque; Urografin; Urografin 310M†; ***USA:*** Angiovist 282; Angiovist 292; Cystografin; Gastrografin; Hypaque; Hypaque-M; MD-60; MD-Gastroview; Reno-M; Renografin; Renovist; Urovist.

Multi-ingredient: ***Canad.:*** Sinografin; ***USA:*** Sinografin.

Ferristene (17904-e)

Ferristene *(USAN)*.

$C_8H_{11}NO_3S,(Fe_2O_3)_{0.725}$.

CAS — 155773-56-1.

Iron ferrite crystals carried on monosized spheres of cross-linked poly(ammonium styrenesulfonate).

Ferristene 100 mg contains approximately 23.4 mg Fe.

Adverse Effects and Precautions

Nausea, vomiting, and constipation or loose stools may occur. Ferristene should not be used in patients with gastro-intestinal obstruction or perforation and should be used with care in patients prone to developing these conditions.

Uses and Administration

Ferristene is a superparamagnetic agent used orally for contrast enhancement in magnetic resonance imaging (p.1002) of the abdomen. It is usually given in a dose of 400 to 800 mL of a suspension containing 0.117 mg of iron per mL.

Preparations

Proprietary Preparations (details are given in Part 3)
Ger.: Abdoscan; ***Norw.:*** Abdoscan; ***Swed.:*** Abdoscan; ***Switz.:*** Abdoscan; ***UK:*** Abdoscan.

Ferumoxides (17059-y)

Ferumoxides *(BAN, USAN)*.

AMI-25.

$(Fe_2O_3)_m(FeO)_n$.

CAS — 119683-68-0.

Ferumoxides is a superparamagnetic agent used intravenously for contrast enhancement in magnetic resonance imaging (p.1002) of the liver.

Preparations

Proprietary Preparations (details are given in Part 3)
Fr.: Endorem; ***Ger.:*** Endorem; ***Ital.:*** Endorem; ***Neth.:*** Endorem; ***Spain:*** Endorem; ***Swed.:*** Endorem; ***Switz.:*** Endorem; ***USA:*** Feridex.

Ferumoxsil (17060-g)

Ferumoxsil *(BAN, USAN)*.

AMI-121.

Ferumoxsil is a superparamagnetic agent used orally for contrast enhancement in magnetic resonance imaging (p.1002) of the gastro-intestinal tract. It is usually given in a dose of 600 to 900 mL of a suspension containing 0.175 mg of iron per mL.

Preparations

Proprietary Preparations (details are given in Part 3)
Aust.: Lumirem; ***Fr.:*** Lumirem; ***Ger.:*** Lumirem; ***Ital.:*** Lumirem; ***Neth.:*** Lumirem; ***Swed.:*** Lumirem; ***Switz.:*** Lumirem.

Gadobenic Acid (15276-g)

Gadobenic Acid *(BAN, rINN)*.

B-19036; Gd-BOPTA. [2-(Benzyloxymethyl)-6-(carboxylatomethyl-κ*O*)-3,9-bis(carboxymethyl-κ*O*)-3,6,9-triazaundecanedioato-$κ^3N^{3,6,9}κ^2O^{1,11}$] gadolinium (III).

$C_{22}H_{28}GdN_3O_{11}$ = 667.7.

CAS — 113662-23-0.

Gadobenate Dimeglumine (17562-v)

Gadobenate Dimeglumine *(USAN)*.

B-19036/7. Dihydrogen [(±)-4-carboxy-5,8,11-tris(carboxymethyl)-1-phenyl-2-oxa-5,8,11-triaza-tridecan-13-oato(5-)]gadolinate(2-) compound with 1-deoxy-1-(methylamino)-D-glucitol (1:2).

$C_{22}H_{28}GdN_3O_{11},2C_7H_{17}NO_5$ = 1058.1.

CAS — 127000-20-8.

Gadobenic acid is an ionic paramagnetic agent investigated, as gadobenate dimeglumine, for contrast enhancement in magnetic resonance imaging (p.1002).

Gadodiamide (14637-q)

Gadodiamide *(BAN, rINN)*.

GdDTPA-BMA; S-041. Aqua[6-carboxylatomethyl-3,9-bis(methylcarbamoylmethyl-κ-*O*)-3,6,9-triazaundecanedioato-$κ^3$-N^3,N^6,N^9-$κ^3$-O^1,O^6,O^{11}(3-)gadolinium(III)]; A complex of gadolinium with diethylenetriamine penta-acetic acid bis-methylamide.

$C_{16}H_{28}GdN_5O_9,xH_2O$ = 591.7 (anhydrous).

CAS — 131410-48-5 (anhydrous gadodiamide); 122795-43-1 (gadodiamide hydrate).

NOTE. Anhydrous Gadodiamide is *USAN*.

Adverse Effects and Precautions

As for Gadopentetic Acid, below.

Pharmacokinetics

Gadodiamide is rapidly distributed into extracellular fluid. About 96% of a dose is excreted unchanged in the urine within 24 hours. An elimination half-life of approximately 70 minutes has been reported. Gadodiamide is not bound to plasma proteins.

Uses and Administration

Gadodiamide is a nonionic paramagnetic agent used for contrast enhancement in magnetic resonance imaging (p.1002) of cranial and spinal structures.

Gadodiamide is available as a solution containing 287 mg (0.5 mmol) per mL. The usual dose in adults is 0.2 mL (0.1 mmol) per kg body-weight intravenously.

Preparations

Proprietary Preparations (details are given in Part 3)
Aust.: Omniscan; ***Austral.:*** Omniscan; ***Belg.:*** Omniscan; ***Canad.:*** Omniscan; ***Ger.:*** Omniscan; ***Ital.:*** Omniscan; ***Neth.:*** Omniscan†; ***Norw.:*** Omniscan; ***Spain:*** Omniscan; ***Swed.:*** Omniscan; ***Switz.:*** Omniscan; ***UK:*** Omniscan; ***USA:*** Omniscan.

Gadopentetic Acid (3798-d)

Gadopentetic Acid *(BAN, rINN)*.

Gadolinium-DTPA. {*N*′,*N*″-Bis(carboxymethyl)-*N*′,*N*″-[(acetato)iminodiethylene]diglycinato-*O*,-*O*′,*O*″,*N*,-*N*′,*N*″}gadolinium(3+); A complex of gadolinium with diethylenetriamine penta-acetic acid.

$C_{14}H_{20}GdN_3O_{10}$ = 547.6.

CAS — 80529-93-7.

Meglumine Gadopentetate (10657-h)

Dimeglumine Gadopentetate; Gadopentetate Dimeglumine *(USAN)*; Gadopentetate Meglumine; SH-L-451-A. The di(*N*-methylglucamine) salt of gadopentetic acid.

$C_{14}H_{20}GdN_3O_{10},(C_7H_{17}NO_5)_2$ = 938.0.

CAS — 86050-77-3.

Adverse Effects

There may be headache, nausea, vomiting, and transient sensations of heat or cold or taste disturbances following injection of gadopentetate. Rarely, convulsions, hypotension, allergic or anaphylactoid reactions, and shock may occur. Paraesthesias, dizziness, and localised pain have also been reported. Transient elevations of serum iron and bilirubin values have been observed.

Hypersensitivity. A report of anaphylactic shock in a patient following the intravenous administration of meglumine gadopentetate.[1] The patient had a history of pollen allergy and had experienced anaphylactic shock when given an iodine-based contrast agent intravenously 2 months earlier.

1. Tardy B, *et al.* Anaphylactic shock induced by intravenous gadopentetate dimeglumine. *Lancet* 1992; **339**: 494.

Precautions

Gadopentetate should be given with care to patients with severe renal impairment, epilepsy, hypotension, and a history of hypersensitivity, asthma, or other allergic respiratory disorders. Care should be taken to avoid extravasation. Gadopentetate may interfere with tests of serum iron or bilirubin concentrations.

Myasthenia gravis. A report of acute deterioration of myasthenia gravis in a patient after magnetic resonance imaging of the brain using gadopentetate as the contrast medium.[1]

1. Nordenbo AM, Somnier FE. Acute deterioration of myasthenia gravis after intravenous administration of gadolinium-DTPA. *Lancet* 1992; **340:** 1168.

Pharmacokinetics

Gadopentetate is rapidly distributed into extracellular space following intravenous injection. An elimination half-life of 1.6 hours has been reported. It is not metabolised and about 90% of a dose is excreted in the urine within 24 hours. A small amount is distributed into breast milk. Gadopentetate is removed by haemodialysis.

Uses and Administration

Gadopentetic acid is an ionic paramagnetic agent used, as meglumine gadopentetate, for contrast enhancement in magnetic resonance imaging (p.1002) of cranial and spinal structures, of the whole body, and of the gastro-intestinal tract; it may also be employed for the evaluation of renal function.

Meglumine gadopentetate is used intravenously for cranial, spinal, and whole body imaging as a solution containing 469.01 mg (0.5 mmol) per mL. The usual dose in adults, children, and neonates is 0.2 mL (0.1 mmol) per kg body-weight intravenously. For cranial and spinal imaging, a further dose of 0.2 mL (0.1 mmol) per kg may be given within 30 minutes if necessary; in adults this second dose may be 0.4 mL (0.2 mmol) per kg. For whole body imaging in adults and children over 2 years, a dose of 0.4 mL (0.2 mmol) per kg may be needed in some cases to produce adequate contrast and in special circumstances a dose of 0.6 mL (0.3 mmol) per kg may be used in adults.

Meglumine gadopentetate is administered orally and rectally for gastro-intestinal imaging. A solution containing 9.38 mg per mL is diluted before use (100 mL with 900 mL of water) and doses in the range or 100 to 1000 mL of this diluted solution are used in adults depending upon the organ or tissue being investigated.

Preparations

USP 23: Gadopentetate Dimeglumine Injection.

Proprietary Preparations (details are given in Part 3)
Aust.: Magnevist; ***Canad.:*** Magnevist; ***Fr.:*** Magnevist; ***Ger.:*** Magnevist; ***Ital.:*** Magnevist; ***Neth.:*** Magnevist; ***Norw.:*** Magnevist; ***Spain:*** Magnevist; Magnograf; ***Swed.:*** Magnevist; ***Switz.:*** Magnevist; ***UK:*** Magnevist; ***USA:*** Magnevist.

Gadoteric Acid (6479-s)

Gadoteric Acid *(BAN, rINN).*

ZK-112004. Hydrogen [1,4,7,10-tetraazacyclododecane-1,4,7,10-tetraaceto(4−)]gadolinate(1−); Hydrogen [1,4,7,10-tetrakis(carboxylatomethyl)-1,4,7,10-tetra-azacyclododecane-κ⁴N]gadolinate(1−).

$C_{16}H_{25}GdN_4O_8$ = 558.6.

CAS — 72573-82-1.

Meglumine Gadoterate (17390-n)

Gadoteric acid is an ionic paramagnetic contrast medium with actions similar to those of gadopentetic acid (above). It is used, as meglumine gadoterate, for contrast enhancement in cranial, spinal, and hepatic magnetic resonance imaging (p.1002).

Meglumine gadoterate is available as a solution containing 377 mg (0.5 mmol) per mL. The usual dose in adults and children is 0.2 mL (0.1 mmol) per kg body-weight by intravenous injection.

Preparations

Proprietary Preparations (details are given in Part 3)
Belg.: Dotarem; ***Fr.:*** Dotarem; ***Ital.:*** Dotarem; ***Neth.:*** Dotarem; ***Swed.:*** Dotarem; ***Switz.:*** Dotarem.

Gadoteridol (15277-q)

Gadoteridol *(BAN, USAN, rINN).*

SQ-32692. (±)-[10-(2-Hydroxypropyl)-1,4,7,10-tetraazacyclododecane-1,4,7-triacetato(3−)]gadolinium.

$C_{17}H_{29}GdN_4O_7$ = 558.7.

CAS — 120066-54-8.

Adverse Effects and Precautions

As for Gadopentetic Acid, above.

Hypersensitivity. Vasovagal response and anaphylactoid reaction has been reported during intravenous use of gadoteridol.[1]

1. Shellock FG, *et al.* Adverse reaction to intravenous gadoteridol. *Radiology* 1993; **189:** 151–2.

Pharmacokinetics

About 94% of a dose of gadoteridol is excreted unchanged in the urine within 24 hours. An elimination half-life of about 1.57 hours has been reported.

Uses and Administration

Gadoteridol is a nonionic paramagnetic agent used for contrast enhancement in magnetic resonance imaging (p.1002) of cranial and spinal structures.

Gadoteridol is available as a solution containing 279.3 mg (0.5 mmol) per mL. The usual adult dose is 0.2 mL (0.1 mmol) per kg body-weight intravenously; an additional dose of up to 0.4 mL (0.2 mmol) per kg may be given approximately 30 minutes after the first if necessary.

Preparations

Proprietary Preparations (details are given in Part 3)
Canad.: Prohance; ***Ger.:*** Prohance; ***Ital.:*** Prohance; ***Neth.:*** Prohance; ***Swed.:*** Prohance†; ***Switz.:*** Prohance; ***UK:*** Prohance; ***USA:*** Prohance.

Galactose (12778-b)

D-Galactopyranose; D-Galactose; Galactosum.

$C_6H_{12}O_6$ = 180.2.

CAS — 59-23-4.

Pharmacopoeias. In *Eur.* (see p.viii).

A white, crystalline or finely granulated powder. Freely **soluble** or soluble in water; very slightly soluble in alcohol.

Galactose is a naturally occurring monosaccharide used as an ultrasound contrast medium (p.1002). It is administered intravenously or transcervically as a microbubble-microparticle suspension to enhance ultrasound images of the heart or female genital tract, respectively. Palmitic acid may be included to stabilise the microbubbles.

The clearance of galactose following intravenous administration has been used as a measure of liver function.

Study of the effect of concentration, pH, elevated temperature, and autoclaving on the stability of galactose solutions.[1]

1. Bhargava VO, *et al.* Stability of galactose in aqueous solutions. *Am J Hosp Pharm* 1989; **46:** 104–8.

Preparations

Proprietary Preparations (details are given in Part 3)
Aust.: Echovist; ***Fr.:*** Echovist; ***Ger.:*** Echovist; Levovist; ***Ital.:*** Levovist; ***Neth.:*** Echovist; Levovist; ***Norw.:*** Echovist; ***S.Afr.:*** Echovist; ***Swed.:*** Echovist; Levovist; ***Switz.:*** Echovist; Levovist; ***UK:*** Echovist; Levovist.

Iobitridol (17092-j)

Iobitridol *(BAN, rINN).*

N,N′-Bis(2,3-dihydroxypropyl)-5-[2-(hydroxymethyl)hydracrylamido]-2,4,6-triiodo-N,N′-dimethylisophthalamide; N,N′-Bis(2,3-dihydroxypropyl)-5-(3-hydroxy-2-hydroxymethylpropionamido)-2,4,6-tri-iodo-N,N′-dimethylisophthalamide.

$C_{20}H_{28}I_3N_3O_9$ = 835.2.

CAS — 136949-58-1.

Iobitridol is an iodinated nonionic monomeric contrast medium used parenterally for a wide range of radiographic diagnostic procedures (p.1002).

Preparations

Proprietary Preparations (details are given in Part 3)
Fr.: Xenetix; ***Ger.:*** Xenetix; ***Ital.:*** Xenetix; ***Neth.:*** Xenetix; ***Swed.:*** Xenetix; ***Switz.:*** Xenetix.

Iocetamic Acid (1561-s)

Iocetamic Acid *(BAN, USAN, pINN).*

DRC-1201; MP-620. N-Acetyl-N-(3-amino-2,4,6-tri-iodophenyl)-2-methyl-β-alanine; 2-[N-(3-Amino-2,4,6-tri-iodophenyl)acetamidomethyl]-propionic acid.

$C_{12}H_{13}I_3N_2O_3$ = 614.0.

CAS — 16034-77-8.

Pharmacopoeias. In *US.*

Iocetamic acid contains approximately 62% of I.

Adverse Effects and Precautions

As for Iopanoic Acid, p.1007.

Pharmacokinetics

Iocetamic acid is variably absorbed from the gastro-intestinal tract. It is conjugated in the liver with glucuronic acid, and is excreted in the bile and concentrated in the gallbladder; about 62% of a dose is excreted in the urine within 48 hours.

Uses and Administration

Iocetamic acid is an iodinated ionic monomeric contrast medium and is used mainly for cholecystography (p.1002). A dose of 3.0 or 4.5 g is given by mouth 10 to 15 hours before examination. If visualisation is unsuccessful a further dose may be given on the evening of the first examination, and the examination repeated on the following day.

Preparations

USP 23: Iocetamic Acid Tablets.

Proprietary Preparations (details are given in Part 3)
Ger.: Cholebrine†; ***Ital.:*** Colebrin†; ***Neth.:*** Cholebrine; ***Spain:*** Colebrina†; ***Swed.:*** Cholebrin; ***USA:*** Cholebrine.

Iodamide (1523-m)

Iodamide *(BAN, USAN, rINN).*

Ametriodinic Acid; B-4130; SH-926. α,5-Diacetamido-2,4,6-tri-iodo-*m*-toluic acid; 3-Acetamido-5-acetamidomethyl-2,4,6-tri-iodobenzoic acid.

$C_{12}H_{11}I_3N_2O_4$ = 627.9.

CAS — 440-58-4.

Pharmacopoeias. In *Jpn.*

Iodamide contains approximately 60.6% of I.

Meglumine Iodamide (1524-b)

Iodamide Meglumine *(USAN).* The N-methylglucamine salt of iodamide.

$C_{12}H_{11}I_3N_2O_4,C_7H_{17}NO_5$ = 823.2.

CAS — 18656-21-8.

Meglumine iodamide contains approximately 46.3% of I.

Sodium Iodamide (1562-w)

Iodamide Sodium.

$C_{12}H_{10}I_3N_2NaO_4$ = 649.9.

CAS — 10098-82-5.

Sodium iodamide contains approximately 58.6% of I.

Iodamide is an iodinated ionic monomeric contrast medium given by intravenous or local administration in a variety of radiographic diagnostic procedures (p.1002).

It is given as a 65% solution of the meglumine salt, as an approximately 53% concentration of the sodium salt, or as a mixture of the sodium and meglumine salts. The dose varies according to the procedure and route of administration. A 24% solution of the meglumine salt has been used for contrast enhancement in computed tomography of the brain.

Preparations

Proprietary Preparations (details are given in Part 3)
Aust.: Uromiro; ***Ger.:*** Uromiro†; ***Ital.:*** Isteropac ER; Opacist ER; Uromiro 24%; Uromiro 300 Sodico; Uromiro 340; ***Neth.:*** Urombrine†; ***Switz.:*** Isteropac; Opacist ER; Uromiro; ***UK:*** Sodium Uromiro†; Uromiro 300†; Uromiro 340†; ***USA:*** Renovue.

Iodipamide (1525-v)

Iodipamide *(BAN).*

Adipiodone *(rINN).* 3,3′-Adipoyldiaminobis(2,4,6-tri-iodobenzoic acid).

$C_{20}H_{14}I_6N_2O_6$ = 1139.8.

CAS — 606-17-7.

Pharmacopoeias. In *Chin., Jpn, Pol.,* and *US.*

A white, practically odourless, crystalline powder. Very slightly **soluble** in water, in chloroform, and in ether; slightly soluble in alcohol. Iodipamide contains approximately 66.8% of I.

Meglumine Iodipamide (1563-e)

Dimeglumine Iodipamide; Iodipamide Meglumine *(BANM).* The di(N-methylglucamine) salt of iodipamide.

$C_{20}H_{14}I_6N_2O_6,(C_7H_{17}NO_5)_2$ = 1530.2.

CAS — 3521-84-4.

Meglumine iodipamide contains approximately 49.8% of I. **Incompatibilities** have been reported with some antihistamines.

Adverse Effects, Treatment, and Precautions

See under the diatrizoates, p.1003. The incidence of adverse effects may be increased following rapid administration.

Iodipamide may show some uricosuric activity.

Effects on the liver. Of 149 patients who received the dose of iodipamide recommended by the manufacturer 13 developed elevated serum aspartate aminotransferase (SGOT) values; of 126 who received twice the dose, 23 developed elevated values.[1] Hepatotoxicity has also been reported[2-4] on isolated occasions in patients given meglumine iodipamide.

1. Scholz FJ, *et al.* Hepatotoxicity in cholangiography. *JAMA* 1974; **229:** 1724.
2. Stillman AE. Hepatotoxic reaction to iodipamide meglumine injection. *JAMA* 1974; **228:** 1420–1.
3. Sutherland LR, *et al.* Meglumine iodipamide (Cholografin) hepatotoxicity. *Ann Intern Med* 1977; **86:** 437–9.
4. Imoto S. Meglumine hepatotoxicity. *Ann Intern Med* 1978; **88:** 129.

Pharmacokinetics

Meglumine iodipamide is rapidly distributed in extracellular fluid following slow intravenous injection and is reported to be extensively bound to plasma protein. It appears in the bile ducts within about 10 to 15 minutes after injection, with peak opacity at about 40 to 80 minutes, and reaches the gallbladder by about 1 hour, peak opacification occurring after about 2 hours. About 80 to 95% is excreted unchanged in the faeces; small amounts are excreted unchanged in urine. A terminal half-life of about 2 hours has been reported.

Uses and Administration

Iodipamide is an iodinated ionic dimeric contrast medium that is used as its meglumine salt for cholecystography and cholangiography (p.1002).

It is administered by slow intravenous injection as a solution containing 52% of the meglumine salt over an average of 10 minutes. The usual dose of meglumine iodipamide used is about 10 g. Alternatively, up to 15 g of meglumine iodipamide may be given by infusion as a 6% or 10.3% solution over 30 to 60 minutes.

Preparations

BP 1998: Meglumine Iodipamide Injection;
USP 23: Iodipamide Meglumine Injection.

Proprietary Preparations (details are given in Part 3)
Belg.: Transbilix; ***Canad.:*** Cholografin; ***Fr.:*** Transbilix; ***USA:*** Cholografin.

Multi-ingredient: ***Canad.:*** Sinografin; ***USA:*** Sinografin.

Iodised Oil (1564-l)

Ethiodized Oil.

CAS — 8001-40-9 (iodised oil); 8008-53-5 (ethiodized oil injection).

An iodine addition product of the ethyl esters of the fatty acids obtained from poppy-seed oil. It contains about 35 to 39% of combined iodine.

Because of its solvent action on polystyrene, iodised oil injection should not be administered in plastic syringes made with polystyrene.

Adverse Effects and Precautions

The risk of hypersensitivity reactions or iodism is greater after the use of iodised oil than after water-soluble iodinated contrast media such as the diatrizoates. Pulmonary oil embolism is reported to be relatively frequent following lymphography but is not usually severe; however, hypotension, tachycardia, and pulmonary oedema and infarction may occur rarely and deaths have been reported in patients with pulmonary disease. Chemical pneumonitis, oedema, granuloma formation, and goitre have occurred.

Great care should be taken to avoid vascular structures, because of the danger of oil embolism; it should not therefore be used in areas affected by haemorrhage or local trauma. Iodised oil should be used with care in patients with thyroid dysfunction or a history of allergic reactions. The administration of iodised oil may interfere with thyroid-function tests for several months.

The use of oily contrast media for hysterosalpingography was considered dangerous and unnecessary.[1] Oil embolism and pelvic adhesions had occurred. In the presence of unsuspected pelvic tuberculosis there have been violent reactions with pelvic abscess formation. Several patients had been seen with bilateral tubal occlusion following an original investigation, using iodised oil, which had shown tubal patency.

1. Wright FW, Stallworthy J. Female sterility produced by investigation. *Br Med J* 1973; **3:** 632.

Pharmacokinetics

Iodised oil may persist in the body for several weeks or months after administration. It is only slowly absorbed from most body sites, although absorption from the peritoneal cavity is stated to be relatively rapid. It is reported to be slowly metabolised to fatty acids and iodine.

Uses and Administration

Iodised oil is an iodinated contrast medium which is used mainly for lymphography although it has also been used in various other radiographic diagnostic procedures (p.1002). It has been used for hysterosalpingography but water-soluble agents are preferred. The dose is dependent upon the procedure. The fluid injection of iodised oil is unsuitable for use in bronchography.

Because it is slowly metabolised to release iodine, iodised oil is used in the management of iodine deficiency (p.1494).

Malignant neoplasms. Injection of iodised oil into the hepatic artery is followed by selective and long-lasting retention within hepatic carcinomas and used with computed tomography is considered to be more sensitive than other imaging techniques.[1] The sensitivity of this method also enables the imaging of very small satellite nodules, which if undetected are responsible for high early rates of recurrence after resection. Iodised oil has also been used to provide targeted delivery of lipophilic antineoplastics or radioactive iodine to hepatic[1-3] or breast tumours.[4]

1. Anonymous. Lipiodol computed tomography for small hepatocellular carcinomas. *Lancet* 1991; **337:** 333–4.
2. Novell R, *et al.* Ablation of recurrent primary liver cancer using ^{131}I-lipiodol. *Postgrad Med J* 1991; **67:** 393–5.
3. Group d'Etude et de Traitement du Carcinome Hépatocellulaire. A comparison of Lipiodol chemoembolization and conservative treatment for unresectable hepatocellular carcinoma. *N Engl J Med* 1995; **332:** 1256–61.
4. Novell JR, *et al.* Targeted therapy for recurrent breast carcinoma with regional 'Lipiodol'/epirubicin infusion. *Lancet* 1990; **336:** 1383.

Preparations

BP 1998: Iodised Oil Fluid Injection;
USP 23: Ethiodized Oil Injection.

Proprietary Preparations (details are given in Part 3)
Aust.: Lipiodol; ***Austral.:*** Lipiodol; ***Belg.:*** Lipiodol; ***Fr.:*** Lipiodol; ***Ger.:*** Lipiodol; ***Ital.:*** Lipiodol; ***Neth.:*** Lipiodol; ***Norw.:*** Lipiodol; ***UK:*** Lipiodol; ***USA:*** Ethiodol.

Iodixanol (2807-d)

Iodixanol (*BAN, USAN, rINN*).

2-5410-3A. 5,5′-[(2-Hydroxytrimethylene)bis(acetylimino)]bis[*N,N*′-bis(2,3-dihydroxypropyl)-2,4,6-triiodoisophthalamide].

$C_{35}H_{44}I_6N_6O_{15} = 1550.2.$

CAS — 92339-11-2.

Iodixanol contains approximately 49.1% of I.

Adverse Effects, Treatment, and Precautions

See under the diatrizoates, p.1003.

Pharmacokinetics

Iodixanol is rapidly distributed into extracellular fluid following intravenous injection. It is not bound to plasma proteins. It is not metabolised and about 97% of a dose is excreted in the urine within 24 hours. A terminal elimination half-life of about 2 hours has been reported. Iodixanol is removed by dialysis.

Uses and Administration

Iodixanol is an iodinated nonionic dimeric contrast medium that is used for angiography and urography and for contrast enhancement during computed tomography (p.1002).

Iodixanol is given by injection as a solution usually containing between 150 and 320 mg of iodine per mL. The dose and strength used vary according to the procedure and route of injection.

References.

1. Spencer CM, Goa KL. Iodixanol: a review of its pharmacodynamic and pharmacokinetic properties and diagnostic use as an x-ray contrast medium. *Drugs* 1996; **52:** 899–927.

Preparations

Proprietary Preparations (details are given in Part 3)
Aust.: Visipaque; ***Canad.:*** Visipaque; ***Fr.:*** Visipaque; ***Ger.:*** Visipaque; ***Ital.:*** Visipaque; ***Neth.:*** Visipaque; ***Norw.:*** Visipaque; ***Spain:*** Visipaque; ***Swed.:*** Visipaque; ***Switz.:*** Visipaque; ***UK:*** Visipaque; ***USA:*** Visipaque.

Iodoxamic Acid (1527-q)

Iodoxamic Acid (*BAN, USAN, rINN*).

B-10610; SQ-21982. 3,3′-(4,7,10,13-Tetraoxahexadecanedioyldiamino)bis(2,4,6-tri-iodobenzoic acid).

$C_{26}H_{26}I_6N_2O_{10} = 1287.9.$

CAS — 31127-82-9.

Iodoxamic acid contains approximately 59.1% of I.

Meglumine Iodoxamate (1567-z)

Meglumine Iodoxamate (*BANM*).

Dimeglumine Iodoxamate; Iodoxamate Meglumine (*USAN*). The di(*N*-methylglucamine) salt of iodoxamic acid.

$C_{26}H_{26}I_6N_2O_{10},(C_7H_{17}NO_5)_2 = 1678.3.$

CAS — 51764-33-1.

Meglumine iodoxamate contains approximately 45.4% of I.

Iodoxamic acid is an iodinated ionic dimeric contrast medium that has been used as the meglumine salt for cholecystography and cholangiography (p.1002).

Preparations

Proprietary Preparations (details are given in Part 3)
Aust.: Endobil; ***Ger.:*** Endomirabil†; ***Irl.:*** Endobil; ***Ital.:*** Endobil†; ***Neth.:*** Endobil†; ***Switz.:*** Endobil†; ***UK:*** Endobil†.

Ioglicic Acid (10491-t)

Ioglicic Acid (*BAN, USAN, rINN*).

SH-H-200-AB. 5-Acetamido-2,4,6-tri-iodo-*N*-(methylcarbamoylmethyl)isophthalamic acid.

$C_{13}H_{12}I_3N_3O_5 = 671.0.$

CAS — 49755-67-1.

Ioglicic acid contains approximately 56.7% of I.

Meglumine Ioglicate (11450-a)

Ioglicate Meglumine. The *N*-methylglucamine salt of ioglicic acid.

$C_{13}H_{12}I_3N_3O_5,C_7H_{17}NO_5 = 866.2.$

Meglumine ioglicate contains approximately 44.0% of I.

Sodium Ioglicate (12855-n)

Ioglicate Sodium.

$C_{13}H_{11}I_3N_3NaO_5 = 692.9.$

Sodium ioglicate contains approximately 54.9% of I.

Ioglicic acid is an iodinated ionic monomeric contrast medium that has been given by injection, as the meglumine and sodium salts, for urography, angiography, and related procedures (p.1002).

Preparations

Proprietary Preparations (details are given in Part 3)
Aust.: Rayvist 350; ***Ger.:*** Rayvist†; ***Ital.:*** Rayvist†; ***Switz.:*** Rayvist.

Iohexol (12856-h)

Iohexol (*BAN, USAN, rINN*).

Iohexolum; Win-39424. *N,N*′-Bis(2,3-dihydroxypropyl)-5-[*N*-(2,3-dihydroxypropyl)acetamido]-2,4,6-tri-iodoisophthalamide.

$C_{19}H_{26}I_3N_3O_9 = 821.1.$

CAS — 66108-95-0.

Pharmacopoeias. In *Eur.* (see p.viii), *Int.*, and *US.*

Iohexol contains approximately 46.4% of I.

A white to off-white, hygroscopic, odourless powder. Very **soluble** in water; freely or very soluble in methyl alcohol; practically insoluble in ether, in chloroform, and in dichloromethane. **Store** in airtight containers. **Protect** from light.

Adverse Effects and Precautions

See under the diatrizoates, p.1003.

Additional neurological adverse effects may occur when nonionic iodinated contrast media such as iohexol are used for myelography. These include severe headache, backache, neck stiffness, dizziness, and leg or sciatic-type pain. Convulsions, aseptic meningitis, and mild and transitory perceptual aberrations, such as visual and speech disturbances, and confusion, may occur occasionally; rarely, more severe mental disturbances have occurred. Urinary retention has also been reported.

Effects on the nervous system. Encephalopathy which developed in a 48-year-old man with sciatica within 9 hours of iohexol administration for lumbar myelography had largely resolved 48 hours after the myelogram; complete resolution took 4 days.[1] However, recovery was slow in a patient who developed paraplegia and areflexia in the legs after a similar procedure. Five months later the patient still complained of paraesthesia in her legs and could not stand without support.[2]

1. Donaghy M, *et al.* Encephalopathy after iohexol myelography. *Lancet* 1985; **ii:** 887.
2. Noda K, *et al.* Prolonged paraplegia after iohexol myelography. *Lancet* 1991; **337:** 681.

Pharmacokinetics

Following intravascular administration, 90% or more of iohexol is eliminated unchanged in the urine within 24 hours. An elimination half-life of approximately 2 hours in patients with normal renal function has been reported. Protein binding in blood is reported to be very low.

Uses and Administration

Iohexol is an iodinated nonionic monomeric contrast medium that is used by injection and locally for a wide range of diagnostic procedures including myelography, angiography, urography, arthrography, and visualisation of the gastro-intestinal tract and body cavities (p.1002). Iohexol is also used to produce contrast enhancement during computed tomography.

Iohexol is usually available as solutions containing 30.2 to 75.5% of iohexol (equivalent to 140 to 350 mg of iodine per mL) and the dose and strength used vary according to the procedure and the route of administration.

Preparations

USP 23: Iohexol Injection.

Proprietary Preparations (details are given in Part 3)
Aust.: Omnipaque; ***Austral.:*** Omnipaque; ***Belg.:*** Omnipaque; ***Canad.:*** Omnipaque; ***Fr.:*** Omnipaque; ***Ger.:*** Accupaque; Omnipaque; ***Ital.:*** Omnipaque; ***Neth.:*** Omnipaque†; ***Norw.:*** Omnipaque; ***Spain:*** Omnigraf; Omnitrast; ***Swed.:*** Omnipaque; ***Switz.:*** Omnipaque; ***UK:*** Omnipaque; ***USA:*** Omnipaque.

Iomeprol (2865-w)

Iomeprol (*BAN, USAN, rINN*).

N,N′-Bis(2,3-dihydroxypropyl)-2,4,6-triiodo-5-(*N*-methylglycolamido)-isophthalamide.

$C_{17}H_{22}I_3N_3O_8 = 777.1.$

CAS — 78649-41-9.

Iomeprol contains approximately 49% of I.

Iomeprol is an iodinated nonionic monomeric contrast medium that is used for a wide range of radiographic procedures (p.1002).

Preparations

Proprietary Preparations (details are given in Part 3)
Aust.: Iomeron; ***Belg.:*** Iomeron; ***Fr.:*** Iomeron; ***Ger.:*** Imeron; ***Ital.:*** Iomeron; ***Jpn:*** Iomeron; ***Neth.:*** Iomeron; ***Spain:*** Iomeron; ***Swed.:*** Iomeron.

Iopamidol (14037-g)

Iopamidol *(BAN, USAN, rINN).*

B-15000; Iopamidolum; SQ-13396. *N,N'*-Bis[2-hydroxy-1-(hydroxymethyl)ethyl]-2,4,6-tri-iodo-5-lactamidoisophthalamide.

$C_{17}H_{22}I_3N_3O_8$ = 777.1.

CAS — 60166-93-0; 62883-00-5.

Pharmacopoeias. In *Eur.* (see p.viii) and *US.*

Iopamidol contains approximately 49% of I. A white to off-white, practically odourless powder. Freely or very **soluble** in water; very slightly to sparingly soluble in methyl alcohol; practically insoluble in alcohol, in chloroform, and in dichloromethane. **Protect** from light.

Adverse Effects and Precautions

As for the diatrizoates, p.1003. For the adverse effects relating to the use of iopamidol for myelography, see under Iohexol, p.1006.

Effects on the nervous system. Reports of serious neurological sequelae to lumbar myelography with iopamidol.

1. Wallers K, *et al.* Severe meningeal irritation after intrathecal injection of iopamidol. *Br Med J* 1985; **291:** 1688.
2. Robinson C, Fon G. Adverse reaction to iopamidol. *Med J Aust* 1986; **144:** 553.
3. Bell JA, McIlwaine GG. Postmyelographic lateral rectus palsy associated with iopamidol. *Br Med J* 1990; **300**: 1343–4.
4. Mallat Z, *et al.* Aseptic meningoencephalitis after iopamidol myelography. *Lancet* 1991; **338**: 252.
5. Bain PG, *et al.* Paraplegia after iopamidol myelography. *Lancet* 1991; **338**: 252–3.

Uses and Administration

Iopamidol is an iodinated nonionic monomeric contrast medium used by injection for a variety of radiographic procedures including angiography, arthrography, myelography, and urography (p.1002). Iopamidol is also used for contrast enhancement during computed tomography.

Iopamidol is usually available as solutions containing 26.1 to 75.5% of iopamidol (equivalent to 128 to 370 mg of iodine per mL) and the dose and strength used vary according to the procedure and route of administration.

Iopamidol has also been administered orally or by enema for visualisation of the gastro-intestinal tract.

Preparations

USP 23: Iopamidol Injection.

Proprietary Preparations (details are given in Part 3)
Aust.: Gastromiro; Jopamiro; ***Canad.:*** Isovue; ***Fr.:*** Iopamiron; ***Ger.:*** Iopamiro†; Solutrast; ***Irl.:*** Gastromiro; Niopam; ***Ital.:*** Gastromiro; Iopamiro; ***Neth.:*** Iopamiro†; ***Norw.:*** Iopamiro; ***Spain:*** Iopamiro; ***Swed.:*** Iopamiro; ***Switz.:*** Iopamiro; ***UK:*** Niopam; ***USA:*** Isovue.

Iopanoic Acid (1570-w)

Iopanoic Acid *(BAN, rINN).*

Acidum Iopanoicum; Iodopanoic Acid. 2-(3-Amino-2,4,6-tri-iodobenzyl)butyric acid.

$C_{11}H_{12}I_3NO_2$ = 570.9.

CAS — 96-83-3.

Pharmacopoeias. In *Chin., Eur.* (see p.viii), *Int., Jpn,* and *US.*

A white to yellowish white powder, with a faint characteristic odour. It contains approximately 66.7% of I. Practically **insoluble** in water; soluble in alcohol, in chloroform, in ether, in methyl alcohol, and in aqueous solutions of alkali hydroxides and carbonates. **Store** in airtight containers. Protect from light.

Adverse Effects

Gastro-intestinal disturbances such as nausea, vomiting, abdominal cramp, and diarrhoea are reported to occur in up to 40% of patients but are usually mild and transient. Mild stinging or burning on micturition, and skin rashes and flushing have occurred occasionally. Acute renal failure, thrombocytopenia, and hypersensitivity reactions have been reported.

Iopanoic acid has potent uricosuric and anticholinesterase effects.

Precautions

Iopanoic acid is contra-indicated in severe hepatic or renal disease; doses higher than 3 g should not be given to patients with renal impairment. It should not be used in the presence of acute gastro-intestinal disorders that may impair absorption. It should be used with caution in patients with a history of hypersensitivity to iodine or to other contrast media, severe hyperthyroidism, hyperuricaemia, or cholangitis. In the light of its cholinergic action premedication with atropine has been suggested in some countries for patients with coronary heart disease. The administration of iodine-containing contrast media may interfere with thyroid-function tests and with some blood and urine tests.

Pharmacokinetics

Iopanoic acid is variably absorbed from the gastro-intestinal tract and is strongly and extensively bound to plasma protein. It is conjugated in the liver to the glucuronide and excreted largely in the bile and the remainder (about one-third of the dose) in the urine. It appears in the gallbladder about 4 hours after a dose is taken and maximum concentrations occur after about 17 hours. About 50% of a dose is excreted in 24 hours, but elevated protein-bound iodine concentrations may persist for several months.

Uses and Administration

Iopanoic acid is an iodinated ionic monomeric contrast medium used for cholecystography and cholangiography (p.1002). Usual doses of 3 g are given by mouth with plenty of water about 10 to 14 hours before X-ray examination. For repeat examinations an additional 3 g may be administered on the same day. Alternatively, repeat examination may be carried out after an interval of 5 to 7 days with a single 6 g dose. No more than 6 g of iopanoic acid should be taken during any 24-hour period, and doses over 3 g should be avoided in renal impairment. Adequate visualisation is achieved in the majority of patients with a single dose.

For the visualisation of biliary calculi 1 g may be given three times daily after relatively fat-free meals for 4 days and X-ray examination carried out on the morning of the 5th day in the fasting patient.

Reviews.

1. Berk RN, *et al.* Oral cholecystography with iopanoic acid. *N Engl J Med* 1974; **290:** 204–10.

Preparations

BP 1998: Iopanoic Acid Tablets;
USP 23: Iopanoic Acid Tablets.

Proprietary Preparations (details are given in Part 3)
Austral.: Telepaque; ***Belg.:*** Telepaque†; ***Canad.:*** Telepaque; ***Irl.:*** Telepaque†; ***Ital.:*** Cistobil; ***Spain:*** Biliopaco†; Colegraf; Neocontrast; ***Switz.:*** Cistobil; ***UK:*** Telepaque; ***USA:*** Telepaque.

Iopentol (2172-b)

Iopentol *(BAN, USAN, rINN).*

Compound 5411. *N,N'*-Bis(2,3-dihydroxypropyl)-5-[*N*-(2-hydroxy-3-methoxypropyl)acetamido]-2,4,6-tri-iodoisophthalamide.

$C_{20}H_{28}I_3N_3O_9$ = 835.2.

CAS — 89797-00-2.

Iopentol contains approximately 45.6% of I.

Iopentol is an iodinated nonionic monomeric contrast medium that is used for a variety of radiographic procedures including enhancement of computed tomography (p.1002).

Preparations

Proprietary Preparations (details are given in Part 3)
Aust.: Imagopaque; ***Fr.:*** Ivepaque; ***Ger.:*** Imagopaque; ***Ital.:*** Imagopaque; ***Norw.:*** Imagopaque; ***Spain:*** Imagopaque; ***Switz.:*** Imagopaque.

Iophendylate (1571-e)

Iophendylate *(BAN).*

Iofendylate *(rINN)*; Ethyl Iodophenylundecanoate; Ethyl Iodophenylundecylate; Iodophendylate. A mixture of stereoisomers of ethyl 10-(4-iodophenyl)undecanoate.

$C_{19}H_{29}IO_2$ = 416.3.

CAS — 99-79-6; 1320-11-2.

Pharmacopoeias. In *Chin.* and *US.*

A colourless to pale yellow viscous liquid, odourless or with a faint ethereal odour, darkening on prolonged exposure to air, and containing about 30.5% of I. Very slightly **soluble** in water; freely soluble in alcohol, in chloroform, and in ether. **Store** in airtight containers. Protect from light.

Polystyrene was soluble in iophendylate and syringes made from polystyrene were rapidly attacked.[1] Syringes made from polypropylene appeared to be unaffected.

1. Irving JD, Reynolds PV. Disposable syringe danger. *Lancet* 1966; **i:** 362.

Iophendylate is an iodinated ionic monomeric contrast medium that was formerly used mainly for myelography (p.1002); it was also formerly used for examination of the third and fourth ventricles, and to visualise the fetus in the amniotic sac prior to intra-uterine blood transfusion. However, serious side-effects including allergy, arachnoiditis, and aseptic meningitis have occurred with its use and it has been superseded by nonionic media such as iohexol (p.1006).

Adverse effects associated with iophendylate have included chronic urticaria and intermittent anaphylaxis in a man who underwent myelography 17 years earlier.[1] After removal of about 8 mL of iophendylate from the spinal canal the patient remained almost totally asymptomatic. Focal seizures, which developed in a 30-year-old woman 4 months after a myelogram, were believed to be associated with retention of a preparation of iophendylate.[2]

1. Lieberman P, *et al.* Chronic urticaria and intermittent anaphylaxis. *JAMA* 1976; **236:** 1495–7.
2. Greenberg MK, Vance SC. Focal seizure disorder complicating iodophendylate myelography. *Lancet* 1980; **i:** 312–13.

Preparations

BP 1998: Iofendylate Injection;
USP 23: Iophendylate Injection.

Iopodic Acid (10912-n)

Ipodic Acid. 3-(3-Dimethylaminomethyleneamino-2,4,6-tri-iodophenyl)propionic acid.

$C_{12}H_{13}I_3N_2O_2$ = 598.0.

CAS — 5587-89-3.

Calcium Iopodate (1553-s)

Calcium Ipodate; Ipodate Calcium. Calcium 3-(3-dimethylaminomethyleneamino-2,4,6-tri-iodophenyl)propionate.

$(C_{12}H_{12}I_3N_2O_2)_2Ca$ = 1234.0.

CAS — 1151-11-7.

Pharmacopoeias. In *US.*

A fine, white or off-white, odourless, crystalline powder, containing approximately 61.7% of I. Slightly **soluble** in water, in alcohol, and in methyl alcohol; soluble 1 in 2.6 of chloroform. **Store** in airtight containers.

Sodium Iopodate (1585-k)

Sodium Iopodate *(rINN).*

Ipodate Sodium *(USAN)*; NSC-106962; Sodium Ipodate *(BAN)*. Sodium 3-(3-dimethylaminomethyleneamino-2,4,6-tri-iodophenyl)propionate.

$C_{12}H_{12}I_3N_2NaO_2$ = 619.9.

CAS — 1221-56-3.

Pharmacopoeias. In *Jpn* and *US.*

A fine, white or off-white, odourless, crystalline powder, containing approximately 61.4% of I. **Soluble** 1 in less than 1 of water, 1 in 2 of alcohol, 1 in 2 of dimethylacetamide, and 1 in 3.5 of dimethylformamide and of dimethyl sulphoxide; very slightly soluble in chloroform; freely soluble in methyl alcohol. **Store** in airtight containers.

Adverse Effects and Precautions

As for Iopanoic Acid, above. Effects on the gastro-intestinal tract may be less with iopodate salts than with iopanoic acid.

Pharmacokinetics

The iopodate salts are absorbed from the gastro-intestinal tract following oral or rectal administration, and almost completely metabolised. Protein binding to plasma proteins is reported to be high. Elimination is by the renal and hepatic routes; about half of an oral dose is stated to be excreted in the urine within 24 hours.

Uses and Administration

Iopodic acid is an iodinated ionic monomeric contrast medium given by mouth as the calcium and sodium salts for cholecystography and cholangiography (p.1002). Calcium iopodate is administered as a freshly-prepared suspension; the sodium salt is normally given as capsules. Following administration, optimal visualisation of the bile ducts usually occurs after 1 to 3 hours and that of the gallbladder after 10 to 12 hours.

For routine cholecystography they are given by mouth in a dose of 3 g of either salt in the evening, 10 to 12 hours before the examination; in fractionated oral cholecystography this may be followed by a second similar dose the following day, 3 hours before examination. In rapid cholecystography a single dose of 3 or 6 g may be given.

For cholangiography, a single dose of 6 g may be given.

Preparations

USP 23: Ipodate Calcium for Oral Suspension; Ipodate Sodium Capsules.

Proprietary Preparations (details are given in Part 3)
Aust.: Biloptin; ***Canad.:*** Oragrafin†; ***Fr.:*** Solubiloptine†; ***Ger.:*** Biloptin; Solu-Biloptin†; ***Ital.:*** Biloptin†; ***S.Afr.:*** Biloptin; ***Spain:*** Solu-Biloptin†; ***Switz.:*** Biloptin; ***UK:*** Biloptin; Solu-Biloptin; ***USA:*** Bilivist; Oragrafin.

Iopromide (18651-j)

Iopromide *(BAN, USAN, rINN).*

ZK-35760. *N,N'*-Bis(2,3-dihydroxypropyl)-2,4,6-tri-iodo-5-(2-methoxyacetamido)-*N*-methylisophthalamide.

$C_{18}H_{24}I_3N_3O_8$ = 791.1.

CAS — 73334-07-3.

Iopromide contains approximately 48.1% of I.

Adverse Effects and Precautions

See under the diatrizoates, p.1003.

Uses and Administration

Iopromide is an iodinated nonionic monomeric contrast medium that is used for angiography, urography, arthrography, and the visualisation of body cavities (p.1002). It is also used for contrast enhancement during computed tomography, and to check functioning of a dialysis shunt.

Iopromide is administered locally and by injection. It is usually available as solutions containing 31.2 to 76.9% of iopromide (equivalent to 150 to 370 mg of iodine per mL) and the dose and strength used vary according to the procedure and route of administration.

Preparations

Proprietary Preparations (details are given in Part 3)
Aust.: Ultravist; ***Austral.:*** Ultravist; ***Belg.:*** Ultravist; ***Canad.:*** Ultravist; ***Fr.:*** Ultravist; ***Ger.:*** Ultravist; ***Ital.:*** Ultravist; ***Neth.:*** Ultravist; ***Norw.:*** Ultravist; ***S.Afr.:*** Ultravist; ***Spain:*** Clarograf; Ultravist; ***Swed.:*** Ultravist; ***Switz.:*** Ultravist; ***UK:*** Ultravist; ***USA:*** Ultravist.

Iopydol (1573-y)

Iopydol *(BAN, USAN)*.

1-(2,3-Dihydroxypropyl)-3,5-di-iodo-4-pyridone.

$C_8H_9I_2NO_3$ = 421.0.

CAS — 5579-92-0.

Iopydol contains approximately 60.3% of I.

Iopydol is an iodinated contrast medium used in conjunction with iopydone for bronchography (p.1002).

Preparations

Proprietary Preparations (details are given in Part 3)
Multi-ingredient: ***Belg.:*** Hytrast†; ***Canad.:*** Hytrast†; ***Fr.:*** Hytrast; ***Ger.:*** Hytrast; ***Ital.:*** Hytrast†; ***Neth.:*** Hytrast†.

Iopydone (1574-j)

Iopydone *(BAN, USAN)*.

3,5-Di-iodo-4-pyridone.

$C_5H_3I_2NO$ = 346.9.

CAS — 5579-93-1.

Iopydone contains approximately 73.2% of I.

Iopydone is an iodinated contrast medium used in conjunction with iopydol for bronchography (p.1002).

Preparations

Proprietary Preparations (details are given in Part 3)
Multi-ingredient: ***Belg.:*** Hytrast†; ***Canad.:*** Hytrast†; ***Fr.:*** Hytrast; ***Ger.:*** Hytrast; ***Ital.:*** Hytrast†; ***Neth.:*** Hytrast†.

Iothalamic Acid (1530-h)

Iothalamic Acid *(BAN, USAN)*.

Iotalamic Acid *(rINN)*; Acidum Iotalamicum; Methalamic Acid; MI-216. 5-Acetamido-2,4,6-tri-iodo-*N*-methylisophthalamic acid.

$C_{11}H_9I_3N_2O_4$ = 613.9.

CAS — 2276-90-6.

Pharmacopoeias. In *Chin., Eur.* (see p.viii), *Jpn,* and *US.*

A white or almost white, odourless powder. Slightly **soluble** in water and in alcohol; practically insoluble in ether; dissolves in dilute solutions of alkali hydroxides. It contains approximately 62% of I.
Protect from light.

Meglumine Iothalamate (1531-m)

Meglumine Iothalamate *(BANM)*.

Iothalamate Meglumine. The *N*-methylglucamine salt of iothalamic acid.

$C_{11}H_9I_3N_2O_4,C_7H_{17}NO_5$ = 809.1.

CAS — 13087-53-1.

Meglumine iothalamate contains approximately 47.1% of I.

Sodium Iothalamate (1575-z)

Sodium Iothalamate *(BANM)*.

Iothalamate Sodium.

$C_{11}H_8I_3N_2NaO_4$ = 635.9.

CAS — 17692-74-9; 1225-20-3.

Sodium iothalamate contains approximately 59.9% of I.

Adverse Effects, Treatment, and Precautions

As for the diatrizoates, p.1003.

In 40 patients who underwent phlebography with 60% meglumine iothalamate minor adverse reactions were common despite the use of saline flushing and muscle contraction to clear the veins after examination.[1] The commonest effect was pain at the site of injection, or in the calf and foot; 15 patients of those who had pain in the calf or foot were found to have venous thrombosis. Serious complications to phlebography appear to be rare but can cause serious morbidity; examination of 200 case notes and a retrospective study involving 3060 patients revealed 4 cases of necrosis in the skin of the foot and gangrene of the foot in 2.

1. Thomas ML, MacDonald LM. Complications of ascending phlebography of the leg. *Br Med J* 1978; **ii:** 317–18.

Pharmacokinetics

Following intravascular administration the iothalamates are rapidly distributed; suitable concentrations for urography reach the urinary tract within 3 to 8 minutes of a bolus intravenous injection. Protein binding of both the sodium and meglumine salts is reported to be low. The iothalamates are eliminated by the kidneys. In patients with normal renal function more than 90% of the dose injected is excreted in urine within 24 hours. Small amounts are reported to be excreted via the bile in the faeces. The iothalamates are removed by peritoneal dialysis and haemodialysis.

Uses and Administration

Iothalamic acid is an iodinated ionic monomeric contrast medium with actions similar to the diatrizoates (p.1004). It is given locally and by injection for a wide range of radiographic procedures, including angiography, arthrography, cholangiography, urography, and for contrast enhancement during computed tomography (p.1002); oral or rectal administration has been used to visualise the gastro-intestinal tract.

Iothalamic acid is usually available as solutions containing up to 80% of sodium iothalamate or up to 60% of meglumine iothalamate. The dose and strength used vary according to the procedure and route of administration. A mixture of the two salts is often preferred to minimise side-effects.

Iothalamates are not suitable for injection into the subarachnoid space.

Preparations

BP 1998: Meglumine Iotalamate Injection; Sodium Iotalamate Injection;
USP 23: Iothalamate Meglumine and Iothalamate Sodium Injection; Iothalamate Meglumine Injection; Iothalamate Sodium I 125 Injection; Iothalamate Sodium Injection.

Proprietary Preparations (details are given in Part 3)
Austral.: Cardio-Conray†; Conray 280; Conray 325†; Conray 420; Gastro-Conray†; ***Belg.:*** Contrix; ***Canad.:*** Conray; Cysto-Conray; ***Fr.:*** Contrix†; ***Ger.:*** Conray 30†; Conray 60†; Conray 70†; Conray 80†; Conray EV†; Conray FL†; ***Ital.:*** Angio-Conray; Conray 24%; Conray 36%; Conray 400; Conray 60%; ***Spain:*** Sombril†; Vascoray†; ***UK:*** Conray 280; Conray 325; Conray 420; ***USA:*** Angio-Conray; Conray; Cysto-Conray; Vascoray.

Iotrolan (3807-p)

Iotrolan *(BAN, USAN, rINN)*.

Iotrol; Iotrolum; ZK-39482. *N,N',N'',N'''*-Tetrakis(2,3-dihydroxy-1-hydroxymethylpropyl)-2,2',4,4',6,6'-hexaiodo-5,5'-(*N,N'*-dimethylmalonyldi-imino)di-isophthalamide.

$C_{37}H_{48}I_6N_6O_{18}$ = 1626.2.

CAS — 79770-24-4.

Iotrolan contains approximately 46.8% of I.

Adverse Effects and Precautions

As for the diatrizoates, p.1003. For the adverse effects relating to the use of iotrolan for myelography, see under Iohexol, p.1006.

Uses and Administration

Iotrolan is an iodinated nonionic dimeric contrast medium that is given locally or by injection for a wide range of diagnostic procedures, including myelography, lymphography, arthrography, hysterosalpingography, cholangiopancreatography, and for visualisation of the mammary ducts and the gastro-intestinal tract (p.1002). It is also used for contrast enhancement during computed tomography.

Iotrolan is usually available as solutions containing 51.3% or 64.1% of iotrolan (equivalent to 240 mg or 300 mg of iodine per mL, respectively) and the dose and strength used vary according to the procedure and route of administration.

Preparations

Proprietary Preparations (details are given in Part 3)
Aust.: Isovist; ***Canad.:*** Osmovist; ***Ger.:*** Isovist; ***Ital.:*** Isovist; ***Neth.:*** Isovist; ***Norw.:*** Isovist; ***S.Afr.:*** Isovist; ***Swed.:*** Isovist; ***Switz.:*** Isovist; ***UK:*** Isovist; ***USA:*** Osmovist†.

Iotroxic Acid (12859-v)

Iotroxic Acid *(BAN, USAN, rINN)*.

SH-213AB. 3,3'-(3,6,9-Trioxaundecanedioyldi-imino)bis(2,4,6-tri-iodobenzoic acid).

$C_{22}H_{18}I_6N_2O_9$ = 1215.8.

CAS — 51022-74-3.

Pharmacopoeias. In *Int.* and *Jpn.*

Iotroxic acid contains approximately 62.6% of I.

Meglumine Iotroxate (12860-r)

Meglumine Iotroxate *(BANM)*.

Dimeglumine Iotroxate; Iotroxate Meglumine; Meglumine Iotroxinate. The di(*N*-methylglucamine)salt of iotroxic acid.

$C_{22}H_{18}I_6N_2O_9,2C_7H_{17}NO_5$ = 1606.2.

CAS — 68890-05-1.

Meglumine iotroxate contains approximately 47.4% of I.

Adverse Effects, Treatment, and Precautions

See under the diatrizoates, p.1003.

Uses and Administration

Iotroxic acid is an iodinated ionic dimeric contrast medium that is used intravenously as the meglumine salt for cholecystography and cholangiography (p.1002).

Meglumine iotroxate is given by intravenous infusion in a dose equivalent to about 5 g of iodine usually as a 10.5% solution. The infusion should be administered over not less than 15 minutes.

Preparations

Proprietary Preparations (details are given in Part 3)
Aust.: Biliscopin; ***Ger.:*** Biliscopin; ***Ital.:*** Chologram†; ***Neth.:*** Biliscopin†; ***Spain:*** Bilisegrol; ***Swed.:*** Biliscopin; ***Switz.:*** Biliscopin; ***UK:*** Biliscopin.

Ioversol (2494-f)

Ioversol *(BAN, USAN, rINN)*.

MP-328. *N,N'*-Bis(2,3-dihydroxypropyl)-5-[*N*-(2-hydroxyethyl)glycolamido]-2,4,6-tri-iodoisophthalamide.

$C_{18}H_{24}I_3N_3O_9$ = 807.1.

CAS — 87771-40-2.

Pharmacopoeias. In *US.*

Ioversol contains approximately 47.2% of I.

Adverse Effects, Treatment, and Precautions

See under the diatrizoates, p.1003.

Uses and Administration

Ioversol is an iodinated nonionic monomeric contrast medium used by injection in angiography and urography (p.1002). It is also used for contrast enhancement during computed tomography. It is usually available as a solution containing 34 to 74% (equivalent to 160 to 350 mg of iodine per mL). The dose and strength used vary according to the procedure and route of administration.

Preparations

USP 23: Ioversol Injection.

Proprietary Preparations (details are given in Part 3)
Aust.: Optiray; ***Austral.:*** Optiray; ***Belg.:*** Optiray; ***Canad.:*** Optiray; ***Fr.:*** Optiray; ***Ital.:*** Optiray; ***Spain:*** Optiray; ***Swed.:*** Optiray†; ***Switz.:*** Optiray; ***USA:*** Optiray.

Ioxaglic Acid (12861-f)

Ioxaglic Acid *(BAN, USAN, rINN)*.

P-286. *N*-(2-Hydroxyethyl)-2,4,6-tri-iodo-5-[2',4',6'-tri-iodo-3'-(*N*-methylacetamido)-5'-methylcarbamoylhippuramido]isophthalamic acid.

$C_{24}H_{21}I_6N_5O_8$ = 1268.9.

CAS — 59017-64-0.

Pharmacopoeias. In *Fr.* and *US.*

Ioxaglic acid contains approximately 60% of I.

Meglumine Ioxaglate (15337-m)

Meglumine Ioxaglate *(BANM)*.

Ioxaglate Meglumine *(USAN)*; MP-302 (with sodium ioxaglate). The *N*-methylglucamine salt of ioxaglic acid.

$C_{24}H_{21}I_6N_5O_8,C_7H_{17}NO_5$ = 1464.1.

CAS — 59018-13-2.

Meglumine ioxaglate contains approximately 52% of I.

Sodium Ioxaglate (15338-b)

Sodium Ioxaglate *(BANM)*.

Ioxaglate Sodium *(USAN)*; MP-302 (with meglumine ioxaglate).

$C_{24}H_{20}I_6N_5NaO_8$ = 1290.9.

CAS — 67992-58-9.

Sodium ioxaglate contains approximately 59% of I.

Adverse Effects, Treatment, and Precautions

See under the diatrizoates, p.1003.

Pharmacokinetics

Following intravascular administration, ioxaglates are rapidly distributed throughout the extracellular fluid. Protein binding is reported to be very low. About 90% of a dose is excreted unchanged in the urine within 24 hours. An elimination half-life of about 90 minutes has been reported, which may be prolonged in renal impairment. Ioxaglates cross the placenta and are distributed into breast milk. They are removed by haemodialysis and peritoneal dialysis.

Uses and Administration

Ioxaglic acid is an iodinated ionic dimeric contrast medium given locally and by injection as a combined solution of its meglumine and sodium salts for a wide range of diagnostic procedures, including angiography, arthrography, hysterosalpingography, and urography (p.1002). It is also used for contrast enhancement during computed tomography.

The dose and strength used depend upon the procedure and route of administration. Commonly used solutions contain 39.30% of meglumine ioxaglate and 19.65% of sodium ioxaglate (equivalent to 320 mg of iodine per mL) or 24.56% of meglumine ioxaglate and 12.28% of sodium ioxaglate (equivalent to 200 mg of iodine per mL).

Ioxaglate is unsuitable for myelography and should not be given by the subarachnoid or epidural routes.

Preparations

USP 23: Ioxaglate Meglumine and Ioxaglate Sodium Injection.

Proprietary Preparations (details are given in Part 3)
Aust.: Hexabrix; ***Austral.:*** Hexabrix; ***Belg.:*** Hexabrix; ***Canad.:*** Hexabrix; ***Fr.:*** Hexabrix; ***Ger.:*** Hexabrix; ***Ital.:*** Hexabrix; ***Neth.:*** Hexabrix; ***Norw.:*** Hexabrix; ***Spain:*** Hexabrix; ***Swed.:*** Hexabrix; ***Switz.:*** Hexabrix; ***UK:*** Hexabrix; ***USA:*** Hexabrix.

Ioxilan (6484-g)

Ioxilan *(USAN, rINN).*

N-(2,3-Dihydroxypropyl)-5-[*N*-(2,3-dihydroxypropyl)acetamido]-*N′*-(2-hydroxyethyl)-2,4,6-triidoisophthalamide.

$C_{18}H_{24}I_3N_3O_8$ = 791.1.

CAS — 107793-72-6.

Pharmacopoeias. In *US.*

Ioxilan contains approximately 48.1% of I. A white to off-white, practically odourless powder. **Soluble** in water and in methyl alcohol. **Protect** from light.

Ioxilan is an iodinated nonionic monomeric contrast medium used for various radiographic procedures including enhancement of computed tomography (p.1002). It is given by injection.

Preparations

USP 23: Ioxilan Injection.

Ioxitalamic Acid (1532-b)

Ioxitalamic Acid *(rINN).*

AG-58107; Ioxithalamic Acid. 5-Acetamido-*N*-(2-hydroxyethyl)-2,4,6-tri-iodoisophthalamic acid.

$C_{12}H_{11}I_3N_2O_5$ = 643.9.

CAS — 28179-44-4.

Pharmacopoeias. In *Fr.*

Ioxitalamic acid contains approximately 59.1% of I.

Meglumine Ioxitalamate (1533-v)

Ioxitalamate Meglumine. The *N*-methylglucamine salt of ioxitalamic acid.

$C_{12}H_{11}I_3N_2O_5,C_7H_{17}NO_5$ = 839.2.

CAS — 29288-99-1.

Meglumine ioxitalamate contains approximately 45.4% of I.

Sodium Ioxitalamate (1576-c)

Ioxitalamate Sodium.

$C_{12}H_{10}I_3N_2NaO_5$ = 665.9.

CAS — 33954-26-6.

Sodium ioxitalamate contains approximately 57.2% of I.

Ioxitalamic acid is an iodinated ionic monomeric contrast medium with actions similar to those of the diatrizoates (p.1003). It is used as its meglumine and sodium salts locally and by injection for a wide range of diagnostic procedures, including angiography, cholangiography, hysterosalpingography, and urography (p.1002). It may be given by mouth or rectally for visualisation of the gastro-intestinal tract. It is also used for contrast enhancement during computed tomography.

Ethanolamine ioxitalamate has also been used.

Preparations

Proprietary Preparations (details are given in Part 3)
Aust.: Telebrix; ***Belg.:*** Telebrix; Telebrix Gastro; Telebrix Hystero; ***Canad.:*** Telebrix; ***Fr.:*** Telebrix 12; Telebrix 30; Telebrix 35; Telebrix Gastro; Telebrix Hystero; Vasobrix†; ***Ger.:*** Telebrix Gastro; Telebrix N 180; Telebrix N 30 g†; Telebrix N 350†; ***Ital.:*** Telebrix 12†; Telebrix 30; Telebrix 38; ***Neth.:*** Telebrix 12; Telebrix 30; Telebrix 350; Telebrix 38†; Telebrix Gastro; Telebrix Polyvidone; ***Switz.:*** Telebrix 12†; Telebrix 30†; Telebrix 38†; Telebrix Gastro.

Mangafodipir Trisodium (5032-c)

Mangafodipir Trisodium *(BANM, rINNM).*

MnDPDP (mangafodipir); S-095 (managafodipir); WIN-59010-2 (mangafodipir). Trisodium trihydrogen (*OC*-6-13)-{[*N,N*-′-ethylenebis(*N*-{[3-hydroxy-5-(hydroxymethyl)-2-methyl-4-pyridyl]methyl}glycine) 5,5′-bis(phosphato)](8-)} manganate(6-); Trisodium trihydrogen (*OC*-6-13)-*N,N′*-ethane-1,2-diylbis{N-[2-methyl-3-oxido-κ*O*-5-(phosphonatooxymethyl)-4-pyridylmethyl]glycinato(*O,N*)}manganate(II).

$C_{22}H_{27}MnN_4Na_3O_{14}P_2$ = 757.3.

CAS — 155319-91-8 (mangafodipir); 140678-14-4 (mangafodipir trisodium).

Mangafodipir trisodium is a paramagnetic agent used intravenously for contrast enhancement in magnetic resonance imaging (p.1002) of the liver.

Preparations

Proprietary Preparations (details are given in Part 3)
Swed.: Teslascan; ***USA:*** Teslascan.

Metrizamide (1578-a)

Metrizamide *(BAN, USAN, rINN).*

Win-39103. 2-[3-Acetamido-2,4,6-tri-iodo-5-(*N*-methylacetamido)benzamido]-2-deoxy-D-glucose.

$C_{18}H_{22}I_3N_3O_8$ = 789.1.

CAS — 31112-62-6 (metrizamide); 55134-11-7 (metrizamide, glucopyranose form).

Metrizamide contains approximately 48.2% of I.

Adverse Effects and Precautions

As for the diatrizoates, p.1003. For the adverse effects relating to the use of metrizamide for myelography, see under Iohexol, p.1006.

References to adverse effects with metrizamide.

1. Davis CE, *et al.* Persistent movement disorder following metrizamide myelography. *Arch Neurol* 1982; **39:** 128.
2. Kwentus JA, *et al.* Manic syndrome after metrizamide myelography. *Am J Psychiatry* 1984; **141:** 700–2.
3. Elliott RL, *et al.* Prolonged delirium after metrizamide myelography. *JAMA* 1984; **252:** 2057–8.
4. Wade JB, *et al.* Neuropsychological implications of metrizamide myelography. *Lancet* 1986; **ii:** 102–3.
5. Dan NG. Intracranial subdural haematoma after metrizamide myelography. *Med J Aust* 1984; **140:** 289–90.

Pharmacokinetics

Following intrathecal administration metrizamide diffuses upwards through the CSF and enters the extracellular fluid of the brain. Most of a dose is eliminated from the CSF within several hours. It enters the blood and is eliminated primarily in urine; in patients with normal renal function 60% or more of an intrathecal dose is excreted in urine within 48 hours. Small amounts are excreted in bile. Metrizamide is not significantly bound to plasma proteins. It has been reported to be distributed into breast milk.

Uses and Administration

Metrizamide is an iodinated nonionic monomeric contrast medium used in myelography, angiography, intravenous urography, and arthrography (p.1002). It is also used for contrast enhancement during computed tomography. The dose and strength used depend upon the procedure and route of administration.

Preparations

Proprietary Preparations (details are given in Part 3)
Austral.: Amipaque†; ***Canad.:*** Amipaque†; ***Spain:*** Amipaque†; ***USA:*** Amipaque.

Metrizoic Acid (1534-g)

3-Acetamido-2,4,6-tri-iodo-5-(*N*-methylacetamido)benzoic acid.

$C_{12}H_{11}I_3N_2O_4$ = 627.9.

CAS — 1949-45-7.

Metrizoic acid contains approximately 60.6% of I.

Meglumine Metrizoate (1535-q)

Metrizoate Meglumine. The *N*-methylglucamine salt of metrizoic acid.

$C_{12}H_{11}I_3N_2O_4,C_7H_{17}NO_5$ = 823.2.

CAS — 7241-11-4.

Meglumine metrizoate contains approximately 46.3% of I.

Sodium Metrizoate (1579-t)

Sodium Metrizoate *(BAN, rINN).*

Metrizoate Sodium *(USAN)*; NSC-107431.

$C_{12}H_{10}I_3N_2NaO_4$ = 649.9.

CAS — 7225-61-8.

Sodium metrizoate contains approximately 58.6% of I.

Metrizoic acid is an iodinated ionic monomeric contrast medium with actions similar to those of the diatrizoates (p.1003). It is used as the meglumine and sodium salts, often together with calcium metrizoate and magnesium metrizoate, for a variety of diagnostic procedures including angiography, cholangiography, and hysterosalpingography (p.1002).

Preparations

Proprietary Preparations (details are given in Part 3)
Belg.: Isopaque; ***Norw.:*** Isopaque Cysto; ***Spain:*** Angiocontrast 370†; ***Swed.:*** Isopaque Amin†; Isopaque Cysto; ***UK:*** Isopaque 350†; Isopaque Amin 200†; Isopaque Cerebral 280†; Isopaque Coronar 370†; Isopaque Cysto 100.

Perflenapent (7208-k)

Perflenapent *(USAN, rINN).*

Dodecafluoropentane.

C_5F_{12} = 288.0.

CAS — 678-26-2.

Perflenapent is a fluorocarbon ultrasound contrast medium (p.1002) used with perflisopent (below) for echocardiography.

Perflisopent (20110-g)

Perflisopent *(USAN, rINN).*

Nonafluoro-2-(trifluoromethyl)butane.

C_5F12 = 288.0.

CAS — 594-91-2.

Perflisopent is a fluorocarbon ultrasound contrast medium (p.1002) used with perflenapent (above) for echocardiography.

Propyliodone (1582-j)

Propyliodone *(rINN).*

Propyliodonum. Propyl 1,4-dihydro-3,5-di-iodo-4-oxo-1-pyridylacetate.

$C_{10}H_{11}I_2NO_3$ = 447.0.

CAS — 587-61-1.

Pharmacopoeias. In *Br., Int.,* and *US.*

A white or almost white, crystalline powder, odourless or almost odourless, containing approximately 56.8% of I.

BP **solubilities** are: practically insoluble in water; slightly soluble in alcohol and in chloroform; very slightly soluble in ether. USP solubilities are: practically insoluble in water; soluble in acetone, in alcohol, and in ether. The BP aqueous suspension has a pH of 6.0 to 7.5.

Store in airtight containers. Protect from light.

Adverse Effects

Propyliodone may give rise to transient pyrexia, sometimes associated with malaise and aching of the joints, especially with the aqueous suspension, lasting 48 hours and sometimes accompanied by coughing. In a few cases, dyspnoea, atelectasis, or pneumonia have occurred. Hypersensitivity reactions may occur rarely.

Precautions

Propyliodone should be used with great care where there is hypersensitivity to iodine and is contra-indicated in patients with severe heart disease. It should also be used with caution in patients with asthma, bronchiectasis, or pulmonary emphysema, or in whom pulmonary function is otherwise reduced. If bilateral examination of the bronchial tract is necessary in such patients an interval of several days should elapse between the examinations. Use of an excessive volume or too-rapid administration may result in lobar collapse.

The administration of iodine-containing contrast media may interfere with thyroid-function tests.

Pharmacokinetics

After instillation into the lungs some propyliodone may be expectorated and swallowed but the remainder is absorbed into the blood. It is rapidly hydrolysed and is excreted in the urine as di-iodopyridone acetate. Approximately 50% of the administered dose is reported to be eliminated in the urine within 3 days.

Uses and Administration

Propyliodone is an iodinated contrast medium that has been used for bronchography (p.1002) as either a 50% aqueous suspension or as a 60% oily suspension.

Preparations

BP 1998: Propyliodone Injection; Propyliodone Oily Injection;
USP 23: Propyliodone Injectable Oil Suspension.

Proprietary Preparations (details are given in Part 3)
Swed.: Dionosil†; ***USA:*** Dionosil Oily.

Sodium Tyropanoate (1586-a)

Sodium Tyropanoate *(BAN, rINN).*

NSC-107434; Tyropanoate Sodium *(USAN)*; Win-8851-2. Sodium 2-(3-butyramido-2,4,6-tri-iodobenzyl)butyrate.

$C_{15}H_{17}I_3NNaO_3$ = 663.0.

CAS — 27293-82-9 (tyropanoic acid); 7246-21-1 (sodium tyropanoate).

Pharmacopoeias. In *US.*

A white odourless hygroscopic powder containing approximately 57.4% of I. **Soluble** in water, in alcohol, and in dimethylformamide; very slightly soluble in acetone and in ether. **Store** in airtight containers. Protect from light.

Sodium tyropanoate is an iodinated ionic monomeric contrast medium with actions similar to those of iopanoic acid (p.1007) used for cholecystography and cholangiography (p.1002). It is given by mouth in a usual dose of 3 g.

Preparations

USP 23: Tyropanoate Sodium Capsules.

Proprietary Preparations (details are given in Part 3)
USA: Bilopaque.

Corticosteroids

The adrenal cortex synthesises a number of steroids, which may be divided into corticosteroids, based on a 21-carbon nucleus, and sex corticoids, primarily androgens, based on a 19-carbon nucleus. The corticosteroids are traditionally divided into those with predominantly glucocorticoid actions, of which cortisol (hydrocortisone) is the most important endogenous example, and those which are primarily mineralocorticoid, of which aldosterone is much the most important.

The endogenous glucocorticoids are under regulatory control from the hypothalamus and pituitary, via the releasing hormones corticorelin (p.1244) and corticotrophin or ACTH (see p.1244). In return the glucocorticoids act to inhibit production and release of these releasing hormones by a negative feedback mechanism. The system is known collectively as the hypothalamic-pituitary-adrenal (HPA) axis. Aldosterone secretion, by contrast, is under the control of the renin-angiotensin system.

The main **mineralocorticoid** actions are on fluid and electrolyte balance. They enhance sodium reabsorption in the kidney and hence expand the extracellular fluid volume, and they enhance renal excretion of potassium and H^+.

The **glucocorticoid** actions are wide-ranging. They have potent anti-inflammatory and immunosuppressive effects, at least partly through inhibition of the release of various cytokines, and it is primarily these that are made use of clinically (see p.1015). They also have profound metabolic effects: blood glucose concentrations are maintained or increased by a decrease in peripheral glucose utilization and an increase in gluconeogenesis; glycogen deposition, protein breakdown, and lipolysis are increased, and effects on calcium uptake and excretion lead to a decrease in body calcium stores. Glucocorticoids play a facilitative or permissive role in the function of many other active endogenous substances, and have effects on the function of cardiovascular system, kidneys, skeletal muscle and CNS.

Many synthetic congeners and derivatives of the corticosteroids are available. The main corticosteroids used systemically are hydroxy compounds (alcohols). They are relatively insoluble in water and the sodium salt of the phosphate or succinate ester is generally used to provide water-soluble forms for injections or solutions. Such esters are readily hydrolysed in the body.

Various structure-activity relationships are understood for the corticosteroids and have been made use of in the development of new compounds. The presence of a hydroxyl group at position 11 seems to be essential for glucocorticoid activity, while a hydroxyl at position 21 is required for mineralocorticoid activity. Fluorination at position 9 enhances both mineralocorticoid and glucocorticoid activity. Substitution at carbon 16 (as in betamethasone, dexamethasone, or triamcinolone) virtually eliminates mineralocorticoid activity. Esterification of corticosteroids at the 17 or 21 positions with fatty acids generally increases the topical activity. The formation of cyclic acetonides at the 16 and 17 positions further increases topical anti-inflammatory activity, usually without increasing systemic glucocorticoid activity.

In the medical and pharmacological literature the names of unesterified corticosteroids have frequently been used indiscriminately for both the unesterified and esterified forms and it is not always apparent to which form reference is being made. The unesterified form is sometimes qualified by the phrase 'free alcohol'.

Adverse Effects of Corticosteroids

The adverse effects of corticosteroids may result from unwanted mineralocorticoid or glucocorticoid actions, or from inhibition of the hypothalamic-pituitary-adrenal axis.

Mineralocorticoid adverse effects are manifest in the retention of sodium and water, with oedema and hypertension, and in the increased excretion of potassium with the possibility of hypokalaemic alkalosis. In susceptible patients, cardiac failure may be induced. Disturbances of electrolyte balance are common with the naturally occurring corticosteroids, such as cortisone and hydrocortisone, but are less frequent with many synthetic glucocorticoids, which have little or no mineralocorticoid activity.

Adverse **glucocorticoid** effects lead to mobilisation of calcium and phosphorus, with osteoporosis and spontaneous fractures; muscle wasting and nitrogen depletion; and hyperglycaemia with accentuation or precipitation of the diabetic state. The insulin requirements of diabetic patients are increased. Increased appetite is often reported.

Impaired tissue repair and immune function can lead to delayed wound healing, and increased susceptibility to infection. Increased susceptibility to all kinds of infection, including septicaemia, tuberculosis, fungal infections, and viral infections, has been reported in patients on corticosteroid therapy. Infections may also be masked by the anti-inflammatory, analgesic, and antipyretic effects of glucocorticoids. Recent attention has focussed on the increased severity of varicella, with a possible fatal outcome in non-immune patients receiving systemic corticosteroid therapy.

Other adverse effects include amenorrhoea, hyperhidrosis, skin thinning, ocular changes including development of glaucoma and cataract, mental and neurological disturbances, benign intracranial hypertension, acute pancreatitis, and avascular necrosis of bone. An increase in the coagulability of the blood may lead to thrombo-embolic complications. Peptic ulceration has been reported but reviews of the literature do not always agree that corticosteroids are responsible for an increased incidence.

The negative feedback effects of glucocorticoids on the hypothalamic-pituitary-adrenal (HPA) axis may lead to adrenal atrophy, in some cases after therapy for as little as 7 days. This produces secondary adrenocortical insufficiency, which may become manifest following overly rapid withdrawal of treatment or be precipitated by some stress such as infection or trauma. Patients vary considerably in the degree and duration of adrenal suppression following a given course of corticosteroid, but adrenal atrophy may persist for months or years, and withdrawal should be gradual in those who have been treated for any length of time (see also Withdrawal, below). High doses of corticosteroids administered during pregnancy may cause fetal or neonatal adrenal suppression. Although the precise mechanism is uncertain, growth retardation may follow the administration of even relatively small doses of corticosteroids to children.

Large doses of corticosteroids, or of corticotrophin, may produce Cushingoid symptoms typical of hyperactivity of the adrenal cortex, with moon-face, sometimes with hirsutism, buffalo hump, flushing, increased bruising, ecchymoses, striae, and acne (see also Cushing's Syndrome, p.1236). Rapid intravenous administration of large doses of corticosteroids may cause cardiovascular collapse.

Hypersensitivity reactions have occurred with corticosteroids, mainly when administered topically.

Adverse effects occur, in general, fairly equally with all systemic corticosteroid preparations and their incidence rises steeply if dosage increases much above physiological values, traditionally considered to be about 7.5 mg daily of prednisolone or its equivalent (see under Uses and Administration, below, for equivalent doses of other corticosteroids). Short courses at high dosage for emergencies appear to cause fewer side-effects than prolonged courses with lower doses.

Most topically applied corticosteroids may, under certain circumstances, be absorbed in sufficient amounts to produce systemic effects. The topical application of corticosteroid preparations to the eyes has produced corneal ulcers, raised intra-ocular pressure, and reduced visual function. Application of corticosteroids to the skin has led to loss of skin collagen and subcutaneous atrophy; local hypopigmentation of deeply pigmented skins has been reported following both the intradermal injection and topical application of potent corticosteroids.

Intrathecal administration (including inadvertent intrathecal administration after attempted epidural injection) has been associated with arachnoiditis.

Adrenal suppression. The inhibition of hypothalamic-pituitary-adrenocortical function associated with corticosteroid administration may persist for a year or more after treatment is withdrawn and may cause acute adrenocortical insufficiency with circulatory collapse during stress. The degree of suppression depends on a number of factors, including length of treatment, time of day of administration, type of corticosteroid preparation used, route of administration, dose administered, and dosing interval. In general, suppression of secretion of adrenocorticotrophic hormone and atrophy of the adrenal gland become progressively more definite as doses of corticosteroid exceed physiological amounts (see under Uses and Administration, below), and as the duration of therapy increases (significant suppression is likely in patients receiving more then 3 weeks of therapy). It is less when the corticosteroid is given as a single dose in the morning, and even less if this morning dose is given on alternate days or less frequently. In patients taking high enough doses of corticosteroids to suppress the adrenals the dose should be increased during any form of stress (for example, illness or surgery), and those treated within the last 2 or 3 months should be restarted on therapy. Where the interval since treatment is greater than 3 months, resumption of treatment depends on clinical assessment of signs of adrenocortical insufficiency.

To avoid precipitating acute adrenocortical insufficiency, withdrawal of corticosteroid treatment should be carried out gradually, differing regimens being used according to the disease being treated and the duration of therapy. Examples of withdrawal regimens that have been used are described under Withdrawal, below.

Adrenal suppression may occur after very short courses of high-dose therapy and since many patients undergoing such therapy will be under continuing stress when the drugs are stopped, gradual withdrawal of corticosteroids over 5 to 7 days is preferable.

It should also be remembered that corticosteroid-induced adrenal suppression has been associated not only with systemic therapy, but has followed topical application of corticosteroid preparations, particularly those containing potent corticosteroids. Adrenal suppression has also been associated with the use of inhalants, and the topical application of eye drops, eye ointments, and nasal preparations.

This topic has been reviewed by Helfer and Rose.[1]

1. Helfer EL, Rose LI. Corticosteroids and adrenal suppression: characterising and avoiding the problem. *Drugs* 1989; **38:** 838–45.

Effects on bones and joints. Corticosteroid-induced **avascular necrosis** of bone is an uncommon but disabling complication of therapy.[1-3] The incidence may vary in patients with different disease states; alcoholics, and patients with collagen disease (especially systemic lupus erythematosus) may have increased susceptibility.[3,4] There may be a relationship with corticosteroid dose: even short courses of high-dose corticosteroids may be associated with its development.[1-3] There is also a report of avascular necrosis associated with topical application of corticosteroids.[5]

Corticosteroids may also produce **osteoporosis.** A review[6] of data obtained from studies published between 1970 and 1990 established that osteoporosis is a common consequence of long-term treatment with corticosteroids, occurring in approximately 50% of patients. Bone loss is more rapid during the early stages of therapy and is most rapid in areas of the skeleton containing the greatest proportion of trabecular bone such as the spine, hip, distal radius, pelvis, and ribs.

Reviews and guidelines[7-9] on the prevention and management of corticosteroid-induced osteoporosis suggest that the dose should be minimised, as doses above 7.5 mg of prednisolone or prednisone (or the equivalent) are associated with more significant bone loss and increased fracture risk. Alternate-day therapy, although desirable for its reduced effect on the hypothalamic-pituitary-adrenal axis, does not reduce the risk of bone loss. Patients should maintain an adequate intake of calcium and vitamin D, should take regular exercise, and avoid smoking and excessive alcohol intake. Hormone replacement therapy is advocated in postmenopausal women. In high risk patients in whom hormone replacement therapy is inappropriate or contra-indicated the prophylactic use of bisphosphonates, calcitriol, or calcitonin should be considered. A thiazide diuretic may be helpful in controlling hypercalciuria in patients not receiving calcitriol. Whether some corticosteroids have reduced effects on the bone is unclear.[10]

1. Nixon JE. Early diagnosis and treatment of steroid induced avascular necrosis of bone. *Br Med J* 1984; **288:** 741–4.
2. Anonymous. Transplant osteonecrosis. *Lancet* 1985; **i:** 965–6.
3. Capell H. Selected side-effects: 5. steroid therapy and osteonecrosis. *Prescribers' J* 1992; **32:** 32–4.
4. Knight A. Images in clinical medicine: corticosteroid osteonecrosis. *N Engl J Med* 1995; **333:** 130.
5. McLean CJ, *et al.* Cataracts, glaucoma, and femoral avascular necrosis caused by topical corticosteroid ointment. *Lancet* 1995; **345:** 330.
6. Lukert BP, Raisz LG. Glucocorticoid-induced osteoporosis: pathogenesis and management. *Ann Intern Med* 1990; **112:** 352–64.
7. Picado C, Luengo M. Corticosteroid-induced bone loss: prevention and management. *Drug Safety* 1996; **15:** 347–59.
8. Anonymous. Corticosteroid-induced osteoporosis. *Drug Ther Bull* 1996; **34:** 84–6.
9. American College of Rheumatology Task Force on Osteoporosis Guidelines. Recommendations for the prevention and treatment of glucocorticoid-induced osteoporosis. *Arthritis Rheum* 1996; **39:** 1791–1801.
10. Eastell R. Management of corticosteroid-induced osteoporosis. *J Intern Med* 1995; **237:** 439–47.

Effects on carbohydrate and protein metabolism. Corticosteroids produce glucose intolerance[1-4] and protein catabolism.[5,6]

1. Hurel SJ, Taylor R. Drugs and glucose tolerance. *Adverse Drug React Bull* 1995; (Oct.): 659–62.
2. Landy HJ, *et al.* The effect of chronic steroid therapy on glucose tolerance in pregnancy. *Am J Obstet Gynecol* 1988; **159:** 612–15.
3. O'Byrne S, Feely J. Effects of drugs on glucose tolerance in non-insulin-dependent diabetics (part I). *Drugs* 1990; **40:** 6–18.
4. Bruno A, *et al.* Serum glucose, insulin and C-peptide response to oral glucose after intravenous administration of hydrocortisone and methylprednisolone in man. *Eur J Clin Pharmacol* 1994; **46:** 411–5.
5. Brownlee KG, *et al.* Catabolic effect of dexamethasone in the preterm baby. *Arch Dis Child* 1992; **67:** 1–4.
6. Van Goudoever JB, *et al.* Effect of dexamethasone on protein metabolism in infants with bronchopulmonary dysplasia. *J Pediatr* 1994; **124:** 112–18.

Effects on the cardiovascular system. Corticosteroids have recognised cardiovascular effects arising from induced changes to electrolyte balance and enhancement of vascular reactivity. Some references to reports of hypertension[1-3] and myocardial thickening[4] in preterm infants are given below.

1. Greenough A, *et al.* Dexamethasone and hypertension in preterm infants. *Eur J Pediatr* 1992; **151:** 134–5.
2. Emery EF, Greenough A. Effect of dexamethasone on blood pressure—relationship to postnatal age. *Eur J Pediatr* 1992; **151:** 364–6.
3. Marinelli KA, *et al.* Effects of dexamethasone on blood pressure in premature infants with bronchopulmonary dysplasia. *J Pediatr* 1997; **130:** 594–602.
4. Evans N. Cardiovascular effects of dexamethasone in the preterm infant. *Arch Dis Child* 1994; **70:** F25–30.

Effects on the cerebrovascular system. Despite being used in high doses to treat benign intracranial hypertension, corticosteroids may also occasionally cause this disorder. Children receiving long-term therapy are mainly affected, an increase in dosage often being responsible. Symptoms usually subside when dosage is reduced.[1]

1. Gibberd B. Drug-induced benign intracranial hypertension. *Prescribers' J* 1991; **31:** 118–21.

Effects on the eyes. Ocular adverse effects of corticosteroids include raised intra-ocular pressure. Most reports implicate prolonged topical administration to the eye or face.[1-3] Young children (less than 8 years of age) may be at increased risk.[4] Increases in intra-ocular pressure appear to be less marked in patients receiving systemic corticosteroids.[5] However, there is evidence of an increased risk in patients receiving inhaled corticosteroids.[6] Again, prolonged or high-dose administration seems to be generally implicated. A recent study in elderly patients has also demonstrated a dose-related increase in the risk of raised intra-ocular pressure or open-angle glaucoma.[7]

Topical administration of corticosteroids to patients with ocular herpes simplex infection can alleviate the symptoms but allow the infection to develop with the risk of irreversible corneal scarring[1] that may lead to loss of vision, or even loss of the eye. Warnings have been sounded about the ocular risks of applying corticosteroid ointments to skin near the eyes.[8]

Cataract formation is another risk from corticosteroid use and some references to case reports are given below;[2,3,9-11] this hazard is associated with systemic corticosteroid absorption. Again, there is evidence that cataract formation may also be associated with use of inhaled corticosteroids.[12,14] Individual susceptibility to this effect appears to vary, but it may be more important than dosage and duration of treatment. Again, children may be more likely to develop cataract than adults.[5]

Systemic corticosteroid use has also been associated with damage to the retinal pigment epithelial barrier, predisposing the patient to serous retinal detachment.[13]

1. Anonymous. Avoiding eye damage from topical corticosteroids. *Drug Ther Bull* 1987; **25:** 29–30.
2. Butcher JM, *et al.* Bilateral cataracts and glaucoma induced by long term use of steroid eye drops. *Br Med J* 1994; **309:** 43.
3. McLean CJ, *et al.* Cataracts, glaucoma, and femoral avascular necrosis caused by topical corticosteroid ointment. *Lancet* 1995; **345:** 330.
4. Lam DSC, *et al.* Accelerated ocular hypertensive response to topical steroids in children. *Br J Ophthalmol* 1997; **81:** 422–3.
5. Rennie IG. Clinically important ocular reactions to systemic drug therapy. *Drug Safety* 1993; **9:** 196–211.
6. Garbe E, *et al.* Inhaled and nasal glucocorticoids and the risks of ocular hypertension or open-angle glaucoma. *JAMA* 1997; **277:** 722–7.
7. Garbe E, *et al.* Risk of ocular hypertension or open-angle glaucoma in elderly patients on oral glucocorticoids. *Lancet* 1997; **350:** 979–82.
8. Chong NHV. Glaucoma induced by steroids. *Br Med J* 1994; **309:** 343.
9. Allen MB, *et al.* Steroid aerosols and cataract formation. *Br Med J* 1989; **299:** 432–3.
10. Karim AKA, *et al.* Steroid aerosols and cataract formation. *Br Med J* 1989; **299:** 918.
11. Ghanchi F. Young patients on inhaled steroids and cataract. *Lancet* 1993; **342:** 1306–7.
12. Cumming RG, *et al.* Use of inhaled corticosteroids and the risk of cataracts. *N Engl J Med* 1997; **337:** 8–14.
13. Polak BCP, *et al.* Diffuse retinal pigment epitheliopathy complicating systemic corticosteroid treatment. *Br J Ophthalmol* 1995; **79:** 922–5.
14. Garbe E, *et al.* Association of inhaled corticosteroid use with cataract extraction in elderly patients. *JAMA* 1998; **280:** 539–43.

Effects on the gastro-intestinal tract. It has long been considered that treatment with corticosteroids might lead to peptic ulcers. Some years ago a review of the data then available suggested that since an ulcer developed in 1% of control patients not receiving steroids, the 2% incidence for patients receiving steroids did not warrant the prophylactic use of anti-ulcer drugs in all patients.[1] Others have found little evidence of an increased risk of peptic ulcer produced by corticosteroids alone although there is some increase in risk associated with the concomitant use of corticosteroids and NSAIDs.[2] It has been suggested that it might be prudent to avoid such combination therapy whenever possible.[3]

Doubt has therefore been cast on the prophylactic value of anti-ulcer therapy given concomitantly with corticosteroids.[1,4] If an ulcer does develop and there is good reason to continue with steroid therapy then corticosteroids may be continued along with some form of ulcer therapy.[1]

There have been several reports of corticosteroids being associated with gastro-intestinal perforation.[5-8] There is a risk that the anti-inflammatory properties of corticosteroids may mask the signs of perforation and delay diagnosis with potentially fatal results.

1. Spiro HM. Is the steroid ulcer a myth? *N Engl J Med* 1983; **309:** 45–7.
2. Piper JM, *et al.* Corticosteroid use and peptic ulcer disease: role of nonsteroidal anti-inflammatory drugs. *Ann Intern Med* 1991; **114:** 735–40.
3. Guslandi M, Tittobello A. Steroid ulcers: a myth revisited. *Br Med J* 1992; **304:** 655–6.
4. Marcus P, McCauley DL. Steroid therapy and H_2-receptor antagonists: pharmacoeconomic implications. *Clin Pharmacol Ther* 1997; **61:** 503–8.
5. Arsura EL. Corticosteroid-associated perforation of colonic diverticula. *Arch Intern Med* 1990; **150:** 1337–8.
6. Ng PC, *et al.* Gastroduodenal perforation in preterm babies treated with dexamethasone for bronchopulmonary dysplasia. *Arch Dis Child* 1991; **66:** 1164–6.
7. O'Neil EA, *et al.* Dexamethasone treatment during ventilator dependency: possible life threatening gastrointestinal complications. *Arch Dis Child* 1992; **67:** 10–11.
8. Epstein A, *et al.* Perforation of colon diverticula during corticosteroid therapy for pemphigus vulgaris. *Ann Pharmacother* 1993; **27:** 979–80.

Effects on growth. Corticosteroids impair normal growth in children when given systemically, and although alternate day therapy may reduce the effect on growth it does not abolish it. Recent concerns have centred on the possible effects of inhaled corticosteroids on growth.[1,2] Some studies have not found an effect of inhaled corticosteroids on growth, and in general this appears to be so when doses are modest, even if treatment is prolonged.[1,3,4] Others have found that inhaled corticosteroids, particularly in high doses, do appear to have some effect on growth parameters,[3,5-7] but it is unclear whether this has long-term effects on the child's ultimate height, and the alternative in children requiring such high-dose therapy is likely to be an oral corticosteroid, with its consequent effects.

1. Allen DB, *et al.* A meta-analysis of the effect of oral and inhaled corticosteroids on growth. *J Allergy Clin Immunol* 1994; **93:** 967–76.
2. Hanania NA, *et al.* Adverse effects of inhaled corticosteroids. *Am J Med* 1995; **98:** 196–208.
3. Wolthers OD, Pedersen S. Controlled study of linear growth in asthmatic children during treatment with inhaled glucocorticosteroids. *Pediatrics* 1992; **89:** 839–42.
4. Volovitz B, *et al.* Growth and pituitary-adrenal function in children with severe asthma treated with inhaled budesonide. *N Engl J Med* 1993; **329:** 1703–8.
5. Wolthers OD, Pedersen S. Short term growth during treatment with inhaled fluticasone propionate and beclomethasone dipropionate. *Arch Dis Child* 1993; **68:** 673–6.
6. Todd G, *et al.* Growth and adrenal suppression in asthmatic children treated with high-dose fluticasone propionate. *Lancet* 1996; **348:** 27–9.
7. McCowan C, *et al.* Effect of asthma and its treatment on growth: four year follow up of cohort of children from general practices in Tayside, Scotland. *Br Med J* 1998; **316:** 668–72.

Effects on immune response. Owing to their immunosuppressant effect administration of corticosteroids in doses greater than those required for physiological replacement therapy is associated with increased susceptibility to infection, aggravation of existing infection, and activation of latent infection. An additional problem is that the anti-inflammatory effect of corticosteroids may mask symptoms until the infection has progressed to an advanced stage; the altered response of the body may also permit the bizarre spread of infections, frequently in aberrant forms, such as disseminated parasitic infections. The risk is greater in patients receiving high doses, or associated therapy with other immunosuppressants such as cytotoxic agents, and in those who are already debilitated. Children receiving high doses of corticosteroids are at special risk from childhood ailments, such as chickenpox, but vaccination with living organisms is contra-indicated since infection may be induced (killed vaccines or toxoids may be given but the response may be reduced). This increased susceptibility to infection coupled with masking of symptoms may also be caused by topical or local corticosteroid therapy. Thus, topical application to the skin has led to unusual changes such as atypical ringworm infection. Fungal infections, generally restricted to the upper respiratory tract, are associated with corticosteroid inhalations. Severe damage to the eye has followed the ocular use of corticosteroids in herpetic infections, and a similar generalised spread of herpes infection may follow application to the mouth in the presence of herpes infection.

Conversely, the effect of corticosteroids on the symptoms and course of some infections may be life-saving (see Uses and Administration, below). Before embarking on a long-term course of corticosteroid therapy general measures for the reduction of risk of infection include a diligent search for active or quiescent infection and, where appropriate, prevention or eradication of the infection before starting, or concurrent administration of chemoprophylaxis during corticosteroid treatment.

Effects on lipid metabolism. Glucocorticoids have potent effects on lipid metabolism, facilitating the effects of growth hormone and endogenous stimulants of lipolysis. As a result they increase both high- and low-density lipoprotein cholesterol concentrations in the blood.

Hydroxychloroquine has been reported to counter the effects of corticosteroids on lipid metabolism in patients with rheumatoid arthritis or systemic lupus erythematosus—see p.432.

On prolonged administration glucocorticoids also have a dramatic effect on body fat distribution, resulting in the characteristic Cushingoid appearance of moon face, and increased fat at the back of the neck and supraclavicular area.

Effects on mental state. Reviews and reports of the effects of corticosteroids on mental state[1-6] suggest a causative link between corticosteroid therapy, particularly in high doses, and certain cases of mental disturbance. These disturbances have included psychosis, euphoria, and depression. Impairment of memory has been associated with pulsed intravenous methylprednisolone.[7]

1. Mitchell DM, Collins JV. Do corticosteroids really alter mood? *Postgrad Med J* 1984; **60:** 467–70.
2. Sultzer DL, Cummings JL. Drug-induced mania—causative agents, clinical characteristics and management: a retrospective analysis of the literature. *Med Toxicol Adverse Drug Exp* 1989; **4:** 127–43.
3. d'Orbán PT. Steroid-induced psychosis. *Lancet* 1989; **ii:** 694.
4. Wolkowitz OM, Rapaport M. Long-lasting behavioral changes following prednisone withdrawal. *JAMA* 1989; **261:** 1731–2.
5. Anonymous. Drugs that cause psychiatric symptoms. *Med Lett Drugs Ther* 1993; **35:** 65–70.
6. Patten SB, Love EJ. Drug-induced depression: incidence, avoidance and management. *Drug Safety* 1994; **10:** 203–19.
7. Oliveri RL, *et al.* Pulsed methylprednisolone induces a reversible impairment of memory in patients with relapsing-remitting multiple sclerosis. *Acta Neurol Scand* 1998; **97:** 366–9.

Effects on the neonate. Various adverse effects have been reported in premature neonates given corticosteroids, see under Dexamethasone, p.1037.

Effects on the nervous system. Paraesthesia and irritation, most commonly occurring in the anogenital region, have been associated with the intravenous administration of dexamethasone sodium phosphate[1] and hydrocortisone sodium phosphate,[2] but not with hydrocortisone sodium succinate.[2] Further comments and discussions on this topic are listed below.[3-5] Also listed below are references to epidural lipomatosis with severe neurological complications following systemic corticosteroid therapy.[6,7]

1. Czerwinski AW, *et al.* Effects of a single, large, intravenous injection of dexamethasone. *Clin Pharmacol Ther* 1972; **13:** 638–42.
2. Novak E, *et al.* Anorectal pruritus after intravenous hydrocortisone sodium succinate and sodium phosphate. *Clin Pharmacol Ther* 1976; **20:** 109–12.
3. Anonymous. Which form of intravenous hydrocortisone. *Drug Ther Bull* 1979; **17:** 71–2.
4. Thomas VL. More on dexamethasone-induced perineal irritation. *N Engl J Med* 1986; **314:** 1643.
5. Allan SG, Leonard RCF. Dexamethasone antiemesis and side-effects. *Lancet* 1986; **i:** 1035.
6. Butcher DL, Sahn SA. Epidural lipomatosis: a complication of corticosteroid therapy. *Ann Intern Med* 1979; **90:** 60.
7. George WE, *et al.* Medical management of steroid-induced epidural lipomatosis. *N Engl J Med* 1983; **308:** 316–19.

Effects on the pancreas. Acute pancreatitis has been associated with corticosteroid use,[1-3] although evidence supporting the association has been challenged on a number of grounds, both clinical and experimental.[2]

1. Nakashima Y, Howard JM. Drug-induced acute pancreatitis. *Surg Gynecol Obstet* 1977; **145:** 105–9.
2. Banerjee AK, *et al.* Drug-induced acute pancreatitis: a critical review. *Med Toxicol Adverse Drug Exp* 1989; **4:** 186–98.
3. Felig DM, Topazian M. Corticosteroid-induced pancreatitis. *Ann Intern Med* 1996; **124:** 1016.

Effects on the skin. Topical corticosteroids are associated with a number of local adverse effects on the skin, principally due to their antiproliferative effects on keratinocytes and fibroblasts (leading to skin thinning and atrophy), and to possible interference with the skin flora (leading to increased risk of superinfection or opportunistic infection).[1] Skin thinning is more likely if corticosteroids are applied under occlusion (this is especially true of halogenated corticosteroids which are more resistant to inactivation by enzymes in the epidermis). Striae, which occur usually in intertriginous areas such as axillae and groin where skin is thin, moist, and occluded, are the most readily appreciable manifestation of skin atrophy, and are irreversible, unlike more minor degrees of atrophy. Other local adverse effects include telangiectasias and purpura. The balance between benefit and the likelihood of local or systemic adverse effects following topical application of corticosteroids will depend on the chemical structure of the drug (i.e. its lipophilicity and resistance to enzymic degradation), the formulation of the vehicle, the way in which it is applied, and the nature of the skin to be treated.[1]

Skin thinning and purpura have also been reported in patients receiving inhaled corticosteroids.[2,3]

The adverse skin effects arising from systemic corticosteroids also include striae and skin thinning as well as acneiform eruptions. Somewhat counter-intuitively a case-control study has suggested an increased risk of Stevens-Johnson syndrome or toxic epidermal necrolysis in patients receiving corticosteroids, particularly in the period shortly after beginning therapy.[4]

1. Mori M, *et al.* Topical corticosteroids and unwanted local effects: improving the benefit/risk ratio. *Drug Safety* 1994; **10:** 406–12.
2. Shuttleworth D, *et al.* Inhaled corticosteroids and skin thinning. *Br J Dermatol* 1990; **122:** 268.
3. Capewell S, *et al.* Purpura and dermal thinning associated with high dose inhaled corticosteroids. *Br Med J* 1990; **300:** 1548–51.
4. Roujeau J-C, *et al.* Medication use and the risk of Stevens-Johnson syndrome or toxic epidermal necrolysis. *N Engl J Med* 1995; **333:** 1600–7.

Effects on the voice. Dysphonia may be associated with inhaled corticosteroids.[1-5] Although oropharyngeal candidiasis may be one possible cause of such hoarseness, most patients with dysphonia are reported not to have candidiasis.[5]

1. Anonymous. Inhaled steroids and dysphonia. *Lancet* 1984; **i:** 375–6.
2. Dash CH, Pover GM. Inhaled steroids and dysphonia. *Lancet* 1984; **i:** 458.
3. Campbell IA. Inhaled steroids and dysphonia. *Lancet* 1984; **i:** 744.
4. Streeton JA. Inhaled steroids and dysphonia. *Lancet* 1984; **i:** 963.
5. Crompton GK. Local adverse effects of inhaled corticosteroids. *Prescribers' J* 1995; **35:** 225.

Hypersensitivity and anaphylaxis. There have been occasional reports of hypersensitivity reactions, and sometimes anaphylaxis, caused by corticosteroids. Reactions have occurred with any route, although the topical route is mainly involved. It has been observed that the incidence of hypersensitivity is increasing[1] and it has been suggested that a lack of response in chronic eczema might be due to a reaction to the corticosteroid treatment.[1]

1. Dooms-Goossens A. Sensitivity to corticosteroids: consequences for anti-inflammatory therapy. *Drug Safety* 1995; **13:** 123–9.

Tumour lysis syndrome. Reports of corticosteroid-induced tumour lysis syndrome.[1-3]

1. Sparano J, *et al.* Increasing recognition of corticosteroid-induced tumour lysis syndrome in non-Hodgkin's lymphoma. *Cancer* 1990; **65:** 1072–3.
2. Smith RE, Stoiber TR. Acute tumor lysis syndrome in prolymphocytic leukemia. *Am J Med* 1990; **88:** 547–8.
3. Haller C, Dhadly M. The tumor lysis syndrome. *Ann Intern Med* 1991; **114:** 808–9.

Treatment of Adverse Effects of Corticosteroids

The adverse effects of corticosteroids are nearly always due to their use in excess of normal physiological requirements. They should be treated symptomatically, where possible the dosage being reduced or the drug slowly withdrawn.

The treatment of acute adrenocortical insufficiency in corticosteroid-treated patients, whether due to accidental abrupt withdrawal of the corticosteroid or the inability of the patient's adrenals to cope with the increased stress of infection or accidental or surgical trauma, is described under Adrenocortical Insufficiency, p.1017.

For mention of the various drugs tried for prophylaxis and treatment of corticosteroid-induced osteoporosis, see Effects on Bones and Joints, under Adverse Effects, above.

Withdrawal of Corticosteroids

The use of pharmacological doses of corticosteroids suppresses the endogenous secretion of corticotrophin by the anterior pituitary, with the result that the adrenal cortex becomes atrophied. Sudden withdrawal or reduction in dosage, or an increase in corticosteroid requirements associated with the stress of infection or accidental or surgical trauma, may then precipitate acute adrenocortical insufficiency; deaths have followed the abrupt withdrawal of corticosteroids. For the emergency treatment of acute adrenal insufficiency caused by abrupt withdrawal of corticosteroids, see under Adrenocortical Insufficiency, p.1017.

In some instances, withdrawal symptoms may involve or resemble a clinical relapse of the disease for which the patient has been undergoing treatment. Other effects that may occur during withdrawal or change of corticosteroid therapy include benign intracranial hypertension with headache and vomiting and papilloedema caused by cerebral oedema. Latent rhinitis or eczema may be unmasked.

Duration of treatment and dosage are important factors in determining suppression of the pituitary-adrenal response to stress on cessation of corticosteroid treatment, and individual liability to suppression is also important.

Following short courses at moderate doses it may be appropriate to withdraw corticosteroids without tapering the dose (see below). However, after high-dose or prolonged therapy, withdrawal should be gradual, the rate depending upon the individual patient's response, the dose, the disease being treated, and the duration of therapy. Recommendations for initial reduction, stated in terms of prednisolone, have varied from as little as steps of 1 mg monthly to 2.5 to 5 mg every 2 to 7 days. Provided the disease is unlikely to relapse the dose of systemic corticosteroid may be reduced rapidly to physiological values; dose reduction should then be slower to allow recovery of pituitary-adrenal function. Symptoms attributable to over-rapid withdrawal should be countered by resuming a higher dose and continuing the reduction at a slower rate. The administration of corticotrophin does not help to re-establish adrenal responsiveness.

This gradual withdrawal of corticosteroid therapy permits a return of adrenal function adequate for daily needs, but years may sometimes be required for the return of function necessary to meet the stress of infection, surgical operations, or trauma. On such occasions patients with a history of recent corticosteroid withdrawal should be protected by means of supplementary corticosteroid therapy as described under Precautions, below.

In the UK, the Committee on Safety of Medicines recommends that moderate dosage with corticosteroids (up to 40 mg daily of prednisolone, or equivalent), for up to 3 weeks, may be stopped without tapering provided that the original disease is unlikely to relapse, although prophylactic cover may be required for any stress within a week of finishing the course.[1] However, it should be borne in mind that individuals vary widely in their response to corticosteroids and their ability to tolerate withdrawal. Gradual withdrawal should be considered, even after shorter courses, if higher doses are given, or in patients with other risk factors for adrenocortical insufficiency, including those who have had repeated courses of systemic corticosteroids, those who receive a course within one year of finishing long-term corticosteroid therapy, or those who regularly take doses in the evening, when their suppressive effect is greater. Withdrawal should not be abrupt in any patient who receives systemic corticosteroids for more than 3 weeks.[1]

How dose reduction is carried out depends largely on the likelihood of relapse of the original disease. If this is unlikely, the dose of systemic corticosteroid may be reduced rapidly to physiological values (traditionally considered to be 7.5 mg of prednisolone daily or equivalent). It should then be reduced more slowly to allow the hypothalamic-pituitary-adrenal axis to recover.[1] Where disease relapse is a possibility even the initial reduction may need to be more cautious. Long-term treatment may require withdrawal over many months (such as a reduction of 1 mg in the daily dose of prednisolone every 3 to 4 weeks).

In reviews of the inhibition of hypothalamic-pituitary-adrenocortical function associated with corticosteroid administration, further regimens for corticosteroid withdrawal are described.[2-4] For example, patients who have been treated for weeks or months may have their daily dose of prednisolone reduced by 2.5 to 5 mg every 2 or 3 days, or, for those on longer-term treatment, the reduction may be more gradual at a rate of 2.5 mg every 1 to 3 weeks and possibly less. When the dose has reached 10 mg daily decrements may be made with 1-mg tablets. Another approach may be to convert daily therapy gradually into alternate-day therapy by progressively reducing the amount of corticosteroid received on every second day, and once alternate-day therapy is established the dose may be further reduced until, for example, a dose of 1 mg on alternate days for one week is attained.

1. Committee on Safety of Medicines/Medicines Control Agency. Withdrawal of systemic corticosteroids. *Current Problems* 1998; **24:** 5–7.
2. Anonymous. Corticosteroids and hypothalamic-pituitary-adrenocortical function. *Br Med J* 1980; **280:** 813–14.
3. Helfer EL, Rose LI. Corticosteroids and adrenal suppression: characterising and avoiding the problem. *Drugs* 1989; **38:** 838–45.
4. Page RC. How to wean a patient off corticosteroids. *Prescribers' J* 1997; **37:** 11–16.

Precautions for Corticosteroids

Corticosteroids should only be used systemically with great caution in the presence of congestive heart failure, recent myocardial infarction, or hypertension, in patients with diabetes mellitus, epilepsy (but see below for use in infantile seizures), glaucoma, hypothyroidism, liver failure, osteoporosis, peptic ulceration, psychoses or severe affective disorders, and renal impairment. Children may be at increased risk of some adverse effects; in addition, corticosteroids may cause growth retardation, and prolonged administration is rarely justified. The elderly too may be at greater risk from adverse effects.

Corticosteroids are usually contra-indicated in the presence of acute infections uncontrolled by appropriate antimicrobial chemotherapy. Similarly, patients already receiving corticosteroid therapy are more susceptible to infection, the symptoms of which, moreover, may be masked until an advanced stage has been reached. Patients with active or doubtfully quiescent tuberculosis should not be given corticosteroids except, very rarely, as adjuncts to treatment with antitubercular drugs. Patients with quiescent tuberculosis should be observed closely and should receive chemoprophylaxis if corticosteroid therapy is prolonged.

The risks of chickenpox and probably of severe herpes zoster are increased in non-immune patients receiving therapeutic doses of systemic corticosteroids, and patients should avoid close personal contact with either infection. Passive immunisation is recommended for non-immune patients who do come into contact with chickenpox. Similar precautions apply to measles. Live vaccines should not be given to patients receiving high-dose systemic corticosteroid therapy nor for at least 3 months afterwards; killed vaccines or toxoids may be given although the response may be attenuated.

During prolonged courses of corticosteroid therapy, patients should be examined regularly. Sodium intake may need to be reduced and calcium and potassium supplements may be necessary. Monitoring of the fluid intake and output, and daily weight records may give early warning of fluid retention. Back pain may signify osteoporosis. Children are at special risk from raised intracranial pressure. Patients should carry cards (and preferably also wear bracelets) giving full details of their corticosteroid therapy; they and their relatives should be fully conversant with the implications of their therapy and the precautions to be taken.

Measures to compensate for the adrenals' inability to respond to stress (see Withdrawal, above) include increasing the dose to cover minor intercurrent illnesses or trauma such as surgery (with intramuscular administration to cover vomiting). For details of dosages used, see Uses and Administration, below.

Rapid intravenous injection of massive doses of corticosteroids may sometimes cause cardiovascular collapse and injections should therefore be given slowly or by infusion.

Many drugs have been reported to interfere with certain assay procedures for corticosteroids in body fluids and corticosteroids themselves may interfere with or alter the results of assays for some endogenous substances or drugs.

The risk of systemic absorption should always be considered when applying corticosteroids topically. They should not be applied with an occlusive dressing to large areas of the body. Long-term topical use is best avoided, especially in children. Also they should not be used for the treatment of ulcerative conditions, nor of rosacea, and should not be used indiscriminately for pruritus. Occasionally they may be used with the addition of a suitable antimicrobial substance in the treatment of infected skin but there is a risk of sensitivity reactions occurring.

Caution is required when corticosteroids are used locally to treat eye disorders (see under Uses and Administration, p.1021).

A report of two cases of Cushing's syndrome associated with inappropriately prolonged use of corticosteroid nasal drops in children.[1] Such drops should not be prescribed on a repeat prescription basis. See also Adrenal Suppression, under Adverse Effects, above.

1. Findlay CA, *et al.* Childhood Cushing's syndrome induced by betamethasone nose drops, and repeat prescriptions. *Br Med J* 1998; **317:** 739–40.

Contraception. There are some isolated case reports of contraceptive failure in women using intra-uterine devices and receiving corticosteroid therapy.[1-3]

1. Zerner J, *et al.* Failure of an intrauterine device concurrent with administration of corticosteroids. *Fertil Steril* 1976; **27:** 1467–8.
2. Inkeles DM, Hansen RI. Unexpected pregnancy in a woman using an intrauterine device and receiving steroid therapy. *Ann Ophthalmol* 1982; **14:** 975.
3. Buhler M, Papiernik E. Successive pregnancies in women fitted with intrauterine devices who take anti-inflammatory drugs. *Lancet* 1983; **i:** 483.

Porphyria. In a review[1] of drug-induced porphyrias and comments on the conflicting evidence concerning corticosteroids it was noted that a report suggesting that corticosteroids may have a role in treating the acute attack together with many reports attesting to their safety, contrasted with their repeated incrimination as the offending agent in producing such episodes. It was considered that as corticosteroids may be life-saving, they should be used if really indicated.

1. Moore MR, Disler PB. Drug-induction of the acute porphyrias. *Adverse Drug React Acute Poisoning Rev* 1983; **2:** 149–89.

Pregnancy and breast feeding. Studies have shown that corticosteroids administered to pregnant women did not have adverse effects on the fetus in terms of psychological development[1] or growth and general health factors.[2] However, there has been an isolated report[3] wherein the topical administration of triamcinolone to a pregnant woman for treatment of eczema was considered to have caused fetal growth retardation. In another study[4] of 11 women with placenta praevia given intramuscular betamethasone 12 mg repeated 24 hours later, there were two cases of constriction of the ductus arteriosus; neither case was severe.

Early studies in *animals* have demonstrated an increase in fetal cleft palate following maternal ingestion of high corticosteroid doses, and cortisone has been used widely as a tool for the investigation of mechanisms responsible for cleft lip and palate. With doses used in clinical practice, however, the risk appears to be low. In an analysis of several hundred cases reported in the literature[5] it was concluded that the incidence of cleft palate in exposed children was slightly higher than in a random sample, but that in the small selected group studied, this higher incidence might be fallacious. Although an increased incidence of malformations in the children of asthmatic mothers given prednisolone 2.5 to 30 mg daily during pregnancy was noted,[6] others[7] have suggested that the outcome might have been worse in untreated asthmatic mothers. Moreover, no significant increase in the risk of fetal or maternal complications was found in a study of asthmatic mothers given prednisolone 2.5 to 20 mg daily.[8] More recently, no evidence of a teratogenic effect for corticosteroids was noted in a comparison of the maternal drug histories of the mothers of 764 infants born with anomalies of the CNS and 764 controls,[9] and in another study[10] there were no striking differences in birth-weight and frequency of 'small for dates' infants born to mothers who received systemic corticosteroids during pregnancy for pemphigoid gestationis and those who did not.

Fears concerning the administration of corticosteroids during late pregnancy relate to their direct adverse effects on the fetus. These involve the known side-effects of corticosteroids, such as increased risk of infection and adrenal insufficiency. No such adverse effects were noted in the infants of 70 exposed pregnancies,[8] although there have been individual reports.[11,12] The potential dangers of maternal diabetogenic effects have been demonstrated in a study of metabolic changes induced in diabetic women by salbutamol (used in the prevention of premature labour) which could be exacerbated by concomitant administration of dexamethasone (used to promote maturation of the fetal lung) with consequent danger to the fetus.[13]

A review[14] by the Committee on Safety of Medicines in the UK concluded that there was no convincing evidence that corticosteroids caused an increased incidence of congenital abnormality. Prolonged or repeated administration during pregnancy did increase the risk of intra-uterine growth retardation but this did not seem to be a problem following short-term treatment. It was noted that the ability of different corticosteroids to cross the placenta varied very markedly. It was also remarked that sufficient prednisolone was distributed into breast milk (see p.1048) that infants of mothers receiving 40 mg or more daily should be monitored for signs of adrenal suppression; it was not known if this applied to other corticosteroids.

1. Schmand B, *et al.* Psychological development of children who were treated antenatally with corticosteroids to prevent respiratory distress syndrome. *Pediatrics* 1990; **86:** 58–64.
2. Doyle LW, *et al.* Antenatal steroid therapy and 5-year outcome of extremely low birth weight infants. *Obstet Gynecol* 1989; **73:** 743–6.
3. Katz VL, *et al.* Severe symmetric intrauterine growth retardation associated with the topical use of triamcinolone. *Am J Obstet Gynecol* 1990; **162:** 396–7.
4. Wasserstrum N, *et al.* Betamethasone and the human fetal ductus arteriosus. *Obstet Gynecol* 1989; **74:** 897–900.
5. Popert AJ. Pregnancy and adrenocortical hormones: some aspects of their interaction in rheumatic diseases. *Br Med J* 1962; **1:** 967–72.
6. Warrell DW, Taylor R. Outcome for the foetus of mothers receiving prednisolone during pregnancy. *Lancet* 1968; **i:** 117–18.
7. Scott JK. Foetal risk with maternal prednisolone. *Lancet* 1968; **i:** 208.
8. Schatz M, *et al.* Corticosteroid therapy for the pregnant asthmatic patient. *JAMA* 1975; **233:** 804–7.
9. Winship KA, *et al.* Maternal drug histories and central nervous system anomalies. *Arch Dis Child* 1984; **59:** 1052–60.
10. Holmes RC, Black MM. The fetal prognosis in pemphigoid gestationis (herpes gestationis). *Br J Dermatol* 1984; **110:** 67–72.
11. Grajwer LA, *et al.* Neonatal subclinical adrenal insufficiency: result of maternal steroid therapy. *JAMA* 1977; **238:** 1279–80.
12. Evans TJ, *et al.* Congenital cytomegalovirus infection after maternal renal transplantation. *Lancet* 1975; **i:** 1359–60.
13. Gündoğdu AS, *et al.* Comparison of hormonal and metabolic effects of salbutamol infusion in normal subjects and insulin-requiring diabetics. *Lancet* 1979; **ii:** 1317–21.
14. Committee on Safety of Medicines/Medicines Control Agency. Systemic corticosteroids in pregnancy and lactation. *Current Problems* 1998; **24:** 9.

Septic shock. Some manufacturers recommend that corticosteroids should not be given to patients with septic shock; for references to the controversial use of high-dose corticosteroids in septic shock see under Septic Shock, in Uses and Administration, below.

Sickle-cell disease. Sickle-cell crisis was reported to have been precipitated by corticosteroids in 2 patients with sickle C disease.[1] The crises in these patients were considered to have started with ischaemic necrosis of the bone marrow leading to fat embolism, cerebral hypoxia, and coma.

For mention of the use of corticosteroids in sickle-cell crisis see under Sickle-cell Disease, in Uses and Administration, below.

1. Huang JC, *et al.* Sickling crisis, fat embolism, and coma after steroids. *Lancet* 1994; **344:** 951–2.

Tooth erosion. The increased incidence of tooth erosion seen in patients with asthma might be related to the pH of inhaled powder (but not aerosol) formulations.[1] Beclomethasone dipropionate and fluticasone had pHs of 4.76 as powder formulations, whereas the aerosols were well above the pH of 5.5 at which tooth substance begins to dissolve. Budesonide was less acidic in its powder formulation (pH 6.47).

1. O'Sullivan EA, Curzon MEJ. Drug treatments for asthma may cause erosive tooth damage. *Br Med J* 1998; **317:** 820.

Varicella. A number of cases of fatal or near fatal chickenpox have been reported in patients receiving corticosteroids.[1-3] Although mostly associated with systemic use, severe disseminated varicella and staphylococcal pericarditis have been reported in an infant following a single application of a potent topical corticosteroid cream.[4] Guidelines issued by the UK Committee on Safety of Medicines state that all patients taking systemic corticosteroids for purposes other than replacement, and who have not had chickenpox, should be regarded as being at risk, irrespective of the dose or duration of treatment.[2,5] Passive immunisation with varicella-zoster immunoglobulin should be given to non-immune patients who are receiving corticosteroids, or who have received them within the last 3 months, if they are exposed to chickenpox. Passive immunisation should preferably be given within 3 days and not later than 10 days from exposure.[2]

1. Rice P, *et al.* Near fatal chickenpox during prednisolone treatment. *Br Med J* 1994; **309:** 1069–70.
2. Committee on Safety of Medicines/Medicines Control Agency. Severe chickenpox associated with systemic corticosteroids. *Current Problems* 1994; **20:** 1–2.
3. Dowell SF, Breese JS. Severe varicella associated with steroid use. *Pediatrics* 1993; **92:** 223–8.
4. Brumund MR, *et al.* Disseminated varicella and staphylococcal pericarditis after topical steroids. *J Pediatr* 1997; **131:** 162–3.
5. Ellender D, *et al.* Severe chickenpox during treatment with corticosteroids. *Br Med J* 1995; **310:** 327.

Interactions

Concurrent administration of barbiturates, carbamazepine, phenytoin, primidone, or rifampicin may enhance the metabolism and reduce the effects of corticosteroids. Concurrent administration of corticosteroids with potassium-depleting diuretics, such as thiazides or frusemide, may cause excessive potassium loss. There may be an increased incidence of gastro-intestinal bleeding and ulceration when corticosteroids are given with NSAIDs. Response to anticoagulants may be altered by corticosteroids and requirements of antidiabetic agents and antihypertensives may be increased. Corticosteroids may decrease serum concentrations of salicylates and may decrease the effect of antimuscarinics in myasthenia gravis.

Analgesics. For the effect of corticosteroids on salicylates see Aspirin, p.17.

Antibacterials. Rifampicin reduces the activity of corticosteroids[1-8] by accelerating their metabolism, and a similar effect would be expected with other rifamycins. There is limited evidence that the macrolide antibacterials triacetyloleandomycin,[9-11] and perhaps erythromycin,[12] may inhibit the metabolism of methylprednisolone, but not of prednisolone.[10] Dosage reduction should be carried out as necessary if triacetyloleandomycin and methylprednisolone are used concurrently. There is no evidence of a clinically significant interaction between these macrolides and other corticosteroids.

For reference to corticosteroids lowering plasma concentrations of isoniazid and enhancing its renal clearance, see p.219.

1. Edwards OM, *et al.* Changes in cortisol metabolism following rifampicin therapy. *Lancet* 1974; **ii:** 549–51.
2. Maisey DN, *et al.* Rifampicin and cortisone replacement therapy. *Lancet* 1974; **ii:** 896–7.
3. Steenbergen GJ, Pfaltzgraff RE. Treatment of neuritis in borderline leprosy with rifampicin and corticosteroids—a pilot trial. *Lepr Rev* 1975; **46:** 115–18.
4. Buffington GA, *et al.* Interaction of rifampin and glucocorticoids: adverse effect on renal allograft function. *JAMA* 1976; **236:** 1958–60.
5. Hendrickse W, *et al.* Rifampicin-induced non-responsiveness to corticosteroid treatment in nephrotic syndrome. *Br Med J* 1979; **1:** 306.
6. van Marle W, *et al.* Concurrent steroid and rifampicin therapy. *Br Med J* 1979; **1:** 1020.
7. Jopline WH, Pettit JHS. Interaction between rifampicin, steroids and oral contraceptives. *Lepr Rev* 1979; **50:** 331–2.
8. McAllister WAC, *et al.* Rifampicin reduces effectiveness and bioavailability of prednisolone. *Br Med J* 1983; **286:** 923–5.
9. Szefler SJ, *et al.* The effect of troleandomycin on methylprednisolone elimination. *J Allergy Clin Immunol* 1980; **66:** 447–51.
10. Szefler SJ, *et al.* Steroid-specific and anticonvulsant interaction aspects of troleandomycin-steroid therapy. *J Allergy Clin Immunol* 1982; **69:** 455–60.
11. Kamada AK, *et al.* Glucocorticoid reduction with troleandomycin in chronic severe asthmatic children: implication for future trials and clinical application. *J Allergy Clin Immunol* 1992; **89:** 285.
12. LaForce CF, *et al.* Inhibition of methylprednisolone elimination in the presence of erythromycin therapy. *J Allergy Clin Immunol* 1983; **72:** 34–9.

Anticoagulants. For the various effects of corticosteroids on anticoagulants, see under Warfarin Sodium, p.968.

Antiepileptics. Reduced efficacy of corticosteroids has been noted in asthmatic, arthritic, renal transplant, and other patients who also received phenytoin or phenobarbitone,[1-3] and the clearance of corticosteroids has also been reported to be markedly increased by concurrent administration of carbamazepine.[3] Induction of microsomal liver enzymes by the antiepileptic drug, resulting in enhanced metabolism of the corticosteroid is believed to be the underlying mechanism. Different corticosteroids appear to be affected to different degrees, but the disease state, doses, and other determinants such as diet, sex, and other drugs administered may also be contributory factors. An increase in the dosage of the corticosteroids may be necessary in order to maintain the desired therapeutic response.[1]

1. Brooks SM, *et al.* Adverse effects of phenobarbital on corticosteroid metabolism in patients with bronchial asthma. *N Engl J Med* 1972; **286:** 1125–8.
2. Nation RL, *et al.* Pharmacokinetic drug interactions with phenytoin (part II). *Clin Pharmacokinet* 1990; **18:** 131–50.
3. Bartoszek M, *et al.* Prednisolone and methylprednisolone kinetics in children receiving anticonvulsant therapy. *Clin Pharmacol Ther* 1987; **42:** 424–32.

Antifungals. Ketoconazole increases serum-methylprednisolone concentrations and enhances methylprednisolone's adrenal suppressive effects.[1,2] A 50% reduction in intravenous methylprednisolone dose was suggested during concomitant ketoconazole therapy.[2] A similar effect was not evident when prednisone was given by mouth[3] although some workers[4] found that ketoconazole reduced the total clearance of prednisolone given intravenously and of prednisone given by mouth.

1. Glynn AM, *et al.* Effects of ketoconazole on methylprednisolone pharmacokinetics and cortisol secretion. *Clin Pharmacol Ther* 1986; **39:** 654–9.
2. Kandrotas RJ, *et al.* Ketoconazole effects on methylprednisolone disposition and their joint suppression of endogenous cortisol. *Clin Pharmacol Ther* 1987; **42:** 465–70.
3. Ludwig EA, *et al.* Steroid-specific effects of ketoconazole on corticosteroid disposition: unaltered prednisolone elimination. *DICP Ann Pharmacother* 1989; **23:** 858–61.
4. Zürcher RM, *et al.* Impact of ketoconazole on the metabolism of prednisolone. *Clin Pharmacol Ther* 1989; **45:** 366–72.

Antineoplastics and immunosuppressants. It has been suggested that mutual inhibition of metabolism occurs between cyclosporin and corticosteroids, and may increase the plasma concentrations of either drug.[1,2] A review[3] cited studies supporting this conclusion but also mentioned studies which showed that cyclosporin did not significantly decrease clearance of prednisolone[4] and that corticosteroids did not change or decreased cyclosporin concentrations.[5,6] Some of these conflicting results may be due to differences in the methods used to measure cyclosporin concentrations.

For reference to single doses of prednisone inhibiting the activation of cyclophosphamide (but longer-term treatment increasing its activation) see Cyclophosphamide, p.517.

1. Klintmalm G, Säwe J. High dose methylprednisolone increases plasma cyclosporin levels in renal transplant recipients. *Lancet* 1984; **i:** 731.
2. Ost L. Effects of cyclosporin on prednisolone metabolism. *Lancet* 1984; **i:** 451.
3. Yee GC, McGuire TR. Pharmacokinetic drug interactions with cyclosporin (part II). *Clin Pharmacokinet* 1990; **19:** 400–15.
4. Frey FJ, *et al.* Evidence that cyclosporine does not affect the metabolism of prednisolone after renal transplantation. *Transplantation* 1987; **43:** 494–8.
5. Ptachcinski RJ, *et al.* Cyclosporine - high-dose steroid interaction in renal transplant recipients: assessment by HPLC. *Transplant Proc* 1987; **19:** 1728–9.
6. Hricik DE, *et al.* Association of the absence of steroid therapy with increased cyclosporine blood levels in renal transplant recipients. *Transplantation* 1990; **49:** 221–3.

Antivirals. As mentioned under Indinavir, p.614, it is suggested that corticosteroids such as dexamethasone and prednisolone may reduce plasma concentrations of HIV-protease inhibitors, and corticosteroid plasma concentrations may in turn be increased.

Lipid regulating drugs. Addition of colestipol to the therapy of a patient with hypopituitarism receiving maintenance therapy with hydrocortisone resulted in headaches, ataxia, and lethargy.[1] Mental status returned to normal within hours of an intravenous dose of hydrocortisone 100 mg, and colestipol was subsequently withdrawn uneventfully.

1. Neki KE, Aron DC. Hydrocortisone-colestipol interaction. *Ann Pharmacother* 1993; **27:** 980–1.

Neuromuscular blockers. For reference to corticosteroids antagonising the neuromuscular blocking effects of pancuronium, see under Atracurium, p.1306.

Sex hormones. Reviews[1,2] discussing several reports of an enhanced effect of corticosteroids in women also receiving oestrogens or oral contraceptives and commenting that the dose of corticosteroids in some cases may need to be reduced.

1. Shenfield GM. Drug interactions with oral contraceptive preparations. *Med J Aust* 1986; **144:** 205–10.
2. Back DJ, Orme ML'E. Pharmacokinetic drug interactions with oral contraceptives. *Clin Pharmacokinet* 1990; **18:** 472–84.

Smoking. There was a report of an appreciable and consistent increase in plasma corticosteroids after cigarette smoking in man.[1] However, a review concerning the clinical importance of smoking and drug interactions[2] concluded that in the majority of examples, including corticosteroids, there was little evidence of a recognisable hazard from the interaction.

1. Kershbaum A, *et al.* Effect of smoking and nicotine on adrenocortical secretion. *JAMA* 1968; **203:** 275–8.
2. D'Arcy PF. Tobacco smoking and drugs: a clinically important interaction? *Drug Intell Clin Pharm* 1984; **18:** 302–7.

Sympathomimetics. Studies in 21 asthmatic patients suggested that the plasma half-life of dexamethasone was decreased when it was administered with ephedrine.[1] More significantly, concomitant administration of corticosteroids with beta$_2$-adrenoceptor stimulants may potentiate any hypokalaemic effects.[2]

1. Brooks SM, *et al.* The effects of ephedrine and theophylline on dexamethasone metabolism in bronchial asthma. *J Clin Pharmacol* 1977; **17:** 308–18.
2. Committee on Safety of Medicines. β_2 agonists, xanthines and hypokalaemia. *Current Problems 28* 1990.

Thalidomide. In a double-blind crossover study of thalidomide in the treatment of severe chronic erythema nodosum leprosum,[1] the dose of prednisolone necessary to suppress symptoms was considerably reduced in 9 of 10 patients while they were receiving thalidomide 300 mg daily and there has been a comment[2] that prednisolone should not be given with thalidomide.

1. Waters MFR. An internally-controlled double blind trial of thalidomide in severe erythema nodosum leprosum. *Lepr Rev* 1971; **42:** 26–42.
2. WHO, Regional Office for the Western Pacific. Final report on the first regional working group on leprosy, Manila, Philippines, 7–12 December, 1978. *Lepr Rev* 1979; **50:** 326–9.

Xanthines. For the effect of corticosteroids on theophylline, see p.769.

Pharmacokinetics of Corticosteroids

Corticosteroids, are, in general, readily absorbed from the gastro-intestinal tract. They are also absorbed from sites of local administration. When administered by topical application, particularly under an occlusive dressing or when the skin is broken, or as a rectal enema, sufficient corticosteroid may be absorbed to give systemic effects; this is also a possibility with other local routes of administration such as inhalation. Water-soluble forms of corticosteroids are given by intravenous injection for a rapid response; more prolonged effects are achieved using lipid-soluble forms of corticosteroids by intramuscular injection.

Corticosteroids are rapidly distributed to all body tissues. They cross the placenta and may be excreted in small amounts in breast milk.

Most corticosteroids in the circulation are extensively bound to plasma proteins, mainly to globulin and less so to albumin. The corticosteroid-binding globulin (transcortin) has high affinity but low binding capacity, while the albumin has low affinity but large binding capacity. The synthetic corticosteroids are less extensively protein bound than hydrocortisone (cortisol). They also tend to have longer half-lives.

Corticosteroids are metabolised mainly in the liver but also in other tissues, and are excreted in the urine. The slower metabolism of the synthetic corticosteroids with their lower protein-binding affinity may account for their increased potency compared with the natural corticosteroids.

Reviews.

1. Begg EJ, *et al.* The pharmacokinetics of corticosteroid agents. *Med J Aust* 1987; **146:** 37–41.
2. McGhee CNJ. Pharmacokinetics of ophthalmic corticosteroids. *Br J Ophthalmol* 1992; **76:** 681–4.

Uses and Administration of Corticosteroids

The corticosteroids are used in physiological doses for replacement therapy in adrenal insufficiency. Pharmacological doses are used when palliative anti-inflammatory or immunosuppressant effects are required. Before instituting therapy the benefits and risks of corticosteroids should be considered; where appropriate, local rather than systemic therapy should be used. The lowest dose of corticosteroids that is effective should be used for the shortest possible duration of time; high doses may be needed for life-threatening situations.

The effects of different corticosteroids vary qualitatively as well as quantitatively, and it may not be possible to substitute one for another in equal therapeutic amounts without provoking side-effects. Thus, whereas cortisone and hydrocortisone have very appreciable mineralocorticoid (or sodium-retaining) properties relative to their glucocorticoid (or anti-inflammatory) properties, prednisolone and prednisone have considerably less, and others, such as betamethasone and dexamethasone, have none or virtually none. In contrast, the mineralocorticoid properties of fludrocortisone are so pronounced that its glucocorticoid effects are considered to have no clinical significance.

As a rough guide, the approximate **equivalent doses** of the main corticosteroids in terms of their glucocorticoid (or anti-inflammatory) properties alone, are:

- betamethasone 0.75 mg
- cortisone acetate 25 mg
- dexamethasone 0.75 mg
- hydrocortisone 20 mg
- methylprednisolone 4 mg
- prednisolone 5 mg
- prednisone 5 mg
- triamcinolone 4 mg.

The mineralocorticoid properties of corticosteroids (see p.1010) are rarely employed. Exceptions include the treatment of primary adrenocortical insufficiency, in which both mineralocorticoid and glucocorticoid replacement is necessary, usually in the form of fludrocortisone with hydrocortisone (for details, see p.1017). The mineralocorticoid properties of fludrocortisone are also employed to maintain blood pressure in patients with orthostatic hypotension (see p.1040).

The anti-inflammatory and immunosuppressant glucocorticoid properties of corticosteroids (see p.1010) are used to suppress the clinical manifestations of disease in a wide range of disorders considered to have inflammatory or immunological components. For these purposes, the synthetic analogues with their considerably reduced mineralocorticoid properties linked with enhanced glucocorticoid properties, are preferred. Despite the existence of very powerful synthetic glucocorticoids with virtually no mineralocorticoid activity, the hazards of inappropriately high glucocorticoid therapy are such that the less powerful prednisolone and prednisone are the glucocorticoids of choice for most conditions, since they allow for a greater margin of safety. There is little to choose between prednisolone and prednisone; prednisolone is usually recommended in the UK since it exists in a metabolically active form, whereas prednisone is inactive and must be converted into its active form by the liver; hence, particularly in some liver disorders, bioavailability of prednisone is less reliable (but see under Precautions of Prednisolone, p.1048).

Because the therapeutic effects of corticosteroids seem to be of longer duration than the metabolic effects, intermittent treatment with corticosteroids has been used to allow the metabolic rhythm of the body to become re-established while maintaining the therapeutic effects. Regimens of intermittent therapy have usually consisted of short courses of treatment or of the administration of single doses on alternate days. Such alternate-day therapy, however, is only appropriate for corticosteroids with a relatively short duration of action and small mineralocorticoid effect, such as prednisolone, and only in certain disease states. Corticosteroids are also given in single daily doses at times coinciding with maximum or minimum function of the adrenal cortex in order to obtain the desired effect on the adrenals.

Doses of corticosteroids higher than those required for physiological replacement will eventually lead to some degree of adrenal suppression, the extent depending on the dose given, and the route, frequency, time, and duration of administration. The adrenal glands are traditionally considered to have a daily output equivalent to approximately 20 mg of hydrocortisone (cortisol), but individual blood-cortisol concentrations may vary widely, and can increase up to tenfold or more during stress. Therefore, during periods of stress or trauma, such as during and after surgery and when suffering from intercurrent infections, the corticosteroid dosage of patients must be increased. Intramuscular or intravenous injection of hydrocortisone 100 mg (usually as the sodium succinate) with the premedication and repeated every 8 hours has been used in patients on long-term corticosteroid therapy undergoing surgical procedures. This dose is generally tapered off over 5 days to reach a typical maintenance dose of 20 to 30 mg of hydrocortisone daily. Whether such a standardised regimen is always appropriate, however, has been questioned—see Surgery, under Administration, below.

Although the empirical use of a corticosteroid is appropriate in a life-threatening situation, generally it is advisable not to begin corticosteroid therapy until a definite diagnosis has been made, for otherwise symptoms may be masked to such an extent that a true diagnosis becomes extremely difficult to make and the disease may reach an advanced stage before detection.

Systemic therapy is indicated in a wide variety of conditions. Where possible the oral route is preferred but parenteral administration may be used if the disease is severe or an emergency arises. Intravenous therapy is generally employed for intensive emergency treatment as the onset of action is relatively fast although intramuscular injections, often formulated as longer-acting depot preparations, may also be used to provide subsequent cover. Examples of conditions treated with systemic corticosteroids include:

- as an adjunct to adrenaline in life-threatening allergic reactions such as angioedema or anaphylaxis (see p.816)
- some blood disorders, including auto-immune haemolytic anaemia (p.702) and idiopathic thrombocytopenic purpura (p.1023)
- selected connective tissue and muscle disorders, such as Behçet's syndrome (p.1018), polymyalgia rheumatica (p.1027), polymyositis (p.1027), systemic lupus erythematosus (p.1029), and the vasculitic syndromes (p.1031)
- some cases of rheumatoid arthritis, where recent evidence suggests there may be value in early treatment of active disease (see p.1028)
- some inflammatory eye disorders, particularly those affecting the posterior chamber
- inflammatory gastro-intestinal disorders, such as Crohn's disease and ulcerative colitis, although administration by the rectal route may be preferred in some circumstances (see p.1171)
- infections accompanied by a severe inflammatory component provided that appropriate anti-infective chemotherapy is also given and that the benefits of corticosteroid therapy outweigh the possible risk of disseminated infection; examples of conditions where corticosteroid may be considered include helminthic infections, the Herxheimer reaction, and tuberculous meningitis
- selected kidney disorders including lupus nephritis (p.1029) and various glomerular disorders (p.1021)
- selected liver disorders, including auto-immune chronic active hepatitis (p.1019)
- some neurological disorders such as infantile seizures and subacute demyelinating polyneuropathy; also in cerebral oedema (p.1019), including that associated with malignancy
- some respiratory disorders, such as asthma (see p.745, although inhaled corticosteroids are preferred to oral therapy for prophylaxis), interstitial lung disease (p.1024), pulmonary sarcoid (p.1028), and neonatal respiratory distress syndrome (p.1025)
- severe skin disorders such as pemphigus and pemphigoid (p.1075).

Glucocorticoids are also used in conjunction with antineoplastic agents in regimens for the management of malignant disease as described under Antineoplastics and Immunosuppressants, p.470. They are also given to reduce immune responses after organ transplantations, often in conjunction with other immunosuppressants (see p.498).

Corticosteroids are not now considered useful in patients with aspiration syndromes, stroke, or septic shock, although they have been used in these conditions.

Intra-articular injection in the absence of infection and with full aseptic precautions, may be used, for example, in the treatment of rheumatoid arthritis (p.2), osteoarthritis (p.2), and ankylosing spondylitis (p.4). Either hydrocortisone acetate or one of the esters of the synthetic corticosteroids are used. It should be noted that there have been several reports of joint damage after the intra-articular injection of corticosteroids into load-bearing joints.

Topical application often produces dramatic suppression of skin diseases, such as eczema, infantile eczema, atopic dermatitis, dermatitis herpetiformis, contact dermatitis, seborrhoeic dermatitis, neurodermatitis, some forms of psoriasis, and intertrigo, in which inflammation is a prominent feature. However, the disease may return or be exacerbated when corticosteroids are withdrawn and this appears to be a particular problem in some of the forms of psoriasis. Occasionally, corticosteroids may be used with the addition of a suitable antimicrobial substance, such as neomycin, in the treatment of infected skin. For comments on the topical application of preparations containing a corticosteroid and neomycin, see Neomycin Sulphate, p.229.

Intralesional injection sometimes hastens the resolution of chronic skin lesions such as lichen planus, lichen simplex, and keloids.

Topical application to the eye in inflammatory and traumatic disorders has led to dramatic results, but the occurrence of herpetic and fungal infections of the cornea and other serious complications are considerable obstacles and eye drops containing corticosteroids, should be used under strict ophthalmic supervision with regular checks of intra-ocular pressure. Care is also required when corticosteroids are given by **subconjunctival injection** in inflammatory eye disorders.

Ear drops containing corticosteroids are used in the treatment of otitis externa (see p.134).

Inhalational therapy is widely used in the prophylaxis of asthma (see p.745).

Nasal application is also used in the prophylaxis and treatment of allergic and non-allergic rhinitis (see p.400).

Rectal administration, by either suppository or enema, may be employed for some corticosteroids.

Administration

It has long been known that the diurnal rhythm of the adrenal cortex leads to about 70% of the daily secretion being made between midnight and 9 am.[1] In the treatment of adrenal cortical hyperplasia a dose of hydrocortisone given at night will be nearly twice as suppressive as the same dose given during the day. However, in treating allergic or collagen disease when suppression of adrenal cortical activity is best avoided a dose of hydrocortisone at about 8 am is indicated. When reducing corticosteroid dosage after treatment, a single dose given at 8 am will be most beneficial and will not inhibit corticotrophin secretion. Also, for similar reasons,[2] when used for replacement therapy corticosteroids are given in unequal doses during the day (two-thirds of the daily dose in the morning, and one-third at night).

1. Demos CH, *et al.* A modified (once a day) corticosteroid dosage regimen. *Clin Pharmacol Ther* 1964; **5:** 721–7.
2. Aronson JK. Chronopharmacology: reflections on time and a new text. *Lancet* 1990; **335:** 1515–16.

Epidural route. A detailed review and discussion[1] concerning the epidural use of corticosteroids in sciatica concluded that the reported clinical complications were uncommon but that the efficacy was unproven. A subsequent study[2] suggested that although epidural injection of methylprednisolone acetate produced short-term improvement in pain and sensory deficit, treatment resulted in no functional benefit and did not reduce the need for surgery.

Although the authors of the first review felt that appropriate clinical studies were needed, it should be noted that inadvertent intrathecal administration of corticosteroids has resulted in severe neurological complications.

1. Bogduk N, Cherry D. Epidural corticosteroid agents for sciatica. *Med J Aust* 1985; **143:** 402–6.
2. Carette S, *et al.* Epidural corticosteroid injections for sciatica due to herniated nucleus pulposus. *N Engl J Med* 1997; **336:** 1634–40.

Inhalational therapy. The majority of patients taking inhaled corticosteroids for asthma only require low doses. A discussion on high-dose inhaled corticosteroids in asthma therapy,[1] published in 1987, concluded that improvement in asthma control could be achieved in patients with severe or chronic asthma when the dose was increased. In some patients dependent upon oral corticosteroids significant reductions in the oral dose could be made by increasing the inhaled dose.[1] Some doubt has been cast on this view by a more recent multicentre study which found that high doses of inhaled beclomethasone dipropionate, given via a spacer device, were no better at permitting a reduction in oral corticosteroid dosage than were low doses.[2] Another study found that although increasing the inhaled doses of beclomethasone or fluticasone did improve pulmonary function, the changes were insufficiently great to be of much clinical significance.[3] However, accepted guidelines for the treatment of asthma include instructions to increase the dose of inhaled corticosteroid should the standard dose not produce improvement (see p.745), and in clinical practice improved asthma control can often be achieved by increasing the dose.

Different inhaled corticosteroids differ in their potency, though there is little evidence of a difference in efficacy at recommended doses.[4] Of those widely available by inhalation, flunisolide is less potent than beclomethasone while budesonide is more potent, and fluticasone more potent still. The ability to use fewer inhalations with more potent drugs might enhance compliance.[4] For inhaled corticosteroids to be effective in the prophylaxis of asthma they must be taken regularly and patient compliance is important.

Efficient delivery to the bronchial tree is crucial and a number of different devices are available for administration. The pressurised aerosol inhaler remains the most convenient and acceptable if the patient's technique is satisfactory. However, many patients, especially children, find that administration by inhalation is made much easier by fitting a spacer device to the inhaler.[5] Such a device is recommended when high doses are to be inhaled, to prevent oropharyngeal deposition and subsequent systemic absorption. However, the type of spacer used and the method of use may dramatically alter the amount of drug available for inhalation. The drug should be introduced into the spacer by single actuations, each followed by inhalation, with the delay between actuation of the inhaler and inhalation from the spacer kept to a minimum. In some spacers static electricity accumulates, and the build up of charge reduces drug delivery: this can be controlled by washing and drying the spacer in air before beginning use.[6]

Changes in formulation of the propellant, to remove chlorofluorocarbons, may also affect drug availability; it is reported to be increased, requiring dose reduction with new formulations.[7]

1. Smith MJ. The place of high-dose inhaled corticosteroids in asthma therapy. *Drugs* 1987; **33:** 423–9.
2. Hummel S, *et al.* Comparison of oral-steroid sparing by high-dose and low-dose inhaled steroid in maintenance treatment of severe asthma. *Lancet* 1992; **340:** 1483–7.
3. Boe J, *et al.* High-dose inhaled steroids in asthmatics: moderate efficacy gain and suppression of the hypothalamic-pituitary-adrenal axis. *Eur Respir J* 1994; **7:** 2179–84.
4. Kelly HW. Comparison of inhaled corticosteroids. *Ann Pharmacother* 1998; **32:** 220–32.
5. Keeley D. Large volume plastic spacers in asthma. *Br Med J* 1992; **305:** 598–9.
6. O'Callaghan C, Barry P. Spacer devices in the treatment of asthma. *Br Med J* 1997; **314:** 1061–2.
7. Legge A. Shift to CFC-free inhalers may require change in doses. *Br Med J* 1997; **315:** 1179.

Intra-articular route. Intra-articular and periarticular injection of corticosteroids is an established treatment for a variety of joint and soft-tissue lesions.[1,2] Pain and inflammation associated with rheumatoid and juvenile chronic arthritis, crystal arthropathies such as gout, and osteoarthritis can be alleviated by injection of a suitable corticosteroid, and in some cases the benefits may be quite prolonged. The longer-acting esters methylprednisolone acetate, triamcinolone acetonide, and triamcinolone hexacetonide are generally preferred. In some cases these may be combined with a local anaesthetic and a short-acting soluble corticosteroid for more rapid relief and to reduce the risk of a post-injection flare. Accurate injection technique is essential, and vigorous skin cleansing and an aseptic technique are required to avoid the introduction of infection into the joint; pre-existing joint infection is a contra-indication to corticosteroid injection. Intra-articular injections may be repeated if necessary but it has been suggested that a single joint should not be injected more than 3 or 4 times a year.

Periarticular injection is also employed in various soft tissue disorders such as bursitis, capsulitis (painful shoulder syndromes), epicondylitis, tenosynovitis, and carpal tunnel syndrome. Particular care is required when injecting to avoid injection directly into a tendon, which may cause the tendon to rupture. A shorter-acting corticosteroid such as hydrocortisone acetate may be more suitable for extra-articular lesions.

1. Anonymous. Articular and periarticular corticosteroid injections. *Drug Ther Bull* 1995; **33:** 67–70.
2. Caldwell JR. Intra-articular corticosteroids: guide to selection and indications for use. *Drugs* 1996; **52:** 507–14.

Surgery. The appropriate glucocorticoid supplementation for patients receiving corticosteroids who undergo surgery has been discussed by Salem and colleagues,[1] who considered that some current recommendations were excessive, in the light of what was known about the adrenal stress response to surgery. They suggested that for minor surgery 25 mg of hydrocortisone or its equivalent pre-operatively was adequate; where surgical stress was likely to be moderate, 50 to 75 mg of hydrocortisone or its equivalent daily in divided doses for 1 to 2 days was suggested. For major surgical stress, a target of 100 to 150 mg of hydrocortisone or its equivalent should be given daily in divided doses for 2 to 3 days, although less might be given if the

Table 1. Guide to potencies of topical corticosteroids.

Very potent	Potent	Moderately potent	Mild
Clobetasol propionate 0.05%	Amcinonide 0.1%	Alclometasone dipropionate 0.05%	Fluocinolone acetonide 0.0025%
Diflucortolone valerate 0.3%	Beclomethasone dipropionate 0.025%	Betamethasone valerate 0.025%	Hydrocortisone 0.5% and 1%
Fluocinolone acetonide 0.2%	Betamethasone benzoate 0.025%	Clobetasone butyrate 0.05%	Hydrocortisone acetate 1%
Halcinonide 0.1%	Betamethasone dipropionate 0.05%	Desoxymethasone 0.05%	Methylprednisolone acetate 0.25%
Halobetasol propionate 0.05%	Betamethasone valerate 0.1%	Flumethasone pivalate 0.02%	
	Budesonide 0.025%	Fluocinolone acetonide 0.00625% and 0.01%	
	Desonide 0.05%	Fluocortin butyl 0.75%	
	Desoxymethasone 0.25%	Fluocortolone preparations (hexanoate with pivalate, each 0.1% and hexanoate with either free alcohol or pivalate, each 0.25%)	
	Diflorasone diacetate 0.05%		
	Diflucortolone valerate 0.1%		
	Fluclorolone acetonide 0.025%	Fluandrenolone 0.0125%	
	Fluocinolone acetonide 0.025%	Hydrocortisone aceponate 0.1%	
	Fluocinonide 0.05%	Prednicarbate 0.25%	
	Fluprednidene acetate 0.1%		
	Hydrocortisone butyrate 0.1%		
	Methyprednisolone aceponate 0.1%		
	Mometasone furoate 0.1%		
	Triamcinolone acetonide 0.1%		

patient's pre-operative glucocorticoid dose was low. Furthermore, these authors considered that the practice of gradually reducing postoperative coverage over several days was not supported by evidence except in cases of high-dose glucocorticoid administration for prolonged periods.

1. Salem M, *et al.* Perioperative glucocorticoid coverage: a reassessment 42 years after emergence of a problem. *Ann Surg* 1994; **219:** 416–25.

Topical application. Guidelines[1,2] for the correct use of topical corticosteroids recommend that an appropriately potent preparation to bring the skin disorder under control should be used. Some recommend use of the lowest potency which will control the disorder, while others have advocated starting treatment with a more potent preparation, treatment may then be continued with a less potent preparation and with less frequent application, once control is obtained. The most potent topical corticosteroids are generally reserved for recalcitrant dermatoses. Once the skin has healed, treatment should be tailed off. Particular care is necessary in the use of topical corticosteroids in children, and the more potent preparations are contra-indicated in infants under 1 year of age, although potent preparations may be needed briefly in older children. It has been suggested that a 'steroid holiday' of at least 2 weeks be considered in children after each 2 or 3 weeks of daily topical therapy to allow thinned epidermis to restore itself and maintain its barrier function.[3]

Care is also necessary in applying corticosteroids to certain anatomical sites such as the face and flexures; some advocate using only hydrocortisone 0.5 or 1% on the face. Patients should be advised that topical corticosteroids should be applied sparingly in thin layers, by smoothing gently into the skin preferably after a bath, and that no benefit is gained from more frequent than twice daily application or by vigorous rubbing.

In a study to determine the requirement of topical corticosteroids,[4] 16 adult patients with eczema were treated with a variety of topical preparations until substantial clearing had occurred (up to 10 days). Results indicated that the mean requirement of preparation, regardless of potency or vehicle, was 6.86 g per m^2 body-surface area. Using this value the calculated quantities of topical corticosteroid to the nearest 5 g required for twice daily application for one week for the whole body, arms and legs only, and trunk only respectively were as follows:

- 6 months of age, 35 g, 20 g, and 15 g
- 1 year, 45 g, 25 g, and 15 g
- 4 years, 60 g, 35 g, and 20 g
- 8 years, 90 g, 50 g, and 35 g
- 12 years, 120 g, 65 g, and 45 g
- 16 years, 155 g, 85 g, and 55 g
- adult (70-kg male), 170 g, 90 g, and 60 g.

Calculated quantities for the same application schedule for an adult (70-kg male) for individual portions of the body were: face and neck, 10 g; one arm, 15 g; one leg, 30 g; hands and feet, 10 g.

Table 1 on p.1016 is a guide to the potency of topical corticosteroids. There may be some degree of overlap between these groups and, not surprisingly, there are minor variations to this classification. For example, some authorities consider fluocinolone acetonide 0.2% to be potent rather than very potent and halcinonide 0.1% to be potent rather than very potent.

It has been suggested, however, that the advent of non-fluorinated double esters such as hydrocortisone and methylprednisolone aceponates, or prednicarbate, has resulted in corticosteroids whose topical anti-inflammatory potency is not as closely related to their potential atrophic effects on skin, and that a classification taking both into account would be desirable.[5,6]

1. Miller JA, Munro DD. Topical corticosteroids: clinical pharmacology and therapeutic use. *Drugs* 1980; **19:** 119–34.
2. Savin JA. Some guidelines to the use of topical corticosteroids. *Br Med J* 1985; **290:** 1607–8.
3. Hepburn D, *et al.* Topical steroid holiday. *Pediatrics* 1995; **95:** 455.
4. Maurice PDL, Saihan EM. Topical steroid requirement in inflammatory skin conditions. *Br J Clin Pract* 1985; **39:** 441–2.
5. Mori M, *et al.* Topical corticosteroids and unwanted local effects: improving the benefit/risk ratio. *Drug Safety* 1994; **10:** 406–12.
6. Schäfer-Korting M, *et al.* Topical glucocorticoids with improved risk-benefit ratio: rationale of a new concept. *Drug Safety* 1996; **14:** 375–85.

Acute respiratory distress syndrome

Acute respiratory distress syndrome (ARDS) is characterised by areas of lung damage leading to decreased compliance, pulmonary oedema associated with increased capillary and alveolar permeability, and refractory hypoxaemia. Diffuse pulmonary infiltrates are seen on radiography, and patients exhibit dyspnoea, tachypnoea, or both. Diagnosis is primarily clinical, and there has been some disagreement as to what should be included in the syndrome;[1] it is now seen as forming the most severe end of a spectrum of symptoms due to lung inflammation and increased permeability known as acute lung injury.[2-4] ARDS is sometimes considered to refer to 'adult respiratory distress syndrome' but it is not confined to adult patients.

ARDS may be caused by a variety of pulmonary or systemic insults but is particularly frequent in patients with sepsis; because of an association with failure of other organs it has been suggested that it represents the pulmonary component of multiple organ failure syndrome.[5] A wide variety of inflammatory mediators have been implicated in its pathogenesis but evidence suggests that recruitment of neutrophils by interleukin-8 plays an important role.[6,7]

Management. Therapy for ARDS is essentially supportive and despite improving understanding of the pathogenesis, mortality rates have remained around 60%. Mechanical ventilation is necessary in most cases, and circulatory support may require fluids, cardiac inotropic agents, and vasodilators. Optimum management may include diuretics and fluid restriction provided that cardiac output and oxygen delivery are maintained.[3] Because of the association with sepsis antibiotic therapy may be important, but studies of anti-endotoxin antibodies have produced disappointing results.[4]

Numerous drugs have been proposed for the management of ARDS, but, although case reports are often encouraging, none has been conclusively shown to improve mortality in controlled trials. Among the drugs which have proved disappointing in this regard are acetylcysteine,[8] alprostadil,[9,10] pulmonary surfactants,[11-13] and nitric oxide[14] (which may, however, improve oxygenation to some degree). Corticosteroids do not appear to reduce acute mortality,[3-5] although they may be tried in the later phases of the syndrome (5 or more days from onset) to try to prevent fibroproliferative lung changes.[3,18] Good results have been reported with inhaled epoprostenol,[15,16] and there is evidence that ketoconazole may prevent development of ARDS in patients considered at risk,[17] but these results await confirmation from larger controlled studies.

1. Rocker GM, *et al.* Diagnostic criteria for adult respiratory distress syndrome: time for reappraisal. *Lancet* 1989; **i:** 120–3.
2. Bernard GR, *et al.* The American-European Consensus Conference on ARDS: definitions, mechanisms, relevant outcomes, and clinical trial coordination. *Am J Respir Crit Care Med* 1994; **149:** 818–24.
3. Kollef MH, Schuster DP. The acute respiratory distress syndrome. *N Engl J Med* 1995; **332:** 27–37.
4. Bigatello LM, Zapol WM. New approaches to acute lung injury. *Br J Anaesth* 1996; **77:** 99–109.
5. Weinberger SE. Recent advances in pulmonary medicine (part 2). *N Engl J Med* 1993; **328:** 1462–70.
6. Repine JE. Scientific perspectives on adult respiratory distress syndrome. *Lancet* 1992; **339:** 466–9.
7. Donnelly SC, *et al.* Interleukin-8 and development of adult respiratory distress syndrome in at-risk patient groups. *Lancet* 1993; **341:** 643–7.
8. Jepsen S, *et al.* Antioxidant treatment with N-acetylcysteine during adult respiratory distress syndrome: a prospective, randomized, placebo-controlled study. *Crit Care Med* 1992; **20:** 918–23.
9. Bone RC, *et al.* Randomized double-blind, multicenter study of prostaglandin E_1 in patients with the adult respiratory distress syndrome. *Chest* 1989; **96:** 114–19.
10. Abraham E, *et al.* Liposomal prostaglandin E_1, in acute respiratory distress syndrome: a placebo-controlled, randomized, double-blind, multicenter clinical trial. *Crit Care Med* 1996; **24:** 10–15.
11. Haslam PL, *et al.* Surfactant replacement therapy in late-stage adult respiratory distress syndrome. *Lancet* 1994; **343:** 1009–11.
12. Weg JG, *et al.* Safety and potential efficacy of an aerosolized surfactant in human sepsis-induced adult respiratory distress syndrome. *JAMA* 1994; **272:** 1433–8.
13. Anzueto A, *et al.* Aerosolized surfactant in adults with sepsis-induced acute respiratory distress syndrome. *N Engl J Med* 1996; **334:** 1417–21.
14. Dellinger RP, *et al.* Effects of inhaled nitric oxide in patients with acute respiratory distress syndrome: results of a randomized phase II trial. *Crit Care Med* 1998; **26:** 15–23.
15. Walmrath D, *et al.* Aerosolised prostacyclin in adult respiratory distress syndrome. *Lancet* 1993; **342:** 961–2.
16. Walmrath D, *et al.* Direct comparison of inhaled nitric oxide and aerosolized prostacyclin in acute respiratory distress syndrome. *Am J Respir Crit Care Med* 1996; **153:** 991–6.
17. Yu M, Tomasa G. A double-blind, prospective, randomized trial of ketoconazole, a thromboxane synthetase inhibitor, in the prophylaxis of the adult respiratory distress syndrome. *Crit Care Med* 1993; **21:** 1635–42.
18. Meduri GU, *et al.* Effect of prolonged methylprednisolone therapy in unresolving acute respiratory distress syndrome: a randomized controlled trial. *JAMA* 1998; **280:** 159–65.

Adrenal hyperplasia, congenital

See Congenital Adrenal Hyperplasia, below.

Adrenocortical insufficiency

The major function of the adrenal cortex is the production of glucocorticoid and mineralocorticoid hormones, of which cortisol (hydrocortisone) and aldosterone respectively are the most important. Glucocorticoid production is regulated by the hypothalamic-pituitary-adrenal axis, being stimulated by the release of ACTH (adrenocorticotrophic hormone; corticotrophin) from the pituitary, while mineralocorticoid production is primarily controlled by the renin-angiotensin system.

Adrenocortical insufficiency is defined as inadequate production of endogenous corticosteroids. It may be primary (Addison's disease), due to destruction of the adrenal cortex by some cause; or secondary, due to hypothalamic or pituitary disease, or corticosteroid therapy which suppresses ACTH release. Diagnosis can be difficult, even with the aid of hormone tests such as the tetracosactrin stimulation test.

Clinical manifestations of adrenocortical insufficiency are usually seen once about 90% of the adrenal cortex is destroyed. Weight loss, anorexia, weakness, and fatigue may be accompanied by gastro-intestinal symptoms such as abdominal pain, nausea, vomiting, and diarrhoea, as well as electrolyte abnormalities (hyponatraemia, hyperkalaemia), salt craving, and postural hypotension. In acute cases, abdominal pain and rigidity, fever, volume depletion, hypotension, and shock may occur. Hyperpigmentation, especially of skin creases, exposed areas, and scars is a distinguishing feature of primary, but not secondary, insufficiency. Hypoglycaemia is more likely in secondary deficiency due to lack of growth hormone, and failure of other pituitary hormones usually accompanies secondary adrenocortical insufficiency.

Treatment. In **acute insufficiency** treatment should be with intravenous hydrocortisone as the sodium succinate, sodium phosphate or other readily soluble ester: the usual dose is the equivalent of 100 mg every 6 to 8 hours for 24 hours. Volume depletion, dehydration, hypotension and hypoglycaemia should be corrected with intravenous saline and glucose, and precipitating factors, such as infection, should be dealt with appropriately. Provided no complications occur, the dosage of hydrocortisone can be tapered over 4 or 5 days to maintenance therapy by mouth.

For chronic insufficiency the usual dosage of **maintenance** or **replacement therapy** is hydrocortisone 20 to 30 mg by mouth, preferably divided unequally, e.g. 30 mg as 20 mg in the morning and 10 mg in the evening, in an attempt to mimic the natural pattern of secretion. Other corticosteroids have been used, including cortisone acetate, prednisolone, prednisone, and dexamethasone, but offer no advantage over hydrocortisone. Patients with primary insufficiency also require additional mineralocorticoid replacement with fludrocortisone, usually in a dose of 0.1 mg daily. Mineralocorticoid replacement is not usually necessary in secondary insufficiency.

Corticosteroid cover. An increase in replacement therapy is required during periods of stress. In mild infection, a doubling of the maintenance dose of hydrocortisone may be appropriate but for major infection, or severe stress such as surgery, parenteral therapy is required. It is generally considered safer to overestimate rather than underestimate the appropriate cover. The usual cover for operations is based on the observation that major stress does not normally lead to the secretion of more than 300 mg of cortisol in 24 hours, and comprises hydrocortisone 100 mg (usually as the sodium succinate) by intramuscular or intravenous injection before surgery, repeated every 8 hours for 24 hours. In the absence of complications the dose can be halved every 24 hours until a normal maintenance dose is reached on the 5th postoperative day.

AIDS

For the use of corticosteroids in AIDS patients with *Pneumocystis carinii* pneumonia, see p.1026.

Alopecia

The management of alopecia (p.1073) is often difficult. In alopecia areata intralesional corticosteroids, most commonly triamcinolone, will induce hair growth although they are not suitable when more than 50% of the scalp is involved.[1] Regrowth is confined to the site of injection and therefore patchy, although soon concealed by spontaneous growth from uninjected regions. Some atrophy of the scalp is inevitable. Topical corticosteroids are mostly reported to be ineffective although some consider them beneficial; the use of systemic corticosteroids is controversial, given their adverse effects and a lack of evidence that they alter the long-term prognosis.

1. Shapiro J. Alopecia areata: update on therapy. *Dermatol Clin* 1993; **11:** 35–46.

Anaemias

For reference to the use of immunosuppressants, including corticosteroid-containing regimens, as an alternative to bone-marrow transplantation in the management of aplastic anaemia, see p.701; for the use of corticosteroids in haemolytic anaemias, including cold haemagglutinin disease, see p.702.

Anaphylactic shock

For the use of corticosteroids in the management of anaphylactic shock, see p.816. Intravenous corticosteroids are given following initial treatment with adrenaline as part of the management of anaphylaxis; their effects are delayed, and they are not suited for immediate relief, but early administration may help prevent deterioration after primary treatment has been given.

Aspiration syndromes

For a review of the management of aspiration syndromes, including reference to the probable lack of value of corticosteroids, see p.1168.

Asthma

The cornerstones of current asthma therapy, as discussed in more detail on p.745, are the beta$_2$-adrenoceptor agonists and the corticosteroids. Drug therapy for chronic asthma is managed by a stepwise approach. Patients requiring only occasional relief from symptoms may be managed with an inhaled short-acting beta$_2$ agonist when required. An inhaled corticosteroid such as beclomethasone dipropionate, budesonide, or fluticasone may be added to therapy if symptomatic relief is required more than once daily. Regular use is important since corticosteroids take several hours to exert an effect in asthma. If control is still inadequate, the dose of inhaled corticosteroid may be increased and given by means of a large volume spacer device, or a long-acting beta$_2$ agonist or theophylline, and possibly cromoglycate or nedocromil, may be added to therapy. Severe asthma may require regular bronchodilator therapy as well as high-dose inhaled corticosteroids, while in the most severe cases, regular oral corticosteroids may also be required. A short 'rescue' course of oral corticosteroid may be needed at any stage for an acute exacerbation. Corticosteroids should be used cautiously in children because of possible adverse effects on growth. While increasing the dose of inhaled corticosteroid is part of this schedule of treatment, it has proved difficult to demonstrate the benefits in controlled studies (see above).

Acute severe asthma (status asthmaticus) is potentially life-threatening and is treated with inhaled oxygen and beta$_2$ agonists, as well as systemic corticosteroids; ipratropium bromide, and intravenous xanthine or beta$_2$ agonist may need to be added. Once lung function is stabilised the patient can be discharged on a regimen of oral and inhaled corticosteroids, inhaled or nebulised beta$_2$ agonists as required, and oral theophylline, long-acting beta$_2$ agonists, or inhaled ipratropium bromide as necessary.

Behçet's syndrome

Behçet's syndrome (or Behçet's disease) is a recurrent multifocal disorder most prevalent in Japan and the countries of the Mediterranean and Middle East, although it is also found elsewhere.

The clinical features include oral and genital ulceration, various types of skin lesion, arthritis, thrombo-embolic disorders and aneurysms, ocular lesions (particularly uveitis, hypopyon, and iridocyclitis leading eventually to blindness), and CNS involvement (meningomyelitis, dementia, extrapyramidal symptoms, and paralysis, sometimes fatal). Gastro-intestinal disturbances and involvement of other body systems have been reported. However, the complete gamut of symptoms is unlikely in a single patient, and the disease has been classified into mucocutaneous, arthritic, neurological, and ocular forms depending on the predominant symptoms. Diagnosis is made difficult by the protean nature of the syndrome, but oral and genital ulceration, ocular involvement, and skin lesions are considered the major signs of involvement.[1]

A large number of drugs have been tried for Behçet's syndrome. Where possible topical treatment of local lesions should be attempted before embarking on systemic therapy. Topical application of a tetracycline is considered the treatment of choice for oral ulceration,[1] while ocular involvement may be treated with corticosteroid eye drops and a mydriatic initially[1,2] (except in patients with marked posterior segment involvement, who require systemic therapy from the outset).[2]

Corticosteroids remain the first-line systemic treatment for Behçet's syndrome although their use is less favoured in some countries, notably Japan,[3] than in others. Prednisone or prednisolone is given by mouth, usually in doses of up to 60 mg initially, which is reduced to a minimum effective maintenance dose as the patient responds. Corticosteroids are believed to be most useful for early active disease.[1]

Long-term maintenance with corticosteroids poses problems of toxicity and various cytotoxic immunosuppressants have been tried for disease control, either alone or as steroid-sparing agents to permit a reduction in the dosage of concomitant corticosteroid therapy. Agents that have reportedly had some success include azathioprine,[4] chlorambucil,[1,2] cyclophosphamide,[3] and cyclosporin.[5] Such therapy carries its own risks of toxicity, including the possibility of the development of malignancy with long-term use, which must be weighed against its value in delaying the most crippling symptoms of Behçet's syndrome, eye disease and blindness.

An alternative is the use of colchicine. This is reportedly beneficial in the treatment of cutaneous and ocular lesions,[2,6] although evidence suggests that cyclosporin is more effective.[5] Colchicine has been used in combination with systemic and topical corticosteroids in acute exacerbations, followed by colchicine maintenance;[7] colchicine with aspirin has also been recommended to prevent acute exacerbations,[8] and colchicine with benzathine penicillin has reportedly been found effective.[9]

Other agents that have been tried include dapsone, interferon alfa-2b (for ocular disease), levamisole, omega-3 fatty acids, oxpentifylline, stanozolol (for vascular symptoms), and thalidomide, which may be particularly useful for refractory ulceration.[10] Sulphasalazine has been given for colitis associated with Behçet's syndrome (although it should be noted that some definitions of the syndrome exclude patients with inflammatory bowel disease), and mesalazine has been applied topically to cutaneous lesions in one patient with some success. Controlled studies of these agents are mostly lacking.

1. Arbesfeld SJ, Kurban AK. Behçet's disease: new perspectives on an enigmatic syndrome. *J Am Acad Dermatol* 1988; **19:** 767–79.
2. Benezra D, Cohen E. Treatment and visual prognosis in Behçet's disease. *Br J Ophthalmol* 1986; **70:** 589–92.
3. Oniki S, *et al.* Immunosuppressive treatment of Behçet's disease with cyclophosphamide. *Jpn J Ophthalmol* 1976; **20:** 32–40.
4. Yazici H, *et al.* A controlled trial of azathioprine in Behçet's syndrome. *N Engl J Med* 1990; **322:** 281–5.
5. Masuda K, *et al.* Double-masked trial of cyclosporin versus colchicine and long-term open study of cyclosporin in Behçet's disease. *Lancet* 1989; **i:** 1093–6.
6. Miyachi Y, *et al.* Colchicine in the treatment of the cutaneous manifestations of Behçet's disease. *Br J Dermatol* 1981; **104:** 67–9.
7. Rakover Y, *et al.* Behcet disease: long-term follow-up of three children and review of the literature. *Pediatrics* 1989; **83:** 986–92.
8. Wechsler B, Piette JC. Behçet's disease. *Br Med J* 1992; **304:** 1199–1200.
9. Çalgüneri M, *et al.* Effect of prophylactic benzathine penicillin on mucocutaneous symptoms of Behçet's disease. *Dermatology* 1996; **192:** 125–8.
10. Hamuryudan V, *et al.* Thalidomide in the treatment of the mucocutaneous lesions of the Behçet syndrome; a randomized, double-blind, placebo-controlled trial. *Ann Intern Med* 1998; **128:** 443–50.

Bell's palsy

Bell's palsy is a condition thought to be caused by herpes simplex virus 1.[1] It affects the facial nerves and results in facial muscle weakness and paralysis. It is often accompanied by pain and lachrymation. Untreated, over 80% of all patients recover completely or almost so, while in a smaller number facial weakness persists; complete failure of motor recovery is very rare.

Prednisone dramatically relieves the pain of Bell's palsy.[2] The suggested dose for adults is 1 mg per kg bodyweight daily in divided doses morning and evening; if the paralysis remains incomplete after 5 or 6 days the prednisone is gradually withdrawn over the next 5 days but if the paralysis is complete the initial dosage should be continued for another 10 days and then gradually withdrawn. The benefits of corticosteroids in this condition have never been established by a large controlled trial,[3,4] although a systematic review of 4 smaller studies suggested an increased rate of complete recovery with corticosteroid treatment.[5]

1. Murakami S, *et al.* Bell palsy and herpes simplex virus: identification of viral DNA in endoneurial fluid and muscle. *Ann Intern Med* 1996; **124:** 27–30.
2. Adour KK. Current concepts in neurology: diagnosis and management of facial paralysis. *N Engl J Med* 1982; **307:** 348–51.
3. Karis R. Facial paralysis. *N Engl J Med* 1982; **307:** 1647.
4. Staal A, *et al.* Facial paralysis. *N Engl J Med* 1982; **307:** 1647.
5. Williamson IG, Whelan TR. The clinical problem of Bell's palsy: is treatment with steroids effective? *Br J Gen Pract* 1996; **46:** 743–7.

Bites and stings

Corticosteroids (prednisone 100 mg daily) have been recommended for the stabilisation of erythrocyte membranes in the management of systemic envenomation by the brown recluse spider (*Loxosceles reclusa*).[1] They have also been given following stings by some species of scorpion, although their value is not certain.[1] Corticosteroids are considered to have no place in snake venom poisoning.[2] Topical corticosteroids may be useful for mild itching of healing skin after some types of jelly fish sting, while systemic corticosteroids have been used for delayed hypersensitivity reactions.[3]

1. Binder LS. Acute arthropod envenomation: incidence, clinical features and management. *Med Toxicol Adverse Drug Exp* 1989; **4:** 163–73.
2. Nelson BK. Snake envenomation: incidence, clinical presentation and management. *Med Toxicol* 1989; **4:** 17–31.
3. Fenner PJ, Williamson JA. Worldwide deaths and severe envenomation from jelly fish stings. *Med J Aust* 1996; **165:** 658–61.

Bone cysts

Methylprednisolone acetate 40 to 200 mg injected into unicameral bone cysts under brief general anaesthesia stimulates bone formation to obliterate the cyst or promote sufficient healing to prevent further fractures.[1] A single injection is sufficient for healing in 10 to 25% of cysts; only rarely will greater than 4 injections be needed. (Systemic corticosteroids are, of course, generally associated with bone loss rather than bone formation—see Effects on Bones and Joints, p.1011).

1. Weinert CR. Administering steroids in unicameral bone cysts. *West J Med* 1989; **150:** 684–5.

Brain injury

See under Spinal Cord Injury, p.1029.

Bronchopulmonary dysplasia

Bronchopulmonary dysplasia is the major cause of chronic lung disease (defined as the need for supplementary oxygen more than 28 days after birth) in neonates. It is considered to comprise 4 radiographically distinct stages: stage 1 is effectively indistinguishable from neonatal respiratory distress syndrome (see p.1025), with which it is usually associated. A 'bubbly' appearance of the lung is seen in radiographs of advanced disease. Bronchopulmonary dysplasia is invariably associated with prolonged mechanical ventilation, but it is uncertain whether it plays a causative role, or whether the disease develops anyway in infants with respiratory failure severe enough to need prolonged ventilation.[1]

Treatment. Corticosteroids,[2-9] usually in the form of intravenous dexamethasone, have been widely used in premature infants with bronchopulmonary dysplasia, or who are considered to be at high risk of it (the borderline between treatment and prophylaxis in studies in these mechanically-ventilated infants is not always clear[6]). Dexamethasone has been reported to improve pulmonary outcome, allowing more rapid weaning from mechanical ventilation, and in some studies was reported to improve neurological outcome as well.[3] However, some investigators consider its benefits in the long term inadequately established.[6,8,10] Many studies have favoured an initial dose of 0.5 mg per kg bodyweight daily intravenously, tapered over a period of days to weeks, but it is not always clear if this is expressed in terms of the base or one of its esters,[11] and in any case regimens have varied between studies and the optimum has yet to be determined.[12] Despite suggestions that beginning therapy shortly after birth might minimise lung injury, evidence suggests that early therapy offers no advantage,[10,13] and may be more hazardous.[10] Meta-analysis has suggested that while beginning dexamethasone at any time between birth and 14 days of age reduced the risk of chronic lung disease, mortality was only reduced in the group who began treatment between 7 and 14 days of age.[25] Results from a small study indicate that nebulised beclomethasone may also produce benefit.[14]

Additional therapy is essentially supportive, including fluid restriction, nutritional supplementation, bronchodilators, and diuretics. In general, diuretics are indicated for episodes of associated cardiac failure but their long-term value is uncertain; if used, consideration should be given to a calcium-sparing regimen.[12] Improved pulmonary status has been reported with oral or parenteral frusemide in established dysplasia;[15,16] results with hydrochlorothiazide and spironolactone are more ambiguous.[17,18] Benefit has been reported following administration of nebulised frusemide,[19,20] although others have not seen an improvement in more severely affected children.[21] Anaemia in infants with bronchopulmonary dysplasia has benefited from erythropoietin.[22] Although vitamin A deficiency has been implicated in the pathogenesis of bronchopulmonary dysplasia, vitamin A supplementation has not been found to produce overall benefit.[23] However, there is some preliminary evidence that treatment with alpha$_1$-proteinase inhibitor may be of value.[24]

1. Bancalari E, *et al.* Bronchopulmonary dysplasia: clinical presentation. *J Pediatr* 1979; **95:** 819–23.
2. Mammel MC, *et al.* Controlled trial of dexamethasone therapy in infants with bronchopulmonary dysplasia. *Lancet* 1983; **i:** 1356–8.
3. Cummings JJ, *et al.* A controlled trial of dexamethasone therapy in preterm infants with bronchopulmonary dysplasia. *N Engl J Med* 1989; **320:** 1505–10.
4. Kazzi NJ, *et al.* Dexamethasone effects on the hospital course of infants with bronchopulmonary dysplasia who are dependent on artificial ventilation. *Pediatrics* 1990; **86:** 722–7.
5. Collaborative Dexamethasone Trial Group. Dexamethasone therapy in neonatal chronic lung disease: an international placebo-controlled trial. *Pediatrics* 1991; **88:** 421–7.
6. Kari MA, *et al.* Dexamethasone treatment in preterm infants at risk for bronchopulmonary dysplasia. *Arch Dis Child* 1993; **68:** 566–9.
7. Durand M, *et al.* Effects of early dexamethasone therapy on pulmonary mechanics and chronic lung disease in very low birth weight infants: a randomized, controlled trial. *Pediatrics* 1995; **95:** 584–90.
8. Jones R, *et al.* Controlled trial of dexamethasone in neonatal chronic lung disease: a 3-year follow-up. *Pediatrics* 1995; **96:** 897–906.
9. Rastogi A, *et al.* A controlled trial of dexamethasone to prevent bronchopulmonary dysplasia in surfactant-treated infants. *Pediatrics* 1996; **98:** 204–10.
10. Papile L-A, *et al.* A multicenter trial of two dexamethasone regimens in ventilator-dependent premature infants. *N Engl J Med* 1998; **338:** 1112–18.
11. Jones RAK, Grant AM. The "dose" question. *Pediatrics* 1992; **90:** 781.
12. Report of a Joint Working Group of the British Association of Perinatal Medicine and the Research Unit of the Royal College of Physicians. Development of audit measures and guidelines for good practice in the management of neonatal respiratory distress syndrome. *Arch Dis Child* 1992; **67:** 1221–7.
13. Tapia JL, *et al.* The effect of early dexamethasone administration on bronchopulmonary dysplasia in preterm infants with respiratory distress syndrome. *J Pediatr* 1998; **132:** 48–52.
14. LaForce WR, Brudno DS. Controlled trial of beclomethasone dipropionate by nebulization in oxygen- and ventilator-dependent infants. *J Pediatr* 1993; **122:** 285–8.
15. Rush MG, *et al.* Double-blind, placebo-controlled trial of alternate-day furosemide therapy in infants with chronic bronchopulmonary dysplasia. *J Pediatr* 1990; **117:** 112–18.
16. Stefano JL, Bhutani VK. Role of furosemide therapy after booster-packed erythrocyte transfusions in infants with bronchopulmonary dysplasia. *J Pediatr* 1990; **117:** 965–8.
17. Engelhardt B, *et al.* Effect of spironolactone-hydrochlorothiazide on lung function in infants with chronic bronchopulmonary dysplasia. *J Pediatr* 1989; **114:** 619–24.
18. Albersheim SG, *et al.* Randomized, double-blind, controlled trial of long-term diuretic therapy for bronchopulmonary dysplasia. *J Pediatr* 1989; **115:** 615–20.
19. Rastogi A, *et al.* Nebulized furosemide in infants with bronchopulmonary dysplasia. *J Pediatr* 1994; **125:** 976–9.
20. Prabhu VG, *et al.* Pulmonary function changes after nebulised and intravenous frusemide in ventilated premature infants. *Arch Dis Child* 1997; **77:** F32–5.
21. Kugelman A, *et al.* Pulmonary effect of inhaled furosemide in ventilated infants with severe bronchopulmonary dysplasia. *Pediatrics* 1997; **99:** 71–5.
22. Ohls RK, *et al.* A randomized double-blind, placebo-controlled trial of recombinant erythropoietin in treatment of the anemia of bronchopulmonary dysplasia. *J Pediatr* 1993; **123:** 996–1000.
23. Pearson E, *et al.* Trial of vitamin A supplementation in very low birth weight infants at risk for bronchopulmonary dysplasia. *J Pediatr* 1992; **121:** 420–7.
24. Stiskal JA, *et al.* α_1-Proteinase inhibitor therapy for the prevention of chronic lung disease of prematurity: a randomized, controlled trial. *Pediatrics* 1998; **101:** 89–94.
25. Bhuta T, Ohlsson A. Systematic review and meta-analysis of early postnatal dexamethasone for prevention of chronic lung disease. *Arch Dis Child Fetal Neonatal Ed* 1998; **79:** F26–F33.

Cerebral oedema

Corticosteroids (usually dexamethasone) play an important role in the treatment of cerebral oedema caused by malignancy and dexamethasone is advocated for the cerebral oedema associated with high-altitude disorders (see p.787). Corticosteroids have also been used for the management of raised intracranial pressure in patients with head injuries or stroke, but despite earlier small studies showing them to be beneficial in some patients, more recent evidence shows that survival and neurological outcome is not improved in these conditions. Current opinion is therefore that corticosteroids are not useful in head injuries or stroke and that their adverse effects may outweigh any possible benefit.[1-5] The management of raised intracranial pressure and the usual agents used to treat it are discussed on p.796.

1. Sila CA, Furlan AJ. Drug treatment of stroke: current status and future prospects. *Drugs* 1988; **35:** 468–76.
2. Anonymous. A fresh look at some old stroke treatments. *Pharm J* 1990; **244:** 202.
3. Lyons MK, Meyer FB. Cerebrospinal fluid physiology and the management of increased intracranial pressure. *Mayo Clin Proc* 1990; **65:** 684–707.
4. Woster PS, LeBlanc KL. Management of elevated intracranial pressure. *Clin Pharm* 1990; **9:** 762–72.
5. Jeevaratnam DR, Menon DK. Survey of intensive care of severely head injured patients in the United Kingdom. *Br Med J* 1996; **312:** 944–7.

Chronic active hepatitis

Chronic hepatitis is characterised by liver cell necrosis and inflammation which persists for more than 6 to 12 months. Probably the most serious form is chronic active hepatitis in which inflammatory infiltrates (mononuclear and plasma cells) are found within and around the portal areas, with piecemeal necrosis of adjacent liver cells, and in severe cases bands of necrotic tissue between portal tracts or to the central vein (bridging necrosis). Symptoms are essentially non-specific and include fatigue, malaise, fever, anorexia, jaundice and raised serum aminotransferase values; biopsy is required for accurate diagnosis. The causes of chronic active hepatitis vary and may include: infection with hepatitis viruses; adverse effects of drugs such as isoniazid, methyldopa, or nitrofurantoin; or, particularly in women, an apparently idiopathic form, autoimmune hepatitis.

Treatment with corticosteroids is widely used in patients with autoimmune hepatitis.[1,2] A moderate initial dose of 20 to 30 mg of prednisolone or prednisone daily is usually given although higher doses have been used,[3] and is then slowly tapered over several months to the minimum required for maintenance. Daily maintenance therapy appears more effective than alternate day regimens. Patients who respond (as shown by a return of serum aminotransferase values to the normal or near normal range and a reduction in the inflammatory processes on biopsy) usually require prolonged treatment; although some patients remain in remission for months to years after withdrawal, relapse generally occurs, and therapy should be reinstated when the disease becomes active again.[1]

Combined treatment including azathioprine is frequently given; such treatment is at least as effective as a corticosteroid alone,[2] can produce[4,5] and maintain[6,7] remission, and permits a reduction in corticosteroid dosage in a group of patients who will require long-term drug treatment.[1] There has been some dispute about the value of azathioprine alone, but combined therapy has generally been found to be superior.[4] However azathioprine has been used alone in high doses to maintain remission.[7]

In contrast to the fairly extensive experience with azathioprine there has been little reported use of cyclosporin in this condition. However, in a patient hypersensitive to azathioprine, in whom prednisone alone was unable to control disease and produced severe side-effects, addition of cyclosporin produced marked improvement and permitted a reduction in steroid dosage to tolerable amounts.[8] The patient had remained asymptomatic on this regimen for 2 years. Cyclosporin may thus offer an alternative in severe disease where corticosteroids alone or with azathioprine cannot suffice. Some investigators have also used cyclophosphamide successfully,[3] and tacrolimus is under investigation.[9]

As an alternative to prolonged use of corticosteroid maintenance therapy, penicillamine has been tried, the dose of penicillamine being gradually increased over several months to a suitable maintenance dose as the dosage of corticosteroid is tapered off.

It is generally agreed that immunosuppression is not suitable in patients with viral chronic active hepatitis.[1,10] However, combination therapy has been reported to produce benefit in patients positive for HBsAg,[4] and Czaja and colleagues[11] have reported that patients with chronic active hepatitis of unknown cause, at least some of whom may have hepatitis C,[10] respond as well to corticosteroids or combined therapy as patients with proven autoimmune disease.

1. Krawitt EL. Autoimmune hepatitis. *N Engl J Med* 1996; **334:** 897–903.
2. Stavinoha MW, Soloway RD. Current therapy of chronic liver disease. *Drugs* 1990; **39:** 814–40.
3. Meyer zum Büschenfelde KH, Lohse AW. Autoimmune hepatitis. *N Engl J Med* 1995; **333:** 1004–5.
4. Giusti G, *et al.* Immunosuppressive therapy in chronic active hepatitis (CAH): a multicentric retrospective study on 867 patients. *Hepatogastroenterology* 1984; **31:** 24–9.
5. Vegnente A, *et al.* Duration of chronic active hepatitis and the development of cirrhosis. *Arch Dis Child* 1984; **59:** 330–5.
6. Stellon AJ, *et al.* Randomised controlled trial of azathioprine withdrawal in autoimmune chronic active hepatitis. *Lancet* 1985; **i:** 668–70.
7. Johnson PJ, *et al.* Azathioprine for long-term maintenance of remission in autoimmune hepatitis. *N Engl J Med* 1995; **333:** 958–63.
8. Mistilis SP, *et al.* Cyclosporin, a new treatment for autoimmune chronic active hepatitis. *Med J Aust* 1985; **143:** 463–5.
9. Van Thiel DH, *et al.* Tacrolimus: a potential new treatment for autoimmune chronic active hepatitis: results of an open-label preliminary trial. *Am J Gastroenterol* 1995; **90:** 771–6.
10. Gitnick G. Cryptogenic versus autoimmune chronic hepatitis: to split or to lump? *Mayo Clin Proc* 1990; **65:** 119–21.
11. Czaja AJ, *et al.* Clinical features and prognostic implications of severe corticosteroid-treated cryptogenic chronic active hepatitis. *Mayo Clin Proc* 1990; **65:** 23–30.

Chronic obstructive pulmonary disease

Corticosteroids play some part in the symptomatic and palliative management of chronic obstructive pulmonary disease (p.747), although there is controversy as to their value. Most patients do not respond to corticosteroids but in about 10% of those receiving maximal bronchodilator therapy a short course of oral corticosteroid therapy can improve airflow further. Some patients require maintenance doses; these should preferably be given by inhalation but fewer patients respond to inhaled corticosteroids.

Churg-Strauss syndrome

The Churg-Strauss syndrome is sometimes classified with polyarteritis nodosa (see p.1027), although, unlike the latter, pulmonary manifestations are relatively common in Churg-Strauss syndrome. Patients commonly have a history of allergic disease (rhinitis, sinusitis, and asthma), and intractable asthma and eosinophilia together with granulomatous vasculitis characterise the syndrome.

Treatment is similar to that of polyarteritis nodosa, being based on systemic corticosteroids and, where necessary, cyclophosphamide.[1-3] When cyclophosphamide is used, administration as intravenous pulse therapy is coming to be preferred to continuous oral administration,[3] as it has been shown to reduce adverse effects.[4] Azathioprine has been used but has been largely superseded by cyclophosphamide.[1] Interferon alfa may also be of benefit.[5]

1. Taylor HG, Samanta A. Treatment of vasculitis. *Br J Clin Pharmacol* 1993; **35:** 93–104.
2. Guillevin L, *et al.* Treatment of polyarteritis nodosa and Churg-Strauss syndrome: a meta-analysis of 3 prospective controlled trials including 182 patients over 12 years. *Ann Med Interne (Paris)* 1992; **143:** 405–16.
3. Guillevin L, Lhote F. Classification and management of necrotising vasculitides. *Drugs* 1997; **53:** 805–16.
4. Chow C-C, *et al.* Allergic granulomatosis and angiitis (Churg-Strauss syndrome): response to 'pulse' intravenous cyclophosphamide. *Ann Rheum Dis* 1989; **48:** 605–8.
5. Tatsis E, *et al.* Interferon-α treatment of four patients with the Churg-Strauss syndrome. *Ann Intern Med* 1998; **129:** 370–4.

Cogan's syndrome

Corticosteroids are useful in the treatment of Cogan's syndrome, a condition characterised by non-syphilitic interstitial keratitis and audiovestibular symptoms including deafness.[1,2] The deafness, although often irreversible, may respond to systemic corticosteroids initiated within 2 weeks of onset of symptoms (prednisolone or prednisone, at least 1.5 mg per kg body-weight daily for 2 weeks is advised) and ocular involvement benefits from topical corticosteroid therapy. Improvement in ocular symptoms has also been seen with sodium cromoglycate eye drops.[3] For patients with severe Cogan's syndrome including large-vessel vasculitis, corticosteroids have been used in conjunction with other immunosuppressants such as cyclosporin and cyclophosphamide.[4]

1. Anonymous. Cogan's syndrome. *Lancet* 1991; **337:** 1011–12.
2. Vollertsen RS, *et al.* Cogan's syndrome: 18 cases and a review of the literature. *Mayo Clin Proc* 1986; **61:** 344–61.
3. Carter F, Nabarro J. Cromoglycate for Cogan's syndrome. *Lancet* 1987; **i:** 858.
4. Allen NB, *et al.* Use of immunosuppressive agents in the treatment of severe ocular and vascular manifestations of Cogan's syndrome. *Am J Med* 1990; **88:** 296–301.

Congenital adrenal hyperplasia

Congenital adrenal hyperplasia comprises a heterogeneous group of disorders due to inherited defects of steroid synthesis in the adrenal gland, the most frequent of which are defects involving 21-hydroxylase or 11-β-hydroxylase. Defective enzyme production blocks the formation of cortisol and aldosterone; the pituitary produces increased amounts of ACTH in an attempt to compensate, but this results in excessive adrenal androgen production. Presentation varies from virilisation and abnormal genital formation at birth to mild cryptic forms that may be detected only later in life. Salt-losing forms (due to lack of aldosterone or the accumulation of precursors with antagonist activity) may lead to hyperkalaemia, acidosis, and dehydration. Patients with 11-β-hydroxylase defect are also prone to hypertension.

Neonates with **salt-losing forms** of congenital adrenal hyperplasia require urgent treatment. Treatment usually consists of a mineralocorticoid, fludrocortisone, and a glucocorticoid (usually hydrocortisone) in regimens similar to those for adrenocortical insufficiency (see p.1017).[1-3] Saline infusion or addition of salt to the feed is required initially.

Even where salt-losing symptoms are not overt or marked, control is reportedly better with a mineralocorticoid added to therapy, rather than with hydrocortisone alone,[1] and it has been recommended that children with salt-losing congenital adrenal hyperplasia should continue to receive combined therapy at least until adult life.[2] Careful titration of dosage is important to avoid growth retardation and toxicity, and potent synthetic glucocorticoids such as betamethasone and dexamethasone are probably inappropriate in infants and children with the condition, even in the non-salt-losing form. An alternative approach is the use of flutamide and testolactone to block androgenic effects, together with a reduced dose of hydrocortisone.[4]

Patients with **non-salt-losing congenital adrenal hyperplasia** may be adequately managed with glucocorticoids alone, and in mild late-onset forms a single dose daily in the late evening (when its suppressive effect on ACTH production is greatest) may be sufficient. In adults who do not require mineralocorticoid treatment betamethasone or dexamethasone may be useful because of their lack of mineralocorticoid actions.

Surgical correction may be necessary in females with masculinised external genitalia. Administration of a glucocorticoid to pregnant women whose offspring are considered at risk has been tried in an attempt to prevent virilisation:[5-7] dexamethasone is preferred to hydrocortisone because of a lack of placental degradation.[6]

1. Hughes IA, *et al.* Continuing the need for mineralocorticoid therapy in salt-losing congenital adrenal hyperplasia. *Arch Dis Child* 1979; **54:** 350–5.
2. Griffiths KD, *et al.* Plasma renin activity in the management of congenital adrenal hyperplasia. *Arch Dis Child* 1984; **59:** 360–5.
3. Young MC, Hughes IA. Response to treatment of congenital adrenal hyperplasia in infancy. *Arch Dis Child* 1990; **65:** 441–4.
4. Merke DP, Cutler GB. New approaches to the treatment of congenital adrenal hyperplasia. *JAMA* 1997; **277:** 1073–6.
5. David M, Forest MG. Prenatal treatment of congenital adrenal hyperplasia resulting from 21-hydroxylase deficiency. *J Pediatr* 1984; **105:** 799–803.
6. Evans MI, *et al.* Pharmacologic suppression of the fetal adrenal gland in utero: attempted prevention of abnormal external genital masculinization in suspected congenital adrenal hyperplasia. *JAMA* 1985; **253:** 1015–20.
7. Anonymous. Prenatal treatment of congenital adrenal hyperplasia. *Lancet* 1990; **335:** 510–11.

Corneal graft rejection

In a study[1] of 48 patients treated for corneal graft rejection with hourly prednisolone acetate 1% eye drops for up to 2 weeks followed by tapering of the dose, half received additional treatment with intravenous methylprednisolone 500 mg as a single injection (pulse therapy) and the other half received oral prednisolone 60 to 80 mg daily for up to 2 weeks, followed by tapering doses over 4 to 6 weeks. Both treatments were equally effective with 79.2% and 62.5% of grafts surviving with pulse and oral therapy respectively. Pulse therapy was better in patients who presented early (within 8 days), with a graft survival rate of 92.3% compared with that of 54.5% following oral therapy. There was no difference in graft survival rates in patients who presented late. Subsequent rejection episodes affected successfully-treated grafts in 26.3% of those treated with the methylprednisolone pulse and 66.7% of those treated with oral prednisolone.

For discussions of the role of corticosteroids in other forms of organ and tissue grafting, see Organ and Tissue Transplantation, p.498.

1. Hill JC, *et al.* Corticosteroids in corneal graft rejection: oral versus single pulse therapy. *Ophthalmology* 1991; **98:** 329–33.

Croup

Croup is an acute syndrome of upper respiratory tract inflammation (laryngotracheobronchitis) associated with viral infection, usually by parainfluenza virus although other viruses may also produce the syndrome. It is characterised by harsh, barking cough, stridor, and hoarseness, most usually occurring at night in children aged 6 months to 4 years.[1,2]

Traditional home management has revolved around the inhalation of steam, despite a lack of evidence for effectiveness, but symptoms may be sufficiently alarming to result in presentation to a hospital.

In severe croup there is clear evidence that treatment with a systemic corticosteroid reduces symptoms and decreases the need for intubation.[3-5] Nebulised budesonide has also been reported to be effective,[6-8] and of similar efficacy to inhalation of nebulised adrenaline;[9] however despite the theoretical attraction of this route, studies have failed to find any significant difference in effectiveness between nebulised budesonide 2 mg and oral dexamethasone 0.6 mg per kg body-weight,[10] or combination therapy with both,[11] and another study found 0.6 mg per kg of dexamethasone given intramuscularly to be more effective than 4 mg of nebulised budesonide.[16] In contrast, others have found that addition of nebulised budesonide to oral dexamethasone produced more rapid improvement than the latter alone.[12] Studies have also shown a significant benefit from corticosteroids in children with mild to moderate croup,[10,13] and although the use of such potent drugs in children with a mild, largely self-limiting condition has been questioned,[14] a review of the risks and benefits concluded that oral dexamethasone 0.15 mg per kg, or nebulised budesonide 2 mg were the treatment of choice in mild to moderate croup while oral prednisolone 1 mg per kg should be given for croup requiring intubation.[2] However, nebulised adrenaline is probably the drug of choice where rapid relief of obstructive symptoms is required.[15]

1. Doull I. Corticosteroids in the management of croup. *Br Med J* 1995; **311:** 1244.
2. Yates RW, Doull IJM. A risk-benefit assessment of corticosteroids in the management of croup. *Drug Safety* 1997; **16:** 48–55.
3. Kairys SW, *et al.* Steroid treatment of laryngotracheitis: a meta-analysis of the evidence from randomized trials. *Pediatrics* 1989; **83:** 683–93.
4. Freezer NJ, *et al.* Steroids in croup: do they increase the incidence of successful extubation? *Anaesth Intensive Care* 1990; **18:** 224–8.
5. Geelhoed GC. Sixteen years of croup in a Western Australian teaching hospital: effects of routine steroid treatment. *Ann Emerg Med* 1996; **28:** 621–6.
6. Klassen TP, *et al.* Nebulized budesonide for children with mild-to-moderate croup. *N Engl J Med* 1994; **331:** 285–9.
7. Husby S, *et al.* Treatment of croup with nebulised steroid (budesonide): a double blind, placebo controlled study. *Arch Dis Child* 1993; **68:** 352–5.
8. Godden CW, *et al.* Double blind placebo controlled trial of nebulised budesonide for croup. *Arch Dis Child* 1997; **76:** 155–8.
9. Fitzgerald D, *et al.* Nebulized budesonide is as effective as nebulized adrenaline in moderately severe croup. *Pediatrics* 1996; **97:** 722–5.
10. Geelhoed GC, MacDonald WBG. Oral and inhaled steroids in croup: a randomized placebo-controlled trial. *Pediatr Pulmonol* 1995; **20:** 355–61.
11. Klassen TP, *et al.* Nebulized budesonide and oral dexamethasone for treatment of croup: a randomized controlled trial. *JAMA* 1998; **279:** 1629–32.
12. Klassen TP, *et al.* The efficacy of nebulized budesonide in dexamethasone-treated outpatients with croup. *Pediatrics* 1996; **97:** 463–6.
13. Geelhoed GC, *et al.* Efficacy of a small single dose of oral dexamethasone for outpatient croup: a double blind placebo controlled clinical trial. *Br Med J* 1996; **313:** 140–2.
14. Macfarlane PI, Suri S. Steroids in the management of croup. *Br Med J* 1996; **312:** 510.
15. Anonymous. Inhaled budesonide and adrenaline for croup. *Drug Ther Bull* 1996; **34:** 23–4.
16. Johnson DW, *et al.* A comparison of nebulised budesonide, intramuscular dexamethasone, and placebo for moderately severe croup. *N Engl J Med* 1998; **339:** 498–503.

Cystic fibrosis

Corticosteroids have been used by mouth or by inhalation in the management of the inflammatory response of the lungs in cystic fibrosis (see p.119).

Deafness

For references to the use of corticosteroids in the treatment of deafness associated with Cogan's syndrome, see above.

Dermatomyositis

For references to the treatment of dermatomyositis with corticosteroids, see Polymyositis and Dermatomyositis, p.1027.

Eczema

Several treatments may be used in the management of atopic eczema (p.1073) but topical corticosteroids are the mainstay. The least potent preparation that is effective should be used, combined with regular use of an emollient; in mild to moderate disease the topical corticosteroid is only given for 1 to 2 weeks at a time. Most children with mild to moderate eczema respond to treatment with a mildly potent preparation such as 1% hydrocortisone ointment. For older children and adults with refractory disease, a more potent topical corticosteroid should be considered for long enough to bring the disease under control, followed by a weaker preparation as the condition improves.

The use of systemic corticosteroids is a treatment of last resort in resistant severe eczema, usually for short periods to control the disease, and very rarely for maintenance.

Epidermolysis bullosa

High-dose oral corticosteroids may be tried to control blistering in severe forms of epidermolysis bullosa (p.1074).

Epilepsy

Corticosteroids and corticotrophin have been commonly used to treat **infantile spasms**[1] since they have generally been unresponsive to conventional antiepileptics. A recent study[2] indicated that high-dose corticotrophin was preferable to prednisone. However, as discussed on p.335, corticotrophin and corticosteroids are associated with frequent and severe adverse effects, and there is controversy over whether they have a better effect on long-term outcome than antiepileptics.

It has been suggested that high doses of corticosteroids may produce a response in epilepsia partialis continua (a form of **status epilepticus**) refractory to standard antiepileptics (see p.337).

1. Robinson RO. Seizures and steroids. *Arch Dis Child* 1985; **60:** 94–5.
2. Baram TZ, *et al.* High-dose corticotropin (ACTH) versus prednisone for infantile spasms: a prospective, randomized, blinded study. *Pediatrics* 1996; **97:** 375–9.

Erythema multiforme

In the management of erythema multiforme systemic corticosteroids may be considered in severe reactions (see p.1074).

Eye disorders

Topical corticosteroids have transformed the management of inflammatory disease of the anterior segment of the eye and it should be noted that their proper use may be sight-saving but that their inappropriate use is potentially blinding.[1] The dangers include the conversion of a simple dendritic herpes simplex epithelial lesion into an extensive amoeboid ulcer with the likelihood of permanent corneal scarring and loss of vision and also the risk of potentiation of bacterial and fungal infections. Other dangers include the development of open-angle glaucoma and cataracts. Topical steroids are used by ophthalmologists in herpes simplex keratitis but always under appropriate antiviral cover and their use requires considerable experience. Topical corticosteroids should never be given for an undiagnosed red eye and many consultant ophthalmic surgeons believe that general practitioners should never initiate therapy without an ophthalmic opinion.

Further studies and discussions on the inappropriate use of corticosteroids to treat eye disorders are listed below.[2-10]

1. St Clair Roberts D. Steroids, the eye, and general practitioners. *Br Med J* 1986; **292:** 1414–15.
2. Lavin MJ, Rose GE. Use of steroid eye drops in general practice. *Br Med J* 1986; **292:** 1448–50.
3. Claoué CMP, Stevenson KE. Incidence of inappropriate treatment of herpes simplex keratitis with topical steroids. *Br Med J* 1986; **292:** 1450–1.
4. Livingstone A. Steroids, the eye, and general practitioners. *Br Med J* 1986; **292:** 1737.
5. Lawrence M. Steroids, the eye, and general practitioners. *Br Med J* 1986; **292:** 1737–8.
6. Trevor-Roper P. Steroids, the eye, and general practitioners. *Br Med J* 1986; **292:** 1738.
7. Jay B. Steroids, the eye, and general practitioners. *Br Med J* 1986; **293:** 205.
8. Rose GE, Lavin MJ. Steroids, the eye, and general practitioners. *Br Med J* 1986; **293:** 205.
9. O'Day DM. Corticosteroids: an unresolved debate. *Ophthalmology* 1991; **98:** 845–6.
10. Stern GA, Buttross M. Use of corticosteroids in combination with antimicrobial drugs in the treatment of infectious corneal disease. *Ophthalmology* 1991; **98:** 847–53.

Giant cell arteritis

Giant cell arteritis (temporal arteritis; cranial arteritis) is a vasculitic disorder which is frequently associated with polymyalgia rheumatica (p.1027). It occurs mainly in persons over 50 years of age of European, particularly Scandinavian, extraction and is more common in women than men. It is characterised by inflammatory, granulomatous lesions with giant mononuclear cell infiltrates affecting large and medium sized arteries, particularly those supplying the neck and extracranial structures of head and arms. Symptoms vary but may include headache, scalp tenderness, claudication of the jaw, swelling and absence of pulse in the temporal artery, fever, weight loss, malaise, anaemia, visual disturbances, and irreversible blindness. About a third of all patients also exhibit polymyalgia rheumatica.

Treatment is with corticosteroids,[1-5] and early diagnosis and treatment is desirable to reduce the risk of sudden blindness. Most regimens have involved high initial doses of corticosteroid to control the disease followed by reduction to a maintenance dose, but both initial and maintenance doses have varied considerably. The current view seems to be that prednisolone 40 mg daily by mouth initially is adequate in uncomplicated cases without visual symptoms;[2,5,6] this can be reduced after one month to 30 mg daily, after a further month to 20 mg daily, and then more gradually to 10 mg daily or less depending on the patient's response.[2]

Patients presenting with visual symptoms should receive at least 60 mg of prednisolone daily, and one suggested regimen in this group is hydrocortisone 250 mg intravenously at first followed by prednisolone 80 mg by mouth daily for 3 days; the daily prednisolone dose is then reduced to 60 mg for 3 days, then 40 mg for 4 days, and subsequently decreased by 5 mg per week until a maintenance dose of 10 mg daily is reached.[1,2] Some ophthalmologists recommend 80 mg (or 1 mg per kg body-weight) of prednisolone daily as an initial dose in all patients with giant cell arteritis;[5,7] in patients with overt anterior ischaemic optic neuropathy an initial 1-g intravenous infusion of methylprednisolone has also been suggested, followed by high-dose oral corticosteroids.[7]

Maintenance treatment is usually required for at least 2 years. While a small number require indefinite treatment, most patients should be able to discontinue treatment within 4 to 5 years;[8] however relapses are not uncommon.

Because of the need for prolonged corticosteroid therapy side-effects are common, and their management may be the most difficult aspect of treatment.[2,8] Azathioprine has been added to corticosteroid therapy for its modest 'steroid-sparing' effect,[9] and there is evidence of similar benefit from the use of low-dose methotrexate.[10] Other cytotoxic immunosuppressants do not appear to be used. The prognosis is excellent in adequately-treated patients, as the life expectancy of patients with giant cell arteritis is the same as the general population.[11]

1. Clearkin LG, Watts MT. Ocular involvement in giant cell arteritis. *Br J Hosp Med* 1990; **43:** 373–6.
2. Taylor HG, Samanta A. Treatment of vasculitis. *Br J Clin Pharmacol* 1993; **35:** 93–104.
3. Pountain G, Hazleman B. Polymyalgia rheumatica and giant cell arteritis. *Br Med J* 1995; **310:** 1057–9.
4. Zilko PJ. Polymyalgia rheumatica and giant cell arteritis. *Med J Aust* 1996; **165:** 438–42.
5. Swannell AJ. Polymyalgia rheumatica and temporal arteritis: diagnosis and management. *Br Med J* 1997; **314:** 1329–32.
6. Kyle V, Hazleman BL. Treatment of polymyalgia rheumatica and giant cell arteritis I: steroid regimens in the first two months. *Ann Rheum Dis* 1989; **48:** 658–61.
7. Ferris J, Lamb R. Polymyalgia rheumatica and giant cell arteritis. *Br Med J* 1995; **311:** 455.
8. Kyle V, Hazleman BL. Stopping steroids in polymyalgia rheumatica and giant cell arteritis. *Br Med J* 1990; **300:** 344–5.
9. De Silva M, Hazleman BL. Azathioprine in giant cell arteritis/polymyalgia rheumatica: a double blind study. *Ann Rheum Dis* 1986; **45:** 136–8.
10. Hernández-García C, *et al.* Methotrexate treatment in the management of giant cell arteritis. *Scand J Rheumatol* 1994; **23:** 295–8.
11. Matteson EL, *et al.* Long-term survival of patients with giant cell arteritis in the American College of Rheumatology giant cell arteritis classification criteria cohort. *Am J Med* 1996; **100:** 193–6.

Glomerular kidney disease

Glomerular disease accounts for a considerable proportion of all kidney disease. Various forms of primary glomerular disease (glomerulopathy) are known, and are discussed below; in addition, numerous systemic diseases, (connective-tissue disorders such as systemic lupus erythematosus as well as malignancy and conditions such as diabetes), may result in secondary glomerular disorders. Despite the various potential causes it is thought that many of these diseases act by common immunological mechanisms to damage the glomerulus, either by accumulation of antigen-antibody complexes (immune-complex nephritis) or more rarely by the formation of antibodies to the glomerular basement membrane (anti-GBM nephritis).

Since the kidney can respond in only a limited number of ways to glomerular damage certain common presentations are seen, regardless of aetiology, including **acute glomerulonephritis** (acute nephritis syndrome), which is marked by haematuria and proteinuria of abrupt onset, usually with impaired renal function (a decrease in glomerular filtration rate), salt and water retention, and hypertension; and the **nephrotic syndrome**, which is marked by severe proteinuria, hypoalbuminaemia, and oedema. Other, less dramatic presentations of glomerular disease are asymptomatic proteinuria or microscopic haematuria; alternatively, glomerular disease may be one of the many potential causes of chronic renal failure. Appropriate management of these conditions depends to a considerable extent on the underlying disease.

MANAGEMENT OF PRIMARY GLOMERULAR DISEASE.

Minimal change nephropathy (MCN; minimal change disease). This condition occurs mainly in children, the highest incidence being at 2 to 4 years, and is the main cause of childhood nephrotic syndrome. It also accounts for about 20% of adult cases of nephrotic syndrome.[1] It is treated with a corticosteroid. Regimens vary somewhat but a suggested regimen for adults has been 60 mg prednisolone daily by mouth for 4 days, reduced to 40 mg daily until remission occurs (which in 90% of patients will be within 3 weeks) and then tapered off.[1] In children, initial doses of 60 mg prednisolone or prednisone per m^2 body-surface area daily have been used,[2] which may be given for anything up to 4 weeks before switching to 40 mg per m^2 given on alternate days for a further 4 weeks, and then tapered off. A recent modification to the children's dose is to give 60 mg of prednisolone per m^2 daily until there is a response when the dose is reduced to 40 mg per m^2 on alternate days for the next 4 weeks. If there is no response within 4 weeks' treatment with the 60 mg per m^2 dose then the corticosteroid should be withdrawn and the child considered to be steroid resistant.[3]

Relapse is common and occurs in about 60% of cases; relapses usually respond to a further course of corticosteroids, but if a third relapse occurs cyclophosphamide 2 to 3 mg per kg body-weight daily for 8 weeks may be added to a course of corticosteroid therapy.[1,2,4]

Prognosis is relatively good, even in those patients who relapse repeatedly, with no evidence of deterioration in renal function,[4] and the potential adverse effects of therapy must be considered. Pulsed intravenous methylprednisolone, followed by low-dose oral prednisone, has been suggested as an alternative to conventional oral doses of corticosteroids in an attempt to reduce adverse effects.[5] Cytotoxic immunosuppressants are reserved for relapsing or steroid-dependent cases because of their potential for severe toxicity, including carcinogenesis; cyclophosphamide appears to be preferred to chlorambucil because it is perceived as entailing a somewhat lower risk, although both are effective.

A minority of patients have minimal change disease resistant to corticosteroids: cyclosporin has been added successfully in both adults[6] and children[7] with this rare form of the disease but must be used with caution because of its own potential for nephrotoxicity. A report of responses to pefloxacin in a few patients[8] has not been confirmed by other groups.[9,10]

Focal glomerulosclerosis. Focal glomerulosclerosis is a sclerosing lesion affecting parts of the glomeruli which occurs in some patients who otherwise have symptoms characteristic of minimal change nephropathy, and some authorities do not regard it as a distinct disease. It is common in abusers of diamorphine and has also been linked with the nephropathy that can occur in patients with AIDS. Treatment is similar to that for minimal change nephropathy but only about 20% of cases respond to corticosteroids; addition of a cytotoxic immunosuppressant such as cyclophosphamide improves the prospect of remission. In patients who fail to respond, progression to renal failure may occur over several years, but renal transplantation may not be helpful as disease can recur in the transplanted kidney. A report of response to pefloxacin in a patient with focal glomerulosclerosis[8] has not been confirmed in other series,[9,10] but responses to cyclosporin have been seen.[6,7]

Membranous nephropathy (membranous glomerulonephritis). This is a disease predominately of adults, in whom it is the single most important cause of the nephrotic syndrome, accounting for about 50% of cases. It is characterised by diffuse thickening of the glomerular basement membrane following subepithelial deposition of immune complexes. Unlike minimal change nephropathy, whose treatment is fairly well established, treatment of membranous nephropathy is a contentious area. The course of disease is variable and often slow, with some spontaneous remissions, which makes the benefits of treatment difficult to demonstrate and the use of potentially toxic drugs difficult to justify. Cyclophosphamide or chlorambucil combined with a corticosteroid appears to produce some clinical improvement, and stabilisation of progressive disease;[11-13] it is not clear if corticosteroids alone are effective.[14-16] Cyclosporin alone has been tried in a few patients and was associated with complete or partial remission in about half;[17] a small controlled study has also reported benefits.[18] Treatment of any kind tends to be reserved for patients with progressive renal dysfunction.[19]

Mesangiocapillary glomerulonephritis (MCGN; membranoproliferative glomerulonephritis; MPGN). Mesangiocapillary glomerulonephritis comprises 2 separate diseases, known as type I and type II, which both occur in children and young adults and usually result in nephrotic syndrome, although about 20% of cases present with acute glomerulonephritis. Both forms show proliferation of mesangial cells and thickening of glomerular walls with formation of deposits (in type I disease due to immune complexes) in capillary walls and basement membranes. There is no established treatment regimen: some improvement or stabilisation of renal function may occur with corticosteroids and cytotoxic immunosuppressants, but about half of all patients develop end-stage renal failure within 15 to 20 years (type I disease) or 6 to 10 years (type II disease). Antiplatelet agents and anticoagulants have also been tried but as with other therapies there is little evidence of benefit, and some centres do not recommend any specific therapy, although prednisolone and cyclophosphamide may be offered to those with a rapidly progressive course.[20]

IGA nephropathy (Berger's disease) is the commonest cause of primary glomerular disease in developed countries, and is most common in young men. It results in focal, segmental proliferative glomerulonephritis associated with mesangial formation of immune deposits largely composed of IgA. The usual presentation is acute glomerulonephritis with gross haematuria, often during or just after viral upper-respiratory-tract infection. Some patients develop rapidly progressive disease similar to idiopathic rapidly progressive glomerulonephritis, with renal failure within 6 months, but in many others the syndrome is benign, and requires only observation. No form of therapy has been unequivocally shown to be of value, but control of associated hypertension is considered important. Corticosteroids and cytotoxic immunosuppressants may be tried in severe rapidly progressive disease;[21-23] mycophenolate mofetil has been reported to be effective in 2 patients.[24] Some promising results have been seen with the use of n-3 fatty acids from fish oil,[25] and there is also a report of benefit with normal immunoglobulin.[26]

Idiopathic rapidly progressive glomerulonephritis (RPGN). Although rapidly progressive glomerulonephritis (crescentic glomerulonephritis) may be a feature of other forms of glomerular disease such as IgA nephropathy (see above) or Goodpasture's syndrome (see below) it also occurs in an idiopathic form. The disease is characterised by the formation of glomerular crescents associated with leakage of fibrin from damaged capillaries, and loss of renal function is very rapid, sometimes with renal failure within weeks. Oral corticosteroids are of little value alone, but pulsed intravenous methylprednisolone followed by oral prednisone or prednisone and cyclophosphamide over several months has produced some impressive responses;[27,28] an alternative is the use of intensive plasma exchange together with a corticosteroid and cytotoxic immunosuppressants.[29] However controlled trials of these therapies are lacking.

Goodpasture's syndrome. Goodpasture's syndrome is a form of anti-GBM nephritis in which rapidly progressive glomerulonephritis is accompanied by pulmonary haemorrhage due to reaction of the same antibody responsible for the renal symptoms with the membranes of the alveoli. It is a disease predominately of young males. Pulmonary haemorrhage responds to high dose oral prednisolone or prednisone, or pulsed intravenous methylprednisolone, but corticosteroids are of little value in controlling renal lesions, which requires vigorous plasma exchange therapy with corticosteroids and cyclophosphamide on a daily or alternate day basis for several weeks, until antibody is no longer detectable and disease progression has halted; it is important to begin therapy before renal damage becomes irreversible.

MANAGEMENT OF SECONDARY GLOMERULAR DISEASE.

Post-infectious glomerulonephritis. The classical form of post-infectious glomerulonephritis is post-streptococcal glomerulonephritis, which produces an immune-complex- mediated acute glomerulonephritis, but glomerular disease may follow other bacterial infections, as well as protozoal infections such as malaria (malaria-associated nephrotic syndrome is familiar in endemic regions) and viral infections such as AIDS (see Focal Glomerulosclerosis, above). In most cases no additional treatment beyond appropriate management of infection and general supportive care is warranted, and corticosteroids and cytotoxic immunosuppressants are not generally used and may in some cases be harmful.[30] Nonetheless, delayed progressive renal disease may occur in a minority of patients, and has prompted efforts to treat.

Other secondary glomerulopathies. Where glomerular disease is secondary to other diseases (connective tissue disorders such as systemic lupus erythematosus, the vasculitides, Henoch-Schönlein purpura, thrombotic thrombocytopenic purpura, or others such as rheumatoid arthritis, amyloidosis, neoplasia, sickle-cell disease, gout, or diabetes mellitus) most treatment is directed at the underlying disease. In addition, symptomatic management such as the use of sodium restriction for the oedema of nephrotic syndrome may be appropriate; diuretics should be used cautiously because of the risk of hypovolaemia.[2] Proteinuria of various causes may respond to the use of ACE inhibitors or NSAIDs,[1,31] although care is required in patients with renal artery stenosis or renal failure respectively. Associated hypertension and hypercholesterolaemia should be treated symptomatically, and anticoagulants may be required for associated coagulation disorders (it has been suggested that warfarin may be more appropriate than heparin, although both have been used[31]). Renal toxicity can arise from various drug treatments and this should also be treated symptomatically.

1. Boulton-Jones M. Management of nephrotic syndrome. *Prescribers' J* 1993; **33:** 96–102. Correction. *ibid.*; 176.
2. Melvin T, Bennett W. Management of nephrotic syndrome in childhood. *Drugs* 1991; **42:** 30–51.
3. Report of a Workshop by the British Association for Paediatric Nephrology and Research Unit, Royal College of Physicians. Consensus statement on management and audit potential for steroid responsive nephrotic syndrome. *Arch Dis Child* 1994; **70:** 151–7.
4. Trompeter RS, *et al.* Long-term outcome for children with minimal-change nephrotic syndrome. *Lancet* 1985; **i:** 368–70.
5. Imbasciati E, *et al.* Controlled trial of methylprednisolone pulses and low dose oral prednisone for the minimal change nephrotic syndrome. *Br Med J* 1985; **291:** 1305–8.
6. Nyrop M, Olgaard K. Cyclosporin A treatment of severe steroid resistant nephrotic syndrome in adults. *J Intern Med* 1990; **227:** 65–8.
7. Niaudet P, *et al.* Steroid-resistant idiopathic nephrotic syndrome and ciclosporin. *Nephron* 1991; **57:** 481.
8. Pruna A, *et al.* Pefloxacin as first-line treatment in nephrotic syndrome. *Lancet* 1992; **340:** 728–9.
9. Geffriaud-Riconard C, *et al.* Inefficacy and toxicity of pefloxacin in focal and segmental glomerulosclerosis with steroid-resistant nephrotic syndrome. *Lancet* 1993; **341:** 1475.
10. Aigrain EJ, *et al.* Side-effects of pefloxacin in idiopathic nephrotic syndrome. *Lancet* 1993; **342:** 438–9.
11. Mathieson PW, *et al.* Prednisolone and chlorambucil treatment in idiopathic membranous nephropathy with deteriorating renal function. *Lancet* 1985; **ii:** 869–72.
12. Ponticelli C, *et al.* A 10-year follow-up of a randomized study with methylprednisolone and chlorambucil in membranous nephropathy. *Kidney Int* 1995; **48:** 1600–4.
13. Bruns FJ, *et al.* Sustained remission of membranous glomerulonephritis after cyclophosphamide and prednisone. *Ann Intern Med* 1991; **114:** 725–30.
14. Cattran DC, *et al.* A randomized controlled trial of prednisone in patients with idiopathic membranous nephropathy. *N Engl J Med* 1989; **320:** 210–15.
15. Ponticelli C, *et al.* Methylprednisolone plus chlorambucil as compared with methylprednisolone alone for the treatment of idiopathic membranous nephropathy. *N Engl J Med* 1992; **327:** 599–603.
16. Falk RJ, *et al.* Treatment of progressive membranous glomerulopathy: a randomized trial comparing cyclophosphamide and corticosteroids with corticosteroids alone. *Ann Intern Med* 1992; **116:** 438–45.
17. Rostoker G, *et al.* Cyclosporin in idiopathic steroid-resistant membranous glomerulonephritis. *Lancet* 1989; **ii:** 975–6.
18. Cattran DC, *et al.* A controlled trial of cyclosporine in patients with progressive membranous nephropathy. *Kidney Int* 1995; **47:** 1130–5.
19. Lewis EJ. Idiopathic membranous nephropathy—to treat or not to treat? *N Engl J Med* 1993; **329:** 127–9.
20. Mason PD, Pusey CD. Glomerulonephritis: diagnosis and treatment. *Br Med J* 1994; **309:** 1557–63. Correction. *ibid* 1995; **310:** 116.
21. Goumenos D, *et al.* Can immunosuppressive drugs slow the progression of IgA nephropathy? *Nephrol Dial Transplant* 1995; **10:** 1173–81.
22. Faedda R, *et al.* Immunosuppressive treatment of Berger's disease. *Clin Pharmacol Ther* 1996; **60:** 561–7.
23. Kobayashi Y, *et al.* Steroid therapy during the early stage of progressive IgA nephropathy: a 10-year follow-up study. *Nephron* 1996; **72:** 237–42.
24. Nowack R, *et al.* Mycophenolate mofetil for systemic vasculitis and IgA nephropathy. *Lancet* 1997; **349:** 774.
25. Donadio JV, *et al.* A controlled trial of fish oil in IgA nephropathy. *N Engl J Med* 1994; **331:** 1194–9.
26. Rostoker G, *et al.* High-dose immunoglobulin therapy for severe IgA nephropathy and Henoch-Schönlein purpura. *Ann Intern Med* 1994; **120:** 476–84.
27. Bolton WK, Sturgill BC. Methylprednisolone therapy for acute crescentic rapidly progressive glomerulonephritis. *Am J Nephrol* 1989; **9:** 368–75.
28. Bruns FJ, *et al.* Long-term follow-up of aggressively treated idiopathic rapidly progressive glomerulonephritis. *Am J Med* 1989; **86:** 400–6.
29. Gianviti A, *et al.* Retrospective study of plasma exchange in patients with idiopathic rapidly progressive glomerulonephritis and vasculitis. *Arch Dis Child* 1996; **75:** 186–90.
30. Adeniyi A, *et al.* A controlled trial of cyclophosphamide and azathioprine in Nigerian children with the nephrotic syndrome and poorly selective proteinuria. *Arch Dis Child* 1979; **54:** 204–7.
31. Alaniz C, *et al.* Pharmacologic management of adult idiopathic nephrotic syndrome. *Clin Pharm* 1993; **12:** 429–39.

Graves' ophthalmopathy

As discussed under Hyperthyroidism, p.1489, patients with moderate to severe ophthalmopathy may be treated with high-dose systemic corticosteroids or with orbital radiotherapy, which appear to be equally effective. It has also been reported that concomitant therapy with a corticosteroid can prevent the transient exacerbation of Graves' ophthalmopathy that may be caused by radioiodine treatment in hyperthyroid patients.[1]

1. Bartalena L, *et al.* Relation between therapy for hyperthyroidism and the course of Graves' ophthalmopathy. *N Engl J Med* 1998; **338:** 73–8.

Haemangioma

Haemangiomas are benign vascular neoplasms of the skin which may enlarge dramatically before regressing spontaneously. Although no treatment is normally required, occasional complications due to ocular or visceral involvement, or associated thrombocytopenia due to platelet trapping (the Kasabach-Merritt syndrome), may merit treatment, generally with corticosteroids. Response is variable.[1-6] There has been a recent report of 2 infants responding to vincristine after corticosteroids had failed.[7] Interferon alfa has also been tried,[8] as has phototherapy with a pulsed dye laser.[9]

1. Evans J, *et al.* Haemangioma with coagulopathy: sustained response to prednisone. *Arch Dis Child* 1975; **50:** 809–12.
2. Sloan GM, *et al.* Intralesional corticosteroid therapy for infantile hemangiomas. *Plast Reconstr Surg* 1989; **83:** 459–66.
3. Morrell AJ, Willshaw HE. Normalisation of refractive error after steroid injection for adnexal haemangiomas. *Br J Ophthalmol* 1991; **75:** 301–5.
4. David TJ, *et al.* Haemangioma with thrombocytopenia (Kasabach-Merritt syndrome). *Arch Dis Child* 1983; **58:** 1022–3.
5. Enjoiras O, *et al.* Management of alarming hemangiomas in infancy: a review of 25 cases. *Pediatrics* 1990; **85:** 491–8.
6. Sadan N, Wolach B. Treatment of hemangiomas of infants with high doses of prednisone. *J Pediatr* 1996; **128:** 141–6.
7. Payarols JP, *et al.* Treatment of life-threatening infantile hemangiomas with vincristine. *N Engl J Med* 1995; **333:** 69.
8. Ezekowitz RAB, *et al.* Interferon alfa-2a therapy for life-threatening hemangiomas of infancy. *N Engl J Med* 1992; **326:** 1456–63. Correction. *ibid.* 1995; **333:** 595–6.
9. Barlow RJ, *et al.* Treatment of proliferative haemangiomas with the 585 nm pulsed dye laser. *Br J Dermatol* 1996; **34:** 700–4.

Headache

Corticosteroids have a limited role in the management of some types of headache. Although their long-term use is not considered desirable, short courses of prednisolone or prednisone in doses of 20 to 40 mg daily can be an effective alternative to standard drugs such as ergotamine in the prevention of cluster headache attacks during cluster periods (p.443). Corticosteroids have also been used for the emergency treatment of prolonged severe attacks of migraine (p.443) refractory to other drugs.

Herpes infections

Although corticosteroids alone are contra-indicated for most forms of ocular herpes simplex infection (p.597), which should be treated with a topical antiviral such as aciclovir, a combination of corticosteroid and antiviral may be useful in some cases.

Hypercalcaemia

For a description of the treatment of hypercalcaemia, including the specific role of corticosteroids, see p.1148.

Hypersensitivity vasculitis

Hypersensitivity vasculitis is usually associated with an antigenic stimulus, either exogenous such as a drug or microbe, or endogenous such as an immune complex associated with connective tissue disease. The term covers a heterogeneous group of disorders, many of which are associated with some underlying disease process (including infections, malignant neoplasms and disorders such as rheumatoid arthritis or systemic lupus erythematosus), as well as vasculitis of less clear aetiology such as Henoch-Schönlein purpura, a disease typically seen in prepubertal males. There is a suggestion that such a broad grouping is inappropriate, and that the term 'hypersensitivity vasculitis' should not be used;[1] however, at present it continues to be employed in the literature.

Hypersensitivity vasculitis is characterised by small vessel involvement (arterioles and venules), particularly of the skin, and skin manifestations such as purpura, rashes, and urticaria predominate. Neutrophil debris is typically present around the vessel (**leucocytoclastic vasculitis**). However other organ systems may also be involved: in **Henoch-Schönlein purpura**, the skin lesions are associated with arthralgia, abdominal pain and other gastro-intestinal symptoms, and glomerulonephritis (usually without impairment of renal function).

The prognosis is typically much better in hypersensitivity vasculitis than in the other major vasculitic syndromes, and most cases resolve spontaneously. Where a recognised antigenic stimulus is present it should be removed if possible, e.g. by withdrawal of a drug or by appropriate antibiotic therapy of infection. Hypersensitivity vasculitis generally responds less well to conventional drug therapy than other vasculitic syndromes. Nonetheless, where disease persists or results in organ dysfunction, a corticosteroid should be given, typically prednisone or prednisolone 60 mg, or 1 mg per kg body-weight, by mouth daily, tapered rapidly until therapy can be discontinued. Plasmapheresis has also been used, but the use of cytotoxic immunosuppressants is less well established. Anecdotal reports of excellent responses to dapsone in Henoch-Schönlein purpura exist.[2] Other drugs that have been tried include danazol,[3] oxpentifylline,[4] the latter sometimes in conjunction with dapsone,[4] and normal immunoglobulin.[5]

1. Jennette JC, *et al.* Nomenclature of systemic vasculitides: proposal of an international consensus conference. *Arthritis Rheum* 1994; **37:** 187–92.
2. Hoffbrand BI. Dapsone in Henoch-Schönlein purpura—worth a trial. *Postgrad Med J* 1991; **67:** 961–2.
3. Lee YJ, *et al.* Danazol for Henoch-Schönlein purpura. *Ann Intern Med* 1993; **118:** 827.
4. Nürnberg W, *et al.* Synergistic effects of pentoxifylline and dapsone in leucocytoclastic vasculitis. *Lancet* 1994; **343:** 491.
5. Rostoker G, *et al.* High-dose immunoglobulin therapy for severe IgA nephropathy and Henoch-Schönlein purpura. *Ann Intern Med* 1994; **120:** 476–84.

Idiopathic thrombocytopenic purpura

Idiopathic thrombocytopenic purpura (ITP; sometimes referred to as autoimmune thrombocytopenic purpura[1]) is an autoimmune bleeding disorder characterised by the development of antibodies to the body's own platelets, with consequent sequestration and destruction of platelets. Both acute and chronic forms are seen; the acute form, which is usually self-limiting and follows viral or other infection, is the usual form in children, whereas chronic and sometimes more serious disease is more likely in adults, particularly young or middle-aged women. Patients develop petechiae, ecchymoses, and epistaxis, and women may develop menorrhagia; death due to haemorrhage is not unknown.

Treatment. There is a reluctance to treat the acute form because of its self-limiting nature. However, in an emergency such as major acute bleeding or intracranial haemorrhage exchange transfusion or massive doses of allogeneic platelets, high dose methylprednisolone, and intravenous normal immunoglobulin may be given.[1-5]

For both adults and children with mild thrombocytopenia (counts of 20 to 30 000 per mm^3 or more) and no severe bruising or haemorrhage, no treatment is required.[2-6] In many cases the platelet count will return to normal or remain in a safe range despite the lack of therapy, and spontaneous remission can occur, even after a period of years.[7]

Where treatment is required in chronic disease, corticosteroids are the mainstay of therapy in adults.[2-4,8] Prednisolone (or prednisone) 1 mg per kg body-weight daily is often used, continued until response occurs (sometimes not for a week or more[1]) and then tapered down. If there is no response within 3 weeks the drug should be gradually discontinued as it is unlikely to be effective. About 70 to 80% of adult patients with chronic disease exhibit some response, although not always a sufficient one, but most will relapse when the drug is withdrawn and may require long-term low-dose maintenance, perhaps using alternate day administration.[2] Good responses have also been reported with the use of high-dose oral or intravenous methylprednisolone for 3 to 7 days,[9-12] (this has also been tried in children with the acute form[13]) and pulsed treatment with high-dose dexamethasone looks promising,[6,14] although it is not clear how great the benefits will be in children.[15-17] Use of corticosteroids for ITP in children is in any case controversial. Some consider low daily doses of prednisolone (0.25 mg per kg) to be as effective as higher ones,[3] while others consider high doses (prednisone 4 mg per kg) to be necessary.[18,19] Some centres consider that corticosteroids are of at best temporary benefit in children.[20]

In patients with chronic disease and bleeding symptoms who fail to respond to first-line therapy, splenectomy should be considered.[2-6,8,20] About 70% of patients will respond but the operative and postoperative risks (notably of sepsis) must be considered, particularly in children.

Responses can also be achieved with intravenous normal immunoglobulin, which in practice is often preferred to corticosteroids for initial drug therapy in children.[21] An increase in platelet count is usually achievable with doses of 400 mg per kg daily for 5 days although the effect may be transient; some patients refractory to these doses respond to high-dose therapy (800 mg to 1 g per kg daily).[2] Response is often achievable even in patients refractory to other therapies, but treatment must be repeated periodically. It is perhaps most useful when acute symptoms supervene, because of its rapid activity, and it is recommended that it be reserved for patients with acute severe bleeding, as preoperative prophylaxis in patients with severe thrombocytopenia, or for patients with bleeding symptoms refractory to corticosteroids.[3-6] Again, some centres have not found it valuable in children.[20] An alternative to normal immunoglobulin in rhesus-positive patients may be the use of anti-D immunoglobulin,[22] although there are conflicting views as to its effectiveness.[8,19,22-25] A response to normal immunoglobulin has been reported to be a good predictor of benefit from splenectomy.[26]

Various other second-line drugs have been tried in the minority of patients with refractory chronic disease, but few have been well evaluated. Generally,[27-30] but not universally,[31] good results have been reported with danazol, particularly in older patients. It may have advantages for long-term maintenance, and is a potential alternative to splenectomy, at least in selected patients.[29,30] It can be used as a 'steroid-sparing' agent, permitting reduction in corticosteroid maintenance doses.[29]

Antineoplastic and immunosuppressive drugs have been tried in refractory disease, but their potential toxicity has meant that they have often been reserved for older patients, as a treatment of last resort. Cyclophosphamide or azathioprine have been given by mouth in doses of 50 to 150 mg daily; responses to cyclophosphamide generally occur within 8 weeks but for azathioprine several months' treatment is generally necessary before response can be assessed.[2,6] High-dose cyclophosphamide has also been tried in refractory, life-threatening disease.[6] Although some patients have responded to intravenous injection of vincristine, responses have tended to be partial and inadequate, and somewhat better results have been achieved with infusions of platelets incubated with vinblastine or vincristine to encourage binding and permit selective drug delivery to the macrophages responsible for platelet destruction.[32-34] Although the developers of this technique have reported long-lasting remission in 38% of patients,[34] enthusiasm elsewhere appears to be muted.[2,35] Combination chemotherapy (cyclophosphamide and prednisone plus vincristine, vincristine and procarbazine, or etoposide) has produced prolonged remission in a few patients,[6,36] but such aggressive treatment would be difficult to justify in most cases.

Other reports of benefit exist for colchicine,[37-39] heparin,[40] and ascorbic acid,[41] the latter having at least the advantage that it is relatively non-toxic, but such therapies remain experimental.

Thrombopoietin can now be produced and this may offer a future new approach to treatment.[42]

Tranexamic acid may be helpful in the symptomatic management of menorrhagia, although hysterectomy is occasionally necessary.

In pregnancy. Particular problems arise in the management of ITP in pregnancy, since antiplatelet antibodies can cross the placenta and produce thrombocytopenia in the fetus. The risk is greater when disease exists before pregnancy than when it develops in the course of pregnancy.

If therapy is considered necessary the mother may be given prednisolone or normal immunoglobulin, with platelet infusions for more serious, unresponsive symptoms.[2] A course of intravenous immunoglobulin before delivery is useful in protecting against postpartum complications. Treatment may be required for the neonate[2] if there are complications or the platelet count falls below 50 000 per mm^3. Delivery by caesarean section may be considered.[4]

1. Karpatkin S. Autoimmune (idiopathic) thrombocytopenic purpura. *Lancet* 1997; **349:** 1531–6.
2. Provan AB. Management of adult idiopathic thrombocytopenic purpura. *Prescribers' J* 1992; **32:** 193–200.
3. Eden OB, Lilleyman JS. Guidelines for management of idiopathic thrombocytopenic purpura. *Arch Dis Child* 1992; **67:** 1056–8.
4. The American Society of Hematology ITP Practice Guideline Panel. Diagnosis and treatment of idiopathic thrombocytopenic purpura: recommendations of the American Society of Hematology. *Ann Intern Med* 1997; **126:** 319–26.
5. Gillis S. The thrombocytopenic purpuras: recognition and management. *Drugs* 1996; **51:** 942–53.
6. McMillan R. Therapy for adults with refractory chronic immune thrombocytopenic purpura. *Ann Intern Med* 1997; **126:** 307–14.
7. Tait RC, Evans DIK. Late spontaneous recovery of chronic thrombocytopenia. *Arch Dis Child* 1993; **68:** 680–1.
8. Stasi R, *et al.* Long-term observation of 208 adults with chronic idiopathic thrombocytopenic purpura. *Am J Med* 1995; **98:** 436–42.
9. von dem Borne AEGK, *et al.* High dose intravenous methylprednisolone or high dose intravenous gammaglobulin for autoimmune thrombocytopenia. *Br Med J* 1988; **296:** 249–50.
10. Özsoylu Ş, *et al.* Megadose methylprednisolone for chronic idiopathic thrombocytopenic purpura. *Lancet* 1990; **336:** 1078–9.
11. Akoğlu T, *et al.* Megadose methylprednisolone pulse therapy in adult idiopathic thrombocytopenic purpura. *Lancet* 1991; **337:** 56.
12. Özsoylu S. Mega-dose methylprednisolone for chronic idiopathic thrombocytopenic purpura. *Lancet* 1991; **337:** 1611–12.
13. Albayrak D, *et al.* Acute immune thrombocytopenic purpura: a comparative study of very high oral doses of methylprednisolone and intravenously administered immune globulin. *J Pediatr* 1994; **125:** 1004–7.
14. Andersen JC. Response of resistant idiopathic thrombocytopenic purpura to pulsed high-dose dexamethasone therapy. *N Engl J Med* 1994; **330:** 1560–4.
15. Adams DM, *et al.* High-dose oral dexamethasone therapy for chronic childhood idiopathic thrombocytopenic purpura. *J Pediatr* 1996; **128:** 281–3.
16. Borgna-Pignatti C, *et al.* A trial of high-dose dexamethasone therapy for chronic idiopathic thrombocytopenic purpura in childhood. *J Pediatr* 1997; **130:** 13–16.
17. Kühne T, *et al.* Platelet and immune responses to oral cyclic dexamethasone therapy in childhood chronic immune thrombocytopenic purpura. *J Pediatr* 1997; **130:** 17–24.
18. Blanchette VS, *et al.* A prospective, randomized trial of high-dose intravenous immune globulin G therapy, oral prednisone therapy, and no therapy in childhood acute immune thrombocytopenia purpura. *J Pediatr* 1993; **123:** 989–95.
19. Blanchette V, *et al.* Randomised trial of intravenous immunoglobulin G, intravenous anti-D, and oral prednisone in childhood acute immune thrombocytopenic purpura. *Lancet* 1994; **344:** 703–7.
20. Reid MM. Chronic idiopathic thrombocytopenic purpura: incidence, treatment, and outcome. *Arch Dis Child* 1995; **72:** 125–8.
21. Bolton-Maggs PHB, Moon I. Assessment of UK practice for management of acute childhood idiopathic thrombocytopenic purpura against published guidelines. *Lancet* 1997; **350:** 620–3.
22. Anonymous. Rho(D) immune globulin iv for prevention of Rh isoimmunization and for treatment of ITP. *Med Lett Drugs Ther* 1996; **38:** 6–8.
23. Andrew M, *et al.* A multicenter study of the treatment of childhood chronic idiopathic thrombocytopenic purpura with anti-D. *J Pediatr* 1992; **120:** 522–7.
24. Zunich KM, *et al.* Intravenous anti-D immunoglobulin for childhood acute immune thrombocytopenic purpura. *Lancet* 1995; **346:** 1363–4.
25. Blanchette V, Wang E. Intravenous anti-D immunoglobulin for childhood acute immune thrombocytopenic purpura. *Lancet* 1995; **346:** 1364–5.
26. Law C, *et al.* High-dose intravenous immune globulin and the response to splenectomy in patients with idiopathic thrombocytopenic purpura. *N Engl J Med* 1997; **336:** 1494–8.
27. Buelli M, *et al.* Danazol for the treatment of idiopathic thrombocytopenic purpura. *Acta Haematol (Basel)* 1985; **74:** 97–8.
28. Mylvaganam R, *et al.* Very low dose danazol in idiopathic thrombocytopenic purpura and its role as an immune modulator. *Am J Med Sci* 1989; **298:** 215–20.
29. Ahn YS, *et al.* Long-term danazol therapy in autoimmune thrombocytopenia: unmaintained remission and age-dependent response in women. *Ann Intern Med* 1989; **111:** 723–9.
30. Edelmann DZ, *et al.* Danazol in non-splenectomized patients with refractory idiopathic thrombocytopenic purpura. *Postgrad Med J* 1990; **66:** 827–30.

31. McVerry BA, *et al.* The use of danazol in the management of chronic immune thrombocytopenic purpura. *Br J Haematol* 1985; **61:** 145–8.
32. Ahn YS, *et al.* The treatment of idiopathic thrombocytopenia with vinblastine-loaded platelets. *N Engl J Med* 1978; **298:** 1101–7.
33. Agnelli G, *et al.* Vinca-loaded platelets. *N Engl J Med* 1984; **311:** 599.
34. Ahn YS, *et al.* Vinca-loaded platelets. *N Engl J Med* 1984; **311:** 599–600.
35. Rosse WF. Whatever happened to vinca-loaded platelets? *N Engl J Med* 1984; **310:** 1051–2.
36. Figueroa M, *et al.* Combination chemotherapy in refractory immune thrombocytopenic purpura. *N Engl J Med* 1993; **328:** 1226–9.
37. Strother SV, *et al.* Colchicine therapy for refractory idiopathic thrombocytopenic purpura. *Arch Intern Med* 1984; **144:** 2198–2200.
38. Jim RTS. Therapeutic use of colchicine in thrombocytopenia. *Hawaii Med J* 1986; **45:** 221–6.
39. Baker RI, Manoharan A. Colchicine therapy for idiopathic thrombocytopenic purpura—an inexpensive alternative. *Aust N Z J Med* 1989; **19:** 412–13.
40. Shen ZX, *et al.* Thrombocytopoietic effect of heparin given in chronic immune thrombocytopenic purpura. *Lancet* 1995; **346:** 220–1.
41. Cohen HA, *et al.* Treatment of chronic idiopathic thrombocytopenic purpura with ascorbate. *Clin Pediatr (Phila)* 1993: **32:** 300–2.
42. Schick BP. Hope for treatment of thrombocytopenia. *N Engl J Med* 1994; **331:** 875–6.

Infections

Although long-term corticosteroid therapy has an adverse effect on the body's response to infection (see Effects on Immune Response, under Adverse Effects, p.1012), the judicious use of corticosteroids, usually on a short-term basis, and in conjunction with appropriate chemotherapeutic agents, may have a beneficial effect on the symptoms of selected acute infections, and may on occasions be life-saving. Guidelines have been published concerning a number of infections and whether corticosteroids should be employed or not.[1]

For further comment on the use of corticosteroids in ocular herpes infections, infectious mononucleosis, leishmaniasis, leprosy, meningitis, *Pneumocystis carinii* pneumonia in AIDS patients, septic shock, and tuberculosis, see under the relevant headings in this section.

1. McGowan JE, *et al.* Report by the Working Group on Steroid Use, Antimicrobial Agents Committee, Infectious Diseases Society of America: Guidelines for the use of systemic glucocorticoids in the management of selected infections. *J Infect Dis* 1992; **165:** 1–13.

Infectious mononucleosis

In a short discussion on the use of corticosteroids in infectious mononucleosis (glandular fever) it was considered that although all cases would respond promptly to therapy, only patients with an unduly prolonged infection and those with an exceptionally severe sore throat that interferes with either respiratory function or eating should be treated with a corticosteroid.[1] Most experts would use corticosteroids in patients with severe thrombocytopenia, haemolytic anaemia, encephalitis, pericarditis, or myocarditis associated with infection by the Epstein-Barr virus. Doses of prednisone may be 80 mg initially decreasing gradually, and withdrawn after 14 days. Prednisone is very safe in infectious mononucleosis but the theoretical risk of impairing immunity is a concern as there might be an increased risk of Epstein-Barr virus-related tumours in later life.[1] Others have also expressed a relatively negative view of the value of corticosteroids.[2]

For a general discussion of infectious mononucleosis and its treatment, see Epstein-Barr Virus Infections, p.597.

1. Sheagren JN. Corticosteroids for treatment of mononucleosis and aphthous stomatitis. *JAMA* 1986; **256:** 1051.
2. McGowan JE, *et al.* Report by the Working Group on Steroid Use, Antimicrobial Agents Committee, Infectious Diseases Society of America: Guidelines for the use of systemic glucocorticoids in the management of selected infections. *J Infect Dis* 1992; **165:** 1–13.

Inflammatory bowel disease

For a discussion of the treatment of inflammatory bowel disease, including the role of corticosteroids, see p.1171. Together with aminosalicylates, the corticosteroids form the mainstay of treatment for active ulcerative colitis and Crohn's disease. In moderate to severe acute disease systemic corticosteroids are indicated for initial management, either orally or in the most severe cases intravenously. Doses are high initially and are gradually reduced as symptoms resolve. Poorly absorbed or rapidly metabolised corticosteroids such as beclomethasone, budesonide, fluticasone, or tixocortol are under investigation in the hope of producing local improvement without systemic effects. In patients with disease confined to the distal colon or rectum, local topical therapy with suppositories or enemas of corticosteroids or of mesalazine may be more appropriate.

Interstitial lung disease

The interstitial lung diseases represent a heterogeneous group of inflammatory disorders which have in common thickening of the interstitial walls between alveoli. In some cases, particularly in the early stages, this is due to accumulation of inflammatory cells in the interstitium, and control of inflammation can reverse the changes; however, when fibrotic changes to the alveolar walls take place these are usually irreversible. The causes of interstitial lung disease are numerous and include pneumoconioses due to inhalation of inorganic dusts (as in asbestosis and silicosis); extrinsic allergic alveolitis due to inhalation of, usually, organic antigens (as in farmers' lung, bird fanciers' lung, and many similar occupational disorders); cryptogenic fibrosing alveolitis (idiopathic pulmonary fibrosis); adverse effects of drugs such as bleomycin; sarcoidosis; lung disease associated with collagen vascular disorders such as rheumatoid arthritis and systemic lupus erythematosus, or with the vasculitides; histiocytic syndromes; and pulmonary eosinophilic syndromes.

The symptoms of interstitial lung diseases are usually insidious and non-specific, and may include dyspnoea of varying severity, usually first noticed on exertion, cough, and fatigue; fine crackling sounds (rales) on breathing and finger clubbing occur in some forms. If disease progresses respiratory failure becomes more severe, and eventually may prove fatal.

Where a causative agent can be identified, initial treatment is to prevent exposure but where inflammation persists, or where the causation is uncertain, corticosteroids are the mainstay of treatment (despite a lack of controlled trials for efficacy),[1-3] in an attempt to control inflammation and preserve as much normal tissue as possible. The management of cryptogenic fibrosing alveolitis is discussed in a little more detail below.

Cryptogenic fibrosing alveolitis (idiopathic pulmonary fibrosis). Cryptogenic fibrosing alveolitis is a form of interstitial lung disease of uncertain origin, associated with alveolitis and thickening of the interstitial walls by oedema, cellular exudate, and fibrosis. The clinical course is variable but the mean survival is only 3 to 5 years.[2,4,5]

Initial therapy is usually with prednisolone or prednisone by mouth, in a fairly high dose such as 1 mg per kg body-weight, or 60 mg, daily for 1 to 2 months, subsequently tapered cautiously to a maintenance dose of 0.25 mg per kg, or 10 to 15 mg, daily. About 10 to 20% of patients show some improvement with oral corticosteroids, particularly those with early disease and hence less extensive fibrosis. However, in patients with few or stable symptoms physicians may prefer to withhold treatment until symptoms become severe.[3,5] Stabilisation of disease or decrease in rate of functional decline is considered a favourable response. Corticosteroid therapy is usually continued lifelong; attempts at withdrawal should be gradual and cautious and if clinical deterioration ensues aggressive therapy with corticosteroids and cytotoxic immunosuppressants should be reinstituted immediately.[4] Azathioprine or cyclophosphamide may be useful in permitting a reduction or substitution of corticosteroid dosage. Combined therapy with either drug plus corticosteroids has been shown to improve survival compared with corticosteroids alone.[6] Cyclosporin has been tried in a few patients, with some evidence of benefit.[6] Because of a proposed role for glutathione deficiency in the inflammatory process of cryptogenic fibrosing alveolitis aerosol inhalation of glutathione has been tried in a few patients with beneficial biochemical results, although no clinical effects were reported.[7] There is also some evidence that colchicine may be as effective as corticosteroids in the management of these patients,[8] although controlled trials are needed to confirm the benefits of treatment.

In patients in whom other options fail, lung transplantation may be considered.[6]

1. Crystal RG, *et al.* Interstitial lung diseases of unknown cause: disorders characterized by chronic inflammation of the lower respiratory tract. *N Engl J Med* 1984; **310:** 154–66 and 235–44.
2. Trembath PW. Corticosteroid therapy in respiratory disorders. *Med J Aust* 1985; **143:** 607–9.
3. Johnston IDA, *et al.* British Thoracic Society study of cryptogenic fibrosing alveolitis: current presentation and initial management. *Thorax* 1997; **52:** 38–44.
4. Panos RJ, *et al.* Clinical deterioration in patients with idiopathic pulmonary fibrosis: causes and assessment. *Am J Med* 1990; **88:** 396–404.
5. Chan-Yeung M, Müller NL. Cryptogenic fibrosing alveolitis. *Lancet* 1997; **350:** 651–6.
6. Nicod LP. Recognition and treatment of idiopathic pulmonary fibrosis. *Drugs* 1998; **55:** 555–62.
7. Borok Z, *et al.* Effect of glutathione aerosol on oxidant-antoxidant imbalance in idiopathic pulmonary fibrosis. *Lancet* 1991; **338:** 215–16.
8. Douglas WW, *et al.* Colchicine versus prednisolone as treatment of usual interstitial pneumonia. *Mayo Clin Proc* 1997; **72:** 201–9.

Juvenile osteopetrosis

Osteopetrosis is a rare set of heterogeneous disorders characterised by an increase in bone density, generally due to a failure of the osteoclasts to resorb mineralised bone. In the severe forms there is reduction in the bone marrow space, leading to anaemia, hepatosplenomegaly, and nerve compression which may produce blindness and deafness; early death often results.

Bone marrow transplantation may be curative if a suitable donor can be found.[1] Corticosteroids are used palliatively. Benefit has been reported in 3 of 4 children treated with prednisone 1 mg per kg body-weight daily by mouth, together with phosphate supplements and a low-calcium diet.[2] Some patients have also benefited from the use of high-dose calcitriol, again with a low-calcium diet.[3]

Another study, in 14 patients, found that treatment with interferon gamma-1b, at a dose of 1.5 µg per kg body-weight three times weekly in those under 10 kg, or 50 µg per m^2 body-surface area three times weekly in heavier patients, increased bone resorption.[4] In 11 who received this treatment for 18 months there was stabilisation or improvement in clinical condition and a reduction in the frequency of serious infection.

1. Gerritsen EJ, *et al.* Bone marrow transplantation for autosomal recessive osteopetrosis: a report from the Working Party on Inborn Errors of the European Bone Marrow Transplantation Group. *J Pediatr* 1994; **125:** 896–902.
2. Dorantes LM, *et al.* Juvenile osteopetrosis: effects on blood and bone of prednisone and a low calcium, high phosphate diet. *Arch Dis Child* 1986; **61:** 666–70.
3. Key LL, Ries WL. Osteopetrosis: the pharmaco-physiologic basis of therapy. *Clin Orthop* 1993; **294:** 85–9.
4. Key LL, *et al.* Long-term treatment of osteopetrosis with recombinant human interferon gamma. *N Engl J Med* 1995; **332:** 1594–9.

Leishmaniasis

Corticosteroids may be required to control severe inflammation in patients with mucocutaneous leishmaniasis (p.575), although pentavalent antimony is the drug used for initial treatment.

Leprosy

Type I lepra (reversal) reactions in patients with leprosy (p.128) frequently respond to high-dose corticosteroids started immediately (for example 40 to 60 mg of prednisolone daily) and given for several days.[1] Doses may be reduced over several weeks or months. Corticosteroids may also be used for type II reactions.

Corticosteroid treatment of nerve function impairment should be started within 6 months of onset, as the earlier that treatment is started, the more likely it is that function will be restored. A standardised regimen employing a usual adult dose of 40 mg daily of prednisolone for 4 weeks, tapered over the following 12 weeks, has been successfully employed in the field management of acute nerve function impairment,[2] as has a regimen employing 30 mg of prednisone for 2 weeks tapered down with a minimum duration of 10 weeks.[3]

1. WHO. WHO expert committee on leprosy. *WHO Tech Rep Ser 874* 1998.
2. Croft RP, *et al.* Field treatment of acute nerve function impairment in leprosy using a standardized corticosteroid regimen—first year's experience with 100 patients. *Lepr Rev* 1997; **68:** 316–25.
3. Bernink EHM, Voskens JEJ. Study on the detection of leprosy reactions and the effect of prednisone on various nerves, Indonesia. *Lepr Rev* 1997; **68:** 225–32.

Lichen

Lichen planus (p.1075) is generally controlled with corticosteroids applied topically, or occasionally, injected intralesionally; systemic corticosteroids are very occasionally used for severe erosive lichen planus.[1,2] However, some consider a short course of prednisolone given by mouth in a moderately high dose (prednisolone 30 mg daily for 10 days) to be effective and safe in mild or moderately severe lichen planus.[3]

The use of topically applied corticosteroids in the treatment of lichen sclerosus (a degenerative disease of upper dermal connective tissue, particularly around the genitals) has been discussed.[4-6] It is considered that relief from vulvar pruritus is obtained in most cases with a potent corticosteroid preparation in conjunction with an antiseptic, but there is disagreement over the optimal frequency of application, some advocating once daily application[5] and others preferring three times daily.[4,6]

1. Anonymous. Treatment of oral lichen planus. *Lancet* 1990; **336:** 913–14.
2. Edwards L. Vulvar lichen planus. *Arch Dermatol* 1989; **125:** 1677–80.
3. Kellett JK, Ead RD. Treatment of lichen planus with a short course of oral prednisolone. *Br J Dermatol* 1990; **123:** 550–1.
4. Shrank AB. *Br Med J* 1990; **301:** 228.
5. Neill S. Treatment for lichen sclerosus. *Br Med J* 1990; **301:** 555.
6. Shrank AB. Treatment for lichen sclerosus. *Br Med J* 1990; **301:** 555–6.

Liver disorders

Corticosteroids are considered to be useful in chronic active hepatitis (p.1019). There is some disagreement over the benefit from corticosteroid therapy in alcoholic liver disease with hepatic encephalopathy,[1-6] and they do not appear to be of benefit in acute liver failure.[7] Corticosteroid therapy may however be of benefit in sclerosing cholangitis.[8]

For the view that corticosteroids should not be used in the management of primary biliary cirrhosis as they may exacerbate bone disease, see p.497.

1. Black M, Tavill AS. Corticosteroids in severe alcoholic hepatitis. *Ann Intern Med* 1989; **110:** 677–80.
2. Imperiale TF, McCullough AJ. Do corticosteroids reduce mortality from alcoholic hepatitis? A meta-analysis of the randomized trials. *Ann Intern Med* 1990; **113:** 299–307.
3. Thomson AD, *et al.* Alcoholic liver disease. *Gut* 1991; (suppl): S97–103.
4. Ramond M-J, *et al.* A randomized trial of prednisolone in patients with severe alcoholic hepatitis. *N Engl J Med* 1992; **326:** 507–12.
5. Wrona SA, Tankanow RM. Corticosteroids in the management of alcoholic hepatitis. *Am J Hosp Pharm* 1994; **51:** 347–53.
6. Christensen E, Gluud C. Glucocorticoids are ineffective in alcoholic hepatitis: a meta-analysis adjusting for confounding variables. *Gut* 1995; **37:** 113–18.
7. Caraceni P, Van Thiel DH. Acute liver failure. *Lancet* 1995; **345:** 163–9.
8. Lindor KD, *et al.* Advances in primary sclerosing cholangitis. *Am J Med* 1990; **89:** 73–80.

Male infertility

Immunosuppressive treatment with corticosteroids is given for male infertility due to low-grade autoimmune orchitis.[1] Examples of regimens after which pregnancy has been successfully achieved in female partners include oral methylprednisolone 96 mg daily for 7 days beginning on day 21 of the partner's menstrual cycle[2] and oral prednisolone 20 mg twice daily on days 1 to 10 of the partner's menstrual cycle plus 5 mg on days 11 and 12.[3] However, there is a lack of evidence from substantial controlled trials of benefit from corticosteroid therapy in men with autoimmune causes of infertility.

For a discussion of male and female infertility and its management, see Infertility, p.1239.

1. Haidl G, Schill W-B. Guidelines for drug treatment of male infertility. *Drugs* 1991; **41:** 60–8.
2. Shulman JF, Shulman S. Methylprednisolone treatment of immunologic infertility in the male. *Fertil Steril* 1982; **38:** 591–9.
3. Hendry WF, *et al.* Comparison of prednisolone and placebo in subfertile men with antibodies to spermatozoa. *Lancet* 1990; **335:** 85–8.

Malignant neoplasms

Corticosteroids are extensively prescribed in malignant disease for the relief of pain, nerve compression, or raised intracranial pressure; to alleviate dyspnoea, effusion, or hypercalcaemia; to counteract adverse effects of other therapies such as antineoplastic-induced nausea and vomiting or radiation-induced inflammation; and in the management of anorexia and to improve mood and sense of well-being.[1] In addition they may form part of multidrug anticancer regimens such as MOPP (see p.481) which play an important role in the management of malignant neoplasms. For discussion of the management of individual malignancies, including numerous mentions of the role of corticosteroids, see under Choice of Antineoplastic, p.476.

1. Twycross R. The risks and benefits of corticosteroids in advanced cancer. *Drug Safety* 1994; **11:** 163–78.

Meningitis

Corticosteroids may be given as adjuncts to antibacterial therapy in bacterial meningitis (p.130), in the hope of moderating any neurological sequelae; there is some evidence that dexamethasone, especially if given early, may reduce the risk of deafness in children with Haemophilus meningitis, although evidence of benefit in pneumococcal and meningococcal meningitis is scanty.

Mouth ulceration

Local treatment of mouth ulcers (p.1172) often involves a topical corticosteroid, the treatment being most effective if given early, before the ulcer develops fully. Systemic corticosteroids have occasionally been given where there is severe underlying disease.

Multiple sclerosis

Corticosteroids are often employed in the management of multiple sclerosis. Oral corticosteroids such as prednisolone or prednisone have been widely used to hasten recovery from acute exacerbations, but there is a trend towards the use of high-dose intravenous methylprednisolone. There are indications that high-dosage oral methylprednisolone or intravenous dexamethasone may also be effective.[1,6,7] Some[1,4] recommend the use of high-dose intravenous methylprednisolone followed by a tapering course of oral prednisone. There have been promising signs that corticosteroids given to patients with acute optic neuritis might reduce the rate of development of multiple sclerosis,[5] but a recent study using methylprednisolone in patients with chronic progressive disease found that initial improvement was not sustained.[3] For a discussion of the management of multiple sclerosis, including the role of corticosteroids, see p.620.

1. van Oosten BW, *et al.* Multiple sclerosis therapy: a practical guide. *Drugs* 1995; **49:** 200–12.
3. Cazzato G, *et al.* Double-blind, placebo-controlled, randomized, crossover trial of high-dose methylprednisolone in patients with chronic progressive form of multiple sclerosis. *Eur Neurol* 1995; **35:** 193–8.
5. Beck RW, *et al.* The effect of corticosteroids for acute optic neuritis on the subsequent development of multiple sclerosis. *N Engl J Med* 1993; **329:** 1764–9.
4. Weinstock-Guttman B, Cohen JA. Newer versus older treatments for relapsing-remitting multiple sclerosis. *Drug Safety* 1996; **14:** 121–30.
6. Barnes D, *et al.* Randomised trial of oral and intravenous methylprednisolone in acute relapses of multiple sclerosis. *Lancet* 1997; **349:** 902–6.
7. Sellebjerg F, *et al.* Double-blind, randomized, placebo-controlled study of oral, high-dose methylprednisolone in attacks of MS. *Neurology* 1998; **51:** 529–34.

Muscular dystrophies

Muscular dystrophies are a range of inherited myopathies in which there is progressive degeneration of muscle fibres and associated muscle weakness. They may be classified according to the mode of inheritance. The most common type is the fatal recessive X-linked **Duchenne muscular dystrophy** (DMD) in which there is a deficiency in the structural muscle protein dystrophin. There is no effective therapy that affects the ultimate outcome of the various muscular dystrophies. Management is mainly through the use of physiotherapy, supports, and surgery. Drug treatment has been tried for symptomatic management, but generally the number of patients studied has been small. However, prednisone given in doses of up to 2 mg per kg bodyweight daily has been effective in increasing muscle strength in children and slowing the progression of Duchenne muscular dystrophy;[1-5] improvement does not appear to be sustained to the same degree with alternate day therapy.[4] It has been suggested that the failure of azathioprine to produce any beneficial effect when used alone or added to prednisone treatment might indicate that prednisone's effectiveness is not due to immunosuppression.[5] There have also been reports of benefit in small numbers of patients given cyclosporin; evidence to support the use of most other drugs is either conflicting or unconvincing. The possible use of gene therapy is being studied.

1. DeSilva S, *et al.* Prednisone treatment in Duchenne muscular dystrophy: long-term benefit. *Arch Neurol* 1987; **44:** 818–22.
2. Mendell JR, *et al.* Randomized double-blind six-month trial of prednisone in Duchenne's muscular dystrophy. *N Engl J Med* 1989; **320:** 1592–7.
3. Griggs RC, *et al.* Prednisone in Duchenne dystrophy: a randomized, controlled trial defining the time course and dose response. *Arch Neurol* 1991; **48:** 383–8.
4. Fenichel GM, *et al.* A comparison of daily and alternate-day prednisone therapy in the treatment of Duchenne muscular dystrophy. *Arch Neurol* 1991; **48:** 575–9.
5. Griggs RC, *et al.* Duchenne dystrophy: randomized, controlled trial of prednisone (18 months) and azathioprine (12 months). *Neurology* 1993; **43:** 520–7.

Myasthenia gravis

Corticosteroids are the main immunosuppressants used in the management of myasthenia gravis (p.1388), and are used in patients who are seriously ill prior to thymectomy or insufficiently improved after thymectomy, as well as in those who are unsuitable for surgical treatment.

Nasal polyps

Nasal polyps are outgrowths of the nasal mucosa, typically pale, smooth, translucent, and round or pear-shaped.[1,2] They are often associated with a history of rhinitis (p.400) or asthma (p.745); patients typically present with obstruction, loss of smell, and often rhinorrhoea and postnasal drip.

Corticosteroids are extremely effective in reducing polyp size, either by intranasal or systemic administration. In the former case beginning with betamethasone sodium phosphate nasal drops, and subsequently maintaining the reduction with an intranasal spray such as beclomethasone, budesonide, or fluticasone, has been suggested.[1] Alternatively prednisone, prednisolone, or dexamethasone can be given by mouth: suggested regimens have included prednisone 60 mg daily, tapered over 10 or 14 days and followed by intranasal corticosteroids,[2] or dexamethasone 12, 8, and 4 mg daily, each for 3 days.[1] Surgery may be necessary where there is marked obstruction, and most patients require it at some point,[1] although polyps usually recur. Pre-operative administration of systemic corticosteroids may help reduce recurrence.[2]

1. Lund VJ. Diagnosis and treatment of nasal polyps. *Br Med J* 1995; **311:** 1411–14.
2. Slavin RG. Nasal polyps and sinusitis. *JAMA* 1997; **278:** 1849–54.

Nausea and vomiting

Corticosteroids, usually in the form of dexamethasone, play an important adjuvant role in combination antiemetic regimens (see p.1172) used to combat the effects of moderately to severely emetogenic cancer chemotherapy: they have been shown to enhance the effects of both metoclopramide- and ondansetron-based regimens. Dexamethasone is probably the most effective single agent available against delayed emesis at present.

Neonatal intraventricular haemorrhage

For the suggestion that antenatal corticosteroids may reduce the incidence of intraventricular haemorrhage in neonates, see p.709.

Neonatal respiratory distress syndrome

Neonatal respiratory distress syndrome is a condition of increasing respiratory distress occurring at, or shortly after, birth and marked by cyanosis, tachypnoea, expiratory grunting and sternal retraction. Symptoms increase in severity with progressive collapse of the lung (atelectasis), leakage of plasma into alveolar spaces, and the formation of hyaline membranes, until death occurs or slow recovery takes place from about the 2nd to 4th day. The syndrome affects primarily premature infants and its incidence increases with the degree of prematurity; severe problems are most likely in those delivered before 30 weeks' gestation. Symptoms are thought to be at least partly due to inadequate amounts of surfactant in the premature lung resulting in high internal surface tension and increased risk of alveolar collapse, but in very immature infants other factors, possibly including impaired sodium and fluid absorption from the lung, may play a role.[1]

Treatment. The optimum treatment is prevention, and UK guidelines[2] recommend the administration of betamethasone or dexamethasone twice daily by intramuscular injection for 2 days to women in whom delivery before 32 weeks of gestation is likely. Results are best if treatment is given more than 24 hours but less than 7 days before delivery. Similar recommendations apply elsewhere. In the USA, for example, antenatal corticosteroid treatment is recommended for women between 24 and 34 weeks of pregnancy who show signs of premature delivery.[3] An overview of studies of antenatal corticosteroid therapy suggests that it may reduce the risk of respiratory distress syndrome by about 50% overall;[4] the risk of death, and of periventricular haemorrhage and necrotising enterocolitis is also reduced. Delaying delivery with beta$_2$ agonists may be considered to increase the time available for management with antenatal corticosteroids.[2] Reported benefit from adding protirelin to antenatal corticosteroids has not been borne out by 2 large multicentre studies.[5-7] The earlier of these studies actually found neonatal outcome and maternal morbidity to be worse in those who also received protirelin,[5,6] but this conclusion has been questioned.[8,9]

In infants born with the syndrome rapid supportive care is required, which may include correction of metabolic acidosis, circulatory support, oxygen supplementation, and assisted ventilation, although there is a lack of consensus about the most appropriate method for these.[2] It has been suggested that ventilation using a helium-oxygen mixture gives better results than a nitrogen-oxygen mix.[10] Another alternative may be the use of partial liquid ventilation with the fluorocarbon compound perflubron.[11] Studies with nitric oxide indicate that it might be useful as a pulmonary vasodilator in infants with the respiratory distress syndrome.[12-14] The majority of infants survive the acute episode with careful management, although complications of ventilation may subsequently develop, including bronchopulmonary dysplasia (see p.1018), retinopathy of prematurity (p.1370), and cerebral palsy.

Since deficiency of surfactant is considered to play an important role in the neonatal respiratory distress syndrome, the use of surfactant replacement therapy has been intensively investigated, and is now accepted as reducing the risk of death from the disease and the development of pneumothorax and other lung complications.[2,15,16] Both natural and synthetic surfactants have been used: although both are effective there is some evidence that results are better with the preparations of natural origin.[17,18] Natural surfactants of differing origins may also vary in their properties: poractant,[19] or a surfactant of calf-lung origin,[20] have both been reported to give better responses than beractant. Surfactant is given by endotracheal tube directly into the infant lung,[21] although other means of administration, such as nebulisers, are reportedly under investigation.[22] Usual doses have varied from 50 to 200 mg per kg body-weight[21] repeated up to four times, but the optimum has yet to be determined. One large study found that a dose of 100 mg per kg, repeated twice, was as effective as 200 mg per kg followed by up to four further doses of 100 mg per kg.[23] Another found that 3 doses, given at 12-hour intervals with the first dose shortly after birth were more effective than the first dose alone in improving physiological findings and mortality rates in low birth-weight infants.[24]

There has been debate as to whether 'prophylactic' early therapy, given immediately after birth to all infants deemed at risk of the syndrome, or delayed therapy given 2 or more hours after birth to infants who have developed symptoms, is the more appropriate,[2,25] but in the light of the large OSIRIS study,[26] and a later systematic review of other studies,[27] both of which found in favour of early intervention, treatment should be started as soon as possible after birth for maximum benefit.

1. Barker PM, *et al.* Decreased sodium ion absorption across nasal epithelium of very premature infants with respiratory distress syndrome. *J Pediatr* 1997; **130:** 373–7.
2. Report of a Joint Working Group of the British Association of Perinatal Medicine and the Research Unit of the Royal College of Physicians. Development of audit measures and guidelines for good practice in the management of neonatal respiratory distress syndrome. *Arch Dis Child* 1992; **67:** 1221–7.
3. NIH Consensus Development Panel on the Effect of Corticosteroids for Fetal Maturation on Perinatal Outcomes. Effect of corticosteroids for fetal maturation on perinatal outcomes. *JAMA* 1995; **273:** 413–18.
4. Crowley PA. Antenatal corticosteroid therapy: a meta-analysis of the randomized trials, 1972 to 1994. *Am J Obstet Gynecol* 1995; **173:** 322–35.
5. ACTOBAT Study Group. Australian collaborative trial of antenatal thyrotropin-releasing hormone (ACTOBAT) for prevention of neonatal respiratory disease. *Lancet* 1995; **345:** 877–82.
6. Crowther CA, *et al.* Australian Collaborative Trial of antenatal thyrotropin-releasing hormone: adverse effects at 12-month follow-up. *Pediatrics* 1997; **99:** 311–17.
7. Ballard RA, *et al.* Antenatal thyrotropin-releasing hormone to prevent lung disease in preterm infants. *N Engl J Med* 1998; **338:** 493–8.
8. Moya FR, Maturana A. Thyrotropin-releasing hormone for prevention of neonatal respiration disease. *Lancet* 1995; **345:** 1572–3.
9. McCormick MC. The credibility of the ACTOBAT follow-up study. *Pediatrics* 1997; **99:** 476–8.
10. Elleau C, *et al.* Helium-oxygen mixture in respiratory distress syndrome: a double-blind study. *J Pediatr* 1993; **122:** 132–6.
11. Leach CL, *et al.* Partial liquid ventilation with perflubron in premature infants with severe respiratory distress syndrome. *N Engl J Med* 1996; **335:** 761–7.
12. Peliowski A, *et al.* Inhaled nitric oxide for premature infants after prolonged rupture of the membranes. *J Pediatr* 1995; **126:** 450–3.
13. The Neonatal Inhaled Nitric Oxide Study Group. Inhaled nitric oxide in full-term and nearly full-term infants with hypoxic respiratory failure. *N Engl J Med* 1997; **336:** 597–604. Correction. *ibid.;* **337:** 434.
14. Skimming JW, *et al.* Nitric oxide inhalation in infants with respiratory distress syndrome. *J Pediatr* 1997; **130:** 225–30.
15. Schwartz RM, *et al.* Effect of surfactant on morbidity, mortality, and resource use in newborn infants weighing 500 to 1500 g. *N Engl J Med* 1994; **330:** 1476–80.
16. Walti H, Monset-Couchard M. A risk-benefit assessment of natural and synthetic exogenous surfactants in the management of neonatal respiratory distress syndrome. *Drug Safety* 1998; **18:** 321–37.
17. Halliday HL. Natural vs synthetic surfactants in neonatal respiratory distress syndrome. *Drugs* 1996; **51:** 226–37.
18. Hudak ML, *et al.* A multicenter randomized, masked comparison trial of natural versus synthetic surfactant for the treatment of respiratory distress syndrome. *J Pediatr* 1996; **128:** 396–406.
19. Speer CP, *et al.* Randomised clinical trial of two treatment regimens of natural surfactant preparations in neonatal respiratory distress syndrome. *Arch Dis Child* 1995; **72:** F8–F13.
20. Bloom BT, *et al.* Randomized double-blind multicenter trial of Survanta (SURV) and Infasurf (IS). *Pediatr Res* 1994; **35:** 326.
21. Jobe AH. Pulmonary surfactant therapy. *N Engl J Med* 1993; **328:** 861–8.
22. Anonymous. Surfactant for babies. *Lancet* 1992; **340:** 1387.
23. Halliday HL, *et al.* Multicentre randomised trial comparing high and low dose surfactant regimens for the treatment of respiratory distress syndrome (the Curosurf 4 trial). *Arch Dis Child* 1993; **69:** 276–80.
24. Corbet A, *et al.* Double-blind, randomized trial of one versus three prophylactic doses of synthetic surfactant in 826 neonates weighing 700 to 1100 grams: effects on mortality rate. *J Pediatr* 1995; **126:** 969–78.
25. Dunn MS. Surfactant replacement therapy: prophylaxis or treatment? *Pediatrics* 1993; **92:** 148–50.
26. The OSIRIS Collaborative Group (Open Study of Infants at high risk of or with Respiratory Insufficiency—the role of surfactant). Early versus delayed neonatal administration of a synthetic surfactant—the judgement of OSIRIS. *Lancet* 1992; **340:** 1363–9.
27. Morley CJ. Systematic review of prophylactic vs rescue surfactant. *Arch Dis Child* 1997; **77:** F70–4.

Optic neuropathies

Improvement in vision was reported in patients with auto-immune optic neuropathy following 5 to 7 days' treatment with high doses of intravenous methylprednisolone (1 to 2 g daily) or oral prednisolone (80 to 400 mg daily).[1] In some patients, recurrent visual loss required repeated high-dose intravenous methylprednisolone, an increase in oral prednisolone dosage, or additional immunosuppressants, but in many patients visual benefits were maintained even when treatment was withdrawn. Visual recovery has also been reported in patients with optic neuritis of unknown aetiology receiving intravenous methylprednisolone 250 or 500 mg every 6 hours for 3 to 7 days.[2] One study has found oral prednisone alone (1 mg per kg body-weight daily for 14 days) to be ineffective whereas intravenous methylprednisolone (1 g daily for 3 days) followed by oral prednisone (1 mg per kg daily for 11 days) was beneficial in the treatment of acute optic neuritis.[3]

1. Kupersmith MJ, *et al.* Autoimmune optic neuropathy: evaluation and treatment. *J Neurol Neurosurg Psychiatry* 1988; **51:** 1381–6.
2. Spoor TC, Rockwell DL. Treatment of optic neuritis with intravenous megadose corticosteroids: a consecutive series. *Ophthalmology* 1988; **95:** 131–4.
3. Beck RW, *et al.* A randomized, controlled trial of corticosteroids in the treatment of acute optic neuritis. *N Engl J Med* 1992; **326:** 581–8.

Organ and tissue transplantation

For a discussion of organ and tissue transplantation, including the role of corticosteroids, see under Choice of Immunosuppressant, p.498.

Osteoarthritis

In contrast to rheumatoid arthritis, systemic corticosteroids are not considered to have a place in the management of osteoarthritis; intra-articular or peri-articular injection, although controversial, may be of some help in patients with localised inflammation. Such injections should be given only infrequently. For mention of the use of corticosteroids in osteoarthritis, see p.2.

Pain

Corticosteroids have produced improvement, often substantial, in neurogenic pain, including pain due to nerve damage and sympathetically maintained pain, and are widely used in conditions such as chronic low back pain and cancer pain. Dexamethasone, methylprednisolone, and prednisolone have been used for pain management, sometimes in the form of long-acting depot injections administered locally. The exact mechanism of action of corticosteroids in analgesia is not clear but may involve relief of pressure on nervous tissue by reduction of inflammation and oedema.

For discussions of pain and its management, see p.4.

Pancreatitis

Corticosteroids are generally contra-indicated for pancreatitis (p.1613), but a response has been reported in 2 patients with acute episodes of pancreatitis caused by sarcoidosis.[1]

For a discussion of the management of sarcoidosis, see below.

1. McCormick PA, *et al.* Pancreatitis in sarcoidosis. *Br Med J* 1985; **290:** 1472–3.

Pemphigus and pemphigoid

Systemic corticosteroids are the mainstay of management of pemphigus and pemphigoid (see p.1075). Initially high doses are used to control blistering and doses up to 400 mg of prednisolone daily have been suggested, although most dermatologists attempt to keep the dose below 120 mg daily. Adjuvant therapy with an immunosuppressant such as azathioprine, cyclophosphamide, or gold may be used.[1] Maintenance treatment must be individualised to every patient but in general the dose of prednisolone should be reduced by 50% every 2 to 3 weeks. When the daily dose has been lowered to 80 mg daily it is desirable to convert gradually to alternate-day therapy. During this period topical therapy with potent corticosteroids is useful and is also a valuable first-line treatment for early relapses. A combined corticosteroid-antibiotic preparation also reduces the chance of infection. Therapy for mucous membranes is also based on the use of corticosteroids, applied topically, sucked as lozenges, or possibly inhaled. High dose oral prednisolone and oral cyclophosphamide have also been found effective in relieving inflammation in patients with ocular cicatricial pemphigoid, although they may not completely prevent cicatrisation.[2]

With the aim of reducing adverse effects, corticosteroids have been administered in lower initial doses by mouth (prednisolone 45 to 60 mg daily)[3] or by intravenous pulse therapy (dexamethasone 136 mg given over 1 to 2 hours daily for 3 days, repeated at least monthly, with intravenous cyclophosphamide 500 mg infused on day 1);[4] pemphigus responded to both of these regimens.

Bullous pemphigoid has responded to high potency corticosteroids applied topically.[5]

1. Carson PJ, *et al.* Influence of treatment on the clinical course of pemphigus vulgaris. *J Am Acad Dermatol* 1996; **34:** 645–52.
2. Elder MJ, *et al.* Role of cyclophosphamide and high dose steroid in ocular cicatricial pemphigoid. *Br J Ophthalmol* 1995; **79:** 264–6.
3. Ratnam KV, *et al.* Pemphigus therapy with oral prednisolone regimens. *Int J Dermatol* 1990; **29:** 363–7.
4. Kaur S, Kanwar AJ. Dexamethasone–cyclophosphamide pulse therapy in pemphigus. *Int J Dermatol* 1990; **29:** 371–4.
5. Westerhof W. Treatment of bullous pemphigoid with topical clobetasol propionate. *J Am Acad Dermatol* 1989; **20:** 458–61.

Pneumocystis carinii pneumonia

The management of *Pneumocystis carinii* pneumonia (PCP; p.370) is primarily with either co-trimoxazole or pentamidine. In patients with moderate or severe attacks, adjuvant therapy with high-dose oral or intravenous corticosteroids reduces both the risk of respiratory failure and the risk of death.[1]

1. Miller RF, *et al.* Pneumocystis carinii infection: current treatment and prevention. *J Antimicrob Chemother* 1996; **37** (suppl B): 33–53.

Polyarteritis nodosa and microscopic polyangiitis

Polyarteritis nodosa is considered the prototype of systemic necrotising vasculitis. It may occur at any age but is more common in white patients and in men. It is characterised by inflammation throughout the arterial wall with fibrinoid necrosis of the arterial media, particularly in medium-sized vessels, partial occlusion of the vessel due to proliferation of the intima (possibly leading to thrombosis and infarction), fibrosis, and the formation of aneurysms. Microscopic polyangiitis, in which small vessels are primarily involved, with frequent renal and pulmonary involvement, has been seen as part of the spectrum of polyarteritis nodosa but is now considered an entity in its own right, although patients may have features of both. Antineutrophil cytoplasmic antibodies (ANCA) are common in patients with microscopic polyangiitis but not in classic polyarteritis nodosa.

Symptoms vary depending on the vessels affected but most patients have fever, weight loss, myalgia, and arthralgia. Gastro-intestinal involvement may be marked by mouth ulceration, diarrhoea, visceral pain, haemorrhage, or sometimes infarction of the bowel, while involvement of liver can lead to hepatomegaly or hepatic necrosis and pancreatic involvement may simulate pancreatitis. Renal involvement may present as acute glomerulonephritis and renal failure or as nephrotic syndrome; like pulmonary involvement it is a feature particularly of microscopic polyarteritis, and associated with a poor prognosis. Skin lesions, peripheral neuropathies, alterations in mental function, convulsions, episcleritis or scleritis and retinal vasculitis, ischaemic heart disease, heart failure, Raynaud's phenomenon, and hypertension are among other potential symptoms. If untreated, death, usually due to renal or cardiac involvement, has been recorded in about 90% of patients within 5 years.

Classic polyarteritis nodosa may respond to treatment with a corticosteroid given alone, typically prednisone or prednisolone in a dose of 40 to 60 mg daily; however, although the benefits of adding a cytotoxic to the regimen have been queried,[1,2] a combined regimen with cyclophosphamide is often preferred.[1,3,4] In patients with microscopic polyangiitis a combined regimen is recommended. One suggested regimen is prednisone or prednisolone 1 mg per kg body-weight together with cyclophosphamide 2 mg per kg, both daily by mouth, for initial induction of remission.[5] The corticosteroid dose is gradually tapered to about 10 mg daily or less over 6 months; once disease remission is established azathioprine is substituted for cyclophosphamide. There is a trend towards the use of shorter courses of cyclophosphamide, and to the use of intravenous pulsed cyclophosphamide rather than oral administration, in an attempt to reduce adverse effects.[5] Mycophenolate mofetil has been tried in a few patients as an alternative to cyclophosphamide in combination therapy after initial induction.[6]

A monoclonal anti-CD4 antibody, campath-1H, has produced benefit in a patient with a systemic vasculitis (not identified as polyarteritis nodosa) refractory to standard therapy[7] and it may be that monoclonal antibodies will prove useful in this disease; results in microscopic polyarteritis are encouraging (see below). Polyarteritis nodosa may be associated with hepatitis B infection; the vasculitis responds in most cases to treatment with antiviral agents and plasma exchange.[3]

Campath-1H and other anti-CD4 monoclonal antibodies have been used successfully in patients with microscopic polyarteritis unresponsive to conventional treatment.[8] Another therapy that has been tried in this group and produced clinical improvement is high dose intravenous normal immunoglobulin,[5] but with ambiguous results.

Vasodilators such as calcium channel blockers, inhibitors of platelet activation, or agents that improve blood flow may be useful to improve local ischaemia.[9] Skin lesions in a patient with cutaneous polyarteritis nodosa have reportedly responded to oral oxpentifylline.[10]

1. Taylor HG, Samanta A. Treatment of vasculitis. *Br J Clin Pharmacol* 1993; **35:** 93–104.
2. Conn DL. Role of cyclophosphamide in treatment of polyarteritis nodosa? *J Rheumatol* 1991; **18:** 489–90.
3. Guillevin L, *et al.* Treatment of polyarteritis nodosa and Churg-Strauss syndrome: a meta-analysis of 3 prospective controlled trials including 182 patients over 12 years. *Ann Med Interne (Paris)* 1992; **143:** 405–16.
4. Guillevin L, *et al.* Longterm follow up after treatment of polyarteritis nodosa and Churg-Strauss angiitis with comparison of steroids, plasma exchange and cyclophosphamide to steroids and plasma exchange: a prospective randomized trial of 71 patients. *J Rheumatol* 1991; **18:** 567–74.
5. Savage COS, *et al.* Primary systemic vasculitis. *Lancet* 1997; **349:** 553–8.
6. Nowack R, *et al.* Mycophenolate mofetil for systemic vasculitis and IgA nephropathy. *Lancet* 1997; **349:** 774.
7. Mathieson PW, *et al.* Monoclonal-antibody therapy in systemic vasculitis. *N Engl J Med* 1990; **323:** 250–4.
8. Lockwood CM, *et al.* Long-term remission of intractable systemic vasculitis with monoclonal antibody therapy. *Lancet* 1993; **341:** 1620–2.
9. Conn DL. Update on systemic necrotizing vasculitis *Mayo Clin Proc* 1989; **64:** 535–43.
10. Calderón MJ, *et al.* Successful treatment of cutaneous PAN with pentoxifylline. *Br J Dermatol* 1993; **128:** 706–7.

Polychondritis

Relapsing polychondritis is a rare systemic disease which results in inflammation and destruction of cartilage in various parts of the body, most seriously in the respiratory system (e.g. nose, larynx, and trachea). Airway narrowing and obstruction due to loss of cartilaginous support results, and may be complicated by pneumonia: fatalities have resulted. Relatively high doses of corticosteroid may improve symptoms in active disease, but do not appear to retard progression. Methotrexate may be of value in reducing corticosteroid requirements.[4] Dapsone,[1] and CD4 antibodies[2,3] have also been tried.

1. Espinoza LR, *et al.* Immune complex-mediated renal involvement in relapsing polychondritis. *Am J Med* 1981; **71:** 181–3.
2. van der Lubbe PA, *et al.* Anti-CD4 monoclonal antibody for relapsing polychondritis. *Lancet* 1991; **337:** 1349.
3. Choy EHS, *et al.* Chimaeric anti-CD4 monoclonal antibody for relapsing polychondritis. *Lancet* 1991; **338:** 450.
4. Trentham DE, Le CH. Relapsing polychondritis. *Ann Intern Med* 1998; **129:** 114–22.

Polymyalgia rheumatica

Polymyalgia rheumatica is a rheumatic disorder of uncertain aetiology. It occurs mainly in persons over 50 years of age of European, especially Scandinavian, extraction and is more common in women than in men. The disease is characterised by myalgia and severe morning stiffness in the neck and shoulder girdle and in the hips and pelvic girdle, which may spread in more advanced cases to the muscles of the thighs, chest, and arms. Stiffness and pain are worse after periods of inactivity. There may be some joint involvement; other symptoms include fatigue, weight loss, and fever, and anaemia and raised erythrocyte sedimentation rate are seen. In some patients polymyalgia rheumatica is associated with giant cell arteritis (p.1021).

Treatment. Although NSAIDs may improve the symptoms of polymyalgia rheumatica they do not control the disease process, and corticosteroids are preferred;[1-7] in particular, corticosteroid therapy is essential where giant cell arteritis is present.

The usual initial dose is prednisolone or prednisone 10 to 20 mg daily by mouth, depending on the severity of symptoms; higher doses are needed where giant cell arteritis is also present, particularly if there are ophthalmic symptoms (see p.1021). After 2 to 3 months a reduction in dosage is usually possible provided symptoms are well controlled. Dosage reduction should be gradual: one suggestion is a reduction of 0.5 to 1 mg every 3 or 4 weeks if dosage levels are low (10 mg daily) or 2.5 to 5 mg weekly at higher doses (40 to 50 mg daily).[1] Most patients in large studies are taking 6 to 7.5 mg daily at one year.[3]

Maintenance therapy may need to be prolonged. Although about a third to a half of all patients may be able to have corticosteroids withdrawn within about 2 years,[5] maintenance can be required for considerably longer periods ranging from 4 to 8 years or more.[1,8] Intramuscular methylprednisolone has also been found to be effective in polymyalgia rheumatica; because the cumulative dose with prolonged therapy is lower it has been suggested that this has advantages over the use of oral corticosteroids.[9] Relapse is not uncommon and is most likely within one year of corticosteroid withdrawal.[5,6] It may be associated with arteritic symptoms,[1] but arteritic relapses are unusual in patients whose original presentation was pure polymyalgia.[5,8] Methotrexate or azathioprine may be used for their steroid-sparing effect in patients in whom withdrawal is difficult.[5,6]

1. Hart FD. Polymyalgia rheumatica: its correct diagnosis and treatment. *Drugs* 1987; **33:** 280–87.
2. Anonymous. The management of polymyalgia rheumatica and giant cell arteritis. *Drug Ther Bull* 1993; **31:** 65–8.
3. Kyle V. Polymyalgia rheumatica. *Prescribers' J* 1997; **37:** 138–44.
4. Pountain G, Hazleman B. Polymyalgia rheumatica and giant cell arteritis. *Br Med J* 1995; **310:** 1057–9.
5. Swannell AJ. Polymyalgia rheumatica and temporal arteritis: diagnosis and management. *Br Med J* 1997; **314:** 1329–32.
6. Zilko PJ. Polymyalgia rheumatica and giant cell arteritis. *Med J Aust* 1996; **165:** 438–42.
7. Salvarani C, *et al.* Polymyalgia rheumatica. *Lancet* 1997; **350:** 43–7.
8. Kyle V, Hazelman BL. Stopping steroids in polymyalgia rheumatica and giant cell arteritis. *Br Med J* 1990; **300:** 344–5.
9. Dasgupta B, *et al.* An initially double-blind controlled 96 week trial of depot methylprednisolone against oral prednisolone in the treatment of polymyalgia rheumatica. *Br J Rheumatol* 1998; **37:** 189–95.

Polymyositis and dermatomyositis

The term polymyositis has been used to describe several types of rare idiopathic inflammatory muscle disorders (myopathies).

The cardinal symptom of polymyositis is symmetrical progressive muscle weakness, usually starting in the shoulder girdle and neck, and pelvic girdle. Onset is usually gradual over a period of months, and accompanied by mild pain and tenderness, although more rapidly evolving disease with intense muscle pain is known. With progression, weakness may prevent the patient from moving their limbs, and muscle atrophy and contracture can develop. Dysphagia, pulmonary aspiration, and hypoventilation may occur, and some patients develop fibrosing alveolitis; pulmonary involvement, especially aspiration pneumonia, can be fatal. ECG abnormalities, usually asymptomatic, are common, and some patients develop Raynaud's syndrome. Primary disease may be associated with skin rashes, in which case it is known as dermatomyositis. Purplish scaly rashes on knees, elbows, and knuckles, and a characteristic purplish ('heliotrope') coloration and oedema of the eyelids may occur. A childhood form known as juvenile dermatomyositis exists, in which additional signs include vasculitis and subcutaneous calcium deposition (calcinosis cutis), and gastro-intestinal haemorrhage and perforation may occur.

Treatment. Patients with active disease require bed rest, with the head elevated in patients at risk of aspiration. Physiotherapy to maintain muscle tone and avoid the development of contractures may be required.

Initial drug therapy is based on corticosteroids.[1-4] The usual choice is oral prednisone or prednisolone 40 to 60 mg, or 1 to 2 mg per kg body-weight, daily. This usually produces improvement within one to two months. The dose may then be gradually tapered off to the minimum required for disease control; some patients with well controlled disease may be satisfactorily maintained on an alternate-day regimen. Maintenance therapy may need to be prolonged (it is considered unwise to attempt discontinuation until disease has been controlled for at least a year[1]) and a reduction in corticosteroid dosage to the minimum is therefore desirable, but too early or too rapid a reduction may lead to relapse.

Up to 25% of patients do not respond to corticosteroids, or develop unacceptable adverse effects,[1] and in these cases the second-line agents are cytotoxic immunosuppressants.[1-4] There is considerable experience with the use of methotrexate, by mouth or intravenously, usually at weekly intervals; it may be combined with corticosteroids, permitting a reduction in corticosteroid dose. Azathioprine may also be given with corticosteroids, again permitting a reduction in corticosteroid dosage, and the combination has also been shown to be superior to a corticosteroid alone for long-term maintenance (although this was only apparent after more than a year of therapy).[5]

Some authorities consider that corticosteroid therapy should be combined with a cytotoxic immunosuppressant such as azathioprine or methotrexate from the outset of treatment. There is some evidence that methotrexate may be superior to azathioprine in patients unresponsive to prednisone alone.[6]

The role of other agents is less well defined. Opinions differ as to the value of cyclophosphamide,[1-4,7] although it may have a role in disease associated with lung fibrosis,[2,3] while chlorambucil and mercaptopurine have produced benefit in individual cases but have not been formally assessed. There have been reports of cyclosporin producing a response in refractory disease.[8,9]

Normal immunoglobulin has also produced responses,[10,11] but remains an experimental therapy at present.

Cutaneous symptoms in patients with dermatomyositis do not always respond satisfactorily to corticosteroids, but hydroxychloroquine is reputed to be of benefit in patients with rash,[12] probably due to a photoprotective effect.[13] Calcinosis, which can cause considerable morbidity, is particularly difficult to treat although there is an intriguing report of almost complete clearance in a child given aluminium hydroxide.[14] Low-dose warfarin has also been proposed for calcinosis.[15]

1. Oddis CV, Medsger TA. Current management of polymyositis and dermatomyositis. *Drugs* 1989; **37:** 382–90.
2. Kaye SA, Isenberg DA. Treatment of polymyositis and dermatomyositis. *Br J Hosp Med* 1994; **52:** 463–8.
3. Plotz PH, *et al.* Myositis: immunologic contributions to understanding cause, pathogenesis, and therapy. *Ann Intern Med* 1995; **122:** 715–24.
4. Bunch TW. Polymyositis: a case history approach to the differential diagnosis and treatment. *Mayo Clin Proc* 1990; **65:** 1480–97.
5. Bunch TW. Prednisone and azathioprine for polymyositis: long-term followup. *Arthritis Rheum* 1981; **24:** 45–8.
6. Joffe MM, *et al.* Drug therapy of the idiopathic inflammatory myopathies: predictors of response to prednisone, azathioprine, and methotrexate and a comparison of their efficacy. *Am J Med* 1993; **94:** 379–87.
7. Bombardieri S, *et al.* Cyclophosphamide in severe polymyositis. *Lancet* 1989; **i:** 1138–9.
8. Heckmatt J, *et al.* Cyclosporin in juvenile dermatomyositis. *Lancet* 1989; **i:** 1063–6.
9. Lueck CJ, *et al.* Cyclosporin in the management of polymyositis and dermatomyositis. *J Neurol Neurosurg Psychiatry* 1991; **54:** 1007–8.
10. Cherin P, *et al.* Efficacy of intravenous gammaglobulin therapy in chronic refractory polymyositis and dermatomyositis: an open study with 20 adult patients. *Am J Med* 1991; **91:** 162–8.
11. Dalakas MC, *et al.* A controlled trial of high-dose intravenous immune globulin infusions as treatment for dermatomyositis. *N Engl J Med* 1993; **329:** 1993–2000.
12. Woo TY, *et al.* Cutaneous lesions of dermatomyositis are improved by hydroxychloroquine. *J Am Acad Dermatol* 1984; **10:** 592–600.
13. Cox NH. Amyopathic dermatomyositis, photosensitivity and hydroxychloroquine. *Br J Dermatol* 1995; **132:** 1016–17.
14. Wang W-J, *et al.* Calcinosis cutis in juvenile dermatomyositis: remarkable response to aluminium therapy. *Arch Dermatol* 1988; **124:** 1721–2.
15. Berger RG, Hadler NM. Treatment of calcinosis universalis secondary to dermatomyositis or scleroderma with low dose warfarin. *Arthritis Rheum* 1983; **26** (suppl): S11.

Polyneuropathies

A report of 10 patients with subacute demyelinating polyneuropathy who obtained a beneficial response to corticosteroid therapy.[1] In one patient the response was initially slight, but became dramatic when azathioprine was added. Prednisone was given in initial single daily doses of 40 to 150 mg, until definite clinical improvement was obtained, and followed by a single-dose alternate-day regimen. In reviewing different forms of polyneuropathy, including the Guillain-Barré syndrome (p.1524), and their response to corticosteroid therapy, it was concluded that subacute demyelinating neuropathy appeared to be a distinct and clinically identifiable entity in which corticosteroid therapy is indicated. High-dose intravenous methylprednisolone has proved ineffective in patients with Guillain-Barré syndrome.[2,3]

1. Oh SJ. Subacute demyelinating polyneuropathy responding to corticosteroid treatment. *Arch Neurol* 1978; **35:** 509–16.
2. Hughes RAC. Ineffectiveness of high-dose intravenous methylprednisolone in Guillain-Barré syndrome. *Lancet* 1991; **338:** 1142.
3. Guillain-Barré Syndrome Steroid Trial Group. Double-blind trial of intravenous methylprednisolone in Guillain-Barré syndrome. *Lancet* 1993; **341:** 586–90.

Postoperative ocular inflammation

Corticosteroid eye drops are used to control the inflammatory response commonly observed following cataract surgery;[1] prednisolone is usually used but dexamethasone may be necessary if the inflammation is severe.

Corticosteroids should only be used with care and for short periods for topical control of postoperative ocular inflammation, as discussed on p.66.

1. Noble BA. *Br Med J* 1986; **292:** 1578.

Pregnancy

For a review of the effects of corticosteroids during pregnancy, see under Precautions, p.1013. However, corticosteroids may appropriately be given during pregnancy to promote fetal maturation where there is a risk of premature delivery (see Neonatal Respiratory Distress Syndrome, above), and in those maternal conditions serious enough to require administration of systemic corticosteroids, the risk to both mother and offspring of discontinuing therapy is often greater than that of corticosteroid administration during pregnancy.

Primary biliary cirrhosis

For the view that corticosteroids should not be used in the management of primary biliary cirrhosis as they may exacerbate bone disease, see p.497.

Psoriasis

Reviews of psoriasis (p.1075) and its management[1-5] list topical corticosteroids as being first-line agents in the treatment of some forms of the disease. However, the adverse effects of corticosteroids, including in some cases exacerbation of psoriasis, or a rebound after treatment is stopped, mean that topical corticosteroid therapy is a problematic first-line choice for the treatment of psoriasis and most UK dermatologists now reserve it for special circumstances. In the USA it has been reported to be the most widely used treatment for psoriasis.[3]

Intralesional injection of corticosteroids has been used for small, localised, recalcitrant plaques of psoriasis but caution is required to avoid skin atrophy or depigmentation.[1] Systemic corticosteroids are not generally recommended, but have been used for short periods in extreme or rare cases; there is a risk of systemic adverse effects and of rebound psoriasis occurring on stopping therapy.[2]

1. Menter A, Barker JNWN. Psoriasis in practice. *Lancet* 1991; **338:** 231–4.
2. Williams REA, *et al.* Workshop of the Research Unit of the Royal College of Physicians of London. Guidelines for management of patients with psoriasis. *Br Med J* 1991; **303:** 829–35.
3. Greaves MW, Weinstein GD. Treatment of psoriasis. *N Engl J Med* 1995; **332:** 581–8.
4. Anonymous. The management of psoriasis. *Drug Ther Bull* 1996; **34:** 17–19.
5. Weller PA. Psoriasis. *Med J Aust* 1996; **165:** 216–21.

Pyoderma gangrenosum

A systemic corticosteroid is one of the treatments that has been tried in pyoderma gangrenosum (p.1076). Six of eight patients with severe refractory pyoderma gangrenosum responded favourably to treatment with high-dose systemic corticosteroid pulse therapy;[1] none had serious complications. However, pulse therapy needs very careful use and monitoring, as it is not without adverse effects.[2] Healing of superficial granulomatous pyoderma has occurred following intralesional injection of triamcinolone,[3,4] oral administration of prednisolone,[3,4] and following long-term topical corticosteroids.[4]

1. Prystowsky JH, *et al.* Present status of pyoderma gangrenosum: review of 21 cases. *Arch Dermatol* 1989; **125:** 57–64.
2. Callen JP. Pyoderma gangrenosum. *Lancet* 1998; **351:** 581–5.
3. Quimby SR, *et al.* Superficial granulomatous pyoderma: clinicopathologic spectrum. *Mayo Clin Proc* 1989; **64:** 37–43.
4. Hardwick N, Cerio R. Superficial granulomatous pyoderma: a report of two cases. *Br J Dermatol* 1993; **129:** 718–22.

Respiratory disorders

Although corticosteroids have been employed in the management of many forms of respiratory disorder, their use has frequently been on an empirical and uncontrolled basis, and evidence of benefit is often somewhat mixed. Thus, while an established role exists for corticosteroids in the management of asthma (see p.745) and probably in croup (see p.1020) they are no longer used in aspiration syndromes (see p.1168) and their role in interstitial lung disorders (see p.1024 and under Sarcoidosis, below) and in respiratory distress syndrome (see p.1017 and p.1025) is uncertain. Other disorders in which they have been tried with varying success include chronic obstructive pulmonary disease (see p.747), fat embolism syndrome,[1] acute eosinophilic pneumonia[2] and pulmonary eosinophilia,[3] diffuse alveolar haemorrhage,[4] and 'ice hockey lung' (due to nitrogen dioxide).[5]

1. Van Besouw J-P, Hinds CJ. Fat embolism syndrome. *Br J Hosp Med* 1989; **42:** 304–11.
2. Anonymous. Acute eosinophilic pneumonia. *Lancet* 1990; **335:** 947.
3. Anonymous. Pulmonary eosinophilia. *Lancet* 1990; **335:** 512.
4. Metcalf JP, *et al.* Corticosteroids as adjunctive therapy for diffuse alveolar hemorrhage associated with bone marrow transplantation. *Am J Med* 1994; **96:** 327–34.
5. Anonymous. Ice hockey lung: NO_2 poisoning. *Lancet* 1990; **335:** 1191.

Retinal vasculitis

In the treatment of retinal vasculitis, corticosteroids are the most useful drugs for the management of inflammation and its sequelae when vision is compromised.[1] For uniocular disease treatment with orbital floor injection of corticosteroids such as methylprednisolone acetate may be possible. For bilateral disease systemic therapy is required, with additional immunosuppressant cover if relapse occurs despite high-dose corticosteroid therapy.

1. Anonymous. Retinal vasculitis. *Lancet* 1989; **i:** 823–4.

Rheumatoid arthritis

The use of corticosteroids in rheumatoid arthritis (p.2) is controversial. Systemic corticosteroids can suppress symptoms of the disease, but their usefulness is limited by their adverse effects and they have usually been reserved for severe rapidly progressing disease unresponsive to therapy with NSAIDs and disease modifying antirheumatic drugs (DMARDs). However, recent results indicate that there may be advantages to the early use of low doses of corticosteroids in active disease. They may also be used temporarily to control disease activity during initiation of therapy with DMARDs, or in disease accompanied by severe extra-articular effects. Intra-articular injection of corticosteroids may be used when an acute flare affects one or two individual joints but should be given infrequently.

Intra-articular injections of corticosteroids have also been given in ankylosing spondylitis (see Spondyloarthropathies, p.4).

Rhinitis

For a brief description of rhinitis and a discussion of its management including the use of corticosteroids, see p.400.

Sarcoidosis

Sarcoidosis is a disorder involving the development of multiple granulomas in a variety of organs, which may subsequently resolve or progress to chronic fibrosis.[1] Almost any organ can be affected, but manifestations in lymph nodes, lungs, skin, joints, and eyes are common. The disease is frequently asymptomatic, and since it usually regresses spontaneously estimating the incidence is difficult, but it appears to vary considerably in different countries. It is most often seen in young adults and is slightly more common in female than male and in black than white patients.

Symptoms vary enormously, depending on the organ affected, and as already mentioned it is often asymptomatic. Lymphadenopathy, some decrease in pulmonary function, dyspnoea, and cough may mark lung and lymph node involvement. Skin manifestations include erythema nodosum, macular or papular lesions due to granuloma formation in the skin, and violaceous plaques on fingers, nose, ears, and cheeks known as lupus pernio. Arthropathy, with painful joint swellings, may be associated with erythema nodosum and fever in acute presentations; bone lesions are most common in fingers and toes. Involvement of the nervous system may be particularly difficult to diagnose because of its protean manifestations. Involvement of the eyes is usually manifest as uveitis although other symptoms include keratoconjunctivitis sicca. Symptomatic disease involving the gastro-intestinal tract, liver, pancreas, heart, or kidneys is rare, although asymptomatic involvement may occur.

In addition to symptoms directly due to the disease, sarcoidosis is often associated with hypercalcaemia and hypersensitivity to the effects of vitamin D (for discussion of the symptoms of hypercalcaemia, see p.1148). Other biochemical abnormalities include raised serum concentrations of angiotensin-converting enzyme (ACE), and there are abnormalities of some aspects of immune function.

Diagnosis of sarcoidosis is problematic because of its multiple manifestations and the fact that it is so often clinically silent. It is often detected by accident, when radiography is performed for other reasons, but biopsy is often needed to help confirm the disease. The Kveim test, in which an antigen derived from patients with sarcoidosis (see p.1593) is given intradermally and produces a delayed reaction in patients with the disease, is now rarely used because of its perceived lack of precision, although some workers still consider it useful.[2]

Treatment. Asymptomatic disease requires no therapy, and since spontaneous remission can occur, corticosteroids, which are the usual therapy,[1] are generally reserved for patients in whom the disease is interfering with the function of a vital organ or for patients with hypercalcaemia (see p.1148). NSAIDs alone may be adequate to control the fever and arthropathy of acute disease. Where corticosteroids are called for a typical regimen is prednisolone or prednisone 30 to 40 mg daily by mouth, the dose being reduced after several weeks as the patient improves. Therapy should be continued (at the minimum effective maintenance dose) for 12 to 18 months before any attempt is made to withdraw it.[3] Some workers favour alternate-day administration, usually beginning at 40 mg every other day.[4] There is some evidence[5] that relapse may be more likely following withdrawal of corticosteroids than in patients who do not receive corticosteroid therapy, but this may simply reflect the natural course of disease in this group. There also remains some dispute about the value of corticosteroids in pulmonary disease: although they produce symptomatic relief they do not appear to alter the course of the disease or avert fibrotic changes.[3] Inhaled corticosteroids have been investigated in pulmonary sarcoidosis, in an attempt to permit earlier treatment with fewer systemic adverse effects.[6] In patients with ocular disease corticosteroid drops and ointment are used for anterior uveitis; resistant cases, or patients with posterior uveitis, require systemic corticosteroids. Skin lesions usually respond to corticosteroids but the high doses that may be required for suppression of lupus pernio may produce changes in appearance as disfiguring as the disease.[3]

Other agents have occasionally been used in sarcoidosis but are very much second-line. In patients in whom corticosteroids are not effective or not tolerated cytotoxic immunosuppressants such as methotrexate, chlorambucil, azathioprine, or cyclosporin have been given, with variable results.[1,3] Methotrexate has perhaps been most useful, having been found to be effective in low doses (up to 22.5 mg weekly) by mouth in refractory cutaneous sarcoidosis,[7] and with reports of benefit from intramuscular administration in nervous system involvement.[8] The antimalarials have also been tried as adjuncts or alternatives to corticosteroid therapy,[9-11] and there is evidence that they reduce the effects of the disease on calcium metabolism[9,10,12] as well as reports of benefit in cutaneous disease.[11,13,14] Other reports of benefit in cutaneous sarcoidosis have involved allopurinol,[15] thalidomide,[16] and tranilast,[17] while there is report of response to melatonin in 2 patients with refractory sarcoidosis.[18]

1. Newman LS, *et al.* Sarcoidosis. *N Engl J Med* 1997; **336:** 1224–34. Correction. *ibid.*; **337:** 139.
2. du Bois RM, *et al.* Moratorium on Kveim test. *Lancet* 1993; **342:** 173.
3. Muthiah MM, Macfarlane JT. Current concepts in the management of sarcoidosis. *Drugs* 1990; **40:** 231–7.
4. DeRemee RA. Sarcoidosis. *Mayo Clin Proc* 1995; **70:** 177–81.
5. Gottlieb JE, *et al.* Outcome in sarcoidosis: the relationship of relapse to corticosteroid therapy. *Chest* 1997; **111:** 623–31.
6. Spiteri MA. Inhaled corticosteroids in pulmonary sarcoidosis. *Postgrad Med J* 1991; **67:** 327–9.
7. Webster GF, *et al.* Methotrexate therapy in cutaneous sarcoidosis. *Ann Intern Med* 1989; **111:** 538–9.
8. Soriano FG, *et al.* Neurosarcoidosis: therapeutic success with methotrexate. *Postgrad Med J* 1990; **66:** 142–3.
9. DeSimone DP, *et al.* Granulomatous infiltration of the talus and abnormal vitamin D and calcium metabolism in a patient with sarcoidosis: successful treatment with hydroxychloroquine. *Am J Med* 1989; **87:** 694–6.
10. O'Leary TJ, *et al.* The effects of chloroquine on serum 1,25-dihydroxyvitamin D and calcium metabolism in sarcoidosis. *N Engl J Med* 1986; **315:** 727–30.
11. Zic JA, *et al.* Treatment of cutaneous sarcoidosis with chloroquine: review of the literature. *Arch Dermatol* 1991; **127:** 1034–40.
12. Adams JS, *et al.* Effective reduction in the serum 1,25-dihydroxy-vitamin D and calcium concentration in sarcoidosis-associated hypercalcemia with short-course chloroquine therapy. *Ann Intern Med* 1989; **111:** 437–8.
13. Spiteri MA, *et al.* Lupus pernio: a clinico-radiological study of thirty-five cases. *Br J Dermatol* 1985; **112:** 315–22.
14. Jones E, Callen JP. Hydroxychloroquine is effective therapy for control of cutaneous sarcoidal granulomas. *J Am Acad Dermatol* 1990; **23:** 487–9.
15. Brechtel B, *et al.* Allopurinol: a therapeutic alternative for disseminated cutaneous sarcoidosis. *Br J Dermatol* 1996; **135:** 307–9.
16. Carlesimo M, *et al.* Treatment of cutaneous and pulmonary sarcoidosis with thalidomide. *J Am Acad Dermatol* 1995; **32:** 866–9.
17. Yamada H, *et al.* Treatment of cutaneous sarcoidosis with tranilast. *J Dermatol* 1995; **22:** 149–52.
18. Cagnoni ML, *et al.* Melatonin for treatment of chronic refractory sarcoidosis. *Lancet* 1995; **346:** 1229–30.

Sciatica

For mention of the use of epidural corticosteroid injections to treat sciatica, and doubts about the extent of benefit, see Administration, Epidural Route, p.1016.

Scleritis

Scleritis and episcleritis are inflammatory diseases of the sclera often associated with various systemic diseases. Episcleritis tends to be a benign superficial condition but treatment can be difficult and it tends to recur. The use of topical corticosteroids and topical NSAIDs are sometimes of temporary benefit. Scleritis is a rarer more deep-seated inflammation. Initial treatment of non-necrotising scleritis is with NSAIDs; high dose systemic corticosteroids (usually prednisolone 60 to 80 mg daily) have been used successfully in many patients unresponsive to NSAIDs.[1,2] If necessary, to reduce any attendant adverse effects, corticosteroids have been given by orbital floor injection (methylprednisolone acetate 40 mg)[1] or at a reduced systemic dosage with an additional immunosuppressant such as cyclosporin.[2] Cyclosporin may also be of value alone in severe or unresponsive disease.[3] Necrotising scleritis requires treatment with high-dose corticosteroids often with another immunosuppressant.[1,2]

1. Hakin KN, *et al.* Use of orbital floor steroids in the management of patients with uniocular non-necrotising scleritis. *Br J Ophthalmol* 1991; **75:** 337–9.
2. Hakin KN, *et al.* Use of cyclosporin in the management of steroid-dependent non-necrotising scleritis. *Br J Ophthalmol* 1991; **75:** 340–1.
3. Wakefiled D, McCluskey P. Cyclosporin therapy for severe scleritis. *Br J Ophthalmol* 1989; **73:** 743–6.

Seborrhoeic dermatitis

Topical corticosteroids are used, together with an antifungal imidazole, in the management of seborrhoeic dermatitis (p.1076).

Septic shock

Although early studies reported both beneficial[1] and detrimental[2] effects, current opinion appears to be that corticosteroids are ineffective in septic shock[2,3] and may worsen secondary infection.[4-7]

1. Sprung CL, *et al.* The effects of high-dose corticosteroids in patients with septic shock: a prospective, controlled study. *N Engl J Med* 1984; **311:** 1137–43.
2. Bone RC, *et al.* A controlled clinical trial of high-dose methylprednisolone in the treatment of severe sepsis and septic shock. *N Engl J Med* 1987; **317:**
3. The Veterans Administration Systemic Sepsis Cooperative Study Group. Effect of high-dose glucocorticoid therapy on mortality in patients with clinical signs of systemic sepsis. *N Engl J Med* 1987; **317:** 659–65.
4. Anonymous. No evidence that corticosteroids help in septic shock. *Drug Ther Bull* 1990; **28:** 74–5.
5. Rackow EC, Astiz ME. Pathophysiology and treatment of septic shock. *JAMA* 1991; **266:** 548–54.
6. Cohen J, Glauser MP. Septic shock: treatment. *Lancet* 1991; **338:** 736–9.
7. McGowan JE, *et al.* Report by the Working Group on Steroid Use, Antimicrobial Agents Committee, Infectious Diseases Society of America: Guidelines for the use of systemic glucocorticoids in the management of selected infections. *J Infect Dis* 1992; **165:** 1–13.

Sickle-cell disease

A recent study[1] has suggested that a short course of high-dose methylprednisolone might be a useful adjunct in controlling pain in sickle-cell crisis (p.11). However, the use of corticosteroids in sickle-cell disease (p.703) is problematic; apart from the usual adverse effects, including the risk of exacerbating underlying infection, corticosteroid therapy has been reported to provoke sickle-cell crisis in patients with sickle C disease—see under Precautions, p.1014.

1. Griffin TC, *et al.* High-dose intravenous methylprednisolone therapy for pain in children and adolescents with sickle cell disease. *N Engl J Med* 1994; **330:** 733–7.

Skin disorders

For some guidelines to the use of topical application of corticosteroids in skin disorders, see under Administration, p.1017. For discussion of the use of corticosteroids in individual skin disorders see under the relevant headings in this section.

Spinal cord injury

Results of a multicentre placebo-controlled study in the USA[1] indicated that high-dose intravenous corticosteroids resulted in improvements in neurological function if given within 8 hours of spinal cord injury. Methylprednisolone was given in an initial dose of 30 mg per kg body-weight followed by 5.4 mg per kg per hour for 23 hours. A subsequent study found that although this regimen was adequate if begun within 3 hours of injury, better results were obtained by continuing methylprednisolone for 48 hours in patients in whom therapy commenced 3 to 8 hours after injury.[2] The lazaroid tirilazad, given for 48 hours, had some benefit in this study, although it was less effective than 48 hours treatment with methylprednisolone in the doses used.

In contrast, these is little evidence that corticosteroids or tirilazad are of any value in acute traumatic brain injury.[3,4]

1. Bracken MB, *et al.* A randomized, controlled trial of methylprednisolone or naloxone in the treatment of acute spinal-cord injury: results of the Second National Acute Spinal Cord Injury Study. *N Engl J Med* 1990; **322:** 1405–11.
2. Bracken MB, *et al.* Administration of methylprednisolone for 24 or 48 hours or tirilazad mesylate for 48 hours in the treatment of acute spinal cord injury: results of the third National Acute Spinal Cord Injury Randomized Controlled Trial. *JAMA* 1997; **277:** 1597–1604.
3. Alderson P, Roberts I. Corticosteroids in acute traumatic brain injury: systematic review of randomised controlled trials. *Br Med J* 1997; **314:** 1855–9.
4. Newell DW, *et al.* Corticosteroids in acute traumatic brain injury. *Br Med J* 1998; **316:** 396.

Systemic lupus erythematosus

Systemic lupus erythematosus (SLE) is an auto-immune disease of unknown aetiology characterised by autoantibodies which participate in the mediation of tissue damage affecting joints, skin, kidney, CNS, and other organs. It is far more common in women than in men, the evidence suggesting that male hormones have a protective effect, and peak onset is usually in women in their 20s and 30s.

The commonest symptom in patients with SLE is arthralgia or arthritis; fatigue, fever, weight loss, rashes (characteristically a so-called 'butterfly rash' on the cheeks and bridge of the nose), CNS involvement including personality changes, anaemia, nephritis, and pulmonary symptoms (notable pleurisy) are also frequent, while other symptoms include myalgia, alopecia, Raynaud's syndrome, convulsions, coma, stroke, pneumonitis, pericarditis, myocarditis with tachycardia, leucopenia, thrombocytopenia, coagulation disorders (both thrombosis and haemorrhage), hepatomegaly, splenomegaly, and lymphadenopathy. Thrombotic symptoms and recurrent abortion may represent an 'antiphospholipid antibody syndrome' due to antibodies against phospholipids, which occurs in about a third of all patients with SLE but may also occur independently.[1]

Management. The management of patients with SLE must be adjusted individually depending on the manifestations of disease and their severity. Since the disease is characterised by exacerbation and remission careful monitoring of the patient and appropriate treatment of symptoms as and when they occur are required. Treatment is largely empirical and symptomatic, and there have been few controlled studies.

In addition to any specific treatment, patients require emotional support, extensive rest, and avoidance where possible of stimuli that may provoke disease exacerbation, including ultraviolet light, certain drugs or foods rich in psoralens, infections, and psychological stress.

Mild disease may require no treatment, or may be managed simply with NSAIDs for muscular and joint symptoms.[2] In more severe, but non-life-threatening disease chloroquine or, more often, hydroxychloroquine is effective, particularly for cutaneous and joint manifestations,[3,4] although disease flare may occur on withdrawal.[5] Retinoids such as acitretin have also been shown to be of use in some patients.[6]

Many patients require treatment with corticosteroids at some point, although in such patients they can be a major cause of morbidity.[4,7] It is usual to employ a corticosteroid when treatment with NSAIDs or antimalarials has failed, or when life or vital organs are threatened.[2] They are usually employed in high doses (1 mg or more of prednisone or prednisolone per kg body-weight daily, sometimes preceded by a course of intravenous methylprednisolone) for life-threatening manifestations such as high fever, severe thrombocytopenia, coma, seizures, or involvement of a major organ such as the kidney[3] (see also Lupus Nephritis, below). Non-life-threatening symptoms which fail to respond to other measures will usually respond to lower corticosteroid doses (not more than 0.5 mg of prednisolone or prednisone per kg daily). Once a response is achieved the dose should be tapered to the lowest required to control symptoms, ideally in the form of alternate-day dosage.[3] Raising the maintenance corticosteroid dose temporarily to counteract any increases in the concentration of antibodies to double-stranded DNA may reduce the number of relapses,[8] but the design and conclusions of this study are open to criticism.

Prolonged corticosteroid therapy, particularly at the higher doses, is associated with adverse effects such as aseptic bone necrosis and an increased susceptibility to infection, and other agents have been added to corticosteroid therapy in an attempt to lower the corticosteroid dose but maintain disease control. In particular the immunosuppressant azathioprine has been used for its steroid-sparing effect;[2,9] immunosuppressants such as cyclophosphamide are considered to pose more of a risk of long-term toxicity but cyclophosphamide has been used with some success to treat severe acute organ involvement in patients with disease refractory to corticosteroids alone.[10-14] Recent results have suggested that methotrexate, too, may be helpful in some patients, such as those with joint disease.[15] The antimalarials may also be combined with corticosteroid therapy, and in addition to a steroid-sparing effect there is a suggestion that hydroxychloroquine may counter the adverse effects of corticosteroids on serum-lipid profiles.[2,16]

Thrombotic symptoms due to antiphospholipid antibodies require adequate long-term anticoagulation with warfarin or low-dose aspirin, and it should be borne in mind that stroke and related CNS symptoms will not respond to corticosteroids. In patients with other severe CNS symptoms that fail to respond to corticosteroids intravenous cyclophosphamide may be helpful,[11,14] but response is unpredictable. Intravenous immunoglobulin has been used as an adjunct in CNS lupus, although its role is unclear; it may also be used in the management of thrombocytopenic symptoms.[17]

In patients with severe and potentially fatal symptoms plasma exchange may provide temporary benefit by removing circulating antibodies.

Lupus nephritis. Renal disease is probably the best studied symptom of systemic lupus erythematosus. Almost all patients develop some renal involvement, with clinical nephritis in up to 75%. Usual manifestations of renal disease include hypertension, oedema, proteinuria or frank nephrotic syndrome, and oliguria; more severe disease is usually associated with focal or diffuse proliferative glomerulonephritis on biopsy.[18,19]

Patients with active disease (worsening renal function, proteinuria, and urinary sediment) require aggressive treatment to prevent irreversible renal damage. It is generally accepted that the combination of a cytotoxic immunosuppressant drug with a corticosteroid is more effective than the use of corticosteroids alone in controlling nephritis and the risk of end-stage renal failure, although corticosteroids alone may be used for less severe disease.[17,20]

One suggested outline for treatment in severe active disease is to begin with pulsed intravenous methylprednisolone as 3 doses of 1g, followed by prednisone by mouth (initially 0.8 to 1 mg per kg daily, gradually reduced to 0.4 mg per kg daily) accompanied if necessary by cyclophosphamide or azathioprine. Provided disease activity is controlled subsequent maintenance can be reduced to alternate-day prednisone.[18] An alternative approach is to begin therapy with intermittent intravenous cyclophosphamide[21-23] (which one recent study has suggested may be more effective than pulsed methylprednisolone[24]) and maintain patients with low-dose oral prednisone plus intravenous cyclophosphamide every 3 months. Cyclosporin has also been investigated, but is viewed with caution because of its nephrotoxicity,[18] and suggestions of a lack of effect in severe active disease.[19]

Pregnancy. Although symptoms of SLE do not appear to be exacerbated in most patients during pregnancy,[25,26] it is considered advisable that pregnancy be deferred until the disease is in remission or controlled by therapy since complications are more likely in active disease.[25] Cyclophosphamide or methotrexate are contra-indicated in pregnancy because of the risk of teratogenesis but corticosteroids, azathioprine, and hydroxychloroquine may be used if necessary:[2,27] the risks of miscarriage, still-birth, growth retardation, or preterm delivery due to the disease are considered greater than the risks to the fetus of continued therapy. The use of low-dose aspirin (75 mg daily) has been recommended in women with renal involvement or a history of pre-eclampsia or fetal growth retardation;[27] it should also be given to women with antiphospholipid antibodies, together with subcutaneous heparin in those with a history of thrombosis.[27,28] The use of high-dose prednisone, with or without aspirin, to suppress antiphospholipid antibodies, while reportedly effective in some women with bad obstetric histories,[29,30] has been found by others to be of no benefit,[31] and is probably not justified in those lacking a history of fetal loss.[25] (Warfarin prophylaxis, which appears effective in other patients with the antiphospholipid antibody syndrome,[32] is unsuited to pregnant women because of the teratogenic effects of warfarin.[33])

Postpartum exacerbation is well recognised,[25,27] and some workers favour prophylactic corticosteroid cover during the puerperium. A small proportion of neonates born to mothers with lupus exhibit a neonatal lupus syndrome,[34] manifesting most seriously as heart block which may require a permanent pacemaker.

1. Hughes GRV. The antiphospholipid syndrome: ten years on. *Lancet* 1993; **342:** 341–4.
2. Anonymous. Systemic lupus erythematosus. *Drug Ther Bull* 1996; **34:** 20–3.
3. Lockshin MD. Therapy for systemic lupus erythematosus. *N Engl J Med* 1991; **324:** 189–91.
4. Hay EM, Snaith ML. Systemic lupus erythematosus and lupus-like syndromes. *Br Med J* 1995; **310:** 1257–61.
5. The Canadian Hydroxychloroquine Study Group. A randomized study of the effect of withdrawing hydroxychloroquine sulfate in systemic lupus erythematosus. *N Engl J Med* 1991; **324:** 150–4.
6. Ruzicka T, *et al.* Treatment of cutaneous lupus erythematosus with acitretin and hydroxychloroquine. *Br J Dermatol* 1992; **127:** 513–18.
7. Mills JA. Systemic lupus erythematosus. *N Engl J Med* 1994; **330:** 1871–9.
8. Bootsma H, *et al.* Prevention of relapses in systemic lupus erythematosus. *Lancet* 1995; **345:** 1595–9. Correction. *ibid.*; **346:** 516.
9. Callen JP, *et al.* Azathioprine: an effective corticosteroid-sparing therapy for patients with recalcitrant cutaneous lupus erythematosus or with recalcitrant cutaneous leukocytoclastic vasculitis. *Arch Dermatol* 1991; **127:** 515–22.
10. Sigal LH. Chronic inflammatory polyneuropathy complicating SLE: successful treatment with monthly oral pulse cyclophosphamide. *J Rheumatol* 1989; **16:** 1518–19.
11. Fricchione GL, *et al.* Electroconvulsive therapy and cyclophosphamide in combination for severe neuropsychiatric lupus with catatonia. *Am J Med* 1990; **88:** 442–3.
12. Boumpas DT, *et al.* Intermittent cyclophosphamide for the treatment of autoimmune thrombocytopenia in systemic lupus erythematosus. *Ann Intern Med* 1990; **112:** 674–7.
13. Barr WG, *et al.* Plasmapheresis and pulse cyclophosphamide in systemic lupus erythematosus. *Ann Intern Med* 1988; **108:** 152–3.
14. Neuwelt CM, *et al.* Role of intravenous cyclophosphamide in the treatment of severe neuropsychiatric systemic lupus erythematosus. *Am J Med* 1995; **98:** 32–41.
15. Wilson K, Abeles M. A 2 year, open ended trial of methotrexate in systemic lupus erythematosus. *J Rheumatol* 1994; **21:** 1674–7.
16. Hodis HN, *et al.* The lipid, lipoprotein, and apolipoprotein effects of hydroxychloroquine in patients with systemic lupus erythematosus. *J Rheumatol* 1993; **20:** 661–5.
17. Boumpas DT, *et al.* Systemic lupus erythematosus: emerging concepts. *Ann Intern Med* 1995; **122:** 940–50 and **123:** 42–53.
18. Ponticelli C. Current treatment recommendations for lupus nephritis. *Drugs* 1990; **40:** 19–30.
19. Dhillon VB, *et al.* Lupus nephritis: a review. *Postgrad Med J* 1989; **65:** 336–43.
20. Venables PJW. Diagnosis and treatment of systemic lupus erythematosus. *Br Med J* 1993; **307:** 663–6.
21. Austin HA, *et al.* Therapy of lupus nephritis: controlled trial of prednisone and cytotoxic drugs. *N Engl J Med* 1986; **314:** 614–19.
22. McCune WJ, *et al.* Clinical and immunologic effects of monthly administration of intravenous cyclophosphamide in severe systemic lupus erythematosus. *N Engl J Med* 1988; **318:** 1423–31.
23. Lehman TJA, *et al.* Intermittent intravenous cyclophosphamide therapy for lupus nephritis. *J Pediatr* 1989; **114:** 1055–60.
24. Boumpas DT, *et al.* Controlled trial of pulse methylprednisolone versus two regimens of pulse cyclophosphamide in severe lupus nephritis. *Lancet* 1992; **340:** 741–5.
25. Anonymous. Systemic lupus erythematosus in pregnancy. *Lancet* 1991; **338:** 87–8.
26. Yell JA, Burge SM. The effect of hormonal changes on cutaneous disease in lupus erythematosus. *Br J Dermatol* 1993; **129:** 18–22.
27. Hunt BJ, Lakasing L. Management of pre-existing disorders in pregnancy: connective-tissue disorders. *Prescribers' J* 1997; **37:** 54–60.
28. Hughes GRV, Khamashta MA. The antiphospholipid syndrome. *J R Coll Physicians Lond* 1994; **28:** 301–4.
29. Lubbe WF, *et al.* Fetal survival after prednisone suppression of maternal lupus-anticoagulant. *Lancet* 1983; **i:** 1361–3.
30. Branch DW, *et al.* Obstetric complications associated with the lupus anticoagulant. *N Engl J Med* 1985; **313:** 1322–6.
31. Laskin CA, *et al.* Prednisone and aspirin in women with autoantibodies and unexplained recurrent fetal loss. *N Engl J Med* 1997; **337:** 148–53.
32. Khamashta MA, *et al.* The management of thrombosis in the antiphospholipid-antibody syndrome. *N Engl J Med* 1995; **332:** 993–7.
33. Lockshin MD. Answers to the antiphospholipid-antibody syndrome? *N Engl J Med* 1995; **332:** 1025–7.
34. Anonymous. Neonatal lupus syndrome. *Lancet* 1987; **ii:** 489–90.

Takayasu's arteritis

Takayasu's arteritis is a vasculitis of the aorta and its branches seen particularly in young women and in Oriental patients. It is characterised by vasculitis followed by fibrosis, leading to stenosis or occlusion of the vessel. Symptoms vary depending on the anatomical site, but include constitutional symptoms such as fever, malaise, and arthralgia, syncope, dyspnoea, palpitations, loss of pulses, intermittent claudication, and visual disturbances.

Active inflammatory disease may respond to corticosteroids: doses of 1 mg per kg body-weight daily of prednisone, tapered after one month in patients who respond, have been suggested.[1] In patients who do not respond, low-dose oral cyclophosphamide has been added, although opinions vary as to the necessity of cytotoxic agents in these patients.[1,2] Widely varying estimates of mortality and aggressiveness exist for Takayasu's arteritis, and in the absence of large controlled studies it is difficult to assess the benefits of drug therapy. The course may be very prolonged, and minimising the maintenance dosage (e.g. by alternate-day corticosteroid therapy) is important to avoid adverse effects.[3]

Surgical reconstruction of affected vessels has been carried out in patients at risk of ischaemic compromise.[4] Angioplasty has been tried.

1. Shelhamer JH, *et al.* Takayasu's arteritis and its therapy. *Ann Intern Med* 1985; **103:** 121–6.
2. Hall S, Hunder GG. Treatment of Takayasu's arteritis. *Ann Intern Med* 1986; **104:** 288.
3. Taylor HG, Samanta A. Treatment of vasculitis. *Br J Clin Pharmacol* 1993; **35:** 93–104.
4. Kerr GS, *et al.* Takayasu arteritis. *Ann Intern Med* 1994; **120:** 919–29.

Tuberculosis

The use of corticosteroids in tuberculosis (p.146) is controversial.[1-3] They should never be given to patients with active disease without protective chemotherapy cover, and must be used with caution in patients with dormant disease as it may be reactivated. Administration of corticosteroids in pulmonary tuberculosis is to be avoided except in life-threatening disease. WHO suggests that corticosteroids may be useful adjuvants to antituberculous therapy in selected conditions including tuberculous meningitis, pericarditis, pleural effusion, or laryngitis, or tuberculosis of the renal tract, adrenocortical insufficiency due to adrenal gland tuberculosis, massive lymph node enlargement, or to control drug hypersensitivity. They are also likely to be of benefit in patients with HIV infection and the above conditions.[4]

1. Horne NW, ed. *Modern drug treatment of tuberculosis.* 7th ed. London: The Chest, Heart and Stroke Association, 1990.
2. McGowan JE, *et al.* Report by the Working Group on Steroid Use, Antimicrobial Agents Committee, Infectious Diseases Society of America: Guidelines for the use of systemic glucocorticoids in the management of selected infections. *J Infect Dis* 1992; **165:** 1–13.
3. Alzeer AH, FitzGerald JM. Corticosteroids and tuberculosis: risks and use as adjunct therapy. *Tubercle Lung Dis* 1993; **74:** 6–11.
4. WHO. *TB/HIV: a clinical manual.* Geneva: WHO, 1996.

Urticaria and angioedema

Oral antihistamines are the mainstay of treatment for urticaria (p.1076). Severe attacks may require a short course of oral corticosteroid therapy.

When angioedema affecting the larynx (laryngeal oedema) is present, the patients should be treated with adrenaline as an allergic emergency (see under Anaphylactic Shock, p.816).

Uveitis

Uveitis is inflammation of the uveal tract of the eye which comprises the choroid, ciliary body, and the iris. It is usually idiopathic but may be secondary to infection, allergy, or inflammatory disorders with an autoimmune component.

In anterior uveitis, also referred to as iridocyclitis, there is inflammation of the iris (iritis) and the ciliary body (cyclitis). It tends to be acute and self-limiting and is likely to be associated with infection. The iris becomes spongy and hyperaemic and exudates may result in adhesions between the iris and the lens (posterior synechiae). Chronic anterior uveitis is associated with formation of cataracts and glaucoma. Posterior uveitis can be acute or chronic and may just affect the choroid (choroiditis) or may also involve the retina (chorioretinitis). It is more likely to be an autoimmune condition.

The treatment of uveitis has been reviewed.[1-4]

Corticosteroids given topically and, when necessary, systemically are the mainstay of treatment for anterior uveitis. Cycloplegics and mydriatics such as atropine, cyclopentolate, and homatropine are used adjunctively to rest the ciliary body and iris, diminish hyperaemia, and to prevent the formation of posterior synechiae. Antibacterials should be used to treat any infection.

Treatment of posterior uveitis is less satisfactory since gross damage to the retina often occurs before the condition can be controlled. Corticosteroids are usually required given either as periocular injections or as high-dose systemic therapy. A suggested protocol[4] involves the use of high-dose systemic corticosteroids to control active disease; long-term control is then maintained primarily with low-dose cyclosporin, corticosteroids being tapered to a low dose or eventually withdrawn. Certain patients may require an additional immunosuppressant, usually azathioprine although methotrexate or cyclophosphamide may be considered. Other immunosuppressants being studied include tacrolimus.

Visual impairment in chronic uveitis is often the result of macular oedema and is not necessarily prevented by immunosuppressants. Short-term treatment with acetazolamide is considered to have produced some encouraging results in reducing chronic uveitic macular oedema but its long-term efficacy or efficacy with low-dose corticosteroids remains to be determined.[5] Although systemic and topical NSAIDs have been shown to reduce cystoid macular oedema in post cataract extraction (see p.66) their role in the treatment of macular oedema associated with uveitis is less clear.

1. Herman DC. Endogenous uveitis: current concepts of treatment. *Mayo Clin Proc* 1990; **65:** 671–83.
2. Lightman S. Uveitis: management. *Lancet* 1991; **338:** 1501–4.
3. Anglade E, Whitcup SM. The diagnosis and management of uveitis. *Drugs* 1995; **49:** 213–23.
4. Dick AD, *et al.* Immunosuppressive therapy for chronic uveitis: optimising therapy with steroids and cyclosporin A. *Br J Ophthalmol* 1997; **81:** 1107–12.
5. Dick AD. The treatment of chronic uveitic macular oedema. *Br J Ophthalmol* 1994; **78:** 1–2.

Vasculitic syndromes

Vasculitis may be defined as inflammation of the blood vessel wall, and the term has been applied in describing a wide range of diseases involving blood vessels of various sizes and types. Vasculitis may occur as part of a systemic disease such as rheumatoid arthritis or systemic lupus erythematosus, or may itself be the primary disorder, and symptoms may vary from superficial cutaneous disease, with purpura and urticaria, to progressive and fatal systemic vasculitides such as Wegener's granulomatosis. In some forms of vasculitis, such as giant cell arteritis, mononuclear giant cells may be seen, while in granulomatous vasculitis the mononuclear cells form granulomata adjacent to the damaged vessel wall. Necrotising vasculitis is used to describe inflammation associated with necrosis of the media, the middle part of the vessel wall, while polyarteritis implies inflammation of the full thickness of an arterial wall.

Because of the heterogeneous nature of this group of diseases and the degree of overlap which exists between some of them, and between them and other diseases, classification has been difficult. Classification has often been based on the size of the affected vessel, as well as the presence or absence of granulomata and antineutrophil cytoplasmic antibodies (ANCA), and whether the vasculitis is primary or secondary. Of the major primary vasculitic syndromes, giant cell arteritis (p.1021) and Takayasu's arteritis (p.1030) are examples of large vessel disease; classic polyarteritis nodosa (p.1027) affects medium-sized vessels; Churg-Strauss syndrome (p.1019), microscopic polyangiitis (p.1027), and Wegener's granulomatosis (below) are diseases of small or medium-sized vessels; the so-called 'hypersensitivity vasculitides', including Henoch-Schönlein purpura, are small vessel diseases (p.1022), though usually limited in extent.

Treatment depends on the type of vasculitis, its severity, and prognosis. Treatment of the systemic vasculitides has revolved around corticosteroids and cyclophosphamide; other cytotoxic immunosuppressants, normal immunoglobulins, NSAIDs, anticoagulants, dapsone, and colchicine have been tried in various forms of disease.

Vitiligo

For mention that topical corticosteroids are sometimes effective in inducing repigmentation in patients with vitiligo, see Pigmentation Disorders, p.1075.

Waldenström's macroglobulinaemia

Where treatment is required, the usual management of Waldenström's macroglobulinaemia is with chlorambucil (see p.496), although other agents have been tried. For example, two patients with Waldenström's macroglobulinaemia resistant to other treatment responded to dexamethasone given in 30-day cycles at a dosage of 40 mg daily for 4 days.[1]

1. Jane SM, Salem HH. Treatment of resistant Waldenstrom's macroglobulinemia with high dose glucocorticosteroids. *Aust N Z J Med* 1988; **18:** 77–8.

Wegener's granulomatosis

Wegener's granulomatosis is a form of granulomatous vasculitis which occurs more frequently in men and in white patients. It is characterised by necrotising vasculitis of small arteries and veins, accompanied by granuloma formation, and affecting particularly the respiratory tract and kidneys. It is usually associated with antineutrophil cytoplasmic antibodies (ANCA). Symptoms include rhinorrhoea, sinusitis, cough and dyspnoea (signs of pulmonary infiltration which is seen in the majority of patients at presentation); renal manifestations include haematuria, proteinuria, uraemia, and oedema of the lower limbs due to a focal glomerulonephritis which can progress to crescentic glomerulonephritis and rapidly progressive renal failure. Other organ systems may be involved, with effects similar to those of polyarteritis nodosa (see p.1027). If untreated, the disease is invariably fatal.

Treatment is with a combination regimen based on cyclophosphamide with a corticosteroid. A standard regimen has been low-dose (1 to 2 mg per kg body-weight daily) oral cyclophosphamide, together with prednisolone or prednisone 1 mg per kg daily by mouth initially, subsequently tapered to an alternate-day regimen and eventually discontinued.[1,2] Cyclophosphamide is usually continued for at least a year before considering gradual discontinuation but there is a trend in Europe towards the use of shorter courses of cyclophosphamide.[3] Regimens similar to the standard regimen, but substituting azathioprine for cyclophosphamide once remission is achieved (usually after 4 to 6 months) and continuing with low dose corticosteroids concomitantly have been employed. Standard treatment regimens produce improvement or remissions in about 90% of patients.[1,4] Relapses may subsequently occur in about half, and require re-treatment; prompt intensification of treatment when serum ANCA concentrations begin to rise may avert relapse.[5] There is evidence from controlled study that addition of co-trimoxazole to maintenance regimens reduces the incidence of relapse.[6]

Despite the success of regimens based on low-dose oral cyclophosphamide there is considerable concern about their toxicity, particularly since prolonged administration may be necessary. Intermittent high-dose intravenous ('pulse') cyclophosphamide has been suggested as an alternative to the oral regimen with fewer adverse effects,[7] but results in practice seem to have been variable.[8,9] Other agents, such as methotrexate, have been tried and addition of low-dose weekly methotrexate to a corticosteroid may be a possible treatment option.[10,11] Cyclosporin has been reported to reverse acute renal failure in 2 patients with Wegener's granulomatosis, as well as controlling fulminant symptoms unresponsive to cyclophosphamide and corticosteroids in one of them.[12] Etoposide has also been successfully used to induce remission in cyclophosphamide-resistant disease.[13] Other agents which have been investigated include high-dose intravenous immunoglobulin,[14] and mycophenolate mofetil,[15] while anti-CD4 monoclonal antibodies have proved useful in patients with microscopic polyarteritis, which has some similarities to Wegener's granulomatosis, but the role of such investigational regimens remains to be determined.

1. Fauci AS, *et al.* Wegener's granulomatosis: prospective clinical and therapeutic experience with 85 patients for 21 years. *Ann Intern Med* 1983; **98:** 76–85.
2. Hoffman GS, *et al.* Wegener granulomatosis: an analysis of 158 patients. *Ann Intern Med* 1992; **116:** 488–98.
3. Savage COS, *et al.* Primary systemic vasculitis. *Lancet* 1997; **349:** 553–8.
4. Rottem M, *et al.* Wegener granulomatosis in children and adolescents: clinical presentation and outcome. *J Pediatr* 1993 **122:** 26–31.
5. Tervaert JWC, *et al.* Prevention of relapses in Wegener's granulomatosis by treatment based on antineutrophil cytoplasmic antibody titre. *Lancet* 1990; **336:** 709–11.
6. Stegeman CA, *et al.* Trimethoprim-sulfamethoxazole (co-trimoxazole) for the prevention of relapses of Wegener's granulomatosis. *N Engl J Med* 1996; **335:** 16–20.
7. Cupps TR. Cyclophosphamide: to pulse or not to pulse? *Am J Med* 1990; **89:** 399–402.
8. Hoffman GS, *et al.* Treatment of Wegener's granulomatosis with intermittent high-dose intravenous cyclophosphamide. *Am J Med* 1990; **89:** 403–10.
9. Reinhold-Keller E, *et al.* Influence of disease manifestation and antineutrophil cytoplasmic antibody titre on the response to pulse cyclophosphamide therapy in patients with Wegener's granulomatosis. *Arthritis Rheum* 1994; **37:** 919–24.
10. Sneller MC. Wegener's granulomatosis. *JAMA* 1995; **273:** 1288–91.
11. Gottlieb BS, *et al.* Methotrexate treatment of Wegener granulomatosis in children. *J Pediatr* 1996; **129:** 604–7.
12. Gremmel F, *et al.* Cyclosporin in Wegener granulomatosis. *Ann Intern Med* 1988; **108:** 491.
13. D'Cruz D, *et al.* Response of cyclophosphamide-resistant Wegener's granulomatosis to etoposide. *Lancet* 1992; **340:** 425–6.
14. Jayne DRW, *et al.* Treatment of systemic vasculitis with pooled intravenous immunoglobulin. *Lancet* 1991; **337:** 1137–9.
15. Nowack R, *et al.* Mycophenolate mofetil for systemic vasculitis and IgA nephropathy. *Lancet* 1997; **349:** 774.

Alclometasone Dipropionate (12338-m)

Alclometasone Dipropionate *(BANM, USAN, rINNM).*

Sch-22219. 7α-Chloro-11β,17α,21-trihydroxy-16α-methylpregna-1,4-diene-3,20-dione 17,21-dipropionate.

$C_{28}H_{37}ClO_7$ = 521.0.

CAS — 67452-97-5 (alclometasone); 66734-13-2 (alclometasone dipropionate).

Pharmacopoeias. In US.

Store in airtight containers.

Alclometasone dipropionate is a corticosteroid used topically for its glucocorticoid activity (p.1010) in the treatment of various skin disorders. It is usually employed as a cream or ointment containing 0.05%.

When applied topically, particularly to large areas, when the skin is broken, or under occlusive dressings, corticosteroids may be absorbed in sufficient amounts to cause systemic effects (p.1010). The effects of topical corticosteroids on the skin are described on p.1012.

Skin disorders. For recommendations concerning the correct use of corticosteroids on the skin, and a rough guide to the clinical potencies of topical corticosteroids, see Corticosteroids, Administration, p.1017.

Preparations

USP 23: Alclometasone Dipropionate Cream; Alclometasone Dipropionate Ointment.

Proprietary Preparations (details are given in Part 3)
Austral.: Logoderm; ***Belg.:*** Modraderm†; ***Fr.:*** Aclosone; ***Ger.:*** Delonal; ***Irl.:*** Modrasone; ***Ital.:*** Legederm; ***Neth.:*** Aclosone; ***S.Afr.:*** Aclosone; ***Swed.:*** Legederm; ***Switz.:*** Delonal; ***UK:*** Modrasone; ***USA:*** Aclovate.

Aldosterone (1061-l)

Aldosterone *(BAN, rINN).*

Electrocortin. 11β,18-Epoxy-18,21-dihydroxypregn-4-ene-3,20-dione.

$C_{21}H_{28}O_5$ = 360.4.

CAS — 52-39-1.

Adverse Effects

Aldosterone has very pronounced mineralocorticoid actions and little effect on carbohydrate metabolism. It may therefore exhibit the mineralocorticoid adverse effects described for the corticosteroids in general (p.1010).

Uses and Administration

Aldosterone is the main mineralocorticoid (p.1010) secreted by the adrenal cortex. It has no significant glucocorticoid (anti-inflammatory) properties.

Aldosterone has been given by intramuscular or intravenous injection, in association with a glucocorticoid, in the treatment of primary adrenocortical insufficiency (p.1017) but synthetic mineralocorticoids such as fludrocortisone (p.1040), which can be given by mouth, are usually preferred. It is also used as the sodium succinate.

Preparations

Proprietary Preparations (details are given in Part 3)
Ger.: Aldocorten†.
Multi-ingredient: *Ital.:* Sinsurrene.

Amcinonide (12351-d)

Amcinonide *(BAN, USAN, rINN)*.

Amcinopol; CL-34699. 16α,17α-Cyclopentylidenedioxy-9α-fluoro-11β,21-dihydroxypregna-1,4-diene-3,20-dione 21-acetate.

$C_{28}H_{35}FO_7$ = 502.6.
CAS — 51022-69-6.
Pharmacopoeias. In US.

Amcinonide is a corticosteroid used topically for its glucocorticoid activity (p.1010) in the treatment of various skin disorders. It is usually employed as a cream, lotion, or ointment containing 0.1%.

When applied topically, particularly to large areas, when the skin is broken, or under occlusive dressings, corticosteroids may be absorbed in sufficient amounts to cause systemic effects (p.1010). The effects of topical corticosteroids on the skin are described on p.1012.

Skin disorders. For recommendations concerning the correct use of corticosteroids on the skin, and a rough guide to the clinical potencies of topical corticosteroids, see Corticosteroids, Administration, p.1017.

Preparations

USP 23: Amcinonide Cream; Amcinonide Ointment.

Proprietary Preparations (details are given in Part 3)
Belg.: Amicla; Cycloderm†; *Canad.:* Cyclocort; *Fr.:* Penticort; *Ger.:* Amciderm; *Ital.:* Amcinil; Penticort†; *Neth.:* Amicla†; *USA:* Cyclocort.
Multi-ingredient: *Fr.:* Penticort Neomycine.

Beclomethasone Dipropionate

(1062-y)

Beclomethasone Dipropionate *(BANM, USAN)*.

Beclometasone Dipropionate *(rINNM)*; Beclometasoni Dipropionas; 9α-Chloro-16β-methylprednisolone Dipropionate; Sch-18020W. 9α-Chloro-11β,17α,21-trihydroxy-16β-methylpregna-1,4-diene-3,20-dione 17,21-dipropionate.

$C_{28}H_{37}ClO_7$ = 521.0.
CAS — 4419-39-0 (beclomethasone); 5534-09-8 (beclomethasone dipropionate).

Pharmacopoeias. In *Chin., Eur.* (see p.viii), *Int.*, and *Jpn.*
US allows either the anhydrous or monohydrate form. *Br.* includes a separate monograph for the monohydrate.

A white to creamy-white odourless crystalline powder. Ph. Eur. **solubilities** are: practically insoluble in water; freely soluble in acetone; sparingly soluble in alcohol. (The BP states that the monohydrate has similar solubilities but is also freely soluble in chloroform.) USP solubilities are: very slightly soluble in water; very soluble in chloroform; freely soluble in acetone and in alcohol. **Protect** from light.

Adverse Effects, Treatment, Withdrawal, and Precautions

As for corticosteroids in general (p.1010).

Adrenal suppression may occur in some patients treated with high-dose long-term inhalation therapy for asthma. It has been stated that in the majority of patients no significant suppression is likely to occur when total daily doses of less than 1.5 mg are employed (but see under Adrenal Suppression, below).

When applied topically, particularly to large areas, when the skin is broken, or under occlusive dressings, corticosteroids may be absorbed in sufficient amounts to cause systemic effects.

Adrenal suppression. The problem of adrenal suppression with corticosteroids is discussed on p.1011. Listed below are some references and correspondence concerning adrenal suppression due to beclomethasone inhalation therapy,[1-9] in some cases occurring with doses below 1.5 mg daily.[7] However, one study found that function of the hypothalamic-pituitary-adrenal axis remained normal in most patients at beclomethasone doses below 3 mg daily.[10]

1. Grant IWB, Crompton GK. Becloforte inhaler. *Br Med J* 1983; **286:** 644–5.
2. Slessor IM. Becloforte inhaler. *Br Med J* 1983; **286:** 645.
3. Ebden P, Davies BH. High-dose corticosteroid inhalers for asthma. *Lancet* 1984; **ii:** 576.
4. Law CM, *et al.* Nocturnal adrenal suppression in asthmatic children taking inhaled beclomethasone dipropionate. *Lancet* 1986; **i:** 942–4.
5. Brown HM. Nocturnal adrenal suppression in children inhaling beclomethasone dipropionate. *Lancet* 1986; **i:** 1269.
6. Littlewood JM, *et al.* Growth retardation in asthmatic children treated with inhaled beclomethasone dipropionate. *Lancet* 1988; **i:** 115–16.
7. Maxwell DL, Webb J. Adverse effects of inhaled corticosteroids. *Br Med J* 1989; **298:** 827–8.
8. Priftis K, *et al.* Adrenal function in asthma. *Arch Dis Child* 1990; **65:** 838–40.
9. Tabachnik E, Zadik Z. Diurnal cortisol secretion during therapy with inhaled beclomethasone dipropionate in children with asthma. *J Pediatr* 1991; **118:** 294–7.
10. Brown PH, *et al.* Large volume spacer devices and the influence of high dose beclomethasone dipropionate on hypothalamo-pituitary-adrenal axis function. *Thorax* 1993; **48:** 233–8.

Candidiasis. Results of a study involving 229 asthmatic children indicated that the presence of a sore throat or a hoarse voice was not related to the presence of *Candida* or to treatment with inhaled beclomethasone.[1] The occurrence of only one clinical case of oral candidiasis in 129 of the children receiving beclomethasone confirmed previous observations that it is an uncommon finding in children compared with the reported incidence of between 4.5 and 13% in adults. The incidence of colonisation with *Candida* was greater in those children who received steroids than in those who did not but was not affected by either the dose used or type of inhaler employed.

1. Shaw NJ, Edmunds AT. Inhaled beclomethasone and oral candidiasis. *Arch Dis Child* 1986; **61:** 788–90.

Effects on the bones. The adverse effects of corticosteroids in general on bones are discussed on p.1011.

Studies in healthy subjects have shown that beclomethasone dipropionate can suppress bone metabolism.[1-3] High-dose inhalation therapy (2000 μg daily) for 2 weeks resulted in a decrease in serum-osteocalcin concentrations.[1] Continuation of treatment for 4 weeks produced a more marked decrease in bone metabolism (using serum alkaline phosphatase activity and urinary hydroxyproline-creatinine ratio as markers).[2] Doses ranging from 400 to 2000 μg daily also decreased serum osteocalcin, with a dose-dependent effect up to 1400 μg daily.[3] Another study found that markers of collagen turnover, but not osteocalcin, were reduced by beclomethasone or budesonide 800 μg daily in mildly asthmatic children.[4] Results are difficult to interpret since osteocalcin concentrations are reduced in patients with asthma regardless of treatment,[5] and it is uncertain whether bone loss does occur in practice; one study in children found no evidence of reduced bone mineralisation or increased resorption,[5] whereas another noted reduced leg growth after beclomethasone but not after fluticasone.[6]

1. Pouw EM, *et al.* Beclomethasone inhalation decreases serum osteocalcin concentrations. *Br Med J* 1991; **302:** 627–8.
2. Ali N, *et al.* Beclomethasone and osteocalcin. *Br Med J* 1991; **302:** 1080.
3. Teelucksingh S, *et al.* Inhaled corticosteroids, bone formation and osteocalcin. *Lancet* 1991; **338:** 60–1.
4. Birkebæk NH, *et al.* Bone and collagen turnover during treatment with inhaled dry powder budesonide and beclomethasone dipropionate. *Arch Dis Child* 1995; **73:** 524–7.
5. König P, *et al.* Bone metabolism in children with asthma treated with inhaled beclomethasone dipropionate. *J Pediatr* 1993; **122:** 219–26.
6. Wolthers OD, Pedersen S. Short term growth during treatment with inhaled fluticasone propionate and beclomethasone dipropionate. *Arch Dis Child* 1993; **68:** 673–6.

Effects on the lungs. References to the development of pulmonary eosinophilia in patients treated with inhaled beclomethasone.

1. Paterson IC, *et al.* Pulmonary eosinophilia after substitution of aerosol for oral corticosteroid therapy. *Br J Dis Chest* 1975; **69:** 217–22.
2. Hudgel DW, Spector SL. Pulmonary infiltration with eosinophilia: recurrence in an asthmatic patient treated with beclomethasone dipropionate. *Chest* 1977; **72:** 359–60.
3. Klotz LR, *et al.* The use of beclomethasone dipropionate inhaler complicated by the development of an eosinophilic pneumonia reaction. *Ann Allergy* 1977; **39:** 133–6.
4. Mollura JL, *et al.* Pulmonary eosinophilia in a patient receiving beclomethasone dipropionate aerosol. *Ann Allergy* 1979; **42:** 326–9.

Hypersensitivity. Reports of asthmatic responses to beclomethasone dipropionate inhalations, possibly associated with materials used in their formulation, or with the containers.

1. Maddern PJ, *et al.* Adverse reaction after aerosol inhalation. *Med J Aust* 1978; **1:** 274.
2. Godin J, Malo JL. Acute bronchoconstriction caused by Beclovent and not Vanceril. *Clin Allergy* 1979; **9:** 585–9.
3. Clark RJ. Exacerbation of asthma after nebulised beclomethasone dipropionate. *Lancet* 1986; **ii:** 574–5.
4. Beasley R, *et al.* Benzalkonium chloride and bronchoconstriction. *Lancet* 1986; **ii:** 1227.

Reformulation. Reformulation of some metered-dose inhalers to use a chlorofluorocarbon (CFC)-free propellant has resulted in a change of efficacy: one CFC-free product is reported to be effective at approximately half the dose[1] required with the standard product (see Uses and Administration, below). However, this dose reduction may not apply to all CFC-free formulations of beclomethasone.

1. Davies RJ, Donnell D. HFA-beclomethasone (BDP) extrafine aerosol improves therapeutic index. *Thorax* 1997; **52** (suppl 6): A58.

Interactions

The interactions of corticosteroids in general are described on p.1014.

Pharmacokinetics

For a brief outline of the pharmacokinetics of corticosteroids, see p.1014. Beclomethasone is stated to be readily absorbed from sites of local application, and rapidly distributed to all body tissues. It is metabolised principally in the liver, but also in other tissues including gastro-intestinal tract and lung; enzymatic hydrolysis rapidly produces the monopropionate (which has some glucocorticoid activity), and, more slowly, the free alcohol, which is virtually devoid of activity. Only a small proportion of an absorbed dose is excreted in urine, the remainder being excreted in the faeces mainly as metabolites.

Uses and Administration

Beclomethasone dipropionate is a corticosteroid with mainly glucocorticoid activity (p.1010) that is stated to exert a topical effect on the lungs without significant systemic activity at recommended doses (but see under Adrenal Suppression in Adverse Effects, above). It is used by inhalation, generally from a metered-dose aerosol, for the prophylaxis of the symptoms of asthma (see below).

In the UK the adult dosage of the **conventional aerosol** is usually 400 μg daily, inhaled in 2 to 4 divided doses for maintenance treatment; if necessary, 600 to 800 μg may be inhaled daily initially, subsequently adjusted according to the patient's response. In patients with severe asthma or in those showing only a partial response to standard inhalation doses, high-dose inhalation therapy may be considered; doses of 1 mg daily (250 μg four times daily or 500 μg twice daily) may be used and may be increased to 1.5 to 2 mg daily (500 μg three or four times daily) if necessary; a maximum of 2 mg daily should not be exceeded. In children, 50 or 100 μg may be inhaled 2 to 4 times daily according to the response or alternatively, 100 or 200 μg may be inhaled twice daily.

Although beclomethasone dipropionate is generally inhaled in aerosol form, inhalation capsules or disks containing **powder for inhalation** are available for patients who experience difficulty in using the aerosol. Owing to differences in the relative bioavailability to the lungs of the preparations a 100-μg dose from an inhalation capsule or disk is approximately equivalent in activity to a 50-μg dose from a conventional aerosol. Recommended maintenance doses of beclomethasone dipropionate from inhalation capsules or disks are therefore 200 μg inhaled 3 or 4 times daily or 400 μg inhaled twice daily for adults, and 100 μg inhaled 2 to 4 times daily or 200 μg inhaled twice daily for children. Up to 800 μg twice daily may be inhaled if necessary in adults requiring high-dose therapy.

In some countries beclomethasone dipropionate is now available as a **CFC-free aerosol**. Because of changes in formulation, the dose required from such inhalers may be *lower* than that from a conventional aerosol: typical UK doses range from 100 to 200 μg daily in mild asthma to 400 to 800 μg daily in severe asthma, given as 2 divided doses.

Inhalation of **nebulised** beclomethasone dipropionate has also been used in the management of asthma in children.

Beclomethasone dipropionate is also used as a **nasal spray** in the prophylaxis and treatment of allergic and non-allergic rhinitis (p.400). Usual doses are 100 μg in each nostril twice daily or 50 μg in each nostril 3 or 4 times daily; a total of 400 μg daily should not generally be exceeded. The nasal spray is also used in the prevention of recurrence of nasal polyps following surgical removal (p.1025).

Beclomethasone dipropionate is also used **topically** in the treatment of various skin disorders. It is generally applied as a cream or ointment containing 0.025%. Beclomethasone salicylate has also been used topically.

Adenoidal hypertrophy. Although normally managed by surgery (or if less severe simply by symptomatic relief) adenoidal hypertrophy in children was reported to respond to aqueous nasal beclomethasone 336 μg daily in an 8-week crossover study.[1] Improvements in adenoidal obstruction and symptom scores were enhanced in a subsequent 16-week follow-on study using 168 μg daily.

1. Demain JG, Goetz DW. Pediatric adenoidal hypertrophy and nasal airway obstruction: reduction with aqueous nasal beclomethasone. *Pediatrics* 1995; **95:** 355–64.

Asthma. Corticosteroids, together with the beta$_2$-adrenoceptor agonists, form one of the cornerstones of the management of asthma (p.745). Patients requiring only occasional relief from symptoms may be managed with an inhaled short-acting beta$_2$ agonist, and an inhaled corticosteroid such as beclomethasone is added if symptomatic relief is needed more than once daily. The dose of inhaled corticosteroid is increased in more severe asthma, often together with the addition of other agents.

The use of high-dose beclomethasone dipropionate inhalation therapy in the control of asthma symptoms has been regarded as having the advantages of controlling asthma not responsive to lower doses and allowing reduction or avoidance of systemic corticosteroid treatment.[1-3] The inhalation of beclomethasone dipropionate as a nebulised solution has been found to be useful in the management of severe asthma in children aged 2 years or under previously unresponsive to other drugs.[4] Also nebulised beclomethasone dipropionate was found to be effective in the management of recurrent episodes of bronchopulmonary obstruction following bronchiolitis in children under 2 years of age.[5] However, there have been less encouraging reports wherein nebulised beclomethasone dipropionate, although more effective than saline in preschool children, produced a response less than that usually observed with inhalation of beclomethasone from an aerosol or capsules,[6] or no benefit at all was seen.[7] This may have been due to beclomethasone somehow failing to reach the lungs.[8] In preschool children able to use a spacer device with a metered aerosol, intermittent therapy with high-dose beclomethasone dipropionate, administered at the first sign of symptoms, was beneficial in modifying the severity of acute episodic asthma.[9]

High-dose regimens may pose problems of compliance if beclomethasone must be inhaled several times daily. However, one study[10] has indicated that once-daily inhalation was as effective as the same dose divided into 2 daily inhalations in short-term control of moderate asthma. Also there are doubts that increasing the dose of inhaled beclomethasone brings about increased benefits.[11]

Beclomethasone dipropionate has been used successfully with salbutamol in the management of asthma. A metered aerosol containing both these agents might be useful in patients unable to cope with two separate inhalers although it has the disadvantage that the fixed ratio of the two components prevents flexible dosage adjustment required for individual patients.[12]

1. Anonymous. High-dose corticosteroid inhalers for asthma. *Lancet* 1984; **ii:** 23.
2. Anonymous. Inhaled corticosteroids: are higher doses better? *Drug Ther Bull* 1986; **24:** 1–2.
3. Cox JM, Mowers RM. Beclomethasone dipropionate in chronic asthma. *DICP Ann Pharmacother* 1989; **23:** 597–8.
4. Pedersen W, Prahl P. Jet-nebulized beclomethasone dipropionate in the management of bronchial asthma: topical steroids for asthmatic children younger than 4 years. *Allergy* 1987; **42:** 272–5.
5. Carlsen KH, *et al.* Nebulised beclomethasone dipropionate in recurrent obstructive episodes after acute bronchiolitis. *Arch Dis Child* 1988; **63:** 1428–33.
6. Storr J, *et al.* Nebulised beclomethasone dipropionate in preschool asthma. *Arch Dis Child* 1986; **61:** 270–3.
7. Webb MSC, *et al.* Nebulised beclomethasone dipropionate suspension. *Arch Dis Child* 1986; **61:** 1108–10.
8. Clarke SW. Nebulised beclomethasone dipropionate suspension: commentary. *Arch Dis Child* 1986; **61:** 1110.
9. Wilson NM, Silverman M. Treatment of acute, episodic asthma in preschool children using intermittent high dose inhaled steroids at home. *Arch Dis Child* 1990; **65:** 407–10.
10. Gagnon M, *et al.* Comparative safety and efficacy of single or twice daily administration of inhaled beclomethasone in moderate asthma. *Chest* 1994; **105:** 1732–7.
11. Boe J, *et al.* High-dose inhaled steroids in asthmatics: moderate efficacy gain and suppression of the hypothalamic-pituitary-adrenal axis. *Eur Respir J* 1994; **7:** 2179–84.
12. Anonymous. Ventide—a useful combination? *Drug Ther Bull* 1986; **24:** 13.

Cough. In children with recurrent cough (p.1052) inhalation of beclomethasone 200 μg twice daily from a conventional aerosol or salbutamol 200 μg twice daily had no effect on cough frequency or severity.[1]

1. Chang AB, *et al.* A randomised, placebo controlled trial of inhaled salbutamol and beclomethasone for recurrent cough. *Arch Dis Child* 1998; **79:** 6–11.

Inflammatory bowel disease. Beclomethasone 0.5 mg administered nightly as an enema was as effective as betamethasone 5 mg enemas in the treatment of acute attacks of distal ulcerative colitis.[1] Although betamethasone produced slightly superior histological improvement and faster disappearance of blood from the stools, systemic adverse effects observed with betamethasone therapy were absent in patients treated with beclomethasone.

For a review of the management of inflammatory bowel disease, including the role of corticosteroids, see p.1171.

1. Halpern Z, *et al.* A controlled trial of beclomethasone versus betamethasone enemas in distal ulcerative colitis. *J Clin Gastroenterol* 1991; **13:** 38–41.

Skin disorders. For recommendations concerning the correct use of corticosteroids on the skin, and a rough guide to the clinical potencies of topical corticosteroids, see Corticosteroids, Administration, p.1017.

Preparations

BP 1998: Beclometasone Cream; Beclometasone Nasal Spray; Beclometasone Ointment; Beclometasone Pressurised Inhalation.

Proprietary Preparations (details are given in Part 3)
Aust.: Beconase; Becotide; ***Austral.:*** Aldecin; Becloforte; Beconase AQ; Beconase†; Becotide; Respocort; ***Belg.:*** Aldecin; Beconase; Becotide; ***Canad.:*** Beclodisk; Becloforte; Beclovent; Beconase; Gen-Beclo; Propaderm; Vancenase; Vanceril; ***Fr.:*** Aldecine†; Beclojet; Beconase; Becotide; Prolair; Spir; ***Ger.:*** AerOBec; Beclomet; Beclorhinol; Becloturmant; Beconase Aquosum; Beconase†; Bronchocort; Sanasthmax; Sanasthmyl; Viarox; ***Irl.:*** AeroBec; Becodisks; Beconase; Becotide; ***Ital.:*** Becotide; Becotide A; Bronco-Turbinal; Cleniderm; Clenil; Menaderm Simplex; Propaderm†; Rino Clenil; Turbinal; ***Neth.:*** AeroBec; Aldecin†; Becloforte; Beconase; Becotide; Clenil†; Rino Clenil†; Viarin†; ***Norw.:*** Becotide; Viarox†; ***S.Afr.:*** AeroBec; Beceze; Beclate; Becloforte; Becodisks; Beconase; Becotide; Clenil; Propaderm†; Rinaze; Ventnaze; Ventzone; Viarox; ***Spain:*** Beclo Asma; Beclo Rino; Becloforte; Beclosona; Beconase; Becotide; Betsuril; Broncivent; Decasona; Dereme; Dermisone Beclo; Menaderm Simple; Novahaler; ***Swed.:*** Becotide; ***Switz.:*** Aldecin; Becloforte; Becodisk; Beconase†; Beconasol; Becotide; ***UK:*** AeroBec; Asmabec; Beceze; Beclazone; Beclo Aqua; Becloforte; Becodisks; Beconase; Becotide; Filair; Nasal Spray for Hayfever; Nasal-Bec; Nasobec; Propaderm; Qvar; Zonivent; ***USA:*** Beclovent; Beconase; Beconase AQ; Vancenase; Vanceril.

Multi-ingredient: ***Aust.:*** Duospirel; Ventide; ***Canad.:*** Propaderm-C†; ***Fr.:*** Ventide†; ***Ital.:*** Clenil Compositum; Menaderm; Recto Menaderm†; Ventolin Flogo; ***S.Afr.:*** Propaderm-C†; ***Spain:*** Aerosoma†; Butosol; Menaderm; Menaderm Clio; Menaderm Otologico; Recto Menaderm; Venoflavan†; ***Switz.:*** Beclonarin; Ventolin plus†; ***UK:*** Ventide.

Bendacort (6589-z)

AF-2071; Cortazac; Hydrocortisone Bendazac.
$C_{37}H_{42}N_2O_7$ = 626.7.
CAS — 53716-43-1.

Bendacort is the 21-ester of hydrocortisone with bendazac (p.21). It has been applied topically in the management of various skin disorders as a 3% cream or ointment.

Skin disorders. For recommendations concerning the correct use of corticosteroids on the skin, see Corticosteroids, Administration, p.1017.

Preparations

Proprietary Preparations (details are given in Part 3)
Ital.: Versacort†.

Betamethasone (1063-j)

Betamethasone *(BAN, USAN, rINN).*

Betadexamethasone; Betamethasonum; Flubenisolone; Flubenisolonum; 9α-Fluoro-16β-methylprednisolone; β-Methasone; NSC-39470; Sch-4831. 9α-Fluoro-11β,17α,21-trihydroxy-16β-methylpregna-1,4-diene-3,20-dione.
$C_{22}H_{29}FO_5$ = 392.5.
CAS — 378-44-9.

Pharmacopoeias. In *Chin.*, *Eur.* (see p.viii), *Int.*, *Jpn*, and *US.*

A white to practically white, odourless crystalline powder. Ph. Eur. states that it is practically **insoluble** in water (USP has soluble 1 in 5300 of water); soluble 1 in 65 of alcohol, 1 in 15 of warm alcohol, 1 in 325 of chloroform, and 1 in 3 of methyl alcohol; sparingly soluble in acetone, in dehydrated alcohol, and in dioxan; very slightly soluble in ether and in dichloromethane. **Protect** from light.

Betamethasone Acetate (1064-z)

Betamethasone Acetate *(BANM, rINNM).*

Betamethasoni Acetas. Betamethasone 21-acetate.
$C_{24}H_{31}FO_6$ = 434.5.
CAS — 987-24-6.

Pharmacopoeias. In *Eur.* (see p.viii) and *US.*

A white to creamy-white odourless crystalline powder. It shows polymorphism. Betamethasone acetate 1.1 mg is approximately equivalent to 1 mg of betamethasone. Ph. Eur. states that it is practically insoluble in water (USP has soluble 1 in 2000 of water); soluble 1 in 9 of alcohol, and 1 in 16 of chloroform; freely soluble in acetone; soluble in dichloromethane. **Store** in airtight containers. Protect from light.

Betamethasone Benzoate (1065-c)

Betamethasone Benzoate *(BANM, USAN, rINNM).*

W-5975. Betamethasone 17α-benzoate.
$C_{29}H_{33}FO_6$ = 496.6.
CAS — 22298-29-9.

Pharmacopoeias. In *US.*

A white to practically white, practically odourless powder. Betamethasone benzoate 1.3 mg is approximately equivalent to 1 mg of betamethasone. Practically **insoluble** in water; soluble in alcohol, in chloroform, and in methyl alcohol. **Store** in airtight containers.

Betamethasone Dipropionate (1066-k)

Betamethasone Dipropionate *(BANM, USAN, rINNM).*

Betamethasoni Dipropionas; Sch-11460. Betamethasone 17α,21-dipropionate.
$C_{28}H_{37}FO_7$ = 504.6.
CAS — 5593-20-4.

NOTE. Compounded preparations of clotrimazole and betamethasone dipropionate in USP 23 may be represented by the name Co-climasone.

Pharmacopoeias. In *Eur.* (see p.viii), *Jpn*, and *US.*

A white or creamy-white odourless crystalline powder. Betamethasone dipropionate 1.3 mg is approximately equivalent to 1 mg of betamethasone. Practically **insoluble** in water; sparingly soluble in alcohol; freely soluble in acetone, in dichloromethane, and in chloroform. **Protect** from light.

Betamethasone Sodium Phosphate (1067-a)

Betamethasone Sodium Phosphate *(BANM, rINNM).*

Betamethasone Disodium Phosphate; Betamethasoni Natrii Phosphas. Betamethasone 21-(disodium phosphate).
$C_{22}H_{28}FNa_2O_8P$ = 516.4.
CAS — 360-63-4 (betamethasone phosphate); 151-73-5 (betamethasone sodium phosphate).

NOTE. BET is a code approved by the BP for use on single unit doses of eye drops containing betamethasone sodium phosphate where the individual container may be too small to bear all the appropriate labelling information.

Pharmacopoeias. In *Eur.* (see p.viii), *Jpn*, and *US.*

A white or almost white, odourless, very hygroscopic powder. Betamethasone sodium phosphate 1.3 mg is approximately equivalent to 1 mg of betamethasone.

Soluble 1 in 2 of water, 1 in 470 of alcohol; freely soluble in methyl alcohol; practically insoluble in acetone, in chloroform, in dichloromethane, and in ether. A 1% solution in water has a pH of 7.5 to 9.0. **Store** in airtight containers. Protect from light.

Betamethasone Valerate (1068-t)

Betamethasone Valerate *(BANM, USAN, rINNM).*

Betamethasoni Valeras. Betamethasone 17α-valerate.
$C_{27}H_{37}FO_6$ = 476.6.
CAS — 2152-44-5.

Pharmacopoeias. In *Eur.* (see p.viii), *Int.*, *Jpn*, and *US.*

A white to almost-white, odourless crystalline powder. Betamethasone valerate 1.2 mg is approximately equivalent to 1 mg of betamethasone.

Practically **insoluble** in water; soluble 1 in 16 of alcohol, 1 in less than 10 of chloroform, and 1 in 400 of ether; freely soluble in acetone and in dichloromethane. **Store** in airtight containers. Protect from light.

Adverse Effects, Treatment, Withdrawal, and Precautions

As for corticosteroids in general (see p.1010).

The effects of betamethasone on sodium and water retention are less than those of prednisolone or prednisone and approximately equal to those of dexamethasone.

When applied topically, particularly to large areas, when the skin is broken, or under occlusive dressings, corticosteroids may be absorbed in sufficient amounts to cause systemic effects.

Anosmia. A report of anosmia occurring in two patients following the use of nasal drops containing betamethasone and neomycin sulphate.[1] The anosmia was complete and, in one patient, showed no sign of resolving one year later. The reaction was thought to be due to thiomersal present in the drops as a preservative, although it was noted that neomycin could exert a toxic effect on the olfactory mucosa and that there have been several reports of anosmia associated with the use of betamethasone alone.

1. Whittet HB, *et al.* Anosmia due to nasal administration of corticosteroid. *Br Med J* 1991; **303:** 651.

Interactions

The interactions of corticosteroids in general are described on p.1014.

Pharmacokinetics

For a brief outline of the pharmacokinetics of corticosteroids, see p.1014.

Uses and Administration

Betamethasone is a corticosteroid with mainly glucocorticoid activity, as described under Corticosteroids, p.1010; 750 µg of betamethasone is equivalent in anti-inflammatory activity to about 5 mg of prednisolone. It has been used, either in the form of the free alcohol or in one of the esterified forms, in the treatment of conditions for which corticosteroid therapy is indicated (p.1015), except adrenal-deficiency states for which hydrocortisone with supplementary fludrocortisone is preferred. Its virtual lack of mineralocorticoid properties makes betamethasone particularly suitable for treating conditions in which water retention would be a disadvantage.

For administration by mouth betamethasone or betamethasone sodium phosphate is used; the usual dose, expressed in terms of betamethasone, ranges from 0.5 to 5 mg daily.

For parenteral administration the sodium phosphate ester may be given intravenously by injection or infusion or intramuscularly by injection in doses equivalent to 4 to 20 mg of betamethasone. It may also be given by local injection into soft tissues in doses equivalent to 4 to 8 mg of betamethasone. Suggested doses in children, as a slow intravenous injection, are, in infants aged up to 1 year the equivalent of 1 mg of betamethasone; children aged 1 to 5 years, 2 mg; 6 to 12 years, 4 mg. Doses may be repeated 3 or 4 times in 24 hours if necessary, depending on the condition being treated and the clinical response. The sodium phosphate ester is also sometimes used in conjunction with the acetate or dipropionate esters, which have a slower and more prolonged action.

Betamethasone sodium phosphate is also used in the topical treatment of allergic and inflammatory conditions of the eyes, ears, or nose, usually as drops or ointment containing 0.1%.

For topical application in the treatment of various skin disorders the benzoate, dipropionate, and valerate esters of betamethasone are extensively used; the usual concentrations available are 0.025% of betamethasone benzoate, 0.05% of betamethasone dipropionate, and 0.025 or 0.1% of betamethasone valerate.

Betamethasone valerate has also been used by inhalation for the prophylaxis of the symptoms of asthma.

Other esters of betamethasone which have occasionally been used include the butyrate propionate, phosphate, salicylate (cortobenzolone), and valeroacetate.

Betamethasone adamantoate has been used in veterinary practice.

Inflammatory bowel disease. For a comparison of betamethasone and beclomethasone enemas in the treatment of ulcerative colitis, see under Beclomethasone, p.1033. Corticosteroids are one of the mainstays of treatment of inflammatory bowel disease, the general management of which is discussed on p.1171.

Skin disorders. For recommendations concerning the correct use of corticosteroids on the skin, and a rough guide to the clinical potencies of topical corticosteroids, see Corticosteroids, Administration, p.1017.

PSORIASIS. A comparative multicentre study of calcipotriol 0.005% and betamethasone valerate 0.1% solutions in patients with psoriasis of the scalp found the corticosteroid to be markedly more effective.[1] However, a comparison of calcipotriol and betamethasone valerate creams (0.005% and 0.1% respectively) in chronic plaque psoriasis of the body found no difference in effectiveness.[2] The indications for topical corticosteroids in psoriasis are generally considered to be limited by dermatologists in the UK, because of the adverse effects, a point made in the discussion of psoriasis and its treatment on p.1075.

1. Klaber MR, *et al.* Comparative effects of calcipotriol solution (50 µg/ml) and betamethasone 17-valerate (1 mg/ml) in the treatment of scalp psoriasis. *Br J Dermatol* 1994; **131:** 678–83.
2. Molin L, *et al.* Comparative efficacy of calcipotriol (MC 903) cream and betamethasone 17-valerate cream in the treatment of chronic plaque psoriasis: a randomized, double-blind, parallel group multicentre study. *Br J Dermatol* 1997; **136:** 89–93.

Preparations

BP 1998: Betamethasone and Clioquinol Cream; Betamethasone and Clioquinol Ointment; Betamethasone Eye Drops; Betamethasone Injection; Betamethasone Sodium Phosphate Tablets; Betamethasone Tablets; Betamethasone Valerate Cream; Betamethasone Valerate Lotion; Betamethasone Valerate Ointment; Betamethasone Valerate Scalp Application;
USP 23: Betamethasone Benzoate Gel; Betamethasone Cream; Betamethasone Dipropionate Cream; Betamethasone Dipropionate Lotion; Betamethasone Dipropionate Ointment; Betamethasone Dipropionate Topical Aerosol; Betamethasone Sodium Phosphate and Betamethasone Acetate Injectable Suspension; Betamethasone Sodium Phosphate Injection; Betamethasone Syrup; Betamethasone Tablets; Betamethasone Valerate Cream; Betamethasone Valerate Lotion; Betamethasone Valerate Ointment; Clotrimazole and Betamethasone Dipropionate Cream.

Proprietary Preparations (details are given in Part 3)

Aust.: Betnesol; Betnovate; Celestan; Diproderm; Diproforte; Diprophos; Solu-Celestan; ***Austral.:*** Betnovate; Celestone Chronodose; Celestone M; Celestone V; Celestone†; Diprosone; ***Belg.:*** Betnelan-V; Betnesol; Celestone; Celestone Chronodose; Diprolene; Diprosone; ***Canad.:*** Beben; Betacort; Betaderm; Betnesol; Betnovate; Celestoderm; Celestone; Celestone Soluspan; Diprolene Glycol; Diprosone; Ectosone; Occlucort; Prevex B; Rholosone†; Rhoprolene†; Rhoprosone†; Rivasone; Rolene; Rosone; Taro-Sone; Topilene; Topisone; Valisone; ***Fr.:*** Betnesol; Betneval; Celestene; Celestene Chronodose; Celestoderm; Diprolene; Diprosone; ***Ger.:*** Beta-Stulln; Betacort†; BetaCreme; Betagalen; Betam-Ophtal; BetaSalbe; Betnesol; Betnesol-V; Betnesol-WL†; Betnesol†; Celestamine N; Celestan solubile; Celestan-V; Celestan†; Cordes Beta; Diprosis; Diprosone; durabetason†; Euvaderm; ***Irl.:*** Betacap; Betnelan; Betnesol; Betnovate; Diprosone; ***Ital.:*** Beben; Bedermin†; Bentelan; Beta 21; Celestoderm-V; Celestone; Celestone Cronodose; Diprosone; Ecoval; Minisone†; P 10†; Paucisone†; ***Neth.:*** Betnelan; Betnesol; Celestoderm; Celestone; Celestone Chronodose; Diprolene; Diprosone; ***Norw.:*** Betnovat; Betoid; Celeston†; ***S.Afr.:*** Betnelan†; Betnesol; Betnovate; Celestoderm-V; Celestone; Celestone Soluspan; Diprolene; Diprosone; Lenasone; Lenovate; Persivate; Steromien; Topivate; ***Spain:*** Betamatil; Betnovate; Celestoderm; Celestoderm-V; Celestone; Celestone Cronodose; Diproderm; Tuplix†; ***Swed.:*** Betapred; Betnovat; Betoid; Celeston; Celeston valerat; Celeston†; Diproderm; ***Switz.:*** Betnesol; Betnovate; Celestoderm-V; Celestone; Celestone Chronodose; Diprolene; Diprosone; ***UK:*** Betacap; Betnelan; Betnesol; Betnovate; Betnovate RD (Ready Diluted); Bettamousse; Diprosone; Vista-Methasone; ***USA:*** Alphatrex; B-S-P†; Beta-Val; Betatrex; Cel-U-Jec; Celestone; Celestone Soluspan; Diprolene; Diprosone; Maxivate; Psorion; Selestoject†; Teladar; Uticort†; Valisone.

Multi-ingredient: ***Aust.:*** Betnesol-N; Betnovate-C; Betnovate-N; Celestamin; Diprogenta; Diprosalic; ***Austral.:*** Celestone VG; ***Belg.:*** Betnelan-VC; Betnelan-VN; Celestamine-F†; Diprophos; Diprosalic; Fucicort; Garasone; Lotriderm; ***Canad.:*** Betnovate-N†; Celestone S†; Diprogen; Diprosalic; Garasone; Lotriderm; Valisone-G; ***Fr.:*** Betnesalic; Betneval-Neomycine; Celestamine; Diprosalic; Diprosept; Diprosone Neomycine; Diprostene; Gentasone; ***Ger.:*** Betadermic; Betagentam; Betamethason Plus; Betnesalic; Betnesol-VN†; Betnesol†; Celestamine; Celestan Depot; Diprogenta; Diprosalic; Diprosone Depot; durabetagent†; Euvaderm; Euvaderm N; Fenistil Plus†; Fucicort; Lotricomb; Ralena†; Sulmycin mit Celestan-V; ***Irl.:*** Betnesol-N; Betnovate-C; Betnovate-N; Diprosalic; Diprosone Duopack†; Fucibet; Lotriderm; Vista-Methasone N; ***Ital.:*** Alfaflor; Antibioticoedermin B†; Apsor; Beben Clorossina; Bentelan†; Betabioptal; Biorinil; Brumeton Colloidale S; Deltavagin; Dermatar; Diproform; Diprogenta; Diprorecto†; Diprosalic; Ecoval con Neomicina; Eubetal; Eubetal Antibiotico; Fluororinil; Gentalyn Beta; Micomplex†; Micutrin Beta; Rinojet; Stranoval; Viobeta; Visublefarite; Visumetazone Antibiotico; Visumidriatic Antiflogistico; ***Neth.:*** Betnelan Clioquinol†; Betnelan Neomycine†; Celestoderm met Garamycin†; Celestoderm met Neomycine; Celestoform; Diprosalic; ***Norw.:*** Betnovat med Chinoform; Celeston; Diprosalic; ***S.Afr.:*** Betnesol-N; Betnovate-C; Betnovate-N†; Celestamine; Celestoderm-V with Garamycin; Diprogenta; Diprosalic; Garasone†; Lotriderm; Quadriderm; ***Spain:*** Alergical; Beta Micoter; Betamatil con Neomicina; Betamida; Betartrinovo; Bronsal; Celesemine; Celestoderm Gentamicina; Celestone S; Clotrasone; Cuatroderm; Diprogenta; Diprosalic; Fucibet; Nasotic Oto; Otocusi Enzimatico†; Ramatocina†; Resorborina; Sclane; Visublefarite; ***Swed.:*** Betnovat med Chinoform; Betnovat med neomycin; Celeston bifas; Celeston valerat comp.; Celeston valerat med chinoform; Celeston valerat med gentamicin; Diprosalic; ***Switz.:*** Betnesalic; Betnovate-C; Betnovate-N; Celestamine; Diprogenta; Diprophos; Diprosalic; Fucicort; Ophtasone; Quadriderm; Triderm; ***UK:*** Betnesol-N; Betnovate Rectal Ointment; Betnovate-C; Betnovate-N; Diprosalic; Fucibet; Lotriderm; Vipsogal; Vista-Methasone N; ***USA:*** Lotrisone.

Budesonide (12463-p)

Budesonide *(BAN, USAN, rINN).*

S-1320. An epimeric mixture of the α- and β-propyl forms of 16α,17α-butylidenedioxy-11β,21-dihydroxypregna-1,4-diene-3,20-dione.

$C_{25}H_{34}O_6$ = 430.5.

CAS — 51333-22-3 (11β,16α); 51372-29-3 (11β,16α(R)); 51372-28-2 (11β,16α(S)).

Pharmacopoeias. In Eur. (see p.viii).

A white or almost white, crystalline powder. Practically **insoluble** in water; sparingly soluble in alcohol; freely soluble in dichloromethane.

Adverse Effects, Treatment, Withdrawal, and Precautions

As for corticosteroids in general (see p.1010).

Inhalation of large amounts of budesonide over a short period may produce adrenal suppression.

When applied topically, particularly to large areas, when the skin is broken, or under occlusive dressings, corticosteroids may be absorbed in sufficient amounts to cause systemic effects.

Effects on the bones. For mention of a reduction in markers of collagen turnover in mildly asthmatic children receiving budesonide by inhalation, see under Adverse Effects of Beclomethasone, p.1032.

Effects on the nervous system. Psychotic behaviour has been reported following use of inhaled budesonide.[1-3]

1. Meyboom RHB, de Graff-Breederveld N. Budesonide and psychic side effects. *Ann Intern Med* 1988; **109:** 683.
2. Lewis LD, Cochrane GM. Psychosis in a child inhaling budesonide. *Lancet* 1983; **ii:** 634.
3. Connett G, Lenney W. Inhaled budesonide and behavioural disturbances. *Lancet* 1991; **338:** 634–5.

Hypersensitivity. Contact dermatitis has been reported to topical or intranasal budesonide.[1]

1. Quintiliani R. Hypersensitivity and adverse reactions associated with the use of newer intranasal corticosteroids for allergic rhinitis. *Curr Ther Res* 1996; **57:** 478–88.

Pharmacokinetics

For a brief outline of the pharmacokinetics of corticosteroids, see p.1014. Budesonide is rapidly and almost completely absorbed following administration by mouth, but has poor systemic availability due to extensive first-pass metabolism in the liver. The major metabolites, 6-β-hydroxybudesonide and 16-α-hydroxyprednisolone have less than 1% of the glucocorticoid activity of unchanged budesonide. Budesonide is reported to have a terminal half-life of about 4 hours.

Uses and Administration

Budesonide is a corticosteroid with mainly glucocorticoid activity (p.1010). It is used by inhalation in the management of asthma (p.745), in usual doses of 400 µg daily in 2 divided doses, from a metered-dose aerosol; in severe asthma the dosage may be increased up to a total of 1.6 mg daily. Maintenance doses may be less than 400 µg daily but should not be below 200 µg daily. A suggested dose for children is 50 to 400 µg inhaled twice daily. Budesonide is also available for the management of asthma in the form of a dry powder inhaler; doses are 200 to 800 µg daily, increased to 1.6 mg daily in adults if necessary. Patients for whom administration of budesonide from a pressurised inhaler or dry powder formulation is unsatisfactory may use a nebulised solution. The usual adult dosage by this method is 1 to 2 mg inhaled twice daily. This may be increased if asthma is severe. Maintenance doses are 0.5 to 1 mg inhaled twice daily. For children between 3 months and 12 years of age, a suggested initial dose is 0.5 to 1 mg twice daily with a maintenance dose of 0.25 to 0.5 mg twice daily.

Budesonide is also given by inhalation as a nebulised solution in the management of childhood croup (p.1020). The usual dose is 2 mg, as a single inhaled dose or 2 doses of 1 mg, given 30 minutes apart.

Budesonide is used topically in the treatment of various skin disorders, as a cream or ointment containing 0.025%.

Budesonide is also used as a nasal spray for the prophylaxis and treatment of rhinitis (p.400), and in the management of nasal polyps (p.1025). It is used for rhinitis in a usual initial dose of 200 μg into each nostril once daily, subsequently reduced to the lowest dose adequate to control symptoms which may be 100 μg into each nostril daily. Alternatively, the initial dose may be 100 μg into each nostril twice daily. The latter dose is given for up to three months in the treatment of nasal polyps.

Local formulations of budesonide have been used in the management of inflammatory bowel disease (see below). It is given in active Crohn's disease in doses of 9 mg daily for up to 8 weeks, as modified-release capsules used for their topical effect on the gastro-intestinal tract. The dosage should be reduced 2 to 4 weeks before discontinuing budesonide therapy. An enema solution containing 0.002% is also available; it is administered at night for 4 weeks in the treatment of ulcerative colitis.

General references.

1. Brogden RN, McTavish D. Budesonide: an updated review of its pharmacological properties, and therapeutic efficacy in asthma and rhinitis. *Drugs* 1992; **44:** 375–407 and 1012.

Administration. INHALATIONAL ROUTE. Although budesonide is administered by nebuliser, evidence suggests that the administration device has a considerable effect on the dose actually received. One study in 6 children aged up to 30 months found that about 75% of the nominal dose was deposited in the nebuliser system,[1] while a study in 126 older children indicated that maintenance doses of budesonide could be halved when the dose was given by dry powder inhaler rather than nebuliser, without any loss of asthma control.[2] Although oropharyngeal deposition is thought to play a role in the systemic effects of inhaled corticosteroids, another study[3] indicated that only about 20% of the systemically available drug appeared to be derived from oropharyngeal deposition following inhalation from a dry powder inhaler.

1. Carlsen KCL, *et al.* How much nebulised budesonide reaches infants and toddlers? *Arch Dis Child* 1992; **67:** 1077–9.
2. Agertoft L, Pedersen S. Importance of the inhalation device on the effect of budesonide. *Arch Dis Child* 1993; **69:** 130–3.
3. Pedersen S, *et al.* The influence of orally deposited budesonide on the systemic availability of budesonide after inhalation from a Turbuhaler. *Br J Clin Pharmacol* 1993; **36:** 211–14.

Cystic fibrosis. Cystic fibrosis (p.119) is associated with bronchial hyper-responsiveness; a small study[1] has suggested that inhalation of budesonide 1600 μg daily for 6 weeks improves hyper-responsiveness slightly and leads to improvement in cough and dyspnoea.

1. Van Haren EHJ, *et al.* The effects of the inhaled corticosteroid budesonide on lung function and bronchial hyperresponsiveness in adult patients with cystic fibrosis. *Respir Med* 1995; **89:** 209–14.

Inflammatory bowel disease. Budesonide has been given as an enema for the treatment of distal ulcerative colitis, in which context its potency, high aqueous solubility, and low systemic availability are advantageous.[1,2] It is also available as a modified-release oral dosage form in the management of active Crohn's disease,[3-5,9] and has been investigated for its potential in delaying relapse in quiescent disease,[6,7,10] although any benefit appears short-term. Oral budesonide has also been tried as an alternative to conventional systemic corticosteroids in ulcerative colitis.[8]

For a discussion of inflammatory bowel disease, in which rectal and oral corticosteroid therapy is one of the mainstays of management, and the possible benefits of newer corticosteroids with low systemic bioavailability, see p.1171.

1. Sachar DB. Budesonide for inflammatory bowel disease: is it a magic bullet? *N Engl J Med* 1994; **331:** 873–4.
2. Spencer CM, McTavish D. Budesonide: a review of its pharmacological properties and therapeutic efficacy in inflammatory bowel disease. *Drugs* 1995; **50:** 854–72.
3. Greenberg GR, *et al.* Oral budesonide for active Crohn's disease. *N Engl J Med* 1994; **331:** 836–41.
4. Rutgeerts P, *et al.* A comparison of budesonide with prednisolone for active Crohn's disease. *N Engl J Med* 1994; **331:** 842–5.
5. Campieri M, *et al.* Oral budesonide is as effective as oral prednisolone in active Crohn's disease. *Gut* 1997; **41:** 209–14.
6. Greenberg GR, *et al.* Oral budesonide as maintenance treatment for Crohn's disease: a placebo-controlled dose-ranging study. *Gastroenterology* 1996; **110:** 45–51.
7. Löfberg R, *et al.* Budesonide prolongs time to relapse in ileal and ileocaecal Crohn's disease: a placebo controlled one year study. *Gut* 1996; **39:** 82–6.
8. Keller R, *et al.* Oral budesonide therapy for steroid-dependent ulcerative colitis: a pilot trial. *Aliment Pharmacol Ther* 1997; **11:** 1047–52.
9. Thomsen OØ, *et al.* A comparison of budesonide and mesalamine for active Crohn's disease. *N Engl J Med* 1998; **339:** 370–4.
10. Gross V, *et al.* Low dose oral pH modified release budesonide for maintenance of steroid induced remission in Crohn's disease. *Gut* 1998; **42:** 493–6.

Skin disorders. For recommendations concerning the correct use of corticosteroids on the skin, and a rough guide to the clinical potencies of topical corticosteroids, see Corticosteroids, Administration, p.1017.

Preparations

Proprietary Preparations (details are given in Part 3)

Aust.: Entocort; Pulmicort; Rhinocortol; ***Austral.:*** Budamax; Entocort; Pulmicort; Rhinocort; ***Belg.:*** Preferid; Pulmicort; Rhinocort; ***Canad.:*** Entocort; Pulmicort; Rhinocort; ***Fr.:*** Pulmicort; ***Ger.:*** Pulmicort; Topinasal†; ***Irl.:*** Entocort; Preferid; Pulmicort; Rhinocort; ***Ital.:*** Bidien; Preferid; Pulmaxan; ***Neth.:*** Entocort; Preferid; Pulmicort; Rhinocort; ***Norw.:*** Entocort; Preferid; Pulmicort; Rhinocort; ***S.Afr.:*** Budeflam; Entocord; Inflammide; Pulmicort; Rhinocort; ***Spain:*** Demotest; Neo Rinactive; Olfex; Pulmicort; Pulmictan; Rhinocort; Ribusol; Rinactive; ***Swed.:*** Entocort; Preferid†; Pulmicort; Rhinocort; ***Switz.:*** Entocort; Preferid; Pulmicort; Rhinocort; ***UK:*** Entocort; Preferid†; Pulmicort; Rhinocort; ***USA:*** Pulmicort; Rhinocort.

Ciprocinonide (3439-d)

Ciprocinonide (*USAN, rINN*).

RS-2386. (6α,11β,16α)-21-[(cyclopropylcarbonyl)oxy]-6,9-difluoro-11-hydroxy-16,17-[(1-methylethylidene)-bis(oxy)]-pregna-1,4-diene-3,20-dione.

$C_{28}H_{34}F_2O_7$ = 520.6.

CAS — 58524-83-7.

Ciprocinonide is a derivative of fluocinolone acetonide (p.1041) which has been applied topically in combination with fluocinonide and procinonide in the management of various skin disorders.

Skin disorders. For recommendations concerning the correct use of corticosteroids on the skin, see Corticosteroids, Administration, p.1017.

Preparations

Proprietary Preparations (details are given in Part 3)

Multi-ingredient: ***Canad.:*** Trisyn.

Clobetasol Propionate (1069-x)

Clobetasol Propionate (*BANM, USAN, rINNM*).

CCI-4725; GR-2/925. 21-Chloro-9α-fluoro-11β,17α-dihydroxy-16β-methylpregna-1,4-diene-3,20-dione 17-propionate.

$C_{25}H_{32}ClFO_5$ = 467.0.

CAS — 25122-41-2 (clobetasol); 25122-46-7 (clobetasol propionate).

Pharmacopoeias. In Br. and US.

A white or almost white crystalline powder. Practically **insoluble** in water; sparingly soluble in alcohol and in dehydrated alcohol; freely soluble in acetone and in dichloromethane; soluble in methyl alcohol, in chloroform, in dimethyl sulphoxide, and in dioxan. **Store** in airtight containers. Protect from light.

Clobetasol propionate is a corticosteroid used topically for its glucocorticoid activity (p.1010) in the treatment of various skin disorders. It is usually employed as a cream, ointment, or scalp application containing 0.05%.

When applied topically, particularly to large areas, when the skin is broken, or under occlusive dressings, corticosteroids may be absorbed in sufficient amounts to cause systemic effects (p.1010). The effects of topical corticosteroids on the skin are described on p.1012.

Skin disorders. For recommendations concerning the correct use of corticosteroids on the skin, and a rough guide to the clinical potencies of topical corticosteroids, see Corticosteroids, Administration, p.1017.

Preparations

BP 1998: Clobetasol Cream; Clobetasol Ointment;
USP 23: Clobetasol Propionate Cream; Clobetasol Propionate Ointment; Clobetasol Propionate Topical Solution.

Proprietary Preparations (details are given in Part 3)

Aust.: Dermovate; ***Belg.:*** Dermovate; ***Canad.:*** Dermasone; Dermovate; ***Fr.:*** Dermoval; ***Ger.:*** Dermoxin; Dermoxinale; Karison; ***Irl.:*** Dermovate; ***Ital.:*** Clobesol; ***Neth.:*** Dermovate; ***Norw.:*** Dermovat; ***S.Afr.:*** Dermovate; Dovate; ***Spain:*** Clovate; Decloban; ***Swed.:*** Dermovat; ***Switz.:*** Dermovate; ***UK:*** Dermovate; ***USA:*** Cormax; Temovate.

Multi-ingredient: ***Switz.:*** Dermovate-NN; ***UK:*** Dermovate-NN.

Clobetasone Butyrate (1070-y)

Clobetasone Butyrate (*BANM, USAN, rINNM*).

CCI-5537; Clobetasoni Butyras; GR-2/1214. 21-Chloro-9α-fluoro-17α-hydroxy-16β-methylpregna-1,4-diene-3,11,20-trione 17-butyrate.

$C_{26}H_{32}ClFO_5$ = 479.0.

CAS — 54063-32-0 (clobetasone); 25122-57-0 (clobetasone butyrate).

Pharmacopoeias. In Eur. (see p.viii).

A white or almost white powder. Practically **insoluble** in water; slightly soluble in alcohol; freely soluble in acetone and in dichloromethane. **Protect** from light.

Clobetasone butyrate is a corticosteroid used topically for its glucocorticoid effects (p.1010) in the treatment of various skin disorders. It is usually employed as a cream or ointment containing 0.05%. It is also used for inflammatory eye disorders, as eye drops containing 0.1%.

When applied topically, particularly to large areas, when the skin is broken, or under occlusive dressings, corticosteroids may be absorbed in sufficient amounts to cause systemic effects (p.1010). The effects of topical corticosteroids on the skin are described on p.1012. Prolonged application to the eye of preparations containing corticosteroids has caused raised intra-ocular pressure and reduced visual function.

Skin disorders. For recommendations concerning the correct use of corticosteroids on the skin, and a rough guide to the clinical potencies of topical corticosteroids, see Corticosteroids, Administration, p.1017.

Preparations

BP 1998: Clobetasone Cream; Clobetasone Ointment.

Proprietary Preparations (details are given in Part 3)

Aust.: Emovate; ***Belg.:*** Eumovate; ***Canad.:*** Eumovate; ***Ger.:*** Emovate; ***Irl.:*** Eumovate; ***Ital.:*** Clobet; Eumovate; Visucloben; ***Neth.:*** Emovate; ***Norw.:*** Cloptison; ***S.Afr.:*** Eumovate; ***Spain:*** Cortoftal; Emovate; Vistaran†; ***Swed.:*** Emovat; ***Switz.:*** Cloptison; Emovate; ***UK:*** Cloburate; Eumovate.

Multi-ingredient: ***Ital.:*** Visucloben Antibiotico; Visucloben Decongestionante; ***Switz.:*** Cloptison-N; ***UK:*** Cloburate-N†; Trimovate.

Clocortolone Pivalate (12584-k)

Clocortolone Pivalate (*USAN, rINNM*).

CL-68; Clocortolone Trimethylacetate; SH-863. 9α-Chloro-6α-fluoro-11β,21-dihydroxy-16α-methylpregna-1,4-diene-3,20-dione 21-pivalate.

$C_{27}H_{36}ClFO_5$ = 495.0.

CAS — 4828-27-7 (clocortolone); 34097-16-0 (clocortolone pivalate).

Pharmacopoeias. In US.

A white to yellowish-white odourless powder. **Soluble** in acetone; freely soluble in chloroform and in dioxan; sparingly soluble in alcohol; slightly soluble in ether. **Store** in airtight containers. Protect from light.

Clocortolone pivalate is a corticosteroid used topically for its glucocorticoid activity (p.1010), as a 0.1% cream or ointment, in the treatment of various skin disorders. Clocortolone hexanoate has been used in combination with the pivalate. Clocortolone trimethylacetate is also used.

When applied topically, particularly to large areas, where the skin is broken, or under occlusive dressings, corticosteroids may be absorbed in sufficient amounts to cause systemic effects (p.1010). The effects of topical corticosteroids on the skin are described on p.1012.

Skin disorders. For recommendations concerning the correct use of corticosteroids on the skin, see Corticosteroids, Administration, p.1017.

Preparations

USP 23: Clocortolone Pivalate Cream.

Proprietary Preparations (details are given in Part 3)

Aust.: Glimbal; ***Ital.:*** Lenent†; ***USA:*** Cloderm.

Multi-ingredient: ***Ger.:*** Corto-Tavegil; Crino-Kaban N; Kaban; Kabanimat; Procto-Kaban.

Cloprednol (1071-j)

Cloprednol (*BAN, USAN, rINN*).

RS-4691. 6-Chloro-11β,17α,21-trihydroxypregna-1,4,6-triene-3,20-dione.

$C_{21}H_{25}ClO_5$ = 392.9.

CAS — 5251-34-3.

Cloprednol is a corticosteroid with mainly glucocorticoid activity (p.1010); 2.5 mg of cloprednol is equivalent in anti-inflammatory activity to about 5 mg of prednisolone. Cloprednol has been given by mouth in various disorders for which corticosteroid therapy is helpful (p.1015), in usual doses ranging from 1.25 to 12.5 mg daily.

Preparations

Proprietary Preparations (details are given in Part 3)
Ger.: Syntestan; ***Ital.:*** Cloradryn; ***Switz.:*** Novacort†.

Cortisone Acetate (1072-z)

Cortisone Acetate *(BANM, rINNM).*

Compound E Acetate; Cortisoni Acetas; 11-Dehydro-17-hydroxycorticosterone Acetate. 17α,21-Dihydroxypregn-4-ene-3,11,20-trione 21-acetate.

$C_{23}H_{30}O_6$ = 402.5.

CAS — 53-06-5 (cortisone); 50-04-4 (cortisone acetate).

Pharmacopoeias. In *Chin., Eur.* (see p.viii), *Jpn, Pol.,* and *US.*

A white or almost white, odourless, crystalline powder. It exhibits polymorphism. Practically **insoluble** in water; soluble 1 in 350 of alcohol, 1 in 75 of acetone, 1 in 4 of chloroform, and 1 in 30 of dioxan; slightly soluble in ether and in methyl alcohol; freely soluble in dichloromethane. **Protect** from light.

Adverse Effects, Treatment, Withdrawal, and Precautions

As for corticosteroids in general (see p.1010).

Interactions

The interactions of corticosteroids in general are described on p.1014.

Pharmacokinetics

For a brief outline of the pharmacokinetics of corticosteroids, see p.1014.

Cortisone acetate is readily absorbed from the gastro-intestinal tract and the cortisone is rapidly converted in the liver to its active metabolite, hydrocortisone (cortisol). The biological half-life of cortisone itself is only about 30 minutes. Absorption of cortisone acetate from intramuscular sites is considerably slower than following oral administration.

Uses and Administration

Cortisone is a corticosteroid secreted by the adrenal cortex. It has glucocorticoid activity (p.1010), as well as appreciable mineralocorticoid activity; 25 mg of cortisone acetate is equivalent in anti-inflammatory activity to about 5 mg of prednisolone.

Cortisone acetate is rapidly effective when given by mouth, and more slowly by intramuscular injection.

Cortisone acetate has been used mainly for replacement therapy in adrenocortical insufficiency (p.1017), but hydrocortisone (p.1043) is generally preferred since cortisone itself is inactive and must be converted by the liver to hydrocortisone, its active metabolite and hence, in some liver disorders the activity of cortisone is less reliable.

Cortisone acetate has been used in the treatment of many of the allergic and inflammatory disorders for which corticosteroid therapy is helpful (p.1015) but prednisolone or other synthetic glucocorticoids are generally preferred. Doses of cortisone acetate employed have generally ranged from about 25 to 300 mg daily by mouth or by intramuscular injection.

Preparations

BP 1998: Cortisone Tablets;
USP 23: Cortisone Acetate Injectable Suspension; Cortisone Acetate Tablets.

Proprietary Preparations (details are given in Part 3)
Aust.: Cortone; ***Austral.:*** Cortate; ***Belg.:*** Adreson; ***Canad.:*** Cortone; ***Irl.:*** Cortisyl†; ***Ital.:*** Cortone; ***Neth.:*** Adreson†; ***Norw.:*** Cortone; ***S.Afr.:*** Cortogen; ***Spain:*** Altesona; ***Swed.:*** Cortal; Cortone; ***UK:*** Cortelan†; Cortistab†; Cortisyl; ***USA:*** Cortone.

Multi-ingredient: ***Ital.:*** Dutimelan; ***Spain:*** Antiblefarica; Blefarida; Gingilone; ***Switz.:*** Septicortin.

Cortivazol (1073-c)

Cortivazol *(USAN, pINN).*

H-3625; MK-650; NSC-80998. 11β,17α,21-Trihydroxy-6,16α-dimethyl-2′-phenyl-2′H-pregna-2,4,6-trieno[3,2-c]pyrazol-20-one 21-acetate.

$C_{32}H_{38}N_2O_5$ = 530.7.

CAS — 1110-40-3.

Cortivazol is a corticosteroid with mainly glucocorticoid activity (p.1010); 300 μg of cortivazol is equivalent in anti-inflammatory activity to about 5 mg of prednisolone. It is given in the treatment of musculoskeletal and joint disorders by intra-articular, periarticular, or epidural injection in doses of about 1.25 to 3.75 mg, according to the size of the joint, usually at intervals of one to three weeks. It has also been given by mouth.

Preparations

Proprietary Preparations (details are given in Part 3)
Fr.: Altim.

Deflazacort (12627-l)

Deflazacort *(BAN, USAN, rINN).*

Azacort; DL-458-IT; L-5458; MDL-458; Oxazacort. 11β,21-Dihydroxy-2′-methyl-5′βH-pregna-1,4-dieno[17,16-*d*]oxazole-3,20-dione 21-acetate.

$C_{25}H_{31}NO_6$ = 441.5.

CAS — 14484-47-0.

Deflazacort is a corticosteroid with mainly glucocorticoid activity (p.1010); 6 mg of deflazacort is reportedly equivalent in anti-inflammatory activity to about 5 mg of prednisolone (but see Action, below).

Deflazacort is used for its anti-inflammatory properties in conditions responsive to corticosteroid therapy (p.1015). It is given by mouth in initial doses of up to 120 mg daily; usual maintenance doses are 3 to 18 mg daily. Doses of 0.25 to 1.5 mg per kg body-weight have been used in children.

References.

1. Elli A, *et al.* Deflazacort versus 6-methylprednisolone in renal transplantation: immunosuppressive activity and side effects. *Transplant Proc* 1990; **22:** 1689–90.
2. Gray RES, *et al.* A double-blind study of deflazacort and prednisone in patients with chronic inflammatory disorders. *Arthritis Rheum* 1991; **34:** 287–95.
3. Loftus J, *et al.* Randomized, double-blind trial of deflazacort versus prednisone in juvenile chronic (or rheumatoid) arthritis: a relatively bone-sparing effect of deflazacort. *Pediatrics* 1991; **88:** 428–36.
4. Visco G, *et al.* Prevention of side-effects of interferon. *Lancet* 1991; **337:** 741.
5. Eberhardt R, *et al.* Long-term therapy with the new glucocorticosteroid deflazacort in rheumatoid arthritis: double-blind controlled randomized 12-months study against prednisone. *Arzneimittelforschung* 1994; **44:** 642–7.
6. Ferraris JR, *et al.* Effect of therapy with a new glucocorticoid, deflazacort, on linear growth and growth hormone secretion after renal transplantation. *J Pediatr* 1992; **121:** 809–13.
7. Markham A, Bryson HM. Deflazacort: a review of its pharmacological properties and therapeutic efficacy. *Drugs* 1995; **50:** 317–33.

Action. Although it has been suggested that deflazacort produces fewer adverse effects than some conventional corticosteroids such as prednisolone, a study in healthy subjects found that the ratio of efficacy for deflazacort compared with prednisolone was higher than the 1.2 : 1 previously assumed,[1] implying that lower effective doses of deflazacort had been used in such comparisons. All systemic corticosteroids may produce clinically significant adverse reactions (see also p.1010) which are primarily dependent on dose and duration of use.

1. Babadjanova G, *et al.* Comparison of the pharmacodynamic effects of deflazacort and prednisolone in healthy subjects. *Eur J Clin Pharmacol* 1996; **51:** 53–7.

Preparations

Proprietary Preparations (details are given in Part 3)
Ger.: Calcort; ***Ital.:*** Deflan; Flantadin; ***Spain:*** Dezacor; Zamene; ***Switz.:*** Calcort; ***UK:*** Calcort.

Deoxycortone Acetate (1075-a)

Deoxycortone Acetate *(BANM).*

Desoxycortone Acetate *(rINNM)*; Cortin; Decortone Acetate; 11-Deoxycorticosterone Acetate; Desoxycorticosterone Acetate; Desoxycortoni Acetas. 21-Hydroxypregn-4-ene-3,20-dione 21-acetate.

$C_{23}H_{32}O_4$ = 372.5.

CAS — 64-85-7 (deoxycortone); 56-47-3 (deoxycortone acetate).

Pharmacopoeias. In *Eur.* (see p.viii), *Pol.,* and *US.*

Colourless crystals or white or creamy-white, odourless crystalline powder. Practically **insoluble** in water; sparingly soluble in alcohol; Ph. Eur. states that it is soluble in acetone where the USP has sparingly soluble; freely soluble in dichloromethane; sparingly soluble in dioxan; slightly soluble in propylene glycol and in vegetable oils. **Protect** from light.

Deoxycortone Pivalate (1074-k)

Deoxycortone Pivalate *(BANM).*

Desoxycortone Pivalate *(rINNM)*; Deoxycorticosterone Pivalate; Deoxycorticosterone Trimethylacetate; Deoxycortone Trimethylacetate; Desoxycorticosterone Pivalate; Desoxycorticosterone Trimethylacetate. 21-Hydroxypregn-4-ene-3,20-dione 21-pivalate.

$C_{26}H_{38}O_4$ = 414.6.

CAS — 808-48-0.

Pharmacopoeias. In *US.*

A white or creamy-white, odourless crystalline powder. **Protect** from light.

Deoxycortone is a corticosteroid secreted by the adrenal cortex and has primarily mineralocorticoid activity (p.1010). It has no significant glucocorticoid action.

Deoxycortone, as the acetate or pivalate, has been used in the treatment of adrenocortical insufficiency (p.1017) as an adjunct to cortisone or hydrocortisone. For this purpose, however, fludrocortisone given by mouth is now usually preferred.

Deoxycortone acetate is given by intramuscular injection as an oily solution, in doses of up to 10 mg once or twice daily. The pivalate has also been used, as an intramuscular depot injection every 4 weeks, and deoxycortone acetate has also been given by subcutaneous implant.

Deoxycortone has also been administered as its enanthate, phenylpropionate, and sodium hemisuccinate esters.

Preparations

USP 23: Desoxycorticosterone Acetate Injection; Desoxycorticosterone Acetate Pellets.

Proprietary Preparations (details are given in Part 3)
Aust.: Cortiron; Percorten†; ***Fr.:*** Syncortyl; ***Ital.:*** Cortiron; ***Switz.:*** Cortisteron.

Multi-ingredient: ***Ger.:*** Docabolin†; ***Ital.:*** Sinsurrene; ***Spain:*** Docabolina†.

Deprodone (6900-g)

Deprodone *(BAN, rINN).*

11β,17α-Dihydroxypregna-1,4-diene-3,20-dione.

$C_{21}H_{28}O_4$ = 344.4.

CAS — 20423-99-8 (deprodone); 20424-00-4 (deprodone propionate).

Deprodone is a corticosteroid that has been used topically as the propionate.

Desonide (1076-t)

Desonide *(BAN, USAN, rINN).*

D2083; Desfluorotriamcinolone Acetonide; 16-Hydroxyprednisolone 16,17-Acetonide; Prednacinolone Acetonide. 11β,21-Dihydroxy-16α,17α-isopropylidenedioxypregna-1,4-diene-3,20-dione.

$C_{24}H_{32}O_6$ = 416.5.

CAS — 638-94-8.

Desonide is a corticosteroid used topically for its glucocorticoid activity (p.1010) in the treatment of various skin disorders. It is usually employed as a cream or ointment containing 0.05%. The pivalate and the sodium phosphate esters have also been used.

When applied topically, particularly to large areas, when the skin is broken, or under occlusive dressings, corticosteroids may be absorbed in sufficient amounts to cause systemic effects (p.1010). The effects of topical corticosteroids on the skin are described on p.1012.

Skin disorders. For recommendations concerning the correct use of corticosteroids on the skin, and a rough guide to the clinical potencies of topical corticosteroids, see Corticosteroids, Administration, p.1017.

Preparations

Proprietary Preparations (details are given in Part 3)
Belg.: Sterax; ***Canad.:*** Desocort; Tridesilon; ***Fr.:*** Locapred; Locatop; Tridesonit; ***Ger.:*** Sterax; Topifug†; Tridesilon†; ***Ital.:*** PR 100; Prenacid; Reticus; ***Norw.:*** Apolar; ***Spain:*** Sine Fluor†; ***Swed.:*** Apolar; ***Switz.:*** Locapred; Sterax; ***USA:*** DesOwen; Tridesilon.

Multi-ingredient: ***Fr.:*** Cirkan a la Prednacinolone; ***Ital.:*** Desonix†; PR 100-Cloressidina; Reticus Antimicotico†; ***Norw.:*** Apolar med dekvalon; ***USA:*** Tridesilon†.

Desoxymethasone (1077-x)

Desoxymethasone *(BAN)*.

Desoximetasone *(USAN, rINN)*; A-41-304; HOE-304; R-2113. 9α-Fluoro-11β,21-dihydroxy-16α-methylpregna-1,4-diene-3,20-dione.

$C_{22}H_{29}FO_4$ = 376.5.

CAS — 382-67-2.

Pharmacopoeias. In *US.*

A white or almost white, odourless, crystalline powder. Practically **insoluble** in water; freely soluble in alcohol, in acetone, and in chloroform.

Desoxymethasone is a corticosteroid used topically for its glucocorticoid activity (p.1010) in the treatment of various skin disorders. It is usually employed as a cream, gel, lotion, or ointment; concentrations used range from 0.05 to 0.25%.

When applied topically, particularly to large areas, when the skin is broken, or under occlusive dressings, corticosteroids may be absorbed in sufficient amounts to cause systemic effects (p.1010). The effects of topical corticosteroids on the skin are described on p.1012.

Adverse effects. A photosensitivity reaction occurred in a patient treated for psoriasis with topical desoxymethasone; rechallenge led to a recurrence.[1] The patient was also receiving propranolol hydrochloride.

1. Stierstorfer MB, Baughman RD. Photosensitivity to desoximetasone emollient cream. *Arch Dermatol* 1988; **124:** 1870–1.

Skin disorders. For recommendations concerning the correct use of corticosteroids on the skin, and a rough guide to the clinical potencies of topical corticosteroids, see Corticosteroids, Administration, p.1017.

Preparations

USP 23: Desoximetasone Cream; Desoximetasone Gel; Desoximetasone Ointment.

Proprietary Preparations (details are given in Part 3)
Aust.: Topisolon; ***Belg.:*** Ibaril†; Topicorte; ***Canad.:*** Topicort; ***Fr.:*** Topicorte; ***Ger.:*** Topisolon; ***Irl.:*** Topisolon; ***Ital.:*** Flubason; Topicort†; ***Neth.:*** Ibaril; Topicorte; ***Norw.:*** Ibaril; ***S.Afr.:*** Topisolon†; ***Spain:*** Flubason; ***Swed.:*** Ibaril; ***Switz.:*** Topisolon; ***UK:*** Stiedex LP; Stiedex†; ***USA:*** Topicort.

Multi-ingredient: ***Aust.:*** Topisolon mit Salicylsaure; ***Fr.:*** Topifram; ***Ger.:*** Topisolon; ***Ital.:*** Topicort Composto†; ***Norw.:*** Ibaril med salicylsyre; ***Swed.:*** Ibaril med salicylsyra; ***Switz.:*** Topisalen†; ***UK:*** Stiedex.

Dexamethasone (1084-t)

Dexamethasone *(BAN, rINN)*.

Desamethasone; Dexametasone; Dexamethasonum; 9α-Fluoro-16α-methylprednisolone; Hexadecadrol. 9α-Fluoro-11β,17α,21-trihydroxy-16α-methylpregna-1,4-diene-3,20-dione.

$C_{22}H_{29}FO_5$ = 392.5.

CAS — 50-02-2.

Pharmacopoeias. In *Eur.* (see p.viii), *Int., Jpn, Pol.,* and *US.*

A white or almost white odourless crystalline powder. Practically **insoluble** in water; sparingly soluble in alcohol, in dehydrated alcohol, in acetone, in dioxan, and in methyl alcohol; slightly soluble in chloroform and in dichloromethane; very slightly soluble in ether. **Protect** from light.

Dexamethasone Acetate (1079-f)

Dexamethasone Acetate *(BANM, USAN, rINNM)*.

Dexamethasoni Acetas. Dexamethasone 21-acetate.

$C_{24}H_{31}FO_6$ = 434.5.

CAS — 1177-87-3 (anhydrous); 55812-90-3 (monohydrate).

Pharmacopoeias. In *Chin.* and *Eur.* (see p.viii).
Int. and *US* allow the anhydrous form or the monohydrate.

A white to off-white, odourless crystalline powder. It exhibits polymorphism. Dexamethasone acetate 1.1 mg is approximately equivalent to 1 mg of dexamethasone. Practically **insoluble** in water; freely soluble in acetone, in alcohol, in dioxan, and in methyl alcohol; slightly soluble in dichloromethane. **Protect** from light.

Dexamethasone Isonicotinate (1080-z)

Dexamethasone Isonicotinate *(BANM, rINNM)*.

Dexamethasone 21-isonicotinate.

$C_{28}H_{32}FNO_6$ = 497.6.

CAS — 2265-64-7.

Dexamethasone isonicotinate 1.3 mg is approximately equivalent to 1 mg of dexamethasone.

Dexamethasone Phosphate (18485-c)

Dexamethasone Phosphate *(BANM, rINNM)*.

Dexamethasone 21-(dihydrogen phosphate).

$C_{22}H_{30}FO_8P$ = 472.4.

CAS — 312-93-6.

Dexamethasone phosphate 1.2 mg is approximately equivalent to 1 mg of dexamethasone.

Dexamethasone Sodium Metasulphobenzoate (1083-a)

Dexamethasone Sodium Metasulphobenzoate *(BANM)*.

Dexamethasone Sodium Metasulfobenzoate *(rINNM)*. Dexamethasone 21-(sodium *m*-sulphobenzoate).

$C_{29}H_{32}FNaO_9S$ = 598.6.

CAS — 3936-02-5.

Dexamethasone sodium metasulphobenzoate 1.5 mg is approximately equivalent to 1 mg of dexamethasone.

Dexamethasone Sodium Phosphate (1078-r)

Dexamethasone Sodium Phosphate *(BANM, rINNM)*.

Dexamethasone Phosphate Sodium; Dexamethasoni Natrii Phosphas; Sodium Dexamethasone Phosphate. Dexamethasone 21-(disodium orthophosphate).

$C_{22}H_{28}FNa_2O_8P$ = 516.4.

CAS — 2392-39-4.

NOTE. DSP is a code approved by the BP for use on single unit doses of eye drops containing dexamethasone sodium phosphate where the individual container may be too small to bear all the appropriate labelling information.

Pharmacopoeias. In *Chin., Eur.* (see p.viii), *Int.,* and *US.*

A white or slightly yellow, very hygroscopic, crystalline powder; odourless or with a slight odour of alcohol. It exhibits polymorphism. Dexamethasone sodium phosphate 1.3 mg is approximately equivalent to 1 mg of dexamethasone and 1.1 mg of dexamethasone sodium phosphate is approximately equivalent to 1 mg of dexamethasone phosphate.

Soluble 1 in 2 of water; slightly soluble in alcohol; practically insoluble in chloroform, in dichloromethane, and in ether; very slightly soluble in dioxan. The Ph. Eur. states that a 1% solution in water has a pH of 7.5 to 9.5; the USP cites a pH of between 7.5 and 10.5. **Store** in airtight containers. Protect from light.

Adverse Effects, Treatment, Withdrawal, and Precautions

As for corticosteroids in general (see p.1010).

It has little or no effect on sodium and water retention.

When applied topically, particularly to large areas, when the skin is broken, or under occlusive dressings, corticosteroids may be absorbed in sufficient amounts to cause systemic effects.

Effects on the nerves. Paraesthesia and irritation, most commonly occurring in the anogenital region, have been associated with the intravenous administration of dexamethasone sodium phosphate[1] and hydrocortisone sodium phosphate,[2] but not with hydrocortisone sodium succinate.[2] Further comments and discussions on this topic are listed below.[3-5]

Neurological complications have occurred with corticosteroid-induced epidural lipomatosis, see p.1012.

1. Czerwinski AW, *et al.* Effects of a single, large, intravenous injection of dexamethasone. *Clin Pharmacol Ther* 1972; **13:** 638–42.
2. Novak E, *et al.* Anorectal pruritus after intravenous hydrocortisone sodium succinate and sodium phosphate. *Clin Pharmacol Ther* 1976; **20:** 109–12.
3. Anonymous. Which form of intravenous hydrocortisone. *Drug Ther Bull* 1979; **17:** 71–2.
4. Thomas VL. More on dexamethasone-induced perineal irritation. *N Engl J Med* 1986; **314:** 1643.
5. Allan SG, Leonard RCF. Dexamethasone antiemesis and side-effects. *Lancet* 1986; **i:** 1035.

Neonates. The adverse effects of corticosteroids on the fetus are discussed on p.1013.

Adverse effects noted in premature neonates with bronchopulmonary dysplasia receiving dexamethasone treatment to enable weaning from assisted ventilation have included hypertension,[1-3] often accompanied by bradycardia,[1,2] gastroduodenal perforation,[4,5] ulceration and thinning of the gastric wall,[4] development of a catabolic state,[6] renal calcification,[7] and transient myocardial hypertrophy.[8-10] There is some evidence of a suppressive effect on motor activity and spontaneous movement.[11] Whether, as has been suggested, corticosteroid therapy can lead to an increase in severe retinopathy of prematurity, remains uncertain.[12-14]

1. Ohlsson A, Heyman E. Dexamethasone-induced bradycardia. *Lancet* 1988; **ii:** 1074.
2. Puntis JWL, *et al.* Dexamethasone-induced bradycardia. *Lancet* 1988; **ii:** 1372.
3. Marinelli KA, *et al.* Effects of dexamethasone on blood pressure in premature infants with bronchopulmonary dysplasia. *J Pediatr* 1997; **130:** 594–602.
4. Ng PC, *et al.* Gastroduodenal perforation in preterm babies treated with dexamethasone for bronchopulmonary dysplasia. *Arch Dis Child* 1991; **66:** 1164–6.
5. Smith H, Sinha S. Gastrointestinal complications associated with dexamethasone treatment. *Arch Dis Child* 1992; **67:** 667.
6. Macdonald PD, *et al.* A catabolic state in dexamethasone treatment of bronchopulmonary dysplasia. *Arch Dis Child* 1990; **65:** 560–1.
7. Kamitsuka MD, Peloquin D. Renal calcification after dexamethasone in infants with bronchopulmonary dysplasia. *Lancet* 1991; **337:** 626.
8. Werner JC, *et al.* Hypertrophic cardiomyopathy associated with dexamethasone therapy for bronchopulmonary dysplasia. *J Pediatr* 1992; **120:** 286–91.
9. Bensky AS, *et al.* Cardiac effects of dexamethasone in very low birth weight infants. *Pediatrics* 1996; **97:** 818–21.
10. Skelton R, *et al.* Cardiac effects of short course dexamethasone in preterm infants. *Arch Dis Child* 1998; **78:** F133–F137.
11. Bos AF, *et al.* Qualitative assessment of general movements in high-risk preterm infants with chronic lung-disease requiring dexamethasone therapy. *J Pediatr* 1998; **132:** 300–6.
12. Sobel DB, Philip AGS. Prolonged dexamethasone therapy reduces the incidence of cryotherapy for retinopathy of prematurity in infants of less than 1 kilogram birth weight with bronchopulmonary dysplasia. *Pediatrics* 1992; **90:** 529–33.
13. Batton DG, *et al.* Severe retinopathy of prematurity and steroid exposure. *Pediatrics* 1992; **90:** 534–6.
14. Ehrenkranz RA. Steroids, chronic lung disease, and retinopathy of prematurity. *Pediatrics* 1992; **90:** 646–7.

Interactions

The interactions of corticosteroids in general are described on p.1014.

Antiepileptics. As described on p.356, dexamethasone may decrease or increase plasma concentrations of phenytoin. Like other enzyme-inducing drugs, phenytoin also has the potential to increase the metabolism of dexamethasone.

Pharmacokinetics

For a brief outline of the pharmacokinetics of corticosteroids, see p.1014.

Dexamethasone is readily absorbed from the gastro-intestinal tract. Its biological half-life in plasma is about 190 minutes. Binding of dexamethasone to plasma proteins is less than for most other corticosteroids. Up to 65% of a dose is excreted in urine within 24 hours. Clearance in premature neonates is reported to be proportional to gestational age, with a reduced elimination rate in the most premature. It crosses the placenta.

Uses and Administration

Dexamethasone is a corticosteroid with mainly glucocorticoid activity (p.1010); 750 µg of dexamethasone is equivalent in anti-inflammatory activity to about 5 mg of prednisolone.

It has been used, either in the form of the free alcohol or in one of the esterified forms, in the treatment of conditions for which corticosteroid therapy is indicated (p.1015), except adrenocortical insufficiency for which hydrocortisone with supplementary fludrocortisone is preferred. Its lack of mineralocorticoid properties makes dexamethasone particularly suitable for treating conditions where water retention would be a disadvantage.

For administration by mouth dexamethasone is used in usual initial doses of 0.5 to 10 mg daily. Dexamethasone is also used by mouth in the dexamethasone suppression tests for the diagnosis of Cushing's syndrome (for further details see under Diagnosis and Testing, below).

For parenteral administration in intensive therapy or in emergencies, the sodium phosphate ester may be given intravenously by injection or infusion or intramuscularly by injection; doses are sometimes expressed in terms of the free alcohol, the phosphate, or the sodium phosphate and confusion has sometimes arisen in the literature because of these variations. Initial doses used, expressed in terms of dexamethasone phosphate, range from about 0.5 to 20 mg daily (about 0.4 to 16.7 mg of dexamethasone). Intravenous doses of the equivalent of 2 to 6 mg of dexamethasone per kg body-weight given slowly over a minimum period of several minutes have been suggested for the treatment of severe shock. These high doses may be repeated within 2 to

6 hours and this treatment should be continued only until the patients' condition is stable and usually for no longer than 48 to 72 hours. Alternatively, the initial intravenous injection may be followed immediately by the same dose administered by intravenous infusion.

Dexamethasone sodium phosphate is also used in the treatment of cerebral oedema caused by malignancy. An initial intravenous dose of the equivalent of 10 mg of the phosphate is usually given followed by 4 mg intramuscularly every 6 hours; a response is usually obtained after 12 to 24 hours and dosage may be reduced after 2 to 4 days, and gradually discontinued over 5 to 7 days. A much higher dosage schedule has also been suggested for use in cerebral oedema in patients with inoperable brain tumours; initial doses of the equivalent of 50 mg of phosphate intravenously have been given on the first day together with 8 mg intravenously every 2 hours reduced gradually over several days to a maintenance dose of 2 mg two or three times daily.

The sodium phosphate ester is given by intra-articular, intralesional, intramuscular, or soft-tissue injection. For intra-articular injection doses equivalent to 0.8 to 4 mg of dexamethasone phosphate are employed depending upon the size of the joint. For soft-tissue injection doses of 2 to 6 mg are used. Injections are repeated every 3 to 5 days to every 2 to 3 weeks.

Dexamethasone acetate may be given by intramuscular injection in conditions where corticosteroid treatment is indicated but a prompt response of short duration is not required; doses are the equivalent of 8 to 16 mg of dexamethasone, repeated, if necessary, every 1 to 3 weeks. The acetate may also be administered locally by intra-articular or soft-tissue injection in doses equivalent to 4 to 16 mg of dexamethasone, repeated, if necessary, every 1 to 3 weeks, or by intralesional injection in doses equivalent to 0.8 to 1.6 mg.

For ophthalmic disorders or for topical application in the treatment of various skin disorders, either dexamethasone or its esters may be employed; concentrations are often expressed in terms of dexamethasone or dexamethasone phosphate and are commonly 0.05 to 0.1% for eye drops or ointments and 0.1% for topical skin preparations.

Dexamethasone sodium phosphate is also used by inhalation for the management of the symptoms of asthma (p.745) and related bronchospastic disorders unresponsive to other therapy. The initial dose is equivalent to 300 μg of dexamethasone phosphate or about 250 μg of dexamethasone inhaled three or four times daily, slowly reduced according to the patients' response to the minimum amount necessary to control the asthma.

For allergic rhinitis and other allergic or inflammatory nasal conditions (p.400), a nasal spray containing dexamethasone isonicotinate or dexamethasone sodium phosphate is available; the acetate, phosphate, and sodium metasulphobenzoate have also been employed.

Dexamethasone has been administered intravenously and orally for the prevention of nausea and vomiting induced by cancer chemotherapy (see below).

Other esters of dexamethasone which have occasionally been used include the hemisuccinate, linoleate, palmitate, pivalate, propionate, sodium succinate, tebutate, and valerate.

The phenpropionate and troxundate esters have been used in veterinary medicine.

Alcohol withdrawal syndrome. Dexamethasone was reported to be effective in a patient with benzodiazepine-resistant delirium tremens[1] and resolved symptoms of alcohol withdrawal syndrome resistant to other treatments in another 110 patients.[2] The usual management of the alcohol withdrawal syndrome is discussed on p.1099.

1. Fischer DK, *et al.* Efficacy of dexamethasone in benzodiazepine-resistant delirium tremens. *Lancet* 1988; **i:** 1340–1.
2. Pol S, *et al.* Dexamethasone for alcohol withdrawal. *Ann Intern Med* 1991; **114:** 705–6.

Blood disorders. High-dose pulsed dexamethasone therapy has been found useful in some patients with idiopathic thrombocytopenic purpura (p.1023), although results have been variable in children.

Cerebral oedema. Corticosteroids, usually dexamethasone, play an important role in the treatment of cerebral oedema in malignancy, and dexamethasone is advocated for the cerebral oedema associated with high-altitude disorders (see below). They have also been tried in head injury and stroke, but are considered not to be useful.[1-4] The management of raised intracranial pressure, and the usual drugs used in its treatment, are discussed further on p.796.

1. Sila CA, Furlan AJ. Drug treatment of stroke: current status and future prospects. *Drugs* 1988; **35:** 468–76.
2. Anonymous. A fresh look at some old stroke treatments. *Pharm J* 1990; **244:** 202.
3. Lyons MK, Meyer FB. Cerebrospinal fluid physiology and the management of increased intracranial pressure. *Mayo Clin Proc* 1990; **65:** 684–707.
4. Woster PS, LeBlanc KL. Management of elevated intracranial pressure. *Clin Pharm* 1990; **9:** 762–72.

Congenital adrenal hyperplasia. Because of its lack of mineralocorticoid properties, dexamethasone has little advantage in the salt-losing form of congenital adrenal hyperplasia (p.1020), in which mineralocorticoid therapy must be given, and its potency means that dose titration to avoid toxicity can be difficult in infants and children, even with the non-salt-losing form. However, it may be useful in adults with forms of the syndrome that do not require mineralocorticoid replacement. It has also been given antenatally to the mother to prevent virilisation of female fetuses.

Diagnosis and testing. CUSHING'S SYNDROME. Dexamethasone has been used to differentiate Cushing's disease (adrenal hyperplasia caused by defects of pituitary origin) from other forms of Cushing's syndrome (caused by ectopic ACTH secretion from non-pituitary tumours or by cortisol secretion from adrenal tumours). The dexamethasone suppression test first proposed by Liddle[1] involved the administration of dexamethasone in low doses of 500 μg four times daily by mouth for 8 doses followed by higher doses of 2 mg again four times daily for 8 doses. In the low-dose tests the urinary excretion of cortisol and 17-hydroxycorticosteroids is suppressed in healthy persons but not in patients and in the high-dose tests the excretion is still not suppressed in those with Cushing's syndrome but is partially suppressed in those with Cushing's disease. Because this test usually involves patients being admitted to hospital for urine collection over a number of days and because false-negative responses are reported to be fairly frequent, more rapid and reliable tests have been sought. Kennedy *et al.*[2] have used the low-dose test in conjunction with the measurement of serum-cortisol concentrations and the excretion of free cortisol in urine over 24 hours and considered it to be a reliable method for screening for Cushing's syndrome. In the UK a single dose of 1 mg of dexamethasone given at night is often used and is considered sufficient to inhibit corticotrophin secretion for 24 hours in most subjects. Another variation of the test has been reported by Tyrrell *et al.*[3] who administered a single dose of dexamethasone 8 mg at night and measured plasma-cortisol concentrations the next day; again they also concluded this test (known as the overnight high-dose dexamethasone suppression test) to be a practical and reliable alternative for the differential diagnosis of Cushing's syndrome. A recent review of the diagnostic tests used in Cushing's syndrome[4] concluded that, together with measurement of plasma-ACTH concentrations by radio-immunoassay, the overnight high-dose dexamethasone suppression test may become the test of choice for differential diagnosis.

Further variations in the dexamethasone suppression test have included administration of a continuous intravenous infusion of dexamethasone at a rate of 1 mg per hour for 7 hours, with hourly measurement of blood-cortisol concentrations.[5] Initial results indicate that this variation produces a lower number of false-positive diagnoses than the test using oral dexamethasone. Other alternatives are a combined low-dose dexamethasone suppression test and corticotropin-releasing hormone (corticorelin) test,[6] or combination of a dexamethasone suppression test with a metyrapone test.[7]

For a discussion of Cushing's disease and its management, see p.1236.

1. Liddle GW. Tests of pituitary-adrenal suppressibility in the diagnosis of Cushing's syndrome. *J Clin Endocrinol Metab* 1960; **20:** 1539–60.
2. Kennedy L, *et al.* Serum cortisol concentrations during low dose dexamethasone suppression test to screen for Cushing's syndrome. *Br Med J* 1984; **289:** 1188–91.
3. Tyrrell JB, *et al.* An overnight high-dose dexamethasone suppression test for rapid differential diagnosis of Cushing's syndrome. *Ann Intern Med* 1986; **104:** 180–6.
4. Kaye TB, Crapo L. The Cushing syndrome: an update on diagnostic tests. *Ann Intern Med* 1990; **112:** 434–44.
5. Biemond P, *et al.* Continuous dexamethasone infusion for seven hours in patients with the Cushing syndrome: a superior differential diagnostic test. *Ann Intern Med* 1990; **112:** 738–42.
6. Yanovski JA, *et al.* Corticotropin-releasing hormone stimulation following low-dose dexamethasone administration: a new test to distinguish Cushing's syndrome from pseudo-Cushing's states. *JAMA* 1993; **269:** 2232–8.
7. Avgerinos PC, *et al.* The metyrapone and dexamethasone suppression tests for the differential diagnosis of the adrenocorticotropin-dependent Cushing syndrome: a comparison. *Ann Intern Med* 1994; **121:** 318–27.

DEPRESSION. Comments[1] by the Health and Public Policy Committee of the American College of Physicians concerning the dexamethasone suppression test for depression (p.271). The test is based on the premise that endogenously depressed patients have shown pituitary-adrenal axis abnormalities but has been found to have a low sensitivity for detecting depression. It is of unproven value and is not recommended as a screening test for melancholic depression (endogenous depression).

1. Young M, Schwartz JS. The dexamethasone suppression test for the detection, diagnosis, and management of depression. *Ann Intern Med* 1984; **100:** 307–8.

High-altitude disorders. Dexamethasone is effective in the prevention of symptoms of acute mountain sickness (p.787), since mild cerebral oedema may contribute to them, but it is not generally considered suitable for prophylaxis because of concern about its adverse effects. In the treatment of acute severe mountain sickness, which may involve the development of pulmonary and cerebral oedema, the mandatory treatment is immediate descent, and drug therapy is primarily adjunctive, to facilitate descent or maintain the patient until descent is possible. Under these circumstances dexamethasone and oxygen form the mainstays of treatment. Some references to the use of dexamethasone for acute mountain sickness are given below.

1. Ferrazzini G, *et al.* Successful treatment of acute mountain sickness with dexamethasone. *Br Med J* 1987; **294:** 1380–2.
2. Ellsworth AJ, *et al.* A randomized trial of dexamethasone and acetazolamide for acute mountain sickness prophylaxis. *Am J Med* 1987; **83:** 1024–30.
3. Montgomery AB, *et al.* Effects of dexamethasone on the incidence of acute mountain sickness at two intermediate altitudes. *JAMA* 1989; **261:** 734–6.
4. Levine BD, *et al.* Dexamethasone in the treatment of acute mountain sickness. *N Engl J Med* 1989; **321:** 1707–13.
5. Keller H-R, *et al.* Simulated descent v dexamethasone in treatment of acute mountain sickness: a randomised trial. *Br Med J* 1995; **310:** 1232–5.

Hirsutism. Unbound testosterone concentrations were consistently elevated in 32 hirsute women; when concentrations were suppressed to normal by dexamethasone 0.5 to 1 mg at night hirsutism was generally improved or ceased to progress after 8 to 10 months of treatment.[1] Other studies have shown only a modest improvement[2] or no improvement at all[3] in hirsutism when treated with dexamethasone.

The mainstay of drug treatment for hirsutism tends to be an anti-androgen such as cyproterone or spironolactone (p.1441). Although low dose corticosteroids can suppress adrenal androgen production, careful consideration of the risks and benefits is advisable, especially since therapy for hirsutism may have to be given long-term.

1. Paulson JD, *et al.* Free testosterone concentration in serum: elevation is the hallmark of hirsutism. *Am J Obstet Gynecol* 1977; **128:** 851–7.
2. Carmina E, Lobo RA. Peripheral androgen blockade versus glandular androgen suppression in the treatment of hirsutism. *Obstet Gynecol* 1991; **78:** 845.
3. Rittmaster RS, Thompson DL. Effect of leuprolide and dexamethasone on hair growth and hormone levels in hirsute women: the relative importance of the ovary and the adrenal in the pathogenesis of hirsutism. *J Clin Endocrinol Metab* 1990; **70:** 1096–1102.

Malaria. Corticosteroids, especially dexamethasone, have been used in cerebral malaria (p.422) in the belief that their anti-inflammatory effect would reduce cerebral oedema.[1] However, studies have shown that cerebral oedema does not play a significant role in the pathophysiology of cerebral malaria and, indeed, double-blind studies using both moderate doses (2 mg per kg body-weight) and high doses (11 mg per kg) of dexamethasone intravenously over 48 hours found no reduction in death rates. Thus it is now considered that corticosteroids have no place in the treatment of cerebral malaria.

1. WHO. Practical chemotherapy of malaria: report of a WHO scientific group. *WHO Tech Rep Ser 805* 1990.

Malignant neoplasms. Dexamethasone has been used in some regimens for the treatment of malignancy, for example in acute lymphoblastic leukaemia (p.478) and multiple myeloma (p.494). For discussions of the management of various malignancies, including the role of corticosteroids, see under p.476.

Meningitis. There is some evidence of benefit from the adjunctive use of dexamethasone in bacterial meningitis (p.130), at least in those cases due to *Haemophilus influenzae*, particularly in reducing deafness. Dexamethasone has been recommended as adjunctive treatment in Haemophilus meningitis, when it should be given with or before the antibacterial. However, the topic is controversial, and it is by no means certain that any benefit exists in other forms of bacterial meningitis.

References.

1. Prasad K, Haines T. Dexamethasone treatment for acute bacterial meningitis: how strong is the evidence for routine use? *J Neurol Neurosurg Psychiatry* 1995; **59:** 31–7.
2. McIntyre PB, *et al.* Dexamethasone as adjunctive therapy in bacterial meningitis: a meta-analysis of randomized clinical trials since 1988. *JAMA* 1997; **278:** 925–31.

Nausea and vomiting. Dexamethasone has antiemetic properties of its own, particularly against delayed vomiting induced by cancer chemotherapy (p.1172), but is more frequently used in combination antiemetic regimens, notably with metoclopramide or the 5-HT_3 antagonists such as ondansetron. Typical dosage regimens have been dexamethasone 8 mg by intravenous injection immediately before chemotherapy followed by 4 mg by mouth every 6 hours, or 8 mg by mouth every 6 hours in combination with ondansetron for more severely emetogenic chemotherapy.

Opportunistic mycobacterial infections. Dexamethasone in doses of 1 to 4 mg daily was associated with weight gain, reduction in fever, and an improved sense of well-being in 5 patients with HIV and disseminated *Mycobacterium avium* complex infection.[1] Combination antimycobacterial therapy for opportunistic mycobacterial infections (p.133) was also given. Similar results have been noted by others.[2]

1. Wormser GP, *et al.* Low-dose dexamethasone as adjunctive therapy for disseminated Mycobacterium avium complex infections in AIDS patients. *Antimicrob Agents Chemother* 1994; **38:** 2215–17.
2. Dorman SE, *et al.* Adjunctive corticosteroid therapy for patients whose treatment for disseminated Mycobacterium avium complex infection has failed. *Clin Infect Dis* 1998; **26:** 682–6.

Respiratory disorders. Corticosteroids such as dexamethasone are given antenatally to mothers at risk of premature delivery in order to hasten fetal lung maturation and help prevent *neonatal respiratory distress syndrome* (p.1025) and *bronchopulmonary dysplasia* (p.1018); once it has occurred, dexamethasone has been reported to improve pulmonary outcome and assist weaning from mechanical ventilation in infants with bronchopulmonary dysplasia.

Dexamethasone is also one of the agents of choice for the management of severe *croup* (see p.1020). However, it appears to be of little value in *bronchiolitis*[1,2] (for discussion of the management of bronchiolitis associated with respiratory syncytial virus infection see p.602).

1. Roosevelt G, *et al.* Dexamethasone in bronchiolitis: a randomised controlled trial. *Lancet* 1996; **348:** 292–5.
2. Klassen TP, *et al.* Dexamethasone in salbutamol-treated inpatients with acute bronchiolitis: a randomized controlled trial. *J Pediatr* 1997; **130:** 191–6.

Retinopathy of prematurity. For a suggestion that dexamethasone might be helpful in the prophylaxis of retinopathy of prematurity, see p.1370.

Skin disorders. For recommendations concerning the correct use of corticosteroids on the skin, and a rough guide to the clinical potencies of topical corticosteroids, see Corticosteroids, Administration, p.1017.

Status epilepticus. Dexamethasone is used in some patients with status epilepticus (for example when associated with cerebral neoplasms) as mentioned on p.337.

Preparations

BP 1998: Dexamethasone Tablets;
USP 23: Dexamethasone Acetate Injectable Suspension; Dexamethasone Elixir; Dexamethasone Gel; Dexamethasone Ophthalmic Suspension; Dexamethasone Sodium Phosphate Cream; Dexamethasone Sodium Phosphate Inhalation Aerosol; Dexamethasone Sodium Phosphate Injection; Dexamethasone Sodium Phosphate Ophthalmic Ointment; Dexamethasone Sodium Phosphate Ophthalmic Solution; Dexamethasone Tablets; Dexamethasone Topical Aerosol; Neomycin and Polymyxin B Sulfates and Dexamethasone Ophthalmic Ointment; Neomycin and Polymyxin B Sulfates and Dexamethasone Ophthalmic Suspension; Neomycin Sulfate and Dexamethasone Sodium Phosphate Cream; Neomycin Sulfate and Dexamethasone Sodium Phosphate Ophthalmic Ointment; Neomycin Sulfate and Dexamethasone Sodium Phosphate Ophthalmic Solution; Tobramycin and Dexamethasone Ophthalmic Ointment; Tobramycin and Dexamethasone Ophthalmic Suspension.

Proprietary Preparations (details are given in Part 3)
Aust.: Decadron†; Dexabene; Fortecortin; ***Austral.:*** Decadron; Dexmethsone; Maxidex; ***Belg.:*** Aacidexam; Decadron; Dexa-Sol†; Maxidex; Oradexon†; ***Canad.:*** Decadron; Dexasone; Diodex; Hexadrol Phosphate; Maxidex; Ocudex†; RO-Dexsone†; Spersadex†; ***Fr.:*** Auxisone†; Cebedex; Decadron; Dectancyl; Maxidex; Soludecadron; ***Ger.:*** afpred-DEXA; Anemul mono; Auxiloson; Cortidexason; Cortisumman; Decadron Phosphat; Decadron†; Dexa in der Ophtiole; Dexa Loscon mono; Dexa-Allvoran; Dexa-Brachialin N; dexa-clinit; Dexa-Effekton; Dexa-ratiopharm; Dexa-sine; Dexabene; Dexaflam N; Dexahexal; Dexamed†; Dexamethason-mp; Dexamonozon; Dexamonozon N; Dexapos; Fortecortin; Isopto Dex; Lipotalon; Predni-F-Tablinen; Sokaral†; Solutio Cordes Dexa N; Spersadex; Totocortin; Tuttozem N; ***Irl.:*** Decadron; Maxidex; ***Ital.:*** Decadron; Decofluor†; Dermadex; Desalark; Deseronil†; Eta Cortilen; Firmalone†; Luxazone; Megacort; Situalin; Soldesam; Visumetazone; ***Jpn:*** Limethason; Methaderm†; Voalla; ***Neth.:*** Decadron; Decadron Depot†; Maxidex†; Oradexon; ***Norw.:*** Decadron; Isopto Maxidex; Spersadex; ***S.Afr.:*** Decadron; Decasone; Maxidex; Oradexon; Spersadex; ***Spain:*** Artrosone†; Decadran; Dexaplast†; Fortecortin; Fosfodexa†; Maxidex; Solone†; ***Swed.:*** Decadron; Dexacortal; Isopto Maxidex; ***Switz.:*** Decadron; Dexalocal; Fortecortin; Maxidex; Mephamesone; Millicortene; Oradexon; Spersadex; ***UK:*** Decadron; Maxidex; ***USA:*** Aeroseb-Dex; Ak-Dex; Alba Dex; Baldex†; Dalalone; Decaderm in Estergel†; Decaject; Decaspray†; Dexacort; Dexameth; Dexasone; Dexone; Hexadrol; Maxidex; Solurex.

Multi-ingredient: ***Aust.:*** Ambene; Clinit; Decadron mit Neomycin†; Dexa-Rhinospray; Dexasalyl†; Doxiproct mit Dexamethason†; Endomethazone; Multodrin; Rheumesser; Uromont; ***Austral.:*** Otodex; Sofradex; Tobispray†; ***Belg.:*** De Icin; De Icol; Decadron avec Neomycine; Dexa-Rhinospray; Dexa-Sol Sofframycine†; Maxitrol; Neodexon; Percutalgine; Polaronil; Polydexa; Tobradex; ***Canad.:*** Dioptrol; Maxitrol; NeoDecadron; Sofracort; Tobradex; ***Fr.:*** Auricularum; Cebedexacol; Chibro-Cadron; Corticetine; Dexaderme Kefrane†; Dexagrane; Dexapolyfra†; Frakidex; Maxidrol; Optidex†; Percutalgine; Pimafucort†; Polydexa; Polydexa a la Phenylephrine; Ster-Dex; ***Ger.:*** Aknichthol Dexa†; Aquapred†; Baycuten; Chibro-Cadron; Corti Biciron N; Cortidexason comp; Cortidexason-S†; Corto-Tavegil; Dexa Biciron; Dexa Loscon†; Dexa Polyspectran N; Dexa-Biofenicol-N†; Dexa-Gentamicin; Dexa-Phlogont L; Dexa-Rhinospray N; Dexa-Siozwo N; Dexabiotan in der Ophtiole†; Dexacrinin; Dexamed†; Dexamytrex; Dexasalyl; Dexatopic†; Dispadex comp; DoloTendin; Duodexa N; Ell-Cranell; Incut†; Isopto Max; Lokalison-antimikrobiell Creme N; Magopsor; Millicorten-Vioform; Nasicortin†; Nystalocal; Otobacid N; Otriven-Millicorten†; Rheumasit; Solupen-D; Spersadex Comp; Spersadexolin; Supertendin 2000 N; Supertendin 3000†; Supertendin-Depot N; Ultra-Demoplas; Uro-Stilloson; ***Irl.:*** Dexa-Rhinaspray; Maxitrol; Otomize; Sofradex; ***Ital.:*** Antimicotico; Aurizone†; Corti-Arscolloid; Dermadex Chinolinico†; Dermadex Neomicina†; Desagamma K†; Desalfa; Desamix Effe; Desamix-Neomicina; Dexatopic†; Dexoline; Doxiproct Plus; Eta Biocortilen; Eta Biocortilen VC; Fluorobioptal; Fluorocortisol K†; Kanaderm†; Kanazone; Lasoproct; Luxazone Eparina; Meclocil Desa†; Nasicortin; Neo-Cortofen; Neo-Cortofen "Antrax"†; Neodes†; Rinedrone; Situalin Antibiotico; Tobradex; Uretral†; Visumetazone Antistaminico; Visumetazone Decongestionante; ***Neth.:*** Decadron met neomycine; Dexamytrex; Dexatopic; Maxitrol†; Sofradex; Tobradex†; ***Norw.:*** Maxitrol; Sofradex; Spersadex med kloramfenikol; ***S.Afr.:*** Covomycin-D; Maxitrol; Sofradex; Spersadex Comp; Spersadexoline; Tobradex; ***Spain:*** Amplidermis; Broncoformo Muco Dexa; Clor Hemi; Cortison Chemicetina†; Cresophene; Cusispray†; Dalamon; Decadran Neomicina; Dexa Fenic; Dexa Tavegil; Dexa Vasoc; Dexabronchisan†; Dexafenicol; Dexam Constric; Dexatopic†; Hem Antih; Hongosan; Icol; Inzitan; Liquipom Dexa Antib; Liquipom Dexa Const; Liquipom Dexamida; Maxitrol; Neodexa; Neodexaplast†; Neurocatavin Dexa; Neurodavur Plus; Neurosido†; Oftalmol Dexa; Oftalmotrim Dexa; Otix; Oto Vitna†; Ozopulmin Antiasmatico†; Percutalin; Phonal; Resorborina; Rino Dexa; Rino Vitna†; Rinoblanco Dexa Antibio; Sabanotropico; Sedionbel†; Sedofarin; Talkosona; Vasodexa; Wasserdermina†; ***Swed.:*** Decadron cum neomycin; Sofradex; ***Switz.:*** Chronocorte; Clinit†; Corticetine; Creme antikeloides; Cresophene; Decadron a la neomycine†; Dexa Loscon†; Dexa-Rhinospray†; Dexalocal-F; Dexasalyl; Dexolan; Doxiproct Plus; Frakidex; Maxitrol; Nystalocal; Otospray; Pigmanorm; Polydexa; Pulpomixine; Sebo-Psor; Septomixine; Sofradex; Spersadex Comp; Spersadexoline; Tobradex; ***UK:*** Dexa-Rhinaspray Duo; Dexa-Rhinaspray†; Maxitrol; Otomize; Sofradex; ***USA:*** Ak-Neo-Dex; Ak-Trol; Dexacidin; Dexasporin; Infectrol†; Maxitrol; Neo-Dexair; Neo-Dexameth; NeoDecadron; Poly-Dex; Storz-N-D; Storz-N-P-D; Tobradex.

Dichlorisone Acetate (12645-j)

Dichlorisone Acetate *(rINNM).*

Diclorisone Acetate. 9α,11β-Dichloro-17α,21-dihydroxypregna-1,4-diene-3,20-dione 21-acetate.

$C_{23}H_{28}Cl_2O_5$ = 455.4.

CAS — 7008-26-6 (dichlorisone); 79-61-8 (dichlorisone acetate).

Dichlorisone acetate is a corticosteroid used topically for its glucocorticoid activity (p.1010) in the treatment of various skin disorders. It is usually employed as a cream or ointment containing 0.25 to 1%.

When applied topically, particularly to large areas, when the skin is broken, or under occlusive dressings, corticosteroids may be absorbed in sufficient amounts to cause systemic effects (see p.1010). The effects of topical corticosteroids on the skin are described on p.1012.

Skin disorders. For recommendations concerning the correct use of corticosteroids on the skin, see Corticosteroids, Administration, p.1017.

Preparations

Proprietary Preparations (details are given in Part 3)
Ital.: Astroderm†; ***Spain:*** Dermaren; Dicloderm Forte.

Diflorasone Diacetate (12651-l)

Diflorasone Diacetate *(BANM, USAN, rINNM).*

U-34865. 6α,9α-Difluoro-11β,17α,21-trihydroxy-16β-methylpregna-1,4-diene-3,20-dione 17,21-diacetate.

$C_{26}H_{32}F_2O_7$ = 494.5.

CAS — 2557-49-5 (diflorasone); 33564-31-7 (diflorasone diacetate).

Pharmacopoeias. In US.

A white to pale yellow, crystalline powder. Practically **insoluble** in water; soluble in acetone and in methyl alcohol; sparingly soluble in ethyl acetate; slightly soluble in toluene; very slightly soluble in ether. **Store** in airtight containers.

Diflorasone diacetate is a corticosteroid used topically for its glucocorticoid activity (p.1010) in the treatment of various skin disorders. It is usually employed as a cream or ointment containing 0.05%.

When applied topically, particularly to large areas, when the skin is broken, or under occlusive dressings, corticosteroids may be absorbed in sufficient amounts to cause systemic effects (p.1010). The effects of topical corticosteroids on the skin are described on p.1012.

Skin disorders. For recommendations concerning the correct use of corticosteroids on the skin, and a rough guide to the clinical potencies of topical corticosteroids, see Corticosteroids, Administration, p.1017.

Preparations

USP 23: Diflorasone Diacetate Cream; Diflorasone Diacetate Ointment.

Proprietary Preparations (details are given in Part 3)
Canad.: Florone; ***Ger.:*** Florone; ***Ital.:*** Dermaflor; Sterodelta; ***Spain:*** Bexilona†; Fulixan†; Murode; Vincosona; ***Swed.:*** Soriflor†; ***USA:*** Florone; Maxiflor; Psorcon.

Diflucortolone Valerate (1087-f)

Diflucortolone Valerate *(BANM, rINNM).*

6α,9α-Difluoro-11β,21-dihydroxy-16α-methylpregna-1,4-diene-3,20-dione 21-valerate.

$C_{27}H_{36}F_2O_5$ = 478.6.

CAS — 2607-06-9 (diflucortolone); 59198-70-8 (diflucortolone valerate); 15845-96-2 (diflucortolone pivalate).

NOTE. Diflucortolone and Diflucortolone Pivalate are *USAN.*

Pharmacopoeias. In Br.

A white to creamy white crystalline powder. Practically **insoluble** in water; slightly soluble in methyl alcohol, freely soluble in dichloromethane and in dioxan; sparingly soluble in ether. **Protect** from light.

Diflucortolone valerate is a corticosteroid used topically for its glucocorticoid activity (p.1010) in the treatment of various skin disorders. It is usually employed as a cream or ointment containing 0.1% or 0.3%.

When applied topically, particularly to large areas, when the skin is broken, or under occlusive dressings, corticosteroids may be absorbed in sufficient amounts to cause systemic effects (p.1010). The effects of topical corticosteroids on the skin are described on p.1012.

Skin disorders. For recommendations concerning the correct use of corticosteroids on the skin, and a rough guide to the clinical potencies of topical corticosteroids, see Corticosteroids, Administration, p.1017.

Preparations

BP 1998: Diflucortolone Cream; Diflucortolone Oily Cream; Diflucortolone Ointment.

Proprietary Preparations (details are given in Part 3)
Aust.: Neriforte; Nerisona; ***Belg.:*** Nerisona; ***Canad.:*** Nerisone; ***Fr.:*** Nerisone; ***Ger.:*** Nerisona; Temetex†; ***Irl.:*** Nerisone†; ***Ital.:*** Cortical; Dermaval; Dervin; Dicortal†; Flu-Cortanest; Nerisona; Temetex; ***Neth.:*** Nerisona; ***S.Afr.:*** Nerisone; ***Spain:*** Claral; Temetex†; ***Switz.:*** Nerifort†; Nerisona; Temetex†; ***UK:*** Nerisone.

Multi-ingredient: ***Aust.:*** Neriquinol; Travocort; ***Belg.:*** Travocort; ***Canad.:*** Nerisalic; ***Fr.:*** Nerisalic; Nerisone C; ***Ger.:*** Nerisona C; Travocort; ***Irl.:*** Travocort; ***Ital.:*** Corti-Fluoral; Dermaflogil; Dermobios; Dermobios Oto†; Impetex; Nerisona C; Travocort; ***S.Afr.:*** Travocort; ***Spain:*** Claral Plus; Temetex Compositum†; ***Switz.:*** Temetex C†; Travocort.

Difluprednate (12652-y)

Difluprednate *(USAN, rINN).*

CM-9155; W-6309. 6α,9α-Difluoro-11β,17α,21-trihydroxypregna-1,4-diene-3,20-dione 21-acetate 17-butyrate.

$C_{27}H_{34}F_2O_7$ = 508.6.

CAS — 23674-86-4.

Difluprednate is a corticosteroid used topically for its glucocorticoid activity (p.1010) in the treatment of various skin disorders. It has usually been employed as a cream, gel, or ointment; concentrations used range from 0.02 to 0.05%.

When applied topically, particularly to large areas, when the skin is broken, or under occlusive dressings, corticosteroids may be absorbed in sufficient amounts to cause systemic effects (p.1010). The effects of topical corticosteroids on the skin are described on p.1012.

Skin disorders. For recommendations concerning the correct use of corticosteroids on the skin, see Corticosteroids, Administration, p.1017.

Preparations

Proprietary Preparations (details are given in Part 3)
Fr.: Epitopic; ***Jpn:*** Myser.

Fluclorolone Acetonide (1088-d)

Fluclorolone Acetonide *(BAN, rINN)*.

Flucloronide *(USAN)*; RS-2252. 9α,11β-Dichloro-6α-fluoro-21-hydroxy-16α,17α-isopropylidenedioxypregna-1,4-diene-3,20-dione.

$C_{24}H_{29}Cl_2FO_5$ = 487.4.

CAS — 3693-39-8.

Fluclorolone acetonide is a corticosteroid used topically for its glucocorticoid activity (p.1010) in the treatment of various skin disorders. It has been employed as a cream or ointment containing 0.025 to 0.2%.

When applied topically, particularly to large areas, when the skin is broken, or under occlusive dressings, corticosteroids may be absorbed in sufficient amounts to cause systemic effects (p.1010). The effects of topical corticosteroids on the skin are described on p.1012.

Skin disorders. For recommendations concerning the correct use of corticosteroids on the skin, and a rough guide to the clinical potencies of topical corticosteroids, see Corticosteroids, Administration, p.1017.

Preparations

Proprietary Preparations (details are given in Part 3)
Austral.: Topilar†; ***Fr.:*** Topilar†; ***Spain:*** Cutanit; ***UK:*** Topilar†.

Fludrocortisone Acetate (1089-n)

Fludrocortisone Acetate *(BANM, rINNM)*.

Fludrocortisoni Acetas; 9α-Fluorohydrocortisone 21-Acetate. 9α-Fluoro-11β,17α,21-trihydroxypregn-4-ene-3,20-dione 21-acetate.

$C_{23}H_{31}FO_6$ = 422.5.

CAS — 127-31-1 (fludrocortisone); 514-36-3 (fludrocortisone acetate).

Pharmacopoeias. In *Chin., Eur.* (see p.viii), *Int., Pol.,* and *US.*

A white to pale yellow, odourless or almost odourless, hygroscopic crystals or crystalline powder. Practically **insoluble** in water; sparingly soluble in alcohol, in dehydrated alcohol, and in chloroform; slightly soluble in ether. **Protect** from light.

Adverse Effects, Treatment, Withdrawal, and Precautions

Fludrocortisone acetate has glucocorticoid actions about 10 times as potent as hydrocortisone and mineralocorticoid effects more than 100 times as potent. Adverse effects are mainly those due to mineralocorticoid activity, as described on p.1010.

When applied topically, particularly to large areas, when the skin is broken, or under occlusive dressings, corticosteroids may be absorbed in sufficient amounts to cause systemic effects.

Interactions

The interactions of corticosteroids in general are described on p.1014.

Pharmacokinetics

For a brief outline of the pharmacokinetics of corticosteroids, see p.1014.

Fludrocortisone is readily absorbed from the gastrointestinal tract. The plasma half-life is about 3.5 hours or more, but fludrocortisone exhibits a more prolonged biological half-life of 18 to 36 hours.

Uses and Administration

Fludrocortisone is a corticosteroid with glucocorticoid and highly potent mineralocorticoid activity as described under Corticosteroids, p.1010.

Fludrocortisone acetate is given by mouth to provide mineralocorticoid replacement in primary adrenocortical insufficiency (p.1017), together with glucocorticoids. It is used in a suggested dose range of 50 to 300 μg daily.

Fludrocortisone acetate may also be given concomitantly with glucocorticoid therapy in doses of up to 200 μg daily in the salt-losing form of congenital adrenal hyperplasia (p.1020).

It is also given by mouth in the management of severe orthostatic hypotension (see below).

Fludrocortisone acetate has been applied topically to the skin, eye, and ear in the treatment of various disorders. It has been employed as an ingredient of cream, ointment, gel, or drops, usually in a concentration of 0.1%.

Administration. A study of fludrocortisone requirements in 10 patients with Addison's disease indicated that dosage was often inadequate.[1] Nine were initially on fludrocortisone 50 to 100 μg daily in addition to cortisone or hydrocortisone; 5 were also taking thyroxine for an associated auto-immune thyroid disease; one, who had detectable levels of aldosterone, was not initially receiving fludrocortisone. All the patients had evidence of sodium and water depletion and initiation of fludrocortisone 300 μg daily, with downwards adjustments, demonstrated that most patients required 200 μg daily. Two patients elected to remain on 300 μg daily, but in most this dose caused pronounced sodium and water retention. The patient with detectable aldosterone levels required 50 μg daily. Eight of the 10 patients felt better on the higher fludrocortisone doses while 2 felt no change.

1. Smith SJ, *et al.* Evidence that patients with Addison's disease are undertreated with fludrocortisone. *Lancet* 1984; **i:** 11–14.

Hypoaldosteronism. A discussion on hyporeninaemic hypoaldosteronism.[1] Traditionally a mineralocorticoid such as fludrocortisone acetate has been used to reduce the hyperkalaemia and acidosis. Unfortunately pharmacological rather than physiological doses are often needed and these may not always be effective.

1. Williams GH. Hyporeninemic hypoaldosteronism. *N Engl J Med* 1986; **314:** 1041–2.

Neurally mediated hypotension. Fludrocortisone is reported to be one of the standard drugs used in the management of neurally mediated hypotension (see p.790).

Orthostatic hypotension. Orthostatic (postural) hypotension[1-5] is a fall in blood pressure that occurs upon rising abruptly to an erect position, although it may also occur following a period of prolonged standing. Characteristic symptoms include lightheadedness, dizziness, blurred vision, weakness in the limbs, and syncope.

The causes of orthostatic hypotension are wide-ranging and include autonomic dysfunction, such as in the Shy-Drager syndrome, diabetes mellitus, and Parkinson's disease, circulating volume depletion, phaeochromocytoma, and Addison's disease. Orthostatic hypotension may also occur following a period of prolonged bed rest or following meals.

Orthostatic hypotension may result from the adverse effects of a range of drugs, such as antihypertensives, diuretics, tricyclic antidepressants, phenothiazines, and MAOIs.

In mild cases **nonpharmacological treatment** alone may be adequate. This includes increasing salt intake if not contraindicated, maintaining adequate hydration, the use of elastic stockings to improve venous return and increase cardiac output, and elevating the head of the bed to reduce early morning symptoms. Drug-induced orthostatic hypotension should be treated by withdrawing the agent or by dose reduction.

Pharmacological treatment. No pharmacological treatment is entirely satisfactory: responses and tolerance vary greatly between patients. Fludrocortisone acetate is usually tried first; it increases sodium retention and thus plasma volume. Most reports indicate some response in about 80% of patients, but hypokalaemia, fluid retention, and supine hypertension may limit its use. In patients who fail to respond adequately an NSAID (usually indomethacin) may be tried, alone or in combination with fludrocortisone. In patients with overt autonomic failure a beta blocker with some partial agonist activity, such as xamoterol or pindolol, may be tried although they are potentially dangerous.

Sympathomimetics may be useful in some patients with autonomic failure; the direct acting agents such as phenylephrine or midodrine usually proving more consistently effective than the indirect such as ephedrine, but even so, responses tend to vary with the degree of denervation. Patients with central neurological abnormalities may respond to desmopressin, while drugs such as ergotamine or dihydroergotamine may be useful for resistant disease.

Other drugs that have been tried include metoclopramide, which may be useful for autonomic symptoms in patients with diabetes mellitus, fluoxetine, octreotide, yohimbine, clonidine, and in patients with concurrent anaemia, erythropoietin. Caffeine has been tried in postprandial hypotension but its value in all but the mildest cases is dubious.[5] The use of MAOIs (which given alone can induce orthostatic hypotension) with a sympathomimetic to induce a pressor reaction is controversial. Most of these drugs have potentially serious adverse effects and few are well evaluated.

1. Ahmad RAS, Watson RDS. Treatment of postural hypotension: a review. *Drugs* 1990; **39:** 74–85.
2. Tonkin AL, Wing LMH. Hypotension: assessment and management. *Med J Aust* 1990; **153:** 474–85.
3. Schoenberger JA. Drug-induced orthostatic hypotension. *Drug Safety* 1991; **6:** 402–7.
4. Stumpf JL, Mitrzyk B. Management of orthostatic hypotension. *Am J Hosp Pharm* 1994; **51:** 648–60.
5. Mathias CJ. Orthostatic hypotension. *Prescribers' J* 1995; **35:** 124–32.

Skin disorders. For recommendations concerning the correct use of corticosteroids on the skin, see Corticosteroids, Administration, p.1017.

Preparations

BP 1998: Fludrocortisone Tablets;
USP 23: Fludrocortisone Acetate Tablets.

Proprietary Preparations (details are given in Part 3)
Aust.: Astonin H; ***Austral.:*** Florinef; ***Canad.:*** Florinef; ***Ger.:*** Astonin H; ***Irl.:*** Florinef; ***Neth.:*** Florinef; ***Norw.:*** Florinef; ***S.Afr.:*** Florinef; ***Spain:*** Astonin; ***Swed.:*** Florinef; ***Switz.:*** Florinef; ***UK:*** Florinef; ***USA:*** Florinef.

Multi-ingredient: ***Belg.:*** Fungispec†; Panotile; ***Fr.:*** Blephaseptyl†; Panotile; ***Ger.:*** Panotile N; ***Neth.:*** Panotile; ***Spain:*** Fludronef; Panotile; ***Switz.:*** Blephaseptyl†; Panotile.

Flumethasone Pivalate (1091-a)

Flumethasone Pivalate *(BANM, USAN)*.

Flumetasone Pivalate *(rINNM)*; Flumethasone Trimethylacetate; NSC-107680. Flumethasone 21-pivalate.

$C_{27}H_{36}F_2O_6$ = 494.6.

CAS — 2002-29-1.

Pharmacopoeias. In *Eur.* (see p.viii), *Pol.,* and *US.*

A white to off-white crystalline powder. It exhibits polymorphism. Practically **insoluble** in water; soluble 1 in 89 of alcohol, 1 in 350 of chloroform, and 1 in 2800 of ether; slightly soluble in methyl alcohol; slightly or very slightly soluble in dichloromethane. **Store** in airtight containers. Protect from light.

Flumethasone pivalate is a corticosteroid used topically for its glucocorticoid activity (p.1010) in the treatment of various skin disorders. It is usually employed as a 0.02% cream, ointment, or lotion.

Flumethasone pivalate is also used in ear drops in a concentration of 0.02% with clioquinol 1%.

When applied topically, particularly to large areas, when the skin is broken, or under occlusive dressings, corticosteroids may be absorbed in sufficient amounts to cause systemic effects (p.1010). The effects of topical corticosteroids on the skin are described on p.1012.

Skin disorders. For recommendations concerning the correct use of corticosteroids on the skin, and a rough guide to the clinical potencies of topical corticosteroids, see Corticosteroids, Administration, p.1017.

Preparations

USP 23: Flumethasone Pivalate Cream.

Proprietary Preparations (details are given in Part 3)
Belg.: Locacortene; ***Canad.:*** Locacorten; ***Ger.:*** Cerson; Locacorten; Lorinden†; ***Ital.:*** Locorten; ***Neth.:*** Locacorten; ***Norw.:*** Locacorten†; ***Spain:*** Locortene; ***Swed.:*** Locacorten†; ***Switz.:*** Locacorten.

Multi-ingredient: ***Aust.:*** Locacorten mit Neomycin; Locacorten Tar; Locacorten Vioform; Locasalen; ***Austral.:*** Locacorten Vioform; ***Belg.:*** Locacortene Tar; Locacortene Vioforme; Locasalen; ***Canad.:*** Locacorten Vioform; Locasalen; ***Fr.:*** Locacortene Vioforme†; Locacortene†; Locasalene†; Psocortene†; ***Ger.:*** Locacorten Vioform; Locasalen; Lorinden T; ***Ital.:*** Locorten; Locorten Neomicina†; Locorten Tar; Locorten Vioformio; Losalen; Nelog†; Vasosterone Oto; ***Neth.:*** Locacorten Vioform; Locasalen; ***Norw.:*** Locacorten Vioform; Locasalen; Logamel†; ***S.Afr.:*** Locacorten Tar†; Locacorten Vioform; ***Spain:*** Locortene Vioformo; Logamel†; Losalen; ***Swed.:*** Locacorten Tar†; Locacorten Vioform; Locasalen†; ***Switz.:*** Locacorten c. Neomycin†; Locacorten Tar; Locacorten Triclosan; Locacorten Vioform†; Locasalen; Logamel†; ***UK:*** Locorten Vioform.

Flunisolide (1092-t)

Flunisolide *(BAN, USAN, rINN)*.

RS-3999; RS-1320 (acetate). 6α-Fluoro-11β,21-dihydroxy-16α,17α-isopropylidenedioxypregna-1,4-diene-3,20-dione.

$C_{24}H_{31}FO_6$ = 434.5.

CAS — 3385-03-3 (flunisolide); 77326-96-6 (flunisolide hemihydrate); 4533-89-5 (flunisolide acetate).

Pharmacopoeias. In *US* which specifies the hemihydrate.

A white to creamy-white crystalline powder. Practically **insoluble** in water; soluble in acetone; sparingly soluble in chloroform; slightly soluble in methyl alcohol.

Adverse Effects, Treatment, Withdrawal, and Precautions

As for corticosteroids in general (see p.1010).

Flunisolide is reported to have little systemic adverse effect when administered by inhalation or the nasal route in usual doses.

Reformulation of flunisolide nasal spray to contain less propylene glycol and a lower molecular weight polyethylene glycol (400 instead of 4000) resulted in a lower incidence of nasal burning and stinging in patients receiving flunisolide by this method for the management of rhinitis.[1]

1. Nielsen NH, *et al.* A new formulation of flunisolide for intranasal application reduces side effects. *Allergy* 1989; **44:** 233–4.

Interactions

The interactions of corticosteroids in general are described on p.1014.

Pharmacokinetics

For a brief outline of the pharmacokinetics of corticosteroids, see p.1014. Flunisolide is reported to undergo extensive first-pass metabolism, with only 20% of the dose available systemically if it is given by mouth. The major metabolite, 6β-hydroxyflunisolide has some glucocorticoid activity; it has a half-life of about 4 hours. Only small amounts of flunisolide are absorbed following intranasal administration.

References.

1. Chaplin MD, *et al.* Flunisolide metabolism and dynamics of a metabolite. *Clin Pharmacol Ther* 1980; **27:** 402–13.
2. Möllmann H, *et al.* Pharmacokinetic/pharmacodynamic evaluation of systemic effects of flunisolide after inhalation. *J Clin Pharmacol* 1997; **37:** 893–903.

Uses and Administration

Flunisolide is a corticosteroid with glucocorticoid activity used as a nasal spray for the prophylaxis and treatment of allergic rhinitis (p.400). It is used in a usual initial dose of 50 μg into each nostril two or three times daily, subsequently reduced to the lowest dose adequate to control symptoms which may be as little as 25 μg into each nostril daily. Children over 5 years of age may be given 25 μg into each nostril up to three times daily. In the USA a dose of 50 μg into each nostril twice daily has also been permitted in children.

Flunisolide is also used by inhalation from a metered-dose aerosol in the management of asthma (p.745). The usual adult dosage is 500 μg inhaled twice daily. In severe asthma the dosage may be increased but should not exceed a total of 2 mg daily. A suggested dose for children over 5 years of age is 500 μg inhaled twice daily.

Preparations

USP 23: Flunisolide Nasal Solution.

Proprietary Preparations (details are given in Part 3)
Aust.: Pulmilide; Syntaris; ***Austral.:*** Rhinalar†; ***Belg.:*** Broncort; Syntaris; ***Canad.:*** Bronalide; Rhinalar; Rhinaris-F†; ***Fr.:*** Bronilide; Nasalide; ***Ger.:*** Inhacort; Syntaris; ***Irl.:*** Syntaris; ***Ital.:*** Gibiflu; Lunibron-A; Lunis; Nisolid; Syntaris; ***Neth.:*** Syntaris; ***Norw.:*** Flunitec; Lokilan; ***S.Afr.:*** Syntaris; ***Swed.:*** Lokilan Nasal; ***Switz.:*** Broncort; Bronilide†; Syntaris; ***UK:*** Syntaris; ***USA:*** AeroBid; Nasalide; Nasarel.

Fluocinolone Acetonide (1093-x)

Fluocinolone Acetonide *(BANM, USAN, rINN).*

6α,9α-Difluoro-16α-hydroxyprednisolone Acetonide; Fluocinoloni Acetonidum; NSC-92339. 6α,9α-Difluoro-11β,21-dihydroxy-16α,17α-isopropylidenedioxypregna-1,4-diene-3,20-dione.

$C_{24}H_{30}F_2O_6$ = 452.5.

CAS — 67-73-2.

Pharmacopoeias. In *Eur.* (see p.viii), *Jpn,* and *Pol. Br.* has a separate monograph for the dihydrate; *US* allows either the anhydrous form or the dihydrate.

A white or almost white, odourless, crystalline powder. Practically **insoluble** in water; the USP substance is stated to be soluble 1 in 45 of alcohol, 1 in 25 of chloroform, and 1 in 350 of ether; soluble in methyl alcohol. Ph. Eur. states that the acetonide is soluble in acetone and in dehydrated alcohol, and practically insoluble in petroleum spirit; the BP stipulates that the acetonide dihydrate is freely soluble in acetone, soluble in dehydrated alcohol, sparingly soluble in dichloromethane or in methyl alcohol, and practically insoluble in hexane. **Protect** from light.

Fluocinolone acetonide is a corticosteroid used topically for its glucocorticoid activity (p.1010) in the treatment of various skin disorders. It is usually employed as a cream, gel, lotion, ointment, or scalp application; usual concentrations used range from 0.0025 to 0.025%. Fluocinolone acetonide has also been used topically in the treatment of inflammatory eye, ear, and nose disorders.

When applied topically, particularly to large areas, when the skin is broken, or under occlusive dressings, corticosteroids may be absorbed in sufficient amounts to cause systemic effects (p.1010). The effects of topical corticosteroids on the skin are described on p.1012.

Formulation. The potency of fluocinolone acetonide varied with the formulation in a study[1] involving different Synalar topical preparations, the gel, ointment, and cream. The cream was the most potent followed by the gel, and then the ointment. Surprisingly dilution of preparation did not reduce the potency.

1. Gao HY, Li Wan Po A. Topical formulations of fluocinolone acetonide: are creams, gels and ointments bioequivalent and does dilution affect activity? *Eur J Clin Pharmacol* 1994; **46:** 71–5.

Skin disorders. For recommendations concerning the correct use of corticosteroids on the skin, and a rough guide to the clinical potencies of topical corticosteroids, see Corticosteroids, Administration, p.1017.

Preparations

BP 1998: Fluocinolone Cream; Fluocinolone Ointment;
USP 23: Fluocinolone Acetonide Cream; Fluocinolone Acetonide Ointment; Fluocinolone Acetonide Topical Solution; Neomycin Sulfate and Fluocinolone Acetonide Cream.

Proprietary Preparations (details are given in Part 3)
Aust.: Synalar; ***Belg.:*** Synalar; ***Canad.:*** Derma-Smoothe†; Fluoderm; Synalar; Synamol†; ***Fr.:*** Synalar; ***Ger.:*** Flucinar; Jellin; Jellisoft; ***Irl.:*** Synalar; ***Ital.:*** Alfa-Fluorone; Alfabios; Boniderma; Coderma†; Cortalar†; Cortamide; Cortiplastol†; Dermaisom†; Dermaplus†; Dermobeta; Dermofil†; Dermolin; Doricum Semplice†; Esacinone; Esilon†; Fluocinil†; Fluocit†; Fluodermol†; Fluomix Same; Fluovitef; Isnaderm†; Leniderm†; Localyn; Localyn SV; Neoderm Ginecologico; Omniderm; Radiocin†; Sterolone; Straderm†; Topifluor†; Ultraderm; ***Neth.:*** Synalar†; ***Norw.:*** Synalar; ***S.Afr.:*** Cortoderm; Fluoderm†; Synalar; ***Spain:*** Alvadermo Fuerte; Anatopic; Co Fluocin Fuerte; Cortiespec; Elasven†; Fluocid Forte; Fluocortan; Fluodermo Fuerte; Gelidina; Intradermo Corticosteroi†; Oxidermiol Fuerte; Synalar; ***Swed.:*** Synalar; ***Switz.:*** Synalar; ***UK:*** Synalar; ***USA:*** Derma-Smoothe/FS; Fluonid; Flurosyn; FS; Synalar; Synemol.

Multi-ingredient: ***Aust.:*** Myco-Synalar; Procto-Synalar; Synalar N; ***Belg.:*** Neo-Synalar†; Procto-Synalar; Synalar Bi-Ophtalmic†; Synalar Bi-Otic; ***Canad.:*** Synalar Bi-Otic†; ***Fr.:*** Antibio-Synalar; Synalar Neomycine; ***Ger.:*** Jellin polyvalent; Jellin-Neomycin; Jellisoft-Neomycin; Myco-Jellin†; Procto-Jellin; ***Irl.:*** Synalar C; Synalar N; ***Ital.:*** Alfa-Fluorone; Cortanest Plus; Doricum; Fluomicetina; Lauromicina; Localyn; Localyn-Neomicina; Mecloderm F; Meclutin; Nefluan; Proctolyn; ***Neth.:*** Synalar + DBO†; Synalar Bi-Otic; ***Norw.:*** Synalar med Chinoform; ***S.Afr.:*** Synalar C; Synalar N; ***Spain:*** Abrasone; Alergical; Anasilpiel†; Artrodesmol Extra; Bazalin; Creanolona; Flodermol; Fluo Fenic; Fluo Vasoc; Intradermo Cort Ant Fung; Midacina; Myco-Synalar; Neo Analsona; Neo Synalar; Otomidrin; Poxider; Synalar Nasal; Synalar Neomicina; Synalar Otico; Synalar Rectal; Synobel; Vinciseptil Otico; ***Swed.:*** Synalar med Chinoform†; ***Switz.:*** Myco-Synalar; Procto-Synalar N; Synalar N; ***UK:*** Synalar C; Synalar N; ***USA:*** Neo-Synalar†.

Fluocinonide (1094-r)

Fluocinonide *(BAN, USAN, rINN).*

Fluocinolide; Fluocinolone Acetonide 21-Acetate; NSC-101791. 6α,9α-Difluoro-11β,21-dihydroxy-16α,17α-isopropylidenedioxypregna-1,4-diene-3,20-dione 21-acetate.

$C_{26}H_{32}F_2O_7$ = 494.5.

CAS — 356-12-7.

Pharmacopoeias. In *Br., Chin., Jpn,* and *US.*

A white to cream-coloured crystalline powder with not more than a slight odour. Practically **insoluble** in water; sparingly soluble in acetone; the BP states that it is slightly, and the USP sparingly, soluble in chloroform; slightly soluble in alcohol, in dehydrated alcohol, in methyl alcohol, and in dioxan; very slightly soluble in ether. **Protect** from light.

Fluocinonide is a corticosteroid used topically for its glucocorticoid activity (p.1010) in the treatment of various skin disorders. It is usually employed as a cream, gel, lotion, ointment, or scalp application containing 0.05%.

When applied topically, particularly to large areas, when the skin is broken, or under occlusive dressings, corticosteroids may be absorbed in sufficient amounts to cause systemic effects (p.1010). The effects of topical corticosteroids on the skin are described on p.1012.

Skin disorders. For recommendations concerning the correct use of corticosteroids on the skin, and a rough guide to the clinical potencies of topical corticosteroids, see Corticosteroids, Administration, p.1017.

Preparations

BP 1998: Fluocinonide Cream; Fluocinonide Ointment;
USP 23: Fluocinonide Cream; Fluocinonide Gel; Fluocinonide Ointment; Fluocinonide Topical Solution.

Proprietary Preparations (details are given in Part 3)
Aust.: Topsym; Topsymin F; ***Belg.:*** Lidex; ***Canad.:*** Lidemol†; Lidex; Lyderm; Tiamol; Topsyn†; ***Fr.:*** Topsyne; ***Ger.:*** Topsym; ***Irl.:*** Metosyn; ***Ital.:*** Flu-21; Topsyn; ***Neth.:*** Topsyne; ***Norw.:*** Metosyn; ***Spain:*** Cusigel; Klariderm; Novoter; ***Switz.:*** Topsym; Topsymin; ***UK:*** Metosyn; ***USA:*** Fluonex; Lidex; Vasoderm.

Multi-ingredient: ***Aust.:*** Topsym polyvalent; ***Canad.:*** Lidecomb†; Trisyn; ***Fr.:*** Topsyne Neomycine; ***Ger.:*** Topsym polyvalent; ***Ital.:*** Combiderm†; Proctonide†; Topsyn Neomicina†; ***Spain:*** Abrasone Rectal; Novoter Gentamicina; ***Switz.:*** Topsym polyvalent; ***UK:*** Vipsogal.

Fluocortin Butyl (12761-a)

Fluocortin Butyl *(BAN, USAN, rINNM).*

SH-K-203. Butyl 6α-fluoro-11β-hydroxy-16α-methyl-3,20-dioxopregna-1,4-dien-21-oate.

$C_{26}H_{35}FO_5$ = 446.6.

CAS — 33124-50-4 (fluocortin); 41767-29-7 (fluocortin butyl).

Fluocortin butyl is a corticosteroid which has been used topically for its glucocorticoid activity (p.1010) in the treatment of various skin disorders. It has usually been employed as a cream or ointment containing 0.75%. Fluocortin butyl has also been used in the form of a dry powder nasal inhalation for the management of allergic rhinitis (p.400) in usual doses of 0.5 mg inhaled into each nostril 2 to 4 times daily.

When applied topically, particularly to large areas, when the skin is broken, or under occlusive dressings, corticosteroids may be absorbed in sufficient amounts to cause systemic effects (p.1010). The effects of topical corticosteroids on the skin are described on p.1012.

Skin disorders. For recommendations concerning the correct use of corticosteroids on the skin, and a rough guide to the clinical potencies of topical corticosteroids, see Corticosteroids, Administration, p.1017.

Preparations

Proprietary Preparations (details are given in Part 3)
Belg.: Varlane; ***Ger.:*** Lenen; Vaspit; ***Ital.:*** Vaspit; ***Spain:*** Vaspit.

Multi-ingredient: ***Ger.:*** Bi-Vaspit.

Fluocortolone (1095-f)

Fluocortolone *(BAN, USAN, rINN).*

6α-Fluoro-16α-methyl-1-dehydrocorticosterone; SH-742. 6α-Fluoro-11β,21-dihydroxy-16α-methylpregna-1,4-diene-3,20-dione.

$C_{22}H_{29}FO_4$ = 376.5.

CAS — 152-97-6.

Fluocortolone Hexanoate (1096-d)

Fluocortolone Hexanoate *(BANM, rINNM).*

Fluocortolone Caproate *(USAN)*; SH-770. Fluocortolone 21-hexanoate.

$C_{28}H_{39}FO_5$ = 474.6.

CAS — 303-40-2.

Pharmacopoeias. In *Br.*

An odourless or almost odourless, white to creamy-white, crystalline powder. Practically **insoluble** in water and in ether; very slightly soluble in alcohol and in methyl alcohol; sparingly soluble in chloroform; slightly soluble in acetone and in dioxan. **Protect** from light.

Fluocortolone Pivalate (1097-n)

Fluocortolone Pivalate *(BANM, rINNM).*

Fluocortolone Trimethylacetate; Fluocortoloni Pivalas. Fluocortolone 21-pivalate.

$C_{27}H_{37}FO_5$ = 460.6.

CAS — 29205-06-9.

Pharmacopoeias. In *Eur.* (see p.viii).

A white or almost white crystalline powder. Practically **insoluble** in water; sparingly soluble in alcohol; freely soluble in dichloromethane and in dioxan. **Protect** from light.

Fluocortolone and its esters are corticosteroids mainly used topically for their glucocorticoid activity (p.1010) in the treatment of various skin disorders. They are usually employed as a cream or ointment; concentrations usually used are 0.25% of the hexanoate with 0.25% of either the free alcohol or pivalate ester. The pivalate and hexanoate esters have also been used together in ointments or suppositories for the treatment of anorectal disorders.

Fluocortolone free alcohol has been given by mouth for its systemic effects, in usual doses of 5 to 100 mg daily.

When applied topically, particularly to large areas, when the skin is broken, or under occlusive dressings, corticosteroids may be absorbed in sufficient amounts to cause systemic effects (p.1010). The effects of topical corticosteroids on the skin are described on p.1012.

Skin disorders. For recommendations concerning the correct use of corticosteroids on the skin, and a rough guide to the clinical potencies of topical corticosteroids, see Corticosteroids, Administration, p.1017.

Preparations

BP 1998: Fluocortolone Cream; Fluocortolone Ointment.

Proprietary Preparations (details are given in Part 3)
Aust.: Omnilan; Ultralan; ***Ger.:*** Syracort†; Ultralan; ***Ital.:*** Ultralan; ***Spain:*** Ultralan M; Ultralan†.

Multi-ingredient: ***Aust.:*** Pilison; Ultralan; Ultraproct; Ultraquinol; ***Austral.:*** Ultralan†; Ultraproct; ***Belg.:*** Ultralan†; Ultraproct; ***Fr.:*** Myco-Ultralan; Ultralan; Ultraproct; ***Ger.:*** Doloproct; Ultralan; Ultralan-crinale; Ultraproct; ***Irl.:*** Ultradil†; Ultralan†; Ultraproct; ***Ital.:*** Dermocur†; Eczecur†; Mycocur†; Proctocort†; Ultradil†; Ultralan; Ultraproct; ***Neth.:*** Ultralan; Ultraproct†; ***Spain:*** Ultralan†; Ultraproct†; ***Swed.:*** Ultralanum†; ***Switz.:*** Ultralan; Ultraproct; ***UK:*** Ultradil Plain†; Ultralanum Plain; Ultraproct.

Fluorometholone (1098-h)

Fluorometholone *(BAN, rINN).*

U-17323 (acetate). 9α-Fluoro-11β,17α-dihydroxy-6α-methylpregna-1,4-diene-3,20-dione.

$C_{22}H_{29}FO_4$ = 376.5.

CAS — 426-13-1.

Pharmacopoeias. In *Br., Jpn,* and *US.*

A white to yellowish-white, odourless crystalline powder. Practically **insoluble** in water; soluble 1 in 200 of alcohol and 1 in 2200 of chloroform; slightly soluble in dehydrated alcohol; slightly or very slightly soluble in ether. **Store** in airtight containers. Protect from light.

Fluorometholone Acetate (14792-a)

Fluorometholone Acetate *(BANM, USAN, rINNM).*

U-17323. 9α-Fluoro-11β,17α-dihydroxy-6α-methylpregna-1,4-diene-3,20-dione 17-acetate.

$C_{24}H_{31}FO_5$ = 418.5.

CAS — 3801-06-7.

Fluorometholone acetate 1.1 mg is approximately equivalent to 1 mg of fluorometholone.

Fluorometholone is a corticosteroid employed for its glucocorticoid activity (p.1010), usually as eye drops containing 0.1%, in the treatment of allergic and inflammatory conditions of the eye. Fluorometholone acetate has been used similarly.

Fluorometholone has also been used topically in the treatment of various skin disorders.

Prolonged application to the eye of preparations containing corticosteroids has caused raised intra-ocular pressure and reduced visual function. When applied topically, particularly to large areas, when the skin is broken, or under occlusive dressings, corticosteroids may be absorbed in sufficient amounts to cause systemic effects (p.1010). The effects of topical corticosteroids on the skin are described on p.1012.

Adverse effects. A report of posterior subcapsular cataract formation in 3 patients following the application of fluorometholone paste (0.25%) to the skin.[1] Amounts applied were about 1 g daily for 2 years for the treatment of psoriasis in 1 patient and ichthyosis in the others.

1. Costagliola C, *et al.* Cataracts associated with long-term topical steroids. *Br J Dermatol* 1989; **120:** 472–3.

Skin disorders. For recommendations concerning the correct use of corticosteroids on the skin, see Corticosteroids, Administration, p.1017.

Preparations

BP 1998: Fluorometholone Eye Drops;
USP 23: Fluorometholone Cream; Fluorometholone Ophthalmic Suspension; Neomycin Sulfate and Fluorometholone Ointment; Tobramycin and Fluorometholone Acetate Ophthalmic Suspension.

Proprietary Preparations (details are given in Part 3)
Aust.: Flarex; ***Austral.:*** Flarex; Flucon; FML; ***Belg.:*** Flucon; FML; ***Canad.:*** Flarex; FML; FML Liquifilm; ***Fr.:*** Flucon; ***Ger.:*** Efflumidex; Isopto Flucon; ***Irl.:*** FML; ***Ital.:*** Flarex; Fluaton; Flumetol Semplice; ***Neth.:*** Flarex†; Flucon†; FML Liquifilm†; ***S.Afr.:*** Flucon; FML; ***Spain:*** FML; Isopto Flucon; ***Switz.:*** Flarex; Flucon†; FML; ***UK:*** FML Liquifilm; ***USA:*** Flarex; Fluor-Op; FML.

Multi-ingredient: ***Canad.:*** FML Neo Liquifilm†; ***Ger.:*** Efemolin; Efflumycin; ***Irl.:*** FML Neo†; ***Ital.:*** Efemoline; Flumetol; Flumetol Antibiotico; Gentacort; Loticort†; ***S.Afr.:*** Efemoline; FML Neo; ***Spain:*** Bexicortil; Cortisdin Urea; FML Neo; ***Switz.:*** Efemoline; FML Neo; Infectoflam; ***UK:*** FML Neo Liquifilm; ***USA:*** FML-S.

Fluprednidene Acetate (1100-m)

Fluprednidene Acetate *(BANM, rINNM).*

Fluprednylidene 21-Acetate. 9α-Fluoro-11β,17α,21-trihydroxy-16-methylenepregna-1,4-diene-3,20-dione 21-acetate.

$C_{24}H_{29}FO_6$ = 432.5.

CAS — 2193-87-5 (fluprednidene); 1255-35-2 (fluprednidene acetate).

Fluprednidene acetate is a corticosteroid used topically for its glucocorticoid activity (p.1010) in the treatment of various skin disorders. It is usually employed as a cream, lotion, or ointment containing 0.1%.

When applied topically, particularly to large areas, when the skin is broken, or under occlusive dressings, corticosteroids may be absorbed in sufficient amounts to cause systemic effects (p.1010). The effects of topical corticosteroids on the skin are described on p.1012.

Skin disorders. For recommendations concerning the correct use of corticosteroids on the skin, and a rough guide to the clinical potencies of topical corticosteroids, see Corticosteroids, Administration, p.1017.

Preparations

Proprietary Preparations (details are given in Part 3)
Aust.: Decoderm; ***Belg.:*** Decoderm; ***Ger.:*** Decoderm; Vobaderm†; ***Neth.:*** Decoderm; ***Norw.:*** Corticoderm; ***Spain:*** Decoderm; ***Swed.:*** Corticoderm; ***Switz.:*** Decoderm.

Multi-ingredient: ***Aust.:*** Decoderm compositum; Decoderm trivalent; Mycocort†; Sali-Decoderm; ***Belg.:*** Decoderm Comp; ***Ger.:*** Candio E comp N; Crinohermal fem neu; Decoderm Comp; Decoderm tri; Decoderm trivalent†; Sali-Decoderm; Vobaderm Plus†; ***Spain:*** Decoderm Trivalente; ***Swed.:*** Corticoderm comp†; ***Switz.:*** Candio E†; Crinohermal FEM†; Decoderm bivalent; Decoderm compositum†; Decoderm trivalent†.

Fluprednisolone (1101-b)

Fluprednisolone *(BAN, USAN, rINN).*

6α-Fluoroprednisolone; NSC-47439; U-7800. 6α-Fluoro-11β,17α,21-trihydroxypregna-1,4-diene-3,20-dione.

$C_{21}H_{27}FO_5$ = 378.4.

CAS — 53-34-9 (fluprednisolone); 23257-44-5 (fluprednisolone valerate).

Fluprednisolone is a corticosteroid with mainly glucocorticoid activity (p.1010); 2 mg of fluprednisolone is roughly equivalent in anti-inflammatory activity to 5 mg of prednisolone. It is given by mouth in the management of a variety of conditions requiring systemic glucocorticoid therapy (p.1015), in usual doses ranging from 2 to 32 mg daily.

Preparations

Proprietary Preparations (details are given in Part 3)
Aust.: Isopredon.

Flurandrenolone (1102-v)

Flurandrenolone *(BAN).*

Fludroxycortide *(rINN)*; 33379; Fluorandrenolone; 6α-Fluoro-16α-hydroxyhydrocortisone 16,17-Acetonide; Flurandrenolide *(USAN)*. 6α-Fluoro-11β,21-dihydroxy-16α,17α-isopropylidenedioxypregn-4-ene-3,20-dione.

$C_{24}H_{33}FO_6$ = 436.5.

CAS — 1524-88-5.

Pharmacopoeias. In *US.*

An odourless, white to off-white, fluffy, crystalline powder. Practically **insoluble** in water and in ether; soluble 1 in 72 of alcohol, 1 in 10 of chloroform, and 1 in 25 of methyl alcohol. **Store** at a temperature not exceeding 8° in airtight containers. Protect from light.

Flurandrenolone is a corticosteroid used topically for its glucocorticoid activity (p.1010) in the treatment of various skin disorders. It is usually employed as a cream or ointment containing 0.0125% or a lotion containing 0.05%. It is also used as a polyethylene tape with an adhesive containing 4 μg of flurandrenolone per cm^2 of tape.

When applied topically, particularly to large areas, when the skin is broken, or under occlusive dressings, corticosteroids may be absorbed in sufficient amounts to cause systemic effects (p.1010). The effects of topical corticosteroids on the skin are described on p.1012.

Skin disorders. For recommendations concerning the correct use of corticosteroids on the skin, and a rough guide to the clinical potencies of topical corticosteroids, see Corticosteroids, Administration, p.1017.

Preparations

USP 23: Flurandrenolide Cream; Flurandrenolide Lotion; Flurandrenolide Ointment; Flurandrenolide Tape; Neomycin Sulfate and Flurandrenolide Cream; Neomycin Sulfate and Flurandrenolide Lotion; Neomycin Sulfate and Flurandrenolide Ointment.

Proprietary Preparations (details are given in Part 3)
Canad.: Drenison; ***Ger.:*** Sermaka; ***Irl.:*** Haelan; ***Ital.:*** Drenison†; ***Spain:*** Drenison; ***UK:*** Haelan; ***USA:*** Cordran.

Multi-ingredient: ***Ger.:*** Sermaform†; Sermaka N†; ***Ital.:*** Drenison con Neomicina†; ***Spain:*** Drenison Neomicina; ***UK:*** Haelan-C†.

Fluticasone Propionate (14742-p)

Fluticasone Propionate *(BANM, USAN, rINNM).*

CCI-18781. S-Fluoromethyl 6α,9α-difluoro-11β,17α-dihydroxy-16α-methyl-3-oxoandrosta-1,4-diene-17β-carbothioate 17-propionate.

$C_{25}H_{31}F_3O_5S$ = 500.6.

CAS — 80474-14-2.

Pharmacopoeias. In *Br.*

A white or almost white crystalline powder. Practically **insoluble** in water; slightly soluble in alcohol; freely soluble in dimethylformamide; sparingly soluble in acetone and in dichloromethane.

Adverse Effects, Treatment, Withdrawal, and Precautions

As for corticosteroids in general (see p.1010). Hypersensitivity reactions have occurred.

Inhalation of large amounts of fluticasone propionate may produce systemic effects in some patients (see below). When administered by nasal spray in doses used clinically, fluticasone propionate is reported to have little or no systemic effect.

When applied topically, particularly to large areas, when the skin is broken, or under occlusive dressings, corticosteroids may be absorbed in sufficient amounts to cause systemic effects.

Adrenal suppression. Despite the fact that inhaled fluticasone is generally thought to lack systemic effects at therapeutic doses, a study in 25 healthy subjects[1] indicated that fluticasone propionate as single inhaled doses of 250, 500, and 1000 μg did produce a reduction in plasma cortisol, indicating suppression of the hypothalamic-pituitary-adrenal axis to some degree. Others have also found evidence of adrenal suppression with fluticasone,[2-4] particularly at high doses, and the effect may be more marked with repeated than with single doses.[4-6] Conflicting claims have been made concerning the risk of clinical effects, for example on growth.[7-9]

1. Grahnén A, *et al.* An assessment of the systemic activity of single doses of inhaled fluticasone propionate in healthy volunteers. *Br J Clin Pharmacol* 1994; **38:** 521–5.
2. Clark DJ, *et al.* Comparative systemic bioactivity of inhaled budesonide and fluticasone propionate in asthmatic children. *Br J Clin Pharmacol* 1996; **42:** 264P.
3. Rohatagi S, *et al.* Dynamic modeling of cortisol reduction after inhaled administration of fluticasone propionate. *J Clin Pharmacol* 1996; **36:** 938–41.
4. Clark DJ, Lipworth BJ. Adrenal suppression with chronic dosing of fluticasone propionate compared with budesonide in adult asthmatic patients. *Thorax* 1997; **52:** 55–8.
5. Lönnebo A, *et al.* An assessment of the systemic effects of single and repeated doses of inhaled fluticasone propionate and inhaled budesonide in healthy volunteers. *Eur J Clin Pharmacol* 1996; **49:** 459–63.
6. Wilson AM, *et al.* Adrenal suppression with high doses of inhaled fluticasone propionate and triamcinolone acetonide in healthy voluteers. *Eur J Clin Pharmacol* 1997; **53:** 33–7.
7. Todd G, *et al.* Growth and adrenal suppression in asthmatic children treated with high-dose fluticasone propionate. *Lancet* 1996; **348:** 27–9.
8. Whitaker K, *et al.* Effect of fluticasone on growth in children with asthma. *Lancet* 1996; **348:** 63–4.
9. Cade A, *et al.* High-dose inhaled steroids in asthmatic children. *Lancet* 1996; **348:** 819.

Interactions

The interactions of corticosteroids in general are described on p.1014.

Pharmacokinetics

For a brief outline of the pharmacokinetics of corticosteroids, see p.1014.

Fluticasone propionate is poorly absorbed from the gastro-intestinal tract and undergoes extensive first-pass metabolism; oral bioavailability is reported to be only about 1%.

References.

1. Falcoz C, *et al.* Oral bioavailability of fluticasone propionate in healthy subjects. *Br J Clin Pharmacol* 1996; **41:** 459P–460P.
2. Mackie AE, *et al.* Pharmacokinetics of intravenous fluticasone propionate in healthy subjects. *Br J Clin Pharmacol* 1996; **41:** 539–42.

Uses and Administration

Fluticasone propionate is a corticosteroid with mainly glucocorticoid activity (p.1010).

Fluticasone propionate is stated to exert a topical effect on the lungs without significant systemic effects at usual doses, due to its low systemic bioavailability (but see above). It is used by inhalation for the prophylaxis of the symptoms of asthma. Initial doses in the UK range from 100 to 250 μg twice daily in mild asthma to 500 to 1000 μg twice daily in severe asthma, adjusted according to response. Children over 4 years of age may be given initial doses of 50 to 100 μg twice daily.

Fluticasone propionate is administered by nasal spray in the prophylaxis and treatment of allergic rhinitis. The usual dose is 100 μg into each nostril once daily, increased if necessary to 100 μg into each nostril twice daily. Children over 4 years of age may be given half these doses.

It is applied topically in the treatment of various skin disorders. Creams and ointments containing 0.05% and 0.005% respectively are available.

Asthma. Corticosteroids, together with the $beta_2$-adrenoceptor agonists, form one of the cornerstones of the management of asthma (p.745). Patients requiring only occasional relief from symptoms may be managed with an inhaled short-acting $beta_2$ agonist, and an inhaled corticosteroid such as fluticasone is added if symptomatic relief is needed more than once daily. The dose of inhaled corticosteroid is increased in more severe asthma, often together with the addition of other agents.

Some references to the use of fluticasone propionate for asthma are given below,[1-5] including one to a study indicating that increasing the dose of inhaled fluticasone did not produce increased benefit.[4]

1. Gustafsson P, *et al.* Comparison of the efficacy and safety of inhaled fluticasone propionate 200 μg/day with inhaled beclomethasone dipropionate 400 μg/day in mild and moderate asthma. *Arch Dis Child* 1993; **69:** 206–11.
2. Holliday SM, *et al.* Inhaled fluticasone propionate: a review of its pharmacodynamic and pharmacokinetic properties, and therapeutic use in asthma. *Drugs* 1994; **47:** 318–31.
3. Anonymous. Fluticasone propionate for asthma prophylaxis. *Drug Ther Bull* 1994; **32:** 25–7.
4. Boe J, *et al.* High-dose inhaled steroids in asthmatics: moderate efficacy gain and suppression of the hypothalamic-pituitary-adrenal (HPA) axis. *Eur Respir J* 1994; **7:** 2179–84.
5. Anonymous. Fluticasone propionate for chronic asthma. *Med Lett Drugs Ther* 1996; **38:** 83–4.

Inflammatory bowel disease. Fluticasone propionate, administered by mouth, was reported to be useful in the treatment of Crohn's disease,[1] ulcerative colitis,[2] and coeliac disease.[3] The dose was 5 mg four times daily but in one study,[2] higher doses were thought necessary.

Corticosteroids with low bioavailability, which might be able to exert topical anti-inflammatory actions on the gut without producing systemic adverse effects, are currently under investigation in the management of inflammatory bowel disease, as discussed on p.1171.

1. Carpani de Kaski M, *et al.* Fluticasone propionate in Crohn's disease. *Gut* 1991; **32:** 657–61.
2. Hawthorne AB, *et al.* Fluticasone propionate versus prednisolone in the treatment of active ulcerative colitis: a multicentre study. *Gut* 1991; **32:** A560–1.
3. Mitchison HC, *et al.* A pilot study of fluticasone propionate in untreated coeliac disease. *Gut* 1991; **32:** 260–5.

Rhinitis. For a discussion of the management of rhinitis, including the use of corticosteroids, see p.400. Some further references to the use of fluticasone in rhinitis are given below.

1. Grossman J, *et al.* Fluticasone propionate aqueous nasal spray is safe and effective for children with seasonal allergic rhinitis. *Pediatrics* 1993; **92:** 594–9.
2. Scadding GK, *et al.* Effect of short-term treatment with fluticasone propionate nasal spray on the response to nasal allergen challenge. *Br J Clin Pharmacol* 1994; **38:** 447–51.
3. Banov CH, *et al.* Once daily intranasal fluticasone propionate is effective for perennial allergic rhinitis. *Ann Allergy* 1994; **73:** 240–6.
4. Darnell R, *et al.* A double-blind comparison of fluticasone propionate aqueous nasal spray, terfenadine tablets and placebo in the treatment of patients with seasonal allergic rhinitis to grass pollen. *Clin Exp Allergy* 1994; **24:** 1144–50.
5. Van Bavel J, *et al.* Intranasal fluticasone propionate is more effective than terfenadine tablets for seasonal allergic rhinitis. *Arch Intern Med* 1994; **154:** 2699–2704.
6. Anonymous. Fluticasone propionate nasal spray for allergic rhinitis. *Med Lett Drugs Ther* 1995; **37:** 5–6.
7. Wiseman LR, Benfield P. Intranasal fluticasone propionate: a reappraisal of its pharmacology and clinical efficacy in the treatment of rhinitis. *Drugs* 1997; **53:** 885–907.

Skin disorders. For recommendations concerning the correct use of corticosteroids on the skin, see Corticosteroids, Administration, p.1017.

Preparations

BP 1998: Fluticasone Cream; Fluticasone Ointment.

Proprietary Preparations (details are given in Part 3)
Aust.: Cutivate; Flixonase; Flixotide; ***Austral.:*** Flixotide; ***Belg.:*** Flixotide; ***Canad.:*** Flonase; Flovent; ***Ger.:*** Atemur; Flutide; Flutivate; ***Irl.:*** Flixonase; Flixotide; ***Ital.:*** Flixonase; Flixotide; Fluspiral; ***Neth.:*** Cutivate; Flixonase; Flixotide; ***Norw.:*** Flutide; Flutivate; ***S.Afr.:*** Cutivate; Flixonase; Flixotide; ***Swed.:*** Flutide; Flutivate; ***Switz.:*** Axotide; Cutivate; Flutinase; ***UK:*** Cutivate; Flixonase; Flixotide; ***USA:*** Cutivate; Flonase; Flovent.

Formocortal (1103-g)

Formocortal *(BAN, USAN, rINN)*.

Fl-6341; Fluoroformylon. 3-(2-Chloroethoxy)-9α-fluoro-11β,21-dihydroxy-16α,17α-isopropylidenedioxy-20-oxopregna-3,5-diene-6-carbaldehyde 21-acetate.

$C_{29}H_{38}ClFO_8$ = 569.1.

CAS — 2825-60-7.

Formocortal is a corticosteroid that has been used for its glucocorticoid activity (see p.1010) in the treatment of inflammatory eye disorders as eye drops and eye ointments containing 0.05%.

Prolonged application to the eye of preparations containing corticosteroids has caused raised intra-ocular pressure and reduced visual function. (For further discussion of the effect of corticosteroids on the eye, see p.1011.)

Preparations

Proprietary Preparations (details are given in Part 3)
Ital.: Formoftil.

Multi-ingredient: ***Ital.:*** Formomicin.

Halcinonide (1104-q)

Halcinonide *(BAN, USAN, rINN)*.

Alcinonide; SQ-18566. 21-Chloro-9α-fluoro-11β-hydroxy-16α,17α-isopropylidenedioxypregn-4-ene-3,20-dione.

$C_{24}H_{32}ClFO_5$ = 455.0.

CAS — 3093-35-4.

Pharmacopoeias. In Chin. and US.

A white to off-white, odourless crystalline powder. Practically **insoluble** in water; soluble in acetone and in chloroform; slightly soluble in alcohol and in ether.

Halcinonide is a corticosteroid used topically for its glucocorticoid activity (p.1010) in the treatment of various skin disorders. It is usually employed as a 0.1% cream, lotion, or ointment.

When applied topically, particularly to large areas, when the skin is broken, or under occlusive dressings, corticosteroids may be absorbed in sufficient amounts to cause systemic effects (p.1010). The effects of topical corticosteroids on the skin are described on p.1012.

Skin disorders. For recommendations concerning the correct use of corticosteroids on the skin, and a rough guide to the clinical potencies of topical corticosteroids, see Corticosteroids, Administration, p.1017.

Preparations

USP 23: Halcinonide Cream; Halcinonide Ointment; Halcinonide Topical Solution.

Proprietary Preparations (details are given in Part 3)
Aust.: Halog; ***Austral.:*** Halciderm; ***Canad.:*** Halog; ***Fr.:*** Halog; ***Ger.:*** Halcimat†; Halog; ***Ital.:*** Halciderm; ***Neth.:*** Halciderm†; ***Norw.:*** Halog; ***Spain:*** Halog; ***Switz.:*** Betacortone; Halciderm†; ***UK:*** Halciderm; ***USA:*** Halog.

Multi-ingredient: ***Canad.:*** Halcicomb†; ***Fr.:*** Halog Neomycine; ***Ger.:*** Halog Tri; ***Ital.:*** Anfocort; Halciderm; Halciderm Combi; ***Switz.:*** Betacortone; Betacortone S; Halciderm comp†; Halciderm†.

Halobetasol Propionate (12198-q)

Halobetasol Propionate *(USAN)*.

Ulobetasol Propionate *(rINNM)*; BMY-30056; CGP-14458. 21-Chloro-6α,9-difluoro-11β,17-dihydroxy-16β-methylpregna-1,4-diene-3,20-dione 17-propionate.

$C_{25}H_{31}ClF_2O_5$ = 485.0.

CAS — 98651-66-2 (halobetasol); 66852-54-8 (halobetasol propionate).

Halobetasol propionate is a corticosteroid that is used topically for its glucocorticoid activity (p.1010) in the treatment of various skin disorders. It is usually employed as cream or ointment containing 0.05%.

When applied topically, particularly to large areas, when the skin is broken, or under occlusive dressings, corticosteroids may be absorbed in sufficient amounts to cause systemic effects (p.1010). The effects of topical corticosteroids on the skin are described on p.1012.

Skin disorders. For recommendations concerning the correct use of corticosteroids on the skin, and a rough guide to the clinical potencies of topical corticosteroids see Corticosteroids, Administration, p.1017.

Preparations

Proprietary Preparations (details are given in Part 3)
Aust.: Miracorten; ***Canad.:*** Ultravate; ***Switz.:*** Miracorten; ***USA:*** Ultravate.

Halometasone (16830-n)

Halometasone *(rINN)*.

C-48401-Ba; Halomethasone. 2-Chloro-6α,9-difluoro-11β,17,21-trihydroxy-16α-methylpregna-1,4-diene-3,20-dione.

$C_{22}H_{27}ClF_2O_5$ = 444.9.

CAS — 50629-82-8.

Halometasone is a corticosteroid used topically for its glucocorticoid activity (p.1010) in the treatment of various skin disorders. It is usually employed as a cream or ointment containing 0.05% of halometasone monohydrate.

When applied topically, particularly to large areas, when the skin is broken, or under occlusive dressings, corticosteroids may be absorbed in sufficient amounts to cause systemic effects (p.1010). The effects of topical corticosteroids on the skin are described on p.1012.

Skin disorders. For recommendations concerning the correct use of corticosteroids on the skin, see Corticosteroids, Administration, p.1017.

Preparations

Proprietary Preparations (details are given in Part 3)
Aust.: Sicorten; ***Belg.:*** Sicorten; ***Ger.:*** Sicorten; ***Neth.:*** Sicorten; ***Spain:*** Sicorten; ***Switz.:*** Sicorten.

Multi-ingredient: ***Ger.:*** Sicorten Plus; ***S.Afr.:*** Sicorten Plus†; ***Spain:*** Sicorten Plus; ***Switz.:*** Sicorten Plus.

Hydrocortamate Hydrochloride (1105-p)

Hydrocortamate Hydrochloride *(rINNM)*.

Ethamicort; Hydrocortisone Diethylaminoacetate Hydrochloride. 11β,17α,21-Trihydroxypregn-4-ene-3,20-dione 21-diethylaminoacetate hydrochloride.

$C_{27}H_{41}NO_6,HCl$ = 512.1.

CAS — 76-47-1 (hydrocortamate); 125-03-1 (hydrocortamate hydrochloride).

Hydrocortamate hydrochloride is a corticosteroid that has been used topically for its glucocorticoid activity (p.1010) in the treatment of various skin disorders.

When applied topically, particularly to large areas, when the skin is broken, or under occlusive dressings, corticosteroids may be absorbed in sufficient amounts to cause systemic effects (p.1010). The effects of topical corticosteroids on the skin are described on p.1012.

Skin disorders. For recommendations concerning the correct use of corticosteroids on the skin, see Corticosteroids, Administration, p.1017.

Preparations

Proprietary Preparations (details are given in Part 3)

Multi-ingredient: ***Ital.:*** Cortanest; Etamicina†.

Hydrocortisone (1138-k)

Hydrocortisone *(BAN, rINN)*.

Anti-inflammatory Hormone; Compound F; Cortisol; Hydrocortisonum; 17-Hydroxycorticosterone; NSC-10483. 11β,17α,21-Trihydroxypregn-4-ene-3,20-dione.

$C_{21}H_{30}O_5$ = 362.5.

CAS — 50-23-7.

Pharmacopoeias. In *Chin., Eur.* (see p.viii), *Int., Jpn, Pol.,* and *US.*

A white or almost white, odourless, crystalline powder. It exhibits polymorphism. Practically **insoluble** to very slightly soluble in water; soluble 1 in 40 of alcohol and 1 in 80 of acetone; slightly soluble in chloroform and in dichloromethane; very slightly soluble in ether. **Protect** from light.

Hydrocortisone Acetate (1107-w)

Hydrocortisone Acetate *(BANM, rINNM)*.

Cortisol Acetate; Hydrocortisoni Acetas. Hydrocortisone 21-acetate.

$C_{23}H_{32}O_6$ = 404.5.

CAS — 50-03-3.

NOTE. HCOR is a code approved by the BP for use on single unit doses of eye drops containing hydrocortisone acetate where the individual container may be too small to bear all the appropriate labelling information.

Pharmacopoeias. In *Chin., Eur.* (see p.viii), *Int., Jpn, Pol.,* and *US.*

An odourless, white or almost white, crystalline powder. Hydrocortisone acetate 112 mg is approximately equivalent to 100 mg of hydrocortisone.

Practically **insoluble** in water; soluble 1 in 230 of alcohol and 1 in 200 of chloroform; slightly soluble in dehydrated alcohol and in dichloromethane. **Protect** from light.

Hydrocortisone Butyrate (1108-e)

Hydrocortisone Butyrate *(BANM, USAN, rINNM).*

Cortisol Butyrate. Hydrocortisone 17α-butyrate.

$C_{25}H_{36}O_6$ = 432.5.

CAS — 13609-67-1.

Pharmacopoeias. In *Jpn* and *US.*

A white to practically white, practically odourless crystalline powder. Hydrocortisone butyrate 119 mg is approximately equivalent to 100 mg of hydrocortisone.

Practically **insoluble** in water; slightly soluble in ether; soluble in acetone, in alcohol, and in methyl alcohol; freely soluble in chloroform.

Hydrocortisone Cypionate (1109-l)

Hydrocortisone Cypionate *(BANM).*

Hydrocortisone Cipionate *(rINNM)*; Cortisol Cypionate; Hydrocortisone Cyclopentylpropionate. Hydrocortisone 21-(3-cyclopentylpropionate).

$C_{29}H_{42}O_6$ = 486.6.

CAS — 508-99-6.

Hydrocortisone Hemisuccinate (1110-v)

Hydrocortisone Hemisuccinate *(rINNM).*

Cortisol Hemisuccinate; Hydrocortisone Hydrogen Succinate *(BANM)*; Hydrocortisone Succinate; Hydrocortisoni Hydrogenosuccinas. Hydrocortisone 21-(hydrogen succinate).

$C_{25}H_{34}O_8$ = 462.5.

CAS — 2203-97-6 (anhydrous); 83784-20-7 (monohydrate).

Pharmacopoeias. In *Eur.* (see p.viii) and *Jpn. US* allows the anhydrous form or the monohydrate.

A white or almost white, hygroscopic crystalline powder. Hydrocortisone hemisuccinate 128 mg is approximately equivalent to 100 mg of hydrocortisone.

Practically **insoluble** in water; freely soluble in acetone and in dehydrated alcohol. It dissolves in dilute solutions of alkali carbonates or hydroxides. **Store** in airtight containers. Protect from light.

Hydrocortisone Sodium Phosphate (1111-g)

Hydrocortisone Sodium Phosphate *(BANM, rINNM).*

Cortisol Sodium Phosphate. Hydrocortisone 21-(disodium orthophosphate).

$C_{21}H_{29}Na_2O_8P$ = 486.4.

CAS — 6000-74-4.

Pharmacopoeias. In *Br., Jpn,* and *US.*

A white or light yellow, odourless or almost odourless, hygroscopic powder. Hydrocortisone sodium phosphate 134 mg is approximately equivalent to 100 mg of hydrocortisone. **Soluble** 1 in 1.5 of water; slightly soluble in alcohol; practically insoluble in dehydrated alcohol, in chloroform, in dioxan, and in ether. A 0.5% solution in water has a pH of 7.5 to 9.0. **Store** in airtight containers. Protect from light.

Hydrocortisone Sodium Succinate (1112-q)

Hydrocortisone Sodium Succinate *(BANM, rINNM).*

Cortisol Sodium Succinate. Hydrocortisone 21-(sodium succinate).

$C_{25}H_{33}NaO_8$ = 484.5.

CAS — 125-04-2.

Pharmacopoeias. In *Int., It., Jpn., Pol.,* and *US.*

A white or almost white, odourless, hygroscopic, amorphous solid. Hydrocortisone sodium succinate 134 mg is approximately equivalent to 100 mg of hydrocortisone.

Very **soluble** in water and in alcohol; very slightly soluble in acetone; practically insoluble in chloroform. **Store** in airtight containers. Protect from light.

Hydrocortisone Valerate (1106-s)

Hydrocortisone Valerate *(BANM, USAN, rINNM).*

Cortisol Valerate. Hydrocortisone 17-valerate.

$C_{26}H_{38}O_6$ = 446.6.

CAS — 57524-89-7.

Pharmacopoeias. In *US.*

Hydrocortisone valerate 123 mg is approximately equivalent to 100 mg of hydrocortisone.

Adverse Effects, Treatment, Withdrawal, and Precautions

As for corticosteroids in general (see p.1010).

When applied topically, particularly to large areas, when the skin is broken, or under occlusive dressings, corticosteroids may be absorbed in sufficient amounts to cause systemic effects.

Effects on fluid and electrolyte balance. A report of marked hypokalaemia and hypomagnesaemia associated with high dose intravenous hydrocortisone therapy in an alcoholic patient with suspected immune thrombocytopenia.[1] Cardiac arrhythmias developed, and prolonged infusion of magnesium and potassium was required to restore normal plasma concentrations.

1. Ramsahoye BH, *et al.* The mineralocorticoid effects of high dose hydrocortisone. *Br Med J* 1995; **310:** 656–7.

Effects on the nerves. For reports and comments on paraesthesia or perineal irritation associated with the administration of hydrocortisone sodium phosphate intravenously, see p.1012.

Hypersensitivity and anaphylaxis. Reviews, discussions, and reports of hypersensitivity reactions and anaphylaxis associated with the intravenous administration of hydrocortisone.[1-6] Topical application of hydrocortisone can also result in hypersensitivity.[7]

1. Chan CS, *et al.* Hydrocortisone-induced anaphylaxis. *Med J Aust* 1984; **141:** 444–6.
2. Seale JP. Anaphylactoid reaction to hydrocortisone. *Med J Aust* 1984; **141:** 446.
3. Corallo CE, Sosnin M. Bronchospasm, tachycardia following intravenous hydrocortisone. *Aust J Hosp Pharm* 1985; **15:** 103–4.
4. Al Mahdy H, Hall M. Anaphylaxis and hydrocortisone. *Ann Intern Med* 1988; **108:** 487–8.
5. Fulcher DA, Katelaris CH. Anaphylactoid reaction to intravenous hydrocortisone sodium succinate: a case report and literature review. *Med J Aust* 1991; **154:** 210–14.
6. Kawane H. Anaphylactoid reaction to intravenous hydrocortisone sodium succinate. *Med J Aust* 1991; **154:** 782.
7. Wilkinson SM, *et al.* Hydrocortisone: an important cutaneous allergen. *Lancet* 1991; **337:** 761–2.

Interactions

The interactions of corticosteroids in general are described on p.1014.

Pharmacokinetics

For a brief account of the pharmacokinetics of corticosteroids, see p.1014.

Hydrocortisone is readily absorbed from the gastro-intestinal tract and peak blood concentrations are attained in about an hour. The biological half-life is about 100 minutes. It is more than 90% bound to plasma proteins. Following intramuscular injection, the absorption of the water-soluble sodium phosphate and sodium succinate esters is rapid, while absorption of hydrocortisone free alcohol and its lipid-soluble esters is slower. Absorption of hydrocortisone acetate after intra-articular or soft-tissue injection is also slow. Hydrocortisone is absorbed through the skin, particularly in denuded areas.

Hydrocortisone is metabolised in the liver and most body tissues to hydrogenated and degraded forms such as tetrahydrocortisone and tetrahydrocortisol. These are excreted in the urine, mainly conjugated as glucuronides, together with a very small proportion of unchanged hydrocortisone.

Uses and Administration

Hydrocortisone is a corticosteroid with both glucocorticoid and to a lesser extent mineralocorticoid activity (p.1010). As cortisol it is the most important of the predominantly glucocorticoid steroids secreted by the adrenal cortex. Hydrocortisone is used, usually in combination with a more potent mineralocorticoid, for replacement therapy in adrenocortical insufficiency (p.1017). It may also be used for its glucocorticoid properties in other conditions for which corticosteroid therapy is indicated (p.1015) but drugs with fewer mineralocorticoid effects tend to be preferred for the long-term systemic therapy of auto-immune and inflammatory disease.

For administration by mouth hydrocortisone free alcohol is usually used and sometimes the cypionate ester is also employed.

For replacement therapy in acute or chronic adrenocortical insufficiency the normal requirement is 20 or 30 mg daily (usually 20 mg is taken in the morning and 10 mg in the early evening, to mimic the circadian rhythm of the body). Additional sodium chloride may be required if there is defective aldosterone secretion, but mineralocorticoid activity is usually supplemented by fludrocortisone acetate by mouth. Similar regimens have also been used to correct glucocorticoid deficiency in the salt-losing form of congenital adrenal hyperplasia (p.1020).

Hydrocortisone may be given intravenously, by slow injection or infusion, in the form of a water-soluble derivative such as hydrocortisone sodium succinate or hydrocortisone sodium phosphate when a rapid effect is required in emergencies: such conditions are acute adrenocortical insufficiency caused by Addisonian or post-adrenalectomy crises, by the abrupt accidental withdrawal of therapy in corticosteroid-treated patients, or by the inability of the adrenal glands to cope with increased stress in such patients; certain allergic emergencies; acute severe asthma (status asthmaticus—see also p.745); and shock. The usual dose is the equivalent of 100 to 500 mg of hydrocortisone, repeated 3 or 4 times in 24 hours, according to the severity of the condition and the patient's response. Children up to 1 year of age may be given 25 mg, those aged 1 to 5 years 50 mg, and those aged 6 to 12 years 100 mg. Fluids and electrolytes should be given as necessary to correct any associated metabolic disorder. Similar doses to those specified above may also be given intramuscularly but the response is likely to be less rapid than that observed following intravenous administration. Corticosteroids are considered to be of secondary value in anaphylactic shock because of their relatively slow onset of action, but they may be a useful adjunct to adrenaline to prevent further deterioration in severely affected patients; hydrocortisone sodium succinate may be given by intravenous injection in a dose equivalent to 100 to 300 mg of hydrocortisone.

In patients with adrenal deficiency states supplementary corticosteroid therapy may be necessary during some surgical operations and hydrocortisone sodium succinate or sodium phosphate may be given intramuscularly or intravenously before surgery. The equivalent of hydrocortisone 100 mg may be given with the premedication and repeated every 8 hours. This dose is generally tapered off over 5 days to reach a maintenance dose of 20 to 30 mg per 24 hours.

For local administration by injection into soft tissues hydrocortisone in the form of the sodium phosphate or sodium succinate esters is usually employed; doses in terms of hydrocortisone are usually 100 to 200 mg. For intra-articular injection hydrocortisone acetate is usually used in doses of 5 to 50 mg depending upon the size of the joint.

For topical application in the treatment of various skin disorders hydrocortisone and the acetate, buteprate, butyrate, and valerate esters are normally employed in creams, ointments, or lotions. Concentrations usually used have ranged from 0.1 to 2.5%. Although it is considered that hydrocortisone has fewer side-effects on the skin and is less liable to cause adrenal suppression than the more potent topical corticosteroids (see p.1017 for a rough guide to the clinical potencies of topical corticosteroids), it should be borne in mind, especially in view of the availability of 'over-the-counter' hydrocortisone preparations in many countries, that this property may be considerably modified both by the type of formulation or vehicle used and by the type of esterification present; other factors that may also influence the degree of absorption include the site of application, use of an occlusive dressing, the degree of skin damage, and the size of the area to which the preparation is applied.

Hydrocortisone or its esters are also available in a variety of other dosage forms including those for ophthalmic, aural, dental, and rectal application, for use in allergic and inflammatory disorders.

Other esters of hydrocortisone which have occasionally been used include the aceponate and glycyrrhetinate. Esters such as the aceponate may show modified topical activity.

Preparations

BP 1998: Hydrocortisone Acetate and Neomycin Ear Drops; Hydrocortisone Acetate and Neomycin Eye Drops; Hydrocortisone Acetate and Neomycin Eye Ointment; Hydrocortisone Acetate Cream; Hydrocortisone Acetate Injection; Hydrocortisone Acetate Ointment; Hydrocortisone and Clioquinol Cream; Hydrocortisone and Clioquinol Ointment; Hydrocortisone and Neomycin Cream; Hydrocortisone Cream; Hydrocortisone Ointment; Hydrocortisone Sodium Phosphate Injection; Hydrocortisone Sodium Succinate Injection;

USP 23: Chloramphenicol and Hydrocortisone Acetate for Ophthalmic Suspension; Chloramphenicol, Polymyxin B Sulfate, and Hydrocortisone Acetate Ophthalmic Ointment; Clioquinol and Hydrocortisone Cream; Clioquinol and Hydrocortisone Ointment; Colistin and Neomycin Sulfates and Hydrocortisone Acetate Otic Suspension; Hydrocortisone Acetate Cream; Hydrocortisone Acetate Injectable Suspension; Hydrocortisone Acetate Lotion; Hydrocortisone Acetate Ointment; Hydrocortisone Acetate Ophthalmic Ointment; Hydrocortisone Acetate Ophthalmic Suspension; Hydrocortisone and Acetic Acid Otic Solution; Hydrocortisone Butyrate Cream; Hydrocortisone Cream; Hydrocortisone Enema; Hydrocortisone Gel; Hydrocortisone Injectable Suspension; Hydrocortisone Lotion; Hydrocortisone Ointment; Hydrocortisone Sodium Phosphate Injection; Hydrocortisone Sodium Succinate for Injection; Hydrocortisone Tablets; Hydrocortisone Valerate Cream; Neomycin and Polymyxin B Sulfates and Hydrocortisone Acetate Cream; Neomycin and Polymyxin B Sulfates and Hydrocortisone Acetate Ophthalmic Suspension; Neomycin and Polymyxin B Sulfates and Hydrocortisone Ophthalmic Suspension; Neomycin and Polymyxin B Sulfates and Hydrocortisone Otic Solution; Neomycin and Polymyxin B Sulfates and Hydrocortisone Otic Suspension; Neomycin and Polymyxin B Sulfates, Bacitracin Zinc, and Hydrocortisone Acetate Ophthalmic Ointment; Neomycin and Polymyxin B Sulfates, Bacitracin Zinc, and Hydrocortisone Ointment; Neomycin and Polymyxin B Sulfates, Bacitracin Zinc, and Hydrocortisone Ophthalmic Ointment; Neomycin and Polymyxin B Sulfates, Bacitracin, and Hydrocortisone Acetate Ointment; Neomycin and Polymyxin B Sulfates, Bacitracin, and Hydrocortisone Acetate Ophthalmic Ointment; Neomycin and Polymyxin B Sulfates, Gramicidin, and Hydrocortisone Acetate Cream; Neomycin Sulfate and Hydrocortisone Acetate Cream; Neomycin Sulfate and Hydrocortisone Acetate Lotion; Neomycin Sulfate and Hydrocortisone Acetate Ointment; Neomycin Sulfate and Hydrocortisone Acetate Ophthalmic Ointment; Neomycin Sulfate and Hydrocortisone Acetate Ophthalmic Suspension; Neomycin Sulfate and Hydrocortisone Cream; Neomycin Sulfate and Hydrocortisone Ointment; Neomycin Sulfate and Hydrocortisone Otic Suspension; Oxytetracycline Hydrochloride and Hydrocortisone Acetate Ophthalmic Suspension; Oxytetracycline Hydrochloride and Hydrocortisone Ointment; Polymyxin B Sulfate and Hydrocortisone Otic Solution.

Proprietary Preparations (details are given in Part 3)

Aust.: Colifoam; Ekzemsalbe; Hydrocortone; Hydroderm; Locoidon; Schericur; ***Austral.:*** Adacor†; Colifoam; Corlan†; Cortaid†; Cortef; Cortic; Derm-Aid; Dermacort†; Efcortelan†; Egocort Cream; Hycor; Hysone; Nordicort; Sigmacort; Siguent Hycor; Solu-Cortef; Squibb-HC; ***Belg.:*** Buccalsone; Colifoam; Cortril; Cremicort-H; Locoid; Pannocort; Sential Hydrocortisone†; Solu-Cortef; ***Canad.:*** A-Hydrocort; Aquacort; Barriere-HC; Cortacet; Cortamed; Cortate; Cortef; Cortenema; Corticreme; Cortifoam; Cortiment; Cortoderm; Emo-Cort; Hycort; Hyderm; Hydrosone; Lanacort; Novo-Hydrocort; Prevex HC; Rectocort; Sarna HC; Solu-Cortef; Texacort; Westcort; ***Fr.:*** Colofoam; Efficort; Hydracort; Locoid; Proctocort; ***Ger.:*** Alfason; Colifoam; Cordes H†; Dermo Posterisan; Ebenol; Ekzesin†; Ficortril; Glycocortison; Hydrocort; Hydrocort Mild; Hydroderm; Laticort; Latimit; Munitren H; Pandel; Posterine Corte; Remederm HC; Retef; Sagittacortin; Sanatison Mono; Soventol Hydrocortison; Velopural; ***Irl.:*** Colifoam; Corlan; Cortopin; Dioderm; Efcortelan Soluble†; Hc45; Hydrocortisyl; Hydrocortone; Locoid; Mildison; Solu-Cortef; ***Ital.:*** Algicortis†; Colifoam; Cortaid; Cortidro; Dermocortal; Flebocortid; Foille Insetti; Idracemi; Idrocortigamma†; Lanacort; Lenirit; Locoidon; Paro; Rapicort; Sintotrat; Solu-Cortef; Urecortyn†; ***Neth.:*** Buccalsone; Hydro-Adreson; Locoid; Mildison; Solu-Cortef; ***Norw.:*** Apocortal; Colifoam; Locoid; Mildison; Solu-Cortef; ***S.Afr.:*** Colifoam; Covocort; Cutaderm; Dilucort; Locoid; Mylocort; Procutan; Skincalm†; Solu-Cortef; Stopitch; ***Spain:*** Actocortina; Ceneo; Crema Transcutan Astier†; Derminovag; Dermosa Hidrocortisona; Hidroaltesona; Isdinium; Lactisona; Oralsone; Scalpicin Capilar; Schericur; Suniderma; Supralef; ***Swed.:*** Amberin†; Colifoam; Ficortril; Locoid; Locoid Crelo; Mildison; Solu-Cortef; Solu-Glyc†; Uniderm; ***Switz.:*** Alfacortone; Colifoam; Dermacalm†; Glycocortisone H; Hydrocortone; Locoid; Sanadermil; Solu-Cortef; ***UK:*** Colifoam; Corlan; Dermacort; Dioderm; Efcortelan; Efcortelan Soluble†; Efcortesol; Hc45; Hydrocortistab; Hydrocortisyl; Hydrocortone; Jungle Formula Sting Relief Cream; Lanacort; Locoid; Mildison; Solu-Cortef; Zenoxone; ***USA:*** A-Hydrocort; Acticort; Aeroseb-HC†; Ala-Cort; Anucort-HC; Anuprep HC†; Anusol-HC; Aquanil HC; Bactine; CaldeCort†; Carmol HC; Cetacort; Cort-Dome; CortaGel†; Cortaid; Cortef; Cortef Feminine Itch; Cortenema; Corticaine; Cortifair†; Cortifoam; Cortizone; Delcort; Dermacort; Dermarest Dri-Cort; Dermol HC; Dermolate; Gynecort; Hemril-HC; Hi-Cor; Hycort; Hydrocortone; HydroTex; Hytone; Lanacort; Locoid; Massengill Medicated; Maximum Strength Dermarest Dricort; Maximum Strength KeriCort-10; Neutrogena T/Scalp; no more itchies†; Nutracort; Orabase HCA; Pandel; Penecort; Preparation H Hydrocortisone; Procort; Proctocort; S-T Cort; Solu-Cortef; Synacort; Tegrin-HC; Texacort; U-Cort; Westcort.

Multi-ingredient: ***Aust.:*** Calmurid HC; Cortison Kemicetin; Daktacort; Ecomytrin-Hydrocortison; Endomethazone; Hydoftal; Hydrocortimycin; Hydrodexan; Ichtho-Cortin; Otosporin; Systrason; Terra-Cortril; Terra-Cortril mit Gentamicin; Terra-Cortril mit Polymyxin B-Sulfat; Tropoderm; ***Austral.:*** Anusol-HC†; Chlorocort; Hydroform; Hydrozole; Proctocort†; Proctosedyl; Vioform-Hydrocortisone†; Xyloproct; ***Belg.:*** Alphaderm; Daktacort; Dolanal†; Eoline; Onctose a l'Hydrocortisone; Otosporin; Pimafucort; Sulfo-Selenium; Terra-Cortril; Xyloproct; ***Canad.:*** Actinac; Anodan-HC; Anugesic-HC; Anusol-HC; Calmurid HC; Coly-Mycin Otic†; Cortisporin; Diospor HC; Hemcort HC; Neo-Cortef; Ophthocort; Pentamycetin-HC; Pramox HC; Proctofoam-HC; Proctosedyl; Proctosone; Sential†; Sopamycetin/HC†; Ti-U-Lac HC; Uremol-HC; Vanoxide-HC†; Vioform-Hydrocortisone; VoSoL HC; ***Fr.:*** Actidilon Hydrocortisone†; Anti-Hemorroidaires; Bacicoline; Cortneo†; Cutisan a l'Hydrocortisone†; Daktacort; Dermiclone†; Dermocalm; Dulcicortine†; Madecassol Neomycine Hydrocortisone; Onctose Hydrocortisone; Soframycine Hydrocortisone; ***Ger.:*** Achromycin†; Antiprurit; Anusol + H†; Bykomycin F†; Calmurid HC; Canesten HC; Corti Jaikal; Corti-Flexiole; Corti-Refobacin†; Daktar-Hydrocortison†; Dermaethyl-H†; Efisol-H†; Ekzemex†; Ficortril Lotio m. Neomycin†; Fucidine H†; Fucidine plus; Hydrodexan; Ichthocortin; Kolpicortin†; Novifort; Nubral 4 HC; Nystaderm Comp; Otosporin; Pantocrinale; Pigmanorm; Pimafucort; Pimarektal†; Poloris HC; Polycid N†; Polyspectran HC; Polyspectran OS†; Posterisan forte; Proctofoam-HC†; Psoil†; Tampovagan C-N N†; Terracortril; Topoderm N; Xylocain†; ***Irl.:*** Actinac; Alphaderm; Alphosyl HC; Anugesic-HC; Anusol-HC; Calmurid HC; Canesten HC; Cortucid†; Daktacort; Eurax-Hydrocortisone; Fucidin H; Genticin HC†; Gentisone HC; Hydrocal; Locoid C; Multifungin H†; Neo-Cortef; Nystaform-HC; Otosporin; Perinal; Proctofoam-HC; Proctosedyl; Quinocort; Terra-Cortril; Terra-Cortril Nystatin; Timodine; Vioform-Hydrocortisone; Xyloproct; ***Ital.:*** Antiemorroidale Milanfarma†; Argisone; Cort-Inal; Cortilen TC†; Cortison Chemicetina; Daktacort†; Emorril; Epartisone†; Flogosone†; Idracemi; Idracemi Eparina; Idrocet; Idroneomicil; Kinogen; Mictasone; Mixotone; Mobilat; Molidex†; Nasomixin; Neocortigamma†; Neocortovol†; Oftalmosporin†; Otobiotic†; Pimafucort†; Pomata Midy HC; Preparazione Antiemorroidaria; Proctidol; Proctosedyl; Proctosoll; Reumacort; Sinrinal†; Sinsurrene; Vasosterone; Vasosterone Antibiotico; Vasosterone Collirio; Xyloproct; ***Neth.:*** Alphacortison; Bacicoline-B; Calmurid HC; Daktacort; Otosporin; Pimafucort; Proctofoam-HC†; Proctosedyl; Terra-Cortril Gel Steraject met polymyxine-B; Terra-Cortril met polymyxine-B; Terra-Cortril†; Xyloproct; ***Norw.:*** Corticyklin†; Cortikinol†; Daktacort; Ecomytrin-Hydrocortison†; Locoidol; Proctosedyl; Salvizol med Hydrocortison†; Terra-Cortril; Terra-Cortril Polymyxin B; Xyloproct; ***S.Afr.:*** Anusol-HC; Chloramex H†; Corti-Flexiole†; Daktacort; Fucidin H; Locoid C†; Manoderm†; Nasomixin; Neoderm; Otoseptil†; Otosporin; Proctofoam; Proctosedyl; Quinoderm-H; Terra-Cortril; Viocort; ***Spain:*** Afta; Alantomicina Complex; Anginovag; Antiblef Eczem; Antihemorr; Antihemorroidal; Bacisporin; Brentan; Cilinafosal Hidrocort; Cohortan; Cohortan Antibiotico; Cortenema; Cortison Chemicet Topica; Dermisone Hidroc Neomic†; Dermo Hubber; Detraine; Ecomitrin†; Euraxil Hidrocort; Ginesona†; Gingilone Comp†; Grietalgen Hidrocort; Grinal Hidrocortisona†; Halibut Hidrocortisona; Hemodren Compuesto; Hemorrane; Hepro; Heridasone†; Hidroc Cloranf; Hidroc Neomic; Indertal†; Leuco Hubber; Milrosina Hidrocort†; Milrosina Nistatina; Nasal Rovi†; Nasokey†; Neo Bacitrin Hidrocortis; Neo Hubber; Neo Visage; Oftalmo; Ophtacortine†; Oralsone B C; Oto Difusor; Oto Neomicin Calm; Oto Vitna†; Otogen Hydrocortisona†; Otosporin; Polirino†; Puodermina Hidrocor†; Rino Vitna†; Rinocusi Descong†; Roberfarin; Terra-Cortril; Tisuderma; Tyroneomicin; Xilorroidal†; ***Swed.:*** Calmuril-Hydrokortison; Chloromycetin Hydrocortison†; Cortimyk; Daktacort; Ecomytrin-Hydrocortison†; Fenuril-Hydrokortison; Fucidin-Hydrocortison; Proctosedyl; Sterosan-Hydrocortisone†; Terracortril; Terracortril med polymyxin B; Xyloproct; ***Switz.:*** Antiprurit†; Bacicoline†; Calmurid HC; Cortifluid N; Cortimycine; Cortiphenol H†; Daktacort; Dermacalm-d; Ecomytrin-Hydrocortison†; Endomethasone; Eurax-Hydrocortisone†; Haemocortin; Hydrocortisone comp; Neo-Hydro; Otosporin; Proctosedyl†; Quinoderm Hydrocortisone†; Rocanal Permanent Gangrene; Terracortril; ***UK:*** Actinac; Alphaderm; Alphosyl HC; Anugesic-HC; Anusol-HC; Calmurid HC; Canesten HC; Carbo-Cort†; Chloromycetin Hydrocortisone; Cobadex; Daktacort; Econacort; Epifoam†; Eurax-Hydrocortisone; Fucidin H; Genticin HC†; Gentisone HC; Gregoderm; Hydrocal†; Locoid C; Neo-Cortef; Nystaform-HC; Otosporin; Perinal; Proctocream HC; Proctofoam-HC; Proctosedyl; Quinocort; Quinoderm with Hydrocortisone†; Sential HC†; Tarcortin; Terra-Cortril; Terra-Cortril Nystatin; Terra-Cortril†; Timodine; Tri-Cicatrin†; Uniroid; Uniroid-HC; Vioform-Hydrocortisone; Xyloproct; ***USA:*** 1 + 1-F; AA-HC Otic; Acetasol HC; Ak-Spore HC; Ala-Quin; Albaform HC; Analpram-HC; AntibiOtic; Anumed HC; Bacticort; Chloromycetin Hydrocortisone; Cipro HC Otic; Coly-Mycin S Otic; Coracin; Corque; Cortatrigen; Cortic; Corticaine; Cortisporin; Cortisporin-TC; Dermtex HC with Aloe; Drotic†; Ear-Eze; EarSol-HC; Emergent-Ez; Enzone; Epifoam; Fungoid HC; HC Derma-Pax; Hysone; Iodo-Cortifair†; Lacticare-HC; LazerSporin-C; Lida-Mantle-HC; Mantadil†; Neo-Cortef†; Neotricin HC; Octicair; Ophthocort†; Oti-Med; Otic-Care; Oticin HC; OtiTricin; Otobiotic; Otocort; Otomar-HC; Otomycin-HPN; Otosporin; Pedi-Cort V; Pediotic; Pramosone; Proctocream HC; Proctofoam-HC; Pyocidin-Otic†; Scalpicin; Terra-Cortril; Tri-Otic; UAD Cream or Lotion†; UAD-Otic; Vanoxide-HC; Vioform-Hydrocortisone†; VoSoL HC; Vytone; Zone-A†; Zoto-HC.

Isoflupredone Acetate (12869-q)

Isoflupredone Acetate *(BANM, USAN, rINNM).*

9α-Fluoroprednisolone Acetate; U-6013. 9α-Fluoro-11β,17α,21-trihydroxypregna-1,4-diene-3,20-dione 21-acetate.

$C_{23}H_{29}FO_6$ = 420.5.

CAS — 338-95-4 (isoflupredone); 338-98-7 (isoflupredone acetate).

Isoflupredone acetate is a corticosteroid that has been employed for its glucocorticoid activity (p.1010) as an ingredient of topical preparations for the treatment of allergic rhinitis.

Isoflupredone is also employed in veterinary medicine.

Preparations

Proprietary Preparations (details are given in Part 3)

Multi-ingredient: ***Belg.:*** Deltarhinol.

Loteprednol Etabonate (14750-p)

Loteprednol Etabonate *(BANM, USAN, rINNM).*

CDDD-5604; HGP-1; Loteprednol Ethyl Carbonate; P-5604. (11β,17α)-17-[(Ethoxycarbonyl)oxy]-11-hydroxy-3-oxoandrosta-1,4-diene-17-carboxylic acid chloromethyl ester.

$C_{24}H_{31}ClO_7$ = 467.0.

CAS — 129260-79-3 (loteprednol); 82034-46-6 (loteprednol etabonate).

Loteprednol etabonate is a corticosteroid used for its glucocorticoid activity (p.1010) in the topical management of inflammatory and allergic disorders of the eye. It is usually employed as eye drops containing 0.2 or 0.5%.

Prolonged application to the eye of preparations containing corticosteroids has caused raised intra-ocular pressure and reduced visual function.

Preparations

Proprietary Preparations (details are given in Part 3)

USA: Alrex; Lotemax.

Medrysone (1113-p)

Medrysone *(USAN, pINN).*

11β-Hydroxy-6α-methylprogesterone; Medrisona; NSC-63278; U-8471. 11β-Hydroxy-6α-methylpregn-4-ene-3,20-dione.

$C_{22}H_{32}O_3$ = 344.5.

CAS — 2668-66-8.

Medrysone is a corticosteroid employed for its glucocorticoid activity (see p.1010) in the topical treatment of allergic and inflammatory conditions of the eye. It is usually given as 1% eye drops.

Prolonged application to the eye of preparations containing corticosteroids has caused raised intra-ocular pressure and reduced visual function.

Preparations

Proprietary Preparations (details are given in Part 3)

Aust.: HMS Liquifilm†; ***Austral.:*** HMS Liquifilm; ***Canad.:*** HMS Liquifilm†; ***Ger.:*** Ophtocortin; Spectramedryn; ***Ital.:*** Medriusar†; ***Neth.:*** HMS Liquifilm†; ***S.Afr.:*** HMS; ***Spain:*** Liquipom Medrisone; ***Switz.:*** HMS; ***USA:*** HMS.

Multi-ingredient: ***Ital.:*** Medramil; Oftisone†; ***Spain:*** Mevaso†; Mirantal.

Meprednisone (1114-s)

Meprednisone *(USAN, rINN).*

16β-Methylprednisone; NSC-527579; Sch-4358. 17α,21-Dihydroxy-16β-methylpregna-1,4-diene-3,11,20-trione.

$C_{22}H_{28}O_5$ = 372.5.

CAS — 1247-42-3.

Pharmacopoeias. In US.

Store at a temperature not exceeding 40° in airtight containers. Protect from light.

Meprednisone is a corticosteroid with mainly glucocorticoid activity, as described under Corticosteroids, p.1010. It has been given by mouth as either the free alcohol or the acetate and by injection as the sodium hemisuccinate.

Methylprednisolone (1115-w)

Methylprednisolone *(BAN, rINN).*
6α-Methylprednisolone; Methylprednisolonum; NSC-19987.
11β,17α,21-Trihydroxy-6α-methylpregna-1,4-diene-3,20-dione.
$C_{22}H_{30}O_5$ = 374.5.
CAS — 83-43-2.
Pharmacopoeias. In *Eur.* (see p.viii), *Jpn*, and *US.*

A white or almost white odourless crystalline powder. It exhibits polymorphism.

Practically **insoluble** in water; soluble 1 in 100 of alcohol, 1 in 800 of chloroform, and 1 in 800 of ether; slightly soluble in acetone and in dichloromethane; sparingly soluble in dioxan and in methyl alcohol. **Store** in airtight containers. Protect from light.

Methylprednisolone Acetate (1116-e)

Methylprednisolone Acetate *(BANM, rINNM).*
Methylprednisoloni Acetas. Methylprednisolone 21-acetate.
$C_{24}H_{32}O_6$ = 416.5.
CAS — 53-36-1.
Pharmacopoeias. In *Eur.* (see p.viii) and *US.*

A white or almost white, odourless crystalline powder. Methylprednisolone acetate 44 mg is approximately equivalent to 40 mg of methylprednisolone. **Soluble** 1 in 1500 of water; soluble 1 in 400 of alcohol, 1 in 250 of chloroform, and 1 in 1500 of ether; sparingly soluble in acetone and in methyl alcohol; soluble in dioxan. **Store** in airtight containers. Protect from light.

Methylprednisolone Hemisuccinate (1117-l)

Methylprednisolone Hemisuccinate *(BANM, rINNM).*
Methylprednisoloni Hydrogenosuccinas. Methylprednisolone 21-(hydrogen succinate).
$C_{26}H_{34}O_8$ = 474.5.
CAS — 2921-57-5.
Pharmacopoeias. In *Eur.* (see p.viii) and *US.*

A white or almost white, odourless or almost odourless hygroscopic solid. Methylprednisolone hemisuccinate 51 mg is approximately equivalent to 40 mg of methylprednisolone.

Ph. Eur. states that it is practically **insoluble** in water; slightly soluble in acetone and in dehydrated alcohol; practically insoluble in ether. It dissolves in dilute solutions of alkali hydroxides. The USP, however, states that it is very slightly soluble in water; freely soluble in alcohol; soluble in acetone. **Store** in airtight containers. Protect from light.

Methylprednisolone Sodium Succinate (1118-y)

Methylprednisolone Sodium Succinate *(BANM, rINNM).*
Methylprednisolone 21-(sodium succinate).
$C_{26}H_{33}NaO_8$ = 496.5.
CAS — 2375-03-3.
Pharmacopoeias. In *US.*

A white or almost white, odourless, hygroscopic, amorphous solid. Methylprednisolone sodium succinate 53 mg is approximately equivalent to 40 mg of methylprednisolone.

Soluble 1 in 1.5 of water, and 1 in 12 of alcohol; very slightly soluble in acetone; practically insoluble in chloroform and in ether. **Store** in airtight containers. Protect from light.

Stability. An American preparation of methylprednisolone sodium succinate injection (Solu-Medrol) was considered to be stable for 7 days when diluted in water for injection and stored in glass vials at 4°. When stored under similar conditions at 22°, it was considered to be stable for 24 hours.[1]

1. Nahata MC, *et al.* Stability of diluted methylprednisolone sodium succinate injection at two temperatures. *Am J Hosp Pharm* 1994; **51:** 2157–9.

Adverse Effects, Treatment, Withdrawal, and Precautions

As for corticosteroids in general (see p.1010). Rapid intravenous administration of large doses has been associated with cardiovascular collapse.

Methylprednisolone may be slightly less likely than prednisolone to cause sodium and water retention.

When applied topically, particularly to large areas, when the skin is broken, or under occlusive dressings, corticosteroids may be absorbed in sufficient amounts to cause systemic effects.

References to various adverse effects associated with intravenous administration of methylprednisolone in high-dose pulse therapy[1-11] and to adverse effects following intra-articular[12] and intranasal administration.[13] Epidural administration (or more particularly inadvertent intrathecal administration during attempted epidural placement) may be associated with serious adverse effects including arachnoiditis and aseptic meningitis, although the degree of risk is uncertain.[14]

1. Newmark KJ, *et al.* Acute arthralgia following high-dose intravenous methylprednisolone therapy. *Lancet* 1974; **ii:** 229.
2. Bailey RR, Armour P. Acute arthralgia after high-dose intravenous methylprednisolone. *Lancet* 1974; **ii:** 1014.
3. Bennett WM, Strong D. Arthralgia after high-dose steroids. *Lancet* 1975; **i:** 332.
4. Moses RE, *et al.* Fatal arrhythmia after pulse methylprednisolone therapy. *Ann Intern Med* 1981; **95:** 781–2.
5. Oto A, *et al.* Methylprednisolone pulse therapy and peritonitis. *Ann Intern Med* 1983; **99:** 282.
6. Suchman AL, *et al.* Seizure after pulse therapy with methyl prednisolone. *Arthritis Rheum* 1983; **26:** 117.
7. Ayoub WT, *et al.* Central nervous system manifestations after pulse therapy for systemic lupus erythematosus. *Arthritis Rheum* 1983; **26:** 809–10.
8. Williams AJ, *et al.* Disseminated aspergillosis in high dose steroid therapy. *Lancet* 1983; **i:** 1222.
9. Barrett DF. Pulse methylprednisolone therapy. *Lancet* 1983; **ii:** 800.
10. Baethge BA, Lidsky MD. Intractable hiccups associated with high-dose intravenous methylprednisolone therapy. *Ann Intern Med* 1986; **104:** 58–9.
11. Gardiner PVG, Griffiths ID. Sudden death after treatment with pulsed methylprednisolone. *Br Med J* 1990; **300:** 125.
12. Black DM, Filak AT. Hyperglycemia with non-insulin-dependent diabetes following intraarticular steroid injection. *J Fam Pract* 1989; **28:** 462–3.
13. Johns KJ, Chandra SR. Visual loss following intranasal corticosteroid injection. *JAMA* 1989; **261:** 2413.
14. Rodgers PT, Connelly JF. Epidural administration of methylprednisolone for back pain. *Am J Hosp Pharm* 1994; **51:** 2789–90.

Interactions

The interactions of corticosteroids in general are described on p.1014.

Pharmacokinetics

For a brief outline of the pharmacokinetics of corticosteroids, see p.1014.

Methylprednisolone is fairly rapidly distributed following administration, with a plasma half-life of 3.5 hours or more. The tissue half-life is reported to range from 18 to 36 hours.

Methylprednisolone acetate is absorbed from joints over a week but is more slowly absorbed following deep intramuscular injection.

References.

1. Ferry JJ, *et al.* Pilot study of the pharmacokinetics of methylprednisolone after single and multiple intravenous doses of methylprednisolone sodium succinate and methylprednisolone suleptanate to healthy volunteers. *J Clin Pharmacol* 1994; **34:** 1109–15.
2. Lawson GJ, *et al.* Methylprednisolone-hemisuccinate and its metabolites in serum, urine and bile from two patients with acute graft rejection. *Br J Clin Pharmacol* 1995; **39:** 176–8.
3. Tornatore KM, *et al.* Repeated assessment of methylprednisolone pharmacokinetics during chronic immunosuppression in renal transplant recipients. *Ann Pharmacother* 1995; **29:** 120–4.
4. Rohatagi S, *et al.* Pharmacokinetics of methylprednisolone and prednisolone after single and multiple oral administration. *J Clin Pharmacol* 1997; **37:** 916–25.

Uses and Administration

Methylprednisolone is a corticosteroid with mainly glucocorticoid activity, as described under Corticosteroids, p.1010; 4 mg of methylprednisolone is equivalent in anti-inflammatory activity to about 5 mg of prednisolone.

It is used, either in the form of the free alcohol or in one of the esterified forms, in the treatment of conditions for which corticosteroid therapy is indicated (see p.1015) except adrenocortical-deficiency states, for which hydrocortisone with supplementary fludrocortisone is preferred.

For administration by mouth, methylprednisolone is usually given in an initial dosage range of 4 to 48 mg daily but higher initial doses of up to 100 mg or more daily may be used in acute severe disease.

For parenteral administration in intensive or emergency therapy, methylprednisolone sodium succinate may be administered by intramuscular or intravenous injection or by intravenous infusion. The intravenous route is preferred for its more rapid effect in emergency therapy. The usual initial intramuscular or intravenous dose ranges from the equivalent of 10 to 500 mg of methylprednisolone daily. Large intravenous doses (over 250 mg) should normally be given slowly over at least 30 minutes; doses up to 250 mg should be given over at least 5 minutes. High doses should generally not be given for prolonged periods; emergency treatment should only be given until the patient is stabilised. High doses given intermittently for a limited period have sometimes been known as 'pulse therapy' (see under Administration, below) and in graft rejection (see p.498) 1 g has been given daily for up to 3 days. In intensive therapy of acute spinal cord injury (p.1029) initial doses of the equivalent of up to 30 mg per kg body-weight of methylprednisolone have been given by bolus intravenous injection over 15 minutes and followed, after a 45-minute pause, by intravenous infusion of 5.4 mg per kg per hour over 24 hours or longer. For slow intravenous infusion methylprednisolone sodium succinate is dissolved in an appropriate volume of glucose 5% or sodium chloride 0.9% or sodium chloride 0.9% and glucose 5%.

Parenteral doses in children have varied considerably, depending on the condition: a range of 1 to 30 mg of methylprednisolone per kg body-weight daily has been suggested, by the intravenous or intramuscular routes. A total dose of 1 g daily should not normally be exceeded.

Methylprednisolone acetate may be administered by intramuscular injection for a prolonged systemic effect, the dose varying from 40 mg every 2 weeks to 120 mg weekly.

For intra-articular injection and for injection into soft tissues methylprednisolone acetate as an aqueous suspension is employed. The dose by intra-articular injection varies from 4 to 80 mg according to the size of the affected joint. The acetate may also be administered by intralesional injection in doses of 20 to 60 mg.

For use in the treatment of various skin disorders methylprednisolone acetate may be applied topically, usually in concentrations of 0.25 to 1%. The aceponate, which may exhibit modified topical activity, has also been applied as a 0.1% cream or ointment.

Other esters of methylprednisolone which have occasionally been used include the cypionate and the suleptanate.

General references.

1. Cronstein BN. Clinical use of methylprednisolone sodium succinate: a review. *Curr Ther Res* 1995; **56:** 1–15.

Administration. For short-term intensive therapy or in certain emergency situations a technique of corticosteroid administration known as 'pulse therapy' has been employed. Methylprednisolone has often been used in this manner and typically high doses of about 1 g intravenously have been given, usually daily or on alternate days, or weekly, for a limited number of doses; the most common regimen appears to be 1 g daily for 3 days.

Blood disorders. Methylprednisolone is one of the corticosteroids that have been used in the management of haemangioma and the Kasabach-Merritt syndrome[1] (for further discussion of the management of haemangiomas, see p.1022). There is also a report of benefit from very high-dose therapy in a few patients with refractory red cell aplasia due to Blackfan-Diamond anaemia.[2]

1. Özsoylu Ş, *et al.* Megadose methylprednisolone therapy for Kasabach-Merritt syndrome. *J Pediatr* 1996; **129:** 947.
2. Bernini JC, *et al.* High-dose intravenous methylprednisolone therapy for patients with Diamond-Blackfan anemia refractory to conventional doses of prednisone. *J Pediatr* 1995; **127:** 654–9.

IDIOPATHIC THROMBOCYTOPENIC PURPURA. High dose methylprednisolone may be employed as part of the emergency management of acute idiopathic thrombocytopenic purpura, for example when major acute bleeding or intracranial haemorrhage supervene, and has also been used by mouth or intravenously in the management of the chronic form, although prednisolone or prednisone are more frequently used for oral therapy. For discussion of the management of idiopathic thrombocytopenic purpura, including the use of methylprednisolone, see p.1023. Some references are given below.

1. von dem Borne AEGKR, *et al.* High dose intravenous methylprednisolone or high dose intravenous gammaglobulin for autoimmune thrombocytopenia. *Br Med J* 1988; **296:** 249–50.
2. Özsoylu S, *et al.* Megadose methylprednisolone for chronic idiopathic thrombocytopenic purpura. *Lancet* 1990; **336:** 1078–9.
3. Akoğlu T, *et al.* Megadose methylprednisolone pulse therapy in adult idiopathic thrombocytopenic purpura. *Lancet* 1991; **337:** 56.
4. Özsoylu S. Mega-dose methylprednisolone for chronic idiopathic thrombocytopenic purpura. *Lancet* 1991; **337:** 1611–12.

Bone disorders. For mention of injection of methylprednisolone into bone cysts to stimulate bone formation, see p.1018.

Glomerular kidney disease. For a discussion of the various forms of glomerular kidney disease and their management, including the use of methylprednisolone, see p.1021. Some references to the use of methylprednisolone are given below.

1. Imbasciati E, *et al.* Controlled trial of methylprednisolone pulses and low dose oral prednisone for the minimal change nephrotic syndrome. *Br Med J* 1985; **291:** 1305–8.
2. Bolton WK, Sturgill BC. Methylprednisolone therapy for acute crescentic rapidly progressive glomerulonephritis. *Am J Nephrol* 1989; **9:** 368–75.
3. Bruns FJ, *et al.* Long-term follow-up of aggressively treated idiopathic rapidly progressing glomerulonephritis. *Am J Med* 1989; **86:** 400–6.
4. Ponticelli C, *et al.* A randomized trial of methylprednisolone and chlorambucil in idiopathic membranous nephropathy. *N Engl J Med* 1989; **320:** 8–13.
5. Ponticelli C, *et al.* Methylprednisolone plus chlorambucil as compared with methylprednisolone alone for the treatment of idiopathic membranous nephropathy. *N Engl J Med* 1992; **327:** 599–603.

Multiple sclerosis. Methylprednisolone is one of the corticosteroids used in multiple sclerosis, the management of which is discussed further on p.620.

Polymyalgia rheumatica. For mention of the use of methylprednisolone to treat polymyalgia rheumatica, see p.1027.

Rheumatoid arthritis. Methylprednisolone administered in intravenous pulses has been reported to be effective in the treatment of rheumatoid arthritis.[1-6] Some studies have shown this treatment to be of greatest benefit when given concomitantly with a disease modifying antirheumatic drug (DMARD) such as gold,[1,3,6] although some showed the addition of methylprednisolone to existing therapy to have no extra benefit.[5] A comparatively low dose of 100 mg was found to be as effective as 1000 mg in one study.[2] Monthly administration of methylprednisolone by deep intramuscular injection was also an effective adjunct to gold therapy.[7] In general, however, the use of corticosteroids in rheumatoid arthritis is controversial. Systemic corticosteroids can suppress symptoms of the disease, but their usefulness is limited by their adverse effects and they are usually reserved for severe rapidly progressing disease unresponsive to conventional therapy, to control disease activity during initiation of therapy with a DMARD, or in disease accompanied by severe extra-articular effects. Intra-articular injection has been used for joints affected by an acute flare but should be given infrequently.

For a discussion of the management of rheumatoid arthritis, including the use of corticosteroids, see p.2.

1. Smith MD, *et al.* The clinical and immunological effects of pulse methylprednisolone therapy in rheumatoid arthritis I: clinical effects. *J Rheumatol* 1988; **15:** 229–32.
2. Igelhart IW, *et al.* Intravenous pulsed steroids in rheumatoid arthritis: a comparative dose study. *J Rheumatol* 1990; **17:** 159–62.
3. Smith MD, *et al.* Pulse methylprednisolone therapy in rheumatoid arthritis: unproved therapy, unjustified therapy, or effective adjunctive treatment? *Ann Rheum Dis* 1990; **49:** 265–7.
4. Kapisinszky N, Keszthelyi B. High dose intravenous methylprednisolone pulse therapy in patients with rheumatoid arthritis. *Ann Rheum Dis* 1990; **49:** 567–8.
5. Hansen TM, *et al.* Double blind placebo controlled trial of pulse treatment with methylprednisolone combined with disease modifying drugs in rheumatoid arthritis. *Br Med J* 1990; **301:** 268–70.
6. Walters HT, Cawley MID. Combined suppressive drug treatment in severe refractory rheumatoid disease: an analysis of the relative effects of parenteral methylprednisolone, cyclophosphamide and sodium aurothiomalate. *Ann Rheum Dis* 1988; **47:** 924–9.
7. Corkill MM, *et al.* Intramuscular depot methylprednisolone induction of chrysotherapy in rheumatoid arthritis: a 24-week randomized controlled trial. *Br J Rheumatol* 1990; **29:** 274–9.

Skin disorders. For recommendations concerning the correct use of corticosteroids on the skin, and a rough guide to the clinical potencies of topical corticosteroids, see Corticosteroids, Administration, p.1017.

Systemic lupus erythematosus. Pulsed intravenous methylprednisolone is used in the management of lupus nephritis, alone or combined with immunosuppressants. For a discussion of the management of systemic lupus erythematosus including the role of methylprednisolone, see p.1029.

Vertigo. In a double-blind study, 9 of 10 patients treated with methylprednisolone 32 mg by mouth on day one followed by 16 mg twice daily for 3 days and then tapered off and stopped after 8 days showed improvement in symptoms of acute vestibular vertigo.[1] Three of 10 patients receiving placebo improved initially, and 7 improved after transferring to methylprednisolone treatment. However, corticosteroids are not one of the usual classes of drugs employed in the treatment of vertigo (p.401), which usually depends on antihistamines or phenothiazines for its management.

1. Ariyasu L, *et al.* The beneficial effect of methylprednisolone in acute vestibular vertigo. *Arch Otolaryngol Head Neck Surg* 1990; **116:** 700–3.

Preparations

BP 1998: Methylprednisolone Acetate Injection; Methylprednisolone Tablets;
USP 23: Methylprednisolone Acetate Cream; Methylprednisolone Acetate for Enema; Methylprednisolone Acetate Injectable Suspension; Methylprednisolone Sodium Succinate for Injection; Methylprednisolone Tablets; Neomycin Sulfate and Methylprednisolone Acetate Cream.

Proprietary Preparations (details are given in Part 3)

Aust.: Advantan; Depo-Medrol; Promedrol; Solu-Medrol; Urbason; ***Austral.:*** Advantan; Depo-Medrol; Medrol†; Solu-Medrol; ***Belg.:*** Advantan; Depo-Medrol; Medrol; Solu-Medrol; ***Canad.:*** Depo-Medrol; Medrol; Medrol Veriderm; Solu-Medrol; ***Fr.:*** Depo-Medrol; Medrol; Solu-Medrol; ***Ger.:*** Advantan; Depo-Medrate; Medrate; Metypred; Metysolon; Predni-M-Tablinen; Urbason; ***Irl.:*** Depo-Medrone; Medrone; Solu-Medrone; ***Ital.:*** Advantan; Asmacortone; Avancort; Caberdelta M†; Depo-Medrol; Emmetipi; Esametone; Firmacort; Medrol; Medrol Veriderm†; Mega-Star†; Metilbetasone Solubile; Prednilen†; Reactenol†; Sieropresol†; Solu-Medrol; Summicort†; Urbason†; ***Neth.:*** Depo-Medrol; Medrol†; Solu-Medrol; ***Norw.:*** Depo-Medrol; Medrol; Solu-Medrol; ***S.Afr.:*** Advantan; Depo-Medrol; Medrol; Metypresol; Solu-Medrol; ***Spain:*** Adventan; Depo Moderin; Solu Moderin; Urbason; ***Swed.:*** Depo-Medrol; Depo-Medrone†; Medrol; Medrone†; Solu-Medrol; Solu-Medrone†; ***Switz.:*** Advantan; Depo-Medrol; Medrol; Promedrol; Solu-Medrol; Urbason; ***UK:*** Depo-Medrone; Medrone; Solu-Medrone; ***USA:*** A-Methapred; Adlone; D-Med; depMedalone; Depo-Medrol; Depo-Predate†; Depoject; Depopred; Duralone; M-Prednisol; Medralone; Medrol; Medrol Acetate†; Solu-Medrol.

Multi-ingredient: ***Aust.:*** Depo-Medrol mit Lidocain; ***Austral.:*** Medrol Acne Lotion†; Neo-Medrol; ***Belg.:*** Depo-Medrol + Lidocaine; ***Canad.:*** Depo-Medrol with Lidocaine; Medrol Acne Lotion; Neo-Medrol Acne; Neo-Medrol Veriderm; ***Ger.:*** Medrate Akne-Lotio†; Neo-Medrate Akne-Lotio†; ***Irl.:*** Depo-Medrone with Lidocaine; Neo-Medrone; ***Ital.:*** Depo-Medrol + Lidocaina; Medrol Lozione Antiacne; Neo-Medrol Lozione Antiacne†; Neo-Medrol Veriderm; ***Neth.:*** Depo-Medrol + Lidocaine; ***Norw.:*** Depo-Medrol cum Lidocain; ***S.Afr.:*** Depo-Medrol with Lidocaine; Neo-Medrol; ***Spain:*** Artrivia Prednisolona†; Moderin Acne; Neo Moderin; ***Swed.:*** Depo-Medrol cum Lidokain; Depo-Medrone med lidokain†; ***Switz.:*** Depo-Medrol Lidocaine; Neo-Medrol†; ***UK:*** Depo-Medrone with Lidocaine; Neo-Medrone†.

Mometasone Furoate (11466-m)

Mometasone Furoate *(BANM, USAN, rINNM).*

Sch-32088. 9α,21-Dichloro-11β,17-dihydroxy-16α-methylpregna-1,4-diene-3,20-dione 17-(2-furoate).

$C_{27}H_{30}Cl_2O_6$ = 521.4.

CAS — 105102-22-5 (mometasone); 83919-23-7 (mometasone furoate).

Pharmacopoeias. In *US.*

A white or nearly white powder. Practically **insoluble** in water; freely soluble in acetone and in dichloromethane.

Mometasone furoate is a corticosteroid used topically for its glucocorticoid activity (see p.1010) in the treatment of various skin disorders. It is usually employed as a cream, ointment, or lotion containing 0.1%.

It is also given as a 0.05% nasal suspension of mometasone furoate monohydrate in the treatment and prophylaxis of the symptoms of allergic rhinitis (p.400); the usual dose is the equivalent of 100 μg of mometasone furoate in each nostril once daily, increased if necessary to 200 μg in each nostril daily. Once symptoms are controlled a dose of 50 μg in each nostril daily may be effective for maintenance.

When applied topically, particularly to large areas, when the skin is broken, or under occlusive dressings, corticosteroids may be absorbed in sufficient amounts to cause systemic effects (see p.1010). The effects of topical corticosteroids on the skin are described on p.1012.

References.

1. Prakash A, Benfield P. Topical mometasone: a review of its pharmacological properties and therapeutic use in the treatment of dermatological disorders. *Drugs* 1998; **55:** 145–63.

Skin disorders. For recommendations concerning the correct use of corticosteroids on the skin, see Corticosteroids, Administration, p.1017.

Preparations

USP 23: Mometasone Furoate Cream; Mometasone Furoate Ointment; Mometasone Furoate Topical Solution.

Proprietary Preparations (details are given in Part 3)

Aust.: Elocon; ***Austral.:*** Elocon; Novasone; ***Belg.:*** Elocom; ***Canad.:*** Elocom; ***Ger.:*** Ecural; ***Irl.:*** Elocon; ***Ital.:*** Altosone; Elocon; ***Neth.:*** Elocon; ***Norw.:*** Elocon; ***S.Afr.:*** Elocon; ***Spain:*** Elica; Elocom; ***Swed.:*** Elocon; Nasonex; ***Switz.:*** Elocom; ***UK:*** Elocon; Nasonex; ***USA:*** Elocon; Nasonex.

Paramethasone Acetate (1119-j)

Paramethasone Acetate *(BANM, USAN, rINNM).*

6α-Fluoro-16α-methylprednisolone 21-Acetate. 6α-Fluoro-11β,17α,21-trihydroxy-16α-methylpregna-1,4-diene-3,20-dione 21-acetate.

$C_{24}H_{31}FO_6$ = 434.5.

CAS — 53-33-8 (paramethasone); 1597-82-6 (paramethasone acetate).

Pharmacopoeias. In *Fr.* and *US.*

A white to creamy-white, fluffy, odourless, crystalline powder. Practically **insoluble** in water; soluble 1 in 50 of chloroform and 1 in 40 of methyl alcohol; soluble in ether. **Store** in airtight containers.

Paramethasone acetate is a corticosteroid with predominantly glucocorticoid activity (p.1010); 2 mg of paramethasone is equivalent in anti-inflammatory activity to about 5 mg of prednisolone. It has been used in the treatment of conditions in which corticosteroid therapy is indicated (see p.1015) except adrenal-deficiency states for which hydrocortisone with supplementary fludrocortisone is preferred. Doses of up to 40 mg by intramuscular injection every 48 hours have been suggested. Paramethasone acetate has also been administered by intra-articular injection; a mixture of the acetate and the disodium phosphate has been given by intramuscular or intralesional injection. Paramethasone acetate has also been given by mouth.

Preparations

USP 23: Paramethasone Acetate Tablets.

Proprietary Preparations (details are given in Part 3)

Belg.: Depodillar†; Dillar†; ***Fr.:*** Dilar; ***Ger.:*** Monocortin†; ***Neth.:*** Depodillar†; ***Spain:*** Cortidene; Triniol†; ***Switz.:*** Monocortin†; ***USA:*** Haldrone†.

Multi-ingredient: ***Spain:*** Triniol.

Prednicarbate (2367-z)

Prednicarbate *(USAN, rINN).*

HOE-777; S-77-0777. 11β,17,21-Trihydroxypregna-1,4-diene-3,20-dione 17-(ethyl carbonate) 21-propionate.

$C_{27}H_{36}O_8$ = 488.6.

CAS — 73771-04-7.

Prednicarbate is a corticosteroid used topically for its glucocorticoid activity (see p.1010) in the treatment of various skin disorders. It has usually been employed as a cream, ointment, or lotion, containing 0.1 to 0.25%.

When applied topically, particularly to large areas, when the skin is broken, or under occlusive dressings, corticosteroids may be absorbed in sufficient amounts to cause systemic effects (see p.1010). The effects of topical corticosteroids on the skin are described on p.1012.

References.

1. Schäfer-Korting M, *et al.* Prednicarbate activity and benefit/risk ratio in relation to other topical glucocorticoids. *Clin Pharmacol Ther* 1993; **54:** 448–56.

Skin disorders. For recommendations concerning the correct use of corticosteroids on the skin, and a rough guide to the clinical potencies of topical corticosteroids, see Corticosteroids, Administration, p.1017.

Preparations

Proprietary Preparations (details are given in Part 3)

Aust.: Prednitop; ***Ger.:*** Dermatop; ***Ital.:*** Dermatop; ***Spain:*** Batmen; Peitel; ***Switz.:*** Prednitop; ***USA:*** Dermatop.

Prednisolamate Hydrochloride (1120-q)

Prednisolamate Hydrochloride *(BANM, rINNM).*

Prednisolone 21-Diethylaminoacetate Hydrochloride. 11β,17α,21-Trihydroxypregna-1,4-diene-3,20-dione 21-diethylaminoacetate hydrochloride.

$C_{27}H_{39}NO_6$,HCl = 510.1.

CAS — 5626-34-6 (prednisolamate).

Prednisolamate hydrochloride has the general properties of prednisolone (see p.1048) and has been used in some countries as a water-soluble form of prednisolone for intravenous injection and as an ointment.

Preparations

Proprietary Preparations (details are given in Part 3)

Multi-ingredient: ***Ital.:*** Etaproctene†.

Prednisolone (1129-c)

Prednisolone *(BAN, rINN)*.

1,2-Dehydrohydrocortisone; Deltahydrocortisone; Δ^1-Hydrocortisone; Metacortandralone; NSC-9120; Prednisolonum. 11β,17α,21-Trihydroxypregna-1,4-diene-3,20-dione.

$C_{21}H_{28}O_5$ = 360.4.

CAS — 50-24-8 (anhydrous); 52438-85-4 (sesquihydrate).

Pharmacopoeias. In *Chin., Eur.* (see p.viii), *Int., Jpn.*, and *Pol. US* allows the anhydrous form or the sesquihydrate.

An odourless, white or almost white, crystalline, hygroscopic powder; it shows polymorphism. Very slightly **soluble** in water; soluble 1 in 30 of alcohol, 1 in 50 of acetone, and 1 in 180 of chloroform; soluble in dioxan and in methyl alcohol; slightly soluble in dichloromethane. **Protect** from light.

Prednisolone Acetate (1122-s)

Prednisolone Acetate *(BANM, rINNM)*.

Prednisoloni Acetas. Prednisolone 21-acetate.

$C_{23}H_{30}O_6$ = 402.5.

CAS — 52-21-1.

Pharmacopoeias. In *Chin., Eur.* (see p.viii), *Int., Jpn, Pol.*, and *US*.

An odourless, white or almost white, crystalline powder. Prednisolone acetate 11 mg is approximately equivalent to 10 mg of prednisolone.

Practically **insoluble** in water; soluble 1 in 120 of alcohol; slightly soluble in acetone, in dichloromethane, and in chloroform. **Protect** from light.

Prednisolone Hemisuccinate (1128-z)

Prednisolone Hemisuccinate *(BANM, rINNM)*.

Prednisolone 21-(hydrogen succinate).

$C_{25}H_{32}O_8$ = 460.5.

CAS — 2920-86-7.

Pharmacopoeias. In *Jpn* and *US*.

A fine, creamy-white, almost odourless powder with friable lumps. Prednisolone hemisuccinate 128 mg is approximately equivalent to 100 mg of prednisolone.

Soluble 1 in 4170 of water, 1 in 6.3 of alcohol, 1 in 1064 of chloroform, and 1 in 248 of ether; soluble in acetone. **Store** in airtight containers.

Prednisolone Hexanoate (1123-w)

Prednisolone Hexanoate *(BANM, rINNM)*.

Prednisolone Caproate. Prednisolone 21-hexanoate.

$C_{27}H_{38}O_6$ = 458.6.

Prednisolone hexanoate 127 mg is approximately equivalent to 100 mg of prednisolone.

Prednisolone Pivalate (1124-e)

Prednisolone Pivalate *(BANM, rINNM)*.

Prednisolone Trimethylacetate; Prednisoloni Pivalas. Prednisolone 21-pivalate.

$C_{26}H_{36}O_6$ = 444.6.

CAS — 1107-99-9.

Pharmacopoeias. In *Eur.* (see p.viii) and *Pol.*

A white, or almost white, crystalline powder. Prednisolone pivalate 123 mg is approximately equivalent to 100 mg of prednisolone.

Practically **insoluble** in water; slightly soluble in alcohol; soluble in dichloromethane. **Protect** from light.

Prednisolone Sodium Metasulphobenzoate (1125-l)

Prednisolone Sodium Metasulphobenzoate *(rINNM)*.

Prednisolone Metasulphobenzoate Sodium *(BANM)*; R-812. Prednisolone 21-(sodium *m*-sulphobenzoate).

$C_{28}H_{31}NaO_9S$ = 566.6.

CAS — 630-67-1.

Prednisolone sodium metasulphobenzoate 157 mg is approximately equivalent to 100 mg of prednisolone.

Prednisolone Sodium Phosphate (1126-y)

Prednisolone Sodium Phosphate *(BANM, rINNM)*.

Prednisoloni Natrii Phosphas. Prednisolone 21-(disodium orthophosphate).

$C_{21}H_{27}Na_2O_8P$ = 484.4.

CAS — 125-02-0.

NOTE. PRED is a code approved by the BP for use on single unit doses of eye drops containing prednisolone sodium phosphate where the individual container may be too small to bear all the appropriate labelling information.

Pharmacopoeias. In *Eur.* (see p.viii) and *US*.

A white or slightly yellow hygroscopic crystalline powder or friable granules, odourless or with a slight odour. Prednisolone sodium phosphate 27 mg is approximately equivalent to 20 mg of prednisolone.

Soluble 1 in 4 of water and 1 in 13 of methyl alcohol; slightly soluble to very slightly soluble in alcohol; slightly soluble in chloroform; very slightly soluble in acetone and in dioxan. Ph. Eur. states that a 5% solution in water has a pH of 7.5 to 9.0; the USP specifies that a 1% solution has a pH of 7.5 to 10.5. **Store** in airtight containers. Protect from light.

Prednisolone Sodium Succinate (16319-s)

Prednisolone Sodium Succinate *(BANM, rINNM)*.

Prednisolone Sodium Hemisuccinate. 11β,17α,21-Trihydroxypregna-1,4-diene-3,20-dione 21-(sodium succinate).

$C_{25}H_{31}NaO_8$ = 482.5.

CAS — 1715-33-9.

Pharmacopoeias. *US* includes Prednisolone Sodium Succinate for Injection.

Prednisolone sodium succinate 134 mg is approximately equivalent to 100 mg of prednisolone. A creamy white powder with friable lumps; it may have a slight odour. The pH of the reconstituted USP injection is between 6.7 and 8.0.

Prednisolone Steaglate (1127-j)

Prednisolone Steaglate *(BAN, rINN)*.

Prednisolone 21-stearoylglycolate.

$C_{41}H_{64}O_8$ = 684.9.

CAS — 5060-55-9.

Prednisolone steaglate 190 mg is approximately equivalent to 100 mg of prednisolone.

Prednisolone Tebutate (1121-p)

Prednisolone Tebutate *(BANM, rINNM)*.

Prednisolone Butylacetate; Prednisolone 21-*tert*-Butylacetate; Prednisolone Tertiary-butylacetate. Prednisolone 21-(3,3-dimethylbutyrate).

$C_{27}H_{38}O_6,H_2O$ = 476.6.

CAS — 7681-14-3 (anhydrous).

Pharmacopoeias. In *US*.

A white to slightly yellow hygroscopic powder, odourless or with a characteristic odour. Prednisolone tebutate 132 mg is approximately equivalent to 100 mg of prednisolone.

Very slightly **soluble** in water; freely soluble in chloroform and in dioxan; soluble in acetone; sparingly soluble in alcohol and in methyl alcohol. **Store** at a temperature not exceeding 8° in an atmosphere of nitrogen in airtight containers.

Adverse Effects, Treatment, Withdrawal, and Precautions

As for corticosteroids in general (see p.1010).

Owing to its less pronounced mineralocorticoid activity prednisolone is less likely than cortisone or hydrocortisone to cause sodium retention, electrolyte imbalance, and oedema.

Hepatic impairment. Conversion of prednisone to prednisolone has been reported to be impaired in chronic active liver disease.[1,2] However, although plasma-prednisolone concentrations were found to be more predictable after administration of prednisolone than of prednisone to a group of healthy subjects,[3] no difference was noted in patients with chronic active hepatitis, in whom impaired elimination of prednisolone compensated for any impaired conversion of prednisone. A review of the pharmacokinetics of prednisone and prednisolone[4] concluded that fear of inadequate conversion of prednisone into prednisolone was not justified.

1. Powell LW, Axelsen E. Corticosteroids in liver disease: studies on the biological conversion of prednisone to prednisolone and plasma protein binding. *Gut* 1972; **13:** 690–6.
2. Madsbad S, *et al.* Impaired conversion of prednisone to prednisolone in patients with liver cirrhosis. *Gut* 1980; **21:** 52–6.
3. Davis M, *et al.* Prednisone or prednisolone for the treatment of chronic active hepatitis? A comparison of plasma availability. *Br J Clin Pharmacol* 1978; **5:** 501–5.
4. Frey BM, Frey FJ. Clinical pharmacokinetics of prednisone and prednisolone. *Clin Pharmacokinet* 1990; **19:** 126–46.

Inflammatory bowel disease. Symptoms recurred in a patient with Crohn's disease on changing from conventional to enteric-coated tablets of prednisolone.[1] This was not an isolated occurrence in the authors' unit, and it was advocated that only non-enteric coated prednisolone tablets should be used in Crohn's disease, and that the enteric-coated form be used with caution in any condition characterised by diarrhoea or a rapid transit time.

1. Beattie RM, Walker-Smith JA. Use of enteric coated prednisolone in Crohn's disease. *Arch Dis Child* 1994; **71:** 282.

Interactions

The interactions of corticosteroids in general are described on p.1014.

Pharmacokinetics

For a brief outline of the pharmacokinetics of corticosteroids, see p.1014.

Prednisolone and prednisone are both readily absorbed from the gastro-intestinal tract, but whereas prednisolone already exists in a metabolically active form, prednisone must be converted in the liver to its active metabolite, prednisolone. In general, this conversion is rapid so this difference is of little consequence when seen in the light of intersubject variation in the pharmacokinetics of prednisolone itself; bioavailability also depends on the dissolution rates of the tablet formulations. As discussed under Hepatic Impairment, above, the possibility of reduced corticosteroid concentrations following administration of prednisone to patients with liver disease does not seem to be a problem in practice. Following intramuscular administration the sodium phosphate ester of prednisolone is rapidly absorbed whereas the acetate, in the suspension form, is only slowly absorbed.

Peak plasma concentrations of prednisolone are obtained 1 or 2 hours after administration by mouth, and it has a usual plasma half-life of 2 to 4 hours. Its initial absorption, but not its overall bioavailability, is affected by food.

Prednisolone is extensively bound to plasma proteins, although less so than hydrocortisone (cortisol). The volume of distribution, and also the clearance are reported to increase with an increase from low to moderate doses; at very high doses, clearance appears to become saturated.

Prednisolone is excreted in the urine as free and conjugated metabolites, together with an appreciable proportion of unchanged prednisolone. Prednisolone crosses the placenta and small amounts are excreted in breast milk.

Prednisolone has a biological half-life lasting several hours, intermediate between those of hydrocortisone (cortisol) and the longer-acting glucocorticoids, such as dexamethasone. It is this intermediate duration of action which makes it suitable for the alternate-day administration regimens which have been found to reduce the risk of adrenocortical insufficiency, yet provide adequate corticosteroid coverage in some disorders.

General reviews of the pharmacokinetics of prednisolone[1,2] and some references to its pharmacokinetics in healthy subjects[3] and in various disease states.[4-8]

1. Begg EJ, *et al.* The pharmacokinetics of corticosteroid agents. *Med J Aust* 1987; **146:** 37–41.
2. Frey BM, Frey FJ. Clinical pharmacokinetics of prednisone and prednisolone. *Clin Pharmacokinet* 1990; **19:** 126–46.
3. Rohatagi S, *et al.* Pharmacokinetics of methylprednisolone and prednisolone after single and multiple oral administration. *J Clin Pharmacol* 1997; **37:** 916–25.
4. Berghouse LM, *et al.* Plasma prednisolone levels during intravenous therapy in acute colitis. *Gut* 1982; **23:** 980–3.
5. Shaffer JA, *et al.* Absorption of prednisolone in patients with Crohn's disease. *Gut* 1983; **24:** 182–6.
6. Reece PA, *et al.* Prednisolone protein binding in renal transplant patients. *Br J Clin Pharmacol* 1985; **20:** 159–62.
7. Frey FJ, *et al.* Altered metabolism and decreased efficacy of prednisolone and prednisone in patients with hyperthyroidism. *Clin Pharmacol Ther* 1988; **44:** 510–21.
8. Miller PFW, *et al.* Pharmacokinetics of prednisolone in children with nephrosis. *Arch Dis Child* 1990; **65:** 196–200.

Distribution into breast milk. Concentrations of prednisone and prednisolone in human milk 120 minutes after prednisone 10 mg by mouth were found to be 26.7 ng and 1.6 ng per mL.[1] In seven lactating women volunteers given a single 5-mg dose of tritium-labelled prednisolone by mouth, a mean of 0.14% of the radioactivity from the dose was recovered per litre of milk during the following 48 to 61 hours.[2]

1. Katz FH, Duncan BE. Entry of prednisone into human milk. *N Engl J Med* 1975; **293:** 1154.
2. McKenzie SA, *et al.* Secretion of prednisolone into breast milk. *Arch Dis Child* 1975; **50:** 894–6.

Uses and Administration

Prednisolone is a corticosteroid with mainly glucocorticoid activity (p.1010); 5 mg of prednisolone is equivalent in anti-inflammatory activity to about 25 mg of cortisone acetate. In general, prednisolone, either in the form of the free alcohol or in one of the esterified forms, is the drug of choice in the UK for conditions in which routine systemic corticosteroid therapy is indicated (see p.1015), except adrenocortical-deficiency states for which hydrocortisone with supplementary fludrocortisone is preferred. The more potent pituitary-suppressant properties of a glucocorticoid such as dexamethasone may, however, be required for the diagnosis and management of conditions associated with adrenal hyperplasia.

For administration by mouth prednisolone is usually used although prednisolone sodium phosphate or prednisolone steaglate are also employed; the usual dose, expressed in terms of prednisolone, is about 5 to 60 mg daily in divided doses, as a single daily dose after breakfast, or as a double dose on alternate days. Alternate-day early-morning dosage regimens produce less suppression of the hypothalamic-pituitary axis but may not always provide adequate control. Enteric-coated tablets of prednisolone are also available (for the view that these should not be employed in patients with inflammatory bowel disease see above).

For parenteral administration the sodium phosphate ester is normally employed and may be given intravenously by injection or infusion or intramuscularly by injection; doses appear to have been variously expressed in terms of prednisolone, prednisolone phosphate, or prednisolone sodium phosphate but are generally within the range of 4 to 60 mg daily. An aqueous suspension of prednisolone acetate is also used intramuscularly to give a prolonged effect with doses of 25 to 100 mg of the acetate being given once or twice weekly. The sodium succinate ester has also been given parenterally.

For intra-articular injection the acetate, sodium phosphate, and tebutate esters are used. Suggested doses are 5 to 25 mg of prednisolone acetate, 2 to 30 mg of prednisolone phosphate (for the sodium phosphate ester), and 4 to 40 mg of prednisolone tebutate. The sodium phosphate and tebutate esters are also given by intralesional injection and by injection into soft tissue.

Prednisolone acetate and prednisolone sodium phosphate are also used in the topical treatment of allergic and inflammatory conditions of the eyes or ears, usually as drops containing 0.5% or 1%. Prednisolone has also been used topically as the free alcohol and as the hemisuccinate, pivalate, and sodium metasulphobenzoate esters.

For rectal use prednisolone sodium metasulphobenzoate or prednisolone sodium phosphate are often employed. Retention enemas containing the equivalent of 20 mg of prednisolone per 100 mL, rectal foam containing the equivalent of 20 mg of prednisolone per dose, or suppositories containing the equivalent of 5 mg of prednisolone are available. Prednisolone has also been used rectally as the free alcohol and as the acetate and hexanoate esters.

Other esters of prednisolone which have occasionally been used include the palmitate and sodium tetrahydrophthalate.

Many references listed in the Uses and Administration section of the introduction to this chapter concern the use of prednisolone and prednisone (see p.1015).

Preparations

BP 1998: Enteric-coated Prednisolone Tablets *(Gastro-resistant Prednisolone Tablets)*; Prednisolone Enema; Prednisolone Sodium Phosphate Eye Drops; Prednisolone Tablets;
USP 23: Chloramphenicol and Prednisolone Ophthalmic Ointment; Gentamicin and Prednisolone Acetate Ophthalmic Ointment; Gentamicin and Prednisolone Acetate Ophthalmic Suspension; Neomycin and Polymyxin B Sulfates and Prednisolone Acetate Ophthalmic Suspension; Neomycin Sulfate and Prednisolone Acetate Ointment; Neomycin Sulfate and Prednisolone Acetate Ophthalmic Ointment; Neomycin Sulfate and Prednisolone Acetate Ophthalmic Suspension; Neomycin Sulfate and Prednisolone Sodium Phosphate Ophthalmic Ointment; Neomycin Sulfate, Sulfacetamide Sodium, and Prednisolone Acetate Ophthalmic Ointment; Prednisolone Acetate Injectable Suspension; Prednisolone Acetate Ophthalmic Suspension; Prednisolone Cream; Prednisolone Sodium Phosphate Injection; Prednisolone Sodium Phosphate Ophthalmic Solution; Prednisolone Sodium Succinate for Injection; Prednisolone Syrup; Prednisolone Tablets; Prednisolone Tebutate Injectable Suspension; Sulfacetamide Sodium and Prednisolone Acetate Ophthalmic Ointment; Sulfacetamide Sodium and Prednisolone Acetate Ophthalmic Suspension.

Proprietary Preparations (details are given in Part 3)

Aust.: Aprednislon; Kuhlprednon; Prednihexal; Solu-Dacortin; Ultracortenol; ***Austral.:*** Adnisolone†; Delta-Cortef†; Deltasolone†; Panafcortelone; Predmix; Predsol; Solone; Sterofrin; ***Belg.:*** Deltacortril; Pred Forte; Prednicortelone; Solu-Dacortine; ***Canad.:*** Diopred; Inflamase; Ophtho-Tate; Pediapred; Pred Forte; Pred Mild; RO-Predphate†; ***Fr.:*** Hydrocortancyl; Solucort; Solupred; ***Ger.:*** Decaprednil; Decortin H; Decortin-H-KS†; Deltacortril†; Dontisolon D; duraprednisolon; hefasolon; Inflanefran; Klismacort; Linola-H N; Linola-H-Fett N; Prectal; Prednabene; Predni; Predni-Coelin†; Predni-H; Predni-POS; Prednihexal; Prednisolut; Scherisolon†; Solu-Decortin-H; Ultracorten-H†; Ultracortenol; ***Irl.:*** Deltacortril; Precortisyl†; Pred Forte; Pred Mild; Predenema; Predfoam; Prednesol; Predsol; ***Ital.:*** Cortisolone†; Deltacortilen†; Deltidrosol†; Itacortone†; Meticortelone; Soludacortin; ***Neth.:*** Di-Adreson-F; Pred Forte†; Ultracortenol; ***Norw.:*** Pred-Clysma; Ultracortenol; ***S.Afr.:*** Capsoid; Lenisolone; Meticortelone; Pred Forte†; Pred Mild; Predeltilone†; Predsol; Prelone; ***Spain:*** Dacortin H; Estilsona; Normonsona; Solu Dacortin H; ***Swed.:*** Precortalon aquosum; Pred-Clysma; Prednicort†; Sintisone†; Ultracortenol; ***Switz.:*** Corti-Clyss; Hexacortone; Pred Forte; Pred Mild; Predni-Helvacort; Solu-Dacortine; Spiricort; Ultracortene-H; Ultracortenol; ***UK:*** Deltacortril; Deltastab; Precortisyl; Pred Forte; Predenema; Predfoam; Prednesol; Predsol; ***USA:*** Ak-Pred; Articulose-50; Delta-Cortef; Econopred; Hydeltra-TBA†; Hydeltrasol; Inflamase; Key-Pred; Key-Pred-SP; Pediapred; Pred; Predaject†; Predalone; Predate†; Predcor; Prednisol; Prelone.

Multi-ingredient: ***Aust.:*** Alpicort†; Blephamide; Conjunctin-S†; Delta-Hadensa; Delta-Tomanol; Phoscortil; Scheriproct; ***Austral.:*** Blephamide; Prednefrin; Scheriproct; ***Belg.:*** Cetapred†; Hemosedan; Isopto Cetapred; Predmycin; Scheriproct; Sofrasolone; Viscocort; ***Canad.:*** Blephamide; Dioptimyd; Metimyd; Vasocidin; ***Fr.:*** Colicort; Cortifra†; Cortisal; Deliproct; Derinox; Desocort; Martisol†; Tergynan; ***Ger.:*** Adeptolon; Alferm; Alpicort; Alpicort F; Anumedin; Aquapred; Berlicetin-Ohrentropfen; Bismolan H; Blefcon; Blephamide; Blephamide N Liquifilm; Corti-Dynexan; Crinohermal P†; Dexa-Phlogont L; Dontisolon M Mundheilpaste†; Dontisolon M Zylinderampullen†; Heliomycort†; Hepathrombin-Procto†; Imazol comp; Inflanegent; Leioderm P; Linola-H-compositum N; Linoladiol-H N; Lygal; Mycinopred†; NeyChondrin "N" (Revitorgan-Dilutionen "N" Nr. 68); NeyNormin "N" (Revitorgan-Dilutionen "N" Nr. 65); NeyTumorin "N" (Revitorgan-Dilutionen Nr. 66); Positex†; Predni aquos. in der Ophtiole†; Prednitracin; Pruriderm ultra†; Scheriproct; Thesit P; Tyzine compositum†; Ultra-Demoplas; Virunguent-P; ***Irl.:*** Blephamide†; Scheriproct; ***Ital.:*** Bio-Delta Cortilen; Deltamidrina; Dutimelan; Prednigamma†; Rexidina Otoiatrica†; Solprene; ***Neth.:*** Predmycin-P Liquifilm†; ***Norw.:*** Scheriproct; ***S.Afr.:*** Blephamide; Pred G; Scheriproct; ***Spain:*** Alergical; Anafilaxol B†; Antigrietun; Bronquiasmol†; Cortivel; Fungusol Prednisona†; Indosolona†; Kanapomada; Lidrone; Nasopomada; Otogen Prednisolona†; Otonina; Poly Pred; Predni Azuleno; Proctium; Rinobanedif; Rinosular†; Rinovel; Ruscus; Scheriproct; Teolixir Compositum; Yodocortison†; ***Swed.:*** Blefcon; Metimyd; Scheriproct N; ***Switz.:*** Alpicort; Alpicort F; Blephamide; Calpred; Cetapred†; Crinohermal P†; Derinox; Desocort†; Dontisolon M†; Imacort; Isopto Cetapred†; Locaseptil-Neo; Locaseptil†; Mycinopred; Nystacortone; Pred G; Prednitracin; Premandol; Scheriproct; Varecort†; Virunguent-P†; ***UK:*** Predsol-N; Scheriproct; ***USA:*** Ak-Cide; Blephamide; Cetapred; Isopto Cetapred; Metimyd; Optimyd; Poly-Pred; Pred G; Sulphrin†; Sulster; Vasocidin.

Prednisone (1131-w)

Prednisone *(BAN, rINN)*.

Δ^1-Cortisone; 1,2-Dehydrocortisone; Deltacortisone; Deltadehydrocortisone; Metacortandracin; NSC-10023; Prednisonum. 17α,21-Dihydroxypregna-1,4-diene-3,11,20-trione.

$C_{21}H_{26}O_5$ = 358.4.

CAS — 53-03-2.

Pharmacopoeias. In *Eur.* (see p.viii). *US* allows the anhydrous form or the monohydrate.

A white or almost white, odourless, crystalline powder. It shows polymorphism. Practically **insoluble** to very slightly soluble in water; soluble 1 in 150 of alcohol and 1 in 200 of chloroform; slightly soluble in dioxan, in methyl alcohol, and in dichloromethane. **Protect** from light.

Prednisone Acetate (1130-s)

Prednisone Acetate *(BANM, rINNM)*.

Prednisone 21-acetate.

$C_{23}H_{28}O_6$ = 400.5.

CAS — 125-10-0.

Pharmacopoeias. In *Chin.* and *Pol.*

Prednisone acetate 11 mg is approximately equivalent to 10 mg of prednisone.

Prednisone is a biologically inert corticosteroid which is converted to the predominantly glucocorticoid corticosteroid prednisolone in the liver. It has the same chemical relationship to prednisolone as cortisone has to hydrocortisone. The indications and dosage of prednisone for oral use are exactly the same as those for prednisolone (see p.1049, and the chapter introduction, p.1015).

In the UK prednisolone has historically been preferred to prednisone, on the grounds that it does not require conversion to the active substance, but in practice this is rarely significant (see p.1048), and in some countries, such as the USA, prednisone is the drug of choice for many of the conditions in which routine systemic corticosteroid therapy is indicated.

Many references listed in the Uses and Administration section of the introduction to this chapter concern the use of prednisone and prednisolone (see p.1015).

Preparations

BP 1998: Prednisone Tablets;
USP 23: Prednisone Oral Solution; Prednisone Syrup; Prednisone Tablets.

Proprietary Preparations (details are given in Part 3)
Austral.: Adasone†; Deltasone†; Panafcort; Sone; ***Belg.:*** Prednicort; ***Canad.:*** Deltasone; Winpred; ***Fr.:*** Cortancyl; ***Ger.:*** Decortin; Predni-Tablinen; Predniment†; Rectodelt; Ultracorten†; ***Irl.:*** Decortisyl†; ***Ital.:*** Decorton†; Deltacortene; ***S.Afr.:*** Meticorten; Panafcort; Predeltin†; Trolic; ***Spain:*** Dacortin; ***Swed.:*** Deltison; ***UK:*** Decortisyl†; ***USA:*** Deltasone; Liquid Pred; Meticorten; Orasone; Panasol-S; Prednicen-M†; Sterapred.

Multi-ingredient: ***Aust.:*** Fluorex Plus; Oleomycetin-Prednison; ***Canad.:*** Metreton; ***Ger.:*** Oleomycetin-Prednison; ***Ital.:*** Demicina†; ***Spain:*** Anafilaxol†; Biocortison†; Coliriocilina Prednisona; Combiflexona†; Fiacin; Hemorrane; Kanafosal Predni; Prednis Neomic.

Prednylidene (1132-e)

Prednylidene *(BAN, rINN)*.

16-Methyleneprednisolone. 11β,17α,21-Trihydroxy-16-methylenepregna-1,4-diene-3,20-dione.

$C_{22}H_{28}O_5$ = 372.5.

CAS — 599-33-7.

Prednylidene is a corticosteroid that has been used for its glucocorticoid activity similarly to prednisolone (see p.1048). It has been given by mouth and by injection as the diethylaminoacetate hydrochloride.

Preparations

Proprietary Preparations (details are given in Part 3)
Ger.: Decortilen; ***Swed.:*** Dacortilen†.

Procinonide (6449-m)

Procinonide *(USAN, rINN)*.

RS-2362. (6α,11β,16α)-6,9-Difluoro-11-hydroxy-16,17-[(1-methylethylidene)bis(oxy)]-21-(1-oxopropoxy)-pregna-1,4-diene-3,20-dione.

$C_{27}H_{34}F_2O_7$ = 508.6.

CAS — 58497-00-0.

Procinonide is a derivative of fluocinolone acetonide (p.1041) which has been applied topically in combination with fluocinonide and ciprocinonide in the management of various skin disorders.

When applied topically, particularly to large areas, when the skin is broken, or under occlusive dressings, corticosteroids may be absorbed in sufficient amounts to cause systemic effects (p.1010). The effects of topical corticosteroids on the skin are described on p.1012.

Skin disorders. For recommendations concerning the correct use of corticosteroids on the skin, see Corticosteroids, Administration, p.1017.

Preparations

Proprietary Preparations (details are given in Part 3)
Multi-ingredient: ***Canad.:*** Trisyn.

Rimexolone (5646-d)

Rimexolone *(BAN, USAN, rINN)*.

Org-6216. 11β-Hydroxy-16α,17α-dimethyl-17β-propionylandrosta-1,4-dien-3-one.

$C_{24}H_{34}O_3$ = 370.5.

CAS — 49697-38-3.

Pharmacopoeias. In *US.*

A white or off-white powder. Freely **soluble** in chloroform; sparingly soluble in methyl alcohol.

Rimexolone is a corticosteroid applied topically to the eye for its glucocorticoid activity (see p.1010) in the treatment of uveitis (p.1030) and postoperative inflammation. It is used as a 1% suspension.

Prolonged application to the eye of preparations containing corticosteroids has caused raised intra-ocular pressure and reduced visual function.

Rimexolone has also been investigated as an intra-articular injection in the treatment of rheumatoid arthritis.

References.

1. van Vliet-Daskalopoulou E, *et al.* Intra-articular rimexolone in the rheumatoid knee: a placebo-controlled, double-blind, multicentre trial of three doses. *Br J Rheumatol* 1987; **26:**450–3.
2. Derendorf H, *et al.* Pharmacokinetics of rimexolone after intra-articular administration. *J Clin Pharmacol* 1990; **30:** 476–9.
3. Foster CS, *et al.* Efficacy and safety of rimexolone 1% ophthalmic suspension vs 1% prednisolone acetate in the treatment of uveitis. *Am J Ophthalmol* 1996; **122:** 171–82.
4. Assil KK, *et al.* Control of ocular inflammation after cataract extraction with rimexolone 1% ophthalmic suspension. *J Cataract Refract Surg* 1997; **23:** 750–7.

Preparations

USP 23: Rimexolone Ophthalmic Suspension.

Proprietary Preparations (details are given in Part 3)
Canad.: Vexol; ***USA:*** Vexol.

Suprarenal Cortex (1133-l)

Suprarenal cortex contains a number of steroid compounds the most active of which are corticosterone, dehydrocorticosterone, hydrocortisone, cortisone, and aldosterone. It has been prepared from the adrenal glands of oxen.

Suprarenal cortex was formerly used for the treatment of adrenocortical insufficiency. It has largely been superseded by hydrocortisone and other corticosteroids (see p.1017), but in some countries it is still administered by intramuscular injection in the management of adrenocortical insufficiency.

Suprarenal cortex is an ingredient of a wide range of preparations, often together with other organ extracts or vitamins, promoted for indications ranging from asthenia to liver disorders.

Preparations

Proprietary Preparations (details are given in Part 3)
Aust.: Cortiglanden; ***Fr.:*** Cortine Naturelle; ***Ital.:*** Cort 2000†; Cortelan†; Cortepacitina†; Cortidin†; Master Cortex 200†; Mencortex†; Novacort†; Solcort†; Supracort†; Tomcor†; Ultracort†; ***Spain:*** Pleocortex.

Multi-ingredient: ***Aust.:*** Flexurat; Mobilat; ***Belg.:*** Cromaton; Mobilat; ***Canad.:*** Heracline; Revitonus C; ***Ger.:*** Arthrodeformat P; Conjunctisan-B; Flexurat; Mastu NH†; Mobilat; ***Ital.:*** Adinepar†; Beta-Cortex B12†; Bio-Rex†; Biocortex†; Biocortone Vit†; Bioepar†; Cebran†; Citicortex†; Cortepar B12†; Cortevit 100†; Cortigen B6†; Cortiplex Forte†; Cromacort†; Cromex†; Disintox Cortex†; Emazian Cortex†; Emonucleosina Cortex†; Endoepacort B12†; Exepin Cortex†; Fegacorten†; Fitepar Cortex†; Folincortex†; Folinemic Cortex†; Glutacortin†; Lesten†; Liverasten†; Mencortex B6†; NE 300†; Neo-Cromaton Cortex†; Nucleo-Cortex†; P-Cortin†; Protidepar 100†; Redinon Cortex†; Ribocort B12†; Ricortex†; Rossocorten†; Rubrocortex†; Stasten C†; Surrenovis†; Vitalion†; ***Spain:*** Cromaton Cortex†; Hepatoclamar†; Movilat; Neurocatavin Dexa; Pleocortex B6; Rubrocortin; ***Switz.:*** Mobilat.

Tixocortol Pivalate (13356-y)

Tixocortol Pivalate *(BANM, USAN, rINNM)*.

JO-1016. 11β,17α-Dihydroxy-21-mercaptopregn-4-ene-3,20-dione 21-pivalate.

$C_{26}H_{38}O_5S$ = 462.6.

CAS — 61951-99-3 (tixocortol); 55560-96-8 (tixocortol pivalate).

Tixocortol pivalate is a corticosteroid with mainly glucocorticoid activity, as described under Corticosteroids, p.1010. It is used as buccal, nasal, throat, and rectal preparations. It is reported to undergo rapid first-pass metabolism, primarily in the liver, and to have minimal systemic effect.

Preparations

Proprietary Preparations (details are given in Part 3)
Belg.: Rhinovalon; ***Canad.:*** Reactovalone†; Rectovalone; ***Fr.:*** Pivalone; Rectovalone; ***Ger.:*** tiovalon†; ***Neth.:*** Pivalone†; Rectovalone; ***Spain:*** Rectovalone; Tiovalone; ***Switz.:*** Pivalone.

Multi-ingredient: ***Belg.:*** Rhinovalon Neomycine; ***Fr.:*** Dontopivalone; Oropivalone Bacitracine; Pivalone Neomycine; Thiovalone; ***Switz.:*** Oro-Pivalone; Pivalone compositum.

Triamcinolone (1134-y)

Triamcinolone *(BAN, rINN)*.

9α-Fluoro-16α-hydroxyprednisolone; Fluoxiprednisolonum. 9α-Fluoro-11β,16α,17α,21-tetrahydroxypregna-1,4-diene-3,20-dione.

$C_{21}H_{27}FO_6$ = 394.4.

CAS — 124-94-7.

Pharmacopoeias. In *Eur.* (see p.viii), *Jpn, Pol.,* and *US.*

A white or almost white, odourless, slightly hygroscopic, crystalline powder. It exhibits polymorphism. Practically **insoluble** or very slightly soluble in water; slightly soluble in alcohol and in methyl alcohol; very slightly soluble in chloroform and in ether; practically insoluble in dichloromethane. **Protect** from light.

Triamcinolone Acetonide (1137-c)

Triamcinolone Acetonide *(BANM, rINNM)*.

CL-61965 (triamcinolone acetonide sodium phosphate); CL-106359 (triamcinolone acetonide sodium phosphate); Triamcinoloni Acetonidum. 9α-Fluoro-11β,21-dihydroxy-16α,17α-isopropylidenedioxypregna-1,4-diene-3,20-dione.

$C_{24}H_{31}FO_6$ = 434.5.

CAS — 76-25-5 (triamcinolone acetonide); 1997-15-5 (triamcinolone acetonide sodium phosphate); 989-96-8 (triamcinolone acetonide 21-(dihydrogen phosphate)).

NOTE. Triamcinolone Acetonide Sodium Phosphate is *USAN.*

Pharmacopoeias. In *Eur.* (see p.viii), *Jpn, Pol.,* and *US.*

Chin. includes Triamcinolone Acetonide Acetate.

A white or cream-coloured, almost odourless, crystalline powder. It exhibits polymorphism. Triamcinolone acetonide 11 mg is approximately equivalent to 10 mg of triamcinolone.

Practically **insoluble** in water; sparingly soluble in alcohol, in dehydrated alcohol, in chloroform, or in methyl alcohol; very slightly soluble in ether. **Protect** from light.

Triamcinolone Diacetate (1136-z)

Triamcinolone Diacetate *(BANM, rINNM)*.

Triamcinolone 16α,21-diacetate.

$C_{25}H_{31}FO_8$ = 478.5.

CAS — 67-78-7.

Pharmacopoeias. In *US.*

A white to off-white, almost odourless, fine crystalline powder. Triamcinolone diacetate 12 mg is approximately equivalent to 10 mg of triamcinolone.

Practically **insoluble** in water; soluble 1 in 13 of alcohol, 1 in 80 of chloroform, and 1 in 40 of methyl alcohol; slightly soluble in ether.

Triamcinolone Hexacetonide (1135-j)

Triamcinolone Hexacetonide *(BAN, USAN, rINN)*.

CL-34433; TATBA; Triamcinolone Acetonide 21-(3,3-Dimethylbutyrate); Triamcinoloni Hexacetonidum. 9α-Fluoro-11β,21-dihydroxy-16α,17α-isopropylidenedioxypregna-1,4-diene-3,20-dione 21-(3,3-dimethylbutyrate).

$C_{30}H_{41}FO_7$ = 532.6.

CAS — 5611-51-8.

Pharmacopoeias. In *Eur.* (see p.viii) and *US.*

A white to cream-coloured crystalline powder. Triamcinolone hexacetonide 14 mg is approximately equivalent to 10 mg of triamcinolone.

Practically **insoluble** in water; sparingly soluble in dehydrated alcohol; soluble in chloroform; sparingly or slightly soluble in methyl alcohol. **Protect** from light.

Adverse Effects, Treatment, Withdrawal, and Precautions

As for corticosteroids in general (see p.1010). High doses of triamcinolone may have a greater tendency to produce proximal myopathy. Its effects on sodium and water retention are less than those of prednisolone.

When applied topically, particularly to large areas, when the skin is broken, or under occlusive dressings, corticosteroids may be absorbed in sufficient amounts to cause systemic effects.

Hypersensitivity. Local reactions to topical triamcinolone preparations have been attributed to the content of ethylenediamine.[1,2] However, there have also been reports of anaphylactic shock following intra-articular[3] or intramuscular[4] injection of triamcinolone acetonide.

1. Wright S, Harman RRM. Ethylenediamine and piperazine sensitivity. *Br Med J* 1983; **287:** 463–4.
2. Freeman S. Allergy to Kenacomb cream. *Med J Aust* 1986; **145:** 361.
3. Larsson L. Anaphylactic shock after ia administration of triamcinolone acetonide in a 35-year-old female. *Scand J Rheumatol* 1989; **18:** 441–2.
4. Gonzalo FE, *et al.* Anaphylactic shock caused by triamcinolone acetonide. *Ann Pharmacother* 1994; **28:** 1310.

Pharmacokinetics

For a brief outline of the pharmacokinetics of corticosteroids, see p.1014.

Triamcinolone is reported to have a half-life in plasma of about 2 to over 5 hours. It is bound to plasma albumin to a much smaller extent than hydrocortisone.

The acetonide, diacetate, and hexacetonide esters of triamcinolone are only very slowly absorbed from injection sites.

References to the pharmacokinetics of triamcinolone and its esters.

1. Möllmann H, *et al.* Pharmacokinetics of triamcinolone acetonide and its phosphate ester. *Eur J Clin Pharmacol* 1985; **29:** 85–9.
2. Derendorf H, *et al.*. Pharmacokinetics and pharmacodynamics of glucocorticoid suspensions after intra-articular administration. *Clin Pharmacol Ther* 1986; **39:** 313–17.
3. Derendorf H, *et al.* Pharmacokinetics of triamcinolone acetonide after intravenous, oral, and inhaled administration. *J Clin Pharmacol* 1995; **35:** 302–5.

Uses and Administration

Triamcinolone is a corticosteroid with mainly glucocorticoid activity (p.1010); 4 mg of triamcinolone is equivalent in anti-inflammatory activity to about 5 mg of prednisolone. It is used, either in the form of the free alcohol or in one of the esterified forms, in the treatment of conditions for which corticosteroid therapy is indicated (see p.1015), except adrenocortical insufficiency for which hydrocortisone with supplementary fludrocortisone is preferred.

For administration by mouth triamcinolone is used in doses of 4 to 48 mg daily although daily doses over 32 mg are seldom indicated.

For parenteral administration the acetonide or diacetate esters are used in doses of about 40 mg by intramuscular injection. They are usually given as suspensions to provide a prolonged systemic effect. A dose of 40 to 100 mg of the acetonide may provide symptomatic control throughout the pollen season for hay fever sufferers; for the diacetate, a 40-mg dose is administered weekly.

For intra-articular injection triamcinolone acetonide, diacetate, and hexacetonide have all been used. Doses for these esters have been in the range of 2.5 to 40 mg, 3 to 48 mg, and 2 to 30 mg respectively, depending upon the size of the joint injected.

For topical application in the treatment of various skin disorders triamcinolone acetonide is used, usually in creams, lotions, or ointments containing 0.1% although concentrations ranging from 0.025 to 0.5% have been employed. Several topical preparations also contain an antibiotic. Triamcinolone esters are also commonly used by intralesional or intradermal injection in the treatment of some inflammatory skin disorders such as keloids. Suggested doses for the various esters have been: acetonide, 1 to 3 mg per site with no more than 5 mg injected into any one site or not more than 30 mg in total if several sites of injection are used; diacetate, a total of 5 mg in divided doses into small lesions or up to a total of 48 mg in divided doses into large lesions with no more than 12.5 mg injected into any one site or 25 mg injected into any one lesion; hexacetonide, up to 500 μg per square inch (approximately 80 μg per cm^2) of affected skin.

Triamcinolone acetonide is also used by inhalation for the control of asthma in a usual dose of about

200 μg by metered-dose inhaler three or four times daily; the dose should not exceed 1600 μg daily.

In the prophylaxis and treatment of allergic rhinitis triamcinolone acetonide may be administered by a nasal spray in a usual dose of 2 sprays (110 μg) into each nostril once daily.

Other esters of triamcinolone which have occasionally been used include the acetonide dipotassium phosphate, acetonide hemisuccinate, aminobenzal benzamidoisobutyrate, and benetonide. Another derivative of triamcinolone, flupamesone has also been used.

Asthma. Intramuscular triamcinolone acetonide has been reported to be more effective than oral low-dose prednisone in controlling exacerbations in patients with severe, chronic, life-threatening asthma,[1] although this conclusion is controversial.[2-7]

Corticosteroids, together with the $beta_2$-adrenoceptor agonists, form one of the cornerstones of the management of asthma (p.745). Inhaled corticosteroids are added to therapy with a short-acting $beta_2$ agonist if symptom relief with the latter is needed more than once daily, although corticosteroids with reduced systemic activity are generally preferred to triamcinolone. Systemic corticosteroids are reserved for the most severe cases, and for the management of acute severe asthma attacks (status asthmaticus).

1. Ogirala RG, *et al.* High-dose intramuscular triamcinolone in severe, chronic, life-threatening asthma. *N Engl J Med* 1991; **324:** 589–9. Correction. *ibid.*; 1380.
2. Salmeron S, *et al.* Intramuscular triamcinolone in severe asthma. *N Engl J Med* 1991; **325:** 429–30.
3. Nicholas SS. Intramuscular triamcinolone in severe asthma. *N Engl J Med* 1991; **325:** 430.
4. Kidney JC, *et al.* Intramuscular triamcinolone in severe asthma. *N Engl J Med* 1991; **325:** 430.
5. Capewell S, McLeod DT. Intramuscular triamcinolone in severe asthma. *N Engl J Med* 1991; **325:** 430.
6. Ogirala RG, *et al.* Intramuscular triamcinolone in severe asthma. *N Engl J Med* 1991; **325:** 431.
7. Capewell S, McLeod D. Injected corticosteroids in refractory asthma. *Lancet* 1991; **338:** 1075–6.

Rhinitis. Triamcinolone is effective when given intranasally for the relief of allergic rhinitis,[1,2] either as a conventional aerosol formulation or a newer, aqueous formulation. For a discussion of rhinitis and its management, including the role of corticosteroids, see p.400.

1. Grubbe R, *et al.* Intranasal therapy with once-daily triamcinolone acetonide aerosol versus twice-daily beclomethasone dipropionate aqueous spray in patients with perennial allergic rhinitis. *Curr Ther Res* 1996; **57:** 825–38.
2. Jeal W, Faulds D. Triamcinolone acetonide: a review of its pharmacological properties and therapeutic efficacy in the management of allergic rhinitis. *Drugs* 1997; **53:** 257–80.

Skin disorders. For recommendations concerning the correct use of corticosteroids on the skin, and a rough guide to the clinical potencies of topical corticosteroids, see Corticosteroids, Administration, p.1017.

Preparations

BP 1998: Triamcinolone Acetonide Injection; Triamcinolone Cream; Triamcinolone Dental Paste; Triamcinolone Ointment; Triamcinolone Tablets;
USP 23: Neomycin Sulfate and Triamcinolone Acetonide Cream; Neomycin Sulfate and Triamcinolone Acetonide Ophthalmic Ointment; Nystatin and Triamcinolone Acetonide Cream; Nystatin and Triamcinolone Acetonide Ointment; Nystatin, Neomycin Sulfate, Gramicidin, and Triamcinolone Acetonide Cream; Nystatin, Neomycin Sulfate, Gramicidin, and Triamcinolone Acetonide Ointment; Triamcinolone Acetonide Cream; Triamcinolone Acetonide Dental Paste; Triamcinolone Acetonide Injectable Suspension; Triamcinolone Acetonide Lotion; Triamcinolone Acetonide Ointment; Triamcinolone Acetonide Topical Aerosol; Triamcinolone Diacetate Injectable Suspension; Triamcinolone Diacetate Syrup; Triamcinolone Hexacetonide Injectable Suspension; Triamcinolone Tablets.

Proprietary Preparations (details are given in Part 3)
Aust.: Delphicort; Lederspan; Solu-Volon; Volon; Volon A; ***Austral.:*** Aristocort; Kenacort-A; Kenacort†; Kenalog in Orabase; Kenalone; ***Belg.:*** Albicort; Delphi; Kenacort; Kenacort Solubile; Kenacort-A; Ledercort; Lederspan; ***Canad.:*** Aristocort; Aristospan; Azmacort; Kenalog; Kenalog in Orabase; Nasacort; Oracort; Scheinpharm Triamcine-A; Triaderm; ***Fr.:*** Hexatrione; Kenacort; Tedarol†; Tibicorten†; ***Ger.:*** Arutrin; Berlicort; Delphicort; Delphimix; Extracort; Extracort N; Kenalog; Kortikoid-ratiopharm; Lederlon; Tri-Anemul; Triam; Triam-Injekt; Triamoral; TriamCreme; Triamgalen; Triamhexal; TriamSalbe; Volon; Volon A; Volonimat; Volonimat N; ***Irl.:*** Adcortyl; Adcortyl in Orabase; Kenacort-A†; Kenacort†; Kenalog; Lederspan; ***Ital.:*** Aftab; Albacort Idrodispersibile†; Ipercortis; Kenacort-A; Kenacort†; Ledercort; Taucorten†; Tibicorten†; Tricortale†; ***Neth.:*** Albicort; Delphi; Kenacort-A; Kenacort-A Solubile†; Kenacort†; Ledercort; Lederspan; ***Norw.:*** Kenacort-T; Ledercort†; Lederspan; ***S.Afr.:*** Kenalog in Orabase; Ledercort; Lederspan; Nasacor; ***Spain:*** Alcorten†; Flutenal; Ledercort; Proctosteroid; Trigon Depot; ***Swed.:*** Kenacort-T; Kenacort†; Ledercort†; Lederspan; ***Switz.:*** Corticotherapique†; Kenacort; Kenacort-A; Kenacort-A Solubile; Ledercort; Respicort†; Triamcort; ***UK:*** Adcortyl; Adcortyl in Orabase; Kenalog; Ledercort; Lederspan; Nasacort; ***USA:*** Amcort; Aristocort; Aristospan; Articulose LA; Atolone; Azmacort; Cinalone 40†; Cinonide 40†; Delta-Tritex; Flutex; Kenacort; Kenaject; Kenalog; Kenalog in Orabase; Kenonel; Nasacort; Oralone Dental; Tac; Tri-Kort; Triacet; Triam; Triam-A; Triamcinair†; Triamolone; Triamonide; Triderm; Trilog; Trilone; Tristoject; Trymex†.

Multi-ingredient: ***Aust.:*** Aureocort; Ledermix; Mycostatin V; Neo-Delphicort; Pevisone; Steros-Anal; Volon A antibiotikahaltig; Volon A-Zinklotion; ***Austral.:*** Aristocomb; Kenacomb; Otocomb Otic; ***Belg.:*** Albicort Compositum; Albicort Oticum; Kenoidal†; Ledercort†; Mycolog; Pevisone; Trianal; ***Canad.:*** Aristoform†; Aureocort†; Kenacomb; Triacomb; Viaderm-KC; ***Fr.:*** Cidermex; Corticotulle Lumiere; Kenalcol; Localone; Mycolog; Pevisone; ***Ger.:*** Ampho-Moronal V; Ampho-Moronal V N†; Aureodelf; Corticotulle Lumiere; Epipevisone; Extracort Rhin sine; Extracort Tinktur N; Korticoid c. Neomycin-ratiopharm†; Moronal V; Moronal V N†; Moronal†; mykoproct sine; mykoproct†; Polcortolon TC; Steros-Anal; Ultexiv; Volon A antibiotikahaltig N; Volon A Tinktur N; Volon A-Rhin neu; Volon A-Schuttelmix; Volonimat Plus N; ***Irl.:*** Audicort; Aureocort; Kenacomb; Ledermix; ***Ital.:*** Assocort; Aureocort; Dirahist; Kataval; Neo-Audiocort; Pevisone; Sprayrin†; Tibicorten F†; ***Neth.:*** Albicort Compositum; Kenalog; Mycolog; Trianal; ***Norw.:*** Kenacort-T comp; Kenacutan; Pevisone; ***S.Afr.:*** Kenacomb; Ledermix; Pevisone; Trialone; ***Spain:*** Aldo Otico; Aldoderma; Anasilpiel; Anso; Cemalyt; Crema Glaan Corticoide†; Cremsol; Deltasiton; Flutenal Gentamicina; Flutenal Sali; Interderm; Nesfare Antibiotico; Positon; Pulverodil†; Tododermil Compuesto; Tododermil Simple†; Triaformo†; Tricin†; Trigon Rectal; Trigon Topico; ***Swed.:*** Kenacombin Novum; Kenacombin†; Kenacort-T comp; Kenacort-T med Graneodin†; Kenacutan; Pevisone; ***Switz.:*** Kenacort-A; Ledermix; Mycolog; Neo Amphocort†; Pevisone; Steros-Anal†; ***UK:*** Adcortyl with Graneodin; Audicort; Aureocort; Ledermix; Nystadermal; Pevaryl TC; Tri-Adcortyl; ***USA:*** Myco-Biotic II; Myco-Triacet II; Mycogen II; Mycolog-II; Myconel; Mytrex; NGT; Tri-Statin II.

Cough Suppressants Expectorants Mucolytics and Nasal Decongestants

This chapter describes those drugs that are used mainly as cough suppressants, expectorants, or mucolytics, and sympathomimetics primarily used for the relief of nasal congestion. Other drugs used in cough include antihistamines (p.397), bronchodilators (p.745 and p.453), and local anaesthetics (p.1281). Compounds with a demulcent action such as glycerol (p.1585) and sucrose (p.1357) are also used, as are various hydrating inhalations.

Cough suppressants. The cough suppressants described in this chapter have either a central or a peripheral action on the cough reflex or a combination of both. Centrally acting cough suppressants increase the threshold of the cough centre in the brain to incoming stimuli whereas those acting peripherally decrease the sensitivity of the receptors in the respiratory tract. Some drugs have an indirect peripheral mechanism of action and may alter mucociliary factors, exert a local analgesic or anaesthetic action on the receptors, protect the receptors from irritant stimuli, or act as bronchodilators.

Centrally acting cough suppressants structurally related to morphine and included in this chapter, such as dextromethorphan, have little or no analgesic action. Those that also have an analgesic action such as codeine or diamorphine are described in the chapter on Analgesics, p.1.

Expectorants. The expectorants described in this chapter are reported to increase the volume of secretions in the respiratory tract and therefore to facilitate their removal by ciliary action and coughing. Some, such as small doses of ipecacuanha and squill, ammonium salts, some volatile oils, and various iodide compounds are traditionally believed to achieve this by a reflex irritant effect on the gastric mucosa.

Mucolytics. The mucolytics described in this chapter alter the structure of mucus to decrease its viscosity and therefore facilitate its removal by ciliary action or expectoration.

Acetylcysteine, carbocisteine, methyl cysteine, and stepronin all have thiol groups; if this group is free as in acetylcysteine it may be substituted for disulphide bonds in mucus and therefore break the mucus chains. However, drugs such as carbocisteine with 'protected' thiol groups cannot act by this mechanism and their exact mode of action is unclear. Thiol groups are also involved in the mechanism of action of some of these drugs when they are used in the treatment of poisoning.

Deoxyribonucleases such as dornase alfa act as mucolytics by hydrolysing the accumulated extracellular DNA from decaying neutrophils that contributes to the viscous respiratory secretions of cystic fibrosis.

Sympathomimetics. Some sympathomimetics described in this chapter are employed, systemically (e.g. phenylephrine, p.1066) or locally (e.g. naphazoline, p.1064), for their alpha agonist actions to produce vasoconstriction of the nasal mucosa, thus relieving congestion. Others (e.g. ephedrine, p.1059) have both alpha and beta agonist actions. The beta agonist actions confer upon them bronchodilating properties, but they have been superseded as bronchodilators by the more selective $beta_2$ agonists such as salbutamol (p.758). The value of bronchodilators in non-asthmatic cough has not been confirmed.

Cough

Cough is characterised by forced expiration against a closed glottis, which suddenly opens to expel air and unwanted material from the respiratory tract. It may be voluntary as well as involuntary.

It is an important physiological protective mechanism, but may also occur as a symptom of an underlying disorder. Treatment of the disorder often alleviates the cough, but there are times when symptomatic treatment is appropriate. The treatment chosen depends on whether the cough is productive or non-productive.

A *non-productive cough* may be considered as serving no useful purpose for the patient. For example, the symptoms of the common cold often include a non-productive cough, and cough suppressants may provide some relief to the patient, particularly if administered at night. Pholcodine and dextromethorphan are commonly employed as cough suppressants and are considered to have fewer adverse effects than codeine which is also widely used. However, there is little evidence that cough suppressants such as codeine, dextromethorphan, or pholcodine are effective in severe cough. Cough suppressants containing codeine or similar opioids are not generally recommended for administration to children, and should be avoided altogether in those under 1 year of age.

A potent cough suppressant such as morphine is needed for the relief of *intractable cough in terminal illness*. The use of such a potent opioid is not otherwise considered appropriate for cough.

A *productive cough* is characterised by the presence of sputum and may be associated with conditions such as chronic bronchitis, bronchiectasis, or cystic fibrosis. Cough suppressants should not be used to treat such a cough which is considered to be a useful protective mechanism.

Expectorants have been used for productive cough on the grounds that increasing the volume of secretions in the respiratory tract enables them to be more easily removed by ciliary action and coughing. However, clinical evidence of their efficacy is lacking, and many authorities consider them to be of no value other than as a placebo. Commonly used expectorants include ammonium salts, guaiphenesin, ipecacuanha, and sodium citrate. Iodides have also been used but there has been concern over their safety for prolonged administration in respiratory disorders and because of their potential for thyroid suppression; in particular, it has been recommended that they should not be given to children, adolescents, pregnant women, or patients with goitre.

Mucolytics have been shown to affect sputum viscosity and structure and patients have reported alleviation of their symptoms, but no consistent improvement has been demonstrated in lung function. Commonly used mucolytics include acetylcysteine, bromhexine, carbocisteine, and methyl cysteine. Dornase alfa is also available, in particular for patients with cystic fibrosis. In theory mucolytics may disrupt the gastric mucosal barrier and caution has been recommended in patients with a history of peptic ulceration.

Other drugs are also employed in the treatment of cough.

- *Sedating antihistamines* such as diphenhydramine are frequently employed as cough suppressants in compound preparations. Suggested mechanisms of action have included reduction in cholinergic nerve transmission, or cough suppression as a result of their sedative effects. Antihistamines reduce nasal secretions and may be of value in treating cough caused by postnasal drip, particularly if associated with allergic rhinitis (see p.400). However, they should not be used to treat a productive cough because they may cause formation of viscid mucus plugs. Their sedative effects are a disadvantage for daytime use but may be a short-term advantage for night coughs.
- *Bronchodilators* such as $beta_2$ agonists or antimuscarinics alleviate cough associated with bronchospasm. However, they have no proven benefit in other forms of cough, and they are not recommended for use in non-asthmatic patients.
- *Demulcents* may be considered as indirect peripherally acting cough suppressants. Their action may involve provision of a protective coating over sensory receptors in the pharynx. Demulcents include glycerol, honey, liquorice, and sucrose syrups.
- *Hydrating agents* liquefy mucus and also have a demulcent effect. Hydration may be achieved simply by inhaling warm moist air. The addition of substances such as menthol, benzoin, or volatile oils is unlikely to provide any additional benefit but may encourage the use of such inhalations. Inhalation aerosols of water, sodium bicarbonate, sodium chloride, surfactants such as tyloxapol, and proteolytic enzymes such as chymotrypsin and trypsin, have also been used for their reported hydrating or mucolytic effects on respiratory secretions.
- *Local anaesthetics* such as lignocaine or bupivacaine have been administered by inhalation in severe intractable cough, including cough caused by malignant neoplasms. Cough suppression is produced by an indirect peripheral action on sensory receptors, but as all protective pulmonary reflexes may be lost and bronchospasm may be induced, such treatment should be used with care. There may also be temporary loss of the swallowing reflex.

Cough and cold preparations containing various combinations of cough suppressants and expectorants, together with sympathomimetics, antihistamines, or analgesics are available. Some of these combinations such as a cough suppressant and an expectorant are illogical and there is little evidence to support their efficacy. As with many combinations, doses of individual drugs may be inadequate or inappropriate, and the large number of ingredients may expose the patient to unnecessary adverse effects.

Some references to cough and its management are listed below.

1. Fuller RW, Jackson DM. Physiology and treatment of cough. *Thorax* 1990; **45:** 425–30.
2. Pratter MR, *et al.* An algorithmic approach to chronic cough. *Ann Intern Med* 1993; **119:** 977–83.
3. Irwin RS, *et al.* Appropriate use of antitussives and protussives: a practical review. *Drugs* 1993; **46:** 80–91.

Nasal congestion

Nasal congestion is frequently a symptom of conditions such as rhinitis, treatment of which (as discussed on p.400) can include the use of antihistamines, sympathomimetics, corticosteroids, antimuscarinics, and cromoglycate or nedocromil.

Sympathomimetics are also widely employed as nasal decongestants to provide symptomatic relief of the common cold. They are used for their alpha adrenergic effects, which produce vasoconstriction, redistributing local blood flow to reduce oedema of the nasal mucosa thus improving ventilation, drainage, and nasal stuffiness. Sympathomimetics such as ephedrine, phenylephrine, oxymetazoline, and xylometazoline can be applied topically as nasal drops or sprays. Those such as phenylpropanolamine and pseudoephedrine are given by mouth.

Topical application of sympathomimetics has been associated with rebound congestion, particularly if use has been prolonged, as vasodilatation becomes prominent and the effects of vasoconstriction subside. Use is therefore restricted to periods of not more than 7 consecutive days. Administration by mouth is not associated with such rebound congestion, but is of doubtful value and more likely to be associated with systemic side-effects and a higher risk of drug interactions.

The benefits of *antihistamines* in nasal congestion other than that associated with allergic rhinitis are doubtful, particularly by topical application.

Inhalations of warm moist air are also useful in the treatment of nasal congestion associated with the common cold. As in the case of cough (see above) the addition of substances such as menthol, benzoin, or volatile oils may encourage the use of such inhalations.

Acetylcysteine (3701-r)

Acetylcysteine *(BAN, USAN, rINN)*.

5052; Acetylcysteinum; NSC-111180. *N*-Acetyl-L-cysteine.

$C_5H_9NO_3S$ = 163.2.

CAS — 616-91-1.

Pharmacopoeias. In *Chin., Eur.* (see p.viii), and *US.*

A white crystalline powder with a slight acetic odour. **Soluble** 1 in 5 of water and 1 in 4 of alcohol; practically insoluble in chloroform, in dichloromethane, and in ether. A 1% solution in water has a pH of 2.0 to 2.8.

Incompatible with some metals, with rubber, and with oxygen and oxidising substances. Some antibiotics including amphotericin, ampicillin sodium, erythromycin lactobionate, and some tetracyclines are either physically incompatible with or may be inactivated on mixture with acetylcysteine.

A change in colour of solutions of acetylcysteine to light purple does not indicate significant impairment of safety or efficacy. **Store** in airtight containers. Protect from light.

Acetylcysteine Sodium (15577-t)

$C_5H_8NNaO_3S$ = 185.2.
CAS — 19542-74-6.

Adverse Effects

Hypersensitivity reactions have been reported in patients receiving acetylcysteine, including bronchospasm, angioedema, rashes and pruritus; hypotension, or occasionally hypertension, may occur. Other adverse effects reported with acetylcysteine include flushing, nausea and vomiting, fever, syncope, sweating, arthralgia, blurred vision, disturbances of liver function, acidosis, convulsions, and cardiac or respiratory arrest. Haemoptysis, rhinorrhoea, and stomatitis have been associated with inhalation of acetylcysteine.

The most common symptoms of patients experiencing anaphylactoid reactions after the intravenous use of acetylcysteine in the treatment of paracetamol poisoning are rash and pruritus; other features have included flushing, nausea or vomiting, angioedema, tachycardia, bronchospasm, hypotension, and hypertension;[1,2] ECG abnormalities associated with an anaphylactoid reaction have also been reported in one patient.[3] One group estimated that when acetylcysteine was administered correctly the frequency of the anaphylactoid response was between 0.3% and 3% whereas of 15 patients who had received an overdose they found that 11 had experienced an anaphylactoid reaction.[4] Intradermal testing and study of plasma-acetylcysteine concentrations in patients who developed reactions to acetylcysteine suggests a 'pseudo-allergic' rather than an immunological reaction,[5,6] although symptoms consistent with a serum sickness-like illness developed following exposure to acetylcysteine in one patient.[7] It has been suggested that generalised reactions to acetylcysteine can be treated with intravenous injection of an antihistamine;[8] infusion of acetylcysteine should be temporarily stopped but can usually be restarted at a slower rate without further reaction.

Symptoms following overdosage with acetylcysteine have been similar to those of anaphylaxis but have been more severe; hypotension appears to be especially prominent;[4] additional symptoms have included respiratory depression, haemolysis, disseminated intravascular coagulation, and renal failure but some of these may have been due to paracetamol poisoning.[1] Death has occurred in 3 patients who received an overdosage of acetylcysteine while being treated for paracetamol poisoning[1,9] but the role of acetylcysteine in this outcome was unclear in 2 of these patients.[1]

1. Mant TGK, *et al.* Adverse reactions to acetylcysteine and effects of overdose. *Br Med J* 1984; **289:** 217–19.
2. Dawson AH, *et al.* Adverse reactions to N-acetylcysteine during treatment for paracetamol poisoning. *Med J Aust* 1989; **150:** 329–31.
3. Bonfiglio MF, *et al.* Anaphylactoid reaction to intravenous acetylcysteine associated with electrocardiographic abnormalities. *Ann Pharmacother* 1992; **26:** 22–5.
4. Sunman W, *et al.* Anaphylactoid response to intravenous acetylcysteine. *Lancet* 1992; **339:** 1231–2.
5. Bateman DN, *et al.* Adverse reactions to N-acetylcysteine. *Hum Toxicol* 1984; **3:** 393–8.
6. Donovan JW, *et al.* Adverse reactions of N-acetylcysteine and their relation to plasma levels. *Vet Hum Toxicol* 1987; **29:** 470.
7. Mohammed S, *et al.* Serum sickness-like illness associated with N-acetylcysteine therapy. *Ann Pharmacother* 1994; **28:** 285.
8. Bateman DN. Adverse reactions to antidotes. *Adverse Drug React Bull* 1988; (Dec.): 496–9.
9. Anonymous. Death after N-acetylcysteine. *Lancet* 1984; **i:** 1421.

Precautions

Acetylcysteine should be used with caution in asthmatic patients. It should also be used with caution in patients with a history of peptic ulceration, both because drug-induced nausea and vomiting may increase the risk of gastro-intestinal haemorrhage in patients predisposed to the condition, and because of a theoretical risk that mucolytics may disrupt the gastric mucosal barrier.

Asthma. Reports of bronchospasm precipitated in two asthmatic patients[1] and severe asthma and respiratory arrest in another[2] after intravenous treatment with acetylcysteine.

1. Ho SW-C, Beilin LJ. Asthma associated with N-acetylcysteine infusion and paracetamol poisoning: report of two cases. *Br Med J* 1983; **287:** 876–7.
2. Reynard K, *et al.* Respiratory arrest after N-acetylcysteine for paracetamol overdose. *Lancet* 1992; **340:** 675.

Pharmacokinetics

Acetylcysteine is rapidly absorbed from the gastro-intestinal tract and peak plasma concentrations have been obtained in a number of studies about 0.5 to 1 hour after oral administration of doses of 200 to 600 mg.[1] Some studies indicate dose-dependent pharmacokinetics with peak concentrations, the time taken to reach peak concentrations, and bioavailability increasing with increasing doses.[2] Acetylcysteine may be present in plasma as the parent compound or as various oxidised metabolites such as *N*-acetylcystine, *N,N*-diacetylcystine, and cysteine either free or bound to plasma proteins by labile disulphide bonds or as a fraction incorporated into protein peptide chains.[3] In one study about 50% was in a covalently protein-bound form 4 hours after administration.[4] Oral bioavailability is low and mean values have ranged from 4 to 10% depending on whether total acetylcysteine or just the reduced forms are measured.[4,5] It has been suggested that acetylcysteine's low oral bioavailability may be due to metabolism in the gut wall and first-pass metabolism in the liver.[4,5] Renal clearance may account for about 30% of total body clearance.[5] Following intravenous administration mean terminal half-lives have been calculated to be 1.95 and 5.58 hours for reduced and total acetylcysteine respectively; the terminal half-life of total acetylcysteine was 6.25 hours after oral administration.[4]

1. Holdiness MR. Clinical pharmacokinetics of N-acetylcysteine. *Clin Pharmacokinet* 1991; **20:** 123–34.
2. Borgström L, Kågedal B. Dose dependent pharmacokinetics of N-acetylcysteine after oral dosing to man. *Biopharm Drug Dispos* 1990; **11:** 131–6.
3. De Caro L, *et al.* Pharmacokinetics and bioavailability of oral acetylcysteine in healthy volunteers. *Arzneimittelforschung* 1989; **39:** 383–6.
4. Olsson B, *et al.* Pharmacokinetics and bioavailability of reduced and oxidized N-acetylcysteine. *Eur J Clin Pharmacol* 1988; **34:** 77–82.
5. Borgström L, *et al.* Pharmacokinetics of N-acetylcysteine in man. *Eur J Clin Pharmacol* 1986; **31:** 217–22.

Uses and Administration

Acetylcysteine is a mucolytic that reduces the viscosity of secretions probably by the splitting of disulphide bonds in mucoproteins. This action is greatest at a pH of 7 to 9 and the pH may have been adjusted in commercial preparations with sodium hydroxide. It is sometimes stated that acetylcysteine sodium is used, although the dose is expressed in terms of acetylcysteine.

Acetylcysteine is also able to promote the detoxification of an intermediate paracetamol metabolite, and has a key role in the management of paracetamol overdosage.

Acetylcysteine is used for its **mucolytic** activity in respiratory disorders associated with acute cough. Administration can be by nebulisation of 3 to 5 mL of a 20% solution or 6 to 10 mL of a 10% solution through a face mask or mouthpiece 3 to 4 times daily. If necessary 1 to 10 mL of a 20% solution or 2 to 20 mL of a 10% solution may be given by nebulisation every 2 to 6 hours. It can also be given by direct endotracheal instillation of 1 to 2 mL of a 10 to 20% solution as often as every hour. Mechanical suction of the liquefied secretions may be necessary, and nebulisers containing metal or rubber components should not be used.

Acetylcysteine has been given by mouth in doses of 200 mg three times daily as granules dissolved in water. Children aged up to 2 years may be given 200 mg daily, and those aged 2 to 7 years 200 mg twice daily.

In the treatment of **dry eye** associated with abnormal mucus production, acetylcysteine is administered topically usually as a 5% solution with hypromellose, 1 to 2 drops being given 3 to 4 times daily. Higher concentrations have been used in some centres.

Acetylcysteine is given by intravenous infusion or by mouth in the treatment of **paracetamol poisoning**. In the UK, an initial dose of 150 mg per kg body-weight of acetylcysteine in 200 mL of glucose 5% is given intravenously over 15 minutes, followed by an intravenous infusion of 50 mg per kg in 500 mL of glucose 5% over the next 4 hours and then 100 mg per kg in one litre over the next 16 hours. The volume of intravenous fluids should be modified for children. In the USA, acetylcysteine is given by mouth in an initial dose of 140 mg per kg as a 5% solution followed by 70 mg per kg every 4 hours for an additional 17 doses. Acetylcysteine is reported to be most effective when administered within 8 hours of paracetamol overdosage, with the protective effect diminishing after this time. However, later initiation of treatment with acetylcysteine (up to and beyond 24 hours) may still be of benefit (see below).

Aspergillosis. Although not one of the standard therapies discussed on p.367, local instillation of acetylcysteine into the cavity containing the fungus ball has been used to treat aspergilloma.[1] There is some evidence *in vitro* that acetylcysteine has inhibitory properties against *Aspergillus* and *Fusarium* spp.[2]

1. Kauffman CA. Quandary about treatment of aspergillomas persists. *Lancet* 1996; **347:** 1640.
2. De Lucca AJ, *et al.* N-Acetylcysteine inhibits germination of conidia and growth of Aspergillus spp. and Fusarium spp. *Antimicrob Agents Chemother* 1996; **40:** 1274–6.

Cystic fibrosis. Mucolytics such as acetylcysteine are generally not considered to be effective in treating the pulmonary manifestations of cystic fibrosis (p.119). Some references to the use of acetylcysteine in cystic fibrosis are listed below.[1,2]

Meconium ileus equivalent (bowel obstruction due to abnormally viscid contents of the terminal ileum and right colon[3]) in patients with cystic fibrosis has largely disappeared with the use of pancreatic enzymes but may occur when insufficient doses are given;[4] mild cases may be treated with acetylcysteine.[4] Doses of 10 mL of a 20% solution of acetylcysteine have been given by mouth 4 times daily together with 100 mL of a 10% solution of acetylcysteine administered as an enema up to 4 times a day depending on the degree of the obstruction.[3]

1. Stanfanger G, *et al.* The clinical effect and the effect on the ciliary motility of oral N-acetylcysteine in patients with cystic fibrosis and primary ciliary dyskinesia. *Eur Respir J* 1988; **1:** 161–7.
2. Ratjen F, *et al.* A double-blind placebo controlled trial with oral ambroxol and N-acetylcysteine for mucolytic treatment in cystic fibrosis. *Eur J Pediatr* 1985; **144:** 374–8.
3. Hanly JG, Fitzgerald MX. Meconium ileus equivalent in older patients with cystic fibrosis. *Br Med J* 1983; **286:** 1411–13.
4. David TJ. Cystic fibrosis. *Arch Dis Child* 1990; **65:** 152–7.

Dry eye. Topical mucolytics such as acetylcysteine are among the treatments mentioned for dry eye on p.1470.

HIV infection and AIDS. The cysteine-containing peptide glutathione is involved in intracellular defence mechanisms, and it has been shown that low glutathione concentrations are associated with poorer survival in HIV-infected patients.[1] Since acetylcysteine can replenish glutathione, it has been suggested[2,3] that it may have a role in the treatment of AIDS (p.599). *In-vitro* studies indicate that acetylcysteine can suppress HIV expression,[4,5] and there has been a suggestion from observational data that acetylcysteine supplements can improve survival in HIV-infected individuals.[1] However, an attempt to use acetylcysteine supplementation to reduce the frequency of adverse reactions to co-trimoxazole in HIV-infected patients was not successful.[6]

1. Herzenberg LA, *et al.* Glutathione deficiency is associated with impaired survival in HIV disease. *Proc Natl Acad Sci U S A* 1997; **94:** 1967–72.
2. Staal FJT, *et al.* Glutathione deficiency and human immunodeficiency virus infection. *Lancet* 1992; **339:** 909–12.
3. Roederer M, *et al.* N-acetylcysteine: potential for AIDS therapy. *Pharmacology* 1993; **46:** 121–9.
4. Roederer M, *et al.* Cytokine-stimulated human immunodeficiency virus replication is inhibited by N-acetyl-L-cysteine. *Proc Natl Acad Sci U S A* 1990; **87:** 4884–8.
5. Kalebic T, *et al.* Suppression of human immunodeficiency virus expression in chronically infected monocytic cells by glutathione, glutathione ester, and N-acetylcysteine. *Proc Natl Acad Sci U S A* 1991; **88:** 986–90.
6. Åkerlund B, *et al.* N-acetylcysteine treatment and the risk of toxic reactions to trimethoprim-sulphamethoxazole in primary Pneumocystis carinii prophylaxis in HIV-infected patients. *J Infect* 1997; **35:** 143–7.

Liver disorders. As well as being effective in the management of paracetamol-induced liver damage (p.72), acetylcysteine has produced beneficial effects in patients with acute liver failure[1] when used alone or in combination with epoprostenol. It may also prevent the development of tissue hypoxia in patients with acute liver failure who are receiving vasopressors.[2] Intravenous infusion of acetylcysteine has not been shown to be of any benefit when added to therapy in patients undergoing orthotopic liver transplantation,[3] however.

1. Harrison PM, *et al.* Improvement by acetylcysteine of hemodynamics and oxygen transport in fulminant hepatic failure. *N Engl J Med* 1991; **324:** 1852–7.
2. Caraceni P, Van Thiel DH. Acute liver failure. *Lancet* 1995; **345:** 163–9.
3. Bromley PN, *et al.* Effects of intraoperative N-acetylcysteine in orthotopic liver transplantation. *Br J Anaesth* 1995; **75:** 352–4.

Myocardial infarction. There is limited evidence suggesting that addition of intravenous acetylcysteine to thrombolytic therapy in patients with acute myocardial infarction (p.791) may be of benefit,[1,2] and would reward further investigation.

1. Arstall MA, *et al.* N-Acetylcysteine in combination with nitroglycerin and streptokinase for the treatment of evolving acute myocardial infarction: safety and biochemical effects. *Circulation* 1995; **92:** 2855–62.
2. Šochman J, *et al.* Infarct size limitation: acute N-acetylcysteine defense (ISLAND trial): preliminary analysis and report after the first 30 patients. *Clin Cardiol* 1996; **19:** 94–100.

Nitrate tolerance. Acetylcysteine appears to be able to potentiate the peripheral and coronary effects of glyceryl trinitrate.[1,2] While some studies[3-6] suggest that it can reverse tolerance to nitrates in patients with coronary heart disease or heart failure, others have failed to demonstrate any benefit.[7] There may be a specific subgroup of responders.[6] The various attempts at overcoming nitrate tolerance are discussed on p.875.

1. Elkayam U. Tolerance to organic nitrates: evidence, mechanisms, clinical relevance, and strategies for prevention. *Ann Intern Med* 1991; **114:** 667–77.
2. Horowitz JD, *et al.* Combined use of nitroglycerin and N-acetylcysteine in the management of unstable angina pectoris. *Circulation* 1988; **77:** 787–94.
3. Packer M, *et al.* Prevention and reversal of nitrate tolerance in patients with congestive heart failure. *N Engl J Med* 1987; **317:** 799–804.
4. May DC, *et al.* In vivo induction and reversal of nitroglycerin tolerance in human coronary arteries. *N Engl J Med* 1987; **317:** 805–9.
5. Boesgaard S, *et al.* Preventive administration of intravenous N-acetylcysteine and development of tolerance to isosorbide dinitrate in patients with angina pectoris. *Circulation* 1992; **85:** 143–9.
6. Pizzulli L, *et al.* N-acetylcysteine attenuates nitroglycerin tolerance in patients with angina pectoris and normal left ventricular function. *Am J Cardiol* 1997; **79:** 28–33.
7. Hogan JC, *et al.* Chronic administration of N-acetylcysteine fails to prevent nitrate tolerance in patients with stable angina pectoris. *Br J Clin Pharmacol* 1990; **30:** 573–7.

Poisoning and toxicity. ANTINEOPLASTICS. Although not widely used, acetylcysteine has been given to patients receiving oxazaphosphorine antineoplastic agents such as cyclophosphamide and ifosfamide to protect against urinary-tract toxicity. Early studies[1] suggested that acetylcysteine given orally afforded some protection without affecting antitumour activity. For a discussion of the effects that oxazaphosphorine antineoplastics have on the bladder and their management, see under Effects on the Bladder in the Adverse Effects and Treatment of Cyclophosphamide, p.516.

Acetylcysteine has also been tried for the prophylaxis of cardiotoxicity associated with doxorubicin (see p.529).

1. Morgan LR, *et al.* Protective effect of N-acetylcysteine on the urotoxicity produced by oxazaphosphorine without interference with anticancer activity. *Eur J Cancer Clin Oncol* 1982; **18:** 113–14.

CARBON TETRACHLORIDE. The treatment of carbon tetrachloride poisoning is discussed on p.1376. Reports suggest that prompt intravenous therapy with acetylcysteine may help to minimise hepatorenal damage in acute poisoning with carbon tetrachloride.[1,2] It could be used in addition to supportive therapy when the initial dosage regimen should be that used for paracetamol poisoning but as carbon tetrachloride has a much longer half-life than paracetamol, the duration of treatment may need to be increased.[3]

1. Ruprah M, *et al.* Acute carbon tetrachloride poisoning in 19 patients: implications for diagnosis and treatment. *Lancet* 1985; **i:** 1027–9.
2. Mathieson PW, *et al.* Survival after massive ingestion of carbon tetrachloride treated by intravenous infusion of acetylcysteine. *Hum Toxicol* 1985; **4:** 627–31.
3. Meredith TJ, *et al.* Diagnosis and treatment of acute poisoning with volatile substances. *Hum Toxicol* 1989; **8:** 277–86.

PARACETAMOL. Acetylcysteine is the antidote of choice for paracetamol overdosage (see p.72). It is most effective when administered during the first 8 hours following ingestion of the overdose. It was previously thought to be of no benefit if begun more than 15 hours after the overdose and it was thought it might aggravate the risk of hepatic encephalopathy, but late administration has now been shown to be safe[1] with beneficial results being observed in patients whose treatment was initiated beyond 15 hours.[1-3] Furthermore, acetylcysteine reduced morbidity and mortality in patients who had already developed fulminant hepatic failure.[4] The manufacturers state that clinical experience indicates that acetylcysteine can still be of benefit when administered up to 24 hours after paracetamol overdose, although expert guidance from specialist poison centres should be sought for patients presenting after 24 hours.

Methods of acetylcysteine administration vary. The intravenous route is favoured in the UK, despite possible anaphylactic reaction, mainly because of concerns over the effects of vomiting and activated charcoal on oral absorption.[5] In the USA the oral route is usually used, despite the unpleasant odour and taste of acetylcysteine solutions, with no evident reduction in effect by charcoal.[6]

1. Parker D, *et al.* Safety of late acetylcysteine treatment in paracetamol poisoning. *Hum Exp Toxicol* 1990; **9:** 25–7.
2. Smilkstein MJ, *et al.* Efficacy of oral N-acetylcysteine in the treatment of acetaminophen overdose: analysis of the National Multicenter Study (1976 to 1985). *N Engl J Med* 1988; **319:** 1557–62.
3. Harrison PM, *et al.* Improved outcome of paracetamol-induced fulminant hepatic failure by late administration of acetylcysteine. *Lancet* 1990; **335:** 1572–3.
4. Keays R, *et al.* Intravenous acetylcysteine in paracetamol induced fulminant hepatic failure: a prospective controlled trial. *Br Med J* 1991; **303:** 1026–9.
5. Vale JA, Proudfoot AT. Paracetamol (acetaminophen) poisoning. *Lancet* 1995; **346:** 547–52.
6. Bowden CA, Krenzelok EP. Clinical applications of commonly used contemporary antidotes: a US perspective. *Drug Safety* 1997; **16:** 9–47.

Respiratory disorders. Acetylcysteine has been used as a mucolytic in a variety of respiratory disorders associated with productive cough (p.1052). Although there is controversy as to the benefits of mucolytics in treating chronic bronchitis (see p.747), acetylcysteine administered by mouth may reduce the number of acute exacerbations.[1] Cough and ease of expectoration may be improved[2] but the effect on sputum viscosity and purulence has been inconsistent.[2,3] Repeated bronchoalveolar lavage with heparin and acetylcysteine to remove proteinaceous material in patients with alveolar proteinosis may prolong survival.[4] Administration of acetylcysteine by nebulisation has relieved severe recurrent atelectasis during mechanical ventilation in premature infants.[5] It has been suggested that intravenous acetylcysteine may also be of use in acute respiratory distress syndrome (ARDS—p.1017),[6] possibly due to its action as a free radical scavenger,[6,7] but this has yet to be clearly demonstrated.

See above for the use of acetylcysteine in the management of cystic fibrosis.

1. Boman G, *et al.* Oral acetylcysteine reduces exacerbation rate in chronic bronchitis: report of a trial organized by the Swedish Society for Pulmonary Diseases. *Eur J Respir Dis* 1983; **64:** 405–15.
2. Jackson IM, *et al.* Efficacy and tolerability of oral acetylcysteine (Fabrol®) in chronic bronchitis: a double-blind placebo controlled study. *J Int Med Res* 1984; **12:** 198–206.
3. Tattersall AB, *et al.* Acetylcysteine (Fabrol) in chronic bronchitis—a study in general practice. *J Int Med Res* 1983; **11:** 279–84.
4. Morrison HM, Stockley RA. The many uses of bronchoalveolar lavage. *Br Med J* 1988; **296:** 1758.
5. Amir J, *et al.* Acetylcysteine for severe atelectasis in premature infants. *Clin Pharm* 1985; **4:** 255.
6. Bernard GR. Potential of N-acetylcysteine as treatment for the adult respiratory distress syndrome. *Eur Respir J* 1990; **3** (suppl 11): 496S–498S.
7. Skolnick A. Inflammation-mediator blockers may be weapons against sepsis syndrome. *JAMA* 1990; **263:** 930–1.

Preparations

BP 1998: Acetylcysteine Injection;
USP 23: Acetylcysteine and Isoproterenol Hydrochloride Inhalation Solution; Acetylcysteine Solution.

Proprietary Preparations (details are given in Part 3)
Aust.: ACC; Aeromuc; Cimelin; Cimexyl; Fluimucil; Mucobene; Mucomyst; Mucret; Pulmovent; Siccoral; Solvomed; ***Austral.:*** Mucomyst; Parvolex; ***Belg.:*** Lysomucil; Lysox; Mucofim†; Mucolair; Mucolator; Mucomyst; Pectomucil; ***Canad.:*** Mucomyst; Parvolex; ***Fr.:*** Broncoclar; Codotussyl Expectorant; Exomuc; Fluimucil; Genac; Humex Expectorant; Mucolator; Mucomyst; Solmucol; Tixair; ***Ger.:*** ACC; Acemuc; Acetyst; Azubronchin; Bisolvon NAC; Bromuc; Broncho-Fips; Cordes Granulat†; Durabronchal; Fluimucil; Frekatuss†; Jenacysteine; Lindocetyl†; Mentopin; Muciteran; Muco Sanigen; Muco-Perasthman N; Mucocedyl; Mucolyticum "Lappe"†; Mucret; Myxofat; NAC; Neo-Fluimucil†; Optipect; Pulmicret; Sigamucil; Siran; Stas Akut; Tamuc; Tussiverlan; Vitenur†; ***Irl.:*** Alveolex; Fabrol†; Parvolex; ***Ital.:*** Brunac; Fluimucil; Hidonac; Mucisol; Mucomist†; Solmucol; Tirocular; ***Mon.:*** Euronac; ***Neth.:*** Bisolbruis; Dampo Mucopect; Fluimucil; Mucocil; Mucomyst; ***Norw.:*** Bronkyl; Mucomyst; ***S.Afr.:*** ACC200; Parvolex; Solmucol; ***Spain:*** Fluimucil; ***Swed.:*** Fabrol†; Mucomyst; Viskoferm; ***Switz.:*** Acemucol; Bisolapid; Dynamucil; Ecomucyl; Fluimucil; L-Cimexyl; Muco-Mepha; Mucofluid; Neo Expectan; Robitussin Expectorant; Secresol; Siran†; Solmucol; ***UK:*** Fabrol†; Parvolex; ***USA:*** Mucomyst; Mucosil.

Multi-ingredient: ***Fr.:*** Rhinofluimucil; ***Ger.:*** Rinofluimucil-S; ***Irl.:*** Ilube; ***Ital.:*** Rinofluimucil; ***Spain:*** Flubiotic; Nuvapen Mucolitico Retard†; Rinofluimucil; ***Switz.:*** Rinofluimucil; ***UK:*** Ilube.

Acetyldihydrocodeine Hydrochloride (12311-z)

4,5-Epoxy-3-methoxy-9a-methylmorphinan-6-yl acetate hydrochloride.

$C_{20}H_{25}NO_4,HCl = 379.9.$
CAS — 3861-72-1 (acetyldihydrocodeine).

Acetyldihydrocodeine hydrochloride is an opioid derivative related to dihydrocodeine (p.34). It is used as a centrally acting cough suppressant for non-productive cough (p.1052) and has been given by mouth in a daily dose of 20 to 50 mg; no more than 20 mg should be taken as a single dose.

Preparations

Proprietary Preparations (details are given in Part 3)
Belg.: Acetylcodone.

Adamexine (3900-v)

Adamexine *(rINN).*

α-(1-Adamantylmethylamino)-4′,6′-dibromo-2-acetotoluidide.

$C_{20}H_{26}Br_2N_2O = 470.2.$
CAS — 54785-02-3.

Adamexine is a derivative of bromhexine (p.1055). It has been used as a mucolytic in the treatment of respiratory disorders associated with productive cough (p.1052) in doses of 20 mg by mouth three times daily.

Preparations

Proprietary Preparations (details are given in Part 3)
Spain: Adamucol†; Broncostyl.

Alloclamide Hydrochloride (5603-l)

Alloclamide Hydrochloride *(rINNM).*

CE-264. 2-Allyloxy-4-chloro-*N*-(2-diethylaminoethyl)benzamide hydrochloride.

$C_{16}H_{23}ClN_2O_2,HCl = 347.3.$
CAS — 5486-77-1 (alloclamide); 5107-01-7 (alloclamide hydrochloride).

Alloclamide hydrochloride is a cough suppressant.

Preparations

Proprietary Preparations (details are given in Part 3)
Multi-ingredient: ***Spain:*** Tuselin Expectorante.

Ambroxol Hydrochloride (16360-w)

Ambroxol Hydrochloride *(rINNM).*

NA-872 (ambroxol). *trans*-4-(2-Amino-3,5-dibromobenzylamino)cyclohexanol hydrochloride.

$C_{13}H_{18}Br_2N_2O,HCl = 414.6.$
CAS — 18683-91-5 (ambroxol); 15942-05-9 (ambroxol hydrochloride).

Pharmacopoeias. In *Ger.* and *It.*

Ambroxol is a metabolite of bromhexine and has similar actions and uses (see p.1055). It is administered as the hydrochloride and a daily dose of 30 to 120 mg has been given by mouth in 2 to 3 divided doses. Similar doses have been given by inhalation, injection, or rectally.

Ambroxol acefyllinate has been used similarly.

Adverse effects. HYPERSENSITIVITY. A report[1] of contact allergy to ambroxol, but not bromhexine, in one patient.

1. Mancuso G, Berdondini RM. Contact allergy to ambroxol. *Contact Dermatitis* 1989; **20:** 154.

Pharmacokinetics. References to pharmacokinetic studies of ambroxol.

1. Hammer R, *et al.* Speziesvergleich in pharmakokinetik und metabolismus von NA 872 Cl ambroxol bei ratte, kaninchen, hund und mensch. *Arzneimittelforschung* 1978; **28:** 899–903.
2. Jauch R, *et al.* Ambroxol, untersuchungen zum stoffwechsel beim menschen und zum quantitativen nachweis in biologischen proben. *Arzneimittelforschung* 1978; **28:** 904–11.
3. Vergin H, *et al.* Untersuchungen zur pharmakokinetik und bioäquivalenz unterscheidlicher darreichungsformen von ambroxol. *Arzneimittelforschung* 1985; **35:** 1591–5.

Respiratory disorders. There are reports of ambroxol being used in a variety of respiratory disorders including chronic bronchitis (mixed results[1-3]), cystic fibrosis (ineffective[4]), and infant respiratory distress syndrome (may be of value for prophylaxis[5,6]). However, it is not among the agents usually considered for the management of these disorders as discussed on p.747, p.119, and p.1025 respectively.

Inhalation of ambroxol aerosol has also produced beneficial effects in a patient with alveolar proteinosis who refused alveolar lavage.[7]

The management of cough, including the use of mucolytics in productive cough, is discussed on p.1052.

1. Olivieri D, *et al.* Ambroxol for the prevention of chronic exacerbations: long-term multicenter trial: protective effect of ambroxol against winter semester exacerbations: a double-blind study versus placebo. *Respiration* 1987; **51** (suppl 1): 42–51.
2. Alcozer G, *et al.* Prevention of chronic bronchitis exacerbations with ambroxol (Mucosolvan Retard): an open, long-term, multicenter study in 5,635 patients. *Respiration* 1989; **55** (suppl 1): 84–96.
3. Guyatt GH, *et al.* A controlled trial of ambroxol in chronic bronchitis. *Chest* 1987; **92:** 618–20.
4. Ratjen F, *et al.* A double-blind placebo controlled trial with oral ambroxol and N-acetylcysteine for mucolytic treatment in cystic fibrosis. *Eur J Pediatr* 1985; 144: 374–8.
5. Henahan J. Expectorant promising for treating infant respiratory distress syndrome. *JAMA* 1983; **249:** 2425–6.
6. Wauer RR, *et al.* The antenatal use of ambroxol (bromhexine metabolite VIII) to prevent hyaline membrane disease: a controlled double-blind study. *Int J Biol Res Pregnancy* 1982; **3:** 84–91.
7. Diaz JP, *et al.* Response to surfactant activator (ambroxol) in alveolar proteinosis. *Lancet* 1984; **i:** 1023.

Uricosuric action. A study[1] was carried out in 48 young male healthy volunteers to examine the uricosuric effect of ambroxol. The minimum effective dose for lowering plasma-uric acid concentrations was found to be between 250 mg and 500 mg daily given in 2 divided doses. Although these doses are much higher than those used to treat bronchopulmonary disease, doses as high as 1 g daily were well tolerated.

1. Oosterhuis B, *et al.* Dose-dependent uricosuric effect of ambroxol. *Eur J Clin Pharmacol* 1993; **44:** 237–41.

Preparations

Proprietary Preparations (details are given in Part 3)
Aust.: Ambrobene; Ambrolan†; Broxol; Mucosolvan; Sekretovit; ***Belg.:*** Surbronc; ***Fr.:*** Muxol; Surbronc; ***Ger.:*** Ambril; Ambro-Puren; Ambrobeta; Ambrohexal; Ambrolos; Antussan; Bisolvon AM; Bronchopront; Bronchowern; Contac Husten-Trunk; Dignobroxol; duramucal; Expit; Farmabroxol; Flavamed Hustentabletten†; frenopect; Gelopol†; Jenabroxol; Larylin Husten-Heissgetrank; Larylin Hustenpastillen-losend; Larylin Hustensaft-losend; Lindoxyl; Logomed Husten; Mibrox†; Muco-Aspecton; Muco-Fips; Muco-Tablinen; Mucobroxol; Mucoclear†; Mucophlogat; Mucosolvan; Mucotablin; Mucovent†; neo-bronchol; Nymix Mucolytikum; Pect Hustenloser; Pulmonal S; Sigabroxol; Stas-Hustenloser; Therapin Hustenloser†; Tussipect A†; Tusso; tusso-basan†; ***Ital.:*** Ambromucil; Amobronc; Atus; Broncomnes; Broxol; Chinson†; Fluibron; Fluixol; Lisopulm; Muciclar; Mucobron; Mucosolvan; Secretil; Surfactal; Surfolase; Tauxolo; Viscomucil; ***Spain:*** Ambrolitic; Dinobroxol; Motosol; Mucibron; Mucosan; Naxpa; ***Switz.:*** Abramen†; Fluibron; Mucabrox; Mucosolvon.

Multi-ingredient: ***Aust.:*** Mucospas; Mucotectan; Vibrabron; ***Ger.:*** Ambrodoxy; Ambroxol AL comp; Ambroxol comp; Amdox-Puren; Azudoxat comp; Broncho-Euphyllin; Doxam; Doximucol; Doxy Comp; Doxy Lindoxyl; Doxy Plus; Doxyduramucal; Doxy-Wolff Mucolyt; Doxysolvat; Jenabroxol comp; Mibrox comp†; Mucotectan; Sagittamuc; Sigamuc; Spasmo-Mucosolvan; Terelit.

Amidephrine Mesylate (2043-a)

Amidephrine Mesylate *(BANM, USAN).*

Amidefrine Mesilate *(rINN)*; 5190; MJ-5190. 3-(1-Hydroxy-2-methylaminoethyl)methanesulphonanilide methanesulphonate.

$C_{10}H_{16}N_2O_3S,CH_4O_3S = 340.4.$

CAS — 3354-67-4 (amidephrine); 1421-68-7 (amidephrine mesylate).

Amidephrine mesylate is a sympathomimetic with alpha-adrenergic activity similar to that of phenylephrine (p.1066). It is used for its vasoconstrictor properties in the local treatment of nasal congestion.

Preparations

Proprietary Preparations (details are given in Part 3)
Aust.: Fentrinol.

Ammonium Acetate (2003-w)

$CH_3CO_2NH_4 = 77.08.$

CAS — 631-61-8 (ammonium acetate); 8013-61-4 (ammonium acetate solution).

Pharmacopoeias. *Br.* includes Strong Ammonium Acetate Solution.

Ammonium Bicarbonate (2004-e)

Ammonium Bicarbonate *(BAN).*

503. Ammonium hydrogen carbonate.

$NH_4HCO_3 = 79.06.$

CAS — 1066-33-7.

Pharmacopoeias. In *Br.*

A fine, white, slightly hygroscopic, crystalline powder, white crystals, or glassy colourless solid, with a slightly ammoniacal odour. It volatilises rapidly at 60° with dissociation into ammonia, carbon dioxide, and water; volatilisation takes place slowly at ordinary temperatures if slightly moist.

Freely **soluble** in water; practically insoluble in alcohol. **Store** at a temperature not exceeding 15°.

NOTE. The BP directs that when Ammonium Carbonate is prescribed or demanded Ammonium Bicarbonate be supplied.

Ammonium Carbonate (2005-l)

503; Carbonato de Amonio.

CAS — 8000-73-5.

Pharmacopoeias. In *Fr.* and *It.* Also in *USNF.*

A white powder or hard white or translucent masses with an ammoniacal odour, consisting of a variable mixture of ammonium bicarbonate and ammonium carbamate, $NH_2.CO_2.NH_4$. It yields 30 to 34% of NH_3. On exposure to air it loses ammonia and carbon dioxide, becoming opaque, and is finally converted into friable porous lumps or a white powder of ammonium bicarbonate. **Soluble** 1 in 4 of water. It is decomposed by hot water. A solution in water is alkaline to litmus. **Store** at a temperature not exceeding 30° in airtight containers. Protect from light.

NOTE. The BP directs that Ammonium Bicarbonate be supplied when Ammonium Carbonate is prescribed or demanded.

Ammonium Chloride (2006-y)

510; Ammonii Chloridum; Ammonium Chloratum; Cloruro de Amonio; Muriate of Ammonia; Sal Ammoniac.

$NH_4Cl = 53.49.$

CAS — 12125-02-9.

NOTE. The food additive number 380 is used for ammonium citrate.

Pharmacopoeias. In *Chin., Eur.* (see p.viii), *Pol.,* and *US.*

Odourless, hygroscopic, white, crystalline powder or colourless crystals. Each g represents 18.69 mmol of chloride.

Freely **soluble** in water and in glycerol, and more so in boiling water; sparingly soluble in alcohol. A 5% solution in water has a pH of 4.6 to 6.0. **Store** in airtight containers.

Adverse Effects and Treatment

Ammonium salts are irritant to the gastric mucosa and may produce nausea and vomiting particularly in large doses. Large doses of ammonium chloride may cause a profound acidosis and hypokalaemia which should be treated symptomatically. Intravenous administration of ammonium chloride may cause pain and irritation at the site of injection, which may be decreased by slowing the rate of infusion.

Excessive doses of ammonium salts, particularly if administered by rapid intravenous injection, may give rise to hepatic encephalopathy due to the inability of the liver to convert the increased load of ammonium ions to urea.

Precautions

Ammonium salts are contra-indicated in the presence of impaired hepatic or renal function.

Pharmacokinetics

Ammonium chloride is absorbed from the gastro-intestinal tract. The ammonium ion is converted into urea in the liver; the anion thus liberated into the blood stream and extracellular fluid causes a metabolic acidosis and decreases the pH of the urine; this is followed by transient diuresis.

Uses and Administration

Ammonium chloride is used as an expectorant in productive cough (p.1052). Other ammonium salts which have been used similarly include the acetate, bicarbonate, camphorate, carbonate, citrate, and glycyrrhizinate.

The administration of ammonium chloride produces a transient diuresis and a mild acidosis. It may be used in the treatment of severe metabolic alkalosis (p.1147). It is administered usually as a 1 to 2% solution by slow intravenous infusion, in a dosage depending on the severity of the alkalosis. A concentrated solution of ammonium chloride may be diluted by sodium chloride injection.

Ammonium chloride may also be used to maintain the urine at an acid pH in the treatment of some urinary-tract disorders, or in forced acid diuresis procedures to aid the excretion of basic drugs, such as amphetamines, in severe cases of overdosage. It is usually given by mouth, often as enteric-coated tablets, in a dose of 1 to 2 g every four to six hours, although 4 g every two hours has been given in forced acid diuresis procedures.

Ammonium chloride has been promoted for self administration as a diuretic, for example in premenstrual water retention; a dose of 1 g three times daily for up to 6 days has been suggested, but such use is generally considered inappropriate.

Preparations

BP 1998: Ammonia and Ipecacuanha Mixture; Ammonium Chloride Mixture; Aromatic Ammonia Solution; Aromatic Ammonia Spirit *(Sal Volatile Spirit)*; Strong Ammonium Acetate Solution; White Liniment *(White Embrocation)*;
USP 23: Ammonium Chloride Delayed-release Tablets; Ammonium Chloride Injection; Aromatic Ammonia Spirit; Potassium Gluconate, Potassium Citrate, and Ammonium Chloride Oral Solution.

Proprietary Preparations (details are given in Part 3)
Fr.: Chlorammonic; ***Jpn:*** Glycyron; Neo-Minophagen C; ***Spain:*** Apir Cloruro Amonico; ***Switz.:*** Chloramon.

Multi-ingredient: numerous preparations are listed in Part 3.

Benproperine (12427-b)

Benproperine *(rINN).*

ASA-158/5 (benproperine phosphate). 1-[2-(2-Benzylphenoxy)-1-methylethyl]piperidine.

$C_{21}H_{27}NO = 309.4.$

CAS — 2156-27-6.

Benproperine is used as a cough suppressant in non-productive cough (p.1052). It is reported to have a peripheral and central action and has been given by mouth in usual doses of 25 to 50 mg two to four times daily as the embonate or the phosphate.

Preparations

Proprietary Preparations (details are given in Part 3)
Ger.: Tussafug; ***Ital.:*** Blascorid†; ***Switz.:*** Tussafug.

Benzonatate (5605-j)

Benzonatate *(BAN, rINN).*

Benzononatine; KM-65. 3,6,9,12,15,18,21,24,27-Nonaoxaoctacosyl 4-butylaminobenzoate.

$C_{13}H_{18}NO_2(OCH_2CH_2)_nOCH_3$, where *n* has an average value of 8.

CAS — 104-31-4 (where n = 8).

Pharmacopoeias. In *US.*

A clear, pale yellow, viscous liquid with a faint characteristic odour. **Soluble** 1 in less than 1 of water, alcohol, chloroform, and ether. **Store** in airtight containers. Protect from light.

Adverse Effects

Headache, dizziness, gastro-intestinal disturbances, nasal congestion, hypersensitivity, pruritus and skin rash have been reported. There may be drowsiness. Benzonatate has local anaesthetic properties and may produce numbness of the mouth, tongue, and pharynx. CNS stimulation and convulsions may occur in overdosage followed by CNS depression.

Uses and Administration

Benzonatate is a cough suppressant used in non-productive cough (p.1052). It is stated to act peripherally and is related to amethocaine (p.1285) and has a local anaesthetic action on mucosa. It is given by mouth in a dose of 100 mg three times daily; up to 600 mg daily in divided doses may be given if necessary. Benzonatate is reported to act within about 20 minutes and its effects are reported to last for 3 to 8 hours.

Preparations

USP 23: Benzonatate Capsules.

Proprietary Preparations (details are given in Part 3)
USA: Tessalon.

Bibenzonium Bromide (5640-k)

Bibenzonium Bromide *(BAN, rINN).*

Diphenetholine Bromide; ES-132. [2-(1,2-Diphenylethoxy)ethyl]trimethylammonium bromide.

$C_{19}H_{26}BrNO = 364.3.$

CAS — 59866-76-1 (bibenzonium); 15585-70-3 (bibenzonium bromide).

Bibenzonium bromide is a cough suppressant used in non-productive cough (p.1052) which is stated to have a central action. It has been given by mouth in a dose of 30 mg two to three times daily.

Preparations

Proprietary Preparations (details are given in Part 3)
Aust.: Lysbex; ***Ital.:*** Lysobex†.

Bromhexine (11273-k)

Bromhexine *(BAN, rINN).*

Bromexina. 2-Amino-3,5-dibromobenzyl(cyclohexyl)methylamine.

$C_{14}H_{20}Br_2N_2 = 376.1.$

CAS — 3572-43-8.

Bromhexine Hydrochloride (2008-z)

Bromhexine Hydrochloride *(BANM, USAN, rINNM).*

Bromhexini Hydrochloridum; Cloridrato de Bromexina; NA-274.

$C_{14}H_{20}Br_2N_2,HCl = 412.6.$

CAS — 611-75-6.

Pharmacopoeias. In *Chin., Eur.* (see p.viii), *Jpn,* and *Pol.*

A white or almost white crystalline powder. Very slightly **soluble** in water; slightly soluble in alcohol and in dichloromethane. **Protect** from light.

Stability studies of bromhexine and identification of its degradation products.[1] It is estimated that under normal storage conditions bromhexine is stable for 10 years and aqueous solutions for 5 years.

1. Göber B, *et al.* Zur stabilität von bromhexin und zur struktur seiner abbauprodukte. *Pharmazie* 1988; **43:** 23–6.

Adverse Effects

Gastro-intestinal side-effects may occur occasionally with bromhexine and a transient rise in serum aminotransferase values has been reported. Other reported adverse effects include headache, dizziness, sweating, and skin rashes. Inhalation of bromhexine has occasionally produced cough or bronchospasm in susceptible subjects.

Precautions

Since mucolytics may disrupt the gastric mucosal barrier bromhexine should be used with care in patients with a history of peptic ulceration. Care is also advisable in asthmatic patients.

Clearance of bromhexine or its metabolites may be reduced in patients with severe hepatic or renal impairment.

Pharmacokinetics

Bromhexine hydrochloride is rapidly absorbed from the gastro-intestinal tract and undergoes extensive first-pass metabolism in the liver: its oral bioavailability is stated to be only about 20%. It is widely distributed to body tissues. About 85 to 90% of a dose is excreted in the urine mainly as metabolites. Ambroxol (p.1054) is a metabolite of bromhexine. Bromhexine is highly bound to plasma proteins. It has a terminal elimination half-life of up to about 12 hours. Bromhexine crosses the blood-brain barrier and small amounts cross the placenta.

Administration of bromhexine hydrochloride by mouth to healthy subjects produced peak plasma concentrations after about 1 hour.[1] Only small amounts were excreted unchanged in the urine with a half-life of about 6.5 hours.

1. Bechgaard E, Nielsen A. Bioavailability of bromhexine tablets and preliminary pharmacokinetics in humans. *Biopharm Drug Dispos* 1982; **3:** 337–44.

Uses and Administration

Bromhexine is a mucolytic used in the treatment of respiratory disorders associated with productive cough (p.1052). Bromhexine is usually given by mouth in a dose of 8 to 16 mg of the hydrochloride three times daily. It has also been given by deep intramuscular or slow intravenous injection or inhaled as an aerosol solution.

Bromhexine has also been used orally and topically in the treatment of dry eye associated with abnormal mucus production (see below).

Dry eye. Bromhexine has been used orally in the treatment of dry eye (p.1470) in Sjögren's syndrome but results have been conflicting,[1-3] and it appears to have no effect on tear secretion in healthy subjects.[4] It has also been tried topically.

1. Frost-Larsen K, *et al.* Sjögren's syndrome treated with bromhexine: a randomised clinical study. *Br Med J* 1978; **1:** 1579–81.
2. Tapper-Jones LM, *et al.* Sjögren's syndrome treated with bromhexine: a reassessment. *Br Med J* 1980; **280:** 1356.
3. Prause JU, *et al.* Lacrimal and salivary secretion in Sjögren's syndrome: the effect of systemic treatment with bromhexine. *Acta Ophthalmol (Copenh)* 1984; **62:** 489–97.
4. Avisar R, *et al.* Oral bromhexine has no effect on tear secretion in healthy subjects. *Ann Pharmacother* 1996; **30:** 1498.

Respiratory-tract infection. USE WITH AN ANTIBACTERIAL. Bromhexine has been shown to enhance the penetration of erythromycin into bronchial secretions[1] and although bromhexine is often administered with other antibiotics as an adjuvant in the treatment of respiratory infections, few controlled studies appear to have been conducted to determine if any additional benefit is obtained. However, among those studies that have been carried out one reported that bromhexine improved the response to cephalexin[2] and another that it improved the response to amoxycillin.[3]

1. Bergogne-Berezin E, *et al.* Etude de l'influence d'un agent mucolytique (bromhexine) sur le passage de l'érythromycine dans les sécrétions bronchiques. *Therapie* 1979; **34:** 705–11.
2. Boraldi F, Palmieri B. Antibiotic and mucolytic therapy in elderly patients with different cases of bronchopulmonary diseases. *Curr Ther Res* 1983; **33:** 686–91.
3. Roa CC, Dantes RB. Clinical effectiveness of a combination of bromhexine and amoxicillin in lower respiratory tract infection: a randomized controlled trial. *Arzneimittelforschung* 1995; **45:** 267–72.

Preparations

Proprietary Preparations (details are given in Part 3)
Aust.: Bisolvon; ***Austral.:*** Bisolvon; Dur-Elix; ***Belg.:*** Bisolvon; Bromex; ***Fr.:*** Bisolvon; ***Ger.:*** Aparsonin N; Bisolvon; Bisolvon F†; Dakryo Biciron†; Hustentabs-ratiopharm; Lubrirhin; Omniapharm; Ophtosol†; ***Irl.:*** Bisolvon; ***Ital.:*** Bisolvon; Broncokin; ***Neth.:*** Bisolvon; Darolan Slijmplossende; Famel Broomhexine; ***Norw.:*** Bisolvon; ***S.Afr.:*** Bisolvon; Bronkese; ***Spain:*** Bisolvon; ***Swed.:*** Bisolvon; ***Switz.:*** Bisolvon; Broncodil†; Metasolvens; Solvolin.

Multi-ingredient: numerous preparations are listed in Part 3.

Brovanexine Hydrochloride (5170-m)

Brovanexine Hydrochloride *(rINNM)*.

4-(Acetyloxy)-*N*-[2,4-dibromo-6-[(cyclohexylmethylamino)methyl]phenyl]-3-methoxybenzamide monohydrochloride.

$C_{24}H_{29}Br_2ClN_2O_4$ = 604.8.

CAS — 54340-61-3 (brovanexine); 54340-60-2 (brovanexine hydrochloride).

Brovanexine is a derivative of bromhexine (above) and is administered as the hydrochloride, usually as an adjunct to antibacterials in preparations for the treatment of respiratory-tract infections.

Preparations

Proprietary Preparations (details are given in Part 3)

Multi-ingredient: ***Spain:*** Amoxidel Bronquial; Bronquimucil; Eupen Bronquial.

Butamyrate Citrate (5606-z)

Butamyrate Citrate *(BANM)*.

Butamirate Citrate *(USAN, rINNM)*; Abbott-36581; HH-197. 2-(2-Diethylaminoethoxy)ethyl 2-phenylbutyrate dihydrogen citrate.

$C_{18}H_{29}NO_3,C_6H_8O_7$ = 499.6.

CAS — 18109-80-3 (butamyrate); 18109-81-4 (butamyrate citrate).

Butamyrate citrate is a cough suppressant used in non-productive cough (p.1052) and stated to have a central action. It has been given by mouth in usual doses of 5 to 10 mg three to five times daily; modified-release tablets containing 50 mg have been given 2 or 3 times daily.

Preparations

Proprietary Preparations (details are given in Part 3)
Belg.: Sinecod; ***Ger.:*** Sinecod†; ***Ital.:*** Butiran; Sinecod Tosse Sedativo; ***Spain:*** Sinecod†; ***Switz.:*** Sinecod.

Multi-ingredient: ***Switz.:*** Hicoseen.

Butethamate Citrate (2045-x)

Butethamate Citrate *(BANM)*.

Butetamate Citrate *(rINNM)*; Butethamate Dihydrogen Citrate. 2-Diethylaminoethyl 2-phenylbutyrate citrate.

$C_{16}H_{25}NO_2,C_6H_8O_7$ = 455.5.

CAS — 14007-64-8 (butethamate); 13900-12-4 (butethamate citrate).

Butethamate citrate is reported to be an antispasmodic and bronchodilator and has been used alone or in combination with other agents for the symptomatic treatment of coughs and other associated respiratory-tract disorders.

Preparations

Proprietary Preparations (details are given in Part 3)
Ger.: Pertix†; ***Irl.:*** CAM.

Multi-ingredient: ***Aust.:*** Coldadolin; Influbene; Panax; ***Ger.:*** Anaesthesetten N†; Antibex†; Pertix-S†; Pertix†; Resedorm†; ***Ital.:*** Pertix†; ***Spain:*** Fluidin Mucolitico; ***Switz.:*** Bronchotussine; Dragees contre la toux no 536; Influbene†; Panax†.

Butopiprine Hydrobromide (12481-w)

Butopiprine Hydrobromide *(rINNM)*.

LD-2351. 2-Butoxyethyl α-phenyl-1-piperidineacetate hydrobromide.

$C_{19}H_{29}NO_3,HBr$ = 400.4.

CAS — 55837-15-5 (butopiprine); 60595-56-4 (butopiprine hydrobromide).

Butopiprine hydrobromide has been used as a cough suppressant.

Preparations

Proprietary Preparations (details are given in Part 3)
Spain: Laucalon†.

Calcium Iodide (4573-j)

CaI_2 = 293.9.

CAS — 10102-68-8.

Calcium iodide has been used by mouth in expectorant mixtures. The limitations of iodides as expectorants are discussed on p.1052. The actions of the iodides are discussed under Iodine (p.1493).

Preparations

Proprietary Preparations (details are given in Part 3)

Multi-ingredient: ***Ger.:*** durajod†; ***Ital.:*** Tussiprene†; ***USA:*** Calcidrine; Norisodrine with Calcium Iodide.

Caramiphen Edisylate (18490-y)

Caramiphen Edisylate *(BANM)*.

Caramiphen Edisilate *(rINNM)*. 2-Diethylaminoethyl 1-phenylcyclopentane-1-carboxylate ethane-1,2-disulphonate.

$C_{38}H_{60}N_2O_{10}S_2$ = 769.0.

CAS — 77-22-5 (caramiphen); 125-86-0 (caramiphen edisylate); 125-85-9 (caramiphen hydrochloride).

Caramiphen is a centrally acting cough suppressant used as the edisylate in combination products for coughs (p.1052). Caramiphen was originally used as the hydrochloride similarly to benzhexol (p.457) for its antimuscarinic actions.

Preparations

Proprietary Preparations (details are given in Part 3)

Multi-ingredient: ***USA:*** Ordrine AT Extended-Release; Rescaps-D SR; Tuss-Allergine Modified TD; Tuss-Genade Modified; Tuss-Ornade†; Tussogest Extended-Release.

Carbocisteine (577-s)

Carbocisteine *(BAN, rINN)*.

AHR-3053; Carbocisteinum; Carbocysteine *(USAN)*; LJ-206. *S*-Carboxymethyl-L-cysteine.

$C_5H_9NO_4S$ = 179.2.

CAS — 2387-59-9; 638-23-3 (carbocisteine, L-form).

Pharmacopoeias. In *Eur.* (see p.viii) and *Jpn.*

A white crystalline powder. Practically **insoluble** in water, in alcohol, and in ether; dissolves in dilute mineral acids and in dilute solutions of alkali hydroxides. A 1% suspension in water has a pH of 2.8 to 3.0. **Protect** from light.

The UK manufacturer states that mixture of carbocisteine with pholcodine linctus causes precipitation of carbocisteine from solution but provides no information on whether this **incompatibility** is with the pholcodine or some component of the formulation used.

Carbocisteine Sodium (11293-r)

Carbocisteine Sodium *(BANM, rINNM)*.

Carbocysteine Sodium.

CAS — 49673-84-9 (carbocisteine sodium, L-form).

Adverse Effects and Precautions

Nausea and gastric discomfort, gastro-intestinal bleeding, and skin rash have occasionally occurred with carbocisteine.

Since mucolytics may disrupt the gastric mucosal barrier carbocisteine should be used with caution in patients with a history of peptic ulceration.

Effects on endocrine function. A report[1] of transient hypothyroidism associated with the administration of carbocisteine in a patient with compromised thyroid function.

1. Wiersinga WM. Antithyroid action of carbocisteine. *Br Med J* 1986; **293:** 106.

Pharmacokinetics

Carbocisteine is rapidly and well absorbed from the gastro-intestinal tract with peak plasma concentrations occurring 90 to 120 minutes after an oral dose. It appears to penetrate into lung tissue and respiratory mucus. Carbocisteine is excreted in the urine as unchanged drug and metabolites. Acetylation, decarboxylation, and sulphoxidation have been identified as the major metabolic pathways. Sulphoxidation may be governed by genetic polymorphism.

References.

1. Karim EFIA, *et al.* An investigation of the metabolism of S-carboxymethyl-L-cysteine in man using a novel HPLC-ECD method. *Eur J Drug Metab Pharmacokinet* 1988; **13:** 253–6.

For reference to polymorphic metabolism of carbocisteine and its use in determination of sulphoxidation phenotype, see under Uses and Administration, below.

Uses and Administration

Carbocisteine is used for its mucolytic activity in respiratory disorders associated with productive cough (p.1052). It is given by mouth in a dose of 750 mg three times daily, reduced by one-third when a response is obtained. Children aged 2 to 5 years may be given 62.5 to 125 mg four times daily and those aged 6 to 12 years 250 mg three times daily. Carbocisteine is also administered by mouth as the sodium and lysine salts.

Chronic bronchitis. Administration of carbocisteine 750 mg three times daily for up to 6 months has been reported to produce some improvements in lung function in patients with chronic bronchitis[1,2] but appears to have no effect on the number of acute exacerbations.[1] Carbocisteine may also produce some beneficial effects on sputum rheology.[2,3] The value of mucolytic therapy in bronchitis is controversial, as discussed on p.747.

1. Grillage M, Barnard-Jones K. Long-term oral carbocisteine therapy in patients with chronic bronchitis: a double blind trial with placebo control. *Br J Clin Pract* 1985; **39:** 395–8.
2. Aylward M, *et al.* Clinical evaluation of carbocisteine (Mucolex) in the treatment of patients with chronic bronchitis: a double-blind trial with placebo control. *Clin Trials J* 1985; **22:** 36–44.
3. Braga PC, *et al.* Identification of subpopulations of bronchitic patients for suitable therapy by a dynamic rheological test. *Int J Clin Pharmacol Res* 1989; **IX:** 175–82.

Determination of sulphoxidation phenotype. Carbocisteine has been reported to undergo polymorphic sulphoxidation[1] and to be used to determine poor from extensive sulphoxidiser phenotypes.[2] However, some workers have reported that they have failed to confirm that carbocisteine sulphoxidation is polymorphic[3] while others have found that results could be influenced by dietary intake.[4] There has also been discussion on the protocol used to determine phenotype and the clinical status of poor sulphoxidisers.[2,5]

1. Mitchell SC, Waring RH. Deficiency of sulfoxidation of S-carboxymethyl-L-cysteine. *Pharmacol Ther* 1989; **43:** 237–49.
2. Küpfer A, Idle JR. False positives with current carbocisteine protocol for sulphoxidation phenotyping. *Lancet* 1990; **335:** 1107.
3. Meese CO, *et al.* Polymorphic sulphoxidation of carbocisteine. *Lancet* 1990; **336:** 693–4.
4. Karim EFIA, *et al.* The influence of diet on drug metabolism studies of S-carboxymethyl-L-cysteine. *Int J Pharmaceutics* 1989; **52:** 155–8.
5. Waring RH, Mitchell SC. Carbocisteine sulphoxidation phenotype. *Lancet* 1990; **335:** 1527.

Preparations

Proprietary Preparations (details are given in Part 3)
Belg.: Bronchathiol; Mucosteine; Pulmoclase; Rhinathiol Mucolyticum; Romilar Mucolyticum; Siroxyl; ***Fr.:*** Bronchathiol; Bronchocyst; Bronchokod; Broncoclar; Broncorinol Expectorant; Codotussyl Expectorant; Drill Expectorant; Fluditec; Fluvic; Hexafluid; Humex Expectorant; Medibronc; Muciclar; Mucoplexil; Rhinathiol; ***Ger.:*** Mucopront; Pectox; Pulmoclase†; Sedotussin Muco; Transbronchin; ***Irl.:*** Exputex; Mucodyne; Mucogen; Mucolex; Pulmoclase; Viscolex; ***Ital.:*** Broncomucil; Bronx; Carbocit; Fluifort; Lisil; Lisomucil; Mucocis; Mucojet; Mucolase; Mucosol†; Mucotreis; Reomucil; Sinecod Tosse Fluidificante; Solfomucil; Solucis; Superthiol; ***Neth.:*** Dampo "Solvopect"; Mucodyne; Pulmoclase; Rami Slijmoplossende; Rhinathiol; Siroxyl†; ***S.Afr.:*** Acuphlem; Arcanacysteine; Betaphlem; Bronchette†; Carbo-Syrup†; Carbospect; Co-Flem; Corbar M; Dynaphlem†; Flemex; Flemgo; Flemlite; Ilvicaps†; Ilvispect†; Lessmusec; Medphlem; Mucocaps; Mucoflem; Mucoless; Mucolinct; Mucopan; Mucopront†; Mucosirop; Mucosol†; Mucospect; Rinofan†; ***Spain:*** Actithiol; Anatac; Mucovital; Pectox; Viscoteina; ***Switz.:*** Mephathiol; Mucoseptal; Pectox; Rhinathiol; Tussantiol; ***UK:*** Mucodyne.

Multi-ingredient: ***Fr.:*** Acnaveen; Rhinathiol Promethazine; ***Ital.:*** Broncofluid; Duplamox Mucolitico†; Libexin Mucolitico; Lisomucil Teofillina†; Polimucil; Sebaveen; ***Spain:*** Actithiol Antihist; Amoxtiol; Ampiorus Balsamico†; Bronquicisteina; Eduprim Mucolitico; Electopen Balsam†; Fluidin Mucolitico; Pectoral Funk Antitus; Pectox Ampicilina; Tilfilin; Tuselin Expectorante; ***Switz.:*** Rhinathiol Promethazine; Triofan.

Chlophedianol Hydrochloride (5608-k)

Chlophedianol Hydrochloride *(BANM, USAN).*

Clofedanol Hydrochloride *(rINNM)*; SL-501. 2-Chloro-α-(2-dimethylaminoethyl)benzyl alcohol hydrochloride.

$C_{17}H_{20}ClNO,HCl = 326.3.$

CAS — 791-35-5 (chlophedianol); 511-13-7 (chlophedianol hydrochloride).

Pharmacopoeias. In *Jpn.*

Chlophedianol hydrochloride is a centrally acting cough suppressant for non-productive cough (p.1052) that has been given by mouth in doses of 25 to 30 mg three to four times daily.

Preparations

Proprietary Preparations (details are given in Part 3)
Canad.: Ulone; ***Ital.:*** Tigonal†; ***Spain:*** Gentos.

Multi-ingredient: ***Ital.:*** Soltux†; ***Spain:*** Xibornol Prodes.

Clobutinol Hydrochloride (5609-a)

Clobutinol Hydrochloride *(rINNM).*

KAT-256. 2-(4-Chlorobenzyl)-3-(dimethylaminomethyl)butan-2-ol hydrochloride.

$C_{14}H_{22}ClNO,HCl = 292.2.$

CAS — 14860-49-2 (clobutinol); 1215-83-4 (clobutinol hydrochloride).

Clobutinol hydrochloride is a centrally acting cough suppressant for non-productive cough (p.1052) given by mouth in doses of 40 to 80 mg three times daily; doses of 20 mg have been given by subcutaneous, intramuscular, or intravenous injection.

Preparations

Proprietary Preparations (details are given in Part 3)
Aust.: Silomat; ***Belg.:*** Silomat; ***Fr.:*** Silomat; ***Ger.:*** Mentopin Hustenstiller; Nullatuss; Rofatuss; Silomat; Stas-Hustenstiller N; Tussamed; ***Ital.:*** Silomat-Fher; ***Spain:*** Lomisat†.

Multi-ingredient: ***Fr.:*** Silomat; ***Ital.:*** Silomat Compositum†; ***S.Afr.:*** Silomat DA; ***Spain:*** Lomisat Compositum†; ***Swed.:*** Silomat Compositum†.

Clonazoline Hydrochloride (14173-j)

Clonazoline Hydrochloride *(rINNM).*

2-[(4-Chloro-1-naphthyl)methyl]-2-imidazoline hydrochloride.

$C_{14}H_{13}ClN_2,HCl = 281.2.$

CAS — 17692-28-3 (clonazoline); 23593-08-0 (clonazoline hydrochloride).

Clonazoline hydrochloride is a sympathomimetic with effects similar to those of naphazoline (p.1064) used for its vasoconstrictor activity in the local treatment of nasal congestion (p.1052)

Preparations

Proprietary Preparations (details are given in Part 3)

Multi-ingredient: ***Ital.:*** Localyn.

Cloperastine Fendizoate (9885-n)

Cloperastine Fendizoate *(pINNM).*

Cloperastine Hydroxyphenylbenzoyl Benzoic Acid; Cloperastine Phendizoate.

$C_{20}H_{24}ClNO,C_{20}H_{14}O_4 = 648.2.$

CAS — 85187-37-7.

Cloperastine Hydrochloride (5610-e)

Cloperastine Hydrochloride *(pINNM).*

1-[2-(4-Chlorobenzhydryloxy)ethyl]piperidine hydrochloride.

$C_{20}H_{24}ClNO,HCl = 366.3.$

CAS — 3703-76-2 (cloperastine); 14984-68-0 (cloperastine hydrochloride).

Cloperastine fendizoate 177 mg is approximately equivalent to 100 mg of cloperastine hydrochloride.

Cloperastine is primarily a centrally acting cough suppressant used for non-productive cough (p.1052). It also has some antihistaminic action. The hydrochloride has been given by mouth as tablets in usual doses of 10 to 20 mg three times daily. Cloperastine fendizoate is used in oral liquid preparations in equivalent doses.

Preparations

Proprietary Preparations (details are given in Part 3)
Belg.: Novotossil; Sekin; ***Ital.:*** Cloel; Clofend; Nitossil; Politosse; Risoltuss; Seki; ***Jpn:*** Hustazol; ***Spain:*** Flutox; Sekisan.

Cloroqualone (13396-r)

Cloroqualone *(rINN).*

Edicloqualone. 3-(2,6-Dichlorophenyl)-2-ethyl-4(3*H*)-quinazolinone.

$C_{16}H_{12}Cl_2N_2O = 319.2.$

CAS — 25509-07-3.

Cloroqualone has been given by mouth as a cough suppressant.

Preparations

Proprietary Preparations (details are given in Part 3)

Multi-ingredient: ***Fr.:*** Eutuxal†.

Cocillana (2009-c)

Grape Bark; Guapi Bark; Huapi Bark.

CAS — 1398-77-2.

Pharmacopoeias. In *Br.*

The dried bark of *Guarea rusbyi* and closely related species (Meliaceae) containing not less than 3.5% of alcohol (60%)-soluble extractive.

Cocillana is used as an expectorant similarly to ipecacuanha (p.1062). It has been used in large doses as an emetic.

Preparations

Proprietary Preparations (details are given in Part 3)

Multi-ingredient: ***Canad.:*** Alsidrine; Bronchosyl; ***Ital.:*** Broncosedina; ***S.Afr.:*** Cocilix†; Cocillana Co; Corbar; ***Swed.:*** Cocillana-Etyfin.

Coltsfoot (5612-y)

Coughwort; Farfara; Huflattich; Tussilage.

Pharmacopoeias. Chin. and *Swiss* include Coltsfoot Flower. A monograph for Coltsfoot Leaf is included in *Aust.*

The leaves and flowers of coltsfoot (*Tussilago farfara*) have been used for their demulcent and supposed expectorant properties in the treatment of cough and other mild respiratory disorders. However, there has been some concern about potential hepatotoxicity and carcinogenicity due to the content of pyrrolizidine alkaloids.

In a review of the actions and uses of coltsfoot Berry[1] has pointed out that given the potential risks of long-term use or use in pregnancy, and the availability of other demulcent herbs, the use of coltsfoot preparations to treat throat irritations can no longer be considered appropriate.

1. Berry M. Coltsfoot. *Pharm J* 1996; **256:** 234–5.

Preparations

Proprietary Preparations (details are given in Part 3)

Multi-ingredient: ***Aust.:*** Puhlmann-Tee†; ***Fr.:*** Mediflor Tisane Pectorale d'Alsace†; ***Ger.:*** Bronchangin†; Bronchostad†; Dr. Klinger's Bergischer Krautertee, Husten- u. Bronchial-tee†; Orbis Husten- und Bronchial-tee†; Pro-Pecton Balsam†; Pro-Pecton Codein Hustentropfen†; Pro-Pecton Forte Hustensaft†; Pro-Pecton Hustensaft†; Pro-Pecton Hustentropfen†; Thymitussin†; ***Switz.:*** Viola Pommade a l'huile d'amandes†; ***UK:*** Antibron.

Creosote (2010-s)

Creasote; Creosotal (creosote carbonate); Wood Creosote.

CAS — 8021-39-4 (creosote); 8001-59-0 (creosote carbonate).

Pharmacopoeias. In *Belg.* and *Jpn.*

A liquid consisting of a mixture of guaiacol, cresol, and other phenols obtained from wood tar. Commercial creosote used for timber preservation is obtained from coal tar.

Creosote possesses disinfectant properties and has been used as an expectorant. It has also been used as the carbonate and as lactocreosote.

Adverse effects are similar to those of Phenol, p.1121.

Preparations

Proprietary Preparations (details are given in Part 3)

Multi-ingredient: ***Aust.:*** Famel cum Codein; Famel cum Ephedrin; ***Austral.:*** Waterbury's Compound†; ***Belg.:*** Pinthym†; ***Fr.:*** Sirop Famel†; ***Ital.:*** Creosolactol Adulti†; Creosolactol Bambini†; Famel; ***Neth.:*** Famel; ***Spain:*** Dentikrisos; Sanaden Reforzado; ***Switz.:*** Famel; ***UK:*** Catarrh Pastilles; Famel Catarrh & Throat Pastilles; Famel Original; Penetrol; Potter's Pastilles.

Dextromethorphan (5634-t)

Dextromethorphan *(BAN, pINN).*

(+)-3-Methoxy-9a-methylmorphinan; (9*S*,13*S*,14*S*)-6,18-Dideoxy-7,8-dihydro-3-*O*-methylmorphine.

$C_{18}H_{25}NO = 271.4.$

CAS — 125-71-3.

Pharmacopoeias. In *US.*

A practically white to slightly yellow odourless crystalline powder. Dextromethorphan 7.3 mg is approximately equivalent to 10 mg of dextromethorphan hydrobromide. Practically **insoluble** in water; freely soluble in chloroform. **Store** in airtight containers.

Dextromethorphan Hydrobromide (5613-j)

Dextromethorphan Hydrobromide *(BANM, pINNM).*

Dextromethorphani Hydrobromidum. Dextromethorphan hydrobromide monohydrate.

$C_{18}H_{25}NO,HBr,H_2O = 370.3.$

CAS — 125-69-9 (anhydrous dextromethorphan hydrobromide); 6700-34-1 (dextromethorphan hydrobromide monohydrate).

Pharmacopoeias. In *Eur.* (see p.viii), *Int.*, *Jpn*, and *US.*

A white or almost white crystalline powder, with a faint odour.

Soluble 1 in 65 of water; freely soluble in alcohol and in chloroform; and practically insoluble in ether. A 1% solution in water has a pH of 5.2 to 6.5. **Store** in airtight containers and protect from light.

Adverse Effects and Treatment

Adverse effects with dextromethorphan appear to be rare and may include dizziness and gastro-intestinal disturbances. Excitation, confusion, and respiratory depression may occur after overdosage. Dextromethorphan has been subject to abuse, but there is little evidence of dependence of the morphine type.

General references.

1. Bem JL, Peck R. Dextromethorphan: an overview of safety issues. *Drug Safety* 1992; **7:** 190–9.

Effects on the skin. A report[1] of a fixed-drug reaction in one patient following ingestion of 30 mg of dextromethorphan. Oral provocation with dextromethorphan produced a positive reaction but the results of topical application tests were negative.

1. Stubb S, Reitamo S. Fixed-drug eruption due to dextromethorphan. *Arch Dermatol* 1990; **126:** 970–1.

Overdosage. Reports[1,2] of overdosage of dextromethorphan hydrobromide in children and reversal of toxicity with intravenous naloxone.

1. Shaul WL, *et al.* Dextromethorphan toxicity: reversal by naloxone. *Pediatrics* 1977; **59:** 117–19.
2. Katona B, Wason S. Dextromethorphan danger. *N Engl J Med* 1986; **314:** 993.

Precautions

Dextromethorphan should not be given to patients at risk of developing respiratory failure. Caution is needed in patients with a history of asthma and it should not be given during an acute attack.

For doubts about the use of dextromethorphan as an antitussive in children see Cough, under Uses and Administration, below.

Abuse. Some individual reports of abuse.

1. Fleming PM. Dependence on dextromethorphan hydrobromide. *Br Med J* 1986; **293:** 597.
2. Orrell MW, Campbell PG. Dependence on dextromethorphan hydrobromide. *Br Med J* 1986; **293:** 1242–3.
3. Walker J, Yatham LN. Benylin (dextromethorphan) abuse and mania. *Br Med J* 1993; **306:** 896.

Interactions

Severe and sometimes fatal reactions have been reported following administration of dextromethorphan to patients receiving MAOIs. Dextromethorphan is primarily metabolised by the cytochrome P450 isoform CYP2D6; the possibility of interactions with inhibitors of this enzyme, including amiodarone, fluoxetine, haloperidol, paroxetine, propafenone, quinidine, and thioridazine, should be borne in mind.

Antiarrhythmics. *Quinidine* can increase serum concentrations of dextromethorphan markedly and some patients have experienced symptoms of dextromethorphan toxicity when the two agents have been used together.[1] *Amiodarone* also appears to be able to increase serum concentrations of dextromethorphan.[2]

1. Zhang Y, *et al.* Dextromethorphan: enhancing its systemic availability by way of low-dose quinidine-mediated inhibition of cytochrome P4502D6. *Clin Pharmacol Ther* 1992; **51:** 647–55.
2. Funck-Brentano C, *et al.* Influence of amiodarone on genetically determined drug metabolism in humans. *Clin Pharmacol Ther* 1991; **50:** 259–66.

Antidepressants. A patient receiving *fluoxetine* experienced visual hallucinations after she began taking dextromethorphan.[1] The hallucinations were similar to those she had had 12 years earlier with lysergide. She had previously taken dextromethorphan alone without any adverse reactions. A serotonergic syndrome, including confusion, tremor, hypertension and tachycardia, myoclonus, and rigidity, has been reported in a patient who took a cold-remedy including dextromethorphan while receiving *paroxetine*.[2]

1. Achamallah NS. Visual hallucinations after combining fluoxetine and dextromethorphan. *Am J Psychiatry* 1992; **149:** 1406.
2. Skop BP, *et al.* The serotonin syndrome associated with paroxetine, an over-the-counter cold remedy, and vascular disease. *Am J Emerg Med* 1994; **12:** 642–4.

Pharmacokinetics

Dextromethorphan is rapidly absorbed from the gastro-intestinal tract. It is metabolised in the liver and excreted in the urine as unchanged dextromethorphan and demethylated metabolites including dextrorphan (p.1571), which has some cough suppressant activity.

The *O*-demethylation of dextromethorphan and the hydroxylation of debrisoquine appear to be under common polymorphic control[1-3] and dextromethorphan is being used as an alternative to debrisoquine for the phenotyping of oxidative metabolism.[4] Results suggest that non-invasive determinations can be made using samples of urine or saliva.[5,6] Dextromethorphan has also been suggested as a tool to investigate *N*-demethylation, an alternate metabolic pathway for this drug.[7]

1. Schmid B, *et al.* Polymorphic dextromethorphan metabolism: co-segregation of oxidative O-demethylation with debrisoquin hydroxylation. *Clin Pharmacol Ther* 1985; **38:** 618–24.
2. Küpfer A, *et al.* Pharmacogenetics of dextromethorphan in man. *Xenobiotica* 1986; **16:** 421–33.
3. Mortimer Ö, *et al.* Dextromethorphan: polymorphic serum pattern of the O-demethylated and didemethylated metabolites in man. *Br J Clin Pharmacol* 1989; **27:** 223–7.
4. Belec L, *et al.* Extensive oxidative metabolism of dextromethorphan in patients with almitrine neuropathy. *Br J Clin Pharmacol* 1989; **27:** 387–90.
5. Hildebrand M, *et al.* Determination of dextromethorphan metabolizer phenotype in healthy volunteers. *Eur J Clin Pharmacol* 1989; **36:** 315–18.
6. Hou Z-Y, *et al.* Salivary analysis for determination of dextromethorphan metabolic phenotype. *Clin Pharmacol Ther* 1991; **49:** 410–19.
7. Jones DR, *et al.* Determination of cytochrome P450 3A4/5 activity in vivo with dextromethorphan N-demethylation. *Clin Pharmacol Ther* 1996; **60:** 374–84.

Uses and Administration

Dextromethorphan hydrobromide is a cough suppressant used for the relief of non-productive cough; it has a central action on the cough centre in the medulla. Although structurally related to morphine, dextromethorphan has no classical analgesic properties and little sedative activity.

Dextromethorphan hydrobromide is reported to act within half an hour of administration by mouth and to exert an effect for up to 6 hours. It is given by mouth in doses of 10 to 20 mg every 4 hours, or 30 mg every 6 to 8 hours, to a usual maximum of 120 mg in 24 hours. Children aged 6 to 12 years may be given 5 to 10 mg every 4 hours or 15 mg every 6 to 8 hours to a maximum of 60 mg in 24 hours, and children aged 2 to 6 years 2.5 to 5 mg every 4 hours, or 7.5 mg every 6 to 8 hours, to a maximum of 30 mg in 24 hours. (But see also Cough, below.)

Dextromethorphan polistirex (a dextromethorphan and sulphonated diethenylbenzene-ethenylbenzene copolymer complex) is used in modified-release oral preparations. The dosage of dextromethorphan polistirex, expressed as dextromethorphan hydrobromide, is 60 mg every 12 hours; children aged 6 to 12 years may be given 30 mg every 12 hours; children aged 2 to 6 years may be given 15 mg every 12 hours. Dextrorphan (p.1571), the *O*-demethylated metabolite of dextromethorphan also has cough suppressant properties.

Cough. Equal doses of dextromethorphan hydrobromide and codeine phosphate appeared to be of similar efficacy in reducing the frequency of chronic cough (p.1052) when compared in adults in a double-blind crossover study but dextromethorphan had a greater effect than codeine on cough intensity.[1] However, it has been reported in further studies that these agents were little more effective than placebo in suppressing night-time cough in children.[2,3] The American Academy of Pediatrics has commented[4] that there is no good evidence for the antitussive efficacy of dextromethorphan in children, that dosage guidelines are derived from (possibly inappropriate) extrapolation from effects in adults, and that adverse effects have been reported.

There is also some evidence that genetic polymorphism in cytochrome CYP2D6, and hence variations in metabolism, may have a significant influence on the antitussive efficacy of dextromethorphan.[5]

1. Matthys H, *et al.* Dextromethorphan and codeine: objective assessment of antitussive activity in patients with chronic cough. *J Int Med Res* 1983; **11:** 92–100.
2. Gadomski A, Horton L. The need for rational therapeutics in the use of cough and cold medicine in infants. *Pediatrics* 1992; **89:** 774–6.
3. Taylor JA, *et al.* Efficacy of cough suppressants in children. *J Pediatr* 1993; **122:** 799–802.
4. American Academy of Pediatrics Committee on Drugs. Use of codeine- and dextromethorphan-containing cough remedies in children. *Pediatrics* 1997; **99:** 918–20.
5. Wright CE, *et al.* CYP2D6 polymorphism and the anti-tussive effect of dextromethorphan in man. *Thorax* 1997; **52** (suppl 6): A73.

Neurological disorders. Dextromethorphan appears to have anticonvulsant activity and may have neuroprotective effects in cerebral ischaemia.[1] These effects may be related to its activity as an antagonist of *N*-methyl-D-aspartate (NMDA) receptors or to interaction with σ-receptors. It is being studied in the treatment of Parkinson's disease,[2] amyotrophic lateral sclerosis[3] (see Motor Neurone Disease, p.1625), and for its potential protective action in stroke and acute brain injury. Its NMDA-antagonist properties are also being investigated in the management of neuropathic pain, such as in diabetic neuropathy,[4] and for the treatment of nonketotic hyperglycinaemia.[5,6]

1. Tortella FC, *et al.* Dextromethorphan and neuromodulation: old drug coughs up new activities. *Trends Pharmacol Sci* 1989; **10:** 501–7.
2. Bonuccelli U, *et al.* Dextromethorphan and parkinsonism. *Lancet* 1992; **340:** 53.
3. Hollander D, *et al.* High-dose dextromethorphan in amyotrophic lateral sclerosis: phase I safety and pharmacokinetic studies. *Ann Neurol* 1994; **36:** 920–4.
4. Nelson KA, *et al.* High-dose oral dextromethorphan versus placebo in painful diabetic neuropathy and postherpetic neuralgia. *Neurology* 1997; **48:** 1212–18.
5. Alemzadeh R, *et al.* Efficacy of low-dose dextromethorphan in the treatment of nonketotic hyperglycinemia. *Pediatrics* 1996; **97:** 924–6.
6. Hamosh A, *et al.* Long-term use of high-dose benzoate and dextromethorphan for the treatment of nonketotic hyperglycinemia. *J Pediatr* 1998; **132:** 709–13.

Preparations

USP 23: Acetaminophen, Dextromethorphan Hydrobromide, Doxylamine Succinate, and Pseudoephedrine Hydrochloride Oral Solution; Dextromethorphan Hydrobromide Syrup; Guaifenesin, Pseudoephedrine Hydrochloride, and Dextromethorphan Hydrobromide Capsules; Terpin Hydrate and Dextromethorphan Hydrobromide Elixir.

Proprietary Preparations (details are given in Part 3)
Aust.: Wick Formel 44; Wick Formel 44 Plus Hustenstiller; ***Belg.:*** Akindex; Benylin Antitussivum; Bronchosedal; Dexir; Pectofree†; Rhinathiol Antitussivum; Romilar Antitussivum; Touxium; Tussipect; Vicks Vaposyrup Antitussif; ***Canad.:*** Balminil DM; Benylin DM; Broncho-Grippol-DM; Bronchopan DM; Buckley's DM; Calmylin #1; Centratuss DM; Contac Coughcaps†; Cough Suppressant Syrup DM; Cough Syrup; Cough Syrup DM; Delsym; DM Cough Syrup; DM Sans Sucre; Drixoral; Drixoral Cough; Formula 44; Koffex DM; Pharmilin-DM; Pharminil DM; Robidex†; Robitussin Pediatric; Sedatuss DM; Sirop DM; Sucrets Cough Control; Syrup DM; Triaminic DM; ***Fr.:*** Akindex; Atuxane; Capsyl; Dexir; Drill toux seche; Nodex; Tuxium; Vicks Toux Seche; Vicks Vaposyrup toux seche; ***Ger.:*** Arpha Hustensirup†; NeoTussan; Rheila Hustenstiller†; Tuss Hustenstiller; Wick Formel 44 plus Husten-Pastillen S; Wick Formel 44 plus Husten-Stiller; Wick Kinder Formel 44 Husten-Stiller; ***Irl.:*** Benylin Non-Drowsy Dry Coughs; Delsym; Robitussin Cough Soother; ***Ital.:*** Aricodil; Bechilar; Bronchenolo; Canfodion†; Fluprim Tosse; Formitrol; Gocce Sedative Della Tosse†; Metorfan; Sanabronchiol; Sedotus†; Simatus†; Torax†; Tussycalm; Valatux; Vicks Tosse Pastiglie; Vicks Tosse Sedativo; ***Neth.:*** Benylin-Dextromethorfanhydrobromide; Dampo bij droge hoest; Darolan Hoestprikkeldempende; Tosion Retard; Vicks Vaposiroop; ***S.Afr.:*** Benylin DM; Benylin Solid; ***Spain:*** Benylin Antitusivo; Cinfatos; Formulatus; Humex; Pastillas Dr Andreu; Robitussin DM Antitusivo; Romilar; Siepex; Tosfriol; Tusitinas; Tusorama; Valdatos; ***Swed.:*** Tussidyl; ***Switz.:*** Bexine; Calmerphan-L; Calmesine; Dextrocalmine; Pulmofor; ***UK:*** Benylin Non-Drowsy Dry Coughs; Contac Coughcaps; Covonia for Children; Franolyn Sedative; Meltus Cough Control; Nirolex for Dry Coughs; Owbridges for Dry Tickly Coughs†; Robitussin for Dry Coughs; Robitussin Junior; Vicks Childrens Vaposyrup†; Vicks Vaposyrup for dry coughs; ***USA:*** Benylin Adult; Benylin DM; Benylin Pediatric; Children's Hold†; Congespirin†; Creo-Terpin; Delsym; Drixoral Cough; Hold DM; Pertussin; Robitussin Cough Calmers; Robitussin Pediatric; Scot-Tussin DM Cough Chasers; Silphen DM; St. Joseph Cough Suppressant; Sucrets 4-Hour Cough; Sucrets Cough Control; Suppress; Trocal; Vicks Dry Hacking Cough.

Multi-ingredient: numerous preparations are listed in Part 3.

Dimemorfan Phosphate (5615-c)

Dimemorfan Phosphate *(rINNM)*.

AT-17. (+)-3,9a-Dimethylmorphinan phosphate.

$C_{18}H_{25}N,H_3PO_4$ = 353.4.

CAS — 36309-01-0 (dimemorfan); 36304-84-4 (dimemorfan phosphate).

Pharmacopoeias. In *Jpn.*

Dimemorfan phosphate is a centrally acting cough suppressant used for non-productive cough (p.1052). It is given by mouth in doses of 10 to 20 mg three or four times daily.

Preparations

Proprietary Preparations (details are given in Part 3)
Ital.: Gentus; Tusben; ***Jpn:*** Astomin; ***Spain:*** Dastosin.

Dimethoxanate Hydrochloride (5616-k)

Dimethoxanate Hydrochloride *(BANM, rINNM)*.

2-(2-Dimethylaminoethoxy)ethyl phenothiazine-10-carboxylate hydrochloride.

$C_{19}H_{22}N_2O_3S,HCl$ = 394.9.

CAS — 477-93-0 (dimethoxanate); 518-63-8 (dimethoxanate hydrochloride).

Dimethoxanate hydrochloride is a centrally acting cough suppressant used for non-productive cough (p.1052). It is given by mouth in usual doses of 37.5 mg 3 or 4 times daily.

Preparations

Proprietary Preparations (details are given in Part 3)
Belg.: Cotrane; ***Ital.:*** Cothera†.

Multi-ingredient: ***S.Afr.:*** Cothera Compound†.

Domiodol (12678-d)

Domiodol *(USAN, pINN)*.

MG-13608. 2-Iodomethyl-1,3-dioxolan-4-ylmethanol.

$C_5H_9IO_3$ = 244.0.

CAS — 61869-07-6.

Domiodol has been used for its mucolytic properties in the relief of productive cough (p.1052).

The actions of the iodides are discussed under Iodine, p.1493.

Preparations

Proprietary Preparations (details are given in Part 3)
Ital.: Mucolitico Maggioni.

Dornase Alfa (3717-g)

Dornase Alfa *(BAN, rINN)*.

Deoxyribonuclease; Desoxyribonuclease; DNase I; rhDNase. Deoxyribonuclease I (human recombinant).

$C_{1321}H_{1995}N_{339}O_{396}S_9$ = 29249.6.

CAS — 143831-71-4; 132053-08-8.

An enzyme derived from cloned human pancreatic deoxyribonuclease I and having the same amino acid sequence and glycosylation pattern as human deoxyribonuclease I.

Adverse Effects

Common adverse effects with dornase alfa aerosol include pharyngitis and hoarseness of the voice. Occasionally laryngitis, conjunctivitis, and skin rashes and urticaria have been reported. There may be a transient decline in pulmonary function on beginning therapy with dornase alfa.

Uses and Administration

Dornase alfa acts as a mucolytic by hydrolysing DNA that has accumulated in sputum from decaying neutrophils. It is used as a nebulised solution in patients with cystic fibrosis; in the UK the manufacturers limit its indication to patients with a forced vital capacity greater than 40% of predicted value and to patients over 5 years of age but in the USA it may also be given for advanced disease (FVC less than 40%) and to younger children. The usual dose is 2500 U (2.5 mg) of dornase alfa given once daily via a jet nebuliser. This dose may be given twice daily to patients over 21 years of age.

Bovine deoxyribonuclease has been used similarly. It has also been used topically, often with plasmin, as a debriding agent in a variety of inflammatory and infected lesions. Bovine deoxyribonuclease has also been given by injection.

Asthma. There is a report of the use of dornase alfa to liquefy a mucus plug and relieve an attack of acute severe asthma (p.745) in an 8-year-old child.[1]

1. Greally P. Human recombinant DNase for mucus plugging in status asthmaticus. *Lancet* 1995; **346:** 1423–4.

Chronic bronchitis. A large phase III study of dornase alfa in patients hospitalised for acute exacerbations of chronic bronchitis (p.747) was halted prematurely because of a non-significant trend to increased mortality in patients given dornase.[1]

1. Hudson TJ. Dornase in treatment of chronic bronchitis. *Ann Pharmacother* 1996; **30:** 674–5.

Cystic fibrosis. There is good evidence that inhalation therapy with dornase alfa can produce modest but useful improvement in lung function in some patients with cystic fibrosis.[1-4] Most studies have concentrated on patients with mild or moderate disease (forced vital capacity at least 40% of the predicted value) in whom FEV_1 and forced vital capacity have shown improvements generally of the order of 5 to 10%,[1-3] and in whom more prolonged therapy (24 weeks) has been shown to reduce the risk of exacerbations of respiratory infections, and hence the need for intravenous antibiotic therapy.[3] Recent evidence has shown that benefit may also occur in patients with more severe disease.[4] Studies differ as to whether subjective symptoms such as dyspnoea and general well-being are improved by dornase alfa.

It is also clear that only a minority of patients, perhaps about one-third,[5] benefit from the drug, and at present there is no way of identifying responders other than a therapeutic trial.[6] It is also unclear whether longer-term therapy can alter the underlying pathophysiology of the disease and retard or prevent the progressive decline in lung function (which is in any case low in optimally-treated patients[7]), although there are reasons to think that this might be the case.[8,9]

Given the high cost of therapy, which is not entirely recouped by savings in acute care, there has been some controversy about the appropriate use of dornase alfa:[10-13] it seems to be generally felt that it should be reserved for specialist use in cystic fibrosis clinics, but that patients should not be denied a trial where appropriate. Most responders with mild to moderate impairment of lung function will show improvements within 2 weeks, although in more severely affected patients a 6-week trial is advocated.[6,7]

For a broader discussion of the therapy of cystic fibrosis see p.119.

1. Ramsey BW, *et al.* Efficacy and safety of short-term administration of aerosolized recombinant human deoxyribonuclease in patients with cystic fibrosis. *Am Rev Respir Dis* 1993; **148:** 145–51.
2. Ranasinha C, *et al.* Efficacy and safety of short-term administration of aerosolised recombinant human DNase I in adults with stable stage cystic fibrosis. *Lancet* 1993; **342:** 199–202.
3. Fuchs H, *et al.* Effect of aerosolized recombinant human DNase on exacerbations of respiratory symptoms and on pulmonary function in patients with cystic fibrosis. *N Engl J Med* 1994; **331:** 637–42.
4. McCoy K, *et al.* Effects of 12-week administration of dornase alfa in patients with advanced cystic fibrosis lung disease. *Chest* 1996; **110:** 889–95.
5. Davis PB. Evolution of therapy for cystic fibrosis. *N Engl J Med* 1994; **331:** 672–3.
6. Conway SP, Littlewood JM. rhDNase in cystic fibrosis. *Br J Hosp Med* 1997; **57:** 371–2.
7. Conway SP. Recombinant human DNase (rhDNase) in cystic fibrosis: is it cost effective? *Arch Dis Child* 1997; **77:** 1–3.
8. Shah PL, *et al.* Two years experience with recombinant human DNase 1 in the treatment of pulmonary disease in cystic fibrosis. *Respir Med* 1995; **89:** 499–502.
9. Costello CM, *et al.* Effect of nebulised recombinant DNase on neutrophil elastase load in cystic fibrosis. *Thorax* 1996; **51:** 619–23.
10. Anonymous. Dornase alfa for cystic fibrosis. *Drug Ther Bull* 1995; **33:** 15–16.
11. Spencer D, Weller P. Dornase-alfa for cystic fibrosis. *Lancet* 1995; **345:** 1307.
12. Bush A, *et al.* Dornase alfa for cystic fibrosis. *Br Med J* 1995; **310:** 1533.
13. Robert G, *et al.* Dornase alfa for cystic fibrosis. *Br Med J* 1995; **311:** 813.

Preparations

Proprietary Preparations (details are given in Part 3)
Aust.: Pulmozyme; ***Austral.:*** Pulmozyme; ***Belg.:*** Pulmozyme; ***Canad.:*** Pulmozyme; ***Fr.:*** Pulmozyme; ***Ger.:*** Pulmozyme; ***Irl.:*** Pulmozyme; ***Ital.:*** Pulmozyme; ***Neth.:*** Pulmozyme; ***Norw.:*** Pulmozyme; ***S.Afr.:*** Pulmozyme; ***Spain:*** Pulmozyme; ***Swed.:*** Pulmozyme; ***Switz.:*** Pulmozyme; ***UK:*** Pulmozyme; ***USA:*** Pulmozyme.

Multi-ingredient: ***Aust.:*** Fibrolan; ***Austral.:*** Elase; ***Canad.:*** Elase; Elase-Chloromycetin; ***Fr.:*** Elase; ***Ger.:*** Fibrolan; Fibrolan mit Chloromycetin†; ***Ital.:*** Derinase Plus; Elase; ***Neth.:*** Elase; ***Spain:*** Parkelase; Parkelase Chloromycetin; ***Switz.:*** Fibrolan; ***USA:*** Elase; Elase-Chloromycetin.

Dropropizine (12680-k)

Dropropizine *(BAN, rINN)*.

UCB-1967. 3-(4-Phenylpiperazin-1-yl)propane-1,2-diol.

$C_{13}H_{20}N_2O_2$ = 236.3.

CAS — 17692-31-8.

Levodropropizine (5399-n)

Levodropropizine *(rINN)*.

DF-526; Levdropropizine. The (−)-(*S*)-isomer of dropropizine.

$C_{13}H_{20}N_2O_2$ = 236.3.

CAS — 99291-25-5.

Dropropizine is a cough suppressant reported to have a peripheral action in non-productive cough (p.1052). It is given by mouth in a dose of 30 mg three to four times daily. Levodropropizine, the (−)-(*S*)-isomer of dropropizine, is claimed to produce fewer CNS effects and is used similarly by mouth in a dose of 60 mg up to three times daily.

References.

1. Bossi R, *et al.* Antitussive activity and respiratory system effects of levodropropizine in man. *Arzneimittelforschung* 1988; **38:** 1159–62.
2. Allegra L, Bossi R. Clinical trials with the new antitussive levodropropizine in adult bronchitic patients. *Arzneimittelforschung* 1988; **38:** 1163–6.

Preparations

Proprietary Preparations (details are given in Part 3)
Belg.: Catabex; ***Ger.:*** Larylin Husten-Stiller Pastillen; Larylin Hustensirup N; ***Ital.:*** Danka; Domutussina†; Levotuss; Rapitux; Ribex Tosse; Salvituss; ***Spain:*** Tusofren.

Multi-ingredient: ***Belg.:*** Catabex Expectorans; ***Fr.:*** Catabex; ***Ger.:*** Larylin Hustenloser†; ***Ital.:*** Elisir Terpina; Guaiacalcium Complex; Ribexen con Espettorante; Tiocalmina; Tussamag Complex.

Elecampane (16013-j)

Alant; Aunée; Inula.

Pharmacopoeias. In *Chin.* (which also includes various other species of *Inula*) and *Fr.*

Elecampane is the root of *Inula helenium* (Compositae). It has been used in herbal preparations for the treatment of cough for its supposed expectorant and cough suppressant properties. It is also used as a flavouring in foods and alcoholic beverages.

Elecampane contains sesquiterpene lactones including alantolactone (alant camphor; elecampane camphor; inula camphor; helenin), which was formerly employed in the treatment of worm infections, and has also been an ingredient of some cough preparations.

Preparations

Proprietary Preparations (details are given in Part 3)

Multi-ingredient: ***Belg.:*** Euphon; ***Fr.:*** Marrubene Codethyline; Mediflor Tisane Digestive No 3; Mediflor Tisane Hepatique No 5; Tisanes de l'Abbe Hamon no 15; Tisanes de l'Abbe Hamon no 18†; Tossarel; ***Ger.:*** Diureticum-Medice†; Phytpulmon†; ***Spain:*** Digestonico Solucion†; ***Switz.:*** Boldoflorine; Hederix; Melior†; ***UK:*** Catarrh-eeze; Cough-eeze; Horehound and Aniseed Cough Mixture; Vegetable Cough Remover.

Ephedra (2054-r)

Ma-huang.

Pharmacopoeias. In *Chin., Ger.,* and *Jpn.*

Ephedra consists of the dried young branches of *Ephedra sinica, E. equisetina,* and *E. gerardiana* (including *E. nebrodensis*) (Ephedraceae), containing not less than 1.25% of alkaloids, calculated as ephedrine. (*Jpn P.* specifies not less than 0.6%). *Chin. P.* also includes Radix Ephedrae, prepared from the roots of *E. sinica* or *E. intermedia.*

The action of ephedra is due to the presence of ephedrine (p.1059) and pseudoephedrine (p.1068). It has been used chiefly as a source of these alkaloids.

For reference to the adverse effects of herbal products containing ephedra see under Adverse Effects in Ephedrine, below.

Preparations

Proprietary Preparations (details are given in Part 3)

Multi-ingredient: ***Canad.:*** Herbal Cold Relief; ***Ger.:*** B 10-Strath†; Cardaminol†; Cardibisana; Cefedrin N; Repursan ST; Silphoscalin†.

Ephedrine (2055-f)

Ephedrine *(BAN)*.

Efedrina; Ephedrina; (−)-Ephedrine; Ephedrinum. (1*R*,2*S*)-2-Methylamino-1-phenylpropan-1-ol.

$C_{10}H_{15}NO$ = 165.2.

CAS — 299-42-3 (anhydrous ephedrine); 50906-05-3 (ephedrine hemihydrate).

Pharmacopoeias. In *Eur.* (see p.viii), *Int.,* and *US* which have specifications, in either the same monograph or in separate monographs, for anhydrous ephedrine and for ephedrine hemihydrate.

An alkaloid obtained from species of *Ephedra,* or prepared synthetically. It may exist in a hemihydrate form or as the anhydrous substance. Colourless crystals or white crystalline powder. The m.p. varies according to the moisture content; Ph. Eur. specifies that the undried substance (hemihydrate) melts at about 42° and the anhydrous substance at about 36°.

Both forms of ephedrine are **soluble** 1 in 20 of water and 1 in 0.2 of alcohol; soluble in chloroform and soluble or freely soluble in ether; moderately and slowly soluble in liquid paraffin, the solution becoming turbid if the water content of ephedrine exceeds 1%. Ephedrine decomposes on exposure to light. **Store** at a temperature not exceeding 8° in airtight containers. Protect from light.

Ephedrine Hydrochloride (2057-n)

Ephedrine Hydrochloride *(BANM)*.

Ephedrinae Hydrochloridum; Ephedrine Chloride; Ephedrini Hydrochloridum; Ephedrinium Chloratum; *l*-Ephedrinum Hydrochloricum.

$C_{10}H_{15}NO,HCl$ = 201.7.

CAS — 50-98-6.

Pharmacopoeias. In *Chin., Eur.* (see p.viii), *Int., Jpn, Pol.,* and *US. Eur.* also includes the racemic form (racephedrine hydrochloride).

Odourless colourless crystals or white crystalline powder. **Soluble** 1 in 3 of water and 1 in 14 of alcohol; practically insoluble in ether. **Protect** from light.

Ephedrine Sulphate (2058-h)

Ephedrine Sulphate *(BANM)*.

Ephedrine Sulfate.

$(C_{10}H_{15}NO)_2,H_2SO_4$ = 428.5.

CAS — 134-72-5.

Pharmacopoeias. In *Int.* and *US.*

Fine white odourless crystals or powder. It darkens on exposure to light. **Soluble** 1 in 1.3 of water and 1 in 90 of alcohol. **Protect** from light.

Adverse Effects

The commonest adverse effects of ephedrine are tachycardia, anxiety, restlessness, and insomnia. Tremor, dry mouth, impaired circulation to the extremities, hypertension, and cardiac arrhythmias may also occur.

Injection of ephedrine during labour can cause fetal tachycardia.

Paranoid psychosis, delusions, and hallucinations may also follow ephedrine overdosage. Prolonged administration has no cumulative effect, but tolerance with dependence has been reported.

For the adverse effects of sympathomimetics in general, see p.951.

Toxicity has been reported from the self-administration of ephedrine-containing dietary supplements or herbal stimulants, usually based on ephedra (ma huang) and marketed for a variety of purposes including weight loss and as an alternative to illegal drugs of abuse. Adverse effects have included myocardial infarction, stroke, convulsions, and psychotic reactions;[1-3] a number of fatalities have been reported. In the USA restrictions upon the ephedrine content of such preparations, and appropriate warning labelling, have been proposed.[4]

1. Anonymous. Adverse events associated with ephedrine-containing products—Texas, December 1993-September 1995. *JAMA* 1996; **276:** 1711–12.
2. Doyle H, Kargin M. Herbal stimulant containing ephedrine has also caused psychosis. *Br Med J* 1996; **313:** 756.
3. Cockings JGL, Brown MA. Ephedrine abuse causing acute myocardial infarction. *Med J Aust* 1997; **167:** 199–200.
4. Anonymous. FDA proposes constraints on ephedrine dietary supplements. *Am J Health-Syst Pharm* 1997; **54:** 1578.

Precautions

Ephedrine should be given with care in patients with hyperthyroidism, diabetes mellitus, ischaemic heart disease, hypertension, or renal impairment or angle-closure glaucoma. In patients with prostatic enlargement, ephedrine may increase difficulty with micturition.

For the precautions to be observed with sympathomimetics in general, see p.951.

Interactions

Administration of ephedrine may cause a hypertensive crisis in patients receiving an MAOI (including an RIMA); the possibility of such an interaction following intranasal use of ephedrine should also be borne in mind. For additional warnings see under phenelzine (p.305) and moclobemide (p.299). Ephedrine should be avoided or used with care in patients undergoing anaesthesia with cyclopropane, halothane, or other volatile anaesthetics. An increased risk of arrhythmias may occur if given to patients receiving cardiac glycosides, quinidine, or tricyclic antidepressants, and there is an increased risk of vasoconstrictor or pressor effects in patients receiving ergot alkaloids or oxytocin.

For the interactions of the sympathomimetics in general, see p.951.

Pharmacokinetics

Ephedrine is readily and completely absorbed from the gastro-intestinal tract. It is resistant to metabolism by monoamine oxidase and is largely excreted unchanged in the urine, together with small amounts of metabolites produced by hepatic metabolism. Ephedrine has been variously reported to have a plasma half-life ranging from 3 to 6 hours depending on urinary pH; elimination is enhanced and half-life accordingly shorter in acid urine.

References.

1. Welling PG, *et al.* Urinary excretion of ephedrine in man without pH control following oral administration of three commercial ephedrine sulfate preparations. *J Pharm Sci* 1971; **60:** 1629–34.
2. Sever PS, *et al.* The metabolism of (−)-ephedrine in man. *Eur J Clin Pharmacol* 1975; **9:** 193–8.
3. Pickup ME, *et al.* The pharmacokinetics of ephedrine after oral dosage in asthmatics receiving acute and chronic treatment. *Br J Clin Pharmacol* 1976; **3:** 123–34.

Uses and Administration

Ephedrine is a sympathomimetic (see p.951) with direct and indirect effects on adrenergic receptors. It has alpha- and beta-adrenergic activity and has pronounced stimulating effects on the central nervous system. It has a more prolonged though less potent action than adrenaline. In therapeutic doses it raises the blood pressure by increasing cardiac output and also by inducing peripheral vasoconstriction. Tachycardia may occur but is less frequent than with adrenaline. Ephedrine also causes bronchodilatation, reduces intestinal tone and motility, relaxes the bladder wall while contracting the sphincter muscle but relaxes the detrusor muscle of the bladder and usually reduces the activity of the uterus. It has a stimulant action on the respiratory centre. It dilates the pupil but does not affect the light reflexes. After ephedrine has been used for a short while, tachyphylaxis may develop.

Ephedrine salts are used, either alone or in conjunction with other drugs, in the symptomatic relief of nasal congestion (p.1052). They may be given by mouth or topically as nasal drops or sprays. Ephedrine salts have sometimes been used in motion sickness in conjunction with hyoscine or an antihistamine and have been tried for postoperative nausea and vomiting (p.1172).

Ephedrine salts have been given parenterally to combat a fall in blood pressure during spinal anaesthesia. Ephedrine is of little value in hypotensive crises due to shock, circulatory collapse, or haemorrhage. It is no longer generally advocated for orthostatic hypotension.

Ephedrine salts have been used as a bronchodilator, but the more beta$_2$-selective sympathomimetics, such as salbutamol, are now preferred.

Other uses of ephedrine salts include diabetic neuropathic oedema, when this treatment may provide marked relief. They have also been used in micturition disorders.

Ephedrine and its salts may be administered by mouth in usual doses of up to 60 mg three times a day. Nasal drops or sprays usually contain ephedrine 0.5%; a 0.25% strength may be used for infants and young children. Ephedrine salts can also be given by oral inhalation.

To reverse hypotension induced by spinal or epidural anaesthesia, a solution containing ephedrine hydrochloride 3 mg per mL is given by slow intravenous injection in doses of 3 to 6 mg (or at most 9 mg) repeated every 3 to 4 minutes as required; the maximum total dose is 30 mg. Ephedrine salts have also been given by intramuscular or subcutaneous injection.

Several other salts of ephedrine have been given including the camsylate and the tannate. Racephedrine hydrochloride has also been used.

Diabetic neuropathic oedema. Ephedrine, in doses of 30 mg three or four times daily was given to 3 type 1 diabetics who had severe neuropathy associated with intractable oedema of the feet and lower legs; a fourth, similar patient was given 60 mg three times daily. Ephedrine produced a rapid decrease in weight and a diminution of oedema. Sodium excretion was also increased and peripheral diastolic flow was reduced. No side-effects were noted and there was no significant change in blood pressure in any of the patients, including one with a history of hypertension. All 4 patients continued on ephedrine for 12 to 15 months, and the effects were sustained with no sign of tachyphylaxis, perhaps because patients with autonomic neuropathy have depleted catecholamine stores and ephedrine is probably acting mainly as a direct-acting sympathomimetic.[1]

For a discussion of diabetic neuropathy and its management see p.315.

1. Edmonds ME, *et al.* Ephedrine: a new treatment for diabetic neuropathic oedema. *Lancet* 1983; **i:** 548–51.

Micturition disorders. Ephedrine salts have been used in nocturnal enuresis (p.453), although other treatments are usually preferred, and have been tried in patients with stress incontinence (p.454) but the value of such treatment is not clear.

Spinal anaesthesia. Several sympathomimetics such as ephedrine and phenylephrine have been advocated for parenteral use in the correction of hypotension developing during local anaesthesia.

Spinal or epidural block is associated with a greater risk of hypotension developing than many other forms of nerve block as mentioned on p.1281 and ephedrine has been used[1,2] although not always successfully[3] for the correction of such hypotension; it has also been used for prophylaxis.[4] However, it should be noted that one of the most important ways of preventing or minimising hypotension is by making sure the patient is adequately hydrated before induction of anaesthesia.

1. Hall PA, *et al.* Spinal anaesthesia for Caesarean section: comparison of infusions of phenylephrine and ephedrine. *Br J Anaesth* 1994; **73:** 471–4.
2. Thomas DG, *et al.* Randomized trial of bolus phenylephrine or ephedrine for maintenance of arterial pressure during spinal anaesthesia for Caesarean section. *Br J Anaesth* 1996; **76:** 61–5.
3. Critchley LAH, *et al.* Hypotension during subarachnoid anaesthesia: haemodynamic effects of ephedrine. *Br J Anaesth* 1995; **74:** 373–8.
4. Sternlo J-E, *et al.* Prophylactic im ephedrine in bupivacaine spinal anaesthesia. *Br J Anaesth* 1995; **74:** 517–20.

Preparations

BP 1998: Ephedrine Elixir; Ephedrine Hydrochloride Tablets; Ephedrine Nasal Drops;
USP 23: Ephedrine Sulfate and Phenobarbital Capsules; Ephedrine Sulfate Capsules; Ephedrine Sulfate Injection; Ephedrine Sulfate Nasal Solution; Ephedrine Sulfate Syrup; Ephedrine Sulfate Tablets; Theophylline, Ephedrine Hydrochloride, and Phenobarbital Tablets.

Proprietary Preparations (details are given in Part 3)
Ger.: Endrine mild†; Endrine†; ***Ital.:*** Rino Pumilene†; ***Mon.:*** Stopasthme†; ***UK:*** CAM; CAM Bronchodilator Mixture; Secron; ***USA:*** Kondon's Nasal; Pretz-D; Resp; Vicks Vatronol†.

Multi-ingredient: numerous preparations are listed in Part 3.

Eprazinone Hydrochloride (12696-h)

Eprazinone Hydrochloride *(rINNM)*.

CE-746. 3-[4-(β-Ethoxyphenethyl)piperazin-1-yl]-2-methylpropiophenone dihydrochloride.

$C_{24}H_{32}N_2O_2,2HCl = 453.4$.

CAS — 10402-90-1 (eprazinone); 10402-53-6 (eprazinone hydrochloride).

Eprazinone hydrochloride has been variously described as having mucolytic or expectorant properties (p.1052) as well as a direct relaxant action on bronchial smooth muscle. It is given by mouth in doses of 50 to 100 mg three times daily. It has also been administered rectally.

Effects on the skin. A report[1] of a skin eruption associated with the oral administration of eprazinone.

1. Faber M, *et al.* Eprazinonexanthem mit subkornealer pustelbildung. *Hautarzt* 1984; **35:** 200–3.

Overdosage. Symptoms in two 22-month-old children who received an overdose of 800 mg of eprazinone included somnolence, ataxia, and seizures.[1]

1. Merigot P, *et al.* Les convulsions avec trois antitussifs dérivés substitutés de la pipérazine: (zipéprol, éprazinone, éprozinol). *Ann Pediatr (Paris)* 1985; **32:** 504–11.

Preparations

Proprietary Preparations (details are given in Part 3)
Aust.: Eftapan; ***Belg.:*** Isilung; ***Fr.:*** Mucitux; ***Ger.:*** Eftapan; ***Ital.:*** Mucitux†; ***Jpn:*** Resplen†.

Multi-ingredient: ***Aust.:*** Eftapan Tetra; ***Ger.:*** Eftapan Doxy†; Eftapan Tetra†.

Erdosteine (2948-y)

Erdosteine *(rINN)*.

(±)-({[(Tetrahydro-2-oxo-3-thienyl)carbamoyl]methyl}thio)acetic acid.

$C_8H_{11}NO_4S_2 = 249.3$.

CAS — 84611-23-4.

Erdosteine is a mucolytic that is used in the treatment of disorders of the respiratory tract characterised by productive cough (p.1052) It is given by mouth in doses of 300 mg twice daily.

References to erdosteine[1] and its use in the management of chronic obstructive pulmonary disease[2] (for controversy about the value of mucolytic therapy in this disorder see p.747).

1. Dechant KL, Noble S. Erdosteine. *Drugs* 1996; **52:** 875–81.
2. Marchioni CF, *et al.* Evaluation of efficacy and safety of erdosteine in patients affected by chronic bronchitis during an infective exacerbation phase and receiving amoxycillin as basic treatment (ECOBES, European Chronic Obstructive Bronchitis Erdosteine Study). *Int J Clin Pharmacol Ther* 1995; **33:** 612–18.

Preparations

Proprietary Preparations (details are given in Part 3)
Fr.: Edirel; Vectrine; ***Switz.:*** Mucofor.

Eriodictyon (2012-e)

Mountain Balm; Yerba Santa.

CAS — 8013-08-9.

The dried leaves of *Eriodictyon californicum* (Hydrophyllaceae).

Eriodictyon has been used as an expectorant. It has also been used to mask the taste of bitter drugs.

Preparations

Proprietary Preparations (details are given in Part 3)

Multi-ingredient: *Ger.:* Mistelan†; *Ital.:* Broncosedina.

Etafedrine Hydrochloride (2059-m)

Etafedrine Hydrochloride *(BANM, USAN, rINNM).*

Ethylephedrine Hydrochloride. (−)-2-(Ethylmethylamino)-1-phenylpropan-1-ol hydrochloride.

$C_{12}H_{19}NO,HCl = 229.7.$

CAS — 7681-79-0 (etafedrine); 48141-64-6 ((−)-etafedrine); 5591-29-7 (etafedrine hydrochloride).

Etafedrine hydrochloride is a sympathomimetic related to ephedrine (p.1059). It is used for its bronchodilator effects in combination with other agents for the relief of cough and associated respiratory-tract disorders.

Preparations

Proprietary Preparations (details are given in Part 3)

Multi-ingredient: *Canad.:* Calmydone; Mercodol with Decapryn; *Ger.:* Ditenate†; *S.Afr.:* Nethaprin Dospan; Nethaprin Expectorant.

Ethyl Cysteine Hydrochloride (16008-k)

Ethyl L-2-amino-3-mercaptopropionate hydrochloride.

$C_5H_{11}NO_2S,HCl = 185.7.$

CAS — 3411-58-3 (ethyl cysteine); 868-59-7 (ethyl cysteine hydrochloride).

Pharmacopoeias. In *Jpn.*

Ethyl cysteine hydrochloride is a mucolytic used in the treatment of disorders of the respiratory tract associated with productive cough.

Preparations

Proprietary Preparations (details are given in Part 3)
Fr.: Fludixan†.

Ethyl Orthoformate (5618-t)

Ether de Kay; Triethoxymethane. Triethyl orthoformate.

$C_7H_{16}O_3 = 148.2.$

CAS — 122-51-0.

Pharmacopoeias. In *Fr.*

Ethyl orthoformate is a cough suppressant (see p.1052). It is reported to be a respiratory antispasmodic and is administered by mouth or rectally.

Preparations

Proprietary Preparations (details are given in Part 3)
Belg.: Aethone†; *Fr.:* Aethone†.

Multi-ingredient: *Switz.:* Rectoquintyl; Rectoquintyl-Promethazine.

Fedrilate (5619-x)

Fedrilate *(rINN).*

Fedrilatum; UCB-3928. 1-Methyl-3-morpholinopropyl perhydro-4-phenylpyran-4-carboxylate.

$C_{20}H_{29}NO_4 = 347.4.$

CAS — 23271-74-1.

Fedrilate is a cough suppressant used for non-productive cough (p.1052) which has been given by mouth as the maleate in doses of 50 mg three to six times daily.

Preparations

Proprietary Preparations (details are given in Part 3)
S.Afr.: Corbar S; Dykatuss "S"†.

Multi-ingredient: *Ger.:* Duotal†.

Fenoxazoline Hydrochloride (2064-d)

Fenoxazoline Hydrochloride *(rINNM).*

2-(2-Isopropylphenoxymethyl)-2-imidazoline hydrochloride.

$C_{13}H_{18}N_2O,HCl = 254.8.$

CAS — 4846-91-7 (fenoxazoline); 21370-21-8 (fenoxazoline hydrochloride).

Fenoxazoline hydrochloride is a sympathomimetic with effects similar to those of naphazoline (p.1064) used for its vasoconstrictor properties in the symptomatic treatment of nasal congestion (p.1052). It is applied topically, usually as a 0.1% solution up to 3 times daily using a nasal spray.

Fominoben Hydrochloride (5620-y)

Fominoben Hydrochloride *(rINNM).*

PB-89. 3′-Chloro-2′-[*N*-methyl-*N*-(morpholinocarbonylmethyl)aminomethyl]benzanilide hydrochloride.

$C_{21}H_{24}ClN_3O_3,HCl = 438.3.$

CAS — 18053-31-1 (fominoben); 24600-36-0 (fominoben hydrochloride).

Fominoben hydrochloride is a centrally acting cough suppressant (see p.1052) which is also reported to have respiratory stimulant properties. It is given in doses of 160 mg up to three times daily by mouth; it has also been given by slow intravenous injection.

Preparations

Proprietary Preparations (details are given in Part 3)
Ger.: Noleptan†; *Ital.:* Terion†; *Spain:* Tosifar.

Multi-ingredient: *Ger.:* Broncho-Noleptan†.

Glaucine (19251-g)

Boldine Dimethyl Ether; DL-832 (*dl*-glaucine phosphate); *dl*-Glaucine; MDL-832 (*dl*-glaucine phosphate). DL-1,2,9,10-Tetramethoxyaporphine.

$C_{21}H_{25}NO_4 = 355.4.$

CAS — 5630-11-5 (dl-glaucine); 73239-87-9 (dl-glaucine phosphate); 475-81-0 (d-glaucine); 5996-06-5 (d-glaucine hydrobromide).

Glaucine is a centrally acting cough suppressant used in non-productive cough (p.1052) which has been studied as the phosphate.

d-Glaucine has been used as the hydrobromide and the hydrochloride as a cough suppressant in eastern Europe. It has been obtained from *Glaucium flavum* (Papaveraceae).

References.

1. Redpath JBS, Pleuvry BJ. Double-blind comparison of the respiratory and sedative effects of codeine phosphate and (±)-glaucine phosphate in human volunteers. *Br J Clin Pharmacol* 1982; **14:** 555–8.
2. Rühle KH, *et al.* Objective evaluation of dextromethorphan and glaucine as antitussive agents. *Br J Clin Pharmacol* 1984; **17:** 521–4.
3. Gastpar H, *et al.*. Efficacy and tolerability of glaucine as an antitussive agent. *Curr Med Res Opin* 1984; **9:** 21–7.

Guacetisal (12801-w)

Guacetisal *(rINN).*

Acetylsalicylic Acid Guaiacol Ester. *o*-Methoxyphenyl salicylate acetate.

$C_{16}H_{14}O_5 = 286.3.$

CAS — 55482-89-8.

Guacetisal has been used in respiratory disorders as an expectorant (see p.1052). It has also been used as an antipyretic to reduce fever (p.1). Doses of 500 mg have been administered by mouth two to three times daily. It has also been administered rectally.

Preparations

Proprietary Preparations (details are given in Part 3)
Ital.: Balsacetil; Broncaspin; Guaiaspir; Guajabronc; Prontomucil.

Guaiacol (2016-z)

Guajacol; Methyl Catechol.

CAS — 90-05-1 (guaiacol); 553-17-3 (guaiacol carbonate); 60296-02-8 (calcium guaiacolglycolate); 4112-89-4 (guaiacol phenylacetate).

Pharmacopoeias. In *Belg., Fr.,* and *Swiss. Fr.* also includes Guaiacol Carbonate.

The main constituent of guaiacol is 2-methoxyphenol, $CH_3O.C_6H_4.OH = 124.1.$

Guaiacol has disinfectant properties and has been used as an expectorant for productive cough (p.1052).

Adverse effects are similar to those of phenol (p.1121).

A wide range of salts and derivatives of guaiacol have been used similarly including the carbonate, cinnamate, ethylglycolate, calcium and sodium glycolates, phenylacetate, and phenylbutyrate. See also Guaiphenesin, p.1061 and Potassium Guaiacolsulfonate, p.1068.

Preparations

Proprietary Preparations (details are given in Part 3)
Ger.: Anastil; *Ital.:* Resina Carbolica Dentilin.

Multi-ingredient: *Austral.:* Waterbury's Compound†; *Belg.:* Baume Dalet; Ebexol†; Eucalyptine Le Brun; Eucalyptine Pholcodine Le Brun; Inalpin; Inopectol†; *Canad.:* Analgesic Balm; Creo-Rectal; Demo-Cineol; Dentalgar; Gouttes Dentaires; Omni-Tuss; Pastilles Valda; Sedatuss; Valda; *Fr.:* Baume Dalet; Bi-Qui-Nol; Biocalyptol; Bronchodermine; Bronchorectine au Citral; Campho-Pneumine; Essence Algerienne; Eucalyptine Le Brun; Eucalyptine Pholcodine; Gaiarsol; Pulmoserum; Rectophedrol; Sirop Boin; Valda; *Ger.:* Anastil†; Cobed†; Dalet-Balsam; Pertix†; Transpulmin†; Zynedo-B†; Zynedo-K†; *Irl.:* Pulmo Bailly; Valda†; *Ital.:* Auricovit†; Biopulmin†; Bronco Valda†; Eucaliptina; Fosfoguaiacol; Glicocinnamina†; Guaiadomus†; Katasma Balsamico†; Lactocol; Lipobalsamo; Otocaina†; Otormon F (Femminile)†; *S.Afr.:* Cocilix†; *Spain:* Bimoxi Mucolitico†; Bronco Aseptilex; Bronco Aseptilex Fuerte; Broncolitic†; Bronquimar; Bronquimar Vit A; Edusan Fte Rectal; Eucalyptospirine; Eucalyptospirine Lact; Maboterpen; Pulmo Grey Balsam; Tos Mai; *Switz.:* Bronchodermine†; Bronchorectine†; Carmol "blanche"†; Liberol; Rectoseptal-Neo Pholcodine; Rectoseptal-Neo simple; Spirogel; *UK:* Dragon Balm; Pulmo Bailly; Valda; *USA:* Methagual.

Guaietolin (12795-v)

Guaietolin *(rINN).*

Glycerylguethol; Glyguetol. 3-(2-Ethoxyphenoxy)propane-1,2-diol.

$C_{11}H_{16}O_4 = 212.2.$

CAS — 63834-83-3.

Guaietolin is an analogue of guaiphenesin which is used as an expectorant (see p.1052). It has been given by mouth in doses of 300 mg two to three times daily.

Preparations

Proprietary Preparations (details are given in Part 3)
Fr.: Guethural.

Guaimesal (1749-r)

Guaimesal *(rINN).*

(±)-2-(*o*-Methoxyphenoxy)-2-methyl-1,3-benzodioxan-4-one.

$C_{16}H_{14}O_5 = 286.3.$

CAS — 81674-79-5.

Guaimesal is reported to have expectorant and antipyretic properties and has been given by mouth in a usual dose of 500 mg two to three times daily as an adjunct in the treatment of respiratory tract disorders. It has also been administered rectally in suppositories.

Guaimesal has been reported to improve fever, cough frequency and intensity, and sputum viscosity in patients with acute or chronic bronchitis.[1] However, as stated in the discussion on the management of cough (p.1052) mucolytics are generally considered to have little effect on lung function and their use in chronic obstructive pulmonary disease is controversial (p.747).

1. Jager EGH. Double-blind, placebo-controlled clinical evaluation of guaimesal in outpatients. *Clin Ther* 1989; **11:** 341–62.

Preparations

Proprietary Preparations (details are given in Part 3)
Ital.: Bronteril.

Guaiphenesin (2018-k)

Guaiphenesin *(BAN).*

Guaifenesin *(USAN, rINN);* Glyceryl Guaiacolate; Glycerylguayacolum; Guaiacol Glycerol Ether; Guaiacyl Glyceryl Ether; Guaifenesina; Guaifenesinum; Guajacolum Glycerolatum. *(RS)*-3-(2-Methoxyphenoxy)propane-1,2-diol.

$C_{10}H_{14}O_4 = 198.2.$

CAS — 93-14-1.

Pharmacopoeias. In *Eur.* (see p.viii), *Jpn,* and *US.*

A white or slightly grey crystalline powder, odourless or with a slight characteristic odour. **Soluble** 1 in 60 to 70 of water; soluble in alcohol, in chloroform, and in propylene glycol; sparingly soluble in glycerol; slightly soluble in ether. **Store** in airtight containers.

Adverse Effects and Precautions

Gastro-intestinal discomfort, nausea, and vomiting have occasionally been reported with guaiphenesin, particularly in very large doses.

Pharmacokinetics

Guaiphenesin is absorbed from the gastro-intestinal tract. It is metabolised and excreted in the urine.

Uses and Administration

Guaiphenesin is reported to increase the volume and reduce the viscosity of tenacious sputum and is used as an expectorant for productive cough. It has been given by mouth in doses of 200 to 400 mg every 4 hours. Children aged 6 to 12 years may be given 100 to 200 mg every 4 hours, and children aged 2 to 6 years 50 to 100 mg every 4 hours. It has been used similarly as the calcium salt.

Infertility. Guaiphenesin given by mouth may improve fertility in women with infertility (p.1239) related to the quality of their cervical mucus.[1]

1. Check JH, *et al.* Improvement of cervical factor with guaifenesin. *Fertil Steril* 1982; **37:** 707–8.

Respiratory disorders. An FDA review of preparations available 'over the counter' concluded that guaiphenesin was an effective expectorant.[1] The use of expectorants for productive cough is discussed on p.1052.

1. Thomas J. Guaiphenesin—an old drug now found to be effective. *Aust J Pharm* 1990; **71:** 101–3.

Uricosuric action. Although guaiphenesin may lower serum-urate concentrations in patients with hyperuricaemia[1] its effect in these patients and in healthy subjects is not considered to be clinically significant.[2]

1. Ramsdell CM, *et al.* Uricosuric effect of glyceryl guaiacolate. *J Rheumatol* 1974; **1:** 114–16.
2. Matheson CE, *et al.* The effect of acute guaifenesin administration on serum uric acid. *Drug Intell Clin Pharm* 1982; **16:** 332–4.

Preparations

USP 23: Dyphylline and Guaifenesin Elixir; Dyphylline and Guaifenesin Tablets; Guaifenesin and Codeine Phosphate Syrup; Guaifenesin and Pseudoephedrine Hydrochloride Capsules; Guaifenesin Capsules; Guaifenesin Syrup; Guaifenesin Tablets; Guaifenesin, Pseudoephedrine Hydrochloride, and Dextromethorphan Hydrobromide Capsules; Theophylline and Guaifenesin Capsules; Theophylline and Guaifenesin Oral Solution.

Proprietary Preparations (details are given in Part 3)
Aust.: Guafen; Myoscain; Resyl; Wick Formel 44 Plus Hustenloser; ***Austral.:*** Robitussin EX; Robitussin†; ***Belg.:*** Vicks Vaposyrup Expectorant; ***Canad.:*** Balminil Expectorant; Benylin-E; Calmylin Expectorant; Cough Syrup Expectorant; Expectorant Cough Formula; Expectorant Cough Syrup; Expectorant Syrup; Koffex Expectorant; Resyl†; Robitussin; Sirop Expectorant; ***Fr.:*** Vicks Vaposyrup Expectorant; ***Ger.:*** Fagusan N; guafrenon†; Gufen N; Larylin†; Nephulon G; Wick Formel 44 plus Husten-Loser; Wick Kinder Formel 44 Husten-Loser; ***Irl.:*** Robitussin Expectorant; ***Ital.:*** Broncovanil; Idropulmina; Resyl; Robitussin†; Vicks Tosse Fluidificante; ***S.Afr.:*** Dimetapp Cough Expectorant†; ***Spain:*** Fluidin; Formulaexpec; Lactocol Expectorante; Robitussin; ***Swed.:*** Resyl; Robitussin†; ***Switz.:*** Bronchol; Resyl; ***UK:*** Benylin Childrens Chesty Coughs; Childrens Chesty Cough Syrup; Do-Do Expectorant Linctus; Expulin Chesty Cough; Famel Expectorant; Famel Honey & Lemon Cough Pastilles†; Jackson's All Fours; Owbridges for Chesty Coughs; Robitussin for Chesty Coughs; Tixylix Chesty Cough; Vicks Vaposyrup for chesty coughs; ***USA:*** Anti-Tuss; Breonesin; Diabetic Tussin EX; Duratuss-G; Fenesin; Gee-Gee; Genatuss; GG-Cen; Glyate; Glycotuss; Glytuss; Guaifenex LA; Halotussin; Humibid; Hytuss; Liquibid; Medi-Tuss†; Monafed; Muco-Fen; Muco-Fen-LA; Mytussin; Naldecon Senior EX; Numobid; Organidin; Pneumomist; Respa-GF; Robitussin; Scot-Tussin Cough Formula†; Scot-Tussin Expectorant; Siltussin; Sinumist-SR; Touro Ex; Tusibron; Uni-tussin.

Multi-ingredient: numerous preparations are listed in Part 3.

Guethol (15580-j)

2-Ethoxyphenol.

$C_8H_{10}O_2$ = 138.2.

CAS — 94-71-3.

Guethol carbonate has been used as an expectorant for productive cough (p.1052) in doses of 170 to 340 mg given 2 or 3 times daily; the nicotinate has also been used in respiratory-tract disorders.

Preparations

Proprietary Preparations (details are given in Part 3)
Fr.: Guethural.

Multi-ingredient: ***Fr.:*** Bronchospray.

Helicidine (13455-c)

Helixinum.

Helicidine is a mucoglycoprotein from the snail *Helix pomatia* that has been used as a cough suppressant.

Preparations

Proprietary Preparations (details are given in Part 3)
Switz.: Helicidine†.

Indanazoline Hydrochloride (11418-a)

Indanazoline Hydrochloride *(rINNM).*

$C_{12}H_{15}N_3$,HCl = 237.7.

CAS — 56601-85-5.

Indanazoline is a sympathomimetic with effects similar to those of naphazoline (p.1064). It is used as the hydrochloride for its vasoconstrictor effect in the management of nasal congestion (p.1052). It is given as nasal drops or as a nasal spray in a concentration equivalent to indanazoline 0.1%.

Preparations

Proprietary Preparations (details are given in Part 3)
Ger.: Farial.

Iodinated Glycerol (4576-k)

Iodinated Glycerol *(BAN, USAN).*

Iodopropylidene Glycerol.

$C_6H_{11}IO_3$ = 258.1.

CAS — 5634-39-9.

An isomeric mixture of iodinated dimers of glycerol.

Iodinated glycerol has been used as an expectorant. It is a methyl derivative of domiodol (p.1058). The limitations of iodides as expectorants are discussed under Cough on p.1052. The actions of iodides and iodine compounds are discussed under Iodine p.1493. Prolonged use of iodinated glycerol has been associated with hypothyroidism and severe skin eruptions; gastro-intestinal disturbances and hypersensitivity reactions have also occurred. Administration of iodinated glycerol to *animals* has resulted in the development of malignant neoplasms.

There have been reports of thyroid dysfunction (both hyperthyroidism and hypothyroidism) following administration of iodinated glycerol to previously euthyroid patients. It was recommended that base-line thyroid function tests should be carried out before commencing treatment with iodinated glycerol;[1] it should be withdrawn if abnormal results are obtained during use.

1. Gittoes NJL, Franklyn JA. Drug-induced thyroid disorders. *Drug Safety* 1995; **13:** 46–55.

Chronic bronchitis. References[1,2] to the use of iodinated glycerol in patients with chronic bronchitis. Although these studies reported some benefits the use of mucolytics or expectorants in chronic obstructive pulmonary disease is controversial, as mentioned on p.747.

1. Repsher LH. Treatment of stable chronic bronchitis with iodinated glycerol: a double-blind, placebo-controlled trial. *J Clin Pharmacol* 1993; **33:** 856–60.
2. Petty TL. The National Mucolytic Study: results of a randomized, double-blind, placebo-controlled study of iodinated glycerol in chronic obstructive bronchitis. *Chest* 1990; **97:** 75–83.

Preparations

Proprietary Preparations (details are given in Part 3)
Canad.: Organidin†; ***USA:*** Iophen; Par Glycerol; R-Gen.

Multi-ingredient: ***Canad.:*** Tussi-Organidin†; ***Ger.:*** Mucolytisches Expectorans†; ***Ital.:*** Golamed Oral; Mucantil; ***Spain:*** Mucorama; Mucorama TS; Respiroma; ***USA:*** Theo-Organidin†; Tusso-DM†.

Ipecacuanha (2020-e)

Ipecac; Ipecacuanha Root; Ipecacuanhae Radix.

CAS — 8012-96-2.

Pharmacopoeias. In *Eur.* (see p.viii), *Int., Jpn,* and *US.*
Eur., Jpn, and *US* also include a monograph for Prepared Ipecacuanha (Ipecacuanhae Pulvis Normatus) or a similar standardised form.

The dried underground organs of *Cephaelis ipecacuanha* (= *Uragoga ipecacuanha*) (Rubiaceae), known in commerce as Matto Grosso ipecacuanha or of *C. acuminata,* (= *U. granatensis*), known in commerce as Costa Rica ipecacuanha, or of a mixture of both species. It contains not less than 2% of total alkaloids, calculated as emetine. USP specifies not less than 2% of ether-soluble alkaloids of which not less than 90% is emetine and cephaeline; the content of cephaeline varies from an amount equal to, to an amount not more than 2.5 times, that of emetine.

Prepared Ipecacuanha (BP) is finely powdered ipecacuanha adjusted with powdered ipecacuanha of lower alkaloidal strength or powdered lactose to contain 1.9 to 2.1% of total alkaloids, calculated as emetine. **Powdered Ipecac** (USP) contains 1.9 to 2.1% of ether-soluble alkaloids, with emetine and cephaeline content as for Ipecacuanha.

Ipecacuanha has a slight odour. Prepared ipecacuanha should be **stored** in airtight containers. Ipecacuanha and prepared ipecacuanha should be protected from light.

NOTE. The BP directs that when Ipecacuanha, Ipecacuanha Root, or Powdered Ipecacuanha is prescribed, Prepared Ipecacuanha shall be dispensed.

Adverse Effects

Large doses of ipecacuanha have an irritant effect on the gastro-intestinal tract, and persistent bloody vomiting or bloody diarrhoea may occur. Mucosal erosions of the entire gastro-intestinal tract have been reported. The absorption of emetine, which is most likely if vomiting does not occur after the administration of emetic doses of ipecacuanha, may give rise to adverse effects on the heart, such as conduction abnormalities or myocardial infarction. These, combined with dehydration due to vomiting may cause vasomotor collapse followed by death.

There have been several reports of chronic abuse of ipecacuanha to induce vomiting in eating disorders; cardiotoxicity and myopathy have occurred and may be a result of accumulation of emetine.

There have also been several reports of ipecacuanha poisoning due to the unwitting substitution of Ipecac Fluidextract (USP XVI) for Ipecac Syrup (USP); the fluidextract was about 14 times the strength of the syrup.

References.

1. Manno BR, Manno JE. Toxicology of ipecac: a review. *Clin Toxicol* 1977; **10:** 221–42.

Prolonged vomiting has been reported in 17% of patients given ipecacuanha in the treatment of poisoning and may lead to gastric rupture, Mallory-Weiss tears of the oesophagogastric junction, cerebrovascular events, and pneumomediastinum and pneumoperitoneum.[1]

1. Bateman DN. Adverse reactions to antidotes. *Adverse Drug React Bull* 1988; **133:** (Dec.): 496–9.

Hypersensitivity. Allergy, characterised by rhinitis, conjunctivitis, and chest tightness, due to inhalation of ipecacuanha dust in packers of ipecacuanha tablets.[1]

1. Luczynska CM, *et al.* Occupational allergy due to inhalation of ipecacuanha dust. *Clin Allergy* 1984; **14:** 169–75.

Treatment of Adverse Effects

After acute overdose of ipecacuanha, activated charcoal is given to delay absorption followed if necessary by gastric lavage. Prolonged vomiting can be controlled by the injection of antiemetics. Fluid and electrolyte imbalance should be corrected and facilities should be available to correct any cardiac effects and subsequent shock.

After the withdrawal of ipecacuanha following chronic abuse, recovery may be prolonged due to the slow elimination of emetine.

Precautions

Ipecacuanha should not be used as an emetic in patients whose condition increases the risk of aspiration or in patients who have taken substances, such as corrosive compounds or petroleum products, that might be especially dangerous if aspirated. Ipecacuanha should not be given to patients in shock or to those at risk from seizures either as a result of their condition or from compounds, such as strychnine, that have been ingested. Patients with cardiovascular disorders are at risk if ipecacuanha is absorbed.

Abuse. Ipecac Syrup has been abused by patients with eating disorders to induce vomiting.[1] Adverse effects of repeated vomiting, such as metabolic complications, aspiration pneumonitis, parotid enlargement, dental abnormalities, and oesophagitis or haematemesis due to mucosal lacerations (the Mallory-Weiss syndrome) may be observed. Cardiotoxicity may occur and fatalities have been reported including one patient who had ingested 90 to 120 mL of ipecac syrup daily for 3 months.[2] It has been suggested that cardiac effects and myopathy following the prolonged abuse of Ipecac Syrup may be due to the long-term accumulation of emetine[3,4] but some workers have expressed doubts.[5]

Cardiomyopathy has also been reported in children to whom ipecacuanha had been administered to produce factitious illness (Munchausen's syndrome by proxy);[6,7] fatalities have occurred.

1. Harris RT. Bulimarexia and related serious eating disorders with medical complications. *Ann Intern Med* 1983; **99:** 800–7.
2. Adler AG, *et al.* Death resulting from ipecac syrup poisoning. *JAMA* 1980; **243:** 1927–8.
3. Palmer EP, Guay AT. Reversible myopathy secondary to abuse of ipecac in patients with major eating disorders. *N Engl J Med* 1985; **313:** 1457–9.
4. Pope HG, *et al.* The epidemiology of ipecac abuse. *N Engl J Med* 1986; **314:** 245–6.
5. Isner JM. Effects of ipecac on the heart. *N Engl J Med* 1986; **314:** 1253.
6. Goebel J, *et al.* Cardiomyopathy from ipecac administration in Munchausen syndrome by proxy. *Pediatrics* 1993; **92:** 601–3.
7. Schneider DJ, *et al.* Clinical and pathologic aspects of cardiomyopathy from ipecac administration in Munchausen's syndrome by proxy. *Pediatrics* 1996; **97:** 902–6.

Interactions

The action of ipecacuanha may be delayed or diminished if it is given with or after charcoal; antiemetics may also diminish its effect (but see below).

Antiemetics. Although poisoning due to agents with antiemetic effects is a theoretical contra-indication to the use of an emetic, few problems occur in practice, and emesis usually occurs satisfactorily.[1]

1. Henry J, Volans G. ABC of poisoning: preventing absorption. *Br Med J* 1984; **289:** 304–5.

Food. Concomitant administration of milk had been believed to impair the emetic efficacy of ipecacuanha but there was no significant difference in the time to onset of vomiting, the duration of vomiting, or the number of episodes in 250 children who were given ipecac syrup with milk compared with 250 given ipecac syrup with clear fluids.[1]

1. Klein-Schwartz W, *et al.* The effect of milk on ipecac-induced emesis. *J Toxicol Clin Toxicol* 1991; **29:** 505–11.

Uses and Administration

Ipecacuanha is used as an expectorant in productive cough (p.1052) in doses of 0.02 to 0.06 mL of Ipecacuanha Liquid Extract (BP) (about 0.4 to 1.2 mg of total alkaloids) and 0.3 to 1 mL of Ipecac Syrup (USP) (about 0.4 to 1.4 mg of total alkaloids).

Ipecacuanha is also used in larger doses as an emetic (but see below). Vomiting usually occurs within 30 minutes of administration by mouth of an emetic dose due to an irritant effect on the gastro-intestinal tract and a central action on the chemoreceptor trigger zone. Doses are usually followed by a copious drink of water or fruit juice; in young children this may be given before the dose. Adults may be given doses of 21 to 42 mg of total alkaloids represented by 15 to 30 mL of Paediatric Ipecacuanha Emetic Mixture (BP) or of Ipecac Syrup (USP). Children aged 6 months to 1 year may be given 7 to 14 mg of total alkaloids, represented by 5 to 10 mL of Paediatric Ipecacuanha Emetic Mixture (BP) or of Ipecac Syrup (USP); older children may be given 21 mg, represented by 15 mL of Paediatric Ipecacuanha Emetic Mixture (BP) or of Ipecac Syrup (USP). Doses may be repeated once only after 20 to 30 minutes if emesis has not occurred.

Ipecacuanha (Ipeca) is used in homoeopathic medicine.

Emesis induction in acute poisoning. It would seem logical to empty the stomach after a poison has been ingested, but the benefits of any procedure designed to achieve this must be weighed against its limitations (it will be of little value if the patient presents late) and the risk of complications. Standard practice in the management of poisoning (p.972) has varied widely, with different procedures favoured at different times and in different countries.

Two techniques of stomach emptying have been very widely employed: emesis induction, with ipecacuanha as the emetic of choice; and gastric lavage. Gastric lavage with a suitable bore tube is perhaps more effective than ipecacuanha,[1] and has tended to be preferred in life-threatening overdose of drugs that can produce rapid loss of consciousness.[2] However there is a risk that it may propel stomach contents beyond the pylorus and thus enhance absorption in some cases.[3]

Ipecacuanha has often been advocated for use in children, in whom gastric lavage may be particularly traumatic, although it is also used in adults. Some workers in the UK do not recommend the use of ipecacuanha syrup outside the hospital since it can occasionally cause protracted vomiting and because some parents, despite instructions, have administered it inappropriately in a moment of panic.[4] However, in the USA, where it is widely advocated that ipecacuanha syrup should be kept in homes with young children, a study of over 24 000 cases of paediatric poisoning concluded that the benefits of early administration at home outweighed the risks.[5] Like gastric lavage, ipecacuanha is sometimes thought to be ineffective when given more than 4 hours after ingestion of toxic agents but its lack of serious adverse effects have led to its general acceptance up to 6 hours after ingestion.[6] A retrospective study[7] in paediatric cases of paracetamol poisoning showed favourable results on reduction of paracetamol absorption when ipecacuanha was administered within 90 minutes of ingestion, but the benefits of emesis on absorption decreased rapidly with time.

Because of the limitations of both methods of gastric emptying a number of studies have addressed the question of whether either is appropriate. Such studies have indicated that the administration of activated charcoal alone, without gastric emptying, is as effective as a combination of both methods.[8-10] This appears to be the case even in severely poisoned patients or those who present within an hour of overdose (in whom gastric emptying is most effective).[10] In consequence there appears to be a trend away from the use of emesis induction or gastric lavage.

1. Auerbach PS, *et al.* Efficacy of gastric emptying: gastric lavage versus emesis induced with ipecac. *Ann Emerg Med* 1986; **15:** 692–8.
2. Krenzelok EP. Selection of a gastric decontamination method for poisoning emergencies. *Clin Pharm* 1989; **8:** 294–5.
3. Saetta JP, *et al.* Gastric emptying procedures in the self-poisoned patient: are we forcing gastric content beyond the pylorus? *J R Soc Med* 1991; **84:** 274–6.
4. Henry J, Volans G. ABC of poisoning: preventing absorption. *Br Med J* 1984; **289:** 304–5.
5. Chafee-Bahamon C, *et al.* Risk assessment of ipecac in the home. *Pediatrics* 1985; **75:** 1105–9.
6. Henry J, Volans G. ABC of poisoning: problems in children. *Br Med J* 1984; **289:** 486–9.
7. Bond GR, *et al.* Influence of time until emesis on the efficacy of decontamination using acetaminophen as a marker in a paediatric population. *Ann Emerg Med* 1993; **22:** 1403–1407.
8. Albertson TE, *et al.* Superiority of activated charcoal alone compared with ipecac and activated charcoal in the treatment of acute toxic ingestions. *Ann Emerg Med* 1989; **18:** 56–9.
9. Merigian KS, *et al.* Prospective evaluation of gastric emptying in the self-poisoned patient. *Am J Emerg Med* 1990; **8:** 479–83.
10. Pond SM, *et al.* Gastric emptying in acute overdose: a prospective randomised controlled trial. *Med J Aust* 1995; **163:** 345–9.

Preparations

BP 1998: Ammonia and Ipecacuanha Mixture; Ipecacuanha Liquid Extract; Ipecacuanha Tincture; Paediatric Ipecacuanha Emetic Mixture;
USP 23: Ipecac Syrup; Powdered Ipecac.

Proprietary Preparations (details are given in Part 3)
Aust.: Ipetitrin; ***Belg.:*** Bromofotyl†; ***Switz.:*** Orpec; ***UK:*** Fennings Little Healers.

Multi-ingredient: ***Austral.:*** Alophen†; Emidote APF†; Prodalix Forte Cough Linctus†; ***Belg.:*** Folcodex; Phenergan Expectorant; Sinetus†; Solucamphre; ***Canad.:*** Bronchisaft; ***Fr.:*** Elixir Contre La Toux Weleda; Humex; Pastilles Monleon; Polypirine; Premidan Adult†; Premidan Infant†; Pulmofluide Ephedrine†; Sirop Pectoral adulte; ***Ger.:*** Expectorans Solucampher†; Monapax mit Dihydrocodein†; Pectolitan mit Codein†; ***Irl.:*** Ipesil; ***Neth.:*** Abdijsiroop (Akker-Siroop)†; Phenergan Expectorant†; ***S.Afr.:*** Efcod†; Efcospect†; Expectco†; Linctus Tussi Infans; Misfans†; ***Spain:*** Alofedina; Buco Regis; Encialina; Fenergan Expectorante; Pectoral Brum; Pulmosepta†; Toscal; Toscal Compuesto; Tuselin Expectorante; ***Switz.:*** Aloinophen; Bromocod N; Bronchalin; Bronchofluid; Cimex Sirop contre la toux; Demo elixir pectoral; Demo gouttes contre la toux; Demo pates pectorales; Demo sirop contre la toux; Demotussil; Dipect†; Escogripp†; Gouttes contre la toux "S"; Hustex†; Neo-Codion Adultes†; Neo-Codion Enfants†; Neo-Codion N; Patussol; Phenergan Expectorant; Sirop antitussif Wyss a base de codeine; Sirop Wyss contre la toux; Solucamphre; Spedro; Thymodrosin; ***UK:*** Buttercup Syrup (Blackcurrant flavour); Buttercup Syrup (Honey and Lemon flavour); Cough-eeze; ES Bronchial Mixture; Galloway's Cough Syrup; Hill's Balsam Expectorant Pastilles; Hill's Balsam Junior Expectorant; Hills Balsam Extra Strong; Honey & Molasses; Jackson's Children's Cough Pastilles; Lemsip Linctus†; Liqufruta Cough Medicine; Mu-Cron Junior; Throaties Family Cough Linctus; Vegetable Cough Remover; ***USA:*** Dasin†; Poison Antidote Kit; Quelidrine; Tusquelin.

Isoaminile (9888-b)

Isoaminile *(BAN, rINN).*

4-Dimethylamino-2-isopropyl-2-phenylpentanonitrile.

$C_{16}H_{24}N_2$ = 244.4.
CAS — 77-51-0.

Pharmacopoeias. In Br.

A colourless or slightly yellow, oily liquid with an amine-like odour. Practically **insoluble** in water; freely soluble in alcohol, in acetone, in chloroform, in ether, and in methyl alcohol; dissolves in dilute acids.

Isoaminile Citrate (5622-z)

Isoaminile Citrate *(BANM, rINNM).*

4-Dimethylamino-2-isopropyl-2-phenylvaleronitrile dihydrogen citrate.

$C_{16}H_{24}N_2,C_6H_8O_7$ = 436.5.
CAS — 126-10-3; 28416-66-2.

Isoaminile is a centrally acting cough suppressant which has actions and uses similar to dextromethorphan hydrobromide (p.1057). Isoaminile is usually given by mouth as the citrate but the cyclamate has also been used. A usual dose of the citrate is 40 mg given three times daily.

Preparations

Proprietary Preparations (details are given in Part 3)
Aust.: Peracon; ***Belg.:*** Peracan†; ***Ger.:*** Peracon; ***Ital.:*** Sedotosse†; ***S.Afr.:*** Peracon; ***UK:*** Dimyril†.

Multi-ingredient: ***S.Afr.:*** Peracon Expectorant.

Letosteine (12893-q)

Letosteine *(pINN).*

2-[2-(Ethoxycarbonylmethylthio)ethyl]thiazolidine-4-carboxylic acid.

$C_{10}H_{17}NO_4S_2$ = 279.4.
CAS — 53943-88-7.

Letosteine is a mucolytic that has been used in the treatment of respiratory disorders associated with productive cough (p.1052) in a dose of 50 mg by mouth three times daily.

Preparations

Proprietary Preparations (details are given in Part 3)
Fr.: Viscotiol; ***Ital.:*** Letoclar†; Letofort; Viscotiol; ***Spain:*** Broluidan.

Levmetamfetamine (17746-y)

l-Deoxyephedrine; Lesoxyephedrine; *l*-Methamphetamine; *l*-Methylamphetamine. (*R*)-*N*,α-Dimethylbenzeneethanamine; (−)-(*R*)-*N*,α-Dimethylphenethylamine.

$C_{10}H_{15}N$ = 149.2.
CAS — 33817-09-3.

Pharmacopoeias. In US.

Levmetamfetamine is the *laevo* isomer of methylamphetamine (p.1482) and is used topically in the treatment of nasal congestion (p.1052).

Preparations

Proprietary Preparations (details are given in Part 3)
USA: Vicks Vapor Inhaler.

Levopropoxyphene Napsylate (5623-c)

Levopropoxyphene Napsylate *(BANM, USAN).*

Levopropoxyphene Napsilate *(rINNM)*; 29866. (1*R*,2*S*)-1-Benzyl-3-dimethylamino-2-methyl-1-phenylpropyl propionate naphthalene-2-sulphonate monohydrate.

$C_{22}H_{29}NO_2,C_{10}H_8O_3S,H_2O$ = 565.7.
CAS — 2338-37-6 (levopropoxyphene); 5714-90-9 (anhydrous levopropoxyphene napsylate); 55557-30-7 (levopropoxyphene napsylate monohydrate).

Levopropoxyphene napsylate has been used as a centrally acting cough suppressant for non-productive cough (p.1052). Unlike the dextro isomer, dextropropoxyphene, levopropoxyphene has little or no analgesic activity. It has also been given as the dibudinate.

Preparations

Proprietary Preparations (details are given in Part 3)
Ger.: Sotornit†.

Marrubium (11837-j)

Andornkraut; Herba Marrubii; White Horehound.

Pharmacopoeias. In Aust. and Fr.

Marrubium is the flower or leaf of *Marrubium vulgare* (Labiatae). It is used for its supposed expectorant properties in herbal preparations for the treatment of cough. It has also been used as a flavouring.

Preparations

Proprietary Preparations (details are given in Part 3)
Ger.: Angocin Bronchialtropfen.

Multi-ingredient: ***Aust.:*** Asthmatee; Gallen- und Lebertee; Krautertee Nr 28; Krautertee Nr 7; St Radegunder Leber-Galle-Tee; ***Austral.:*** Verbascum Complex; ***Fr.:*** Elixir Contre La Toux Weleda; Marrubene Codethyline; Mediflor Tisane Hypotensive†; Tisanes de l'Abbe Hamon no 15; Tossarel; ***Ger.:*** Gastro-Vial†; Neo-Codion†; Toxorephan†; ***Ital.:*** Broncosedina; ***Spain:*** Iodocafedrina†; Stomosan; ***Switz.:*** Bronchosan; Hederix; Neo-Codion†; Tisane hepatique et biliaire "H"†; ***UK:*** Catarrh; Catarrh Tablets; Catarrh-eeze; Chest Mixture; Cough Elixir; Cough-eeze; Herb and Honey Cough Elixir; Honey & Molasses; Horehound and Aniseed Cough Mixture; Vegetable Cough Remover.

Menglytate (11608-n)

Menglytate *(rINN).*

Menthol Ethylglycolate. *p*-Menth-3-yl ethoxyacetate.

$C_{14}H_{26}O_3$ = 242.4.
CAS — 579-94-2.

Menglytate is an ingredient of a number of preparations promoted for the treatment of cough.

Preparations

Proprietary Preparations (details are given in Part 3)
Multi-ingredient: ***Aust.:*** Expigen; ***Ital.:*** Coryfin C; Neo Borocillina Balsamica; Neo Borocillina Tosse Compresse; Neo Borocillina Tosse Gocce†; Neo Borocillina Tosse Sciroppo.

Methoxyphenamine Hydrochloride (2081-n)

Methoxyphenamine Hydrochloride *(BANM, rINNM).*

Methoxiphenadrin Hydrochloride; Mexyphamine Hydrochloride. 2-Methoxy-*N*α-dimethylphenethylamine hydrochloride.

$C_{11}H_{17}NO,HCl$ = 215.7.
CAS — 93-30-1 (methoxyphenamine); 5588-10-3 (methoxyphenamine hydrochloride).

Methoxyphenamine is a sympathomimetic with effects similar to those of ephedrine (p.1059), given by mouth as the hydrochloride. It is used as a bronchodilator and in combination with other ingredients for the relief of cough and nasal congestion.

Preparations

Proprietary Preparations (details are given in Part 3)
Ital.: Euspirol†.

Multi-ingredient: ***Austral.:*** Orthoxicol Cough Suppressant For Children†; Orthoxicol Cough Suppressant†; Orthoxicol Expectorant (with antihistamine)†; Orthoxicol Expectorant†; Orthoxicol Nasal Relief with Antihistamine†; Orthoxicol Nasal Relief†; Orthoxicol†; ***Belg.:*** Orthoxicol; ***Irl.:*** Casacol; Orthoxicol†; ***S.Afr.:*** Orthoxicol.

Methyl Cysteine Hydrochloride (607-f)

Methyl Cysteine Hydrochloride *(BANM).*

Mecysteine Hydrochloride *(rINNM)*; Methylcysteine Hydrochloride. Methyl L-2-amino-3-mercaptopropionate hydrochloride.

$C_4H_9NO_2S,HCl = 171.6.$

CAS — 2485-62-3 (methyl cysteine); 18598-63-5 (methyl cysteine hydrochloride); 5714-80-7 (methyl cysteine hydrochloride).

Adverse Effects and Precautions

Nausea and heartburn have occasionally been reported. Since mucolytics may disrupt the gastric mucosal barrier methyl cysteine hydrochloride should be used with caution in patients with a history of peptic ulceration.

Uses and Administration

Methyl cysteine hydrochloride is used as a mucolytic in respiratory disorders associated with productive cough (p.1052). It is given by mouth in a dose of 100 to 200 mg three or four times daily before meals reduced to 200 mg twice daily after 6 weeks. Children over 5 years of age may be given 100 mg three times daily. It has also been administered by inhalation.

Respiratory disorders. Methyl cysteine hydrochloride given by mouth has reduced symptoms of cough in patients with chronic bronchitis (p.747) or other respiratory disorders but its effect on sputum production and pulmonary function has been variable.[1,2]

1. Aylward M, *et al.* Clinical therapeutic evaluation of methylcysteine hydrochloride in patients with chronic obstructive bronchitis: a balanced double-blind trial with placebo control. *Curr Med Res Opin* 1978; **5:** 461–71.
2. Sahay JN, *et al.* The effect of methyl cysteine (Visclair) in respiratory diseases: a pilot study. *Clin Trials J* 1982; **19:** 137–43.

Preparations

Proprietary Preparations (details are given in Part 3)
Irl.: Visclair; ***Ital.:*** Actiol†; ***UK:*** Visclair.

Multi-ingredient: ***Ital.:*** Broncometil†; Donatiol.

Methyl Diacetylcysteinate (13491-x)

Methyl Dacisteine. Methyl N,S-diacetyl-L-cysteinate.

$C_8H_{13}NO_4S = 219.3.$

CAS — 19547-88-7.

NOTE. Dacisteine is *rINN.*

Like acetylcysteine (p.1052), methyl diacetylcysteinate has been used as a mucolytic in respiratory disorders associated with productive cough (p.1052). It has been given by mouth in a dose of 600 mg daily, divided into 3 or 4 doses.

Preparations

Proprietary Preparations (details are given in Part 3)
Fr.: Mucothiol; ***Ital.:*** Mucothiol.

Methylephedrine Hydrochloride (2083-m)

Methylephedrine Hydrochloride *(BANM).*

2-Dimethylamino-1-phenylpropan-1-ol hydrochloride.

$C_{11}H_{17}NO,HCl = 215.7.$

CAS — 552-79-4 (methylephedrine, −); 1201-56-5 (methylephedrine, ±); 38455-90-2 (methylephedrine hydrochloride, −); 942-46-1 (methylephedrine hydrochloride, ±); 18760-80-0 (methylephedrine hydrochloride, ±).

Pharmacopoeias. Jpn includes the (±)-form, *dl*-Methylephedrine Hydrochloride.

Methylephedrine hydrochloride is a sympathomimetic with effects similar to those of ephedrine (p.1059). It has been used as a bronchodilator and is given by mouth in combination preparations for the relief of cough and nasal congestion.

Preparations

Proprietary Preparations (details are given in Part 3)

Multi-ingredient: ***Aust.:*** Tussoretardin; ***Ger.:*** Ilvico†; Keldrin†; Tussoretard†; ***S.Afr.:*** Ilvico; ***Switz.:*** Tossamine plus.

Metyzoline Hydrochloride (6183-c)

Metyzoline Hydrochloride *(BANM).*

Metizoline Hydrochloride *(USAN, rINNM)*; EX-10-781; RMI-10482A. 2-(2-Methylbenzo[*b*]thienylmethyl)-2-imidazoline hydrochloride.

$C_{13}H_{14}N_2S,HCl = 266.8.$

CAS — 17692-22-7 (metyzoline); 5090-37-9 (metyzoline hydrochloride).

Metyzoline hydrochloride is a sympathomimetic with effects similar to those of naphazoline (p.1064) used for its vasoconstrictor activity in the treatment of nasal congestion. It is given as a 0.05% nasal spray.

Preparations

Proprietary Preparations (details are given in Part 3)
Ital.: Eunasin.

Moguisteine (11023-f)

Moguisteine *(rINN).*

Ethyl (±)-2-[(o-methoxyphenoxy)methyl]-β-oxo-thiazolidine-propionate.

$C_{16}H_{21}NO_5S = 339.4.$

CAS — 119637-67-1.

Moguisteine has been investigated as a cough suppressant. It is reported to have a peripheral mechanism of action.

References.

1. Aversa C, *et al.* Clinical trial of the efficacy and safety of moguisteine in patients with cough associated with chronic respiratory diseases. *Drugs Exp Clin Res* 1993; **19:** 273–9.
2. Fasciolo G, *et al.* Efficacy and safety of moguisteine in comparison with levodropropizine in patients with cough associated with chronic obstructive pulmonary disease, lung cancer, or pulmonary fibrosis. *Curr Ther Res* 1994; **55:** 251–61.

Morclofone (14231-p)

Morclofone *(rINN).*

Dimeclofenone; Morclophon. 4′-Chloro-3,5-dimethoxy-4-(2-morpholinoethoxy)benzophenone.

$C_{21}H_{24}ClNO_5 = 405.9.$

CAS — 31848-01-8 (morclofone); 31848-02-9 (morclofone hydrochloride).

Morclofone is a centrally acting cough suppressant used for non-productive cough (p.1052) by mouth in doses of 150 mg four to six times daily. It has also been given as the hydrochloride.

Preparations

Proprietary Preparations (details are given in Part 3)
Ital.: Plausitin; ***Switz.:*** Nitux.

Naphazoline (9504-a)

Naphazoline *(BAN, rINN).*

2-(1-Naphthylmethyl)-2-imidazoline.

$C_{14}H_{14}N_2 = 210.3.$

CAS — 835-31-4.

Naphazoline Hydrochloride (2085-v)

Naphazoline Hydrochloride *(BANM, rINNM).*

Naphazolini Hydrochloridum.

$C_{14}H_{14}N_2,HCl = 246.7.$

CAS — 550-99-2.

Pharmacopoeias. In *Eur.* (see p.viii), *Jpn*, and *US.*

A white or almost white, odourless, crystalline powder. Freely **soluble** in water; soluble or freely soluble in alcohol; very slightly soluble in chloroform; practically insoluble in ether. A 1% solution in water has a pH of 5.0 to 6.6. **Store** in airtight containers. Protect from light.

Naphazoline Nitrate (2086-g)

Naphazoline Nitrate *(BANM, rINNM).*

Naphazolini Nitras; Naphazolinium Nitricum; Naphthizinum.

$C_{14}H_{14}N_2,HNO_3 = 273.3.$

CAS — 5144-52-5.

Pharmacopoeias. In *Eur.* (see p.viii), *Jpn*, and *Pol.*

A white or almost white, crystalline powder. Sparingly **soluble** in water; soluble in alcohol; practically insoluble in ether. A 1% solution in water has a pH of 5.0 to 6.5. **Protect** from light.

Adverse Effects, Treatment, and Precautions

After local use of naphazoline transient irritation may occur. Rebound congestion may occur after frequent or prolonged use. Systemic effects, including nausea, headache, and dizziness have occurred after local administration. Overdosage or accidental administration by mouth may cause depression of the central nervous system with marked reduction of body temperature and bradycardia, sweating, drowsiness, and coma, particularly in children; it should be used with great caution, if at all, in infants and young children. Liberation of pigment granules from the iris may occur after ocular administration of naphazoline, especially in high doses to elderly patients. Hypertension may be followed by rebound hypotension. Treatment of side-effects is symptomatic.

For the adverse effects of sympathomimetics in general, and precautions to be observed, see p.951.

Interactions

Since naphazoline is absorbed through the nasal mucosa interactions may follow topical application. An authoritative source in the UK considers that all sympathomimetic nasal decongestants are liable to cause a hypertensive crisis if used during treatment with an MAOI. For the interactions of sympathomimetics in general, see p.951.

Pharmacokinetics

Systemic absorption has been reported following topical application of solutions of naphazoline. It is not used systemically, but it is readily absorbed from the gastro-intestinal tract.

Uses and Administration

Naphazoline is a sympathomimetic (p.951) with marked alpha-adrenergic activity. It is a vasoconstrictor with a rapid and prolonged action in reducing swelling and congestion when applied to mucous membranes.

Naphazoline and its salts are used for the symptomatic relief of nasal congestion (p.1052). Solutions containing 0.05 to 0.1% of the hydrochloride or the nitrate may be applied topically as nasal drops or a spray usually up to once every 6 hours. Children over 6 years of age have used a preparation containing 0.025%.

Solutions containing up to 0.1% of naphazoline hydrochloride have been instilled into the eye as a conjunctival decongestant.

Naphazoline acetate has also been used in nasal preparations.

Preparations

USP 23: Naphazoline Hydrochloride Nasal Solution; Naphazoline Hydrochloride Ophthalmic Solution.

Proprietary Preparations (details are given in Part 3)
Aust.: Aconex; Coldan; Isoftal; Privin; Rhinon; Rhinoperd; ***Austral.:*** Albalon; Clear Eyes; Naphcon; Optazine; ***Belg.:*** Albalon; Naphcon†; Neusinol; Priciasol; Vasocedine; ***Canad.:*** Ak-Con; Albalon Liquifilm; Allergy Drops; Clear Eyes; Diopticon; Naphcon Forte; Opcon†; Privine†; Red Away; Rhino-Mex-N; RO-Naphz; Vasocon; ***Ger.:*** Piniol; Privin; Proculin; Rhinex; Vistalbalon; ***Irl.:*** Albalon†; ***Ital.:*** Alfa†; Collirio Alfa; Desamin Same; Imidazyl; Imizol; Iridina Due; Naftazolina; Pupilla; Ran†; Rinazina; Rino Naftazolina; Rinoftal†; Transpulmina Rino†; Virginiana Gocce Verdi; ***Neth.:*** Albalon Liquifilm†; ***S.Afr.:*** Albalon; Murine Clear Eyes; ***Spain:*** Alfa; Miraclar; Privina; Vasoconstrictor Pensa; ***Swed.:*** Rimidol; ***Switz.:*** Albalon; Minha; ***UK:*** Murine; ***USA:*** Ak-Con; Albalon; Allerest; Allergy Drops; Allersol; Clear Eyes; Comfort Eye Drops; Degest; Nafazair; Naphcon; Privine; Vasocon.

Multi-ingredient: ***Aust.:*** Coldistan; Coldophthal; Histophtal; Luuf-Nasenspray; Ophtaguttal; Rectosan; Rhinodrin; Rhinon; Rhinoperd comp; ***Austral.:*** Albalon-A Liquifilm; Antistine-Privine; In A Wink; Naphcon-A; Optazine A†; Optrex Medicated; ***Belg.:*** Deltarhinol; Diphenhydramine Constrictor; Naphcon-A†; Neofenox; Sofraline; Sofrasolone; Zincfrin Antihistaminicum; ***Canad.:*** Albalon-A Liquifilm; Blue Collyrium; Collyre Bleu; Cooper AR; Diopticon A; Naphcon-A; Onrectal; Opcon-A; Rhino-Mex; Vasocon-A; Zincfrin-A; ***Fr.:*** Collyre Bleu; Derinox; Frazoline; Soframycine Naphazoline; ***Ger.:*** Alformin†; Antistin-Privin; Aquapred†; Bisrenin; Boro-Hexamin†; Borocarpin-N†; Borocarpin†; Combiamid; Dexa-Siozwo N; Diabenyl-Rhinex; Diabenyl†; duraforte†; duraultra; duraultra forte†; Idril; Konjunktival Thilo; Lensch†; Oculosan N; Ophtalmin; Ophtocain; Ophtomydrol†; Ophtopur-N; Proculens N†; Prothanon†; Rhinosovil; Siozwo N; Siozwo†; Solupen-D; Solupen†; Stipo; Syncarpin; Tele-Stulln; ***Ital.:*** Adrenosin Composto†; Alfaflor; Antisettico Astringente Sedativo; Antistin-Privina; Citroftalmina VC; Collirio Alfa Antistaminico; Corizzina; Deltarinolo; Fenox; Fotofil; Genalfa; Idroneomicil; Imidazyl Antistaminico; Indaco;

Lucisan; Oftalmil; Oftalzina; Pupilla Antistaminico; Rinocidina; Rinospray; Rinovit Nube; Vapor Sol†; Zinc-Imizol; Zincoimidazyl†; *Norw.:* Antistin-Privin†; *S.Afr.:* Albalon-A; Antistin-Privin; Covomycin; Covosan; ENT; Fenox; Nasdro; Oculosan; Universal Nasal Drops; Wink; Zincfrin-A†; *Spain:* Alergoftal; Centilux; Clo Zinc; Coliriocilina Adren Astr; Dexa Vasoc; Epistaxol; Euboral; Fluo Vasoc; Kanafosal; Kanafosal Predni; Lidrone; Nasal Rovi†; Oftalmol Dexa; Oftalmol Ocular; Ojosbel; Ojosbel Azul; Polirino†; Rinosular†; Rinovel; Vasocon Ant; Vasoconstr; Zolina; *Swed.:* Antasten-Privin; *Switz.:* Antistin-Privin; Collyre Alpha; Collyre Bleu Laiter; Derinox; Gouttes nasales N; Napharzol†; Oculosan; Optazine; Zincfrin-A†; *UK:* Optrex Clear Eyes; Optrex Eye Dew; Vasocon-A†; *USA:* 4-Way Fast Acting; Ak-Con-A; Antazoline-V; Clear Eyes ACR; Estivin; Maximum Strength Allergy Drops; Muro's Opcon; Nafazair A; Naphazole-A; Naphazoline Plus; Naphcon-A; Naphoptic-A; Opcon-A; Vaso-Clear; VasoClear A; Vasocon-A.

Used as an adjunct in: Fr.: Xylocaine; *Spain:* Anest Compuesto; Anestesico.

Neltenexine (13828-g)

Neltenexine *(rINN)*.

4′,6′-Dibromo-α-[(*trans*-4-hydroxycyclohexyl)amino]-2-thiophene-carboxy-*o*-toluidide.

$C_{18}H_{20}Br_2N_2O_2S$ = 488.2.

CAS — 99453-84-6.

Neltenexine is a mucolytic that is given by mouth as the monohydrate, in usual doses of 37.4 mg three times daily, in patients with respiratory disorders associated with productive cough (p.1052) . Neltenexine has also been given rectally as the hydrochloride.

Preparations

Proprietary Preparations (details are given in Part 3)
Ital.: Alveoten; Muco4; Tenoxol.

Nepinalone (13829-q)

Nepinalone *(rINN)*.

(±)-3,4-Dihydro-1-methyl-1-(2-piperidinoethyl)-2(1*H*)-naphthalenone.

$C_{18}H_{25}NO$ = 271.4.

CAS — 22443-11-4.

Nepinalone has been used as the hydrochloride as a cough suppressant in non-productive cough (p.1052). Doses of nepinalone hydrochloride 10 mg have been given three times daily by mouth.

Preparations

Proprietary Preparations (details are given in Part 3)
Ital.: Nepituss; Placatus; Tussolvina.

Nesosteine (19564-d)

Nesosteine *(rINN)*.

CO-1177 (nesosteine sodium). *o*-(3-Thiazolidinylcarbonyl)benzoic acid.

$C_{11}H_{11}NO_3S$ = 237.3.

CAS — 84233-61-4 (nesosteine); 84210-62-8 (nesosteine sodium).

Nesosteine has been investigated as the sodium salt for its mucolytic actions.

References.

1. Siquet J. Clinical trial with a new mucolytic agent (CO1177) in the treatment of patients with chronic bronchitis. *Acta Ther* 1985; **11:** 61–7.
2. Mbuyamba P. Clinical trial with CO-1177: a preliminary report. *Int J Clin Pharmacol Res* 1986; **VI:** 119–21.
3. Braga PC, *et al.* Preliminary data on the action of nesosteine, a mucomodifying drug, on mucociliary transport. *J Int Med Res* 1987; **15:** 57–61.
4. Braga PC, *et al.* Rheological profile of nesosteine: a new mucoactive agent. *Int J Clin Pharmacol Res* 1989; **IX:** 77–83.

Nicocodine (10339-e)

Nicocodine *(BAN, rINN)*.

6-Nicotinoylcodeine; 3-*O*-Methyl-6-*O*-nicotinoylmorphine.

$C_{24}H_{24}N_2O_4$ = 404.5.

CAS — 3688-66-2.

Nicocodine is an opioid related to codeine (p.26). It has been used as the hydrochloride for its central cough suppressant effects in non-productive cough (p.1052). Nicocodine hydrochloride is given by mouth in doses of 5 to 7.5 mg up to three times daily.

Preparations

Proprietary Preparations (details are given in Part 3)
Aust.: Tusscodin.

Normethadone Hydrochloride (13033-k)

Normethadone Hydrochloride *(BANM, rINNM)*.

Desmethylmethadone Hydrochloride; Hoechst-10582 (normethadone); Phenyldimazone Hydrochloride. 6-Dimethylamino-4,4-diphenylhexan-3-one hydrochloride.

$C_{20}H_{25}NO,HCl$ = 331.9.

CAS — 467-85-6 (normethadone); 847-84-7 (normethadone hydrochloride).

Normethadone is closely related to methadone (p.53). The hydrochloride is given by mouth as a cough suppressant in non-productive cough.

References.

1. Gourlay GK, Coulthard K. The role of naloxone infusions in the treatment of overdoses of long half-life narcotic agonists: application to nor-methadone. *Br J Clin Pharmacol* 1983; **15:** 269–72.

Preparations

Proprietary Preparations (details are given in Part 3)
Multi-ingredient: *Canad.:* Cophylac.

Noscapine (5625-a)

Noscapine *(BAN, rINN)*.

Narcotine; L-α-Narcotine; Noscapinum; NSC-5366. (3*S*)-6,7-Dimethoxy-3-[(5*R*)-5,6,7,8-tetrahydro-4-methoxy-6-methyl-1,3-dioxolo[4,5-*g*]isoquinolin-5-yl]phthalide.

$C_{22}H_{23}NO_7$ = 413.4.

CAS — 128-62-1.

Pharmacopoeias. In *Eur.* (see p.viii), *Int.*, *Jpn*, and *US.*

Noscapine is an alkaloid obtained from opium. It occurs as colourless crystals or as a fine white or practically white crystalline powder.

Practically **insoluble** in water at 20°, very slightly soluble at 100°; slightly soluble in alcohol and in ether; soluble in acetone; freely soluble in chloroform; dissolves in strong acids although the base may be precipitated on dilution with water. **Protect** from light.

Noscapine Camsylate (12514-m)

Camphoscapine. Noscapine camphor-10-sulphonate.

$C_{22}H_{23}NO_7,C_{10}H_{16}O_4S$ = 645.7.

CAS — 25333-79-3.

Noscapine Hydrochloride (5626-t)

Noscapine Hydrochloride *(BANM, rINNM)*.

Narcotine Hydrochloride; Noscapini Hydrochloridum; Noscapinium Chloride.

$C_{22}H_{23}NO_7,HCl,H_2O$ = 467.9.

CAS — 912-60-7 (anhydrous noscapine hydrochloride).

Pharmacopoeias. In *Eur.* (see p.viii), *Int.*, and *US* (all with H_2O); in *Jpn* (with xH_2O).

Colourless crystals or a white crystalline powder; hygroscopic. Freely **soluble** in water and in alcohol; practically insoluble in ether. A 2% solution in water has a pH not below 3.0. Aqueous solutions may deposit the base on standing. **Protect** from light.

Adverse Effects and Precautions

As for Dextromethorphan, p.1057. Hypersensitivity reactions have been reported.

The CSM in the UK have stood by their recommendation[1] that products containing noscapine should be contra-indicated in women of child-bearing potential (because of potential mutagenic effects[2]) after criticism that the decision was based solely on the results of *in-vitro* work.[3]

1. Asscher AW, Fowler LK. Papaveretum in women of childbearing potential. *Br Med J* 1991; **303:** 648.
2. Committee on Safety of Medicines. Genotoxicity of papaveretum and noscapine. *Current Problems 31* 1991.
3. Allen S, *et al.* Papaveretum in women of child bearing potential. *Br Med J* 1991; **303:** 647.

Interactions

Noscapine should not be given concomitantly with alcohol or other CNS depressants.

Pharmacokinetics

References to the pharmacokinetics of noscapine.

1. Karlsson MO, *et al.* Pharmacokinetics of oral noscapine. *Eur J Clin Pharmacol* 1990; **39:** 275–9.
2. Karlsson MO, Dahlstrom B. Serum protein binding of noscapine: influence of a reversible hydrolysis. *J Pharm Pharmacol* 1990; **42:** 140–3.

Uses and Administration

Noscapine is a centrally acting cough suppressant that has actions and uses similar to those of dextromethorphan hydrobromide (p.1058). It is given by mouth in a dose of up to 50 mg three times a day. It has also been given as the camsylate, embonate, and the hydrochloride.

Preparations

Proprietary Preparations (details are given in Part 3)
Belg.: Noscaflex; *Ger.:* Capval; Lyobex retard†; *Neth.:* Finipect; Roter Noscapect†; *S.Afr.:* Nitepax; *Spain:* Tuscalman; *Swed.:* Nipaxon; *Switz.:* Tussanil N.

Multi-ingredient: *Aust.:* Pneumopect†; Tuscalman; *Belg.:* Noscaflex; Rosils; Sinetus†; *Fr.:* Broncho-Tulisan Eucalyptol; Tussisedal; *Ger.:* Tussoretard†; *Ital.:* Difmetus Compositum; Difmetus†; Ribelfan; Tuscalman; *S.Afr.:* Degoran†; *Spain:* Tuscalman†; *Swed.:* Spasmofen; *Switz.:* Brosoline-Rectocaps; Hederix; No Grip; Noscalin†; Noscorex; Tossamine; Tossamine plus; Tuscalman; Tussanil Compositum.

Oxeladin Citrate (5627-x)

Oxeladin Citrate *(BANM, rINNM)*.

2-(2-Diethylaminoethoxy)ethyl 2-ethyl-2-phenylbutyrate dihydrogen citrate.

$C_{20}H_{33}NO_3,C_6H_8O_7$ = 527.6.

CAS — 468-61-1 (oxeladin); 52432-72-1 (oxeladin citrate).

Oxeladin citrate has been given by mouth as a centrally acting cough suppressant for non-productive cough (p.1052). It has been reported to be mutagenic *in vitro*, and many preparations have since been withdrawn.

Preparations

Proprietary Preparations (details are given in Part 3)
Belg.: Paxeladine†; *Fr.:* Paxeladine; *Ger.:* Dorex-retard†; *Ital.:* Pectamol†; *Norw.:* Pectamol.

Multi-ingredient: *Fr.:* Paxeladine Noctee; *Ger.:* Dorex Hustensaft N mit Oxeladin†; Kontagripp-RR†; Kontagripp†; Toramin N†; Tussinfantum†; *Ital.:* Tussiflex.

Oxolamine (14838-c)

Oxolamine *(rINN)*.

683-M. 5-[2-(Diethylamino)ethyl]-3-phenyl-1,2,4-oxadiazole.

$C_{14}H_{19}N_3O$ = 245.3.

CAS — 959-14-8.

Oxolamine Citrate (13067-b)

Oxolamine Citrate *(rINNM)*.

AF-438; SKF-9976.

$C_{14}H_{19}N_3O,C_6H_8O_7$ = 437.4.

CAS — 1949-20-8.

Oxolamine Phosphate (14238-z)

Oxolamine Phosphate *(rINNM)*.

CAS — 1949-19-5.

Oxolamine is a cough suppressant with a predominantly peripheral action that has been used for non-productive cough (p.1052). Doses of 100 to 200 mg have been given by mouth as the citrate or phosphate. It has also been given as the tannate.

Hallucinations in children have been reported after its use.

References.

1. McEwen J, *et al.* Hallucinations in children caused by oxolamine citrate. *Med J Aust* 1989; **150:** 449–52.

Preparations

Proprietary Preparations (details are given in Part 3)
Austral.: Bredon†; *Ital.:* Gantrimex; Perebron; Tussibron; *Spain:* Perebron.

Multi-ingredient: *Ital.:* Broncopiam†; Fargepirina†; Pulmotrim†; Temoxa†; Uniplus; Upsa Plus; *Spain:* Bequipecto; Dimayon; Pectoral Funk Antitus.

Oxymetazoline Hydrochloride

(2093-v)

Oxymetazoline Hydrochloride *(BANM, USAN, rINNM)*.

H-990; Oxymetazolini Hydrochloridum; Sch-9384.

$C_{16}H_{24}N_2O,HCl$ = 296.8.

CAS — 2315-02-8.

Pharmacopoeias. In *Eur.* (see p.viii) and *US.*

A white or practically white, hygroscopic, crystalline powder. **Soluble** 1 in 6.7 of water, 1 in 3.6 of alcohol, and 1 in 862 of chloroform; practically insoluble in ether. A 5% solution in water has a pH of 4.0 to 6.5. **Store** in airtight containers.

Adverse Effects and Precautions

As for Naphazoline, p.1064.

After local use of oxymetazoline transient irritation may occur. Rebound congestion may occur after frequent or prolonged nasal use. Systemic effects have occurred after local administration.

Porphyria. Oxymetazoline has been associated with clinical exacerbations of porphyria and is considered unsafe in porphyric patients.[1]

1. Moore MR, McColl KEL. *Porphyria: drug lists*. Glasgow: Porphyria Research Unit, University of Glasgow, 1991.

Interactions

Since oxymetazoline is absorbed through the mucosa interactions may follow topical application. An authoritative source in the UK considers that all sympathomimetic nasal decongestants are liable to cause a hypertensive crisis if used during treatment with an MAOI. For the interactions of sympathomimetics in general, see p.951.

Uses and Administration

Oxymetazoline is a direct-acting sympathomimetic (p.951) with marked alpha-adrenergic activity. It is a vasoconstrictor which reduces swelling and congestion when applied to mucous membranes. It acts within a few minutes and the effect lasts for up to 12 hours. It is used as the hydrochloride for the symptomatic relief of nasal congestion (p.1052). A 0.05% solution of oxymetazoline hydrochloride is applied topically as nasal drops or a spray to each nostril usually twice daily as required.

A 0.025% solution of oxymetazoline hydrochloride may be instilled into the eye as a conjunctival decongestant.

Hypersensitivity. Anaphylactic reactions are usually treated with adrenaline (p.816), but occasions do arise when it is not always readily available. One patient who had suffered previous reactions to aspirin or ibuprofen that had been treated with corticosteroid and adrenaline suffered another attack following a dose of ketoprofen.[1] She was able to relieve the symptoms, including the potentially fatal upper airways obstruction, by pumping 12 inhalations of oxymetazoline nasal solution into each nostril.

1. Kim KT, *et al.* Use of non-prescription decongestant to abort anaphylaxis. *Lancet* 1993; **341:** 439. Correction. *ibid.*; 704.

Preparations

USP 23: Oxymetazoline Hydrochloride Nasal Solution; Oxymetazoline Hydrochloride Ophthalmic Solution.

Proprietary Preparations (details are given in Part 3)
Aust.: Nasivin; ***Austral.:*** Coldrex Nasal Spray†; Dimetapp 12 Hour Nasal; Drixine Nasal; Ordov Sinudec; ***Belg.:*** Nesivine; Vicks Sinex; ***Canad.:*** Dristan; Drixoral; Duration†; Nafrine; Ocuclear; Vicks Sinex; Visine Workplace; ***Fr.:*** Aturgyl; Iliadine†; ***Ger.:*** Nasivin gegen Schnupfen; Nasivinetten gegen Schnupfen; Vistoxyn; Wick Sinex; ***Irl.:*** Afrazine†; Dristan; Vicks Sinex; ***Ital.:*** Actifed Nasale; Nasivin; Oxilin; Rino Calyptol; ***Neth.:*** Dampo; Nasivin; Nezeril†; Oxylin Liquifilm†; ***Norw.:*** Iliadin; Rhinox; ***S.Afr.:*** Advil NS†; Afrin†; Drixine; Iliadin; Nose-X†; Oxylin; Sinustop†; ***Spain:*** Alerfrin; Descongestan; Egarone Oximetazolina; Humoxal; Idasal Nebulizador; Inalintra; Nasaltex†; Nasovalda; Nebulicina; Oftinal; Respibien; Respir; Rinocorin; Rinodif; Rinofol†; Sinust†; Tioclin†; Utabon; ***Swed.:*** Iliadin; Nasin; Nezeril; Zolin; ***Switz.:*** Nasivine; Nasivinetten; Vistoxyn; ***UK:*** Afrazine; Dristan; Sudafed Nasal Spray; ***USA:*** 12 Hour Sinarest; 4-Way Long Lasting; Afrin; Allerest 12 Hour Nasal; Cheracol Nasal; Chlorphed-LA; Dristan 12-hr Nasal Decongestant Spray; Dristan Long Lasting; Duramist Plus; Duration; Genasal; Maximum Strength Nasal Decongestant; Nasal Relief; Neo-Synephrine 12 Hour; Nostrilla; NTZ Long Acting Nasal; Ocuclear; Twice-A-Day; Vicks Sinex 12-Hour; Visine LR.

Multi-ingredient: ***Aust.:*** Wick Sinex; ***Austral.:*** Euky Bear Nasex; Vasylox; Vicks Sinex; ***Fr.:*** Sinex; ***Ger.:*** Larylin Nasenspray N; Nasicortin†; ***Ital.:*** Nasicortin; Triaminic; Vicks Sinex; ***Neth.:*** Vicks Sinex; ***S.Afr.:*** Nazene-Z; ***Spain:*** Antirrinum; Corilisina; Egarone; Orto Nasal; Respir Balsamico; Vicks Spray; ***Switz.:*** Vicks Sinex; ***UK:*** Vicks Sinex.

Pentoxyverine (11490-m)

Pentoxyverine *(rINN)*.

Carbetapentane. 2-[2-(Diethylamino)ethoxy]ethyl 1-phenylcyclopentanecarboxylate.

$C_{20}H_{31}NO_3$ = 333.5.

CAS — 77-23-6.

Pentoxyverine Citrate (5607-c)

Pentoxyverine Citrate *(rINNM)*.

Carbetapentane Citrate; UCB-2543.

$C_{20}H_{31}NO_3,C_6H_8O_7$ = 525.6.

CAS — 23142-01-0.

Pharmacopoeias. In *Chin.* and *Jpn.*

Pentoxyverine Hydrochloride (9884-d)

Carbetapentane Hydrochloride.

$C_{20}H_{31}NO_3,HCl$ = 369.9.

CAS — 1045-21-2.

Pentoxyverine is a centrally acting cough suppressant used for non-productive cough (p.1052). Doses of 25 to 50 mg of the citrate have usually been given by mouth up to four times daily. The hydrochloride and the tannate are also given by mouth. The base has been administered rectally in doses of 20 mg once or twice daily.

Preparations

Proprietary Preparations (details are given in Part 3)
Aust.: Sedotussin; ***Austral.:*** Nyal Dry Cough; ***Belg.:*** Tuclase; ***Fr.:*** Atussil†; ***Ger.:*** Germapect†; Pertix; Sedotussin; Tussa-Tablinen; ***Ital.:*** Tuclase; ***Neth.:*** Balsoclase; Tuclase; ***Norw.:*** Toclase; ***Swed.:*** Toclase.

Multi-ingredient: ***Aust.:*** Tussoretardin; ***Austral.:*** Vicks Cough Syrup; Vicks Decongestive Cough Syrup†; ***Belg.:*** Balsoclase; ***Canad.:*** Vicks Cough Syrup; ***Fr.:*** Atussil-Eucalyptol†; Vicks Sirop†; ***Ger.:*** Sedotussin Expectorans; Sedotussin plus; ***Ital.:*** Vicks Pectoral†; ***Neth.:*** Balsoclase Compositum; Balsoclase-E; ***S.Afr.:*** Dykatuss Expectorant†; ***Switz.:*** Sedotussin; ***USA:*** Cophene-X; Rentamine Pediatric; Rynatuss; Tri-Tannate Plus Pediatric.

Phenylephrine (9512-a)

Phenylephrine *(BAN, rINN)*.

Fenilefrina; Phenylephrinum; *m*-Synephrine. (*S*)-1-(3-Hydroxyphenyl)-2-methylaminoethanol.

$C_9H_{13}NO_2$ = 167.2.

CAS — 59-42-7.

NOTE. Synephrine has been used as a synonym for oxedrine. Care should be taken to avoid confusion between the two compounds.

Pharmacopoeias. In *Eur.* (see p.viii).

A white or almost white crystalline powder. Slightly **soluble** in water and in alcohol; sparingly soluble in methyl alcohol. It dissolves in dilute mineral acids and in solutions of alkali hydroxides. **Store** in airtight containers. Protect from light.

Phenylephrine Acid Tartrate (9511-k)

Phenylephrine Bitartrate; Phenylephrine Tartrate *(BANM)*.

$C_9H_{13}NO_2,C_4H_6O_6$ = 317.3.

CAS — 13998-27-1.

Phenylephrine Hydrochloride (2094-g)

Phenylephrine Hydrochloride *(BANM, rINNM)*.

Mesatonum; Metaoxedrini Chloridum; Phenylephrini Hydrochloridum.

$C_9H_{13}NO_2,HCl$ = 203.7.

CAS — 61-76-7.

NOTE. PHNL is a code approved by the BP for use on single unit doses of eye drops containing phenylephrine hydrochloride where the individual container may be too small to bear all the appropriate labelling information. PHNCYC is a similar code approved for eye drops containing phenylephrine hydrochloride and cyclopentolate hydrochloride.

Pharmacopoeias. In *Chin., Eur.* (see p.viii), *Jpn,* and *US.*

White or almost white, odourless crystals or crystalline powder. Freely **soluble** in water and in alcohol. **Store** in airtight containers. Protect from light.

Incompatibility. Phenylephrine is stated to be incompatible with the local anaesthetic butacaine.

Adverse Effects and Precautions

For the adverse effects of sympathomimetics in general, and precautions for their use, see p.951. Phenylephrine has a longer duration of action than noradrenaline and an excessive vasopressor response may cause a prolonged rise in blood pressure. It induces tachycardia or reflex bradycardia and should therefore be avoided in severe hyperthyroidism and used with caution in severe ischaemic heart disease.

Since phenylephrine is absorbed through the mucosa systemic effects may follow application to the eyes or the nasal mucosa. In particular, phenylephrine 10% eye drops should be avoided or only used with extreme caution in infants and the elderly since they can have powerful systemic effects.

Excessive or prolonged use of phenylephrine nasal drops can lead to rebound congestion.

Phenylephrine hydrochloride is irritant and may cause local discomfort at the site of application; extravasation of the injection may even cause local tissue necrosis.

Effects on the cardiovascular system. Systemic side-effects have occurred following the use of phenylephrine eye drops, particularly at a strength of 10%, and after the use of phenylephrine nasal drops.

Hypertension[1] and hypertension with pulmonary oedema[2] have been described in infants after the use of phenylephrine 10% eye drops and hypertension has occurred in an infant after phenylephrine was also given intranasally with pseudoephedrine orally.[3] The specific problem of eye drops and neonatal blood pressure has also been reviewed.[4] Hypertension with arrhythmias has been reported in an 8-year-old child[5] and in an adult[6] after phenylephrine 10% eye drops had been used. Details have also been published on a series of 32 patients who experienced systemic cardiovascular reactions after the administration of phenylephrine 10% solutions to the eye.[7]

Despite there being some evidence to suggest that the incidence of such reactions is low[8] there is a reasonable body of opinion that has advocated the use of lower concentrations[1,7] and use with caution in susceptible patients such as those with cardiovascular disorders or the elderly.[7] A reduction in the eye-drop volume has been found to produce adequate mydriasis and may reduce systemic absorption and the risk of adverse cardiovascular effects.[9,10]

1. Borromeo-McGrail V, *et al.* Systemic hypertension following ocular administration of 10% phenylephrine in the neonate. *Pediatrics* 1973; **51:** 1032–6.
2. Matthews TG, *et al.* Eye-drop induced hypertension. *Lancet* 1977; **ii:** 827.
3. Saken R, *et al.* Drug-induced hypertension in infancy. *J Pediatr* 1979; **95:** 1077–9.
4. Anonymous. Babies' blood pressure raised by eye drops. *Br Med J* 1974; **1:** 2–3.
5. Vaughan RW. Ventricular arrhythmias after topical vasoconstrictors. *Anesth Analg* 1973; **52:** 161–5.
6. Lai Y-K. Adverse effect of intraoperative phenylephrine 10%: case report. *Br J Ophthalmol* 1989; **73:** 468–9.
7. Fraunfelder FT, Scafidi AF. Possible adverse effects from topical ocular 10% phenylephrine. *Am J Ophthalmol* 1978; **85:** 447–53.
8. Brown MM, *et al.* Lack of side effects from topically administered 10% phenylephrine eyedrops: a controlled study. *Arch Ophthalmol* 1980; **98:** 487–9.
9. Craig EW, Griffiths PG. Effect on mydriasis of modifying the volume of phenylephrine drops. *Br J Ophthalmol* 1991; **75:** 222–3.
10. Wheatcroft S, *et al.* Reduction in mydriatic drop size in premature infants. *Br J Ophthalmol* 1993; **77:** 364–5.

Effects on mental function. Hallucinations and paranoid delusions have been reported in a patient following excessive use of a nasal spray containing phenylephrine 0.5%.[1] Mania has also followed the use of high doses by mouth.[2]

1. Snow SS, *et al.* Nasal spray 'addiction' and psychosis: a case report. *Br J Psychiatry* 1980; **136:** 297–9.
2. Waters BGH, Lapierre YD. Secondary mania associated with sympathomimetic drug use. *Am J Psychiatry* 1981; **138:** 837–40.

Hypersensitivity. Cross-sensitivity to phenylephrine has been reported in a patient hypersensitive to pseudoephedrine.[1]

1. Buzo-Sanchez G, *et al.* Stereoisomeric cutaneous hypersensitivity. *Ann Pharmacother* 1997; **31:** 1091.

Interactions

For the interactions of sympathomimetics in general, see p.951.

Phenylephrine is less liable than adrenaline and noradrenaline to induce ventricular fibrillation if used as a pressor agent during anaesthesia with inhalational anaesthetics such as cyclopropane and halothane; nevertheless, caution is necessary. Since phenylephrine is absorbed through the mucosa interactions may also follow topical application, particularly in patients receiving an MAOI (including an RIMA). For additional warnings see under phenelzine (p.305) and moclobemide (p.299).

Cardiovascular drugs. Hypertensive reactions have been reported in a patient stabilised on *debrisoquine* when given phenylephrine by mouth,[1] in patients receiving *reserpine* or *guanethidine* when given phenylephrine eye drops,[2] and a fatal reaction occurred in a patient receiving *propranolol* and *hydrochlorothiazide* also after the instillation of phenylephrine eye drops.[3]

1. Aminu J, *et al.* Interaction between debrisoquine and phenylephrine. *Lancet* 1970; **ii:** 935–6.
2. Kim JM, *et al.* Hypertensive reactions to phenylephrine eyedrops in patients with sympathetic denervation. *Am J Ophthalmol* 1978; **85:** 862–8.
3. Cass E, *et al.* Hazards of phenylephrine topical medication in persons taking propranolol. *Can Med Assoc J* 1979; **120:** 1261–2.

Pharmacokinetics

Phenylephrine has low oral bioavailability owing to irregular absorption and first-pass metabolism by monoamine oxidase in the gut and liver. When injected subcutaneously or intramuscularly it takes 10 to 15 minutes to act; subcutaneous and intramuscular injections are effective for up to about one hour and up to about two hours respectively. Intravenous injections are effective for about 20 minutes.

Systemic absorption follows topical administration.

Uses and Administration

Phenylephrine hydrochloride is a sympathomimetic (p.951) with mainly direct effects on adrenergic receptors. It has predominantly alpha-adrenergic activity and is without significant stimulating effects on the central nervous system at usual doses. Its pressor activity is weaker than that of noradrenaline (p.924) but of longer duration. After injection it produces peripheral vasoconstriction and increased arterial pressure; it also causes reflex bradycardia. It reduces blood flow to the skin and to the kidneys.

Phenylephrine and its salts are most commonly used either topically or by mouth for the symptomatic relief of nasal congestion (p.1052). They are frequently included in preparations intended for the relief of cough and cold symptoms. For nasal congestion, a 0.25 to 0.5% solution may be instilled as nasal drops or a spray into each nostril every 4 hours as required, or phenylephrine hydrochloride may be given by mouth in doses of about 5 to 20 mg three or four times daily.

In ophthalmology, phenylephrine hydrochloride is employed as a mydriatic (p.454) in concentrations of up to 10%; generally solutions containing 2.5% or 10% are employed but systemic absorption can occur (see Adverse Effects, above) and the 10% strength, in particular, should be used with caution. The mydriatic effect can last several hours. Solutions stronger than 2% may cause intense irritation and a local anaesthetic other than butacaine (which is incompatible) should be instilled into the eye a few minutes beforehand.

Ocular solutions containing lower concentrations (up to 0.25% phenylephrine hydrochloride) are used as a conjunctival decongestant.

Phenylephrine has been used parenterally in the treatment of hypotensive states (see p.790), such as those encountered during circulatory failure or spinal anaesthesia. For hypotension, an initial dose of phenylephrine hydrochloride 2 to 5 mg may be given as a 1% solution subcutaneously or intramuscularly with further doses of 1 to 10 mg if necessary, according to response. A dose of 100 to 500 μg by slow intravenous injection as a 0.1% solution, repeated as necessary after at least 15 minutes, has also been employed. In severe hypotensive states, 10 mg in 500 mL of glucose 5% or sodium chloride 0.9% has been infused intravenously, initially at a rate of up to 180 μg per minute, reduced, according to the response, to 30 to 60 μg per minute.

Phenylephrine hydrochloride has also been given by intravenous injection to stop paroxysmal supraventricular tachycardia but other agents are preferred (see Cardiac Arrhythmias, p.782). The initial dose is usually not greater than 500 μg given as a 0.1% solution with subsequent doses gradually increased up to 1 mg if necessary.

Phenylephrine hydrochloride has been used as a vasoconstrictor with local anaesthetics.

Phenylephrine has also been used as the acid tartrate to prolong the bronchodilator effects of isoprenaline when administered by inhalation. However, isoprenaline is now little used by this route.

Phenylephrine tannate has also been employed.

Priapism. For reference to phenylephrine in low dosage and dilute solution being given by intracavernosal injection to reverse priapism, see under Alprostadil, p.1413.

Preparations

BP 1998: Phenylephrine Eye Drops; Phenylephrine Injection;
USP 23: Antipyrine, Benzocaine, and Phenylephrine Hydrochloride Otic Solution; Isoproterenol Hydrochloride and Phenylephrine Bitartrate Inhalation Aerosol; Phenylephrine Hydrochloride Injection; Phenylephrine Hydrochloride Nasal Jelly; Phenylephrine Hydrochloride Nasal Solution; Phenylephrine Hydrochloride Ophthalmic Solution; Procaine and Phenylephrine Hydrochlorides Injection.

Proprietary Preparations (details are given in Part 3)
Aust.: Prefrin Liquifilm; Visadron; ***Austral.:*** Albalon Relief; Decongestant Eye Drops†; Decongestant Nasal Spray†; Isopto Frin; Neo-Synephrine; Nyal Decongestant; Prefrin; Visopt; ***Belg.:*** Isopto Frin; Neo-Synephrine; Spraydil†; Visadron; ***Canad.:*** Dionephrine; Mydfrin; Neo-Synephrine; Novahistine; Prefrin Liquifilm; ***Fr.:*** Auristan; Nycto†; ***Ger.:*** Mydrial; Neo-Synephrine†; Neosynephrin-POS; Visadron; Vistosan; ***Irl.:*** Fenox†; Isopto Frin; Prefrin†; ***Ital.:*** Isonefrine; Neo-Synephrine; Optistin†; Visadron; ***Neth.:*** Boradrine; Visadron†; ***S.Afr.:*** Fenox†; Naphensyl; Prefrin; ***Spain:*** ADA; Analux; Boraline; Disneumon Pernasal; Mirazul; Neo Lacrim; Pulverizador Nasal; Rin Up†; Visadron; Vistafrin; ***Swed.:*** Neo-Synephrine; ***Switz.:*** Gouttes nasales; Neo-Synephrine†; ***UK:*** Fenox; Isopto Frin; ***USA:*** AH-chew D; Ak-Dilate; Ak-Nefrin; Alconefrin; Children's Nostril; Eye Drops Extra; Isopto Frin; Mydfrin; Neo-Synephrine; Neofrin; Nostril; Phenoptic; Prefrin Liquifilm; Relief; Rhinall; Ricobid D; Sinex; Storzfen.

Multi-ingredient: numerous preparations are listed in Part 3.

Phenylpropanolamine (18492-z)

Phenylpropanolamine *(BAN, rINN).*

(±)-Norephedrine. (1*RS*,2*SR*)-2-Amino-1-phenylpropan-1-ol.

$C_9H_{13}NO$ = 151.2.

CAS — 14838-15-4.

Phenylpropanolamine Hydrochloride (2095-q)

Phenylpropanolamine Hydrochloride *(BANM, rINNM).*

Mydriatin; Phenylpropanolamini Hydrochloridum.

$C_9H_{13}NO,HCl$ = 187.7.

CAS — 154-41-6.

Pharmacopoeias. In *Eur.* (see p.viii) and *US. US* also includes phenylpropanolamine bitartrate.

A white or almost white crystalline powder, with a slight aromatic odour. **Soluble** 1 in 1.1 of water, 1 in 7.4 of alcohol, and 1 in 4100 of chloroform; practically insoluble in dichloromethane and ether. A 3% solution in water has a pH of 4.2 to 5.5. **Store** in airtight containers. Protect from light.

Adverse Effects and Precautions

As for Ephedrine, p.1059.

Severe hypertensive episodes have followed phenylpropanolamine ingestion (see below). As with other indirect-acting sympathomimetics such as ephedrine tolerance to the therapeutic effects of phenylpropanolamine has been reported with prolonged administration.

An extensive and detailed review of adverse effects attributed to phenylpropanolamine.[1]

Phenylpropanolamine exists in four isomeric forms: *d*- and *l*-norephedrine and *d*- and *l*-norpseudoephedrine. Of the isomers, *d*-norpseudoephedrine is the most potent stimulant of the CNS and is contained in European phenylpropanolamine preparations; however, in North America only the racemic mixture of *d,l*-norephedrine is used. This consideration of the isomers present in a given preparation may partly explain why many of the adverse drug reactions reported in Europe describe an alteration of mental status whereas those in North America are more often compatible with hypertension. In Australia the isomer involved in adverse reaction reports has never been conclusively determined but it may be *l*-norephedrine.

Since the isomers of phenylpropanolamine present in proprietary preparations vary worldwide the literature review concentrated on North American cases. The majority of products available were decongestants or cough or cold remedies; a small number were promoted as diet aids.

The data suggested that over-the-counter products were more likely to be associated with an adverse reaction than a prescription medication; this may be because such OTC products were more likely to be overused and to be considered innocuous by the patient. It was also likely that drug interactions rather than 'true overdosages', were involved in many of the adverse events, particularly as many OTC preparations contain other ingredients.

The adverse reactions varied widely ranging from headache and elevated blood pressure to cardiopulmonary arrest, intracranial haemorrhage, and death. Mild reactions included blurred vision, dizziness, anxiety, agitation, tremor, confusion, and hypersensitivity reaction. Severe reactions also included hypertensive crisis with hypertensive encephalopathy, seizures, arrhythmias, psychosis, and acute tubular necrosis. One unifying theme of many of the severe cases was that high blood pressure or symptoms suggestive of this were the presenting feature; an acute, persistent, severe headache was also noted in many cases.

It was pointed out that overall phenylpropanolamine was relatively safe. Although billions of doses were consumed annually, few cases of adverse drug reactions had been reported.

It was believed that certain groups may be at particular risk of adverse reactions to phenylpropanolamine: persons with elevated blood pressure, overweight persons (who are likely to be both hypertensive and to use diet aids), patients with eating disorders (who tend to abuse substances including diet aids), and the elderly (who may be multiple drug takers and likely to be hypertensive and at risk already of a stroke).

1. Lake CR, *et al.* Adverse drug effects attributed to phenylpropanolamine: a review of 142 case reports. *Am J Med* 1990; **89:** 195–208.

Interactions

For the interactions of sympathomimetics in general, see p.951. For a comment that drug interactions were likely to have been involved in many adverse events associated with phenylpropanolamine see under Adverse Effects and Precautions, above. Hypertensive crisis is a particular risk in patients receiving MAOIs.

Antipsychotics. A 27-year-old woman with schizophrenia and T-wave abnormality of the heart, who had responded to thioridazine 100 mg daily with procyclidine 2.5 mg twice daily, died from ventricular fibrillation within 2 hours of taking a single dose of a preparation reported to contain chlorpheniramine maleate 4 mg with phenylpropanolamine hydrochloride 50 mg (Contac C), concurrently with thioridazine.[1]

1. Chouinard G, *et al.* Death attributed to ventricular arrhythmia induced by thioridazine in combination with a single Contac C capsule. *Can Med Assoc J* 1978; **119:** 729–31.

Bromocriptine. There have been isolated reports[1,2] of severe hypertension, with headache and convulsions, in patients receiving bromocriptine concomitantly with phenylpropanolamine.

1. Kulig K, *et al.* Bromocriptine-associated headache: possible life-threatening sympathomimetic interaction. *Obstet Gynecol* 1991; **78:** 941–3.
2. Chan JCN, *et al.* Postpartum hypertension, bromocriptine, and phenylpropanolamine. *Drug Invest* 1994; **8:** 254–6.

Indomethacin. A 27-year-old woman who had been taking D-phenylpropanolamine [sic.] 85 mg daily for some months, experienced severe hypertension when she also took indomethacin 25 mg. It was considered that the inhibition of prostaglandin synthesis by indomethacin might have caused enhancement of the sympathomimetic effect of phenylpropanolamine.[1]

1. Lee KY, *et al.* Severe hypertension after ingestion of an appetite suppressant (phenylpropanolamine) with indomethacin. *Lancet* 1979; **i:** 1110–11.

Pharmacokinetics

Phenylpropanolamine is readily and completely absorbed from the gastro-intestinal tract, peak plasma concentrations being achieved about an hour or two after oral administration. It undergoes some metabolism in the liver, to an active hydroxylated metabolite, but the majority of a dose (up to 80 to 90%) is excreted unchanged in the urine within 24 hours. The half-life has been reported to be about 3 to 5 hours.

References.

1. Scherzinger SS, *et al.* Steady state pharmacokinetics and dose-proportionality of phenylpropanolamine in healthy subjects. *J Clin Pharmacol* 1990; **30:** 372–7.
2. Simons FER, *et al.* Pharmacokinetics of the orally administered decongestants pseudoephedrine and phenylpropanolamine in children. *J Pediatr* 1996; **129:** 729–34.

Uses and Administration

Phenylpropanolamine is a largely indirect-acting sympathomimetic (p.951) with an action similar to that of ephedrine (p.1060) but less active as a CNS stimulant.

Phenylpropanolamine is given by mouth as the hydrochloride for the symptomatic treatment of nasal congestion (p.1052). It is frequently used in mixed preparations for the relief of cough and cold symptoms.

In the management of nasal congestion, phenylpropanolamine hydrochloride is given in usual doses of up to 25 mg three or four times daily by mouth; a dose of 150 mg daily should not be exceeded. Modified-release preparations are also available.

Other uses of phenylpropanolamine include the control of urinary incontinence in some patients (see p.454). It has also been used to suppress appetite in the management of obesity although the usual treatment is outlined on p.1476.

Phenylpropanolamine polistirex (a phenylpropanolamine and sulphonated diethenylbenzene-ethenylbenzene copolymer complex) is also used as are phenylpropanolamine bitartrate and phenylpropanolamine sulphate.

Preparations

USP 23: Phenylpropanolamine Hydrochloride Capsules; Phenylpropanolamine Hydrochloride Extended-release Capsules; Phenylpropanolamine Hydrochloride Extended-release Tablets; Phenylpropanolamine Hydrochloride Oral Solution; Phenylpropanolamine Hydrochloride Tablets.

Proprietary Preparations (details are given in Part 3)
Aust.: Kontexin; ***Ger.:*** Fasupond; ***Irl.:*** Procol; ***Norw.:*** Monydrin; Rinexin; ***S.Afr.:*** Restaslim; ***Swed.:*** Monydrin; Rinexin; ***Switz.:*** Dexatrim; Fugoa N†; Kontexin; ***UK:*** Procol; ***USA:*** Acutrim; Amfed TD†; Appedrine; Control; Dexatrim; Diet Plan with Diadax†; Diet-Aid†; Phenoxine; Phenyldrine; Propagest; Spray-U-Thin; Stay Trim; Unitrol.

Multi-ingredient: numerous preparations are listed in Part 3.

Pholcodine (5602-e)

Pholcodine *(BAN, rINN)*.

Folcodina; Pholcodinum. 3-*O*-(2-Morpholinoethyl)morphine monohydrate.

$C_{23}H_{30}N_2O_4,H_2O = 416.5$.

CAS — 509-67-1 (anhydrous pholcodine).

Pharmacopoeias. In Eur. (see p.viii).

Colourless crystals or a white or almost white crystalline powder. Sparingly **soluble** in water; freely soluble in alcohol and in acetone; slightly soluble in ether; dissolves in dilute mineral acids.

Adverse Effects and Precautions

As for Dextromethorphan, p.1057. Constipation or drowsiness have been reported occasionally.

Interactions

Concomitant administration of pholcodine with alcohol or other CNS depressants may increase the effects on the CNS.

Uses and Administration

Pholcodine is a centrally acting cough suppressant that has actions and uses similar to those of dextromethorphan (p.1058). It is administered by mouth in a usual dose of 5 to 10 mg three or four times daily; children over 5 years of age may be given 2.5 to 5 mg three or four times daily and children 1 to 5 years, 2 to 2.5 mg three times daily. The citrate has also been used. Pholcodine polistirex (a pholcodine and sulphonated diethenylbenzene-ethenylbenzene copolymer complex) is used in modified-release preparations.

Cough. Although pholcodine appears to possess antitussive activity in cough (p.1052), it was considered by a reviewer from Wellcome[1] that there was little evidence from well-controlled studies to confirm its efficacy or support the claim that it is more active than codeine. The majority of studies have been conducted using combination preparations of pholcodine, have not been adequately controlled, or have been in subjects with artificially induced cough. Unlike codeine, there is little or no metabolism of pholcodine to morphine[2,3] and this may contribute to its lack of analgesic activity, morphine-like side-effects, and addictive potential.[1] Pholcodine has a much longer elimination half-life than codeine and data suggest that the current dosing frequency could possibly be reduced to once or twice daily.[1]

1. Findlay JWA. Pholcodine. *J Clin Pharm Ther* 1988; **13:** 5–17.
2. Findlay JWA, *et al.* Comparative disposition of codeine and pholcodine in man after single oral doses. *Br J Clin Pharmacol* 1986; **22:** 61–71.
3. Maurer HH, Fritz CF. Metabolism of pholcodine in man. *Arzneimittelforschung* 1990; **40:** 564–6.

Preparations

BP 1998: Pholcodine Linctus; Strong Pholcodine Linctus.

Proprietary Preparations (details are given in Part 3)
Austral.: Actuss; Adaphol†; Duro-Tuss; Ordov Dry Tickly Cough; Pholcolin†; Pholtrate; Tussinol; ***Belg.:*** Bromofotyl†; ***Fr.:*** Respilene; Sirop Des Vosges Caze; ***Irl.:*** Expulin Dry Cough; Pholcolin; ***Norw.:*** Tuxi; ***S.Afr.:*** Pholcolinct; ***UK:*** Benylin Childrens Dry Coughs; Evaphol; Expulin Dry Cough; Famel Linctus†; Galenphol; Pavacol-D; Pholcomed; Tixylix Daytime.

Multi-ingredient: ***Austral.:*** Decongestant Cough Elixir Junior†; Difflam Anti-Inflammatory Cough Lozenges; Duro-Tuss Cough Lozenges; Duro-Tuss Decongestant; Duro-Tuss Expectorant; Junicol Junior†; Junicol V†; Phensedyl; Tixylix; ***Belg.:*** Antigrip†; Broncal; Bronchalene; Broncho-pectoralis; Eucalyptine Pholcodine Le Brun; Folcodex; Folex; Pectocalmine Baby†; Pholco-Mereprine; Quintex Pediatrique; ***Fr.:*** Biocalyptol; Bronchalene; Broncorinol toux seches; Clarix; Codotussyl; Denoral; Dimetane; Eucalyptine Pholcodine; Hexapneumine; Humex; Isomyrtine; Lyptocodine; Pholcones; Pholcones Bismuth-Quinine†; Pholcones Guaiphenesine-Quinine†; Premidan Adult†; Premidan Infant†; Pulmofluide Enfants†; Quintopan Enfant; Sirop Adrian a la pholcodine adulte†; Sirop Adrian a la pholcodine enfant†; Trophires; ***Irl.:*** Expulin; Expulin Childrens Cough; Tixylix; ***Norw.:*** Tuxidrin; ***S.Afr.:*** Bronchilate†; Bronchistop; Contra-Coff; Docsed; Folcofen; Pholtex; Procof; Respinol Compound; Tixylix; ***Spain:*** Caltoson Balsamico; Homocodeina Timol†; Trophires; ***Switz.:*** Pecto-Baby; Phol-Tussil; Phol-Tux; Pholprin†; Rectoseptal-Neo Pholcodine; Tussiplex; ***UK:*** Cold Relief Daytime; Cold Relief Night-Time; Copholco†; Copholcoids†; Davenol†; Day Cold Comfort; Expulin; Expulin Paediatric; Hill's Balsam Adult Suppressant; Night Cold Comfort; Phensedyl Plus; Tixylix Cough & Cold; Tixylix Night-Time; Triolinctus†.

Pipazethate Hydrochloride (5629-f)

Pipazethate Hydrochloride *(BANM)*.

Pipazetate Hydrochloride *(rINNM)*; D-254 (pipazethate); Piperestazine Hydrochloride; SKF-70230-A (pipazethate); SQ-15874 (pipazethate). 2-(2-Piperidinoethoxy)ethyl pyrido[3,2-*b*][1,4]benzothiazine-10-carboxylate hydrochloride.

$C_{21}H_{25}N_3O_3S,HCl = 436.0$.

CAS — 2167-85-3 (pipazethate); 6056-11-7 (pipazethate hydrochloride).

NOTE. Pipazethate is *USAN*.

Pipazethate hydrochloride is a centrally acting cough suppressant which also has some peripheral actions in non-productive cough (p.1052). It has been given by mouth, in usual doses of 20 to 40 mg three times daily, and rectally.

A healthy 4-year-old child became somnolent and agitated, with convulsions, followed by coma, after swallowing an unknown number of tablets containing pipazethate; cardiac arrhythmias also developed.[1]

1. da Silva OA, Lopez M. Pipazethate—acute childhood poisoning. *Clin Toxicol* 1977; **11:** 455–8.

Preparations

Proprietary Preparations (details are given in Part 3)
Aust.: Selvigon; ***Ger.:*** Selvigon Hustensaft; ***Ital.:*** Selvjgon.

Piperidione (5630-z)

NU-1510. 3,3-Diethylpiperidine-2,4-dione.

$C_9H_{15}NO_2 = 169.2$.

CAS — 77-03-2.

Piperidione has been given by mouth as a centrally acting cough suppressant.

Preparations

Proprietary Preparations (details are given in Part 3)
Ital.: Tusseval†.

Multi-ingredient: ***Ital.:*** Bechicon†.

Poppy Capsule (6260-y)

Dormideiras; Fruit du Pavot; Fruto de Adormidera; Mohnfrucht; Papaveris Capsula; Poppy Heads.

Pharmacopoeias. In Chin.

The dried fruits of *Papaver somniferum* (Papaveraceae), collected before dehiscence has occurred, containing about very small amounts of morphine with traces of other opium alkaloids.

Poppy capsule is mildly sedative and has been used as a liquid extract or syrup in cough mixtures.

Preparations

Proprietary Preparations (details are given in Part 3)

Multi-ingredient: ***Belg.:*** Sedemol†; Sulfa-Sedemol†; Tisane Pectorale; Tisane pour Dormir; ***Fr.:*** Mediflor Tisane Pectorale d'Alsace†.

Potassium Guaiacolsulfonate (2022-y)

Sulfogaiacol *(rINN)*; Kalium Guajacolsulfonicum; Potassium Guaiacolsulphonate. Potassium hydroxymethoxybenzenesulphonate hemihydrate.

$C_7H_7KO_5S,\frac{1}{2}H_2O = 251.3$.

CAS — 1321-14-8 (anhydrous potassium guaiacolsulfonate); 78247-49-1 (potassium guaiacolsulfonate hemihydrate).

Pharmacopoeias. In US. Also in *Aust., Belg., Fr., Jpn, Neth.,* and *Pol.,* none of which specifies hemihydrate.

Potassium guaiacolsulfonate should be **protected** from light.

Potassium guaiacolsulfonate is used as an expectorant for productive cough (p.1052). Calcium guaiacolsulfonate has been used similarly.

Preparations

Proprietary Preparations (details are given in Part 3)
Aust.: Pectosorin; ***Ital.:*** Bron†; Pulmovirolo; Silborina†; Tioguaialina.

Multi-ingredient: numerous preparations are listed in Part 3.

Prednazoline (15332-r)

Prednazoline *(rINN)*.

Prednisolone-Fenoxazoline Compound. 11β,17α,21-Trihydroxypregna-1,4-diene-3,20-dione 21-(dihydrogen phosphate) compound with 2-(2-isopropylphenoxymethyl)-2-imidazoline.

$C_{21}H_{29}O_8P,C_{13}H_{18}N_2O = 658.7$.

CAS — 6693-90-9.

Prednazoline has the general properties of prednisolone (p.1048) and of fenoxazoline (p.1061) and is used locally in the form of a 0.25% nasal spray in the treatment of pharyngitis, rhinitis, and sinusitis.

Preparations

Proprietary Preparations (details are given in Part 3)
Fr.: Deturgylone.

Prenoxdiazine Hydrochloride (5631-c)

Prenoxdiazine Hydrochloride *(rINNM)*.

HK-256; Prenoxdiazin Hydrochloride. 3-(2,2-Diphenylethyl)-5-(2-piperidinoethyl)-1,2,4-oxadiazole hydrochloride.

$C_{23}H_{27}N_3O,HCl = 397.9$.

CAS — 47543-65-7 (prenoxdiazine); 37671-82-2 (prenoxdiazine hybenzate); 982-43-4 (prenoxdiazine hydrochloride).

Prenoxdiazine hydrochloride is used as a peripherally acting cough suppressant for non-productive cough (p.1052). It has been given by mouth in doses of 100 to 200 mg three or four times daily. Prenoxdiazine hybenzate is also used.

Preparations

Proprietary Preparations (details are given in Part 3)
Ital.: Libexin†; ***Switz.:*** Libexine; Mephaxine.

Multi-ingredient: ***Ger.:*** Lomapect†; ***Ital.:*** Broncofluid; Libexin Mucolitico; ***Switz.:*** Libexine Compositum; Mephaxine Compositum.

Pseudoephedrine (9514-x)

Pseudoephedrine *(BAN, rINN)*.

d-Ψ-Ephedrine; *d*-Isoephedrine. (+)-(1*S*,2*S*)-2-Methylamino-1-phenylpropan-1-ol.

$C_{10}H_{15}NO = 165.2$.

CAS — 90-82-4.

An alkaloid obtained from *Ephedra* spp.

Pseudoephedrine Hydrochloride (2098-w)

Pseudoephedrine Hydrochloride *(BANM, USAN, rINNM)*.

$C_{10}H_{15}NO,HCl = 201.7$.

CAS — 345-78-8.

Pharmacopoeias. In Eur. (see p.viii) and US.

White or off-white crystals or crystalline powder; odourless or almost odourless. Very or freely **soluble** in water; soluble 1 in 3.6 of alcohol, 1 in 91 of chloroform, and 1 in 7000 of ether; sparingly soluble in dichloromethane. A 5% solution in water has a pH of 4.6 to 6.0. **Store** in airtight containers. Protect from light.

Pseudoephedrine Sulphate (2099-e)

Pseudoephedrine Sulphate *(BANM, rINNM)*.

Pseudoephedrine Sulfate *(USAN)*; Sch-4855.

$(C_{10}H_{15}NO)_2,H_2SO_4 = 428.5$.

CAS — 7460-12-0.

Pharmacopoeias. In US.

White odourless crystals or crystalline powder. Freely **soluble** in alcohol. A 5% solution in water has a pH of 5.0 to 6.5. **Store** in airtight containers. Protect from light.

Adverse Effects and Precautions

As for Ephedrine, p.1059. The commonest adverse effects of pseudoephedrine include tachycardia, anxiety, restlessness, and insomnia; skin rashes and urinary retention have occasionally occurred. Hallucinations have been reported rarely, particularly in children.

In 34 healthy males given pseudoephedrine 120 or 150 mg, as a modified-release preparation, twice daily for 7 days mean plasma concentrations were about 450 and 510 ng per mL respectively. Side-effects (dry mouth, anorexia, insomnia, anxiety, tension, restlessness, tachycardia, palpitations) were common; there was some evidence of tachyphylaxis.[1]

1. Dickerson J, *et al.* Dose tolerance and pharmacokinetic studies of L(+) pseudoephedrine capsules in man. *Eur J Clin Pharmacol* 1978; **14:** 253–9.

Effects on mental function. Reports[1-3] of adverse mental effects associated with a preparation containing pseudoephedrine and triprolidine (Actifed).

1. Leighton KM. Paranoid psychosis after abuse of Actifed. *Br Med J* 1982; **284:** 789–90.
2. Sankey RJ, *et al.* Visual hallucinations in children receiving decongestants. *Br Med J* 1984; **288:** 1369.
3. Stokes MA. Visual hallucinations in children receiving decongestants. *Br Med J* 1984; **288:** 1540.

Effects on the skin. Recurrent pseudo-scarlatina has been described in one female patient and attributed, on some occasions at least, to ingestion of pseudoephedrine.[1] Further fixed drug eruptions associated with pseudoephedrine have been reported.[2-4] In one woman, an erythematous macular rash developed 5 and a half hours after a challenge dose of pseudoephedrine 60 mg by mouth; other symptoms, which mimicked the effects of toxic shock syndrome, included nausea and vomiting, fever, orthostatic hypotension, light-headedness, fatigue, and desquamation of the skin on her palms and soles.[3] However, considering the frequent use of pseudoephedrine in over-the-counter medications, associated drug eruptions generally appear to be rare.[2]

1. Taylor BJ, Duffill MB. *Br J Dermatol* 1988; **118:** 827–9.
2. Camisa C. Fixed drug reactions to pseudoephedrine hydrochloride. *Br J Dermatol* 1989; **120:** 857–8.
3. Cavanah DK, Ballas ZK. Pseudoephedrine reaction presenting as recurrent toxic shock syndrome. *Ann Intern Med* 1993; **119:** 302–3.
4. Hauken M. Fixed drug eruption and pseudoephedrine. *Ann Intern Med* 1994; **120:** 442.

Epileptogenic effect. A report of a child who suffered a generalised seizure after ingesting a large quantity of pseudoephedrine hydrochloride tablets was believed to be the first report of convulsions associated with overdose of a preparation containing the drug as a single ingredient.[1]

1. Clark RF, Curry SC. Pseudoephedrine dangers. *Pediatrics* 1990; **85:** 389–90.

Interactions

As for Ephedrine, p.1060.

Antacids. The absorption rate of pseudoephedrine hydrochloride was increased by the concomitant administration of aluminium hydroxide mixture but was decreased by the administration of kaolin; in the latter case adsorption may have competed with absorption.[1]

1. Lucarotti RL, *et al.* Enhanced pseudoephedrine absorption by concurrent administration of aluminium hydroxide gel in humans. *J Pharm Sci* 1972; **61:** 903–5.

Pharmacokinetics

Pseudoephedrine is readily absorbed from the gastro-intestinal tract. It is resistant to metabolism by monoamine oxidase and is largely excreted unchanged in the urine together with small amounts of its hepatic metabolite. It has a half-life of about 5 to 8 hours; elimination is enhanced and half-life accordingly shorter in acid urine. Small amounts are distributed into breast milk.

References.

1. Kuntzman RG, *et al.* The influence of urinary pH on the plasma half-life of pseudoephedrine in man and dog and a sensitive assay for its determination in human plasma. *Clin Pharmacol Ther* 1971; **12:** 62–7.
2. Lai CM, *et al.* Urinary excretion of chlorpheniramine and pseudoephedrine in humans. *J Pharm Sci* 1979; **68:** 1243–6.
3. Yacobi A, *et al.* Evaluation of sustained-action chlorpheniramine-pseudoephedrine dosage form in humans. *J Pharm Sci* 1980; **69:** 1077–81.
4. Simons FER, *et al.* Pharmacokinetics of the orally administered decongestants pseudoephedrine and phenylpropanolamine in children. *J Pediatr* 1996; **129:** 729–34.

Breast feeding. A study of concentrations of pseudoephedrine and triprolidine in plasma and breast milk of 3 lactating mothers for up to 48 hours after ingestion of a preparation containing pseudoephedrine hydrochloride 60 mg with triprolidine hydrochloride 2.5 mg. Concentrations of pseudoephedrine in milk were consistently higher than in plasma; the half-life in both fluids was between 4.2 and 7.0 hours. Assuming a generous milk secretion of 500 mL over 12 hours it was calculated that the excreted dose was the equivalent of 250 to 330 μg of pseudoephedrine base, or 0.5 to 0.7% of the dose ingested by the mothers. Triprolidine did not appear to be concentrated in breast milk. The amounts of pseudoephedrine and triprolidine distributed into breast milk were probably not high enough to warrant cessation of breast feeding.[1]

1. Findlay JWA, *et al.* Pseudoephedrine and triprolidine in plasma and breast milk of nursing mothers. *Br J Clin Pharmacol* 1984; **18:** 901–6.

Uses and Administration

Pseudoephedrine is a direct- and indirect-acting sympathomimetic (p.951). It is a stereoisomer of ephedrine (p.1059) and has a similar action, but has been stated to have less pressor activity and fewer CNS effects.

Pseudoephedrine and its salts are given by mouth for the symptomatic relief of nasal congestion (p.1052). They are commonly combined with other ingredients in preparations intended for the relief of cough and cold symptoms.

Pseudoephedrine hydrochloride or sulphate are generally given in doses of 60 mg three to four times daily by mouth. Suggested oral doses for children are: 2 to 5 years, 15 mg three times daily; 6 to 12 years, 30 mg three or four times daily. Modified-release preparations are also available; a usual adult dose is 120 mg every 12 hours.

Some patients with urinary incontinence may gain some benefit from pseudoephedrine, see p.454. It has also been given in the management of some forms of priapism (p.903).

Pseudoephedrine polistirex (a pseudoephedrine and sulphonated diethenylbenzene-ethenylbenzene copolymer complex) has also been used as has pseudoephedrine tannate.

Preparations

BP 1998: Pseudoephedrine Tablets;
USP 23: Acetaminophen and Pseudoephedrine Hydrochloride Tablets; Acetaminophen, Dextromethorphan Hydrobromide, Doxylamine Succinate, and Pseudoephedrine Hydrochloride Oral Solution; Acetaminophen, Diphenhydramine Hydrochloride, and Pseudoephedrine Hydrochloride Tablets; Brompheniramine Maleate and Pseudoephedrine Sulfate Syrup; Chlorpheniramine Maleate and Pseudoephedrine Hydrochloride Oral Solution; Dexbrompheniramine Maleate and Pseudoephedrine Sulfate Oral Solution; Diphenhydramine and Pseudoephedrine Capsules; Guaifenesin and Pseudoephedrine Hydrochloride Capsules; Guaifenesin, Pseudoephedrine Hydrochloride, and Dextromethorphan Hydrobromide Capsules; Ibuprofen and Pseudoephedrine Hydrochloride Tablets; Pseudoephedrine Hydrochloride Extended-release Tablets; Pseudoephedrine Hydrochloride Syrup; Pseudoephedrine Hydrochloride Tablets; Triprolidine and Pseudoephedrine Hydrochlorides Syrup; Triprolidine and Pseudoephedrine Hydrochlorides Tablets.

Proprietary Preparations (details are given in Part 3)

Austral.: Demazin Sinus; Dimetapp Daytime†; Drixora†; Logicin Sinus; Orthoxicol Infant; Sinutab Sinus Relief†; Sudafed; Tixylix Daytime; ***Belg.:*** Nasa-12; Sudafed†; ***Canad.:*** Balminil Decongestant; Benylin Decongestant†; Congest Aid; Congest-Eze; Contac C Nondrowsy; Decongestant Tablets; Drixoral ND; Durafedrin†; Eltor; Maxenal†; Nasal & Sinus Relief; Pseudofrin; Robidrine; Sudafed; Sudodrin; Tantafed; Triaminic; Triaminic Pediatric Drops; ***Fr.:*** Drill rhinites; Rhinalair; Sudafed; ***Irl.:*** Galpseud; Sudafed; ***Ital.:*** Narixan; Sudafed; ***S.Afr.:*** Acunaso; Drilix; Drixora; Monofed; Sinumed; Sudafed; Symptofed; ***Spain:*** Sudafed†; ***Switz.:*** Otrinol; ***UK:*** Bronalin Decongestant; Decongestant Tablets; Galpseud; Sudafed; ***USA:*** Afrin; AlleRid†; Allermed; Cenafed; Congestion Relief; Decofed; Decorin; DeFed; Dorcol Children's Decongestant; Drixoral Non-Drowsy Formula; Dynafed Pseudo; Efidac; Genaphed; Halofed; Mini Thin Pseudo; Myfedrine; Novafed†; PediaCare Infant's Decongestant; Pseudo; Pseudo-Gest; Seudotabs; Silfedrine; Sinustat†; Sinustop Pro; Sudafed; Sudex†; Triaminic AM Decongestant Formula.

Multi-ingredient: numerous preparations are listed in Part 3.

Senega Root (2025-c)

Polígala Raíz; Polygalae Radix; Rattlesnake Root; Seneca Snakeroot; Senega.

CAS — 1260-04-4 (polygalic acid).

Pharmacopoeias. In *Eur.* (see p.viii) and *Jpn. Jpn* also describes Powdered Senega Root.

The dried and usually fragmented root and root crown of *Polygala senega* or certain closely related species of *Polygala* or a mixture of these. **Protect** from light and humidity.

Senega root has been used as an expectorant in preparations given by mouth for respiratory-tract disorders.

Polygala amara is a related species that is used similarly.

Preparations

Proprietary Preparations (details are given in Part 3)

Multi-ingredient: ***Aust.:*** Bronchiplant; Bronchiplant light; Tussimont; ***Austral.:*** ASA Tones; Nyal Bronchitis; Senamon†; Senega and Ammonia; ***Belg.:*** Tux; ***Canad.:*** Bronchial; Bronchozone; Wampole Bronchial Cough Syrup; ***Fr.:*** Broncorinol toux seches; Dinacode; Dinacode avec codeine; Neo-Codion; Passedyl; Polery; Premidan Adult†; Pulmothiol†; Quintopan Adult; Sirop Pectoral adulte; Tuberol†; ***Ger.:*** Asthma 6-N; Silphoscalin†; ***S.Afr.:*** Cocilix†; ***Spain:*** Broncovital; Bronquiasmol†; Combitorax; Iodocafedrina†; Pastillas Pectoral Kely; Pulmofasa; Pulmofasa Antihist; ***Swed.:*** Cocillana-Etyfin; Senega†; ***Switz.:*** Bronchocodin; Bronchofluid; Expectoran avec codeine†; Expectoran Codein; Expectoran†; Foral; GEM†; Hederix; Makatussin; Makatussin forte; Melior†; Neo-Codion N†; Neo-Codion Nourrissons†; Patussol; Pectocalmine; Pectoral N; Phol-Tux; Radix†; Sirop antitussif Wyss a base de codeine; Sirop Wyss contre la toux; ***UK:*** Antibron; Chest Mixture.

Sfericase (926-j)

AI-794.

Sfericase is a proteolytic enzyme from *Bacillus sphaericus* which has been studied as a mucolytic for productive cough (p.1052) in respiratory disorders.

References.

1. Yoshida K. Sfericase, a novel proteolytic enzyme. *Int J Clin Pharmacol Ther Toxicol* 1983; **21:** 439–46.
2. Itoh K, *et al.* Clinical effects of proteinase, sfericase (AI-794), on chronic bronchitis and similar diseases–review of proper dosage with multi-institutional double-blind tests. *Int J Clin Pharmacol Ther Toxicol* 1984; **22:** 32–8.
3. Miyoshi Y, *et al.* Clinical results of sfericase (AI-794) in chronic parasinusitis. *Int J Clin Pharmacol Ther Toxicol* 1984; **22:** 73–80.

Sobrerol (13239-p)

Cyclidrol; Sobrerolo. *p*-Menth-6-ene-2,8-diol.

$C_{10}H_{18}O_2$ = 170.2.

CAS — 498-71-5.

Pharmacopoeias. In *It.*

Sobrerol is a mucolytic which is used in respiratory disorders characterised by productive cough (p.1052). Doses of up to 800 mg have been given by mouth daily in divided doses. Sobrerol has also been administered by injection, inhalation, or rectally.

Pharmacokinetics. The pharmacokinetics of sobrerol after oral or intravenous administration has been studied in patients with acute exacerbations of chronic bronchitis.[1] Sobrerol was rapidly absorbed from the gastro-intestinal tract and rapidly distributed. Thirteen and 23% of the dose was excreted in the urine as unchanged drug, glucuronidated sobrerol, and hydrated carvone after intravenous and oral administration respectively. Sobrerol was shown to accumulate in bronchial mucus.

1. Braga PC, *et al.* Pharmacokinetics of sobrerol in chronic bronchitis: comparison of serum and bronchial mucus levels. *Eur J Clin Pharmacol* 1983; **24:** 209–15.

Respiratory disorders. References.

1. Bellussi L, *et al.* Evaluation of the efficacy and safety of sobrerol granules in patients suffering from chronic rhinosinusitis. *J Int Med Res* 1990; **18:** 454–9.
2. Bellussi L, *et al.* Sobrerol in the treatment of secretory otitis media in childhood. *J Int Med Res* 1989; **17:** 277–86.
3. Azzollini E, *et al.* Sobrerol (Sobrepim®) administered dropwise to children with acute hypersecretory bronchopulmonary disease: a controlled trial v bromhexine. *Clin Trials J* 1990; **27:** 241–9.

Preparations

Proprietary Preparations (details are given in Part 3)
Ital.: Sobrepin; Sopulmin; ***Spain:*** Sobrepin.

Multi-ingredient: ***Ital.:*** Fluental; Polimucil; Sobrepin Antibiotico†; Sobrepin Respiro†; Soltux†; ***Spain:*** Sobrepin Amoxi†.

Sodium Dibunate (5632-k)

Sodium Dibunate *(BAN, rINN)*.

L-1633. Sodium 2,6-di-*tert*-butylnaphthalene-1-sulphonate.

$C_{18}H_{23}NaO_3S$ = 342.4.

CAS — 14992-59-7 (sodium dibunate).

Sodium dibunate is a cough suppressant used in non-productive cough (p.1052). It is claimed to have central and peripheral actions and has been given by mouth in usual doses of 30 mg three to four times daily. Chlorcyclizine dibunate (naftoclizine) has also been administered by mouth or rectally.

Preparations

Proprietary Preparations (details are given in Part 3)
Belg.: Becantex†; ***Ital.:*** Bechisan†; ***Neth.:*** Bexedyl†.

Multi-ingredient: ***Belg.:*** Becantex; Ebexol†; ***Canad.:*** Balminil Suppositoires; ***Ger.:*** Cito-Guakalin†; Ephepect-Blocker-Pastillen N; Makatussin†; ***Ital.:*** Sedobex; ***Neth.:*** Bexedyl Expectorans†; ***Spain:*** Super Koki†.

Squill (2026-k)

Bulbo de Escila; Cebolla Albarrana; Cila; Meerzwiebel; Scilla; Scillae Bulbus; Scille; White Squill.

Pharmacopoeias. In Br. and Ger.

The dried sliced bulb of *Drimia maritima* (Liliaceae), with the membranous outer scales removed, and containing not less than 68% of alcohol (60%)-soluble extractive.

Store at a temperature not exceeding 25° in a dry place.

Indian Squill (2027-a)

Urginea.

Pharmacopoeias. In Br.

The bulb of *Drimia indica* (Liliaceae), with the outer membranous scales removed, usually sliced and dried. **Store** at a temperature not exceeding 25° in a dry place.

Adverse Effects, Treatment, and Precautions

The adverse effects of squill and Indian squill in large doses include nausea, vomiting, and diarrhoea. As squill and Indian squill contain cardiac glycosides they can cause similar adverse effects to digoxin (p.849).

Abuse. Reports of cardiac glycoside toxicity and myopathy associated with the abuse of linctuses which have contained opiates and squill.[1-5]

1. Kennedy M. Cardiac glycoside toxicity: an unusual manifestation of drug addiction. *Med J Aust* 1981; **2:** 686–9.
2. Kilpatrick C, *et al.* Myopathy with myasthenic features possibly induced by codeine linctus. *Med J Aust* 1982; **2:** 410.
3. Seow SSW. Abuse of APF linctus codeine and cardiac glycoside toxicity. *Med J Aust* 1984; **140:** 54.
4. Thurston D, Taylor K. Gee's Linctus. *Pharm J* 1984; **233:** 63.
5. Smith W, *et al.* Wenckebach's phenomenon induced by cough linctus. *Br Med J* 1986; **292:** 868.

Uses and Administration

Squill and Indian squill are used as expectorants in productive cough (p.1052) and have been given in doses of 30 to 250 mg, as the oxymel, elixir, tincture, or vinegar. Preparations containing squill are used in some countries in the treatment of cardiovascular disorders.

Red squill has been used as a rodenticide (p.1410).

A history[1] of the use of squill.

1. Court WE. Squill – energetic diuretic. *Pharm J* 1985; **235:** 194–7.

Preparations

BP 1998: Squill Liquid Extract; Squill Oxymel.

Proprietary Preparations (details are given in Part 3)
Ger.: Digitalysat Scilla-Digitaloid; Scillamiron†; Scillase N.

Multi-ingredient: ***Austral.:*** Nyal Bronchitis; ***Canad.:*** Bronco Asmol; ***Fr.:*** Humex; Polypirine; ***Ger.:*** Befelka Herz-Dragees†; Cefascillan N; Cor-loges; Cor-Vel N; Diureticum-Medice†; Entwasserungs-Tee†; Gelsadon†; Hevert-Entwasserungs-Tee; Hocura-Diureticum†; Miroton; Miroton N; Nephrisan P; Raufuncton N; Szillosan forte; Szillosan†; Urodil N†; Urodil S†; Venopyronum N triplex; ***Irl.:*** Ipesil; ***S.Afr.:*** Cocilix†; Cocillana Co; Contra-Coff; Linctus Tussi Infans; Misfans†; Tusselix†; ***UK:*** Balm of Gilead; Buttercup Syrup; Catarrh Pastilles; Catarrh Tablets; Chest Mixture; Collins Elixir Pastilles; ES Bronchial Mixture; Fisherman's Friend Honey Cough Syrup†; Galloway's Cough Syrup; Honey & Molasses; Jackson's Children's Cough Pastilles; Lobelia Compound; Sanderson's Throat Specific.

Stepronin (980-x)

Stepronin *(rINN)*.

2-(α-Thenoylthio)-propionylglycine; Tiofacic. *N*-(2-Mercaptopropionyl)glycine 2-thiophenecarboxylate.

$C_{10}H_{11}NO_4S_2$ = 273.3.

CAS — 72324-18-6 (stepronin); 78126-10-0 (stepronin sodium).

Stepronin has been reported to have mucolytic actions in productive cough (p.1052), and has also been used in the treatment of liver disorders. It is reported to be metabolised to tiopronin (p.997). Stepronin is mainly used as the sodium and lysinate salts.

Preparations

Proprietary Preparations (details are given in Part 3)
Ital.: Broncoplus; Masor; Mucodil; Tiase†; Tioten; Valase†.

Tasuldine (2769-w)

Tasuldine *(pINN)*.

2-[(3-Pyridylmethyl)thio]pyrimidine.

$C_{10}H_9N_3S$ = 203.3.

CAS — 88579-39-9.

Tasuldine has been studied as an expectorant and mucolytic.

References.

1. Dorow P, *et al.* Influence of tasuldine and acetylcysteine on mucociliary clearance in patients with chronic airways obstruction. *Arzneimittelforschung* 1986; **36:** 131–3.

Telmesteine (14665-e)

Telmesteine *(rINN)*.

(−)-3-Ethyl hydrogen (*R*)-3,4-thiazolidinedicarboxylate.

$C_7H_{11}NO_4S$ = 205.2.

CAS — 122946-43-4.

Telmesteine is used as a mucolytic (p.1052) in the treatment of respiratory-tract disorders in doses of 300 mg two or three times daily.

Preparations

Proprietary Preparations (details are given in Part 3)
Ital.: Muconorm; Reolase.

Terpin Hydrate (2029-x)

Terpin Hydrate *(BANM)*.

Terpene Hydrate; Terpinol. *p*-Menthane-1,8-diol monohydrate; 4-Hydroxy-α,α,4-trimethylcyclohexanemethanol monohydrate.

$C_{10}H_{20}O_2,H_2O$ = 190.3.

CAS — 80-53-5 (anhydrous terpin); 2451-01-6 (terpin monohydrate).

Pharmacopoeias. In Fr., Swiss, and US.

Colourless lustrous crystals or white powder with a slight odour. It effloresces in dry air. **Soluble** 1 in 200 of water, 1 in 35 of boiling water, 1 in 13 of alcohol, 1 in 3 of boiling alcohol, and 1 in 140 of chloroform and of ether. A 1% solution in hot water is neutral to litmus. **Store** in airtight containers.

If crystals form in terpin hydrate elixir, they may be redissolved by warming the closed container of solution in warm water and then gently shaking it.

Terpin hydrate has been stated to increase bronchial secretion directly and is used as an expectorant in productive cough (p.1052). It has been given by mouth in doses of up to 200 mg every 4 hours.

Nausea, vomiting, or abdominal pain may follow the ingestion of terpin hydrate on an empty stomach.

Terpin hydrochloride has also been used.

Preparations

USP 23: Terpin Hydrate and Codeine Elixir; Terpin Hydrate and Dextromethorphan Hydrobromide Elixir; Terpin Hydrate Elixir.

Proprietary Preparations (details are given in Part 3)
Fr.: Terpine des Monts-Dore.

Multi-ingredient: ***Belg.:*** Balsoclase; Tri-Cold; ***Canad.:*** Pastilles Valda; Valda; ***Fr.:*** Bronchodermine; Bronchorectine au Citral; Bronpax; Codotussyl†; Marrubene Codethyline; Passedyl; Pulmofluide Enfants†; Pulmofluide Ephedrine†; Pulmofluide Simple; Pulmoll; Pulmothiol†; Pulveol†; Tercodine†; Terpine Gonnon; Terpone; Tossarel; ***Ger.:*** Nasalgon†; Ozothin; Sedotussin Expectorans; Tetra-Ozothin†; ***Irl.:*** Coldrex; ***Ital.:*** Bromoterpina†; Chymoser Balsamico†; Elisir Terpina; Glicocinnamina†; Guaiadomus†; Neo Borocillina Balsamica; Sedopulmina†; Tionamil; Tussiflex; Vapor Sol†; ***Neth.:*** Balsoclase Compositum; ***S.Afr.:*** Cocilix†; Degoran†; Dykatuss Expectorant†; Tusselix†; ***Spain:*** Pastillas Juanola; Pastillas Pectoral Kely; Prontal†; Terponil; ***Switz.:*** Bromocod N; Bronchodermine†; Bronchorectine†; Libexine Compositum; Mephaxine Compositum; Rectoseptal-Neo bismuthe; Rectoseptal-Neo Pholcodine; Rectoseptal-Neo simple; Sedotussin; Spedro; ***UK:*** Cabdrivers Adult Linctus; Coldrex; Copholco†; Copholcoids†.

Tetrahydrozoline Hydrochloride (2108-t)

Tetrahydrozoline Hydrochloride *(BANM)*.

Tetryzoline Hydrochloride *(rINNM)*. 2-(1,2,3,4-Tetrahydro-1-naphthyl)-2-imidazoline hydrochloride.

$C_{13}H_{16}N_2,HCl$ = 236.7.

CAS — 84-22-0 (tetrahydrozoline); 522-48-5 (tetrahydrozoline hydrochloride).

Pharmacopoeias. In US.

A white odourless solid. **Soluble** 1 in 3.5 of water and 1 in 7.5 of alcohol; very slightly soluble in chloroform; practically insoluble in ether. **Store** in airtight containers.

Tetrahydrozoline is a sympathomimetic with effects similar to those of naphazoline (p.1064). It is used as the hydrochloride for its vasoconstrictor effect in the symptomatic relief of nasal congestion (p.1052). A 0.1% solution is instilled into each nostril as nasal drops or a spray three to four times daily as necessary; it should not be used more often than every 3 hours. Children aged 2 to 6 years of age may be given 2 to 3 drops of a 0.05% solution in each nostril.

Solutions of tetrahydrozoline hydrochloride containing 0.05% are used as a conjunctival decongestant.

Other salts of tetrahydrozoline including the nitrate, phosphate, and sulphate have been used similarly.

Preparations

USP 23: Tetrahydrozoline Hydrochloride Nasal Solution; Tetrahydrozoline Hydrochloride Ophthalmic Solution.

Proprietary Preparations (details are given in Part 3)
Austral.: Visine; ***Belg.:*** Visine; ***Canad.:*** Eye Drops; RO-Eye Drops; Visine; ***Fr.:*** Constrilia; ***Ger.:*** Caltheon; Cleer†; Diabenyl T; Exrhinin; Rhinopront; Tyzine; Vasopos N; Vidiseptal EDO Sine; Yxin; ***Ital.:*** Demetil; Octilia; Rinobios†; Stilla Decongestionante; Vasorinil; Visine; ***Jpn:*** Narbel†; ***Neth.:*** Constrilia†; Visine†; ***Spain:*** Vispring; ***Switz.:*** Constrilia†; Demo collyre No 2†; Rhinopront Top; Stilla†; Tyzine; Visine; ***USA:*** Eyesine; Geneye Extra; Mallazine; Optigene 3; Soothe; Tetrasine; Tyzine; Visine†.

Multi-ingredient: ***Austral.:*** In A Wink Allergy; Murine Sore Eyes; Visine Allergy; Visine Revive; ***Canad.:*** Collyrium; Visine Allergy; Visine Moisturizing; ***Ger.:*** Allergopos N; Berberil N; Efemolin; Spersadexolin; Spersallerg; Tyzine compositum†; ***Ital.:*** Aldrisone VC†; Biorinil; Cromozil; Desonix†; Dexoline; Efemoline; Eta Biocortilen VC; Etaproctene†; Flumetol; Ischemol A; Medramil; Tetramil; Vasosterone; Vasosterone Antibiotico; Vasosterone Collirio; Visublefarite; Visucloben Decongestionante; Visumetazone Antibiotico; Visumetazone Decongestionante; Visumicina; Visustrin; ***Norw.:*** Spersallerg; ***S.Afr.:*** Efemoline; Gemini; Oculoforte; Spersadexoline; Spersallerg; ***Spain:*** Dexam Constric; Medrivas; Medrivas Antib; Mevaso†; Oftalmo†; Tivitis; Vasodexa; Visublefarite; ***Switz.:*** Collypan; Efemoline; Oculosan forte; Spersadexoline; Spersallerg; ***USA:*** Collyrium Fresh; Geneye AC Allergy†; Murine Plus; Tetrasine Extra; Visine Allergy Relief; Visine Moisturizing.

Thebacon Hydrochloride (6261-j)

Thebacon Hydrochloride *(BANM, rINNM)*.

Acethydrocodone Hydrochloride; Acetyldihydrocodeinone Hydrochloride; Dihydrocodeinone Enol Acetate Hydrochloride. 6-*O*-Acetyl-7,8-dihydro-3-*O*-methyl-6,7-didehydromorphine hydrochloride; (−)-(5*R*)-4,5-Epoxy-3-methoxy-9a-methylmorphin-6-en-6-yl acetate hydrochloride.

$C_{20}H_{23}NO_4,HCl$ = 377.9.

CAS — 466-90-0 (thebacon); 20236-82-2 (thebacon hydrochloride).

Thebacon hydrochloride is a centrally acting cough suppressant used for non-productive cough (p.1052). It has actions similar to those of codeine (p.26) but stated to be approximately 4 times more potent. It has been given by mouth in divided doses up to a maximum of 20 mg daily.

Preparations

Proprietary Preparations (details are given in Part 3)
Belg.: Acedicone.

Tipepidine Hybenzate (13352-s)

Tipepidine Hibenzate *(rINNM)*; AT-327 (tipepidine); CR-662 (tipepidine). 3-[Di(2-thienyl)methylene]-1-methylpiperidine 2-(4-hydroxybenzoyl)benzoate.

$C_{15}H_{17}NS_2,C_{14}H_{10}O_4$ = 517.7.

CAS — 5169-78-8 (tipepidine); 31139-87-4 (tipepidine hybenzate).

Pharmacopoeias. In Jpn.

Tipepidine hybenzate is a cough suppressant used for non-productive cough (p.1052) which is claimed also to have an expectorant action. It has been given by mouth in doses of 50 to 100 mg three times a day.

Report[1] of generalised convulsions associated with the administration of therapeutic doses of tipepidine hybenzate by mouth in one patient.

1. Cuomo RM. On the possible convulsive activity of an antitussive piperidinic derivative ('tipepidina ibenzato') in man. *Acta Neurol (Napoli)* 1982; **37:** 110–16.

Preparations

Proprietary Preparations (details are given in Part 3)
Jpn: Asverin; ***Spain:*** Asvelik.

Tolu Balsam (287-f)

Balsamum Tolutanum; Baume de Tolu.

CAS — 9000-64-0; 8017-09-2.

Pharmacopoeias. In *It., Swiss,* and *US.*

A balsam obtained from *Myroxylon balsamum* (=*M. toluiferum*) (Leguminosae). It is a brownish-yellow or brown plastic solid when fresh, but becomes brittle when old, dried, or exposed to cold temperatures. It has an aromatic and vanilla-like odour.

Practically **insoluble** in water and petroleum spirit; soluble in alcohol, in chloroform, and in ether, but sometimes leaving some insoluble residues or turbidity. **Store** at a temperature not exceeding 40° in airtight containers.

Tolu balsam is considered to have very mild antiseptic properties and some expectorant action but is mainly used in the form of a syrup to flavour cough mixtures. However, Tolu Syrup (BP) no longer contains tolu balsam but is based on cinnamic acid (p.1111).

Preparations

USP 23: Compound Benzoin Tincture.

Tramazoline Hydrochloride (2109-x)

Tramazoline Hydrochloride (*BANM, USAN, rINNM*).

2-(5,6,7,8-Tetrahydro-1-naphthylamino)-2-imidazoline hydrochloride.

$C_{13}H_{17}N_3,HCl = 251.8.$

CAS — 1082-57-1 (tramazoline); 3715-90-0 (tramazoline hydrochloride).

Tramazoline hydrochloride is a sympathomimetic with effects similar to those of naphazoline (p.1064). It is used to provide symptomatic relief of nasal congestion (p.1052). It is given as a metered-dose nasal spray in doses of 120 μg into each nostril 3 or 4 times daily; dosage has been increased temporarily to 6 times daily in severe cases.

Tramazoline hydrochloride has also been used in eye drops as a conjunctival decongestant.

Preparations

Proprietary Preparations (details are given in Part 3)

Austral.: Rhinaspray†; Spray-Tish; ***Belg.:*** Rhinospray; ***Ger.:*** Biciron; Ellatun; Rhinospray; ***Ital.:*** Ringogutt Spray-Fher; ***Neth.:*** Bisolnasal; Rhinospray†; ***Spain:*** Rhinospray.

Multi-ingredient: ***Aust.:*** Dexa-Rhinospray; Rhinospray Plus; ***Austral.:*** Tobispray†; ***Belg.:*** Dexa-Rhinospray; ***Ger.:*** Cimporhin†; Dexa Biciron; Dexa-Rhinospray N; Oxy Biciron; ***Irl.:*** Dexa-Rhinaspray; ***Ital.:*** Ringogutt Antiallergico Spray; Ringogutt Eucalipto-Fher; ***Switz.:*** Dexa-Rhinospray†; Lurgyl†; ***UK:*** Dexa-Rhinaspray Duo; Dexa-Rhinaspray†.

Tuaminoheptane Sulphate (2112-z)

Tuaminoheptane Sulphate (*BANM, rINNM*).

$(C_7H_{17}N)_2,H_2SO_4 = 328.5.$

CAS — 6411-75-2.

Tuaminoheptane is a volatile sympathomimetic (p.951) that has been used as the sulphate for the symptomatic relief of nasal congestion. Tuaminoheptane has also been employed in the form of the carbonate.

Preparations

Proprietary Preparations (details are given in Part 3)

Multi-ingredient: ***Fr.:*** Rhinofluimucil; ***Ger.:*** Rinofluimucil-S; ***Ital.:*** Otomicetina; Rinofluimucil; ***Spain:*** Rinofluimucil; ***Switz.:*** Rinofluimucil.

Tymazoline Hydrochloride (2113-c)

Tymazoline Hydrochloride (*BANM*).

2-Thymyloxymethyl-2-imidazoline Hydrochloride. 2-(2-Isopropyl-5-methylphenoxymethyl)-2-imidazoline hydrochloride.

$C_{14}H_{20}N_2O,HCl = 268.8.$

CAS — 24243-97-8 (tymazoline); 28120-03-8 (tymazoline hydrochloride).

Pharmacopoeias. In *Pol.*

Tymazoline is a sympathomimetic (p.951) that is used as the hydrochloride for its local vasoconstrictor effect in the symptomatic relief of nasal congestion (p.1052). A 0.05% solution is administered into each nostril by nasal spray every 4 hours as necessary.

Preparations

Proprietary Preparations (details are given in Part 3)

Fr.: Pernazene.

Xylometazoline Hydrochloride

(2114-k)

Xylometazoline Hydrochloride (*BANM, rINNM*).

2-(4-*tert*-Butyl-2,6-dimethylbenzyl)-2-imidazoline hydrochloride.

$C_{16}H_{24}N_2,HCl = 280.8.$

CAS — 526-36-3 (xylometazoline); 1218-35-5 (xylometazoline hydrochloride).

Pharmacopoeias. In *Eur.* (see p.viii), *Pol.*, and *US.*

A white to off-white odourless or almost odourless crystalline powder. Ph. Eur. **solubilities** are: freely soluble in water, in alcohol, and in methyl alcohol; practically insoluble in ether. USP solubilities are: soluble 1 in 35 of water; freely soluble in alcohol; sparingly soluble in chloroform; practically insoluble in ether. A 5% solution in water has a pH of 5.0 to 6.6. **Store** in airtight containers. Protect from light.

Adverse Effects and Precautions

As for Naphazoline, p.1064.

Interactions

Since xylometazoline is absorbed through the mucosa interactions may follow topical application. An authoritative source in the UK considers that all sympathomimetic nasal decongestants are liable to cause a hypertensive crisis if used during treatment with an MAOI. For the interactions of sympathomimetics in general, see p.951.

Uses and Administration

Xylometazoline is a direct-acting sympathomimetic (p.951) with marked alpha-adrenergic activity. It is a vasoconstrictor which reduces swelling and congestion when applied to mucous membranes. The effect begins within 5 to 10 minutes of application and lasts for up to 10 hours.

Xylometazoline is used as the hydrochloride for the symptomatic relief of nasal congestion (p.1052). A 0.1% solution of xylometazoline hydrochloride is applied topically as nasal drops or a spray into each nostril two or three times daily. A 0.05% solution is used once or twice daily for children less than 12 years of age but is not recommended for infants of less than 3 months of age; 1 or 2 drops of the solution are instilled into each nostril.

A 0.05% solution of xylometazoline hydrochloride may be instilled into the eye as a conjunctival decongestant.

Preparations

BP 1998: Xylometazoline Nasal Drops;
USP 23: Xylometazoline Hydrochloride Nasal Solution.

Proprietary Preparations (details are given in Part 3)

Aust.: Olynth; Otrivin; ***Austral.:*** Otrivin; ***Belg.:*** Otrivine; Rhinidine; ***Canad.:*** Certified Decongestant; Decongestant Nasal Spray; Decongestant Nose Drops; Novahistex†; Otrivin; Vaporisateur Nasal Decongestionnant; ***Ger.:*** Balkis; Dorenasin; Gelonasal; Idril N†; Imdin S; Imidin N; Logomed Nasen-Tropfen; Mentopin Nasenspray; Nasan; Nasengel; Nasengel AL; Nasenspray AL; Nasenspray E; Nasenspray K; Nasentropfen AL; Nasentropfen E; Nasentropfen K; Olynth; Otalgicin; Otriven; Otriven gegen Schnupfen; Rapako xylo; Rhino-stas; schnupfen endrine; Snup†; Stas Nasentropfen; Therapin Schnupfentropfen/spray†; ViviRhin S; Xylo; Xylo-Comod; ***Irl.:*** Otrivine; ***Ital.:*** Neo-Rinoleina; Otrivin; ***Neth.:*** Otrivin; ***Norw.:*** Otrivin; Zymelin; ***S.Afr.:*** Otrivin; Sinutab; ***Spain:*** Desconasal; Otrivin; Rationasal; ***Swed.:*** Nasoferm; Otrivin; ***Switz.:*** Nasben; Olynth; Otrivin; Rinosedin; ***UK:*** Otrivine; ***USA:*** Otrivin.

Multi-ingredient: ***Aust.:*** Lomusol comp; ***Austral.:*** Allergy Eyes; Sinex†; ***Belg.:*** Lomusol plus Xylometazoline; ***Canad.:*** Ophtrivin-A; ***Ger.:*** Lomupren compositum; Otriven-Millicorten†; Vividrin comp; ***Irl.:*** Otrivine-Antistin; Rynacrom Compound; ***Ital.:*** Iodosan Nasale Contact†; Nasalemed; Respiro; Rinos; Tririnol; ***Spain:*** Rinoblanco Dexa Antibio; ***Swed.:*** Otrivin Menthol; ***Switz.:*** Lomusol-X; Muco-Trin; Nospilin†; Triofan; ***UK:*** Otrivine-Antistin; Resiston One; Rynacrom Compound.

Zipeprol Hydrochloride (5633-a)

Zipeprol Hydrochloride (*rINNM*).

CERM-3024. α-(α-Methoxybenzyl)-4-(β-methoxyphenethyl)-1-piperazineethanol dihydrochloride.

$C_{23}H_{32}N_2O_3,2HCl = 457.4.$

CAS — 34758-83-3 (zipeprol); 34758-84-4 (zipeprol hydrochloride).

Zipeprol is a centrally acting cough suppressant which is stated to have a peripheral action on bronchial spasm. It is given by mouth as the hydrochloride in doses of 150 to 300 mg daily in divided doses. Zipeprol has also been administered rectally. There have been reports of abuse and overdosage producing neurological symptoms.

Abuse and overdosage. Severe neurological symptoms have been reported in young adults following habitual abuse of zipeprol for euphoria. Patients have presented with generalised seizures, followed by coma.[1] One patient who ingested 750 mg of zipeprol had several opisthotonic crises and developed cerebral oedema.[2] Symptoms of overdosage in children have included restlessness, somnolence, ataxia, choreic movements, forced deviation of the head and eyes, generalised seizures, respiratory depression, and coma.[1,3]

Dependence and withdrawal symptoms similar to those produced by opioids have been reported.[4] WHO has assessed zipeprol to have a moderate potential for dependence and liability for abuse.[5] Although zipeprol is a weak opioid agonist at high doses its toxicity and hallucinogenic and other psychotropic effects constitute a significant element in its abuse, and the public health and social problems associated with such abuse were considered substantial.

1. Moroni C, *et al.* Overdosage of zipeprol, a non-opioid antitussive agent. *Lancet* 1984; **i:** 45.
2. Perraro F, Beorchia A. Convulsions and cerebral oedema associated with zipeprol abuse. *Lancet* 1984; **i:** 45–6.
3. Merigot P, *et al.* Les convulsions avec trois antitussifs dérivés substitués dé la pipérazine (zipépról, éprazinone, éprozinol). *Ann Pediatr (Paris)* 1985; **32:** 504–11.
4. Mallaret MP, *et al.* Zipeprol: primary dependence in an unaddicted patient. *Ann Pharmacother* 1995; **29:** 540.
5. WHO. WHO expert committee on drug dependence: twenty-ninth report. *WHO Tech Rep Ser 856* 1995.

Preparations

Proprietary Preparations (details are given in Part 3)

Ital.: Antituxil-Z†; Bechizolo†; Broncozina†; Respirase†; Zitoxil; ***Spain:*** Respirex†; ***Switz.:*** Mirsol.

Dermatological Drugs

The skin is subject to a very wide range of lesions. Some may be characteristic of specific systemic diseases and fade as the disease regresses. Some are caused by specific local infections and are best treated by the appropriate antimicrobial (see bacterial skin infections, p.142, and fungal skin infections, p.371). The skin is also subject to damage from environmental hazards. Exposure to solar radiation is associated with malignant neoplasms of the skin (see p.492). Many skin disorders are side-effects of therapeutic and other agents, ranging from mild hypersensitivity to the life-threatening Stevens-Johnson syndrome or toxic epidermal necrolysis (see Drug-induced Skin Reactions, below). There also remains a wide range of skin disorders whose aetiology is poorly understood.

The distribution and morphological description of the skin lesion (its shape, colour, and surface characteristics) are important in the diagnosis of skin disorders. There are many terms used to describe skin lesions:

- abscess–a collection of pus in a cavity
- bulla (or blister)–a fluid-filled circumscribed lesion larger than 0.5 cm in diameter
- comedo–a plug of keratin and sebum in a pilosebaceous follicle
- ecchymosis–an extravasation of blood into the skin
- erythema–red coloration due to vascular dilatation
- fissure–a slit through the whole thickness of the skin
- horn–a thickening of the skin that is taller than it is broad
- keratosis–a horny thickening of the skin
- lichenification–hard, thickened skin with increased markings
- macule–an area of altered colour or texture with no elevation above the surface of the surrounding skin
- nodule–a dome-shaped or spherical-shaped, solid lesion, usually more than 0.5 cm in diameter and depth
- papilloma–a nipple-like mass
- papule–a raised solid lesion, usually less than 0.5 cm in diameter
- petechia–a pinhead-sized macule of blood in the skin
- plaque–a raised, flat-topped, circumscribed lesion, usually larger than 2 cm in diameter but with no substantial depth
- purpura–a macule of blood in the skin, larger than a petechia
- pustule–an accumulation of pus in the skin
- scale–a flat plate or flake of stratum corneum
- stria–a streak-like, linear, atrophic lesion, pink, purple, or white in colour
- telangiectasia–a visible dilatation of small cutaneous blood vessels
- vesicle–a fluid-filled circumscribed lesion less than 0.5 cm in diameter
- wheal–an elevated, white, compressible area of oedema often surrounded by a red flare.

This chapter describes the drugs used in the management of skin disorders and the treatment of some of the commoner skin disorders. The pharmacology of many of the drugs used in dermatology is often poorly understood. Treatment may include topical and/or systemic drug therapy. Physical methods such as cryotherapy, UV radiation, radiotherapy, and surgery also have a role.

Drugs with a traditional place in the treatment of skin disorders include coal tar, dithranol, ichthammol, and urea, as well as keratolytics such as benzoyl peroxide and salicylic acid. Vitamin D analogues such as calcipotriol, photosensitisers such as the psoralen methoxsalen and the vitamin A analogues, retinoids (such as acitretin, isotretinoin, and tretinoin) have an important role in certain skin disorders.

Agents with primarily a protective function include calamine, starch, talc, titanium dioxide, and zinc oxide. Some agents, for example ammonium lactate and sodium pidolate, have humectant properties and are used in topical moisturising preparations.

Drugs used to increase pigmentation include dihydroxyacetone, methoxsalen, and trioxsalen. Those used to reduce pigmentation include hydroquinone, mequinol, and monobenzone. Other agents used to protect against sunlight are described under Sunscreens, p.1486.

For agents that are applied topically, the vehicle and formulation may be as important as the active drug, and some cream and ointment bases are used alone for their protective properties. Adverse effects occurring with topical preparations may sometimes be attributed to constituents of the vehicle such as stabilisers and preservatives. The choice of formulation depends on the skin condition being treated and the area affected. Lotions and gels are useful for hairy areas. Creams (oil-in-water emulsions) have cooling and emollient effects, are readily absorbed by the skin, and are used for acute and exudative conditions. Ointments (water-in-oil emulsions) are more occlusive than creams and are particularly suitable for chronic dry lesions. Pastes (powder incorporated in an ointment basis) are less occlusive than ointments and are useful for their protective properties and for their use on circumscribed lesions. Other less frequently used formulations include applications, collodions, and dusting powders. Typical quantities of preparations required per week for twice daily application to specific areas of an adult are given in Table 1, below.

Table 1. Typical quantities of preparations required per week for twice daily application to an adult.

	Creams and Ointments	Lotions
Face	15 to 30 g	100 mL
Both hands	25 to 50 g	200 mL
Scalp	50 to 100 g	200 mL
Both arms or both legs	100 to 200 g	200 mL
Trunk	400 g	500 mL
Groins and genitalia	15 to 25 g	100 mL

NOTE. These quantities do *not* apply to corticosteroid preparations.

Acne

Acne is a disorder of the pilosebaceous follicle; common features include increased sebum production, follicular keratinisation, colonisation by *Propionibacterium acnes*, and localised inflammation. The initial lesions are noninflamed comedones that form in the pilosebaceous follicles. These comedones may be open (blackheads) or closed (whiteheads). Closed comedones may develop into inflamed lesions, such as papules, pustules, or nodules. The most common form of acne is acne vulgaris. It is common in teenagers and while by their mid-20s the majority of cases have resolved, a few people still require treatment in their 30s and 40s. Skin areas typically affected are the face, shoulders, upper chest, and back. Acne may also occur in late middle age and in the elderly (late onset acne) and in infants (infantile acne). Certain drugs, including androgens, corticosteroids, corticotrophin, hormonal contraceptives containing androgenic progestogens such as levonorgestrol, isoniazid, lithium, methoxsalen, and some antiepileptics may produce an acneiform rash, as may substances such as tars, oils, and oily cosmetics.

Mild acne is characterised by blackheads and whiteheads, with some papules and pustules. In moderate acne, the papules and pustules are more widespread, and there may be mild scarring. Severe acne is characterised by the presence of nodular abscesses or cysts in addition to widespread pustules and papules, and may lead to extensive scarring.

Treatment aims to reduce the bacterial population of the pilosebaceous follicles, reduce the rate of sebum production, reduce inflammation, and remove the keratinised layer blocking the follicles. Drugs used include keratolytics and antibacterials. If topical preparations are not effective, oral preparations may be required. Response to therapy is commonly slow and long-term treatment is usually necessary.[1-6]

Mild acne is treated topically, in particular with benzoyl peroxide, antibacterials, or retinoids. Abrasives have been used but their effectiveness is doubtful, and preparations based on sulphur or salicylic acid are considered by some to be obsolete; the effectiveness of degreasing agents has also been questioned. Topical corticosteroids, despite their presence in some compound preparations, should not be used. Benzoyl peroxide is probably the most widely used first-line drug. Azelaic acid is an alternative to benzoyl peroxide.

Topical antibacterials may also be used as first-line treatment or following ineffective benzoyl peroxide application. Tetracycline, clindamycin, and erythromycin are generally available as solutions for topical use, and appear to be roughly equivalent in efficacy. However, development of resistance by the skin flora may be a problem; combination therapy with benzoyl peroxide and erythromycin has been reported to be helpful in preventing the selection of resistant mutants. It has also been recommended that courses of topical antibacterials be restricted to 10 to 12 weeks, repeated if necessary after a few weeks, and that concomitant treatment with different oral and topical drugs or rotation be avoided.[7]

The retinoids, isotretinoin and tretinoin, appear to be equally effective when used topically. Tazarotene is a recently-introduced retinoid for topical use. Some dermatologists consider a topical retinoid to be the treatment of choice for mild to moderate comedonal acne. Topical retinoids and antibacterials may be used together, since antibacterials are more effective for inflammation and retinoids for comedones; retinoids may also be alternated with benzoyl peroxide. Adapalene, a naphthoic acid derivative, has recently been introduced for the topical treatment of acne. Nicotinamide is also used topically.

Moderate acne is best treated with oral antibacterials. Topical drugs may also be used as adjunctive treatment. Of the oral antibacterials tetracyclines appear to be the drugs of choice. Tetracycline, doxycycline, or oxytetracycline may be used. Minocycline has also been reported to be effective; however, it may cause skin pigmentation and may be associated rarely with immunologically mediated reactions. Alternatives to the tetracyclines include erythromycin and trimethoprim. All oral antibacterials have to be administered for at least 3 months; the maximal response is thought to occur after 3 to 4 months, although in some cases treatment for 2 or more years may be necessary. Again, resistance may be a problem.

Women with moderate acne who also require oral contraception may be treated with a combined oral contraceptive containing a non-androgenic progestogen.

Severe acne is usually treated with oral isotretinoin. Where it cannot be used, high doses of oral antibacterials may be considered. In women with hormonal disturbances, the anti-androgen cyproterone with ethinyloestradiol (available as a combination preparation) or a combined (non-androgenic) contraceptive may be effective. Spironolactone used for its anti-androgenic properties has been advocated for women in whom oestrogens are contra-indicated.

Topical drugs, particularly antibacterials, described above under mild acne, may be used as adjunctive treatment.

1. Healy E, Simpson N. Acne vulgaris. *Br Med J* 1994; **308:** 831–3.
2. Sykes NL, Webster GF. Acne: a review of optimum treatment. *Drugs* 1994; **48:** 59–70.
3. Sharpe GR. Prescribing for acne vulgaris. *Prescribers' J* 1995; **35:** 53–8.
4. Leyden JJ. Therapy for acne vulgaris. *N Engl J Med* 1997; **336:** 1156–62.
5. Livingstone C. Acne. *Pharm J* 1997; **259:** 725–7.
6. Brown SK, Shalita AR. Acne vulgaris. *Lancet* 1998; **351:** 1871–6.
7. Eady EA, *et al.* Antibiotic resistant propionibacteria in acne: need for policies to modify antibiotic usage. *Br Med J* 1993; **306:** 555–6.

Alopecia

Alopecia (hair loss) has many causes. The most common form, male-pattern alopecia, is androgen-related. Alopecia may also be congenital, be associated with systemic disorders, severe emotional and physical stress, or skin disorders, or be due to nutritional deficiencies. Some drugs may cause alopecia; examples include antineoplastics, beta blockers, diazoxide, heparin, verapamil, and warfarin. In some cases there is destruction of the hair follicles (scarring) resulting in permanent hair loss. If the hair follicles remain intact (nonscarring alopecia) then treatment of the underlying condition or removal of the suspected drug may produce hair regrowth. For a discussion of the management of chemotherapy-induced alopecia, see under Treatment of the Adverse Effects of Antineoplastics, p.474. Drug treatment may be tried in alopecia areata and male-pattern alopecia, although it is often not successful.

Alopecia areata is an auto-immune disorder in which there is a loss of hair in sharply defined areas of skin that normally bear hair. The affected area can vary in size from about 1 cm^2 to the whole scalp (alopecia totalis) or all body hair (alopecia universalis).

Small or isolated patches of alopecia areata may not need treatment and in many patients hair regrows within a few months. If loss of hair becomes a problem cosmetically, treatment may be offered but is often not totally satisfactory. Several treatment options have been tried.[1] Among these are corticosteroids, which may be given by intralesional injection; photochemotherapy with ultraviolet A radiation (PUVA) with either systemic or topical psoralens; topical minoxidil; and allergic sensitisation with topical diphencyprone.

Male-pattern alopecia (androgenetic alopecia or male-pattern baldness)[2,3] involves recession of the hairline in the frontal region of the scalp or loss of hair at the vertex. It is usually associated with increasing age in men. A similar pattern of hair loss occurs in women with elevated androgen concentrations; hair loss associated with increasing age in women with normal androgen concentrations is usually much more diffuse. Topical minoxidil is more effective in male-pattern alopecia than it is in the areata forms of alopecia, but is still, at best, only modestly effective. Because of the role of androgens in this condition anti-androgens and 5α-reductase inhibitors, such as finasteride, may also be tried. Finasteride is restricted to use in males.

1. Shapiro J. Alopecia areata: update on therapy. *Dermatol Clin* 1993; **11:** 35–46.
2. Bergfeld WF. Androgenetic alopecia: an autosomal dominant disorder. *Am J Med* 1995; **98** (suppl 1A): 95S–98S.
3. Sinclair R. Male pattern androgenetic alopecia. *Br Med J* 1998; **317:** 865–9.

Burns

Burns may be caused by chemicals or heat. Initial treatment of burns is irrigation with cold water for 10 to 15 minutes. This limits the skin damage in burns caused by heat and removes the causative agent in chemical burns. Sodium bicarbonate solution is then used on acid burns and acetic acid solution on alkaline burns. The major problems associated with burns are hypovolaemic shock, inhalation injury, and infection.[1]

Hypovolaemic shock (p.798) may develop if burns involve at least 15 to 20% of the body-surface area. After a burn, fluid accumulates rapidly in the wound area due to increased permeability of the microcirculation and this loss of fluid from the circulation produces hypovolaemic shock.

Inhalation injury producing airway oedema is mainly a result of exposure to toxic gases. Endotracheal intubation is required until the oedema subsides.

Prevention of infection is an important part of burn wound management. Micro-organisms proliferate rapidly in burn wounds, especially those severe enough to impair immune function and sepsis remains the major fatal complication of burns. Burn wounds should be cleansed with normal saline (see Wounds and Ulcers, below). This may be all that is required for very minor burn wounds; a non-adherent dressing, such as paraffin tulle, may be used if necessary. Topical antibacterials, such as silver sulphadiazine and mafenide acetate, may be applied as required. Removal of devitalised tissue is also an essential element of management. Infections require aggressive systemic treatment (see under Skin Infections, p.142).

Full thickness burn wounds require skin grafting. This is performed as soon as possible after stabilisation of the patient. Skin grafting may also be considered for deep partial thickness wounds. If the area to be grafted is very extensive, the grafting procedure may have to be in stages (at intervals of about a week) as sufficient autologous skin becomes available. Alternatively, temporary skin substitutes may be used to supplement autologous skin and allow wound closure in one stage. In severely burnt children growth hormone has reduced donor-site healing times to allow earlier reharvest.

1. Monafo WW. Initial management of burns. *N Engl J Med* 1996; **335:** 1581–6.

Darier's disease

Darier's disease (keratosis follicularis) is an uncommon inherited keratinisation disorder (see below) and is characterised by groups of horny papules over the body. These may become irritated and/or infected, exudative, and crusted. Severity varies greatly; mild disease may require the use of emollients only while more severe cases are treated with keratolysis using topical agents such as salicylic acid or tretinoin, or the oral retinoids acitretin, etretinate, or isotretinoin. Cyclosporin and topical fluorouracil have also been tried.

Dermatitis herpetiformis

Dermatitis herpetiformis is a rare blistering disorder of the subepidermal tissue in which the vesicles and papules are intensely irritant and pruritic. The knees, elbows, buttocks, shoulders, scalp, and face are areas typically affected. The disease presents usually during early to middle adult life and is a chronic condition, although there may be periods of remission that last several months. In many patients there is also a mild gastro-intestinal absorptive defect characterised by gluten hypersensitivity (gluten enteropathy). Skin lesions can be suppressed by dapsone; the sulphonamides sulphamethoxypyridazine or sulphapyridine have been used as alternatives to dapsone.[1,2] A gluten-free diet may improve both gastro-intestinal symptoms and the skin disorder.[3]

1. Fine J-D. Management of acquired bullous skin diseases. *N Engl J Med* 1995; **333:** 1475–84.
2. Garioch JJ. Dermatitis herpetiformis and its management. *Prescribers' J* 1996; **36:** 141–5.
3. Garioch JJ, *et al.* 25 years' experience of a gluten-free diet in the treatment of dermatitis herpetiformis. *Br J Dermatol* 1994; **131:** 541–5.

Drug-induced skin reactions

Drugs are a frequent cause of adverse skin reactions. The skin reaction may mimic a spontaneously occurring skin disorder and is therefore included in the differential diagnosis of most skin diseases. Alternatively, the drug may produce quite specific changes. The reaction can develop after the first dose or after a period of sensitisation. Pigmentation changes or effects on hair may take some months to become apparent.

Reactions range from mild rashes to severe life-threatening reactions including angioedema with urticaria (see below), Stevens-Johnson syndrome, and toxic epidermal necrolysis. **Stevens-Johnson syndrome** (see also Erythema Multiforme, below) is a severe, blistering skin reaction also affecting the mucous membranes of the oropharynx, eyes, and genitalia and accompanied sometimes by fever, pain, and malaise. **Toxic epidermal necrolysis** (Lyell's syndrome or scalded skin syndrome) is a more severe form of the reaction where considerable amounts of the epidermis may be shed. Sulphonamides, carbamazepine, and allopurinol are among the many drugs that have been associated with both these reactions. Other serious skin reactions include a hypersensitivity syndrome, serum sickness, and vasculitis. **Hypersensitivity syndrome** is a severe, idiosyncratic reaction which includes rash and fever, and often hepatitis, arthralgias, lymphadenopathy, and haematological abnormalities. It tends to have a relatively late and slow onset. Some antiepileptics and sulphonamides cause this syndrome, as well as allopurinol, dapsone, and gold salts. **Serum sickness** is manifest as rash, fever, arthralgia and arthritis and typically develops 8 to 14 days after administration of serum preparations and vaccines. **Vasculitic reactions** may occur 7 to 21 days after beginning therapy with drugs such as allopurinol, penicillins, and sulphonamides (see Hypersensitivity Vasculitis, p.1022). The vasculitis usually affects small vessels of the lower extremities producing purpura, although it can also affect vessels in the kidney, liver, and gastro-intestinal tract, in which case it may be life-threatening.

Maculo-papular exanthematic eruptions are probably the most frequent drug-induced skin reaction. Drugs commonly causing these rashes include carbamazepine, chlorpromazine, nitrofurantoin, penicillins, and sulphonamides. **Urticaria** (below) is also frequently drug-induced. **Photosensitivity** rashes where the skin reaction is confined to light-exposed areas may be phototoxic or photoallergic in nature. Phototoxic reactions occur in many patients and are dose-dependent, while photoallergic reactions affect only a few individuals. Amiodarone produces a phototoxic reaction in many patients. Some drugs cause **pigmentary changes** (see Pigmentation Disorders, below). Chlorpromazine can cause both photosensitivity and pigmentary changes. **Acneiform eruptions** may be produced by a number of drugs (see Acne, above). Some drugs produce skin reactions resembling **pemphigus** and **pemphigoid** (see below). Most of the drugs implicated contain a thiol group or metabolism of the drug generates a thiol group. Examples include captopril, penicillamine, penicillins, piroxicam, and rifampicin. **Fixed-drug eruptions** are inflammatory patches that appear at the same sites each time the drug is taken. Numerous drugs may be responsible including dapsone, sulphonamides, and tetracycline.

The majority of drug-induced adverse skin reactions are mild. However, severe reactions necessitate rapid withdrawal of the suspected drug. In some cases, this may mean stopping several drugs. In most cases the skin reaction will be resolved by symptomatic treatment. Readministration of the offending drug may establish whether the skin eruption is drug-induced, although reactions after rechallenge may be more severe and therefore rechallenge should not be performed after a serious reaction.

General references.

1. Smith AG. Important cutaneous adverse drug reactions. *Adverse Drug React Bull* 1994; **167:** 631–4.
2. Roujeau JC, Stern RS. Severe adverse cutaneous reactions to drugs. *N Engl J Med* 1994; **331:** 1272–85.
3. Wolkenstein P, Revuz J. Drug-induced severe skin reactions: incidence, management and prevention. *Drug Safety* 1995; **13:** 56–68.

Eczema

The term eczema is used for a variety of skin conditions characterised by epidermal inflammation. The term dermatitis is used synonymously with eczema, although dermatitis may sometimes be used in a broader sense to describe any skin inflammation. There are many different types of eczema and they may be categorised as exogenous or endogenous depending on the cause. Examples of exogenous eczemas include allergic, irritant, and photosensitivity eczema. Endogenous eczemas include atopic, discoid (nummular), gravitational, and seborrhoeic eczema. However, this classification is not always helpful, as there may be many different causes of eczema, both endogenous and exogenous in an individual patient. The areas of skin affected vary in the different types of eczema, but the skin lesions share certain common features. In acute eczema the skin is typically red and inflamed with papules, vesicles, and blisters. In chronic eczema the skin may show the same features but be more scaly, pigmented, and thickened. Two of the most common forms of eczema are atopic eczema and seborrhoeic dermatitis. The management of seborrhoeic dermatitis is described below.

Atopic eczema predominantly affects infants and children although adults may also suffer. The skin is itchy and there is a chronic or relapsing dermatitis in which the face and neck and flexures of the elbows and knees are involved most often and are excoriated and lichenified.

General principles for the management of **atopic eczema** may also be applied to other eczematous skin disorders. Cure of atopic eczema is said to be unrealistic, but good control can be achieved with proper management. The following **guidelines** are those agreed at a joint meeting of the British Association of Dermatologists and the Research Unit of the Royal College of Physicians of London.[1]

First line treatment. Regular bathing using soap substitutes is important to cleanse and hydrate the skin; soaps and detergents should be avoided as these remove the natural lipid from the skin. Suitable bath oils should be used to maintain skin hydration. Emollients should be applied liberally to the whole body at least twice a day, especially after bathing, and more frequently throughout the day to hands and face.

Overt secondary bacterial infections are treated with systemic antibacterials (see Skin Infections, p.142). Topical antibacterials are not generally used as they should be restricted to limited areas and patients with eczema often have widespread bacterial infection.

Topical corticosteroids are the mainstay of treatment for atopic eczema. To minimise potential side-effects preparations should not be applied more than twice daily, the minimum strength should be used to control the disease, and the age of patient, site of eczema, and extent of disease should be considered when selecting the appropriate preparation. For most patients with mild to moderate eczema 1% hydrocortisone for periods of one to two weeks is adequate. In adults and older children with severe atopic eczema or a flare-up of mild to moderate eczema more potent preparations may be required for short periods to control the disease. Wet wrap bandaging may be useful especially in younger children. In adults, mild to moderately potent corticosteroids are unlikely to cause systemic or local adverse effects. More potent preparations should be used with caution for short periods only. In general only 1% hydrocortisone should be used on the face and in flexures as absorption is increased in these areas. Ointment bases are usually preferred to cream bases since the occlusive effect of ointments produces better penetration of the corticosteroid. Impermeable or semipermeable films may sometimes be used on the palms and soles, or on limited very thickened lichenified areas, to enhance absorption.

Ichthammol and coal tar preparations are widely used. Ichthammol is less irritant than coal tar and may be used as an ointment or paste bandages especially on lichenified areas. Coal tar is used in a variety of topical preparations and may be added to the bath water.

A sedating antihistamine may be used short term for severe pruritus associated with relapse or at night-time if scratching disturbs sleep or occurs while asleep. Large doses may be required in children. Non-sedating antihistamines are ineffective in eczema. Patients whose eczema fails to respond to these first line treatments, even under specialist supervision, require further measures.

Second line treatment. PUVA, that is photochemotherapy with psoralen (P) [generally methoxsalen] and ultraviolet A (UVA), and to a lesser extent phototherapy with UVB have been useful in selected patients. However, potential long-term adverse effects such as premature ageing and skin malignancy need to be considered. There has been much research into the role of allergens such as house dust mites and certain food allergens in atopic eczema, although at present measures to eradicate house dust mites are not recommended and dietary restriction should only be tried in those patients with suspected food allergy.

Third line treatment. In patients with resistant severe atopic eczema systemic corticosteroids may be required for short periods to control the disease and very occasionally it may be necessary to use systemic corticosteroids for maintenance therapy if all other forms of treatment are unsuccessful. It is especially important to avoid systemic corticosteroids during rapid adolescent growth. Various other drugs have been tried in resistant eczema. Azathioprine and cyclosporin may be tried in selected patients. Evening primrose oil has also been tried although evidence in favour of a useful therapeutic effect is poor. Other drugs at an experimental stage include Chinese herbal medicines (hepatotoxicity has been reported), interferons, tacrolimus, and thymopentin.

1. McHenry PM, *et al.* Management of atopic eczema. *Br Med J* 1995; **310:** 843–7.

Epidermolysis bullosa

Epidermolysis bullosa consists of a group of similar congenital disorders characterised by severe blistering of the skin. Sometimes the mucosae, especially of the mouth and oesophagus, are also affected. The blistering may be caused by various structural and metabolic defects and occurs at different levels in the skin in the different forms (simple, junctional, and dystrophic). Blistering can follow even minor trauma or can arise spontaneously. In some patients blistering and scarring can cause marked tissue loss of the affected areas and the most severe forms are fatal in early infancy due to infection of the blisters. Milder forms may be managed by avoiding trauma and keeping blisters clean and dry, but there is no truly effective treatment for the severe forms. High dose oral corticosteroids may be needed. Phenytoin has been tried, but was unsuccessful in a controlled study. Thalidomide has also been tried.

There is also an acquired form of the disease, epidermolysis bullosa acquisita, and it too is difficult to treat;[1] corticosteroids and immunosuppressants may be tried. Individual patients have responded to high-dose intravenous immunoglobulins or extracorporeal photochemotherapy (oral methoxsalen followed by removal of blood and UV irradiation of leucocytes outside the body before reinfusion).[2,3]

1. Fine J-D. Management of acquired bullous skin diseases. *N Engl J Med* 1995; **333:** 1475–84.
2. Miller JL, *et al.* Remission of severe epidermolysis bullosa acquisita induced by extracorporeal photochemotherapy. *Br J Dermatol* 1995; **133:** 467–71.
3. Gordon KB, *et al.* Treatment of refractory epidermolysis bullosa acquisita with extracorporeal photochemotherapy. *Br J Dermatol* 1997; **136:** 415–20.

Erythema multiforme

Erythema multiforme is an inflammatory reaction of the skin in which the lesions are maculopapules which may become annular and blister. Areas typically affected are the hands, forearms, elbows, knees, and feet. It is usually associated with a precipitating trigger such as infection (notably herpes simplex infection); it may also be associated with drug use, neoplastic disease, or collagen or inflammatory diseases. In severe forms there is also blistering of the mucous membranes (usually of the mouth). This form has been termed the Stevens-Johnson syndrome, although it has been suggested that erythema multiforme with mucosal involvement and the Stevens-Johnson syndrome represent two distinct clinical entities.[1] Erythema multiforme occurs predominantly after infections whereas the Stevens-Johnson syndrome is mainly a drug-induced reaction. The Stevens-Johnson syndrome itself seems to be part of a spectrum of skin reactions with life-threatening toxic epidermal necrolysis being the more severe form (see Drug-induced Skin Reactions, above).

As erythema multiforme is usually an acute reaction of relatively short duration, symptomatic treatment as for burns (see above) may be all that is required. If severe reactions occur systemic corticosteroids may be considered. In some patients erythema multiforme may become a recurrent disorder although this is not common. A review[2] of the treatment of this recurrent form has suggested that where there is a clearly defined association with herpes simplex infection, a 5-day course of oral aciclovir at the start of the infection will often be successful in preventing the subsequent skin lesions. If this fails, a 6-month course of oral aciclovir may be tried, even if the association with herpes is not obvious. If long-term aciclovir fails, then dapsone or antimalarials may be given, with the final choice being azathioprine.

1. Assier H, *et al.* Erythema multiforme with mucous membrane involvement and Stevens-Johnson syndrome are clinically different disorders with distinct causes. *Arch Dermatol* 1995; **131:** 539–43.
2. Schofield JK, *et al.* Recurrent erythema multiforme: clinical features and treatment in a large series of patients. *Br J Dermatol* 1993; **128:** 542–5.

Hyperhidrosis

Hyperhidrosis (excessive sweating) can affect the hands, feet, and axillae. No cause can usually be established although it may be secondary to an underlying endocrinological or inflammatory disorder.[1]

Drug therapy should be tried initially but is often ineffective in severe cases. Aluminium salts, such as aluminium chloride or aluminium chlorohydrate in alcoholic solvents applied topically, may be successful in milder forms. Antimuscarinics such as diphemanil methylsulphate, glycopyrronium bromide, or hyoscine hydrobromide also applied topically may provide some relief. Side-effects of antimuscarinics administered by mouth generally preclude their use by this route, although there is a recent report of oral propantheline bromide being used successfully to control excessive sweating in 2 patients with spinal cord injuries. Intradermal or subcutaneous injection of botulinum A toxin has produced promising results in a few patients with severe resistant palmar hyperhidrosis. Formaldehyde and glutaraldehyde solutions have been employed for hyperhidrosis affecting the feet but are not very effective and are not usually recommended.

When drug therapy fails to provide adequate relief surgery may be attempted. Subcutaneous curettage or excision of skin bearing the eccrine glands has been employed but minimally invasive techniques, notably endoscopic transthoracic sympathectomy, are now available; the latter offers a simple and effective management for severe localised upper limb hyperhidrosis.

1. Quraishy MS, Giddings AEB. Treating hyperhidrosis. *Br Med J* 1993; **306:** 1221–2.

Ichthyosis

Ichthyosis is a term used for generalised noninflammatory dry scaling or keratinisation disorders (see below). There are several different forms of ichthyosis and severity and incidence varies. They are generally inherited disorders. Emollients, including urea, should be employed and provide relief to the dry skin by coating the skin surface with an oily film thus preventing evaporation of water. If scaling is more severe topical keratolytics are of benefit. Typically, drugs such as salicylic acid or urea are used. In the severest forms of ichthyosis oral retinoids may be necessary where emollients and topical keratolytics fail to provide adequate relief. Acitretin, etretinate, and isotretinoin have all been used. A few patients are reported to have responded to topical calcipotriol.

Keratinisation disorders

Keratinisation is the process whereby basal epidermal cells are transformed into dead cells of the stratum corneum from where they are shed. The process takes about fourteen days and shedding normally balances production so that the thickness of the stratum corneum does not alter. Keratinisation disorders (keratoses) are characterised by reduced shedding and the formation of scale at the skin surface. A scale is an aggregate of horn cells that have failed to separate horizontally and hyperkeratosis is an exaggeration of this failure in which there is also a vertical build up of the horn cells. Keratinisation disorders include Darier's disease and ichthyosis (see above). Certain inflammatory skin disorders, such as psoriasis (see below), also show enhanced epidermal proliferation.

Lichen planus

Lichen planus is an inflammatory skin disorder with itchy papular lesions arising usually on the extremities. The nails and oral or buccal mucosa and rarely the genital mucosa may also be affected. Its cause is uncertain although sufferers do have a higher incidence of auto-immune disease than normal. Some drugs can produce lichenoid reactions; examples include mepacrine, methyldopa, penicillamine, and sodium aurothiomalate.

In most patients lichen planus remits spontaneously and, if mild and localised, little or no treatment is needed. For more generalised mild disease topical corticosteroids may be useful for relieving pruritus and intralesional corticosteroids can be employed for hypertrophic and hyperkeratotic lesions.[1,2] Mucosal lesions are usually asymptomatic and require no treatment; symptomatic mucosal lesions may be treated with corticosteroid pastes or lozenges. Cyclosporin mouthwashes have been tried for oral mucosal lesions, with variable results. In severe forms systemic therapy may be necessary. Corticosteroids, cyclosporin, and retinoids such as acitretin, etretinate, and isotretinoin have been successfully employed by the oral route. Other treatments tried have included griseofulvin, antimalarials, and oral photochemotherapy with PUVA.

1. Anonymous. Treatment of oral lichen planus. *Lancet* 1990; **336:** 913–14.
2. Oliver GF, Winkelmann RK. Treatment of lichen planus. *Drugs* 1993; **45:** 56–65.

Pemphigus and pemphigoid

Pemphigus and pemphigoid are severe, disabling, and potentially fatal blistering skin diseases. They are distinct disorders although both have an auto-immune basis. There are several types of pemphigus. Pemphigus vulgaris is the most common, although all types are rare. In pemphigus vulgaris the blistering is intra-epidermal and can occur anywhere on the skin surface or on the mucous membranes. It is a chronic, progressive disorder requiring prolonged treatment. Pemphigoid is also known as bullous pemphigoid and occurs mainly in elderly persons. The blistering is subepidermal and affects the skin but rarely the mucous membranes. Pemphigoid is usually a self-limiting disorder and treatment can often be stopped after a couple of years.

The treatment of the blistering in both pemphigus and pemphigoid follows a similar pattern. Wet dressings and general treatment as for burns (see above) are commonly employed. Systemic corticosteroids are given to control the blistering and high doses initially are usually required. The doses suggested have varied enormously; the usual range is equivalent to about 60 to 100 mg daily of prednisolone by mouth although up to 400 mg daily has been suggested. However, there is some controversy about the appropriate corticosteroid dosage for initial therapy, since one study has indicated that the highest doses are associated with a poorer prognosis.[1] Maintenance therapy with corticosteroids at lower oral doses or topically may then follow. Intralesional corticosteroids may be useful for isolated lesions. Blistering of the oral mucous membranes may be treated with corticosteroid lozenges, and dinoprostone has also been reported to be effective.

Various therapies have been used as adjuncts or occasionally as alternatives to treatment with corticosteroids.[2-4] However, due to the rarity of the diseases, few controlled studies have been performed. Immunosuppressive therapy, usually with azathioprine, cyclophosphamide, or methotrexate, may be combined with a corticosteroid to improve disease control and permit a reduction in corticosteroid dosage. Systemic gold therapy has been used similarly. However, it has been suggested that evidence for the steroid-sparing effect of these drugs is lacking, and that they should be reserved for patients who cannot tolerate corticosteroids or in whom corticosteroids are contra-indicated.[3] Cyclosporin has been tried in a few patients with refractory pemphigus, with some apparent benefit, and high-dose intravenous immunoglobulin has been given to permit reduction of corticosteroid therapy to maintenance doses in pemphigus and pemphigoid. Some patients with bullous pemphigoid respond to dapsone. Plasmapheresis (plasma exchange) may be tried in severe, unresponsive pemphigus.

There have also been a number of reports suggesting that a tetracycline (often minocycline) alone or in combination with nicotinamide, may be useful in controlling the lesions of various types of pemphigus and pemphigoid.

1. Mourellou O, *et al.* The treatment of pemphigus vulgaris: experience with 48 patients seen over an 11-year period. *Br J Dermatol* 1995; **133:** 83–7.
2. Fine J-D. Management of acquired bullous skin diseases. *N Engl J Med* 1995; **333:** 1475–84.
3. Bystryn J-C, Steinman NM. The adjuvant therapy of pemphigus: an update. *Arch Dermatol* 1996; **132:** 203–12.
4. Carson PJ, *et al.* Influence of treatment on the clinical course of pemphigus vulgaris. *J Am Acad Dermatol* 1996; **34:** 645–52.

Pigmentation disorders

The pigment melanin is produced in melanocytes in the basal layer of the epidermis. Its production is under pituitary control but is also influenced by other endocrine secretions. Melanin is a complex polymer, and is synthesised from the amino acid, dihydroxyphenylalanine.

Decreased pigmentation (hypopigmentation) and excessive pigmentation (hyperpigmentation) can occur and may be either generalised or localised.

The commonest form of generalised hypopigmentation results in albinism. Affected individuals are extremely sensitive to solar irradiation and must use sunscreens regularly.

A common form of localised hypopigmentation is **vitiligo**. Sharply defined areas of depigmentation are seen and may spread so that total depigmentation eventually occurs or may persist in the localised form. There is no totally effective treatment, although some therapies may offer a degree of benefit. Oral or topical photochemotherapy with psoralens (PUVA) is currently considered to be the best treatment.[1,2] Topical corticosteroids are sometimes effective at inducing repigmentation. Dihydroxyacetone produces a brown staining of the skin which may be cosmetically acceptable. Experimental drug therapy for re-inducing pigment has included UVA light therapy with either khellin or phenylalanine; oral levamisole, alone or with topical corticosteroids, has also been reported to be of benefit. If the vitiligo affects a large proportion of the body (more than 50%), and if PUVA is ineffective at inducing repigmentation, an option is to consider inducing depigmentation in the remaining normal skin in order to match the lighter vitiligous areas. Depigmentation may be induced by drugs such as hydroquinone or monobenzone, its monobenzylether. This leaves the patients permanently needing to use topical sunscreens in order to avoid damage caused by solar exposure.

Hyperpigmentation can be caused by increased amounts of the pigment melanin or other substances such as iron in the skin. Generalised hyperpigmentation may be seen in Addison's disease, acanthosis nigricans, and primary haemochromatosis; other causes may include cirrhosis, chronic renal failure, and glycogen storage disease. Darkening of the skin can also occur in patients taking certain drugs due to a deposition of the drug-melanin complex in the skin. Notable examples include amiodarone, minocycline, and phenothiazines. Localised hyperpigmentation is seen in chloasma (melasma) in which there is facial involvement and is encountered most commonly in pregnancy. A number of compounds have been used basically as bleaching agents in hyperpigmentary disorders, and of these hydroquinone has been used most often; monobenzone is not recommended. A beneficial response to topical tretinoin in patients with chloasma has been described.

1. Antoniou C, Katsambas A. Guidelines for the treatment of vitiligo. *Drugs* 1992; **43:** 490–8.
2. British Photodermatology Group. British Photodermatology Group guidelines for PUVA. *Br J Dermatol* 1994; **130:** 246–55.

Pruritus

Pruritus (itching) is a common symptom of many skin disorders as well as of several systemic diseases, and may be extremely distressing. The exact pathophysiology of itching is unclear, and different inflammatory mediators may be associated with itching in different disorders; the CNS is also thought to play a role in the perception of itch. Some drugs also cause pruritus. Treatment of the underlying disorder or removal of the offending agent are important, but symptomatic treatment of pruritus may also be necessary. Calamine and crotamiton are commonly used topical agents, as are preparations containing phenol or agents such as menthol that cause capillary dilatation with a subsequent sensation of cold and analgesia. Local anaesthetics are sometimes included in topical preparations. However, they are only marginally effective and can very occasionally cause sensitisation. Topical capsaicin has also been used. Emollients may be useful where dry skin is a contributory factor and topical corticosteroids also relieve pruritus. Sedating antihistamines given by mouth are commonly employed to relieve more generalised pruritus and are used to control the severe itching associated with dermatoses such as atopic eczema (see above). Doxepin, a tricyclic antidepressant with very potent antihistaminic activity, has been used topically for the relief of pruritus associated with dermatitis, although its efficacy is questioned by some. Bile acid binding resins, such as cholestyramine, are used to relieve pruritus associated with the deposition in dermal tissue of excess bile acids in patients with partial biliary obstruction or primary biliary cirrhosis. There are reports of cholestatic pruritus also responding to ondansetron. Central opioid receptors modulate itch and opioid antagonists such as nalmefene have been reported to relieve pruritus. Numerous other drugs including cimetidine and propofol have been of benefit in some patients. PUVA (see under Methoxsalen, p.1088) may be helpful in some pruritic skin conditions including aquagenic pruritus.

Psoriasis

Psoriasis is a chronic inflammatory skin disorder characterised by enhanced epidermal proliferation leading to erythema, scaling, and thickening of the skin. There are several types of psoriasis including guttate, flexural, pustular, and erythrodermic, but chronic plaque psoriasis (psoriasis vulgaris) is the most common form. In chronic plaque psoriasis the areas most commonly affected are the extensor sides of the knees, elbows, and hands, and the sacrum. There is no cure and treatment is therefore suppressive, either inducing a remission or reducing the amount of psoriasis to a tolerable level.

The treatment of psoriasis has been the subject of a number of reviews.[1-4,6]

Topical drugs are the treatment of first choice for chronic plaque psoriasis. Mild conditions may be managed with the use of emollients alone but dithranol, coal tar, or calcipotriol are the usual active treatments for mild to moderate forms. Unfortunately dithranol stains the skin and clothes and as it is irritant careful adjustment of the strength and duration of application needs to be made. It has traditionally been applied overnight in the form of ointments or pastes but newer short-contact regimens and creams are more suitable for home therapy. Coal tar is used either as crude extracts or refined products and although the refined products may be more aesthetically acceptable they may also be less effective. Salicylic acid enhances the rate of loss of surface scale and is included in many combination preparations with dithranol or coal tar. Calcipotriol, a vitamin D analogue, has the advantage of being odourless and nonstaining. Tacalcitol, another vitamin D analogue, and tazarotene, a topical retinoid, have recently been introduced. Topical corticosteroids are effective but they may lead to dermal atrophy, tachyphylaxis, systemic toxicity, and may precipitate unstable and pustular psoriasis. Although UK dermatologists tend to reserve their use for special circumstances, they are reported to be the most widely used treatment in the USA.[1] Guttate psoriasis is sometimes associated with streptococcal infection and patients may require antimicrobial treatment. Patients unresponsive to one topical drug may respond to another and alternatives should be tried before considering more aggressive management. Topical drugs are often used in combination.

Phototherapy with UVB light is effective used alone for chronic plaque or guttate psoriasis but also enhances the effectiveness of calcipotriol, coal tar, or dithranol. Commercially available sunbeds, which emit UVA light are not recommended as they are rarely effective and induce skin ageing and fragility.

Psoriasis refractory to topical therapy may respond to **systemic drugs**. Systemic treatment may also be indicated for extensive chronic plaque psoriasis in elderly or infirm patients, for generalised pustular or erythrodermic psoriasis, or for severe psoriatic arthritis (see p.4). The administration of oral or topical psoralens such as methoxsalen with UVA light (PUVA) is generally considered to be the systemic treatment of first choice and guidelines for PUVA have been published.[5] Psoralens have also been used with UVB light.

Immunosuppressants such as methotrexate are useful for severe refractory psoriasis, the aim of treatment being to bring psoriasis under control, enabling a return to other modes of treatment rather than to induce remission. Cyclosporin is also used in severe refractory psoriasis and may be employed either to induce a remission or in low-dose maintenance therapy to prevent relapse. Retinoids, such as acitretin are effective and combination with PUVA may allow a reduction in doses and associated toxicity for each therapy. Hydroxyurea has also been tried.

Many anecdotal cases have been reported of psoriasis improving when patients are given drug therapy for other concomitant disease. The value of such drugs can be difficult to establish particularly due to the chronic relapsing and recurring nature of psoriasis.

1. Greaves MW, Weinstein GD. Treatment of psoriasis. *N Engl J Med* 1995; **332:** 581–8.
2. Weller PA. Psoriasis. *Med J Aust* 1996; **165:** 216–21.
3. Gawkrodger DJ (ed.). Current management of psoriasis. *J Dermatol Treat* 1997; **8:** 27–55.
4. Stern RS. Psoriasis. *Lancet* 1997; **350:** 349–53.
5. British Photodermatology Group. British Photodermatology Group guidelines for PUVA. *Br J Dermatol* 1994; **130:** 246–55.
6. Livingstone C. Psoriasis. *Pharm J* 1997; **259:** 890–2.

Pyoderma gangrenosum

Pyoderma gangrenosum is a rare serious ulcerative skin disorder often associated with systemic diseases such as inflammatory bowel disease, rheumatoid arthritis, or myeloproliferative disorders. Initially an acutely inflamed nodule is present which progresses very rapidly to large ulcers. Any area of the body may be involved, but the legs, buttocks, and face are frequent sites.

Treatment essentially consists of cleansing and dressings for the ulcers and appropriate therapy for any underlying disease. When necessary high doses of systemic corticosteroids have been given. There have also been reports in small numbers of patients of benefit with sulphonamides, dapsone, azathioprine, cyclosporin, tacrolimus, colchicine, and nicotine chewing gum.

A related but less severe form of the disease, superficial granulomatous pyoderma has responded to intralesional or oral corticosteroids.

General references.

1. Callen JP. Pyoderma gangrenosum. *Lancet* 1998; **351:** 581–5.

Rosacea

Rosacea is a chronic inflammatory condition mainly affecting the face. Phases of this disorder include flushing episodes, persistent erythema and telangiectasia, a papulopustular phase, and rarely rhinophyma (nasal hypertrophy and deformity).[1] The precise cause remains unclear. It has been proposed that the different phases of rosacea have different aetiologies.[1] For example, the papulopustular phase might be associated with the mite, *Demodex folliculorum*.[2]

The inflammatory episodes of rosacea (papules, swelling, and pustules) are responsive to treatment, but the underlying erythema and telangiectasia usually persist. Surgery is required for rhinophyma.[1] Oral antibacterials have been the treatment of choice, tetracycline being the most commonly used, although metronidazole or erythromycin may also be employed. Long-term treatment is usually necessary. In resistant cases of rosacea, isotretinoin may be tried. Topical antibacterials, in particular metronidazole gel, provide an effective alternative to oral drugs. Topical metronidazole and clindamycin generally improve the inflammatory episodes of rosacea, although other features may not respond. Topical corticosteroids should not be used since they exacerbate the condition.

1. Rebora A. The red face: rosacea. *Clin Dermatol* 1993; **11:** 225–34.
2. Forton F, Seys B. Density of Demodex folliculorum in rosacea: a case-control study using standardized skin-surface biopsy. *Br J Dermatol* 1993; **128:** 650–9.

Seborrhoeic dermatitis

Seborrhoeic dermatitis is a common eczematous skin disorder (see Eczema above) in which erythematous pruritic patches of skin may become either scaly or exudative and crusted. Scaling lesions are the type most commonly observed. In some cases, known as seborrhoeic folliculitis, there may also be follicular papules or pustules. Seborrhoeic dermatitis occurs in regions of the body where sebaceous glands are plentiful, such as the scalp, face, and chest, although the condition is not associated with increased sebum production. The cause of seborrhoeic dermatitis is unknown, although it might be related to overgrowth with *Malassezia ovalis* (*Pityrosporum ovale*), a normal commensal yeast.

Treatment is suppressive rather than curative. Topical preparations containing an imidazole antifungal such as clotrimazole, ketoconazole, or miconazole, usually together with hydrocortisone may be effective and are the main drugs used. If unsuccessful keratolytics such as salicylic acid or tars may be used. Shampoos containing pyrithione zinc or selenium sulphide are commonly used for scalp involvement. Topical lithium succinate has been tried.

Dandruff due to normal shedding of scalp skin (pityriasis capitis) is treated similarly to seborrhoeic dermatitis of the scalp.

Urticaria and angioedema

Urticaria (also known as nettlerash or hives) is characterised by circumscribed, elevated, erythematous, and usually pruritic areas of oedema (wheals) involving the superficial portion of the dermis. Individual lesions arise suddenly, often within a few minutes, and may last up to 24 hours. When subcutaneous or submucosal tissues are involved, causing swelling of the eyelids, lips, tongue, larynx, or genitalia, it is called angioedema. Urticaria and angioedema are caused by the release of inflammatory mediators from mast cells and basophils.

There are various types of urticaria including dermographism (linear wheal formation on scratching or stroking) and cholinergic urticaria evoked by such triggers as exercise, heat, and emotion and characterised by small papulous wheals surrounded by an erythematous flare. Chronic urticaria is arbitrarily defined as continuous or recurrent lesions of at least 6-weeks' duration. Although urticaria may be caused by an allergy, it often has a non-allergic mechanism. Urticaria occurs as an adverse effect of many drugs, for example aspirin and many antibacterials. In severe, acute urticaria, wheals may cover most of the skin surface. In chronic urticaria only a few wheals may develop each day. Angioedema may be dangerous if there is laryngeal oedema and is treated as an allergic emergency.

The **management** of urticaria and angioedema has been reviewed.[1-3] Avoidance of unnecessary exposure to known allergens is of prime importance in the management of urticaria, although in the majority of chronic cases no trigger factor can be found. Severe, acute urticaria or angioedema is treated as for anaphylaxis (p.816).

Topical treatment of urticaria is rarely effective except for mild cases. Calamine, menthol, and crotamiton have cooling or antipruritic effects. Topical corticosteroids are of no value; topical antihistamines are not very effective and carry a slight risk of sensitisation.

Most patients with urticaria derive some benefit from oral antihistamines, especially in the relief of pruritus. A non-sedating antihistamine is the first line of treatment. Sedating antihistamines are useful at bedtime. If such antihistamines (H_1-receptor antagonists) are only partly successful their combination with an H_2-receptor antagonist may be tried; cimetidine or ranitidine, administered alone or in combination with an H_1-receptor antagonist, have shown benefit in certain types of urticaria, especially those associated with cold or angioedema. The routine use of H_2-antagonists in urticaria is controversial, but in practice their addition to conventional treatment can be tried in resistant cases. Little additional benefit has been found with combination therapy in dermographic urticaria.[4]

The tricyclic antidepressant doxepin has H_1- and H_2-receptor antagonist properties and has sometimes been effective in patients with urticaria.

Addition of a sympathomimetic such as terbutaline or a calcium-channel blocker such as nifedipine has also been suggested for patients unresponsive to treatment with an H_1-receptor antagonist alone, but results have varied.

A short course of an oral corticosteroid may be indicated for patients refractory to other measures. A number of other drugs including danazol, stanozolol, dapsone, sulphasalazine, and immunosuppressants, have reportedly produced benefit in limited numbers of patients, but such therapies are largely employed empirically.

1. Ormerod AD. Urticaria: recognition, causes, and treatment. *Drugs* 1994; **48:** 717–30.
2. Greaves MW. Chronic urticaria. *N Engl J Med* 1995; **332:** 1767–72.
3. Greaves MW, Sabroe RA. Allergy and the skin: urticaria. *Br Med J* 1998; **316:** 1147–50.
4. Sharpe GR, Shuster S. In dermographic urticaria H_2 receptor antagonists have a small but therapeutically irrelevant additional effect compared with H_1 antagonists alone. *Br J Dermatol* 1993; **129:** 575–9.

Warts

Warts are caused by human papillomaviruses. The lesions present in several different forms and can affect any skin site although the hands, feet, and anogenital areas are most frequently affected. Plantar warts on the soles of the feet are sometimes called verrucas. Anogenital warts are known as condylomata acuminata. Warts do disappear spontaneously but as they may not do so for months or years patients often seek treatment.

There is no specific antiviral therapy against the human papillomavirus.[1-3] Treatment relies on some form of local tissue destruction. Non-pharmacological techniques include surgical excision, electrocauterisation, or laser therapy. Cryotherapy (tissue freezing) may be performed with liquid nitrogen or solid carbon dioxide. Chemical destruction with acids (acetic acid, lactic acid, nitric acid, salicylic acid, or trichloroacetic acid), silver nitrate, potassium hydroxide, formaldehyde or glutaraldehyde, or podophyllum resin or its derivatives (podophyllotoxin) is another option. Podophyllum resin or podophyllotoxin are possibly used more frequently than other forms of drug therapy in anogenital warts. Intralesional injection of cytotoxics such as bleomycin or fluorouracil also destroys the wart and may be employed in severe or resistant cases. Fluorouracil may also be applied topically. Interferons have antiviral, antiproliferative, and immunomodulatory actions and have thus been investigated in the management of warts; some studies, especially those involving intralesional administration, have demonstrated benefit. Imiquimod has recently been introduced for the topical treatment of anogenital warts. Other drugs with immunomodulatory effects, such as cimetidine, have been tried in a few patients.

1. Phelps WC, Alexander KA. Antiviral therapy for human papillomaviruses: rationale and prospects. *Ann Intern Med* 1995; **123:** 368–82.
2. Beutner KR, Ferenczy A. Therapeutic approaches to genital warts. *Am J Med* 1997; **102** (suppl 5A): 28–37.
3. Centers for Disease Control. 1998 Guidelines for treatment of sexually transmitted diseases. *MMWR* 1998; **47** (RR-1): 88–95.

Wounds and ulcers

The management of wounds (and ulcers) requires understanding of the wound healing process and any underlying factors that may have contributed to the skin damage. Wounds may be the result of mechanical injury, burns, or chemical injury. Ulcers are often the result of various underlying disorders. Common ulcers include decubitus, leg, and neuropathic ulcers. Decubitus ulcers (bedsores, pressure sores) occur in patients with extended immobility when prolonged pressure on the skin over a bony prominence produces localised ischaemia. Leg ulcers may result from venous incompetence or be ischaemic in origin, and patients with peripheral neuropathy, such as diabetics or those with leprosy, may develop neuropathic ulcers due to repetitive inadvertent injury. Some wounds, especially ulcers, are very slow to heal and are the cause of much discomfort and disablement.

Healing mechanisms are essentially the same regardless of the cause of the damage and may be considered in three phases: an immediate haemostatic phase, an early granulation and re-epithelialisation phase, and a later phase of dermal repair and remodelling. The haemostatic processes involve formation of a platelet plug and fibrin clot, as described under Haemostasis, p.704. The early granulation and re-epithelialisation phase takes place up to about 21 days after injury depending on wound size and site. Platelet-derived growth factors stimulate fibroblasts to produce granulation tissue, comprising a collagen matrix well-supplied with capillary vessels, and growth of epidermal cells leading to re-epithelialisation of the wound surface. The collagen matrix undergoes strengthening during the dermal repair and remodelling phase and there is a reduction in vascularity. This phase can continue for up to 2 years after injury.

Several factors are important for efficient wound healing. Adequate supplies of nutrients, especially vitamin C and zinc (which are often given as supplements) and oxygen are needed. A good blood supply is thus essential. Clinical infection, either systemic or local, due to contamination by environmental microbes, causes tissue damage and delays healing. The process of wound repair requires many cellular and acellular factors, such as platelets and growth factors, and deficiencies in these may also be responsible for delayed healing. Thus, the patient's age, systemic conditions, concomitant drugs, nutritional status, and congenital deficiencies all influence the rate of healing.

Local **wound management** includes cleansing, removal of exudate, and prevention of microbial contamination. There are many preparations available to treat wounds and the choice will depend on the size, location, type, and cause of the wound, on the presence of infection, and on the particular stage of healing. As the wound heals, different preparations will be required. Wounds may be described as superficial, partial thickness, or full thickness. Superficial wounds are limited to epithelial tissue and heal rapidly by regeneration of epithelial cells. Partial thickness wounds involve the dermis and include some blood vessel damage, and therefore wound repair is a longer process. Full thickness wounds extend to the subcutaneous fat layer at least and healing requires synthesis of new connective tissue.

Wound **cleansing** is required to remove any dirt or foreign body and to **remove exudate** and slough (pus and necrotic tissue). This helps to prevent infection and aids healing. Commonly used cleansing solutions are sodium chloride 0.9%, hypochlorite, hydrogen peroxide, povidone-iodine, and chlorhexidine. However, some antiseptics and hypochlorites might be associated with delayed wound healing, especially with prolonged use, as they delay collagen production and cause inflammation. Also, many antiseptics are inactivated by organic material. Sodium chloride solution may be all that is required for routine cleansing of non-infected wounds. Many of the cleansing solutions also help to remove slough. Other wound management preparations more specifically directed at removing slough include dextranomer, hydrogels, hydrocolloids, and enzyme preparations such as a mixture of streptokinase and streptodornase. Dextranomer, hydrogels, and hydrocolloids cause debridement by their occlusive, rehydrating properties. Surgical debridement is a fast and efficient way of removing necrotic tissue. Wounds may produce large volumes of exudate as a result of inflammatory reactions, especially during the first few days. Hydrocolloid and alginate preparations and foam dressings are effective moisture absorbers.

All wounds are colonised by bacteria to some extent and there is no evidence that this superficial **infection** affects healing. However, infection with *Pseudomonas aeruginosa* may delay healing and silver sulphadiazine is used especially in burns. Acetic acid has also been used. Infections are treated systemically if there are indications of clinical infection such as sudden pain, cellulitis, and increased discharge (for systemic management of bacterial skin infections see p.142).

Wound **dressings** and packing preparations help to protect the wound and provide the correct environment for wound healing. Some also help by absorbing exudate. Superficial wounds usually only require a low-adherent dressing. Alginates may be used for exuding wounds. Traditional dry dressings such as cotton wool, gauze, and lint are not used for partial or full thickness cavity wounds since they shed fibres, adhere to the wound, and cause wound dehydration. Hydrogels, hydrocolloids, polysaccharides, cadexomer-iodine, alginates, and foam dressings are all effective cavity wound preparations.

Activated charcoal is very effective at reducing offensive odours from **malodorous wounds** as are sugar pastes. Sugar may exert its antibacterial effect by competing for water present in the cells of bacteria. Metronidazole is active against anaerobic bacteria that are associated with the pungent smell and is used topically for deodorising malodorous tumours (but not wounds because of the risk of inducing resistance).

In addition to the use of wound preparations, there may be other measures that aid healing of specific wounds or ulcers. Measures that aid the return of fluid from the leg, such as flexing the ankles, elevation, and use of compression bandages are beneficial in **venous ulcers**. The bioflavonoids, given orally, may improve venous insufficiency and therefore also aid healing. Systemic drugs that improve the supply of oxygen to tissues, for example oxpentifylline, may be useful in ischaemic and venous ulcers. Topical and systemic ketanserin has been investigated in a few patients and may be beneficial in wounds and ulcers where there is impaired blood flow. Vascular surgery may be necessary in the management of some ulcers caused by ischaemia. In **decubitus ulcers**, relief of pressure is the most important measure in management. The management of **burns** and **chemical burns** is described above. Some wounds may require skin grafting. Certain cytokines, such as becaplermin and molgramostim, and a replacement human skin are being investigated in non-healing ulcers and wounds.

General references.

1. Anonymous. Healing of cavity wounds. *Lancet* 1991; **337:** 1010–1.
2. Anonymous. Leg ulcers. In: Buxton PK, ed. *ABC of Dermatology.* London: BMJ Publishing Group, 1993: 35–8.
3. Turner T. Wound management: the healing process. *Pharm J* 1993; **250:** 735–7.
4. Morgan D. Wound management: which dressing? *Pharm J* 1993; **250:** 738–43.
5. Thomas S. Wound management: bandages and bandaging. *Pharm J* 1993; **250:** 744–5.
6. Vohra RK, McCollum CN. Pressure sores. *Br Med J* 1994; **309:** 853–7.
7. Douglas WS, Simpson NB. Guidelines for the management of chronic venous leg ulceration: report of a multidisciplinary workshop. *Br J Dermatol* 1995; **132:** 446–52.
8. Smith DM. Pressure ulcers in the nursing home. *Ann Intern Med* 1995; **123:** 433–42.
9. Cooke ED, Nicolaides AN. Management of leg ulcers. *Prescribers' J* 1997; **37:** 61–8.
10. Angle N, Bergan JJ. Chronic venous ulcer. *Br Med J* 1997; **314:** 1019–23.
11. Warren K, Bennett G. Wound care. *Prescribers' J* 1998; **38:** 115–22.
12. Grey JE, Harding KG. The chronic non-healing wound: how to make it better. *Hosp Med* 1998; **59:** 557–63.

Abrasive Agents (10099-e)

Aluminium Oxide (12348-v)

Al_2O_3 = 102.0.

CAS — 1344-28-1.

Pumice (1631-q)

Lapis Pumicis; Pierre Ponce Granulée; Pumex; Pumex Granulatus; Pumice Stone.

CAS — 1332-09-8.

Pharmacopoeias. In Fr. and US.

Pumice is a substance of volcanic origin consisting chiefly of complex silicates of aluminium, potassium, and sodium. Odourless, very light, hard, rough, porous greyish masses or gritty, greyish powder. Practically **insoluble** in water and not attacked by acids.

The USP recognises 3 grades of powdered pumice: (1) superfine (=pumice flour)—not less than 97% passes through a No. 200 [US] sieve; (2) fine—not less than 95% passes through a No. 150 sieve and not more than 75% through a No. 200 sieve; (3) coarse—not less than 95% passes through a No. 60 sieve and not more than 5% through a No. 200 sieve.

Abrasive agents such as fused synthetic aluminium oxide or powdered pumice have been used either as adjuncts in the treatment of acne (p.1072) or for the removal of hard skin. Pumice has also been used as a dental abrasive and as a filtering medium. Other agents used as an abrasive for acne include polyethylene granules.

Preparations

Proprietary Preparations (details are given in Part 3)

Austral.: Brasivol; Ionax Scrub; ***Canad.:*** Brasivol; ***Fr.:*** Brasivol†; Ionax Scrub; ***Ger.:*** Brasivil; ***Irl.:*** Ionax Scrub; ***S.Afr.:*** Brasivol†; Ionax Scrub†; ***UK:*** Brasivol; Ionax Scrub; ***USA:*** Brasivol.

Multi-ingredient: ***Canad.:*** Ancatropine Gel†; Pernox; Topol with Fluoride†; ***Ital.:*** Neo Zeta-Foot; Zeta-Foot†; ***Neth.:*** Suspensie Tegen Overmatig Maagzuur†; ***S.Afr.:*** Magagel; Pedimed; ***Switz.:*** Cliniderm; ***USA:*** Pernox.

Acitretin (19160-m)

Acitretin *(BAN, USAN, rINN).*

Etretin; Ro-10-1670. *(all-trans)*-9-(4-Methoxy-2,3,6-trimethylphenyl)-3,7-dimethyl-2,4,6,8-nonatetraenoic acid; (2*E*,4*E*,6*E*,8*E*)-9-(4-Methoxy-2,3,6-trimethylphenyl)-3,7-dimethylnona-2,4,6,8-tetraenoic acid.

$C_{21}H_{26}O_3$ = 326.4.

CAS — 55079-83-9.

Adverse Effects and Precautions

As for Isotretinoin, p.1084.

Acitretin has a relatively short half-life, but etretinate, which has a much longer half-life, has been detected in the plasma of some patients receiving acitretin. Recommendations vary slightly in different countries but pregnancy should be avoided for at least 2 to 3 years after treatment has been withdrawn (see also under Pregnancy, below) and patients should not donate blood for at least 1 to 3 years after cessation of therapy. Female patients should avoid alcohol during treatment with acitretin and for 2 months after stopping treatment (see under Interactions, below).

Effects on the musculoskeletal system. For reference to severe myopathy occurring during therapy with acitretin, see under Isotretinoin, p.1084.

Effects on the skin. For mention of the phototoxic potential of acitretin, see under Isotretinoin, p.1085.

Pregnancy. In the UK the manufacturers of acitretin recommend that pregnancy should be avoided for at least 2 years (3 years in the US) after withdrawal of therapy since etretinate, which is teratogenic and has a much longer half-life than acitretin, has been detected in the plasma of some patients receiving acitretin. It has been pointed out that plasma-etretinate concentrations are a poor indication of total body stores; one study[1] has indicated that there may be substantial concentrations of etretinate in the fatty tissues of women who have received acitretin.

1. Sturkenboom MCJM, *et al.* Inability to detect plasma etretinate and acitretin is a poor predictor of the absence of these teratogens in tissue after stopping acitretin treatment. *Br J Clin Pharmacol* 1994; **38:** 229–35.

Interactions

As for Isotretinoin, p.1085.

Etretinate has been detected in the plasma of some patients receiving acitretin and acitretin is also a metabolite of etretinate; therefore interactions associated with etretinate (see p.1082) may also apply to acitretin. Concurrent ingestion of acitretin and alcohol has been associated with etretinate formation.

Pharmacokinetics

Acitretin is absorbed from the gastro-intestinal tract and peak plasma concentrations have been obtained 1 to 6 hours after oral administration. Oral bioavailability may be increased by administration with food. Acitretin is highly bound to plasma proteins. It is metabolised to 13-*cis*-acitretin. Etretinate (p.1082) has also been detected in the plasma of some patients following administration of acitretin. The elimination half-life of acitretin is approximately 2 days but account should always be taken of the fact that the half-life of etretinate is much longer, being about 120 days. Acitretin is excreted in bile and urine.

General references.

1. Larsen FG, *et al.* Pharmacokinetics and therapeutic efficacy of retinoids in skin diseases. *Clin Pharmacokinet* 1992; **23:** 42–61.

Renal impairment. The pharmacokinetics of acitretin are reported to be altered in patients with chronic renal failure but neither acitretin nor its 13-cis metabolite are removed by haemodialysis.[1]

1. Stuck AE, *et al.* Pharmacokinetics of acitretin and its 13-cis metabolite in patients on haemodialysis. *Br J Clin Pharmacol* 1989; **27:** 301–4.

Uses and Administration

Acitretin is a retinoid. It is a metabolite of etretinate (p.1082). Acitretin is used by mouth in the treatment of severe psoriasis resistant to other forms of therapy and in severe congenital ichthyosis and Darier's disease (keratosis follicularis).

It is given in an initial daily dose of 25 or 30 mg with food for 2 to 4 weeks. The daily dosage is adjusted thereafter according to clinical response and adverse effects; optimal results are usually obtained with 25 to 50 mg given daily for a further 6 to 8 weeks but some patients may require up to 75 mg daily. For the treatment of Darier's disease a starting dose of 10 mg may be appropriate, adjusted thereafter according to response. In Darier's disease and congenital ichthyosis treatment may be required for more than 3 months but a daily dosage of 50 mg should not be exceeded. In the UK, the manufacturer recommends that continuous treatment should not last longer than 6 months for any indication.

Acitretin is not generally considered suitable for use in children, but if deemed necessary a dose of 0.5 mg per kg body-weight daily or occasionally up to 1 mg per kg daily has been suggested, but the maximum daily dose should not exceed 35 mg.

Administration in children. Acitretin is not generally considered suitable for use in children. A review of its use in 29 children with severe inherited disorders of keratinisation[1] reported that acitretin is an effective and safe treatment in children provided that the minimal effective dose is used and that side-effects are carefully monitored.

1. Lacour M, *et al.* An appraisal of acitretin therapy in children with inherited disorders of keratinization. *Br J Dermatol* 1996; **134:** 1023–9.

Skin disorders. Acitretin is used alone or with PUVA or UVB in psoriasis[1] (p.1075). Studies have shown that use with PUVA or UVB light may increase efficacy and allow a reduction in the exposure to radiation required. It is also used in keratinisation disorders such as severe forms of ichthyosis[2,3] (p.1074) and Darier's disease (keratosis follicularis)[4] (p.1073). Benefit has been reported in various other skin disorders.[5-9]

1. Gollnick HPM. Oral retinoids—efficacy and toxicity in psoriasis. *Br J Dermatol* 1996; **135** (suppl 49): 6–17.
2. Bruckner-Tuderman L, *et al.* Acitretin in the symptomatic therapy for severe recessive X-linked ichthyosis. *Arch Dermatol* 1988; **124:** 529–32.
3. Steijlen PM, *et al.* Acitretin in the treatment of lamellar ichthyosis. *Br J Dermatol* 1994; **130:** 211–14.
4. van Dooren-Greebe RJ, *et al.* Acitretin monotherapy in Darier's disease. *Br J Dermatol* 1989; **121:** 375–9.
5. Laurberg G, *et al.* Treatment of lichen planus with acitretin: a double-blind, placebo-controlled study in 65 patients. *J Am Acad Dermatol* 1991; **24:** 434–7.
6. Lucker GPH, *et al.* Treatment of palmoplantar lichen nitidus with acitretin. *Br J Dermatol* 1994; **130:** 791–3.
7. Lassus A, Geiger J-M. Acitretin and etretinate in the treatment of palmoplantar pustulosis: a double-blind comparative trial. *Br J Dermatol* 1988; **119:** 755–9.
8. Ruzicka T, *et al.* Efficiency of acitretin in the treatment of cutaneous lupus erythematosus. *Arch Dermatol* 1988; **124:** 897–902.
9. Yuan Z-f, *et al.* Use of acitretin for the skin complications in renal transplant recipients. *N Z Med J* 1995; **108:** 255–6.

Preparations

Proprietary Preparations (details are given in Part 3)
Aust.: Neotigason; ***Austral.:*** Neotigason; ***Belg.:*** Neotigason; ***Canad.:*** Soriatane; ***Fr.:*** Soriatane; ***Ger.:*** Neotigason; ***Irl.:*** Neotigason; ***Neth.:*** Neotigason; ***Norw.:*** Neotigason; ***S.Afr.:*** Neotigason; ***Spain:*** Neotigason; ***Swed.:*** Neotigason; ***Switz.:*** Neotigason; ***UK:*** Neotigason; ***USA:*** Soriatane.

Adapalene (14937-t)

Adapalene *(BAN, USAN, rINN)*.

CD-271. 6-[3-(1-Adamantyl)-4-methoxyphenyl]-2-naphthoic acid.

$C_{28}H_{28}O_3$ = 412.5.

CAS — 106685-40-9.

Adverse Effects

Adapalene is a skin irritant. Topical application may cause transitory stinging and a feeling of warmth at the site of application.

Precautions

As for Tretinoin, p.1094.

Pregnancy. Anophthalmia and agenesis of the optic chiasma were found in a fetus following termination of pregnancy in a woman who had applied adapalene 0.1% topically for the month before pregnancy until 13 weeks' gestation.[1]

1. Autret E, *et al.* Anophthalmia and agenesis of optic chiasma associated with adapalene gel in early pregnancy. *Lancet* 1997; **350:** 339.

Uses and Administration

Adapalene is a naphthoic acid derivative and retinoid analogue with actions similar to those of tretinoin (p.1094). Adapalene is used in topical treatment of mild to moderate acne (p.1072) where comedones, papules, and pustules predominate.

Adapalene is applied once daily at night as a 0.1% gel to skin that has been cleansed and dried. Some patients may require less frequent applications. Other topical preparations that may cause irritation should not be used concurrently. If concurrent treatment with topical antibacterials or benzoyl peroxide is required, these should be applied with an interval of 12 hours between application of adapalene.

There may be apparent exacerbations of the acne during early treatment and a therapeutic response may not be evident for 8 to 12 weeks.

References.

1. Brogden RN, Goa KL. Adapalene: a review of its pharmacological properties and clinical potential in the management of mild to moderate acne. *Drugs* 1997; **53:** 511–19.

Preparations

Proprietary Preparations (details are given in Part 3)
Aust.: Differin; ***Austral.:*** Differin; ***Canad.:*** Differin; ***Fr.:*** Differine; ***Ger.:*** Differin; ***Irl.:*** Differin; ***Ital.:*** Differin; ***S.Afr.:*** Differin; ***Spain:*** Differine; ***Swed.:*** Differin; ***Switz.:*** Differin; ***UK:*** Differin; ***USA:*** Differin.

Alcloxa (1591-z)

Alcloxa *(USAN, rINN)*.

ALCA; Aluminium Chlorhydroxyallantoinate; RC-173. Chlorotetrahydroxy[(2-hydroxy-5-oxo-2-imidazolin-4-yl)urea-to]dialuminium.

$C_4H_9Al_2ClN_4O_7$ = 314.6.

CAS — 1317-25-5.

Alcloxa is an astringent and keratolytic related to allantoin (p.1078). It is present in multi-ingredient preparations intended for various skin and gastro-intestinal disorders.

Preparations

Proprietary Preparations (details are given in Part 3)
Multi-ingredient: ***Austral.:*** Z-Acne†; ***Fr.:*** Posebor†; Ulfon; ***Ital.:*** Aseptil; ***UK:*** Dermidex; ***USA:*** Gentz†.

Aldioxa (1592-c)

Aldioxa *(USAN, rINN)*.

ALDA; Aluminium Dihydroxyallantoinate; Dihydroxyaluminum Allantoinate; RC-172. Dihydroxy[(2-hydroxy-5-oxo-2-imidazolin-4-yl)ureato]aluminium.

$C_4H_7AlN_4O_5$ = 218.1.

CAS — 5579-81-7.

Pharmacopoeias. In *Jpn.*

Aldioxa is an astringent and keratolytic related to allantoin (p.1078). It is present in multi-ingredient preparations intended for various skin and gastro-intestinal disorders.

Preparations

Proprietary Preparations (details are given in Part 3)
Multi-ingredient: ***Austral.:*** ZeaSorb; ***Belg.:*** Rikosol Silicone†; ***Canad.:*** ZeaSorb; ***Fr.:*** Ulfon; ZeaSorb; ***Ger.:*** ZeaSorb; ***Irl.:*** ZeaSorb; ***Ital.:*** Rikospray; ***S.Afr.:*** Rikerspray†; ZeaSorb†; ***UK:*** Cetanorm; ZeaSorb.

Allantoin (1593-k)

Allantoin *(BAN, USAN)*.

Glyoxyldiureide. 5-Ureidohydantoin; 5-Ureidoimidazolidine-2,4-dione; 2,5-Dioxoimidazolidin-4-ylurea.

$C_4H_6N_4O_3$ = 158.1.

CAS — 97-59-6.

Pharmacopoeias. In *Eur.* (see p.viii).

A white crystalline powder. Slightly **soluble** in water; very slightly soluble in alcohol.

Allantoin is an astringent and keratolytic. It is present in multi-ingredient preparations intended for various skin disorders and is also used for its astringent properties in preparations for the treatment of haemorrhoids and other anorectal disorders.

In the USA the FDA decided that allantoin should be removed from lotions indicated for psoriasis as it was considered to be ineffective.[1]

1. Anonymous. Nonprescription drug review gains momentum. *WHO Drug Inf* 1991; **5:** 62.

Preparations

Proprietary Preparations (details are given in Part 3)
Canad.: Soothex.

Multi-ingredient: ***Aust.:*** Alphosyl; Contractubex; Rheumex; Riker Silicone-Spray; Sunsan-Heillotion; Ulcurilen; ***Austral.:*** Alphosyl; Blistex Medicated Lip Ointment; Blistex Sun Block Lip Balm†; Blistik†; First Aid Antiseptic Powder†; Hemocane; Lipguard†; Macro Natural Vitamin E Cream; Medi Creme; Medi Pulv; Mediderm†; Paxyl; Septacene†; SoloSite; Solyptol; ***Belg.:*** Activante†; Alphosyl; ***Canad.:*** Actinac; Alphosyl; AVC/Dienestrol†; Blistex Lip Ointment; Bye Bye Burn; Dermolan†; Le Stick a Levres; Phenoris; Tanac; ***Fr.:*** Alphosyl; Aveenoderm; Cicatryl; Clearasil Lotion†; Fadiamone; Genola; ***Ger.:*** Adebilan†; Alferm; Chlortesin-N†; Contractubex; Elbozon†; Ellsurex; Essaven Tri-Complex; HAEMO-Exhirud; Hydro Cordes; Leukona-Wundsalbe; Lipo Cordes; Magocrus†; Magopsor; Mederma†; Poloris; Poloris HC; Psoriasis-Salbe M; Rectosellan N†; Retterspitz Gelee; Retterspitz Heilsalbe; Ulcurilen N; Vulneral†; Vulnostad†; Wund- und Brand-Gel Eu Rho; ***Irl.:*** Actinac; Alphosyl; Alphosyl HC; Pedamed†; ***Ital.:*** Aflogine; Alphosyle; Angstrom Viso/Labbra Alta Protezione; Balta-Crin Tar; Dermogamma†; Flebogamma†; Herbatar; Herbatar Plus; Katosilver; Xerial; ***S.Afr.:*** Alphosyl; Arola Rosebalm; Masse†; ***Spain:*** Alantomicina; Alantomicina Complex; Alphosyl; Amplidermis; Antigrietun; Balneogel; Cortenema; Egarone; Hepro; Polaramine Topico; ***Swed.:*** Alphosyl; ***Switz.:*** Alphastria; Alphosyl; Alumagall; Carmol "thermogene"†; Contractubex; Demo-Rhinil†; Demosept; Dolorex Neo; Gorgonium; Hepathrombine; Keli-med; Lenidern†; Lyman; Optrex; Stomaqualine†; Teerol-H; Unatol; Wulnasin†; ***UK:*** Actinac; Alphosyl; Alphosyl HC; Anodesyn; Cold Sore Ointment†; Modantis; Sunspot; ***USA:*** Alasulf; Benegyn†; Blistex; Blistex Lip Balm; Deltavac; DIT1-2; Dr Dermi-Heal; Herpecin-L; Ionax Astringent; Orabase Lip; Tanac; Tanac Dual Core; Triple Care Protective Cream; Unicare†.

Aluminium Chloride (297-n)

Aluminii Chloridum Hexahydricum; Aluminium Chloratum; Aluminum Chloride; Cloreto de Aluminio; Cloruro de Aluminio. Aluminium chloride hexahydrate.

$AlCl_3,6H_2O$ = 241.4.

CAS — 7446-70-0 (anhydrous aluminium chloride); 7784-13-6 (aluminium chloride hexahydrate).

Pharmacopoeias. In *Eur.* (see p.viii) and *US.*

Deliquescent white or slightly yellow crystalline powder or colourless crystals. **Soluble** 1 in 0.9 of water and 1 in 4 of alcohol; soluble in glycerol. **Store** in airtight containers.

Adverse Effects

Aluminium chloride may cause irritation especially if applied to damp skin; this is attributed to the formation of hydrochloric acid.

Uses and Administration

Aluminium chloride has astringent properties and is used in a 20% alcoholic solution as an antiperspirant in the treatment of hyperhidrosis (p.1074). It is applied to dry skin usually at bedtime and is washed off in the morning before the sweat glands are fully active.

References.

1. Scholes KT, *et al.* Axillary hyperhidrosis treated with alcoholic solution of aluminium chloride hexahydrate. *Br Med J* 1978; **2:** 84–5.

Preparations

BP 1998: Aluminium Chloride Solution.

Proprietary Preparations (details are given in Part 3)
Austral.: Driclor; Hidrosol†; Odaban; ***Fr.:*** Driclor; Etiaxil†; ***Ger.:*** Albron-Saar; Mallebrin Konzentrat; ***Irl.:*** Anhydrol Forte; ***Switz.:*** Etiaxil; Mallebrin†; Racestyptine; ***UK:*** Anhydrol Forte; Driclor; Odaban; ***USA:*** Certain Dri; Drysol.

Multi-ingredient: ***Aust.:*** Racestyptin; ***Ger.:*** Gargarisma; Sepso†; ***Switz.:*** Deca; Racestyptine; ***USA:*** Stypto-Caine; Xerac AC.

Aluminium Chlorohydrate (298-h)

Aluminium Chlorhydrate; Aluminium Chloride Hydroxide Hydrate; Aluminum Chlorhydroxide; Aluminium Chloride Hydroxide Hydrate; Aluminum Chlorohydrate *(USAN)*; Aluminum Hydroxychloride; Basic Aluminium Chloride.

$Al_2(OH)_5Cl,xH_2O$.

CAS — 1327-41-9 (anhydrous).

Pharmacopoeias. In *US.*

US includes a range of compounds based on aluminium chlorohydrate. These are:
aluminium dichlorohydrate and sesquichlorohydrate
the polyethylene glycol (macrogol) complexes and propylene glycol complexes of aluminium chlorohydrex, aluminium dichlorohydrex, and aluminium sesquichlorohydrex;
the tri-, tetra-, penta-, and octachlorohydrates of aluminium zirconium and their respective glycine derivatives.

Aluminium chlorohydrate is used similarly to aluminium chloride in hyperhidrosis (p.1074). Single-ingredient products for hyperhidrosis generally have a concentration of 19%.

Aluminium chlorohydrate is also included in a variety of dermatological preparations for its astringent and antiperspirant properties.

Preparations

USP 23: Aluminum Chlorohydrate Solution; Aluminum Dichlorohydrate Solution; Aluminum Sesquichlorohydrate Solution; Aluminum Zirconium Octachlorohydrate Solution; Aluminum Zirconium Octachlorohydrex Gly Solution; Aluminum Zirconium Pentachlorohydrate Solution; Aluminum Zirconium Pentachlorohydrex Gly Solution; Aluminum Zirconium Tetrachlorohydrate Solution; Aluminum Zirconium Tetrachlorohydrex Gly Solution; Aluminum Zirconium Trichlorohydrate Solution; Aluminum Zirconium Trichlorohydrex Gly Solution.

Proprietary Preparations (details are given in Part 3)
Canad.: Roll-On; Scholl Dry Antiperspirant Foot Spray; ***Fr.:*** pM; ***Ger.:*** Phosphonorm; Primamed; ***Ital.:*** Spirial Antitraspirante; ***Mon.:*** Dermagor; ***Swed.:*** Biopac†; ***Switz.:*** Alopon; Gelsica; Phosphonorm; Sansudor; ***UK:*** Chiron Barrier Cream; ***USA:*** Dr Scholl's Super Deodorant Foot Powder†.

Multi-ingredient: ***Aust.:*** Sulgan 99; ***Austral.:*** Action†; Medrol Acne Lotion†; Nappy-Mate; Neo-Medrol; ***Canad.:*** Athletes Foot Antifungal; Medrol Acne Lotion; Neo-Medrol Acne; ***Ger.:*** Ansudor; Epipak; Hydonan†; Medrate Akne-Lotio†; Myxal†; Neo-Medrate Akne-Lotio†; ***Irl.:*** Neo-Medrone; ***Ital.:*** Medrol Lozione Antiacne; Neo-Medrol Lozione Antiacne†; ***S.Afr.:*** Neo-Medrol; ***Spain:*** Hongosan; Moderin Acne; Sudermin†; ***Switz.:*** Neo-Medrol†; Stomaqualine†; ***UK:*** Hands Dry†; ***USA:*** Ostiderm; Pedi-Pro.

Ammonium Lactate (19210-x)

Ammonium Lactate *(USAN)*.

BMS-186091.

$C_3H_9NO_3 = 107.1$.

CAS — 52003-58-4.

Ammonium lactate is a humectant applied as a lotion containing 12% lactic acid neutralised with ammonium hydroxide. It is used in the treatment of dry scaly conditions of the skin including ichthyosis.

Preparations

Proprietary Preparations (details are given in Part 3)
Canad.: Lac-Hydrin; ***Fr.:*** Lactagel; ***Ital.:*** Keratotal; ***USA:*** Am Lactin; Lac-Hydrin.

Multi-ingredient: ***Fr.:*** Ichtyosoft; Lactar; ***Ital.:*** Alfa Acid; Herbatar Plus.

Azelaic Acid (14036-v)

Azelaic Acid *(USAN, rINN)*.

Anchoic acid; Lepargylic acid; ZK-62498. Nonanedioic acid; Heptane-1,7-dicarboxylic acid.

$C_9H_{16}O_4 = 188.2$.

CAS — 123-99-9.

Adverse Effects and Precautions

Topical application of azelaic acid may produce a transient skin irritation that disappears on continued treatment. In a few patients the irritation may persist requiring reduced frequency of application or temporary suspension of treatment. There have been rare reports of hypopigmentation and photosensitivity. Azelaic acid should not be applied to the eyes, mouth, or other mucous membranes.

Uses and Administration

Azelaic acid inhibits the growth of *Propionibacterium* spp. and reduces keratinisation. It is used in the topical treatment of mild to moderate inflammatory acne (p.1072). It has also been tried in hyperpigmentary skin disorders such as melasma, and in malignant melanoma.

In the treatment of acne azelaic acid is applied twice daily for up to 6 months as a 20% cream. Improvement usually occurs within four weeks.

References.

1. Fitton A, Goa KL. Azelaic acid: a review of its pharmacological properties and therapeutic efficacy in acne and hyperpigmentary skin disorders. *Drugs* 1991; **41:** 780–98.

Preparations

Proprietary Preparations (details are given in Part 3)
Aust.: Skinoren; ***Austral.:*** Skinoren; ***Belg.:*** Skinoren; ***Fr.:*** Skinoren; ***Ger.:*** Skinoren; ***Ital.:*** Skinoren; ***Norw.:*** Skinoren; ***S.Afr.:*** Skinoren; ***Spain:*** Skinoren; Zeliderm; ***Swed.:*** Skinoren; ***Switz.:*** Skinoren; ***UK:*** Skinoren; ***USA:*** Azelex.

Multi-ingredient: ***Ital.:*** Neocutis.

Becaplermin (2718-f)

Becaplermin *(BAN, USAN, rINN)*.

RWJ-60235. Recombinant human platelet-derived growth factor B.

CAS — 165101-51-9.

Becaplermin is a platelet-derived growth factor that is applied topically as a 0.01% gel in the management of diabetic skin ulcers.

References.

1. Anonymous. Platelet-derived growth factor for diabetic ulcers. *Med Lett Drugs Ther* 1998; **40:** 73–4.
2. Wieman TJ, *et al.* Efficacy and safety of a topical gel formulation of recombinant human platelet-derived growth factor-BB (becaplermin) in patients with chronic neuropathic diabetic ulcers: a phase III randomized placebo-controlled double-blind study. *Diabetes Care* 1998; **21:** 822–7.

Preparations

Proprietary Preparations (details are given in Part 3)
USA: Regranex.

Bentoquatam (5759-s)

Bentoquatam *(USAN)*.

Quaternium 18-bentonite.

CAS — 1340-69-8.

Bentoquatam, described as an organoclay compound, is a barrier preparation that is applied topically as a 5% lotion to prevent allergic contact dermatitis caused by poison ivy, poison oak, or poison sumac. The lotion is applied in a sufficient quantity to form a visible coating 15 minutes before possible contact with the plants. If continued protection is required the lotion may be re-applied every 4 hours or at any time if the visible coating is removed.

Preparations

Proprietary Preparations (details are given in Part 3)
USA: Ivy Block.

Benzoyl Peroxide (5905-m)

Benzoyl Peroxide *(USAN)*.

Benzoylis Peroxidum; NSC-675. Dibenzoyl peroxide.

$C_{14}H_{10}O_4 = 242.2$.

CAS — 94-36-0 (anhydrous benzoyl peroxide).

Pharmacopoeias. Eur. (see p.viii) and *US* include hydrous benzoyl peroxide.

The Ph. Eur. specifies that Hydrous Benzoyl Peroxide (Benzoylis Peroxidum Cum Aqua) contains not less than 70% and not more than 77% of anhydrous benzoyl peroxide and not less than 20% of water. The USP specifies not less than 65% and not more than 82% of anhydrous benzoyl peroxide with a water content of about 26%. It rapidly loses water on exposure to air and may explode if the water content is too low.

The hydrous form is a white amorphous or granular powder with a characteristic odour. Practically **insoluble** to sparingly soluble in water; slightly to sparingly soluble in alcohol; soluble in acetone, chloroform, and ether; soluble in dichloromethane with separation of water.

Store at 2° to 8° in a container that has been treated to reduce static charges and that has a device for the release of excess pressure. Unused material should not be returned to its original container but should be destroyed by the addition of sodium hydroxide solution (10%). Destruction can be considered to be complete if the addition of a crystal of potassium iodide does not result in the release of free iodine. Protect from light.

CAUTION. *Benzoyl peroxide may explode if subjected to grinding, percussion, or heat. Hydrous benzoyl peroxide containing water to reduce the risk of explosion may still explode if exposed to temperatures higher than 60° or cause fires in the presence of reducing substances.*

Adverse Effects and Precautions

Application of benzoyl peroxide may produce an initial stinging effect. Skin dryness may also occur. Contact sensitisation has been reported in some patients using preparations containing benzoyl peroxide. Caution is required when applying it near the eyes, the mouth and other mucous membranes, and to the neck and other sensitive areas. Patients should be alerted to benzoyl peroxide's bleaching property.

Body odour. A report of an unusual unpleasant body odour in one patient attributed to the topical use of benzoyl peroxide.[1]

1. Molberg P. Body odor from topical benzoyl peroxide. *N Engl J Med* 1981; **304:** 1366.

Carcinogenicity. There has been concern at the implications of some *animal* studies showing benzoyl peroxide to possess some tumour-promoting activity.[1] However, one retrospective survey in Canada concluded that there was no indication that the normal use of benzoyl peroxide in the treatment of acne was associated with an increased risk of facial cancer.[2]

1. Jones GRN. Skin cancer: risk to individuals using the tumour promoter benzoyl peroxide for acne treatment. *Hum Toxicol* 1985; **4:** 75–8.
2. Hogan DJ, *et al.* A study of acne treatments as risk factors for skin cancer of the head and neck. *Br J Dermatol* 1991; **125:** 343–8.

Hypersensitivity. When used in the treatment of leg ulcers benzoyl peroxide appears to induce contact hypersensitivity frequently[1] but there is some uncertainty over its sensitising potential when used in the treatment of acne. Like some other acne treatments benzoyl peroxide can produce irritation but this usually resolves on continued use.[2] Patch testing[3,4] in some studies suggests that up to 76% of patients may be hypersensitive to benzoyl peroxide but this does not appear to correlate either with the clinical irritation produced during treatment or the reported incidence of hypersensitivity.[2,4] In one study 25% of patients were deemed to be hypersensitive from patch testing but only 2 of 44 patients developed clinical hypersensitivity.[4] However, there has been concern that hypersensitivity to benzoyl peroxide may be mistaken for irritation or worsening of the acne.[3]

1. Vena GA, *et al.* Contact dermatitis to benzoyl peroxide. *Contact Dermatitis* 1982; **8:** 338.
2. Cunliffe WJ, Burke B. Benzoyl peroxide: lack of sensitization. *Acta Derm Venereol (Stockh)* 1982; **62:** 458–9.
3. Leyden JJ, Kligman AM. Contact sensitization to benzoyl peroxide. *Contact Dermatitis* 1977; **3:** 273–5.
4. Rietschel RL, Duncan SH. Benzoyl peroxide reactions in an acne study group. *Contact Dermatitis* 1982; **8:** 323–6.

Pharmacokinetics

Work *in vitro* and in *animals*[1] suggests that although there is some absorption of benzoyl peroxide following topical application, any absorbed drug appears to be metabolised in the skin to benzoic acid and rapidly excreted in the urine.

1. Yeung D, *et al.* Benzoyl peroxide: percutaneous penetration and metabolic disposition II: effect of concentration. *J Am Acad Dermatol* 1983; **9:** 920–4.

Uses and Administration

Benzoyl peroxide has mild keratolytic properties. Its antimicrobial action is probably due to its oxidising effect and activity has been reported against *Staphylococcus epidermidis* and *Propionibacterium acnes*. It is used mainly in the treatment of acne (below), usually in topical preparations containing 2.5 to 10%, sometimes in conjunction with other antimicrobials. It has been used similarly in the treatment of fungal skin infections such as tinea pedis (p.371) although other drugs are usually preferred. A 20% lotion has been applied every 8 to 12 hours in the treatment of decubitus or stasis ulcers. Strengths are expressed as anhydrous benzoyl peroxide although it is usually employed in a hydrous form for safety (see above).

Benzoyl peroxide is also used as a bleaching agent in the food industry and as a catalyst in the plastics industry.

Acne. Benzoyl peroxide applied topically in concentrations of up to 10% is probably the most widely used first-line drug in the management of mild acne (p.1072). Early studies in *animals* found benzoyl peroxide to be sebosuppressive[1] but later studies demonstrated that sebum excretion rises during the first few months of treatment,[2,3] probably due to the comedolytic action of benzoyl peroxide, and remains at a stable level thereafter. Benzoyl peroxide has been shown to have a significant inhibitory effect on skin microflora, with reductions in surface and follicular micro-organisms within 48 hours of beginning treatment, but clinical improvement took several more days to appear.[4] Benzoyl peroxide has also been used in combination therapy with topical erythromycin when it has been reported to be helpful in preventing the selection of antibiotic-resistant mutants.[5,6]

1. Gloor M, *et al.* Cytokinetic studies on the sebo-suppressive effect of drugs using the example of benzoyl peroxide. *Arch Dermatol Res* 1980; **267:** 97–9.
2. Cunliffe WJ, *et al.* Topical benzoyl peroxide increases the sebum excretion rate in patients with acne. *Br J Dermatol* 1983; **109:** 577–9.

3. Pierard-Franchimont C, *et al.* Topical benzoyl peroxide increases the sebum excretion rate. *Br J Dermatol* 1984; **110:** 506.
4. Bojar RA, *et al.* The short-term treatment of acne vulgaris with benzoyl peroxide: effects on the surface and follicular cutaneous microflora. *Br J Dermatol* 1995; **132:** 204–8.
5. Eady EA, *et al.* Effects of benzoyl peroxide and erythromycin alone and in combination against antibiotic-sensitive and -resistant skin bacteria from acne patients. *Br J Dermatol* 1994; **131:** 331–6.
6. Eady EA, *et al.* The effects of acne treatment with a combination of benzoyl peroxide and erythromycin on skin carriage of erythromycin-resistant propionibacteria. *Br J Dermatol* 1996; **134:** 107–13.

Preparations

BP 1998: Benzoyl Peroxide Cream; Benzoyl Peroxide Gel; Benzoyl Peroxide Lotion; Potassium Hydroxyquinoline Sulphate and Benzoyl Peroxide Cream;
USP 23: Benzoyl Peroxide Gel; Benzoyl Peroxide Lotion; Erythromycin and Benzoyl Peroxide Topical Gel.

Proprietary Preparations (details are given in Part 3)
Aust.: Akneroxid; Benzaknen; PanOxyl; Scherogel; Ultra-Clear-A-Med; ***Austral.:*** Acnacyl†; Benzac; Brevoxyl; Clearasil Ultra Medication; Neutrogena Acne Mask; Oxy; PanOxyl; Skitz†; Topex†; ***Belg.:*** Akneroxid; Benzac; Pangel; Scherogel; Tinagel; ***Canad.:*** Acetoxyl; Acnomel BP 5; Benoxyl; Benzac; Benzagel; Clearasil B.P. Plus; Dermacne; Dermoxyl; Desquam-X; H_2Oxyl; Loroxide; Neutrogena Acne Mask; Neutrogena On-The-Spot Acne Lotion; Oxy; Oxyderm; PanOxyl; Solugel; ***Fr.:*** Cutacnyl; Eclaran; Effacne; Pannogel; PanOxyl; ***Ger.:*** Akne-Aid-Lotion mild†; Aknederm Oxid; Aknefug-oxid†; Akneroxid; Benzaknen; Benzoyt; Cordes BPO; H_2 Oxyl†; Klinoxid; Logomed Akne-Gel†; Marduk; Oxy Fissan; PanOxyl; Sanoxit; Scherogel; ***Irl.:*** Acnecide; Benoxyl; PanOxyl; ***Ital.:*** Benoxid; Benzac; Benzomix; Clearasil Ultra; Delta 80; PanOxyl; Reloxyl; Samil-O_2†; Scherogel; ***Neth.:*** Akneroxid; Benzac; Peauline†; Tinagel†; ***Norw.:*** Basiron; PanOxyl; ***S.Afr.:*** Benoxyl; Benzac-AC; PanOxyl; ***Spain:*** Acne-Aid†; Aldoacne; Benoxygel; Clearamed; Oxiderma; Oxytoko†; PanOxyl; Peroxacne; Peroxiben; Scherogel†; Stop Espinilla Normaderm; ***Swed.:*** Basiron; Clearamed†; Mytolac†; Stioxyl; ***Switz.:*** Acnefuge; Akneroxid; Aknex; Basiron; Benzac; Desanden; Effacne; H_2Oxyl†; Ledoxid Acne; Lubexyl; PanOxyl; ***UK:*** Acetoxyl†; Acnecide; Acnegel†; Benoxyl; Benzagel†; Clearasil Max 10; Mediclear; Nericur; Oxy; PanOxyl; Ultra Clearasil†; Valderma Active†; ***USA:*** Ambi 10; Ben-Aqua; Benoxyl; Benzac; Benzagel; Benzashave; Blemerase; Brevoxyl; Buf-Oxal†; Clear By Design; Clearasil; Cuticura†; Del Aqua; Dermoxyl†; Desquam; Exact; Fostex; Loroxide; Neutrogena Acne Mask; Oxy; PanOxyl; Peroxin; Persa-Gel; Theroxide†; Triaz; Vanoxide; Xerac BP†.

Multi-ingredient: ***Austral.:*** Clearasil Extra Strength†; ***Belg.:*** Acnidazil; Benzamycin; ***Canad.:*** Persol; Sulfoxyl; Vanoxide-HC†; ***Fr.:*** Uvacnyl†; ***Ger.:*** Acnidazil; ***Irl.:*** Benzamycin; Quinoderm; ***Ital.:*** Acnidazil; Delta 80 Plus; Katoxyn; ***Neth.:*** Acnecure; Acnidazil; ***S.Afr.:*** Acneclear; Acnidazil; Benzamycine; Quinoderm-H; Quinoderm†; ***Switz.:*** Acne Creme Plus; Acnidazil; Quinoderm; Quinoderm Hydrocortisone†; ***UK:*** Acnidazil; Benzamycin; Quinoderm; Quinoderm with Hydrocortisone†; Quinoped; ***USA:*** Benzamycin; Sulfoxyl; Vanoxide-HC.

Calamine (1598-f)

Prepared Calamine.

Pharmacopoeias. In *Br.*, *Chin.*, *Int.*, and *US.*

The BP describes calamine as a basic zinc carbonate coloured with ferric oxide whereas the USP describes as zinc oxide with a small proportion of ferric oxide.

Calamine is an amorphous, impalpable, pink or reddish-brown powder, the colour depending on the variety and amount of ferric oxide present and the process by which it is incorporated. Practically **insoluble** in water; it dissolves with effervescence in hydrochloric acid.

Calamine has mild astringent and antipruritic actions and is used as a dusting-powder, cream, lotion, or ointment in a variety of skin conditions.

Preparations

BP 1998: Aqueous Calamine Cream; Calamine and Coal Tar Ointment *(Compound Calamine Ointment)*; Calamine Lotion; Calamine Ointment;
USP 23: Calamine Lotion; Phenolated Calamine Lotion.

Proprietary Preparations (details are given in Part 3)
USA: Calamox.

Multi-ingredient: ***Austral.:*** Animine; Ansene†; Bronz†; Calaband; Caladryl; Calistaflex†; Dermalife Plus; Quinaband; Septacene†; Ungvita; ***Canad.:*** Aveeno Anti-Itch; Caladryl; Calamine Antihistamine; Calmasol†; Ivarest†; Noivy; ***Irl.:*** Caladryl; Hydrocal; RBC; Vasogen; ***Neth.:*** Caladryl; ***S.Afr.:*** Beracal†; Biohist; Caladryl; Calasthetic; Histamed; Lacto Calamine; Pasta Prura†; ***Spain:*** Caladryl; Poliglicol Anti Acne; Talco Antihistam Calber; Talquissar; Talquistina; ***UK:*** Cal-A-Cool†; Calaband; Caladryl; Eczederm†; Hydrocal†; Lacto Calamine; Quinaband; RBC; Swarm; Vasogen; ***USA:*** Aveeno Anti-Itch; Caladryl; Calamatum; Calamycin; Dome-Paste; Ivarest; RA Lotion; Resinol; Rhuli Spray.

Calcipotriol (10943-p)

Calcipotriol *(BAN, rINN).*

Calcipotriene *(USAN)*; MC-903. (5Z,7E,22E,24S)-24-Cyclopropyl-9,10-secochola-5,7,10(19),22-tetraene-1α,3β,24-triol.
$C_{27}H_{40}O_3$ = 412.6.
CAS — 112828-00-9; 112965-21-6.

Adverse Effects and Precautions

The most frequent adverse effect associated with calcipotriol is skin irritation and it should not therefore be applied to the facial area. Symptoms may include burning, itching, erythema, and dry skin, but discontinuation of therapy is seldom necessary. Aggravation of psoriasis may occur. Hypercalcaemia that is rapidly reversible on withdrawal has occurred during treatment with calcipotriol and it should not be used in patients with disorders of calcium metabolism. Other adverse effects include skin atrophy and photosensitivity.

Effects on calcium homoeostasis. Calcipotriol is a vitamin D derivative and therefore has the potential to cause hypercalcaemia and hypercalciuria. Up to December 1993, when about 150 000 patients in the UK had been treated with calcipotriol, the UK Committee on Safety of Medicines had received 6 reports of hypercalcaemia and 2 of hypercalciuria.[1] Three of the patients with hypercalcaemia either had used doses in excess of the recommended maximum (see Uses and Administration, below) or had pustular or exfoliative psoriasis. Hypercalcaemia and hypercalciuria were reversible on withdrawal of calcipotriol. A study[2] investigating the effect of calcipotriol on urine calcium excretion found that use of the maximum recommended dose for four weeks produced increased urine calcium excretion, and the authors suggested that patients requiring the maximum dose of calcipotriol should be monitored for hypercalciuria before and during treatment. A review[3] of the effects of vitamin D analogues on calcium homoeostasis concluded that patients with unstable psoriasis are at particular risk of toxicity from calcipotriol and that measurement of urine calcium excretion is a more sensitive indicator of toxicity than serum-calcium concentrations.

1. Committee on Safety of Medicines/Medicines Control Agency. Dovonex ointment (calcipotriol). *Current Problems* 1994; **20:** 3.
2. Berth-Jones J, *et al.* Urine calcium excretion during treatment of psoriasis with topical calcipotriol. *Br J Dermatol* 1993; **129:** 411–14.
3. Bourke JF, *et al.* Vitamin D analogues in psoriasis: effects on systemic calcium homeostasis. *Br J Dermatol* 1996; **135:** 347–54.

Uses and Administration

Calcipotriol is a vitamin D_3 derivative. *In vitro* it appears to induce differentiation and to suppress proliferation of keratinocytes.

Calcipotriol is used in a cream or ointment for the management of mild to moderate plaque psoriasis and as a solution in the management of scalp psoriasis; the concentration of calcipotriol used is 0.005%. In adults, applications should be made once or twice daily. No more than 100 g of cream or ointment and no more than 60 mL of scalp solution should be applied in one week. If used in combination the limit is 60 g of cream or ointment together with 30 mL of scalp solution or 30 g of cream or ointment with 60 mL of scalp solution.

In children, the cream or ointment may be applied twice daily. No more than 50 g of cream or ointment should be applied in one week in children aged 6 to 12 years; not more than 75 g per week should be applied in children over 12-years-old.

Skin disorders. Topical drugs are the treatment of first choice for chronic plaque psoriasis (p.1075). Calcipotriol, dithranol, and coal tar are commonly used for mild to moderate forms of the disorder. Calcipotriol has been shown to be effective[1] and has the advantages of being odourless and non-staining. Its efficacy in children[2] and during long-term[3] use has also been demonstrated. A study comparing calcipotriol ointment with coal tar for chronic plaque psoriasis[4] found rapid improvement within the first 2 weeks of treatment with calcipotriol, whereas improvement with tar occurred only after 4 weeks. When solutions of calcipotriol and betamethasone were compared for mild to moderate scalp psoriasis,[5] calcipotriol produced a satisfactory response, but betamethasone was more effective and was associated with less irritation of the scalp and face. Combination of calcipotriol with other antipsoriatic drugs may be beneficial; combination with betamethasone was more effective than treatment with calcipotriol alone in one study[6] and in another,[7] addition of calcipotriol to treatment with acitretin improved efficacy.

Beneficial results with calcipotriol have also been reported in pityriasis rubra pilaris[8] and congenital ichthyoses.[9]

1. Murdoch D, Clissold SP. Calcipotriol: a review of its pharmacological properties and therapeutic use in psoriasis vulgaris. *Drugs* 1992; **43:** 415–29.
2. Darley CR, *et al.* Safety and efficacy of calcipotriol ointment (Dovonex®) in treating children with psoriasis vulgaris. *Br J Dermatol* 1996; **135:** 390–3.
3. Ellis JP, *et al.* Long-term treatment of chronic plaque psoriasis with calcipotriol ointment in patients unresponsive to short-contact dithranol. *Eur J Clin Res* 1995; **7:** 247–57.
4. Tham SN, *et al.* A comparative study of calcipotriol ointment and tar in chronic plaque psoriasis. *Br J Dermatol* 1994; **131:** 673–7.
5. Klaber MR, *et al.* Comparative effects of calcipotriol solution (50 μg/mL) and betamethasone 17-valerate solution (1 mg/mL) in the treatment of scalp psoriasis. *Br J Dermatol* 1994; **131:** 678–83.
6. Ruzicka T, Lorenz B. Comparison of calcipotriol monotherapy and a combination of calcipotriol and betamethasone valerate after 2 weeks' treatment with calcipotriol in the topical therapy of psoriasis vulgaris: a multicentre, double-blind, randomized study. *Br J Dermatol* 1998; **138:** 254–8.
7. van de Kerkhof PCM, *et al.* The effect of addition of calcipotriol ointment (50 μg/g) to acitretin therapy in psoriasis. *Br J Dermatol* 1998; **138:** 84–9.
8. van de Kerkhof PCM, Steijlen PM. Topical treatment of pityriasis rubra pilaris with calcipotriol. *Br J Dermatol* 1994; **130:** 675–8.
9. Lucker GPH, *et al.* Effect of topical calcipotriol on congenital ichthyoses. *Br J Dermatol* 1994; **131:** 546–50.

Preparations

Proprietary Preparations (details are given in Part 3)
Aust.: Psorcutan; ***Austral.:*** Daivonex; ***Belg.:*** Daivonex; ***Canad.:*** Dovonex; ***Fr.:*** Daivonex; ***Ger.:*** Daivonex; Psorcutan; ***Irl.:*** Dovonex; ***Ital.:*** Daivonex; Psorcutan; ***Neth.:*** Daivonex; ***Norw.:*** Daivonex; ***S.Afr.:*** Dovonex; ***Spain:*** Daivonex; ***Swed.:*** Daivonex; ***Switz.:*** Daivonex; ***UK:*** Dovonex; ***USA:*** Dovonex.

Centella (1600-d)

Herba Centellae; Hydrocotyle; Indian Pennywort.
CAS — 18449-41-7 (madecassic acid); 464-92-6 (asiatic acid); 16830-15-2 (asiaticoside).
Pharmacopoeias. In *Chin.*

The fresh and dried leaves and stems of *Centella asiatica* (=*Hydrocotyle asiatica*) (Umbelliferae). It contains madecassic acid, asiatic acid, and asiaticoside.

Centella has been used topically and by mouth in the management of wounds, ulcers, and keloid scars. Contact dermatitis has been reported.

The names gotu kola, gotu cola, and gota kola are used for *Centella asiatica* in herbal medicine. Centella is also used in homoeopathic medicine.

References.

1. Santucci B, *et al.* Contact dermatitis due to Centelase®. *Contact Dermatitis* 1985; **12:** 39.

Preparations

Proprietary Preparations (details are given in Part 3)
Aust.: Collaven; Madecassol; ***Belg.:*** Madecassol; ***Canad.:*** Cothilyne; Madecassol†; ***Fr.:*** Madecassol; Madecassol Tulgras; Marticassol†; ***Ital.:*** Centellase; ***Neth.:*** Madecassol†; ***Spain:*** Blastoestimulina; ***Switz.:*** Madecassol.

Multi-ingredient: ***Austral.:*** Zestabs†; ***Fr.:*** Madecassol Neomycine Hydrocortisone; ***Ger.:*** Emdecassol†; ***Ital.:*** Angioton; Fluiven; Neomyrt Plus; ***Spain:*** Blastoestimulina.

Cerous Nitrate (12550-q)

Cerium Nitrate.
$Ce(NO_3)_3$ = 326.1.
CAS — 10108-73-3.

Cerous nitrate has been used topically in conjunction with silver sulphadiazine in the treatment of burns.

Preparations

Proprietary Preparations (details are given in Part 3)

Multi-ingredient: ***Belg.:*** Flammacerium; ***Fr.:*** Flammacerium; ***Neth.:*** Flammacerium.

Crilanomer (2788-y)

Crilanomer *(rINN).*
Acrylonitrile-starch Copolymer; ZK-94006. A starch polymer with acrylonitrile.
CAS — 37291-07-9.

Crilanomer is a starch copolymer used as a hydrogel wound dressing in the management of wounds.

Preparations

Proprietary Preparations (details are given in Part 3)
Austral.: Intrasite; ***Fr.:*** Intrasite; ***S.Afr.:*** Intrasite.

Crotamiton (1603-m)

Crotamiton *(BAN, rINN).*

Crotam; Crotamitonum. *N*-Ethyl-*N*-*o*-tolylcrotonamide; *N*-Ethylcrotono-*o*-toluidide; *N*-Ethyl-*N*-(2-methylphenyl)-2-butenamide.

$C_{13}H_{17}NO = 203.3.$

CAS — 483-63-6.

Pharmacopoeias. In *Eur.* (see p.viii) and *US.*

A colourless or pale yellow oily liquid with a faint amine-like odour. It solidifies partly or completely at low temperatures and it must be completely liquefied by warming before use. The Ph. Eur. specifies that it is predominantly the (*E*)-isomer, with not more than 15% of the (*Z*)-isomer. USP specifies a mixture of *cis*- and *trans*-isomers.

Slightly **soluble** in water; miscible with or soluble in alcohol; soluble in methyl alcohol. **Store** in small airtight containers. Protect from light.

Adverse Effects and Precautions

Applied topically, crotamiton occasionally causes irritation. There have been rare reports of hypersensitivity reactions. Crotamiton should not be used in the presence of acute exudative dermatitis. It should not be applied near the eyes, mouth, or other mucous membranes or on excoriated skin.

Ingestion of crotamiton may cause burning and irritation of oral, oesophageal, and gastric mucosa with nausea, vomiting, and abdominal pain.

Overdosage. A report of a 23-year-old woman who developed tonic-clonic seizures requiring treatment with diazepam after ingestion of a crotamiton emulsion.[1] Other hospital treatment included gastric lavage, activated charcoal, and metoclopramide. Crotamiton was detected in serum at a concentration of 34 μg per mL and was also detectable with several metabolites in the urine. Reference was also made to a report of a 2½-month-old child who had developed pallor and cyanosis after excessive dermal application of a crotamiton cream.

1. Meredith TJ, *et al.* Crotamiton overdose. *Hum Exp Toxicol* 1990; **9:** 57.

Uses and Administration

Crotamiton is an acaricide and has been used in the treatment of scabies as a 10% cream or lotion but other more effective drugs are usually preferred (p.1401). It is applied, after first bathing and drying, to the whole of the body surface below the chin, particular attention being paid to body folds and creases. A second application should be applied 24 hours later but it may need to be used once daily up to a total of 5 days to be effective. Appropriate measures should be taken to avoid re-infection especially from contaminated clothing and bed-linen. Some recommend the concurrent treatment of close contacts and household members to prevent re-infection.

Crotamiton is also used as an antipruritic (p.1075). One application may be effective for 6 to 10 hours.

Pruritus. A double-blind study in 31 patients[1] found that 10% crotamiton lotion was no more effective an antipruritic than its vehicle.

1. Smith EB, *et al.* Crotamiton lotion in pruritus. *Int J Dermatol* 1985; **23:** 684–5.

Preparations

BP 1998: Crotamiton Cream; Crotamiton Lotion;
USP 23: Crotamiton Cream.

Proprietary Preparations (details are given in Part 3)
Aust.: Eurax; ***Austral.:*** Eurax; ***Belg.:*** Eurax; ***Canad.:*** Eurax; ***Fr.:*** Eurax; ***Ger.:*** Crotamitex; Euraxil; ***Irl.:*** Eurax; ***Ital.:*** Eurax; ***Norw.:*** Eurax; ***S.Afr.:*** Eurax; ***Spain:*** Euraxil; ***Swed.:*** Eurax†; ***Switz.:*** Eurax; ***UK:*** Eurax; ***USA:*** Eurax.

Multi-ingredient: ***Fr.:*** Acarcid; ***Irl.:*** Eurax-Hydrocortisone; ***Spain:*** Euraxil Hidrocort; ***Switz.:*** Eurax-Hydrocortisone†; ***UK:*** Eurax-Hydrocortisone.

Dextranomer (1604-b)

Dextranomer *(BAN, rINN).*

Dextran cross-linked with epichlorohydrin (1-chloro-2,3-epoxypropane); Dextran 2,3-dihydroxypropyl 2-hydroxy-1,3-propanediyl ether.

CAS — 56087-11-7.

Precautions

Dextranomer should not be used in deep wounds or cavities from which its removal cannot be assured, nor should it be used on dry wounds. Care should be exercised when paste formulations of dextranomer are used near the eyes.

Spillage may render surfaces very slippery.

Implantation studies in *animals* indicated that entrapment of dextranomer beads in wounds was unlikely to initiate granuloma formation or chronic inflammation.[1] Most beads were apparently unchanged 3 years after implantation.

1. Falk J, Tollerz G. Chronic tissue response to implantation of Debrisan®: an experimental study. *Clin Ther* 1977; **1:** 185–91.

Uses and Administration

The action of dextranomer depends upon its ability to absorb up to 4 times its weight of fluid, including dissolved and suspended material of molecular weight up to about 5000.

Dextranomer is used for the cleansing of exudative and infected wounds, including burns and ulcers, and for preparation for skin grafting. The management of burns and wounds are discussed on p.1073 and p.1076, respectively.

The wound is cleansed with sterile water or saline and allowed to remain wet; dextranomer in the form of spherical beads is sprinkled on to a depth of at least 3 to 6 mm and covered with a sterile dressing. Occlusive dressings are not recommended as they may lead to maceration around the wound. The dextranomer can be renewed up to 5 times daily (usually once or twice daily), before the layer has become saturated with exudate; the old layer is washed off with a stream of sterile water or saline before renewal. All dextranomer must be removed before skin grafting. Dextranomer may also be applied as a paste (either ready-made or prepared by mixing 4 parts of the dextranomer beads with 1 part glycerol) or a paste-containing absorbent pad which need only be changed twice daily to every 2 days according to the rate of wound exudation.

Cadexomer-iodine (p.1105) has similar properties of absorption and releases iodine.

Preparations

Proprietary Preparations (details are given in Part 3)
Aust.: Debrisorb; ***Austral.:*** Debrisan†; ***Belg.:*** Debrisan; ***Canad.:*** Debrisan; ***Fr.:*** Debrisan; ***Ger.:*** Debrisorb; ***Irl.:*** Debrisan; ***Ital.:*** Debrisan; ***Neth.:*** Debripad†; Debrisan; ***S.Afr.:*** Debrisan; ***Swed.:*** Debrisan; ***Switz.:*** Debrisan; ***UK:*** Debrisan; ***USA:*** Debrisan; Envisan†.

Multi-ingredient: ***UK:*** Debrisan.

Dihydroxyacetone (1605-v)

DHA; Ketotriose. 1,3-Dihydroxypropan-2-one.

$C_3H_6O_3 = 90.08.$

CAS — 96-26-4.

Pharmacopoeias. In *US.*

A white to off-white crystalline powder. Freely **soluble** in water; the monomeric form is freely soluble in alcohol and in ether; the dimeric form is soluble in alcohol and sparingly soluble in ether. The pH of a 5% solution in water is between 4.0 and 6.0. **Store** in airtight containers below 15°.

Adverse Effects and Precautions

Skin irritation from dihydroxyacetone occurs rarely; rashes and allergic dermatitis have been reported. Contact with eyes, abraded skin, and clothing should be avoided.

Uses and Administration

Application to the skin of preparations containing dihydroxyacetone slowly produces a brown coloration similar to that caused by exposure to the sun, probably due to a reaction with the amino acids of the skin.

A single application may give rise to a patchy appearance; progressive darkening of the skin results from repeated use until a point is reached when no further darkening takes place. If the treatment is stopped the colour starts to fade after about 2 days and disappears completely within 8 to 14 days as the external epidermal cells are lost by normal attrition.

Preparations containing up to 8% (but usually 5%) of dihydroxyacetone have been used to camouflage vitiligo (see Pigmentation Disorders, p.1075) or to produce an artificial suntan. Some preparations include sunscreens since dihydroxyacetone gives no protection against sunburn.

Preparations

Proprietary Preparations (details are given in Part 3)
Austral.: Le Tan Fast; Le Tan Self Tan; Vitadye; ***Canad.:*** Vitadye†; ***Fr.:*** Euvitil†; ***USA:*** Chromelin Complexion Blender.

Multi-ingredient: ***Austral.:*** Le Tan Fast Plus; ***USA:*** QT.

Diphencyprone (4896-w)

2,3-Diphenylcyclopropenone-1.

Diphencyprone has been applied as a contact sensitiser for the treatment of alopecia. It has also been tried in warts.

Adverse effects. Diphencyprone is considered to lack serious adverse effects but some patients may not be able to tolerate the induced hypersensitivity reaction and there have been reports of generalised urticaria following the use of diphencyprone.[1,2] Allergy to diphencyprone has been reported in medical and nursing staff in spite of taking protective precautions during its application.[3] One patient who received diphencyprone treatment for warts developed in addition palpitations due to ventricular extrasystoles.[2] Vitiligo has also been reported in patients treated with diphencyprone[4-6] and it has been suggested that this might be due to unmasking of subclinical vitiligo.[4,5] Erythema multiforme-like eruptions were associated with the topical application of diphencyprone in 3 patients.[7]

1. Tosti A, *et al.* Contact urticaria during topical immunotherapy. *Contact Dermatitis* 1989; **21:** 196–7.
2. Lane PR, Hogan DJ. Diphencyprone. *J Am Acad Dermatol* 1988; **19:** 364–5.
3. Shah M, *et al.* Hazards in the use of diphencyprone. *Br J Dermatol* 1996; **134:** 1151–65.
4. Hatzis J, *et al.* Vitiligo as a reaction to topical treatment with diphencyprone. *Dermatologica* 1988; **177:** 146–8.
5. Duhra P, Foulds IS. Persistent vitiligo induced by diphencyprone. *Br J Dermatol* 1990; **123:** 415–16.
6. Henderson CA, Ilchyshyn A. Vitiligo complicating diphencyprone sensitization therapy for alopecia universalis. *Br J Dermatol* 1995; **133:** 496–7.
7. Perret CM, *et al.* Erythema multiforme-like eruptions: a rare side effect of topical immunotherapy with diphenylcyclopropenone. *Dermatologica* 1990; **180:** 5–7.

Alopecia. Diphencyprone has been used with varying degrees of success in the treatment of various forms of alopecia (p.1073) including areata, totalis, and universalis.[1-6] While some workers have achieved good results in adults[1-3] and children[4,7] others have obtained little benefit using diphencyprone.[5] Induction of a delayed (type IV) hypersensitivity reaction after application of diphencyprone appears to be an integral part of successful treatment.[8] Sensitisation has been achieved by applying a 2% solution of diphencyprone in acetone to a small area of scalp but this may be repeated if necessary beneath plastic occlusion if adequate sensitisation is not produced.[3] Thereafter, weaker concentrations of 0.01 to 2% are applied and gradually increased in strength to produce erythema and pruritus for 36 hours post-therapy; treatment is repeated weekly. Only one side of the scalp is treated until the optimum concentration is found, in order to prevent a widespread adverse reaction. One group of patients who achieved total regrowth of hair were able to discontinue treatment with diphencyprone for a mean of 15 months without relapse[9] and another group maintained satisfactory hair growth for a mean follow-up period of 19.8 months.[10]

1. MacDonald Hull S, Norris JF. Diphencyprone in the treatment of long-standing alopecia areata. *Br J Dermatol* 1988; **119:** 367–74.
2. Monk B, Williams HC. Topical diphencyprone therapy in alopecia totalis. *Br J Dermatol* 1988; **119** (suppl 33)**:** 16.
3. MacDonald Hull S, Cunliffe WJ. Successful treatment of alopecia areata using the contact allergen diphencyprone. *Br J Dermatol* 1991; **124:** 212–13.
4. MacDonald Hull S, *et al.* Alopecia areata in children: response to treatment with diphencyprone. *Br J Dermatol* 1991; **125:** 164–8.
5. Ashworth J, *et al.* Allergic and irritant contact dermatitis compared in the treatment of alopecia totalis and universalis: a comparison of the value of topical diphencyprone and tretinoin gel. *Br J Dermatol* 1989; **120:** 397–401.
6. Hoting E, Boehm A. Therapy of alopecia areata with diphencyprone. *Br J Dermatol* 1992; **127:** 625–9.
7. Schuttelaar M-L, *et al.* Alopecia areata in children: treatment with diphencyprone. *Br J Dermatol* 1996; **135:** 581–5.
8. MacDonald Hull S, *et al.* Alopecia areata treated with diphencyprone: is an allergic response necessary? *Br J Dermatol* 1990; **122:** 716–17.
9. van der Steen PHM, *et al.* Topical immunotherapy for alopecia areata: re-evaluation of 139 cases after an additional follow-up period of 19 months. *Dermatology* 1992; **184:** 198–201.
10. Gordon PM, *et al.* Topical diphencyprone for alopecia areata: evaluation of 48 cases after 30 months' follow-up. *Br J Dermatol* 1996; **134:** 869–71.

Dipyrithione (3520-c)

Dipyrithione *(USAN, rINN).*

OMDS. 2,2′-Dithiodipyridine 1,1′-dioxide.

$C_{10}H_8N_2O_2S_2 = 252.3.$

CAS — 3696-28-4.

Dipyrithione is reported to have antibacterial and antifungal properties and is included in preparations for the treatment of dandruff.

Preparations

Proprietary Preparations (details are given in Part 3)
Multi-ingredient: ***Switz.:*** Crimanex.

Dithiosalicylic Acid (13417-w)

2-Hydroxybenzenecarbodithioic acid.

$C_7H_6OS_2 = 170.3.$

CAS — 527-89-9.

Dithiosalicylic acid has been used in multi-ingredient preparations used topically for the treatment of acne and seborrhoeic dermatitis.

Preparations

Proprietary Preparations (details are given in Part 3)
Multi-ingredient: ***Fr.:*** Sacnel†; ***Ital.:*** Sacnel.

Dithranol (1606-g)

Dithranol *(BAN, rINN).*

Anthralin; Dioxyanthranol; Dithranolum. 1,8-Dihydroxyanthrone; 1,8-Dihydroxy-9(10*H*)-anthracenone.

$C_{14}H_{10}O_3$ = 226.2.

CAS — 1143-38-0 (dithranol); 16203-97-7 (dithranol triacetate).

Pharmacopoeias. In *Chin., Eur.* (see p.viii), and *US.*

A yellow to yellowish-brown, odourless, crystalline powder. Practically **insoluble** in water; slightly soluble in alcohol, in ether, and in glacial acetic acid; soluble in chloroform and in dichloromethane; soluble to sparingly soluble in acetone; dissolves in dilute solutions of alkali hydroxides. The filtrate from a suspension in water is neutral to litmus. **Store** at a temperature of 8° to 15° in airtight containers. Protect from light.

CAUTION. *Dithranol is a powerful irritant and should be kept away from the eyes and tender parts of the skin.*

Stability. The stability of dithranol has been studied in a number of bases and vehicles.[1,2] The weaker preparations of dithranol may be the least stable.[1] Salicylic acid is included in dithranol preparations as an antoxidant and its inclusion in pastes also containing zinc oxide prevents their discoloration due to the inactivation of dithranol by zinc oxide.[3] However, zinc oxide or starch can be omitted from dithranol pastes without loss of effectiveness provided stiffness is maintained.[3] Addition of ascorbic or oxalic acid may improve dithranol's stability in 'Unguentum Merck' but salicylic acid appears to be ineffective.[1] The effect of salicylic acid on the instability of dithranol in yellow soft paraffin is variable[1,2] and its inclusion has been questioned as it can be irritant and percutaneous absorption can be significant.[1] Dithranol is relatively stable in white soft paraffin.[1]

The application of any type of heat and contact with metal spatulas should be avoided during the manufacture of dithranol pastes[4] and if milling facilities are not available dithranol can be incorporated into Lassar's paste by dissolving it first in chloroform.[3]

1. Green PG, *et al.* The stability of dithranol in various bases. *Br J Dermatol* 1985; **113** (suppl 29): 26.
2. Lee RLH. Stability of dithranol (anthralin) in various vehicles. *Aust J Hosp Pharm* 1987; **17:** 254–8.
3. Comaish S, *et al.* Factors affecting the clearance of psoriasis with dithranol (anthralin). *Br J Dermatol* 1971; **84:** 282–9.
4. *PSGB Lab Report P/79/1* 1979.

Adverse Effects and Precautions

Dithranol may cause a burning sensation especially on perilesional skin. Patients with fair skin may be more sensitive than those with dark skin. It is irritant to the eyes and mucous membranes. Use on the face, skin flexures, and genitals should be avoided. Hands should be washed after use.

Dithranol should not be used for acute or pustular psoriasis or on inflamed skin. It stains skin, hair, some fabrics, plastics, and enamel. Staining of bathroom ware may be less of a problem with creams than ointments. Stains on skin and hair disappear on cessation of treatment although such disappearance may be slow.

Uses and Administration

Dithranol is used in the treatment of subacute and chronic psoriasis usually in one of two ways. *Conventional treatment* is commonly started with an ointment or paste containing 0.1% dithranol (0.05% in very fair patients) applied for a few hours; the strength is gradually increased as necessary to 0.5%, occasionally to 1%, and the duration of contact extended to overnight periods or longer. The preparation is sparingly and accurately applied to the lesions only. If, on initial treatment, lesions spread or excessive irritation occurs, the concentration of dithranol or the frequency of application should be reduced; if necessary, treatment should be stopped. After each treatment period the patient should bathe or shower to remove any residual dithranol.

For *short-contact therapy* dithranol is usually applied in a soft basis to the lesions for up to 60 minutes daily, before being washed off. As with conventional treatment the strength used is gradually increased from 0.1% to 2% but strengths up to 5% have been used. Surrounding unaffected skin may be protected by white soft paraffin.

Treatment for psoriasis should be continued until the skin is entirely clear. Intermittent courses may be needed to maintain the response. Treatment schedules often involve coal tar and UV irradiation (preferably UVB) before the application of dithranol (see below). Salicylic acid is included in many topical preparations of dithranol.

A cream containing dithranol triacetate 1% has been used similarly to dithranol in conventional treatment of psoriasis.

Psoriasis. Dithranol used alone or with coal tar with or without ultraviolet light continues to be one of the drugs of first-line treatment for psoriasis (p.1075). It is particularly suited to the treatment of stable chronic plaque psoriasis but unlike coal tar, is irritant to healthy skin and care is required to ensure that it is only applied to lesions. Treatment with dithranol is therefore more feasible when the plaques are large or few in number. Concomitant use of coal tar may help to reduce the irritant effects of dithranol without affecting efficacy. Traditional treatment with dithranol is time consuming and more suitable for use on hospital inpatients. Dithranol formulated in stiff preparations such as Lassar's paste to minimise spreading to perilesional skin is left on overnight covered with a suitable dressing and washed off the next day. Treatment is usually initiated with a concentration of 0.1% (0.05% in fair-skinned patients) and gradually increased according to the response and irritation produced. Cream formulations may be less effective but are more suitable for domestic use. Dithranol is also used with UVB phototherapy and there have been many modifications of the original Ingram's regimen in which dithranol is applied after bathing in a tar bath and exposure to ultraviolet light. Inpatient stays of up to 3 weeks may be required but long periods of remission can be obtained. However, short-contact therapy in which concentrations of up to 5% of dithranol are applied daily for up to 1 hour are more suitable for use on an outpatient basis and there appears to be little reduction in efficacy; irritation and staining may also be reduced.

Preparations

BP 1998: Dithranol Cream; Dithranol Ointment; Dithranol Paste; *USP 23:* Anthralin Cream; Anthralin Ointment.

Proprietary Preparations (details are given in Part 3)
Austral.: Dithrocream; ***Canad.:*** Anthraforte; Anthranol; Anthrascalp; ***Fr.:*** Anthranol†; Dithrasis†; ***Irl.:*** Dithrocream; Micanol; ***Ital.:*** Psoriderm; ***Neth.:*** Psoricreme; ***Norw.:*** Micanol; ***S.Afr.:*** Anthranol†; ***Spain:*** Anthranol; ***Swed.:*** Amitase†; Micanol; ***UK:*** Alphodith†; Anthranol†; Dithrocream; Exolan†; Micanol; ***USA:*** Anthra-Derm; Dritho-Scalp; Drithocreme; Micanol; Miconal.

Multi-ingredient: ***Aust.:*** Anthraderm; Psoradexan; ***Austral.:*** Dithrasal; Psorin†; ***Fr.:*** Anaxeryl; ***Ger.:*** Plesial†; Psoradexan; Psoralon MT; Psorispray†; StieLasan†; Warondo Psoriasissalbe†; ***Irl.:*** Psoradrate; ***Ital.:*** Pentagamma†; ***Spain:*** Lapices Epiderm Metadier; Psorantral; ***Switz.:*** Psoradexan; Psoralon MT†; ***UK:*** Dithrolan†; Psoradrate†; Psorin.

Ethyl Lactate (16638-n)

$C_5H_{10}O_3$ = 118.1.

CAS — 97-64-3.

Ethyl lactate has been applied topically in the treatment of acne vulgaris. It is reported to lower the pH within the skin thereby exerting a bactericidal effect.

Ethyl lactate is also used in the flavouring of foods.

Preparations

Proprietary Preparations (details are given in Part 3)
Multi-ingredient: ***UK:*** Tri-Ac†.

Etretinate (1609-s)

Etretinate *(BAN, USAN, rINN).*

Ro-10-9359. Ethyl 3-methoxy-15-apo-φ-caroten-15-oate; Ethyl (*all-trans*)-9-(4-methoxy-2,3,6-trimethylphenyl)-3,7-dimethylnona-2,4,6,8-tetra-enoate.

$C_{23}H_{30}O_3$ = 354.5.

CAS — 54350-48-0.

Adverse Effects and Precautions

As for Isotretinoin, p.1084.

Donation of blood should be avoided for at least 2 years after cessation of treatment. The period of time during which pregnancy must be avoided following cessation of treatment has not been determined; detectable plasma-etretinate concentrations have been reported nearly 3 years after stopping treatment.

In addition to the references cited below under the various headings, further references to the adverse effects of etretinate can be found in Isotretinoin, p.1084, under Effects on the Blood, Eyes, Liver, Musculoskeletal System, Serum Lipids, and the Skin as well as under Vasculitic Syndromes.

Carcinogenicity. A report of 2 patients developing lymphomas while receiving etretinate[1] prompted a report of 3 other malignancies in patients taking etretinate.[2]

1. Woll PJ, *et al.* Lymphoma in patients taking etretinate. *Lancet* 1987; **ii:** 563–4.
2. Harrison PV. Retinoids and malignancy. *Lancet* 1987; **ii:** 801.

Effects on the cardiovascular system. The Italian Ministry of Health recommended[1] that the electrocardiogram, blood lipids, and clotting factors should be monitored before and throughout treatment with etretinate as there had been rare suspected cases of myocardial ischaemia and infarction reported in treated patients.

1. Anonymous. Reports from regulatory agencies: etretinate. *WHO Drug Inf* 1987; **1:** 29.

Effects on the kidneys. A report of impaired renal function associated with etretinate in one patient.[1] It was noted that in manufacturer-sponsored studies the mean serum-creatinine concentration had been raised in patients receiving etretinate.

1. Horber FF, *et al.* Impaired renal function and hypercalcaemia associated with etretinate. *Lancet* 1984; **ii:** 1093.

Oedema. A report of generalised oedema following treatment with etretinate.[1] Five other cases had been reported in the literature and rechallenge in 4 patients had provoked a recurrence.

1. Allan S, Christmas T. Severe edema associated with etretinate. *J Am Acad Dermatol* 1988; **19:** 140.

Interactions

As for Isotretinoin, p.1085.

Methotrexate. The risk of developing hepatotoxicity may be increased by concomitant administration of etretinate and methotrexate (see Interactions under Methotrexate, p.549).

Warfarin. Etretinate has been reported to reduce the therapeutic efficacy of warfarin (see Interactions under Warfarin, p.968).

Pharmacokinetics

The mean bioavailability of etretinate is about 40% following oral administration but there is a large interindividual variation. Absorption can be increased by administration with milk or fatty food. Etretinate undergoes significant first-pass metabolism and plasma concentrations of the active carboxylic acid metabolite, acitretin (p.1077), may be detected before those of the parent drug; acitretin may itself be metabolised to etretinate (p.1077). Both etretinate and acitretin are extensively bound to plasma protein. Etretinate appears to accumulate in adipose tissue after repeated dosing and has a prolonged elimination half-life of about 120 days; detectable serum concentrations have been observed up to 3 years after the discontinuation of therapy. Up to 75% of a dose is excreted in the faeces mainly as unchanged drug. Etretinate is also excreted in the urine as metabolites. Etretinate crosses the placenta and is distributed into breast milk.

References.

1. Brazzell RK, Colburn WA. Pharmacokinetics of the retinoids isotretinoin and etretinate. *J Am Acad Dermatol* 1982; **6:** 643–51.
2. Rollman O, Vahlquist A. Retinoid concentrations in skin, serum and adipose tissue of patients treated with etretinate. *Br J Dermatol* 1983; **109:** 439–47.
3. Colburn WA, *et al.* Effect of meals on the kinetics of etretinate. *J Clin Pharmacol* 1985; **25:** 583–9.
4. Lucek RW, Colburn WA. Clinical pharmacokinetics of the retinoids. *Clin Pharmacokinet* 1985; **10:** 38–62.
5. DiGiovanna JJ, *et al.* Etretinate: persistent serum levels after long-term therapy. *Arch Dermatol* 1989; **125:** 246–51.

Uses and Administration

Etretinate is a retinoid and is a derivative of tretinoin (p.1093). It has been given by mouth for the treatment of severe, extensive psoriasis that has not responded to other treatment, especially generalised and palmo-plantar pustular psoriasis. It has also been used in severe congenital ichthyosis, and severe Darier's disease (keratosis follicularis) as well as other disorders of keratinisation. Acitretin (p.1077) is now preferred to etretinate.

Therapy has generally been begun at a dosage of 0.75 to 1 mg per kg body-weight daily in divided doses by mouth. A maximum dose of 1.5 mg per kg daily should not be exceeded (some sources have suggested a maximum of 75 mg daily). Erythrodermic psoriasis may respond to lower initial doses of 0.25 mg per kg per day, increased at weekly intervals by 0.25 mg per kg per day until optimal response occurs. Following the initial response, generally after 8 to 16 weeks of therapy, maintenance doses of 0.5 to 0.75 mg per kg daily have been given. Therapy should be discontinued once lesions have sufficiently resolved.

Preparations

Proprietary Preparations (details are given in Part 3)
Austral.: Tigason†; ***Canad.:*** Tegison†; ***Fr.:*** Tigason†; ***Ger.:*** Tigason†; ***Irl.:*** Tigason†; ***Ital.:*** Tigason; ***S.Afr.:*** Tigason†; ***Spain:*** Tigason†; ***Swed.:*** Tigason†; ***Switz.:*** Tigason†; ***UK:*** Tigason†; ***USA:*** Tegison.

Fumaric Acid (1310-y)

297; Allomalenic Acid; Boletic Acid. *trans*-Butenedioic acid.
$C_2H_2(CO_2H)_2$ = 116.1.
CAS — 110-17-8 (fumaric acid); 624-49-7 (dimethyl fumarate).
Pharmacopoeias. In *Pol.* Also in *USNF.*

White odourless granules or crystalline powder. Slightly **soluble** in water and ether; soluble in alcohol; very slightly soluble in chloroform.

Uses and Administration

Fumaric acid and some of its derivatives have been used in the treatment of psoriasis and other skin disorders.

Fumaric acid is also used as an acidifier and flavouring agent in foods.

Skin disorders. Fumaric acid, its sodium salts, and derivatives such as dimethyl fumarate, monoethyl fumarate (ethyl hydrogen fumarate), and octyl hydrogen fumarate have been used in the treatment of psoriasis (p.1075) and other skin disorders both topically and systemically. Dimethyl fumarate appears to be the most active compound given orally but combination with various salts of monoethyl fumarate has been claimed to improve efficacy.[1-4] However, there have been reports of acute renal failure associated with treatment and the German Federal Office of Health has expressed the opinion that the available evidence did not establish the value of fumaric acid derivatives in psoriasis or other skin disorders.[5] Other adverse effects with oral therapy have included disturbances of liver function,[3,6] gastro-intestinal effects,[2-4,6,7] and flushing.[2-4,6,7]

1. van Loenen AC, *et al.* Fumaarzuurtherapie: van fictie tot werkelijkheid? *Pharm Weekbl* 1989; **124:** 894–900.
2. Kolbach DN, Nieboer C. Fumaric acid therapy in psoriasis: a long-term retrospective study on the effect of fumaric acid combination (FAC-EC) therapy and dimethyl-fumaric acid ester (DMFAE) monotherapy. *Br J Dermatol* 1990; **123:** 534–5.
3. Nugteren-Huying WM, *et al.* Fumaric acid therapy for psoriasis: a randomized, double-blind, placebo-controlled study. *J Am Acad Dermatol* 1990; **22:** 311–12.
4. Altmeyer PJ, *et al.* Antipsoriatic effect of fumaric acid derivatives: results of a multicenter double-blind study in 100 patients. *J Am Acad Dermatol* 1994; **30:** 977–81.
5. Anonymous. Fumaric acid derivatives and nephrotoxicity. *WHO Drug Inf* 1990; **4:** 28.
6. Nieboer C, *et al.* Systemic therapy with fumaric acid derivates: new possibilities in the treatment of psoriasis. *J Am Acad Dermatol* 1989; **20:** 601–8.
7. Mrowietz U, *et al.* Treatment of psoriasis with fumaric acid esters: results of a prospective multicentre study. *Br J Dermatol* 1998; **138:** 456–60.

Preparations

Proprietary Preparations (details are given in Part 3)
Ger.: Psoriasis-Solution; Psoriasis-Tabletten.

Multi-ingredient: *Austral.:* Pro-PS; ***Ger.:*** Fumaderm; Psoriasis-Bad; Psoriasis-Salbe M.

Glycolic Acid (8922-v)

Hydroxyacetic Acid. Hydroxyethanoic acid.
$C_2H_4O_3$ = 76.05.

Glycolic acid is an organic acid that has been used in topical preparations for hyperpigmentation and photodamaged skin.

Preparations

Proprietary Preparations (details are given in Part 3)
Canad.: Neostrata.

Multi-ingredient: *Ital.:* Acnesan.

Hydroquinone (1612-b)

Hydrochinonum; Quinol. 1,4-Benzenediol.
$C_6H_6O_2$ = 110.1.
CAS — 123-31-9.

NOTE. Do not confuse with Hydroquinine (p.1589).
Pharmacopoeias. In *Belg.* and *US.*

Fine white needle crystals which darken on exposure to light and air. **Soluble** 1 in 17 of water, 1 in 4 of alcohol, 1 in 51 of chloroform, and 1 in 16.5 of ether. **Store** in airtight containers. Protect from light.

Adverse Effects, Treatment, and Precautions

Hydroquinone may cause transient erythema and a mild burning sensation. High concentrations or prolonged use may produce hyperpigmentation especially on areas of skin exposed to sunlight. Occasionally hypersensitivity has occurred and some recommend skin testing before use. Hydroquinone should not be applied to abraded or sunburnt skin. It should not be used to bleach eyelashes or eyebrows and contact with the eyes should be avoided as it may produce staining and corneal opacities. The systemic effects of hydroquinone and their treatment are similar to those of phenol (see p.1121) but tremors and convulsions may also occur.

Effects on the liver. Toxic hepatitis in a radiographer was attributed to occupational exposure to hydroquinone fumes from the developing medium used in the darkroom.[1] However, it has been pointed out[2] that hydroquinone is not volatile under normal conditions of use and that surveillance of 879 people engaged in the manufacture and use of hydroquinone from 1942 to 1990 found no association between toxic hepatitis and hydroquinone exposure.

1. Nowak AK, *et al.* Darkroom hepatitis after exposure to hydroquinone. *Lancet* 1995; **345:** 1187.
2. O'Donaghue JL, *et al.* Hydroquinone and hepatitis. *Lancet* 1995; **346:** 1427–8.

Effects on the skin. The incidence of exogenous ochronosis (blue-black hyperpigmentation) in a survey of black South African patients was found to be 15% in males and 42% in females with 69% of affected individuals admitting to using hydroquinone-containing preparations.[1] This was considered to be more consistent with a toxic side-effect of a drug with a low therapeutic index, rather than an idiosyncratic reaction. The data revealed that even preparations with hydroquinone 2% or less with a sunscreen produced ochronosis. Ochronosis usually became apparent after about 6 months application of hydroquinone and, once established, was probably irreversible. Patients may initially use skin lighteners for cosmetic purposes but once ochronosis develops they may fall into the 'skin lightener trap' as they use other hydroquinone preparations to remove the disfigurement.[1] The problems caused by over-the-counter skin-lightening creams in countries such as the UK have also been highlighted.[2] Reversible brown discoloration of the nails has also been reported following the use of skin lighteners containing hydroquinone.[3]

1. Hardwick N, *et al.* Exogenous ochronosis: an epidemiological study. *Br J Dermatol* 1989; **120:** 229–38.
2. Williams H. Skin lightening creams containing hydroquinone. *Br Med J* 1992; **305:** 903–4.
3. Mann RJ, Harman RRM. Nail staining due to hydroquinone skin-lightening creams. *Br J Dermatol* 1983; **108:** 363–5.

Uses and Administration

Hydroquinone increases melanin excretion from melanocytes and may also prevent its production. Hydroquinone is used topically as a depigmenting agent for the skin in hyperpigmentation conditions such as chloasma (melasma), freckles, and lentigines (small macules that resemble freckles). It may be several weeks before any effect is apparent but depigmentation may last for 2 to 6 months after discontinuation. Application of hydroquinone should be discontinued if there is no improvement after 2 months of treatment. Hydroquinone should be applied twice daily only to intact skin which should be protected from sunlight to reduce repigmentation. Concentrations of 2 to 4% are commonly employed. Hydroquinone preparations often include a sunscreen or a sunblocking basis.

Hydroquinone is also used as an antoxidant for ether and in photographic developers.

Pigmentation disorders. Hydroquinone is modestly effective for hyperpigmentation (see Pigmentation Disorders, p.1075) but successful treatment depends upon diligent long-term use by carefully instructed patients as well as protection from sun exposure.[1] Preparations containing hydroquinone 2% are less effective than those containing 4%.[2] Supplemental use of topical corticosteroids, salicylic acid, or tretinoin may improve results and once the desired effect has been achieved the use of hydroquinone alone may be sufficient for maintenance.[1] Hydroquinone 2% with tretinoin 0.05 to 0.1% has produced good results but preparations containing hydroquinone 5% with or without tretinoin and corticosteroids have been reported to be highly irritant.[2] However, even with the most careful management most patients only experience partial improvement.[1]

1. Engasser PG, Maibach HI. Cosmetics and dermatology: bleaching creams. *J Am Acad Dermatol* 1981; **5:** 143–7.
2. Pathak MA, *et al.* Treatment of melasma with hydroquinone. *J Invest Dermatol* 1981; **76:** 324.

Preparations

USP 23: Hydroquinone Cream; Hydroquinone Topical Solution.

Proprietary Preparations (details are given in Part 3)
Canad.: African Gold; Banishing Cream; Eldopaque; Eldoquin; Esoterica Regular; Jouvence; Nadinola; Neostrata HQ; Porcelana; Ultraquin Plain; ***Fr.:*** Aida; Creme des 3 Fleurs d'Orient; ***Ital.:*** Discromil; Epocler; ***UK:*** Esoterica; ***USA:*** Eldopaque; Eldoquin; Esoterica Sensitive Skin; Melanex; Melpaque HP; Melquin HP; Neostrata AHA; Porcelana; Solaquin.

Multi-ingredient: *Austral.:* Superfade; ***Canad.:*** Esoterica; Porcelana with Sunscreen; Skinicles; Solaquin; Ultraquin; ***Fr.:*** Melanex Duo; ***Ger.:*** Pigmanorm; ***Switz.:*** Pigmanorm; ***USA:*** Ambi Skin Tone; Esoterica Facial; Nuquin HP; Porcelana with Sunscreen; Solaquin Forte; Viquin Forte.

Ichthammol (1615-q)

Ichthammol *(BAN).*

Ammonii Sulfogyrodalas; Ammonio Sulfoittiolato; Ammonium Bithiolicum; Ammonium Bitumenosulfonicum; Ammonium Bituminosulphonate; Ammonium Ichthosulphonate; Ammonium Sulfobituminosum; Ammonium Sulpho-Ichthyolate; Bithiolate Ammonique; Bithyol; Bituminol; Ichthammolum; Ichthosulphol; Ichthyol; Ichthyolammonium.
CAS — 8029-68-3.
Pharmacopoeias. In *Chin., Eur.* (see p.viii), *Jpn, Pol.,* and *US.*

Ichthammol is a reddish-brown to almost black viscous liquid with a strong characteristic empyreumatic odour. It consists mainly of the ammonium salts of the sulphonic acids of an oily substance prepared from the destructive distillation of a bituminous schist or shale, together with ammonium sulphate and water. The Ph. Eur. specifies not less than 4.5% and not more than 7.0% of total ammonia, not less than 10.5% of organically combined sulphur, calculated on the dried material, and not more than 20% of the total sulphur in the form of sulphates. The USP specifies that it yields not less than 10.0% of total sulphur and not less than 2.5% of ammonia.

Miscible with water and with glycerol; slightly soluble in alcohol, in ether, in fatty oils, and in liquid paraffin; forms homogeneous mixtures with wool fat and soft paraffin. **Incompatible** with wool alcohols.

Light Ammonium Bituminosulphonate (Ammoniumbituminosulfonat Hell) is produced from the light distillate fraction of shale oil.

Ammoniumsulfobital, an ammonium bituminosulphonate similar to ichthammol but with a low sulphur content, is commercially available as Tumenol Ammonium.

Ichthammol has slight bacteriostatic properties and is used in a wide range of topical preparations, for a variety of skin disorders; it has also been used in suppositories for anorectal disorders. Ichthammol is often used with zinc oxide in medicated bandages for chronic eczema (p.1073). Ichthammol may be slightly irritant to the skin and there have been rare reports of hypersensitivity.

Preparations

BP 1998: Zinc and Ichthammol Cream;
USP 23: Ichthammol Ointment.

Proprietary Preparations (details are given in Part 3)
Aust.: Ichtho-Bad; Ichtholan; Ichtopur; ***Austral.:*** Egoderm Cream; ***Ger.:*** Ichtho-Bad; Ichtholan; Ichtholan Spezial; Ichthyol; Schwarze-Salbe; Thiobitum; ***Spain:*** Adnexol†; Jabon de Ictiol†; ***Switz.:*** Ichtho-Bad; Ichtholan.

Multi-ingredient: *Aust.:* Aknemycin compositum; Delta-Hadensa; Hadensa; Ichth-Oestren; Inotyol; ***Austral.:*** Acnederm; Egoderm Ointment; Icthaband; ***Belg.:*** Inotyol; Zinc-Ichtyol; ***Canad.:*** Boil Ease; Ictholin; ***Fr.:*** Aloplastine Ichthyolee†; Anaxeryl; Gelictar de Charlieu†; Inotyol; Oxythyol; ***Ger.:*** Aknemycin; Crinohermal P†; Crinohermal†; Dreisalan†; Hoemarin Derma; Lugro†; Protitis†; Rheumichthol Bad; Robusanon†; Sebohermal†; Warondo-Flechtensalbe†; Warondo-Wundsalbe†; ***Ital.:*** Antiemorroidali; Bal Tar; Dermatar; Essaproct†; Ichthopaste; Inotyol; Sebohermal†; ***Norw.:*** Inotyol; ***S.Afr.:*** Antipeol; ***Spain:*** Aknederm†; Antihemorroidal†; Hadensa; Ictiomen; Inotyol†; Lamnotyl; Queratil; ***Swed.:*** Inotyol; ***Switz.:*** Aknemycin; Crinohermal FEM†; Crinohermal P†; Crinohermal†; Epithelial†; Escothyol†; Furodermal; Furodermil; Phlogidermil; Riccomycine; Riccovitan; Vulnat†; ***UK:*** Antipeol; Ichthopaste; Icthaband; St James Balm; ***USA:*** Boil Ease; Boyol Salve; Medicone Derma.

Ictasol (6045-g)

Ictasol *(USAN).*

Ichthyol-Natrium Hell; Light Sodium Bituminosulphonate; Natrium Sulfobituminosum Decoloratum.
$C_{28}H_{36}Na_2O_6S_3$ = 610.8.
CAS — 12542-33-5.

Sodium bituminosulphonate is obtained by the destructive distillation of certain bituminous schists, sulphonation of the distillate, and neutralisation of the product with sodium hydroxide. Ictasol is a sodium bituminosulphonate produced from the light distillate fraction of shale oil.

Ictasol has similar properties to ichthammol (p.1083) and is used in a wide range of preparations for a variety of skin disorders.

Preparations

Proprietary Preparations (details are given in Part 3)
Aust.: Ichthraletten; Lavichthol; Solutio Cordes; ***Ger.:*** Aknichthol Creme; Crino Cordes N; Dermichthol; Ichthoderm; Ichtholan T; Ichthosin; Ichthraletten; Leukichtan N; Solutio Cordes; ***Switz.:*** Ichtholan T†; Ichthraletten.

Multi-ingredient: *Aust.:* Aknichthol; Crino Cordes; Ichthalgan forte; Ichtho-Bellol; Ichtho-Cadmin; Ichtho-Cortin; Leukichtan; Pelvichthol; ***Fr.:*** Ichtyosoft; ***Ger.:*** Aknederm Neu; Aknichthol Dexa†; Aknichthol N; Ichthalgan; Ichtho-Bellol; Ichtho-Bellol compositum S; Ichtho-Cadmin†; Ichtho-Himbin†; Ichthocortin;

Ichthoseptal; Ichthospasmin N†; Pelvichthol N; *Switz.:* Aknichthol N; Ichtho-Cadmin†.

Isotretinoin (1616-p)

Isotretinoin *(BAN, USAN, rINN).*

Isotretinoinum; 13-*cis*-Retinoic Acid; Ro-4-3780. (13*Z*)-15-Apo-β-caroten-15-oic acid; (2*Z*,4*E*,6*E*,8*E*)-3,7-Dimethyl-9-(2,6,6-trimethylcyclohex-1-enyl)nona-2,4,6,8-tetraenoic acid.

$C_{20}H_{28}O_2$ = 300.4.

CAS — 4759-48-2.

Pharmacopoeias. In *Eur.* (see p.viii) and *US.*

A yellow or light orange, crystalline powder or yellow crystals. Practically **insoluble** in water; sparingly soluble to slightly soluble in alcohol; sparingly soluble in ether, in isopropyl alcohol, and in macrogol 400; soluble in chloroform and in dichloromethane. **Store** in airtight containers at a temperature not exceeding 25°. Protect from light. The Ph. Eur. recommends that the contents of an opened container be used as soon as possible and that any unused part be protected by an atmosphere of an inert gas. The USP specifies that all the contents should be stored under an atmosphere of an inert gas.

Adverse Effects

The adverse effects of isotretinoin and other oral retinoids are similar to those of vitamin A (see p.1358) and are generally reversible and dose-related. The most common are dryness of the mucous membranes and of the skin with scaling, fragility, and erythema, especially of the face, cheilitis, pruritus, epistaxis, conjunctivitis, dry sore mouth, and palmo-plantar exfoliation. Corneal opacities, dry eyes, visual disturbances, skeletal hyperostosis, and musculoskeletal symptoms may also occur. Elevation of serum triglycerides, hepatic enzymes, erythrocyte sedimentation rate, and blood glucose have been reported. Other effects have included hair thinning, photosensitivity, changes in skin pigmentation, paronychia, gastro-intestinal symptoms, headache, drowsiness, sweating, mood changes, psychotic symptoms, depression, suicidal behaviour, benign intracranial hypertension, seizures, vasculitis, and an association with skin infections and an inflammatory bowel syndrome.

Isotretinoin and other retinoids are teratogenic.

When isotretinoin is applied topically the adverse effects are similar to those of tretinoin (see p.1094).

General references.

1. David M, *et al.* Adverse effects of retinoids. *Med Toxicol* 1988; **3:** 273–88.
2. Keefe M. Adverse reactions profile: retinoids. *Prescribers' J* 1995; **35:** 71–6.

Effects on the blood. Thrombocytopenia has been reported in 2 patients receiving etretinate and in one patient treated with isotretinoin.[1] There has also been a report of agranulocytosis associated with isotretinoin therapy in a 16-year-old boy.[2] Leucocytosis[3,4] and multiple thrombosis[5] have been reported in patients who received tretinoin by mouth for treatment of acute promyelocytic leukaemia.

1. Naldi L, *et al.* Etretinate therapy and thrombocytopenia. *Br J Dermatol* 1991; **124:** 395.
2. Waisman M. Agranulocytosis from isotretinoin. *J Am Acad Dermatol* 1988; **18:** 395–6.
3. Toh CH, Winfield DA. All-trans retinoic acid and side-effects. *Lancet* 1992; **339:** 1239–40.
4. Frankel SR, *et al.* The "retinoic acid syndrome" in acute promyelocytic leukemia. *Ann Intern Med* 1992; **117:** 292–6.
5. Forjaz De Lacerda J, *et al.* Multiple thrombosis in acute promyelocytic leukaemia after tretinoin. *Lancet* 1993; **342:** 114–15.

Effects on the eyes. Corneal opacities and papilloedema are among the more serious effects of isotretinoin on the eye but they are usually reversible if therapy is discontinued; papilloedema can result from benign intracranial hypertension[1,2] and patients receiving concomitant treatment with tetracyclines are particularly at risk.[2] Oral retinoids appear to interfere with retinal function[3] and there have been reports of alterations in colour sense,[4] poor night vision, and photophobia.[5] However, a 1-year follow-up failed to find any evidence of ocular toxicity attributable to etretinate in patients who had received long-term treatment and one patient who had toxic optic neuropathy due to methotrexate was able to continue treatment with etretinate.[6]

Ectropion has been associated with etretinate therapy in one patient.[7]

1. Fraunfelder FT, *et al.* Adverse ocular reactions possibly associated with isotretinoin. *Am J Ophthalmol* 1985; **100:** 534–7.
2. Gibberd B. Drug-induced benign intracranial hypertension. *Prescribers' J* 1991; **31:** 118–21.
3. Brown RD, Grattan CEH. Visual toxicity of synthetic retinoids. *Br J Ophthalmol* 1989; **73:** 286–8.
4. Weber U, *et al.* Abnormal retinal function associated with long-term etretinate? *Lancet* 1988; **i:** 235–6.
5. Weleber RG, *et al.* Abnormal retinal function associated with isotretinoin therapy for acne. *Arch Ophthalmol* 1986; **104:** 831–7.
6. Pitts JF, *et al.* Etretinate and visual function: a 1-year follow-up study. *Br J Dermatol* 1991; **125:** 53–5.
7. Brenner S, *et al.* Ectropion: an adverse effect of etretinate therapy for psoriasis. *DICP Ann Pharmacother* 1990; **24:** 1007.

Effects on the liver. Transient slight elevations of serum concentrations of liver enzymes are common with etretinate, but there have been few reports of acute hepatitis[1,2] or cholestatic jaundice.[3] In one patient, acute hepatitis progressed to chronic active hepatitis, despite cessation of etretinate therapy[4] but studies examining serial liver biopsies from patients receiving long-term etretinate have failed to show any significant chronic liver damage.[5-7] The manufacturers have reported instances of hepatic fibrosis, necrosis, and/or cirrhosis.

In a recent overview it was considered that some form of hepatotoxicity may be seen in up to 20% of patients treated with etretinate and significant liver disease is thought to occur in 1%.[8]

Isotretinoin may also cause mild elevations of liver enzymes and the manufacturers state that jaundice and hepatitis have occurred rarely. There is also a report of fatty liver.[9]

1. Foged EK, Jacobsen FK. Side effects due to RO 10-9359 (Tigason). *Dermatologica* 1982; **164:** 395–403.
2. Weiss VC, *et al.* Hepatotoxic reactions in a patient treated with etretinate. *Arch Dermatol* 1984; **120:** 104–6.
3. Gavish D, *et al.* Cholestatic jaundice, an unusual side effect of etretinate. *J Am Acad Dermatol* 1985; **13:** 669–70.
4. Weiss VC, *et al.* Chronic active hepatitis associated with etretinate therapy. *Br J Dermatol* 1985; **112:** 591–7.
5. Glazer SD, *et al.* Ultrastructural survey and tissue analysis of human livers after a 6-month course of etretinate. *J Am Acad Dermatol* 1984; **10:** 632–8.
6. Foged E, *et al.* Histologic changes in the liver during etretinate treatment. *J Am Acad Dermatol* 1984; **11:** 580–3.
7. Roenigk HH, *et al.* Serial liver biopsies in psoriatic patients receiving long-term etretinate. *Br J Dermatol* 1985; **112:** 77–81.
8. Boyd AS. An overview of the retinoids. *Am J Med* 1989; **86:** 568–74.
9. Taylor AEM, Mitchison H. Fatty liver following isotretinoin therapy. *Br J Dermatol* 1991; **124:** 505–6.

Effects on the musculoskeletal system. An ossification disorder resembling diffuse skeletal hyperostosis, with myalgia, arthralgia, and stiffness was first reported by Pittsley in patients who had taken large doses of isotretinoin for prolonged periods.[1] Premature closure of the epiphyses in a child treated with isotretinoin has also been described.[2] DiGiovanna later found radiographic evidence of extraspinal tendon and ligament calcification in patients who had received long-term therapy with etretinate[3] and there were reports of spinal hyperostosis from other workers[4] and one of spinal cord compression.[5] Gilbert *et al.*[6] were unable to find radiographic skeletal changes after 6 to 18 months of treatment with etretinate but Wilson *et al.*[7] found that hyperostosis was fairly common in patients taking moderately prolonged therapy and they recommended that radiological examinations should be carried out every 12 months in patients taking etretinate. However, they were unable to find any clear association between these effects and the total dose or duration of treatment. Others have found evidence of changes after 4 months in patients who had taken isotretinoin 1 mg per kg body-weight daily and recommended that radiological examinations should be made every 6 months in patients receiving isotretinoin for more than a year.[8] However, another study found that although 12% of patients receiving isotretinoin 0.5 mg per kg had evidence of hyperostoses this was not clinically significant in any patient.[9] Tangrea *et al.* suggested that monitoring beyond the treatment period might be unnecessary as calcifications and hyperostosis in patients who had received isotretinoin for 3 years had neither progressed nor improved 10 to 24 months after the end of treatment; additionally no new hyperostoses had developed during that period.[10] Of 25 patients treated with acitretin for a mean of 5 years one had abnormal calcification thought to be caused by the drug;[11] therapy with acitretin was continued with no further side-effects. The authors recommended radiological examinations after twelve months of treatment and then every second year. A study in 135 patients[12] who had received oral retinoids for a mean of 30 months could establish no relationship between spinal abnormalities and prolonged oral retinoid treatment and the authors suggested that spinal abnormalities only occur sporadically in predisposed patients.

There have also been individual reports of hypercalciuria[7] or hypercalcaemia[13-15] associated with oral retinoid therapy. Oral retinoids may also cause muscle damage;[16,17] myositis has been reported with tretinoin[18] and severe myopathy with acitretin.[19]

1. Pittsley RA, Yoder FW. Retinoid hyperostosis: skeletal toxicity associated with long-term administration of 13-cis-retinoic acid for refractory ichthyosis. *N Engl J Med* 1983; **308:** 1012–14.
2. Milstone LM, *et al.* Premature epiphyseal closure in a child receiving oral 13-cis-retinoic acid. *J Am Acad Dermatol* 1982; **7:** 663–6.
3. DiGiovanna JJ, *et al.* Extraspinal tendon and ligament calcification associated with long-term therapy with etretinate. *N Engl J Med* 1986; **315:** 1177–82.
4. Archer CB, *et al.* Spinal hyperostosis and etretinate. *Lancet* 1987; **i:** 741.
5. Tfelt-Hansen P, *et al.* Spinal cord compression after long-term etretinate. *Lancet* 1989; **ii:** 325–6.
6. Gilbert M, *et al.* Lack of skeletal radiographic changes during short-term etretinate therapy for psoriasis. *Dermatologica* 1986; **172:** 160–3.
7. Wilson DJ, *et al.* Skeletal hyperostosis and extraosseous calcification in patients receiving long-term etretinate (Tigason). *Br J Dermatol* 1988; **119:** 597–607.
8. Török L, *et al.* Bone-scintigraphic examinations in patients treated with retinoids: a prospective study. *Br J Dermatol* 1989; **120:** 31–6.
9. Carey BM, *et al.* Skeletal toxicity with isotretinoin therapy: a clinico-radiological evaluation. *Br J Dermatol* 1988; **119:** 609–14.
10. Tangrea JA, *et al.* Isotretinoin and the axial skeleton. *Lancet* 1992; **340:** 495–6.
11. Mørk N-J, *et al.* Skeletal side-effects of 5 years' acitretin treatment. *Br J Dermatol* 1996; **134:** 1156–7.
12. Van Dooren-Greebe RJ, *et al.* Prolonged treatment with oral retinoids in adults: no influence on the frequency and severity of spinal abnormalities. *Br J Dermatol* 1996; **134:** 71–6.
13. Valentic JP, *et al.* Hypercalcemia associated with oral isotretinoin in the treatment of severe acne. *JAMA* 1983; **250:** 1899–1900.
14. Horber FF, *et al.* Impaired renal function and hypercalcaemia associated with etretinate. *Lancet* 1984; **ii:** 1093.
15. Akiyama H, *et al.* Hypercalcaemia due to all-trans retinoic acid. *Lancet* 1992; **339:** 308–9.
16. Hodak E, *et al.* Muscle damage induced by isotretinoin. *Br Med J* 1986; **293:** 425–6.
17. David M, *et al.* Electromyographic abnormalities in patients undergoing long-term therapy with etretinate. *J Am Acad Dermatol* 1988; **19:** 273–5.
18. Miranda N, *et al.* Myositis with tretinoin. *Lancet* 1994; **334:** 1096.
19. Lister RK, *et al.* Acitretin-induced myopathy. *Br J Dermatol* 1996; **134:** 989–90.

Effects on the respiratory system. There have been reports of exercise-induced wheezing,[1] eosinophilic pleural effusion,[2] and worsening asthma[3] associated with isotretinoin therapy. The USA manufacturers have records of adverse effects on the lung including worsening asthma, recurrent pneumothorax, interstitial fibrosis, and pulmonary granuloma.[4] A study of healthy subjects confirmed that lung function tests could deteriorate after treatment with isotretinoin.[4]

1. Fisher DA. Exercise-induced bronchoconstriction related to isotretinoin therapy. *J Am Acad Dermatol* 1985; **13:** 524.
2. Bunker CB, *et al.* Isotretinoin and eosinophilic pleural effusion. *Lancet* 1989; **i:** 435–6.
3. Sabroe RA, *et al.* Bronchospasm induced by isotretinoin. *Br Med J* 1996; **312:** 886.
4. Bunker CB, *et al.* Isotretinoin and the lung. *Br J Dermatol* 1991; **125** (suppl 38): 29.

Effects on serum lipids. The oral retinoids induce dose-dependent changes in serum lipids. There can be increases in very-low-density-lipoprotein cholesterol with smaller increases in low-density-lipoprotein cholesterol and reductions in high-density-lipoprotein cholesterol.[1] These effects appear to be unrelated to age or sex. They occur early during treatment and are usually reversible within a few weeks of discontinuation. Overall, the effect of isotretinoin is much greater than that of etretinate. Although the total cholesterol and triglyceride concentrations may remain within normal limits, types IIb and IV hyperlipidaemias are not uncommon among patients receiving oral retinoids. There has been a report of pancreatitis associated with hypertriglyceridaemia in patients treated with isotretinoin.[2]

Retinoids should be used with caution in patients with pre-existing hypertriglyceridaemia or in those at risk of developing hypertriglyceridaemia.[1] Concomitant administration of fish oil containing eicosapentaenoic acid has been reported to attenuate retinoid-induced increases in serum-cholesterol and serum-triglyceride concentrations.[3]

1. Henkin Y, *et al.* Secondary dyslipidemia: inadvertent effects of drugs in clinical practice. *JAMA* 1992; **267:** 961–8.
2. Flynn WJ, *et al.* Pancreatitis associated with isotretinoin-induced hypertriglyceridemia. *Ann Intern Med* 1987; **107:** 63.
3. Marsden JR. Effect of dietary fish oil on hyperlipidaemia due to isotretinoin and etretinate. *Hum Toxicol* 1987; **6:** 219–22.

Effects on sexual function. Ejaculatory failure has been reported in 3 men to be associated with isotretinoin treatment.[1] A possible mechanism could be an effect on the goblet cells of the seminal vesicles, an effect similar to the general reduction in body secretions which leads to dry mucous membranes.

1. Coleman R, MacDonald D. Effects of isotretinoin on male reproductive system. *Lancet* 1994; **344:** 198.

Effects on the skin, hair, and nails. Apart from the more common adverse effects of oral retinoids on the skin and hair (see above), there have been isolated reports of granulomatous lesions,[1,2] precipitation or exacerbation of erythroderma,[3,4] palmo-plantar eruptions,[5] prurigo-like eruptions,[6] scalp folliculitis,[7] pyoderma gangrenosum,[7,8] palmo-plantar stickiness,[9] curling hair,[10] and chloasma (melasma).[11] There has been a report of fatal toxic epidermal necrolysis associated with etretinate.[12] Acne fulminans has been reported as a complication of isotretinoin treatment[13] although there have also been cases of acne fulminans being treated successfully with isotretinoin.[14] For other reports of acne fulminans and eruptions associated with vasculitic syndromes, see below.

Oral retinoids have been associated with paronychia and other forms[15] of nail dystrophy.

1. Lane PR, Hogan DJ. Granulomatous lesions appearing during isotretinoin therapy. *Can Med Assoc J* 1984; **130:** 550.
2. Williamson DM, Greenwood R. Multiple pyogenic granulomata occurring during etretinate therapy. *Br J Dermatol* 1983; **109:** 615–17.
3. Wantzin GL, Thomsen K. A new cutaneous side effect of isotretinoin. *J Am Acad Dermatol* 1985; **13:** 665.
4. Levin J, Almeyda J. Erythroderma due to etretinate. *Br J Dermatol* 1985; **112:** 373.
5. David M, *et al.* Palmoplantar eruption associated with etretinate therapy. *Acta Derm Venereol (Stockh)* 1986; **66:** 87–9.
6. Boer J, Smeenk G. Nodular prurigo-like eruptions induced by etretinate. *Br J Dermatol* 1987; **116:** 271–4.
7. Hughes BR, Cunliffe WJ. Development of folliculitis and pyoderma gangrenosum in association with abdominal pain in a patient following treatment with isotretinoin. *Br J Dermatol* 1990; **122:** 683–7.
8. Gangaram HB, *et al.* Pyoderma gangrenosum following treatment with isotretinoin. *Br J Dermatol* 1997; **136:** 636–7.
9. Penneys NS, Hernandez D. A sticky problem with etretinate. *N Engl J Med* 1991; **325:** 521.
10. van der Pijl JW, *et al.* Isotretinoin and azathioprine: a synergy that makes hair curl? *Lancet* 1996; **348:** 622–3.
11. Burke H, Carmichael AJ. Reversible melasma associated with isotretinoin. *Br J Dermatol* 1996; **135:** 862.
12. McIvor A. Fatal toxic epidermal necrolysis associated with etretinate. *Br Med J* 1992; **304:** 548.
13. Huston NR, Mules R. Acne fulminans with severe myalgia precipitated by isotretinoin therapy. *N Z Med J* 1985; **36:** 821.
14. Darley CR, *et al.* Acne fulminans with arthritis in identical twins treated with isotretinoin. *J R Soc Med* 1984; **77:** 328–30.
15. Dharmagunawardena B, Charles-Holmes R. Median canaliform dystrophy following isotretinoin therapy. *Br J Dermatol* 1997; **137:** 658–9.

PHOTOTOXICITY. *In vitro* photohaemolysis studies demonstrated that tretinoin and isotretinoin have a phototoxic potential while etretinate has none.[1] However, acitretin the major metabolite of etretinate had a phototoxic potential greater than that of tretinoin. The apparently low incidence of photosensitivity suggested that an idiosyncrasy is responsible. Patients should use appropriate photoprotection against UVA and UVB wavebands.

1. Ferguson J, Johnson BE. Photosensitivity due to retinoids: clinical and laboratory studies. *Br J Dermatol* 1986; **115:** 275–83.

Effects on taste. Almost complete loss of taste has been reported in a patient given isotretinoin 0.6 mg per kg bodyweight daily by mouth for 20 weeks.[1] Sense of taste was recovered approximately six months after isotretinoin was discontinued. Up to September 1994 the Committee on Safety of Medicines in the UK knew of 5 cases of taste changes, including 4 reports of loss of taste.

1. Halpern SM, *et al.* Loss of taste associated with isotretinoin. *Br J Dermatol* 1996; **134:** 378.

Overdosage. Apart from vague abdominal discomfort there were no other symptoms or significant abnormalities in a 15-year-old who was treated with gastric lavage 1.5 hours after ingestion of 350 mg of isotretinoin.[1] There was a similar outcome in the 2 other cases of isotretinoin overdosage reported in the literature.

1. Hepburn NC. Deliberate self-poisoning with isotretinoin. *Br J Dermatol* 1990; **122:** 840–1.

Vasculitic syndromes. The manufacturer of isotretinoin and etretinate has received isolated reports of vasculitis associated with the use of these oral retinoids; Wegener's granulomatosis has also been reported following the use of isotretinoin.[1,2] The precise mechanism underlying these effects is unknown; in some patients there may have been a direct toxic effect as symptoms developed shortly after the start of treatment, in other patients the onset was long-delayed and in some may have been triggered by the incidental use of antibiotics. Erythema nodosum and acne fulminans associated with circulating immune complexes had previously been reported after the use of isotretinoin.[3]

1. Dwyer JM, *et al.* Vasculitis and retinoids. *Lancet* 1989; **ii:** 494–6.
2. Anonymous. Retinoids and necrotizing vasculitis. *WHO Drug Inf* 1989; **3:** 187.
3. Kellett JK, *et al.* Erythema nodosum and circulating immune complexes in acne fulminans after treatment with isotretinoin. *Br Med J* 1985; **290:** 820.

Precautions

Isotretinoin is teratogenic and should not be used in pregnant patients. It is advisable for female patients to commence using contraceptive measures one month before starting isotretinoin treatment. Pregnancy should be avoided during treatment and for 1 month after treatment has been withdrawn. Patients receiving isotretinoin should not donate blood during, or for 1 month after cessation of therapy. (NOTE. Pregnancy or blood donation must be avoided for *much* longer periods in patients taking acitretin or etretinate.) Isotretinoin is contra-indicated in patients with hepatic and renal impairment, hyperlipidaemias, hypervitaminosis A, and in breast-feeding mothers. Isotretinoin should be used with care in patients with a history of depression and patients receiving isotretinoin should be monitored for signs of depressive illness.

Liver function and fasting blood lipids should be measured at the start of therapy, after the first month, and thereafter as appropriate. Blood glucose should be monitored throughout treatment in patients who either have, or are predisposed to, diabetes mellitus. Some recommend routine radiological evaluation in patients receiving long-term therapy (see under Effects on the Musculoskeletal System, above). Patients may experience a reduced tolerance to contact lenses.

Excessive exposure to sunlight and UV light should be avoided.

When applied topically the precautions described under tretinoin (see p.1094) should be adopted.

Advice that patients receiving retinoids should not use wax depilation following reports of facial and leg erosions.[1-3] It has been suggested[3] that wax depilation should be avoided for up to 2 months following cessation of isotretinoin treatment.

1. Romo ME. Isotretinoin and wax epilation. *Br J Dermatol* 1991; **124:** 393–7.
2. Holmes SC, Thomson J. Isotretinoin and skin fragility. *Br J Dermatol* 1995; **132:** 165.
3. Woollons A, Price ML. Roaccutane and wax epilation: a cautionary tale. *Br J Dermatol* 1997; **137:** 839–40.

Pregnancy. The problem of prescribing oral retinoids to women of child-bearing potential has been discussed by Mitchell[1] and Chan *et al.*[2] Intra-uterine exposure to isotretinoin has caused spontaneous abortion and a characteristic pattern of fetal malformations involving craniofacial, cardiac, thymic, and central nervous system structures.[3,4] Some infants have also shown subnormal intelligence and other neuropsychological impairments.[5] The risk of malformation appears to be high at all therapeutic doses of isotretinoin even when the duration of exposure is short.[6] Despite warnings on the use of retinoids during pregnancy and the need for adequate contraception in women of child-bearing potential and other strict guidelines on their use, intra-uterine exposure to retinoids has still occurred.[7] Isotretinoin has a relatively short half-life and it has been recommended that conception should be avoided for at least one month after the end of treatment. A survey of women who conceived after the use of isotretinoin (64% within one month of discontinuation of treatment) suggested that the incidence of spontaneous abortion or congenital malformations was no greater than in the general population.[8] However, patients taking oral retinoids with longer half-lives must avoid conception for much longer periods; at least two years (3 years in the US) is recommended if patients are taking acitretin although the period of time for patients taking etretinate has not been established. Malformations similar to those associated with isotretinoin have been reported in infants conceived within one year of stopping etretinate.[9,10]

1. Mitchell AA. Oral retinoids: what should the prescriber know about their teratogenic hazards among women of child-bearing potential? *Drug Safety* 1992; **7:** 79–85.
2. Chan A, *et al.* Oral retinoids and pregnancy. *Med J Aust* 1996; **165:** 164–7.
3. Lammer EJ, *et al.* Retinoic acid embryopathy. *N Engl J Med* 1985; **313:** 837–41.
4. Rosa F. Isotretinoin dose and teratogenicity. *Lancet* 1987; **ii:** 1154.
5. Adams J. High incidence of intellectual deficits in 5-year-old children exposed to isotretinoin 'in utero'. *Teratology* 1990; **41:** 614.
6. Dai WS, *et al.* Epidemiology of isotretinoin exposure during pregnancy. *J Am Acad Dermatol* 1992; **26:** 599–606.
7. Stern RS. When a uniquely effective drug is teratogenic: the case of isotretinoin. *N Engl J Med* 1989; **320:** 1007–9.
8. Dai WS, *et al.* Safety of pregnancy after discontinuation of isotretinoin. *Arch Dermatol* 1989; **125:** 362–5.
9. Grote W, *et al.* Malformation of fetus conceived 4 months after termination of maternal etretinate treatment. *Lancet* 1985; **i:** 1276.
10. Lammer EJ. Embryopathy in infant conceived one year after termination of maternal etretinate. *Lancet* 1988; **ii:** 1080–1.

Interactions

Concomitant use of isotretinoin and vitamin A (including dietary supplements) should be avoided because of additive toxic effects. Tetracyclines should be avoided as their use with isotretinoin has been associated with the development of benign intracranial hypertension.

Carbamazepine. For the effect of isotretinoin on carbamazepine, see p.342.

Pharmacokinetics

Isotretinoin is absorbed from the gastro-intestinal tract and absorption may be increased by administration with food. Peak plasma concentrations have been obtained 1 to 4 hours after oral administration. Oral bioavailability is low possibly due to metabolism in the gut wall and first-pass metabolism in the liver. Isotretinoin is highly bound to plasma proteins. It is metabolised in the liver to its major metabolite 4-oxo-isotretinoin; there is also some isomerisation of isotretinoin to tretinoin. Isotretinoin, tretinoin, and their metabolites undergo enterohepatic recycling. The terminal elimination half-life of isotretinoin is 10 to 20 hours. Equal amounts of a dose appear in the faeces, mainly as unchanged drug, and in the urine as metabolites.

Isotretinoin crosses the placenta.

References.

1. Brazzell RK, Colburn WA. Pharmacokinetics of the retinoids isotretinoin and etretinate. *J Am Acad Dermatol* 1982; **6:** 643–51.
2. Khoo K-C, *et al.* Pharmacokinetics of isotretinoin following a single oral dose. *J Clin Pharmacol* 1982; **22:** 395–402.
3. Colburn WA, *et al.* Food increases the bioavailability of isotretinoin. *J Clin Pharmacol* 1983; **23:** 534–9.
4. Colburn WA, *et al.* Pharmacokinetics of isotretinoin and its major blood metabolite following a single oral dose to man. *Eur J Clin Pharmacol* 1983; **24:** 689–94.
5. Brazzell RK, *et al.* Pharmacokinetics of isotretinoin during repetitive dosing to patients. *Eur J Clin Pharmacol* 1983; **24:** 695–702.
6. Lucek RW, Colburn WA. Clinical pharmacokinetics of the retinoids. *Clin Pharmacokinet* 1985; **10:** 38–62.
7. Kraft JC, *et al.* Embryonic retinoid concentrations after maternal intake of isotretinoin. *N Engl J Med* 1989; **321:** 262.
8. Larsen FG, *et al.* Pharmacokinetics and therapeutic efficacy of retinoids in skin diseases. *Clin Pharmacokinet* 1992; **23:** 42–61.

Uses and Administration

Isotretinoin is a retinoid. It is the *cis* configuration of tretinoin (p.1093) which is the acid form of vitamin A (p.1358). It is given by mouth for the treatment of severe acne that has not responded to other measures; it is also applied topically in milder forms of acne. It is not indicated for uncomplicated adolescent acne. Isotretinoin has also been tried in a number of other skin disorders and in some forms of neoplastic disease.

The initial oral daily dose of isotretinoin for acne is 0.5 to 1 mg per kg body-weight, given with food once daily or in two divided doses and adjusted after 4 weeks according to response and side-effects. Acute exacerbation of acne is occasionally seen during the initial period, but usually subsides within 7 to 10 days on continued treatment. Patients intolerant to the initial dose may be able to continue treatment at 0.1 to 0.2 mg per kg daily. Doses up to 2 mg per kg daily are permitted in some countries for patients whose disease is very severe or primarily on the body instead of the face. Treatment should continue for 12 to 20 weeks or until the total cyst count has decreased by over 70%. Improvement may continue for several months after cessation of treatment; prolonged remissions can occur. It is recommended that repeat courses should not normally be given but occasionally they may be required. However, since acne may continue to improve following discontinuation of isotretinoin, there must be at least a 2-month drug-free period before initiating repeat treatment.

For the topical treatment of acne a gel containing 0.05% of isotretinoin is applied sparingly once or twice daily. A therapeutic response may not be evident for 6 to 8 weeks.

General reviews.

1. Orfanos CE, *et al.* Current use and future potential role of retinoids in dermatology. *Drugs* 1997; **53:** 358–88.

Apart from its established role in the treatment of acne (below), isotretinoin has been used in other skin disorders including the keratinisation disorders Darier's disease (p.1073) and ichthyosis (p.1074); lichen planus (p.1075); rosacea[1] (p.1076); and some neoplastic disorders (below).

1. Ertl GA, *et al.* A comparison of the efficacy of topical tretinoin and low-dose oral isotretinoin in rosacea. *Arch Dermatol* 1994; **130:** 319–24.

Acne. The retinoids play an important role in the treatment of acne (p.1072). Severe conglobate and nodulocystic acne unresponsive to other therapy including systemic antibacterials is the main indication for oral isotretinoin therapy. Administration of isotretinoin produces a dose-related reduction in sebum excretion with a subsequent reduction in levels of *Propionibacterium acnes*, inflammation, and cyst formation.[1] A skin reaction with the appearance of papulopustules frequently occurs after 2 to 4 weeks of therapy but this rapidly clears with continued treatment. Although sebum excretion may approach pretreatment levels after discontinuation of therapy most patients remain free of their disease after a single course and long-term remissions lasting months or years have been obtained.[2,3] Men under 25 appear to be more prone to relapse than older men or women.[4] To avoid relapse long-term therapy of up to 5 months' duration is required. Improvement may continue for several months after cessation of therapy and at least 2 months should elapse before determining whether further treatment is necessary. Approximately 10% of patients relapse and may require further treatment with antibacterials; repeat courses of isotretinoin are not usually recommended but may occasionally be required. Use of isotretinoin with antibacterials or anti-androgens does not markedly improve efficacy but if concomitant antibacterial therapy is contemplated then erythromycin is preferred as use with tetracyclines can produce benign intracranial hypertension. Isotretinoin has also been used for the treatment of acne associated with immunosuppressive therapy in transplant recipients.[5,6] Variable results have been obtained when using isotretinoin topically[7,8] and it appears to interact with the epidermis in a different manner to other retinoids.[9]

1. Jones DH. The role and mechanism of action of 13-cis-retinoic acid in the treatment of severe (nodulocystic) acne. *Pharmacol Ther* 1989; **40:** 91–106.
2. Layton AM, *et al.* Isotretinoin for acne vulgaris—10 years later: a safe and successful treatment. *Br J Dermatol* 1993; **129:** 292–6.
3. Lehucher-Ceyrac D, Weber-Buisset MJ. Isotretinoin and acne in practice: a prospective analysis of 188 cases over 9 years. *Dermatology* 1993; **186:** 123–8.
4. Orfanos CE, *et al.* The retinoids: a review of their clinical pharmacology and therapeutic use. *Drugs* 1987; **34:** 459–503.
5. Tam M, Cooper A. The use of isotretinoin in a renal transplant patient with acne. *Br J Dermatol* 1987; **116:** 463.
6. Bunker CB, *et al.* Isotretinoin treatment of severe acne in post-transplant patients taking cyclosporine. *J Am Acad Dermatol* 1990; **22:** 693–4.
7. Harms M, *et al.* Isotretinoin ineffective topically. *Lancet* 1985; **i:** 398.
8. Chalker DK, *et al.* Efficacy of topical isotretinoin 0.05% gel in acne vulgaris: results of a multicenter, double-blind investigation. *J Am Acad Dermatol* 1987; **17:** 251–4.
9. Hirschel-Scholz S, *et al.* Isotretinoin differs from other synthetic retinoids in its modulation of human cellular retinoic acid binding protein (CRABP). *Br J Dermatol* 1989; **120:** 639–44.

Neoplastic disorders. Retinoids including isotretinoin have been studied in the treatment of various neoplastic or preneoplastic disorders. Encouraging results were reported in a pilot study[1] of isotretinoin in juvenile chronic myelogenous leukaemia (p.480). [Note that oral tretinoin (p.1094) is used in acute promyelocytic leukaemia.]

Benefit in cutaneous neoplastic disease (p.492) has been noted in patients with squamous cell carcinoma (when given with calcitriol)[2] and with T-cell lymphomas, including mycosis fungoides[3-5] (p.482), although in patients with advanced disease[6] treated with isotretinoin rather than acitretin (which had been used in some of the previous successes) no benefit, and even deterioration, occurred. The comment[7] was also made that the two retinoids do not share a similar therapeutic profile.

There is some evidence that retinoids may be useful in preventing the development of squamous cell carcinoma[8,9] (for example in patients with oral leucoplakia, p.509, who are at increased risk of developing cancer of the mouth) and other neoplasms.[10]

1. Castleberry RP, *et al.* A pilot study of isotretinoin in the treatment of juvenile chronic myelogenous leukaemia. *N Engl J Med* 1994; **331:** 1680–4.
2. Majewski S, *et al.* Combination of isotretinoin and calcitriol for precancerous and cancerous skin lesions. *Lancet* 1994; **344:** 1510–11.
3. Knobler RM, *et al.* Treatment of cutaneous T cell lymphoma with a combination of low-dose interferon alfa-2b and retinoids. *J Am Acad Dermatol* 1991; **24:** 247–52.
4. Thomsen K, *et al.* Retinoids plus PUVA (RePUVA) and PUVA in mycosis fungoides, plaque stage: a report from the Scandinavian Mycosis Fungoides Group. *Acta Derm Venereol (Stockh)* 1989; **69:** 536–8.
5. French LE, *et al.* Remission of cutaneous T-cell lymphoma with combined calcitriol and acitretin. *Lancet* 1994: **344:** 686–7.
6. Thomsen K. Cutaneous T-cell lymphoma and calcitriol and isotretinoin treatment. *Lancet* 1995; **345:** 1583.
7. French LE, Saurat J-H. Treatment of cutaneous T-cell lymphoma by retinoids and calcitriol. *Lancet* 1995; **346:** 376.
8. Hong WK, *et al.* Prevention of second primary tumors with isotretinoin in squamous-cell carcinoma of the head and neck. *N Engl J Med* 1990; **323:** 795–801.
9. Lippman SM, *et al.* Comparison of low-dose isotretinoin with beta carotene to prevent oral carcinogenesis. *N Engl J Med* 1993; **328:** 15–20.
10. De Palo G, Formelli F. Risks and benefits of retinoids in the chemoprevention of cancer. *Drug Safety* 1995; **13:** 245–56.

Preparations

Proprietary Preparations (details are given in Part 3)
Aust.: Roaccutan; ***Austral.:*** Accure; Isotrex; Roaccutane; ***Belg.:*** Roaccutane; ***Canad.:*** Accutane; Isotrex; ***Fr.:*** Isotrex; Roaccutane; ***Ger.:*** Isotrex; Roaccutan; ***Irl.:*** Isotrex; Roaccutane; ***Ital.:*** Isotrex; Roaccutan; ***Neth.:*** Roaccutane; ***S.Afr.:*** Isotrex; Roaccutane; ***Spain:*** Roacutan; ***Switz.:*** Roaccutane; ***UK:*** Isotrex; Roaccutane; ***USA:*** Accutane.

Multi-ingredient: ***UK:*** Isotrexin.

Keluamid (13467-x)

Keluamid has been used in topical preparations for the treatment of seborrhoeic dermatitis and other scaling skin disorders.

Preparations

Proprietary Preparations (details are given in Part 3)
Fr.: Kelual†.

Multi-ingredient: ***Fr.:*** Kelual†; Sabal.

Lithium Succinate (19412-q)

$C_4H_6O_4.xLi$.
CAS — 16090-09-8.

Lithium succinate is reported to have anti-inflammatory properties and is used as an 8% ointment, usually in combination with zinc sulphate. It is applied twice daily initially in the treatment of seborrhoeic dermatitis (p.1076). It should be used with caution in patients with psoriasis as it may exacerbate their condition.

References.

1. Gould DJ, *et al.* A double-blind, placebo-controlled, multicentre trial of lithium succinate ointment in the treatment of seborrheic dermatitis. *J Am Acad Dermatol* 1992; **26:** 452–7.
2. Cuelenaere C, *et al.* Use of topical lithium succinate in the treatment of seborrhoeic dermatitis. *Dermatology* 1992; **184:** 194–7.

Preparations

Proprietary Preparations (details are given in Part 3)

Multi-ingredient: ***Ger.:*** Efadermin; ***Irl.:*** Efalith; ***Switz.:*** Efalith; ***UK:*** Efalith.

Lonapalene (719-q)

Lonapalene *(USAN, rINN)*.

RS-43179. 6-Chloro-2,3-dimethoxy-1,4-naphthalenediol diacetate.

$C_{16}H_{15}ClO_6 = 338.7$.
CAS — 91431-42-4.

Lonapalene is a 5-lipoxygenase inhibitor studied for the topical treatment of psoriasis.

References.

1. Lassus A, Forsstrom S. A dimethoxynaphthalene derivative (RS-43179 gel) compared with 0.025% fluocinolone acetonide gel in the treatment of psoriasis. *Br J Dermatol* 1985; **113:** 103–6.
2. Black AK, *et al.* Pharmacologic and clinical effects of lonapalene (RS 43179), a 5-lipoxygenase inhibitor, in psoriasis. *J Invest Dermatol* 1990; **95:** 50–4.

Mequinol (1619-e)

Mequinol *(rINN)*.

Hydroquinone Monomethyl Ether; *p*-Hydroxyanisole. 4-Methoxyphenol.

$C_7H_8O_2 = 124.1$.
CAS — 150-76-5.

Mequinol is used similarly to hydroquinone (p.1083), in concentrations of up to 20%, in the treatment of hyperpigmentation (see Pigmentation Disorders, p.1075).

A report of severe reversible irregular hypopigmentation of the hands, arms, neck, and legs in a West Indian woman who applied a bleaching wax containing mequinol for 2 to 3 months to lighten the colour of her skin.[1]

1. Boyle J, Kennedy CTC. British cosmetic regulations inadequate. *Br Med J* 1984; **288:** 1998–9.

Preparations

Proprietary Preparations (details are given in Part 3)
Aust.: Leucobasal; ***Fr.:*** Any; Clairodermyl; Creme des 3 Fleurs d'Orient; Leucodinine B; ***Spain:*** Novo Dermoquinona; ***Switz.:*** Leucobasal.

Ammoniated Mercury (1620-b)

Aminomercuric Chloride; Hydrargyri Aminochloridum; Hydrargyrum Amidochloratum; Hydrargyrum Ammoniatum; Hydrargyrum Praecipitatum Album; Mercuric Ammonium Chloride; Mercury Amide Chloride; Mercury Aminochloride; White Precipitate.

$NH_2HgCl = 252.1$.
CAS — 10124-48-8.

NOTE. 'White Precipitate' has also been used as a name for Precipitated Mercurous Chloride.

Pharmacopoeias. In *US.*

A white odourless amorphous powder or pulverulent pieces which are stable in air, but darken on exposure to light. Practically **insoluble** in water and alcohol; readily soluble in warm hydrochloric, nitric, and acetic acids. **Protect** from light.

Ammoniated mercury was formerly used topically in the treatment of skin infections and psoriasis but the use of such mercurial preparations is generally deprecated. Frequent or prolonged application to large areas or to broken skin or mucous membranes can cause mercury poisoning (see p.1601) and use on infants has produced acrodynia (pink disease). Ammoniated mercury is also a potent sensitiser and can produce allergic reactions.

Of 60 patients who were found to have nephrotic syndrome, 32 had used skin-lightening creams containing 5 to 10% of ammoniated mercury.[1] Concentrations of mercury in the urine of these patients were up to 250 ng per mL compared with a usual upper limit of 80 ng per mL. Of 26 patients followed up for up to 2 years, 13 had no remission or response to treatment; 6 of these had used skin-lighteners.

1. Barr RD, *et al.* Nephrotic syndrome in adult Africans in Nairobi. *Br Med J* 1972; **2:** 131–4.

Preparations

USP 23: Ammoniated Mercury Ointment; Ammoniated Mercury Ophthalmic Ointment.

Proprietary Preparations (details are given in Part 3)

Multi-ingredient: ***USA:*** Emersal; Unguentum Bossi.

Mesulphen (1622-g)

Mesulphen *(BAN)*.

Mesulfen *(pINN)*; Dimethyldiphenylene Disulphide; Dimethylthianthrene. It consists mainly of 2,7-dimethylthianthrene.

$C_{14}H_{12}S_2 = 244.4$.
CAS — 135-58-0.

Pharmacopoeias. In *Aust.*

Jpn includes thianthol, a mixture of 2,7-dimethylthianthrene and ditolyl disulphide.

Mesulphen has been used as a parasiticide and antipruritic in a range of skin disorders including acne, scabies, and seborrhoea. Sensitivity to mesulphen has occasionally been reported.

Preparations

Proprietary Preparations (details are given in Part 3)
Ger.: Citemul S; ***Ital.:*** Shampoo Potenziato Cruz Verde Allo Zolfo Organico†; ***Switz.:*** Soufrol.

Multi-ingredient: ***Aust.:*** Tineafax.

Methoxsalen (1623-q)

Methoxsalen *(BAN)*.

Ammoidin; 8-Methoxypsoralen; Metoxaleno; Xanthotoxin. 9-Methoxyfuro[3,2-g]chromen-7-one; 9-Methoxy-7*H*-furo[3,2-g][1]benzopyran-7-one.

$C_{12}H_8O_4 = 216.2$.
CAS — 298-81-7.

Pharmacopoeias. In *Jpn* and *US.*

A constituent of the fruits of *Ammi majus*. It occurs as white to cream-coloured, odourless, fluffy, needle-like crystals. Practically **insoluble** in water; sparingly soluble in boiling water and in ether; freely soluble in chloroform; soluble in boiling alcohol, and in acetone, acetic acid, and propylene glycol. **Protect** from light.

Adverse Effects

Methoxsalen given orally commonly causes nausea and less frequently mental effects including insomnia, nervousness, and depression.

Photochemotherapy or PUVA (see under Uses and Administration, below) may cause pruritus and mild transient erythema. Other effects include oedema, dizziness, headache, vesiculation, bulla formation, onycholysis, acneform eruption, and severe skin pain. Overexposure to sunlight or UVA radiation may produce severe burns in patients being treated with psoralens. PUVA can produce premature ageing of the skin. Hypertrichosis and pigmentation alterations of skin or nails have also been reported. PUVA may be associated with an increased risk of malignant neoplasms of the skin.

Carcinogenicity. See under Effects on the Blood and Effects on the Skin, below.

Effects on the blood. There have been isolated reports of leukaemia[1] or a preleukaemic condition[2] developing in elderly patients after up to one year of PUVA therapy.

1. Hansen NE. Development of acute myeloid leukaemia in a patient with psoriasis treated with oral 8-methoxypsoralen and longwave ultraviolet light. *Scand J Haematol* 1979; **22:** 57–60.
2. Wagner J, *et al.* Preleukaemia (haemopoietic dysplasia) developing in a patient with psoriasis treated with 8-methoxypsoralen and ultraviolet light (PUVA) treatment. *Scand J Haematol* 1978; **21:** 299–304.

Effects on the eyes. Free methoxsalen has been detected in the lens of the eye for at least 12 hours after oral administration[1] although it may become integrated into the structure of the lens and cataracts may occur in patients who fail to wear suitable eye protection for 12 to 24 hours after therapy.[2] However, provided that eye protection is used there appears to be no significant dose-dependent increase in the risk of cataract formation, although a higher risk of developing nuclear sclerosis and posterior subcapsular opacities has been noted in patients who have received more than 100 treatments.[3] Other ocular effects include dose-related transient visual-field defects reported in 3 patients receiving PUVA therapy.[4] Psoralens may also increase the sensitivity of the retina to visible light.[5]

1. Lerman S, *et al.* Potential ocular complications from PUVA therapy and their prevention. *J Invest Dermatol* 1980; **74:** 197–9.
2. Woo TY, *et al.* Lenticular psoralen photoproducts and cataracts of a PUVA-treated psoriatic patient. *Arch Dermatol* 1985; **121:** 1307–8.
3. Stern RS, *et al.* Ocular findings in patients treated with PUVA. *J Invest Dermatol* 1985; **85:** 269–73.
4. Fenton DA, Wilkinson JD. Dose-related visual-field defects in patients receiving PUVA therapy. *Lancet* 1983; **i:** 1106.
5. Souêtre E, *et al.* 5-Methoxypsoralen increases the sensitivity of the retina to light in humans. *Eur J Clin Pharmacol* 1989; **36:** 59–61.

Effects on the hair. Hypertrichosis was noticed in 15 of 23 female patients receiving PUVA therapy compared with 2 of 14 patients treated with UVA alone.[1]

1. Rampen FHJ. Hypertrichosis in PUVA-treated patients. *Br J Dermatol* 1983; **109:** 657–60.

Effects on the immune system. PUVA therapy appears to have immunosuppressive effects and inhibits lymphocytes, polymorphonuclear leucocytes, and Langerhans' cells.[1-3] It is capable of inducing antinuclear antibody formation and a syndrome similar to systemic lupus syndrome has developed during treatment.[4,5] An immunological basis has also been suspected for the development of nephrotic syndrome in one patient who received PUVA therapy.[6]

See also Hypersensitivity, below.

1. Farber EM, *et al.* Long-term risks of psoralen and UV-A therapy for psoriasis. *Arch Dermatol* 1983; **119:** 426–31.
2. Morison WL, *et al.* Abnormal lymphocyte function following long-term PUVA therapy for psoriasis. *Br J Dermatol* 1983; **108:** 445–50.
3. Chang A, *et al.* PUVA and UVB inhibit the intra-epidermal accumulation of polymorphonuclear leukocytes. *Br J Dermatol* 1988; **119:** 281–7.
4. Bruze M, *et al.* Fatal connective tissue disease with antinuclear antibodies following PUVA therapy. *Acta Derm Venereol (Stockh)* 1984; **64:** 157–60.
5. Bruze M, Ljunggren B. Antinuclear antibodies appearing during PUVA therapy. *Acta Derm Venereol (Stockh)* 1985; **65:** 31–6.
6. Lam Thuon Mine LTK, *et al.* Nephrotic syndrome after treatment with psoralens and ultraviolet A. *Br Med J* 1983; **287:** 94–5.

Effects on the skin. MALIGNANT NEOPLASMS. Squamous cell carcinoma, basal cell carcinoma, keratoacanthoma, actinic keratosis, Bowen's disease, and malignant melanoma have all been reported during or after cessation of PUVA.[1-3] There have been several large long-term follow-up studies to assess the risk of **non-melanoma** skin cancer in patients receiving PUVA therapy. Early studies from Europe found no clear evidence that PUVA was independently carcinogenic but did find that previous treatment with arsenic, methotrexate, or ionising radiation increased the incidence of skin tumours.[4] Studies from the USA have found an increase in the incidence of basal cell carcinoma and squamous cell carcinoma independent of other treatment,[5] which was dose-related in some studies.[6] Male genitalia appeared to be particularly susceptible.[7] It has been suggested that the differences between the findings might be due to the fact that in Europe higher and fewer doses are used and the median total dose employed may be only 29% of that used in the USA.[8] However, more recent studies from northern Europe have also found a dose-related increase in the risk of developing squamous cell carcinomas.[9,10] One small series suggested that about 50% of the recipients of high-dose PUVA went on to develop squamous cell carcinomas or premalignant lesions.[11] While some European workers have findings that confirm the increased susceptibility of the male genitalia[12] others have failed to find any such evidence.[13] A few patients have gone on to develop metastatic disease.[14,15]

Previously, there had been only a few anecdotal reports of **malignant melanomas** occurring in patients who had received PUVA. However, a recent prospective study[16] study in 1380 patients with psoriasis who were first treated with PUVA in 1975 or 1976 found that the risk of melanoma increases about 15 years after the first treatment with PUVA and that the risk was increased especially in patients who had received 250 treatments or more. The authors suggested that long-term PUVA should therefore be used with caution, especially in younger patients. The comment has also been made[17] that patients receiving long-term therapy should be followed up carefully and that such therapy should not be used in patients at risk for melanoma.

There has also been a suggestion that PUVA may increase the risk of some internal cancers.[10]

1. Reshad H, *et al.* Cutaneous carcinoma in psoriatic patients treated with PUVA. *Br J Dermatol* 1984; **110:** 299–305.
2. Kemmett D, *et al.* Nodular malignant melanoma and multiple squamous cell carcinomas in a patient treated by photochemotherapy for psoriasis. *Br Med J* 1984; **289:** 1498.
3. Suurmond D, *et al.* Skin cancer and PUVA maintenance therapy for psoriasis. *Br J Dermatol* 1985; **113:** 485–6.
4. Henseler T, *et al.* Skin tumors in the European PUVA study. *J Am Acad Dermatol* 1987; **16:** 108–16.
5. Forman AB, *et al.* Long-term follow-up of skin cancer in the PUVA-48 cooperative study. *Arch Dermatol* 1989; **125:** 515–19.
6. Stern RS, *et al.* Non-melanoma skin cancer occurring in patients treated with PUVA five to ten years after first treatment. *J Invest Dermatol* 1988; **91:** 120–4.
7. Stern RS, *et al.* Genital tumors among men with psoriasis exposed to psoralens and ultraviolet A radiation (PUVA) and ultraviolet B radiation. *N Engl J Med* 1990; **322:** 1093–7.
8. Mosely H, Ferguson J. Photochemotherapy: a reappraisal of its use in dermatology. *Drugs* 1989; **38:** 822–37.
9. Bruynzeel I, *et al.* 'High single-dose' European PUVA regimen also causes an excess of non-melanoma skin cancer. *Br J Dermatol* 1991; **124:** 49–55.
10. Lindelöf B, *et al.* PUVA and cancer: a large-scale epidemiological study. *Lancet* 1991; **338:** 91–3.
11. Lever LR, Farr PM. Skin cancers or premalignant lesions occur in half of high-dose PUVA patients. *Br J Dermatol* 1994; **131:** 215–19.
12. Perkins W, *et al.* Cutaneous malignancy in males treated with photochemotherapy. *Lancet* 1990; **336:** 1248.
13. Wolff K, Hönigsmann H. Genital carcinomas in psoriasis patients treated with photochemotherapy. *Lancet* 1991; **337:** 439.
14. Lewis FM, *et al.* Metastatic squamous-cell carcinoma in patient receiving PUVA. *Lancet* 1994; **344:** 1157.
15. Stern RS. Metastatic squamous cell cancer after psoralen photochemotherapy. *Lancet* 1994; **344:** 1644–5.
16. Stern RS, *et al.* Malignant melanoma in patients treated for psoriasis with methoxsalen (psoralen) and ultraviolet A radiation (PUVA). *N Engl J Med* 1997; **336:** 1041–5.
17. Wolff K. Should PUVA be abandoned? *N Engl J Med* 1997; **336:** 1090–1.

NON-MALIGNANT SKIN DISORDERS. Toxic pustuloderma, marked by erythema and superficial pustular lesions, has been reported in a patient given PUVA therapy for mycosis fungoides.[1] Another effect sometimes associated with PUVA is severe skin pain;[2,3] the pain may respond to treatment with topical capsaicin.[3]

1. Yip J, *et al.* Toxic pustuloderma due to PUVA treatment. *Br J Dermatol* 1991; **125:** 401–2.
2. Burrows NP, *et al.* PUVA-induced skin pain. *Br J Dermatol* 1993; **129:** 504.
3. Burrows NP, Norris PG. Treatment of PUVA-induced skin pain with capsaicin. *Br J Dermatol* 1994; **131:** 584–5.

Hypersensitivity. Hypersensitivity reactions to methoxsalen and PUVA therapy occur rarely but there have been reports of drug-induced fever,[1] bronchoconstriction,[2] and contact dermatitis.[3]

1. Tóth Kása I, Dobozy A. Drug fever caused by PUVA treatment. *Acta Derm Venereol (Stockh)* 1985; **65:** 557–8.
2. Ramsay B, Marks JM. Bronchoconstriction due to 8-methoxypsoralen. *Br J Dermatol* 1988; **119:** 83–6.
3. Takashima A, *et al.* Allergic contact and photocontact dermatitis due to psoralens in patients with psoriasis treated with topical PUVA. *Br J Dermatol* 1991; **124:** 37–42.

Precautions

Methoxsalen should not be given to patients with diseases associated with light sensitivity such as porphyria, although it is used with care to decrease some patients' sensitivity to sunlight. Other contra-indications include aphakia, melanoma or a history of melanoma, and invasive squamous cell carcinoma. It is generally recommended that PUVA therapy should not be used in children. Methoxsalen should be used with caution in patients with hepatic insufficiency. It is recommended that unless specific treatment is required male genitalia should be shielded during PUVA therapy.

Patients should not sunbathe for 24 hours before and 48 hours after PUVA treatment. They should avoid exposure to sun, even through glass or cloud cover for at least 8 hours after methoxsalen ingestion and patients should wear wrap-around UVA absorbing glasses for 24 hours after ingestion. Photosensitivity is more prolonged following topical application and treated skin should be protected from exposure to sunlight for at least 12 to 48 hours. It has been recommended that patients should undergo an ophthalmic examination, and that measurements of antinuclear antibody titre and hepatic function be carried out before, and at intervals after, commencing therapy. Patients should also receive regular examinations for signs of premalignant or malignant skin lesions.

Interactions

Methoxsalen should be used with caution if other drugs known to cause photosensitivity are used concurrently because of an increased risk of phototoxicity.

Food. Some foods, for example, celery, parsnip, and parsley, contain psoralens and consumption of large quantities may increase the risk of phototoxicity with methoxsalen. A patient[1] who had consumed a large quantity of celery soup the evening before and two hours before undergoing PUVA therapy for atopic eczema developed severe phototoxicity following the treatment which was attributed to the additive effects of methoxsalen and psoralens contained in the celery.

1. Boffa MJ, *et al.* Celery soup causing severe phototoxicity during PUVA therapy. *Br J Dermatol* 1996; **135:** 334.

Phenytoin. Failure of PUVA treatment due to abnormally low serum concentrations of methoxsalen in a patient with epilepsy was probably a result of induction of hepatic enzymes by phenytoin.[1]

1. Staberg B, Hueg B. Interaction between 8-methoxypsoralen and phenytoin. *Acta Derm Venereol (Stockh)* 1985; **65:** 553–5.

Pharmacokinetics

When taken by mouth methoxsalen is well but variably absorbed from the gastro-intestinal tract and there is considerable interindividual variation in peak serum concentrations. Depending on the oral formulation used increased photosensitivity is present 1 hour after a dose, reaches a peak at about 1 to 4 hours, and disappears after about 8 hours. Methoxsalen is highly protein bound. It appears to be preferentially taken up by epidermal cells. It also diffuses into the lens of the eye. Methoxsalen is almost completely metabolised. Approximately 95% of a dose is excreted in the urine within 24 hours. Photosensitivity after topical application may persist for several days, reaching a peak after about 2 days.

References.

1. de Wolff FA, Thomas TV. Clinical pharmacokinetics of methoxsalen and other psoralens. *Clin Pharmacokinet* 1986; **11:** 62–75.

Uses and Administration

Methoxsalen, a psoralen, is a photosensitiser markedly increasing skin reactivity to long-wavelength ultraviolet radiation (320 to 400 nm), an effect used in photochemotherapy or PUVA [psoralen (P) and high-intensity long-wavelength UVA irradiation]. In the presence of UVA, methoxsalen bonds with DNA inhibiting DNA synthesis and cell division, and can lead to cell injury. Recovery from the cell injury may be followed by increased melanisation of the epidermis. Methoxsalen may also increase pigmentation by an action on melanocytes.

PUVA is used to treat idiopathic vitiligo and severe, recalcitrant, disabling psoriasis not adequately responsive to conventional topical therapy. It may also be useful in selected cases of atopic eczema and polymorphic light eruptions and may be used in T-cell lymphomas such as mycosis fungoides.

Methoxsalen is given both by mouth and applied topically in PUVA regimens. Differing oral dosage forms of methoxsalen may exhibit significantly varying bioavailabilities and times to onset of photosensitisation. The UVA exposure dose should generally be based on prior measurement of the minimal phototoxic dose although it can be calculated with regard to the skin type of the patient if phototoxic dose testing cannot be carried out.

To repigment **vitiliginous** areas, methoxsalen is given in a dose of up to 600 μg per kg body-weight by mouth 2 to 4 hours before measured periods of exposure to UVA twice a week, at least 48 hours apart. Methoxsalen may also be applied topically to repigment small, well-defined vitiliginous lesions. Preparations containing up to 1% have been used but dilution to 0.1 or 0.01% may be necessary to avoid adverse cutaneous effects. The surrounding skin should be protected by an opaque sunscreen. Some suggest that the treated area should be exposed to UVA immediately after application while others recommend waiting up to 2 hours. After exposure the lesions should be washed and protected from light; protection may be necessary for up to 48 hours or longer. Treatment is repeated usually once weekly. Significant repigmentation may not appear until after six to nine months of treatment.

For the treatment of **psoriasis** a similar schedule is used to that outlined above for vitiligo. A dose of up to 600 μg per kg by mouth 2 hours before UVA is usually given twice a week although increased frequencies, but with at least 48-hour intervals between doses, have been suggested. If there is no response or only minimal response after the fifteenth PUVA treatment some suggest that the dosage may be increased, once only, by 10 mg for the remainder of the course of treatment. Methoxsalen may also be used topically with UVA exposure for the treatment of psoriasis. For direct application to affected areas of skin a preparation containing approximately 0.1% (or diluted to 0.01% if necessary to avoid adverse cutaneous effects) is applied 30 minutes before UVA exposure. Alternatively the patient may soak affected areas or take a whole-body bath in methoxsalen-containing solutions containing 3.75 mg per litre; the soak or bath should be for 15 minutes and be followed immediately by UVA exposure. Baths are generally given two or three times a week.

Psoralen itself has also been used.

Administration. The dose of methoxsalen is usually calculated on the basis of body-weight. This method of dose calculation produces a considerable difference between the doses received by heavy and light patients. A study in 41 patients with psoriasis[1] suggested that using methoxsalen 25 mg per m^2 body-surface gave more consistent plasma concentrations and may reduce the potential for burning in heavy patients and prevent underdosing in light patients undergoing PUVA therapy.

1. Sakuntabhai A, *et al.* Calculation of 8-methoxypsoralen dose according to body surface area in PUVA treatment. *Br J Dermatol* 1995; **133:** 919–23.

PUVA. PUVA, which utilises a combination of oral or topically applied psoralens and ultraviolet A irradiation, has been used in a wide range of disorders and guidelines have been published by the British Photodermatology Group[1] which are summarised as follows.

Indications for PUVA in chronic plaque **psoriasis** include severe extensive psoriasis unresponsive to conventional topical therapies, relapse within 3 to 6 months of successful topical treatment, or patient refusal of topical treatment if UVB phototherapy has failed (see p.1075 for a discussion of the various treatments of psoriasis). Initial UVA exposure should preferably be determined on the basis of prior measurement of the minimal phototoxic dose rather than on the skin type. Increases in UVA irradiation are then calculated as a percentage of previous doses. Methoxsalen in a dose of 600 μg per kg body-weight by mouth given 2 hours before UVA exposure is the widely accepted standard regimen. Alternatively, 5-methoxypsoralen 1.2 mg per kg, again 2 hours before UVA exposure, can be given and appears to be almost free of the adverse reactions such as nausea, pruritus, and erythema induced by methoxsalen. However, until the clinical efficacy of 5-methoxypsoralen has been clearly demonstrated, methoxsalen should remain the psoralen of choice for most clinical situations. Alternatives to oral PUVA are baths or soaks using methoxsalen or trioxsalen. For whole-body bathing or hand and foot soaks a concentration of methoxsalen 3.75 mg per litre is utilised with the patient bathing for 15 minutes followed by immediate exposure to UVA; treatment is given 2 or 3 times each week. For trioxsalen a concentration of about 330 μg per litre is used for a 10-minute whole-body bath or a 30-minute hand and foot soak again followed by immediate UVA exposure; whole-body baths are used 2 or 3 times weekly and hand and foot soaks are given 3 times each week. Methoxsalen may also be applied topically to the affected areas. A concentration of approximately 0.1% (or 0.01% if erythema occurs) is employed and applied 30 minutes before UVA exposure. PUVA treatment should be discontinued as soon as clearance is achieved and maintenance PUVA after routine clearance should be avoided. A combination of PUVA with acitretin (300 to 700 μg per kg by mouth) or etretinate (0.5 to 1 mg per kg by mouth) may be considered in patients who have reached 50 treatment sessions or relapsed within 6 months of PUVA. PUVA and methotrexate are effective for severe psoriasis but should be reserved for such cases because of the possible increased risk of skin cancer.

Oral PUVA twice weekly with methoxsalen 600 μg per kg or 5-methoxypsoralen 1.2 mg per kg has been effective in many patients with **vitiligo** (see Pigmentation Disorders, p.1075). If patches are large and well demarcated topical application of methoxsalen 0.15% may be preferable.

In **mycosis fungoides** PUVA is an effective symptomatic treatment for early disease and a useful adjunct for late-stage disease but optimal regimens have not been established (see below).

PUVA is effective for atopic **eczema** (p.1073) but clearance is less certain than for psoriasis, twice the number of treatments may be needed, and relapse is more frequent. It should therefore be reserved for severe disease unresponsive to conventional treatments. Optimal regimens have not been established.

In **polymorphic light eruptions** PUVA is effective in up to 90% of patients but is only indicated in those who are frequently or severely affected despite the regular use of high-protection broad-spectrum sunscreens. Several arbitrary regimens are in use.

Variable results have also been reported in a variety of other disorders but data has been insufficient to establish precise guidelines. Such disorders include actinic prurigo, alopecia areata, aquagenic pruritus, chronic actinic dermatitis, graft-versus-host disease, granuloma annulare, lichen planus, nodular prurigo, pityriasis lichenoides, localised scleroderma, solar urticaria, and urticaria pigmentosa. In most cases relapse occurs in the absence of maintenance therapy and PUVA should usually only be tried as a last resort.

Extracorporeal photochemotherapy (a technique in which oral methoxsalen is given, followed by removal of blood and UV irradiation of leucocytes outside the body before reinfusion) has been used successfully in a patient with severe epidermolysis bullosa acquisita[2] and in another patient with chronic graft-versus-host disease.[3]

1. British Photodermatology Group. British Photodermatology Group guidelines for PUVA. *Br J Dermatol* 1994; **130:** 246–55.
2. Miller JL, *et al.* Remission of severe epidermolysis bullosa acquisita induced by extracorporeal photochemotherapy. *Br J Dermatol* 1995; **133:** 467–71.
3. Konstantinow A, *et al.* Chronic graft-versus-host disease: successful treatment with extracorporeal photochemotherapy: a follow-up. *Br J Dermatol* 1996; **135:** 1007–8.

NEOPLASTIC AND MYELOPROLIFERATIVE DISORDERS. PUVA therapy is considered to be effective in the treatment of the early stages of cutaneous T-cell lymphomas,[1,2] a range of diseases including mycosis fungoides and Sèzary syndrome (see also p.482), as well as most adult T-cell lymphomas, but its long-term role is controversial as no data exist to show that it improves life expectancy.[3] Encouraging results, with few side-effects, have been obtained with extracorporeal PUVA therapy in otherwise resistant cutaneous T-cell lymphomas;[4] after oral administration of the psoralen the patient's leucocytes are isolated by leucopheresis and exposed to UVA extracorporeally after which they are returned to the patient.

PUVA therapy has also been used to control cutaneous lesions in a patient with histiocytosis X of the Letterer-Siwe type.[5]

1. Briffa DV, *et al.* Photochemotherapy in mycosis fungoides: a study of 73 patients. *Lancet* 1980; **ii:** 49–53.
2. Logan RA, *et al.* Photochemotherapy for cutaneous T-cell lymphoma—the St John's experience. *Br J Dermatol* 1986; **115** (suppl 30): 17–18.
3. Moseley H, Ferguson J. Photochemotherapy: a reappraisal of its use in dermatology. *Drugs* 1989; **38:** 822–37.
4. Edelson R, *et al.* Treatment of cutaneous T-cell lymphoma by extracorporeal photochemotherapy. *N Engl J Med* 1987; **316:** 297–303.
5. Neumann C, *et al.* Histiocytosis X in an elderly patient: ultrastructure and immunocytochemistry after PUVA photochemotherapy. *Br J Dermatol* 1988; **119:** 385–91.

Preparations

USP 23: Methoxsalen Capsules; Methoxsalen Topical Solution.

Proprietary Preparations (details are given in Part 3)
Aust.: Geralen; Oxsoralen; ***Austral.:*** Oxsoralen; ***Belg.:*** Mopsoralen; Oxsoralon; ***Canad.:*** Oxsoralen; Ultramop; ***Fr.:*** Meladinine; ***Ger.:*** Meladinine; ***Irl.:*** Deltasoralen; ***Ital.:*** Oxsoralen; ***Neth.:*** Geroxalen; Meladinine†; Oxsoralen†; ***Norw.:*** Geroxalen; ***S.Afr.:*** Oxsoralen; ***Spain:*** Oxsoralen; ***Switz.:*** Meladinine; ***UK:*** Puvasoralen; ***USA:*** Oxsoralen.

5-Methoxypsoralen (12944-h)

Bergapten. 4-Methoxy-7*H*-furo[3,2-*g*]chromen-7-one.
$C_{12}H_8O_4$ = 216.2.
CAS — 484-20-8.

5-Methoxypsoralen is an ingredient of bergamot oil.

5-Methoxypsoralen is a photosensitiser with actions similar to those of methoxsalen (p.1086). It may be given by mouth in the PUVA therapy (p.1088) of psoriasis and vitiligo.

5-Methoxypsoralen is included in some cosmetic suntan preparations to enhance tanning but because of its potential phototoxicity this is considered unwise by some authorities. Photosensitivity caused by 5-methoxypsoralen is sometimes known as Berloque dermatitis.

References.

1. Tanew A, *et al.* 5-Methoxypsoralen (Bergapten) for photochemotherapy: bioavailability, phototoxicity, and clinical efficacy in psoriasis of a new drug preparation. *J Am Acad Dermatol* 1988; **18:** 333–8.
2. Treffel P, *et al.* A new micronized 5-methoxypsoralen preparation. *Acta Derm Venereol (Stockh)* 1992; **72:** 65–7.
3. Ehrsson H, *et al.* Food-induced increase in bioavailability of 5-methoxypsoralen. *Eur J Clin Pharmacol* 1994; **46:** 375–7.

Preparations

Proprietary Preparations (details are given in Part 3)
Fr.: Psoraderm 5; ***Switz.:*** Psoraderm 5.

Monobenzone (1624-p)

Monobenzone (*rINN*).

Hydroquinone Monobenzyl Ether. 4-Benzyloxyphenol.
$C_{13}H_{12}O_2$ = 200.2.
CAS — 103-16-2.
Pharmacopoeias. In *US.*

A white odourless, crystalline powder. Practically **insoluble** in water; soluble 1 in 14.5 of alcohol, 1 in 29 of chloroform, 1 in 14 of ether; soluble in acetone. **Store** at a temperature not exceeding 30° in airtight containers. Protect from light.

Adverse Effects and Precautions

Monobenzone may cause skin irritation and sensitisation. In some patients, this may be transient and need not necessitate withdrawal of the drug. In other patients, an eczematous sensitisation may occur. Excessive depigmentation may occur even beyond the areas under treatment and may produce unsightly patches.

Monobenzone can produce permanent depigmentation and should not be used as a substitute for hydroquinone.

Uses and Administration

Monobenzone has actions similar to those of hydroquinone (p.1083) but in some patients it also produces extensive and selective destruction of melanocytes. It is used locally for final, permanent depigmentation of normal skin in extensive vitiligo (see Pigmentation Disorders, p.1075). Monobenzone is not recommended for freckling, chloasma, or hyperpigmentation following skin inflammation or due to photosensitisation following the use of certain perfumes. It has no effect on melanomas or pigmented naevi.

For vitiligo monobenzone is applied in the form of a cream containing up to 20% to the affected parts two or three times daily until a satisfactory response is obtained, and thereafter as necessary, usually about twice weekly. Excessive exposure to sunlight should be avoided during treatment. The results are variable. Depigmentation only becomes apparent when the preformed melanin pigments have been lost with the normal sloughing of the stratum corneum and this may take several months. If, however, no improvement is noted after 4 months, treatment should be abandoned.

Preparations

USP 23: Monobenzone Cream.

Proprietary Preparations (details are given in Part 3)
Austral.: Aloquin†; ***Belg.:*** Leucodinine†; ***Canad.:*** Benoquin; ***Ger.:*** Depigman†; ***Ital.:*** Dermochinona†; ***USA:*** Benoquin.

Motretinide (12980-g)

Motretinide (*USAN, rINN*).

Ro-11-1430. (*all-trans*)-*N*-Ethyl-9-(4-methoxy-2,3,6-trimethylphenyl)-3,7-dimethyl-2,4,6,8-nonatetraenamide.
$C_{23}H_{31}NO_2$ = 353.5.
CAS — 56281-36-8.

Motretinide is a retinoid structurally related to acitretin (p.1077). Motretinide is used topically in the treatment of acne (p.1072). It is applied in preparations containing 0.1%.

Preparations

Proprietary Preparations (details are given in Part 3)
Switz.: Tasmaderm.

Piroctone Olamine (6387-v)

Piroctone Olamine *(USAN, rINNM).*

1-Hydroxy-4-methyl-6-(2,4,4-trimethylpentyl)-2(1*H*)-pyridone compound with 2-aminoethanol (1:1).

$C_{14}H_{23}NO_2.C_2H_7NO = 298.4.$

CAS — 50650-76-5 (piroctone); 68890-66-4 (piroctone olamine).

Piroctone olamine has been used in shampoos for the treatment of dandruff.

Preparations

Proprietary Preparations (details are given in Part 3)
Fr.: Cystelle Antipelliculaire; Ultrex Shampooing Antipelliculaire d'Entretien†; *Ital.:* Olamin P.

Multi-ingredient: *Fr.:* Biolan Tar; Sabal; *Ital.:* Shamday Antiforfora; Sideck Shampoo Antiforfora†.

Podophyllum (7523-v)

American Mandrake; May Apple Root; Podoph.; Podophyllum Rhizome.

CAS — 568-53-6 (α-peltatin); 518-29-6 (β-peltatin).

Pharmacopoeias. In *US.*

The dried rhizomes and roots of *Podophyllum peltatum* (Berberidaceae). It yields not less than 5% of resin.

Indian Podophyllum (7524-g)

Ind. Podoph.; Indian Podophyllum Rhizome.

Pharmacopoeias. Chin. includes a monograph for the fruits only.

The dried fruits or rhizomes and roots of *Podophyllum emodi* (=*P. hexandrum*) (Berberidaceae).

Podophyllum Resin (7525-q)

Podoph. Resin; Podophylli Resina; Podophyllin.

CAS — 8050-60-0.

Pharmacopoeias. In *Aust., Int., Swiss,* and *US* (all from podophyllum only). In *Br.* from Indian podophyllum.

The BP specifies the resin obtained from the dried rhizomes and roots of *Podophyllum hexandrum (P. emodi)* (Indian podophyllum). It should contain not less than 50% of total aryltetralin lignans, calculated as podophyllotoxin.

The USP specifies the powdered mixture of resins obtained by percolation of the dried rhizomes and roots of *P. peltatum* with alcohol and precipitation with acidified water. It should contain not less than 40% and not more than 50% of hexane-insoluble matter.

An amorphous caustic powder, varying in colour from light brown to greenish-yellow or brownish-grey, with a characteristic odour. On exposure to light or to temperatures above 25° it becomes darker in colour.

Partly **soluble** in hot water but precipitated again on cooling; soluble in alcohol with a slight opalescence; partly soluble in chloroform, ether, and dilute ammonia solution. A solution in alcohol is acid to litmus. **Store** in a cool place in airtight containers. Protect from light.

CAUTION. *Podophyllum resin is strongly irritant to the skin, eyes, and mucous membranes and requires careful handling.*

Podophyllotoxin (10037-x)

Podophyllotoxin *(BAN).*

Podofilox *(USAN).* (5*R*,5a*R*,8a*R*,9*R*)-5,5a,6,8,8a,9-Hexahydro-9-hydroxy-5-(3,4,5-trimethoxyphenyl)furo[3′4′:6,7]naphtho[2,3-*d*]-1,3-dioxol-6-one.

$C_{22}H_{22}O_8 = 414.4.$

CAS — 518-28-5.

Adverse Effects

Podophyllum is very irritant, especially to the eyes and mucous membranes. It can also cause severe systemic toxicity after ingestion or topical application, which is usually reversible but has been fatal. Symptoms of toxicity include nausea, vomiting, abdominal pain, and diarrhoea; there may be thrombocytopenia, leucopenia, renal failure, and hepatotoxicity. Central effects are delayed in onset and prolonged in duration and include acute psychotic reactions, hallucinations, confusion, dizziness, stupor, ataxia, hypotonia, seizures, and coma. EEG changes may persist for several days. Peripheral and autonomic neuropathies develop later and may result in paraesthesias, reduced reflexes, muscle weakness, tachycardia, apnoea, orthostatic hypotension, paralytic ileus, and urinary retention. Neuropathy may improve but full recovery is unusual.

Carcinogenicity. A report of the transformation of a condyloma acuminatum into an invasive squamous cell carcinoma after treatment with podophyllum 25% in alcohol.[1]

1. Svindland HB. Malignant transformation of condyloma acuminatum after treatment with podophyllin. *Eur J Sex Transm Dis* 1984; **1:** 165–7.

Poisoning. Reports and reviews of podophyllum toxicity.[1-4] A few of the cases followed consumption of herbal preparations containing podophyllum. Death has occurred following ingestion of 10 g of podophyllum.

1. Cassidy DE, *et al.* Podophyllum toxicity: a report of a fatal case and a review of the literature. *J Toxicol Clin Toxicol* 1982; **19:** 35–44.
2. Dobb GJ, Edis RH. Coma and neuropathy after ingestion of herbal laxative containing podophyllin. *Med J Aust* 1984; **140:** 495–6.
3. Holdright DR, Jahangiri M. Accidental poisoning with podophyllin. *Hum Exp Toxicol* 1990; **9:** 55–6.
4. Chan TYK, Critchley JAJH. Usage and adverse effects of Chinese herbal medicines. *Hum Exp Toxicol* 1996; **15:** 5–12.

Precautions

Podophyllum should not be used during pregnancy or breast feeding or in children.

The risk of systemic toxicity after topical application is increased by the treatment of large areas with excessive amounts for prolonged periods, by the treatment of friable, bleeding, or recently biopsied warts, and by inadvertent application to normal skin or mucous membranes.

Uses and Administration

Podophyllum resin has an antimitotic action and is used principally as a topical treatment for anogenital warts (condylomata acuminata). It is applied as a 15% (Indian podophyllum) or up to a 25% solution (American podophyllum) in alcohol or compound benzoin tincture, left on the warts for 1 to 6 hours, and then washed off. This procedure is carried out once a week and, if unsuccessful after about 4 weeks, an alternative treatment should be tried. A preparation containing podophyllotoxin 0.5% in alcohol or a 0.15% podophyllotoxin cream is used similarly. They are applied twice daily for 3 days but not washed off. Treatment may be repeated at weekly intervals for up to a total of 5 weeks of treatment. Podophyllum resin has been used on external genital, perianal, and intra-meatal warts, but should not be used on cervical or urethral warts. Only a small area or number of warts should be treated at any one time. Care must be taken to avoid application to healthy tissue. Podophyllum resin is also used with other keratolytics for the removal of plantar warts.

When taken by mouth podophyllum resin has a drastic purging action and it is highly irritant to the intestinal mucosa and produces violent peristalsis. It has been superseded by less toxic laxatives.

Podophyllum has been used in homoeopathic medicine.

Anogenital warts. Podophyllum preparations are one of the treatment choices for anogenital warts caused by human papillomavirus infection (condylomata acuminata) (p.1076).

Paints containing 10% or 25% of podophyllum resin appear to be equally effective for the treatment of external anogenital warts.[1] However, preparations containing podophyllotoxin 0.5%, the major active constituent of podophyllum resin, appear to be initially more effective[2] and unlike podophyllum, are suitable for self-treatment in both men and women.[3,4]

1. Simmons PD. Podophyllin 10% and 25% in the treatment of ano-genital warts: a comparative double-blind study. *Br J Vener Dis* 1981; **57:** 208–9.
2. Anonymous. Painting penile warts. *Drug Ther Bull* 1990; **28:** 63–4.
3. Beutner KR, *et al.* Patient-applied podofilox for treatment of genital warts. *Lancet* 1989; **i:** 831–4.
4. Greenberg MD, *et al.* A double-blind, randomized trial of 0.5% podofilox and placebo for the treatment of genital warts in women. *Obstet Gynecol* 1991; **77:** 735–9.

Preparations

BP 1998: Compound Podophyllin Paint;
USP 23: Podophyllum Resin Topical Solution.

Proprietary Preparations (details are given in Part 3)
Aust.: Condylox; *Austral.:* Condyline; Wartec†; *Belg.:* Condyline; *Canad.:* Condyline; Podofilm; Wartec; *Fr.:* Condyline; *Ger.:* Condylox; Wartec; *Irl.:* Warticon; *Ital.:* Condyline; *Neth.:* Condyline; *Norw.:* Condyline; Wartec; *S.Afr.:* Wartec; *Spain:* Condelone; Wartec; *Swed.:* Condyline; Wartec; *Switz.:* Condyline; Warix; *UK:* Condyline; Warticon; *USA:* Condylox; Pod-Ben-25†; Podocon; Podofin.

Multi-ingredient: *Austral.:* Posalfilin; Salicylin-P†; Wart-Off†; Wartkil†; *Belg.:* Carters; Sanicolax; *Canad.:* Canthacur-PS; Cantharone Plus; *Ger.:* Unguentum Lymphaticum; *Irl.:* Posalfilin; *S.Afr.:* Posalfilin; *Spain:* Alofedina; Laxo Vian; Pildoras Zeninas; *UK:* Posalfilin; Vericap†; *USA:* Cantharone Plus†; Verrex†; Verrusol†.

Polyphloroglucinol Phosphate (13148-v)

Polyphloroglucin Phosphate. Poly[benzene-1,3,5-triol mono(dihydrogen phosphate)].

$(C_6H_7O_6P)_n = 206.1 \times n.$

CAS — 51202-77-8.

Polyphloroglucinol phosphate has an inhibitory effect on hyaluronidase and has been applied topically in the treatment of wounds and pruritic skin disorders.

Preparations

Proprietary Preparations (details are given in Part 3)
Aust.: Dealyd.

Polyprenoic Acid (2035-a)

E-5166; Polyprenic Acid. (all-*E*)-3,7,11,15-Tetramethyl-2,4,6,10,14-hexadecapentaenoic acid.

$C_{20}H_{30}O_2 = 302.5.$

CAS — 81485-25-8.

Polyprenoic acid is a retinoid being studied in the treatment of psoriasis, keratoderma, and liver and bladder cancers.

References.

1. Muto Y, *et al.* Prevention of second primary tumors by an acyclic retinoid, polyprenoic acid, in patients with hepatocellular carcinoma. *N Engl J Med* 1996; **334:** 1561–7.

Prezatide Copper Acetate (16788-z)

Prezatide Copper Acetate *(USAN, rINN).*

PC-1020 (prezatide copper). Hydrogen [N^2-(*N*-glycyl-L-histidyl)-L-lysinato][N^2-(*N*-glycyl-L-histidyl)-L-lysinato(2–)]cuprate(1–) diacetate.

$C_{28}H_{46}CuN_{12}O_8.2C_2H_4O_2 = 862.4.$

CAS — 130120-57-9.

Prezatide copper acetate is a copper containing tripeptide which has been investigated as a wound-healing agent and in inflammatory bowel disease.

Pyrithione Zinc (1633-s)

Pyrithione Zinc *(BAN, USAN, rINN).*

Zinc 2-Pyridinethiol 1-Oxide; Zinc Pyridinethione. Bis[1-hydroxypyridine-2(1*H*)-thionato]zinc.

$C_{10}H_8N_2O_2S_2Zn = 317.7.$

CAS — 13463-41-7.

Pyrithione zinc has bacteriostatic and fungistatic properties. It is used similarly to selenium sulphide (p.1091) in usual concentrations of 1 to 2% in the control of seborrhoeic dermatitis and dandruff (p.1076). It is an ingredient of some proprietary shampoos. It has also been used in the treatment of pityriasis versicolor.

Pyrithione magnesium has also been used.

Peripheral neuritis with paraesthesia and muscle weakness in one patient was associated with the prolonged use of a shampoo containing pyrithione zinc 2%.[1] The muscle weakness had disappeared 3 months after stopping the shampoo and 2 years later the paraesthesia had improved by about 75%.

Studies in *animals* had found signs of neurotoxicity following oral administration of pyrithione zinc but whereas absorption following topical application was found to be 13% for pyrithione sodium it was less than 1% for pyrithione zinc.[2]

1. Beck JE. Zinc pyrithione and peripheral neuritis. *Lancet* 1978; **i:** 444.
2. Parekh CK. Zinc pyrithione and peripheral neuritis. *Lancet* 1978, **i:** 940.

Preparations

Proprietary Preparations (details are given in Part 3)
Aust.: Desquaman; *Austral.:* Dan-Gard; Dandruff Control Pert 2 in 1; *Canad.:* Anti-Dandruff Shampoo; Avant Garde Shampoo; Dan-Gard; Dandruff Treatment Shampoo; Hair and Scalp; Head & Shoulders; Keep Clear Anti-Dandruff Shampoo; Lander Dandruff Control; No-Name Dandruff Treatment; Out of Africa; Pert Plus;

Satinique Anti-Dandruff; Sebulon; Shaklee Dandruff Control; Shampooing Anti-Pelliculaire; ZNP; ZP 11; ***Fr.:*** Hermal; Ultrex†; ZNP; ***Ger.:*** Desquaman N; ***Ital.:*** Rivescal ZPT; Shampoo SDE Zinc; ZNP; ***Switz.:*** Desquaman†; ***USA:*** DHS Zinc; Head & Shoulders; Sebulon†; Theraplex Z; TVC-2 Dandruff Shampoo; Zincon; ZNP.

Multi-ingredient: ***Austral.:*** Fongitar; ***Canad.:*** Dan-Tar Plus; Multi-Tar Plus; Polytar AF; X-Seb Plus; Z-Plus; ***Fr.:*** Fongitar†; ***Ital.:*** Aminotril; Fongitar; Kevis Shampoo Antiforfora; Omadine; ***Switz.:*** Crinotar; Sebo Shampooing; Soufrol ZNP; Squa-med; ***UK:*** Polytar AF; ***USA:*** X-Seb Plus.

Pyrogallol (1634-w)

Pyrogallic Acid. Benzene-1,2,3-triol.

$C_6H_6O_3$ = 126.1.

CAS — 87-66-1.

Pharmacopoeias. In *Aust., Fr.,* and *Pol.*

Pyrogallol was formerly used topically in the treatment of psoriasis and parasitic skin diseases, but application over large areas or denuded surfaces is dangerous and may produce systemic effects similar to phenol poisoning (see p.1121); methaemoglobinaemia, haemolysis, and kidney damage may also occur.

Pyrogallol stains the skin and hair black.

Pyroxylin (1636-l)

Pyroxylin *(rINN).*

Algodão-Polvora; Cellulose Nitrate; Colloxylinum; Fulmicoton; Gossypium Collodium; Kollodiumwolle; Pyroxylinum; Soluble Guncotton.

CAS — 9004-70-0.

Pharmacopoeias. In *Aust., Br., Jpn,* and *US.*

A nitrated cellulose of variable composition consisting chiefly of cellulose tetranitrate $(C_{12}H_{16}N_4O_{18})_n$. It is prepared by treating defatted wood pulp or cotton linters with a mixture of nitric and sulphuric acids. It occurs as white to light yellow cuboid granules or fibrous material resembling cotton wool but harsher to the touch and more powdery. It is highly flammable.

Soluble in acetone and in glacial acetic acid. **Store** in well-closed containers, loosely packed, protected from light, and at a temperature not exceeding 15°, remote from fire. The container should be suitably designed to disrupt should the internal pressure reach or exceed 1400 kPa. It should be kept moistened with not less than 25% of industrial methylated spirit or isopropyl alcohol. The amount of damping fluid must not be allowed to fall below 25% w/w; should this happen, the material should be either rewetted or used immediately for the preparation of Collodion. When kept in well-closed containers and exposed to light, it decomposes with the evolution of nitrous vapours, leaving a carbonaceous residue.

CAUTION. *Dry pyroxylin is explosive and sensitive to ignition by impact or friction and should be handled carefully.*

Pyroxylin is used in the preparation of collodions which are applied to the skin for the protection of small cuts and abrasions. Collodions are also used as vehicles for the application of drugs when prolonged local action is required.

Preparations

BP 1998: Collodion; Flexible Collodion;
USP 23: Collodion; Flexible Collodion.

Proprietary Preparations (details are given in Part 3)
Multi-ingredient: ***Spain:*** Curacallos Pedykur†.

Resorcinol (1637-y)

m-Dihydroxybenzene; Dioxybenzolum; Resorcin; Resorcinolum. Benzene-1,3-diol.

$C_6H_6O_2$ = 110.1.

CAS — 108-46-3.

Pharmacopoeias. In *Chin., Eur.* (see p.viii), *Pol.,* and *US.*

Colourless, white, practically white, or slightly pinkish-grey, acicular crystals or crystalline powder with a characteristic odour. M.p. 109° to 112°. It may become red on exposure to air and light.

Soluble 1 in 1 of water, 1 in 1 of alcohol; freely soluble in ether, and glycerol; slightly soluble in chloroform. A 5% solution in water is neutral or acid to litmus.

Incompatible with ferric salts. **Protect** from light.

Resorcinol Monoacetate (1638-j)

Resorcin Acetate. 3-Acetoxyphenol.

$C_8H_8O_3$ = 152.1.

CAS — 102-29-4.

Pharmacopoeias. In *US.*

Resorcinol monoacetate is a pale yellow or amber viscous liquid with a faint characteristic odour. Sparingly **soluble** in water; soluble in alcohol and most organic solvents. A saturated solution in water is acid to litmus. **Store** in airtight containers. Protect from light.

Adverse Effects, Treatment, and Precautions

Resorcinol is a mild irritant and may result in skin sensitisation. It should not be applied to large areas of the body, for prolonged periods, or in high concentrations, especially in children, as it is absorbed through intact skin as well as broken skin and may interfere with thyroid function or produce methaemoglobinaemia. Resorcinol may produce hyperpigmentation in patients with dark skins and may darken light-coloured hair. Systemic toxic effects of resorcinol are similar to those of phenol and are treated similarly (see p.1121) but convulsions may occur more frequently.

Resorcinol could cause green discoloration of the urine.[1]

1. Karlstrand J. The pharmacist and the ostomate. *J Am Pharm Assoc* 1977; **NS17:** 735–8.

Uses and Administration

Resorcinol has keratolytic properties and has been used in topical preparations for the treatment of acne (p.1072) and seborrhoeic skin conditions (p.1076) usually in combination with sulphur, although other treatments are generally preferred.

Resorcinol has also been used in preparations for the treatment of anorectal disorders often complexed with bismuth compounds (see Haemorrhoids, p.1170).

Resorcinol monoacetate has been used similarly but may provide a milder action with a longer duration.

Preparations

BPC 1973: Magenta Paint;
USP 23: Carbol-Fuchsin Topical Solution; Compound Resorcinol Ointment; Resorcinol and Sulfur Lotion.

Proprietary Preparations (details are given in Part 3)
USA: Castel.

Multi-ingredient: ***Aust.:*** Apotheker Bauer's Huhneraugentinktur; Wisamt; ***Austral.:*** Acne-Ban†; Egomycol; Eskamel; Seborrol; ***Belg.:*** Nestosyl; Pelarol†; Synthol; ***Canad.:*** Acne-Aid; Acnomel; Clearasil Acne Cream; Clearskin 2 Tinted Blemish; Lanacane Medicated Cream; Mazon Medicated Cream; Night Cast S†; Rezamid†; Sebo Concept D/A; Vagisil; ***Fr.:*** Anaxeryl; Bain de Bouche Lipha†; Balsofletol†; Eau Precieuse Depensier; Myscat†; Nestosyl; Osmotol; Synthol; ***Ger.:*** Akne-Aid-Creme†; Akne-Medice Kombipackung†; Clabin†; Crinohermal P†; Crinohermal†; Jaikal; Lugro†; Sebohermal†; Skin-Aid†; Wisamt N†; ***Irl.:*** Anugesic-HC; Eskamel†; ***Ital.:*** Anusol; Betullosin†; Blefarolin; Dermogamma†; Labocaina; Loticort†; Rinantipiol; Sebohermal†; Zincosin†; ***S.Afr.:*** Anugesic; Anusol-HC; Eskamel†; Rectosan 'A'†; ***Spain:*** Acnisdin; Acnomel†; Acnosan; Aknederm†; Anti-Acne; Antiseptico Dent Donner†; Dentafijal†; Dermomycose; Frikton†; Juveacne†; Lucil†; Milrosina; Milrosina Hidrocort†; Poliglicol Anti Acne; Regal; Resorborina; Resorpil†; Synthol†; ***Switz.:*** Clabin; Crinohermal P†; Crinohermal†; Euproctol; Lotio decapans; Synthol†; ***UK:*** Eskamel; ***USA:*** Acnomel; Bensulfoid; Bicozene; Castaderm; Dermarest; Fungi-Nail; Neo-Castaderm†; Night Cast Special Formula†; R/S Lotion; RA Lotion; Resinol; Rezamid; Sulforcin; Vagisil; Yeast-Gard Maximum Strength Formula†.

Ro-13-6298 (518-r)

Ethyl *p*-[(*E*)-2-(5,6,7,8-tetrahydro-5,5,8,8-tetramethyl-2-naphthyl)-1-propenyl] benzoate.

$C_{26}H_{32}O_2$ = 376.5.

CAS — 71441-09-3.

Ro-13-6298 is an arotinoid studied in psoriasis and other keratinisation disorders.

References.

1. Gollnick H. New indications and new retinoids. *Dermatologica* 1987; **175** (suppl 1): 182–95.
2. Orfanos CE, *et al.* The retinoids: a review of their clinical pharmacology and therapeutic use. *Drugs* 1987; **34:** 459–503.
3. Saurat J-H, *et al.* Arotinoid acid (Ro 13-7410): a pilot study in dermatology. *Dermatologica* 1988; **176:** 191–9.
4. Boyd AS. An overview of the retinoids. *Am J Med* 1989; **86:** 568–74.

Salicylic Acid (2701-y)

Acido Ortóxibenzoico; Acidum Salicylicum; Salizylsäure. 2-Hydroxybenzoic acid.

$C_7H_6O_3$ = 138.1.

CAS — 69-72-7.

Pharmacopoeias. In *Chin., Eur.* (see p.viii), *Int., Jpn, Pol.,* and *US.*

White or colourless acicular crystals or a white fluffy crystalline powder. The synthetic form is white and odourless but if prepared from natural methyl salicylate it may have a slightly yellow or pink tint, and a faint, mint-like odour.

Soluble 1 in 460 of water, 1 in 15 of boiling water, 1 in 3 of alcohol, 1 in 3 of ether, and 1 in 45 of chloroform. Sparingly soluble in dichloromethane. **Protect** from light.

Adverse Effects and Precautions

Salicylic acid is a mild irritant and application of salicylic acid preparations to the skin may cause dermatitis. Salicylic acid is readily absorbed through the skin and symptoms of acute systemic salicylate poisoning (see Aspirin, p.16) have been reported after excessive application of salicylic acid to large areas of the body; several deaths have occurred, mainly in children. To minimise absorption following topical application salicylic acid should not be used for prolonged periods, in high concentrations, on large areas of the body, or on inflamed or broken skin. Contact with mouth, eyes, and other mucous membranes should be avoided. It should also be used with care on the extremities of patients with impaired peripheral circulation or diabetes.

There has been a report that application of 2% salicylic acid in a cream base before phototherapy delayed or reduced the clearance of psoriatic lesions when compared with the use of the base alone.[1] It was suggested that salicylic acid might have been acting as a photoprotective agent[1] but a later study[2] failed to confirm this. However, emulsifying ointment was found to have such an effect and it was recommended that it should not be used before phototherapy or in phototesting procedures.[2]

1. Kristensen B, Kristensen O. Salicylic acid and ultraviolet B for psoriasis. *Lancet* 1989; **ii:** 1109–10.
2. Cox NH, Sharpe G. Emollients, salicylic acid, and ultraviolet erythema. *Lancet* 1990; **335:** 53–4.

Uses and Administration

Salicylic acid has keratolytic properties and is applied topically in the treatment of hyperkeratotic and scaling skin conditions such as dandruff and seborrhoeic dermatitis (p.1076), ichthyosis (p.1074), psoriasis (p.1075), and acne (p.1072). Initially a concentration of about 2% is used, increased to about 6% if necessary, though a wider range of concentrations has been used. It is often used in conjunction with other drugs, notably coal tar.

Preparations containing up to 60% salicylic acid have been used as a caustic for the removal of plantar warts (p.1076), corns, or calluses.

Salicylic acid also possesses fungicidal properties and is used topically in the treatment of dermatophyte skin infections (see p.371).

Preparations

BP 1998: Coal Tar and Salicylic Acid Ointment; Compound Benzoic Acid Ointment *(Whitfield's Ointment)*; Dithranol Paste; Salicylic Acid Collodion; Salicylic Acid Ointment; Zinc and Salicylic Acid Paste *(Lassar's Paste)*;
BPC 1973: Salicylic Acid and Sulphur Ointment;
USP 23: Benzoic and Salicylic Acids Ointment; Salicylic Acid Collodion; Salicylic Acid Gel; Salicylic Acid Plaster; Salicylic Acid Topical Foam; Zinc Oxide and Salicylic Acid Paste.

Proprietary Preparations (details are given in Part 3)
Aust.: Squamasol; ***Austral.:*** Clear Away; Clearasil Medicated Wipes; Egocappol†; Ionil Scalp Cleanser; Isophyl†; John Plunkett's Sunspot Cream†; Johnson's Clean & Clear Skin Balancing Moisturiser; Salact; Sunspot; ***Belg.:*** Sicombyl; ***Canad.:*** Acnex; Acnomel Acne Mask; Anti-Acne Control Formula; Anti-Acne Spot Treatment; Blemish Control; Callus Salve; Clean & Clear Deep Cleaning Astringent; Clean & Clear Invsible Blemish; Clear Away; Clear Pore Treatment; Clearasil Clearstick; Clearasil Pads; Compound W; Compound W Plus; Duoforte; Fostex Medicated Cleansing; Freezone; Ionil; Keralyt; Mosco; Mudd Acne; Neutrogena Healthy Scalp Anti-Dandruff; Nova Perfecting Lotion; Occlusal; Off-Ezy; Oil-Free Acne Wash; Oxy Control; Oxy Deep Pore; Oxy Night Watch; Oxy Power Pads; P & S; Propa PH; Salac; Salseb; Scholl 2-Drop Corn Remedy; Scholl Corn Salve; Scholl Corn, Callus Plaster Preparation; Scholl Wart Remover; Scholl Zino; Sebcur; Soluver; Ten-O-Six; Trans-Plantar; Trans-Ver-Sal; Wart Remover; X-Seb; ***Fr.:*** Clearasil Gel soin de nuit†; Coricide le Diable; Coricides feuille de saule†; Feuille de Saule; Pommade Mo Cochon; Septisol; Transvercid; Verrucosal; ***Ger.:*** Cornina Hornhaut; Cornina Huhneraugen; Efasit N; Gehwol Schalpaste; Guttaplast; Gyan†; Humopin N; Lygal N; Psorimed; Radikal-Salicylcollodicum†; Rheumagutt-Bad N†; Schrundensalbe - Dermicyl; Sophtal-POS N; Squamasol; Urgo-N Huhneraugenpflaster; Verrucid; ***Irl.:*** Acnisal; Compound W; Freezone; Occlusal; Vericaps; ***Ital.:*** Trans-Ver-Sal; ***Neth.:*** Formule W; ***S.Afr.:*** Ionil†; Jiffy Corn Plasters†; ***Spain:*** Callicida Globodermis; Callicida Gras; Callicida Salve; Callofin; Unguento Morryth; Urgocall; ***Swed.:*** Salsyvase; ***UK:*** Acnisal; Biactol Antibacterial Double Action Pads†; Callous Removers; Carnation; Clearasil Dual Action Pads; Clearasil Nightclear; Compound V; Compound W; Corn Removers; Corn Solvent†; Freezone; Noxacorn†; Occlusal; Pickles Foot Ointment; SCR; Verruca Treatment; Verrugon; Verucca Removal System; Verucca Treatment†; Wartex; ***USA:*** Clearasil Clearstick; Clearasil Medicated Astringent†; Compound W; DHS Sal; Dr Scholl's Callus Removers; Dr Scholl's Clear Away; Dr Scholl's Corn Removers; Dr Scholl's Corn/Callus Remover; Dr Scholl's Wart Remover; Duofilm; Duoplant; Fostex Acne Medication

Cleansing; Freezone; Gordofilm; Hydrisalic†; Ionil; Ionil Plus; Keralyt; Listerex†; Mediplast; Mosco; Occlusal; Off-Ezy; Oxy Night Watch; P & S; Panscol; Paplex Ultra†; Propa PH; PROPApH; Psor-a-set; Sal-Acid; Sal-Clens; Sal-Plant; Salac; Salactic Film; Sebucare; Stri-Dex Clear; Sulfoam; Trans-Ver-Sal AdultPatch; Trans-Ver-Sal PediaPatch; Trans-Ver-Sal PlantarPatch; Viranol†; Wart Remover; Wart-Off; X-Seb.

Multi-ingredient: numerous preparations are listed in Part 3.

Sebacic Acid (13225-h)

Decanedioic acid; Octane-1,8-dicarboxylic acid.

$C_{10}H_{18}O_4$ = 202.2.

CAS — 111-20-6.

Sebacic acid is an emollient included in preparations used to protect damaged skin.

Diisopropyl sebacate ($C_{16}H_{30}O_4$ = 286.4) has been used in skin moisturising preparations.

Preparations

Proprietary Preparations (details are given in Part 3)

Multi-ingredient: ***Canad.:*** Domol†.

Selenium Sulphide (1639-z)

Selenii Disulfidum; Selenium Disulphide; Selenium Sulfide.

SeS_2 = 143.1.

CAS — 7488-56-4.

Pharmacopoeias. In *Eur.* (see p.viii) and *US.*

A bright orange to reddish-brown powder with a faint odour of hydrogen sulphide. Practically **insoluble** in water; soluble 1 in 161 of chloroform and 1 in 1667 of ether; practically insoluble in most other organic solvents. Selenium sulphide may discolour metals.

Adverse Effects and Treatment

Topical application of selenium sulphide can produce irritation of the conjunctiva, scalp, and skin, especially in the genital area and skin folds. Oiliness or dryness of scalp or hair, hair discoloration, and hair loss have been reported.

Selenium sulphide can be highly toxic when taken by mouth. Only traces of selenium sulphide are absorbed through intact skin but prolonged use on broken skin has resulted in systemic toxicity.

Treatment of poisoning is symptomatic.

Systemic toxicity. A woman with excoriated eruptions on her scalp developed weakness, anorexia, abdominal pain, vomiting, tremors, sweating, a metallic taste in her mouth, and a garlic-like smell on her breath after using a shampoo containing selenium sulphide two to three times a week for 8 months.[1] All symptoms subsided 10 days after withdrawal of the shampoo.

1. Ransone JW, *et al.* Selenium sulfide intoxication. *N Engl J Med* 1961; **264:** 384–5.

Precautions

To minimise absorption selenium sulphide should not be applied to mucous membranes, inflamed or broken skin, or to extensive areas of the skin. Contact with the eyes should be avoided.

Selenium sulphide shampoos should not be used within 48 hours of applying hair colours or permanent waving preparations.

Uses and Administration

Selenium sulphide has antifungal and antiseborrhoeic properties. It is used as a shampoo in the treatment of dandruff (pityriasis capitis) and seborrhoeic dermatitis of the scalp (p.1076). Five to 10 mL of a suspension containing 2.5% of selenium sulphide is applied to the wet scalp; the hair is rinsed and the application repeated; the suspension should remain in contact with the scalp for 2 to 3 minutes each time. The hair should be well rinsed after the treatment and all traces of the suspension removed from the hands and nails. Applications are usually made twice weekly for 2 weeks, then once weekly for 2 weeks and then only when necessary. Shampoos containing 1% are also used.

Selenium sulphide is also used as a 2.5% lotion in the treatment of pityriasis versicolor (p.371). The lotion may be applied to the affected areas with a small amount of water and allowed to remain for 10 minutes before thorough rinsing. This procedure is repeated once daily for about 7 to 14 days. Alternatively undiluted 2.5% lotion may be applied at bedtime and washed off in the morning on 3 separate occasions at 3-day intervals.

Selenium sulphide has also been used as an adjunct to the systemic treatment of tinea capitis (see Dermatophytoses, p.371).

Preparations

BP 1998: Selenium Sulphide Scalp Application;
USP 23: Selenium Sulfide Lotion.

Proprietary Preparations (details are given in Part 3)
Aust.: Selsun; Selukos; STOI-X†; ***Austral.:*** Selsun; ***Belg.:*** Selsun; ***Canad.:*** Selsun; Versel; ***Fr.:*** Selegel; Selepain†; Selsun; ***Ger.:*** Selsun; Selukos; ***Irl.:*** Lenium; Selsun; ***Ital.:*** Selsun Blu; ***Neth.:*** Selsun-R; ***Norw.:*** Selsun; Selukos; ***S.Afr.:*** Selsun†; ***Spain:*** Abbottselsun; Bioselenium; Caspiselenio; ***Swed.:*** Selsun; Selukos; ***Switz.:*** Sebo-Lenium†; Selsun; ***UK:*** Lenium; Selsun; ***USA:*** Exsel; Head & Shoulders Intensive Treatment; Selsun.

Multi-ingredient: ***Belg.:*** Sulfo-Selenium; ***Fr.:*** Blephaseptyl†; ***Ger.:*** Ellsurex; ***Ital.:*** Node Tar; Selsun Trattamento†; ***Spain:*** Sebumselen; Sulfiselen; ***Switz.:*** Blephaseptyl†; Ektoselene.

Sodium Pidolate (13256-s)

Sodium Pidolate (*pINNM*).

NaPCA; Sodium Pyroglutamate; Sodium Pyrrolidone Carboxylate. Sodium 5-oxopyrrolidine-2-carboxylate.

$C_5H_7NNaO_3$ = 152.1.

CAS — 28874-51-3 (DL-sodium pidolate); 54571-67-4 (L-sodium pidolate).

Sodium pidolate is used as a humectant. It is applied topically as a cream or lotion often in mixed preparations in the treatment of dry skin disorders.

Preparations

Proprietary Preparations (details are given in Part 3)
UK: Humiderm.

Multi-ingredient: ***Austral.:*** Dermadrate; DermaVeen Moisturising; DermaVeen Shower and Bath; Lacticare†; ***Canad.:*** Lacticare; ***Fr.:*** Lacticare†; ***Irl.:*** Hydromol; Lacticare; ***Ital.:*** Angstrom Viso/Labbra Alta Protezione; Detoxergon†; ***S.Afr.:*** Lacticare†; ***UK:*** Hydromol Cream; Lacticare.

Squaric Acid Dibutylester (3919-c)

Quadratic Acid Dibutylester. The dibutyl ester of 3,4-dihydroxy-3-cyclobutene-1,2-dione.

$C_{12}H_{18}O_4$ = 226.3.

CAS — 2892-51-5 (squaric acid).

Squaric acid dibutylester has been tried similarly to diphencyprone (p.1081) as a contact sensitiser in the treatment of alopecia.

References.

1. Van der Steen PHM, *et al.* Topical immunotherapy for alopecia areata: re-evaluation of 139 cases after an additional follow-up period of 19 months. *Dermatology* 1992; **184:** 198–201.

Sulphur (1643-e)

Azufre; Enxôfre; Schwefel; Soufre; Sulfur.

S = 32.066.

CAS — 7704-34-9.

Pharmacopoeias. In *Chin., Eur.* (see p.viii), *Jpn, Pol.,* and *US.* Some have monographs for Precipitated Sulphur (Milk of Sulphur), Sublimed Sulphur (Flowers of Sulphur), or both. Some specify it is only for external use.

Sulphur for External Use (Ph. Eur.) is a yellow powder. The size of most of the particles is not greater than 20 μm. Practically **insoluble** in water; soluble in carbon disulphide; slightly soluble in vegetable oils. **Protect** from light.

Precipitated Sulfur (USP 23) is a very fine pale yellow, odourless, amorphous or microcrystalline powder. Practically **insoluble** in water; slowly and usually incompletely soluble 1 in 2 of carbon disulphide; soluble 1 in 100 of olive oil; very slightly soluble in alcohol.

Sublimed Sulfur (USP 23) is a fine yellow, crystalline powder with a faint odour. Practically **insoluble** in water or alcohol; sparingly soluble in olive oil.

Colloidal sulphur has a smaller particle size than either precipitated or sublimed sulphur. It is sulphur in an aqueous medium containing a colloid such as albumin or gelatin.

WARNING. *Sulphur has been used for the illicit preparation of explosives or fireworks; care is required with its supply.*

Adverse Effects and Precautions

Topical application of sulphur can cause skin irritation and dermatitis has been reported following repeated application. Contact with the eyes, mouth, and other mucous membranes should be avoided. Contact with sulphur can discolour certain metals such as silver, and concomitant application of sulphur and topical mercurial compounds can lead to the generation of hydrogen sulphide which has a foul odour and may stain the skin black.

Uses and Administration

Sulphur is a keratolytic, a mild antiseptic, a mild antifungal, and a parasiticide. It has been widely employed, in the form of lotions, creams, or ointments, usually in combination with other agents, in concentrations of up to 10% in the treatment of acne, dandruff, seborrhoeic conditions, scabies, and superficial fungal infections, though there are more convenient and effective preparations.

Lotions of precipitated sulphur with lead acetate have been used to darken grey hair.

Sulphur was also formerly used as a mild irritant laxative.

Sulphur is used in homoeopathic medicine.

General references.

1. Lin AN, *et al.* Sulfur revisited. *J Am Acad Dermatol* 1988; **18:** 553–8.

Preparations

BPC 1973: Salicylic Acid and Sulphur Ointment;
USP 23: Resorcinol and Sulfur Lotion; Sulfur Ointment.

Proprietary Preparations (details are given in Part 3)
Aust.: Sulfosol; ***Canad.:*** Acne Blemish Cream; Postacne; Pureness Blemish Control; ***Ger.:*** Loscon†; Schwefel-Diasporal; Sulfopino; ***Ital.:*** Acqua di Sirmione; Eudermal Sapone Allo Zolfo pH 5; Nosebo; Royal Zolfo†; Veriderm; ***USA:*** Acne Lotion 10; Bensulfoid†; Liquimat; Sastid; Sulmasque; Xerac†.

Multi-ingredient: numerous preparations are listed in Part 3.

Sulphurated Lime (1645-y)

Calcium Sulphide; Calx Sulphurata; Sulfurated Lime.

CAS — 8028-82-8 (sulphurated lime solution).

Sulphurated lime is a mixture containing calcium sulphate and not less than 50% of calcium sulphide (CaS), prepared by heating calcium sulphate. Sulphurated lime solution (Vleminckx's solution) is an aqueous solution containing calcium polysulphides and calcium thiosulphate prepared by boiling sublimed sulphur with calcium hydroxide in water.

Sulphurated lime has been used topically as sulphurated lime solution for acne, scabies, seborrhoeic dermatitis, and pustular infections such as boils and carbuncles. A similar solution known as 'lime-sulphur' is used as a fungicide in horticulture.

An impure grade of calcium sulphide (Hepar Sulphuris; Hepar Sulph.) is used in homoeopathic medicine.

NOTE. The titles Hepar Sulfuris and Hepar Sulph are also applied to Sulphurated Potash (see below).

Preparations

Proprietary Preparations (details are given in Part 3)
Canad.: Vlemasque†.

Sulphurated Potash (1646-j)

Foie de Soufre; Hepar Sulfuris; Kalii Sulfidum; Liver of Sulphur; Potassa Sulphurata; Schwefelleber; Sulfurated Potash.

CAS — 39365-88-3.

NOTE. The title Hepar Sulphuris is used in homoeopathic medicine for an impure grade of calcium sulphide—see Sulphurated Lime, above.

Pharmacopoeias. In *US.*

A mixture composed chiefly of potassium polysulphides and potassium thiosulphate, containing not less than 12.8% of sulphur as sulphide. Irregular, liver-brown pieces rapidly changing to greenish-yellow on exposure to air. It has an odour of hydrogen sulphide.

Almost completely **soluble** 1 in 2 of water. Alcohol dissolves only the sulphides. A 10% solution in water is alkaline to litmus. **Incompatible** with acids. **Store** in small airtight containers.

Sulphurated potash has been used in the treatment of acne and other skin disorders usually in the form of a lotion with zinc sulphate.

Sulphurated potash is used in homoeopathic medicine when it is known as Hepar Sulph.

Preparations

USP 23: White Lotion.

Proprietary Preparations (details are given in Part 3)
Ger.: Schwefelbad Saar.

Multi-ingredient: ***Aust.:*** Leukona-Sulfomoor-Bad; ***Ger.:*** Leukona-Sulfomoor-Bad N.

Tacalcitol (15404-r)

Tacalcitol *(BAN, rINN)*.

1α,24-Dihydroxycholecalciferol; 1α,24-Dihydroxyvitamin D_3.
(+)-(5Z,7E,24R)-9,10-Secocholesta-5,7,10(19)-triene-1α,3β,24-triol monohydrate.

$C_{27}H_{44}O_3,H_2O = 434.7$.

CAS — 57333-96-7 (anhydrous tacalcitol); 93129-94-3 (tacalcitol monohydrate).

Adverse Effects and Precautions

As for Calcipotriol, p.1080. Paraesthesia may also occur. Tacalcitol may be applied to the face, but care should be taken to avoid the eyes. Tacalcitol may be degraded by UV radiation (see Uses and Administration, below).

Uses and Administration

Tacalcitol is a vitamin D_3 derivative. *In vitro* it appears to induce differentiation and to suppress proliferation of keratinocytes.

Tacalcitol is used as the monohydrate in an ointment for the management of plaque psoriasis (p.1075); the concentration used is equivalent to 0.0004% of tacalcitol. Applications are made once daily and no more than 5 g of ointment should be applied each day. Normally no more than two 12-week courses of treatment should be required in one year.

Tacalcitol may be degraded by UV radiation and therefore if combined with UV therapy, the radiation should be given in the morning and tacalcitol applied at bedtime. Patients exposed to sunlight should also apply tacalcitol at bedtime rather than during the day.

General reviews.

1. Peters DC, Balfour JA. Tacalcitol. *Drugs* 1997; **54:** 265–71.

Preparations

Proprietary Preparations (details are given in Part 3)
Ger.: Curatoderm; ***Switz.:*** Curatoderm; ***UK:*** Curatoderm.

Purified Talc (1647-z)

553(b); Powdered Talc; Purified French Chalk; Talc; Talcum; Talcum Purificatum.

CAS — 14807-96-6.

Pharmacopoeias. In Chin., Eur. (see p.viii), Int., Jpn, Pol., and US.

A purified native hydrated magnesium silicate, approximating to the formula $Mg_6(Si_2O_5)_4(OH)_4$; it may contain varying amounts of aluminium silicate and iron. A very fine, light, homogeneous, white or almost white, or greyish-white, odourless, impalpable, and unctuous crystalline powder, which adheres readily to the skin. Purified talc should be free from microscopic asbestos fibres.

Practically **insoluble** in water, in alcohol, and in dilute solutions of mineral acids or of alkali hydroxides.

Adverse Effects and Precautions

Contamination of wounds or body cavities with talc is liable to cause granulomas and it should not be used for dusting surgical gloves.

Inhalation of talc can cause respiratory irritation. Prolonged exposure to talc may produce pneumoconiosis.

Talc is liable to be heavily contaminated with bacteria, including *Clostridium tetani, Cl. welchii,* and *Bacillus anthracis.* When used in dusting-powders or to treat pneumothorax and pleural effusions, it should be sterilised.

Abuse. Pulmonary granulomas occurring after intravenous or intranasal drug abuse have been associated with the presence of talc as a filler in the abused preparations.[1,2]

1. Schwartz IS, Bosken C. Pulmonary vascular talc granulomatosis. *JAMA* 1986; **256:** 2584.
2. Johnson DC, *et al.* Foreign body pulmonary granulomas in an abuser of nasally inhaled drugs. *Pediatrics* 1991; **88:** 159–61.

Carcinogenicity. A review by a working group of the International Agency for Research on Cancer (IARC) concluded that there was inadequate evidence to confirm whether purified talc was carcinogenic in humans but there was sufficient evidence to confirm that talc containing asbestiform fibres was carcinogenic to man.[1] There have been suggestions of a link between the use of talc and ovarian cancer[2] but although a case-controlled study suggested an approximate doubling of the risk among women after perineal use of talc the working group noted that information was not available on the asbestos content of the talcs.[1]

1. IARC/WHO. Silica and some silicates. *IARC monographs on the evaluation of the carcinogenic risk of chemicals to humans* 42 1987.

Young RC. Cosmetic talc and ovarian cancer. *Lan-* 49–51.

Effects on the lungs. Inhalation of talc can cause respiratory irritation. Campos *et al.*[1] report that acute respiratory failure developed in 4 patients out of a total of 338 in whom pleurodesis for benign or malignant effusions was performed using insufflated talc in conjunction with thoracoscopy. Three of the 4 patients died. Talc crystals were found in the bronchoalveolar lavage of all 4 patients and on necropsy of one patient talc crystals were found in almost every organ.

For other effects on the lungs, see under Abuse, above and Infant Skin Care, below.

1. Campos JRM, *et al.* Respiratory failure due to insufflated talc. *Lancet* 1997; **349:** 251–2.

Infant skin care. The routine use of non-medicated powders in the skin care of infants can be hazardous and their use should be discouraged.[1,2] Talc acts as a pulmonary irritant and inhalation of baby powders by infants has caused severe respiratory difficulties and several deaths have been reported. Careful respiratory monitoring is indicated in children suspected of inhaling talcum powder as the onset of symptoms may be delayed for several hours.[1] There have also been reports of umbilical granulomas resulting from contamination of umbilical stumps with talcum powder used for skin care.[2]

1. Pairaudeau PW, *et al.* Inhalation of baby powder: an unappreciated hazard. *Br Med J* 1991; **302:** 1200–1.
2. Sparrow SA, Hallam LA. Talc granulomas. *Br Med J* 1991; **303:** 58.

Uses and Administration

Purified talc is used in massage and as a dusting-powder to allay irritation and prevent chafing. It is usually mixed with starch, to increase absorption of moisture, and zinc oxide. Talc used in dusting-powders or as talc poudrage should be sterilised. Purified talc is used as a lubricant and diluent in making tablets and capsules and to clarify liquids.

Talc poudrage has been used to treat recurrent spontaneous pneumothorax and pleural effusions (see under Malignant Effusions, Choice of Antineoplastic, p.484).

References.

1. Eselin J, Thompson DF. Talc in the treatment of malignant pleural effusion. *DICP Ann Pharmacother* 1991; **25:** 1187–9.
2. Vaughan LM, Bishop TD. Sterilization of talc USP for intrapleural use. *Ann Pharmacother* 1994; **28:** 1309–10.
3. Kennedy L, Sahn SA. Talc pleurodesis for the treatment of pneumothorax and pleural effusion. *Chest* 1994; **106:** 1215–22.

Preparations

BP 1998: Talc Dusting Powder.

Proprietary Preparations (details are given in Part 3)

Multi-ingredient: *Aust.:* Cutimix; Herposicc; Prurimix; Rombay; ***Belg.:*** Aloplastine; Baseler Haussalbe; ***Canad.:*** Bebia; ***Fr.:*** Aloplastine; Aloplastine Acide†; Aloplastine Ichthyolee†; Bebia; Denisoline; ***Ger.:*** Granugen†; ***Spain:*** Amniolina; Ictiomen; Pomada Infantil Vera; Talco Antihistam Calber; Talquissar; Talquistina; Tegunal; ***USA:*** ZBT.

Tars and Tar Oils (15703-s)

Birch Tar Oil (1652-l)

Birkenteer; Goudron de Bouleau; Oleum Betulae Albae; Oleum Betulae Empyreumaticum; Oleum Betulae Pyrolignēum; Oleum Rusci; Pix Betulae; Pyroleum Betulae.

Birch tar oil is obtained by the destructive distillation of the wood and bark of the silver birch, *Betula verrucosa* (= *B. pendula; B. alba*), and the birch, *B. pubescens* (Betulaceae); the distillate is allowed to stand and the oily upper layer separated from the residual tar.

Cade Oil (1595-t)

Alquitrán de Enebro; Goudron de Cade; Juniper Tar; Juniper Tar Oil; Kadeöl; Oleum Cadinum; Oleum Juniperi Empyreumaticum; Pix Cadi; Pix Juniperi; Pix Oxycedri; Pyroleum Juniperi; Pyroleum Oxycedri; Wacholderteer.

Pharmacopoeias. In Swiss and US.

Cade oil is obtained by the destructive distillation of the branches and wood of *Juniperus oxycedrus* (Pinaceae). It is a dark brown thick liquid with an empyreumatic odour. It contains guaiacol, ethylguaiacol, creosol, and cadinene. Very slightly **soluble** in water; soluble 1 in 9 of alcohol; soluble 1 in 3 of ether leaving only a slight flocculent residue; partially soluble in petroleum spirit; miscible with amyl alcohol, chloroform, and glacial acetic acid. **Store** in airtight containers. Avoid exposure to excessive heat. Protect from light.

Coal Tar (1650-w)

Alcatrão Mineral; Alquitrán de Hulla; Brea de Hulla; Crude Coal Tar; Goudron de Houille; Oleum Lithanthracis; Pix Carbon.; Pix Carbonis; Pix Lithanthracis; Pix Mineralis; Pyroleum Lithanthracis; Steinkohlenteer.

Pharmacopoeias. In Aust., Br., Fr., Int., Port., and US.

Coal tar is obtained by the destructive distillation of bituminous coal at temperatures in the range of 900° to 1100°. It may be processed further either by extraction with alcohol and suitable dispersing agents and maceration times or by fractional distillation with or without the use of suitable organic solvents.

A thick, nearly black, viscous liquid with a strong characteristic penetrating odour. On exposure to air it gradually becomes more viscous. It burns in air with a luminous sooty flame.

Slightly **soluble** in water; partly soluble in alcohol, acetone, chloroform, ether, carbon disulphide, methyl alcohol, volatile oils, and petroleum spirit. A saturated solution in water is alkaline to litmus. **Store** in airtight containers.

Incompatible with wool alcohols. Prepared coal tar is commercial coal tar heated at 50° for 1 hour. Alcoholic solutions of coal tar or prepared coal tar prepared with the aid of polysorbate have been referred to as Liquor Picis Carbonis and Liquor Carbonis Detergens.

Tar (1648-c)

Alquitrán Vegetal; Brea de Pino; Goudron Végétal; Nadelholzteer; Pine Tar; Pix Abietinarum; Pix Liquida; Pix Pini; Pyroleum Pini; Wood Tar.

NOTE. It is known in commerce as Stockholm tar.

Pharmacopoeias. In Aust. and Br.
Aust. also includes beech tar.

Tar is obtained by the destructive distillation of the wood of various trees of the family Pinaceae. It is a dark brown or nearly black viscous semi-liquid with a characteristic empyreumatic odour; it is heavier than water. Tar has an acid reaction which it imparts to water when shaken with it, and it may thereby be distinguished from coal tar, which has an alkaline reaction. **Soluble** in alcohol, chloroform, ether, and in fixed and volatile oils.

When stored for some time tar separates into a layer which is granular in character due to minute crystallisation of catechol, resin acids, etc. and a surface layer of a syrupy consistence.

Adverse Effects and Precautions

Tars and tar oils may cause irritation and acne-like eruptions of the skin and should not be applied to inflamed or broken skin. They should be used with caution on the face, skin flexures, or on the genitalia. Hypersensitivity reactions are rare but wood tars are more likely to cause sensitisation than coal tar. However, unlike wood tars, coal tar has a photosensitising action. Preparations of refined tar products appear to be less likely than crude tars to stain the skin, hair, and clothing.

Depending on their composition the systemic effects of tars and tar oils are similar to those for phenol (see p.1121).

Carcinogenicity. Although Stern *et al.*[1] found an increased risk of skin carcinoma in 59 patients with psoriasis who had had very high exposures to tar and/or UV radiation, Pittelkow *et al.*[2] found no such evidence in 260 patients followed for a mean of 20 years and Jones *et al.*[3] noted that long-term topical tar therapy alone was not associated with an increase in malignancy in 719 patients. Relatively high systemic absorption of polycyclic aromatic hydrocarbons, which are potential carcinogens, has, however, been reported after use of a coal-tar shampoo.[4]

1. Stern RS, *et al.* Skin carcinoma in patients with psoriasis treated with topical tar and artificial ultraviolet radiation. *Lancet* 1980; **i:** 732–5.
2. Pittelkow MR, *et al.* Skin cancer in patients with psoriasis treated with coal tar. *Arch Dermatol* 1981; **117:** 465–8.
3. Jones SK, *et al.* Further evidence of the safety of tar in the management of psoriasis. *Br J Dermatol* 1985; **113:** 97–101.
4. van Schooten F-J, *et al.* Dermal uptake of polycyclic aromatic hydrocarbons after hairwash with coal-tar shampoo. *Lancet* 1994; **344:** 1505–6.

Extemporaneous preparation. Concern about the possible carcinogenic potential of coal tar (see above) led the Health and Safety Executive in the UK to recommend that chemical gloves, as opposed to disposable surgeon's gloves, should be worn during the extemporaneous preparation of formulations containing coal tar.[1]

1. Anonymous. Chemical protection gloves recommended for coal tar ointments. *Pharm J* 1997; **259:** 757.

Uses and Administration

Tars and tar oils can reduce the thickness of the epidermis. They are antipruritic and may be weakly antiseptic. They are used topically in eczema (p.1073), psoriasis (below), dandruff, seborrhoeic dermatitis (p.1076), and other skin disorders though coal tar preparations have largely replaced the use of wood tars. Ultraviolet (UVB) light increases the efficacy of coal tar in the treatment of psoriasis.

Some wood tars, including creosote (p.1057) have been used in expectorant preparations. Tar has also been used in homoeopathic medicine.

Following their review of products for safety and efficacy the FDA ruled that cade oil or tar should not be used in nonprescription shampoos[1] and that tar should no longer be included in nonprescription expectorants.[2]

1. Anonymous. Nonprescription drug review gains momentum. *WHO Drug Inf* 1991; **5:** 62.
2. Anonymous. FDA announces standards for nonprescription sleep-aid products and expectorants. *Clin Pharm* 1989; **8:** 388.

Psoriasis. Coal tar has long been employed in the treatment of psoriasis (p.1075) and used alone or with dithranol and/or ultraviolet light it continues to be one of the drugs of first choice. It is particularly suited to the treatment of stable chronic plaque psoriasis. Its mode of action is unknown but after an initial transient increase in epidermal proliferation it can produce a reduction in the thickness of viable epidermis. *Animal* studies suggest that isoquinoline and analogous ingredients of coal tar may contribute to the anti-psoriatic activity. Crude tar preparations are considered to be safe even if rather messy and unpleasant; refined products may be more aesthetically acceptable and less likely to stain skin, hair, and clothing although some consider them to be less effective. There appears to be little evidence to support the use of one strength over another but treatments usually start with concentrations equivalent to 0.5 to 1.0% of crude coal tar with the concentration being increased as necessary every few days up to a maximum of 10%. Coal tar may not clear psoriasis as fast as other agents but extended periods of remission can be obtained with its use. The Goeckerman regimen utilises the enhanced efficacy obtained when coal tar is applied before exposure to ultraviolet (UVB) light. The mechanism for this effect is not known but it does not appear to be due to the photosensitising action of coal tar. In most regimens the coal tar is applied 2 hours before exposure to UVB light. In Ingram's regimen and its modifications the use of coal tar and UVB light is followed by topical treatment with dithranol. It has been suggested that the irritant effects of dithranol treatment are reduced by concomitant treatment with coal tar without loss of efficacy.

References.

1. Rotstein H, Baker C. The treatment of psoriasis. *Med J Aust* 1990; **152:** 153–64.
2. Menter A, Barker JNWN. Psoriasis in practice. *Lancet* 1991; **338:** 231–4.
3. Foreman MI, *et al.* Isoquinoline is a possible anti-psoriatic agent in coal tar. *Br J Dermatol* 1985; **112:** 323–8.
4. Williams REA, *et al.*. Workshop of the Research Unit of the Royal College of Physicians of London; Department of Dermatology, University of Glasgow; British Association of Dermatologists. Guidelines for management of patients with psoriasis. *Br Med J* 1991; **303:** 829–35.

Preparations

BP 1998: Calamine and Coal Tar Ointment *(Compound Calamine Ointment)*; Coal Tar and Salicylic Acid Ointment; Coal Tar and Zinc Ointment; Coal Tar Paste; Coal Tar Solution; Strong Coal Tar Solution; Zinc and Coal Tar Paste *(White's Tar Paste)*;
USP 23: Coal Tar Ointment; Coal Tar Topical Solution; Compound Resorcinol Ointment.

Proprietary Preparations (details are given in Part 3)
Austral.: Alpha Keri Tar; Alphosyl; Dermatar; Formicare Bath†; Formicare Shower†; Formicare Skin Gel†; Formicare Skin Wash†; Ionil-T Plus; Linotar; Neutrogena T/Gel; Psorigel; ***Canad.:*** Balnetar; Bebitar†; Estar; Ionil-T; Ionil-T Plus; Mazon Medicated Soap; Neutrogena T/Gel; Pentrax; Psoriasol; Psorigel; Robatar; Spectro Tar; T/Gel†; Tar Doak; Targel; Tarseb; Tegrin; Tersa-Tar; Zetar; ***Fr.:*** Caditar; Carbo-Dome†; Cosmetar-S; Ramet Cade; Ultrex a l'Huile de Cade†; ***Ger.:*** Basiter; Berniter; Hoepixin Bad N; Pixfix; Sebopona flussig mit Teer†; Teer-Linola-Fett; Teerseife "Blucher-Schering" flussig†; ***Irl.:*** Baltar; Clinitar; Pentrax; Psoriderm; Psorigel; ***Ital.:*** Konor; Meditar; Polytar; Shampoo SDE Tar; Tarmed; Tarphosyl†; ***Norw.:*** Soraderm; ***S.Afr.:*** L.P.C. Shampoo†; Linotar; Psorigel; ***Spain:*** Psoriasdin; Tarisdin Cutaneo†; ***Swed.:*** Basotar†; ***Switz.:*** Teerol; ***UK:*** Alphosyl 2 in 1; Baltar†; Carbo-Dome; Clinitar; Exorex; Pentrax; Psoriderm; Psorigel; T/Gel; ***USA:*** Advanced Formula Tegrin; AquaTar; Balnetar; Creamy Tar; Cutar; DHS Tar; Doctar; Duplex T; Estar; Fototar; Iocon; Ionil-T Plus; MG217 Dual; MG217 Medicated; Neutrogena T/Derm; Neutrogena T/Gel; Oxipor VHC; Pentrax; Pentrax Gold; Polytar; Protar Protein; Psorigel; PsoriNail; Taraphilic; Tegrin; Tegrin Medicated; Theraplex T; Zetar.

Multi-ingredient: ***Aust.:*** Alphosyl; Alpicort†; Balneum Hermal mit Teer; Locacorten Tar; ***Austral.:*** Alpha Keri Tar; Alphosyl; Eczema Cream; Egopsoryl TA; Fongitar; Formicare Skin Relief†; Ionil-T; Neutrogena T/Sal; Pinetarsol; Polytar; Psor-asist; Psorin†; QV Tar†; Sebitar; Tarband; ***Belg.:*** Alphosyl; Locacortene Tar; Pelarol†; ***Canad.:*** Alphosyl; Boil Ease; Dan-Tar Plus; Denorex; Doak-Oil; Mazon Medicated Cream; Mazon Medicated Shampoo; Medi-Dan; Multi-Tar Plus; Oxipor; P & S Plus; Polytar; Polytar AF; Sebcur/T; Sebutone; SJ Liniment; Spectro Tar; Tardan; Targel SA; X-Seb T; X-Seb T Plus; X-Tar; ***Fr.:*** Alphosyl; Anaxeryl; Biolan Cad†; Biolan Tar; Coalgel†; Coaltar Saponine le Beuf; Cystelle Shampooing Cheveux Gras; Fongitar†; Gelictar de Charlieu†; Glyco-Thymoline; Ionax T; Laccoderme a l'huile de cade†; Laccoderme goudron de houille†; Lactar; Mysca†; Phytocoltar†; Polytar†; Psocortene†; S-Coaltar; Salycad†; ***Ger.:*** Aknefug-liquid N; Balneum mit Teer†; Dermaethyl-H†; Dermaethyl†; Dexacrinin; Discmigon; Hoepixin N; Lorinden T; Poloris; Poloris HC; Polytar; Psoriasis-Salbe M; Psorigerb N; Psorispray†; Sulfotar†; Vobaderm Plus†; ***Irl.:*** Alphosyl; Alphosyl HC; Balneum with Tar; Capasal; Cocois; Denorex; Gelcotar; Genisol; Ionil-T; Oxipor†; Polytar; Polytar Emollient; Polytar Plus; Pragmatar; ***Ital.:*** Alphosyle; Balta-Crin Tar; Coltapaste†; Fongitar; Genisol; Herbatar; Herbatar Plus; Ionil-T; Locorten Tar; Neo-Cortofen "Antrax"†; Node Tar; Pentagamma†; Pentrax; Rivescal Tar; Soluzione Composta Alcoolica Saponosa di Coaltar; ***Neth.:*** Denorex; Resdan Rx†; ***S.Afr.:*** Alphosyl; Ionil-T†; Locacorten Tar†; Pasta Prura†; Polytar; Tritar†; ***Spain:*** Alphosyl; Bazalin; Deltasiton; Emolytar; Mercufila Coaltar†; Polytar; Quinortar; Tarisdin; ***Swed.:*** Alphosyl; Locacorten Tar†; ***Switz.:*** Acne-Med†; Alphosyl; Bain extra-doux dermatologique; Crinotar; Jonil T; Locacorten Tar; Polytar†; Teerol-H; ***UK:*** Alphosyl; Alphosyl HC; Balneum with Tar†; Capasal; Carbo-Cort†; Cocois; Coltapaste; Denorex; Gelcosal; Gelcotar; Genisol†; Ionil-T; Pixol†; Polytar AF; Polytar Emollient; Polytar Liquid; Polytar Plus; Pragmatar; Psorin; Snowfire; Tarband; Tarcortin; Tardrox†; Varicose Ointment; ***USA:*** Boil Ease; Denorex; Ionil-T; Medotar; MG217 Medicated; Neutrogena T/Sal; P & S Plus; Sal-Oil-T; Sebex-T; Sebutone†; SLT; Tarlene; Tarsum; Unguentum Bossi; X-Seb T; X-Seb T Plus.

Tazarotene (15710-p)

Tazarotene *(BAN, USAN, rINN)*.

AGN-190168. Ethyl 6-[(4,4-dimethylthiochroman-6-yl)ethynyl]nicotinate.

$C_{21}H_{21}NO_2S$ = 351.5.

CAS — 118292-40-3.

Adverse Effects and Precautions

As for Tretinoin, p.1094.

Tazarotene is fetotoxic and teratogenic in *animals*. Experience in human pregnancy is very limited.

A 57-year-old man with diabetes and recalcitrant psoriasis on the trunk and limbs developed acute dermatitis[1] in the genital area two weeks after starting treatment with topical tazarotene 0.1%. The affected areas became ulcerated over the next few days. It was suspected that accidental contact with the tazarotene that had been applied to the truncal psoriasis was responsible.

1. Wollina U. Genital ulcers in a psoriasis patient using topical tazarotene. *Br J Dermatol* 1998; **138:** 713–14.

Uses and Administration

Tazarotene is a retinoid used for the topical treatment of mild to moderate acne (p.1072) and plaque psoriasis (p.1075). Tazarotene is a prodrug that is de-esterified in the skin to its active form, tazarotenic acid. The mode of action of tazarotenic acid in acne and psoriasis is unknown but it appears to modulate cell proliferation and differentiation.

In the treatment of psoriasis, tazarotene is applied as a 0.05% or 0.1% gel once daily in the evening. In the UK it is recommended that tazarotene should not be used in patients with psoriasis affecting more than 10% of the body surface; in the USA, it may be used on psoriasis involving up to 20% of the body surface.

In the treatment of acne, tazarotene is applied as a 0.1% gel once daily in the evening.

There may be exacerbation of acne during early treatment or of psoriasis at any time during treatment.

General reviews.

1. Foster RH, *et al.* Tazarotene. *Drugs* 1998; **55:** 705–11.

Preparations

Proprietary Preparations (details are given in Part 3)

Swed.: Zorac; ***UK:*** Zorac; ***USA:*** Tazorac.

Thioglycollic Acid (15327-n)

Mercaptoacetic acid.

$C_2H_4O_2S$ = 92.12.

CAS — 68-11-1.

Calcium Thioglycollate (1599-d)

Calcium Mercaptoacetate. Calcium mercaptoacetate trihydrate.

$C_2H_2CaO_2S,3H_2O$ = 184.2.

CAS — 814-71-1.

Thioglycollic acid is used, usually as the calcium salt, in depilatory preparations. Thioglycollates are also used in hair waving or straightening products together with potassium bromate as the neutraliser. There have been reports of skin reactions associated with the use of thioglycollates.

Thioxolone (1654-j)

Thioxolone *(BAN)*.

Tioxolone *(rINN)*; OL-110. 6-Hydroxy-1,3-benzoxathiol-2-one; 4-Hydroxy-1,3-benzoxathiol-2-one.

$C_7H_4O_3S$ = 168.2.

CAS — 4991-65-5.

Pharmacopoeias. In *Pol.*

Thioxolone has been used topically in the treatment of various skin and scalp disorders.

Preparations

Proprietary Preparations (details are given in Part 3)
Ital.: Wasacne†; ***Swed.:*** Camyna†.

Multi-ingredient: ***Ger.:*** Dexa Loscon†; Loscon; Psoil†; ***Switz.:*** Dexa Loscon†.

Titanium Dioxide (1655-z)

CI Pigment White 6; Colour Index No. 77891; E171; Titanii Dioxidum; Titanium Oxide.

TiO_2 = 79.87.

CAS — 13463-67-7.

Pharmacopoeias. In *Eur.* (see p.viii), *Jpn*, and *US.*

A white or almost white odourless powder.

Practically **insoluble** in water and dilute mineral acids; dissolves slowly in hot sulphuric acid; dissolves in hydrofluoric acid; it is rendered soluble by fusion with potassium bisulphate and alkali hydroxides or carbonates. A 10% suspension in water is neutral to litmus.

Titanium dioxide has an action on the skin similar to that of zinc oxide (p.1096) and has similar uses. Titanium peroxide and titanium salicylate are used in combination with titanium dioxide for napkin rash. Titanium dioxide reflects ultraviolet light and is used in sunscreens. It is also an ingredient of some cosmetics. It is used to pigment and opacify hard gelatin capsules and tablet coatings and as a delustring agent for regenerated cellulose and other man-made fibres. Specially purified grades may be used in food colours.

Preparations

Proprietary Preparations (details are given in Part 3)
Austral.: Sunsense Low Irritant; UV Triplegard Low Allergenic; ***Canad.:*** Baby Block; Life Brand Natural Source; Marcelle Protective Block; Neutrogena Sunblocker; Presun; Special Defense Sun Block; Sunblock; ***UK:*** Coppertone Sunstick; ***USA:*** Hawaiian Tropic Protective Tanning; Neutrogena Chemical-Free; TI Baby Natural; TI Screen Natural.

Multi-ingredient: numerous preparations are listed in Part 3.

Tretinoin (1656-c)

Tretinoin *(BAN, USAN, rINN)*.

NSC-122758; Retinoic Acid; Tretinoinum; Vitamin A Acid. *all-trans*-Retinoic acid; 15-Apo-β-caroten-15-oic acid; 3,7-Dimethyl-9-(2,6,6-trimethylcyclohex-1-enyl)nona-2,4,6,8-*all-trans*-tetraenoic acid.

$C_{20}H_{28}O_2$ = 300.4.

CAS — 302-79-4.

Pharmacopoeias. In *Eur.* (see p.viii) and *US.*

A yellow to light-orange crystalline powder.

Practically **insoluble** in water; slightly soluble in alcohol and chloroform; sparingly soluble in ether; soluble in dichloromethane. It is very sensitive to light, heat, and air, especially in solution.

Store at a temperature not greater than 25° in airtight containers. Protect from light. The Ph. Eur. recommends that the contents of an opened container should be used as soon as possible and any unused portion should be protected by an atmosphere of an inert gas. The USP specifies that all the contents should preferably be stored under an atmosphere of an inert gas.

Adverse Effects

Tretinoin is a skin irritant. Topical application may cause transitory stinging and a feeling of warmth and in normal use it produces some erythema and peeling similar to that of mild sunburn. Sensitive individuals may experience oedema, blistering, and crusting of the skin. Excessive application can cause severe erythema, peeling, and discomfort with no increase in efficacy. Photosensitivity may occur. Temporary hypopigmentation and hyperpigmentation have been reported.

Oral administration of tretinoin may produce similar adverse effects to those of isotretinoin (see p.1084). Cardiac arrhythmias may also occur.

Carcinogenicity. Studies in *mice* suggested that tretinoin could enhance photocarcinogenesis.[1] However, other studies refuted this[2] and evidence indicates that topical tretinoin is not carcinogenic in humans.

1. Epstein JH. Chemicals and photocarcinogenesis. *Australas J Dermatol* 1977; **18:** 57–61.
2. Epstein JH. All-trans-retinoic acid and cutaneous cancers. *J Am Acad Dermatol* 1986; **15:** 772–8.

Effects on the blood. For reports of leucocytosis and multiple thrombosis occurring in patients given oral tretinoin for the treatment of acute promyelocytic leukaemia, see Isotretinoin, p.1084.

Effects on the endocrine system. Symptoms typical of the premenstrual syndrome followed by vaginal bleeding in a 64-year-old woman were reported to be associated with the topical application of tretinoin[1] but others doubted a causal relationship.[2]

1. Meurehg CC, Xóchitl Amelio P. Vaginal bleeding and tretinoin cream. *Ann Intern Med* 1990; **113:** 483.
2. Worobec SM, *et al.* Topical tretinoin and vaginal bleeding. *Ann Intern Med* 1991, **114:** 97.

Effects on the musculoskeletal system. For a report of myositis occurring in a patient receiving oral tretinoin, see Isotretinoin, p.1084.

Effects on the nervous system. Oral retinoids may produce neurotoxic adverse effects. Children seem to be particularly sensitive to the CNS effects of tretinoin.[1,2] Neurotoxicity (ataxia, dysarthria, and headache) has been reported in a woman with liver impairment using topical tretinoin 0.025% for acne.[3]

1. Warrell RP, *et al.* Acute promyelocytic leukemia. *N Engl J Med* 1993; **329:** 177–89.
2. Mahmoud HH, *et al.* Tretinoin toxicity in children with acute promyelocytic leukaemia. *Lancet* 1993; **342:** 1394–5.
3. Bernstein AL, Leventhal-Rochon JL. Neurotoxicity related to the use of topical tretinoin (Retin-A). *Ann Intern Med* 1996; **124:** 227–8.

Retinoic acid syndrome. A syndrome consisting primarily of fever and respiratory distress developed in 9 of 35 patients between 2 and 21 days after starting induction therapy with oral tretinoin for suspected acute promyelocytic leukaemia.[1] Other symptoms included weight gain, oedema of the lower extremities, pleural or pericardial effusions, and episodic hypotension. Symptoms were life-threatening in 5 patients, 3 of whom subsequently died of multi-system failure. Leucocytosis was frequently, although not invariably, associated with development of the syndrome. Experience showed that early treatment with high-dose corticosteroids should be given to these patients irrespective of the leucocyte count.

A review[2] of this syndrome, known as the 'retinoic acid syndrome', reported that it occurs in about 25% of patients with acute promyelocytic leukaemia treated with tretinoin and that the median time to onset is 10 to 12 days after the start of treatment; the severity of the syndrome varies greatly. A high leucocyte count at diagnosis or a rapidly-increasing count on initiation of therapy increase the likelihood of the syndrome occurring. Close monitoring of leucocyte counts and clinical signs is recommended with the initiation of high-dose intravenous corticosteroids, and possibly the use of antineoplastic drugs, if symptoms appear or the leucocyte count increases rapidly.

1. Frankel SR, *et al.* The "retinoic acid syndrome" in acute promyelocytic leukemia. *Ann Intern Med* 1992; **117:** 292–6.
2. Fenaux P, De Botton S. Retinoic acid syndrome: recognition, prevention and management. *Drug Safety* 1998; **18:** 273–9.

Precautions

Tretinoin is contra-indicated in pregnancy and in breast-feeding mothers.

Contact of tretinoin with the eyes, mouth, or other mucous surfaces should be avoided. It should not be applied to eczematous, sunburnt, or abraded skin an[d] [s]hould not be applied at the same time as other [topical] treatment, especially with keratolytics. Ex[posure to] UV light and excessive exposure to sun[light should] be avoided.

Absorption does not seem to occur to any great extent with topical use. When tretinoin is given by mouth the precautions described under isotretinoin (see p.1085) should be adopted.

Tretinoin should not be applied at the same time as other topical treatment. The use of depilatory products should also be avoided. Erosions of the skin occurred in 2 patients after the use of wax depilation on facial areas also being treated topically with tretinoin.[1]

1. Goldberg NS, Zalka AD. Retin-A and wax epilation. *Arch Dermatol* 1989; **125:** 1717.

Pregnancy. Although there have been isolated reports[1-4] of congenital abnormalities in infants born to mothers who used tretinoin 0.05% topically before and during pregnancy, studies involving 215 women[5] and 94 women,[6] respectively showed no increased risk for major congenital disorders in infants who had been exposed in the first trimester.

1. Camera G, Pregliasco P. Ear malformation in baby born to mother using tretinoin cream. *Lancet* 1992; **339:** 687.
2. Lipson AH, *et al.* Multiple congenital defects associated with maternal use of topical tretinoin. *Lancet* 1993; **341:** 1352–3.
3. Navarre-Belhassen C, *et al.* Multiple congenital malformations associated with topical tretinoin. *Ann Pharmacother* 1998; **32:** 505–6.
4. Colley SMJ, *et al.* Topical tretinoin and fetal malformations. *Med J Aust* 1998; **168:** 467.
5. Jick SS, *et al.* First trimester topical tretinoin and congenital disorders. *Lancet* 1993; **341:** 1181–2.
6. Shapiro L, *et al.* Safety of first-trimester exposure to topical tretinoin: prospective cohort study. *Lancet* 1997; **350:** 1143–4.

Interactions

As for Isotretinoin, p.1085.

Tretinoin is metabolised by microsomal liver enzymes therefore there is a potential for interaction between oral tretinoin and inhibitors or inducers of these enzymes.

Minoxidil. Percutaneous absorption of minoxidil is enhanced by tretinoin as a result of increased stratum corneum permeability.[1]

1. Ferry JJ, *et al.* Influence of tretinoin on the percutaneous absorption of minoxidil from an aqueous topical solution. *Clin Pharmacol Ther* 1990; **47:** 439–46.

Pharmacokinetics

Following oral administration tretinoin is well absorbed from the gastro-intestinal tract and peak plasma concentrations are obtained after 1 to 2 hours. Oral bioavailability is about 50%. Tretinoin is highly bound to plasma proteins. It undergoes metabolism in the liver. Metabolites include isotretinoin, 4-oxo-*trans*-retinoic acid, and 4-oxo-*cis*-retinoic acid. The terminal elimination half-life of tretinoin is 0.5 to 2 hours. Tretinoin is excreted in the bile and the urine.

References.

1. Regazzi MB, *et al.* Clinical pharmacokinetics of tretinoin. *Clin Pharmacokinet* 1997; **32:** 382–402.

Uses and Administration

Tretinoin is a retinoid and is the acid form of vitamin A (p.1358).

Tretinoin is used primarily in the topical treatment of acne vulgaris in which comedones, papules, and pustules predominate. It appears to stimulate mitosis and turnover of follicular epithelial cells and reduce their cohesiveness thereby facilitating the extrusion of existing comedones and preventing the formation of new ones. It also appears to have a thinning effect on the stratum corneum. Tretinoin is applied as a cream, gel, or alcoholic solution, usually containing 0.01 to 0.10%. The skin should be cleansed to remove excessive oiliness and dried 15 to 30 minutes before applying tretinoin lightly, once or twice daily according to response and irritation; some patients may require less frequent applications. Other topical preparations (including skin moisturisers) should not be applied at the same time as an application of tretinoin, and caution is required if other local irritants are used concurrently but applications of tretinoin can be alternated with applications of benzoyl peroxide with an interval of 12 or 24 hours between each application. There may be apparent exacerbations of the acne during early treatment and a therapeutic response may not be evident for 6 to 8 weeks. When the condition has resolved maintenance therapy should be less frequent.

A preparation containing tretinoin 0.05% is available for the treatment of mottled hyperpigmentation, roughness, and fine wrinkling of photodamaged skin. It is applied once daily at night. Effects may not be seen until about 6 months after starting treatment.

Tretinoin is also used in attempts to induce remission in acute promyelocytic leukaemia. A daily dose of 45 mg per m^2 body-surface is given by mouth in 2 divided doses. Treatment is continued until remission occurs or 90 days of treatment have been given.

General reviews.

1. Orfanos CE, *et al.* Current use and future potential role of retinoids in dermatology. *Drugs* 1997; **53:** 358–88.

Neoplastic disorders. A number of retinoids have been shown to act against leukaemic cells. Their mode of action is not precisely understood, but it involves induction of differentiation in neoplastic cells.[1] Tretinoin given by *mouth* has produced complete remissions in more than 80% of patients with **acute promyelocytic leukaemia.**[2-8] However the duration of remission is short unless consolidation, usually with an anthracycline- and cytarabine-based regimen, is given subsequently; prolonged maintenance with tretinoin is unhelpful and resistance may develop. The combination of tretinoin followed by chemotherapy has been shown to result in improved survival compared with chemotherapy alone.[6,7,9] Combination of tretinoin with a colony-stimulating factor may improve response.[10] A life-threatening syndrome has developed in some patients who have received oral tretinoin for acute promyelocytic leukaemia (see under Adverse Effects, above). Children seem particularly sensitive to the adverse effects of oral tretinoin on the CNS (see also under Adverse Effects, above). For a discussion of the overall treatment of acute promyelocytic leukaemia, see under Acute Non-lymphoblastic Leukaemia, p.479.

Tretinoin has also been tried for the *topical* treatment of various neoplastic and related **skin disorders**. Some beneficial effects have been reported in the treatment of actinic keratoses, basal cell carcinoma, metastatic melanoma, and dysplastic naevi.[11-13] It also appears to be of use for the treatment of warts and solar keratoses in organ transplant recipients.[14]

1. Warrell RP, *et al.* Acute promyelocytic leukemia. *N Engl J Med* 1993; **329:** 177–89.
2. Warrell RP, *et al.* Differentiation therapy of acute promyelocytic leukemia with tretinoin (all-trans-retinoic acid). *N Engl J Med* 1991; **324:** 1385–93.
3. Huang M-E, *et al.* Use of all-trans retinoic acid in the treatment of acute promyelocytic leukemia. *Blood* 1988; **72:** 567–72.
4. Castaigne S, *et al.* All-trans retinoic acid as a differentiation therapy for acute promyelocytic leukemia I: clinical results. *Blood* 1990; **76:** 1704–9.
5. Degos L, *et al.* Treatment of first relapse in acute promyelocytic leukaemia with all-trans retinoic acid. *Lancet* 1990; **336:** 1440–1.
6. Fenaux P, *et al.* Tretinoin with chemotherapy in newly diagnosed acute promyelocytic leukaemia. *Lancet* 1994; **343:** 1033.
7. Frankel SR, *et al.* All-trans retinoic acid for acute promyelocytic leukemia: results of the New York study. *Ann Intern Med* 1994; **120:** 278–86.
8. Gillis JC, Goa KL. Tretinoin: a review of its pharmacodynamic and pharmacokinetic properties and use in the management of acute promyelocytic leukaemia. *Drugs* 1995; **50:** 897–923.
9. Tallman MS, *et al.* All-trans-retinoic acid in acute promyelocytic leukemia. *N Engl J Med* 1997; **337:** 1021–8.
10. Usuki K, *et al.* Filgrastim combined with tretinoin in acute promyelocytic leukaemia. *Lancet* 1994; **343:** 803–4.
11. Meyskens FL, *et al.* Role of topical tretinoin in melanoma and dysplastic nevi. *J Am Acad Dermatol* 1986; **15:** 822–5.
12. Peck GL. Topical tretinoin in actinic keratosis and basal cell carcinoma. *J Am Acad Dermatol* 1986; **15:** 829–35.
13. Edwards L, Jaffe P. The effect of topical tretinoin on dysplastic nevi: a preliminary trial. *Arch Dermatol* 1990; **126:** 494–9.
14. Euvrard S, *et al.* Topical retinoids for warts and keratoses in transplant recipients. *Lancet* 1992; **340:** 48–9.

Skin disorders. Topical treatment with tretinoin has been tried with varying success in a wide range of cutaneous conditions. Its use in acne (p.1072) is well established. Some benefit has also been reported in rosacea[1] (p.1076), in keratinisation disorders such as Darier's disease (p.1073), in pigmentation disorders (p.1075) such as chloasma,[2] and in some neoplastic disorders (above).

A number of studies suggest that tretinoin can reverse some of the skin changes associated with chronic exposure to sunlight.[3-12] However, the effects seen during treatment are transient and the skin reverts to its pretreatment state once application stops.[13] One study found that several changes taken as indicative of an antiphoto-ageing effect, such as thickening of the skin and epidermis and an increase in the blood supply were not specific to topically applied retinoids and could equally be produced by the use of an abrasive preparation.[14]

1. Ertl GA, *et al.* A comparison of the efficacy of topical tretinoin and low-dose oral isotretinoin in rosacea. *Arch Dermatol* 1994; **130:** 319–24.
2. Griffiths CEM, *et al.* Topical tretinoin (retinoic acid) improves melasma: a vehicle-controlled, clinical trial. *Br J Dermatol* 1993; **129:** 415–21.
3. Weiss JS, *et al.* Topical tretinoin improves photoaged skin: a double-blind vehicle-controlled study. *JAMA* 1988; **259:** 527–32.
4. Leyden JJ, *et al.* Treatment of photodamaged facial skin with topical tretinoin. *J Am Acad Dermatol* 1989; **21:** 638–44.
5. Lever L, *et al.* Topical retinoic acid for treatment of solar damage. *Br J Dermatol* 1990; **122:** 91–8.
6. Berardesca E, *et al.* In vivo tretinoin-induced changes in skin mechanical properties. *Br J Dermatol* 1990; **122:** 525–9.
7. Woodley DT, *et al.* Treatment of photoaged skin with topical tretinoin increases epidermal-dermal anchoring fibrils: a preliminary report. *JAMA* 1990; **263:** 3057–9.
8. Weinstein GD, *et al.* Topical tretinoin for treatment of photodamaged skin: a multicenter study. *Arch Dermatol* 1991; **127:** 659–65.
9. Rafal ES. Topical tretinoin (retinoic acid) treatment for liver spots associated with photodamage. *N Engl J Med* 1992; **326:** 368–74.
10. Griffiths CEM, *et al.* Restoration of collagen formation in photodamaged human skin by tretinoin (retinoic acid). *N Engl J Med* 1993; **329:** 530–5.
11. Popp C, *et al.* Pretreatment of photoaged forearm skin with topical tretinoin accelerates healing of full-thickness wounds. *Br J Dermatol* 1995; **132:** 46–53.
12. Gilchrest BA. A review of skin ageing and its medical therapy. *Br J Dermatol* 1996; **135:** 867–75.
13. Anonymous. Tretinoin for sun-aged skin. *Drug Ther Bull* 1996; **34:** 55–6.
14. Marks R, *et al.* The effects of an abrasive agent on normal skin and on photoaged skin in comparison with topical tretinoin. *Br J Dermatol* 1990; **123:** 457–66.

Preparations

BP 1998: Tretinoin Gel; Tretinoin Solution;
USP 23: Tretinoin Cream; Tretinoin Gel; Tretinoin Topical Solution.

Proprietary Preparations (details are given in Part 3)
Aust.: Airol; Eudyna; Retin-A; ***Austral.:*** Airol†; Retin-A; Re-Trieve; Stieva-A; Vesanoid; ***Belg.:*** Acid A Vit†; ***Canad.:*** Renova; Retin-A; Retisol-A; Stieva-A; Vesanoid; Vitinoin; ***Fr.:*** Aberel; Effederm; Locacid; Retacnyl; Retin-A; Retinova; Retitop; Tretinoine Kefrane; Vesanoid; ***Ger.:*** Airol†; Cordes VAS; Epi-Aberel; Eudyna; Vesanoid; ***Irl.:*** Retin-A; ***Ital.:*** Airol; Relastef†; Retin-A; Vesanoid; ***Neth.:*** Acid A Vit†; Vesanoid; ***Norw.:*** Aberela; Airol†; Vesanoid; ***S.Afr.:*** Airol†; Retin-A; Vesanoid; ***Spain:*** Dermojuventus; Retirides; ***Swed.:*** Aberela; Dermairol†; Retinova; Vesanoid; ***Switz.:*** Airol; Retin-A; Vesanoid; ***UK:*** Retin-A; Retinova; Vesanoid; ***USA:*** Avita; Renova; Retin-A; Vesanoid.

Multi-ingredient: ***Aust.:*** Keratosis forte; ***Canad.:*** Stievamycin; ***Fr.:*** Antibio-Aberel; ***Ger.:*** Balisa VAS†; Carbamid + VAS; Clinesfar; Pigmanorm; Ureotop + VAS; ***Ital.:*** Apsor; ***Spain:*** Acnisdin Retinoico; Loderm Retinoico; ***Switz.:*** Creme Carbamide + VAS; Pigmanorm; Sebo-Psor; Tretinoine; Verra-med.

Trioxsalen (1657-k)

Trioxsalen *(USAN)*.

Trioxysalen *(rINN)*; NSC-71047; 4,5′,8-Trimethylpsoralen. 2,5,9-Trimethyl-7*H*-furo[3,2-g][1]benzopyran-7-one.

$C_{14}H_{12}O_3$ = 228.2.

CAS — 3902-71-4.

Pharmacopoeias. In US.

A white to off-white or greyish, odourless, crystalline solid. Practically **insoluble** in water; soluble 1 in 1150 of alcohol, 1 in 84 of chloroform, 1 in 43 of dichloromethane, and 1 in 100 of methyl isobutyl ketone. **Protect** from light.

Trioxsalen, a psoralen, is a photosensitiser used similarly to methoxsalen in photochemotherapy or PUVA therapy (p.1088).

Trioxsalen is used in idiopathic vitiligo to enhance pigmentation or increase the tolerance to sunlight in selected patients. In vitiligo a dose of 10 mg daily is given by mouth 2 to 4 hours before exposure to sunlight or ultraviolet radiation; prolonged therapy may be necessary. To increase tolerance to sunlight a dose of 10 mg daily is given 2 hours before exposure; treatment should not be continued for longer than 14 days.

Trioxsalen may also be used topically in the PUVA treatment of psoriasis.

Preparations

USP 23: Trioxsalen Tablets.

Proprietary Preparations (details are given in Part 3)
Austral.: Trisoralen; ***Canad.:*** Trisoralen; ***Ital.:*** Trisoralen; ***S.Afr.:*** Trisoralen†; ***USA:*** Trisoralen.

Triphenyl Antimony Sulphide (11585-w)

Triphenylstibinsulfid.

$C_{18}H_{15}SbS$ = 385.1.

CAS — 3958-19-8.

Triphenyl antimony sulphide has been applied topically for the treatment of a range of skin disorders including seborrhoea, acne, eczema, and minor fungal infections.

Preparations

Proprietary Preparations (details are given in Part 3)
Aust.: Sulfoform†; ***Ger.:*** Sulfoform†.

Multi-ingredient: ***Ger.:*** Sulfoform†.

Urea (2361-s)

Carbamide; Ureia; Ureum. Carbonic acid diamide.

$NH_2.CO.NH_2$ = 60.06.

CAS — 57-13-6.

Pharmacopoeias. In *Aust., Br., Chin., Cz., Eur.* (see p.viii), *Fr., Ger., Hung., Jpn, Neth., Pol., Port., Swiss,* and *US.*

Colourless, transparent, slightly hygroscopic, odourless or almost odourless, prismatic crystals, or white crystalline powder or pellets. May gradually develop a slight odour of ammonia on prolonged standing.

Very **soluble** in water; soluble in alcohol; practically insoluble in chloroform, in dichloromethane, and in ether.

Solutions in water are neutral to litmus.

Urea can cause haemolysis when mixed with blood and should never be added to whole blood for transfusion or given through the same set by which blood is being infused.

Adverse Effects and Precautions

As for Mannitol, p.900.

Urea is reported to be more irritant than mannitol.

The intravenous administration of urea may cause venous thrombosis or phlebitis at the site of injection and only large veins should be used for infusion.

Urea should not be infused into veins of the lower limbs of elderly subjects. Rapid intravenous injection of solutions of urea can cause haemolysis; the risk is reduced by using glucose or invert sugar solutions as diluent. Extreme care is essential to prevent accidental extravasation of urea infusions. Extravasation may cause sloughing or necrosis. Thrombosis may occur independently of extravasation.

Urea should not be administered with whole blood.

Topical applications may be irritant to sensitive skin.

In infants and neonates. High plasma-urea concentrations have been reported[1,2] in neonates following topical application of emollient creams containing urea. Since there was no evidence of dehydration[2,3] absorption of urea through the skin was the likely cause. Garty[4] has observed raised plasma-urea concentrations in infants with erythematous skin conditions who had not been treated with urea cream and he attributed this to dehydration due to increased insensible water loss through the damaged skin. Atherton and Harper have commented[5] that topical application of any systemically active agent to neonates is undesirable.

1. Beverley DW, Wheeler D. High plasma urea concentrations in collodion babies. *Arch Dis Child* 1986; **61:** 696–8.
2. Oudesluys-Murphy AM, van Leeuwen M. High plasma urea concentrations in collodion babies. *Arch Dis Child* 1987; **62:** 212.
3. Beverley DW, Wheeler D. High plasma urea concentration in babies with lamellar ichthyosis. *Arch Dis Child* 1986; **61:** 1245–6.
4. Garty BZ. High plasma urea concentration in babies with lamellar ichthyosis. *Arch Dis Child* 1986; **61:** 1245–6.
5. Atherton DJ, Harper JI. High plasma urea concentrations in collodion babies. *Arch Dis Child* 1987; **62:** 212.

Pregnancy. There have been reports of women suffering coagulopathy associated with urea administered for termination of pregnancy.[1,2]

1. Grundy MFB, Craven ER. Consumption coagulopathy after intra-amniotic urea. *Br Med J* 1976; **2:** 677–8.
2. Burkman RT, *et al.* Coagulopathy with midtrimester induced abortion: association with hyperosmolar urea administration. *Am J Obstet Gynecol* 1977; **127:** 533–6.

Pharmacokinetics

Urea is fairly rapidly absorbed from the gastro-intestinal tract but causes gastro-intestinal irritation. Urea is distributed into extracellular and intracellular fluids including lymph, bile, CSF, and blood. It is reported to cross the placenta, and penetrate the eye. It is excreted unchanged in the urine.

Uses and Administration

Urea is an osmotic agent similar to mannitol (p.901). It is mainly applied topically in the treatment of ichthyosis and hyperkeratotic skin disorders (p.1074). It has been used intravenously in the treatment of acute increases in intracranial pressure (p.796), due to cerebral oedema, and to decrease intra-ocular pressure in acute glaucoma (p.1387), but has been largely superseded by mannitol. Urea has also been given intra-amniotically for the termination of pregnancy (p.1412).

When applied topically urea has hydrating and keratolytic properties. In the management of ichthyosis and other dry skin disorders it is applied in creams or lotions containing 10 to 25% urea. A preparation containing 40% may be used for nail destruction.

For the reduction of raised intracranial or intra-ocular pressure, urea is given intravenously, as an infusion of a 30% solution in glucose 5 to 10% or invert sugar 10%, at a rate not exceeding 4 mL per minute, in a dose of 0.5 to 1.5 g per kg body-weight to a maximum of 2.0 g per kg daily. For children under 2 years a dose of 0.1 g per kg has been suggested. Rebound increases in intracranial and intra-ocular pressure may occur after about 12 hours.

Solutions of urea 40 to 50% have been given by intra-amniotic injection for the termination of pregnancy.

Urea labelled with carbon-13 is used in the *in vivo* diagnosis of *Helicobacter pylori* infection. A single 100-mg dose of ^{13}C-urea is taken by mouth, and a breath sample taken 30 minutes later; an excess of carbon-13 in the sample, compared with a baseline sample, indicates infection, which may predispose to peptic ulcer disease (p.1174).

Preparations

BP 1998: Urea Cream;
USP 23: Urea for Injection.

Proprietary Preparations (details are given in Part 3)
Aust.: Basodexan; Excipial U; Nubral; ***Austral.:*** Aquacare-HP; Aquacare†; Aquadrate†; Hamilton Skin Cream; Nutraplus; Urecare; Urederm; ***Canad.:*** Aqua Care†; Calmurid; Dermaflex; Nutraplus†; Onyvul†; Rhodurea†; Ti-U-Lac; Ultra Mide; Uree; Uremol; Urisec; Velvelan; ***Fr.:*** Anti-Dessechement†; Nutra Nutraplus; ***Ger.:*** Balisa†; Basodexan; Elacutan; Hyanit N; Laceran; Nubral; Onychomal; Ureotop; ***Irl.:*** Aquadrate; Nutraplus; ***Neth.:*** Alphadrate; Calmurid; ***S.Afr.:*** Eulactol†; Nutraplus†; ***Swed.:*** Calmuril; Caress; Fenuril; ***Switz.:*** Basodexan†; Excipial U; Nutraplus; ***UK:*** Aquadrate; Nutraplus; ***USA:*** Aquacare; Atrac-Tain; Carmol; Dr Scholl's Smooth Touch Deep Moisturizing Cream†; Gormel; Lanaphilic; Nutraplus; Ultra Mide; Ureacin; Ureaphil.

Multi-ingredient: ***Aust.:*** Aleot; Calmurid; Calmurid HC; Hydrodexan; Ichth-Oestren; Keratosis; Keratosis forte; Mirfulan; Mykozem; Psoradexan; ***Austral.:*** Aussie Tan Skin Moisturiser; Calmurid; Dermadrate; Psor-asist; ***Belg.:*** Alphaderm; Calmurid; ***Canad.:*** Amino-Cerv; Calmurid HC; Hydrophil; Sential†; Ti-U-Lac HC; Uremol-HC; ***Fr.:*** Amycor Onychoset; Keratosane; ***Ger.:*** Balisa VAS†; Brand- u. Wundgel-Medice N; Calmurid; Calmurid HC; Carbamid + VAS; Condilan†; Fungidexan; Grune Salbe "Schmidt" N; Hydrodexan; Jacosulfon†; Kelofibrase; Mirfulan; Mycospor Nagelset; Nubral 4 HC; Oestrugol N; Optiderm; Prolugol-liquid N†; Psoradexan; Psorigerb N; Remederm; Thrombimed†; Ureata S; Ureotop + VAS; ***Irl.:*** Alphaderm; Calmurid; Calmurid HC; Psoradrate; ***Ital.:*** Gel Tar†; Hidro Tar 30†; Optiderm; Otocaina†; Verunec 3; Xerial; ***Neth.:*** Alphacortison; Calmurid HC; Symbial; ***Norw.:*** Mycospor Carbamid; ***S.Afr.:*** Covancaine; ***Spain:*** Cortisdin Urea; Kanapomada; Mycospor Onicoset; ***Swed.:*** Calmuril-Hydrokortison; Fenuril-Hydrokortison; Mycosporan-Karbamid; ***Switz.:*** Acne Gel; Betacortone; Calmurid; Calmurid HC; Creme antikeloides; Creme Carbamide; Creme Carbamide + VAS; Kerasal; Klyx Magnum; Optiderm; Psoradexan; Sebo Creme; Sebo-Psor; Squa-med; Tretinoine; Turexan Capilla; Turexan Lotion; Undex†; ***UK:*** Alphaderm; Antipeol; Balneum Plus; Calmurid; Calmurid HC; Cymex; Psoradrate†; Sential E†; Sential HC†; St James Balm; ***USA:*** Amino-Cerv; Dayto Sulf; Fostex Medicated Cleansing Bar†; Panafil; Panafil-White.

Xenysalate Hydrochloride (1658-a)

Xenysalate Hydrochloride *(BANM, rINNM)*.

Biphenamine Hydrochloride *(USAN)*. 2-Diethylaminoethyl 3-phenylsalicylate hydrochloride; 2-Diethylaminoethyl 2-hydroxy-3-phenylbenzoate hydrochloride.

$C_{19}H_{23}NO_3,HCl$ = 349.9.

CAS — 3572-52-9 (xenysalate); 5560-62-3 (xenysalate hydrochloride).

Xenysalate hydrochloride has antibacterial and antifungal properties and has been used for the control of seborrhoeic dermatitis of the scalp.

Preparations

Proprietary Preparations (details are given in Part 3)
Fr.: Sebaklen.

Zinc Carbonate (1659-t)

Zinc Carbonate *(USAN)*.

$ZnCO_3$ = 125.4.

CAS — 3486-35-9.

Basic Zinc Carbonate (11593-w)

NOTE. The names zinc carbonate, hydrated zinc carbonate, zinc subcarbonate, and zinc carbonate hydroxide have all been applied to basic zinc carbonate of varying composition occurring naturally or produced by the reaction of a soluble zinc salt with sodium carbonate.

Pharmacopoeias. In *US.*

Basic zinc carbonate corresponds to $3Zn(OH)_2.2ZnCO_3$ containing the equivalent of not less than 70% ZnO. **Store** in airtight containers.

Zinc carbonate is mildly astringent and protective to the skin and is used topically, mainly in the form of calamine (p.1080), in a variety of skin conditions. In the USA the name calamine is used for zinc oxide (rather than zinc carbonate) with a small proportion of ferric oxide.

Preparations

Proprietary Preparations (details are given in Part 3)
Multi-ingredient: ***Fr.:*** Pygmal; ***Spain:*** Neo Visage.

Zinc Oxide (1660-l)

Blanc de Zinc; Flores de Zinc; Zinci Oxidum; Zinci Oxydum; Zincum Oxydatum.

ZnO = 81.39.

CAS — 1314-13-2.

NOTE. 'Zinc White' is a commercial form of zinc oxide for use as a pigment.

Pharmacopoeias. In *Chin., Eur.* (see p.viii), *Int., Jpn, Pol.,* and *US.*

A white or faintly yellowish-white, odourless, amorphous, soft powder, free from grittiness. It gradually absorbs carbon dioxide from air.

Practically **insoluble** in water and in alcohol; it dissolves in dilute mineral acids.

Black discoloration has been reported when zinc oxide and glycerol are in contact in the presence of light.

Uses and Administration

Zinc oxide is mildly astringent and is used topically as a soothing and protective application in eczema and slight excoriations, in wounds, and for haemorrhoids. It is also used with coal tar (p.1093) or ichthammol (p.1083) in the treatment of eczema. Zinc oxide reflects ultraviolet radiation and is used in sunscreens.

In the USA the name calamine is used for zinc oxide with a small proportion of ferric oxide.

Zinc oxide is used as the basis for the production of a number of dental cements. Mixed with phosphoric acid it forms a hard material composed largely of zinc phosphate; mixed with clove oil or eugenol, it is used as temporary dental filling.

For further details of zinc and its salts, see p.1373.

Complications of dental use. Solitary aspergillosis of the maxillary sinus in 29 of 30 patients was associated with zinc oxide from overfilled teeth.[1] Treatment consisted of removal of the fungal ball containing the zinc oxide; no antifungal treatment was necessary. Zinc oxide has been shown to accelerate the growth of *Aspergillus fumigatus.*

1. Beck-Mannagetta J, *et al.* Solitary aspergillosis of maxillary sinus, a complication of dental treatment. *Lancet* 1983; **ii:** 1260.

Preparations

BP 1998: Aqueous Calamine Cream; Calamine and Coal Tar Ointment *(Compound Calamine Ointment)*; Calamine Lotion; Coal Tar and Zinc Ointment; Coal Tar Paste; Compound Aluminium Paste *(Baltimore Paste)*; Compound Zinc Paste; Dithranol Paste; Hexachlorophene Dusting Powder *(Zinc and Hexachlorophene Dusting Powder)*; Zinc and Castor Oil Ointment; Zinc and Coal Tar Paste *(White's Tar Paste)*; Zinc and Ichthammol Cream; Zinc and Salicylic Acid Paste *(Lassar's Paste)*; Zinc Cream; Zinc Ointment;

USP 23: Calamine Lotion; Coal Tar Ointment; Compound Resorcinol Ointment; Zinc Oxide and Salicylic Acid Paste; Zinc Oxide Ointment; Zinc Oxide Paste.

Proprietary Preparations (details are given in Part 3)

Austral.: Curash Anti-Rash; Prickly Heat Powder; Zinc Cream White; Zincaband; Zink'N'Swim; Zink'N'Swim Fluorescent; ***Canad.:*** Babys Own Ointment; Diaper Rash; Herisan; Infazinc; Neoderm; Pate d'Unna; Prevex Diaper Rash Cream; Zinaderm; Zincoderm; Zincofax; ***Fr.:*** Lanofene; Oxyplastine; Senophile; ***Ger.:*** Desitin; Fissan-Zinkschuttelmixtur†; Lotio Artesan†; Robuvalen; St. Jakobs-Balsam Mono; Weiche Zinkpaste; ***Irl.:*** Coltapaste; Viscopaste PB7; ***Ital.:*** Biogena Baby†; Gelocast; Oz; Pangamma†; Varicex; Viscopaste PB7; Zinco All' Acqua; Zincotape; Zincotex; ***Neth.:*** Zinkolie; Zinkzalf; ***S.Afr.:*** Johnson's Baby Nappy Rash Ointment; Viscopaste PB7; ***Spain:*** Anticongestiva; ***Swed.:*** Mezinc†; Salvstrumpa; Zincaband; ***Switz.:*** Oxyplastine; ***UK:*** Protective Healing Cream†; Steripaste; Viscopaste PB7; Zincaband; Zipzoc; ***USA:*** Borofax; Daily Care; Diaparene Diaper Rash; Flanders Buttocks; Nupercainal.

Multi-ingredient: numerous preparations are listed in Part 3.

Zinc Phenolsulphonate (17036-g)

Zinc 4-Hydroxybenzenesulphonate. Zinc *p*-hydroxybenzenesulphonate.

$C_{12}H_{10}O_8S_2Zn$ = 411.7.

CAS — 127-82-2.

Zinc phenolsulphonate has astringent properties and has been used in multi-ingredient preparations applied topically for the treatment of a variety of disorders.

Preparations

Proprietary Preparations (details are given in Part 3)

Multi-ingredient: ***Austral.:*** BFI; ***Ital.:*** Antisettico Astringente Sedativo; Citroftalmina; Citroftalmina VC; Oftalmil; Zincosin†; ***Spain:*** Antiseptico Dent Donner†; Regal; ***Switz.:*** Medi-Kord; ***USA:*** BFI.

Disinfectants and Preservatives

This chapter describes those antimicrobial agents which are used for chemical methods of disinfection, antisepsis, preservation, and sterilisation. There is some overlap between these procedures and some agents may be used as both disinfectants and preservatives. Iodine (p.1493) is also used for its disinfectant properties.

Definition of terms. There is often confusion between the terms disinfectant and antiseptic.

- The term **disinfectant** is applied to a chemical agent which destroys or inhibits the growth of pathogenic micro-organisms in the non-sporing or vegetative state; disinfectants do not necessarily kill all micro-organisms, but reduce them to a level which is harmful neither to health nor the quality of perishable goods. The term is applicable to agents used to treat inanimate objects and materials and may also be applied to agents used to treat the skin and other body membranes and cavities
- An **antiseptic** is a disinfectant which is used on skin and other living tissues thereby limiting or preventing infection
- **Sterilisation** is the total removal or destruction of all living micro-organisms; a few disinfectants (such as ethylene oxide) are capable of producing sterility under suitable conditions but, in general, sterility is produced by heat or radiation methods, with filtration being employed for some heat-labile materials. Sterilisation by heating with a bactericide is no longer a recommended practice
- A **preservative** is one of a number of chemical agents which are included in preparations to prevent deterioration from oxidation **(antoxidants)** or to kill or inhibit the growth of micro-organisms inadvertently introduced during manufacture or use **(antimicrobial preservatives)**.

Use of disinfectants. Disinfectants are used in hospitals, industrial establishments, public buildings, on farms, and in the home for control and prevention of infection.

The choice of disinfectant depends on the purpose for which it is employed and the likely contaminating organisms. In addition to vegetative bacteria, many common disinfectants could be expected to kill some fungi and lipid-containing viruses. Gram-negative bacteria, mycobacteria, and bacterial spores are generally more resistant to disinfectants, and some disinfectants are less effective against non-lipid enveloped viruses, for example the enteroviruses including polio and coxsackie. Prions are generally resistant to many disinfectants (see Disinfection in Creutzfeldt-Jakob Disease, below). Other factors affecting the effectiveness of disinfectants include the contact time, concentration of the disinfectant, the pH of the system, the number and accessibility of the contaminating microorganisms, and the presence of interfering substances including lipids, organic matter, rubber and plastics. Aqueous solutions of disinfectants, particularly quaternary ammonium compounds (such as benzalkonium chloride and cetrimide), chlorhexidine, and phenols, may be susceptible to contamination with micro-organisms. To reduce this risk many preparations are provided for clinical use in a sterile form for single use.

Uses of preservatives. Antimicrobial preservatives are used in sterile preparations such as eye drops and multidose injections to maintain sterility during use. They may also be added to aqueous injections that cannot be sterilised in their final containers and have to be prepared using aseptic precautions, unless the volume to be injected as a single dose exceeds 15 mL. Antimicrobial preservatives are also used in cosmetics, foods, and non-sterile pharmaceutical products such as oral liquids and creams to prevent microbial spoilage. They are not used indiscriminately, and preparations that should *not* contain preservatives include those for injection into the CSF, eye, or heart. Generally, the antimicrobial preservatives that may be added to foods, animal feeding stuffs, and cosmetics are controlled.

Preservatives used as antoxidants may be classified in 3 groups. *True antoxidants*, or anti-oxygens, probably inhibit oxidation by reacting with free radicals blocking the chain reaction. Examples are the alkyl gallates, butylated hydroxyanisole, butylated hydroxytoluene, nordihydroguaiaretic acid, and the tocopherols (see Vitamin E Substances, p.1369). The second group consists of *reducing agents*; these substances have a lower redox potential than the drug or adjuvants which they are intended to protect and are therefore more readily oxidised. Reducing agents may act also by reacting with free radicals. Examples are ascorbic acid (p.1365) and the potassium and sodium salts of sulphurous acid (see Sulphites and Sulphur Dioxide). The third group consists of *antoxidant synergists* which usually have little antoxidant effect themselves but probably enhance the action of antoxidants in the first group by reacting with heavy-metal ions which catalyse oxidation. Examples of synergists are citric acid (p.1564), edetic acid and its salts (p.980), lecithin (p.1595) and tartaric acid (p.1634).

General guidelines for the use of disinfectants.

1. Committee on Health Care Issues, American Neurological Association. Precautions in handling tissues, fluids, and other contaminated materials from patients with documented or suspected Creutzfeldt-Jakob disease. *Ann Neurol* 1986; **19:** 75–7.
2. WHO. Guidelines on sterilization and disinfection methods effective against human immunodeficiency virus (HIV). *WHO AIDS Series 2* 1989.
3. BMA. *A code of practice for sterilisation of instruments and control of cross-infection.* London: BMA, 1989.
4. Ayliffe GAJ, *et al. Hospital-acquired infection: principles and prevention.* London: Wright, 1990.
5. Ayliffe GAJ, *et al. Chemical disinfection in hospitals.* 2nd ed. London: PHLS, 1993.
6. Advisory Committee on Dangerous Pathogens. *Precautions for work with human and animal transmissible spongiform encephalopathies.* London: HMSO, 1994.
7. Advisory Committee on Dangerous Pathogens. *Protection against blood-borne infections in the workplace: HIV and hepatitis.* London: HMSO, 1995.
8. Rutala WA. APIC guideline for selection and use of disinfectants. *Am J Infect Control* 1996; **24:** 313–42.

Contact lens care

Wearers of contact lenses are at increased risk of corneal infections. Factors that predispose the cornea to infection include surface abrasions which may occur during normal wear, accidental trauma during insertion of a lens, and anoxia. In addition, the lens may provide a medium for introducing pathogens into the eye, especially if handling, cleaning, and disinfecting procedures are not adhered to. The most common pathogens are bacteria, in particular *Pseudomonas aeruginosa, Serratia marcescens, Staphylococcus aureus, Staph. epidermidis,* and *Streptococcus pneumoniae.* Fungi rarely cause lens-related keratitis, although contamination of soft (hydrogel) lenses has been reported. *Acanthamoeba* can cause rare but serious corneal infections (p.573) mainly associated with soft contact lens wear. These protozoa are resistant to some commonly used disinfection systems and can colonise lens storage cases.

Lens care systems for rigid lenses typically entail cleansing and disinfection stages. Daily cleansing with solutions containing surfactants and sometimes mild abrasives can substantially reduce microbial contamination as well as removing organic material which can compromise the activity of the disinfection stage. Cleansing solutions frequently contain substances which are irritant to the eye and should be removed by rinsing and soaking the lens. Soaking solutions also maintain lens hydration, disinfect the lens, and prevent contamination during storage. Although not intended for introduction into the eye, soaking solutions should be non-irritant. Commonly used disinfectants include benzalkonium chloride and chlorhexidine. Thiomersal is also used but has been associated with a high incidence of hypersensitivity reactions. Wetting or rewetting solutions are used to improve the comfort of the lens and, since they are applied to the eye, must be non-irritant. They commonly contain hypromellose, hydroxyethylcellulose, polyvinyl alcohol, or povidone, although a simple sodium chloride 0.9% solution may be used.

Soft contact lenses contain a high proportion of water and are liable to absorb substances from solution. For this reason some disinfectants, notably benzalkonium chloride, are not suitable for inclusion in solutions for soft lenses. Soft lenses may be disinfected by heating in a suitable unit, usually in isotonic saline solution, but this can shorten the life of the lens by denaturing the polymer or causing deposits of denatured protein, minerals, or preservatives from the saline solution. Stabilised hydrogen peroxide is suitable for cold disinfection of soft lenses and is particularly useful for preventing *Acanthamoeba* infections. However, it is irritant to the cornea and must be neutralised before the lens is inserted into the eye. Other suitable disinfectants for soft lenses include chlorhexidine and polyhexanide. Cleansers for soft lenses may contain surfactants or enzymes such as papain or pancreatin which remove protein deposits.

Disinfection in Creutzfeldt-Jakob disease

Creutzfeldt-Jakob disease is a transmissible spongiform encephalopathy believed to be caused by infection of the nervous system with prions. The agent causing Creutzfeldt-Jakob disease (CJD) is resistant to many disinfection procedures including ultraviolet irradiation, alcohol, eusol, formaldehyde, and iodine.[1] Although no sterilisation procedure can be guaranteed to be completely effective under all circumstances,[2-4] those usually recommended are autoclaving at 132° for at least 30 minutes[5] or at 134 to 138° for 18 minutes,[5,6] immersion in 1N sodium hydroxide[7,8] (also in combination with autoclaving at 121° for 30 minutes[5]), or in sodium hypochlorite 0.5%[9] for 1 hour. The Department of Health in the UK recommend that neurosurgical and ophthalmic instruments should be destroyed if used in patients with confirmed or suspected CJD.[6] Suggested prophylaxis for individuals after accidental exposure to human prions involves immediate decontamination of intact skin sites with sodium hypochlorite or sodium hydroxide solutions followed by copious rinsing; if skin penetration has occurred, surgical excision of the site of inoculation combined with a course of systemic corticosteroids is proposed.[10]

1. Patterson WB, *et al.* Occupational hazards to hospital personnel. *Ann Intern Med* 1985; **102:** 658–80.
2. Russell AD, *et al. Principles and practice of disinfection, preservation, and sterilization.* 2nd ed. Oxford: Blackwell, 1992.
3. Taylor DM, Bell JE. Prevention of iatrogenic transmission of Creutzfeldt-Jakob disease. *Lancet* 1993; **341:** 1543–4.
4. Taylor DM. Inactivation of SE agents. *Br Med Bull* 1993; **49:** 810–21.
5. Rutala WA. APIC guideline for selection and use of disinfectants. *Am J Infect Control* 1996; **24:** 313–42.
6. Wight AL. Prevention of iatrogenic transmission of Creutzfeldt-Jakob disease. *Lancet* 1993; **341:** 1543.
7. Committee on Health Care Issues, American Neurological Association. Precautions in handling tissues, fluids, and other contaminated materials from patients with documented or suspected Creutzfeldt-Jakob disease. *Ann Neurol* 1986; **19:** 75–7.
8. Brown P, *et al.* Sodium hydroxide decontamination of Creutzfeldt-Jakob disease virus. *N Engl J Med* 1984; **310:** 727.
9. Brown P, *et al.* Chemical disinfection of Creutzfeldt-Jakob disease virus. *N Engl J Med* 1982; **306:** 1279–81.
10. Aguzzi A, Collinge J. Post-exposure prophylaxis after accidental prion inoculation. *Lancet* 1997; **350:** 1519–20.

Disinfection of endoscopes

Whenever possible, medical equipment which comes into intimate contact with the body should be heat sterilised, but some equipment, notably endoscopes, will not withstand high temperatures. Low-temperature steam and formaldehyde or ethylene oxide will achieve sterilisation, but may not be practical in a clinical setting. Satisfactory chemical disinfection of endoscopes and other heat-sensitive instruments relies on initial thorough cleansing of the instrument and choice of an appropriate disinfectant which should be rapidly active against a wide range of pathogens including vegetative bacteria, bacterial spores, mycobacteria, and viruses. The disinfectant should not damage the instrument or discolour the optical components, and it should not leave a toxic residue. It is usually necessary to rinse the instrument with sterile water or alcohol after disinfection.[1-3]

Glutaraldehyde 2% is commonly used.[2] To achieve sterilisation, immersion in glutaraldehyde 2% for 3 hours is necessary, but high-level disinfection, achieved by immersion for 10 to 20 minutes, is usually considered adequate for most endoscopes.[2,4,5] Immersion for a minimum of 20 minutes is required for elimination of tubercle bacilli, but immersion for 4 minutes may be adequate for gastroscopes, except for use on immunocompromised patients. Other recommended specific immersion times are 60 minutes for bronchoscopes before use on immunocompromised patients,[1] and 90 to 120 minutes after bronchoscopy on known or suspected infections with *Mycobacterium avium* complex.[2]

A disadvantage of glutaraldehyde is that it is irritant and may cause sensitisation. In addition, glutaraldehyde-resistant strains of *M. chelonae* have been isolated from endoscope disinfecting equipment.[6] Alternative disinfectants include peracetic acid, chlorine dioxide, and superoxidised water.[5] Other alternatives include peroxygen compounds, a quaternary ammonium compound followed by alcohol, succinic dialdehyde, povidone-iodine, and alcohol 70%.[2,5,7,8] However, peracetic acid and chlorine dioxide produce irritant fumes, peroxygen-containing compounds and quaternary ammonium compounds have questionable activity against mycobacteria and viruses, and alcohol and povidone-iodine have a number of practical limitations.[5,9]

1. Woodcock A, *et al.* Bronchoscopy and infection control. *Lancet* 1989; **ii:** 270–1.
2. Ayliffe GAJ, *et al. Chemical disinfection in hospitals.* 2nd ed. London: PHLS, 1993.
3. Ryan CK, Potter GD. Disinfectant colitis: rinse as well as you wash. *J Clin Gastroenterol* 1995; **21:** 6–9.
4. American Society for Gastrointestinal Endoscopy. Reprocessing of flexible gastrointestinal endoscopes. *Gastrointest Endosc* 1996; **43:** 540–6.
5. British Society of Gastroenterology Working Party. Cleaning and disinfection of equipment for gastrointestinal endoscopy. *Gut* 1998; **42:** 585–93.
6. Griffiths PA, *et al.* Glutaraldehyde-resistant Mycobacterium chelonae from endoscope washer disinfectors. *J Appl Microbiol* 1997; **82:** 519–26.
7. Axon ATR, Cotton PB. Endoscopy and infection. *Gut* 1983; **24:** 1064–6.
8. Fraise AP. Disinfection in endoscopy. *Lancet* 1995; **346:** 787–8.
9. Ridgway GL. Decontamination of fibreoptic endoscopes. *J Hosp Infect* 1985; **6:** 363–8.

Disinfection of water

Travellers to regions of the world where water is not disinfected at source should be advised to boil or chemically sterilise water for drinking, cleaning teeth, and washing fruit and vegetables. Chlorine-releasing disinfectants including chloramine, halazone, sodium dichloroisocyanurate, and sodium hypochlorite are commonly used. Iodine-releasing disinfectants such as tetraglycine hydroperiodide or iodine itself are also sometimes used. Organic material suspended in the water may reduce the available halogen concentration, and cloudy water should be filtered or allowed to settle and decanted before treatment. Emergency treatment of drinking water with lemon juice has been suggested during epidemics of waterborne gastro-enteritis.[1] Chlorine-releasing disinfectants are also used for recreational and therapeutic bathing pools, often in combination with ozone.[2]

Legionnaires' disease (p.128) is commonly transmitted via cooling water in air conditioning systems or hot water supplies. Hyperchlorination has been attempted to eradicate the organism from contaminated water sources but has been largely ineffective[3,4] and is no longer recommended. Other disadvantages of using chlorine-based systems at these temperatures and concentrations are corrosion of the plumbing system[4] and the production of potentially carcinogenic byproducts.[5] Effective disinfection can be achieved by raising the water temperature, ultraviolet light, and copper-silver ionisation.

1. D'Aquino M, Teves SA. Lemon juice as a natural biocide for disinfecting drinking water. *Bull Pan Am Health Organ* 1994; **28:** 324–30.
2. Dadswell JV. Managing swimming, spa, and other pools to prevent infection. *Commun Dis Rep* 1996; **6** (review 2): R37–R40.
3. Kurtz JB, *et al.* Legionella pneumophila in cooling water systems: report of a survey of cooling towers in London and a pilot trial of selected biocides. *J Hyg (Camb)* 1982; **88:** 369–81.
4. Helms CM, *et al.* Legionnaires' disease associated with a hospital water system: a five-year progress report on continuous hyperchlorination. *JAMA* 1988; **259:** 2423–7.
5. Morris RD, *et al.* Chlorination, chlorination by-products, and cancer: a meta-analysis. *Am J Public Health* 1992; **82:** 955–63.

Injection site and catheter care

The need to disinfect the skin before injection is controversial.[1] Routine skin preparation of the injection site by swabbing with antiseptic has been reported to be both ineffective and unnecessary.[2,3] Central venous and arterial catheters, however, require the application of strict aseptic technique and injection site antisepsis to reduce the chance of infection.[4] Disinfection of catheter insertion sites with aqueous chlorhexidine 2% has been reported to be associated with fewer local and systemic infections than site preparation with either 10% povidone-iodine solution or 70% isopropyl alcohol,[5] although this has been challenged.[6] A subsequent study reported lower rates of catheter colonisation and catheter-related infection with an alcoholic solution of chlorhexidine 0.25% and benzalkonium chloride 0.025% than with povidone-iodine 10%.[7] In a study in preterm infants, technique had greater influence on bacterial counts at injection sites than the antiseptic used; chlorhexidine 0.5% in isopropyl alcohol and aqueous povidone-iodine 10% were equally effective, but cleansing with alcoholic chlorhexidine for 30 seconds or for two 10-second periods was more effective than cleansing for 5 or 10 seconds.[8]

The use of catheters impregnated with antiseptics has also been studied. Failure of chlorhexidine-coated catheters to prevent catheter-related infections in a study in patients in intensive care was attributed to inactivation of the chlorhexidine by the gamma radiation sterilisation used.[9] A study in patients undergoing central venous catheterisation found that, while the use of catheters coated with chlorhexidine and silver sulphadiazine reduced bacterial growth at the catheter tip, it had no effect on the incidence of catheter-related bacteraemia.[10] A more favourable result was reported with similarly impregnated catheters in another study: bacteraemia was about one-fifth of that seen in control patients.[11]

1. Ayliffe GAJ, *et al. Chemical disinfection in hospitals.* 2nd ed. London: PHLS, 1993.
2. Dann TC. Routine skin preparation before injection: an unnecessary procedure. *Lancet* 1969; **ii:** 96–8.
3. Liauw J, Archer GJ. Swabaholics? *Lancet* 1995; **345:** 1648.
4. Shepherd A, Williams N. Care of long-term central venous catheters. *Br J Hosp Med* 1994; **51:** 598–602.
5. Maki DG, *et al.* Prospective randomised trial of povidone-iodine, alcohol, and chlorhexidine for prevention of infection associated with central venous and arterial catheters. *Lancet* 1991; **338:** 339–43.
6. Segura M, Sitges-Serra A. Intravenous catheter sites and sepsis. *Lancet* 1991; **338:** 1218.
7. Mimoz O, *et al.* Prospective, randomized trial of two antiseptic solutions for prevention of central venous or arterial catheter colonization and infection in intensive care unit patients. *Crit Care Med* 1996; **24:** 1818–23.
8. Malathi I, *et al.* Skin disinfection in preterm infants. *Arch Dis Child* 1993; **69:** 312–16.
9. Sherertz RJ, *et al.* Gamma radiation-sterilized, triple-lumen catheters coated with a low concentration of chlorhexidine were not efficacious at preventing catheter infections in intensive care unit patients. *Antimicrob Agents Chemother* 1996; **40:** 1995–7.
10. Heard SO, *et al.* Influence of triple-lumen central venous catheters coated with chlorhexidine and silver sulfadiazine on the incidence of catheter-related bacteremia. *Arch Intern Med* 1998; **158:** 81–7.
11. Maki DG, *et al.* Prevention of central venous catheter-related bloodstream infection by use of an antiseptic-impregnated catheter: a randomized, controlled trial. *Ann Intern Med* 1997; **127:** 257–66.

Wound disinfection

Antiseptic preparations are widely used to treat or prevent superficial infections, but their usefulness on broken skin and wounds has been questioned.[1] Antiseptic solutions are commonly used to clean wounds (p.1076) but are of doubtful value. Chlorine-releasing antiseptic solutions are generally regarded as irritant and although there is little direct evidence in patients there is concern that they may delay wound healing. Cetrimide,[2] chloramine,[3] hydrogen peroxide 3%,[4] iodophores,[4] and sodium hypochlorite solutions[2] are all reported to be cytotoxic to *in vitro* or in *animal* models. Long term or repeated use of these antiseptics for wound toilet should probably be avoided. Chlorhexidine is relatively non-toxic.[2,3]

1. Brown CD, Zitelli JA. A review of topical agents for wounds and methods of wounding: guidelines for wound management. *J Dermatol Surg Oncol* 1993; **19:** 732–7.
2. Thomas S, Hay NP. Wound cleansing. *Pharm J* 1985; **2:** 206.
3. Brennan SS, *et al.* Antiseptic toxicity in wounds healing by secondary intention. *J Hosp Infect* 1986; **8:** 263–7.
4. Lineweaver W, *et al.* Topical antimicrobial toxicity. *Arch Surg* 1985; **120:** 267–70.

Acridine Derivatives (12107-e)

A group of quinoline antimicrobial dyes structurally related to acridine.

Acriflavine (2201-c)

Acriflavinium Chloride *(rINN)*; Acriflavine Hydrochloride. A mixture of 3,6-diamino-10-methylacridinium chloride hydrochloride and 3,6-diaminoacridine dihydrochloride.

CAS — 8063-24-9; 65589-70-0.

NOTE. Distinguish from euflavine.

Pharmacopoeias. In *Aust. Swiss* includes separate monographs for the hydrochloride and the dihydrochloride.

Aminacrine Hydrochloride (2204-t)

Aminacrine Hydrochloride *(BANM, USAN)*.

Aminoacridine Hydrochloride *(rINNM)*; NSC-7571. 9-Aminoacridine hydrochloride monohydrate.

$C_{13}H_{10}N_2,HCl,H_2O = 248.7.$

CAS — 90-45-9 (aminacrine); 134-50-9 (aminacrine hydrochloride, anhydrous).

Ethacridine Lactate (2243-m)

Ethacridine Lactate *(rINNM)*.

Acrinol; Aethacridinium Lacticum; Lactoacridine. 6,9-Diamino-2-ethoxyacridine lactate.

$C_{15}H_{15}N_3O,C_3H_6O_3 = 343.4.$

CAS — 442-16-0 (ethacridine); 1837-57-6 (ethacridine lactate).

Pharmacopoeias. In *Pol.* and *Swiss*; in *Aust., Ger.,* and *Jpn* as monohydrate.

Euflavine (2245-v)

Neutral Acriflavine; Neutroflavin. A mixture of 3,6-diamino-10-methylacridinium chloride and 3,6-diaminoacridine monohydrochloride. The latter is usually present to the extent of between 30 and 40%.

CAS — 68518-47-8.

NOTE. Distinguish from acriflavine.

Proflavine Hemisulphate (2271-q)

Proflavine Hemisulphate *(pINNM)*.

Neutral Proflavine Sulphate. 3,6-Diaminoacridine sulphate dihydrate.

$(C_{13}H_{11}N_3)_2,H_2SO_4,2H_2O = 552.6.$

CAS — 92-62-6 (proflavine).

The acridine derivatives are slow-acting antiseptics. They are bacteriostatic against many Gram-positive bacteria but less effective against Gram-negative bacteria. They are ineffective against spores. Their activity is increased in alkaline solutions and is not reduced by tissue fluids.

The acridine derivatives have been used for the treatment of infected wounds or burns and for skin disinfection although they have been largely superseded by other antiseptics or suitable antibacterials (p.142). Prolonged treatment may delay healing. They have also been used for the treatment of local ear, oropharyngeal, and genito-urinary infections.

Aminacrine hydrochloride which is reported to be non-staining has been used most recently as eye drops in the treatment and prophylaxis of superficial eye infections.

Ethacridine lactate has been included in some preparations for the treatment of diarrhoea. It has also been given by extra-amniotic injection for the termination of pregnancy (p.1412) but other methods are usually preferred.

Hypersensitivity to acridine derivatives has been reported.

Preparations

BPC 1973: Proflavine Cream *(Flavine Cream)*.

Proprietary Preparations (details are given in Part 3)

Austral.: Aminopt; ***Ger.:*** Biseptol simplex; Gelastypt M†; Metifex; Neochinosol; Panflavin; Rivanol; Urocridin; ***UK:*** Burn-aid†.

Multi-ingredient: ***Aust.:*** Dermowund; Tebege-Tannin; Tonexol; ***Austral.:*** Calistaflex†; Mac†; Medijel; ***Canad.:*** AVC/Dienestrol†; ***Fr.:*** Chromargon; Pyorex; ***Ger.:*** Anaesthesin-Rivanol; Biseptol compositum†; Cholosom†; Nordapanin N; Otolitan N mit Rivanol; Perflamint†; Stas Halstabletten†; Tannacomp; Tectivit†; ***Irl.:*** Aidex†; ***S.Afr.:*** Achromide; Daromide†; Masse†; Vagarsol; ***Spain:*** Antigrietun; Bucodrin; Hepro; ***Switz.:*** Anginol; Flavangin; Haemocortin; Haemolan; Tonexol†; Tyrothricin; ***UK:*** Bonjela; Medijel; ***USA:*** Alasulf; Benegyn†; Deltavac; DIT1-2; Vagisec Plus†.

Alcohol (551-f)

Aethanolum; Alcool; Ethanol; Ethanol (96 per cent); Ethanolum; Ethyl Alcohol.

C_2H_5OH = 46.07.

CAS — 64-17-5.

Pharmacopoeias. In *Chin., Eur.* (see p.viii), *Int., Jpn, Pol.,* and *US.*

Eur. specifies under Ethanol (96 per cent) not less than 95.1% and not more than 96.9% v/v; 92.6 to 95.2% w/w of C_2H_5OH. *US* specifies under Alcohol not less than 94.9% and not more than 96.0% v/v; 92.3 to 93.8% w/w of C_2H_5OH.

In *Martindale* the term alcohol is used for alcohol 95 or 96% v/v.

A mixture of ethyl alcohol and water. A clear, colourless, mobile, volatile, hygroscopic liquid with a characteristic spirituous odour and burning taste; readily flammable, burning with a smokeless blue flame.

Miscible with water (with rise of temperature and contraction of volume), with chloroform, with ether, with glycerol, and with almost all other organic solvents. **Store** at 8° to 15° away from fire in airtight containers. Protect from light.

Anhydrous Ethanol (Ph. Eur.) (Absolute Alcohol; Dehydrated Alcohol) contains not less than 99.5% v/v or 99.2% w/w of C_2H_5OH.

Dehydrated Alcohol (USP 23) contains not less than 99.5% v/v or 99.2% w/w of C_2H_5OH (sp. gr. not more than 0.7964 at 15.56°).

Dilute Ethanols (BP 1998) includes several **dilute alcohols** containing between 20 and 90% v/v of C_2H_5OH, and one of these, ethanol (90%), is also known as rectified spirit.

Diluted Alcohol (USNF 18) contains 48.4 to 49.5% v/v or 41 to 42% w/w of C_2H_5OH and is prepared by mixing equal volumes of Alcohol (USP 23) and water.

Alcoholic strength is expressed as a percentage by volume of alcohol. It was previously often expressed in terms of *proof spirit*. Proof spirit contained about 57.1% v/v or 49.2% w/w of C_2H_5OH, and was defined as 'that which at the temperature of 51° F weighs exactly twelve-thirteenths of an equal measure of distilled water'. Spirit of such a strength that 100 volumes contained as much ethyl alcohol as 160 volumes of proof spirit was described as '60 OP' (over proof). Spirit of which 100 volumes contained as much alcohol as 40 volumes of proof spirit was described as '60 UP' (under proof). An alternative method of indicating spirit strength was used on the labels of alcoholic beverages in the UK when the strength was given as a number of degrees, proof spirit being taken as 100°. In the USA alcoholic strength is expressed in degrees, the value of which is equal to twice the percentage by volume. Thus 70° proof (old UK system) is equivalent to 40% v/v, and therefore to 80° proof (USA system).

Adverse Effects

Adverse effects of alcohol arise chiefly from the intake of alcoholic beverages. The concentration of alcohol in the blood producing a state of intoxication varies between individuals. At low to moderate concentrations alcohol acts as an apparent stimulant; depression of cortical function causes loss of judgement, emotional lability, muscle incoordination, visual impairment, slurred speech, and ataxia. Hangover effects may include nausea, headache, dizziness, and tremor. Alcohol depresses medullary action; lethargy, amnesia, hypothermia, hypoglycaemia (especially in children), stupor, coma, respiratory depression, cardiomyopathy, hypertension or hypotension, and cardiovascular collapse may occur. The median lethal blood-alcohol concentration is generally estimated to be approximately 400 to 500 mg per 100 mL. Death may occur at lower blood-alcohol concentrations due to inhalation of vomit during unconsciousness.

Chronic excessive consumption of alcohol may cause damage to many organs, particularly the brain and the liver. Brain damage may lead to Wernicke-Korsakoff syndrome. Fat deposits may occur in the liver and there may be a reduction in various blood-cell counts. Nutritional diseases may occur due to inadequate diet. High alcohol consumption has been associated with pancreatitis, and an increased risk of cardiovascular disease, although moderate consumption may have a protective effect against ischaemic heart disease.

Alcohol consumption has also been associated with an increased risk of some types of cancer.

The term 'alcoholism' may be used to denote dependence on alcohol, which is of the barbiturate-alcohol type (see p.641) and usually involves tolerance to other sedatives and anaesthetics. Following prolonged periods of excessive alcohol consumption, a drop in blood-alcohol concentration may precipitate a withdrawal syndrome characterised by tremor, agitation, feelings of dread, nausea, vomiting, and sweating; hallucinations, seizures, and delirium tremens may also develop.

A fetal alcohol syndrome has been identified in which infants born to some alcoholic mothers have characteristic features and abnormalities. There have been some reports of the syndrome and other adverse effects on the fetus being associated with moderate alcohol intake in pregnancy; it is generally suggested that alcohol is best avoided during pregnancy.

Frequent application of alcohol to the skin produces irritation and dry skin.

Reviews of the adverse effects of alcohol.

1. Adinoff B, *et al.* Acute ethanol poisoning and the ethanol withdrawal syndrome. *Med Toxicol* 1988; **3:** 172–96.
2. Charness ME, *et al.* Ethanol and the nervous system. *N Engl J Med* 1989; **321:** 442–54.
3. Edwards G, Peters TJ, eds. Alcohol and alcohol problems. *Br Med Bull* 1994; **50:** 1–230.
4. Lieber CS. Medical disorders of alcoholism. *N Engl J Med* 1995; **333:** 1058–65.
5. Sherlock S. Alcoholic liver disease. *Lancet* 1995; **345:** 227–9.
6. Cowie MR. Alcohol and the heart. *Br J Hosp Med* 1997; **57:** 457–60.
7. Hills KS, Westaby D. Alcohol and the liver. *Br J Hosp Med* 1997; **57:** 517–21.
8. Scheepers BDM. Alcohol and the brain. *Br J Hosp Med* 1997; **57:** 548–51.
9. Marshall EJ, Alan F. Psychiatric problems associated with alcohol misuse and dependence. *Br J Hosp Med* 1997; **58:** 44–6.
10. O'Connor PG, Schottenfeld RS. Patients with alcohol problems. *N Engl J Med* 1998; **338:** 592–601.

Effects on the skin. A 70% solution of alcohol, containing povidone-iodine, caused partial thickness chemical burns when held under pressure against the skin of 3 young children.[1] Other adverse effects on the skin reported with the topical application of alcohols have included necrosis occurring following skin cleansing of preterm neonates with methylated spirits[2,3] and haemorrhagic skin necrosis due to the alcohol content of chlorhexidine in spirit used as a disinfectant in umbilical artery catheterisation in preterm infants.[4]

See also Adverse Effects of Isopropyl Alcohol, p.1118.

1. Dickinson JC, Bailey BN. Chemical burns beneath tourniquets. *Br Med J* 1988; **297:** 1513.
2. Harpin V, Rutter N. Percutaneous alcohol absorption and skin necrosis in a preterm infant. *Arch Dis Child* 1982; **57:** 477–9.
3. Murch S, Costelloe K. Hyperosmolality related to propylene glycol in an infant. *Br Med J* 1990; **301:** 389.
4. Al-Jawad ST. Percutaneous alcohol absorption and skin necrosis in a preterm infant. *Arch Dis Child* 1983; **58:** 395–6.

Treatment of Adverse Effects

In acute poisoning the patient should be kept warm and given supportive and symptomatic care. The use of intravenous infusions of fructose to treat severe alcohol poisoning is not recommended as they may produce metabolic disturbances. Haemodialysis is of value in severe alcoholic poisoning.

The management of the alcohol withdrawal syndrome and long-term abstinence following withdrawal are discussed below.

Alcohol withdrawal and abstinence. The alcohol withdrawal syndrome presents in the early stages as a classical hyperadrenergic state with tremor, tachycardia, sweating, and hypertension. Sometimes this is accompanied by mild disorientation, anxiety, impaired concentration, depression, agitation, and gastro-intestinal symptoms. Insomnia, nightmares, and transient hallucinations can also be present. The condition may be self-limiting without the need for therapeutic intervention or it may progress to the severe and potentially fatal condition of delirium tremens (DTs), often characterised by delirium, disorientation, and hallucinations. In some cases generalised tonic-clonic seizures occur within 24 hours of alcohol withdrawal and are followed by delirium tremens.

Withdrawal. The general management of the alcohol withdrawal syndrome has been the subject of many reviews and discussions.[1-6] In most cases symptoms do not require treatment and disappear within a few days but more severe cases may require managed withdrawal from alcohol to avoid complications.

Sedatives are commonly used to reduce the symptoms of alcohol withdrawal and, if administered promptly, can prevent progression to seizures and delirium tremens. *Benzodiazepines* are usually the drugs of first choice. Longer-acting drugs such as chlordiazepoxide or diazepam may be more effective against withdrawal seizures and provide smoother withdrawal while shorter-acting ones such as lorazepam or oxazepam have a smaller risk of producing oversedation and may be more suitable for use in the elderly, and, since they do not rely on hepatic enzymes for their metabolism, for patients with liver disease. Benzodiazepines should be given in short courses only, to prevent the development of dependence. Some advocate that benzodiazepine dosage should be adjusted according to the severity of symptoms with special care being paid to patients with a history of withdrawal seizures, comorbid conditions, or those using sedative or hypnotic medication. This reduces the amount of drug required and the duration of treatment but entails regular monitoring by trained nursing staff. For mild to moderate symptoms standard anxiolytic or muscle-relaxing oral doses of benzodiazepines may be sufficient. For severe symptoms or for the treatment of delirium tremens higher doses and use of the intravenous route may be required. *Chlormethiazole* appears to be an effective alternative to the benzodiazepines but although widely used in Europe it is not available in the US. Some centres use phenobarbitone but *barbiturates* are generally not recommended for the treatment of alcohol withdrawal syndrome.

Antipsychotics are not usually recommended for use in the control of symptoms of alcohol withdrawal since they do not reduce delirium tremens and some may reduce the seizure threshold. However, they might be considered for use as an adjunct in patients requiring treatment of marked agitation or hallucinations.

The generalised tonic-clonic seizures associated with alcohol withdrawal are usually self-limiting and patients who experience only one or two seizures do not usually require any specific treatment beyond continuing therapy with benzodiazepines or chlormethiazole. For recurrent seizures or status epilepticus (p.337) diazepam may be given intravenously. Other types of seizure may be associated with head trauma or pre-existing seizure disorders (p.335) and should be treated accordingly. Other *antiepileptics* such as carbamazepine have been tried in the treatment of alcohol withdrawal seizures and may be of use as adjuncts in controlling other symptoms of alcohol withdrawal syndrome. As benzodiazepines are effective in preventing withdrawal seizures other prophylactic drugs are not usually indicated.

Beta blockers can reduce symptoms of autonomic overactivity such as tachycardia, hypertension, tremor, and agitation but because they can mask these symptoms of withdrawal and do not prevent the development of more serious complications they should not be used alone. Some beta blockers such as propranolol which penetrate the CNS may produce CNS effects which complicate therapy. The $alpha_2$-adrenergic receptor agonist *clonidine* may be of similar benefit as an adjunct.

Other drugs that have been reported to be of benefit in alcohol withdrawal syndrome include nitrous oxide and gamma-hydroxybutyric acid.

It is essential that in all cases of alcohol withdrawal syndrome hypoglycaemia, dehydration, electrolyte disturbances (in particular magnesium), and vitamin deficiencies be corrected. It is usually recommended that all patients should be given thiamine because of their increased risk of developing Wernicke's encephalopathy (p.1361). It should be noted that intravenous administration of glucose solutions before thiamine may precipitate Wernicke's encephalopathy in thiamine-deficient patients. However, hydration should be undertaken with care as alcoholics may be more prone to develop cerebral oedema. The management of cerebral oedema is discussed under Raised Intracranial Pressure on p.796.

Abstinence. Once the initial acute withdrawal of alcohol is achieved treatment may be required to maintain long-term abstinence. Pharmacotherapy should only be used as an adjunct to psychotherapy and supportive care. Drugs used to modify alcohol seeking behaviour either sensitise the patient to alcohol (aversive drugs) or reduce or alleviate the craving for alcohol. The main agents used for aversive therapy are *disulfiram* and *calcium carbimide*. A patient who ingests alcohol after taking an adequate dose of one of these drugs will experience a severe and unpleasant reaction (see p.1573). However, the deterrent value of aversive drugs, and their potential toxicity, has long been a matter of debate. Such treatment is likely to be of little use unless it is undertaken with the willing cooperation of the patient and is used with psychotherapy and even then there is no evidence that it has any effect on the long-term course of alcoholism.

Of those drugs which have been reported to reduce alcohol craving *acamprosate* and *naltrexone* have been the most promising as adjuncts for management of alcohol dependence and have been shown to improve abstinence and reduce relapse rates. Whether benefit is maintained long-term after treatment is stopped is unclear. *Other drugs* tried with varying benefit include tiapride, selective serotonin reuptake inhibitors, gammahydroxybutyric acid, and bromocriptine. Use of antidepressants may improve outcome in patients with concomitant depression.

References.

1. McMicken DB, Freedland ES. Alcohol-related seizures: pathophysiology, differential diagnosis, evaluation, and treatment. *Emerg Med Clin North Am* 1994; **12:** 1057–79.

2. Lohr RH. Treatment of alcohol withdrawal in hospitalized patients. *Mayo Clin Proc* 1995; **70:** 777–82.
3. Erstad BL, Cotugno CL. Management of alcohol withdrawal. *Am J Health-Syst Pharm* 1995; **52:** 697–709.
4. Hall W, Zador D. The alcohol withdrawal syndrome. *Lancet* 1997; **349:** 1897–1900.
5. Mayo-Smith MF. American Society of Addiction Medicine Working Group on Pharmacological Management of Alcohol Withdrawal. Pharmacological management of alcohol withdrawal: a meta-analysis and evidence-based practice guideline. *JAMA* 1997; **278:** 144–51.
6. Saitz R, O'Malley SS. Pharmacotherapies for alcohol abuse: withdrawal and treatment. *Med Clin North Am* 1997; **81:** 881–907.

Precautions

Women and the elderly may be more susceptible to the adverse effects of alcohol ingestion. Alcohol may aggravate peptic ulcer or impaired liver function. Ingestion of alcohol during pregnancy or by nursing mothers is not advisable. Excessive alcohol intake should be avoided in patients with diabetes mellitus or epilepsy. In chronic alcoholics there may be tolerance to the effects of other CNS depressants including general anaesthetics.

All processes requiring judgement and coordination are affected by alcohol and these include the driving of any form of transport and the operating of machinery. It is an offence in many countries for motorists to drive when the blood-alcohol concentration is above a stated value. The alcohol concentration in urine and expired air can be used to estimate the blood-alcohol concentration.

It should be remembered that alcohol may be present in a number of pharmaceutical preparations such as elixirs and mouthwashes, and that children may be particularly susceptible to its hypoglycaemic effects.

Porphyria. Alcohol has been associated with acute attacks of porphyria and is considered unsafe in patients with acute porphyria.[1]

1. Moore MR, McColl KEL. *Porphyria: drug lists*. Glasgow: Porphyria Research Unit, University of Glasgow, 1991.

Interactions

Reports of interactions between alcohol and other drugs are not consistent, possibly because acute alcohol intake may inhibit drug metabolism while chronic alcohol intake may enhance the induction of drug-metabolising enzymes in the liver. Alcoholic beverages containing tyramine may cause reactions when taken by patients receiving MAOIs. Alcohol may enhance the acute effects of drugs which depress the central nervous system, such as hypnotics, antihistamines, opioid analgesics, antiepileptics, antidepressants, antipsychotics, and sedatives. Unpleasant reactions, similar to those occurring with disulfiram (see p.1573), may occur when alcohol is taken concomitantly with chlorpropamide, mepacrine, metronidazole and other nitroimidazoles, the nitrofuran derivatives furazolidone and nifuratel, procarbazine, and some cephalosporins.

Alcohol may cause hypoglycaemic reactions in patients receiving sulphonylurea antidiabetics or insulin, and may cause orthostatic hypotension in patients taking drugs with vasodilator action. It may enhance the hypotensive effects of antihypertensives and has also increased the sedative effect of indoramin. Alcohol may increase gastric bleeding caused by analgesics and may have a variable effect on oral anticoagulants. It may decrease the antidiuretic effect of vasopressin.

Interactions involving alcohol have been reviewed.[1-3]

The effects of *paracetamol* poisoning may be exacerbated by prolonged alcohol use (see p.72).

When taken concomitantly with alcohol *verapamil*[4] has been reported to cause an increase in peak blood-alcohol concentrations of approximately 17%. Such an interaction may extend the toxic effects of alcohol and raise its blood concentration above the legal limit for driving.[5] Increased blood-alcohol concentrations have also been reported in patients receiving *cycloserine*.[6] Alcohol has also been reported to interact with *nifedipine*,[7] resulting in increased blood concentrations of nifedipine.

The existence of an interaction between H_2-receptor antagonists and alcohol is controversial and has not been established. While some studies suggest that *cimetidine*[8-10] and *nizatidine*[10] can increase peak blood concentrations of alcohol the effects of *ranitidine*[9,11] have been variable; *famotidine* appears to have no significant effect.[9] Recent studies report that any interaction between H_2-receptor antagonists and alcohol is minor and unlikely to be of clinical importance.[12-15]

1. McInnes GT. Interactions that matter: alcohol. *Prescribers' J* 1985; **25:** 87–90.
2. Lieber CS. Interaction of alcohol with other drugs and nutrients: implications for the therapy of alcoholic liver disease. *Drugs* 1990; **40** (suppl 3): 23–44.
3. Fraser AG. Pharmacokinetic interactions between alcohol and other drugs. *Clin Pharmacokinet* 1997; **33:** 79–90.
4. Schumock G, *et al.* Verapamil inhibits ethanol elimination. *Pharmacotherapy* 1989; **9:** 184–5.
5. Anonymous. Does verapamil increase the effects of alcohol? *Pharm J* 1990; **244:** 14.
6. Glass F, *et al.* Beobachtungen und untersuchungen über die gemeinsame wirkung von alkohol und D-cycloserin. *Arzneimittelforschung* 1965; **15:** 684–8.
7. Qureshi S, *et al.* Nifedipine-alcohol interaction. *JAMA* 1990; **264:** 1660–1.
8. Caballeria J, *et al.* Effects of cimetidine on gastric alcohol dehydrogenase activity and blood ethanol levels. *Gastroenterology* 1989; **96:** 388–92.
9. DiPadova C, *et al.* Effects of ranitidine on blood alcohol levels after ethanol ingestion: comparison with other H_2-receptor antagonists. *JAMA* 1992; **267:** 83–6.
10. Holt S, *et al.* Evidence for an interaction between alcohol and certain H_2 receptor antagonists. *Gut* 1991; **32:** A1220.
11. Toon S, *et al.* Lack of effect of high dose ranitidine on the postprandial pharmacokinetics of alcohol. *Gut* 1992; **33** (suppl): S10.
12. Raufman J-P, *et al.* Histamine-2 receptor antagonists do not alter serum ethanol levels in fed, nonalcoholic men. *Ann Intern Med* 1993; **118:** 488–94.
13. Levitt MD. Do histamine-2 receptor antagonists influence the metabolism of ethanol? *Ann Intern Med* 1993; **118:** 564–5.
14. Kleine M-W, Ertl D. Comparative trial in volunteers to investigate possible ethanol-ranitidine interaction. *Ann Pharmacother* 1993; **27:** 841–5.
15. Gugler R. H_2-antagonists and alcohol: do they interact? *Drug Safety* 1994; **10:** 271–80.

Pharmacokinetics

Alcohol is rapidly absorbed from the gastro-intestinal tract and is distributed throughout the body fluids. It readily crosses the placenta. Alcohol vapour can be absorbed through the lungs. Absorption through intact skin is said to be negligible.

The rate of absorption of alcohol from the gastro-intestinal tract may be modified by such factors as the presence of food, the concentration of alcohol, and the period of time during which it is ingested. Some alcohol is reported to be metabolised by the gastric mucosa.

Alcohol is mainly metabolised in the liver; it is converted by alcohol dehydrogenase to acetaldehyde and is then further oxidised to acetate. A hepatic microsomal oxidising system is also involved. About 90 to 98% of alcohol is oxidised and the remainder is excreted unchanged by the kidneys and the lungs and also in breast milk, sweat, and other secretions.

The rate of metabolism may be accelerated following repeated excessive intake and by certain substances including insulin.

The pharmacokinetics of alcohol have been reviewed by Holford.[1] A study by Frezza and others,[2] showing that gastric oxidation of alcohol was reduced in women compared with men leading to women having increased blood-alcohol concentrations, stimulated considerable correspondence. Seitz *et al.*[3] demonstrated that only women under the age of 50 years have lower alcohol dehydrogenase activity than men, and that in elderly women the activity was not significantly less than in men. Phillips[4] pointed out that acetaldehyde may be more toxic than alcohol and that reduced first-pass metabolism in women may lessen their risk of toxic liver effects. The study by Frezza has also been criticised on pharmacokinetic grounds[5,6] and on the basis that men and women display differences in social drinking patterns.[7] In reply Frezza *et al.*[8] refute some of these criticisms but point out that other factors, such as sex-related differences in tissue vulnerability, may contribute to differences in the severity of medical problems related to drinking.

1. Holford NHG. Clinical pharmacokinetics of ethanol. *Clin Pharmacokinet* 1987; **13:** 273–92.
2. Frezza M, *et al.* High blood alcohol levels in women: the role of decreased gastric alcohol dehydrogenase activity and first-pass metabolism. *N Engl J Med* 1990; **322:** 95–9.
3. Seitz HK, *et al.* High blood alcohol levels in women. *N Engl J Med* 1990; **323:** 58.
4. Phillips M. High blood alcohol levels in women. *N Engl J Med* 1990; **323:** 58.
5. Sweeney GD. High blood alcohol levels in women. *N Engl J Med* 1990; **323:** 58–9.
6. Zedeck MS. High blood alcohol levels in women. *N Engl J Med* 1990; **323:** 59.
7. York JL. High blood alcohol levels in women. *N Engl J Med* 1990; **323:** 59–60.
8. Frezza M, *et al.* High blood alcohol levels in women. *N Engl J Med* 1990; **323:** 60–1.

Uses and Administration

Alcohol has bactericidal activity and is used to disinfect skin prior to injection, venepuncture, or surgical procedures. It is also used to disinfect hands and clean surfaces. A concentration of 70%, often as methylated spirits (p.1119), is commonly employed for disinfection. Alcohol should not be used for disinfection of surgical or dental instruments because of its low efficacy against bacterial spores.

Alcohol also has anhidrotic, rubefacient, and astringent and haemostatic properties. It is sometimes used for its skin-cooling properties and to harden the skin. It is an ingredient of several topical preparations used for skin disorders.

Alcohol is widely used as a solvent and preservative in pharmaceutical preparations.

Alcohol may be used as a neurolytic in the management of severe and chronic pain. Intrathecal injection of alcohol has also been used for the intractable pain of spasticity (p.1303).

Alcohol is given intravenously in the treatment of acute poisoning from ethylene glycol (p.1577) and methyl alcohol (p.1379).

Alcohol is also used in sclerotherapy.

Disinfection. VIRUSES. Hanson *et al.*[1] reported 70% alcohol to be ineffective against HIV dried onto sterile glass coverslips in the presence of 10% serum. However, de Jong and van Klingeren[2] pointed out that HIV in suspension was very sensitive to 70% alcohol and that in practice, the poor penetrating power of alcohol was compensated for by removal of visible contamination from surfaces prior to disinfection. Another study[3] showed that inactivation of dried HIV by 70% alcohol was slow, especially in the presence of a high concentration of protein, and that high titres of virus required a 2-minute full immersion period in alcohol.

WHO has published guidelines on sterilisation and disinfection methods effective against HIV[4] which state that alcohols are not considered suitable for dealing with contaminated surfaces because of their limited penetration of organic residues and rapid evaporation but that for disinfection of living tissues, alcohol 70% is effective.

1. Hanson PJV, *et al.* Chemical inactivation of HIV on surfaces. *Br Med J* 1989; **298:** 862–4.
2. de Jong JC, van Klingeren B. Chemical inactivation of HIV on surfaces. *Br Med J* 1989; **298:** 1646–7.
3. van Bueren J, *et al.* Inactivation of HIV on surfaces by alcohol. *Br Med J* 1989; **299:** 459.
4. WHO. Guidelines on sterilization and disinfection methods effective against human immunodeficiency virus (HIV). *WHO AIDS Series 2* 1989.

Pain. The neurolytic use of alcohol to produce destructive nerve block (p.6) has produced variable results, and some consider the risk of complications outweighs the benefits. However, alcohol has been injected into the pituitary gland for relief of severe pain of the head and neck;[1,2] doses of 1 mL of absolute alcohol have been used.[1] It may be useful in coeliac plexus block, and has been injected into the muscle sheath to relieve painful muscle spasms in patients with multiple sclerosis.[1] Alcohol 50 to 100% may be used for peripheral or central nerve block in terminally ill patients with pain that does not respond to drug therapy;[3] the block produced by alcohol may occasionally last up to 2 years, even longer than that produced by phenol.

1. Lloyd JW. Use of anaesthesia: the anaesthetist and the pain clinic. *Br Med J* 1980; **281:** 432–4.
2. Lipton S. Pain relief in active patients with cancer: the early use of nerve blocks improves the quality of life. *Br Med J* 1989; **298:** 37–8.
3. Hardy, PAJ. The role of the pain clinic in the management of the terminally ill. *Br J Hosp Med* 1990; **43:** 142–6.

Prostatectomy. Intravascular absorption of irrigating solutions during transurethral resection of the prostate can be monitored by measuring breath-alcohol concentrations resulting from alcohol added to the solution before use.[1]

1. Anonymous. Monitoring TURP. *Lancet* 1991; **338:** 606–7.

Sclerotherapy. Alcohol has been used successfully as a sclerosant in a variety of conditions including aldosterone-producing adenoma,[1] parathyroid adenomas,[2] thyroid nodules,[3,4] advanced rectal cancer,[5] hepatocellular carcinoma,[6,7] dysphagia associated with oesophagastric cancer,[8,9] hepatic cyst,[10] and gallbladder obstruction.[11] It has also been used in the sclerotherapy of oesophageal varices[12,13] although the safety of this procedure has been questioned following a report of complications developing in 13 of 17 patients, 2 of whom died.[14] Other conditions in which alcohol has been used include bleeding from ruptured hepatomas[15] and from peptic ulcers,[16] and obstructive cardiomyopathies[17] resistant to usual treatment (see p.785).

Other sclerosants used in varicose veins and oesophageal varices are discussed on p.1576.

1. Mathias CJ, *et al.* Therapeutic venous infarction of an aldosterone producing adenoma (Conn's tumour). *Br Med J* 1984; **288:** 1416–17.
2. Verges B, *et al.* Percutaneous ethanol injection of parathyroid adenomas in primary hyperparathyroidism. *Lancet* 1991; **337:** 1421–2.
3. Monzani F, *et al.* Autonomous thyroid nodule and percutaneous ethanol injection. *Lancet* 1991; **337:** 743.
4. Bennedbaek FN, Hegedüs L. Alcohol sclerotherapy for benign solitary solid cold thyroid nodules. *Lancet* 1995; **346:** 1227.
5. Payne-James J, *et al.* Advanced rectal cancer. *Br Med J* 1990; **300:** 746.
6. Sheu J-C, *et al.* Intratumor injection of absolute ethanol under ultrasound guidance for the treatment of small hepatocellular carcinoma. *Hepatogastroenterology* 1987; **34:** 255–61.
7. Salmi A. Percutaneous alcohol injection of hepatocellular carcinoma. *Ann Intern Med* 1989; **110:** 494.
8. Payne-James JJ, *et al.* Use of ethanol-induced tumor necrosis to palliate dysphagia in patients with esophagogastric cancer. *Gastrointest Endosc* 1990; **36:** 43–6.
9. Stanners AJ, *et al.* Alcohol injection for palliation of malignant oesophageal disease. *Lancet* 1993; **341:** 767.
10. Bean WJ, Rodan BA. Hepatic cysts: treatment with alcohol. *Am J Roentg* 1985; **144:** 237–41.
11. Asfar S, *et al.* Percutaneous sclerosis of gallbladder. *Lancet* 1989; **ii:** 387.
12. Sarin SK, *et al.* Endoscopic sclerotherapy using absolute alcohol. *Gut* 1985; **26:** 120–4.
13. Hassall E, *et al.* Sclerotherapy for extrahepatic portal hypertension in childhood. *J Pediatr* 1989; **115:** 69–74.
14. Bhargava DK, *et al.* Endoscopic sclerotherapy using absolute alcohol. *Gut* 1986; **27:** 1518.
15. Chung SCS, *et al.* Injection of alcohol to control bleeding from ruptured hepatomas. *Br Med J* 1990; **301:** 421.
16. Lin HJ, *et al.* Heat probe thermocoagulation and pure alcohol injection in massive peptic ulcer haemorrhage: a prospective, randomised controlled trial. *Gut* 1990; **31:** 753–7.
17. Sigwart U. Non-surgical myocardial reduction for hypertrophic obstructive cardiomyopathy. *Lancet* 1995; **346:** 211–14.

Preparations

USP 23: Alcohol in Dextrose Injection; Rubbing Alcohol.

Proprietary Preparations (details are given in Part 3)
Fr.: Curethyl; Pharmadose alcool; ***Ger.:*** AHD 2000; Amphisept E; Fugaten; Manusept HD; Sterillium Virugard; ***Ital.:*** Resina Carbolica Dentilin; ***Spain:*** Alcohten; ***Switz.:*** Amphisept; ***UK:*** Brushtox; ***USA:*** Alcare; Alco-Gel; Kleen-Handz.

Multi-ingredient: numerous preparations are listed in Part 3.

Alkyl Gallates (12172-x)

Dodecyl Gallate (6645-q)

E312; Lauryl Gallate; Laurylum Gallicum. Dodecyl 3,4,5-trihydroxybenzoate.

$C_{19}H_{30}O_5$ = 338.4.

CAS — 1166-52-5.

Pharmacopoeias. In *Aust.*, *Br.*, and *Fr.*

A white or creamy-white, odourless or almost odourless powder. Practically **insoluble** in water; freely soluble in alcohol, in acetone, in ether, and in methyl alcohol; sparingly soluble in arachis oil, in chloroform, and in propylene glycol. **Protect** from light. Avoid contact with metals.

Ethyl Gallate (6647-s)

Ethyl 3,4,5-trihydroxybenzoate.

$C_9H_{10}O_5$ = 198.2.

CAS — 831-61-8.

Pharmacopoeias. In *Br.*

A white to creamy-white, odourless or almost odourless, crystalline powder. Slightly **soluble** in water; freely soluble in alcohol and in ether; practically insoluble in arachis oil. **Protect** from light. Avoid contact with metals.

Octyl Gallate (6654-p)

E311. Octyl 3,4,5-trihydroxybenzoate.

$C_{15}H_{22}O_5$ = 282.3.

CAS — 1034-01-1.

Pharmacopoeias. In *Br.* and *Fr.*

A white or creamy-white, odourless or almost odourless powder. Practically **insoluble** in water; freely soluble in alcohol, in acetone, in ether, and in propylene glycol; very soluble in methyl alcohol; sparingly soluble in arachis oil and in chloroform. **Protect** from light. Avoid contact with metals.

Propyl Gallate (6664-w)

E310; Propylis Gallas; Propylum Gallicum. Propyl 3,4,5-trihydroxybenzoate.

$C_{10}H_{12}O_5$ = 212.2.

CAS — 121-79-9.

Pharmacopoeias. In *Eur.* (see p.viii) and *Pol.* Also in *USNF.*

A white or almost white crystalline powder with a slight characteristic odour. Slightly or very slightly **soluble** in water; freely soluble in alcohol and in ether; dissolves in dilute solutions of alkali hydroxides. **Store** in airtight containers. Avoid contact with metals. Protect from light.

Adverse Effects and Precautions

The alkyl gallates may cause contact sensitivity and skin reactions.

Effects on the blood. Methaemoglobinaemia associated with the antoxidants (butylated hydroxyanisole, butylated hydroxytoluene, and propyl gallate) used to preserve the oil in a soybean infant feed formula has been reported.[1] Propyl gallate was suspected of being the most likely cause because its chemical structure is similar to pyrogallol, a methaemoglobinaemia inducer.

1. Nitzan M, *et al.* Infantile methemoglobinemia caused by food additives. *Clin Toxicol* 1979; **15:** 273–80.

Uses

The alkyl esters of gallic acid (3,4,5-trihydroxybenzoic acid) have antoxidant properties and are used as preservatives in pharmaceuticals and cosmetics. Alkyl gallates are also used as antoxidants in foods and are useful in preventing deterioration and rancidity of fats and oils. They are used in concentrations of 0.001 to 0.1%.

To improve acceptability and efficacy, the alkyl gallates are frequently used in combination with other antoxidants such as butylated hydroxyanisole or butylated hydroxytoluene and with sequestrants and synergists such as citric acid.

The alkyl gallates have also been reported to have limited antimicrobial activity.

Alkylaryltrialkylammonium Chloride (16344-w)

Alkylaryltrialkylammonium chloride is a quaternary ammonium disinfectant with properties similar to those of other cationic surfactants (see Cetrimide, p.1105).

Preparations

Proprietary Preparations (details are given in Part 3)
UK: Resistone QD.

Alkylaryltrimethylammonium Chloride (16340-g)

Alkylaryltrimethylammonium chloride is a quaternary ammonium disinfectant with properties similar to those of other cationic surfactants (see Cetrimide, p.1105).

Preparations

Proprietary Preparations (details are given in Part 3)
UK: Gloquat C.

Ambazone (2203-a)

Ambazone *(BAN, rINN).*

Ambazonum. 4-Amidinohydrazonocyclohexa-1,4-dien-3-one thiosemicarbazone monohydrate.

$C_8H_{11}N_7S,H_2O$ = 255.3.

CAS — 539-21-9 (anhydrous ambazone); 6011-12-7 (ambazone monohydrate).

Ambazone is an antiseptic which has been used in the form of lozenges for minor infections of the mouth and pharynx.

Preparations

Proprietary Preparations (details are given in Part 3)
Ger.: Iversal†.

Multi-ingredient: ***Ger.:*** Iversal-A cum anaesthetico†.

Aminoquinuride Hydrochloride (11245-y)

Aminoquinuride Hydrochloride *(rINNM).*

1,3-Bis(4-amino-2-methyl-6-quinolyl)urea dihydrochloride.

$C_{21}H_{20}N_6O,2HCl$ = 445.3.

CAS — 3811-56-1 (aminoquinuride); 5424-37-3 (aminoquinuride hydrochloride).

Aminoquinuride hydrochloride is an antiseptic that has been used in topical preparations for the treatment of mouth and skin disorders.

Preparations

Proprietary Preparations (details are given in Part 3)

Multi-ingredient: ***Aust.:*** Herviros; ***Ger.:*** Dontisolon M Mundheilpaste†; Dontisolon M Zylinderampullen†; Herviros; Polyfen†; ***Ital.:*** Loticort†; ***Switz.:*** Dontisolon M†.

Amylmetacresol (2205-x)

Amylmetacresol *(BAN, rINN).*

6-Pentyl-*m*-cresol; 5-Methyl-2-pentylphenol.

$C_{12}H_{18}O$ = 178.3.

CAS — 1300-94-3.

Pharmacopoeias. In *Br.*

A clear or almost clear liquid or a solid crystalline mass with a characteristic odour, colourless or slightly yellow when freshly prepared; it darkens on keeping. F.p. about 22°. Practically **insoluble** in water; soluble in alcohol, in ether, and in fixed and volatile oils. **Protect** from light.

Amylmetacresol is a phenolic antiseptic used chiefly as an ingredient of lozenges in the treatment of minor infections of the mouth and throat.

Preparations

Proprietary Preparations (details are given in Part 3)
Ital.: Benagol Collutorio; Mac†; ***UK:*** Antiseptic Throat Lozenges.

Multi-ingredient: ***Aust.:*** Coldangin; Neo-Angin; ***Austral.:*** Sore Throat Chewing Gum; Strepsils; Strepsils Anaesthetic†; Strepsils Plus; ***Belg.:*** Strepsils; Strepsils Menthol; Strepsils Vit C; ***Fr.:*** Strepsils; Strepsils Menthol Eucalyptus†; Strepsils Miel-Citron; Strepsils Vitamine C; Strepsilspray Lidocaine; ***Ger.:*** Neo-Angin N; ***Irl.:*** Strepsils; Strepsils Dual Action; Strepsils Vitamin C; ***Ital.:*** Benagol; Benagol Mentolo-Eucaliptolo; Benagol Vitamina C; ***Neth.:*** Strepsils; Strepsils Menthol en Eucalyptus; Strepsils Sinaasappel en Vitamine C; ***S.Afr.:*** Strepsils; Strepsils Eucalyptus Menthol; Strepsils Orange-C; Strepsils Plus; Strepsils Soothing Honey & Lemon; ***Spain:*** Angiseptina†; Strepsils; Strepsils con Vitamina C; ***Swed.:*** Strepsils; ***Switz.:*** Neo-Angin au miel et citron; Neo-Angin avec vitamin C exempt de sucre; Neo-Angin exempt de sucre; ***UK:*** Antiseptic Lozenges; Antiseptic Throat Lozenges; Mac; Strepsils; Strepsils Dual Action; Strepsils with Vitamin C.

Ascorbyl Palmitate (6633-m)

Ascorbylis Palmitas; E304; Vitamin C Palmitate. L-Ascorbic acid 6-hexadecanoate; L-Ascorbic acid 6-palmitate; 3-Oxo-L-gulofuranolactone 6-palmitate.

$C_{22}H_{38}O_7$ = 414.5.

CAS — 137-66-6.

Pharmacopoeias. In *Eur.* (see p.viii). Also in *USNF.*

A white to yellowish-white powder with a characteristic odour. Ph. Eur. **solubilities** are: practically insoluble in water; freely soluble in alcohol and in methyl alcohol; practically insoluble in dichloromethane and in fatty oils. USNF solubilities are: very slightly soluble in water, chloroform, ether, and vegetable oils; soluble 1 in 125 of alcohol. **Store** at 8° to 15° in airtight containers, protected from light.

Ascorbyl palmitate is an antoxidant used as a preservative in pharmaceutical products and foods. It is often used in combination with alpha tocopherol (p.1369), and this combination shows marked synergy.

Benzalkonium Chloride (2206-r)

Benzalkonium Chloride *(BAN, rINN).*

Benzalconio Cloruro; Benzalkonii Chloridum; Benzalkonium Chloratum; Cloreto de Benzalconio.

CAS — 8001-54-5.

Pharmacopoeias. In *Eur.* (see p.viii), *Int.*, *Jpn*, and *Pol.* Also in *USNF. Chin.* includes benzalkonium bromide. Some pharmacopoeias also have a monograph for Benzalkonium Chloride Solution.

A mixture of alkylbenzyldimethylammonium chlorides of the general formula $[C_6H_5.CH_2.N(CH_3)_2.R]Cl$, in which R represents a mixture of the alkyls having chain lengths from C_8 to C_{18}. The Ph. Eur. specifies that it contains not less than 95% and not more than 104% of alkylbenzyldimethylammonium chlorides, calculated as $C_{22}H_{40}ClN$ with reference to the anhydrous substance. The USNF specifies not less than 40% of the $C_{12}H_{25}$ compound, calculated on the anhydrous substance, not less than 20% of the $C_{14}H_{29}$ compound, and not less than 70% of the 2 compounds together.

A white or yellowish-white powder, thick gel, or gelatinous pieces with a mild aromatic odour; hygroscopic and unctuous. It forms a clear molten mass on heating. The Ph. Eur. specifies that it contains not more than 10% of water; the USNF specifies not more than 15%. Very **soluble** in water and alcohol; the anhydrous form is soluble 1 in 100 of ether. A solution in water is usually slightly alkaline and foams strongly when shaken. **Store** in airtight containers.

Incompatible with soaps and other anionic surfactants, citrates, iodides, nitrates, permanganates, salicylates, silver salts, and tartrates. Incompatibilities have been demonstrated with ingredients of some commercial rubber mixes or plastics. Incompatibilities have also been reported with other substances including aluminium, cotton dressings, fluorescein sodium, hydrogen peroxide, kaolin, hydrous wool fat, and some sulphonamides.

Adverse Effects, Treatment, and Precautions

As for Cetrimide, p.1105.

Catheters and cannulas. For reference to benzalkonium chloride used in the manufacturing process of heparin-bonded catheters interfering with determination of serum concentrations of sodium and potassium, see under Precautions for Heparin, p.881.

Effects on the eyes. Benzalkonium chloride is one of the most disruptive ophthalmic additives to the stability of the lipid film and to corneal epithelial membranes; it has been shown to be toxic to the eyes of *rabbits* but less so to the eyes of humans.[1] Toxicity experiments have tended to be carried out using relatively high concentrations of benzalkonium chloride[2] but deleterious effects on the tear film and corneoconjunctival surface have been noted in patients receiving regular long-term treatment for glaucoma with eye drops preserved with benzalkonium chloride in usual concentrations.[3,4] However, the use of preservatives in eye drops should generally be avoided and the formulation of such preparations in single-dose containers is desirable.[1,2] Benzalkonium chloride is not suitable for use in solutions employed in storing and washing hydrophilic soft contact lenses, as it can bind to the lenses and may later produce ocular toxicity when the lenses are worn.[5]

1. Burstein NL. The effects of topical drugs and preservatives on the tears and corneal epithelium in dry eye. *Trans Ophthalmol Soc U K* 1985; **104:** 402–9.
2. Burstein NL. Corneal cytotoxicity of topically applied drugs, vehicles and preservatives. *Surv Ophthalmol* 1980; **25:** 15–30.
3. Herreras JM, *et al.* Ocular surface alteration after long-term treatment with an antiglaucomatous drug. *Ophthalmology* 1992; **99:** 1082–8.
4. Kuppens EVMJ, *et al.* Effect of timolol with and without preservative on the basal tear turnover in glaucoma. *Br J Ophthalmol* 1995; **79:** 339–42.
5. Gasset AR. Benzalkonium chloride toxicity to the human cornea. *Am J Ophthalmol* 1977; **84:** 169–71.

Effects on the respiratory tract. A hypersensitivity reaction in one patient to benzalkonium chloride used as a preservative in nose drops was confirmed by challenge which produced nasal congestion and irritation of the eyes and throat lasting 48 hours.[1] Benzalkonium chloride used as a preservative in nebulised solutions of anti-asthma agents has been reported to cause dose-related bronchoconstriction especially in asthmatic patients[2] and has been associated with the precipitation of respiratory arrest in one patient.[3]

1. Hillerdal G. Adverse reaction to locally applied preservatives in nose drops. *ORL J Otorhinolaryngol Relat Spec* 1985; **47:** 278–9.
2. Committee on Drugs, American Academy of Pediatrics. "Inactive" ingredients in pharmaceutical products: update. *Pediatrics* 1997; **99:** 268–78.
3. Boucher M, *et al.* Possible association of benzalkonium chloride in nebulizer solutions with respiratory arrest. *Ann Pharmacother* 1992; **26:** 772–4.

Uses and Administration

Benzalkonium chloride is a quaternary ammonium antiseptic and disinfectant with actions and uses similar to those of the other cationic surfactants (see Cetrimide, p.1105). It is also used as an antimicrobial preservative for pharmaceutical products. Benzalkonium bromide and benzalkonium saccharinate have also been used.

Solutions of benzalkonium chloride 0.01 to 0.1% are used for cleansing skin, mucous membranes, and wounds. More dilute solutions of 0.005% are suitable for irrigation of deep wounds. A 0.02 to 0.05% solution has been used as a vaginal douche. An aqueous solution containing 0.005 to 0.02% has been used for irrigation of the bladder and urethra and a 0.0025 to 0.005% solution for retention lavage of the bladder.

Creams containing benzalkonium chloride are used in the treatment of napkin rash and other dermatoses.

A 0.2 to 0.5% solution has been used as a shampoo in seborrhoeic dermatitis.

Lozenges containing benzalkonium chloride are used for the treatment of superficial infections of the mouth and throat.

A 0.01 to 0.02% solution of benzalkonium chloride is used as a preservative for some eye drops. It is not suitable for eye drops containing local anaesthetics as it accelerates their dehydrating effect. Because some rubbers are incompatible with benzalkonium chloride the BPC 1973 recommended that, unless the suitability has been established, silicone rubber teats be used on eye drop containers. Benzalkonium chloride is used for disinfecting rigid contact lenses (p.1097) but is unsuitable as a preservative in solutions for washing and storing hydrophilic soft contact lenses (see also Adverse Effects, above).

Benzalkonium chloride is also used as a spermicide.

Solutions of 0.13% are used for disinfection and storage of surgical instruments, sometimes with the addition of sodium nitrite to inhibit rust.

Action. The antibacterial effect of benzalkonium chloride 0.003% was enhanced by 0.175% of benzyl alcohol, phenylpropanol, or phenethyl alcohol.[1] For the use of phenethyl alcohol with benzalkonium chloride as a preservative for ophthalmic solutions, see Phenethyl Alcohol, p.1121.

1. Richards RME, McBride RJ. Enhancement of benzalkonium chloride and chlorhexidine acetate activity against Pseudomonas aeruginosa by aromatic alcohols. *J Pharm Sci* 1973; **62:** 2035–7.

Catheter-related sepsis. Benzalkonium chloride has been investigated[1] for incorporation into catheters to reduce catheter-related sepsis (p.1098).

1. Tebbs SE, Elliott TSJ. A novel, antimicrobial central venous catheter impregnated with benzalkonium chloride. *J Antimicrob Chemother* 1993; **31:** 261–71.

Disinfection. VIRUSES. Benzalkonium chloride inactivates HIV and HSV *in vitro*.[1,2] This property may contribute to the prevention of sexually transmitted disease when benzalkonium is used as a spermicide.[1]

1. Wainberg MA, *et al.* Inactivation of human immunodeficiency virus type 1 in tissue culture fluid and in genital secretions by the spermicide benzalkonium chloride. *J Clin Microbiol* 1990; **28:** 156–8.
2. Jennings R, Clegg A. The inhibitory effect of spermicidal agents on replication of HSV-2 and HIV-1 in-vitro. *J Antimicrob Chemother* 1993; **32:** 71–82.

Preparations

USNF 18: Benzalkonium Chloride Solution.

Proprietary Preparations (details are given in Part 3)
Austral.: Cetal Concentrate; Dettol Fresh; ***Belg.:*** Cedium; Pansteryl; ***Canad.:*** Arkonsol; Zephiran; ***Fr.:*** Comprimes Gynecologiques Pharmatex; Pharmatex; Sparaplaie NA; ***Ger.:*** Baktonium; Killavon†; Laudamonium; Lysoform Killavon; Quartamon†; Rheila Stringiet N; Sagrotan Med; Zephirol†; ***Irl.:*** Roccal; ***Ital.:*** 3D Tipo P-Disinfettante†; Alfa C; Bluesteril; Ceroxmed Steril; Citrosil; Citrosil Sapoplus; Citrosil Spray; Colli; D-Pronto-Disinfettante Analcolico†; Detergil; Di-Mill; Diseptil; Disintyl; Display; Distasil; Disteril; Elialconio†; Eso Deterferri; Eso Ferri; Esoform Deterferri; Esoform Sanacasa†; Esosan; Euronormol-Disinfettante Concentrato Profumato†; Germicidin; Germozero Plus; Geyderm; Gola†; Helis; Hygienist Pavimenti e Piastrelle; Iridina Light; Iriflor†; Lacribase; Lozione Vittoria; Neo-Desogen; Norica; Polisan; Quack†; Sanaform; Sangen Medical; Sapocitrosil†; Sebogel†; Sguardi; Sincosan; Sirigen; Steramin; Steramina G; Sterilix; Stilla Delicato; Streptosil L PMC; Video; Zefirol; ***S.Afr.:*** Oraldettes†; ***Spain:*** Armil; Benzalc; Crema Contracepti Lanzas; Mini Ovulo Lanzas; Novamina; Tearisol†; ***Switz.:*** Benzaltex†; ***UK:*** Bradosol; Capitol†; Dettol Fresh; Roccal; Zensyls; ***USA:*** Bacti-Cleanse; Benza; Mycocide NS; no more germies†; Zephiran.

Multi-ingredient: ***Aust.:*** Aleot; Cleanomed; Cutasept; Dequonal; Dermaspray; Dr Schmidgall Halsweh†; Nasimild†; Tyrothricin comp; ***Austral.:*** Animine; Clean Skin Face Wash; Diaguard†; Drapolex†; Gum-Ese; Oilatum Plus; Paxyl; Solyptol; Virasolve; ***Belg.:*** Dermaspray; ***Canad.:*** Amino-Cerv; Bactine; Family Medicated First Aid Treatment; Medi-Dan; Medi-Quik; Murine Supplemental Tears; Orajel Mouth Aid; Protectaid; Tanac; ***Fr.:*** Acarcid; Biseptine; Dermaspray†; Euvanol; Frekaderm; Humex; Kenalcol; Pharmatex; Rhinofluimucil; ***Ger.:*** Afid Plus; Aknelan Milch†; Altego†; Baccalin; Bacillocid rasant; Bacillocid Spezial; Baktobod; Baktobod N; Buraton 25†; Cutasept; Demykosan S†; Demykosan†; Dequonal; Dorithricin; Dynexan A; Freka-Derm; Freka-Sept 80; Hexaquart L; Hexaquart S; Incidin Extra; Incidin perfekt; Incidur Spray; Indulfan plus; Kohrsolin FF; Mikrobac; Neo-Angin; Pimarektal†; Quatohex; Sekusept Extra N; Sekusept forte; Septolit; Skinman Soft; Tegodor F†; Tegodor forte†; Tegodor†; Tegofektol†; Terralin; Teta-Aktiv†; Thesit; Ultrasol-F; Ultrasol-K†; Ultrasol-S; ***Irl.:*** Conotrane; Drapolene; Emulsiderm; Mycil; Torbetol; ***Ital.:*** Agena; Agipiu; Alfa-Fluorone; Alquat†; Antalgola Plus†; Antalgola†; AZ 15 Gengidentifricio; Barrycidal; Benzogen Ferri; Betaform Habitat; Cedril; Cedril Strumenti; Cedril Tintura†; Cepacol; Citrosil Alcolico Azzuro; Citrosil Alcolico Bruno; Citrosil Alcolico Incolore; Citrosil Nubesan; Collyria; Combisan Plus†; Conta-Lens Wetting; Dentaton Antisettico; Emoplast; Eso Ferri Alcolico; Eso Ferri Alcolico Plus; Eso S 80; Esoalcolico Incolore; Esoform 92; Esoform Alcolico; Esoform Ferri; Esoform Ferri Alcolico; Hamamilla; Herbe; Hexaquart L†; Incidin Spezial; Indulfan; Linea F; Lycia Luminique; Neo-Emocicatrol; Neofen†; Oradyne-Z; Otazul; Pupilla Light; Sangen Casa; Silvana; Simp; Simpottantacinque; Sterosan; T 10 Sapone Chirurgico†; T 21†; Tannovit†; Tirs; Zincometil; ***Mon.:*** Akila spray; ***Neth.:*** Dermaspray†; ***Spain:*** Aerospray Antialergico†; Afta; Alcohcan; Alcopac Reforzado; Anafilaxol†; Avril; Biseptidine†; Corilisina; Curine; Dermo H Infantil; Desinvag; Egarone; Ginejuvent; Gradin Del D Andreu; Gramicidin†; Hemostatico Antisep Asen; Lindemil; Neospray†; Odamida; Otogen Calmante; Pental Forte; Phonal; Pomada Heridas; Resorborina; Sebumselen; Talkosona; Topicaina; Topicaina Miro†; Tulgrasum Cicatrizante; Vigencial; ***Switz.:*** Dequonal; Frekaderm; Jonil T; ***UK:*** Beechams Throat-Plus; Bumps 'n Falls; Callusolve†; Cetanorm; Conotrane; Dermol; Dettol; Drapolene; Emulsiderm; Germolene; Germoloids; Medi-Tissue; Mycil; Neo; Oilatum Plus; Pennine†; Sunspot; Tegodor; ***USA:*** Amino-Cerv; Bactine Antiseptic; Cetylcide†; Medi-Quik; Orajel Mouth Aid; Oxyzal; Tanac; Tanac Dual Core; Yeast-Gard Advanced Sensitive Formula†; Zonite.

Benzethonium Chloride (2207-f)

Benzethonium Chloride *(BAN, rINN)*.

Benzethonii Chloridum; Diisobutylphenoxyethoxyethyldimethylbenzylammonium chloride. Benzyldimethyl(2-{2-[4-(1,1,3,3-tetramethylbutyl)phenoxy]ethoxy}ethyl)ammonium chloride.

$C_{27}H_{42}ClNO_2$ = 448.1.

CAS — 121-54-0.

Pharmacopoeias. In *Eur.* (see p.viii), *Jpn*, and *US*.

White crystals or a white or yellowish-white powder with a mild odour. **Soluble** 1 in less than 1 of water, alcohol, and chloroform, and 1 in 6000 of ether; freely soluble in dichloromethane. An aqueous solution foams copiously when shaken and a 1% solution in water is slightly alkaline to litmus. **Store** in airtight containers. Protect from light. **Incompatible** with soaps and other anionic surfactants.

Benzethonium chloride is a quaternary ammonium antiseptic with actions and uses similar to those of other cationic surfactants (see Cetrimide, p.1105). It is also used as a vaginal spermicide.

Benzethonium chloride produced mild skin irritation at a concentration of 5% but not lower, was not considered to be a sensitiser, and was considered to be safe at a concentration of 0.5% in cosmetics applied to the skin and at a maximum concentration of 0.02% in cosmetics used in the eye area.[1]

1. The Expert Panel of the American College of Toxicology. Final report on the safety assessment of benzethonium chloride and methylbenzethonium chloride. *J Am Coll Toxicol* 1985; **4:** 65–106.

Preparations

USP 23: Benzethonium Chloride Tincture; Benzethonium Chloride Topical Solution.

Proprietary Preparations (details are given in Part 3)
Canad.: Skin Cleanser & Deodorizer; Vi-Medin†; ***Ital.:*** Ribex Gola; ***S.Afr.:*** Johnson's Antiseptic Powder.

Multi-ingredient: ***Austral.:*** Summer's Eve Feminine; ***Belg.:*** Neo-Golaseptine†; ***Canad.:*** Antiseptic Ointment; Antiseptic Skin Cream; Buro Derm; Buro-Sol; Dermoplast; MRX; Protecto; Skin Shield; VoSoL; VoSoL HC; ***Fr.:*** Ta-Ro-Cap†; ***Ger.:*** Brand- u. Wundgel-Medice N; Dexamed†; Mediosept†; Thrombimed†; Vulnostad†; ***Ital.:*** Barrycidal; Borossigeno Plus Stomatologico; Cedril; Cedril Strumenti; Cedril Tintura†; Milupa Neo†; Neo Topico Giusto; Sangen Casa; T 21†; ***S.Afr.:*** Dermoplast†; ***Spain:*** Eupnol; Halibut; Halibut Hidrocortisona; Isdinex; Pental Col†; Tegunal; ***Switz.:*** Angidine; Cemaquin†; Rhinocure; Rhinocure Simplex; Tyrocombine; Tyrothricine + Gramicidine; Undex†; ***UK:*** Lanasting†; ***USA:*** AA-HC Otic; Acetasol; Acetasol HC; Aerocaine; Aerotherm; Americaine; Americaine First Aid; Americaine Otic; Skin Shield; Triple Care Cleanser; Vagisil; VoSoL; VoSoL HC.

Benzoates (11730-m)

Benzoic Acid (6634-b)

Acidum Benzoicum; Benzoesäure; Dracylic Acid; E210.

$C_6H_5.CO_2H$ = 122.1.

CAS — 65-85-0.

Pharmacopoeias. In *Chin.*, *Eur.* (see p.viii), *Int.*, *Jpn*, *Pol.*, and *US*.

Colourless or white crystals or white scales, needles, or crystalline powder; odourless or with a slight characteristic odour. **Soluble** 1 in 300 of water, 1 in 3 of alcohol, 1 in 5 of chloroform, and 1 in 3 of ether; freely soluble in fatty oils. The Ph. Eur. has soluble in boiling water while the USP has freely volatile in steam. M.p. 121° to 124°. The USP provides similar figures (121° to 123°) as the congealing range.

Incompatibilities are described under Sodium Benzoate, below.

Sodium Benzoate (6666-l)

E211; Natrii Benzoas; Natrium Benzoicum; Sodii Benzoas.

$C_6H_5.CO_2Na$ = 144.1.

CAS — 532-32-1.

Pharmacopoeias. In *Chin.*, *Eur.* (see p.viii), *Jpn*, and *Pol.* Also in *USNF.*

A white, odourless or practically odourless, granular or crystalline slightly hygroscopic powder or flakes. **Soluble** 1 in 2 of water, 1 in 75 of alcohol, and 1 in 50 of alcohol 90%. Benzoic acid and its salts are **incompatible** with quaternary compounds, calcium salts, ferric salts, and salts of heavy metals. Their activity is also diminished by nonionic surfactants or due to absorption by kaolin. They are relatively inactive above a pH of about 5.

Adverse Effects and Precautions

The benzoates can cause hypersensitivity reactions, but there have also been reports of non-immunological contact urticaria. The acid can be irritant to skin, eyes, and mucous membranes.

Infants given large doses of sodium benzoate have suffered vomiting. Symptoms of overdosage reported in this group have been restricted to vomiting and irritability.

Premature infants have been reported to be at risk of metabolic acidosis and kernicterus.

Hypersensitivity. Respiratory reactions to benzoates may occur, especially in patients susceptible to aspirin-induced asthma.[1,2] Urticarial reactions have also been associated with these compounds,[3,4] though at a lower incidence[5] and they can be non-immunological.[6] However, these reports have to be balanced against a controlled study[7] that showed no difference in the incidence of urticaria or atopic symptoms between patients given benzoic acid and those given lactose placebo.

Erythema multiforme has been observed in several patients.[8] Anaphylactoid reactions have been reported in two patients.[9,10]

1. Rosenhall L. Evaluation of intolerance to analgesics, preservatives and food colorants with challenge tests. *Eur J Respir Dis* 1982; **63:** 410–19.
2. Settipane GA. Aspirin and allergic diseases: a review. *Am J Med* 1983; **74** (suppl): 102–9.
3. Michaëlsson G, Juhlin L. Urticaria induced by preservatives and dye additives in food and drugs. *Br J Dermatol* 1973; **88:** 525–32.
4. Warin RP, Smith RJ. Challenge test battery in chronic urticaria. *Br J Dermatol* 1976; **94:** 401–6.
5. Wüthrich B, Fabro L. Acetysalicylsäure-und lebensmitteladditiva-intoleranz bei urtikaria, asthma bronchiale und chronischer rhinopathie. *Schweiz Med Wochenschr* 1981; **III:** 1445–50.
6. Nethercott JR, *et al.* Airborne contact urticaria due to sodium benzoate in a pharmaceutical manufacturing plant. *J Occup Med* 1984; **26:** 734–6.
7. Lahti A, Hannuksela M. Is Benzoic acid really harmful in cases of atopy and urticaria? *Lancet* 1981; **ii:** 1055.
8. Lewis MAO, *et al.* Recurrent erythema multiforme: a possible role of foodstuffs. *Br Dent J* 1989; **166:** 371–3.
9. Moneret-Vautrin DA, *et al.* Anaphylactoid reaction to general anaesthesia: a case of intolerance to sodium benzoate. *Anaesth Intensive Care* 1982; **10:** 156–7.
10. Michils A, *et al.* Anaphylaxis with sodium benzoate. *Lancet* 1991; **337:** 1424–5.

Neonates. Serious metabolic disturbances in premature neonates given intravenous fluids with benzyl alcohol as a preservative have been attributed to the accumulation of the benzoic acid metabolite of the benzyl alcohol (see p.1104). This risk led to the recommendation that Caffeine and Sodium Benzoate Injection (USP), which has been given as a respiratory stimulant, should not be used in neonates.[1]

Benzoates can also displace bound bilirubin from albumin putting neonates at risk of kernicterus.[2] However, sodium benzoate has been tried in the treatment of some neonatal metabolic disorders (see under Uses and Administration, below).

1. Edwards RC, Voegeli CJ. Inadvisability of using caffeine and sodium benzoate in neonates. *Am J Hosp Pharm* 1984; **41:** 658.
2. Schiff D, *et al.* Fixed drug combinations and the displacement of bilirubin from albumin. *Pediatrics* 1971: **48:** 139–41.

Pharmacokinetics

The benzoates are absorbed from the gastro-intestinal tract and conjugated with glycine in the liver to form hippuric acid which is rapidly excreted in the urine.

Neonates. References.

1. Green TP, *et al.* Disposition of sodium benzoate in newborn infants with hyperammonemia. *J Pediatr* 1983; **102:** 785–90.

Uses and Administration

Benzoates have antibacterial and antifungal properties. Their antimicrobial activity is due to the undissociated benzoic acid and is therefore pH-dependent. They are relatively inactive above a pH of about 5.

They are used as preservatives in pharmaceutical formulations including oral preparations; benzoic acid and sodium benzoate are typically employed in concentrations of up to 0.1%. They are used as preservatives in foods, (and are also present naturally in some foods), and at a higher concentration in cosmetics.

Benzoic acid 6% with salicylic acid 3%, as Compound Benzoic Acid Ointment (BP 1998), has a long history of use as an antifungal (see Skin Infections, p.371). Benzoic acid has also been employed in desloughing preparations and has been given as a urinary antiseptic.

An injection of caffeine and sodium benzoate has been used as a CNS stimulant, but see above for a caution against its use in neonates.

Sodium benzoate is used as part of the treatment of hyperammonaemia that occurs in inborn errors of the urea cycle. It has also been reported to be effective in reducing plasma-glycine concentrations in nonketotic hyperglycinaemia (p.1633), although it may not be effective in preventing mental retardation.

Sodium benzoate is a common ingredient of cough preparations.

Hyperammonaemia. The dose of sodium benzoate used for treatment of hyperammonaemia (p.1334) has generally been 250 mg per kg body-weight daily by intravenous infusion.[1-3]

1. Maestri NE, *et al.* Long-term survival of patients with argininosuccinate synthetase deficiency. *J Pediatr* 1995; **127:** 929–35.
2. Maestri NE, *et al.* Long-term treatment of girls with ornithine transcarbamylase deficiency. *N Engl J Med* 1996; **335:** 855–9.
3. Zammarchi E, *et al.* Neonatal onset of hyperornithinemia-hyperammonemia-homocitrullinuria syndrome with favorable outcome. *J Pediatr* 1997; **131:** 440–3.

Preparations

BP 1998: Benzoic Acid Solution; Compound Benzoic Acid Ointment *(Whitfield's Ointment)*; Tolu-flavour Solution;
USP 23: Benzoic and Salicylic Acids Ointment; Caffeine and Sodium Benzoate Injection.

Proprietary Preparations (details are given in Part 3)
USA: Drazoic.

Multi-ingredient: ***Aust.:*** Acerbine; Aplexil; Bisolvotin; Expigen; Mycopol; ***Austral.:*** Egomycol; Mycozol; ***Belg.:*** Bronchobel; Bronchosedal; Colimax; Dermacide†; Kamfeine; Normogastryl; Pelarol†; Pholco-Mereprine; Rectoplexil; Tercinol†; Toplexil; Tux; ***Canad.:*** Mouthrinse; MRX; Plax; Sea Breeze; ***Fr.:*** Asthmalgine; Asthmasedine†; Bronchalene; Bronchalene Nourisson; Broncorinol toux seches; Bronpax; Campho-Pneumine Aminophylline†; Campho-Pneumine†; Camphodionyl; Codotussyl; Curibronches†; Dermacide; Desbly†; Dimetane; Dinacode; Dinacode avec codeine; Ephydion; Germose; Glyco-Thymoline; Gynescal; Humex; Marrubene Codethyline; Neo-Codion; Nican†; Ozothine; Paregorique; Passedyl; Pastaba†; Pecto 6†; Pneumaseptic; Pneumogeine; Pneumopan; Polaramine Pectoral; Polery; Pulmofluide Enfants†; Pulmofluide Ephedrine†; Pulmofluide Simple; Pulmonase; Pulmosodyl; Pulmospir†; Pulmothiol†; Quintopan Adult; Rectoplexil; Rhinamide; Silomat; Sirop Pectoral adulte; Sirop Pectoral enfant; Terpine Gonnon†; Theralene Pectoral Nourrisson; Toplexil; Tossarel; Tuberol†; Uraseptine Rogier†; ***Ger.:*** Aplexil†; Bronchitussin SC†; Kytta-Nagelsalbe†; Sagrosept; Soledum Hustensaft N†; ***Irl.:*** Aserbine†; ***Ital.:*** Borocaina; Bronchised†; Broncobeta†; Chymoser Balsamico†; Cort-Inal; Creosolactol Bambini†; Dentinale; Guaiacalcium Complex; Guaiadomus†; Neo Borocillina; Sedobex; Sedocalcio; Timolene†; Tiocosol; Tionamil; Xival†; ***Neth.:*** Toplexil; ***S.Afr.:*** Aserbine; ***Spain:*** Acerbiol; Bronco Sergo; Broncoformo Muco Dexa; Broncomicin Bals; Broncovital; Bronquiasmol†; Bronquidiazina CR; Bronquimar; Diptol Antihist†; Efralen†; Etermol Antitusivo; Iodocafedrina†; Lomisat Compositum†; Maboterpen; Mentobox; Neumopectolina; Pastillas Pectoral Kely; Pazbronquial; Pectoral Brum; Pulmo Menal; Pulmofasa; Pulmofasa Antihist; Tos Mai; ***Switz.:*** Acerbine; Bronchalin; Bronchocodin; Demo pates pectorales; Dinacode N; Foral; GEM†; Marciderm†; Melior†; Nasobol; Neo-Codion Enfants†; Neo-Codion N†; Neo-Codion Nourrisons†; Nican; Phol-Tussil; Phol-Tux; Saintbois nouvelle formule; Sirop pectoral DP1; Sirop pectoral DP2; Spedro; Toplexil; ***UK:*** Antiseptic Throat Pastilles; Aserbine; Eczema Ointment; Hemocane; Malatex†; Melissin; Sanderson's Throat Specific; Toepedo; ***USA:*** Atrosept; Cystex; Dolsed; Feminique; Prosed/DS; Summer's Eve Disposable; Trac Tabs 2X; UAA; Ucephan; Uridon Modified; Urised.

Benzododecinium Bromide (2208-d)

Benzyldodecyldimethylammonium bromide.
$C_{21}H_{38}BrN$ = 384.4.
CAS — 10328-35-5 (benzododecinium); 7281-04-1 (benzododecinium bromide); 139-07-1 (benzododecinium chloride).

NOTE. Benzododecinium Chloride is *rINN.*
Pharmacopoeias. In *Fr.*

Benzododecinium bromide is a quaternary ammonium antiseptic with properties similar to those of other cationic surfactants (see Cetrimide, p.1105). It is used in mouthwashes and nasal sprays and solutions for the treatment of minor infections. It is also used as a spermicide. Benzododecinium chloride has also been used.

Preparations

Proprietary Preparations (details are given in Part 3)
Austral.: TAGG.

Multi-ingredient: ***Fr.:*** Arpha†; Genola; Humex; Prorhinel; Sedacollyre; ***Ger.:*** Prorhinel; ***Ital.:*** Larilon; ***Switz.:*** Azulene†; Kemerhinose; Prorhinel.

Benzoxonium Chloride (11594-e)

Benzoxonium Chloride *(rINN).*
Benzyldodecylbis(2-hydroxyethyl)ammonium chloride.
$C_{23}H_{42}ClNO_2$ = 400.0.
CAS — 19379-90-9.

Benzoxonium chloride is a quaternary ammonium antiseptic used for disinfection of the skin and mucous membranes. It is also used for instrument disinfection.

Preparations

Proprietary Preparations (details are given in Part 3)
Belg.: Orofar; ***Ital.:*** Bactofen; Bialcol; Sinecod Bocca; ***Switz.:*** Merfen nouveau.

Multi-ingredient: ***Belg.:*** Orofar Lidocaine; ***Ger.:*** Dexa Loscon†; Includal†; Loscon; Myxal†; ***Ital.:*** Halciderm; ***Spain:*** Cohortan; Cohortan Antibiotico; ***Switz.:*** Halciderm†; Orofar; Vita-Merfen (nouveau).

Benzyl Alcohol (554-h)

Benzyl Alcohol *(rINN).*
Alcohol Benzylicus; Alcool Benzylique; Benzenemethanol; Phenylcarbinol; Phenylmethanol.
$C_6H_5.CH_2OH$ = 108.1.
CAS — 100-51-6.

Pharmacopoeias. In *Eur.* (see p.viii), *Int., Jpn,* and *Pol.* Also in *USNF.*

A clear, colourless, oily, refractive liquid with a slightly aromatic odour. **Soluble** or sparingly soluble in water; freely soluble in alcohol (50%); miscible with alcohol, chloroform, ether, and fatty and essential oils. It is neutral to litmus.

Benzyl alcohol oxidises to produce benzaldehyde and benzoic acid and oxidation may take place slowly on exposure to air. Benzaldehyde may also be produced on autoclaving. The Ph. Eur. has a limit of not more than 0.05% of benzaldehyde and 0.1% of other related substances for benzyl alcohol intended for use in the manufacture of a parenteral dosage form. **Store** in completely filled airtight containers and prevent exposure to excessive heat. Protect from light. Benzyl alcohol is **incompatible** with oxidising agents and strong acids. The antimicrobial activity may be reduced by nonionic surfactants and benzyl alcohol may be lost from solutions stored in polyethylene containers.

Adverse Effects and Precautions

There have been a few reports of hypersensitivity reactions to benzyl alcohol when used as a preservative.

The pure alcohol is irritant and requires handling with care; ingestion or inhalation can cause nausea, vomiting, diarrhoea, headache, vertigo, and CNS depression. However, concentrations of benzyl alcohol normally used for preservation are not associated with such effects.

There have been some instances of neurotoxic effects in patients given intrathecal injections that contained benzyl alcohol.

A fatal toxic syndrome in premature infants was attributed to benzyl alcohol present as a preservative in solutions used to flush intravenous catheters. This has led to restriction on the use of benzyl alcohol in neonates, see below.

Effects on the lungs. Severe bronchitis and haemoptysis was reported in a patient with obstructive pulmonary disease who, over a period of 2 years, had inhaled salbutamol nebuliser solution diluted with a bacteriostatic sodium chloride solution containing benzyl alcohol.[1]

1. Reynolds RD. Nebulizer bronchitis induced by bacteriostatic saline. *JAMA* 1990; **264:** 35.

Effects on the nervous system. Rapid development of flaccid areflexic paraplegia, total anaesthesia below the groin, and radicular abdominal pain occurred in a 64-year-old man following a lumbar intrathecal injection of cytarabine which contained 1.5% benzyl alcohol.[1] The patient recovered fully after 100 mL of CSF was replaced with sodium chloride injection (0.9%) and 40 mg of methylprednisolone. Intrathecal injections of cytarabine dissolved in sterile distilled water before and after the episode of paraplegia caused no neurologic symptoms. On reviewing 20 other cases of paraparesis associated with methotrexate or cytarabine intrathecal injections, benzyl alcohol had been used as a preservative in 7. Of the 7, 4 developed neurotoxicity immediately; in the other 3 it did not develop until 6 to 48 hours after administration. The duration varied. One patient did not improve, one made a partial recovery, a third took 6 weeks to recover, another took 5 days; yet 2 patients recovered within 1½ to 2½ hours while the final patient experienced only transient effects.

1. Hahn AF, *et al.* Paraparesis following intrathecal chemotherapy. *Neurology* 1983; **33:** 1032–8.

Hypersensitivity. Some reports of hypersensitivity reactions to benzyl alcohol.

1. Grant JA, *et al.* Unsuspected benzyl alcohol hypersensitivity. *N Engl J Med* 1982; **306:** 108.
2. Shmunes E. Allergic dermatitis to benzyl alcohol in an injectable solution. *Arch Dermatol* 1984; **120:** 1200–1.
3. Wilson JP, *et al.* Parenteral benzyl alcohol-induced hypersensitivity reaction. *Drug Intell Clin Pharm* 1986; **20:** 689–91.

Neonates. During 1981 and 1982 reports were published from 2 centres in the USA[1-3] of 20 deaths in low-birth-weight neonates attributed to the use of benzyl alcohol as a preservative in solutions used to flush their umbilical catheters and in some cases also to dilute their medication. The neonates suffered a toxic syndrome whose features included metabolic acidosis, symptoms of progressive encephalopathy, intracranial haemorrhage, and respiratory depression with gasping.

These deaths prompted the FDA[4] to recommend that benzyl alcohol should not be used in such flushing solutions; sodium chloride injection (0.9%) without preservative should be used instead. The FDA had also advised against the use of benzyl alcohol or any preservative in fluids being used for the dilution or reconstitution of medicines for the newborn.

Those reporting the deaths[2,3] considered that the toxic syndrome could have been caused by the accumulation of the benzoic acid metabolite of benzyl alcohol, which could not be handled effectively by the immature liver; given the very low weight of the neonates they would have been receiving a high dose of benzyl alcohol. In commenting on the problem, the American Academy of Pediatrics[5] agreed that the FDA's warning was warranted, but pointed out that there was no evidence from controlled studies to confirm that benzyl alcohol was responsible.

1. Gershanik JJ, *et al.* The gasping syndrome: benzyl alcohol (BA) poisoning? *Clin Res* 1981; **29:** 895A.
2. Brown WJ, *et al.* Fatal benzyl alcohol poisoning in a neonatal intensive care unit. *Lancet* 1982; **i:** 1250.
3. Gershanik J, *et al.* The gasping syndrome and benzyl alcohol poisoning. *N Engl J Med* 1982; **307:** 1384–8.
4. Anonymous. Benzyl alcohol may be toxic to newborns. *FDA Drug Bull* 1982; **12:** 10–11.
5. American Academy of Pediatrics. Benzyl alcohol: toxic agent in neonatal use. *Pediatrics* 1983; **72:** 356–7.

Pharmacokinetics

Benzyl alcohol is metabolised to benzoic acid. This is conjugated with glycine in the liver to form hippuric acid which is excreted in the urine. Benzaldehyde and benzoic acid are degradation products *in vitro*.

Uses

Benzyl alcohol is used as an antimicrobial preservative. It is bacteriostatic mainly against Gram-positive organisms and some fungi. It is used in a range of pharmaceutical preparations in concentrations up to 2%. Concentrations of 5% or more are employed when it is used as a solubiliser. Benzyl alcohol is also used as a preservative in foods and cosmetics.

In addition to its antiseptic properties, diluted benzyl alcohol possesses weak local anaesthetic and antipruritic activity and this is the reason for its inclusion in some preparations.

Preparations

Proprietary Preparations (details are given in Part 3)
Canad.: Babys Own Teething Gel; Zilactin.

Multi-ingredient: ***Aust.:*** Dermaspray; ***Austral.:*** Coso; ***Belg.:*** Dermaspray; ***Canad.:*** Foille; ***Fr.:*** Biseptine; Dermaspray†; Vicks Pastilles†; Vicks Soulagil†; Vicks vitamine C pastilles†; ***Ger.:*** Spitacid; Varicocid†; ***Irl.:*** Sudocrem; ***Ital.:*** Antimicotico†; Borocaina; Foille; Foille Sole; ***Neth.:*** Dermaspray†; ***Spain:*** Acerbiol; ***UK:*** Lanasting†; Sudocrem; ***USA:*** Anusol; Cepacol Throat; Florida Sunburn Relief; Itch-X; Medadyne†; MouthKote O/R; Rhuli Gel; Step 2; TiSol; Topic.

Used as an adjunct in: ***Jpn:*** Panpurol.

Biclotymol (16535-k)

Biclotymol *(rINN)*.
2,2′-Methylenebis(6-chlorothymole).
$C_{21}H_{26}Cl_2O_2$ = 381.3.
CAS — 15686-33-6.

Biclotymol is a phenolic antiseptic which is used as lozenges and sprays in mouth and throat infections. It is also an ingredient of cough preparations.

Preparations

Proprietary Preparations (details are given in Part 3)
Fr.: Hexadreps; Hexapock†; Hexaspray.
Multi-ingredient: ***Fr.:*** Hexalyse; Hexapneumine.

Bisdequalinium Diacetate (2209-n)

R-199. 1,1′-Decamethylene-*NN*′-decamethylenebis(4-amino-2-methylquinolinium acetate).
$C_{44}H_{64}N_4O_4$ = 713.0.
CAS — 3785-44-2.

Bisdequalinium diacetate is a bisquaternary quinolinium antiseptic with properties similar to those of other quinolinium cationic surfactants (see Dequalinium Chloride, p.1112). It has been applied topically in the treatment of a variety of minor skin infections.

Preparations

Proprietary Preparations (details are given in Part 3)
Multi-ingredient: ***Ger.:*** Lensch†.

Brilliant Green (2211-a)

CI Basic Green 1; Colour Index No. 42040; Diamond Green G; Emerald Green; Ethyl Green; Malachite Green G; Solid Green; Viride Nitens. 4-(4-Diethylaminobenzhydrylidene)cyclohexa-2,5-dien-1-ylidenediethylammonium hydrogen sulphate.
$C_{27}H_{34}N_2O_4S$ = 482.6.
CAS — 633-03-4.

NOTE. The name Emerald Green has also been used to denote copper acetoarsenite.

Brilliant green is a triphenylmethane antiseptic dye with actions similar to those of crystal violet (p.1111). Its activity is greatly reduced in the presence of serum.

A gel containing brilliant green 0.5% with lactic acid has been used in the treatment of skin ulcers.

An alcoholic solution of brilliant green 0.5% and crystal violet 0.5% (Bonney's Blue) has been used for disinfecting the skin, but concern at evidence of *animal* carcinogenicity with crystal violet has led to the decline of such paints. However, a solution of the two disinfectants may be used for marking incisions prior to surgery.

There have been occasional reports of sensitivity to brilliant green.

For a report of necrotic skin reactions following application of a 1% solution of brilliant green to stripped skin, see under the Adverse Effects of Crystal Violet, p.1111.

Preparations

Proprietary Preparations (details are given in Part 3)
Multi-ingredient: ***UK:*** Variclene†.

Bromchlorophen (11596-y)

Bromchlorophene; Bromochlorophane. 2,2′-Methylenebis[6-bromo-4-chlorophenol].
$C_{13}H_8Br_2Cl_2O_2$ = 426.9.
CAS — 15435-29-7.

Bromchlorophen is a halogenated bisphenol antiseptic more active against Gram-positive than Gram-negative bacteria. It is used for disinfection of the hands and skin.

Preparations

Proprietary Preparations (details are given in Part 3)
Multi-ingredient: ***Ger.:*** Dibromol.

Bromsalans (2289-k)

CAS — 55830-61-0.

A series of brominated salicylanilides which possess antimicrobial activity.

Dibromsalan (2290-w)

Dibromsalan *(USAN, pINN)*.
NSC-20527. 4′,5-Dibromosalicylanilide; 5-Bromo-*N*-(4-bromophenyl)-2-hydroxybenzamide.
$C_{13}H_9Br_2NO_2$ = 371.0.
CAS — 87-12-7.

Metabromsalan (2291-e)

Metabromsalan *(USAN, pINN)*.
NSC-526280. 3,5-Dibromosalicylanilide; 3,5-Dibromo-2-hydroxy-*N*-phenylbenzamide.
$C_{13}H_9Br_2NO_2$ = 371.0.
CAS — 2577-72-2.

Tribromsalan (2213-x)

Tribromsalan *(BAN, USAN, rINN)*.
ET-394; NSC-20526; TBS. 3,4′,5-Tribromosalicylanilide; 3,5-Dibromo-*N*-(4-bromophenyl)-2-hydroxybenzamide.
$C_{13}H_8Br_3NO_2$ = 449.9.
CAS — 87-10-5.

Bromsalans have antibacterial and antifungal activity and were used in medicated soaps, but there have been many reports of photosensitivity arising from this use.

Preparations

Proprietary Preparations (details are given in Part 3)
Ital.: Bergamon Sapone.

Bronopol (6636-g)

Bronopol *(BAN, rINN)*.
2-Bromo-2-nitropropane-1,3-diol.
$C_3H_6BrNO_4$ = 200.0.
CAS — 52-51-7.
Pharmacopoeias. In *Br.* and *Pol.*

White or almost white crystals or crystalline powder, odourless or almost odourless. Freely **soluble** in water and in alcohol; slightly soluble in glycerol and in liquid paraffin. A 1% solution in water has a pH of 5 to 7. **Protect** from light.

Incompatibilities. Activity can be diminished by sodium metabisulphite, sodium thiosulphate, cysteine hydrochloride, and compounds with a thiol group. Increases in temperature affect stability as do increases in pH above 8. Incompatibility with unprotected aluminium affects packaging.

Creams and shampoos containing bronopol 0.01% as a preservative were found to contain free nitrite and, as a result of amines present in the preparations, nitrosamines.[1] Antioxidants complexed the free nitrite to varying extents and inhibited nitrosamine formation. Alpha tocopherol had a similar inhibitory effect to butylated hydroxytoluene and ascorbate but a lower effect on nitrite complexation, suggesting that it might act directly on the nitrosation reaction. It was recommended that nitrosamine formation could be reduced in preparations containing amines and bronopol by limiting the bronopol concentration to 0.01% and inclusion of alpha tocopherol 0.2% or butylated hydroxytoluene 0.05%.

1. Dunnett PC, Telling GM. Study of the fate of bronopol and the effects of antioxidants on N-nitrosamine formation in shampoos and skin creams. *Int J Cosmet Sci* 1984; **6:** 241–7.

Adverse Effects

Bronopol may be irritant when applied topically.

Pharmacokinetics

Bronopol is absorbed following topical administration.

Uses

Bronopol is active against a wide range of bacteria, including *Pseudomonas aeruginosa*, but is less active against moulds and yeasts. Bronopol is used as a preservative in shampoos, cosmetics, and both topical and oral pharmaceutical preparations; concentrations in pharmaceutical preparations range from 0.01 to 0.1%, with the usual concentration being 0.02%.

Butylated Hydroxyanisole (6638-p)

Butylated Hydroxyanisole *(BAN)*.
BHA; Butilidrossianisolo; Butylhydroxyanisole; Butylhydroxyanisolum; E320. 2-*tert*-Butyl-4-methoxyphenol; 2-(1,1-dimethylethyl)-4-methoxyphenol.
$C_{11}H_{16}O_2$ = 180.2.
CAS — 25013-16-5.
Pharmacopoeias. In *Eur.* (see p.viii), *Int.*, and *Pol.* Also in *USNF.*

A white, yellowish, or slightly pinkish crystalline powder or a yellowish-white waxy solid with an aromatic odour. The Ph. Eur. specifies not more than 10% of 3-(1,1-dimethylethyl)-4-methoxyphenol.

Practically **insoluble** in water; soluble 1 in 4 of alcohol, 1 in 2 of chloroform, and 1 in 1.2 of ether; freely soluble in propylene glycol and in fatty oils; very soluble in dichloromethane; it dissolves in dilute solutions of alkali hydroxides. **Protect** from light.

Incompatible with oxidising agents and ferric salts. Traces of metals can cause loss of activity.

Adverse Effects

Butylated hydroxyanisole can be irritant to the eyes, skin, and mucous membranes and can cause depigmentation. There are reports of delayed (type IV) hypersensitivity reactions and non-immunogenic skin reactions.

Effects on the blood. For a report of methaemoglobinaemia associated with the antoxidants (butylated hydroxyanisole, butylated hydroxytoluene, and propyl gallate) used to preserve the oil in a soybean infant feed, see under Adverse Effects in Alkyl Gallates (p.1101).

Pharmacokinetics

Butylated hydroxyanisole is absorbed from the gastro-intestinal tract, then metabolised and conjugated, and excreted in the urine; less than 1% is excreted in the urine as unchanged drug within 24 hours of ingestion.

Uses

Butylated hydroxyanisole is an antoxidant with some antimicrobial activity. It is used as a preservative in cosmetics and foods as well as pharmaceutical preparations, particularly to delay or prevent oxidative rancidity of fats and oils in concentrations of up to 0.02%; higher concentrations have been used for essential oils. It is also used to prevent the loss of activity of oil-soluble vitamins.

Commercial supplies of butylated hydroxyanisole employed in food technology consist of mixtures of the 2-*tert* and 3-*tert* isomers.

To improve efficacy, butylated hydroxyanisole is frequently used in combination with other antoxidants such as butylated hydroxytoluene or an alkyl gallate and with sequestrants or synergists such as citric acid.

In the UK the Food Advisory Committee has recommended that the use of butylated hydroxyanisole and butylated hydroxytoluene should no longer be permitted as additives for infant formulas as they are no longer required for the economic manufacture of vitamin A and vitamin A esters.[1]

1. MAFF. Food Advisory Committee: report on the review of the use of additives in foods specially prepared for infants and young children. *FdAC/REP/12*. London: HMSO, 1992.

Butylated Hydroxytoluene (6639-s)

Butylated Hydroxytoluene *(BAN)*.

BHT; Butylhydroxitoluenum; Butylhydroxytoluene; E321. 2,6-Di-*tert*-butyl-*p*-cresol.

$C_{15}H_{24}O$ = 220.4.

CAS — 128-37-0.

Pharmacopoeias. In *Eur.* (see p.viii), *Int.*, and *Pol.* Also in *USNF.*

Colourless crystals or white or yellowish-white crystalline powder, odourless or with a faint odour. Practically **insoluble** in water; soluble 1 in 4 of alcohol and about 1 in 1 of chloroform and of ether; very soluble in acetone; practically insoluble in propylene glycol; freely soluble in vegetable oils. **Incompatible** with oxidising agents and ferric salts. Traces of metals can cause loss of activity.

Adverse Effects

As for Butylated Hydroxyanisole, p.1104.

A 22-year-old woman experienced severe epigastric cramping, nausea and vomiting, and generalised weakness, followed by dizziness, confusion, and a brief loss of consciousness after ingesting 4 g of butylated hydroxytoluene on an empty stomach. She recovered following conservative treatment which was given 2 days later. The antoxidant had been taken as an unauthorised remedy for genital herpes simplex.[1]

1. Shlian DM, Goldstone J. Toxicity of butylated hydroxytoluene. *N Engl J Med* 1986; **314:** 648–9.

Effects on the blood. For a report of methaemoglobinaemia associated with the antoxidants (butylated hydroxyanisole, butylated hydroxytoluene, and propyl gallate) used to preserve the oil in a soybean infant feed formula, see under Adverse Effects in Alkyl Gallates (p.1101).

Pharmacokinetics

Butylated hydroxytoluene is readily absorbed from the gastro-intestinal tract. It is excreted in the urine mainly as glucuronide conjugates of oxidation products.

Uses

Butylated hydroxytoluene is an antoxidant with similar uses to Butylated Hydroxyanisole, p.1105.

Cadexomer-Iodine (15334-d)

Cadexomer-iodine *(BAN)*.

Cadexomer Iodine *(USAN)*. 2-Hydroxymethylene cross-linked (1→4)-α-D-glucan carboxymethyl ether containing iodine.

CAS — 94820-09-4.

Adverse Effects and Precautions

As for Povidone-Iodine, p.1123. Some patients have experienced stinging and erythema following application of cadexomer-iodine to their ulcers. Free iodine is released during exposure of cadexomer-iodine preparations to wound exudate and absorption of iodine may occur. Prolonged treatment with cadexomer-iodine should be used with caution in patients with thyroid disorders.

Uses and Administration

Cadexomer-iodine, like povidone-iodine (p.1124), is an iodophore that releases iodine. It is used for its absorbent and antiseptic properties in the management of venous leg ulcers and pressure sores. It is applied as a powder, ointment, or paste containing iodine 0.9%; the manufacturer suggests sufficient powder or ointment should be applied to form a layer about 3 mm thick. Treatment should not usually be continued for more than 3 months.

Beneficial results were reported with cadexomer-iodine in patients with chronic infected venous ulcers (p.1076) unresponsive to previous treatments.[1,2] In another study cadexomer-iodine did not improve the healing rate.[3]

1. Skog E, *et al.* A randomized trial comparing cadexomer iodine and standard treatment in the out-patient management of chronic venous ulcers. *Br J Dermatol* 1983; **109:** 77–83.
2. Ormiston MC, *et al.* Controlled trial of Iodosorb in chronic venous ulcers. *Br Med J* 1985; **291:** 308–10.
3. Moss C, *et al.* Controlled trial of Iodosorb in chronic venous ulcers. *Br Med J* 1985; **291:** 902.

Preparations

Proprietary Preparations (details are given in Part 3)
Aust.: Iodosorb; ***Fr.:*** Iodosorb†; ***Ger.:*** Essasorb†; Iodosorb; ***Ital.:*** Iodosorb; ***Spain:*** Iodosorb; ***Swed.:*** Iodosorb; ***Switz.:*** Iodosorb; ***UK:*** Iodoflex; Iodosorb; ***USA:*** Iodosorb†.

Cetalkonium Chloride (2214-r)

Cetalkonium Chloride *(BAN, USAN, rINN)*.

NSC-32942. Benzylhexadecyldimethylammonium chloride.

$C_{25}H_{46}ClN$ = 396.1.

CAS — 122-18-9.

Cetalkonium chloride is a quaternary ammonium antiseptic with actions and uses similar to those of other cationic surfactants (see Cetrimide, p.1105). It is used in a variety of topical preparations in the treatment of minor infections of the eye, mouth, and throat. Cetalkonium bromide has also been used.

Preparations

Proprietary Preparations (details are given in Part 3)
Multi-ingredient: ***Aust.:*** Mundisal; ***Austral.:*** Bonjela; ***Canad.:*** Bionet; Emercol; ***Fr.:*** Pansoral; ***Ger.:*** Biseptol compositum†; Mundisal; ***Irl.:*** Bonjela; ***S.Afr.:*** AAA; ***Spain:*** Topicaina Miro†; ***Switz.:*** Deca; Mundisal; Pansoral; ***UK:*** AAA; Bonjela; ***USA:*** Babee.

Cethexonium Bromide (2215-f)

Hexadecyl(2-hydroxycyclohexyl)dimethylammonium bromide.

$C_{24}H_{50}BrNO$ = 448.6.

CAS — 6810-42-0 (cethexonium); 1794-74-7 (cethexonium bromide); 58703-78-9 (cethexonium chloride).

NOTE. Cethexonium Chloride is *rINN*.

Cethexonium bromide is a quaternary ammonium antiseptic with properties similar to those of other cationic surfactants (see Cetrimide, p.1105). It is used in preparations for the local treatment of minor infections of the eye, nose, and throat.

Preparations

Proprietary Preparations (details are given in Part 3)
Fr.: Biocidan.
Multi-ingredient: ***Fr.:*** Biocidan.

Cetrimide (2216-d)

Cetrimide *(BAN, rINN)*.

Cetrimidum.

CAS — 1119-97-7 (trimethyltetradecylammonium bromide); 1119-94-4 (dodecyltrimethylammonium bromide); 8044-71-1 (cetrimide).

NOTE. The name cetrimonium bromide was often formerly applied to cetrimide. Cetrimonium bromide is hexadecyltrimethylammonium bromide.

Pharmacopoeias. In *Eur.* (see p.viii) and *Int.*

Cetrimide consists chiefly of trimethyltetradecylammonium bromide (= tetradonium bromide) together with smaller amounts of dodecyltrimethylammonium bromide and hexadecyltrimethylammonium bromide (= cetrimonium bromide, p.1106).

A white to almost white, voluminous, free-flowing powder. Freely **soluble** in water and alcohol; practically insoluble in ether. A 2.0% solution in water foams strongly on shaking. **Incompatible** with soaps and other anionic surfactants, bentonite, iodine, phenylmercuric nitrate, and alkali hydroxides. Aqueous solutions react with metals. The antimicrobial activity of quaternary ammonium compounds may be diminished through absorption, or through combination with organic matter, or by reducing pH.

Strong Cetrimide Solution (BP 1998) contains 20 to 40% cetrimide and up to 10% alcohol or isopropyl alcohol, or both, as a preservative; alcohol may be replaced by industrial methylated spirit.

Adverse Effects and Treatment

If ingested, cetrimide and other quaternary ammonium compounds cause nausea and vomiting; strong solutions may cause oesophageal damage and necrosis. They have depolarising muscle relaxant properties and toxic symptoms include dyspnoea and cyanosis due to paralysis of the respiratory muscles, possibly leading to asphyxia. Depression of the CNS (sometimes preceded by excitement and convulsions), hypotension, coma, and death may also occur. Accidental intra-uterine or intravenous administration may cause haemolysis.

At the concentrations used on the skin, solutions of cetrimide and other quaternary compounds do not generally cause irritation, but some patients become hypersensitive to cetrimide after repeated applications. Cetrimide powder is reported to be irritant. There have been rare reports of burns with concentrated solutions of cetrimide. Treatment of poisoning is symptomatic; demulcents may be given if necessary but emesis and lavage should be avoided, particularly if concentrated solutions have been ingested. CNS stimulants and cholinesterase inhibitors are reported not to reverse paralysis due to cetrimide intoxication although sympathomimetics have been tried.

The fatal dose of quaternary ammonium compounds was estimated to be 1 to 3 g.[1]

1. Arena JM. Poisonings and other health hazards associated with use of detergents. *JAMA* 1964; **190:** 56–8.

Adverse effects following irrigation with cetrimide solutions in the treatment of hydatid cysts have included chemical peritonitis,[1] methaemoglobinaemia with cyanosis,[2] and metabolic acidosis.[3]

1. Gilchrist DS. Chemical peritonitis after cetrimide washout in hydatid-cyst surgery. *Lancet* 1979; **ii:** 1374.
2. Baraka A, *et al.* Cetrimide-induced methaemoglobinaemia after surgical excision of hydatid cyst. *Lancet* 1980; **ii:** 88–9.
3. Momblano P, *et al.* Metabolic acidosis induced by cetrimonium bromide. *Lancet* 1984; **ii:** 1045.

Precautions

Prolonged and repeated applications of cetrimide to the skin are inadvisable as hypersensitivity may occur. Contact with the eyes, brain, meninges, and middle ear should be avoided. Cetrimide should not be used in body cavities or as an enema.

Solutions of quaternary ammonium compounds should not be used for disinfection of soft contact lenses.

Aqueous solutions of cetrimide or other quaternary ammonium disinfectants may be susceptible to contamination with micro-organisms. To reduce this risk, a sterilised preparation should be used or, where necessary, solutions must be freshly prepared at the recommended concentration and appropriate measures should be taken to prevent contamination during storage or dilution.

Cetrimide powder is irritant; it has been recommended that the nose and mouth should be protected by a mask when working with the powder[1] and eyes should be protected by goggles.

1. Jacobs JY. Work hazards from drug handling. *Pharm J* 1984; **233:** 195–6.

Uses and Administration

Cetrimide is a quaternary ammonium antiseptic with actions and uses typical of cationic surfactants. These surfactants dissociate in aqueous solution into a relatively large and complex cation, which is responsible for the surface activity, and a smaller inactive anion. In addition to emulsifying and detergent properties, quaternary ammonium compounds have bactericidal activity against Gram-positive and, at a higher concentration, against some Gram-negative bacteria. Some *Pseudomonas* spp. are particularly resistant as are strains of *Mycobacterium tuberculosis*. They are ineffective against bacterial spores, have variable antifungal activity, and are effective against some viruses.

Quaternary ammonium compounds are most effective in neutral or slightly alkaline solution and their bactericidal activity is appreciably reduced in acid media; their activity is enhanced by alcohols.

Like other quaternary ammonium compounds, notably benzalkonium chloride, cetrimide has been employed for cleansing skin, wounds (but see under Wound Disinfection, p.1098), and burns. For these purposes it has been used as a 0.1 to 1.0% aqueous solution, generally prepared by dilution of a more concentrated solution, or as a cream containing 0.5%. However, a mixture of cetrimide with chlorhexidine (p.1107) has often been preferred to cetrimide alone. This combination is also used in a lotion for acne, (p.1072).

Solutions containing up to 10% of cetrimide have been used as shampoos to remove the scales in seborrhoeic dermatitis (p.1076).

Cetrimide solution 0.5 or 1% has been used as a scolicide to irrigate hydatid cysts during surgery (see Echinococcosis, p.94) but systemic adverse effects have been reported (see above).

Cetrimide and benzalkonium chloride are also used as preservatives in cosmetics and pharmaceutical formulations including eye drops and in disinfecting solutions for hard contact lenses; neither compound should be used for disinfection of soft contact lenses.

Quaternary ammonium compounds are not reliable agents for sterilising surgical instruments and heat-labile articles.

Cetrimide is also present in some emulsifying preparations such as Cetrimide Emulsifying Ointment (BP 1998).

Preparations

BP 1998: Cetrimide Cream; Cetrimide Emulsifying Ointment; Cetrimide Solution.

Proprietary Preparations (details are given in Part 3)
Austral.: Cetavlon†; Cetoderm†; ***Canad.:*** Resdan; Savlon; ***Fr.:*** Asepto 7; Cetavlon; ***Irl.:*** Cetavlex; Cetavlon†; Cradocap†; Vesagex; ***Ital.:*** Cetavlon†; Germozero Hospital; ***Neth.:*** Cetavlon; ***S.Afr.:*** Cetavlon; ***Spain:*** Cetavlon; ***UK:*** Bactrian; Bansor; Cetavlex; Cetavlon†; Cradocap; Medi-Prep; Vesagex.

Multi-ingredient: ***Aust.:*** Xylonor; ***Austral.:*** Acnederm Wash; Ansene L†; Ansene†; Cetal Instrument Disinfectant; Cross Prep; Dermocaine; Dimethicream; Drapolex†; Formicare Skin Relief†; Hamilton Skin Repair Cream; Hibicet; Medi Creme; Mediderm†; Microshield Antiseptic; Pro-PS; Savlon Antiseptic; Savlon Hospital Concentrate†; Septimide†; Soov Bite; Soov Burn; Soov Cream; ***Belg.:*** Lemocin; ***Canad.:*** Savlodil; Savlon Hospital Concentrate; ***Fr.:*** Rectoquotane; ***Irl.:*** Ceanel; Drapolene; Hibicet; Morsep†; RBC; Savlodil†; Savlon†; Siopel; Torbetol; ***Ital.:*** Baxidin; Cetrisan; Citroen Alcolico Strumenti†; Citroen Alcolico†; Farvicett; Hibicet; Iketoncid; Panseptil; Savlodil†; Savlon†; Steridol; ***Neth.:*** Cetavlex†; Hibicet concentraat; Hibicet verdunning; ***S.Afr.:*** Benzet; Bronchilate†; Bronchistop; Ceanel; Hibicet; Meditussi; Orocaine; Savloclens†; Savlodil†; Savlon; Siopel; Trochain; Virobis†; ***Spain:*** Lidrone; Savlon†; ***Switz.:*** GEM†; ***UK:*** Ceanel; Cetanorm; Cetriclens†; Cymex; Dermidex; Drapolene; Hibicet Hospital Concentrate; Lypsyl Cold Sore Gel; Modantis; Morsep†; Neo; Quinoderm Antibacterial Face Wash; RBC; Savlon Cream; Savlon Liquid; Savlon Nappy Rash Cream†; Siopel; Steripod Yellow; Steriwipe†; Tisept; Torbetol; Travasept; ***USA:*** Scadan.

Cetrimonium Bromide (16343-s)

Cetrimonium Bromide *(rINN)*.

Cetyltrimethylammonium Bromide; CTAB. Hexadecyltrimethylammonium bromide.

$C_{19}H_{42}BrN = 364.4$.

CAS — 57-09-0 (cetrimonium bromide); 6899-10-1 (cetrimonium); 112-02-7 (cetrimonium chloride).

NOTE. Cetrimonium Chloride is *BAN*.
The name cetrimonium bromide was formerly applied to cetrimide.

Cetrimonium bromide is a quaternary ammonium antiseptic with actions and uses similar to those of other cationic surfactants (see Cetrimide, p.1105). Cetrimonium chloride and cetrimonium tosylate are also used.

Preparations

Proprietary Preparations (details are given in Part 3)
Belg.: Aseptiderm; ***Ital.:*** Golaval; Neo-Intol; Senol; ***Switz.:*** Turisan.

Multi-ingredient: ***Aust.:*** Lemocin; Xylestesin; ***Belg.:*** Cetavlex; HAC; Hacdil-S; ***Canad.:*** Bye Bye Burn; Clearasil Sensitive Skin Cleanser; ***Fr.:*** Eryteal; Nostril†; ***Ger.:*** Lemocin; ***Ital.:*** Aflogine; Golamixin; Leucorsan; Neofen†; Xylestesina†; Xylonor; ***Spain:*** Diformiltricina; Hongosan; Topicaina; Xylonor; ***Switz.:*** Desitur; Largal ultra; Lemocin; Sebo Lotion†; Septivon N; Turexan Capilla; Xylestesin; Xylonor.

Cetyldimethylethylammonium Bromide

(18468-z)

Ethylhexadecyldimethylammonium bromide.

$C_{20}H_{44}BrN = 378.5$.

Cetyldimethylethylammonium bromide is a quaternary ammonium disinfectant with properties similar to those of other cationic surfactants (see Cetrimide, p.1105). It has been used for the disinfection of instruments and hard surfaces.

Preparations

Proprietary Preparations (details are given in Part 3)
Multi-ingredient: ***USA:*** Cetylcide†.

Cetylpyridinium Chloride (2217-n)

Cetylpyridinium Chloride *(BAN, rINN)*.

Cetylpyridinii Chloridum. 1-Hexadecylpyridinium chloride monohydrate.

$C_{21}H_{38}ClN,H_2O = 358.0$.

CAS — 7773-52-6 (cetylpyridinium); 123-03-5 (cetylpyridinium chloride, anhydrous); 6004-24-6 (cetylpyridinium chloride, monohydrate).

Pharmacopoeias. In *Eur.* (see p.viii) and *US.*

A white unctuous powder with a slight characteristic odour. Ph. Eur. solubilities are: **soluble** in water, foaming strongly on shaking; soluble in alcohol; very slightly soluble in ether. USP solubilities are: soluble 1 in 4.5 of water and of chloroform, and 1 in 2.5 of alcohol; slightly soluble in ether. **Incompatible** with soaps and other anionic surfactants.

Cetylpyridinium chloride is a quaternary pyridinium antiseptic with actions and uses similar to those of other cationic surfactants (see Cetrimide, p.1105). It is used chiefly as lozenges or solutions for the treatment of minor infections of the mouth and throat. It is also used topically for the treatment of skin and eye infections.

Mouth infections. Periodontitis and gingivitis can be prevented by control of plaque formation (p.132). Use of a mouthwash containing cetylpyridinium chloride 0.05% (three times a day)[1] or 0.1% (twice a day)[2] has been shown to reduce plaque accumulation.

1. Holbeche JD, *et al.* A clinical trial of the efficacy of a cetylpyridinium chloride-based mouthwash: effect on plaque accumulation and gingival condition. *Aust Dent J* 1975; **20:** 397–404.
2. Ashley FP, *et al.* The effect of a 0.1% cetylpyridinium chloride mouthrinse on plaque and gingivitis in adult subjects. *Br Dent J* 1984; **157:** 191–6.

Preparations

USP 23: Cetylpyridinium Chloride Lozenges; Cetylpyridinium Chloride Topical Solution.

Proprietary Preparations (details are given in Part 3)
Aust.: Dobendan; Halset; ***Austral.:*** Actifed Antiseptic†; Cepacol Antibacterial; Cepacol Mint; Cepacol Regular; Lemsip Lozenges; ***Canad.:*** Benylin Sore Throat Lozenges†; Cepacol; Emereze Plus; Mouthwash; Rince Bouche Antiseptique; Throat Lozenges; ***Fr.:*** Novoptine†; ***Ger.:*** Dobendan; Dobendan X; Formamint N†; Frubizin; Halset†; Halstabletten-ratiopharm†; ***Irl.:*** Merocets; ***Ital.:*** Alsol; Bat; Borocaina Gola; Bronchenolo; Cetilsan; Citroen Disinfettante†; Citroen Towel†; Exil; Farin Gola; Fluprim-Gola†; Getderm Sepsi†; Geyderm Sepsi; Gola Sel†; Golacetin; Helios†; Herbagola; Johnson's Penaten Crema Disinfettante; Neo Coricidin Gola; Neo Formitrol; Neo Gola Sel†; No-Alcool Sella†; Pronto G†; Ragaden; Sorbocetil†; Sterinet; ***Norw.:*** Pyrisept; ***S.Afr.:*** Cepacol; Denti Gum C†; Medi-Keel A†; Universal Throat Lollies; ***Spain:*** Angifonil; Formamint†; Tirocetil†; ***Switz.:*** Novoptine†; ***UK:*** Dettol†; Merocets; Search; Tyrocane Junior†; ***USA:*** Cepacol; Scope.

Multi-ingredient: ***Aust.:*** Coldistan; Dentinox; Focusan; Paididont; Riker Silicone-Spray; Tetesept; Tyrosolvin; ***Austral.:*** Actifed Anaesthetic; Adacol†; Cepacaine; Cepacol Anaesthetic; Cepacol Cough and Sore Throat; Difflam Anti-inflammatory Antiseptic Mouth Gel; Difflam Anti-Inflammatory Cough Lozenges; Difflam Anti-inflammatory Lozenges; Duro-Tuss Cough Lozenges; Gentlees; ***Canad.:*** Balminil Lozenges; Cepacol Anesthetic; Cepacol with Fluoride; Emercol; Emercrene No 4; Green Antiseptic Mouthwash & Gargle; Kank-A; Mouthrinse; Mouthwash & Gargle; Mouthwash Mint/Peppermint; Oral-B Anti-Bacterial with Fluoride; Scope with Oraseptate; Throat Lozenges; ***Fr.:*** Alodont; Broncorinol maux de gorge; Vicks Soulagil†; ***Ger.:*** Anginetten†; Bioget; Broncho-Tyrosolvetten; Chinomint Plus†; Dexamed†; Dolo-Dobendan; Dori; Ekzemex†; Emser Pastillen echt "Stark"†; Enzym-Tyrosolvetten†; Frubienzym; Frubizin Forte; Hexetidin comp.†; Imposit N; Larylin Hustenloser†; Mandro-Angin†; Medicreme†; Nordathricin N; Psilo-Balsam N; Sorot-comp†; Stas Halsschmerz; Therapin Halstabletten†; Thrombimed†; Tonsilase dolo; Tonsilase†; Tussipect; Tyrosolvetten; Tyrosolvetten-C; Tyrosur; Wick Sulagil; Wund- und Brand-Gel Eu Rho; ***Irl.:*** AAA; Anbesol; Listermint with Fluoride; Merocaine; Vicks Original Cough Syrup for Chesty Coughs; ***Ital.:*** Bo-Gum; Carefluor†; Cepral; Citroen Action 2 Collutorio†; Citroen Action 2 Dentrificio†; Delta 80 Plus; Neo Cepacol Collutorio; Neo Cepacol Pastiglie; Neo-Stomygen; Neoperborina Gola†; Oral-B Collutorio per la Protezione di Denti e Gengive; Oraseptic Gola; Rikospray; Rinosil; Vicks Cetamium Vit/C†; Vicks Gola†; Zeta-Bat†; ***Neth.:*** Agre-Gola; Focusan†; ***Norw.:*** Aselli; Focusan†; ***S.Afr.:*** Cepacaine; Cepacol; Cepacol Cough Discs; Cetoxol; Colphen; Denti Gum CF†; Medi-Keel A; Rikerspray†; Vagarsol; ***Spain:*** Alcohocel; Babysiton; Capota; Noquema; Pastillas Vicks Limon†; Pastillas Vicks Mentol†; Silidermil; Vicks Formula 44; Xylonibsa; ***Swed.:*** Bafucin; ***Switz.:*** Alodont nouvelle formule; Angina MCC; DemoAngina†; Flavangin; Focusan†; Larocal†; Lidazon; Mebucaine; Nasex; Neo-Angin Lido; Novomint N; Otothricinol; Tyrosolvin†; Vicks Formel 44; Wulnasin†; ***UK:*** Anbesol; Calgel; De Witt's Lozenges; Dentinox Teething Gel; Listermint; Listermint with Fluoride Mouthwash; Macleans Mouthguard; Medilave†; Meltus Expectorant; Merocaine; Merocet; Merothol; Merovit†; Oragard; Reach†; Rinstead Teething Gel; Tyrocane†; Ulcaid†; Vicks Expectorant; ***USA:*** Cepacol Anesthetic; Cepacol Maximum Strength; Cepacol Maximum Strength Sore Throat; Cepacol Regular Strength; Cepacol Throat; Cylex; Massengill Disposable; MouthKote O/R; MouthKote P/R; Orajel Mouth Aid.

Chloramine (2218-h)

Tosylchloramide Sodium *(rINN)*; Chloramidum; Chloramine T; Chloraminum; Cloramina; Mianin; Natrium Sulfaminochloratum; Tosylchloramidum Natricum. Sodium *N*-chlorotoluene-*p*-sulphonimidate trihydrate.

$C_7H_7ClNNaO_2S,3H_2O = 281.7$.

CAS — 127-65-1 (anhydrous).

NOTE. The name Chloramin is applied to a preparation of chlorpheniramine maleate.

Pharmacopoeias. In *Eur.* (see p.viii). *Pol.* includes chloramine B.

White or slightly yellow crystalline powder. It contains about 25% w/w of 'available chlorine' (see p.1110). Freely **soluble** in water; soluble in alcohol; practically insoluble in ether. A 5% solution in water has a pH of 8 to 10. **Store** in airtight containers at a temperature of 8° to 15°. Protect from light.

Adverse Effects and Treatment

Vomiting, cyanosis, circulatory collapse, frothing at the mouth, and respiratory failure can occur within a few minutes of chloramine ingestion. Fatalities have occurred. Chloramine in tap water has caused methaemoglobinaemia and haemolysis in patients undergoing dialysis. Bronchospasm has occurred after inhalation.

Treatment of adverse effects is similar to that for Sodium Hypochlorite, p.1125.

Uses and Administration

Chloramine is an organic chlorine-releasing compound with the general properties of chlorine (p.1109). It is stable at an alkaline pH although it is much more active in acid media. It is more slowly active than hypochlorite solutions.

Chloramine is used for the treatment of minor wound infections and as a skin and hard surface disinfectant. It is also used for the treatment of drinking water (p.1098). It was formerly used as a spermicide.

Chloramine B (chlorogenium; sodium *N*-chlorobenzenesulphonimidate sesquihydrate) has been used similarly to chloramine.

Preparations

Proprietary Preparations (details are given in Part 3)
Belg.: Chlorazol; Dercusan; ***Fr.:*** Hydroclonazone; ***Ger.:*** Clorina; Trichlorol; ***Ital.:*** Cloromi-T; Dermedal; Disinclor; Euclorina; Germozero; Halamid†; Minachlor; Ottoclor; Seroclorina†; Steridrolo; ***Spain:*** Clorina.

Chlorbutol (6640-h)

Chlorbutol *(BAN)*.

Chlorobutanol *(rINN)*; Acetone-Chloroforme; Alcohol Trichlorisobutylicus; Chlorbutanol; Chlorbutanolum; Chloretone; Chlorobutanolum; Trichlorbutanolum. 1,1,1-Trichloro-2-methylpropan-2-ol.

$C_4H_7Cl_3O = 177.5$.

CAS — 57-15-8 (anhydrous chlorbutol); 6001-64-5 (chlorbutol hemihydrate).

Pharmacopoeias. In *Chin.* (with $\frac{1}{2}H_2O$). In *Int.* and *USNF* (anhydrous or with $\frac{1}{2}H_2O$).
Eur. (see p.viii) has separate monographs for anhydrous and hemihydrate. *Jpn* permits up to 6% of water.

Colourless or white crystals or a white crystalline powder with a characteristic, somewhat camphoraceous odour. It sublimes readily. It melts at about 76° to 78° for the hemihydrate and about 95° for the anhydrous form. Both anhydrous and hemihydrated forms are: **soluble** 1 in 125 of water, 1 in 1 of alcohol, and 1 in 10 of glycerol; freely or very soluble in ether, in chloroform, and in volatile oils. **Store** at 8° to 15° in airtight containers.

Incompatibilities. The activity of chlorbutol can be adversely affected by the presence of other compounds as well as by the packaging material. There may be sorption onto substances like magnesium trisilicate, bentonite, carmellose,[1] polyethylene,[2,3] or polyhydroxy-ethylmethacrylate that has been used in soft contact lenses.[4] Increasing heat[2,3] or pH[5,6] can reduce stability and activity.

1. Yousef RT, *et al.* Effect of some pharmaceutical materials on the bactericidal activities of preservatives. *Can J Pharm Sci* 1973; **8:** 54–6.
2. Friesen WT, Plein EM. The antibacterial stability of chlorobutanol stored in polyethylene bottles. *Am J Hosp Pharm* 1971; **28:** 507–12.
3. Holdsworth DG, *et al.* Fate of chlorbutol during storage in polyethylene dropper containers and simulated patient use. *J Clin Hosp Pharm* 1984; **9:** 29–39.
4. Richardson NE, *et al.* The interaction of preservatives with polyhydroxy-ethylmethacrylate (polyHEMA). *J Pharm Pharmacol* 1978; **30:** 469–75.
5. Nair AD, Lach JL. The kinetics of degradation of chlorobutanol. *J Am Pharm Assoc (Sci)* 1959; **48:** 390–5.
6. Patwa NV, Huyck CL. Stability of chlorobutanol. *J Am Pharm Assoc* 1966; **NS6:** 372–3.

Adverse Effects

Acute poisoning with chlorbutol may produce CNS depression with weakness, loss of consciousness, and depressed respiration. Delayed (type IV) hypersensitivity reactions have been reported rarely.

Effects on the cardiovascular system. Rapid falls in arterial blood pressure were observed following injections of heparin with chlorbutol in patients undergoing coronary bypass.[1] No fall in blood pressure was seen in patients who received preservative-free heparin injection.

1. Bowler GMR, *et al.* Sharp fall in blood pressure after injection of heparin containing chlorbutol. *Lancet* 1986; **i:** 848–9.

Effects on mental function. The sedative effects of chlorbutol have been reported to be a problem in a patient dependent on large doses (0.9 to 1.5 g daily with salicylamide 1.8 to 3.0 g daily)[1] and in another patient given high doses of morphine in an infusion preserved with chlorbutol.[2]

1. Borody T, *et al.* Chlorbutol toxicity and dependence. *Med J Aust* 1979; **i:** 288.
2. DeChristoforo R, *et al.* High-dose morphine infusion complicated by chlorobutanol-induced somnolence. *Ann Intern Med* 1983; **98:** 335–6.

Hypersensitivity. A delayed, cellular type of hypersensitivity reaction to chlorbutol used to preserve heparin injection following subcutaneous injection has been reported.[1] Pruritus from intranasal desmopressin has been reported as due to the chlorbutol preservative.[2]

1. Dux S, *et al.* Hypersensitivity reaction to chlorbutanol-preserved heparin. *Lancet* 1981; **i:** 149.
2. Itabashi A, *et al.* Hypersensitivity to chlorobutanol in DDAVP solution. *Lancet* 1982; **i:** 108.

Uses and Administration

Chlorbutol has antibacterial and antifungal properties and it is used at a concentration of 0.5% as a preservative in injections and in eye drops as well as cosmetics.

Chlorbutol has been used as a mild sedative and local analgesic but other compounds are preferred. It has been used in preparations for inflammatory and painful conditions of the ear and oropharynx.

Preparations

Proprietary Preparations (details are given in Part 3)

Multi-ingredient: ***Aust.:*** Aleot; DDD; Nautisan; ***Austral.:*** Acne-Ban†; Benzotol†; Cerumol; ***Belg.:*** Givalex; ***Canad.:*** Aurisan; Balminil Nasal Ointment; Cerumol; Gouttes pour Mal d'Oreilles; Oralgar; Outgro; ***Fr.:*** Alodont; Angispray; Balsamorhinol; Biphedrine Aqueuse†; Ciella; Eludril; Givalex; Optrex; ***Ger.:*** Alsol†; Givalex; ***Irl.:*** Cerumol; Karvol; Monphytol; ***Ital.:*** Fialetta Odontalgica Dr Knapp; Otocaina†; Paf; Respiro; ***S.Afr.:*** Cerumol; Karvol; ***Spain:*** Cloraseptic; Eludril; Otocerum; ***Switz.:*** Alodont nouvelle formule; Cerumenol; Demo baume; Dental-Phenjoca; Eludril; Emoform†; Spirogel; ***UK:*** Aezodent; Cerumol; Cetanorm; DDD; Dermidex; Eludril; Frador; Karvol; Monphytol; Wax Aid†; ***USA:*** Outgro.

Chlorhexidine (12118-j)

Chlorhexidine *(BAN, rINN).*

CAS — 55-56-1.

Chlorhexidine Acetate (2220-t)

Chlorhexidine Acetate *(BANM, rINNM).*

Chlorhexidine Diacetate; Chlorhexidini Diacetas. 1,1′-Hexamethylenebis[5-(4-chlorophenyl)biguanide] diacetate.

$C_{22}H_{30}Cl_2N_{10},2C_2H_4O_2 = 625.6.$

CAS — 56-95-1.

Pharmacopoeias. In *Chin., Eur.* (see p.viii), *Int.*, and *Pol.*

A white or almost white microcrystalline powder. Sparingly **soluble** in water; soluble in alcohol; slightly soluble in glycerol and in propylene glycol.

Stability and incompatibilities are discussed under Chlorhexidine Hydrochloride, below.

Chlorhexidine Gluconate (2221-x)

Chlorhexidine Gluconate *(BANM, USAN, rINNM).*

Chlorhexidine Digluconate. 1,1′-Hexamethylenebis[5-(4-chlorophenyl)biguanide] digluconate.

$C_{22}H_{30}Cl_2N_{10},2C_6H_{12}O_7 = 897.8.$

CAS — 18472-51-0.

Pharmacopoeias. Eur. (see p.viii) and *Pol.* include Chlorhexidine Gluconate Solution which contains 19 to 21% of chlorhexidine gluconate.

The Ph. Eur. solution is an almost colourless or pale yellowish liquid. **Miscible** with water; soluble in alcohol and in acetone. A 5% v/v dilution in water has a pH of 5.5 to 7.0.

Protect from light.

NOTE. Commercial 5% concentrate contains a nonionic surfactant to prevent precipitation on dilution with hard water and is not suitable for use in body cavities or for disinfection of instruments containing cemented glass components; dilutions of the 20% concentrate should be used for this purpose. Dilutions of commercial concentrated solutions may be **sterilised** by autoclaving.

Stability and incompatibilities are discussed under Chlorhexidine Hydrochloride, below.

Chlorhexidine Hydrochloride (2222-r)

Chlorhexidine Hydrochloride *(BANM, USAN, rINNM).*

AY-5312; Chlorhexidine Dihydrochloride; Chlorhexidini Dihydrochloridum. 1,1′-Hexamethylenebis[5-(4-chlorophenyl)biguanide] dihydrochloride.

$C_{22}H_{30}Cl_2N_{10},2HCl = 578.4.$

CAS — 3697-42-5.

Pharmacopoeias. In *Eur.* (see p.viii), *Int.*, and *Jpn.*

A white or almost white crystalline powder. Sparingly **soluble** in water and in propylene glycol; very slightly soluble in alcohol.

Chlorhexidine and its salts are stable at normal storage temperatures but when heated may decompose with the production of trace amounts of 4-chloroaniline. Chlorhexidine hydrochloride is less readily decomposed than chlorhexidine acetate and may be heated at 150° for 1 hour without appreciable production of 4-chloroaniline. Aqueous solutions of chlorhexidine salts decompose with the formation of trace amounts of 4-chloroaniline. This decomposition is increased by heating and alkaline pH.

Incompatibilities. Chlorhexidine salts are incompatible with soaps and other anionic materials. Activity may be reduced in the presence of suspending agents such as alginates and tragacanth, insoluble powders such as kaolin, and insoluble compounds of calcium, magnesium, and zinc. Chlorhexidine acetate is incompatible with potassium iodide. At a concentration of 0.05%, chlorhexidine salts are incompatible with borates, bicarbonates, carbonates, chlorides, citrates, nitrates, phosphates, and sulphates, forming salts of low solubility which may precipitate out of solution. At dilutions of 0.01% or more, these salts are generally soluble. Insoluble salts may form in hard water. Chlorhexidine salts are inactivated by cork.

Fabrics which have been in contact with chlorhexidine solution may develop a brown stain if bleached with a hypochlorite. A peroxide bleach may be used instead.

References to incompatibilities with suspending agents and insoluble solids.[1-3]

1. McCarthy TJ. The influence of insoluble powders on preservatives in solution. *J Mond Pharm* 1969; **12:** 321–8.
2. Yousef RT, *et al.* Effect of some pharmaceutical materials on the bactericidal activities of preservatives. *Can J Pharm Sci* 1973; **8:** 54–6.
3. McCarthy TJ, Myburgh JA. The effect of tragacanth gel on preservative activity. *Pharm Weekbl* 1974; **109:** 265–8.

Adverse Effects and Treatment

Skin sensitivity to chlorhexidine has occasionally been reported. Strong solutions may cause irritation of the conjunctiva and other sensitive tissues. The use of chlorhexidine dental gel and mouthwash has been associated with reversible discoloration of the tongue, teeth, and silicate or composite restorations. Transient taste disturbances and a burning sensation of the tongue may occur on initial use. Oral desquamation and occasional parotid gland swelling have been reported with the mouthwash. If desquamation occurs, 50% dilution of the mouthwash with water and less vigorous rinsing may allow continued use.

The main consequence of ingestion is mucosal irritation and systemic toxicity is rare (see Poisoning, below). Haemolysis has been reported following accidental intravenous administration. Gastric lavage with demulcents has been suggested following acute ingestion.

Effects on the eyes. Report of 4 cases of corneal damage due to contact with chlorhexidine gluconate, that was being used for pre-operative preparation of facial skin.[1]

1. Tabor E, *et al.* Corneal damage due to eye contact with chlorhexidine gluconate. *JAMA* 1989; **261:** 557–8.

Effects on the nose. Temporary hyposmia in some patients after transsphenoidal pituitary adenoma operation was assumed to be caused by pre-operative disinfection of the nasal cavity with chlorhexidine gluconate solution.[1]

1. Yamagishi M, *et al.* Impairment of olfactory epithelium treated with chlorhexidine digluconate (Hibitane). *Pract Otol* 1985; **78:** 399–409.

Hypersensitivity. Severe hypersensitivity reactions including anaphylactic shock have been reported following topical applications of chlorhexidine,[1-4] and from the use of chlorhexidine-containing lubricants for urinary catheterisation or cystoscopy.[5] There is concern that similar reactions may occur with chlorhexidine-impregnated medical devices including intravenous catheters and implanted surgical mesh.[6] Occupational asthma has been attributed to an alcoholic chlorhexidine spray.[7]

1. Cheung J, O'Leary JJ. Allergic reaction to chlorhexidine in an anaesthetised patient. *Anaesth Intensive Care* 1985; **13:** 429–39.
2. Okano M, *et al.* Anaphylactic symptoms due to chlorhexidine gluconate. *Arch Dermatol* 1989; **125:** 50–2.
3. Evans RJ. Acute anaphylaxis due to topical chlorhexidine acetate. *Br Med J* 1992; **304:** 686.
4. Chisholm DG, *et al.* Intranasal chlorhexidine resulting in an anaphylactic circulatory arrest. *Br Med J* 1997; **315:** 785.
5. Visser LE, *et al.* Anafylaxie door chloorhexidine na cystoscopie of urethrale catheterisatie. *Ned Tijdschr Geneeskd* 1994; **138:** 778–80.
6. Anonymous. Hypersensitivity to chlorhexidine-impregnated medical devices. *JAMA* 1998; **279:** 1684.
7. Waclawski ER, *et al.* Occupational asthma in nurses caused by chlorhexidine and alcohol aerosols. *Br Med J* 1989; **298:** 929–30.

Poisoning. Reports of adverse effects following ingestion of chlorhexidine salts include a neonate who developed multiple episodes of cyanosis and bradycardia;[1] the infant's mother had sprayed chlorhexidine onto her breasts to prevent mastitis. On the other hand an 89-year-old woman only experienced mild giddiness, unusual laughter, and an increased appetite for her lunch after drinking 30 mL of a solution containing chlorhexidine gluconate 4% and isopropyl alcohol 4% thinking it was her breakfast fruit juice.[2] There has also been a report of a patient who developed gastritis after ingesting a pre-operative skin preparation containing chlorhexidine gluconate 4% after using it as a mouthwash.[3] Another subject experienced much more serious effects in a suicide attempt after drinking about 150 mL of chlorhexidine gluconate solution, corresponding to about 30 g of the pure substance.[4] Besides pharyngeal oedema and necrotic oesophageal lesions, the patient had very high aminotransferase concentrations which rose to 30 times normal 5 days after ingestion and were still 8 times normal one week later. After one month the aspartate aminotransferase (SGOT) was returning to normal while the alanine aminotransferase (SGPT) was still 3 times normal. Six months after ingestion the aminotransferase levels were normal. A liver biopsy performed soon after the peak in aminotransferase levels showed diffuse fatty degeneration and lobular hepatitis suggesting that chlorhexidine was absorbed from the gastro-intestinal tract in a concentration high enough to produce liver necrosis.

1. Quinn MW, Bini RM. Bradycardia associated with chlorhexidine spray. *Arch Dis Child* 1989; **64:** 892–3.
2. Emerson D, Pierce C. A case of a single ingestion of 4% Hibiclens. *Vet Hum Toxicol* 1988; **30:** 583.
3. Roche S, *et al.* Chlorhexidine-induced gastritis. *Postgrad Med J* 1991; **67:** 210–11.
4. Massano G, *et al.* Striking aminotransferase rise after chlorhexidine self-poisoning. *Lancet* 1982; **i:** 289.

Precautions

Since chlorhexidine is irritant it is recommended that it should not be used on the brain, meninges, middle ear, or other sensitive tissues. Contact with the eye should be avoided except for dilute solutions expressly for use in the eyes. Chlorhexidine may be adsorbed by some soft contact lenses and may cause eye irritation. Syringes and needles that have been immersed in chlorhexidine solutions should be thoroughly rinsed with sterile water or saline before use.

Aqueous solutions of chlorhexidine salts may be susceptible to contamination with micro-organisms. To reduce this risk, a sterilised preparation should be used or, where necessary, solutions must be freshly prepared at the recommended concentration and appropriate measures should be taken to prevent contamination during storage or dilution.

Aqueous solutions of chlorhexidine used for instrument storage should contain sodium nitrite 0.1% to inhibit metal corrosion, and should be changed every 7 days.

Haemorrhagic skin necrosis associated with umbilical artery catheterisation in extremely pre-term infants was attributed to damage by the alcohol from the use of chlorhexidine 0.5% in spirit 70% as a disinfectant.[1]

For reference to the percutaneous absorption of chlorhexidine following topical use in neonates and infants, see Pharmacokinetics, below.

1. Rutter N. Percutaneous alcohol absorption and skin necrosis in a preterm infant. *Arch Dis Child* 1983; **58:** 396.

Contamination. *Pseudomonas pickettii* septicaemia developed in 6 patients following the use of aqueous chlorhexidine 0.05%, prepared with contaminated twice-distilled water, for skin disinfection prior to venepuncture and it was considered that unsterilised 0.05% solutions should not be used for such skin preparation.[1] Positive blood cultures of *Burkholderia (formerly Pseudomonas) cepacia* were found in 2 patients following inappropriate use of a chlorhexidine handwash for the same purpose.[2] Further studies showed that the handwash supported pseudomonal growth only when diluted.[3]

1. Kahan A, *et al.* Is chlorhexidine an essential drug? *Lancet* 1984; **ii:** 759–60.
2. Gosden PE, Norman P. Pseudobacteraemia associated with contaminated skin cleansing agent. *Lancet* 1985; **ii** 671–2.
3. Norman P, *et al.* Pseudobacteraemia associated with contaminated skin cleansing agent. *Lancet* 1986; **i:** 209.

Oral hygiene. As toothpastes may contain anionic surfactants such as sodium lauryl sulphate, which are incompatible with chlorhexidine, it has been recommended that at least 30 minutes should be allowed to elapse between the use of toothpaste and oral chlorhexidine preparations.[1]

1. Barkvoll P, *et al.* Interaction between chlorhexidine digluconate and sodium lauryl sulfate in vivo. *J Clin Periodontol* 1989; **16:** 593–5.

Pharmacokinetics

Chlorhexidine is poorly absorbed from the gastro-intestinal tract and skin.

Neonates. Occasional reports of the percutaneous absorption of chlorhexidine in neonates and infants include a study in which chlorhexidine was detected in low concentrations in the venous blood of 5 of 24 infants after washing them with a preparation containing chlorhexidine gluconate 4% (Hibiscrub); no adverse effects were observed.[1] Low concentrations have been found in the venous blood of neonates following the topical use of a powder containing chlorhexidine 1%.[2] Percutaneous absorption of chlorhexidine was reported in pre-term neonates (but not full-term infants) treated with chlorhexidine 1% in alcohol for neonatal cord care; no such absorption occurred when a dusting powder containing chlorhexidine 1% and zinc oxide 3% was used.[3]

1. Cowen J, *et al.* Absorption of chlorhexidine from the intact skin of newborn infants. *Arch Dis Child* 1979; **54:** 379–83.
2. Alder VG, *et al.* Comparison of hexachlorophane and chlorhexidine powders in prevention of neonatal infection. *Arch Dis Child* 1980; **55:** 277–80.
3. Aggett PJ, *et al.* Percutaneous absorption of chlorhexidine in neonatal cord care. *Arch Dis Child* 1981; **56:** 878–91.

Uses and Administration

Chlorhexidine is a bisbiguanide antiseptic and disinfectant which is bactericidal or bacteriostatic against a wide range of Gram-positive and Gram-negative bacteria. It is more effective against Gram-positive than Gram-negative bacteria, and some species of *Pseudomonas* and *Proteus* have low susceptibility. It is relatively ineffective against mycobacteria. Chlorhexidine inhibits some viruses and is active against some fungi. It is inactive against bacterial spores at room temperature. Chlorhexidine is most active at a neutral or slightly acid pH. Combinations of chlorhexidine with cetrimide (p.1105) or in alcoholic solution are used to enhance the efficacy.

Chlorhexidine is formulated as lotions, washes, and creams for disinfection and cleansing of skin and wounds (p.1076), and as oral gels and mouthwashes for mouth infections including candidiasis and to reduce dental plaque accumulation. It has also been used in combination with neomycin to eliminate nasal carriage of staphylococci (p.144) and for disinfection of contact lenses, although it may not be suitable for use with some soft lenses (see p.1097 and above). It has been suggested for use for the treatment of Acanthamoeba keratitis in combination with propamidine isethionate and in spermicides to prevent transmission of HIV infection (p.601).

For pre-operative skin disinfection and hand-washing, chlorhexidine is used as a 0.5% solution of the acetate or gluconate in alcohol (70%) or as a 2 or 4% detergent solution of the gluconate. For disinfection of wounds, burns, or other skin damage or disorders chlorhexidine is used as a 0.05% aqueous solution of the gluconate, as a tulle dressing impregnated with chlorhexidine acetate 0.5%, or as a cream or powder containing chlorhexidine gluconate 1%. Preparations containing chlorhexidine acetate or gluconate 0.015% and cetrimide 0.15% are also used for cleansing and disinfection of skin and wounds. In obstetrics, chlorhexidine gluconate is used as a 0.05% aqueous solution or a 1% cream. The cream is also used as a barrier against bacterial hand infection.

Chlorhexidine gluconate is used in a 1% dental gel and 0.1 to 0.2% mouthwash for the prevention of plaque and the prevention and treatment of gingivitis and in the treatment of oral candidiasis. A slow-release formulation for insertion into periodontal pockets is also available.

A 0.02% solution may be used as a bladder irrigation in some urinary-tract infections. A gel containing 0.25% chlorhexidine gluconate and lignocaine hydrochloride has been used in catheterisation and cystoscopy.

For the emergency disinfection of clean instruments a 2-minute immersion in chlorhexidine acetate or gluconate 0.5% in alcohol (70%) is used; for the storage and disinfection of clean instruments a 30-minute immersion in a 0.05% aqueous solution containing 0.1% sodium nitrite to inhibit metal corrosion is used.

As an antimicrobial preservative, chlorhexidine is used at a concentration of 0.01% of the acetate or gluconate in eye drops.

Acanthamoeba infections. As discussed on p.573, the optimal antiamoebic therapy for *Acanthamoeba* keratitis has yet to be determined. Propamidine isethionate is commonly used, usually in combinations including a biguanide. Chlorhexidine gluconate 0.02% with propamidine isethionate 0.1% has been suggested.[1] However, concern has been expressed over the possible toxicity of chlorhexidine at this concentration on the cornea.[2]

Chlorhexidine is also an effective disinfectant against *Acanthamoeba* cysts and most bacteria found in contact lens storage cases.[1]

Chlorhexidine has also been used to treat skin lesions associated with disseminated *Acanthamoeba* infection[3] as an adjunct to systemic therapy (see p.573).

1. Seal DV. Acanthamoeba keratitis. *Br Med J* 1994; **308:** 1116–17.
2. Elder MJ, Dart JKG. Chemotherapy for acanthamoeba keratitis. *Lancet* 1995; **345:** 791–2.
3. Slater CA, *et al.* Brief report: successful treatment of disseminated Acanthamoeba infection in an immunocompromised patient. *N Engl J Med* 1994; **331:** 85–7.

Contraception. Bisbiguanides of the chlorhexidine type are reported to have the ability to diffuse into cervical mucus and render it impenetrable to sperm at concentrations as low as 1 mg per mL.[1] Higher concentrations of chlorhexidine structurally modify the mucus, producing a barrier to both the entry of sperm and chlorhexidine. The potency of chlorhexidine in inhibiting sperm motility *in vitro* is identical to that of nonoxinol 9,[1] but unlike spermicides containing nonoxinol 9, which tend to trickle out, the clearance of chlorhexidine from the vagina is delayed.[2] Chlorhexidine also has potential for reducing transmission of HIV infection as it does not disrupt the vaginal epithelium and has activity *in vitro* against the HIV virus in low concentrations.[2]

For a review of contraception, including the view that spermicides are not a particularly effective method unless combined with other means of contraception, see Choice of Contraceptive Method, p.1434.

1. Pearson RM. Update on vaginal spermicides. *Pharm J* 1985; **234:** 686–7.
2. Anonymous. Multipurpose spermicides. *Lancet* 1992; **340:** 211–13.

Disinfection. Viable bacterial counts on the hands were reduced by a mean of 97.9% by the application of 0.5% chlorhexidine gluconate in 95% alcohol.[1] The reduction was not so substantial with 0.5% chlorhexidine gluconate in water (65.1% reduction in bacterial count) or 4% chlorhexidine gluconate detergent solution (86.7%). Hand disinfection with chlorhexidine gluconate 4% appeared to be more effective than the use of isopropyl alcohol 60% and soap in preventing nosocomial infections in a study conducted in intensive care units but this may have been partly due to better compliance with hand-washing instructions when using chlorhexidine.[2] In another study,[3] pre-operative total body bathing with 4% chlorhexidine detergent did not decrease the risk of wound infection in patients compared with bathing in detergent alone.

Chlorhexidine 1% nasal cream failed to control an epidemic of methicillin-resistant *Staphylococcus aureus* in a neurosurgical ward[4] and handwashing with chlorhexidine soap failed to control an outbreak of infection with *Staph. aureus* resistant to methicillin and gentamicin in a neonatal intensive care unit.[5] The organisms were subsequently eradicated by the use of nasal mupirocin and hexachlorophane handwashing, respectively.

1. Lowbury EJL, *et al.* Preoperative disinfection of surgeons' hands: use of alcoholic solutions and effects of gloves on skin flora. *Br Med J* 1974; **4:** 369–72.
2. Doebbeling BN, *et al.* Comparative efficacy of alternative hand-washing agents in reducing nosocomial infections in intensive care units. *N Engl J Med* 1992; **327:** 88–93.
3. The European Working Party on Control of Hospital Infections. A comparison of the effects of preoperative whole-body bathing with detergent alone and with detergent containing chlorhexidine gluconate on the frequency of wound infections after clean surgery. *J Hosp Infect* 1988; **11:** 310–20.
4. Duckworth G. New method for typing Staphylococcus aureus resistant to methicillin. *Br Med J* 1986; **293:** 885.
5. Reboli AC, *et al.* Epidemic methicillin-gentamicin-resistant Staphylococcus aureus in a neonatal intensive care unit. *Am J Dis Child* 1989; **143:** 34–9.

CHLAMYDIA. Chlorhexidine 0.0625% or 0.0313% formulated as a gel was active against strains of *Chlamydia trachomatis* immediately on exposure.[1] More dilute gels were effective after 120 minutes. The activity was not affected by adjustments of pH between 4 and 8.

1. Lampe MF, *et al.* Susceptibility of Chlamydia trachomatis to chlorhexidine gluconate gel. *Antimicrob Agents Chemother* 1998; **42:** 1726–30.

INJECTION SITE AND CATHETER CARE. See p.1098.

SPORES. Although chlorhexidine is inactive against spores at room temperature, a solution of chlorhexidine 0.5% was reported to be sporicidal after 5 minutes at 100°.[1] The author suggests that chlorhexidine might perhaps be used in an emergency when an autoclave breaks down or in countries or situations where steam pressure sterilisation was impossible.

1. Fowler AW. Is chlorhexidine an essential drug? *Lancet* 1984; **ii:** 760.

VIRUSES. Chlorhexidine gluconate at concentrations down to 0.2% inactivated HIV *in vitro*.[1]

1. Harbison MA, Hammer SM. Inactivation of human immunodeficiency virus by Betadine products and chlorhexidine. *J Acquir Immune Defic Syndr* 1989; **2:** 16–20.

Endocarditis. Antiseptics applied immediately before dental procedures may reduce postextraction bacteraemia. Chlorhexidine mouthwash or gel may be used as an adjunct to antibacterial prophylaxis in dental patients at risk of bacterial endocarditis.[1,2] The protective cover required for such patients is discussed in detail on p.120.

1. Dajani AS, *et al.* Prevention of bacterial endocarditis: recommendations by the American Heart Association. *JAMA* 1997; **277:** 1794–1801.
2. Simmons NA, *et al.* Antibiotic prophylaxis and infective endocarditis. *Lancet* 1992; **339:** 1292–3.

Mouth disorders. Chlorhexidine mouthwashes and gels are used to prevent accumulation of dental plaque (see Mouth Infections, p.132). Studies have generally shown chlorhexidine mouthwash 0.1% to 0.2% used 2 or 3 times daily to be effective in reducing plaque accumulation and gingivitis,[1-4] and to be superior to other disinfectant mouthwashes.[5] Its effect against subgingival plaque bacteria is enhanced by phenoxyethanol.[6] However, a 1% gel used nightly as a toothpaste was not more effective than placebo in reducing gingivitis in children.[7] Other studies have shown that chlorhexidine reduces gingivitis by 60 to 90% but its use is limited by its unpleasant taste and staining properties; special circumstances in which chlorhexidine is helpful include management of acute gingivitis, control of periodontal involvement in immunocompromised patients, and promotion of healing after periodontal treatment.[8]

Chlorhexidine gluconate may be useful in controlling secondary bacterial infections of aphthous ulcers (see Mouth Ulceration, p.1172). Local application of chlorhexidine has been reported to reduce the incidence[9] and duration and severity[10] of recurrent ulcers, although one study showed no benefit compared with placebo.[11]

Chlorhexidine may be a useful adjunct to antifungal treatment of oral candidiasis[12] (p.367).

For precautions to be observed when using chlorhexidine with other oral hygiene preparations, see above.

1. Flötra L, *et al.* A 4-month study on the effect of chlorhexidine mouth washes on 50 soldiers. *Scand J Dent Res* 1972; **80:** 10–17.
2. O'Neil TCA, Figures KH. The effects of chlorhexidine and mechanical methods of plaque control on the recurrence of gingival hyperplasia in young patients taking phenytoin. *Br Dent J* 1982; **152:** 130–3.
3. de la Rosa M, *et al.* The use of chlorhexidine in the management of gingivitis in children. *J Periodontol* 1988; **59:** 387–9.
4. O'Neil TCA. The use of chlorhexidine mouthwash in the control of gingival inflammation. *Br Dent J* 1976; **141:** 276–80.
5. Brecx M, *et al.* Efficacy of Listerine, Meridol and chlorhexidine mouthrinses on plaque, gingivitis and plaque bacteria vitality. *J Clin Periodontol* 1990; **17:** 292–7.
6. Wilson M, *et al.* Effect of phenoxyethanol, chlorhexidine and their combination on subgingival plaque bacteria. *J Antimicrob Chemother* 1990; **25:** 921–9.
7. Hoyos DF, *et al.* The effect of chlorhexidine gel on plaque and gingivitis in children. *Br Dent J* 1977; **142:** 366–9.
8. Greene JC, *et al.* Preventive dentistry II: periodontal diseases, malocclusion, trauma, and oral cancer. *JAMA* 1990; **263:** 421–5.
9. Hunter L, Addy M. Chlorhexidine gluconate mouthwash in the management of minor aphthous ulceration. *Br Dent J* 1987; **162:** 106–10.
10. Addy M, *et al.* Management of recurrent aphthous ulceration: a trial of chlorhexidine gluconate gel. *Br Dent J* 1976; **141:** 118–20.
11. Matthews RW, *et al.* Clinical evaluation of benzydamine, chlorhexidine, and placebo mouthwashes in the management of recurrent aphthous stomatitis. *Oral Surg Oral Med Oral Pathol* 1987; **63:** 189–91.
12. Hay KD. Candidosis of the oral cavity: recognition and management. *Drugs* 1988; **36:** 633–42.

Obstetric use. Cleansing of the birth canal with chlorhexidine gluconate 0.25% has not been shown to reduce perinatal transmission of HIV except when membranes were ruptured for more than 4 hours before delivery,[1] although it has been reported to reduce neonatal morbidity and mortality from other neonatal infections in Africa.[2] In Swedish hospitals, flushing the vagina every 6 hours during labour with chlorhexidine acetate 0.2% reduced the incidence of transmission of group B streptococci but a reduction in neonatal morbidity was not demonstrated.[3,4] Comparable results have been reported with the use of chlorhexidine gluconate 1% obstetric cream at each examination during labour.[5]

1. Biggar RJ, *et al.* Perinatal intervention trial in Africa: effect of a birth canal cleansing intervention to prevent HIV transmission. *Lancet* 1996; **347:** 1647–50.
2. Taha TE, *et al.* Effect of cleansing the birth canal with antiseptic solution on maternal and newborn morbidity and mortality in Malawi: clinical trial. *Br Med J* 1997; **315:** 216–20.
3. Burman LG, *et al.* Prevention of excess neonatal morbidity associated with group B streptococci by vaginal chlorhexidine disinfection during labour. *Lancet* 1992; **340:** 65–9.
4. Burman LG, Tullus K. Vaginal chlorhexidine disinfection during labour. *Lancet* 1992; **340:** 791–2.
5. Lindemann R, *et al.* Vaginal chlorhexidine disinfection during labour. *Lancet* 1992; **340:** 792.

Peritoneal dialysis. The addition of chlorhexidine to ambulatory dialysis fluid containing high concentrations of chloride ions was not recommended as precipitation of chlorhexidine was likely.[1] In contrast, lavage with aqueous solutions of chlorhexidine had been shown to be both acceptable and very effective for controlling peritoneal sepsis.

1. Denton GW. Chlorhexidine: a WHO essential drug. *Lancet* 1984; **ii:** 517.

Urinary-tract infection. Chlorhexidine solutions have been used in the management of catheter-related bladder infections and for urinary catheter maintenance. Twice-daily bladder irrigation with chlorhexidine acetate 0.02% did not produce a reduction in urinary bacterial counts in geriatric patients with indwelling catheters, and there was a tendency for overgrowth of *Proteus* spp. in patients given chlorhexidine.[1] In patients undergoing prostatectomy, intermittent pre-operative bladder irrigation with chlorhexidine gluconate 0.05% reduced the incidence of bacteraemia and severe wound infection although urinary infections were eradicated in only 3 of the 13 patients treated.[2]

Addition of chlorhexidine to catheter drainage bags was not shown to reduce the frequency of urinary infections[3] but infection rates were reduced by combining this technique with the use of a catheter lubricant containing chlorhexidine, disinfection of the urethral meatus, and aseptic nursing procedures.[4] The use of lubricating gel containing chlorhexidine did not reduce the risk of urinary-tract infections associated with short-term catheterisation.[5]

A study *in vitro* suggested that chlorhexidine was less effective against *Escherichia coli* growing in biofilms than in suspension.[6]

The treatment of urinary-tract infections is discussed on p.149.

1. Davies AJ, *et al.* Does instillation of chlorhexidine into the bladder of catheterized geriatric patients help reduce bacteriuria? *J Hosp Infect* 1987; **9:** 72–5.
2. Adesanya AA, *et al.* The use of intermittent chlorhexidine bladder irrigation in the prevention of post-prostatectomy infective complications. *Int Urol Nephrol* 1993; **25:** 359–67.
3. Gillespie WA, *et al.* Does the addition of disinfectant to urine drainage bags prevent infection in catheterised patients? *Lancet* 1983; **i:** 1037–9.
4. Southampton Infection Control Team. Evaluation of aseptic techniques and chlorhexidine on the rate of catheter-associated urinary-tract infection. *Lancet* 1982; **i:** 89–91.
5. Schiøtz HA. Antiseptic catheter gel and urinary tract infection after short-term postoperative catheterization in women. *Arch Gynecol Obstet* 1996; **258:** 97–100.
6. Stickler D, *et al.* Activity of antiseptics against Escherichia coli growing as biofilms on silicone surfaces. *Eur J Clin Microbiol Infect Dis* 1989; **8:** 974–8.

Preparations

BP 1998: Chlorhexidine Irrigation Solution; Lidocaine and Chlorhexidine Gel.

Proprietary Preparations (details are given in Part 3)
Aust.: Angisan; Chlorhexamed; Hexidin; Hibident; Kleenocid; Plak Out; Sorbifen; ***Austral.:*** Anti-Plaque Chewing Gum; Bactigras; Body Lotion; Bush Formula; Catheter Preparation; Chlorohex; Clorhexitulle; Hexol; Hibiclens; Hibitane; Novaclens†; Novacol†; Novatane†; Plaqacide; Savacol Mouth and Throat Rinse; Savacol Throat Lozenges†; Savlon Medicated Powder†; Trisdine†; ***Belg.:*** Chlorhexamed†; Corsodyl; Golaseptine†; Hibident; Hibidil; Hibigel†; Hibiguard; Hibiscrub; Hibitane; Mefren Incolore; Mefren Pastilles; Pixidin; Rotersept†; Sterilon; Uro-Tainer; ***Canad.:*** Bactigras; Baxedin; Chlorhexseptic; Hexifoam†; Hibidil; Hibitane; Oro-Clense; Peridex; Rouhex-G; Spectro Gram; Stanhexidine; ***Fr.:*** Chlorhex-a-myl†; Collunovar; Corsodyl; Elgydium; Elugel; Equation†; Hibident†; Hibidil; Hibiscrub; Hibisprint; Hibitane; Lauvir†; Merfene; Plurexid; Prexidine; Rhino-Blache†; Septeal; Urgospray†; Vitacontact†; ***Ger.:*** Bactigras; Chlorhexamed; Cidegol C; Corsodyl; Frubilurgyl; Hansamed Spray; Hibiclens†; Lemocin CX; Mentopin Gurgellosung; Rotersept†; ***Irl.:*** Corsodyl; Hibidil†; Hibiscrub; Hibitane; Hydrex; Rotersept; ***Ital.:*** Aseptil Liquido†; Broxodin; Clorexident; Clorosan; Contact; Corsodyl; Cyteal†; D-Seb; Dempol; Dentosan Parodontale; Eburos; Effetre; Ekuba; Esoform Mani; Eurosan-Antisettico Battericida†; Germozero Hospital; Golasan; Golasol; Hibidil†; Hibiscrub; Hibitane†; Lenil; Lenixil; Lyasin; N32 Collutorio; Neomercurochromo; Neoxene; Neoxinal; Odontoxina; Oralsan; Percyl†; Plak Out; Rimargen†; Sanoral; Triseptil; Vaxidina; ***Neth.:*** Cefasept†; Corsodyl; Hibident†; Hibigel†; Hibiscrub; Hibitane; Roter Keel†; Sterilon; Urogliss-S; ***Norw.:*** Corsodyl; Eksplorasjonskrem†; Hexidin; Hibiscrub; Hibitane; ***S.Afr.:*** Bactigras; Hibident†; Hibidil†; Hibiscrub; Hibitane; Orosept; ***Spain:*** Cristalcrom; Cristalmina; Curafil; Cuvefilm; Deratin; Elgydium†; Hibimax; Hibiscrub; Hibitane†; Menalmina; Odol Med Dental; Sterilon; Urgospray†; ***Swed.:*** Cervitec; Corsodyl; Descutan; Hibiscrub; Hibitane; ***Switz.:*** Chlorhexamed; Chlorohex; Chlorohex-U†; Collunovar; Corsodyl; Dentohexine; Gleitmittel; Hibidil; Hibiscrub; Hibitane; Merfen nouveau; Sterilon†; ***UK:*** Acriflex; Bactiglens†; Bactigras; Cepton; Chlorasept; Chlorohex; Clorhexitulle; Corsodyl; CX Powder; Elgydium; Hibiscrub; Hibitane; Hydrex; Periochip; pHiso-MED; Rotersept†; Savlon Wound Wash; Serotulle; Spotoway; Sterexidine; Steripod Pink; Uniscrub; Unisept; Uriflex C; ***USA:*** Betasept; Biopatch; Dyna-Hex; Exidine; Hibiclens; Hibistat; Luroscrub†; Peridex; Periochip.

Multi-ingredient: ***Aust.:*** Bepanthen plus; Cathejell; Cathejell mit Lidocain; Dermaspray; Endosgel; Hansamed†; Hermalind†; Hermasept; Instillagel; Salbei-Halspastillen; Uromont; Vitawund; ***Austral.:*** Adacol†; Ansene L†; Cetal Instrument Disinfectant; Cleansing Lotion; Cross Prep; Derma Care†; Difflam Dental†; Difflam-C; Egomycol; First Aid Antiseptic Powder†; Hemocane; Hexidin; Hibicet; Hibicol; Hibitane; Lip-Sed†; Lipguard†; Medi Creme; Medi Pulv; Mediderm†; Microshield Antiseptic; Microshield Handrub; Microshield Tincture; Nasalate; Oralife Peppermint; Paraderm Plus; Pro-PS; Savlon Antiseptic; Savlon Hospital Concentrate†; Septimide†; Silvazine; Soov Cream; Steri-Sal II†; Tuscodin†; Xylocaine Jelly with Hibitane; ***Belg.:*** Cetavlex; Dermaspray; Endosgel†; HAC; Hacdil-S; Hibitane; Instillagel†; Medica; Neo-Cutigenol; Sedasept; Triga†; Vita-Merfen; ***Canad.:*** Clearasil Sensitive Skin Cleanser; Flamazine C; Ic-Gel; Savlodil; Savlon Hospital Concentrate; Spectro Tar; ***Fr.:*** Antalyre; Biseptine; Cantalene; Chlorispray; Clearasil Lotion†; Collu-Blache†; Collupressine; Collustan; Cyteal; Dacryne; Dermaspray†; Desocort; Dontopivalone; Drill; Dulcidrine†; Eludril; Isodril; Nostril†; Parodium; Sophtal; Spitaderm; Thiovalone; Visiodose; ***Ger.:*** Desmanol; Dexatopic†; Doretonsin†; Endosgel; Hansamed Balsam†; Hermalind; Hexoraletten N; Hibitane Hautdesinfiziens†; Instillagel; Nystalocal; Skinman Intensiv; Skinsept F; Skinsept Mucosa; Spitaderm†; Trachisan; Uro-Stilloson; ***Irl.:*** Hibicet; Hibisol; Instillagel; Mycil; Naseptin; Norgotin†; Nystaform; Nystaform-HC; Pedamed†; Savlodil†; Savlon†; ***Ital.:*** Anadermin; Baxidin; Cetrisan; Clorexan; Clorexident Ortodontico; Dentaton Antisettico; Dentosan "Pagni" Collutorio†; Dentosan Mese†; Dentosan Ortodontico Collutorio; Dexatopic†; Ekuba†; Eso Ferri Plus; Eso S 80; Esoform Maniferri; Farvicett; Ferrisept†; Handexin; Hibicet; Jalovis; Larilon; Levaknel; Medical Pic; Neo-Destomygen; Panseptil; PR 100-Cloressidina; Rexidina Otoiatrica†; Rikosilver†; Savlodil†; Savlon†; Simp; Simpottantacinque; Spitaderm; Steridol; Trust†; Videorelax; ***Mon.:*** Akila mains et peau; ***Neth.:*** Cetavlex†; Dermaspray†; Dexatopic; Hibicet concentraat; Hibicet verdunning; Hibisol; Medicanol†; Urogliss; ***Norw.:*** Bacimycin; Citanest; ***S.Afr.:*** Andolex-C; Dermoswab†; Hibicet; Naseptin; Orochlor; Savloclens†; Savlodil†; Savlon; ***Spain:*** Angicola†; Antirrinum; Biseptidine†; Bucometasona; Bucospray; Cavum Pediatrico†; Cloraseptic; Dexatopic†; Drill; Eludril; Faringesic; Hibitane; Mastiol; Menalcol; Piorreol†; Salvesept; Savlon†; ***Swed.:*** Instillagel; ***Switz.:*** Adro-derm; Antebor N; Auristan†; Bepanthene Plus; Cathejell-N; Cathejell†; Collu-Blache; Collunosol-N; Demosept; DermaSept-d†; DermaSept†; Desocort†; Eludril; Endosgel; Eubucal†; Galamila; Gelee lubrifiante simple; Hibital; Instillagel; Kamillosan; Lidohex; Lurgyl†; Neo-Urtisan; Nystacortone; Nystalocal; Rexophtal; Rhinipan; Secalan; Trachisan; Vita-Hexin; Vita-Merfen (nouveau); ***UK:*** Cetriclens†; Clearasil Medicated Lotion; Dermol; Eludril; Germolene; Germoloids; Hibicet Hospital Concentrate; Hibisol; Instillagel; Medi-Swab H; Medi-Wipe; Mycil; Naseptin; Nystaform; Nystaform-HC; Nystaform†; Primahex; Quinoderm Antibacterial Face Wash; Savlon Cream; Savlon Liquid; Sterets H; Steripod Yellow; Steriwipe†; Tisept; Torbetol; Travasept; Tri-Ac Medicated Cleanser†; Xylocaine; ***USA:*** BactoShield; Periogard.

Chlorinated Lime (2223-f)

Bleaching Powder; Cal Clorada; Calcaria Chlorata; Calcii Hypochloris; Calcium Hypochlorite; Calcium Hypochlorosum; Calx Chlorata; Calx Chlorinata; Chloride of Lime; Chlorkalk; Chlorure de Chaux; Cloruro de Cal.

CAS — 7778-54-3.

Pharmacopoeias. In *Br., Chin., Jpn,* and *Swiss.*

A dull white powder with a characteristic odour, containing not less than 30% w/w of 'available chlorine' (see p.1110). It becomes moist and gradually decomposes in air, carbon dioxide being absorbed and chlorine evolved. Partly **soluble** in water and alcohol.

Adverse Effects, Treatment, and Precautions

As for Sodium Hypochlorite, p.1125.

Uses and Administration

Chlorinated lime is a disinfectant and antiseptic with the general properties of chlorine (p.1109).

Its action is rapid but brief, the 'available chlorine' soon being exhausted by combination with organic material. It is used to disinfect faeces, urine, and other organic material, and as a cleansing agent for lavatories, drains, and effluents.

Chlorinated lime is used in the preparation of Surgical Chlorinated Soda Solution (BPC 1973) (Dakin's Solution) which has been employed as a wound disinfectant, and Chlorinated Lime and Boric Acid Solution (BP 1993), (Eusol), which has been used as a disinfectant lotion and wet dressing, sometimes with equal parts of liquid paraffin. However, such solutions are irritant when applied undiluted, and are no longer recommended for use in this way. In addition, there is some evidence that such chlorine-releasing solutions may delay wound healing (see Disinfection, Wounds, under Uses and Administration of Chlorine, p.1110).

References.

1. Bloomfield SF, Sizer TJ. Eusol BPC and other hypochlorite formulations used in hospital. *Pharm J* 1985; **235:** 153–5 and 157.
2. Greenblo K, *et al.* T-eusol: modified eusol without boric acid. *Pharm J* 1985; **235:** 267.

Preparations

BPC 1973: Surgical Chlorinated Soda Solution *(Dakin's Solution).*

Chlorine (2224-d)

925; 926 (chlorine dioxide).

Cl_2 = 70.9054.

CAS — 7782-50-5.

A greenish-yellow gas with a suffocating odour; commonly available as a pressurised liquid.

Adverse Effects and Treatment

Chlorine gas is irritant and corrosive producing inflammation, burns, and necrosis. Inhalation may result in coughing, choking, headache, dyspnoea, dizziness, expectoration of frothy white sputum (which may be blood stained), a burning chest pain, and nausea. Bronchospasm, laryngeal oedema, acute pulmonary oedema with cyanosis, and hypoxia may occur. There may be vomiting and development of acidosis. Death may result from hypoxia.

Some of the toxicity of chlorine may be due to its dissolution in tissue water to produce hydrochloric acid and hypochlorite. Following exposure to chlorine, conjunctivitis may require a topical anaesthetic and frequent irrigations of water or saline. Respiratory distress should be treated with inhalations of humidified oxygen and bronchodilators; mechanical ventilation may be required. Corticosteroids have been given in an attempt to minimise pulmonary damage. Acidosis may require the intravenous use of sodium bicarbonate or other suitable alkalising agent.

Experience gained from 186 cases of acute chlorine exposure indicated that medical support was required for only a short time even when exposure was repeated;[1] late sequelae were not observed, even in patients with abnormal respiratory function tests or blood gases on admission. Another report on 76 children with chlorine poisoning revealed that the longest period of hospitalisation was 12 hours.[2] There have been reports of deliberate inhalation of chlorine,[3,4] in one instance for pleasure,[3] leading to severe adverse effects. Some individuals may be unduly insensitive to chlorine-induced irritation and workers should be warned that concentrations of chlorine which can be tolerated for short periods without undue discomfort can still cause serious injury which may not be immediately apparent.[4]

1. Barret L, Faure J. Chlorine poisoning. *Lancet* 1984; **i:** 561–2.
2. Fleta J, *et al.* Intoxication of 76 children by chlorine gas. *Hum Toxicol* 1986; **5:** 99–100.
3. Rafferty P. Voluntary chlorine inhalation: a new form of self-abuse? *Br Med J* 1980; **281:** 1178–9.
4. Dewhurst F. Voluntary chlorine inhalation. *Br Med J* 1981; **282:** 565–6.

Effects on the eyes. Eye examinations performed on 50 subjects immediately before and after swimming in a chlorinated pool (chlorine range 1.0 to 1.5 ppm) showed that 68% had symptoms of corneal oedema and 94% had corneal epithelial erosions. No subject experienced a measurable decrease in visual acuity.[1]

1. Haag JR, Gieser RG. Effects of swimming pool water on the cornea. *JAMA* 1983; **249:** 2507–8.

Precautions

The antimicrobial activity of chlorine disinfectants is diminished by the presence of organic material and by increasing pH. Hypochlorite solutions may delay wound healing (see Disinfection: Wounds under Uses and Administration, below).

Uses and Administration

Chlorine is a disinfectant with a rapid potent brief bactericidal action. It is capable of killing most bacteria, and some fungi, yeasts, algae, viruses, and protozoa. It is slowly active against spores.

It is used as liquid chlorine for the treatment of water (p.1098), but for most other purposes it is used in the form of hypochlorites, organic and inorganic chloramines, chlorinated hydantoins, chlorinated isocyanurates, and similar oxidising compounds capable of releasing chlorine. In the presence of water these compounds produce hypochlorous acid (HOCl) and hypochlorite ion (OCl^-) and it is generally considered that the lethal action on organisms is due to chlorination of cell protein or enzyme systems by nonionised hypochlorous acid, although the hypochlorite ion may also contribute.

The activity of most of the compounds decreases with increase of pH, the activity of solutions of pH 4 to 7 being greater than those of higher pH values. However, stability is usually greater at an alkaline pH.

The potency of chlorine disinfectants is expressed in terms of **available chlorine**. This is based on the concept of chlorine gas (Cl_2) as the reference substance. Two atoms of chlorine (2 × Cl) yield in water only one molecule of hypochlorous acid (on which activity is based), while hypochlorites and chloramines yield one molecule of hypochlorous acid for each atom of chlorine as shown in the following equations:

$$Cl_2+H_2O \leftrightarrow HOCl+H^++Cl^-$$

$$NaOCl+H_2O \leftrightarrow HOCl+NaOH$$

Thus the assayed chlorine in such compounds has to be multiplied by 2 to produce 'available chlorine'. The term 'active chlorine' has been used confusingly for either 'available chlorine' (Cl_2) or 'combined chlorine' (Cl).

Because they have relatively low residual toxicity, chlorine compounds are useful for the disinfection of relatively clean impervious surfaces, such as babies' feeding bottles, baths, and food and dairy equipment. A concentration of 100 to 300 ppm of 'available chlorine' is used; a detergent may be added to ensure wetting of the surface. Solutions containing 10 000 ppm 'available chlorine' are used to disinfect surfaces contaminated with spilled blood or body fluids; this strength is effective against viruses including human immunodeficiency virus (HIV) and hepatitis B virus. Solutions containing 1000 ppm 'available chlorine' are recommended for minor surface contamination and as part of general good hygiene practice.

On a large scale, chlorine gas is used to disinfect public water supplies. On a smaller scale, the use of chlorine compounds is more convenient and sodium hypochlorite, chloramine, chlorinated lime, chlorine dioxide, and halazone are used. After satisfying the chlorine demand (the amount of chlorine needed to react with organic matter and other substances), a free-residual content of 0.2 to 0.4 ppm 'available chlorine' should be maintained, though more is required for alkaline waters with a pH of 9 or more. For the disinfection of potentially contaminated water a concentration of 1 ppm is recommended. Excessive residual chlorine may be removed by adding a little citric acid or sodium thiosulphate.

For use in small swimming pools, sodium or calcium hypochlorite may be added daily to maintain a free-residual 'available chlorine' concentration of 1 to 3 ppm. Chloramine, chlorinated lime, and the isocyanurates (see Sodium Dichloroisocyanurate, p.1124) may also be used. To minimise irritation of the eyes, maintain disinfectant activity, prevent precipitation of salts, and prevent metal corrosion, a pH of 7.2 to 7.8 should be maintained.

Solutions of chlorine-releasing compounds are also used in wound desloughing and disinfection (but see below).

Disinfection. CREUTZFELDT-JAKOB DISEASE. See p.1097.

INSTRUMENTS. Chlorine dioxide solutions are being assessed as an alternative to glutaraldehyde for the disinfection of endoscopes (p.1097). They are rapidly sporicidal, but their compatibility with endoscope and processing components has yet to be determined.[1] Needles and syringes should not usually be sterilised chemically. However, use of full strength domestic bleach (approximately 5% sodium hypochlorite, about 2% of 'available chlorine') is reported to be effective for the cleaning by intravenous drug users of needles and syringes as a last resort in the absence of sterile equipment; a 30-second contact time was required.[2,3] A 1 in 10 dilution of bleach was not effective after 5 minutes' exposure.[3]

1. Fraise AP. Disinfection in endoscopy. *Lancet* 1995; **346:** 787–8.
2. Donoghoe MC, Power R. Household bleach as disinfectant for use by injecting drug users. *Lancet* 1993; **341:** 1658.
3. Watters JK, *et al.* Household bleach as disinfectant for use by injecting drug users. *Lancet* 1993; **342:** 742–3.

WORMS. Sodium hypochlorite in aqueous solution at a concentration of 3.75% (or greater) is an effective ovicide for *Echinococcus*.[1]

1. Craig PS, Macpherson CNL. Sodium hypochlorite as an ovicide for Echinococcus. *Ann Trop Med Parasitol* 1988; **82:** 211–13.

WOUNDS. Hypochlorite solutions are now generally considered to be too irritant for use in the management of wounds (p.1076). Studies suggest that they may delay wound healing if repeatedly applied to open wounds.[1,2] It has been suggested that they may still be of use in debriding burns or necrotic chronic wounds,[3] but any benefit that might be seen from the desloughing of necrotic tissue might be produced by damage of the superficial cell layer leading to separation[4] or from tissue hydration produced by wet dressing packs.[5]

See also p.1098.

1. Thomas S, Hay NP. Wound healing. *Pharm J* 1985; **235:** 206.
2. Lineweaver W, *et al.* Topical antimicrobial toxicity. *Arch Surg* 1985; **120:** 267–70.
3. Leaper DJ. Eusol. *Br Med J* 1992; **304:** 930–1.
4. Anonymous. Local applications to wounds—I: cleansers, antibacterials, debriders. *Drug Ther Bull* 1991; **29:** 93–5.
5. Thomas S. Milton and the treatment of burns. *Pharm J* 1986; **236:** 128–9.

Chloroacetamide (18953-v)

Chloracetamide. 2-Chloroacetamide.

$C_2H_4ClNO = 93.51.$

CAS — 79-07-2.

Chloroacetamide is a preservative that has been used in topical pharmaceutical preparations and cosmetics.

N-(3-Chloroallyl)hexaminium Chloride (5579-v)

Quaternium-15. 1-(3-Chloroallyl)-3,5,7-triaza-1-azoniaadamantane chloride.

$C_9H_{16}Cl_2N_4 = 251.2.$

CAS — 4080-31-3.

N-(3-Chloroallyl)hexaminium chloride is an antimicrobial preservative used in pharmaceutical preparations and cosmetics. Skin reactions have been reported.

Chlorocresol (2226-h)

Chlorocresol *(USAN, rINN).*

Chlorkresolum; Parachlorometacresol; PCMC. *p*-Chloro-*m*-cresol; 4-Chloro-3-methylphenol.

$C_7H_7ClO = 142.6.$

CAS — 59-50-7.

Pharmacopoeias. In *Eur.* (see p.viii) and *Int.* Also in *USNF.*

Colourless or almost colourless crystals or white crystalline powder with a characteristic nontarry odour; it is volatile in steam. M.p. 63° to 67°. **Soluble** 1 in 260 of water; more soluble in hot water; soluble 1 in 0.4 of alcohol; soluble or freely soluble in ether and in fatty oils; soluble in terpenes and in solutions of alkali hydroxides. Solutions in water acquire a yellowish colour on exposure to light and air. **Store** in airtight containers. Protect from light. The antimicrobial activity of chlorocresol may be diminished through incompatibility (see below), through adsorption, through increasing pH, or through combination with organic matter (including oils and fats) or nonionic surfactants.

Incompatibilities. Chlorocresol has long been recognised to be incompatible with a range of compounds including: codeine phosphate, diamorphine hydrochloride, papaveretum, quinine hydrochloride,[1] methylcellulose,[2] and nonionic surfactants such as cetomacrogol 1000[3] and polysorbate 80.[4]

1. McEwan JS, Macmorran GH. The compatibility of some bactericides. *Pharm J* 1947; **158:** 260–2.
2. Harris WA. The inactivation of cationic antiseptics by bentonite suspensions. *Australas J Pharm* 1961; **42:** 583–8.
3. *PSGB Lab Report P/70/15* 1970.
4. Yousef RT, *et al.* Effect of some pharmaceutical materials on the bactericidal activities of preservatives. *Can J Pharm Sci* 1973; **8:** 54–6.

Adverse Effects, Treatment, and Precautions

As for Phenol, p.1121.

Chlorocresol is less toxic than phenol. Sensitisation reactions may follow application to the skin and hypersensitivity has occurred following systemic administration of injections containing chlorocresol as a preservative.

Uses and Administration

Chlorocresol is a potent chlorinated phenolic disinfectant and antiseptic. It has bactericidal activity against Gram-positive and Gram-negative bacteria and is effective against fungi but has little activity against bacterial spores except at high temperatures. It is more active in acid than in alkaline solution.

Chlorocresol is used in various preparations for disinfection of the skin and wounds. It is also used as a preservative in creams and other preparations for external use which contain water.

Chlorocresol is used as a preservative in aqueous injections issued in multidose containers. It may also be added to aqueous preparations that cannot be sterilised in their final containers and have to be prepared using aseptic precautions. Concentrations of 0.1% have generally been used. Injections prepared with chlorocresol should not be injected into the CSF, the eye, or the heart. Also such injections should generally not be administered in volumes greater than 15 mL. Sterilisation by heating with a bactericide such as chlorocresol in no longer a recommended practice.

Preparations

BPC 1973: Proflavine Cream.

Proprietary Preparations (details are given in Part 3)
UK: Wright's Vaporizing Fluid.

Multi-ingredient: ***Aust.:*** Ulcurilen; ***Austral.:*** Curatin; ***Belg.:*** Helipur†; Ivisol†; ***Fr.:*** Cicatryl; Cyteal; ***Ger.:*** Aru-Sept-Spray†; Bacillotox; Bomix; Grotanat; Helipur; Lysolin†; Ulcurilen N; Velicin†; ***Irl.:*** Anbesol; Valderma; ***Ital.:*** Gevisol†; Helipur; Hygienist; ***Spain:*** Fungusol; Fungusol Prednisona†; ***UK:*** Anbesol; Cymex; Valderma Cream.

Chlorothymol (2227-m)

Monochlorothymol. 6-Chlorothymol; 4-Chloro-2-isopropyl-5-methylphenol.

$C_{10}H_{13}ClO$ = 184.7.

CAS — 89-68-9.

Chlorothymol is a chlorinated phenolic antiseptic used as an ingredient of preparations for hand and skin disinfection and topical treatment of fungal infections. It has also been used in preparations for anorectal disorders, cold symptoms, and mouth disorders.

Preparations

Proprietary Preparations (details are given in Part 3)
Ital.: Pioral Pasta.

Multi-ingredient: ***Austral.:*** Alcos-Anal†; ***Ger.:*** Onymyken S†; ***Ital.:*** Labocaina; Traumicid; Vagisil; ***Neth.:*** Rhinocaps; ***USA:*** Medadyne†.

Chloroxylenol (2228-b)

Chloroxylenol *(BAN, USAN, rINN).*

Parachlorometaxylenol; PCMX. 4-Chloro-3,5-xylenol; 4-Chloro-3,5-dimethylphenol.

C_8H_9ClO = 156.6.

CAS — 88-04-0.

Pharmacopoeias. In Br. and US.

White or cream-coloured crystals or crystalline powder with a characteristic odour; volatile in steam. Very slightly **soluble** in water; freely soluble in alcohol; soluble in ether, in terpenes, and in fixed oils; dissolves in solutions of alkali hydroxides. **Incompatibility** has been reported with nonionic surfactants and methylcellulose. The antimicrobial activity of chloroxylenol may be diminished through combination with organic matter.

Adverse Effects and Precautions

Chloroxylenol in the recommended dilutions is generally non-irritant but skin sensitivity has occurred. There have been isolated reports of poisoning.

Aqueous solutions of chloroxylenol may be susceptible to contamination with micro-organisms. To reduce this risk, solutions must be freshly prepared at the recommended concentration and appropriate measures should be taken to prevent contamination during storage or dilution.

Reports of fatal[1] or severe[2,3] self-poisoning with chloroxylenol solution.

1. Meek D, *et al.* Fatal self-poisoning with Dettol. *Postgrad Med J* 1977; **53:** 229–31.
2. Joubert P, *et al.* Severe Dettol (chloroxylenol and terpineol) poisoning. *Br Med J* 1978; **1:** 890.
3. Chan TYK, *et al.* Chemical gastro-oesophagitis, upper gastrointestinal haemorrhage and gastroscopic findings following Dettol poisoning. *Hum Exp Toxicol* 1995; **14:** 18–19.

Uses and Administration

Chloroxylenol is a chlorinated phenolic antiseptic which is bactericidal against most Gram-positive bacteria but less active against staphylococci and Gram-negative bacteria, and is often inactive against *Pseudomonas* spp. Its activity against *Ps. aeruginosa* appears to be increased by the addition of edetic acid. It is inactive against bacterial spores.

Chloroxylenol Solution (BP 1998) is used for skin and wound disinfection, and chloroxylenol is used in a variety of other topical formulations.

Preparations

BP 1998: Chloroxylenol Solution *(Roxenol).*

Proprietary Preparations (details are given in Part 3)
Austral.: Dettol Classic; ***Belg.:*** Dettol; ***Ital.:*** Neomercurochromo; ***UK:*** Dettol; Prinsyl; ***USA:*** Micro-Guard†; Sween Prep†.

Multi-ingredient: ***Aust.:*** Dolothricin; ***Austral.:*** Dettol; Solyptol; ZeaSorb; ***Canad.:*** Acne-Aid; Antiseptic Ointment; Iba-Cide; ZeaSorb; ***Ger.:*** Akne-Aid-Creme†; Bacillotox; Gehwol Fungizid; Gehwol Fungizid Creme N; Skin-Aid†; ZeaSorb; ***Irl.:*** Dettol; ZeaSorb; ***Ital.:*** Foille Sole; Vironox; ***S.Afr.:*** Respisniffers; ZeaSorb†; ***UK:*** Dettol; Rinstead; Skintex; TCP; Waxwane; ZeaSorb; ***USA:*** Calamycin; Comfortine; Cortic; Dermacoat; Foille; FungiNail; Gordochom; Lobana Peri-Garde; Otomar-HC; Pedi-Pro; TriOtic; Triple Care Extra Protective Cream; Unguentine Plus; Zoto-HC.

Cinnamic Acid (6641-m)

Cinnamylic Acid. *trans*-3-Phenylpropenoic acid.

$C_6H_5.CH:CH.CO_2H$ = 148.2.

CAS — 621-82-9.

Pharmacopoeias. In Br.

Colourless crystals with a faint balsamic odour. Very slightly **soluble** in water; freely soluble in alcohol, soluble in chloroform and in ether.

Cinnamic acid has preservative properties. It is used with benzoic acid and other substances to simulate the flavour of tolu.

Preparations

BP 1998: Tolu-flavour Solution.

Proprietary Preparations (details are given in Part 3)

Multi-ingredient: ***Switz.:*** Spirogel; ***UK:*** Hemocane; Sanderson's Throat Specific.

Clorophene (2230-r)

Clorophene *(USAN).*

Clorofene *(pINN)*; Clorfene; NSC-59989; Septiphene. 2-Benzyl-4-chlorophenol.

$C_{13}H_{11}ClO$ = 218.7.

CAS — 120-32-1.

Clorophene is a chlorinated phenolic antiseptic stated to be active against a wide range of bacteria, fungi, protozoa, and viruses. It is used as a skin disinfectant. Clorophene sodium has also been used.

Preparations

Proprietary Preparations (details are given in Part 3)
Ger.: Akne-Pyodron Kur†; Akne-Pyodron lokal†.

Multi-ingredient: ***Belg.:*** Helipur†; Ivisol†; Neo-Sabenyl; ***Fr.:*** Frekaderm; ***Ger.:*** Aru-Sept-Spray†; Bacillotox; Bomix; Freka-Derm; Freka-Sept 80; Grotanat; Helipur; ***Ital.:*** Helipur; Hygienist; ***Switz.:*** Frekaderm.

Cresol (2231-f)

Cresolum Crudum; Cresylic Acid; Kresolum Venale; Tricresol; Trikresolum. Methylphenol.

C_7H_8O = 108.1.

CAS — 1319-77-3; 95-48-7 (o-cresol); 108-39-4 (m-cresol); 106-44-5 (p-cresol).

Pharmacopoeias. In Aust., Br., Chin., Fr., It., and Jpn. Also in US-NF.

NOTE. Some grades of mixed cresols may be equivalent to Tar Acids (p.1126).

A colourless, yellowish to pale brownish-yellow, or pinkish liquid, becoming darker with age or on exposure to light, with a characteristic odour resembling phenol, but more tarry. It consists of a mixture of cresol isomers and other phenols obtained from coal tar or petroleum. **Soluble** 1 in 50 of water, usually forming a cloudy solution; freely soluble in alcohol, in ether, in chloroform, and in fixed and volatile oils; dissolves in solutions of alkali hydroxides; miscible with glycerol. A saturated solution in water is neutral or slightly acid to litmus. **Store** in airtight containers. Protect from light.

Cresol is a disinfectant with a similar action to phenol (p.1121); suitable precautions should be taken to prevent absorption through the skin.

It has been used as Cresol and Soap Solution (Lysol) as a general disinfectant but it has been largely superseded by other, less irritant, phenolic disinfectants. Cresol has been used in dentistry, alone or in combination with formaldehyde, but is caustic to the skin and unsuitable for skin and wound disinfection. The cresols have been widely used in disinfectants for domestic and hospital use.

Poisoning. A 52-year-old man who swallowed approximately 100 mL of a petroleum distillate containing cresol 12% suffered acute intravascular haemolytic anaemia with massive haemoglobinuria; this was probably due to cresol intoxication.[1]

1. Côté M-A, *et al.* Acute Heinz-body anaemia due to severe cresol poisoning: successful treatment with erythrocytapheresis. *Can Med Assoc J* 1984; **130:** 1319–22.

Preparations

Proprietary Preparations (details are given in Part 3)
Ital.: Creolina.

Multi-ingredient: ***Austral.:*** Formo-Cresol Mitis; ***Canad.:*** Gernel; ***Fr.:*** Eau Precieuse Depensier; ***Spain:*** Empapol; Neodesfila; Riosol F†; Tifell; ***USA:*** Cresylate.

Crystal Violet (2232-d)

Methylrosanilinium Chloride *(rINN)*; CI Basic Violet 3; Colour Index No. 42555; Gentian Violet; Hexamethylpararosaniline Chloride; Kristallviolett; Methylrosaniline Chloride; Pyoctaninum Caeruleum; Viola Crystallina. 4-[4,4′Bis(dimethylamino)benzhydrylidene]cyclohexa-2,5-dien-1-ylidenedimethylammonium chloride.

$C_{25}H_{30}ClN_3$ = 408.0.

CAS — 548-62-9.

Pharmacopoeias. In Chin., Fr., and US.

Aust. and *Jpn* include mixtures of hexamethylpararosaniline hydrochloride with the tetramethyl- and pentamethyl- compounds.

The name methyl violet—CI Basic Violet 1; Colour Index No. 42535—has been used as a synonym for crystal violet, but is applied to a mixture of the hydrochlorides of the higher methylated pararosanilines consisting principally of the tetramethyl-, pentamethyl-, and hexamethyl- compounds.

Dark green powder or greenish, glistening crystals with a metallic lustre; odourless or almost odourless. Sparingly **soluble** in water; soluble 1 in 10 of alcohol and 1 in 15 of glycerol; also soluble in chloroform; practically insoluble in ether.

Incompatibilities. The antimicrobial activity of crystal violet may be diminished through incompatibilities (see below), decreasing pH, or through combination with organic matter.

The antibacterial activity of crystal violet was inhibited in suspensions of bentonite with which it formed a stable complex.[1]

1. Harris WA. The inactivation of cationic antiseptics by bentonite suspensions. *Australas J Pharm* 1961; **42:** 583–8.

Adverse Effects and Precautions

Topical application of crystal violet can produce irritation and ulceration of mucous membranes. Ingestion of crystal violet during prolonged or frequent treatment for oral candidiasis has resulted in oesophagitis, laryngitis, and tracheitis; ingestion may also cause nausea, vomiting, diarrhoea, and abdominal pain. In the UK it is recommended that crystal violet should not be applied to mucous membranes or open wounds. Contact with the eyes or broken skin should be avoided. Crystal violet may stain skin and clothing.

Animal carcinogenicity has restricted its use.

Carcinogenicity. Crystal violet has been shown *in vitro* to be capable of interacting with DNA of living cells,[1] and has demonstrable carcinogenicity in *mice*.[2]

1. Rosenkranz HS, Carr HS. Possible hazard in use of gentian violet. *Br Med J* 1971; **3:** 702–3.
2. MAFF Food Advisory Committee. Final report on the review of the Colouring Matter in Food Regulations 1973: FdAC/REP/4. London: HMSO, 1987.

Effects on the skin and mucous membranes. Necrotic skin reactions have been reported following the use of topical 1% aqueous solutions of crystal violet;[1] areas affected include the submammary folds, gluteal fold, genitalia, and toe-webs. Similar reactions were observed in 2 patients following use of 1% crystal violet or brilliant green on stripped skin.[1] Oral ulceration developed in all of 6 neonates treated with aqueous crystal violet 0.5 or 1% for oral candidiasis.[2]

In the UK it is recommended that crystal violet should not be applied to mucous membranes or open wounds.

1. Björnberg A, Mobacken H. Necrotic skin reactions caused by 1% gentian violet and brilliant green. *Acta Derm Venereol (Stockh)* 1972; **52:** 55–60.
2. Horsfield P, *et al.* Oral irritation with gentian violet. *Br Med J* 1976; **2:** 529.

Effects on the urinary tract. Severe haemorrhagic cystitis rapidly occurred in a 32-year-old woman after accidental injection through the urethra of a solution of crystal violet 1% and alcohol 2%.[1] Severe cystitis was also reported following instillation into the bladder of a solution containing crystal violet and brilliant green 1:1 (Bonney's blue).[2]

1. Walsh C, Walsh A. Haemorrhagic cystitis due to gentian violet. *Br Med J* 1986; **293:** 732.
2. Christmas TJ, *et al.* Bonney's blue. *Lancet* 1988; **ii:** 459–60.

Porphyria. Crystal violet has been associated with clinical exacerbations of porphyria and is considered unsafe in porphyric patients.[1]

1. Moore MR, McColl KEL. *Porphyria: drug lists.* Glasgow: Porphyria Research Unit, University of Glasgow, 1991.

Uses and Administration

Crystal violet is a triphenylmethane antiseptic dye effective against some Gram-positive bacteria, particularly *Staphylococcus* spp., and some pathogenic fungi such as *Candida* spp. It is much less active against Gram-negative bacteria and ineffective against acid-fast bacteria and bacterial spores. Its activity increases as pH increases.

Crystal violet has been applied topically as a 0.25 to 2.0% aqueous solution or as a cream for the treatment of bacterial and fungal infections, but in the UK its use is now restricted to application to unbroken skin because of concern over *animal* carcinogenicity. However, it may be used as a 0.5% solution with brilliant green 0.5% (Bonney's blue) for skin marking prior to surgery.

In the UK, crystal violet is no longer permitted for use in foods.

Trypanosomiasis. Crystal violet is used in some countries to prevent the transmission of American trypanosomiasis (p.578) by blood transfusion.[1] In areas where the proportion of blood donors seropositive for *Trypanosoma cruzi* is high, emergency blood supplies positive for *T. cruzi* can be made safe by the addition of crystal violet 125 mg per 500 mL of blood and storing it for 24 hours at 4°;[2] it appears to work for most but not all strains of *T. cruzi in vitro*.[1] There is no evidence that crystal violet at such doses produces any side-effects apart from transient blue staining of the skin and mucosa.[2] It has been suggested that addition of sodium ascorbate can markedly reduce the amount of crystal violet required.[3]

1. Gutteridge WE. Existing chemotherapy and its limitations. *Br Med Bull* 1985; **41:** 162–8.

2. WHO. Control of Chagas disease: report of a WHO expert committee. *WHO Tech Rep Ser 811* 1991.
3. Chagas' Disease. In: *Tropical diseases: progress in research, 1989–1990.* Tenth programme report of the UNDP/World Bank/WHO Special Programme for Research and Training in Tropical Diseases (TDR). Geneva: WHO, 1991: 69–77.

Preparations

USP 23: Gentian Violet Cream; Gentian Violet Topical Solution.

Proprietary Preparations (details are given in Part 3)
Spain: Viogencianol†; ***USA:*** Genapax†.

Multi-ingredient: ***Fr.:*** Antiseptique-Calmante; ***Ger.:*** Robusanon†; ***Ital.:*** Violgen; ***Spain:*** Vigencial.

Dehydroacetic Acid (6642-b)

Methylacetopyronone. 3-Acetyl-6-methyl-2*H*-pyran-2,4(3*H*)-dione (keto form); 3-Acetyl-4-hydroxy-6-methyl-2*H*-pyran-2-one (enol form).

$C_8H_8O_4$ = 168.1.

CAS — 520-45-6 (keto form); 771-03-9 (enol form).

A white or nearly white crystalline powder; odourless or practically odourless. Very slightly **soluble** in water; sparingly soluble in alcohol; freely soluble in acetone; soluble in aqueous solutions of fixed alkalis. M.p. 109° to 111°.

Sodium Dehydroacetate (6668-j)

The sodium salt of 3-acetyl-6-methyl-2*H*-pyran-2,4(3*H*)-dione.

$C_8H_7NaO_4$ = 190.1.

CAS — 4418-26-2.

Pharmacopoeias. In *USNF.*

A white or practically white, odourless powder. Freely **soluble** in water, glycerol, and propylene glycol.

Incompatibilities. Activity may be reduced by alkaline pH or interaction with nonionic surfactants.

Dehydroacetic acid and sodium dehydroacetate have some antifungal activity and have been used in the preservation of cosmetics.

Dequalinium Chloride (2234-h)

Dequalinium Chloride *(BAN, rINN).*

BAQD-10; Decalinium Chloride; Decaminum. *N,N*-Decamethylenebis(4-amino-2-methylquinolinium chloride).

$C_{30}H_{40}Cl_2N_4$ = 527.6.

CAS — 6707-58-0 (dequalinium); 522-51-0 (dequalinium chloride); 4028-98-2 (dequalinium acetate); 16022-70-1 (dequalinium salicylate).

Pharmacopoeias. In *Br.* and *Ger.*

A creamy-white odourless or almost odourless powder. Slightly **soluble** in water; soluble in boiling water; slightly soluble in propylene glycol. **Incompatible** with soaps and other anionic surfactants, with phenol, and with chlorocresol.

Dequalinium chloride is a bisquaternary quinolinium antiseptic, bactericidal against many Gram-positive and Gram-negative bacteria, and effective against fungi. The action is little affected by the presence of serum. It is mainly used in the form of lozenges in the treatment of minor infections of the mouth and throat. It has been applied topically in the treatment of skin and vaginal infections.

Dequalinium salicylate and undecenoate are also used.

Preparations

Proprietary Preparations (details are given in Part 3)
Aust.: Dequadin; Dequavagyn; Evazol; Sorot; Tonsillol; ***Austral.:*** Dequadin†; ***Belg.:*** Anginol; ***Canad.:*** Dequadin; ***Ger.:*** Efisol S; Evazol; Fluomycin N; Gurgellosung-ratiopharm; Maltyl; Phyllettent†; Soor-Gel; Sorot; ***Irl.:*** Dequadin; Labosept; ***Ital.:*** Decabis†; Dequadin; Dequosangola; Faringina; Formocillina al Dequalinium†; Osangin; Pastiglie al Pumilene†; Pumilsan; ***Neth.:*** Gargilon; ***S.Afr.:*** Dequadin†; ***Spain:*** Dequadin; Dequin†; Leuco Dibios†; ***Switz.:*** Decatylene; Grocreme†; Pastilles pour la gorge no 535; ***UK:*** Dequadin; Labosept.

Multi-ingredient: ***Aust.:*** Dequafungan; Dequalinetten; Dequonal; Eucillin; Fluorex Plus; Tetesept; ***Austral.:*** Dequadin Mouth Ulcer Paint†; ***Belg.:*** Bucco-Spray; Buccosan; Dequalinium; Laryngarsol; ***Fr.:*** Eufosyl†; Humex Kinaldine; Oroseptol; Oroseptol Lysozyme; Vicks Soulagil†; ***Ger.:*** Alformin†; Anginettent†; Bakteriostat "Herbrand"; Corti-Dynexan; De-menthasin; Dequonal; Dynexan MHP†; Efisol-H†; Ephepect-Blocker-Pastillen N; eusept†; Hamoagil†; Inspirol Halsschmerztabletten; Jasimenth CN; Mederma†; Mycatox; Neo-Pyodron; Otolitan N farblos; Sirinal†; Sirit†; Sorot-comp†; Stas Halsschmerz; Tyrosirinal†; Wick Sulagil; ***Irl.:*** Dequacaine; ***Ital.:*** Ferrisept†; Golosan†; Neoperborina Gola†; Rinospray; Sterox†; Transpulmina Gola; Transpulmina Gola Nebulizzatore†; Tririnol; ***Norw.:*** Apolar med dekvalon; Salvizol med Hydrocortison†; ***S.Afr.:*** Dequadin Mouth Paint; Dequamed†; ***Spain:*** Anginovag; Roberfarin; Sedofarin; ***Switz.:*** Anginova Nouvelle formule; Arbid-top; Decasept; Decatylene Neo; Delica-Sol†; Dequonal; Diabetosan†; Gramipan; Neo-Bucosin; Rhinipan; Stomaqualine†; Tyroqualine; ***UK:*** Dequacaine.

Dibromopropamidine Isethionate (2236-b)

Dibromopropamidine Isethionate *(BANM).*

Dibrompropamidine Isetionate *(rINNM).* 3,3′-Dibromo-4,4′-trimethylenedioxydibenzamidine bis(2-hydroxyethanesulphonate).

$C_{17}H_{18}Br_2N_4O_2,2C_2H_6O_4S$ = 722.4.

CAS — 496-00-4 (dibromopropamidine); 614-87-9 (dibromopropamidine isethionate).

Pharmacopoeias. In *Br.*

A white or almost white, odourless or almost odourless, crystalline powder. Freely **soluble** in water; sparingly soluble in alcohol; soluble in glycerol; practically insoluble in chloroform, in ether, in fixed oils, and in liquid paraffin. A 5% solution in water has a pH of 5 to 7.

Dibromopropamidine isethionate is an aromatic diamidine antiseptic similar to propamidine (p.1124). It is bactericidal against Gram-positive bacteria but is less active against Gram-negative bacteria and spore-forming organisms. It also has antifungal properties. It is available as topical preparations for the local treatment of minor eye and skin infections.

Preparations

Proprietary Preparations (details are given in Part 3)
Austral.: Brolene; Brulidine; ***Irl.:*** Brolene; Brulidine; ***Norw.:*** Brulidine; ***UK:*** Brolene; Brulidine; Golden Eye Ointment; Pickles Antiseptic Cream.

Multi-ingredient: ***Austral.:*** Phenergan†; ***S.Afr.:*** Phenergan†; ***UK:*** Healthy Feet; Nosor Nose Balm; Soleze; Swarm.

Dichlordimethylhydantoin (2237-v)

1,3-Dichloro-5,5-dimethylhydantoin; 1,3-Dichloro-5,5-dimethylimidazolidine-2,4-dione.

$C_5H_6Cl_2N_2O_2$ = 197.0.

CAS — 118-52-5.

It contains about 72% w/w of 'available chlorine' (see p.1110).

Dichlordimethylhydantoin is a disinfectant used as a source of chlorine, for sterilising food and dairy equipment and as a bleach.

Bromochlorodimethylhydantoin ($C_5H_6N_2O_2BrCl$=241.5) is a bromine-releasing compound used for the disinfection of swimming-pool water.

Dichlorobenzyl Alcohol (2238-g)

Dichlorophenylcarbinol. 2,4-Dichlorobenzyl alcohol.

$C_7H_6Cl_2O$ = 177.0.

CAS — 1777-82-8.

Dichlorobenzyl alcohol is an antiseptic used chiefly as an ingredient of lozenges in the treatment of minor infections of the mouth and throat.

Preparations

Proprietary Preparations (details are given in Part 3)
Ital.: Neo Borocillina Collutorio; Neo Borocillina Spray.

Multi-ingredient: ***Aust.:*** Coldangin; Neo-Angin; Sulgan 99; ***Austral.:*** Actifed Anaesthetic; Ayrton's Antiseptic; Sore Throat Chewing Gum; Strepsils; Strepsils Anaesthetic†; Strepsils Plus; ***Belg.:*** Neofenox; Strepsils; Strepsils Menthol; Strepsils Vit C; ***Fr.:*** Strepsils; Strepsils Menthol Eucalyptus†; Strepsils Miel-Citron; Strepsils Vitamine C; Strepsilspray Lidocaine; ***Ger.:*** Neo-Angin N; Rapidosept†; ***Irl.:*** Strepsils; Strepsils Dual Action; Strepsils Vitamin C; ***Ital.:*** Arscolloid; Benagol; Benagol Mentolo-Eucaliptolo; Benagol Vitamina C; Bio-Arscolloid; Corti-Arscolloid; Neo Borocillina; Neo Borocillina Balsamica; Neo Borocillina C; Neo Borocillina Tosse Compresse; Oraseptic Gola; ***Neth.:*** Strepsils; Strepsils Menthol en Eucalyptus; Strepsils Sinaasappel en Vitamine C; ***S.Afr.:*** Strepsils; Strepsils Eucalyptus Menthol; Strepsils Orange-C; Strepsils Plus; Strepsils Soothing Honey & Lemon; ***Spain:*** Angiseptina†; Strepsils; Strepsils con Vitamina C; ***Swed.:*** Bafucin; Strepsils; ***Switz.:*** DemoAngina†; Demosept; Lidazon; Neo-Angin au miel et citron; Neo-Angin avec vitamin C exempt de sucre; Neo-Angin exempt de sucre; Sulgan; ***UK:*** Antiseptic Throat Lozenges; Strepsils; Strepsils Dual Action; Strepsils with Vitamin C.

Didecyldimethylammonium Chloride (11329-k)

N-Decyl-*N,N*-demethyl-l-decanaminium chloride.

$C_{22}H_{48}ClN$ = 362.1.

Didecyldimethylammonium chloride is a quaternary ammonium disinfectant used in preparations for disinfection of the skin and mucous membranes. It is also used to disinfect instruments and surfaces.

Preparations

Proprietary Preparations (details are given in Part 3)
Ger.: Gercid forte†; ***Ital.:*** Gram 2†.

Multi-ingredient: ***Belg.:*** Melsitt†; ***Fr.:*** Amphosept BV; Aniospray; Bacterianos D; Chlorispray; Hexanios G+R; Instrunet liquid†; Ultrasep; ***Ger.:*** Baccalin; Bacillocid rasant; Demykosan S†; Demykosan†; Desoform; Freka nol†; Fugisept; Gercid†; Hexaquart L; Hexaquart S; Kohrsolin FF; Lysoformin 3000; Lysoformin spezial; Melsept SF; Melsitt; Quatohex; Tegodor F†; Ultrasol-K†; ***Ital.:*** Alquat†; Cedril; Cedril Strumenti; Cedril Tintura†; Hexaquart L†; Melsept SF; Neo Intol Plus†; Neofen†; T 21†.

Dodicin (11358-f)

Dodicin *(BAN).*

Dodecyldi(aminoethyl) glycine. 3,6,9-Triazahenicosanoic acid.

$C_{18}H_{39}N_3O_2$ = 329.5.

CAS — 6843-97-6 (dodicin); 59079-49-1 (dodicin sodium); 18205-85-1 (dodicin hydrochloride).

Dodicin is an ampholytic surfactant with bactericidal and fungicidal properties. It is also active against some viruses. It is used mainly for surface disinfection. The hydrochloride is also used.

Preparations

Proprietary Preparations (details are given in Part 3)
Ger.: Tego 103 S†; ***Ital.:*** Dinosan†; Sanatot†; Tego 103 G†; Tego Spray†; ***UK:*** Tego 103 G†.

Multi-ingredient: ***Ger.:*** Tego 103 G†; Tego Spray†.

Domiphen Bromide (2242-h)

Domiphen Bromide *(BAN, USAN, rINN).*

NSC-39415; PDDB; Phenododecinium Bromide. Dodecyldimethyl-2-phenoxyethylammonium bromide.

$C_{22}H_{40}BrNO$ = 414.5.

CAS — 13900-14-6 (domiphen); 538-71-6 (domiphen bromide).

Pharmacopoeias. In *Br.* and *Chin.*

Colourless or faintly yellow crystalline flakes. Freely **soluble** in water and in alcohol; soluble in acetone. **Incompatible** with soaps and other anionic surfactants.

Domiphen bromide is a quaternary ammonium antiseptic with actions and uses similar to those of other cationic surfactants (see Cetrimide p.1105). Lozenges containing domiphen bromide are used in the treatment of minor infections of the mouth and throat.

Preparations

Proprietary Preparations (details are given in Part 3)
Canad.: Antiseptique Pastilles; Bronchodex Pastilles; Oraseptic; ***Irl.:*** Bradosol†; ***Ital.:*** Bradoral; ***Switz.:*** Neo-Bradoral†.

Multi-ingredient: ***Aust.:*** Bepanthen; Bradosol; ***Canad.:*** Mouthwash & Gargle; Mouthwash Mint/Peppermint; Nupercainal; Scope with Oraseptate; ***Fr.:*** Fluoselgine; ***Ital.:*** Golamed Oral; Iodosan Nasale Contact†; Nasalemed; ***Switz.:*** Bradoral†; ***UK:*** Bradosol Plus.

Ethylene Oxide (2244-b)

Oxirane.

C_2H_4O = 44.05.

CAS — 75-21-8.

A colourless flammable gas at room temperature and atmospheric pressure. Mixtures of ethylene oxide with oxygen or air are explosive but the risk can be reduced by the addition of carbon dioxide or fluorocarbons.

Adverse Effects and Precautions

Ethylene oxide irritates the eyes and respiratory tract and may also cause nausea and vomiting, diarrhoea, headache, vertigo, CNS depression, dyspnoea, and pulmonary oedema. Liver and kidney damage and haemolysis may occur. Fatalities have occurred. Excessive exposure of the skin to liquid or solution causes burns, blistering, irritation, and dermatitis; percutaneous absorption may lead to systemic effects.

Many materials including plastics and rubber adsorb ethylene oxide. If such materials are being sterilised with ethylene oxide all traces of the gas must be removed before the materials can be used; removal may be by ventilation or more active means. Hypersensitivity reactions, including anaphylaxis, have been associated with ethylene oxide-contaminated materials. Ethylene oxide may also react with materials being sterilised to produce substances such as ethylene chlorohydrin (with chloride) or ethylene glycol (with water); these may contribute to any toxicity.

Pharmaceutical manufacturers within the European Union have been advised to use ethylene oxide only when there is no alternative. Ethylene oxide has been shown to have carcinogenic and mutagenic properties and there is evidence of increased risk of neoplasms following occupational exposure.

Carcinogenicity. Exposure of workers to ethylene oxide has been associated with the development of lymphatic and haematopoietic cancer. However, epidemiological studies have not consistently shown an excess of cases among workers exposed to ethylene oxide, and excesses that have been seen have been small[1-4] although a trend towards increased risk related to cumulative exposure has been reported.[2,4]

1. Hogstedt C, *et al.* Epidemiologic support for ethylene oxide as a cancer-causing agent. *JAMA* 1986; **255:** 1575–8.
2. Steenland K, *et al.* Mortality among workers exposed to ethylene oxide. *N Engl J Med* 1991; **324:** 1402–7.
3. Hagmar L, *et al.* An epidemiological study of cancer risk among workers exposed to ethylene oxide using hemoglobin adducts to validate environmental exposure assessments. *Int Arch Occup Environ Health* 1991; **63:** 271–7.
4. Stayner L, *et al.* Exposure-response analysis of cancer mortality in a cohort of workers exposed to ethylene oxide. *Am J Epidemiol* 1993; **138:** 787–98.

Effects on the nervous system. Four men exposed to ethylene oxide at a concentration of greater than 700 ppm developed neurological disorders. One experienced headaches, nausea, vomiting, and lethargy followed by major motor seizures. The others experienced headaches, limb numbness and weakness, increased fatigue, trouble with memory and thought processes, and slurred speech. Three also developed cataracts, and one required bilateral cataract extractions.[1]

1. Jay WM, *et al.* Possible relationship of ethylene oxide exposure to cataract formation. *Am J Ophthalmol* 1982; **93:** 727–32.

Hypersensitivity. Anaphylactoid reactions in dialysis patients have resulted from the use of dialysis equipment sterilised with ethylene oxide.[1-3] There have also been reports of hypersensitivity[4] and anaphylactoid[5] reactions in plateletpheresis donors caused by residues of ethylene oxide in components of apheresis kits. The most common adverse reactions reported have been dyspnoea, wheezing, urticaria, flushing, headache, and hypotension, but acute severe bronchospasm, circulatory collapse, cardiac arrest, and death have also occurred. It was noted[6] that where severe, sometimes fatal, anaphylactoid reactions have occurred at the beginning of dialysis, ethylene oxide has almost universally been implicated, although exposure to cuprammonium cellulose (cuprophane) dialysis membranes may also have been involved.

It has been reported that there may be an increased risk of ethylene oxide-induced anaphylactic shock in children undergoing surgery for spina bifida.[7] Such children might be at increased risk of sensitisation and anaphylaxis, and came into frequent contact with ethylene oxide through multiple operations and catheterisations.

Occupational asthma and contact dermatitis have been attributed to residual ethylene oxide in surgical gloves.[8]

1. Bommer J, *et al.* Anaphylactoid reactions in dialysis patients: role of ethylene-oxide. *Lancet* 1985; **ii:** 1382–5.
2. Rumpf KW, *et al.* Association of ethylene-oxide-induced IgE antibodies with symptoms in dialysis patients. *Lancet* 1985; **ii:** 1385–7.
3. Röckel A, *et al.* Ethylene oxide hypersensitivity in dialysis patients. *Lancet* 1986; **i:** 382–3.
4. Leitman SF, *et al.* Allergic reactions in healthy plateletpheresis donors caused by sensitization to ethylene oxide gas. *N Engl J Med* 1986; **315:** 1192–6.
5. Muylle L, *et al.* Anaphylactoid reaction in platelet-pheresis donor with IgE antibodies to ethylene oxide. *Lancet* 1986; **ii:** 1225.
6. Nicholls A. Ethylene oxide and anaphylaxis during haemodialysis. *Br Med J* 1986; **292:** 1221–2.
7. Moneret-Vautrin DA, *et al.* High risk of anaphylactic shock during surgery for spina bifida. *Lancet* 1990; **335:** 865–6.
8. Verraes S, Michel O. Occupational asthma induced by ethylene oxide. *Lancet* 1995; **346:** 1434–5.

Pregnancy. A study, by Hemminki *et al.*,[1] of female hospital sterilising staff in all general hospitals in Finland showed that the incidence of spontaneous abortion (analysed according to employment at the time of conception and corrected for maternal age, parity, decade of pregnancy, smoking, and consumption of alcohol and coffee) was significantly increased in those exposed to ethylene oxide during pregnancy compared with those not so exposed. This study provoked criticism,[2,3] and Hemminki *et al.*[4] conceded that the study was not large enough to compare abortion rates and known ethylene oxide concentrations.

1. Hemminki K, *et al.* Spontaneous abortions in hospital staff engaged in sterilising instruments with chemical agents. *Br Med J* 1982; **285:** 1461–3.
2. Gordon JE, Meinhardt TJ. Spontaneous abortions in hospital sterilising staff. *Br Med J* 1983; **286:** 1976.
3. Austin SG. Spontaneous abortions in hospital sterilising staff. *Br Med J* 1983; **286:** 1976.
4. Hemminki K, *et al.* Spontaneous abortions in hospital sterilising staff. *Br Med J* 1983; **286:** 1976–7.

Pharmacokinetics

Ethylene oxide gas is rapidly absorbed through the lungs and distributed throughout the body. Percutaneous absorption can occur from aqueous solutions. It is rapidly metabolised by hydrolysis or conjugation with glutathione.

References.

1. Föst U, *et al.* Distribution of ethylene oxide in human blood and its implications for biomonitoring. *Hum Exp Toxicol* 1991; **10:** 25–31.

Uses

Ethylene oxide is a bactericidal and fungicidal gaseous disinfectant which is effective against most micro-organisms, including viruses. It is also sporicidal. It is used for the gaseous sterilisation of heat-labile pharmaceutical and surgical materials that cannot be sterilised by other means.

Ethylene oxide forms explosive mixtures with air; this may be overcome by using mixtures containing 10% ethylene oxide in carbon dioxide, or by removing at least 95% of the air from the apparatus before admitting either ethylene oxide or a mixture of 90% ethylene oxide in carbon dioxide. Alternatively, non-flammable mixtures of dichlorodifluoromethane and trichlorofluoromethane with 9 to 12% w/w of ethylene oxide have been employed, but restrictions on the release of fluorocarbons or CFCs limit their use.

Effective sterilisation by ethylene oxide depends on exposure time, temperature, humidity, the amount and type of microbial contamination, and the partial pressure of the ethylene oxide in the exposure chamber. The material being sterilised must be permeable to ethylene oxide if occluded micro-organisms are present. The bactericidal action is accelerated by increase of temperature; a temperature of about 55° can be used for most thermolabile materials.

Moisture is essential for sterilisation by ethylene oxide. In practice, dry micro-organisms need to be rehydrated before ethylene oxide can be effective; humidification is normally carried out under vacuum prior to introduction of ethylene oxide. Relative humidities of 40 to 60% are used. Control of physical factors does not assure sterility, and the process should be monitored usually by employing standardised suspensions of aerobic spores such as those of *Bacillus subtilis* var. *niger.*

Formaldehyde Solution (2246-g)

Formaldehydi Solutio.

NOTE. The names formalin and formol have been used for formaldehyde solution but in some countries Formalin is a trade mark.

Pharmacopoeias. In *Eur.* (see p.viii), *Jpn*, and *US.*

Formaldehyde Solution (Ph. Eur.) contains 34.5 to 38% w/w of CH_2O (= 30.03) with methyl alcohol as a stabilising agent to delay polymerisation of the formaldehyde to solid paraformaldehyde. Formaldehyde Solution (USP 23) contains not less than 36.5% or 37.0% w/w (depending on the packaging) of CH_2O with methyl alcohol.

Formaldehyde solution is a clear, colourless, or practically colourless liquid with a characteristic, pungent, irritating odour. **Miscible** with water and with alcohol. **Store** at a temperature between 15° and 25° in airtight containers. Protect from light. A slight white deposit of paraformaldehyde may form on keeping, especially if the solution is kept in a cold place.

Incompatibilities. Formaldehyde reacts with protein and this may diminish its antimicrobial activity.

NOTE. Formaldehyde solution is sometimes known simply as formaldehyde and this has led to confusion in interpreting the strength and the form in which formaldehyde is being used. In practice formaldehyde is available as formaldehyde solution which is diluted before use, the percentage strength being expressed in terms of formaldehyde solution rather than formaldehyde (CH_2O). For example, in the UK formaldehyde solution 3% consists of 3 volumes of Formaldehyde Solution (BP 1998) diluted to 100 volumes with water and thus contains 1.02 to 1.14% w/w of formaldehyde (CH_2O); it is *not* prepared by diluting Formaldehyde Solution (BP 1998) to arrive at a solution containing 3% w/w of formaldehyde (CH_2O).

Adverse Effects and Precautions

Concentrated formaldehyde solutions applied to the skin cause whitening and hardening. Contact dermatitis and sensitivity reactions have occurred after the use of conventional concentrations and after contact with residual formaldehyde in resins.

Ingestion of formaldehyde solution causes intense pain, with inflammation, ulceration, and necrosis of mucous membranes. There may be vomiting, haematemesis, blood-stained diarrhoea, haematuria, and anuria; metabolic acidosis, vertigo, convulsions, loss of consciousness, and circulatory failure may occur. Death has occurred after the ingestion of the equivalent of about 30 mL of formaldehyde solution. If the patient survives 48 hours, recovery is probable. Formaldehyde vapour is irritant to the eyes, nose, and upper respiratory tract, and may cause coughing, dysphagia, spasm and oedema of the larynx, bronchitis, pneumonia, and rarely, pulmonary oedema. Asthma has been reported after repeated exposure.

General references.

1. Health and Safety Executive. Formaldehyde. *Toxicity Review 2.* London: HMSO, 1981.
2. Formaldehyde. *Environmental Health Criteria 89.* Geneva: WHO, 1989.
3. Formaldehyde health and safety guide. *IPCS Health and Safety Guide 57.* Geneva: WHO, 1991.

Carcinogenicity. There is controversy as to the risk formaldehyde presents as a carcinogen. Studies on the occupational exposure of medical personnel[1] and industrial workers[2-4] to formaldehyde have generally concluded that although the risk is small or non-existent, the possibility that formaldehyde is a human carcinogen cannot be excluded. Reanalyses of such studies have led to different interpretations of the results, with some workers concluding that the risk of cancer from formaldehyde is greater than originally thought,[5-7] while others maintain that the risk is small,[8] and that follow-up of large cohorts exposed to high concentrations for long periods is required to detect such a risk.[9] In the meantime, USA regulatory authorities still consider formaldehyde to be a probable human carcinogen.[10]

1. Kreiger N. Formaldehyde and nasal cancer mortality. *Can Med Assoc J* 1983; **128:** 248–9.
2. Acheson ED, *et al.* Formaldehyde in the British chemical industry. *Lancet* 1984; **i:** 611–16.
3. Acheson ED, *et al.* Formaldehyde process workers and lung cancer. *Lancet* 1984; **i:** 1066–7.
4. Gérin M, *et al.* Cancer risks due to occupational exposure to formaldehyde: results of a multi-site case-control study in Montreal. *Int J Cancer* 1989; **44:** 53–8.
5. Sterling T, Arundel A. Formaldehyde and lung cancer. *Lancet* 1985; **ii:** 1366.
6. Infante PF, Schneiderman MA. Formaldehyde, lung cancer, and bronchitis. *Lancet* 1986; **i:** 436–7.
7. Sterling TD, Weinkam JJ. Reanalysis of lung cancer mortality in a National Cancer Institute study on mortality among industrial workers exposed to formaldehyde. *J Occup Med* 1988; **30:** 895–901.
8. Gardner MJ, *et al.* Formaldehyde and lung cancer. *Lancet* 1985; **ii:** 1366–7.
9. Gardner MJ, *et al.* Formaldehyde, lung cancer, and bronchitis. *Lancet* 1986; **i:** 437–8.
10. Council on Scientific Affairs of the American Medical Association. Formaldehyde. *JAMA* 1989; **261:** 1183–7.

Effects on the blood. Haemolysis during chronic haemodialysis was due to formaldehyde eluted from filters.[1]

1. Orringer EP, Mattern WD. Formaldehyde-induced hemolysis during chronic hemodialysis. *N Engl J Med* 1976; **294:** 1416–20.

Effects on the urinary tract. Adverse effects of intravesical instillation of formaldehyde solutions in the treatment of haemorrhagic cystitis have included dysuria, suprapubic pain, ureteric and bladder fibrosis, hydronephrosis, vesicoureteral reflux, and fatal acute renal failure.[1] Intraperitoneal spillage through a fistula, leading to adverse systemic effects, has also occurred.[2] See also Haemorrhagic Cystitis under Uses, below.

Breysse *et al.*[3] report four patients exposed to high levels of atmospheric formaldehyde who developed membranous nephropathy, and suggest that there may be genetic susceptibility for this effect.

1. Melekos M, Lalos J. Intravesical instillation of formalin and its complications. *Urology* 1983; **21:** 331–2.
2. Capen CV, *et al.* Intraperitoneal spillage of formalin after intravesical instillation. *Urology* 1982; **19:** 599–601.
3. Breysse P, *et al.* Membranous nephropathy and formaldehyde exposure. *Ann Intern Med* 1994; **120:** 396–7.

Hypersensitivity. Hypersensitivity to formaldehyde has had several manifestations. Effects on the skin have included acute exacerbation of eczema after injection of hepatitis B vaccine, containing up to 20 μg of formaldehyde per mL.[1] In another case formaldehyde sensitivity was characterised by pruritus, burning, and redness within minutes of exposure to sunlight.[2] Painful, enlarged, and haemorrhagic gingival margins have occurred following the use of a toothpaste containing a solution of formaldehyde.[3] There is conflicting evidence of the respiratory effects of formaldehyde: although a low concentration has been reported not to trigger an asthma attack in patients with severe bronchial hyperresponsiveness,[4] occupational asthma has been documented.[5] More severe manifestations of hypersensitivity include seven cases of shock of possible toxic or anaphylactic aetiology, which occurred following the use of formaldehyde solutions during surgical removal of hydatid cysts.[6]

For mention of an allergic response to root canal paste containing paraformaldehyde, see p.1121.

1. Ring J. Exacerbation of eczema by formalin-containing hepatitis B vaccine in formaldehyde-allergic patients. *Lancet* 1986; **ii:** 522–3.
2. Shelley WB. Immediate sunburn-like reaction in a patient with formaldehyde photosensitivity. *Arch Dermatol* 1982; **118:** 117–18.
3. Laws IM. Toothpaste formulations. *Br Dent J* 1984; **156:** 240.
4. Harving H, *et al.* Low concentrations of formaldehyde in bronchial asthma: a study of exposure under controlled conditions. *Br Med J* 1986; **293:** 310.
5. Heard BE. Low concentrations of formaldehyde in bronchial asthma. *Br Med J* 1986; **293:** 821.
6. Galland MC, *et al.* Risques thérapeutiques de l'utilisation des solutions de formol dans le traitement chirurgical des kystes hydatiques du foie. *Therapie* 1980; **35:** 443–6.

Treatment of Adverse Effects

Contaminated skin should be washed with soap and water. After ingestion water, milk, charcoal, and/or demulcents should be given; gastric lavage and emesis should be avoided. Assisted ventilation may be required and shock should be alleviated appropriately. Acidosis, resulting from metabolism of formaldehyde to formic acid, may require the intravenous administration of sodium bicarbonate or sodium lactate. The use of haemodialysis has been suggested.

Uses and Administration

Formaldehyde solution is a bactericidal disinfectant also effective against fungi and many viruses. It is slowly effective against bacterial spores but its sporicidal effect is greatly increased by increase in temperature.

- *Formaldehyde solution is usually used diluted and it is important to note that the strength of preparations is given in terms of the content of formaldehyde solution and not in terms of the final concentration of formaldehyde* (see NOTE, above).

Formaldehyde solution is used in the disinfection of blankets and bedding and in the disinfection of the membranes in dialysis equipment. It is important to ensure that there are no traces of formaldehyde on any equipment before it is used. Formaldehyde solution is also used in combination with succinic dialdehyde for instrument disinfection.

When applied to the unbroken skin, formaldehyde solution hardens the epidermis, renders it tough and whitish, and produces a local anaesthetic effect. Formaldehyde solution 3% v/v has been used for the treatment of warts on the palms of the hands and soles of the feet. Sweating of the feet may be treated by the application of formaldehyde solution in glycerol or alcohol but such applications are liable to produce sensitisation reactions and other treatments are regarded as more effective (see Hyperhidrosis, p.1074).

After surgical removal of hydatid cysts, diluted formaldehyde solution has been used for irrigating the cavities to destroy scolices but other larvicides are preferred (see Echinococcosis, p.94). It is generally too irritant for use on mucous membranes but it has been used in mouthwashes and pastes as an antiseptic and hardening agent for the gums. In dentistry it has been used in endodontic treatment.

Formaldehyde solution in concentrations of up to 10% v/v in saline is used as a preservative for pathological specimens. It is not suitable for preserving urine for subsequent examination. Formaldehyde solution has been used for the inactivation of viruses in vaccine production.

Formaldehyde gas has little penetrating power and readily polymerises and condenses on surfaces and its effectiveness depends on it dissolving in a film of moisture before acting on micro-organisms; in practice a relative humidity of 80 to 90% is necessary. Formaldehyde gas is used for the disinfection of rooms and cabinets. The gas may be produced from 500 mL of undiluted formaldehyde solution by boiling with 1 litre of water or by addition of potassium permanganate or by heating a formaldehyde-containing solid such as paraformaldehyde (p.1121). Formaldehyde gas is used in combination with low-temperature steam for the sterilisation of heat-sensitive items.

Other compounds which are thought to act by releasing formaldehyde include noxythiolin (p.1120), taurolidine (p.257), and hexamine (p.216).

Disinfection. VIRUSES. Formaldehyde solution 0.1% v/v was too slow in action to be recommended for the inactivation of HIV.[1] However, Nye and Patou[2] have found a higher concentration of formaldehyde effective in inactivating HIV in CSF samples.

1. Spire B, *et al.* Inactivation of lymphadenopathy associated virus by chemical disinfectants. *Lancet* 1984; **ii:** 899–901.
2. Nye P, Patou G. Treatment of cerebrospinal fluid with formalin from patients infected with human immunodeficiency virus before diagnostic microscopy. *J Clin Pathol* 1987; **40:** 119.

Haemorrhagic cystitis. Formaldehyde has been used for local therapy of haemorrhagic cystitis although there has been debate about the most appropriate regimen. The Fair regimen[1] for the intravesical administration of formaldehyde solution in haemorrhagic cystitis involves passive irrigation of the bladder with formaldehyde solution 1% v/v 500 to 1000 mL for a total of 10 minutes, the bladder subsequently being emptied and washed out with one litre of distilled water. Stronger concentrations of formaldehyde solution and other methods can be used if bleeding does not stop.[2] In a review of 118 patients treated with solutions of formaldehyde for intractable haematuria, the authors felt that this was probably the most effective treatment, but also probably the most dangerous.[3] More concentrated instillations, containing formaldehyde solution 5 to 10% seem to be generally viewed as unnecessary, and associated with an increased risk of complications which militates against their use.[4-7] Instillation of intravesical alum (p.1547) has successfully controlled bleeding without complications and Smith *et al.* concluded that alum was a safe and effective treatment for intractable bladder bleeding and should replace formaldehyde solution, no matter how dilute. Instillation of prostaglandins such as alprostadil (p.1413) or carboprost trometamol (p.1414) has also been used.

1. Fair WR. Formalin in the treatment of massive bladder hemorrhage: techniques, results, and complications. *Urology* 1974; **3:** 573–6.
2. Anonymous. Haemorrhagic cystitis after radiotherapy. *Lancet* 1987; **i:** 304–6.
3. Godec CJ, Gleich P. Intractable hematuria and formalin. *J Urol (Baltimore)* 1983; **130:** 688–91.
4. Bullock N, Whitaker RH. Massive bladder haemorrhage. *Br Med J* 1985; **291:** 1522–3.
5. Donahue LA, Frank IN. Intravesical formalin for haemorrhagic cystitis: analysis of therapy. *J Urol (Baltimore)* 1989; **141:** 809–12.
6. Murray JA, *et al.* Massive bladder haemorrhage. *Br Med J* 1986; **292:** 57.
7. Smith PJB, *et al.* Massive bladder haemorrhage. *Br Med J* 1986; **292:** 412.

Warts. Formaldehyde solution 3% v/v has been applied for the treatment of warts (p.1076), in conjunction with the removal of scale and dead tissue by scraping.[1] However, in another study the efficacy of formaldehyde solution was no better than the use of an inert agent.[2]

1. Vickers CFH. Treatment of plantar warts in children. *Br Med J* 1961; **2:** 743–5.
2. Anderson I, Shirreffs E. The treatment of plantar warts. *Br J Dermatol* 1963; **75:** 29–32.

Preparations

Proprietary Preparations (details are given in Part 3)

Ger.: Lysoform; ***Irl.:*** Veracur; ***Spain:*** Diformil; Lysoform†; ***UK:*** Emoform†; Veracur; ***USA:*** Lazerformaldehyde.

Multi-ingredient: ***Austral.:*** Formo-Cresol Mitis; ***Belg.:*** Angi C†; Melsitt†; ***Canad.:*** British Army Foot Powder; Duoplant; ***Fr.:*** Aniospray; Arthrodont; Bacterianos D; Chlorispray; Emoform; Ephydrol; Incidine; Instrunet liquid†; Parodium; Surfalyse†; Veybirol-Tyrothyricine; ***Ger.:*** Aseptisol; Buraton 10 F; Buraton 25†; Buraton†; Demykosan†; Desoform; Gigasept; Gigasept FF; Incidin GG†; Incidin perfekt; Incidin Spezial; Indulfan plus; Lysetol V; Lysoformin; Melsept; Melsitt; Minutil; Pfefferminz-Lysoform; Sekusept forte; Sporcid; Tegodor forte†; Tegodor†; Tegofektol†; Tegoment†; Tegosinol†; Ultrasol-F; Ultrasol-S; ***Ital.:*** Melsept; ***Spain:*** Antiseptico Dent Donner†; Diformiltricina; Elixir Dental Formahina†; Gargaril Sulfamida†; Gargaril†; Sudosin; Tifell; Viberol Tirotricina; ***Switz.:*** Emoform†; ***UK:*** Tegodor.

Glutaraldehyde (2248-p)

Glutaral *(USAN, rINN)*; Glutaric Dialdehyde; Pentanedial. Pentane-1,5-dial.

$C_5H_8O_2$ = 100.1.

CAS — 111-30-8.

Pharmacopoeias. Solutions of glutaraldehyde are included in *Br., Chin.*, and *US*.

Glutaraldehyde is a liquid. **Soluble** in water and alcohol.

Glutaral Concentrate (USP 23) contains 50 to 52% w/w of glutaraldehyde and has a pH between 3.7 and 4.5; Glutaral Disinfectant Solution (USNF 18) has a pH between 2.7 and 3.7. They should be **stored** at a temperature not exceeding 40° in airtight containers, protected from light.

Glutaraldehyde Solution (BP 1998) contains 9.2 to 10.5% w/v of glutaraldehyde; Strong Glutaraldehyde Solution (BP 1998) contains 47 to 53% w/w of glutaraldehyde. They should be **stored** at a temperature not exceeding 15°.

Adverse Effects

As for Formaldehyde Solution, p.1113.

In a brief review of the occupational hazards of glutaraldehyde Burge[1] noted that several studies showed adverse effects, including nausea, headache, airway obstruction, asthma, rhinitis, eye irritation, and dermatitis, occurring among medical personnel exposed to glutaraldehyde, generally at concentrations below the recommended limits. Skin reactions were due to hypersensitivity or a direct irritant effect. Burge concluded that when using glutaraldehyde workers should take suitable precautions to protect the skin, and should avoid inhaling the vapour.

The risk of occupational exposure to glutaraldehyde vapour may be higher in warm climates.[2]

There has also been a report of accidental ocular contact with glutaraldehyde due to leakage of glutaraldehyde solution retained in an anaesthesia mask; moderate chemical conjunctivitis ensued.[3]

1. Burge PS. Occupational risks of glutaraldehyde. *Br Med J* 1989; **299:** 342.
2. Mwaniki DL, Guthua SW. Occupational exposure to glutaraldehyde in tropical climates. *Lancet* 1992; **340:** 1476–7.
3. Murray WJ, Ruddy MP. Toxic eye injury during induction of anaesthesia. *South Med J* 1985; **78:** 1012–13.

Effects on the gastro-intestinal tract. Insufficient rinsing of a glutaraldehyde 2% solution from flexible sigmoidoscopes after disinfection appeared to be responsible for an outbreak of fever and gastro-intestinal symptoms including abdominal cramps, bloody diarrhoea, and nausea and vomiting in patients undergoing sigmoidoscopy.[1]

1. Durante L, *et al.* Investigation of an outbreak of bloody diarrhea: association with endoscopic cleaning solution and demonstration of lesions in an animal model. *Am J Med* 1992; **92:** 476–80.

Uses and Administration

Glutaraldehyde is a bactericidal disinfectant which is rapidly effective against Gram-positive and Gram-negative bacteria. It is also effective against *Mycobacterium tuberculosis*, some fungi, and viruses, including hepatitis B virus and HIV, and is slowly effective against bacterial spores. Aqueous solutions show optimum activity between pH 7.5 and 8.5; such solutions are chemically stable for about 14 days. Solutions at lower pH values are more stable.

A 2% aqueous solution buffered to a pH of about 8 (activated glutaraldehyde; alkaline glutaraldehyde) is used for the sterilisation of endoscopic and dental instruments, rubber or plastic equipment, and for other equipment which cannot be sterilised by heat. Glutaraldehyde is non-corrosive towards most materials. Complete immersion in the solution for 10 to 20 minutes is sufficient for rapid disinfection of thoroughly cleansed instruments but exposure for up to 10 hours may be necessary for sterilisation.

A 10% gel is applied twice daily for the treatment of warts (p.1076); a 5% or 10% solution may also be used. Glutaraldehyde should not be used for facial or anogenital warts. Glutaraldehyde has also been used topically for treating hyperhidrosis of the palms and soles, although other agents are generally preferred (see p.1074).

Disinfection. ENDOSCOPES. For reference to the use of glutaraldehyde for disinfection of endoscopes, see p.1097.

See also below under Viruses.

VIRUSES. Glutaraldehyde 1% and 2% in alkaline solution inactivated HIV in 10% serum dried onto sterile coverslips within 1 (cell-free HIV) or 2 (cell-associated HIV) minutes.[1] Similar results were obtained with a 2% solution using HIV in neat serum. However, a 1% solution failed to inactivate the virus in neat serum within 15 minutes. It should be noted that use for 14 days can reduce the strength of 2% alkaline glutaraldehyde to almost 1%, and that protein should be removed before disinfection. Another study, on the elimination of HIV from fibreoptic endoscopes with glutaraldehyde 2% highlighted the importance of cleaning equipment with detergent prior to disinfection with glutaraldehyde.[2] In this latter study cleaning followed by disinfection for 2 minutes was effective in decontaminating the 5 endoscopes tested indicating that the guidelines recommended by the British Society of Gastroenterologists of cleaning followed by 4 minutes disinfection in glutaraldehyde carried a reasonable margin of safety against HIV.

WHO guidelines on sterilisation and disinfection methods against HIV recommend alkaline glutaraldehyde 2% for the disinfection of medical or surgical instruments (30-minute immersion).[3]

1. Hanson PJV, *et al.* Glutaraldehyde and endoscopic disinfection: a cautionary tale. *Gut* 1989; **30:** A704.
2. Hanson PJV, *et al.* Elimination of high titre HIV from fibreoptic endoscopes. *Gut* 1990; **31:** 657–9.
3. WHO. Guidelines on sterilization and disinfection methods effective against human immunodeficiency virus (HIV). *WHO AIDS Series 2* 1989.

Preparations

BP 1998: Glutaraldehyde Solution; Strong Glutaraldehyde Solution;
USNF 18: Glutaral Disinfectant Solution;
USP 23: Glutaral Concentrate.

Proprietary Preparations (details are given in Part 3)
Austral.: Diswart; Glutarall; ***Belg.:*** Aldetex†; ***Canad.:*** Glutacide†; Sonacide; ***Fr.:*** Cidex; Endosporine†; Sekucid; Sporicidine†; Steranios; Verutal; ***Ger.:*** Cidex; Korsolex-Endo-Disinfectant; Sekumatic FD; ***Irl.:*** Glutarol; Verucasep; ***Ital.:*** Asporin 2; Cidex; Diba; Eso Cem; Eso H1; Esoform HP†; Esoxid; Ferriseptil; H1; Sporacid; Sporex; Sporicidin; ***Switz.:*** Glutarol; ***UK:*** ASEP; Cidex; Glutarol; Novaruca†; Verucasep†; ***USA:*** Cidex.

Multi-ingredient: ***Belg.:*** Melsitt†; ***Fr.:*** Aniospray; Bacterianos D; Chlorispray; Incidine; Instrunet liquid†; Surfalyse†; Ultrasep; ***Ger.:*** Aerodesin; Altego†; Aseptisol; Bacillocid rasant; Bacillocid Spezial; Bacillol plus; Baktobod; Buraton 10 F; Demykosan S†; Demykosan†; Desoform; Helipur H plus; Incidin perfekt; Incidin Spezial; Incidur; Incidur Spray; Indulfan plus; Kohrsolin; Kohrsolin FF; Kohrsolin iD; Korsolex FF; Lysetol FF; Lysetol V; Lysoformin; Lysoformin 3000; Melsept; Melsept SF; Melsitt; Minutil; Mucocit A†; Pursept N†; Sekusept Extra N; Sekusept forte; Tegodor F†; Tegodor forte†; Tegodor†; Tegofektol†; Tegoment†; Tegosinol†; Ultra-scope†; Ultrasol-F; Ultrasol-S; Ultrasol-spezial†; ***Ital.:*** Alquat†; Asporin 0.5; Combisan Plus†; Diaril; Eso Din; Esoform 92; Iketoncid; Incidin Spezial; Melsept; Melsept SF; Sekucid; Sekugerm; Sekumatic D; Tegodor†; Tegoment†; ***Mon.:*** Akila spray; ***UK:*** Tegodor.

Glyoxal (11603-t)

Ethanedial; Oxalaldehyde. 1,2-Ethanedione.
$C_2H_2O_2$ = 58.04.
CAS — 107-22-2.

Glyoxal is an aldehyde used for the disinfection of medical and surgical instruments.

Preparations

Proprietary Preparations (details are given in Part 3)
Multi-ingredient: ***Belg.:*** Meliseptol†; ***Fr.:*** Aniospray; Bacterianos D; Incidine; Instrunet liquid†; Surfalyse†; ***Ger.:*** Antifect; Baktobod; Baktobod N; Buraton 10 F; Buraton 25†; Buraton†; Demykosan S†; Demykosan†; Desoform; Freka nol†; Fugisept; Helipur H plus; Incidin GG†; Incidin perfekt; Incidin Spezial; Incidur; Indulfan plus; Lysoformin 3000; Meliseptol; Melsept; Melsept SF; Minutil; Mucocit A†; Pursept A; Pursept N†; Sekusept forte; Sporcid; Tegodor forte†; Tegoment†; Tegosinol†; Ultra-scope†; Ultrasol-F; Ultrasol-S; Ultrasol-spezial†; ***Ital.:*** Incidin Spezial; Indulfan; Melsept; Melsept SF; Melsept Spray; Sekugerm; Tegoment†.

Halazone (2249-s)

Halazone *(pINN)*.
Pantocide. 4-(Dichlorosulphamoyl)benzoic acid.
$C_7H_5Cl_2NO_4S$ = 270.1.
CAS — 80-13-7.
Pharmacopoeias. In *Pol.* and *US.*

A white crystalline powder with a characteristic odour of chlorine, containing about 52% of 'available chlorine' (see p.1110). **Soluble** 1 in more than 1000 of water and chloroform, 1 in more than 2000 of ether, and 1 in 140 of alcohol; soluble in glacial acetic acid. It dissolves in aqueous solutions of alkali hydroxides and carbonates with the formation of a salt. **Store** in airtight containers. Protect from light.

Halazone is a disinfectant with the general properties of chlorine (p.1109) in aqueous solution and is used for the disinfection of drinking water (p.1098). One tablet containing 4 mg of halazone, stabilised with sodium carbonate and sodium chloride, is sufficient to treat about a litre of water in about 30 minutes to 1 hour, more being required for heavily contaminated water. The taste of residual chlorine may be removed by adding sodium thiosulphate.

Preparations

USP 23: Halazone Tablets for Solution.

Proprietary Preparations (details are given in Part 3)
Ital.: Clordispenser; Steridrolo a rapida idrolisi.

Multi-ingredient: ***Spain:*** Cloritines.

Hexachlorophane (2250-h)

Hexachlorophane *(BAN)*.
Hexachlorophene *(rINN)*; G-11. 2,2′-Methylenebis(3,4,6-trichlorophenol).
$C_{13}H_6Cl_6O_2$ = 406.9.
CAS — 70-30-4.
Pharmacopoeias. In *Aust., Br.,* and *US.*

A white or pale buff crystalline powder which is odourless or has a slight phenolic odour.

Practically **insoluble** in water; freely soluble in alcohol; very soluble in acetone and in ether; soluble in chloroform; dissolves in dilute solutions of alkali hydroxides. **Store** in airtight containers. Protect from light.

Incompatibilities. The activity of hexachlorophane may be reduced in the presence of blood or other organic material. It retains some activity in the presence of soap.

Hexachlorophane's activity has been reported to be reduced by alkaline media and by nonionic surfactants such as polysorbate 80.[1] It is extremely sensitive to iron, and to avoid discoloration due to traces of this metal in hexachlorophane detergent solutions, it is advisable to incorporate a sequestrant such as disodium edetate.[2]

1. Walter G, Gump W. Effect of pH on hexachlorophene. *Soap Chem Spec* 1963; **39:** 55–6.
2. Bell M. Hexachlorophene-based skin cleansers. *Specialities* 1965; **1:** 16–18.

Adverse Effects and Treatment

Following ingestion, anorexia, nausea, vomiting, diarrhoea, abdominal cramps, dehydration, shock, and confusion may occur. Convulsions and death may follow. CNS stimulation, convulsions, and death have also occurred after absorption of hexachlorophane from burns and damaged skin. There have been reports showing that hexachlorophane can be absorbed through the skin of infants in amounts sufficient to produce spongy lesions of the brain, sometimes fatal.

Photosensitivity and skin sensitisation have occasionally occurred after repeated use of hexachlorophane.

Treatment of adverse effects is as for Phenol, p.1121.

Effects on the respiratory system. Asthma developed in a 43-year-old nurse after long-term exposure to hexachlorophane powder.[1]

1. Nagy L, Orosz M. Occupational asthma due to hexachlorophene. *Thorax* 1984; **39:** 630–1.

Precautions

Hexachlorophane should not be applied to mucous membranes, large areas of skin, or to burnt, damaged, or denuded skin and should not be used vaginally, applied under occlusive dressings, or applied to areas affected by dermatoses. It should be used with caution on infants, especially premature and low birth-weight neonates. Its use is advised against in pregnancy.

Preparations of hexachlorophane are liable to contamination, especially with Gram-negative bacteria.

Neonates. Spongiform encephalopathy has occurred in neonates who have been treated topically with hexachlorophane.[1] Neonates with a birth-weight of 1.4 kg or less appear to be most susceptible, whereas those weighing over 2 kg were not considered to be at risk.[1,2] Also most of the reports have involved hexachlorophane applied in a concentration of 3%. This concentration appears to be used in some areas for the control of neonatal staphylococcal infection when other measures are not effective; in the UK the concentration that is now used for this purpose is 0.33%.

1. Anonymous. Hexachlorophene today. *Lancet* 1982; **i:** 87–8.
2. Plueckhahn VD, Collins RB. Hexachlorophene emulsions and antiseptic skin care of newborn infants. *Med J Aust* 1976; **1:** 815–19.

Pregnancy. Hexachlorophane is absorbed from the skin and crosses the placenta, but whether it has produced teratogenic effects is subject to debate.[1,2] However, it is considered best to avoid its use during pregnancy.

1. Halling H. Suspected link between exposure to hexachlorophene and malformed infants. *Ann N Y Acad Sci* 1979; **320:** 426–35.
2. Baltzar B, *et al.* Pregnancy outcome among women working in Swedish hospitals. *N Engl J Med* 1979; **300:** 627–8.

Pharmacokinetics

Hexachlorophane is absorbed from the gastro-intestinal tract following accidental ingestion, and through intact and denuded skin. Percutaneous absorption may be significant in premature infants and through damaged skin. Hexachlorophane crosses the placenta.

Uses and Administration

Hexachlorophane is a chlorinated bisphenol antiseptic with a bacteriostatic action against Gram-positive organisms, but much less effective against Gram-negative organisms. It is more active at pH 5 to 6.

Hexachlorophane is mainly used in soaps and creams in a concentration of 0.23 to 3% and is an ingredient of various preparations used for skin disorders. After repeated use of these preparations for several days there is a marked diminution of the bacterial flora due to accumulation of hexachlorophane in the skin. This residual effect is rapidly lost after washing with unmedicated soap or alcohol.

A preparation containing 3% is used for the disinfection of the hands of surgeons and other healthcare personnel. Thorough rinsing is recommended before drying. Hexachlorophane may be applied as a 0.33% dusting powder to the umbilical cord stump for the control of staphylococcal infection in the newborn. However, care is necessary when using hexachlorophane in neonates.

Hexachlorophane sodium has also been used.

Disinfection. Eradication of an outbreak of infection with methicillin-resistant *Staphylococcus aureus* in a neonatal intensive care unit was achieved by use of hexachlorophane soap for hand washing. Previous infection-control measures including the use of chlorhexidine had failed.[1] For a discussion of staphylococcal infections and their treatment, see p.144.

1. Reboli AC, *et al.* Epidemic methicillin-gentamicin-resistant Staphylococcus aureus in a neonatal intensive care unit. *Am J Dis Child* 1989; **143:** 34–9.

Preparations

BP 1998: Hexachlorophene Dusting Powder *(Zinc and Hexachlorophene Dusting Powder)*;
USP 23: Hexachlorophene Cleansing Emulsion *(Hexachlorophene Detergent Lotion)*; Hexachlorophene Liquid Soap.

Proprietary Preparations (details are given in Part 3)
Canad.: Hexaphenyl; Sapoderm; ***Ger.:*** Aknefug simplex; ***S.Afr.:*** Lotocreme†; ***Spain:*** Jabon Antiseptico Asens; ***UK:*** Dermalex; Ster-Zac; ***USA:*** pHisoHex; Septisol.

Multi-ingredient: ***Belg.:*** Hemosedan; Pulvo 47; ***Canad.:*** pHisoHex; ***Fr.:*** Acnestrol; ***Ger.:*** Aknefug-Emulsion N; Mediphon†; Pulvicrus†; Robusanon†; ***Irl.:*** Torbetol; ***Ital.:*** pHisoHex†; Solfofil†; ***Spain:*** Cresophene; Neo Visage; S 13†; Solarcaine; ***Switz.:*** Acerbine; Varecort†.

Hexamidine Isethionate (2251-m)

Hexamidine Isetionate *(rINNM)*. 4,4′-(Hexamethylenedioxy)dibenzamidine bis(2-hydroxyethanesulphonate).
$C_{20}H_{26}N_4O_2,2C_2H_6O_4S$ = 606.7.
CAS — 3811-75-4 (hexamidine); 659-40-5 (hexamidine isethionate).

NOTE. The name Hexamidinum has also been used for primidone.

Pharmacopoeias. In *Fr.*

Hexamidine isethionate has antibacterial and antifungal properties and is available in a variety of preparations for the local treatment of minor infections.

Acanthamoeba keratitis. Hexamidine was suggested[1] as a possible alternative to propamidine for the treatment of *Acanthamoeba* keratitis (p.573).

1. Perrine D, *et al.* Amoebicidal efficiencies of various diamidines against two strains of Acanthamoeba polyphaga. *Antimicrob Agents Chemother* 1995; **39:** 339–42.

Preparations

Proprietary Preparations (details are given in Part 3)
Belg.: Hexomedine; Ophtamedine; ***Fr.:*** Desomedine; Hexomedine; ***Ger.:*** Hexomedin N; Laryngomedin N; ***Neth.:*** Hexomedine; ***Spain:*** Hexomedin; ***Switz.:*** Desomedine; Hexomedine.

Multi-ingredient: ***Austral.:*** Medi Creme; Medi Pulv; ***Belg.:*** Colludol; ***Fr.:*** Amygdospray; Blephaseptyl†; Collucalmyl†; Colludol†; Colluspir†; Cyteal; Dermster†; Hexo-Imotryl; Hexomedine; Oromedine; Oroseptol; Otomide; Posebor†; Pulvo 47; ***Ger.:*** Hexomedin transkutan†; Imazol; Imazol comp; Pulvo; ***Spain:*** Tantum; ***Switz.:*** Blephaseptyl†; Imacort; Imazol.

Hexetidine (2587-b)

Hexetidine *(BAN, rINN).*

Hexetidinum. 5-Amino-1,3-bis(2-ethylhexyl)hexahydro-5-methylpyrimidine.

$C_{21}H_{45}N_3$ = 339.6.

CAS — 141-94-6.

Pharmacopoeias. In *Eur.* (see p.viii).

An oily, colourless or slightly yellow liquid. Very slightly **soluble** in water; very soluble in alcohol, in acetone, and in dichloromethane. Dissolves in dilute mineral acids. **Protect** from light.

Adverse Effects

Allergic contact dermatitis and alterations in taste and smell have occasionally been reported.

Uses and Administration

Hexetidine is a bactericidal and fungicidal antiseptic. It is used for minor infections of mucous membranes, and in particular as a 0.1% mouthwash for local infections and oral hygiene.

Mouth ulceration. A mouthwash containing 0.1% hexetidine was no more effective than placebo in the management of patients with aphthous ulceration (p.1172) and provided no additional benefits to oral hygiene or gingival health.[1] It has been suggested that antiseptic mouthwashes might be helpful, since secondary bacterial infection can delay healing of aphthous ulcers.

1. Chadwick B, *et al.* Hexetidine mouthrinse in the management of minor aphthous ulceration and as an adjunct to oral hygiene. *Br Dent J* 1991; **171:** 83–7.

Preparations

Proprietary Preparations (details are given in Part 3)
Aust.: Gurfix; Hexatin; Hexoral; Isozid-H; Kleenosept; ***Belg.:*** Collu-Hextril†; Hextril; ***Canad.:*** Steri/Sol; ***Fr.:*** Collu-Hextril; Hexifrice†; Hexigel†; Hextril; ***Ger.:*** Doreperol N; Hexoral; Mallebrin Fertiglosung†; Stas Gurgellosung; ***Irl.:*** Oraldene; ***Ital.:*** Oraseptic; ***Neth.:*** Hextril; ***S.Afr.:*** Oraldine; ***Spain:*** Oraldine; Oralspray; ***Switz.:*** Drossadin; Hexigel; Hextril; Vagi-Hex; ***UK:*** Oraldene.

Multi-ingredient: ***Belg.:*** Givalex; ***Fr.:*** Angispray; Givalex; Nifluril; ***Ger.:*** Anginasin N; De-menthasin; Givalex; Hexetidin comp.†; Neo-Angin; ***Spain:*** Abrasone Rectal; Anso; Mentamida.

Hexylresorcinol (782-j)

Esilresorcina; Hexylresorc. 4-Hexylbenzene-1,3-diol.

$C_{12}H_{18}O_2$ = 194.3.

CAS — 136-77-6.

Pharmacopoeias. In *Aust., Br., It., Swiss,* and *US.*

White or almost white needles, crystalline powder, plates, or plate aggregates composed of needle masses with a pungent odour. It acquires a brownish-pink tint on exposure to light and air. M.p. 62° to 68°. Very slightly **soluble** in water; freely soluble in alcohol, in chloroform, in ether, in glycerol, and in fixed oils; practically insoluble in petroleum spirit. **Store** in airtight containers. Protect from light. **Incompatible** with alkalis and oxidising agents.

Hexylresorcinol is a phenolic antiseptic which is used topically for the treatment of minor infections of the skin and mucous membranes. It is also used in vaginal spermicidal preparations.

High concentrations of hexylresorcinol are irritant and corrosive to skin and mucous membranes. Alcoholic solutions are vesicant.

It was formerly used as an anthelmintic.

Preparations

USP 23: Hexylresorcinol Lozenges.

Proprietary Preparations (details are given in Part 3)
Austral.: Nyal Medithroat Anaesthetic Lozenges; ***Canad.:*** Antiseptic Sore Throat Lozenges; Bradosol; Bronchodex Pastilles Antiseptiques; Soothe Aid; Sucrets; Throat Lozenges; ***UK:*** Mac Extra; Strepsils Extra; ***USA:*** ST 37; Sucrets Sore Throat.

Multi-ingredient: ***Canad.:*** Listerine†; ***Fr.:*** Genola; ***Ger.:*** Akne-Medice Kombipackung†; Animbo-N†; Bergauf†; Dermaethyl-H†; Dermaethyl†; Dexamed†; Hexamon N; Mycatox; Mycatox N†; Onymyken S†; Para Muc†; ***Ital.:*** Golamed Due; ***UK:*** Beechams Throat-Plus.

Hydrogen Peroxide (13871-s)

Hydrogenii Peroxidum.

H_2O_2 = 34.01.

CAS — 7722-84-1.

Aqueous solutions of hydrogen peroxide gradually decompose on standing and if allowed to become alkaline. Decomposition is increased by light, agitation, and heat. Incompatibility may also produce decomposition. Hydrogen peroxide solutions are **incompatible** with reducing agents, including organic matter and oxidisable substances, and with some metals, metallic salts, alkalis, iodides, permanganates, and other stronger oxidising agents. Solutions are comparatively stable in the presence of a slight excess of acid. Strong solutions are considered to be more stable than weak solutions.

Solutions of hydrogen peroxide should be **stored** in airtight containers at 15° to 30° (but see Hydrogen Peroxide Solution (30 per cent), below). Solutions should not be stored for long periods. Those not containing a stabiliser should be stored at a temperature not exceeding 15°. Protect from light.

Hydrogen Peroxide Solution (3 per cent)

(5901-f)

Dilute Hydrogen Peroxide Solution; Hydrogen Peroxide Solution (10-volume); Hydrogen Peroxide Topical Solution; Oxydol.

Pharmacopoeias. In *Chin., Eur.* (see p.viii), *Jpn, Pol.,* and *US.*

An aqueous solution containing 2.5 to 3.5% w/w of H_2O_2 corresponding to about 10 times its volume of available oxygen. It may contain a suitable stabilising agent. The USP permits up to 0.05% of a suitable preservative or preservatives.

A clear, colourless liquid; odourless or having an odour resembling ozone. It is acid to litmus.

Hydrogen Peroxide Solution (6 per cent)

(5902-d)

Hydrog. Perox. Soln; Hydrogen Dioxide Solution; Hydrogen Peroxide Solution; Hydrogen Peroxide Solution (20-volume); Liq. Hydrog. Perox.; Liquor Hydrogenii Peroxidi; Solución de Bióxido de Hidrogeno; Soluté Officinal d'Eau Oxygénée; Wasserstoffsuperoxydlösung.

Pharmacopoeias. In *Br.*

A clear, colourless aqueous solution containing 5 to 7% w/v of H_2O_2 corresponding to about 20 times its volume of available oxygen. It may contain a suitable stabilising agent.

NOTE. The BP directs that when Hydrogen Peroxide is prescribed or demanded, Hydrogen Peroxide Solution (6 per cent) be dispensed or supplied.

Hydrogen Peroxide Solution (27 per cent)

(5903-n)

Hydrogenii Peroxidum; Perossido D'Idrogeno Soluzione; Solutio Hydrogenii Peroxydati; Strong Hydrog. Perox. Soln; Strong Hydrogen Peroxide Solution.

Pharmacopoeias. In *Aust.* and *It.*

A clear, colourless aqueous solution containing 26 to 28% w/w of H_2O_2, corresponding to about 100 times its volume of available oxygen. It may contain a suitable stabilising agent.

Hydrogen Peroxide Solution (30 per cent)

(5904-h)

Hydrogen Peroxide Concentrate; Hydrogen Peroxide Solution (100-volume).

Pharmacopoeias. In *Chin., Eur.* (see p.viii), and *Pol. US* specifies 29 to 32%.

A clear, colourless aqueous solution containing 29 to 31% w/w of H_2O_2 corresponding to about 110 times its volume of available oxygen. It may contain a suitable stabilising agent. The USP permits up to 0.05% of a suitable preservative or preservatives. It is acid to litmus. **Store** in partially-filled containers having a small vent in the closure, at a temperature of 8° to 15°. Protect from light.

Adverse Effects and Precautions

Strong solutions of hydrogen peroxide produce irritating 'burns' on the skin and mucous membranes with a white eschar, but the pain disappears in about an hour. Continued use of hydrogen peroxide as a mouthwash may cause reversible hypertrophy of the papillae of the tongue.

It is dangerous to inject or instil hydrogen peroxide into closed body cavities from which the released oxygen has no free exit. Colonic lavage with solutions of hydrogen peroxide has been followed by gas embolism, rupture of the colon, proctitis, ulcerative colitis, and gangrene of the intestine.

Closed body cavities. Liberation of oxygen during the use of hydrogen peroxide in surgical procedures has resulted in oxygen embolism and local emphysema.[1-3] Gas embolism has also been reported after accidental ingestion of hydrogen peroxide solution.[4] Local damage to the colonic and rectal mucosa has followed the use of hydrogen peroxide 3% as an enema[5] and from residual hydrogen peroxide following disinfection of endoscopes.[6]

1. Sleigh JW, Linter SPK. Hazards of hydrogen peroxide. *Br Med J* 1985; **291:** 1706.
2. Saïssy JM, *et al.* Risques de l'irrigation au peroxyde d'hydrogène en chirurgie de guerre. *Ann Fr Anesth Reanim* 1994; **13:** 749–53.
3. Konrad C, *et al.* Pulmonary embolism and hydrogen peroxide. *Can J Anaesth* 1997; **44:** 338–9.
4. Rackoff WR, Merton DF. Gas embolism after ingestion of hydrogen peroxide. *Pediatrics* 1990; **85:** 593–4.
5. Auroux J, *et al.* Rectocolite aiguë iatrogène après lavement à l'eau oxygénée. *Rev Geriatr* 1997; **22:** 21–4.
6. Ryan CK, Potter GD. Disinfectant colitis: rinse as well as you wash. *J Clin Gastroenterol* 1995; **21:** 6–9.

Effects on the eyes. Hydrogen peroxide, in a concentration as low as 30 ppm, caused damage to human corneal epithelial cells *in vitro*; concentrations of 70 to 100 ppm caused cell death within minutes.[1]

1. Tripathi BJ, Tripathi RC. Hydrogen peroxide damage to human corneal epithelial cells in vitro: implications for contact lens disinfection systems. *Arch Ophthalmol* 1989; **107:** 1516–19.

Effects on the mouth. Use of hydrogen peroxide 3% as a mouthwash has been reported to cause mouth ulceration.[1]

1. Rees TD, Orth CF. Oral ulcerations with use of hydrogen peroxide. *J Periodontol* 1986; **57:** 689–92.

Intravascular administration. Intravenous administration of hydrogen peroxide solutions as unconventional therapy for AIDS or cancer has resulted in severe acute haemolysis.[1,2] Haemolysis was also reported following contamination of haemodialysis fluid with hydrogen peroxide.[3]

1. Hirschtick RE, *et al.* Death from an unconventional therapy for AIDS. *Ann Intern Med* 1994; **120:** 694.
2. Jordan KS, *et al.* A 39-year-old man with acute hemolytic crisis secondary to intravenous injection of hydrogen peroxide. *J Emerg Nurs* 1991; **17:** 8–10.
3. Gordon SM, *et al.* Hemolysis associated with hydrogen peroxide at a pediatric dialysis center. *Am J Nephrol* 1990; **10:** 123–7.

Uses and Administration

Hydrogen peroxide is an oxidising agent used as an antiseptic, disinfectant, and deodorant. It has weak antibacterial activity and is also effective against viruses, including HIV. It also has a mild haemostatic action. It owes its antiseptic action to its ready release of oxygen when applied to tissues, but the effect lasts only as long as the oxygen is being released and is of short duration; in addition the antimicrobial effect of the liberated oxygen is reduced in the presence of organic matter. The mechanical effect of effervescence is probably more useful for wound cleansing than the antimicrobial action (but see p.1098).

Hydrogen peroxide solutions are used to cleanse wounds and ulcers in concentrations of up to 6%; creams containing 1% or 1.5% stabilised hydrogen peroxide are also used. Although hydrogen peroxide alone is not considered effective on intact skin, it is used in combination with other antiseptics for the disinfection of hands, skin, and mucous membranes. Injection into closed body cavities is dangerous (see above). Adhering and blood-soaked dressings may be released by the application of a solution of hydrogen peroxide.

A 1.5% solution of hydrogen peroxide has been used as a mouthwash in the treatment of acute stomatitis and as a deodorant gargle. A suitable solution can be prepared by diluting 15 mL of hydrogen peroxide 6% in half a tumblerful of warm water. An oral gel has also been used.

Hydrogen peroxide ear drops have been used for the removal of wax. Such ear drops were prepared by diluting a 6% solution of hydrogen peroxide with 3 parts of water preferably just before use.

Hydrogen peroxide 3% is used for disinfecting soft contact lenses.

Immersion for 30 minutes in hydrogen peroxide 6% has been suggested for disinfecting cleaned equipment.

For bleaching hair and delicate fabrics hydrogen peroxide 6% should be diluted with an equal volume of water.

Strong solutions (27 per cent and 30 per cent) of hydrogen peroxide are used for the preparation of weaker solutions and should not be applied to tissues undiluted.

Hydrogen peroxide and other peroxides have many industrial uses as bleaching and oxidising agents.

Disinfection. CONTACT LENSES. Hydrogen peroxide 3% is particularly useful for disinfecting soft contact lenses (p.1097) and lens storage cases since it is effective against *Acanthamoeba* spp. However, it is irritant to the cornea (see under Adverse Effects, above) and requires inactivating with sodium pyruvate, catalase, or sodium thiosulphate before the lenses are used.

DIALYSIS EQUIPMENT. A disinfectant containing hydrogen peroxide and peracetic acid (Renalin) was not completely effective in killing *Mycobacterium chelonae* in high-flux dialysers. This possibly led to infection of 5 dialysis patients.[1] For a report of haemolysis following inadvertent contamination of dialysis fluid with hydrogen peroxide, see Intravascular Administration, under Adverse Effects and Precautions, above.

1. Lowry PW, *et al.* Mycobacterium chelonae infection among patients receiving high-flux dialysis in a hemodialysis clinic in California. *J Infect Dis* 1990; **161:** 85–90.

ENDOSCOPES. Peroxygen compounds have been suggested for disinfection of endoscopes as an alternative to glutaraldehyde (p.1097). Hydrogen peroxide solution 3% is fully effective against oocysts of *Cryptosporidium* and immersion for 30 minutes at room temperature has been recommended.[1] However, it has been pointed out that hydrogen peroxide damages external surfaces, particularly rubbers and plastics of the insertion tubes, and thus is not ideal for such purposes.[2] Other peroxygen-containing compounds have been assessed for disinfecting endoscopes but their activity against enteroviruses and mycobacteria may be inadequate.[3,4] Residual hydrogen peroxide solution can cause mucosal damage (see above) and endoscopes should be thoroughly rinsed before use.

1. Casemore DP, *et al.* Cleaning and disinfection of equipment for gastrointestinal flexible endoscopy: interim recommendations of a working party of the British Society of Gastroenterology. *Gut* 1989; **30:** 1156.
2. Weller IVD, *et al.* Reply. *Gut* 1989; **30:** 1156–7.
3. Tyler R, *et al.* Virucidal activity of disinfectants: studies with the poliovirus. *J Hosp Infect* 1990; **15:** 339–45.
4. Broadley SJ, *et al.* Antimycobacterial activity of 'Virkon'. *J Hosp Infect* 1993; **23:** 189–97.

Mouth ulceration and infection. The use of antiseptic mouthwashes may be helpful in the management of mouth ulcers (p.1172), although the use of hydrogen peroxide 3% is not advisable. However, application of a 1.5% solution to individual ulcers in combination with a topical corticosteroid may be useful. For oral candidal infections, specific antifungals are recommended (see p.367), and a hydrogen peroxide denture cleaner was not effective in either preventing reinfection or in reducing mucosal inflammation in a study of 49 patients.[1] See also Adverse Effects on the Mouth, above.

1. Walker DM, *et al.* The treatment of denture-induced stomatitis: evaluation of two agents. *Br Dent J* 1981; **151:** 416–19.

Preparations

BP 1998: Hydrogen Peroxide Mouthwash;
USP 23: Hydrogen Peroxide Topical Solution.

Proprietary Preparations (details are given in Part 3)
Aust.: Aosept; Austrosept; Hioxyl; Lensan A; Lensept; Les Yeux 1; Persol; Titmus Losung 1; ***Austral.:*** Aosept; Lensept†; Soft Mate Consept 1; Soft Mate Hydrogen Peroxide†; ***Ger.:*** Omnicare†; ***Irl.:*** Crystacide; Hioxyl; ***Spain:*** Oximen; ***Swed.:*** Microcid; ***UK:*** Crystacide; Hioxyl; Peroxyl; ***USA:*** Oxysept; Peroxyl.

Multi-ingredient: ***Aust.:*** Omnicare; Oxy-Care; Oxysept; Oxysept Comfort; Septicon; Soft Mate Consept 1; ***Austral.:*** Omnicare; Oxysept; ***Canad.:*** UltraCare; ***Fr.:*** Aosept†; Spitaderm; ***Ger.:*** Oxysept; Oxysept Comfort; Oxysept Light†; Peresal; Skinsept F; Skinsept Mucosa; Spitaderm†; ***Ital.:*** Esoform 7 mc; Esoform 70 mc; Peresal; Spitaderm; ***Mon.:*** Akila mains et peau; ***Spain:*** Oxitimol†; ***USA:*** Aosept; Lensept; MiraSept; Renalin Dialyzer Reprocessing Concentrate; Soft Mate Consept; UltraCare.

The symbol † denotes a preparation no longer actively marketed

Hydroxybenzoates (11734-q)

Parabens.

Benzyl Hydroxybenzoate (6635-v)

Benzyl Parahydroxybenzoate; Benzylparaben. Benzyl 4-hydroxybenzoate.

$C_{14}H_{12}O_3$ = 228.2.
CAS — 94-18-8.
Pharmacopoeias. In *Br.* and *Int.*

A white to creamy-white, odourless or almost odourless, crystalline powder. Practically **insoluble** in water; freely soluble in alcohol and in ether. It dissolves in solutions of alkali hydroxides. M.p. about 112°. **Incompatibilities** are described under Sodium Propyl Hydroxybenzoate, below.

Butyl Hydroxybenzoate (6637-q)

Butyl Parahydroxybenzoate; Butylis Parahydroxybenzoas; Butylis Paraoxybenzoas; Butylparaben. Butyl 4-hydroxybenzoate.

$C_{11}H_{14}O_3$ = 194.2.
CAS — 94-26-8.
Pharmacopoeias. In *Eur.* (see p.viii) and *Jpn.* Also in *USNF.*

Small colourless crystals or a white or almost white crystalline powder. Very slightly **soluble** in water and in glycerol; freely soluble in alcohol, in acetone, in ether, in methyl alcohol, and in propylene glycol. M.p. 68° to 72°. **Incompatibilities** are described under Sodium Propyl Hydroxybenzoate, below.

Ethyl Hydroxybenzoate (6648-w)

Aethylum Hydroxybenzoicum; E214; Ethyl Parahydroxybenzoate; Ethylis Parahydroxybenzoas; Ethylis Paraoxybenzoas; Ethylparaben. Ethyl 4-hydroxybenzoate.

$C_9H_{10}O_3$ = 166.2.
CAS — 120-47-8.
Pharmacopoeias. In *Chin.*, *Eur.* (p.viii), *Int.*, *Jpn.*, and *Pol.* Also in *USNF.*

Small colourless crystals or a white or almost white crystalline powder. Slightly or very slightly **soluble** in water; freely soluble in alcohol, in ether, in methyl alcohol, and in propylene glycol; slightly soluble in glycerol. M.p. 115° to 118°. **Incompatibilities** are described under Sodium Propyl Hydroxybenzoate, below.

Methyl Hydroxybenzoate (6651-v)

E218; Metagin; Methyl Parahydroxybenzoate; Methylis Oxybenzoas; Methylis Parahydroxybenzoas; Methylis Paraoxibenzoas; Methylparaben *(USAN)*; Metilparabeno. Methyl 4-hydroxybenzoate.

$C_8H_8O_3$ = 152.1.
CAS — 99-76-3.
Pharmacopoeias. In *Eur.* (see p.viii), *Int.*, *Jpn*, and *Pol.* Also in *USNF.*

Colourless crystals or a white crystalline powder. Ph. Eur. **solubilities** are: very slightly soluble in water; freely soluble in alcohol, and in methyl alcohol. USNF solubilities include: soluble 1 in 400 of water, 1 in 50 of water at 80°, 1 in 3 of alcohol, and 1 in 10 of ether; freely soluble in methyl alcohol. M.p. 125° to 128°. **Incompatibilities** are described under Sodium Propyl Hydroxybenzoate, below.

Propyl Hydroxybenzoate (6665-e)

E216; Propagin; Propyl Parahydroxybenzoate; Propylis Oxybenzoas; Propylis Parahydroxybenzoas; Propylis Paraoxibenzoas; Propylparaben *(USAN)*. Propyl 4-hydroxybenzoate.

$C_{10}H_{12}O_3$ = 180.2.
CAS — 94-13-3.
Pharmacopoeias. In *Eur.* (see p.viii), *Int.*, *Jpn*, and *Pol.* Also in *USNF.*

Small colourless crystals or a white crystalline powder. **Soluble** 1 in 2500 of water, 1 in 400 of boiling water, 1 in 1.5 of alcohol, and 1 in 3 of ether; freely soluble in methyl alcohol. M.p. 95° to 99°. **Incompatibilities** are described under Sodium Propyl Hydroxybenzoate, below.

Sodium Butyl Hydroxybenzoate (6667-y)

Sodium Butyl Parahydroxybenzoate; Sodium Butylparaben.

$C_{11}H_{13}NaO_3$ = 216.2.
CAS — 36457-20-2.
Pharmacopoeias. In *Br.*

A white, odourless or almost odourless, hygroscopic powder. Freely **soluble** in water and in alcohol. A 0.1% solution in water has a pH of 9.5 to 10.5. **Incompatibilities** are described under Sodium Propyl Hydroxybenzoate, below.

Sodium Methyl Hydroxybenzoate (6674-l)

E219; Methylis Parahydroxybenzoas Natricum; Methylparaben Sodium *(USAN)*; Sodium Methyl Parahydroxybenzoate; Sodium Methylparaben; Soluble Methyl Hydroxybenzoate.

$C_8H_7NaO_3$ = 174.1.
CAS — 5026-62-0.
Pharmacopoeias. In *Eur.* (see p.viii). Also in *USNF.*

A white, hygroscopic, crystalline powder. Freely **soluble** in water; sparingly soluble in alcohol; practically insoluble in dichloromethane and in fixed oils. A 0.1% solution has a pH of 9.5 to 10.5. **Store** in airtight containers. **Incompatibilities** are described under Sodium Propyl Hydroxybenzoate, below.

Sodium Propyl Hydroxybenzoate (6676-j)

E217; Propylis Parahydroxybenzoas Natricum; Propylparaben Sodium *(USAN)*; Sodium Propyl Parahydroxybenzoate; Sodium Propylparaben; Soluble Propyl Hydroxybenzoate.

$C_{10}H_{11}NaO_3$ = 202.2.
CAS — 35285-69-9.
Pharmacopoeias. In *Eur.* (see p.viii). Also in *USNF.*

A white, hygroscopic, crystalline powder. Freely **soluble** in water; sparingly soluble in alcohol; practically insoluble in fixed oils and in dichloromethane. A 0.1% solution in water has a pH of 9.5 to 10.5. **Store** in airtight containers.

Incompatibilities. The activity of hydroxybenzoates can be adversely affected by the presence of other excipients or active ingredients. There may be adsorption onto substances like magnesium trisilicate, aluminium magnesium silicate, talc, polysorbate 80,[1,2] carmellose sodium,[3] or plastics.[4] Nonionic surfactants can reduce hydroxybenzoate activity,[5] as may essential oils.[6] Other incompatibilities that have been reported include atropine,[7] iron,[4] sorbitol,[8] weak alkalis,[4] and strong acids.[4] Syrup preserved with hydroxybenzoates is incompatible with a range of compounds.[9,10] Methyl hydroxybenzoate 0.1% was reported[11] to be a poor preservative in insulin preparations, especially soluble insulin preparations. Increasing heat or pH can reduce stability and activity;[12] freeze-drying may also lead to a loss of activity.[13]

1. Yousef RT, *et al.* Effect of some pharmaceutical materials on the bactericidal activities of preservatives. *Can J Pharm Sci* 1973; **8:** 54–6.
2. Allwood MC. The adsorption of esters of p-hydroxybenzoic acid by magnesium trisilicate. *Int J Pharmaceutics* 1982; **11:** 101–7.
3. Fawcett JP, *et al.* Binding of parabens to sodium carboxymethylcellulose in oral liquid formulations. *Aust J Hosp Pharm* 1996; **26:** 552–4.
4. Rieger MM. Methylparaben. In: Wade A, Weller PJ, eds. *Handbook of pharmaceutical excipients.* 2nd ed. Washington and London: American Pharmaceutical Association and The Pharmaceutical Press, 1994: 310–13.
5. Yamaguchi M, *et al.* Antimicrobial activity of butylparaben in relation to its solubilization behavior by nonionic surfactants. *J Soc Cosmet Chem* 1982; **33:** 297–307.
6. Chemburkar PB, Joslin RS. Effect of flavoring oils on preservative concentrations in oral liquid dosage forms. *J Pharm Sci* 1975; **64:** 414–17.
7. Deeks T. Oral atropine sulphate mixtures. *Pharm J* 1983; **230:** 481.
8. Runesson B, Gustavii K. Stability of parabens in the presence of polyols. *Acta Pharm Suec* 1986; **23:** 151–62.
9. *PSGB Lab Report P/79/2* 1979.
10. *PSGB Lab Report P/80/1* 1980.
11. Allwood MC. The effectiveness of preservatives in insulin injections. *Pharm J* 1982; **229:** 340.
12. Sunderland VB, Watts DW. Kinetics of the degradation of methyl, ethyl and n-propyl 4-hydroxybenzoate esters in aqueous solution. *Int J Pharmaceutics* 1984; **19:** 1–15.
13. Flora KP, *et al.* The loss of paraben preservatives during freeze drying. *J Pharm Pharmacol* 1980; **32:** 577–80.

Adverse Effects and Precautions

Hypersensitivity reactions occur with the hydroxybenzoates. Generally these are of the delayed type, appearing as contact dermatitis. Immediate reactions with urticaria and bronchospasm have occurred rarely.

Hypersensitivity. Immediate hypersensitivity reactions have been reported following the injection of preparations containing hydroxybenzoates.[1,2] Delayed contact dermatitis occurs more frequently, usually after topical application but has also occurred after oral administration of an ester or of *p*-hydroxybenzoic acid.[3-5] The North American Contact Dermatitis Group[6] provided an incidence of 3%, while another review[7] of a large number of patients gave an incidence of 2.2%. However, subjects with healthy skin exposed to hydroxybenzoates, for example in cosmetics, are considered to have a much lower incidence of reactions.[8] Unusually, patients who have reacted to a hydroxybenzoate with a contact dermatitis appear to be able to apply that preservative to another unaffected site and yet not suffer a reaction; this has been termed the paraben paradox.[9]

Hypersensitivity reactions have occurred in patients given local anaesthetics containing hydroxybenzoates[1,10] and cross-sensitivity between the two groups of drugs has been proposed.[1]

1. Aldrete JA, Johnson DA. Allergy to local anaesthetics. *JAMA* 1969; **207:** 356–7.
2. Nagel JE, *et al.* Paraben allergy. *JAMA* 1977; **237:** 1594–5.
3. Michäelsson G, Juhlin L. Urticaria induced by preservatives and dye additives in food and drugs. *Br J Dermatol* 1973; **88:** 525–32.
4. Warin RP, Smith RJ. Challenge test battery in chronic urticaria. *Br J Dermatol* 1976; **94:** 401–6.
5. Kaminer Y, *et al.* Delayed hypersensitivity reaction to orally administered methylparaben. *Clin Pharm* 1982; **1:** 469–70.
6. North American Contact Dermatitis Group. Epidemiology of contact dermatitis in North America 1972. *Arch Dermatol* 1973; **108:** 537–40.
7. Moore J. Final report on the safety assessment of methylparaben, ethylparaben, propylparaben, and butylparaben. *J Am Coll Toxicol* 1984; **3:** 147–209.
8. Fisher AA. Cosmetic dermatitis. Part II; reactions to some commonly used preservatives. *Cutis* 1980; **26:** 136–7, 141–2, 147–8.
9. Fisher AA. Cortaid cream dermatitis and the "paraben paradox". *J Am Acad Dermatol* 1982; **6:** 116–7.
10. Lederman DA, *et al.* An unusual skin reaction following local anesthetic injection: review of the literature and report of four cases. *Oral Surg* 1980; **49:** 28–33.

Neonates. An *in-vitro* study on serum from neonates with hyperbilirubinaemia indicated that methyl hydroxybenzoate at a concentration of 200 µg per mL of serum increased the concentration of free unconjugated bilirubin and interfered with the binding of bilirubin to serum proteins. Methyl hydroxybenzoate was present in an injection of gentamicin sulphate at a concentration of 1.3 to 1.8 mg per mL. Neither gentamicin nor propyl hydroxybenzoate had a significant effect on bilirubin.[1]

1. Loria CJ, *et al.* Effect of antibiotic formulations in serum protein: bilirubin interaction of newborn infants. *J Pediatr* 1976; **89:** 479–82.

Pharmacokinetics

Neonates. Methyl hydroxybenzoate present in an injectable preparation of gentamicin was excreted in the urine of preterm infants following intramuscular injection to a variable extent and mainly in the conjugated form.[1] *p*-Hydroxybenzoic acid was detected as a metabolite. The injection contained 3.6 mg of methyl hydroxybenzoate, 400 µg of propyl hydroxybenzoate, and 80 mg of gentamicin. Propyl hydroxybenzoate was also detected in the urine samples.

1. Hindmarsh KW, *et al.* Urinary excretion of methylparaben and its metabolites in preterm infants. *J Pharm Sci* 1983; **72:** 1039–41.

Uses

The hydroxybenzoate preservatives (parabens) are alkyl esters of *p*-hydroxybenzoic acid with antibacterial and antifungal properties. They are active over a broad pH range (4 to 8), though are generally more active in acidic solutions. Activity increases with increasing alkyl chain length but aqueous solubility decreases, although this may be overcome by employing the more soluble sodium salts as long as the pH of the preparation is not increased. Activity may also be increased by combining two hydroxybenzoates with short alkyl chains. Another way of increasing activity is to use a hydroxybenzoate with propylene glycol.

Hydroxybenzoates are used as preservatives in pharmaceutical preparations in concentrations of up to 0.25%. Methyl hydroxybenzoate and propyl hydroxybenzoate are used together in some preparations. There have been reports of the hydroxybenzoates not being satisfactory preservatives for ophthalmic preparations because of their relative lack of efficacy against some Gram-negative bacteria, particularly *Pseudomonas aeruginosa*. The hydroxybenzoate preservatives are widely used in cosmetics and are also used for food preservation.

Hydroxybenzoates are also used for treating skin infections.

Preparations

Proprietary Preparations (details are given in Part 3)
UK: Dorant†.

Multi-ingredient: *Austral.:* Mycoderm; Steri-Soft†; *Fr.:* Nisapulvol; Nisaseptol; Nisasol; *Ger.:* Iversal-A cum anaesthetico†; Trachitol; *Spain:* Doctodermis.

Imidurea (18353-b)

N,N″-Methylenebis{*N*′-[3-(hydroxymethyl)-2,5-dioxo-4-imidazolidinyl]urea}.

$C_{11}H_{16}N_8O_8$ = 388.3.

CAS — 39236-46-9.

Pharmacopoeias. In *USNF.*

A white, odourless, tasteless powder. **Soluble** in water and glycerol; sparingly soluble in propylene glycol; practically insoluble in most organic solvents. **Store** in airtight containers.

Imidurea is used as an antimicrobial preservative in topical pharmaceutical and cosmetic preparations.

Iodoform (4577-a)

Tri-iodomethane.

CHI_3 = 393.7.

CAS — 75-47-8.

Pharmacopoeias. In *Aust., It.,* and *Jpn.*

Iodoform slowly releases iodine (p.1493) when applied to the tissues and has a mild antiseptic action. Bismuth subnitrate and iodoform paste has been applied to wounds and abscesses. Sterile gauze impregnated with the paste has also been used for packing cavities after oral and otorhinological surgery.

Adverse effects on the nervous system. Encephalopathy has been associated with the use of bismuth iodoform paraffin paste (BIPP) for the packing of wound cavities after surgery to the head and neck,[1] although there is some debate as to whether the bismuth or the iodoform component is responsible.[1,2] However, encephalopathy has been reported after application of iodoform gauze without bismuth.[3,4]

1. Wilson APR. The dangers of BIPP. *Lancet* 1994; **344:** 1313–14.
2. Farrell RWR. Dangers of bismuth iodoform paraffin paste. *Lancet* 1994; **344:** 1637–8.
3. Roy P-M, *et al.* Dangers of bismuth iodoform paraffin paste. *Lancet* 1994; **344:** 1708.
4. Yamasaki K, *et al.* Delirium and a subclavian abscess. *Lancet* 1997; **350:** 1294.

Preparations

BPC 1954: Bismuth Subnitrate and Iodoform Paste *(BIPP)*; Compound Iodoform Paint *(Whitehead's Varnish).*

Proprietary Preparations (details are given in Part 3)
Ger.: Jodoform.

Multi-ingredient: *Spain:* Alvogil; *Switz.:* Alvogyl; Pate Iodoforme du Prof Dr Walkhoff; *UK:* OxBipp.

Isopropyl Alcohol (555-m)

Alcohol Isopropylicus; Dimethyl Carbinol; Isopropanol; 2-Propanol; Secondary Propyl Alcohol. Propan-2-ol.

$(CH_3)_2CHOH$ = 60.10.

CAS — 67-63-0.

Pharmacopoeias. In *Eur.* (see p.viii), *Int., Jpn, Pol.,* and *US.*

A clear, colourless, mobile, volatile, flammable liquid with a characteristic spirituous odour. **Miscible** with water, with alcohol, with chloroform, and with ether. **Store** in a cool place in airtight containers. Protect from light.

Adverse Effects, Treatment, and Precautions

Isopropyl alcohol is considered to be more toxic than ethyl alcohol (p.1099), and the symptoms of intoxication appear to be similar, except that isopropyl alcohol has no initial euphoric action and gastritis, haemorrhage, pain, nausea, and vomiting are more prominent. The lethal dose by mouth is reported to be about 250 mL; however, toxic symptoms may be produced by as little as 20 mL. Ketoacidosis and ketonuria commonly occur due to the presence of the major metabolite, acetone, in the circulation. Inhalation of isopropyl alcohol vapour has been reported to produce coma.

Application of isopropyl alcohol to the skin may cause dryness and irritation; suitable precautions should be taken to prevent absorption through the skin.

Treatment of adverse effects is as for Alcohol, p.1099.

General references.

1. 2-Propanol. *Environmental Health Criteria 103.* Geneva: WHO, 1990.

Neonates. Reports of chemical skin burns caused by the topical application of isopropyl alcohol in premature infants.[1,2]

1. Schick JB, Milstein JM. Burn hazard of isopropyl alcohol in the neonate. *Pediatrics* 1981; **68:** 587–8.
2. Weintraub Z, Iancu TC. Isopropyl alcohol burns. *Pediatrics* 1982; **69:** 506.

Rectal absorption. A report of intoxication and raised serum-creatinine concentrations due to absorption of isopropyl alcohol following its use as a rectal douche.[1]

1. Barnett JM, *et al.* Intoxication after an isopropyl alcohol enema. *Ann Intern Med* 1990; **113:** 638–9.

Pharmacokinetics

Isopropyl alcohol is readily absorbed from the gastro-intestinal tract but there appears to be little absorption through intact skin. The vapour may be absorbed through the lungs. Isopropyl alcohol is metabolised more slowly than ethyl alcohol and about 15% of an ingested dose is metabolised to acetone.

For a report of rectal absorption of isopropyl alcohol, see above.

Uses and Administration

Isopropyl alcohol is an antiseptic with bactericidal properties similar to those of alcohol (p.1100). It is used for pre-operative skin cleansing in concentrations of about 60 to 70%, and is an ingredient of preparations used for disinfection of hands and surfaces. Its marked degreasing properties may limit its usefulness in preparations used repeatedly. It is also used as a solvent, especially in cosmetics and perfumes, and as a vehicle for other disinfectant compounds. Propyl alcohol (p.1124) is also used as an antiseptic.

Disinfection. VIRUSES. WHO has published guidelines on sterilisation and disinfection methods effective against HIV[1] which state that alcohols are not considered suitable for dealing with contaminated surfaces because of their limited penetration of organic residues and rapid evaporation but that for disinfection of living tissues, isopropyl alcohol 70% is effective.

1. WHO. Guidelines on sterilization and disinfection methods effective against human immunodeficiency virus (HIV). *WHO AIDS Series 2* 1989.

Preparations

USP 23: Azeotropic Isopropyl Alcohol; Isopropyl Rubbing Alcohol.

Proprietary Preparations (details are given in Part 3)
Canad.: Alcojel; Alko Isol; Duonalc; Friction Rub; ***UK:*** Alcowipe; Medi-Swab; Sterets.

Multi-ingredient: numerous preparations are listed in Part 3.

Isothiazolinones (9492-q)

Methylchloroisothiazolinone (10323-m)

5-Chloro-2-methyl-3(2*H*)-isothiazolone; 5-Chloro-2-methyl-4-isothiazolin-3-one.

CAS — 26172-55-4.

Methylisothiazolinone (5495-n)

2-Methyl-3(2*H*)-isothiazolone; 2-Methyl-4-isothiazolin-3-one.

CAS — 2682-20-4.

A mixture of isothiazolinones consisting of methylchloroisothiazolinone and methylisothiazolinone in a ratio of approximately 3:1 is used as a preservative in industry and in cosmetic products. The mixture is often referred to as Kathon CG, one of its proprietary names.

Isothiazolinones may cause contact dermatitis and local irritation.

Hypersensitivity. There have been several reports of allergic contact dermatitis arising from the use of isothiazolinones in cosmetics.[1-4] One review lists incidences ranging from 0.4 to 8.4%[4] and considers that the risks are reduced when these preservatives are used in 'rinse-off' preparations such as shampoos at low concentrations. Maximum concentrations permitted within the EEC have been progressively reduced from 50 to 30 and then 15 ppm.[2,5] Irritant reactions can also occur,[1,3] and occupational asthma has been reported.[6]

1. Björkner B, *et al.* Contact allergy to the preservative Kathon CG. *Contact Dermatitis* 1986; **14:** 85–90.
2. De Groot AC, Bos JD. Preservatives in the European standard series for epicutaneous testing. *Br J Dermatol* 1987; **116:** 289–92.
3. Fransway AF. Sensitivity to Kathon CG: findings in 365 consecutive patients. *Contact Dermatitis* 1988; **19:** 342–7.
4. De Groot AC, Herxheimer A. Isothiazolinone preservative: cause of a continuing epidemic of cosmetic dermatitis. *Lancet* 1989; **i:** 314–16.
5. Anonymous. *Lancet* 1989; **i:** 910. (Comment on Fransway AF. Isothiazolinone sensitivity. *ibid.*)
6. Bourke SJ, *et al.* Occupational asthma in an isothiazolinone manufacturing plant. *Thorax* 1997; **52:** 746–8.

Preparations

Proprietary Preparations (details are given in Part 3)

Multi-ingredient: *Switz.:* Saltrates.

Magenta (2254-g)

Aniline Red; Basic Fuchsin; Basic Magenta; CI Basic Violet 14; Colour Index No. 42510; Fuchsine.

CAS — 569-61-9 (pararosaniline hydrochloride); 632-99-5 (rosaniline hydrochloride).

Pharmacopoeias. In *US.*

A mixture of the hydrochlorides of pararosaniline {4-[(4-aminophenyl)(4-iminocyclohexa-2,5-dien-1-ylidene)-methyl]aniline} and rosaniline {4-[(4-aminophenyl)(4-

iminocyclohexa-2,5-dien-1-ylidene)methyl]-2-methylaniline}. The dried material contains not less than 88% of rosaniline hydrochloride ($C_{20}H_{20}ClN_3$ = 337.8).

Glistening greenish crystals, or a dark green powder with a bronze-like lustre, having not more than a faint odour. **Soluble** in water, alcohol, and amyl alcohol; insoluble in ether.

Magenta is a triphenylmethane antiseptic dye effective against Gram-positive bacteria and some fungi. Magenta paint (Castellani's paint) was formerly used in the treatment of superficial dermatophytoses (see Skin Infections, p.371). Decolorised magenta solution (Schiff reagent) is used as a test for the presence of aldehydes.

Concerns about possible carcinogenicity have restricted the use of magenta.

The handling of magenta was not thought to induce carcinogenesis but its actual manufacture may produce tumours.[1] Magenta was also considered to be unsafe for use in food.[2]

1. Glashan RW. Changes in compensation for occupationally induced bladder cancer. *Br Med J* 1984; **288:** 1181–2.
2. FAO/WHO. Specifications for the identity and purity of food additives and their toxicological evaluation: food colours and some antimicrobials and antoxidants: eighth report of the joint FAO/WHO expert committee on food additives. *WHO Tech Rep Ser 309* 1965.

Preparations

BPC 1973: Magenta Paint *(Castellani's Paint; Fuschine Paint)*; ***USP 23:*** Carbol-Fuchsin Topical Solution.

Magnesium Peroxide (5906-b)

Magnesium Perhydrolum.

CAS — 1335-26-8; 14452-57-4.

Pharmacopoeias. In *Aust., Fr., Ger., Neth.,* and *Swiss,* most of which specify about 25% of MgO_2 (6.5% available oxygen).

Magnesium peroxide is used as an antiseptic. It is also an ingredient of preparations for gastro-intestinal disorders.

Preparations

Proprietary Preparations (details are given in Part 3)
Aust.: Ozovit; ***Ger.:*** Ozovit.

Multi-ingredient: ***Fr.:*** Ektogan; ***Ger.:*** Bismulcid†; Dystomin E†; Fidozon†; ***Ital.:*** Carbonesia; Ektogan; ***Switz.:*** Geli-Stop†; Magenpulver Hafter.

Malachite Green (2255-q)

Aniline Green; China Green; CI Basic Green 4; Colour Index No. 42000; Diamond Green B; Viride Malachitum. [4-(4-Dimethylaminobenzhydrylidene)cyclohexa-2,5-dienylidene]dimethylammonium chloride.

CAS — 569-64-2.

Malachite green is a triphenylmethane antiseptic dye with actions similar to those of brilliant green (p.1104). It has been used for skin disinfection.

Mecetronium Ethylsulphate (3820-v)

Mecetronium Ethylsulphate *(BAN).*

Mecetronium Etilsulfate *(rINN)*; Mecetronium Ethylsulfate *(USAN)*. Ethylhexadecyldimethylammonium ethyl sulphate.

$C_{22}H_{49}NO_4S$ = 423.7.

CAS — 3006-10-8.

Mecetronium ethylsulphate is a quaternary ammonium antiseptic with actions and uses similar to those of other cationic surfactants (see Cetrimide, p.1105). It is active against bacteria, including mycobacteria; fungi; and viruses, including hepatitis B virus. It is used in alcoholic solution for disinfection of the skin and hard surfaces.

Preparations

Proprietary Preparations (details are given in Part 3)

Multi-ingredient: ***Fr.:*** Sterillium; ***Ger.:*** Bacillol; D1 Handedesinfektion†; Sterillium.

Mercurobutol (13488-h)

Mercurobutol *(rINN).*

L-542. 4-*tert*-Butyl-2-chloro-mercuriphenol.

$C_{10}H_{13}ClHgO$ = 385.3.

CAS — 498-73-7.

Pharmacopoeias. In *Fr.*

Mercurobutol is an organic mercurial antiseptic with antifungal properties. It has been used in the treatment of infections of the skin and mucous membranes.

Preparations

Proprietary Preparations (details are given in Part 3)
Fr.: Mercryl Lauryle; ***Spain:*** Mercryl Lauryle.

Mercurochrome (2256-p)

Merbromin *(rINN)*; Disodium 2,7-dibromo-4-hydroxymercurifluorescein; Mercurescéine Sodique; Mercurodibromofluorescein. The disodium salt of [2,7-dibromo-9-(2-carboxyphenyl)-6-hydroxy-3-oxo-3*H*-xanthen-5-yl]hydroxymercury.

$C_{20}H_8Br_2HgNa_2O_6$ = 750.7.

CAS — 129-16-8.

NOTE. The use of the name Mercurochrome is limited; in some countries it is a trade-mark.

Pharmacopoeias. In *Fr., It.,* and *Jpn.*

Incompatible with acids, most alkaloidal salts, many local anaesthetics, metals, and sulphides. Activity may be reduced in the presence of organic material.

Adverse Effects, Treatment, and Precautions

As for Mercury, p.1601.

Reports of mercurochrome toxicity have included contact dermatitis[1] and epidermal cell toxicity.[2] A fatality has occurred following transcutaneous absorption of mercurochrome during treatment of infected omphalocele (umbilical hernia)[3,4] and death due to shock, with aplastic anaemia, has followed application to surgical wounds and decubitus areas.[5] Extensive absorption following ingestion has also been reported.[6]

1. Camarasa G. Contact dermatitis from mercurochrome. *Contact Dermatitis* 1976; **2:** 120.
2. Anonymous. Topical antiseptics and antibiotics. *Med Lett Drugs Ther* 1977; **19:** 83–4.
3. Yeh T-F, *et al.* Mercury poisoning from mercurochrome therapy of infected omphalocele. *Lancet* 1978; **i:** 210.
4. Yeh TF, *et al.* Mercury poisoning from mercurochrome therapy of an infected omphalocele. *Clin Toxicol* 1978; **13:** 463–7.
5. Slee PHTJ, *et al.* A case of Merbromin (mercurochrome) intoxication possibly resulting in aplastic anemia. *Acta Med Scand* 1979; **205:** 463–6.
6. Magarey JA. Absorption of mercurochrome. *Lancet* 1993; **342:** 1424.

Uses and Administration

Mercurochrome is a mercurial antiseptic that has been used for disinfection of skin and wounds.

Preparations

Proprietary Preparations (details are given in Part 3)
Belg.: Medichrom; Stellachrome†; ***Fr.:*** Pharmadose mercurescéine; Soluchrom; ***Ger.:*** Mercuchrom; ***Ital.:*** Cromocur†; Pronto Red†; ***Spain:*** Cinfacromin; Cromer Orto; Logacron; Mercromina; Mercroverk†; Mercurin; Mercurio Rojo†; Mercurobromo; Mercutina Brota; Pintacrom; Super Cromer Orto.

Multi-ingredient: ***Belg.:*** Angichrome†; ***S.Afr.:*** Achromide; Daromide†; Ung Vernleigh; ***Spain:*** Argentocromo; Mercrotona.

Methylated Spirits (557-v)

CAS — 8013-52-3 (ethyl alcohol-methyl alcohol mixture; industrial methylated spirit).

Three classes of methylated spirits are listed under the UK Methylated Spirits Regulations, 1987 (SI 1987: No. 2009): industrial methylated spirits, mineralised methylated spirits, and denatured ethanol (denatured alcohol).

Industrial Methylated Spirits is defined as 95 parts by volume of spirits mixed with wood naphtha 5 parts by volume. (See under Methyl Alcohol, p.1379, for a description of wood naphtha). Mineralised methylated spirits is spirits mixed with wood naphtha 9.5 parts by volume and crude pyridine 0.5 parts by volume, and to every 2000 litres of this mixture is added 7.5 litres of mineral naphtha (petroleum oil) and 3 g of synthetic organic dyestuff (methyl violet). This is the only variety that may be sold in Great Britain for general use. Denatured ethanol is 999 parts by volume of spirits (of a strength not less than 85%) mixed with 1 part by volume of tertiary butyl alcohol, and to this mixture is added Bitrex (denatonium benzoate) 10 mg per litre.

Industrial Methylated Spirit (BP 1998) (Industrial Methylated Spirits; IMS) is a mixture of 19 volumes of ethyl alcohol of an appropriate strength with 1 volume of approved wood naphtha. Two strengths are available containing 99% and 95% v/v alcohol (also known as 74 OP and 66 OP respectively). It is a colourless, clear, mobile, volatile liquid with an odour which is spirituous and of wood naphtha.

Industrial Methylated Spirit (Ketone-free) (BP 1998) is a mixture of the same strength as Industrial Methylated Spirit (BP 1998), but is substantially free from ketones, containing not more than the equivalent of 500 ppm of acetone.

As Industrial Methylated Spirit may contain small amounts of acetone it should not be used for the preparation of iodine solutions, since an irritating compound is formed by reaction between iodine and acetone; for such preparations Industrial Methylated Spirit (Ketone-free) should be used.

Adverse Effects

As for Alcohol, p.1099, and Methyl Alcohol, p.1379. Adverse effects are due chiefly to consumption of methylated spirits rather than its topical use as a disinfectant.

Uses and Administration

Industrial methylated spirit, in a concentration of about 70%, is the usual form in which alcohol (p.1099) is used for disinfection. It is applied externally for its astringent action, but mucous membranes and excoriated skin surfaces must be protected. It may be used for skin preparation before injection.

Methylated spirits may be used in the form of Surgical Spirit, a mixture of methyl salicylate (0.5% v/v), diethyl phthalate (2% v/v), and castor oil (2.5% v/v) in industrial methylated spirit.

Preparations

BP 1998: Surgical Spirit.

Methylbenzethonium Chloride (2258-w)

Methylbenzethonium Chloride *(BAN, rINN).*

Benzyldimethyl-2-{2-[4-(1,1,3,3-tetramethylbutyl)-*o*-tolyloxy]ethoxy}ethylammonium chloride monohydrate.

$C_{28}H_{44}ClNO_2,H_2O$ = 480.1.

CAS — 25155-18-4 (anhydrous methylbenzethonium chloride); 1320-44-1 (methylbenzethonium chloride monohydrate).

Pharmacopoeias. In *US.*

White hygroscopic crystals with a mild odour. **Soluble** 1 in 0.8 of water, 1 in 0.9 of alcohol, 1 in 0.7 of ether, and 1 in more than 10 000 of chloroform. Solutions are neutral or slightly alkaline to litmus. **Store** in airtight containers.

Methylbenzethonium chloride is a quaternary ammonium disinfectant and antiseptic with actions and uses similar to those of other cationic surfactants (see Cetrimide, p.1105). It is used topically for minor infections or irritation of the skin.

Leishmaniasis. Topical treatment of cutaneous leishmaniasis (p.575) with methylbenzethonium chloride 5 or 12% and paromomycin sulphate is listed among treatments producing a promising response.

Preparations

USP 23: Methylbenzethonium Chloride Lotion; Methylbenzethonium Chloride Ointment; Methylbenzethonium Chloride Topical Powder.

Proprietary Preparations (details are given in Part 3)
Ital.: Benzibel; ***USA:*** Diaparene Cradol†; Diaparene†; Puri-Clens.

Multi-ingredient: ***Ger.:*** Magocrus†; ***Ital.:*** Traumicid; ***USA:*** Acnotex; Dermasept Antifungal; Diaparene Peri-Anal†; Drytex; Finac; Medadyne†; Orasept.

Miripirium Chloride (2260-b)

Miripirium Chloride *(rINN).*

Myristyl-gamma-picolinium Chloride. 4-Methyl-1-tetradecylpyridinium chloride.

$C_{20}H_{36}ClN$ = 326.0.

CAS — 7631-49-4 (miripirium); 2748-88-1 (miripirium chloride).

Miripirium chloride is used as an antimicrobial preservative in some pharmaceutical products.

Hypersensitivity. Two patients displayed delayed hypersensitivity reactions to retrobulbar injection of methylprednisolone acetate suspension (Depo-Medrol).[1] Intradermal testing confirmed sensitivity to methylprednisolone and to miripirium chloride, included as a preservative in the formulation.

1. Mathias CGT, Robertson DB. Delayed hypersensitivity to a corticosteroid suspension containing methylprednisolone. *Arch Dermatol* 1985; **121:** 258–61.

Miristalkonium Chloride (2259-e)

Miristalkonium Chloride *(BAN, rINN).*

Myristylbenzalkonium Chloride. Benzyldimethyltetradecylammonium chloride.

$C_{23}H_{42}ClN$ = 368.0.

CAS — 139-08-2.

Miristalkonium chloride is a quaternary ammonium antiseptic with actions and uses similar to those of other cationic surfactants (see Cetrimide, p.1105). It is used in creams and lotions for disinfection of the skin and has been an ingredient of sprays used for treatment of minor infections of the mouth and throat. It is also used as a vaginal spermicide.

Preparations

Proprietary Preparations (details are given in Part 3)
Fr.: Alpagelle.

Multi-ingredient: *Fr.:* Laccoderme Dalibour†; Sterlane; *Ital.:* Eburdent F.

Monalazone Disodium (12972-g)

Monalazone Disodium *(rINN)*.

Disodium 4-(*N*-chlorosulphamoyl)benzoate.

$C_7H_4ClNNa_2O_4S$ = 279.6.

CAS — 61477-95-0.

Monalazone disodium is an antiseptic closely related structurally to halazone (p.1115) and is used as a vaginal disinfectant and spermicide.

Preparations

Proprietary Preparations (details are given in Part 3)
Belg.: Speton†; *Ger.:* Malun N†; *Spain:* Sperlisin†.

Multi-ingredient: *Ger.:* Malun†.

Monothioglycerol (6652-g)

α-Monothioglycerol; Thioglycerol. 3-Mercaptopropane-1,2-diol.

$C_3H_8O_2S$ = 108.2.

CAS — 96-27-5.

Pharmacopoeias. In USNF.

A colourless or pale yellow, viscous, hygroscopic liquid with a slight odour of sulphide. Freely **soluble** in water; miscible with alcohol; practically insoluble in ether. A 10% solution in water has a pH of 3.5 to 7. **Store** in airtight containers.

Monothioglycerol is used as an antoxidant preservative in pharmaceutical preparations. It has some antimicrobial activity.

Nitromersol (2261-v)

5-Methyl-2-nitro-7-oxa-8-mercurabicyclo[4.2.0]octa-1,3,5-triene.

$C_7H_5HgNO_3$ = 351.7.

CAS — 133-58-4.

Pharmacopoeias. In US.

A brownish-yellow to yellow odourless powder or granules. Very slightly **soluble** in water, in alcohol, in acetone, in chloroform, and in ether; soluble in solutions of alkalis and of ammonia with the formation of salts. **Store** in airtight containers. Protect from light. **Incompatible** with metals and sulphides. Its antimicrobial activity may be diminished in the presence of organic material.

Adverse Effects, Treatment, and Precautions

As for Mercury, p.1601.

Nitromersol occasionally gives rise to hypersensitivity reactions.

Uses and Administration

Nitromersol is a mercurial antiseptic effective against some bacteria. It is not effective against spores or acid-fast bacteria. It has been used for superficial skin infections and for disinfection of the skin prior to surgical treatment as a 0.5% alcohol-acetone-aqueous solution.

Preparations

USP 23: Nitromersol Topical Solution.

Proprietary Preparations (details are given in Part 3)
Austral.: Metaphen†.

Multi-ingredient: *Austral.:* Butesin Picrate; Cold Sore Balm†; Dental Ointment†.

Nordihydroguaiaretic Acid (6653-q)

NDGA. 4,4′-(2,3-Dimethyltetramethylene)bis(benzene-1,2-diol).

$C_{18}H_{22}O_4$ = 302.4.

CAS — 500-38-9.

Nordihydroguaiaretic acid has been used as an antoxidant preservative. Allergic contact dermatitis has been reported.

Nordihydroguaiaretic acid has been reported to have antimicrobial as well as antoxidant activity.[1]

1. Shih AL, Harris ND. Antimicrobial activity of selected antioxidants. *Cosmet Toilet* 1980; **95:** 75–9.

Noxythiolin (2262-g)

Noxythiolin *(BAN)*.

Noxytiolin *(rINN)*. 1-Hydroxymethyl-3-methyl-2-thiourea.

$C_3H_8N_2OS$ = 120.2.

CAS — 15599-39-0.

Stability. Aqueous solutions of noxythiolin 1% and 2.5% were unstable and the manufacturer recommended that they should be stored for no longer than 7 days in glass containers between 2° and 10°. It was found that these solutions could be stored safely in polypropylene containers under the same conditions. There was no adsorption of noxythiolin or of its degradation products (N-methylthiourea and formaldehyde).[1]

1. McCafferty DF, *et al.* Stability of noxythiolin solutions stored in plastic and glass containers. *J Clin Hosp Pharm* 1984; **9:** 241–7.

Adverse Effects

When given initially by irrigation for the treatment of the purulent infected bladder there may be an intense reaction with a burning sensation and the passage of large fibrin clumps. Administration of a local anaesthetic such as amethocaine hydrochloride with noxythiolin, may control the pain.

A pervasive sweet breath odour characteristic of decaying vegetables has been noted in patients treated with peritoneal dialysis fluid containing noxythiolin.[1] The odour was attributed to unidentified sulphur metabolites.

1. Stewart WK, Fleming LW. Use your nose. *Lancet* 1983; **i:** 426.

Uses and Administration

Noxythiolin is an antiseptic with wide antibacterial and antifungal actions. It may act by slowly releasing formaldehyde in solution.

For instillation into, or irrigation of, the peritoneal cavity or other body cavities, a 0.5 to 2.5% solution is used. Solutions of noxythiolin should be warmed to 37° prior to instillation or irrigation. Treatment is usually for 3 to 7 days, modified or repeated thereafter as required. The normal total daily amount used in adults should not exceed 5 g for instillation or 10 g for continuous irrigation.

Although noxythiolin has generally been thought to act, at least in part, by slowly releasing formaldehyde into solution Gorman *et al.*[1] reported that much smaller amounts are released than have previously been reported and that the antimicrobial effects of noxythiolin solutions cannot be attributed solely to the presence of formaldehyde. There is evidence *in vitro* that noxythiolin might reduce the adherence of microorganisms to epithelial surfaces.[2]

1. Gorman SP, *et al.* Formaldehyde release from noxythiolin solutions. *Pharm J* 1984; **234:** 62–3.
2. Anderson L, *et al.* Clinical implications of the microbial antiadherence properties of noxythiolin. *J Pharm Pharmacol* 1985; **37** (suppl): 64P.

Infections of the pleural cavity. Three patients with pleural empyema or pneumonectomy space infection were treated by irrigation of the cavity with noxythiolin 1% in normal saline for 3 hours, followed by drainage for 1 hour, the cycle being repeated 4-hourly. Infection was eradicated within 21 days in all 3 patients.[1]

1. Rosenfeldt FL, *et al.* Comparison between irrigation and conventional treatment for empyema and pneumonectomy space infection. *Thorax* 1984; **36:** 272–7.

Preparations

Proprietary Preparations (details are given in Part 3)
Fr.: Noxyflex; *Irl.:* Noxyflex S; *UK:* Noxyflex S.

Octaphonium Chloride (2263-q)

Octaphonium Chloride *(BAN)*.

Octafonium Chloride *(rINN)*; Phenoctide. Benzyldiethyl-2-[4-(1,1,3,3-tetramethylbutyl)phenoxy]ethylammonium chloride monohydrate.

$C_{27}H_{42}ClNO,H_2O$ = 450.1.

CAS — 15687-40-8; 78-05-7 (both anhydrous octaphonium chloride).

Octaphonium chloride is a quaternary ammonium antiseptic with actions and uses similar to those of other cationic surfactants (see Cetrimide, p.1105).

Preparations

Proprietary Preparations (details are given in Part 3)

Multi-ingredient: *UK:* Germolene.

Octenidine Hydrochloride (19599-e)

Octenidine Hydrochloride *(BANM, USAN, rINNM)*.

Win-41464 (octenidine); Win-41464-2 (octenidine hydrochloride); Win-41464-6 (octenidine saccharin). 1,1′,4,4′-Tetrahydro-*N,N*′-dioctyl-1,1′-decamethylenedi-(4-pyridylideneamine) dihydrochloride.

$C_{36}H_{62}N_4,2HCl$ = 623.8.

CAS — 71251-02-0 (octenidine); 70775-75-6 (octenidine hydrochloride).

NOTE. Octenidine Saccharin is *USAN.*

Octenidine hydrochloride is a bispyridine bactericidal antiseptic with some antiviral and antifungal activity. It has been used for skin and mucous membrane disinfection.

Preparations

Proprietary Preparations (details are given in Part 3)

Multi-ingredient: *Aust.:* Octenisept; *Ger.:* Neo Kodan; Octenisept; *Switz.:* Octenidermt†; Octenisept.

Orthophenylphenol (6661-q)

2-Biphenylol; E231; E232 (sodium-o-phenylphenol); 2-Hydroxybiphenyl; o-Hydroxydiphenyl.

$C_{12}H_{10}O$ = 170.2.

CAS — 90-43-7.

Orthophenylphenol is a phenolic disinfectant with antimicrobial properties similar to those of chloroxylenol (p.1111). It is used for disinfection of skin, hands, and hard surfaces. It also has many industrial uses as a preservative for a wide range of materials, particularly against moulds and rots. Sodium-*o*-phenylphenol has been used similarly.

Preparations

Proprietary Preparations (details are given in Part 3)
Fr.: Instrunet mains†; *Ger.:* Amocid; Manusept; *Ital.:* Crescom; Esofenol 60; Germozero Plus; Helix I; Neo Esoformolo.

Multi-ingredient: *Austral.:* Winseptic†; *Belg.:* Helipur†; *Canad.:* G-Nol†; *Fr.:* Frekaderm; *Ger.:* Bacillotox; Bomix; Freka-Derm; Freka-Sept 80; Grotanat; Helipur; Incidin Extra; Kodan Spray F†; Kodan Tinktur Forte; Lysolin†; Primasept Med; Velicin†; *Ital.:* Esofenol Ferri; Helipur; Hygienist; Neo Intol Plus†; Primasept M†; Sangen Casa; *Switz.:* Frekaderm; Stellisept; *USA:* Lubraseptic Jelly†.

Oxychlorosene (2264-p)

Oxychlorosene *(USAN)*.

Monoxychlorosene.

$C_{20}H_{34}O_3S,HOCl$ = 407.0.

CAS — 8031-14-9 (oxychlorosene); 52906-84-0 (oxychlorosene sodium).

NOTE. Oxychlorosene Sodium is *USAN.*

The hypochlorous acid complex of a mixture of the phenyl sulphonate derivatives of aliphatic hydrocarbons.

Oxychlorosene is a chlorine-releasing antiseptic with the general properties of chlorine, p.1109.

A 0.4% solution of the sodium salt of oxychlorosene has been used for cleansing wounds (although chlorine-releasing antiseptics are generally regarded as too irritant for this purpose—see under Chlorine, p.1110) and pre-operative skin preparation; a 0.2% solution has been used in urological and ophthalmological disinfection.

Disinfection. VIRUSES. At the concentration of virus likely to be found in clinical specimens, HIV was inactivated by oxychlorosene sodium 4 mg per mL, the concentration recommended for clinical use.[1]

1. Klein RJ, *et al.* Inactivation of human immunodeficiency, herpes simplex, and vaccinia viruses by sodium oxychlorosene. *Lancet* 1987; **i:** 281–2.

Preparations

Proprietary Preparations (details are given in Part 3)
Canad.: Clorpactin; *USA:* Clorpactin WCS-90; Clorpactin XCB†.

Parachlorophenol (2265-s)

4-Chlorophenol.

C_6H_5ClO = 128.6.

CAS — 106-48-9.

Pharmacopoeias. In Aust., Swiss, and US. US also includes camphorated parachlorophenol.

White or pink crystals with a characteristic phenolic odour. M.p. about 42°. Sparingly **soluble** in water and liquid paraffin; very soluble in alcohol, chloroform, ether, glycerol, and fixed and volatile oils; soluble in melted soft paraffin. A 1% solution in water is acid to litmus. **Store** in airtight containers. Protect from light.

Parachlorophenol is a chlorinated phenolic disinfectant and antiseptic with similar properties to phenol (p.1121). Camphorated parachlorophenol has been used in dentistry in the treatment of infected root canals.

Preparations

USP 23: Camphorated Parachlorophenol.

Proprietary Preparations (details are given in Part 3)

Multi-ingredient: *Ital.:* Esofenol Ferri; *Spain:* Cresophene; *Switz.:* Cresophene; Pate Iodoforme du Prof Dr Walkhoff; Solution ChKM du Prof Dr Walkhoff.

Paraformaldehyde (2266-w)

Paraform; Paraformic Aldehyde; Polymerised Formaldehyde; Polyoxymethylene; Trioxyméthylène.

$(CH_2O)_n$.

CAS — 30525-89-4.

Pharmacopoeias. In *Aust., Jpn,* and *Swiss.*

Adverse Effects, Treatment, and Precautions

As for Formaldehyde Solution, p.1113. There have been reports of allergic reactions and nerve damage associated with the dental use of paraformaldehyde as a root canal sealant; it should not extrude beyond the apex.

Uses and Administration

Paraformaldehyde is a disinfectant and antiseptic with the properties and uses of formaldehyde (p.1114) and is used as a source of formaldehyde. For disinfecting rooms it has been vapourised by heating. Tablets prepared for disinfecting rooms by vaporisation should be coloured by the addition of a suitable blue dye.

Paraformaldehyde has been used in lozenges for the treatment of minor throat infections. In dentistry, it has been used as an obtundent for sensitive dentine and as an antiseptic in mummifying pastes and for root canals.

Preparations

Proprietary Preparations (details are given in Part 3)

Multi-ingredient: ***Aust.:*** Umadren; ***Austral.:*** Gartech; ***Fr.:*** Gynescal; ***Ital.:*** Devigen†; Esoform 7 mc; Esoform 70 mc; ***Switz.:*** Asphaline; Caustinerf forte; Rocanal Permanent Gangrene; Rocanal Permanent Vital.

Peracetic Acid (13094-q)

Acetyl Hydroperoxide; Peroxyacetic Acid.

$C_2H_4O_3$ = 76.05.

CAS — 79-21-0.

Peracetic acid is a strong oxidising disinfectant which is corrosive to the skin. It is active against many micro-organisms including bacteria, spores, fungi, and viruses. It is used for disinfecting medical equipment including dialysers and endoscopes. It is used in the food industry and for disinfecting sewage sludge, and has been used as a spray for sterilisation of laboratories.

Disinfection. References to the use of peracetic acid to disinfect endoscopes.[1,2] Peracetic acid is a possible alternative to glutaraldehyde for such use (see p.1097).

For use of peracetic acid with hydrogen peroxide in the disinfection of dialysis equipment, see under Hydrogen Peroxide, p.1117.

1. Bradley CR, *et al.* Evaluation of the Steris system 1 peracetic acid endoscope processor. *J Hosp Infect* 1995; **29:** 143–51.
2. Middleton AM, *et al.* Disinfection of bronchoscopes, contaminated in vitro with Mycobacterium tuberculosis, Mycobacterium avium-intracellulare and Mycobacterium chelonae in sputum, using stabilized, buffered peracetic acid solution ('Nu-Cidex'). *J Hosp Infect* 1997; **37:** 137–43.

Preparations

Proprietary Preparations (details are given in Part 3)

Multi-ingredient: ***Ger.:*** Peresal; ***Ital.:*** Peresal; ***USA:*** Renalin Dialyzer Reprocessing Concentrate.

Phenethyl Alcohol (6656-w)

Phenethyl Alcohol *(BAN).*

Benzyl Carbinol; Phenethanolum; Phenylethyl alcohol. 2-Phenylethanol.

$C_6H_5.CH_2.CH_2OH$ = 122.2.

CAS — 60-12-8.

Pharmacopoeias. In *Pol.* and *US.*

A colourless liquid with a rose-like odour. **Soluble** 1 in 60 of water, 1 in less than 1 of alcohol, chloroform, ether, benzyl benzoate, and diethyl phthalate; slightly soluble in liquid paraffin; very soluble in glycerol, propylene glycol, and fixed oils. **Store** in a cool, dry place in airtight containers. Protect from light.

Incompatible with oxidising agents and proteins. Activity may be reduced by nonionic surfactants or by adsorption onto low density polyethylene containers.

Phenethyl alcohol is more active against Gram-negative than Gram-positive bacteria. It is used as a preservative in ophthalmic and parenteral solutions at a concentration of 0.25 to 0.5%, in conjunction with another bactericide, and up to 1% in topical preparations. It is also used as an antiseptic in topical products in concentrations of up to 7.5%. It is also used as a component of flavouring essences and perfumes.

Phenethyl alcohol may cause eye irritation.

Antimicrobial activity may be enhanced by the addition of phenethyl alcohol to solutions preserved with benzalkonium chloride, chlorhexidine acetate, phenylmercuric nitrate, chlorocresol, or chlorbutol.[1]

1. Richards RME, McBride RJ. The preservation of ophthalmic solutions with antibacterial combinations. *J Pharm Pharmacol* 1972; **24:** 145–8.

Preparations

Proprietary Preparations (details are given in Part 3)

Multi-ingredient: ***Austral.:*** Sebirinse; ***Canad.:*** Sclerodex†; ***Irl.:*** Ceanel; ***S.Afr.:*** Ceanel; ***UK:*** Ceanel.

Phenol (2268-l)

Carbolic Acid; Fenol; Phenolum; Phenyl Hydrate; Phenylic Acid. Hydroxybenzene.

$C_6H_5.OH$ = 94.11.

CAS — 108-95-2.

Pharmacopoeias. In *Chin., Eur.* (see p.viii), *Jpn, Pol.,* and *US. Aust., Br., Swiss,* and *US* also include a monograph for Liquefied Phenol.

Colourless or faintly pink or faintly yellow deliquescent needle-shaped crystals or crystalline masses, darkening on keeping, with a characteristic odour. USP permits the addition of a suitable stabilising agent. F.p. not less than 39.5°.

Soluble 1 in 15 of water; very soluble in alcohol, in chloroform, in dichloromethane, in ether, in glycerol, and in fixed and volatile oils; soluble 1 in 70 of liquid paraffin. A solution of 1 g in 15 mL water is clear and is neutral or acid to litmus. **Store** in airtight containers. Protect from light. **Incompatible** with alkaline salts and nonionic surfactants. The antimicrobial activity of phenol may be diminished through increasing pH or through combination with blood and other organic matter.

When phenol is to be mixed with collodion, fixed oils, or paraffins, melted phenol should be used, and not Liquefied Phenol. (Liquefied Phenol (BP 1998) is an aqueous mixture containing phenol 77 to 81.5% w/w in purified water. Liquefied Phenol (USP 23) contains not less than 89% by weight of phenol.)

Phenol should not be used to preserve preparations that are to be freeze-dried.

Adverse Effects

When ingested, phenol causes extensive local corrosion, with pain, nausea, vomiting, sweating, and diarrhoea. Excitation may occur initially but it is quickly followed by unconsciousness. There is depression of the CNS, with cardiac arrhythmias, and circulatory and respiratory failure which may lead to death. Acidosis may develop and occasionally there is haemolysis and methaemoglobinaemia with cyanosis. The urine may become green. Pulmonary oedema and myocardial damage may develop, and damage to the liver and kidneys may lead to organ failure.

Severe or fatal poisoning may occur from the absorption of phenol from unbroken skin or wounds and suitable precautions should be taken to prevent absorption. Applied to skin, phenol causes blanching and corrosion, sometimes with little pain. Aqueous solutions as dilute as 10% may be corrosive.

Toxic symptoms may also arise through absorption of phenol vapour by the skin or lungs. Phenol throat spray may cause local oedema.

Cresols and other phenolic substances have similar effects.

Effects on the heart. A 10-year-old boy developed life-threatening premature ventricular complexes during the application of a solution of phenol 40% and croton oil 0.8% in hexachlorophane soap and water for chemical peeling of a giant hairy naevus.[1] Cardiac arrhythmias have been reported following the use of phenol for chemical face peeling.[2] They were also observed in 3 of 16 children who received phenol 5% as a neurolytic.[3]

1. Warner MA, Harper JV. Cardiac dysrhythmias associated with chemical peeling with phenol. *Anesthesiology* 1985; **62:** 366–7.
2. Botta SA, *et al.* Cardiac arrhythmias in phenol face peeling: a suggested protocol for prevention. *Aesthetic Plast Surg* 1988; **12:** 115–17.
3. Morrison JE, *et al.* Phenol motor point blocks in children: plasma concentrations and cardiac dysrhythmias. *Anesthesiology* 1991; **75:** 359–62.

Effects on the kidneys. A 41-year-old man developed acute renal failure due to cutaneous absorption of phenol after falling into a shallow vat of industrial solvent containing 40% phenol in dichloromethane. No ingestion occurred. Other symptoms included 50% body-surface burns, cold extremities, nausea, vomiting, and respiratory distress. The patient required haemodialysis for 3 weeks; some abnormalities of renal function remained one year later.[1]

1. Foxall PJD, *et al.* Acute renal failure following accidental cutaneous absorption of phenol: application of NMR urinalysis to monitor the disease process. *Hum Toxicol* 1989; **9:** 491–6.

Effects on sexual function. A report[1] of 3 patients who developed urinary symptoms and impotence which lasted up to one year after each receiving phenol 5% in arachis oil sclerotherapy for haemorrhoids.

1. Bullock N. Impotence after sclerotherapy of haemorrhoids: case reports. *Br Med J* 1997; **314:** 419.

Effects on the throat. Acute life-threatening epiglottitis occurred in a 49-year-old woman following the use of a throat spray containing the equivalent of 1.4% phenol. The reaction may have been anaphylactic or due to a direct toxic effect of the spray.[1] In the UK the Committee on Safety of Medicines[2] reported in 1990 that it had received 4 reports (probably including the one detailed above) of oedema of the epiglottis and/or larynx leading to respiratory difficulties. While the incidence was rare, the effects were severe; one patient died and 2 survived only after emergency hospital treatment.

1. Ho S-L, Hollinrake K. Acute epiglottitis and Chloraseptic. *Br Med J* 1989; **298:** 1584.
2. Committee on Safety of Medicines. Chloraseptic throat spray and oedema of the epiglottis and larynx. *Current Problems 28* 1990.

Treatment of Adverse Effects

If phenol has been swallowed, activated charcoal may be useful. Some sources suggest the cautious use of gastric lavage although this is generally inappropriate following ingestion of corrosive substances.

If phenol has been spilled on the skin removal of contaminated clothing and excess phenol should be followed by washing of the skin with copious amounts of water, then a vegetable oil. Macrogol 300 and eucalyptus oil have also been used.

Contamination of the eyes should be treated by flooding with water only for at least ten minutes.

The patient should be kept warm and given supportive treatment.

Precautions

Solutions containing phenol should not be applied to large areas of skin or large wounds since sufficient phenol may be absorbed to give rise to toxic symptoms. Phenol should not be used as a throat spray in patients with epiglottitis, or in children aged under 6 years.

Pharmacokinetics

Phenol is absorbed from the gastro-intestinal tract and through skin and mucous membranes. It is metabolised to phenylglucuronide and phenyl sulphate, and small amounts are oxidised to catechol and quinol which are mainly conjugated. The metabolites are excreted in the urine; on oxidation to quinones they may tint the urine green.

Uses and Administration

Phenol is an antiseptic and disinfectant effective against vegetative Gram-positive and Gram-negative bacteria, mycobacteria, and some fungi, but only very slowly effective against spores. It is also active against certain viruses. Phenol is more active in acid solution.

Aqueous solutions up to 1% are bacteriostatic while stronger solutions are bactericidal.

A 0.5 to 1% solution has been used for its local anaesthetic effect to relieve itching.

A 1.4% solution is used for pain or irritation of the mouth and throat. Weak concentrations have also been used topically for disinfection. A 5% solution has been used as a disinfectant for excreta.

Oily Phenol Injection (BP 1998), up to 10 mL has been injected into the tissues around internal haemorrhoids as an analgesic sclerosing agent, but alternative procedures may be preferred. Aqueous phenol has also used been as a sclerosant in the treatment of hydroceles.

Solutions of phenol in glycerol have been administered intrathecally for the alleviation of spasticity (p.1303) or injected intrathecally or into soft-tissue structures for the treatment of chronic low-back pain. Other types of severe intractable pain may be relieved by injecting aqueous phenol close to motor nerves. Aqueous phenol has been used for chemical sympathectomy in peripheral vascular disorders and for the treatment of urinary incontinence.

Liquefied phenol has been used in the treatment of ingrowing toenails.

Chemical face peeling. References to the use of phenol in chemical face peeling.[1,2] For a report of adverse cardiac effects associated with phenol being used for skin peeling, see Effects on the Heart under Adverse Effects, above.

1. Baker TJ, *et al.* Chemical face peeling for facial wrinkling. *JAMA* 1974; **228:** 898–9.
2. Ariagno RP, Briggs DR. Chemexfoliation as an adjunct to facial rejuvenation. *Trans Am Acad Ophthalmol Otolaryngol* 1975; **80:** 536–9.

Ingrowing toenail. Liquefied phenol ablation has been performed as an alternative to surgical avulsion in the treatment of ingrowing toenails.[1-5] Cauterisation with phenol 88% has also been successfully used to treat ingrowing toenails and onychogryphosis.[6]

1. Shepherdson A. Nail matrix phenolization: a preferred alternative to surgical excision. *Practitioner* 1977; **219:** 725–8.
2. Cameron PF. Ingrowing toenails: an evaluation of two treatments. *Br Med J* 1981; **283:** 821–2.
3. Morkane AJ, *et al.* Segmental phenolization of ingrowing toenails: a randomized controlled study. *Br J Surg* 1984; **71:** 526–7.
4. Sykes PA, Kerr R. Treatment of ingrowing toenails by surgeons and chiropodists. *Br Med J* 1988; **297:** 335–6.
5. Leahy AL, *et al.* Ingrowing toenails: improving treatment. *Surgery* 1990; **107:** 566–7.
6. Andrew T, Wallace WA. Nail bed ablation—excise or cauterise? A controlled study. *Br Med J* 1979; **1:** 1539.

Pain. The neurolytic use of phenol to produce destructive nerve block (p.6) has produced variable results, and some consider the risk of complications outweighs the benefits.

Sclerotherapy. HAEMORRHOIDS. Sclerotherapy with oily phenol injection has been used to treat haemorrhoids (p.1170). The technique for preventing mucosal prolapse is to inject 2 to 5 mL of a 5% solution of phenol in arachis oil into the submucous space above each of the 3 principal haemorrhoids.[1] Rather than causing the haemorrhoidal veins to thrombose, the injection works by producing submucosal fibrosis, fixing the mucosa to the underlying muscle. Other techniques for mucosal fixation such as rubber band ligation or perhaps infra-red coagulation are more effective and associated with fewer complications.[2-5]

1. Alexander-Williams J. The management of piles. *Br Med J* 1982; **285:** 1137–9.
2. Gartell PC, *et al.* A randomised clinical trial to compare rubber band ligation with phenol injection in the treatment of haemorrhoids. *Gut* 1984; **25:** A563.
3. Ambrose NS, *et al.* Prospective randomised trial of injection therapy against photocoagulation therapy in first and second degree haemorrhoids. *Gut* 1984; **25:** A563–4.
4. Johanson JF, Rimm A. Optimal nonsurgical treatment of hemorrhoids: a comparative analysis of infrared coagulation, rubber band ligation, and injection sclerotherapy. *Am J Gastroenterol* 1992; **87:** 1601–6.
5. MacRae HM, McLeod RS. Comparison of hemorrhoidal treatment modalities: a meta-analysis. *Dis Colon Rectum* 1995; **38:** 687–94.

Spasmodic torticollis. Intramuscular phenol was reported[1] to have produced improvement in 2 patients with moderately severe spasmodic torticollis who had not responded adequately to other therapies. Response was maintained by re-injection every 6 months. For a discussion of the management of dystonias such as spasmodic torticollis, see under Levodopa on p.1141.

1. Massey JM. Treatment of spasmodic torticollis with intramuscular phenol injection. *J Neurol Neurosurg Psychiatry* 1995; **58:** 258–9.

Urinary incontinence. Although injection of phenol into the pelvic plexus to produce partial denervation has been used in the management of severe intractable urge incontinence (p.454) its use has been largely abandoned. Some patients, especially those with detrusor hyperreflexia, have derived benefit[1,2] but overall efficacy can be poor and benefits short-lived.[3]

1. Ewing R, *et al.* Subtrigonal phenol injection therapy for incontinence in female patients with multiple sclerosis. *Lancet* 1983; **i:** 1304–5.
2. Blackford HN, *et al.* Results of transvesical infiltration of the pelvic plexuses with phenol in 116 patients. *Br J Urol* 1984; **56:** 647–9.
3. Rosenbaum TP, *et al.* Trans-trigonal phenol failed the test of time. *Br J Urol* 1990; **66:** 164–9.

Preparations

BP 1998: Liquefied Phenol; Oily Phenol Injection; Phenol and Glycerol Injection;
BPC 1973: Magenta Paint;
USP 23: Carbol-Fuchsin Topical Solution; Liquefied Phenol; Phenolated Calamine Lotion.

Proprietary Preparations (details are given in Part 3)
Austral.: Summer's Eve Disposable; ***Canad.:*** Chloraseptic Sore Throat Spray; P & S; ***Irl.:*** Vicks Chloraseptic; ***S.Afr.:*** Chloraseptic†; Medi-Keel A; Septosol; ***Spain:*** Jabon Fenicado†; ***USA:*** Cheracol Sore Throat; P & S; Ulcerease; Vicks Children's Chloraseptic; Vicks Chloraseptic.

Multi-ingredient: numerous preparations are listed in Part 3.

Phenoxyethanol (6657-e)

Ethyleneglycol Monophenylether; Phenoxyaethanol; Phenoxyethanolum; β-Phenoxyethyl Alcohol. 2-Phenoxyethanol.

$C_8H_{10}O_2$ = 138.2.

CAS — 122-99-6.

Pharmacopoeias. In *Eur.* (see p.viii).

A colourless slightly viscous liquid. Slightly **soluble** in water, in arachis oil and in olive oil; miscible with acetone, alcohol, and glycerol. **Incompatibilities.** The activity of phenoxyethanol may be reduced by interaction with nonionic surfactants and possibly by adsorption onto polyvinyl chloride.

Phenoxyethanol is effective against strains of *Pseudomonas aeruginosa* but less so against other Gram-negative and Gram-positive bacteria. It has been used as a preservative in cosmetics and topical pharmaceuticals at a concentration of 0.5 to 1%. It is often used in combination with other preservatives, commonly hydroxybenzoates, to obtain a wider spectrum of antimicrobial activity.

Phenoxyethanol is used in concentrations of about 2% as an antiseptic for minor infections of skin, wounds, and mucous membranes. Aqueous solutions may be prepared by shaking the phenoxyethanol with hot water until dissolved, then adjusting to final volume when cool. Preparation of the solution can be aided by propylene glycol.

Phenoxypropanol and chlorophenoxyethanol are related compounds used in topical preparations.

Preparations

Proprietary Preparations (details are given in Part 3)
Canad.: Clearasil Face Wash; Lanohex; ***Fr.:*** Clearasil Face Wash†; ***Irl.:*** Biactol Antibacterial Facewash; ***UK:*** Biactol Liquid; Clearasil Medicated Face Wash.

Multi-ingredient: ***Aust.:*** Octenisept; ***Austral.:*** Dermocaine; Medidermt†; ***Belg.:*** Solubeol; ***Ger.:*** Octenisept; Terralin; ***Ital.:*** Fitostimoline; Florigien; ***S.Afr.:*** Tantol Skin Cleanser; ***Spain:*** Pentoderm†; ***Switz.:*** Octenisept; ***UK:*** Phytocil†.

Phenylmercuric Salts (12171-t)

Phenylmercuric Acetate (6658-l)

Phenylhydrargyri Acetas; PMA. (Acetato)phenylmercury.

$C_8H_8HgO_2$ = 336.7.

CAS — 62-38-4.

Pharmacopoeias. In *Aust.*, *Fr.*, and *Pol.* Also in *USNF.*

A white or creamy-white, odourless, crystalline powder or small prisms or leaflets. **Soluble** 1 in 180 of water, 1 in 225 of alcohol, 1 in 6.8 of chloroform, and 1 in 200 of ether; soluble in acetone. **Store** in airtight containers. Protect from light. **Incompatibilities** are described under Phenylmercuric Nitrate, below.

Phenylmercuric Borate (6659-y)

Phenylmercuric Borate (*rINN*).

Hydrargyrum Phenyloboricum; Phenomerborum; Phenylhydrargyri Boras.

$C_6H_5HgOH, C_6H_5HgOB(OH)_2$ = 633.2 or $C_6H_5HgOH, C_6H_5HgBO_2$ = 615.2.

CAS — 8017-88-7 ($C_{12}H_{13}BHg_2O_4$); *6273-99-0* ($C_{12}H_{11}BHg_2O_3$); *102-98-7* ($C_6H_7BHgO_3$).

Pharmacopoeias. In *Eur.* (see p.viii) and *Pol.*

A compound consisting of equimolecular proportions of phenylmercuric orthoborate and phenylmercuric hydroxide ($C_{12}H_{13}BHg_2O_4$) or of the dehydrated form (metaborate, $C_{12}H_{11}BHg_2O_3$) or a mixture of the two compounds. Colourless shiny crystals or a white or slightly yellowish crystalline powder; Slightly **soluble** in water and in alcohol. **Protect** from light. **Incompatibilities** are described under Phenylmercuric Nitrate, below.

Phenylmercuric Nitrate (6660-g)

Basic Phenylmercury Nitrate; Phenylhydrargyri Nitras; PMN. Nitratophenylmercury.

$C_6H_5HgOH, C_6H_5HgNO_3$ = 634.4.

CAS — 8003-05-2 ($C_6H_5HgOH, C_6H_5HgNO_3$); *55-68-5* ($C_6H_5HgNO_3$).

Pharmacopoeias. In *Eur.* (see p.viii), *Int.*, and *Pol.* Also in *USNF.*

A mixture of phenylmercuric nitrate and phenylmercuric hydroxide. A white or pale yellow, crystalline powder. Slightly or very slightly **soluble** in water and in alcohol; slightly soluble in hot water and in glycerol; more soluble in the presence of nitric acid or alkali hydroxides; dissolves in fatty oils. A saturated solution in water is acid to litmus. **Store** in airtight containers. Protect from light.

Incompatibilities. The activity of phenylmercuric salts may be reduced by interaction with compounds such as kaolin, magnesium trisilicate, starch, and talc.[1,2] Disodium edetate and sodium thiosulphate can also produce inactivation.[3] Sodium metabisulphite can lead to precipitation,[3] or chemical destruction,[4] but it can also produce increased activity.[3] Other incompatibilities include bromides, iodides (chlorides to a lesser extent), metals, and ammonia and its salts.[5] There can be adsorption onto rubber and some plastics[5,6] although sorption by low density polyethylene can be inhibited by phosphate ions.[7] Some filters, though not membrane filters, used for sterilisation removed considerable amounts of phenylmercuric nitrate from solution.[8] The pH may also affect activity.[9]

1. Yousef RT, *et al.* Effect of some pharmaceutical materials on the bactericidal activities of preservatives. *Can J Pharm Sci* 1973; **8:** 54–6.
2. Horn NR, *et al.* Interactions between powder suspensions and selected quaternary ammonium and organomercurial preservatives. *Cosmet Toilet* 1980; **95:** 69–73.
3. Richards RME, Reary JME. Changes in antibacterial activity of thiomersal and PMN on autoclaving with certain adjuvants. *J Pharm Pharmacol* 1972; **24** (suppl): 84P–89P.
4. Collins AJ, *et al.* Incompatibility of phenylmercuric acetate with sodium metabisulphite in eye drop formulations. *J Pharm Pharmacol* 1985; **37** (suppl): 123P.
5. Allwood MC. Phenylmercuric nitrate. In: Wade A, Weller PJ, eds. *Handbook of pharmaceutical excipients.* 2nd ed. Washington and London: American Pharmaceutical Association and The Pharmaceutical Press, 1994: 346–9.
6. Aspinall JA, *et al.* The effect of low density polyethylene containers on some hospital-manufactured eyedrop formulations. *J Clin Hosp Pharm* 1980; **5:** 21–9.
7. Aspinall JE, *et al.* The effect of low density polyethylene containers on some hospital-manufactured eyedrop formulations II. Inhibition of the sorption of phenylmercuric acetate. *J Clin Hosp Pharm* 1983; **8:** 233–40.
8. Naido NT, *et al.* Preservative loss from ophthalmic solutions during filtration sterilisation. *Aust J Pharm Sci* 1972; **NS1:** 16–18.
9. Wessels JMC, Adema DMM. Some data on the relationship between fungicidal protection and pH. In: Walters AH, Elphick JJ, eds. *Biodeterioration of materials.* Amsterdam: Elsevier, 1968: 517–23.

Adverse Effects and Precautions

While the adverse effects of inorganic mercury (p.1601) should be taken into account when considering the adverse effects of phenylmercuric compounds, there is little evidence of systemic toxicity arising from their use. They are irritant to the skin and may give rise to erythema and blistering. Hypersensitivity reactions have been reported. Topical application to eyes has been associated with mercurialentis and atypical band keratopathy; prolonged use of eye drops containing phenylmercuric preservatives is not recommended.

Effects on the eyes. References to primary atypical band keratopathy and pigmentation of the anterior capsule of the lens (mercurialentis) associated with the prolonged use of eye drops containing phenylmercuric preservative.

1. Kennedy RE, *et al.* Further observations on atypical band keratopathy in glaucoma patients. *Trans Am Ophthalmol Soc* 1974; **72:** 107–22.
2. Garron LK, *et al.* A clinical pathologic study of mercurialentis medicamentosus. *Trans Am Ophthalmol Soc* 1976; **74:** 295–320.
3. Brazier DJ, Hitchings RA. Atypical band keratopathy following long-term pilocarpine treatment. *Br J Ophthalmol* 1989; **73:** 294–6.

Uses

Phenylmercuric salts have antibacterial and antifungal properties. They are primarily bacteriostatic compounds although they also have a slow bactericidal action. Their activity has been reported to be pH dependent.

Phenylmercuric compounds are used as preservatives in cosmetic, ophthalmic, or pharmaceutical preparations and as antiseptics. They have also been used as spermicides.

When employed as a preservative in eye drops, a concentration of 0.002% is usually used; in injection solutions the concentration is 0.001%.

Picloxydine (2269-y)

Picloxydine *(BAN, rINN).*

1,1′-[Piperazine-1,4-diylbis(formimidoyl)]bis[3-(4-chlorophenyl)guanidine].

$C_{20}H_{24}Cl_2N_{10}$ = 475.4.

CAS — 5636-92-0.

Picloxydine is a biguanide disinfectant with properties similar to those of chlorhexidine (p.1107). It has been used in eye drops as the dihydrochloride for the treatment of superficial infections of the eye. It is also used as a surface disinfectant in combination with quaternary ammonium compounds.

Preparations

Proprietary Preparations (details are given in Part 3)
Fr.: Vitabact; *Switz.:* Vitabact.

Polyhexanide (13146-m)

Polyhexanide *(BAN).*

Polihexanide *(rINN)*; ICI-9073; Polyhexamethylene Biguanide Hydrochloride. Poly(1-hexamethylenebiguanide hydrochloride).

$(C_8H_{17}N_5,HCl)_n$ = 219.7×*n*.

CAS — 32289-58-0.

Polyhexanide has antibacterial and antiamoebic activity. It is used as a surface disinfectant and for disinfecting soft contact lenses (p.1097). It has been tried in the treatment of *Acanthamoeba* keratitis (p.573).

Preparations

Proprietary Preparations (details are given in Part 3)
Switz.: Lavasept.

Multi-ingredient: *Fr.:* Ampholysine Plus†; Hexanios G+R; Novospray; *Ger.:* Complete; Teta-Aktiv†; Teta-S.

Polynoxylin (2270-g)

Polynoxylin *(BAN, rINN).*

Poly{[bis(hydroxymethyl)ureylene]methylene}.

$(C_4H_8N_2O_3)_n$.

CAS — 9011-05-6.

Polynoxylin is a condensation product of formaldehyde and urea. It is an antiseptic with antibacterial and antifungal actions and, like noxythiolin (p.1120), may act by the release of formaldehyde. It is available in a variety of preparations for the local treatment of minor infections, usually at a concentration of 10%.

Preparations

Proprietary Preparations (details are given in Part 3)
Aust.: Anaflex; *Austral.:* Ponoxylan†; *S.Afr.:* Ponoxylan†; *Spain:* Larex†; Noxylin†; *Switz.:* Anaflex†; *UK:* Anaflex.

Potassium Nitrate (13155-b)

E252; Kalii Nitras; Kalium Nitricum; Nitre; Saltpetre.

KNO_3 = 101.1.

CAS — 7757-79-1.

Pharmacopoeias. In *Aust., Belg., Br., Pol., Swiss,* and *US.*

Colourless crystals or a white crystalline powder. Freely **soluble** in water; very soluble in boiling water; practically insoluble in alcohol; soluble in glycerol. **Store** in airtight containers.

CAUTION. *Potassium nitrate has been used for the illicit preparation of explosives or fireworks; care is required with its supply.*

The name saltpetre has been used as a generic term for a number of potassium- and sodium-based preservatives used in food manufacture. For a report of poisoning when a mixture of sodium nitrate and sodium nitrite was supplied for saltpetre, see p.1125.

Adverse Effects

After ingestion potassium nitrate may be reduced to nitrite in the gastro-intestinal tract by the action of bacteria and ingestion of large amounts can therefore cause methaemoglobinaemia. Gastro-intestinal disturbances, vertigo, headache, flushing of the skin, hypotension, irregular pulse, cyanosis, convulsions, and collapse may occur. The toxic dose varies greatly; 15 g may prove fatal but much larger doses have been taken without serious effects. Poisoning has frequently been reported in infants given water from wells contaminated with nitrates.

For reference to nitrites as precursors of nitrosamines and the potential role of nitrosamines as carcinogens, see p.995.

Concern has been expressed regarding the concentrations of nitrates and nitrites in the public drinking water supply. In the UK a maximum nitrate concentration of 50 mg per litre and a maximum nitrite concentration of 0.1 mg per litre have been set for drinking water.[1]

1. MAFF. Nitrate, nitrite and N-nitroso compounds in food: second report. *Food Surveillance Paper 32.* London: HMSO, 1992.

Uses and Administration

Potassium nitrate is used as a preservative in foods. It is also included in dentrifices to reduce the pain of hypersensitive teeth. When taken by mouth in dilute solution, it acts as a diuretic and was formerly used for this purpose.

Preparations

USP 23: Potassium Nitrate Solution.

Proprietary Preparations (details are given in Part 3)
USA: Denquel; Mint Sensodyne.

Multi-ingredient: *Austral.:* Mackenzies Menthoids; Oral-B Sensitive; Thermodent; *Belg.:* Escouflaire; *Canad.:* Sensodyne-F; *Switz.:* Grafco†; *UK:* AVOCA; *USA:* Promise†; Sensitivity Protection Crest; Sensodyne-F.

Potassium Permanganate (5907-v)

Kalii Permanganas; Kalium Hypermanganicum; Kalium Permanganicum; Pot. Permang.

$KMnO_4$ = 158.0.

CAS — 7722-64-7.

Pharmacopoeias. In *Chin., Eur.* (see p.viii), *Jpn, Pol.,* and *US.*

Dark purple or almost black crystals or granular powder, almost opaque by transmitted light and with a blue metallic lustre by reflected light. It decomposes in contact with certain organic substances. **Soluble** in cold water and freely soluble in boiling water. An acidified solution in water is readily reduced by hydrogen peroxide, by easily oxidisable substances, and by organic matter. **Incompatible** with iodides, reducing agents, and most organic substances.

CAUTION. *Potassium permanganate may be explosive if it is brought into contact with organic or other readily oxidisable substances. It has been used for the illicit preparation of fireworks; care is required with its supply.*

Adverse Effects and Treatment

The crystals and concentrated solutions of potassium permanganate are caustic and even fairly dilute solutions are irritant to tissues and stain skin brown.

Symptoms of poisoning following ingestion of potassium permanganate should be treated symptomatically; they include nausea, vomiting of a brownish coloured material, corrosion, oedema, and brown coloration of the buccal mucosa, gastro-intestinal haemorrhage, liver and kidney damage, and cardiovascular depression. The fatal dose is probably about 10 g and death may occur up to 1 month from the time of poisoning.

The insertion into the vagina of potassium permanganate for its supposed abortifacient action causes corrosive burns, severe vaginal haemorrhage, and perforation of the vaginal wall, leading to peritonitis. Vascular collapse may occur.

Case reports of adverse effects following ingestion of potassium permanganate.

1. Mahomedy MC, *et al.* Methaemoglobinaemia following treatment dispensed by witch doctors: two cases of potassium permanganate poisoning. *Anaesthesia* 1975; **30:** 190–3.
2. Kochhar R, *et al.* Potassium permanganate induced oesophageal stricture. *Hum Toxicol* 1986; **5:** 393–4.
3. Southwood T, *et al.* Ingestion of potassium permanganate crystals by a three-year-old boy. *Med J Aust* 1987; **146:** 639–40.
4. Middleton SJ, *et al.* Haemorrhagic pancreatitis—a cause of death in severe potassium permanganate poisoning. *Postgrad Med J* 1990; **66:** 657–8.
5. Young RJ, *et al.* Fatal acute hepatorenal failure following potassium permanganate ingestion. *Hum Exp Toxicol* 1996; **15:** 259–61.

Uses and Administration

Potassium permanganate possesses oxidising properties which in turn confer disinfectant and deodorising properties. It is also astringent. Though bactericidal *in vitro* its clinical value as a bactericide is minimised by its rapid reduction in the presence of body fluids.

Solutions are used as cleansing applications to wounds, ulcers, or abscesses and as wet dressings and in baths in eczematous conditions and acute dermatoses especially where there is secondary infection. It is often prepared as a 0.1% solution in water to be diluted 1 in 10 before use to provide a 0.01% (1 in 10 000) solution. Solutions have also been used in bromhidrosis, in mycotic infections such as athlete's foot, and in poison ivy dermatitis.

Potassium permanganate is added to formaldehyde solution to produce formaldehyde vapour for the disinfection of rooms and cabinets (see p.1114).

Preparations

Proprietary Preparations (details are given in Part 3)
UK: Permitabs.

Povidone-Iodine (4580-y)

Povidone-Iodine *(BAN).*

Iodinated Povidone; Polyvidone-Iodine; Polyvinylpyrrolidone-Iodine Complex; Povidonum Iodinatum; PVP-Iodine.

CAS — 25655-41-8.

Pharmacopoeias. In *Chin., Eur.* (see p.viii), *Jpn,* and *US.*

A complex of iodine with povidone containing 9 to 12% of available iodine calculated on the dried basis. Yellowish-brown or reddish-brown amorphous powder with a slight characteristic odour. It loses not more than 8% of its weight on drying. **Soluble** in water and alcohol; practically insoluble in acetone, carbon tetrachloride, chloroform, ether, and petroleum spirit. A 10% solution in water has a pH of 1.5 to 5.0. **Store** in airtight containers. Protect from light.

Incompatibilities. Antimicrobial activity may be reduced at high pH.

Incompatibilities. Dermatological reactions, described as second- and third-degree burns, were observed in 4 patients in whom wounds were covered with a povidone-iodine soaked bandage secured to the skin by compound benzoin tincture. It was suggested that an interaction had occurred resulting in a more acidic pH.[1]

A mixture of povidone-iodine solution and hydrogen peroxide [brown bubbly] has caused explosions.[2]

1. Schillaci LJ, *et al.* Reduced pH associated with mixture of povidone-iodine and compound tincture of benzoin. *Am J Hosp Pharm* 1983; **40:** 1694–5.
2. Dannenberg E, Peebles J. Betadine-hydrogen peroxide irrigation solution incompatibility. *Am J Hosp Pharm* 1978; **35:** 525.

Adverse Effects and Precautions

Povidone-iodine can cause hypersensitivity reactions and irritation of the skin and mucous membranes, although severe reactions are rare and povidone-iodine is considered to be less irritant than iodine.

The application of povidone-iodine to severe burns or to large areas otherwise denuded of skin may produce the systemic adverse effects associated with iodine (p.1493) such as metabolic acidosis, hypernatraemia, and impairment of renal function. Hyperthyroidism or hypothyroidism may occur following ingestion of large quantities. Hypothyroidism has occurred in neonates both as a result of absorption of iodine from povidone-iodine applied to the neonate and also to the mother during pregnancy or breast feeding.

Regular or prolonged use should be avoided in patients with thyroid disorders or those receiving lithium therapy.

Acidosis. There have been a number of reports of acidosis in patients whose burns were treated topically with povidone-iodine.[1,2] Fatal metabolic acidosis[3] and seizures[4] have been reported following mediastinal irrigation with povidone-iodine.

1. Pietsch J, Meakins JL. Complications of povidone-iodine absorption in topically treated burn patients. *Lancet* 1976; **i:** 280–2.
2. Scoggin C, *et al.* Hypernatraemia and acidosis in association with topical treatment of burns. *Lancet* 1977; **i:** 959.
3. Glick PL, *et al.* Iodine toxicity in a patient treated by continuous povidone-iodine mediastinal irrigation. *Ann Thorac Surg* 1985; **39:** 478–80.
4. Zec N, *et al.* Seizures in a patient treated with continuous povidone-iodine mediastinal irrigation. *N Engl J Med* 1992; **326:** 1784.

Hypersensitivity. Anaphylaxis was associated with vaginal application of povidone-iodine solution.[1]

1. Waran KD, Munsick RA. Anaphylaxis from povidone-iodine. *Lancet* 1995; **345:** 1506.

Neonates. Hypothyroidism has been reported in premature and very low birth-weight infants following the use of povidone-iodine for routine antisepsis,[1,2] and hyperthyroidism in a full-term infant following mediastinal lavage.[3]

Perinatal vaginal use of povidone-iodine may also cause neonatal thyroid dysfunction.[4]

1. Parravicini E, *et al.* Iodine, thyroid function, and very low birth weight infants. *Pediatrics* 1996; **98:** 730–4.
2. Linder N, *et al.* Topical iodine-containing antiseptics and subclinical hypothyroidism in preterm infants. *J Pediatr* 1997; **131:** 434–9.
3. Bryant WP, Zimmerman D. Iodine-induced hyperthyroidism in a newborn. *Pediatrics* 1995; **95:** 434–6. Correction. *ibid.*; **96:** 779.
4. l'Allemand D, *et al.* Iodine-induced alterations of thyroid function in newborn infants after prenatal and perinatal exposure to povidone iodine. *J Pediatr* 1983; **102:** 935–8.

Uses and Administration

Povidone-iodine is an iodophore which is used as a disinfectant and antiseptic mainly for the treatment of contaminated wounds and pre-operative preparation of the skin and mucous membranes as well as for the disinfection of equipment.

Iodophores are loose complexes of iodine and carrier polymers. Solutions of povidone-iodine gradually release iodine to exert an effect against bacteria, fungi, viruses, protozoa, cysts, and spores; povidone-iodine is thus less potent than preparations containing free iodine but it is less toxic.

A wide variety of topical formulations is available, the majority containing about 4 to 10% of povidone-iodine; a 1% mouthwash has been used for oral infections and topical powders containing 0.5 to 5% povidone-iodine have been tried in the treatment and prevention of wound infection. For vaginal application povidone-iodine has also been used as pessaries containing 200 mg.

Preparations

BP 1998: Povidone-Iodine Solution;
USP 23: Povidone-Iodine Cleansing Solution; Povidone-Iodine Ointment; Povidone-Iodine Topical Aerosol Solution; Povidone-Iodine Topical Solution.

Proprietary Preparations (details are given in Part 3)
Aust.: Betaisodona; Betasan; Betaseptic; Braunol; Braunovidon; Wundesin; ***Austral.:*** Betadine; EDP-Evans Dermal Powder; Iodine Tri-Test†; Isodine; Microshield PVP; Microshield PVP-S; Minidine; Novadine†; Nyal Cold Sore†; Nyal Medithroat Gargle; Orodine†; Savlon Antiseptic; Stoxine†; Viodine; Viraban; ***Belg.:*** Braunol; Iodex Buccal; Iodex Dermique; Iso-Betadine; ***Canad.:*** Betadine; Massengill Medicated; Proviodine; ***Fr.:*** Betadine; Poliodine; ***Ger.:*** Amyderm S†; Batticon S†; Betaisodona; Braunol; Braunovidon; Freka-cid; Inadine; Jodobac; Logomed Desinfektions-Salbe; Polydona; Poysept; Sepso J; SP Betaisodona; Traumasept; ***Irl.:*** Betadine; Braunol; Braunosan; Braunovidon; Disadine DP†; Inadine; ***Ital.:*** Betadermyl†; Betadine; Betaseptic; Braunol; Braunosan†; Braunovidon†; Destrobac; Esoform Jod 10; Euroiod-Disinfettante Iodoforo Analcolico†; Evadermin; Gammadin; Garze Disinfettanti alla Pomata Betadine; Golasept; Inadine; Iodocid; Iodoril†; Iodoscrub†; Iodosteril†; Iodoten; Jodocur; Jodogard; Paniodal; Paniodine; Poviderm; ***Jpn:*** Isodine; ***Neth.:*** Betadermyl†; Betadine; ***S.Afr.:*** Betadine; Dermadine; Podine; Septadine; ***Spain:*** Betadine; Betaseptic†; Betatul; Braunoderm; Braunol; Ioden†; Iodina; Kaput; Meniodina†; Orto Dermo P; Povidona Yodada; Solucionic; Topionic; Topionic Gin†; ***Swed.:*** Inadine†; ***Switz.:*** Betadine; Braunol; Braunosan; Braunosan H Plus; Braunovidon; Demosept Jod†; Destrobac; Jodoplex; Rocanal Imediat; ***UK:*** Betadine; Betasept†; Brush Off; Cold Sore Lotion†; Inadine; Savlon Dry; Videne; ***USA:*** ACU-dyne; Aerodine; Betadine; Biodine; Efodine; Femidine; Iodex; Mallisol; Massengill Medicated; Minidyne; Operand; Polydine; Povidex; Summer's Eve Medicated; Yeast-Gard Medicated.

Multi-ingredient: ***Aust.:*** Braunoderm; ***Austral.:*** Microshield PVP Plus; Novasrub†; ***Belg.:*** Braunoderm; ***Canad.:*** Metadyne; ***Ger.:*** Betaseptic; Braunoderm; ***Irl.:*** Braunoderm; ***Ital.:*** Braunoderm; Diafen†; ***Spain:*** Yodocortison†; ***Switz.:*** Betaseptic; Braunoderm; ***UK:*** Codella; ***USA:*** Anbesol; Orasol; ProTech.

Propamidine Isethionate (2272-p)

Propamidine Isethionate *(BANM)*.

Propamidine Isetionate *(rINNM)*; M&B-782. 4,4′-Trimethylenedioxydibenzamidine bis(2-hydroxyethanesulphonate).

$C_{17}H_{20}N_4O_2,2C_2H_6O_4S$ = 564.6.
CAS — 104-32-5 (propamidine); 140-63-6 (propamidine isethionate).

Propamidine isethionate is an aromatic diamidine antiseptic which is active against Gram-positive bacteria, but less active against Gram-negative bacteria and spore-forming organisms. It also has antifungal properties and is active against *Acanthamoeba*. Ophthalmic solutions containing 0.1% of propamidine isethionate are used for the treatment of conjunctivitis and blepharitis.

Acanthamoeba keratitis. The optimal regimen for the treatment of *Acanthamoeba* keratitis (p.573) has yet to be determined. Propamidine isethionate 0.1% is commonly used, usually in conjunction with neomycin[1,2] or a neomycin-polymyxin-gramicidin combination,[3] plus chlorhexidine gluconate,[4] or polyhexanide.[5] However, reported resistance of some strains of *Acanthamoeba* to propamidine has prompted the suggestion that it should be replaced by another diamidine such as hexamidine.[6]

1. Wright P, *et al.* Acanthamoeba keratitis successfully treated medically. *Br J Ophthalmol* 1985; **69:** 778–82.
2. Varga JH, *et al.* Combined treatment of Acanthamoeba keratitis with propamidine, neomycin, and polyhexamethylene biguanide. *Am J Ophthalmol* 1993; **115:** 466–70.
3. Moore MB, McCulley JP. Acanthamoeba keratitis associated with contact lenses: six consecutive cases of successful management. *Br J Ophthalmol* 1989; **73:** 271–5.
4. Seal DV. Chlorhexidine or polyhexamethylene biguanide for acanthamoeba keratitis. *Lancet* 1995; **345:** 136.
5. Kilvington S. Chemotherapy for acanthamoeba keratitis. *Lancet* 1995; **345:** 792.
6. Perrine D, *et al.* Amoebicidal efficiencies of various diamidines against two strains of Acanthamoeba polyphaga. *Antimicrob Agents Chemother* 1995; **39:** 339–42.

Preparations

Proprietary Preparations (details are given in Part 3)
Austral.: Brolene; ***Irl.:*** Brolene; ***UK:*** Brolene; Golden Eye Drops.

Propiolactone (2273-s)

Propiolactone *(BAN, USAN, rINN)*.

BPL; NSC-21626; 2-Oxetanone; Propanolide; β-Propiolactone. Propiono-3-lactone.

$C_3H_4O_2$ = 72.06.
CAS — 57-57-8.

Propiolactone vapour is an irritant, mutagenic, possibly carcinogenic disinfectant which is very active against most micro-organisms including viruses. It is rather less effective against bacterial spores.

Propiolactone vapour has been used for the gaseous sterilisation of pharmaceutical and surgical materials and for disinfecting large enclosed areas. It has low penetrating power. Propiolactone liquid has also been used.

Disinfection. VIRUSES. Propiolactone has been used to treat blood products including those contaminated with HIV[1,2] and hepatitis C (parenteral non-A non-B) virus.[3]

1. Ball MJ, Griffiths D. Effect on chemical analyses of beta-propiolactone treatment of whole blood and plasma. *Lancet* 1985; **i:** 1160–1.
2. Anonymous. Guidelines for work with HIV. *Lancet* 1986; **ii:** 174–5.
3. Prince AM, *et al.* Inactivation of the Hutchinson strain of non-A, non-B hepatitis virus by combined use of β-propiolactone and ultraviolet irradiation. *J Med Virol* 1985; **16:** 119–25.

Propyl Alcohol (561-n)

Normal Propyl Alcohol; Primary Propyl Alcohol; Propanol; Propanolum. Propan-1-ol.

$CH_3.CH_2.CH_2OH$ = 60.10.
CAS — 71-23-8.

Adverse Effects and Treatment

As for Alcohol, p.1099; propyl alcohol is considered more toxic.

References.

1. 1-Propanol. *Environmental Health Criteria 102.* Geneva: WHO, 1990.

Uses and Administration

Propyl alcohol is an antiseptic with properties similar to those of alcohol (p.1100), used in preparations for disinfection of the hands, skin, surfaces, and instruments. Isopropyl alcohol (p.1118) is also used as an antiseptic.

Ritiometan (2979-x)

Ritiometan *(rINN)*.

(Methylidynetrithio)triacetic acid.

$C_7H_{10}O_6S_3$ = 286.3.
CAS — 34914-39-1.

Ritiometan has been used as the magnesium salt in an aerosol preparation for the treatment of infections of the nose and throat.

Preparations

Proprietary Preparations (details are given in Part 3)
Fr.: Necyrane.

Scarlet Red (2274-w)

Biebrich Scarlet R Medicinal; CI Solvent Red 24; Colour Index No. 26105; Fat Ponceau R; Rubrum Scarlatinum; Scharlachrot; Sudan IV. 1-[4-(o-Tolylazo)-o-tolylazo]naphth-2-ol.

$C_{24}H_{20}N_4O$ = 380.4.
CAS — 85-83-6.

Pharmacopoeias. In *Aust.*

Scarlet red is an antiseptic dye which has been used topically. It can be irritant.

Sodium Azide (16985-x)

N_3Na = 65.01.
CAS — 26628-22-8.

Adverse Effects and Precautions

Acute poisoning with sodium azide may cause life-threatening hypotension, tachycardia, convulsions, and severe headache. Fatalities have been reported. Solutions containing sodium azide must not be disposed of into drain pipelines containing copper, lead or brass since highly explosive heavy metal azides may be produced.

References to acute poisoning with sodium azide.

1. Edmonds OP, Bourne MS. Sodium azide poisoning in five laboratory technicians. *Br J Ind Med* 1982; **39:** 308–9.
2. Klein-Schwartz W, *et al.* Three fatal sodium azide poisonings. *Med Toxicol Adverse Drug Exp* 1989; **4:** 219–27.
3. Anonymous. Sodium azide contamination of hemodialysis water supplies. *JAMA* 1989; **261:** 2603.

Uses

Sodium azide has been used as an antimicrobial preservative in laboratory reagents, serum samples, and dialysis equipment.

Sodium Diacetate (6669-z)

E262. Sodium hydrogen diacetate.

$CH_3COONa,CH_3COOH(+xH_2O)$.
CAS — 126-96-5 (anhydrous sodium diacetate).

Sodium diacetate is used as a preservative in foods, particularly as an inhibitor of moulds and rope-forming micro-organisms in bread.

Sodium Dichloroisocyanurate (2276-l)

Sodium Dichloro-s-triazinetrione; Sodium Troclosene. 1,3-Dichloro-1,3,5-triazine-2,4,6(1*H*,3*H*,5*H*)-trione sodium.

$C_3Cl_2N_3NaO_3$ = 219.9.
CAS — 2893-78-9.

It contains about 65% of 'available chlorine' (see p.1110).

Sodium dichloroisocyanurate is a disinfectant with the general properties of chlorine (p.1109) and sodium hypochlorite (p.1124) but it remains active as pH increases from 6 to 10 and is reported to be less susceptible to inactivation by organic material. It is used for disinfecting hard surfaces, babies' feeding bottles, and food and dairy equipment, for treating water (p.1098), for soft contact lens care (p.1097), and in various commercial bleach detergents and scouring powders as a relatively stable source of chlorine.

Dichloroisocyanuric acid ($C_3HCl_2N_3O_3$ = 198.0), potassium dichloroisocyanurate (potassium troclosene; troclosene potassium, $C_3Cl_2KN_3O_3$ = 236.1), and trichloroisocyanuric acid (symclosene, $C_3Cl_3N_3O_3$ = 232.4) are similarly used.

Preparations

Proprietary Preparations (details are given in Part 3)
Aust.: Polyrinse Desinfektionssystem; ***Austral.:*** Milton Anti-Bacterial; Puritabs; Softab; ***Fr.:*** Milton; Polycare; Solusteril; ***Irl.:*** Aquatabs; Klorsept; Milton; Sterinova; ***Ital.:*** Dialster; Presept; ***UK:*** Milton; Presept.

Multi-ingredient: ***Irl.:*** Klor-Kleen.

Sodium Formaldehyde Sulphoxylate (6671-s)

Sodium Formaldehyde Sulfoxylate. Sodium hydroxymethanesulphinate dihydrate.

$CH_3NaO_3S,2H_2O$ = 154.1.
CAS — 149-44-0 (anhydrous sodium formaldehyde sulphoxylate); 6035-47-8 (sodium formaldehyde sulphoxylate, dihydrate).

Pharmacopoeias. In *Pol.* Also in *USNF.*

White crystals or hard white masses with an alliaceous odour. The USNF allows a suitable stabiliser, such as sodium carbonate. **Soluble** 1 in 3.4 of water, 1 in 510 of alcohol, 1 in 175 of chloroform, and 1 in 180 of ether. A 2% solution in water has a pH of 9.5 to 10.5. **Store** at 15° to 30°. Protect from light.

Sodium formaldehyde sulphoxylate is an antoxidant used as a preservative in pharmaceuticals. It has been used in the treatment of acute mercury poisoning (p.1602).

Preparations

Proprietary Preparations (details are given in Part 3)
Multi-ingredient: ***Fr.:*** Arthrodont.

Sodium Hypochlorite (2277-y)

$NaOCl,5H_2O$ = 164.5.
CAS — 7681-52-9.

Pharmacopoeias. Br., Fr., Jpn, Port., and *US* include sodium hypochlorite solutions.

Sodium hypochlorite pentahydrate contains about 43% of 'available chlorine' (see p.1110); anhydrous sodium hypochlorite contains about 95%.

Incompatibilities. The antimicrobial activity of hypochlorites is rapidly diminished in the presence of organic material; it is also pH dependent being greater in acid pH although hypochlorites are more stable at alkaline pH.

CAUTION. *Sodium hypochlorite solutions should not be mixed with solutions of strong acids or ammonia; the subsequent reactions release chlorine gas and chloramine gas, respectively.*

Stability. The stability of sodium hypochlorite solutions increases with pH, solutions of pH 10 or more being most stable.[1] Stability studies have shown that solutions providing 0.04 to 0.12% 'available chlorine' stored in amber glass bottles at room temperature could carry a 23-month expiry date.[2]

1. Bloomfield SF, Sizer TJ. Eusol BPC and other hypochlorite formulations used in hospitals. *Pharm J* 1985; **235:** 153–5 and 157.
2. Fabian TM, Walker SE. Stability of sodium hypochlorite solutions. *Am J Hosp Pharm* 1982; **39:** 1016–17.

Adverse Effects

Hypochlorite solutions release hypochlorous acid upon contact with gastric juice and acids, and ingestion causes irritation and corrosion of mucous membranes with pain and vomiting, oedema of the pharynx and larynx, and, rarely, perforation of the oesophagus and stomach. A fall in blood pressure, delirium, and coma may occur. Inhalation of hypochlorous fumes causes coughing and choking and may cause severe respiratory tract irritation and pulmonary oedema. Hypochlorite solutions may be irritating to the skin.

A patient who accidentally received an intravenous infusion of 150 mL of a 1% solution of sodium hypochlorite experienced a slow heart rate, mild hypotension, and increased respiratory rate. The slow heart rate persisted for 3 days but other parameters returned to normal after symptomatic treatment.[1]

1. Marroni M, Menichetti F. Accidental intravenous infusion of sodium hypochlorite. *DICP Ann Pharmacother* 1991; **25:** 1008–9.

For comment on the adverse effects of hypochlorite solutions on wound healing, see Disinfection: Wounds under Uses and Administration of Chlorine, p.1110.

Effects on the blood. An acute haemolytic crisis was reported in a child who had swum for about 4 hours in an indoor pool containing very high concentrations of sodium hypochlorite.[1] The child was subsequently found to have glucose-6-phosphate dehydrogenase deficiency.

1. Ong SJ, Kearney B. Local swimming pool and G-6-PD deficiency. *Med J Aust* 1994; **161:** 226–7.

Treatment of Adverse Effects

If sodium hypochlorite solution is ingested, water, milk, or other demulcents should be given; antacids and sodium thiosulphate 1 to 2.5% solution may be of value. If spilled on skin, washing with copious amounts of water is recommended.

Precautions

Topically applied hypochlorites may dissolve blood clots and cause bleeding.

Uses and Administration

Sodium hypochlorite is a disinfectant and antiseptic with the brief and rapid actions of chlorine (see p.1110). Powders and solutions are commonly used for the rapid disinfection of hard surfaces, food and dairy equipment, babies' feeding bottles, excreta, and water (p.1098). Solutions for use as domestic bleaches contain about 5% of hypochlorite. Only diluted solutions containing up to 0.5% of 'available chlorine' are suitable for use on the skin and in wounds (but see Wound Disinfection, p.1098).

Labarraque's Solution contains sodium hypochlorite with sodium chloride and an alkali and Eau de Javel is a potassium hypochlorite solution.

Preparations

BP 1998: Dilute Sodium Hypochlorite Solution; Strong Sodium Hypochlorite Solution;
USP 23: Sodium Hypochlorite Solution; Sodium Hypochlorite Topical Solution.

Proprietary Preparations (details are given in Part 3)
Austral.: Milton Anti-Bacterial; ***Belg.:*** Dakincooper; ***Canad.:*** Hygeol; ***Fr.:*** Dakin; Milton; ***Ger.:*** Maranon H; ***Irl.:*** Milton; ***Ital.:*** Milton; Naclon; Tiutol KF†; ***UK:*** Chlorasol; Milton.

Multi-ingredient: ***Fr.:*** Amukine.

Sodium Nitrate (13254-q)

E251; Natrii Nitras; Natrium Nitricum.
$NaNO_3$ = 84.99.
CAS — 7631-99-4.

NOTE. Crude sodium nitrate is known as Chile Saltpetre.
Pharmacopoeias. In *Pol.*

CAUTION. *Sodium nitrate has been used for the illicit preparation of explosives or fireworks; care is required with its supply.*

Sodium nitrate has similar actions to potassium nitrate (p.1123) and is used as a preservative in foods, particularly in meat products.

Crude sodium nitrate is used as a fertiliser.

Poisoning. A report[1] of 3 patients who developed cyanosis and methaemoglobinaemia after eating sausages which had been preserved mistakenly with a mixture of sodium nitrate and sodium nitrite rather than with potassium nitrate (saltpetre). The name saltpetre is used as a generic term for a number of potassium- or sodium-based preservatives used in food manufacture.

1. Kennedy N, *et al.* Faulty sausage production causing methaemoglobinaemia. *Arch Dis Child* 1997; **76:** 367–8.

Sodium Perborate (5908-g)

Natrii Perboras; Sod. Perbor.
$NaBO_2,H_2O_2,3H_2O$ = 153.9.
CAS — 7632-04-4 (anhydrous sodium perborate); 10042-94-1 (sodium perborate hydrate).

NOTE. Sodium Perborate Monohydrate is *USAN.*
Pharmacopoeias. In *Br.*

Odourless or almost odourless, colourless prismatic crystals or a white powder, stable in crystalline form. Sparingly **soluble** in water, with some decomposition. **Store** in airtight containers.

Adverse Effects

Frequent use of toothpowders containing sodium perborate may cause blistering and oedema. Hypertrophy of the papillae of the tongue has also been reported. The effects of swallowed sodium perborate are similar to those of boric acid (p.1554).

Uses and Administration

Sodium perborate is a mild disinfectant and deodorant. It readily releases oxygen in contact with oxidisable matter and has been used in aqueous solutions for purposes similar to weak solutions of hydrogen peroxide.

Sodium perborate has also been used, with calcium carbonate, as a toothpowder. A freshly prepared solution is used as a mouthwash.

The less soluble $NaBO_2,H_2O_2$ known as sodium perborate monohydrate is used similarly.

Preparations

Proprietary Preparations (details are given in Part 3)
Canad.: Amosan; ***Irl.:*** Bocasan; ***Ital.:*** Kavosan; Sekusept N; ***UK:*** Bocasan; ***USA:*** Amosan.

Multi-ingredient: ***Austral.:*** Amosan; ***Belg.:*** Sulfaryl; ***Fr.:*** Bactident; Hydralin; Mucosodine†; ***Ger.:*** Sekusept; ***Ital.:*** Borossigeno Plus Stomatologico; Gineosepta†; ***Switz.:*** Saltrates Rodell; ***USA:*** Trichotine.

Sorbates (12173-r)

Potassium Sorbate (6663-s)

E202; Kalii Sorbas. Potassium (*E,E*)-hexa-2,4-dienoate.
$C_6H_7KO_2$ = 150.2.
CAS — 590-00-1; 24634-61-5;.
Pharmacopoeias. In *Eur.* (see p.viii). Also in *USNF.*

White or almost white crystals, granules, or powder with a characteristic odour. Ph. Eur. **solubilities** are: very soluble in water; slightly soluble in alcohol. USNF solubilities are: soluble 1 in 4.5 of water and 1 in 35 of alcohol; very slightly soluble in chloroform and in ether. **Store** at a temperature not exceeding 40° in airtight containers. Protect from light. **Incompatibility** is discussed under Sorbic Acid, below.

Sorbic Acid (6679-k)

Acidum Sorbicum; E200. (*E,E*)-Hexa-2,4-dienoic acid.
$C_6H_8O_2$ = 112.1.
CAS — 22500-92-1.
Pharmacopoeias. In *Eur.* (see p.viii) and *Pol.* Also in *USNF.*

A free-flowing, white or almost white, crystalline powder with a characteristic odour. Ph. Eur. **solubilities** are: slightly soluble in water; freely soluble in alcohol and in ether. USNF solubilities are: soluble 1 in 1000 of water, 1 in 10 of alcohol, 1 in 8 of dehydrated alcohol, 1 in 15 of chloroform, 1 in 30 of ether, 1 in 8 of methyl alcohol, and 1 in 19 of propylene glycol. **Store** at a temperature not exceeding 40° in airtight containers. Protect from light.

Incompatibility. Sorbic acid can be inactivated by oxidation and to some extent by nonionic surfactants and plastics. Activity of the sorbates may be reduced by increases in pH.[1]

1. Weller PJ. Potassium sorbate. In: Wade A, Weller PJ, eds. *Handbook of pharmaceutical excipients.* 2nd ed. Washington and London: American Pharmaceutical Association and The Pharmaceutical Press, 1994: 390–1.

Adverse Effects and Precautions

The sorbates can be irritant and have caused contact dermatitis.

Hypersensitivity. References to allergic-type skin reactions[1] and non-allergic irritant-type reactions[2,3] with potassium sorbate or sorbic acid.

1. Saihan EM, Harman RRM. Contact sensitivity to sorbic acid in 'Unguentum Merck'. *Br J Dermatol* 1978; **99:** 583–4.
2. Soschin D, Leyden JJ. Sorbic acid-induced erythema and edema. *J Am Acad Dermatol* 1986; **14:** 234–41.
3. Fisher AA. Erythema limited to the face due to sorbic acid. *Cutis* 1987; **40:** 395–7.

Uses

Potassium sorbate and sorbic acid possess antifungal, and to a lesser extent antibacterial, activity. They are relatively ineffective above a pH of about 6.5. They are used as preservatives in pharmaceutical preparations in concentrations of up to 0.2%, in enteral formulas, foods, and in cosmetic preparations.

Sozoiodol Sodium (11613-r)

Sozoiodole Sodium. Sodium 2,6-diiodophenol-4-sulphonate.
$C_6H_3I_2NaO_4S$ = 448.0.
CAS — 554-71-2 (sozoiodolic acid); 515-44-6 (anhydrous sozoiodol sodium).

Sozoiodol Zinc (11614-f)

Sozoiodole Zinc. Zinc di(2,6-diiodophenol-4-sulphonate).
$C_{12}H_6I_4O_8S_2Zn$ = 915.3.
CAS — 547-41-1 (anhydrous sozoiodol zinc).

Sozoiodol contains iodine and the sodium and zinc salts have been used for their disinfectant properties.

Preparations

Proprietary Preparations (details are given in Part 3)
Multi-ingredient: ***Ger.:*** Animbo-Tinktur†; ***Ital.:*** Rinoleina Adulti†; Rinoleina Bambini†; ***Switz.:*** Euproctol.

Sulphites and Sulphur Dioxide

(12174-f)

Potassium Bisulphite (16966-k)

E228; Potassium Bisulfite; Potassium Hydrogen Sulphite.
$KHSO_3$ = 120.2.
CAS — 7773-03-7.

Potassium Metabisulphite (6662-p)

Dipotassium Pyrosulphite; E224; Potassium Metabisulfite; Potassium Pyrosulphite.
$K_2S_2O_5$ = 222.3.
CAS — 16731-55-8.
Pharmacopoeias. In *Fr.* Also in *USNF.*

White or colourless, crystals, crystalline powder, or granules, usually with an odour of sulphur dioxide. **Soluble** in water; practically insoluble in alcohol. Gradually oxidises in air to the sulphate. **Store** in well-filled airtight containers. **Incompatibility** is discussed under Sulphur Dioxide, below.

Sodium Bisulphite (9880-t)

E222; Sodium Bisulfite; Sodium Hydrogen Sulphite.
$NaHSO_3$ = 104.1.
CAS — 7631-90-5.
Pharmacopoeias. In *Jpn* which has Sodium Bisulfite, described as consisting of the acid sulphite ($NaHSO_3$ = 104.1) and the metabisulphite in varying proportions.

Sodium Metabisulphite (6673-e)

Disodium Pyrosulphite; E223; Natrii Disulfis; Natrii Metabisulfis; Sodium Disulphite; Sodium Metabisulfite; Sodium Pyrosulphite.
$Na_2S_2O_5$ = 190.1.
CAS — 7681-57-4.
Pharmacopoeias. In *Chin., Eur.* (see p.viii), *Jpn,* and *Pol.* Also in *USNF.*

Colourless or white crystals or a white or yellowish crystalline powder with an odour of sulphur dioxide. On exposure to air and moisture, it is slowly oxidised to the sulphate with disintegration of the crystals. Freely **soluble** in water; slightly soluble in alcohol; freely soluble in glycerol. A 5% solution in water has a pH of 3.5 to 5.0. **Store** at a temperature not exceeding 40° in well-filled airtight containers. Protect from light. **Incompatibility** is discussed under Sulphur Dioxide, below.

Sodium Sulphite (6678-c)

Anhydrous Sodium Sulphite; E221; Exsiccated Sodium Sulphite; Natrii Sulfis Anhydricus; Natrii Sulfis Siccatus; Natrii Sulphis; Sodium Sulfite.

Na_2SO_3 = 126.0.

CAS — 7757-83-7.

Pharmacopoeias. In *Eur.* (see p.viii), *Jpn,* and *Pol.*

Eur. and *Pol.* also include Sodium Sulphite Heptahydrate.

A white powder (anhydrous) or colourless crystals (heptahydrate). Freely **soluble** in water; very slightly soluble in alcohol. Anhydrous sodium sulphite should be **stored** in airtight containers. **Incompatibility** is discussed under Sulphur Dioxide, below.

Sulphur Dioxide (6680-w)

E220; Sulfur Dioxide.

SO_2 = 64.06.

CAS — 7446-09-5.

Pharmacopoeias. In *USNF.*

A colourless non-flammable gas with a strong suffocating odour characteristic of burning sulphur. It condenses readily under pressure to a colourless liquid which boils at about −10° and has a wt per mL of about 1.5 g. **Soluble** 36 in 1 of water and 114 in 1 of alcohol by vol. at 20° and normal pressure; soluble in chloroform and in ether. **Store** in cylinders. It is usually packaged under pressure in liquid form.

Incompatibilities. Sulphite antoxidants can react with sympathomimetics such as adrenaline leading to their inactivation.[1] Measures need to be taken to prevent such a reaction if sulphites have to be used. Cisplatin is another compound that can be inactivated.[2] Phenylmercuric nitrate may be inactivated or its activity enhanced.[3,4] Sulphites are reported to react with chloramphenicol.[1] Hydrogen peroxide generation has been reported on exposure to light of amino acid solutions containing sulphites.[5] When used in foods there can be a noticeable taste and a reduction in thiamine content.[6] Stability is affected by air and moisture,[7] and there is decomposition at very low pH.[7] There can be adsorption on to rubber closures.[8]

1. Higuchi T, Schroeter LC. Reactivity of bisulfite with a number of pharmaceuticals. *J Am Pharm Assoc (Sci)* 1959; **48:** 535–40.
2. Garren KW, Repta AJ. Incompatibility of cisplatin and Reglan Injectable. *Int J Pharmaceutics* 1985; **24:** 91–9.
3. Richards RME, Reary JME. Changes in antibacterial activity of thiomersal and PMN on autoclaving with certain adjuvants. *J Pharm Pharmacol* 1972; **24** (suppl): 84P–89P.
4. Collins AJ, *et al.* Incompatibility of phenylmercuric acetate with sodium metabisulphite in eye drop formulations. *J Pharm Pharmacol* 1985; **37** (suppl): 123P.
5. Brawley V, *et al.* Effect of sodium metabisulfite on hydrogen peroxide production in light-exposed pediatric parenteral amino acid solutions. *Am J Health-Syst Pharm* 1998; **55:** 1288–92.
6. FAO/WHO. Evaluation of the toxicity of a number of antimicrobials and antioxidants: sixth report of the joint FAO/WHO expert committee on food additives. *WHO Tech Rep Ser 228* 1962.
7. Stewart JT. Sodium metabisulfite. In: Wade A, Weller PJ, eds. *Handbook of pharmaceutical excipients.* 2nd ed. Washington and London: American Pharmaceutical Association and The Pharmaceutical Press, 1994: 451–3.
8. Schroeter LC. Sulfurous acid salts as pharmaceutical antioxidants. *J Pharm Sci* 1961; **50:** 891–901.

Adverse Effects and Precautions

Gastric irritation due to liberation of sulphurous acid can follow ingestion of sodium metabisulphite and other sulphites. Large doses of sulphites may cause gastro-intestinal upsets, respiratory or circulatory failure, and central nervous system disturbances.

Concentrated solutions of salts of sulphurous acid are irritant to skin and mucous membranes.

Sulphur dioxide is highly irritant to the eyes, skin, and mucous membranes. Inhalation results in irritation of the respiratory tract which may lead to bronchoconstriction and pulmonary oedema; very high concentrations may cause respiratory arrest and asphyxia. Contact with liquid sulphur dioxide results in acid burns.

Allergic reactions including anaphylaxis and deaths have been reported.

Hypersensitivity. Hypersensitivity reactions including bronchospasm, anaphylaxis, and some deaths have occurred in subjects, especially those with a history of asthma or atopic allergy, exposed to sulphites used as preservatives in foods.[1] These reactions have led to restrictions by the FDA on such use.[2] There have been case reports of reactions to sulphites in drugs;[3-7] such reports are considered to be few in number and the FDA has not extended the restriction on sulphites in foods to apply to their use in drugs since it was felt that in certain medications there was no suitable alternative to a sulphite.[2] It was even accepted that adrenaline recommended for use in treating allergic reactions could itself contain sulphite and that its presence should not preclude use of the adrenaline preparation even in sulphite-sensitive patients.[2]

1. Anonymous. Sulfites in drugs and food. *Med Lett Drugs Ther* 1986; **28:** 74–5.
2. Anonymous. Warning for prescription drugs containing sulfites. *FDA Drug Bull* 1987; **17:** 2–3.
3. Baker GJ, *et al.* Bronchospasm induced by metabisulphite-containing foods and drugs. *Med J Aust* 1981; **ii:** 614–17.
4. Twarog FJ, Leung DYM. Anaphylaxis to a component of isoetharine (sodium bisulfite). *JAMA* 1982; **248:** 2030–1.
5. Koepke JW, *et al.* Dose-dependent bronchospasm from sulfites in isoetharine. *JAMA* 1984; **251:** 2982–3.
6. Mikolich DJ, McCloskey WW. Suspected gentamicin allergy could be sulfite sensitivity. *Clin Pharm* 1988; **7:** 269.
7. Deziel-Evans LM, Hussey WC. Possible sulfite sensitivity with gentamicin infusion. *DICP Ann Pharmacother* 1989; **23:** 1032–3.

Pharmacokinetics

Sulphites and metabisulphites are oxidised in the body to sulphate and excreted in the urine. Any sulphurous acid or sulphur dioxide is also converted to sulphate.

Uses

Sulphur dioxide and the sulphites which produce sulphur dioxide and sulphurous acid are strong reducing agents and are used as antoxidants. Concentrations of the sulphites in pharmaceutical preparations have ranged from 0.01 to 1.0%. At higher concentrations and preferably at an acid pH sulphur dioxide and the sulphites exhibit antimicrobial activity.

Sulphur dioxide and the sulphites are used in the food industry as antoxidants, antimicrobial preservatives, and anti-browning agents. They are used in wine making where tabletted sodium metabisulphite is commonly known as Campden Tablets. Concentrations of sulphites above 500 ppm impart a noticeable unpleasant taste to preparations. There is concern at the risk of severe allergic reactions arising from the use of sulphites in foods (see Hypersensitivity, above).

Tar Acids (2279-z)

Tar acids are phenolic substances derived from the distillation of coal tar or petroleum fractions. The lowest boiling fraction of coal tar, distilling at 188° to 205°, consists of mixed cresol isomers. The middle fraction, known as 'cresylic acids', distils at 205° to 230° and consists of cresols and xylenols. The 'high-boiling tar acids', distilling at 230° to 290°, consist mainly of alkyl homologues of phenol, with naphthalenes and other hydrocarbons. Cresol is described on p.1111.

Black Fluids are homogeneous solutions of coal-tar acids, or similar acids derived from petroleum, or any mixture of these, with or without hydrocarbons and with a suitable emulsifying agent. **White Fluids** are finely dispersed emulsions of coal-tar acids, or similar acids derived from petroleum, or any mixture of these, with or without hydrocarbons. **Modified Black Fluids** and **Modified White Fluids** may contain, as an addition, any other active ingredients, but if these are used, the type and amount must be disclosed, if required.

Adverse Effects and Treatment

As for Phenol, p.1121.

Tar acids are generally very irritant and corrosive to the skin, even when diluted to concentrations used for disinfection.

A report of fatal self-poisoning in a 59-year-old man following the ingestion of approximately 250 mL of a xylenol-containing disinfectant (Stericol Hospital Disinfectant).[1]

1. Watson ID, *et al.* Fatal xylenol self-poisoning. *Postgrad Med J* 1986; **62:** 411–12.

Uses

Tar acids are phenolic disinfectants used in the preparation of a range of fluids of varied activity used for household and general disinfection purposes.

Hydrocarbons are often used to enhance the activity of the tar acids in disinfectant fluids; they also help to reduce crystallisation of phenols.

Preparations

Proprietary Preparations (details are given in Part 3)
UK: Clearsol; Cresolox; Printol; Sterilite; Sudol.

Tertiary Butylhydroquinone (9873-x)

TBHQ. 2-*tert*-butylhydroquinone.

$C_{10}H_{14}O_2$ = 166.2.

CAS — 1948-33-0.

Tertiary butylhydroquinone is an antoxidant preservative used in foods. It has some antimicrobial activity.

Tetrabromocresol (16356-j)

3,4,5,6-Tetrabromo-*o*-cresol.

$C_7H_4Br_4O$ = 423.7.

Tetrabromocresol is a brominated phenolic antiseptic. It is used for hand disinfection and is applied topically for the treatment of fungal infections of the skin.

Preparations

Proprietary Preparations (details are given in Part 3)

Multi-ingredient: ***Austral.:*** Pedoz; ***Belg.:*** Desderman†; ***Ger.:*** Desderman; Gehwol Fungizid; Gehwol Fungizid Creme N.

Tetraglycine Hydroperiodide (17597-c)

$C_{16}H_{42}I_7N_8O_{16}$ = 1490.9.

CAS — 7097-60-1.

Tetraglycine hydroperiodide is an iodine-based disinfectant used in the treatment of drinking water (p.1098).

Preparations

Proprietary Preparations (details are given in Part 3)
USA: Potable Aqua.

Thiomersal (2281-s)

Thiomersal *(BAN, rINN).*

Mercurothiolate; Mercurothiolate Sodique; Sodium Ethyl Mercurithiosalicylate; Thimerosal; Thiomersalate. Sodium (2-carboxyphenylthio)ethylmercury.

$C_9H_9HgNaO_2S$ = 404.8.

CAS — 54-64-8.

Pharmacopoeias. In *Br., Fr., It., Pol., Swiss,* and *US.*

A light cream-coloured crystalline powder with a slight characteristic odour. **Soluble** 1 in 1 of water and 1 in 12 of alcohol; practically insoluble in ether. A 1% solution in water has a pH of 6 to 8. **Store** in airtight containers. Protect from light.

Incompatible with acids, metal ions, and iodine. It forms precipitates with many alkaloids. The rate of oxidation of thiomersal in solution is greatly increased by traces of copper ions. In slightly acid solution thiomersal may be precipitated as the corresponding acid which undergoes slow decomposition with the formation of insoluble products. The activity of thiomersal may also be reduced by boric acid, edetic acid, or sodium thiosulphate or the presence of blood or organic matter. Thiomersal may be adsorbed by plastic or rubber packaging materials.

References to incompatibilities.

1. Richards RME, Reary JME. Changes in antibacterial activity of thiomersal and PMN on autoclaving with certain adjuvants. *J Pharm Pharmacol* 1972; **24** (suppl): 84P–89P.
2. Reader MJ. Influence of isotonic agents on the stability of thimerosal in ophthalmic formulations. *J Pharm Sci* 1984; **73:** 840–1.
3. Morton DJ. EDTA reduces antimicrobial efficacy of thiomersal. *Int J Pharmaceutics* 1985; **23:** 357–8.

Adverse Effects, Treatment, and Precautions

As for Mercury, p.1601.

Hypersensitivity reactions occasionally occur. Allergic conjunctivitis has been reported.

Appropriate measures should be taken to prevent contamination of thiomersal preparations during storage or dilution.

Serious adverse effects have followed parenteral and topical use of thiomersal. Six poisonings (5 fatal) resulted from the use of 1000 times the normal concentration of thiomersal in a preparation of chloramphenicol for intramuscular injection.[1] Thiomersal used in topical antiseptic preparations was found to be toxic to epidermal cells.[2] Following the death of 10 of 13 children as a result of treatment of omphaloceles (umbilical hernia) with a tincture of thiomersal, it was recommended that organic mercurial disinfectants be heavily restricted or withdrawn from hospital use as absorption occurred readily through intact membranes.[3]

1. Axton JHM. Six cases of poisoning after a parenteral organic mercurial compound (Merthiolate). *Postgrad Med J* 1972; **48:** 417–21.
2. Anonymous. Topical antiseptics and antibiotics: organic mercurials. *Med Lett Drugs Ther* 1977; **19:** 83.
3. Fagan DG, *et al.* Organ mercury levels in infants with omphaloceles treated with organic mercurial antiseptic. *Arch Dis Child* 1977; **52:** 962–4.

Hypersensitivity. The safety of thiomersal as a preservative for vaccines, eye and nose drops, and contact lens solutions has been questioned.[1] False positive reactions to old tuberculin have been attributed to the presence of thiomersal[2] and there have been reports of severe reactions to vaccines preserved with thiomersal.[3,4] Delayed hypersensitivity reactions have been associated with the use of thiomersal in contact lens solutions.[5] In one clinic, 7 of 116 patients with chronic blepharitis, who had never worn contact lenses, were found to be already sensitised to thiomersal.[1] Furthermore there has been an isolated report of acute laryngeal obstruction in a patient previously sensitised to thiomersal who used a throat spray preserved with thiomersal.[6]

1. Seal D, *et al.* The case against thiomersal. *Lancet* 1991; **338:** 316–16.
2. Hansson H, Möller H. Intracutaneous test reactions to tuberculin containing merthiolate as a preservative. *Scand J Infect Dis* 1971; **3:** 169–72.
3. Cox NH, Morley WN. Vaccination reactions and thiomersal. *Br Med J* 1987; **294:** 250.
4. Noel I, *et al.* Hypersensitivity to thiomersal in hepatitis B vaccine. *Lancet* 1991; **338:** 705.
5. Wilson LA, *et al.* Delayed hypersensitivity to thiomersal in soft contact lens wearers. *Ophthalmology* 1981; **88:** 804–9.
6. Maibach H. Acute laryngeal obstruction presumed secondary to thiomersal (merthiolate) delayed hypersensitivity. *Contact Dermatitis* 1975; **1:** 221–2.

Interactions

Nine patients using a contact lens solution containing 0.004% thiomersal developed varying degrees of ocular irritation after taking oral tetracyclines concurrently. Exposure to either the tetracyclines or thiomersal alone did not cause the response.[1]

1. Crook TG, Freeman JJ. Reactions induced by the concurrent use of thimerosal and tetracycline. *Am J Optom Physiol Opt* 1983; **60:** 759–61.

Uses and Administration

Thiomersal is a bacteriostatic and fungistatic mercurial antiseptic that has been applied topically usually in a concentration of 0.1%.

Thiomersal, 0.01 to 0.02%, is used as a preservative in biological and pharmaceutical products. It has also been used to preserve solutions used in the care of contact lenses (p.1097).

Preparations

USP 23: Thimerosal Tincture; Thimerosal Topical Aerosol; Thimerosal Topical Solution.

Proprietary Preparations (details are given in Part 3)
Fr.: Vitaseptol; ***Ital.:*** Merthiolate†; ***S.Afr.:*** Merthiolate; ***Spain:*** Merthiolate†; Topicaldermo†; ***USA:*** Aeroaid; Mersol.

Multi-ingredient: ***Austral.:*** Hexidin; Steri-Sal II†; ***Fr.:*** Collyrex; Dermachrome; ***Spain:*** Deltacina; Proskin; Tintu. Mertiolato Asens.

Thymol (2282-w)

Acido Timico; Isopropylmetacresol; Thymolum; Timol. 2-Isopropyl-5-methylphenol.
$C_{10}H_{14}O = 150.2.$
CAS — 89-83-8.
Pharmacopoeias. In *Eur.* (see p.viii), *Jpn,* and *Pol.* Also in *USNF.*

Colourless, often large, crystals or white crystalline powder with an aromatic thyme-like odour. The melting range is 48° to 52°; when melted it remains liquid at a considerably lower temperature.

Ph. Eur. **solubilities** are: very slightly soluble in water; very soluble in alcohol, and in ether; freely soluble in volatile and in fixed oils; sparingly soluble in glycerol; dissolves in dilute solutions of alkali hydroxides. USNF solubilities are: soluble 1 in 1000 of water, 1 in 1 of alcohol, 1 in 1 of chloroform, 1 in 1.5 of ether, and 1 in 2 of olive oil; soluble in glacial acetic acid and in fixed and volatile oils. **Store** in airtight containers. Protect from light. **Incompatibilities.** The antimicrobial activity of thymol is diminished through combination with protein.

Adverse Effects, Treatment, and Precautions

As for Phenol, p.1121.

When ingested, thymol is less toxic than phenol. It is irritant to the gastric mucosa. Fats and alcohol increase absorption and aggravate the toxic symptoms.

Appropriate measures should be taken to avoid contamination of thymol preparations during storage or dilution.

Contact allergy to a heparinoid cream was due to an allergen formed by the reaction between thymol and the degradation products of a triazine derivative, both present as preservatives.[1]

1. Smeenk G, *et al.* Contact allergy to a reaction product in Hirudoid cream: an example of compound allergy. *Br J Dermatol* 1987; **116:** 223–31.

Uses and Administration

Thymol is a phenolic antiseptic with antibacterial and antifungal activity. It is more powerful than phenol but its use is limited by its low solubility in water, irritancy, and susceptibility to protein.

Thymol is used chiefly as a deodorant in mouthwashes and gargles such as Compound Thymol Glycerin (BP 1988), an aqueous mixture of thymol 0.05% and glycerol 10% with colouring and flavouring, which is diluted with about 3 times its volume of warm water before use. Thymol has been used topically in the treatment of skin disorders and is also inhaled, with other volatile substances, for colds, coughs, and associated respiratory disorders.

Thymol (0.01%) is added as an antoxidant to halothane, trichloroethylene, and tetrachloroethylene.

Thymol iodide is used in preparations for dental hygiene.

Preparations

Proprietary Preparations (details are given in Part 3)
Ger.: Medophyll; ***Ital.:*** Resina Carbolica Dentilin; ***Switz.:*** Intrasol.

Multi-ingredient: ***Aust.:*** Alpicort†; Criniton; DDD; Kinder Luuf; Luuf Balsam; Pe-Ce; Recessan; Resol; Spasmo Claim; Thrombocid; Wick Vaporub; ***Austral.:*** BFI; Gartech; Logicin Chest Rub; Sigma Relief Chest Rub†; SM-33; ***Belg.:*** Balsoclase; Borostyrol; Dentophar; Pelarol†; Perubore; Vicks Vaporub; ***Canad.:*** Antiseptic Mouthwash; Boil Ease; Buckley's White Rub; Carboseptol; Listerine; Mouthwash Antiseptic & Gargle; Nasal Jelly; Pastilles Valda; Thermo-Gel; Valda; Vap Air; Vaporisateur Medicamente; Vaporizing Ointment; ***Fr.:*** Balseptol†; Borostyrol; Glyco-Thymoline; Ophtalmine; Oxy-thymoline†; Perubore; Stom-Antiba†; Tuberol†; Valda; Vicks Pastilles†; Vicks Vaporub; Vicks vitamine C pastilles†; ***Ger.:*** Adebilan†; Alferm; Animbo-Tinktur†; Bormelin†; Cobed†; Criniton; Customed; DDD; Denosol; Influsanbalm†; Kamistad†; Lyobalsam N ohne Menthol†; Lyobalsam N†; Mycatox N†; Oestrugol N; Optipect†; Parodontal F5 med; Prolugol-liquid N†; Pulmotin-N; Pumilen-Balsam†; Pumilen-N; Retterspitz Ausserlich; Retterspitz Gelee; Retterspitz Heilsalbe; Retterspitz Quick; Risocon†; Salviathymol N; Sedotussin Expectorans; Thymitussin†; Zynedo-B†; Zynedo-K†; ***Irl.:*** Karvol; Listerine; Valda†; ***Ital.:*** Eucalipto Composto; Florigien; Golosan†; Neoperborina Gola†; Pinselina Dr. Knapp; Rinoleina Adulti†; Rinoleina Bambini†; Rinos; Rinostil; Salonpas; ***Neth.:*** Vicks Vaporub; ***S.Afr.:*** Karvol; Oramond†; ***Spain:*** Cloroboral; Co Bucal; Homocodeina Timol†; Kneipp Balsamo; Mentobox†; Mentol Sedans Sulfamidad†; Oxitimol†; Pastillas Vicks Mentol†; Piorlis; Pomada Balsamica; Sudosin; Thrombocid; Vicks Vaporub; ***Swed.:*** Vicks Vaporub; ***Switz.:*** Adrectal; Asphaline; Borostyrol N; Butaparin; Cresophene; Demovarin; Dental-Phenjoca; Endomethasone; Furodermal; Huile analgesique "Polar-Bar"; Perubare; Rapura; Roliwol; Sedasept; Sedotussin; Spirogel; Stix†; Thrombocid; Tumarol; Vicks Vaporub; ***UK:*** Boots Vapour Rub; Chloraseptic†; DDD; Dragon Balm; Eftab; Karvol; Listerine Antiseptic Mouthwash; Potter's Pastilles; Valda; ***USA:*** BFI; Boil Ease; Cool-Mint Listerine; FreshBurst Listerine; Listerine; Massengill; Phenaseptic†; Vicks Menthol Cough Drops; Zonite.

Toloconium Methylsulphate (13361-w)

Toloconium Metilsulfate *(rINN).* Trimethyl[1-(*p*-tolyl)dodecyl]ammonium methylsulphate.
$C_{23}H_{43}NO_4S = 429.7.$
CAS — 552-92-1.

Toloconium methylsulphate is a quaternary ammonium antiseptic which has been used for disinfection of skin, mucous membranes, and surgical instruments.

Preparations

Proprietary Preparations (details are given in Part 3)
Ital.: Desogen; ***Switz.:*** Desogene†.

Triclocarban (2286-j)

Triclocarban *(USAN, rINN).*
NSC-72005; TCC; 3,4,4′-Trichlorocarbanilide. 1-(4-Chlorophenyl)-3-(3,4-dichlorophenyl)urea.
$C_{13}H_9Cl_3N_2O = 315.6.$
CAS — 101-20-2.

Adverse Effects and Precautions

When subjected to prolonged high temperatures triclocarban can decompose to form toxic chloroanilines, which can be absorbed through the skin and cause methaemoglobinaemia. Mild photosensitivity has been seen in patch testing.

Uses and Administration

Triclocarban is an anilide antiseptic. It is bacteriostatic against Gram-positive organisms in high dilutions but is less effective against Gram-negative organisms and some fungi. It is used in antiperspirants and soaps for disinfection of skin and mucous membranes.

Preparations

Proprietary Preparations (details are given in Part 3)
Belg.: Solubacter†; ***Fr.:*** Cutisan; Nobacter; Solubacter; ***Irl.:*** Valderma; ***Ital.:*** Citrosil Sapone; Procutene†; Sangen Sapone Disinfettante; ***Spain:*** Genoface†; ***UK:*** Valderma Soap; ***USA:*** Cuticura.

Multi-ingredient: ***Canad.:*** Bebia Antiseptic Soap†; ***Fr.:*** Cutisan a l'Hydrocortisone†; Septivon; ***Ger.:*** Ansudor; ***Spain:*** Cusiter; ***Switz.:*** Septivon N; Undex†.

Triclosan (2287-z)

Triclosan *(BAN, USAN, rINN).*
CH-3565; Cloxifenol. 5-Chloro-2-(2,4-dichlorophenoxy)phenol; 2,4,4′-Trichloro-2′-hydroxydiphenyl ether.
$C_{12}H_7Cl_3O_2 = 289.5.$
CAS — 3380-34-5.
Pharmacopoeias. In *US.*

A fine whitish crystalline powder. Practically **insoluble** in water; soluble in alcohol, in acetone, and in methyl alcohol; slightly soluble in petroleum spirit. M.p. about 57°. **Store** in airtight containers. Protect from light.

Triclosan is a chlorinated bisphenol antiseptic, effective against Gram-positive and most Gram-negative bacteria but with variable or poor activity against *Pseudomonas* spp. It is also active against fungi. It is used in soaps, creams and solutions in concentrations of up to 2% for disinfection of the hands and wounds and for disinfection of the skin prior to surgery, injections, or venepuncture. It is also used in oral hygiene products and in preparations for acne. There have been isolated reports of contact dermatitis.

Reports of control of methicillin-resistant *Staphylococcus aureus* (MRSA) infection in surgical units involving handwashing and bathing with triclosan.[1-3] Triclosan resistance has been reported.[4,5]

1. Bartzokas CA, *et al.* Control and eradication of methicillin-resistant Staphylococcus aureus on a surgical unit. *N Engl J Med* 1984; **311:** 1422–5.
2. Bartzokas CA. Eradication of resistant Staphylococcus aureus on a surgical unit. *N Engl J Med* 1985; **312:** 858–9.
3. Brady LM, *et al.* Successful control of endemic MRSA in a cardiothoracic surgical unit. *Med J Aust* 1990; **152:** 240–5.
4. Cookson BD, *et al.* Transferable resistance to triclosan in MRSA. *Lancet* 1991; **337:** 1548–9.
5. Sasatsu M, *et al.* Triclosan-resistant Staphylococcus aureus. *Lancet* 1993; **341:** 756. Correction. *ibid.* **342:** 248.

Preparations

Proprietary Preparations (details are given in Part 3)
Austral.: Dettol Liquid Wash; Gamophen; Johnson's Clean & Clear Foaming Facial Wash; Johnson's Clean & Clear Medicated Cleansing Bar; Liquid Soap Pre-Op; Microshield T; Neutrogena Acne Skin Cleanser; Novaderm†; Oxy Skin Wash; Phisohex Face Wash; Sapoderm; Softwash; Solyptol; ***Canad.:*** Adasept; Clean & Clear Antibacterial Foam Cleanser; Oxy Gentle; Oxy Medicated Soap; Promani; Tersaseptic; ***Ital.:*** Dermico†; Dermo-Steril; Geroderm; Ippi Verde; Irgaman; Lactacyd Antibatterico; Till; ***Switz.:*** Cliniderm; Lipo Sol; Procoutol; Shampooing extra-doux; ***UK:*** Aquasept; Clearasil Medicated Moisturiser; Clearasil Soap; Dettol†; Gamophen; Oxy Facial Wash; Ster-Zac; Triclosept†; ***USA:*** Ambi 10; Clearasil Daily Face Wash; no more germies†; Oxy Medicated Soap; Septi-Soft; Septisol; Stri-Dex Antibacterial Cleansing; Stridex Face Wash.

Multi-ingredient: ***Austral.:*** Clearasil Acne Treatment Cream; Clearasil Medicated Foam†; Dettol; Microshield PVP Plus; Novasrub†; Oilatum Plus; Z-Acne†; ***Canad.:*** Adasept; Bebia Antiseptic Soap†; Clearasil Acne Cream; Dermolan†; Solarcaine; Tersac; ***Fr.:*** Clearasil Cream†; ***Ger.:*** Rutisept Extra; Sicorten Plus; ***Irl.:*** Dettol; ***Ital.:*** Angstrom Viso/Labbra Alta Protezione; Dermogamma†; Dopo Pik; Geroderm Zolfo; Lenisun†; Levaknel; Neolog†; Plax; Steril Zeta; ***Norw.:*** Logamel†; ***S.Afr.:*** Sicorten Plus†; Tantol Skin Cleanser; ***Spain:*** Anti-Acne; Logamel†; Poliglicol Anti Acne; Sicorten Plus; ***Switz.:*** Acne Creme; Acne Gel; Acne Lotion; Acnidazil†; Antebor N; Clearasil†; Keroderm; Locacorten Triclosan; Logamel†; Pixor Stick Anti-acne N; Saltrates; Sebo Creme; Sebo Shampooing; Sicorten Plus; Sulgan; Teerol-H; Tretinoine; Turexan Emulsion; Undex†; ***UK:*** Actibrush; Clearasil Treatment Cream; Dentyl pH; Dettol; Germolene; Manusept; Oilatum Plus; Oxy Clean Facial Scrub; Oxy Cleanser; Oxy Duo Pads; Solarcaine; TCP; ***USA:*** Clearasil Antibacterial; Oxy ResiDon't†; Solarcaine.

Urea Hydrogen Peroxide (5910-d)

Carbamide Peroxide; Hydroperite; Urea Peroxide.
$NH_2.CO.NH_2,H_2O_2 = 94.07.$
CAS — 124-43-6.
Pharmacopoeias. In *US.*

Store in airtight containers at a temperature not exceeding 40°. Protect from light.

Urea hydrogen peroxide consists of hydrogen peroxide and urea in equimolecular proportions. It is used for the extemporaneous preparation of hydrogen peroxide. It has been employed for infections of the ear, mouth, and skin and for softening ear wax.

Preparations

USP 23: Carbamide Peroxide Topical Solution.

Proprietary Preparations (details are given in Part 3)
Austral.: Ear Clear; ***Canad.:*** Murine; ***Irl.:*** Exterol; ***Ital.:*** Debrox; Dermoxyl; Ginoxil; ***UK:*** Exterol; Otex; ***USA:*** Auro; Debrox; ERO; Gly-Oxide; Mollifene; Murine; Orajel Perioseptic; Proxigel.

Zinc Peroxide (5912-h)

CAS — 1314-22-3.

The action of zinc peroxide is similar to that of hydrogen peroxide (p.1116). Applied locally it has been used for disinfecting and deodorising burns, wounds and various ulcers and lesions.

Preparations

Proprietary Preparations (details are given in Part 3)
Canad.: Neoderm.

Multi-ingredient: ***Fr.:*** Bioxyol; Ektogan; ***Ital.:*** Ektogan; ***Switz.:*** Baume†.

Dopaminergics

Dopamine is a key neurotransmitter in the CNS; in particular, striatal dopamine depletion is associated with the clinical condition of parkinsonism. Dopamine also inhibits prolactin release from the pituitary and is believed to be the prolactin-release inhibiting factor (PRIF or PIF); its deficiency here is associated with conditions characterised by hyperprolactinaemia.

Accordingly, drugs which replenish central dopamine or which themselves can act as stimulants of dopamine receptors (dopamine agonists), may alleviate the symptoms of parkinsonism (see below), hyperprolactinaemia (p.1238), and related disorders.

At least 5 subtypes of dopamine receptor are thought to exist: D_1 receptors, which appear to stimulate adenylate cyclase activity; D_2 receptors, which activate various systems including inhibition of adenylate cyclase activity; D_3, D_4, and D_5 receptors have been less well studied. D_2 receptors have been implicated in the pathophysiology of parkinsonism and schizophrenia.

Dopaminergics, or drugs that enhance their actions, described in this chapter include:

- levodopa, which is converted by decarboxylation into dopamine in the body, and which, unlike dopamine itself, can penetrate the blood-brain barrier hence supplying a source of dopamine to the brain
- the peripheral dopa-decarboxylase inhibitors, benserazide and carbidopa, which have no antiparkinsonian action of their own but enhance the action of levodopa
- apomorphine, which is structurally related to dopamine and acts as a dopamine agonist
- the adamantanamines, amantadine and memantine, which may augment dopaminergic activity
- the ergot derivatives, bromocriptine, cabergoline, lysuride, and pergolide, which act as dopamine agonists
- the specific monoamine oxidase type B inhibitor, selegiline, which enhances the action of dopamine and levodopa
- the catechol-*O*-methyltransferase inhibitors (COMT-inhibitors), entacapone and tolcapone, which enhance the action of levodopa
- various other non-ergot dopamine agonists, such as naxagolide, piribedil, pramipexole, quinagolide, and ropinirole.

Parkinsonism

The syndrome of parkinsonism is characterised by tremor, rigidity, akinesia or bradykinesia, and loss of postural reflexes. It may be classified into primary (idiopathic) parkinsonism, usually referred to as Parkinson's disease (formerly paralysis agitans); secondary (acquired) parkinsonism, including postencephalitic parkinsonism, drug-induced parkinsonism, and symptoms associated with manganese poisoning; and 'parkinsonism-plus' syndromes where parkinsonism is a feature of other degenerative diseases of the CNS, such as progressive supranuclear palsy and multiple system atrophy. 'Arteriosclerotic parkinsonism' has been used to describe parkinsonism associated with cerebrovascular disease although this may be confusing since vascular brain damage is not a cause of Parkinson's disease. The term parkinsonism is often used for the idiopathic form, that is, Parkinson's disease.

In parkinsonism there is reduced dopamine activity in the brain. Parkinson's disease and postencephalitic parkinsonism have been attributed primarily to depletion of striatal dopamine in the basal ganglia as a result of the loss of neurones in the substantia nigra. Striatal dopamine deficiency results in loss of the normal functional balance between dopaminergic and cholinergic activity and treatment aims to increase the former and/or decrease the latter.

The cause of Parkinson's disease is not established although environmental and genetic factors superimposed on a background of neuronal loss related to ageing has been postulated. Great interest was aroused by the discovery that MPTP (1-methyl-4-phenyl-1,2,3,6-tetrahydropyridine), a contaminant of an illicitly produced pethidine analogue MPPP (1-methyl-4-phenyl-4-propionoxypiperidine), caused irreversible parkinsonism which had a pathology similar to that of Parkinson's disease and likewise responded to treatment with levodopa. *Animal* studies revealed that MPTP was converted by monoamine oxidase B to the neurotoxic methylphenylpyridinium ion which was selectively concentrated in dopaminergic neurones in the substantia nigra. Of those biochemical mechanisms proposed as possibly being involved in the pathogenesis of Parkinson's disease the most prominent has been the oxidant stress hypothesis. Proponents of this theory have postulated that free radicals produced during normal metabolism of dopamine in the brain by monoamine oxidase B might be neurotoxic to dopaminergic neurones in the substantia nigra. This has led to concern over the possibility that administration of levodopa, by increasing the supply of dopamine, might therefore exacerbate neurodegeneration and hasten the progression of Parkinson's disease but compelling evidence of such an effect is lacking.

Drug-induced parkinsonism can arise from depletion of presynaptic dopamine as occurs with drugs such as reserpine and tetrabenazine or from blockade of postsynaptic dopamine receptors in the striatum by antipsychotics and some antiemetics such as metoclopramide. It is generally reversible on drug withdrawal or dose reduction and may sometimes disappear gradually despite continuous drug therapy. Although the use of levodopa to overcome antipsychotic-induced blockade of dopamine receptors might appear rational, it has generally been reported to be ineffective or to increase psychiatric symptoms. For a discussion of the treatment of drug-induced parkinsonism see under Extrapyramidal Disorders in Adverse Effects of Chlorpromazine, p.650.

There is no cure for Parkinson's disease. Although the possibility of using drug therapy to slow the chronic progressive neurodegeneration associated with Parkinson's disease is being investigated no drug so far has a proved neuroprotective effect. Treatment is palliative and symptomatic and consists mainly of drug therapy supplemented when necessary with physical treatment such as physiotherapy and speech therapy. Surgery is occasionally used and there is growing interest in the use of transplantation and electrical devices for the control of tremor.

Drugs used in Parkinson's disease. Drug therapy consists largely of the use of dopaminergics or antimuscarinics in an attempt to restore the normal balance between dopaminergic and cholinergic activity. Dopaminergics may act by direct replacement of dopamine, by delaying the metabolism of endogenous dopamine, by stimulation of dopamine receptors directly, or by enhancement of release of endogenous dopamine. Drugs with differing actions are often used together to achieve optimum control of symptoms.

- *Levodopa* is converted by decarboxylation into dopamine, and unlike dopamine, can penetrate the blood-brain barrier hence supplying a source of dopamine to the brain. Levodopa is usually given with a decarboxylase inhibitor such as *benserazide* or *carbidopa*. These drugs are unable to penetrate the blood-brain barrier and therefore prevent only extracerebral conversion of levodopa to dopamine. This allows effective concentrations of dopamine to be achieved in the brain with lower doses of levodopa and also reduces unwanted effects such as nausea and vomiting and cardiovascular effects associated with peripheral formation of dopamine. Catechol-*O*-methyltransferase inhibitors, such as *entacapone* and *tolcapone*, inhibit another enzyme involved in the metabolism of levodopa and dopamine and when given concomitantly with levodopa and a decarboxylase inhibitor can help to stabilise patients, especially those experiencing end-of-dose deterioration.

The majority of patients respond initially to levodopa and its use has improved the quality and duration of life. However, after 2 or more years, benefit is reduced as the disease progresses and late complications emerge. Apart from dyskinesias and psychiatric effects, a major problem with long-term levodopa treatment is the appearance of fluctuations in mobility, the two predominant forms being 'end-of-dose' deterioration ('wearing-off' effect) and the 'on-off' phenomenon (see Complications of Treatment, below). Thus, although it is generally agreed that levodopa, given with a peripheral decarboxylase inhibitor such as carbidopa or benserazide, is currently the most effective treatment for Parkinson's disease, views differ as to the best time to start treatment and the dosage to employ in order to limit the long-term complications. Those who consider that these long-term effects reflect severity of the disease favour the early use of levodopa, whereas those implicating cumulative exposure to levodopa advocate later use.

- *Selegiline* is a selective inhibitor of monoamine oxidase type B, an enzyme involved in the metabolism of dopamine in the brain. Used with levodopa in severe parkinsonism it has a dose-sparing effect and is of use in patients experiencing fluctuations in mobility. Although early treatment with selegiline may delay the need for levodopa there is no evidence that it has a favourable effect on the long-term course of the disease. Whether any benefit obtained is due to a symptomatic or neuroprotective effect is unclear. Used alone, selegiline produces few side-effects but when used with levodopa it can provoke or worsen dyskinesias or psychiatric symptoms and doubts have been expressed on the safety of long-term use.
- *Bromocriptine* and similar dopamine agonists such as *cabergoline*, *lysuride*, *pergolide*, *pramipexole*, and *ropinirole* act by direct stimulation of remaining postsynaptic dopamine receptors. Some neurologists use dopamine agonists early in treatment in an attempt to delay therapy with levodopa but as their efficacy often decreases after a few years others reserve them for adjunctive use when levodopa is no longer effective alone or cannot be tolerated. They are sometimes useful in reducing 'off' periods with levodopa and in ameliorating fluctuations of mobility in the later stages of the disease. *Apomorphine* is a potent dopamine agonist, but it needs to be given parenterally. Although this restricts its use, it has a role in stabilising patients who suffer unpredictable 'on-off' effects. It is also used in the differential diagnosis of parkinsonism syndromes.
- *Antimuscarinics* are considered to have a weak antiparkinsonian effect compared with levodopa. They may reduce tremor but have little effect on bradykinesia. They may be of use alone or with other drugs in the initial treatment of patients with mild symptoms, especially when tremor is pronounced, or later as an adjunct to levodopa such as in patients with refractory tremor or dystonias. Antimuscarinic side-effects occur frequently and can limit their use. However, some side-effects can ameliorate complications associated with Parkinson's disease; dry mouth may be an advantage in patients with sialorrhoea. There appear to be no important differences in the efficacy of antimuscarinics for Parkinson's disease but some patients may tolerate one drug better than another. Those commonly used for Parkinson's disease include *benzhexol, benztropine, orphenadrine,* and *procyclidine*.
- *Amantadine* is a weak dopamine agonist with some antimuscarinic activity although its activity as an antagonist of *N*-methyl-D-aspartate may also have a beneficial effect in Parkinson's disease. It has mild antiparkinsonian effects compared with levodopa but is relatively free from side-effects. It can improve bradykinesia as well as tremor and rigidity but only a small proportion of patients derive much benefit. It is used similarly to antimuscarinics in early disease when symptoms are mild, but tolerance to its effects can occur rapidly.

Choice and implementation of drug treatment. There is no consensus on when to initiate treatment with *levodopa* or whether to use other drugs before levodopa. Many neurologists delay initial treatment with levodopa as they believe early use may increase the likelihood of problems such as dyskinesias and fluctuations in mobility and may accelerate the loss of dopaminergic neurones. In the early stages of the disease if symptoms are mild drug therapy may not be required. Some have initiated treatment with *selegiline* immediately, but there have been doubts over whether it has a neuroprotective effect, as postulated, and also over long-term safety. When symptoms become troublesome but are still relatively mild *amantadine* or an *antimuscarinic* may be started; antimuscarinics are useful when tremor predominates but are generally more suitable for younger patients. As the disease progresses some neurologists may advocate a trial of a *dopamine agonist* in an attempt to delay the introduction of levodopa. For most patients treatment with levodopa eventually becomes necessary.

The usual practice is to start with small doses of levodopa, together with a peripheral decarboxylase inhibitor, and increase slowly to a dose which reduces disability to an acceptable level. Variations in response and diminishing effectiveness over the years necessitate careful adjustment of the size and form of the dose and the schedule of administration.

Complications of treatment. Fluctuations in mobility have been reported in more than half of patients on levodopa after 5 years of therapy. They generally proceed through predictable **'end-of-dose'** deterioration to the **'on-off'** phenomenon with marked very sudden swings from mobility to immobility. The cause of the fluctuations is not known, but multiple factors including desensitisation of dopamine receptors, interference with the response to dopamine by other levodopa metabolites such as 3-*O*-methyldopa, fluctuating plasma concentrations, and erratic transport of levodopa from blood to the brain have been suggested. It appears that as the disease progresses the capacity of the nigrostriatal dopaminergic system to synthesise and store dopamine, and to act as a buffer in maintaining dopamine brain concentrations, declines. Dopamine concentrations therefore become more dependent on levodopa administration and the pattern of response will come to reflect more closely the rise and fall in levodopa concentrations. Eventually the effect of various factors which produce even small changes in plasma concentrations of levodopa will progressively become more pronounced.

Approaches to the management of 'end-of-dose' fluctuations include more frequent administration of smaller doses and the use of modified-release preparations. Addition of selegiline or partial replacement of levodopa with a dopamine agonist with a more prolonged action are also used.

Various attempts have been made to overcome the 'on-off' phenomenon. Those speculating that long-term treatment results in altered dopamine receptor sensitivity have used controlled withdrawal of levodopa for short periods ('drug holidays') but it is a dangerous procedure of doubtful value and no longer recommended.

Others have linked the 'on-off' phenomenon to variable plasma concentrations although, since transfer of levodopa into the brain involves active transport mechanisms, concentrations in plasma may not necessarily reflect those in the brain. Continuous intravenous infusion of levodopa has been shown to reduce fluctuations in mobility which suggests that dopamine receptors are still sensitive but this is not practical for day-to-day management. However, there is evidence that some patients may benefit from modified-release formulations of levodopa with a decarboxylase inhibitor. As levodopa competes with amino acids for uptake into the brain attempts to lessen fluctuations in dopamine brain concentrations have included taking levodopa on an empty stomach and also delaying most of a day's protein consumption until the evening. Addition of selegiline or a dopamine agonist may also help to reduce 'on-off' phenomena. If fluctuations remain a problem subcutaneous apomorphine is often effective.

Other complication of treatment with levodopa may include **dyskinesia** which may respond to dosage adjustment or partial replacement of levodopa with a dopamine agonist. Some patients with Parkinson's disease may experience **severe pain** and **dystonia** and it has been considered that measures to increase 'on' periods will reduce or eliminate pain in most patients.

Patients with Parkinson's disease can suffer from a range of **psychiatric effects** due to the adverse effects of drug therapy and to disease progression. It has been recommended that if patients develop psychotic reactions the use of antiparkinsonian drugs should be manipulated before resorting to the use of antipsychotics. Although antipsychotics are usually contra-indicated because they can exacerbate parkinsonism, atypical antipsychotics such as clozapine have been tried with benefit for psychiatric problems. **Nausea and vomiting** induced by dopaminergics may be minimised by introducing the drug gradually and administering the dose with food but if this is ineffective or apomorphine is being used these effects can be controlled by the antiemetic domperidone. Domperidone does not readily cross the blood-brain barrier and therefore acts mainly as a peripheral dopamine antagonist. Tolerance to the nausea usually develops after a few weeks and domperidone may be withdrawn.

References.

1. Marsden CD. Parkinson's disease. *Lancet* 1990; **335:** 948–52.
2. Clough CG. Parkinson's disease: management. *Lancet* 1991; **337:** 1324–7.
3. Marsden CD. Parkinson's disease. *Postgrad Med J* 1992; **68:** 538–43.
4. Calne DB. Treatment of Parkinson's disease. *N Engl J Med* 1993; **329:** 1021–7.
5. Montastruc JL, *et al.* Current status of dopamine agonists in Parkinson's disease management. *Drugs* 1993; **46:** 384–93.
6. Mizuno Y, *et al.* Potential of neuroprotective therapy in Parkinson's disease. *CNS Drugs* 1994; **1:** 45–56.
7. Bodagh IYO, Robertson DRC. A risk-benefit assessment of drugs used in the management of Parkinson's disease. *Drug Safety* 1994; **11:** 94–103.
8. Mizuno Y, *et al.* Practical guidelines for the drug treatment of Parkinson's disease. *CNS Drugs* 1994; **1:** 410–26.
9. Quinn N. Drug treatment of Parkinson's disease. *Br Med J* 1995; **310:** 575–9.
10. Harder S, *et al.* Concentration-effect relationship of levodopa in patients with Parkinson's disease. *Clin Pharmacokinet* 1995; **29:** 243–56.
11. Giron LT, Koller WC. Methods of managing levodopa-induced dyskinesias. *Drug Safety* 1996; **14:** 365–74.
12. Ahlskog JE. Treatment of early Parkinson's disease: are complicated strategies justified? *Mayo Clin Proc* 1996; **71:** 659–70.
13. Mendis T, *et al.* Drug-induced psychosis in Parkinson's disease: a review of management. *CNS Drugs* 1996; **5:** 166–74.
14. Andrew AJ. Drug treatment of Parkinson's disease in the 1990s. *Drugs* 1997; **53:** 195–205.
15. Gottwald MD, *et al.* New pharmacotherapy for Parkinson's disease. *Ann Pharmacother* 1997; **31:** 1205–17.
16. Olanow CW, Koller WC, eds. An algorithm (decision tree) for the management of Parkinson's disease: treatment guidelines. *Neurology* 1998; **50** (suppl 3): S1–S57.
17. Lang AE, Lozano AM. Parkinson's disease. *N Engl J Med* 1998; **339:** 1044–53 and 1130–43.
18. Bhatia K, *et al.* Guidelines for the management of Parkinson's disease. *Hosp Med* 1998; **59:** 469–80.

Amantadine Hydrochloride (9852-z)

Amantadine Hydrochloride *(BANM, USAN, pINNM).*

1-Adamantanamine Hydrochloride; Amantadini Hydrochloridum; EXP-105-1; NSC-83653. Tricyclo[3.3.1.1^{3,7}]dec-1-ylamine hydrochloride.

$C_{10}H_{17}N,HCl$ = 187.7.

CAS — 768-94-5 (amantadine); 665-66-7 (amantadine hydrochloride).

Pharmacopoeias. In *Chin., Eur.* (see p.viii), *Jpn,* and *US.*

A white or almost white crystalline powder. It sublimes on heating. **Soluble** 1 in 2.5 of water, 1 in 5.1 of alcohol, 1 in 18 of chloroform, and 1 in 70 of macrogol 400; practically insoluble in ether. A 20% solution in water has a pH of 3.0 to 5.5.

Amantadine Sulphate (4542-q)

$(C_{10}H_{17}N)_2,SO_4$ = 398.6.

CAS — 31377-23-8.

Adverse Effects

Most side-effects associated with amantadine therapy appear to be dose-related and relatively mild; some resemble those of antimuscarinic drugs. They may be reversed by withdrawing therapy but many resolve despite continuation.

Livedo reticularis, sometimes associated with ankle oedema, is quite common in patients given amantadine long-term. Mild CNS effects such as nervousness, inability to concentrate, dizziness, insomnia, nightmares, headache, and changes in mood may occur. Psychotic reactions, hallucinations, and confusion have been reported, especially in the elderly, patients with impaired renal function, and those also receiving antimuscarinic drugs.

Other side-effects reported have included orthostatic hypotension, urinary retention, slurred speech, ataxia, lethargy, nausea, anorexia, vomiting, dry mouth, constipation, skin rash, diaphoresis, photosensitisation, and blurred vision. There have been isolated reports of congestive heart failure, palpitations, leucopenia, neutropenia, facial dyskinesias, oculogyric episodes, and convulsions.

Effects on the cardiovascular system. Congestive heart failure has been associated with amantadine;[1] in this report the patient had been receiving combined treatment with amantadine, levodopa, and orphenadrine for 4 years. Others have considered that while amantadine sometimes causes ankle oedema, an association between amantadine and heart failure is not proven.[2] Livedo reticularis, a mottled blue discoloration of the skin due to prominence of the normal pattern of venous drainage, has been reported[2] to occur in about 50% of all elderly patients given amantadine 100 to 300 mg daily for 2 to 6 weeks and was associated with oedema in 5 to 10%. Both livedo and oedema have usually been confined to the legs and may result from the catecholamine-releasing action of amantadine in certain vascular beds; the oedema was unlikely to be due to heart failure. Angina, dyspnoea, pulmonary congestion, or distension of neck veins has also been reported[2] in 4 of 89 parkinsonian patients treated with amantadine; only 2 of these 4 had had ankle oedema before heart failure developed. No patient had been observed in whom heart failure seemed due directly to amantadine.

See also under Overdosage, below.

1. Vale JA, Maclean KS. Amantadine-induced heart-failure. *Lancet* 1977; **i:** 548.
2. Parkes JD, *et al.* Amantadine-induced heart-failure. *Lancet* 1977; **i:** 904.

Effects on electrolytes. For a report of a patient who developed hyponatraemia when given amantadine or levodopa, see under Effects on Kidney Function in Levodopa, p.1137.

Effects on the eyes. Superficial punctate keratitis and corneal abrasion with loss of visual acuity was observed in both eyes of a 64-year-old man about 3 weeks after starting treatment with amantadine 100 mg daily.[1] Symptoms resolved on discontinuation of amantadine but recurred when re-treatment with amantadine was attempted.

1. Nogaki H, Morimatsu M. Superficial punctate keratitis and corneal abrasion due to amantadine hydrochloride. *J Neurol* 1993; **240:** 388–9.

Effects on mental function. It has been suggested[1] that the ability of amantadine and memantine to cause psychotic disturbances in patients with Parkinson's disease might be related to their action as *N*-methyl-D-aspartate antagonists.

1. Riederer P, *et al.* Pharmacotoxic psychosis after memantine in Parkinson's disease. *Lancet* 1991; **338:** 1022–3.

Overdosage. A patient with postencephalitic parkinsonism who had taken an estimated 2.8 g of amantadine hydrochloride in a suicide attempt suffered an acute toxic psychosis with disorientation, visual hallucinations, and aggressive behaviour.[1] Convulsions did not occur, possibly because he had been receiving phenytoin which was continued. The patient was treated with hydration and chlorpromazine and recovered in 4 days.

A 2-year-old child who had ingested 600 mg of amantadine hydrochloride developed symptoms of acute toxicity, including agitation and dystonic posturing, despite emesis with 'syrup of ipecac'.[2] She responded immediately to a trial of physostigmine 500 μg intravenously, repeated after 10 minutes. Her pupils remained moderately dilated until about 20 hours after the ingestion; thereafter she made a full recovery.

Cardiac arrest developed 4 hours after a 37-year-old woman ingested 2.5 g of amantadine hydrochloride and was treated successfully.[3] However, ventricular arrhythmias, including torsade de pointes, continued over the ensuing 48 hours and may have been exacerbated by administration of isoprenaline and dopamine. The patient was subsequently stabilised with lignocaine by intravenous infusion, but died of respiratory failure 10 days after admission.

1. Fahn S, *et al.* Acute toxic psychosis from suicidal overdosage of amantadine. *Arch Neurol*, 1971; **25:** 45–8.
2. Berkowitz CD. Treatment of acute amantadine toxicity with physostigmine. *J Pediatr* 1979; **95:** 144–5.
3. Sartori M, *et al.* Torsade de pointe: malignant cardiac arrhythmia induced by amantadine poisoning. *Am J Med* 1984; **77:** 388–91.

Precautions

Amantadine is usually contra-indicated in severe renal disease and in patients with a history of epilepsy or other seizure disorders or gastric ulceration. It should be used with caution in patients with cardiovascular or liver disease, impaired renal function, recurrent eczema, or psychosis. Care should be taken in all elderly patients, who may be more sensitive to antimuscarinic effects, and in whom renal clearance is likely to be reduced.

Amantadine should not be used during pregnancy; toxicity has been reported in *animal* studies. It is also distributed into breast milk and the manufacturer has reported that adverse effects have occurred in infants being breast fed by mothers taking amantadine.

In common with other drugs having antimuscarinic properties amantadine may cause blurred vision or impair alertness; patients so affected should not drive or operate machinery. Treatment with amantadine should not be stopped abruptly in parkinsonian patients since they may experience a sudden marked clinical deterioration. There have been isolated reports of neuroleptic malignant syndrome associated with abrupt withdrawal of amantadine, especially in patients receiving concomitant treatment with antipsychotics.

Antiviral resistance. See under Influenza in Uses and Administration, below.

Pregnancy. A complex cardiovascular lesion occurred in an infant whose mother had taken amantadine hydrochloride 100 mg daily during the first 3 months of pregnancy.[1] Amantadine has been reported to be embryotoxic and teratogenic in *rats* given high doses[1] and it is recommended that it should not be used in pregnancy.[2]

1. Nora JJ, *et al.* Cardiovascular maldevelopment associated with maternal exposure to amantadine. *Lancet* 1975; **ii:** 607.
2. Anonymous. Safety of antimicrobial drugs in pregnancy. *Med Lett Drugs Ther* 1985; **27**: 93–5.

Renal impairment. Soung and colleagues found evidence of extremely limited excretion of amantadine in 12 patients who were either anephric or had negligible renal function, and who received a single dose of 100 mg of amantadine hydrochloride.[1] Only small amounts were removed by dialysis. They suggested that amantadine should be given with caution to patients requiring maintenance haemodialysis. It should be remembered that a single dose may provide adequate plasma concentrations for many days.[1] Dosage regimens based on creatinine clearance[2] or fixed doses at extended intervals[3] have been published. However both regimens have been criticised, and a conservative approach to amantadine dosage in these patients recommended.[4] The need for caution in using amantadine in patients with renal impairment is highlighted by a report of a patient with end-stage renal disease who progressed from delirium to coma after receiving amantadine 100 mg twice daily for 3 days.[5]

1. Soung L-S, *et al.* Amantadine hydrochloride pharmacokinetics in hemodialysis patients. *Ann Intern Med* 1980; **93:** 46–9.
2. Horadam VW, *et al.* Pharmacokinetics of amantadine hydrochloride in subjects with normal and impaired renal function. *Ann Intern Med* 1981; **94:** 454–8.
3. Wu MJ, *et al.* Amantadine hydrochloride pharmacokinetics in patients with impaired renal function. *Clin Nephrol* 1982; **17:** 19–23.
4. Aoki FY, Sitar DS. Clinical pharmacokinetics of amantadine hydrochloride. *Clin Pharmacokinet* 1988; **14:** 35–51.
5. Macchio GJ, *et al.* Amantadine-induced coma. *Arch Phys Med Rehabil* 1993; **74:** 1119–20.

Withdrawal. Neuroleptic malignant syndrome occurred in a patient being treated for heat stroke when all his medication, including antipsychotics and amantadine, was withdrawn.[1] It is suggested that dopamine agonists should not be discontinued in patients with hyperpyrexia at risk from this syndrome.

1. Simpson DM, Davis GC. Case report of neuroleptic malignant syndrome associated with withdrawal from amantadine. *Am J Psychiatry* 1984; **141:** 796–7.

Interactions

Amantadine may enhance the adverse effects of antimuscarinics and the dose of these drugs should be reduced when amantadine is given concomitantly; side-effects of levodopa may also be exacerbated.

The manufacturer recommends that amantadine should be used with caution in patients receiving drugs with CNS stimulant properties. The rate of excretion of amantadine may be reduced by drugs that raise urinary pH.

Antiarrhythmics. Quinine and quinidine have been reported to reduce the renal clearance of amantadine in healthy male, but not female subjects.[1] Patients taking these drugs concomitantly should be observed for signs of amantadine toxicity.

1. Gaudry SE, *et al.* Gender and age as factors in the inhibition of renal clearance of amantadine by quinine and quinidine. *Clin Pharmacol Ther* 1993; **54:** 23–7.

Antimalarials. See under Antiarrhythmics, above.

Diuretics. A patient with Parkinson's disease, previously stabilised on amantadine hydrochloride 300 mg daily, developed symptoms of amantadine toxicity, including ataxia, myoclonus, and confusion, 7 days after starting treatment with triamterene in association with hydrochlorothiazide (Dyazide).[1] It was postulated that the effect was due to reduction of the tubular secretion of amantadine.

1. Wilson TW, Rajput AH. Amantadine-Dyazide interaction. *Can Med Assoc J* 1983; **129:** 974–5.

MAOIs. Hypertension occurred about 48 hours after starting treatment with phenelzine sulphate in a patient already receiving amantadine.[1]

1. Jack RA, Daniel DG. Possible interaction between phenelzine and amantadine. *Arch Gen Psychiatry* 1984; **41:** 726.

Pharmacokinetics

Amantadine hydrochloride is readily absorbed from the gastro-intestinal tract; peak concentrations in the plasma appear within about 4 hours. It is mainly excreted unchanged in the urine by glomerular filtration and tubular secretion although small amounts of an acetylated metabolite have also been detected in urine; the plasma elimination half-life is reported to be about 11 to 15 hours in patients with normal renal function but is significantly prolonged in the elderly and in patients with renal impairment. The rate of elimination may be increased by acidification of the urine. Amantadine crosses the placenta and the blood-brain barrier. It is also distributed into breast milk. Plasma protein binding is reported to be about 67%.

References.

1. Aoki FY, Sitar DS. Clinical pharmacokinetics of amantadine hydrochloride. *Clin Pharmacokinet* 1988; **14:** 35–51.

Uses and Administration

Amantadine is a weak dopamine agonist with some antimuscarinic activity; it is also an antagonist of *N*-methyl-D-aspartate receptors. Amantadine has mild antiparkinsonian activity and is used in the management of parkinsonism, mainly in early disease when symptoms are mild. It may improve akinesia, rigidity, and tremor but tolerance can develop.

Amantadine is also an antiviral that inhibits replication of influenza type A virus. Variable activity has been reported *in vitro* against other viruses. It is used prophylactically against infection with influenza type A virus and to ameliorate symptoms when administered during the early stages of infection.

Amantadine has also been used in the management of herpes zoster.

Amantadine is usually given by mouth as the hydrochloride and the doses below are expressed in terms of the hydrochloride. Amantadine sulphate has been used similarly to the hydrochloride; it has been given by mouth or by intravenous infusion.

In parkinsonism, treatment is usually started with 100 mg daily and is increased to 100 mg twice daily after a week or more. Doses of up to 400 mg daily have occasionally been used.

In the treatment of influenza 100 mg is usually given daily for about 5 days. For the prophylaxis of influenza the same dose is given for as long as protection from infection is required, this may be for about 6 weeks. If amantadine is being given in conjunction with influenza vaccination then it is usually only given for up to 3 weeks after vaccination. In herpes zoster, treatment with 100 mg twice daily may be given for 14 days; if pain persists treatment may be continued for a further 14 days.

A daily dose of less than 100 mg or 100 mg given at intervals greater than one day have been recommended for patients over 65 years of age. The dosage of amantadine should be reduced in patients with renal impairment.

Administration. Amantadine sulphate has been used successfully in doses of up to 600 mg daily by intravenous infusion in the management of akinetic crisis in patients with Parkinson's disease.[1]

1. Gadoth N, *et al.* I.V. amantadine sulfate for extrapyramidal crisis. *Clin Pharm* 1985; **4:** 146.

Chronic granulomatous disease. Beneficial results have been reported[1] with amantadine 25 mg twice daily by mouth in a child of 4 years 9 months with chronic granulomatous disease.

1. Warner JO. Amantadine in chronic granulomatous disease. *Lancet* 1985; **ii:** 447.

Extrapyramidal disorders. Amantadine has been used as an alternative to antimuscarinics[1] in the short-term management of drug-induced extrapyramidal symptoms (p.650). See also Parkinsonism, below.

1. König P, *et al.* Amantadine versus biperiden: a double-blind study of treatment efficacy in neuroleptic extrapyramidal movement disorders. *Neuropsychobiology* 1996; **33:** 80–4.

Hiccup. Amantadine[1] has been reported to have produced beneficial results in patients with intractable hiccups (p.655).

1. Askenasy JJM, *et al.* Persistent hiccup cured by amantadine. *N Engl J Med* 1988; **318:** 711.

Influenza. Amantadine is used similarly to rimantadine (p.624) in the prophylaxis and symptomatic treatment of influenza (p.601). Amantadine can reduce the duration of influenza A symptoms when given within 48 hours of the onset of symptoms and may be considered for treatment in high-risk individuals.[1] Treatment and prophylaxis failures may be due to the rapid emergence of drug-resistant viruses.[2] Vaccination is usually the method of choice for prophylaxis of influenza but amantadine may be indicated in addition to vaccination in certain individuals or when vaccination is contra-indicated.

1. Nicholson KG, Wiselka MJ. Amantadine for influenza A. *Br Med J* 1991; **302:** 425–6.
2. Belshe RB, *et al.* Resistance of influenza A virus to amantadine and rimantadine: results of one decade of surveillance. *J Infect Dis* 1989; **159:** 430–5.

Neuroleptic malignant syndrome. Amantadine has been tried[1-3] in the treatment of the neuroleptic malignant syndrome (p.651).

1. McCarron MM, *et al.* A case of neuroleptic malignant syndrome successfully treated with amantadine. *J Clin Psychiatry* 1982; **43:** 381–2.
2. Amdurski S, *et al.* A therapeutic trial of amantadine in haloperidol-induced malignant neuroleptic syndrome. *Curr Ther Res* 1983; **33:** 225–9.
3. Woo J, *et al.* Neuroleptic malignant syndrome successfully treated with amantadine. *Postgrad Med J* 1986; **62:** 809–10.

Parkinsonism. Amantadine's mechanism of action in parkinsonism (p.1128) is unclear but may be due to its antimuscarinic activity and alterations in dopamine release and reuptake. It has also been suggested that amantadine's action as a non-competitive antagonist of *N*-methyl-D-aspartate may have a beneficial effect.[1,2] It has mild antiparkinsonian activity compared with levodopa but is relatively free from side-effects. It can improve bradykinesia as well as tremor and rigidity and is used in a similar manner to antimuscarinics mainly in the treatment of patients with early Parkinson's disease when symptoms are mild. However few patients obtain much benefit and tolerance to its effects can occur.

1. Laing P. Stroke treatment. *Lancet* 1991; **337:** 1601.
2. Greenamyre JT, O'Brien CF. N-Methyl-D-aspartate antagonists in the treatment of Parkinson's disease. *Arch Neurol* 1991; **48:** 977–81.

Withdrawal syndromes. COCAINE. Despite some earlier promising results more recent studies[1,2] have failed to confirm the value of amantadine in the management of the symptoms of cocaine withdrawal (p.1291). Any benefit appeared to decline after a few weeks of treatment.

1. Kosten TR, *et al.* Pharmacotherapy for cocaine-abusing methadone-maintained patients using amantadine or desipramine. *Arch Gen Psychiatry* 1992; **49:** 894–8.
2. Kampman K, *et al.* Amantadine in the early treatment of cocaine dependence: a double-blind, placebo-controlled trial. *Drug Alcohol Depend* 1996; **41:** 25–33.

Preparations

BP 1998: Amantadine Capsules; Amantadine Oral Solution;
USP 23: Amantadine Hydrochloride Capsules; Amantadine Hydrochloride Syrup.

Proprietary Preparations (details are given in Part 3)

Aust.: Hofcomant; PK-Merz; Symmetrel†; Virucid; ***Austral.:*** Antadine†; Symmetrel; ***Belg.:*** Amantan; Mantadix; ***Canad.:*** Endantadine; Symmetrel; ***Fr.:*** Mantadix; ***Ger.:*** Amixx; Contenton†; Grippin-Merz; Infectogripp†; PK-Merz; Symmetrel†; Tregor; Viregyt; ***Irl.:*** Symmetrel; ***Ital.:*** Mantadan; ***Neth.:*** Symmetrel; ***Norw.:*** Symmetrel†; ***S.Afr.:*** Antadine†; Symmetrel; ***Swed.:*** Symmetrel†; Virofral; ***Switz.:*** PK-Merz; Symmetrel; ***UK:*** Symmetrel; ***USA:*** Symadine†; Symmetrel.

Apomorphine Hydrochloride

(4543-p)

Apomorphine Hydrochloride *(BANM)*.

Apomorphini Hydrochloridum; Cloridrato de Apomorfina. 6aβ-Aporphine-10,11-diol hydrochloride hemihydrate; (R)-10,11-Dihydroxy-6a-aporphine hydrochloride hemihydrate; (6aR)-5,6,6a,7-Tetrahydro-6-methyl-4H-dibenzo[de,g]quinoline-10,11-diol hydrochloride hemihydrate.

$C_{17}H_{17}NO_2,HCl,\frac{1}{2}H_2O = 312.8.$

CAS — 58-00-4 (apomorphine); 314-19-2 (apomorphine hydrochloride, anhydrous); 41372-20-7 (apomorphine hydrochloride, hemihydrate).

Pharmacopoeias. In *Chin., Eur.* (see p.viii), *Pol.*, and *US.*

Odourless white or faintly yellow to green-tinged greyish crystals or crystalline powder, the green tinge becoming more pronounced on exposure to air and light. **Soluble** 1 in 50 of water and 1 in 20 of water at 80°; soluble 1 in 50 of alcohol; very slightly soluble in ether and in chloroform. A 1% solution in water has a pH of 4.0 to 5.0. Aqueous solutions decompose on storage and should not be used if they turn green or brown or contain a precipitate. **Store** in airtight containers. Protect from light. The USP requires that containers should be small, and, where they contain apomorphine hydrochloride for immediate use in compounding prescriptions, that they should contain not more than 350 mg.

Adverse Effects

Apomorphine usually produces nausea and vomiting when given in therapeutic doses but these effects can be controlled by treatment with domperidone. Apomorphine may induce dyskinesias during 'on' periods in patients with parkinsonism and these may be severe enough to require discontinuation of therapy. Transient sedation can be common during the first few weeks of treatment. Transient postural hypotension may also occur infrequently. Apomorphine can produce neuropsychiatric disturbances including personality changes, confusion, and visual hallucinations. Signs of CNS stimulation including euphoria, lightheadedness, restlessness, tremor, tachycardia, and tachypnoea occur less frequently. Increased salivation and perspiration have also been reported. Eosinophilia has occurred rarely. The use of apomorphine with levodopa may cause haemolytic anaemia and treatment may need to be discontinued if this cannot be satisfactorily controlled through dosage adjustment. Induration, nodule formation, and panniculitis, sometimes leading to ulceration often develops at the site of subcutaneous injection.

Overdosage with apomorphine can produce persistent vomiting, respiratory depression, bradycardia, hypotension, and coma; death may occur.

Akinesia. A 60-year-old man who was being investigated for parkinsonian symptoms became totally immobile and mute 15 minutes after receiving apomorphine 4 mg subcutaneously.[1] He remained conscious but was drowsy and sweating. Similar profound akinesia occurred on rechallenge with 2- and 6-mg doses. A diagnosis of probable striato-nigral degeneration was made as the patient had previously shown no improvement after administration of levodopa but the mechanism of the idiosyncratic reaction to apomorphine was unclear.

1. Jenkins JR, Pearce JMS. Paradoxical akinetic response to apomorphine in parkinsonism. *J Neurol Neurosurg Psychiatry* 1992; **55:** 414–15.

Effects on the heart. A 67-year-old man developed palpitations with cold perspiration and chest pain, in addition to asthenia, salivation, nausea and vomiting, 5 minutes after receiving 3 mg apomorphine subcutaneously. An ECG demonstrated atrial fibrillation with a ventricular frequency of 140 beats per minute.[1]

1. Stocchi F, *et al.* Transient atrial fibrillation after subcutaneous apomorphine bolus. *Mov Disord* 1996; **11:** 584–5.

Effects on mental function. Severe confusion, hallucinations, and acute psychosis were reported by Ruggieri *et al.* in 4 of 6 parkinsonian patients given subcutaneous apomorphine.[1] Three of the 4 had previously experienced mental disturbances while receiving lysuride. However, other studies have failed to note effects on mental function in parkinsonian patients given apomorphine[2,3] and Poewe *et al.* suggest that the risk of psychosis in patients with no history of confusion or hallucinations is low.

1. Ruggieri S, *et al.* Side-effects of subcutaneous apomorphine in Parkinson's disease. *Lancet* 1989; **i:** 566.
2. Stibe CMH, *et al.* Subcutaneous apomorphine in parkinsonian on-off oscillations. *Lancet* 1988; **i:** 403–6.
3. Poewe W, *et al.* Side-effects of subcutaneous apomorphine in Parkinson's disease. *Lancet* 1989; **i:** 1084–5.

Hypersensitivity. Allergic reactions including contact dermatitis, severe rhinitis, and respiratory distress have been reported in 2 workers who came into contact with apomorphine powder.[1] Contact allergy has also been reported in a patient who developed a swollen nose and lips after intranasal use of apomorphine.[2] Skin testing in all these cases[1,2] gave a positive reaction to apomorphine. Biopsy of subcutaneous nodules, which develop at the site of infection in most patients using apomorphine subcutaneously, has not been able to clarify what type of reaction was responsible for the development of panniculitis.[3] Although the nodules may slowly resolve the sites are often unsuitable for reuse as absorption from them is unpredictable; concern has been expressed that this may limit long-term use of apomorphine.[3]

1. Dahlquist I. Allergic reactions to apomorphine. *Contact Dermatitis* 1977; **3:** 349–50.
2. van Laar T, *et al.* Nasolabiale allergische reactie op intranasale toediening van apomorfine bij de ziekte van Parkinson. *Ned Tijdschr Geneeskd* 1992; **136** (suppl 47): 26–7.
3. Acland KM, *et al.* Panniculitis in association with apomorphine infusion. *Br J Dermatol* 1998; **138:** 480–2.

Oedema. A report of severe reversible oedema of the lower limbs in a patient receiving subcutaneous apomorphine.[1] Oedema recurred when apomorphine was reintroduced, but to a lesser extent.

1. Vermersch P. Severe oedema after subcutaneous apomorphine in Parkinson's disease. *Lancet* 1989; **ii:** 802.

Stomatitis. Stomatitis, severe enough to warrant discontinuation of treatment, occurred in 4 of 8 patients after 2 to 6 months of therapy with sublingual apomorphine.[1]

1. Montastruc JL, *et al.* Sublingual apomorphine in Parkinson's disease: a clinical and pharmacokinetic study. *Clin Neuropharmacol* 1991; **14:** 432–7.

Treatment of Adverse Effects

Domperidone is usually given to control nausea and vomiting when apomorphine is used in the management of Parkinson's disease. Pretreatment with domperidone for at least 3 days is advised before starting treatment with apomorphine. Usually domperidone can be withdrawn gradually over several weeks to 6 months although some patients may need to continue treatment indefinitely.

In overdosage an opioid antagonist such as naloxone has been given to treat excessive vomiting and CNS and respiratory depression.

References.

1. Bonuccelli U, *et al.* Naloxone partly counteracts apomorphine side effects. *Clin Neuropharmacol* 1991; **14:** 442–9.

Precautions

Apomorphine should not be given to patients with respiratory or CNS depression, hypersensitivity to opioids, neuropsychiatric problems, or dementia. It is not suitable for use in patients who have an 'on' response to levodopa marred by severe dyskinesia, hypotonia, or psychiatric effects.

It should be used with caution in patients prone to nausea and vomiting or when vomiting is likely to pose a risk. Apomorphine should also be used with care in patients with pulmonary, cardiovascular, or endocrine disease or with renal impairment. Extra care is needed during initiation of treatment in elderly or debilitated patients and in those with a history of postural hypotension. Periodic monitoring of hepatic, renal, haemopoietic, and cardiovascular function has been advised and it is recommended that patients receiving apomorphine and levodopa together should be screened for haemolytic anaemia before starting treatment and then every 6 months.

Patients who develop anaemia, or those who have continuing confusion, or hallucinations during treatment with apomorphine require observation and dosage adjustment under specialist supervision; treatment may need to be discontinued.

Interactions

The therapeutic effects of apomorphine may be antagonised by antipsychotics and other drugs that act as CNS dopamine inhibitors.

Pharmacokinetics

Following subcutaneous administration apomorphine is reported to be well absorbed, and to be metabolised in the liver. Apomorphine undergoes extensive first-pass hepatic metabolism when given by mouth and oral bioavailability is low. It is excreted in urine, mainly as metabolites.

Uses and Administration

Apomorphine is a morphine derivative with structural similarities to dopamine. It is a dopamine D_2-receptor agonist used in the diagnosis and management of parkinsonism, especially in the control of the 'on-off' effect.

The optimal dose of apomorphine in the management of 'off' periods in parkinsonism should be established individually under specialist care. At least 3 days of pretreatment with the antiemetic domperidone is advised before administration of apomorphine. After withholding antiparkinsonian therapy overnight to provoke an 'off' period, test doses of apomorphine hydrochloride ranging from 1.5 to 7 mg or occasionally 10 mg are given subcutaneously at intervals of 40 minutes in an increasing regimen to determine the lowest dose producing a response. Once the patient's normal antiparkinsonian therapy is re-established, this dose of apomorphine hydrochloride is given at the first signs of an 'off' period. The dose and frequency of administration is further adjusted according to response; patients typically require 3 to 30 mg daily in divided doses but individual injections should not be greater than 10 mg. Patients who require more than 10 injections per day or those whose overall control of symptoms remains unsatisfactory with intermittent injections may benefit from continuous subcutaneous infusion. The infusion is started at a rate of 1 mg per hour and this may be increased in steps of 0.5 mg per hour at intervals of not less than 4 hours up to a maximum rate of 4 mg per hour. It is advised that infusions should only be given during waking hours and that the infusion site should be changed every 12 hours; 24-hour infusions are not advised unless there are severe night-time symptoms. Patients usually need to supplement the infusion with intermittent bolus injections but the recommended maximum total daily dose given by infusion and/or injection is 100 mg.

Apomorphine stimulates the chemoreceptor trigger zone in the brain and can produce emesis within a few minutes of administration. However the use of apomorphine for the induction of emesis in poisoning is considered dangerous owing to the risk of inducing protracted vomiting and shock and is not recommended.

Erectile dysfunction. Apomorphine is among a wide range of drugs that have been tried in the management of erectile dysfunction (p.1614) with some beneficial results. It has been given subcutaneously[1] or by sublingual administration.[2]

1. Segraves RT, *et al.* Effect of apomorphine on penile tumescence in men with psychogenic impotence. *J Urol (Baltimore)* 1991; **145:** 1174–5.
2. Heaton JPW, *et al.* Recovery of erectile function by the oral administration of apomorphine. *Urology* 1995; **45:** 200–6.

Parkinsonism. Although apomorphine has produced benefit in Parkinson's disease (p.1128) when given orally, the high doses required to overcome extensive first-pass hepatic metabolism (up to 1.4 g daily in one study[1]), were associated with uraemia. The use of apomorphine in Parkinson's disease has therefore been limited by the need for parenteral administration. The current main use of apomorphine in Parkinson's disease is for the stabilisation of patients with 'on-off' fluctuations unresponsive to other dopamine agonists. It is usually given subcutaneously either by injection or infusion but a review[2] of the use of apomorphine in Parkinson's disease also discusses studies of rectal, sublingual, and intranasal administration. Of these, the intranasal route was considered to be the most promising alternative route.

1. Cotzias GC, *et al.* Treatment of Parkinson's disease with aporphines. *N Engl J Med* 1976; **294:** 567–72.
2. Corboy DL, *et al.* Apomorphine for motor fluctuations and freezing in Parkinson's disease. *Ann Pharmacother* 1995; **29:** 282–8.

DIAGNOSIS. There have been a number of reports of the use of subcutaneous apomorphine in the differential diagnosis of parkinsonian syndromes, to distinguish forms responsive to dopaminergics, such as idiopathic Parkinson's disease, from other parkinsonian syndromes such as Wilson's disease, corticobasal degeneration, and diffuse Lewy body dementia, which are unresponsive to, or made worse by, dopaminergics.[1-4] Some consider that oral challenge with levodopa is still the best test of dopaminergic responsiveness[5] but testing with apomorphine has proved of value in re-assessing patients who have become less responsive to levodopa.[1,4] In most cases testing has involved administration of a series of increasing doses of subcutaneous apomorphine hydrochloride, usually starting with 1 mg and increasing up to about 5 mg or until central adverse effects supervene; the patient's motor function is assessed at various times after each dose and a suitable interval allowed between doses. Patients should be pretreated with domperidone before the test to prevent nausea and vomiting.

1. Barker R, *et al.* Subcutaneous apomorphine as a diagnostic test for dopaminergic responsiveness in parkinsonian syndromes. *Lancet* 1989; **i:** 675.
2. Oertel WH, *et al.* Apomorphine test for dopaminergic responsiveness. *Lancet* 1989; **i:** 1262–3.
3. Frankel JP, *et al.* Use of apomorphine to test for dopamine responsiveness in Wilson's disease. *Lancet* 1989; **ii:** 801–2.
4. Hughes AJ, *et al.* Apomorphine test to predict dopaminergic responsiveness in parkinsonian syndromes. *Lancet* 1990; **336:** 32–4.
5. Steiger MJ, Quinn NP. Levodopa challenge test in Parkinson's disease. *Lancet* 1992; **339:** 751–2.

Preparations

USP 23: Apomorphine Hydrochloride Tablets.

Proprietary Preparations (details are given in Part 3)
Austral.: Apomine; ***Fr.:*** Apokinon; ***UK:*** Britaject.

Benserazide Hydrochloride (4544-s)

Benserazide Hydrochloride *(BANM, rINNM).*

Benserazidi Hydrochloridum; Ro-4-4602 (benserazide); Serazide Hydrochloride. DL-Serine 2-(2,3,4-trihydroxybenzyl)hydrazide hydrochloride; 2-Amino-3-hydroxy-2′-(2,3,4-trihydroxybenzyl)propionohydrazide hydrochloride.

$C_{10}H_{15}N_3O_5,HCl = 293.7$.

CAS — 322-35-0 (benserazide); 14919-77-8 (benserazide hydrochloride); 14046-64-1 (benserazide hydrochloride).

NOTE. Benserazide is *USAN*.
Compounded preparations of benserazide hydrochloride and levodopa in proportions, by weight, of 1 part of benserazide and 4 parts of levodopa have the British Approved Name Co-beneldopa.

Pharmacopoeias. In *Chin., Eur.* (see p.viii), and *Jpn.*

A white or yellowish-white or orange-white crystalline powder. Benserazide hydrochloride 28.5 mg is approximately equivalent to 25 mg of benserazide. Freely **soluble** in water; slightly soluble in dehydrated alcohol; sparingly soluble in acetone. A 1% solution in water has a pH of 4.0 to 5.0. **Protect** from light.

Solubility. Benserazide is unstable in a neutral, alkaline, or strongly acidic medium.[1]

1. Schwartz DE, Brandt R. Pharmacokinetic and metabolic studies of the decarboxylase inhibitor benserazide in animals and man. *Arzneimittelforschung* 1978; **28:** 302–7.

Adverse Effects and Precautions

Developmental abnormalities of the *rat* skeleton have been reported with benserazide by Theiss and Schärer,[1] but Ziegler *et al.* found no evidence of any disorder involving bone metabolism in man.[2] Nevertheless the manufacturers have recommended that benserazide should not be given to patients under 25 years of age or to pregnant women.

1. Theiss E, Schärer K. Toxicity of L-dopa and a decarboxylase inhibitor in animal experiments. In: de Ajuriaguerra J, Gauthier G, eds. *Monoamines Noyaux Gris Centraux et Syndrome de Parkinson*. Geneva: Georg, 1971: 497–504.
2. Ziegler WH, *et al.* Toxicity of L-dopa and a dopa decarboxylase inhibitor in humans. In: de Ajuriaguerra J, Gauthier G, eds. *Monoamines Noyaux Gris Centraux et Syndrome de Parkinson*. Geneva: Georg, 1971: 505–16.

Pharmacokinetics

Pharmacokinetic and metabolic studies of benserazide in *animals* and man.[1,2] Following oral administration to parkinsonian patients benserazide was rapidly absorbed to the extent of about 58%, simultaneous administration of levodopa tending to increase this slightly. It was rapidly excreted in the urine in the form of metabolites, mostly within the first 6 hours; 85% of urinary excretion had occurred within 12 hours. Benserazide is predominantly metabolised in the gut and appears to protect levodopa against decarboxylation primarily in the gut, but also in the rest of the organism, mainly by way of its metabolite trihydroxybenzylhydrazine. Benserazide did not cross the blood-brain barrier in *rats*.

1. Schwartz DE, *et al.* Pharmacokinetics of the decarboxylase benserazide in man: its tissue distribution in the rat. *Eur J Clin Pharmacol* 1974; **7:** 39–45.
2. Schwartz DE, Brandt R. Pharmacokinetic and metabolic studies of the decarboxylase inhibitor benserazide in animals and man. *Arzneimittelforschung* 1978; **28:** 302–7.

Uses and Administration

Benserazide hydrochloride is a peripheral decarboxylase inhibitor with actions similar to those of carbidopa (p.1136) and is used similarly as an adjunct to levodopa in the treatment of parkinsonism (p.1128). For details of administration and dosage, see Levodopa, p.1140.

References.

1. Dingemanse J, *et al.* Pharmacodynamics of benserazide assessed by its effects on endogenous and exogenous levodopa pharmacokinetics. *Br J Clin Pharmacol* 1997; **44:** 41–8.

Preparations

Proprietary Preparations (details are given in Part 3)

Multi-ingredient: ***Aust.:*** Madopar; ***Austral.:*** Madopar; ***Belg.:*** Prolopa; ***Canad.:*** Prolopa; ***Fr.:*** Modopar; ***Ger.:*** Madopar; ***Irl.:*** Madopar; ***Ital.:*** Madopar; ***Neth.:*** Madopar; ***Norw.:*** Madopar; ***S.Afr.:*** Madopar; ***Spain:*** Madopar; ***Swed.:*** Madopark; ***Switz.:*** Madopar; ***UK:*** Madopar.

Bromocriptine Mesylate (4546-e)

Bromocriptine Mesylate *(BANM, USAN).*

Bromocriptine Mesilate *(rINNM)*; Bromocriptina Mesilato; Bromocriptine Methanesulphonate; Bromocriptini Mesilas; Bromocryptine Mesylate; 2-Bromo-α-ergocryptine Mesylate; 2-Bromoergocryptine Monomethanesulfonate; CB-154 (bromocriptine); Mesilato de Bromocriptina. (5′S)-2-Bromo-12′-hydroxy-2′-(1-methylethyl)-5′-(2-methylpropyl)-ergotaman-3′,6′,18-trione methanesulphonate.

$C_{32}H_{40}BrN_5O_5,CH_4O_3S = 750.7$.

CAS — 25614-03-3 (bromocriptine); 22260-51-1 (bromocriptine mesylate).

Pharmacopoeias. In *Eur.* (see p.viii), *Jpn,* and *US.*

A white or slightly coloured fine crystalline powder; odourless or almost odourless. Bromocriptine mesylate 2.87 mg is approximately equivalent to 2.5 mg of bromocriptine. Practically **insoluble** in water; soluble in alcohol; sparingly soluble in dichloromethane; freely soluble in methyl alcohol. A 1% solution in a mixture of 2 parts methyl alcohol to 8 of water has a pH of 3.1 to 3.8. **Store** in airtight containers at a temperature not exceeding −15°. Protect from light.

Adverse Effects

Nausea is the most common side-effect at the beginning of treatment with bromocriptine, but vomiting, dizziness, and orthostatic hypotension may also occur. Syncope has followed initial doses of bromocriptine.

Side-effects are generally dose-related and may therefore be more frequent with the higher doses that have been used in the treatment of parkinsonism and acromegaly. Reduction of the dosage of bromocriptine, followed in a few days by a more gradual increase, may alleviate many side-effects. Nausea may be diminished by taking bromocriptine with food.

Bromocriptine is a vasoconstrictor; digital vasospasm, induced by cold, and leg cramps have been reported. Other cardiovascular effects have included erythromelalgia, prolonged severe hypotension, arrhythmias, and exacerbation of angina. Very rarely hypertension, myocardial infarction, seizures or stroke (both sometimes preceded by severe headache or visual disturbances), and mental disorders have been reported in postpartum women given bromocriptine.

The use of ergot derivatives such as bromocriptine has been associated with retroperitoneal fibrosis, pleural thickening and effusions, and pericarditis and pericardial effusions.

Other side-effects reported include headache, nasal congestion, drowsiness, dry mouth, constipation, diarrhoea, and altered liver-function tests. Dyskinesias have occurred in patients suffering from parkinsonism. Gastro-intestinal bleeding has been reported in acromegalic patients. Psychosis, with hallucinations, delusions, and confusion, occurs particularly when high doses are used to treat parkinsonism, but has also been reported with low doses.

In 27 published studies of bromocriptine in the treatment of Parkinson's disease, 217 of the 790 patients given bromocriptine had adverse effects.[1] Mental changes were noted in 90 patients, dyskinesia in 20, orthostatic hypotension in 40, and gastro-intestinal effects in 40. The fewest adverse effects (9%) occurred with low-dose bromocriptine, more occurred with high-dose bromocriptine (27%) or with low-dose bromocriptine with levodopa (26%), and the most occurred with high-dose bromocriptine and levodopa (32%). However, those on high doses had more advanced disease and might be more susceptible to mental changes and dyskinesias.

An analysis by the manufacturer of published reports on patients treated with bromocriptine for 1 to 10 years concluded that in general, side-effects noted were no different from those associated with short-term treatment.[2]

1. Lieberman AN, Goldstein M. Bromocriptine in Parkinson disease. *Pharmacol Rev* 1985; **37:** 217–27.
2. Weil C. The safety of bromocriptine in long-term use: a review of the literature. *Curr Med Res Opin* 1986; **10:** 25–51.

Effects on the blood. Severe leucopenia and mild thrombocytopenia developed in a 23-year-old woman after treatment with bromocriptine 7.5 to 10 mg daily for about 3 months.[1]

1. Giampietro O, *et al.* Severe leukopenia and mild thrombocytopenia after chronic bromocriptine (CB-154) administration. *Am J Med Sci* 1981; **281:** 169–72.

Effects on the cardiovascular system. Asymptomatic hypotension occurs in many subjects given bromocriptine.[1] However, faintness and dizziness, sometimes accompanied by nausea and vomiting, are common at the start of treatment with bromocriptine and these symptoms rather than an anaphylactic type of reaction are likely to account for the collapse that occurs in a few sensitive patients. Two of 53 patients with Parkinson's disease fainted after an initial dose of 1.25 or 2.5 mg, but the exact incidence of shock-like syndromes is difficult to assess; the manufacturers have stated that 22 of over 10 000 subjects given bromocriptine have had hypotension and collapse, mainly at the start of treatment. It is essential to warn all patients starting treatment of the possibility of fainting. The initial dose should not exceed 1.25 to 2.5 mg and should be taken with food and in bed. If fainting does occur recovery is usually rapid and spontaneous. Tolerance to side-effects such as hypotension and nausea may develop rapidly.

Hypertension, seizures, stroke, and myocardial infarction have been associated with bromocriptine therapy, notably in postpartum women.[2-4] A study involving 1813 women suggested that the risk of postpartum hypertension was increased in women who experienced pregnancy-induced hypertension and that this risk was further increased in those who took bromocriptine for suppression of lactation.[5] A case-controlled study[6] involving 43 of the women who had had postpartum seizures while taking bromocriptine found that while the initial risk of seizures appeared to be lower in patients taking bromocriptine there was a small positive association with seizures occurring more than 72 hours after delivery.

Although a causal relationship between the use of bromocriptine and these adverse effects in postpartum women has not been established the manufacturer recommends that bromocriptine should not be used postpartum or in the puerperium in women with high blood pressure, coronary artery disease, or symptoms or history of serious mental disorders. It is also recommended that when bromocriptine is used in postpartum women blood pressure should be carefully monitored, especially during the first few days and if hypertension, unremitting headache, or signs of CNS toxicity develop treatment should be discontinued immediately.

1. Parkes D. Side effects of bromocriptine. *N Engl J Med* 1980; **302:** 749–50.
2. Anonymous. Postpartum hypertension, seizures, strokes reported with bromocriptine. *FDA Drug Bull* 1984; **14:** 3.
3. Ruch A, Duhring JL. Postpartum myocardial infarction in a patient receiving bromocriptine. *Obstet Gynecol* 1989; **74:** 448–51.
4. Larrazet F, *et al.* Possible bromocriptine-induced myocardial infarction. *Ann Intern Med* 1993; **118:** 199–200.
5. Watson DL, *et al.* Bromocriptine mesylate for lactation suppression: a risk for postpartum hypertension? *Obstet Gynecol* 1989; **74:** 573–6.
6. Rothman KJ, *et al.* Bromocriptine and puerperal seizures. *Epidemiology* 1990; **1:** 232–8.

Effects on the ears. Audiometric evidence of bilateral sensorineural hearing loss was reported in 3 patients receiving bromocriptine 15 or 20 mg daily for chronic hepatic encephalopathy.[1] Hearing improved when the dose was reduced to 10 mg daily.

1. Lanthier PL, *et al.* Bromocriptine-associated ototoxicity. *J Laryngol Otol* 1984; **98:** 399–404.

Effects on the eyes. Blurred vision and diplopia has been reported in several patients receiving bromocriptine.[1] There is a report of reversible myopia developing in a patient with hyperprolactinaemia given bromocriptine.[2]

In a patient with progressive visual loss due to compression of the optic chiasm by a large pituitary tumour, administration of bromocriptine caused total visual loss within hours.[3] Vision slowly returned to normal when the patient was placed in the supine position; the most likely cause of the visual loss was thought to be orthostatic hypotension with resultant decrease in perfusion pressure to the visual system.

Bromocriptine has been reported to cause visual cortical disturbances.[4] In some cases blurred vision and transient cortical blindness have preceded seizures and strokes (see Effects on the Cardiovascular System, above).

1. Calne DB, *et al.* Long-term treatment of parkinsonism with bromocriptine. *Lancet* 1978; **i:** 735–7.
2. Manor RS, *et al.* Myopia during bromocriptine treatment. *Lancet* 1981; **i:** 102.
3. Couldwell WT, Weiss MH. Visual loss associated with bromocriptine. *Lancet* 1992; **340:** 1410–11.
4. Lane RJM, Routledge PA. Drug-induced neurological disorders. *Drugs* 1983; **26:** 124–47.

Effects on electrolytes. There have been isolated reports of severe hyponatraemia associated with the use of bromocriptine.[1,2]

1. Marshall AW, *et al.* Bromocriptine-associated hyponatraemia in cirrhosis. *Br Med J* 1982; **285:** 1534–5.
2. Damase-Michel C, *et al.* Hyponatraemia in a patient treated with bromocriptine. *Drug Invest* 1993; **5:** 285–7.

Effects on mental state. Psychotic reactions to high doses of bromocriptine are well known in patients with parkinsonism.[1] However, mania has been associated with the use of bromocriptine post partum[2,3] and Pearce and Pearce state that psychological symptoms may occur with doses of only 2.5 to 5 mg daily.[4] They also note that, unlike the relatively mild and transient symptoms associated with levodopa, bromocriptine produces a severe psychosis in which the patient is violent and aggressive, suffering from intense delusions which are often hostile and violent; complete withdrawal of bromocriptine may still leave a residue of severe psychotic illness persisting for 1 to 3 weeks. Psychosis associated with low doses of bromocriptine has often occurred in patients with a history of psychotic illness or considerable changes in behaviour and mood prior to treatment.[5-7] Drug-related psychotic reactions have also been reported in patients with no psychiatric history;[8,9] 8 of 600 patients given bromocriptine or lysuride for the treatment of acromegaly or prolactinoma developed symptoms including anxiety, depression, auditory hallucinations, delusions, hyperactivity, disinhibition, euphoria, and insomnia and 4 had received doses only previously associated with psychosis in susceptible patients.[9]

1. Calne DB, *et al.* Long-term treatment of parkinsonism with bromocriptine. *Lancet* 1978; **i:** 735–7.
2. Vlissides DN, *et al.* Bromocriptine-induced mania? *Br Med J* 1978; **1:** 510.
3. Brook NM, Cookson IB. Bromocriptine-induced mania? *Br Med J* 1978; **1:** 790.
4. Pearce I, Pearce JMS. Bromocriptine in parkinsonism. *Br Med J* 1978; **1:** 1402–4.
5. Pearson KC. Mental disorders from low-dose bromocriptine. *N Engl J Med* 1981; **305:** 173.
6. Le Feuvre CM, *et al.* Bromocriptine-induced psychosis in acromegaly. *Br Med J* 1982; **285:** 1315.
7. Procter AW, *et al.* Bromocriptine induced psychosis in acromegaly. *Br Med J* 1983; **286:** 50. Correction. *ibid.*; 311.
8. Einarson TR, Turchet EN. Psychotic reaction to low-dose bromocriptine. *Clin Pharm* 1983; **2:** 273–4.
9. Turner TH, *et al.* Psychotic reactions during treatment of pituitary tumours with dopamine agonists. *Br Med J* 1984; **289:** 1101–3.

Effects on the nervous system. A report of 2 cases of cerebrospinal-fluid rhinorrhoea associated with the use of bromocriptine following partial surgical resection of prolactinoma.[1]

For reference to seizures associated with the use of bromocriptine in postpartum women, see under Effects on the Cardiovascular System, above.

1. Baskin DS, Wilson CB. CSF rhinorrhea after bromocriptine for prolactinoma. *N Engl J Med* 1982; **306:** 178.

Effects on the respiratory tract. Interstitial lung disease, with dyspnoea, chest pain, cough, and pulmonary fibrosis was reported in a patient following administration of relatively high doses of bromocriptine (62 mg daily) for Parkinson's disease.[1] Respiratory symptoms largely resolved on withdrawal of the drug, although functional respiratory changes and moderate dyspnoea persisted after 6 months. A review of the literature revealed a number of other reports of pleuropulmonary fibrosis associated with relatively high doses of bromocriptine. Although the incidence of this effect did not seem to be high, similar cases continue to be reported.[2,3]

1. Vergeret J, *et al.* Fibrose pleuro-pulmonaire et bromocriptine. *Sem Hop Paris* 1984; **60:** 741–4.
2. Kinnunen E, Viljanen A. Pleuropulmonary involvement during bromocriptine treatment. *Chest* 1988; **94:** 1034–6.
3. Macak IA, *et al.* Bromocriptine-induced pulmonary disease. *Can J Hosp Pharm* 1991; **44:** 37–8, xxiv.

Effects on sexual function. Severe hypersexuality has been reported in a middle-aged man receiving bromocriptine and levodopa for Parkinson's disease.[1] About 3 years after the onset of hypersexuality he developed paranoid-hallucinatory psychoses which subsided on the reduction of dosage. It was apparent that addictive abuse of dopaminergic drugs had occurred. Clitoral tumescence and increased libido has been noted in a woman receiving bromocriptine to suppress lactation[2] but there has been a report of sexual dissatisfaction and decreased libido in 3 women receiving bromocriptine for hyperprolactinaemia.[3]

1. Vogel HP, Schiffter R. Hypersexuality—a complication of dopaminergic therapy in Parkinson's disease. *Pharmacopsychiatry* 1983; **16:** 107–10.
2. Blin O, *et al.* Painful clitoral tumescence during bromocriptine therapy. *Lancet* 1991; **337:** 1231–2.
3. Saleh AK, Moussa MAA. Sexual dysfunction in women due to bromocriptine. *Br Med J* 1984; **289:** 228.

Effects on the urinary tract. Constant dribbling urinary incontinence developed in a woman receiving bromocriptine 2.5 mg daily for a recurrent pituitary growth; symptoms resolved on discontinuing the drug and recurred on rechallenge.[1] Bromocriptine has been shown to have two effects, one on the bladder outflow tract and one on the detrusor muscle, that could predispose to urinary incontinence.[2]

1. Sandyk R, Gillman MA. Urinary incontinence in patient on long-term bromocriptine. *Lancet* 1983; **ii:** 1260–1.
2. Caine M. Bromocriptine and urinary incontinence. *Lancet* 1984; **i:** 228.

Hypersensitivity. A report of an allergic reaction due to bromocriptine in a 26-year-old woman being treated for a prolactin-secreting microadenoma.[1] The patient reacted similarly to lysuride and treatment was continued with quinagolide.

1. Merola B, *et al.* Allergy to ergot-derived dopamine agonists. *Lancet* 1992; **339:** 620.

Oedema. Oedema poorly responsive to diuretics has been reported[1] in a patient given bromocriptine as part of treatment for prolactinoma. The oedema improved on substitution of pergolide but worsened with higher doses. Oedema resolved when treatment was changed to quinagolide. The reaction was considered to be idiosyncratic since enquiries by the author of the report had revealed only one similar case.

1. Blackard WG. Edema—an infrequently recognized complication of bromocriptine and other ergot dopaminergic drugs. *Am J Med* 1993; **94:** 445.

Overdosage. The most striking symptom in two children aged 2 and 2½ years who accidentally ingested an estimated 25 and 7.5 mg of bromocriptine respectively, was lethargy with altered mental status.[1] The first child vomited and became sleepy. On admission he was markedly lethargic, but combative when disturbed, and also had hypotension, shallow breathing, dilated pupils, and hyperreflexic lower extremities. Nasogastric lavage was promptly performed and activated charcoal and then magnesium citrate administered. Blood pressure and ECG were monitored and glucose and sodium chloride solution infused. The other child vomited, became lethargic, and had dilated pupils. Ipecacuanha was administered and activated charcoal followed by magnesium citrate given by nasogastric tube. Both children recovered completely.

1. Vermund SH, *et al.* Accidental bromocriptine ingestion in childhood. *J Pediatr* 1984; **105:** 838–40.

Withdrawal syndromes. Transient galactorrhoea and hyperprolactinaemia occurred in a young woman after withdrawal of bromocriptine therapy for Parkinson's disease.[1] It was suggested the effects were due to a rebound phenomenon. There has been a report of hyperthermia following withdrawal of treatment with levodopa/carbidopa and bromocriptine.[2]

1. Pentland B, Sawers JSA. Galactorrhoea after withdrawal of bromocriptine. *Br Med J* 1980; **281:** 716.
2. Figà-Talamanca L, *et al.* Hyperthermia after discontinuance of levodopa and bromocriptine therapy: impaired dopamine receptors a possible cause. *Neurology* 1985; **35:** 258–61.

Precautions

Patients with hyperprolactinaemia should be investigated for the possibility of a pituitary tumour before treatment with bromocriptine. Annual gynaecological examinations (or every 6 months for postmenopausal women) are recommended. Treatment of women with hyperprolactinaemic amenorrhoea results in ovulation; such patients should be advised to use contraceptive measures other than an oral contraceptive. Acromegalic patients should be checked for symptoms of peptic ulceration before therapy and should immediately report symptoms of gastro-intestinal discomfort during therapy.

Bromocriptine should be given with caution to patients with cardiovascular disease or a history of psychotic disorders. It is contra-indicated in patients with hypersensitivity to bromocriptine or other ergot alkaloids and in patients with hypertensive disorders during pregnancy or with hypertension postpartum or in the puerperium. It should not be used postpartum or in the puerperium in women with high blood pressure, coronary artery disease, or serious mental disorders. Blood pressure should be monitored carefully, especially during the first few days in postpartum women. Treatment in postpartum women should be discontinued immediately if hypertension, unremitting headache, or signs of CNS toxicity develop. Hypotensive reactions may be disturbing in some patients during the first few days of treatment. Patients who drive or operate machinery should be warned of the possibility of dizziness and fainting during the first few days of treatment.

Patients on long-term, high-dose therapy should be monitored for signs of retroperitoneal fibrosis and bromocriptine withdrawn if fibrotic changes are diagnosed or suspected.

Porphyria. Bromocriptine was considered to be unsafe in patients with acute porphyria because it has been shown to be porphyrinogenic in *animals* or *in-vitro* systems.[1]

1. Moore MR, McColl KEL. *Porphyria: drug lists.* Glasgow: Porphyria Research Unit, University of Glasgow, 1991.

Pregnancy. Details of various surveys of the effect of the use of bromocriptine during pregnancy have been published by the manufacturer.[1,2] The first survey was based on spontaneous reporting of all pregnancies between 1973 and 1980 in women who had taken bromocriptine after conception.[1] Information was obtained on 1410 pregnancies in 1335 women, the majority of whom had been treated for hyperprolactinaemic conditions, while in 256 pregnancies pituitary tumours and acromegaly were the primary diagnosis. Bromocriptine was generally taken at some time in the first 8 weeks after conception, the mean duration of treatment being 21 days. In 4 patients bromocriptine was not prescribed until late in pregnancy and in 9 with acromegaly and pituitary microadenoma it was taken continuously throughout gestation. There were 157 (11.1%) spontaneous abortions, 12 (0.9%) extrauterine pregnancies, 2 patients with 3 hydatidiform moles (0.2%), and an incidence of twin pregnancies of 1.8%. Major congenital abnormalities were detected in 12 (1%) infants at birth and minor abnormalities in 31 (2.5%). A second survey,[2] which consisted of formal monitoring of the use of bromocriptine at 33 clinics between 1979 and 1980, collected data on a further 743 pregnancies in 668 women and had similar findings. The incidence rates reported in these surveys were comparable with those quoted for normal populations and the data indicate that the use of bromocriptine in the treatment of women with infertility is not associated with an increased risk of abortion, multiple pregnancy, or congenital abnormalities. Furthermore, follow-up, for up to 9 years, of 546 children exposed to bromocriptine *in utero* found no evidence that bromocriptine had any adverse effect on postnatal development.[2] Nevertheless, since the risk of abortion is not increased by interruption of treatment, it is still recommended that bromocriptine therapy be stopped as soon as pregnancy is confirmed unless there is a definite indication for its continuation.

See also Pregnancy under Hyperprolactinaemia and Prolactinomas under Uses and Administration, below.

1. Turkalj I, *et al.* Surveillance of bromocriptine in pregnancy. *JAMA* 1982; **247:** 1589–91.
2. Krupp P, Monka C. Bromocriptine in pregnancy: safety aspects. *Klin Wochenschr* 1987; **65:** 823–7.

Interactions

Dopamine antagonists such as the phenothiazines, butyrophenones, thioxanthenes, and metoclopramide (but see below) might be expected to reduce the prolactin-lowering and the antiparkinsonian effect of bromocriptine. Domperidone might reduce the prolactin-lowering effect. Concomitant administration of octreotide and bromocriptine increases the bioavailability of bromocriptine.

Alcohol. Mention of alcohol intolerance in 5 of 73 patients receiving bromocriptine 10 to 60 mg daily for the treatment of acromegaly.[1]

Gastro-intestinal side-effects with low doses of bromocriptine were markedly reduced in 2 women when they abstained from alcohol.[2]

1. Wass JAH, *et al.* Long-term treatment of acromegaly with bromocriptine. *Br Med J* 1977; **1:** 875–8.
2. Ayres J, Maisey MN. Alcohol increases bromocriptine's side effects. *N Engl J Med* 1980; **302:** 806.

Antibacterials. Drowsiness, dystonia, choreoathetoid dyskinesias, and visual hallucinations occurred when *josamycin* was given to a patient receiving bromocriptine.[1]

The systemic bioavailability of a single oral dose of bromocriptine 5 mg was markedly increased in 5 healthy subjects following treatment with *erythromycin estolate* 250 mg four times daily for 4 days;[2] clearance of bromocriptine decreased by 70.6% and peak plasma concentrations of bromocriptine were more than 4 times higher than following the same dose before erythromycin administration.

1. Montastruc JL, Rascol A. Traitement de la maladie de Parkinson par doses élevées de bromocriptine: interaction possible avec la josamycine. *Presse Med* 1984; **13:** 2267–8.
2. Nelson MV, *et al.* Pharmacokinetic evaluation of erythromycin and caffeine administered with bromocriptine in normal subjects. *Clin Pharmacol Ther* 1990; **47:** 166.

Antifungals. The response to bromocriptine was blocked in a patient who was also receiving *griseofulvin.*[1]

1. Schwinn G, *et al.* Metabolic and clinical studies on patients with acromegaly treated with bromocriptine over 22 months. *Eur J Clin Invest* 1977; **7:** 101–7.

Antipsychotics. Serum concentrations of prolactin rose and visual fields deteriorated following administration of *thioridazine* to a 40-year-old man receiving bromocriptine therapy for a large prolactinoma.[1]

For a discussion of the effect of bromocriptine on patients receiving antipsychotics, see under Antiparkinsonian Drugs in Chlorpromazine on p.653.

1. Robbins RJ, *et al.* Interactions between thioridazine and bromocriptine in a patient with a prolactin-secreting pituitary adenoma. *Am J Med* 1984; **76:** 921–3.

Metoclopramide. A study[1] in 10 patients with Parkinson's disease given single doses of bromocriptine 12.5 to 100 mg found that pretreatment with metoclopramide 60 mg had no consistent effect upon plasma concentrations of bromocriptine or growth hormone and no consistent effect upon clinical response.

1. Price P, *et al.* Plasma bromocriptine levels, clinical and growth hormone responses in parkinsonism. *Br J Clin Pharmacol* 1978; **6:** 303–9.

Sympathomimetics. There have been isolated reports[1,2] of severe hypertension, with headache and life-threatening complications, in patients receiving bromocriptine concomitantly with *isometheptene mucate* or *phenylpropanolamine*.

1. Kulig K, *et al.* Bromocriptine-associated headache: possible life-threatening sympathomimetic interaction. *Obstet Gynecol* 1991; **78:** 941–3.
2. Chan JCN, *et al.* Postpartum hypertension, bromocriptine and phenylpropanolamine. *Drug Invest* 1994; **8:** 254–6.

Pharmacokinetics

Only about 30% of an oral dose of bromocriptine is absorbed from the gastro-intestinal tract, and due to extensive first-pass metabolism the bioavailability is only about 6%. It is metabolised in the liver, mainly by hydrolysis to lysergic acid and peptides, and excreted chiefly in faeces via the bile, with small amounts in urine. It has been reported to be 90 to 96% bound to serum albumin *in vitro*.

In a study involving 10 patients with Parkinson's disease, single doses of bromocriptine 12.5, 25, 50, and 100 mg resulted in very variable peak plasma concentrations ranging from 1.3 to 5.3, 1.4 to 3.5, 2.6 to 19.7, and 6.5 to 24.6 ng per mL respectively, 30 to 210 minutes (mean 102 minutes) after dosage.[1] After 4 hours plasma concentrations were about 75% of the peak values. Clinical improvement was evident within 30 to 90 minutes of a dose with peak effect at about 130 minutes and in most patients improvement persisted throughout the 4-hour study period. Peak clinical response, peak fall in blood pressure, and peak rise in plasma concentrations of growth hormone occurred about 30, 60, and 70 minutes respectively after peak plasma-bromocriptine concentrations but there was no significant relationship between them. There was however a significant relationship between plasma concentrations and concurrent changes in clinical response compared with pretreatment scores. Dyskinesias occurred within 90 to 180 minutes of dosage in 5 of 10 patients.

Bromocriptine is well absorbed from standard oral tablets placed in the vagina and plasma concentrations sufficient to lower plasma prolactin concentrations have been achieved using this route.[2,3]

1. Price P, *et al.* Plasma bromocriptine levels, clinical and growth hormone responses in parkinsonism. *Br J Clin Pharmacol* 1978; **6:** 303–9.
2. Vermesh M, *et al.* Vaginal bromocriptine: pharmacology and effect on serum prolactin in normal women. *Obstet Gynecol* 1988; **72:** 693–8.
3. Katz E, *et al.* Successful treatment of a prolactin-producing pituitary macroadenoma with intravaginal bromocriptine mesylate: a novel approach to intolerance of oral therapy. *Obstet Gynecol* 1989; **73:** 517–20.

Uses and Administration

Bromocriptine, an ergot derivative (p.1576), is a dopamine D_2-agonist. It inhibits the secretion of prolactin (p.1259) from the anterior pituitary and is used in the treatment of prolactinoma and in endocrinological disorders associated with hyperprolactinaemia, including amenorrhoea, galactorrhoea, hypogonadism, and infertility in both men and women. Bromocriptine is also used to suppress puerperal lactation for medical reasons; it is not recommended for the routine suppression of physiological lactation or for the treatment of post-partum breast pain and engorgement that may be adequately relieved with simple analgesics and breast support. Growth-hormone secretion may be suppressed by bromocriptine in some patients with acromegaly. Because of its dopaminergic activity bromocriptine is also used in the management of Parkinson's disease.

Bromocriptine is usually administered by mouth as the mesylate; doses are expressed in terms of the base. It should be taken with food.

For the prevention of puerperal lactation bromocriptine 2.5 mg is given on the day of delivery followed by 2.5 mg twice daily for 14 days. The risk of hypotension and, more rarely, hypertension must be borne in mind and it has been recommended that bromocriptine should not be given until at least 4 hours after delivery. For the suppression of established lactation it is given in a dose of 2.5 mg daily for 2 to 3 days subsequently increased to 2.5 mg twice daily for 14 days.

For the treatment of other conditions the dose of bromocriptine is usually increased gradually as follows: an initial dose of 1 to 1.25 mg at night, increased to 2 to 2.5 mg at night after 2 to 3 days, and subsequently increased by 1 to 2.5 mg at intervals of 2 to 3 days to a dose of 2.5 mg twice daily. Any further increments should be made in a similar manner.

In the treatment of hypogonadism and galactorrhoea syndromes and infertility bromocriptine is introduced gradually as described above. Most of the patients with hyperprolactinaemia respond to 7.5 mg daily but up to 30 mg daily may be required. In patients known to have prolactinomas the dose is increased gradually up to 5 mg every 6 hours but occasionally patients may require up to 30 mg daily. Infertile patients without raised serum concentrations of prolactin are usually given 2.5 mg twice daily.

In cyclical benign breast and menstrual disorders bromocriptine is introduced gradually up to a usual dosage of 2.5 mg twice daily.

Bromocriptine may be used as an adjunct to surgery and radiotherapy to reduce growth-hormone concentrations in plasma in acromegalic patients. It is introduced gradually up to a dose of 2.5 mg twice daily and may then be increased further by 2.5 mg every 2 to 3 days if necessary up to 5 mg every 6 hours, according to response.

In Parkinson's disease bromocriptine has been used alone, although it is usually given as an adjunct to levodopa treatment. It should be introduced gradually and during this period patients already receiving levodopa can have their levodopa dosage decreased gradually until an optimal response is achieved. A suggested initial dose is 1 to 1.25 mg of bromocriptine at night during week 1, increased to 2 to 2.5 mg at night for week 2, 2.5 mg twice daily for week 3, and for week 4, 2.5 mg three times daily; the dose may be increased thereafter by 2.5 mg every 3 to 14 days depending on response. Most patients require doses within the range of 10 to 40 mg daily.

Bromocriptine mesylate has also been given intramuscularly as a depot injection for disorders associated with hyperprolactinaemia.

Acromegaly. Dopaminergics can produce a paradoxical reduction in growth hormone secretion and bromocriptine has been used in acromegaly (p.1235) as adjunctive therapy to surgery and/or radiotherapy to reduce circulating growth hormone levels. While it is less effective than octreotide, it can be given orally and is therefore more convenient to administer.

Cushing's syndrome. There have been occasional reports of benefit with the use of bromocriptine in the treatment of Cushing's syndrome (p.1236). Atkinson *et al.*[1] reported that remission of ACTH-dependent Cushing's syndrome was maintained for 6 years by bromocriptine 2.5 mg twice daily in a patient who had initially received pituitary irradiation. However, in a later review Atkinson reported that they had recently found that bromocriptine did not effectively reduce ACTH secretion following bilateral adrenalectomy.[2]

1. Atkinson AB, *et al.* Six year remission of ACTH-dependent Cushing's syndrome using bromocriptine. *Postgrad Med J* 1985; **61:** 239–42.
2. Atkinson AB. The treatment of Cushing's syndrome. *Clin Endocrinol (Oxf)* 1991; **34:** 507–13.

Hyperprolactinaemia and prolactinomas. Prolactinomas (prolactin-secreting pituitary adenomas) are among the commonest causes of hyperprolactinaemia. Raised serum-prolactin concentrations may result in reduced gonadotrophin production, which in turn may suppress gonadal function. Consequences may include oligomenorrhoea or amenorrhoea, and infertility in either sex. Galactorrhoea may also result from high prolactin levels and can occur in men as well as women.

Dopamine is the major inhibitory factor in the hypothalamus and directly inhibits the secretion of prolactin. Bromocriptine, a dopamine agonist, has historically been the first choice of treatment in many centres for the treatment of hyperprolactinaemia secondary to a prolactinoma although cabergoline is now preferred by some. Bromocriptine is extremely effective in controlling elevated circulating prolactin concentrations and restoring gonadal function; although it is rarely curative, it may produce considerable shrinkage of the adenoma.[1-5]

The sensitivity of hyperprolactinaemia to bromocriptine therapy can vary considerably between patients and this is reflected in the wide range of oral doses required to reduce prolactin concentrations to normal levels. Although methods such as initiating therapy with gradually increasing doses can minimise adverse effects it has been reported that about 5 to 10% of patients are unable to tolerate bromocriptine by mouth;[6] various other routes of administration have therefore been investigated. Bromocriptine is well absorbed from standard oral tablets placed in the vagina and appears to be both effective in lowering prolactin concentrations and well tolerated when given by this route.[7] However, limitations are considered to be the relatively short duration of action and the relatively low dose that can be administered.[6] Of the various injectable depot formulations that have been tried, one preparation given intramuscularly in a dose of 50 to 250 mg monthly has been found to be effective and well tolerated in long-term studies;[8,9] it is reported to be used in some centres to initiate treatment for macroprolactinomas.[6]

For discussions of the management of hyperprolactinaemia and associated disorders see p.1238 (hyperprolactinaemia), p.1236 (amenorrhoea), p.1239 (hypogonadism), p.1614 (erectile dysfunction), and p.1239 (infertility).

1. Prescott RWG, *et al.* Hyperprolactinaemia in men—response to bromocriptine therapy. *Lancet* 1982; **i:** 245–8.
2. Hancock KW, *et al.* Long term suppression of prolactin concentrations after bromocriptine induced regression of pituitary prolactinomas. *Br Med J* 1985; **290:** 117–8.
3. Grossman A, Besser GM. Prolactinomas. *Br Med J* 1985; **290:** 182–4.
4. Liuzzi A, *et al.* Low doses of dopamine agonists in the long-term treatment of macroprolactinomas. *N Engl J Med* 1985; **313:** 656–9.
5. Ho KY, Thorner MO. Therapeutic applications of bromocriptine in endocrine and neurological diseases. *Drugs* 1988; **36:** 67–82.
6. Ciccarelli E, Camanni F. Diagnosis and drug therapy of prolactinoma. *Drugs* 1996; **51:** 954–65.
7. Ginsburg J, *et al.* Vaginal bromocriptine. *Lancet* 1991; **338:** 1205–6.
8. Ciccarelli E, *et al.* Long term therapy of patients with macroprolactinoma using repeatable injectable bromocriptine. *J Clin Endocrinol Metab* 1993; **76:** 484–8.
9. Ciccarelli E, *et al.* Double blind randomized study using oral or injectable bromocriptine in patients with hyperprolactinaemia. *Clin Endocrinol (Oxf)* 1994; **40:** 193–8.

PREGNANCY. Pregnancy and the hyperprolactinaemic woman has been discussed.[1] The continuous administration of bromocriptine throughout pregnancy has been advocated in women with macroadenomas, but the effects on the developing fetus are not yet known and such therapy cannot be recommended. However, existing information is reassuring and discovery of pregnancy at an advanced stage in a woman taking bromocriptine does not justify therapeutic abortion. If symptomatic tumour enlargement occurs during pregnancy reinstitution of bromocriptine is probably less harmful to the mother and child than surgery.

See also under Precautions, above.

1. Molitch ME. Pregnancy and the hyperprolactinemic woman. *N Engl J Med* 1985; **312:** 1364–70.

Lactation inhibition. Because of its effects on prolactin, bromocriptine is a potent suppressor of lactation and has been widely used for the prevention of lactation in women who choose not to breast feed postpartum. However, bromocriptine has been associated with severe adverse effects in some women receiving it, and its use to suppress a physiological state has been criticised (see p.1240). Consequently, the manufacturers in a number of countries recommend that bromocriptine should only be used to suppress puerperal lactation for medical reasons; it is also not recommended for the treatment of postpartum breast pain and engorgement that may be adequately relieved with simple analgesics and breast support.

Mastalgia. Since mastalgia (p.1443) can improve spontaneously treatment should rarely be considered unless pain has been present for about 6 months. Bromocriptine is one of the drugs that may be used to treat mastalgia.[1,2] It may improve symptoms in up to about 50% of patients with cyclical mastalgia, but is less effective in the non-cyclical form.[3,4] Adverse effects can be severe in some patients.

1. Gateley CA, Mansel RE. Management of the painful and nodular breast. *Br Med Bull* 1991; **47:** 284–94.
2. Anonymous. Cyclical breast pain—what works and what doesn't. *Drug Ther Bull* 1992; **30:** 1–3.
3. Pye JK, *et al.* Clinical experience of drug treatments for mastalgia. *Lancet* 1985; **ii:** 373–7.
4. Mansel RE, Dogliotti L. European multicentre trial of bromocriptine in cyclical mastalgia. *Lancet* 1990; **335:** 190–3.

Neuroleptic malignant syndrome. Bromocriptine has been used in doses of up to 30 mg daily,[1-5] usually alone or with dantrolene, in the treatment of neuroleptic malignant syndrome (p.651) although some workers have not found it to be of use.[6]

1. Mueller PS, *et al.* Neuroleptic malignant syndrome: successful treatment with bromocriptine. *JAMA* 1983; **249:** 386–8.
2. Dhib-Jalbut S, *et al.* Treatment of the neuroleptic malignant syndrome with bromocriptine. *JAMA* 1983; **250:** 484–5.
3. Clarke CE, *et al.* Clinical spectrum of neuroleptic malignant syndrome. *Lancet* 1988; **ii:** 969–70.
4. Guerrero RM, Shifrar KA. Diagnosis and treatment of neuroleptic malignant syndrome. *Clin Pharm* 1988; **7:** 697–701.
5. Lo TCM, *et al.* Neuroleptic malignant syndrome: another medical cause of acute abdomen. *Postgrad Med J* 1989; **65:** 653–5.
6. Rosebush PI, *et al.* The treatment of neuroleptic malignant syndrome: are dantrolene and bromocriptine useful adjuncts to supportive care? *Br J Psychiatry* 1991; **159:** 709–12.

Parkinsonism. While some neurologists use dopamine agonists such as bromocriptine early in the treatment of parkinsonism (p.1128), in an attempt to delay therapy with levodopa, others reserve them for adjunctive use when levodopa is no longer effective alone or cannot be tolerated. They are sometimes useful in reducing 'off' periods with levodopa and in ameliorating other fluctuations of mobility in the later stage of the disease.

References.

1. Temlett JA, *et al.* Adjunctive therapy with bromocriptine in Parkinson's disease. *S Afr Med J* 1990; **78:** 680–5.
2. Hely MA, *et al.* The Sydney Multicentre Study of Parkinson's disease: a randomised, prospective five year study comparing low dose bromocriptine with low dose levodopa-carbidopa. *J Neurol Neurosurg Psychiatry* 1994; **57:** 903–10.
3. Montastruc JL, *et al.* A randomised controlled study comparing bromocriptine to which levodopa was later added, with levodopa alone in previously untreated patients with Parkinson's disease: a five year follow up. *J Neurol Neurosurg Psychiatry* 1994; **57:** 1034–8.
4. Giménez-Roldán S, *et al.* Early combination of bromocriptine and levodopa in Parkinson's disease: a prospective randomized study of two parallel groups over a total follow-up period of 44 months including an initial 8-month double-blind stage. *Clin Neuropharmacol* 1997; **20:** 67–76.
5. Ogawa N, *et al.* Nationwide multicenter prospective study on the long-term effects of bromocriptine for Parkinson's disease: final report of a ten-year follow-up. *Eur Neurol* 1997; **38** (suppl 2): 37–49.

Polycystic ovary syndrome. Up to one-third of women with the polycystic ovary syndrome (p.1240) have mild basal hyperprolactinaemia without evidence of a pituitary tumour. Bromocriptine 5 mg daily for up to 2 years was given to 34 women with polycystic ovary syndrome and either normal or increased prolactin levels; none had monthly menses. Improved menstrual patterns were achieved in 28 women and 24 developed monthly menses.[1] Gonadotrophin, prolactin, and dehydroepiandrosterone sulphate levels before treatment were not significantly different in responders and nonresponders. Prolactin levels were uniformly depressed in both groups.

1. Pehrson JJ, *et al.* Bromocriptine, sex steroid metabolism, and menstrual patterns in the polycystic ovary syndrome. *Ann Intern Med* 1986; **105:** 129–30.

Restless legs syndrome. The aetiology of restless legs syndrome (see under Parasomnias, p.639) is obscure and treatment has largely been empirical. Bromocriptine showed some benefit in one small study.[1]

1. Walters AS, *et al.* A double-blind randomized crossover trial of bromocriptine and placebo in restless legs syndrome. *Ann Neurol* 1988: **24:** 455–8.

Withdrawal syndromes. ALCOHOL. Studies of the efficacy of bromocriptine as an aid in the maintenance of abstinence from alcohol (p.1099) have yielded conflicting results.[1-4] However, it has been suggested[3] that response to bromocriptine might be linked to a specific genotype of the D_2 dopamine receptor.

1. Dongier M, *et al.* Bromocriptine in the treatment of alcohol dependence. *Alcohol Clin Exp Res* 1991; **15:** 970–7.
2. Naranjo CA, *et al.* Long-acting bromocriptine (B) does not reduce relapse in alcoholics. *Clin Pharmacol Ther* 1995; **57:** 161.
3. Lawford BR, *et al.* Bromocriptine in the treatment of alcoholics with the D_2 dopamine receptor A1 allele. *Nat Med* 1995; **1:** 337–41.
4. Powell BJ, *et al.* A double-blind, placebo-controlled study of nortriptyline and bromocriptine in male alcoholics subtyped by comorbid psychiatric disorders. *Alcohol Clin Exp Res* 1995; **19:** 462–8.

Preparations

BP 1998: Bromocriptine Capsules; Bromocriptine Tablets;
USP 23: Bromocriptine Mesylate Capsules; Bromocriptine Mesylate Tablets.

Proprietary Preparations (details are given in Part 3)
Aust.: Antipark†; Broman; Bromed; Cehapark; Maylaktin†; Parlodel; Umprel; ***Austral.:*** Bromolactin; Kripton; Parlodel; ***Belg.:*** Parlodel; ***Canad.:*** Parlodel; ***Fr.:*** Bromo-Kin; Parlodel; ***Ger.:*** kirim; Pravidel; ***Irl.:*** Parlodel; ***Ital.:*** Parlodel; Serocryptin†; ***Jpn:*** Parlodel; ***Neth.:*** Parlodel; ***Norw.:*** Parlodel; ***S.Afr.:*** Parlodel; ***Spain:*** Lactismine†; Parlodel; ***Swed.:*** Pravidel; ***Switz.:*** Parlodel; Serocryptin; ***UK:*** Parlodel; ***USA:*** Parlodel.

Budipine (1967-p)

Budipine *(rINN).*
1-*tert*-Butyl-4,4-diphenylpiperidine.
$C_{21}H_{27}N = 293.4$.
CAS — 57982-78-2.

Budipine is a phenylpiperidine derivative under investigation for the treatment of tremor associated with parkinsonism.

References.

1. Spieker S, *et al.* Tremorlytic activity of budipine: a quantitative study with long-term tremor recordings. *Clin Neuropharmacol* 1995; **18:** 266–72.

Cabergoline (2841-h)

Cabergoline *(BAN, USAN, rINN).*
FCE-21336. 1-[(6-Allylergolin-8β-yl)carbonyl]-1-[3-(dimethylamino)propyl]-3-ethylurea; (8*R*)-6-Allyl-*N*-[3-(dimethylamino)propyl]-*N*-(ethylcarbamoyl)ergoline-8-carboxamide.
$C_{26}H_{37}N_5O_2 = 451.6$.
CAS — 81409-90-7.

Adverse Effects and Precautions

As for Bromocriptine, p.1132, although patients unable to tolerate bromocriptine may tolerate cabergoline (and *vice versa*).

The manufacturer recommends that conception should be avoided for at least one month after treatment.

Effects on the respiratory system. Report[1] of a patient who developed pleuropulmonary disease 16 months after starting treatment with cabergoline. The patient had previously received bromocriptine for 10 years and had had a normal chest X-ray at the time of transfer to treatment with cabergoline. Two other cases of pleural effusion/pulmonary fibrosis, occurring after 10 to 11 months of treatment, have also been described.[2] One patient had modest pre-treatment lung alterations attributed to previous bromocriptine treatment. Withdrawal was associated with improvement in both cases.

1. Bhatt MH, *et al.* Pleuropulmonary disease associated with dopamine agonist therapy. *Ann Neurol* 1991; **30:** 613–16.
2. Geminiani G, *et al.* Cabergoline in Parkinson's disease complicated by motor fluctuations. *Mov Disord* 1996; **11:** 495–500.

Oedema. Three cases of lower limb oedema following chronic treatment with cabergoline have been reported.[1] In one case the oedema was severe enough to necessitate withdrawal of therapy.

1. Geminiani G, *et al.* Cabergoline in Parkinson's disease complicated by motor fluctuations. *Mov Disord* 1996; **11:** 495–500.

Interactions

As for Bromocriptine, p.1133.

Pharmacokinetics

Cabergoline is absorbed from the gastro-intestinal tract and extensively metabolised to several metabolites, which do not appear to contribute to its pharmacological activity. Plasma protein binding has been estimated to be about 40%. Cabergoline is mainly eliminated via the faeces; a small proportion is excreted in the urine.

Pharmacokinetic studies of cabergoline have been hampered by lack of an assay method sensitive enough to detect plasma concentrations of cabergoline following therapeutic doses. However, the plasma elimination half-life of cabergoline has been estimated indirectly to be 63 to 68 hours in healthy volunteers and 79 to 115 hours in patients with hyperprolactinaemia.[1]

1. Rains CP, *et al.* Cabergoline: a review of its pharmacological properties and therapeutic potential in the treatment of hyperprolactinaemia and inhibition of lactation. *Drugs* 1995; **49:** 255–79.

Uses and Administration

Cabergoline, an ergot derivative, is a dopamine D_2-agonist with actions and uses similar to those of bromocriptine (p.1134). It is a potent and long-lasting inhibitor of prolactin secretion and is given by mouth in the management of disorders associated with hyperprolactinaemia. It is also used to suppress puerperal lactation for medical reasons; it is not recommended for the routine suppression of physiological lactation or for the treatment of postpartum breast pain and engorgement that may be adequately relieved with simple analgesics and breast support. Cabergoline is also used in the management of Parkinson's disease.

To inhibit physiological lactation, cabergoline is given as a single 1-mg dose on the first day postpartum. For suppression of established lactation, the dose is 0.25 mg every 12 hours for 2 days. In the treatment of disorders associated with hyperprolactinaemia, the initial dose of cabergoline is 0.5 mg per week. The dose is then increased at monthly intervals by 0.5 mg per week according to response. The weekly dose may be administered on a single occasion or divided into 2 doses on separate days; doses over 1 mg should be given as divided doses. The usual dose is 1 mg per week but up to 4.5 mg has been used.

In Parkinson's disease, cabergoline is used as an adjunct in patients experiencing 'on-off' fluctuations in control with levodopa treatment alone. It should be introduced gradually and during this period the dose of levodopa may be reduced gradually until an optimal response is achieved. A suggested initial dose of cabergoline is 1 mg as a single daily dose given with meals. The dose may be increased in increments of 0.5 or 1 mg at intervals of 7 or 14 days. The recommended therapeutic dose range is 2 to 6 mg daily.

General references.

1. Rains CP, *et al.* Cabergoline: a review of its pharmacological properties and therapeutic potential in the treatment of hyperprolactinaemia and inhibition of lactation. *Drugs* 1995; **49:** 255–79.

Acromegaly. Dopamine agonists have been used in acromegaly (p.1235) as adjuvants to surgery or radiotherapy to reduce circulating growth hormone concentrations, although they are less effective than the somatostatin analogue octreotide. However, a small study comparing cabergoline with depot bromocriptine and quinagolide failed to find evidence of its effectiveness (see p.1143).

Hyperprolactinaemia and prolactinomas. Dopamine agonists are widely used for the treatment of hyperprolactinaemia secondary to a prolactinoma (see p.1238). Although bromocriptine has historically been the first choice for this indication some centres now reportedly prefer cabergoline,[1] which appears to be more effective and better tolerated.[2]

References.[1-7]

1. Webster J. A comparative review of the tolerability profiles of dopamine agonists in the treatment of hyperprolactinaemia and inhibition of lactation. *Drug Safety* 1996; **14:** 228–38. Correction. *ibid.*, 342.
2. Pascal-Vigneron V, *et al.* Amenorrhée hyperprolactinémique: traitement par cabergoline versus bromocriptine. *Presse Med* 1995; **24:** 753–7.
3. Falsetti L, *et al.* Cabergoline treatment in hyperprolactinaemic women. *J Obstet Gynaecol* 1991; **11:** 68–71.
4. Webster J, *et al.* Dose-dependent suppression of serum prolactin by cabergoline in hyperprolactinaemia: a placebo controlled, double blind, multicentre study. *Clin Endocrinol (Oxf)* 1992; **37:** 534–41.
5. Ferrari C, *et al.* Cabergoline in the long-term therapy of hyperprolactinemic disorders. *Acta Endocrinol (Copenh)* 1992; **126:** 489–94.
6. Webster J, *et al.* The efficacy and tolerability of long-term cabergoline therapy in hyperprolactinaemic disorders: an open, uncontrolled, multicentre study. *Clin Endocrinol (Oxf)* 1993; **39:** 323–9.
7. Webster J,*et al.* A comparison of cabergoline and bromocriptine in the treatment of hyperprolactinemic amenorrhea. *N Engl J Med* 1994; **331:** 904–9.

Lactation inhibition. A single 1-mg dose of cabergoline was found to be as effective as bromocriptine 2.5 mg given twice daily for 14 days for preventing puerperal lactation in a double-blind multicentre study involving 272 women.[1] It has been suggested that cabergoline would be a better choice than bromocriptine for lactation inhibition.[2] However, as discussed on p.1240, the routine use of dopaminergics such as bromocriptine or cabergoline is not recommended for the suppression of physiological lactation.

1. European Multicentre Study Group for Cabergoline in Lactation Inhibition. Single dose cabergoline versus bromocriptine in inhibition of puerperal lactation: randomised, double blind, multicentre study. *Br Med J* 1991; **302:** 1367–71.
2. Webster J. A comparative review of the tolerability profiles of dopamine agonists in the treatment of hyperprolactinaemia and inhibition of lactation. *Drug Safety* 1996; **14:** 228–38. Correction. *ibid.*; 342.

Parkinsonism. Cabergoline is used as a long-acting dopamine agonist in Parkinson's disease (see p.1128). While some neurologists use dopamine agonists early in treatment in an attempt to delay therapy with levodopa others reserve them for use when levodopa is no longer effective or cannot be tolerated. They are sometimes useful in reducing 'off' periods with levodopa and in ameliorating other fluctuations of mobility in the later stages of the disease.

References.

1. Inzelberg R, *et al.* Double-blind comparison of cabergoline and bromocriptine in Parkinson's disease patients with motor fluctuations. *Neurology* 1996; **47:** 785–8.
2. Geminiani G, *et al.* Cabergoline in Parkinson's disease complicated by motor fluctuations. *Mov Disord* 1996; **11:** 495–500.
3. Hutton JT, *et al.* Multicenter, placebo-controlled trial of cabergoline taken once daily in the treatment of Parkinson's disease. *Neurology* 1996; **46:** 1062–5.
4. Marsden CD. Clinical experience with cabergoline in patients with advanced Parkinson's disease treated with levodopa. *Drugs* 1998; **55** (suppl 1): 17–22.
5. Rinne UK, *et al.* Early treatment of Parkinson's disease with cabergoline delays the onset of motor complications: results of a double-blind levodopa controlled trial. *Drugs* 1998; **55** (suppl 1): 23–30.

Preparations

Proprietary Preparations (details are given in Part 3)
Aust.: Dostinex; ***Austral.:*** Dostinex; ***Belg.:*** Dostinex; ***Ger.:*** Dostinex; ***Irl.:*** Dostinex; ***Ital.:*** Dostinex; ***Neth.:*** Dostinex; ***Norw.:*** Dostinex; ***Spain:*** Dostinex; ***Swed.:*** Cabaser; Dostinex; ***Switz.:*** Dostinex; ***UK:*** Cabaser; Dostinex; ***USA:*** Dostinex.

Carbidopa (4547-l)

Carbidopa *(BAN, USAN, rINN)*.

Carbidopum; α-Methyldopa Hydrazine; MK-486. (+)-2-(3,4-Dihydroxybenzyl)-2-hydrazinopropionic acid monohydrate; (−)-L-α-Hydrazino-3,4-dihydroxy-α-methylhydrocinnamic acid monohydrate.

$C_{10}H_{14}N_2O_4,H_2O = 244.2$.

CAS — 28860-95-9 (anhydrous); 38821-49-7 (monohydrate).

NOTE. The synonym MK-485 has been used for the racemic mixture.

Compounded preparations of carbidopa and levodopa have the British Approved Name Co-careldopa; the proportions are expressed in the form *x/y* where *x* and *y* are the strengths in milligrams of carbidopa and levodopa respectively.

Compounded preparations of carbidopa and levodopa in USP 23 may be represented by the name Co-careldopa.

Pharmacopoeias. In Eur. (see p.viii), Int., Jpn, and US.

A white to yellowish white, odourless or almost odourless powder. Slightly **soluble** in water and in methyl alcohol; very slightly soluble to practically insoluble in alcohol; freely soluble in 3M hydrochloric acid; practically insoluble in acetone, in chloroform, in dichloromethane, and in ether; dissolves in dilute solutions of mineral acids. **Protect** from light.

Adverse Effects

Hypersensitivity. Henoch-Schönlein purpura which developed in a 68-year-old patient being treated for Parkinson's disease appeared to be due to either carbidopa or an excipient of the preparation containing the carbidopa (Sinemet).[1]

1. Niedermaier G, Briner V. Henoch-Schönlein syndrome induced by carbidopa/levodopa. *Lancet* 1997; **349:** 1071–2.

Pharmacokinetics

Carbidopa is rapidly but incompletely absorbed from the gastro-intestinal tract. It is rapidly excreted in the urine both unchanged and in the form of metabolites. It does not cross the blood-brain barrier. In *rats*, carbidopa has been reported to cross the placenta and to be distributed into breast milk.

Uses and Administration

Carbidopa is a peripheral decarboxylase inhibitor with little or no pharmacological activity when given alone in usual doses. It inhibits the peripheral decarboxylation of levodopa to dopamine and as, unlike levodopa, it does not cross the blood-brain barrier, effective brain concentrations of dopamine are produced with lower doses of levodopa. At the same time reduced peripheral formation of dopamine reduces peripheral side-effects, notably nausea and vomiting, and cardiac arrhythmias, although the dyskinesias and adverse mental effects associated with levodopa therapy tend to develop earlier. Contrary to its effect in patients on levodopa alone, pyridoxine does not inhibit the response to levodopa in patients also receiving a peripheral decarboxylase inhibitor.

In the treatment of parkinsonism it is given with levodopa to enable a lower dosage of the latter to be used and a more rapid response to be obtained, and to decrease side-effects. For details of administration and dosage, see Levodopa, p.1140.

Carbidopa also inhibits the peripheral decarboxylation of the serotonin precursor oxitriptan (p.301).

General references.

1. Pinder RM, *et al.* Levodopa and decarboxylase inhibitors: a review of their clinical pharmacology and use in the treatment of parkinsonism. *Drugs* 1976; **11:** 329–77.
2. Boshes B. Sinemet and the treatment of parkinsonism. *Ann Intern Med* 1981; **94:** 364–70.

Preparations

BP 1998: Co-careldopa Tablets;
USP 23: Carbidopa and Levodopa Tablets.

Proprietary Preparations (details are given in Part 3)
USA: Lodosyn.

Multi-ingredient: ***Aust.:*** Sinemet; ***Austral.:*** Kinson; Sinacarb; Sinemet; ***Belg.:*** Sinemet; ***Canad.:*** Apo-Levocarb; Sinemet; ***Fr.:*** Sinemet; ***Ger.:*** Isicom; Nacom; Striaton; ***Irl.:*** Half Sinemet; Sinemet; ***Ital.:*** Sinemet; ***Neth.:*** Sinemet; ***Norw.:*** Sinemet; ***S.Afr.:*** Carbilev; Sinemet; ***Spain:*** Sinemet; ***Swed.:*** Sinemet; ***Switz.:*** Sinemet; ***UK:*** Half Sinemet; Sinemet; ***USA:*** Sinemet.

Droxidopa (3676-y)

Droxidopa *(rINN)*.

L-*threo*-3,4-Dihydroxyphenylserine. (−)-*threo*-3-(3,4-Dihydroxyphenyl)-L-serine.

$C_9H_{11}NO_5 = 213.2$.

CAS — 23651-95-8.

Droxidopa is a precursor of noradrenaline that is used in the treatment of parkinsonism and some forms of orthostatic hypotension. The racemic form (DL-*threo*-3,4-dihydroxyphenylserine) has been studied for similar uses.

References.

1. Iida N, *et al.* Treatment of dialysis-induced hypotension with L-threo-3, 4-dihydroxyphenylserine. *Nephrol Dial Transplant* 1994; **9:** 1130–5.

Preparations

Proprietary Preparations (details are given in Part 3)
Jpn: Dops.

Entacapone (15430-d)

Entacapone *(BAN, rINN)*.

OR-611. (*E*)-α-Cyano-*N,N*-diethyl-3,4-dihydroxy-5-nitrocinnamamide; (*E*)-2-Cyano-3-(3,4-dihydroxy-5-nitrophenyl)-*N,N*-diethylacrylamide.

$C_{14}H_{15}N_3O_5 = 305.3$.

CAS — 130929-57-6.

Adverse Effects

The most frequent adverse effects produced by entacapone relate to increased dopaminergic activity and occur most commonly at the start of treatment; reduction of the levodopa dosage may reduce the severity and frequency of such effects. Adverse effects may include nausea, vomiting, abdominal pain, constipation, diarrhoea, dry mouth, and dyskinesias. A decrease in haemoglobin has been observed in some patients treated for more than 6 months. Increases in liver enzyme values have been reported rarely. Entacapone may produce a harmless reddish-brown discoloration of the urine.

Precautions

Entacapone is contra-indicated in patients with phaeochromocytoma and in patients with a previous history of neuroleptic malignant syndrome or nontraumatic rhabdomyolysis; it should not be used in patients with hepatic impairment. Use with levodopa may cause dizziness and orthostatic hypotension; if affected patients should not drive or operate machinery. Treatment with entacapone should not be stopped abruptly; when necessary withdrawal should be made gradually, increasing the dose of levodopa as required.

Interactions

Entacapone should be used with caution or not at all in patients receiving other drugs metabolised by catechol-*O*-methyltransferase (COMT) including adrenaline, apomorphine, dobutamine, dopamine, isoprenaline, methyldopa, noradrenaline, and rimiterol.

Entacapone may aggravate levodopa-induced orthostatic hypotension and should be used cautiously in patients who are taking other drugs which may cause orthostatic hypotension.

Entacapone may form chelates with iron preparations in the gastro-intestinal tract; the two drugs should be taken at least 2 to 3 hours apart.

Pharmacokinetics

There are large intra- and interindividual variations in the absorption of entacapone. Peak plasma concentrations are achieved about one hour after oral administration. Entacapone undergoes extensive first-pass metabolism and oral bioavailability is about 35%. Absorption is not affected significantly by food. Entacapone is extensively bound to plasma proteins. It is eliminated mainly in the faeces with about 10 to 20% being excreted in the urine, mainly as glucuronide conjugates.

Entacapone is rapidly absorbed from the gastro-intestinal tract and bioavailability following oral administration has been reported to range from 29 to 46%. It does not cross the blood-brain barrier. Over half of a dose appears in the faeces with smaller amounts being excreted in the urine as glucuronides of entacapone and its (Z)-isomer. Elimination half-lives of about 1.6 to 3.4 hours have been reported for entacapone.

References.

1. Wikberg T, *et al.* Identification of major metabolites of the catechol-O-methyltransferase inhibitor entacapone in rats and humans. *Drug Metab Dispos* 1993; **21:** 81–92.
2. Keränen T, *et al.* Inhibition of soluble catechol-O-methyltransferase and single-dose pharmacokinetics after oral and intravenous administration of entacapone. *Eur J Clin Pharmacol* 1994; **46:** 151–7.

Uses and Administration

Entacapone is a peripheral inhibitor of catechol-*O*-methyltransferase (COMT) an enzyme involved in the metabolism of dopamine and levodopa. It is used as an adjunct to combination preparations of levodopa and dopa decarboxylase inhibitors, in patients with Parkinson's disease and 'end-of-dose' motor fluctuations who cannot be stabilised on levodopa combinations alone. Entacapone is given by mouth in a dosage of 200 mg at the same time as each dose of levodopa, up to a maximum of 200 mg ten times daily. It is often necessary to gradually reduce the dosage of levodopa by about 10 to 30% within the first few weeks after starting treatment with entacapone.

Parkinsonism. As a peripheral inhibitor of catechol-*O*-methyltransferase (COMT) entacapone extends the duration and effect of levodopa when given concomitantly.[1] In studies[2-5] in patients with Parkinson's disease and levodopa-related fluctuations in disability it has prolonged the response to levodopa and permitted the dosage of levodopa to be reduced.

1. Nutt JG. Catechol-O-methyltransferase inhibitors for treatment of Parkinson's disease. *Lancet* 1998; **351:** 1221–2.
2. Nutt JG, *et al.* Effect of peripheral catechol-O-methyl transferase inhibition on the pharmacokinetics and pharmacodynamics of levodopa in parkinsonian patients. *Neurology* 1994; **44:** 913–19.
3. Ruottinen HM, Rinne UK. Entacapone prolongs levodopa response in a one month double blind study in parkinsonian patients with levodopa related fluctuations. *J Neurol Neurosurg Psychiatry* 1996; **60:** 36–40.
4. Ruottinen HM, Rinne UK. A double-blind pharmacokinetic and clinical dose-response study of entacapone as an adjuvant to levodopa therapy in advanced Parkinson's disease. *Clin Neuropharmacol* 1996; **19:** 283–96.
5. Parkinson Study Group. Entacapone improves motor fluctuations in levodopa-treated Parkinson's disease patients. *Ann Neurol* 1997; **42:** 747–55.

Preparations

Proprietary Preparations (details are given in Part 3)
UK: Comtess.

Lazabemide (15902-c)

Lazabemide *(USAN, rINN)*.

Ro-19-6327; Ro-19-6327/000. *N*-(2-Aminoethyl)-5-chloropicolinamide.

$C_8H_{10}ClN_3O = 199.6$.

CAS — 103878-84-8.

Lazabemide is a reversible inhibitor of monoamine oxidase type B that is under investigation in the management of parkinsonism.

References.

1. Parkinson Study Group. A controlled trial of lazabemide (Ro 19-6327) in levodopa-treated Parkinson's disease. *Arch Neurol* 1994; **51:** 342–7.
2. The Parkinson Study Group. Effect of lazabemide on the progression of disability in early Parkinson's disease. *Ann Neurol* 1996; **40:** 99–107.
3. Dingemanse J, *et al.* Pharmacokinetics and pharmacodynamics of single and multiple doses of the MAO-B inhibitor lazabemide in healthy subjects. *Br J Clin Pharmacol* 1997; **43:** 41–7.

Levodopa (4541-g)

Levodopa *(BAN, USAN, rINN).*

Dihydroxyphenylalanine; L-Dopa; 3-Hydroxy-L-tyrosine; Laevo-dopa; Levodopum. (−)-3-(3,4-Dihydroxyphenyl)-L-alanine.

$C_9H_{11}NO_4$ = 197.2.

CAS — 59-92-7.

NOTE. Compounded preparations of levodopa and benserazide hydrochloride in proportions, by weight, corresponding to 4 parts of levodopa and 1 part of benserazide have the British Approved Name Co-beneldopa.

Compounded preparations of carbidopa and levodopa have the British Approved Name Co-careldopa; the proportions are expressed in the form *x/y* where *x* and *y* are the strengths in milligrams of carbidopa and levodopa respectively.

Compounded preparations of carbidopa and levodopa in USP 23 may be represented by the name Co-careldopa.

Pharmacopoeias. In *Chin., Eur.* (see p.viii), *Int., Jpn,* and *US.*

A white or slightly cream-coloured, odourless, crystalline powder. In the presence of moisture it is rapidly oxidised by atmospheric oxygen and darkens.

Slightly **soluble** in water; freely soluble in 1M hydrochloric acid but sparingly soluble in 0.1M hydrochloric acid; practically insoluble in alcohol, and in ether. A 1% suspension in water has a pH of 4.5 to 7.0. **Store** in airtight containers. Protect from light. The USP recommends storage at a temperature not exceeding 40°.

Stability. A warning that extemporaneously prepared oral liquid dosage forms may be unstable and manufacturers' formulations should be used where possible.[1] An extemporary formula is available for levodopa syrup. Water dispersible formulations of levodopa with benserazide are available in some countries but a method that can be used by patients to prepare daily solutions of levodopa with carbidopa has been suggested by Giron and Koller.[2] One litre of a solution in potable water may be prepared with ten crushed standard tablets of levodopa 100 mg with carbidopa 25 mg and 2 g of ascorbic acid added to stabilise the levodopa.

1. Walls TJ, *et al.* Problems with inactivation of drugs used in Parkinson's disease. *Br Med J* 1985; **290:** 444–5.
2. Giron LT, Koller WC. Methods of managing levodopa-induced dyskinesias. *Drug Safety* 1996; **14:** 365–74.

Adverse Effects

Gastro-intestinal effects, notably nausea, vomiting, and anorexia are common early in treatment with levodopa, particularly if the dosage is increased too rapidly. Gastro-intestinal bleeding has been reported in patients with a history of peptic ulcer disease.

The commonest cardiovascular effect is orthostatic hypotension, which is usually asymptomatic, but may be associated with faintness and dizziness. Cardiac arrhythmias have been reported and hypertension has occasionally occurred.

Psychiatric symptoms occur in a high proportion of patients, especially the elderly, and include agitation, anxiety, euphoria, nightmares, and insomnia, or sometimes drowsiness and depression. More serious effects, usually requiring a reduction in dosage or withdrawal of levodopa, include aggression, paranoid delusions, hallucinations, delirium, severe depression, with or without suicidal behaviour, and unmasking of psychoses. Psychotic reactions are more likely in patients with postencephalitic parkinsonism or a history of mental disorders.

Abnormal involuntary movements or dyskinesias are the most serious dose-limiting adverse effects of levodopa and are very common at the optimum dose required to control parkinsonism; their frequency increases with duration of treatment. Involuntary movements of the face, tongue, lips, and jaw often appear first and those of the trunk and extremities later. Severe generalised choreoathetoid and dystonic movements may occur after prolonged administration. Muscle twitching and blepharospasm may be early signs of excessive dosage. Exaggerated respiratory movements and exacerbated oculogyric crises have been reported in patients with postencephalitic parkinsonism. Re-emergence of bradykinesia and akinesia, in the form of 'end-of-dose' deterioration and the 'on-off' phenomenon, in patients with parkinsonism is a complication of long-term treatment, but may be due to progression of the disease rather than to levodopa (see also under Parkinsonism, p.1128).

A positive response to the direct Coombs' test may occur, usually without evidence of haemolysis although auto-immune haemolytic anaemia has occasionally been reported. Transient leucopenia has occurred rarely. The effects of levodopa on liver and kidney function are generally slight. Levodopa may cause discoloration of the urine; reddish at first then darkening on standing. Other body fluids may also be discoloured.

Some of the adverse effects reported may not be attributable directly to levodopa, but rather to the concomitant use of antimuscarinics, to increased mobility, or to the unmasking of underlying conditions as parkinsonism improves. Concomitant administration of a peripheral decarboxylase inhibitor may reduce the severity of peripheral symptoms such as gastro-intestinal and cardiovascular effects, but central effects such as dyskinesias and mental disturbances may occur earlier in treatment.

The major adverse effects of levodopa are dyskinesia in 75% of patients and psychiatric disturbances in 25%.[1] Nausea and vomiting in 40 to 50% are gradually tolerated and hypotension in 25 to 30% is generally asymptomatic. Other adverse effects include cardiac arrhythmias, particularly atrial and ventricular ectopic beats and less commonly atrial flutter and fibrillation; palpitations and flushing often accompanied by excessive sweating; hypertension; polyuria, incontinence, and urinary retention, although antimuscarinic drugs often contribute to problems with micturition; and dark coloration of the urine and saliva. Rare adverse effects include abdominal pain, constipation, and diarrhoea; mydriasis, blurred vision, diplopia, and precipitation of glaucoma; headache; stridor; tachypnoea; and paraesthesias.

1. Calne DB, Reid JL. Antiparkinsonian drugs: pharmacological and therapeutic aspects. *Drugs* 1972; **4:** 49–74.

Abnormal coloration. Black pigmentation of ribs cartilage has been noted at necropsy in patients treated with levodopa.[1,2] Abnormal pigmentation is generally not seen at other sites[2] but there have been isolated reports[2,3] of patients who also had pigmentation of the intervertebral discs. Although the pigmentation appears to be irreversible it was considered to be probably harmless.[2] It has been suggested that the pigmentation was due to deposition of dihydroxyphenylalanine (DOPA) in the cartilage.[1] It is known that DOPA will readily auto-oxidise *in vitro* in the presence of oxygen to a black pigment and this can also happen *in vivo* since black urine is a well known side-effect of levodopa therapy. Dark sweat and pigmentation of the skin and teeth are also side-effects known to the manufacturers of levodopa.

See also Effects on Skin and Hair, below.

1. Connolly CE, *et al.* Black cartilage associated with levodopa. *Lancet* 1986; **i:** 690.
2. Rausing A, Rosén U. Black cartilage after therapy with levodopa and methyldopa. *Arch Pathol Lab Med* 1994; **118:** 531–5.
3. Keen CE. *Br Med J* 1998; **316:** 240.

Dysgeusia. A change in taste sensation was reported[1] in one study by 23 of 514 patients treated with levodopa in association with a decarboxylase inhibitor; 2 of the 23 had total loss of taste initially. The altered taste was often described as insipid, metallic, or plastic, was first observed 3 to 32 weeks after beginning treatment, and lasted for 2 to 40 weeks. In an earlier report 22 of 100 patients receiving levodopa alone had experienced changes in taste.[2]

1. Siegfried J, Zumstein H. Changes in taste under L-DOPA therapy. *Z Neurol* 1971; **200:** 345–8.
2. Barbeau A. L-DOPA therapy: past, present and future. *Ariz Med* 1970; **27:** 1–4.

Effects on the blood. Reports of effects of levodopa on the blood are mostly confined to individual case reports. One study in 365 patients, receiving levodopa in a mean daily dosage of 4.04 g, found that 32 developed a positive direct Coombs' test, the majority after between 3 and 12 months of therapy, but none developed haemolytic anaemia.[1] However, occasional cases of auto-immune haemolytic anaemia have been reported;[2-4] in one case dosage reduction and concurrent administration of a peripheral decarboxylase inhibitor largely abolished haemolysis,[3] but in another report haemolysis recurred on re-institution of levodopa with carbidopa and required corticosteroid treatment.[4] A case of severe acute non-haemolytic anaemia related to levodopa therapy has also been reported.[5]

Although levodopa is widely stated to produce leucopenia in some patients, there are few published reports. However transient minor decreases in total leucocyte counts were reported by Barbeau *et al.* in 3 of 80 patients receiving levodopa.[6]

There is also a report of severe thrombocytopenia in a patient who had received levodopa for 3 years;[7] the condition was apparently an auto-immune response and responded to prednisone therapy.

1. Joseph C. Occurrence of positive Coombs test in patients treated with levodopa. *N Engl J Med* 1972; **286:** 1401–2.
2. Territo MC, *et al.* Autoimmune hemolytic anemia due to levodopa therapy. *JAMA* 1973; **226:** 1347–8.
3. Lindström FD, *et al.* Dose-related levodopa-induced haemolytic anaemia. *Ann Intern Med* 1977; **86:** 298–300.
4. Bernstein RM. Reversible haemolytic anaemia after levodopa-carbidopa. *Br Med J* 1979; **1:** 1461–2.
5. Alkalay I, Zipoli T. Levodopa-induced acute non-hemolytic anemia. *Ann Allergy* 1977; **39:** 191.
6. Barbeau A. L-Dopa therapy in Parkinson's disease: a critical review of nine years' experience. *Can Med Assoc J* 1969; **101:** 791–800.
7. Wanamaker WM, *et al.* Thrombocytopenia associated with long-term levodopa therapy. *JAMA* 1976; **235:** 2217–19.

Effects on the cardiovascular system. There have been conflicting reports on the effects of peripheral decarboxylase inhibitors on orthostatic hypotension attributed to levodopa therapy. Calne *et al.*[1] found supine and erect systolic blood pressure to be significantly higher in parkinsonian patients given levodopa in association with carbidopa than in those receiving levodopa alone and suggested that the peripheral actions of dopamine contribute to levodopa-induced hypotension. However, Leibowitz and Lieberman[2] found no change in the incidence and degree of orthostatic hypotension after levodopa in association with carbidopa and, similarly, no difference in the frequency of ventricular arrhythmias.

See also Effects on Kidney Function, below and under Precautions, below.

1. Calne DB, *et al.* Action of L-α-methyldopahydrazine on the blood pressure of patients receiving levodopa. *Br J Pharmacol* 1972; **44:** 162–4
2. Leibowitz M, Lieberman A. Comparison of dopa decarboxylase inhibitor (carbidopa) combined with levodopa and levodopa alone on the cardiovascular system of patients with Parkinson's disease. *Neurology* 1975; **25:** 917–21.

Effects on electrolytes. See under Effects on Kidney Function, below.

Effects on the endocrine system. Single doses of levodopa cause an increase in plasma concentrations of glucose, insulin, and glucagon, as well as of growth hormone, when given to healthy subjects[1] and there has been concern over the potential endocrine effects of levodopa therapy in patients with Parkinson's disease.[2] A study of carbohydrate metabolism in 24 patients with Parkinson's disease indicated that these patients had abnormally low rates of glucose utilisation when untreated, apparently due to impaired insulin release, and this was not altered when levodopa therapy was given.[3] However, a similar study completed by 19 patients[2] noted increased impairment of glucose utilisation following levodopa therapy for 1 year with a delayed hypersecretion of insulin in response to a glucose load similar to the metabolic changes of acromegaly. It was considered that patients receiving levodopa for parkinsonism should be monitored for evidence of diabetes mellitus or frank acromegaly.[2]

Postmenopausal bleeding occurred in varying degrees in 12 of 47 women treated with levodopa.[4] In one case bleeding was severe enough to warrant interrupting treatment and subsequent dosage reduction.

For the effects of levodopa on pituitary function, see under Uses, below.

1. Rayfield EJ, *et al.* L-Dopa stimulation of glucagon secretion in man. *N Engl J Med* 1975; **293:** 589–91.
2. Sirtori CR, *et al.* Metabolic responses to acute and chronic L-dopa administration in patients with parkinsonism. *N Engl J Med* 1972; **287:** 729–33.
3. Van Woert MH, Mueller PS. Glucose, insulin, and free fatty acid metabolism in Parkinson's disease treated with levodopa. *Clin Pharmacol Ther* 1971; **12:** 360–7.
4. Wajsbort J. Post-menopausal bleeding after L-dopa. *N Engl J Med* 1972; **286:** 784.

Effects on the eyes. Both miosis[1] and mydriasis[2] have been reported with levodopa.

For a report of the exacerbation of oculogyric crises by levodopa, see Extrapyramidal Effects, below.

1. Spiers ASD, *et al.* Miosis during L-dopa therapy. *Br Med J* 1970; **2:** 639–40.
2. Weintraub MI, *et al.* Pupillary effects of levodopa therapy: development of anisocoria in latent Horner's syndrome. *N Engl J Med* 1970; **283:** 120–3.

Effects on the gastro-intestinal tract. Although gastro-intestinal bleeding has more commonly been reported in patients with a history of peptic ulceration there is a rare report[1] of acute melaena and non-specific gastritis associated with levodopa therapy in a 56-year-old man without any previous evidence of a gastric disorder.

See also Dysgeusia, above.

1. Riddoch D. Gastritis and L-dopa. *Br Med J* 1972; **1:** 53–4.

Effects on kidney function. Administration of levodopa 1 to 2 g to 7 patients with idiopathic or postencephalitic Parkinson's disease produced significant increments in renal plasma flow, glomerular filtration rate, and sodium and potassium excretion.[1] It was considered that the natriuretic effects could contribute to the orthostatic hypotension commonly noted in patients receiving levodopa. There is a report of a patient who developed hyponatraemia when treated with levodopa with carbidopa.[2] The patient had previously had a similar reaction when given amantadine. On each occasion symptoms disappeared when dopaminergic medication was withdrawn and recurred on rechallenge. Inappropriate secretion of antidiuretic hormone was suggested as a possible mechanism.

Levodopa has also been reported to have a kaliuretic effect, resulting in hypokalaemia, in some parkinsonian patients;[3] the effect could be prevented by concomitant administration of a peripheral dopa decarboxylase inhibitor.

1. Finlay GD, *et al.* Augmentation of sodium and potassium excretion, glomerular filtration rate and renal plasma flow by levodopa. *N Engl J Med* 1971; **284:** 865–70.
2. Lammers GJ, Roos RAC. Hyponatraemia due to amantadine hydrochloride and L-dopa/carbidopa. *Lancet* 1993; **342:** 439.
3. Granérus A-K, *et al.* Kaliuretic effect of L-dopa treatment in parkinsonian patients. *Acta Med Scand* 1977; **201:** 291–7.

Effects on mental function. Psychiatric complications were the single commonest reason for stopping levodopa treatment in a 6-year follow-up study of 178 patients with idiopathic Parkinson's disease.[1] Within 2 years levodopa was withdrawn because of toxic confusional states (21 patients), paranoid psychosis (6), unipolar depression (2), and mania (1). The incidence of visual hallucinations increased as treatment continued but, as with toxic confusional states, patients generally improved when levodopa was withdrawn. Before treatment 40 patients had suffered severe depression and levodopa produced sustained improvement in only 2. After 6 years, 20 of the 81 patients remaining were moderately or severely depressed and were rarely improved by withdrawal or reduction in dosage of levodopa. Increasing dementia affected 26 of the 81 patients after 6 years; withdrawal of levodopa in 5 failed to improve cognitive disabilities, but increased parkinsonism.

Another study[2] reported that 141 of 400 patients being treated for Parkinson's disease developed mental disorders. In this study certain acute states, particularly anxiety, on-off hallucinations, and fits of delirium were linked to treatment with levodopa, whereas dementia and depression were not.

Sleep-related complaints have occurred and were reported by 74 of 100 patients with Parkinson's disease.[3] All 74 were on levodopa and the prevalence of symptoms increased with the duration of treatment. Symptoms included insomnia, excessive daytime somnolence, altered dream phenomena, nocturnal vocalisation, involuntary myoclonic movements, and rarely, sleep walking. Sleep fragmentation, which includes insomnia and somnolence, was the most common symptom overall. It has been suggested[4] that in patients with mild to moderate disease levodopa and dopamine agonists could cause sleep disruption. However, these drugs produce beneficial effects on nocturnal disabilities in patients with more severe disease.

1. Shaw KM, *et al.* The impact of treatment with levodopa on Parkinson's disease. *Q J Med* 1980; **49:** 283–93.
2. Rondot P, *et al.* Mental disorders in Parkinson's disease after treatment with L-Dopa. *Adv Neurol* 1984; **40:** 259–69.
3. Nausieda PA, *et al.* Psychiatric complications of levodopa therapy of Parkinson's disease. *Adv Neurol* 1984; **40:** 271–7.
4. van Hilten B, *et al.* Sleep disruption in Parkinson's disease: assessment by continuous activity monitoring. *Arch Neurol* 1994; **51:** 922–8.

Effects on respiration. Respiratory crises, including attacks of gasping, panting, sniffing, puffing, and breath-holding, occurred in 12 of 25 patients with postencephalitic parkinsonism during treatment with levodopa.[1] A further 8 developed respiratory and phonatory tics, including sudden deep breaths, yawns, coughs, giggles, sighing, grunting, and moaning. All 20 patients also suffered tachypnoea, bradypnoea, and asymmetrical movement of both sides of the chest, paradoxical diaphragmatic movements, and reversal of inspiratory and expiratory phases. The induction of respiratory crises may be prompt or greatly delayed; 3 patients only developed crises after more than 9 months of treatment with levodopa. Crises were readily precipitated by psychophysiological arousals such as rage and exertion. Most of the patients who developed marked respiratory disorders had shown slight irregularities of respiratory rhythm, rate, and force before receiving levodopa.

In another report a distressing dose-related irregularity in the rate and depth of breathing occurred when a patient with Parkinson's disease was given levodopa with benserazide.[2] The respiratory abnormality was completely suppressed by concomitant administration of tiapride, with no reduction in the beneficial effect of levodopa.

1. Sacks OW, *et al.* Side-effects of L-dopa in postencephalitic parkinsonism. *Lancet* 1970; **i:** 1006.
2. De Keyser J, Vincken W. L-Dopa-induced respiratory disturbance in Parkinson's disease suppressed by tiapride. *Neurology* 1985; **35:** 235–7.

Effects on sexual function. An increase in libido, over and above the effects of improved mobility and well-being, has been reported in parkinsonian patients receiving levodopa. Barbeau *et al.* noted increased libido but no improvement in sexual performance in 4 of 80 patients;[1] Brown *et al.* reported a moderate increase in sexual interest in 4 of 7 male patients.[2] Extreme hypersexuality has been reported only rarely: Vogel and Schiffter reported severe hypersexuality in a patient receiving levodopa and bromocriptine who may have been abusing the drugs.[3] Hypersexual behaviour and hypergenitalism has also been reported in a pre-pubertal boy given levodopa for behaviour disturbances.[4]

1. Barbeau A. L-Dopa therapy in Parkinson's disease: a critical review of nine years' experience. *Can Med Assoc J* 1969; **101:** 791–9.
2. Brown E, *et al.* Sexual function and affect in parkinsonian men treated with L-dopa. *Am J Psychiatry* 1978; **135:** 1552–5.
3. Vogel HP, Schiffter R. Hypersexuality—a complication of dopaminergic therapy in Parkinson's disease. *Pharmacopsychiatry* 1983; **16:** 107–10.
4. Korten JJ, *et al.* Undesirable prepubertal effects of levodopa. *JAMA* 1973; **226:** 355.

Effects on the skin and hair. Two women who were given levodopa, up to 3 g daily, developed diffuse alopecia in addition to other adverse effects.[1] Repigmentation of hair has occurred in a white-bearded man after being treated with levodopa 1.5 g daily for 8 months.[2]

See also Melanoma, under Precautions, below.

1. Marshall A, Williams MJ. Alopecia and levodopa. *Br Med J* 1971; **2:** 47.
2. Grainger KM. Pigmentation in Parkinson's disease treated with levodopa. *Lancet* 1973; **i:** 97–8.

Extrapyramidal effects. Choreiform movements were the major dose-limiting complication of long-term treatment with levodopa in a follow-up study of 178 patients with idiopathic Parkinson's disease, 81 of whom were still taking levodopa after 6 years.[1] Dyskinesias usually appeared in the first year and became more severe and generalised with time. Certain distinctive patterns of involuntary movements occurred as follows: peak-dose movements affected 65 of the 81 patients and were dose-related. Movements were usually choreic, affecting the face and limbs, but dystonic and ballistic movements were also seen; characteristically they began 20 to 90 minutes after an oral dose and lasted from 10 minutes to 4 hours with a tendency to be more severe mid-way through the interdose period; biphasic movements presenting as 2 distinct episodes of chorea or dystonia within each interdose period occurred in only 3 patients; early morning and 'end-of-dose' dystonia was present in 15 patients after 6 years of treatment with levodopa, but rarely developed during the first 3 years; nocturnal myoclonus occurred in 12 patients. The frequency, intensity, and complexity of spontaneous fluctuations in performance were greatly enhanced by long-term levodopa therapy. Two clinically distinct types of fluctuation, 'end-of-dose' deterioration and the 'on-off' phenomenon, were related to treatment. 'End-of-dose' deterioration or the 'wearing-off' effect affected 52 patients after 6 years of treatment and was characterised by progressive reduction in the duration of benefit from each dose together with a gradual return of nocturnal and early morning disability in some patients. The 'on-off' phenomenon affected 14 patients who experienced completely unpredictable swings from relative mobility, usually accompanied by involuntary movements, to periods of profound bradykinesia and hypotonia. In addition, 'freezing episodes' and abrupt falls became increasingly common and affected 50 patients after 6 years compared with 33 before therapy.

1. Shaw KM, *et al.* The impact of treatment with levodopa on Parkinson's disease. *Q J Med* 1980; **49:** 283–93.

OCULOGYRIC CRISIS. After initial remission, oculogyric crises in 5 of 25 patients with postencephalitic parkinsonism recurred and were subsequently severely exacerbated during treatment with levodopa.[1] One patient, who previously had not had oculogyric crises, developed severe crises in the fourth month of therapy with levodopa. During these crises forced gaze deviation was always accompanied by severe neurological and mental symptoms, some of which were scarcely tolerable.

1. Sacks OW, Kohl M. L-Dopa and oculogyric crises. *Lancet* 1970; **ii:** 215–16.

Gout. There have been a number of reports of elevated serum-uric acid concentrations in patients receiving levodopa, but some of these are of doubtful significance since levodopa has been shown to give falsely-elevated uric acid concentrations by colorimetric methods.[1] However, hyperuricaemia as measured by more specific methods,[2,3] with a few cases of overt gout,[2,3] has also been reported.

1. Cawein MJ, Hewins J. False rise in serum uric acid after L-dopa. *N Engl J Med* 1969; **281:** 1489–90.
2. Honda H, Gindin RA. Gout while receiving levodopa for parkinsonism. *JAMA* 1972; **219:** 55–7.
3. Calne DB, Fermaglich J. Gout induced by L-dopa and decarboxylase inhibitors. *Postgrad Med J* 1976; **52:** 232–3.

Hypersensitivity. Reports of hypersensitivity reactions to levodopa have included a vasculitis characterised by neuromyopathy, periarteriolitis with eosinophilia,[1] and a lupus-like auto-immune syndrome.[2]

1. Wolf S, *et al.* Neuromyopathy and periarteriolitis in a patient receiving levodopa. *Arch Intern Med* 1976; **136:** 1055–7.
2. Massarotti G, *et al.* Lupus-like autoimmune syndrome after levodopa and benserazide. *Br Med J* 1979; **2:** 553.

Overdosage. Adverse effects following ingestion of 80 to 100 g of levodopa over a 12-hour period by a parkinsonian patient included hypertension initially, followed by hypotension of a few hours' duration, sinus tachycardia, and symptomatic postural hypotension for more than a week.[1] Marked confusion, agitation, insomnia, and restlessness were the most prominent clinical symptoms and did not disappear completely for over a week; severe anorexia and insomnia persisted for 2 to 3 weeks. After the overdose the patient had virtually no signs of parkinsonism and received no levodopa or antimuscarinic medication for 6 days; rigidity and akinesia began to recur on the fourth day.

1. Hoehn MM, Rutledge CO. Acute overdose with levodopa: clinical and biochemical consequences. *Neurology* 1975; **25:** 792–4.

Withdrawal syndromes. There are several reports implicating the withdrawal of levodopa in the development of a syndrome resembling the neuroleptic malignant syndrome,[1-4] characterised by fever, muscle rigidity, profuse sweating, tachycardia, tachypnoea, and elevated muscle enzyme values.[1] Several fatalities have occurred.[1,2] It has been suggested that the neuroleptic malignant syndrome is associated with blockade of dopamine receptors in the striatum, leading to increased rigidity and heat production, and in the hypothalamus, resulting in impaired thermoregulation[5] and it seems reasonable that withdrawal of levodopa, a dopaminergic agonist, might have a similar effect in patients with depleted central dopamine concentrations. It is thus recommended that extreme caution be taken if using a 'drug holiday' to manage fluctuations in response to levodopa (see under Parkinsonism, p.1128).

Fever, extrapyramidal symptoms and raised creatine kinase concentrations, resembling a very mild form of the neuroleptic malignant syndrome, have also been reported in parkinsonian patients exposed to stress such as dehydration or infection but without any change in medication.[6]

1. Friedman JH, *et al.* A neuroleptic malignantlike syndrome due to levodopa therapy withdrawal. *JAMA* 1985; **254:** 2792–5.
2. Sechi GP, *et al.* Fatal hyperpyrexia after withdrawal of levodopa. *Neurology* 1984; **34:** 249–51.
3. Figà-Talamanca L, *et al.* Hyperthermia after discontinuance of levodopa and bromocriptine therapy: impaired dopamine receptors a possible cause. *Neurology* 1985; **35:** 258–61.
4. Gibb WRG, Griffith DNW. Levodopa withdrawal syndrome identical to neuroleptic malignant syndrome. *Postgrad Med J* 1986; **62:** 59–60.
5. Henderson VW, Wooten GF. Neuroleptic malignant syndrome: a pathogenetic role for dopamine receptor blockade? *Neurology* 1981; **31:** 132–7.
6. Mezaki T, *et al.* Benign type of malignant syndrome. *Lancet* 1989; **i:** 49–50.

Treatment of Adverse Effects

Reduction in dosage reverses most of the side-effects of levodopa. Nausea and vomiting may be diminished by increasing the dose of levodopa gradually, and/or by taking with or after meals, although taking levodopa on a full stomach may lead to lower plasma concentrations. Gastro-intestinal effects may also be reduced by giving an antiemetic such as cyclizine hydrochloride or domperidone but not a phenothiazine (see under Interactions, below). Administration with a peripheral decarboxylase inhibitor reduces peripheral but not central side-effects. Orthostatic hypotension may respond to the use of elastic stockings.

If acute overdosage occurs the stomach should be emptied by lavage and supportive measures instituted. Pyridoxine may reverse some effects of levodopa (see under Interactions, below) but its value in overdosage has not been established; it does not reverse the effects of levodopa given with a peripheral decarboxylase inhibitor.

Nausea and vomiting. For reference to the use of domperidone in the management of nausea and vomiting associated with levodopa in patients with Parkinson's disease, see under Uses and Administration, p.1191.

Psychosis. Atypical antipsychotics such as clozapine (p.660) have been tried in the management of psychosis occurring as a complication of parkinsonism and of drugs like levodopa used in its treatment.

Precautions

Levodopa is contra-indicated in patients with angle-closure glaucoma and should be used with caution in open-angle glaucoma. Caution is also required in patients with cardiovascular disease, pulmonary disease, endocrine disorders, psychiatric disturbances, osteomalacia, or a history of peptic ulceration. Periodic evaluations of hepatic, psychiatric, haematological, renal, and cardiovascular functions have been advised.

Since an association between levodopa and activation of malignant melanoma has been suspected (although not confirmed), it is generally recommended that levodopa should not be given to patients with (or with a history of) the disease or with skin disorders suggestive of it.

Parkinsonian patients who benefit from levodopa therapy should be warned to resume normal activities gradually to avoid the risk of injury. Treatment with levodopa should not be stopped abruptly.

Levodopa inhibits prolactin secretion and may therefore interfere with lactation.

Food interferes with the absorption of levodopa, though levodopa is usually given with or immediately after meals to reduce nausea and vomiting. However, patients experiencing the 'on-off' phenomenon may benefit from administration on an empty stomach (see under Parkinsonism, p.1128).

Abuse. Several cases of abuse of levodopa in patients with Parkinson's disease have been reported.[1,2] Patients had progressively increased the dosage of levodopa to obtain psychotropic effects such as euphoria despite accompanying dystonia and other extrapyramidal adverse effects. Discontinuation often led to craving, drug-seeking behaviour, and mood disturbances such as depression, features resembling a psychological dependence syndrome.

1. Nausieda PA. Sinemet "abusers". *Clin Neuropharmacol* 1985; **8:** 318–27.
2. Soyka M, Huppert D. L-dopa abuse in a patient with former alcoholism. *Br J Addict* 1992; **87:** 117–18.

Cardiovascular disorders. A high incidence of cardiovascular side-effects was reported in early studies of levodopa, although both Parkinson's disease and heart disease are common in the elderly and adverse cardiac effects of levodopa may be less prevalent than was first thought. A study in 40 patients[1] concluded that, apart from those with severe postural hypotension or unstable coronary disease, levodopa may be used safely in parkinsonian patients with heart disease. Others[2] noted that levodopa and bromocriptine cause cardiac arrhythmias in less than 1% of all patients, the incidence for levodopa in association with a decarboxylase inhibitor being lower still. Nevertheless, caution is advised in patients with cardiovascular disease.

1. Jenkins RB, *et al.* Levodopa therapy of patients with parkinsonism and heart disease. *Br Med J* 1972; **3:** 512–14.
2. Parkes JD, *et al.* Amantadine-induced heart failure. *Lancet* 1977; **i:** 904.

Diabetes mellitus. For reference to concern over the potential of levodopa to impair glucose utilisation, see Effects on the Endocrine System under Adverse Effects, above.

Melanoma. There has been concern over the effects of levodopa on melanoma in view of the ability of malignant melanoma cells to convert levodopa to melanin and isolated reports of melanoma developing or being exacerbated during levodopa therapy continue to appear.[1] However, in a survey of 1099 patients with primary cutaneous malignant melanoma only one had taken levodopa.[2] It was concluded that levodopa therapy is not an important factor in the induction of malignant melanoma. Furthermore, administration of levodopa in daily doses of up to 4 g with carbidopa to 17 patients with metastatic melanoma failed to provide any evidence that levodopa accelerated the progression of the disease.[3]

For a report of antineoplastic chemotherapy used for the treatment of melanoma reducing the efficacy of levodopa, see under Interactions, below.

1. Haider SA, Thaller VT. Lid melanoma and parkinsonism. *Br J Ophthalmol* 1992; **76:** 246–7.
2. Sober AJ, Wick MM. Levodopa therapy and malignant melanoma. *JAMA* 1978; **240:** 554–5.
3. Gurney H, *et al.* The use of L-dopa and carbidopa in metastatic malignant melanoma. *J Invest Dermatol* 1991; **96:** 85–7.

Pregnancy. Levodopa alone and with carbidopa has been associated with fetal abnormalities in *animals* given high doses; no teratogenic effect has been noted with carbidopa alone. However, 2 women with parkinsonism who received levodopa with carbidopa or levodopa alone throughout their pregnancies gave birth to normal infants.[1]

1. Cook DG, Klawans HL. Levodopa during pregnancy. *Clin Neuropharmacol* 1985; **8:** 93–5.

Withdrawal. For adverse effects associated with withdrawal of levodopa, see under Adverse Effects, above.

Interactions

The therapeutic or adverse effects of levodopa may be affected by interactions with a variety of drugs. Mechanisms may include effects on catecholamine metabolising enzymes, neurotransmitters, or receptor sites, effects on the endocrine system, and effects on gastro-intestinal absorption. Drugs which modify gastric emptying may affect the absorption of levodopa.

Antibacterials. A study[1] in 7 healthy subjects showed that administration of *spiramycin* with levodopa and carbidopa resulted in reduced plasma-levodopa concentrations and an increase in its peripheral metabolism.

A hypertensive reaction and severe tremor occurred when *isoniazid* was given to a patient receiving levodopa;[2] it was not certain whether isoniazid was acting as an MAOI.

1. Brion N, *et al.* Effect of a macrolide (spiramycin) on the pharmacokinetics of L-dopa and carbidopa in healthy volunteers. *Clin Neuropharmacol* 1992; **15:** 229–35.
2. Morgan JP. Isoniazid and levodopa. *Ann Intern Med* 1980; **92:** 434.

Antidepressants. BUPROPION. Caution has been advised with bupropion because of reports of a higher incidence of adverse effects during concomitant use with levodopa.

MAOIS. Administration of levodopa with non-specific MAOIs such as *phenelzine, pargyline, nialamide*, or *tranylcypromine* may cause dangerous hypertension;[1-4] it is recommended that levodopa should not be given within at least 14 days of stopping an MAOI. Teychenne *et al.*[5] found that hypertensive reactions to levodopa with the MAOI *tranylcypromine* were inhibited by carbidopa, but the manufacturers of preparations containing levodopa with carbidopa or benserazide still contra-indicate the concomitant use of MAOIs. There has also been a warning that hypertensive crises may occur if levodopa is used with *moclobemide*, an MAO type A inhibitor. *Selegiline*, an MAO type B inhibitor, is used to enhance the antiparkinsonian effect of levodopa, see p.1145.

1. Hunter KR, *et al.* Monoamine oxidase inhibitors and L-dopa. *Br Med J* 1970; **3:** 388.
2. Hodge JV. Use of monoamine oxidase inhibitors. *Lancet* 1965; **i:** 764–5.
3. Friend DG, *et al.* The action of L-dihydroxyphenylalanine in patients receiving nialamide. *Clin Pharmacol Ther* 1965; **6:** 362–6.
4. Sharpe J, *et al.* Idiopathic orthostatic hypotension treated with levodopa and MAO inhibitor: a preliminary report. *Can Med Assoc J* 1972; **107:** 296–300.
5. Teychenne PF, *et al.* Interactions of levodopa with inhibitors of monoamine oxidase and L-aromatic amino acid decarboxylase. *Clin Pharmacol Ther* 1975; **18:** 273–7.

TRICYCLIC ANTIDEPRESSANTS. Although tricyclic antidepressants have been used safely with levodopa[1] hypertensive crises have occurred in patients receiving *amitriptyline* or *imipramine* and levodopa with carbidopa.[2,3] Imipramine has been reported to impair the rate of levodopa absorption,[4] presumably due to its antimuscarinic properties (for the effect of antimuscarinics on the absorption of levodopa, see below).

1. Hunter KR, *et al.* Use of levodopa with other drugs. *Lancet* 1970; **ii:** 1283–5.
2. Rampton DS. Hypertensive crisis in a patient given Sinemet, metoclopramide, and amitriptyline. *Br Med J* 1977; **2:** 607–8.
3. Edwards M. Adverse interaction of levodopa with tricyclic antidepressants. *Practitioner* 1982; **226:** 1447–8.
4. Morgan JP, *et al.* Imipramine-mediated interference with levodopa absorption from the gastrointestinal tract in man. *Neurology* 1975; **25:** 1029–34.

TRYPTOPHAN. See Amino Acids under Nutritional Agents, below.

Antiepileptics. *Phenytoin* has been shown to diminish the therapeutic effect of levodopa in patients with parkinsonism or chronic manganese poisoning.[1] The mechanism of the interaction was considered uncertain.

1. Mendez JS. Diphenylhydantoin: blocking of levodopa effects. *Arch Neurol* 1975; **32:** 44–6.

Antihypertensives. Concurrent administration of levodopa with *guanethidine* may cause increased hypotension.[1] *Clonidine* has been reported to inhibit the therapeutic effect of levodopa, possibly by stimulating central alpha adrenoceptors.[2] *Methyldopa* and levodopa may enhance each other's therapeutic or adverse effects, although there has been mention of the inhibitory effect of methyldopa on the therapeutic response to levodopa.[3,4]

1. Hunter KR, *et al.* Use of levodopa with other drugs. *Lancet* 1970; **ii:** 1283–5.
2. Shoulson I, Chase TN. Clonidine and the anti-parkinsonian response to L-dopa or piribedil. *Neuropharmacology* 1976; **15:** 25–7.
3. Cotzias GC, *et al.* L-Dopa in Parkinson's syndrome. *N Engl J Med* 1969; **281:** 272.
4. Kofman O. Treatment of Parkinson's disease with L-dopa: a current appraisal. *Can Med Assoc J* 1971; **104:** 483–7.

Antimuscarinics. Antimuscarinic antiparkinsonian drugs may enhance the therapeutic effects of levodopa but by delaying gastric emptying they may reduce its absorption.[1]

1. Algeri S, *et al.* Effect of anticholinergic drugs on gastro-intestinal absorption of L-dopa in rats and in man. *Eur J Pharmacol* 1976; **35:** 293–9.

Antineoplastics. A patient with Parkinson's disease noted[1] that the efficacy of levodopa was reduced each time he received *dacarbazine* for the treatment of melanoma. As serum-dopamine concentrations were unchanged it was suggested[1] that dacarbazine might compete with levodopa at the blood-brain barrier.

1. Merello M, *et al.* Impaired levodopa response in Parkinson's disease during melanoma therapy. *Clin Neuropharmacol* 1992; **15:** 69–74.

Antipsychotics. The therapeutic effects of levodopa may be diminished by CNS dopamine inhibitors including phenothiazine derivatives[1] such as *prochlorperazine*.[2] Butyrophenones such as *haloperidol* and thioxanthenes such as *flupenthixol* might be expected to have a similar effect due to their antidopaminergic properties.

1. Yahr MD, Duvoisin RC. Drug therapy of parkinsonism. *N Engl J Med* 1972; **287:** 20–4.
2. Duvoisin RC. Diphenidol for levodopa induced nausea and vomiting. *JAMA* 1972; **221:** 1408.

Anxiolytics. Reversible deterioration of parkinsonism has been reported in patients receiving levodopa who were given *benzodiazepines* such as *diazepam*,[1,2] *nitrazepam*[1] (although the evidence was equivocal), or *chlordiazepoxide*.[3] In one case parkinsonian symptoms resolved without alteration in the medication.[1]

1. Hunter KR, *et al.* Use of levodopa with other drugs. *Lancet* 1970; **ii:** 1283–5.
2. Wodak J, *et al.* Review of 12 months' treatment with L-dopa in Parkinson's disease, with remarks on unusual side effects. *Med J Aust* 1972; **2:** 1277–82.
3. Yosselson-Superstine S, Lipman AG. Chlordiazepoxide interaction with levodopa. *Ann Intern Med* 1982; **96:** 259–60.

Baclofen. Adverse effects including hallucinations, confusion, headache, and nausea and worsening of symptoms have been reported[1,2] in patients with Parkinson's disease taking levodopa when given baclofen.

1. Skausig OB, Korsgaard S. Hallucinations and baclofen. *Lancet* 1977; **i:** 1258.
2. Lees AJ, *et al.* Baclofen in Parkinson's disease. *J Neurol Neurosurg Psychiatry* 1978; **41:** 707–8.

Gastro-intestinal drugs. ANTACIDS. Some studies have suggested that administration of an antacid before a dose of levodopa enhances the absorption of levodopa, apparently by enhancing gastric emptying and reducing metabolism of levodopa in the stomach.[1,2] This was particularly marked in one case report in a patient with prolonged gastric emptying time.[1] However, another study in 8 patients with presumably normal gastric motility, only 3 of whom had Parkinson's disease, found no significant increase in overall absorption of levodopa when given with an antacid although there was some evidence of increased absorption in one or two of the patients.[3]

1. Rivera-Calimlim L, *et al.* L-Dopa treatment failure: explanation and correction. *Br Med J* 1970; **4:** 93–4.
2. Pocelinko R, *et al.* The effect of an antacid on the absorption and metabolism of levodopa. *Clin Pharmacol Ther* 1972; **13:** 149.
3. Leon AS, Spiegel HE. The effect of antacid administration on the absorption and metabolism of levodopa. *J Clin Pharmacol* 1972; **12:** 263–7.

ANTIEMETICS. *Metoclopramide* accelerates gastric emptying and has been reported to increase the rate of levodopa absorption.[1] Berkowitz and McCallum[2] noted the importance of timing since levodopa delayed gastric emptying and metoclopramide antagonised this effect. *Domperidone* has been reported to increase the bioavailability of levodopa slightly.[3]

1. Morris JGL, *et al.* Plasma dopa concentrations after different preparations of levodopa in normal subjects. *Br J Clin Pharmacol* 1976; **3:** 983–90.
2. Berkowitz DM, McCallum RW. Interaction of levodopa and metoclopramide on gastric emptying. *Clin Pharmacol Ther* 1980; **27:** 414–20.
3. Shindler JS, *et al.* Domperidone and levodopa in Parkinson's disease. *Br J Clin Pharmacol* 1984; **18:** 959–62.

PROKINETICS. Maximum plasma concentrations of levodopa are increased by concomitant administration of *cisapride*.[1]

See also Metoclopramide and Domperidone, under Antiemetics, above.

1. Neira WD, *et al.* The effects of cisapride on plasma L-dopa levels and the clinical response in Parkinson's disease. *Mov Disord* 1995; **10:** 66–70.

General anaesthetics. The general anaesthetics *cyclopropane* and *halothane* lower the threshold for ventricular arrhythmias to sympathomimetic amines, including dopamine, and should probably not be used within 6 to 8 hours of the administration of levodopa.[1,2] However, it has been suggested that levodopa can safely be taken before surgery when given with a decarboxylase inhibitor.[3]

1. Goldberg LI, Whitsett TL. Cardiovascular effects of levodopa. *Clin Pharmacol Ther* 1971; **12:** 376–82.
2. Bianchine JR, Sunyapridakul L. Interactions between levodopa and other drugs: significance in the treatment of Parkinson's disease. *Drugs* 1973; **6:** 364–88.
3. Anonymous. Surgery and long-term medication. *Drug Ther Bull* 1984; **22:** 73–6.

Nutritional agents. AMINO ACIDS. Daniel *et al.* reported that transport of levodopa into the brain is subject to competition from chemically related L-amino acids, especially the other aromatic amino acids *phenylalanine, tyrosine, tryptophan*, and *histidine*.[1] Later, Nutt *et al.* demonstrated that a high-protein diet or the large neutral amino acids phenylalanine, *leu-*

cine, or *isoleucine* reduced the therapeutic effect of levodopa given by intravenous infusion to parkinsonian patients and concluded that alterations in the absorption and transport of levodopa may contribute to the fluctuating responses seen in Parkinson's disease, the so-called 'on-off' phenomenon[2] (see also under Parkinsonism, p.1128). Other reported interactions with amino acids include *methionine*-antagonism of the therapeutic effect of levodopa in parkinsonism[3] and *tryptophan*-reduced blood concentrations of levodopa.[4]

1. Daniel PM, *et al.* Do changes in blood levels of other aromatic aminoacids influence levodopa therapy? *Lancet* 1976; **i:** 95.
2. Nutt JG, *et al.* The "on-off" phenomenon in Parkinson's disease: relation to levodopa absorption and transport. *N Engl J Med* 1984; **310:** 483–8.
3. Pearce LA, Waterbury LD. L-methionine: a possible levodopa antagonist. *Neurology* 1974; **24:** 640–1.
4. Weitbrecht W-U, Weigel K. Der Einflußvon L-Tryptophan auf die L-Dopa-Resorption. *Dtsch Med Wochenschr* 1976; **101:** 20–2.

IRON SALTS. Levodopa forms complexes with iron salts and administration with ferrous sulphate has reduced bioavailability of levodopa by about 50% in healthy subjects.[1] Administration of ferrous sulphate to 9 patients with Parkinson's disease receiving levodopa with carbidopa reduced the area under the curve by 30% and greater than 75% for levodopa and carbidopa respectively. Although this was associated with deterioration in some patients' disability the average reduction in efficacy of therapy did not achieve statistical significance.[2]

1. Campbell NRC, Hasinoff BB. Iron supplements: a common cause of drug interactions. *Br J Clin Pharmacol* 1991; **31:** 251–5.
2. Campbell NRC, *et al.* Sinemet-ferrous sulphate interaction in patients with Parkinson's disease. *Br J Clin Pharmacol* 1990; **30:** 599–605.

PYRIDOXINE. The enzyme responsible for the decarboxylation of levodopa, L-amino acid decarboxylase, is dependent on pyridoxine and pyridoxine supplements have been reported to enhance the peripheral metabolism of levodopa to dopamine leaving less available to cross the blood-brain barrier for central conversion to dopamine;[1-4] pyridoxine therefore inhibits the action of levodopa but this can be stopped by concurrent administration of a peripheral decarboxylase inhibitor.[3,4]

1. Carter AB. Pyridoxine and parkinsonism. *Br Med J* 1973; **4:** 236.
2. Leon AS, *et al.* Pyridoxine antagonism of levodopa in parkinsonism. *JAMA* 1971; **218:** 1924–7.
3. Cotzias GC, Papavasiliou PS. Blocking the negative effects of pyridoxine on patients receiving levodopa. *JAMA* 1971; **215:** 1504–5.
4. Yahr MD, Duvoisin RC. Pyridoxine, levodopa, and L-α-methyldopa hydrazine regimen in parkinsonism. *JAMA* 1971; **216:** 2141.

Papaverine. Antagonism of the beneficial effects of levodopa in parkinsonism has been reported when patients were also given papaverine,[1,2] and it was recommended that the combination should be avoided.

1. Duvoisin RC. Antagonism of levodopa by papaverine. *JAMA* 1975; **231:** 845.
2. Posner DM. Antagonism of levodopa by papaverine. *JAMA* 1975; **233:** 768.

Penicillamine. Isolated case reports suggest that penicillamine increases plasma-levodopa concentrations.[1]

1. Mizuta E, *et al.* Effect of D-penicillamine on pharmacokinetics of levodopa in Parkinson's disease. *Clin Neuropharmacol* 1993; **16:** 448–50.

Sympathomimetics. It has been suggested that sympathomimetics such as *adrenaline* or *isoprenaline* may enhance the cardiac side-effects of levodopa.[1]

1. Goldberg LI, Whitsett TL. Cardiovascular effects of levodopa. *Clin Pharmacol Ther* 1971; **12:** 376–82.

Pharmacokinetics

Levodopa is rapidly absorbed from the gastro-intestinal tract by an active transport system. Most absorption takes place in the small intestine; absorption is very limited from the stomach, and since decarboxylation may take place in the stomach wall, delays in gastric emptying may reduce the amount of levodopa available for absorption.

Levodopa is rapidly decarboxylated by the enzyme aromatic L-amino acid decarboxylase, mostly in the gut, liver, and kidney, to dopamine, which is metabolised in turn, principally to dihydroxyphenylacetic acid (DOPAC) and homovanillic acid (HVA). Other routes of metabolism include *O*-methylation, transamination, and oxidation, producing a variety of minor metabolites including noradrenaline and 3-*O*-methyldopa; the latter may accumulate in the CNS due to its relatively long half-life. The plasma half-life of levodopa itself is reported to be about 1 to 3 hours.

Unlike dopamine, levodopa is actively transported across the blood-brain barrier, but because of the extent of peripheral decarboxylation very little is available to enter the CNS unless it is given in association with a peripheral decarboxylase inhibitor. In the presence of a peripheral decarboxylase inhibitor the major route of metabolism of levodopa becomes the formation of 3-*O*-methyldopa by the enzyme catechol-*O*-methyltransferase.

About 80% of an oral dose of levodopa is excreted in the urine within 24 hours, mostly as dihydroxyphenylacetic and homovanillic acids. Only small amounts of levodopa are excreted unchanged in the faeces.

General references.

1. Nutt JG, Fellman JH. Pharmacokinetics of levodopa. *Clin Neuropharmacol* 1984; **7:** 35–49.
2. Cedarbaum JM. Clinical pharmacokinetics of anti-parkinsonian drugs. *Clin Pharmacokinet* 1987; **13:** 141–78.
3. Robertson DRC, *et al.* The effect of age on the pharmacokinetics of levodopa administered alone and in the presence of carbidopa. *Br J Clin Pharmacol* 1989; **28:** 61–9.
4. Robertson DRC, *et al.* The influence of levodopa on gastric emptying in man. *Br J Clin Pharmacol* 1990; **29:** 47–53.

Uses and Administration

Levodopa, a naturally occurring amino acid, is the immediate precursor of the neurotransmitter dopamine. The actions of levodopa are mainly those of dopamine (p.861).

Unlike dopamine, levodopa can readily enter the CNS and is used in the treatment of conditions, such as Parkinson's disease, which are associated with depletion of dopamine in the brain. Levodopa is rapidly decarboxylated so that very little unchanged drug is available to cross the blood-brain barrier for central conversion into dopamine. Consequently levodopa is usually given together with a peripheral decarboxylase inhibitor such as benserazide (p.1132) or carbidopa (p.1136) to increase the proportion of levodopa that can enter the brain. This enables the dosage of levodopa to be reduced and may diminish peripheral side-effects, such as nausea and vomiting and cardiac arrhythmias, by blocking the peripheral production of dopamine. It may also provide a more rapid response at the start of therapy.

The majority of patients with Parkinson's disease are benefited by levodopa, but after 2 or more years improvement in disability is gradually lost as the disease progresses and fluctuations in mobility emerge. Postencephalitic parkinsonism responds to levodopa, but a higher incidence of side-effects has been reported than in the idiopathic form so smaller doses are generally used. Levodopa has also been used to control the neurological symptoms of chronic manganese poisoning, which resemble those of parkinsonism. It is not generally considered beneficial in drug-induced parkinsonism.

Levodopa has an effect on pituitary function as a result of its conversion to dopamine. It may enhance growth-hormone secretion and has been used diagnostically as a provocative test for growth-hormone deficiency. Levodopa also inhibits prolactin secretion.

Response to levodopa varies considerably between patients. **Treatment of parkinsonism** should commence with small doses increased gradually, ideally to a dose which improves mobility without incurring side-effects. Levodopa should be taken with or after meals, although in later disease, it may be preferable to administer on an empty stomach (see Precautions, above). Once established, maintenance doses may need to be reduced as the patient ages. When given **without a peripheral decarboxylase inhibitor** (which is rare) a suggested initial dose is 125 mg twice daily by mouth increased gradually every 3 to 7 days, according to response, to up to 8 g daily in divided doses. The intervals between doses should be adjusted to meet individual needs; many patients find 4 or 5 divided doses daily to be satisfactory although some may require smaller, more frequent doses in order to control fluctuations in mobility. Maximum improvement may take up to 6 months or longer to occur.

When given **with a peripheral decarboxylase inhibitor** lower doses of levodopa are employed. As high central dopamine concentrations can be achieved more quickly, both beneficial and adverse effects tend to occur more rapidly than with levodopa alone and patients should be monitored carefully. In those already receiving levodopa the drug should be discontinued and benserazide or carbidopa with levodopa started on the following day or after 24 hours if the patient was receiving a modified-release preparation of levodopa.

Benserazide hydrochloride is usually given with levodopa in the ratio of 1 part of benserazide base to 4 parts of levodopa (co-beneldopa) and doses below for co-beneldopa are expressed in terms of the levodopa component. An initial dose for *patients not previously treated with levodopa* is levodopa 50 mg three or four times daily by mouth increased gradually in increments of levodopa 100 mg once or twice weekly, according to response. For some elderly patients, an initial dose of levodopa 50 mg once or twice daily, increased by 50 mg every third or fourth day, may be suitable. If the disease is at an advanced stage, the initial starting dose may be increased to levodopa 100 mg three times daily. Maintenance doses usually lie within the range of levodopa 400 to 800 mg daily in divided doses. It is rarely necessary to exceed levodopa 600 mg daily; if optimal improvement has not been achieved after several weeks at the average dose, further increases may be made with caution; it is rarely necessary to give more than 1 g of levodopa daily. The initial dose of levodopa given with benserazide in *patients previously treated with levodopa* should be about 10 to 15% of the dose previously being taken, thus levodopa 300 mg would be appropriate for a patient previously taking levodopa 2 g daily. For *patients previously treated with other levodopa/dopa decarboxylase inhibitor combinations* an initial dose is levodopa 50 mg given three or four times daily. *Modified-release capsules containing benserazide* 25 mg with levodopa 100 mg are available to reduce fluctuations in response to conventional preparations. For patients not already receiving levodopa the initial dose is one capsule three times daily adjusted every 2 to 3 days according to response; it is recommended that initial dosages should not exceed 600 mg of levodopa daily. For patients already receiving a conventional preparation of levodopa with benserazide, initially one capsule should be substituted for every 100 mg of levodopa and should be given at the same dosage frequency as before; increases in dosage can then be made every 2 to 3 days according to response. An average of 50% more levodopa may be required compared with previous therapy and titration may take up to 4 weeks. Supplementary doses of a conventional preparation of benserazide with levodopa may also be required with the first morning dose.

Full inhibition of peripheral dopa decarboxylase is reported to be achieved by 70 to 100 mg of **carbidopa** daily. Tablets of carbidopa with levodopa (co-careldopa) are available in the ratio of 1 to 4 and 1 to 10 which allows dosage adjustments of either drug for individual patients. Doses of carbidopa are expressed in terms of the anhydrous base. A suggested initial dose for *patients not previously treated with levodopa* is carbidopa 25 mg with levodopa 100 mg three times daily by mouth, increased gradually, in increments of carbidopa 12.5 mg with levodopa 50 mg or carbidopa 25 mg with levodopa 100 mg every day or on alternate days, as necessary. The usual maintenance dosage range is carbidopa 75 to 200 mg with levodopa 0.75 to 2 g daily in divided doses. Carbidopa doses greater than 200 mg daily are not generally exceeded. The initial dose of levodopa given with carbidopa in *patients previously treated with levodopa* should be about 20 to 25% of the dose previously being taken, thus for patients taking less than 1.5 g of levodopa daily a suggested initial dose is carbidopa 25 mg with levodopa 100 mg given three or four times daily; a suggested initial dose for patients taking more than 1.5 g of levodopa daily is carbidopa 25 mg with levodopa 250 mg given three or four times daily. *Modified-release tablets containing carbidopa* with levodopa in the ratio of 1 to 4 are available to reduce fluctuations in response to conventional preparations. For patients not already receiving levodopa therapy, or for those currently receiving levodopa alone, the initial dose is carbidopa 50 mg with levodopa 200 mg twice daily adjusted according to response at intervals of not less than 3 days. It is recommended that for patients who are not already receiving levodopa initial dosages should not exceed 600 mg of levodopa daily. For patients already receiving a conventional preparation of carbidopa with levodopa, the initial dose of the modified-release preparation should provide a similar amount of levodopa per day, but the dosing intervals should be prolonged by 30 to 50% at intervals ranging from 4 to 12 hours. The initial substitution dose of the modified-release preparation should provide not more than 10% more levodopa than was previously given for doses of levodopa greater than 900 mg daily. Doses and intervals may then be altered according to clinical response, allowing at least 3 days between adjustments. Up to 30% more levodopa may be required in the modified-release preparation than was previously administered in the conventional preparation. Average maintenance doses of modified-release preparations lie within the range of carbidopa 100 mg with levodopa 400 mg to carbidopa 400 mg with levodopa 1.6 g. Supplementary doses of a conventional preparation of carbidopa with levodopa may be required in some patients.

Chorea. Levodopa usually exacerbates Huntington's disease. It was formerly used as a diagnostic agent to attempt to identify presymptomatic patients at risk of developing Huntington's chorea by provoking chorea. However, this practice has been abandoned, partly because of the distress caused, and also because of false negative results.[1] More accurate non-provocative testing based on genetic markers for the disease is now feasible (see p.636).

1. Marsden CD. Basal ganglia disease. *Lancet* 1982; **ii:** 1141–6.

Drug-induced extrapyramidal disorders. The management of drug-induced extrapyramidal disorders is discussed under the Adverse Effects of Chlorpromazine on p.650. Although the use of dopamine agonists, especially levodopa, to overcome antipsychotic-induced blockade of dopamine receptors might appear rational, levodopa has generally been reported to be ineffective or to increase psychiatric symptoms.

Dysphagia. Results of a small study[1] have suggested that levodopa may improve the impaired swallowing reflex in patients with basal ganglia infarctions and thereby help to prevent aspiration pneumonia in these patients.

1. Kobayashi H, *et al.* Levodopa and swallowing reflex. *Lancet* 1996; **348:** 1320–1.

Dystonias. Dystonias and their management have been reviewed.[1-3] A dystonia is a syndrome of sustained muscle contractions, frequently causing twisting and repetitive movements or abnormal postures; it may also have additional myoclonic or tremulous components. Typically it starts as a focal dystonia localised in one part of the body and to begin with may appear only during a specific motor act (action dystonia). If the syndrome is progressive the dystonias may become apparent at rest and spread first to more than one part of the body (segmental dystonia) and may eventually affect most or all of the body (generalised dystonia). Progression of the dystonia appears to be related to age of onset. Dystonia beginning in childhood usually starts in the legs and progresses to become segmental or generalised. Whereas in adults the dystonia usually starts in other parts of the body and rarely becomes generalised. Examples of focal dystonias are blepharospasm (affecting the eye and surrounding facial muscles), writer's cramp (hand and arm), spasmodic torticollis (neck), spasmodic dysphonia, or dystonic dysphagia (larynx or pharynx), and leg dystonias. Some dystonias are symptomatic, and may be associated with metabolic disorders such as Wilson's disease or Lesch-Nyhan syndrome; with neurological disorders such as Huntington's disease; or with other causes including head trauma, manganese or carbon disulphide toxicity, or the side-effects of antipsychotics or antiparkinsonian agents. However, in the majority of cases the disease is idiopathic.

There are no cures for most types of dystonia, but symptomatic relief is possible in many patients. It has been suggested that all children and adolescents presenting with dystonia, particularly starting in the legs, should first be given a trial with levodopa.[2] A suggested regimen is to gradually build up to a dose of levodopa 200 mg with carbidopa 50 mg given three times daily and to maintain this dose for three months; if there is no useful response in this period the drug is withdrawn. Where there is benefit it is usually dramatic and is sustained as long as the drug is taken, which may be more than 10 years in some cases, in general without the long-term problems associated with levodopa for parkinsonism (see p.1128).

In children and adolescents who fail to respond to levodopa an antimuscarinic such as benzhexol is second choice. Side-effects are minimised by starting with a low dose which is then gradually increased. General experience indicates that about half of all children and adolescents benefit from antimuscarinics; adults tolerate the drug less well and only about a fifth of adult patients with focal dystonia benefit.

In patients who do not respond to levodopa or high-dose antimuscarinics other drugs may be used. Many benefit from benzodiazepines such as diazepam; a few have responded to baclofen or carbamazepine. Antipsychotics are sometimes useful but carry the risk of inducing tardive dyskinesia. Tetrabenazine carries less risk of tardive dyskinesia but may induce depression. In very severe dystonia combination therapy may be required: tetrabenazine with pimozide and benzhexol is sometimes effective.

The response in patients with adult onset focal dystonia is usually poor. However, the use of botulinum A toxin can produce relief in blepharospasm, spasmodic torticollis, and spasmodic dysphonia, and is under investigation for writer's cramp and other occupational dystonias. Local injections into the affected muscles produce weakness over the next week or so, thereby reducing or abolishing dystonic spasms. The effect lasts some 2 to 4 months.

Further details of blepharospasm and its management can be found under Botulinum A Toxin, on p.1311. For a discussion of the management of antipsychotic-induced dystonic reactions, see under Extrapyramidal Disorders in the Adverse Effects of Chlorpromazine, p.650.

1. Anonymous. Dystonia: underdiagnosed and undertreated? *Drug Ther Bull* 1988; **26:** 33–6.
2. Marsden CD, Quinn NP. The dystonias. *Br Med J* 1990; **300:** 139–44.
3. Williams A. Consensus statement for the management of focal dystonias. *Br J Hosp Med* 1993; **50:** 655–9.

Neuroleptic malignant syndrome. There have been isolated reports[1-4] that levodopa used alone or with bromocriptine has been successful in the treatment of patients with neuroleptic malignant syndrome (p.651). However, bromocriptine is usually preferred when a dopaminergic is required for the treatment of this condition.

1. Knezevic W, *et al.* Neuroleptic malignant syndrome. *Med J Aust* 1984; **140:** 28–30.
2. Clarke CE, *et al.* Clinical spectrum of neuroleptic malignant syndrome. *Lancet* 1988; **ii:** 969–70.
3. Lo TCN, *et al.* Neuroleptic malignant syndrome: another medical cause of acute abdomen. *Postgrad Med J* 1989; **65:** 653–5.
4. Shoop SA, Cernek PK. Carbidopa/levodopa in the treatment of neuroleptic malignant syndrome. *Ann Pharmacother* 1997; **31:** 119.

Parasomnias. The aetiology of *restless legs syndrome* and *periodic movements in sleep* is obscure and treatment has been largely empirical (p.639). Few of the treatments tried in these often co-existent disorders have been studied in a controlled manner but small controlled studies[1-4] have reported beneficial effects such as improved sleep quality and reduced leg movements from levodopa used with a decarboxylase inhibitor. Most patients received a bedtime dose of 50 to 200 mg of levodopa with possible additional doses during the night.

Levodopa has also been reported to have been of benefit in a study of 10 patients with *sleep bruxism*.[5]

1. von Scheele C. Levodopa in restless legs. *Lancet* 1986; **ii:** 426–7.
2. Brodeur C, *et al.* Treatment of restless legs syndrome and periodic movements during sleep with L-dopa: a double-blind controlled study. *Neurology* 1988; **38:** 1845–8.
3. Kaplan PW, *et al.* A double-blind, placebo-controlled study of the treatment of periodic limb movements in sleep using carbidopa/levodopa and propoxyphene. *Sleep* 1993; **16:** 717–23.
4. Trenkwalder C, *et al.* L-dopa therapy of uremic and idiopathic restless legs syndrome: a double-blind crossover trial. *Sleep* 1995; **18:** 681–8.
5. Lobbezoo F, *et al.* The effect of the catecholamine precursor L-dopa on sleep bruxism: a controlled clinical trial. *Mov Disord* 1997; **12:** 73–8.

Parkinsonism. Parkinson's disease is characterised by reduced dopaminergic activity in the brain. However, administration of dopamine is not a practical treatment as dopamine cannot penetrate the blood-brain barrier. Levodopa which is converted by decarboxylation into dopamine can penetrate the blood-brain barrier and is therefore used to provide a source of dopamine in the brain. Levodopa is usually given with a dopa-decarboxylase inhibitor such as benserazide or carbidopa. These drugs are unable to penetrate the blood-brain barrier and therefore prevent only extracerebral conversion of levodopa to dopamine. This allows effective concentrations of dopamine to be achieved in the brain with lower doses of levodopa and also reduces unwanted effects such as nausea and vomiting and cardiovascular effects associated with peripheral formation of dopamine.

Levodopa is the mainstay in the treatment of Parkinson's disease (p.1128) but opinion varies on when it should be used in the course of the disease. Most patients respond to levodopa initially but after a few years benefit may be reduced. There may be problems with dyskinesias and psychiatric effects and fluctuations in mobility necessitating careful dosage adjustment or the use of adjunctive drugs. Those who consider that long-term complications reflect the progressing severity of the disease favour early use of levodopa, whereas those who regard them as being due to cumulative exposure to levodopa advocate later use. The various methods used for the pharmacokinetic optimisation of levodopa administration as Parkinson's disease progresses have been discussed in detail and include timing of administration, the use of modified-release formulations, oral solutions (see above) and dispersible formulations for immediate absorption, the timing of food intake, and the use of other drugs to increase the absorption of levodopa.

References.

1. Giron LT, Koller WC. Methods of managing levodopa-induced dyskinesias. *Drug Safety* 1996; **14:** 365–74.
2. Contin M, *et al.* Pharmacokinetic optimisation in the treatment of Parkinson's disease. *Clin Pharmacokinet* 1996; **30:** 463–81.

Pituitary and hypothalamic disorders. DIAGNOSIS AND TESTING. Diminished growth-hormone reserve is one of the earliest functional abnormalities in anterior pituitary failure and, since dopamine is believed to stimulate growth-hormone secretion, the administration of levodopa has been used as a provocative test for the diagnosis of growth-hormone deficiency.[1,2] Levodopa 500 mg has been given by mouth after an overnight fast and serum concentrations of growth hormone measured hourly at 0 to 3 hours; children may be given 10 mg per kg body-weight to a maximum of 500 mg. Transient nausea, vomiting, vertigo, and hypotension may occur and the patient should be kept recumbent during the test. A normal response is an increase in serum concentration of growth hormone of more than 5 ng per mL or to a level of more than 10 ng per mL, although 10 to 15% of normal subjects may not respond. However, there is some dispute as to whether stimulated growth hormone secretion tests are superior to measurements of circulating somatomedins in detecting growth hormone deficiency.[3-5] For a discussion of the management of growth retardation, including the problems of accurate diagnosis, see p.1237.

1. Abboud CF. Laboratory diagnosis of hypopituitarism. *Mayo Clin Proc* 1986; **61:** 35–48.
2. Müller EE, *et al.* Involvement of brain catecholamines and acetylcholine in growth hormone deficiency states: pathophysiological, diagnostic and therapeutic implications. *Drugs* 1991; **41:** 161–77.
3. Hoffmann DM, *et al.* Diagnosis of growth-hormone deficiency in adults. *Lancet* 1994; **343:** 1064–8. Correction. *ibid.*, **344:** 206.
4. de Boer H, *et al.* Diagnosis of growth hormone deficiency in adults. *Lancet* 1994; **343:** 1645–6.
5. Rosenfeld RG, *et al.* Diagnostic controversy: the diagnosis of childhood growth hormone deficiency revisited. *J Clin Endocrinol Metab* 1995; **80:** 1532–40.

Preparations

BP 1998: Co-careldopa Tablets; Levodopa Capsules; Levodopa Tablets;
USP 23: Carbidopa and Levodopa Tablets; Levodopa Capsules; Levodopa Tablets.

Proprietary Preparations (details are given in Part 3)

Aust.: Ceredopa; ***Canad.:*** Larodopa†; ***Fr.:*** Larodopa†; ***Ger.:*** Dopaflex; ***Irl.:*** Larodopa†; ***Ital.:*** Larodopa†; ***Neth.:*** Eldopal†; ***S.Afr.:*** Larodopa†; ***UK:*** Brocadopa†; Larodopa; ***USA:*** Dopar; Larodopa.

Multi-ingredient: ***Aust.:*** Madopar; Sinemet; ***Austral.:*** Kinson; Madopar; Sinacarb; Sinemet; ***Belg.:*** Prolopa; Sinemet; ***Canad.:*** Apo-Levocarb; Prolopa; Sinemet; ***Fr.:*** Modopar; Sinemet; ***Ger.:*** Isicom; Madopar; Nacom; NeyDop "N" (Revitorgan-Dilutionen "N" Nr. 97); Striaton; ***Irl.:*** Half Sinemet; Madopar; Sinemet; ***Ital.:*** Madopar; Sinemet; ***Neth.:*** Madopar; Sinemet; ***Norw.:*** Madopar; Sinemet; ***S.Afr.:*** Carbilev; Madopar; Sinemet; ***Spain:*** Madopar; Sinemet; ***Swed.:*** Madopark; Sinemet; ***Switz.:*** Madopar; Sinemet; ***UK:*** Half Sinemet; Madopar; Sinemet; ***USA:*** Sinemet.

Lysuride Maleate (1510-r)

Lysuride Maleate *(BANM)*.

Lisuride Maleate *(rINNM)*; Methylergol Carbamide Maleate. 3-(9,10-Didehydro-6-methylergolin-8α-yl)-1,1-diethylurea hydrogen maleate; 8-Decarboxamido-8-(3,3-diethylureido)-D-lysergamide maleate.

$C_{20}H_{26}N_4O,C_4H_4O_4$ = 454.5.

CAS — 18016-80-3 (lysuride); 19875-60-6 (lysuride maleate).

Adverse Effects and Precautions

As for Bromocriptine, p.1132. Infusion of lysuride in parkinsonian patients has been associated with severe psychiatric adverse effects.

Effects on the respiratory tract. A report[1] of a woman with Parkinson's disease who developed bilateral pleural effusions after taking lysuride 4 mg daily for about 17 months. Her condition improved on discontinuation of lysuride.

1. Bhatt MH, *et al.* Pleuropulmonary disease associated with dopamine agonist therapy. *Ann Neurol* 1991; **30:** 613–16.

Porphyria. Lysuride maleate was considered to be unsafe in patients with acute porphyria because it has been shown to be porphyrinogenic in *animals* or *in-vitro* systems.[1]

1. Moore MR, McColl KEL. *Porphyria: drug lists.* Glasgow: Porphyria Research Unit, University of Glasgow, 1991.

Interactions

As for Bromocriptine, p.1133.

Pharmacokinetics

Plasma concentrations varied widely following a single oral dose of lysuride maleate 300 µg in 11 patients with Parkinson's disease.[1] Absorption was rapid and the mean plasma elimination half-life was 2.2 hours. Only a mean of 0.05% of the dose was excreted unchanged in the urine in 24 hours. The mean oral bioavailability of lysuride maleate has been reported[2] to be 10% after a 100-µg dose and 22% after a 300-µg dose.

A single dose of lysuride 25 µg given by intravenous, intramuscular, or subcutaneous injection reduced plasma-prolactin concentrations by up to 60% in 11 of 12 healthy subjects, the effect lasting for about 10 hours.[3] Plasma concentrations after intravenous administration fell in 2 phases with half-lives of 14 minutes and 1.5 hours respectively. Peak plasma concentrations following subcutaneous and intramuscular injection were obtained after 12 and 15 minutes respectively.

1. Burns RS, *et al.* Disposition of oral lisuride in Parkinson's disease. *Clin Pharmacol Ther* 1984; **35:** 548–56.
2. Hümpel M, *et al.* Radioimmunoassay of plasma lisuride in man following intravenous and oral administration of lisuride hydrogen maleate; effect on plasma prolactin level. *Eur J Clin Pharmacol* 1981; **20:** 47–51.
3. Krause W, *et al.* The pharmacokinetics and pharmacodynamics of lisuride in healthy volunteers after intravenous, intramuscular, and subcutaneous injection. *Eur J Clin Pharmacol* 1991; **40:** 399–403.

Uses and Administration

Lysuride maleate, an ergot derivative, is a dopamine D_2-agonist with actions and uses similar to those of bromocriptine (p.1132). It is also reported to have serotonergic activity. It is used similarly in the management of Parkinson's disease and has been used in disorders associated with hyperprolactinaemia. It is also used to suppress puerperal lactation for medical reasons; it is not recommended for the routine suppression of physiological lactation or for the treatment of postpartum breast pain and engorgement that may be adequately relieved with simple analgesics and breast support.

In the management of Parkinson's disease lysuride has been given alone or added to treatment in patients experiencing 'on-off' fluctuations in control with levodopa. It is normally given by mouth; doses should be taken with food. Initially 200 µg is taken at bedtime and additional doses of 200 µg may be added, at intervals of a week, first at midday and then in the morning; further increases are made, until an optimum response is obtained, by adding 200 µg each week using the same sequence of increases, starting with the bedtime dose; dosage should not normally exceed 5 mg daily in divided doses.

Lysuride maleate is given for the prophylaxis of migraine in some countries in usual doses of up to 25 µg three times daily.

Hyperprolactinaemia and prolactinomas. Dopamine agonists have been widely used for the treatment of hyperprolactinaemia secondary to a prolactinoma (p.1238). Lysuride has been used as an alternative to bromocriptine. There is a report of plasma-prolactin concentrations being reduced to normal in 4 female patients with macroprolactinomas given lysuride 400 to 800 µg daily for 2 years.[1] Subsequent dosage reduction in 3 was followed by a rise in prolactin values. In the fourth patient prolactin remained in the normal range when the dose was progressively reduced from 400 to 50 µg daily, although complete withdrawal was followed by an increase in prolactin concentration within 3 months.

Vaginal administration of lysuride is being studied in an attempt to avoid adverse effects associated with oral therapy. In a study[2] involving 40 women with hyperprolactinaemia a 200-µg standard oral tablet placed in the vagina at night produced a similar reduction in prolactin concentrations to that obtained with 400 µg taken orally and was better tolerated.

1. Liuzzi A, *et al.* Low doses of dopamine agonists in the long-term treatment of macroprolactinomas. *N Engl J Med* 1985; **313:** 656–9.
2. Tasdemir M, *et al.* Vaginal lisuride for hyperprolactinaemia. *Lancet* 1995; **346:** 1362.

Lactation inhibition. Lysuride is used in some countries for the prevention of puerperal lactation (p.1240). However, the routine use of dopaminergics is not recommended for the suppression of physiological lactation.

References.

1. Venturini PL, *et al.* Effects of lisuride and bromocriptine on inhibition of lactation and on serum prolactin levels: comparative double-blind study. *Eur J Obstet Gynecol Reprod Biol* 1981; **11:** 395–400.

Migraine. Although lysuride is used in some countries for the prophylaxis of migraine (p.443) it is not usually considered to be the drug of choice or even one of the main alternatives.

Parkinsonism. While some neurologists use dopamine agonists such as lysuride early in the treatment of parkinsonism (p.1128) in an attempt to delay therapy with levodopa others reserve them for adjunctive use when levodopa is no longer effective alone or cannot be tolerated. They are sometimes useful in reducing 'off' periods with levodopa and in ameliorating other fluctuations in mobility in the later stages of the disease.

References.

1. Rinne UK. Lisuride, a dopamine agonist in the treatment of early Parkinson's disease. *Neurology* 1989; **39:** 336–9.

ADMINISTRATION. Lysuride has been of benefit when administered by continuous intravenous or subcutaneous infusion in patients experiencing fluctuations in mobility with levodopa therapy[1-3] but severe psychiatric effects have been associated with the use of these routes.[3]

1. Obeso JA, *et al.* Intravenous lisuride corrects oscillations of motor performance in Parkinson's disease. *Ann Neurol* 1986; **19:** 31–5.
2. Obeso JA, *et al.* Lisuride infusion pump: a device for the treatment of motor fluctuations in Parkinson's disease. *Lancet* 1986; **i:** 467–70.
3. Critchley P, *et al.* Psychosis and the lisuride pump. *Lancet* 1986; **i:** 349.

Preparations

Proprietary Preparations (details are given in Part 3)
Aust.: Dopergin; Prolacam; ***Belg.:*** Dopergine†; ***Fr.:*** Arolac; Dopergine; ***Ger.:*** Cuvalit; Dopergin; ***Ital.:*** Cuvalit†; Dopergin; ***Neth.:*** Dopergin; ***Spain:*** Dopergin; ***Switz.:*** Dopergin; ***UK:*** Revanil.

Memantine Hydrochloride (11453-r)

Memantine Hydrochloride *(rINNM)*.

1-Amino-3,5-dimethyladamantane Hydrochloride; D-145 (memantine); 3,5-Dimethyl-l-adamantanamine hydrochloride; DMAA (memantine). 3,5-Dimethyltricyclo[3.3.1.1.^{3,7}]decan-l-amine hydrochloride.

$C_{12}H_{21}N,HCl$ = 215.8.

CAS — 19982-08-2 (memantine).

Memantine is a derivative of amantadine (p.1129) and is likewise an antagonist of *N*-methyl-D-aspartate receptors. It has been given as the hydrochloride in the treatment of parkinsonism (p.1128) and central spasticity (p.1303), and has also been used in dementia (p.1386), brain injury, or comatose states. It is given by mouth in usual doses of up to 30 mg of the hydrochloride daily in divided doses.

Memantine hydrochloride is also given by slow intravenous injection for cerebral spasticity.

References.

1. Ditzler K. Efficacy and tolerability of memantine in patients with dementia syndrome: a double-blind, placebo controlled trial. *Arzneimittelforschung* 1991; **41:** 773–80.
2. Görtelmeyer R, Erbler H. Memantine in the treatment of mild to moderate dementia syndrome: a double-blind placebo-controlled study. *Arzneimittelforschung* 1992; **42:** 904–13.

Preparations

Proprietary Preparations (details are given in Part 3)
Ger.: Akatinol.

Metergoline (1511-f)

Metergoline *(BAN, rINN)*.

FI-6337; MCE; Methergoline. Benzyl (8S,10S)-(1,6-dimethylergolin-8-ylmethyl)carbamate.

$C_{25}H_{29}N_3O_2$ = 403.5.

CAS — 17692-51-2.

Metergoline, an ergot derivative, is a dopamine agonist with actions and uses similar to those of bromocriptine (p.1132). It is also a serotonin antagonist. Metergoline has been used similarly to bromocriptine in disorders associated with hyperprolactinaemia and to inhibit lactation. In some countries it is also used in the prophylaxis of migraine and other vascular headaches.

Hyperprolactinaemia and prolactinomas. Dopamine agonists have been widely used for the treatment of hyperprolactinaemia secondary to a prolactinoma (p.1238). There is a report of metergoline being tried in patients intolerant of bromocriptine.[1] In this report metergoline lowered plasma-prolactin concentrations, although not to normal, in 3 men and 8 women with hyperprolactinaemia. Galactorrhoea was abolished and/or a regular menstrual cycle established in 5 of the women. Prolactin concentrations and symptoms were unchanged in 3 further women with normoprolactinaemic galactorrhoea. Initial doses of 2 mg daily were increased over 2 weeks to 4 mg three times daily and at monthly re-assessment the dose was increased up to 24 mg daily in divided doses, according to response.

1. Casson IF, *et al.* Intolerance of bromocriptine: is metergoline a satisfactory alternative? *Br Med J* 1985; **290:** 1783–4.

Lactation inhibition. Metergoline has been tried for the prevention of puerperal lactation (p.1240) in doses of 8 to 12 mg daily for 5 days.[1,2] However the routine use of dopaminergics is not recommended for the suppression of physiological lactation.

1. Delitala G, *et al.* Metergoline in the inhibition of puerperal lactation. *Br Med J* 1977; **1:** 744–6.
2. Crosignani PG, *et al.* Suppression of puerperal lactation by metergoline. *Obstet Gynecol* 1978; **51:** 113–15.

Migraine. Although metergoline is used in some countries for the prophylaxis of migraine (p.443) it is not usually considered to be the drug of choice or even one of the main alternatives.

Preparations

Proprietary Preparations (details are given in Part 3)
Ger.: Liserdol; ***Ital.:*** Liserdol; ***S.Afr.:*** Liserdol; ***Switz.:*** Liserdol.

Naxagolide Hydrochloride (10334-g)

Naxagolide Hydrochloride *(USAN, rINNM)*.

Dopazinol Hydrochloride; L-647339; MK-458; PHNO (naxagolide); (+)-4-Propyl-9-hydroxynaphthoxazine hydrochloride. (+)-(4a*R*,10b*R*)-3,4,4a,5,6,10b-Hexahydro-4-propyl-2*H*-naphth[1,2*b*]-1,4-oxazin-9-ol hydrochloride.

$C_{15}H_{21}NO_2,HCl$ = 283.8.

CAS — 88058-88-2 (naxagolide); 99705-65-4 (naxagolide hydrochloride).

Naxagolide is a dopamine D_2-agonist that has been investigated in the management of Parkinson's disease.

References.

1. Koller WC, *et al.* Effect of MK-458 (HPMC) in Parkinson's disease previously untreated with dopaminergic drugs: a double-blind, placebo-controlled multicenter study. *Clin Neuropharmacol* 1991; **14:** 322–9.
2. Cutler NR, *et al.* Pharmacokinetics and dose proportionality of D_2-agonist MK-458(HPMC) in parkinsonism. *Clin Pharmacokinet* 1992; **22:** 223–30.

Pergolide Mesylate (13095-p)

Pergolide Mesylate *(BANM, USAN)*.

Pergolide Mesilate *(rINNM)*; LY-127809. 8β-Methylthiomethyl-6-propylergoline methanesulphonate; Methyl (8*R*,10*R*)-6-propylergolin-8-ylmethyl sulphide mesylate.

$C_{19}H_{26}N_2S,CH_4O_3S$ = 410.6.

CAS — 66104-22-1 (pergolide); 66104-23-2 (pergolide mesylate).

Adverse Effects and Precautions

As for Bromocriptine, p.1132. Other reported adverse effects include rash and fever and abnormal liver function tests. Abrupt withdrawal of pergolide may precipitate hallucinations and confusion, and withdrawal should be undertaken gradually.

An increased incidence of uterine neoplasms has been reported in *rodents* given high doses of pergolide mesylate.

Interactions

As for Bromocriptine, p.1133.

Pharmacokinetics

Pergolide mesylate is absorbed from the gastro-intestinal tract. It is reported to be about 90% bound to plasma proteins. It is excreted mainly in the urine in the form of metabolites.

Uses and Administration

Pergolide mesylate, an ergot derivative, is a dopamine agonist with actions and uses similar to those of bromocriptine (p.1132) but in contrast to bromocriptine it has agonist properties both at D_2 and to a lesser extent at D_1 receptors. It is used similarly in the management of Parkinson's disease usually as an adjunct to levodopa therapy to reduce 'end-of-dose' or 'on-off' fluctuations in response. It should be introduced gradually and during this period patients already receiving levodopa can have their levodopa dosage decreased gradually until an optimum response is achieved. The initial dose is the equivalent of 50 µg of pergolide daily for the first 2 days, increased gradually by 100 or 150 µg every third day over the next 12 days of therapy. Further increases of 250 µg may then be made every third day until an optimum response is achieved. A usual maintenance dose is 3 mg daily given in three divided doses but doses of up to 5 mg daily have been used.

Acromegaly. Dopaminergics can produce a paradoxical reduction in growth hormone secretion and may be used in the treatment of acromegaly as adjunctive therapy to surgery and/or radiotherapy to reduce circulating growth hormone levels, although they are less effective than octreotide (p.1235). While bromocriptine is the main dopamine agonist used pergolide has also been tried.[1]

1. Kleinberg DL, *et al.* Pergolide for the treatment of pituitary tumors secreting prolactin or growth hormone. *N Engl J Med* 1983; **309:** 704–9.

Hyperprolactinaemia and prolactinomas. Dopamine agonists are widely used for the treatment of hyperprolactinaemia secondary to a prolactinoma (p.1238). Pergolide has been suggested as an alternative to bromocriptine in this condition.

Studies[1-3] of pergolide mesylate in patients with hyperprolactinaemia indicate that single doses reduce serum-prolactin concentrations for more than 24 hours. In most patients, the effective daily dose was between 50 and 150 µg daily. Adverse effects were similar to those seen with bromocriptine, although some patients who could not take bromocriptine were able to tolerate pergolide (and *vice versa*). However, pergolide has reportedly lost favour for this indication because of reports of an increased incidence of uterine neoplasms in *animals*.

1. Franks S, *et al.* Treatment of hyperprolactinaemia with pergolide mesylate: acute effects and preliminary evaluation of long-term treatment. *Lancet* 1981; **ii:** 659–61.
2. Franks S, *et al.* Effectiveness of pergolide mesylate in long-term treatment of hyperprolactinaemia. *Br Med J* 1983; **286:** 1177–9.
3. Kleinberg DL, *et al.* Pergolide for the treatment of pituitary tumors secreting prolactin or growth hormone. *N Engl J Med* 1983; **309:** 704–9.

Parkinsonism. While some neurologists use dopamine agonists such as pergolide early in the treatment of parkinsonism (p.1128) in an attempt to delay therapy with levodopa, others reserve them for adjunctive use when levodopa is no longer effective alone or cannot be tolerated. They are sometimes useful in reducing 'off' periods with levodopa and in ameliorating other fluctuations in mobility in the later stages of the disease. Pergolide has a relatively long duration of action compared with other dopamine agonists commonly used. Although the duration of the clinical anti-parkinsonian effect of pergolide remains to be determined, studies suggest it is of the order of 5 to 8 hours. Depending on the dose used the response to other dopamine agonists in late parkinsonism is 1 to 4 hours for levodopa, 2 to 4 hours for lysuride, and 4 to 6 hours for bromocriptine.

References.

1. Anonymous. Pergolide (Celance)—a third dopamine agonist. *Drug Ther Bull* 1991; **29:** 79.
2. Markham A, Benfield P. Pergolide: a review of its pharmacology and therapeutic use in Parkinson's disease. *CNS Drugs* 1997; **7:** 328–40.

Tourette's syndrome. Pergolide is being studied in the management of Tourette's syndrome (p.636). A preliminary study[1] has produced encouraging results.

1. Lipinski JF, *et al.* Dopamine agonist treatment of Tourette disorder in children: results of an open-label trial of pergolide. *Mov Disord* 1997; **12:** 402–7.

Preparations

Proprietary Preparations (details are given in Part 3)
Aust.: Parkotil†; Permax; ***Austral.:*** Permax; ***Belg.:*** Permax; ***Canad.:*** Permax; ***Ger.:*** Parkotil; ***Irl.:*** Celance; ***Ital.:*** Nopar; ***Neth.:*** Permax; ***S.Afr.:*** Permax; ***Spain:*** Pharken; ***UK:*** Celance; ***USA:*** Permax.

Piribedil (4551-p)

Piribedil *(rINN).*

ET-495; EU-4200. 2-(4-Piperonylpiperazin-1-yl)pyrimidine.

$C_{16}H_{18}N_4O_2$ = 298.3.

CAS — 3605-01-4.

Piribedil is a non-ergot dopamine agonist that has been given by mouth in the treatment of parkinsonism and in circulatory disorders. Piribedil mesylate has been given by injection for similar indications.

Adverse effects reported include nausea and vomiting, dizziness, hallucinations, confusion, drowsiness, hypothermia, dyskinesias, and occasional changes in liver function.

Parkinsonism. The antiparkinsonian actions of piribedil have been discussed briefly in a review[1] of the status of dopamine agonists in the management of Parkinson's disease (p.1128). Piribedil is a dopamine D_2-agonist while its metabolite is reported to act on D_1 receptors. It has been mainly used as an adjunct to levodopa therapy and appears to act more on tremor than on other symptoms of Parkinson's disease, although it was noted that most of the evidence for this came from uncontrolled studies.

1. Montastruc JL, *et al.* Current status of dopamine agonists in Parkinson's disease management. *Drugs* 1993; **46:** 384–93.

Preparations

Proprietary Preparations (details are given in Part 3)
Fr.: Trivastal; ***Ger.:*** Trivastal; ***Ital.:*** Trivastan.

Pramipexole (5570-t)

Pramipexole *(BAN, USAN, rINN).*

SUD919CL2Y; U-98528E. (*S*)-2-Amino-4,5,6,7-tetrahydro-6-(propylamino)benzothiazole.

$C_{10}H_{17}N_3S$ = 211.3.

CAS — 104632-26-0.

Adverse Effects and Precautions

As for Bromocriptine, p.1132. Pramipexole should be administered with caution to patients with renal impairment.

Interactions

As for Bromocriptine, p.1133. Cimetidine is reported to reduce the renal clearance of pramipexole.

Pharmacokinetics

Pramipexole is readily absorbed from the gastro-intestinal tract and peak plasma concentrations have been reached within about 2 hours in fasting patients and in about 3 hours when given with food. Oral bioavailability is reported to be about 90%. Pramipexole is widely distributed throughout the body and its protein binding is low. Metabolism is minimal and more than 90% of a dose is excreted via renal tubular secretion unchanged into the urine. Elimination half-lives of 8 to 12 hours have been reported.

References.

1. Wright CE, *et al.* Steady-state pharmacokinetic properties of pramipexole in healthy volunteers. *J Clin Pharmacol* 1997; **37:** 520–5.

Uses and Administration

Pramipexole is a dopamine D_2-agonist with actions similar to those of bromocriptine (p.1134).

For parkinsonism the initial dose is 125 µg given three times daily increased to 250 µg three times daily in the second week. Thereafter the daily dose is increased by 750 µg at weekly intervals to a maximum of 4.5 mg daily. The dosage should be reduced in patients with renal impairment. Use with levodopa may necessitate a reduction in the dosage of levodopa.

References.

1. Kasper S, *et al.* Pramipexole as adjunct to haloperidol in schizophrenia: safety and efficacy. *Eur Neuropsychopharmacol* 1997; **7:** 65–70.
2. Parkinson Study Group. Safety and efficacy of pramipexole in early Parkinson disease: a randomized dose-ranging study. *JAMA* 1997; **278:** 125–30.
3. Lieberman A, *et al.* Clinical evaluation of pramipexole in advanced Parkinson's disease: results of a double-blind, placebo-controlled, parallel-group study. *Neurology* 1997; **49:** 162–8.
4. Shannon KM, *et al.* Efficacy of pramipexole, a novel dopamine agonist, as monotherapy in mild to moderate Parkinson's disease. *Neurology* 1997; **49:** 724–8.
5. Guttman M. International Pramipexole-Bromocriptine Study Group. Double-blind comparison of pramipexole and bromocriptine treatment with placebo in advanced Parkinson's disease. *Neurology* 1997; **49:** 1060–5.
6. Lin S-C, *et al.* Effect of pramipexole in treatment of resistant restless legs syndrome. *Mayo Clin Proc* 1998; **73:** 497–500.

Preparations

Proprietary Preparations (details are given in Part 3)
USA: Mirapex.

Quinagolide Hydrochloride (17700-f)

Quinagolide Hydrochloride *(BANM, rINNM).*

CV-205-502 (quinagolide); SD2-CV-205-502 (quinagolide). (±)-*N*,*N*-Diethyl-*N*′-[(3*R**,4a*R**,10a*S**)-1,2,3,4,4a,5,10,10a-octahydro-6-hydroxy-1-propylbenzo[*g*]quinolin-3-yl]sulfamide hydrochloride.

$C_{20}H_{33}N_3O_3S,HCl$ = 432.0.

CAS — 87056-78-8 (quinagolide); 94424-50-7 (quinagolide hydrochloride).

Adverse Effects and Precautions

As for Bromocriptine, p.1132, although some patients unable to tolerate bromocriptine may tolerate quinagolide (and *vice versa*).

Interactions

As for Bromocriptine, p.1133.

Pharmacokinetics

Quinagolide is rapidly absorbed from the gastro-intestinal tract and undergoes extensive first-pass metabolism to the *N*-desethyl analogue which is biologically active and the *N,N*-didesethyl analogue. Approximately equal amounts of a dose appear in the urine and the faeces; it is excreted in the urine as sulphate or glucuronide conjugates of quinagolide and its metabolites and in the faeces as the unconjugated forms. Protein binding has been reported to be about 90%. The elimination half-life of quinagolide at steady state is about 17 hours.

Uses and Administration

Quinagolide is a non-ergot dopamine D_2-agonist that has actions and uses similar to those of bromocriptine (p.1132). It is used as the hydrochloride in the treatment of disorders associated with hyperprolactinaemia.

Quinagolide hydrochloride is given in single daily doses with food at bedtime. The initial dose is 25 µg daily for 3 days increasing thereafter at 3-day intervals in steps of 25 µg until the optimal response is achieved, which is usually within the range of 75 to 150 µg daily. If doses greater than 300 µg daily are required, increases should be made in steps of 75 to 150 µg daily at intervals of not less than 4 weeks.

Quinagolide has also been investigated in the treatment of acromegaly, lactation inhibition, and Parkinson's disease.

Acromegaly. Dopaminergics can produce a paradoxical reduction in growth hormone secretion and may be used in the treatment of acromegaly as adjunctive therapy to surgery and/or radiotherapy to reduce circulating growth hormone levels, although they are less effective than octreotide (see p.1235). Bromocriptine is the main dopamine agonist used, but quinagolide has been tried and results of an open study[1] in which quinagolide was administered to 17 patients with acromegaly suggest that quinagolide has a more prolonged effect on suppression of growth hormone secretion than bromocriptine. However, it was ineffective in bromocriptine-resistant patients. In another study involving 34 patients, quinagolide was more effective than either cabergoline or a depot preparation of bromocriptine in normalising circulating growth hormone and insulin-like growth factor.[2]

1. Chiodini PG, *et al.* CV 205-502 in acromegaly. *Acta Endocrinol (Copenh)* 1993; **128:** 389–93.
2. Colao A, *et al.* Effect of different dopaminergic agents in the treatment of acromegaly. *J Clin Endocrinol Metab* 1997; **82:** 518–23.

Hyperprolactinaemia and prolactinomas. Dopamine agonists are widely used for the treatment of hyperprolactinaemia secondary to a prolactinoma (see p.1238). Quinagolide has been tried as an alternative in patients unresponsive to or intolerant of bromocriptine.

References.

1. Vance ML, *et al.* Treatment of prolactin-secreting pituitary macroadenomas with the long-acting non-ergot dopamine agonist CV 205-502. *Ann Intern Med* 1990; **112:** 668–73.
2. Shoham Z, *et al.* CV 205-502—effectiveness, tolerability, and safety over 24-month study. *Fertil Steril* 1991; **55:** 501–6.
3. Rasmussen C, *et al.* Clinical response and prolactin concentration in hyperprolactinemic women during and after treatment for 24 months with the new dopamine agonist, CV 205-502. *Acta Endocrinol (Copenh)* 1991; **125:** 170–6.
4. Verhelst JA, *et al.* Acute and long-term effects of once-daily oral bromocriptine and a new long-acting non-ergot dopamine agonist, quinagolide, in the treatment of hyperprolactinemia: a double-blind study. *Acta Endocrinol (Copenh)* 1991; **125:** 385–91.
5. van der Heijden PFM, *et al.* CV205-502, a new dopamine agonist, versus bromocriptine in the treatment of hyperprolactinaemia. *Eur J Obstet Gynecol Reprod Biol* 1991; **40:** 111–18.
6. Vilar L, Burke CW. Quinagolide efficacy and tolerability in hyperprolactinaemic patients who are resistant to or intolerant of bromocriptine. *Clin Endocrinol (Oxf)* 1994; **41:** 821–6.

Lactation inhibition. A small preliminary study[1] has suggested that quinagolide is of similar efficacy to bromocriptine for prevention of puerperal lactation. However, the routine use of dopaminergics is not recommended for the suppression of physiological lactation (see p.1240).

1. van der Heijden PFM, *et al.* Lactation inhibition by the dopamine agonist CV 205-502. *Br J Obstet Gynaecol* 1991; **98:** 270–6.

Parkinsonism. Quinagolide has been studied[1] for use as a dopamine agonist in Parkinson's disease (p.1128). While some neurologists use such dopamine agonists early in treatment in an attempt to delay therapy with levodopa others reserve them for use when levodopa is no longer effective or cannot be tolerated. They are sometimes useful in reducing 'off' periods with levodopa and in ameliorating other fluctuations of mobility in the later stages of the disease.

1. Olanow CW, *et al.* CV 205-502: safety, tolerance to, and efficacy of increasing doses in patients with Parkinson's disease in a double-blind, placebo crossover study. *Clin Neuropharmacol* 1989; **12:** 490–7.

Preparations

Proprietary Preparations (details are given in Part 3)
Aust.: Norprolac; ***Fr.:*** Norprolac; ***Ger.:*** Norprolac; ***Neth.:*** Norprolac; ***Norw.:*** Norprolac; ***S.Afr.:*** Norprolac; ***Spain:*** Norprolac; ***Swed.:*** Norprolac; ***Switz.:*** Norprolac; ***UK:*** Norprolac.

Ropinirole Hydrochloride (17393-b)

Ropinirole Hydrochloride *(BANM, USAN, pINNM).*

SKF-101468 (ropinirole); SKF-0101468-A (ropinirole hydrochloride). 4-[2-(Dipropylamino)ethyl]-2-indolinone hydrochloride.

$C_{16}H_{24}N_2O,HCl$ = 296.8.

CAS — 91374-21-9 (ropinirole); 91374-20-8 (ropinirole hydrochloride).

Adverse Effects and Precautions

As for Bromocriptine, p.1132. It should not be used in patients with hepatic or severe renal impairment.

Interactions

As for Bromocriptine, p.1133. In addition, high doses of oestrogens can increase plasma concentrations of ropinirole and dosage adjustments may be necessary if oestrogen therapy is started or withdrawn during treatment with ropinirole. Ropinirole is metabolised by the cytochrome P450 isoenzyme CYP1A2 and there is therefore the potential for interactions between ropinirole and other drugs that are metabolised similarly or are enzyme inducers.

Pharmacokinetics

Ropinirole is rapidly absorbed from the gastro-intestinal tract and mean peak plasma concentrations have been achieved 1.5 hours after oral administration; the rate of absorption, but not the extent, may be reduced if taken with food. Bioavailability is reported to be about 50%. Plasma protein binding of ropinirole is low (10 to 40%).

Ropinirole is metabolised primarily by the cytochrome P450 isoenzyme CYP1A2 and excreted in the urine as metabolites. A mean elimination half-life of about 6 hours has been reported for ropinirole.

References.

1. Taylor AC, *et al.* Linear pharmacokinetics of ropinirole in patients with Parkinson's disease. *Br J Clin Pharmacol* 1998; **45:** 204P.
2. Brefel C, *et al.* Effect of food on the pharmacokinetics of ropinirole in parkinsonian patients. *Br J Clin Pharmacol* 1998; **45:** 412–15.

Uses and Administration

Ropinirole is a non-ergot dopamine D_2-agonist with similar actions to those of bromocriptine (p.1132). It is given by mouth as the hydrochloride in the management of Parkinson's disease, either alone or as an adjunct to levodopa. It should be introduced gradually and during this period patients already receiving levodopa can have their levodopa dosage decreased gradually until an optimal response is achieved. The concurrent dose of levodopa may be reduced by about 20%. The daily dosage of ropinirole should be given in three divided doses, preferably with food. The initial daily dose is 750 μg increased at weekly intervals in steps of 750 μg daily until the optimal response is achieved, which is usually within the range of 3 to 9 mg daily, although higher doses may be required if used with levodopa. If doses greater than 3 mg daily are required the weekly increments may be made in steps of up to 3 mg. The daily dosage should not exceed 24 mg.

Reviews.

1. Tulloch IF. Pharmacologic profile of ropinirole: a nonergoline dopamine agonist. *Neurology* 1997; **49** (suppl 1): S58–S62.

Parkinsonism. While some neurologists use dopamine agonists such as ropinirole early in the treatment of parkinsonism (p.1128) in an attempt to delay therapy with levodopa others reserve them for adjunctive use when levodopa is no longer effective alone or cannot be tolerated. They are sometimes useful in reducing 'off' periods with levodopa and in ameliorating other fluctuations of mobility in the later stage of the disease.

References.

1. Rascol O, *et al.* A placebo-controlled study of ropinirole a new D_2 agonist, in the treatment of motor fluctuations of L-DOPA-treated parkinsonian patients. *Adv Neurol* 1996; **69:** 531–4.
2. Adler CH, *et al.* The Ropinirole Study Group. Ropinirole for the treatment of early Parkinson's disease. *Neurology* 1997; **49:** 393–9.
3. Rascol O, *et al.* Ropinirole in the treatment of early Parkinson's disease: a 6-month interim report of a 5-year levodopa-controlled study. *Mov Disord* 1998; **13:** 39–45.
4. Korczyn AD, *et al.* Ropinirole versus bromocriptine in the treatment of early Parkinson's disease: a 6-month interim report of a 3-year study. *Mov Disord* 1998; **13:** 46–51.

Preparations

Proprietary Preparations (details are given in Part 3)
Fr.: Requip; ***Irl.:*** Requip; ***Ital.:*** Requip; ***Neth.:*** Requip; ***Swed.:*** Requip; ***UK:*** Requip; ***USA:*** Requip.

Selegiline Hydrochloride (13228-v)

Selegiline Hydrochloride *(BANM, USAN, rINNM).*

Deprenyl; L-Deprenyl. (−)-(*R*)-*N*,α-Dimethyl-*N*-(prop-2-ynyl)phenethylamine hydrochloride; (*R*)-Methyl(α-methylphenethyl)prop-2-ynylamine hydrochloride.

$C_{13}H_{17}N,HCl$ = 223.7.

CAS — 14611-51-9 (selegiline); 2079-54-1 (selegiline hydrochloride); 14611-52-0 (selegiline hydrochloride).

Pharmacopoeias. In *Eur.* (see p.viii) and *US.*

A white or almost white, odourless crystalline powder. Freely **soluble** in water, in chloroform, and in methyl alcohol; slightly soluble in acetone. A 2% solution in water has a pH of 3.5 to 4.5. **Store** in airtight containers. Protect from light.

Adverse Effects

Selegiline is often given as an adjunct to levodopa therapy and many of the adverse effects reported can be attributed to enhanced levodopa activity; dosage of levodopa may have to be reduced. Adverse effects have included hypotension, chest pain, nausea, vomiting, diarrhoea, confusion, dizziness, psychosis, depression, hallucinations, agitation, dry mouth, liver enzyme disturbances, difficulty in micturition, skin reactions, myopathy, and increased dyskinesias. The amphetamine metabolites of selegiline may cause insomnia; evening doses should be avoided.

For reference to a study which observed an increased mortality rate in patients with Parkinson's disease taking selegiline and levodopa compared with those taking levodopa alone, see under Parkinsonism in Uses and Administration, below.

Effects on carbohydrate metabolism. Profound hypoglycaemia developed in a 70-year-old man after selegiline was added to his existing medication for Parkinson's disease.[1] Hypoglycaemia was accompanied by hyperinsulinaemia and resolved 1 week after discontinuation of selegiline.

1. Rowland MJ, *et al.* Hypoglycemia caused by selegiline, an antiparkinsonian drug: can such side effects be predicted? *J Clin Pharmacol* 1994; **34:** 80–5.

Precautions

Selegiline should be used with caution in patients with peptic ulceration, uncontrolled hypertension, arrhythmias, angina, or psychosis.

Interactions

Selegiline is less likely than non-selective MAOIs, such as phenelzine, to interact with tyramine in food; such hypertensive reactions have been reported rarely at usual doses but the manufacturer has warned that its selectivity is lost at higher doses and it must be assumed that selegiline can usually only be used safely without dietary restrictions at doses of up to 10 mg daily. For dietary restrictions applicable to patients taking MAOIs, see p.304.

Even when given in therapeutic doses life-threatening interactions can occur between selegiline and pethidine. Serious reactions, sometimes fatal, have also been reported when selegiline has been used with tricyclic antidepressants or selective serotonin reuptake inhibitors (SSRIs). The manufacturer recommends that 14 days should elapse between discontinuation of selegiline and starting treatment with tricyclic antidepressants or SSRIs. Conversely, selegiline should not be given to patients who have recently received these antidepressants; at least 5 weeks should elapse between discontinuing fluoxetine and starting treatment with selegiline.

Although selegiline (a selective inhibitor of MAO type B) is less likely than non-selective MAOIs to interact with tyramine in food, like other MAOIs it can produce life-threatening reactions when given with *pethidine*.[1] The manufacturers (Somerset, USA) have stated that there has been a report of hypertensive crisis in a patient taking recommended doses of selegiline and *ephedrine*.

Although there have been studies in which patients with parkinsonism have received selegiline with *selective serotonin reuptake inhibitors (SSRIs)* such as fluoxetine[2] or paroxetine[3] (apparently without any problems) there have been reports of reactions[4-6] such as shivering and sweating, hypertension, hyperactivity, and ataxia occurring when selegiline and fluoxetine have been used together. The FDA noted[7] that reactions similar to those between SSRIs and non-selective MAOIs had also been reported in patients taking selegiline with paroxetine or sertraline.

Severe reactions, sometimes fatal, have also occurred in patients taking selegiline and *tricyclic antidepressants*.[7]

There has been a report[8] of a patient receiving the non-selective MAOI *iproniazid* who experienced severe orthostatic hypotension when given selegiline. A study[9] of selegiline and the reversible MAOI *moclobemide* administered concomitantly to healthy subjects showed that the two drugs together markedly increased the pressor response to tyramine compared with the effects of each drug used alone. The authors concluded that dietary restriction of tyramine-containing foods would be necessary if these two drugs were to be used together.

1. Zornberg GL, *et al.* Severe adverse interaction between pethidine and selegiline. *Lancet* 1991; **337:** 246. Correction. *ibid.*; 440.
2. Waters CH. Fluoxetine and selegiline—lack of significant interaction. *Can J Neurol Sci* 1994; **21:** 259–61.
3. Toyama SC, Iacono RP. Is it safe to combine a selective serotonin reuptake inhibitor with selegiline? *Ann Pharmacother* 1994; **28:** 405–6.
4. Suchowersky O, de Vries JD. Interaction of fluoxetine and selegiline. *Can J Psychiatry* 1990; **35:** 571–2.
5. Jermain DM, *et al.* Potential fluoxetine-selegiline interaction. *Ann Pharmacother* 1992; **26:** 1300.

6. Montastruc JL, *et al.* Pseudophaeochromocytoma in parkinsonian patient treated with fluoxetine plus selegiline. *Lancet* 1993; **341:** 555.
7. Anonymous. Eldepryl and antidepressant interaction. *FDA Med Bull* 1995; **25** (Feb.): 6.
8. Pare CMB, *et al.* Attempts to attenuate the 'cheese effect': combined drug therapy in depressive illness. *J Affective Disord* 1985; **9:** 137–41.
9. Korn A, *et al.* Tyramine pressor sensitivity in healthy subjects during combined treatment with moclobemide and selegiline. *Eur J Clin Pharmacol* 1996; **49:** 273–8.

Pharmacokinetics

Selegiline is readily absorbed from the gastro-intestinal tract from conventional preparations and crosses the blood-brain barrier. It undergoes extensive first-pass metabolism in the liver to produce at least 5 metabolites, including *l*-(−)-desmethylselegiline (norselegiline), *l*-(−)-*N*-methylamphetamine and *l*-(−)-amphetamine. Concentrations of selegiline metabolites are greatly reduced following administration of the oral lyophilisate preparation, the majority of which undergoes absorption through the buccal mucosa. It is excreted as metabolites mainly in the urine and approximately 15% appears in the faeces.

References.

1. Heinonen EH, *et al.* Pharmacokinetic aspects of l-deprenyl (selegiline) and its metabolites. *Clin Pharmacol Ther* 1994; **56:** 742–9.
2. Mahmood I, *et al.* Clinical pharmacokinetics and pharmacodynamics of selegiline: an update. *Clin Pharmacokinet* 1997; **33:** 91–102.

Uses and Administration

Selegiline is an irreversible selective inhibitor of monoamine oxidase type B, an enzyme involved in the metabolic degradation of dopamine in the brain. It enhances the effects of levodopa and is used in Parkinson's disease as an adjunct to levodopa therapy, usually when fluctuations in mobility have become a problem, but see below. Selegiline may also be given alone in early Parkinson's disease in an attempt to delay the need for levodopa therapy.

Selegiline hydrochloride is given by mouth as conventional preparations such as tablets or oral liquid, or as oral lyophilisate tablets. The dose of the conventional preparations is 10 mg daily, either as a single dose in the morning or in 2 divided doses of 5 mg at breakfast and lunchtime. The initial dose of the oral lyophilisate tablets is 1.25 mg daily before breakfast; patients already receiving 10 mg of conventional preparations can be transferred to 1.25 mg of the oral lyophilisate. Addition of selegiline to levodopa therapy may enable the dosage of levodopa to be reduced by about 20 to 50%. To avoid initial confusion and agitation, particularly in the elderly, it may be appropriate for the conventional preparations to start treatment with a dose of 2.5 mg daily.

Other conditions in which selegiline has been tried include dementia and depression.

Some references to the actions of selegiline.

1. Youdim MBH, Finberg JPM. Pharmacological actions of l-deprenyl (selegiline) and other selective monoamine oxidase B inhibitors. *Clin Pharmacol Ther* 1994; **56:** 725–33.
2. Lange KW, *et al.* Biochemical actions of l-deprenyl (selegiline). *Clin Pharmacol Ther* 1994; **56:** 734–41.

Dementia. The hypothesis that neurodegeneration in Alzheimer's disease (p.1386) might be due to free radical formation has led to drugs such as selegiline being tried as antioxidant therapy. However, the value of selegiline in Alzheimer's disease remains unclear.

Double-blind studies[1,2] indicate that selegiline 10 mg daily may produce beneficial effects in patients with Alzheimer's disease but it has been suggested that improvements in mood and cognitive function may be due to a reduction in tension and depression.[3] A 15-month study in Alzheimers's patients with mild cognitive impairment showed selegiline 10 mg daily to have little effect,[4] although the authors pointed out that those with more severe dementia have shown more response in other studies. The conclusion of a later study[5] that selegiline 10 mg daily slowed progression in patients with moderate disease has been criticised[6] on the grounds that any effect was only evident after statistical adjustment to the original analysis.

1. Piccinin GL, *et al.* Neuropsychological effects of L-deprenyl in Alzheimer's type dementia. *Clin Neuropharmacol* 1990; **13:** 147–63.
2. Mangoni A, *et al.* Effects of a MAO-B inhibitor in the treatment of Alzheimer disease. *Eur Neurol* 1991; **31:** 100–107.
3. Anonymous. Drugs for Alzheimer's disease. *Drug Ther Bull* 1990; **28:** 42–4.
4. Burke WJ, *et al.* L-Deprenyl in the treatment of mild dementia of the Alzheimer type: results of a 15-month trial. *J Am Geriatr Soc* 1993; **41:** 1219–25.
5. Sano M, *et al.* A controlled trial of selegiline, alpha-tocopherol, or both as treatment for Alzheimer's disease. *N Engl J Med* 1997; **336:** 1216–22.
6. Pincus MM. Alpha-tocopherol and Alzheimer's disease. *N Engl J Med* 1997; **337:** 572.

Depression. Selegiline is a monoamine oxidase inhibitor and there are reports of it producing improvement in depression.[1-3] However at the dosage level usually required to produce an antidepressant effect the specificity of selegiline is reported to be lost and it has been suggested that the efficacy of selegiline as an antidepressant might depend on inhibition of monoamine oxidase A rather than inhibition of monoamine oxidase B alone. Such a loss of specificity would mean that patients taking selegiline for depression would need to observe the dietary restrictions applicable to non-selective MAOIs.

1. Mendlewicz J, Youdim MBH. L-Deprenil, a selective monoamine oxidase type B inhibitor, in the treatment of depression: a double-blind evaluation. *Br J Psychiatry* 1983; **142:** 508–11
2. Mann JJ, *et al.* A controlled study of the antidepressant efficacy and side-effects of (−)-deprenyl. *Arch Gen Psychiatry* 1989; **46:** 45–50.
3. Sunderland T, *et al.* High-dose selegiline in treatment-resistant older depressive patients. *Arch Gen Psychiatry* 1994; **51:** 607–15.

Narcoleptic syndrome. Controlled studies[1,2] in a small number of patients suggested that selegiline 20 to 40 mg daily has a beneficial effect on symptoms of narcolepsy and cataplexy (p.1476); at such a dosage a low-tyramine diet is considered necessary.

1. Hublin C, *et al.* Selegiline in the treatment of narcolepsy. *Neurology* 1994; **44:** 2095–2101.
2. Mayer G, *et al.* Selegeline hydrochloride treatment in narcolepsy: a double-blind, placebo-controlled study. *Clin Neuropharmacol* 1995; **18:** 306–19.

Parkinsonism. As a selective monoamine oxidase type B inhibitor, selegiline reduces the metabolism of dopamine and thereby enhances its actions. It reduces levodopa's 'end-of-dose' effect and has a dose-sparing effect. Some have used it in an attempt to delay the need for levodopa. It has been postulated that progression of Parkinson's disease (p.1128) might be due to free radicals, generated during the metabolism of dopamine, having a cytotoxic effect on dopaminergic neurones in the substantia nigra. It has been suggested that selegiline might therefore slow disease progression by reducing the formation of free radicals generated by oxidation of dopamine by monoamine oxidase type B. In one large early study,[1] the DATATOP study, selegiline monotherapy delayed the need to start levodopa in patients with early Parkinson's disease. These findings were corroborated by other smaller studies.[2,3] There has been much debate over whether the benefit was due to a neuroprotective or symptomatic effect. Reanalysis of the DATATOP data by independent workers[4,5] and findings of other studies[6] support a symptomatic effect. Subsequent studies involving DATATOP patients have also been consistent with a symptomatic effect; any benefit produced by selegiline appeared to be less pronounced as the duration of treatment increased[7] and was lost completely long-term.[8,9] A later study[10] designed to minimise any symptomatic effect has cast doubt on whether the delay in progression of the signs and symptoms of Parkinson's disease obtained with selegiline is entirely due to a symptomatic effect.

Studies of the addition of levodopa to selegiline therapy[6,11,12] indicate that selegiline permits a modest reduction in the dosage requirements of levodopa. An interim analysis of a study of the early addition of selegiline to levodopa has also suggested that selegiline might stabilise the long-term daily levodopa dosage.[13]

However, the use of selegiline in Parkinson's disease has been questioned after one UK study[11] found an unexpected increase in mortality in patients taking levodopa with selegiline compared with those taking levodopa alone. No difference in mortality had been detected at the 3-year follow-up[14] but after an average follow-up of 5.6 years[11] mortality was 60% higher in the group receiving selegiline. The study has been criticised on many grounds including the fact that mortality was very high in both arms of the study[15] and has been the subject of much debate.[16,17] The authors of the study[11] had stated that they would advise the study patients to withdraw selegiline therapy. Analysis of follow-up data[18] until the selegiline arm of the study was terminated (average 6.8 years) found an excess mortality of about 35%, a figure calculated[19] to be no longer significant. However, because of the premature termination of the study such results were considered[20] to be biased. Whether any excess in mortality is causally related to selegiline is still unclear. Some consider that changes in prescribing practice based on this study are not warranted.[16] Others[20] have made a cautious recommendation not to start combination treatment in patients with newly diagnosed Parkinson's disease but consider that there is little evidence to advise patients who have been using selegiline with levodopa for years without problem to change their treatment. An evaluation of mortality among patients taking antiparkinsonian drugs (using the UK General Practice Research Database) provided evidence against there being substantial excess mortality associated with the use of selegiline.[21]

1. The Parkinson Study Group. Effect of deprenyl on the progression of disability in early Parkinson's disease. *N Engl J Med* 1989; **321:** 1364–71.
2. Tetrud JW, Langston JW. The effect of deprenyl (selegiline) on the natural history of Parkinson's disease. *Science* 1989; **245:** 519–22.
3. Allain H, *et al.* Selegiline in de novo parkinsonian patients: the French selegiline multicenter trial (FSMT). *Acta Neurol Scand* 1991; **84** (suppl 136): 73–8.
4. Schulzer M, *et al.* The antiparkinson efficacy of deprenyl derives from transient improvement that is likely to be symptomatic. *Ann Neurol* 1992; **32:** 795–8.
5. Ward CD. Does selegiline delay progression of Parkinson's disease? A critical re-evaluation of the DATATOP study. *J Neurol Neurosurg Psychiatry* 1994; **57:** 217–20.
6. Brannan T, Yahr MD. Comparative study of selegiline plus L-dopa–carbidopa versus L-dopa–carbidopa alone in the treatment of Parkinson's disease. *Ann Neurol* 1995; **37:** 95–8.
7. The Parkinson Study Group. Effects of tocopherol and deprenyl on the progression of disability in early Parkinson's disease. *N Engl J Med* 1993; **328:** 176–83.
8. Parkinson Study Group. Impact of deprenyl and tocopherol treatment on Parkinson's disease in DATATOP subjects not requiring levodopa. *Ann Neurol* 1996; **39:** 29–36.
9. Parkinson Study Group. Impact of deprenyl and tocopherol treatment on Parkinson's disease in DATATOP patients requiring levodopa. *Ann Neurol* 1996; **39:** 37–45.
10. Olanow CW, *et al.* The effect of deprenyl and levodopa on the progression of Parkinson's disease. *Ann Neurol* 1996; **38:** 771–7.
11. Parkinson's Disease Research Group of the United Kingdom. Comparison of therapeutic effects and mortality data of levodopa and levodopa combined with selegiline in patients with early, mild Parkinson's disease. *Br Med J* 1995; **311:** 1602–7.
12. Myllylä VV, *et al.* Early selegiline therapy reduces levodopa dose requirement in Parkinson's disease. *Acta Neurol Scand* 1995; **91:** 177–82.
13. Larsen JP, Boas J. Norwegian-Danish Study Group. The effects of early selegiline therapy on long-term treatment and parkinsonian disability: an interim analysis of a Norwegian-Danish 5-year study. *Mov Disord* 1997; **12:** 175–82.
14. Parkinson's Disease Research Group in the United Kingdom. Comparisons of the therapeutic effects of levodopa, levodopa and selegiline, and bromocriptine in patients with early, mild Parkinson's disease: three year interim report. *Br Med J* 1993; **307:** 467–72.
15. Olanow CW, *et al.* Patients taking selegiline may have received more levodopa than necessary. *Br Med J* 1996; **312:** 702–3.
16. Ahlskog JE. Treatment of early Parkinson's disease: are complicated strategies justified? *Mayo Clin Proc* 1996; **71:** 659–70.
17. Mizuno Y, Kondo T. Mortality associated with selegiline in Parkinson's disease: what do the available data mean? *Drug Safety* 1997; **16:** 289–94.
18. Ben-Shlomo Y, *et al.* Investigation by Parkinson's Disease Research Group of United Kingdom into excess mortality seen with combined levodopa and selegiline treatment in patients with early, mild Parkinson's disease: further results of randomised trial and confidential inquiry. *Br Med J* 1998; **316:** 1191–6.
19. Abrams KR. Monitoring randomised controlled trials. *Br Med J* 1998; **316:** 1183–4.
20. Breteler MMB. Selegiline, or the problem of early termination of clinical trials. *Br Med J* 1998; **316:** 1182–3.
21. Thorogood M, *et al.* Mortality in people taking selegiline: observational study. *Br Med J* 1998; **317:** 252–4.

Preparations

USP 23: Selegiline Hydrochloride Tablets.

Proprietary Preparations (details are given in Part 3)
Aust.: Amboneural; Cognitiv; Jumex; Regepar; ***Austral.:*** Eldepryl; Selgene; ***Belg.:*** Eldepryl; ***Canad.:*** Eldepryl; ***Fr.:*** Deprenyl; ***Ger.:*** Amindan; Antiparkin; Deprenyl; Movergan; Selegam; Selepark; ***Irl.:*** Clondepryl; Eldepryl; ***Ital.:*** Egibren; Jumex; Seledat; Selpar; ***Neth.:*** Eldepryl; ***Norw.:*** Eldepryl; ***S.Afr.:*** Eldepryl; ***Spain:*** Plurimen; ***Swed.:*** Eldepryl; ***Switz.:*** Jumexal; ***UK:*** Centrapryl; Eldepryl; Stilline; Vivapryl; Zelapar; ***USA:*** Carbex; Eldepryl.

Talipexole Hydrochloride (2990-z)

Talipexole Hydrochloride (*rINNM*).

Alefexole Hydrochloride; B-HT-920. 6-Allyl-2-amino-5,6,7,8-tetrahydro-4*H*-thiazolo[4,5-*d*]azepine dihydrochloride.

$C_{10}H_{15}N_3S,2HCl = 282.2.$

CAS — 101626-70-4 (talipexole); 36085-73-1 (talipexole hydrochloride).

Talipexole hydrochloride is a dopamine D_2-agonist that is used in the management of parkinsonism. It is also under investigation in the treatment of schizophrenia.

References.

1. Mizuno Y, *et al.* Preliminary study of B-HT 920, a novel dopamine agonist, for the treatment of Parkinson's disease. *Drug Invest* 1993; **5:** 186–92.
2. Ohmori T, *et al.* B-HT 920, a dopamine D2 agonist, in the treatment of negative symptoms of chronic schizophrenia. *Biol Psychiatry* 1993; **33:** 687–93.

Terguride (3639-p)

Terguride *(rINN)*.

1,1-Diethyl-3-(6-methylergolin-8α-yl) urea.

$C_{20}H_{28}N_4O$ = 340.5.

CAS — 37686-84-3.

Terguride, an ergot derivative, is a partial dopamine agonist with general properties similar to those of bromocriptine (p.1132). It is used in the treatment of disorders related to hyperprolactinaemia. It is also being investigated in the management of parkinsonism.

References.

1. Krause W, *et al.* Pharmacokinetics and endocrine effects of terguride in healthy subjects. *Eur J Clin Pharmacol* 1990; **38:** 609–15.
2. Baronti F, *et al.* Partial dopamine agonist therapy of levodopa-induced dyskinesias. *Neurology* 1992; **42:** 1241–3.

Tolcapone (15928-m)

Tolcapone *(BAN, USAN, rINN)*.

Ro-40-7592. 3,4-Dihydroxy-4′-methyl-5-nitrobenzophenone; 3,4-Dihydroxy-5-nitrophenyl(4-methylphenyl)methanone.

$C_{14}H_{11}NO_5$ = 273.2.

CAS — 134308-13-7.

Adverse Effects

The most common adverse effects associated with tolcapone are diarrhoea, nausea, anorexia, dyskinesia, and sleep disorders. Increases in liver enzyme values have occurred and hepatitis, sometimes fatal, has been reported. Tolcapone and its metabolites can produce a yellow intensification in the colour of urine.

Effects on the liver. A report of acute liver failure associated with tolcapone;[1] the patient died in hepatic coma.

1. Assal F, *et al.* Tolcapone and fulminant hepatitis. *Lancet* 1998; **352:** 958.

Precautions

Tolcapone should not be given to patients with hepatic impairment or raised liver enzymes values. Liver enzyme levels should be monitored when starting treatment with tolcapone and then every 2 weeks for the first year of therapy, every 4 weeks for the next 6 months, and then every 8 weeks thereafter. If the dose is to be increased to 200 mg three times daily liver enzyme monitoring should take place before increasing the dose and then re-initiated at the frequency above. Tolcapone should be discontinued if liver enzyme levels exceed the upper limit of normal or if signs or symptoms suggestive of the onset of hepatic failure occur. Tolcapone should not be reintroduced to patients who have developed evidence of hepatic injury while receiving tolcapone. Tolcapone should be administered with caution to patients with severe renal impairment.

Tolcapone should be withdrawn gradually if a substantial clinical benefit is not obtained within the first 3 weeks of treatment; abrupt withdrawal or dose reduction should be avoided.

Elderly. A report of confusion in 3 elderly patients with severe Parkinson's disease associated with addition of tolcapone to antiparkinsonian therapy.[1] It was suggested that a starting dose of tolcapone 100 mg daily might be more suitable in frail patients with severe disease. It was noted[2] that a reduction in levodopa dosage is generally recommended when tolcapone is given to patients such as these, who were receiving 500 to 600 mg of levodopa daily.

1. Henry C, Wilson JA. Catechol-O-methyltransferase inhibitors in Parkinson's disease. *Lancet* 1998; **351:** 1965–6.
2. Harper J, Vieira B. Catechol-O-methyltransferase inhibitors in Parkinson's disease. *Lancet* 1998; **352:** 578.

Interactions

Tolcapone may influence the pharmacokinetics of drugs metabolised by catechol-*O*-methyltransferase; concomitant administration should be undertaken with care. Increased concentrations of benserazide and its active metabolite have been reported during concomitant administration. The manufacturer advises that non-selective MAOIs should not be used with tolcapone.

Pharmacokinetics

Tolcapone is rapidly absorbed from the gastro-intestinal tract and maximum plasma concentrations have been obtained within 2 hours of administration by mouth; food delays and decreases the absorption. Absolute bioavailability is reported to be about 65%. Tolcapone is more than 99% bound to plasma proteins and is not widely distributed into body tissues. It is extensively metabolised, mainly by conjugation to the inactive glucuronide, but methylation by catechol-*O*-methyltransferase to 3-*O*-methyltolcapone and metabolism by cytochrome P450 enzymes also occurs. About 60% of a dose is excreted in the urine with the remainder appearing in the faeces. The elimination half-life has been reported to be about 2 hours. The clearance of unbound tolcapone may be reduced by 50% in patients with moderate cirrhotic liver disorders.

References.

1. Dingemanse J, *et al.* Integrated pharmacokinetics and pharmacodynamics of the novel catechol-O-methyltransferase inhibitor tolcapone during first administration to humans. *Clin Pharmacol Ther* 1995; **57:** 508–17.
2. Jorga KM, *et al.* Effect of liver impairment on the pharmacokinetics of tolcapone and its metabolites. *Clin Pharmacol Ther* 1998; **63:** 646–54.

Uses and Administration

Tolcapone is a peripheral inhibitor of catechol-*O*-methyltransferase (COMT), an enzyme involved in the metabolism of dopamine and levodopa. It is used as an adjunct to levodopa and dopa decarboxylase inhibitor combinations in the management of Parkinson's disease for patients who cannot be stabilised on these levodopa combinations or for those who experience 'end-of-dose' deterioration. Because of the risk of hepatotoxicity the FDA in the USA restricted its use to when other adjunctive therapy was ineffective or contra-indicated. In Europe, tolcapone was withdrawn from the market in November 1998.

The usual recommended dosage of tolcapone is 100 mg given three times daily; up to a maximum of 200 mg three times daily may be considered if the clinical benefit justifies the increased risk of hepatotoxicity. The first dose of the day should be taken at the same time as the levodopa preparation. Most patients already taking more than 600 mg of levodopa daily will require a reduction in their dosage of levodopa.

Reviews.

1. Spencer CM, Benfield P. Tolcapone. *CNS Drugs* 1996; **5:** 475–81.

Parkinsonism. Tolcapone is a reversible peripheral inhibitor of catechol-*O*-methyltransferase (COMT), an enzyme involved in the metabolism of levodopa and dopamine.[1] It appears to differ from entacapone by being a more potent COMT inhibitor in the periphery and by penetrating into the brain (although the significance of any central effects of COMT inhibition are not known).[1] When given to patients with Parkinson's disease (p.1128) and levodopa-related fluctuations in disability or 'end-of-dose' effects it has prolonged the clinical benefit obtained with levodopa and allowed the total daily dosage of levodopa to be reduced.[2,3] Benefit has also been reported[4] when added to levodopa therapy in patients with stable Parkinson's disease.

1. Nutt JG. Catechol-O-methyltransferase inhibitors for treatment of Parkinson's disease. *Lancet* 1998; **351:** 1221–2.
2. Kurth MC, *et al.* Tolcapone improves motor function and reduces levodopa requirement in patients with Parkinson's disease experiencing motor fluctuations: a multicenter, double-blind, randomized, placebo-controlled trial. *Neurology* 1997; **48:** 81–7.
3. Rajput AH, *et al.* Tolcapone improves motor function in parkinsonian patients with the "wearing-off" phenomenon: a double-blind placebo-controlled, multicenter trial. *Neurology* 1997; **49:** 1066–71.
4. Waters CH, *et al.* Tolcapone Stable Study Group. Tolcapone in stable Parkinson's disease: efficacy and safety of long-term treatment. *Neurology* 1997; **49:** 665–71.

Preparations

Proprietary Preparations (details are given in Part 3)
Irl.: Tasmar†; ***Swed.:*** Tasmar†; ***UK:*** Tasmar†; ***USA:*** Tasmar.

Electrolytes

Electrolytes are used to correct disturbances in fluid and electrolyte homoeostasis or acid-base balance and to re-establish osmotic equilibrium of specific ions. The osmotic effects of solutions may be expressed in terms of osmolality which is defined as the 'molal' concentration in moles (or osmoles) per kg of solvent, or in terms of osmolarity which is the 'molar' concentration in moles (or osmoles) per litre of solution. In clinical practice, solute concentrations are measured per litre of solution and are expressed as millimoles (mmol) per litre or sometimes as milliequivalents (mEq) per litre. Milliequivalents are converted to millimoles by dividing by the valency of the ion. Positively charged ions are known as *cations* and include calcium, magnesium, potassium, and sodium ions. Negatively charged ions are known as *anions* and include bicarbonate, chloride, and phosphate ions. The ions principally involved in fluid and electrolyte homoeostasis and acid-base balance are sodium, chloride, bicarbonate, and potassium. Calcium, phosphate, and magnesium have a central role in the formation of bone mineral.

Acid-base Balance

Within the body, acid is mostly produced during cellular respiration in the form of carbon dioxide. Small amounts of various non-volatile acids are generated via metabolism, including lactic acid, uric acid, keto acids and some inorganic acids such as sulphuric and phosphoric acids. However, for normal tissue function, the pH of the body needs to be held within a narrow range. The pH of arterial blood is normally maintained between about 7.38 and 7.42 by means of compensatory respiratory, renal, and buffering mechanisms.

The most important buffer system in the extracellular fluid is the bicarbonate-carbonic acid system. Bicarbonate and hydrogen ions are in equilibrium with carbonic acid which is in turn in equilibrium with carbon dioxide in the body fluid, as expressed by:

$$H^+ + HCO_3^- \leftrightarrow H_2CO_3 \leftrightarrow CO_2 + H_2O$$

A normal plasma-bicarbonate concentration in adults is in the range of 20 to 30 mmol per litre and arterial partial pressure of carbon dioxide (P_aCO_2) is normally 4.7 to 5.7 kPa (31 to 43 mmHg).

Ultimately, excess acid must be removed from the body and base regenerated. P_aCO_2 is under respiratory control with carbon dioxide being excreted by the lungs. Plasma-bicarbonate concentrations are regulated by the kidneys, where bicarbonate is actively regenerated or reabsorbed. Organic acids such as lactic acid may be eliminated by metabolism; and other non-volatile acids, such as the inorganic acids of phosphate and sulphate, are excreted via the kidneys with simultaneous regeneration of bicarbonate.

The relationship between plasma pH, P_aCO_2, and bicarbonate is defined by the Henderson-Hasselbalch equation which is used to assess acid-base balance. For clinical purposes, this equation becomes

$$pH = pK_{CO_2} + \log\left(\frac{C_{HCO_3}}{\alpha \times P_aCO_2}\right)$$

where pH is the plasma pH, pK_{CO_2} is the carbonic acid dissociation constant (6.1), C_{HCO_3} is the plasma-bicarbonate concentration, α is a value representing carbon dioxide solubility, and P_aCO_2 is the arterial partial pressure of carbon dioxide. Disorders of acid-base balance may be due to a change in plasma-bicarbonate concentrations (metabolic) or to a change in P_aCO_2 (respiratory), although mixed disorders do occur.

The 4 major acid-base disturbances are:

- metabolic acidosis caused by a decrease in the plasma-bicarbonate concentration
- metabolic alkalosis caused by an increase in the plasma-bicarbonate concentration
- respiratory acidosis caused by hypoventilation and a raised P_aCO_2
- respiratory alkalosis caused by hyperventilation and a reduced P_aCO_2.

A further measure that may provide useful information in the assessment of metabolic acidosis is the plasma anion gap. This is the difference in ionic charge between the principal plasma cation (sodium) and anions (chloride and bicarbonate), and provides an estimation of unmeasured serum anions, which include inorganic and organic acids.

Metabolic acidosis. Metabolic acidosis, characterised by a low plasma-bicarbonate concentration and a tendency towards a fall in arterial pH, is the most frequent acid-base abnormality.

Metabolic acidosis with a normal anion gap is usually caused by excessive losses of bicarbonate from the gastro-intestinal tract (as in severe diarrhoeas) or failure of the kidneys to reabsorb or regenerate adequate bicarbonate (as in the renal tubular acidoses). Ingestion of acidifying salts such as ammonium chloride, which generate hydrochloric acid, can also result in this type of acidosis. Metabolic acidosis characterised by an increased anion gap is often due to a reduction in the renal excretion of inorganic acids such as phosphates and sulphates as in renal failure (uraemic acidosis), or to the net accumulation of organic acids as, for example, in lactic acidosis or diabetic ketoacidosis.

Metabolic acidosis is diagnosed and monitored by measurement of serum electrolytes, arterial pH, and P_aCO_2. There is often hyperventilation with reduced cardiac function, constriction of peripheral veins, inhibition of the hepatic metabolism of lactate, and impairment of consciousness.

The main aim of **treatment** is to manage any underlying disorder, and in some cases this will be sufficient to enable the body's homoeostatic mechanisms to correct the acid-base imbalance. The advantages of more active treatment of the acidosis must be balanced against the risks, including over-alkalinisation, and in consequence such therapy tends to be reserved for more persistent or severe cases.

The usual alkalinising agent is sodium bicarbonate. It may be given by mouth to replace bicarbonate losses in various chronic metabolic acidoses such as uraemic acidosis or renal tubular acidosis. Potassium bicarbonate may be preferred if the acidosis is associated with potassium deficiency. Potassium citrate and sodium citrate have also been used. More severe and acute cases (particularly where arterial pH is below 7.1) may require intravenous sodium bicarbonate therapy. Intravenous sodium bicarbonate has a role in acute metabolic acidoses attributable to severe renal failure, severe secretory diarrhoeas, and renal tubular acidosis. Although hypertonic solutions have been used, for example, in patients with circulatory overload, roughly isotonic bicarbonate solutions are otherwise preferred; arterial pH and plasma bicarbonate should be raised a little at a time and the patient's response monitored.

Although the role of bicarbonate is accepted in the forms of metabolic acidosis mentioned, its use in the treatment of metabolic acidosis with concomitant tissue hypoxia, particularly lactic acidosis, is controversial.[1,2] The administration of bicarbonate generates carbon dioxide which, if not appropriately eliminated, due to poor tissue perfusion or impaired ventilation or both, diffuses rapidly into the cells exacerbating intracellular acidosis. In addition, in metabolic acidosis associated with organic acids such as lactic acid, there is a risk of over-alkalinisation due to the metabolism of the acid after correction of the arterial pH.

For similar reasons, the use of sodium bicarbonate in advanced cardiac life support is no longer routine, although current guidelines permit consideration of its use to correct acidosis if the resuscitation effort is prolonged (see p.779).

The role of bicarbonate in the management of diabetic ketoacidosis is also limited, although it may be appropriate in certain situations—see p.316.

Because of concerns about the effects of bicarbonate other agents have been investigated for the treatment of metabolic acidosis, including trometamol (THAM) and sodium dichloroacetate.[1,2] Alkalinising agents that have to be metabolised to bicarbonate before they have an effect, such as sodium lactate, are not generally used as many patients with acute acidosis have impaired metabolic activity, particularly of lactate.

Peritoneal dialysis, haemodialysis, or haemofiltration is required for refractory metabolic acidosis associated with acute renal failure (p.1152).

1. Arieff AI. Indications for use of bicarbonate in patients with metabolic acidosis. *Br J Anaesth* 1991; **67:** 165–77.
2. Adrogué HJ, Madias NE. Management of life-threatening acid-base disorders. *N Engl J Med* 1998; **338:** 26–34. Correction. *ibid.* 1999; **340:** 247.

Metabolic alkalosis. Metabolic alkalosis with an increased plasma-bicarbonate concentration and a sustained elevation in arterial pH results from excessive renal reabsorption and/or regeneration of bicarbonate. It is commonly seen with volume contraction (chloride depletion), potassium depletion, or mineralocorticoid excess, and may occur with excessive alkali intake as in the milk-alkali syndrome. If the metabolic alkalosis is severe, cardiac arrhythmias and hypoventilation may develop and there can be symptoms of concomitant hypokalaemia such as muscle weakness.

Treatment is generally aimed at the underlying disturbances.[1] Correcting volume depletion by administration of a chloride salt often obviates the need for other treatment; sodium chloride is normally used. However, potassium chloride may also be required if there is potassium depletion, particularly if this is severe. Rarely, direct acidification by the administration of ammonium chloride, dilute hydrochloric acid, or acidifying salts such as lysine hydrochloride or arginine hydrochloride may be required if the alkalosis is severe.

1. Adrogué HJ, Madias NE. Management of life-threatening acid-base disorders. *N Engl J Med* 1998; **338:** 107–11.

Calcium Homoeostasis

The adult body contains about 1.2 kg of calcium, of which approximately 99% is incorporated into the skeleton where its primary role is structural. The remaining 1% is found in body tissues and fluids and is essential for normal nerve conduction, muscle activity, and blood coagulation.

The concentration of calcium in plasma is normally kept within a narrow range (total calcium about 2.15 to 2.60 mmol per litre) by homoeostatic mechanisms involving parathyroid hormone, calcitonin, and vitamin D. Normally about 47% of calcium in plasma is in the ionised physiologically active form (giving a usual range of about 1.00 to 1.25 mmol per litre), about 6% is complexed with anions such as phosphate or citrate, and the remainder is bound to proteins, principally albumin. If the plasma-albumin concentration is raised (as in dehydration) or reduced (as is common in malignancy) it will affect the proportion of ionised calcium. Thus, the total plasma-calcium concentration is commonly adjusted for plasma albumin.

Hypercalcaemia. Hypercalcaemia, an increase in plasma-calcium concentration above the normal range, is most commonly due to primary hyperparathyroidism or malignant disease.[1,2] Rare causes of hypercalcaemia include vitamin D intoxication, granulomatous diseases such as sarcoidosis, prolonged immobility, acute renal failure, thiazide diuretics, and excess calcium carbonate ingestion (milk-alkali syndrome).[1]

Mild asymptomatic hypercalcaemia is often associated with a plasma-concentration elevated above the normal but below 3.00 mmol per litre. Severe symptomatic hypercalcaemia is broadly correlated with a plasma-calcium concentration of more than 3.50 mmol per litre.

Symptoms of hypercalcaemia include thirst, polyuria, anorexia, constipation, muscle weakness, fatigue, and confusion. In severe cases, there may be nausea and vomiting; cardiac arrhythmias may develop but are rare. Extreme hypercalcaemia may result in coma and death. Chronic hypercalcaemia can lead to interstitial nephritis and calcium renal calculi.

Mild asymptomatic hypercalcaemia does not require specific **treatment** and is best corrected by increasing oral fluid intake and treating any identified underlying disease. Patients with severe hypercalcaemia and/or significant symptoms require immediate therapy to reduce plasma-calcium concentrations independent of the cause.[2,3] The first step is rehydration with intravenous sodium chloride 0.9% to restore the intravascular volume and to promote calcium diuresis. Frusemide or other loop diuretics may assist in promoting the renal excretion of calcium but only in the presence of adequate volume expansion and control of other electrolyte losses. Large doses, for example 80 to 100 mg of frusemide administered intravenously every one to two hours, may be required. Thiazide diuretics should be avoided as they increase the renal tubular reabsorption of calcium. Peritoneal dialysis or haemodialysis with calcium-free dialysate should be considered in patients with renal failure for whom urinary excretion of calcium is inadequate. In life-threatening hypercalcaemia, more specific immediate therapy is generally required in addition to saline.[2,3] Calcitonins are likely to be first choice in this situation as they have a rapid onset of action. However, their effect is moderate and generally short-lived, and drugs with a more sustained effect may also be required. Most experience has been gained in the treatment of hypercalcaemia of malignancy (see below) using drugs that inhibit bone resorption such as bisphosphonates. Corticosteroids have been used to prolong the efficacy of calcitonin. Intravenous phosphates have been used to rapidly lower plasma-calcium concentrations but can cause soft tissue calcification resulting in serious adverse effects such as irreversible renal damage and hypotension, and are best avoided. Another drug that has been used for the emergency treatment of hypercalcaemia is trisodium edetate.

Choice of subsequent therapy is likely to depend on the specific cause.

1. Boyle I, Ralston S. Treatment of hypercalcaemia. *Prescribers' J* 1990; **30:** 180–6.
2. Bushinsky DA, Monk RD. Calcium. *Lancet* 1998; **352:** 306–11.
3. Bilezikian JP. Management of acute hypercalcemia. *N Engl J Med* 1992; **326:** 1196–1203.

HYPERCALCAEMIA OF MALIGNANCY. About 10% of patients with cancer develop hypercalcaemia of malignancy, which is typically severe and progressive.[1-4] The condition is generally thought to be due to either the production of parathyroid hormone-related protein by a tumour (humoral hypercalcaemia of malignancy) or to the release of bone-resorbing factors (osteoclast-activating factors), which include cytokines such as tumour necrosis factor, growth factors, and interleukin-1, from the site of bone metastases (local osteolytic hypercalcaemia of malignancy). Humoral hypercalcaemia is frequently associated with squamous cell carcinomas of the lung and head and neck whereas local osteolytic hypercalcaemia tends to occur with breast cancer or myeloma.[2,5]

The bisphosphonate pamidronate has been widely used and is considered by many to be the drug of choice[1-5] for **treating** hypercalcaemia once the patient has been adequately rehydrated (see above). It is given as a single dose, adjusted according to initial plasma-calcium concentrations, by slow intravenous infusion and although it may be 24 to 48 hours before calcium concentrations start to decrease, the effects can last for 20 to 30 days: regular infusions at intervals of 2 to 3 weeks can be given to maintain normocalcaemia. Clodronate has also been given, administered by intravenous infusion and then by mouth or by intermittent infusion. Etidronate, administered by intravenous infusion on 3 successive days, has been found to reduce hypercalcaemia but has been reported to be less effective than pamidronate[6] and to have a shorter duration of action. Subsequent oral therapy with daily doses of etidronate can prolong the period of normocalcaemia but may cause osteomalacia. There is some evidence that the bisphosphonates may be less effective for humoral than for osteolytic hypercalcaemia.[7]

Plicamycin, a cytotoxic antibiotic with particular activity against osteoclasts, has been used to obtain a rapid (within 24 hours) and sustained reduction in plasma-calcium concentrations in severe hypercalcaemia. However, it is highly toxic and safer drugs such as the bisphosphonates and calcitonins are generally preferred. Gallium nitrate also inhibits bone resorption; initial studies in patients with hypercalcaemia associated with malignancy have indicated beneficial effects but clinical experience is limited; again, the bisphosphonates are likely to be preferred.[3,4]

Corticosteroids are useful in hypercalcaemia associated with steroid-sensitive haematological malignancies such as lymphoma or myeloma. In addition they may be useful to overcome renal tubular resistance to calcitonin[8] (see above) but otherwise are not usually effective.[9] There have been individual reports of beneficial results using somatostatin analogues such as octreotide for the treatment of hypercalcaemia of malignancy.

1. Anonymous. Treating cancer-associated hypercalcaemia. *Drug Ther Bull* 1990; **28:** 85–7.
2. Hall TG, Schaiff RAB. Update on the medical treatment of hypercalcemia of malignancy. *Clin Pharm* 1993; **12:** 117–25.
3. Chisholm MA, *et al.* Acute management of cancer-related hypercalcemia. *Ann Pharmacother* 1996; **30:** 507–13.
4. Watters J, *et al.* The management of malignant hypercalcaemia. *Drugs* 1996; **52:** 837–48.
5. Mundy GR, Guise TA. Hypercalcemia of malignancy. *Am J Med* 1997; **103:** 134–45.
6. Ralston SH, *et al.* Comparison of three intravenous bisphosphonates in cancer-associated hypercalcaemia. *Lancet* 1989; **ii:** 1180–82.
7. Gurney H, *et al.* Parathyroid hormone-related protein and response to pamidronate in tumour-induced hypercalcaemia. *Lancet* 1993; **341:** 1611–13.
8. Hosking DJ, *et al.* Potentiation of calcitonin by corticosteroids during the treatment of the hypercalcaemia of malignancy. *Eur J Clin Pharmacol* 1990; **38:** 37–41.
9. Percival RC, *et al.* Role of glucocorticoids in management of malignant hypercalcaemia. *Br Med J* 1984; **389:** 287.

HYPERPARATHYROIDISM. Excess secretion of parathyroid hormone in primary hyperparathyroidism is characterised by hypercalcaemia, which is most frequently asymptomatic, and by hypophosphataemia. Oral phosphates have been used to control hypercalcaemia, and oral bisphosphonates are being investigated. However, in the long term, hypercalcaemia associated with primary hyperparathyroidism appears to be best managed by parathyroidectomy (p.733). Symptomatic hypocalcaemia may occur after surgery, requiring short-term treatment with calcium supplements and vitamin D.

VITAMIN D-MEDIATED HYPERCALCAEMIA. Hypercalcaemia can occur because of increased gastro-intestinal absorption of calcium mediated by the active metabolite of vitamin D, 1,25-dihydroxycholecalciferol (calcitriol).[1] This may be a feature of diseases associated with increased vitamin D sensitivity or increased vitamin D production, or may occur due to excess vitamin D administration. For example, granulomatous diseases such as sarcoidosis (p.1028) are associated with unregulated production of 1,25-dihydroxycholecalciferol. Hypercalcaemia due to vitamin D administration is most commonly seen in patients with renal failure receiving vitamin D analogues such as ergocalciferol (p.1367).

Treatment of severe hypercalcaemia requires prompt rehydration regardless of the cause (see above). Where hypercalcaemia is due to vitamin D administration, the vitamin D analogue should be discontinued until normocalcaemia is achieved. Corticosteroids effectively reduce gastro-intestinal absorption of calcium, and these may be used intravenously as adjuncts to rehydration in severe hypercalcaemia, and orally for milder hypercalcaemia or longer term therapy. Oral sodium cellulose phosphate, which binds calcium in the gastro-intestinal tract, and a low-calcium diet may also be considered. Oral chloroquine phosphate has been used in hypercalcaemia associated with sarcoidosis.

1. Adams JS. Vitamin D metabolite-mediated hypercalcemia. *Endocrinol Metab Clin North Am* 1989; **18:** 765–78.

Hypocalcaemia. Hypocalcaemia, a decrease in plasma-calcium concentration below the normal range, may be due to impaired or reduced absorption of calcium from the gastro-intestinal tract as with vitamin D deficiency disorders (see Osteomalacia, p.730) and chronic renal failure (see Renal Osteodystrophy, p.732). Alternatively, it may be due to deficient parathyroid hormone secretion and/or action as in hypoparathyroidism (p.733) and hypomagnesaemia (see below). Excessive phosphate administration is also a cause of hypocalcaemia (see below). Rarely, hypocalcaemia may follow repeated infusions of citrate ions, for example, during transfusions utilising citrated blood, as the citrate complexes with the calcium ion. Respiratory alkalosis due to hyperventilation can also lead to depression of ionised plasma-calcium concentrations.

Where symptoms of hypocalcaemia occur, they are typically associated with increased neuromuscular excitability; paraesthesias can occur and in more severe cases, carpopedal spasm, muscle cramps, tetany, and convulsions may develop.[1-3] Other symptoms include ECG changes and mental disturbances such as irritability and depression. Prolonged hypocalcaemia can lead to dental defects, cataract formation, and in children can result in mental retardation.

In patients with hypocalcaemia due to an underlying disease, long-term management should be aimed at **treating** this disease. Vitamin D supplements are widely used to enhance calcium absorption and correct vitamin D deficiency disorders and hypoparathyroidism. Oral supplements of calcium salts are often also given. Acute hypocalcaemia or hypocalcaemic tetany require emergency treatment with calcium salts administered intravenously.

1. Lebowitz MR, Moses AM. Hypocalcemia. *Semin Nephrol* 1992; **12:** 146–58.
2. Reber PM, Heath H. Hypocalcemic emergencies. *Med Clin North Am* 1995; **79:** 93–106.
3. Bushinsky DA, Monk RD. Calcium. *Lancet* 1998; **352:** 306–11.

Magnesium Homoeostasis

Magnesium is an essential body cation which is involved in numerous enzymatic reactions and physiological processes including energy transfer and storage, skeletal development, nerve conduction, and muscle contraction. Over half of the magnesium in the body is found in bone, about 40% is present in muscle and soft tissue, and only about 1% is present in the extracellular fluid. A normal concentration for magnesium in plasma is from about 0.7 to 1.0 mmol per litre.

Magnesium homoeostasis appears to be primarily regulated by the kidney where magnesium is extensively reabsorbed. Bone may act as a magnesium reservoir to reduce plasma-magnesium fluctuations. Magnesium is actively absorbed from the gastro-intestinal tract and this is enhanced to some extent by 1,25-dihydroxycholecalciferol (calcitriol).

Hypermagnesaemia. Hypermagnesaemia is an increase in the plasma concentration of magnesium above the normal range, as may follow excessive parenteral administration of salts such as magnesium sulphate. Hypermagnesaemia due to oral magnesium intake is uncommon as the kidneys are able to excrete a relatively large magnesium load. However, it may occur in patients with impaired renal function taking large amounts of magnesium, for example, in antacids or laxatives.

Symptoms of hypermagnesaemia include nausea, vomiting, CNS and respiratory depression, hyporeflexia, muscle weakness, and cardiovascular effects including peripheral vasodilatation, hypotension, bradycardia, and cardiac arrest.

Treatment of mild hypermagnesaemia is usually limited to restricting magnesium intake. In severe hypermagnesaemia, ventilatory and circulatory support may be required. Slow intravenous administration of 10 to 20 mL of calcium gluconate 10% is recommended to reverse the effects on cardiovascular and respiratory systems. If renal function is normal, adequate fluids should be given to promote renal magnesium clearance. This may be increased by the use of frusemide. Haemodialysis using a magnesium-free dialysis solution effectively removes magnesium, and this may be necessary in patients with renal impairment, or for whom other methods prove ineffective.

Hypomagnesaemia. Hypomagnesaemia, a plasma-magnesium concentration below the normal range, may result from a reduced magnesium intake as in dietary deficiency or malabsorption syndromes. Alternatively, it may be due to excessive magnesium loss either via the kidney because of inadequate reabsorption or more often from the gut, for example, during chronic diarrhoea. Drugs that may cause renal magnesium wasting include aminoglycosides, cisplatin (p.514), and diuretics.

Hypomagnesaemia is closely associated with other electrolyte disturbances, especially hypocalcaemia (see above) and hypokalaemia (see below), and rarely occurs alone. Specific symptoms are therefore difficult to determine but may include anorexia, nausea, weakness, neuromuscular dysfunction such as tetany, tremor, and muscle fasciculations, and rarely seizures. Cardiac arrhythmias may occur, but the relative contribution of hypomagnesaemia and hypokalaemia to these is uncertain.

Magnesium salts can be given by mouth for the **treatment** of chronic or asymptomatic magnesium deficiency.[1,2] Parenteral therapy may be preferred in patients with poor gastro-intestinal absorption of magnesium or who are unable to tolerate oral supplements (usually because they cause diarrhoea); magnesium sulphate can be given by intravenous or intramuscular injection. In acute symptomatic hypomagnesaemia, rapid replacement therapy with intravenous magnesium salts may be necessary. Renal function and plasma-magnesium concentrations should be monitored.

1. Whang R, *et al.* Magnesium homeostasis and clinical disorders of magnesium deficiency. *Ann Pharmacother* 1994; **28:** 220–6.
2. Weisinger JR, Bellorín-Font E. Magnesium and phosphorus. *Lancet* 1998; **352:** 391–6.

Phosphate Homoeostasis

Phosphate is an essential bone mineral; about 80% of phosphorus in an adult body is incorporated into the skeleton as a calcium salt where it is required to give rigidity. The remainder is present in the soft tissues and is involved in several metabolic and enzymatic reactions including energy storage and transfer.

Phosphate exists in body fluids mainly as the divalent HPO_4^{2-} ion (about 80%) or monovalent $H_2PO_4^-$ ion (about 20%). Phosphate measurements are usually expressed as inorganic phosphorus to avoid confusion with the anion content. A normal range for phosphorus in plasma in adults is about 0.85 to 1.45 mmol per litre, but as only a small proportion of body phosphate is found in the extracellular fluid, plasma-phosphorus levels may not always reflect total body stores or predict replacement needs.

Phosphate concentrations in plasma are primarily regulated by renal excretion; parathyroid hormone reduces the renal tubular reabsorption of phosphate. Intestinal absorption of phosphate is enhanced by the vitamin D metabolite, 1,25-hydroxycholecalciferol.

Hyperphosphataemia. Hyperphosphataemia, an abnormally raised plasma-phosphorus concentration, is usually associated with renal failure and may lead to renal osteodystrophy (p.732). Hyperphosphataemia may also be a consequence of release of phosphate from cells; this may occur in conditions of cell breakdown such as in haemolysis or rhabdomyolysis, during chemotherapy when it may be part of the tumour lysis syndrome, or as a result of acidoses. Hypoparathyroidism may also lead to hyperphosphataemia due to decreased levels of parathyroid hormone (see p.733). Other causes include excessive phosphate administration during treatment of hypophosphataemia, overuse of phosphate enemas or oral phosphate bowel preparations, and excessive vitamin D intake.

Hyperphosphataemic symptoms include those of associated hypocalcaemia (see above). Complexation with calcium may lead to metastatic calcification.

The **treatment** of hyperphosphataemia[1] usually involves control of the relevant underlying condition, and the use of low-phosphate diets, and if necessary oral phosphate-binding agents, such as calcium acetate or carbonate or aluminium hydroxide. Haemodialysis has been used to correct hyperphosphataemia due to oral phosphate administration in renal failure.

1. Weisinger JR, Bellorín-Font E. Magnesium and phosphorus. *Lancet* 1998; **352:** 391–6.

Hypophosphataemia. Hypophosphataemia, a reduction in plasma-phosphorus concentrations below the normal range, may be due to insufficient absorption of phosphate or increased renal clearance as in primary hyperparathyroidism, vitamin D deficiency, or X-linked familial hypophosphataemia. An increased cell uptake of phosphate can also result in hypophosphataemia, as for example, in chronic respiratory alkalosis and related disorders including alcoholism, hepatic failure, and septicaemia. As phosphate is widely available in most foods, dietary deficiency is rare though it may occur in infants of low birth-weight fed exclusively on human breast milk (p.1160). The absorption of phosphate from the gastro-intestinal tract can be reduced if phosphate-binding antacids are taken in large amounts.

Hypophosphataemia is usually asymptomatic but clinical symptoms become apparent when plasma-phosphorus concentrations fall below 0.3 mmol per litre.[1-3] Symptoms include neuromuscular dysfunction such as muscle weakness and paraesthesias, convulsions, cardiomyopathy, respiratory failure, and haematological abnormalities. Prolonged hypophosphataemia can result in rickets or osteomalacia (p.730).

Treatment of hypophosphataemia primarily involves correction of any underlying disease. Milk or oral phosphate supplements may be appropriate if a phosphate deficiency is identified or in certain disorders such as X-linked hypophosphataemic rickets. Intravenous phosphate administration may be required for severe hypophosphataemia, but this should be used cautiously to avoid hypocalcaemia and metastatic calcification.[2,3] Consideration should be given to correcting concomitant electrolyte disturbances such as hypomagnesaemia.

1. Larner AJ. Clinical applicability of inorganic phosphate measurements. *Br J Hosp Med* 1992; **48:** 748–53.
2. Lloyd CW, Johnson CE. Management of hypophosphatemia. *Clin Pharm* 1988; **7:** 123–8.
3. Weisinger JR, Bellorín-Font E. Magnesium and phosphorus. *Lancet* 1998; **352:** 391–6.

Potassium Homoeostasis

Potassium is predominantly an intracellular cation, primarily found in muscle; only about 2% is present in the extracellular fluid. It is essential for numerous metabolic and physiological processes including nerve conduction, muscle contraction, and acid-base regulation. A normal concentration of potassium in plasma is about 3.5 to 5.0 mmol per litre, but factors influencing transfer between intracellular and extracellular fluids such as acid-base disturbances can distort the relationship between plasma concentrations and total body stores. The body content of potassium is primarily regulated by renal glomerular filtration and tubular secretion. Aldosterone enhances the renal secretion of potassium and several other factors such as sodium excretion, dietary potassium intake, and plasma pH can modulate the excretion of potassium by the kidney. Insulin, beta$_2$ agonists, and aldosterone, and increases in plasma pH, can promote the cellular uptake of potassium. The passage of potassium into the cells and retention against the concentration gradient requires active transport via the Na^+/K^+ ATPase enzyme.

Hyperkalaemia. Hyperkalaemia, an abnormally raised plasma-potassium concentration, can occur if the potassium intake is increased, if the renal excretion decreases as in renal failure or adrenocortical insufficiency, or if there is a sudden efflux of potassium from the intracellular stores, for example, in acidosis or cell destruction due to tissue trauma, burns, haemolysis, or rhabdomyolysis. Hyperkalaemia may also be induced by drugs such as the potassium-sparing diuretics or ACE inhibitors. Usually the renal mechanisms for potassium excretion adapt readily to an increased potassium load and hyperkalaemia due to increased dietary intake is rare unless renal function is also impaired.

Hyperkalaemia predominantly results in disruption of cardiac function, but skeletal muscle function may also be affected. Symptoms include ECG abnormalities, ventricular arrhythmias, cardiac arrest, and also neuromuscular dysfunction such as muscle weakness and paralysis.[1-4]

Treatment involves the administration of calcium to counteract the negative effects of hyperkalaemia on cardiac excitability, the use of agents such as insulin or sodium bicarbonate to promote the transfer of potassium from the extracellular to the intracellar fluid compartment, and enhanced potassium excretion with exchange resins or dialysis.[1-4] The methods employed depend largely on the severity of the hyperkalaemia and critically, any associated ECG changes. Hyperkalaemia associated with a plasma concentration of potassium above 6.0 to 7.0 mmol per litre or with ECG changes is usually considered a medical emergency.

If cardiac manifestations of hyperkalaemia are present, then first-line therapy should be with a calcium salt administered intravenously; 10 to 30 mL of calcium gluconate 10% may be given by slow intravenous injection, the dosage being titrated and adjusted based on ECG improvement.

Calcium will not, however, reduce the plasma-potassium concentration. In moderate to severe hyperkalaemia, insulin, together with glucose to prevent hypoglycaemia, may be given intravenously in order to reduce the potassium concentration by stimulating the uptake of potassium by cells. Insulin is administered as a rapid-acting soluble insulin and typical doses are 5 to 15 units with 50 mL of glucose 50% given slowly over 5 to 15 minutes. Doses may need to be repeated as necessary. Alternatively or additionally, sodium bicarbonate may be employed to correct acidosis and promote cellular uptake of potassium; usual doses are in the order of 50 to 100 mL of a 4.2% solution (equivalent to 25 to 50 mmol) given intravenously.

The beta$_2$ agonist, salbutamol, administered intravenously or by a nebuliser, has also been found to enhance the cellular uptake of potassium and reduce plasma-potassium concentrations.[1,3,5,6] However, some clinicians prefer to avoid beta$_2$ agonists because of fears that large doses may induce cardiac arrhythmias.[7]

After the plasma-potassium concentration has been reduced in the immediate term by enhancing cellular potassium uptake, treatments are often required that will remove excess potassium from the body over the longer term. Cation exchange resins such as calcium or sodium polystyrene sulphonate can be given orally or rectally and, after about 1 to 2 hours, will begin to remove potassium from the body. Haemodialysis removes potassium from the body very effectively and is particularly useful in patients with acute renal failure, hypervolaemia, hypernatraemia, or severe hyperkalaemia. Peritoneal dialysis is effective in some patients.

1. Anonymous. Hyperkalaemia—silent and deadly. *Lancet* 1989; **i:** 1240.
2. Saxena K. Clinical features and management of poisoning due to potassium chloride. *Med Toxicol Adverse Drug Exp* 1989; **4:** 429–43.
3. Anonymous. Potassium disorders and cardiac arrhythmias. *Drug Ther Bull* 1991; **29:** 73–5.
4. Vaughan RS. Potassium in the perioperative period. *Br J Anaesth* 1991; **67:** 194–200.
5. Allon M, *et al.* Nebulized albuterol for acute hyperkalemia in patients on hemodialysis. *Ann Intern Med* 1989; **110:** 426–9.
6. McClure RJ, *et al.* Treatment of hyperkalaemia using intravenous and nebulised salbutamol. *Arch Dis Child* 1994; **70:** 126–8.
7. Halperin ML, Kamel KS. Potassium. *Lancet* 1998; **352:** 135–40.

HYPERKALAEMIC PERIODIC PARALYSIS. Hyperkalaemic periodic paralysis is an inherited disorder in which sudden increases in plasma-potassium concentrations cause muscle paralysis. An acute attack may require intravenous calcium gluconate and insulin with glucose (see above). Inhalation of a $beta_2$ agonist such as salbutamol has been used to treat or abort attacks.[1] Diuretics such as acetazolamide or the thiazides are used prophylactically to reduce the frequency of attacks.

1. Wang P, Clausen T. Treatment of attacks in hyperkalaemic familial periodic paralysis by inhalation of salbutamol. *Lancet* 1976; **i:** 221–3.

Hypokalaemia. Chronic hypokalaemia, a prolonged reduction of the plasma concentration of potassium, usually indicates a reduction in total body potassium. It may result from an inadequate intake, or gastrointestinal losses, for example in patients with secretory diarrhoeas, or from excessive renal losses as in hyperaldosteronism, Cushing's syndrome, or chronic metabolic alkalosis. Thiazides or loop diuretics increase urinary-potassium losses. Other drugs, notably corticosteroids and some antibacterials such as gentamicin, also have this effect. Hypokalaemia can also be caused by an increased cellular uptake of potassium rather than excess body losses. This may occur with drugs such as $beta_2$ agonists or xanthines, during insulin therapy, acute alkalosis, or possibly be induced by catecholamines after myocardial infarction. Hypokalaemia secondary to hypomagnesaemia can occur (see above).

Hypokalaemia results in neuromuscular disturbances ranging from muscle weakness to paralysis and respiratory insufficiency and can also cause rhabdomyolysis, ECG abnormalities, and ileus. Chronic hypokalaemia may lead to renal tubular damage (hypokalaemic nephropathy). Hypokalaemia increases the risk of digoxin toxicity.

Treatment involves correcting any underlying disorder and replacement therapy with potassium salts. Oral potassium supplements are generally preferred but in severe hypokalaemia associated with cardiac arrhythmias, paralysis or diabetic ketoacidosis, parenteral therapy may be necessary. Potassium salts, usually potassium chloride, may be given by intravenous infusion but must be administered slowly to avoid causing hyperkalaemia and associated cardiac toxicity; plasma-potassium concentrations should be closely monitored and ECG monitoring may be required. The choice of salt for oral potassium replacement depends on co-existing acid-base and electrolyte disturbances. Potassium chloride is generally the drug of choice for the treatment of hypokalaemia in patients with metabolic alkalosis with hypochloraemia, whereas a salt such as the bicarbonate may be preferred in patients with hyperchloraemic acidosis as in some renal tubular acidoses. Hypokalaemia secondary to hypomagnesaemia requires magnesium replacement therapy.

References.

1. Anonymous. Potassium disorders and cardiac arrhythmias. *Drug Ther Bull* 1991; **29:** 73–5.
2. Vaughan RS. Potassium in the perioperative period. *Br J Anaesth* 1991; **67:** 194–200.
3. Halperin ML, Kamel KS. Potassium. *Lancet* 1998; **352:** 135–40.
4. Gennari FJ. Hypokalemia. *N Engl J Med* 1998; **339:** 451–8.

BARTTER'S SYNDROME. Bartter's syndrome is thought to result from an inherited defect in the thick ascending limb of the loop of Henle. Patients exhibit hyperplasia of the juxtaglomerular cells, hypokalaemia and metabolic alkalosis, and excess aldosterone, prostaglandin, and renin production. Symptoms are primarily those of the hypokalaemia, including muscle weakness; polyuria and enuresis, and growth retardation in children, can occur. In contrast to other hyperreninaemic states, patients do not have hypertension or oedema.

Treatment rarely completely corrects hypokalaemia. Potassium supplementation may be given, while a cyclo-oxygenase inhibitor such as indomethacin,[1,2] or an ACE inhibitor such as captopril,[3,4] can produce benefit. Spironolactone and propranolol have also been tried.[4] Magnesium sulphate may be given by depot injection if there is hypomagnesaemia.[4]

1. Littlewood JM, *et al.* Treatment of childhood Bartter's syndrome with indomethacin. *Lancet* 1976; **ii:** 795.
2. Sechi LA, *et al.* Abnormalities of erythrocyte sodium transport systems in Bartter's syndrome. *Am J Nephrol* 1992; **12;** 137–43.
3. Jest P, *et al.* Angiotensin-converting enzyme inhibition as a therapeutic principle in Bartter's syndrome. *Eur J Clin Pharmacol* 1991; **41:** 303–5.
4. Crowe P, *et al.* Bartter's syndrome in two generations of an Irish family. *Postgrad Med J* 1993; **69:** 791–6.

DIURETIC-INDUCED HYPOKALAEMIA. Reduced potassium concentrations may result from the use of potassium-losing diuretics, particularly thiazides and loop diuretics. Clinically significant hypokalaemia is unlikely at the doses used in hypertension and the routine use of potassium supplements is no longer recommended. However, the concomitant administration of a potassium-sparing diuretic such as amiloride or, less usually, a potassium supplement may be necessary in patients at risk of hypokalaemia (see also p.885).

HYPOKALAEMIC PERIODIC PARALYSIS. Hypokalaemic periodic paralysis is an inherited disorder in which episodes of paralysis appear to be associated with a shift in potassium from the extracellular to the intracellular fluid resulting in hypokalaemia. Therapy has included the use of potassium supplements; acetazolamide has been found to reduce the frequency and severity of attacks.[1]

1. Griggs RC, *et al.* Acetazolamide treatment of hypokalemic periodic paralysis: prevention of attacks and improvement of persistent weakness. *Ann Intern Med* 1970; **73:** 39–48.

Sodium Homoeostasis

Sodium is the principal cation in the extracellular fluid and is responsible for the maintenance of the extracellular fluid volume and osmolality. In addition, sodium is also involved in nerve conduction, muscle contraction, acid-base balance, and cell nutrient uptake. A normal concentration of sodium in plasma would be expected to be within 135 to 145 mmol per litre.

Sodium homoeostasis is complex and closely associated with fluid balance. The osmolality and volume of the extracellular fluid are tightly regulated. Small changes in osmolality (plasma-sodium concentrations) are corrected by alteration of extracellular volume. This balance of plasma osmolality is achieved by the secretion or suppression of antidiuretic hormone (ADH; vasopressin), which primarily controls water excretion by the kidney. A tendency towards hyponatraemia suppresses ADH secretion and promotes renal loss of water; an increase in ADH secretion increases water reabsorption by the renal distal tubules. Changes in extracellular volume will also affect ADH release independently of osmolality. In addition, changes in extracellular volume result in modulation of the renal excretion of sodium.

Total body sodium content is regulated by renal sodium excretion, which can vary widely depending on dietary intake. Various mechanisms are involved in controlling renal sodium excretion including the renin-angiotensin system, glomerular filtration rate, and natriuretic factors. A reduction in extracellular fluid volume leads to the production of angiotensin II which stimulates the secretion of aldosterone. Aldosterone promotes the reabsorption of sodium ions by the distal tubules. There may be significant effects on sodium homoeostasis if adrenal insufficiency or mineralocorticoid excess disturb this mechanism.

Hypernatraemia. Hypernatraemia is an abnormal rise in the plasma-sodium concentration with a simultaneous rise in plasma osmolality. It is generally associated with volume depletion when water intake is less than water losses through renal or extrarenal routes. The causes include impaired thirst, as in coma or essential hypernatraemia, osmotic diuresis (solute diuresis), as in diabetic ketoacidosis or after mannitol administration, and excessive water losses, either from the kidney, as in diabetes insipidus, or extrarenally, for example, because of excessive sweating or diarrhoea.

Hypernatraemia can also occur following excessive oral sodium intake (but this is uncommon) and after inappropriate use of intravenous sodium chloride.

The clinical manifestations of hypernatraemia are caused by the effect of increased plasma osmolality on the brain and include somnolence, confusion, respiratory paralysis, and coma. CNS symptoms are more severe when hypernatraemia develops rapidly. In the presence of volume depletion, other symptoms such as hypotension, tachycardia, and various symptoms of circulatory insufficiency may occur concomitantly. A high volume of dilute urine is seen in patients with abnormal renal water conservation, whereas a low volume of concentrated urine is expected in patients with impaired thirst or excessive extrarenal water loss.

Treatment of hypernatraemia usually requires water replacement and oral administration of water may be sufficient for some patients. In more severe conditions, glucose 5% may be administered by slow intravenous infusion. Alternatively, some recommend the use of sodium chloride 0.9%. Care is required as too rapid correction can induce cerebral oedema, particularly in chronic conditions.

If the total body sodium is too high, loop diuretics may be used to increase sodium excretion with fluid losses being replaced by an infusion of glucose 5% and potassium chloride. It has also been suggested that dialysis may be necessary if there is significant renal impairment, if the patient is moribund, or if the serum-sodium concentration is greater than 200 mmol per litre.

For the treatment of hypernatraemia associated with some specific causes see diabetes insipidus (p.1237), diabetic ketoacidosis (p.316), and sodium chloride overdose (p.1162).

Hyponatraemia. Hyponatraemia, an abnormal fall in the plasma-sodium concentration, usually with a simultaneous fall in the plasma osmolality, is a frequent electrolyte disturbance that occurs with many different diseases including heart failure, cirrhosis, adrenocortical insufficiency, hyperglycaemia, and AIDS.

The kidney is able to conserve sodium and sodium depletion due to low salt intake is rare. Sodium depletion may occur if there are abnormal losses, either from the gut as a consequence of repeated diarrhoea and/or vomiting or from the kidney, for example, due to various renal disorders or the overuse of diuretics (p.886).

The most common cause of hyponatraemia is dilution. This may result from excessive fluid intake, for example, due to the ingestion of large volumes of water as in patients with primary polydipsia (psychogenic polydipsia). More frequently, however, it is a result of reduced water excretion, for example in impaired renal function or the syndrome of inappropriate secretion of antidiuretic hormone (SIADH) which is discussed on p.1241. Postoperative hyponatraemia is a frequent complication which may be exacerbated by the inappropriate intravenous administration of hypotonic, or even isotonic,[1] fluids.

Hyponatraemia due to sodium depletion in the presence of volume contraction may cause postural hypotension and circulatory insufficiency. Dilutional hyponatraemia can be asymptomatic but headache, confusion, nausea, vomiting, somnolence, and weakness may occur. If severe, cerebral oedema is present, and respiratory arrest, convulsions, and coma may ensue. CNS symptoms are more common when the condition is acute.

Therapy is guided by the rate of development and degree of hyponatraemia, accompanying symptoms, and the state of water balance, and should also take into account the underlying cause. Mild asymptomatic hyponatraemia does not usually require specific therapy. Chronic mild to moderate sodium depletion, such as occurs in salt-losing bowel or renal disease, may be treated with oral sodium chloride supplements while ensuring adequate fluid intake.

When there is substantial volume depletion, volume replacement is necessary and intravenous sodium chloride 0.9% is often used.

Chronic dilutional hyponatraemia, which is often asymptomatic, can generally be managed by correcting the underlying disease; water restriction may also be necessary and drugs that interfere with the action of ADH such as demeclocycline or lithium carbonate may be useful in SIADH.[2,3] Frusemide plus oral sodium chloride supplements have also been used (p.1241).

Acute symptomatic hyponatraemia (water intoxication) is generally associated with plasma-sodium concentrations below 120 mmol per litre and requires more aggressive therapy. This involves the intravenous administration of hypertonic or isotonic sodium chloride, often in conjunction with a loop diuretic such as frusemide, especially if fluid overload is likely to be a problem.[2,3] The aim is to render the patient asymptomatic with a plasma-sodium concentration of 120 to 130 mmol per litre; the plasma-sodium concentration should not be corrected to normal values nor should hypernatraemia be allowed to develop.[2,3] Plasma-sodium concentrations and the total-body-water volume should be monitored throughout.

A rare neurological syndrome known as central pontine myelinolysis (osmotic demyelination) has been associated with the over-rapid correction of symptomatic hyponatraemia, particularly if the condition is well established, and it has been recommended that the plasma-sodium concentration should be increased at a rate not exceeding 0.5 mmol per litre per hour[4,5] in these patients, though the best correction rate is debatable.[3,6] Some have suggested an initial prompt increase in plasma sodium of about 10% or 10 mmol per litre, followed by correction at a rate not exceeding 1.0 to 1.5 mmol per litre per hour or 15 mmol per litre per 24 hours.[7] However, the association of hyponatraemia with central pontine myelinolysis is controversial and some authorities do not consider the rate of correction to be a factor in hyponatraemic brain injury.[3]

1. Steele A, *et al.* Postoperative hyponatremia despite near-isotonic saline infusion: a phenomenon of desalination. *Ann Intern Med* 1997; **126:** 20–5.
2. Swales JD. Management of hyponatraemia. *Br J Anaesth* 1991; **67:** 146–53.
3. Arieff AI. Management of hyponatraemia. *Br Med J* 1993; **307:** 305–8.
4. Cluitmans FHM, Meinders AE. Management of severe hyponatremia : rapid or slow correction? *Am J Med* 1990; **88:** 161–6.
5. Laureno R, Karp BI. Myelinolysis after correction of hyponatremia. *Ann Intern Med* 1997; **126:** 57–62.
6. Stems RH. The treatment of hyponatremia: first, do no harm. *Am J Med* 1990; **88:** 557–60.
7. Kumar S, Berl T. Sodium. *Lancet* 1998; **352:** 220–8.

Dialysis Solutions (3276-x)

Pharmacopoeias. In *Eur.* (see p.viii), which includes separate monographs for solutions for haemodialysis, haemofiltration, and peritoneal dialysis.

Dialysis and filtration solutions are solutions of electrolytes formulated in concentrations similar to those of extracellular fluid or plasma. They always contain sodium and chloride and bicarbonate or a bicarbonate precursor. In addition, they often contain calcium and magnesium, and rarely potassium. Glucose may be added as an osmotic agent. These solutions allow the removal of water and metabolites and the replacement of electrolytes.

In *haemodialysis*, the exchange of ions between the solution and the patient's blood is made across a semi-permeable membrane, primarily by diffusion. Excess fluid is removed by ultrafiltration achieved by a pressure gradient. Membranes are either derived from cellulose (e.g. cuprophane) or are synthetic. Bicarbonate rather than a bicarbonate precursor is increasingly preferred as the bicarbonate source in haemodialysis since the problems of precipitation of calcium and magnesium have been overcome by changes in dialysis technique. Acetate is still used in some dialysers, but is thought to have vasodilatory and cardiodepressant actions, and may not be converted to bicarbonate fast enough for high-flux haemodialysis or in patients with liver disease. Haemodialysis solutions are provided in a sterile concentrated form for dilution with water before use; this water need not be sterile.

In *peritoneal dialysis*, the exchange is made across the membranes of the peritoneal cavity primarily by diffusion. Excess fluid is removed by ultrafiltration achieved by the use of osmotic agents such as glucose. The problems of calcium bicarbonate precipitation have not yet been overcome, and lactate is generally used as the bicarbonate precursor. Peritoneal dialysis solutions must be sterile and apyrogenic.

In *haemofiltration*, blood is filtered rather than dialysed. Metabolites are removed by convective transport, and excess water by hydrostatic ultrafiltration. Fluid and electrolytes are replaced by direct intravenous infusion of haemofiltration solution. Most haemofiltration solutions use acetate as the bicarbonate source. Haemofiltration solutions must be sterile and apyrogenic.

References.

1. Carlsen DB, Wild ST. Grams to milliequivalents: a concise guide to adjusting hemodialysate composition. *Adv Renal Replacement Ther* 1996; **3:** 261–5.
2. Zucchelli P, Santoro A. How to achieve optimal correction of acidosis in end-stage renal failure patients. *Blood Purif* 1995; **13:** 375–84.
3. Passlick-Deetjen J, Kirchgessner J. Bicarbonate: the alternative buffer for peritoneal dialysis. *Perit Dial Int* 1996; **16** (suppl 1): S109–S113.
4. Pastan S, Bailey J. Dialysis therapy. *N Engl J Med* 1998; **338:** 1428–37.

Adverse Effects

Adverse effects occurring during *haemodialysis* include nausea, vomiting, hypotension, muscle cramps, and air embolus. Effects related to vascular access include infection, thrombosis, and haemorrhage. Adverse effects occurring during *haemofiltration* are similar to those for haemodialysis.

The most common adverse effects associated with *peritoneal dialysis* include peritonitis, hernias, hyperglycaemia, protein malnutrition, and catheter complications.

Long-term complications in dialysed patients, some of which may relate to renal failure itself, include haemodialysis-related amyloidosis, acquired cystic kidney disease, and accelerated atherosclerosis. Dialysis dementia is a special hazard of aluminium overload. Long-term peritoneal dialysis results in progressive structural changes to the peritoneal membrane ultimately resulting in dialysis failure.

Aluminium overload. Accumulation of aluminium in patients on dialysis may result in dialysis dementia, anaemia, and aluminium-related bone disease (see also p.1547). Sources of aluminium include the water used for preparation of dialysis fluids and aluminium-containing phosphate binders used in treating renal osteodystrophy (p.732). It is therefore important that water used for the preparation of dialysis fluids has a low aluminium concentration; Ph. Eur. specifies a limit of aluminium of 10 μg per litre. Non-aluminium-containing phosphate binders such as calcium acetate or calcium carbonate may be preferred for long-term therapy. Aluminium overload in patients on dialysis has been treated with desferrioxamine (p.977).

Copper toxicity. Liver and haematological toxicity has occurred as a result of absorption of copper from dialysis fluids (p.1338).

Haemodialysis-induced cramp. Muscle cramps commonly occur during haemodialysis procedures, and are often associated with hypotension as a result of inappropriate volume removal. In addition, they may be exacerbated by cellulose-derived membranes or the use of acetate as a bicarbonate precursor. Sodium chloride tablets (p.1163), intravenous sodium chloride 0.9%, intravenous hypertonic glucose (p.1344), and quinine (p.442) have been used in the prevention or treatment of haemodialysis-induced cramp.

Hypersensitivity. The use of ethylene oxide for the disinfection of dialysis equipment has been associated with severe, sometimes fatal, anaphylactic reactions (p.1113).

Infections. Patients undergoing haemodialysis are at risk of infections from microbial contamination of dialysis fluid, and from inadequate care of vascular access sites. Maximum microbial counts and limits for endotoxins have been specified for water used in dialysis fluids. Bicarbonate-based dialysis solutions are more susceptible to microbial growth than acetate-based solutions.

Peritonitis is common in patients receiving peritoneal dialysis. The risk of infection may be minimised by using disconnect systems, good aseptic technique, and by good care of catheters. Treatment of bacterial peritonitis requires intraperitoneal administration of antibacterials, which are usually added to the dialysis fluid. Guidelines for treating peritonitis in patients on continuous ambulatory peritoneal dialysis have been published (see p.136).

Dialysis equipment should be regularly disinfected with agents such as formaldehyde (p.1114) or ethylene oxide (p.1113), but for mention of ethylene oxide anaphylactoid reactions, see p.1113.

Metabolic complications. The high concentrations of glucose in peritoneal dialysis solutions required to form an osmotic gradient can lead to weight gain, hyperglycaemia, hyperlipidaemia, and increased protein loss. Alternative osmotic agents such as icodextrin (p.1339) and amino acid-based solutions are being investigated.

Precautions

Peritoneal dialysis is not appropriate for patients with abdominal sepsis, previous abdominal surgery, or severe inflammatory bowel disease.

Haemodialysis should be used with caution in patients with unstable cardiovascular disease or active bleeding. During haemodialysis and haemofiltration, heparin (p.882) or epoprostenol (p.1418) are required to prevent clotting of the blood in the extracorporeal circuit.

Dialysis solutions should be warmed to body temperature with dry heat because wet heat carries a risk of microbial contamination.

Interactions

The effects of dialysis and filtration procedures on drug concentrations in the body can be complex. Because of the differences between the dialysis techniques, more drug may be removed by one technique than another. In general, drugs of low molecular weight, high water solubility, low volume of distribution, low protein binding, and high renal clearance are most extensively removed by dialysis. For example, aminoglycosides are extensively removed by dialysis procedures, and extra doses may be needed to replace losses, usually guided by serum-drug concentrations. Specific drug dosage adjustments for dialysis procedures may be employed where these are known. For drugs where the effect of dialysis is unknown, it is usual to give maintenance doses after dialysis. The ability of dialysis to remove some drugs has been used in the treatment of overdosage (see below).

Dialysis-induced changes in fluids and electrolytes have the potential to alter the effects of some drugs. For example, hypokalaemia predisposes to digoxin toxicity.

In patients undergoing peritoneal dialysis, drugs such as insulin and antibacterials may be added to the dialysis fluid. Consideration should be given to the possibility of adsorption of drugs onto the PVC bags.

References.

1. Aronson JK. The principles of prescribing in renal failure. *Prescribers' J* 1992; **32:** 220–31.
2. Bennett WM, *et al. Drug Prescribing in renal failure: dosing guidelines for adults.* 3rd ed. Philadelphia: American College of Physicians, 1994.
3. Cotterill S. Antimicrobial prescribing in patients on haemofiltration. *J Antimicrob Chemother* 1995; **36:** 773–80.

Uses and Administration

Dialysis and filtration procedures are used as part of renal replacement therapy in renal failure to correct electrolyte imbalance, correct fluid overload, and remove metabolites. They also have a limited role in the treatment of overdosage and poisoning. There are a number of techniques, and the choice between them will depend in part on the condition to be treated, the clinical state of the patient, patient preference, and availability. The two main techniques are haemodialysis and peritoneal dialysis, and a third less frequently used technique is haemofiltration.

Haemodialysis is more efficient than peritoneal dialysis at clearing small molecules such as urea, whereas peritoneal dialysis may be better at clearing larger molecules. Haemodialysis is considered to be less physiological than peritoneal dialysis as it involves periods of high clearance spaced between periods of no clearance.

Haemodialysis is usually performed intermittently, often 3 times a week, a typical session taking 3 to 5 hours. More recently high-flux dialysers have been developed which have reduced the time required for dialysis sessions. Haemodialysis is usually carried out in a dialysis centre, and less commonly at home.

Peritoneal dialysis may be performed continuously or intermittently. Continuous ambulatory peritoneal dialysis (CAPD) is the most commonly used technique. Patients remain mobile, except during exchanges, and can carry out the procedure themselves. There is always dialysis solution in the peritoneal cavity, and this is drained and replaced 3 to 5 times a day. Continuous cycle peritoneal dialysis (CCPD) is similar, except that exchanges are carried out automatically overnight, and patients do not have to carry out any exchanges during the day. Intermittent peritoneal dialysis (IPD) requires the patient to be connected to a dialysis machine for 12 to 24 hours 2 to 4 times a week. During this time, dialysis solution is pumped into and out of the peritoneal cavity, with a dwell time of about 10 to 20 minutes.

Haemofiltration is usually performed as a continuous technique and, as it is not portable, its principal use is in intensive care units. It may also be used intermittently as an adjunct to haemodialysis in patients with excess fluid weight gain. Continuous arteriovenous or venovenous haemodiafiltration (CAVHD or CVVHD) combines dialysis and filtration by perfusing the filtrate side of the haemofiltration membrane with peritoneal dialysis fluid.

Assessing serum concentrations of urea or creatinine before the next dialysis session is not a good measure of the adequacy of the dialysis, therefore various other measures have been developed including the urea reduction ratio and urea kinetic modelling. The use of such measures is more established for haemodialysis than for peritoneal dialysis.

Acute renal failure. Acute renal failure is characterised by a rapid decline in kidney function, and has a variety of causes.[1-3] It is often classified by origin as *prerenal* (e.g. due to hypovolaemia such as that associated with shock, burns, or dehydration; congestive heart failure; or renal artery obstruction), *renal* (such as acute tubular necrosis or interstitial nephritis of various causes, including nephrotoxic drugs and infections), or *postrenal* (acute urinary tract obstruction). The prognosis depends on the underlying disease, which should be identified and treated if possible, but the mortality may still be as high as 60%, particularly in patients who become oliguric, and after surgery or trauma. Management is essentially supportive in the hope that renal function will recover. Complications of acute renal failure include extracellular volume overload and hyponatraemia, hyperkalaemia, metabolic acidosis, hyperphosphataemia and hypocalcaemia. Those complications requiring urgent treatment, often including the use of dialysis, are severe hyperkalaemia (p.1149), pulmonary oedema, pericarditis, and severe metabolic acidosis (p.1147). The use of dialysis before clinical signs of uraemia is a matter of debate since it does not appear to hasten recovery *per se*,[1] but all save the shortest episodes of acute renal failure will require some form of renal replacement therapy with dialysis or filtration. Intermittent haemodialysis and peritoneal dialysis are both used, but the newer haemofiltration techniques have theoretical advantages in terms of volume control and cardiovascular stability, and are increasingly preferred.[2,4,5]

Numerous drugs have been tried in attempts to attenuate renal injury or hasten recovery in patients with acute tubular necrosis due to ischaemia or nephrotoxins.[1] These include drugs to increase renal blood flow (e.g. low-dose dopamine, atrial natriuretic peptide, or prostaglandins), drugs to increase urine flow and protect the epithelial cells (mannitol and loop diuretics, calcium channel blockers), or the use of chelating agents or antidotes against specific nephrotoxins. Consistent clinical benefit has not, however, been demonstrated.

Acute renal failure is reversible in about 95% of patients who survive the complications. A few patients who survive acute renal failure will require long-term dialysis or renal transplantation (p.499).

1. Brady HR, Singer GG. Acute renal failure. *Lancet* 1995; **346:** 1533–40.
2. Morgan AG. The management of acute renal failure. *Br J Hosp Med* 1996; **55:** 167–70.
3. Evans JHC. Acute renal failure in children. *Br J Hosp Med* 1994; **52:** 159–61.
4. McCarthy JT. Renal replacement therapy in acute renal failure. *Curr Opin Nephrol Hypertens* 1996; **5:** 480–4.
5. Joy MS, *et al.* A primer on continuous renal replacement therapy for critically ill patients. *Ann Pharmacother* 1998; **32:** 362–75.

Chronic renal failure. Chronic renal failure is the irreversible, usually progressive, loss of renal function that eventually results in end-stage renal disease (ESRD) and the need for renal replacement therapy (dialysis or renal transplantation). The rate of decline in renal function is generally constant for each patient and is usually monitored by measuring serum-creatinine concentrations as an indirect index of the glomerular filtration rate (GFR). In its early stages when the patient is asymptomatic, progressive loss of renal function is described as diminished renal reserve or chronic renal insufficiency. When the limits of renal reserve have been exceeded and symptoms become apparent, it is termed chronic renal failure or overt renal failure. When renal function is diminished to such an extent that life is no longer sustainable (GFR less than 5 mL per minute), the condition is termed ESRD or uraemia. Many diseases can lead to ESRD, the most common being diabetes (p.315), glomerulonephritis (p.1021), and hypertension (p.788).

The management of patients with chronic renal failure prior to ESRD involves measures to conserve renal function and compensate for renal insufficiency. Methods to slow the progression of renal failure include the treatment of hypertension, reduction of proteinuria with dietary protein restriction (p.1331) or in some cases ACE inhibitors (p.809), or both, and the reduction of hyperlipidaemia (p.1265). Anaemia (p.719) and renal osteodystrophy (p.732) often require active treatment. Nephrotoxic drugs, including NSAIDs, should be avoided.

The choice between haemodialysis, peritoneal dialysis, and organ transplantation is considered, and the patient prepared, before it is actually required. In patients for whom transplantation is the preferred option, dialysis may still be required while waiting for a kidney. Kidney transplantation is discussed on p.499. There are differences between countries in the choice of dialysis technique for patients with ESRD. For example, in-centre haemodialysis is used in about 80% of patients in the USA, whereas CAPD is used in over 50% of patients in the UK. Overall survival appears to be similar between the 2 techniques, but more patients on CAPD will eventually require haemodialysis.

Unlike renal transplant patients, dialysis patients still require replacement therapy with hormones that are usually produced by the kidney. Thus, recombinant erythropoietin (p.718) and hydroxylated vitamin D analogues (p.1368) are commonly administered.

References.

1. Klahr S. Chronic renal failure: management. *Lancet* 1991; **338:** 423–7.
2. NIH. Morbidity and mortality of dialysis. *NIH Consens Statement* 1993; **11:** 1–33.
3. The Renal Association. *Treatment of adult patients with renal failure: recommended standards and audit measures.* London: Royal College of Physicians of London, 1995.
4. Steinman TI. Kidney protection: how to prevent or delay chronic renal failure. *Geriatrics* 1996; **51:** 28–35.
5. Friedman AL. Etiology, pathophysiology, diagnosis, and management of chronic renal failure in children. *Curr Opin Pediatr* 1996; **8:** 148–51.
6. Gokal R, Mallick N. Continuous ambulatory peritoneal dialysis. *Prescribers' J* 1992; **32:** 251–6.
7. Walker R. General management of end stage renal disease. *Br Med J* 1997; **315:** 1429–32.

Electrolyte disturbances. Haemodialysis with magnesium-free dialysis solution has been used to remove magnesium from the body in severe hypermagnesaemia (p.1148). Similarly, haemodialysis, and sometimes peritoneal dialysis, has been used in treating hypercalcaemia (p.1148), hyperkalaemia (p.1149), hypernatraemia (p.1150), and hyperphosphataemia (p.1149).

Overdosage and poisoning. Haemodialysis, or less often peritoneal dialysis, can be used to remove some substances from the body after overdosage or poisoning. Substances most readily removed have a low molecular weight, low volume of distribution, low protein binding, high water solubility, and high renal clearance. Examples of agents for which haemodialysis may have a role in the treatment of severe overdosage include alcohol (p.1099), methyl alcohol (p.1379), lithium (p.292), and salicylates such as aspirin (p.16). Dialysis may be particularly important when poisoning with these agents is complicated by renal failure.

Preparations

Ph. Eur.: Solutions for Haemodialysis; Solutions for Haemofiltration; Solutions for Peritoneal Dialysis.

Proprietary Preparations (details are given in Part 3)

Multi-ingredient: ***Aust.:*** Acetat-Haemodialyse; Dianeal; HAMFL; Hamofiltrasol; Peritofundin; ***Austral.:*** Dianeal; ***Fr.:*** Dialysol Acide; Dialysol Bicarbonate; Dialytan H; DPCA 2; ***Ital.:*** Nutrineal PD2; ***Spain:*** CAPD; Dialisol; Dianeal; DPCA†; Nutrineal PD4; Sol Dial Perit†; ***Swed.:*** Altracart II; BiCart; Bicbag; Biorenal; Biosol A; Biosol B; Dianeal; Diasol†; Dicalys 11; Duolys A; Duolys B; Extraneal; Gambrolys; Gambrosol; Haemovex; Hemofiltrasol; Hemofiltrationslosning 401; Lockolys; Nutrineal PD4; Peritolys med glukos†; Schiwalys Hemofiltration; Spectralys Hemofiltration 05, 23†; Spectralys Hemofiltration 19, 20†; Sterilys B 84†; ***Switz.:*** Clear-Flex Formula; Dianeal; DPCA; Gambrosol; HF; Nutrineal PD4; ***UK:*** Dialaflex Solutions†; Diambulate Solutions†; Dianeal; Difusor†; Nutrineal PD4; ***USA:*** Dialyte; Dianeal†; Inpersol†.

Oral Rehydration Solutions (3277-r)

Oral rehydration solutions have 4 main constituents:

- electrolytes—typically sodium chloride and potassium chloride
- a bicarbonate source to correct or prevent metabolic acidosis, such as sodium bicarbonate or sodium citrate
- water to replace fluid losses
- a carbohydrate source to maximise absorption of fluid and electrolytes—typically glucose, although cereal-based formulations have also been tried.

They are most commonly available as oral powders (oral rehydration salts) that are reconstituted with water before use, but effervescent tablets and ready-to-use oral solutions are also available.

The composition of oral rehydration solutions varies, particularly in sodium content. For example, in the UK the sodium content of oral rehydration solutions ranges from 50 to 60 mmol per litre, whereas the WHO formulation contains 90 mmol of sodium per litre. High sodium concentrations may be particularly appropriate for secretory diarrhoeas such as cholera. For discussion of modified formulations of oral rehydration solutions in the treatment of diarrhoea, including the use of cereal-based and low osmolarity preparations, see oral rehydration therapy under Diarrhoea on p.1168.

Adverse Effects

Vomiting can occur after administration of oral rehydration solution, and may be an indication that it was administered too quickly. If vomiting occurs, administration should be halted for 10 minutes then resumed in smaller, more frequent, amounts.

The risk of hypernatraemia or overhydration after administration of oral rehydration solutions is low in patients with normal renal function. Overdosage of oral rehydration solutions in patients with renal impairment may lead to hypernatraemia and hyperkalaemia.

Precautions

Oral rehydration salts or effervescent tablets should be reconstituted only with water and at the volume stated. Fresh drinking water is generally appropriate, but freshly boiled and cooled water is preferred when the solution is for infants or when drinking water is not available. The solution should not be boiled after it is prepared. Other ingredients such as sugar should not be added. Unused solution should be stored in a refrigerator and discarded 24 hours after preparation.

Oral rehydration solutions are not appropriate for patients with gastro-intestinal obstruction, oliguric or anuric renal failure, or when parenteral rehydration therapy is indicated as in severe dehydration or intractable vomiting.

Uses and Administration

Oral rehydration solutions are used for oral replacement of electrolytes and fluids in patients with dehydration, particularly that associated with acute diarrhoea of various aetiologies (p.1168).

The dosage of oral rehydration solutions should be tailored to the individual based on body-weight and the stage and severity of the condition. The initial aim of treatment is to rehydrate the patient, and, subsequently, to maintain hydration by replacing any further losses due to continuing diarrhoea and vomiting and normal losses from respiration, sweating, and urination.

For adults, 200 to 400 mL of oral rehydration solution for every loose motion has been suggested. The dosage for children is 200 mL for every loose motion, and for infants is 1 to 1.5 times their usual feed volume. Normal feeding can continue after the initial fluid deficit has been corrected. Breast feeding should continue between administrations of oral rehydration solution.

Preparations

BP 1998: Oral Rehydration Salts;
USP 23: Oral Rehydration Salts;
WHO/UNICEF: Oral Rehydration Salts.

Proprietary Preparations (details are given in Part 3)

Aust.: Elodrink†; Elotrans; Eloverlan†; Milupa GES; Normhydral†; Normolyt; Oralpadon; ***Austral.:*** Gastrolyte; Gastrolyte-R; Repalyte; ***Canad.:*** Gastrolyte; Lytren; Lytren RHS; Pedialyte; Rehydralyte; ***Fr.:*** Adiaril; Alhydrate; Caril; Carogil; Gallialite†; GES 45; Lytren; ***Ger.:*** D-Iso; Elotrans; Isolyt; Oralpadon; Saltadol; Santalyt; ***Irl.:*** Dioralyte; Electrolade†; Elotrans†; Rapolyte; Rehidrat; ***Ital.:*** Alhydrate; Amidral†; Dicodral; Medidral†; Milupa GES; Pedialyte; Reidrax; Sodioral; Soluzione Darrow; ***Neth.:*** Dioralyte; ***Norw.:*** Gem; ***S.Afr.:*** Darrow-Liq; Darrowped; Electrona; Electropak; Enterolyte; Hemapep†; Hydrol; Kaostatex; Medipect†; Pectolin†; Pectrolyte; Rehidrat; Resalt; Scriptolyte; ***Spain:*** Bebesales; Didrica; Huberlitren; Oral Rehidr Sal Farmasur; Oralesper; Reemplazante Intesti; Sueroral; Sueroral Hiposodico; ***Switz.:*** Elotrans; GES 45; Normolytoral; Oralpadon; Servidrat†; ***UK:*** Diocalm Replenish; Dioralyte; Dioralyte Relief; Dycol†; Electrolade; Gluco-lyte†; Rapolyte†; Rehidrat; ***USA:*** Infalyte; Kao Lectrolyte; Naturalyte; Pedialyte; Rehydralyte; Resol.

Bicarbonate (3269-r)

Bicarbonate is an alkalinising agent administered as bicarbonate-containing salts (sodium or potassium bicarbonate) or bicarbonate-producing salts (acetate, citrate, or lactate salts). Allowance should be made for the effect of the cation. Bicarbonate-producing or bicarbonate-containing solutions have been reported to be **incompatible** with a wide range of drugs. In many cases this incompatibility is a function of the alkaline nature of the bicarbonate solution. Precipitation of insoluble carbonates may occur as may production of gaseous carbon dioxide when the bicarbonate ion is reduced by acidic solutions.

Potassium Bicarbonate (1178-h)

501; Kalii Hydrogenocarbonas; Monopotassium Carbonate; Potassium Hydrogen Carbonate.
$KHCO_3$ = 100.1.
CAS — 298-14-6.
Pharmacopoeias. In *Eur.* (see p.viii), *Pol.*, and *US.*

Colourless, odourless, transparent prisms or white granular powder. Each g of potassium bicarbonate represents approximately 10 mmol of potassium and of bicarbonate. Potassium bicarbonate 2.56 g is approximately equivalent to 1 g of potassium.

Freely **soluble** in water; practically insoluble in alcohol. It is gradually converted to potassium carbonate on heating. The pH of a 5% solution in water is not more than 8.6.

Potassium Citrate (1180-t)

E332; Kalii Citras; Tripotassium Citrate. Tripotassium 2-hydroxypropane-1,2,3-tricarboxylate monohydrate.
$C_6H_5K_3O_7,H_2O$ = 324.4.
CAS — 866-84-2 (anhydrous potassium citrate); 6100-05-6 (potassium citrate monohydrate).
Pharmacopoeias. In *Chin.*, *Eur.* (see p.viii), *Int.*, and *US.*

Transparent, odourless, hygroscopic crystals or a white granular powder. It is deliquescent in moist air.

Each g of potassium citrate (anhydrous) represents approximately 9.8 mmol of potassium and 3.26 mmol of citrate. Each g of potassium citrate (monohydrate) represents approximately 9.3 mmol of potassium and 3.08 mmol of citrate. Potassium citrate (monohydrate) 2.77 g is approximately equivalent to 1 g of potassium.

Soluble 1 in 1 of water and 1 in 2.5 of glycerol; practically insoluble in alcohol. **Store** in airtight containers.

Sodium Acetate (1189-v)

262; Natrii Acetas; Natrium Aceticum.
$CH_3.CO_2Na,3H_2O$ = 136.1.
CAS — 127-09-3 (anhydrous sodium acetate); 6131-90-4 (sodium acetate trihydrate).
Pharmacopoeias. In *Eur.* (see p.viii), *Jpn*, *Pol.*, and *US.*
US also allows the anhydrous form.

Colourless transparent crystals or a white granular crystalline powder or white flakes, odourless or with a slight odour of acetic acid. It effloresces in warm dry air.

Each g of sodium acetate (anhydrous) represents approximately 12.2 mmol of sodium and of acetate. Each g of sodium acetate (trihydrate) represents approximately 7.3 mmol of sodium and of acetate. Sodium acetate (anhydrous) 3.57g is approximately equivalent to 1g of sodium. Sodium acetate (trihydrate) 5.92g is approximately equivalent to 1 g of sodium.

Soluble 1 in 0.8 of water, 1 in 0.6 of boiling water, and 1 in 19 of alcohol. A 5% solution in water has a pH of 7.5 to 9.0. **Store** in airtight containers.

Sodium Acid Citrate (1192-d)

Disodium Hydrogen Citrate; E331; Natrium Citricum Acidum.
$C_6H_6Na_2O_7,1\frac{1}{2}H_2O$ = 263.1.
CAS — 144-33-2.
Pharmacopoeias. In *Br.*

A white odourless or almost odourless powder. Each g of sodium acid citrate (sesquihydrate) represents approximately 7.6 mmol of sodium and 3.8 mmol of citrate. Sodium acid citrate (sesquihydrate) 5.72g is approximately equivalent to 1 g of sodium.

Freely **soluble** in water; practically insoluble in alcohol. A 3% solution in water has a pH of 4.9 to 5.2.

Sodium Bicarbonate (1190-r)

500; Baking Soda; Monosodium Carbonate; Natrii Bicarbonas; Natrii Hydrogenocarbonas; Sal de Vichy; Sodium Acid Carbonate; Sodium Hydrogen Carbonate.
$NaHCO_3$ = 84.01.
CAS — 144-55-8.
Pharmacopoeias. In *Chin.*, *Eur.* (see p.viii), *Int.*, *Jpn*, *Pol.*, and *US.*

A white crystalline powder. Each g of sodium bicarbonate (anhydrous) represents approximately 11.9 mmol of sodium and of bicarbonate. Sodium bicarbonate 3.65 g is approximately equivalent to 1 g of sodium. When heated or in moist air it decomposes, and is converted progressively into sodium carbonate.

Soluble 1 in 12 of water; practically insoluble in alcohol. A solution in water is alkaline to litmus; alkalinity increases on standing, agitation, or heating.

Sodium Citrate (1193-n)

E331; Natrii Citras; Trisodium Citrate. Trisodium 2-hydroxypropane-1,2,3-tricarboxylate dihydrate.
$C_6H_5Na_3O_7,2H_2O$ = 294.1.
CAS — 68-04-2 (anhydrous sodium citrate); 6132-04-3 (sodium citrate dihydrate).
Pharmacopoeias. In *Chin.*, *Eur.* (see p.viii), *Int.*, *Jpn*, and *Pol. Int.* and *US* specify anhydrous or dihydrate.

White granular crystals or crystalline powder; slightly deliquescent in moist air.

Each g of sodium citrate (anhydrous) represents approximately 11.6 mmol of sodium and 3.9 mmol of citrate. Each g of sodium citrate (dihydrate) represents approximately 10.2 mmol of sodium and 3.4 mmol of citrate. Sodium citrate (anhydrous) 3.74g is approximately equivalent to 1g of sodium. Sodium citrate (dihydrate) 4.26g is approximately equivalent to 1g of sodium.

Soluble 1 in 1.5 of water and 1 in 0.6 of boiling water; practically insoluble in alcohol. Sterilised solutions when stored may cause separation of particles from glass containers and solutions containing such particles must not be used. **Store** in airtight containers.

Sodium Lactate (1194-h)

E325. Sodium 2-hydroxypropionate.
$C_3H_5NaO_3$ = 112.1.
CAS — 72-17-3.
Pharmacopoeias. Chin., *Eur.* (see p.viii), and *US* include preparations of sodium lactate.

Each g of sodium lactate (anhydrous) represents approximately 8.9 mmol of sodium and of lactate. Sodium lactate (anhydrous) 4.88 g is approximately equivalent to 1 g of sodium.

Sodium Lactate Solution (Ph. Eur.) is a clear, colourless, slightly syrupy liquid; **miscible** with water and with alcohol. It has a pH of 6.5 to 9.0. Sodium Lactate Solution (USP) is a similar preparation, with a pH between 5.0 and 9.0. It should be **stored** in airtight containers.

Adverse Effects and Treatment

Excessive administration of bicarbonate or other compounds that are metabolised to form the bicarbonate anion may lead to hypokalaemia and metabolic alkalosis, especially in patients with impaired renal function. Symptoms may include mood changes, tiredness, shortness of breath, muscle weakness, and irregular heartbeat. Muscle hypertonicity, twitching, and tetany may develop especially in hypocalcaemic patients. Treatment of metabolic alkalosis associated with bicarbonate overdose consists mainly of appropriate correction of fluid and electrolyte balance. Replacement of calcium, chloride, and potassium ions may be of particular importance.

Excessive doses of *sodium salts* may also lead to sodium overloading and hyperosmolality (p.1162). Administration of sodium bicarbonate by mouth can cause stomach cramps, belching, and flatulence. Extravasation of irritant hypertonic sodium bicarbonate solutions resulting in tissue necrosis at the injection site has been reported following intravenous administration.

Excessive doses of *potassium salts* may lead to hyperkalaemia (p.1161). Oral administration of potassium salts can cause gastro-intestinal adverse effects, and tablet formulations may cause contact irritation due to high local concentrations of potassium.

Excessive oral administration of *citrate salts* may have a laxative effect.

Effects on the gastro-intestinal tract. In addition to minor gastro-intestinal effects (see above), spontaneous rupture of the stomach, although an exceedingly rare event, has been reported on several occasions following ingestion of sodium bicarbonate. The bicarbonate was believed to have resulted in the rapid production of enough carbon dioxide to rupture a stomach already distended with food.[1]

1. Mastrangelo MR, Moore EW. Spontaneous rupture of the stomach in a healthy adult man after sodium bicarbonate ingestion. *Ann Intern Med* 1984; **101:** 649.

Effects on mental state. Lactate infusions have been reported to induce feelings of anxiety, especially in patients with anxiety states, and have been used as a pharmacological model in the evaluation of mechanisms involved in clinical anxiety.[1] There has also been a report[2] of a patient receiving oral lactate (as calcium lactate) who was suffering from panic disorder associated with agoraphobia; when lactate was discontinued, the patient reported a reduction in panic intensity without a decrease in the frequency of attacks.

1. Lader M, Bruce M. States of anxiety and their induction by drugs. *Br J Clin Pharmacol* 1986; **22:** 251–61.
2. Robinson D, *et al.*. Possible oral lactate exacerbation of panic disorder. *Ann Pharmacother* 1995; **29:** 539–40.

Epileptogenic effect. Alkalosis may precipitate seizures; however, absence seizures have also been reported to be associated with sodium bicarbonate administration in a child in whom the serum pH was normal.[1]

1. Reif S, *et al.* Absence seizures associated with bicarbonate therapy and normal serum pH. *JAMA* 1989; **262:** 1328–9.

Precautions

It is generally recommended that bicarbonate, or agents that form the bicarbonate anion after metabolism, should not be administered to patients with metabolic or respiratory alkalosis, hypocalcaemia, or hypochlorhydria. During treatment of acidosis, frequent monitoring of serum-electrolyte concentrations and acid-base status is essential.

Sodium-containing salts should be administered extremely cautiously to patients with heart failure, oedema, renal impairment, hypertension, eclampsia, or aldosteronism (see Sodium, p.1162).

Potassium-containing salts should be administered with considerable care to patients with renal or adrenocortical insufficiency, cardiac disease, or other conditions that may predispose to hyperkalaemia (see Potassium, p.1161).

Abuse. High doses of bicarbonate have been taken by athletes to enhance performance in endurance sports by buffering hydrogen ions produced in conjunction with lactic acid.[1] Bicarbonates have also been used to alkalinise the urine and prolong the half-life of basic drugs, notably sympathomimetics and stimulants, thereby avoiding detection; however, such a practice may enhance toxicity.

1. Kennedy M. Drugs and athletes—an update. *Adverse Drug React Bull* 1994; (Dec): 639–42.

Interactions

Alkalinisation of the urine by bicarbonate or bicarbonate precursors leads to increased renal clearance of acidic drugs such as salicylates and barbiturates. Conversely, urinary alkalinisation prolongs the half-life of basic drugs and may result in toxicity (see also under Abuse, above).

The concomitant use of *potassium-containing salts* with drugs that increase serum-potassium concentrations such as ACE inhibitors and potassium-sparing diuretics should generally be avoided (p.1161). *Citrate salts* taken by mouth can enhance the absorption of aluminium from the gastro-intestinal tract (see p.1177 under Aluminium Hydroxide). Patients with impaired renal function are particularly susceptible to aluminium accumulation and citrate-containing oral preparations, including many effervescent or dispersible tablets, are best avoided by patients with renal failure taking aluminium-containing compounds.

Pharmacokinetics

Administration of bicarbonate, such as sodium bicarbonate, by mouth causes neutralisation of gastric acid with the production of carbon dioxide. Bicarbonate not involved in that reaction is absorbed and in the absence of a deficit of bicarbonate in the plasma, bicarbonate ions are excreted in the urine, which is rendered alkaline, and there is an accompanying diuresis.

Acetates such as potassium acetate and sodium acetate, citrates such as potassium citrate, sodium acid citrate, and sodium citrate, and lactates such as sodium lactate are metabolised, after absorption, to bicarbonate.

Uses and Administration

Bicarbonate-providing salts are alkalinising agents used for a variety of purposes including the correction of metabolic acidosis, alkalinisation of the urine, and use as antacids.

When an alkalinising agent is indicated for treating acute or chronic **metabolic acidosis** (p.1147), the usual agent used is sodium bicarbonate. In conditions when acute metabolic acidosis is associated with tissue hypoxia, such as *cardiac arrest* and *lactic acidosis*, the role of alkalinising agents such as sodium bicarbonate is controversial (see p.1147, and for guidelines on advanced cardiac life support, p.779). Sodium lactate has been given as an alternative to sodium bicarbonate in acute metabolic acidosis, but is no longer recommended because of the risk of precipitating lactic acidosis. In *chronic hyperchloraemic acidosis* associated with potassium deficiency, potassium bicarbonate may be preferred to sodium bicarbonate. The citrate salts of potassium or sodium have also been used as alternatives to sodium bicarbonate in treating chronic metabolic acidosis resulting from *renal disorders*. Sodium bicarbonate, lactate and acetate, and potassium acetate are used as bicarbonate sources in *dialysis fluids* (p.1151).

The dose of bicarbonate required for the treatment of acidotic states must be calculated on an individual basis, and is dependent on the acid-base balance and electrolyte status of the patient. In the treatment of moderate acidosis bicarbonate has been given by mouth and doses providing 57 mmol (4.8 g sodium bicarbonate) or more daily may be required. In acute acidosis, sodium bicarbonate has been given intravenously by continuous infusion usually with a 1.26% (150 mmol per litre) solution or by slow intravenous injection of a stronger (hypertonic) solution of up to 8.4% (1000 mmol per litre) sodium bicarbonate (but see the discussion on metabolic acidosis, p.1147). For the correction of acidosis during advanced cardiac life support procedures, doses of 50 mmol of sodium bicarbonate (50 mL of an 8.4% solution) may be given intravenously to adults. Frequent monitoring of serum-electrolyte concentrations and acid-base status is essential during treatment of acidosis.

Sodium bicarbonate may be employed in the management of **hyperkalaemia** (p.1149) to promote the intracellular uptake of potassium and correct associated acidosis.

Sodium bicarbonate, sodium citrate, and potassium citrate cause **alkalinisation of the urine**. They may therefore be given to relieve discomfort in mild *urinary-tract infections* (p.149) and to prevent the development of uric acid renal calculi in the initial stages of *uricosuric* therapy for hyperuricaemia in chronic gout (for example, see Probenecid, p.394). In both cases, they are administered with a liberal fluid intake, usually by mouth, in divided doses of up to about 10 g daily. Sodium bicarbonate has also been used with a diuretic in the treatment of *acute poisoning* from weakly acidic drugs such as phenobarbitone and salicylates to enhance their excretion, but this process, which is known as 'forced alkaline diuresis', is generally no longer recommended.

When administered by mouth, sodium bicarbonate and potassium bicarbonate neutralise acid secretions in the gastro-intestinal tract and sodium bicarbonate in particular is therefore frequently included in **antacid** preparations (p.1167). To relieve *dyspepsia* doses of about 1 to 5 g of sodium bicarbonate in water have been taken when required. Sodium citrate has been widely employed as a 'clear' (non-particulate) antacid, usually with an H_2-receptor antagonist, for the *prophylaxis of acid aspiration* associated with anaesthesia (p.1168). Sodium bicarbonate is also used in various preparations for *double-contrast radiography* where production of gas (carbon dioxide) in the gastro-intestinal tract is necessary. Similarly, solutions containing sodium bicarbonate or citrate have been used to treat acute *oesophageal impaction* (p.1174).

Sodium bicarbonate and sodium or potassium citrate are used as buffering or alkalinising agents in *pharmaceutical formulation*. Sodium bicarbonate and anhydrous sodium citrate are used in effervescent tablet formulations.

Individual salts also have **other specific uses**. A 5% solution of sodium bicarbonate can be administered as ear drops to soften and remove *ear wax*. Sodium bicarbonate injection has been used to treat *extravasation of anthracycline antineoplastics* (p.474) although as mentioned in Adverse Effects, above, hypertonic solutions may themselves cause necrosis.

Sodium citrate has anti-clotting properties and is employed, as sodium acid citrate, with other agents in solutions for the anticoagulation and preservation of blood for *transfusion* purposes. Similarly, sodium citrate 3% irrigation may be useful for the dissolution of *blood clots in the bladder* as an alternative to sodium chloride 0.9%. Enemas containing sodium citrate are given rectally as *osmotic laxatives*. Sodium citrate is also a common ingredient in *cough* mixtures.

Eye disorders. Sodium citrate eye drops have been employed in the management of certain ocular injuries. It has been suggested that corneal epithelial defects due to chemical weapon injuries and lasting for more than one week or those accompanied by limbal ischaemia require intensive topical therapy with eye drops of sodium citrate 10% and of potassium ascorbate 10%. Such therapy is said to prevent late corneal melting and to permit the continuation of local corticosteroid therapy as necessary.[1] The two types of eye drops are given in alternate doses and are believed to act by mopping up free oxygen radicals after chemical burns.[2]

Sodium bicarbonate is also used in the management of blepharitis, an inflammation of the margin of the eyelids that may be caused by a variety of conditions. It may be allergic in nature or associated with seborrhoea of the scalp. Infection of the eyelids can produce ulcerative blepharitis, a condition characterised by the formation of yellow crusts which may glue the eyelashes together. Parasites occasionally cause blepharitis. The condition is first treated by cleaning the eyes and eyelids with sodium bicarbonate solution or a suitable bland eye lotion; simple eye ointment or diluted baby shampoo can also be used to soften crusts to aid removal. If an infection is present suitable antibiotic eye drops or ointment may be used once the crusts have been removed (p.122). Long-term management consists of daily cleansing of the lid margins with a bland eye lotion.

1. Wright P. Injuries due to chemical weapons. *Br Med J* 1991; **302:** 239.
2. Anonymous. Citrate/ascorbate eye-drops for chemical weapons injuries. *Pharm J* 1991; **246:** 145.

Osteoporosis. Potassium bicarbonate administered by mouth in a dose of 1 to 2 mmol per kg body-weight daily for 18 days in 18 postmenopausal women was found to improve calcium and phosphorus balance, reduce bone resorption and increase its formation.[1] However, elderly subjects with renal impairment might be at risk of hyperkalaemia with the doses used and long-term studies would be required before this emerged as an effective treatment or preventative strategy for postmenopausal osteoporosis (p.731).[2]

1. Sebastian A, *et al.* Improved mineral balance and skeletal metabolism in postmenopausal women treated with potassium bicarbonate. *N Engl J Med* 1994, **330:** 1776–81.
2. Sebastian A, Morris RC. Improved mineral balance and skeletal metabolism in postmenopausal women treated with potassium bicarbonate. *N Engl J Med* 1994; **331:** 279.

Renal calculi. Citrate forms soluble complexes with calcium, thereby reducing urinary saturation of stone-forming calcium salts. Potassium citrate has a hypocalciuric effect when given by mouth, probably due to enhanced renal calcium absorption. Urinary calcium excretion is unaffected by sodium citrate, since the alkali-mediated hypocalciuric effect is offset by a sodium-linked calciuresis.[1] An uncontrolled study has demonstrated that potassium citrate may be beneficial in reducing the rate of stone formation in patients with hypocitraturia.[2] As mentioned in Uses above, sodium bicarbonate or sodium or potassium citrate may also be employed for their alkalinising action, as an adjunct to a liberal fluid intake, to prevent development of uric acid renal calculi during uricosuric therapy.

Other causes of renal calculi and their treatment are discussed on p.888.

Urinary alkalinisation with sodium bicarbonate, sodium citrate, or potassium citrate may be useful in the management of cystine stone formation in patients with cystinuria (p.991).

1. Anonymous. Citrate for calcium nephrolithiasis. *Lancet* 1986; **i:** 955.
2. Pak CYC, Fuller C. Idiopathic hypocitraturic calcium-oxalate nephrolithiasis successfully treated with potassium citrate. *Ann Intern Med* 1986; **104:** 33–7.

Preparations

BP 1998: Alkaline Gentian Mixture; Aromatic Magnesium Carbonate Mixture; Compound Magnesium Trisilicate Oral Powder; Compound Sodium Bicarbonate Tablets *(Soda Mint Tablets)*; Compound Sodium Chloride Mouthwash; Kaolin and Morphine Mixture; Kaolin Mixture; Magnesium Trisilicate Mixture; Potassium Citrate Mixture; Sodium Bicarbonate Ear Drops; Sodium Bicarbonate Eye Lotion; Sodium Bicarbonate Intravenous Infusion; Sodium Citrate Eye Drops; Sodium Citrate Irrigation Solution; Sodium Citrate Tablets; Sodium Lactate Intravenous Infusion;
BPC 1968: Effervescent Potassium Tablets;
Ph. Eur.: Anticoagulant Acid-Citrate-Glucose Solutions (ACD); Anticoagulant Citrate-Phosphate-Glucose Solution (CPD);
USP 23: Anticoagulant Citrate Dextrose Solution; Anticoagulant Citrate Phosphate Dextrose Adenine Solution; Anticoagulant Citrate Phosphate Dextrose Solution; Anticoagulant Sodium Citrate Solution; Half-strength Lactated Ringer's and Dextrose Injection; Lactated Ringer's and Dextrose Injection; Lactated Ringer's Injection; Magnesium Carbonate and Sodium Bicarbonate for Oral Suspension; Modified Lactated Ringer's and Dextrose Injection; Potassium and Sodium Bicarbonates and Citric Acid Effervescent Tablets for Oral Solution; Potassium Bicarbonate and Potassium Chloride Effervescent Tablets for Oral Solution; Potassium Bicarbonate and Potassium Chloride for Effervescent Oral Solution; Potassium Bicarbonate Effervescent Tablets for Oral Solution; Potassium Chloride in Lactated Ringer's and Dextrose Injection; Potassium Chloride, Potassium Bicarbonate, and Potassium Citrate Effervescent Tablets for Oral Solution; Potassium Citrate And Citric Acid Oral Solution; Potassium Citrate Extended-release Tablets; Potassium Gluconate and Potassium Citrate Oral Solution; Potassium Gluconate, Potassium Citrate, and Ammonium Chloride Oral Solution; Sodium Acetate Injection; Sodium Acetate Solution; Sodium Bicarbonate Injection; Sodium Bicarbonate Oral Powder; Sodium Bicarbonate Tablets; Sodium Citrate and Citric Acid Oral Solution; Sodium Lactate Injection; Sodium Lactate Solution; Tricitrates Oral Solution; Trikates Oral Solution.

Proprietary Preparations (details are given in Part 3)

Aust.: Bullrich Salz; ***Austral.:*** Citralka†; Sodibic; ***Canad.:*** Brioschi; Eno; K-Lyte; Polycitra-K; ***Fr.:*** Soludial; ***Ger.:*** Alkala T; Kalitrans; Kohlensaurebad Bastian; Natron†; Nephrotrans; ***Irl.:*** Cystopurin; ***Ital.:*** Citrosodina; Kation; ***Norw.:*** Kajos; ***S.Afr.:*** Nitrocit; ***Spain:*** Acalka; Plurisalina; ***Swed.:*** Kajos; ***Switz.:*** Nephrotrans; ***UK:*** Cymalon; Cystemme; Cystitis Treatment†; Cystocalm; Cystoleve; Cystopurin; Urisal†; ***USA:*** Bell/ans; Citra pH; K-Lyte; Neut; Urocit-K.

Multi-ingredient: numerous preparations are listed in Part 3.

Calcium (1151-j)

Ca = 40.078.

Calcium is a cation administered as various calcium-containing salts. Calcium salts have been reported to be **incompatible** with a wide range of drugs. Complexes may form resulting in the formation of a precipitate.

Calcium Acetate (1152-z)

E263.
$C_4H_6CaO_4$ = 158.2.
CAS — 62-54-4.
Pharmacopoeias. In *Br.* and *US.*

A white, odourless or almost odourless, hygroscopic crystalline powder. Each g of calcium acetate (anhydrous) represents approximately 6.3 mmol of calcium. Calcium acetate (anhydrous) 3.95 g is approximately equivalent to 1 g of calcium.

Freely **soluble** in water; slightly soluble in alcohol and in methyl alcohol; practically insoluble in acetone and in dehydrated alcohol. The BP states that a 5% solution in water has a pH of 7.2 to 8.2 and the USP states that a 5% solution in water has a pH of 6.3 to 9.6. **Store** in airtight containers.

Calcium Chloride (1154-k)

509; Calcii Chloridum; Calcium Chloratum; Calcium Chloride Dihydrate; Cloreto de Cálcio; Cloruro de Calcio.
$CaCl_2,2H_2O$ = 147.0.
CAS — 10043-52-4 (anhydrous calcium chloride); 7774-34-7 (calcium chloride hexahydrate); 10035-04-8 (calcium chloride dihydrate).
Pharmacopoeias. In *Chin., Eur.* (see p.viii), *Jpn,* and *US.*
Eur. also specifies the hexahydrate. *Pol.* only specifies the hexahydrate.

The dihydrate occurs as a white, hygroscopic, odourless, crystalline powder or granules. Each g of calcium chloride (dihydrate) represents approximately 6.8 mmol of calcium and 13.6 mmol of chloride. Calcium chloride (dihydrate) 3.67 g is approximately equivalent to 1 g of calcium.

Ph. Eur. **solubilities** are: freely soluble in water; soluble in alcohol. USP solubilities are: soluble 1 in 0.7 of water, 1 in 0.2 of boiling water, 1 in 4 of alcohol, and 1 in 2 of boiling alcohol. A 5% solution in water has a pH of 4.5 to 9.2. **Store** in airtight containers.

The hexahydrate is a white crystalline mass or colourless crystals. It melts above about 29°. Very **soluble** in water; freely soluble in alcohol. Each g of calcium chloride (hexahydrate) represents approximately 4.56 mmol of calcium and 9.13 mmol of chloride. Calcium chloride (hexahydrate) 5.47 g is approximately equivalent to 1 g of calcium.

Calcium Citrate (3275-t)

Tricalcium Citrate. Tricalcium 2-hydroxypropane-1,2,3-tricarboxylate tetrahydrate.
$C_{12}H_{10}Ca_3O_{14},4H_2O$ = 570.5.
CAS — 5785-44-4.
Pharmacopoeias. In *Aust.* and *US.*

A white, odourless, crystalline powder. Each g of calcium citrate (tetrahydrate) represents approximately 5.3 mmol of calcium and 3.5 mmol of citrate. Calcium citrate (tetrahydrate) 4.74 g is approximately equivalent to 1 g of calcium.

Slightly **soluble** in water; practically insoluble in alcohol; freely soluble in diluted 3N hydrochloric acid and in diluted 2N nitric acid.

Calcium Glubionate (1156-t)

Calcium Glubionate *(USAN, rINN).*

Calcium Gluconate Lactobionate Monohydrate; Calcium Gluconogalactogluconate Monohydrate. Calcium D-gluconate lactobionate monohydrate.
$(C_{12}H_{21}O_{12},C_6H_{11}O_7)Ca,H_2O$ = 610.5.
CAS — 31959-85-0 (anhydrous calcium glubionate); 12569-38-9 (calcium glubionate monohydrate).
Pharmacopoeias. US includes Calcium Glubionate Syrup.

Each g of calcium glubionate (monohydrate) represents approximately 1.6 mmol of calcium. Calcium glubionate (monohydrate) 15.2 g is approximately equivalent to 1 g of calcium.

Calcium Gluceptate (1157-x)

Calcium Glucoheptonate *(pINN).*
$C_{14}H_{26}CaO_{16}$ = 490.4.
CAS — 17140-60-2 (anhydrous calcium gluceptate); 29039-00-7 (anhydrous calcium gluceptate).
Pharmacopoeias. In *Fr.,* and *US* which allows anhydrous or with varying amounts of water of hydration.

Calcium gluceptate is the calcium salt of the alpha-epimer of glucoheptonic acid or is a mixture of the alpha- and beta-epimers. A white to faintly yellow amorphous powder. It is stable in air, but the hydrous forms may lose part of their water of hydration on standing. Each g of calcium gluceptate (anhydrous) represents approximately 2 mmol of calcium. Calcium gluceptate (anhydrous) 12.2 g is approximately equivalent to 1 g of calcium.

Freely **soluble** in water; practically insoluble in alcohol and in many other organic solvents. A 10% solution in water has a pH of 6 to 8.

Calcium Gluconate (1158-r)

578; Calcii Gluconas; Calcium Glyconate. Calcium D-gluconate monohydrate.
$C_{12}H_{22}CaO_{14},H_2O$ = 448.4.
CAS — 299-28-5 (anhydrous calcium gluconate); 18016-24-5 (calcium gluconate monohydrate).
Pharmacopoeias. In *Chin., Eur.* (see p.viii), *Int., Jpn,* and *Pol.* Also in *US* as the anhydrous or the monohydrate form.
Calcium borogluconate is included in *Aust.* and as an injection in *BP(Vet).*

A white, odourless, crystalline or granular powder. Each g of calcium gluconate (monohydrate) represents approximately 2.2 mmol of calcium. Calcium gluconate (monohydrate) 11.2 g is approximately equivalent to 1 g of calcium.

Soluble 1 in 30 of water and 1 in 5 of boiling water; practically insoluble in alcohol.

Calcium Glycerophosphate (1931-t)

Calcii Glycerophosphas; Calcium Glycerinophosphate.
$C_3H_7CaO_6P(+xH_2O)$ = 210.1.
CAS — 27214-00-2 (anhydrous calcium glycerophosphate).
Pharmacopoeias. In *Eur.* (see p.viii).

A white hygroscopic powder. Sparingly **soluble** in water; practically insoluble in alcohol. It loses not more than 12% of its weight on drying. Each g of calcium glycerophosphate (anhydrous) represents approximately 4.8 mmol of calcium. Calcium glycerophosphate (anhydrous) 5.24 g is approximately equivalent to 1 g of calcium.

Calcium Lactate (1160-z)

Calcii Lactas; E327. Calcium 2-hydroxypropionate.
$C_6H_{10}CaO_6,xH_2O$ = 218.2 (anhydrous); 308.3 (pentahydrate); 272.3 (trihydrate).
CAS — 814-80-2 (anhydrous calcium lactate); 41372-22-9 (hydrated calcium lactate); 5743-47-5 (calcium lactate pentahydrate); 63690-56-2 (calcium lactate pentahydrate).
Pharmacopoeias. In *Chin., Eur.* (see p.viii), *Jpn, Pol.,* and *US.*
Eur. has separate monographs for the pentahydrate and the trihydrate. *Port.* also includes the hexahydrate. *US* allows anhydrous or hydrous forms.

A white or almost white, practically odourless, crystalline or granular powder. Each g of calcium lactate (trihydrate) represents approximately 3.7 mmol of calcium. Each g of calcium lactate (pentahydrate) represents approximately 3.2 mmol of calcium. Calcium lactate (pentahydrate) 7.7 g and calcium lactate (trihydrate) 6.8 g are approximately equivalent to 1 g of calcium.

Soluble 1 in 20 of water; freely soluble in boiling water; very slightly soluble, or practically insoluble in alcohol. The pentahydrate effloresces on exposure to air and becomes anhydrous when heated at 120°. **Store** in airtight containers.

Calcium Lactate Gluconate (16157-q)

$Ca_5(C_3H_5O_3)_6,(C_6H_{11}O_7)_4,2H_2O$ = 1551.4.

Each g of calcium lactate gluconate (dihydrate) represents approximately 3.2 mmol of calcium. Calcium lactate gluconate (dihydrate) 7.74 g is approximately equivalent to 1 g of calcium.

Calcium Lactobionate (16158-p)

Calcium Lactobionate Dihydrate. Calcium 4-*O*-β-D-galactopyranosyl-D-gluconate dihydrate.
$C_{24}H_{42}CaO_{24},2H_2O$ = 790.7.
CAS — 110638-68-1.
Pharmacopoeias. In *US.*

Each g of calcium lactobionate (dihydrate) represents approximately 1.3 mmol of calcium. Calcium lactobionate (dihydrate) 19.7 g is approximately equivalent to 1 g of calcium. A 5% solution in water has a pH of 5.4 to 7.4.

Calcium Laevulinate (1161-c)

Calcii Levulinas; Calcium Laevulate; Calcium Levulinate; Lévulinate Calcique. Calcium 4-oxovalerate dihydrate.
$C_{10}H_{14}CaO_6,2H_2O$ = 306.3.
CAS — 591-64-0 (anhydrous calcium laevulinate); 5743-49-7 (calcium laevulinate dihydrate).
Pharmacopoeias. In *Eur.* (see p.viii) and *US.*

A white crystalline or amorphous powder with a faint odour suggestive of burnt sugar. Each g of calcium laevulinate (dihydrate) represents approximately 3.3 mmol of calcium. Calcium laevulinate (dihydrate) 7.64 g is approximately equivalent to 1 g of calcium.

Freely **soluble** in water; slightly soluble or very slightly soluble in alcohol; practically insoluble in chloroform and in ether. The USP states that a 10% solution in water has a pH of 7.0 to 8.5; Ph. Eur. requires a pH of 6.8 to 7.8.

Calcium Hydrogen Phosphate (1159-f)

Calcii et Hydrogenii Phosphas; Calcii Hydrogenophosphas; Calcium Hydrophosphoricum; Calcium Monohydrogen Phosphate; Dibasic Calcium Phosphate; Dicalcium Orthophosphate; Dicalcium Phosphate; E341. Calcium hydrogen orthophosphate dihydrate.
$CaHPO_4,2H_2O$ = 172.1.
CAS — 7757-93-9 (anhydrous calcium hydrogen phosphate); 7789-77-7 (calcium hydrogen phosphate dihydrate).
Pharmacopoeias. In *Eur.* (see p.viii), *Jpn, Pol.,* and *US,* which include specifications for the anhydrous substance, the dihydrate form, or both.

A white, odourless, crystalline powder. Each g of calcium hydrogen phosphate (dihydrate) represents approximately 5.8 mmol of calcium and of phosphate. Calcium hydrogen phosphate (dihydrate) 4.29 g is approximately equivalent to 1 g of calcium. Practically **insoluble** in cold water and in alcohol; dissolves in dilute hydrochloric and nitric acids.

Calcium Phosphate (1162-k)

Calcium Orthophosphate; Fosfato Tricalcico; Phosphate Tertiaire de Calcium; Precipitated Calcium Phosphate; Tribasic Calcium Phosphate; Tricalcii Phosphas; Tricalcium Phosphate.
CAS — 7758-87-4 ($Ca_3(PO_4)_2$); 12167-74-7 ($Ca_5(OH)(PO_4)_3$).
Pharmacopoeias. In *Eur.* (see p.viii) and *Pol.* Also in *USNF.*

A white or almost white, odourless, amorphous powder. Calcium phosphate is not a clearly defined chemical entity but is a mixture of calcium phosphates that has been most frequently described as tricalcium diorthophosphate, $Ca_3(PO_4)_2$ (=310.2), or calcium hydroxide phosphate, $Ca_5(OH)(PO_4)_3$ (=502.3). Ph. Eur. specifies that it consists of a mixture of calcium phosphates and contains 35 to 40% of Ca. The USNF specifies that it consists of a variable mixture of calcium phosphates having the approximate composition $10CaO.3P_2O_5.H_2O$ (=1004.6) and contains 34 to 40% of Ca.

Practically **insoluble** in water and in alcohol. It dissolves in dilute mineral acids.

Calcium Pidolate (12511-d)

Calcium Pidolate *(pINNM).*

Calcium Pyroglutamate. Calcium 5-oxopyrrolidine-2-carboxylate.
$Ca(C_5H_6NO_3)_2$ = 296.3.
CAS — 31377-05-6.

Each g of calcium pidolate (anhydrous) represents approximately 3.4 mmol of calcium. Calcium pidolate (anhydrous) 7.39 g is approximately equivalent to 1 g of calcium.

Calcium Sodium Lactate (1164-t)

$2C_3H_5NaO_3,(C_3H_5O_3)_2Ca,4H_2O$ = 514.4.
Pharmacopoeias. In *Br.*

A white deliquescent powder or granules with a slight characteristic odour. Each g of calcium sodium lactate (tetrahydrate) represents approximately 1.9 mmol of calcium and 3.9 mmol of sodium and of lactate. Calcium sodium lactate (tetrahydrate) 12.8 g is approximately equivalent to 1 g of calcium.

Soluble in water and in boiling alcohol; practically insoluble in ether.

Adverse Effects and Treatment

Administration of some calcium salts by mouth can cause gastro-intestinal irritation; calcium chloride is generally considered to be the most irritant of the commonly used calcium salts.

Injection of calcium salts can also produce irritation and in particular intramuscular or subcutaneous injection can cause local reactions including sloughing or necrosis of the skin; solutions of calcium chloride are extremely irritant and should not be injected intramuscularly or subcutaneously. Soft-tissue calcification has also followed the use of calcium salts parenterally.

Excessive amounts of calcium salts may lead to hypercalcaemia. This complication is usually associated with the parenteral route of administration, but can occur after oral administration, usually in patients with renal failure or who are taking vitamin D concurrently. Symptoms of hypercalcaemia may include anorexia, nausea, vomiting, constipation, abdominal pain, muscle weakness, mental disturbances, polydipsia, polyuria, nephrocalcinosis, renal calculi, and, in severe cases, cardiac arrhythmias and coma. Too rapid intravenous injection of calcium salts may also lead to many of the symptoms of hypercalcaemia as well as a chalky taste, hot flushes, and peripheral vasodilatation. Mild asymptomatic hypercalcaemia will usually resolve on stopping administration of calcium and other contributory drugs such as vitamin D (see also Vitamin D-mediated Hypercalcaemia, p.1148). If hypercalcaemia is severe, urgent treatment is required as outlined on p.1148.

Precautions

Solutions of calcium salts, particularly calcium chloride, are irritant, and care should be taken to prevent extravasation during intravenous injection. Calcium salts should be given cautiously to patients with impaired renal function, or diseases associated with elevated vitamin D concentrations such as sarcoidosis. In addition, they should generally be avoided in patients with calcium renal calculi, or a history of renal calculi. Calcium chloride, because of its acidifying nature, is unsuitable for the treatment of hypocalcaemia caused by renal insufficiency or in patients with respiratory acidosis or failure.

Plasma-calcium concentrations should be monitored closely in patients with renal insufficiency and during parenteral administration and if large doses of vitamin D are used concurrently.

Interactions

Hypercalcaemia has occurred when calcium salts are coadministered with thiazide diuretics or vitamin D. Vitamin D increases the gastro-intestinal absorption of calcium and thiazide diuretics decrease its urinary excretion. Plasma-calcium concentrations should be monitored in patients receiving the drugs concurrently.

Bran decreases the gastro-intestinal absorption of calcium, and may therefore decrease the efficacy of calcium supplements.

Calcium enhances the effects of digitalis glycosides on the heart and may precipitate digitalis intoxication; parenteral calcium therapy is best avoided in patients receiving cardiac glycosides. Citrate salts increase the absorption of aluminium from the gastro-intestinal tract (p.1177), therefore patients with renal failure taking aluminium phosphate should avoid taking calcium citrate. Calcium salts reduce the absorption of a number of other drugs such as bisphosphonates, fluoride, some fluoroquinolones, and tetracyclines; administration should be separated by at least 3 hours.

Pharmacokinetics

Calcium is absorbed predominantly from the small intestine by active transport and passive diffusion. About one-third of ingested calcium is absorbed although this can vary depending upon dietary factors and the state of the small intestine; also absorption is increased in calcium deficiency and during periods of high physiological requirement such as during childhood or pregnancy and lactation. 1,25-Dihydroxycholecalciferol (calcitriol), a metabolite of vitamin D, enhances the active phase of absorption.

Excess calcium is predominantly excreted renally. Unabsorbed calcium is eliminated in the faeces, together with that secreted in the bile and pancreatic juice. Minor amounts are lost in the sweat, skin, hair, and nails. Calcium crosses the placenta and is distributed into breast milk.

Human Requirements

Calcium is the most abundant mineral in the body and is an essential body electrolyte. However, defining individual calcium requirements has proved difficult and guidelines vary widely by country and culture. Some authorities have adopted a factorial approach. For example, in the UK the dietary reference value (DRV) represents the apparent calcium requirements of healthy people under the prevailing dietary circumstances. The amount of calcium absorbed varies according to several factors including the requirements of the body, but is normally only about 30 to 40% of the dietary intake.

The richest dietary sources of calcium are milk and milk products. Significant amounts can also be consumed in green leafy vegetables, fortified flour, and hard water.

In the United Kingdom dietary reference values (see p.1332) have been published for calcium.[1] In the USA recommended dietary allowances (RDA) had been set,[2] and have recently been replaced by dietary reference intakes (see p.1332).[3] In the UK the estimated average requirement (EAR) for adults is 525 mg (13.1 mmol) daily and the reference nutrient intake (RNI) for adults is 700 mg (17.5 mmol) daily; these figures are based on a mean absorption of calcium of 30% from mixed diets. In the USA the traditional RDA was 800 mg daily for adults aged over 25 years; this figure was based on an absorption rate of 40%. Under the new dietary reference intakes, adequate intakes (AI) for calcium have been set, which are higher in some age groups than the previous RDAs.[3] For adults aged up to 50 years the AI is 1 g daily, and for those 51 years or older, it is 1.2 g daily.[3]

1. DoH. Dietary reference values for food energy and nutrients for the United Kingdom: report of the panel on dietary reference values of the committee on medical aspects of food policy. *Report on health and social subjects 41*. London: HMSO, 1991.
2. Subcommittee on the tenth edition of the RDAs, Food and Nutrition Board, Commission on Life Sciences, National Research Council. *Recommended dietary allowances*. 10th ed. Washington, DC: National Academy Press, 1989.
3. Standing Committee on the Scientific Evaluation of Dietary Reference Intakes of the Food and Nutrition Board. *Dietary Reference Intakes for calcium, phosphorus, magnesium, vitamin D, and fluoride*. Washington, DC: National Academy Press, 1997.

Uses and Administration

Calcium salts are used in the management of **hypocalcaemia** (p.1148) and **calcium deficiency states** resulting from dietary deficiency or ageing (see also Osteoporosis, p.731). Doses may be expressed in terms of mmol or mEq of calcium, mass (mg) of calcium, or mass of calcium salt (for comparative purposes, see Table 1, below).

Table 1. Some calcium salts and their calcium content.

Calcium salt	Calcium content per g		
	mg	mmol	mEq
Calcium acetate (anhydrous)	253	6.3	12.6
Calcium carbonate	400	10.0	20.0
Calcium chloride (dihydrate)	273	6.8	13.6
Calcium citrate (tetrahydrate)	211	5.3	10.5
Calcium glubionate (monohydrate)	66	1.6	3.3
Calcium gluceptate (anhydrous)	82	2.0	4.1
Calcium gluconate (monohydrate)	89	2.2	4.5
Calcium glycerophosphate (anhydrous)	191	4.8	9.5
Calcium lactate (anhydrous)	184	4.6	9.2
Calcium lactate (trihydrate)	147	3.7	7.3
Calcium lactate (pentahydrate)	130	3.2	6.5
Calcium lactate gluconate (dihydrate)	129	3.2	6.4
Calcium lactobionate (dihydrate)	51	1.3	2.5
Calcium laevulinate (dihydrate)	131	3.3	6.5
Calcium hydrogen phosphate (dihydrate)	233	5.8	11.6
Calcium phosphate [$10CaO.3P_2O_5.H_2O$]	399	10.0	19.9
Calcium pidolate (anhydrous)	135	3.4	6.7
Calcium sodium lactate (tetrahydrate)	78	1.9	3.9

In simple deficiency states calcium salts may be given by mouth, usually in doses of 10 to 50 mmol (400 mg to 2 g) of calcium daily adjusted to the individual patient's requirements.

In severe acute hypocalcaemia or hypocalcaemic tetany parenteral administration is necessary, generally by slow intravenous injection or continuous infusion of calcium chloride or calcium gluconate (see also Administration, below). A typical dose is 2.25 mmol of calcium by slow intravenous injection, either repeated as required, or followed by continuous intravenous infusion of about 9 mmol daily. 2.25 mmol of calcium is provided by 10 mL of calcium gluconate 10%. Calcium gluceptate and calcium glycerophosphate with calcium lactate have been given by the intramuscular route; the chloride and gluconate are unsuitable for this route because of their irritancy. The intravenous route is used in children.

Intravenous calcium salts are also used to reverse the toxic cardiac effects of potassium in the emergency treatment of severe **hyperkalaemia** (p.1149), and as an antidote to magnesium in severe **hypermagnesaemia** (p.1148). For these indications, 2.25 to 4.5 mmol of calcium (10 to 20 mL of calcium gluconate 10%) is commonly used.

Individual calcium salts have specific uses. Calcium carbonate or acetate are effective phosphate binders and are given by mouth to reduce phosphate absorption from the gut in patients with **hyperphosphataemia**; this is particularly relevant to patients with chronic renal failure in order to prevent the development of renal osteodystrophy (p.732). The initial dose of calcium carbonate is 2.5 g daily titrated to a maximum of 17 g daily. The initial dose of calcium acetate is 3 or 4 g daily; most patients require 6 to 12 g daily.

Calcium carbonate, administered by mouth, is also widely used for its **antacid** properties (p.1167).

The calcium salts discussed here also have *pharmaceutical uses*. Calcium carbonate is employed as a diluent in capsules and tablets and as a buffer and dissolution aid in dispersible tablets. Other applications include its use as a basis for some dental formulations. Calcium phosphate is also used as a diluent for solid dose forms and sometimes as a disintegrant and anticaking agent. Calcium hydrogen phosphate is another tablet or capsule diluent and is employed for its abrasive properties in toothpastes.

Calcium phosphate (Calcarea Phosphorica; Calc. Phos.) is used in homoeopathic medicine.

Administration. Views have been expressed that calcium chloride rather than calcium gluconate is the calcium salt of choice for parenteral preparations.[1,2] This opinion is based on the fact that the body's retention of calcium chloride is greater and more predictable than its retention of calcium gluconate and that the increase in extracellular ionised calcium concentration is unpredictable for the gluconate.

It should, however, be remembered that calcium chloride is considered to be the most irritant of the calcium salts in general use (see under Adverse Effects, above).

Calcium gluconate has also been administered by the intraperitoneal route[3] for the treatment of chronic hypocalcaemia after parathyroidectomy in a patient undergoing continuous ambulatory peritoneal dialysis, resulting in improved systemic bioavailability compared with oral and intravenous administration.

1. Worthley LIG, Phillips PJ. Intravenous calcium salts. *Lancet* 1980; **ii:** 149.
2. Broner CW, *et al.* A prospective, randomized, double-blind comparison of calcium chloride and calcium gluconate therapies for hypocalcemia in critically ill children. *J Pediatr* 1990; **117:** 986–9.
3. Stamatakis MK, Seth SK. Treatment of chronic hypocalcemia with intraperitoneal calcium. *Am J Health-Syst Pharm* 1995; **52:** 201–3.

Bites and stings. Calcium gluconate 10% solution has been administered intravenously as an alternative to the use of conventional muscle relaxants for neurotoxic spider envenomation (p.1534). Mention has been made of such use of calcium in the management of *Latrodectus mactans* (black widow spider) envenomation.[1] Although the precise mechanism of action of calcium in the alleviation of neuromuscular symptoms is unknown it is believed to be due to the replenishment of calcium stores in the sarcoplasmic reticulum of muscle depleted by stimulation.

1. Binder LS. Acute arthropod envenomation: incidence, clinical features and management. *Med Toxicol Adverse Drug Exp* 1989; **4:** 163–73.

Bone disease. Calcium is essential for the development and maintenance of normal bone, and calcium salts may be indicated in the treatment of some bone disorders associated with calcium deficiency, such as certain types of osteomalacia and rickets (p.730). Doses of 1 to 3 g of calcium daily are used in osteomalacia.

Oral calcium supplements can also be used as an adjunct in the management of osteoporosis (p.731).

Fluoride toxicity. Inorganic fluoride is corrosive to skin and mucous membranes and acute intoxication disrupts many physiological systems and severe burns and profound hypocalcaemia may ensue. Absorption of the fluoride can be prevented by conversion to an insoluble form such as calcium fluoride and thus irrigation of skin (or gastric lavage as appropriate) with lime water, milk, or a 1% solution of calcium gluconate is recommended. Immediate treatment should also consist of 10 mL of calcium gluconate 10% intravenously repeated after one hour; 30 mL should be given if tetany is present. In the short term affected skin and tissue should be injected with a 10% solution of calcium gluconate at a dose of 0.5 mL per cm^2 and burned skin treated with a calcium gluconate 2.5% gel.[1]

See also under Hydrofluoric Acid, p.1589.

1. McIvor ME. Acute fluoride toxicity: pathophysiology and management. *Drug Safety* 1990; **5:** 79–85.

Hypertension. Two recent meta-analyses report that calcium supplementation results in a small reduction in systolic, but not diastolic, blood pressure.[1,2] Both studies concluded that the effect was too small to support the use of calcium supplementation for preventing or treating hypertension (p.788), but the authors of the second study considered it possible that calcium supplementation might have beneficial effects on blood pressure in those with an inadequate intake.[2]

1. Allender PS, *et al.* Dietary calcium and blood pressure: a meta-analysis of randomized clinical trials. *Ann Intern Med* 1996; **124:** 825–31.
2. Bucher HC, *et al.* Effects of dietary calcium supplementation on blood pressure: a meta-analysis of randomized controlled trials. *JAMA* 1996; **275:** 1016–22.

PREGNANCY. A meta-analysis of 14 trials involving 2459 women concluded that calcium supplementation during pregnancy reduced systolic and diastolic blood pressure and the incidence of pre-eclampsia and hypertension.[1] However, inclusion criteria for this meta-analysis have been criticised.[2] Moreover, results from a double-blind, placebo-controlled trial in a total of 4589 women indicated that calcium supplementation during normal pregnancy did not prevent pre-eclampsia, pregnancy-associated hypertension without pre-eclampsia, and a number of other related disorders.[3]

For discussions of hypertension in pregnancy and eclampsia and pre-eclampsia, see p.788 and p.338, respectively.

1. Bucher HC, *et al.* Effect of calcium supplementation on pregnancy-induced hypertension and preeclampsia: a meta-analysis of randomized controlled trials. *JAMA* 1996; **275:** 1113–17. Correction. *ibid.*; **276:** 1388.
2. Various. Effects of calcium supplementation on pregnancy-induced hypertension. *JAMA* 1996; **276:** 1386–7.
3. Levine RJ, *et al.* Trial of calcium to prevent preeclampsia. *N Engl J Med* 1997; **337:** 69–76.

Preparations

BP 1998: Calcium Chloride Intravenous Infusion; Calcium Gluconate Injection; Calcium Gluconate Tablets; Calcium Lactate Tablets; Effervescent Calcium Gluconate Tablets;
BPC 1973: Calcium with Vitamin D Tablets;
USP 23: Aluminum Sulfate and Calcium Acetate Tablets for Topical Solution; Calcium Acetate Tablets; Calcium Chloride Injection; Calcium Glubionate Syrup; Calcium Gluceptate Injection; Calcium Gluconate Injection; Calcium Gluconate Tablets; Calcium Lactate Tablets; Calcium Levulinate Injection; Calcium with Vitamin D Tablets; Dibasic Calcium Phosphate Tablets; Half-strength Lactated Ringer's and Dextrose Injection; Lactated Ringer's and Dextrose Injection; Lactated Ringer's Injection; Modified Lactated Ringer's and Dextrose Injection; Potassium Chloride in Lactated Ringer's and Dextrose Injection.

Proprietary Preparations (details are given in Part 3)
Aust.: Calcilin; ***Austral.:*** Calcium-Sandoz†; Celloids CP 57; DCP 340†; Nephrex; Sandocal; ***Belg.:*** Calcium-Sandoz; ***Canad.:*** Cal Gel; Calais; Calciject†; Calcimax; Calcium-Sandoz; H-F Antidote†; Nu-Cal; Topol†; ***Fr.:*** Calcium Corbiere; Calcium-Sandoz; Ostram; ***Ger.:*** Calcedon†; Calcipot; Calcitrans†; Calcium-Sandoz; Cerasorb; Dobo 600†; Dreisacal†; RMS; Spuman c. Acid. lactic. 5%†; ***Irl.:*** Calcium-Sandoz; ***Ital.:*** Calcioporf†; Calcium-Sandoz; Rubrocalcium; ***Neth.:*** Calcium-Sandoz; ***Norw.:*** Calcium-Sandoz; Phos-Ex; ***S.Afr.:*** Calcium-Sandoz; Glucal†; ***Spain:*** Calbion; Calcio 20 Emulsion; Calcium-Sandoz; Ibercal; Ostram; Royen; ***Swed.:*** Calcium-Sandoz; Phos-Ex; ***Switz.:*** Calcium-Sandoz; ***UK:*** Calcium-Sandoz; Ostram; Phosex; ***USA:*** Calphron; Citracal; Neo-Calglucon; Phos-Ex†; PhosLo; Posture; Prelief.

Multi-ingredient: numerous preparations are listed in Part 3.

Used as an adjunct in: ***Swed.:*** Deltison.

Magnesium (1170-k)

Mg = 24.305.

Magnesium is a cation administered as various magnesium-containing salts. Magnesium salts have been reported to be **incompatible** with a wide range of drugs.

Magnesium Acetate (1171-a)

$C_4H_6MgO_4,4H_2O$ = 214.5.
CAS — 142-72-3 (anhydrous magnesium acetate); 16674-78-5 (magnesium acetate tetrahydrate).
Pharmacopoeias. In *Br.*

Odourless or almost odourless colourless crystals or a white crystalline powder. Each g of magnesium acetate (tetrahydrate) represents approximately 4.7 mmol of magnesium and the equivalent of bicarbonate. Magnesium acetate (tetrahydrate) 8.83 g is approximately equivalent to 1 g of magnesium.

Freely **soluble** in water and in alcohol. A 5% solution in water has a pH of 7.5 to 8.5.

Magnesium Ascorbate (12907-x)

$(C_6H_7O_6)_2Mg$ = 374.5.
CAS — 15431-40-0.

Each g of magnesium ascorbate (anhydrous) represents approximately 2.7 mmol of magnesium. Magnesium ascorbate (anhydrous) 15.4 g is approximately equivalent to 1 g of magnesium.

Magnesium Aspartate (600-z)

Magnesium aminosuccinate tetrahydrate.
$C_8H_{12}MgN_2O_8,4H_2O$ = 360.6.
CAS — 7018-07-7.
Pharmacopoeias. In *Ger.* and *It.*
Ger. specifies the racemic salt ((*RS*)-aspartate) whereas *It.* makes no statement regarding the isomer. *Ger.* also includes the dihydrate form of the (*S*)-aspartate.

Each g of magnesium aspartate (tetrahydrate) represents approximately 2.8 mmol of magnesium. Magnesium aspartate (tetrahydrate) 14.8 g is approximately equivalent to 1 g of magnesium.

Magnesium Chloride (1172-t)

Chlorure de Magnésium Cristallisé; Cloreto de Magnésio; Magnesii Chloridum Hexahydricum; Magnesium Chloratum.
$MgCl_2,6H_2O$ = 203.3.
CAS — 7786-30-3 (anhydrous magnesium chloride); 7791-18-6 (magnesium chloride hexahydrate).
Pharmacopoeias. In *Eur.* (see p.viii), which also includes Magnesium Chloride 4.5-Hydrate, *Pol.*, and *US.*

Colourless, odourless, deliquescent or hygroscopic crystals or flakes. Each g of magnesium chloride (hexahydrate) represents approximately 4.9 mmol of magnesium and 9.8 mmol of chloride. Magnesium chloride (hexahydrate) 8.36 g is approximately equivalent to 1 g of magnesium.

Very **soluble** in water; freely soluble in alcohol. A 5% solution in water has a pH of 4.5 to 7.0. **Store** in airtight containers.

Magnesium Gluceptate (12909-f)

Magnesium Glucoheptonate.
$C_{14}H_{26}MgO_{16}$ = 474.7.

Each g of magnesium gluceptate (anhydrous) represents approximately 2.1 mmol of magnesium. Magnesium gluceptate (anhydrous) 19.5 g is approximately equivalent to 1 g of magnesium.

Magnesium Gluconate (1203-w)

Magnesium D-gluconate hydrate.
$C_{12}H_{22}MgO_{14}$ $(+xH_2O)$ = 414.6 (anhydrous).
CAS — 3632-91-5 (anhydrous magnesium gluconate); 59625-89-7 (magnesium gluconate dihydrate).
Pharmacopoeias. In *US* which allows either anhydrous or the dihydrate.

Colourless odourless crystals or a white powder or granules. Each g of magnesium gluconate (anhydrous) represents approximately 2.4 mmol of magnesium. Magnesium gluconate (anhydrous) 17.1 g is approximately equivalent to 1 g of magnesium. Freely **soluble** in water; very slightly soluble in alcohol; practically insoluble in ether. A 5% solution in water has a pH of 6.0 to 7.8.

Magnesium Glycerophosphate (1938-m)

Magnesium Glycerinophosphate.
$C_3H_7MgO_6P$ $(+xH_2O)$ = 194.4 (anhydrous).
CAS — 927-20-8 (anhydrous magnesium glycerophosphate).

Each g of magnesium glycerophosphate (anhydrous) represents approximately 5.1 mmol of magnesium. Magnesium glycerophosphate (anhydrous) 8 g is approximately equivalent to 1 g of magnesium.

Magnesium Lactate (12911-c)

Magnesium 2-hydroxypropionate.
$C_6H_{10}MgO_6$ = 202.4.
CAS — 18917-93-6.

Each g of magnesium lactate (anhydrous) represents approximately 4.9 mmol of magnesium. Magnesium lactate (anhydrous) 8.33 g is approximately equivalent to 1 g of magnesium.

Magnesium Phosphate (703-f)

Tribasic Magnesium Phosphate; Trimagnesium Phosphate.
$Mg_3(PO_4)_2,5H_2O$ = 352.9.
CAS — 7757-87-1 (anhydrous magnesium phosphate); 10233-87-1 (magnesium phosphate pentahydrate).
Pharmacopoeias. In *US.*
Ger. includes Dibasic Magnesium Phosphate Trihydrate (Magnesium Hydrogen Phosphate Trihydrate).

A white odourless powder. Practically **insoluble** in water; readily soluble in dilute mineral acids.

Each g of magnesium phosphate (pentahydrate) represents approximately 8.5 mmol of magnesium and 5.7 mmol of phosphate. Magnesium phosphate (pentahydrate) 4.84 g is approximately equivalent to 1 g of magnesium.

Magnesium Pidolate (12912-k)

Magnesium Pidolate (*pINNM*).
Magnesium Pyroglutamate. Magnesium 5-oxopyrrolidine-2-carboxylate.
$(C_5H_6NO_3)_2Mg$ = 280.5.
CAS — 62003-27-4.

Each g of magnesium pidolate (anhydrous) represents approximately 3.6 mmol of magnesium. Magnesium pidolate (anhydrous) 11.5 g is approximately equivalent to 1 g of magnesium.

Magnesium Sulphate (1174-r)

518; Epsom Salts; Magnesii Sulfas; Magnesium Sulfate; Magnesium Sulfuricum Heptahydricum; Sal Amarum; Sel Anglais; Sel de Sedlitz.
$MgSO_4,7H_2O$ = 246.5.
CAS — 7487-88-9 (anhydrous magnesium sulphate); 10034-99-8 (magnesium sulphate heptahydrate).
Pharmacopoeias. In *Chin.*, *Eur.* (see p.viii), *Jpn*, *Pol.*, and *US.*
US allows the dried form, the monohydrate, or the heptahydrate form.
Dried Magnesium Sulphate (Dried Epsom Salts) is included in *Aust.*, *Br.*, and *Pol.*

Magnesium sulphate (heptahydrate) is a white crystalline powder or brilliant, colourless crystals. It effloresces in warm dry air. Each g of magnesium sulphate (heptahydrate) represents approximately 4.1 mmol of magnesium. Magnesium sulphate (heptahydrate) 10.1 g is approximately equivalent to 1 g of magnesium. **Soluble** 1 in 0.8 of water and 1 in 0.5 of boiling water; freely but slowly soluble 1 in 1 of glycerol; sparingly soluble or practically insoluble in alcohol. A 5% solution in water has a pH of 5.0 to 9.2.

Dried magnesium sulphate is a white odourless or almost odourless powder, prepared by drying magnesium sulphate (heptahydrate) at 100° until it has lost about 25% of its weight; it contains 62 to 70% of $MgSO_4$. Freely **soluble** in water; more rapidly soluble in hot water.

Adverse Effects

Excessive parenteral administration of magnesium salts leads to the development of hypermagnesaemia, important signs of which are loss of deep tendon reflexes and respiratory depression, both due to neuromuscular blockade. Other symptoms of hypermagnesaemia may include nausea, vomiting, flushing of the skin, thirst, hypotension due to peripheral vasodilatation, drowsiness, confusion, muscle weakness, bradycardia, coma, and cardiac arrest.

Hypermagnesaemia is uncommon after oral administration of magnesium salts except in the presence of renal impairment. Ingestion of magnesium salts may cause gastro-intestinal irritation and watery diarrhoea.

Effects on the gastro-intestinal tract. Although oral magnesium salts stimulate peristalsis, paralytic ileus has occurred in a woman receiving an intravenous infusion of magnesium sulphate for premature labour; magnesium concentrations were within the normal range.[1] See also Pregnancy, under Precautions, below.

1. Hill WC, *et al.* Maternal paralytic ileus as a complication of magnesium sulfate tocolysis. *Am J Perinatol* 1985; **2:** 47–8.

Hypersensitivity. Hypersensitivity reactions characterised by urticaria have been described in 2 women after receiving magnesium sulphate intravenously.[1]

1. Thorp JM, *et al.* Hypersensitivity to magnesium sulfate. *Am J Obstet Gynecol* 1989; **161:** 889–90.

Treatment of Adverse Effects

The management of hypermagnesaemia is reviewed on p.1148.

A patient with supralethal hypermagnesaemia was successfully treated using assisted ventilation, calcium chloride administered intravenously, and forced diuresis with mannitol infusions.[1]

1. Bohman VR, Cotton DB. Supralethal magnesemia with patient survival. *Obstet Gynecol* 1990; **76:** 984–6.

Precautions

Parenteral magnesium salts should generally be avoided in patients with heart block or severe renal impairment. They should be used with caution in less severe degrees of renal impairment and in patients with myasthenia gravis. Patients should be monitored for clinical signs of excess magnesium (see above), particularly when being treated for conditions not associated with hypomagnesaemia such as eclampsia. An intravenous preparation of a calcium salt should be available in case of toxicity. When used for hypomagnesaemia, serum-magnesium concentrations should be monitored.

Magnesium crosses the placenta. When used in pregnant women, fetal heart rate should be monitored and administration within 2 hours of delivery should be avoided.

Oral magnesium salts should be used cautiously in patients with impaired renal function. Administration with food may decrease the incidence of diarrhoea. Chronic diarrhoea due to long-term administration may result in electrolyte imbalance.

Hepatic disorders. Severe hypermagnesaemia and hypercalcaemia developed in 2 patients with hepatic encephalopathy following the administration of magnesium sulphate enemas; both patients died, one during and one after asystole. It was recommended that patients with liver disease who might develop renal impairment, or in whom renal failure is established, should not be prescribed enemas containing magnesium for treatment of hepatic encephalopathy as serious magnesium toxicity can occur, which may contribute to death.[1]

1. Collinson PO, Burroughs AK. Severe hypermagnesaemia due to magnesium sulphate enemas in patients with hepatic coma. *Br Med J* 1986; **293:** 1013–14.

Pregnancy. The meconium-plug syndrome (abdominal distention and failure to pass meconium) has been described in 2 neonates who were hypermagnesaemic after their mothers had received magnesium sulphate for eclampsia.[1] It was believed that the hypermagnesaemia may have depressed the function of intestinal smooth muscle. See also Effects on the Gastro-intestinal Tract, above.

In a study in 12 women with pre-eclampsia there was a decrease in short-term fetal heart rate variability when women were administered intravenous magnesium sulphate; however, although variability is considered a sign of fetal well-being the decrease was considered clinically insignificant.[2]

1. Sokal MM, *et al.* Neonatal hypermagnesemia and the meconium-plug syndrome. *N Engl J Med* 1972; **286:** 823–5.
2. Atkinson MW, *et al.* The relation between magnesium sulfate therapy and fetal heart rate variability. *Obstet Gynecol* 1994; **83:** 967–70.

Interactions

Parenteral administration of magnesium sulphate potentiates the effects of neuromuscular blockers such as tubocurarine, suxamethonium, and vecuronium (p.1307). The neuromuscular blocking effects of parenteral magnesium and aminoglycoside antibacterials may be additive. Similarly, parenteral magnesium sulphate and nifedipine have been reported to have additive effects (p.919).

Oral magnesium salts decrease the absorption of tetracyclines and bisphosphonates, and administration should be separated by a number of hours.

Pharmacokinetics

Approximately one third to one half of magnesium is absorbed from the small intestine following oral administration and even soluble magnesium salts are generally very slowly absorbed. The fraction of magnesium absorbed increases if magnesium intake decreases. In plasma, about 25 to 30% of magnesium is protein bound. Parenterally administered magnesium salts are excreted mainly in the urine, and orally administered magnesium salts are eliminated in the urine (absorbed fraction) and the faeces (unabsorbed fraction). Small amounts are distributed into breast milk. Magnesium crosses the placenta.

Human Requirements

Magnesium is the second most abundant cation in intracellular fluid and is an essential body electrolyte which is a cofactor in numerous enzyme systems.

The body is very efficient in maintaining magnesium concentrations by regulating absorption and renal excretion and symptoms of deficiency are rare. It is therefore difficult to establish a daily requirement.

Foods rich in magnesium include nuts, unmilled grains, and green vegetables.

In the United Kingdom dietary reference values (DRV)[1] and in the United States recommended daily allowances (RDA)[2] have been published for magnesium. In the UK the estimated average requirement (EAR) is 200 mg (or 8.2 mmol) daily for adult females and 250 mg (or 10.3 mmol) daily for adult males; the reference nutrient intake (RNI) is 270 mg (or 10.9 mmol) daily for adult females and 300 mg (or 12.3 mmol) daily for adult males; no increment is recommended during pregnancy but an increment of 50 mg (or 2.1 mmol) daily in the RNI is advised during lactation. In the USA under the new dietary reference intakes an EAR of 330 to 350 mg daily has been set in adult males and 255 to 265 mg daily in adult females; the corresponding RDAs are 400 to 420 mg and 310 to 320 mg daily.[2] An increase in RDA to 350 to 360 mg is recommended during pregnancy but the standard RDA is considered adequate during lactation.

1. DoH. Dietary reference values for food energy and nutrients for the United Kingdom: report of the panel on dietary reference values of the committee on medical aspects of food policy. *Report on health and social subjects 41.* London: HMSO, 1991.
2. Standing Committee on the Scientific Evaluation of Dietary Reference Intakes of the Food and Nutrition Board. *Dietary Reference Intakes for calcium, phosphorus, magnesium, vitamin D, and fluoride.* Washington, DC: National Academy Press, 1997.

Uses and Administration

Magnesium salts have a variety of actions and uses. Many are given as a source of magnesium ions in the treatment of **magnesium deficiency and hypomagnesaemia** (p.1149). Doses may be expressed in terms of mmol or mEq of magnesium, mass (mg) of magnesium, or mass of magnesium salt (for comparative purposes, see Table 2, below).

In simple deficiency states magnesium salts may be given by mouth in doses of up to 50 mmol of magnesium daily adjusted according to individual requirements. Salts that are, or have been, employed include magnesium aspartate, magnesium chloride, magnesium gluceptate, magnesium gluconate, magnesium glycerophosphate, magnesium lactate, magnesium laevulinate, magnesium orotate, and magnesium pidolate. In acute or severe hypomagnesaemia, magnesium may be given parenterally most usually as the chloride or sulphate. A suggested regimen is to administer 35 to 75 mmol of magnesium by slow intravenous infusion (in glucose 5%) on the first day followed by 25 mmol daily until the hypomagnesaemia is corrected; up to a total of 160 mmol may be required. Alternatively, magnesium sulphate has been given by intramuscular or slow intravenous injection. Careful monitoring of plasma-magnesium and other electrolyte concentrations is essential. Doses should be reduced in renal impairment. Other salts which are, or have been, used parenterally include magnesium acetate, magnesium ascorbate, magnesium aspartate hydrochloride, magnesium laevulinate, and magnesium pidolate.

Table 2. Some magnesium salts and their magnesium content.

Magnesium salt	Magnesium content per g		
	mg	mmol	mEq
Magnesium acetate (tetrahydrate)	113	4.7	9.3
Magnesium ascorbate (anhydrous)	65	2.7	5.3
Magnesium aspartate (tetrahydrate)	67	2.8	5.5
Magnesium chloride (hexahydrate)	120	4.9	9.8
Magnesium gluceptate (anhydrous)	51	2.1	4.2
Magnesium gluconate (anhydrous)	59	2.4	4.8
Magnesium glycerophosphate (anhydrous)	125	5.1	10.3
Magnesium lactate (anhydrous)	120	4.9	9.9
Magnesium phosphate (pentahydrate)	207	8.5	17.0
Magnesium pidolate (anhydrous)	87	3.6	7.1
Magnesium sulphate (heptahydrate)	99	4.1	8.1

Several magnesium salts such as the carbonate, hydroxide, oxide, and trisilicate are widely used for their **antacid** properties (p.1167). Magnesium salts also act as **osmotic laxatives** (see Constipation, p.1168); the salts generally used for this purpose are magnesium sulphate (an oral dose of 5 to 10 g in 250 mL of water being administered for rapid bowel evacuation) and magnesium hydroxide (p.1198).

Parenterally administered magnesium sulphate has some specific uses. It is used for the emergency treatment of some **arrhythmias** such as torsade de pointes (p.782) and those associated with hypokalaemia (p.1150). The usual dose is 2 g of magnesium sulphate (8 mmol of magnesium) administered intravenously over 10 to 15 minutes.

Parenteral magnesium sulphate is also used for the prevention of recurrent seizures in pregnant women with **eclampsia** (see below). A variety of dosage regimens have been used and debate continues as to which is most appropriate. Typically an intravenous loading dose of 4 g of magnesium sulphate (16 mmol of magnesium) is administered over up to 20 minutes. This is then followed by either an infusion of 1 g (4 mmol magnesium) per hour or deep intramuscular administration of 5 g (20 mmol magnesium) into each buttock then 5 g intramuscularly every 4 hours. Should seizures recur under either regimen, then an additional intravenous dose of 2 to 4 g can be administered. It is essential to monitor for signs of hypermagnesaemia, and to stop magnesium administration should this occur. Doses should be reduced in renal impairment.

The use of magnesium sulphate in **acute myocardial infarction** and **premature labour** is discussed below.

Dried magnesium sulphate has been used in the form of Magnesium Sulphate Paste (BP 1998) as an application to inflammatory skin conditions such as boils and carbuncles, but prolonged or repeated use may damage the surrounding skin.

General references.

1. McLean RM. Magnesium and its therapeutic uses: a review. *Am J Med* 1994; **96:** 63–76.

Anaesthesia. Magnesium sulphate has been used to prevent the undesirable haemodynamic response sometimes associated with intubation (p.1302).

Eclampsia and pre-eclampsia. For many years magnesium sulphate has been the preferred treatment in the USA for seizures associated with eclampsia (p.338) and studies have shown it to be more effective than phenytoin[1-3] or diazepam,[2] as well as causing fewer adverse effects.

A commentary[4] on 2 of these studies thought that magnesium sulphate offered considerable advantages. It produced a rapid effect and did not cause sedation in the mother or the infant. It was also considered to have a wide safety margin with the added security of calcium gluconate being an easily available antidote should overdose occur. Subsequently a meta-analysis[5] of 9 randomised trials reinforced this favourable view. Thus many in the UK now consider magnesium sulphate to be the preferred drug for the treatment of eclampsia. Magnesium sulphate may also be used for prophylaxis in pre-eclampsia, but some uncertainty remains about the degree of benefit; nonetheless, it appears to be more effective than phenytoin.[5] (For a recent study that raised some concerns about the effects of *early* use of magnesium sulphate on the fetus, see Premature Labour, below).

1. Dommisse J. Phenytoin sodium and magnesium sulphate in the management of eclampsia. *Br J Obstet Gynaecol* 1990; **97:** 104–9.
2. The Eclampsia Trial Collaborative Group. Which anticonvulsant for women with eclampsia: evidence from the Collaborative Eclampsia Trial. *Lancet* 1995; **345:** 1455–63. Correction. *ibid.*; **346:** 258.
3. Lucas MJ, *et al.* A comparison of magnesium sulfate with phenytoin for the prevention of eclampsia. *N Engl J Med* 1995; **333:** 201–5.
4. Saunders N, Hammersley B. Magnesium for eclampsia. *Lancet* 1995; **346:** 788–9.
5. Chien PFW, *et al.* Magnesium sulphate in the treatment of eclampsia and pre-eclampsia: an overview of the evidence from randomised trials. *Br J Obstet Gynaecol* 1996; **103:** 1085–91.

Hypokalaemia. Potassium and magnesium homoeostasis are linked, and hypokalaemia with increased urine potassium excretion may occur in patients with hypomagnesaemia. In this situation, correction of potassium deficit usually requires concomitant magnesium administration. Administration of magnesium sulphate at doses greater than those required to correct hypomagnesaemia has been associated with greater improvements in potassium balance than doses just sufficient to correct hypomagnesaemia.[1]

1. Hamill-Ruth RJ, McGory R. Magnesium repletion and its effect on potassium homeostasis in critically ill adults: results of a double-blind, randomized, controlled trial. *Crit Care Med* 1996; **24:** 38–45.

Myocardial infarction. Magnesium has an important physiological role in maintaining the ion balance in muscle including the myocardium. Administration of magnesium might have an antiarrhythmic effect and might protect the myocardium against reperfusion injury including myocardial stunning (delayed recovery of myocardial contractility function). Intravenous magnesium salts have been used for cardiac arrhythmias and in an overview of studies in patients with suspected myocardial infarction their administration, generally within 12 hours of the onset of chest pain, had reduced mortality.[1] The beneficial effect on mortality appeared to be confirmed by the LIMIT-2 study[2] in which 8 mmol of magnesium was given by intravenous injection before thrombolysis and followed by a maintenance infusion of 65 mmol over the following 24 hours. Benefit was confirmed at follow-up an average of 2.7 years later;[3] however, there was no evidence of an antiarrhythmic effect. These beneficial effects were not borne out by the larger ISIS-4 study,[4] and although there were slight differences in the magnesium regimen and its timing which might have played a part in these contradictory results, at present the routine use of magnesium in myocardial infarction (p.791) cannot be recommended.

Patients with acute myocardial infarction may have magnesium deficiency and long-term treatment with oral magnesium has been tried, but in one study was associated with an increased risk of adverse cardiac events and could not be recommended for secondary prevention.[5]

1. Teo KK, *et al.* Effects of intravenous magnesium in suspected acute myocardial infarction: overview of randomised trials. *Br Med J* 1991; **303:** 1499–1503.
2. Woods KL, *et al.* Intravenous magnesium sulphate in suspected acute myocardial infarction: results of the second Leicester Intravenous Magnesium Intervention Trial (LIMIT-2). *Lancet* 1992; **339:** 1553–8.
3. Woods KL, Fletcher S. Long-term outcome after intravenous magnesium sulphate in suspected acute myocardial infarction: the second Leicester Intravenous Magnesium Intervention Trial (LIMIT-2). *Lancet* 1994; **343:** 816–19.
4. Fourth International Study of Infarct Survival Collaborative Group. ISIS–4: a randomised factorial trial assessing early oral captopril, oral mononitrate, and intravenous magnesium sulphate in 58 050 patients with suspected acute myocardial infarction. *Lancet* 1995; **345:** 669–85.
5. Galløe AM, *et al.* Influence of oral magnesium supplementation on cardiac events among survivors of an acute myocardial infarction. *Br Med J* 1993; **307:** 585–7.

Porphyria. Magnesium sulphate is one of the drugs that has been used for seizure prophylaxis in patients with porphyria (p.339) who continue to experience convulsions while in remission.

Premature labour. Magnesium sulphate has been given intravenously to suppress initial uterine contractions in the management of premature labour[1-5] and has been found to possess similar efficacy to beta$_2$ agonists (see Salbutamol, p.760). Other magnesium salts have also sometimes been given by mouth. Retrospective observational studies have also found a lower incidence of cerebral palsy in children with birth weights of less than 1500 g when mothers were treated with magnesium sulphate for pre-eclampsia, eclampsia or premature labour.[6,7] However, increased total paediatric mortality was noted in an interim analysis of a recent trial of antenatal magnesium sulphate in preterm labour,[8] and the trial was subsequently discontinued. Although they considered the safety of magnesium sulphate well established in gestation at term, the authors cautioned against the use of magnesium sulphate in very preterm labour.

1. Martin RW, *et al.* Comparison of oral ritodrine and magnesium gluconate for ambulatory tocolysis. *Am J Obstet Gynecol* 1988; **158:** 1440–3.
2. Weiner CP, *et al.* The therapeutic efficacy and cost-effectiveness of aggressive tocolysis for premature labor associated with premature rupture of the membranes. *Am J Obstet Gynecol* 1988; **159:** 216–22.
3. Wilkins IA, *et al.* Efficacy and side effects of magnesium sulfate and ritodrine as tocolytic agents. *Am J Obstet Gynecol* 1988; **159:** 685–9.
4. Ridgway LE, *et al.* A prospective randomized comparison of oral terbutaline and magnesium oxide for the maintenance of tocolysis. *Am J Obstet Gynecol* 1990; **163:** 879–82.
5. Dudley D, *et al.* Long-term tocolysis with intravenous magnesium sulfate. *Obstet Gynecol* 1989; **73:** 373–8.
6. Nelson KB, Grether JK. Can magnesium sulfate reduce the risk of cerebral palsy in very low birthweight infants? *Pediatrics* 1995; **95:** 263–9.
7. Schendel DE, *et al.* Prenatal magnesium sulfate exposure and the risk for cerebral palsy or mental retardation among very low-birth-weight children aged 3 to 5 years. *JAMA* 1996; **276:** 1805–10.
8. Mittendorf R, *et al.* Is tocolytic magnesium sulphate associated with increased total paediatric mortality? *Lancet* 1997; **350:** 1517–18.

Pulmonary hypertension of the newborn. Preliminary studies have suggested that intravenous magnesium sulphate may be effective in treating persistent pulmonary hypertension of the newborn, as mentioned on p.796.

Respiratory disorders. Magnesium sulphate, administered intravenously over 20 minutes in doses of 1.2 g to patients with acute exacerbations of chronic obstructive pulmonary disease (p.747) who had received inhaled salbutamol, appeared to have moderate efficacy.[1]

Infusion or inhalation of magnesium has been reported to be of benefit in some patients with asthma (p.745) but results have been conflicting.[2-5]

1. Skorodin MS, *et al.* Magnesium sulfate in exacerbations of chronic obstructive pulmonary disease. *Arch Intern Med* 1995; **155:** 496–500.
2. Skobeloff EM, *et al.* Intravenous magnesium sulfate for the treatment of acute asthma in the emergency department. *JAMA* 1989; **262:** 1210–13.
3. Green SM, Rothrack SG. Intravenous magnesium for acute asthma: failure to decrease emergency treatment duration or need for hospitalization. *Ann Emerg Med* 1992; **21:** 260–5.
4. Ciarallo L, *et al.* Intravenous magnesium therapy for moderate to severe pediatric asthma: results of a randomized, placebo-controlled trial. *J Pediatr* 1996; **129:** 809–14.
5. Hill J, Britton J. Dose-response relationship and time-course of the effect of inhaled magnesium sulphate on airflow in normal and asthmatic subjects. *Br J Clin Pharmacol* 1995; **40:** 539–44.

Preparations

BP 1998: Magnesium Sulphate Injection; Magnesium Sulphate Mixture; Magnesium Sulphate Paste *(Morison's Paste)*;
USP 23: Magnesium Gluconate Tablets; Magnesium Sulfate in Dextrose Injection; Magnesium Sulfate Injection.

Proprietary Preparations (details are given in Part 3)
Aust.: Cormagnesin; Emgecard; FX Passage; Magnesium Diasporal; Magvital; Mg 5-Longoral; Solumag; Ultra-Mag; ***Austral.:*** Celloids MP 65; Magmin; ***Belg.:*** Magnespasmyl; Ultra-Mg; ***Canad.:*** Mag 2; Maglucate; Magnolex; Magnorol; ***Fr.:*** Efimag; Ionimag; Mag 2; Magnespasmyl; Magnogene; Megamag; Solumag; Spasmag; Top Mag; ***Ger.:*** Basti-Mag; Cormagnesin; FX Passage; Lasar mono†; Magium; Magnaspart; Magnerot A; Magnerot Ampullen†; Magnerot Classic; Magnesiocard; Magnesium Diasporal; Magnesium Tonil; Magnetrans†; Magnorbin; Magtrom; metamagnesol; Mg 5-Granulat; Mg 5-Longoral; Mg 5-Sulfat; Mg-nor; Nourymag; ***Ital.:*** Actimag; Mag 2; Solumag; ***Neth.:*** Andrews Laxeerzout†; ***S.Afr.:*** Magnesit; Slow-Mag; ***Spain:*** Actimag; Mag 2; Magnesioboi; Magneston†; Sulmetin; ***Switz.:*** Mag 2; Mag-Min; Magnesiocard; Magnesium Biomed; Magnesium Diasporal; Magnespasmyl; Magnogene; Magvital; Mg 5-Granoral; Mg 5-Longoral; Mg 5-Oraleff; Mg 5-Sulfat; ***USA:*** Almora; Mag-G; Mag-Tab SR; Magonate; Magtrate; Slow-Mag.

Multi-ingredient: numerous preparations are listed in Part 3.

Phosphate (2898-t)

Phosphate is an anion administered as various potassium or sodium salts. Phosphates are **incompatible** with calcium salts; the mixing of calcium and phosphate salts can lead to the formation of insoluble calcium-phosphate precipitates. Incompatibility has also been reported with magnesium salts.

Dibasic Potassium Phosphate (1184-d)

Dikalii Phosphas; Dipotassium Hydrogen Phosphate; Dipotassium Phosphate; E340; Potassium Phosphate. Dipotassium hydrogen orthophosphate.

K_2HPO_4 = 174.2.
CAS — 7758-11-4.

Pharmacopoeias. In *Eur.* (see p.viii) and *US.*

Colourless or white, hygroscopic granular powder. Each g of dibasic potassium phosphate represents approximately 11.5 mmol of potassium and 5.7 mmol of phosphate. Freely or very **soluble** in water; very slightly soluble in alcohol. A 5% solution in water has a pH of 8.5 to 9.6. **Store** in airtight containers.

Monobasic Potassium Phosphate (1183-f)

E340; Kalii Dihydrogenophosphas; Monopotassium Phosphate; Potassium Acid Phosphate; Potassium Biphosphate; Potassium Dihydrogen Phosphate. Potassium dihydrogen orthophosphate.

KH_2PO_4 = 136.1.
CAS — 7778-77-0.

Pharmacopoeias. In *Eur.* (see p.viii). Also in *USNF.*

Colourless crystals or a white odourless granular or crystalline powder. Each g of monobasic potassium phosphate represents approximately 7.3 mmol of potassium and of phosphate. Freely **soluble** in water; practically insoluble in alcohol. A 1% solution in water has a pH of about 4.5. **Store** in airtight containers.

Dibasic Sodium Phosphate (1196-b)

Dinatrii Phosphas; Disodium Hydrogen Phosphate; Disodium Phosphate; E339; Natrii Phosphas; Sodium Phosphate. Disodium hydrogen orthophosphate.

Na_2HPO_4,xH_2O.

CAS — 7558-79-4 (anhydrous dibasic sodium phosphate); 10028-24-7 (dibasic sodium phosphate dihydrate); 7782-85-6 (dibasic sodium phosphate heptahydrate); 10039-32-4 (dibasic sodium phosphate dodecahydrate).

Pharmacopoeias. In *Eur.* (see p.viii), *Jpn, Pol.*, and *US.* The pharmacopoeias may specify one or more states of hydration; monographs and specifications can be found for the anhydrous form (Na_2HPO_4 =142.0), the dihydrate ($Na_2HPO_4,2H_2O$ =178.0), the heptahydrate ($Na_2HPO_4,7H_2O$ =268.1), and the dodecahydrate ($Na_2HPO_4,12H_2O$ =358.1), although not necessarily all will be found in any one pharmacopoeia.

The Ph. Eur. has monographs for the dihydrate and dodecahydrate forms. It specifies for the dihydrate: a white or almost white powder or colourless crystals; for the dodecahydrate: colourless, transparent, very efflorescent crystals. The USP has a monograph for the anhydrous, dihydrate, heptahydrate, and dodecahydrate forms. It specifies for the dried substance: a white powder that readily absorbs moisture; and for the heptahydrate: a colourless or white, granular or caked salt that effloresces in warm, dry air.

Each g of dibasic sodium phosphate (anhydrous) represents approximately 14.1 mmol of sodium and 7.0 mmol of phosphate. Each g of dibasic sodium phosphate (dihydrate) represents approximately 11.2 mmol of sodium and 5.6 mmol of phosphate. Each g of dibasic sodium phosphate (heptahydrate) represents approximately 7.5 mmol of sodium and 3.7 mmol of phosphate. Each g of dibasic sodium phosphate (dodecahydrate) represents approximately 5.6 mmol of sodium and 2.8 mmol of phosphate.

Ph. Eur. **solubilities** for the dihydrate are soluble in water; practically insoluble in alcohol; and for the dodecahydrate: very soluble in water; practically insoluble in alcohol. USP solubilities are for the dried substance: soluble 1 in 8 of water; insoluble in alcohol; and for the heptahydrate: freely soluble in water; very slightly soluble in alcohol. **Store** in airtight containers.

Monobasic Sodium Phosphate (1195-m)

E339; Natrii Dihydrogenophosphas; Natrium Phosphoricum Monobasicum; Sodium Acid Phosphate; Sodium Biphosphate; Sodium Dihydrogen Phosphate. Sodium dihydrogen orthophosphate.

NaH_2PO_4,xH_2O.

CAS — 7558-80-7 (anhydrous monobasic sodium phosphate); 10049-21-5 (monobasic sodium phosphate monohydrate); 13472-35-0 (monobasic sodium phosphate dihydrate); 10028-24-7 (monobasic sodium phosphate dihydrate).

Pharmacopoeias. In *Eur.* (see p.viii) and *Pol.* (with $2H_2O$); in *Chin.* (with $1H_2O$). *Br.* also includes monographs for the anhydrous and monohydrate forms. *US* permits the anhydrous, monohydrate, and dihydrate forms.

The BP specifies for the anhydrous form: white, slightly deliquescent crystals or granules; and for the monohydrate and dihydrate: colourless crystals or a white powder. The USP specifies: odourless colourless crystals or white crystalline powder; slightly deliquescent.

Each g of monobasic sodium phosphate (anhydrous) represents approximately 8.3 mmol of sodium and of phosphate. Each g of monobasic sodium phosphate (monohydrate) represents approximately 7.2 mmol of sodium and of phosphate. Each g of monobasic sodium phosphate (dihydrate) represents approximately 6.4 mmol of sodium and of phosphate.

BP **solubilities** are: very soluble in water; very slightly soluble in alcohol. USP solubilities are: freely soluble in water; practically insoluble in alcohol.

A 5% solution of the monohydrate form in water has a pH of 4.2 to 4.5.

Tribasic Sodium Phosphate (14285-f)

E339; Trisodium Orthophosphate; Trisodium Phosphate.

Na_3PO_4 = 163.9.

CAS — 7601-54-9.

Each g of tribasic sodium phosphate (anhydrous) represents approximately 18.3 mmol of sodium and 6.1 mmol of phosphate.

Adverse Effects and Treatment

Excessive administration of intravenous phosphate causes hyperphosphataemia, particularly in patients with renal failure. Hyperphosphataemia leads in turn to hypocalcaemia, which may be severe, and to ectopic calcification, particularly in patients with initial hypercalcaemia. Tissue calcification may cause hypotension and organ damage and result in acute renal failure. Hyperphosphataemia, hypocalcaemia, and tissue calcification are rare after oral or rectal phosphate administration (but see also below).

Adverse effects that may occur with the use of oral phosphates include nausea, vomiting, diarrhoea, and abdominal pain. When oral phosphates are being used for indications other than their laxative effects, diarrhoea may necessitate a reduction in dosage. When administered rectally for bowel evacuation, sodium phosphates may cause local irritation.

Phosphates are administered as the potassium or sodium salts or both; therefore, additional electrolyte disturbances that may be expected on excessive administration include hyperkalaemia, and hypernatraemia and dehydration.

Treatment of adverse effects involves withdrawal of phosphate, general supportive measures, and correction of serum-electrolyte concentrations, especially calcium. Measures to remove excess phosphate such as oral phosphate binders and haemodialysis may be required (see also p.1149).

Effects on electrolytes. Although less common than after intravenous therapy, hyperphosphataemia, accompanied by hypocalcaemia or other severe electrolyte disturbances and resulting in tetany[1,2] and even death,[2] has been reported on a number of occasions following the use of phosphate enemas. Similar effects have also been reported with the use of oral phosphate laxatives.[3,4] Infants or children,[2,5] and those with renal impairment,[1,4] have often been the subjects of these adverse effects. Soft tissue calcification appears to occur rarely with oral phosphate, but nephrocalcinosis has been reported in children with hypophosphataemic rickets treated with calcitriol and phosphate supplements, and was found to be associated with the phosphate dose.[6]

1. Haskell LP. Hypocalcaemic tetany induced by hypertonic-phosphate enema. *Lancet* 1985; **ii:** 1433.
2. Martin RR, *et al.* Fatal poisoning from sodium phosphate enema: case report and experimental study. *JAMA* 1987; **257:** 2190–2.
3. Peixoto Filho AJ, Lassman MN. Severe hyperphosphatemia induced by a phosphate-containing oral laxative. *Ann Pharmacother* 1996; **30:** 141–3.
4. Adverse Drug Reactions Advisory Committee. Electrolyte disturbances with oral phosphate bowel preparations. *Aust Adverse Drug React Bull* 1997; **16:** 2.
5. McCabe M, *et al.* Phosphate enemas in childhood: cause for concern. *Br Med J* 1991; **302:** 1074.
6. Verge CF, *et al.* Effects of therapy in X-linked hypophosphatemic rickets. *N Engl J Med* 1991; **325:** 1843–8.

Local toxicity. Rectal gangrene has been associated with the use of phosphate enemas in elderly patients and was believed to be due to a direct necrotising effect of the phosphate on the rectum.[1]

1. Sweeney JL, *et al.* Rectal gangrene: a complication of phosphate enema. *Med J Aust* 1986; **144:** 374–5.

Precautions

Phosphates should not generally be administered to patients with severely impaired renal function. They should be avoided in patients who may have low serum-calcium concentrations, as these may decrease further, and in patients with infected phosphate renal calculi. Potassium phosphates should be avoided in patients with hyperkalaemia and sodium phosphates should generally be avoided in patients with congestive heart failure, hypertension, and oedema. Serum electrolytes and renal function should be monitored during therapy, particularly if phosphates are administered parenterally.

Oral or rectal sodium phosphate preparations for bowel evacuation should not be used in patients with gastro-intestinal obstruction, inflammatory bowel disease, and conditions where there is likely to be increased colonic absorption. They should be used cautiously in elderly and debilitated patients, and in those with pre-existing electrolyte disturbances.

Interactions

Oral phosphate supplements should not be administered concomitantly with aluminium, calcium, or magnesium salts as these will bind phosphate and reduce its absorption. Vitamin D increases the gastro-intestinal absorption of phosphates and therefore increases the potential for hyperphosphataemia.

Hyperphosphataemia, hypocalcaemia, and hypernatraemia are more likely to occur with phosphate enemas or oral laxatives if these are administered to patients receiving diuretics or other drugs that may affect serum electrolytes. The risk of ectopic calcification may be increased by concurrent use of calcium supplements or calcium-containing antacids.

The risk of hyperkalaemia is increased if potassium phosphates are coadministered with drugs that can increase serum-potassium concentrations.

Pharmacokinetics

Approximately two-thirds of ingested phosphate is absorbed from the gastro-intestinal tract. Excess phosphate is predominantly excreted in the urine, the remainder being excreted in the faeces.

References.

1. Larson JE, *et al.* Laxative phosphate poisoning: pharmacokinetics of serum phosphorus. *Hum Toxicol* 1986; **5:** 45–9.

Human Requirements

Phosphorus requirements are usually regarded to be equal to those of calcium.

Most foods contain adequate amounts of phosphate, particularly meat and dairy products, hence deficiency is virtually unknown except in certain disease states, in patients receiving total parenteral nutrition, or in those who have received phosphate-binding agents for prolonged periods; further details see under Hypophosphataemia, p.1149.

In the United Kingdom dietary reference values (DRV)[1] and in the United States dietary reference intakes including recommended dietary allowances (RDA)[2] have been published for phosphorus. In the UK the reference nutrient intake (RNI) for adults is approximately 550 mg (17.5 mmol) daily; no additional amount is recommended for pregnancy although an additional amount of about 440 mg (14.3 mmol) daily is advised during lactation. In the USA the RDA is 1250 mg daily for those aged 9 to 18 years and 700 mg daily in adults; no increase in RDA is recommended during pregnancy and lactation.

1. DoH. Dietary reference values for food energy and nutrients for the United Kingdom: report of the panel on dietary reference values of the committee on medical aspects of food policy. *Report on health and social subjects 41.* London: HMSO, 1991.
2. Standing Committee on the Scientific Evaluation of Dietary Reference Intakes of the Food and Nutrition Board. *Dietary Reference Intakes for calcium, phosphorus, magnesium, vitamin D, and fluoride.* Washington, DC: National Academy Press, 1997.

Uses and Administration

Phosphates are used in the management of **hypophosphataemia** caused by phosphate deficiency or hypophosphataemic states (p.1149). Doses of up to 100 mmol of phosphate daily may be given by mouth. The intravenous route is seldom necessary, but a dose of up to 9 mmol of monobasic potassium phosphate may be given over 12 hours and repeated every 12 hours as necessary for severe hypophosphataemia (see also below). Plasma-electrolyte concentrations, especially phosphate and calcium, and renal function should be carefully monitored. Reduced doses may be necessary in patients with impaired renal function. Phosphate supplements are used in total parenteral nutrition regimens; typical daily requirements are 20 to 30 mmol of phosphate.

Phosphates act as mild osmotic **laxatives** (p.1167) when administered by mouth as dilute solutions or by the rectal route. Phosphate enemas or concentrated oral solutions are used for bowel cleansing prior to surgery or endoscopy procedures. Preparations typically combine monobasic and dibasic sodium phosphates but the composition and dosage do vary slightly. Phosphate enemas act within 2 to 5 minutes, whereas the oral solutions act within 30 minutes to 6 hours.

Phosphates have also been employed for **other uses**. They lower the pH of urine and have been given as adjuncts to urinary antimicrobials that depend on an acid urine for their activity. Phosphates have also been employed for the prophylaxis of calcium renal calculi; the phosphates reduce urinary excretion of calcium thus preventing calcium deposition. A suggested dose for both uses is 7.4 mmol of phosphate four times daily by mouth.

Butafosfan (1-butylamino-1-methylethylphosphinic acid) and the sodium salt of toldimfos (4-dimethylamino-*O*-tolylphosphinic acid) are used as phosphorus sources in veterinary medicine.

Hypercalcaemia. Intravenous phosphates have been used to lower plasma-calcium concentrations in hypercalcaemic emergencies (p.1148), but because of their potential to cause serious adverse effects other drugs are now preferred. Oral phosphates may be used to prevent gastro-intestinal absorption of calcium in the treatment of hypercalcaemia.

Hypophosphataemia. Phosphate salts are given in the management of hypophosphataemia when a phosphate deficiency is identified, as discussed in Uses and Administration, above. Intravenous phosphates are associated with serious adverse effects if hypophosphataemia is over-corrected, and the rise in serum-phosphorus concentration cannot be predicted from a given dose. Consequently, it has been recommended that intravenous phosphate be used cautiously in the treatment of severe hypophosphataemia.[1-4] However, some advocate a more aggressive fixed-dose regimen in critically ill patients.[5]

1. Vannatta JB, *et al.* Efficacy of intravenous phosphorus therapy in the severely hypophosphataemic patient. *Arch Intern Med* 1981; **141:** 885–7.
2. Anonymous. Treatment of severe hypophosphatemia. *Lancet* 1981; **ii:** 734.
3. Lloyd CW, Johnson CE. Management of hypophosphatemia. *Clin Pharm* 1988; **7:** 123–8.
4. Coyle S, *et al.* Treatment of hypophosphataemia. *Lancet* 1992; **340:** 977.
5. Perreault MM, *et al.* Efficacy and safety of intravenous phosphate replacement in critically ill patients. *Ann Pharmacother* 1997; **31:** 683–8.

Osteomalacia. Vitamin D deficiency, or its abnormal metabolism, is the most usual cause of osteomalacia and rickets (p.730); however, phosphate depletion may also contribute, and phosphate supplementation may be given as appropriate.

RICKETS OF PREMATURITY. Dietary deficiency of phosphorus is unusual, but can occur in small premature infants fed exclusively on human breast milk. The phosphate intake in these infants appears to be inadequate to meet the needs of bone mineralisation, and hypophosphataemic rickets can develop. It has been proposed that this condition, variably called metabolic bone disease of prematurity, or rickets of prematurity, could be prevented by giving phosphorus supplements to very low-birth-weight babies (less than about 1000 g) fed on breast milk alone.[1] A suggested regimen is to add 10 to 15 mg of phosphorus per 100 mL of feed (as buffered sodium phosphate) until the infant reached 2000 g. Concomitant calcium and vitamin D supplementation are also recommended.[1] A placebo-controlled study[2] in infants weighing less than 1250 g at birth confirmed that phosphate supplements (50 mg daily) could prevent the development of the bone defects of rickets of prematurity.

1. Brooke OG, Lucas A. Metabolic bone disease in preterm infants. *Arch Dis Child* 1985; **60:** 682–5.
2. Holland PC, *et al.* Prenatal deficiency of phosphate, phosphate supplementation, and rickets in very-low-birthweight infants. *Lancet* 1990; **335:** 697–701. Correction. *ibid.*; 1408–9.

Preparations

BP 1998: Phosphates Enema;
Ph. Eur.: Anticoagulant Citrate-Phosphate-Glucose Solution (CPD);
USP 23: Anticoagulant Citrate Phosphate Dextrose Adenine Solution; Anticoagulant Citrate Phosphate Dextrose Solution; Methenamine and Monobasic Sodium Phosphate Tablets; Potassium

Phosphates Injection; Sodium Phosphates Enema; Sodium Phosphates Injection; Sodium Phosphates Oral Solution.

Proprietary Preparations (details are given in Part 3)
Austral.: Celloids PP 85; Celloids SP 96; ***Neth.:*** Fleet Klysma†; ***UK:*** New Era Calm & Clear; ***USA:*** K-Phos Original.

Multi-ingredient: ***Aust.:*** Clysmol; Klysma Salinisch; Prepacol; Reducto; Relaxyl; ***Austral.:*** Cal-Alkyline; Celloid Compounds Magcal Plus; Celloid Compounds Sodical Plus; Duo Celloids PPIP; Duo Celloids PPMP; Duo Celloids SPCF; Duo Celloids SPCP; Duo Celloids SPIP; Duo Celloids SPMP; Duo Celloids SP-PC; Duo Celloids SPPP; Duo Celloids SPPS; Duo Celloids SPS; Duo Celloids SPSS; Fleet Phospho-Soda; Fleet Ready-to-Use; Gingo A; Ginkgo Plus Herbal Plus Formula 10; Lifesystem Herbal Plus Formula 11 Ginkgo; Lifesystem Herbal Plus Formula 2 Valerian; Magcal Plus†; Magnesium Plus; ML 20; Phosphate-Sandoz; Sodical Plus†; Travad; Valerian Plus Herbal Plus Formula 12; ***Belg.:*** Fleet Enema; Fleet Phospho-Soda; Lavement au Phosphate; Normogastryl; Practo-Clyss; Prepacol; ***Canad.:*** Citrocarbonate; Enemol; Fleet Enema; Fleet Phospho-Soda; Gent-L-Tip; Normo Gastryl; Phosphate-Sandoz; PMS-Phosphates; ***Fr.:*** Azym; Bactident; Digedryl; Dologastrine†; Gastrilax; Hepargitol; Leuco-4†; Normacol Lavement; Normogastryl; Ortho-Gastrine†; Oxyboldine; Phosphocholine†; Phosphoneuros; Phosphore-Sandoz; Prefagyl; Prepacol; Soker; Solugastryl†; Triphosmag; Uromil; ***Ger.:*** Eupronerv†; Fluor-Gel†; Hanooxygen†; Isogutt; Klistier; Klysma Salinisch; Klyxenema salinisch†; Lecicarbon; Liquisorb K†; Practo-Clyss; Prepacol; Reducto-spezial; Sepdelen 7†; Somnium†; Stomasal†; ***Irl.:*** Fleet; Fletchers Phosphate Enema; Phosphate-Sandoz; ***Ital.:*** Clisflex; Clisma Bieffe Medital†; Clisma Evacuante; Clisma Fleet; Clisma-Lax; Digestivo Dr. Ragionieri†; Enemac; Fosfo-Soda Fleet; Non Acid; Phospho-Lax; Phospho-Soda Fleet†; Ra-Cliss; ***Neth.:*** Colex; ***S.Afr.:*** Fosenema†; Lenolax; Phosphate-Sandoz; Sabax Fosenema; ***Spain:*** Acetuber; Alcalinos Gelos; Boldosal; Darmen Salt; Enema Casen; Eupeptina; Ibsesal†; Lebersal; Normogastryl; ***Switz.:*** Clisma Fleet†; Freka-Clyss; Lecicarbon; Normogastryl; Practo-Clyss; Reducto-special; ***UK:*** Carbalax; Fleet Phospho-Soda; Fleet Ready-to-Use; Fletchers Phosphate Enema; Juno Junipah; Phosphate-Sandoz; ***USA:*** Fleet Enema; Fleet Phospho-Soda; K-Phos MF; K-Phos Neutral; K-Phos No.2; Neutra-Phos; Neutra-Phos-K; pHos-pHaid†; Summer's Eve Post-Menstrual; Thiacide†; Urimar-T; Uro-Phosphate; Urogesic Blue; Uroqid-Acid.

Potassium (1176-d)

K = 39.0983.

Potassium salts covered in this section are those principally given as a source of potassium ions, but consideration should also be given to the effect of the anion. Phosphate salts of potassium are covered under Phosphate, p.1159, and the bicarbonate and citrate salts under Bicarbonate, p.1153.

Potassium Acetate (1177-n)

E261; Kalii Acetas.

$CH_3.CO_2K$ = 98.14.

CAS — 127-08-2.

Pharmacopoeias. In *Eur.* (see p.viii), *Pol.*, and *US.*

Colourless crystals or a white crystalline powder; odourless or with a faint acetous odour. It is deliquescent in moist air. Each g of potassium acetate (anhydrous) represents approximately 10.2 mmol of potassium. Potassium acetate (anhydrous) 2.51 g is approximately equivalent to 1 g of potassium. **Soluble** 1 in 0.5 of water, 1 in 0.2 of boiling water, and 1 in 3 of alcohol. A 5% solution in water has a pH of 7.5 to 9.0. **Store** in airtight containers.

Potassium Chloride (1179-m)

508; Cloreto de Potássio; Kalii Chloridum; Kalium Chloratum.

KCl = 74.55.

CAS — 7447-40-7.

Pharmacopoeias. In *Chin., Eur.* (see p.viii), *Int., Jpn, Pol.*, and *US.*

Odourless, colourless, cubical, elongated, or prismatic crystals or white crystalline or granular powder. Each g of potassium chloride represents approximately 13.4 mmol of potassium. Potassium chloride 1.91 g is approximately equivalent to 1 g of potassium. **Soluble** 1 in 2.8 of water, and 1 in 2 of boiling water; practically insoluble in alcohol and in dehydrated alcohol.

Potassium Gluconate (1181-x)

577. Potassium D-gluconate.

$CH_2OH.[CH(OH)]_4.CO_2K$ = 234.2.

CAS — 299-27-4 (anhydrous potassium gluconate); 35398-15-3 (potassium gluconate monohydrate).

Pharmacopoeias. In *Fr.*

US permits anhydrous or the monohydrate.

A white or yellowish-white, odourless, crystalline powder or granules. Each g of potassium gluconate (anhydrous) represents approximately 4.3 mmol of potassium. Each g of potassium gluconate (monohydrate) represents approximately 4 mmol of potassium. Potassium gluconate (anhydrous) 5.99 g and potassium gluconate (monohydrate) 6.45 g are each approximately equivalent to 1 g of potassium. **Soluble** 1 in 3 of water and 1 in 2.5 of glycerol; practically insoluble in dehydrated alcohol, in chloroform, and in ether. A solution in water is slightly alkaline. **Store** in airtight containers.

Potassium Sulphate (1185-n)

515; Kalium Sulfuricum; Potassii Sulphas; Tartarus Vitriolatus.

K_2SO_4 = 174.3.

CAS — 7778-80-5.

Pharmacopoeias. In *Aust., Jpn*, and *Swiss.*

Each g of potassium sulphate represents approximately 11.5 mmol of potassium. Potassium sulphate 4.46 g is approximately equivalent to 1 g of potassium.

Potassium Tartrate (1187-m)

E336.

$C_4H_4K_2O_6,\frac{1}{2}H_2O$ = 235.3.

CAS — 921-53-9 (anhydrous potassium tartrate).

Each g of potassium tartrate (hemihydrate) represents approximately 8.5 mmol of potassium. Potassium tartrate (hemihydrate) 6.02 g is approximately equivalent to 1 g of potassium.

Adverse Effects

Excessive administration of potassium may lead to the development of hyperkalaemia, especially in patients with renal impairment. Symptoms include paraesthesia of the extremities, muscle weakness, paralysis, cardiac arrhythmias, heart block, cardiac arrest, and mental confusion. Cardiac toxicity is of particular concern after intravenous administration.

Pain or phlebitis may occur during intravenous administration via the peripheral route, particularly at higher concentrations.

Nausea, vomiting, diarrhoea, and abdominal cramps may occur following oral administration of potassium salts. There have been numerous reports of gastro-intestinal ulceration, sometimes with haemorrhage and perforation or with the late formation of strictures, after the use of enteric-coated tablets of potassium chloride. Ulceration has also occurred after the use of sustained-release tablets.

Treatment of Adverse Effects

The treatment of hyperkalaemia discussed on p.1149 also applies when hyperkalaemia occurs during potassium therapy. However, in mild hyperkalaemia that has developed on long-term treatment, discontinuation of the potassium supplement and other drugs that may increase plasma-potassium concentrations, and avoidance of foods with a high potassium content may be sufficient to correct the hyperkalaemia.

In cases of acute oral overdosage of potassium supplements, the stomach should be emptied by gastric lavage in addition to the measures described on p.1149.

References.

1. Saxena K. Clinical features and management of poisoning due to potassium chloride. *Med Toxicol Adverse Drug Exp* 1989; **4:** 429–43.

Precautions

Potassium salts should be administered with considerable care to patients with cardiac disease or conditions predisposing to hyperkalaemia such as renal or adrenocortical insufficiency, acute dehydration, or extensive tissue destruction as occurs with severe burns. Excessive use of potassium-containing salt substitutes or potassium supplements may lead to accumulation of potassium especially in patients with renal insufficiency. Regular monitoring of clinical status, serum electrolytes, and the ECG is advisable in patients receiving potassium therapy, particularly those with cardiac or renal impairment.

Liquid or effervescent preparations are preferred to solid dosage forms for oral administration; use of the former, with or after food, may reduce gastric irritation. Solid oral dosage forms of potassium salts should not be administered to patients with gastro-intestinal ulceration or obstruction. They should be given with caution to patients in whom passage through the gastro-intestinal tract may be delayed, as in pregnant patients. Treatment should be discontinued if severe nausea, vomiting, or abdominal distress develops.

Potassium chloride should not be used in patients with hyperchloraemia.

Direct injection of potassium chloride concentrates intended for dilution before use may cause instant death.

Interactions

Potassium supplements should be used with caution, if at all, in patients receiving drugs that increase serum-potassium concentrations. These include potassium-sparing diuretics, ACE inhibitors, and cyclosporin, and drugs that contain potassium such as the potassium salts of penicillin. Similarly, the concomitant use of potassium-containing salt substitutes for flavouring food should be avoided. Antimuscarinics delay gastric emptying and consequently may increase the risk of gastro-intestinal adverse effects in patients receiving solid oral dosage forms of potassium.

Pharmacokinetics

Potassium salts other than the phosphate, sulphate, and tartrate are generally readily absorbed from the gastro-intestinal tract. Potassium is excreted mainly by the kidneys; it is secreted in the distal tubules in exchange for sodium or hydrogen ions. The capacity of the kidneys to conserve potassium is poor and some urinary excretion of potassium continues even when there is severe depletion. Some potassium is excreted in the faeces and small amounts may also be excreted in sweat.

Human Requirements

Potassium is an essential body electrolyte. However, requirements are difficult to determine and have been estimated from the amount accumulated during growth and reported urinary and faecal excretion.

Over 90% of dietary potassium is absorbed from the gastro-intestinal tract. Potassium is particularly abundant in vegetables, potatoes, and fruit.

In the United Kingdom dietary reference values (DRV)[1] have been estimated for potassium. The reference nutrient intake (RNI) for adults is 3.5 g (90 mmol) daily. In the United States, no recommended dietary allowance (RDA) has been established for potassium. However a daily intake of 1.6 to 2 g (40 to 50 mmol) is considered adequate for adults.

1. DoH. Dietary reference values for food energy and nutrients for the United Kingdom: report of the panel on dietary reference values of the committee on medical aspects of food policy. *Report on health and social subjects 41.* London: HMSO, 1991.

Uses and Administration

Potassium salts in this section are used for the prevention and treatment of potassium depletion and/or **hypokalaemia** (p.1150) and in the prevention of **diuretic-induced hypokalaemia** (p.885). Doses may be expressed in terms of mmol or mEq of po-

Table 3. Some potassium salts and their potassium content.

Potassium salt	Potassium content per g		
	mg	mmol	mEq
Potassium acetate (anhydrous)	398	10.2	10.2
Potassium bicarbonate	391	10.0	10.0
Potassium chloride	524	13.4	13.4
Potassium citrate (anhydrous)	383	9.8	9.8
Potassium citrate (monohydrate)	361	9.3	9.3
Potassium gluconate (anhydrous)	167	4.3	4.3
Potassium gluconate (monohydrate)	155	4.0	4.0
Potassium sulphate (anhydrous)	224	11.5	11.5
Potassium tartrate (hemihydrate)	166	8.5	8.5

tassium, mass (mg) of potassium, or mass of potassium salt (for comparative purposes see Table 3, above). Treatment should be monitored by plasma-potassium estimations because of the risk of inducing hyperkalaemia, especially where there is renal impairment.

Potassium chloride is probably the most commonly used potassium salt; this is because hypochloraemic alkalosis, which is often associated with hypokalaemia, can be corrected by the chloride ions. If a metabolic acidosis, such as occurs in renal tubular acidosis, accompanies the hypokalaemia an alkalinising salt such as potassium acetate, potassium bicarbonate, or potassium citrate may be preferable (see p.1147). Other salts that are or have been employed in the management of potassium deficiency include potassium ascorbate, potassium aspartate, potassium benzoate, potassium gluceptate, potassium gluconate and potassium tartrate. Typical doses for the prevention of hypokalaemia may be up to 50 mmol daily and similar doses may be adequate in mild potassium deficiency. However, higher doses may be needed in more severe deficiency. Patients with renal impairment should receive correspondingly lower doses. Oral treatment is used for prophylaxis and is also suitable for treating most cases of hypokalaemia. Potassium salts by mouth are more irritating than the corresponding sodium salts; they should be taken with or after meals with plenty of fluid and liquid preparations are preferable.

Intravenous administration of a potassium salt may be required in severe acute hypokalaemia. This is normally carried out by infusing a solution containing 20 mmol of potassium in 500 mL over 2 to 3 hours under ECG control. A recommended maximum dose is 2 to 3 mmol of potassium per kg bodyweight in 24 hours. Higher concentrations have been given when an infusion pump has been employed (see Administration below). Adequate urine flow must be ensured and careful monitoring of plasma-potassium and other electrolyte concentrations is essential. Potassium chloride is the salt most commonly employed and solutions intended for intravenous use that are in a concentrated form (such as 1.5 or 2 mmol per mL) *must* be diluted to the appropriate concentration before administration. There should be careful and thorough mixing when adding concentrated potassium chloride solutions to infusion fluids. Potassium chloride is also available as premixed infusions with sodium chloride and/or glucose containing 10 to 40 mmol of potassium per litre. Potassium acetate is also given intravenously.

Amongst **other uses**, the phosphate, sulphate, and tartrate salts of potassium have been given by mouth as osmotic laxatives (p.1167).

Some potassium salts are used as sodium-free condiments when sodium intake must be restricted.

Potassium chloride is sometimes used as a capsule and tablet diluent.

Administration. The standard concentration and rate of administration of potassium chloride for infusion is discussed in Uses and Administration, above. However, higher concentrations (200 or 300 mmol per litre) and faster infusion rates have been used, via an infusion pump, for cases of severe symptomatic hypokalaemia, especially with fluid overload.[1,2]

There has been controversy regarding the preferred route of administration of these higher concentrations of potassium chloride, as discussed by Kruse and Carlson.[1] The central route avoids the problems of pain and phlebitis when potassium is given peripherally. However, it has been suggested that high concentrations of potassium administered centrally may carry a greater risk of cardiac toxicity if the infusion is carried directly to the heart.

Use of lignocaine has improved tolerability of peripheral administration of potassium chloride.[2]

1. Kruse JA, Carlson RW. Rapid correction of hypokalemia using concentrated intravenous potassium chloride infusions. *Arch Intern Med* 1990; **150:** 613–17.
2. Pucino F, *et al.* Patient tolerance to intravenous potassium chloride with and without lidocaine. *Drug Intell Clin Pharm* 1988; **22:** 676–9.

Diabetic ketoacidosis. As discussed on p.316 potassium replacement is given in diabetic ketoacidosis to prevent the hypokalaemia induced by the administration of insulin.

Hypertension. A meta-analysis[1] has reported that potassium supplementation results in reductions of both systolic and diastolic blood pressure. The size of the effect in hypertensive patients was sufficiently great to suggest a possible role in the treatment of hypertension (p.788); effects in normotensive subjects were less marked but consistent with a role for potassium supplementation in preventing hypertension.

1. Whelton PK, *et al.* Effects of oral potassium on blood pressure: meta-analysis of randomized controlled clinical trials. *JAMA* 1997; **277:** 1624–32.

Termination of pregnancy. Solutions of potassium chloride are used to reduce fetal numbers in multifetal pregnancies[1,2] by abolishing the fetal cardiac activity. The solution is injected into the thorax of the fetus without affecting the others which are allowed to continue to term.

1. Wapner RJ, *et al.* Selective reduction of multifetal pregnancies. *Lancet* 1990; **335:** 90–3.
2. Berkowitz RL, *et al.* The current status of multifetal pregnancy reduction. *Am J Obstet Gynecol* 1996; **174:** 1265–72.

Preparations

BP 1973: Strong Potassium Chloride Solution;
BP 1998: Bumetanide and Slow Potassium Tablets; Effervescent Potassium Chloride Tablets; Potassium Chloride and Glucose Intravenous Infusion; Potassium Chloride and Sodium Chloride Intravenous Infusion; Potassium Chloride, Sodium Chloride and Glucose Intravenous Infusion; Slow Potassium Chloride Tablets; Sterile Potassium Chloride Concentrate;
USP 23: Half-strength Lactated Ringer's and Dextrose Injection; Lactated Ringer's and Dextrose Injection; Lactated Ringer's Injection; Modified Lactated Ringer's and Dextrose Injection; Potassium Acetate Injection; Potassium Bicarbonate and Potassium Chloride Effervescent Tablets for Oral Solution; Potassium Bicarbonate and Potassium Chloride for Effervescent Oral Solution; Potassium Chloride Extended-release Capsules; Potassium Chloride Extended-release Tablets; Potassium Chloride for Injection Concentrate; Potassium Chloride for Oral Solution; Potassium Chloride in Dextrose and Sodium Chloride Injection; Potassium Chloride in Dextrose Injection; Potassium Chloride in Lactated Ringer's and Dextrose Injection; Potassium Chloride in Sodium Chloride Injection; Potassium Chloride Oral Solution; Potassium Chloride, Potassium Bicarbonate, and Potassium Citrate Effervescent Tablets for Oral Solution; Potassium Gluconate and Potassium Chloride for Oral Solution; Potassium Gluconate and Potassium Chloride Oral Solution; Potassium Gluconate and Potassium Citrate Oral Solution; Potassium Gluconate Elixir; Potassium Gluconate Tablets; Potassium Gluconate, Potassium Citrate, and Ammonium Chloride Oral Solution; Trikates Oral Solution.

Proprietary Preparations (details are given in Part 3)
Aust.: Micro-Kalium; Rekawan; ***Austral.:*** Celloids PC 73; Celloids PS 29; K-San†; Kay Ciel†; KSR; Slow-K; Span-K; ***Belg.:*** Chloropotassuril; Kalium Durettes; Ultra-K; ***Canad.:*** Apo-K; K-10; K-Dur; K-Long†; K-Lor; K-Lyte/Cl; K-Med 900†; Kalium Durules; Kaochlor; Kaon; Micro-K; Roychlor; Slow-K; ***Fr.:*** Diffu-K; Kaleorid; Microkaleorid†; Nati-K; Potassion†; ***Ger.:*** Kalinor-retard P; Kalitrans retard; Kalium-Duriles; KCl-retard; Rekawan; ***Irl.:*** Kay-Cee-L; Leo K†; Slow-K; ***Ital.:*** K-Flebo; Kadalex; Lento-Kalium; ***Neth.:*** Kalium Durettes; Slow-K; ***Norw.:*** Kaleorid; Kalilente†; Kalinorm; ***S.Afr.:*** Micro-K†; Plenish-K; Slow-K; Swiss-Kal SR; ***Spain:*** Boi K; Boi K Aspartico; Miopotasio†; Potasion; ***Swed.:*** K-MIC†; Kaleorid; Kalilente†; Kalipor†; Kalitabs; Kalium Duretter; Kalium Retard; ***Switz.:*** Kaliglutol; Plus Kalium retard; ***UK:*** Kay-Cee-L; Leo K†; Nu-K†; Slow-K; ***USA:*** Cena-K; Gen-K; K + 10; K + 8; K + Care; K-Dur; K-G Elixir; K-Lease; K-Lor; K-Lyte/Cl; K-Norm; K-Tab; Kaochlor; Kaon; Kaon-Cl; Kato†; Kay Ciel; Kaylixir; Klor-Con; Klorvess; Klotrix; Micro-K; Potasalan; Rum-K; Slow-K; Ten-K.

Multi-ingredient: numerous preparations are listed in Part 3.

Sodium (1188-b)

Na = 22.98977.

Sodium chloride is the principal sodium salt used as a source of sodium ions. Sodium salts used chiefly as sources of bicarbonate ions, such as the acetate, bicarbonate, citrate, and lactate, are covered under Bicarbonate, p.1153. Phosphate salts of sodium are covered under Phosphate, p.1159.

Sodium Chloride (1191-f)

Chlorure de Sodium; Cloreto de Sódio; Natrii Chloridum; Salt.

NaCl = 58.44.

CAS — 7647-14-5.

NOTE. An aqueous solution of sodium chloride 0.9% is often known as physiological saline.

SALINE is a code approved by the BP for use on single unit doses of eye drops containing sodium chloride 0.9% where the individual container may be too small to bear all the appropriate labelling information. HECL is a similar code approved for hydroxyethylcellulose and sodium chloride eye drops.

Pharmacopoeias. In *Chin., Eur.* (see p.viii), *Int., Jpn, Pol.*, and *US.*

Colourless cubic crystals or white crystalline powder. Each g of sodium chloride represents approximately 17.1 mmol of sodium and of chloride. Sodium chloride 2.54 g is approximately equivalent to 1 g of sodium.

Soluble 1 in 2.8 of water; 1 in 2.7 of boiling water; and 1 in 10 of glycerol; slightly soluble in alcohol; practically insoluble in dehydrated alcohol. A 0.9% solution in water is iso-osmotic, and thus in most cases isotonic with serum and lachrymal secretions.

Solutions of some sodium salts, including sodium chloride, when stored, may cause separation of solid particles from glass containers and solutions containing such particles must not be used.

Adverse Effects

Adverse effects of sodium salts are attributable to electrolyte imbalances from excess sodium; there may also be effects due to the specific anion.

Retention of excess sodium in the body usually occurs when there is defective renal sodium excretion. This leads to the accumulation of extracellular fluid to maintain normal plasma osmolality, which may result in pulmonary and peripheral oedema and their consequent effects.

Hypernatraemia (a rise in plasma osmolality) is usually associated with inadequate water intake, or excessive water losses (see p.1150). It rarely occurs after therapeutic doses of sodium chloride, but has occurred with the use of hypertonic saline for induction of emesis or for gastric lavage and after errors in the formulation of infant feeds. Hypernatraemia may also occur after inappropriate intravenous administration of hypertonic saline.

The most serious effect of hypernatraemia is dehydration of the brain which causes somnolence and confusion progressing to convulsions, coma, respiratory failure, and death. Other symptoms include thirst, reduced salivation and lachrymation, fever, tachycardia, hypertension, headache, dizziness, restlessness, irritability, and weakness.

Gastro-intestinal effects associated with acute oral ingestion of hypertonic solutions or excessive amounts of sodium chloride include nausea, vomiting, diarrhoea, and abdominal cramps.

Excessive administration of chloride salts may cause a loss of bicarbonate with an acidifying effect.

Intra-amniotic injection of hypertonic solutions of sodium chloride, which has been used for abortion induction, has been associated with serious adverse effects including disseminated intravascular coagulation, renal necrosis, cervical and uterine lesions, haemorrhage, pulmonary embolism, pneumonia, and death.

General references.

1. Moder KG, Hurley DL. Fatal hypernatremia from exogenous salt intake: report of a case and review of the literature. *Mayo Clin Proc* 1990; **65:** 1587–94.

Treatment of Adverse Effects

In patients with mild sodium excess, oral administration of water and restriction of sodium intake is sufficient. However, in the event of recent acute oral overdose of sodium chloride, induction of emesis or gastric lavage should be carried out along with general symptomatic and supportive treatment. Serum-sodium concentrations should be measured, and if severe hypernatraemia is present this should be treated (see p.1150).

Precautions

Sodium salts should be administered with caution to patients with hypertension, heart failure, peripheral or pulmonary oedema, impaired renal function, pre-eclampsia, or other conditions associated with sodium retention.

When sodium supplements are administered by mouth, adequate water intake should be maintained. Sustained-release tablets should not be administered to patients with gastro-intestinal disorders associated with strictures or diverticula because of the risk of obstruction.

Pharmacokinetics

Sodium chloride is well absorbed from the gastro-intestinal tract. Excess sodium is predominantly excreted by the kidney, and small amounts are lost in the faeces and sweat.

Human Requirements

The body contains about 4 mol (92 g) of sodium of which about one third is found in the skeleton and approximately half is present in the extracellular fluid.

The body can adapt to a wide range of intakes by adjustment of renal excretion through physical and hormonal factors. Loss through the skin is significant only if excessive sweating occurs. Sodium requirements may be increased with exercise or exposure to high ambient temperatures in the short term, until the body adjusts.

Sodium is widely available in foods and is also added as salt during processing, cooking, and at the table. Dietary deficiency of sodium is therefore extremely rare and more concern has been expressed that current intakes are excessive. Restriction of sodium intake, by limiting the amount of culinary salt consumed, may be a useful aid in the management of some patients with hypertension (p.788).

In the United Kingdom dietary reference values (DRV)[1] have been published for sodium. The reference nutrient intake (RNI) for adults is 1.6 g of sodium (70 mmol) daily, which is about 4 g of sodium chloride. In the USA, it has been recommended that daily intakes of sodium be limited to 2.4 g (6 g of sodium chloride) or less.[2] Dietary intake is often in excess of these recommendations, and may be a factor in essential hypertension,[3] and osteoporosis.[4]

1. DoH. Dietary reference values for food energy and nutrients for the United Kingdom: report of the panel on dietary reference values of the committee on medical aspects of food policy. *Report on health and social subjects 41*. London: HMSO, 1991.
2. Subcommittee on the tenth edition of the RDAs, Food and Nutrition Board, Commission on Life Sciences, National Research Council. *Recommended dietary allowances*. 10th ed. Washington, DC: National Academy Press, 1989.
3. Midgley JP, *et al.* Effect of reduced dietary sodium on blood pressure: a meta-analysis of randomized controlled trials. *JAMA* 1996; **275:** 1590–7.
4. Devine A, *et al.* A longitudinal study of the effect of sodium and calcium intakes on regional bone density in postmenopausal women. *Am J Clin Nutr* 1995; **62:** 740–5.

Uses and Administration

Sodium chloride is used in the management of deficiencies of sodium and chloride ions in salt-losing conditions (p.1150). Sodium chloride solutions are used as a source of sodium chloride and water for hydration. Doses may be expressed in terms of mEq or mmol of sodium, mass (mg) of sodium, or mass of sodium salt. For comparative purposes, see Table 4.

Table 4. Some sodium salts and their sodium content.

Sodium salt	Sodium content per g		
	mg	mmol	mEq
Sodium acetate (anhydrous)	280	12.2	12.2
Sodium acetate (trihydrate)	169	7.3	7.3
Sodium acid citrate	175	7.6	7.6
Sodium bicarbonate	274	11.9	11.9
Sodium chloride	394	17.1	17.1
Sodium citrate (anhydrous)	267	11.6	11.6
Sodium citrate (dihydrate)	235	10.2	10.2
Sodium lactate	205	8.9	8.9

A suggested oral replacement dose of sodium chloride in **chronic salt-losing conditions** is about 1 to 2 g (approximately 17 to 34 mmol of sodium) three times daily depending on individual needs either with food or as a solution; doses of up to 12 g daily may be necessary in severe cases. Oral supplements are also used for the prevention of muscle cramps during routine haemodialysis.

Glucose facilitates the absorption of sodium from the gastro-intestinal tract, and solutions containing sodium chloride and glucose usually with additional electrolytes (see p.1152) are used for oral rehydration in acute diarrhoea (p.1168).

The concentration and dosage of sodium chloride solutions for intravenous use is determined by several factors including the age, weight, and clinical condition of the patient and in particular the patients' hydration state. Serum-electrolyte concentrations should be carefully monitored.

In severe sodium depletion, 2 to 3 litres of sodium chloride 0.9% (isotonic; iso-osmotic) may be given over 2 to 3 hours and thereafter at a slower rate. If there is combined water and sodium depletion a 1 to 1 mixture of sodium chloride 0.9% and glucose 5% may be appropriate. Although hypertonic sodium chloride solutions may be used in certain patients with severe acute dilutional hyponatraemia, over-rapid correction may have severe neurological adverse effects—see p.1150. Solutions containing 1.8 to 5% are available.

In **hypernatraemia** with volume depletion (p.1150), sodium chloride 0.9% may be used to maintain plasma-sodium concentrations with expanding fluid volume. Sodium chloride 0.9% (or rarely, in marked hypernatraemia, 0.45%) is used for fluid replacement in diabetic ketoacidosis (p.316).

Among its **other uses**, sodium chloride solution 0.9%, being isotonic, is a useful fluid for sterile irrigations, for example, of the eye or bladder, and general skin or wound cleansing. The 0.9% concentration is also widely used as a vehicle or diluent for the parenteral administration of other drugs. Nasal drops of sodium chloride 0.9% are used to relieve nasal congestion. A mouthwash containing sodium chloride is also available for oral hygiene.

Sodium chloride solutions should *not* be used to induce emesis; this practice is dangerous and deaths from resulting hypernatraemia have been reported.

Sodium chloride (Natrium muriaticum; Nat. Mur.) is used in homoeopathic medicine. It is also sometimes used as an excipient in capsules and tablets.

Catheters and cannulas. For reference to sodium chloride 0.9% being used to maintain the patency of catheters and cannulas, and to its equivalent efficacy to heparin, see Catheters and Cannulas under Uses and Administration of Heparin, p.882.

Termination of pregnancy. Trans-abdominal intra-amniotic instillation of sodium chloride 20% (maximum volume 200 to 250 mL) has been used for the termination of second-trimester pregnancy. However, serious adverse effects have occurred (see above), and other methods are generally preferred (p.1412).

Preparations

BP 1998: Compound Sodium Chloride Mouthwash; Potassium Chloride and Sodium Chloride Intravenous Infusion; Potassium Chloride, Sodium Chloride and Glucose Intravenous Infusion; Sodium Chloride and Glucose Intravenous Infusion; Sodium Chloride Eye Drops; Sodium Chloride Eye Lotion; Sodium Chloride Intravenous Infusion; Sodium Chloride Irrigation Solution; Sodium Chloride Solution; Sodium Chloride Tablets;
USP 23: Bacteriostatic Sodium Chloride Injection; Dextrose and Sodium Chloride Injection; Fructose and Sodium Chloride Injection; Half-strength Lactated Ringer's and Dextrose Injection; Inulin in Sodium Chloride Injection; Lactated Ringer's and Dextrose Injection; Lactated Ringer's Injection; Mannitol in Sodium Chloride Injection; Modified Lactated Ringer's and Dextrose Injection; Potassium Chloride in Dextrose and Sodium Chloride Injection; Potassium Chloride in Lactated Ringer's and Dextrose Injection; Potassium Chloride in Sodium Chloride Injection; Sodium Chloride and Dextrose Tablets; Sodium Chloride Inhalation Solution; Sodium Chloride Injection; Sodium Chloride Irrigation; Sodium Chloride Ophthalmic Ointment; Sodium Chloride Ophthalmic Solution; Sodium Chloride Tablets; Sodium Chloride Tablets for Solution.

Proprietary Preparations (details are given in Part 3)
Aust.: Otrisal; Polyrinse-Aufnahmelosung; Uro-Pract; ***Austral.:*** Bausch & Lomb Saline Plus; Bausch & Lomb Sensitive Eyes Saline; Narium; Slow-Sodium; Softwear; ***Belg.:*** Naaprep; Physiologica; Physiorhine; Uro-Tainer; ***Canad.:*** Cordema†; EFA Steri; Lens Plus Buffered Saline Solution; Muro 128; Physium; Salinex; Thalaris; ***Fr.:*** Gingivyl†; Hydralarm†; Larmes Artificielles; Physiologica; Physiomer; Physiosoin; Physiospir†; Polyrinse; Selgine; Serophy; Unilarm; Uro 3000; Versol; Vesirig; Vitasol†; ***Ger.:*** Adsorbonac; Biosteril†; Freka-Drainjet; Isotone Kochsalz; Rhinomer; Uro-Pract N; ***Irl.:*** Slow-Sodium; ***Ital.:*** Adsorbonac; Libenar; ***Spain:*** Antiedema; Apir Clorurado; Apiroflex Clorurado Simp†; Estericlean; Fisiologica; Fisiologico Betafar; Fisiologico Bieffe M; Fisiologico Braun; Fisiologico Mein; Fisiologico Vitulia; Flebobag Fisio; Fleboplast Fisio; Lavaflac; Libenar; Liberanas; Meinvenil Fisiologico; Plast Apyr Fisio Irrigac; Plast Apyr Fisiologico; Respitol; Solucion Fisio Nasal; Suero Fisio Andal Farm†; Suero Fisio Hayem Rapide†; Suero Fisio Vitulia†; Suero Fisiologico†; ***Swed.:*** Lisal†; Tresal; ***Switz.:*** Amuchina†; Drossa-Nose†; Naaprep; Nasben soft; Nose Fresh; Physiologica; Rhinomer; Serophy; Triomer; ***UK:*** Irriclens; Labmist; Normasol; Rhinomer; Slow-Sodium; Sterac; Sterijet; Steripod Blue; Topiclens†; Uriflex S; Uro-Tainer M; ***USA:*** Adsorbonac; Afrin Moisturizing Saline Mist; Ak-NaCl; Ayr Saline; Breathe Free; Broncho Saline; Dristan Saline Spray; HuMist Nasal Mist; Irigate; Marlin Salt System; Muro 128; Muroptic; NaSal; Nasal Moist; Ocean; Pretz; Salinex; SeaMist; Soft Rinse 250; Your Choice.

Multi-ingredient: numerous preparations are listed in Part 3.

Gases

This chapter includes monographs on gases with medical or pharmaceutical uses and applications (such as oxygen, carbon dioxide, helium, and nitrogen) as well as those where the medical interest lies primarily in management of their toxicity or adverse effects (such as carbon monoxide or hydrogen sulphide). Also included are some compressed and liquefied gases used as refrigerants and aerosol propellants. Nitric oxide gas is under investigation in bronchopulmonary disorders and is discussed in Cardiovascular Drugs (p.923). Other gases with medical uses can be found in Disinfectants and Preservatives (p.1097) and General Anaesthetics (p.1219).

Refrigerants and Aerosol Propellants

A number of compressed and liquefied gases are used as refrigerants and as aerosol propellants; these include nitrogen, nitrous oxide, carbon dioxide, propane, and the butanes. Chlorofluorocarbons (CFCs) were widely used but because of environmental hazards their general use has been severely restricted and they are being phased out in medicine and pharmacy. Hydrogenated chlorofluorocarbons (hydrochlorofluorocarbons) and nonchlorinated fluorocarbons (hydrofluorocarbons) are being developed as alternatives, although neither are devoid of environmental effects.

The evaporation of halogenated hydrocarbon propellants produces an intense cold that numbs the tissues, and they have been used as topical analgesics (p.7).

Refrigerants and aerosol propellants have been subject to deliberate abuse. Inhalation of high concentrations of halogenated hydrocarbons for their euphoriant effect may result in CNS depression, cardiac arrhythmias, respiratory depression, and death. Propane and butane can act as simple asphyxiants. Heat can cause the decomposition of halogenated hydrocarbons into irritant and toxic gases such as hydrogen chloride and phosgene.

Reviews have covered the toxicity and adverse effects that may occur as a consequence of the deliberate abuse of aerosol propellants[1-3] as well as the hazards associated with occupational exposure.[4] Further references relevant to the toxicity of individual agents are given in the monographs.

1. Volatile substance abuse—an overview. *Hum Toxicol* 1989; **8:** 255–344.
2. Ashton CH. Solvent abuse. *Br Med J* 1990; **300:** 1356–6.
3. Anderson HR. Increase in deaths from deliberate inhalation of fuel gases and pressurised aerosols. *Br Med J* 1990; **301:** 41.
4. Matthews G. Toxic gases. *Postgrad Med J* 1989; **65:** 224–32.

Bromochlorodifluoromethane (18869-s)

$CBrClF_2$ = 165.4.

Bromochlorodifluoromethane has been employed as a fire-extinguishing agent.

Reports of toxicity following the misuse or abuse of fire extinguishers containing bromochlorodifluoromethane.[1,2]

1. Steadman C, *et al.* Abuse of fire-extinguishing agent and sudden death in adolescents. *Med J Aust* 1984; **141:** 115–17.
2. Lerman Y, *et al.* Fatal accidental inhalation of bromochlorodifluoromethane (Halon 1211). *Hum Exp Toxicol* 1991; **10:** 125–8.

Butane (18361-b)

n-Butane.

C_4H_{10} = 58.12.

CAS — 106-97-8.

Pharmacopoeias. In *USNF.*

A colourless, flammable, explosive gas. It is supplied compressed in metal cylinders which should be stored in a cool place free from materials of a flammable nature.

Butane is used as an aerosol propellant (see above). It is widely used as a fuel.

Reports of toxicity associated with the abuse of butane.[1-3]

1. Gunn J, *et al.* Butane sniffing causing ventricular fibrillation. *Lancet* 1989; **i:** 617.
2. Siegel E, Wason S. Sudden death caused by inhalation of butane and propane. *N Engl J Med* 1990; **323:** 1638.
3. Roberts MJD, *et al.* Asystole following butane gas inhalation. *Br J Hosp Med* 1990; **44:** 294.

Carbon Dioxide (5202-a)

Carbonei Dioxidum; Carbonei Dioxydum; Carbonic Acid Gas; Carbonic Anhydride; E290.

CO_2 = 44.01.

CAS — 124-38-9.

Pharmacopoeias. In *Chin., Eur.* (see p.viii), *Jpn,* and *US.*

A colourless odourless gas which does not support combustion. It is supplied liquefied under pressure in metal cylinders. National standards are usually in operation for the labelling and marking of such cylinders. It is about 1½ times as heavy as air. A solution in water has weakly acid properties.

Soluble 1 in about 1 of water by volume at normal temperature and pressure.

Adverse Effects

Above a concentration of 6%, carbon dioxide gives rise to headache, dizziness, mental confusion, palpitations, hypertension, dyspnoea, increased depth and rate of respiration, and depression of the central nervous system. Concentrations of about 30% may produce convulsions. Higher concentrations are depressant; inhalation of 50% carbon dioxide is reported to produce central effects similar to anaesthetics. The inhalation of high concentrations may produce respiratory acidosis.

Abrupt withdrawal of carbon dioxide after prolonged inhalation commonly produces pallor, hypotension, dizziness, severe headache, and nausea or vomiting.

Uses and Administration

Carbon dioxide has been added to the oxygen in certain types of pump oxygenators to maintain the carbon dioxide content of the blood.

Although carbon dioxide stimulates respiration, it is seldom used for this purpose. Treatment of carbon monoxide poisoning with carbon dioxide/oxygen mixtures is discouraged due to the risk of respiratory acidosis.

Inhalation of carbon dioxide has been tried for relief of intractable hiccup (p.655). Carbonated vehicles are useful for masking the unpleasant taste of some medicinal preparations.

Solid carbon dioxide, or 'dry ice' has a temperature of −80° and has been used to treat warts (p.1076) and naevi by cryotherapy.

Carbon dioxide may be used as the insufflating gas for laparoscopy.

Carbon Monoxide (12525-g)

CO = 28.01.

CAS — 630-08-0.

A colourless, odourless, tasteless, highly flammable gas.

Adverse Effects

Carbon monoxide is produced by incomplete combustion of organic materials and is highly toxic when inhaled; infants, small children, and elderly people are particularly susceptible. Although, the number of cases of poisoning in countries like the UK has fallen as the availability of coal gas has declined and as changes have been made to motor vehicles to improve their exhaust fumes, carbon monoxide is still a major cause of poisoning. Common sources of carbon monoxide include poorly maintained and ventilated heating systems and improperly burnt fuel in domestic fires.

When inhaled, carbon monoxide combines with haemoglobin in the blood to form carboxyhaemoglobin which is unable to transport oxygen; the symptoms of carbon monoxide poisoning are largely due to anoxia. The skin and tissues turn a classic cherry red in patients poisoned with carbon monoxide although this is seen most often after death.

Unconsciousness may occur suddenly or may be preceded by dizziness, weakness, nausea, vomiting, headache, skin lesions, excessive sweating, pyrexia, increased respiration, mental dullness and confusion, visual disturbances, convulsions, hypotension, tachycardia or other cardiac arrhythmias, myocardial ischaemia, and possibly myocardial infarction; there may be involuntary defaecation and urination. Death may result from respiratory failure, pulmonary oedema, cardiovascular failure, or cerebral damage. Neurological and psychiatric sequelae may develop in the survivors of severe poisoning and therefore a prolonged follow-up of such patients is advised. The lethal concentration of carboxyhaemoglobin in the blood is about 50% or more. Concentrations over 1000 ppm of carbon monoxide in inspired air may be fatal in 1 hour.

Smoking during pregnancy may be hazardous to the fetus due to high maternal blood concentration of carboxyhaemoglobin.

General references.

1. Carbon Monoxide. *Environmental Health Criteria 13.* Geneva: WHO, 1979.
2. Meredith T, Vale A. Carbon monoxide poisoning. *Br Med J* 1988; **296:** 77–9.

Treatment of Adverse Effects

The patient should be removed from the contaminated atmosphere and an effective airway established. Oxygen (100%) should be given until blood carboxyhaemoglobin concentration has fallen below dangerous levels (usually 5%). Hyperbaric oxygen therapy is recommended by most authorities, especially in pregnant patients or in severe poisoning (if the patient is, or has been, unconscious; if the carboxyhaemoglobin concentration exceeds 40%; if there are neurological symptoms or cardiac complications). Management is then usually symptomatic and supportive with attention being given to the possible need to treat or correct any cardiovascular disorders, metabolic acidosis, or cerebral oedema.

References.

1. Anonymous. Treatment of carbon monoxide poisoning. *Drug Ther Bull* 1988; **26:** 77–9.
2. Van Hoesen KB, *et al.* Should hyperbaric oxygen be used to treat the pregnant patient for acute carbon monoxide poisoning: a case report and literature review. *JAMA* 1989; **261:** 1039–43. Correction. *ibid.* 1990; **263:** 2750.
3. Gorman DF. Problems and pitfalls in the use of hyperbaric oxygen for the treatment of poisoned patients. *Med Toxicol Adverse Drug Exp* 1989; **4:** 393–9.
4. Langford RM, Armstrong RF. Algorithm for managing injury from smoke inhalation. *Br Med J* 1989; **299:** 902–5.
5. Crawford R, *et al.* Carbon monoxide poisoning in the home: recognition and treatment. *Br Med J* 1990; **301:** 977–9.
6. Ely EW, *et al.* Warehouse workers' headache: emergency evaluation and management of 30 patients with carbon monoxide poisoning. *Am J Med* 1995; **98:** 145–55.
7. Ernst A, Zibrak JD. Carbon monoxide poisoning. *N Engl J Med* 1998; **339:** 1603–8.

Uses

Carbon monoxide has been used in low concentrations as a tracer gas in measurements of lung function. Carbon monoxide labelled with carbon-11 may also be employed to assess the blood volume.

Chlorofluorocarbons (10497-h)

CFCs.

Dichlorodifluoromethane (5206-f)

CFC-12; Difluorodichloromethane; Propellant 12; Refrigerant 12.

CCl_2F_2 = 120.9.

CAS — 75-71-8.

Pharmacopoeias. In *USNF.*

A colourless non-flammable gas with a faint ethereal odour. It is supplied under compression in metal cylinders.

Dichlorotetrafluoroethane (5207-d)

Cryofluorane (*rINN*); CFC-114; Propellant 114; Refrigerant 114; Tetrafluorodichloroethane. 1,2-Dichloro-1,1,2,2-tetrafluoroethane.

$C_2Cl_2F_4$ = 170.9.

CAS — 76-14-2.

Pharmacopoeias. In *USNF.*

A colourless non-flammable gas with a faint ethereal odour. It is supplied under compression in metal cylinders.

Trichlorofluoromethane (5208-n)

CFC-11; Fluorotrichloromethane; Propellant 11; Refrigerant 11; Trichloromonofluoromethane.

CCl_3F = 137.4.

CAS — 75-69-4.

Pharmacopoeias. In *USNF.*

A clear, colourless, non-flammable, volatile liquid with a faint ethereal odour; it is a gas above 24°. It is usually supplied under compression in metal cylinders.

Chlorofluorocarbons are used as refrigerants and as aerosol propellants (p.1164). They may also be used as a spray for topical anaesthesia, the intense cold produced by the rapid evaporation of the spray making the tissues insensitive.

Preparations

Proprietary Preparations (details are given in Part 3)
Aust.: Pharmaethyl; ***Ger.:*** Provotest; ***USA:*** Gebauer "114" Spray.

Multi-ingredient: ***Austral.:*** Derm-Freeze; Frezan†; ***Fr.:*** Dynacold; ***UK:*** Deep Freeze; ***USA:*** Aerofreeze; Fluori-Methane; Fluro-Ethyl.

Dimethyl Ether (6963-r)

Dimethyl Oxide; Methoxymethane; Oxybismethane.

C_2H_6O = 46.07.
CAS — 115-10-6.

Dimethyl ether is used as a refrigerant, aerosol propellant (see p.1164), and topical anaesthetic.

Preparations

Proprietary Preparations (details are given in Part 3)

Multi-ingredient: ***Austral.:*** Histofreezer; ***Fr.:*** Histofreezer; ***UK:*** PR Freeze Spray; Ralgex Freeze Spray.

Helium (5203-t)

He = 4.002602.
CAS — 7440-59-7.
Pharmacopoeias. In *US.*

A colourless odourless tasteless gas which is not combustible and does not support combustion. It is usually supplied under compression in metal cylinders. National standards are usually in operation for the labelling and marking of such cylinders.

As helium is less dense than nitrogen, breathing a mixture of 80% helium and 20% oxygen requires less effort than breathing air. Thus mixtures containing the desired concentration of oxygen ('Heliox') have been used in patients with respiratory disorders. Due to the low solubility of helium, mixtures of helium and oxygen are used by divers or others working under high pressure to prevent the development of decompression sickness (caisson disease); they are preferred to compressed air since they do not cause nitrogen narcosis. Helium has been employed in pulmonary function testing.

Breathing helium increases vocal pitch and causes voice distortion.

Hydrochlorofluorocarbons (10495-d)

HCFCs.

Chlorodifluoroethane (17661-p)

Propellant 142b; Refrigerant 142b. 1-Chloro-1,1-difluoroethane.

$C_2H_3ClF_2$ = 100.5.
CAS — 75-68-3.

Chlorodifluoromethane (17662-s)

Propellant 22; Refrigerant 22.

$CHClF_2$ = 86.47.
CAS — 75-45-6.

Hydrochlorofluorocarbons are used as refrigerants and as aerosol propellants (p.1164).

Hydrofluorocarbons (10513-s)

Fluorocarbons; HFAs; HFCs; Hydrofluroalkanes.

Difluoroethane (17663-w)

Ethylene Fluoride; HFC 152a; Propellant 152a; Refrigerant 152a. 1,1-Difluoroethane.

$C_2H_4F_2$ = 66.05.
CAS — 75-37-6.

Norflurane (15021-g)

Norflurane *(BAN, USAN, rINN).*

Fluorocarbon 134a; GR-106642X; HFA-134a; HFC-134a; Propellant 134a; Refrigerant 134a. 1,1,1,2-Tetrafluoroethane.

$C_2H_2F_4$ = 102.0.
CAS — 811-97-2.

Hydrofluorocarbons are used as refrigerants and as aerosol propellants (p.1164). As they are nonchlorinated fluorocarbons, it is believed that they will have a less detrimental effect on the environment than the chlorinated fluorocarbons.

References.

1. Denyer LH, *et al.* GR106642X, a non-chlorinated propellant for use in metered-dose inhalers: safety, tolerability and pharmacokinetics in healthy volunteers. *Br J Clin Pharmacol* 1994; **38:** 509P.
2. Taggart SCO, *et al.* GR106642X: a new, non-ozone depleting propellant for inhalers. *Br Med J* 1995; **310:** 1639–40.

Hydrogen Sulphide (12832-k)

Sulphuretted Hydrogen.

H_2S = 34.08.
CAS — 7783-06-4.

A colourless flammable gas with a characteristic odour.

Adverse Effects

Hydrogen sulphide poisoning is a common industrial hazard and is encountered in such places as chemical works, mines, sewage works, and stores of decomposing protein. Concentrations of 0.1 to 0.2% in the atmosphere may be fatal in a few minutes. At concentrations of about 0.005% and above hydrogen sulphide causes anosmia and its unpleasant odour is no longer detectable. Pulmonary irritation, oedema, and respiratory failure usually occur after acute poisoning; prolonged exposure to low concentrations may give rise to severe conjunctivitis with photophobia and corneal opacity, irritation of the respiratory tract, cough, nausea, vomiting and diarrhoea, pharyngitis, headache, dizziness, and lassitude. There are some similarities to poisoning with cyanides.

General references.

1. Hydrogen Sulfide. *Environmental Health Criteria 19.* Geneva: WHO, 1981.

Treatment of Adverse Effects

The patient should be removed from the contaminated atmosphere and an effective airway established. Some authorities have advocated oxygen by mask or hyperbaric oxygen therapy. Inhalation of amyl nitrite or parenteral therapy with sodium nitrite have been suggested. The conjunctival sacs should be carefully washed out if eye irritation is severe. Management is then usually symptomatic and supportive.

References.

1. Gorman DF. Problems and pitfalls in the use of hyperbaric oxygen for the treatment of poisoned patients. *Med Toxicol Adverse Drug Exp* 1989; **4:** 393–9.

Uses

Hydrogen sulphide is widely employed in many industrial processes.

Isobutane (18352-m)

2-Methylpropane.

C_4H_{10} = 58.12.
Pharmacopoeias. In *USNF.*

A colourless, flammable, explosive gas. It is usually supplied under compression in metal cylinders which should be stored in a cool place free from materials of a flammable nature.

Isobutane is used as an aerosol propellant (p.1164).

Nitrogen (5204-x)

Azote; Nitrogenium.

N_2 = 28.01348.
CAS — 7727-37-9.

Pharmacopoeias. In *Eur.* (see p.viii) and *Jpn.*
USNF has two monographs: Nitrogen (not less than 99% by volume of N_2) and Nitrogen 97 Percent (not less than 97% by volume of N_2).

A colourless, odourless, tasteless gas which is non-flammable and does not support combustion. It is usually supplied under compression in metal cylinders. National standards are usually in operation for the labelling and marking of such cylinders.

Adverse Effects

Nitrogen narcosis has been reported from nitrogen breathed at high pressure as in deep-water diving. Under high pressure, nitrogen dissolves in blood and lipid. If decompression is too rapid, nitrogen effervesces from body stores producing gas emboli and leading to the syndrome of decompression sickness.

Uses and Administration

Nitrogen is used as a diluent for pure oxygen or other active gases and as an inert gas to replace air in containers holding oxidisable substances. Liquid nitrogen is used as a cryotherapeutic agent for the removal of warts (p.1076) and for preservation of tissues and organisms.

Oxygen (5201-k)

Ossigeno; Oxygenium; Sauerstoff.

O_2 = 31.9988.
CAS — 7782-44-7.

Pharmacopoeias. In *Chin., Eur.* (see p.viii), *Jpn,* and *US.*
US also includes Oxygen 93 Percent (90 to 96% by volume of O_2).
Eur. and *US* also include Medical Air (a mixture of oxygen and nitrogen). *Eur.* specifies 20.4 to 21.4% oxygen. *US* specifies 19.5 to 23.5% oxygen.

A colourless odourless tasteless gas. Oxygen intended for aviation or mountain rescue must have a sufficiently low moisture content to avoid blocking of valves by freezing.

Oxygen is usually supplied under compression in metal cylinders. National standards are usually in operation for the labelling and marking of such cylinders.

Adverse Effects

Oxygen toxicity depends upon both the inspired pressure (a function of concentration and barometric pressure) and the duration of exposure, the safe duration decreasing as the pressure increases. At lower pressures of up to 2 atmospheres absolute pulmonary toxicity occurs before CNS toxicity; at higher pressures, the reverse applies. Symptoms of pulmonary toxicity include a decrease in vital capacity, cough, and substernal distress. Symptoms of CNS toxicity include nausea, mood changes, vertigo, twitching, convulsions, and loss of consciousness.

In a review of hyperbaric oxygen therapy[1] the following were mentioned as potential complications: barotrauma (ear or sinus trauma, tympanic membrane rupture, or rarely pneumothorax or air embolism); oxygen toxicity (CNS toxicity or pulmonary toxicity); and reversible visual changes.

1. Grim PS, *et al.* Hyperbaric oxygen therapy. *JAMA* 1990; **263:** 2216–20.

Retinopathy of prematurity. In the 1940s and 1950s an epidemic of retinopathy of prematurity, affecting perhaps 10 000 babies, was believed to have been caused by excessive administration of oxygen to the neonates. This resulted in the use of oxygen being reduced or curtailed and the incidence of the condition fell dramatically. However, in the 1970s and later an unexpected resurgence of retinopathy of prematurity occurred (probably *not* due to excessive oxygen administration). It is now believed that oxygen plays only a minor part and that retinopathy of prematurity is a multifactorial condition that affects the most immature and sick children.[1,2] The increased incidence may reflect the improved survival of these very premature neonates.

1. Anonymous. Retinopathy of prematurity. *Lancet* 1991; **337:** 83–4.
2. Holmström G. Retinopathy of prematurity. *Br Med J* 1993; **307:** 694–5.

Precautions

Any fire or spark is highly dangerous in the presence of increased oxygen concentrations especially when oxygen is used under pressure.

Metal cylinders containing oxygen should be fitted with a reducing valve by which the rate of flow can be controlled. It is important that the reducing valve should be free from all traces of oil or grease, as otherwise a violent explosion may occur. Combustible material soaked in liquid oxygen is potentially explosive and the low temperature of liquid oxygen may cause unsuitable equipment to become brittle and crack. Liquid oxygen should not be allowed to come into contact with the skin as it produces severe 'cold burns'.

High concentrations of oxygen should be avoided in patients whose respiration is dependent upon hypoxic drive, otherwise carbon dioxide retention and respiratory depression may ensue.

Uses and Administration

Oxygen is given by inhalation to correct hypoxaemia in conditions causing respiratory failure (below) and in conditions where the oxygen content of the air breathed is inadequate such as in high-altitude disorders (p.787). Oxygen is of value in the treatment of poisoning with a number of substances, including carbon monoxide (p.1164), cyanides (p.1407), and dichloromethane (p.1377). It provides enhanced oxygenation in inhalation injury. Oxygen is also given by inhalation to subjects working in pressurised spaces and to divers to reduce the concentration of nitrogen inhaled. It is used as a diluent of volatile and gaseous anaesthetics.

Oxygen is usually administered by means of nasal prongs or via a face mask; these can usually deliver concentrations of up to 60%. Tight-fitting anaesthetic-type masks, or delivery via an endotracheal tube or oxygen tent can provide higher concentrations of up to 100%. Face masks are commonly employed for domiciliary oxygen therapy when flow rates are 2 or 4 litres per minute. Oxygen is commonly supplied compressed in metal cylinders although oxygen concentrators produce oxygen-enriched air and are useful for domiciliary therapy, especially in patients using large quantities of oxygen. Oxygen may also be supplied at low temperature in insulated containers as liquid oxygen.

In respiratory failure in conditions not usually associated with retention of carbon dioxide, such as pneumonia, pulmonary oedema, or fibrosing alveolitis, oxygen should be administered in high concentrations (usually 40 to 100%). Concentrations of 40 to 60% should be used in acute severe asthma even though carbon dioxide retention may have increased as the patient's condition deteriorated. High concentrations of oxygen should always be reduced as soon as possible to the lowest concentration needed to correct hypoxaemia in order to prevent development of any associated oxygen toxicity including increased carbon dioxide retention. High concentrations of oxygen should be administered in carbon monoxide poisoning and treatment with hyperbaric oxygen considered.

In respiratory failure associated with chronic obstructive pulmonary disease (conditions such as chronic bronchitis and emphysema) oxygen is usually administered to give an inspired concentration of up to 28%. High concentrations are to be avoided as they may enhance carbon-dioxide retention and narcosis.

Oxygen at a pressure greater than 1 atmosphere absolute, i.e. hyperbaric oxygen therapy (below), is administered by enclosing the patient in a special high-pressure chamber. It is used to correct hypoxaemia in poisoning by carbon monoxide, as an adjunct in the treatment of severe anaerobic infections, especially gas gangrene, and for the treatment of decompression sickness and gas emboli.

General references.

1. Naylor-Shepherd MF, *et al.* Oxygen homeostasis: theory, measurement, and therapeutic implications. *DICP Ann Pharmacother* 1990; **24:** 1195–1203.
2. Gribbin HR. Management of respiratory failure. *Br J Hosp Med* 1993; **49:** 461–77.
3. Tarpy SP, Celli BR. Long-term oxygen therapy. *N Engl J Med* 1995; **333:** 710–14.
4. Bateman NT, Leach RM. ABC of oxygen: acute oxygen therapy. *Br Med J* 1998; **317:** 798–801.
5. Rees PJ, Dudley F. ABC of oxygen: oxygen therapy in chronic lung disease. *Br Med J* 1998; **317:** 871–4.
6. Rees PJ, Dudley F. ABC of oxygen: provision of oxygen at home. *Br Med J* 1998; **317:** 935–8.
7. Treacher DF, Leach RM. ABC of oxygen: oxygen transport: basic principles. *Br Med J* 1998; **317:** 1302–6.
8. Leach RM, Treacher DF. ABC of oxygen: oxygen transport: tissue hypoxia. *Br Med J* 1998; **317:** 1370–3.

Cluster headache. Inhalation of 100% oxygen can provide rapid and effective treatment of cluster headache attacks but as mentioned on p.443, practical difficulties associated with its use result in other drugs being preferred. References.

1. Fogan L. Treatment of cluster headache: a double-blind comparison of oxygen v air inhalation. *Arch Neurol* 1985; **42:** 362–3.

Hyperbaric oxygen therapy. The use of hyperbaric oxygen therapy, which involves the intermittent inhalation of 100% oxygen under a pressure of greater than 1 atmosphere, has been the subject of reviews.[1-3] In the 1960s hyperbaric therapy was used for disorders such as *myocardial infarction, stroke, senility,* and *cancer* but clinical studies and experience have shown little benefit and enthusiasm has since waned. There are, however, other disorders for which the evidence supporting the efficacy of hyperbaric oxygen is much stronger.

Hyperbaric oxygen is a safe and effective primary therapy for *decompression sickness* and *air or gas embolism.* The effect is achieved through the mechanical reduction in bubble size in the blood brought about by an increase in ambient pressure; the increased oxygenation of blood due to the additional pressure employed for these conditions (often 6 rather than 2 or 3 atmospheres) is also beneficial.

In severe *carbon monoxide poisoning* hyperbaric oxygen remains the preferred treatment (for further references see under Carbon Monoxide, p.1164) although its mechanism of action is said to be poorly understood; one explanation is that it stops lipid peroxidation which in turn spares neuronal cell membranes.

Hyperbaric oxygen is employed as adjunctive therapy in *clostridial infections (gas gangrene)* (p.123). Early treatment appears to reduce systemic toxic reactions (probably by inhibiting the production of alpha toxin by the anaerobic bacteria, *Clostridium*) thus enabling patients to tolerate surgery more readily; additionally there is a clearer demarcation of viable and nonviable tissue. Necrotising fasciitis (p.132) is another infection in which hyperbaric oxygen therapy may be useful.

There is some evidence that hyperbaric oxygen may be useful in other types of *wounds.* In an *acute crush injury* therapy may reduce oedema via vasoconstriction and reverse ischaemia by increased oxygen delivery. In *problem wounds* therapy may increase the tissue oxygen tension and stimulate angioneogenesis but it is emphasised that it is adjunctive therapy and not a replacement for meticulous local care. Other wounds in which therapy may be beneficial include thermal burns and compromised skin grafts and flaps. The management of burns and wounds is described on p.1073 and p.1076, respectively.

Radiation therapy can damage normal adjacent tissue resulting in tissue hypoxia and eventual cell death. Hyperbaric oxygen therapy appears to aid in salvaging such tissue by stimulating angioneogenesis in marginally viable tissue and has been demonstrated to be beneficial in osteoradionecrosis, radiation-induced cystitis,[4] and other radiation-damaged soft tissue.

One of the applications not covered by the above reviews is *multiple sclerosis* (p.620). The use of hyperbaric oxygen therapy in this condition has been a matter of debate for many years and continues to be controversial. Some workers have reported benefit, especially in bladder and bowel function or in cerebellar function.[5] Others have been unable to substantiate any useful long-term effect[6] and a review of the many therapeutic options available in multiple sclerosis concluded that there was no convincing evidence that hyperbaric oxygen therapy was successful.[7]

1. Grim PS, *et al.* Hyperbaric oxygen therapy. *JAMA* 1990; **263:** 2216–20.
2. Tibbles PM, Edelsberg JS. Hyperbaric-oxygen therapy. *N Engl J Med* 1996; **334:** 1642–8.
3. Leach RM, *et al.* ABC of oxygen: hyperbaric oxygen therapy. *Br Med J* 1998; **317:** 1140–3.
4. Bevers RFM, *et al.* Hyperbaric oxygen treatment for haemorrhagic radiation cystitis. *Lancet* 1995; **346:** 803–5.
5. James PB, Webster CJ. Long-term results of hyperbaric oxygen therapy in multiple sclerosis. *Lancet* 1989; **ii:** 327.
6. Kindwall EP, *et al.* Treatment of multiple sclerosis with hyperbaric oxygen: results of a national registry. *Arch Neurol* 1991; **48:** 195–9.
7. Webb HE. Multiple sclerosis: therapeutic pessimism. *Br Med J* 1992; **304:** 1260–1.

Respiratory failure. Respiratory failure occurs when the arterial plasma partial pressure of oxygen (P_aO_2) and of carbon dioxide (P_aCO_2) cannot be maintained within normal physiological limits.[1] Respiratory failure can be classified into 2 types both of which are characterised by a low P_aO_2 (hypoxaemia). However, in type I the P_aCO_2 is normal or low whereas in type II, referred to as ventilatory failure, P_aCO_2 is raised (hypercapnia). Some conditions, for example asthma, can produce either type of respiratory failure.

Management of respiratory failure primarily involves administration of oxygen to reverse hypoxaemia, and specific therapy for any underlying condition. Respiratory stimulants may be considered in some situations.

Treatment of type I respiratory failure consists of the administration of oxygen in high concentrations. Nasal prongs and certain face masks can provide concentrations of up to 60% but if concentrations higher than this are needed (such as up to 100%) then tight-fitting anaesthetic-type masks or methods of delivery such as by endotracheal intubation have to be employed.

In type II respiratory failure both high and low concentrations are used according to need.

Patients with *acute severe asthma* (p.745) should usually be given oxygen at high concentrations of 40 to 60%. Low controlled concentrations of oxygen (24 to 28%) are used in the management of respiratory failure in patients with chronic respiratory disorders such as *chronic obstructive pulmonary disease* (p.747) the aim being to improve hypoxaemia without increasing hypercapnia and respiratory acidosis. Patients with exacerbations of chronic ventilatory failure already have an increased central drive to the respiratory muscles and therefore respiratory stimulants such as doxapram have a limited role but may be indicated for short-term use if hypercapnia worsens as a result of the administration of oxygen. Respiratory stimulants may be considered in the management of *postanaesthetic hypoventilation.* Although naloxone can reverse respiratory depression caused by opioid analgesics careful dosage adjustment is required as it can also abolish analgesia. Specific antagonists such as naloxone and flumazenil are also used to treat hypoventilation associated with opioid and benzodiazepine overdosage, respectively. If oxygen therapy fails to raise P_aO_2 in respiratory failure and there is worsening hypercapnia and respiratory acidosis the use of artificial ventilation should be considered.

Severe respiratory failure in *neonates* may require the technique of extracorporeal membrane oxygenation (ECMO) where blood is removed from the neonate, oxygenated, and re-injected in a continuous circuit that also removes carbon dioxide.[2]

1. Gribbin HR. Management of respiratory failure. *Br J Hosp Med* 1993; **49:** 461–77.
2. Barrington KJ, Finer NN. Care of near term infants with respiratory failure. *Br Med J* 1997; **315:** 1215–18.

Preparations

Proprietary Preparations (details are given in Part 3)
Multi-ingredient: *UK:* Entonox.

Propane (16196-j)

Dimethylmethane; Propyl Hydride.
C_3H_8 = 44.10.
CAS — 74-98-6.
Pharmacopoeias. In *USNF.*

A colourless, flammable, explosive gas. It is usually supplied under compression in metal cylinders which should be stored in a cool place free from materials of a flammable nature.

Propane is used as a refrigerant and as an aerosol propellant (see p.1164). It is also widely used as a fuel.

Reports of toxicity associated with the abuse or misuse of propane.[1,2]

1. James NK, Moss ALH. Cold injury from liquid propane. *Br Med J* 1989; **299:** 950–1.
2. Siegel E, Wason S. Sudden death caused by inhalation of butane and propane. *N Engl J Med* 1990; **323:** 1638.

Preparations

Proprietary Preparations (details are given in Part 3)
Multi-ingredient: *Austral.:* Histofreezer; *Fr.:* Histofreezer.

Gastro-intestinal Drugs

This chapter describes the principal drugs used in the treatment of gastro-intestinal disorders, and the choice of treatment for some of the main disorders.

Gastro-intestinal Drug Groups

Antacids

Antacids are basic compounds which neutralise hydrochloric acid in the gastric secretions. They are used in the symptomatic management of gastro-intestinal disorders associated with gastric hyperacidity such as dyspepsia, gastro-oesophageal reflux disease, and peptic ulcer disease (below).

Antacids do not reduce the volume of hydrochloric acid secreted and elevation of the gastric pH may actually promote an increase in acid and pepsin secretion. However, this is usually minor and short-lived except after large doses of calcium carbonate. They are normally given between meals and at bedtime when symptoms will usually occur; the presence of food in the stomach can prolong the neutralising activity. Some authorities calculate doses as mEq or mmol of acid-neutralising capacity, but the relationship between neutralising capacity and beneficial effect is not straightforward. Other factors, including formulation (liquid preparations are more effective than solids) and duration of action (relatively insoluble antacids are longer acting) are also important.

Aluminium salts tend to produce constipation and to delay gastric emptying, while magnesium salts have the reverse effect; a combination of the two may reduce adverse gastro-intestinal effects. Another advantage of combined antacid formulations is that a slow-acting antacid such as aluminium hydroxide may be combined with a more rapidly acting drug such as magnesium hydroxide to improve the onset and duration of effect. Alternatively, complexes containing both aluminium and magnesium may be used, such as almasilate, hydrotalcite, and magaldrate. Other drugs which may be combined with antacid formulations include simethicone, to act as a defoaming agent to reduce excess gas in the stomach, and alginates, which may be useful in gastro-oesophageal reflux disease by forming a gel or foam on the surface of the stomach contents which impedes reflux and protects the oesophageal mucosa from acid attack.

Calcium carbonate and sodium bicarbonate are both rapidly acting but have disadvantages: calcium carbonate is usually reserved for short-term treatment because of the risks of rebound acid secretion and metabolic alkalosis, while sodium bicarbonate is absorbed and is contra-indicated in patients who must control sodium intake (e.g. in heart failure, hypertension, renal failure, cirrhosis, or pregnancy).

Antacids may interact with numerous other drugs, affecting the rate and extent of their absorption, and in some cases their renal elimination. Changes in gastric pH affect the dissolution of other drugs, and together with altered gastric emptying can markedly influence absorption. Aluminium compounds in particular are noted for their propensity to adsorb other drugs and to form insoluble complexes that are not absorbed. Antacids which alter urinary pH will affect renal clearance of drugs that are weak acids or bases. Several mechanisms may play a part in any particular interaction.

Among the drugs whose absorption or bioavailability may be significantly affected by concomitant oral administration with an antacid are various antibacterials including ethambutol, isoniazid, nitrofurantoin, quinolones, and tetracyclines; benzodiazepines; some corticosteroids; fluoride; iron; indomethacin; ketoconazole; phenothiazines; phenytoin; phosphate; ranitidine; theophylline; valproate; and vitamin A. For further details see under the individual drugs affected.

Interactions can be minimised by giving antacids and other medication 2 to 3 hours apart.

Antacids in this chapter include aluminium salts (p.1177), magnesium salts (p.1198), and calcium carbonate (p.1182).

Antidiarrhoeals

Antidiarrhoeals are used as adjuncts in the symptomatic treatment of diarrhoea (see below), although the main aim in the management of *acute* diarrhoea is the correction of fluid and electrolyte depletion with rehydration therapy; this is especially important in infants and young children and antidiarrhoeals are not generally recommended for this age group. Their use is also limited in *chronic* diarrhoea since treatment aimed at the underlying disorder will often alleviate the diarrhoea.

Described in this chapter are drugs which reduce intestinal motility such as diphenoxylate and loperamide, and adsorbents such as attapulgite and kaolin.

Antiemetics

Antiemetics are a diverse group of drugs used to treat or prevent nausea and vomiting, including that associated with cancer therapy, anaesthesia, and motion sickness (see below).

The choice of drug depends partly on the cause of nausea and vomiting. For example, hyoscine or an antihistamine are used in motion sickness whereas dopamine antagonists and 5-HT_3 antagonists are ineffective. Conversely, nausea and vomiting associated with cancer chemotherapy is often hard to control and special regimens have been devised including the use of metoclopramide in high doses, dexamethasone, and, more recently, the 5-HT_3 antagonists.

Antiemetics described in this chapter include: the dopamine antagonists metoclopramide and domperidone; the 5-HT_3 antagonists ondansetron and granisetron; the cannabinoid nabilone; and miscellaneous substances such as ginger.

Anti-ulcer drugs

Anti-ulcer drugs are used in the treatment and prophylaxis of peptic ulcer disease (below); some are also employed in other disorders associated with gastric hyperacidity. Several types of drug are employed, as described below, but they are used, broadly, either for their antisecretory action on the production of gastric acid, or for their cytoprotective or mucosal protectant properties. Antacids (see above) also play an adjuvant role in the symptomatic treatment of peptic ulceration while antibacterial therapy aimed at *Helicobacter pylori* is increasingly important.

Antisecretory drugs may be divided into:

- *Histamine H_2-receptor antagonists* (H_2-antagonists), which act by blocking histamine H_2-receptors on gastric parietal cells, thereby antagonising the normal stimulatory effect of endogenous histamine on gastric acid production. Those described in this chapter include cimetidine, famotidine, nizatidine, and ranitidine.
- *Proton-pump inhibitors*, which act by blocking the enzyme system responsible for active transport of protons into the gastro-intestinal lumen, namely the hydrogen/potassium adenosine triphosphatase (H^+/K^+ ATPase) of the gastric parietal cell, also known as the 'proton pump'. Those described in this chapter include lansoprazole, omeprazole, and pantoprazole.
- *Selective antimuscarinics*, which block cholinergic stimulation of gastric acid production with fewer adverse effects than standard antimuscarinics (p.453), but have already largely been superseded. Pirenzepine (p.467) is an example.
- *Prostaglandin analogues*, which inhibit gastric acid secretion by a direct action on the parietal cell and may also inhibit gastrin release and possess cytoprotective properties. Misoprostol (p.1419) is an example.

Cytoprotective drugs (mucosal protectants) also play a role in the management of peptic ulcer disease. They may be divided into:

- *Chelates or complexes*, which coat the gastric mucosa preferentially at sites of ulceration by forming an adherent complex with proteins. Those described in this chapter include sucralfate and tripotassium dicitratobismuthate (which also has an antibacterial role in regimens aimed at eradicating *Helicobacter pylori*).
- *Miscellaneous drugs* include liquorice and its derivatives, such as carbenoxolone, which act by stimulating the synthesis of protective mucus.

Antacids, particularly those containing aluminium or bismuth, may also exert cytoprotective effects, possibly by stimulating production of protective endogenous prostaglandins. Prostaglandins themselves may possess cytoprotective properties in addition to their antisecretory effects (see above).

Laxatives

Laxatives (purgatives or cathartics) promote defaecation and are used in the treatment of constipation (below) and for bowel evacuation before investigational procedures, such as endoscopy or radiological examination, or before surgery.

Laxatives are frequently employed for self-medication and may sometimes be abused. Abuse of laxatives is a well-known phenomenon that may occasionally lead to toxicity.

Laxatives may be classified according to their mode of action. There is, however, a degree of overlap between the various groups and in some cases the precise mechanisms of action are not fully understood. Many traditionally used laxatives have fallen from use owing to the violence of their action or their adverse effect profile.

- *Bulk laxatives* (bulk-forming laxatives or bulking agents) cause retention of fluid and an increase in faecal mass resulting in stimulation of peristalsis. Owing to their hydrophilic nature, bulk laxatives may also be used to control acute diarrhoea and to regulate the consistency of effluent in colostomy patients. Those described in this chapter include bran, ispaghula, psyllium, and sterculia.
- *Stimulant laxatives* (contact laxatives) act by directly stimulating nerve endings in the colonic mucosa, thereby increasing intestinal motility. It is this group of laxatives which is most commonly associated with abuse. Those described in this chapter include bisacodyl, cascara, phenolphthalein, senna, and sodium picosulphate.
- *Osmotic laxatives* act by increasing intestinal osmotic pressure thereby promoting retention of fluid within the bowel. Those described in this chapter include saline laxatives such as magnesium carbonate, magnesium citrate, magnesium hydroxide, and sodium sulphate (for magnesium sulphate and sodium phosphate see p.1157 and p.1159 respectively). Lactulose may also be classified as an osmotic laxative because its breakdown products exert a similar effect. Also included in this group are the hyperosmotic laxatives such as glycerol (p.1585) and sorbitol (p.1354).
- *Faecal softeners* (emollient laxatives) are claimed to act by decreasing surface tension and increasing penetration of intestinal fluid into the faecal mass. Those described in this chapter include docusate (which is also believed to have a stimulant action). For the lubricant laxative liquid paraffin see p.1382.

Prokinetic drugs

Prokinetic drugs stimulate the motility of the gastro-intestinal tract. Gastro-intestinal smooth muscle exhibits intrinsic motor activity which is modified by autonomic innervation, local reflexes, and gastro-intestinal hormones to produce peristaltic waves which move the gut contents from stomach to anus and segmentations which encourage digestion. Prokinetic drugs may act at various points within this complex system to enhance gastro-intestinal movement. Those described in this chapter include metoclopramide, cisapride, and domperidone. Other drugs with prokinetic properties include parasympathomimetics such as bethanechol (p.1389) or neostigmine (p.1394), and the macrolide antibiotic erythromycin (p.204).

Management of Gastro-intestinal Disorders

The management of some gastro-intestinal disorders is discussed below.

Aspiration syndromes

Regurgitation and aspiration of gastric contents (Mendelson's syndrome) is an important cause of morbidity and mortality associated with anaesthesia, especially in obstetrics and in emergency surgery.[1] Chemical pneumonitis and respiratory distress result from the acid aspiration, the risk of which is increased by the drugs given as adjuncts to anaesthesia such as opioid analgesics and atropine. Apart from good anaesthetic technique, including a prohibition on oral intake before elective procedures, efforts to **prevent** or reduce the problem have focussed mainly on increasing the pH of gastric contents to above 2.5, so that if aspiration occurs the damage is less. Other measures include enhancing gastric emptying.

The *histamine H_2-receptor antagonists* decrease gastric acid secretion and may decrease gastric fluid volume. However, although they are valuable in elective procedures they do not affect the pH of fluid already in the stomach; they must therefore be given some time before anaesthesia which limits their value in emergency procedures.[1] Cimetidine is considered effective in most patients, although where more prolonged reduction of acidity is required H_2-antagonists with a longer duration of action such as ranitidine or famotidine may be preferred. Nizatidine has the advantage of a relatively rapid onset of action.[2]

The *proton-pump inhibitors*, have also been tried, but results have been variable. Combination with a prokinetic drug may produce better results.[3]

Because of the lack of effect of antisecretory drugs on the pH of existing gastric fluid they may be combined with *antacids* to neutralise gastric acidity. Although magnesium trisilicate has been extensively used[4] without apparent problems particulate antacids are potentially toxic to the lung, which is why soluble antacids such as sodium citrate have been widely employed. An effervescent formulation of sodium citrate with cimetidine has been reported to raise gastric pH above 2.5 in more than 98% of patients undergoing caesarean section.[5] Sodium bicarbonate, given alone, has also been reported to be effective for three hours or more.[6]

A third component of prophylactic regimens for acid aspiration may be use of a *prokinetic drug* such as metoclopramide or cisapride. These increase gastric emptying and thereby decrease the volume of stomach contents, and also increase pressure at the lower oesophageal sphincter. The ability of metoclopramide to reverse the effects of opioids on gastric emptying appears to depend on the route of administration: 10 mg given intravenously after opioid analgesia is reported to be effective in promoting gastric emptying,[7,8] whereas the same dose intramuscularly is not.[8,9] In contrast, cisapride is effective when given intramuscularly.[10]

If aspiration occurs, pulmonary damage may result within seconds; **treatment** has included removal of any particulate matter, and measures to maintain the airway and ensure adequate oxygenation. Corticosteroids have been used but are no longer considered helpful.[11]

1. Anonymous. Routine H_2-receptor antagonists before elective surgery? *Lancet* 1989; **i:** 1363–4.
2. Popat MT, *et al.* Comparison of the effects of oral nizatidine and ranitidine on gastric volume and pH in patients undergoing gynaecological laparoscopy. *Anaesthesia* 1991; **46:** 816–19.
3. Orr DA, *et al.* Effects of omeprazole, with and without metoclopramide, in elective obstetric anaesthesia. *Anaesthesia* 1993; **48:** 114–19.
4. Sweeney BL, Wright I. The use of antacids as a prophylaxis against Mendelson's syndrome in the United Kingdom: a survey. *Anaesthesia* 1986; **41:** 419–22.
5. Ormezzano X, *et al.* Aspiration pneumonitis prophylaxis in obstetric anaesthesia: comparison of effervescent cimetidine–sodium citrate mixture and sodium citrate. *Br J Anaesth* 1990; **64:** 503–6.
6. Acosta F, *et al.* Efficiency of sodium bicarbonate as an antacid. *Br J Anaesth* 1995; **74** (suppl 1): 60.
7. Murphy DF, *et al.* Effect of metoclopramide on gastric emptying before elective and emergency caesarean section. *Br J Anaesth* 1984; **56:** 1113–16.
8. McNeill MJ, *et al.* Effect of iv metoclopramide on gastric emptying after opioid premedication. *Br J Anaesth* 1990; **64:** 450–2.
9. Nimmo WS, *et al.* Narcotic analgesics and delayed gastric emptying during labour. *Lancet* 1975; **i:** 890–3.
10. Rowbotham DJ, *et al.* Comparison of the effect of cisapride and metoclopramide on morphine-induced delay in gastric emptying. *Br J Clin Pharmacol* 1988; **26:** 741–6.
11. Ryan DW. Pulmonary aspiration: high dose steroids should be abandoned. *Br Med J* 1984; **289:** 51.

Constipation

The pattern of normal defaecation is extremely variable. Constipation may be considered to occur if there is a change in that pattern, e.g. a reduced frequency of defaecation, a hardening of the stool, a reduction in stool volume, or a feeling of incomplete evacuation.[1] It is of serious clinical concern when faecal impaction is likely. Constipation can be a symptom of a range of disorders or of drug toxicity[2] and the necessary attention to these underlying causes can resolve it. Constipation can also reflect a change in lifestyle.

An increase in fibre intake, preferably through a high-fibre diet, will help to relieve constipation in the majority of patients[3] without the need for laxatives. Laxatives are often taken unnecessarily and their regular use can lead to problems of abuse, but when dietary modification is difficult or unacceptable a *bulk laxative* may be appropriate.[3,4] The choice of bulk laxative includes bran, ispaghula, methylcellulose and related compounds, psyllium, or sterculia. Bulk laxatives generally have an effect after 1 to 3 days and are of particular value in those with small hard stools; a gradual increase in dose is advisable to avoid flatulence and distention.[1] They may not be the first choice for elderly patients who are frail or immobile since the resulting soft faeces may result in faecal incontinence.[5]

If constipation fails to respond to an increase in fibre intake or use of a bulk laxative, a *stimulant laxative* may be given. Many traditional stimulant laxatives have fallen from use due to adverse effects, and their prolonged use or abuse may irreversibly damage colonic nerves and muscles.[1,4] Provided appropriate stimulant laxatives are used infrequently and at the minimal effective dose, however, they are unlikely to cause significant harm.[4] Commonly used stimulant laxatives include anthraquinone-containing drugs such as senna, and diphenylmethane derivatives such as bisacodyl or sodium picosulphate. Stimulant laxatives have a more rapid onset of action than bulk laxatives, usually proving effective within 6 to 12 hours.[1] Combined preparations are also available, and a combination of senna and fibre has been found to be more effective than lactulose in elderly patients with chronic constipation.[6]

Osmotic laxatives such as magnesium carbonate, magnesium hydroxide, and magnesium sulphate, have a very rapid action, and are alternatives to the stimulant laxatives, but the resultant watery stool, urgency, and occasional incontinence may limit their usefulness.[4] Lactulose and sorbitol have a similar, but slower, action. Prolonged use of all osmotic laxatives should be avoided.[1]

Other laxatives include surfactants such as docusates which are relatively ineffective alone but are often combined with a stimulant laxative,[1] and may be of value in patients with haemorrhoids or anal fissures, or those in whom straining is potentially hazardous (such as the elderly or those with existing cardiovascular disease). Liquid paraffin is no longer recommended owing to its adverse effects, which include anal seepage and the risks of granulomatous disease of the gastro-intestinal tract or of lipoid pneumonia on aspiration.[1] Stimulation of the bowel with cisapride or the cholecystokinin antagonist loxiglumide has been tried.

Rectal administration of laxatives using enemas or suppositories is appropriate in patients requiring rapid relief from constipation. Enemas, which usually combine osmotic and stimulant laxatives, are generally easier for patients to retain than suppositories.[1] Phosphate enemas should be used with caution in patients with renal impairment because of the risks of absorption of significant amounts of phosphate.[1] Glycerol may be administered rectally as suppositories to promote faecal evacuation, and usually acts within 15 to 30 minutes; its action is probably due to an osmotic effect although it may have additional stimulant, lubricating, or faecal-softening properties. Bisacodyl suppositories also have a rapid stimulant effect on the bowel.[1] Faecal impaction may be treated with a laxative enema; should that fail manual disimpaction is necessary.[1,2,4]

1. Bateman DN. Management of constipation. *Prescribers' J* 1991; **31:** 7–15.
2. Moriarty KJ, Irving MH. Constipation. *Br Med J* 1992; **304:** 1237–40.
3. Taylor R. Management of constipation 1: high fibre diets work *Br Med J* 1990; **300:** 1063–4.
4. Spiller R. Management of constipation 2: when fibre fails *Br Med J* 1990; **300:** 1064–5.
5. Ardron ME, Main ANH. Management of constipation. *Br Med J* 1990; **300:** 1400.
6. Passmore AP, *et al.* Chronic constipation in long stay elderly patients: a comparison of lactulose and a senna-fibre combination. *Br Med J* 1993; **307:** 769–71.

Decreased gastro-intestinal motility

Decreased gastro-intestinal motility may occur in any part of the gastro-intestinal tract, with symptoms depending on the site. It is of varying aetiology and often secondary to some other disorder, such as infection, metabolic or electrolyte disturbance (for example in gastroparesis due to diabetic neuropathy—see also p.315), or insult to the gastro-intestinal tract (for example, paralytic or adynamic ileus is frequently a consequence of abdominal surgery and is a serious adverse effect of some drugs).

Acute loss of gastro-intestinal motility is often self-limiting once the underlying cause has been treated. Provided the ability of gastro-intestinal smooth muscle to contract has not been lost, however, prokinetic drugs such as metoclopramide, cisapride, or domperidone, or other drugs capable of stimulating functional contraction including erythromycin or parasympathomimetics such as neostigmine or bethanechol, may be employed.

Drugs are less successful in chronic conditions such as chronic intestinal pseudo-obstruction where neuromuscular function of the gastro-intestinal tract has some intrinsic abnormality.

Diarrhoea

Diarrhoea is characterised by liquid stools, increased stool weight, and frequency of defaecation. Although diarrhoea is commonly associated with infection, it may also result from the accumulation of nonabsorbed osmotically active solutes in the gastro-intestinal lumen, such as in lactase deficiency, or from the gastro-intestinal effects of secretory stimuli, other than the enterotoxins from an infection. It may also occur when intestinal motility or morphology is altered.

Acute diarrhoea may lead to excessive water and electrolyte loss and dehydration, and is potentially life-threatening in infants. *Oral rehydration therapy* (ORT) to correct fluid and electrolyte depletion forms the basis of treatment for acute diarrhoea[1-7] and an oral rehydration solution containing essential electrolytes (sodium, potassium, chloride, and bicarbonate or citrate) and glucose is indicated regardless of the age of the patient or the cause of the diarrhoea. A rehydration phase, which involves the replenishment of fluid and electrolytes lost through the diarrhoea, is followed by a maintenance phase to replace continuing losses. Oral rehydration therapy does not stop diarrhoea, which usually continues for a limited period. Oral rehydration therapy may need to be modified if the diarrhoea is associated with malnutrition.[8] (Malnourished children may also benefit from zinc supplementation in acute diarrhoea;[9,10] vitamin A supplementation may also be important in reducing mortality—see p.1359.) The rationale for the composition of oral rehydration solutions is that glucose promotes the active transport of electrolytes, the absorption of which theoretically increases in efficiency as the ratio of carbohydrate to sodium approaches 1:1.[4] WHO recommends a solution containing 90 mmol of sodium per litre and 111 mmol of glucose per litre; this type of preparation is used predominantly in developing countries where diarrhoeas are commonly bacterial in origin. Once initial rehydration has been achieved extra water may be added to the preparation to make a solution containing about 60 mmol of sodium per litre for maintenance. In developed countries viral diarrhoeas, which are associated with less electrolyte loss, are more common. Commercial preparations available in the UK therefore usually provide 35 to 60 mmol of sodium per litre and 90 to 200 mmol of glucose per litre; those with a low sodium content tend to have a higher glucose content to render the solution isotonic.[3] There is now some evidence to suggest that solutions of reduced sodium content and osmolarity may be preferable to conventional WHO solutions, even in developing countries.[11,12] Other areas of debate include the necessity for inclusion of citrate or bicarbonate, and whether cereal-based rather than glucose-based rehydration solutions would be preferable.[13-16] There is considerable evidence that cereal-based solutions tend to produce more rapid resolution of diarrhoea, although one study has suggested that the reduction in stool output is temporary,[17] and another found that a glucose-based solution was equally effective when combined with early re-introduction of feeding.[14] A review of clinical trials concluded that a rice-based rehydration solution should be recommended for patients with cholera, but that there was no reason to change from WHO's glucose-based formulation for children with non-cholera diarrhoea.[18]

Home remedies[2,7] which have been used for oral rehydration include coconut water, rice water, soups, weak tea, and solutions of various salts and sugars; these may be of value when more conventional oral rehydration solutions are unavailable. The use of cordials and soft drinks with low pH and high osmolality, however, may exacerbate diarrhoea and infant deaths have been associated with their use for rehydration.[19]

Severe dehydration associated with acute diarrhoea (greater than 10% loss of body-weight), requires *intravenous rehydration therapy* preferably with Ringer's lactate solution.[2,7] Intravenous therapy is also needed for patients who are unable to drink.

Oral rehydration therapy should be combined with *dietary measures*, particularly in children, to avoid malnutrition owing to low food intake during the illness, and as mentioned above, may need to be modified if the diarrhoea is associated with malnutrition. Breast feeding should be continued throughout rehydration therapy.[19,20] In the case of cows' milk formula feeds dilution has been advocated[20,21] but may not be necessary.[22] Withholding food during diarrhoea in both adults and children is not recommended:[2] feeding may decrease stool output and shorten the duration of diarrhoea.[6]

Oral rehydration therapy prevents dehydration, but does not necessarily shorten the duration of the diarrhoea, and patients therefore frequently desire the symptomatic relief provided by drug therapy. Use of such therapy should be balanced against the risk that it may distract from the need for oral rehydration therapy and may have undesirable side-effects. WHO considers that antidiarrhoeal drug therapy is of limited value, does not reduce fluid and electrolyte loss, may delay the expulsion of causative micro-organisms, and should never be used in children.[23]

The main groups of antidiarrhoeal drugs are adsorbents such as attapulgite, kaolin, and pectin, and drugs which reduce intestinal motility such as diphenoxylate, loperamide, and codeine. Bulk laxatives such as methylcellulose have also been used for symptomatic treatment because of their absorptive capacity. Bismuth salicylate is another compound used in diarrhoea. The calmodulin inhibitor zaldaride is also reported to be effective in providing symptomatic relief.

Antibacterial and antiprotozoal drugs have been used for infective diarrhoeas, including the prophylaxis and treatment of travellers' diarrhoea (see Gastro-enteritis, p.123 and p.574), but their overuse encourages the development of resistance. Prophylactic use should be reserved for adults who are not in good health spending up to 3 weeks in areas where clean food and water cannot be obtained, or when it is important that travel not be interrupted.

Chronic diarrhoea may be associated with underlying disease and therefore symptomatic relief is less appropriate than treatment of the disease itself. For example, cholestyramine will reduce the diarrhoea associated with bile acid malabsorption. Where the disease process responsible for chronic diarrhoea cannot be satisfactorily suppressed, however, symptomatic relief may be appropriate, for example in diabetic diarrhoea (see p.315).

1. WHO Diarrhoeal Diseases Control Programme/Fédération Internationale Pharmaceutique. *The treatment of acute diarrhoea: information for pharmacists*. Geneva: (WHO/CDD/SER/87.11).
2. WHO. *The management and prevention of diarrhoea: practical guidelines*. 3rd ed. Geneva: WHO, 1993.
3. Elliott EJ, *et al*. Sodium content of oral rehydration solutions: a reappraisal. *Gut* 1989; **30:** 1610–21.
4. Avery ME, Snyder JD. Oral therapy for acute diarrhea: the underused simple solution. *N Engl J Med* 1990; **323:** 891–4.
5. Balistreri WF. Oral rehydration in acute infantile diarrhoea. *Am J Med* 1990; **88** (suppl 6A): 30S–33S.
6. American Academy of Pediatrics. Practice parameter: the management of acute gastroenteritis in young children. *Pediatrics* 1996; **97:** 424–35.
7. Sack DA. Use of oral rehydration therapy in acute watery diarrhoea: a practical guide. *Drugs* 1991; **41:** 566–73.
8. Golden MHN, Briend, A. Treatment of malnutrition in refugee camps. *Lancet* 1993; **342:** 360.
9. Roy SK, *et al*. Randomised controlled trial of zinc supplementation in malnourished Bangladeshi children with acute diarrhoea. *Arch Dis Child* 1997; **77:** 196–200.
10. Ruel MT, *et al*. Impact of zinc supplementation on morbidity from diarrhea and respiratory infections among rural Guatemalan children. *Pediatrics* 1997; **99:** 808–13.
11. International Study Group on Reduced-osmolarity ORS Solutions. Multicentre evaluation of reduced-osmolarity oral rehydration salts solution. *Lancet* 1995; **345:** 282–5.
12. Santosham M, *et al*. A double-blind clinical trial comparing World Health Organization oral rehydration solution with a reduced osmolarity solution containing equal amounts of sodium and glucose. *J Pediatr* 1996; **128:** 45–51.
13. Gore SM, *et al*. Impact of rice-based oral rehydration solution on stool output and duration of diarrhoea: metaanalysis of 13 clinical trials. *Br Med J* 1992; **304:** 287–91.
14. Fayad IM, *et al*. Comparative efficacy of rice-based and glucose-based oral rehydration salts plus early reintroduction of food. *Lancet* 1993; **342:** 772–5.
15. Bang A. Towards better oral rehydration. *Lancet* 1993; **342:** 755–6.
16. Islam A, *et al*. Is rice-based oral rehydration therapy effective in young infants? *Arch Dis Child* 1994; **71:** 19–23.
17. Molina S, *et al*. Clinical trial of glucose-oral rehydration solution (ORS), rice dextrin-ORS, and rice flour-ORS for the management of children with acute diarrhea and mild or moderate dehydration. *Pediatrics* 1995; **95:** 191–7.
18. Bhan MK, *et al*. Clinical trials of improved oral rehydration salt formulations: a review. *Bull WHO* 1994; **72:** 945–55.
19. Elliott EJ. Viral diarrhoeas in childhood. *Br Med J* 1992; **305:** 1111–12.
20. Jelliffe DB, Jelliffe EFP. *Dietary management of young children with acute diarrhoea*. 2nd ed. Geneva: WHO, 1991.
21. Kleinman RE. We have the solution: now what's the problem? *Pediatrics* 1992; **90:** 113–15.
22. Chew F, *et al*. Is dilution of cows' milk formula necessary for dietary management of acute diarrhoea in infants aged less than 6 months? *Lancet* 1993; **341:** 194–7.
23. WHO. *The rational use of drugs in the management of acute diarrhoea in children*. Geneva: WHO, 1990.

Diverticular disease

Diverticula are small hernias or pouches of mucosa which develop through the muscular wall of the gut (especially the colon) or other hollow organs; they increase in prevalence with increasing age. Diverticular disease (the presence of colonic diverticula) is usually asymptomatic, but may be associated with symptoms of abdominal pain and altered bowel habit (diverticulosis). Occasionally there may be severe life-threatening complications such as inflammation and necrosis of diverticula (diverticulitis), perforation, fistula formation, obstruction, or haemorrhage.[1,2]

In uncomplicated diverticular disease, treatment is with a high-fibre diet, gradually supplemented if necessary with a bulk laxative such as bran or ispaghula,[1,2] to ease constipation, but such supplements may not relieve the other symptoms of diverticular disease. Antispasmodics such as antimuscarinics or mebeverine may be useful in relieving pain due to muscle spasm.[1]

Diverticulitis requires treatment with broad-spectrum antibiotics and fluid support; analgesia may be needed for severe pain. If peritonitis or abscess develops, surgical intervention may be necessary. Surgical resection is usually considered when fistula, perforation, or obstruction are present.[1,2]

1. Jones DJ. Diverticular disease. *Br Med J* 1992; **304:** 1435–7.
2. Cook TA, Mortensen NJM. Diverticular disease of the colon. *Prescribers' J* 1997; **37:** 213–19.

Dumping syndrome

The word dumping in this context is used to describe the unnaturally rapid transport of gastric contents to the small intestine. The dumping syndrome is an important cause of morbidity following gastro-intestinal surgery, and is thought to be due to the destruction of normal regulatory mechanisms in the upper gastro-intestinal tract.[1-3] Early dumping begins within 10 to 30 minutes of the ingestion of a meal (typically, symptoms are precipitated by hyperosmolar, carbohydrate-rich food) and comprises gastro-intestinal symptoms (fullness, abdominal pain, nausea and vomiting, explosive diarrhoea) and vasomotor symptoms (sweating, weakness, dizziness, flushing, and palpitations). The effects are thought to be due to fluid shifts from the intravascular space to the bowel lumen. Some patients experience late dumping, 1 to 4 hours after a meal, which comprises only the vasomotor symptoms and appears to be due to reactive hypoglycaemia following high carbohydrate concentrations in the small intestine.

The mainstays of therapy are dietary modifications, taking small frequent meals low in carbohydrate, followed by liquids 30 minutes later. Attempts to slow or reduce carbohydrate absorption have involved the use of dietary fibre (guar gum or pectin) or α-glucosidase inhibitors such as acarbose; acarbose and pectin have also been tried in combination.[4] However, such agents may themselves cause gastro-intestinal disturbances and they do not seem to be helpful in most patients.[2] More recently, beneficial results with somatostatin have led to the use of its longer-acting analogue, octreotide.[2,3,5] Octreotide substantially reduces the symptoms of both early and late dumping, probably by slowing gastric emptying and by inhibiting the release of gastro-intestinal mediators (peptide hormones such as neurotensin), and prevents hyperinsulinaemia and subsequent reactive hypoglycaemia. It may be given up to 2 hours before a meal.

In the minority of patients who do not respond to medical therapy surgery may be required.[1,2]

1. Eagon JC, *et al*. Postgastrectomy syndromes. *Surg Clin North Am* 1992; **72:** 445–65.
2. Carvajal SH, Mulvihill SJ. Postgastrectomy syndromes: dumping and diarrhea. *Gastroenterol Clin North Am* 1994; **23:** 261–79.
3. Lamers CBHW, *et al*. Octreotide, a long-acting somatostatin analog, in the management of postoperative dumping syndrome: an update. *Dig Dis Sci* 1993; **38:** 359–64.
4. Speth PAJ, *et al*. Effect of acarbose, pectin, a combination of acarbose with pectin, and placebo on postprandial reactive hypoglycaemia after gastric surgery. *Gut* 1983; **24:** 799–802.
5. Farthing MJG. Octreotide in dumping and short bowel syndromes. *Digestion* 1993; **54** (suppl 1): 47–52.

Dyspepsia

Dyspepsia, also commonly known as indigestion, is a frequent but ill-defined disorder primarily associated with epigastric discomfort or pain. It may be a symptom of specific diseases such as peptic ulcer disease, gastro-oesophageal reflux disease, gastric carcinoma, chronic pancreatitis, or gallstones. However, in many patients there is no identifiable systemic disease, in which case it is known as non-ulcer dyspepsia or functional dyspepsia.

A number of reviews and recommendations have addressed the subject of dyspepsia,[1-8] but despite the frequency with which the disorder occurs, definitive treatment guidelines have yet to be established. The initial management of non-ulcer dyspepsia usually includes advice to avoid alcohol, smoking, and aggravating foods, and to eat small regular meals to aid digestion. Results of studies of drugs for non-ulcer dyspepsia have been variable and difficult to evaluate since the condition tends to be self-limiting, and there is often a large placebo response.

Antacids or *histamine H_2-antagonists* are usually the first drugs to be tried. Antacids frequently give symptomatic relief, and are widely used for self-medication. Studies of H_2-antagonists in non-ulcer dyspepsia have been largely disappointing, but they are often tried, especially for symptoms of reflux. Most authorities consider that a short course of drug therapy may be given to younger patients (under 40 to 45 years of age) lacking obvious symptoms of organic disease before any investigation needs to be performed. However, the use of H_2-antagonists can mask the symptoms of gastric carcinoma, and in older patients who are at greater risk, early investigation may be desirable.

Alternatively, prokinetic drugs such as metoclopramide or cisapride may be given, particularly if an underlying gastro-intestinal motility disorder is suspected. Meta-analysis has suggested that prokinetic therapy may be more effective than an H_2-antagonist in non-ulcer dyspepsia.[9] Other approaches to drug therapy include the use by some people of an insoluble bismuth salt, and the administration of antimuscarinics to relieve spasm. It is not clear whether *Helicobacter pylori* plays any role in the pathology of non-ulcer dyspepsia, but eradication in *H. pylori*-positive patients has been suggested on the grounds that it will benefit patients with undiagnosed peptic ulcer disease and reduce the need for endoscopy.[8]

1. Talley NJ, Phillips SF. Non-ulcer dyspepsia: potential causes and pathophysiology. *Ann Intern Med* 1988; **108:** 865–79.
2. Colin-Jones DG, *et al.* Management of dyspepsia: report of a working party. *Lancet* 1988; **i:** 576–9.
3. Brown C, Rees WDW. Dyspepsia in general practice. *Br Med J* 1990; **300:** 829–30.
4. Heading RC. More deliberations on dyspepsia. *Lancet* 1991; **337:** 1535–6.
5. Bernersen B, *et al.* Is Helicobacter pylori the cause of dyspepsia? *Br Med J* 1992; **304:** 1276–9.
6. Holtmann G, Talley NJ. Functional dyspepsia: current treatment recommendations. *Drugs* 1993; **45:** 918–30.
7. Whitaker MJ, *et al.* Controversy and consensus in the management of upper gastrointestinal disease in primary care. *Int J Clin Pract* 1997; **51:** 239–43.
8. Agréus L, Talley N. Challenges in managing dyspepsia in general practice. *Br Med J* 1997; **315:** 1284–8.
9. Finney JS, *et al.* Meta-analysis of antisecretory and gastrokinetic compounds in functional dyspepsia. *J Clin Gastroenterol* 1998; **26:** 312–20.

Gastro-intestinal spasm

Pain or discomfort of the gastro-intestinal tract may be associated with spasm of the smooth muscle of the gut; such pain and spasm may be associated with the irritable bowel syndrome (below), dyspepsia (above), or diverticular disease (above). Antispasmodic drugs have traditionally been used in patients thought to have gastro-intestinal spasm, and have mainly been of two groups: antimuscarinics such as propantheline, and direct smooth muscle relaxants such as mebeverine; use of antimuscarinics, in particular, has tended to be limited by concern about their adverse effects.

Colic is a general term used to describe spasmodic or griping pain, usually of the viscera (see p.8), and when not otherwise qualified is often understood to refer to pain in the gastro-intestinal tract. Infantile colic is common in children up to about four months of age[1] and tends to be managed by nonpharmacological measures and assessment of the feeding technique. Traditional remedies such as gripe water, which contains essential oils of dill or fennel and is mildly carminative, are of dubious efficacy, and antimuscarinic antispasmodics, although effective[5] may be associated with adverse effects, and are no longer considered appropriate. Simethicone suspension, given before feeds, has sometimes been tried,[2] but has been found to be no better than a placebo.[3] It has been reported that sucrose, given as a 12% solution, improves infant colic.[4]

1. Illingworth RS. Infantile colic revisited. *Arch Dis Child* 1985; **60:** 981–5.
2. Sethi KS, Sethi JK. Simethicone in the management of infant colic. *Practitioner* 1988; **232:** 508.
3. Metcalf TJ, *et al.* Simethicone in the treatment of infant colic: a randomized, placebo-controlled, multicenter trial. *Pediatrics* 1994; **94:** 29–34.
4. Markestad T. Use of sucrose as a treatment for infant colic. *Arch Dis Child* 1997; **76:** 356–8.
5. Lucassen PLBJ, *et al.* Effectiveness of treatments for infantile colic: systematic review. *Br Med J* 1998; **316:** 1563–9.

Gastro-oesophageal reflux disease

Gastro-oesophageal reflux disease (reflux oesophagitis) results from the reflux of gastric or duodenal contents into the oesophagus. Symptoms include heartburn, acid regurgitation, and dysphagia (difficulty in swallowing); oesophageal inflammation, ulceration, and stricture formation may occur. Protracted reflux over several years can lead to the development of Barrett's oesophagus (columnar epithelial metaplasia) which is a risk factor for malignancy.

In the management of gastro-oesophageal reflux disease, simple measures such as weight loss, raising the head of the bed, and avoidance of alcohol, smoking, and aggravating foods such as fats can provide considerable relief of symptoms.[1-4] (In some cases the effectiveness of these interventions has not been shown in controlled trials.[14]) Drugs that reduce gastro-oesophageal sphincter tone and hence exacerbate reflux are best avoided: such drugs include calcium-channel blockers, nitrates, theophylline, benzodiazepines, and antimuscarinics.[1]

Antacids are used for mild disease and as adjuncts to other therapies. Alginate-containing antacids are said to form an alkaline 'raft' that floats on the surface of the stomach contents to impede reflux and protect the oesophageal mucosa; they are more effective than simple antacids for symptomatic relief.[14]

Should more vigorous therapy be needed suppression of gastric acid secretion is a likely next step. In the first instance, particularly in patients with more moderate degrees of oesophagitis, this is likely to be with a *histamine H_2-antagonist* such as cimetidine or ranitidine.[3,4] Although H_2-antagonists have been found to relieve symptoms and reduce antacid consumption, rates of oesophageal healing depend on the severity of the disease and duration of therapy. If symptoms have not resolved within 2 to 3 months of treatment, an increased dosage may be tried. Alternatively, a *prokinetic drug* such as metoclopramide or cisapride may improve gastro-oesophageal sphincter function and accelerate gastric emptying. The value of prokinetic drugs in the treatment of gastro-oesophageal reflux disease is not clear, and their adverse effects may be a problem. The most consistent reports of benefit seem to be with cisapride, alone[5] or combined with an H_2-antagonist.[6,7]

However, a better alternative for resistant disease, or for initial therapy in patients with more severe disease, may be treated with a *proton pump inhibitor* such as omeprazole or lansoprazole. Some commentators note that proton pump inhibitors are increasingly seen as first-line drugs, even in milder disease.[3,8,14]

Regardless of the type of initial therapy, relapse is common. Maintenance with H_2-antagonists has generally been disappointing although some patients respond. A proton pump inhibitor is more effective.[3,4,9] Another approach is to use a combination for maintenance and in a recent comparison omeprazole with cisapride provided more effective maintenance than ranitidine or cisapride alone or in combination.[10]

In patients who have a poor response to drug therapy, or in those with complications such as oesophageal stricture or ulceration, surgery to re-establish gastro-oesophageal competence may be considered.[11,12]

In **infants**, gastro-oesophageal reflux is common but usually resolves spontaneously with increasing age and requires no treatment. Occasionally, it may be associated with complications such as failure to thrive, oesophagitis, and pulmonary symptoms of acid regurgitation but may be managed by upright positioning and the use of thickened foods; drug therapy is controversial. It has been suggested that where drug therapy is needed, an alginate-antacid combination may be appropriate initially, and if necessary cisapride to improve gastric motility.[13] Some favour the combination of cisapride with an antisecretory drug.[15] However, the risk of cardiotoxicity makes the use of cisapride in infants extremely problematic (see p.1187).

1. Katz PO. Pathogenesis and management of gastroesophageal reflux disease. *J Clin Gastroenterol* 1991; **13** (suppl 2): S6–S15.
2. Hixson LJ, *et al.* Current trends in the pharmacotherapy for gastroesophageal reflux disease. *Arch Intern Med* 1992; **152:** 717–23.
3. Klinkenberg-Knol EC, *et al.* Pharmacological management of gastro-oesophageal reflux disease. *Drugs* 1995; **49:** 695–710.
4. Anonymous. The medical management of gastro-oesophageal reflux. *Drug Ther Bull* 1996; **34:** 1–4.
5. Toussaint J, *et al.* Healing and prevention of relapse of reflux oesophagitis by cisapride. *Gut* 1991; **32:** 1280–5.
6. Galmiche JP, *et al.* Combined therapy with cisapride and cimetidine in severe reflux oesophagitis: a double blind controlled trial. *Gut* 1988; **29:** 675–81.
7. Inauen W, *et al.* Effects of ranitidine and cisapride on acid reflux and oesophageal motility in patients with reflux oesophagitis: a 24 hour ambulatory combined pH and manometry study. *Gut* 1993; **34:** 1025–31.
8. Skoutakis VA, *et al.* Comparative role of omeprazole in the treatment of gastroesophageal reflux disease. *Ann Pharmacother* 1995; **29:** 1252–62.
9. Hallerbäck B, *et al.* Omeprazole or ranitidine in long-term treatment of reflux esophagitis. *Gastroenterology* 1994; **107:** 1305–11.
10. Vigneri S, *et al.* A comparison of five maintenance therapies for reflux esophagitis. *N Engl J Med* 1995; **333:** 1106–10.
11. Taylor TV, Holt S. Antireflux surgery: a time for reappraisal. *Br Med J* 1990; **300:** 1603–4.
12. Richter JE. Surgery for reflux disease—reflections of a gastroenterologist. *N Engl J Med* 1992; **326:** 825–7.
13. Anonymous. Managing childhood gastro-oesophageal reflux. *Drug Ther Bull* 1997; **35:** 77–80.
14. Galmiche JP, *et al.* Treatment of gastro-oesophageal reflux disease in adults. *Br Med J* 1998; **316:** 1720–3.
15. Faubion WA, Zein NN. Gastroesophageal reflux in infants and children. *Mayo Clin Proc* 1998; **73:** 166–73.

Haemorrhoids

Haemorrhoids ('piles') are venous swellings of the tissues around the anus: those above the dentate line (the point where the modified skin of the outer anal canal becomes gut epithelium), which usually protrude into the anal canal, are termed internal haemorrhoids, while those below this point are called external haemorrhoids. Due to internal pressure, internal haemorrhoids tend to congest, bleed, and eventually prolapse; with external haemorrhoids painful thrombosis may develop.

Initial treatment of internal haemorrhoids involves a high-fibre diet and avoidance of straining at stool, so bulk laxatives and faecal softeners may be indicated. Small bleeding haemorrhoids may be injected with a sclerosing agent such as oily phenol injection, but rubber band ligation, or perhaps a technique such as infrared coagulation, is more effective and associated with fewer complications.[1,2] More severe and prolonged prolapse generally requires surgery. Surgical excision to remove the clot is used for thrombosed external haemorrhoids.

An enormous range of mainly topical drug treatments is available for symptomatic relief, but in many cases their value is at best unproven.

Topical preparations are usually made up in a lubricating or emollient base. Local anaesthetics may be included to relieve pain, and corticosteroids may be used where infection is not present: preparations containing either group of drugs are intended only for short-term use. Inclusion of antibiotics is thought to be of little value and may encourage the development of resistant organisms. Some preparations include heparinoids. Other agents frequently included for their soothing properties include various bismuth salts, zinc oxide, hamamelis, resorcinol, and peru balsam.

Bioflavonoids and various derivatives of aesculus may also be included in topical preparations; they have also been given systemically in some countries as have some other compounds such as calcium dobesilate and tribenoside, presumably for their supposed action on venous capillary walls.

Other agents which have been employed in the treatment of haemorrhoids include ficaria ('pilewort') and combinations of yeast extract with shark-liver oil.

1. Johanson JF, Rimm A. Optimal nonsurgical treatment of hemorrhoids: a comparative analysis of infrared coagulation, rubber band ligation, and injection sclerotherapy. *Am J Gastroenterol* 1992; **87:** 1601–6.
2. MacRae HM, McLeod RS. Comparison of hemorrhoidal treatment modalities: a meta-analysis. *Dis Colon Rectum* 1995; **38:** 687–94.

Hepatic encephalopathy

Hepatic encephalopathy (portal systemic encephalopathy) is a metabolically related dysfunction of the brain associated with abnormalities of liver function. It may be acute, as in patients with fulminant hepatic failure, or chronic, with acute episodes precipitated by some triggering factor, as in patients with cirrhosis or other chronic liver disease.

Treatment is aimed at identifying any precipitating factor and correcting it, and at decreasing the production of possible toxins in the gut. Precipitating factors include infection, increased protein load due to gastro-intestinal haemorrhage or high protein intake, alcohol abuse, electrolyte imbalance, and certain drugs (notably anxiolytics, hypnotics, and diuretics).

Restriction of dietary protein intake is a mainstay of treatment, but in the long-term, care must be taken to provide adequate protein to avoid muscle wasting and reduced host defence to infection; there is some evidence that vegetable protein is better tolerated than animal protein.[1] The administration of branched-chain amino acids by infusion or as dietary supplements has been tried but their value is uncertain;[1] a meta-analysis of studies on parenteral nutrition with branched-chain amino acids in hepatic encephalopathy indicated improved mental recovery but the adverse effects and impact on mortality were unclear.[2]

Active drug treatment is generally initiated with bowel cleansing by means of a magnesium sulphate enema, especially if the patient is constipated. Lactulose is subsequently the treatment of choice in many cases, particularly in the elderly, the constipated, and those with renal impairment. It reduces colonic pH and absorption of ammonia and aromatic amino acids. Alternatively, locally active antibacterials have been given to reduce the colonic flora. Neomycin is the traditional drug but adverse effects such as ototoxicity and nephrotoxicity may be a problem, particularly if used long-term. Metronidazole[1,3] or vancomycin[4] have been substituted in some patients, but these too have a potential for severe toxicity. A combination of lactulose and neomycin[1] or metronidazole may be tried in patients who fail to respond to single-drug therapy. The lactulose analogue lactitol is also effective,[5,6] and is reportedly more palatable than lactulose. Another approach which has been tried, apparently with some success, in low grade chronic recurrent encephalopathy, is the oral ingestion of *Enterococcus faecium* SF68, in an attempt to produce a more favourable bowel flora.[7]

Investigational therapy has also attempted to affect cerebral function directly. Flumazenil, a benzodiazepine antagonist, has produced beneficial responses in some patients,[8,9] but others have failed to respond.[10,11] Liver transplantation (p.500) is the ultimate therapy for end-stage cirrhosis, acute liver failure, or patients with severe refractory hepatic encephalopathy.[1]

1. Riordan SM, Williams R. Treatment of hepatic encephalopathy. *N Engl J Med* 1997; **337:** 473–9.
2. Naylor CD, *et al.* Parenteral nutrition with branched-chain amino acids in hepatic encephalopathy: a meta-analysis. *Gastroenterology* 1989; **97:** 1033–42.
3. Morgan MH, *et al.* Treatment of hepatic encephalopathy with metronidazole. *Gut* 1982; **23:** 1–7.
4. Tarao K, *et al.* Successful use of vancomycin hydrochloride in the treatment of lactulose resistant chronic hepatic encephalopathy. *Gut* 1990; **31:** 702–6.
5. Riggio O, *et al.* Lactitol in prevention of recurrent episodes of hepatic encephalopathy in cirrhotic patients with portal-systemic shunt. *Dig Dis Sci* 1989; **34:** 823–9.
6. Cammà C, *et al.* Lactitol in treatment of chronic hepatic encephalopathy: a meta-analysis. *Dig Dis Sci* 1993; **38:** 916–22.
7. Loguercio C, *et al.* Long-term effects of Enterococcus faecium SF68 versus lactulose in the treatment of patients with cirrhosis and grade 1-2 hepatic encephalopathy. *J Hepatol* 1995; **23:** 39–46.
8. Grimm G, *et al.* Improvement of hepatic encephalopathy treated with flumazenil. *Lancet* 1988; **ii:** 1392–4.
9. Basile AS, *et al.* The pathogenesis and treatment of hepatic encephalopathy: evidence for the involvement of benzodiazepine receptor ligands. *Pharmacol Rev* 1991; **43:** 27–71.
10. Sutherland LR, Minuk GY. Ro 15-1788 and hepatic failure. *Ann Intern Med* 1988; **108:** 158.
11. Klotz U, Walker S. Flumazenil and hepatic encephalopathy. *Lancet* 1989; **i:** 155–6.

Inflammatory bowel disease

Inflammatory bowel disease covers chronic non-specific inflammatory conditions of the gastro-intestinal tract, of which the two major forms are **Crohn's disease** and **ulcerative colitis.**

Crohn's disease is characterised by thickened areas of the gastro-intestinal wall, with inflammation extending through all layers, deep ulceration and fissuring of the mucosa, and the presence of granulomas; affected areas may occur in any part of the gastro-intestinal tract, interspersed with areas of relatively normal tissue; the terminal ileum is frequently involved. Symptoms depend on the site of disease but may include abdominal pain, diarrhoea, fever, weight loss, and rectal bleeding. Extra-intestinal manifestations may include joint inflammation, skin lesions, mouth ulcers, and liver disorders.

In ulcerative colitis, disease is confined to the colon and rectum, inflammation is superficial but continuous over the affected area, and granulomas are rare. In mild disease, the rectum alone may be affected (proctitis); in severe disease, ulceration is extensive and much of the mucosa may be lost, with an increased risk of toxic dilatation of the colon, a potentially life-threatening complication. Symptoms include diarrhoea and rectal bleeding. The extra-intestinal manifestations are similar to those of Crohn's disease.

Although there are important differences between Crohn's disease and ulcerative colitis which affect their management, the broad principles of treatment, and the drugs used, are similar. A corticosteroid or an aminosalicylate is the first choice in active disease. Corticosteroids have the broadest activity, and are the drugs of choice in more severe disease, dose and route varying with disease severity. For Crohn's disease an elemental diet may be as effective although diet plays a lesser role in ulcerative colitis. The aminosalicylate derivatives may be used to treat mild active disease but are of particular value for maintenance treatment of ulcerative colitis; the role of maintenance treatment in Crohn's disease is not well established. Immunosuppressant therapy may be helpful in chronic active disease.

Active disease. Oral sulphasalazine, a **5-aminosalicylate** derivative (5-aminosalicylic acid linked to sulphasalazine), has been a mainstay in the treatment of active disease for many years. It is of value in producing remission of mild-to-moderate ulcerative colitis and in Crohn's disease affecting the colon, but has produced equivocal results in Crohn's ileitis.[1-4]

The discovery that the 5-aminosalicylate component of sulphasalazine was active led to the development of numerous derivatives, including mesalazine (5-aminosalicylic acid itself in slow-release or enteric-coated form), olsalazine (2 molecules of 5-aminosalicylic acid joined by an azo bond), and a variety of forms in which the active moiety was joined to inert carriers, such as balsalazide. All the above have been shown to be effective in *active ulcerative colitis*, and may be better tolerated than sulphasalazine, since many of the latter's adverse effects are due to its sulphonamide portion. However, in patients who can tolerate sulphasalazine, the newer drugs have no demonstrable advantage,[5] and there is some suggestion that their actions are not the same as those of sulphasalazine.[6] Nevertheless, the risk of adverse effects on starting treatment with sulphasalazine has led to increasing use of the newer derivatives.

Similarly in Crohn's disease mesalazine has been useful in patients with colonic disease and there has been a report of benefit in patients with higher intestinal involvement.[7]

The other major group of drugs used in the treatment of *active ulcerative colitis* and *Crohn's disease* (including ileal disease) is the **corticosteroids**, and in *moderate to severe acute disease* systemic corticosteroids are indicated for initial management.[4,8] Oral prednisolone or prednisone is often used; in the most severe cases hydrocortisone or methylprednisolone may be given intravenously. Dosage is high initially, and is reduced gradually as symptoms improve, but adverse effects remain a problem, hence the interest in poorly absorbed or rapidly metabolised corticosteroids such as beclomethasone, budesonide, fluticasone, or tixocortol. Oral budesonide is effective in inducing remission in Crohn's disease,[9-12] and is probably comparable in effect to conventional corticosteroids;[12] although some suggest that it may be slightly less effective,[11] adverse effects are reduced. It appears to be more effective than mesalazine in inducing remission of Crohn's disease affecting the ileum or colon or both.[34]

In patients with disease confined to the *distal colon* or *rectum*, local topical therapy may be appropriate. Suppositories of prednisolone or mesalazine may be suitable in *mild proctitis*. However, *proctocolitis* involving more of the distal colon is usually treated with enemas of corticosteroids or of mesalazine. Meta analysis has suggested that rectal mesalazine is more effective than rectal corticosteroids in the management of distal ulcerative colitis.[13] Combined oral and rectal mesalazine may be more effective for ulcerative colitis that either alone.[14,15] Systemic corticosteroids are reserved for patients who fail to respond to topical therapy.

Other drugs used in active inflammatory bowel disease include **immunosuppressants**. The majority of studies have been with azathioprine, or its metabolite mercaptopurine. Although these have a slow onset of action, they are of benefit in patients with *Crohn's disease*, particularly if complicated by fistulas, and may be useful in *refractory ulcerative colitis*. Some of the best results have been seen in patients already receiving corticosteroids, and the immunosuppressants have a valuable steroid-sparing effect. Results with cyclosporin have been rather disappointing.[16] Low-dose methotrexate appears to be useful in active Crohn's disease,[17] and probably in ulcerative colitis.[17,18]

There is a limited role for **metronidazole** in inflammatory bowel disease; it has improved the *perineal manifestations of Crohn's disease*. Other antibiotics may be given empirically; ciprofloxacin is reported to have gained favour, despite a lack of evidence from controlled studies,[4] and has been given with metronidazole,[19] although the combination is not very well tolerated. Rifabutin, in combination with a macrolide (clarithromycin or azithromycin) may also be of benefit.[20]

A wide variety of **other drugs** have been tried in active inflammatory bowel disease, including immunoglobulins, interferons, short-chain fatty acids, heparin, factor XIII, chloroquine, omega-3 triglycerides, aminosalicylic acid (4-aminosalicylic acid as opposed to 5-aminosalicylic acid), omeprazole, camostat mesylate, and ketotifen. Interest in the possible role of tumour necrosis factor has led to studies of tumour necrosis factor antibodies, and benefit has been reported with infliximab.[21] Thalidomide, a tumour necrosis factor inhibitor, has also been tried with some benefit,[22] but another such inhibitor, oxpentifylline, was ineffective.[23] Preliminary results, based on the observation that ulcerative colitis is rare in smokers, have suggested that nicotine, supplied via transdermal patch, may have benefit in active disease,[24] although it is ineffective for maintenance.[25] Rectal administration of nicotine is under investigation.

Antidiarrhoeals should be used with caution[4] and avoided completely in severe disease because of the risk of toxic megacolon.[26] Correction of nutritional deficiencies may be necessary in severe disease; some patients have responded to fixed formula diets, but the value of parenteral nutrition to provide "bowel rest" is a matter of debate. Nonetheless in Crohn's disease an elemental diet is as effective as corticosteroid therapy,[4] the chief problem being patient compliance. Diet appears to play only a modest role in the management of ulcerative colitis.

Maintenance of remission. Treatment in patients who achieve remission depends on disease type. The 5-aminosalicylates are of value in the maintenance of remission in *ulcerative colitis*, and are widely used for this purpose, particularly when the danger of relapse is high, although some consider that maintenance treatment offers no advantage over treatment of acute attacks alone. Maintenance for *Crohn's disease* is not well established.[27,28] Results of aminosalicylate maintenance have been conflicting, although some workers consider them encouraging,[27] and it appears that mesalazine can reduce postsurgical recurrence of Crohn's disease.[29] Meta-analysis suggests that overall benefit is unimpressive.[30] It is generally agreed that conventional corticosteroids have no role in the maintenance of remission of either condition; although there is limited evidence that budesonide may prolong the time to relapse in patients with Crohn's disease,[32] low-dose budesonide appears ineffective for this indication.[35] Azathioprine and mercaptopurine have been used for maintenance treatment in Crohn's disease, although it has been suggested that they be withdrawn after four years.[31] A controlled diet, excluding foods that precipitated symptoms, has been reported to maintain remission in patients with Crohn's disease brought to remission by an elemental diet.[33]

Surgery. In patients with ulcerative colitis in whom medical therapy is inadequate surgical colectomy is curative, and may avoid the risks of long-term corticosteroid therapy and the increased risk of bowel cancer to which patients with inflammatory bowel disease are subject. Formation of an ileoanal pouch, which acts as a reservoir for the ileal contents, avoids the necessity for a standard ileostomy and maintains a degree of continence in suitable patients. Curative surgery is not possible in Crohn's disease, since recurrence elsewhere in the gut is almost inevitable, but resection of the affected area becomes necessary in many patients during the course of their illness.

1. Summers RW, *et al.* National cooperative Crohn's disease study: results of drug treatment. *Gastroenterology* 1979; **77:** 847–69.
2. Malchow H, *et al.* European cooperative Crohn's disease study (ECCDS): results of drug treatment. *Gastroenterology* 1984; **86:** 249–66.
3. van Hees PAM, *et al.* Effect of sulphasalazine in patients with active Crohn's disease: a controlled double-blind study. *Gut* 1981; **22:** 404–9.
4. Hanauer SB. Inflammatory bowel disease. *N Engl J Med* 1996; **334:** 841–8.
5. Sutherland LR, *et al.* Sulfasalazine revisited: a meta-analysis of 5-aminosalicylic acid in the treatment of ulcerative colitis. *Ann Intern Med* 1993; **118:** 540–9.
6. Hayllar J, Bjarnason I. Sulphasalazine in ulcerative colitis: in memoriam? *Gut* 1991; **32:** 462–3.
7. Singleton JW, *et al.* Mesalamine capsules for the treatment of active Crohn's disease: results of a 16-week trial. *Gastroenterology* 1993; **104:** 1293–1301.
8. Hanauer SB, Stathopoulos G. Risk-benefit assessment of drugs used in the treatment of inflammatory bowel disease. *Drug Safety* 1991; **6:** 192–219.
9. Greenberg GR, *et al.* Oral budesonide for active Crohn's disease. *N Engl J Med* 1994; **331:** 836–41.
10. Rutgeerts P, *et al.* A comparison of budesonide with prednisolone for active Crohn's disease. *N Engl J Med* 1994; **331:** 842–5.
11. Anonymous. Controlled-release budesonide in Crohn's disease. *Drug Ther Bull* 1997; **35:** 30–1.
12. Campieri M, *et al.* Oral budesonide is as effective as oral prednisolone in active Crohn's disease. *Gut* 1997; **41:** 209–14.
13. Marshall JK, Irvine EJ. Rectal corticosteroids versus alternative treatments in ulcerative colitis: a meta-analysis. *Gut* 1997; **40:** 775–81.
14. d'Albasio G, *et al.* Combined therapy with 5-aminosalicylic acid tablets and enemas for maintaining remission in ulcerative colitis: a randomized double-blind study. *Am J Gastroenterol* 1997; **92:** 1143–7.

15. Safdi M, *et al.* A double-blind comparison of oral versus rectal mesalamine versus combination therapy in the treatment of distal ulcerative colitis. *Am J Gastroenterol* 1997; **92:** 1867–71.
16. Feagan BG, McDonald JWD. Cyclosporin in Crohn's disease. *Lancet* 1997; **349:** 1328.
17. Egan LJ, Sandborn WJ. Methotrexate for inflammatory bowel disease: pharmacology and preliminary results. *Mayo Clin Proc* 1996; **71:** 69–80.
18. Kozarek RA. Methotrexate for refractory Crohn's disease: preliminary answers to definitive questions. *Mayo Clin Proc* 1996; **71:** 104–5.
19. Prantera C, *et al.* An antibiotic regimen for the treatment of active Crohn's disease: a randomized, controlled clinical trial of metronidazole plus ciprofloxacin. *Am J Gastroenterol* 1996; **91:** 328–32.
20. Gui GPH, *et al.* Two-year-outcomes analysis of Crohn's disease treated with rifabutin and macrolide antibiotics. *J Antimicrob Chemother* 1997; **39:** 393–400.
21. Targan SR, *et al.* A short-term study of chimeric monoclonal antibody cA2 to tumor necrosis factor α for Crohn's disease. *N Engl J Med* 1997; **337:** 1029–35.
22. Wettstein AR, Meagher AP. Thalidomide in Crohn's disease. *Lancet* 1997; **350:** 1445–6.
23. Bauditz J, *et al.* Treatment with tumour necrosis factor inhibitor oxpentifylline does not improve corticosteroid dependent chronic active Crohn's disease. *Gut* 1997; **40:** 470–4.
24. Pullan RD, *et al.* Transdermal nicotine for active ulcerative colitis. *N Engl J Med* 1994; **330:** 811–15.
25. Thomas GAO, *et al.* Transdermal nicotine as maintenance therapy for ulcerative colitis. *N Engl J Med* 1995; **332:** 988–92.
26. Mils PR. Management of ulcerative colitis. *Prescribers' J* 1993; **33:** 1–7.
27. Stark ME, Tremaine WJ. Maintenance of symptomatic remission in patients with Crohn's disease. *Mayo Clin Proc* 1993; **68:** 1183–90.
28. Greenberger NJ, Miner PB. Is maintenance therapy effective in Crohn's disease? *Lancet* 1994; **344:** 900–1.
29. McLeod RS, *et al.* Prophylactic mesalamine treatment decreases postoperative recurrent of Crohn's disease. *Gastroenterology* 1995; **109:** 404–13.
30. Cammà C, *et al.* Mesalamine in the maintenance treatment of Crohn's disease: a meta-analysis adjusted for confounding variables. *Gastroenterology* 1997; **113:** 1465–73.
31. Bouhnik Y, *et al.* Long-term follow-up of patients with Crohn's disease treated with azathioprine or 6-mercaptopurine. *Lancet* 1996; **347:** 215–19.
32. Löfberg R, *et al.* Budesonide prolongs time to relapse in ileal and ileocaecal Crohn's disease: a placebo controlled one year study. *Gut* 1996; **39:** 82–6.
33. Riordan AM, *et al.* Treatment of active Crohn's disease by exclusion diet: East Anglian Multicentre Controlled Trial. *Lancet* 1993; **342:** 1131–4.
34. Thomsen OØ, *et al.* A comparison of budesonide and mesalamine for active Crohn's disease. *N Engl J Med* 1998; **339:** 370–4.
35. Gross V, *et al.* Low dose oral pH modified release budesonide for maintenance of steroid induced remission in Crohn's disease. *Gut* 1998; **42:** 493–6.

Irritable bowel syndrome

Irritable bowel syndrome is a functional bowel disorder of abdominal pain and altered bowel habit;[1-7] pain is characteristically relieved by defaecation and may be associated with increase or decrease in stool frequency. There may be abdominal bloating. The value of drug therapy is difficult to demonstrate, given the heterogeneity of symptoms and the high rate of response to placebo.[8] Primary treatment comprises counselling and when necessary dietary modification.[3,4] Drug therapy may bring some benefit if directed at individual symptoms.[7]

In patients in whom *diarrhoea* is predominant, loperamide is the drug of choice;[3,4] it is preferred to other opioid antidiarrhoeal drugs because it does not pass the blood-brain barrier. Alternatively, cholestyramine may be of benefit.[3,4]

The mainstay of treatment in *constipation-predominant* forms of the syndrome is bran or ispaghula to increase dietary fibre.[3,4] Fibre supplementation should be gradual to avoid bloating.[4] A report that bran may exacerbate symptoms of irritable bowel syndrome[9] has been queried.[10] An osmotic laxative or stool softener may be added in patients who fail to respond to fibre, but stimulant laxatives should be avoided.[3,4] Sodium phosphate enemas may be useful for bowel retraining.[3] Although prokinetic drugs such as metoclopramide or domperidone do not show activity on the lower bowel,[4] cisapride has been suggested to be of benefit in constipation-predominant irritable bowel syndrome;[4] however, others consider it ineffective in moderate to severe constipation.[3] An antimuscarinic, given before meals, may be beneficial in patients with episodes of abdominal *pain* after eating.[3] Alternatives include mebeverine,[3,4] or peppermint oil,[3,4] although the ability of the latter to relieve pain has been questioned.[11] Analgesic use needs to be minimised.

Many other drugs have been tried in the irritable bowel syndrome, including activated charcoal, cromoglycate, naloxone, ondansetron, calcium-channel blockers, simethicone, leuprorelin, octreotide, and cholecystokinin antagonists, with variable results.[3,4,8] Patients whose symptoms are associated with mild or masked depression may obtain substantial benefit from antidepressant therapy; a depressed patient with bowel frequency may benefit from a tricyclic antidepressant, whose antimuscarinic effects slow intestinal transit, while one with constipation may be better with a serotonin re-uptake inhibitor, such as paroxetine. There is no evidence to support the use of benzodiazepines in the irritable bowel syndrome.[3,4]

1. Christensen J. Pathophysiology of the irritable bowel syndrome. *Lancet* 1992; **340:** 1444–7.
2. Jones R, Lydeard S. Irritable bowel syndrome in the general population. *Br Med J* 1992; **304:** 87–90.
3. Pattee PL, Thompson WG. Drug treatment of the irritable bowel syndrome. *Drugs* 1992; **44:** 200–6.
4. Weber FH, McCallum RW. Clinical approaches to irritable bowel syndrome. *Lancet* 1992; **340:** 1447–52.
5. Lynn RB, Friedman LS. Irritable bowel syndrome. *N Engl J Med* 1993; **329:** 1940–5.
6. Farthing MJG. Irritable bowel, irritable body, or irritable brain? *Br Med J* 1995; **310:** 171–5.
7. Maxwell PR, *et al.* Irritable bowel syndrome. *Lancet* 1997; **350:** 1691–5.
8. Klein KB. Controlled treatment trials in the irritable bowel syndrome: a critique. *Gastroenterology* 1988; **95:** 232–41.
9. Francis CY, Whorwell PJ. Bran and irritable bowel syndrome: time for reappraisal. *Lancet* 1994; **344:** 39–40.
10. Thompson WG. Doubts about bran. *Lancet* 1994; **344:** 3.
11. Nash P, *et al.* Peppermint oil does not relieve the pain of irritable bowel syndrome. *Br J Clin Pract* 1986; **40:** 292–3.

Mouth ulceration

Ulceration of the oral mucosa (aphthous ulcer or aphthous stomatitis) may be idiopathic and self-limiting, but it may also be caused by mechanical trauma, nutritional deficiencies, drug reactions, or underlying disease.

Where ulceration is due to minor trauma frequent use of a warm saline or compound thymol glycerin mouthwash may be all that is required to relieve discomfort and swelling. Often, however, more active treatment is required. Pain relief may be obtained with local anaesthetics or analgesics but their effectiveness in oral ulceration is limited by their relatively short duration of action when applied topically. Salicylates are widely used, mainly as choline salicylate gel, although they themselves have the potential for local irritation and ulceration. Benzydamine spray or mouthwash may also be helpful although one study found it no more useful than placebo.[1] Lignocaine, as a gel or lozenges, may be of value in pain that has not responded to other measures. Local treatment often involves a topical corticosteroid which is most effective if applied early before the ulcer develops fully. Pellets or lozenges of hydrocortisone allowed to dissolve next to an ulcer, or triamcinolone in an oral paste formulation may be used, although the paste may sometimes be difficult to apply. Mouthwash formulations have been employed particularly when ulceration is widespread in the mouth and a dexamethasone mouthwash has been used effectively.[2] The healing properties of carbenoxolone have also been employed as a gel or mouthwash.

Mechanical protection may be provided by a paste or powder of carmellose sodium, although application may be difficult.

Use of an antiseptic mouthwash such as chlorhexidine or povidone-iodine may be helpful, since secondary bacterial infection can delay healing, but one study found placebo to be as effective as chlorhexidine.[1] Tetracyclines, used as mouthwashes, reportedly reduce ulcer pain and duration,[2-4] but their potential for adverse effects if swallowed must be borne in mind, and their acidity may damage tooth enamel if poorly formulated.[2] Topical application of a tetracycline has been considered the treatment of choice for oral ulceration associated with Behçet's syndrome (p.1018). Use of hydrogen peroxide 3% is inadvisable, as it can cause ulceration, but application of a 1.5% solution to individual ulcers in combination with a topical corticosteroid may be helpful in producing resolution.[2]

A wide variety of other drugs have been tried in aphthous ulceration. Systemic antihistamines have not been found useful,[2] and evidence of value for topical sodium cromoglycate is at best equivocal.[5,6] Sucralfate may be of benefit,[7] and amlexanox is also used. Drugs such as levamisole and thalidomide, although possibly beneficial,[8,9] are unlikely to be suitable in most cases because of their adverse effects, although thalidomide is used, for example, for aphthous stomatitis in patients with AIDS.[10] Oxpentifylline, which, like thalidomide, inhibits tumour necrosis factor production, has been used in patients with minor recurrent aphthous ulceration.[11] Systemic corticosteroids are generally reserved for cases with severe underlying disease. Because anxiety appears to contribute to the development of lesions benzodiazepine anxiolytics have been prescribed where this appears to be a factor,[2] but their use is limited by the need to avoid dependence.

1. Matthews RW, *et al.* Clinical evaluation of benzydamine, chlorhexidine, and placebo mouthwashes in the management of recurrent aphthous stomatitis. *Oral Surg Oral Med Oral Pathol* 1987; **63:** 189–91.
2. Burgess JA, *et al.* Pharmacological management of recurrent oral mucosal ulceration. *Drugs* 1990; **39:** 54–65.
3. Graykowski EA, *et al.* Recurrent aphthous stomatitis: clinical, therapeutic, histopathologic and hypersensitivity aspects. *JAMA* 1966; **196:** 129–36.
4. Henricsson V, Axéll T. Treatment of recurrent aphthous ulcers with Aureomycin mouth rinse or Zendium dentifrice. *Acta Odontol Scand* 1985; **43:** 47–52.
5. Kowolik MJ, *et al.* Di-sodium cromoglycate in the treatment of recurrent aphthous ulceration. *Br Dent J* 1978; **144:** 384–5.
6. Potts AJC, *et al.* Sodium cromoglycate toothpaste in the management of aphthous ulceration. *Br Dent J* 1984; **156:** 250–1.
7. Rattan J, *et al.* Sucralfate suspension as a treatment of recurrent aphthous stomatitis. *J Intern Med* 1994; **236:** 341–3.
8. Miller MF. Use of levamisole in recurrent aphthous stomatitis. *Drugs* 1980; **20:** 131–6.
9. Jenkins JS, *et al.* Thalidomide in severe orogenital ulceration. *Lancet* 1984; **ii:** 1424–6.
10. Jacobson JM, *et al.* Thalidomide for the treatment of oral aphthous ulcers in patients with human immunodeficiency virus infection. *N Engl J Med* 1997; **336:** 1487–93.
11. Pizarro A, *et al.* Treatment of recurrent aphthous stomatitis with pentoxifylline. *Br J Dermatol* 1995; **133:** 659–60.

Nausea and vomiting

Vomiting follows stimulation of the vomiting centre in the medulla of the brain, and closely associated with this centre is the chemoreceptor trigger zone (CTZ) which is sensitive to many drugs and to certain metabolic disturbances. Stimulation of the vomiting centre also occurs following actions on other areas such as the vestibular apparatus of the ear in motion sickness, the cerebral cortex in psychogenic vomiting, and multiple peripheral receptors. In adults vomiting is almost invariably preceded by a sensation of nausea.

As well as being a symptom of gastro-intestinal disease, nausea and vomiting occurs in many conditions including motion sickness, other vestibular disorders such as Ménière's disease, and migraine; it is common in early pregnancy.

Nausea and vomiting are side-effects of numerous drugs, but may be a particular problem with antineoplastics, anaesthetics, opioid analgesics, and the dopaminergic antiparkinsonian drugs levodopa and bromocriptine. It is also a side-effect of radiotherapy.

In situations where it can be anticipated, such as motion sickness, surgery, and cancer therapy, antiemetic drugs are given prophylactically, but if this fails they may need to be given therapeutically. Vomiting of unknown origin should ideally not be treated until the underlying cause has been found. If vomiting is prolonged, dehydration, hypokalaemia, and alkalosis may occur and replacement of fluid and electrolytes may be necessary, especially in young children and the elderly.

Cancer chemotherapy. Nausea and vomiting are common side-effects of cancer chemotherapy[1,2] and for many patients represent a major drawback to treatment.[3] Once experienced, anticipatory vomiting may occur at the sight of medical staff or a needle and this problem may be severe enough in some cases to hinder or prevent further treatment.

Antineoplastic or cytotoxic drugs may induce vomiting by both a central action on the chemoreceptor trigger zone and a peripheral action on the gastro-intestinal tract. The cerebral cortex is probably responsible for anticipatory vomiting. Mechanisms involving 5-HT_3-receptors are important in the pathogenesis of *acute cisplatin-associated vomiting*, whereas different mechanisms are probably involved in *delayed emesis*.

The emetic potential of antineoplastics varies in terms of severity and incidence. Vomiting may be *very severe* with cisplatin, dacarbazine, dactinomycin, mustine, high-dose cyclophosphamide, and streptozocin, and occurs in most patients. *Moderate* vomiting is likely with drugs such as doxorubicin and more modest doses of cyclophosphamide, as well as with high-dose methotrexate, while others such as the vinca alkaloids, fluorouracil, lower doses of methotrexate, chlorambucil, bleomycin, and etoposide *rarely* cause significant vomiting. Emetogenicity may depend to some extent on the dose, route, and schedule of administration. Some combination therapy has resulted in a higher incidence of vomiting than would be expected from the constituents.

The *onset and duration* of vomiting also varies from drug to drug. After cisplatin the onset may be between 4 and 8 hours following a dose, while the duration may be up to 48 hours or occasionally even longer; a persistent feeling of nausea, and sometimes vomiting, lasting for several days may also occur, and requires prolonged antiemetic therapy. After mustine, vomiting may begin within a half to 2 hours, whereas after cyclophosphamide there may be a latent interval of 9 to 18 hours, but in both cases vomiting is generally less prolonged than with cisplatin. *Acute emesis* (that occurring within 24 hours of chemotherapy) has generally been easier to control than *delayed emesis* (that occurring more than 24 hours after chemotherapy).

MANAGEMENT. It is important that effective antiemetic prophylaxis is given from the first course of chemotherapy, to avoid subsequent problems with anticipatory vomiting. With the antiemetic drugs now available it should be possible to control *acute emesis*; *delayed emesis* is more resistant. A variety of drugs has been used in antiemetic regimens including:

- dopamine antagonists such as metoclopramide, domperidone, droperidol, and some phenothiazines
- corticosteroids such as dexamethasone
- 5-HT_3 antagonists such an ondansetron
- cannabinoids such as nabilone
- benzodiazepines such as lorazepam
- antihistamines such as diphenhydramine.

The choice depends on the emetogenicity of the cancer chemotherapy regimen, as well as factors such as the age of the patient. Route of administration and dosage also depend on how emetogenic the chemotherapy is likely to be.

High-dose **metoclopramide** has been one of the most commonly used antiemetics and the standard against which others have been assessed. Plasma concentrations above 850 ng per mL were found to protect against *cisplatin-induced emesis*,[4] but extrapyramidal adverse effects are more frequent at high doses, especially in patients under 30 years of age. Metoclopramide is usually given by continuous intravenous infusion for *highly emetogenic regimens*, sometimes followed by oral administration for several days. It may not provide complete protection, but dexamethasone enhances its effectiveness.[5] Metoclopramide has also been combined with lorazepam[6] and with diphenhydramine;[7] diphenhydramine reduces the risk of extrapyramidal effects.

Dexamethasone is effective on its own against *moderately emetogenic chemotherapy*, but is usually given with other antiemetics such as metoclopramide or ondansetron, especially against *highly emetogenic regimens*. It may be administered intravenously or orally, and at present is probably the most effective single drug against delayed emesis. Its mechanism of action may involve central inhibition of prostaglandin synthesis. A combination of metoclopramide and dexamethasone is more effective than dexamethasone alone against *cisplatin-induced delayed emesis*,[8] but many patients still experience delayed symptoms.[9]

Ondansetron is more effective than metoclopramide in protecting against *acute cisplatin-induced nausea and vomiting*[10,11] and does not cause extrapyramidal effects. It is given intravenously or orally. In common with metoclopramide, the effectiveness of ondansetron against *highly emetogenic chemotherapy* is improved by dexamethasone.[12,13] Ondansetron with dexamethasone has been shown to be more effective than metoclopramide with dexamethasone[14] or than metoclopramide with dexamethasone and diphenhydramine[15] and is better tolerated. For *delayed emesis after cisplatin*, ondansetron appears to be inferior to dexamethasone. For *moderately emetogenic chemotherapy* the advantage of ondansetron over other antiemetics is less clear. Intravenous ondansetron or dexamethasone were both effective in controlling *acute emesis* in one outpatient study but dexamethasone proved more effective in controlling *delayed emesis*.[16] Oral ondansetron was effective when compared with placebo,[17] but less so than dexamethasone intravenously with metoclopramide by mouth.[18] Combining ondansetron with the dopamine antagonist **metopimazine**, both taken by mouth, was more effective than ondansetron alone against *acute* and *delayed emesis* in another study of outpatients with breast cancer receiving *moderately emetogenic chemotherapy*.[19]

Experience with other 5-HT_3 antagonists, such as **granisetron** and **tropisetron**, is more limited. Their effects appear comparable with those of ondansetron,[20-22] and are similarly improved by combination with dexamethasone.[23,24]

Of the other antiemetics that have been advocated in patients undergoing cancer chemotherapy, **domperidone** has been given orally or rectally to patients receiving *moderately emetogenic chemotherapy*; it may be less likely than metoclopramide to cause extrapyramidal reactions. The butyrophenone **droperidol** has been given intramuscularly or intravenously, but is little used now. **Lorazepam** is a short-acting benzodiazepine with sedative and amnestic properties, used in antiemetic regimens (for example, lorazepam with dexamethasone) and may help to prevent *anticipatory nausea and vomiting*. **Nabilone** might be more effective than prochlorperazine (see below), but side-effects are more frequent. **Phenothiazines** are used less often than previously, but may still have a place in the management of outpatients receiving *low to moderately emetogenic chemotherapy*. Prochlorperazine is the most widely used phenothiazine and can be given orally, rectally, or by injection; it is less sedating than chlorpromazine, but severe dystonic reactions are more likely, especially in young children.

Motion sickness. Motion sickness has been described as a normal reaction to stimuli that occur during passive transportation and to which the individual is not adapted. The term embraces all forms of travel sickness including sea sickness, car sickness, train sickness, and air sickness. It is a type of vertigo in which autonomic symptoms predominate, therefore signs and symptoms include pallor, sweating, increased salivation, yawning, malaise, and hyperventilation.

MANAGEMENT. The aim is to *prevent* motion sickness and antiemetics are more effective if given prophylactically rather than after nausea and vomiting has developed. The principal drugs used are the antimuscarinic hyoscine and some of the centrally acting antihistamines. Antiemetic drugs *not* effective against motion sickness include dopamine antagonists such as metoclopramide, domperidone, and chlorpromazine and 5-HT_3 receptor antagonists such as ondansetron.

For short-term protection against motion sickness **hyoscine hydrobromide** by mouth is often the drug of choice. It is taken about 30 minutes before a journey followed by a further dose after 6 hours if necessary. Transdermal administration of hyoscine from modified-release systems markedly prolongs the duration of action, but they need to be applied to the skin several hours before travelling.

The **antihistamines** may be slightly less effective than hyoscine against motion sickness, but are often better tolerated. They are usually given by mouth and include cinnarizine, cyclizine, dimenhydrinate, meclozine, and promethazine; all have similar efficacy, but differ in onset and duration of action and in the extent of side-effects such as drowsiness. Non-sedating antihistamines (e.g. astemizole and terfenadine) penetrate poorly into the CNS and do not appear to be effective against motion sickness.

It has been reported that **ginger** prevents the gastro-intestinal symptoms of motion sickness,[25] but in one study[26] it had no prophylactic effect.

Once motion sickness has developed gastric motility is inhibited and it may be preferable to administer antiemetics intramuscularly rather than by mouth. The intramuscular route has been used in the US space programme for antiemetic sickness medication. In one study promethazine appeared to be the drug of choice for intramuscular use; a 25-mg dose had a duration of action of 12 hours.[27]

Postoperative nausea and vomiting. Postoperative nausea and vomiting is a common and distressing side-effect of anaesthesia and surgery; it may sometimes be more of a problem than pain, especially in day-case surgery.[28-30] The incidence depends on many factors, including the type of anaesthetic, the type and duration of operation, and the sex of the patient (women are more at risk than men). Patients with a history of postoperative vomiting or of motion sickness may be more susceptible.

MANAGEMENT. The aim is prevention and most studies have been directed at this rather than treatment. Routine antiemetic prophylaxis is not necessary in all surgical patients since less than 30% are said to experience postoperative nausea and vomiting.

A popular choice of antiemetic is **metoclopramide** which has been used in both treatment and prevention of postoperative nausea and vomiting; when given prophylactically, results have been variable. **Droperidol** has also been widely used. Phenothiazines such as **perphenazine** and **prochlorperazine** have been used extensively over the years to manage postoperative emesis, especially that associated with opioid analgesics; their duration of action is shorter than that of commonly used opioids therefore repeated dosing may be necessary. Nonetheless, one comparative study of metoclopramide, perphenazine, droperidol, and ondansetron in women undergoing major gynaecological surgery concluded that perphenazine was the drug of choice for routine intravenous antiemetic prophylaxis in this group.[31] Antimuscarinics such as **atropine** or **hyoscine hydrobromide** may be given as part of preoperative medication to reduce salivary and bronchial secretions and to prevent bradycardia; they also have antiemetic activity but again their duration of action is shorter than that of morphine. Transdermal hyoscine has also been tried, but results have been variable. The antihistamine **cyclizine** is also given as a supplement to opioids for premedication and has been effective in postoperative nausea and vomiting. **Promethazine** has also been used for prevention and treatment, but has marked sedative effects. There is a report of a reduced incidence of postoperative vomiting in children given premedication with **clonidine**.[32] **Ginger** has been reported to be similar in efficacy to metoclopramide in preventing postoperative nausea and vomiting,[33] although a lack of effect has also been reported.[34] Variable results have also been reported with **ephedrine**.[35,36] Intravenous **propofol** is reported to be effective in the treatment of established postoperative nausea and vomiting.[37]

Much recent research has focussed on the 5-HT_3-receptor antagonists, and **ondansetron** has been shown to be effective in the treatment and prophylaxis of postoperative nausea and vomiting when compared with placebo;[38-40] comparative studies have indicated that ondansetron is at least as effective as metoclopramide[41,42] or droperidol.[43,44] However a review[45] of several large studies noted that although effective in treatment, it needs to be given to about 4 patients for every 1 in whom further postoperative nausea or vomiting is prevented. **Granisetron,**[46] **dolasetron,**[47] and **tropisetron**[48] have also been tried.

There is less experience with combined antiemetic regimens for postoperative emesis, although ondansetron or granisetron combined with dexamethasone is reportedly more effective than the 5-HT_3-receptor antagonist alone.[49-51] Ondansetron has also been combined with droperidol for the prophylaxis of postoperative emesis.[52]

Pregnancy. Nausea and vomiting or 'morning sickness' is common in the first trimester of pregnancy, but generally does not require drug therapy. Dietary modification such as the taking of small frequent carbohydrate meals often helps. On rare occasions short-term treatment with an antihistamine such as promethazine may be required if vomiting is severe. There have been anecdotal reports of ondansetron being used successfully in life-threatening hyperemesis gravidarum unresponsive to conventional treatment,[53] although a double-blind pilot study found it to be no more effective than promethazine.[54] There is also some evidence that pyridoxine can reduce nausea in pregnancy.[55] For reference to the controversy that has surrounded the risk to the fetus of antiemetic therapy during pregnancy, see under the Precautions of Antihistamines, p.398.

Radiotherapy. With the modification of dosage levels, vomiting is less of a problem than in the early days of radiotherapy, but it depends to some extent on the area of the body irradiated and the type of radiation used. Dopamine antagonists or 5-HT_3-receptor antagonists are given.

1. Grunberg SM, Hesketh PJ. Control of chemotherapy-induced emesis. *N Engl J Med* 1993; **329:** 1790–6.
2. Nicholson M, Leonard RCF. Adverse effects of cancer chemotherapy: an overview of techniques for avoidance/minimisation. *Drug Safety* 1992; **7:** 316–22.

3. Coates A, *et al.* On the receiving end—patient perception of the side-effects of cancer chemotherapy. *Eur J Cancer Clin Oncol* 1983; **19:** 203–8.
4. Warrington PS, *et al.* Optimising antiemesis in cancer chemotherapy: efficacy of continuous versus intermittent infusion of high dose metoclopramide in emesis induced by cisplatin. *Br Med J* 1986; **293:** 1334–7. Correction. *ibid.*; 1540.
5. Allan SG, *et al.* Dexamethasone and high dose metoclopramide: efficacy in controlling cisplatin induced nausea and vomiting. *Br Med J* 1984; **289:** 878–9.
6. Gordon CJ, *et al.* Metoclopramide versus metoclopramide and lorazepam: superiority of combined therapy in the control of cisplatin-induced emesis. *Cancer* 1989; **63:** 578–82.
7. Kris MG, *et al.* Improved control of cisplatin-induced emesis with high-dose metoclopramide and with combinations of metoclopramide, dexamethasone, and diphenhydramine: results of consecutive trials in 255 patients. *Cancer* 1985; **55:** 527–34.
8. Kris MG, *et al.* Controlling delayed vomiting: double-blind, randomised trial comparing placebo, dexamethasone alone, and metoclopramide plus dexamethasone in patients receiving cisplatin. *J Clin Oncol* 1989; **7:** 108–14.
9. Italian Group for Antiemetic Research. Cisplatin-induced delayed emesis: patterns and prognostic factors during three subsequent cycles. *Ann Oncol* 1994; **5:** 585–9.
10. Marty M, *et al.* Comparison of the 5-hydroxytryptamine$_3$ (serotonin) antagonist ondansetron (GR 38032F) with high-dose metoclopramide in the control of cisplatin-induced emesis. *N Engl J Med* 1990; **322:** 816–21.
11. De Mulder PHM, *et al.* Ondansetron compared with high-dose metoclopramide in prophylaxis of acute and delayed cisplatin-induced nausea and vomiting: a multicenter, randomized, double-blind, crossover study. *Ann Intern Med* 1990; **113:** 834–40.
12. Smith DB, *et al.* Comparison of ondansetron and ondansetron plus dexamethasone as antiemetic prophylaxis during cisplatin-containing chemotherapy. *Lancet* 1991; **338:** 487–90.
13. Smyth JF, *et al.* Does dexamethasone enhance control of acute cisplatin induced emesis by ondansetron? *Br Med J* 1991; **303:** 1423–6.
14. Weissbach L. Ondansetron. *Lancet* 1991; **338:** 753.
15. Italian Group for Antiemetic Research. Ondansetron + dexamethasone vs metoclopramide + dexamethasone + diphenhydramine in prevention of cisplatin-induced emesis. *Lancet* 1992; **340:** 96–9.
16. Jones AL, *et al.* Comparison of dexamethasone and ondansetron in the prophylaxis of emesis induced by moderately emetogenic chemotherapy. *Lancet* 1991; **338:** 483–7.
17. Beck TM, *et al.* Efficacy of oral ondansetron in the prevention of emesis in outpatients receiving cyclophosphamide-based chemotherapy. *Ann Intern Med* 1993; **118:** 407–13.
18. Levitt M, *et al.* Ondansetron compared with dexamethasone and metoclopramide as antiemetics in the chemotherapy of breast cancer with cyclophosphamide, methotrexate, and fluorouracil. *N Engl J Med* 1993; **328:** 1081–4.
19. Herrstedt J, *et al.* Ondansetron plus metopimazine compared with ondansetron alone in patients receiving moderately emetogenic chemotherapy. *N Engl J Med* 1993; **328:** 1076–80.
20. Jantunen IT, *et al.* 5-HT$_3$ receptor antagonists in the prophylaxis of acute vomiting induced by moderately emetogenic chemotherapy—a randomised study. *Eur J Cancer* 1993; **29A:** 1669–72.
21. Noble A, *et al.* A double-blind randomised, crossover comparison of granisetron and ondansetron in 5-day fractionated chemotherapy: assessment of efficacy, safety and patient preference. *Eur J Cancer* 1994; **30A:** 1083–8.
22. Ruff P, *et al.* Ondansetron compared with granisetron in the prophylaxis of cisplatin-induced acute emesis: a multicentre, double-blind, randomised, parallel-group study *Oncology* 1994; **51:** 113–18.
23. The Italian Group for Antiemetic Research. Dexamethasone, granisetron, or both for the prevention of nausea and vomiting during chemotherapy for cancer. *N Engl J Med* 1995; **332:** 1–5.
24. Bruntsch U, *et al.* Prevention of chemotherapy-induced nausea and vomiting by tropisetron (Navoban) alone or in combination with other antiemetic agents. *Semin Oncol* 1994; **21**(suppl 9): 7–11.
25. Mowrey DB, Clayson DE. Motion sickness, ginger, and psychophysics. *Lancet* 1982; **i:** 655–7.
26. Stewart JJ, *et al.* Effects of ginger on motion sickness susceptibility and gastric function. *Pharmacology* 1991; **42:** 111–20.
27. Wood CD, *et al.* Effectiveness and duration of intramuscular antimotion sickness medications. *J Clin Pharmacol* 1992; **32:** 1008–12.
28. Rowbotham DJ, Smith G, eds. Supplement on postoperative nausea and vomiting. *Br J Anaesth* 1992; **69**(suppl 1): 1S–68S.
29. Watcha MF, White PF. Postoperative nausea and vomiting: its etiology, treatment, and prevention. *Anesthesiology* 1992; **77:** 162–84.
30. Sung Y-F. Risks and benefits of drugs used in the management of postoperative nausea and vomiting. *Drug Safety* 1996; **14:** 181–97.
31. Desilva PHDP, *et al.* The efficacy of prophylactic ondansetron, droperidol, perphenazine, and metoclopramide in the prevention of nausea and vomiting after major gynecologic surgery. *Anesth Analg* 1995; **81:** 139–43.
32. Mikawa K, *et al.* Oral clonidine premedication reduces vomiting in children after strabismus surgery. *Can J Anaesth* 1995; **42:** 977–81.
33. Phillips S, *et al.* Zingiber officinale (ginger)—an antiemetic for day case surgery. *Anaesthesia* 1993; **48:** 715–17.
34. Arfeen Z, *et al.* A double-blind randomized controlled trial of ginger for the prevention of postoperative nausea and vomiting. *Anaesth Intensive Care* 1995; **23:** 449–52.
35. Rothenberg DM, *et al.* Efficacy of ephedrine in the prevention of postoperative nausea and vomiting. *Anesth Analg* 1991; **72:** 58–61.
36. Liu Y-C, *et al.* Comparison of antiemetic effect among ephedrine, droperidol and metoclopramide in pediatric inguinal hernioplasty. *Acta Anaesthesiol Sin* 1992; **32:** 37–42.
37. Gan TJ, *et al.* Determination of plasma concentrations of propofol associated with 50% reduction in postoperative nausea. *Anesthesiology* 1997; **87:** 779–84.
38. Kenny GNC, *et al.* Efficacy of orally administered ondansetron in the prevention of postoperative nausea and vomiting: a dose ranging study. *Br J Anaesth* 1992; **68:** 466–70.
39. Scuderi P, *et al.* Treatment of postoperative nausea and vomiting after outpatient surgery with the 5-HT3 antagonist ondansetron. *Anesthesiology* 1993; **78:** 15–20.
40. McKenzie R, *et al.* Comparison of ondansetron versus placebo to prevent postoperative nausea and vomiting in women undergoing ambulatory gynecologic surgery. *Anesthesiology* 1993; **78:** 21–8.
41. Malins AF, *et al.* Nausea and vomiting after gynaecological laparoscopy: comparison of premedication with oral ondansetron, metoclopramide and placebo. *Br J Anaesth* 1994; **72:** 231–3.
42. Diemunsch P, *et al.* Ondansetron compared with metoclopramide in the treatment of established postoperative nausea and vomiting. *Br J Anaesth* 1997; **79:** 322–6.
43. Gan TJ, *et al.* Double-blind comparison of ondansetron, droperidol and saline in the prevention of postoperative nausea and vomiting. *Br J Anaesth* 1994; **72:** 544–7.
44. Alexander R, Seingry D. Comparison of ondansetron, droperidol and saline for prevention of nausea and vomiting with patient controlled analgesia following orthopaedic surgery. *Br J Anaesth* 1994; **72**(suppl 1): 121.
45. Tramèr MR, *et al.* A quantitative systematic review of ondansetron in treatment of established postoperative nausea and vomiting. *Br Med J* 1997; **314:** 1088–92.
46. Fujii Y, *et al.* Reduction of postoperative nausea and vomiting with granisetron. *Can J Anaesth* 1994; **41:** 291–4.
47. Kovac AL, *et al.* Treatment of postoperative nausea and vomiting with single intravenous doses of dolasetron mesylate: a multicenter trial. *Anesth Analg* 1997; **85:** 546–52.
48. Zomers PJW, *et al.* Tropisetron for postoperative nausea and vomiting in patients after gynaecological surgery. *Br J Anaesth* 1993; **71:** 677–80.
49. McKenzie R, *et al.* Comparison of ondansetron with ondansetron plus dexamethasone in the prevention of postoperative nausea and vomiting. *Anesth Analg* 1994; **79:** 961–4.
50. López-Olaondo L, *et al.* Combination of ondansetron and dexamethasone in the prophylaxis of postoperative nausea and vomiting. *Br J Anaesth* 1996; **76:** 835–40.
51. Fujii Y, *et al.* Granisetron-dexamethasone combination reduces postoperative nausea and vomiting. *Can J Anaesth* 1995; **42:** 387–90.
52. Koivuranta M, *et al.* The anti-emetic efficacy of a combination of ondansetron and droperidol. *Anaesthesia* 1997; **52:** 863–8.
53. World MJ. Ondansetron and hyperemesis gravidarum. *Lancet* 1993; **341:** 185.
54. Sullivan CA, *et al.* A pilot study of intravenous ondansetron for hyperemesis gravidarum. *Am J Obstet Gynecol* 1996; **174:** 1565–8.
55. Vutyavanich T, *et al.* Pyridoxine for nausea and vomiting of pregnancy: a randomized, double-blind, placebo-controlled trial. *Am J Obstet Gynecol* 1995; **173:** 881–4.

Oesophageal motility disorders

A variety of oesophageal disorders, many due to disturbances in oesophageal motility, may produce non-cardiac chest pain, similar to that of angina pectoris, from which they must be differentiated.

Achalasia. Achalasia is obstruction caused by failure of the lower oesophageal sphincter to relax and permit passage of food into the stomach. It is accompanied by dilatation and abnormal peristalsis in the oesophagus, which acts as a reservoir for the unassimilated matter; symptoms include dysphagia and sometimes pain. The treatment of choice is mechanical dilation of the sphincter,[1] or if necessary surgery. Some studies have found a calcium-channel blocker such as nifedipine to be of benefit,[2-6] but results of other studies conflict.[7] Isosorbide dinitrate has been reported to be more effective than nifedipine, but to produce more adverse effects.[3] More recently, injection of botulinum toxin into the lower oesophageal sphincter has been found to be effective.[8,9] Such an approach has been recommended in patients thought to be at risk from mechanical dilation or surgery,[10] although the choice is less clear in patients with uncomplicated achalasia.

Impaction. The ingestion of an effervescent solution or carbonated drink may be all that is necessary to release an impacted bolus in the oesophagus.[11-13] Removal by endoscopy will be required should the effervescent solution not be effective.

Oesophageal spasm. Oesophageal spasm, although frequently asymptomatic, can produce dysphagia and pain. Treatment of diffuse oesophageal spasm, or its variant 'nutcracker oesophagus' which is characterised by high amplitude peristalsis in the oesophagus, is often ineffective. Antimuscarinics, nitrates, and calcium-channel blockers have been tried in an attempt to relax the smooth muscle, but results are often disappointing: experience with nifedipine in patients with nutcracker oesophagus suggests that decrease in oesophageal pressure may not correlate with reduction in pain.[1]

1. Richter JE, *et al.* Esophageal chest pain: current controversies in pathogenesis, diagnosis, and therapy. *Ann Intern Med* 1989; **110:** 66–78.
2. Bortolotti M, Labò G. Clinical and manometric effects of nifedipine in patients with esophageal achalasia. *Gastroenterology* 1981; **80:** 39–44.
3. Gelfond M, *et al.* Isosorbide dinitrate and nifedipine treatment of achalasia: a clinical, manometric and radionuclide evaluation. *Gastroenterology* 1982; **83:** 963–9.
4. Traube M, *et al.* Effects of nifedipine in achalasia and in patients with high-amplitude peristaltic esophageal contractions. *JAMA* 1984; **252:** 1733–6.
5. Román FJ, *et al.* Effects of nifedipine in achalasia and patients with high-amplitude peristaltic esophageal contractions. *JAMA* 1985; **253:** 2046.
6. Coccia G, *et al.* Prospective clinical and manometric study comparing pneumatic dilatation and sublingual nifedipine in the treatment of oesophageal achalasia. *Gut* 1991; **32:** 604–6.
7. Robertson CS, *et al.* Quantitative assessment of the response to therapy in achalasia of the cardia. *Gut* 1989; **30:** 768–73.
8. Pasricha PJ, *et al.* Intrasphincteric botulinum toxin for the treatment of achalasia. *N Engl J Med* 1995; **332:** 774–8. Correction. *ibid.*; **333:** 75.
9. Cuillière C, *et al.* Achalasia: outcome of patients treated with intrasphincteric injection of botulinum toxin. *Gut* 1997; **41:** 87–92.
10. Cohen S, Parkman HP. Treatment of achalasia—from whalebone to botulinum toxin. *N Engl J Med* 1995; **332:** 815–16.
11. Campbell N, Sykes P. Non-endoscopic relief of oesophageal obstruction. *Lancet* 1986; **ii:** 1405.
12. John DG, *et al.* Non-endoscopic relief of oesophageal obstruction. *Lancet* 1987; **i:** 107.
13. Mohammed SH, Hegedüs V. Non-endoscopic relief of oesophageal obstruction. *Lancet* 1987; **i:** 393.

Peptic ulcer disease

Peptic ulceration is a common condition consisting of a distinct break in the gastro-intestinal mucosa, usually of the stomach or duodenum, although it may occur in the oesophagus, jejunum, or ileum. The resulting duodenal ulcers are rarely malignant but gastric ulcers are more commonly associated with malignancy. Gastric ulcers are often more refractory to drug therapy and may require more prolonged treatment to achieve healing than duodenal ulcers; however, recurrence after healing is less common than with duodenal ulcer.

The aetiology of peptic ulcer disease is probably multifactorial but the bacterium *Helicobacter pylori* appears to play an important role.[1] Abnormalities of normal mucosal defence mechanisms, and, in the case of gastric ulcer, reflux of duodenal contents into the stomach or delayed gastric emptying may also be involved. Other factors include emotional stress, smoking, alcohol, and drugs such as nonsteroidal anti-inflammatory drugs or corticosteroids.

Peptic ulcer disease usually presents as dyspeptic pain, sometimes associated with nausea, vomiting, anorexia, heartburn, or bloating. Patients may develop complications such as bleeding, obstruction, or perforation.

Certain simple measures such as bed rest, dietary modification, and cessation of smoking, may accelerate ulcer healing, but these play an adjuvant role, and the basis of treatment is pharmacological.[2,3] Treatment has traditionally been aimed at neutralising or inhibiting acid activity. Many drugs have been used including antacids, antisecretory drugs, and mucosal protectants such as sucralfate, and have broadly similar efficacy, but once healing is achieved relapse is common. However, with the acceptance of the significance of *H. pylori* infection, combined antibacterial and antisecretory therapy is increasingly recommended as the first line of treatment. Surgical treatment is still employed in patients with acute complications such as perforation, haemorrhage, obstruction, or pyloric stenosis, or in patients with recurrent or intractable ulcer disease, or where there is suspicion of malignancy.

Anti-Helicobacter therapy. The causal role of *H. pylori* in chronic gastritis and duodenal ulcer is now widely accepted.[1,4,5] Eradication of *H. pylori* during healing of duodenal ulcer decreases the incidence of relapse.[6,7] Studies have demonstrated that only 5 to 10% of patients experience relapse within one year of healing if they have undergone *H. pylori* eradication, compared with around 85% of patients who have not,[8] and the benefits appear to be maintained for at least 7 years after treatment.[7] A reduction in the incidence of relapse of benign gastric ulcer has also been demonstrated.[6,9]

The best eradication regimen has not yet been established, and the number of regimens being tried is continually increasing. The first successful and widely used regimens comprised so-called **'triple therapy'** with a bismuth compound (usually tripotassium dicitratobismuthate) and two antibacterials, one a nitroimidazole (metronidazole or tinidazole). A fairly standard regimen is tripotassium dicitratobismuthate with metronidazole and tetracycline hydrochloride, all given for 2 weeks. Variations include the use of an alternative bismuth compound,[10] or the substitution of amoxycillin for tetracycline (although this may be less effective).[11] One-week courses may also be effective.[10] Such a regimen can produce eradication of *H. pylori* in over 80% of patients. However, problems with compliance caused by its complexity and adverse effects, and problems with metronidazole resistance, mean that the benefits may not be so great in clinical practice.[12] Because of these problems there has been a trend in favour of modified triple therapies containing omeprazole, a nitroimidazole, and either amoxycillin or clarithromycin. Such regimens probably only require to be given for 1 week in most cases,[13,14] and consensus seems to be moving in their favour as the current optimal therapy.[15,16] The variants containing clarithromycin may be somewhat more effective than those that do not, although clarithromycin resistance is a problem.[4,17] Very high eradication rates (98%) have been reported from initial studies of the OTC regimen (omeprazole, tinidazole, and clarithromycin) given for as little as 7 days.[18]

Modified regimens using a histamine H_2-receptor antagonist rather than a proton pump inhibitor, together with two antibacterials (for example, ranitidine with amoxycillin and metronidazole) also appear to be effective,[19,20] but a 2-week regimen seems to be required.[4] Another alternative is the use of ranitidine bismutrex, a complex of ranitidine and a bismuth salt, with amoxycillin or clarithromycin, for 2 weeks; some authorities consider a second antibacterial should be added.[4]

Further variations have been tried. A **dual therapy** of omeprazole with amoxycillin or clarithromycin has been used,[17,21] and has the advantage that it is less complex than triple therapy, but there seems to be agreement that it is also less effective.[16] Pretreatment with omeprazole appears to reduce efficacy.[21] Some studies have investigated **quadruple therapy** in which omeprazole is added to a conventional bismuth-based triple therapy regimen, but while some have found this to be superior to triple therapy,[22] others have not.[23] Other proton pump inhibitors, such as lansoprazole, are under investigation as part of anti-Helicobacter regimens and appear to be effective,[24] but experience is limited.

In the longer term, **immunisation** against *H. pylori* is a possibility. Studies in *animals* suggest that an oral vaccine may be able to eradicate active infection[25] as well as protecting against infective challenge.

Other therapy. Historically, treatment of gastric and duodenal ulcers has relied on drugs which neutralise or inhibit acid activity, of which the **histamine H_2-receptor antagonists** (H_2-antagonists) have probably been the most widely used. Single oral doses of cimetidine 800 mg, ranitidine 300 mg, nizatidine 300 mg, and famotidine 40 mg are approximately equivalent in effect. Healing rates achieved with H_2-antagonists in duodenal ulcer generally range from 70 to 90% after 4 weeks of treatment and may be even greater after 8 weeks.[26-29] Gastric ulcers tend to heal more slowly and may require 12 weeks' treatment, but similar healing rates can eventually be achieved. The view that overnight control of gastric acidity is as effective in producing ulcer healing as 24-hour control has led to the use of a reduced single daily dose given at bedtime, thereby reducing adverse effects and improving compliance.[28]

Omeprazole and other **proton pump inhibitors** such as lansoprazole or pantoprazole produce profound and sustained inhibition of gastric acid secretion. A single daily dose of omeprazole is sufficient to provide effective suppression of gastric acid for a 24-hour period,[30] thus aiding patient compliance. Healing rates approaching 100% have been achieved in duodenal ulcers after 2 to 4 weeks of treatment with omeprazole, with slightly lower rates of 70 to 90% achieved in gastric ulcer after 4 weeks of treatment.[3,31,32] Lansoprazole[33] and pantoprazole[34,35] appear to be comparable to omeprazole in efficacy. Although response is more rapid than with other antisecretory drugs, overall healing rates may not differ greatly. However, omeprazole does heal ulcers resistant to a standard course of H_2-antagonist therapy, and has been the treatment of choice in such situations.[2,26]

An **antacid** may be used at the start of antisecretory therapy to provide relief from acid already secreted.[31] Antacids act by neutralisation of acid rather than by preventing secretion; however, aluminium-containing ones may also have a cytoprotective effect via formation of aluminium complexes.[3,36] Although seldom employed as primary therapy since the advent of H_2-antagonists, antacids have been shown to heal duodenal ulcers at a rate comparable to that of H_2-antagonists;[2,3] gastric ulcers may be more resistant.[2] However, the high doses traditionally employed (despite some suggestion that low-dose regimens might be effective[37]) are unpleasant to take.

Numerous other drugs have been tried in peptic ulcer disease. The **prostaglandins** inhibit gastric acid secretion by a direct action on the parietal cells and also have mucosal protectant properties. Analogues of alprostadil, such as misoprostol, are effective in promoting ulcer healing. They have a role in prevention of ulceration induced by nonsteroidal anti-inflammatory drugs (see below). The antimuscarinics have also been used to treat peptic ulceration, notably the M_1-selective antimuscarinic **pirenzepine** which blocked cholinergic stimulation of gastric acid secretion but had few classical antimuscarinic adverse effects at clinically effective doses. The sucrose-aluminium complex **sucralfate** appears to act via a direct cytoprotective effect by binding to proteins in the ulcer base to form a barrier to acid attack, by forming complexes with pepsin, and by stimulating endogenous prostaglandin synthesis in the gastro-intestinal mucosa.[3]

Maintenance or intermittent treatment of relapse. Long-term healing of peptic ulceration can be obtained in many patients given anti-Helicobacter therapy. Where this is not given, peptic ulcer disease is characterised by episodes of relapse and remission and, after withdrawal of therapy, up to 90% of patients with duodenal ulcer and 50% or more of those with gastric ulcer will experience a recurrence of the disease within 12 months.[3,30] Continued maintenance treatment with half the healing dose of an **H_2-antagonist** or **sucralfate** has been shown to reduce this rate of relapse in duodenal ulcer, although some have argued that maintenance with full healing doses of H_2-antagonists or sucralfate might be preferable.[38] Maintenance therapy with once-daily **omeprazole** is also effective.[39]

Even with continuous maintenance therapy some 20% of patients with duodenal ulcer treated with non-antibacterial therapy will experience relapse,[27,30] and there has been debate as to whether complete withdrawal of therapy once healing occurs followed by standard courses of treatment at relapse (intermittent therapy) might not be preferable.[29,30,40,41] Where it is considered that maintenance therapy is not absolutely necessary, therapy at relapse is usually given with **omeprazole** or an **H_2-antagonist** at the full healing dose.

NSAID-induced ulceration. If peptic ulceration develops during treatment with nonsteroidal anti-inflammatory drugs (NSAIDs) the NSAID should be withdrawn if possible. If this can be done, the ulcer may be treated conventionally, with anti-Helicobacter therapy if *H. pylori* is present, but otherwise with an antisecretory drug or a mucosal protectant.[4,5] If NSAIDs are continued, H_2-antagonists are less effective than in idiopathic disease.[42] Some evidence of a protective effect has been demonstrated with ranitidine[43] and some evidence of both duodenal and gastric protection has been demonstrated with high-dose famotidine;[44] however, omeprazole appears to be more effective than an H_2-antagonist.[45] The ulcerogenic effects of NSAIDs have been attributed to inhibition of prostaglandin synthesis and of mucosal cell proliferation and the ulcers they cause may differ from non-iatrogenic ulcers in their pathology and prognosis. Synthetic analogues of alprostadil (prostaglandin E_1) such as **misoprostol**, or of dinoprostone (prostaglandin E_2) have been suggested for the treatment of this condition.[3,26,42,46,47] Misoprostol seems to reduce the incidence of ulcer complications in patients receiving NSAIDs,[48-50] but omeprazole is as effective[51] and is better tolerated and associated with fewer relapses. It is not clear whether eradication of *H. pylori* infection reduces the occurrence of NSAID-induced ulcer,[52,62] and despite a European guideline indicating that eradication should be considered in planned or existing NSAID therapy[15] some doubt the benefits of such a policy.[53]

Stress ulceration. Stress ulceration may occur in the stomach or the duodenum following major physical trauma such as burns or surgery, or after severe sepsis or illness.[29] H_2-antagonists are widely used for the prevention of stress ulceration in high-risk patients in intensive care units although some[54] consider pirenzepine more effective in neurosurgical patients and those with head trauma. It is thought that raising the gastric pH to above 4 by use of intravenously administered H_2-antagonists is effective for prevention of stress ulcer formation.[27,29] Continuous intravenous administration is superior to intermittent administration.[27,29] However, the rise in gastric pH which results from such use may predispose patients to nosocomial pneumonia due to bacterial overgrowth in the stomach and retrograde colonisation of the pharynx.[27,29] Meta-analysis has indicated that sucralfate may be as effective as an H_2-antagonist in reducing bleeding, and is associated with lower rates of pneumonia and mortality.[55] However it remains a matter of debate whether all patients in intensive care should receive prophylaxis or just those considered at high risk.

Bleeding ulcer. Peptic ulceration is responsible for about 50% of all cases of upper gastro-intestinal bleeding. Although many patients cease to bleed without a specific intervention, the condition is potentially life-threatening and in severe cases prompt resuscitation with intravenous fluids and blood may be required. Endoscopic therapy has substantially improved management of patients with severe bleeding or at high risk of rebleeding. Lesions may be treated by thermal methods or by injection sclerotherapy. Repeated endoscopic injection of a fibrin glue may be more effective than sclerotherapy.[56] Adrenaline is often used for its vasoconstrictor properties and may be combined with local heat coagulation[57] or thrombin.[58] If such therapy fails to stop bleeding, or rebleeding occurs, further endoscopic therapy may be considered, but otherwise patients require surgery.

There is little evidence that treatment with H_2-antagonists or omeprazole is useful in the acute management of bleeding, and evidence of value for tranexamic acid is ambiguous. However, once haemorrhage has been controlled, long-term treatment with an antisecretory drug to promote healing and reduce the risk of rebleeding is often given, particularly in frail and elderly patients. Eradication of *H. pylori* is generally recommended, using an appropriate regimen.[59-61]

1. Marshall BJ. Helicobacter pylori: the etiologic agent for peptic ulcer. *JAMA* 1995; **274:** 1064–6.
2. Weir DG. Peptic ulceration. *Br Med J* 1988; **296:** 195–200.
3. Hixson LJ, *et al.* Current trends in the pharmacotherapy for peptic ulcer disease. *Arch Intern Med* 1992; **152:** 726–32.
4. Soll AH. Medical treatment of peptic ulcer disease: practice guidelines. *JAMA* 1996; **275:** 622–9.
5. Ching CK, Lam SK. Drug therapy of peptic ulcer disease. *Br J Hosp Med* 1995; **54:** 101–6.
6. Sung JJY, *et al.* Antibacterial treatment of gastric ulcers associated with Helicobacter pylori. *N Engl J Med* 1995; **332:** 139–42.
7. Forbes GM, *et al.* Duodenal ulcer treated with Helicobacter pylori eradication: seven-year follow-up. *Lancet* 1994; **343:** 258–60.
8. Anonymous. Helicobacter pylori infection—when and how to treat. *Drug Ther Bull* 1993; **31:** 13–15.
9. Axon ATR, *et al.* Randomised double blind controlled study of recurrence of gastric ulcer after treatment for eradication of Helicobacter pylori infection. *Br Med J* 1997; **314:** 565–8.
10. Hosking SW, *et al.* Duodenal ulcer healing by eradication of Helicobacter pylori without anti-acid treatment: randomised controlled trial. *Lancet* 1994; **343:** 505–10.
11. Chiba N, *et al.* Eradication of Helicobacter pylori—meta-analysis to determine optimal therapy. *Gut* 1991; **32:** A1220–A1221.
12. Cottrill MRB. The prevalence of Helicobacter pylori infection in patients receiving long-term H2-receptor antagonists in general practice: clinical and financial consequences of eradication using omeprazole plus amoxycillin or triple therapy. *Br J Med Econ* 1994; **7:** 35–41.
13. Bell GD, *et al.* Rapid eradication of Helicobacter pylori infection. *Aliment Pharmacol Ther* 1995; **9:** 41–6.
14. Labenz J, *et al.* One week low-dose triple therapy for the eradication of Helicobacter pylori infection. *Eur J Gastroenterol Hepatol* 1995; **7:** 9–11.
15. The European Helicobacter Pylori Study Group. Current European concepts in the management of Helicobacter pylori infection: the Maastricht consensus report. *Gut* 1997; **41:** 8–13.
16. Rauws EAJ, van der Hulst RWM. The management of H pylori infection. *Br Med J* 1998; **316:** 162–3.
17. Markham A, McTavish D. Clarithromycin and omeprazole: as Helicobacter pylori eradication therapy in patients with H. pylori-associated gastric disorders. *Drugs* 1996; **51:** 161–78.
18. Bazzoli F, *et al.* Short-term low-dose triple therapy for the eradication of Helicobacter pylori. *Eur J Gastroenterol Hepatol* 1994; **6:** 773–7.
19. Hentschel E, *et al.* Effect of ranitidine and amoxycillin plus metronidazole on the eradication of Helicobacter pylori and the recurrence of duodenal ulcer. *N Engl J Med* 1993; **328:** 308–12.
20. Holtmann G, *et al.* Proton-pump inhibitors or H_2-receptor antagonists for Helicobacter pylori eradication—a meta-analysis. *Lancet* 1996; **347:** 763.
21. Labenz J, *et al.* Omeprazole plus amoxicillin: efficacy of various treatment regimens to eradicate Helicobacter pylori. *Am J Gastroenterol* 1993; **88:** 491–5.
22. de Boer W, *et al.* Effect of acid suppression on efficacy of treatment for Helicobacter pylori infection. *Lancet* 1995; **345:** 817–20.
23. Phull PS, *et al.* One week treatment for Helicobacter pylori infection: a randomised study of quadruple therapy versus triple therapy. *J Antimicrob Chemother* 1995; **36:** 1085–8.
24. Schütze K, Hentschel E. Duodenal ulcer healing after 7-day treatment: a pilot study with lansoprazole, amoxicillin and clarithromycin. *Z Gastroenterol* 1995; **33:** 651–3.

25. Telford JL, Ghiara P. Prospects for the development of a vaccine against Helicobacter pylori. *Drugs* 1996; **52:** 799–804.
26. Colin-Jones DG. Acid suppression: how much is needed? *Br Med J* 1990; **301:** 564–5.
27. Lipsy RJ, *et al.* Clinical review of histamine$_2$ receptor antagonists. *Arch Intern Med* 1990; **150:** 745–51.
28. Deakin M, Williams JG. Histamine H_2-receptor antagonists in peptic ulcer disease: efficacy in healing peptic ulcers. *Drugs* 1992; **44:** 709–19.
29. Feldman M, Burton ME. Histamine$_2$-receptor antagonists: standard therapy for acid-peptic diseases. *N Engl J Med* 1990; **323:** 1672–80 and 1749–55.
30. Bardhan KD. Treatment of duodenal ulceration: reflections, recollections, and reminiscences. *Gut* 1989; **30:** 1647–55.
31. Siepler JK, *et al.* Selecting drug therapy for patients with duodenal ulcers. *Clin Pharm* 1990; **9:** 463–7.
32. Maton PN. Omeprazole. *N Engl J Med* 1991; **324:** 965–75.
33. Ekström P, *et al.* Lansoprazole versus omeprazole in active duodenal ulcer: a double-blind, randomized, comparative study. *Scand J Gastroenterol* 1995; **30:** 210–15.
34. Rehner M, *et al.* Comparison of pantoprazole versus omeprazole in the treatment of acute duodenal ulceration—a multicentre study. *Aliment Pharmacol Ther* 1995; **9:** 411–16.
35. Witzel L, *et al.* Pantoprazole versus omeprazole in the treatment of acute gastric ulcers. *Aliment Pharmacol Ther* 1995; **9:** 19–24.
36. Grim WM. Explaining the cytoprotective properties of an antacid. *Drug Invest* 1990; **2:** 59.
37. Sewing K-F. Efficacy of low-dose antacids in the treatment of peptic ulcers: pharmacological explanation? *J Clin Gastroenterol* 1991; **13** (suppl 1): S134–S138.
38. Bolin TD. Sucralfate maintenance therapy in duodenal ulcer disease: a review. *Am J Med* 1989; **86** (suppl 6A): 148–51.
39. Lauritsen K, *et al.* Omeprazole 20 mg three days a week and 10 mg daily in prevention of duodenal ulcer relapse. *Gastroenterology* 1991; **100:** 663–9.
40. Wormsley KG. Maintenance treatment with H_2 receptor antagonists in patients with peptic ulcer disease: reduces morbidity in a significant minority of patients. *Br Med J* 1988; **297:** 1392 and 1394.
41. Howden CW. Maintenance treatment with H_2 receptor antagonists in patients with peptic ulcer disease: rarely justified in terms of cost or patient benefit. *Br Med J* 1988; **297:** 1393–4.
42. Hawkey CJ. Non-steroidal anti-inflammatory drugs and peptic ulcers. *Br Med J* 1990; **300:** 278–84. Correction. *ibid.*; 764.
43. Robinson M, *et al.* Ranitidine prevents duodenal ulcers associated with non-steroidal anti-inflammatory drug therapy. *Aliment Pharmacol Ther* 1991; **5:** 143–50.
44. Taha AS, *et al.* Famotidine for the prevention of gastric and duodenal ulcers caused by nonsteroidal antiinflammatory drugs. *N Engl J Med* 1996; **334:** 1435–9.
45. Yeomans ND, *et al.* A comparison of omeprazole with ranitidine for ulcers associated with nonsteroidal antiinflammatory drugs. *N Engl J Med* 1998; **338:** 719–26.
46. Ballinger A. Prevention of peptic ulceration in patients receiving NSAIDs. *Br J Hosp Med* 1993; **49:** 767–72.
47. Walt RP. Misoprostol for the treatment of peptic ulcer and antiinflammatory-drug-induced gastroduodenal ulceration. *N Engl J Med* 1992; **327:** 1575–80.
48. Silverstein FE, *et al.* Misoprostol reduces serious gastrointestinal complications in patients with rheumatoid arthritis receiving nonsteroidal anti-inflammatory drugs: a randomized, double-blind, placebo-controlled trial. *Ann Intern Med* 1995; **123:** 241–9.
49. Raskin JB, *et al.* Misoprostol dosage in the prevention of nonsteroidal anti-inflammatory drug-induced gastric and duodenal ulcers: a comparison of three regimens. *Ann Intern Med* 1995; **123:** 344–50.
50. Champion GD, *et al.* NSAID-induced gastrointestinal damage: epidemiology, risk and prevention with an evaluation of the role of misoprostol. An Asia-Pacific perspective and consensus. *Drugs* 1997; **53:** 6–19.
51. Hawkey CJ, *et al.* Omeprazole compared with misoprostol for ulcers associated with nonsteroidal antiinflammatory drugs. *N Engl J Med* 1998; **338:** 727–34.
52. Chan FKL, *et al.* Randomised trial of eradication of Helicobacter pylori before non-steroidal anti-inflammatory drug therapy to prevent peptic ulcers. *Lancet* 1997; **350:** 975–9.
53. Hawkey CJ, *et al.* Helicobacter pylori, NSAIDs, and peptic ulcers. *Lancet* 1998; **351:** 61.
54. Tryba M, Cook D. Current guidelines on stress ulcer prophylaxis. *Drugs* 1997; **54:** 581–96.
55. Cook DJ, *et al.* Stress ulcer prophylaxis in critically ill patients: resolving discordant meta-analyses. *JAMA* 1996; **275:** 308–14.
56. Rutgeerts P, *et al.* Randomised trial of single and repeated fibrin glue compared with injection of polidocanol in treatment of bleeding peptic ulcer. *Lancet* 1997; **350:** 692–6.
57. Chung SSC, *et al.* Randomised comparison between adrenaline injection alone and adrenaline injection plus heat probe treatment for actively bleeding ulcers. *Br Med J* 1997; **314:** 1307–11.
58. Kubba AK, *et al.* Endoscopic injection for bleeding peptic ulcer: a comparison of adrenaline alone with adrenaline plus human thrombin. *Gastroenterology* 1996; **111:** 623–8.
59. Panos MZ, Walt RP. Current management of bleeding peptic ulcer: a review. *Drugs* 1993; **46:** 269–80.
60. Laine L, Peterson WL. Bleeding peptic ulcer. *N Engl J Med* 1994; **331:** 717–27.
61. Jaspersen D, *et al.* Omeprazole-amoxycillin therapy for eradication of Helicobacter pylori in duodenal ulcer bleeding: preliminary results of a pilot study. *J Gastroenterol* 1995; **30:** 319–21.
62. Hawkey CJ, *et al.* Randomised controlled trial of Helicobacter pylori eradication in patients on non-steroidal anti-inflammatory drugs: HELP NSAIDs study. *Lancet* 1998; **352:** 1016–21.

Zollinger-Ellison syndrome

Zollinger-Ellison syndrome is characterised by the presence of a gastrin-producing tumour (gastrinoma) in the pancreas, which leads to hypersecretion of gastric acid and consequent peptic ulcer disease, often with complications such as perforation or bleeding, diarrhoea, or malabsorption.

Initial treatment is aimed at controlling this hypersecretion with an antisecretory drug. Giving enough medication just to control symptoms is not considered adequate, and it is important that acid secretion is reduced below 10 mmol per hour.[1] Once the symptoms have been controlled the tumour can be investigated for surgical removal. When complete removal is not possible then antisecretory therapy is continued indefinitely. Omeprazole (or perhaps lansoprazole) is the drug of choice;[1-3] it profoundly reduces acid secretion with once-daily administration, although relatively high doses of omeprazole are required compared with those used in other conditions.

A histamine H_2-receptor antagonist (H_2-antagonist) such as cimetidine or ranitidine may be used as an alternative to omeprazole,[1] and as with omeprazole doses are higher than those used for other patients. H_2-antagonists have been administered intravenously to control acute acid hypersecretion.

Drug treatment may be combined with vagotomy to reduce acid secretion and to allow lower doses of antisecretory drugs to be used.

The somatostatin analogue octreotide has also been used successfully to treat Zollinger-Ellison syndrome.[4]

For discussion of the treatment of secretory neoplasms in general, including gastrinomas, see under Choice of Antineoplastic, p.477.

1. Maton PN. Zollinger-Ellison syndrome: recognition and management of acid hypersecretion. *Drugs* 1996; **52:** 33–44.
2. Lloyd-Davies KA, *et al.* Omeprazole in the treatment of Zollinger-Ellison syndrome: a 4-year international study. *Aliment Pharmacol Ther* 1988; **2:** 13–32.
3. Maton PN, *et al.* Long-term efficacy and safety of omeprazole in patients with Zollinger-Ellison syndrome: a prospective study. *Gastroenterology* 1989; **97:** 827–36.
4. Mozell EJ, *et al.* Long-term efficacy of octreotide in the treatment of Zollinger-Ellison syndrome. *Arch Surg* 1992; **127:** 1019–26.

Aceglutamide Aluminium (12307-t)

Aceglutamide Aluminium (*rINNM*).

Aceglutamide Aluminum (*USAN*); KW-110. Pentakis (N^2-acetyl-L-glutaminato)tetrahydroxytrialuminium.

$C_{35}H_{59}Al_3N_{10}O_{24}$ = 1084.8.

CAS — 12607-92-0.

Aceglutamide aluminium, a complex of aceglutamide with aluminium hydroxide, is an antacid with general properties similar to those of aluminium hydroxide (p.1177). It is given by mouth in usual doses of 700 mg three or four times daily.

Preparations

Proprietary Preparations (details are given in Part 3)
Jpn: Glumal; ***Spain:*** Glumal.

Acetorphan (14912-w)

(±)-*N*-{2-[(Acetylthio)methyl]-1-oxo-3-phenylpropyl}glycine phenylmethyl ester; *N*-[(*R*,*S*)-3-acetylthio-2-benzylpropanoyl]glycine benzyl ester.

$C_{21}H_{23}NO_4S$ = 385.5.

CAS — 81110-73-8.

Acetorphan is an enkephalinase inhibitor given by mouth in doses of 100 mg three times daily for the symptomatic management of acute diarrhoea (p.1168).

The *S*-form of acetorphan (sinorphan, ecadotril) is reported to be under investigation as an antihypertensive.

References.

1. Baumer P, *et al.* Effects of acetorphan, an enkephalinase inhibitor, on experimental and acute diarrhoea. *Gut* 1992; **33:** 753–8.

Preparations

Proprietary Preparations (details are given in Part 3)
Fr.: Tiorfan.

Acetoxolone Aluminium (3931-l)

Aluminium Acetylglycyrrhetinate. (3-(Acetyloxy)-11-oxoolean-12-en-29-oic acid aluminium complex (3:1)).

$C_{96}H_{141}AlO_{15}$ = 1562.1.

CAS — 6277-14-1 (acetoxolone); 29728-34-5 (acetoxolone aluminium).

Acetoxolone aluminium is a derivative of carbenoxolone. It has been given in a dose of 200 to 300 mg daily by mouth in the treatment of peptic ulcer disease (p.1174) and other gastro-intestinal disorders.

Preparations

Proprietary Preparations (details are given in Part 3)
Ital.: Oriens†.

Multi-ingredient: ***Ital.:*** Sinulene†.

Albumin Tannate (293-x)

Albutannin; Tannin Albuminate.

CAS — 9006-52-4.

Pharmacopoeias. In *Aust.* and *Jpn.*

Albumin tannate, a compound of tannin with albumin, is given by mouth for its astringent properties in the treatment of diarrhoea (p.1168). It is stated to liberate tannic acid (p.1634) in the gastro-intestinal tract.

Preparations

Proprietary Preparations (details are given in Part 3)
Aust.: Tannalbin; ***Austral.:*** Tannalbin†; ***Ger.:*** Albutannin†; Tannalbin; ***Neth.:*** Entosorbine-N; Tannalbin; Tendosimol†; ***Spain:*** Cunticina.

Multi-ingredient: ***Aust.:*** Neoplex; ***Belg.:*** Tanalone; ***Ger.:*** Diaront NN†; Kontabletten†; Neoplex†; Tannacomp; ***Spain:*** Cunticina Adultos†; Cunticina Infantil†; Demusin; Kolotanino†; Neodemusin†; Salitanol Estreptomicina; Salvacolina; ***Switz.:*** Geli-Stop†.

Alexitol Sodium (712-d)

Alexitol Sodium (*BAN, rINN*).

Sodium poly(hydroxyaluminium) carbonate-hexitol complex.

CAS — 66813-51-2.

Alexitol sodium is an antacid with general properties similar to those of aluminium hydroxide (p.1177). It is given in doses of 360 to 720 mg by mouth.

Preparations

Proprietary Preparations (details are given in Part 3)
Irl.: Actal; ***Ital.:*** Actal†; ***S.Afr.:*** Actan; ***UK:*** Actal.

Multi-ingredient: ***UK:*** Magnatol.

Alizapride Hydrochloride (16020-y)

Alizapride Hydrochloride (*rINNM*).

N-(1-Allyl-2-pyrrolidinylmethyl)-6-methoxy-1*H*-benzotriazole-5-carboxamide hydrochloride.

$C_{16}H_{21}N_5O_2$,HCl = 351.8.

CAS — 59338-93-1 (alizapride); 59338-87-3 (alizapride hydrochloride).

Alizapride 50 mg is approximately equivalent to alizapride hydrochloride 55.8 mg.

Adverse Effects and Precautions

Alizapride hydrochloride may be expected to have the adverse effects and precautions of metoclopramide hydrochloride (see p.1200).

Some of the adverse effects that have been reported when alizapride hydrochloride has been used in patients receiving emetic cytotoxic therapy include diarrhoea, sweating, dizziness, hypotension, extrapyramidal symptoms, and isolated cases of convulsions and arrhythmia.

Pharmacokinetics

Alizapride is well absorbed from the gastro-intestinal tract. It is mainly excreted unchanged in the urine and has an elimination half-life of about 3 hours.

Uses and Administration

Alizapride hydrochloride is a substituted benzamide which is used to control nausea and vomiting (p.1172) associated with a variety of disorders. Alizapride hydrochloride is given in usual doses equivalent to 100 to 300 mg of alizapride daily in divided doses by mouth; children have been given 5 mg per kg body-weight daily. It is also given by intravenous or intramuscular injection in doses equivalent to 50 to 200 mg of alizapride daily, and has been given rectally by suppository.

For patients receiving cancer chemotherapy usual daily doses equivalent to alizapride 2 to 5 mg per kg body-weight have been administered intravenously or intramuscularly in 2 divided doses, one 30 minutes before and one 4 to 8 hours after cytotoxic drug administration. For highly emetic cytotoxic regimens requiring doses above 5 mg of alizapride per kg it may be given by intravenous infusion over 15 minutes every 2 hours for 5 doses, starting 30 minutes before cytotoxic administration. It has been recommended that the total dose given with a course of chemotherapy does not exceed 4.5 g.

Preparations

Proprietary Preparations (details are given in Part 3)
Belg.: Litican; ***Fr.:*** Plitican; ***Ger.:*** Vergentan; ***Ital.:*** Limican; Nausilen; ***Neth.:*** Litican; ***Spain:*** Liticum†; Pesalin†; ***Switz.:*** Plitican.

Almagate (19021-z)

Almagate *(BAN, USAN, rINN).*

LAS-3876. Aluminium trimagnesium carbonate heptahydroxide dihydrate.

$AlMg_3(CO_3)(OH)_7,2H_2O = 315.0.$

CAS — 66827-12-1 (almagate); 72526-11-5 (anhydrous almagate).

Almagate is a hydrated aluminium-magnesium hydroxycarbonate. It is an antacid (p.1167) that is given in doses of 1 to 1.5 g by mouth.

Preparations

Proprietary Preparations (details are given in Part 3)
Spain: Almax; Deprece; Obetine.

Almasilate (15333-f)

Almasilate *(BAN, rINN).*

Aluminium Magnesium Silicate Hydrate; Magnesium Aluminosilicate Hydrate; Magnesium Aluminum Silicate Hydrate.

$Al_2O_3.MgO.2SiO_2,xH_2O = 262.4$ (anhydrous).

CAS — 71205-22-6; 50958-44-6.

Almasilate is an artificial form of aluminium magnesium silicate hydrate. It is an antacid (p.1167) that is given in doses of up to about 1 g by mouth.

A hydrated native aluminium magnesium silicate (p.1471) is used as a suspending, thickening, and stabilising agent in pharmaceutical preparations. Attapulgite (p.1178) is another native form.

Preparations

Proprietary Preparations (details are given in Part 3)
Aust.: Gelusil; ***Ger.:*** Gelusil; Lac 4 n; Megalac; Simagel; ***Spain:*** Alubifar; Alufilm†; Alyma†; Mosil†; Sinegastrin; ***Switz.:*** Gelusil.

Multi-ingredient: ***Aust.:*** Gastripan; ***Ger.:*** Gelusil-Lac; Gelusil-LacQuick†; Neo-Pyodron; Ultilac N; ***Ital.:*** Belsar†; ***Spain:*** Dolcopin; Sedo Alufilm†; ***Switz.:*** Gelusil-Lac.

Aloes (7501-f)

Acibar.

CAS — 8001-97-6; 67479-27-0 (aloe gum).

Pharmacopoeias. In *Chin., Eur.* (see p.viii), *Jpn,* and *US.*

The residue obtained by evaporating the juice of the leaves of various species of *Aloe* (Liliaceae).

The Ph. Eur. describes Barbados Aloes (Curaçao aloes) obtained from *Aloe barbadensis* (= *A. vera*) containing not less than 28% of hydroxyanthracene derivatives, calculated as anhydrous barbaloin and Cape Aloes (*Aloe capensis*) obtained mainly from *Aloe ferox* and its hybrids containing not less than 18% of hydroxyanthracene derivatives, calculated as anhydrous barbaloin.

Aloe (USP 23) is Cape Aloe or Curaçao Aloe, yielding not less than 50% of water-soluble extractive.

Barbados aloes is dark brown masses, slightly shiny or opaque with a conchoidal fracture, or a brown powder. Cape aloes is similar, but tinged with green. Barbados and Cape aloes are partly **soluble** in boiling water, soluble in hot alcohol, and practically insoluble in ether. **Store** in airtight containers. Protect from light.

Adverse Effects and Precautions

As for Senna, p.1212, although aloes has a more drastic and irritant action.

Uses and Administration

Aloes is an anthraquinone stimulant laxative but other less toxic drugs are generally preferred.

It is used in homoeopathic medicine.

Aloe vera. Aloe vera gel is a mucilaginous preparation obtained from the leaves of *Aloe vera* (=*A. barbadensis*) once all the sap has drained away.[1] It is widely used in cosmetics and toiletries for a reported moisturising and revitalising action. There are also claims for the beneficial and even curative properties of aloe vera gel in the self-treatment of medical conditions such as acne, haemorrhoids, psoriasis, anaemia, arthritis, burns, cancer, depression, diabetes, glaucoma, multiple sclerosis, peptic ulcer, tuberculosis, and even blindness.[1,2] Evidence to support these claims is lacking.

1. Marshall JM. Aloe vera gel: what is the evidence? *Pharm J* 1990; **244:** 360–2.
2. Hecht A. The overselling of aloe vera. *FDA Consumer* 1981; **15** (July-Aug.): 26–9.

Contraception. A combination of zinc acetate with lyophilised aloe barbadensis has been reported to be an effective spermicide, and has been proposed as a vaginal contraceptive.[1] More usual approaches to contraception are discussed on p.1434.

1. Fahim MS, *et al.* Zinc acetate and lyophilized aloe barbadensis as vaginal contraceptive. *Contraception* 1996; **53:** 231–6.

Preparations

BP 1998: Compound Benzoin Tincture *(Friars' Balsam)*;
USP 23: Compound Benzoin Tincture.

Proprietary Preparations (details are given in Part 3)
Fr.: Vulcase; ***Ger.:*** Aristo L; Dr. Janssens Teebohnen; Krauterlax A; Laxatan†; Leo-Pillen†; ***Switz.:*** Elixir Rebleuten; ***UK:*** Forehead-C; ***USA:*** Dermaide.

Multi-ingredient: numerous preparations are listed in Part 3.

Aloglutamol (12343-d)

2-Amino-2-hydroxymethylpropane-1,3-diol gluconate dihydroxyaluminate.

$C_{10}H_{24}AlNO_{12} = 377.3.$

Aloglutamol is an antacid (p.1167) that is given in doses of 0.5 to 1 g by mouth.

Preparations

Proprietary Preparations (details are given in Part 3)
Ital.: Altris†; Tasto†; ***Spain:*** Pyreses.

Aloin (7502-d)

Aloin *(BAN).*

CAS — 5133-19-7; 8015-61-0; 1415-73-2 (barbaloin).

Aloin is an anthraquinone laxative. Like aloes it is very irritant and other less toxic laxatives are generally preferred. The use of aloin as a flavouring in alcoholic beverages is restricted by law in the UK.

Preparations

Proprietary Preparations (details are given in Part 3)
UK: Beechams Pills†; Calsalettes.

Multi-ingredient: ***Austral.:*** Alophen†; Ford Pills; Slimrite†; ***Belg.:*** Sanicolax; ***Canad.:*** Agarol†; Aid-Lax; Alsiline; Bicholate; Carters Little Pills; Laxa; Thunas Bilettes; Triolax; ***Fr.:*** Neo-Boldolaxine†; ***Ger.:*** Boldo "Dr. Eberth"†; ***Irl.:*** Alophen; ***Ital.:*** Boldina He; Cuscutine; Enteroton Lassativo†; Grani di Vals; ***Spain:*** Alofedina; Laxante Bescansa Aloico; Laxante Geve†; Takata; ***Switz.:*** Ajaka; Carter Petites Pilules; ***UK:*** Alophen; Carters; Dual-Lax Extra Strong.

Alosetron (10697-w)

Alosetron *(BAN, rINN).*

GR-68755X. 2,3,4,5-Tetrahydro-5-methyl-2-[(5-methylimidazol-4-yl)methyl]-1*H*-pyrido[4,3-*b*]indol-1-one.

$C_{17}H_{18}N_4O = 294.4.$

CAS — 122852-42-0.

Alosetron is a 5-HT_3-receptor antagonist with general properties similar to those of ondansetron (p.1206). It is under investigation in the treatment of irritable bowel syndrome and is also being investigated for schizophrenia and other mental disorders.

Basic Aluminium Carbonate (9518-n)

Aluminium Hydroxycarbonate; Basic Aluminum Carbonate *(USAN).*

A combination of aluminium hydroxide and aluminium carbonate.

Basic aluminium carbonate gel is an antacid with general properties similar to those of aluminium hydroxide (below). Doses are given in terms of the equivalent amount of aluminium hydroxide; a dose equivalent to about 1 g of aluminium hydroxide is usually taken.

Basic aluminium carbonate may also be given by mouth as a phosphate binder in the treatment of hyperphosphataemia. For a discussion of the choice of phosphate binders, see Renal Osteodystrophy, p.732.

Preparations

Proprietary Preparations (details are given in Part 3)
Fr.: Lithiagel; ***USA:*** Basaljel.

Multi-ingredient: ***Fr.:*** Dextoma.

Aluminium Glycinate (671-q)

Basic Aluminium Aminoacetate; Dihydroxyaluminum Aminoacetate. (Glycinato-*N,O*)dihydroxyaluminium hydrate.

$C_2H_6AlNO_4(+xH_2O) = 135.1$ (anhydrous).

CAS — 13682-92-3 (anhydrous); 41354-48-7 (hydrate).

Pharmacopoeias. In *Br.* and *US.*

A white or almost white, odourless or almost odourless, powder. The BP specifies 34.5 to 38.5% of Al_2O_3 calculated on the dried substance, and not more than 12% loss of weight on drying. The USP specifies not more than 14.5% loss on drying. Practically **insoluble** in water and organic solvents; dissolves in dilute mineral acids and solutions of alkali hydroxides. A 4% suspension in water has a pH of 6.5 to 7.5.

Aluminium glycinate is an antacid with general properties similar to those of aluminium hydroxide (below). It has been given in doses of up to 1 g by mouth.

Preparations

USP 23: Dihydroxyaluminum Aminoacetate Capsules; Dihydroxyaluminum Aminoacetate Magma; Dihydroxyaluminum Aminoacetate Tablets.

Proprietary Preparations (details are given in Part 3)
Canad.: Robalate†.

Multi-ingredient: ***Aust.:*** Acidrine; Gastripan; ***Belg.:*** Acidrine; Alucid; Normacidine; ***Fr.:*** Acidrine; Gastralgine; Polysilane Reglisse†; Triglysal†; ***Ger.:*** Acidrine; para sanol†; Stomaform†; ***Ital.:*** Acidrine; Anacidase†; Gastrostop; Gefarnil Compositum†; Placacid†; ***Neth.:*** Polysilane Comp†; ***Spain:*** Digestinas Super; Digestinas†; Gastroglutal; Jorkil; Meteoril; Natrocitral; PH 3 Compuesto†; Salvacolina NN†; Secrepat; Triglysal†; Voxaletas†.

Used as an adjunct in: ***Aust.:*** Ambene N; Gaurit; ***Austral.:*** Bufferin†; ***Canad.:*** Bufferin; ***Ger.:*** Fensum N†; ***Ital.:*** Aspirina 03; ***Switz.:*** Bonidon; ***UK:*** Askit; ***USA:*** Buffex.

Aluminium Hydroxide (673-s)

Aluminii Oxidum Hydricum; Aluminum Hydroxide; Wasserhaltiges Aluminiumoxid.

CAS — 21645-51-2 [Al(OH)₃].

NOTE. Compounded preparations of magnesium hydroxide and aluminium hydroxide have the British Approved Name Co-magaldrox; the proportions are expressed in the form *x/y* where *x* and *y* are the strengths in milligrams per unit dose of magnesium hydroxide and aluminium hydroxide respectively.

Pharmacopoeias. In *Chin., Eur.* (see p.viii), *Int., Jpn, Pol.,* and *US.*

Hydrated Aluminium Oxide (Ph. Eur.) [Dried Aluminium Hydroxide; Dried Aluminium Hydroxide Gel] contains the equivalent of 47 to 60% Al_2O_3. It is a white amorphous powder. Practically **insoluble** in water; dissolves in dilute mineral acids and in solutions of alkali hydroxides. **Store** in airtight containers at a temperature not exceeding 30°.

Aluminum Hydroxide Gel (USP 23) is a suspension of amorphous aluminium hydroxide in which there is a partial substitution of carbonate for hydroxide. It is a white viscous suspension from which small amounts of clear liquid may separate on standing. It has a pH of between 5.5 and 8.0.

Dried Aluminum Hydroxide Gel (USP 23) is an amorphous form of aluminium hydroxide in which there is a partial substitution of carbonate for hydroxide. It contains the equivalent of not less than 76.5% of $Al(OH)_3$ and may contain varying quantities of basic aluminium carbonate and bicarbonate. In the labelling requirements the USP states that 1 g of dried aluminum hydroxide gel is equivalent to 765 mg of $Al(OH)_3$. It is a white, odourless, tasteless, amorphous powder. Practically **insoluble** in water and in alcohol; soluble in dilute mineral acids and in solutions of alkali hydroxides. A 4% aqueous dispersion has a pH of not more than 10.0. **Store** in airtight containers.

Algeldrate (*USAN, pINN*) is defined as a hydrated aluminium hydroxide with the general formula of $Al(OH)_3,xH_2O$.

Adverse Effects and Precautions

Aluminium hydroxide in common with other aluminium compounds is astringent and may cause constipation; large doses can cause intestinal obstruction.

Excessive doses, or even normal doses in patients with low-phosphate diets, may lead to phosphate depletion accompanied by increased bone resorption and hypercalciuria with the risk of osteomalacia.

Aluminium salts are not, in general, well absorbed from the gastro-intestinal tract, and systemic effects are therefore rare in patients with normal renal function. However, care is necessary in patients with chronic renal impairment, since osteomalacia or adynamic bone disease, encephalopathy, dementia, and microcytic anaemia, have been associated with aluminium accumulation in patients with chronic renal failure who received large doses of aluminium hydroxide as a phosphate-binding agent. Similar adverse effects have also been associated with the aluminium content of dialysis fluids.

Aluminium hydroxide used as an adjuvant in adsorbed vaccines has been associated with the formation of granulomas.

References to aluminium toxicity in dialysis patients and the possible association between aluminium ingestion and Alzheimer's disease are included under aluminium (see p.1547).

Aluminium accumulation does not generally appear to be significant in patients with normal renal function taking therapeutic doses of aluminium-containing antacids and there is little evidence that aluminium containing antacids are a risk factor for Alzheimer's disease.[1] Elevated plasma-aluminium concentrations have been reported in infants with normal renal function given aluminium-containing antacids but there were no obvious signs of toxicity.[2] However, aluminium accumulation resulting in osteomalacia or encephalopathy with seizures and dementia has been reported in children with renal failure treated with aluminium-containing phosphate binders.[3-7] Aluminium-containing antacids should therefore be used with caution in patients with chronic renal failure, especially in children.

Oral citrate salts increase the absorption of aluminium from the gastro-intestinal tract[8] and patients with renal failure taking aluminium compounds should avoid citrate-containing preparations, which include many effervescent or dispersible tablets.[9,10] Ascorbic acid has also been reported to enhance aluminium absorption.[11]

1. Flaten TP, *et al.* Mortality from dementia among gastroduodenal ulcer patients. *J Epidemiol Community Health* 1991; **45:** 203–6.
2. Tsou VM, *et al.* Elevated plasma aluminum levels in normal infants receiving antacids containing aluminum. *Pediatrics* 1991; **87:** 148–51.
3. Pedersen S, Nathan E. Water treatment and dialysis dementia. *Lancet* 1982; **ii:** 1107.
4. Griswold WR, *et al.* Accumulation of aluminum in a nondialyzed uremic child receiving aluminum hydroxide. *Pediatrics* 1983; **71:** 56–8.
5. Randall ME. Aluminium toxicity in an infant not on dialysis. *Lancet* 1983; **i:** 1327–8.
6. Sedman AB, *et al.* Encephalopathy in childhood secondary to aluminum toxicity. *J Pediatr* 1984; **105:** 836–8.
7. Andreoli SP, *et al.* Aluminum intoxication from aluminum-containing phosphate binders in children with azotemia not undergoing dialysis. *N Engl J Med* 1984; **310:** 1079–84.
8. Walker JA, *et al.* The effect of oral bases on enteral aluminum absorption. *Arch Intern Med* 1990; **150:** 2037–9.
9. Mees EJD, Basçi A. Citric acid in calcium effervescent tablets may favour aluminium intoxication. *Nephron* 1991; **59:** 322.
10. Main J, Ward MK. Potentiation of aluminium absorption by effervescent analgesic tablets in a haemodialysis patient. *Br Med J* 1992; **304:** 1686.
11. Domingo JL, *et al.* Effect of ascorbic acid on gastrointestinal aluminium absorption. *Lancet* 1992; **338:** 1467.

Interactions

As outlined on p.1167, aluminium compounds used as antacids interact with many other drugs, both by alterations in gastric pH and emptying, and by direct adsorption and formation of complexes that are not absorbed. Interactions can be minimised by giving the antacid and any other medication 2 to 3 hours apart.

Pharmacokinetics

Aluminium hydroxide, given by mouth, slowly reacts with the hydrochloric acid in the stomach to form soluble aluminium chloride, some of which is absorbed. The presence of food or other factors which decrease gastric emptying prolongs the availability of aluminium hydroxide to react and may increase the amount of aluminium chloride formed. About 0.1 to 0.5 mg of the cation is reported to be absorbed from standard daily doses of an aluminium-containing antacid, leading to about a doubling of usual aluminium concentrations in the plasma of patients with normal renal function.

Absorbed aluminium is eliminated in the urine, and patients with renal failure are therefore at particular risk of accumulation (especially in bone and the CNS), and aluminium toxicity.

The aluminium compounds remaining in the gastro-intestinal tract, which account for most of a dose, form insoluble, poorly absorbed aluminium salts in the intestines including hydroxides, carbonates, phosphates and fatty acid derivatives, which are excreted in the faeces.

Uses and Administration

Aluminium hydroxide is used as an antacid (p.1167). It is given in doses of up to about 1 g by mouth. Aluminium hydroxide raises gastric pH more slowly than calcium or magnesium antacids and passage through an empty stomach may be too rapid for it to exert any significant acid-neutralising effect. In order to compensate for this and to reduce the constipating effects, aluminium hydroxide is often given in association with a magnesium-containing antacid, such as magnesium oxide or magnesium hydroxide.

Aluminium hydroxide binds phosphate in the gastro-intestinal tract to form insoluble complexes and reduces phosphate absorption. It is thus used to treat hyperphosphataemia in patients with chronic renal failure (see Renal Osteodystrophy, p.732). With this use the dose must be adjusted to the individual patient's requirement but up to about 10 g a day by mouth may be given in divided doses.

Aluminium hydroxide is also used as an adjuvant in adsorbed vaccines.

Polymyositis and dermatomyositis. Corticosteroids form the basis of the management of polymyositis (p.1027) but the calcinosis that may occur in dermatomyositis does not always respond well. Aluminium hydroxide 1.68 to 2.24 g daily produced clinical improvement with complete clearing of most calcified nodules after 1 year in a patient with calcinosis cutis complicating juvenile dermatomyositis.[1] The calcified masses are made up of hydroxyapatite and amorphous calcium phosphate and reduction in phosphate absorption by aluminium hydroxide probably helped to reverse their formation.

1. Wang W-J, *et al.* Calcinosis cutis in juvenile dermatomyositis: remarkable response to aluminium hydroxide therapy. *Arch Dermatol* 1988; **124:** 1721–2.

Preparations

BP 1998: Aluminium Hydroxide Oral Suspension; Aluminium Hydroxide Tablets; Co-magaldrox Oral Suspension; Co-magaldrox Tablets; Compound Magnesium Trisilicate Tablets *(Aluminium Hydroxide and Magnesium Trisilicate Tablets)*;
USP 23: Alumina and Magnesia Oral Suspension; Alumina and Magnesia Tablets; Alumina and Magnesium Carbonate Oral Suspension; Alumina and Magnesium Carbonate Tablets; Alumina and Magnesium Trisilicate Oral Suspension; Alumina and Magnesium Trisilicate Tablets; Alumina, Magnesia, and Calcium Carbonate Oral Suspension; Alumina, Magnesia, and Calcium Carbonate Tablets; Alumina, Magnesia, and Simethicone Oral Suspension; Alumina, Magnesia, and Simethicone Tablets; Alumina, Magnesia, Calcium Carbonate, and Simethicone Tablets; Alumina, Magnesium Carbonate, and Magnesium Oxide Tablets; Aluminum Hydroxide Gel; Aspirin, Alumina, and Magnesia Tablets; Aspirin, Alumina, and Magnesium Oxide Tablets; Aspirin, Codeine Phosphate, Alumina, and Magnesia Tablets; Dried Aluminum Hydroxide Gel; Dried Aluminum Hydroxide Gel Capsules; Dried Aluminum Hydroxide Gel Tablets.

Proprietary Preparations (details are given in Part 3)
Aust.: Anti-Phosphat; *Austral.:* Alu-Tab; Amphojel; Amphotabs†; *Belg.:* Aldrox†; *Canad.:* Alu-Tab; Alugel; Amphojel; Basaljel; *Fr.:* Urfadyn†; *Ger.:* Alu-Cap†; Aludrox; Antacidum OPT; Anti-Phosphat; Gastrocaps A; *Irl.:* Aludrox; *Ital.:* Alucol†; Aludyal†; Diplogel; *S.Afr.:* Alukon; Amphojel; *Spain:* Alugelibys; Dialumet†; Pepsamar; *Switz.:* Alu-Phar†; Anti-Phosphate; Gastracol; *UK:* Alu-Cap; Aludrox; *USA:* ALternaGEL; Alu-Cap; Alu-Tab; Amphojel; Dialume; Nephrox.

Multi-ingredient: numerous preparations are listed in Part 3.

Aluminium Hydroxide-Magnesium Carbonate Co-dried Gel (674-w)

F-MA 11.

A co-precipitate of aluminium hydroxide and magnesium carbonate dried to contain a proportion of water for antacid activity.

Aluminium hydroxide-magnesium carbonate co-dried gel is an antacid with general properties similar to those of aluminium hydroxide (above) and magnesium carbonate (p.1198). It is given in doses of about 400 to 800 mg by mouth.

Preparations

Proprietary Preparations (details are given in Part 3)
Austral.: Almacarb†; Dijene†; *Norw.:* Link; *Swed.:* Link; *UK:* Dijex; Gastrils.

Multi-ingredient: *Austral.:* Algicon; Simeco†; *Belg.:* Barexal; Gastropulgite; Nozid; Syngel; *Canad.:* Algicon†; Amphojel Plus; Diovol; Diovol Plus; Gastrinol; Gastrocalm; Maalox HRF; Thunas Hyperacidity Tablets; *Fr.:* Algicon†; Gastropulgite; *Ger.:* Azulon compositum Homburg†; Colina Spezial; Distra-cid†; Duoventrinetten N; Gastropulgit; *Irl.:* Algicon; Andursil†; Polycrol†; *Ital.:* Belsar†; *Neth.:* Algicon; Rigoletten; *Norw.:* Algicon; *S.Afr.:* Tac-id-4; *Swed.:* Algicon†; *Switz.:* Anacidol; Andursil; Combacid; Gastropulgite; Refluxine; Regla pH; Syntrogel-4†; *UK:* Algicon; Aludrox; Simeco; *USA:* Duracid†; Maalox Heartburn Relief.

Used as an adjunct in: Ger.: Amuno M†.

Aluminium Phosphate (676-l)

Aluminum Phosphate.

CAS — 7784-30-7 ($AlPO_4$).

Pharmacopoeias. In *Fr.* and *Pol.*
Br. includes Dried Aluminium Phosphate. *US* includes Aluminum Phosphate Gel.

Dried Aluminium Phosphate (BP 1998) consists largely of hydrated aluminium orthophosphate and contains not less than 80% of $AlPO_4$. It is a white powder containing some friable aggregates. Practically **insoluble** in water, alcohol, and solutions of alkali hydroxides; soluble in dilute mineral acids. A 4% suspension in water has a pH of 5.5 to 6.5. **Store** at a temperature not exceeding 30°.

Aluminum Phosphate Gel (USP 23) is a 4 to 5% suspension of aluminium phosphate ($AlPO_4$) in water and has a pH of 6.0 to 7.2. It is a white viscous suspension from which small amounts of water separate on standing. It should be stored in airtight containers.

Aluminium phosphate is an antacid with general properties similar to those of aluminium hydroxide (p.1177), but it does not produce phosphate depletion.

Aluminium phosphate is also used as an adjuvant in adsorbed vaccines.

Preparations

USP 23: Aluminum Phosphate Gel.

Proprietary Preparations (details are given in Part 3)
Aust.: Phosphalugel; *Belg.:* Phosphalugel; *Fr.:* Phosphalugel; *Ger.:* Phosphalugel; *Ital.:* Fosfalugel; Fosfidral†; *Spain:* Fosfalumina; Fosfoalugel†; *Switz.:* Phosphalugel.

Multi-ingredient: *Aust.:* Phoscortil; *Fr.:* Isudrine; Lycaon†; Moxydar; *Spain:* Plasmutan†.

Used as an adjunct in: Switz.: Febradolor sans codeine†.

Aluminium Sodium Silicate (677-y)

554; Sodium Aluminium Silicate; Sodium Aluminosilicate; Sodium Silicoaluminate.

CAS — 1344-00-9.

Aluminium sodium silicate is an antacid with general properties similar to those of aluminium hydroxide (p.1177). Aluminium silicate has been used similarly. They are also used as food additives.

Preparations

Proprietary Preparations (details are given in Part 3)
Fr.: Sulfuryl; *Ger.:* Mucal; *Ital.:* Neutralon†.

Multi-ingredient: *Belg.:* Mucal; *Fr.:* Anti-H; Bain Soufre au Sulfuryl; Cerat Inalterable; Mucal; *Ger.:* Enelbin-Paste N; Sulfredox†; Ulgastrin†; *Ital.:* Neutralon Con Belladonna†; *Spain:* Doctogaster; *Switz.:* TRI-OM.

Attapulgite (679-z)

CAS — 1337-76-4; 12174-11-7.

Pharmacopoeias. In *Br.* Activated Attapulgite is included in *Br.*, *It.*, and *US.* Colloidal Activated Attapulgite is included in *US.*

Attapulgite is a purified native hydrated aluminium magnesium silicate essentially consisting of the clay mineral palygorskite. Activated attapulgite is attapulgite which has been carefully heated to increase its adsorptive capacity; it is a light, cream or buff, very fine powder, free or almost free from gritty particles. A 5% suspension in water has a pH of 7.0 to 9.5.

Another native aluminium magnesium silicate is described on p.1471.

Attapulgite is highly adsorbent and is used in a wide range of products including fertilisers, pesticides, and pharmaceuticals. Activated attapulgite is an adsorbent antidiarrhoeal used as an adjunct in the management of diarrhoea (p.1168) in a daily dose of up to 9 g by mouth in divided doses.

Preparations

Proprietary Preparations (details are given in Part 3)
Belg.: Actapulgite; *Canad.:* Fowlers Diarrhea Tablet; Kaopectate; *Fr.:* Actapulgite; Norgagil; *Switz.:* Actapulgite; *USA:* Children's Kaopectate; Diasorb; Donnagel; K-Pek; Kaopectate Advanced Formula; Kaopectate Maximum Strength; Rheaban Maximum Strength.

Multi-ingredient: *Austral.:* Diaguard†; Diarcalm†; Diareze; *Belg.:* Gastropulgite; Mucipulgite; *Canad.:* Diban; Donnagel-PG; *Fr.:* Gastropulgite; Mucipulgite; *Ger.:* Gastropulgit; Neutromil†; *Irl.:* Diocalm; *Ital.:* Streptomagma; *S.Afr.:* Kantrexil; *Spain:* Sorbitoxin†; Terpalate; *Switz.:* Gastropulgite; Mucipulgite; *UK:* Diocalm Dual Action.

Azasetron Hydrochloride (17071-s)

Azasetron Hydrochloride *(rINNM).*

Nazasetron Hydrochloride; Y-25130. (±)-6-Chloro-3,4-dihydro-4-methyl-3-oxo-*N*-3-quinuclidinyl-2*H*-1,4-benzoxazine-8-carboxamide hydrochloride.

$C_{17}H_{20}ClN_3O_3,HCl$ = 386.3.

CAS — 123040-69-7 (azasetron); 141922-90-9 (azasetron hydrochloride).

Azasetron hydrochloride is a highly selective 5-HT_3-receptor antagonist with general properties similar to those of ondansetron (p.1206). It is used as an antiemetic in the management of nausea and vomiting induced by cytotoxic therapy, in usual doses of 10 mg daily by intravenous administration.

Preparations

Proprietary Preparations (details are given in Part 3)
Jpn: Serotone.

Balsalazide Disodium (18555-j)

Balsalazide Disodium *(USAN, rINNM).*

Balsalazide Sodium *(BANM)*; Balsalazine Disodium; BX-661A. 5-[4-(2-Carboxyethylcarbamoyl)phenylazo]salicylic acid, disodium salt, dihydrate.

$C_{17}H_{13}N_3Na_2O_6,2H_2O$ = 437.3.

CAS — 80573-04-2 (balsalazide); 150399-21-6 (balsalazide disodium dihydrate).

Adverse Effects and Precautions

As for Mesalazine, p.1199. If a blood dyscrasia is suspected treatment should be stopped immediately and a blood count performed. Patients or their carers should be told how to recognise signs of blood toxicity and should be advised to seek immediate medical attention if symptoms such as fever, sore throat, mouth ulcers, bruising, or bleeding develop. Balsalazide should not be used in patients with severe hepatic impairment or moderate or severe renal function impairment; care is required in those with lesser degrees of impairment, and in asthma, bleeding disorders, or active peptic ulcer disease.

Effects on fertility. Three men suffered infertility while taking sulphasalazine 2 to 3 g daily;[1] sperm count and motility returned to normal in 2 after taking balsalazide 2 g daily instead of sulphasalazine, and presumably in the third whose wife became pregnant. There was no relapse of their ulcerative colitis.

1. McIntyre PB, Lennard-Jones JE. Reversal with balsalazide of infertility caused by sulphasalazine. *Br Med J* 1984; **288:** 1652–3.

Uses and Administration

Balsalazide, which consists of mesalazine linked to 4-aminobenzoylalanine, is a prodrug of mesalazine with similar properties (p.1200). Balsalazide disodium is given by mouth in the treatment of mild to moderate active ulcerative colitis, in a dose of 2.25 g three times daily.

General references.

1. Prakash A, Spencer CM. Balsalazide. *Drugs* 1998; **56:** 83–9.

Inflammatory bowel disease. A study[1] has suggested that balsalazide 6.75 g by mouth daily was more effective than delayed-release mesalazine (Asacol) 2.4 g daily in producing remission in patients with acute ulcerative colitis (p.1171). Balsalazide also appeared to be better tolerated.

1. Green JRB, *et al.* Balsalazide is more effective and better tolerated than mesalamine in the treatment of acute ulcerative colitis. *Gastroenterology* 1998; **114:** 15–22.

Preparations

Proprietary Preparations (details are given in Part 3)
UK: Colazide.

Batanopride Hydrochloride (10928-s)

Batanopride Hydrochloride *(USAN, pINNM).*

BMY-25801-01. (±)-4-Amino-5-chloro-*N*-[2-(diethylamino)ethyl]-2-[(1-methylacetonyl)oxy]benzamide hydrochloride.

$C_{17}H_{26}ClN_3O_3,HCl$ = 392.3.

CAS — 102670-46-2 (batanopride); 102670-59-7 (batanopride hydrochloride).

Batanopride hydrochloride is a 5-HT_3-receptor antagonist under investigation as an antiemetic for the management of chemotherapy-induced nausea and vomiting.

Benexate Hydrochloride (3666-e)

Benexate Hydrochloride *(rINNM).*

Benzyl salicylate *trans*-4-(guanidinomethyl)cyclohexanecarboxylate hydrochloride.

$C_{23}H_{27}N_3O_4,HCl$ = 445.9.

CAS — 78718-52-2 (benexate); 78718-25-9 (benexate hydrochloride).

Benexate hydrochloride has been used in the management of peptic ulcer disease. It has been given by mouth as the clathrate with β-cyclodextrin, benexate betadex.

Benzquinamide Hydrochloride (6542-d)

Benzquinamide Hydrochloride *(BANM, rINNM).*

NSC-64375 (benzquinamide); P-2647 (benzquinamide). 3-Diethylcarbamoyl-1,3,4,6,7,11b-hexahydro-9,10-dimethoxy-2*H*-benzo[*a*]quinolizin-2-yl acetate hydrochloride.

$C_{22}H_{32}N_2O_5,HCl$ = 441.0.

CAS — 63-12-7 (benzquinamide); 113-69-9 (benzquinamide hydrochloride).

NOTE. Benzquinamide is *USAN.*

Benzquinamide 50 mg is approximately equivalent to benzquinamide hydrochloride 54.5 mg.

Incompatibilities. Benzquinamide hydrochloride has been reported to be incompatible with chlordiazepoxide hydrochloride, diazepam, pentobarbitone sodium, phenobarbitone sodium, quinalbarbitone sodium, and thiopentone sodium. The injection should not be reconstituted with sodium chloride 0.9% solution as precipitation may occur.

Adverse Effects and Precautions

The most common side-effect associated with benzquinamide hydrochloride is drowsiness. Other side-effects reported include antimuscarinic, cardiovascular, and extrapyramidal effects; hypersensitivity reactions such as skin rashes have also occurred.

Intravenous administration may cause a sudden increase in blood pressure and transient arrhythmias; this route should not be used in patients with cardiovascular disease or in those receiving pre-anaesthetic or cardiovascular drugs. Intramuscular administration is preferred.

Extrapyramidal effects. Single cases[1,2] of acute dystonic reactions following benzquinamide administration.

1. Rose TE, Averbuch SD. Acute dystonic reaction due to benzquinamide. *Ann Intern Med* 1975; **83:** 231–2.
2. Grove WR, *et al.* A benzquinamide-induced extrapyramidal reaction. *Drug Intell Clin Pharm* 1976; **10:** 638–9.

Interactions

Because of the risk of additive effects on blood pressure, benzquinamide should be given with caution, and in fractions of the normal dose, to patients receiving pressor agents or other drugs with sympathomimetic action resembling those of adrenaline.

Pharmacokinetics

The bioavailability of benzquinamide is low, and it is normally given by parenteral administration. It is metabolised in the liver and excreted in the urine and bile; less than 10% is excreted as unchanged drug in the urine. The half-life of benzquinamide in plasma is stated to be about 40 minutes. About 58% is bound to plasma protein.

References.

1. Hobbs DC, Connolly AG. Pharmacokinetics of benzquinamide in man. *J Pharmacokinet Biopharm* 1978; **6:** 477–85.

Uses and Administration

Benzquinamide hydrochloride is a benzoquinolizine derivative with antiemetic properties used to control postoperative nausea and vomiting (p.1172).

Benzquinamide hydrochloride is administered by deep intramuscular injection in a dose equivalent to 50 mg of benzquinamide. It acts within about 15 minutes of injection and a second dose of 50 mg may be given 1 hour later if necessary; subsequent doses of 50 mg may be repeated every 3 to 4 hours as necessary. It may also be given by slow intravenous injection in a dose of 25 mg administered over 30 to 60 seconds in selected patients; subsequent doses should be given intramuscularly.

Preparations

Proprietary Preparations (details are given in Part 3)
USA: Emete-con†.

Bisacodyl (7503-n)

Bisacodyl *(BAN, rINN).*

Bisacodylum. 4,4′-(2-Pyridylmethylene)di(phenyl acetate).

$C_{22}H_{19}NO_4$ = 361.4.

CAS — 603-50-9 (bisacodyl); 1336-29-4 (bisacodyl tannex).

NOTE. Bisacodyl Tannex is *USAN.*

Pharmacopoeias. In *Eur.* (see p.viii), *Jpn, Pol.,* and *US.*

A white or almost white crystalline powder. Ph. Eur. **solubilities** are: practically insoluble in water; sparingly soluble in alcohol; soluble in acetone; slightly soluble in ether; dissolves in dilute mineral acids. USP solubilities are: practically insoluble in water; soluble 1 in 210 of alcohol, 1 in 275 of ether and 1 in 2.5 of chloroform; sparingly soluble in methyl alcohol. **Protect** from light.

CAUTION. Avoid inhalation of the powder and contact with eyes, skin, and mucous membranes.

Adverse Effects

Bisacodyl may cause abdominal discomfort such as colic or cramps. When administered rectally it sometimes causes irritation and repeated use may cause proctitis or sloughing of the epithelium. To avoid gastric irritation bisacodyl tablets are enteric-coated. Prolonged use or overdosage can result in diarrhoea with excessive loss of water and electrolytes, particularly potassium; there is also the possibility of developing an atonic non-functioning colon.

Precautions

Bisacodyl should not be given to patients with intestinal obstruction or with undiagnosed abdominal symptoms; care should also be taken in patients with inflammatory bowel disease. The suppositories should be used with caution in patients with rectal fissures or ulcerated haemorrhoids. Prolonged use should be avoided.

Bisacodyl suppositories may cause a profound inflammatory reaction in the rectum and so if used prior to sigmoidoscopy the mucosal appearances are difficult to interpret.[1]

1. Colin-Jones DG. Drug-induced gastrointestinal ulceration and bleeding. *Prescribers' J* 1981; **21:** 209–15.

Pharmacokinetics

Following administration of bisacodyl by mouth or rectally, it is rapidly converted to the active metabolite bis(*p*-hydroxyphenyl)pyridyl-2-methane. Absorption from the gastro-intestinal tract is minimal; the small amount absorbed is excreted in the urine as the glucuronide. Bisacodyl is mainly excreted in the faeces.

Uses and Administration

Bisacodyl is a diphenylmethane stimulant laxative used for the treatment of constipation (p.1168) and for bowel evacuation before investigational procedures or surgery. Its action is mainly in the large intestine and it is usually effective within 6 to 12 hours following administration by mouth and within 15 to 60 minutes following rectal administration.

Bisacodyl is given in usual doses of 5 to 15 mg daily as enteric-coated tablets administered at night or 10 mg as a suppository or enema administered in the morning; doses of up to 20 mg have been given by mouth for complete bowel evacuation, followed if necessary by 10 mg as a suppository the next day. The tablets should be swallowed whole and should not be taken within one hour of milk or antacids.

Children may be given 5 mg by mouth or 5 to 10 mg rectally.

Bisacodyl may be administered with a barium sulphate enema before radiographic examination of the colon. A complex of bisacodyl with tannic acid (bisacodyl tannex) is generally used in a dose equivalent to 1.5 to 3.0 mg of bisacodyl dissolved in 1 litre of barium sulphate suspension. The total dose for one procedure should not exceed 4.5 mg of bisacodyl and no more than 6 mg should be administered in 72 hours.

Preparations

BP 1998: Bisacodyl Suppositories; Bisacodyl Tablets;
USP 23: Bisacodyl Delayed-release Tablets; Bisacodyl Rectal Suspension; Bisacodyl Suppositories.

Proprietary Preparations (details are given in Part 3)
Aust.: Dulcolax; Laxbene; ***Austral.:*** Bisalax; Durolax; Fleet Laxative; ***Belg.:*** Dulcolax; Horton; Mucinum; Purgo-Pil; ***Canad.:*** Bisacolax; Correctol; Dulcolax; Feen-A-Mint; ***Fr.:*** Contalax; Dulcolax; ***Ger.:*** Agaroletten N; Bekunis Bisacodyl; Bisco-Zitron; Darmol Bisacodyl; Drix N; Dulcolax; Florisan N; Laxagetten; Laxanin N; Laxans-ratiopharm; Laxbene; Laxbene N; Laxoberal Bisa; Logomed Abfuhr-Dragees†; Mandrolax; Marienbader Pillen N; Mediolax; Pyrilax; Rhabarex B; Stadalax; Tempolax; Tirgon N; Vinco Forte; Vinco-Abfuhrperlen; ***Irl.:*** Dulcolax; Toilax; ***Ital.:*** Alaxa; Dulcolax; Normalene; ***Neth.:*** Dulcolax; Nourilax†; Toilax†; Zwitsalax/N; ***Norw.:*** Dulcolax; Toilax; ***S.Afr.:*** Capolax†; Dulcolax; Megalax; Perilax†; ***Spain:*** Dulco Laxo; Medesup; ***Swed.:*** Dulcolax; Toilax; ***Switz.:*** Demolaxin; Dulcolax; Ercolax; Laxbene†; Muxol; Prontolax; ***UK:*** Dulcolax; ***USA:*** Bisac-Evac; Bisco-Lax; Clysodrast; Correctol; Dulcagen; Dulcolax; Evac-Q-Kwik Suppository; Feen-A-Mint; Fleet Bisacodyl; Fleet Laxative.

Multi-ingredient: ***Aust.:*** Laxbene; Prepacol; Purgazen; Purigoa; ***Austral.:*** Coloxyl; Durolax X-Pack; Raykit†; ***Belg.:*** Prepacol; Softene; ***Canad.:*** Evac-Q-Kwik; Fruitatives; Royvac Kit; ***Fr.:*** Neo-Boldolaxine†; Pilule Dupuis; Prepacol; ***Ger.:*** Daluwal Forte†; Milkitten Abfuhrdragees†; Milkitten S†; Potsilo; Prepacol; Rheolind†; Tirgon†; Vinco V†; ***Ital.:*** Fisiolax†; ***Spain:*** Bekunis Complex†; Boldolaxin; ***Switz.:*** Aloinophen; Bekunis; Drix; Tavolax; Tirgon†; ***UK:*** Nylax; ***USA:*** Dulcolax Bowel Prep Kit; Tridrate Bowel Evacuant Kit; X-Prep Bowel Evacuant Kit-1; X-Prep Bowel Evacuant Kit-2.

Bismuth Compounds (17157-z)

Bismuth compounds have been used for their astringent and antidiarrhoeal properties in a variety of gastro-intestinal disorders, and have been applied topically in skin disorders and anorectal disorders such as haemorrhoids. Certain salts are active against *Helicobacter pylori* and are used in the treatment of peptic ulcer disease.

Bismuth (5265-w)

Bi = 208.98038.
CAS — 7440-69-9.

A silvery-white crystalline brittle metal with a pinkish tinge.

Bismuth Aluminate (5268-y)

Bismuth Aluminate *(USAN)*.
Aluminum Bismuth Oxide.
$Bi_2(Al_2O_4)_3,10H_2O$ = 952.0.
CAS — 12284-76-3 (anhydrous bismuth aluminate).
Pharmacopoeias. In *Fr.*

Bismuth Citrate (14763-y)

CAS — 813-93-4.

Bismuth Oxide (5271-p)

Bismuth Trioxide.
Bi_2O_3 = 466.0.
CAS — 1304-76-3.

Bismuth Phosphate (18850-r)

$BiPO_4$ = 304.0.
CAS — 10049-01-1.
Pharmacopoeias. In *Fr.*

Bismuth Salicylate (5275-l)

Basic Bismuth Salicylate; Bismuth Oxysalicylate; Bismuth Subsalicylate *(USAN)*.
CAS — 14882-18-9.
Pharmacopoeias. In *Fr., It., Neth.,* and *US.*

A basic salt of varying composition, corresponding approximately to $C_6H_4(OH).CO_2(BiO)$ and containing not less than 56.0% and not more than 59.4% of Bi. It is a fine, odourless, white to off-white microcrystalline powder. Practically **insoluble** in water, in alcohol, and in ether. It reacts with alkalis and mineral acid. **Store** in airtight containers. Protect from light.

Bismuth Subcarbonate (5279-c)

Bismuth Subcarbonate *(USAN)*.
Basic Bismuth Carbonate; Basisches Wismutkarbonat; Bism. Carb.; Bismuth Carbonate; Bismuth Oxycarbonate; Bismuthi Subcarbonas; Bismutylum Carbonicum; Carbonato de Bismutila.
CAS — 5892-10-4 (anhydrous bismuth subcarbonate); 5798-45-8 (bismuth subcarbonate hemihydrate).
Pharmacopoeias. In *Chin., Eur.* (see p.viii), and *US.*

A white or almost white powder.
Practically **insoluble** in water, in alcohol, and in ether; dissolves in mineral acids with effervescence. **Protect** from light.

Bismuth Subgallate (5280-s)

Bismuth Subgallate *(USAN)*.
Basic Bismuth Gallate; Basisches Wismutgallat; Bism. Subgall.; Bismuth Oxygallate; Bismuthi Subgallas.
$C_7H_5BiO_6$ = 394.1.
CAS — 99-26-3.
Pharmacopoeias. In *Fr., Ger., Jpn, Neth., Pol.,* and *US.*

USP specifies 52 to 57% of Bi_2O_3 when dried at 105° for 3 hours. It is an odourless amorphous bright yellow powder. Practically **insoluble** in water, in alcohol, in chloroform, in ether, and in very dilute mineral acids; dissolves readily with decomposition in warm, moderately dilute hydrochloric, nitric, or sulphuric acids; readily dissolves in solutions of alkali hydroxides to form a clear yellow liquid which rapidly becomes deep red. **Store** in airtight containers. Protect from light.

Bismuth Subnitrate (5281-w)

Basic Bismuth Nitrate; Basisches Wismutnitrat; Bism. Subnit.; Bismuth Hydroxide Nitrate Oxide; Bismuth Oxynitrate; Bismuth (Sous-Nitrate de) Lourd; Bismuthi Subnitras; Bismuthyl Nitrate; Magistery of Bismuth; Nitrato de Bismutilo; Subazotato de Bismuto; White Bismuth.
$Bi_5O(OH)_9(NO_3)_4$ = 1462.0.
CAS — 1304-85-4.
Pharmacopoeias. In *Aust., Fr., Ger., Jpn, Pol.,* and *US.*
Fr. also includes Bismuth (Sous-Nitrate de) Léger (Bismuthi Subnitras Levis) which is described as a variable mixture of bismuth hydroxide, carbonate, and subnitrate.

USP specifies not less than 79% of Bi_2O_3 calculated on the dried basis. It is a white slightly hygroscopic powder. Practically **insoluble** in water and in alcohol; readily dissolves in nitric and hydrochloric acids.

Bismuth Tribromphenate (5282-e)

Bismuth Tribromophenate; Bismutum Tribromophenylicum; Bromphenobis; Bromphenol Bismuth; Xeroformium.
CAS — 5175-83-7.

Tripotassium Dicitratobismuthate (3778-t)

Colloidal Bismuth Subcitrate.
CAS — 57644-54-9.

Adverse Effects, Treatment, and Precautions

The bismuth compounds listed above are insoluble or very poorly soluble, and bismuth toxicity does not currently appear to be common with them if they are used as they are now for limited periods. However, excessive or prolonged dosage may produce symptoms of bismuth poisoning, and for this reason long-term systemic therapy is not recommended. Reversible encephalopathy was once a problem in some countries, notably France and Australia, and did not appear to be related to dose or duration of use; bone and joint toxicity had also occurred, sometimes associated with the encephalopathy. This led to restrictions on the use of bismuth salts and a virtual disappearance of these toxic effects.

Nausea and vomiting have been reported. Darkening or blackening of the faeces and tongue may occur due to conversion to bismuth sulphide in the gastro-intestinal tract.

The effects of *acute bismuth intoxication* include gastro-intestinal disturbances, skin reactions, stomatitis, and discoloration of mucous membranes; a characteristic blue line may appear on the gums. There may be renal failure and liver damage.

Other adverse effects may not be related to the bismuth content. With bismuth subnitrate given orally there is a risk of the nitrate being reduced in the intestines to nitrite and the development of methaemoglobinaemia. Absorption of salicylate occurs following the administration of bismuth salicylate by mouth and therefore the adverse effects, treatment of adverse effects, and precautions of aspirin (p.16) should be considered.

Bismuth compounds should not be given to patients with renal impairment.

Acute toxicity. Reviews[1,2] and reports[3-6] of bismuth toxicity. Many of the original reports implicated bismuth subgallate or subnitrate, although toxicity has certainly occurred with other salts. A recent study in patients receiving the subcitrate or the subnitrate for 8 weeks in the treatment of *Helicobacter pylori* infection, showed no evidence of neurological changes compared with a control group.[7]

1. Winship KA. Toxicity of bismuth salts. *Adverse Drug React Acute Poisoning Rev* 1983; **2:** 103–21.
2. Slikkerveer A, de Wolff FA. Pharmacokinetics and toxicity of bismuth compounds. *Med Toxicol Adverse Drug Exp* 1989; **4:** 303–23.
3. Morrow AW. Request for reports: adverse reactions with bismuth subgallate. *Med J Aust* 1973; **1:** 912.
4. Martin-Bouyer G. Intoxications par les sels de bismuth administrés par voie orale: enquête épidémiologique. *Therapie* 1976; **31:** 683–702.
5. Stahl JP, *et al.* Encéphalites au sel insoluble de bismuth: toujours d'actualité. *Nouv Presse Med* 1982; **11:** 3856.
6. Von Bose MJ, Zaudig M. Encephalopathy resembling Creutzfeldt-Jakob disease following oral, prescribed doses of bismuth nitrate. *Br J Psychiatry* 1991; **158:** 278–80.
7. Noach LA, *et al.* Bismuth salts and neurotoxicity: a randomised, single-blind and controlled study. *Hum Exp Toxicol* 1995; **14:** 349–55.

FOLLOWING TOPICAL APPLICATION. Encephalopathy has been associated with the use of bismuth iodoform paraffin paste (BIPP) for the packing of wound cavities after surgery to the head and neck,[1] although there is some debate as to whether the bismuth or the iodoform component is responsible.[1,2]

1. Wilson APR. The dangers of BIPP. *Lancet* 1994; **344:** 1313–14.
2. Roy P-M, *et al.* Dangers of bismuth iodoform paraffin paste. *Lancet* 1994; **344:** 1708.

Overdosage. Bismuth salicylate or tripotassium dicitratobismuthate in recommended doses are rarely associated with serious adverse effects but there are reports of renal failure,[1-3] encephalopathy,[4-6] and neurotoxicity[1] following acute[1-3,5] or chronic[4,6] overdose. Bismuth has been detected in the blood, urine, stools, and kidneys of these patients; a blood concentration of 1.6 µg per mL was found 4 hours after a dose of 9.6 g.[2] Chronic ingestion of clinical doses intermittently over 2 years has been reported to cause paraesthesia, insomnia, and impaired memory.[7] Encephalopathy has not been associated with recommended doses of tripotassium dicitratobismuthate but it has been suggested that if blood-bismuth concentrations exceed 100 ng per mL, bismuth preparations should be discontinued.[8]

The optimal treatment of bismuth overdosage is unknown. Gastric lavage, purgation, and hydration should be considered, even if the patient presents late, as bismuth may be absorbed from the colon.[1,2] Chelating agents may be effective in the early stages following ingestion,[3] and 2,3-dimercapto-1-propane sulphonic acid at a dose of 100 mg three times daily has been reported to increase the renal clearance of bismuth with a reduction in the blood concentration.[4] Haemodialysis may be necessary[1-3] but whether this hastens tissue clearance is uncertain.

Prolonged ingestion of bismuth salicylate in excessive doses by an elderly diabetic was associated with hearing disturbances, vertigo, acid-base abnormalities and mild clotting disturbances.[9] The toxicity was thought to be due to the salicylate component of the drug.

1. Hudson M, *et al.* Reversible toxicity in poisoning with colloidal bismuth subcitrate. *Br Med J* 1989; **299:** 159.
2. Taylor EG, Klenerman P. Acute renal failure after colloidal bismuth subcitrate overdose. *Lancet* 1990; **335:** 670–1.
3. Huwez F, *et al.* Acute renal failure after overdose of colloidal bismuth subcitrate. *Lancet* 1992; **340:** 1298.
4. Playford RJ, *et al.* Bismuth induced encephalopathy caused by tri potassium dicitrato bismuthate in a patient with chronic renal failure. *Gut* 1990; **31:** 359–60.
5. Hasking GJ, Duggan JM. Encephalopathy from bismuth subsalicylate. *Med J Aust* 1982; **2:** 167.
6. Mendelowitz PC, *et al.* Bismuth absorption and myoclonic encephalopathy during bismuth subsalicylate therapy. *Ann Intern Med* 1990; **112:** 140–1.
7. Weller MPI. Neuropsychiatric symptoms following bismuth intoxication. *Postgrad Med J* 1988; **64:** 308–10.
8. Miller JP. Relapse of duodenal ulcer. *Br Med J* 1986; **293:** 1501.
9. Vernace MA, *et al.* Chronic salicylate toxicity due to consumption of over-the-counter bismuth subsalicylate. *Am J Med* 1994; **97:** 308–9.

Interactions

Although bismuth salts such as tripotassium dicitratobismuthate or bismuth salicylate are given with tetracycline as part of triple therapy (see below) they may inhibit the efficacy of tetracyclines taken by mouth and doses of the two drugs should be separated by as long as possible.

Antisecretory drugs. Pretreatment with omeprazole resulted in about a threefold increase in absorption of bismuth from tripotassium dicitratobismuthate in 6 healthy subjects.[1] The mean peak plasma concentration of bismuth following a single dose of 240 mg of tripotassium dicitratobismuthate was increased from 36.7 to 86.7 ng per mL after omeprazole administration, suggesting an increased risk of toxicity from dual therapy. The mechanism was thought to be the reduction in gastric pH produced by the antisecretory drug as similar results had been reported with ranitidine.[2]

1. Treiber G, *et al.* Omeprazole-induced increase in the absorption of bismuth from tripotassium dicitrato bismuthate. *Clin Pharmacol Ther* 1994; **55:** 486–91.
2. Nwokolo. CU, *et al.* The effect of histamine H_2-receptor blockade on bismuth absorption from three ulcer-healing compounds. *Gastroenterology* 1991; **101:** 889–94.

Pharmacokinetics

Poorly soluble bismuth compounds are largely converted to insoluble bismuth oxide, hydroxide, and oxychloride in the stomach. Most of the bismuth compounds included in this monograph are thus only slightly absorbed, with the absorbed portion excreted mainly in the urine. Some bismuth is retained in the bones and tissues and some is excreted in the faeces. Bismuth can cross the placenta.

Following oral administration of tripotassium dicitratobismuthate the plasma concentration reaches steady state after about 4 to 5 weeks of chronic administration. Absorbed bismuth has a plasma half-life of about 5 days and continues to be excreted for about 12 weeks after stopping therapy. Changes in gastric pH may affect absorption—see under Interactions, above.

References.

1. Nwokolo CU, *et al.* The absorption of bismuth from oral doses of tripotassium dicitrato bismuthate. *Aliment Pharmacol Ther* 1989; **3:** 29–39.
2. Froomes PRA, *et al.* Absorption and elimination of bismuth from oral doses of tripotassium dicitrato bismuthate. *Eur J Clin Pharmacol* 1989; **37:** 533–6.
3. Lauritsen K, *et al.* Clinical pharmacokinetics of drugs used in the treatment of gastrointestinal diseases. *Clin Pharmacokinet* 1990; **19:** 11–31 and 94–125.
4. Lacey LF, *et al.* Comparative pharmacokinetics of bismuth from ranitidine bismuth citrate (GR122311X), a novel anti-ulcerant and tripotassium dicitrato bismuthate (TDB). *Eur J Clin Pharmacol* 1994; **47:** 177–80.

Uses and Administration

Some insoluble salts of bismuth have been given by mouth for their supposed antacid action and for their mildly astringent action in various gastro-intestinal disorders, including diarrhoea (p.1168) and dyspepsia (p.1169). Such salts include the aluminate, phosphate, salicylate, subcarbonate, subgallate, subnitrate, and tannate. Bismuth salicylate, which is given as an antidiarrhoeal and weak antacid in doses up to about 4 g daily in divided doses, possesses in addition the properties of the salicylates.

Tripotassium dicitratobismuthate is used for the treatment of peptic ulcer disease. It is active against *Helicobacter pylori* and is used with metronidazole together with either tetracycline or amoxycillin (the regimen known as 'triple therapy'—see p.1174), to eradicate this organism and thereby prevent relapse of duodenal ulcer. Bismuth salicylate is also active against *H. pylori* and has been used as an alternative to tripotassium dicitratobismuthate.

The usual dose of tripotassium dicitratobismuthate in benign gastric and duodenal ulceration is 240 mg twice daily, or 120 mg four times daily by mouth taken before food. Treatment is for a period of 4 weeks, extended to 8 weeks if necessary. Maintenance therapy with tripotassium dicitratobismuthate is not recommended although treatment may be repeated after a drug-free interval of one month.

When used as part of **triple therapy** the usual dose of tripotassium dicitratobismuthate is 120 mg four times daily and the treatment period is usually 2 weeks. Such a triple regimen would involve combination with tetracycline (or amoxycillin) 500 mg four times daily (for a potential interaction between bismuth salts and tetracyclines, see Interactions, above), and metronidazole 400 mg three times daily. However such two-week regimens are increasingly being challenged by one-week regimens which do not include bismuth. Appropriate antisecretory treatment with a histamine H_2-receptor antagonist or a proton pump inhibitor may also be given for ulcer healing.

A complex of bismuth citrate with ranitidine, ranitidine bismutrex (p.1211), is also used in the treatment of peptic ulcer disease.

Some insoluble salts of bismuth have been used topically in the treatment of skin disorders, wounds, and burns. Some have been used as ingredients of ointments or suppositories (sometimes containing more than one bismuth salt) in the treatment of haemorrhoids and other anorectal disorders (p.1170). Bismuth compounds that have been used topically and/or rectally include the dipropylacetate, oxide, subgallate, subnitrate, and tribromphenate; bismuth resorcinol compounds have also been used. For the use of bismuth subnitrate and iodoform paste as a wound dressing, see Iodoform, p.1118.

Bismuth and some of its salts were formerly given mainly by injection, alone or with other agents, in the treatment of syphilis. Numerous other salts and compounds of bismuth have been promoted for various therapeutic purposes. Bismuth glycollylarsanilate was formerly used by mouth as an amoebicide.

Bismuth (Bismuthum) is used in homoeopathic medicine.

Preparations

BPC 1954: Bismuth Subnitrate and Iodoform Paste *(BIPP)*;
USP 23: Compound Resorcinol Ointment; Milk of Bismuth.

Proprietary Preparations (details are given in Part 3)
Austral.: De-Nol; ***Belg.:*** Angimuth†; De-Nol; ***Canad.:*** Bismed; Bismylate; Neo-Laryngobis†; Pepto-Bismol; ***Fr.:*** Amygdorectol; ***Ger.:*** Angass S; Campylotec†; Dermatol; Dignodenum†; Gastripan M†; Jatrox; Noemin N; Telen; Ulcolind Wismut; Ulcumel†; Ulgastrin Bis; Ulkowis; Ultin†; ***Irl.:*** De-Nol; De-Noltab; Ulso†; ***Ital.:*** De-Nol; ***Neth.:*** De-Nol; ***Norw.:*** De-Nol; ***S.Afr.:*** De-Nol; Ulcerone; ***Spain:*** Gastrodenol; Helinol†; Helol; Lacertral†; Rectamigdol†; ***Switz.:*** Amygdorectol; Bismuth Tulasne; De-Nol; ***UK:*** De-Nol; De-Noltab; Pepto-Bismol; ***USA:*** Bismatrol; Devrom; Pepto-Bismol; Pink Biscoat; Stomax.

Multi-ingredient: numerous preparations are listed in Part 3.

Bisoxatin Acetate (12446-q)

Bisoxatin Acetate *(BANM, USAN, rINNM)*.

Bisoxatin Diacetate; Wy-8138. 2,2-Bis(4-hydroxyphenyl)-1,4-benzoxazin-3(2*H*,4*H*)-one diacetate.

$C_{24}H_{19}NO_6$ = 417.4.

CAS — 17692-24-9 (bisoxatin); 14008-48-1 (bisoxatin acetate).

Bisoxatin acetate is a stimulant laxative that has been used in the treatment of constipation (p.1168) in doses of 120 to 180 mg by mouth daily at bedtime.

Preparations

Proprietary Preparations (details are given in Part 3)
Belg.: Wylaxine.

Bran (681-s)

The fibrous outer layers of cereal grains, usually wheat, consisting of the pericarp, testa, and aleurone layer. It contains celluloses, polysaccharides or hemicelluloses, protein, fat, minerals, and moisture and may contain part of the germ or embryo. Bran provides water-insoluble fibre and, depending on the source, may also provide water-soluble fibre.

It comprises about 12% of the weight of the grain and is a byproduct of flour milling. It is available in various grades.

Adverse Effects

Large quantities of bran may temporarily increase flatulence and abdominal distension, and intestinal obstruction may occur rarely. Interference with iron, zinc, and calcium absorption has been reported; calcium phosphate may be added to bran to neutralise phytic acid, which can contribute to such interference.

Diarrhoea. A report of diarrhoea induced by a dramatic increase in fibre intake. Reduction of dietary fibre led to a return to normal bowel habit in 2 to 3 days.[1]

1. Saibil F. Diarrhea due to fiber overload. *N Engl J Med* 1989; **320:** 599.

Intestinal obstruction. Intestinal obstruction associated with excessive bran intake has been reported.[1-3]

1. Allen-Mersh T, De Jode LR. Is bran useful in diverticular disease? *Br Med J* 1982; **284:** 740.
2. Cooper SG, Tracey EJ. Small-bowel obstruction caused by oat-bran bezoar. *N Engl J Med* 1989; **320:** 1148–9.
3. Miller DL, *et al.* Small-bowel obstruction from bran cereal. *JAMA* 1990; **263:** 813–14.

Precautions

Bran is contra-indicated in patients with intestinal obstruction or with undiagnosed abdominal symptoms. Bran should not be eaten dry because of the possibility of oesophageal or intestinal obstruction.

Interactions

Bran can bind to, and reduce the absorption of, a number of drugs including cardiac glycosides and salicylates when given concomitantly by mouth.

Uses and Administration

The main use of bran is as a source of dietary fibre in the management of disorders of the gastro-intestinal tract such as constipation (p.1168), especially in diverticular disease (p.1169) and the irritable bowel syndrome (p.1172). It should always be taken with plenty of fluid.

It is used as the basis for some breakfast cereals.

There is no precise definition for the complex mixture of substances known as dietary fibre. It has been defined as plant polysaccharides and lignin resistant to hydrolysis by the digestive enzymes of man but this covers many substances other than cell wall and related polysaccharides. Non-starch polysaccharides are the major component of the plant cell wall and are used as an index of dietary fibre. They comprise water-soluble fibres such as pectins, gums, and mucilages and water-insoluble fibres such as cellulose; wheat, maize, and rice contain mainly insoluble non-starch polysaccharides whereas oats, barley, and rye have a significant proportion of soluble fibres.

In the United Kingdom dietary reference values (DRV) have been published for non-starch polysaccharides.[1] In the UK it is proposed that adult diets should contain an average for the population of 18 g daily (individual range 12 to 24 g daily) non-starch polysaccharide from a variety of foods whose constituents contain it as a naturally integrated component. Children should receive proportionately less non-starch polysaccharide according to body size. No evidence exists for benefit of intakes of non-starch polysaccharide in excess of 32 g daily, and therefore there is no advantage in exceeding this amount.

1. DOH. Dietary reference values for food energy and nutrients for the United Kingdom: report of the panel on dietary reference values of the committee on medical aspects of food policy. *Report on health and social subjects 41.* London: HMSO, 1991.

Diseases such as colorectal cancer, ischaemic heart disease, diabetes mellitus, and obesity are common in affluent Western civilisation but occur rarely in rural Africa. This difference in disease patterns has been linked to the low fibre intake of Westerners compared with rural Africans. However, there are many other differences in diet and lifestyle, such as a lower intake of fat, protein, and sugar in rural Africans and less exposure to toxins and pollutants, any of which could contribute to the difference. The excessive consumption of energy-rich foods may be more to blame for diseases of Western civilisation than is deficiency of dietary fibre.[1] Furthermore, there is some concern that the use of fibre supplements is not entirely without harmful effects: it has been pointed out that fermentable fibre substrates can stimulate cell proliferation in the colon.[2] However the role of cell proliferation as a marker for the development of colonic cancer is questioned by some authors.[3]

1. Anonymous. The bran wagon. *Lancet* 1987; **i:** 782–3.
2. Wasan HS, Goodlad RA. Fibre-supplemented foods may damage your health. *Lancet* 1996; **348:** 319–20.
3. Hill MJ, Leeds AR. Fibre and colorectal cancer. *Lancet* 1996; **348:** 957.

Preparations

Proprietary Preparations (details are given in Part 3)
Canad.: Fibyrax; ***Fr.:*** Celluson; Doses-O-Son; Infibran; Regison†; ***Ger.:*** Silvapin Weizenkleie-Extrakt†; ***Irl.:*** Trifyba; ***Ital.:*** Crusken; ***Spain:*** Fibralax†; ***Swed.:*** Fibertabletter†; ***Switz.:*** Fibion; ***UK:*** Fybranta†; Proctofibe†; Trifyba.

Bromopride (12454-q)

Bromopride *(rINN)*.

CM-8252; VAL-13081. 4-Amino-5-bromo-*N*-(2-diethylaminoethyl)-*o*-anisamide.

$C_{14}H_{22}BrN_3O_2$ = 344.2.

CAS — 4093-35-0.

Bromopride is a substituted benzamide similar to metoclopramide (p.1200), used in a variety of gastro-intestinal disorders including nausea and vomiting (p.1172) and motility disorders. It is given in a usual dose of 20 to 60 mg daily by mouth in divided doses, or 10 to 20 mg daily by intramuscular or intravenous injection. The hydrochloride is also used.

Preparations

Proprietary Preparations (details are given in Part 3)
Ger.: Cascapride; Viaben†; ***Ital.:*** Opridan; Valopride; ***Spain:*** Valopride†.

Multi-ingredient: *Ger.:* Tri Viaben†.

Buckthorn (7504-h)

Bacca Spinae Cervinae; Espino Cerval; Nerprun; Rhamnus.

Pharmacopoeias. In Fr. and Ger.

The dried ripe fruit of buckthorn, *Rhamnus cathartica* (Rhamnaceae). The bark is occasionally used.

Buckthorn has been used as a laxative.

Preparations

Proprietary Preparations (details are given in Part 3)
Ger.: Laxysat mono.

Multi-ingredient: ***Austral.:*** Neo-Cleanse; ***Canad.:*** Floralaxative; Herbal Laxative; Linoforce†; ***Ger.:*** Presselin Stoffwechseltee†; Salus Abfuhr-Tee Nr. 2; ***UK:*** Herbalene.

Calcium Carbonate (682-w)

Calcii Carbonas; Creta Preparada; E170; Precipitated Calcium Carbonate; Precipitated Chalk.

$CaCO_3$ = 100.1.

CAS — 471-34-1.

Pharmacopoeias. In *Eur.* (see p.viii), *Int., Jpn, Pol.,* and *US.*

A white, odourless, powder.

Practically **insoluble** in water; its solubility in water is increased by the presence of carbon dioxide or ammonium salts; practically insoluble in alcohol; dissolves with effervescence in acetic acid, hydrochloric acid, and nitric acid.

Adverse Effects, Treatment, and Precautions

Calcium carbonate has adverse effects similar to those of other calcium salts (see p.1155). Ingestion may occasionally cause constipation. Flatulence from released carbon dioxide may occur in some patients. High doses or prolonged use may lead to gastric hypersecretion and acid rebound.

Hypercalcaemia (p.1148) can occur as can alkalosis (p.1147) following high doses of calcium carbonate by mouth; they may resolve on reducing the dose. The milk-alkali syndrome, which includes hypercalcaemia and alkalosis together with renal dysfunction, has occasionally occurred, usually in patients taking large doses; patients with renal impairment or dehydration and electrolyte imbalance are predisposed. Calcium carbonate should also be used with caution in patients with a history of renal calculi.

Milk-alkali syndrome. The milk-alkali syndrome of hypercalcaemia, alkalosis and renal impairment was first identified in the 1920s and may still occur in patients who ingest large amounts of calcium and absorbable alkali.[1] Metastatic calcification can develop.[2] For reference to thiazide diuretics increasing the risk of the milk-alkali syndrome in patients taking moderately large doses of calcium carbonate, see p.887.

1. Orwoll ES. The milk-alkali syndrome: current concepts. *Ann Intern Med* 1982; **97:** 242–8.
2. Duthie JS, *et al.* Milk-alkali syndrome with metastatic calcification. *Am J Med* 1995; **99:** 102–3.

Interactions

As outlined on p.1167 antacids, including calcium salts, interact with many other drugs both by alterations in gastric pH and emptying, and by formation of complexes that are not absorbed. Interactions can be minimised by giving the antacid and any other medication 2 to 3 hours apart.

Pharmacokinetics

Calcium carbonate is converted to calcium chloride by gastric acid. Some of the calcium is absorbed from the intestines but about 85% is reconverted to insoluble calcium salts and soaps, and is excreted in the faeces.

Uses and Administration

Calcium carbonate is used as an antacid (p.1167), usually in doses of up to about 1.5 g by mouth. It is often given in association with other antacids, especially magnesium-containing antacids.

It is also used as a calcium supplement in deficiency states (p.1156) and as an adjunct in the treatment of osteoporosis (p.731).

Calcium carbonate binds phosphate in the gastro-intestinal tract to form insoluble complexes and reduces phosphate absorption. It is used to treat hyperphosphataemia in patients with chronic renal failure (see Renal Osteodystrophy, p.732). For this purpose, initial doses of 2.5 g daily by mouth have been given, increased to up to 17 g daily.

A preparation of a native calcium carbonate (Calcarea Carbonica; Calc. Carb.) is used in homoeopathic medicine.

Calcium carbonate is also used as a food additive.

Preparations

USP 23: Alumina, Magnesia, and Calcium Carbonate Oral Suspension; Alumina, Magnesia, and Calcium Carbonate Tablets; Alumina, Magnesia, Calcium Carbonate, and Simethicone Tablets; Aluminum Subacetate Topical Solution; Calcium and Magnesium Carbonates Oral Suspension; Calcium and Magnesium Carbonates Tablets; Calcium Carbonate and Magnesia Tablets; Calcium Carbonate Lozenges; Calcium Carbonate Oral Suspension; Calcium Carbonate Tablets; Calcium Carbonate, Magnesia, and Simethicone Tablets.

Proprietary Preparations (details are given in Part 3)
Aust.: Kalzonorm†; Tetesept Calcium; ***Austral.:*** Andrews Tums Antacid; Cal-Sup; Calcimax†; Caltrate; Effercal-600†; Macro Liquical†; Sandocal; Titralac; ***Belg.:*** Cacit; Calci-Chew; ***Canad.:*** Apo-Cal; Cal-500; Calcite; Calsan; Caltrate; Hi Potency Cal; Mega-Cal†; Neo Cal; Os-Cal; Pharmacal†; Titralac; Tums; ***Fr.:*** Cacit; Calcidia; Calcidose; Calciprat; Calperos; Caltrate; Eucalcic; ***Ger.:*** Calcedon; Calcilos; Calcimagon; Calcitridin; Calcium Dago; Calcium Verla; Calcium-dura; Dreisacarb; Frubiase Calcium; Loscalcon; Ospur; Vivural; ***Irl.:*** Cacit; Calcichew; Remegel; Rennie Rap-Eze; Rowarolan; Setlers Tums; ***Ital.:*** Cacit; Remegel; Top Calcium; ***Mon.:*** Orocal; ***Neth.:*** Cacit; Calci-Chew; ***Norw.:*** Titralac; ***S.Afr.:*** Caltrate; Titralac; ***Spain:*** Caosina; Carbocal; Fortical; Mastical; Natecal 600; ***Swed.:*** Calcitugg; Kalcipos; Kalcitena; ***Switz.:*** Fixateur phospho-calcique; Maxi-calc; ***UK:*** Cacit; Calcichew; Calcidrink; Citrical†; Rap-eze; Remegel; Rennie Gold; Sea-Cal; Setlers; Titralac; Tums; ***USA:*** Alka-Mints; Alkets; Amitone; Antacid; Cal Carb-HD; Cal-Guard; Cal-Plus; Calci-Chew; Calci-Mix; Calciday; Caltrate; Caltrate Jr.; Chooz; Dicarbosil; Equilet; Gencalc; Maalox Antacid; Mallamint; Mylanta; Nephro-Calci; Os-Cal; Oysco; Oyst-Cal; Oyster Shell Calcium; Oystercal; Titralac Extra Strength; Tums.

Multi-ingredient: numerous preparations are listed in Part 3.

Calcium Silicate (683-e)

552.

CAS — 1344-95-2; 10101-39-0 ($CaSiO_3$); 10034-77-2 (Ca_2SiO_4); 12168-85-3 (Ca_3SiO_5).

Pharmacopoeias. In *USNF.*

A naturally occurring mineral, the most common forms being calcium metasilicate ($CaSiO_3$ = 116.2), calcium diorthosilicate (Ca_2SiO_4 = 172.2), and calcium trisilicate (Ca_3SiO_5 = 228.3). It is usually found in hydrated forms containing various amounts of water of crystallisation. Commercial calcium silicate is prepared synthetically. USNF 18 describes calcium silicate as a compound of calcium oxide and silicon dioxide containing not less than 4% of CaO and not less than 45% of SiO_2. A white to off-white free-flowing powder. Practically **insoluble** in water; with mineral acids it forms a gel. A 5% aqueous suspension has a pH of 8.4 to 10.2.

Calcium silicate is used as an antacid (p.1167).

It is also used as an anticaking agent in the preparation of pharmaceuticals and as a food additive.

Preparations

Proprietary Preparations (details are given in Part 3)

Multi-ingredient: ***Belg.:*** Mucal; ***Ger.:*** calcivitase; ***Swed.:*** Relax-it.

Carbenoxolone Sodium (685-y)

Carbenoxolone Sodium *(BANM, USAN, rINNM).*

Disodium Enoxolone Succinate. The disodium salt of 3β-(3-carboxypropionyloxy)-11-oxo-olean-12-en-30-oic acid.

$C_{34}H_{48}Na_2O_7$ = 614.7.

CAS — 5697-56-3 (carbenoxolone); 7421-40-1 (carbenoxolone disodium).

Pharmacopoeias. In Br. and Chin.

A white or pale cream-coloured hygroscopic powder. Freely **soluble** in water; sparingly soluble in alcohol; practically insoluble in chloroform and ether. A 10% solution in water has a pH of 8.0 to 9.2.

CAUTION. *Carbenoxolone sodium powder is irritant to nasal membranes.*

Adverse Effects

Carbenoxolone sodium has mineralocorticoid-like effects and may produce sodium and water retention and hypokalaemia. This may cause or exacerbate hypertension, heart failure, oedema, alkalosis, and muscle weakness and damage. If hypokalaemia is prolonged, renal impairment can occur.

Effects on fluid and electrolyte homoeostasis. Adverse effects associated with carbenoxolone therapy are usually secondary to water and electrolyte disturbances, notably hypokalaemia. Muscle weakness,[1-5] muscle necrosis,[4] myopathy,[1] hypertension,[2] headache,[2] cardiac failure,[2] mental confusion,[4] areflexia,[3] renal tubular dysfunction,[5] and acute tubular necrosis[4] have all been associated with carbenoxolone-induced hypokalaemia. Carbenoxolone-induced hypertension may have precipitated the onset of fatal polyarteritis in a patient predisposed to this condition.[6]

1. Fyfe T, *et al.* Myopathy and hypokalaemia in carbenoxolone therapy. *Br Med J* 1969; **3:** 476.
2. Davies GJ, *et al.* Complications of carbenoxolone therapy. *Br Med J* 1974; **3:** 400–2.
3. Royston A, Prout BJ. Carbenoxolone-induced hypokalaemia simulating Guillain-Barré syndrome. *Br Med J* 1976; **2:** 150–1.
4. Descamps C, *et al.* Rhabdomyolysis and acute tubular necrosis associated with carbenoxolone and diuretic treatment. *Br Med J* 1977; **1:** 272.
5. Dickinson RJ, Swaminathan R. Total body potassium depletion and renal tubular dysfunction following carbenoxolone therapy. *Postgrad Med J* 1978; **54:** 836–7.
6. Sloan J, Weaver JA. A case of polyarteritis developing after carbenoxolone therapy. *Ir Med J* 1968; **1:** 505–7.

Precautions

Carbenoxolone sodium is contra-indicated in patients with hypokalaemia, in pregnancy, in the elderly, and in children. It should be used with caution, if at all, in patients with cardiac disease, hypertension, or impaired hepatic or renal function.

Interactions

Because of the risk of toxicity, carbenoxolone should not be given with digitalis glycosides unless serum-electrolyte concentrations are measured at weekly intervals and measures are taken to avoid hypokalaemia.

Although amiloride or spironolactone relieve sodium and water retention, they should not be used with carbenoxolone as they antagonise the healing properties of carbenoxolone. The hypokalaemia associated with diuretics may be exacerbated by carbenoxolone.

Pharmacokinetics

Carbenoxolone sodium is absorbed from the gastro-intestinal tract. It is highly bound to plasma proteins, mainly albumin. Carbenoxolone is mainly excreted in the faeces via the bile. It appears to undergo enterohepatic circulation.

Uses and Administration

Carbenoxolone sodium is a synthetic derivative of glycyrrhizinic acid (see Liquorice, p.1197). It has been given by mouth in the treatment of peptic ulcer disease (p.1174) and is sometimes given in combination with antacids in gastro-oesophageal reflux disease (p.1170). It appears to act by stimulating the synthesis of protective mucus. The suggested dosage of carbenoxolone sodium in gastro-oesophageal reflux disease is 20 mg three times daily by mouth and 40 mg at night for 6 to 12 weeks, as a preparation also containing antacids and alginic acid.

Carbenoxolone sodium is one of many topical treatments for the symptomatic management of mouth ulceration (p.1172). It is used as a 2% gel or as a 1% mouthwash.

Preparations

Proprietary Preparations (details are given in Part 3)
Aust.: Rowadermat; ***Austral.:*** Bioral; ***Ger.:*** Ulcus-Tablinen†; ***Irl.:*** Biogastrone†; Bioral; Carbosan; Duogastrone†; ***Ital.:*** Gastrausil†; ***S.Afr.:*** Bioral†; ***Spain:*** Sanodin; ***UK:*** Biogastrone†; Bioplex; Bioral.

Multi-ingredient: ***Irl.:*** Pyrogastrone; ***Ital.:*** Gastrausil Complex†; Gastrausil D†; Megast†; ***UK:*** Pyrogastrone.

Casanthranol (7505-m)

Casanthranol *(USAN).*

CAS — 8024-48-4.

Pharmacopoeias. In US.

Prepared from cascara (see below) it contains not less than 20% of total hydroxyanthracene derivatives calculated on the dried basis, of which not less than 80% consists of cascarosides, calculated as cascaroside A.

It is a light tan to brown, amorphous hygroscopic powder. Freely **soluble** in water with some residue; partially soluble in methyl alcohol and hot isopropyl alcohol; practically insoluble in acetone. **Store** in airtight containers at a temperature not exceeding 30°. Protect from light.

Casanthranol is an anthraquinone laxative with general properties similar to those of senna (p.1212). It is given in usual doses of 30 to 60 mg daily by mouth, together with a faecal softener. In severe cases a dose of 90 mg daily, or 60 mg twice daily, may be given.

Preparations

Proprietary Preparations (details are given in Part 3)
Belg.: Cascalax.

Multi-ingredient: ***Canad.:*** Peri-Colace; ***Spain:*** Laxvital; ***USA:*** Black-Draught; D-S-S Plus†; Diocto-K Plus; Dioctolose Plus; Disanthrol; Disolan Forte; Docusoft Plus; DSMC Plus; Genasoft Plus Softgels; Peri-Colace; Peri-Dos Softgels; Pro-Sof Plus; Regulace; Silace-C; Soflax Overnight.

Cascara (7506-b)

Cascara Sagrada; Cascararinde; Chittem Bark; Rhamni Purshianae Cortex; Rhamni Purshiani Cortex; Sacred Bark.

CAS — 8047-27-6; 8015-89-2 (cascara sagrada extract).

Pharmacopoeias. In *Eur.* (see p.viii) and *US.*

The dried bark of *Rhamnus purshianus* (=*Frangula purshiana*) (Rhamnaceae). The Ph. Eur. specifies that it contains not less than 8% of hydroxyanthracene glycosides of which not less than 60% consists of cascarosides, both expressed as cascaroside A and calculated with reference to the dried drug; the USP specifies not less than 7% of total hydroxyanthracene derivatives. **Protect** from light.

Cascara is an anthraquinone stimulant laxative with general properties similar to those of senna (p.1212). It has been used in the treatment of constipation in doses equivalent to up to about 20 to 70 mg of total hydroxyanthracene derivatives daily by mouth.

Preparations

BP 1998: Cascara Dry Extract; Cascara Tablets;
USP 23: Aromatic Cascara Fluidextract; Cascara Sagrada Extract; Cascara Sagrada Fluidextract; Cascara Tablets.

Proprietary Preparations (details are given in Part 3)
Canad.: Le 500 D; ***Fr.:*** Peristaltine; ***Ger.:*** Legapas mono; ***Ital.:*** Bonlax; Brevilax†; Colamin; Sagrada-Lax; ***Switz.:*** Legapas; ***USA:*** LBC-LAX.

Multi-ingredient: numerous preparations are listed in Part 3.

Cassia Pulp (7507-v)

The evaporated aqueous extract of crushed ripe cassia fruits (cassia pods), *Cassia fistula* (Leguminosae).

Cassia pulp has mild laxative properties owing to its content of anthraquinone glycosides.

Preparations

Proprietary Preparations (details are given in Part 3)

Multi-ingredient: ***Ital.:*** Tamarine; ***Spain:*** Pruina; ***Switz.:*** Tamarine.

Cerium Oxalate (12549-j)

CAS — 139-42-4 (cerous oxalate, anhydrous).

Pharmacopoeias. In *Aust.*

Cerium oxalate is used as an antiemetic.

Preparations

Proprietary Preparations (details are given in Part 3)

Multi-ingredient: ***Spain:*** Novonausin.

Cetraxate Hydrochloride (15314-t)

Cetraxate Hydrochloride *(USAN, rINNM).*

DV-1006. 4-(2-Carboxyethyl)phenyl tranexamate hydrochloride; 4-(2-Carboxyethyl)phenyl *trans*-4-aminomethylcyclohexanecarboxylate hydrochloride.

$C_{17}H_{23}NO_4,HCl = 341.8.$

CAS — 34675-84-8 (cetraxate); 27724-96-5 (cetraxate hydrochloride).

Pharmacopoeias. In *Jpn.*

Cetraxate hydrochloride is stated to be a mucosal protectant with actions on gastric microcirculation as well as prostaglandin synthesis and kallikrein. It is used in the treatment of gastritis and peptic ulcer disease (p.1174) in doses of 600 to 800 mg daily.

Preparations

Proprietary Preparations (details are given in Part 3)
Jpn: Neuer.

Chalk (713-n)

Prepared Chalk.

$CaCO_3 = 100.1.$

CAS — 13397-25-6.

Pharmacopoeias. In *Br.*

A native calcium carbonate purified by elutriation. It consists of the calcareous shells and detritus of various foraminifera and contains when dried not less than 97% of $CaCO_3$.

White or greyish-white, odourless or almost odourless, amorphous, earthy, friable masses, usually conical in form, or powder. Practically **insoluble** in water; slightly soluble in water containing carbon dioxide; it absorbs water readily.

Chalk has been used as an adsorbent antidiarrhoeal agent. Calcium carbonate (precipitated chalk) is used as an antacid, see p.1182.

Preparations

BP 1998: Compound Magnesium Trisilicate Oral Powder.

Chlorbenzoxamine Hydrochloride (688-c)

Chlorbenzoxamine Hydrochloride *(rINNM).*

UCB-1474 (anhydrous). 1-[2-(2-Chlorobenzhydryloxy)ethyl]-4-(2-methylbenzyl)piperazine dihydrochloride dihydrate.

$C_{27}H_{31}ClN_2O,2HCl,2H_2O = 544.0.$

CAS — 522-18-9 (chlorbenzoxamine); 5576-62-5 (chlorbenzoxamine hydrochloride, anhydrous).

Chlorbenzoxamine hydrochloride has been used for its antimuscarinic properties in the treatment of peptic ulcer disease.

Preparations

Proprietary Preparations (details are given in Part 3)

Multi-ingredient: ***Ital.:*** Libratar†.

Cimetidine (6117-g)

Cimetidine *(BAN, USAN, rINN).*

Cimetidinum; SKF-92334. 2-Cyano-1-methyl-3-[2-(5-methylimidazol-4-ylmethylthio)ethyl]guanidine.

$C_{10}H_{16}N_6S = 252.3.$

CAS — 51481-61-9 (cimetidine); 70059-30-2 (cimetidine hydrochloride).

Pharmacopoeias. In *Chin., Eur.* (see p.viii), *Int., Jpn, Pol.,* and *US.*

A white to off-white polymorphic crystalline powder, odourless or with a slight odour. Slightly **soluble** in water and chloroform; soluble in alcohol; freely soluble in methyl alcohol; sparingly soluble in isopropyl alcohol; practically insoluble in dichloromethane and in ether. It dissolves in dilute mineral acids. **Store** in airtight containers. Protect from light.

Adverse Effects

Adverse reactions to cimetidine are generally infrequent and are usually reversible following a reduction of dosage or withdrawal of therapy. The commonest side-effects reported have been altered bowel habit, dizziness, tiredness, headache, and rashes.

Reversible confusional states, especially in the elderly or in seriously ill patients such as those with renal failure, have occasionally occurred. Cimetidine has a weak anti-androgenic effect and gynaecomastia and impotence have also occasionally occurred in men receiving relatively high doses for conditions such as the Zollinger-Ellison syndrome.

Other adverse effects which have been reported rarely are hypersensitivity reactions and fever, arthralgia and myalgia, blood disorders including agranulocytosis and thrombocytopenia, interstitial nephritis, hepatotoxicity, and cardiovascular disorders including bradycardia and heart block.

The histamine H_2-receptor antagonists are considered to have a low incidence of minor adverse effects and to produce serious reactions only rarely.[1] In a meta-analysis of 24 double-blind placebo-controlled studies,[2] the incidence of adverse effects among patients receiving cimetidine for acute disorders was not significantly different from that of patients receiving placebo. The most common adverse effects reported by patients taking cimetidine who were followed-up for at least one year[3,4] were diarrhoea, headache, fatigue, skin rash or pruritus, and gynaecomastia. The incidence of adverse effects was dose-related and decreased with length of treatment.[4] No fatal adverse effect of cimetidine could be found in a mortality survey involving 9928 patients taking cimetidine and 9351 controls;[5] although the mortality rate was higher in the cimetidine patients, this was explained by the presence of underlying disease (known or unknown) before starting cimetidine treatment and the use of cimetidine to counter adverse gastric effects of other drugs. Follow-up of 9377 of these cimetidine-treated patients for a further 3 years[6] still revealed no fatal disorder attributable to cimetidine treatment and a steady fall in the excess death rate in cimetidine users was observed with increasing length of follow-up; by the fourth year there was little difference between the observed and expected death rate. Cimetidine still appeared to be safe after 10 years of follow-up.[7]

Further details of the adverse effects that have been reported or proposed are given below.

1. Penston J, Wormsley KG. Adverse reactions and interactions with H_2-receptor antagonists. *Med Toxicol* 1986; **1:** 192–216.
2. Richter JM, *et al.* Cimetidine and adverse reactions: a meta-analysis of randomized clinical trials of short-term therapy. *Am J Med* 1989; **87:** 278–84.
3. Colin Jones DG, *et al.* Post-marketing surveillance of the safety of cimetidine : twelve-month morbidity report. *Q J Med* 1985; **54:** 253–68.
4. Bardhan KD, *et al.* Safety of longterm cimetidine (CIM) treatment: the view from one centre. *Gut* 1990; **31:** A599.
5. Colin-Jones DG, *et al.* Postmarketing surveillance of the safety of cimetidine: 12 month mortality report. *Br Med J* 1983; **286:** 1713–16.
6. Colin-Jones DG, *et al.* Postmarketing surveillance of the safety of cimetidine: mortality during second, third, and fourth years of follow up. *Br Med J* 1985; **291:** 1084–8.
7. Colin-Jones DG, *et al.* Postmarketing surveillance of the safety of cimetidine: 10 year mortality report. *Gut* 1992; **33:** 1280–4.

Carcinogenicity. An association between H_2-receptor antagonists and gastric cancer has been proposed following individual case reports, the finding of tumours in long-term high-dose *animal* studies, and the possibility that nitrites and nitroso compounds may be produced; but such proposals are considered to have little clinical relevance.[1] The excess risk of gastric cancer reported in patients taking cimetidine[2-5] or ranitidine[5] decreases with time and there is no evidence for any long-term persistence of the effect.[5] Also an apparently protective effect has been observed for H_2-antagonist use starting 10 or more years before diagnosis of gastric cancer.[5]

An increased risk of cancers of the gastro-intestinal tract may be explained by initial symptoms resembling those of benign gastro-intestinal disorders, resulting in misdiagnosis and inappropriate cimetidine treatment.[2-4]

The observed excess risk for cancers of the respiratory system is probably related to smoking, since this is causally related to both peptic ulcer and lung cancer and the excess risk does not decline with time.[2-4]

While it would appear that the prolonged clinical use of H_2-receptor antagonists does not induce cancer, further long-term studies into their safety are needed before the possibility of such a risk can be dismissed completely.[6]

1. Penston J, Wormsley KG. H_2-receptor antagonists and gastric cancer. *Med Toxicol* 1986; **1:** 163–8.
2. Colin-Jones DG, *et al.* Postmarketing surveillance of the safety of cimetidine: 12 month mortality report. *Br Med J* 1983; **286:** 1713–16.
3. Colin-Jones DG, *et al.* Postmarketing surveillance of the safety of cimetidine: mortality during second, third, and fourth years of follow up. *Br Med J* 1985; **291:** 1084–8.
4. Møller H, *et al.* Cancer occurrence in a cohort of patients treated with cimetidine. *Gut* 1989; **30:** 1558–62.
5. La Vecchia C, *et al.* Histamine-2-receptor antagonists and gastric cancer risk. *Lancet* 1990; **336:** 355–7.
6. Møller H, *et al.* Use of cimetidine and other peptic ulcer drugs in Denmark 1977–1990 with analysis of the risk of gastric cancer among cimetidine users. *Gut* 1992; **33:** 1166–9.

Effects on the blood. The haematological adverse effects of histamine H_2-receptor antagonists were reviewed by Aymard and colleagues in 1988.[1] They noted that leucopenia, thrombocytopenia, and pancytopenia have all been reported with cimetidine and ranitidine, with neutropenia and agranulocytosis occurring most often. There were also isolated reports of haemolytic anaemia and leucocytosis associated with cimetidine therapy. The review stated that the overall incidence of cimetidine-associated blood cytopenia has been estimated as 2.3 per 100 000 treated patients; the incidence for ranitidine was less and although there were reports with famotidine (see p.1192) the incidence had not been determined.

However, a subsequent case-control study,[2] based on a population of 4.9 million patients concluded that the risk of hospitalisation due to neutropenia in patients receiving a six-week course of cimetidine was no more than 1 in 116 000, while agranulocytosis did not occur in more than 1 in 573 000 patients. Thus if there were an association between cimetidine and neutropenia it would appear to be very small.

1. Aymard J-P, *et al.* Haematological adverse effects of histamine H_2-receptor antagonists. *Med Toxicol* 1988; **3:** 430–48.
2. Strom BL, *et al.* Is cimetidine associated with neutropenia? *Am J Med* 1995; **99:** 282–90.

Effects on bones and joints. Severe arthritic symptoms have been reported in 5 patients receiving cimetidine[1] and there is one report[2] of cimetidine and ranitidine precipitating a reaction clinically identical to gout, but without elevation of uric acid. Further reports of arthritis during cimetidine therapy have been filed with the manufacturer.

1. Khong TK, Rooney PJ. Arthritis associated with cimetidine. *Lancet* 1980; **ii:** 1380.
2. Einarson TR, *et al.* Gout-like arthritis following cimetidine and ranitidine. *Drug Intell Clin Pharm* 1985; **19:** 201–2.

Effects on the cardiovascular system. Bradycardia,[1-4] atrioventricular block,[5,6] tachycardia,[7] and hypotension[4,8] have been reported during cimetidine treatment given by mouth and by intravenous injection or infusion. Although there are studies in patients[9] and healthy subjects[10,11] that have found no significant cardiovascular effects associated with cimetidine treatment, it is likely that a small proportion of patients are more susceptible to the cardiovascular effects of cimetidine and caution is recommended if the drug is given to patients with cardiovascular disease.

See also under Overdosage, below.

1. Jefferys DB, Vale JA. Cimetidine and bradycardia. *Lancet* 1978; **i:** 828.
2. Ligumsky M, *et al.* Cimetidine and arrhythmia suppression. *Ann Intern Med* 1978; **89:** 1008–9.
3. Tanner LA, Arrowsmith JB. Bradycardia and H_2 antagonists. *Ann Intern Med* 1988; **109:** 434–5.
4. Drea EJ, *et al.* Cimetidine-associated adverse reaction. *DICP Ann Pharmacother* 1990; **24:** 581–3.
5. Tordjman T, *et al.* Complete atrioventricular block and long-term cimetidine therapy. *Arch Intern Med* 1984; **144:** 861.
6. Ishizaki M, *et al.* First-degree atrioventricular block induced by oral cimetidine. *Lancet* 1987; **i:** 225–6.
7. Dickey W, Symington M. Broad-complex tachycardia after intravenous cimetidine. *Lancet* 1987; **i:** 99–100.
8. Mahon WA, Kolton M. Hypotension after intravenous cimetidine. *Lancet* 1978; **i:** 828.
9. Jackson G, Upward JW. Cimetidine, ranitidine, and heart rate. *Lancet* 1982; **ii:** 265.
10. Hughes DG, *et al.* Cardiovascular effects of H_2-receptor antagonists. *J Clin Pharmacol* 1989; **29:** 472–7.
11. Hilleman DE, *et al.* Impact of chronic oral H_2-antagonist therapy on left ventricular systolic function and exercise capacity. *J Clin Pharmacol* 1992; **32:** 1033–7.

Effects on the endocrine system. Cimetidine has dose-related mild anti-androgenic properties and reduced sperm counts, and raised serum-prolactin concentrations have been reported in men during cimetidine treatment[1] as have gynaecomastia, breast tenderness, and impotence.[2] Symptoms resolved following withdrawal of cimetidine,[1,2] reduction of the dose,[2] or transfer to ranitidine.[2]

A study by the Boston Collaborative Drug Surveillance Program, using data from 81 535 men in the UK, found that cimetidine was associated with an incidence of 3.29 cases of gynaecomastia per 1000 person years, representing a relative risk 7.2 times greater than that of non-users.[3] The period at highest risk seemed to be between the seventh and twelfth month after starting treatment, and the occurrence was related to dose, with most of the risk associated with doses over 1 g daily. There was no significant risk of gynaecomastia with ranitidine or omeprazole.

1. Wang C, *et al.* Effect of cimetidine on gonadal function in man. *Br J Clin Pharmacol* 1982; **13:** 791–4.
2. Jensen RT, *et al.* Cimetidine-induced impotence and breast changes in patients with gastric hypersecretory states. *N Engl J Med* 1983; **308:** 883–7.
3. García Rodríguez LA, Jick H. Risk of gynaecomastia associated with cimetidine, omeprazole, and other antiulcer drugs. *Br Med J* 1994; **308:** 503–6. Correction. *ibid.*; 819.

Effects on the eyes. Ocular pain, blurred vision, and a rise in intra-ocular pressure occurred in a patient with chronic glaucoma during treatment with cimetidine; subsequently ocular symptoms associated with raised intra-ocular pressure also developed during ranitidine treatment.[1] However, a study in healthy subjects and preliminary results in patients with chronic simple glaucoma suggested that cimetidine had no effect on intra-ocular pressure.[2] A cohort study involving 140 128 patients receiving anti-ulcer therapy, 68 504 of whom received cimetidine, found no evidence that any of the drugs were associated with a major increased risk of vascular or inflammatory disorders of the eye.[3]

1. Dobrilla G, *et al.* Exacerbation of glaucoma associated with both cimetidine and ranitidine *Lancet* 1982; **i:** 1078.
2. Feldman F, Cohen MM. Intraocular pressure and H_2 receptor antagonists. *Lancet* 1982; **i:** 1359.
3. García Rodríguez LA, *et al.* A cohort study of the ocular safety of anti-ulcer drugs. *Br J Clin Pharmacol* 1996; **42:** 213–16.

Effects on the kidneys. Up to the end of 1981 the manufacturers of cimetidine were aware of 20 patients who may have had interstitial nephritis out of an estimated total of 20 million cimetidine-treated patients. On the assumption that only 10% of these adverse effects have been reported, which is a figure consistent with that suggested for a voluntary reporting system, the incidence would be around 1 in 100 000 treated patients. The interstitial nephritis related to cimetidine administration has always been reversed on cessation of therapy.[1]

1. Rowley-Jones D, Flind AC. Cimetidine-induced renal failure. *Br Med J* 1982; **285:** 1422–3.

Effects on the liver. A cohort study[1] involving 108 891 patients who had received cimetidine, ranitidine, famotidine, or omeprazole between 1990 and 1993, found 33 cases meeting the authors' definition of clinically serious liver injury (cholestatic in 8 cases, hepatocellular in 15 and mixed in 10), most of whom presented with jaundice. Of these cases of liver injury, 12 were among current users of cimetidine, compared with 5 among users of ranitidine and 1 omeprazole user. It was estimated that the incidence of hepatotoxicity among patients using cimetidine was 2.3 cases per 10 000 users, and the adjusted relative risk was 5.5 times that of non-users. The relative risk for use of ranitidine or omeprazole was calculated at 1.7 and 2.1 respectively. The risk with cimetidine was greatest at high doses (800 mg daily or above) and at the beginning of therapy.

1. García Rodríguez LA, *et al.* The risk of acute liver injury associated with cimetidine and other acid-suppressing anti-ulcer drugs. *Br J Clin Pharmacol* 1997; **43:** 183–8.

Effects on the muscles. Polymyositis has been reported in a patient taking cimetidine,[1] but it was questioned whether this was a cimetidine-induced reaction.[2,3]

1. Watson AJS, *et al.* Immunologic studies in cimetidine-induced nephropathy and polymyositis. *N Engl J Med* 1983; **308:** 142–5.
2. Hawkins RA, *et al.* Cimetidine and polymyositis. *N Engl J Med* 1983; **309:** 187–8.
3. Watson AJS, *et al.* Cimetidine and polymyositis. *N Engl J Med* 1983; **309:** 188.

Effects on the nervous system. Cimetidine has been associated with a number of adverse neurological effects including confusion,[1-8] bizarre behaviour,[9] reversible brain stem syndrome (with ataxia, dysarthria, visual impairment, deafness, and paraesthesia),[10] coma,[8,11] convulsions,[7] encephalopathy,[12] visual hallucinations,[9,13,14] paranoia,[5] chorea,[15,16] myopathy,[17] and neuropathy.[18,19] These reactions occur mainly in patients who are elderly, critically ill, or with impaired renal or hepatic function, in whom there may be increased penetration of the blood-brain barrier by cimetidine. Single-dose studies in young healthy subjects[20] have found no adverse changes in performance, central nervous function, or subjective assessment of mood after administration of cimetidine 200 or 400 mg by mouth.

There is no clear evidence that cimetidine is a more frequent cause of CNS reactions than ranitidine, famotidine, or nizatidine.[21]

1. Robinson TJ, Mulligan TO. Cimetidine and mental confusion. *Lancet* 1977; **ii:** 719.
2. Spears JB. Cimetidine and mental confusion. *Am J Hosp Pharm* 1978; **35:** 1035.
3. Wood CA, *et al.* Cimetidine and mental confusion. *JAMA* 1978; **239:** 2550–1.
4. McMillen MA, *et al.* Cimetidine and mental confusion. *N Engl J Med* 1978; **298:** 284–5.
5. Kinnell HG, Webb A. Confusion associated with cimetidine. *Br Med J* 1979; **ii:** 1438.
6. Mogelnicki SR, *et al.* Physostigmine reversal of cimetidine-induced mental confusion. *JAMA* 1979; **241:** 826–7.
7. Edmonds ME, *et al.* Cimetidine: does neurotoxicity occur? Report of three cases. *J R Soc Med* 1979; **72:** 172–5.
8. Sonnenblick M, *et al.* Neurological and psychiatric side effects of cimetidine—report of 3 cases with review of the literature. *Postgrad Med J* 1982; **58:** 415–18.
9. Papp KA, Curtis RM. Cimetidine-induced psychosis in a 14-year-old girl. *Can Med Assoc J* 1984; **131:** 1081–4.
10. Cumming WJK, Foster JB. Cimetidine-induced brainstem dysfunction. *Lancet* 1978; **i:** 1096.
11. Levine ML. Cimetidine-induced coma in cirrhosis of the liver. *JAMA* 1978; **240:** 1238.
12. Niv Y, *et al.* Cimetidine and encephalopathy. *Ann Intern Med* 1986; **105:** 977.
13. Agarwal SK. Cimetidine and visual hallucinations. *JAMA* 1978; **240:** 214.
14. Rushton AR. Pseudohypoparathyroidism, cimetidine, and neurologic toxicity. *Ann Intern Med* 1983; **98:** 677.
15. Kushner MJ. Chorea and cimetidine. *Ann Intern Med* 1982; **96:** 126.
16. Lehmann AB. Reversible chorea due to ranitidine and cimetidine. *Lancet* 1988; **ii:** 158.
17. Feest TG, Read DJ. Myopathy associated with cimetidine? *Br Med J* 1980; **281:** 1284–5.
18. Walls TJ, *et al.* Motor neuropathy associated with cimetidine. *Br Med J* 1980; **281:** 974–5.
19. Atkinson AB, *et al.* Neurological dysfunction in two patients receiving captopril and cimetidine. *Lancet* 1980; **ii:** 36–7.
20. Nicholson AN, Stone BM. The H_2-antagonists, cimetidine and ranitidine : studies on performance. *Eur J Clin Pharmacol* 1984; **26:** 579–82.
21. Cantú TG, Korek JS. Central nervous system reactions to histamine-2 receptor blockers. *Ann Intern Med* 1991; **114:** 1027–34.

Effects on the respiratory system. A report[1] of 20 patients who developed work-related respiratory symptoms associated with exposure to cimetidine dust; the effects were most common in those most often exposed.

1. Coutts II, *et al.* Respiratory symptoms related to work in a factory manufacturing cimetidine tablets. *Br Med J* 1984; **288:** 1418.

Effects on the skin. Widespread erythrosis-like lesions in a 36-year-old man were probably induced by cimetidine.[1] There has been a report[2] of a skin eruption clinically consistent with erythema annulare centrifugum developing in a patient after 6 months of treatment with cimetidine; the eruption resolved after withdrawal of cimetidine and reappeared on rechallenge. The condition had not recurred during therapy with ranitidine. Urticarial vasculitis[3] and alopecia[4] have also been associated with cimetidine treatment.

There have been reports of the Stevens-Johnson syndrome during cimetidine treatment in patients with a history of hypersensitivity to penicillin[5] or sulphonamides.[6]

1. Angelini G, *et al.* Cimetidine and erythrosis-like lesions. *Br Med J* 1979; **i:** 1147–8.
2. Merrett AC, *et al.* Cimetidine-induced erythema annulare centrifugum: no cross-sensitivity with ranitidine. *Br Med J* 1981: **283:** 698.
3. Mitchell GG, *et al.* Cimetidine-induced cutaneous vasculitis. *Am J Med* 1983; **75:** 875–6.
4. Khalsa JH, *et al.* Cimetidine-associated alopecia. *Int J Dermatol* 1983; **22:** 202–4.
5. Ahmed AH, *et al.* Stevens-Johnson syndrome during treatment with cimetidine. *Lancet* 1978; **ii:** 433.
6. Guan R, Yeo PPB. Stevens-Johnson syndrome: was it cimetidine? *Aust N Z J Med* 1983; **13:** 182.

Fever. Reports of febrile reactions associated with cimetidine.

1. Ramboer C. Drug fever with cimetidine. *Lancet* 1978; **i:** 330–1.
2. McLoughlin JC, *et al.* Cimetidine fever. *Lancet* 1978; **ii:** 499–500.
3. Corbett CL, Holdsworth CD. Fever, abdominal pain, and leucopenia during treatment with cimetidine. *Br Med J* 1978; **i:** 753–4.
4. Landolfo K, *et al.* Cimetidine-induced fever. *Can Med Assoc J* 1984; **130:** 1580.

Hypersensitivity. Facial oedema,[1] laryngospasm,[1] pruritus,[2,3] rash,[2,3] angioedema[3] and anaphylaxis[4] have been reported in patients receiving cimetidine by mouth or intravenously.

See also under Effects on the Skin, above.

1. Delaunois L. Hypersensitivity to cimetidine. *N Engl J Med* 1979; **300:** 1216.
2. Hadfield WA. Cimetidine and giant urticaria. *Ann Intern Med* 1979; **91:** 128–9.
3. Sandhu BS, Requena R. Hypersensitivity to cimetidine. *Ann Intern Med* 1982; **97:** 138.
4. Knapp AB, *et al.* Cimetidine-induced anaphylaxis. *Ann Intern Med* 1982; **97:** 374–5.

Infection. Treatment with histamine H_2-receptor antagonists may predispose patients to salmonella infection, probably because the decrease in gastric acidity reduces the gastric killing of ingested organisms.[1] The greatest increase in risk was seen in patients over 65 years of age.

Similar increased risk of infection with brucellosis had also been proposed in patients receiving cimetidine,[2] although it was suggested that this might be due to an immunosuppressant effect of cimetidine rather than reduced gastric acidity.[3] (However, cimetidine has generally been thought of as enhancing immune response—see Hypersensitivity and Immunological Disorders, under Uses, below).

1. Neal KR, *et al.* Recent treatment with H_2 antagonists and antibiotics and gastric surgery as risk factors for salmonella infection. *Br Med J* 1994; **308:** 176.
2. Cristiano P, Paradisi F. Can cimetidine facilitate infections by oral route? *Lancet* 1982; **ii:** 45.
3. Thornes RD. Cimetidine and brucellosis. *Lancet* 1982; **ii:** 217.

Lupus. Cimetidine has been reported to induce a lupus erythematosus-like eruption[1] and to exacerbate cutaneous disease activity in a patient with pre-existing systemic lupus erythematosus.[2]

1. Macdonald KJS, Kenicer KJA. Can cimetidine induce lupus erythematosus? *Br Med J* 1984; **288:** 1498.
2. Davidson BL, *et al.* Cimetidine-associated exacerbation of cutaneous lupus erythematosus. *Arch Intern Med* 1982; **142:** 166–7.

Overdosage. Overdosage with cimetidine 5.2 to 20 g, including one patient who took about 12 g daily for 5 days,[1] has not produced serious toxic effects,[1-3] despite plasma concentrations of up to 57 μg per mL (peak plasma concentration after a 200-mg dose is reported to be 1 μg per mL). However, an overdose of about 12 g produced high pulse rate, dilated pupils, speech disturbances, agitation and disorientation in one patient[4] and respiratory depression in another patient who had chronic schizophrenia and was also taking trifluoperazine and hydroxyzine.[5] Also, fatal bradycardia has been reported after overdosage with an unknown amount of cimetidine and diazepam.[6]

Treatment of cimetidine overdosage should consist of gastric lavage or emesis induction, provided that not more than 4 hours have elapsed since ingestion of the drug, followed by supportive measures and symptomatic treatment only. Forced diuresis does not appear to enhance the excretion of cimetidine from the body, and is not recommended.[3]

1. Gill GV. Cimetidine overdose. *Lancet* 1978; **i:** 99.
2. Illingworth RN, Jarvie DR. Absence of toxicity in cimetidine overdosage. *Br Med J* 1979; **i:** 453–4.
3. Meredith TJ, Volans GN. Management of cimetidine overdose. *Lancet* 1979; **ii:** 1367.
4. Nelson PG. Cimetidine and mental confusion. *Lancet* 1977; **ii:** 928.
5. Wilson JB. Cimetidine overdosage. *Br Med J* 1979; **i:** 955.
6. Hiss J, *et al.* Fatal bradycardia after intentional overdose of cimetidine and diazepam. *Lancet* 1982; **ii:** 982.

Parotitis. Recurrent parotitis in a patient when given cimetidine or ranitidine.[1]

1. Caraman P, *et al.* Recurrent parotitis with H_2 receptor antagonists. *Lancet* 1986; **ii:** 1455–6.

Precautions

Before giving cimetidine to patients with gastric ulcers the possibility of malignancy should be considered since cimetidine may mask symptoms and delay diagnosis. It should be given in reduced dosage to patients with impaired renal function.

Intravenous injections of cimetidine should be given slowly and intravenous infusion is recommended in patients with cardiovascular impairment.

Breast feeding. See under Distribution into Breast Milk, below.

Burns. The clearance of cimetidine has been reported to be increased in burn patients, with the increase correlating to the size of the burn.[1] Despite another study which reported a decreased renal clearance (but an increase non-renal clearance) early in the evolution of burn injury,[2] it has been recommended that the dosage of cimetidine be increased in patients with burns, depending on the extent of injury. A requirement for increased dosage has also been noted in paediatric burns patients.[3]

1. Martyn JAJ, *et al.* Increased cimetidine clearance in burn patients. *JAMA* 1985; **253:** 1288–91.
2. Ziemniak JA, *et al.* Cimetidine kinetics during resuscitation from burn shock. *Clin Pharmacol Ther* 1984; **36:** 228–33.
3. Martyn JAJ, *et al.* Alteration by burn injury of the pharmacokinetics and pharmacodynamics of cimetidine in children. *Eur J Clin Pharmacol* 1989; **36:** 361–7.

Hepatic impairment. The bioavailability of cimetidine may be increased in patients with cirrhosis[1,2] and a dosage reduction of up to 40% has been suggested in patients with portal systemic encephalopathy.[3]

An increased resistance to H_2-receptor antagonists has been reported in patients with cirrhosis, see Ranitidine p.1210.

1. Gugler R, *et al.* Altered disposition and availability of cimetidine in liver cirrhotic patients. *Br J Clin Pharmacol* 1982; **14:** 421–30.
2. Cello JP, Øie S. Cimetidine disposition in patients with Laennec's cirrhosis during multiple dosing therapy. *Eur J Clin Pharmacol* 1983; **25:** 223–9.
3. Ziemniak JA, *et al.* Hepatic encephalopathy and altered cimetidine kinetics. *Clin Pharmacol Ther* 1983; **34:** 375–82.

Renal impairment. The clearance of cimetidine is reduced in renal impairment and dosage reduction is recommended (see Uses and Administration, below).

Interactions

Cimetidine may inhibit the hepatic metabolism of many drugs by binding to cytochrome P450. Although many such interactions have been demonstrated, a few are considered clinically significant, notably those with phenytoin, theophylline, lignocaine and other antiarrhythmics, and oral anticoagulants. Reduction in the dosage of some drugs may be required.

Antacids. Single-dose studies of the interaction between cimetidine and antacids[1] have shown reduced bioavailability of cimetidine as well as no interaction. The neutralising capacity of the antacid appears to be a factor in determining whether an interaction occurs and a dose with less than 50 mmol neutralising capacity will have little, if any, effect on cimetidine absorption. There is no evidence that the therapeutic efficacy of cimetidine is reduced and with long-term use of the combination the bioavailability of cimetidine is unlikely to be reduced.

1. Gugler R, Allgayer H. Effects of antacids on the clinical pharmacokinetics of drugs: an update. *Clin Pharmacokinet* 1990; **18:** 210–19.

Antimuscarinics. The antimuscarinic *propantheline* delays gastric emptying and reduces intestinal motility and has been reported to reduce the bioavailability of cimetidine.[1]

1. Kanto J, *et al.* The effect of metoclopramide and propantheline on the gastrointestinal absorption of cimetidine. *Br J Clin Pharmacol* 1981; **11:** 629–31.

Prokinetic drugs. *Metoclopramide* may reduce the bioavailability of cimetidine possibly due to reduction of gastrointestinal transit time.[1-3] A similar interaction has been reported between cimetidine and the prokinetic drug *cisapride*[4] The clinical significance of this interaction is questionable since such combinations may be clinically effective.

1. Gugler R, *et al.* Impaired cimetidine absorption due to antacids and metoclopramide. *Eur J Clin Pharmacol* 1981; **20:** 225–8.
2. Kanto J, *et al.* The effect of metoclopramide and propantheline on the gastrointestinal absorption of cimetidine. *Br J Clin Pharmacol* 1981; **11:** 629–31.
3. Barzaghi N, *et al.* Effects on cimetidine bioavailability of metoclopramide and antacids given two hours apart. *Eur J Clin Pharmacol* 1989; **37:** 409–10.
4. Kirch W, *et al.* Cisapride-cimetidine interactions; enhanced cisapride bioavailability and accelerated cimetidine absorption. *Ther Drug Monit* 1989; **11:** 411–14.

Sucralfate. The manufacturers of the mucosal protectant sucralfate state that it has been shown to reduce the bioavailability of cimetidine, presumably due to binding in the gastrointestinal tract. The effect can be avoided by separating doses of the two drugs by 2 hours, but it is not clear whether the interaction has a clinical significance.

Effects on other drugs. Cimetidine can affect a wide range of drugs[1-4] but these interactions are of clinical significance for only a small number of drugs, particularly those which have a narrow therapeutic index where the risk of toxicity may necessitate adjustment of dosage. The majority of interactions are due to binding of cimetidine to cytochrome P450 in the liver with subsequent inhibition of microsomal oxidative metabolism and increased bioavailability or plasma concentrations of drugs metabolised by these enzymes. Other mechanisms of interaction such as altered absorption, competition for renal tubular secretion, and changes in hepatic blood flow play only a minor role.

Significant or potentially significant interactions have occurred with antiarrhythmics such as lignocaine and procainamide, sulphonylurea and biguanide antidiabetics, antiepileptics such as phenytoin and carbamazepine, chloramphenicol, chlorpromazine, cyclosporin, nifedipine, opioids such as pethidine, suxamethonium, theophylline, tricyclic antidepressants such as amitriptyline, vasopressin, and warfarin and other oral anticoagulants. The plasma concentrations of these and many other drugs which are metabolised by oxidation may need to be monitored, and caution exercised, when cimetidine is given concomitantly. For further information, see under the appropriate drug monographs.

There is a continuing dispute as to whether a significant interaction exists between cimetidine and alcohol. Although cimetidine inhibits alcohol dehydrogenase in the gastric mucosa, the significance of this site for alcohol metabolism is uncertain.[5] Studies have reported both significant increases in blood alcohol,[6,7] and a lack of such increases,[8,9] following pretreatment with cimetidine but such studies are sensitive to variations in design, and the current consensus appears to be that any interaction is unlikely to be of clinical significance.[5,10]

Other H_2-antagonists have less effect on cytochrome P450, if any, than cimetidine and the potential for drug interactions is reduced.

1. Penston J, Wormsley KG. Adverse reactions and interactions with H_2-receptor antagonists. *Med Toxicol* 1986; **i:** 192–216.
2. Somogyi A, Muirhead M. Pharmacokinetic interactions of cimetidine 1987. *Clin Pharmacokinet* 1987; **12:** 321–66.
3. Smith SR, Kendall MJ. Ranitidine versus cimetidine: a comparison of their potential to cause clinically important drug interactions. *Clin Pharmacokinet* 1988; **15:** 44–56.
4. Shinn AF. Clinical relevance of cimetidine drug interactions. *Drug Safety* 1992; **7:** 245–67.
5. Levitt MD. Do histamine-2 receptor antagonists influence the metabolism of ethanol? *Ann Intern Med* 1993; **118:** 564–5.
6. Holt S, *et al.* Evidence for an interaction between alcohol and certain H_2 receptor antagonists. *Gut* 1991; **32:** A1220.
7. DiPadova C, *et al.* Effects of ranitidine on blood alcohol levels after ethanol ingestion: comparison with other H_2-receptor antagonists. *JAMA* 1992; **267:** 83–6.
8. Fraser AG, *et al.* Effects of H_2-receptor antagonists on blood alcohol levels. *JAMA* 1992; **267:** 2469.
9. Raufman J-P, *et al.* Histamine-2 receptor antagonists do not alter serum ethanol levels in fed, nonalcoholic men. *Ann Intern Med* 1993; **118:** 488–94.
10. Hansten PD. Effects of H_2-receptor antagonists on blood alcohol levels. *JAMA* 1992; **267:** 2469.

Pharmacokinetics

Cimetidine is readily absorbed from the gastro-intestinal tract and peak plasma concentrations are obtained about an hour after administration on an empty stomach; a second peak may be seen after about 3 hours. Food delays the rate and may slightly decrease the extent of absorption, with the peak plasma concentration occurring after about 2 hours.

The bioavailability of cimetidine following oral administration is about 60 to 70% because of first-pass metabolism. Cimetidine is widely distributed and has a volume of distribution of about 1 litre per kg and is weakly bound, about 20%, to plasma proteins. The elimination half-life from plasma is about 2 hours and is increased in renal impairment. Cimetidine is partially metabolised in the liver to the sulphoxide and to hydroxymethylcimetidine, but most is excreted unchanged in the urine. Cimetidine crosses the placental barrier and is distributed into breast milk.

Reviews.

1. Somogyi A, Gugler R. Clinical pharmacokinetics of cimetidine. *Clin Pharmacokinet* 1983; **8:** 463–95.
2. Lauritsen K, *et al.* Clinical pharmacokinetics of drugs used in the treatment of gastrointestinal diseases. *Clin Pharmacokinet* 1990; **19:** 11–31 (part I) and 94–125 (part II).
3. Lin JH. Pharmacokinetic and pharmacodynamic properties of histamine H_2-receptor antagonists: relationship between intrinsic potency and effective plasma concentrations. *Clin Pharmacokinet* 1991; **20:** 218–36.
4. Gladziwa U, Klotz U. Pharmacokinetics and pharmacodynamics of H_2-receptor antagonists in patients with renal insufficiency. *Clin Pharmacokinet* 1993; **24:** 319–32.

Children. Renal function is limited in the first few months of life and half-lives of 1.1 to 3.7 hours have been reported for cimetidine in neonates.[1-3] A dosage regimen for neonates based on renal function has been suggested[1] with 15 to 20 mg per kg body-weight daily for full-term neonates, but with lower doses for premature neonates and those with renal dysfunction. However, a dose of 5 to 7 mg per kg may be sufficient to suppress gastric acid secretion in neonates.[3]

In older infants and children maturation of renal function is complete and the clearance of cimetidine is increased compared with that in adults while younger children show higher clearance values than older children. A typical dosage regimen for children is 30 mg per kg daily, in 3 or 4 divided doses.[4] However, even this dose might not produce optimal control of gastric acid.[5]

1. Ziemniak JA, *et al.* The pharmacokinetics and metabolism of cimetidine in neonates. *Dev Pharmacol Ther* 1984; **7:** 30–8.
2. Lloyd CW, *et al.* The pharmacokinetics of cimetidine and metabolites in a neonate. *Drug Intell Clin Pharm* 1985; **19:** 203–5.
3. Stile IL, *et al.* Pharmacokinetic evaluation of cimetidine in newborn infants. *Clin Ther* 1985; **7:** 361–4.
4. Somogyi A, *et al.* Cimetidine pharmacokinetics and dosage requirements in children. *Eur J Pediatr* 1985; **144:** 72–6.
5. Lambert J, *et al.* Efficacy of cimetidine for gastric acid suppression in pediatric patients. *J Pediatr* 1992; **120:** 474–8.

Distribution into breast milk. Cimetidine is reported to be actively transported into breast milk, resulting in a milk:serum ratio 5.5 times higher than that expected with passive diffusion.[1] In one case, where cimetidine was detected in the milk of a nursing mother in concentrations higher than in her plasma, it was calculated that the maximum amount of cimetidine that an infant could ingest assuming an intake of about 1 litre of milk daily and fed at the time of peak concentrations would be about 6 mg.[2]

However, the Committee on Drugs of the American Academy of Pediatrics has pointed out that there was no evidence of signs or symptoms attributable to the drug in the infant in this case,[3] despite 6 months of breast feeding, which explains why cimetidine has been classified as usually compatible with breast feeding.

1. Oo CY, *et al.* Active transport of cimetidine into human milk. *Clin Pharmacol Ther* 1995; **58:** 548–55.
2. Somogyi A, Gugler R. Cimetidine excretion into breast milk. *Br J Clin Pharmacol* 1979; **7:** 627–9.
3. Berlin CM. Cimetidine and breast-feeding. *Pediatrics* 1991; **88:** 1294.

Uses and Administration

Cimetidine is a histamine H_2-receptor antagonist. Accordingly, it inhibits gastric acid secretion and reduces pepsin output; it has also been shown to inhibit other actions of histamine mediated by H_2-receptors. It is used in conditions where inhibition of gastric acid secretion may be beneficial. Such conditions include peptic ulcer disease (p.1174), gastro-oesophageal reflux disease (p.1170), selected cases of persistent dyspepsia (p.1169), pathological hypersecretory states such as the Zollinger-Ellison syndrome (p.1176), stress ulceration, and in patients at risk of acid aspiration (p.1168) during general anaesthesia. Cimetidine may also be used to reduce malabsorption and fluid loss in patients with the short bowel syndrome and to reduce the degradation of enzyme supplements given to patients with pancreatic insufficiency.

Cimetidine may be given by mouth, by the nasogastric route, or parenterally by the intravenous or intramuscular routes; the total daily dose by any route should not normally exceed 2.4 g. Although some formulations are prepared as the hydrochloride, strengths and doses are expressed in terms of the base. When cimetidine is given by mouth, daytime doses should generally be taken with meals.

In the management of benign **gastric** and **duodenal ulceration** a single daily dose of 800 mg by mouth at bedtime is recommended which should be given initially for at least 4 weeks in the case of duodenal and for at least 6 weeks in the case of gastric ulcers. Where appropriate a maintenance dose of 400 mg may then be given once daily at bedtime, or twice daily in the morning and at bedtime. In the US, doses of 300 mg by mouth four times daily have been used.

In **gastro-oesophageal reflux disease** the recommended dose is 400 mg by mouth four times daily (with meals and at bedtime), or 800 mg twice daily, for 4 to 8 weeks. In pathological hypersecretory conditions, such as the **Zollinger-Ellison syndrome**, a dose of 300 or 400 mg by mouth four times daily is normally used, although sometimes higher doses may be necessary.

Doses of 200 to 400 mg by mouth, by nasogastric administration, or parenterally (200 mg only for direct intravenous injection) every 4 to 6 hours are recommended for the management of patients at risk from **stress ulceration** of the upper gastro-intestinal tract. In patients at risk of developing the **acid aspiration syndrome**, a dose of 400 mg by mouth may be given 90 to 120 minutes before the induction of anaesthesia or at the start of labour, and doses of up to 400 mg (by the parenteral route if appropriate, see below) may be repeated at intervals of 4 hours if required.

Doses of up to 200 mg four times daily have been taken for non-ulcer **dyspepsia**; 100 mg at night has been used in the prophylaxis of nocturnal heart burn.

To reduce the degradation of pancreatic enzyme supplements, patients with **pancreatic insufficiency** may be given cimetidine 800 to 1600 mg daily by mouth in 4 divided doses, 60 to 90 minutes before meals.

The usual dose of cimetidine by intravenous injection is 200 mg which should be given slowly over at least 2 minutes and may be repeated every 4 to 6 hours. If a larger dose is required, or if the patient has cardiovascular impairment, intravenous infusion is recommended. For an intermittent intravenous infusion the recommended dose is 400 mg (in 100 mL of sodium chloride 0.9%) given over 30 minutes to 1 hour and repeated every 4 to 6 hours if necessary. For a continuous intravenous infusion the recommended rate is 50 to 100 mg per hour. The usual intramuscular dose is 200 mg which may be repeated at intervals of 4 to 6 hours. In the USA, dosage recommendations for parenteral administration are 300 mg every 6 to 8 hours by intramuscular injection or by slow intravenous injection over at least 5 minutes. The same dosage may be given by intermittent intravenous infusion over 15 to 20 minutes; for continuous intravenous infusion the recommended rate is 37.5 mg per hour, which may be preceded by 150 mg as an intravenous loading dose. However, a rate of 50 mg per hour is recommended for prevention of stress ulceration.

For **children** over one year of age 25 to 30 mg per kg body-weight daily may be given in divided doses, by mouth or parenterally. Under 1 year of age, 20 mg per kg daily in divided doses has been used.

The dosage of cimetidine should be reduced in patients with impaired renal function; suggested doses according to creatinine clearance are: creatinine clearance of 0 to 15 mL per minute, 200 mg twice daily; 15 to 30 mL per minute, 200 mg three times daily; 30 to 50 mL per minute, 200 mg four times daily; over 50 mL per minute, normal dosage. Cimetidine is removed by haemodialysis, but not significantly removed by peritoneal dialysis. Dosage reduction may be required in some patients with hepatic impairment—see Precautions, above.

Carcinoid syndrome. For a discussion of the carcinoid syndrome, including the view that cimetidine in combination with a histamine H_1-antagonist ('antihistamine') may sometimes be useful in patients with a histamine-secreting tumour, see p.477.

Cystic fibrosis. For a review of the management of cystic fibrosis, including mention of the role of cimetidine and other histamine H_2-receptor antagonists, see p.119.

Dapsone toxicity. Cimetidine given with dapsone might reduce the haemolysis and methaemoglobinaemia associated with the latter drug. References supporting this suggestion are given under Dapsone on p.199.

Diagnostic use. Cimetidine blocks renal tubular secretion of creatinine and has been used experimentally to improve the accuracy of estimations of glomerular filtration rate from creatinine clearance in patients with renal disease.[1] Best results were achieved with a bolus dose of 1.2 g and the use of such a high dose was questioned.[2]

1. van Acker BAC, *et al.* Creatinine clearance during cimetidine administration for measurement of glomerular filtration rate. *Lancet* 1992; **340:** 1326–9.
2. Agarwal R. Creatinine clearance with cimetidine for measurement of GFR. *Lancet* 1993; **341:** 188.

Echinococcosis. Cimetidine has been given with albendazole to increase its effect (by inhibiting its metabolism) in the treatment of echinococcosis (p.94).

Eosinophilic fasciitis. Eosinophilic fasciitis is a scleroderma-like syndrome of inflammation of the muscle fascia and associated eosinophilia and hypergammaglobulinaemia. Although it responds well to corticosteroid therapy in most cases, cimetidine has also been tried. The effect of cimetidine on eosinophilic fasciitis is unpredictable with both remission[1-3] and lack of response[4,5] having been reported in a few patients.

1. Solomon G, *et al.* Eosinophilic fasciitis responsive to cimetidine. *Ann Intern Med* 1982; **97:** 547–9.
2. Laso FJ, *et al.* Cimetidine and eosinophilic fasciitis. *Ann Intern Med* 1983; **98:** 1026.
3. Garcia-Morteo O, *et al.* Cimetidine and eosinophilic fasciitis. *Ann Intern Med* 1984; **100:** 318–19.
4. Loftin EB. Cimetidine and eosinophilic fasciitis. *Ann Intern Med* 1983; **98:** 111–12.
5. Herson S, *et al.* Cimetidine in eosinophilic fasciitis. *Ann Intern Med* 1990; **113:** 412–13.

Herpesvirus infections. Although there have been numerous isolated and anecdotal reports of a beneficial response to cimetidine in patients with infections due to various herpes viruses, including genital herpes simplex,[1] infectious mononucleosis,[2,3] and herpes zoster[4-7] some of these reports have been criticised[8,9] mainly on the grounds that the majority of cases of herpes zoster will resolve within 2 to 3 weeks whether any treatment is given or not. Also, a double-blind placebo-controlled study involving 63 patients with herpes zoster[10] found no evidence that cimetidine relieved the pain or accelerated the rate of healing of lesions.

For a discussion of herpesvirus infections and their management, see p.596.

1. Wakefield D. Cimetidine in recurrent genital herpes simplex infection. *Ann Intern Med* 1984; **101:** 882.
2. Goldstein JA. Cimetidine and mononucleosis. *Ann Intern Med* 1983; **99:** 410–11.
3. Goldstein JA. Cimetidine, ranitidine, and Epstein-Barr virus infection. *Ann Intern Med* 1986; **105:** 139.
4. Hayne ST, Mercer JB. Herpes zoster: treatment with cimetidine. *Can Med Assoc J* 1983; **129:** 1284–5.
5. Shandera R. Treatment of herpes zoster with cimetidine. *Can Med Assoc J* 1984; **131:** 279.
6. Mavligit GM, Talpaz M. Cimetidine for herpes zoster. *N Engl J Med* 1984; **310:** 318–19.
7. Arnot RS. Herpes zoster and cimetidine. *Med J Aust* 1984; **141:** 903.
8. Tyrrell DL. Course of herpes zoster. *Can Med Assoc J* 1984; **130:** 1109.
9. Giles KE. Herpes zoster and cimetidine. *Med J Aust* 1985; **142:** 283.
10. Levy DW, *et al.* Cimetidine in the treatment of herpes zoster. *J R Coll Physicians Lond* 1985; **19:** 96–8.

Hypersensitivity and immunological disorders. Studies in *mice* and man have shown that H_2-receptor antagonists have an immunoregulatory effect.[1] T-lymphocyte suppressor cells have histamine H_2 receptors and cimetidine has been reported to reduce activity of these cells, thus enhancing immune response.[1,2] There is also some evidence that it enhances cellular immunity, notably natural killer cell activity.[3] This discovery has led to the investigation of cimetidine in a number of disorders associated with alteration of the immune response including eosinophilic fasciitis, herpesvirus infections, mucocutaneous candidiasis, hypogammaglobulinaemia, and various malignancies.[1,4,5]

Histamine H_2-antagonists have been used in conjunction with H_1-antagonists ('antihistamines') in the management of various allergic conditions, see Food Allergy, p.400 and Rhinitis, p.400.

1. Kumar A. Cimetidine: an immunomodulator. *DICP Ann Pharmacother* 1990; **24:** 289–95.
2. Snyman JR, *et al.* Cimetidine as modulator of the cell-mediated immune response in vivo using the tuberculin skin test as parameter. *Br J Clin Pharmacol* 1990; **29:** 257–60.
3. Katoh J, *et al.* Cimetidine and immunoreactivity. *Lancet* 1996; **348:** 404–5.
4. White WB, Ballow M. Modulation of suppressor-cell activity by cimetidine in patients with common variable hypogammaglobulinemia. *N Engl J Med* 1985; **312:** 198–202.
5. Polizzi B, *et al.* Successful treatment with cimetidine and zinc sulphate in chronic mucocutaneous candidiasis. *Am J Med Sci* 1996; **311:** 189–90.

Malignant neoplasms. Because of its immunomodulatory effects cimetidine has been tried, with very variable results, as an adjuvant in the management of a variety of malignant neoplasms. Perhaps the most interesting results are the reports from a number of small studies of a survival advantage in patients with gastric[1] or colorectal[2,3] cancer who received cimetidine in addition to their antineoplastic therapy. Numerous adjuvant therapies have been tried in malignancies of the gastro-intestinal tract (see p.487) and the large scale studies necessary to determine the place of cimetidine (if any) in the management of these diseases have yet to be carried out.

1. Tønnesen H, *et al.* Effect of cimetidine on survival after gastric cancer. *Lancet* 1988; **ii:** 990–2.
2. Adams WJ, Morris DL. Short-course cimetidine and survival with colorectal cancer. *Lancet* 1994; **344:** 1768–9.
3. Matsumoto S. Cimetidine and survival with colorectal cancer. *Lancet* 1995; **346:** 115.

Mastocytosis. Cimetidine, alone or in combination with a histamine H_1-antagonist ('antihistamine'), has been reported to relieve gastro-intestinal symptoms,[1,2] pruritus, and urticaria[3,4] in patients with mastocytosis.

1. Hirschowitz BI, Groarke JF. Effect of cimetidine on gastric hypersecretion and diarrhea in systemic mastocytosis. *Ann Intern Med* 1979; **90:** 769–71.
2. Linde R, *et al.* Combination H1 and H2 receptor antagonist therapy in mastocytosis. *Ann Intern Med* 1980; **92:** 716.
3. Simon RA. Treatment of systemic mastocytosis. *N Engl J Med* 1980; **302:** 231.
4. Frieri M, *et al.* Comparison of the therapeutic efficacy of cromolyn sodium with that of combined chlorpheniramine and cimetidine in systemic mastocytosis: results of a double-blind clinical trial. *Am J Med* 1985; **78:** 9–14.

Paracetamol toxicity. It has been suggested that cimetidine might be of use in the treatment of paracetamol poisoning (see p.72) because of its inhibition of the cytochrome P450 system. However, there is no current evidence to support the claims of benefit made in some anecdotal reports.

Porphyria. There are reports[1,2] of patients with acute intermittent porphyria (p.983) showing clinical and biochemical improvement during treatment with cimetidine.

1. Baccino E, *et al.* Cimetidine in the treatment of acute intermittent porphyria. *JAMA* 1989; **262:** 3000.
2. Horie Y, *et al.* Clinical usefulness of cimetidine treatment for acute relapse in intermittent porphyria. *Clin Chim Acta* 1995; **234:** 171–5.

Skin disorders. Cimetidine has been used alone[1-8] and in combination with an antihistamine (H_1-receptor antagonist)[5,8,9] in various skin disorders. H_2-antagonists such as cimetidine and ranitidine have produced improvement in certain types of *urticaria*, especially those associated with cold or angioedema. Their routine use in urticaria is controversial, but in practice their addition to conventional treatment can be tried in resistant cases.[10-12] Little additional benefit has been found with combination therapy in dermographic urticaria.[13] Although they may act by antagonism of H_2-receptors on cutaneous blood vessels, other mechanisms of action may be involved.[8] The management of urticaria is discussed further on p.1076. Patients with *pruritus* of various causes may also respond to H_2-antagonists,[1,2,6,7,9] but studies in larger groups of patients have demonstrated no benefit.[3-5,14] For the more usual drugs employed in pruritus, see p.1075.

There are reports of benefit from the use of cimetidine in patients with *viral warts*,[15] but a controlled study failed to show any significant benefit.[16]

1. Easton P, Galbraith PR. Cimetidine treatment of pruritus in polycythemia vera. *N Engl J Med* 1978; **299:** 1134.
2. Hess CE. Cimetidine for the treatment of pruritus. *N Engl J Med* 1979; **300:** 370.
3. Harrison AR, *et al.* Pruritus, cimetidine and polycythemia. *N Engl J Med* 1979; **300:** 433–4.
4. Scott GL, Horton RJ. Pruritus, cimetidine and polycythemia. *N Engl J Med* 1979; **300:** 434. Correction. *ibid.*; 936.
5. Zappacosta AR, Hauss D. Cimetidine doesn't help pruritus of uremia. *N Engl J Med* 1979; **300:** 1280.
6. Schapira DV, Bennett JM. Cimetidine for pruritus. *Lancet* 1979; **i:** 726–7.
7. Aymard JP, *et al.* Cimetidine for pruritus in Hodgkin's disease. *Br Med J* 1980; **280:** 151–2.
8. Theoharides TC. Histamine$_2$ (H_2)-receptor antagonists in the treatment of urticaria. *Drugs* 1989; **37:** 345–55.
9. Deutsch PH. Dermatographism treated with hydroxyzine and cimetidine and ranitidine. *Ann Intern Med* 1984; **101:** 569.
10. Advenier C, Queille-Roussel C. Rational use of antihistamines in allergic dermatological conditions. *Drugs* 1989; **38:** 634–44.
11. Ormerod AD. Urticaria: recognition, causes, and treatment. *Drugs* 1994; **48:** 717–30.
12. Greaves MW. Chronic urticaria. *N Engl J Med* 1995; **332:** 1767–72.
13. Sharpe GR, Shuster S. In dermographic urticaria H_2 receptor antagonists have a small but therapeutically irrelevant additional effect compared with H_1 antagonists alone. *Br J Dermatol* 1993; **129:** 575–9.
14. Raisch DW, *et al.* Evaluation of a non-food and drug administration-approved use of cimetidine: treatment of pruritus resulting from epidural morphine analgesia. *DICP Ann Pharmacother* 1991; **25:** 716–8.
15. Gooptu C, *et al.* Successful treatment of multiple viral warts with cimetidine. *Br J Dermatol* 1997; **137** (suppl 50): 51.
16. Karabulut AA, *et al.* Is cimetidine effective for nongenital warts: a double-blind, placebo-controlled study. *Arch Dermatol* 1997; **133:** 533–4.

Preparations

BP 1998: Cimetidine Injection; Cimetidine Oral Solution; Cimetidine Oral Suspension; Cimetidine Tablets;
USP 23: Cimetidine Tablets.

Proprietary Preparations (details are given in Part 3)
Aust.: Cimetag; Neutromed; Neutronorm; Ulcometin; Ulcostad; ***Austral.:*** Cimetimax; Magicul; Sigmetadine; Tagamet; ***Belg.:*** Nuardin; Tagamet; ***Canad.:*** Novo-Cimetine; Nu-Cimet; Peptol; Tagamet; ***Fr.:*** Stomedine; Tagamet; ***Ger.:*** Altramet; Azucimet; Cime; Cime-Puren; Cimebeta; Cimehexal; Cimemerck; Cimephil; Ci-

met; CimLich; Ciuk; Contracid; duraH2; Gastroprotect; H 2 Blocker; Jenametidin; Sigacimet; Tagagel; Tagamet; Ulcolind H_2; Ulcubloc; Ulkusal; ***Irl.:*** Cedine; Cimagen; Cimeldine; Dyspamet; Galenamet; Pinamet; Tagamet; ***Ital.:*** Biomag; Brumetidina; Citimid; Dina; Eureceptor; Gastromet; Neo Gastrausil; Notul; Stomet; Tagamet; Tametin; Temic; Ulcedin; Ulcestop; Ulcodina; Ulcofalk†; Ulcomedina; Ulcomet†; Ulis; Vagolisal; Valmagen†; ***Neth.:*** Tagamet; ***Norw.:*** Cimal; Gastrobitan; Tagamet; ***S.Afr.:*** Aci-Med; Acidown; Cinadine; Cymi†; Duomet; Hexamet; Lenamet; Secadine; Sonsuur; Tagamet; Ulcim†; Ulmet†; ***Spain:*** Ali Veg; Cinulcus†; Duogastril†; Fremet; Gastro H2; Mansal; Tagamet; ***Swed.:*** Aciloc; Acinil; Cimal†; Tagamet; ***Switz.:*** Malimed; Tagamet; Zimetin†; ***UK:*** Acid-Eze; Acitak; Dyspamet; Galenamet; Peptimax; Phimetin; Tagamet; Ultec; Zita; ***USA:*** Tagamet.

Multi-ingredient: ***Aust.:*** Cimetalgin; ***Irl.:*** Algitec; ***Neth.:*** Aciflux; ***UK:*** Algitec; Tagamet Dual Action†.

Cinitapride (11133-v)

Cinitapride *(rINN)*.

4-Amino-*N*-[1-(3-cyclohexen-1-ylmethyl)-4-piperidyl]-2-ethoxy-5-nitrobenzamide.

$C_{21}H_{30}N_4O_4$ = 402.5.

CAS — 66564-14-5.

Cinitapride is a substituted benzamide used for its prokinetic properties. It is given by mouth as the acid tartrate in doses of 1 mg three times daily before meals in the management of gastroparesis and gastro-oesophageal reflux disease.

Preparations

Proprietary Preparations (details are given in Part 3)
Spain: Blaston; Cidine.

Cisapride (16581-d)

Cisapride *(BAN, USAN, rINN)*.

Cisapridum; R-51619. *cis*-4-Amino-5-chloro-*N*-{1-[3-(4-fluorophenoxy)propyl]-3-methoxy-4-piperidyl}-2-methoxybenzamide monohydrate.

$C_{23}H_{29}ClFN_3O_4,H_2O$ = 484.0.

CAS — 81098-60-4 (anhydrous).

Pharmacopoeias. In *Eur.* (see p.viii) and *Pol.*

A white or almost white powder; it exhibits polymorphism. Practically **insoluble** in water; freely soluble in dimethylformamide; soluble in dichloromethane; sparingly soluble in methyl alcohol. **Protect** from light.

Adverse Effects

The most commonly reported side-effects with cisapride are gastro-intestinal disturbances including abdominal cramps, borborygmi, and diarrhoea. Headache, lightheadedness, dizziness, convulsions, extrapyramidal effects, increased urinary frequency, and tachycardia have also been reported. Cases of arrhythmias, including torsade de pointes, have occurred. There have been a few cases of disturbances in liver function among patients receiving cisapride.

A comparison of data from prescription-event monitoring in over 13 000 recipients of cisapride and from a further 9726 recipients involved in a controlled study showed that diarrhoea, in about 2 to 4% of patients, was the commonest adverse effect reported.[1] Other relatively common adverse effects were headache, abdominal pain, nausea and vomiting, and constipation, all in around 1 to 1.5% of patients. There were 46 reports in the prescription-event monitoring data of increased urinary frequency (plus a further 20 among the controlled study patients), and 5 reports of arrhythmias.

1. Wager E, *et al.* A comparison of two cohort studies evaluating the safety of cisapride: prescription-event monitoring and a large phase IV study. *Eur J Clin Pharmacol* 1997; **52:** 87–94.

Effects on the heart. Seven reports[1] of cardiac effects associated with cisapride were submitted to the WHO Programme for International Drug Monitoring between 1989 and 1991. They included palpitations in 4, tachycardia and hypertension in 1, and extrasystole in 2. Subsequent reports have implicated cisapride in the development of prolonged QT interval and torsade de pointes or ventricular fibrillation or both.[2,3] The US Food and Drug Administration (FDA) had received 57 such reports as of April 1996,[3] of which 4 had proved fatal. Most patients were either receiving other drugs known to impair cisapride metabolism (see Interactions, below) or had other factors predisposing to arrhythmias. In the light of this and of evidence for a direct effect of cisapride on the heart at therapeutic concentrations the UK Committee on Safety of Medicines (CSM) contra-indicated[2] the use of cisapride in patients receiving drugs which could inhibit cisapride metabolism or which also prolong QT interval, as well as in patients with a history of QT interval prolongation, ventricular arrhythmia, or torsade de pointes, or other risk factors for arrhythmia (see Precautions, below). In the light of evidence that children,[5] and neonates[4] (especially of low gestational age) are vulnerable to cisapride-induced QT interval prolongation the CSM also specifically contra-indicated use in premature neonates[2] and noted that there were insufficient data to support use in children up to the age of 12. Warnings have also been issued in the USA.

1. Olsson S, Edwards IR. Tachycardia during cisapride treatment. *Br Med J* 1992; **305:** 748–9.
2. Committee on Safety of Medicines/Medicines Control Agency. Cisapride (Prepulsid): risk of arrhythmias. *Current Problems* 1998; **24:** 11.
3. Wysowski DK, Bacsanyi J. Cisapride and fatal arrhythmia. *N Engl J Med* 1996; **335:** 290–1.
4. Bernardini S, *et al.* Effect of cisapride on QTc interval in neonates. *Arch Dis Child* 1997; **77:** F241–3.
5. Hill SL, *et al.* Proarrhythmia associated with cisapride in children. *Pediatrics* 1998; **101:** 1053–6.

Effects on the respiratory system. Chest tightness, wheezing, and a fall in peak flow rate occurred in a patient with severe brittle asthma following administration of cisapride 10 mg.[1] Four other cases of bronchospasm associated with cisapride use have been discussed in a subsequent report;[2] in 2 of these cases symptoms resolved on withdrawal and recurred on rechallenge.

1. Nolan P, *et al.* Cisapride and brittle asthma. *Lancet* 1990; **336:** 1443.
2. Pillans P. Bronchospasm associated with cisapride. *Br Med J* 1995; **311:** 1472.

Effects on the urinary tract. There had been 12 cases of urinary disturbances associated with use of cisapride[1] reported to the Australian Adverse Drug Reactions Advisory Committee between March 1991 and July 1993. Five reports were of urinary incontinence, 8 involved frequency, and individual reports involved cystitis, hesitancy, and urinary retention. The majority of the cases involved women, and most patients were elderly.

1. Boyd IW, Rohan AP. Urinary disorders associated with cisapride. *Med J Aust* 1994; **160:** 579–80.

Precautions

Cisapride should not be used when stimulation of muscular contractions might adversely affect gastro-intestinal conditions as in gastro-intestinal haemorrhage, obstruction, perforation, or immediately after surgery. Cisapride is contra-indicated in any patient receiving CYP3A4 inhibiting drugs such as macrolide antibiotics, azole antifungals, HIV-protease inhibitors, or nefazodone (see also under Interactions, below). It is similarly contra-indicated in those taking other drugs which prolong the QT interval, in those with a personal or family history of such prolongation, or a previous history of ventricular arrhythmia or torsade de pointes. Furthermore, it should not be given to those with risk factors for arrhythmia including second or third degree atrioventricular block, clinically significant heart disease, uncorrected electrolyte disturbances (particularly hypokalaemia and hypomagnesaemia), and renal or respiratory failure. Use is also contra-indicated in premature infants.

Cisapride should be used with caution and in reduced doses in patients with hepatic or renal impairment.

Care should be taken not to exceed the recommended dose.

Interactions

Cisapride is metabolised by the isoenzyme cytochrome P450 3A4 (CYP3A4), and concomitant administration with drugs which inhibit this enzyme is contra-indicated because it may result in increased plasma concentrations of cisapride, with QT interval prolongation and ventricular arrhythmias. Such an interaction has been reported with ketoconazole, and is possible with other azoles such as itraconazole and miconazole as well as with the macrolides triacetyloleandomycin, erythromycin, and clarithromycin, and with delavirdine or HIV-protease inhibitors such as indinavir. Nefazodone may interact similarly. Cisapride should not be used in patients receiving other medication known to prolong the QT interval, including quinine or halofantrine, terfenadine, astemizole, certain antiarrhythmics such as amiodarone or quinidine, some antidepressants such as amitriptyline, phenothiazine antipsychotics, and sertindole. Cimetidine may enhance cisapride bioavailability.

Antimuscarinics and possibly opioid analgesics may antagonise the gastro-intestinal effects of cisapride. Because cisapride increases intestinal motility it may affect the absorption of other drugs, either diminishing absorption from the stomach or enhancing absorption from the small intestine. Prothrombin times may be increased in some patients receiving oral anticoagulants, and the effects of alcohol and some other CNS depressants may be enhanced.

References.

1. Bedford TA, Rowbotham DJ. Cisapride: drug interactions of clinical significance. *Drug Safety* 1996; **15:** 167–75.

Antidepressants. It has been pointed out[1] that a number of antidepressants, including *fluoxetine, fluvoxamine, nefazodone*, and *sertraline* all appear to markedly inhibit cytochrome P450 3A4, and therefore might interact with cisapride.

1. Caley CF. Cisapride interaction with antidepressants. *Ann Pharmacother* 1996; **30:** 684.

Antimicrobials. As mentioned under Effects on the Heart, above, there are reports of prolonged QT interval and torsade de pointes and/or ventricular fibrillation in patients receiving cisapride concomitantly with drugs which can impair cisapride metabolism (through inhibition of cytochrome P450 3A4). Drugs implicated in the reported incidents are mainly azole antifungals (*fluconazole, itraconazole, ketoconazole*, or *miconazole*) or macrolide antibacterials (*erythromycin* or *clarithromycin*).

H_2-antagonists. *Cimetidine*[1] but not *ranitidine*[2] has been reported to enhance the bioavailability of oral cisapride, possibly by inhibition of cisapride metabolism (cimetidine is an inhibitor of P450 3A4). Cisapride conversely increases the rate of absorption and decreases the oral bioavailability of both cimetidine[1] and ranitidine.[2]

1. Kirch W, *et al.* Cisapride-cimetidine interaction: enhanced cisapride bioavailability and accelerated cimetidine absorption. *Ther Drug Monit* 1989; **11:** 411–14.
2. Rowbotham DJ, *et al.* Effect of single doses of cisapride and ranitidine administered simultaneously on plasma concentrations of cisapride and ranitidine. *Br J Anaesth* 1991; **67:** 302–305.

Pharmacokinetics

Cisapride is readily absorbed from the gastro-intestinal tract, with peak plasma concentrations achieved 1 to 2 hours after a dose by mouth. It undergoes extensive first-pass metabolism in the liver and gut wall, resulting in an absolute bioavailability of 35 to 40%. The main metabolic pathways are oxidative *N*-dealkylation, producing the major metabolite norcisapride, and aromatic hydroxylation. More than 90% of a dose is excreted as metabolites in the urine and faeces in approximately equal amounts. A small amount is distributed into breast milk.

The elimination half-life has been reported to be about 10 hours. Cisapride is about 98% bound to plasma proteins.

References.

1. Meuldermans W, *et al.* Excretion and biotransformation of cisapride in dogs and humans after oral administration. *Drug Metab Dispos* 1988; **16:** 403–9.
2. Hedner T, *et al.* Comparative bioavailability of a cisapride suppository and tablet formulation in healthy volunteers. *Eur J Clin Pharmacol* 1990; **38:** 629–31.
3. Hofmeyr GJ, Sonnendecker EWW. Secretion of the gastrokinetic agent cisapride in human milk. *Eur J Clin Pharmacol* 1986; **30:** 735–6.

Uses and Administration

Cisapride is a substituted benzamide used for its prokinetic properties. It stimulates gastro-intestinal motility probably by increasing the release of acetylcholine in the gut wall at the level of the myenteric plexus, increases the resting tone of the lower oesophageal sphincter, and increases the amplitude of lower oesophageal contractions. Gastric emptying is accelerated and the mouth-to-caecum transit time is reduced. Colonic peristalsis is also increased which decreases colonic transit time.

Cisapride apparently lacks antidopaminergic or direct parasympathomimetic activity and it does not affect prolactin release or gastric secretion. It is reported to be an agonist at serotonin-4 ($5\text{-}HT_4$) receptors.

Cisapride is used principally in the treatment of gastro-oesophageal reflux disease (p.1170), in disorders associated with decreased gastric motility (below), and in non-ulcer dyspepsia (p.1169).

Cisapride is given as the monohydrate, but doses are calculated in terms of the anhydrous substance. It is taken by mouth 15 to 30 minutes before a meal and at bedtime, if necessary.

For **dyspepsia**, 10 mg is given 3 times daily, usually for 4 weeks. In patients with **decreased gastro-intestinal motility**, 10 mg is given 3 or 4 times daily, initially for 6 weeks. For **gastro-oesophageal reflux disease** 10 mg is given 3 or 4 times daily; alternatively, 20 mg twice daily may be given. The usual course is 12 weeks. In the USA, doses of up to 20 mg four times daily have been recommended. A dose of 10 mg twice daily or 20 mg at night may be given for maintenance treatment; the maintenance dose may be increased to 20 mg twice daily if lesions were initially very severe.

In patients with impaired hepatic or renal function the initial dose should be half the usual dose, followed by adjustment depending on clinical response.

Reviews.

1. Barone JA, *et al.* Cisapride: a gastrointestinal prokinetic drug. *Ann Pharmacother* 1994; **28:** 488–500.

Aspiration syndromes. For a discussion of the management of aspiration syndromes, including mention of the role of cisapride, see p.1168.

Constipation. Some benefits have been reported from the use of cisapride in chronic constipation;[1,2] for a discussion of constipation and its conventional management, see p.1168.

1. Müller-Lissner SA, Bavarian Constipation Study Group. Treatment of chronic constipation with cisapride and placebo. *Gut* 1987; **28:** 1033–8.
2. Verheyen K, *et al.* Double-blind comparison of two cisapride dosage regimens with placebo in the treatment of functional constipation: a general-practice multicenter study. *Curr Ther Res* 1987; **41:** 978–85.

Cystic fibrosis. Striking improvements in stool character, weight gain, and sense of well-being have been reported[1] following the use of cisapride in children with cystic fibrosis although these responses were not observed in another study.[2] Gastro-oesophageal reflux is common in infants and young children with cystic fibrosis, but is not the consequence of respiratory or gastro-intestinal complications of the disease; it has responded to treatment with cisapride in a usual dose of 200 μg per kg body-weight by mouth four times daily.[3]

For a discussion of cystic fibrosis and other agents used in its management, see p.119. For a comparative study suggesting that ranitidine relieves the gastro-intestinal symptoms of cystic fibrosis better than cisapride see p.1211.

1. Prinsen JE, Thomas M. Cisapride in cystic fibrosis. *Lancet* 1985; **i:** 512–13.
2. Smith HL, *et al.* Cisapride and cystic fibrosis. *Lancet* 1989; **i:** 338.
3. Malfroot A, Dab I. New insights on gastro-oesophageal reflux in cystic fibrosis by longitudinal follow up. *Arch Dis Child* 1991; **66:** 1339–45.

Decreased gastro-intestinal motility. Some benefit has been reported from the use of cisapride in patients with chronic intestinal pseudo-obstruction[1-3] and also in the acute form.[4,5] For a general discussion of decreased gastro-intestinal motility and its treatment, see p.1168. Cisapride is also employed in diabetic gastroparesis, one of the diabetic complications discussed on p.315.

1. Camilleri M, *et al.* Impaired transit of chyme in chronic intestinal pseudoobstruction: correction by cisapride. *Gastroenterology* 1986; **91:** 619–26.
2. Puntis JWL, *et al.* Cisapride in neonatal short gut. *Lancet* 1986; **ii:** 108–9.
3. Coombs RC, Booth IW. Small intestinal motor activity response to cisapride in children with dysmotility syndromes. *Gut* 1989; **30:** A1473.
4. Vantrappen G. Acute colonic pseudo-obstruction. *Lancet* 1993; **341:** 152–3.
5. Lander A, *et al.* Cisapride reduces neonatal postoperative ileus: randomised placebo controlled trial. *Arch Dis Child* 1997; **77:** F119–22.

Diabetes mellitus. Cisapride has been used as an alternative to metoclopramide in the management of diabetic gastroparesis. For a discussion of diabetic complications, and their management, see p.315.

Preparations

Proprietary Preparations (details are given in Part 3)
Aust.: Prepulsid; Pulsitil; ***Austral.:*** Prepulsid; ***Belg.:*** Cyprid; Prepulsid; ***Canad.:*** Prepulsid; ***Fr.:*** Prepulsid; ***Ger.:*** Alimix; Propulsin; ***Irl.:*** Prepulsid; ***Ital.:*** Alimix; Cipril; Prepulsid; ***Neth.:*** Prepulsid; ***Norw.:*** Prepulsid; ***S.Afr.:*** Prepulsid; ***Spain:*** Arcasin; Fisiogastrol; Kelosal; Kinet; Prepulsid; Trautil; ***Swed.:*** Prepulsid; ***Switz.:*** Prepulsid; ***UK:*** Alimix†; Prepulsid; ***USA:*** Propulsid.

Clebopride Malate (14171-l)

Clebopride Malate *(rINNM)*.

LAS-9273 (clebopride). 4-Amino-*N*-(1-benzyl-4-piperidyl)-5-chloro-*o*-anisamide malate.

$C_{20}H_{24}ClN_3O_2,C_4H_6O_5$ = 508.0.

CAS — 55905-53-8 (clebopride); 57645-91-7 (clebopride malate).

NOTE. Clebopride is *USAN*.

Pharmacopoeias. In *Eur.* (see p.viii).

A white or almost white crystalline powder. Clebopride malate 679 μg is approximately equivalent to clebopride 500 μg. Sparingly **soluble** in water; slightly soluble in dehydrated alcohol; sparingly soluble in methyl alcohol; practically insoluble in dichloromethane. The pH of a 1% solution is 3.8 to 4.2. **Protect** from light.

Clebopride is a substituted benzamide similar to metoclopramide (p.1200), that is used for its antiemetic and prokinetic actions in nausea and vomiting (p.1172) and various other gastro-intestinal disorders.

Clebopride malate is given in a usual dose equivalent to clebopride 0.5 mg by mouth three times daily before meals or 0.5 to 1 mg by intramuscular or intravenous injection for acute symptoms. A dose equivalent to clebopride 15 to 20 μg per kg body-weight daily has been recommended for children.

Preparations

Proprietary Preparations (details are given in Part 3)
Ital.: Cleprid†; Motilex; ***Jpn:*** Clast†; ***Spain:*** Clanzol; Cleboril; Madurase; Vuxolin†.

Multi-ingredient: ***Spain:*** Clanzoflat; Flatoril.

Colocynth (7508-g)

Bitter Apple; Bitter Cucumber; Colocynth Pulp; Colocynthis; Coloquinte; Coloquintidas; Koloquinthen.

NOTE. The synonym Bitter Apple has also been applied to the fruits of *Solanum incanum*.

The dried pulp of the fruit of *Citrullus colocynthis* (Cucurbitaceae).

Colocynth has a drastic purgative and irritant action. It has been superseded by less toxic laxatives.

Colocynth is used in homoeopathic medicine.

Croton Oil (7509-q)

Oleum Crotonis; Oleum Tiglii.

CAS — 8001-28-3.

Pharmacopoeias. Chin. includes fruits of *Croton tiglium*.

An oil expressed from the seeds of *Croton tiglium* (Euphorbiaceae).

Croton oil has such a violent purgative action that it should not now be employed. Externally, it is a powerful counter-irritant and vesicant. It is used in homoeopathic medicine.

Preparations

Proprietary Preparations (details are given in Part 3)

Multi-ingredient: ***Canad.:*** Rheumalan.

Danthron (7510-d)

Danthron *(BAN)*.

Dantron *(rINN)*; Antrapurol; Chrysazin; Dianthon; Dioxyanthrachinonum. 1,8-Dihydroxyanthraquinone.

$C_{14}H_8O_4$ = 240.2.

CAS — 117-10-2.

NOTE. Compounded preparations of danthron and poloxamer 188 have the British Approved Name Co-danthramer; the proportions are expressed in the form *x/y*, where *x* and *y* are the strengths in milligrams of danthron and poloxamer respectively.

Compounded preparations of danthron and docusate sodium in the proportions, by weight, 5 parts to 6 parts have the British Approved Name Co-danthrusate.

Pharmacopoeias. In *Aust.*, *Br.*, and *Neth.*

An orange, odourless or almost odourless, crystalline powder. Practically **insoluble** in water; very slightly soluble in alcohol; soluble in chloroform; slightly soluble in ether; dissolves in solutions of alkali hydroxides.

Adverse Effects and Precautions

As for Senna, p.1212. Danthron may colour the perianal skin pink or red as well as colour the urine. Superficial sloughing of discoloured skin may occur in incontinent patients or children wearing napkins; danthron should not be used in such patients. The mucosa of the large intestine may be discoloured with prolonged use or high dosage.

Some studies have suggested that chronic administration of very high doses of danthron to *rats* and *mice* may be associated with the development of intestinal and liver tumours.

References to adverse effects occurring with danthron-containing laxatives include individual cases of leucopenia with liver damage,[1] greyish-blue skin discoloration,[2] and orange vaginal discharge.[3] There has also been a report of intestinal sarcoma in an 18-year-old girl with a history of prolonged use of a danthron-containing laxative.[4]

1. Tolman KG, *et al.* Possible hepatotoxicity of Doxidan. *Ann Intern Med* 1976; **84:** 290–2.
2. Darke CS, Cooper RG. Unusual case of skin discoloration. *Br Med J* 1978; **1:** 1188–9.
3. Greer IA. Orange periods. *Br Med J* 1984; **289:** 323.
4. Patel PM, *et al.* Anthraquinone laxatives and human cancer: an association in one case. *Postgrad Med J* 1989; **65:** 216–17.

Pharmacokinetics

Unlike most naturally occurring anthraquinones danthron is not a glycoside; it is absorbed from the gastro-intestinal tract in sufficient quantities to produce discoloration of body fluids in some patients. It is excreted in the faeces and the urine, and also in other secretions including breast milk.

Uses and Administration

Danthron is an anthraquinone stimulant laxative. It is given by mouth to treat constipation (p.1168) and is effective within 6 to 12 hours. However, because of concern over *rodent* carcinogenicity its use tends to be restricted now to the elderly, to terminally ill patients, and to those in whom straining would be potentially hazardous.

Danthron is given in doses of 25 to 75 mg when given with poloxamer 188 as co-danthramer, and in doses of 50 to 150 mg when given with docusate sodium as co-danthrusate. Doses are usually given at bedtime. Children have been given danthron 12.5 to 25 mg as co-danthramer or, in those aged 6 to 12 years, 50 mg as co-danthrusate. It should be noted that in some countries danthron is not authorised for use in children below the age of 12 years.

Preparations

BP 1998: Co-danthrusate Capsules.

Proprietary Preparations (details are given in Part 3)

Multi-ingredient: ***Canad.:*** Doss; Regulex-D; ***Irl.:*** Codalax; ***S.Afr.:*** Norilax†; ***UK:*** Ailax; Capsuvac; Codalax; Normax.

Difenoxin Hydrochloride (6220-v)

Difenoxin Hydrochloride *(BANM, rINNM)*.

Difenoxylic Acid Hydrochloride; Diphenoxylic Acid Hydrochloride; McN-JR-15403-11 (difenoxin); R-15403. 1-(3-Cyano-3,3-diphenylpropyl)-4-phenylpiperidine-4-carboxylic acid hydrochloride.

$C_{28}H_{28}N_2O_2,HCl$ = 461.0.

CAS — 28782-42-5 (difenoxin); 35607-36-4 (difenoxin hydrochloride).

NOTE. Difenoxin is *USAN*.

Difenoxin is the principal active metabolite of diphenoxylate (p.1189) and has similar actions and uses. It is given by mouth as the hydrochloride, but doses are in terms of the base.

In the treatment of diarrhoea (p.1168), the usual dose in adults is the equivalent of difenoxin 2 mg initially, followed by 1 mg after each loose stool or every 3 to 4 hours as required, up to a maximum of 8 mg daily.

Preparations of difenoxin usually contain subclinical amounts of atropine sulphate in an attempt to discourage abuse.

Preparations

Proprietary Preparations (details are given in Part 3)
S.Afr.: Dioctin†; Lyspafen†; ***Switz.:*** Lyspafen; ***USA:*** Motofen.

Dihydroxyaluminum Sodium Carbonate (689-k)

Aluminium Sodium Carbonate Hydroxide; Carbaldrate; Dihydroxyaluminium Sodium Carbonate. Sodium (carbonato)dihydroxyaluminate(1-).

CH_2AlNaO_5 = 144.0.

CAS — 12011-77-7; 16482-55-6.

Pharmacopoeias. In *US.*

A fine white odourless powder. It loses not more than 14.5% of its weight on drying. Practically **insoluble** in water and organic solvents; soluble in dilute mineral acids with the evolution of carbon dioxide. A 4% suspension in water has a pH of 9.9 to 10.2. **Store** in airtight containers.

Dihydroxyaluminum sodium carbonate is an antacid (see p.1167) that is given in doses of about 300 to 600 mg by mouth.

Preparations

USP 23: Dihydroxyaluminum Sodium Carbonate Tablets.

Proprietary Preparations (details are given in Part 3)
Aust.: Antacidum; *Ger.:* Kompensan; *Switz.:* Kompensan.

Multi-ingredient: *Ger.:* Kompensan-S; Kompensan-S forte†; *Ital.:* Eugastran†.

Di-isopromine Hydrochloride (3719-p)

Diisopromine Hydrochloride *(rINNM)*. *NN*-Di-isopropyl-3,3-diphenylpropylamine hydrochloride.

$C_{21}H_{29}N,HCl = 331.9.$

CAS — 5966-41-6 (di-isopromine); 24358-65-4 (di-isopromine hydrochloride).

Di-isopromine hydrochloride is an antispasmodic used with sorbitol in various gastro-intestinal disorders.

Preparations

Proprietary Preparations (details are given in Part 3)

Multi-ingredient: *Belg.:* Bilagol; *Fr.:* Megabyl; *S.Afr.:* Agofell.

Diphenidol Hydrochloride (6543-n)

Diphenidol Hydrochloride *(BANM, USAN)*.

Difenidol Hydrochloride *(pINNM)*; SKF-478 (diphenidol); SKF-478-A; SKF-478-J (diphenidol embonate). 1,1-Diphenyl-4-piperidinobutan-1-ol hydrochloride.

$C_{21}H_{27}NO,HCl = 345.9.$

CAS — 972-02-1 (diphenidol); 3254-89-5 (diphenidol hydrochloride); 26363-46-2 (diphenidol embonate).

Pharmacopoeias. In *Chin.* and *Jpn.*

Adverse Effects

Adverse effects of diphenidol hydrochloride include auditory and visual hallucinations, disorientation, and confusion. Drowsiness, restlessness, depression, sleep disturbances, and antimuscarinic effects may occur. Transient hypotension, headache, dizziness, and skin rashes have occasionally been reported.

Precautions

Due to the risk of confusional states diphenidol should only be given to patients under close supervision. It is contra-indicated in anuria and because of weak antimuscarinic activity it should be used cautiously in patients with glaucoma, obstructive lesions of the gastro-intestinal or genito-urinary tracts, or sinus tachycardia.

Pharmacokinetics

Following oral administration diphenidol is well absorbed, and peak blood concentrations are usually achieved in 1.5 to 3 hours. It is excreted primarily in the urine, mostly as metabolites, with about 5 to 10% unchanged drug. The half-life has been stated to be about 4 hours.

Uses and Administration

Diphenidol hydrochloride is an antiemetic which probably acts through the chemoreceptor trigger zone. It is claimed to control vertigo by means of a specific effect on the vestibular apparatus. Diphenidol also has a weak peripheral antimuscarinic action.

It is used in the treatment of some forms of nausea and vomiting such as that associated with surgery, radiotherapy, and cancer chemotherapy. It is also used for the symptomatic treatment of vertigo, nausea and vomiting due to Ménière's disease, and other labyrinthine disturbances. The more usual drugs used in the treatment of nausea and vomiting are discussed on p.1172, while for the management of vertigo see p.401.

The usual dose is the equivalent of 25 mg of diphenidol by mouth every 4 hours; doses of 50 mg every 4 hours may sometimes be required.

Diphenidol has also been given rectally and parenterally.

Preparations

Proprietary Preparations (details are given in Part 3)
USA: Vontrol†.

Diphenoxylate Hydrochloride

(6223-p)

Diphenoxylate Hydrochloride *(BANM, rINNM)*.

Diphenoxylati Hydrochloridum; R-1132. Ethyl 1-(3-cyano-3,3-diphenylpropyl)-4-phenylpiperidine-4-carboxylate hydrochloride.

$C_{30}H_{32}N_2O_2,HCl = 489.0.$

CAS — 915-30-0 (diphenoxylate); 3810-80-8 (diphenoxylate hydrochloride).

NOTE. Compounded preparations of diphenoxylate hydrochloride and atropine sulphate in the proportions, by weight, 100 parts to 1 part have the British Approved Name Co-phenotrope.

Pharmacopoeias. In *Chin., Eur.* (see p.viii), *Int.,* and *US.*

A white or almost white odourless or almost odourless crystalline powder. Slightly or very slightly **soluble** in water; sparingly soluble in alcohol and in acetone; freely soluble in chloroform and in dichloromethane; slightly soluble in isopropyl alcohol; soluble in methyl alcohol; practically insoluble in ether and in petroleum spirit. A saturated solution has a pH of about 3.3. **Protect** from light.

Dependence and Withdrawal

Short-term administration of diphenoxylate with atropine in the recommended dosage carries a negligible risk of dependence, although prolonged use or use of high doses may produce dependence of the morphine type (see p.67).

Adverse Effects

Diphenoxylate is related to the opioid analgesics (p.68), and its adverse effects and their treatment are similar, particularly in overdosage. Reported side-effects include anorexia, nausea and vomiting, abdominal distension or discomfort, paralytic ileus, toxic megacolon, pancreatitis, headache, drowsiness, dizziness, restlessness, euphoria, depression, numbness of the extremities, and hypersensitivity reactions including angioedema, urticaria, pruritus, and swelling of the gums. Signs of overdosage may be delayed and patients should be observed for at least 48 hours after an overdose. Young children are particularly susceptible to the effects of overdosage.

The presence of subclinical doses of atropine sulphate in preparations containing diphenoxylate may give rise to the side-effects of atropine in susceptible individuals or in overdosage—see Atropine Sulphate, p.455.

Precautions

Diphenoxylate hydrochloride should be used with caution in patients with hepatic dysfunction; it is contra-indicated in patients with jaundice. It should also be used with caution in young children because of a greater variability of response in this age group, and is not generally recommended for use in infants. Patients with inflammatory bowel disease receiving diphenoxylate should be carefully observed for signs of toxic megacolon. It has been recommended that diphenoxylate should not be used for the treatment of diarrhoea associated with pseudomembranous colitis or enterotoxin-producing bacteria.

Interactions

Because of the structural relationship of diphenoxylate to pethidine there is a theoretical risk of hypertensive crisis if diphenoxylate is given concomitantly with monoamine oxidase inhibitors. Diphenoxylate may potentiate the effects of other CNS depressants such as alcohol, barbiturates, and some anxiolytics.

Pharmacokinetics

Diphenoxylate hydrochloride is well absorbed from the gastro-intestinal tract. It is rapidly and extensively metabolised in the liver principally to diphenoxylic acid (difenoxin, p.1188) which has antidiarrhoeal activity; other metabolites include hydroxydiphenoxylic acid. It is excreted mainly as metabolites and their conjugates in the faeces; lesser amounts are excreted in urine. It may also be distributed into breast milk.

Uses and Administration

Diphenoxylate hydrochloride is a synthetic derivative of pethidine with little or no analgesic activity; it reduces intestinal motility and is used in the symptomatic treatment of acute and chronic diarrhoea (p.1168). It may also be used to reduce the frequency and fluidity of the stools in patients with colostomies or ileostomies.

In acute diarrhoea the usual initial dose for adults is 10 mg by mouth followed by 5 mg every six hours, later reduced as the diarrhoea is controlled. In the UK diphenoxylate hydrochloride is not recommended for children under 4 years of age. Suggested initial doses for children are: 4 to 8 years, 2.5 mg three times daily; 9 to 12 years, 2.5 mg four times daily; over 12 years, 5 mg three times daily. In the US diphenoxylate is not recommended for children under the age of 2 years and an initial dose of 0.3 to 0.4 mg per kg body-weight (up to an effective maximum of 10 mg) daily in 4 divided doses is suggested for children aged 2 years or over. (For the view that antidiarrhoeal drugs should not be used at all in children, see p.1168.)

Similar initial doses are used for chronic diarrhoea, and subsequently reduced as necessary. If clinical improvement is not observed after 10 days' treatment with the maximum daily dose of 20 mg (in adults) further administration is unlikely to result in any benefit.

Preparations of diphenoxylate usually contain subclinical amounts of atropine sulphate in an attempt to discourage abuse.

Withdrawal syndromes. OPIOID ANALGESICS. Diphenoxylate, in conjunction with a small dose of thioridazine, may be useful[1] in the symptomatic management of diarrhoea associated with opioid withdrawal syndromes (p.67).

1. DOH. *Drug misuse and dependence: guidelines on clinical management.* London: HMSO, 1991.

Preparations

USP 23: Diphenoxylate Hydrochloride and Atropine Sulfate Oral Solution; Diphenoxylate Hydrochloride and Atropine Sulfate Tablets.

Proprietary Preparations (details are given in Part 3)
Austral.: Lofenoxal; Lomotil; *Belg.:* Reasec; *Canad.:* Lomotil; *Fr.:* Diarsed; *Ger.:* Reasec; *Irl.:* Lomotil; *Ital.:* Reasec; *S.Afr.:* Eldox; Lomotil; *Spain:* Protector; *Switz.:* Reasec; *UK:* Diarphen; Lomotil; Lotharin; Tropergen; *USA:* Di-Atro†; Logen; Lomotil; Lonox.

Multi-ingredient: *Spain:* Saleton†.

Docusates (17137-e)

Docusate Calcium (6018-m)

Docusate Calcium *(USAN)*.

Dioctyl Calcium Sulfosuccinate; Dioctyl Calcium Sulphosuccinate. Calcium 1,4-bis(2-ethylhexyl) sulphosuccinate.

$C_{40}H_{74}CaO_{14}S_2 = 883.2.$

CAS — 128-49-4.

Pharmacopoeias. In *US.*

A white amorphous solid with the characteristic odour of octyl alcohol. **Soluble** 1 in 3300 of water; 1 in less than 1 of alcohol, chloroform, or ether; very soluble in macrogol 400, and in maize oil.

Docusate Potassium (6019-b)

Docusate Potassium *(USAN)*.

Dioctyl Potassium Sulfosuccinate; Dioctyl Potassium Sulphosuccinate. Potassium 1,4-bis(2-ethylhexyl) sulphosuccinate.

$C_{20}H_{37}KO_7S = 460.7.$

CAS — 7491-09-0.

Pharmacopoeias. In *US.*

A white amorphous solid with a characteristic odour suggestive of octyl alcohol. Sparingly **soluble** in water; soluble in alcohol and glycerol; very soluble in petroleum spirit.

Docusate Sodium (6020-x)

Docusate Sodium *(BAN, USAN, rINN)*.

Dioctyl Sodium Sulfosuccinate; Dioctyl Sodium Sulphosuccinate; DSS; Sodium Dioctyl Sulphosuccinate. Sodium 1,4-bis(2-ethylhexyl) sulphosuccinate.

$C_{20}H_{37}NaO_7S = 444.6.$

CAS — 577-11-7.

NOTE. Compounded preparations of docusate sodium and danthron in the proportions, by weight, 6 parts to 5 parts have the British Approved Name Co-danthrusate.

Pharmacopoeias. In *Br.* and *US.*

White or almost white hygroscopic waxy masses or flakes with a characteristic odour suggestive of octyl alcohol.

Slowly **soluble** 1 in 70 of water, higher concentrations forming a thick gel; freely soluble in alcohol, in chloroform, in ether, and in glycerol; very soluble in petroleum spirit.

Adverse Effects and Precautions

Adverse effects occur rarely with docusates; diarrhoea, nausea, abdominal cramps, and skin rash have been reported. Anorectal pain or bleeding have occasionally occurred following rectal administration.

Like all laxatives, docusates should not be administered when intestinal obstruction or undiagnosed abdominal symptoms are present; prolonged use should be avoided.

Docusate sodium should not be used to soften ear wax when the ear is inflamed or the ear drum perforated.

Pregnancy. Hypomagnesaemia, manifested by jitteriness, in a neonate was considered to be secondary to maternal hypomagnesaemia caused by the use of docusate sodium by the mother during pregnancy.[1]

1. Schindler AM. Isolated neonatal hypomagnesaemia associated with maternal overuse of stool softener. *Lancet* 1984; **ii:** 822.

Interactions

Docusates may enhance the gastro-intestinal uptake of other drugs, such as liquid paraffin (which should not be given concomitantly). Dosage of anthraquinone laxatives may need to be reduced if given together with docusates. It has also been suggested that concomitant administration of docusates and aspirin increases the incidence of adverse effects on the gastro-intestinal mucosa.

Pharmacokinetics

Docusate salts are absorbed from the gastro-intestinal tract and excreted in bile. Docusate sodium is also distributed into breast milk.

Uses and Administration

Docusates may be administered as the calcium, potassium, or sodium salt and are used as laxatives in the management of constipation (p.1168). They are also used as adjuncts for bowel evacuation before abdominal radiological procedures.

Docusates are anionic surfactants which have been considered to act primarily by increasing the penetration of fluid into the faeces, but may also have other effects on intestinal fluid secretion, and probably act both as stimulants and as faecal softening agents. The effect is usually seen within 1 to 3 days. The usual daily dose by mouth of docusate as one of the above salts is up to 360 mg given in divided doses although docusate sodium has been given in doses of up to 500 mg daily. Suggested doses for children have been up to 150 mg daily.

Docusate sodium is also given rectally as an enema in doses of 50 to 120 mg.

Docusate sodium is also used for softening wax in the ear and as a spermicide.

Ear wax removal. Cerumen or ear wax is a normal secretion of the ceruminous glands present in the lining of the external auditory canal. Excessive accumulation or impaction of ear wax may decrease hearing acuity, and may also produce tinnitus and otalgia.

Syringing of the external auditory canal with warm water is the favoured method for removing wax from the ear; a suitable dispersing agent may be given as ear drops for 7 days beforehand.[1] Such agents may also be used alone for self-medication. Traditionally a fixed oil such as olive oil or almond oil has been favoured;[1] other dispersing agents that have been reported as effective include docusates,[2] peroxides such as hydrogen peroxide or urea hydrogen peroxide,[3] choline salicylate,[4] and an oily solution of paradichlorobenzene and chlorbutol.[4] Glycerol and sodium bicarbonate solution have also been used. However, a comparative study *in vitro* of the efficacy of various wax dispersing agents found the most effective to be water, which had originally been included as a control.[5]

1. Sharp JF, *et al.* Ear wax removal: a survey of current practice. *Br Med J* 1990; **301:** 1251–3.
2. Chen DA, Caparosa RJ. A nonprescription cerumenolytic. *Am J Otol* 1991; **12:** 475–6.
3. Fahmey S, Whitefield M. Multicentre clinical trial of Exterol as a cerumenolytic. *Br J Clin Pract* 1982; **36:** 197–204.
4. Drummer DS, *et al.* A single-blind, randomized study to compare the efficacy of two ear drop preparations ('Audax' and 'Cerumol') in the softening of ear wax. *Curr Med Res Opin* 1992; **13:** 26–30.
5. Andaz C, Whittet HB. An in vitro study to determine efficacy of different wax-dispersing agents. *ORL J Otorhinolaryngol Relat Spec* 1993; **55:** 97–9.

Preparations

BP 1998: Co-danthrusate Capsules; Docusate Tablets;
USP 23: Docusate Calcium Capsules; Docusate Potassium Capsules; Docusate Sodium Capsules; Docusate Sodium Solution; Docusate Sodium Syrup; Docusate Sodium Tablets; Ferrous Fumarate and Docusate Sodium Extended-release Tablets.

Proprietary Preparations (details are given in Part 3)
Austral.: Coloxyl; Waxsol; ***Belg.:*** Norgalax; ***Canad.:*** Calax; Colace; Colax-C; Colax-S; Correctol Stool Softener; Dioctyl; Doxate-C; Doxate-S; Laxagel; Pharmalax†; Regulex; Selax; Silace; Soflax; Surfak; ***Fr.:*** Jamylene; Norgalax; ***Ger.:*** Norgalax; Otitex; Otowaxol; ***Irl.:*** Colace†; Fletchers Enemette; Norgalax; Waxsol; ***Ital.:*** Lambanol†; ***S.Afr.:*** Waxsol NF; ***Spain:*** Tirolaxo; ***Switz.:*** Norgalax; ***UK:*** Dioctyl; Docusol; Fletchers Enemette; Molcer; Norgalax; Soliwax†; Waxsol; ***USA:*** Colace; Correctol Extra Gentle; D-S-S; DC Softgels; Dialose; Diocto-K; Dioeze; Disonate; Docusoft S; DOK; DOS Softgel; Kasof; Modane Soft; Pro-Cal-Sof; Regulax SS; Regutol†; Silace; Soflax Fleet; Sulfalax Calcium; Surfak.

Multi-ingredient: ***Aust.:*** Purigoa; Yal; ***Austral.:*** Coloxyl; Coloxyl with Senna; Migrex Pink†; Migrex Yellow†; Rectalad; ***Belg.:*** Laxavit; Softene; Suppolax†; ***Canad.:*** Calcium Docuphen; Doss; Doxidan; Ex-Lax Light; Fruitatives; Peri-Colace; Phillips Gelcaps; Regulex-D; Senokot-S; ***Fr.:*** Neo-Boldolaxine†; ***Ger.:*** Divinal-Bohnen†; Hepaticum-Divinal†; Potsilo; Protitis†; Regenon A†; Rheolind†; Tirgon†; Yal; ***Ital.:*** Fisiolax†; Ikelax†; Macrolax; Prontoclisma†; Sorbiclis; Verecolene†; ***Norw.:*** Klyx; ***S.Afr.:*** Norilax†; ***Spain:*** Boldolaxin; Damalax; Dermijabon Antiseborreic†; Laxvital; Migraleve; Rovilax†; ***Swed.:*** Emulax; Klyx; ***Switz.:*** Elle-care; Klyx Magnum; Tavolax; Yal; ***UK:*** Audinorm†; Capsuvac; Correctol†; Normax; ***USA:*** Colax; D-S-S Plus†; Dialose Plus; Diocto-K Plus; Dioctolose Plus; Disanthrol; Disolan; Disolan Forte; Disoplex; Docucal-P; Docusoft Plus; Doxidan; DSMC Plus; Ex-Lax Extra Gentle Pills; Feen-a-mint Pills; Femilax; Fostex Medicated Cleansing Bar†; Genasoft Plus Softgels; Gentlax S; Modane Plus; Peri-Colace; Peri-Dos Softgels; Peritinic†; Phillips' Laxative Gelcaps; Phillips' Laxcaps; Pro-Sof Plus; Regulace; Senokot-S; Silace-C; Soflax Overnight; Therevac Plus; Therevac SB; Unilax; Vagisec Plus†; Vagisec†; X-Prep Bowel Evacuant Kit-1.

Used as an adjunct in: ***Spain:*** Glutaferro; ***USA:*** Ferocyl; Ferro-Dok; Ferro-Sequels; Hem Fe†; Hemaspan; Nephron FA; Tabron†; TriHEMIC.

Dolasetron Mesylate (13692-g)

Dolasetron Mesylate *(BANM, USAN).*

Dolasetron Mesilate *(rINNM)*; MDL-73,147EF. (6*R*,8*r*,9a*S*)-3-Oxoperhydro-2*H*-2,6-methanoquinolizin-8-yl indole-3-carboxylate mesylate.

$C_{19}H_{20}N_2O_3,CH_4O_3S$ = 420.5.

CAS — 115956-12-2 (dolasetron); 115956-13-3 (dolasetron mesylate).

Dolasetron is a 5-HT_3-receptor antagonist with general properties similar to those of ondansetron (see p.1206). It is used as the mesylate in the prevention of nausea and vomiting (p.1172) associated with chemotherapy, and in the prevention and treatment of postoperative nausea and vomiting.

For nausea and vomiting associated with chemotherapy dolasetron mesylate may be given by mouth in a dose of 100 mg within 1 hour of treatment. Alternatively it may be given in a dose of 1.8 mg per kg body-weight, or 100 mg, by intravenous injection at a rate of up to 100 mg over 30 seconds within 30 minutes of chemotherapy; the same dose may be diluted to 50 mL with a suitable infusion solution and given intravenously over up to 15 minutes.

When given for the prophylaxis of postoperative nausea and vomiting the recommended dose is 100 mg of dolasetron mesylate by mouth within 2 hours of surgery, or 12.5 mg intravenously approximately 15 minutes before the end of anaesthesia. The same intravenous dose may be given to treat established postoperative nausea and vomiting.

Children may be given dolasetron mesylate 1.8 mg per kg orally (up to 1 hour before chemotherapy) or intravenously (30 minutes before chemotherapy), up to a maximum dose of 100 mg, to prevent chemotherapy-induced nausea and vomiting. For postoperative nausea and vomiting 1.2 mg per kg by mouth, up to a maximum of 100 mg, may be given 2 hours before surgery, or 0.35 mg per kg, up to a maximum of 12.5 mg, may be given intravenously either 15 minutes before the end of anaesthesia or, for treatment, when nausea and vomiting occur.

References.

1. Hunt TL, *et al.* A double-blind, placebo-controlled, dose-ranging safety evaluation of single-dose intravenous dolasetron in healthy male volunteers. *J Clin Pharmacol* 1995; **35:** 705–12.
2. Audhuy B, *et al.* A double-blind, randomised comparison of the anti-emetic efficacy of two intravenous doses of dolasetron mesilate and granisetron in patients receiving high dose cisplatin chemotherapy. *Eur J Cancer* 1996; **32A:** 807–13.
3. Dempsey E, *et al.* Pharmacokinetics of single intravenous and oral doses of dolasetron mesylate in healthy elderly volunteers. *J Clin Pharmacol* 1996; **36:** 903–10.
4. Kovac AL, *et al.* Treatment of postoperative nausea and vomiting with single intravenous doses of dolasetron mesylate: a multicenter trial. *Anesth Analg* 1997; **85:** 546–52.
5. Balfour JA, Goa KL. Dolasetron: a review of its pharmacology and therapeutic potential in the management of nausea and vomiting induced by chemotherapy, radiotherapy or surgery. *Drugs* 1997; **54:** 273–98.

Preparations

Proprietary Preparations (details are given in Part 3)
Austral.: Anzemet; ***USA:*** Anzemet.

Domperidone (6544-h)

Domperidone *(BAN, USAN, rINN).*

Domperidonum; R-33812. 5-Chloro-1-{1-[3-(2-oxobenzimidazolin-1-yl)propyl]-4-piperidyl}benzimidazolin-2-one.

$C_{22}H_{24}ClN_5O_2$ = 425.9.

CAS — 57808-66-9.

Pharmacopoeias. In *Eur.* (see p.viii), which includes a separate monograph for Domperidone Maleate.

Domperidone (Ph. Eur.) is a white or almost white powder. Practically **insoluble** in water; slightly soluble in alcohol and methyl alcohol; soluble in dimethylformamide. **Protect** from light.

Domperidone Maleate (Ph. Eur.) is a white or almost white powder; its exhibits polymorphism. Very slightly soluble in water and in alcohol; sparingly soluble in dimethylformamide; slightly soluble in methyl alcohol. Protect from light.

Adverse Effects

Domperidone does not readily cross the blood-brain barrier and the incidence of central effects such as extrapyramidal reactions or drowsiness may be lower than with metoclopramide (p.1200); however, there have been reports of dystonic reactions. Plasma-prolactin concentrations may also be increased which may lead to galactorrhoea or gynaecomastia.

Domperidone by injection has been associated with convulsions, arrhythmias, and cardiac arrest. Fatalities have restricted administration by this route.

Effects on the cardiovascular system. Sudden death has occurred in cancer patients given domperidone intravenously in high doses.[1-3] Four cancer patients experienced cardiac arrest following high intravenous doses[4] and 2 of 4 similar patients experienced ventricular arrhythmias.[5] Following such reports the manufacturers withdrew the injection from general use in the UK.

1. Joss RA, *et al.* Sudden death in cancer patient on high-dose domperidone. *Lancet* 1982; **i:** 1019.
2. Giaccone G, *et al.* Two sudden deaths during prophylactic antiemetic treatment with high doses of domperidone and methylprednisolone. *Lancet* 1984; **ii:** 1336–7.
3. Weaving A, *et al.* Seizures after antiemetic treatment with high dose domperidone: report of four cases. *Br Med J* 1984; **288:** 1728.
4. Roussak JB, *et al.* Cardiac arrest after treatment with intravenous domperidone. *Br Med J* 1984; **289:** 1579.
5. Osborne RJ, *et al.* Cardiotoxicity of intravenous domperidone. *Lancet* 1985; **ii:** 385.

Effects on the endocrine system. Reports of galactorrhoea with gynaecomastia[1] or mastalgia[2,3] generally associated with raised serum-prolactin concentrations. Gynaecomastia without galactorrhoea has also been reported.[4]

1. Van der Steen M, *et al.* Gynaecomastia in a male infant given domperidone. *Lancet* 1982; **ii:** 884–5.
2. Cann PA, *et al.* Galactorrhoea as side effect of domperidone. *Br Med J* 1983; **286:** 1395–6.
3. Cann PA, *et al.* Oral domperidone: double blind comparison with placebo in irritable bowel syndrome. *Gut* 1983; **24:** 1135–40.
4. Keating JP, Rees M. Gynaecomastia after long-term administration of domperidone. *Postgrad Med J* 1991; **67:** 401–2.

Extrapyramidal effects. Reports of extrapyramidal symptoms, including acute dystonic reactions, in individual patients given domperidone.

1. Sol P, *et al.* Extrapyramidal reactions due to domperidone. *Lancet* 1980; **ii:** 802.
2. Debontridder O. Extrapyramidal reactions due to domperidone. *Lancet* 1980; **ii:** 802. Correction, *ibid.*; 1259.
3. Casteels-Van Daele M, *et al.* Refusal of further cancer chemotherapy due to antiemetic drug. *Lancet* 1984; **i:** 57.

Precautions

Due to similarities in the mode of action, the precautions described under Metoclopramide Hydrochloride (p.1201) should be observed. Domperidone should be used with great caution if given intravenously, because of the risk of arrhythmias, especially in patients predisposed to cardiac arrhythmias or hypokalaemia.

Pharmacokinetics

The systemic bioavailability of domperidone is only about 15% in fasting subjects given a dose by mouth, although this is increased when domperidone is given after food. The low bioavailability is thought to be due to first-pass hepatic and intestinal metabolism. The bioavailability of rectal domperidone is similar to that following oral administration, although peak plasma concentrations are only achieved after about an hour, compared with 30 minutes after a dose by mouth.

Domperidone is more than 90% bound to plasma protein, and has a terminal elimination half-life of about 7.5 hours. It is chiefly cleared from the blood by extensive metabolism. About 30% of an oral dose is excreted in urine within 24 hours, almost entirely as metabolites; the remainder of a dose is excreted in faeces over several days, about 10% as unchanged drug. It does not readily cross the blood-brain barrier.

Small amounts of domperidone are distributed into breast milk, reaching concentrations about one-quarter of those in maternal serum.

References.

1. Meuldermans W, *et al.* On the pharmacokinetics of domperidone in animals and man III: comparative study on the excretion and metabolism of domperidone in rats, dogs and man. *Eur J Drug Metab Pharmacokinet* 1981; **6:** 49–60.
2. Heykants J, *et al.* On the pharmacokinetics of domperidone in animals and man IV: the pharmacokinetics of intravenous domperidone and its bioavailability in man following intramuscular, oral and rectal administration. *Eur J Drug Metab Pharmacokinet* 1981; **6:** 61–70.
3. Hofmeyr GJ, *et al.* Domperidone: secretion in breast milk and effect on puerperal prolactin levels. *Br J Obstet Gynaecol* 1985; **92:** 141–4.

Uses and Administration

Domperidone is a dopamine antagonist with actions and uses similar to those of metoclopramide (p.1202). It is used as an antiemetic for the short-term treatment of nausea and vomiting of various aetiologies (p.1172), including that associated with cancer therapy, and nausea and vomiting associated with levodopa or bromocriptine therapy for parkinsonism (see below). It is not considered suitable for chronic nausea and vomiting, nor for the routine prophylaxis of postoperative vomiting.

Domperidone is also used for its prokinetic actions in disorders of gastro-intestinal motility (p.1168) such as diabetic gastroparesis and has been tried in other gastro-intestinal disorders.

Domperidone is used as the maleate in tablet preparations, but doses are expressed in terms of the base.

It is administered in doses of 10 to 20 mg by mouth or 30 to 60 mg rectally every 4 to 8 hours. In the treatment of nausea and vomiting in parkinsonian patients, therapy may be continued for a maximum of 12 weeks. In children doses of 200 to 400 μg per kg body-weight may be given by mouth every 4 to 8 hours; approximately 2 to 4 mg per kg daily may be given rectally.

Domperidone has been administered parenterally, but such administration has been associated with severe adverse effects (see above).

Parkinsonism. Domperidone is used to control gastro-intestinal effects of dopaminergic drugs in the management of parkinsonism (see p.1128). It may be of use in those patients who experience peripheral effects with levodopa despite the use of peripheral decarboxylase inhibitors and for patients using dopamine agonists such as bromocriptine or apomorphine since peripheral decarboxylase inhibitors are ineffective for preventing the peripheral effects of these drugs. Although domperidone does not readily cross the blood brain barrier there have been isolated reports of extrapyramidal effects associated with its use (see above). Consequently there has been concern over its potential to produce central effects and some consider that domperidone should only be used in patients with parkinsonism when safer antiemetic measures have failed.[1,2] However this view has been contested both by the manufacturers and other workers.[3,4] In a subsequent review of the use of domperidone in Parkinson's disease Parkes[5] considered that domperidone might produce central blockade of the therapeutic effects of levodopa if given at a high oral dosage such as 120 mg daily for prolonged periods but also noted that such high doses were rarely required to control levodopa-induced vomiting. In the UK, domperidone is limited to a maximum of 12 weeks' treatment in nausea and vomiting induced by antiparkinsonian treatment.

1. Leeser J, Bateman DN. Domperidone. *Br Med J* 1985; **290:** 241.
2. Bateman DN. Domperidone. *Br Med J* 1985; **290:** 1079.
3. Lake-Bakaar G, Cameron HA. Domperidone. *Br Med J* 1985; **290:** 241–2.
4. Critchley P, *et al.* Domperidone. *Br Med J* 1985; **290:** 788.
5. Parkes JD. Domperidone and Parkinson's disease. *Clin Neuropharmacol* 1986; **9:** 517–32.

Preparations

Proprietary Preparations (details are given in Part 3)
Aust.: Motilium; ***Austral.:*** Motilium; ***Belg.:*** Motilium; ***Canad.:*** Motilium; ***Fr.:*** Motilium; Peridys; ***Ger.:*** Motilium; ***Irl.:*** Motilium; ***Ital.:*** Digestivo Giuliani; Fobidon; Gastronorm; Mod; Motilium; Peridon; ***Neth.:*** Gastrocure; Motilium; ***S.Afr.:*** Motilium; ***Spain:*** Motilium; Nauzelin; ***Switz.:*** Motilium; ***UK:*** Motilium.

Multi-ingredient: ***Belg.:*** Touristil; ***UK:*** Domperamol.

Dronabinol (3780-y)

Dronabinol *(USAN, rINN).*

NSC-134454; Δ^9-Tetrahydrocannabinol; Δ^9-THC. (6a*R*,10a*R*)-6a,7,8,10a-Tetrahydro-6,6,9-trimethyl-3-pentyl-6*H*-dibenzo[*b,d*]pyran-1-ol.

$C_{21}H_{30}O_2$ = 314.5.

CAS — 1972-08-3.

Pharmacopoeias. In US.

Store at a temperature between 2° and 15° in airtight glass containers in an inert atmosphere. Protect from light.

Adverse Effects and Precautions

Dronabinol may produce adverse effects similar to those of cannabis (see p.1558). The most frequent adverse effects include abdominal pain, nausea and vomiting, dizziness, euphoria, paranoid reactions, and somnolence. See also under Nabilone (p.1203) for adverse effects and precautions associated with the use of cannabinoids as therapeutic agents.

The possibility of dependence similar to that of cannabis should be borne in mind.

The abuse liability of dronabinol was rated as being substantially lower than that of cannabis.[1]

1. WHO. WHO expert committee on drug dependence: twenty-seventh report. *WHO Tech Rep Ser 808* 1991.

Pharmacokinetics

Following oral administration dronabinol is slowly and erratically absorbed from the gastro-intestinal tract; the bioavailability of an oral dose is about 10 to 20%, due to extensive first-pass metabolism. Peak plasma concentrations of dronabinol and its 11-hydroxy metabolite are achieved about 2 to 3 hours after a dose by mouth. It is widely distributed and is extensively protein bound, with a volume of distribution approximately 100 times greater than the plasma volume.

Dronabinol is extensively metabolised; the primary metabolite, 11-hydroxydronabinol is also active, and has an elimination half-life of 15 to 18 hours. The 11-hydroxy metabolite is converted to other, more polar and acidic compounds which are excreted in faeces via the bile, and in the urine. About 50% of an oral dose is recovered in faeces within 72 hours and 10 to 15% in urine. Many of the metabolites have relatively prolonged half-lives of 25 to 36 hours, and accumulation may occur with repeated administration.

Dronabinol is found in breast milk, and should be avoided, where possible, in nursing mothers.

Uses and Administration

Dronabinol, the major psychoactive constituent of cannabis (p.1558), has antiemetic properties and is used for the control of nausea and vomiting associated with cancer chemotherapy (p.1172) in patients who have failed to respond adequately to conventional antiemetics.

The usual initial dose of dronabinol by mouth is 5 mg per m^2 body-surface given 1 to 3 hours before the first dose of the antineoplastic drug with subsequent doses being given every 2 to 4 hours after chemotherapy to a maximum of 4 to 6 doses daily. If necessary, the dose may be increased by increments of 2.5 mg per m^2 to a maximum dose of 15 mg per m^2 if adverse effects permit.

Dronabinol also has appetite-stimulant effects and is used in the treatment of anorexia associated with weight loss in patients with AIDS. For this purpose 2.5 mg may be taken twice daily by mouth, before lunch and supper, reduced to a single 2.5-mg dose in the evening in patients who tolerate the drug poorly. If necessary, and if adverse effects permit, doses may also be increased up to 20 mg daily in divided doses.

General references.

1. Voth EA, Schwartz RH. Medicinal applications of delta-9-tetrahydrocannabinol and marijuana. *Ann Intern Med* 1997; **126:** 791–8.

HIV-associated wasting and diarrhoea. References[1,2] to the management of anorexia in patients with HIV-associated wasting and diarrhoea (p.601) including the use of dronabinol.

1. Struwe M, *et al.* Effect of dronabinol on nutritional status in HIV infection. *Ann Pharmacother* 1993; **27:** 827–31.
2. von Roenn JH. Management of HIV-related bodyweight loss. *Drugs* 1994; **47:** 774–83.

Preparations

USP 23: Dronabinol Capsules.

Proprietary Preparations (details are given in Part 3)
Canad.: Marinol; ***S.Afr.:*** Elevat; ***USA:*** Marinol.

Ebrotidine (3677-j)

Ebrotidine *(rINN).*

p-Bromo-*N*-[(*E*)-({2-[({2-[(diaminomethylene)amino]-4-thiazolyl}methyl)thio]ethyl}amino)methylene]benzenesulfonamide.

$C_{14}H_{17}BrN_6O_2S_3$ = 477.4.

CAS — 100981-43-9.

Ebrotidine is a histamine H_2-receptor antagonist with general properties similar to those of ranitidine (see p.1209), but which also has cytoprotective actions. It is used in peptic ulcer disease in doses of 400 to 800 mg daily by mouth.

References.

1. Patel SS, Wilde MI. Ebrotidine. *Drugs* 1996; **51:** 974–80.
2. Various. Ebrotidine: a new generation H_2-receptor antagonist and gastroprotective agent. *Arzneimittelforschung* 1997; **47:** 427–590.

Preparations

Proprietary Preparations (details are given in Part 3)
Spain: Ebrocit.

Ecabet Sodium (15272-h)

Ecabet Sodium *(rINNM).*

12-Sulphodehydroabietic Acid, Monosodium Salt; TA-2711. Sodium salt of 13-Isopropyl-12-sulphopodocarpa-8,11,13-trien-15-oic acid pentahydrate.

$C_{20}H_{27}NaO_5S,5H_2O$ = 492.6.

CAS — 33159-27-2 (ecabet); 86408-72-2 (ecabet sodium).

Ecabet sodium is a cytoprotective drug used in the treatment of peptic ulcer disease (p.1174). The suggested dose is 1 g of ecabet sodium by mouth twice daily.

Action. Ecabet has been reported by the manufacturers to have an antibacterial action against *Helicobacter pylori* in a study *in vitro*.[1]

1. Shibata K, *et al.* Bactericidal activity of a new antiulcer agent, ecabet sodium, against Helicobacter pylori under acidic conditions. *Antimicrob Agents Chemother* 1995; **39:** 1295–9.

Preparations

Proprietary Preparations (details are given in Part 3)
Jpn: Gastrom.

Enoxolone Aluminium (14505-a)

Enoxolone Aluminium *(BANM, rINNM).*

Aluminium Glycyrrhetate; Aluminium Glycyrrhetinate; Enoxolone Aluminum. 3β-Hydroxy-11-oxo-olean-12-en-30-oic acid, aluminium salt.

$(C_{30}H_{46}O_4)_3.Al$ = 1439.0.

CAS — 4598-66-7.

Enoxolone aluminium is an analogue of carbenoxolone that has been used in preparations for the treatment of peptic ulcer disease and other gastro-intestinal disorders.

Preparations

Proprietary Preparations (details are given in Part 3)

Multi-ingredient: ***Spain:*** Gastroalgine; Terpalate.

Euonymus (7511-n)

Fusain Noir Pourpré; Spindle Tree Bark; Wahoo Bark.

The dried root-bark of *Euonymus atropurpureus* (=*Evonymus atropurpurea*) (Celastraceae).

Euonymus is reported to have laxative, choleretic, and diuretic activity.

Preparations

Proprietary Preparations (details are given in Part 3)

Multi-ingredient: ***Belg.:*** Stago†; ***Fr.:*** Jecopeptol; ***Ger.:*** Ludoxin†; Stomachiagil†; ***UK:*** GB Tablets; Indigestion Mixture.

Famotidine (16598-s)

Famotidine *(BAN, USAN, rINN).*

Famotidinum; L-643341; MK-208; YM-11170. 3-[2-(Diaminomethyleneamino)thiazol-4-ylmethylthio]-*N*-sulphamoylpropionamidine.

$C_8H_{15}N_7O_2S_3$ = 337.4.

CAS — 76824-35-6.

Pharmacopoeias. In Eur. (see p.viii), *Jpn, Pol.,* and *US.*

A white to pale yellowish-white crystalline powder. Very slightly **soluble** in water and in dehydrated alcohol; practically insoluble in acetone, alcohol, chloroform, ether, and ethyl acetate; slightly soluble in methyl alcohol; freely soluble in dimethylformamide and glacial acetic acid. It dissolves in dilute mineral acids. **Protect** from light.

Stability and incompatibility. References.

1. Bullock LS, *et al.* Stability of intravenous famotidine stored in polyvinyl chloride syringes. *DICP Ann Pharmacother* 1989; **23:** 588–90.
2. Keyi X, *et al.* Stability of famotidine in polyvinyl chloride minibags and polypropylene syringes and compatibility of famotidine with selected drugs. *Ann Pharmacother* 1993; **27:** 422–6.
3. Shea BF, Souney PF. Stability of famotidine frozen in polypropylene syringes. *Am J Hosp Pharm* 1990; **47:** 2073–4.
4. Fong PA, Ward J. Visual compatibility of intravenous famotidine with selected drugs. *Am J Hosp Pharm* 1989; **46:** 125–6.
5. Bullock L, *et al.* Stability of famotidine 20 and 50 mg/L in total nutrient admixtures. *Am J Hosp Pharm* 1989; **46:** 2326–9.
6. Montoro JB, *et al.* Stability of famotidine 20 and 40 mg/L in total nutrient admixtures. *Am J Hosp Pharm* 1989; **46:** 2329–32.
7. Shea BF, Souney PF. Stability of famotidine in a 3-in-1 total nutrient admixture. *DICP Ann Pharmacother* 1990; **24:** 232–5.

Adverse Effects

As for Cimetidine, p.1183. However, unlike cimetidine, famotidine is reported to have little or no anti-androgenic effect, although there are isolated reports of gynaecomastia and impotence.

General references.

1. Howden CW, Tytgat GNJ. The tolerability and safety profile of famotidine. *Clin Ther* 1996; **18:** 36–54.

Effects on the blood. Reversible leucopenia and thrombocytopenia occurred in a patient with chronic renal failure receiving famotidine and resolved on discontinuation of the drug.[1]

A review[2] of the safety profile of famotidine noted that as of May 1992 there had been 60 reports of serious blood dyscrasias in patients receiving famotidine, of which 22 were considered possibly related to drug therapy (6 cases of pancytopenia or bone marrow depression, 5 of thrombocytopenia, 4 of leucopenia, 3 of combined leucopenia and thrombocytopenia, and 3 of agranulocytosis).

1. Oymak O, *et al.* Reversible neutropenia and thrombocytopenia during famotidine treatment. *Ann Pharmacother* 1994; **28:** 406–7.
2. Howden CW, Tytgat GNJ. The tolerability and safety profile of famotidine. *Clin Ther* 1996; **18:** 36–54.

Effects on body temperature. Famotidine 20 mg intravenously every 12 hours was associated with hyperpyrexia in a patient with facial and cranial trauma.[1] Rectal temperature in the 24 hours after starting famotidine was 40.5° and remained elevated for the 5 days of famotidine treatment, despite administration of antipyretics. Withdrawal of famotidine resulted in a return to normal temperature within 24 hours.

1. Norwood J, *et al.* Famotidine and hyperpyrexia. *Ann Intern Med* 1990; **112:** 632.

Effects on the cardiovascular system. The evidence for a significant haemodynamic effect of famotidine is conflicting. Famotidine 40 mg daily by mouth reduced cardiac output and stroke volume, measured by noninvasive techniques, compared with placebo, cimetidine, or ranitidine in healthy subjects.[1] Similar effects observed in another study[2] were revised by pretreatment with ranitidine. However, other workers have found that oral famotidine had no effect on exercise capacity or left ventricular systolic function in healthy subjects[3] or that famotidine 20 mg intravenously had no effect on any of the haemodynamic parameters measured in 11 critically ill patients.[4]

1. Hinrichsen H, *et al.* Hemodynamic effects of different H_2-receptor antagonists. *Clin Pharmacol Ther* 1990; **48:** 302–8.
2. Mescheder A, *et al.* Changes in the effects of nizatidine and famotidine on cardiac performance after pretreatment with ranitidine. *Eur J Clin Pharmacol* 1993; **45:** 151–6.
3. Hillermann DE, *et al.* Impact of chronic oral H_2-antagonist therapy of left ventricular systolic function and exercise capacity. *J Clin Pharmacol* 1992; **32:** 1033–7.
4. Heiselman DE, *et al.* Hemodynamic status during famotidine infusion. *DICP Ann Pharmacother* 1990; **24:** 1163–5.

Effects on the endocrine system. There has been a report of hyperprolactinaemia and breast engorgement occurring in one woman during the fourth month of treatment with famotidine 80 mg daily;[1] she had by mistake been given twice the usual maximum dose. Recovery occurred when famotidine was withdrawn. Transient hyperprolactinaemia and galactorrhoea have also been reported in a woman after standard doses (40 mg daily) of famotidine.[2] There have been a few instances of impotence.[3]

1. Delpre G, *et al.* Hyperprolactinaemia during famotidine therapy. *Lancet* 1993; **342:** 868.
2. Güven K. Hyperprolactinemia and galactorrhea with standard-dose famotidine therapy. *Ann Pharmacother* 1995; **29:** 788.
3. Kassianos GC. Impotence and nizatidine. *Lancet* 1989; **i:** 963.

Effects on the liver. Mixed hepatocellular jaundice[1] and acute hepatitis[2] have been associated with famotidine administration; in the latter case the patient subsequently experienced a recurrence when given cimetidine.

1. Ament PW, *et al.* Famotidine-induced mixed hepatocellular jaundice. *Ann Pharmacother* 1994; **28:** 40–2.
2. Hashimoto F, *et al.* Hepatitis following treatments with famotidine and then cimetidine. *Ann Pharmacother* 1994; **28:** 37–9.

Effects on mental function. Convulsions and mental deterioration in 2 elderly patients with renal failure were associated with grossly elevated plasma and cerebrospinal fluid concentrations of the drug.[1] Symptoms resolved within 3 days of withdrawing famotidine.

1. Yoshimoto K, *et al.* Famotidine-associated central nervous system reactions and plasma and cerebrospinal drug concentrations in neurosurgical patients with renal failure. *Clin Pharmacol Ther* 1994; **55:** 693–700.

Effects on the skin. A report of toxic epidermal necrolysis following administration of famotidine.[1]

1. Brunner M, *et al.* Toxic epidermal necrolysis (Lyell syndrome) following famotidine administration. *Br J Dermatol* 1995; **133:** 814–15.

Precautions

As for Cimetidine, p.1185.

Hepatic impairment. For a report of increased resistance to H_2-antagonists in patients with liver cirrhosis, see Ranitidine, p.1210.

Renal impairment. Famotidine is largely excreted unchanged in the urine and in patients with renal impairment clearance is reduced and the elimination half-life increased resulting in increased serum concentrations of famotidine and in some cases clinical sequelae (see Effects on Mental Function, above). The half-life of famotidine in healthy subjects is about 3 hours, but in patients with a creatinine clearance less than 38 mL per minute[1] or those with end-stage renal disease[2] it has been reported to be 19.3 hours and 27.2 hours respectively. A 50% reduction in the dose of famotidine in patients with severe renal failure has therefore been recommended in patients whose creatinine clearance is less than 10 mL per minute. However, it may not be sufficient to adjust the dose only on the basis of creatinine clearance since famotidine is partly eliminated by tubular secretion which may also be diminished.[1]

Haemodialysis does not effectively remove famotidine from the systemic circulation. The proportion removed depends on the type of membrane used; with a high flux polysulphone membrane about 16% is reported to be removed, but only 6% with a cuprophan membrane.[2] Continuous ambulatory peritoneal dialysis is reported to remove about 5% of a dose.[2] Continuous haemofiltration may remove about 16% of a dose;[2] intermittent haemofiltration is reported to remove about 4%[3] or 8%.[2] Dosage supplements of famotidine are not required during or after dialysis or filtration procedures.

1. Inotsume N, *et al.* Pharmacokinetics of famotidine in elderly patients with and without renal insufficiency and in healthy young volunteers. *Eur J Clin Pharmacol* 1989; **36:** 517–20.
2. Gladziwa U, *et al.* Pharmacokinetics and dynamics of famotidine in patients with renal failure. *Br J Clin Pharmacol* 1988; **26:** 315–21.
3. Saima S, *et al.* Hemofiltrability of H_2-receptor antagonist, famotidine, in renal failure patients. *J Clin Pharmacol* 1990; **30:** 159–62.

Interactions

Unlike cimetidine (see p.1185) famotidine does not seem to affect cytochrome P450, and therefore is considered to have little effect on the metabolism of other drugs.

Antacids. Concurrent administration of famotidine 40 mg and a 10 mL dose of antacid containing 800 mg aluminium hydroxide with 800 mg magnesium hydroxide,[1] resulted in a decrease in the bioavailability of famotidine which was considered clinically insignificant. Concurrent administration of famotidine 40 mg and a 30 mL dose of the same antacid resulted in a greater reduction in the absorption of famotidine from the gastro-intestinal tract, but the interaction could be minimised by separating ingestion by 2 hours.[2]

1. Lin JH, *et al.* Effects of antacids and food on absorption of famotidine. *Br J Clin Pharmacol* 1987; **24:** 551–3.
2. Barzaghi N, *et al.* Impaired bioavailability of famotidine given concurrently with a potent antacid. *J Clin Pharmacol* 1989; **29:** 670–2.

Probenecid. Probenecid in a total dose of 1500 mg had a significant effect on the pharmacokinetics of famotidine 20 mg in 8 healthy subjects.[1] The maximum serum concentration of famotidine and the area under the concentration/time curve were significantly increased and renal clearance significantly reduced. These effects were explained by inhibition of the renal tubular secretion of famotidine by probenecid.

1. Inotsume N, *et al.* The inhibitory effect of probenecid on renal excretion of famotidine in young, healthy volunteers. *J Clin Pharmacol* 1990; **30:** 50–6.

Theophylline. Although famotidine is considered not to interfere with the metabolism of other drugs there is a report of a clinically significant interaction with theophylline—see p.770.

Pharmacokinetics

Famotidine is readily but incompletely absorbed from the gastro-intestinal tract with peak concentrations in plasma occurring about 2 hours after administration by mouth. The bioavailability of famotidine following oral administration is about 40 to 45% and is not significantly affected by the presence of food.

The elimination half-life from plasma is reported to be about 3 hours and is prolonged in renal impairment. Famotidine is weakly bound, about 15 to 20%, to plasma proteins. A small proportion of famotidine is metabolised in the liver to famotidine *S*-oxide, but most is excreted unchanged in the urine, in part by active tubular secretion. Famotidine is also found in breast milk.

Reviews.

1. Echizen H, Ishizaki T. Clinical pharmacokinetics of famotidine. *Clin Pharmacokinet* 1991; **21:** 178–94.

Children. Famotidine 300 μg per kg body-weight intravenously was given to 10 children aged 2 to 7 years, after cardiac surgery and before extubation, to prevent aspiration.[1] This dose (equivalent to about 20 mg in adults) induced a rise in the intragastric pH within 1 hour of administration and the pH remained above 3.5 for about 9 hours. The mean elimination half-life was 3.3 hours, similar to the value in healthy adults and it was considered that doses in children need therefore only be adjusted according to body-weight and renal function. The pharmacokinetics of famotidine in children has also been reviewed.[2]

1. Kraus G, *et al.* Famotidine: pharmacokinetic properties and suppression of acid secretion in paediatric patients following cardiac surgery. *Clin Pharmacokinet* 1990; **18:** 77–81.
2. James LP, Kearns GL. Pharmacokinetics and pharmacodynamics of famotidine in paediatric patients. *Clin Pharmacokinet* 1996; **31:** 103–10.

Distribution into breast milk. The peak concentration of famotidine in breast milk which occurred in 8 lactating women 6 hours after an oral dose of 40 mg was similar to the peak plasma concentration which occurred 2 hours after the dose.[1]

1. Courtney TP, *et al.* Excretion of famotidine in breast milk. *Br J Clin Pharmacol* 1988; **26:** 639P.

Enterohepatic recirculation. Some individuals exhibit a second peak in the plasma concentration of famotidine which could be due to enterohepatic recirculation. However, a maximum of 0.43% of a dose of famotidine was excreted in the bile of 2 patients following single doses of 20 mg intravenously or 40 mg by mouth indicating that significant recirculation had not occurred.[1]

1. Klotz U, Walker S. Biliary excretion of H_2-receptor antagonists. *Eur J Clin Pharmacol* 1990; **39:** 91–2.

Uses and Administration

Famotidine is a histamine H_2-receptor antagonist with actions and uses similar to those of cimetidine (see p.1185).

Famotidine may be given by mouth or parenterally by the intravenous route.

In the management of **benign gastric and duodenal ulceration** the dose is 40 mg daily by mouth at bedtime, for 4 to 8 weeks. A dose of 20 mg twice daily has also been given. A maintenance dose of 20 mg at bedtime may be given to prevent the recurrence of duodenal ulceration. In **gastro-oesophageal reflux disease** the recommended dose is 20 mg by mouth twice daily for 6 to 12 weeks. Where gastro-oesophageal reflux disease is associated with oesophageal ulceration, the recommended dosage is 40 mg twice daily for a similar period. For the short-term symptomatic relief of heartburn or non-ulcer **dyspepsia** a dose of 10 mg up to twice daily is suggested. In the **Zollinger-Ellison syndrome** the initial dose by mouth is 20 mg every 6 hours, increased as necessary; doses up to 800 mg daily have been employed.

The usual dose of famotidine by the intravenous route is 20 mg and may be given as a slow injection over at least 2 minutes or as an infusion over 15 to 30 minutes; the dose may be repeated every 12 hours.

The dosage of famotidine should be reduced in patients with impaired renal function. A 50% reduction is suggested for patients whose creatinine clearance is less than 10 mL per minute. Alternatively, the dosage interval may be prolonged to 36 to 48 hours.

Reviews of the actions and uses of famotidine.

1. Berardi RR, *et al.* Comparison of famotidine with cimetidine and ranitidine. *Clin Pharm* 1988; **7:** 271–84.
2. Langtry HD, *et al.* Famotidine: an updated review of its pharmacodynamic and pharmacokinetic properties, and therapeutic use in peptic ulcer disease and other allied diseases. *Drugs* 1989; **38:** 551–90.

Administration. Although famotidine is most usually given as a film-coated tablet an alternative wafer formulation, designed to dissolve on the tongue without the need for water, has also been developed.[1]

Parenteral formulations of famotidine are also available in some countries. Although the manufacturers recommend that intravenous injections be given over at least 2 minutes, a study which compared rapid intravenous injection (over up to 1 minute) with slow intravenous infusion found both to be safe.[2] Continuous infusion has however been reported by others[3] to be more effective in the prevention of stress ulceration than bolus injection.

1. Schwartz JI, *et al.* Novel oral medication delivery system for famotidine. *J Clin Pharmacol* 1995; **35:** 362–7.
2. Fish DN. Safety and cost of rapid iv injection of famotidine in critically ill patients. *Am J Health-Syst Pharm* 1995; **52:** 1889–94.
3. Baghaie AA, *et al.* Comparison of the effect of intermittent administration and continuous infusion of famotidine on gastric pH in critically ill patients: results of a prospective, randomized, crossover study. *Crit Care Med* 1995; **23:** 687–91.

Parkinsonism. A pilot study in 7 patients with Parkinson's disease reported modest clinical improvements, mainly in cognitive symptoms, when famotidine 40 mg twice daily was added to their conventional antiparkinsonian medication;[1] the role of such conventional therapy in the management of parkinsonism is discussed on p.1128.

1. Molinari SP, *et al.* The use of famotidine in the treatment of Parkinson's disease: a pilot study. *J Neural Transm* 1995; **9:** 243–7.

Schizophrenia. There are reports of improvement in schizophrenic symptoms in patients given famotidine.[1-3] The more conventional drugs used in the management of schizophrenia are discussed on p.637.

1. Kaminsky R, *et al.* Effect of famotidine on deficit symptoms of schizophrenia. *Lancet* 1990; **335:** 1351–2.
2. Rosse RB, *et al.* Famotidine adjunctive pharmacotherapy of schizophrenia: a case report. *Clin Neuropharmacol* 1995; **18:** 369–74.
3. Rosse RB, *et al.* An open-label study of the therapeutic efficacy of high-dose famotidine adjuvant pharmacotherapy in schizophrenia: preliminary evidence for treatment efficacy. *Clin Neuropharmacol* 1996; **19:** 341–8.

Preparations

USP 23: Famotidine Tablets.

Proprietary Preparations (details are given in Part 3)
Aust.: Pepcidine; Ulcusan; ***Austral.:*** Amfamox; Pepcid; Pepcidine; ***Belg.:*** Pepcidine; ***Canad.:*** Pepcid; ***Fr.:*** Pepcidac; Pepdine; ***Ger.:*** Ganor; Pepdul; ***Irl.:*** Pepcid; ***Ital.:*** Famodil; Gastridin; Motiax; ***Jpn:*** Gaster; ***Neth.:*** Pepcid; Pepcidin; ***Norw.:*** Famotal; Pepcid; Pepcidin; ***S.Afr.:*** Pepcid; ***Spain:*** Brolin; Confobos; Cronol; Cuantin†; Digervin; Dispromil; Fagastril; Famulcer; Fanosin; Fanox; Gastrion; Gastrodomina; Gastropen; Huberdina†; Ingastri; Invigan; Muclox; Neotul†; Nulcerin; Rubacina; Tairal; Tameran; Tamin; Tipodex; Ulcetrax; Ulgarine; Vagostal; ***Swed.:*** Pepcid; Pepcidin; ***Switz.:*** Pepcidine; ***UK:*** Pepcid; ***USA:*** Pepcid.

Fedotozine (13790-p)

Fedotozine *(rINN)*.

(+)-(*R*)-α-Ethyl-*N*,*N*-dimethyl-α-{[(3,4,5-trimethoxybenzyl)oxy]methyl}benzylamine.

$C_{22}H_{31}NO_4$ = 373.5.

CAS — 123618-00-8.

Fedotozine is a peripherally acting selective agonist of opioid κ-receptors which is under investigation in dyspepsia and the irritable bowel syndrome.

References.

1. Fraitag B, *et al.* Double-blind dose-response multicenter comparison of fedotozine and placebo in treatment of nonulcer dyspepsia. *Dig Dis Sci* 1994; **39:** 1072–7.
2. Read NW, *et al.* Efficacy and safety of the peripheral kappa agonist fedotozine versus placebo in the treatment of functional dyspepsia. *Gut* 1997; **41:** 664–8.

Fig (7512-h)

Carica; Ficus.

Pharmacopoeias. In *Br.* and *Swiss.*

The sun-dried succulent fruit of *Ficus carica* (Moraceae) containing not less than 60% of water-soluble extractive. **Store** in a dry place.

Fig is a mild laxative and demulcent used medicinally as a syrup, usually with other laxatives.

Preparations

Proprietary Preparations (details are given in Part 3)

Multi-ingredient: ***Aust.:*** Frugelletten; Herbelax; Neda Fruchtewurfel; Sinolax-Milder; ***Switz.:*** Dragees aux figues avec du sene; Valverde Dragees laxatives; Valverde Sirop laxatif; ***UK:*** Califig.

Frangula Bark (7513-m)

Alder Buckthorn Bark; Amieiro Negro; Bourdaine; Faulbaumrinde; Frangulae Cortex; Rhamni Frangulae Cortex.

CAS — 8057-57-6 (frangula extract).

Pharmacopoeias. In *Eur.* (see p.viii) and *Pol.*

The dried, whole or fragmented bark of the stems and branches of *Rhamnus frangula* (=*Frangula alnus*) (Rhamnaceae). It contains not less than 7% of glucofrangulins, expressed as glucofrangulin A and calculated with reference to the dried drug. **Protect** from light.

Frangula bark is an anthraquinone stimulant laxative with actions and uses similar to those of senna (p.1212).

It is also used in homoeopathic medicine.

Preparations

Proprietary Preparations (details are given in Part 3)
Ger.: Eupond-F; ***Switz.:*** Emodella; ***UK:*** Inner Fresh Tablets.

Multi-ingredient: numerous preparations are listed in Part 3.

Gefarnate (690-w)

Gefarnate *(BAN, rINN)*.

DA-688; Geranyl Farnesylacetate. A mixture of stereoisomers of 3,7-dimethylocta-2,6-dienyl 5,9,13-trimethyltetradeca-4,8,12-trienoate.

$C_{27}H_{44}O_2$ = 400.6.

CAS — 51-77-4.

Gefarnate is a cytoprotective which has been used in the treatment of peptic ulcer disease (p.1174) and gastritis in doses of 100 to 300 mg daily by mouth.

Preparations

Proprietary Preparations (details are given in Part 3)
Ital.: Farnesil†; Farnisol†; Gefarnil†; Vagogernil†; ***Jpn:*** Gefanil.

Multi-ingredient: ***Ital.:*** Gefarnax†; Gefarnil Compositum†; ***Spain:*** Timulcer†.

Ginger (4653-j)

Gengibre; Gingembre; Ingwer; Zingib.; Zingiber.

Pharmacopoeias. In *Aust., Br., Chin., Ger., Jpn,* and *Swiss.* Also in *USNF.*

The scraped or unscraped rhizome of *Zingiber officinale* (Zingiberaceae), known in commerce as unbleached ginger. It contains not less than 4.5% of alcohol (90%)-soluble extractive and not less than 10% of water-soluble extractive. **Store** in a dry place. Protect from light.

Ginger has carminative properties. It is used as a flavouring agent and has been tried for the prophylaxis of motion sickness and postoperative nausea and vomiting.

It is also used in homoeopathic medicine.

Nausea and vomiting. For a discussion of the management of nausea and vomiting including mention of the role of ginger, see p.1172.

References.

1. Grøntved A, Hentzer E. Vertigo-reducing effect of ginger root: a controlled clinical study. *ORL J Otorhinolaryngol Relat Spec* 1986; **48:** 282–6.
2. Bone ME, *et al.* Ginger root—a new antiemetic: the effect of ginger root on postoperative nausea and vomiting after major gynaecological surgery. *Anaesthesia* 1990; **45:** 669–71.
3. Stewart JJ, *et al.* Effects of ginger on motion sickness susceptibility and gastric function. *Pharmacology* 1991; **42:** 111–20.
4. Phillips S, *et al.* Zingiber officinale (ginger)—an antiemetic for day case surgery. *Anaesthesia* 1993; **48:** 715–17.
5. Arfeen Z, *et al.* A double-blind randomized controlled trial of ginger for the prevention of postoperative nausea and vomiting. *Anaesth Intensive Care* 1995; **23:** 449–52.

Preparations

BP 1998: Aromatic Cardamom Tincture; Strong Ginger Tincture *(Ginger Essence)*; Weak Ginger Tincture.

Proprietary Preparations (details are given in Part 3)
Aust.: Zintona; ***Ger.:*** Zintona; ***Switz.:*** Zintona; ***UK:*** Travel Sickness; Travellers.

Multi-ingredient: ***Aust.:*** Mariazeller; Sanvita Magen; ***Austral.:*** Adenas; Adrenas†; Cal-Alkyline; Digestive Aid; Ginkgo Plus Herbal Plus Formula 10; Herbal Cleanse; Herbal Digestive Formula; Lifesystem Herbal Plus Formula 11 Ginkgo; PC Regulax; PMS Support; PMT Complex; Travelaide; Vitaglow Herbal Laxative†; ***Canad.:*** Chase Kolik Gripe Water; ***Ger.:*** Dr. Maurers Magen-Apotheke†; Fovysat†; Fovysatum†; Gastrosecur; Imbak; JuViton; Majocarmin†; Presselin 214†; Presselin 52 N; Unex Amarum; ***Ital.:*** Cura; Donalg; ***Switz.:*** Padma-Lax; ***UK:*** Herbal Booster; Neo; Super Mega B+C; Travel-Caps.

Granisetron Hydrochloride (15846-n)

Granisetron Hydrochloride *(BANM, USAN, rINNM)*.

BRL-43694A. 1-Methyl-*N*-(9-methyl-9-azabicyclo[3.3.1]non-3-yl)-1*H*-indazole-3-carboxamide hydrochloride.

$C_{18}H_{24}N_4O,HCl$ = 348.9.

CAS — 109889-09-0 (granisetron); 107007-99-8 (granisetron hydrochloride).

Granisetron hydrochloride 1.1 mg is approximately equivalent to 1 mg of granisetron base.

Adverse Effects and Precautions

As for Ondansetron Hydrochloride, p.1206. Headache and constipation are the most frequent adverse effects.

The manufacturer has reported an increased incidence of hepatic neoplasms in *rodents* given very high doses of granisetron for prolonged periods, although the relevance of these results to the clinical situation is undetermined. Although mutagenicity and genotoxicity have not been seen in some tests, others have reported an increased incidence of polyploidy or unscheduled DNA synthesis in exposed cells.

Pharmacokinetics

Granisetron is absorbed following administration by mouth, with peak plasma concentrations occurring about 2 hours after a dose. It has a large volume of distribution of around 200 litres. The pharmacokinetics of granisetron exhibit considerable interindividual variation, and the elimination half-life is reported to be around 3 to 4 hours in healthy subjects but about 9 to 12 hours in cancer patients. It is metabolised in the liver, primarily by 7-hydroxylation, with less than 20% of a dose recovered unchanged in urine, the remainder being excreted in faeces and urine as metabolites.

Uses and Administration

Granisetron hydrochloride is a highly selective 5-HT_3-receptor antagonist with a potent antiemetic action similar to that of ondansetron (p.1207). It is used in the management of nausea and vomiting induced by cancer treatment and for the prevention and treatment of postoperative nausea and vomiting (p.1172). Doses are expressed in terms of the base.

For nausea and vomiting associated with cancer treatment, granisetron hydrochloride is given by intravenous infusion, in a dose equivalent to 3 mg of granisetron base, diluted to a volume of 20 to 50 mL with a suitable infusion solution and infused over 5 minutes; alternatively this dose may be administered in 15 mL of infusion solution and given as a bolus over not less than 30 seconds. For the prophylaxis of nausea and vomiting this dose will suffice in the majority of patients. The dose may be repeated up to twice in 24 hours but all prophylactic administration should be completed before cytotoxic therapy is commenced. Similarly, up to 3 infusions in 24 hours may be administered, at least 10 minutes apart, for the treatment of cytotoxic-induced nausea and vomiting. A dose of 9 mg daily should not be exceeded. In children, intravenous infusion of the equivalent of 40 µg per kg body-weight, up to a maximum total dose of 3 mg, has been recommended, dissolved in 10 to 30 mL of infusion fluid and given over 5 minutes. This dose may be repeated once within 24 hours, but at least 10 minutes after the original infusion.

In the USA, lower doses of the equivalent of 10 µg of granisetron per kg infused over 5 minutes are recommended in both adults and children over 2 years of age, beginning within 30 minutes before chemotherapy.

Granisetron hydrochloride is also given by mouth for chemotherapy-induced nausea and vomiting. The recommended dose is the equivalent of 1 mg of granisetron twice daily during cancer therapy, the first dose being given within one hour before therapy begins, alternatively a single 2-mg dose may be given daily. Children may be given the equivalent of 20 µg of granisetron per kg twice daily for up to 5 days during therapy.

For the prevention of postoperative nausea and vomiting the equivalent of 1 mg of granisetron may be given diluted to 5 mL and administered by slow intravenous injection over 30 seconds. Administration should be completed prior to induction of anaesthesia. The same dose may be given for the treatment of established postoperative nausea and vomiting.

References.

1. Anonymous. Granisetron to prevent vomiting after cancer chemotherapy. *Med Lett Drugs Ther* 1994; **36:** 61–2.
2. Yarker YE, McTavish D. Granisetron: an update of its therapeutic use in nausea and vomiting induced by antineoplastic therapy. *Drugs* 1994; **48:** 761–93.
3. Adams VR, Valley AW. Granisetron: the second serotonin-receptor antagonist. *Ann Pharmacother* 1995; **29:** 1240–51. Correction. *ibid.* 1996; **30:** 1043.

Preparations

Proprietary Preparations (details are given in Part 3)
Aust.: Kytril; ***Belg.:*** Kytril; ***Canad.:*** Kytril; ***Fr.:*** Kytril; ***Ger.:*** Kevatril; ***Irl.:*** Kytril; ***Ital.:*** Kytril; ***Neth.:*** Kytril; ***Norw.:*** Kytril; ***S.Afr.:*** Kytril; ***Spain:*** Kytril; ***Swed.:*** Kytril; ***Switz.:*** Kytril; ***UK:*** Kytril; ***USA:*** Kytril.

Hydrotalcite (691-e)

Hydrotalcite *(BAN, rINN).*

Aluminium magnesium carbonate hydroxide hydrate.

$Mg_6Al_2(OH)_{16}CO_3,4H_2O = 604.0.$

CAS — 12304-65-3.

NOTE. Compounded preparations of simethicone and hydrotalcite have the British Approved Name Co-simalcite; the proportions are expressed in the form *x/y* where *x* and *y* are the strengths in milligrams of simethicone and hydrotalcite respectively.

Pharmacopoeias. In *Br.*

A white or almost white, free-flowing, granular powder. It contains not less than 15.3% and not more than 18.7% w/w of Al_2O_3 and not less than 36.0% and not more than 44.0% w/w of MgO. The ratio of Al_2O_3 to MgO is not less than 0.40 and not more than 0.45. Practically **insoluble** in water; it dissolves in dilute mineral acids with slight effervescence. A 4% suspension in water has a pH of 8.0 to 10.0.

Hydrotalcite is an antacid (see p.1167) that is given in doses of up to about 1 g by mouth.

Preparations

BP 1998: Hydrotalcite Tablets.

Proprietary Preparations (details are given in Part 3)
Aust.: Talcid; ***Fr.:*** Ultacite; ***Ger.:*** Ancid; Talcid; Talidat; ***Irl.:*** Altacite; ***Ital.:*** Idrotal†; ***Neth.:*** Ultacit; ***S.Afr.:*** Altacite; ***Spain:*** Hidralma; Talcid; ***Swed.:*** Altacet; Talcid†; ***UK:*** Altacite.

Multi-ingredient: ***Irl.:*** Altacite Plus; ***UK:*** Altacite Plus.

Infliximab (9898-g)

Infliximab *(rINN).*

cA2; CenTNF.

Infliximab is a chimeric monoclonal antibody to tumour necrosis factor α. It is used in the treatment of refractory Crohn's disease, and is also under investigation in the treatment of rheumatoid arthritis.

References.

1. Elliott MJ, *et al.* Randomised double-blind comparison of chimeric monoclonal antibody to tumour necrosis factor α (cA2) versus placebo in rheumatoid arthritis. *Lancet* 1994; **344:** 1105–10.
2. Elliott MJ, *et al.* Repeated therapy with monoclonal antibody to tumour necrosis factor α (cA2) in patients with rheumatoid arthritis. *Lancet* 1994; **344:** 1125–7.
3. Targan SR, *et al.* A short-term study of chimeric monoclonal antibody cA2 to tumor necrosis factor α for Crohn's disease. *N Engl J Med* 1997; **337:** 1029–35.

Preparations

Proprietary Preparations (details are given in Part 3)
USA: Remicade.

Ipomoea (7514-b)

Ipomoea Root; Mexican Scammony Root; Orizaba Jalap Root; Scammony Root.

The dried root of *Ipomoea orizabensis* (Convolvulaceae).

Ipomoea Resin (7515-v)

Mexican Scammony Resin; Scammony Resin.

CAS — 9000-34-4.

A mixture of glycosidal resins obtained from ipomoea.

Ipomoea resin has a drastic purgative and irritant action. It has been superseded by less toxic laxatives.

Preparations

Proprietary Preparations (details are given in Part 3)

Multi-ingredient: ***Fr.:*** Mucinum; ***Spain:*** Laxante Olan.

Irsogladine Maleate (19528-t)

Irsogladine Maleate *(rINNM).*

MN-1695. 2,4-Diamino-6-(2,5-dichlorophenyl)-S-triazine maleate.

$C_9H_7Cl_2N_5.C_4H_4O_4 = 372.2.$

CAS — 57381-26-7 (irsogladine); 84504-69-8 (irsogladine maleate).

Irsogladine maleate is a cytoprotective drug that is used in the treatment of peptic ulcer disease (p.1174) in a usual dose of 4 mg daily by mouth.

Preparations

Proprietary Preparations (details are given in Part 3)
Jpn: Gaslon N.

Ispaghula (5439-c)

Pharmacopoeias. In *Eur.* (see p.viii). Also in *US* under the title of Plantago Seed.

Ispaghula seed (Ph. Eur.) consists of the dried ripe seeds of *Plantago ovata* (Plantaginaceae) known in commerce as Blond Psyllium or Indian Plantago Seed. **Store** in airtight containers. Protect from light.

Plantago Seed (USP 23) is the cleaned, dried, ripe seed of *Plantago ovata*, or of *Plantago psyllium* (*Plantago afra*), or of *Plantago indica* (*Plantago arenaria*), known in commerce as Spanish Psyllium Seed or French Psyllium Seed.

Ispaghula Husk (5440-s)

Pharmacopoeias. In *Eur.* (see p.viii). Also in *US* under the title of Psyllium Husk.

Ispaghula Husk (Ph. Eur.) consists of the husks of *Plantago ovata*. It loses not more than 12% of its weight on drying. **Store** in airtight containers. Protect from light.

Psyllium Husk (USP 23) is the cleaned, dried seed coat (epidermis), in whole or in powdered form, separated by winnowing and threshing from the seeds of *Plantago ovata*, *Plantago psyllium* (*Plantago afra*), or *Plantago indica* (*Plantago arenaria*).

Psyllium (5452-y)

Flea Seed; Psyllii Semen.

Pharmacopoeias. In *Eur.* (see p.viii) and *Pol.* Also in *US* under the title of Plantago Seed.

Psyllium Seed (Ph. Eur.) consists of the whole dried ripe seed of *Plantago psyllium* (*Plantago afra*) or of *Plantago indica* (*Plantago arenaria*) (Plantaginaceae). **Store** in airtight containers. Protect from light.

Plantago Seed (USP 23) is the cleaned, dried, ripe seed of *Plantago ovata*, *Plantago psyllium*, or *Plantago indica* (*Plantago arenaria*) (see Ispaghula, above).

Adverse Effects and Precautions

Large quantities of ispaghula and other bulk laxatives may temporarily increase flatulence and abdominal distension; hypersensitivity reactions have been reported following ingestion or inhalation. There is a risk of intestinal or oesophageal obstruction and faecal impaction, especially if such compounds are swallowed dry. Therefore, they should always be taken with sufficient fluid and should not be taken immediately before going to bed. They should be avoided by patients who have difficulty swallowing.

Bulk laxatives should not be given to patients with pre-existing faecal impaction, intestinal obstruction, or colonic atony.

Hypersensitivity. Hypersensitivity reactions associated with the ingestion or inhalation of ispaghula or psyllium have been reported;[1-6] symptoms have included rhinitis, urticaria, bronchospasm, and anaphylactic shock. In most patients, sensitisation was thought to have occurred during occupational exposure.

1. Busse WW, Schoenwetter WF. Asthma from psyllium in laxative manufacture. *Ann Intern Med* 1975; **83:** 361–2.
2. Gross R. Acute bronchospasm associated with inhalation of psyllium hydrophilic mucilloid. *JAMA* 1979; **241:** 1573–4.
3. Suhonen R, *et al.* Anaphylactic shock due to ingestion of psyllium laxative. *Allergy* 1983; **38:** 363–5.
4. Zaloga GP, *et al.* Anaphylaxis following psyllium ingestion. *J Allergy Clin Immunol* 1984; **74:** 79–80.
5. Kaplan MJ. Anaphylactic reaction to "Heartwise". *N Engl J Med* 1990; **323:** 1072–3.
6. Lantner RR, *et al.* Anaphylaxis following ingestion of a psyllium-containing cereal. *JAMA* 1990; **264:** 2534–6.

Uses and Administration

Ispaghula, ispaghula husk, and psyllium are bulk laxatives. They absorb water in the gastro-intestinal tract to form a mucilaginous mass which increases the volume of faeces and hence promotes peristalsis. They are used in the treatment of constipation (p.1168), especially in diverticular disease (p.1169) and irritable bowel syndrome (p.1172), and when excessive straining at stool must be avoided, for example following anorectal surgery or in the management of haemorrhoids. The ability to absorb water and increase faecal mass means that they may also be used in the management of diarrhoea (p.1168) and for adjusting faecal consistency in patients with colostomies.

The usual dose is about 3.5 g twice daily by mouth although higher doses have been given. It should be taken dispersed in water or fruit juice immediately after mixing.

The full effect may not be achieved for up to 3 days.

Plantain seed (see p.1208) has been suggested as a substitute for ispaghula.

Ispaghula is also given for mild to moderate hypercholesterolaemia in doses of about 3.5 to 5.25 g twice daily by mouth.

Hyperlipidaemias. Preparations of ispaghula have been reported[1,2] to lower serum-cholesterol concentrations in patients with mild to moderate hypercholesterolaemia. They have also been given in combination with reduced doses of a bile acid binding resin in the treatment of hyperlipidaemia,[3] which is reported to be effective and better tolerated than full doses of the resin alone. However, ispaghula or psyllium should be regarded as adjuncts to dietary modification rather than substitutes for it. For a discussion of the hyperlipidaemias and their management, see p.1265.

1. Anderson JW, *et al.* Cholesterol-lowering effect of psyllium hydrophilic mucilloid for hypercholesterolemic men. *Arch Intern Med* 1988; **148:** 292–6.
2. Bell LP, *et al.* Cholesterol-lowering effects of psyllium hydrophilic mucilloid: adjunct therapy to a prudent diet for patients with mild to moderate hypercholesterolemia. *JAMA* 1989; **261:** 3419–23.
3. Spence JD, *et al.* Combination therapy with colestipol and psyllium mucilloid in patients with hyperlipidemia. *Ann Intern Med* 1995; **123:** 493–9.

Preparations

USP 23: Psyllium Hydrophilic Mucilloid for Oral Suspension.

Proprietary Preparations (details are given in Part 3)
Aust.: Agiolind; Laxans; Metamucil; Pascomucil; ***Austral.:*** Fybogel; Metamucil; Mucilax; Natural Fibre; ***Belg.:*** Colofiber; Fybogel†; Metamucil; Spagulax M†; ***Canad.:*** Fibrepur; Floralax; Karacil; Laxagel; Laxucil; Metamucil; Mucilloid; Natural Source Laxative; Naturcil; Novo-Mucilax; Prodiem Plain; ***Fr.:*** Mucivital; Phytofibre; Spagulax; Transilane; ***Ger.:*** Agiolax; Agiolind†; Bekunis Leicht; Flosa; Flosine; Kneipp Abfuhr Herbagran; Laxiplant Soft; Metamucil; Mucofalk; Pascomucil; Plantocur; ***Irl.:*** Fybogel; Isogel†; Metamucil†; Regulan; ***Ital.:*** Fibrolax; Mucivital; Planten; ***Mon.:*** Psylia; ***Neth.:*** Metamucil; Volcolon; ***Norw.:*** Lunelax; Vi-Siblin; ***S.Afr.:*** Fybogel; Metamucil; ***Spain:*** Biopasal Fibra; Fibramucil; Fybogel; Laxisoft; Metamucil; Naturlix†; Plantaben; Sandilax†; ***Swed.:*** Lunelax; Metamucil†; Vi-Siblin; ***Switz.:*** Bekunis Plantago Granule; Colosoft; Dulconatur; Konsyl; Laxiplant Soft; Metamucil; Mucilar; ***UK:*** Fibre Plus; Fybogel; Fybozest; Isogel; Konsyl; Metamucil†; Regulan; ***USA:*** Alramucil; Alramucil Instant Mix; Effer-Syllium; Fiberall; Hydrocil Instant; Konsyl; Konsyl-D; Maalox Daily Fiber; Metamucil; Modane Bulk; Mylanta Natural Fiber; Perdiem Fiber; Reguloid; Restore; Serutan; Siblin†; Syllact; V-Lax.

Multi-ingredient: ***Aust.:*** Abbiofort; Agiocur; Agiolax; Effersyllium; ***Austral.:*** Agiofibe; Agiolax; Diet Fibre Complex 1500†; Herbal Cleanse; Herbal Laxative; PC Regulax; Plantago Complex†; ***Belg.:*** Agiolax; Spagulax K†; Spagulax L†; Spagulax S†; ***Canad.:*** Prodiem Plus; ***Fr.:*** Agiolax; Imegul; Parapsyllium; Spagulax au Citrate de Potassium; Spagulax au Sorbitol; ***Ger.:*** Agiocur; Agiolax; Kneipplax N; Laxiplant-N†; ***Irl.:*** Fybogel Mebeverine; ***Ital.:*** Agiolax; Fibrolax Complex; Ginolax; Syllamalt†; ***Neth.:*** Agiolax; ***S.Afr.:*** Agiobulk; Agiolax; ***Spain:*** Agiolax; Cenat; ***Swed.:*** Lunelax comp.; Vi-Siblin S; ***Switz.:*** Agiolax; Agiolax mite; Bronchalin; Laxiplant cum Senna; Mucilar Avena; ***UK:*** Fybogel Mebeverine; Manevac; Priory Cleansing Herbs†; ***USA:*** Perdiem; Syllamalt.

Itopride Hydrochloride (15899-j)

Itopride Hydrochloride *(rINNM)*.

HC-803. *N*-{*p*-[2-(Dimethylamino)ethoxy]benzyl}veratramide hydrochloride.

$C_{20}H_{26}N_2O_4$,HCl = 394.9.

CAS — 122898-67-3 (itopride).

Itopride hydrochloride is a substituted benzamide with general properties similar to those of metoclopramide (p.1200). It is used for its prokinetic and antiemetic actions in doses of 50 mg by mouth three times daily before meals.

Preparations

Proprietary Preparations (details are given in Part 3)
Jpn: Ganaton.

Jalap (7516-g)

Jalap Root; Jalap Tuber; Jalapa; Jalapenwurzel; Vera Cruz Jalap.

Pharmacopoeias. In Aust.

The dried tubercles of *Ipomoea purga* (=*Exogonium purga*) (Convolvulaceae).

Jalap Resin (7517-q)

Jalapenharz.

CAS — 9000-35-5.

Pharmacopoeias. In Aust.

A mixture of glycosidal resins obtained by extraction of jalap with alcohol.

Jalap resin has a drastic purgative and irritant action. It has been superseded by less toxic laxatives.

Preparations

Proprietary Preparations (details are given in Part 3)

Multi-ingredient: ***Ger.:*** Mandrogallan†; ***Spain:*** Pildoras Zeninas.

Kaolin (694-j)

559; Bolus Alba; Weisser Ton.

CAS — 1332-58-7.

Pharmacopoeias. In *Chin., Eur.* (see p.viii), *Int., Jpn,* and *US.* Some pharmacopoeias do not differentiate between the heavy and light varieties.

Kaolin is a hydrated aluminium silicate.

Heavy Kaolin (Ph. Eur.) is a purified natural form of variable composition. It is a fine white or greyish-white unctuous powder. Practically **insoluble** in water and in organic solvents.

Light Kaolin (BP 1998) is a native form, freed from most of its impurities by elutriation, and dried. It contains a suitable dispersing agent. It is a light, white, odourless or almost odourless unctuous powder free from gritty particles. Practically **insoluble** in water and in mineral acids.

Light Kaolin (Natural) (BP 1998) is Light Kaolin which does not contain a dispersing agent.

Kaolin (USP 23) is a native form, powdered and freed from gritty particles by elutriation. It is a soft, white or yellowish-white powder or lumps with an earthy or clay-like taste and when moistened with water assumes a darker colour and develops a marked clay-like odour. Practically **insoluble** in water, in cold dilute acids, and in solutions of alkali hydroxides.

NOTE. The BP directs that when Kaolin or Light Kaolin is prescribed or demanded, Light Kaolin must be dispensed or supplied unless it is ascertained that Light Kaolin (Natural) is required.

Light kaolin and light kaolin (natural) are adsorbent antidiarrhoeal agents that have been used as adjuncts to rehydration therapy in the management of diarrhoea (p.1168). They may be taken by mouth in doses of about 2 to 6 g every four hours as required. Kaolin is often given in combination with other antidiarrhoeals, especially pectin.

Externally, light kaolin is used as a dusting-powder. Kaolin is liable to be heavily contaminated with bacteria, and when used in dusting-powders, it should be sterilised.

Light kaolin is also used as a food additive.

Heavy kaolin is used in the preparation of kaolin poultice, which is applied topically with the intention of reducing inflammation and alleviating pain (see p.7).

Kaolin can form insoluble complexes with a number of other drugs in the gastro-intestinal tract and reduce their absorption; concomitant oral administration should be avoided.

Preparations

BP 1998: Kaolin and Morphine Mixture; Kaolin Mixture; Kaolin Poultice.

Proprietary Preparations (details are given in Part 3)
Ital.: Kao-Pront; ***UK:*** Childrens Diarrhoea Mixture.

Multi-ingredient: ***Aust.:*** Munari†; ***Austral.:*** De Witt's Antacid; Diaguard Forte†; Diaguard†; Diarcalm; Donnagel; Glucomagma†; Kaodyne†; Kaofort†; Kaomagma; Kaomagma with Pectin; Kaopectate; ***Belg.:*** Alopate; Kaopectate; Neutroses; ***Canad.:*** Bebia; Diarex; Donnagel-MB†; Donnagel-PG; Donnagel†; Kaomycin†; ***Fr.:*** Anti-H; Antiphlogistine; Bebia; Carbonaphtine Pectinee†; Gastropax; Kaobrol; Kaologeais; Kaomuth; Karayal; Neutroses; Pectipar†; ***Ger.:*** Aruto-Magenpulver-forte†; Aruto-Magenpulver†; Dystomin E†; Kaopectate N†; Kaoprompt-H; Katulcin†; Kontabletten†; Noventerol†; Pektan N†; rohasal; ***Irl.:*** Kaopectate; Pekolin†; ***Ital.:*** Anacidase†; Carbotiol; Gastrosanol†; Katoxyn; Magnesia Bisurata; Neo Zeta-Foot; Neutrose S Pellegrino; Streptomagma; Zeta-Foot†; ***S.Afr.:*** Bipectinol; Biskapect; Chloropect; Collodyne; Diastat†; Enterolyte; Gastropect; Kao; Kaomagma†; Kaomycin†; Kaoneo†; Kaopectin; Kaostatex; Medipect†; Neopect†; Pectikon; Pectin-K; Pectolin†; Pectrolyte; Peterpect†; Plastolin Poultice†; ***Spain:*** Balsamo BOI†; ***Switz.:*** Cicafissan; Decongestine†; Fissan; Kaomycine†; Kaopectate; Neo-Decongestine†; Neutroses; Padma-Lax; Phlogantine†; ***UK:*** Bolus Eucalypti Comp; Codella; Collis Browne's; De Witt's Antacid; Enterosan; Entrocalm; Junior Kao-C; Kaodene; Kaopectate†; KLN; Moorland; Opazimes; ***USA:*** Donnagel-PG†; K-C; Kao-Spen; Kaodene Non-Narcotic; Mexsana; Parepectolin.

Lactitol (19392-t)

Lactitol *(BAN, rINN)*.

E966; β-Galactosido-sorbitol; Lactit; Lactobiosit; Lactositol. 4-*O*-(β-D-Galactopyranosyl)-D-glucitol.

$C_{12}H_{24}O_{11}$ = 344.3.

CAS — 585-86-4.

Pharmacopoeias. In *USNF. Eur.* (see p.viii) includes the monohydrate.

Lactitol Monohydrate (Ph. Eur.) is a white crystalline powder. Very **soluble** in water; slightly soluble in alcohol; practically insoluble in dichloromethane. Lactitol (USNF 18) may be the anhydrous form, the monohydrate, or the dihydrate. Lactitol monohydrate 1.05 g is approximately equivalent to 1 g of anhydrous lactitol. Lactitol dihydrate 1.10 g is approximately equivalent to 1 g of anhydrous lactitol.

Lactitol is a disaccharide analogue of lactulose (p.1195) and has similar actions.

Lactitol monohydrate is used as an oral powder in the management of hepatic encephalopathy (p.1170) and in constipation (p.1168).

In the treatment of hepatic encephalopathy, lactitol monohydrate is given in usual doses of 500 to 700 mg per kg bodyweight daily by mouth in 3 divided doses at meal times. The dose is subsequently adjusted to produce 2 soft stools daily.

In the treatment of constipation, lactitol monohydrate is given in an initial dose of 20 g daily by mouth as a single dose with the morning or evening meal, subsequently adjusted to produce one stool daily. A dose of 10 g daily may be sufficient for many patients.

Doses should be mixed with food or liquid, and 1 to 2 glasses of liquid should be drunk with the meal.

Lactitol is a permitted sweetener in foods.

Preparations

Proprietary Preparations (details are given in Part 3)
Aust.: Floralac; Importal; Portolac†; Pselac; ***Belg.:*** Importal; Portolac; ***Fr.:*** Importal; ***Ger.:*** Importal; Neda Lactiv Importal; ***Ital.:*** Portolac; ***Neth.:*** Importal; ***Norw.:*** Importal; ***S.Afr.:*** Importal; ***Spain:*** Emportal; Oponaf; ***Swed.:*** Importal; ***Switz.:*** Importal; ***UK:*** Importal†.

Multi-ingredient: ***Fr.:*** Fucafibres.

Lactulose (7519-s)

Lactulose *(BAN, USAN, rINN)*.

Lactulosum. 4-*O*-β-D-Galactopyranosyl-D-fructose.

$C_{12}H_{22}O_{11}$ = 342.3.

CAS — 4618-18-2.

Pharmacopoeias. In *Eur.* (see p.viii) and *Jpn. US* only contains specifications for lactulose in solution and concentrate.

A white or almost white crystalline powder. Freely **soluble** in water; sparingly soluble in methyl alcohol; practically insoluble in toluene. Liquid Lactulose (Ph. Eur.) is a clear, viscous liquid, colourless or pale brownish yellow, **miscible** with water. The Ph. Eur. states that it may be a supersaturated solution or may contain crystals which disappear on heating. It contains not less than 62% w/v of lactulose; it may contain lesser amounts of other sugars including lactose, epilactose, galactose, tagatose, and fructose. It may contain a suitable antimicrobial preservative. Lactulose Concentrate (USP 23) is a colourless to amber syrupy liquid, **miscible** with water; the USP states that it should be **stored** in airtight containers preferably at a temperature between 2° and 30°.

Adverse Effects

Lactulose may cause abdominal discomfort associated with flatulence or cramps. Nausea and vomiting have occasionally been reported following high doses. Some consider the taste to be unpleasant. Prolonged use or excessive dosage may result in diarrhoea with excessive loss of water and electrolytes, particularly potassium. Hypernatraemia has been reported.

Precautions

Lactulose should not be given to patients with intestinal obstruction. It should not be used in patients on a low galactose diet and care should be taken in patients with lactose intolerance or in diabetic patients because of the presence of some free galactose and lactose.

There has been a report of severe lactic acidosis developing in a patient with adynamic ileus who was being given lactulose for hepatic encephalopathy.[1]

1. Mann NS, *et al.* Lactulose and severe lactic acidosis. *Ann Intern Med* 1985; **103:** 637.

Pharmacokinetics

Following administration by mouth, lactulose passes essentially unchanged into the large intestine where it is metabolised by saccharolytic bacteria with the formation of simple organic acids, mainly lactic acid and small amounts of acetic and formic acids. The small amount of absorbed lactulose is subsequently excreted unchanged in the urine.

Uses and Administration

Lactulose is a synthetic disaccharide used in the treatment of constipation (p.1168) and in hepatic encephalopathy (p.1170). Lactulose is broken down by colonic bacteria mainly into lactic acid which exerts a local osmotic effect in the colon resulting in increased faecal bulk and stimulation of peristalsis. It may take up to 48 hours before an effect is obtained. When larger doses are given for hepatic encephalopathy the pH in the colon is reduced significantly by this acid production and the absorption of ammonium ions and other toxic nitrogenous compounds is decreased leading to a fall in blood-ammonia concentration and an improvement in mental function.

Lactulose is usually administered as a solution containing approximately 3.35 g of lactulose per 5 mL together with other sugars such as galactose and lactose; an oral powder formulation is also available in some countries. In the treatment of **constipation,** the usual initial dose is 10 to 20 g (15 to 30 mL) given daily by mouth in a single dose or in 2 divided doses; doses up to 40 g (60 mL) daily have been given. The dose is gradually adjusted according to the patient's needs. Children aged 5 to 10 years may be given initial doses of 10 mL twice daily; 1 to 5 years, 5 mL twice daily; under 1 year, 2.5 mL twice daily.

In **hepatic encephalopathy**, 60 to 120 g (90 to 180 mL) is given daily by mouth in 3 or 4 divided doses; initially doses of 20 to 30 g (30 to 45 mL) may be given every 1 to 2 hours. The dose is subsequently adjusted to produce 2 or 3 soft stools each day. Lactulose solution 300 mL mixed with 700 mL of water or physiological saline has been used as a retention enema; the enema is retained for 30 to 60 minutes, repeated every 4 to 6 hours until the patient is able to take oral medication.

References.

1. Clausen MR, Mortensen PB. Lactulose, disaccharides and colonic flora: clinical consequences. *Drugs* 1997; **53:** 930–42.

Bowel decontamination. Lactulose may be useful in the selective decontamination of the gastro-intestinal tract since by lowering colonic pH it alters the bacterial flora. A dose of 30 mL daily for 6 months was reported[1] significantly to reduce the incidence of urinary-tract infections and associated bacteraemia in a study involving 45 elderly patients in long-term hospital care. It may be useful in suppressing faecal excretion of shigella in asymptomatic carriers, although it was ineffective in the treatment of acute infection with *Shigella flexneri*.[2] Lactulose also has anti-endotoxin activity.[3,4] It has also been suggested as an adjunct to controlling infection in neutropenic patients and in intensive care.[5]

1. McCutcheon J, Fulton JD. Lowered prevalence of infection with lactulose therapy in patients in long-term hospital care. *J Hosp Infect* 1989; **13:** 81–6.
2. Levine MM, Hornick RB. Lactulose therapy in shigella carrier state and acute dysentery. *Antimicrob Agents Chemother* 1975; **8:** 581–4.
3. Greve JW, *et al.* Lactulose inhibits endotoxin induced tumour necrosis factor production by monocytes: an in vitro study. *Gut* 1990; **31:** 198–203.
4. Fulton JD. Lactulose as an anti-endotoxin in liver transplantation. *Lancet* 1989; **ii:** 927.
5. Fulton JD, Mack DJ. Selective decontamination of the digestive tract. *Br Med J* 1990; **300:** 192.

Diagnosis and testing. Lactulose has been used to investigate gastro-intestinal disorders. In healthy individuals lactulose is largely unabsorbed from the gastro-intestinal tract, but in coeliac disease there is increased permeability to disaccharides such as lactulose and a paradoxical decrease in the absorption of monosaccharides. This led to the development of the differential sugar absorption test in which 2 sugars are given simultaneously by mouth and the urinary recovery of each is determined; rhamnose or mannitol is commonly used as the monosaccharide component and lactulose or cellobiose as the disaccharide. The permeability to sugars is also abnormal in Crohn's disease[1] and this absorption test has a wide application in the investigation of intestinal disease.[2]

Lactulose is converted by bacteria in the large bowel to short chain fatty acids with the production of small quantities of hydrogen gas. The hydrogen is rapidly absorbed and is exhaled in the breath and measurement of its production is used to quantify intestinal transit time[3] and carbohydrate malabsorption.[4] However, even small doses of lactulose shorten transit time and this limits the value of this test.[3]

1. Wyatt J, *et al.* Intestinal permeability and the prediction of relapse in Crohn's disease. *Lancet* 1993; **341:** 1437–9.
2. Anonymous. Intestinal permeability. *Lancet* 1985; **i:** 256–8.
3. Staniforth DH. Comparison of orocaecal transit times assessed by the lactulose/breath hydrogen and the sulphasalazine/sulphapyridine methods. *Gut* 1989; **30:** 978–82.
4. Rumessen JJ, *et al.* Interval sampling of end-expiratory hydrogen (H_2) concentrations to quantify carbohydrate malabsorption by means of lactulose standards. *Gut* 1990; **31:** 37–42.

Fish odour syndrome. Lactulose may provide some benefit in the fish odour syndrome,[1] a syndrome characterised by a foul body odour arising from impaired hepatic oxidation of trimethylamine derived from the diet.

1. Pike MG, *et al.* Lactulose in trimethylaminuria, the fish-odour syndrome. *Helv Paediatr Acta* 1988; **43:** 345–8.

Preparations

Ph. Eur.: Lactulose Solution;
USP 23: Lactulose Solution.

Proprietary Preparations (details are given in Part 3)
Aust.: Bifiteral; Duphalac; Eugalac; Laevolac; Laktulax†; ***Austral.:*** Actilax; Duphalac; Lac-Dol; ***Belg.:*** Bifiteral; Duphalac; ***Canad.:*** Acilac; Alpha-Lact†; Cephulac; Chronulac; Comalose-R; Duphalac; Gel-Ose†; Gen-Lac; Lactulax; Laxilose; Pharmalose†; Rhodialax†; Rhodialose†; ***Fr.:*** Duphalac; Fitaxal; ***Ger.:*** Bifinorma; Bifiteral; Eugalac; Hektulose†; Hepa-Merz Lact; Hepaticum-Lac-Medice; Kattwilact; Lactocur; Lactofalk; Lactuflor; Lactuverlan; Laevilac S; Laxomundin; Mandrolax Lactu; Natulax; Tulotract; ***Irl.:*** Dulax; Duphalac; Gerelax; Laxose; ***Ital.:*** Biolac EPS; Dia-Colon; Duphalac; Epalat EPS; Epalfen; Lactoger; Laevolac; Lassifar; Laxulac†; Lis; Normase; Osmolac; Sintolatt; Verelait; ***Jpn:*** Monilac; ***Neth.:*** Duphalac; Laxeersiroop†; Legendal; ***Norw.:*** Duphalac; Levolac; ***S.Afr.:*** Duphalac; Lacson; Laevolac; Laxette; ***Spain:*** Belmalax; Duolax; Duphalac; Gatinar; ***Swed.:*** Betulac; Duphalac; Laktipex; Loraga; Tikalac†; ***Switz.:*** Duphalac; Gatinar; Laevolac; Legendal; Rudolac; ***UK:*** Duphalac; Lactugal; Laxose; Regulose; ***USA:*** Cephulac; Cholac; Chronulac; Constilac; Constulose; Duphalac; Enulose; Evalose; Heptalac.

Multi-ingredient: ***Fr.:*** Transulose; ***Ger.:*** Eugalan Topfer forte; Eugalan Topfer forte LC; ***Switz.:*** Dessertase†.

Lansoprazole (9499-j)

Lansoprazole *(BAN, USAN, rINN)*.

A-65006; AG-1749. 2-({3-Methyl-4-(2,2,2-trifluoroethoxy)-2-pyridyl}methyl) sulphinylbenzimidazole.

$C_{16}H_{14}F_3N_3O_2S$ = 369.4.

CAS — 103577-45-3.

Adverse Effects and Precautions

As for Omeprazole, p.1204.

Glossitis (associated in some cases with black tongue or stomatitis) has been reported in a few patients taking lansoprazole as part of a triple therapy regimen for *Helicobacter pylori* elimination in peptic ulcer disease.[1] The effect did not seem to have been reported in patients taking lansoprazole alone.

1. Greco S, *et al.* Glossitis, stomatitis, and black tongue with lansoprazole plus clarithromycin and other antibiotics. *Ann Pharmacother* 1997; **31:** 1548.

Interactions

Antacids and sucralfate may reduce the bioavailability of lansoprazole, and should not be taken within 1 hour of a dose of lansoprazole.

Like omeprazole (p.1205), lansoprazole is thought to be a weak inducer of hepatic cytochrome P450, and may affect the pharmacokinetics of other drugs which are metabolised by this system. The possibility of an interaction with oral contraceptives, phenytoin, theophylline, or warfarin should be borne in mind if given concomitantly (but see also below).

Although it has been reported that repeated administration of lansoprazole induced hepatic microsomal cytochrome P450 sufficiently to increase the clearance of a dose of theophylline by about 19%,[1] others have found that lansoprazole did not significantly affect the relevant cytochrome P450 (CYP1A2).[2] The conclusion of a reviewer was that the potential for interaction with other drugs via this mechanism was limited.[3]

1. Kokufu T, *et al.* Effects of lansoprazole on pharmacokinetics and metabolism of theophylline. *Eur J Clin Pharmacol* 1995; **48:** 391–5.
2. Rizzo N, *et al.* Omeprazole and lansoprazole are not inducers of cytochrome P4501A2 under conventional therapeutic conditions. *Eur J Clin Pharmacol* 1996; **49:** 491–5.
3. Andersson T. Pharmacokinetics, metabolism and interactions of acid pump inhibitors: focus on omeprazole, lansoprazole and pantoprazole. *Clin Pharmacokinet* 1996; **31:** 9–28.

Pharmacokinetics

Lansoprazole is rapidly absorbed after oral administration, with peak plasma concentrations achieved about 1.5 hours after a dose by mouth; bioavailability is reported to be 80% or more even with the first dose, although the drug must be given in an enteric-coated form since lansoprazole is unstable at acid pH. It is extensively metabolised in the liver and excreted primarily in faeces via the bile; only about 15 to 30% of a dose is excreted in urine. The plasma elimination half-life is around 1.4 to 2 hours but the duration of action is much longer. Lansoprazole is about 97% bound to plasma protein. Clearance is decreased in elderly patients, and in liver disease.

References.

1. Hussein Z, *et al.* Age-related differences in the pharmacokinetics and pharmacodynamics of lansoprazole. *Br J Clin Pharmacol* 1993; **36:** 391–8.
2. Flouvat B, *et al.* Single and multiple dose pharmacokinetics of lansoprazole in elderly subjects. *Br J Clin Pharmacol* 1993; **36:** 467–9.
3. Delhotal-Landes B, *et al.* Pharmacokinetics of lansoprazole in patients with renal or liver disease of varying severity. *Eur J Clin Pharmacol* 1993; **45:** 367–71.
4. Delhetal Landes B, *et al.* Clinical pharmacokinetics of lansoprazole. *Clin Pharmacokinet* 1995; **28:** 458–70.
5. Karol MD, *et al.* Lansoprazole pharmacokinetics in subjects with various degrees of kidney function. *Clin Pharmacol Ther* 1997; **61:** 450–8.

Uses and Administration

Lansoprazole is a proton pump inhibitor with actions and uses similar to those of omeprazole (p.1205). It is used in the treatment of peptic ulcer disease and in other conditions where inhibition of gastric acid secretion may be beneficial.

Lansoprazole is given by mouth as an enteric-coated formulation. It is normally taken before food in the morning.

For the relief of acid-related **dyspepsia** lansoprazole may be given in doses of 15 or 30 mg daily by mouth, for 2 to 4 weeks. In the treatment of **gastro-oesophageal reflux disease** the recommended dosage is 30 mg daily by mouth for 4 to 8 weeks; thereafter maintenance therapy can be continued with 15 or 30 mg daily according to response.

Lansoprazole is given for the treatment of **peptic ulcer disease** in doses of 30 mg once daily. Treatment is continued for 4 weeks for duodenal and 8 weeks for gastric ulcer. In the USA a dose of 15 mg daily for 4 weeks has been found to be effective for duodenal ulcer. Lansoprazole 15 mg daily has also been recommended as maintenance therapy for the prevention of relapse of duodenal ulcer. Lansoprazole may be combined with antibacterials in **triple therapy** regimens for the elimination of *Helicobacter pylori*. Effective regimens include lansoprazole 30 mg twice daily combined with clarithromycin 250 mg twice daily and either amoxycillin 1 g twice daily or metronidazole 400 mg twice daily; lansoprazole, amoxycillin, and metronidazole has also been used. In patients with **NSAID-associated ulceration** a dose of 15 or 30 mg daily for 4 to 8 weeks is recommended.

Lansoprazole is also used in the treatment of pathological hypersecretory states such as the **Zollinger-Ellison syndrome**; the initial dose is 60 mg daily, adjusted as required. Doses of up to 90 mg twice daily have been used.

General references.

1. Barradell LB, *et al.* Lansoprazole: a review of its pharmacodynamic and pharmacokinetic properties and its therapeutic efficacy in acid-related disorders. *Drugs* 1992; **44:** 225–50.
2. Spencer CM, Faulds D. Lansoprazole: a reappraisal of its pharmacodynamic and pharmacokinetic properties, and its therapeutic efficacy in acid-related disorders. *Drugs* 1994; **48:** 404–30.
3. Anonymous. Lansoprazole–another proton pump inhibitor. *Drug Ther Bull* 1995; **33:** 36–7.
4. Anonymous. Lansoprazole. *Med Lett Drugs Ther* 1995; **37:** 63–4.
5. Blum RA. Lansoprazole and omeprazole in the treatment of acid peptic disorders. *Am J Health-Syst Pharm* 1996; **53:** 1401–15.
6. Garnett WR. Lansoprazole: a proton pump inhibitor. *Ann Pharmacother* 1996; **30:** 1425–36.
7. Langtry HD, Wilde MI. Lansoprazole: an update of its pharmacological properties and clinical efficacy in the management of acid-related disorders. *Drugs* 1997; **54:** 473–500.

Aspiration syndromes. For a discussion of the management of aspiration syndromes, including reference to the use of proton pump inhibitors such as lansoprazole, see p.1168.

Gastro-oesophageal reflux disease. The first aim of treatment in gastro-oesophageal reflux disease is to reduce acid exposure of the oesophagus and proton pump inhibitors such as lansoprazole may be valuable,[1,2] particularly in more severe or refractory disease although, as discussed on p.1170, they are increasingly being used even in milder cases.

1. Robinson M, *et al.* A comparison of lansoprazole and ranitidine in the treatment of erosive oesophagitis. *Aliment Pharmacol Ther* 1995; **9:** 25–31.
2. Robinson M, *et al.* Effective maintenance treatment of reflux oesophagitis with low-dose lansoprazole: a randomized, double-blind, placebo-controlled trial. *Ann Intern Med* 1996; **124:** 859–67.

Peptic ulcer disease. For a discussion of the management of peptic ulcer disease, including mention of the use of lansoprazole, see p.1174. Some references to the use of lansoprazole are given below.

1. Hawkey CJ, *et al.* Improved symptom relief and duodenal ulcer healing with lansoprazole, a new proton pump inhibitor, compared with ranitidine. *Gut* 1993; **34:** 1458–62.
2. Ekström P, *et al.* Lansoprazole versus omeprazole in active duodenal ulcer: a double-blind, randomized, comparative study. *Scand J Gastroenterol* 1995; **30:** 210–15.
3. Avner DL, *et al.* A comparison of three doses of lansoprazole (15, 30 and 60 mg) and placebo in the treatment of duodenal ulcer. *Aliment Pharmacol Ther* 1995; **9:** 521–8.
4. Schütze K, Hentschel E. Duodenal ulcer healing after 7-day treatment: a pilot study with lansoprazole, amoxicillin and clarithromycin. *Z Gastroenterol* 1995; **33:** 651–3.

Zollinger-Ellison syndrome. For a discussion of the management of the Zollinger-Ellison syndrome, including mention of the role of proton pump inhibitors, see p.1176.

Preparations

Proprietary Preparations (details are given in Part 3)
Aust.: Agopton; ***Austral.:*** Zoton; ***Belg.:*** Dakar; ***Canad.:*** Prevacid; ***Fr.:*** Lanzor; Ogast; ***Ger.:*** Agopton; Lanzor; ***Irl.:*** Zoton; ***Ital.:*** Lansox; Limpidex; Zoton; ***Jpn:*** Takepron; ***Neth.:*** Prezal; ***Norw.:*** Lanzo; ***S.Afr.:*** Lanzor; ***Spain:*** Bamalite; Opiren; ***Swed.:*** Lanzo; ***Switz.:*** Agopton; ***UK:*** Zoton; ***USA:*** Prevacid.

Multi-ingredient: *USA:* Prevpac.

Lidamidine Hydrochloride (16875-j)

Lidamidine Hydrochloride *(USAN, rINNM).*

WHR-1142A. *N*-(2,6-Dimethylphenyl)-*N'*-[imino(methylamino)methyl]urea hydrochloride.

$C_{11}H_{16}N_4O,HCl = 256.7$.

CAS — 66871-56-5 (lidamidine); 65009-35-0 (lidamidine hydrochloride).

Lidamidine hydrochloride is an alpha$_2$-adrenergic receptor stimulant which has been investigated for the management of diarrhoea.

References.

1. Goff JS. Diabetic diarrhoea and lidamidine. *Ann Intern Med* 1984; **101:** 874–5.
2. Gasbarrini G, *et al.* A multicenter double-blind controlled trial comparing lidamidine HCl and loperamide in the symptomatic treatment of acute diarrhoea. *Arzneimittelforschung* 1986; **36:** 1843–5.
3. Edwards C, *et al.* Effect of two new antisecretory drugs on fluid and electrolyte transport in a patient with secretory diarrhoea. *Gut* 1986; **27:** 581–6.
4. Allison MC, *et al.* A double-blind crossover comparison of lidamidine, loperamide and placebo for the control of chronic diarrhoea. *Aliment Pharmacol Ther* 1988; **2:** 347–51.
5. Prior A, *et al.* Double-blind study of an α_2 agonist in the treatment of irritable bowel syndrome. *Aliment Pharmacol Ther* 1988; **2:** 535–9.

Liquorice (2021-l)

Alcaçuz; Glycyrrhiza; Licorice; Liquiritiae Radix; Liquorice Root; Orozuz; Raiz de Regaliz; Süssholzwurzel.

Pharmacopoeias. In *Chin.*, *Eur.* (see p.viii), *Jpn*, and *Pol.* Many allow peeled or unpeeled liquorice.

Liquorice Root (Ph. Eur.) consists of the dried unpeeled roots and stolons of *Glycyrrhiza glabra* (Leguminosae) containing not less than 4% of glycyrrhizinic acid. **Store** in airtight containers. Protect from light.

The dried rhizome and roots of *Glycyrrhiza glabra* are known in commerce as Spanish Licorice and those of *G. glabra* var. *glandulifera* as Russian Licorice.

Adverse Effects

Liquorice has mineralocorticoid-like effects. It may cause sodium and water retention and hypokalaemia which can lead to further adverse effects (see below).

Deglycyrrhizinised liquorice is not usually associated with such adverse effects.

Effects on fluid and electrolyte homoeostasis. Mineralocorticoid effects have been reported following excessive ingestion of liquorice. The liquorice may be ingested in confectionery, soft drinks, medicines, or by chewing tobacco. Adverse effects reported include hypokalaemia,[1-13] hypertension,[1,2,6,9] congestive heart failure,[1] arrhythmias,[13] fatal cardiac arrest,[10] headache,[1] muscle weakness,[1,6,9,13] myopathy,[3,7,8] myoglobinuria,[5] paralysis,[5,11] hyperprolactinaemia,[4] and amenorrhoea.[4] The effects are thought to be due to inhibition of 11-β-hydroxysteroid dehydrogenase (cortisol oxidase) by glycyrrhetinic acid, (a metabolite produced by the hydrolysis of glycyrrhizinic acid), resulting in increased concentrations of cortisol in the body.[12,14,15]

1. Chamberlain TJ. Licorice poisoning, pseudoaldosteronism, and heart failure. *JAMA* 1970; **213:** 1343.
2. Wash LK, Bernard JD. Licorice-induced pseudoaldosteronism. *Am J Hosp Pharm* 1975; **32:** 73–4.
3. Bannister B, *et al.* Cardiac arrest due to liquorice-induced hypokalaemia. *Br Med J* 1977; **2:** 738–9.
4. Werner S, *et al.* Hyperprolactinaemia and liquorice. *Lancet* 1979; **i:** 319.
5. Cumming AMM, *et al.* Severe hypokalaemia with paralysis induced by small doses of liquorice. *Postgrad Med J* 1980; **56:** 526–9.
6. Blachley JD, Knochel JP. Tobacco chewer's hypokalemia: licorice revisited. *N Engl J Med* 1980; **302:** 784–5.
7. Lai F, *et al.* Licorice, snuff, and hypokalemia. *N Engl J Med* 1980; **303:** 463.
8. Nightingale S, *et al.* Anorexia nervosa, liquorice and hypokalaemic myopathy. *Postgrad Med J* 1981; **57:** 577–9.
9. Cereda JM, *et al.* Liquorice intoxication caused by alcohol-free pastis. *Lancet* 1983; **i:** 1442.
10. Haberer JP, *et al.* Severe hypokalaemia secondary to overindulgence in alcohol-free "pastis". *Lancet* 1984; **i:** 575–6.
11. Nielsen I, Pedersen RS. Life-threatening hypokalaemia caused by liquorice ingestion. *Lancet* 1984; **i:** 1305.
12. Farese RV, *et al.* Licorice-induced hypermineralocorticoidism. *N Engl J Med* 1991; **325:** 1223–7.
13. Bauchart J-J, *et al.* Alcohol-free pastis and hypokalaemia. *Lancet* 1995; **346:** 1701.
14. Edwards CRW. Lessons from licorice. *N Engl J Med* 1991; **325:** 1242–3.
15. Teelucksingh S, *et al.* Liquorice. *Lancet* 1991; **337:** 1549.

Uses and Administration

Liquorice is used as a flavouring and sweetening agent. It has demulcent and expectorant properties and has been used in cough preparations. It has ulcer-healing properties which may result from stimulation of mucus synthesis. It also has mild anti-inflammatory and mineralocorticoid properties associated with the presence of glycyrrhizinic acid and its metabolite glycyrrhetinic acid, which is an inhibitor of cortisol metabolism. Liquorice may also possess some antispasmodic and laxative properties.

Deglycyrrhizinised liquorice has a reduced mineralocorticoid activity and has been used, usually in combination with antacids, for the treatment of peptic ulcer disease (p.1174).

Preparations

BP 1998: Liquorice Liquid Extract.

Proprietary Preparations

Multi-ingredient: numerous preparations are listed in Part 3.

Loperamide Hydrochloride (5235-b)

Loperamide Hydrochloride *(BANM, USAN, rINNM).*

Loperamidi Hydrochloridum; R-18553. 4-(4-*p*-Chlorophenyl-4-hydroxypiperidino)-*NN*-dimethyl-2,2-diphenylbutyramide hydrochloride.

$C_{29}H_{33}ClN_2O_2,HCl = 513.5$.

CAS — 53179-11-6 (loperamide); 34552-83-5 (loperamide hydrochloride).

Pharmacopoeias. In *Eur.* (see p.viii), *Int.*, and *US.*

A white to slightly yellow powder. Slightly **soluble** in water and dilute acids; freely soluble in chloroform, isopropyl alcohol, and methyl alcohol; soluble in alcohol. **Protect** from light.

Adverse Effects and Treatment

Abdominal pain or bloating, nausea, constipation, dry mouth, dizziness, fatigue, and hypersensitivity reactions including skin rashes have been reported. Loperamide hydrochloride has been associated with paralytic ileus, particularly in infants and young children, and deaths have been reported. Depression of the CNS, to which children may be more sensitive, may be seen in overdosage, and naloxone hydrochloride (see p.987) has been recommended for its treatment.

Some references to loperamide toxicity covering toxic megacolon[1,2] and severe effects in young children including coma,[3] paralytic ileus with death,[4] and delirium.[5]

1. Brown JW. Toxic megacolon associated with loperamide therapy. *JAMA* 1979; **241:** 501–2.
2. Walley T, Milson D. Loperamide related toxic megacolon in Clostridium difficile colitis. *Postgrad Med J* 1990; **66:** 582.
3. Minton NA, Smith PGD. Loperamide toxicity in a child after a single dose. *Br Med J* 1987; **294:** 1383.
4. Bhutta TI, Tahir KI. Loperamide poisoning in children. *Lancet* 1990; **335:** 363.
5. Schwartz RH, Rodriguez WJ. Toxic delirium possibly caused by loperamide. *J Pediatr* 1991; **118:** 656–7.

Precautions

Loperamide should be used with caution in patients with hepatic dysfunction because of its considerable first-pass metabolism in the liver. It should also be used with caution in young children because of a greater variability of response in this age group, and it is not recommended for use in infants (see Uses and Administration, below).

Loperamide should not be used when inhibition of peristalsis is to be avoided, in particular where ileus or constipation occur, and should be avoided in patients with abdominal distension. Toxic megacolon has occurred in patients with inflammatory bowel disease or pseudomembranous colitis given antidiarrhoeal therapy. Loperamide should not be used alone in patients with dysentery.

Interactions

Co-trimoxazole. Concomitant administration with co-trimoxazole increases the bioavailability of loperamide,[1] apparently by inhibiting its first-pass metabolism.

1. Kamali F, Huang ML. Increased systemic availability of loperamide after oral administration of loperamide and loperamide oxide with cotrimoxazole. *Br J Clin Pharmacol* 1996; **41:** 125–8.

Pharmacokinetics

About 40% of a dose of loperamide is reported to be absorbed from the gastro-intestinal tract to undergo first-pass metabolism in the liver and excretion in the faeces via the bile as inactive conjugate; there is slight urinary excretion. Little intact drug reaches the systemic circulation. The elimination half-life is reported to be about 10 hours.

Uses and Administration

Loperamide hydrochloride is a synthetic opioid analogue which inhibits gut motility and may also reduce gastro-intestinal secretions. It is given by mouth as an antidiarrhoeal drug as an adjunct in the management of acute and chronic diarrhoeas and may also be used in the management of colostomies or ileostomies to reduce the volume of discharge.

In acute diarrhoea the usual initial dose for adults is 4 mg followed by 2 mg after each loose stool to a maximum of 16 mg daily; the usual daily dose is 6 to 8 mg. In the UK, loperamide hydrochloride is not recommended for children under 4 years of age (see also below). Suggested doses for older children are: 4 to 8 years, 1 mg three or four times daily for up to 3 days; 9 to 12 years, 2 mg four times daily for up to 5 days. In the USA, loperamide is not recommended for children under the age of 2 years and an initial dose of 1 mg three times daily is suggested for children aged 2 to 5 years. (For the view that antidiarrhoeal drugs should not be used at all in children with diarrhoea, see p.1168.)

In chronic diarrhoea the usual initial dose for adults is 4 to 8 mg daily in divided doses subsequently adjusted as necessary; doses of 16 mg daily should not be exceeded. If no improvement has been observed after treatment with 16 mg daily for at least 10 days, further administration is unlikely to be of benefit.

Loperamide has also been given as the prodrug, loperamide oxide, which is converted to loperamide in the gastro-intestinal tract. It has been given for acute diarrhoea in doses of 2 to 4 mg initially followed by 1 mg after each loose stool, to a maximum of 8 mg daily.

Diarrhoea. The mainstay of treatment for diarrhoea is rehydration therapy. Antidiarrhoeals like loperamide have a limited role for symptomatic relief in adults with diarrhoea (see the discussion on the management of diarrhoea on p.1168). WHO does not recommend the use of any antidiarrhoeal drug in children with diarrhoea. There have been problems regarding the use of antidiarrhoeals such as loperamide in young children in developing countries. Manufacturers have considered that a lower age limit is acceptable in those countries than is recommended in the UK or USA; even that lower limit is not always observed in practice and there have been reports of serious toxicity in very young children.[1] In response to such reports the manufacturers have withdrawn concentrated drops of loperamide worldwide and the syrup from countries where the WHO have a programme for control of diarrhoeal diseases, but tablets and capsules remain available.[2] In some countries the use of antidiarrhoeals is now restricted by law.

1. Bhutta TI, Tahir KI. Loperamide poisoning in children. *Lancet* 1990; **335:** 363.
2. Gussin RZ. Withdrawal of loperamide drops. *Lancet* 1990; **335:** 1603–4.

References to the use of *loperamide oxide* in diarrhoea.

1. Van Den Eynden B, *et al.* New approaches to the treatment of patients with acute, nonspecific diarrhea: a comparison of the effects of loperamide and loperamide oxide. *Curr Ther Res* 1995; **56:** 1132–41.
2. Hughes IW, *et al.* First-line treatment in acute non-dysenteric diarrhoea: clinical comparison of loperamide oxide, loperamide and placebo. *Br J Clin Pract* 1995; **49:** 181–5.
3. van Outryve M, Toussaint J. Loperamide oxide for the treatment of chronic diarrhoea in Crohn's disease. *J Int Med Res* 1995; **23:** 335–41.

Preparations

USP 23: Loperamide Hydrochloride Capsules; Loperamide Hydrochloride Tablets.

Proprietary Preparations (details are given in Part 3)
Aust.: Arestal; Enterobene; Imodium; ***Austral.:*** Gastro-Stop; Imodium; ***Belg.:*** Imodium; Toriac; ***Canad.:*** Anti-Diarrheal; Diarrhea Relief; Imodium; Loperacap; ***Fr.:*** Altocel; Dyspagon; Imodium; Imossel; Lopelin; Peracel; ***Ger.:*** Aperamid; Azuperamid; Boxolip; D-Stop; Diarstop L†; duralopid; Endiaron; Imodium; Logomed Durchfall-Kapseln; Lop-Dia; Lopalind; Lopedium; Loperamerck; Loperhoe; Lopetrans; Mandros Diarstop; Metifex-L; Sanifug; ***Irl.:*** Arret; Imodium; ***Ital.:*** Blox†; Brek†; Diarstop; Dissenten; Imodium; Lodis; Lopemid; Loperyl; Tebloc; ***Neth.:*** Diacure; Imodium; ***Norw.:*** Imodium; Travello; ***S.Afr.:*** Betaperamide; Gastron; Imodium; Lopedium; Loperastat; Loperol; Norimode†; Prodium; ***Spain:*** Fortasec; Imodium; Imosec; Loperam†; Orulop; Taguinol; ***Swed.:*** Dimor; Imodium; Primodium; Travello; ***Switz.:*** Binaldan; Imodium; Lopimed; ***UK:*** Arret; Diah-Limit; Diareze; Diasorb; Diocalm Ultra; Diocaps; Imodium; Lodiar; LoperaGen; Norimode; Normaloe; ***USA:*** Diar-Aid†; Imodium; Kaopectate II; Maalox Anti-Diarrheal; Neo-Diaral; Pepto Diarrhea Control.

Loxiglumide (3692-y)

Loxiglumide *(rINN)*.

CR-1505. (±)-4-(3,4-Dichlorobenzamido)-*N*-(3-methoxypropyl)-*N*-pentylglutaramic acid.

$C_{21}H_{30}Cl_2N_2O_5$ = 461.4.

CAS — 107097-80-3.

Loxiglumide is a specific cholecystokinin antagonist related to proglumide (see p.1209), and has been investigated in biliary and gastro-intestinal dyskinesias, constipation and irritable bowel syndrome, and pancreatitis.

References.

1. Meyer BM, *et al.* Role of cholecystokinin in regulation of gastrointestinal motor functions. *Lancet* 1989; **ii:** 12–15.
2. Beglinger C, *et al.* Treatment of biliary colic with loxiglumide. *Lancet* 1989; **ii:** 167.
3. Setnikar I, *et al.* Pharmacokinetics and tolerance of repeated oral doses of loxiglumide. *Arzneimittelforschung* 1989; **39:** 1454–9.
4. Meier R, *et al.* Therapeutic effects of loxiglumide, a cholecystokinin antagonist, on chronic constipation in elderly patients: a prospective, randomized, double-blind, controlled trial. *J Gastrointest Mot* 1993; **5:** 129–35.
5. Lieverse RJ, *et al.* Effects of somatostatin and loxiglumide on gallbladder motility. *Eur J Clin Pharmacol* 1995; **47:** 489–92.

Magaldrate (695-z)

Magaldrate *(BAN, USAN, rINN)*.

Aluminum Magnesium Hydroxide Sulfate; AY-5710.

$Al_5Mg_{10}(OH)_{31}(SO_4)_2,xH_2O$ = 1097.3 (anhydrous).

CAS — 74978-16-8.

Pharmacopoeias. In *Br.* and *US.*

A combination of aluminium and magnesium hydroxides (see p.1177 and p.1198 respectively), and sulphates. It contains the equivalent of 90 to 105% of $Al_5Mg_{10}(OH)_{31}(SO_4)_2$, calculated on the dried basis. A white or almost white odourless crystalline powder. Practically **insoluble** in water and alcohol; soluble in dilute mineral acids. It loses between 10 and 20% of its weight on drying at 200° for 4 hours.

Magaldrate is an antacid (see p.1167) that is given in doses of up to about 2 g by mouth. Aluminium magnesium hydroxide has also been used.

Preparations

BP 1998: Magaldrate Oral Suspension;
USP 23: Magaldrate and Simethicone Oral Suspension; Magaldrate and Simethicone Tablets; Magaldrate Oral Suspension; Magaldrate Tablets.

Proprietary Preparations (details are given in Part 3)
Aust.: Riopan; ***Belg.:*** Gastricalm; Riopan; ***Canad.:*** Riopan; ***Ger.:*** Gastrimagal; Gastripan; Gastrostad; Glysan; Hevert-Mag; Logomed Magen; Magalphil; Magasan; Magastron; Magmed; Marax; ProWohl; Riopan; Simaphil; ***Irl.:*** Antacin†; ***Ital.:*** Riopan; ***Neth.:*** Riopan; ***S.Afr.:*** Gastrobon; Riopone; ***Spain:*** Bemolan; Gastromol; Magion; Minoton; ***Switz.:*** Riopan; ***UK:*** Dynese; ***USA:*** Iosopan; Riopan; WinGel†.

Multi-ingredient: ***Austral.:*** Mylanta Plus; ***Canad.:*** Riopan Plus; ***Spain:*** Aci Kestomal†; Compagel; Silargin†; ***UK:*** Bisodol Heartburn; ***USA:*** Iosopan Plus; Lowsium Plus; Riopan Plus.

Magnesium Carbonate (698-a)

504; Magnesii Subcarbonas.

CAS — 546-93-0 (anhydrous); 23389-33-5 (normal, hydrate); 39409-82-0 (basic, hydrate).

Pharmacopoeias. In *Chin., Eur.* (see p.viii), *Jpn, Pol.,* and *US.*

Some pharmacopoeias include a single monograph which permits both the light and heavy varieties while some have 2 separate monographs for the 2 varieties.

Heavy Magnesium Carbonate (Ph. Eur.) and Light Magnesium Carbonate (Ph. Eur.) are hydrated basic magnesium carbonates containing the equivalent of 40 to 45% of MgO. Both are white powders and are practically **insoluble** in water but dissolve in dilute acids with strong effervescence. For the heavy variety 15 g occupies a volume of about 30 mL and for the light variety 15 g occupies a volume of about 180 mL.

Magnesium Carbonate (USP 23) is a basic hydrated magnesium carbonate or a normal hydrated magnesium carbonate containing the equivalent of 40.0 to 43.5% of MgO. It is an odourless bulky white powder or light, white, friable masses. Practically **insoluble** in water and alcohol; dissolves in dilute acids with effervescence.

Magnesium carbonate is an antacid with general properties similar to those of magnesium hydroxide (below) that is given in doses of up to about 500 mg by mouth. When administered by mouth, it reacts with gastric acid to form soluble magnesium chloride and carbon dioxide in the stomach; the carbon dioxide may cause flatulence and eructation. Magnesium carbonate is often given in conjunction with aluminium-containing antacids such as aluminium hydroxide which counteract its laxative effect. Some magnesium is slowly absorbed from the gastro-intestinal tract and excreted in the urine.

Magnesium carbonate is also used as a food additive.

Phosphate binding. Although calcium salts such as the carbonate or acetate, or in some cases aluminium hydroxide, are usually used as phosphate binders in patients with chronic renal failure other drugs have been used to control plasma-phosphate concentrations. For a reference to magnesium carbonate as a phosphate binder, see under Renal Osteodystrophy, p.732.

Preparations

BP 1998: Aromatic Magnesium Carbonate Mixture; Compound Magnesium Trisilicate Oral Powder; Kaolin Mixture; Magnesium Sulphate Mixture; Magnesium Trisilicate Mixture;
USP 23: Alumina and Magnesium Carbonate Oral Suspension; Alumina and Magnesium Carbonate Tablets; Alumina, Magnesium Carbonate, and Magnesium Oxide Tablets; Calcium and Magnesium Carbonates Oral Suspension; Calcium and Magnesium Carbonates Tablets; Magnesium Carbonate and Citric Acid for Oral Solution; Magnesium Carbonate and Sodium Bicarbonate for Oral Suspension; Magnesium Citrate Oral Solution.

Proprietary Preparations (details are given in Part 3)
Aust.: Tetesept Magnesium; ***Belg.:*** Magnezyme†; ***Canad.:*** Cepasium; ***Ger.:*** Palmicol; ***Switz.:*** Magnesium Diasporal.

Multi-ingredient: numerous preparations are listed in Part 3.

Magnesium Citrate (1173-x)

$C_{12}H_{10}Mg_3O_{14}$ = 451.1.

CAS — 3344-18-1.

Pharmacopoeias. In *US.*

Magnesium citrate is an osmotic laxative with general properties similar to those of other magnesium salts (see p.1157). It is used as a bowel evacuant prior to investigational procedures or surgery of the colon. An aqueous solution containing 17.7 g of magnesium citrate, prepared from a sachet of effervescent powder dissolved in 200 mL of water, may be used. Dosages with other preparations have ranged from about 11 to 25 g of magnesium citrate. A high fluid intake and low residue diet are needed in conjunction with such bowel preparation.

Magnesium citrate has also been used as a magnesium supplement in doses of up to about 1.9 g daily by mouth.

Bowel evacuation. For references to the use of magnesium citrate with sodium picosulphate for bowel evacuation, see under Sodium Picosulphate, p.1213.

Preparations

USP 23: Magnesium Citrate for Oral Solution.

Proprietary Preparations (details are given in Part 3)
Aust.: Magnesium Diasporal; ***Canad.:*** Citro-Mag; ***Ger.:*** Magnesium Diasporal; Magnesium Tonil N; ***Switz.:*** Magnesium Diasporal; ***UK:*** Citramag; ***USA:*** Evac-Q-Mag.

Multi-ingredient: ***Aust.:*** Magnofit; ***Austral.:*** Raykit†; ***Belg.:*** Carbobel; ***Canad.:*** Evac-Q-Kwik; Royvac Kit; ***Fr.:*** Citrocholine; ***Ger.:*** Acidovert; Lithurex; Magnerot N; Migranex†; ***Irl.:*** Picolax; ***Spain:*** Salmagne; ***Switz.:*** Magnesium Biomed; ***UK:*** Picolax; Porosis D; ***USA:*** Fleet Prep Kit No. 4; Fleet Prep Kit No. 5; Fleet Prep Kit No. 6; Tridrate Bowel Evacuant Kit.

Magnesium Hydroxide (699-t)

528; Magnesii Hydroxidum; Magnesium Hydrate.

$Mg(OH)_2$ = 58.32.

CAS — 1309-42-8.

NOTE. Compounded preparations of magnesium hydroxide and aluminium hydroxide have the British Approved Name Co-magaldrox; the proportions are expressed in the form *x/y* where *x* and *y* are the strengths in milligrams per unit dose of magnesium hydroxide and aluminium hydroxide respectively.

Pharmacopoeias. In *Eur.* (see p.viii), *Int.,* and *US.*

A fine white amorphous powder. Practically **insoluble** in water and alcohol; dissolves in dilute acids. A solution in water is alkaline to phenolphthalein. **Store** in airtight containers.

Adverse Effects, Treatment, and Precautions

Magnesium hydroxide, in common with other magnesium salts (see p.1157), may cause diarrhoea. Hypermagnesaemia may occur in patients with impaired renal function.

There have been reports of hypermagnesaemia (p.1148) in infants given magnesium-containing antacids.[1,2]

1. Brand JM, Greer FR. Hypermagnesemia and intestinal perforation following antacid administration in a premature infant. *Pediatrics* 1990; **85:** 121–4.
2. Alison LH, Bulugahapitiya D. Laxative induced magnesium poisoning in a 6 week old infant. *Br Med J* 1990; **300:** 125.

Interactions

As outlined on p.1167, antacids, including magnesium salts, interact with many other drugs both by alterations in gastric pH and emptying, and by formation of complexes that are not absorbed. Interactions can be minimised by giving the antacid and any other medications 2 to 3 hours apart.

Uses and Administration

Magnesium hydroxide is an antacid (see p.1167) that is given in doses of up to about 1 g by mouth. It is often given in conjunction with aluminium-containing antacids such as aluminium hydroxide which counteract its laxative effect.

Magnesium hydroxide is also given as a laxative in doses of up to about 5 g by mouth and as a magnesium supplement in deficiency states.

Magnesium hydroxide is also used as a food additive.

Renal calculi. Magnesium salts[1,2] have been used in the prophylaxis of recurrent renal calculi (p.888).

1. Melnick I, *et al.* Magnesium therapy for recurring calcium oxalate urinary calculi. *J Urol (Baltimore)* 1971; **105:** 119–22.
2. Johansson G, *et al.* Biochemical and clinical effects of the prophylactic treatment of renal calcium stones with magnesium hydroxide. *J Urol (Baltimore)* 1980; **124:** 770–4.

Preparations

BP 1998: Co-magaldrox Oral Suspension; Co-magaldrox Tablets; Liquid Paraffin and Magnesium Hydroxide Oral Emulsion *(Emuls. Paraff. Liq. et Mag. Hydrox.; Mist. Mag. Hydrox. et Paraff. Liq.)*; Magnesium Hydroxide Mixture;
USP 23: Alumina and Magnesia Oral Suspension; Alumina and Magnesia Tablets; Alumina, Magnesia, and Calcium Carbonate Oral Suspension; Alumina, Magnesia, and Calcium Carbonate Tablets; Alumina, Magnesia, and Simethicone Oral Suspension; Alumina, Magnesia, and Simethicone Tablets; Alumina, Magnesia, Calcium Carbonate, and Simethicone Tablets; Aspirin, Alumina, and Magnesia Tablets; Aspirin, Codeine Phosphate, Alumina, and Magnesia Tablets; Calcium Carbonate and Magnesia Tablets; Calcium Carbonate, Magnesia, and Simethicone Tablets; Magnesia Tablets; Magnesium Hydroxide Paste; Milk of Magnesia.

Proprietary Preparations (details are given in Part 3)
Canad.: Phillips' Milk of Magnesia; ***Fr.:*** Chlorumagene; ***Irl.:*** Milk of Magnesia; ***Ital.:*** Citrato Espresso S. Pellegrino; Magnesia S Pellegrino; Magnesia Volta; ***S.Afr.:*** Deopens; ***Spain:*** Crema de Magnesia; ***Swed.:*** Emgesan; ***Switz.:*** Chlorumagene; Magnesia S Pellegrino; Milk of Magnesia†; Rivomag†; ***UK:*** Milk of Magnesia; ***USA:*** Phillips' Chewable; Phillips' Milk of Magnesia.

Multi-ingredient: numerous preparations are listed in Part 3.

Magnesium Oxide (702-r)

530; Magnesii Oxidum.

MgO = 40.30.

CAS — 1309-48-4.

Pharmacopoeias. In *Chin., Eur.* (see p.viii), *Int., Jpn, Pol.,* and *US.*

Some pharmacopoeias include a single monograph which permits both the light and heavy varieties while some have 2 separate monographs for the 2 varieties.

Heavy Magnesium Oxide (Ph. Eur.) and Light Magnesium Oxide (Ph. Eur.) (Light Magnesia) are fine white powders and are practically **insoluble** in water yielding solutions that are alkaline to phenolphthalein. Both heavy and light magnesium oxide dissolve in dilute acids with at most slight effervescence. For the heavy variety 15 g occupies a volume of about 30 mL and for the light variety 15 g occupies a volume of about 150 mL.

Magnesium Oxide (USP 23) is either the heavy or light variety. Heavy magnesium oxide is a relatively dense white powder with 5 g occupying a volume of about 10 to 20 mL. Light magnesium oxide is a very bulky white powder with 5 g occupying a volume of about 40 to 50 mL. Both varieties are practically **insoluble** in water and alcohol but soluble in dilute acids. **Store** in airtight containers.

Magnesium oxide is an antacid with general properties similar to those of magnesium hydroxide (p.1198). It is given in doses of up to about 800 mg by mouth. It is often given in conjunction with aluminium-containing antacids such as aluminium hydroxide which counteract its laxative effect.

Magnesium oxide has been employed for its laxative properties in bowel preparation; doses of 3.5 g by mouth are given for this purpose, combined with bisacodyl or sodium picosulphate.

Magnesium oxide is also used as a magnesium supplement in deficiency states, and as a food additive.

Preparations

USP 23: Alumina, Magnesium Carbonate, and Magnesium Oxide Tablets; Aromatic Cascara Fluidextract; Aspirin, Alumina, and Magnesium Oxide Tablets; Citric Acid, Magnesium Oxide, and Sodium Carbonate Irrigation; Magnesium Oxide Capsules; Magnesium Oxide Tablets.

Proprietary Preparations (details are given in Part 3)
Aust.: Magnofit; ***Ger.:*** Dystomin M; Magnesium Diasporal; Magnetrans forte; ***S.Afr.:*** Solumag; ***Swed.:*** Salilax; ***USA:*** Mag-200; Mag-Ox; Maox; Uro-Mag.

Multi-ingredient: numerous preparations are listed in Part 3.

Magnesium Trisilicate (704-d)

553(a); Magnesii Trisilicas; Magnesium Silicate.

CAS — 14987-04-3 (anhydrous); 39365-87-2 (hydrate).

Pharmacopoeias. In *Chin., Eur.* (see p.viii), *Jpn,* and *US.*

A hydrated magnesium silicate corresponding approximately to the formula $2MgO,3SiO_2$, with water of crystallisation. An odourless, white powder free from gritty particles. Practically **insoluble** in water and alcohol. It is readily decomposed by mineral acids.

Magnesium trisilicate is an antacid with general properties similar to those of magnesium hydroxide (p.1198). It is given in doses of up to about 2 g by mouth. When given by mouth it reacts slowly with hydrochloric acid in the gastric secretion to form magnesium chloride and silicon dioxide and is primarily excreted in the faeces as insoluble and soluble magnesium salts. The antacid action is therefore exerted slowly, so that it does not give such rapid symptomatic relief as magnesium carbonate or magnesium hydroxide; passage through the stomach may be too rapid for it to exert a significant acid-neutralising effect. Magnesium trisilicate is often given in conjunction with aluminium-containing antacids such as aluminium hydroxide which counteract its laxative effect.

Magnesium trisilicate is also used as a food additive.

Effects on the kidneys. A 68-year-old man with a history of renal calculus passed a 300-mg stone which was found to consist chiefly of silica.[1] He had been taking the equivalent of 2 g of magnesium trisilicate daily for many years.

1. Joekes AM, *et al.* Multiple renal silica calculi. *Br Med J* 1973; **1:** 146–7.

Preparations

BP 1998: Compound Magnesium Trisilicate Oral Powder; Compound Magnesium Trisilicate Tablets *(Aluminium Hydroxide and Magnesium Trisilicate Tablets)*; Magnesium Trisilicate Mixture; ***USP 23:*** Alumina and Magnesium Trisilicate Oral Suspension; Alumina and Magnesium Trisilicate Tablets; Magnesium Trisilicate Tablets.

Proprietary Preparations (details are given in Part 3)
Ger.: Gastrobin†; Solitab; ***Spain:*** Mabosil; Silimag.

Multi-ingredient: numerous preparations are listed in Part 3.

Manna (604-t)

Manne en Larmes.

Pharmacopoeias. In *Aust. It.* permits other *Fraxinus* species.

The dried exudation from the bark of the European flowering ash, *Fraxinus ornus* (Oleaceae), containing about 40 to 60% of mannitol.

Manna has been used as a laxative.

Preparations

Proprietary Preparations (details are given in Part 3)

Multi-ingredient: ***Aust.:*** Krauterdoktor Entschlackungs-Elixier; Sinolax-Milder; St Radegunder Entschlackungs-Elixier; ***Ger.:*** Infi-tract N; Schwedentrunk; Schwedentrunk mit Ginseng; ***Ital.:*** Certobil; Tamarmanna†.

Mebeverine Hydrochloride (5236-v)

Mebeverine Hydrochloride *(BANM, USAN, pINNM).*

CSAG-144. 4-[Ethyl(4-methoxy-α-methylphenethyl)amino]butyl veratrate hydrochloride.

$C_{25}H_{35}NO_5,HCl$ = 466.0.

CAS — 3625-06-7 (mebeverine); 2753-45-9 (mebeverine hydrochloride).

Pharmacopoeias. In *Br.*

A white or almost white crystalline powder. Very **soluble** in water; freely soluble in alcohol; practically insoluble in ether. A 2% solution in water has a pH of 4.5 to 6.5. **Store** in airtight containers at a temperature not exceeding 30°. Protect from light.

Adverse Effects and Precautions

Although adverse effects appear rare, gastro-intestinal disturbances, dizziness, headache, insomnia, anorexia, and tachycardia have been reported in patients receiving mebeverine. It should be used with care in patients with marked hepatic or renal impairment, and those with cardiac disorders.

A 24-year-old man with cystic fibrosis, prescribed mebeverine hydrochloride for lower abdominal pain and constipation, was found to have a perforated stercoral ulcer with generalised peritonitis.[1] It was suggested that mebeverine produced colonic stasis which predisposed the patient to ulceration,[1] but the manufacturers[2] considered that the concomitant development of constipation and distal intestinal syndrome (meconium ileus equivalent) in this patient precipitated the development of stercoral ulceration. It was recommended[1] that antispasmodics such as mebeverine should not be used for the symptomatic treatment of distal intestinal syndrome in cystic fibrosis.

1. Hassan W, Keaney N. Mebeverine-induced perforated colon in distal intestinal syndrome of cystic fibrosis. *Lancet* 1990; **335:** 1225.
2. Whitehead AM. Perforation of colon in distal intestinal syndrome of cystic fibrosis. *Lancet* 1990; **336:** 446.

Uses and Administration

Mebeverine hydrochloride is an antispasmodic with a direct action on the smooth muscle of the gastro-intestinal tract. It is used in conditions such as the irritable bowel syndrome (p.1172) in doses of 135 mg three times daily by mouth before meals, or 100 mg three or four times daily. The embonate is also used in a dose equivalent to 150 mg of the hydrochloride three times daily.

Preparations

BP 1998: Mebeverine Tablets.

Proprietary Preparations (details are given in Part 3)
Aust.: Colofac; ***Austral.:*** Colese; Colofac; ***Belg.:*** Duspatalin; Spasmonal; ***Fr.:*** Colopriv; Duspatalin; Spasmopriv; ***Ger.:*** Duspatal; ***Irl.:*** Colofac; ***Ital.:*** Duspatal; ***Neth.:*** Duspatal; ***S.Afr.:*** Bevispas; Colofac; ***Spain:*** Duspatalin; ***Switz.:*** Duspatalin; ***UK:*** Colofac; Equilon; Fomac.

Multi-ingredient: ***Irl.:*** Fybogel Mebeverine; ***UK:*** Fybogel Mebeverine.

Mesalazine (16887-a)

Mesalazine *(BAN, rINN).*

5-Aminosalicylic Acid; 5-ASA; Fisalamine; Mesalamine *(USAN).* 5-Amino-2-salicylic acid.

$C_7H_7NO_3$ = 153.1.

CAS — 89-57-6.

NOTE. Distinguish from 4-aminosalicylic acid (Aminosalicylic Acid, p.151) which is used in the treatment of tuberculosis.

Pharmacopoeias. In *Belg.* and *US.*

Light tan to pink needle-shaped crystals, odourless or with a slight characteristic odour. The colour may darken on exposure to air. Slightly **soluble** in water; very slightly soluble in dehydrated alcohol, acetone, and methyl alcohol; practically insoluble in chloroform, ether, butyl alcohol, ethyl acetate, *n*-hexane, dichloromethane, and propyl alcohol; soluble in dilute hydrochloric acid and in dilute alkali hydroxides.

Adverse Effects and Precautions

Headache, gastro-intestinal disturbances, such as nausea, diarrhoea, and abdominal pain, or hypersensitivity reactions may occasionally occur. Some patients may experience exacerbation of symptoms of colitis. There are some reports of nephrotoxicity, pulmonary symptoms, hepatitis, aplastic anaemia, agranulocytosis, leucopenia, neutropenia, thrombocytopenia, myocarditis, pancreatitis, and peripheral neuropathy. A lupus-like syndrome has occurred.

It has been recommended that mesalazine should not be given to patients with impaired renal function or salicylate hypersensitivity, and should be used with caution in the elderly. It is contra-indicated in children under 2 years of age. If a blood dyscrasia is suspected treatment should be stopped immediately and a blood count performed. Patients or their carers should be told how to recognise signs of blood toxicity and should be advised to seek immediate medical attention if symptoms such as fever, sore throat, mouth ulcers, bruising, or bleeding develops.

Many of the adverse effects associated with sulphasalazine therapy have been attributed to the sulphapyridine moiety and most patients unable to tolerate sulphasalazine because of hypersensitivity or adverse reactions can be transferred to mesalazine without adverse effects occurring.[1-4] However, a small number of patients also experience adverse effects whilst taking mesalazine and these are often very similar to those seen with sulphasalazine.[1-4] They may include nausea, abdominal discomfort or pain, exacerbation of diarrhoea, headache, fever, and rashes; mesalazine is not associated with sulphasalazine's adverse effects on sperm.

Mesalazine therapy should be initiated cautiously in patients with a history of sulphasalazine hypersensitivity and it should be withdrawn if signs of sensitivity develop or if there is diarrhoea or rectal bleeding. It has been suggested[2] that patients with a history of sulphasalazine hypersensitivity should be given test doses of mesalazine before starting a full course.

1. Dew MJ, *et al.* Treatment of ulcerative colitis with oral 5-aminosalicylic acid in patients unable to take sulphasalazine. *Lancet* 1983; **ii:** 801.
2. Campieri M, *et al.* 5-Aminosalicylic acid as rectal enema in ulcerative colitis patients unable to take sulphasalazine. *Lancet* 1984; **i:** 403.
3. Donald IP, Wilkinson SP. The value of 5-aminosalicylic acid in inflammatory bowel disease for patients intolerant or allergic to sulphasalazine. *Postgrad Med J* 1985; **61:** 1047–8.
4. Rao SS, *et al.* Clinical experience of the tolerance of mesalazine and olsalazine in patients intolerant of sulphasalazine. *Scand J Gastroenterol* 1987; **22:** 332–6.

Effects on the blood. Although uncommon, mesalazine-associated adverse effects on the blood have been reported, including thrombocytopenia,[1] neutropenia,[2] and fatal aplastic anaemia.[3] In July 1995 the Committee on Safety of Medicines in the UK stated that it had been notified of 49 haematological reactions suspected to be associated with mesalazine,[4] including 5 reports of aplastic anaemia, 1 of agranulocytosis, 11 of leucopenia, and 17 of thrombocytopenia. There had been 3 fatalities. They recommended a blood count and immediate withdrawal of the drug if a dyscrasia was suspected. Antilymphocyte immunoglobulin may be useful in the management of mesalazine-associated aplastic anaemia.[5]

1. Daneshmend TK. Mesalazine-associated thrombocytopenia. *Lancet* 1991; **337:** 1297–8.
2. Wyatt S, *et al.* Filgrastim for mesalazine-associated neutropenia. *Lancet* 1993; **341:** 1476.
3. Abboudi ZH, *et al.* Fatal aplastic anaemia after mesalazine. *Lancet* 1994; **343:** 542.
4. Committee on Safety of Medicines/Medicines Control Agency. Blood dyscrasias and mesalazine. *Current Problems* 1995; **21:** 5–6.
5. Laidlaw ST, Reilly JT. Antilymphocyte globulin for mesalazine-associated aplastic anaemia. *Lancet* 1994; **343:** 981–2.

Effects on the cardiovascular system. Myocarditis associated with chest pain and ECG abnormalities has been reported[1,2] in 2 patients taking mesalazine; 1 patient died in cardiogenic shock.[2] It was suggested that mesalazine or sulphasalazine should be replaced by glucocorticoids if cardiac symptoms arise during treatment.[2] Pericarditis[3,4] together with fever, rash, dyspnoea, pleural and pericardial effusions, and arthritis, has also been described, and is considered to constitute a drug-induced lupus-like syndrome.

1. Agnholt J, *et al.* Cardiac hypersensitivity to 5-aminosalicylic acid. *Lancet* 1989; **i:** 1135.
2. Kristensen KS, *et al.* Fatal myocarditis associated with mesalazine. *Lancet* 1990; **335:** 605.
3. Dent MT, *et al.* Mesalazine induced lupus-like syndrome. *Br Med J* 1992; **305:** 159.
4. Lim AG, Hine KR. Fever, vasculitic rash, arthritis, pericarditis, and pericardial effusion after mesalazine. *Br Med J* 1994; **308:** 113.

Effects on fertility. For a review of the effects of sulphasalazine on male fertility and reversal of these effects on changing therapy to mesalazine, see Sulphasalazine, p.1215.

Effects on the hair. Accelerated hair loss from the scalp occurred in 2 patients receiving mesalazine enemas[1] in whom this reaction did not occur during sulphasalazine treatment. There have been case reports of sulphasalazine causing hair loss[2] as well as improvement in alopecia.[3]

1. Kutty PK, *et al.* Hair loss and 5-aminosalicylic acid enemas. *Ann Intern Med* 1982; **97:** 785–6.
2. Breen EG, Donnelly S. Alopecia associated with sulphasalazine (Salazopyrin). *Br Med J* 1986; **292:** 802.
3. Jawad ASM, Scott DGI. Remission of alopecia universal during sulphasalazine treatment for rheumatoid arthritis. *Br Med J* 1989; **298:** 675.

Effects on the kidneys. The risk of nephrotoxicity may be low for mesalazine and the related compounds sulphasalazine and olsalazine.[1] Even so, adverse effects on the kidneys have occurred and between February 1988 and December 1990 the UK Committee on Safety of Medicines[2] received 9 reports of serious nephrotoxic reactions associated with the use of Asacol, a modified-release mesalazine preparation. The reactions included 4 cases of interstitial nephritis, 3 of severe renal failure, and 2 cases of nephrotic syndrome. A subsequent case report[5] indicated that by September 1998 the number of such reports for mesalazine totalled 104, including 35 cases of interstitial nephritis. The authors considered that monitoring of renal function was required in patients receiving mesalazine. The nephrotic syndrome[3] and interstitial nephritis[4] have also been reported with sulphasalazine.

1. Anonymous. Choosing an oral 5-aminosalicylic acid preparation for ulcerative colitis. *Drug Ther Bull* 1992; **30:** 50–2.
2. Committee on Safety of Medicines. Nephrotoxicity associated with mesalazine (Asacol). *Current Problems 30* 1990.
3. Barbour VM, Williams PF. Nephrotic syndrome associated with sulphasalazine. *Br Med J* 1990; **301:** 818.
4. Dwarakanath AD, *et al.* Sulphasalazine induced renal failure. *Gut* 1992; **33:** 1006–1007.
5. Popoola J, *et al.* Late onset interstitial nephritis associated with mesalazine treatment. *Br Med J* 1998; **317:** 795–7.

Effects on the nervous system. A report of peripheral neuropathy,[1] predominantly affecting the legs, associated with mesalazine treatment. The symptoms resolved on discontinuing the drug. Mononeuritis multiplex was part of the presentation of an eosinophilic reaction attributed to mesalazine in an asthmatic patient;[2] Churg-Strauss syndrome (see p.1019) developed after withdrawal of mesalazine, but the patient subsequently recovered without sequelae.

1. Woodward DK. Peripheral neuropathy and mesalazine. *Br Med J* 1989; **299:** 1224.
2. Morice AH, *et al.* Mesalazine activation of eosinophil. *Lancet* 1997; **350:** 1105.

Effects on the pancreas. Reports of pancreatitis, with abdominal pain and raised serum amylase activity, in 2 patients taking mesalazine.[1,2] The reaction was confirmed by rechallenge in both patients and symptoms resolved on withdrawal of mesalazine. The Committee on Safety of Medicines in the UK had received 15 reports of pancreatitis associated with mesalazine therapy at February 1994.[3]

1. Sachedina B, *et al.* Acute pancreatitis due to 5-aminosalicylate. *Ann Intern Med* 1989; **110:** 490–2.
2. Deprez P, *et al.* Pancreatitis induced by 5-aminosalicylic acid. *Lancet* 1989; **ii:** 445–6.
3. Committee on Safety of Medicines. Drug-induced pancreatitis. *Current Problems* 1994; **20:** 2–3.

Effects on the respiratory system. Pulmonary complications occur rarely with sulphasalazine (see p.1216). It is not known which component of sulphasalazine is responsible although, following a report of alveolitis in a patient with ulcerative colitis given mesalazine,[1] it was concluded that both sulphasalazine and 5-aminosalicylate (mesalazine) could induce hypersensitivity lung disease. Similar cases have since been reported,[2,3] and pulmonary symptoms may also manifest as part of a broader lupus-like syndrome (see Effects on the Cardiovascular System, above).

1. Welte T, *et al.* Mesalazine alveolitis. *Lancet* 1991; **338:** 1273. Correction *ibid.* 1992; **339:** 70.
2. Honeybourne D. Mesalazine toxicity. *Br Med J* 1994; **308:** 533–4.
3. Pascual-Lledó JF, *et al.* Interstitial pneumonitis due to mesalamine. *Ann Pharmacother* 1997; **31:** 499.

Pregnancy. Renal insufficiency in a neonate whose mother received mesalazine during pregnancy was suggested to be due to the drug,[1] although the proposed mechanism, inhibition of prostaglandin synthesis in the neonatal kidney, has been questioned.[2]

1. Colombel J-F, *et al.* Renal insufficiency in infant: side-effect of prenatal exposure to mesalazine? *Lancet* 1994; **344:** 620–1.
2. Marteau P, Devaux CB. Mesalazine during pregnancy. *Lancet* 1994; **344:** 1708–9.

Interactions

Preparations in which the formulation is designed to release mesalazine in the colon should not be given with lactulose or similar drugs which lower pH thereby preventing the release of mesalazine.

Mesalazine may inhibit the metabolism of thiopurine antineoplastics such as azathioprine or mercaptopurine (see p.1216).

Pharmacokinetics

Following oral administration of conventional formulations, mesalazine would be extensively absorbed from the upper gastro-intestinal tract, with little of the drug reaching the colon. Oral preparations are therefore generally formulated to release the drug in the terminal ileum and colon, where it is thought to exert a mainly local action. The specific release characteristics differ somewhat between formulations and this, together with interindividual variation, makes comparison of pharmacokinetic data between studies difficult. Some 20 to 50% of an oral dose is thought to be lost to absorption in healthy subjects, but absorption is lower in patients with active inflammatory bowel disease. Absorption from rectal dosage forms has also varied widely, with factors such as the dose, the formulation, and the pH also playing a role, but mean absorption of around 10 to 20% of a rectal dose has been reported in several studies.

The absorbed portion of mesalazine is almost completely acetylated in the gut wall and in the liver, and the rate of acetylation, and hence the concentration of parent drug and metabolite in the systemic circulation, is independent of the acetylator status. It has been suggested that the metabolite, acetyl-5-aminosalicylic acid, may itself have some activity. The acetylated metabolite is excreted mainly in urine by tubular secretion, together with traces of the parent compound; a clearance of about 3 to 4 mL per minute per kg has been reported for the former.

The elimination half-life of mesalazine is reported to be about 1 hour and it is 40 to 50% bound to plasma proteins; the acetylated metabolite has a half-life of up to 10 hours and is about 80% bound to plasma proteins.

Only negligible quantities of mesalazine cross the placenta. Amounts distributed into breast milk are very small.

Reviews.

1. Klotz U. Clinical pharmacokinetics of sulphasalazine, its metabolites and other prodrugs of 5-aminosalicylic acid. *Clin Pharmacokinet* 1985; **10:** 285–302.

Distribution into breast milk. The concentrations of mesalazine in maternal plasma and breast milk in a lactating woman taking 500 mg three times daily, were 410 and 110 ng per mL respectively.[1] Although it was considered that the amount of mesalazine excreted in breast milk was small and that it was safe during breast feeding,[2,3] maternal use of mesalazine 500 mg suppositories twice daily has been associated with watery diarrhoea in a breast-fed infant.[2]

1. Jenss H, *et al.* 5-Aminosalicylic acid and its metabolite in breast milk during lactation. *Am J Gastroenterol* 1990; **85:** 331.
2. Nelis GF. Diarrhoea due to 5-aminosalicylic acid in breast milk. *Lancet* 1989; **i:** 383.
3. Klotz U, Harings-Kaim A. Negligible excretion of 5-aminosalicylic acid in breast milk. *Lancet* 1993; **342:** 618–19.

Uses and Administration

Mesalazine is an anti-inflammatory drug structurally related to the salicylates and active in inflammatory bowel disease (p.1171); it is considered to be the active moiety of sulphasalazine (p.1215). Its mode of action is uncertain, but may be due, at least in part, to its ability to inhibit local prostaglandin and leukotriene synthesis in the gastro-intestinal mucosa.

Mesalazine is given by mouth or rectally in the management of mild to moderate acute ulcerative colitis or the maintenance of remission, particularly in patients who tolerate sulphasalazine poorly. An oral dose of 400 mg of mesalazine is theoretically equivalent to 1 g of sulphasalazine.

There are several differently formulated oral preparations of mesalazine available, and dosage recommendations vary. For some UK enteric-coated tablets (Asacol and Coltec EC) the usual initial adult dose is 2.4 g daily in divided doses followed by 1.2 to 2.4 g in divided doses daily for maintenance of remission. The dose of another enteric-coated tablet (Salofalk) is 1.5 g daily in divided doses, followed by 0.75 to 1.5 g daily in divided doses for maintenance of remission. Yet another formulation (Pentasa Slow Release tablets) is given in doses of up to 4 g daily in divided doses; for maintenance therapy the dose is adjusted individually from an initial dose of 1.5 g daily.

When given rectally, the suggested dose is 0.75 to 3 g daily in divided doses as suppositories. In the UK, 1 or 2 g has been given daily as an enema formulation, but in the USA an enema containing 4 g of mesalazine has been given.

Administration. Because the release characteristics of different formulations of mesalazine vary, they should not be regarded as interchangeable.[1] This applies even to those formulations (such as Asacol and Coltec EC) where the dosage is apparently similar.[2]

1. Forbes A, Chadwick C. Mesalazine preparations. *Lancet* 1997; **350:** 1329.
2. Benbow AG, Gould I. Mesalazine preparations. *Lancet* 1998; **351:** 68.

Behçet's syndrome. A topical aqueous suspension of mesalazine produced healing of oral and vaginal ulcers in a patient with Behçet's syndrome.[1]

For a discussion of Behçet's syndrome and the many agents tried in its management, see p.1018.

1. Ranzi T, *et al.* Successful treatment of genital and oral ulceration in Behcet's disease with topical 5-aminosalicylic acid (5-ASA). *Br J Dermatol* 1989; **120:** 471–2.

Preparations

Proprietary Preparations (details are given in Part 3)
Aust.: Claversal; Pentasa; Salofalk; ***Austral.:*** Mesasal; ***Belg.:*** Asacol; Claversal; Colitofalk; Pentasa; ***Canad.:*** Asacol; Mesasal; Pentasa; Quintasa; Salofalk; ***Fr.:*** Pentasa; Rowasa; ***Ger.:*** Asacolitin; Claversal; Pentasa; Salofalk; ***Irl.:*** Asacolon; Pentasa; Salofalk; ***Ital.:*** Asacol; Claversal; Pentacol; Pentasa; Salisofar Clismi†; Salofalk; ***Neth.:*** Asacol; Pentasa; Salofalk; ***Norw.:*** Asacol; Mesasal; Pentasa; ***S.Afr.:*** Asacol; ***Spain:*** Claversal; Lixacol; Quintasa; ***Swed.:*** Asacol; Mesasal; Pentasa; ***Switz.:*** Asacol; Pentasa; Salofalk; ***UK:*** Asacol; Coltec†; Pentasa; Salofalk; ***USA:*** Asacol; Pentasa; Rowasa.

Metoclopramide Hydrochloride

(6541-f)

Metoclopramide Hydrochloride *(BANM, USAN, rINNM).*

AHR-3070-C; DEL-1267; Metoclopramidi Hydrochloridum; MK-745. 4-Amino-5-chloro-*N*-(2-diethylaminoethyl)-2-methoxybenzamide hydrochloride monohydrate.

$C_{14}H_{22}ClN_3O_2,HCl,H_2O$ = 354.3.

CAS — 364-62-5 (metoclopramide); 7232-21-5 (metoclopramide hydrochloride, anhydrous); 54143-57-6 (metoclopramide hydrochloride, monohydrate); 2576-84-3 (metoclopramide dihydrochloride, anhydrous).

Pharmacopoeias. In *Eur.* (see p.viii), *Int., Pol.,* and *US.*
Chin., Eur., and *Jpn* include anhydrous metoclopramide.

A white or almost white, odourless or almost odourless, crystalline powder. Metoclopramide hydrochloride 10.5 mg is approximately equivalent to 10.0 mg of the anhydrous substance which is approximately equivalent to 8.9 mg of the anhydrous base. Very **soluble** in water; freely soluble in alcohol; sparingly soluble in chloroform and in dichloromethane; practically insoluble in ether. A 10% solution in water has a pH of 4.5 to 6.0. **Store** in airtight containers. Protect from light.

Incompatibilities. Proprietary preparations of metoclopramide hydrochloride are stated to be incompatible with cephalothin sodium and other cephalosporins, chloramphenicol sodium, and sodium bicarbonate.

Cisplatin, cyclophosphamide, doxorubicin hydrochloride, and methotrexate sodium are stated to be conditionally compatible with metoclopramide hydrochloride but compatibility is dependent upon factors such as the particular formulation, drug concentration, pH, and temperature.

Adverse Effects

Metoclopramide is a dopamine antagonist and may cause extrapyramidal symptoms which usually occur as acute dystonic reactions; these are more common in young patients especially if female. The risk may be reduced by keeping the daily dose below 500 μg per kg body-weight. Parkinsonism and tardive dyskinesia have occasionally occurred, usually during prolonged treatment in elderly patients.

Other adverse effects include restlessness, drowsiness, dizziness, headache, and bowel upsets such as diarrhoea. Hypotension, hypertension, and depression may occur and there are isolated reports of blood disorders, hypersensitivity reactions, neuroleptic malignant syndrome, and urinary incontinence. Disorders of cardiac conduction have been reported with intravenous metoclopramide.

Metoclopramide stimulates prolactin secretion and may cause galactorrhoea or related disorders. Transient increases in plasma-aldosterone concentrations have been reported.

Effects on the blood. There has been a report[1] of agranulocytosis associated with administration of metoclopramide on 2 separate occasions. Both episodes resolved within 2 to 3 weeks of withdrawing metoclopramide. Methaemoglobinaemia[2] has also been reported.

1. Harvey RL, Luzar MJ. Metoclopramide-induced agranulocytosis. *Ann Intern Med* 1988; **108:** 214–15.
2. Grant SCD, *et al.* Methaemoglobinaemia produced by metoclopramide in an adult. *Eur J Clin Pharmacol* 1994; **47:** 89.

Effects on the cardiovascular system. Reports of hypotension,[1] hypertension,[2,3] and supraventricular tachycardia[4] associated with metoclopramide. Bradycardia followed by total heart block,[5] and sinus arrest,[6] have also been reported.

1. Park GR. Hypotension following metoclopramide administration during hypotensive anaesthesia for intracranial aneurysm. *Br J Anaesth* 1978; **50:** 1268–9.
2. Sheridan C, *et al.* Transient hypertension after high doses of metoclopramide. *N Engl J Med* 1982; **307:** 1346.
3. Filibeck DJ, *et al.* Metoclopramide-induced hypertensive crisis. *Clin Pharm* 1984; **3:** 548–9.
4. Bevacqua BK. Supraventricular tachycardia associated with postpartum metoclopramide administration. *Anesthesiology* 1988; **68:** 124–5.
5. Midttun M, Øberg B. Total heart block after intravenous metoclopramide. *Lancet* 1994; **343:** 182–3.
6. Malkoff MD, *et al.* Sinus arrest after administration of intravenous metoclopramide. *Ann Pharmacother* 1995; **29:** 381–3.

Effects on the endocrine system. ALDOSTERONISM. Metoclopramide has been reported to increase plasma-aldosterone concentrations in healthy individuals[1] and in patients with liver cirrhosis and ascites associated with secondary hyperaldosteronism.[2] Increased plasma aldosterone following metoclopramide administration has also been associated with the development of oedema in a patient with congestive heart failure.[3] The metoclopramide-induced aldosterone response was blunted by prior administration of neostigmine.[1]

1. Sommers DK, *et al.* Effect of neostigmine on metoclopramide-induced aldosterone secretion in man. *Eur J Clin Pharmacol* 1989; **36:** 411–13.
2. Mazzacca G, *et al.* Metoclopramide and secondary hyperaldosteronism. *Ann Intern Med* 1983; **98:** 1024–5.
3. Zumoff B. Metoclopramide and edema. *Ann Intern Med* 1983; **98:** 557.

HYPERPROLACTINAEMIA. Hyperprolactinaemia, galactorrhoea, and pituitary adenoma occurred in a 49-year-old woman with reflux oesophagitis who had received metoclopramide for 3 months.[1] Her plasma-prolactin concentrations fell to normal and her symptoms resolved over 4 months following withdrawal of metoclopramide. The pituitary tumour was considered to be incidental to, and not caused by, metoclopramide therapy.

1. Cooper BT, *et al.* Galactorrhoea, hyperprolactinaemia, and pituitary adenoma presenting during metoclopramide therapy. *Postgrad Med J* 1982; **58:** 314–15.

Effects on mental state. There are isolated reports of dose-related delirium, depression, and uncontrollable crying in patients treated with metoclopramide in doses of 40 to 80 mg daily.[1-3] Symptoms resolved on reducing the dose or withdrawing metoclopramide and tolerance could be achieved by gradually increasing the dose.

Insomnia, with or without daytime drowsiness, has also been reported in patients taking metoclopramide 40 mg daily.[4]

1. Bottner RK, Tullio CJ. Metoclopramide and depression. *Ann Intern Med* 1985; **103:** 482.
2. Adams CD. Metoclopramide and depression. *Ann Intern Med* 1985; **103:** 960.
3. Fishbain DA, Rogers A. Delirium secondary to metoclopramide hydrochloride. *J Clin Psychopharmacol* 1987; **7:** 281–2.
4. Saxe TG. Metoclopramide side effects. *Ann Intern Med* 1983; **98:** 674.

Extrapyramidal effects. The Adverse Reactions Register of the Committee on the Safety of Medicines for the years 1967-82 contained 479 reports of extrapyramidal reactions in which metoclopramide was the suspected drug: 455 were for dystonic-dyskinetic reactions, 20 for parkinsonism, and 4 for tardive dyskinesia.[1]

Acute **dystonia** and **dyskinesias** often occur together in patients receiving metoclopramide and show a similar reaction interval and distribution of age and sex.[1] The reactions occur most commonly in children and young adults[1-3] and about 70% of reactions are in females;[1,3] a substantial proportion of reactions are associated with doses in excess of those recommended by the manufacturers.[1,3,4] Symptoms reported include oculogyric crisis,[4,5] opisthotonus,[6] torticollis,[5,7] trismus,[5,7] a tetanus-like reaction,[8] and blue coloration of the tongue;[6] akathisia following the pre-operative use of metoclopramide with droperidol has been reported.[9] The effects usually occur within 72 hours of starting treatment[1] but have been reported within 30 minutes of receiving metoclopramide.[4] They may occur in patients who have previously received metoclopramide without complications[5,8,9] and may be precipitated by other drugs. Although generally self-limiting, deaths have occurred.[1,5] The reactions are readily reversed by an antihistamine such as diphenhydramine,[7] or an antimuscarinic such as benztropine;[4,6] prophylactic use of diphenhydramine has been suggested for patients with a history of extrapyramidal reactions and in those less than 30 years of age.[7,8]

Metoclopramide-associated **parkinsonism** is thought to occur less commonly than the acute dystonias and is seen predominantly in older patients. Symptoms usually appear several months after starting metoclopramide, but may occur within days or not for several years. Withdrawal of metoclopramide usually results in resolution of symptoms, although it may take several months.[1] A study has suggested that metoclopramide-induced parkinsonism (misdiagnosed as idiopathic Parkinson's disease) may be more common in the elderly than generally realised.[10]

Tardive dyskinesia may rarely be associated with metoclopramide administration. The reaction is usually confined to elderly patients following prolonged oral use,[11,12] but it has been reported after short-term high-dose parenteral use as an antiemetic in cancer chemotherapy,[13] and a case has been reported in an 8-year-old child treated with metoclopramide for gastro-oesophageal reflux disease in usual doses.[14] The average duration of treatment before the onset of symptoms was 14 months (range 4 to 44 months) in a report of 11 cases[12] and 26 months (range 8 to 60 months) in a report of 12 cases;[15] some patients did not experience symptoms until after withdrawal of metoclopramide. Tardive dyskinesia is potentially irreversible and its management is difficult.[15] Some patients improve after withdrawal of metoclopramide but symptoms persisting during follow-up periods of up to 3 years have been reported[11,12] The emphasis must be on prevention hence the recommendation that metoclopramide should not be prescribed for the long-term treatment of minor symptoms, especially in elderly patients.[15]

1. Bateman DN, *et al.* Extrapyramidal reactions with metoclopramide. *Br Med J* 1985; **291:** 930–2.
2. Anonymous. Measuring therapeutic risk. *Lancet* 1989; **ii:** 139–40.
3. Adverse Drug Reactions Advisory Committee. Metoclopramide—choose the dose carefully. *Aust Adverse Drug React Bull* 1990; Feb.
4. Tait P, *et al.* Metoclopramide side effects in children. *Med J Aust* 1990; **152:** 387.
5. Pollera CF, *et al.* Sudden death after acute dystonic reaction to high-dose metoclopramide. *Lancet* 1984; **ii:** 460–1.
6. Alroe C, Bowen P. Metoclopramide and prochlorperazine: "the blue-tongue sign". *Med J Aust* 1989; **150:** 724–5.
7. Kris MG, *et al.* Extrapyramidal reactions with high-dose metoclopramide. *N Engl J Med* 1983; **309:** 433–4.
8. Della Valle R, *et al.* Metoclopramide-induced tetanus-like dystonic reaction. *Clin Pharm* 1985; **4:** 102–3.
9. Barnes TRE, *et al.* Acute akathisia after oral droperidol and metoclopramide preoperative medication. *Lancet* 1982; **ii:** 48–9.
10. Avorn J, *et al.* Increased incidence of levodopa therapy following metoclopramide use. *JAMA* 1995; **274:** 1780–2.
11. Grimes JD, *et al.* Long-term follow-up of tardive dyskinesia due to metoclopramide. *Lancet* 1982; **ii:** 563.
12. Wiholm B-E, *et al.* Tardive dyskinesia associated with metoclopramide. *Br Med J* 1984; **288:** 545–7.
13. Breitbart W. Tardive dyskinesia associated with high-dose intravenous metoclopramide. *N Engl J Med* 1986; **315:** 518.
14. Putnam PE, *et al.* Tardive dyskinesia associated with use of metoclopramide in a child. *J Pediatr* 1992; **121:** 983–5.
15. Orme ML'E, Tallis RC. Metoclopramide and tardive dyskinesia in the elderly. *Br Med J* 1984; **289:** 397–8.

Neuroleptic malignant syndrome. Neuroleptic malignant syndrome developed in a 73-year-old man following a single dose of metoclopramide 30 mg.[1] He had generalised muscular rigidity, fever, raised creatine phosphokinase activity, leucocytosis and became unconscious and unresponsive to pain. After an initial improvement on bromocriptine, gradually increased to 5 mg three times daily, his condition deteriorated, he lapsed into a coma, and died.

1. Cassidy T, Bansal SK. Neuroleptic malignant syndrome associated with metoclopramide. *Br Med J* 1988; **296:** 214.

Precautions

Metoclopramide should not be used when stimulation of muscular contractions might adversely affect gastro-intestinal conditions as in gastro-intestinal haemorrhage, obstruction, perforation, or immediately after surgery. There have been reports of hypertensive crises in patients with phaeochromocytoma given metoclopramide, thus its use is not recommended in such patients. It has also been suggested that it should be avoided in patients with epilepsy, because of a risk of increased frequency and severity of seizures.

Children, young patients, and the elderly should be treated with care as they are at increased risk of extrapyramidal reactions; in the UK, use of metoclopramide is severely restricted in patients under 20 years (see Uses and Administration, below). Patients on prolonged therapy should be reviewed regularly. Care should also be taken when metoclopramide is administered to patients with renal impairment or to those at risk of fluid retention as in hepatic impairment. Caution is advisable in patients with a history of mental depression.

Metoclopramide may cause drowsiness or impaired reactions; patients so affected should not drive or operate machinery.

Hepatic impairment. The UK manufacturers recommend that the dose of metoclopramide should be reduced in patients with clinically significant hepatic impairment, although the US manufacturer notes that it has been used safely in patients with advanced liver disease and makes no such recommendation.

Porphyria. Metoclopramide has been associated with episodes of acute porphyria.[1,2] It is probably appropriate to use alternative drugs in patients with porphyria,[3,4] although there is some doubt about the risk with metoclopramide, and some have used it successfully in the management of acute attacks.[4]

1. Doss M, *et al.* Drug safety in porphyria: risks of valproate and metoclopramide. *Lancet* 1981; **ii:** 91.
2. Milo R, *et al.* Acute intermittent porphyria in pregnancy. *Obstet Gynecol* 1989; **73:** 450–2.
3. Gorchein A. Metoclopramide and acute porphyria. *Lancet* 1997; **350:** 1104.
4. Elder GH, *et al.* Metoclopramide and acute porphyria. *Lancet* 1997; **350:** 1104.

Renal impairment. Total clearance of metoclopramide is significantly reduced in patients with renal impairment[1-3] and the elimination half-life is prolonged to up to 19 hours.[2] This may be due to impaired metabolism[1,2] or to an alteration in enterohepatic circulation of metoclopramide.[1] Accumulation of metoclopramide could therefore occur in renal impairment with a possible increased risk of side-effects. Dosage reductions of at least 50% have therefore been recommended in patients with moderate to severe renal impairment.[1,2]

Patients undergoing haemodialysis do not require dosage supplements since relatively little metoclopramide is cleared by this process.[2,3]

1. Bateman DN, *et al.* The pharmacokinetics of single doses of metoclopramide in renal failure. *Eur J Clin Pharmacol* 1981; **19:** 437–41.
2. Lehmann CR, *et al.* Metoclopramide kinetics in patients with impaired renal function and clearance by haemodialysis. *Clin Pharmacol Ther* 1985; **37:** 284–9.
3. Wright MR, *et al.* Effect of haemodialysis on metoclopramide kinetics in patients with severe renal failure. *Br J Clin Pharmacol* 1988; **26:** 474–7.

Interactions

Caution should be observed when using metoclopramide in patients taking other drugs that can also cause extrapyramidal reactions, such as the phenothiazines. Increased toxicity may occur if metoclopramide is used in patients receiving lithium, and caution is advisable with other centrally active drugs including antidepressants, antiepileptics, and sympathomimetics. Antimuscarinics and opioid analgesics antagonise the gastro-intestinal effects of metoclopramide.

The absorption of other drugs may be affected by metoclopramide; it may either diminish absorption from the stomach (as with digoxin) or enhance absorption from the small intestine (for example, with aspirin or paracetamol). It inhibits serum cholinesterase and may prolong suxamethonium-induced neuromuscular blockade (see p.1321). Metoclopramide may also increase prolactin blood-concentrations and therefore interfere with drugs which have a hypoprolactinaemic effect such as bromocriptine. It has been suggested that it should not be given to patients receiving monoamine oxidase inhibitors (MAOIs).

Carbamazepine. For a report of neurotoxicity associated with administration of metoclopramide and carbamazepine, see p.342.

Hydroxyzine. Acute anxiety, rigidity, generalised tremor, opisthotonus, and hypertension developed in a 20-year-old man after administration of metoclopramide 10 mg intravenously and hydroxyzine 100 mg intramuscularly.[1] The side-effects occurred 30 minutes after hydroxyzine administration and it was suggested that hydroxyzine potentiated the onset of the reaction.

1. Fouilladieu JL, *et al.* Possible potentiation by hydroxyzine of metoclopramide's undesirable side effects. *Anesth Analg* 1985; **64:** 1227–8.

Pharmacokinetics

Metoclopramide is rapidly and almost completely absorbed from the gastro-intestinal tract following a dose by mouth, although conditions such as vomiting or impaired gastric motility may reduce absorption. Peak plasma concentrations of metoclopramide occur about 1 to 2 hours after an oral dose. However, it undergoes hepatic first-pass metabolism, which varies considerably between subjects, and hence the absolute bioavailability and the plasma concentrations are subject to wide interindividual variation. On average, the bioavailability of oral metoclopramide is about 75%, but it appears to vary between about 30 and 100%.

Attempts to overcome the problems of oral administration by rectal or intranasal administration have demonstrated that bioavailability is equally variable by these routes, although it may be somewhat better if given intramuscularly.

Metoclopramide is widely distributed in the body, with an apparent volume of distribution of about 3.5 litres per kg. It readily crosses the blood-brain barrier into the CNS. It also freely crosses the placenta, and has been reported to attain concentrations in fetal plasma about 60 to 70% of those in maternal plasma. Concentrations higher than those in maternal plasma may be reached in the breast milk of lactating mothers, particularly in the early puerperium, although concentrations decrease somewhat in the late puerperium.

Elimination of metoclopramide is biphasic, with a terminal elimination half-life of about 4 to 6 hours, although this may be prolonged in renal impairment, with consequent elevation of plasma concentrations. It is excreted in the urine, about 85% of a dose being eliminated in 72 hours, 20 to 30% as unchanged metoclopramide and the remainder as sulphate or glucuronide conjugates, or as metabolites. About 5% of a dose is excreted in faeces via the bile.

Uses and Administration

Metoclopramide hydrochloride is a substituted benzamide used for its prokinetic and antiemetic properties. It stimulates the motility of the upper gastro-intestinal tract without affecting gastric, biliary, or pancreatic secretion and increases gastric peristalsis, leading to accelerated gastric emptying. Duodenal peristalsis is also increased which decreases intestinal transit time. The resting tone of the gastro-oesophageal sphincter is increased and the pyloric sphincter is relaxed. Metoclopramide possesses parasympathomimetic activity as well as being a dopamine-receptor antagonist with a direct effect on the chemoreceptor trigger zone. It may have serotonin-receptor ($5-HT_3$) antagonist properties.

Metoclopramide is used in disorders of decreased gastro-intestinal motility (p.1168) such as gastroparesis or ileus; in gastro-oesophageal reflux disease (p.1170) and dyspepsia (p.1169); and in nausea and vomiting (p.1172) associated with various gastro-intestinal disorders, with migraine, following surgery, and with cancer therapy. Metoclopramide is of no value in the prevention or treatment of motion sickness. It may be used to stimulate gastric emptying during radiographic examinations, to facilitate intubation of the small bowel, and in the management of aspiration syndromes (p.1168).

It is usually given as the hydrochloride with doses expressed as the anhydrous form. In the USA the strength of preparations of the hydrochloride is usually expressed in terms of the base. For most purposes the total daily dose should not exceed 0.5 mg per kg body-weight; dosage reduction is recommended in renal and perhaps hepatic impairment (see Precautions, above). In the UK, metoclopramide hydrochloride monohydrate is administered by mouth in a dose equivalent to 10 mg of anhydrous metoclopramide hydrochloride three times daily but may also be given by intramuscular or slow intravenous injection in the same dosage; in the USA the equivalent of 10 to 15 mg of the base up to four times daily has been given. Single doses should be considered where appropriate and single doses of 10 to 20 mg expressed as anhydrous base or anhydrous hydrochloride have been used.

In the UK the use of metoclopramide is restricted in patients under 20 years of age to severe intractable vomiting of known cause, chemotherapy- or radiotherapy-induced vomiting, as an aid to gastro-intestinal intubation, and in premedication. Suggested doses for those aged 15 to 19 years are 5 mg three times daily for those weighing 30 to 59 kg and 10 mg three times daily for those weighing 60 kg and over; 9 to 14 years, 5 mg three times daily for those weighing 30 kg and over; 5 to 9 years, 2.5 mg three times daily for those weighing 20 to 29 kg; 3 to 5 years, 2 mg two or three times daily for those weighing 15 to 19 kg; 1 to 3 years, 1 mg two or three times daily for those weighing 10 to 14 kg; and under 1 year 1 mg twice daily for those weighing up to 10 kg. Where body-weight is below that specified for a given age group, the dose should reflect the weight rather than the age, so that a lower dose is chosen.

High-dose therapy. High doses are employed in the treatment of the nausea and vomiting associated with cancer chemotherapy often in combination with other agents such as dexamethasone. The loading dose of metoclopramide given before cancer therapy is 2 to 4 mg per kg body-weight administered as a continuous intravenous infusion over 15 to 20 minutes and is followed by a maintenance dose of 3 to 5 mg per kg, again as a continuous intravenous infusion, administered over 8 to 12 hours. Alternatively, initial doses of 1 to 2 mg per kg by intravenous infusion over at least 15 minutes may be given before cancer therapy and repeated every 2 or 3 hours for a further 5 doses. The total dosage by either continuous or intermittent infusion should not normally exceed 10 mg per kg in 24 hours.

The base, the dihydrochloride, and the glycyrrhizinate have also been used.

Metoclopramide has been investigated as a radiosensitiser in patients undergoing radiotherapy for malignant neoplasms.

Hiccup. Metoclopramide has been used with chlorpromazine in protocols for the management of intractable hiccup. For a discussion of hiccup and its management see p.655.

Lactation induction. Metoclopramide has been used for its dopamine antagonist properties to stimulate lactation in women who wish to breast feed and in whom mechanical stimulation of the nipple alone is inadequate. Doses of 10 mg three times daily have been used for this purpose, but should be viewed as adjunctive to mechanical methods and the duration of therapy should probably be limited to 7 to 14 days.[1] For a discussion of lactation inhibition and induction, see p.1240.

1. Anderson PO, Valdés V. Increasing breast milk supply. *Clin Pharm* 1993; **12:** 479–80.

Migraine. Metoclopramide is used in the treatment of migraine (p.443) to alleviate nausea and vomiting and gastric stasis both of which commonly develop as a migraine attack progresses and can lead to poor absorption of oral antimigraine preparations. It may also be given to counteract any exacerbation of nausea and vomiting that may occur when the antimigraine drug ergotamine is used. Metoclopramide is included in some combination analgesic preparations for the treatment of acute attacks of migraine. In a recent study lysine aspirin with metoclopramide was as effective as sumatriptan in the treatment of migraine.[1]

Studies indicate that metoclopramide given intravenously can relieve the pain of migraine attacks;[2,3] this effect may be related to its action as a dopamine antagonist and may be worth trying in patients who require parenteral treatment and do not respond to sumatriptan or dihydroergotamine.

1. Tfelt-Hansen P, *et al.* The effectiveness of combined oral lysine acetylsalicylate and metoclopramide compared with oral sumatriptan for migraine. *Lancet* 1995; **346:** 923–6.
2. Tek DS, *et al.* A prospective, double-blind study of metoclopramide hydrochloride for the control of migraine in the emergency department. *Ann Emerg Med* 1990; **19:** 1083–7.
3. Ellis GL, *et al.* The efficacy of metoclopramide in the treatment of migraine. *Ann Emerg Med* 1993; **22:** 191–5.

Orthostatic hypotension. Metoclopramide has been tried in the management of some patients with orthostatic hypotension, as mentioned on p.1040.

Variceal haemorrhage. Metoclopramide 20 mg intravenously controlled bleeding from oesophageal varices within 15 minutes in 10 of 11 patients compared with 4 of 11 patients given placebo; all patients were treated by sclerotherapy.[1] Lower oesophageal sphincter pressure is increased by metoclopramide, thus reducing blood flow to varices and achieving haemostasis; another study[2] found a combination of metoclopramide and intravenous glyceryl trinitrate to be more effective than glyceryl trinitrate alone in reducing intravariceal pressure.

For a discussion of variceal haemorrhage and its management, see p.1576.

1. Hosking SW, *et al.* Pharmacological constriction of the lower oesophageal sphincter: a simple method of arresting variceal haemorrhage. *Gut* 1988; **29:** 1098–1102.
2. Sarin SK, Saraya A. Effects of intravenous nitroglycerin and nitroglycerin and metoclopramide on intravariceal pressure: a double blind, randomized study. *Am J Gastroenterol* 1995; **90:** 48–53.

Preparations

BP 1998: Metoclopramide Injection; Metoclopramide Oral Solution; Metoclopramide Tablets;
USP 23: Metoclopramide Injection; Metoclopramide Oral Solution; Metoclopramide Tablets.

Proprietary Preparations (details are given in Part 3)
Aust.: Gastro-Timelets; Gastronerton†; Gastrosil; Metogastron; Nausigon; Paspertin; Pertin; ***Austral.:*** Maxolon; Pramin; ***Belg.:*** Dibertil; Primperan; ***Canad.:*** Maxeran; Reglan; ***Fr.:*** Anausin; Primperan; ***Ger.:*** Cerucal; duraclamid†; duraMCP; Gastro-Tablinen†; Gastro-Timelets; Gastronerton; Gastrosil; Gastrotem†; Gastrotranquil; Gastrotrop†; Hyrin; MCP; MCP-ratiopharm; Metoclamid†; Paspertin; Reginerton†; ***Irl.:*** Antimet; Gastrobid Continus; Maxolon; Metocyl; Opram†; Primperan; ***Ital.:*** Anandat†; Citroplus; Clopan; Cronauzan†; Enterosil†; Metocobil†; Nadir†; Plasil; Randum; Regastrol†; Viscal; ***Mon.:*** Prokinyl; ***Neth.:*** Primperan; ***Norw.:*** Afipran; Primperan; ***S.Afr.:*** Abbemetic†; Acumet; Ametic; Betaclopramide; Clinamide†; Clopamon; Contromet; Dynamide†; Gastrocolon†; Gastrotat†; Maxolon; Metalon; Metcon; Perinorm; Primperan†; Prostal; Setin; ***Spain:*** Metagliz; Primperan; ***Swed.:*** Primperan; ***Switz.:*** Gastro-Timelets; Gastrosil; Paspertin; Primperan; ***UK:*** Gastrobid Continus; Gastroflux; Gastromax; Maxolon; Metramid†; Mygdalon; Parmid; Primperan; ***USA:*** Clopra; Intensol; Maxolon; Octamide; Reclomide; Reglan.

Multi-ingredient: ***Aust.:*** Ceolat Compositum; Paspertase; ***Belg.:*** Migpriv; ***Fr.:*** Cephalgan; Migpriv; Primperoxane; ***Ger.:*** Migrane-Neuridal; Migranerton; Paspertase; ***Irl.:*** Paramax; ***Ital.:*** Ede; Essen†; Eugastran†; Geffer; Kilozim†; Megast†; Plasil Enzimatico†; Quanto†; ***Neth.:*** Migrafin; ***Spain:*** Aci Kestomal†; Aero Plus; Aeroflat; Anti Anorex Triple; Edym Sedante; Gastro Gobens; Gastrosindrom†; Hepadigest; Ibsesal†; Jorkil; Liberbil; Metagliz Bismutico; Novo Aerofil Sedante; Paidozim; Primperan Complex; Salcemetic; Sedo Alufilm†; Starlep; Sualyn; Sulmetin†; Surifarm; Suxidina; Timulcer†; ***Switz.:*** Primoxan†; ***UK:*** Migravess; Paramax.

Metopimazine (6545-m)

Metopimazine *(BAN, USAN, rINN)*.

EXP-999; RP-9965. 1-[3-(2-Methylsulphonylphenothiazin-10-yl)propyl]piperidine-4-carboxamide.

$C_{22}H_{27}N_3O_3S_2$ = 445.6.

CAS — 14008-44-7.

Pharmacopoeias. In Fr.

Metopimazine, a phenothiazine dopamine antagonist, is an antiemetic with general properties similar to those of chlorpromazine (p.649). It is used in the treatment of nausea and vomiting, including that associated with cancer chemotherapy (p.1172). It is given in usual doses of 15 to 30 mg daily by mouth, in 2 or 3 divided doses; similar doses have been given by rectum. It has also been given by injection, usually intramuscularly but occasionally by the intravenous route in a dose of 10 to 20 mg daily.

Preparations

Proprietary Preparations (details are given in Part 3)
Belg.: Vogalene; ***Fr.:*** Vogalene; ***Spain:*** Vogalen†.

Mifentidine (19514-y)

Mifentidine *(rINN)*.

N-(*p*-Imidazol-4-ylphenyl)-*N'*-isopropylformamidine.

$C_{13}H_{16}N_4$ = 228.3.

CAS — 83184-43-4.

Mifentidine is a histamine H_2-receptor antagonist with general properties similar to those of cimetidine (p.1183). It is reported to have a long duration of action.

References.

1. Pagani F, *et al.* Pharmacology of mifentidine, a novel H_2-receptor antagonist. *Arzneimittelforschung* 1985; **35:** 451–5.
2. Imbimbo BP, *et al.* Pharmacokinetics of mifentidine after single and multiple oral administration to healthy volunteers. *Br J Clin Pharmacol* 1988; **26:** 407–13.
3. Sabbatini F, *et al.* Comparative study of mifentidine and ranitidine in the short-term treatment of duodenal ulcer. *Eur J Clin Pharmacol* 1990; **39:** 515–17.

Mosapride (15908-f)

Mosapride *(rINN)*.

(±)-4-Amino-5-chloro-2-ethoxy-*N*-{[4-(*p*-fluorobenzyl)-2-morpholinyl]methyl}benzamide.

$C_{21}H_{25}ClFN_3O_3$ = 421.9.

CAS — 112885-41-3.

Mosapride is a substituted benzamide that has been investigated, as the citrate, for its prokinetic actions.

References.

1. Sakashita M, *et al.* Pharmacokinetics of the gastrokinetic agent mosapride citrate after single and multiple oral administrations in healthy subjects. *Arzneimittelforschung* 1993; **43:** 867–72.

Nabilone (843-e)

Nabilone *(BAN, USAN, pINN)*.

Compound 109514; Lilly-109514. (±)-(6a*R*,10a*R*)-3-(1,1-Dimethylheptyl)-6a,7,8,9,10,10a-hexahydro-1-hydroxy-6,6-dimethyl-6*H*-benzo[*c*]chromen-9-one.

$C_{24}H_{36}O_3$ = 372.5.

CAS — 51022-71-0.

Adverse Effects

Nabilone may produce adverse effects similar to those of cannabis (see p.1558). The most common side-effect is reported to be drowsiness; other neurological side-effects that have been observed include confusion, disorientation, dizziness, euphoria, dysphoria, hallucinations, psychosis, mental depression, headache, decreased concentration, blurred vision, sleep disturbances, decreased coordination, and tremors. Adverse cardiovascular reactions that have occurred are postural hypotension and tachycardia. Dry mouth, decreased appetite, and abdominal cramp have also been reported.

The incidence of side-effects is higher with nabilone than with prochlorperazine, but most side-effects are mild or moderate in severity and the severity usually decreases with continued treatment, although occasionally nabilone may need to be discontinued. The most commonly reported side-effects with nabilone at usual therapeutic doses are drowsiness in 4 to 89% of patients, dizziness in 12 to 65%, and dry mouth in 6 to 62%.[1] Postural hypotension is potentially one of the most troublesome adverse effects seen with nabilone and has been observed in around 5% of patients on several occasions. Other side-effects reported include euphoria in 6 to 25% of patients, mood elevation in 7 to 27%, dysphoria in 7 to 23%, depression in 7 to 10%, headache in 9 to 34%, and sleep disturbances in 6 to 18%.

1. Ward A, Holmes B. Nabilone: a preliminary review of its pharmacological properties and therapeutic use. *Drugs* 1985; **30:** 127–44.

Precautions

Nabilone is extensively metabolised and largely excreted in bile, and therefore is not recommended for use in patients with severe liver impairment. It should be administered cautiously to patients with a history of psychosis or depression, or those with hypertension or heart disease.

Because of the possibility of CNS depression patients should be warned not to drive or operate machinery.

The possibility of dependence similar to that of cannabis should be borne in mind.

Interactions

Nabilone has been shown to have an additive CNS depressant effect when given with alcohol, diazepam, or other CNS depressants.

Pharmacokinetics

Nabilone is well absorbed from the gastro-intestinal tract and is rapidly and extensively metabolised; one or more of the metabolites may be active. The major excretory pathway is the biliary system; about 65% of a dose is excreted in the faeces and about 20% in the urine. The elimination half-life of nabilone is about 2 hours, but the half-lives of its combined metabolites are about 35 hours after a dose by mouth.

References.

1. Rubin A, *et al.* Physiologic disposition of nabilone, a cannabinol derivative, in man. *Clin Pharmacol Ther* 1977; **22:** 85–91.

Uses and Administration

Nabilone, a synthetic cannabinoid with antiemetic and anxiolytic properties, is used for the control of nausea and vomiting associated with cancer chemotherapy in patients who have failed to respond adequately to conventional antiemetics (see p.1172).

The usual dose for adults is 1 mg twice daily by mouth initially, increased to 2 mg twice daily if necessary. The first dose should be given the evening before initiation of chemotherapy with the second dose of nabilone being given 1 to 3 hours before the first dose of the antineoplastic. Nabilone may be given throughout each cycle of chemotherapy and for 48 hours after the last dose of chemotherapy, if required. The dose of nabilone should not exceed 6 mg daily.

Multiple sclerosis. There is a report of reduction in spasticity and nocturia, and improvement in mood and well-being, in a patient with multiple sclerosis who received nabilone 1 mg every second day.[1] Given that there are also anecdotal reports of improvement in symptoms in patients with multiple sclerosis who took cannabis, it was suggested that synthetic cannabinoids might be worthy of study in the treatment of spasticity. For a discussion of the various approaches to treatment of multiple sclerosis, see p.620.

1. Martyn CN, *et al.* Nabilone in the treatment of multiple sclerosis. *Lancet* 1995; **345:** 579.

Preparations

Proprietary Preparations (details are given in Part 3)
Canad.: Cesamet; ***Irl.:*** Cesamet; ***UK:*** Cesamet; ***USA:*** Cesamet†.

Niperotidine Hydrochloride (2874-e)

Niperotidine Hydrochloride *(rINNM)*.

Piperonyl Ranitidine Hydrochloride. *N*-[2-({5-[(Dimethylamino)methyl]furfuryl}thio)ethyl]-2-nitro-*N′*-piperonyl-1,1-ethenediamine hydrochloride.

$C_{20}H_{26}N_4O_5S$, HCl = 471.0.

CAS — 84845-75-0 (niperotidine).

Niperotidine hydrochloride is a histamine H_2-receptor antagonist with general properties similar to those of cimetidine (p.1183). Severe hepatic disorders have occurred in patients receiving niperotidine.

Preparations

Proprietary Preparations (details are given in Part 3)
Ital.: Gafir†; Perultid†; Rotil.

Nizatidine (12003-m)

Nizatidine *(BAN, USAN, rINN)*.

LY-139037. 4-[2-(1-Methylamino-2-nitrovinylamino)ethylthiomethyl]thiazol-2-ylmethyl(dimethyl)amine; *N*-[2-(2-Dimethylaminomethylthiazol-4-ylmethylthio)ethyl]-*N′*-methyl-2-nitrovinylidenediamine.

$C_{12}H_{21}N_5O_2S_2$ = 331.5.

CAS — 76963-41-2.

Pharmacopoeias. In US.

Store in airtight containers. Protect from light.

Adverse Effects

As for Cimetidine, p.1183. Some patients taking nizatidine may experience excessive sweating and urticaria; anaemia may also occur.

Nizatidine is considered to have little or no anti-androgenic activity although there are isolated reports of gynaecomastia and impotence.

Effects on the cardiovascular system. Nizatidine has been reported to reduce heart rate in healthy subjects,[1,2] an effect that was not seen when they were pretreated with ranitidine[1] or also given the antimuscarinic pirenzepine.[2]

1. Mescheder A, *et al.* Changes in the effects of nizatidine and famotidine on cardiac performance after pretreatment with ranitidine. *Eur J Clin Pharmacol* 1993; **45:** 151–6.
2. Hinrichsen H, *et al.* Dose-dependent heart rate reducing effect of nizatidine, a histamine H_2-receptor antagonist. *Br J Clin Pharmacol* 1993; **35:** 461–6.

Effects on the endocrine system. A report of reversible impotence with nizatidine 300 mg at night in one patient.[1]

1. Kassianos GC. Impotence and nizatidine. *Lancet* 1989; **i:** 963.

Precautions

As for Cimetidine, p.1185.

Interactions

Unlike cimetidine (p.1185) nizatidine does not seem to affect cytochrome P450, and therefore is considered to have little effect on the metabolism of other drugs.

Pharmacokinetics

Nizatidine is readily and almost completely absorbed from the gastro-intestinal tract. The bioavailability of nizatidine following oral administration exceeds 70% and may be slightly increased by the presence of food. It is widely distributed and is approximately 35% bound to plasma proteins.

The elimination half-life of nizatidine is 1 to 2 hours and is prolonged in renal impairment. Nizatidine is partly metabolised in the liver: nizatidine *N*-2-oxide, nizatidine *S*-oxide, and *N*-2-monodesmethylnizatidine have been identified, the latter having about 60% of the activity of nizatidine.

More than 90% of a dose of nizatidine is excreted in the urine, in part by active tubular secretion, within 12 hours, about 60% as unchanged drug. Less than 6% is excreted in the faeces. Nizatidine is found in breast milk in concentrations much lower than those in plasma.

References.

1. Callaghan JT, *et al.* A pharmacokinetic profile of nizatidine in man. *Scand J Gastroenterol* 1987; **22** (suppl 136): 9–17.
2. Lauritsen K, *et al.* Clinical pharmacokinetics of drugs used in the treatment of gastrointestinal diseases. *Clin Pharmacokinet* 1990; **19:** 11–31 (part I) and 94–125 (part II).
3. Obermeyer BD, *et al.* Secretion of nizatidine into human breast milk after single and multiple doses. *Clin Pharmacol Ther* 1990; **47:** 724–30.

Uses and Administration

Nizatidine is a histamine H_2-receptor antagonist with actions and uses similar to those of cimetidine (see p.1185). It is given by mouth and by intravenous infusion.

In the management of benign gastric and duodenal ulceration a single daily dose of nizatidine 300 mg by mouth at night is recommended, which should be given initially for 4 weeks and may be extended to 8 weeks if necessary; alternatively 150 mg may be given twice daily in the morning and evening. Where appropriate a maintenance dose of 150 mg daily may be given at night. In patients who are unsuited to receive oral therapy nizatidine may be given on a short-term basis by intravenous infusion. Continuous infusion of 10 mg per hour as a 0.2% solution in a suitable infusion fluid such as 0.9% sodium chloride or 5% glucose is recommended; alternatively 100 mg may be diluted in 50 mL of infusion fluid and be given over 15 minutes, three times daily. The total intravenous dose should not exceed 480 mg daily.

In gastro-oesophageal reflux disease a dose of 150 to 300 mg twice daily by mouth is recommended for up to 12 weeks.

The dosage of nizatidine should be reduced in patients with impaired renal function. Suggested doses by mouth according to creatinine clearance are: creatinine clearance of 20 to 50 mL per minute, 150 mg daily for treatment and 150 mg every other day for maintenance therapy; creatinine clearance of less than 20 mL per minute, 150 mg every other day for treatment and 150 mg every third day for maintenance therapy.

Reviews.

1. Price AH, Brogden RN. Nizatidine: a preliminary review of its pharmacodynamic and pharmacokinetic properties, and its therapeutic use in peptic ulcer disease. *Drugs* 1988; **36:** 521–39.

Preparations

USP 23: Nizatidine Capsules.

Proprietary Preparations (details are given in Part 3)
Aust.: Axid†; Ulxit; ***Austral.:*** Tazac; ***Belg.:*** Calmaxid†; Panaxid; ***Canad.:*** Axid; ***Fr.:*** Nizaxid; ***Ger.:*** Gastrax; Nizax; ***Irl.:*** Axid; ***Ital.:*** Cronizat; Nizax; Zanizal; ***Neth.:*** Axid; Naxidine; ***S.Afr.:*** Antizid; Axid; ***Spain:*** Distaxid; Ulcosal; ***Swed.:*** Nizax; ***Switz.:*** Calmaxid; ***UK:*** Axid; Zinga; ***USA:*** Axid.

Olsalazine Sodium (16608-a)

Olsalazine Sodium *(BANM, USAN, rINNM)*.

Azodisal Sodium; CI Mordant Yellow 5; CI No. 14130; CJ-91B; Sodium Azodisalicylate. Disodium 5,5′-azodisalicylate.

$C_{14}H_8N_2Na_2O_6$ = 346.2.

CAS — 6054-98-4.

Adverse Effects and Precautions

The most common side-effect associated with olsalazine sodium is watery diarrhoea. It may resolve with dosage reduction but may be severe enough to require withdrawal of treatment in some patients. Diarrhoea is less likely if the drug is taken after meals. Other gastro-intestinal disturbances such as nausea, abdominal pain, and dyspepsia may occasionally occur, and also headache, arthralgia, and skin rashes. Olsalazine is converted to mesalazine in the colon and although systemic mesalazine concentrations are not as high as with oral mesalazine preparations (see Pharmacokinetics, below), the potential exists for adverse effects of mesalazine (see p.1199) to occur. There have been a few reports of blood dyscrasias.

It has been recommended that olsalazine should not be given to patients with impaired renal function or with a history of salicylate hypersensitivity. If a blood dyscrasia is suspected treatment should be stopped immediately and a blood count performed. Patients or their carers should be told how to recognise signs of blood toxicity and should be advised to seek immediate medical attention if symptoms such as fever, sore throat, mouth ulcers, bruising, or bleeding develop.

In an open study[1] of olsalazine 1 g daily by mouth involving 160 patients with active ulcerative colitis and a history of sulphasalazine intolerance, 103 (64.4%) patients experienced no side-effects; 29 patients reported only minor side-effects: gastro-intestinal disturbances in 22 patients, transient skin rash in 3, and headache, increased salivation, cough, and irritability each in one patient. The most common side-effect was frequent loose stools which affected 25 patients, 20 of whom had to discontinue treatment. This side-effect occurred early in treatment, within 10 hours of the first dose in 13 patients. Severe diarrhoea was more frequent in patients with widespread disease, but the incidence of diarrhoea did not correlate with disease severity.

A subsequent study[2] in healthy subjects has shown that olsalazine has a significant inhibitory effect on water and electrolyte absorption in the small intestine, which may account, at least in part, for the induction of diarrhoea. Patients with extensive colitis have reduced colonic absorptive function and may be less able to assimilate the increased colonic inflow volumes.

1. Sandberg-Gertzén H, *et al.* Azodisal sodium in the treatment of ulcerative colitis: a study of tolerance and relapse-prevention properties. *Gastroenterology* 1986; **90:** 1024–30.
2. Raimundo AH, *et al.* Effects of olsalazine and sulphasalazine on jejunal and ileal water and electrolyte absorption in normal human subjects. *Gut* 1991; **32:** 270–4.

Effects on the blood. As of July 1995, the Committee on Safety of Medicines in the UK had received 4 reports of blood dyscrasias associated with olsalazine, none of them fatal.[1] It was recommended that a blood count be performed and the drug stopped immediately if there was suspicion of a dyscrasia.

1. Committee on Safety of Medicines/Medicines Control Agency. Blood dyscrasias and mesalazine. *Current Problems* 1995; **21:** 5–6.

Effects on the kidneys. A report of nephrotoxicity, characterised by interstitial nephritis, associated with the use of olsalazine.[1] Symptoms resolved on discontinuation of the drug.

1. Wilcox GM, *et al.* Nephrotoxicity associated with olsalazine. *Am J Med* 1996; **100:** 238–40.

Interactions

Prolonged prothrombin times have been reported in patients receiving olsalazine concomitantly with warfarin.

Pharmacokinetics

Very little of an oral dose of olsalazine is absorbed via the upper gastro-intestinal tract, and almost the entire dose reaches its site of action in the colon intact. It is broken down by the colonic bacterial flora into 2 molecules of 5-aminosalicylic acid (mesalazine). Some mesalazine is absorbed and acetylated (see p.1200) but systemic concentrations of mesalazine and its metabolite are reported to be lower than those following comparable doses of mesalazine by mouth, perhaps because there is less release of mesalazine in the small intestine, where absorption is better. Mesalazine concentrations in the colon following a dose of olsalazine are stated to be about 1000 times greater than systemic concentrations, which would imply that olsalazine ought to produce fewer systemic adverse effects at effective doses, although this has not yet been clearly demonstrated.

The small amounts (1 to 2% of the dose or less) of intact olsalazine which are absorbed are excreted mainly in urine; the elimination half-life after an intravenous dose has been calculated at about 1 hour. Some olsalazine is metabolised by sulphate conjugation in the liver: the elimination half-life of the metabolite is reported to be about 7 days.

References.

1. Ryde EM. Pharmacokinetic aspects of drugs targeted for the colon, with special reference to olsalazine. *Acta Pharm Suec* 1988; **25:** 327–8.
2. Laursen LS, *et al.* Disposition of 5-aminosalicylic acid by olsalazine and three mesalazine preparations in patients with ulcerative colitis: comparison of intraluminal colonic concentrations, serum values, and urinary excretion. *Gut* 1990; **31:** 1271–6.

Uses and Administration

Olsalazine consists of two molecules of mesalazine (p.1199) linked with an azo bond. It is activated in the colon where the active mesalazine is released. It is used as the sodium salt in the management of acute mild ulcerative colitis and for the maintenance of remission (see Inflammatory Bowel Disease, p.1171). The usual initial adult dose is 1 g by mouth daily in divided doses and this is gradually increased, if necessary, over one week, to a maximum dose of 3 g daily. The usual dose for the maintenance of remission is 500 mg twice daily. Doses should be taken after meals and a single dose should not exceed 1 g.

References.

1. Anonymous. Olsalazine—a further choice in ulcerative colitis. *Drug Ther Bull* 1990; **28:** 57–8.
2. Anonymous. Olsalazine for ulcerative colitis. *Med Lett Drugs Ther* 1990; **32:** 105–6.
3. Wadworth AN, Fitton A. Olsalazine: a review of its pharmacodynamic and pharmacokinetic properties, and therapeutic potential in inflammatory bowel disease. *Drugs* 1991; **41:** 647–64.

Preparations

Proprietary Preparations (details are given in Part 3)

Aust.: Dipentum; ***Austral.:*** Dipentum; ***Canad.:*** Dipentum; ***Fr.:*** Dipentum; ***Ger.:*** Dipentum; ***Irl.:*** Dipentum; ***Ital.:*** Dipentum; ***Neth.:*** Dipentum; ***Norw.:*** Dipentum; ***S.Afr.:*** Dipentum; ***Spain:*** Rasal; ***Swed.:*** Dipentum; ***Switz.:*** Dipentum; ***UK:*** Dipentum; ***USA:*** Dipentum.

Omeprazole (16938-y)

Omeprazole *(BAN, USAN, rINN)*.

H-168/68; Omeprazolum. 5-Methoxy-2-(4-methoxy-3,5-dimethyl-2-pyridylmethylsulphinyl)benzimidazole.

$C_{17}H_{19}N_3O_3S$ = 345.4.

CAS — 73590-58-6.

Pharmacopoeias. In *Eur.* (see p.viii) and *US.*

A white or almost white powder. Very slightly **soluble** in water; soluble in alcohol, in methyl alcohol, and in dichloromethane. It dissolves in dilute solutions of alkali hydroxides. **Store** in airtight containers at a temperature between 2° and 8°. Protect from light.

Omeprazole Sodium (15383-s)

Omeprazole Sodium *(BANM, USAN, rINNM)*.

$C_{17}H_{18}N_3NaO_3S$ = 367.4.

CAS — 95510-70-6.

Pharmacopoeias. In *Eur.* (see p.viii).

A white or almost white hygroscopic powder. Freely **soluble** in water and in alcohol; soluble in propylene glycol; very slightly soluble in dichloromethane. The pH of a 2% solution is 10.3 to 11.3. **Store** in airtight containers. Protect from light.

Adverse Effects

The adverse effects reported most frequently with omeprazole have been gastro-intestinal disturbances, in particular diarrhoea, skin rashes, and headache; they have sometimes been severe enough to require discontinuation of treatment. Effects on the CNS, including reversible confusional states, agitation, depression, and hallucinations in severely ill patients, have occurred. Other adverse effects reported rarely include arthralgia and myalgia, paraesthesia, aggression, blurred vision, taste disturbances, peripheral oedema, hyponatraemia, blood disorders including agranulocytosis, leucopenia, and thrombocytopenia, interstitial nephritis, and hepatotoxicity.

Early toxicological studies identified carcinoid-like tumours of the gastric mucosa in *rats* given very high doses of omeprazole over long periods; this is reviewed in more detail under Genotoxicity, below.

Effects on the endocrine system. Up to December 1991, the WHO had received 30 reports of impotence or gynaecomastia which might have been due to omeprazole;[1] of these reports 15 were of impotence, 13 of gynaecomastia in men, and 2 of breast enlargement in women.

1. Lindquist M, Edwards IR. Endocrine adverse effects of omeprazole. *Br Med J* 1992; **305:** 451–2.

Effects on the eyes. There have been reports of visual disturbances associated with the use of omeprazole, including 6 cases of irreversible blindness or visual impairment in severely ill patients given the drug intravenously, and 13 cases of visual disturbances associated with oral use.[1] As a result of concern about these effects the availability of intravenous omeprazole has been restricted in Germany; however, the consensus appears to be that a causal link has not been established between omeprazole and these ocular effects. Suggestions that visual (and also auditory[2]) impairment could follow drug-induced vasculitis[2-4] appear to be contentious.[1,5-7] A cohort study involving 140 128 patients receiving antisecretory therapy, 33 988 of whom received omeprazole, found no evidence that any of the drugs used was associated with a major increase in risk of vascular or inflammatory disorders of the eye;[8] however, the statistical power of this study was not high.[9]

1. Creutzfeldt WC, Blum AL. Safety of omeprazole. *Lancet* 1994; **343:** 1098.
2. Schönhöfer PS. Intravenous omeprazole and blindness. *Lancet* 1994; **343:** 665.
3. Schönhöfer PS. Safety of omeprazole and lansoprazole. *Lancet* 1994; **343:** 1369–70.
4. Schönhöfer PS, *et al.* Ocular damage associated with proton pump inhibitors. *Br Med J* 1997; **314:** 1805.
5. Colin-Jones D. Safety of omeprazole and lansoprazole. *Lancet* 1994; **343:** 1369.
6. Lessell S. Omeprazole and ocular damage. *Br Med J* 1998; **316:** 67.
7. Sachs G. Omeprazole and ocular damage. *Br Med J* 1998; **316:** 67–8.
8. García Rodríguez LA, *et al.* A cohort study of the ocular safety of anti-ulcer drugs. *Br J Clin Pharmacol* 1996; **42:** 213–16.
9. Merlo J, Ranstam J. Ocular safety of anti-ulcer drugs. *Br J Clin Pharmacol* 1997; **43:** 449.

Effects on the joints. Beutler and colleagues have reported 5 cases of arthralgia, sometimes associated with swelling of the affected joints, in patients receiving omeprazole,[1] and noted that some reported cases of omeprazole-associated headache were accompanied by arthralgia or myalgia. In another case[2] arthralgia in a patient with a hereditary myopathy receiving omeprazole appeared to represent one aspect of a drug-induced lupus syndrome, being accompanied by malaise, fever, Raynaud's phenomenon, raised antinuclear antibody titres, and anticardiolipin and antihistone antibodies. Symptoms resolved on withdrawal of the drug.

There has also been a report of 2 cases of acute gout associated with omeprazole;[3] in one patient symptoms, which resolved on withdrawal, recurred on rechallenge. However, case control studies have failed to show an increased risk of polyarthralgia[4] or gout[5] associated with omeprazole use.

1. Beutler M, *et al.* Arthralgias and omeprazole. *Br Med J* 1994; **309:** 1620.
2. Sivakumar K, Dalakas MC. Autoimmune syndrome induced by omeprazole. *Lancet* 1994; **344:** 619–20.
3. Kraus A, Flores-Suárez LF. Acute gout associated with omeprazole. *Lancet* 1995; **345:** 461–2.
4. Meier CR, Jick H. Omeprazole, H_2 blockers, and polyarthralgia: case-control study. *Br Med J* 1997; **315:** 1283.
5. Meier CR, Jick H. Omeprazole, other antiulcer drugs and newly diagnosed gout. *Br J Clin Pharmacol* 1997; **44:** 175–8.

Effects on the kidneys. Acute interstitial nephritis developed in two elderly patients receiving omeprazole for the treatment of gastro-oesophageal reflux disease.[1,2] In one patient renal function improved rapidly following discontinuation of the drug but the condition recurred upon rechallenge,[1] while in the other renal function remained severely affected for several months.[2] It was postulated that this adverse effect might have an allergic mechanism.[2] In these cases interstitial nephritis was associated with rash and eosinophilia; however, a further 2 cases of acute interstitial nephritis associated with omeprazole therapy in elderly patients[3,4] did not exhibit these symptoms. In another report, associated rash without eosinophiluria was seen.[5]

1. Ruffenach SJ, *et al.* Acute interstitial nephritis due to omeprazole. *Am J Med* 1992; **93:** 472–3.
2. Christensen PB, *et al.* Renal failure after omeprazole. *Lancet* 1993; **341:** 55.
3. Assouad M, *et al.* Recurrent acute interstitial nephritis on rechallenge with omeprazole. *Lancet* 1994; **344:** 549.
4. Jones B, *et al.* Acute interstitial nephritis due to omeprazole. *Lancet* 1994; **344:** 1017–18.
5. Kuiper JJ. Omeprazole-induced acute interstitial nephritis. *Am J Med* 1993; **95:** 248.

Effects on the liver. For a study suggesting a relatively low incidence of acute liver injury in patients receiving omeprazole see Cimetidine, p.1184.

Effects on the nervous system. A report of ataxia in a patient receiving omeprazole;[1] symptoms resolved on discontinuing the drug.

1. Varona L, *et al.* Gait ataxia during omeprazole therapy. *Ann Pharmacother* 1996; **30:** 192.

Effects on skeletal muscle. Progressive muscular weakness suggestive of myopathy developed in a 78-year-old patient given omeprazole.[1] After 4 weeks of treatment the patient required assistance in walking and rising from squatting. Weakness resolved on withdrawal of the drug, but returned on rechallenge.

1. Garrote FJ, *et al.* Subacute myopathy during omeprazole therapy. *Lancet* 1992; **340:** 672.

Effects on the skin. An extensive blistering erythematous skin rash in an elderly woman given omeprazole[1] was characteristic of acute disseminated epidermal necrosis. The Committee on Safety of Medicines in the UK had received 223 reports of cutaneous reactions to omeprazole up to August 1992, including 6 of erythema multiforme, but none of this severity. Other severe reactions that have been reported include a toxic bullous skin reaction[2] and exfoliative dermatitis.[3]

For a report of urticaria and angioedema possibly associated with the formulation of omeprazole see Hypersensitivity, below. For the association of rash with interstitial nephritis, see Effects on the Kidneys, above.

1. Cox NH. Acute disseminated epidermal necrosis due to omeprazole. *Lancet* 1992; **340:** 857.
2. Stenier C, *et al.* Bullous skin reaction induced by omeprazole. *Br J Dermatol* 1995; **133:** 343–4.
3. Epelde Gonzalo FD, *et al.* Exfoliative dermatitis related to omeprazole. *Ann Pharmacother* 1995; **29:** 82–3.

Genotoxicity. Early toxicological studies in *rats* given high doses of omeprazole over 2 years identified carcinoid tumours of the gastric mucosa associated with complete block of gastric acid secretion leading to hypergastrinaemia and hyperplasia of enterochromaffin-like cells.[1] This has been the main issue concerning the safety of omeprazole in man and has led to restrictions in its use and duration of treatment. Workers at Glaxo developed a new test to detect genotoxicity of antisecretory drugs which indicated that a genotoxic effect of omeprazole could not be discounted.[2] This study was heavily criticised; more established genotoxicity tests have been reported to be negative for omeprazole,[3-5] and other groups have not been able to replicate the findings with the new test.[6] The lowest doses at which the Glaxo workers found a genotoxic effect of omeprazole were 10 to 20 mg per kg bodyweight[2] and the clinical significance of their results was questioned.[3] Although some short-term studies with omeprazole have found slight hypergastrinaemia,[7] long-term studies in patients with Zollinger-Ellison syndrome have found no increase in fasting serum-gastrin concentrations and no evidence of gastric carcinoid tumours.[8,9] More recently there has been a report of gastric polyps developing in 3 of 8 patients after receiving omeprazole 20 or 40 mg daily for one year.[10] Further long-term studies of omeprazole may be needed before a realistic risk assessment can be made.

1. Ekman L, *et al.* Toxicological studies on omeprazole. *Scand J Gastroenterol* 1985; **20** (suppl 108): 53–69.
2. Burlinson B, *et al.* Genotoxicity studies of gastric acid inhibiting drugs. *Lancet* 1990; **335:** 419.
3. Ekman L, *et al.* Genotoxicity studies of gastric acid inhibiting drugs. *Lancet* 1990; **335:** 419–20.
4. Wright NA, Goodlad RA. Omeprazole and genotoxicity. *Lancet* 1990; **335:** 909–10.
5. Helander HF, *et al.* Omeprazole and genotoxicity. *Lancet* 1990; **335:** 910–11.
6. Goodlad RA. Acid suppression and claims of genotoxicity: what have we learned? *Drug Safety* 1994; **10:** 413–19.
7. Lanzon-Miller S, *et al.* Twenty-four-hour intragastric acidity and plasma gastrin concentration before and during treatment with either ranitidine or omeprazole. *Aliment Pharmacol Ther* 1987; **1:** 239–51.
8. Lloyd-Davies KA, *et al.* Omeprazole in the treatment of Zollinger-Ellison syndrome: a 4-year international study. *Aliment Pharmacol Ther* 1988; **2:** 13–32.
9. Maton PN, *et al.* Long-term efficacy and safety of omeprazole in patients with Zollinger-Ellison syndrome: a prospective study. *Gastroenterology* 1989; **97:** 827–36.
10. Graham JR. Gastric polyposis: onset during long-term therapy with omeprazole. *Med J Aust* 1992; **157:** 287–8.

Hypersensitivity. Urticaria, facial angioedema, and bronchospasm in a patient given omeprazole capsules did not recur when the patient was given omeprazole granules and the reaction might have been precipitated by the ingredients of the capsule shell.[1]

1. Haeney MR. Angio-oedema and urticaria associated with omeprazole. *Br Med J* 1992; **305:** 870.

Infection. Oesophageal candidiasis occurred in two elderly patients receiving omeprazole but was successfully treated with antifungal therapy. It was postulated that gastric acid secretion and a degree of physiological reflux of acid into the oesophagus might normally play a protective role in preventing candidal infection.[1] The profound reduction in acid secretion produced by omeprazole may also predispose to gastro-intestinal infection; there is some evidence for an increased risk of campylobacter infection in patients receiving omeprazole,[2] as well as a report of recurrent salmonellal infection.[3]

1. Larner AJ, Lendrum R. Oesophageal candidiasis after omeprazole therapy. *Gut* 1992; **33:** 860–1.
2. Neal KR, *et al.* Omeprazole as a risk factor for campylobacter gastroenteritis: case-control study. *Br Med J* 1996; **312:** 414–15.
3. Wingate DL. Acid reduction and recurrent enteritis. *Lancet* 1990; **335:** 222.

Lupus syndrome. For a report of drug-induced lupus syndrome associated with omeprazole therapy, see Effects on the Joints, above.

Malabsorption. Omeprazole has been reported to result in a substantial reduction in cyanocobalamin (vitamin B_{12}) absorption,[1] probably related to the increase in gastric pH, and indicating a potential risk of vitamin deficiency with long-term therapy.[2]

1. Marcuard SP, *et al.* Omeprazole therapy causes malabsorption of cyanocobalamin (vitamin B_{12}). *Ann Intern Med* 1994; **120:** 211–15.
2. Termanini B, *et al.* Effect of long-term gastric acid suppressive therapy on serum vitamin B_{12} levels in patients with Zollinger-Ellison syndrome. *Am J Med* 1998; **104:** 422–30.

Overdosage. A report of 2 cases of overdosage with omeprazole.[1] The major clinical features were drowsiness, headache (possibly due to a metabolite), and tachycardia. Both patients recovered uneventfully without specific treatment.

1. Ferner RE, Allison TR. Omeprazole overdose. *Hum Exp Toxicol* 1993; **12:** 541–2.

Precautions

Before giving omeprazole to patients with gastric ulcers the possibility of malignancy should be considered since omeprazole may mask symptoms and delay diagnosis. Omeprazole is extensively metabolised in the liver and some sources recommend that dosage should be reduced in hepatic impairment.

Helicobacter infection. Although omeprazole plays an important part in combined therapies to eliminate *Helicobacter pylori* infection, its long-term use alone in *H. pylori*-positive patients with gastro-oesophageal reflux disease was associated with a greatly increased risk of atrophic gastritis.[1] It was suggested that where prolonged maintenance therapy was needed in these patients, those with Helicobacter infection should receive therapy to eliminate the bacterium.

1. Kuipers EJ, *et al.* Atrophic gastritis and Helicobacter pylori infection in patients with reflux esophagitis treated with omeprazole or fundoplication. *N Engl J Med* 1996; **334:** 1018–22.

Interactions

Omeprazole has been reported to inhibit the cytochrome P450 system and alter the metabolism of some other drugs metabolised by these enzymes. It may prolong the elimination of diazepam, phenytoin, and warfarin. The decreased gastric acidity caused by omeprazole may affect the absorption of other drugs given concomitantly.

References.

1. Andersson T. Omeprazole drug interaction studies. *Clin Pharmacokinet* 1991; **21:** 195–212.

Clarithromycin. Studies in healthy subjects have indicated that concurrent administration of omeprazole and clarithromycin results in an approximate 30% increase in peak plasma concentrations of omeprazole, and an increase in its mean half-life from 1.2 to 1.6 hours.[1] At the same time, plasma concentrations of clarithromycin were also modestly increased, as were local concentrations in gastric tissue and mucus. The interaction may contribute to the benefits of combined therapy for *Helicobacter pylori* infection.

1. Gustavson LE, *et al.* Effect of omeprazole on concentrations of clarithromycin in plasma and gastric tissue at steady state. *Antimicrob Agents Chemother* 1995; **39:** 2078–83.

Effects on other drugs. Omeprazole is metabolised primarily by the cytochrome CYP2C19, and therefore may interact with diazepam;[1,2] some metabolism of phenytoin, tolbutamide, and the R-enantiomer of warfarin also takes place by this route, but the effects seen have been minor.[1] (For references to interactions between omeprazole and phenytoin, see p.356.) Although some induction of CYP1A2, which metabolises caffeine and theophylline, has been reported this does not appear to be clinically significant,[3] and omeprazole does not appear to have a significant effect on CYP3A4, which is the most important cytochrome for drug metabolism.[1,4] The potential for metabolic interactions between omeprazole and other drugs is considered very limited.[1] (For a study *in vitro* suggesting that there was an effect of omeprazole on tacrolimus metabolism via CYP3A4, see p.563.)

For a study suggesting that omeprazole reduces the absorption of cyanocobalamin, see Malabsorption, above.

1. Andersson T. Pharmacokinetics, metabolism and interactions of acid pump inhibitors: focus on omeprazole, lansoprazole and pantoprazole. *Clin Pharmacokinet* 1996; **31:** 9–28.
2. Andersson T, *et al.* Effect of omeprazole treatment on diazepam plasma levels in slow versus normal rapid metabolizers of omeprazole. *Clin Pharmacol Ther* 1990; **47:** 79–85.
3. Rizzo N, *et al.* Omeprazole and lansoprazole are not inducers of cytochrome P4501A2 under conventional therapeutic conditions. *Eur J Clin Pharmacol* 1996; **49:** 491–5.
4. Tateishi T, *et al.* Omeprazole does not affect measured CYP3A4 activity using the erythromycin breath test. *Br J Clin Pharmacol* 1995; **40:** 411–12.

Pharmacokinetics

Omeprazole is rapidly absorbed, but to a variable extent, following oral administration. Absorption of omeprazole is not affected by food. Omeprazole is acid-labile and various formulations have been developed in an attempt to improve bioavailability from the gastro-intestinal tract. Consequently, its pharmacokinetics may vary with different formulations of the drug. The absorption of omeprazole, as well as being formulation-dependent, also appears to be dose-dependent, as increasing the dosage above 40 mg has been reported to increase the plasma concentrations in a non-linear fashion.

Bioavailability of omeprazole may be increased in elderly patients, in some ethnic groups such as Chinese, and in patients with impaired hepatic function, but is not markedly affected in patients with renal impairment.

Following absorption, omeprazole is almost completely metabolised in the liver, primarily by cytochrome P450 isoform CYP2C19, and rapidly eliminated, mostly in the urine. Although the elimination half-life from plasma is short, being reported to be about 0.5 to 3 hours, its duration of action with regard to inhibition of acid secretion is much longer allowing it to be used in single daily doses. Omeprazole is highly bound (about 95%) to plasma proteins.

References.

1. Andersson T, *et al.* Pharmacokinetics of various single intravenous and oral doses of omeprazole. *Eur J Clin Pharmacol* 1990; **39:** 195–7.
2. Andersson T, Regårdh C-G. Pharmacokinetics of omeprazole and metabolites following single intravenous and oral doses of 40 and 80 mg. *Drug Invest* 1990; **2:** 255–63.
3. Howden CW. Clinical pharmacology of omeprazole. *Clin Pharmacokinet* 1991; **20:** 38–49.
4. Ching MS, *et al.* Oral bioavailability of omeprazole before and after chronic therapy in patients with duodenal ulcer. *Br J Clin Pharmacol* 1991; **31:** 166–70.
5. Landahl S, *et al.* Pharmacokinetic study of omeprazole in elderly healthy volunteers. *Clin Pharmacokinet* 1992; **23:** 469–76.
6. Andersson T, *et al.* Pharmacokinetics of [^{14}C]omeprazole in patients with liver cirrhosis. *Clin Pharmacokinet* 1993; **24:** 71–8.
7. Jacqz-Aigrain E, *et al.* Pharmacokinetics of intravenous omeprazole in children. *Eur J Clin Pharmacol* 1994; **47:** 181–5.

Uses and Administration

Omeprazole inhibits secretion of gastric acid by irreversibly blocking the enzyme system of hydrogen/potassium adenosine triphosphatase (H^+/K^+ ATPase), the 'proton pump' of the gastric parietal cell. It is used in conditions where inhibition of gastric acid secretion may be beneficial, including aspiration syndromes (p.1168), dyspepsia (p.1169), gastro-oesophageal reflux disease (p.1170), peptic ulcer disease (p.1174), and the Zollinger-Ellison syndrome (p.1176).

Omeprazole may be given by mouth or intravenously as the sodium salt. Intravenous doses are expressed in terms of the base.

For the relief of acid-related **dyspepsia** omeprazole is given in usual doses of 10 or 20 mg daily by mouth for 2 to 4 weeks.

The usual dose for the treatment of **gastro-oesophageal reflux disease** is 20 to 40 mg by mouth once daily for 4 to 12 weeks; thereafter maintenance therapy can be continued with 20 mg once daily. In children, doses in the range 0.7 to 1.4 mg per kg bodyweight daily, up to a maximum daily dose of 40 mg, have been given for 4 to 12 weeks.

In the management of **peptic ulcer disease** a single daily dose of 20 mg by mouth, or 40 mg in severe cases, is given. Treatment is continued for 4 weeks for duodenal ulcer and 8 weeks for gastric ulcer. A dose of 10 to 20 mg once daily may be given for maintenance.

For the eradication of *Helicobacter pylori* in peptic ulceration omeprazole may be combined with antibacterials in dual or triple therapy. Effective **triple therapy** regimens include omeprazole 40 mg daily combined with: amoxycillin 500 mg and metronidazole 400 mg, both three times daily; or with clarithromycin 250 mg and metronidazole 400 mg (or tinidazole 500 mg) both twice daily; or with amoxycillin 1 g and clarithromycin 500 mg both twice daily. These regimens are given for 1 week. Dual therapy regimens such as omeprazole 40 mg daily with amoxycillin 750 mg or 1 g twice daily, or with clarithromycin 500 mg three times daily, are less effective and must be given for 2 weeks.

Doses of 20 mg daily are used in the treatment of ulceration associated with the use of nonsteroidal anti-inflammatory drugs (NSAIDs); a dose of 20 mg daily may also be used for prophylaxis in susceptible patients.

The initial recommended dosage for patients with the **Zollinger-Ellison syndrome** is 60 mg by mouth once daily, but doses up to 120 mg three times daily have been administered. The majority of patients are effectively controlled by doses in the range 20 to 120 mg daily. Doses above 80 mg should be divided and given twice daily; treatment should be continued for as long as is clinically indicated.

Omeprazole is also used for the prophylaxis of **acid aspiration**, in a dose of 40 mg the evening before surgery and a further 40 mg on the day of surgery, 2 to 6 hours before the procedure.

In the UK the manufacturers recommend that the maximum daily dose should be reduced to 20 mg in patients with impaired hepatic function; in some other countries, however, the manufacturers' literature states that no dosage adjustment is required in hepatic impairment.

In patients who are unsuited to receive oral therapy omeprazole sodium may be given on a short-term basis by slow intravenous injection, in a usual dose equivalent to 40 mg of the base, given over at least 2½ minutes. Alternatively the same dose may be infused over a period of 20 to 30 minutes in 100 mL of a suitable infusion fluid. Higher intravenous doses have been given to patients with Zollinger-Ellison syndrome.

Reviews.

1. McTavish D, *et al.* Omeprazole: an updated review of its pharmacology and therapeutic use in acid-related disorders. *Drugs* 1991; **42:** 138–70.
2. Howden CW. Clinical pharmacology of omeprazole. *Clin Pharmacokinet* 1991; **20:** 38–49.
3. Maton PN. Omeprazole. *N Engl J Med* 1991; **324:** 965–75.
4. Wilde MI, McTavish D. Omeprazole: an update of its pharmacology and therapeutic use in acid-related disorders. *Drugs* 1994; **48:** 91–132.

Administration. Omeprazole is given by mouth as capsules containing enteric-coated granules which should be swallowed whole and not crushed or chewed. In patients with swallowing difficulties the manufacturers recommend that the contents of the capsules be mixed with a little fruit juice or yogurt and swallowed.

Asthma. Gastro-oesophageal reflux is a potential exacerbating factor for asthma (p.745), and acid suppressive therapy with omeprazole has been reported to reduce asthma symptoms.

Cystic fibrosis. Omeprazole has been given to patients with cystic fibrosis receiving pancreatic enzyme supplements in order to decrease enzyme inactivation by gastric acid. For reference to this and other aspects of the management of cystic fibrosis see p.119.

Inflammatory bowel disease. There are a few reports of responses to omeprazole 20 mg daily in patients with inflammatory bowel disease.[1,2] Combination of omeprazole with mesalazine has also been tried.[2] For a discussion of inflammatory bowel disease and more usual drugs used for its treatment, see p.1171.

1. Heinzow U, Schlegelberger T. Omeprazole in ulcerative colitis. *Lancet* 1994; **343:** 477.
2. Dickinson JB. Is omeprazole helpful in inflammatory bowel disease? *J Clin Gastroenterol* 1994; **18:** 317–19.

Scleroderma. Gastro-oesophageal reflux is one of the gastro-intestinal manifestations of systemic sclerosis, and proton pump inhibitors such as omeprazole are coming to play a major role in the management of such gastro-intestinal disease.[1] For a discussion of the broader management of the condition see p.501.

1. Williamson DJ. Update on scleroderma. *Med J Aust* 1995; **162:** 599–601.

Preparations

Proprietary Preparations (details are given in Part 3)
Aust.: Antra; Losec; ***Austral.:*** Losec; ***Belg.:*** Logastric; Losec; ***Canad.:*** Losec; ***Fr.:*** Mopral; Zoltum; ***Ger.:*** Antra; Gastroloc; ***Irl.:*** Losec; ***Ital.:*** Antra; Losec; Mepral; Omeprazen; ***Neth.:*** Losec; ***Norw.:*** Losec; ***S.Afr.:*** Losec; ***Spain:*** Audazol; Aulcer; Belmazol; Ceprandal; Elgam; Emeproton; Gastrimut; Indurgan; Losec; Miol; Mopral; Norpramin; Nuclosina; Omapren; Ompranyt; Parizac; Pepticum; Prysma; Sanamidol; Secrepina; Ulceral; Ulcesep; Ulcometion; Zimor; ***Swed.:*** Losec; ***Switz.:*** Antra; ***UK:*** Losec; ***USA:*** Prilosec.

Multi-ingredient: ***Austral.:*** Losec Helicopak.

Ondansetron Hydrochloride (3149-y)

Ondansetron Hydrochloride *(BANM, USAN, rINNM).*

GR-38032 (ondansetron); GR-38032F. ±-1,2,3,4-Tetrahydro-9-methyl-3-(2-methylimidazol-1-ylmethyl)-carbazol-4-one hydrochloride dihydrate.

$C_{18}H_{19}N_3O,HCl,2H_2O = 365.9.$

CAS — 99614-02-5 (ondansetron); 116002-70-1 (ondansetron); 103639-04-9 (ondansetron hydrochloride).

Ondansetron hydrochloride 1.25 mg is approximately equivalent to 1 mg of ondansetron base.

Incompatibility. Ondansetron hydrochloride and dexamethasone sodium phosphate were not compatible when high concentrations were combined in polypropylene syringes.[1] Lower concentrations (up to 0.64 mg per mL of ondansetron and 0.4 mg per mL of dexamethasone phosphate) were stable in 50 mL containers of infusion fluid for 30 days under refrigeration.

1. Hagan RL, *et al.* Stability of ondansetron hydrochloride and dexamethasone sodium phosphate in infusion bags and syringes for 32 days. *Am J Health-Syst Pharm* 1996; **53:** 1431–5.

Adverse Effects and Precautions

Ondansetron hydrochloride may cause headache, a sensation of flushing or warmth in the head and epigastrium, and rarely hypersensitivity reactions. Large bowel transit time may be increased causing constipation. A transient rise in liver enzymes has occasionally occurred. It does not appear to affect plasma prolactin concentrations. Transient visual disturbances such as blurred vision have been reported during rapid administration of intravenous doses.

Dosage restriction is advisable in patients with moderate to severe hepatic impairment.

Administration in hepatic impairment. The manufacturers recommend that the dose of ondansetron should not exceed 8 mg daily in patients with moderate or severe hepatic impairment. When this dose was given intravenously to patients with various degrees of impairment it was found that in those who were severely impaired there was an increase in the area under the plasma concentration/time curve (AUC) and in the terminal plasma half-life and a decrease in plasma clearance.[1] The authors of this study, some of whom were from the manufacturers, considered that the dosing frequency of ondansetron should be restricted to once daily in severe hepatic impairment.

1. Blake JC, *et al.* The pharmacokinetics of intravenous ondansetron in patients with hepatic impairment. *Br J Clin Pharmacol* 1993; **35:** 441–3.

Effects on the cardiovascular system. Ballard and colleagues[1] reported chest pain and/or cardiac arrhythmias in 4 patients (fatal in 2) which might have been associated with ondansetron. This experience led to a change in the management of patients receiving this antiemetic; in 3 subsequent patients who developed severe chest or anginal pain treatment with ondansetron was discontinued.

The manufacturers (Glaxo) had at that time no evidence of a causal relationship between ondansetron and episodes of chest pain and cardiac abnormalities.[2] Administration of ondansetron 32 mg intravenously over 15 minutes produced no clinically important cardiovascular changes in a study in 12 healthy subjects.[3]

1. Ballard HS, *et al.* Ondansetron and chest pain. *Lancet* 1992; **340:** 1107.
2. Palmer JBD, Greenstreet YL. Ondansetron and chest pain. *Lancet* 1992; **340:** 1410.
3. Boike SC, *et al.* Cardiovascular effects of i.v. granisetron at two administration rates and of ondansetron in healthy adults. *Am J Health-Syst Pharm* 1997; **54:** 1172–6.

Effects on the liver. Although disturbances in liver enzyme values have been reported in patients receiving ondansetron, more severe symptoms of liver disorder appear to be very rare; however, there is a report of severe jaundice associated with ondansetron as an antiemetic for chemotherapy.[1] Symptoms did not recur when the patient was given granisetron.

1. Verrill M, Judson I. Jaundice with ondansetron. *Lancet* 1994; **344:** 190–1.

Effects on the nervous system. There has been a report of tonic-clonic movements and frothing at the mouth in one patient 90 minutes after an infusion of ondansetron;[1] the patient responded to diazepam intravenously. The manufacturers had observed 10 patients who developed seizures during initial clinical studies, but considered that all these patients had predisposing factors. The patient who was the subject of this more recent report had no such predisposing factors. Extrapyramidal reactions in patients receiving ondansetron as part of a chemotherapy regimen have also been reported.[2,3]

1. Sargent AI, *et al.* Seizure associated with ondansetron. *Clin Pharm* 1993; **12:** 613–15.
2. Krstenansky PM, *et al.* Extrapyramidal reaction caused by ondansetron. *Ann Pharmacother* 1994; **28:** 280.
3. Mathews HG, Tancil CG. Extrapyramidal reaction caused by ondansetron. *Ann Pharmacother* 1996; **30:** 196.

Hypersensitivity. Anaphylactoid reactions have been reported in patients receiving ondansetron injection. The Food and Drug Administration in the USA stated in October 1993 that it had received 24 reports of such reactions,[1] mostly occurring after the first ondansetron dose of the second or third chemotherapy cycle, and characterised by urticaria, angioedema, hypotension, bronchospasm, and dyspnoea.

Kataja and de Bruijn have since reported on 2 patients in whom a mild hypersensitivity reaction following one $5-HT_3$-receptor antagonist was followed by a more severe reaction after exposure to a second drug of the same class.[2] In the first case severe acute asthma, cyanosis, and loss of consciousness developed after ondansetron in a patient who had previously experienced an asthmatic reaction after tropisetron. The second patient had had pruritus after a tropisetron injection and urticaria after ondansetron, and subsequently developed anaphylactic shock 5 minutes after a further dose of tropisetron. It was recommended that another $5-HT_3$-receptor antagonist should not be given as a replacement to patients who developed a hypersensitivity reaction to a drug of this class.

1. Chen M, *et al.* Anaphylactoid-anaphylactic reactions associated with ondansetron. *Ann Intern Med* 1993; **119:** 862.
2. Kataja V, de Bruijn KM. Hypersensitivity reactions associated with 5-hydroxytryptamine$_3$-receptor antagonists: a class effect? *Lancet* 1996; **347:** 584–5.

Pharmacokinetics

Following oral administration, ondansetron is rapidly absorbed with peak plasma concentration of around 0.03 to 0.04 µg per mL being reported about 1.5 to 2 hours after an oral dose of 8 mg. The absolute bioavailability is about 60%, due mainly to hepatic first-pass metabolism. It is extensively distributed in the body; results *in vitro* suggest that about 70 to 75% of the drug in plasma is protein bound. It is cleared from the systemic circulation predominantly by hepatic metabolism, with less than 5% of a dose being excreted in urine unchanged: clearances of around 6 mL per minute per kg have been reported in young, healthy subjects. In elderly subjects, bioavailability may be somewhat higher (65%) and clearance lower (4 to 5 mL per minute per kg), presumably due to reduced hepatic metabolism. The terminal elimination half-life is about 3 hours in younger subjects, prolonged to 5 hours in the elderly. These differences are not considered sufficient to warrant dosage adjustment; however, in patients with severe hepatic impairment, in whom bioavailability may approach 100% and clearance is markedly slowed, with elimination half-lives of 15 to 32 hours, dosage restriction is advisable (see Administration in Hepatic Impairment, above).

References.

1. Roila F, Del Favero A. Ondansetron clinical pharmacokinetics. *Clin Pharmacokinet* 1995; **29:** 95–109.
2. Figg WD, *et al.* Pharmacokinetics of ondansetron in patients with hepatic insufficiency. *J Clin Pharmacol* 1996; **36:** 206–15.

Uses and Administration

Ondansetron hydrochloride is a highly selective 5-HT_3-receptor antagonist with potent antiemetic activity. It is used in the management of **nausea and vomiting** induced by cytotoxic chemotherapy and radiotherapy, particularly where this is severe or unresponsive to other therapy. It has also been given for postoperative nausea and vomiting. For the treatment of nausea and vomiting, and the important role of ondansetron, see p.1172.

Ondansetron hydrochloride is given by intramuscular or slow intravenous injection, or by mouth; doses are expressed in terms of ondansetron. Ondansetron base is given rectally.

For highly emetogenic chemotherapy the following dose schedules appear to be equally effective: a single dose of 8 mg by slow intravenous or intramuscular injection immediately before treatment; 8 mg by slow intravenous or intramuscular injection immediately before treatment, either followed by a continuous intravenous infusion of 1 mg per hour for up to 24 hours, or by a further two doses of 8 mg two to four hours apart; a single dose of 32 mg given by intravenous infusion over 15 minutes immediately before chemotherapy; a 16-mg suppository rectally, given 1 to 2 hours before treatment. The effects of ondansetron may be enhanced by intravenous administration of dexamethasone before chemotherapy. These regimens should be followed by ondansetron 8 mg orally twice daily, or 16 mg daily as a suppository, for up to 5 days after the end of a course of chemotherapy, to protect against delayed emesis.

For less emetogenic chemotherapy and radiotherapy a dose of 8 mg may be given as a slow intravenous or intramuscular injection immediately before treatment; alternatively 8 mg by mouth or 16 mg rectally can be given 1 to 2 hours before treatment; these regimens are followed by 8 mg by mouth twice daily, or 16 mg rectally, for up to 5 days after the end of a course of chemotherapy.

For children a recommended dose is 5 mg per m^2 body-surface intravenously over 15 minutes immediately before chemotherapy, followed by 4 mg orally every 12 hours for up to 5 days after the end of chemotherapy.

To prevent postoperative nausea and vomiting adults may be given 16 mg by mouth an hour before anaesthesia; alternatively a single dose of 4 mg may be given by intramuscular or slow intravenous injection at induction of anaesthesia. For the treatment of postoperative nausea and vomiting a single 4-mg dose by intramuscular or slow intravenous injection is recommended. Children may be given 0.1 mg per kg body-weight by slow intravenous injection, up to a maximum dose of 4 mg, both for the prevention and treatment of postoperative nausea and vomiting.

In patients with moderate or severe hepatic impairment the manufacturers have recommended that the total daily dose of ondansetron should not exceed 8 mg (see above).

Numerous other 5-HT_3-receptor antagonists similar to ondansetron have been developed. They include: alosetron, azasetron (see p.1179), bemesetron, cilansetron, dolasetron (see p.1190), granisetron (see p.1193), itasetron, ramosetron (see p.1209), tropisetron (see p.1217), and zatosetron, but so far not all have been marketed.

References.

1. Milne RJ, Heel RC. Ondansetron: therapeutic use as an antiemetic. *Drugs* 1991; **41:** 574–95.
2. Chaffee BJ, Tankanow RM. Ondansetron—the first of a new class of antiemetic agents. *Clin Pharm* 1991; **10:** 430–6.
3. Markham A, Sorkin EM. Ondansetron: an update of its therapeutic use in chemotherapy-induced and postoperative nausea and vomiting. *Drugs* 1993; **45:** 931–52.
4. McQueen KD, Milton JD. Multicenter postmarketing surveillance of ondansetron therapy in pediatric patients. *Ann Pharmacother* 1994; **28:** 85–92.
5. Cooke CE, Mehra IV. Oral ondansetron for preventing nausea and vomiting. *Am J Hosp Pharm* 1994; **51:** 762–71.
6. Wilde MI, Markham A. Ondansetron: a review of its pharmacology and preliminary clinical findings in novel applications. *Drugs* 1996; **52:** 773–94.

Administration. A report[1] of the successful use of ondansetron by continuous subcutaneous infusion to control intractable nausea and vomiting. Despite concern about the low pH of ondansetron injection there was no problem with the skin at the infusion site. Rectal administration (using ondansetron tablets) has also been used successfully.[2]

1. Mulvenna PM, Regnard CFB. Subcutaneous ondansetron. *Lancet* 1992; **339:** 1059.
2. Al-Moundhri M, *et al.* Rectal administration of ondansetron in uncontrolled emesis induced by chemotherapy. *Aust N Z J Med* 1995; **25:** 538.

Alcohol dependence. Ondansetron is being studied in the management of alcohol dependence (p.1099). However, in a study by Sellers *et al.*[1] a significant reduction in alcohol consumption was found only in lighter drinkers after subgroup analysis.

1. Sellers EM, *et al.* Clinical efficacy of the 5-HT_3 antagonist ondansetron in alcohol abuse and dependence. *Alcohol Clin Exp Res* 1994; **18:** 879–85.

Mental disorders. Ondansetron has been tried experimentally in a number of mental disorders including schizophrenia[1] and psychosis in patients with parkinsonism.[2] It is also reported to be under investigation in the management of panic attacks. For the more conventional management of schizophrenia and parkinsonism see p.637 and p.1128 respectively, while for the management of anxiety disorders see p.635.

1. White A, *et al.* Ondansetron in the treatment of schizophrenia. *Lancet* 1991; **337:** 1173.
2. Zoldan J, *et al.* Psychosis in advanced Parkinson's disease: treatment with ondansetron, a 5-HT_3 receptor antagonist. *Neurology* 1995; **45:** 1305–8.

Pain. Preliminary results from a small crossover study[1] indicated that ondansetron was more effective than paracetamol in relieving the pain of fibromyalgia, a chronic disorder that responds poorly to conventional analgesics.

1. Hrycaj P, *et al.* Pathogenetic aspects of responsiveness to ondansetron (5-hydroxytryptamine type 3 receptor antagonist) in patients with primary fibromyalgia syndrome—a preliminary study. *J Rheumatol* 1996; **23:** 1418–23.

Pruritus. A report of a response of intractable cholestatic pruritus to intravenous injection of ondansetron[1] was followed by excellent results in 5 patients with liver disease and severe cholestatic pruritus given ondansetron 8 mg by injection, followed in 3 patients by 8 mg twice daily by mouth.[2] For the more usual agents employed in pruritus, see p.1075.

1. Schwörer H, Ramadri G. Improvement of cholestatic pruritus by ondansetron. *Lancet* 1993; **341:** 1277.
2. Raderer M, *et al.* Ondansetron for pruritus due to cholestasis. *N Engl J Med* 1994; **330:** 1540.

Preparations

Proprietary Preparations (details are given in Part 3)
Aust.: Zofran; ***Austral.:*** Zofran; ***Belg.:*** Zofran; ***Canad.:*** Zofran; ***Fr.:*** Zophren; ***Ger.:*** Zofran; ***Irl.:*** Zofran; ***Ital.:*** Zofran; ***Neth.:*** Zofran; ***Norw.:*** Zofran; ***S.Afr.:*** Zofran; ***Spain:*** Datron†; Fixca; Helmine; Yatrox; Zofran; ***Swed.:*** Zofran; ***Switz.:*** Zofran; ***UK:*** Zofran; ***USA:*** Zofran.

Oxyphenisatin (7520-h)

Oxyphenisatin *(BAN).*

Oxyphenisatine *(rINN)*; Dihydroxyphenylisatin. 3,3-Bis(4-hydroxyphenyl)indolin-2-one.

$C_{20}H_{15}NO_3$ = 317.3.

CAS — 125-13-3.

Oxyphenisatin Diacetate (7521-m)

Oxyphenisatin Diacetate *(BANM).*

Oxyphenisatine Acetate *(rINNM)*; Acetphenolisatin; Bisatin; Diacetoxydiphenylisatin; Diacetyldiphenolisatin; Diasatin; Diphesatin; Isaphenin; NSC-59687; Oxyphenisatin Acetate *(USAN)*; Phenlaxine.

$C_{24}H_{19}NO_5$ = 401.4.

CAS — 115-33-3.

Pharmacopoeias. In *Pol.*

Adverse Effects

Liver damage has occurred usually following prolonged use of oxyphenisatin diacetate. Abdominal discomfort such as cramps, nausea and vomiting, or diarrhoea may occur. Other adverse effects which have been reported include sweating, tachycardia, and occasionally syncope.

Effects on the liver. Reports of liver toxicity associated with oxyphenisatin.

1. Reynolds TB, *et al.* Chronic active and lupoid hepatitis caused by a laxative, oxyphenisatin. *N Engl J Med* 1971; **285:** 813–20.
2. Gjone E, Stave R. Liver disease associated with a "non-constipating" iron preparation. *Lancet* 1973; **i:** 421–2.
3. Kotha P, *et al.* Liver damage induced by oxyphenisatin. *Br Med J* 1980; **281:** 1530.

Precautions

As for Bisacodyl, p.1179.

Uses and Administration

Oxyphenisatin is a stimulant laxative with limited indications because of liver toxicity and its use is no longer permitted in some countries.

Oxyphenisatin 50 mg is given rectally in 2 litres of water as an enema for cleansing the large intestine and as an adjunct in barium enema examinations.

Preparations

Proprietary Preparations (details are given in Part 3)
Irl.: Veripaque†; ***UK:*** Veripaque.

Pantoprazole (13840-h)

Pantoprazole *(BAN, USAN, rINN).*

BY-1023; SKF-96022. 5-Difluoromethoxybenzimidazol-2-yl 3,4-dimethoxy-2-pyridylmethyl sulphoxide.

$C_{16}H_{15}F_2N_3O_4S$ = 383.4.

CAS — 102625-70-7.

Adverse Effects and Precautions

As for Omeprazole, p.1204.

In short term trials the most frequent adverse effects reported in patients receiving pantoprazole were diarrhoea, headache, dizziness, pruritus, and skin rash.[1] The effects were rarely so severe as to require withdrawal of treatment.

1. Fitton A, Wiseman L. Pantoprazole: a review of its pharmacological properties and therapeutic use in acid-related disorders. *Drugs* 1996; **51:** 460–82.

Interactions

Like omeprazole, p.1205, pantoprazole is metabolised by the cytochrome P450 isoform CYP2C19, and might be expected to have a similar potential for interaction, but there is little evidence to date of any clinically significant interaction.

Uses and Administration

Pantoprazole is a proton pump inhibitor with actions and uses similar to those of omeprazole (p.1205). It is given by mouth as the sodium salt but doses are calculated in terms of the base. The usual dose for the treatment of peptic ulcer disease or gastro-oesophageal reflux disease is the equivalent of 40 mg of pantoprazole once daily. Treatment is usually given for 2 to 4 weeks for duodenal ulceration, or 4 to 8 weeks for patients with benign gastric ulceration or gastro-oesophageal reflux disease. In exceptional cases doses of the equivalent of 80 mg daily may be given, but a dose of 40 mg daily should not be exceeded in the elderly or those with renal impairment. A dose reduction to 40 mg every other day is recommended in patients with hepatic impairment due to cirrhosis.

Pantoprazole has also been given intravenously, as the sodium salt, in recommended doses of 40 mg daily given over 2 to 15 minutes. Doses should be reduced to 40 mg every other day in hepatic impairment due to cirrhosis.

References.

1. Pue MA, *et al.* Pharmacokinetics of pantoprazole following single intravenous and oral administration to healthy male subjects. *Eur J Clin Pharmacol* 1993; **44:** 575–8.
2. Judmaier G, *et al.* Comparison of pantoprazole and ranitidine in the treatment of acute duodenal ulcer. *Aliment Pharmacol Ther* 1994; **8:** 81–6.
3. Andersson T. Pharmacokinetics, metabolism and interactions of acid pump inhibitors: focus on omeprazole, lansoprazole and pantoprazole. *Clin Pharmacokinet* 1996; **31:** 9–28.
4. Fitton A, Wiseman L. Pantoprazole: a review of its pharmacological properties and therapeutic use in acid-related disorders. *Drugs* 1996; **51:** 460–82.
5. Anonymous. Pantoprazole—a third proton pump inhibitor. *Drug Ther Bull* 1997; **35:** 93–4.

Administration. Administration of the daily dose of pantoprazole in the morning produced a greater increase in gastric pH than administration of the same dose in the evening.[1] Morning dosage was considered the regimen of choice.

1. Müssig S, *et al.* Morning and evening administration of pantoprazole: a study to compare the effect on 24-hour intragastric pH. *Eur J Gastroenterol Hepatol* 1997; **9:** 599–602.

Preparations

Proprietary Preparations (details are given in Part 3)
Aust.: Pantoloc; Zurcal; ***Austral.:*** Somac; ***Belg.:*** Pantozol; Zurcale; ***Fr.:*** Eupantol; Inipomp; ***Ger.:*** Pantozol; Rifun; ***Irl.:*** Protium; ***Ital.:*** Pantecta; Pantopan; Peptazol; ***Neth.:*** Pantozol; ***Norw.:*** Somac; ***S.Afr.:*** Controloc; Pantoloc; ***Spain:*** Anagastra; Pantecta; Ulcotenal; ***Swed.:*** Pantoloc; ***UK:*** Protium.

Pentaerythritol (13090-m)

Tetramethylolmethane. 2,2-Bis(hydroxymethyl)propane-1,3-diol.
$C_5H_{12}O_4$ = 136.1.
CAS — 115-77-5.

Pentaerythritol is an osmotic laxative used in the treatment of constipation in doses of 5 to 15 g daily. The limited role of osmotic laxatives in the management of constipation is discussed on p.1168.

Pentaerythritol tetranitrate (see p.927) is a vasodilator.

Preparations

Proprietary Preparations (details are given in Part 3)
Fr.: Auxitrans; Combeylax†.

Peppermint Leaf (4690-t)

Black Mint (*M. piperita* var. *vulgaris*); Hoja de Menta; Hortelã-Pimenta; Menth. Pip.; Mentha Piperita; Menthae Piperitae Folium; Menthe Poivrée; Peppermint; Pfefferminzblätter; White Mint (*M. piperita* var. *officinalis*).

Pharmacopoeias. In *Eur.* (see p.viii) and *Pol.* Also in *USNF.*
Chin. P. specifies *M. haplocalyx*. *Jpn. P.* specifies *M. arvensis* var. *piperascens*.

The dried leaves of *Mentha × piperita* (Labiatae), containing not less than 1.2% v/w of volatile oil if whole, or not less than 0.9% if cut. It has a characteristic aromatic odour and an aromatic cooling taste. Peppermint in the USNF consists of the dried leaves and flowering tops of *M. piperita*. **Protect** from light.

Peppermint Oil (4691-x)

Essence de Menthe Poivrée; Essência de Hortelã-Pimenta; Menthae Piperitae Aetheroleum; Ol. Menth. Pip.; Oleum Menthae Piperitae; Pfefferminzöl.
CAS — 8006-90-4.

Pharmacopoeias. In *Eur.* (see p.viii) and *Pol.* Also in *USNF.*
Oleum Menthae(*Chin. P.*) is from *M. haplocalyx*. Mentha Oil (*Jpn P.*) is from *M.arvensis* var *piperascens*.

The volatile oil obtained by distillation from the fresh overground parts of *Mentha × piperita* (Labiatae) and rectified if necessary.

It is a colourless, pale yellow, or greenish-yellow oil with the characteristic odour of peppermint and a pungent aromatic cooling taste. It contains menthol, menthone, and menthyl acetate. The Ph. Eur. specifies 2.8 to 10% menthyl acetate, 30 to 50% menthol, and 14 to 32% menthone. The USNF specifies not less than 5% of esters calculated as menthyl acetate and not less than 50% of total menthol, free and as esters.

Miscible with alcohol; **soluble** 1 in 3 of alcohol (70%) with slight opalescence; miscible with ether and with dichloromethane. **Store** at a temperature not exceeding 40° in airtight containers. Protect from light.

The Pharmaceutical Society's Department of Pharmaceutical Sciences found that PVC bottles softened and distorted fairly rapidly in the presence of peppermint oil, which should not be stored or dispensed in such bottles.[1]

1. Department of Pharmaceutical Sciences of the Pharmaceutical Society of Great Britain. Plastic medicine bottles of rigid PVC. *Pharm J* 1973; **210:** 100.

Adverse Effects and Precautions

Peppermint oil can be irritant and may rarely cause hypersensitivity reactions. Reported reactions include erythematous skin rash, headache, bradycardia, muscle tremor, and ataxia. Heartburn has also been reported.

Effects on the cardiovascular system. Idiopathic atrial fibrillation in 2 patients addicted to 'peppermints'. Normal rhythm was restored when peppermint-sucking ceased.[1]

1. Thomas JG. Peppermint fibrillation. *Lancet* 1962; **i:** 222.

Hypersensitivity. Exacerbation of asthma, with wheezing and dyspnoea, associated with the use of paste-based toothpastes containing peppermint or wintergreen as a flavouring.[1]

1. Spurlock BW, Dailey TM. Shortness of (fresh) breath—toothpaste-induced bronchospasm. *N Engl J Med* 1990; **323:** 1845–6.

Interactions

Reactions may be more likely if peppermint oil is taken in conjunction with alcohol. Enteric-coated capsules containing peppermint oil should not be taken immediately after food or with antacids.

Uses and Administration

Peppermint oil is an aromatic carminative which relaxes gastro-intestinal smooth muscle and relieves flatulence and colic. Enteric-coated capsules containing peppermint oil are used for the relief of symptoms of the irritable bowel syndrome or gastro-intestinal spasm secondary to other disorders. Usual doses are 0.2 mL three times daily by mouth, half to one hour before food, increased to 0.4 mL three times daily if necessary.

Peppermint oil is also used as a flavour and with other volatile agents in preparations for respiratory-tract disorders.

Peppermint leaf, the source of the oil, has also been used for its carminative and flavouring properties.

Gastro-intestinal disorders. Any effect of peppermint oil on the irritable bowel syndrome may be through a local action on the gastro-intestinal tract.[1] For a discussion of the management of irritable bowel syndrome, including mention of the role of peppermint oil, see p.1172. Pharmacological studies have shown that menthol, the major constituent of peppermint oil, has properties similar to those of calcium-channel antagonists and inhibits influx of calcium ions through smooth muscle including that in the human gut.[2-4]

The relaxant effect of peppermint oil on the gastro-intestinal tract has been used to reduce colonic spasm during endoscopy by injecting the oil or a diluted suspension of the oil along the biopsy channel of the colonoscope.[5] Addition of peppermint oil to barium enema has also been tried and appears to reduce spasm and reduce the need for intravenous antispasmodics.[6]

1. Anonymous. Hole for the mint. *Lancet* 1988; **i:** 1144–5.
2. Taylor BA, *et al.* Inhibitory effect of peppermint oil on gastrointestinal smooth muscle. *Gut* 1983; **24:** A992.
3. Taylor BA, *et al.* Inhibitory effect of peppermint oil and menthol on human isolated coli. *Gut* 1984; **25:** A1168–9.
4. Taylor BA, *et al.* Calcium antagonist activity of menthol on gastrointestinal smooth muscle. *Br J Clin Pharmacol* 1985; **20:** 293P–4P.
5. Leicester RJ, Hunt RH. Peppermint oil to reduce colonic spasm during endoscopy. *Lancet* 1982; **ii:** 989.
6. Sparks MJW, *et al.* Does peppermint oil relieve spasm during barium enema? *Br J Radiol* 1995; **68:** 841–3.

Preparations

BP 1998: Concentrated Peppermint Emulsion; Peppermint Spirit;
USNF 18: Peppermint Water;
USP 23: Peppermint Spirit.

Proprietary Preparations (details are given in Part 3)
Aust.: Colpermin; Dr Fischer's Minzol; ***Austral.:*** Mintec; ***Canad.:*** Colpermin; ***Ger.:*** China Minze†; Cholaktol forte; Citaethol†; Eu-minz N; Inspirol Heilpflanzenol; Leukona-Mintol; Mentacur; Ni-No-Fluid N; ***Irl.:*** Colpermin; ***Switz.:*** Colpermin; ***UK:*** Colpermin; Kiminto; Mintec.

Multi-ingredient: numerous preparations are listed in Part 3.

Phenolphthalein (7522-b)

Phenolphthalein (*BAN, rINN*).

Dihydroxyphthalophenone; Fenolftaleina; Phenolphthaleinum. 3,3-Bis(4-hydroxyphenyl)phthalide.
$C_{20}H_{14}O_4$ = 318.3.
CAS — 77-09-8.

Pharmacopoeias. In *Aust., Belg., Br., Chin., It., Swiss,* and *US. US* also includes Yellow Phenolphthalein.

A white or yellowish-white, odourless or almost odourless, crystalline or amorphous powder.

Practically **insoluble** in water; soluble 1 in 15 of alcohol and 1 in 100 of ether; dissolves in dilute solutions of alkali hydroxides, and in hot solutions of alkali carbonates, forming a red solution.

Adverse Effects

Hypersensitivity reactions, usually as skin rashes or eruptions, have occurred with phenolphthalein. Abdominal discomfort such as cramps or colic may occasionally occur.

Prolonged use or overdosage can result in diarrhoea with excessive loss of water and electrolytes, particularly potassium; there is also the possibility of developing an atonic non-functioning colon.

Phenolphthalein may cause pink discoloration of alkaline urine.

Tumours have occurred in *rats* and *mice* given very high doses of phenolphthalein; there does not appear to be evidence of carcinogenicity in humans, but phenolphthalein-containing products have been withdrawn in a number of countries because of concerns about long-term safety.

Effects on the skin. Reports of skin reactions associated with phenolphthalein include fixed drug eruptions,[1,2] erythema multiforme reactions,[1,3] and toxic epidermal necrolysis.[4,5]

1. Baer RL, Harris H. Types of cutaneous reactions to drugs. *JAMA* 1967; **202:** 710–13.
2. Savin JA. Current causes of fixed drug eruptions. *Br J Dermatol* 1970; **83:** 546–9.
3. Shelley WB, *et al.* Demonstration of intercellular immunofluorescence and epidermal hysteresis in bullous fixed drug eruption due to phenolphthalein. *Br J Dermatol* 1972; **86:** 118–25.
4. Kar PK, *et al.* Toxic epidermal necrolysis in a patient induced by phenolphthalein. *J Indian Med Assoc* 1986; **84:** 189–93.
5. Artymowicz RJ, *et al.* Phenolphthalein-induced toxic epidermal necrolysis. *Ann Pharmacother* 1997; **31:** 1157–9.

Overdosage. The most likely consequence of phenolphthalein overdosage is excessive purgation, which may require fluid and electrolyte replacement. However, a possible association with acute pancreatitis occurred in a 34-year-old man who inadvertently ingested phenolphthalein 2 g. There was complete recovery with no sequelae from the pancreatitis.[1] Widespread organ failure with disseminated intravascular coagulation, massive liver damage, pulmonary oedema, renal failure, and myocardial damage in a second patient[2] were attributed to self-poisoning with an unknown quantity of phenolphthalein-containing laxative, although the diagnosis was problematic. The patient died despite intensive support.

1. Lambrianides AL, Rosin RD. Acute pancreatitis complicating excessive intake of phenolphthalein. *Postgrad Med J* 1984; **60:** 491–2.
2. Sidhu PS, *et al.* Fatal phenolphthalein poisoning with fulminant hepatic failure and disseminated intravascular coagulation. *Hum Toxicol* 1989; **8:** 381–4.

Precautions

As for Bisacodyl, p.1179.

Pharmacokinetics

Up to 15% of phenolphthalein given by mouth is subsequently excreted in the urine. Enterohepatic circulation occurs and the glucuronide is excreted in the bile. Elimination may take several days.

Uses and Administration

Phenolphthalein is a diphenylmethane stimulant laxative which has been used for the treatment of constipation (p.1168) and for bowel evacuation before investigational procedures or surgery. It usually has an effect within 4 to 8 hours following administration by mouth.

It is usually administered in pills or tablets, and is also available as an emulsion with liquid paraffin. It is usually given in a dose of 30 to 200 mg taken at bedtime; doses of 270 mg daily should not be exceeded. A dose of 260 mg has been used in regimens for bowel evacuation.

Yellow phenolphthalein, an impure form, is used similarly.

Preparations

USP 23: Phenolphthalein Tablets.

Proprietary Preparations (details are given in Part 3)
Austral.: Figsen; Laxettes; ***Belg.:*** Caolax; ***Canad.:*** Alophen†; Espotabs; Ex-Lax; Laxative Pills; Neo-Prunex; ***Fr.:*** Purganol; ***Ger.:*** Darmol; ***Irl.:*** Petrolagar with Phenolphthalein; ***Ital.:*** Bom-Bon†; Confetto†; Euchessina†; Fructine-Vichy†; Neopurghes†; Prunetta†; Purgestol†; ***S.Afr.:*** Laxatone†; ***Spain:*** Laxen Busto; Purgante; ***Switz.:*** Reguletts; ***UK:*** Bonomint; Brooklax; Ex-Lax; Reguletts; Sure-Lax; ***USA:*** Alophen Pills; Espotabs; Evac-Q-Tabs; Evac-U-Gen; Evac-U-Lax; Ex-Lax; Ex-Lax Maximum Relief; Fletchers Childrens Laxative; Lax Pills; Laxative Pills; Medilax; Modane; Phenolax; Prulet.

Multi-ingredient: numerous preparations are listed in Part 3.

Plantain Seed (5448-k)

Pharmacopoeias. In *Jpn.*.
Chin. includes the seeds of *Plantago asiatica* or *P. depressa*.

The seed of *Plantago major* var. *asiatica*.

Plantain seed has been suggested as a substitute for ispaghula.

Plantago major is used in homoeopathic medicine and various forms of traditional medicine.

Preparations

Proprietary Preparations (details are given in Part 3)
Fr.: Sensivision au plantain; ***Ger.:*** Broncho-Sern.

Multi-ingredient: ***Austral.:*** Hamamelis Complex; ***Switz.:*** Kernosan Elixir; Sirop pectoral DP1; Sirop pectoral DP2; Tisane pectorale et bechique Natterman instantee no 9†.

Plaunotol (2366-j)

Plaunotol (*rINN*).

CS-684. (2*Z*,6*E*)-2-[(3*E*)-4,8-Dimethyl-3,7-nonadienyl]-6-methyl-2,6-octadiene-1,8-diol.
$C_{20}H_{34}O_2$ = 306.5.
CAS — 64218-02-6.

Plaunotol is a complex aliphatic alcohol extracted from the Thai medicinal plant plau-noi (*Croton sublyratus* (Euphorbiaceae)). It is reported to possess cytoprotective properties and is used in the treatment of gastritis and peptic ulcer disease in a dose of 240 mg daily by mouth.

Preparations

Proprietary Preparations (details are given in Part 3)
Jpn: Kelnac.

Polaprezinc (15917-d)

Polaprezinc *(rINN)*.

catena-Poly{zinc-μ-[β-alanyl-L-histidinato(2-)-*N*,*N*^{N},*O*:*N*$^\tau$]}.

$(C_9H_{12}N_4O_3Zn)_n$.

CAS — 107667-60-7.

Polaprezinc is a cytoprotective agent which is used in the treatment of peptic ulcer disease.

Polycarbophil (11505-k)

Polycarbophil *(BAN, rINN)*.

CAS — 9003-97-8.

Pharmacopoeias. In *US.*

Polycarbophil Calcium (5008-c)

Polycarbophil Calcium *(BANM, rINNM)*.

AHR-3260B; Calcium Polycarbophil *(USAN)*; Polycarbophilum Calcii; WI-140.

CAS — 9003-97-8 (polycarbophil and calcium salt).

Pharmacopoeias. In *US.*

The calcium salt of polyacrylic acid cross-linked with divinyl glycol. A white to creamy-white powder. Practically **insoluble** in water, common organic solvents, and dilute acids and alkalis. It loses not more than 10% of its weight on drying and contains not less than 18% and not more than 22% of calcium, calculated on the anhydrous basis. **Store** in airtight containers.

Adverse Effects and Precautions

As for Ispaghula, p.1194.

Polycarbophil calcium releases calcium ions in the gastro-intestinal tract and should be avoided by patients who must restrict their calcium intake.

There is a risk of intestinal or oesophageal obstruction and faecal impaction, especially if such bulk laxatives are swallowed dry. Therefore, they should always be taken with sufficient fluid and should not be taken immediately before going to bed. They should be avoided by patients who have difficulty swallowing.

Interactions

The calcium component of polycarbophil calcium may reduce the absorption of tetracyclines from the gastro-intestinal tract; it should be taken at least 1 hour before or 2 hours after the antibiotic.

Uses and Administration

Polycarbophil is used as the calcium salt. It has similar properties to ispaghula (p.1194) and is used as a bulk laxative and for adjusting faecal consistency. Following ingestion calcium ions are replaced by hydrogen ions from gastric acid and the resultant polycarbophil acid exerts a hydrophilic effect in the intestines. The more usual drugs used in the management of constipation are discussed on p.1168, while those used in diarrhoea are discussed on p.1168.

It is given by mouth as chewable tablets in a usual dose of the equivalent of 1 g of polycarbophil up to four times daily, as necessary. Doses should be taken with at least 250 mL of water.

Reviews.

1. Danhof IE. Pharmacology, toxicology, clinical efficacy, and adverse effects of calcium polycarbophil, an enteral hydrosorptive agent. *Pharmacotherapy* 1982; **2:** 18–28.

Preparations

Proprietary Preparations (details are given in Part 3)
Austral.: Replens; ***Canad.:*** Mitrolan†; Replens; ***Fr.:*** Replens; ***Ital.:*** Modula; Pursennid Fibra; Replens; ***S.Afr.:*** Replens; ***Spain:*** Replens; ***UK:*** Replens; ***USA:*** Equalactin; Fiber-Lax; Fiberall; Fibercon; FiberNorm; Konsyl Fiber; Mitrolan; Replens.

Multi-ingredient: ***Ital.:*** Pursennid Complex; ***USA:*** Aquasite.

Potassium Acid Tartrate (1186-h)

E336; Kalium Hydrotartaricum; Potassium Bitartrate *(USAN)*; Potassium Hydrogen Tartrate; Purified Cream of Tartar; Tartarus Depuratus; Weinstein.

$C_4H_5KO_6$ = 188.2.

CAS — 868-14-4.

Pharmacopoeias. In *Aust., Br., Fr.,* and *Neth.*

Colourless or white crystals or white crystalline powder. Slightly **soluble** in water; practically insoluble in alcohol and in ether.

Potassium acid tartrate was used as an osmotic laxative. It is now usually given with sodium bicarbonate as a suppository in a dose of about 1 g for the treatment of constipation (p.1168) and, more commonly, for bowel evacuation before investigational procedures or surgery. Carbon dioxide gas is produced in the rectum which stimulates defaecation within 10 to 30 minutes. Potassium tartrate (see p.1161) was also used as an osmotic laxative.

Potassium acid tartrate is used as a food additive and pharmaceutical aid.

Potassium acid tartrate has been used as an ingredient of preparations for potassium supplementation, although other potassium salts are usually preferred. For the general properties of potassium salts, see p.1161.

Preparations

BPC 1968: Effervescent Potassium Tablets.

Proprietary Preparations (details are given in Part 3)

Multi-ingredient: ***Aust.:*** Lecicarbon; ***Belg.:*** Suppolax†; ***Ital.:*** Potassion; ***Mon.:*** Eductyl; ***Swed.:*** Relaxit; ***USA:*** Ceo-Two; Evac-Q-Sert.

Proglumide (705-n)

Proglumide *(BAN, USAN, rINN)*.

CR-242; W-5219; Xylamide. (±)-4-Benzamido-*N*,*N*-dipropylglutaramic acid.

$C_{18}H_{26}N_2O_4$ = 334.4.

CAS — 6620-60-6.

Pharmacopoeias. In *Jpn.*

Proglumide is a cholecystokinin antagonist with an inhibitory effect on gastric secretion. It is used in the treatment of peptic ulcer disease (p.1174) and other gastro-intestinal disorders in usual doses of 400 mg three or four times daily by mouth before meals; it has also been given by intramuscular or by slow intravenous injection.

Proglumide has been reported to inhibit stimulation of cancer cell lines by gastrin *in vitro* and *vivo*[1] and to inhibit pancreatic cancer growth in experimental models.[2] However, a randomised, controlled study[3] involving 110 patients with gastric carcinoma found that proglumide 800 mg four times daily by mouth produced no significant difference in survival time compared to placebo. Sixteen patients ceased therapy with proglumide due to adverse effects, most commonly nausea, vomiting, or general malaise. Proglumide has a relatively low affinity for the gastrin receptor and also has partial agonist activity and it was concluded that more specific and potent gastrin-receptor antagonists were required to achieve an antineoplastic effect.

1. Morris DL, *et al.* Hormonal control of gastric and colorectal cancer in man. *Gut* 1989; **30:** 425–9.
2. Carter DC. Cancer of the pancreas. *Gut* 1990; **31:** 494–6.
3. Harrison JD, *et al.* The effect of the gastrin receptor antagonist proglumide on survival in gastric carcinoma. *Cancer* 1990; **66:** 1449–52.

Preparations

Proprietary Preparations (details are given in Part 3)
Aust.: Milid; ***Ger.:*** Milid; ***Ital.:*** Milid; ***S.Afr.:*** Milid†.

Prune (7526-p)

Ameixa; Prunus.

The dried ripe fruits of *Prunus domestica* and some other species of *Prunus* (Rosaceae).

Prune has laxative and demulcent properties. It is used as a food.

Preparations

Proprietary Preparations (details are given in Part 3)

Multi-ingredient: ***Austral.:*** Neo-Cleanse; Prolax; ***Canad.:*** Fruitatives; ***Ital.:*** Cruscaprugna Dietetica†; ***S.Afr.:*** Misfans†; ***Spain:*** Jarabe Manzanas Siken; ***Switz.:*** Falqui.

Rabeprazole (17310-p)

Rabeprazole *(BAN, rINN)*.

E-3810 (rabeprazole sodium); LY-307640; Pariprazole. 2-({[4-(3-Methoxypropoxy)-3-methyl-2-pyridyl]methyl}sulfinyl)-1*H*-benzimidazole.

$C_{18}H_{21}N_3O_3S$ = 359.4.

CAS — 117976-89-3 (rabeprazole); 117976-90-6 (rabeprazole sodium).

NOTE. Rabeprazole Sodium is *USAN.*

Rabeprazole is a proton pump inhibitor with properties similar to those of omeprazole (p.1204). Rabeprazole sodium is used in the treatment of peptic ulcer disease and gastro-oesophageal reflux disease in usual doses of 20 mg daily.

References.

1. Prakash A, Faulds D. Rabeprazole. *Drugs* 1998; **55:** 261–7.

Preparations

Proprietary Preparations (details are given in Part 3)
UK: Pariet.

Ramosetron (17443-r)

Ramosetron *(rINN)*.

(−)-(*R*)-1-Methylindol-3-yl 4,5,6,7-tetrahydro-5-benzimidazolyl ketone.

$C_{17}H_{17}N_3O$ = 279.3.

CAS — 132036-88-5.

Ramosetron is a 5-HT_3-receptor antagonist with general properties similar to those of ondansetron (see p.1206). It is used for its antiemetic properties and has been tried in the irritable bowel syndrome.

Ranitidine Hydrochloride (6162-e)

Ranitidine Hydrochloride *(BANM, rINNM)*.

AH-19065; Ranitidini Hydrochloridum. *NN*-Dimethyl-5-[2-(1-methylamino-2-nitrovinylamino)ethylthiomethyl]furfurylamine hydrochloride.

$C_{13}H_{22}N_4O_3S,HCl$ = 350.9.

CAS — 66357-35-5 (ranitidine); 66357-59-3 (ranitidine hydrochloride).

NOTE. Ranitidine is *USAN.*

Pharmacopoeias. In *Chin., Eur.* (see p.viii), and *US.*

A white to pale yellow, practically odourless, crystalline powder sensitive to moisture. It is polymorphic. Freely or very **soluble** in water; moderately soluble in alcohol; very slightly soluble in dichloromethane; freely soluble in methyl alcohol; sparingly soluble in dehydrated alcohol and in chloroform. A 1% solution in water has a pH of 4.5 to 6.0.

Store in airtight containers. Protect from light.

Stability and incompatibility. References.

1. Galante LJ, *et al.* Stability of ranitidine hydrochloride at dilute concentration in intravenous infusion fluids at room temperature. *Am J Hosp Pharm* 1990; **47:** 1580–4.
2. Stewart JT, *et al.* Stability of ranitidine in intravenous admixtures stored frozen, refrigerated, and at room temperature. *Am J Hosp Pharm* 1990; **47:** 2043–6.
3. Chilvers MR, Lysne JM. Visual compatibility of ranitidine hydrochloride with commonly used critical-care medications. *Am J Hosp Pharm* 1989; **46:** 2057–8.
4. Galante LJ, *et al.* Stability of ranitidine hydrochloride with eight medications in intravenous admixtures. *Am J Hosp Pharm* 1990; **47:** 1606–10.
5. Wohlford JG, *et al.* More information on the visual compatibility of hetastarch with injectable critical-care drugs. *Am J Hosp Pharm* 1990; **47:** 297–8.
6. Williams MF, *et al.* In vitro evaluation of the stability of ranitidine hydrochloride in total parenteral nutrition mixtures. *Am J Hosp Pharm* 1990; **47:** 1574–9.
7. Montoro JB, Pou L. Comment on stability of ranitidine hydrochloride in total nutrient admixtures. *Am J Hosp Pharm* 1991; **48:** 2384.
8. Stewart JT, *et al.* Stability of ranitidine hydrochloride and seven medications. *Am J Hosp Pharm* 1994; **51:** 1802–7.
9. Crowther RS, *et al.* In vitro stability of ranitidine hydrochloride in enteral nutrient formulas. *Ann Pharmacother* 1995; **29:** 859–62.

Adverse Effects

As for Cimetidine, p.1183. However, unlike cimetidine, ranitidine has little or no anti-androgenic effect, although there have been isolated reports of gynaecomastia and impotence.

General references.

1. Wormsley KG. Safety profile of ranitidine: a review. *Drugs* 1993; **46:** 976–85.

Carcinogenicity. For a discussion of the possible association between histamine H_2-receptor antagonists and cancer, including mention of a study with ranitidine, see Cimetidine, p.1183.

Effects on the blood. For a discussion of the adverse haematological effects of histamine H_2-receptor antagonists, see Cimetidine, p.1183.

Effects on body temperature. A report[1] of pyrexia associated with ranitidine. Apart from raised temperature the patient was otherwise well; fever resolved on discontinuation and recurred on rechallenge with ranitidine.

1. Kavanagh GM, *et al.* Ranitidine fever. *Lancet* 1993; **341:** 1422.

Effects on bones and joints. See under Cimetidine, p.1183.

Effects on the cardiovascular system. Bradycardia,[1,2] atrioventricular block,[2] and cardiac arrest[3] have been reported rarely during ranitidine therapy; a positive inotropic effect, without significant changes in heart rate or blood pressure, has also been reported in healthy subjects[4] and pretreatment with ranitidine has blocked the cardiac depressant effects seen in some subjects given famotidine or nizatidine.[5] Although studies in critically ill patients[6] and healthy subjects[7,8] have found no adverse haemodynamic effects associated with ranitidine, it is likely that a small proportion of patients are more susceptible to the cardiovascular effects of ranitidine and caution is recommended in patients with cardiovascular disease or renal impairment.

1. Johnson WS, Miller DR. Ranitidine and bradycardia. *Ann Intern Med* 1988; **108:** 493.
2. Tanner LA, Arrowsmith JB. Bradycardia and H_2 antagonists. *Ann Intern Med* 1988; **109:** 434–5.
3. Hart AM. Cardiac arrest associated with ranitidine. *Br Med J* 1989; **299:** 519.
4. Meyer EC, *et al.* Inotropic effects of ranitidine. *Eur J Clin Pharmacol* 1990; **39:** 301–3.
5. Mescheder A, *et al.* Changes in the effects of nizatidine and famotidine on cardiac performance after pretreatment with ranitidine. *Eur J Clin Pharmacol* 1993; **45:** 151–6.
6. Vohra SB, *et al.* The haemodynamic effects of ranitidine injected centrally in optimally resuscitated patients. *Br J Hosp Med* 1989; **42:** 149.
7. Hughes DG, *et al.* Cardiovascular effects of H_2-receptor antagonists. *J Clin Pharmacol* 1989; **29:** 472–7.
8. Hilleman DE, *et al.* Impact of chronic oral H_2-antagonist therapy on left ventricular systolic function and exercise capacity. *J Clin Pharmacol* 1992; **32:** 1033–7.

Effects on the endocrine system. Unlike cimetidine, ranitidine does not bind to androgen receptors and has little, if any, anti-androgenic effect. Studies in males taking ranitidine for the management of duodenal ulcer[1,2] reported no significant changes in the plasma concentrations of testosterone, luteinising hormone, follicle-stimulating hormone, or prolactin after up to 2 years of treatment; no significant changes in sperm concentration, motility, or morphology were noted.[1] There have been isolated reports of gynaecomastia,[3] loss of libido,[4] and impotence[5] associated with ranitidine, but in 9 patients with cimetidine-induced breast changes and impotence, transfer to ranitidine resulted in resolution of these symptoms.[6]

1. Wang C, *et al.* Ranitidine does not affect gonadal function in man. *Br J Clin Pharmacol* 1983; **16:** 430–2.
2. Knigge U, *et al.* Plasma concentrations of pituitary and peripheral hormones during ranitidine treatment for two years in men with duodenal ulcer. *Eur J Clin Pharmacol* 1989; **37:** 305–7.
3. Tosi S, Cagnoli M. Painful gynaecomastia with ranitidine. *Lancet* 1982; **i:** 160.
4. Smith RN, Elsdon-Dew RW. Alleged impotence with ranitidine. *Lancet* 1983; **ii:** 798.
5. Kassianos GC. Impotence and nizatidine. *Lancet* 1989; **i:** 963.
6. Jensen RT, *et al.* Cimetidine-induced impotence and breast changes in patients with gastric hypersecretory states. *N Engl J Med* 1983; **308:** 883–7.

Effects on the eyes. For a report of an increase in intra-ocular pressure associated with ranitidine, see under Cimetidine, p.1184. A cohort study involving 140 128 patients receiving anti-ulcer therapy, 70 389 of whom received ranitidine, found no evidence that any of the drugs studied were associated with a major increased risk of vascular or inflammatory disorders of the eye.[1]

1. García Rodríguez LA, *et al.* A cohort study of the ocular safety of anti-ulcer drugs. *Br J Clin Pharmacol* 1996; **42:** 213–16.

Effects on the liver. There have been some case reports of ranitidine hepatotoxicity.[1] However, as mentioned under Cimetidine, p.1184, the increase in relative risk seen in a large cohort study involving 108 891 patients receiving antisecretory therapy was much less for ranitidine (1.7:1) than for cimetidine.

1. Souza Lima MA. Ranitidine and hepatic injury. *Ann Intern Med* 1986; **105:** 140.

Effects on the nervous system. Ranitidine has been associated with a number of adverse neurological effects including confusion,[1-8] loss of colour vision,[4] aggressiveness,[2,4,6] lethargy,[8] somnolence,[8] disorientation,[8] depression,[8] hallucinations,[1,7-9] and severe headache.[10] As with cimetidine these reactions occur mainly in the elderly, the severely ill, or patients with renal or hepatic impairment. Single-dose studies in young healthy subjects have found no adverse changes in performance, central nervous system function, or subjective assessment of mood after administration of ranitidine 150 or 300 mg by mouth.[11]

1. Hughes JD, *et al.* Mental confusion associated with ranitidine. *Med J Aust* 1983; **2:** 12–13.
2. Silverstone PH. Ranitidine and confusion. *Lancet* 1984; **i:** 1071.
3. Epstein CM. Ranitidine and confusion. *Lancet* 1984; **i:** 1071.
4. De Giacomo C, *et al.* Ranitidine and loss of colour vision in a child. *Lancet* 1984; **ii:** 47.
5. Mani RB, *et al.* H_2-receptor blockers and mental confusion. *Lancet* 1984; **ii:** 98.
6. Mandal SK. Psychiatric side effects of ranitidine. *Br J Clin Pract* 1986; **40:** 260.
7. MacDermott AJ, *et al.* Acute confusional episodes during treatment with ranitidine. *Br Med J* 1987; **294:** 1616.
8. Slugg PH, *et al.* Ranitidine pharmacokinetics and adverse central nervous system reactions. *Arch Intern Med* 1992; **152:** 2325–9.
9. Price W, *et al.* Ranitidine-associated hallucinations. *Eur J Clin Pharmacol* 1985; **29:** 375–6.
10. Epstein CM. Ranitidine. *N Engl J Med* 1984; **310:** 1602.
11. Nicholson AN, Stone BM. The H_2-antagonists, cimetidine and ranitidine: studies on performance. *Eur J Clin Pharmacol* 1984; **26:** 579–82.

Effects on the skin. A report of vasculitic rash occurring in three patients undergoing ranitidine therapy.[1] In each case the rash cleared following withdrawal of the drug.

For further information on the effects of ranitidine on the skin, see under Hypersensitivity, below, and for a lack of effect see under Effects on the Skin in Cimetidine, p.1184.

1. Haboubi N, Asquith P. Rash mediated by immune complexes associated with ranitidine treatment. *Br Med J* 1988; **296:** 897.

Hypersensitivity. Respiratory stridor and an urticarial rash in one patient occurred shortly after taking the first dose of ranitidine;[1] the symptoms responded to adrenaline subcutaneously.

1. Brayko CM. Ranitidine. *N Engl J Med* 1984; **310:** 1601–2.

Meningitis. Aseptic meningitis developed on 3 occasions following administration of ranitidine to a 30-year-old man.[1] In each case symptoms resolved rapidly on withdrawal of the drug.

1. Durand JM, *et al.* Ranitidine and aseptic meningitis. *Br Med J* 1996; **312:** 886. Correction. *ibid.*; 1392.

Parotitis. Recurrent parotitis occurred in a patient when given ranitidine or cimetidine.[1]

1. Caraman P, *et al.* Recurrent parotitis with H_2 receptor antagonists. *Lancet* 1986; **ii:** 1455–6.

Precautions

As for Cimetidine, p.1185.

Cardiovascular disorders. For a caution on the use of ranitidine in patients with cardiovascular disease, see Effects on the Cardiovascular System under Adverse Effects, above.

Hepatic impairment. Sixteen of 27 patients with cirrhosis of the liver and indications for treatment with an H_2-antagonist (peptic ulcer, gastritis, or reflux oesophagitis) failed to respond to ranitidine 300 mg compared with 6 failures from 32 patients without cirrhosis. Famotidine 40 mg was given to 10 of the cirrhotic non-responders and 8 still exhibited no response; 7 of these patients were given cimetidine 800 mg and only 1 responded. In the control group, all 3 patients given famotidine did not respond and only 1 responded when given cimetidine. It was concluded that the incidence of non-response to H_2-antagonists is increased in patients with liver cirrhosis but no explanation could be given for this effect.[1] Interestingly there is an earlier report of patients with cirrhosis demonstrating increased bioavailability and decreased clearance of ranitidine.[2]

1. Walker S, *et al.* Frequent non-response to histamine H_2-receptor antagonists in cirrhotics. *Gut* 1989; **30:** 1105–9.
2. Young CJ, *et al.* Effects of cirrhosis and ageing on the elimination and bioavailability of ranitidine. *Gut* 1982; **23:** 819–23.

Renal impairment. A study in patients with varying degrees of renal impairment[1] found that mean terminal half-life was increased from 2.09 hours in subjects with normal renal function to between 4.23 and 8.45 hours in patients with renal impairment, the degree of prolongation being proportional to the degree of impairment as measured by glomerular filtration rate. As a result of these findings it was recommended that the dose of ranitidine should be halved in patients with a glomerular filtration rate of 20 mL per minute or less. Ranitidine 150 mg daily provided adequate serum concentrations without excessive accumulation in 20 patients undergoing regular haemodialysis.[2] The serum-ranitidine concentrations fell by about 50% during a 4-hour haemodialysis session but less than 3% of the administered dose was removed and supplemental doses after dialysis were considered unnecessary.

1. Dixon JS, *et al.* The effect of renal function on the pharmacokinetics of ranitidine. *Eur J Clin Pharmacol* 1994; **46:** 167–71.
2. Comstock TJ, *et al.* Ranitidine accumulation in patients undergoing chronic hemodialysis. *J Clin Pharmacol* 1988; **28:** 1081–5.

Interactions

Unlike cimetidine (p.1185) ranitidine does not seem to affect cytochrome P450 to any great extent, and therefore is considered to have little effect on the metabolism of other drugs. The absorption of ranitidine is reported to be impaired by the concomitant administration of sucralfate.

A review comparing the drug interactions of ranitidine with those of cimetidine.[1]

1. Smith SR, Kendall MJ. Ranitidine versus cimetidine: a comparison of their potential to cause clinically important drug interactions. *Clin Pharmacokinet* 1988; **15:** 44–56.

Cisapride. Peak plasma concentrations of ranitidine were achieved significantly more rapidly in 12 healthy subjects who took cisapride concomitantly.[1]

1. Rowbotham DJ, *et al.* Effect of single doses of cisapride and ranitidine administered simultaneously on plasma concentrations of cisapride and ranitidine. *Br J Anaesth* 1991; **67:** 302–305.

Pharmacokinetics

Ranitidine is readily absorbed from the gastro-intestinal tract with peak concentrations in plasma occurring about 2 to 3 hours after administration by mouth. Food does not significantly impair absorption of ranitidine. The bioavailability of ranitidine following oral administration is about 50% due to first-pass metabolism. Ranitidine is rapidly absorbed following intramuscular injection and has a bioavailability of about 90 to 100%. The elimination half-life from plasma is around 2 to 3 hours and ranitidine is weakly bound, about 15%, to plasma proteins.

A small proportion of ranitidine is metabolised in the liver to the N-oxide, the S-oxide, and desmethylranitidine; the N-oxide is the major metabolite but accounts for only about 4% of a dose. Approximately 30% of an oral dose and 70% of an intravenous dose is excreted unchanged in the urine by active transport in 24 hours; there is some excretion in the faeces. Clearance is markedly reduced in severe renal impairment. Ranitidine crosses the placental barrier and is distributed into breast milk. It does not readily cross the blood-brain barrier but adverse effects on the CNS have been reported (see above).

Reviews.

1. Lauritsen K, *et al.* Clinical pharmacokinetics of drugs used in the treatment of gastrointestinal diseases. *Clin Pharmacokinet* 1990; **19:** 11–31 and 94–125.

Distribution into breast milk. Pharmacokinetic study in a lactating mother given multiple doses of ranitidine showed higher concentrations in breast milk than in serum; the minimum milk concentration occurred between 1 and 2 hours after maternal drug administration and the highest concentration was towards the end of the 12-hour dosing interval.[1] It was not clear that there were any clinical implications since the dose that would be ingested by the neonate could not be reliably estimated, although it would be reduced if feeding took place 1 to 2 hours after maternal administration.

1. Kearns GL, *et al.* Appearance of ranitidine in breast milk following multiple dosing. *Clin Pharm* 1985; **4:** 322–4.

Enterohepatic recycling. Some individuals exhibit a second peak in the plasma concentration of ranitidine which could be due to enterohepatic recirculation. However, only 0.7 to 2.6% and 0.3 to 1.0% of a dose of ranitidine was excreted into the bile of 3 patients in 24 hours following 50 mg intravenously or 300 mg by mouth indicating that significant recirculation did not occur.[1]

1. Klotz U, Walker S. Biliary excretion of H_2-receptor antagonists. *Eur J Clin Pharmacol* 1990; **39:** 91–2.

Neonatal pharmacokinetics. Blood samples taken from 27 full-term newborn infants given a single intravenous dose of 2.4 mg of ranitidine per kg body-weight revealed the following pharmacokinetic data: elimination half-life, 207.1 minutes; total volume of distribution, 1.52 litres per kg; total plasma clearance, 5.02 mL per kg per minute.[1] None of the infants had renal or hepatic impairment.

1. Fontana M, *et al.* Ranitidine pharmacokinetics in newborn infants. *Arch Dis Child* 1993; **68:** 602–3.

Uses and Administration

Ranitidine is a histamine H_2-receptor antagonist with actions and uses similar to those of cimetidine (p.1185).

Ranitidine may be given by mouth or parenterally by the intravenous or intramuscular routes. Although most preparations contain ranitidine hydrochloride, strengths and doses are expressed in terms of the base.

Depending on the condition being treated the usual dose of ranitidine by mouth is 300 mg once daily or 150 mg twice daily. The usual dose by intramuscular or intravenous injection is 50 mg which may be repeated every 6 to 8 hours; the intravenous injection should be given slowly over not less than 2 minutes and should be diluted to contain 50 mg in 20 mL. For an intermittent intravenous infusion the recommended dose in the UK is 25 mg per hour given for 2 hours which may be repeated every 6 to 8 hours. A rate of 6.25 mg per hour has been suggested for continuous intravenous infusion although higher rates may be employed for conditions such as Zollinger-Ellison syndrome or in patients at risk from stress ulceration (see below). The dosage of ranitidine should be reduced in patients with severely impaired renal function; in the UK the suggested doses for those with several renal impairment are 150 mg daily by mouth or 25 mg for parenteral administration.

In the management of benign **gastric** and **duodenal ulceration** a single daily dose of 300 mg by mouth at bedtime or 150 mg twice daily (in the morning and at bedtime) is recommended, given initially for at least 4 weeks. A dose of 300 mg twice daily may also be used. Where appropriate a maintenance dose of 150 mg daily may be given at bedtime. Ranitidine 150 mg twice daily may be given during therapy with nonsteroidal anti-inflammatory drugs for prophylaxis against duodenal ulceration. A suggested dose for the treatment of peptic ulcer in children is 2 to 4 mg per kg body-weight twice daily to a maximum of 300 mg in 24 hours.

For duodenal ulcer associated with *Helicobacter pylori* infection ranitidine in a usual dose of 300 mg once daily or 150 mg twice daily by mouth may be given in combination with amoxycillin 750 mg and metronidazole 500 mg, both three times daily, for 2 weeks. Therapy with ranitidine should then be continued for a further 2 weeks.

In **gastro-oesophageal reflux disease** the recommended dose is 150 mg twice daily by mouth or 300 mg at bedtime for up to 8 weeks or, if required, 12 weeks. This may be increased to 150 mg four times daily for up to 12 weeks in severe cases. In pathological hypersecretory conditions, such as the **Zollinger-Ellison syndrome**, the initial oral dose is usually 150 mg twice or three times daily and may be increased if necessary; doses of up to 6 g daily have been employed. Alternatively, an intravenous infusion may be given, initially at a rate of 1 mg per kg body-weight per hour; the rate may be increased by increments of 0.5 mg per kg per hour, beginning after 4 hours, if required.

For the management of patients at risk from **stress ulceration** of the upper gastro-intestinal tract parenteral therapy may be employed in the form of slow intravenous injection of a 50-mg priming dose followed by a continuous intravenous infusion of 0.125 to 0.25 mg per kg body-weight per hour. Doses of 150 mg twice daily by mouth may be given once oral feeding is resumed.

In patients at risk of developing the **acid aspiration syndrome** during general anaesthesia, a dose of 150 mg by mouth may be given 2 hours before the induction of anaesthesia and preferably also 150 mg the previous evening. At the start of labour a dose of 150 mg by mouth may be given and may be repeated at intervals of 6 hours if required; alternatively a dose of 50 mg may be given by intramuscular or slow intravenous injection 45 to 60 minutes before the induction of anaesthesia.

In patients with chronic episodic **dyspepsia**, a dose of 150 mg twice daily by mouth for up to 6 weeks may be given. For the short-term symptomatic relief of dyspepsia a dose of 75 mg, repeated if necessary up to a maximum of 4 doses daily, may be taken. Treatment should be restricted to a maximum of 2 weeks' continuous use at one time.

Reviews.

1. Grant SM, *et al.* Ranitidine: an updated review of its pharmacodynamic and pharmacokinetic properties and therapeutic use in peptic ulcer disease and other allied diseases. *Drugs* 1989; **37:** 801–70.

Administration in children. The disposition of ranitidine in children is not significantly different from that in young adults and a dose of 2 mg per kg body-weight (approximately equal to an adult dose of 150 mg) by mouth has been used for the prevention of acid aspiration in children. Doses of 2, 3, or 4 mg per kg every 12 hours by mouth have been used in infants with gastro-oesophageal reflux disease but a regimen of 2 mg per kg every 8 hours was significantly more effective at raising intragastric pH.[1,2] Ranitidine 200 μg per kg per hour, given intravenously for 37 hours, controlled severe gastro-intestinal bleeding in a premature anuric infant, but the dose was considered excessive since accumulation occurred with a plasma-ranitidine concentration of 1390 ng per mL 7 hours after the end of the infusion.[3] Another study in premature infants being treated with dexamethasone for bronchopulmonary dysplasia found that infusion of ranitidine 62.5 μg per kg per hour was sufficient to raise and maintain gastric pH above 4 to help protect against gastro-intestinal bleeding and perforation.[4]

1. Christensen S, *et al.* Effects of ranitidine and metoclopramide on gastric fluid pH and volume in children. *Br J Anaesth* 1990; **65:** 456–60.
2. Sutphen JL, Dillard VL. Effect of ranitidine on twenty-four-hour gastric acidity in infants. *J Pediatr* 1989; **114:** 472–4.
3. Rosenthal M, Miller PW. Ranitidine in the newborn. *Arch Dis Child* 1988; **63:** 88–9.
4. Kelly EJ, *et al.* The effect of intravenous ranitidine on the intragastric pH of preterm infants receiving dexamethasone. *Arch Dis Child* 1993; **69:** 37–9.

Cystic fibrosis. Although cisapride (p.1188) has been successfully used to treat signs of decreased gastro-intestinal motility in patients with cystic fibrosis, a comparative study involving 29 such patients found that ranitidine was more effective than cisapride in improving dyspeptic symptoms and gastric emptying and distension.[1]

For a discussion of cystic fibrosis and its broader management see p.119. Antisecretory drugs are also used in this condition to decrease the inactivation of orally administered pancreatic enzymes.

1. Cucchiara S, *et al.* Ultrasound measurement of gastric emptying time in patients with cystic fibrosis and effect of ranitidine on delayed gastric emptying. *J Pediatr* 1996; **128:** 485–8.

Eczema. Ranitidine 300 mg twice daily by mouth has been reported to be of benefit as an adjuvant to local treatment with corticosteroids and a moisturising ointment in patients with atopic dermatitis.[1] The conventional management of eczema is discussed on p.1073.

1. Veien NK, *et al.* Ranitidine treatment of hand eczema in patients with atopic dermatitis: a double-blind placebo-controlled trial. *J Am Acad Dermatol* 1995; **32:** 1056–7.

Psoriasis. There are reports of improvements in psoriasis following administration of ranitidine,[1-3] although this is a field that is notoriously difficult to evaluate because of the chronic relapsing and remitting nature of the disease, and others have failed to show benefit.[4] For a discussion of psoriasis and the usual drugs used in its management, see p.1075.

1. Witkamp L, *et al.* An open prospective clinical trial with systemic ranitidine in the treatment of psoriasis. *J Am Acad Dermatol* 1993; **28:** 778–81.
2. Smith KC. Ranitidine useful in the management of psoriasis in a patient with acquired immunodeficiency syndrome. *Int J Dermatol* 1994; **33:** 220–1.
3. Kristensen JK, *et al.* Systemic high-dose ranitidine in the treatment of psoriasis: an open prospective clinical trial. *Br J Dermatol* 1995; **133:** 905–8.
4. Çetin L, *et al.* High-dose ranitidine is ineffective in the treatment of psoriasis. *Br J Dermatol* 1997; **137:** 1021–2.

Urticaria. Histamine H_2-receptor antagonists, including ranitidine, have been tried in the management of urticaria as discussed on p.1076.

Preparations

BP 1998: Ranitidine Injection; Ranitidine Oral Solution; Ranitidine Tablets;
USP 23: Ranitidine in Sodium Chloride Injection; Ranitidine Injection; Ranitidine Oral Solution; Ranitidine Tablets.

Proprietary Preparations (details are given in Part 3)
Aust.: Digestosan; Ulsal; Zantac; ***Austral.:*** Rani 2; Zantac; ***Belg.:*** Ranic; Zantac; ***Canad.:*** Novo-Ranidine; Nu-Ranit; Zantac; ***Fr.:*** Azantac; Raniplex; ***Ger.:*** Azuranit; Rani; Rani-nerton; Raniberl; Ranibeta; Ranibloc; Ranicux; Ranidura; Ranimerck; Raniprotect; Ranitic; Sostril; Ulcolind Rani; Zantic; ***Irl.:*** Gertac; Xanomel; Zandine; Zantac; ***Ital.:*** Mauran†; Nodol†; Raniben; Ranibloc; Ranidil; Trigger; Ulcex; Ulkobrin†; Zantac; ***Neth.:*** Zantac; ***Norw.:*** Noktone; Ranacid; Zantac; ***S.Afr.:*** Zantac; ***Spain:*** Coralen; Quantor; Ran H2; Ranidin; Ranilonga; Ranix; Ranuber; Rubiulcer; Tanidina; Terposen; Toriol; Zantac; ***Swed.:*** Artonil; Rani-Q; Zantac; ***Switz.:*** Zantic; ***UK:*** Ranaps; Rantec; Zaedoc; Zantac; ***USA:*** Zantac.

Ranitidine Bismutrex (15497-t)

A complex of ranitidine and bismuth citrate; GR-122311X; Ranitidine Bismuth Citrate *(BAN, USAN)*. *N*-[2-({5-[(Dimethylamino)methyl]furfuryl}thio)-ethyl]-*N'*-methyl-2-nitro-1,1-ethenediamine, compound with bismuth(3+) citrate (1:1).

$C_{13}H_{22}N_4O_3S,C_6H_5BiO_7$ = 712.5.

CAS — 128345-62-0.

Adverse Effects and Precautions

Ranitidine bismutrex would be expected to combine the adverse effects of bismuth compounds (see p.1180) with those of ranitidine (p.1209). Blackening of the tongue and stool, gastro-intestinal disturbances, headache, hypersensitivity reactions (including anaphylaxis), mild anaemia, and altered liver enzyme values have been reported.

Ranitidine bismutrex should not be given to patients with severely impaired renal function. It is not suitable for long-term or maintenance therapy because of the risk of bismuth accumulation.

Pharmacokinetics

Following oral administration, ranitidine bismutrex dissociates into its ranitidine and bismuth components in the stomach. Only about 1% of the bismuth dose administered is absorbed and subsequently slowly excreted, mainly in the urine, with a plasma elimination half-life of at least 5 to 10 days. Some accumulation of bismuth occurs in plasma on repeated dosage with ranitidine bismutrex.

For the pharmacokinetics of ranitidine, see p.1210.

References.

1. Lacey LF, *et al.* Comparative pharmacokinetics of bismuth from ranitidine bismuth citrate (GR122311X), a novel anti-ulcerant and tripotassium dicitrato bismuthate (TDB). *Eur J Clin Pharmacol* 1994; **47:** 177–80.
2. Koch KM, *et al.* Pharmacokinetics of bismuth and ranitidine following single doses of ranitidine bismuth citrate. *Br J Clin Pharmacol* 1996; **42:** 201–5.
3. Koch KM, *et al.* Pharmacokinetics of bismuth and ranitidine following multiple doses of ranitidine bismuth citrate. *Br J Clin Pharmacol* 1996; **42:** 207–11.

Uses and Administration

Ranitidine bismutrex is a complex of ranitidine with bismuth and citrate, which releases ranitidine and bismuth in the gastro-intestinal tract and therefore possesses both the actions of the bismuth compounds (see p.1181) and of ranitidine (p.1210). It is used in the management of peptic ulcer disease (p.1174), and may be given in combination with antibiotics for the eradication of *Helicobacter pylori* infection and the prevention of relapse of duodenal ulcer.

Doses are 400 mg twice daily by mouth; treatment is usually given for 4 to 8 weeks for duodenal ulceration and for 8 weeks for benign gastric ulceration. For duodenal ulceration where *H.pylori* infection is present, ranitidine bismutrex may be combined with amoxycillin 500 mg four times daily, or clarithromycin 250 mg four times daily or 500 mg three times daily. The antibiotic should be given for 2 weeks, and ranitidine bismutrex alone continued for a further 2 weeks.

References.

1. Bardhan KD, *et al.* GR122311X (ranitidine bismuth citrate), a new drug for the treatment of duodenal ulcer. *Aliment Pharmacol Ther* 1995; **9:** 497–506.
2. Peterson WL, *et al.* Ranitidine bismuth citrate plus clarithromycin is effective for healing duodenal ulcers, eradicating H.pylori and reducing ulcer recurrence. *Aliment Pharmacol Ther* 1996; **10:** 251–61.
3. Anonymous. Pylorid, H.pylori and peptic ulcer. *Drug Ther Bull* 1996; **34:** 69–70.

Preparations

Proprietary Preparations (details are given in Part 3)
Aust.: Helirad; Pylorisin; ***Irl.:*** Pylorid; ***Ital.:*** Elicodil; Pylorid; ***Neth.:*** Pylorid; ***UK:*** Pylorid; ***USA:*** Tritec.

Rebamipide (11045-v)

Rebamipide *(rINN)*.

(±)-α-(*p*-Chlorobenzamido)-1,2-dihydro-2-oxo-4-quinolinepropionic acid.

$C_{19}H_{15}ClN_2O_4$ = 370.8.

CAS — 90098-04-7 (was 111911-87-6).

Rebamipide is stated to possess cytoprotective properties and is used in the treatment of peptic ulcer disease (p.1174) and gastritis in usual doses of 100 mg by mouth three times daily.

Preparations

Proprietary Preparations (details are given in Part 3)
Jpn: Mucosta.

Renzapride (3382-f)

Renzapride *(BAN, rINN)*.

BRL-24924A (hydrochloride). (±)-*endo*-4-Amino-*N*-(1-azabicyclo[3.3.1]non-4-yl)-5-chloro-*o*-anisamide.

$C_{16}H_{22}ClN_3O_2$ = 323.8.

CAS — 88721-77-1 (racemate); 112727-80-7.

Renzapride is a substituted benzamide which stimulates gastro-intestinal motility. It has 5-HT_3-receptor antagonist activity.

It is being investigated, mainly as the hydrochloride, in the management of gastro-intestinal disorders.

References.

1. Robertson CS, *et al*. A double-blind dose ranging study of BRL 24924 and metoclopramide on lower oesophageal sphincter pressure in healthy volunteers. *Br J Clin Pharmacol* 1989; **28:** 323–7.
2. Mackie A, *et al*. BRL 24924, a novel prokinetic agent, potentially valuable in diabetic gastroparesis. *Gut* 1989; **30:** A1489.
3. Staniforth DH, Pennick M. Human pharmacology of renzapride: a new gastrokinetic benzamide without dopamine antagonist properties. *Eur J Clin Pharmacol* 1990; **38:** 161–4.
4. Mackie ADR, *et al*. The effects of renzapride, a novel prokinetic agent, in diabetic gastroparesis. *Aliment Pharmacol Ther* 1991; **5:** 135–42.

Rhubarb (7527-s)

Chinese Rhubarb; Rabarbaro; Rhabarber; Rhei Radix; Rhei Rhizoma; Rheum; Rhubarb Rhizome; Ruibarbo.

Pharmacopoeias. In *Chin.*, *Eur.* (see p.viii), *Jpn*, and *Pol. Chin.* also permits *R. tanguticum* and *Jpn* also permits *R. coreanum*. .

The dried underground parts of *Rheum palmatum* or *R. officinale* (Polygonaceae) or hybrids of these species, or mixtures of these, separated from the stem, rootlets, and most of the bark. The Ph. Eur. specifies not less than 2.2% of hydroxyanthracene derivatives, calculated as rhein ($C_{15}H_8O_6$=284.2). **Protect** from light.

Other rhubarbs include Indian rhubarb (Himalayan rhubarb), the dried rhizome and roots of *R. emodi*, *R. webbianum*, or some other species of *Rheum*, and an adulterant of rhubarb known as rhapontic rhubarb (Chinese rhapontica), obtained from *R. rhaponticum*. English rhubarb is derived from *R. rhaponticum* and other species of *Rheum*.

Adverse Effects and Precautions

As for Senna, p.1212.

Uses and Administration

Rhubarb is an anthraquinone stimulant laxative. It also exerts an astringent action due to the presence of tannins.

It is used in homoeopathic medicine when it is known as Rheum.

The leaf-stalks of garden rhubarb (*R.rhaponticum*) are used as a food.

Preparations

BP 1998: Compound Rhubarb Tincture.

Proprietary Preparations

Multi-ingredient: numerous preparations are listed in Part 3.

Roxatidine Acetate Hydrochloride (2430-g)

Roxatidine Acetate Hydrochloride *(BANM, USAN, rINNM)*.

HOE-062 (roxatidine); HOE-760 (roxatidine acetate hydrochloride); TZU-0460 (roxatidine acetate hydrochloride). *N*-{3-[(α-Piperidino-*m*-tolyl)oxy]propyl}glycolamide acetate monohydrochloride.

$C_{17}H_{26}N_2O_3,C_2H_2O,HCl$ = 384.9.

CAS — 97900-88-4 (roxatidine); 78628-28-1 (roxatidine acetate); 93793-83-0 (roxatidine acetate hydrochloride).

Adverse Effects and Precautions

As for Cimetidine, p.1183.

Administration in renal impairment. Preliminary results in 6 patients with chronic renal failure and creatinine clearance less than 20 mL per minute indicated that administration of the recommended dose of roxatidine acetate hydrochloride, 75 mg every other day, was inadequate to maintain gastric pH above 4 for more than 6 hours. Subsequent study in 8 patients showed that a dose of 75 mg daily was well tolerated and effective.[1]

1. Gladziwa U, *et al*. Pharmacokinetics and pharmacodynamics of roxatidine in patients with renal insufficiency. *Br J Clin Pharmacol* 1995; **39:** 161–7.

Interactions

Unlike cimetidine (see p.1185) roxatidine does not appear to affect cytochrome P450, and therefore is considered to have little effect on the metabolism of other drugs.

Pharmacokinetics

Roxatidine acetate hydrochloride is rapidly and almost completely absorbed from the gastro-intestinal tract with peak concentrations in plasma occurring about 1 to 3 hours after administration by mouth. It is rapidly hydrolysed to the active desacetyl metabolite, roxatidine, by esterases in the liver, small intestine, and serum.

Over 90% of a dose is excreted in the urine as roxatidine and other metabolites. The elimination half-life of roxatidine is about 6 hours and is prolonged in renal impairment.

Small amounts of roxatidine have been reported to be distributed into breast milk.

References.

1. Collins JD, Pidgen AW. Pharmacokinetics of roxatidine in healthy volunteers. *Drugs* 1988; **35** (suppl 3): 41–7.
2. Lameire N, *et al*. A pharmacokinetic study of roxatidine acetate in chronic renal failure. *Drugs* 1988; **35** (suppl 3): 48–52.

Uses and Administration

Roxatidine acetate hydrochloride is a histamine H_2-receptor antagonist with actions and uses similar to those of cimetidine (p.1185). It is given by mouth.

In the management of peptic ulcer disease the dose is 150 mg at bedtime or 75 mg twice daily. Where appropriate a maintenance dose of 75 mg at bedtime may be given to prevent the recurrence of duodenal ulcers. In gastro-oesophageal reflux disease the recommended dose is 75 mg twice daily.

The dosage should be reduced in patients with renal impairment. Suggested doses for patients on acute therapy are: creatinine clearance of 20 to 50 mL per minute, 75 mg at bedtime; creatinine clearance of less than 20 mL per minute, 75 mg every 2 days (but see above).

Reviews.

1. Murdoch D. Roxatidine acetate: a review of its pharmacodynamic and pharmacokinetic properties, and its therapeutic potential in peptic ulcer disease and related disorders. *Drugs* 1991; **42:** 240–60.

Preparations

Proprietary Preparations (details are given in Part 3)

Aust.: Roxane†; ***Ger.:*** Roxit; ***Ital.:*** Gastralgin; Neo H2; Roxit; ***Jpn:*** Altat; ***Neth.:*** Roxit; ***S.Afr.:*** Roxit; ***Spain:*** Roxiwas; Sarilen.

Senna (7530-b)

CAS — 8013-11-4 (senna); 81-27-6 (sennoside A); 128-57-4 (sennoside B); 52730-36-6 (sennoside A, calcium salt); 52730-37-7 (sennoside B, calcium salt).

Pharmacopoeias. Senna fruit, from Alexandrian and Tinnevelly senna is included in *Eur.* (see p.viii) and *Int.* Senna leaf, from Alexandrian or Tinnevelly senna or both, is included in *Eur.*, *Int.*, *Jpn*, and *US. US* also includes Sennosides.

In commerce senna obtained from *Cassia senna* (=*C. acutifolia*) (Leguminosae) is known as Alexandrian senna or Khartoum senna and that from *Cassia angustifolia* (Leguminosae) as Tinnevelly senna.

Alexandrian Senna Pods (Alexandrian Senna Fruit) of the Ph. Eur. is the dried fruit of *Cassia senna* containing not less than 3.4% of hydroxyanthracene glycosides calculated as sennoside B. Protect from light. **Store** in airtight containers.

Tinnevelly Senna Pods (Tinnevelly Senna Fruit) of the Ph. Eur. is the dried fruit of *Cassia angustifolia* containing not less than 2.2% of hydroxyanthracene glycosides calculated as sennoside B. Protect from light. **Store** in airtight containers.

Senna Leaf (Ph. Eur.) is the dried leaflets of *Cassia senna*, or of *Cassia angustifolia* or a mixture of both species containing not less than 2.5% of hydroxyanthracene glycosides calculated as sennoside B. Protect from light. Senna (USP 23) is the dried leaflets of *Cassia acutifolia* (=*C. senna*) or *Cassia angustifolia*.

Sennosides (USP 23) is a partially purified natural complex of anthraquinone glucosides found in senna, isolated from *Cassia acutifolia* (=*C. senna*) or *Cassia angustifolia* as calcium salts. It is a brownish powder. **Soluble** 1 in 35 of water, 1 in 2100 of alcohol, 1 in 3700 of chloroform, and 1 in 6100 of ether.

Adverse Effects

Senna may cause mild abdominal discomfort such as colic or cramps. Prolonged use or overdosage can result in diarrhoea with excessive loss of water and electrolytes, particularly potassium; there is also the possibility of developing an atonic non-functioning colon. Anthraquinone derivatives may colour the urine yellowish-brown at acid pH, and red at alkaline pH. Reversible melanosis coli has been reported following chronic use.

Abuse. Prolonged use or abuse of senna laxatives has been associated with reversible finger clubbing,[1-4] hypokalaemia[3] and tetany,[1] hypertrophic osteoarthropathy,[4] intermittent urinary excretion of aspartylglucosamine,[2] hypogammaglobulinaemia,[3] reversible cachexia,[3] and hepatitis.[5]

1. Prior J, White I. Tetany and clubbing in patient who ingested large quantities of senna. *Lancet* 1978; **ii:** 947.
2. Malmquist J, *et al*. Finger clubbing and aspartylglucosamine excretion in a laxative-abusing patient. *Postgrad Med J* 1980; **56:** 862–4.
3. Levine D, *et al*. Purgative abuse associated with reversible cachexia, hypogammaglobulinaemia, and finger clubbing. *Lancet* 1981; **i:** 919–20.
4. Armstrong RD, *et al*. Hypertrophic osteoarthropathy and purgative abuse. *Br Med J* 1981; **282:** 1836.
5. Beuers U, *et al*. Hepatitis after chronic abuse of senna. *Lancet* 1991; **337:** 372–3.

Precautions

Senna should not be given to patients with intestinal obstruction or with undiagnosed abdominal symptoms; care should also be taken in patients with inflammatory bowel disease. Prolonged use should be avoided.

Although anthraquinone derivatives may be distributed into the milk of lactating mothers, following normal dosage the concentration is usually insufficient to affect the nursing infant.

Colonic perforation with faecal peritonitis,[1,2] in one case fatal,[1] has been reported following the use of a senna preparation containing total sennosides 142 mg for bowel preparation prior to barium enema. In 1985, the strength of the UK preparation was halved to contain 72 mg of total sennosides. To reduce the risk of colonic perforation, patients with suspected stricture, inflammatory bowel disease, or impending obstruction should not receive a bowel stimulant.[2]

1. Galloway D, *et al*. Faecal peritonitis after laxative preparation for barium enema. *Br Med J* 1982; **284:** 472.
2. Cave-Bigley D. Faecal peritonitis after laxative preparation for barium enema. *Br Med J* 1982; **284:** 740.

Pharmacokinetics

There is some absorption of anthraquinone laxatives following administration by mouth. Absorbed anthraquinones are metabolised in the liver. Unabsorbed senna is hydrolysed in the colon by bacteria to release the active free anthraquinones. Excretion occurs in the urine and the faeces and also in other secretions including breast milk.

Uses and Administration

Senna is an anthraquinone stimulant laxative which is used to treat constipation (p.1168) and for bowel evacuation before investigational procedures or surgery. The active anthraquinones are liberated into the colon from the sennoside glycosides by colonic bacteria and an effect usually occurs within 6 to 12 hours of administration.

For the treatment of constipation senna is usually administered as tablets, granules, or syrup. It has also been administered rectally as suppositories. In the UK, doses of senna preparations are usually expressed in terms of total sennosides calculated as sennoside B. In the USA, doses are usually expressed in terms of total sennosides and may appear to be slightly larger. In the UK, the usual adult dose is 15 to 30 mg given by mouth as a single dose at bedtime. Children over 6 years of age have been given one-half the adult dose, and those aged 2 to 6 years one-quarter the adult dose. In the USA, the usual adult dose is 12 to 50 mg.

For bowel evacuation in the UK a dose equivalent to 1 mg per kg body-weight of total sennosides (up to 72 mg) was formerly given as a liquid preparation by mouth on the day before the examination; in the USA doses of up to 158 mg are given.

The purified sennosides (sennosides A and B), and their calcium salts (calcium sennoside A and calcium sennoside B) have been used similarly.

Senna is used in homoeopathic medicine.

Preparations

BP 1998: Senna Liquid Extract; Senna Tablets; Standardised Senna Granules;
USP 23: Senna Fluidextract; Senna Syrup; Sennosides Tablets.

Proprietary Preparations (details are given in Part 3)
Aust.: Bekunis; Carilax; Colonorm; Darmol; Dragees Neunzehn Senna; Neda Krautertabletten†; Tara Abfuhrsirup; X-Prep; ***Austral.:*** Bekunis Chocolate†; Bekunis Herbal Tea; Bekunis Instant; Laxettes; Senokot; ***Belg.:*** Darlin; Midro; Prunasine; Pursennide†; Senokot; Transix†; ***Canad.:*** Castoria; Glysennid; Mucinum Herbal†; Senokot; Senolax; X-Prep; ***Fr.:*** Senokot; X-Prep; ***Ger.:*** Bad Heilbrunner Abfuhrtee N extra; Bekunis Instant; Bekunis-Krautertee; Colonorm†; Depuran; Drix Abfuhr-Dragees; Hermes Drix Abfuhr-Tee; Hevertolax Phyto; JuLax S; Kneipp Abfuhr Tee N; Kneipp Worisetten S; Krauterlax-S; Laxativum Truw†; Liquidepur; Maskam Krauter-Tee; Midro Abfuhr; Midro N; Milkitten-Fruchtewurfel†; Neda Fruchtewurfel; Pursennid†; Ramend; Regulax N; Superlaxol†; Vinco†; Worisetten S†; X-Prep; ***Irl.:*** Bekunis; California Syrup of Figs; Senokot; ***Ital.:*** Bekunis†; Depuran†; Falquilax; Neo Confetto Falqui†; Tisana Kelemata; X-Prep; ***Neth.:*** Sennocol; X-Praep; ***Norw.:*** Senokot; X-Prep; ***S.Afr.:*** Depuran; Senokot; Silaxon; X-Prep; ***Spain:*** Depuran; Justelax; Senokot†; X-Prep; ***Swed.:*** Pursennid; ***Switz.:*** Darmol; Demodon N; Senokot†; X-Prep; ***UK:*** Nylax with Senna; Senlax; Senokot; ***USA:*** Black-Draught; Dosaflex; Dosalax; Dr Caldwell Senna Laxative; Ex-Lax Gentle Nature; Fletchers Castoria; Gentlax; Senexon; Senna-Gen; Sennatural; Senokot; Senokotxtra; Senolax†; X-Prep.

Multi-ingredient: numerous preparations are listed in Part 3.

Simethicone (6427-x)

Simethicone *(USAN)*.

Activated Dimethicone; Activated Dimethylpolysiloxane; Antifoam A; Antifoam AF.

CAS — 8050-81-5.

NOTE. Compounded preparations of simethicone and hydrotalcite have the British Approved Name Co-simalcite; the proportions are expressed in the form *x/y* where *x* and *y* are the strengths in milligrams of simethicone and hydrotalcite respectively.

Pharmacopoeias. In *US*.
BP(Vet) includes Silica in Dimeticone Suspension.

A mixture of liquid dimethicones containing finely divided silicon dioxide to enhance the defoaming properties of the silicone. It is a grey, translucent, viscous fluid. Silica in Dimeticone Suspension (BP (Vet) 1998) contains 4.5 to 8.0% w/w of silicon dioxide. Simethicone (USP 23) contains 4 to 7% w/w of silicon dioxide.

Practically **insoluble** in, or immiscible with, water and alcohol; the liquid phase is soluble 1 in 10 of chloroform and of ether leaving a residue of silicon dioxide. **Store** in airtight containers.

Simethicone lowers surface tension and when administered by mouth causes bubbles of gas in the gastro-intestinal tract to coalesce, thus aiding their dispersion.

It is promoted for the relief of flatulence and abdominal discomfort due to excess gastro-intestinal gas; doses of 125 or 250 mg three or four times daily have been given. Doses of 20 to 40 mg of simethicone have been given with feeds to relieve colic in infants.

For many gastro-intestinal disorders, it is given in conjunction with an antacid.

Simethicone is also used as a defoaming agent in radiography or endoscopy of the gastro-intestinal tract.

A brief review of the use of simethicone for gastro-intestinal symptoms concluded that although it is commonly prescribed in combination with an antacid, there is no good evidence that it provides additional benefit. When used alone it probably helps to relieve minor postoperative and postprandial symptoms and it is a useful aid in upper gastro-intestinal endoscopy.[1] Results *in vitro* suggest that simethicone may have inhibitory effects on *Helicobacter pylori*.[2] However, there is no convincing evidence that it is effective for the treatment of eructation, flatulence, or other signs or symptoms of excess gastro-intestinal gas.[3]

The management of dyspepsia and gastro-oesophageal reflux disease are discussed on p.1169 and p.1170. The management of infantile colic with a mention of the role of simethicone is discussed under Gastro-intestinal Spasm on p.1170.

1. Anonymous. Dimethicone for gastrointestinal symptoms? *Drug Ther Bull* 1986; **24:** 21–2.
2. Ansorg R, *et al.* Susceptibility of Helicobacter pylori to simethicone and other non-antibiotic drugs. *J Antimicrob Chemother* 1996; **37:** 45–52.
3. Anonymous. Simethicone for gastrointestinal gas. *Med Lett Drugs Ther* 1996; **38:** 57–8.

Preparations

USP 23: Alumina, Magnesia, and Simethicone Oral Suspension; Alumina, Magnesia, and Simethicone Tablets; Alumina, Magnesia, Calcium Carbonate, and Simethicone Tablets; Calcium Carbonate, Magnesia, and Simethicone Tablets; Magaldrate and Simethicone Oral Suspension; Magaldrate and Simethicone Tablets; Simethicone Capsules; Simethicone Emulsion; Simethicone Oral Suspension; Simethicone Tablets.

Proprietary Preparations (details are given in Part 3)
Aust.: Lefaxin; SAB Simplex; ***Austral.:*** Infacol; Medefoam-2; Mylicon†; Phazyme; ***Belg.:*** Polysilon; ***Canad.:*** Babys Own Infant Drops; Gas-X; Maalox GRF; Ovol; Phazyme; Siligaz; ***Fr.:*** Polysilane†; Siligaz; ***Ger.:*** Absorber HFV; Aegrosan; Busala; Ceolat; Dremisan†; Elugan; Elugan N; Endo-Paractol; Espumisan; Ilio-Funkton; Lefax; Meteosan; SAB Simplex; ***Irl.:*** Infacol; ***Ital.:*** Mylicon; Polisilon; ***Neth.:*** Aeropax†; Carboticon†; Ceolat; Polysilane†; ***Norw.:*** Ceolat; Minifom; Siloxan; ***S.Afr.:*** Telament; ***Spain:*** Aero Red; Enterosilicona; Pergastric; ***Swed.:*** Abulen†; Ceolat; Minifom; ***Switz.:*** Aeropax; Disflatyl; Flatulex; Lefax; Polysilane; SAB Simplex; ***UK:*** Asilone Windcheaters; Dentinox Colic Drops; Infacol; Setlers Wind-eze; ***USA:*** Degas; Extra Strength Mintox Plus; Flatulex; Gas Relief; Gas-X; Maalox Anti-Gas; Major-Con; Mylanta Gas; Mylicon; Phazyme.

Multi-ingredient: numerous preparations are listed in Part 3.

Sodium Picosulphate (7533-q)

Sodium Picosulphate *(BAN)*.

Sodium Picosulfate *(rINN)*; DA-1773; LA-391; Natrii Picosulfas; Picosulphol. Disodium 4,4′-(2-pyridylmethylene)di(phenyl sulphate).

$C_{18}H_{13}NNa_2O_8S_2$ = 481.4.

CAS — 10040-45-6.

Pharmacopoeias. In *Eur.* (see p.viii), *Jpn*, and *Pol.*

A white or almost white crystalline powder. Freely **soluble** in water; slightly soluble in alcohol; practically insoluble in ether.

Adverse Effects

Sodium picosulphate may cause abdominal discomfort such as colic. Prolonged use or overdosage can result in diarrhoea with excessive loss of water and electrolytes, particularly potassium; there is also the possibility of developing an atonic non-functioning colon.

Precautions

Sodium picosulphate should not be given to patients with intestinal obstruction or with undiagnosed abdominal symptoms; care should also be taken in patients with inflammatory bowel disease, although it has been reported to be well tolerated in these patients (see Bowel Evacuation, under Uses, below). Prolonged use should be avoided.

Pharmacokinetics

Like bisacodyl, sodium picosulphate is metabolised by colonic bacteria to the active compound bis(*p*-hydroxyphenyl)pyridyl-2-methane.

Uses and Administration

Sodium picosulphate is a stimulant laxative related to bisacodyl used for the treatment of constipation (p.1168) and for evacuation of the colon before investigational procedures or surgery. When taken by mouth it stimulates bowel movements following metabolism by colonic bacteria. It is usually effective within 10 to 14 hours although when used with magnesium citrate for bowel evacuation an effect may be seen within 3 hours.

It is given by mouth as a solution in doses of 5 to 15 mg as a single dose, usually at bedtime. Doses of 2.5 mg have been given to children aged 2 to 5 years and doses of 2.5 to 5 mg to children aged 5 to 10 years.

For bowel evacuation, a dose of sodium picosulphate 10 mg with magnesium citrate is given in the morning and again in the afternoon of the day before the examination. Doses are reduced in children.

Bowel evacuation. Bowel preparation for double-contrast examination with sodium picosulphate and magnesium citrate (Picolax) was preferred to preparation with senna.[1] Sodium picosulphate with magnesium citrate is a safe and effective bowel cleansing agent in adults[2] and children[3] with inflammatory bowel disease. They tolerate the preparation as well as patients with other colonic disorders with no adverse effect on their disease symptoms. Patients should be kept well hydrated (it may be appropriate to carry out bowel preparation in hospital in frail or elderly patients to avoid the risks of over- or underhydration[4,5]), and this procedure should not be used in suspected toxic dilatation of the colon.

1. Lee JR, Ferrando JR. Variables in the preparation of the large intestine for double contrast barium enema examination. *Gut* 1984; **25:** 69–72.
2. McDonagh AJG, *et al.* Safety of Picolax (sodium picosulphate-magnesium citrate) in inflammatory bowel disease. *Br Med J* 1989; **299:** 776–7.
3. Evans M, *et al.* Safety of Picolax in inflammatory bowel disease. *Br Med J* 1989; **299:** 1101–2.
4. Lewis M, *et al.* Bowel preparation at home in elderly people. *Br Med J* 1997; **314:** 74.
5. Hanning CD. Bowel preparation at home in elderly people. *Br Med J* 1997; **314:** 74.

Preparations

BP 1998: Sodium Picosulfate Oral Powder.

Proprietary Preparations (details are given in Part 3)
Aust.: Agaffin; Guttalax; ***Belg.:*** Fructines; Guttalax; Laxoberon; Obstilax; Picolaxine; ***Fr.:*** Fructines; ***Ger.:*** Abfuhrtropfen; Agiolax Pico; Dulcolax NP; Laxoberal; Mandrolax Pico; Regulax Picosulfat; ***Irl.:*** Laxoberal; ***Ital.:*** Falquigut; Gocce Antonetto; Gocce Lassative Aicardi; Guttalax; Neopax†; Picolax†; ***Neth.:*** Dulcodruppels; Laxoberon†; ***Spain:*** Contumax; Elimin; Evacuol; Gutalax; Laxonol†; Lubrilax; Skilax; ***Swed.:*** Laxoberal; ***Switz.:*** Fructines nouvelle formule; Guttalax; Laxoberon; ***UK:*** Dulcolax Liquid; Laxoberal.

Multi-ingredient: ***Belg.:*** Pilules de Vichy; ***Irl.:*** Picolax; ***Norw.:*** Pico-Salax; ***Swed.:*** Pico-Salax; ***Switz.:*** Laxasan; Pico-Salax; ***UK:*** Picolax.

Sodium Potassium Tartrate (1198-g)

E337; Kalium Natrium Tartaricum; Rochelle Salt; Seignette Salt; Sodii et Potassii Tartras; Tartarus Natronatus.

$C_4H_4KNaO_6,4H_2O$ = 282.2.

CAS — 304-59-6 (anhydrous); 6381-59-5 (tetrahydrate); 6100-16-9 (tetrahydrate).

Pharmacopoeias. In *Aust., Neth., Swiss,* and *US.*

Odourless or almost odourless colourless crystals or white crystalline powder, with a cooling saline taste. It effloresces slightly in warm dry air, the crystals often being coated with a white powder. **Soluble** 1 in 1 of water; practically insoluble in alcohol. **Store** in airtight containers.

Sodium potassium tartrate has been used, in doses of 8 to 16 g, as an osmotic laxative. It is also used as a food additive.

For the general properties of potassium salts, see p.1161, and of sodium salts, see p.1162.

Preparations

BPC 1973: Compound Effervescent Powder.

Proprietary Preparations (details are given in Part 3)

Multi-ingredient: ***Aust.:*** Laxalpin; ***Fr.:*** Romarene; ***Ger.:*** Basofer forte†; Basofer†; Bilisan forte†; Original-Hico-Gallenheil†; Stoffwechseldragees†; ***Spain:*** Samarin Sal de Frutas†; ***UK:*** Jaaps Health Salt.

Anhydrous Sodium Sulphate (1200-q)

Dried Sodium Sulphate; Exsiccated Sodium Sulphate; Natrii Sulfas Anhydricus; Natrium Sulfuricum Siccatum.

Na_2SO_4 = 142.0.

CAS — 7757-82-6.

Pharmacopoeias. In *Chin., Eur.* (see p.viii), *Int.,* and *Pol.*
US includes a single monograph for both the anhydrous form and the decahydrate.

A white odourless hygroscopic powder. Freely **soluble** in water.

Sodium Sulphate (1199-q)

514; Glauber's Salt; Natrii Sulfas Decahydricus; Natrii Sulphas; Natrium Sulfuricum Crystallisatum; Sodium Sulfate; Sodium Sulphate Decahydrate.

$Na_2SO_4,10H_2O$ = 322.2.

CAS — 7727-73-3 (decahydrate).

Pharmacopoeias. In *Chin., Eur.* (see p.viii), *Int.,* and *Pol.*
US includes a single monograph for both the anhydrous form and the decahydrate.

Large colourless odourless transparent crystals or white crystalline powder; effloresces in dry air. It partially dissolves in its own water of crystallisation at about 33°. It loses between 51 and 57% of its weight on drying. Freely **soluble** in water;

soluble in glycerol; practically insoluble in alcohol. **Store** in airtight containers, preferably at a temperature not exceeding 30°.

Sodium sulphate is an osmotic laxative. It is given by mouth in dilute solution, usually with a high molecular weight macrogol, for prompt bowel evacuation before investigational procedures or surgery (see Macrogols, p.1598). It has also been used as a 3.9% solution administered by slow intravenous infusion in the treatment of severe hypercalcaemia.

Sodium sulphate is also used as a diluent for colours in foods.

For the general properties of sodium salts, see p.1162.

Preparations

USP 23: Sodium Sulfate Injection.

Proprietary Preparations (details are given in Part 3)
Austral.: Celloids SS 69; ***UK:*** Fynnon Salt.

Multi-ingredient: ***Austral.:*** Duo Celloids SPSS; Duo Celloids SSMP; Duo Celloids SSPC; Duo Celloids SSS; Liv-Detox; Silybum Complex; ***Belg.:*** Kruschels; Normogastryl; ***Canad.:*** Normo Gastryl; ***Fr.:*** Actisoufre; Arthryl†; Azym; Digedryl; Dologastrine†; Fortrans; Gastrilax; Gastropax; Hepargitol; Hepatorex†; Ionarthrol; Jecobiase; Normogastryl; Ortho-Gastrine†; Oxyboldine; Prefagyl; Solugastryl†; ***Ger.:*** Bagnisan S med Rheumabad†; Original-Hico-Gallenheil†; Sepdelen 7†; Stacho N†; Ulgastrin†; Uricedin†; ***Ital.:*** Argirofedrina; Carbotiol; Sali Chianciano Epatobiliari†; ***Spain:*** Arthrisel†; Boldosal; Darmen Salt; Digestovital; Ibsesal†; Leberetic; Lebersal; Normogastryl; Salcedol; ***Switz.:*** Drix; Normogastryl; Padma-Lax; Thiorubrol; ***UK:*** Juno Junipah; New Era Zief; ***USA:*** Triv.

Sodium Tartrate (1201-p)

E335 (sodium tartrate or monosodium tartrate).

$C_2H_4O_2(CO_2Na)_2,2H_2O = 230.1.$

CAS — 868-18-8 (anhydrous); 6106-24-7 (dihydrate).

Sodium tartrate is used as an osmotic laxative. It is also used as a food additive.

For the general properties of sodium salts, see p.1162.

Preparations

Proprietary Preparations (details are given in Part 3)

Multi-ingredient: ***Belg.:*** Meral†; ***Ger.:*** Sepdelen 7†; ***Spain:*** Sales de Frutas Verkos†; Samarin Sal de Frutas†.

Sterculia (5461-j)

416; Indian Tragacanth; Karaya; Karaya Gum; Sterculia Gum.

CAS — 9000-36-6.

Pharmacopoeias. In Br. and Fr.

Sterculia is the gum obtained from *Sterculia urens* and other species of *Sterculia* (Sterculiaceae). Irregular or vermiform pieces, greyish-white with a brown or pink tinge, with an odour resembling that of acetic acid and containing not less than 14% of volatile acid (or not less than 10% if supplied in powdered form), calculated as acetic acid. Sparingly **soluble** in water, in which it swells to a homogeneous, adhesive, gelatinous mass; practically insoluble in alcohol. **Store** at a temperature not exceeding 25°.

Sterculia has general properties similar to those of ispaghula (p.1194) and is used as a bulk laxative and for adjusting faecal consistency. It is also used as an aid to appetite control in the management of obesity (p.1476). There is a risk of intestinal or oesophageal obstruction and faecal impaction, especially if such compounds are swallowed dry. Therefore they should always be taken with sufficient fluid and should not be taken immediately before going to bed. They should be avoided by patients who have difficulty swallowing.

Sterculia has adhesive properties and is used in the fitting of ileostomy and colostomy appliances and in dental fixative powders.

Sterculia is also used as an emulsifier and stabiliser in foods.

Preparations

BP 1998: Sterculia Granules.

Proprietary Preparations (details are given in Part 3)
Austral.: Hollister Karaya Paste†; ***Belg.:*** Calox; Normacol; ***Canad.:*** Normacol; ***Fr.:*** Decorpa†; Enteromucilage; Inolaxine; Normagil; Normacol; Prefine; ***Ger.:*** Decorpa; Granamon; Purayat†; ***Irl.:*** Normacol; ***S.Afr.:*** Normacol; ***Swed.:*** Inolaxol; ***Switz.:*** Colosan mite; Inolaxine; Normacol; ***UK:*** Normacol; Prefil.

Multi-ingredient: ***Austral.:*** Alvercol; Granocol; Normacol Plus; ***Belg.:*** Normacol Antispasmodique; Normacol Plus; ***Fr.:*** Kaologeais; Karayal; Normacol a la Bourdaine; Normacol a la Dipropyline†; Poly-Karaya; ***Ger.:*** Carbomucil†; Normacol Granulat†; ***Irl.:*** Alvercol; Normacol Plus; ***S.Afr.:*** Alvercol; Normacol Plus; ***Spain:*** Normacol Forte; ***Switz.:*** Colosan; Enterospasmyl N†; Normacol (avec bourdaine); Poly-Karaya; ***UK:*** Alvercol; Normacol Plus.

Sucralfate (707-m)

Sucralfate *(BAN, USAN, rINN).*

Sucrose hydrogen sulphate basic aluminium salt; Sucrose octakis(hydrogen sulphate) aluminium complex; β-D-Fructofuranosyl-α-D-glucopyranoside octakis (hydrogen sulphate) aluminium complex.

$C_{12}H_mAl_{16}O_nS_8$.

CAS — 54182-58-0.

Pharmacopoeias. In Chin., Jpn, and US.

The hydrous basic aluminium salt of sucrose octasulphate. **Store** in airtight containers.

Adverse Effects

Constipation is the most frequently reported adverse effect of sucralfate although other gastro-intestinal effects such as diarrhoea, nausea, or gastric discomfort may occur. Other adverse effects reported have included dry mouth, dizziness, drowsiness, vertigo, skin rashes, pruritus, and back pain.

In patients with renal impairment absorption of aluminium may cause adverse effects (see Administration in Renal Impairment in Precautions, below).

A report of a sucralfate bezoar in a patient given sucralfate in crushed form via a nasogastric tube.[1]

1. Algozzine GJ, *et al.* Sucralfate bezoar. *N Engl J Med* 1983; **309:** 1387.

Precautions

Sucralfate should be administered with caution to patients with renal impairment because of the risk of accumulation of the small amount of aluminium absorbed from the drug.

Administration in renal impairment. Sucralfate under acid conditions can release aluminium ions which may be absorbed systemically. Significant increases in the urinary excretion of aluminium have been observed in healthy subjects given sucralfate 4 g daily,[1,2] reflecting gastro-intestinal absorption of aluminium; aluminium concentrations in serum and urine were significantly higher in patients with chronic renal insufficiency than in subjects with normal renal function.[3] Aluminium toxicity in patients with normal renal function receiving sucralfate would not be expected, but seizures, muscle weakness, bone pain,[1] and severe aluminium encephalopathy[4] have been reported in patients with end-stage renal disease requiring dialysis. Sucralfate should be used with caution in patients with renal impairment, especially if other aluminium-containing agents are also taken.

1. Robertson JA, *et al.* Sucralfate, intestinal aluminium absorption, and aluminium toxicity in a patient on dialysis. *Ann Intern Med* 1989; **111:** 179–81.
2. Allain P, *et al.* Plasma and urine aluminium concentrations in healthy subjects after administration of sucralfate. *Br J Clin Pharmacol* 1990; **29:** 391–5.
3. Burgess E, *et al.* Aluminum absorption and excretion following sucralfate therapy in chronic renal insufficiency. *Am J Med* 1992; **92:** 471–5.
4. Withers DJ, *et al.* Encephalopathy in patient taking aluminium-containing agents, including sucralfate. *Lancet* 1989; **ii:** 674.

Interactions

Sucralfate may interfere with the absorption of other drugs and it has been suggested that there should be an interval of 2 hours between the administration of sucralfate and other concurrent non-antacid medication. Some of the drugs reported to be affected by sucralfate include cimetidine, ranitidine, digoxin, ketoconazole, phenytoin, fluoroquinolone antibacterials, tetracycline, quinidine, theophylline, thyroxine, and possibly warfarin. The recommended interval between sucralfate and antacids is 30 minutes. In the case of enteral feeds the interval is 1 hour.

Pharmacokinetics

Sucralfate is only slightly absorbed from the gastro-intestinal tract following oral administration. However, there can be some release of aluminium ions and of sucrose sulphate and small quantities of sucrose sulphate may be absorbed and excreted, primarily in the urine; some absorption of aluminium may also occur (see Administration in Renal Impairment, above).

Uses and Administration

Sucralfate is a cytoprotective agent which, under acid gastro-intestinal conditions, forms an adherent complex with proteins which coats the gastric mucosa and is reported to have a special affinity for ulcer sites. It also inhibits the action of pepsin and adsorbs bile salts.

Sucralfate is used in the treatment of peptic ulcer disease and chronic gastritis. It is given by mouth and should be taken on an empty stomach before meals and at bedtime. The usual dose is 1 g four times daily or 2 g twice daily for 4 to 8 weeks; if necessary the dose may be increased to a maximum of 8 g daily. If longer-term therapy is required sucralfate may be administered for up to 12 weeks. Where appropriate a maintenance dose of 1 g twice daily may be given to prevent the recurrence of duodenal ulcers.

For prophylaxis of stress ulceration the usual dose of sucralfate is 1 g six times daily; a dose of 8 g daily should not be exceeded.

Sucralfate has also been used to treat mouth ulcers and oral mucositis following radiotherapy.

Action. A study *in vitro* demonstrated that in addition to its other properties, sucralfate had bacteriostatic or bactericidal action against a number of Gram-negative organisms.[1]

1. Bragman SGL, *et al.* Activity of sucralfate (sucrose octa-sulphate), an anti-ulcer agent, against opportunistic Gram-negative bacilli. *J Antimicrob Chemother* 1995; **36:** 703–6.

Diagnostic use. Sucralfate labelled with technetium-99m has been investigated for the detection of active inflammatory bowel disease[1] and oesophageal mucosal ulceration.[2] The labelled sucralfate probably binds to active lesions in a similar way to its binding in peptic ulcer and thus provides a positive scan.

1. Dawson DJ, *et al.* Detection of inflammatory bowel disease in adults and children: evaluation of a new isotopic technique. *Br Med J* 1985; **291:** 1227–30.
2. Mearns AJ, *et al.* Dynamic radionuclide imaging with 99mTc-sucralfate in the detection of oesophageal ulceration. *Gut* 1989; **30:** 1256–9.

Gastro-intestinal bleeding. Sucralfate is an effective drug for the prophylaxis and management of stress-induced gastro-intestinal bleeding in severely ill patients, and may reduce the risk of late-onset pneumonia compared with an H_2-antagonist.[1] For further discussion of stress ulceration and bleeding, including the use of sucralfate, see under Peptic Ulcer Disease, p.1174. In another study,[2] severe gastro-intestinal bleeding resistant to high doses of an H_2-antagonist with pirenzepine was successfully controlled in 10 patients by the addition of sucralfate 12 g every 2 hours given as a suspension via a stomach tube. The dose of sucralfate was subsequently reduced to 4 g every 4 hours. Two of the patients had been receiving sucralfate for prophylaxis when severe bleeding developed. There is also some evidence from another study[3] that sucralfate reduces gastro-intestinal bleeding associated with NSAID administration, although it does not prevent drug-induced gastric erosion.

Sucralfate in a dose of 1 g four times daily has also been used in the treatment of bleeding oesophageal varices.[4] The incidence of oesophageal and gastric variceal rebleeding was 59% in patients given sucralfate compared with 55% in patients treated with sclerotherapy. For further discussion of bleeding oesophageal varices and their management, see p.1576.

1. Prod'hom G, *et al.* Nosocomial pneumonia in mechanically ventilated patients receiving antacid, ranitidine, or sucralfate as prophylaxis for stress ulcer: a randomized controlled trial. *Ann Intern Med* 1994; **120:** 653–62.
2. Tryba M, May B. Acute treatment of severe haemorrhagic gastritis with high-dose sucralfate. *Lancet* 1988; **ii:** 1304.
3. Hudson N, *et al.* Effect of sucralfate on aspirin induced mucosal injury and impaired haemostasis in humans. *Gut* 1997; **41:** 19–23.
4. Burroughs AK, *et al.* Randomised trial of longterm sclerotherapy for variceal rebleeding using the same protocol to treat rebleeding in all patients: final report. *Gut* 1989; **30:** A1506.

Gastro-oesophageal reflux disease. Although sucralfate has been tried for gastro-oesophageal reflux disease the results of studies have been inconsistent.[1,2] As discussed on p.1170, the first aim of treatment is a reduction in exposure of the oesophagus to acid, and therefore antacids or antisecretory agents are chiefly employed.

1. Orlando RC. Sucralfate therapy and reflux esophagitis: an overview. *Am J Med* 1991; **91** (suppl 2A): 123S–124S.
2. Klinkenberg-Knol EC, *et al.* Pharmacological management of gastro-oesophageal reflux disease. *Drugs* 1995; **49:** 695–710.

Mouth ulceration. Sucralfate has been investigated in the treatment and prophylaxis of stomatitis induced by cancer chemotherapy. In a prospective pilot study, 9 of 14 evaluable patients experienced subjective relief from mouth-rinsing at least three times daily with an oral suspension of sucralfate.[1] One patient withdrew from the study because the rinsing procedure aggravated chemotherapy-induced nausea. Side-effects were limited to constipation in a single patient. A randomised, double-blind crossover study[2] in 40 patients found a significant reduction in symptoms among 23 evaluable patients given sucralfate in a similar manner prophylactically. Seven patients withdrew due to aggravation of chemotherapy-induced nausea. No other adverse effects were noted. It was suggested that to overcome this problem, the suspension should have a neutral taste, should not be swallowed after rinsing, and that rinsing should not be commenced until nausea had ceased. A combination of sucralfate suspension with oral fluconazole has also been found to be effective,[3] the fluconazole being added to minimise the risk of *Candida* infection.

Sucralfate has also been reported to be of benefit in patients with recurrent aphthous stomatitis. A double-blind crossover study involving 21 such patients over 2 years found that topical application of sucralfate suspension 4 times daily was superior to treatment with an antacid (aluminium hydroxide with magnesium hydroxide) or placebo.[4] For a review of the management of mouth ulceration, see p.1172.

1. Pfeiffer P, *et al.* A prospective pilot study on the effect of sucralfate mouth-swishing in reducing stomatitis during radiotherapy of the oral cavity. *Acta Oncol* 1990; **29:** 471–3.
2. Pfeiffer P, *et al.* Effect of prophylactic sucralfate suspension on stomatitis induced by cancer chemotherapy: a randomized, double-blind cross-over study. *Acta Oncol* 1990; **29:** 171–3.
3. Allison RR, *et al.* Symptomatic acute mucositis can be minimized or prophylaxed [sic] by the combination of sucralfate and fluconazole. *Cancer Invest* 1995; **13:** 16–22.
4. Rattan J, *et al.* Sucralfate suspension as a treatment of recurrent aphthous stomatitis. *J Intern Med* 1994; **236:** 341–3.

Peptic ulcer disease. For a discussion of the management of peptic ulcer disease, including NSAID-induced and stress ulceration, and mention of the role of sucralfate, see p.1174.

Phosphate binding. For reference to sucralfate as a phosphate binder see under Renal Osteodystrophy, p.732.

Skin ulceration. Sucralfate has reportedly been applied topically with some success to treat bleeding skin ulcers associated with malignancy,[1] and to promote the healing of venous stasis ulcers.[2] It has been suggested that sucralfate promotes angiogenesis by binding to, and preventing degradation of, basic fibroblast growth factor (bFGF).[2] The management of wounds and ulcers is described on p.1076.

1. Regnard CFB. Control of bleeding in advanced cancer. *Lancet* 1991; **337:** 974.
2. Tsakayannis D, *et al.* Sucralfate and chronic venous stasis ulcers. *Lancet* 1994; **343:** 424–5.

Preparations

USP 23: Sucralfate Tablets.

Proprietary Preparations (details are given in Part 3)
Aust.: Sucralan; Sucralbene; Ulcogant; ***Austral.:*** Carafate; SCF; Ulcyte; ***Belg.:*** Ulcogant; ***Canad.:*** Novo-Sucralate; Sulcrate; ***Fr.:*** Keal; Ulcar; ***Ger.:*** duracralfat†; Sucrabest; Sucraphil; Ulcogant; ***Irl.:*** Antepsin; ***Ital.:*** Antepsin; Citogel; Crafilm; Gastrogel; Sucrager; Sucral; Sucralfin; Sucramal; Sucrate; Sugast; Suril; ***Jpn:*** Ulcerlmin; ***Neth.:*** Ulcogant; ***Norw.:*** Antepsin; ***S.Afr.:*** Cralsanic; Ulcefate; Ulcetab†; Ulcetic†; Ulsanic; ***Spain:*** Gastral; Heprone†; Tiblex; Ulcufato; Urbal; ***Swed.:*** Andapsin; Succosa; ***Switz.:*** Gastrogel; Ulcogant; ***UK:*** Antepsin; ***USA:*** Carafate.

Used as an adjunct in: ***Ital.:*** Ketodol.

Sulglycotide (13282-e)

Sulglycotide *(BAN)*.
Sulglicotide *(rINN)*.
CAS — 54182-59-1.

Sulglycotide is a sulphated glycopeptide with cytoprotective properties extracted from pig duodenum. It is used in the treatment of peptic ulcer disease (p.1174) and other gastrointestinal disorders in a usual dose of 600 mg daily by mouth.

References.

1. Luminari M, *et al.* Effectiveness of sulglycotide treatment for active chronic superficial gastritis. *Acta Ther* 1988; **14:** 45–54.
2. Psilogenis M, *et al.* A multicenter double-blind study of sulglycotide versus sucralfate in nonulcer dyspepsia. *Int J Clin Pharmacol Ther Toxicol* 1990; **28:** 369–74.

Preparations

Proprietary Preparations (details are given in Part 3)
Ital.: Gliptide.

Sulisatin Sodium (13283-l)

Sulisatin Sodium *(pINNM)*.

The disodium salt of 3,3-bis(4-hydroxyphenyl)-7-methylindolin-2-one bis(hydrogen sulphate) (ester).

$C_{21}H_{15}NNa_2O_9S_2$ = 535.5.

CAS — 54935-03-4 (sulisatin); 54935-04-5 (sulisatin sodium).

Sulisatin sodium has been used as a stimulant laxative.

Preparations

Proprietary Preparations (details are given in Part 3)
Spain: Laxitex†.

Sulphasalazine (4951-n)

Sulphasalazine *(BAN)*.

Sulfasalazine *(USAN, rINN)*; Salazosulfapyridine; Salicylazosulfapyridine; Sulfasalazinum. 4-Hydroxy-4′-(2-pyridylsulphamoyl)azobenzene-3-carboxylic acid.

$C_{18}H_{14}N_4O_5S$ = 398.4.

CAS — 599-79-1.

Pharmacopoeias. In *Eur.* (see p.viii), *Int., Jpn,* and *US.*

A fine odourless bright yellow to brownish-yellow powder. Practically **insoluble** in water, chloroform, dichloromethane, and ether; soluble 1 in 2900 of alcohol, and 1 in 1500 of methyl alcohol; dissolves in dilute solutions of alkali hydroxides. **Store** in airtight containers. Protect from light.

Adverse Effects and Precautions

Since sulphasalazine is metabolised to sulphapyridine and 5-aminosalicylic acid (mesalazine), its adverse effects, treatment, and precautions are similar to those of sulphonamides (see Sulphamethoxazole, p.254) and of mesalazine (p.1199). Many adverse effects have been attributed to the sulphapyridine moiety and appear to be more common if serum-sulphapyridine concentrations are greater than 50 µg per mL, if the daily dose of sulphasalazine is 4 g or more, or in slow acetylators of sulphapyridine.

The most commonly reported adverse effects include nausea and vomiting, abdominal discomfort, headache, fever, and skin rash.

Adverse effects can be broadly divided into 2 groups. The first is dose-related, dependent on acetylator phenotype, and largely predictable; this group includes nausea and vomiting, headache, haemolytic anaemia, and methaemoglobinaemia. The second group are the hypersensitivity reactions which are essentially unpredictable and usually occur at the start of treatment; this group includes skin rash, aplastic anaemia, hepatic and pulmonary dysfunction, and autoimmune haemolysis.

Oligospermia, reversible on withdrawal of sulphasalazine, has also been reported. Administration of sulphasalazine may result in yellow-orange discoloration of skin, urine, and other body fluids.

Sulphasalazine should not be given to patients with a history of sensitivity to sulphonamides or salicylates. Use in children under 2 years of age is contra-indicated because of the risk of kernicterus.

Blood counts should be performed at the start of therapy and at least once a month for a minimum of the first 3 months of treatment. If a blood dyscrasia is suspected treatment should be stopped immediately and a blood count performed. Patients or their carers should be told how to recognise signs of blood toxicity and should be advised to seek immediate medical attention if symptoms such as fever, sore throat, mouth ulcers, bruising or bleeding develop.

Liver function tests should be carried out at monthly intervals for the first 3 months of treatment; periodic monitoring of kidney function has also been recommended.

Reviews of the adverse effects associated with the administration of sulphasalazine in patients with inflammatory bowel disease[1] or rheumatoid arthritis.[2,3] The type and incidence of adverse effects appears to be similar in both groups of patients.[2] Although most reactions are minor and patients may continue therapy at the same or reduced dosage, some patients discontinue treatment because of adverse effects and in these cases a hyposensitisation regimen may be considered.[1,4,5] Hyposensitisation should not be attempted in patients with a history of a serious adverse effect such as agranulocytosis, toxic epidermal necrolysis, erythema multiforme, frank haemolysis, or a severe hypersensitivity reaction.[1,4,5] An alternative to hyposensitisation in patients with inflammatory bowel disease who cannot tolerate sulphasalazine, is to give the active 5-aminosalicylic acid component without sulphapyridine which is thought to be responsible for many of the adverse effects. Alternatives include mesalazine and olsalazine.

1. Taffet SL, Das KM. Sulfasalazine: adverse effects and desensitization. *Dig Dis Sci* 1983; **28:** 833–42.
2. Amos RS, *et al.* Sulphasalazine for rheumatoid arthritis: toxicity in 774 patients monitored for one to 11 years. *Br Med J* 1986; **293:** 420–3.
3. Farr M, *et al.* Side effect profile of 200 patients with inflammatory arthritides treated with sulphasalazine. *Drugs* 1986; **32** (suppl 1): 49–53.
4. Purdy BH, *et al.* Desensitization for sulfasalazine skin rash. *Ann Intern Med* 1984; **100:** 512–14.
5. Bax DE, Amos RS. Sulphasalazine in rheumatoid arthritis: desensitising the patient with a skin rash. *Ann Rheum Dis* 1986; **45:** 139–40.

Effects on the blood. Blood disorders constitute 19% of all reactions reported with sulphasalazine.[1] As of June 1993 the Committee on Safety of Medicines in the UK was aware of 191 reports of neutropenia, leucopenia, or agranulocytosis (22 fatal), 44 reports of bone marrow depression or aplastic anaemia (13 fatal) and 30 reports of thrombocytopenia (1 fatal).[1]

Although blood dyscrasias were initially thought to be caused by the sulphapyridine moiety, subsequent experience has shown that the aminosalicylates can also cause haematological reactions (see for example Mesalazine, p.1199). The risk of blood dyscrasias with sulphasalazine has been estimated at 0.6 per 1000 in those given the drug for inflammatory bowel disease, but approximately 10 times greater in patients receiving sulphasalazine for rheumatoid arthritis.[2]

Sulphasalazine inhibits folic acid absorption, interferes with its metabolism, and can increase folic acid requirements through haemolysis of red blood cells.[3,4] These effects are not usually significant in patients with inflammatory bowel disease unless there are additional factors causing folate deficiency such as intercurrent illness or an exacerbation of bowel disease.[3,4] However, clinical folate deficiency with macrocytosis, megaloblastic anaemia, or pancytopenia has been reported rarely.[3,4] Macrocytic anaemia associated with sulphasalazine may occur more commonly in patients with rheumatoid arthritis; it was found in 7 of 50 patients within 3 to 4 months of starting treatment with sulphasalazine.[5] The effects of sulphasalazine on folic acid metabolism appear to be dose-related and respond to withdrawal or dosage reduction, and folic acid supplements;[3-5] intravenous folinic acid may sometimes be needed.[4] Although the effects may be potentially serious, they are not a contra-indication to continuing sulphasalazine treatment.[4,5]

Patients with a history of leucopenia associated with administration of gold for rheumatoid arthritis should not be given sulphasalazine since a similar reaction may occur.[6]

1. Committee on Safety of Medicines/Medicines Control Agency. Sulphasalazine and fatal blood dyscrasias. *Current Problems* 1993; **19:** 6.
2. Committee on Safety of Medicines/Medicines Control Agency. Blood dyscrasias and mesalazine. *Current Problems* 1995; **21:** 5–6.
3. Swinson CM, *et al.* Role of sulphasalazine in the aetiology of folate deficiency in ulcerative colitis. *Gut* 1981; **22:** 456–61.
4. Logan ECM, *et al.* Sulphasalazine associated pancytopenia may be caused by acute folate deficiency. *Gut* 1986; **27:** 868–72.
5. Prouse PJ, *et al.* Macrocytic anaemia in patients treated with sulphasalazine for rheumatoid arthritis. *Br Med J* 1986; **293:** 1407.
6. Bliddal H, *et al.* Gold-induced leucopenia may predict a similar adverse reaction to sulphasalazine. *Lancet* 1987; **i:** 390.

Effects on the cardiovascular system. Reports include Raynaud's syndrome with sulphasalazine[1] and myocarditis with sulphasalazine and with mesalazine.[2] Myocarditis leading to fatal cardiogenic shock has been reported in one patient receiving mesalazine and it has been recommended that sulphasalazine or mesalazine should be replaced by glucocorticoids if cardiac symptoms arise.[3]

1. Reid J, *et al.* Raynaud's phenomenon induced by sulphasalazine. *Postgrad Med J* 1980; **56:** 106–7.
2. Agnholt J, *et al.* Cardiac hypersensitivity to 5-aminosalicylic acid. *Lancet* 1989; **i:** 1135.
3. Kristensen KS, *et al.* Fatal myocarditis associated with mesalazine. *Lancet* 1990; **335:** 605.

Effects on contact lenses. Irreversible yellow staining of an extended-wear soft contact lens was associated with administration of sulphasalazine.[1] Staining of gas permeable lenses did not occur.

1. Riley SA, *et al.* Contact lens staining due to sulphasalazine. *Lancet* 1986; **i:** 972.

Effects on fertility. Although successful pregnancies have been reported in the partners of men taking sulphasalazine,[1,2] male infertility is a well recognised complication of sulphasalazine treatment. Untreated inflammatory bowel disease is not associated with abnormal seminal quality or infertility, but oligospermia, reduced sperm motility, and an increase in morphological abnormalities are seen after treatment with sulphasalazine which may lead to infertility.[1-4] Oligospermia has been reported in 86% of men with inflammatory bowel disease treated with sulphasalazine.[1] Seminal characteristics and fertility return to normal within 2 to 3 months of withdrawing sulphasalazine and successful pregnancies have been reported following withdrawal.[1-3] The mechanism involved is thought to be a direct toxic effect on immature and developing spermatozoa, possibly due to the sulphapyridine moiety.[2-4] Improvement in seminal characteristics and successful pregnancies have been reported following substitution of mesalazine for sulphasalazine in patients with ulcerative colitis.[4,5]

1. Birnie GG, *et al.* Incidence of sulphasalazine-induced male infertility. *Gut* 1981; **22:** 452–5.
2. Riley SA, *et al.* Sulphasalazine induced seminal abnormalities in ulcerative colitis: results of mesalazine substitution. *Gut* 1987; **28:** 1008–12.
3. Toovey S, *et al.* Sulphasalazine and male infertility: reversibility and possible mechanism. *Gut* 1981; **22:** 445–51.
4. Ó'Moráin C, *et al.* Reversible male infertility due to sulphasalazine: studies in man and rat. *Gut* 1984; **25:** 1078–84.
5. Cann PA, Holdsworth CD. Reversal of male infertility on changing treatment from sulphasalazine to 5-aminosalicylic acid. *Lancet* 1984; **i:** 1119.

Effects on the gastro-intestinal tract. Sulphasalazine-induced exacerbations of ulcerative colitis have been reported[1,2] and are probably caused by the salicylate moiety rather than sulphapyridine.[3] Other reported effects include a dose-related metallic taste[4] and intestinal villous atrophy.[5]

1. Schwartz AG, *et al.* Sulfasalazine-induced exacerbation of ulcerative colitis. *N Engl J Med* 1982; **306:** 409–12.
2. Ring FA, *et al.* Sulfasalazine-induced colitis complicating idiopathic ulcerative colitis. *Can Med Assoc J* 1984; **131:** 43–5.
3. Shanahan F, Targan S. Sulfasalazine and salicylate-induced exacerbation of ulcerative colitis. *N Engl J Med* 1987; **317:** 455.
4. Ogburn RM. Sulfamethazine-related dysgeusia. *JAMA* 1979; **241:** 837.
5. Smith MA, *et al.* Angioimmunoblastic lymphadenopathy, sulphasalazine exposure and villous atrophy. *Postgrad Med J* 1985; **61:** 337–8.

Effects on the hair. Alopecia occurred on 2 occasions[1] after starting sulphasalazine 2 or 3 g daily in a patient with ulcerative colitis. On both occasions normal hair growth returned after treatment was stopped, and the patient was later successfully desensitised. However, alopecia which developed in another patient during sulphasalazine treatment did not recur on rechallenge.[2] In this case postpartum alopecia was considered to be the cause and these authors doubted whether sulphasalazine causes alopecia at all. Hair loss has been reported in 2 patients receiving mesalazine enemas.[3] However, remission of alopecia universalis has been reported during sulphasalazine treatment of rheumatoid arthritis.[4]

1. Breen EG, Donnelly S. Alopecia associated with sulphasalazine (Salazopyrin). *Br Med J* 1986; **292:** 802.
2. Fich A, Eliakim R. Does sulfasalazine induce alopecia? *J Clin Gastroenterol* 1988; **10:** 466.
3. Kutty PK, *et al.* Hair loss and 5-aminosalicylic acid enemas. *Ann Intern Med* 1982; **97:** 785–6.
4. Jawad ASM, Scott DGI. Remission of alopecia universalis during sulphasalazine treatment for rheumatoid arthritis. *Br Med J* 1989; **298:** 675.

Effects on the kidneys. For reports of nephrotic syndrome and of interstitial nephritis associated with sulphasalazine treatment, see under Adverse Effects of Mesalazine, p.1199.

Effects on the nervous system. There have been individual reports of multiple sclerosis[1] and chorea[2] in patients receiving sulphasalazine. For a report of reversible peripheral neuropathy associated with mesalazine, see p.1200.

1. Gold R, *et al.* Development of multiple sclerosis in patient on long-term sulfasalazine. *Lancet* 1990; **335:** 409–10.
2. Quinn AG, *et al.* Chorea precipitated by sulphasalazine. *Br Med J* 1991; **302:** 1025.

Effects on the pancreas. The Committee on Safety of Medicines in the UK had received 6 reports of pancreatitis associated with sulphasalazine as of February 1994.[1] There had been further reports associated with mesalazine (see p.1200).

1. Committee on Safety of Medicines/Medicines Control Agency. Drug-induced pancreatitis. *Current Problems* 1994; **20:** 2–3.

Effects on the respiratory system. Sulphasalazine-induced pulmonary complications are reported rarely. Most reports include dyspnoea, cough, pulmonary infiltrates, fever, and eosinophilia, usually developing in the first few months of treatment although they may occur after several years.[1,2] Symptoms are generally readily reversible on withdrawal of sulphasalazine, although death due to fibrosing alveolitis has been reported.[1] It is not known which component of sulphasalazine is responsible for these effects (but see Mesalazine p.1200); they have been reported in patients with a history of sensitivity to salicylates, sulphonamides, or with no known sensitivity to these drugs.[1,2]

1. Wang KK, *et al.* Pulmonary infiltrates and eosinophilia associated with sulfasalazine. *Mayo Clin Proc* 1984; **59:** 343–6.
2. Jordan A, Cowan RE. Reversible pulmonary disease and eosinophilia associated with sulphasalazine. *J R Soc Med* 1988; **81:** 233–5.

Lupus. A study in 11 patients with sulphasalazine-induced lupus found that induction of disease was more likely in patients who were slow acetylators of sulphapyridine, and who had HLA haplotypes associated with idiopathic systemic lupus erythematosus (SLE).[1] Furthermore, the risk of developing persistent SLE and lupus nephritis increased with duration of treatment and cumulative dose of sulphasalazine.

1. Gunnarsson I, *et al.* Predisposing factors in sulphasalazine-induced systemic lupus erythematosus. *Br J Rheumatol* 1997; **36:** 1089–94.

Porphyria. Sulphasalazine has been associated with acute attacks of porphyria and is considered unsafe in patients with acute porphyria.[1]

1. Moore MR, McColl KEL. *Porphyria: drug lists.* Glasgow: Porphyria Research Unit, University of Glasgow, 1991.

Pregnancy and breast feeding. Sulphasalazine and its sulphapyridine metabolites readily cross the placenta resulting in similar concentrations in the cord serum and maternal serum at delivery.[1,2] The concentration of the 5-aminosalicylic acid component of sulphasalazine in both cord serum and maternal serum is negligible.[1] There have been isolated reports of congenital abnormalities associated with administration of sulphasalazine during pregnancy including coarctation of the aorta with a ventricular septal defect,[3,4] and genito-urinary disorders.[4] There is also a theoretical risk of kernicterus in the neonate if sulphasalazine is given close to delivery (see p.255). Despite these reports there have been many successful and uncomplicated pregnancies during treatment with sulphasalazine and the general consensus favours continuing sulphasalazine throughout pregnancy when indicated.[1,3-6] The minimum effective dose should be used and since sulphasalazine may precipitate folate deficiency (see Effects on the Blood, above), folic acid supplements are recommended.[7] It has been suggested[8] that sulphasalazine treatment cannot be justified during pregnancy in asymptomatic patients. Both sulphasalazine and its sulphapyridine metabolites have a poor bilirubin displacing capacity and the risk of kernicterus is considered minimal.[2]

Small amounts of sulphasalazine and its sulphapyridine metabolites are excreted in breast milk; the concentrations of sulphasalazine and total sulphapyridine may be up to 30% and 50% of maternal serum concentrations.[1] Bloody diarrhoea in a breast-fed infant whose mother was taking sulphasalazine 3 g daily has been reported.[9] The mother was a slow acetylator with a relatively high blood concentration of sulphapyridine which contributed to the appearance of the drug in the infant's blood. However, continued treatment with sulphasalazine can generally be recommended to breast-feeding mothers of healthy infants.[5]

1. Khan AKA, Truelove SC. Placental and mammary transfer of sulphasalazine. *Br Med J* 1979; **2:** 1553.
2. Järnerot G, *et al.* Placental transfer of sulphasalazine and sulphapyridine and some of its metabolites. *Scand J Gastroenterol* 1981; **16:** 693–7.
3. Hoo JJ, *et al.* Possible teratogenicity of sulfasalazine. *N Engl J Med* 1988; **318:** 1128.
4. Newman NM, Correy JF. Possible teratogenicity of sulphasalazine. *Med J Aust* 1983; **1:** 528–9.
5. Peppercorn MA. Sulfasalazine and related new drugs. *J Clin Pharmacol* 1987; **27:** 260–5.
6. Korelitz BI. Commentary: observations on sulfasalazine in Crohn's disease and ulcerative colitis. *J Clin Pharmacol* 1987; **27:** 265–6.
7. Byron MA. Treatment of rheumatic diseases. *Br Med J* 1987; **294:** 236–8.
8. Donaldson RM. Management of medical problems in pregnancy—inflammatory bowel disease. *N Engl J Med* 1985; **312:** 1616–19.
9. Branski D, *et al.* Bloody diarrhea—a possible complication of sulfasalazine transferred through human breast milk. *J Pediatr Gastroenterol Nutr* 1986; **5:** 316–17.

Interactions

As discussed below, concurrent administration of sulphasalazine with antibacterial therapy may reduce conversion of sulphasalazine to its active metabolite.

Sulphasalazine has been reported to interfere with the absorption of digoxin or folic acid from the gastro-intestinal tract.

Antibacterials. Since sulphasalazine depends for its effects on release of 5-aminosalicylic acid by bacterial metabolism in the gut, any antibiotic which reduces the intestinal microflora may reduce the production of active metabolite. Evidence for this has been seen in patients given rifampicin and ethambutol,[1] or subjects given ampicillin,[2] concurrently with sulphasalazine. However, a decrease in clinical effect does not seem to have been demonstrated.

1. Shaffer JL, Houston JB. The effect of rifampicin on sulphapyridine plasma concentrations following sulphasalazine administration. *Br J Clin Pharmacol* 1985; **19:** 526–8.
2. Houston JB, *et al.* Azo reduction of sulphasalazine in healthy volunteers. *Br J Clin Pharmacol* 1982; **14:** 395–8.

Antineoplastics. Results *in vitro* indicated that sulphasalazine, and to a lesser extent 5-aminosalicylic acid (mesalazine), inhibited the enzyme thiopurine methyltransferase which is important for thiopurine metabolism.[1] In consequence the possibility of a clinically significant interaction between sulphasalazine and *azathioprine* or *mercaptopurine* exists.

1. Szumlanski CL, Weinshilboum RM. Sulphasalazine inhibition of thiopurine methyltransferase: possible mechanism for interaction with 6-mercaptopurine and azathioprine. *Br J Clin Pharmacol* 1995; **39:** 456–9.

Effects on other drugs. For a report that concurrent administration of sulphasalazine reduced the absorption of digoxin, see p.852. For the possible effects of interference by sulphasalazine with absorption of folic acid, see Effects on the Blood, above.

Pharmacokinetics

Following oral administration up to about 15% of a dose of sulphasalazine is absorbed from the small intestine, although some of this is subsequently returned to the intestine in bile via enterohepatic circulation. The great majority of the dose reaches the colon where the azo bond is cleaved by the action of the intestinal flora, producing sulphapyridine and 5-aminosalicylic acid (mesalazine). Results in patients who have undergone colectomy suggest that between 60 and 90% of the total dose is metabolised in this way, but the degree of metabolism depends both on the activity of the intestinal flora and the speed of intestinal transit; colonic metabolism is reduced in patients with diarrhoea (for example, in active inflammatory bowel disease).

The small amount of intact sulphasalazine which is absorbed is extensively protein bound and subsequently excreted unchanged in urine. It crosses the placenta and is found in breast milk.

Following cleavage of the sulphasalazine molecule about 60 to 80% of available sulphapyridine is absorbed and undergoes extensive metabolism by acetylation, hydroxylation, and glucuronidation. Peak steady-state concentrations of sulphapyridine are higher in slow acetylators than fast acetylators after similar doses and the former are 2 to 3 times more likely to experience adverse effects. Some 60% of the original dose of sulphasalazine is excreted in urine as sulphapyridine and its metabolites. Like sulphasalazine, absorbed sulphapyridine crosses the placenta and is found in breast milk.

The 5-aminosalicylic acid (5-ASA) moiety is much less well absorbed. Of the approximately one-third of liberated 5-ASA which is absorbed, almost all is acetylated and is excreted in urine. For further details of the pharmacokinetics of 5-aminosalicylic acid see under Mesalazine, p.1200.

Reviews of the absorption and fate of sulphasalazine.

1. Klotz U. Clinical pharmacokinetics of sulphasalazine, its metabolites and other prodrugs of 5-aminosalicylic acid. *Clin Pharmacokinet* 1985; **10:** 285–302.

Uses and Administration

Sulphasalazine is a compound of a sulphonamide, sulphapyridine, with 5-aminosalicylic acid (mesalazine), which is used in the management of inflammatory bowel diseases. Its activity is generally considered to lie in the 5-aminosalicylic acid moiety, which is released in the colon by bacterial metabolism, although intact sulphasalazine has some anti-inflammatory properties in its own right.

It is used alone or as an adjunct to corticosteroids in the treatment of active ulcerative colitis and is effective in maintaining remission. Sulphasalazine may also be effective in the active treatment of Crohn's disease, particularly of the colon, but it does not appear to be of value in maintaining remissions. In the UK, the usual initial adult dose of sulphasalazine is 1 to 2 g by mouth 4 times daily, although doses over 4 g daily are associated with an increased risk of toxicity. In the US, therefore, the usual dose is 1 g given 3 or 4 times daily, and an initial dose of 500 mg every 6 to 12 hours may be recommended to lessen gastro-intestinal adverse effects. Enteric-coated tablets are also claimed to decrease the adverse gastro-intestinal effects which may be associated with administration of sulphasalazine. The overnight interval between doses should not exceed 8 hours. On remission the dose in patients with ulcerative colitis is gradually reduced to 2 g or less daily and then generally continued indefinitely. For children 2 years of age or older doses should be proportional to body-weight; initially 40 to 60 mg per kg body-weight may be given daily in divided doses reduced to 20 to 30 mg per kg daily for the maintenance of remission.

Sulphasalazine is also given rectally, as suppositories, in a dose of 0.5 to 1 g night and morning, either alone or as an adjunct to treatment by mouth; it may also be given by enema in a dose of 3 g at bedtime.

Sulphasalazine is also used as an antirheumatic drug in the treatment of severe or progressive rheumatoid arthritis. Treatment is usually commenced with a dose of 500 mg daily by mouth, as enteric-coated tablets, for the first week; dosage is then increased by 500 mg each week to a maximum of 3 g daily given in 2 to 4 divided doses.

Ankylosing spondylitis. Sulphasalazine has been reported[1,2] to be effective in the treatment of active ankylosing spondylitis (p.4) in doses of up to 3 g daily by mouth for 6 months. Compared with placebo it produced a greater improvement in a number of clinical and laboratory parameters and allowed a reduction in the dose of NSAIDs. It was administered as enteric-coated tablets and the incidence of side-effects was similar to that for placebo. The improvement with sulphasalazine was significant from the third month of treatment; mesalazine does not appear to be the active component.[1]

1. Dougados M, *et al.* Sulphasalazine in ankylosing spondylitis: a double blind controlled study in 60 patients. *Br Med J* 1986; **293:** 911–14.
2. Nissilä M, *et al.* Sulfasalazine in the treatment of ankylosing spondylitis: a twenty-six-week, placebo-controlled clinical trial. *Arthritis Rheum* 1988; **31:** 1111–16.

Behçet's syndrome. Treatment with prednisolone and codeine phosphate produced only a slight improvement in a patient with Behçet's syndrome with colonic and oesophageal involvement but addition of sulphasalazine gave a clinical and serological remission.[1] A subsequent relapse was successfully treated with the addition of cyclosporin for 6 weeks. For a discussion of Behçet's syndrome and its management, see p.1018.

1. Foster GR. Behçet's colitis with oesophageal ulceration treated with sulphasalazine and cyclosporin. *J R Soc Med* 1988; **81:** 545–6.

Inflammatory bowel disease. Together with corticosteroids sulphasalazine has long been a mainstay of the treatment of inflammatory bowel disease. For a review of the management of Crohn's disease and ulcerative colitis, including mention of the role of sulphasalazine, see p.1171.

COLLAGENOUS COLITIS. Collagenous colitis is a rare condition which presents as persistent watery diarrhoea and is associated with a thickened band of collagen immediately below the surface epithelium of the colonic mucosa. Treatment is largely symptomatic.[1-3] A suggested approach from analysis of data from 163 patients was to try antidiarrhoeal therapy with loperamide initially, and then sulphasalazine if this was ineffective.[3] In unresponsive patients cholestyramine, prednisolone, antibacterials such as metronidazole, or mepacrine, or an immunosuppressant such as methotrexate, might all be tried. Mesalazine and olsalazine seemed to be less effective than sulphasalazine,[3] although they may be useful where sulphasalazine is not tolerated.[3,4]

1. Weldon M. A useful collagenous colitis registry. *Lancet* 1997; **349:** 1410–11.
2. Rams H, *et al.* Collagenous colitis. *Ann Intern Med* 1987; **106:** 108–13.
3. Bohr J, *et al.* Collagenous colitis: a retrospective study of clinical presentation and treatment in 163 patients. *Gut* 1996; **39:** 846–51.
4. O'Mahony S, *et al.* Coeliac disease and collagenous colitis. *Postgrad Med J* 1990; **66:** 238–41.

Measurement of orocaecal transit time. Sulphasalazine has been used to measure orocaecal transit time.[1] Following administration of sulphasalazine by mouth with a test meal, azoreductase-producing flora in the large bowel split the azo link releasing 5-aminosalicylic acid and sulphapyridine; most of the sulphapyridine is absorbed. A series of blood samples are taken and the time at which sulphapyridine appears in the blood indicates the arrival of the test meal in the caecum and thus the orocaecal transit time.

1. Staniforth DH. Comparison of orocaecal transit times assessed by the lactulose/breath hydrogen and the sulphasalazine/sulphapyridine methods. *Gut* 1989; **30:** 978–82.

Psoriasis. In a double-blind placebo-controlled study involving 50 patients with moderate to severe plaque-type psoriasis, sulphasalazine 3 to 4 g daily produced a significantly greater clinical improvement than placebo after 4 weeks of treatment with a further improvement at 8 weeks.[1] After 8 weeks in the 17 sulphasalazine treated patients, there was a marked response in 7, a moderate response in 7, and minimal or no response in 3. Six patients in the sulphasalazine group dropped out during the study due to adverse effects; 4 developed a cutaneous eruption and 2 had nausea. In general, it appears that monotherapy with sulphasalazine is not as effective as is therapy with methotrexate, psoralen plus UV-A, or etretinate. However, in a small proportion of patients (approximately 25%) sulphasalazine is of comparable efficacy to these treatments and is associated with a lower incidence of adverse effects. The more usual drugs used in the management of psoriasis are discussed on p.1075.

See also Psoriatic Arthritis, below.

1. Gupta AK, *et al.* Sulfasalazine improves psoriasis: a double-blind analysis. *Arch Dermatol* 1990; **126:** 487–93.

Psoriatic arthritis. A double-blind placebo-controlled study of sulphasalazine in psoriatic arthritis.[1] The dose of sulphasalazine was initially 500 mg daily, increasing to a maximum maintenance dose of 2 g daily, and was continued for a total of 24 weeks. Overall in the sulphasalazine group there was a good response in 5 patients, a partial response in 7, and a poor or no response in 2; the corresponding figures for the placebo group were 0, 4, and 10. Three patients discontinued sulphasalazine because of adverse reactions and a further three required a reduction in the dose of sulphasalazine. For a discussion of psoriatic arthritis and its management, see under Spondyloarthropathies, p.4.

See also under Psoriasis, above.

1. Farr M, *et al.* Sulphasalazine in psoriatic arthritis: a double-blind placebo-controlled study. *Br J Rheumatol* 1990; **29:** 46–9.

Rheumatoid arthritis. Sulphasalazine was synthesised in the 1940s specifically for the treatment of rheumatoid arthritis (p.2). However, it became more widely used in the management of inflammatory bowel diseases and it was not investigated further for the treatment of rheumatoid arthritis until a number of years later. It is now considered to be a useful disease modifying antirheumatic drug (DMARD) in the treatment of rheumatoid arthritis. Meta-analyses[1,2] of generally short-term comparative studies suggest that sulphasalazine is roughly comparable in efficacy to methotrexate, intramuscular gold (sodium aurothiomalate), and penicillamine, and some rheumatologists now use it as one of the DMARDs of first choice.[3] In an open study[5] of 200 patients with rheumatoid arthritis who were randomly allocated to treatment with sulphasalazine or auranofin, 31% of the sulphasalazine recipients were still taking the drug after 5 years compared with 15% of auranofin recipients. Improvement over baseline was still significant at 5 years for those patients receiving sulphasalazine but not in those treated with auranofin. Combination treatment with sulphasalazine plus methotrexate and hydroxychloroquine has been reported to be more effective than methotrexate alone or sulphasalazine with hydroxychloroquine.[4]

1. Felson DT, *et al.* The comparative efficacy and toxicity of second-line drugs in rheumatoid arthritis. *Arthritis Rheum* 1990; **33:** 1449–61.
2. Capell HA, *et al.* Second line (disease modifying) treatment in rheumatoid arthritis: which drug for which patient? *Ann Rheum Dis* 1993; **52:** 423–8.
3. Rains CP, *et al.* Sulfasalazine: a review of its pharmacological properties and therapeutic efficacy in the treatment of rheumatoid arthritis. *Drugs* 1995; **50:** 137–56.
4. O'Dell JR, *et al.* Treatment of rheumatoid arthritis with methotrexate alone, sulfasalazine and hydroxychloroquine, or a combination of all three medications. *N Engl J Med* 1996; **334:** 1287–91.
5. McEntegart A, *et al.* Sulfasalazine has a better efficacy/toxicity profile than auranofin—evidence from a 5 year prospective, randomized trial. *J Rheumatol* 1996; **23:** 1887–90.

JUVENILE CHRONIC ARTHRITIS. Juvenile chronic arthritis (p.2) is generally managed similarly to rheumatoid arthritis, but there is limited experience with the use of some antirheumatic drugs in children. Sulphasalazine produced significant improvement in 15 of 18 patients with juvenile chronic arthritis treated for 4 to 14 months.[1] A dose of 50 mg per kg bodyweight was used, starting with one-quarter of the total dose increased weekly by increments of one-quarter. Two patients withdrew after 7 and 11 months due to lack of effect and treatment was stopped in one patient because of leucopenia; 5 patients experienced minor side-effects which resolved on reducing the dose. Another prospective study found that 73% of 139 evaluable patients given sulphasalazine experienced some improvement in their symptoms within 12 months.[2]

1. Özdogan H, *et al.* Sulphasalazine in the treatment of juvenile rheumatoid arthritis: a preliminary open trial. *J Rheumatol* 1986; **13:** 124–5.
2. Imundo LF, Jacobs JC. Sulfasalazine therapy for juvenile rheumatoid arthritis. *J Rheumatol* 1996; **23:** 360–6.

Scleroderma. Sulphasalazine has been tried in the management of scleroderma (see p.501).

Preparations

USP 23: Sulfasalazine Delayed-release Tablets; Sulfasalazine Tablets.

Proprietary Preparations (details are given in Part 3)
Aust.: Colo-Pleon†; Salazopyrin; ***Austral.:*** Pyralin; Salazopyrin; Sulazine†; Ulcol†; ***Belg.:*** Salazopyrine; ***Canad.:*** Salazopyrin; SAS; ***Fr.:*** Salazopyrine; ***Ger.:*** Azulfidine; Colo-Pleon; Pleon RA; ***Irl.:*** Salazopyrin; Sulfazine†; ***Ital.:*** Salazopyrin; Salisulf Gastroprotetto†; ***Neth.:*** Salazopyrine; ***Norw.:*** Salazopyrin; ***S.Afr.:*** Salazopyrin; ***Spain:*** Salazopyrina; ***Swed.:*** Salazopyrin; ***Switz.:*** Salazopyrin; ***UK:*** Salazopyrin; Sulazine; Ucine; ***USA:*** Azulfidine.

Tamarind (7534-p)

West Indian Tamarind.

The fruits of *Tamarindus indica* (Leguminosae) freed from the brittle outer part of the pericarp and preserved with sugar or syrup.

Tamarind has been used as a laxative.

Preparations

Proprietary Preparations (details are given in Part 3)

Multi-ingredient: ***Aust.:*** Frugelletten; Neda Fruchtewurfel; ***Belg.:*** Tamarine; ***Fr.:*** Actisane Constipation Occasionnelle; Delabarre; Laxasan; Tamarine; ***Ital.:*** Ortisan; Tamarine; ***Spain:*** Dentomicin; Pruina; ***Switz.:*** Tamarine.

Teprenone (17004-r)

Teprenone *(rINN)*.

E-671. 6,10,14,18-Tetramethyl-5,9,13,17-nonadecatetraen-2-one, mixture of (5*E*,9*E*,13*E*) and (5*Z*,9*E*,13*E*) isomers.

$C_{23}H_{38}O$ = 330.5.

Teprenone is a cytoprotective drug which is used in the treatment of gastritis and peptic ulcer disease (p.1174) in a usual dose of 50 mg three times daily by mouth.

Preparations

Proprietary Preparations (details are given in Part 3)
Jpn: Selbex.

Tritiozine (13383-c)

Tritiozine *(rINN)*.

ISF-2001; Trithiozine. 4-(3,4,5-Trimethoxythiobenzoyl)morpholine.

$C_{14}H_{19}NO_4S$ = 297.4.

CAS — 35619-65-9.

Tritiozine has been used in the treatment of peptic ulcer disease.

Preparations

Proprietary Preparations (details are given in Part 3)
Ital.: Tresanil†.

Tropisetron Hydrochloride (3089-k)

Tropisetron Hydrochloride *(BANM, rINNM)*.

ICS-205-930. 1α*H*,5α*H*-Tropan-3α-yl indole-3-carboxylate hydrochloride.

$C_{17}H_{20}N_2O_2$,HCl = 320.8.

CAS — 89565-68-4 (tropisetron); 105826-92-4 (tropisetron hydrochloride).

Adverse Effects and Precautions

As for Ondansetron Hydrochloride, p.1206. Dizziness, fatigue, and gastro-intestinal disturbances may occur. Visual hallucinations, and an increase in blood pressure in patients with pre-existing hypertension, have been noted at high repeated doses. Seizure threshold may be reduced in susceptible patients.

Adverse effects reported with tropisetron include headache and mild sedation.[1] There have been reports of fever requiring drug withdrawal;[2,3] one patient[3] also experienced mild hypotension, macular rash, joint aches, and cervical lymphadenopathy.

The manufacturer has reported an increased incidence of hepatic neoplasms in *rodents* given high doses of tropisetron for prolonged periods, although the relevance of these results to the clinical situation is undetermined.

1. Leibundgut U, Lancranjan I. First results with ICS 205-930 (5-HT_3 receptor antagonist) in prevention of chemotherapy-induced emesis. *Lancet* 1987; **i:** 1198.
2. Anderson JV, *et al.* Remission of symptoms in carcinoid syndrome with a new 5-hydroxytryptamine M receptor antagonist. *Br Med J* 1987; **294:** 1129.
3. Coupe M. Adverse reaction to 5-HT_3 antagonist ICS 205930. *Lancet* 1987; **i:** 1494.

Pharmacokinetics

Tropisetron is well absorbed following oral administration. Peak plasma concentrations are achieved within 3 hours. It is 71% bound to plasma proteins. Its metabolism is saturable, resulting in nonlinear pharmacokinetics: absolute bioavailability depends on the dose.

Uses and Administration

Tropisetron hydrochloride is a highly selective 5-HT_3-receptor antagonist with a potent antiemetic action similar to that of ondansetron (p.1207) but more prolonged. It is used in the management of nausea and vomiting induced by cytotoxic therapy and in the treatment and prevention of postoperative nausea and vomiting. For a discussion of the management of nausea and vomiting, see p.1172.

Tropisetron hydrochloride is given intravenously, as a slow injection or into a running intravenous infusion, or by mouth; doses are calculated in terms of tropisetron base. For the prophylaxis of nausea and vomiting associated with cytotoxic chemotherapy a single dose equivalent to 5 mg of tropisetron may be given intravenously on the day of treatment, shortly before chemotherapy. Subsequent doses of tropisetron 5 mg daily are given by mouth, at least one hour before food, for a further 5 days.

For the treatment of postoperative nausea and vomiting the equivalent of tropisetron 2 mg may be given by slow intravenous injection, or by infusion over 15 minutes, within 2 hours of the end of anaesthesia. For prophylaxis, the same dose may be given shortly before induction of anaesthesia.

References.

1. van Oosterom AT, Bainco AR. First international symposium on tropisetron. *Drugs* 1992; **43** (suppl 3): 1–44.
2. Lee CR, *et al.* Tropisetron: a review of its pharmacodynamic and pharmacokinetic properties, and therapeutic potential as an antiemetic. *Drugs* 1993; **46:** 925–43.

Anxiety disorders. A dose-dependent anxiolytic effect was reported for tropisetron when studied in patients with generalised anxiety,[1] but clinical evidence for the benefit of $5HT_3$-receptor antagonists in anxiety disorders is lacking.[2]

1. Lecrubier Y, *et al.* A randomized double-blind placebo-controlled study of tropisetron in the treatment of outpatients with generalized anxiety disorder. *Psychopharmacology (Berl)* 1993; **112:** 129–33.
2. Greenshaw AJ, Silverstone PH. The non-antiemetic uses of serotonin 5-HT_3 receptor antagonists: clinical pharmacology and therapeutic applications. *Drugs* 1997; **53:** 20–39.

Preparations

Proprietary Preparations (details are given in Part 3)
Aust.: Navoban; ***Austral.:*** Navoban; ***Belg.:*** Novaban; ***Fr.:*** Navoban; ***Ger.:*** Navoban; ***Irl.:*** Navoban; ***Ital.:*** Navoban; ***Neth.:*** Novaban; ***Norw.:*** Navoban; ***S.Afr.:*** Navoban; ***Spain:*** Navoban; ***Swed.:*** Navoban; ***Switz.:*** Navoban; ***UK:*** Navoban.

Troxipide (2471-z)

Troxipide (*rINN*).

(±)-3,4,5-Trimethoxy-*N*-3-piperidylbenzamide.

$C_{15}H_{22}N_2O_4$ = 294.3.

CAS — 30751-05-4.

Troxipide is used for its cytoprotective properties in the treatment of gastritis and peptic ulcer disease (p.1174) in a usual dose of 300 mg daily by mouth.

Preparations

Proprietary Preparations (details are given in Part 3)
Jpn: Aplace.

Urogastrone (709-v)

Anthelone; EGF-URO; Epidermal Growth Factor; Uroanthelone; Uroenterone.

CAS — 9010-53-1.

A polypeptide first isolated from human urine. Two forms have been identified, β and γ urogastrone. The β form consists of 53 amino acids and is distinguishable from the γ form by an additional terminal arginine residue. The β form is reported to be identical to human epidermal growth factor and this term is widely used in the literature.

Urogastrone inhibits gastric acid secretion and has been tried in the treatment of peptic ulcer disease and other gastro-intestinal disorders but its rapid destruction in the stomach has limited its clinical use.

It is a potent stimulator of cellular proliferation and has also been used as an aid to wound healing.

A review of the discovery, characterisation, physiological roles, and possible clinical use of epidermal growth factor (EGF) and transforming growth factor (TGF).[1]

Human epidermal growth factor is the same substance as the human urinary protein, β-urogastrone. EGF is synthesised as a precursor of 1217 amino acids but the physiologically active polypeptide consists of only 53 amino acids. The amino acid sequence is very similar to that of murine EGF (murodermin). Very few tissues contain significant amounts of EGF but it has effects on many cell types including skin thickening, retardation of hair follicles, cell proliferation in the gastro-intestinal tract, blood vessel development, and effects on the immune and endocrine systems. The exact physiological role of EGF is still a subject of considerable speculation. There is no evidence to suggest that EGF itself is associated with induction, promotion, or invasiveness of tumour cells but α-TGF, a closely related growth factor, is associated with proliferating epithelia and tumour cells.

EGF inhibits release of gastric acid but its rapid destruction in the stomach necessitates large and frequent doses which limit its clinical usefulness. It has also been investigated to aid wound healing, in the treatment of chemotherapy-induced mucositis, and to target cytotoxic agents to tumour cells with EGF receptors. In veterinary practice it has a potential role in the defleecing of sheep and as a growth modulator.

The potential role of epidermal growth factor in obstetrics and gynaecology has also been reviewed.[2]

1. Burgess AW. Epidermal growth factor and transforming growth factor α. *Br Med Bull* 1989; **45:** 401–24.
2. Miyazawa K. Role of epidermal growth factor in obstetrics and gynecology. *Obstet Gynecol* 1992; **79:** 1032–40.

Gastro-intestinal disorders. Intravenous infusion of urogastrone 250 ng per kg body-weight over 1 hour has been reported to reduce the secretion of gastric acid in patients with duodenal ulcer[1] or the Zollinger-Ellison syndrome.[2] Ulcer pain was relieved 30 to 60 minutes after the start of the infusion.[2] The more usual drugs used in the treatment of peptic ulcer disease and the Zollinger-Ellison syndrome are discussed on p.1174 and p.1176. A dose of 100 ng per kg per hour by intravenous infusion has been used with partial success in an infant with microvillous atrophy[3] and was apparently beneficial in an infant with necrotising enteritis.[4]

1. Koffman CG, *et al.* Effect of urogastrone on gastric secretion and serum gastrin concentration in patients with duodenal ulceration. *Gut* 1982; **23:** 951–6.
2. Elder JB, *et al.* Effect of urogastrone in the Zollinger-Ellison syndrome. *Lancet* 1975; **ii:** 424–7.
3. Walker-Smith JA, *et al.* Intravenous epidermal growth factor/urogastrone increases small-intestinal cell proliferation in congenital microvillous atrophy. *Lancet* 1985; **ii:** 1239–40.
4. Sullivan PB, *et al.* Epidermal growth factor in necrotising enteritis. *Lancet* 1991; **338:** 53–4.

Wound healing. The effect on the rate of wound healing of a cream containing silver sulphadiazine plus recombinant human epidermal growth factor (10 μg per mL) was compared with silver sulphadiazine alone in 12 patients each requiring skin grafts at 2 donor sites.[1] The cream containing epidermal growth factor accelerated the rate of epidermal regeneration in all patients and reduced the average time to 100% healing by about 1.5 days. Patients were followed up for a maximum of 1 year after cessation of therapy and no complications or clinical evidence of neoplasia at the healed donor sites occurred.

In contrast, recombinant human epidermal growth factor as an ophthalmic solution containing 30 or 100 μg per mL was investigated in patients who had undergone keratoplasty, but the weaker solution had no effect on the rate of re-epithelialisation, and the more concentrated one was actually associated with slower healing.[2]

The management of wounds and ulcers in general is discussed on p.1076.

1. Brown GL, *et al.* Enhancement of wound healing by topical treatment with epidermal growth factor. *N Engl J Med* 1989; **321:** 76–9.
2. Dellaert MMMJ, *et al.* Influence of topical human epidermal growth factor on postkeratoplasty re-epithelialisation. *Br J Ophthalmol* 1997; **81:** 391–5.

Preparations

Proprietary Preparations (details are given in Part 3)
Switz.: Gentel†.

Zacopride Hydrochloride (2929-w)

Zacopride Hydrochloride (*USAN, rINNM*).

AHR-11190 (zacopride); AHR-11190-B. 4-Amino-5-chloro-*N*-3-quinuclidinyl-*o*-anisamide hydrochloride monohydrate.

$C_{15}H_{20}ClN_3O_2,HCl,H_2O$ = 364.3.

CAS — 90182-92-6 (zacopride); 99617-34-2 (zacopride hydrochloride).

Zacopride is a prokinetic and antiemetic drug with potent 5-HT_3-receptor antagonist properties. It has also been investigated for various mental disorders.

Zaldaride (15934-n)

Zaldaride (*rINN*).

(±)-1-{1-[(4-Methyl-4*H*,6*H*-pyrrolo[1,2-*a*][4,1]benzoxazepin-4-yl)methyl]-4-piperidyl}-2-benzimidazolinone.

$C_{26}H_{28}N_4O_2$ = 428.5.

CAS — 109826-26-8.

Zaldaride is under investigation as the maleate for the treatment of diarrhoea.

Diarrhoea. Studies in patients with travellers' diarrhoea have indicated that zaldaride in doses of 20 mg by mouth as the maleate four times daily is an effective antidiarrhoeal.[1,2] It was somewhat less effective then loperamide when given without a loading dose,[2] but a regimen of 40 mg initially, followed by 20 mg approximately every 6 hours was as effective as loperamide 4 mg initially followed by 2 mg after each unformed stool.[3] Although antidiarrhoeal drugs may be given for symptom control in adults, the mainstay of therapy for diarrhoea should still be fluid and electrolyte replacement as discussed on p.1168.

1. DuPont HL, *et al.* Zaldaride maleate, an intestinal calmodulin inhibitor, in the therapy of travelers' diarrhea. *Gastroenterology* 1993; **104:** 709–15.
2. Okhuysen PC, *et al.* Zaldaride maleate (a new calmodulin antagonist) versus loperamide in the treatment of traveler's diarrhea: randomized, placebo-controlled trial. *Clin Infect Dis* 1995; **21:** 341–4.
3. Silberschmidt G, *et al.* Treatment of travellers' diarrhoea: zaldaride compared with loperamide and placebo. *Eur J Gastroenterol Hepatol* 1995; **7:** 871–5.

Zaltidine Hydrochloride (18696-b)

Zaltidine Hydrochloride (*BANM, USAN, rINNM*).

CP-57361-01. [4-(2-Methyl-1*H*-imidazol-4-yl)thiazol-2-yl]guanidine dihydrochloride.

$C_8H_{10}N_6S,2HCl$ = 295.2.

CAS — 85604-00-8 (zaltidine); 90274-23-0 (zaltidine hydrochloride).

Zaltidine hydrochloride is a histamine H_2-antagonist with general properties similar to those of cimetidine (see p.1183). It is reported to have a long duration of action. Zaltidine has been reported to cause hepatic damage.

References.

1. Laferla G, *et al.* The antisecretory effects of zaltidine, a novel long-acting H_2-receptor antagonist, in healthy volunteers and in subjects with a past history of duodenal ulcer. *Br J Clin Pharmacol* 1986; **22:** 395–9.
2. Farup PG, *et al.* Zaltidine: an effective but hepatotoxic H_2-receptor antagonist. *Scand J Gastroenterol* 1988; **23:** 655–8.

General Anaesthetics

This chapter includes drugs used for the induction and maintenance of general anaesthesia. General anaesthetics are administered either by inhalation or by intravenous or occasionally intramuscular injection (see below).

Injectable	Inhalational
Barbiturate	*Halogenated*
Methohexitone	Chloroform
Thiamylal	Desflurane
Thiopentone	Enflurane
Miscellaneous	Halothane
Alphadolone	Isoflurane
Alphaxolone	Methoxyflurane
Eltanolone	Sevoflurane
Etomidate	Trichloroethylene
Ketamine	*Miscellaneous*
Propanidid	Cyclopropane
Propofol	Anaesthetic Ether
Sodium Oxybate	Nitrous Oxide
Tiletamine	Xenon

Adverse Effects of General Anaesthetics

Adverse effects that may be associated with general anaesthesia include involuntary muscle movements, hiccup, coughing, bronchospasm, laryngospasm, hypotension, cardiac arrhythmias, respiratory depression, emergence reactions, mild hypothermia, and postoperative nausea and vomiting.

Malignant hyperthermia (malignant hyperpyrexia) is a rare but potentially fatal complication of general anaesthesia that may be induced by inhalational anaesthetics (mainly halogenated hydrocarbons). The condition and its management are described under Dantrolene Sodium, p.1314.

Sensitisation of the myocardium to beta-adrenergic stimulation occurs with some anaesthetics.

There has been concern over the possible danger to anaesthetists, dentists, and other personnel from exposure to volatile anaesthetics.

General references.

1. Derrington MC, Smith G. A review of studies of anaesthetic risk, morbidity and mortality. *Br J Anaesth* 1987; **59:** 815–33.
2. Davies CJ, *et al.* Delayed adverse reactions to drugs used in anaesthesia. *Adverse Drug React Bull* 1995 (Apr.); 647–50.
3. Klafta JM, *et al.* Neurological and psychiatric adverse effects of anaesthetics: epidemiology and treatment. *Drug Safety* 1995; **13:** 281–95.
4. Fee JPH, Thompson GH. Comparative tolerability profiles of the inhaled anaesthetics. *Drug Safety* 1997; **16:** 157–70.

Following general anaesthesia many patients will experience drowsiness and impaired mental performance for at least 24 hours. Nausea with or without vomiting occurs in 20 to 40% of postanaesthetic patients; nausea may last for 2 days but vomiting seldom persists beyond the first day. Other adverse effects include anorexia, malaise, fatigue, dizziness, and headache; these have been reported in 6 to 12% of patients. Delirium has been noted in at least 10% of elderly general surgical patients and in up to 50% of patients undergoing hip fracture repair. Sore throat is frequent in patients who have been intubated or have had a throat pack inserted. Dry mouth as a result of premedication can add to the patient's discomfort. Manipulations for the maintenance of a clear airway may result in postoperative jaw pain. Muscle pain, typically involving the neck, shoulders, and upper abdomen, may occur if the neuromuscular blocker suxamethonium has been given. It is usually worse on the second postoperative day and may last up to six days. Shoulder ache after laparoscopy resolves after 24 hours; it is due to accumulation of carbon dioxide under the diaphragm. Backache is common after epidural or spinal anaesthesia. Urinary retention may follow regional block, cystoscopic or gynaecological surgery, or when there is prostatism.

References.

1. Kalmanovitch DVA, Simmons P. Post-anaesthetic complications in the home. *Prescribers' J* 1988; **28:** 124–31.
2. Anonymous. Nausea and vomiting after general anaesthesia. *Lancet* 1989; **i:** 651–2.
3. Anonymous. Following up day case anaesthesia in general practice. *Drug Ther Bull* 1990; **28:** 81–2.
4. Rowbotham DJ, Smith G, eds. Postoperative nausea and vomiting. *Br J Anaesth* 1992; **69** (suppl 1): 1S–68S.
5. O'Keeffe ST, NíChonchubhair Á. Postoperative delirium in the elderly. *Br J Anaesth* 1994; **73:** 673–87.
6. Marcantonio ER, *et al.* A clinical prediction rule for delirium after elective noncardiac surgery. *JAMA* 1994; **271:** 134–9.

Hypersensitivity. Type I hypersensitivity reactions have occurred with general anaesthetics.[1] In most patients the release of histamine and other mediators such as prostaglandins and leukotrienes is of no clinical importance but in a few susceptible individuals anaphylaxis may result. Numerous factors to identify those at risk have been proposed over the years along with suggested modifications for anaesthetic management. Of the drugs used in anaesthesia, neuromuscular blockers are associated with the highest incidence of anaphylaxis; the most commonly implicated is reported to be suxamethonium followed by alcuronium (see under the Adverse Effects of Suxamethonium, p.1320). It has been suggested[2] that routine prophylaxis with histamine H_1- and histamine H_2-receptor antagonists should be considered as part of anaesthetic management but others[3] thought it better to avoid the use of combinations such as thiopentone, suxamethonium, and alcuronium that are well known to cause histamine release.

1. McKinnon RP, Wildsmith JAW. Histaminoid reactions in anaesthesia. *Br J Anaesth* 1995; **74:** 217–28.
2. Lorenz W, *et al.* Incidence and clinical importance of perioperative histamine release: randomised study of volume loading and antihistamines after induction of anaesthesia. *Lancet* 1994; **343:** 933–40.
3. O'Connor B, Edwards ND. Reactions to gelatin plasma expanders. *Lancet* 1994; **344:** 328.

Nausea and vomiting. For a discussion on postoperative nausea and vomiting and its management, see p.1172.

Shivering and its treatment. Postoperative shivering, also referred to as spontaneous postanaesthetic tremor, can occur in up to 65% of patients recovering from general anaesthesia.[1] Although there are some signs of true thermogenic shivering its aetiology and relationship to thermoregulation is unclear.[1,2] Postoperative shivering may be part of a more generalised neurological disturbance associated with anaesthesia.[1] It also occurs following regional anaesthesia, especially when given epidurally, but this is probably produced by different mechanisms.[2] Muscular activity during shivering greatly increases metabolic rate, oxygen consumption, and cardiac output and may cause complications in patients with cardiac or respiratory disorders. It can also strain surgical sutures, raise intra-ocular pressure, and impede haemodynamic monitoring.

Some have questioned whether it is appropriate to suppress postoperative shivering and urge caution before using drug therapy in all hypothermic patients.[2] To avoid inadvertent induction of hypothermia it is important before starting therapy to check the patient's temperature to ensure that the shivering is not an appropriate thermoregulatory response to a low body temperature.[1]

Although the relationship between postoperative shivering, body temperature, and heat loss is unclear, patients may respond to warming their environment and the use of blankets.[1,2] Numerous drugs have been tried for the management of postoperative shivering including the central and respiratory stimulant doxapram[3-5] and the opioid analgesic pethidine.[4] Reviews have discussed[1,2] a number of other opioids that have been tried including morphine, butorphanol, fentanyl, and sufentanil but studies suggest that not all opioids are effective or that some may only be effective when given epidurally. However, this may be due to the use of insufficient doses rather than a true difference between opioids.[6] Tramadol, a recently introduced opioid analgesic, has also been tried.[7] Skeletal muscle relaxants have been used after cardiac surgery in order to reduce cardiovascular stress.[8] Vecuronium might be preferable to pancuronium as it does not increase myocardial work and may be associated with fewer complications.[9] However, as profound neuromuscular block is required to inhibit shivering, repeated or higher doses of vecuronium might be required to prevent recurrence. Other drugs being investigated include clonidine,[10-12] ketanserin,[10] and ketamine.[13]

1. Crossley AWA. Postoperative shivering. *Br J Hosp Med* 1993; **49:** 204–8.
2. Anonymous. Perioperative shivering. *Lancet* 1991; **338:** 547–8.
3. Sarma V, Fry ENS. Doxapram after general anaesthesia: its role in stopping shivering during recovery. *Anaesthesia* 1991; **46:** 460–1.
4. Singh P, *et al.* Double-blind comparison between doxapram and pethidine in the treatment of postanaesthetic shivering. *Br J Anaesth* 1993; **71:** 685–8.
5. Fry ENS. Muscle spasticity. *Anaesthesia* 1990; **45:** 67–8.
6. Alfonsi P, *et al.* Fentanyl, as pethidine, inhibits post anaesthesia shivering. *Br J Anaesth* 1993; **70** (suppl 1): 38.
7. De Witte J, *et al.* Tramadol for treatment of shivering after general anaesthesia. *Br J Anaesth* 1996; **76** (suppl 2): 91–2.
8. Cruise C, *et al.* Comparison of meperidine and pancuronium for the treatment of shivering after cardiac surgery. *Can J Anaesth* 1992; **39:** 563–8.
9. Dupuis J-Y, *et al.* Pancuronium or vecuronium for treatment of shivering after cardiac surgery. *Anesth Analg* 1994; **79:** 472–81.
10. Joris J, *et al.* Clonidine and ketanserin both are effective treatment for postanesthetic shivering. *Anesthesiology* 1993; **79:** 532–9.
11. Steinfath M, *et al.* Clonidine administered intraoperatively prevents postoperative shivering. *Br J Clin Pharmacol* 1995; **39:** 580P–581P.
12. Vanderstappen I, *et al.* The effect of prophylactic clonidine on postoperative shivering. *Anaesthesia* 1996; **51:** 351–5.
13. Sharma DR, Thakur JR. Ketamine and shivering. *Anaesthesia* 1990; **45:** 252–3.

Precautions for General Anaesthetics

Patients with impaired function of the adrenal cortex, for example, those who are being treated, or have recently been treated, with corticosteroids, may experience hypotension with the stress of anaesthesia. Treatment with corticosteroids, pre-operatively and postoperatively, may be necessary. Patients taking other long-term medication such as aspirin, oral anticoagulants, oestrogens, monoamine oxidase inhibitors, and lithium, may require a change in dosage or cessation of therapy before major elective surgery.

Patients with chronic diseases such as diabetes or hypertension may require adjustment to their therapy prior to anaesthesia. Anaesthetics should be used with caution in patients with cardiac, respiratory, renal, or hepatic impairment.

Patients should not undertake hazardous tasks such as driving for at least 24 hours after a general anaesthetic; alcohol should also be avoided.

Intraoperative awareness. The use of neuromuscular blockers has enabled anaesthetic doses to be reduced. However, lack of a reliable method for detecting conscious awareness in patients with complete neuromuscular block has resulted in paralysed patients who have received inadequate anaesthesia being aware during surgery.[1,2] Recommendations to control this problem include premedication with sedative or amnesic drugs, the use of sufficient doses of intravenous induction anaesthetics, the use of effective analgesic techniques during surgery, and, in particular, adequate concentrations of inspired anaesthetic gas. However, even patients given lorazepam or opioids may have some recall and there is no certain way to avoid awareness in paralysed patients. One commentator[3] considered that the routine use of neuromuscular blockers during surgery should be re-assessed since modern anaesthetics and analgesics could provide good operating conditions without paralysis for most major surgical procedures.

1. Brighouse DI, Norman J. To wake in fright. *Br Med J* 1992; **304:** 1327–8.
2. Jones JG. Memory of intraoperative events. *Br Med J* 1994; **309:** 967–8.
3. Ponte J. Neuromuscular blockers during general anaesthesia. *Br Med J* 1995; **310:** 1218–19.

Interactions of General Anaesthetics

Sensitisation of the myocardium to beta-adrenergic stimulation occurs with some anaesthetics and ventricular fibrillation may occur if *sympathomimetics* such as adrenaline and isoprenaline are administered concomitantly. Enhanced hypotensive effects may result when anaesthetics are given with *ACE inhibitors*, *tricyclic antidepressants*, *MAOIs*, *antihypertensives*, *antipsychotics*, or *beta blockers*. The effects of *competitive neuromuscular blockers* may be increased by inhalational anaesthetics. The concurrent use of anaesthetics with other *CNS depressant drugs* such as those used for premedication may produce synergistic effects on the CNS and, in some cases, a smaller dose of general anaesthetic should be given.

Reviews.

1. Wood M. Pharmacokinetic drug interactions in anaesthetic practice. *Clin Pharmacokinet* 1991; **21:** 285–307.
2. Ransom ES, Mueller RA. Safety considerations in the use of drug combinations during general anaesthesia. *Drug Safety* 1997; **16:** 88–103.

Uses of General Anaesthetics

General anaesthetics depress the CNS and cause loss of consciousness associated with an inability to perceive pain. An ideal anaesthetic would produce unconsciousness, analgesia, and muscle relaxation suitable for all surgical procedures and would be metabolically inert and rapidly eliminated. No anaesthetic fulfils all these requirements in safe concentrations and it is customary to employ a number of drugs to achieve the required conditions while minimising the risk of toxicity.

The activity of any anaesthetic is dependent on its ability to reach the brain. With inhalational anaesthetics there has to be a transfer from the alveolar space to the blood, then to the brain; recovery is a function of the removal of the anaesthetic from the brain. With injectable anaesthetics their activity is similarly dependent on their ability to penetrate the blood/brain barrier and recovery in turn is governed by their redistribution and excretion. The potency of inhalational anaesthetics is often expressed in terms of minimum alveolar concentrations, known as MAC values. The MAC of an anaesthetic is the concentration at 1 atmosphere that will produce immobility in 50% of subjects exposed to a noxious stimulus. Values given under the individual monographs are based on the anaesthetic being used without nitrous oxide which can reduce the MAC. Other factors including age, body temperature, and concurrent medication such as opioid analgesics can also affect MAC values.

Anaesthesia. A wide range of drugs is involved in achieving and maintaining conditions suitable for surgery. Conventional general anaesthesia may be divided into a number of stages including:

- premedication
- induction
- muscle relaxation and intubation
- maintenance
- analgesia
- reversal.

A brief outline of the drugs typically used in each stage follows.

For **premedication**, benzodiazepines and various phenothiazines may be given to sedate and relieve *anxiety* in apprehensive patients. Butyrophenones such as droperidol have also been used. The benzodiazepines have useful amnesic and muscle-relaxant properties and short-acting oral analogues are common in current regimens. The phenothiazines and butyrophenones are rarely used now although their antiemetic actions may be useful to control *postoperative vomiting* (see p.1172). Chloral hydrate is still used in some countries for pre-operative sedation. The use of barbiturates has largely ceased. Chlormethiazole has been used to sedate patients before regional anaesthesia. For sedation of children the oral or rectal route is often preferred to injections; drugs used include diazepam and oral trimeprazine.

Antimuscarinics such as atropine, glycopyrronium, and hyoscine are given to inhibit excessive *bronchial* and *salivary secretions* induced by intubation and some anaesthetics for example ketamine and ether. Antimuscarinics are also given as premedicants to reduce the intra-operative bradycardia and hypotension induced by drugs such as suxamethonium, halothane, or propofol or following vagal stimulation. Hyoscine also provides some degree of amnesia.

Opioids, including morphine and its derivatives, papaveretum and pethidine, have been widely used before surgery to reduce anxiety, smooth induction of anaesthesia, reduce overall anaesthetic requirements, and provide pain relief during and after surgery. However, some consider that the routine use of opioids as premedicants is largely traditional and, in view of the high incidence of side-effects, advocate restriction to patients already in pain.

In addition to premedicants with antiemetic properties, patients may be given drugs that further reduce the danger of regurgitation and aspiration of gastric contents (see under Aspiration Syndromes, p.1168). Those favoured include the histamine H_2-receptor antagonists, cimetidine and ranitidine, and the proton-pump inhibitor, omeprazole. Cardiovascular drugs may be required during surgery to control blood pressure and counteract arrhythmias.

The aim of **induction** is to produce anaesthesia rapidly and smoothly. Induction may be achieved with intravenous or inhalational anaesthetics but intravenous induction may be more pleasant for the patient. Intravenous drugs used include the barbiturate thiopentone, the benzodiazepine midazolam, and other anaesthetics such as etomidate, propofol, or ketamine. Small doses of short-acting opioids, for example alfentanil or fentanyl, given before or at induction allow the use of smaller induction doses of thiopentone and technique is particularly suitable for poor-risk patients.

Following induction, **muscle relaxation** with a rapidly acting neuromuscular blocker such as suxamethonium facilitates **intubation** of the patient. Longer acting neuromuscular blockers may then be administered to allow procedures such as abdominal surgery to be carried out under lighter anaesthesia. For more detail see Anaesthesia on p.1302.

Maintenance of anaesthesia may be achieved with an inhalational anaesthetic, an intravenous anaesthetic, or an intravenous opioid, either alone or in combination.

Opioid analgesics may also be given for **analgesia** as supplements during general anaesthesia (see also Balanced Anaesthesia, under Anaesthetic Techniques, below). Long-acting opioids such as morphine or papaveretum are avoided because of problems with postoperative respiratory depression. The short-acting opioids fentanyl and its cogeners alfentanil and sufentanil appear to produce fewer circulatory changes and may be preferred to other opioids, especially in cardiovascular surgery. Various combinations of analgesic techniques, including the use of pre-emptive analgesia, are used or are being investigated for the management of surgical pain (see Postoperative Pain, under Analgesics, on p.11).

At the end of surgery drugs are sometimes administered to accelerate recovery by **reversal** of the effects of the various agents used during anaesthesia. The *neuromuscular block* produced by competitive neuromuscular blockers may be reversed with anticholinesterases such as neostigmine and edrophonium but concomitant administration of atropine or glycopyrronium is required to prevent bradycardia and other muscarinic actions developing. The opioid antagonist naloxone has been given to reverse opioid-induced *respiratory depression*. However, it may antagonise the analgesic effects of the opioids in the control of postoperative pain and the increasing use of short-acting intravenous opioid analgesics should reduce the need for its use. Flumazenil is a benzodiazepine antagonist that is used to reverse the *central sedative effects* of benzodiazepines in anaesthetic procedures.

ANAESTHETIC TECHNIQUES. A balanced combination of drugs with different actions is often used to provide the various components of general anaesthesia including unconsciousness (hypnosis), muscle relaxation, and analgesia. This technique, termed **balanced anaesthesia**, has been reported to minimise intra-operative cardiovascular depression, to facilitate a rapid return of consciousness, and to have a low incidence of postoperative adverse effects such as nausea and vomiting, and excitation. Typically an opioid is included in premedication, and anaesthesia is induced using nitrous oxide and an intravenous barbiturate such as thiopentone. The opioid is then given in small incremental doses to achieve and maintain adequate analgesia during surgery. Opioid analgesics commonly used in this technique include morphine, fentanyl, sufentanil, and alfentanil; buprenorphine and nalbuphine have also been used.

In **total intravenous anaesthesia** (TIVA), induction and maintenance of anaesthesia is achieved with one or more anaesthetics given intravenously. This allows a high inspired oxygen concentrations in situations where hypoxaemia may otherwise occur, and is advantageous in surgery where delivery of inhaled anaesthetic may be difficult (for example in bronchoscopy). Combinations used in TIVA include propofol with alfentanil or fentanyl, and midazolam with alfentanil. Neuromuscular blockers are given to produce muscle relaxation but there can be difficulty in assessing the depth of anaesthesia in patients who are paralysed for mechanical ventilation and there have been reports of awareness during procedures under total intravenous anaesthesia (see also under Intraoperative Awareness in Precautions, above).

Use of a neuroleptic together with an opioid analgesic produces an altered state of consciousness known as **neuroleptanalgesia** in which the patient is calm and indifferent to the surroundings yet is responsive to commands. The technique is useful for diagnostic or therapeutic procedures such as minor surgery, endoscopy, and changing dressings. Neuroleptanalgesia can be converted to **neuroleptanaesthesia** by the concurrent administration of nitrous oxide in oxygen; a muscle relaxant may also be included. Neuroleptanaesthesia is particularly useful if the patient's cooperation is required, as consciousness soon returns once the nitrous oxide is discontinued. The neuroleptic most commonly employed is droperidol and it is usually used with fentanyl although other opioids have also been employed.

Ketamine used alone can produce a state of **dissociative anaesthesia** similar to that of neuroleptanalgesia in which the patient may appear to be awake but is unconscious. Marked analgesia and amnesia are produced, but there may be an increase in muscle tone and emergence reactions. Dissociative anaesthesia is considered suitable for use in various diagnostic procedures, dressing changes, and in minor surgery not requiring muscle relaxation.

Techniques employing **local anaesthetics** are discussed on p.1284.

Alphadolone Acetate (3102-r)

Alphadolone Acetate *(BANM)*.

Alfadolone Acetate *(rINNM)*; GR-2/1574. 3α,21-Dihydroxy-5α-pregnane-11,20-dione 21-acetate.

$C_{23}H_{34}O_5$ = 390.5.

CAS — 14107-37-0 (alphadolone); 23930-37-2 (alphadolone acetate).

Pharmacopoeias. In *BP(Vet)*.

A white to creamy white powder. Practically **insoluble** in water and in petroleum spirit; soluble in alcohol; freely soluble in chloroform.

Alphadolone acetate has been used to enhance the solubility of alphaxalone (below). It possesses some anaesthetic properties and is considered to be about half as potent as alphaxalone.

Alphaxalone (3103-f)

Alphaxalone *(BAN)*.

Alfaxalone *(rINN)*; GR-2/234. 3α-Hydroxy-5α-pregnane-11,20-dione.

$C_{21}H_{32}O_3$ = 332.5.

CAS — 23930-19-0.

Pharmacopoeias. In *BP(Vet)*.

A white to creamy white powder. Practically **insoluble** in water and in petroleum spirit; soluble in alcohol; freely soluble in chloroform.

Alphaxalone was formerly used in combination with alphadolone acetate (above) ['Althesin'], as an intravenous anaesthetic for induction and maintenance of anaesthesia.

Adverse reactions associated with polyethoxylated castor oil (present as a vehicle) led to the general withdrawal of alphaxalone with alphadolone acetate from human use. It is still used in veterinary medicine.

Alphaxalone: alphadolone has been associated with acute attacks of porphyria and is considered unsafe in patients with acute porphyria.[1]

1. Moore MR, McColl KEL. *Porphyria: drug lists.* Glasgow: Porphyria Research Unit, University of Glasgow, 1991.

Chloroform (3104-d)

Chloroformium Anesthesicum; Chloroformum; Chloroformum pro Narcosi. Trichloromethane.

$CHCl_3$ = 119.4.

CAS — 67-66-3.

Pharmacopoeias. In *Aust.*, *Belg.*, *Br.*, and *Chin.*

Some pharmacopoeias include a grade of chloroform, with less stringent standards, which may be used in oral preparations but which must not be used as an anaesthetic.

A colourless volatile liquid with a characteristic odour. The BP specifies that it contains 1.0 to 2.0% v/v of ethyl alcohol; the BP allows amylene 50 μg per mL as an alternative to ethyl alcohol. Not flammable. B.p. about 61°. The addition of the small percentage of alcohol greatly retards the gradual oxidation which occurs when chloroform is exposed to air and light and which results in its becoming contaminated with the very poisonous carbonyl chloride (phosgene) and with chlorine; the alcohol also serves to decompose any carbonyl chloride that may have been formed.

Slightly **soluble** in water; miscible with dehydrated alcohol, ether, fixed and volatile oils, and most other organic solvents. **Store** in airtight containers with glass stoppers or other suitable closures. Protect from light. The BP specifies that the label should state whether it contains ethyl alcohol or amylene.

CAUTION. *Suitable precautions should be taken to avoid skin contact with chloroform as it can penetrate skin and produce systemic toxicity. Care should be taken not to vaporise chloroform in the presence of a flame because of the production of toxic gases.*

Stability. From a study[1] of chloroform losses from chloroform water and from 6 typical BPC mixtures under various conditions of storage the following shelf-lives were recommended: chloroform solutions and non-sedimented mixtures could be stored in well-closed well-filled containers for 2 months at ambient temperatures; when stored in partially-filled containers periodically opened the shelf-life should not exceed 2 weeks; sedimented mixtures could be stored for 2 months in well-closed well-filled containers, but because loss of chloroform could be expected in containers periodically opened such mixtures should be prepared as required or packed in their final containers; for chloroform-containing mixtures in the home a shelf-life of 2 weeks was suggested.

1. Lynch M, *et al.* Chloroform as a preservative in aqueous systems: losses under "in-use" conditions and antimicrobial effectiveness. *Pharm J* 1977; **219:** 507–10.

Storage. It has been recommended[1] that PVC bottles should not be used for storing or dispensing Chloroform and Morphine Tincture, aqueous mixtures containing more than 5% thereof, mixtures or dispersions in which chloroform was present in excess of its aqueous solubility, aqueous mixtures containing chloroform and high concentrations of electrolytes, or Chloroform Water (BP) or mixtures containing it if the period of use would exceed 6 weeks.

1. Anonymous. Plastics medicine bottles of rigid PVC. *Pharm J* 1973; **210:** 100.

Adverse Effects and Precautions

Chloroform is hepatotoxic and nephrotoxic. It depresses respiration and produces hypotension. Cardiac output is reduced and arrhythmias may develop. Poisoning leads to respiratory depression and cardiac arrest; it may take 6 to 24 hours after a dose before appearance of delayed symptoms characterised by abdominal pain, vomiting, and, at a later stage, jaundice.

Liquid chloroform is irritant to the skin and mucous membranes and may cause burns if spilt on them.

In the UK medicinal products are limited to a chloroform content of not more than 0.5% (w/w or v/v as appropriate) of chloroform. Exceptions include supply by a doctor or dentist, or in accordance with his prescription, to a particular patient, supply for external use, and supply for anaesthetic purposes.

In the USA the FDA have banned the use of chloroform in medicines and cosmetics, because of reported carcinogenicity in *animals*. It has also been withdrawn from systemic use in other countries.

The sale within or import into England and Wales and Scotland of food containing any added chloroform is prohibited.

See also Adverse Effects and Precautions for General Anaesthetics, p.1219.

Porphyria. Chloroform has been associated with clinical exacerbations of porphyria and is considered unsafe in porphyric patients.[1]

1. Moore MR, McColl KEL. *Porphyria: drug lists.* Glasgow: Porphyria Research Unit, University of Glasgow, 1991.

Uses and Administration

Chloroform is a volatile halogenated anaesthetic administered by inhalation but because of its toxicity it is seldom used now in anaesthesia.

Chloroform is used as a carminative and as a flavouring agent and preservative. For these purposes it is usually employed as Chloroform Spirit (BP 1998) or Chloroform Water (BP 1998) but doubts have been cast on the safety of the long-term use of chloroform in mixtures.

Externally, chloroform has a rubefacient action.

Chloroform is also used as a solvent.

A historical review of the use of chloroform in clinical anaesthesia.[1]

1. Payne JP. Chloroform in clinical anaesthesia. *Br J Anaesth* 1981; **53:** 11S–15S.

Preparations

BP 1998: Chloroform and Morphine Tincture *(Chlorodyne)*; Chloroform Spirit; Chloroform Water; Double-strength Chloroform Water.

Proprietary Preparations (details are given in Part 3)

Multi-ingredient: ***Belg.:*** Baume Dalet; Dentophar; Dolpyc; Revocyl†; ***Fr.:*** Baume Dalet; Chloridia†; Dolpyc; Eludril; Hepatoum; Kamol; Lao-Dal; Solution Buvable Hepatoum†; Stom-Antiba†; ***UK:*** Copholcoids†; Galloway's Cough Syrup.

Cyclopropane (3105-n)

Cyclopropane *(rINN)*.

Trimethylene.

C_3H_6 = 42.08.

CAS — 75-19-4.

Pharmacopoeias. In *Aust.* and *US.*

A colourless highly flammable gas with a characteristic odour and pungent taste. Freely **soluble** in alcohol; soluble in fixed oils. One volume dissolves in about 2.7 volumes of water at 15°.

It is supplied compressed in metal cylinders. National standards are usually in operation for the labelling and marking of such cylinders.

CAUTION. *Mixtures of cyclopropane with oxygen or air at certain concentrations are explosive. Cyclopropane should not be used in the presence of an open flame or of any electrical apparatus liable to produce a spark. Precautions should be taken against the production of static electrical discharge.*

Adverse Effects and Precautions

Cyclopropane depresses respiration to a greater extent than many other anaesthetics. Laryngospasm, cardiac arrhythmias, or hepatic injury may occur. Cyclopropane increases the sensitivity of the heart to sympathomimetic amines. Malignant hyperthermia has also been reported. Postoperative nausea, vomiting, and headache are frequent.

Cyclopropane should be used with caution in patients with bronchial asthma and cardiovascular disorders. Premedication with atropine may be advisable to reduce vagal tone.

See also Adverse Effects and Precautions for General Anaesthetics, p.1219.

Abuse. A report following-on from a nationwide survey in the USA of four deaths from abuse of volatile anaesthetics in operating rooms.[1] Two of the deaths were attributed to cyclopropane.

1. Bass M. Abuse of inhalation anesthetics. *JAMA* 1984; **251:** 604.

Malignant hyperthermia. One case of malignant hyperthermia associated with cyclopropane.[1]

1. Lips FJ, *et al.* Malignant hyperthermia triggered by cyclopropane during cesarean section. *Anesthesiology* 1982; **56:** 144–6.

Interactions

Care is advised if adrenaline or other sympathomimetics are given during cyclopropane anaesthesia. Potentiation of competitive neuromuscular blockers occurs after cyclopropane administration.

See also Interactions for General Anaesthetics, p.1219.

Uses and Administration

Cyclopropane is an anaesthetic administered by inhalation. It has a minimum alveolar concentration (MAC) value (see p.1220) of 9.2%. It has been used for analgesia and induction and maintenance of anaesthesia. It produces skeletal muscle relaxation, is non-irritant, and induction and recovery are rapid. Because of the risk of explosion, the usual method of administration has been by means of a closed circuit.

Desflurane (11789-f)

Desflurane *(USAN, rINN)*.

I-653. (±)-2-Difluoromethyl 1,2,2,2-tetrafluoroethyl ether.

$C_3H_2F_6O$ = 168.0.

CAS — 57041-67-5.

Pharmacopoeias. In *US.*

Store in airtight containers. Protect from light.

Adverse Effects

As with other halogenated anaesthetics, respiratory depression, hypotension, and arrhythmias may occur. *Animal* studies indicate that desflurane may precipitate malignant hyperthermia in susceptible individuals. Desflurane appears to sensitise the myocardium to sympathomimetics to a lesser extent than halothane or enflurane. Nausea and vomiting have been reported in the postoperative period.

Desflurane is irritant to the airways and may provoke breath holding, apnoea, coughing, increased salivation, and laryngospasm.

See also Adverse Effects of General Anaesthetics, p.1219.

Effects on the blood. The development of carboxyhaemoglobinaemia in patients anaesthetised with volatile anaesthetics is discussed under Precautions, below.

Effects on the cardiovascular system. A review[1] of *animal* and human studies concluded that the cardiorespiratory effects of desflurane were similar to those of isoflurane but that there might be better control of arterial pressure with desflurane during stressful stimuli. One study[2] in patients undergoing coronary artery bypass surgery demonstrated that a state of haemodynamic stability suitable for patients at risk of myocardial ischaemia could be maintained when desflurane was supplemented with the opioid analgesic fentanyl.

1. Warltier DC, Pagel PS. Cardiovascular and respiratory actions of desflurane: is desflurane different from isoflurane? *Anesth Analg* 1992; **75:** S17–S31.
2. Parsons RS, *et al.* Comparison of desflurane and fentanyl-based anaesthetic techniques for coronary artery bypass surgery. *Br J Anaesth* 1994; **72:** 430–8.

Effects on the liver. Although considered to be less hepatotoxic than some other halogenated anaesthetics (see under Adverse Effects of Halothane, p.1224), delayed hepatotoxicity has occurred in a 65-year-old woman following maintenance anaesthesia involving desflurane.[1] She had received halothane on two previous occasions which may have caused sensitisation. Investigation of hepatocellular integrity (by measuring glutathione transferase alpha) in 30 women who had received desflurane indicated a mild subclinical disturbance.[2]

1. Martin JL, *et al.* Hepatotoxicity after desflurane anesthesia. *Anesthesiology* 1995; **83:** 1125–9.
2. Tiainen P, *et al.* Changes in hepatocellular integrity during and after desflurane or isoflurane anaesthesia in patients undergoing breast surgery. *Br J Anaesth* 1998; **80:** 87–9.

Effects on the respiratory tract. The irritant effect of desflurane on the lungs limits its role in the induction of anaesthesia, especially in children. Pre-operative use of nebulised lignocaine 4% failed to alleviate the response.[1]

1. Bunting HE, *et al.* Effect of nebulized lignocaine on airway irritation and haemodynamic changes during induction of anaesthesia with desflurane. *Br J Anaesth* 1995; **75:** 631–3.

Precautions

Desflurane is not recommended for induction of anaesthesia in paediatric patients because of reactions to its pungency. As with other halogenated anaesthetics, patients with known or suspected susceptibility to malignant hyperthermia should not be anaesthetised with desflurane. Desflurane may increase cerebrospinal fluid pressure and should therefore be used with caution in patients with, or at risk from, raised intracranial pressure.

In order to minimise the risk of developing elevated carboxyhaemoglobin levels carbon dioxide absorbents in anaesthetic apparatus should not be allowed to dry out when delivering volatile anaesthetics such as desflurane.

See also Precautions for General Anaesthetics, p.1219.

Significant carboxyhaemoglobinaemia may develop during anaesthesia with volatile anaesthetics given by circle breathing systems containing carbon dioxide absorbents.[1] The effect is only seen when the absorbent (usually barium hydroxide lime) has become excessively dried out.

1. Committe on Safety of Medicines/Medicines Control Agency. Safety issues in anaesthesia: volatile anaesthetic agents and carboxyhaemoglobinaemia. *Current Problems* 1997; **23:** 7.

Interactions

The effects of competitive neuromuscular blockers such as atracurium are enhanced by desflurane (see p.1307). Lower doses of desflurane are required in those receiving opioids, benzodiazepines or other sedatives. Care is advised if adrenaline or other sympathomimetics are given to patients during desflurane anaesthesia.

See also Interactions of General Anaesthetics, p.1219.

References.

1. Dale O. Drug interactions in anaesthesia: focus on desflurane and sevoflurane. *Baillieres Clin Anaesthesiol* 1995; **9:** 105–17.

Pharmacokinetics

Desflurane has a low blood/gas coefficient and following inhalation its absorption, distribution, and elimination are reported to be more rapid than for other halogenated anaesthetics such as isoflurane or halothane. It is excreted mainly unchanged through the lungs. A small amount diffuses through the skin. About 0.02% of administered desflurane is metabolised in the liver and trichloroacetic acid has been detected in the serum and urine of patients given desflurane.

References.

1. Caldwell JE. Desflurane clinical pharmacokinetics and pharmacodynamics. *Clin Pharmacokinet* 1994; **27:** 6–18.

Uses and Administration

Desflurane is a volatile halogenated anaesthetic administered by inhalation. It is structurally similar to isoflurane and has anaesthetic actions similar to those of halothane (p.1225). Desflurane has a minimum alveolar concentration (MAC) value (see p.1220) ranging from about 6% in the elderly to about 11% in infants. It is non-flammable and non-explosive in clinical concentrations but, because of its low boiling-point, it must be delivered by a special vaporiser, preferably within a closed circuit system.

Desflurane is used for induction and maintenance of general anaesthesia (p.1220), but because of its pungency is not recommended for induction in children. Concentrations of 4 to 11% v/v have been used for induction and usually produce surgical anaesthesia in 2 to 4 minutes. Concentrations of 2 to 6% v/v with nitrous oxide or 2.5 to 8.5% v/v in oxygen or oxygen enriched air may be used to maintain anaesthesia. Higher concentrations of desflurane have been used but it is important to ensure adequate oxygenation; concentrations in excess of 17% v/v are not recommended. Recovery from anaesthesia is reported to be more rapid than with other halogenated anaesthetics.

As with other volatile halogenated anaesthetics supplemental neuromuscular blockers may be required.

The characteristics of desflurane have been discussed in a number of reviews.[1-3] Its advantages are considered to include rapid induction and emergence from anaesthesia, and minimal metabolism makes end-organ toxicity unlikely. Emergence from anaesthesia and recovery of psychomotor and cognitive skills with desflurane is more rapid than after anaesthesia with other halogenated volatile anaesthetics such as isoflurane and possibly than after the intravenous anaesthetic propofol. This is considered to be of particular advantage for outpatient treatment, but studies so far have found no difference in time to discharge with desflurane or other general anaesthetics. Furthermore, the incidence of nausea and vomiting with desflurane is significantly greater than after the use of propofol. Desflurane's pungency may also limit its use for induction.

1. Jones RM. Desflurane and sevoflurane: inhalation anaesthetics for this decade? *Br J Anaesth* 1990; **65:** 527–36.
2. Caldwell JE. Desflurane clinical pharmacokinetics and pharmacodynamics. *Clin Pharmacokinet* 1994; **27:** 6–18.
3. Patel SS, Goa KL. Desflurane: a review of its pharmacodynamic and pharmacokinetic properties and its efficacy in general anaesthesia. *Drugs* 1995; **50:** 742–67.

Preparations

Proprietary Preparations (details are given in Part 3)
Aust.: Suprane; ***Belg.:*** Suprane; ***Ger.:*** Suprane; ***Irl.:*** Suprane; ***Ital.:*** Suprane; ***Neth.:*** Suprane; ***Norw.:*** Suprane; ***Spain:*** Suprane; ***Swed.:*** Suprane; ***Switz.:*** Suprane; ***UK:*** Suprane; ***USA:*** Suprane.

Eltanolone (15431-n)

Eltanolone *(rINN)*.

Pregnanolone; ZK-4915. 3α-Hydroxy-5β-pregnan-20-one.

$C_{21}H_{34}O_2$ = 318.5.

CAS — 128-20-1.

Eltanolone, a naturally occurring metabolite of progesterone (p.1459), has been studied for use as an intravenous anaesthetic. It is insoluble in water and has been administered as an emulsion containing soya oil and egg phospholipids.

Enflurane (3106-h)

Enflurane *(BAN, USAN, rINN)*.

Anaesthetic Compound No. 347; Compound 347; Methylflurether; NSC-115944. 2-Chloro-1,1,2-trifluoroethyl difluoromethyl ether; 2-Chloro-1-(difluoromethoxy)-1,1,2-trifluoroethane.

$C_3H_2ClF_5O$ = 184.5.

CAS — 13838-16-9.

Pharmacopoeias. In *Jpn* and *US.*

A clear colourless volatile liquid with a mild sweet odour. Non-flammable. B.p. 55.5° to 57.5°. Slightly **soluble** in water; miscible with organic solvents, fats, and oils. **Store** at a temperature not exceeding 40° in airtight containers. Protect from light.

Adverse Effects

As with other halogenated anaesthetics, respiratory depression, hypotension, and arrhythmias have been reported although the incidence of arrhythmias is lower with enflurane than with halothane. It sensitises the myocardium to sympathomimetics to a lesser extent then halothane. Compared with halothane, enflurane has a stimulant effect on the CNS and convulsions may occur when concentrations of enflurane are high or hypocapnia is present. Malignant hyperthermia has also been reported. Asthma and bronchospasm may occur. There have been reports of elevated serum-fluoride concentrations although resulting renal damage appears to be rare. There have been changes in measurements of hepatic enzymes and a number of reports of liver damage. Shivering, nausea, and vomiting have been reported in the postoperative period.

See also Adverse Effects of General Anaesthetics, p.1219.

Abuse. Report[1] of a fatality in a 29-year-old student nurse anaesthetist who had applied enflurane to the herpes simplex lesions of her lower lip. She was found with an empty 250 mL bottle of enflurane.

1. Lingenfelter RW. Fatal misuse of enflurane. *Anesthesiology* 1981; **55:** 603.

Effects on the blood. The development of carboxyhaemoglobinaemia in patients anaesthetised with volatile anaesthetics is discussed under Precautions, below.

Effects on the kidneys. The nephrotoxicity of volatile anaesthetics has been reviewed.[1] Although enflurane released inorganic fluoride it appeared to be safe in patients with normal renal function. It had also been given to patients with mild to moderate renal impairment without any further deterioration. There was an increase in serum-fluoride concentrations when enflurane was administered to a group of patients who had been receiving isoniazid, but there was no change in kidney function. Pretreatment of patients with a single dose of disulfiram before anaesthesia was found to produce a consistent and almost complete inhibition of enflurane metabolism as shown by substantial reductions in plasma-fluoride concentrations and urinary excretion of fluoride.[2]

1. Mazze RI. Nephrotoxicity of fluorinated anaesthetic agents. *Clin Anaesthesiol* 1983; **1:** 469–83.
2. Kharasch ED, *et al.* Clinical enflurane metabolism by cytochrome P450 2E1. *Clin Pharmacol Ther* 1994; **55:** 434–40.

Effects on the liver. In a review of 58 cases of suspected enflurane hepatitis Lewis *et al.*[1] considered enflurane to be the likely cause of the liver damage in 24. There was biochemical evidence of liver damage in 23 of these cases. Histology reports were available for 15 patients and all showed some degree of hepatocellular necrosis and degeneration.

While the incidence of liver damage from enflurane seemed to be lower than from halothane, the character of the injury was similar.

Another review[2] of the same cases plus an additional 30 (88 in all) came to different conclusions; the main author was a consultant to the manufacturer of enflurane. Of the 88 patients with suspected enflurane hepatitis, 30 were rejected because of insufficient evidence and 43 were considered to have other factors known to produce liver injury. This left 15 possible cases of enflurane hepatitis compared with the 24 identified by Lewis *et al.* While agreeing that in the rare patient unexplained liver damage follows enflurane anaesthesia, it was considered that the incidence was too small to suggest an association. No consistent histological pattern was identified in this study.

See also under Adverse Effects in Halothane, p.1224.

1. Lewis JH, *et al.* Enflurane hepatotoxicity: a clinicopathologic study of 24 cases. *Ann Intern Med* 1983; **98:** 984–92.
2. Eger EI, *et al.* Is enflurane hepatotoxic? *Anesth Analg* 1986; **65:** 21–30.

Effects on respiration. Overall, enflurane is considered to produce more respiratory depression than halothane or isoflurane.[1,2]

1. Quail AW. Modern inhalation anaesthetic agents: a review of halothane, isoflurane and enflurane. *Med J Aust* 1989; **150:** 95–102.
2. Merrett KL, Jones RM. Inhalational anaesthetic agents. *Br J Hosp Med* 1994; **52:** 260–3.

Precautions

Enflurane should be used with caution in patients with convulsive disorders. High concentrations of enflurane may cause uterine relaxation. In order to minimise the risk of developing elevated carboxyhaemoglobin levels, carbon dioxide absorbents in anaesthetic apparatus should not be allowed to dry out when delivering volatile anaesthetics such as enflurane.

As with other halogenated anaesthetics, patients with known or suspected susceptibility to malignant hyperthermia should not be anaesthetised with enflurane.

See also Precautions for General Anaesthetics, p.1219.

Significant carboxyhaemoglobinaemia may develop during anaesthesia with volatile anaesthetics given by circle breathing systems containing carbon dioxide absorbents.[1] The effect is only seen when the absorbent (usually barium hydroxide lime) has became excessively dried out.

1. Committee on Safety of Medicines/Medicines Control Agency. Safety issues in anaesthesia: volatile anaesthetic agents and carboxyhaemoglobinaemia. *Current Problems* 1997; **23:** 7.

Porphyria. Enflurane was considered to be unsafe in patients with acute porphyria because it has been shown to be porphyrinogenic in *animals* or *in-vitro* systems.[1]

1. Moore MR, McColl KEL. *Porphyria: drug lists.* Glasgow: Porphyria Research Unit, University of Glasgow, 1991.

Interactions

Care is advised if adrenaline or other sympathomimetics are given to patients during enflurane anaesthesia. The effects of competitive neuromuscular blockers such as atracurium are enhanced by enflurane (see p.1307).

See also Interactions of General Anaesthetics, p.1219.

Antibacterials. For the effects of *isoniazid* on enflurane defluorination, see Effects on the Kidneys under Adverse Effects, above.

Antidepressants. It appeared likely that the enflurane-induced seizure activity observed in 2 patients could have been enhanced by *amitriptyline*.[1] It may be advisable to avoid the use of enflurane in patients requiring tricyclic antidepressants, especially when the patient has a history of seizures or when hyperventilation or high enflurane concentrations are a desired part of the anaesthetic technique.

1. Sprague DH, Wolf S. Enflurane seizures in patients taking amitriptyline. *Anesth Analg* 1982; **61:** 67–8.

Disulfiram. For the effect of disulfiram on the metabolism of enflurane, see Effects on the Kidneys under Adverse Effects, above.

Neuromuscular blockers. For the effects of enflurane on the neuromuscular blocking effects of neuromuscular blockers, see p.1307.

Pharmacokinetics

Enflurane is absorbed on inhalation. The blood/gas coefficient is low. It is mostly excreted unchanged through the lungs. Up to 10% of administered enflurane is metabolised in the liver, mainly to inorganic fluoride.

Reviews.

1. Dale O, Brown BR. Clinical pharmacokinetics of the inhalational anaesthetics. *Clin Pharmacokinet* 1987; **12:** 145–67.

Uses and Administration

Enflurane is a volatile halogenated anaesthetic administered by inhalation. It is an isomer of isoflurane. It has anaesthetic actions similar to those of halothane (p.1225). Enflurane has a minimum alveolar concentration (MAC) value (see p.1220) ranging from 1.7% in middle age to 2.5% in children. It is employed in the induction and maintenance of anaesthesia (p.1220) and is also used in subanaesthetic doses to provide analgesia in obstetrics and other painful procedures.

Enflurane is administered using a calibrated vaporiser for induction and maintenance of general anaesthesia. To avoid CNS excitement a short-acting barbiturate or other intravenous induction agent is recommended before the inhalation of enflurane. Anaesthesia is induced starting at an enflurane concentration of 0.4% v/v in air, oxygen, or nitrous oxide-oxygen mixtures and increasing by increments of 0.5% v/v every few breaths to a maximum of 4.5%. Anaesthesia may be maintained with a concentration of 0.5 to 3.0% v/v of enflurane in nitrous oxide-oxygen; a concentration of 3.0% v/v should not be exceeded during spontaneous respiration. Although enflurane is reported to possess muscle relaxant properties, neuromuscular blockers may nevertheless be required. Postoperative analgesia may be necessary.

Reviews.

1. Quail AW. Modern inhalational anaesthetic agents: a review of halothane, isoflurane and enflurane. *Med J Aust* 1989; **150:** 95–102.

Pain. Enflurane is used in subanaesthetic doses to provide analgesia in obstetrics and other painful procedures although Tomi *et al.*[1] were unable to confirm that it had an analgesic effect at subanaesthetic concentrations. For a discussion of the use of inhalational analgesics, see p.6.

1. Tomi K, *et al.* Alterations in pain threshold and psychomotor response associated with subanaesthetic concentrations of inhalation anaesthetics in humans. *Br J Anaesth* 1993; **70:** 684–6.

Preparations

Proprietary Preparations (details are given in Part 3)
Aust.: Ethrane; ***Austral.:*** Alyrane; Ethrane; ***Belg.:*** Alyrane; Ethrane; ***Canad.:*** Ethrane; ***Ger.:*** Ethrane; ***Irl.:*** Ethrane; ***Ital.:*** Ethrane†; ***Neth.:*** Alyrane; Ethrane; ***Norw.:*** Efrane; ***S.Afr.:*** Ethrane; ***Spain:*** Ethrane†; ***Swed.:*** Alyrane; Efrane; ***Switz.:*** Ethrane; ***USA:*** Ethrane.

Anaesthetic Ether (3107-m)

Aether ad Narcosin; Aether Anaestheticus; Aether pro Narcosi; Aether Purissimus; Diethyl Ether; Éter Purísimo; Ether; Ether Anesthesicus.

$(C_2H_5)_2O$ = 74.12.

CAS — 60-29-7.

Pharmacopoeias. In *Chin., Eur.* (see p.viii), *Int., Jpn, Pol.,* and *US.*

Anaesthetic ether is diethyl ether to which an appropriate quantity of a non-volatile antoxidant may have been added. The Ph. Eur. and USP state that ether suitable for anaesthesia contains not more than 0.2% of water. The USP also specifies that it contains 96 to 98% of $(C_2H_5)_2O$, the remainder consisting of alcohol and water. It is slowly oxidised by the action of air and light, with the formation of peroxides. A clear, colourless, volatile, highly flammable, and very mobile liquid with a characteristic odour. B.p. 34° to 35°.

Soluble 1 in 12 to 15 of water; miscible with alcohol, chloroform, dichloromethane, petroleum spirit, and fixed and volatile oils. **Store** at a temperature of 8° to 15° in airtight containers. Protect from light. Ether remaining in a partly used container may deteriorate rapidly.

The label should state that it is suitable for use as an anaesthetic. The Ph. Eur. also directs that the name and concentration of the antoxidant used should be specified.

CAUTION. *Ether is very volatile and flammable and mixtures of its vapour with oxygen, nitrous oxide, or air at certain concentrations are explosive. It should not be used in the presence of an open flame or any electrical apparatus liable to produce a spark. Precautions should be taken against the production of static electrical discharge.*

Storage. The Pharmaceutical Society's Department of Pharmaceutical Sciences found that free ether, even in low concentrations, caused softening of PVC bottles and was associated with loss by permeation.[1]

1. Anonymous. Plastics medicine bottles of rigid PVC. *Pharm J* 1973; **210:** 100.

Adverse Effects

Ether has an irritant action on the mucous membrane of the respiratory tract; it stimulates salivation and increases bronchial secretion. Laryngeal spasm may occur. Ether causes vasodilatation which may lead to a severe fall in blood pressure and it reduces blood flow to the kidneys; it also increases capillary bleeding. The bleeding time is unchanged but the prothrombin time may be prolonged. Ether may cause malignant hyperthermia in certain individuals. Alterations in kidney and liver function have been reported. Convulsions occasionally occur. Hyperglycaemia due to gluconeogenesis has been noted.

Recovery is slow from prolonged ether anaesthesia and postoperative vomiting commonly occurs. Acute overdosage of ether is characterised by respiratory failure and cardiac arrest.

Dependence on ether or ether vapour has been reported. Prolonged contact with ether spilt on any tissue produces necrosis.

See also Adverse Effects of General Anaesthetics, p.1219.

Precautions

Ether anaesthesia is contra-indicated in patients with diabetes mellitus, impaired kidney function, raised cerebrospinal fluid pressure, and severe liver disease. Its use is not advisable in hot and humid conditions in patients with fever as convulsions are liable to occur, particularly in children and in patients who have been given atropine.

See also Precautions for General Anaesthetics, p.1219.

Interactions

Ether enhances the action of competitive neuromuscular blockers to a greater degree than most other anaesthetics. Potentiation of the arrhythmogenic effect of sympathomimetics, including adrenaline, by ether is less than that seen with other inhalational anaesthetics.

See also Interactions of General Anaesthetics, p.1219.

Uses and Administration

Ether is an anaesthetic administered by inhalation. It has a minimum alveolar concentration (MAC) value (see p.1220) of 1.92%. Ether is still used in some countries for the induction and maintenance of anaesthesia although it has been replaced in many other countries by the halogenated anaesthetics. It possesses a respiratory stimulant effect in all but the deepest planes of anaesthesia. Ether also possesses analgesic and muscle relaxant properties. Premedication with an antimuscarinic such as atropine is necessary to reduce salivary and bronchial secretions.

Solvent ether is described on p.1378.

Preparations

Proprietary Preparations (details are given in Part 3)
Ital.: OG (Odontalgico Gazzoni)†.

Etomidate (3110-r)

Etomidate *(BAN, USAN, rINN).*

R-16659; R-26490 (sulphate). *R*-(+)-Ethyl 1-(α-methylbenzyl)imidazole-5-carboxylate.

$C_{14}H_{16}N_2O_2$ = 244.3.

CAS — 33125-97-2.

Adverse Effects and Precautions

Excitatory phenomena especially involuntary myoclonic muscle movements, which are sometimes severe, are common following injection of etomidate, but may be reduced by the prior administration of an opioid analgesic. Pain on injection may be reduced by giving the injection into a large vein in the arm, rather than into the hand or, again, by premedication with an opioid analgesic. Convulsions may occur in unpremedicated patients. Hypersensitivity reactions including anaphylaxis have been reported. Etomidate is associated with less hypotension than other agents commonly used for induction.

Because etomidate inhibits adrenocortical function during maintenance anaesthesia (see below) its use is limited to induction of anaesthesia. In addition it should not be used in patients whose adrenocortical function is already reduced or at risk of being reduced.

See also Adverse Effects and Precautions for General Anaesthetics, p.1219.

Effects on the endocrine system. Ledingham and Watt warned[1] that etomidate used for sedation in an intensive care unit was implicated in an increase in mortality. The UK Committee on Safety of Medicines agreed that etomidate could cause a significant fall in circulating plasma-cortisol concentrations, unresponsive to corticotrophin stimulation.[2] As a result of this effect, use of etomidate is restricted to induction of anaesthesia. The manufacturers advise that the postoperative rise in serum-cortisol concentration, which has been observed after thiopentone induction, is delayed for about 3 to 6 hours when etomidate is used for induction.

A study comparing the effects of etomidate with those of methohexitone on the adrenocortical function of neonates of mothers who received these agents for induction of anaesthesia prior to caesarean section indicated that there was no evidence to preclude the use of etomidate in such patients. However, regardless of which anaesthetic agent was used, early feeding was recommended to avoid neonatal hypoglycaemia.[3]

1. Ledingham IM, Watt I. Influence of sedation on mortality in critically ill multiple trauma patients. *Lancet* 1983; **i:** 1270.
2. Goldberg A. Etomidate. *Lancet* 1983; **ii:** 60.
3. Crozier TA, *et al.* Effects of etomidate on the adrenocortical and metabolic adaptation of the neonate. *Br J Anaesth* 1993; **70:** 47–53.

Hypersensitivity. Reactions involving immediate widespread cutaneous flushing or urticaria attributed to etomidate have been described.[1] There have also been reports[2,3] of anaphylactic reactions following injection of etomidate.

1. Watkins J. Etomidate: an 'immunologically safe' anaesthetic agent. *Anaesthesia* 1983; **38** (suppl): 34–8.
2. Sold M, Rothhammer A. Lebensbedrohliche anaphylaktoide reaktion nach etomidat. *Anaesthesist* 1985; **34:** 208–10.
3. Krumholz W, *et al.* Ein fall von anaphylaktoider reaktion nach gabe von etomidat. *Anaesthesist* 1984; **33:** 161–2.

Porphyria. Etomidate was considered to be unsafe inpatients with acute porphyria because it has been shown to be porphyrinogenic in *animals* or *in-vitro* systems.[1]

1. Moore MR, McColl KEL. *Porphyria: drug lists.* Glasgow: Porphyria Research Unit, University of Glasgow, 1991.

Interactions

A reduced dose of etomidate may be necessary in patients who have received antipsychotics, sedatives, or opioids. The hypnotic effect of etomidate has been potentiated by other sedative drugs.

See also Interactions of General Anaesthetics, p.1219.

Calcium channel blockers. Prolonged anaesthesia and Cheyne-Stokes respiration following etomidate injection has been reported in 2 patients given concomitant treatment with *verapamil.*[1]

1. Moore CA, *et al.* Potentiation of etomidate anesthesia by verapamil: a report of two cases. *Hosp Pharm* 1989; **24:** 24–5.

General anaesthetics. For a report of synergy between *propofol* and etomidate, see p.1230.

Pharmacokinetics

After injection, etomidate is rapidly redistributed from the CNS to other body tissues, and undergoes rapid metabolism in the liver and plasma. Pharmacokinetics are complex and have been described by both 2- and 3-compartment models. Etomidate is about 76% bound to plasma protein. It is mainly excreted in the urine, but some is excreted in the bile. It may cross the placenta and is distributed into breast milk.

References.

1. Swerdlow BN, Holley FO. Intravenous anaesthetic agents: pharmacokinetic-pharmacodynamic relationships. *Clin Pharmacokinet* 1987; **12:** 79–110.
2. Esener Z, *et al.* Thiopentone and etomidate concentrations in maternal and umbilical plasma, and in colostrum. *Br J Anaesth* 1992; **69:** 586–8.

Uses and Administration

Etomidate is an intravenous anaesthetic administered for the induction of anaesthesia (p.1220). Anaesthesia is rapidly induced and may last for 6 to 10 minutes with a single usual dose. Recovery is usually rapid without hangover effect. Etomidate has no analgesic activity.

For the induction of anaesthesia, the usual dose is 300 µg of etomidate per kg body-weight given slowly, preferably into a large vein in the arm. Opioid analgesics as premedication reduce myoclonic muscle movements and injection site pain. A neuromuscular blocker is necessary if intubation is required.

Administration in the elderly. One study[1] in elderly patients has demonstrated that although reducing the rate of intravenous administration of etomidate reduces the speed of induction, the dosage required is also reduced. Administration of etomidate 0.2% solution at a rate of 10 mg per minute induced anaesthesia in a mean of 89.6 seconds and required a mean dose of 0.11 mg per kg body-weight. Corresponding values for an administration rate of 40 mg per minute were 47.7 seconds and 0.26 mg per kg respectively.

1. Berthoud MC, *et al.* Comparison of infusion rates of three i.v. anaesthetic agents for induction in elderly patients. *Br J Anaesth* 1993; **70:** 423–7.

Anaesthesia. Etomidate might be useful for induction if rapid tracheal intubation is required with a competitive neuromuscular blocker as it has been shown to reduce the time to onset of block with vecuronium.[1]

1. Gill RS, Scott RPF. Etomidate shortens the onset time of neuromuscular block. *Br J Anaesth* 1992; **69:** 444–6.

Status epilepticus. Anaesthesia in conjunction with assisted ventilation may be instituted to control refractory tonic-clonic status epilepticus (p.337). A short-acting barbiturate such as thiopentone is usually used, but other anaesthetics including etomidate have also been tried[1] for intractable convulsive status epilepticus. However, like a number of other anaesthetics there have been reports of seizures associated with its use in anaesthesia, especially in patients with epilepsy.

1. Yeoman P, *et al.* Etomidate infusions for the control of refractory status epilepticus. *Intensive Care Med* 1989; **15:** 255–9.

Preparations

Proprietary Preparations (details are given in Part 3)
Aust.: Hypnomidate; ***Belg.:*** Hypnomidate; ***Fr.:*** Hypnomidate; ***Ger.:*** Hypnomidate; Radenarcon; ***Neth.:*** Hypnomidate; ***S.Afr.:*** Hypnomidate; ***Spain:*** Hypnomidate; ***Switz.:*** Hypnomidate; ***UK:*** Hypnomidate; ***USA:*** Amidate.

Halothane (3101-x)

Halothane *(BAN, rINN).*

Alotano; Halothanum; Phthorothanum. (*RS*)-2-Bromo-2-chloro-1,1,1-trifluoroethane.

$CHBrCl.CF_3$ = 197.4.

CAS — 151-67-7.

Pharmacopoeias. In *Chin., Eur.* (see p.viii), *Int., Jpn, Pol.,* and *US.*

A clear, colourless, mobile, dense, non-flammable liquid with a characteristic chloroform-like odour. Distillation range 49° to 51°.

Slightly **soluble** in water; miscible with alcohol, dehydrated alcohol, chloroform, ether, trichloroethylene, and fixed oils. In the presence of moisture it reacts with many metals. The USP specifies that it should contain not more than 0.03% of water. Rubber and some plastics deteriorate when in contact with halothane vapour or liquid.

Halothane contains 0.01% w/w of thymol as a stabiliser; some commercial preparations may also contain up to 0.00025% w/w of ammonia. Thymol does not volatilise with halothane and therefore accumulates in the vaporiser. It may give a yellow colour to any remaining liquid; halothane that has discoloured should be discarded.

Store at a temperature not greater than 25° in airtight containers. Protect from light.

Adverse Effects

As with other halogenated anaesthetics, halothane has a depressant action on the cardiovascular system and reduces blood pressure; signs of overdosage are bradycardia and profound hypotension. It is also a respiratory depressant and can cause cardiac arrhythmias; there have been instances of cardiac arrest. The sensitivity of the heart to sympathomimetic amines is increased.

Adverse effects on the liver have limited its use in recent years (see below); these effects range from liver dysfunction to hepatitis and necrosis and are more frequent following repeated use.

Halothane can produce nausea, vomiting, and shivering. Malignant hyperthermia has been reported.

See also Adverse Effects of General Anaesthetics, p.1219.

Abuse. A brief review[1] of abuse of volatile anaesthetics found that of 14 patients who had ingested or sniffed halothane 10 had died. Another patient who had injected halothane intravenously also died. There has also been another report[2] of fatalities resulting from acute pulmonary oedema after intravenous injection of halothane.

1. Yamashita M, *et al.* Illicit use of modern volatile anaesthetics. *Can Anaesth Soc J* 1984; **31:** 76–9.
2. Berman P, Tattersal M. Self-poisoning with intravenous halothane. *Lancet* 1982; **i:** 340.

Effects on the cardiovascular system. The incidence of cardiac arrhythmias is higher with halothane than with enflurane or isoflurane; also the arrhythmogenic threshold with injected adrenaline is lower with halothane than isoflurane or enflurane.

Effects on the kidneys. Renal failure has been reported following halothane anaesthesia,[1,2] sometimes with concurrent liver failure.[2]

1. Cotton JR, *et al.* Acute renal failure following halothane anesthesia. *Arch Pathol Lab Med* 1976; **100:** 628–9.
2. Gelman ML, Lichtenstein NS. Halothane-induced nephrotoxicity. *Urology* 1981; **17:** 323–7.

Effects on the liver. Liver damage has been recognised as an adverse effect of halothane for many years.[1-3]

Two types of hepatotoxicity are recognised; in the first there is a minor disturbance in liver function shown by increases in liver enzyme values (type I). As measured by serum-aminotransferase activity, this type might occur in up to 30% of patients given halothane.[4] A higher percentage of patients may be affected if activity is measured by glutathione S-transferase.[5] Subsequent re-exposure to halothane is not necessarily associated with liver damage.[2,6]

The second type of hepatotoxicity which is rarer involves massive liver cell necrosis (type II); reported incidences range from 1 in 2500 to 1 in 36 000.[2] Type II liver toxicity is characterised by several clinical features: non-specific gastro-intestinal upset, delayed pyrexia, jaundice, eosinophilia, serum auto-antibodies, rash, and arthralgia.[1,3] Biochemical tests of liver function show changes typical of hepatocellular damage; histological features are typified by centrilobular necrosis.[1] Several risk factors for development of serious toxicity have become apparent;[1-3] they include repeated exposure, previous adverse reactions to halothane (jaundice, pyrexia), female gender, obesity, middle age, genetic predisposition, enzyme induction, and a history of drug allergy.

Several theories have been proposed to explain halothane hepatotoxicity. Type I reactions may result from toxic products of halothane metabolism, possibly influenced by genetic factors or from an imbalance between hepatic oxygen supply and demand. Changes in cellular calcium homoeostasis may also be involved. Type II reactions are most likely immune-mediated.[1,2] It has been suggested[4] that cytochrome P450-mediated metabolism of halothane produces a reactive metabolite which binds covalently to proteins in the endoplasmic reticulum of hepatocytes. In susceptible patients it is believed that these metabolite-modified proteins provoke an immune response which is responsible for the liver damage. Recent findings[7,8] have implicated the P450 2E1 isoenzyme as having a major role in the metabolism of halothane and patients with high levels of this isoenzyme may be predisposed to developing immune-medicated liver damage following halothane exposure.

The Committee on Safety of Medicines,[9] after receiving 84 further reports of hepatotoxicity in the UK between 1978 and 1985, issued the following guidelines on precautions to be taken before using halothane:

- a careful anaesthetic history should be taken to determine previous exposure and previous reactions to halothane
- repeated exposure to halothane within a period of at least 3 months should be avoided unless there are overriding clinical circumstances. An opinion has been expressed that the 3-month interval between exposures would be unlikely to prevent hepatotoxicity[2]
- a history of unexplained jaundice or pyrexia in a patient following exposure to halothane is an absolute contra-indication to its future use in that patient.

These guidelines were reiterated in 1997 after the CSM were notified of a further 15 cases of acute liver failure all requiring transplantation.[10]

The problem of patients sensitised to halothane who require subsequent anaesthesia with a volatile anaesthesia has been discussed.[4] Although the incidence of hepatotoxicity produced by enflurane appears to be less than with halothane it is of a similar nature and there have been reports of several patients who apparently had cross-sensitivity to both. Hepatotoxicity with isoflurane appears to be rare and it was suggested that for the majority of patients sensitised to halothane, isoflurane would be likely to be free from hepatotoxic effects. However, there has been a report[11] of a patient who had had two previous exposures to isoflurane and subsequently developed liver function abnormalities after receiving halothane. Hepatotoxicity with desflurane (see p.1221) might also be associated with sensitisation to halothane.

1. Ray DC, Drummond GB. Halothane hepatitis. *Br J Anaesth* 1991; **67:** 84–99.
2. Neuberger JM. Halothane and hepatitis: incidence, predisposing factors and exposure guidelines. *Drug Safety* 1990; **5:** 28–38.
3. Rosenak D, *et al.* Halothane and liver damage. *Postgrad Med J* 1989; **65:** 129–35.
4. Kenna JG, Neuberger JM. Immunopathogenesis and treatment of halothane hepatitis. *Clin Immunother* 1995; **3:** 108–24.
5. Allan LG, *et al.* Hepatic glutathione S-transferase release after halothane anaesthesia: open randomised comparison with isoflurane. *Lancet* 1987; **i:** 771–4.
6. Neuberger J, Williams R. Halothane anaesthesia and liver damage. *Br Med J* 1984; **289:** 1136–9.
7. Kharasch ED, *et al.* Identification of the enzyme responsible for oxidative halothane metabolism: implications for prevention of halothane hepatitis. *Lancet* 1996; **347:** 1367–71.
8. Kenna JC, *et al.* Formation of the $C[F]_3CO$-protein antigens implicated in the pathogenesis of halothane hepatitis is catalyzed in human liver microsomes in vitro by CYP 2E1. *Br J Clin Pharmacol* 1997; **43:** 209.
9. Committee on Safety of Medicines. Halothane hepatotoxicity. *Current Problems 18* 1986.
10. Committe on Safety of Medicines/Medicines Control Agency. Safety issues in anaesthesia: reminder: hepatotoxicity with halothane. *Current Problems* 1997; **23:** 7.
11. Slayter KL, *et al.* Halothane hepatitis in a renal transplant patient previously exposed to isoflurane. *Ann Pharmacother* 1993; **27:** 101.

Precautions

The risk of halothane hepatitis led the Committee on Safety of Medicines in the UK to issue guidelines on its use (see Effects on the Liver, under Adverse Effects, above). It is also recommended that patients be informed of any reactions and that this be done in addition to the updating of the patients' medical records.

Halothane reduces uterine muscle tone during pregnancy and generally its use is not recommended in obstetrics because of the increased risk of postpartum haemorrhage.

Premedication with atropine has been recommended to reduce vagal tone and to prevent bradycardia and severe hypotension.

Allowance may need to be made for any increase in CSF pressure or in cerebral blood flow. Halothane should be used with caution in patients with phaeochromocytoma.

As with other halogenated anaesthetics, patients with known or suspected susceptibility to malignant hyperthermia should not be anaesthetised with halothane.

See also Precautions for General Anaesthetics, p.1219.

Porphyria. Halothane has been associated with acute attacks of porphyria and is considered unsafe in patients with acute porphyria.[1]

1. Moore MR, McColl KEL. *Porphyria: drug lists.* Glasgow: Porphyria Research Unit, University of Glasgow, 1991.

Interactions

Adrenaline and most other sympathomimetics, and theophylline, should be avoided during halothane anaesthesia since they can produce cardiac arrhythmias; the risk of arrhythmias is also increased if halothane is used in patients receiving dopaminergics. The effects of competitive neuromuscular blockers such as atracurium, and of ganglion blockers such as pentolinium, pempidine, and trimetaphan are enhanced by halothane and if required they should be given in reduced dosage. Morphine increases the depressant effects of halothane on respiration. Chlorpromazine also enhances the respiratory depressant effect of halothane. The effects of both ergometrine and oxytocin on the parturient uterus are diminished by halothane.

See also Interactions of General Anaesthetics, p.1219.

Anorectics. For a possible interaction between *fenfluramine* and halothane anaesthesia, see p.1481.

Antiepileptics. For a case of *phenytoin* intoxication associated with halothane anaesthesia, see p.354.

Benzodiazepines. *Midazolam* has been reported to potentiate the anaesthetic action of halothane.[1]

1. Inagaki Y, *et al.* Anesthetic interaction between midazolam and halothane in humans. *Anesth Analg* 1993; **76:** 613–17.

Neuromuscular blockers. For the potentiation of the neuromuscular blockade of neuromuscular blockers such as atracurium by halothane, see p.1307. For increased toxicity during halothane anaesthesia, see suxamethonium p.1321.

Trichloroethane. A report[1] of 2 patients showing evidence of chronic cardiac toxicity following repeated exposure to trichloroethane. In both cases there was circumstantial evidence of a deterioration after routine anaesthetic use of halothane.

1. McLeod AA, *et al.* Chronic cardiac toxicity after inhalation of 1,1,1-trichloroethane. *Br Med J* 1987; **294:** 727–9.

Xanthines. For references to increased cardiotoxicity in patients taking *theophylline* when anaesthetised with halothane, see p.770.

Pharmacokinetics

Halothane is absorbed on inhalation. It has a relatively low solubility in blood and is more soluble in the neutral fats of adipose tissue than in the phospholipids of brain cells. Up to 80% of administered halothane is excreted unchanged through the lungs. Up to 20% is metabolised by the liver by oxidative and, under hypoxic conditions, reductive pathways. Urinary metabolites include trifluoroacetic acid and bromide and chloride salts (oxidative pathway) and fluoride salts (reductive pathway). It diffuses across the placenta and has been detected in breast milk.

Reviews.

1. Dale O, Brown BR. Clinical pharmacokinetics of the inhalational anaesthetics. *Clin Pharmacokinet* 1987; **12:** 145–67.

Uses and Administration

Halothane is a volatile halogenated anaesthetic administered by inhalation. It has a minimum alveolar concentration (MAC) value (see p.1220) ranging from 0.64% in the elderly to 1.08% in infants. It is non-flammable and is not explosive when mixed with oxygen at normal atmospheric pressure. It is not irritant to the skin and mucous membranes and does not produce necrosis when spilt on tissues. It suppresses salivary, bronchial, and gastric secretions and dilates the bronchioles.

Halothane is used for the induction and maintenance of anaesthesia (p.1220) and is given using a vaporiser to provide close control over the concentration of inhaled vapour.

Anaesthesia may be induced with 2 to 4% v/v of halothane in oxygen or mixtures of nitrous oxide and oxygen; induction may also be started at a concentration of 0.5% v/v and increased gradually to the required level. For induction in children a concentration of 1.5 to 2% v/v has been used. It takes up to about 5 minutes to attain surgical anaesthesia and halothane produces little or no excitement in the induction period. The more usual practice is to induce anaesthesia with an intravenous agent. Anaesthesia is maintained with concentrations of 0.5 to 2.0% v/v depending on the flow rate used.

Adequate muscle relaxation is only achieved with deep anaesthesia so a neuromuscular blocker is given to increase muscular relaxation if necessary.

Reviews.

1. Quail AW. Modern inhalational anaesthetic agents: a review of halothane, isoflurane and enflurane. *Med J Aust* 1989; **150:** 95–102.

Preparations

Proprietary Preparations (details are given in Part 3)
Aust.: Fluothane; ***Austral.:*** Fluothane; ***Belg.:*** Fluothane; ***Canad.:*** Fluothane†; ***Fr.:*** Fluothane; ***Ger.:*** Fluothane; ***Irl.:*** Fluothane; ***Ital.:*** Fluothane; ***Neth.:*** Fluothane; ***Norw.:*** Fluothane; ***S.Afr.:*** Fluothane; ***Spain:*** Fluothane; ***Swed.:*** Fluothane; ***Switz.:*** Fluothane; ***UK:*** Fluothane; ***USA:*** Fluothane.

Isoflurane (3113-n)

Isoflurane *(BAN, USAN, rINN)*.

Compound 469. 1-Chloro-2,2,2-trifluoroethyl difluoromethyl ether; 2-Chloro-2-(difluoromethoxy)-1,1,1-trifluoroethane.

$C_3H_2ClF_5O$ = 184.5.

CAS — 26675-46-7.

Pharmacopoeias. In US.

A clear, colourless, volatile liquid with a slight pungent odour. B.p. about 49°. It is non-flammable.

Practically **insoluble** in water; miscible with common organic solvents and with fats and oils. **Store** in airtight containers.

Adverse Effects

As with other halogenated anaesthetics, respiratory depression, hypotension, arrhythmias, and malignant hyperthermia have been reported. Isoflurane differs from halothane and enflurane in that it produces less cardiac depression than either drug and heart rate may be increased. Also isoflurane sensitises the myocardium to sympathomimetics to a lesser extent than halothane and enflurane. The incidence of cardiac arrhythmias is lower with isoflurane than with halothane. Shivering, nausea, and vomiting have been reported in the postoperative period.

Induction with isoflurane is not as smooth as with halothane and this may be connected with its pungency; breath holding, coughing, and laryngospasm may occur.

See also Adverse Effects of General Anaesthetics, p.1219.

Cattermole *et al.*[1] in comparing isoflurane and halothane for outpatient dental anaesthesia in children considered that isoflurane would produce fewer arrhythmias than halothane, but that the ease of induction and the quality of anaesthesia was inferior to that with halothane. McAteer[2] also found a higher incidence of coughing, salivation, and laryngospasm with isoflurane than halothane, but felt that it could be used as an alternative.

Further information on the adverse effects profile of isoflurane can be obtained from the report of and commentaries on an extensive multicentre study of patients undergoing anaesthesia with this agent.[3,4]

1. Cattermole RW, *et al.* Isoflurane and halothane for outpatient dental anaesthesia in children. *Br J Anaesth* 1986; **58:** 385–9.
2. McAteer PM, *et al.* Comparison of isoflurane and halothane in outpatient paediatric dental anaesthesia. *Br J Anaesth* 1986; **58:** 390–3.
3. Forrest JB, *et al.* A multi-centre clinical evaluation of isoflurane. *Can Anaesth Soc J* 1982; **29** (suppl): S1–S69.
4. Levy WJ. Clinical anaesthesia with isoflurane: a review of the multicentre study. *Br J Anaesth* 1984; **56:** 101S–112S.

Effects on the blood. The development of carboxyhaemoglobinaemia in patients anaesthetised with volatile anaesthetics is discussed under Precautions, below.

Effects on the cardiovascular system. Isoflurane is considered to produce less cardiovascular depression than halothane. However, results of a study[1] by one group of workers suggest that while this may be true for young patients, in elderly patients isoflurane appears to have a cardiac depressant effect similar to that of halothane.

1. McKinney MS, *et al.* Cardiovascular effects of isoflurane and halothane in young and elderly adult patients. *Br J Anaesth* 1993; **71:** 696–701.

CEREBRAL BLOOD FLOW. Autoregulation of cerebral blood flow appears to be impaired at higher concentrations of isoflurane. A study[1] in healthy subjects found that increasing isoflurane anaesthesia from a concentration of 1 to 2 MAC increased cerebral blood flow and reduced cerebral oxygen metabolism.

1. Olsen KS, *et al.* Effect of 1 or 2 MAC isoflurane with or without ketanserin on cerebral blood flow autoregulation in man. *Br J Anaesth* 1994; **72:** 66–71.

CORONARY CIRCULATION. Halothane, enflurane, and isoflurane decrease coronary perfusion pressure, coronary blood flow, ventricular function, and myocardial oxygen demand. Halothane and enflurane have a variable effect on coronary vascular resistance, but isoflurane dilates coronary vessels.[1] There has been concern over the potential of isoflurane to produce coronary steal and whether this effect is detrimental in patients with ischaemic heart disease.[2] However, despite conflicting results of individual studies[3-6] a review[7] concluded that isoflurane could be used safely even in high-risk patients with coronary artery disease provided that blood pressure and heart rate were maintained close to base-line levels.

1. Quail AW. Modern inhalational anaesthetic agents: a review of halothane, isoflurane and enflurane. *Med J Aust* 1989; **150:** 95–102.
2. Stoelting RK. Anesthesiology. *JAMA* 1991; **265:** 3103–5.
3. Buffington CW, *et al.* The prevalence of steal-prone coronary anatomy in patients with coronary artery disease: an analysis of the coronary artery surgery study registry. *Anesthesiology* 1988; **69:** 721–7.
4. Inoue K, *et al.* Does isoflurane lead to a higher incidence of myocardial infarction and perioperative death than enflurane in coronary artery surgery? A clinical study of 1178 patients. *Anesth Analg* 1990; **71:** 469–74.
5. Slogoff S, *et al.* Steal-prone coronary anatomy and myocardial ischemia associated with four primary anesthetic agents in humans. *Anesth Analg* 1991; **72:** 22–7.
6. Stühmeier KD, *et al.* Isoflurane does not increase the incidence of intraoperative myocardial ischaemia compared with halothane during vascular surgery. *Br J Anaesth* 1992; **69:** 602–6.
7. Hogue CW, *et al.* Anesthetic-induced myocardial ischemia: the isoflurane-coronary steal controversy. *Coron Artery Dis* 1993; **4:** 413–19.

Effects on the kidneys. See under Metabolism in Pharmacokinetics, below.

Effects on the liver. Of 45 cases of isoflurane-associated hepatotoxicity reported to the FDA between 1981 and 1984 there was some other cause for the liver damage in 29. While isoflurane might have been one of the causes of the damage in the other 16 cases, there was not a reasonable likelihood of an association between isoflurane and postoperative liver impairment.[1] A subsequent case report of hepatic necrosis and death following surgery was possibly attributable to isoflurane.[2]

See also under the Adverse Effects of Halothane, p.1224.

1. Stoelting RK, *et al.* Hepatic dysfunction after isoflurane anesthesia. *Anesth Analg* 1987; **66:** 147–53.
2. Carrigan TW, Straughen WJ. A report of hepatic necrosis and death following isoflurane anesthesia. *Anesthesiology* 1987; **67:** 581–3.

Effects on the nervous system. Seizures associated with induction of anaesthesia with isoflurane have been reported in patients without known neurological abnormalities and not undergoing neurosurgery.[1,2] However, data from a retrospective analysis of patients undergoing intracranial surgery indicated that when convulsions occurred postoperatively in these conditions, it was the neurosurgical procedures rather than the anaesthetics that were responsible.[3]

See also under Status Epilepticus in Uses, below.

1. Poulton TJ, Ellingson RJ. Seizure associated with induction of anesthesia with isoflurane. *Anesthesiology* 1984; **61:** 471–6.
2. Hymes JA. Seizure activity during isoflurane anesthesia. *Anesth Analg* 1985; **64:** 367–8.
3. Christys AR, *et al.* Retrospective study of early postoperative convulsions after intracranial surgery with isoflurane or enflurane anaesthesia. *Br J Anaesth* 1989; **62:** 624–7.

Effects on the respiratory tract. A study[1] conducted mainly in adults found that humidification of anaesthetic mixtures containing isoflurane could reduce respiratory complications such as coughing, laryngospasm, and breath-holding that were usually associated with the use of isoflurane for induction. However, a similar study[2] in children failed to confirm these findings.

1. van Heerden PV, *et al.* Effect of humidification on inhalation induction with isoflurane. *Br J Anaesth* 1990; **64:** 235–7.
2. McAuliffe GL, *et al.* Effect of humidification on inhalation induction with isoflurane in children. *Br J Anaesth* 1994; **73:** 587–9.

Precautions

As with other halogenated anaesthetics, patients with known or suspected susceptibility to malignant hyperthermia should not be anaesthetised with isoflurane. It has been reported to increase the cerebrospinal pressure and should be used with caution in patients with raised intracranial pressure. Isoflurane relaxes the uterine muscle. In order to minimise the risk of developing elevated carboxyhaemoglobin levels, carbon dioxide absorbents in anaesthetic apparatus should not be allowed to dry out when delivering volatile anaesthetics such as isoflurane.

See also Precautions for General Anaesthetics, p.1219.

Significant carboxyhaemoglobinaemia may develop during anaesthesia with volatile anaesthetics given by circle breathing systems containing carbon dioxide absorbents.[1] The effect is only seen when the absorbent (usually barium hydroxide lime) has became excessively dried out.

1. Committee on Safety of Medicines/Medicines Control Agency. Safety issues in anaesthesia: volatile anesthetic agents and carboxyhaemoglobinaemia. *Current Problems* 1997; **23:** 7.

Interactions

The effects of competitive neuromuscular blockers such as atracurium are enhanced by isoflurane (see p.1307). Care is advised if adrenaline and other sympathomimetics are given during isoflurane anaesthesia.

See also Interactions of General Anaesthetics, p.1219.

General anaesthetics. For a report that isoflurane increases serum concentrations of *propofol*, see p.1230.

Pharmacokinetics

Isoflurane is absorbed on inhalation. The blood/gas coefficient is lower than that of enflurane or halothane. It is mostly excreted unchanged through the lungs. About 0.2% of administered isoflurane is metabolised mainly to inorganic fluoride.

Reviews.

1. Dale O, Brown BR. Clinical pharmacokinetics of the inhalational anaesthetics. *Clin Pharmacokinet* 1987; **12:** 145–67.

Metabolism. In 26 patients sedated with isoflurane for 24 hours, plasma fluoride ion concentration increased from a mean of 4.03 nmol per mL to 13.57 nmol per mL in 12 hours after stopping sedation.[1] These fluoride concentrations were considered to be too low to cause clinical renal dysfunction. In 30 patients sedated with isoflurane for up to 127 hours (mean duration was 36 hours), mean plasma fluoride ion concentration increased to 20.01 nmol per mL during sedation and continued rising for 16 hours after discontinuing isoflurane to a maximum mean concentration of 25.34 nmol per mL;[2] thereafter, levels gradually declined to normal values by the fifth day. Despite the increased plasma fluoride ion concentrations, no biochemical or clinical evidence of deterioration in renal function was found. Administration of isoflurane for 34 days to a patient with tetanus who required sedation to facilitate mechanical ventilation resulted in sustained fluoride ion concentrations of 50 nmol per mL and a peak concentration of 87 nmol per mL.[3] Although such concentrations are considered to be potentially nephrotoxic no clinical effect on renal function was found.

1. Kong KL, *et al.* Isoflurane sedation for patients undergoing mechanical ventilation: metabolism to inorganic fluoride and renal effects. *Br J Anaesth* 1990; **64:** 159–62.
2. Spencer EM, *et al.* Plasma inorganic fluoride concentrations during and after prolonged (>24h) isoflurane sedation: effect on renal function. *Anesth Analg* 1991; **73:** 731–7.
3. Stevens JJWM, *et al.* Prolonged use of isoflurane in a patient with tetanus. *Br J Anaesth* 1993; **70:** 107–109.

Uses and Administration

Isoflurane is a volatile halogenated anaesthetic administered by inhalation. It is an isomer of enflurane and has anaesthetic actions similar to those of halothane (p.1225). Isoflurane has a minimum alveolar concentration (MAC) value (see p.1220) ranging from 1.05% in the elderly to 1.87% in infants. It is employed in the induction and maintenance of anaesthesia (p.1220) although induction is more often carried out using an intravenous anaesthetic with isoflurane being given for maintenance. Isoflurane is also used in subanaesthetic doses to provide analgesia in obstetrics and other painful procedures.

Isoflurane is administered using a calibrated vaporiser. If it is used for induction then it is given with oxygen or oxygen and nitrous oxide and induction should start with an isoflurane concentration of 0.5% v/v increased to 1.5 to 3.0% v/v which generally produces surgical anaesthesia within 10 minutes. Its pungency may limit the rate of induction. Anaesthesia may be maintained with a concentration of 1.0 to 2.5% v/v with oxygen and nitrous oxide; 1.5 to 3.5% v/v may be required if used only with oxygen. Isoflurane 0.5 to 0.75% v/v with oxygen and nitrous oxide is suitable to maintain anaesthesia for caesarean section. Although isoflurane is reported to possess muscle relaxant properties, neuromuscular blockers may nevertheless be required. Recovery is rapid.

Reviews.

1. Quail AW. Modern inhalational anaesthetic agents: a review of halothane, isoflurane and enflurane. *Med J Aust* 1989; **150:** 95–102.

Anaesthesia. CAESAREAN SECTION. Isoflurane 0.8% v/v has been found to be a suitable supplement to nitrous oxide-oxygen anaesthesia for patients undergoing caesarean section.[1] It has been suggested[2] that an overpressure technique might be of use to further reduce awareness in such patients. Administration of isoflurane at a concentration of 2% v/v for 5 minutes followed by concentrations of 1.5% v/v for the next 5 minutes and 0.8% v/v thereafter produced higher arterial concentrations of isoflurane in patients undergoing caesarean section than when it was given at a concentration of 1% v/v throughout.[2]

1. Dwyer R, *et al.* Uptake of halothane and isoflurane by mother and baby during Caesarean section. *Br J Anaesth* 1995; **74:** 379–83.
2. McCrirrick A, *et al.* Overpressure isoflurane at Caesarean section: a study of arterial isoflurane concentrations. *Br J Anaesth* 1994; **72:** 122–4.

Pain. Isoflurane is used in subanaesthetic doses to provide analgesia in obstetrics and other painful procedures (see Inhalational Analgesics, p.6) but studies[1,2] have been unable to confirm that it had an analgesic effect at subanaesthetic concentrations. The use of isoflurane 0.2 or 0.25% v/v in a mixture of nitrous oxide 50% v/v and oxygen 50% v/v has been studied.[3,4]

1. Tomi K, *et al.* Alterations in pain threshold and psychomotor response associated with subanaesthetic concentrations of inhalation anaesthetics in humans. *Br J Anaesth* 1993; **70:** 684–6.
2. Roth D, *et al.* Analgesic effect in humans of subanaesthetic isoflurane concentrations evaluated by evoked potentials. *Br J Anaesth* 1996; **76:** 38–42.
3. Wee MYK, *et al.* Isoflurane in labour. *Anaesthesia* 1993; **48:** 369–72.
4. Bryden FM, *et al.* Isoflurane for removal of chest drains after cardiac surgery. *Br J Anaesth* 1994; **73:** 712P–713P.

Sedation. INTENSIVE CARE. The various drugs used to provide sedation in intensive care are discussed on p.638. Isoflurane is not usually considered for such a purpose but in a comparative 24-hour study[1] in 60 patients requiring mechanical ventilation, isoflurane 0.1 to 0.6% v/v in an air-oxygen mixture produced satisfactory sedation for a greater proportion of time than did the continuous infusion of midazolam 0.01 to 0.20 mg per kg body-weight per hour. Patients given isoflurane also recovered more rapidly. Isoflurane has also been used successfully for sedation in a 3-year-old infant admitted to intensive care with pneumonia, a complication of the child's myasthenia gravis.[2] However, there has been some concern over high plasma fluoride concentrations following prolonged use of isoflurane (see under Metabolism in Pharmacokinetics, above).

1. Kong KL, *et al.* Isoflurane compared with midazolam for sedation in the intensive care unit. *Br Med J* 1989; **298:** 1277–80.
2. McBeth C, Watkins TGL. Isoflurane for sedation in a case of congenital myasthenia gravis. *Br J Anaesth* 1996; **77:** 672–4.

Status epilepticus. Anaesthesia in conjunction with assisted ventilation may be instituted to control refractory tonic-clonic status epilepticus (p.337). A short-acting barbiturate such as thiopentone is usually used. Despite there being rare reports of seizures associated with the use of isoflurane in anaesthetic procedures (see under Adverse Effects, above) concentrations of 0.5 to 1% v/v have been used successfully in isolated patients[1,2] to control refractory convulsive status epilepticus. Although some[3] consider that isoflurane-induced coma may be more easy to control than barbiturate-induced coma, the use of isoflurane may be limited by the need for special anaesthetic equipment and continuous EEG monitoring.

1. Meeke RI, *et al.* Isoflurane for the management of status epilepticus. *DICP Ann Pharmacother* 1989; **23:** 579–81.
2. Hilz MJ, *et al.* Isoflurane anaesthesia in the treatment of convulsive status epilepticus. *J Neurol* 1992; **239:** 135–7.
3. Bauer J, Elger CE. Management of status epilepticus in adults. *CNS Drugs* 1994; **1:** 26–44.

Preparations

Proprietary Preparations (details are given in Part 3)
Aust.: Forane; ***Austral.:*** AErrane; Forthane; ***Belg.:*** AErrane; Forene; ***Canad.:*** Forane; ***Fr.:*** Tensocold†; ***Ger.:*** Forene; ***Irl.:*** AErrane; Forane; ***Ital.:*** AErrane; Forane; ***Neth.:*** AErrane; Forene; ***Norw.:*** Forene; ***S.Afr.:*** Forane; Isofor; ***Spain:*** AErrane; Forane; ***Swed.:*** Forene; ***Switz.:*** Forene; ***UK:*** AErrane; Isoflurane; ***USA:*** Forane.

Ketamine Hydrochloride (3114-h)

Ketamine Hydrochloride *(BANM, USAN, rINNM).*

CI-581; CL-369; CN-52372-2; Ketamini Hydrochloridum.

(±)-2-(2-Chlorophenyl)-2-methylaminocyclohexanone hydrochloride.

$C_{13}H_{16}ClNO,HCl = 274.2$.

CAS — 6740-88-1 (ketamine); 1867-66-9 (ketamine hydrochloride).

Pharmacopoeias. In *Chin., Eur.* (see p.viii), *Int., Jpn,* and *US.*

A white crystalline powder with a slight characteristic odour. Ketamine hydrochloride 1.15 mg is approximately equivalent to 1 mg of ketamine base. **Soluble** 1 in 4 of water, 1 in 14 of alcohol, 1 in 60 of dehydrated alcohol and of chloroform, and 1 in 6 of methyl alcohol; practically insoluble in ether. A 10% solution has a pH of 3.5 to 4.1. **Incompatible** with soluble barbiturates. The US manufacturer has recommended that when concomitant administration of diazepam and ketamine is required they should be given separately and not mixed in the same giving equipment. **Protect** from light.

Adverse Effects

Emergence reactions are common during recovery from ketamine anaesthesia and include vivid often unpleasant dreams, confusion, hallucinations, and irrational behaviour. Children and elderly patients appear to be less sensitive. Patients may also experience increased muscle tone, sometimes resembling seizures. Blood pressure and heart rate may be temporarily increased by ketamine; hypotension, arrhythmias, and bradycardia have occurred rarely.

Respiration may be depressed following rapid intravenous injection or with high doses. Apnoea and laryngospasm have occurred. Diplopia and nystagmus may occur. Nausea and vomiting, lachrymation, hypersalivation, and raised intra-ocular and cerebrospinal fluid pressure have also been reported. Transient skin rashes and pain at the site of injection may occur.

See also Adverse Effects of General Anaesthetics, p.1219.

Abuse. Health care workers in the USA were alerted to the dangers associated with the abuse of ketamine as long ago as 1979.[1] Similar concern has been voiced more recently in the UK[2] over the abuse of ketamine at social gatherings where it has been taken intranasally or orally under the names of 'vitamin K', 'super K', or 'special K'. Ketamine produces a state of psychological dissociation resulting in hallucinations and out of body or near death experiences. It can induce a state of helplessness in which the user loses awareness of the environment and this together with severe loss of coordination and pronounced analgesia can put the user at great risk. Furthermore, some users experience a state in which they are unconcerned about whether they live or die. Ketamine has the potential for compulsive repeated use and there have been reports of users self-injecting ketamine several times a day for prolonged periods. There has been a report[3] of an acute dystonic reaction in a 20-year old man following self-administration of ketamine intravenously.

Some[2] suggest that patients seeking medical attention are best placed in a quiet darkened room to recover with diazepam being given for unresponsive panic attacks while others advocate that such patients should be admitted to an intensive care unit for close monitoring.[4]

1. Anonymous. Ketamine abuse. *FDA Drug Bull* 1979; **9:** 24.
2. Jansen KLR. Non-medical use of ketamine. *Br Med J* 1993; **306:** 601–2.
3. Felser JM, Orban DJ. Dystonic reaction after ketamine abuse. *Ann Emerg Med* 1982; **11:** 673–5.
4. Gill PA. Non-medical use of ketamine. *Br Med J* 1993; **306:** 1340.

Effects on the cardiovascular system. Ketamine has been advocated by some for maintaining or increasing cardiovascular performance in selected patients during induction of anaesthesia as it may increase blood pressure and heart rate.[1] However, there have been reports of reduced cardiac and pulmonary performance in severely ill patients[1] and of arrhythmias.[2]

Some of the cardiovascular effects of ketamine may be attenuated by premedication with diazepam[2] or clonidine.[3]

1. Waxman K, *et al.* Cardiovascular effects of anesthetic induction with ketamine. *Anesth Analg* 1980; **59:** 355–8.
2. Cabbabe EB, Behbahani PM. Cardiovascular reactions associated with the use of ketamine and epinephrine in plastic surgery. *Ann Plast Surg* 1985; **15:** 50–2.
3. Tanaka M, Nishikawa T. Oral clonidine premedication attenuates the hypertensive response to ketamine. *Br J Anaesth* 1994; **73:** 758–62.

Effects on the liver. Changes in serum-enzyme levels have occurred following infusion of large doses of ketamine.[1]

1. Dundee JW, *et al.* Changes in serum enzyme levels following ketamine infusions. *Anaesthesia* 1980; **35:** 12–16.

Effects on mental state. Mental disturbances following ketamine anaesthesia may vary in incidence from less than 5% to greater than 30%.[1] See also Abuse, above.

1. White PF, *et al.* Ketamine—its pharmacology and therapeutic uses. *Anesthesiology* 1982; **56:** 119–36.

Effects on the skin. Harlequin-like colour skin changes were reported[1] in a 9-month-old boy during anaesthesia with ketamine 15 mg.

1. Wagner DL, Sewell AD. Harlequin color change in an infant during anesthesia. *Anesthesiology* 1985; **62:** 695.

Malignant hyperthermia. Malignant hyperthermia has been reported in a patient given ketamine.[1]

1. Rasore-Quartino A, *et al.* Forma atipica di ipertermia maligna: osservazione di un caso da ketamina. *Pathologica* 1985; **77:** 609–17.

Precautions

Ketamine is contra-indicated in patients in whom elevation of blood pressure would be a serious hazard including those with hypertension or a history of cerebrovascular accident. Cardiac function should be monitored in patients found to have hypertension or cardiac decompensation. Ketamine should be used with caution in patients with elevated CSF pressure. It can raise intra-ocular pressure and should not be used in the presence of eye injury or increased intra-ocular pressure.

Ketamine does not reliably suppress pharyngeal and laryngeal reflexes and mechanical stimulation of the pharynx should be avoided unless a muscle relaxant is used.

The use of ketamine should be avoided in patients prone to hallucinations or psychotic disorders. Verbal, tactile, and visual stimuli should be kept to a minimum during recovery in an attempt to reduce the risk of emergence reactions.

See also Precautions for General Anaesthetics, p.1219.

Interactions

Inhalational anaesthetics, such as ether and halothane, and other cerebral depressants may prolong the effect of ketamine and delay recovery. Prolonged recovery has also occurred when barbiturates and/or opioids have been given concomitantly with ketamine. It has been recommended that ketamine should not be used in combination with ergometrine.

See also Interactions of General Anaesthetics, p.1219.

For the enhancement of the effect of *tubocurarine* or *atracurium* by ketamine, see p.1307. For a reference to increased cardiovascular adverse effects with *thyroid drugs*, see p.1498. For a reference to seizures and tachycardia attributed to an interaction between ketamine and *theophylline*, see p.770.

Pharmacokinetics

After intravenous bolus administration, ketamine shows a bi- or triexponential pattern of elimination. The alpha phase lasts about 45 minutes with a half-life of 10 to 15 minutes. This first phase, which represents ketamine's anaesthetic action, is terminated by redistribution from the CNS to peripheral tissues and hepatic biotransformation to an active metabolite norketamine. Other metabolic pathways include hydroxylation of the cyclohexone ring and conjugation with glucuronic acid. The beta phase half-life is about 2.5 hours. It is excreted mainly in the urine as metabolites. Ketamine crosses the placenta.

References.

1. Clements JA, Nimmo WS. Pharmacokinetics and analgesic effect of ketamine in man. *Br J Anaesth* 1981; **53:** 27–30.
2. Grant IS, *et al.* Pharmacokinetics and analgesic effects of IM and oral ketamine. *Br J Anaesth* 1981; **53:** 805–9.
3. Nimmo WS, *et al.* The pharmacokinetics of ketamine in children. *Br J Clin Pharmacol* 1982; **14:** 144P.
4. Geisslinger G, *et al.* Pharmacokinetics and pharmacodynamics of ketamine enantiomers in surgical patients using a stereoselective analytical method. *Br J Anaesth* 1993; **70:** 666–71.
5. Malinovsky J-M, *et al.* Ketamine and norketamine plasma concentrations after iv, nasal and rectal administration in children. *Br J Anaesth* 1996; **77:** 203–7.

Uses and Administration

Ketamine is an anaesthetic administered by intravenous injection, intravenous infusion, or intramuscular injection. It produces dissociative anaesthesia characterised by a trance-like state, amnesia, and marked analgesia which may persist into the recovery period. There is often an increase in muscle tone and the patient's eyes may remain open for all or part of the period of anaesthesia. Ketamine is used in anaesthesia for diagnostic or short surgical operations that do not require skeletal muscle relaxation, for the induction of anaesthesia to be maintained with other drugs, and as a supplementary anaesthetic (see p.1220). It is considered to be of particular value in children requiring frequent repeated anaesthesia. Recovery is relatively slow.

Ketamine is administered as the hydrochloride but doses are expressed in terms of the equivalent amount of base. For induction the dose given by *intravenous injection* may range from 1 to 4.5 mg of ketamine per kg body-weight; a dose of 2 mg of ketamine per kg body-weight given intravenously over 60 seconds usually produces surgical anaesthesia within 30 seconds of the end of the injection and lasting for 5 to 10 minutes. The initial *intramuscular* dose may range from 6.5 to 13 mg of ketamine per kg; an intramuscular dose of 10 mg of ketamine per kg usually produces surgical anaesthesia within 3 to 4 minutes lasting for 12 to 25 minutes. For diagnostic or other procedures not involving intense pain an initial intramuscular dose of 4 mg of ketamine per kg has been used. Additional doses may be given for maintenance. For induction by *intravenous infusion* a total dose of 0.5 to 2 mg of ketamine per kg is usually given at an appropriate infusion rate. Maintenance is achieved with 10 to 45μg per kg per minute, the infusion rate being adjusted according to response.

Administration should be preceded by atropine or another suitable antimuscarinic. Diazepam or another benzodiazepine may be given before surgery or as an adjunct to ketamine to reduce the incidence of emergence reactions.

Reviews.

1. Hirota K, Lambert DG. Ketamine: its methanism(s) of action and unusual clinical uses. *Br J Anaesth* 1996; **77:** 441–4.

Administration. Although ketamine hydrochloride is usually given intravenously or intramuscularly, oral[1,2] and rectal[3] administration has been used successfully in children. Intranasal administration of ketamine with midazolam in a neonate requiring anaesthesia has also been reported.[4] Unfortunately the onset of sedation with these three routes is too slow for emergency procedures and therefore a jet-injector of ketamine has been developed[5] to provide non-traumatic, painless, and rapid anaesthesia in children. Preliminary studies show the new technique to be well accepted by children.

1. Tobias JD, *et al.* Oral ketamine premedication to alleviate the distress of invasive procedures in pediatric oncology patients. *Pediatrics* 1992; **90:** 537–41.
2. Gutstein HB, *et al.* Oral ketamine preanesthetic medication in children. *Anesthesiology* 1992; **76:** 28–33.
3. Lökken P, *et al.* Conscious sedation by rectal administration of midazolam or midazolam plus ketamine as alternatives to general anesthesia for dental treatment of uncooperative children. *Scand J Dent Res* 1994; **102:** 274–80.
4. Louon A, *et al.* Sedation with nasal ketamine and midazolam for cryotherapy in retinopathy of prematurity. *Br J Ophthalmol* 1993; **77:** 529–30.
5. Zsigmond EK, *et al.* A new route, jet-injection for anesthetic induction in children–ketamine dose-range finding studies. *Int J Clin Pharmacol Ther* 1996; **34:** 84–8.

ADMINISTRATION IN ASTHMA. The manufacturer states that ketamine is suitable for use in the asthmatic patient, either to minimise the risk of an attack of bronchospasm developing during anaesthesia or in the presence of bronchospasm where anaesthesia cannot be delayed.

References.

1. L'Hommedieu CS, Arens JJ. The use of ketamine for the emergency intubation of patients with status asthmaticus. *Ann Emerg Med* 1987; **16:** 568–71.
2. Jahangir SM, *et al.* Ketamine infusion for postoperative analgesia in asthmatics: a comparison with intermittent meperidine. *Anesth Analg* 1993; **76:** 45–9.

Nonketotic hyperglycinaemia. Ketamine was tried in combination with strychnine in a newborn infant with severe nonketotic hyperglycinaemia and resulted in neurological improvement, although motor development remained unsatisfactory.[1] It was thought that ketamine might act by blocking N-methyl-D-aspartate (NMDA) receptors, which are activated in the CNS by glycine. The management of nonketotic hyperglycinaemia is discussed further on p.1633.

1. Tegtmeyer-Metadorf H, *et al.* Ketamine and strychnine treatment of an infant with nonketotic hyperglycinaemia. *Eur J Pediatr* 1995; **154:** 649–53.

Pain. For a discussion of pain and its management, see p.5. Ketamine has been used for its analgesic action[1-8] and may be of value in neuropathic or other pain unresponsive to opioid analgesics. Subcutaneous, intramuscular, epidural, intrathecal, and oral administration have all been tried.

1. Naguib M, *et al.* Epidural ketamine for postoperative analgesia. *Can Anaesth Soc J* 1986; **33:** 16–21.
2. Oshima E, *et al.* Continuous subcutaneous injection of ketamine for cancer pain. *Can J Anaesth* 1990; **32:** 385–6.
3. Laird D, Lovel T. Paradoxical pain. *Lancet* 1993; **341:** 241.
4. Stannard CF, Porter GE. Ketamine hydrochloride in the treatment of phantom limb pain. *Pain* 1993; **54:** 227–30.
5. Bhattacharya A, *et al.* Subcutaneous infusion of ketamine and morphine for relief of postoperative pain: a double-blind comparative study. *Ann Acad Med Singapore* 1994; **23:** 456–9.
6. Wong C-S, *et al.* Ketamine potentiates analgesic effect of morphine in postoperative epidural pain control. *Reg Anesth* 1996; **21:** 534–41.
7. Gurhani A, *et al.* Analgesia for acute musculoskeletal trauma: low-dose subcutaneous infusion of ketamine. *Anaesth Intensive Care* 1996; **24:** 32–6.
8. Semple D, *et al.* The optimal dose of ketamine for caudal epidural blockade in children. *Anaesthesia* 1996; **51:** 1170–2.

Preparations

BP 1998: Ketamine Injection;
USP 23: Ketamine Hydrochloride Injection.

Proprietary Preparations (details are given in Part 3)
Aust.: Ketalar; ***Austral.:*** Ketalar; ***Belg.:*** Ketalar; ***Canad.:*** Ketalar; ***Fr.:*** Ketalar; ***Ger.:*** Ketanest; Velonarcon; ***Irl.:*** Ketalar; ***Ital.:*** Ketalar; ***Neth.:*** Ketalar; ***Norw.:*** Ketalar; ***S.Afr.:*** Brevinaze; Ketalar†; ***Spain:*** Ketolar; ***Swed.:*** Ketalar; ***Switz.:*** Ketalar; ***UK:*** Ketalar; ***USA:*** Ketalar.

Methohexitone (3115-m)

Methohexitone *(BAN)*.

Methohexital *(rINN)*. (±)-5-Allyl-1-methyl-5-(1-methylpent-2-ynyl)barbituric acid; 1-Methyl-5-(1-methyl-2-pentynyl)-5-(2-propenyl)-2,4,6(1*H*,3*H*,5*H*)-pyrimidinetrione.

$C_{14}H_{18}N_2O_3$ = 262.3.

CAS — 151-83-7; 18652-93-2.

Pharmacopoeias. In US.

A white to faintly yellowish-white crystalline odourless powder. M.p. 92° to 96° with a range not exceeding 3°. Very slightly **soluble** in water; slightly soluble in alcohol, chloroform, and dilute alkalis.

Methohexitone Sodium (3116-b)

Methohexitone Sodium *(BANM)*.

Methohexital Sodium *(rINNM)*; Compound 25398; Enallynymalnatrium.

$C_{14}H_{17}N_2NaO_3$ = 284.3.

CAS — 309-36-4; 22151-68-4; 60634-69-7.

Pharmacopoeias. Br. includes Methohexitone Injection; *US* includes Methohexital Sodium for Injection.

Methohexitone Sodium for Injection (BP 1993) is a sterile mixture of 100 parts by weight of the a-form of methohexitone sodium and 6 parts by weight of dried sodium carbonate included as a buffer. It may also contain auxiliary substances. A 5% solution in water has a pH of 10.6 to 11.6.

Methohexital Sodium for Injection (USP 23) is a similar freeze-dried sterile mixture prepared from an aqueous solution of methohexitone, sodium hydroxide, and sodium carbonate. It is a white to off-white hygroscopic powder. A 5% solution in water has a pH of 10.6 to 11.6.

Solutions of methohexitone sodium are **incompatible** with acidic substances so that, amongst other drugs, a number of antibiotics, neuroleptics, muscle relaxants, antimuscarinics, and analgesics should not be mixed with it. Compounds commonly listed as incompatible include atropine sulphate, pethidine hydrochloride, metocurine iodide, fentanyl citrate, morphine sulphate, pentazocine lactate, silicones, suxamethonium chloride, tubocurarine chloride, and compound sodium lactate injection. Only preservative-free diluents should be used to reconstitute methohexitone sodium; precipitation may occur if a diluent containing a bacteriostatic agent is used.

Solutions in Water for Injections are **stable** for at least 6 weeks at room temperature; however reconstituted solutions should be stored no longer than 24 hours as they contain no bacteriostatic agent. Solutions in glucose or sodium chloride injections are stable only for about 24 hours.

Adverse Effects and Precautions

As for Thiopentone Sodium, p.1233.

Excitatory phenomena are more common and induction less smooth with methohexitone than with thiopentone. Methohexitone should be used with caution, if at all, in patients with a history of epilepsy.

See also Adverse Effects and Precautions for General Anaesthetics, p.1219.

In a study of 4379 administrations of methohexitone in dentistry to 2722 patients using the minimal incremental technique the total dose ranged from 20 mg to 560 mg with a mean of 151 mg, the mean duration of treatment ranged from 8 to 32 minutes.[1] The most frequent complication was restlessness and occurred in 292 administrations; a supplement of diazepam 5 mg did not prevent restlessness. Respiratory complications occurred in 214 administrations and uncontrollable crying during recovery after 73 administrations. Pain along the vein was recorded in 45 cases, with 5 patients developing thrombophlebitis. In 22 administrations jactitations were observed and allergic reaction occurred in 10 administrations.

1. McDonald D. Methohexitone in dentistry. *Aust Dent J* 1980; **25:** 335–42.

Effects on the nervous system. Two case reports of seizures induced by methohexitone in children with seizure disorders.[1] Seizures are considered a rare adverse effect of methohexitone. In 48 000 patients given methohexitone, only 3 developed clonic-type seizures.[2]

A case of a tonic-clonic seizure possibly due to an interaction between paroxetine and methohexitone is discussed below.

1. Rockoff MA, Goudsouzian NG. Seizures induced by methohexital. *Anesthesiology* 1981; **54:** 333–5.
2. Metriyakool K. Seizures induced by methohexital. *Anesthesiology* 1981; **55:** 718.

Pain on injection. Methohexitone is associated with severe pain particularly if veins on the back of the hands are used. The incidence of pain on injection may be reduced by using a forearm vein or by pre-injection with lignocaine.

Rebound anaesthesia. Rebound of anaesthesia with abolition of reflexes and depression of respiration occurred in a 6-year-old boy[1] 100 minutes after anorectal induction with 27.6 mg per kg body-weight methohexitone.

1. Kaiser H, Al-Rafai S. Wie sicher ist die rektale narkoseeinleitung mit methohexital in der kinderanaesthesie? *Anaesthesist* 1985; **34:** 359–60.

Interactions

As for Thiopentone Sodium, p.1233.

Antidepressants. A 42-year-old woman[1] suffered a generalised tonic-clonic seizure immediately after being anaesthetised with methohexitone for the last in a series of six electroconvulsive therapies. She had been receiving *paroxetine* throughout the series. A previous course, without concurrent paroxetine, had been uneventful.

1. Folkerts H. Spontaneous seizure after concurrent use of methohexital anesthesia for electroconvulsive therapy and paroxetine: a case report. *J Nerv Ment Dis* 1995; **183:** 115–16.

Pharmacokinetics

Methohexitone is less lipid soluble than thiopentone but when administered intravenously as the sodium salt concentrations sufficient to produce anaesthesia are attained in the brain within 30 seconds. Methohexitone is also absorbed when given rectally, producing an effect within about 5 to 11 minutes. Recovery from anaesthesia occurs quickly as a result of rapid metabolism and redistribution into other body tissues. Methohexitone does not appear to concentrate in fatty tissues to the same extent as other barbiturate anaesthetics. Protein binding has been reported to be about 73%. Methohexitone is rapidly metabolised in the liver through demethylation and oxidation. The terminal half-life ranges from 1.5 to 6 hours. Methohexitone diffuses across the placenta and has been detected in breast milk.

References.

1. Swerdlow BN, Holley FO. Intravenous anaesthetic agents: pharmacokinetic-pharmacodynamic relationships. *Clin Pharmacokinet* 1987; **12:** 79–110.
2. Le Normand Y, *et al.* Pharmacokinetics and haemodynamic effects of prolonged methohexitone infusion. *Br J Clin Pharmacol* 1988; **26:** 589–94.
3. Redke F, *et al.* Pharmacokinetics and clinical experience of 20-h infusions of methohexitone in intensive care patients with postoperative pyrexia. *Br J Anaesth* 1991; **66:** 53–9.
4. van Hoogdalem EJ, *et al.* Pharmacokinetics of rectal drug administration, part I: general considerations and clinical applications of centrally acting drugs. *Clin Pharmacokinet* 1991; **21:** 11–26.
5. Borgatta L, *et al.* Clinical significance of methohexital, meperidine, and diazepam in breast milk. *J Clin Pharmacol* 1997; **37:** 186–92.

Uses and Administration

Methohexitone is a short-acting barbiturate anaesthetic which has actions similar to those of thiopentone (p.1233) but it is about 2 to 3 times more potent. It is administered as the sodium salt and has similar uses to thiopentone in anaesthesia. Induction of anaesthesia is less smooth than with thiopentone and there may be excitatory phenomena. It has a shorter duration of action than thiopentone and recovery after an induction dose occurs within 5 to 7 minutes although drowsiness may persist for some time.

As with other barbiturate anaesthetics the dose of methohexitone required varies greatly according to the state of the patient and the nature of other drugs being used concurrently (see under Precautions of Thiopentone, p.1233, and Interactions of Thiopentone, p.1233, for further details). Methohexitone sodium is usually given intravenously as a 1% solution. Higher concentrations may markedly increase the incidence of adverse effects. A typical dose for induction of anaesthesia is 50 to 120 mg administered at a rate of approximately 10 mg (1 mL of a 1% solution) every 5 seconds. Doses in children range from 1 to 2 mg per kg body-weight. For the maintenance of general anaesthesia methohexitone sodium may be given in doses of 20 to 40 mg every 4 to 7 minutes as required or it may be administered as a 0.2% solution by continuous intravenous infusion.

Administration in the elderly. It is usually recommended that the dosage of barbiturate anaesthetics is reduced in the elderly. One study[1] in elderly patients has demonstrated that although reducing the rate of intravenous administration reduces the speed of induction, the dosage required is also reduced. Administration of methohexitone sodium 0.5% at a rate of 25 mg per minute induced anaesthesia in a mean of 83.8 seconds and required a mean dose of 0.56 mg per kg body-weight. Corresponding values for an administration rate of 100 mg per minute were 43.6 seconds and 1.00 mg per kg respectively.

1. Berthoud MC, *et al.* Comparison of infusion rates of three i.v. anaesthetic agents for induction in elderly patients. *Br J Anaesth* 1993; **70:** 423–7.

Dental sedation. Some anaesthetics are used as sedatives in dental procedures (see p.638). Methohexitone has been tried for patient-controlled sedation in oral surgery under local anaesthesia.[1] In a group of 42 patients, results with 2.5 mg of methohexitone compared favourably with those obtained in patients receiving 5 mg of propofol on demand, although patients in the methohexitone group experienced a greater degree of postoperative drowsiness.

1. Hamid SK, *et al.* Comparison of patient-controlled sedation with either methohexitone or propofol. *Br J Anaesth* 1996; **77:** 727–30.

Preparations

BP 1998: Methohexital Injection;
USP 23: Methohexital Sodium for Injection.

Proprietary Preparations (details are given in Part 3)
Aust.: Brietal; ***Austral.:*** Brietal; ***Belg.:*** Brietal†; ***Canad.:*** Brietal; ***Fr.:*** Brietal†; ***Ger.:*** Brevimytal; ***Irl.:*** Brietal; ***Neth.:*** Brietal; ***Norw.:*** Brietal; ***S.Afr.:*** Brietal; ***Swed.:*** Brietal; ***Switz.:*** Brietal; ***UK:*** Brietal; ***USA:*** Brevital.

Methoxyflurane (3117-v)

Methoxyflurane *(BAN, USAN, rINN)*.

NSC-110432. 2,2-Dichloro-1,1-difluoro-1-methoxyethane; 2,2-Dichloro-1,1-difluoroethyl methyl ether.

$C_3H_4Cl_2F_2O$ = 165.0.

CAS — 76-38-0.

Pharmacopoeias. In *US.*

A clear, almost colourless, mobile liquid with a characteristic odour. The USP permits a suitable stabiliser.

Soluble 1 in 500 of water; miscible with alcohol, acetone, chloroform, ether, and fixed oils. **Store** in airtight containers at a temperature not exceeding 40°. Protect from light.

Adverse Effects

As with other halogenated anaesthetics respiratory depression, hypotension, and malignant hyperthermia have been reported. Methoxyflurane sensitises the myocardium to sympathomimetics to a lesser extent than halothane; arrhythmias appear to be rare.

Methoxyflurane impairs renal function in a dose-related manner due to the effect of the released fluoride on the distal tubule and may cause polyuric or oliguric renal failure, oxaluria being a prominent feature. Nephrotoxicity is greater with methoxyflurane than with other halogenated anaesthetics because of its slower metabolism over several days resulting in prolonged production of fluoride ions.

There have also been occasional reports of hepatic dysfunction, jaundice, and fatal hepatic necrosis. Headache has been reported by some patients. Cardiac arrest, gastro-intestinal side-effects, delirium, and prolonged postoperative somnolence have been observed.

See also Adverse Effects of General Anaesthetics, p.1219.

Abuse. A 27-year-old nurse suffered from progressive renal disease and painful diffuse and multifocal periostitis which had developed as a probable consequence of intermittent self-exposure to methoxyflurane possibly over a 9-year period.[1] There has also been a report[2] of hepatitis in a 39-year-old physician who repeatedly self-administered subanaesthetic concentrations of methoxyflurane for insomnia. Inhalation of about 2 mL of methoxyflurane had occurred once or twice almost every day for six weeks. A 125 mL bottle of methoxyflurane had been consumed in approximately one month.

1. Klemmer PJ, Hadler NM. Subacute fluorosis: a consequence of abuse of an organofluoride anesthetic. *Ann Intern Med* 1978; **89:** 607–11.
2. Okuno T, *et al.* Hepatitis due to repeated inhalation of methoxyflurane in subanaesthetic concentrations. *Can Anaesth Soc J* 1985; **32:** 53–5.

Precautions

The use of methoxyflurane is limited because of its potential to cause renal toxicity. It should not be used to achieve deep anaesthesia or for surgical procedures expected to last longer than 4 hours. Methoxyflurane is contra-indicated in the presence of renal impairment. Renal function and urine output should be monitored during anaesthesia. As with other halogenated anaesthetics it is advisable not to administer methoxyflurane to patients who have shown signs of liver damage or fever after previous anaesthesia involving halogenated anaesthetics. Patients with known, or suspected, susceptibility to malignant hyperthermia should not be anaesthetised with methoxyflurane. Allowance may need to be made for any increase in CSF pressure or in cerebral blood flow.

There is significant absorption of methoxyflurane by the rubber and soda lime in anaesthetic circuits. Polyvinyl chloride plastics are partially soluble in methoxyflurane.

See also Precautions for General Anaesthetics, p.1219.

Porphyria. Methoxyflurane was considered to be unsafe in patients with acute porphyria because it has been shown to be porphyrinogenic in *animals* or *in-vitro* systems.[1]

1. Moore MR, McColl KEL. *Porphyria: drug lists.* Glasgow: Porphyria Research Unit, University of Glasgow, 1991.

Interactions

Care is advised if adrenaline or other sympathomimetics are given to patients during methoxyflurane anaesthesia. The effects of competitive neuromuscular blockers are enhanced by methoxyflurane. The chronic use of hepatic enzyme-inducing drugs may enhance the metabolism of methoxyflurane thereby increasing the risk of nephrotoxicity. Concurrent use of nephrotoxic drugs with methoxyflurane should be avoided.

See also Interactions of General Anaesthetics, p.1219.

Pharmacokinetics

Methoxyflurane is absorbed on inhalation. The blood/gas coefficient is high. Methoxyflurane is metabolised to a greater extent than other inhalational anaesthetics. About 50 to 70% of absorbed methoxyflurane undergoes metabolism in the liver to free fluoride, oxalic acid, difluoromethoxyacetic acid, and dichloroacetic acid. Methoxyflurane is very soluble in adipose tissue and excretion may be slow. Peak plasma concentrations of fluoride occur 2 to 4 days after administration. Methoxyflurane crosses the placenta.

Uses and Administration

Methoxyflurane is a volatile halogenated anaesthetic administered by inhalation. It has a minimum alveolar concentration (MAC) value (see p.1220) of 0.16%. In recommended concentrations it is non-flammable and not explosive when mixed with oxygen. Methoxyflurane possesses good analgesic properties. It does not produce appreciable skeletal muscle relaxation at the concentrations used. Methoxyflurane does not relax the uterus and has little effect on uterine contractions during labour. It is used mainly for maintenance of anaesthesia (p.1220) and in subanaesthetic doses to provide analgesia in painful procedures (see Inhalational Analgesics, p.6).

Because of its low vapour pressure, induction of anaesthesia with methoxyflurane is slow and anaesthesia is therefore usually induced with an intravenous anaesthetic. For maintenance, a concentration of up to 2% v/v methoxyflurane in oxygen and at least 50% v/v nitrous oxide should be given for not more than 5 minutes and then progressively reduced to the lowest concentration that will maintain adequate anaesthesia. The production of deep anaesthesia with methoxyflurane is not recommended, and a maximum of 4 hours exposure to a concentration of 0.25% v/v or the equivalent total dosage is suggested. Recovery may be prolonged.

Concentrations of 0.3 to 0.8% v/v are used to provide analgesia in a variety of situations. When used for self-administration it is recommended that no more than 15 mL of liquid should be provided.

Preparations

Proprietary Preparations (details are given in Part 3)
Austral.: Penthrane†; ***Ger.:*** Penthrane†; ***USA:*** Penthrane†.

Nitrous Oxide (3119-q)

Azoto Protossido; Dinitrogen Oxide; Dinitrogenii Oxidum; Distickstoffmonoxid; Laughing Gas; Nitrogen Monoxide; Nitrogenii Monoxidum; Nitrogenii Oxidum; Nitrogenium Oxydulatum; Oxyde Nitreux; Oxydum Nitrosum; Protoxyde d'Azote; Stickoxydul.

N_2O = 44.01.

CAS — 10024-97-2.

Pharmacopoeias. In *Chin., Eur.* (see p.viii), *Jpn,* and *US.*

A colourless gas, heavier than air, odourless or almost odourless and tasteless; it supports combustion. One vol. measured at a pressure of 101 kPa dissolves, at 20°, in about 1.5 vol. of water; freely soluble in alcohol; soluble in ether and in oils.

It is supplied compressed in metal cylinders. National standards are usually in operation for the labelling and marking of such cylinders.

Storage. Cylinders containing 50% nitrous oxide and 50% oxygen should be protected from the cold to prevent separation of the gases. Cylinders exposed to temperatures lower than −7° should be rolled at room temperature to ensure mixing or alternatively stored horizontally for 24 hours at a temperature of not less than 10°.

Adverse Effects

The main complications following the use of nitrous oxide are those due to varying degrees of hypoxia. Prolonged administration has been followed by megaloblastic anaemia and peripheral neuropathy. Depression of white cell formation may also occur. There is a risk of increased pressure and volume from the diffusion of nitrous oxide into air-containing cavities. Malignant hyperthermia has been reported rarely. Nitrous oxide has been subject to abuse.

See also Adverse Effects of General Anaesthetics, p.1219.

Reviews.

1. Brodsky JB, Cohen EN. Adverse effects of nitrous oxide. *Med Toxicol* 1986; **1:** 362–74.

Effects on the blood. Nitrous oxide interacts with vitamin B_{12}. This blocks the transmethylation reaction for which vitamin B_{12} is a coenzyme and results in depletion of methionine and tetrahydrofolate. Metabolic consequences have been attributed to depletion of either or both. Interference by nitrous oxide with DNA synthesis prevents production of both leucocytes and red blood cells by the bone marrow. Megaloblastic changes in bone marrow and impaired granulocyte production are found in patients exposed to anaesthetic concentrations of nitrous oxide for 24 hours. In patients with normal bone marrow, stores of mature granulocytes will normally be adequate to prevent leucopenia during exposure for up to 3 days; in patients exposed to nitrous oxide for longer periods of time, leucopenia will develop and exposure for 4 days or longer can result in agranulocytosis. In general, healthy surgical patients can be given nitrous oxide for up to 24 hours without harm. In situations where nitrous oxide is used for more than 24 hours, folinic acid 30 mg twice daily has been given to protect the haematopoietic system. Repeat exposure to nitrous oxide at intervals of less than 3 days will have a cumulative effect on DNA synthesis and megaloblastic marrow changes have been reported following multiple short-term exposure.[1] Depletion of methionine has been implicated in the neurological deficit (see below) seen mainly after chronic use of nitrous oxide. It may also account for the fetotoxicity observed in *rats*, see below.

1. Nunn JF. Clinical aspects of the interaction between nitrous oxide and vitamin B_{12}. *Br J Anaesth* 1987; **59:** 3–13.

Effects on the nervous system. Neurological disorders (mainly myeloneuropathies and neuropathies) have occurred in persons who chronically abuse nitrous oxide. Similar effects have been noted after repeated administration of nitrous oxide in hospitalised patients. These neurological effects are considered to be due to nitrous oxide-induced methionine deficiency (see Effects on the Blood, above).

In patients with undiagnosed subclinical deficiency of vitamin B_{12} (a coenzyme involved in methionine synthesis) neurological manifestations, including those consistent with subacute combined degeneration of the spinal cord, have occurred following a single exposure to nitrous oxide for anaesthesia.[1,2]

1. Schilling RF. Is nitrous oxide a dangerous anesthetic for vitamin B_{12}-deficient subjects? *JAMA* 1986; **255:** 1605–6.
2. Nestor PJ, Stark RJ. Vitamin B_{12} myeloneuropathy precipitated by nitrous oxide anaesthesia. *Med J Aust* 1996; **165:** 174.

Malignant hyperthermia. An 11-year-old girl whose father had died from malignant hyperthermia after anaesthesia developed hyperthermia after anaesthesia with nitrous oxide and oxygen.[1]

1. Ellis FR, *et al.* Malignant hyperpyrexia induced by nitrous oxide and treated with dexamethasone. *Br Med J* 1974; **4:** 270–1.

Precautions

Hypoxic anaesthesia is dangerous and nitrous oxide should always be administered with at least 20 to 30% oxygen. Nitrous oxide diffuses into gas-filled body cavities and care is essential when using it in patients at risk from such diffusion such as those with abdominal distension, occlusion of the middle ear, pneumothorax, or similar cavities in the pericardium or peritoneum. Care is also required in patients during or after air encephalography. Oxygen should be administered during emergence from prolonged anaesthesia with nitrous oxide to prevent diffusion hypoxia where the alveolar oxygen concentration is diminished. See also Precautions for General Anaesthetics, p.1219. In addition to the above precautions, mixtures of equal parts of nitrous oxide and oxygen should not be employed for analgesia in patients with head injuries with impairment of consciousness, maxillo facial injuries, decompression sickness, or those heavily sedated.

Driving. A slight but quantified impairment in driving ability was found up to 30 minutes following 15 minutes' inhalation of nitrous oxide/oxygen mixtures.[1]

1. Moyes DG, *et al.* Driving after anaesthetics. *Br Med J* 1979; **1:** 1425.

Epidural anaesthesia. Nitrous oxide diffuses into gas-filled body cavities and can increase the size of any air bubbles injected into the epidural space to determine placement of the needle in epidural anaesthesia.[1] This could result in uneven spread of the local anaesthetic and produce inadequate analgesia. The volume of air injected should be limited or another technique used to determine placement of the needle if nitrous oxide is to be given subsequently.

1. Stevens R, *et al.* Fate of extradural air bubbles during inhalation of nitrous oxide. *Br J Anaesth* 1994; **72:** 482P–483P.

Hazard to user. A scavenging system and effective ventilation may be necessary to control the nitrous oxide pollution that can occur when this gas is used for analgesia or anaesthesia. Risk areas include, in addition to operating theatres, delivery rooms and dental surgeries.[1-3] Occupational exposure can lead to serious toxicity with bone-marrow and neurological impairment.[2,3] Reduced fertility has been reported in female dental workers exposed to high concentrations of nitrous oxide;[4] such women also appear to have a higher rate of spontaneous abortion.[5] It has been suggested that nitrous oxide can also affect male fertility;[6] in one study a dose-related increase in the incidence of spontaneous abortion was found in the wives of men with occupational exposure to nitrous oxide.[7]

1. Munley AJ, *et al.* Exposure of midwives to nitrous oxide in four hospitals. *Br Med J* 1986; **293:** 1063–4. Correction. *ibid.*: 1280.
2. Sweeney B, *et al.* Toxicity of bone marrow in dentists exposed to nitrous oxide. *Br Med J* 1985; **291:** 567–9.
3. Brodsky JB, *et al.* Exposure to nitrous oxide and neurologic disease among dental professionals. *Anesth Analg* 1981; **60:** 297–301.
4. Rowland AS, *et al.* Reduced fertility among women employed as dental assistants exposed to high levels of nitrous oxide. *N Engl J Med* 1992; **327:** 993–7.
5. Rowland AS, *et al.* Nitrous oxide and fertility. *N Engl J Med* 1993; **328:** 284.
6. Brodsky JB. Nitrous oxide and fertility. *N Engl J Med* 1993; **328:** 284–5.
7. Cohen EN, *et al.* Occupational disease in dentistry and chronic exposure to trace anesthetic gases. *J Am Dent Assoc* 1980; **101:** 21–31.

Pregnancy. Nitrous oxide is fetotoxic in *rats*.[1] However, retrospective reviews,[2] and individual case reports[3] have not shown nitrous oxide anaesthesia to be fetotoxic in man. See also under Hazard to User, above.

1. Lane GA, *et al.* Anesthetics as teratogens: nitrous oxide is fetotoxic, xenon is not. *Science* 1980; **210:** 899–901.
2. Aldridge LM, Tunstall ME. Nitrous oxide and the fetus: a review and the results of a retrospective study of 175 cases of anaesthesia for insertion of Shirodkar suture. *Br J Anaesth* 1986; **58:** 1348–56.
3. Park GR, *et al.* Normal pregnancy following nitrous oxide exposure in the first trimester. *Br J Anaesth* 1986; **58:** 576–7.

Vitamin B_{12} deficiency. For reports of neurological dysfunction associated with the use of nitrous oxide in patients with undiagnosed subclinical vitamin B_{12} deficiency, see Effects on the Nervous System, above.

Interactions

The concurrent administration of nitrous oxide with an inhalational anaesthetic accelerates the uptake of the latter from the lungs. This phenomenon is known as the *second gas effect*. It is due to the disproportionate absorption of nitrous oxide into the blood resulting in an increased alveolar concentration of the second gas.

The use of high doses of opioids such as fentanyl with nitrous oxide may result in a drop in heart rate and cardiac output.

See also Interactions for General Anaesthetics, p.1219.

Methotrexate. Combined use of nitrous oxide and methotrexate may increase the side-effects of methotrexate therapy, see p.549.

Pharmacokinetics

Nitrous oxide is rapidly absorbed on inhalation. The blood/gas partition coefficient is low and most of the inhaled nitrous oxide is rapidly eliminated unchanged through the lungs though small amounts diffuse through the skin.

Reviews of the pharmacokinetics of nitrous oxide.

1. Dale O, Brown BR. Clinical pharmacokinetics of the inhalational anaesthetics. *Clin Pharmacokinet* 1987; **12:** 145–67.

Uses and Administration

Nitrous oxide is an anaesthetic administered by inhalation. It is a weak anaesthetic with a minimum alveolar concentration (MAC) value (see p.1220) of 110%. It has strong analgesic properties, but produces little muscle relaxation. Nitrous oxide must be administered with air or oxygen, otherwise hypoxia will occur although mixtures with air are rarely used now, oxygen being preferred.

Nitrous oxide with oxygen may be used in the induction and maintenance of anaesthesia (p.1220). However, it is now mainly employed as an adjuvant to other inhalational anaesthetics, permitting them to be used at significantly lower concentrations. It is also used, with oxygen, in subanaesthetic concentrations for analgesia in obstetrics and other painful procedures (see Inhalational Analgesics, p.6), and for analgesia and sedation during dental procedures (see p.638).

Induction of anaesthesia may be carried out with about 20 to 30% v/v of oxygen and maintenance with up to 50% v/v of oxygen. Recovery is usually rapid from nitrous oxide anaesthesia.

Nitrous oxide 25 to 50% v/v with oxygen is used for analgesia; cylinders containing premixed nitrous oxide 50% v/v and oxygen 50% v/v are available in some countries.

Alcohol withdrawal syndrome. The symptoms of acute alcohol withdrawal (p.1099) are usually managed with benzodiazepines but nitrous oxide has been reported[1] to reduce symptoms when tried in alcohol withdrawal. In mild to moderate cases a single administration of up to 20 minutes' duration of a nitrous oxide-oxygen mixture in analgesic doses has been employed.

1. Gillman MA, Lichtigfeld FJ. Analgesic nitrous oxide for alcohol withdrawal: a critical appraisal after 10 years' use. *Postgrad Med J* 1990; **66:** 543–6.

Preparations

Proprietary Preparations (details are given in Part 3)
Ger.: Stickoxydul†.

Multi-ingredient: *UK:* Entonox.

Propanidid (3120-d)

Propanidid *(BAN, USAN, rINN).*

Bayer-1420; FBA-1420; TH-2180; WH-5668. Propyl 4-diethylcarbamoylmethoxy-3-methoxyphenylacetate.

$C_{18}H_{27}NO_5$ = 337.4.

CAS — 1421-14-3.

Pharmacopoeias. In *Pol.*

Propanidid has been used as an intravenous anaesthetic for rapid induction and for maintenance of anaesthesia of short duration.

Commercial preparations of propanidid were provided as a liquid in polyethoxylated castor oil. Anaphylactoid reactions associated with the vehicle led to the general withdrawal of propanidid from use.

Propofol (12677-f)

Propofol *(BAN, USAN, rINN).*

Disoprofol; ICI-35868. 2,6-Di-isopropylphenol; 2,6-Bis(1-methylethyl)phenol.

$C_{12}H_{18}O$ = 178.3.

CAS — 2078-54-8.

Adverse Effects

Early studies with propofol employed a preparation formulated with polyethoxylated castor oil. Because of anaphylactoid reactions the preparation was reformulated with a vehicle of soya oil and purified egg phosphatide. Adverse effects with this preparation include pain on injection especially if the injection is into a small vein. Local pain may be reduced by injection into a large vein or by injection of intravenous lignocaine. Apnoea may be frequent; apnoea lasting longer than 60 seconds has been reported to occur in 12% of patients. Cardiovascular effects include a reduction in blood pressure and bradycardia. There have been reports of convulsions and involuntary movements. Fever has occurred. Discoloration of urine has been reported following prolonged use. Anaphylactic-like reactions have been reported. Nausea, vomiting, and headache may occur during recovery.

Children who have received propofol for prolonged sedation have suffered severe reactions and there have been fatalities, see below.

See also Adverse Effects of General Anaesthetics, p.1219.

In May 1989 the UK Committee on Safety of Medicines commented on the 268 reports of adverse reactions to propofol that it had received since propofol was introduced to the UK market, during which period about 2 million patients had been anaesthetised with the drug. Among these reports there were 37 describing seizures (13 of these were in known epileptics), 16 involuntary movements, 10 opisthotonus, 32 anaphylactic reactions, and 13 cardiac arrests. There were also 8 reports of delayed recovery.[1]

In June 1992 the CSM commented again on propofol, this time to warn of the dangers of using it for the sedation of children in intensive care,[2] a use for which it is not licensed in the UK. This prohibition does not apply to its use for the sedation of ventilated adults or to propofol's use as an anaesthetic in children over 3 years of age. The CSM reported that there had been 66 reports worldwide of serious adverse effects in children sedated with propofol and some fatalities had ensued. The children had suffered neurological, cardiac, and renal effects, hyperlipaemia, hepatomegaly, and metabolic acidosis. Five deaths had been reported to the CSM and details of 5 deaths were provided by Parke *et al.*[3] These 5 children[3] were aged 4 weeks to 6 years and doses of propofol ranged from 4 to 10.7 mg per kg body-weight per hour. They developed metabolic acidosis, bradyarrhythmia, and progressive myocardial failure resistant to treatment.

Also in 1992 the CSM pointed to the risk of delayed convulsions with propofol and its particular importance for day-case surgery.[4] While the incidence of convulsions was low (170 reports), 31% of the reports described the convulsions as delayed.

1. Committee on Safety of Medicines. Propofol—convulsions, anaphylaxis and delayed recovery from anaesthesia. *Current Problems 26* 1989.
2. Committee on Safety of Medicines. Serious adverse effects and fatalities in children associated with the use of propofol (Diprivan) for sedation. *Current Problems 34* 1992.
3. Parke TJ, *et al.* Metabolic acidosis and fatal myocardial failure after propofol infusion in children: five case reports. *Br Med J* 1992; **305:** 613–16.
4. Committee on Safety of Medicines. Propofol and delayed convulsions. *Current Problems 35* 1992.

Effects on the cardiovascular system. The main effect of propofol on the cardiovascular system is a fall in both systolic and diastolic blood pressure of 20 to 30%. The compensatory tachycardia seen after a fall in arterial pressure with other intravenous anaesthetics is not usually seen with propofol. Propofol can also decrease systemic vascular resistance, cardiac output, myocardial blood flow, and myocardial oxygen consumption. Bradycardia can occur even in those premedicated with antimuscarinics and can occasionally be profound with asystole developing.[1] Despite these cardiovascular depressant effects propofol in doses of 1.5 to 2.5 mg per kg body-weight does not generally cause unacceptable haemodynamic changes in patients with a healthy cardiovascular system although concern has been expressed regarding its safety in cardiac surgical patients.[2]

Children who have received propofol for continuous sedation in intensive care units have suffered adverse cardiac reactions with bradyarrhythmia, progressive myocardial failure, and death, see above.

1. Tramèr MR, *et al.* Propofol and bradycardia: causation, frequency and severity. *Br J Anaesth* 1997; **78:** 642–51.
2. Ginsberg R, Lippmann M. Haemodynamic effects of propofol. *Br J Anaesth* 1994; **72:** 370–1.

Effects on lipids. Prolonged administration of propofol may be associated with increases in serum triglycerides. In one patient this was believed to have been the cause of necrotising pancreatitis.[1]

1. Metkus AP, *et al.* A firefighter with pancreatitis. *Lancet* 1996; **348:** 1702.

Effects on mental function. There have been anecdotal reports[1] of disinhibited behaviour or sexually orientated hallucinations associated with the use of propofol, but a study using subanaesthetic doses found no evidence that propofol produced euphoria or other mood changes.[2]

1. Canaday BR. Amorous, disinhibited behaviour associated with propofol. *Clin Pharm* 1993; **12:** 449–51.
2. Whitehead C, *et al.* The subjective effects of low-dose propofol. *Br J Anaesth* 1994; **72** (suppl 1): 89.

Effects on the nervous system. See under Precautions, below.

Effects on respiration. See under Precautions, below.

Hypersensitivity. Anaphylactic reactions associated with polyethoxylated castor oil used in propofol preparations had prompted a change to the use of soya oil and egg phosphatide in the formulation. One group of workers have reported a patient who experienced anaphylactic shock when given the reformulated emulsion.[1]

1. Laxenaire MC, *et al.* Anaphylactic shock due to propofol. *Lancet* 1988; **ii:** 739–40.

Infection. Between June 1990 and February 1993 62 cases of postsurgical infections identified in 7 hospitals in the USA were attributed to improper handling of propofol.[1] The infusion was not prepared aseptically and the syringes used in the infusion pumps were reused for several patients. Propofol is formulated as a soybean fat emulsion and the injection contains no antimicrobial preservative although, in the USA, the formulation now contains the microbial-retarding agent, disodium edetate (see under Administration, below). However, either formulation still has the potential to support microbial growth. The UK and USA manufacturers now warn of the importance of aseptic technique in the preparation and administration of propofol. Microbial multiplication did not appear to be clinically significant when propofol infusions were prepared and administered using conventional aseptic techniques.[2]

1. Bennett SN, *et al.* Postoperative infections traced to contamination of an intravenous anesthetic, propofol. *N Engl J Med* 1995; **333:** 147–54.
2. Farrington M, *et al.* Do infusions of midazolam and propofol pose an infection risk to critically ill patients? *Br J Anaesth* 1994; **72:** 415–17.

Malignant hyperthermia. From an *in-vitro* study it was concluded that propofol does not trigger malignant hyperthermia.[1] There is a report of the administration of propofol to 19 patients considered susceptible to malignant hyperthermia; none of the patients showed signs of malignant hyperthermia.[2]

1. Denborough M, Hopkinson KC. Propofol and malignant hyperpyrexia. *Lancet* 1988; **i:** 191.
2. Harrison GG. Propofol in malignant hyperthermia. *Lancet* 1991; **337:** 503.

Pain on injection. The manufacturers have suggested the use of lignocaine to reduce the pain associated with injection of propofol; alternatively, the larger veins in the forearm and antecubital fossa can be used. Studies indicate that alfentanil[1] and metoclopramide[2] might also be effective. It has been suggested[3] that the analgesic action of lignocaine and possibly metoclopramide is due to a pH-lowering effect, rather than to a local anaesthetic action, permitting more propofol to exist in the oily phase of the emulsion. Propofol concentrated in the aqueous phase is believed to be responsible for the pain on injection.

1. Fletcher JE, *et al.* Pretreatment with alfentanil reduces pain caused by propofol. *Br J Anaesth* 1994; **72:** 342–4.
2. Ganta R, Fee JPH. Pain on injection of propofol: comparison of lignocaine with metoclopramide. *Br J Anaesth* 1992; **69:** 316–17.
3. Eriksson M, *et al.* Effect of lignocaine and pH on propofol-induced pain. *Br J Anaesth* 1997; **78:** 502–6.

Urine discoloration. A case report of dark green urine in a 16-year-old during a prolonged infusion of propofol.[1]

1. Bodenham A, *et al.* Propofol infusion and green urine. *Lancet* 1987; **ii:** 740.

Precautions

Propofol should not be given to patients known to be allergic to it. Propofol should be administered with caution to patients with hypovolaemia, epilepsy, lipid metabolism disorders, and the elderly. Since there have been reports of delayed convulsions associated with the use of propofol it is recommended that special care should be taken when propofol is used for day-case surgery. When used in patients with increased intracranial pressure it should be administered slowly to avoid a substantial decrease in mean arterial pressure and a resultant decrease in cerebral perfusion pressure. It is also recommended that propofol should not be used with electroconvulsive therapy. Premedication with an antimuscarinic may be advisable since propofol does not cause vagal inhibition.

Propofol is used to provide continuous sedation for ventilated adult patients under intensive care. Account should be taken of increasing the patient's lipid load. If the duration of sedation is in excess of 3 days, lipid concentrations should be monitored. Children should not be sedated in this manner with propofol (see under Adverse Effects, above). Propofol is not recommended as an anaesthetic in children under 3 years of age. Propofol is not recommended for use in obstetrics including caesarean section. See also Precautions for General Anaesthetics, p.1219.

Effects on the nervous system. The central effects of propofol are as yet unclear. For instance Hodkinson[1] observed epileptic activity on the EEGs of 3 patients given propofol and suggested that it might be useful in ECT, but Simpson *et al.*[2] and Rampton *et al.*[3] found that the duration of seizures was less with propofol anaesthesia than with methohexitone anaesthesia. It has been suggested that propofol should not be used with ECT[4] and this is the advice of the manufacturer.

One group of workers considers that abnormal movements induced by propofol are not associated with cortical seizure activity.[5,6] They appear to be more frequent with low doses of propofol and can be abolished in children by increasing the induction dose of propofol from 3 to 5 mg per kg body-weight.[6]

1. Hodkinson BP, *et al.* Propofol and the electroencephalogram. *Lancet* 1987; **ii:** 1518.
2. Simpson KH, *et al.* Seizure duration after methohexitone or propofol for induction of anaesthesia for electroconvulsive therapy (ECT). *Br J Anaesth* 1987; **59:** 1323P–4P.
3. Rampton AJ, *et al.* Propofol and electroconvulsive therapy. *Lancet* 1988; **i:** 296–7.
4. Anonymous. Addendum: propofol better avoided with ECT at present. *Drug Ther Bull* 1990; **28:** 72.
5. Borgeat A, *et al.* Spontaneous excitatory movements during recovery from propofol anaesthesia in an infant: EEG evaluation. *Br J Anaesth* 1993; **70:** 459–61.
6. Borgeat A, *et al.* Propofol and epilepsy: time to clarify. *Anesth Analg* 1994; **78:** 198–9.

Effects on respiration. The manufacturer has stated[1] that some patients who have received propofol for sedation in regional anaesthesia have experienced bradypnoea or hypoxaemia, or both. A reduction in oxygen saturation has also been noted in other patients sedated for endoscopy.[2] The manufacturer therefore recommends that oxygen saturation should be monitored in all such patients and that oxygen supplementation should be readily available.

1. Arnold BDC. Sedation with propofol during regional anaesthesia. *Br J Anaesth* 1993; **70:** 112.
2. Patterson KW, *et al.* Propofol sedation for outpatient upper gastrointestinal endoscopy: comparison with midazolam. *Br J Anaesth* 1991; **67:** 108–11.

Porphyria. Reports of use of propofol in patients[1-4] with porphyria suggest that propofol is not porphyrinogenic when used for the induction of anaesthesia.

1. McLouglin C. Use of propofol in a patient with porphyria. *Br J Anaesth* 1989; **62:** 114.
2. Meissner PN, *et al.* Propofol as an I.V. anaesthetic induction agent in variegate porphyria. *Br J Anaesth* 1991; **66:** 60–5.
3. Tidmarsh MA, Baigent DF. Propofol in acute intermittent porphyria. *Br J Anaesth* 1992; **68:** 230.
4. Shaw IH, McKeith IG. Propofol and electroconvulsive therapy in a patient at risk from acute intermittent porphyria. *Br J Anaesth* 1998; **80:** 260–2.

Interactions

The concurrent administration of propofol with other CNS depressants including those used in premedication may increase the sedative, anaesthetic, and cardiorespiratory depressant effects of propofol. It is recommended that propofol is administered after opioids so that the dose of propofol can be carefully titrated against the response. The dosage of propofol should be reduced if given with nitrous oxide or halogenated anaesthetics. Although propofol does not potentiate the effects of neuromuscular blockers, bradycardia and asystole have occurred after administration of propofol with atracurium or suxamethonium (but see under Adverse Effects, above for the effects of propofol itself on the cardiovascular system).

See also Interactions of General Anaesthetics, p.1219.

In one study mean blood concentrations of propofol were higher in patients pretreated with *fentanyl* compared with patients maintained only on nitrous oxide.[1] However, Dixon and co-workers[2] were unable to confirm this interaction. Concomitant administration of *halothane* or *isoflurane* has also been reported to increase serum concentrations of propofol.[3] Propofol and *midazolam* have been reported to act synergistically.[4-6] Synergy has also been reported between propofol and *etomidate*.[7] A reduction in the amount of propofol required to provide adequate hypnosis[8] or sedation[9] has been reported after the administration of *bupivacaine*[8] or *lignocaine*.[8,9] Premedication with *clonidine* has been reported[10] to reduce intraoperative requirements of propofol.

1. Cockshott ID, *et al.* Pharmacokinetics of propofol in female patients. *Br J Anaesth* 1987; **59:** 1103–10.
2. Dixon J, *et al.* Study of the possible interaction between fentanyl and propofol using a computer-controlled infusion of propofol. *Br J Anaesth* 1990; **64:** 142–7.
3. Grundmann U, *et al.* Propofol and volatile anaesthetics. *Br J Anaesth* 1994; **72** (suppl 1): 88.
4. Short TG, Chui PT. Propofol and midazolam act synergistically in combination. *Br J Anaesth* 1991; **67:** 539–45.
5. McClune S, *et al.* Synergistic interaction between midazolam and propofol. *Br J Anaesth* 1992; **69:** 240–5.
6. Teh J, *et al.* Pharmacokinetic interactions between midazolam and propofol: an infusion study. *Br J Anaesth* 1994; **72:** 62–5.
7. Drummond GB, Cairns DT. Do propofol and etomidate interact kinetically during induction of anaesthesia? *Br J Anaesth* 1994; **73:** 272P.
8. Ben-Shlomo I, *et al.* Hypnotic effect of iv propofol is enhanced by im administration of either lignocaine or bupivacaine. *Br J Anaesth* 1997; **78:** 375–7.
9. Mallick A, *et al.* Local anaesthesia to the airway reduces sedation requirements in patients undergoing artificial ventilation. *Br J Anaesth* 1996; **77:** 731–4.
10. Guglielminotti J, *et al.* Effects of premedication on dose requirements for propofol: comparison of clonidine and hydroxyzine. *Br J Anaesth* 1998; **80:** 733–6.

Pharmacokinetics

The pharmacokinetics of propofol are best described by a 3-compartment model. After a single bolus dose, two distribution phases are seen. The first phase has a half-life of 2 to 4 minutes. This is followed by a slow distribution phase with a half-life of 30 to 60 minutes. Significant metabolism of propofol occurs during the second phase. The termination of anaesthetic effect after a single intravenous bolus or maintenance infusion is due to extensive redistribution from the brain to other tissues and to metabolic clearance. Propofol is over 95% bound to plasma proteins. It undergoes extensive hepatic metabolism to conjugates which are eliminated in the urine. The terminal half-life ranges from 3 to 12 hours; with prolonged use, the terminal half-life may be longer. The pharmacokinetics of propofol do not appear to be altered by gender, chronic hepatic cirrhosis, or chronic renal impairment. Propofol crosses the placental barrier and is distributed into breast milk.

References.

1. Kanto J, Gepts E. Pharmacokinetic implications for the clinical use of propofol. *Clin Pharmacokinet* 1989; **17:** 308–26.
2. Morgan DJ, *et al.* Pharmacokinetics of propofol when given by intravenous infusion. *Br J Clin Pharmacol* 1990; **30:** 144–8.
3. Jones RDM, *et al.* Pharmacokinetics of propofol in children. *Br J Anaesth* 1990; **65:** 661–7.
4. Saint-Maurice C, *et al.* Pharmacokinetics of propofol in young children after a single dose. *Br J Anaesth* 1989; **63:** 667–70.
5. Servin F, *et al.* Pharmacokinetics of propofol infusions in patients with cirrhosis. *Br J Anaesth* 1990; **65:** 177–83.
6. Gin T, *et al.* Pharmacokinetics of propofol in women undergoing elective caesarean section. *Br J Anaesth* 1990; **64:** 148–53.
7. Gin T, *et al.* Disposition of propofol at caesarean section and in the postpartum period. *Br J Anaesth* 1991; **67:** 49–53.
8. Bailie GR, *et al.* Pharmacokinetics of propofol during and after long term continuous infusion for maintenance of sedation in ICU patients. *Br J Anaesth* 1992; **68:** 486–91.
9. Altmayer P, *et al.* Propofol binding in human blood. *Br J Anaesth* 1994; **72** (suppl 1): 86.
10. Oei-Lim VLB, *et al.* Pharmacokinetics of propofol during conscious sedation using target-controlled infusion in anxious patients undergoing dental treatment. *Br J Anaesth* 1998; **80:** 324–31.

Uses and Administration

Propofol is an anaesthetic given intravenously for the induction and maintenance of anaesthesia (p.1220). It is also used for sedation (p.638) in patients undergoing diagnostic procedures, in those undergoing surgery in conjunction with local or regional anaesthesia, and in ventilated adult patients under intensive care for a period of up to 3 days. When used for anaesthesia, induction is rapid, as is recovery. Propofol has no analgesic activity and supplementary analgesia may be required.

Propofol is available as a 1 or 2% emulsion. The 1% emulsion may be given by intravenous injection or infusion, but the 2% emulsion is for infusion only.

Induction of **anaesthesia** is generally carried out by administering 40 mg of propofol by injection or infusion every 10 seconds; 20 mg every 10 seconds may be used in high-risk patients including elderly, neurosurgical, and debilitated patients. Most adults will be anaesthetised by a dose of 1.5 to 2.5 mg per kg body-weight; elderly patients usually require a dose of 1.0 to 1.5 mg per kg. When used for maintenance propofol is infused at a rate of between 4 to 12 mg per kg per hour (or half this dosage for elderly and debilitated patients); alternatively intermittent bolus injections of 20 to 50 mg may be given; rapid administration of bolus doses should be avoided in high-risk patients. A novel delivery system is also available for the induction and maintenance of anaesthesia in adults. The Diprifusor target-controlled infusion system allows the speed of induction and depth of anaesthesia to be controlled by specifying target blood concentrations of propofol. Initial target concentrations for induction range from 4 to 8 μg per mL. Target concentrations for maintenance are 3 to 6 μg per mL. Children over 3 years of age can be given a dose of 2.5 to 3.5 mg per kg for induction adjusted as necessary; a dose of 9 to 15 mg per kg per hour by intravenous infusion or intermittent bolus injections is suitable for maintenance.

For **sedation** in diagnostic and surgical procedures an initial infusion of 6 to 9 mg per kg per hour may be given for 3 to 5 minutes; alternatively 0.5 to 1.0 mg per kg may be injected slowly over 1 to 5 minutes. An infusion of 1.5 to 4.5 mg per kg per hour may be used for maintenance of sedation. High-risk patients usually require a 20% reduction in the maintenance dose.

For the sedation of ventilated adults propofol can be given by intravenous infusion in a dose of 0.3 to 4.0 mg per kg per hour. If the duration of sedation is in excess of 3 days, lipid concentrations should be monitored.

Propofol is not recommended for sedation in children.

Intravenous infusions and injections of propofol should be prepared using aseptic techniques, see under Administration, below.

Reviews.

1. Langley MS, Heel RC. Propofol: a review of its pharmacodynamic and pharmacokinetic properties and use as an intravenous anaesthetic. *Drugs* 1988; **35:** 334–72.
2. Larijani GE, *et al.* Clinical pharmacology of propofol: an intravenous anesthetic agent. *DICP Ann Pharmacother* 1989; **23:** 743–9.
3. Bryson HM, *et al.* Propofol: an update of its use in anaesthesia and conscious sedation. *Drugs* 1995; **50:** 513–59.
4. Fulton B, Sorkin EM. Propofol: an overview of its pharmacology and a review of its clinical efficacy in intensive care sedation. *Drugs* 1995; **50:** 636–57.

Administration. Propofol is formulated as an oil in water emulsion for injection. Strict aseptic techniques must be maintained when handling propofol as, in some countries including the UK, the parenteral product contains no antimicrobial preservatives and the vehicle can support rapid growth of micro-organisms. Aseptic techniques must also be applied to formulations, such as those available in the USA, that contain the microbial-retarding agent disodium edetate as microbial growth is still possible. An emulsion containing 1% of propofol may be diluted with glucose 5% immediately before administration but it should not be diluted to a concentration of less than 2 mg per mL. An emulsion containing 2 % of propofol should not be diluted. The use of a 5-micron filter needle to withdraw propofol emulsion from an ampoule does not cause significant loss of drug.[1] A reduction in concentration of propofol can occur when the diluted emulsion is run through polyvinyl chloride intravenous tubing.[1] Propofol 1% or 2% may be administered into a running intravenous infusion through a Y-site close to the injection site and under these circumstances it is compatible with glucose 5%, sodium chloride 0.9%, and glucose with sodium chloride intravenous solutions.

1. Bailey LC, *et al.* Effect of syringe filter and I.V. administration set on delivery of propofol emulsion. *Am J Hosp Pharm* 1991; **48:** 2627–30.

Nausea and vomiting. It is commonly believed that propofol is associated with less postoperative nausea and vomiting than some other anaesthetics.[1,2] However, a recent review[3] concluded that any reduction in nausea and vomiting when using propofol anaesthesia may be short term and clinically relevant only for maintenance anaesthesia in procedures with an inherent risk of nausea and vomiting.

There are also reports[4-8] indicating that propofol may have some intrinsic antiemetic action when used in sub-hypnotic doses although a study[9] of the effect of sedative and non-sedative (sub-hypnotic) doses against apomorphine-induced vomiting has suggested that any antiemetic effect is probably due to sedation.

1. McCollum JSC, *et al.* The antiemetic action of propofol. *Anaesthesia* 1988; **43:** 239–40.
2. Woodward WM, *et al.* Comparison of post-operative nausea and vomiting after thiopentone/isoflurane or propofol infusion for 'bat-ear' correction in children. *Br J Anaesth* 1994; **72** (suppl 1): 92.
3. Tramèr M, *et al.* Propofol anaesthesia and postoperative nausea and vomiting: quantitative systematic review of randomized controlled studies. *Br J Anaesth* 1997: **78:** 247–55.
4. Borgeat A, *et al.* Adjuvant propofol for refractory cisplatin-associated nausea and vomiting. *Lancet* 1992; **340:** 679–80.
5. Törn K, *et al.* Effects of sub-hypnotic doses of propofol on the side effects of intrathecal morphine. *Br J Anaesth* 1994; **73:** 411–12.
6. Borgeat A, *et al.* Adjuvant propofol enables better control of nausea and emesis secondary to chemotherapy for breast cancer. *Can J Anaesth* 1994; **41:** 1117–19.
7. Ewalenko P, *et al.* Antiemetic effect of subhypnotic doses of propofol after thyroidectomy. *Br J Anaesth* 1996; **77:** 463–7.
8. Gan TJ, *et al.* Determination of plasma concentrations of propofol associated with 50% reduction in postoperative nausea. *Anesthesiology* 1997; **87:**779–84.
9. Thörn S-E, *et al.* Propofol effects upon apomorphine induced vomiting. *Br J Anaesth* 1994; **72** (suppl 1): 90.

Pruritus. Propofol is one of many drugs that have been tried in the management of pruritus (p.1075). Sub-hypnotic doses of propofol appear to have an antipruritic action. It has been found to be effective in the treatment and prophylaxis of pruritus associated with epidural and intrathecal morphine[1,2] and appears to be able to relieve cholestasis-associated pruritus.[3] It has been suggested that propofol might act by suppression of the spinal transmission of pruritic signals.

1. Borgeat A, *et al.* Subhypnotic doses of propofol relieve pruritus induced by epidural and intrathecal morphine. *Anesthesiology* 1992; **76:** 510–12.
2. Törn K, *et al.* Effects of sub-hypnotic doses of propofol on the side effects of intrathecal morphine. *Br J Anaesth* 1994; **73:** 411–12.
3. Borgeat A, *et al.* Subhypnotic doses of propofol relieve pruritus associated with liver disease. *Gastroenterology* 1993; **104:** 244–7.

Status epilepticus. Anaesthesia in conjunction with assisted ventilation may be instituted to control refractory tonic-clonic status epilepticus (p.337). A short-acting barbiturate such as thiopentone is usually used. Propofol has also been tried although it has caused seizures when used in anaesthesia (see under Precautions, above) and should be given with caution to patients with epilepsy. There appear to be only a few cases reports and small uncontrolled studies of the effectiveness of propofol in status epilepticus,[1] but one review[2] stated that it was widely used for this purpose. It has a rapid onset of action and its effects are maintained while the infusion is maintained; recovery is rapid on discontinuation. However, as it can cause profound respiratory and cerebral depression assisted ventilation and monitoring needs to be provided in the setting of an intensive care unit. There is also the risk of lipid overload with prolonged therapy. It may induce involuntary movements and care is required to distinguish these from seizures. A suggested regimen for management is an initial intravenous bolus of 2 mg per kg body-weight which can be repeated if seizures continue. This may be followed by an infusion of 5 to 10 mg per kg per hour guided by EEG monitoring. The dose should be gradually reduced and the infusion tapered 12 hours after seizure activity is halted. Lower doses should be used in the elderly.

1. Brown LA, Levin GM. Role of propofol in refractory status epilepticus. *Ann Pharmacother* 1998; **32:** 1053–9.
2. Shorvon S. Tonic clonic status epilepticus. *J Neurol Neurosurg Psychiatry* 1993; **56:** 125–34.

Preparations

Proprietary Preparations (details are given in Part 3)
Aust.: Diprivan; ***Austral.:*** Diprivan; ***Belg.:*** Diprivan; ***Canad.:*** Diprivan; ***Fr.:*** Diprivan; ***Ger.:*** Disoprivan; Klimofol; ***Irl.:*** Diprivan; ***Ital.:*** Diprivan; ***Neth.:*** Diprivan; ***Norw.:*** Diprivan; Recofol; ***S.Afr.:*** Diprivan; ***Spain:*** Diprivan; ***Swed.:*** Diprivan; Recofol; ***Switz.:*** Disoprivan; ***UK:*** Diprivan; ***USA:*** Diprivan.

Sevoflurane (13234-m)

Sevoflurane *(BAN, USAN, rINN).*

BAX-3084; MR-654. Fluoromethyl 2,2,2-trifluoro-1-(trifluoromethyl)ethyl ether; 1,1,1,3,3,3-Hexafluoro-2-(fluoromethoxy)-propane.

$C_4H_3F_7O$ = 200.1.

CAS — 28523-86-6.

A clear, colourless, volatile liquid with a light odour. Nonflammable. B.p. 58.5° to 58.9°. **Store** at a temperature not exceeding 40°. Protect from light.

Adverse Effects

As with other halogenated anaesthetics sevoflurane may cause cardiorespiratory depression, hypotension, and malignant hyperthermia. However, the effects of sevoflurane on heart rate have only been seen at higher concentrations and it appears to have little effect on heart rhythm in comparison to other halogenated anaesthetics. Sevoflurane appears to sensitise the myocardium to sympathomimetics to a lesser extent than halothane or enflurane. Other effects seen with sevoflurane include agitation, especially in children, laryngospasm, and increased cough and salivation. Acute renal failure has also been noted. Shivering, nausea, and vomiting have been reported in the postoperative period.

See also Adverse Effects of General Anaesthetics, p.1219.

Effects on the cardiovascular system. The cardiovascular effects of sevoflurane are similar to those of isoflurane (see p.1225) but it does not produce coronary steal. Also sevoflurane produces less tachycardia than isoflurane suggesting that it may be preferable in those predisposed to myocardial ischaemia.

Effects on the kidneys. Investigations[1] of the nephrotoxic potential of sevoflurane have found no evidence of renal function impairment despite peak plasma-fluoride ion concentrations greater than 50 nmol per mL (a level considered to be nephrotoxic with methoxyflurane) being recorded in some patients at the end of sevoflurane anaesthesia.[2] The lack of renal toxicity with sevoflurane may be due to low concentrations of intrarenally generated fluoride ions;[3] in comparison, methoxyflurane defluorination in the kidney is much greater and may contribute to its known nephrotoxicity.

The breakdown of sevoflurane by carbon dioxide absorbents (such as soda lime) results in the formation of pentafluoroisopropenyl fluoromethyl ether (compound A), a nephrotoxic compound in *rats.*[1] However, studies in humans undergoing sevoflurane anaesthesia have detected no renal impairment postoperatively even when compound A was detected in the anaesthetic circuits.

1. Malan TP. Sevoflurane and renal function. *Anesth Analg* 1995; **81:** S39–S45.
2. Kobayashi Y, *et al.* Serum and urinary inorganic fluoride concentrations after prolonged inhalation of sevoflurane in humans. *Anesth Analg* 1992; **74:** 753–7.

3. Kharasch ED, *et al.* Human kidney methoxyflurane and sevoflurane metabolism: intrarenal fluoride production as a possible mechanism of methoxyflurane nephrotoxicity. *Anesthesiology* 1995; **82:** 689–99.

Effects on the liver. There have been signs of hepatotoxicity in *animal* studies but in studies in humans, markers for hepatocellular dysfunction were no greater following sevoflurane anaesthesia than those after halothane[1] or isoflurane.[2] Also the metabolism of sevoflurane differs from other halogenated anaesthetics in such a way that metabolites implicated in liver toxicity are not formed (see Pharmacokinetics, below).

1. Taivainen T, *et al.* Comparison of the effects of sevoflurane and halothane on the quality of anaesthesia and serum glutathione transferase alpha and fluoride in paediatric patients. *Br J Anaesth* 1994; **73:** 590–5.
2. Darling JR, *et al.* Comparison of the effects of sevoflurane with those of isoflurane on hepatic glutathione-S-transferase concentrations after body surface surgery. *Br J Anaesth* 1994; **73:** 268P.

Effects on the nervous system. Clonic and tonic seizure-like movements of the extremities have been reported[1] in a child during induction of anaesthesia using sevoflurane. It was considered that this might have been a result of seizure activity in the CNS or due to myoclonus of the extremities.

1. Adachi M, *et al.* Seizure-like movements during induction of anaesthesia with sevoflurane. *Br J Anaesth* 1992; **68:** 214–15.

Precautions

As with other halogenated anaesthetics, patients with known or suspected susceptibility to malignant hyperthermia should not be anaesthetised with sevoflurane. Although the effects of sevoflurane on cerebral pressure is minimal in normal patients, safety in those with raised intracranial pressure has not been established and therefore sevoflurane should be used with caution.

See also Precautions for General Anaesthetics, p.1219.

Interactions

Care is advised if adrenaline or other sympathomimetics are given during sevoflurane anaesthesia. The effects of competitive neuromuscular blockers such as atracurium are enhanced by sevoflurane (see p.1307). The metabolism, and hence toxicity, of sevoflurane may be increased by drugs or compounds that induce cytochrome P450 isoenzyme CYP2E1 including isoniazid and alcohol.

See also Interactions of General Anaesthetics, p.1219.

References.

1. Dale O. Drug interactions in anaesthesia: focus on desflurane and sevoflurane. *Baillieres Clin Anaesthesiol* 1995; **9:** 105–17.

Pharmacokinetics

Sevoflurane is absorbed on inhalation. The blood/gas coefficient is low. Up to 5% of the absorbed dose of sevoflurane is metabolised in the liver by defluorination to its major metabolites hexafluoroisopropanol (HFIP), inorganic fluoride, and carbon dioxide. HFIP is rapidly conjugated with glucuronic acid and eliminated in the urine. Sevoflurane crosses the placenta.

Uses and Administration

Sevoflurane is a volatile halogenated anaesthetic administered by inhalation. It has a minimum alveolar concentration (MAC) value (see p.1220) ranging from 1.4% in the elderly to 3.3% in neonates. It is employed for the induction and maintenance of general anaesthesia (p.1220). It is non-flammable. Sevoflurane has a nonpungent odour and does not cause respiratory irritation. It also has muscle relaxant properties which may be sufficient for some surgical procedures to be performed without a neuromuscular blocker. However, it possesses no analgesic properties.

Sevoflurane is administered using a calibrated vaporiser. To avoid intra-operative excitement a short-acting barbiturate is recommended before commencing induction which is performed by giving sevoflurane, in concentrations of up to 5% v/v in adults, with oxygen or oxygen and nitrous oxide. Concentrations of up to 7% v/v may be used in children. Induction with sevoflurane is rapid (surgical anaesthesia in less than 2 minutes) and smooth because of its nonpungent odour. Maintenance of anaesthesia is achieved with a concentration of 0.5 to 3.0% v/v with or without nitrous oxide.

Reviews.

1. Patel SS, Goa KL. Sevoflurane: a review of its pharmacodynamic and pharmacokinetic properties and its clinical use in general anaesthesia. *Drugs* 1996; **51:** 658–700.
2. Smith I, *et al.* Sevoflurane—a long-awaited volatile anaesthetic. *Br J Anaesth* 1996; **76:** 435–45.
3. Grounds RM, Newman PJ. Sevoflurane. *Br J Hosp Med* 1997; **57:** 43–6.

Administration. Sevoflurane's relative instability in soda lime has cast doubt over whether it can be used in closed circuit absorber systems. There has also been concern over the safety of sevoflurane if used in such systems. However, the physical characteristics of sevoflurane are such that it can be used with conventional vaporisation techniques.

Preparations

Proprietary Preparations (details are given in Part 3)
Austral.: Sevorane; ***Canad.:*** Sevorane; ***Ger.:*** Sevorane; ***Irl.:*** Sevorane; ***Ital.:*** Sevorane; ***Neth.:*** Sevorane; ***Norw.:*** Sevorane; ***S.Afr.:*** Ultane; ***Swed.:*** Sevorane; ***Switz.:*** Sevorane; ***USA:*** Ultane.

Sodium Oxybate (3121-n)

Sodium Oxybate *(USAN)*.

NSC-84223; Sodium Gamma-hydroxybutyrate; Wy-3478.

Sodium 4-hydroxybutyrate.

$C_4H_7NaO_3$ = 126.1.

CAS — 502-85-2.

Pharmacopoeias. In *Chin.*

Adverse Effects

When used in general anaesthesia side-effects with sodium oxybate include abnormal muscle movements during the induction period and nausea and vomiting. Occasional emergence delirium has been reported. Bradycardia frequently occurs. Respiration may be slowed and hypokalaemia has been reported.

Patients receiving sodium oxybate orally for the management of narcolepsy may experience dizziness, lightheadedness, and confusion; gastro-intestinal effects and enuresis occur occasionally.

See also Adverse Effects of General Anaesthetics, p.1219.

Abuse. Reports[1] of acute poisoning with sodium oxybate following illicit use led the FDA in the USA to issue warnings[2] about its potential for abuse. It is usually supplied illicitly as the sodium salt under a variety of names including GHB or GBH, gammahydroxybutyrate, liquid ecstasy, liquid X, sodium oxybutyrate, and somatomax PM and has been promoted for body building, weight loss, as a psychedelic substance, and as a sleep aid. Adverse effects include vomiting, drowsiness, amnesia, hypotonia, vertigo, respiratory depression, and involuntary movements. Seizure-like activity, bradycardia, hypotension, and respiratory arrest have also been reported. Resolution of symptoms occurs spontaneously over 2 to 96 hours. However, some patients have required hospitalisation and respiratory support and deaths have been reported in both the UK[3] and USA.[4] Severity of symptoms depends on the dose of sodium oxybate and the presence of other drugs such as alcohol, benzodiazepines, cannabis, or amphetamines. Prolonged use of large doses may lead to a withdrawal syndrome on discontinuation.[5]

1. Centers for Disease Control. Multistate outbreak of poisonings associated with illicit use of gamma hydroxy butyrate. *JAMA* 1991; **265:** 447–8.
2. Food and Drug Administration. Warning about GHB. *JAMA* 1991; **265:** 1802.
3. Anonymous. GBH death indicates increasing problem. *Pharm J* 1996; **256:** 441.
4. Centers for Disease Control. Gamma hydroxy butyrate use—New York and Texas, 1995–1996. *JAMA* 1997; **277:** 1511.
5. Galloway GP, *et al.* Physical dependence on sodium oxybate. *Lancet* 1994; **343:** 57.

Effects on electrolyte balance. A report of severe metabolic disorders occurring during therapy with sodium oxybate and tetracosactrin in 4 patients with severe head injuries.[1] The disorders consisted of hypernatraemia, hypokalaemia, and metabolic acidosis.

1. Béal JL, *et al.* Troubles métaboliques induits par l'association gamma-hydroxy butyrate de sodium et tétracosactide chez le traumatisé crânien. *Therapie* 1983; **38:** 569–71.

Precautions

Sodium oxybate should not be given to patients with severe hypertension, bradycardia, conditions associated with defects of cardiac conduction, epilepsy, eclampsia, renal impairment, or alcohol abuse.

See also Precautions for General Anaesthetics, p.1219.

Interactions

Sodium oxybate enhances the effects of opioid analgesics and skeletal muscle relaxants. The action of sodium oxybate may be potentiated by benzodiazepines or antipsychotics.

See also Interactions of General Anaesthetics, p.1219.

Pharmacokinetics

Following oral administration sodium oxybate is absorbed from the gastro-intestinal tract and rapidly metabolised in the liver to carbon dioxide and water. In one study the mean values for the terminal half-life ranged from 20 to 23 minutes. It crosses the blood-brain barrier and the placental barrier.

References.

1. Palatini P, *et al.* Dose-dependent absorption and elimination of gamma-hydroxybutyric acid in healthy volunteers. *Eur J Clin Pharmacol* 1993; **45:** 353–6.

Uses and Administration

Sodium oxybate has hypnotic properties and, in its endogenous form, Gamma hydroxybutyrate (a catabolite of gamma-aminobutyric acid), increases dopamine concentrations in the brain. It is given intravenously to produce anaesthesia (p.1220) usually in conjunction with an opioid analgesic and an antipsychotic. Skeletal muscle relaxants may also be necessary. Sodium oxybate given orally is being investigated for use in narcolepsy.

In general anaesthesia a solution of sodium oxybate equivalent to 20% of the acid is administered slowly by intravenous injection, usually in a dose of 60 mg per kg body-weight; further smaller doses may be required in long procedures. In children up to 100 mg per kg may be necessary.

Alcohol withdrawal syndrome. Gammahydroxybutyric acid has been reported[1] to be effective in reducing symptoms of alcohol withdrawal (p.1099) and to be of use as an aid in the maintenance of abstinence.[2,3] However, following reports of CNS toxicity associated with abuse of gammahydroxybutyric acid its role in the treatment of substance abuse disorders appears questionable.[4]

1. Gallimberti L, *et al.* Gamma-hydroxybutyric acid for treatment of alcohol withdrawal syndrome. *Lancet* 1989; **ii:** 787–9.
2. Gallimberti L, *et al.* Gamma-hydroxybutyric acid in the treatment of alcohol dependence: a double blind study. *Alcohol Clin Exp Res* 1992; **16:** 673–6.
3. Addolorato G, *et al.* Maintaining abstinence from alcohol with γ-hydroxybutyric acid. *Lancet* 1998; **351:** 38.
4. Quinn DI, *et al.* Pharmacokinetic and pharmacodynamic principles of illicit drug use and treatment of illicit drug users. *Clin Pharmacokinet* 1997; **33:** 344–400.

Cerebrovascular disorders. Gammahydroxybutyric acid has been tried as an alternative to barbiturates to reduce intracranial pressure and protect against cerebral ischaemia in patients with head injuries.[1,2] The management of raised intracranial pressure is discussed on p.796.

1. Escuret E, *et al.* Gamma hydroxy butyrate as a substitute for barbiturate therapy in comatose patients with head injuries. *Acta Neurol Scand* 1979; **60** (suppl 72): 38–9.
2. Strong AJ, *et al.* Reduction of raised intracranial pressure (ICP) by gamma-hydroxybutyric acid following severe head injury. *Br J Surg* 1983; **70:** 303.

Narcoleptic syndrome. Central stimulants are the mainstay in the treatment of the sleep attacks of narcolepsy while tricyclic antidepressants are the primary treatment for cataplexy and sleep paralysis (p.1476). Sodium oxybate[1-3] given at night has been reported to improve symptoms of patients with narcoleptic syndrome treated with stimulants during the day.

1. Broughton R, Mamelak M. The treatment of narcolepsy-cataplexy with nocturnal gamma-hydroxybutyrate. *Can J Neurol Sci* 1979; **6:** 1–6.
2. Mamelak M, Webster P. Treatment of narcolepsy and sleep apnea with gammahydroxybutyrate: a clinical and polysomnographic case study. *Sleep* 1981; **4:** 105–111.
3. Scharf MB, *et al.* The effects and effectiveness of γ-hydroxybutyrate in patients with narcolepsy. *J Clin Psychiatry* 1985; **46:** 222–5.

Preparations

Proprietary Preparations (details are given in Part 3)
Fr.: Gamma-OH; ***Ger.:*** Somsanit; ***Ital.:*** Alcover.

Thiamylal Sodium (3122-h)

Sodium 5-allyl-5-(1-methylbutyl)-2-thiobarbiturate.

$C_{12}H_{17}N_2NaO_2S$ = 276.3.

CAS — 77-27-0 (thiamylal); 337-47-3 (thiamylal sodium).

Pharmacopoeias. In *Jpn. US* includes Thiamylal and Thiamylal Sodium for Injection.

Thiamylal Sodium for Injection (USP 23) is a sterile mixture of thiamylal and anhydrous sodium bicarbonate. It is a pale yellow hygroscopic powder with a disagreeable odour. A 5% solution in water has a pH between 10.7 and 11.5.

Thiamylal sodium is a short-acting intravenous barbiturate anaesthetic. It is possibly slightly more potent than thiopentone sodium (p.1233) and has similar actions and uses. It has been used for the production of complete anaesthesia of short duration, for the induction of general anaesthesia, or for inducing a hypnotic state.

Thiamylal sodium has been given as a 2.5% solution, an initial injection of 3 to 6 mL being sufficient to produce short periods of anaesthesia. During induction the rate of injection should be 1 mL every 5 seconds. A continuous intravenous infusion of a 0.3% solution has been used for maintenance.

Preparations

USP 23: Thiamylal Sodium for Injection.

Thiopentone Sodium (3124-b)

Thiopentone Sodium *(BANM)*.

Thiopental Sodium *(rINN)*; Natrium Isopentylaethylthiobarbituricum (cum Natrio Carbonico); Penthiobarbital Sodique; Soluble Thiopentone; Thiomebumalnatrium cum Natrii Carbonate; Thiopental Sodium and Sodium Carbonate; Thiopentalum Natricum; Thiopentalum Natricum et Natrii Carbonas; Thiopentobarbitalum Solubile; Tiopentol Sódico. Sodium 5-ethyl-5-(1-methylbutyl)-2-thiobarbiturate.

$C_{11}H_{17}N_2NaO_2S$ = 264.3.

CAS — 76-75-5 (thiopentone); 71-73-8 (thiopentone sodium).

NOTE. The name thiobarbital has been applied to thiopentone and has also been used to describe a barbiturate of different composition.

Pharmacopoeias. In *Chin., Eur.* (see p.viii), *Int., Jpn,* and *US.* Some include thiopentone sodium with, some without, anhydrous sodium carbonate; some only include a sterile mixture for injection.

A white to yellowish-white hygroscopic crystalline powder, or pale greenish hygroscopic powder with a characteristic alliaceous odour.

Thiopental Sodium and Sodium Carbonate (Ph. Eur.) contains 84 to 87% thiopentone and 10.2 to 11.2% sodium. Its **solubilities** are: freely soluble in water; partly soluble in dehydrated alcohol; practically insoluble in ether. Thiopental Sodium (USP 23) solubilities are: soluble in water and in alcohol; insoluble in ether and in petroleum spirit. Solutions of thiopentone sodium are **incompatible** with acidic and oxidising substances so that, amongst other drugs, a number of antibiotics, muscle relaxants, and analgesics should not be mixed with it. Compounds commonly listed as incompatible include amikacin sulphate, benzylpenicillin salts, cefapirin sodium, codeine phosphate, ephedrine sulphate, fentanyl citrate, glycopyrronium bromide, morphine sulphate, pentazocine lactate, prochlorperazine edisylate, suxamethonium salts, and tubocurarine chloride. Solutions decompose on standing and precipitation occurs on boiling. **Store** in airtight containers. Protect from light.

Loss of thiopentone in polyvinyl chloride and cellulose propionate delivery systems has been reported,[1,2] but in another study,[3] no loss of potency was noted.

1. Kowaluk EA, *et al.* Interactions between drugs and polyvinyl chloride infusion bags. *Am J Hosp Pharm* 1981; **38:** 1308–14.
2. Kowaluk EA, *et al.* Interactions between drugs and intravenous delivery systems. *Am J Hosp Pharm* 1982; **39:** 460–7.
3. Martens HJ, *et al.* Sorption of various drugs in polyvinyl chloride, glass, and polyethylene-lined infusion containers. *Am J Hosp Pharm* 1990; **47:** 369–73.

Adverse Effects and Treatment

As for Phenobarbitone, p.350.

Excitatory phenomena such as coughing, hiccuping, sneezing, and muscle twitching or jerking may occur with any of the barbiturate anaesthetics, particularly during induction, but they occur more frequently with methohexitone than with thiopentone. Laryngeal spasm or bronchospasm may also occur during induction. The intravenous injection of concentrated solutions of thiopentone sodium such as 5% may result in thrombophlebitis. Extravasation of barbiturate anaesthetics may cause tissue necrosis. Intra-arterial injection causes severe arterial spasm with burning pain and may cause prolonged blanching of the forearm and hand and gangrene of digits. Hypersensitivity reactions have been reported. Barbiturate anaesthetics can cause respiratory depression. They depress cardiac output and often cause an initial fall in blood pressure, and overdosage may result in circulatory failure. Postoperative vomiting is infrequent but shivering may occur and there may be persistent drowsiness, confusion, and amnesia. Headache has also been reported.

See also under Adverse Effects of General Anaesthetics, p.1219.

Hypersensitivity. Anaphylactic reactions to thiopentone have been reported[1,2] although such reactions are rare. There has also been a report of haemolytic anaemia and renal failure in association with the development of an anti-thiopentone antibody in a patient who had undergone general anaesthesia induced by thiopentone.[3]

1. Westacott P, *et al.* Anaphylactic reaction to thiopentone: a case report. *Can Anaesth Soc J* 1984; **31:** 434–8.
2. Moneret-Vautrin DA, *et al.* Simultaneous anaphylaxis to thiopentone and a neuromuscular blocker: a study of two cases. *Br J Anaesth* 1990; **64:** 743–5.
3. Habibi B, *et al.* Thiopental-related immune hemolytic anemia and renal failure: specific involvement of red-cell antigen I. *N Engl J Med* 1985; **312:** 353–5. Correction. *ibid.*: 1136.

Intra-arterial injection. Accidental intra-arterial injection of thiopentone sodium produces severe arterial spasm with intense burning pain. Anaesthesia, paresis, paralysis, and gangrene may occur. Therapy has concentrated on dilution of injected thiopentone, prevention and treatment of arterial spasm, prophylaxis of thrombosis, thrombectomy and other measures to sustain good blood flow. There has been a report[1] of the successful use of urokinase intra-arterially in the management of one patient accidentally given thiopentone intra-arterially.

1. Vangerven M, *et al.* A new therapeutic approach to accidental intra-arterial injection of thiopentone. *Br J Anaesth* 1989; **62:** 98–100.

Precautions

Barbiturate anaesthetics are contra-indicated when there is dyspnoea or respiratory obstruction such as in acute severe asthma or when maintenance of an airway cannot be guaranteed. They are also contra-indicated in porphyria.

Barbiturate anaesthetics should be used with caution in shock and dehydration, hypovolaemia, severe anaemia, hyperkalaemia, toxaemia, myasthenia gravis, myxoedema and other metabolic disorders, or in severe renal disease. Caution is also required in patients with cardiovascular disease, muscular dystrophies, adrenocortical insufficiency, or with increased intracranial pressure. Reduced doses are required in the elderly and in severe hepatic disease.

See also Precautions for General Anaesthetics, p.1219.

Interactions

Difficulty may be experienced in producing anaesthesia with the usual dose of barbiturate anaesthetics in patients accustomed to taking alcohol or other CNS depressants; additional anaesthetics may be necessary. Care is required when anaesthetising patients being treated with phenothiazine antipsychotics since there may be increased hypotension. Some phenothiazines, especially promethazine, may increase the incidence of excitatory phenomena produced by barbiturate anaesthetics; cyclizine may possibly have a similar effect. Opioid analgesics can potentiate the respiratory depressant effect of barbiturate anaesthetics and the dose of the anaesthetic may need to be reduced. Concomitant administration of nitrous oxide greatly reduces the dose of barbiturate anaesthetics required for anaesthesia. Reduced doses of thiopentone may be required in patients receiving sulphafurazole.

See also Interactions of General Anaesthetics, p.1219.

Antidepressants. Potentiation of barbiturate anaesthesia may be expected in patients receiving *tricyclic antidepressants* or *MAOIs* (see under Anaesthesia in Precautions for Amitriptyline, p.275 and for Phenelzine, p.304, respectively).

Aspirin. Pretreatment with aspirin, a highly protein-bound drug, has been shown to potentiate thiopentone anaesthesia.[1]

1. Dundee JW, *et al.* Aspirin and probenecid pretreatment influences the potency of thiopentone and the onset of action of midazolam. *Eur J Anaesthesiol* 1986; **3:** 247–51.

Probenecid. Pretreatment with probenecid, a highly protein-bound drug, has been shown to potentiate thiopentone anaesthesia.[1]

1. Dundee JW, *et al.* Aspirin and probenecid pretreatment influences the potency of thiopentone and the onset of action of midazolam. *Eur J Anaesthesiol* 1986; **3:** 247–51.

Pharmacokinetics

Thiopentone is highly lipid soluble and when it is administered intravenously as the sodium salt, concentrations sufficient to produce unconsciousness are achieved in the brain within 30 seconds. Onset of action occurs within 8 to 10 minutes when thiopentone sodium is given rectally but absorption may be unpredictable if a suspension rather than a solution is used. Recovery from anaesthesia is also rapid due to redistribution to other tissues, particularly fat. About 80% of thiopentone may be bound to plasma proteins, although reports show a wide range of figures. Thiopentone is metabolised almost entirely in the liver, but as it is only released slowly from lipid stores this occurs at a very slow rate.

It is mostly metabolised to inactive metabolites but a small amount is desulphurated to pentobarbitone. Repeated or continuous administration can lead to accumulation of thiopentone in fatty tissue and this can result in prolonged anaesthesia and respiratory and cardiovascular depression. Elimination of thiopentone following bolus injection can be described by a triexponential curve. The terminal elimination half-life has been reported to be 10 to 12 hours in adults and about 6 hours in children. However, values of 26 to 28 hours have been reported in obese patients and pregnant patients at term. Thiopentone readily diffuses across the placenta and is distributed into breast milk.

References.

1. Swerdlow BN, Holley FO. Intravenous anaesthetic agents: pharmacokinetic-pharmacodynamic relationships. *Clin Pharmacokinet* 1987; **12:** 79–110.
2. Gaspari F, *et al.* Elimination kinetics of thiopentone in mothers and their newborn infants. *Eur J Clin Pharmacol* 1985; **28:** 321–5.
3. Esener Z, *et al.* Thiopentone and etomidate concentrations in maternal and umbilical plasma, and in colostrum. *Br J Anaesth* 1992; **69:** 586–8.
4. Gedney JA, Ghosh S. Pharmacokinetics of analgesics, sedatives and anaesthetic agents during cardiopulmonary bypass. *Br J Anaesth* 1995; **75:** 344–51.

Uses and Administration

Thiopentone is a short-acting barbiturate anaesthetic. It is usually given for the induction of general anaesthesia (p.1220) but may be used as the sole anaesthetic to maintain anaesthesia for short procedures with minimal painful stimuli. It is also used in anaesthesia as a supplement to other anaesthetics, as a hypnotic in balanced anaesthesia, and for basal anaesthesia or basal narcosis. Thiopentone sodium may also be used in the control of refractory tonic-clonic status epilepticus and in neurosurgical patients to reduce increased intracranial pressure.

Thiopentone does not usually produce excitation and induction of anaesthesia is usually smooth. It has poor muscle relaxant properties and a muscle relaxant must be administered before intubation is attempted. Thiopentone also has poor analgesic properties and small doses may even lower the pain threshold. Recovery from an induction dose may occur within 10 to 30 minutes although drowsiness may persist for some time.

In anaesthesia, the dosage of thiopentone varies greatly according to the state of the patient and the nature of other drugs being used concurrently (see under Precautions above and Interactions above for further details). Thiopentone is usually administered intravenously as the sodium salt as a 2.5% solution but a 5% solution is occasionally used. A typical dose for inducing anaesthesia is 100 to 150 mg injected over 10 to 15 seconds, repeated after 30 to 60 seconds according to response. Some prefer to initiate induction with a test dose of 25 to 75 mg. The UK manufacturer recommends that the total dosage used in pregnant patients should not exceed 250 mg. Children's doses range from 2 to 7 mg per kg bodyweight. When thiopentone is used as the sole anaesthetic, anaesthesia can be maintained by repeat doses as needed or by continuous intravenous infusion of a 0.2 or 0.4% solution. Thiopentone sodium may be given rectally for basal anaesthesia or basal narcosis.

A suggested dose in refractory tonic-clonic status epilepticus is 50 to 125 mg intravenously given as soon as possible after convulsions begin; up to 250 mg may be required over 10 minutes (see also under Status Epilepticus, below).

Recovery is usually rapid after moderate doses, but the patient may remain sleepy or confused for several hours. Large doses, repeated smaller doses, or continuous administration may markedly delay recovery.

References.

1. Russo H, Bressolle F. Pharmacodynamics and pharmacokinetics of thiopental. *Clin Pharmacokinet* 1998; **35:** 95–134.

Administration in the elderly. It is usually recommended that the dosage of barbiturate anaesthetics is reduced in the elderly. One study[1] in elderly patients has demonstrated that although reducing the rate of intravenous administration reduces the speed of induction, the dosage required is also reduced. Administration of thiopentone sodium 2.5% solution at a rate of 125 mg per minute induced anaesthesia in a mean of 90.8 seconds and required a mean dose of 2.8 mg per kg body-weight. Corresponding values for an administration rate of 500 mg per minute were 40.8 seconds and 5 mg per kg respectively.

1. Berthoud MC, *et al.* Comparison of infusion rates of three i.v. anaesthetic agents for induction in elderly patients. *Br J Anaesth* 1993; **70:** 423–7.

Anaesthesia. Some of the adverse effects of the neuromuscular blocker suxamethonium may be reduced when thiopentone is used as part of the anaesthetic regimen. For a suggestion that thiopentone may help to counteract the rise in intra-ocular pressure associated with the use of suxamethonium for intubation, see under Anaesthesia, p.1302. For reports that thiopentone reduces the adverse effects of suxamethonium on muscles, see under Effects on the Muscles in the Adverse Effects of Suxamethonium, p.1319.

Cerebrovascular disorders. Barbiturates are considered to be suitable anaesthetics for use in patients with or at risk of raised intracranial pressure. Barbiturate-induced coma (commonly with pentobarbitone or thiopentone) has been used, both therapeutically and prophylactically, to protect the brain from ischaemia resulting from all kinds of neurological insults including head injury, stroke, Reye's syndrome, and hepatic encephalopathy.[1-3] Rationale includes the ability of barbiturates to reduce intracranial pressure and to reduce metabolic demands of cerebral tissues. While Nussmeier *et al.*[4] showed that thiopentone could protect patients against the neuropsychiatric complications of cardiopulmonary bypass, the Brain Resuscitation Clinical Trial I Study Group[5] found no cerebral benefit from thiopentone in comatose survivors of cardiac arrest. Nor did Eyre and Wilkinson[6] observe any benefit from thiopentone-induced coma in infants with severe birth asphyxia. It is considered that there is no convincing evidence of improvement in neurological outcome to justify the risks of the procedure in conditions causing global ischaemia, although administration of barbiturates without necessarily inducing coma may have a limited role in reduction of raised intracranial pressure refractory to other therapy. Use of barbiturates in the setting of regional cerebral ischaemia, including use during cardiopulmonary bypass to prevent focal neurological complications, remains controversial.[1] For a discussion of the treatment of raised intracranial pressure, including a mention of the use of barbiturates, see p.796.

1. Rogers MC, Kirsch JR. Current concepts in brain resuscitation. *JAMA* 1989; **261:** 3143–7.
2. Lyons MK, Meyer FB. Cerebrospinal fluid physiology and the management of increased intracranial pressure. *Mayo Clin Proc* 1990; **65:** 684–707.
3. Woster PS, LeBlanc KL. Management of elevated intracranial pressure. *Clin Pharm* 1990; **9:** 762–72.
4. Nussmeier NA, *et al.* Neuropsychiatric complications after cardiopulmonary bypass: cerebral protection by a barbiturate. *Anesthesiology* 1986; **64:** 165–70.
5. Abramson NS, *et al.* Randomized clinical study of thiopental loading in comatose survivors of cardiac arrest. *N Engl J Med* 1986; **314:** 397–403.
6. Eyre JA, Wilkinson AR. Thiopentone induced coma after severe birth asphyxia. *Arch Dis Child* 1986; **61:** 1084–9.

Status epilepticus. Anaesthesia in conjunction with assisted ventilation may be instituted to control refractory tonic-clonic status epilepticus (p.337). A short-acting barbiturate such as thiopentone is usually used. A loading dose of 5 mg per kg body-weight given intravenously has been suggested.[1] This may be followed after 30 minutes by an infusion given at a rate of 1 to 3 mg per kg per hour adjusted to maintain a maximum blood concentration of 60 to 100 μg per mL.[1] It has been recommended that administration should be continued for at least 12 hours after seizure activity has ceased and then slowly discontinued.[2]

1. O'Brien MD. Management of major status epilepticus in adults. *Br Med J* 1990; **301:** 918.
2. Bauer J, Elger CE. Management of status epilepticus in adults. *CNS Drugs* 1994; **1:** 26–44.

Preparations

BP 1998: Thiopental Injection;
USP 23: Thiopental Sodium for Injection.

Proprietary Preparations (details are given in Part 3)
Austral.: Pentothal; ***Belg.:*** Nesdonal; Pentothal; ***Canad.:*** Pentothal; ***Fr.:*** Nesdonal†; ***Ger.:*** Trapanal; ***Irl.:*** Intraval Sodium; ***Ital.:*** Farmotal; Pentothal; ***Neth.:*** Nesdonal; ***Norw.:*** Pentothal; ***S.Afr.:*** Intraval Sodium; Sandothal†; ***Spain:*** Pentothal; Tiobarbital Miro; ***Swed.:*** Pentothal; ***Switz.:*** Pentothal; ***UK:*** Intraval Sodium; ***USA:*** Pentothal.

Tiletamine Hydrochloride (13344-s)

Tiletamine Hydrochloride *(BANM, USAN, rINNM).*

CI-634; CL-399; CN-54521-2. 2-Ethylamino-2-(2-thienyl)cyclohexanone hydrochloride.

$C_{12}H_{17}NOS,HCl = 259.8.$

CAS — 14176-49-9 (tiletamine); 14176-50-2 (tiletamine hydrochloride).

Pharmacopoeias. In *US* for veterinary use only.

A white to off-white crystalline powder. Freely **soluble** in water; slightly soluble in chloroform; practically insoluble in ether; soluble in methyl alcohol; freely soluble in 0.1N hydrochloric acid. A 10% solution in water has a pH of 3.0 to 5.0. **Store** in airtight containers.

Tiletamine has similar properties to ketamine (p.1226). It is used as the hydrochloride with zolazepam (p.698) for general anaesthesia in veterinary medicine.

Trichloroethylene (3126-g)

Trichloroethylene *(rINN).*

Trichlorethylene; Trichlorethylenum; Trichloroethene; Trichloroethylenum.

$CHCl:CCl_2 = 131.4.$

CAS — 79-01-6.

Trichloroethylene is non-flammable. Trichloroethylene used for anaesthetic purposes contains thymol 0.01% w/v as a stabiliser and is coloured blue for identification.

Adverse Effects and Precautions

Trichloroethylene increases the rate and decreases the depth of respiration and may be followed by apnoea. The sensitivity of the heart to beta-adrenergic activity may increase, possibly with ventricular arrhythmias.

Acute exposure to trichloroethylene may be followed by dizziness, lightheadedness, lethargy, nausea, and vomiting; hepatic and renal dysfunction may follow. Fatalities have occurred, although temporary unconsciousness is a more common manifestation.

Chronic poisoning may result in visual disturbances, intolerance to alcohol as manifested by transient redness of the face and neck ('degreasers or trichloroethylene flush'), impairment of performance, hearing defects, neuralgia and mild liver dysfunction. Prolonged contact with trichloroethylene can cause dermatitis, eczema, burns, and conjunctivitis.

Dependence has been reported in medical personnel and factory workers who regularly inhale trichloroethylene vapour.

If trichloroethylene is used as an anaesthetic it should not be used in closed-circuit apparatus since there is a reaction with soda lime to produce a toxic end product that may cause cranial nerve paralysis and possibly death.

See also Adverse Effects and Precautions for General Anaesthetics, p.1219.

Reviews of the toxicity of trichloroethylene.

1. Health and Safety Executive. Trichloroethylene. *Toxicity Review* 6. London: HMSO, 1982.
2. Davidson IWF, Beliles RP. Consideration of the target organ toxicity of trichloroethylene in terms of metabolite toxicity and pharmacokinetics. *Drug Metab Rev* 1991; **23:** 493–599.

Abuse. Toxicity associated with inhalation of volatile substances including trichloroethylene has been reviewed.[1,2] Trichloroethylene can damage the kidney, liver, heart, and lung. However, in young healthy subjects, organ toxicity becomes apparent only with intensive and protracted abuse of volatile substances.

1. Marjot R, McLeod AA. Chronic non-neurological toxicity from volatile substance abuse. *Hum Toxicol* 1989; **8:** 301–6.
2. Anonymous. Solvent abuse: little progress after 20 years. *Br Med J* 1990; **300:** 135–6.

Carcinogenicity. The use of trichloroethylene in foods, drugs, and cosmetics was banned by the FDA following studies demonstrating that hepatocellular carcinomas could be induced in *mice* by chronic exposure to very high doses. However, similar effects have not been found in *rats* and larger species and several epidemiologic studies have failed to demonstrate an increased incidence of liver tumours, total mortality or mortality due to cancer in workers exposed to trichloroethylene. Suggestions that the carcinogenicity of trichloroethylene is due to one of its intermediate metabolites, chloral hydrate, have raised concern over the continuing use of chloral hydrate as a medicine. For further details, see p.645.

Effects on the liver. References[1,2] to hepatotoxicity following occupational exposure to trichloroethylene. See also under Carcinogenicity, above.

1. McCunney RJ. Diverse manifestations of trichloroethylene. *Br J Ind Med* 1988; **45:** 122–6.
2. Schattner A, Malnick SDH. Anicteric hepatitis and uveitis in a worker exposed to trichloroethylene. *Postgrad Med J* 1990; **66:** 730–1.

Effects on the skin. A report[1] of scleroderma in 3 patients occupationally exposed to trichloroethylene and, in 2 cases, also to trichloroethane.

1. Flindt-Hansen H, Isager H. Scleroderma after occupational exposure to trichlorethylene and trichlorethane. *Acta Derm Venereol (Stockh)* 1987; **67:** 263–4.

Interactions

The arrhythmogenic effects of trichloroethylene may be potentiated by the concurrent use of sympathomimetics such as adrenaline. Alcohol consumption after chronic exposure to trichloroethylene may result in a reddening of the skin (see under Adverse Effects and Precautions, above).

See also Interactions of General Anaesthetics, p.1219.

Pharmacokinetics

Trichloroethylene is rapidly absorbed by inhalation and ingestion. Percutaneous absorption can occur. Some of the inhaled trichloroethylene is slowly eliminated through the lungs; trichloroethylene is metabolised primarily in the liver, chloral hydrate (see p.645) being the first stable major metabolite formed; most is then metabolised to trichloroethanol and trichloroacetic acid which are excreted in the urine. The latter may be used as an indicator of industrial exposure. Trichloroethylene diffuses across the placenta.

Uses and Administration

Trichloroethylene is a volatile halogenated anaesthetic administered by inhalation. It is used in some countries for the maintenance of light anaesthesia (p.1220) in concentrations of 0.5 to 1.5% v/v but it has weak anaesthetic properties compared to other halogenated anaesthetics and poor muscle relaxant activity. It may also be used to supplement anaesthesia with nitrous oxide-oxygen or halothane. Trichloroethylene is a potent analgesic and is used in subanaesthetic concentrations of about 0.35 to 0.5% v/v to provide analgesia for obstetrics, emergency management of trauma, and other acutely painful procedures (see Inhalational Analgesics, p.6).

Trichloroethylene is used in industry as a solvent for oils and fats, for degreasing metals, and for dry cleaning. It has also been used in typewriter correction fluids but is no longer included in most brands.

Preparations

Proprietary Preparations (details are given in Part 3)

Multi-ingredient: ***Spain:*** Talgo Odontalgico.

Xenon (13865-e)

Xe = 131.29.

Xenon is a non-explosive gas. A mixture of 70% v/v xenon and 30% v/v oxygen has been tried as a general anaesthetic.

References.

1. Lachmann B, *et al.* Safety and efficacy of xenon in routine use as an inhalational anaesthetic. *Lancet* 1990; **335:** 1413–15.
2. Yagi M, *et al.* Analgesic and hypnotic effects of subanaesthetic concentrations of xenon in human volunteers: comparison with nitrous oxide. *Br J Anaesth* 1995; **74:** 670–3.
3. Goto T, *et al.* Emergence times from xenon anaesthesia are independent of the duration of anaesthesia. *Br J Anaesth* 1997; **79:** 595–9.

Hypothalamic and Pituitary Hormones

The pituitary gland or hypophysis in humans is composed of 2 main parts, namely the adenohypophysis and neurohypophysis. The adenohypophysis consists of the anterior lobe and the neurohypophysis of the posterior lobe and the neural stalk, above which lies the hypothalamus. The anterior lobe is linked to the hypothalamus by a portal vascular system but there is no vascular link between the posterior lobe and the hypothalamus.

The following hormones are secreted by the anterior lobe of the **pituitary**: adrenocorticotrophic hormone (corticotrophin); the gonadotrophic hormones, follicle-stimulating hormone and luteinising hormone; growth hormone (somatropin); lactogenic hormone (prolactin); and thyroid-stimulating hormone (thyrotrophin). In some mammals, but apparently not in humans, the pituitary also secretes melanocyte-stimulating hormone. The anterior pituitary hormones are produced independently by specialised cell types known as corticotrophs (producing corticotrophin), gonadotrophs (producing the gonadotrophic hormones), somatotrophs (producing growth hormone), lactotrophs (producers of prolactin) and thyrotrophs (secreting thyrotrophin).

Oxytocin and vasopressin are synthesised in the **hypothalamus**. They become associated with carrier proteins, neurophysins, and are then transported down nerve fibres to the posterior pituitary where they are stored until required. The release of oxytocin and vasopressin appears to be controlled mainly by nervous reflex responses.

The secretion of anterior pituitary hormones, in which the hypothalamus plays a major part, is regulated by a complex interaction between stimulatory and inhibitory neural and hormonal influences. A stylised representation of the hypothalamic-pituitary-endocrine axis is depicted in Figure 1, below. The hypothalamus produces transmitter substances which regulate pituitary secretion. These substances are secreted by hypothalamic neurones called neuroendocrine transducers, and stored in the median eminence of the hypothalamus. On receipt of an appropriate stimulus they are released into the blood of the hypophyseal portal system which carries them to the anterior pituitary. Conventionally these substances are known as factors until their structure and function is reasonably well established, when they may be referred to as hormones.

Hypothalamic releasing factors stimulate release of anterior pituitary hormones into the systemic circulation. Some pituitary hormones such as growth hormone are under a system of double regulation, since the hypothalamus also secretes a release-inhibiting factor (in this case somatostatin). For others, secretion of the releasing factor is controlled by feedback mechanisms involving target organ hormones, pituitary hormones, and perhaps the hypothalamic hormones themselves as well as by excitatory and inhibitory impulses from different parts of the brain.

The major groups of hypothalamic and pituitary hormones and their analogues described in this chapter are summarised in Table 1, p.1236.

Figure 1. A stylised representation of the hypothalamic-pituitary-endocrine axis.

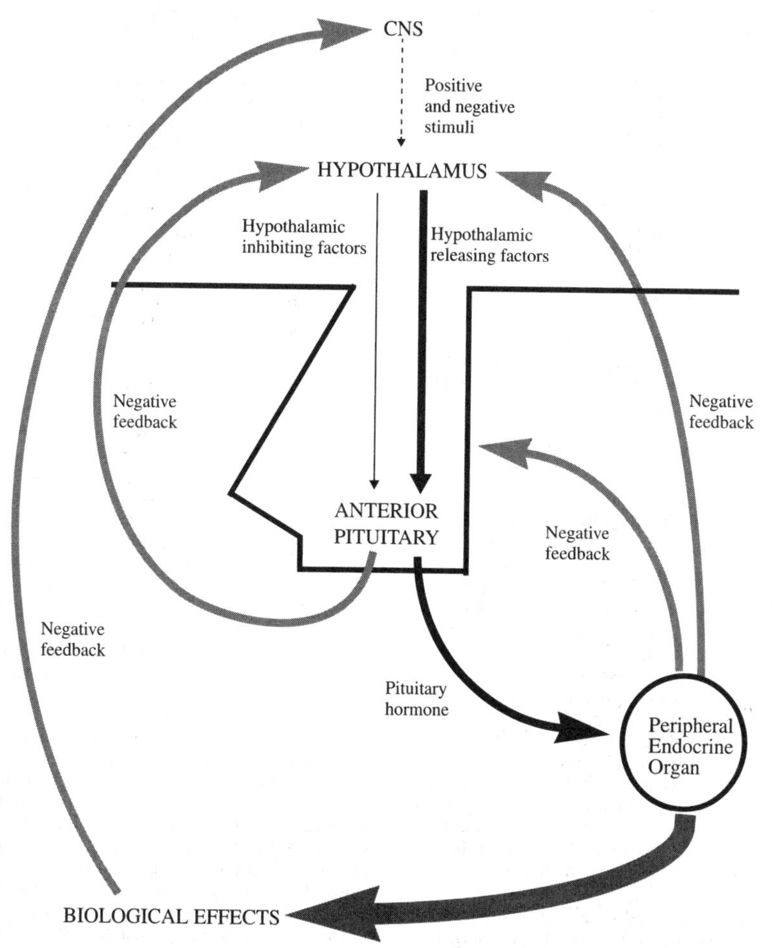

Use of Hypothalamic and Pituitary Hormones

A number of disorders associated with hypothalamic or pituitary dysfunction are discussed below. Some other endocrine disorders which may be due to dysfunction of the hypothalamic-pituitary-endocrine axes include adrenocortical insufficiency (p.1017), and hyperthyroidism (p.1489) or hypothyroidism (p.1490), as well as some of the disorders discussed in the chapter on Sex Hormones (p.1426).

Acromegaly and gigantism

Acromegaly and gigantism are syndromes of excess growth hormone secretion, usually associated with a secretory pituitary adenoma (somatropinoma).[1-4]

Excessive growth hormone secretion in childhood, while the epiphyses of the long bones are open, results in **gigantism**, with a proportional growth spurt and skeletal enlargement. Subsequently skeletal deformities develop, including kyphosis and deformity of the chest wall, as a consequence of osteoporosis. Puberty, with the increase in sex hormone secretion which leads to epiphyseal fusion, may be delayed by concomitant hypogonadism, leading to attainment of an even greater ultimate height. If growth hormone excess persists into adulthood, features of acromegaly may be superimposed on gigantism.

When excess growth hormone secretion develops first in adulthood the condition is known as **acromegaly**. Signs and symptoms tend to develop slowly and may be missed, sometimes for years. Growth hormone concentrations, and hence those of insulin-like growth factor 1 (IGF-1) are elevated, sometimes markedly. The facial features become coarser, the jaw enlarges (prognathism), and hands and feet become enlarged. Peripheral neuropathy and carpal tunnel syndrome due to nerve entrapment, arthropathy, osteoarthritis, and muscle weakness, abnormal glucose tolerance, hypertension and left ventricular hypertrophy are all common, as is nodular goitre. Daytime somnolence may occur due to sleep apnoea. Acromegalics have an increased mortality if left untreated, largely due to cardiovascular disease.

Treatment. As for most pituitary tumours, other than prolactinomas, **surgery** is the mainstay of treatment.[1-5] The success rate varies considerably, depending in part on the definition of cure, but in patients with microadenomas (tumours less than 10 mm in diameter) most achieve growth hormone concentrations below 2.5 μg per litre.[1] However, this is not necessarily accompanied by a fall in IGF-1, and there is now a view that normalisation of IGF-1 concentrations or growth hormone concentrations below about 2 μg per litre, or both, should be required for response to be considered successful.[3-5] Surgery is less successful in patients with large intrasellar or extrasellar tumours, and is associated, even in experienced hands, with about a 30% risk of subsequent hypopituitarism in such cases.[1] In elderly patients with macroadenomas, where surgery may carry considerable risks, drug therapy with octreotide (see below) may be a better option.[4]

Tumour regression induced by **radiotherapy** is a possible alternative to surgery where the latter cannot be performed, or more often is used in patients in whom surgical treatment has failed to lower growth hormone concentrations to acceptable levels.[5] Although it reduces growth hormone concentrations in about 90% of patients and prevents recurrence of tumour in 99% its effects are slow, and it often produces hypopituitarism. Since it may take several years for growth hormone concentrations to fall, **drug therapy** is given until the effects of radiation therapy are satisfactory.[1-5]

Dopaminergic drugs, and in particular bromocriptine, can produce a paradoxical reduction in growth hormone secretion. Bromocriptine has often been tried first in patients requiring drug therapy,[3] but the somatostatin analogue octreotide is more effective than bromocriptine in suppressing growth hormone secretion.[1-5] Although bromocriptine can produce symptomatic improvements in many patients, it reduces growth hormone to concentrations below 5 μg per litre only in about 14%;[1] a similar proportion experience some tumour shrinkage.[3] Another dopaminergic agent, quinagolide, has been reported to produce better results than a depot preparation of bromocriptine, or cabergoline.[6] Reduction in growth hormone concentration below 5 μg per litre, and a reduction in tumour size, have both been reported in up to about half of acromegalic patients given octreotide; 30% of patients may experience a reduction of growth hormone to below 2.5 μg per litre.[1] Reduction in growth hormone concentrations using octreotide has been shown to produce reduction of left ventricular hypertrophy.[7] Octreotide is generally given by injection, which, together with its short half-life limits its usefulness. There is some suggestion that continuous subcutaneous infusion may be more effective in acromegaly than intermittent injection,[8] but good controlled studies are lacking. A sustained-release intramuscular injection is reportedly as effective as the shorter-acting preparation in historical comparisons,[9] and is undoubtedly more convenient. Another analogue of somatostatin, lanreotide, is also available in sustained-release formulation, and appears to be effective in acromegaly,[10,11] with results roughly comparable to those seen with octreotide, although the two do not appear to have been compared directly in a randomised study.

1. Wass JAH. Acromegaly: treatment after 100 years. *Br Med J* 1993; **307:** 1505–6.
2. Levy A, Lightman SL. Diagnosis and management of pituitary tumours. *Br Med J* 1994; **308:** 1087–91.
3. Jaffe CA, Barkan AL. Acromegaly: recognition and treatment. *Drugs* 1994; **47:** 425–45.
4. Acromegaly Therapy Consensus Development Panel. Consensus statement: benefits versus risks of medical therapy for acromegaly. *Am J Med* 1994; **97:** 468–73.
5. Newman CB. Acromegaly. *Curr Ther Endocrinol Metab* 1997; **6:** 47–51.
6. Colao A, *et al.* Effect of different dopaminergic agents in the treatment of acromegaly. *J Clin Endocrinol Metab* 1997; **82:** 518–23.
7. Lim MJ, *et al.* Rapid reduction of left ventricular hypertrophy in acromegaly after suppression of growth hormone hypersecretion. *Ann Intern Med* 1992; **117:** 719–26.
8. Harris AG, *et al.* Continuous versus intermittent subcutaneous infusion of octreotide in the treatment of acromegaly. *J Clin Pharmacol* 1995; **35:** 59–71.
9. Gillis JC, *et al.* Octreotide long-acting release (LAR): a review of its pharmacological properties and therapeutic use in the management of acromegaly. *Drugs* 1997; **53:** 681–99.
10. Boucekkine C, *et al.* Traitement de l'acromégalie par un nouvel analogue de la somatostatine, le lanréotide à action prolongée. *Ann Endocrinol (Paris)* 1994; **55:** 261–9.
11. Caron P, *et al.* Three year follow-up of acromegalic patients treated with intramuscular slow-release lanreotide. *J Clin Endocrinol Metab* 1997; **82:** 18–22.

Table 1. Hypothalamic and pituitary hormones.

Antidiuretic hormones Argipressin Lypressin Desmopressin Felypressin Ornipressin Terlipressin Powdered Pituitary, Posterior Lobe Vasopressin	*Oxytocic hormones* Carbetocin Demoxytocin Oxytocin Powdered Pituitary, Posterior Lobe *Oxytocin antagonists* Atosiban
Corticotrophic hormones Corticotrophin Tetracosactrin *Corticotrophic releasing hormone* Corticorelin	*Somatotrophic hormones* Mecasermin Somatrem Somatropin *Somatotrophic releasing hormones* Sermorelin Somatorelin *Somatotrophic release inhibitors* Lanreotide Octreotide Somatostatin Vapreotide
Gonadotrophic hormones Chorionic Gonadotrophin Follicle-stimulating Hormone Follitropin Alfa Follitropin Beta Luteinising Hormone Menotrophin Urofollitrophin *Gonadotrophic releasing hormones* Buserelin Deslorelin Gonadorelin Goserelin Histrelin Leuprorelin Nafarelin Triptorelin	*Thyrotrophic hormones* Thyrotrophin *Thyrotrophic releasing hormones* Posatirelin Protirelin
Lactotrophic hormones Prolactin	

Amenorrhoea

Amenorrhoea is the absence of menstruation: a break in menstruation of 3 months or more is considered pathological in an adult woman who is not pregnant, lactating, or menopausal. Amenorrhoea occurring from the time of puberty is known as primary, while amenorrhoea developing later in life is referred to as secondary. Pathological amenorrhoea is usually associated with infertility (see also below). Other associated conditions may include mastalgia (p.1443) and hirsutism (p.1441).

The causes of amenorrhoea (or oligomenorrhoea—infrequent and erratic periods) are most often ovarian or hypothalamic/pituitary in origin. Ovarian causes include failure of normal gonadal development, as in Turner's syndrome, below; premature ovarian failure including that due to trauma, drugs, radiotherapy, or autoimmunity; and conditions such as the polycystic ovary syndrome, below. Hypothalamic or pituitary causes include reduced production of gonadotrophins due to inadequate nutrition, excessive exercise, or pituitary trauma (see also Hypogonadism, below); or excess prolactin production (see Hyperprolactinaemia, below). Other causes, including adrenal disorders, thyroid disorders, abnormalities of the vagina or uterus, or testicular feminisation, may be found rarely.

The management of amenorrhoea essentially involves the identification of any underlying disorder and its correction, if possible. When the cause cannot be corrected, oestrogen replacement therapy, usually in the form of an oral contraceptive, is appropriate to minimise the consequences of long-term oestrogen deficiency.

Cryptorchidism

The testes are formed within the abdomen and subsequently descend the inguinal canal to the scrotum. Failure of the testes to descend (cryptorchidism) occurs in about 3 to 6% of newborn males but in many the testes descend during the first year of life decreasing the prevalence to about 1%. In children with cryptorchidism, pathological testicular damage has been noted by the age of 2 years, which may result in subsequent infertility;[1,2] cryptorchidism also significantly increases the risk of testicular cancer. Abnormalities of the testes and anatomical abnormalities such as inguinal hernia may contribute to maldescent, and both primary testicular disease and gonadotrophin deficiency may be associated with cryptorchidism. For discussions of Hypogonadism and Infertility, see below. Cryptorchidism should be distinguished from retractile testes in which the testes develop normally and for which treatment is usually not required.[1]

If sterility is to be avoided, treatment should be carried out preferably before 18 months of age.[2] Surgery remains the treatment with the best success rate but in most clinics boys are referred for surgery only after the failure of hormonal therapy.[3] Meta-analysis suggests that gonadorelin, and probably chorionic gonadotrophin, are more effective than placebo in the treatment of cryptorchidism:[4] success rates of about 20% overall have been reported, although this may be considerably lower when care is taken to exclude retractile testes. The lower the position of the undescended testis, the more likely benefit from hormonal therapy appears to be.[4-6] Results may perhaps be improved by combined therapy with gonadorelin and chorionic gonadotrophin.[5] Chorionic gonadotrophin may also be useful as an adjuvant before surgery, in order to cause a non-palpable testis to become palpable;[7] however, changes suggestive of inflammation in the testis have been reported following such treatment.[6]

1. Palmer JM. The undescended testicle. *Endocrinol Metab Clin North Am* 1991; **20:** 231–40.
2. Cilento BG, *et al.* Cryptorchidism and testicular torsion. *Pediatr Clin North Am* 1993; **40:** 1133–49.
3. Müller J, Skakkebaek NE. Cryptorchidism. *Curr Ther Endocrinol Metab* 1997; **6:** 363–6.
4. Pyörälä S, *et al.* A review and meta-analysis of hormonal treatment of cryptorchidism. *J Clin Endocrinol Metab* 1995; **80:** 2795–9.
5. Nane I, *et al.* Primary gonadotropin releasing hormone and adjunctive human chorionic gonadotropin treatment in cryptorchidism: a clinical trial. *Urology* 1997; **49:** 108–11.
6. Kaleva M, *et al.* Treatment with human chorionic gonadotrophin for cryptorchidism: clinical and histological effects. *Int J Androl* 1996; **19:** 293–8.
7. Polascik TJ, *et al.* Reappraisal of the role of human chorionic gonadotropin in the diagnosis and treatment of the nonpalpable testis: a 10 year-old experience. *J Urol (Baltimore)* 1996; **156:** 804–6.

Cushing's syndrome

Cushing's syndrome is the result of a chronic excess of glucocorticoids. It is commonly divided into those forms independent of ACTH (corticotrophin) secretion (either due to an adrenal tumour secreting cortisol, or to administration of exogenous corticosteroids) and those which are ACTH-dependent (caused by excessive ACTH secretion from a pituitary adenoma—Cushing's disease proper, pituitary hyperplasia, or an ectopic ACTH-secreting tumour elsewhere —usually bronchus or lung cancer). About two-thirds of all cases are due to Cushing's disease, which is 8 times more common in women than men.

Symptoms may develop insidiously over several years and include obesity, particularly of the trunk, rounding of the face, atrophy of the skin leading to striae, poor wound healing, muscle weakness, osteoporosis, hypertension, diabetes mellitus, depression and other psychological disturbances. Hypokalaemia is rare in Cushing's disease but common in other forms of the syndrome. Women may experience hirsutism due to adrenal androgen secretion, and both sexes may develop hypogonadism and loss of libido.

Diagnosis of Cushing's syndrome may be problematic since no test is wholly reliable.[1-3] Where there is suspicion, measurement of urinary cortisol and an overnight low dose dexamethasone suppression test may be carried out, and if either of these is abnormal, further measurement of urinary and blood cortisol, plasma electrolytes and ACTH, and high dose dexamethasone suppression testing may be required. For further discussion of the dexamethasone suppression test, see p.1038. Radiological examination can be important in detecting tumours.[3] Administration of corticorelin may be useful in differentiating between a pituitary, adrenal, or ectopic origin of the disease,[4,5] although sampling of central (petrosal) venous blood may be required[3] (see also p.1244). A diagnostic role has also been suggested for octreotide.[6]

Appropriate **treatment** depends on accurate identification of the cause of the syndrome.[7] The usual treatment in Cushing's disease is transsphenoidal resection of the tumour, which when carried out by an experienced surgeon produces a successful response in the great majority of patients.[3,7] If pituitary surgery fails, bilateral adrenalectomy may be considered (although this has some risks including that of Nelson's syndrome due to hyperactivity of residual pituitary tumour). Patients who undergo such surgery require corticosteroid replacement therapy for life.[7] Pituitary radiotherapy is slower than surgery to take effect, produces a lower remission rate, and is more likely to produce hypopituitarism.[7] It is thus rarely used as first-line therapy in

Cushing's disease. However, excellent results have been reported from the use of pituitary radiotherapy, together with ketoconazole until symptoms regressed, in patients who failed to respond to pituitary surgery,[8] and this may be an alternative to adrenalectomy. Surgery is also the treatment of choice for a resectable adrenal tumour or ectopic ACTH-secreting tumour; even where there is metastasis it may be useful in moderating symptoms.

A number of drugs have been used in patients with Cushing's disease, but their role appears to be mainly adjuvant.[3] Agents aimed at reducing ACTH secretion do not seem to be of much value, and reports of benefit with bromocriptine[9] or cyproheptadine[10] have not been confirmed[7]. There is some evidence that sodium valproate may further reduce cortisol secretion when combined with metyrapone.[11] Agents which inhibit adrenal secretion are more effective.[7] Metyrapone inhibits cortisol synthesis and has been used before surgery,[7] to reduce symptoms and improve wound healing. Metyrapone may also have a role in patients treated with pituitary irradiation, the effects of which are slow to manifest.[3] Aminoglutethimide has been used similarly to metyrapone, but its use appears to be in decline. Mitotane can be effective in controlling symptoms but is poorly tolerated.[7] Other inhibitors of steroid synthesis such as trilostane and ketoconazole have also been tried.[3,7] Ketoconazole has been reported to normalise cortisol secretion and relieve symptoms in a number of patients.[12]

In patients with the ectopic ACTH syndrome in whom surgery is unsuitable or ineffective, chemotherapy aimed at the primary tumour is the treatment of choice but is likely to be only palliative. Metyrapone has been widely used, and ketoconazole has also proved effective in relieving symptoms.[13] Other agents which have been tried include mifepristone,[14-16] octreotide,[6,17] and trilostane.

Surgery is the preferred treatment for an adrenal tumour but although this is usually curative for adrenal adenoma, it is less successful for adrenal carcinoma and in these patients mitotane is widely employed after surgery and can prolong remission.[3,7] Metyrapone,[7] aminoglutethimide,[7] and ketoconazole[18] can also be given to control steroid hypersecretion.

In patients who are successfully treated for Cushing's syndrome adrenocortical replacement therapy (see p.1017) is usually required until the hypothalamic-pituitary-adrenal axis recovers normal function, a process which may take many months.

1. Orth DN. Differential diagnosis of Cushing's syndrome. *N Engl J Med* 1991; **325:** 957–9.
2. Sheaves R. Adrenal profiles. *Br J Hosp Med* 1994; **51:** 357–60.
3. Orth DN. Cushing's syndrome, *N Engl J Med* 1995; **332:** 791–803.
4. Kaye TB, Crapo L. The Cushing syndrome: an update on diagnostic tests. *Ann Intern Med* 1990; **112:** 434–44.
5. Anonymous. CRH test in the 1990s. *Lancet* 1990; **336:** 1416.
6. Woodhouse NJY, *et al.* Acute and long-term effects of octreotide in patients with ACTH-dependent Cushing's syndrome. *Am J Med* 1993; **95:** 305–8.
7. Atkinson AB. The treatment of Cushing's syndrome. *Clin Endocrinol (Oxf)* 1991; **34:** 507–13.
8. Estrada J, *et al.* The long-term outcome of pituitary irradiation after unsuccessful transsphenoidal surgery in Cushing's disease. *N Engl J Med* 1997; **336:** 172–7.
9. Atkinson AB, *et al.* Six year remission of ACTH-dependent Cushing's syndrome using bromocriptine. *Postgrad Med J* 1985; **61:** 239–42.
10. Marek J, *et al.* Cyproheptadine in Cushing's syndrome. *Lancet* 1977; **ii:** 653–4.
11. Nussey SS, *et al.* The combined use of sodium valproate and metyrapone in the treatment of Cushing's syndrome. *Clin Endocrinol (Oxf)* 1988; **28:** 373–80.
12. Angeli A, Frairia R. Ketoconazole therapy in Cushing's disease. *Lancet* 1985; **i:** 821.
13. Shepherd FA, *et al.* Ketoconazole: use in the treatment of ectopic adrenocorticotrophic hormone production and Cushing's syndrome in small-cell lung cancer. *Arch Intern Med* 1985; **145:** 863–4.
14. Nieman LK, *et al.* Successful treatment of Cushing's syndrome with the glucocorticoid antagonist RU 486. *J Clin Endocrinol Metab* 1985; **61:** 536–40.
15. van der Lely A-J, *et al.* Rapid reversal of acute psychosis in the Cushing syndrome with the cortisol-receptor antagonist mifepristone (RU 486). *Ann Intern Med* 1991; **114:** 143–4.
16. Sartor O, Cutler GB. Mifepristone: treatment of Cushing's syndrome. *Clin Obstet Gynecol* 1996; **39:** 506–10.
17. de Herder WW, Lamberts SWJ. Is there a role for somatostatin and its analogs in Cushing's syndrome. *Metabolism* 1996; **45:** 83–5.
18. Contreras P, *et al.* Regression of metastatic adrenal carcinoma during palliative ketoconazole treatment. *Lancet* 1985; **ii:** 151–2.

Delayed puberty

Puberty in boys usually begins between the ages of 9 and 14 years; in girls pubertal development starts about 2 years earlier than in boys and 95% of normal girls in the UK experience menstruation by 15 years of age. Delay beyond these norms should lead to investigation to try and eliminate the possibility of an underlying organic disorder. In addition to the various causes of hypogonadism (see below), some of which may be difficult to diagnose, severe systemic illness such as asthma or diabetes, or hypothyroidism, may cause delay in sexual maturation. Where no apparent cause can be found a family history of delayed maturation may suggest constitutional delayed puberty, in which normal pubertal development can eventually be expected.

Where pubertal delay is secondary to some other condition appropriate management of the precipitating cause is required. In constitutional delayed puberty small doses of oestrogens in girls, or androgens (such as oxandrolone or a testosterone ester) in boys, may be given to promote growth and sexual development if psychological problems are apparent. Care is required as overly aggressive therapy with sex hormones may lead to premature closure of the epiphyses and compromise final adult height. Treatment should be interrupted periodically to see if spontaneous pubertal development has begun. The use of chorionic gonadotrophin or a gonadorelin analogue has no advantage in such patients, although they have a role in hypogonadotrophic hypogonadism, which may be difficult to distinguish from constitutional delay.

Diabetes insipidus

Diabetes insipidus deprives the kidney of its capacity to produce a concentrated urine, resulting in the passage of large volumes of dilute urine (polyuria) and excessive thirst (polydipsia). Patients generally have moderately raised serum-sodium concentrations but are prone to more severe hypernatraemia (p.1150) when fluid is restricted.

The syndrome of diabetes insipidus is caused either by a deficiency in secretion of antidiuretic hormone (ADH; vasopressin) from the posterior pituitary gland (cranial, pituitary, or neurogenic diabetes insipidus), or by a failure in activity of secreted ADH at the renal tubular level (nephrogenic diabetes insipidus). Cranial diabetes insipidus is most commonly idiopathic (although it is now increasingly suspected to have an auto-immune basis) or occurs following surgery or trauma when it may be temporary. Cranial diabetes insipidus more rarely results from primary or secondary neoplasms of the pituitary, pituitary stalk, or hypothalamus, or may be caused by infections and infiltrations of the CNS such as sarcoidosis, eosinophilic granuloma, or encephalitis or meningitis. Alternatively it may form part of the familial DIDMOAD syndrome (diabetes insipidus, diabetes mellitus, optic atrophy, and deafness). Nephrogenic diabetes insipidus may occur as a familial X-linked recessive disorder in male infants, or more commonly secondarily to hypercalcaemia, hypokalaemia, or drug therapy (notably lithium salts and demeclocycline).

The mainstay of diagnosis of diabetes insipidus is measurement of serum and urine osmolality, urine specific gravity, and serum-sodium concentration. If these are found to be normal a formal water deprivation test may be performed in conjunction with careful monitoring of urine volume, osmolality, and body-weight. The test should be discontinued if more than 3 litres of urine is passed or 3% of total body-weight is lost, although this is in any case virtually diagnostic of diabetes insipidus. A dose of ADH in the form of desmopressin is then given to test renal responsiveness—prompt urine concentration is indicative of cranial diabetes insipidus, while failure indicates the nephrogenic form.

Cranial diabetes insipidus is usually treated by replacement therapy with ADH in the form of intranasal desmopressin though tablets are now also available and may be preferred in children; desmopressin has greater antidiuretic efficacy and considerably less vasoconstrictor activity than lypressin or vasopressin itself.

Nephrogenic diabetes insipidus is by definition unresponsive to ADH therapy and water replacement tends to be the mainstay of treatment. Thiazide diuretics, notably hydrochlorothiazide, are given to patients with nephrogenic diabetes insipidus in conjunction with some restriction of sodium intake; the resultant mild sodium depletion enhances proximal renal tubular sodium and water resorption. The co-administration of amiloride has been reported to have an additive effect while also preventing hypokalaemia.

A variety of other drugs have also been tried in the management of diabetes insipidus. Chlorpropamide stimulates ADH secretion and augments the activity of residual ADH in patients with partial cranial disease and as in nephrogenic disease the thiazides may be useful. Clofibrate and carbamazepine have also been found to promote ADH secretion in these patients. Indomethacin and other prostaglandin synthetase inhibitors decrease urine volume in all types of the condition, and the biguanides such as metformin also have this effect in patients with hypokalaemic diabetes insipidus. Combination of indomethacin with a thiazide and desmopressin has been investigated.

Some references to diabetes insipidus and its management are given below.

1. Seckl JR, Dunger DB. Diabetes insipidus: current treatment recommendations. *Drugs* 1992; **44:** 216–24.
2. Knoers N, Monnens LAH. Nephrogenic diabetes insipidus: clinical symptoms, pathogenesis, genetics and treatment. *Pediatr Nephrol* 1992; **6:** 476–82.
3. Singer I, *et al.* The management of diabetes insipidus in adults. *Arch Intern Med* 1997; **157:** 1293–1301.
4. Baylis PH, Cheetham T. Diabetes insipidus. *Arch Dis Child* 1998; **79:** 84–9.

Endometriosis

Gonadorelin analogues are employed in the management of endometriosis (see p.1442) but the need for long-term therapy to prevent recurrence limits their value because of the risk of osteoporosis, and they tend to be reserved for patients unable to tolerate therapy with danazol or progestogens.

Growth retardation

Stature follows a normal (bell-shaped) distribution within the population and there may be some difficulty in deciding at what point short stature becomes abnormal; to some extent this is determined by cultural as well as physiological norms. However, certain disorders are associated with well defined deficiencies of growth which may be severe enough to warrant the description dwarfism. Some forms are associated with disorders of bone or cartilage growth (skeletal dysplasias), and many of these result additionally in disproportionate growth, as in the short-limbs and large head characteristic of achondroplasia. Other important causes of dwarfism include inadequate production of growth hormone (idiopathic growth hormone deficiency), either alone (isolated growth hormone deficiency) or combined with other pituitary hormone deficiencies as part of hypopituitarism; resistance to circulating growth hormone, as in Laron-type dwarfism, where there is a mutation of the growth hormone receptor; or defects in somatomedin synthesis. Some other endocrine causes of short stature include hypothyroidism, Cushing's syndrome, and Turner's syndrome. Severe chronic disease in childhood such as asthma, chronic renal failure, or liver disorders can result in some growth retardation as can inadequate nutrition due to malabsorption syndromes such as coeliac disease.

Endocrine causes of growth retardation are significant because they may generally be treatable by appropriate replacement therapy. Isolated growth hormone deficiency, or growth hormone and gonadotrophin deficiencies, are the commonest congenital forms of hypopituitarism. The deficiency is rarely complete, and since most children with short stature will not have growth hormone deficiency care is required in its diagnosis. Although provocative growth hormone tests, which use non-physiological means to stimulate growth hormone secretion, have long been considered the gold standard for diagnosis of growth hormone deficiency they have a number of limitations and some consider measurement of circulating somatomedins (IGF) or their binding proteins to be more useful.[1] Different assays may give different results, and it has been advised that therapeutic decisions should not be based solely on the results of growth hormone tests.[2]

In children with confirmed growth hormone deficiency replacement therapy is appropriate, and is given with subcutaneous injections of synthetic human growth hormone (somatropin) or its methionyl analogue (somatrem). Treatment improves bone density and growth velocity.[3-6] The greatest increase in the latter occurs in the first year of treatment, and subsequently declines,[3] perhaps due to downregulation of the growth hormone receptor; intermittent[7] or pulsatile[8] administration do not appear to have any advantage in this regard. The extent of the benefit in terms of increase in final height is unclear. A cohort study of French children registered to receive growth hormone between 1973 and 1993 suggested that the eventual outcome was not as good as expected, and treated individuals remained short.[9] However, others are of the opinion that many growth-hormone deficient children achieve their genetic height potential with replacement therapy, and that most attain adult heights significantly greater than untreated children.[2] Increasing the dose or the frequency of administration may improve outcome[10] but the most important prognostic factor is age. For optimum results, treatment should be started as early as possible.[3,9-11] Somatorelin (growth hormone releasing hormone) or its analogue sermorelin have also been tried to boost growth hormone secretion in patients with growth hormone deficiency,[12-14] and improved growth rates have been reported in some children. Another peptide analogue, pralmorelin is also under investigation.[36] There is a report that the effects of releasing hormone can be enhanced by concomitant administration of a beta blocker.[15]

In patients with Laron dwarfism, conventional growth hormone therapy is ineffective because of defects in the growth hormone receptors. However, replacement therapy with mecasermin, the recombinant form of insulin-like growth factor-I, may be of substantial benefit in the treatment of this disorder.[16]

Benefit has been reported from growth hormone therapy in children with chronic renal failure,[17-19] in girls with Turner's syndrome, (see below), and in young children (6 months to 3 years of age) with Down's syndrome,[20] all of which are associated with marked growth retardation. However, the use of growth hormone in short stature other than that due to indisputable growth hormone deficiency, including these disorders, is controversial. Many commentators see such interventions as essentially cosmetic. The treatment of short stature for which no underlying disorder can be identified, in particular, poses problems as the risks and also the benefits in terms of final height are uncertain.[21-25] Guidelines for paediatric endocrinologists issued in the USA[2] suggest that therapy is justifiable in renal insufficiency and in Turner's syndrome, but that evidence of benefit is lacking for other growth disorders including non-growth hormone deficient short stature and growth retardation associated with Down's syndrome. It was considered that growth hormone should not be given to children with constitutional delay of growth.

Although sex hormones have effects on growth they may also cause premature closure of the epiphyses when given to prepubertal or pubertal children, and this has limited their use. Nonetheless, anabolic agents such as testosterone,[26] oxandrolone[27] and fluoxymesterone[28] have been used in boys with constitutional delay of growth associated with delayed puberty (see also above) and oestrogens such as ethinyloestradiol have been reported to increase growth rate in some girls for example with Turner's syndrome.[29]

A number of other agents have been investigated in growth retardation. Clonidine, which can promote GHRH release, has been given to children with growth hormone deficiency as well as to short children without proven deficiency, but results have been contradictory and largely unsatisfactory.[30-32] A possible association of growth with zinc or vitamin A has led to preliminary studies of the benefits of supplementation with these agents.[33,34] Gonadorelin analogues have also been given in combination with growth hormone to short girls without growth hormone deficiency, in an attempt to slow bone maturation and delay puberty, thereby improving adult height.[35]

1. Rosenfeld RG, *et al.* Diagnostic controversy: the diagnosis of childhood growth hormone deficiency revisited. *J Clin Endocrinol Metab* 1995; **80:** 1532–40.
2. Drug and Therapeutics Committee, Lawson Wilkins Pediatric Endocrine Society. Guidelines for the use of growth hormone in children with short stature. *J Pediatr* 1995; **127:** 857–67.
3. Milner RDG, *et al.* Experience with human growth hormone in Great Britain: the report of the MRC working party. *Clin Endocrinol (Oxf)* 1979; **11:** 15–38.
4. Clayton PE, *et al.* Growth hormone state after completion of treatment with growth hormone. *Arch Dis Child* 1987; **62:** 222–6.
5. Leiper AD, *et al.* Growth in children treated for acute lymphoblastic leukaemia. *Lancet* 1988; **i:** 943.
6. Saggese G, *et al.* Effects of long-term treatment with growth hormone on bone and mineral metabolism in children with growth hormone deficiency. *J Pediatr* 1993; **122:** 37–45.
7. Hakeem V, *et al.* Intermittent versus continuous administration of growth hormone treatment. *Arch Dis Child* 1993; **68:** 783–4.
8. Smith PJ, *et al.* Single dose and pulsatile treatment with human growth hormone in growth hormone deficiency. *Arch Dis Child* 1987 **62:** 849–51.
9. Coste J, *et al.* Long term results of growth hormone treatment in France in children of short stature: population, register based study. *Br Med J* 1997; **315:** 708–13.
10. Blethen SL, *et al.* Factors predicting the response to growth hormone (GH) therapy in prepubertal children with GH deficiency. *J Clin Endocrinol Metab* 1993; **76:** 574–9.
11. Smith PJ, *et al.* Contribution of dose and frequency of administration to the therapeutic effect of growth hormone. *Arch Dis Child* 1988; **63:** 491–4.
12. Wit JM, *et al.* Short-term effect on growth of two doses of GRF 1-44 in children with growth hormone deficiency: comparison with growth induced by methionyl-GH administration. *Horm Res* 1987; **27:** 181–9.
13. Ross RJM, *et al.* Treatment of growth hormone deficiency with growth-hormone-releasing hormone. *Lancet* 1987; **i:** 5–8.
14. Smith PJ, Brook CGD. Growth hormone releasing hormone or growth hormone treatment in growth hormone insufficiency? *Arch Dis Child* 1988; **63:** 629–34.
15. Cassorla F, *et al.* The effects of β-1-adrenergic blockade on the growth response to growth hormone (GH)-releasing hormone therapy in GH-deficient children. *J Clin Endocrinol Metab* 1995; **80:** 2997–3001.
16. Laron Z. Somatomedin-1 (insulin-like growth factor-I) in clinical use: facts and potential. *Drugs* 1993; **45:** 1–8.
17. Hokken-Koelega ACS, *et al.* Placebo-controlled, double-blind, cross-over trial of growth hormone treatment in prepubertal children with chronic renal failure. *Lancet* 1991; **338:** 585–90.
18. Fine RN, *et al.* Growth after recombinant human growth hormone treatment in children with chronic renal failure: report of a multicenter randomized double-blind placebo-controlled study. *J Pediatr* 1994; **124:** 374–82.
19. Fine RN. Growth retardation in children with chronic renal insufficiency. *Nephron* 1997; **76:** 125–9.
20. Annerén G, *et al.* Normalized growth velocity in children with Down's syndrome during growth hormone therapy. *J Intellect Disabil Res* 1993; **37:** 381–7.
21. Lantos J, *et al.* Ethical issues in growth hormone therapy. *JAMA* 1989; **261:** 1020–4.
22. Walker JM, *et al.* Treatment of short normal children with growth hormone—a cautionary tale? *Lancet* 1990; **336:** 1331–4.
23. Bierich JR, *et al.* Constitutional delay of growth and adolescence: results of short-term and long-term treatment with GH. *Acta Endocrinol (Copenh)* 1992; **127:** 392–6.
24. Hindmarsh PC, Brook CGD. Final height of short normal children treated with growth hormone. *Lancet* 1996; **348:** 13–16.
25. Kawai M, *et al.* Unfavorable effects of growth hormone therapy on the final height of boys with short stature not caused by growth hormone deficiency. *J Pediatr* 1997; **130:** 205–9.
26. Brown DC, *et al.* A double blind, placebo controlled study of the effects of low dose testosterone undecanoate on the growth of small for age, prepubertal boys. *Arch Dis Child* 1995; **73:** 131–5.
27. Stanhope R, *et al.* Double blind placebo controlled trial of low dose oxandrolone in the treatment of boys with constitutional delay of growth and puberty. *Arch Dis Child* 1988; **63:** 501–5.
28. Strickland AL. Long-term results of treatment with low-dose fluoxymesterone in constitutional delay of growth and puberty and in genetic short stature. *Pediatrics* 1993; **91:** 716–20.
29. Ross JL, *et al.* A preliminary study of the effect of estrogen dose on growth in Turner's syndrome. *N Engl J Med* 1983; **309:** 1104–6.
30. Pintor C, *et al.* Clonidine treatment for short stature. *Lancet* 1987; **i:** 1226–30.
31. Pescovitz OH, Tan E. Lack of benefit of clonidine treatment for short stature in a double-blind, placebo-controlled trial. *Lancet* 1988; **ii:** 874–7.
32. Allen DB. Effects of nightly clonidine administration on growth velocity in short children without growth hormone deficiency: a double-blind, placebo-controlled study. *J Pediatr* 1993; **122:** 32–6.
33. Nakamura T, *et al.* Mild to moderate zinc deficiency in short children: effect of zinc supplementation on linear growth velocity. *J Pediatr* 1993; **123:** 65–9.
34. Evain-Brion D, *et al.* Vitamin A deficiency and nocturnal growth hormone secretion in short children. *Lancet* 1994; **343:** 87–8.
35. Saggese G, *et al.* Combination treatment with growth hormone and gonadotropin-releasing hormone analogs in short normal girls. *J Pediatr* 1995; **126:** 468–73.
36. Mericq V, *et al.* Effects of eight months treatment with graded doses of a growth hormone (GH)-releasing peptide in GH-deficient children. *J Clin Endocrinol Metab* 1998; **83:** 2355–60.

Hyperprolactinaemia

Hyperprolactinaemia is a condition of elevated circulating prolactin concentrations. It occurs for physiological reasons in pregnancy or following mechanical stimulation of the nipple, as in suckling. However, hyperprolactinaemia may also be induced pharmacologically as an adverse effect of drugs such as oestrogens, inhibitors of dopaminergic function such as antipsychotics, or drugs such as histamine H_2 antagonists, opioid analgesics, or methyldopa which interfere with dopamine secretion. Furthermore, pathological hyperprolactinaemia may be associated with prolactin-secreting pituitary adenomas (prolactinomas), damage to the pituitary stalk or hypothalamus (including that caused by non-secreting tumours), or trauma to the chest wall; it may also be associated with disorders such as Cushing's syndrome or hypothyroidism. Prolactinomas are amongst the commonest pathological causes, and so-called idiopathic hyperprolactinaemia, in which no apparent cause is found, may in fact represent undetected microadenoma.

The consequences of hyperprolactinaemia include suppression of ovarian function in women, leading to erratic cycles or amenorrhoea, and infertility (see also above and below); in men, in whom the condition is less common, reduced gonadotrophin production leads to testosterone deficiency, diminished libido, and impotence. Both sexes may develop unwanted milk flow (galactorrhoea), although this depends on the concomitant presence of oestrogens; men may rarely develop gynaecomastia (p.1442) due to the change in oestrogen/androgen balance.

Management of hyperprolactinaemia depends on its cause. Pathological hyperprolactinaemia must be distinguished from physiological, and where it is secondary to another disease this should be managed appropriately; any drug thought likely to be causative should be withdrawn if possible. Some patients are asymptomatic, or are untroubled by their symptoms; whether such patients should be treated has been a matter of some controversy, although the risk of osteoporosis in women with prolonged suppression of ovarian function has been cited as a reason for such treatment.[1]

In many cases hyperprolactinaemia will be secondary to a prolactinoma. These are generally classified as microadenomas (less than 10 mm in size) or macroadenomas (over 10 mm in size); macroadenomas are often associated with prolactin concentrations more than 10 times the normal upper limit and their rapid expansion may result in visual defects and headache. Initially a course of treatment with a dopamine agonist such as bromocriptine, while rarely curative, is extremely effective in controlling hyperprolactinaemia and restoring gonadal function.[2-4] Surgical removal is now rarely indicated, although transsphenoidal decompression may be necessary for macroadenomas despite bromocriptine therapy, and ultimately radiotherapy may also be required.

The most extensively used dopamine agonist has been bromocriptine. Bromocriptine therapy may produce considerable shrinkage of the tumour, although macroadenomas in particular can re-expand, sometimes rapidly, if treatment is stopped, so compliance is important. In microadenomas, however, remission can occur and there is a case for periodic discontinuation after 1 to 2 years of therapy to see if normoprolactinaemia is maintained.[5] The short half-life and the adverse effects of bromocriptine may pose problems, although depot formulations can minimise these. Combination of oral prednisolone with intramuscular depot injection of bromocriptine has been reported to produce a reduced incidence of adverse effects.[6] If a woman becomes pregnant bromocriptine is usually discontinued, although this may pose problems in women with macroadenoma: if symptomatic enlargement of the tumour occurs during pregnancy re-institution of bromocriptine is probably the least harmful option.[7]

More recently a number of alternative dopaminergic drugs have become available, including cabergoline, lysuride, metergoline, quinagolide, and terguride. All of these can suppress prolactin secretion, but it is not clear that most of them offer much advantage over bromocriptine. Quinagolide appears to be of similar efficacy,[8,9] but may possibly be useful in patients intolerant of or unresponsive to other agents.[10] However, cabergoline appears to be both more effective than bromocriptine[11,12] (and probably quinagolide[13]), and better tolerated, and as a result some centres now reportedly use it as first line treatment in many hyperprolactinaemic patients,[14] although bromocriptine may still be favoured (because of greater experience) in women who wish to become pregnant.

1. Klibanski A, Greenspan SL. Increase in bone mass after treatment of hyperprolactinemic amenorrhea. *N Engl J Med* 1986; **315:** 542–6.
2. Ciccarelli E, Camanni F. Diagnosis and drug therapy of prolactinoma. *Drugs* 1996; **51:** 954–65.
3. Andrews DW. Pituitary adenomas. *Curr Opin Oncol* 1997; **9:** 55–60.
4. Molitch ME, *et al.* Therapeutic controversy: management of prolactinomas. *J Clin Endocrinol Metab* 1997; **82:** 996–1000.
5. Hancock KW, *et al.* Long term suppression of prolactin concentrations after bromocriptine induced regression of pituitary prolactinomas. *Br Med J* 1985; **290:** 117–18.

6. Jenkins PJ, *et al.* Oral prednisolone supplement abolishes the acute adverse effects following initiation of depot bromocriptine therapy. *Clin Endocrinol (Oxf)* 1996; **45:** 447–51.
7. Molitch ME. Pregnancy and the hyperprolactinemic woman. *N Engl J Med* 1985; **312:** 1364–70.
8. Verhelst JA, *et al.* Acute and long-term effects of once-daily oral bromocriptine and a new long-acting non-ergot dopamine agonist, quinagolide, in the treatment of hyperprolactinemia: a double-blind study. *Acta Endocrinol (Copenh)* 1991; **125:** 385–91.
9. van der Heijden PFM, *et al.* CV205-502, a new dopamine agonist, versus bromocriptine in the treatment of hyperprolactinaemia. *Eur J Obstet Gynecol Reprod Biol* 1991; **40:** 111–18.
10. Vilar L, Burke CW. Quinagolide efficacy and tolerability in hyperprolactinaemic patients who are resistant to or intolerant of bromocriptine. *Clin Endocrinol (Oxf)* 1994; **41:** 821–6.
11. Webster J, *et al.* A comparison of cabergoline and bromocriptine in the treatment of hyperprolactinemic amenorrhea. *N Engl J Med* 1994; **331:** 904–9.
12. Pascal-Vigneron V, *et al.* Aménorrhée hyperprolactinémique: traitement par cabergoline versus bromocriptine. *Presse Med* 1995; **24:** 753–7.
13. Giusti M, *et al.* A cross-over study with the two novel dopaminergic drugs cabergoline and quinagolide in hyperprolactinemic patients. *J Endocrinol Invest* 1994; **17:** 51–7.
14. Webster J. A comparative review of the tolerability profiles of dopamine agonists in the treatment of hyperprolactinaemia and inhibition of lactation. *Drug Safety* 1996; **14:** 228–38. Correction. *ibid*; 342.

Hypogonadism

Hypogonadism (decreased or absent gonadal function) may occur in both men and women, and may be either primary, due to some dysfunction of the gonads themselves, or secondary, due to hypopituitarism or some other cause of decreased gonadotrophic stimulation.

Causes of ovarian dysfunction are discussed under Ovarian Dysfunction, below. Primary testicular dysfunction may be due to congenital disorders such as Klinefelter's syndrome (associated with an XXY chromosome constitution); the effects of chemotherapy, radiotherapy, infections (particularly mumps), or trauma; and a few other conditions such as testicular degeneration.

Secondary hypogonadism may be due to general hypopituitarism, or to a specific deficiency of gonadotrophin production, or gonadorelin production. Kallmann's syndrome is a congenital disorder of hypogonadotrophic hypogonadism due to gonadorelin deficiency associated with anosmia or hyposmia. The causes of pituitary or hypothalamic failure include neoplasms, trauma, or infiltrative granulomatous diseases such as tuberculosis. Gonadotrophin production may also be suppressed by various drugs (notably exogenous sex steroids and continuous, rather than pulsatile, administration of gonadorelin analogues), by weight loss or inadequate nutrition, by excessive exercise, by severe systemic illness, and by hyperprolactinaemia (see above).

The fundamental treatment for primary hypogonadism is replacement therapy with sex hormones to produce appropriate sexual development and activity and counteract effects such as osteoporosis, but fertility can not usually be restored. In prepubertal children, the induction of secondary sexual characteristics must be balanced against a possible reduction in final height due to stimulation of premature closure of the bone epiphyses. Women may be given an oestrogen with a progestogen (for a discussion on the management of ovarian dysfunction, see below) and men are treated with androgens, often in the form of a long-acting testosterone ester such as the cypionate or enanthate given intramuscularly. The transdermal administration of testosterone is also effective.

The cause of secondary hypogonadism should be determined and managed appropriately if possible. In some cases this may be adequate to restore gonadal function but in other cases sex hormone replacement therapy as in primary hypogonadism will be required. Where there is no fundamental defect in gonadal function the possibility of using a gonadotrophic hormone or stimulating the release of gonadotrophins also exists. In general, however, such therapy is often reserved for patients desiring restoration of fertility, since it is inconvenient and expensive. For a discussion on the management of infertility including the use of agents such as clomiphene, gonadotrophins, and the pulsatile administration of gonadorelin and its analogues in men and women with hypogonadism, see under Infertility, below.

Infertility

Although about one couple in 6 may experience sufficient difficulty in conceiving children to seek medical help, most are subfertile rather than infertile, and may eventually conceive, with or without treatment. A number of possible treatments are available, but which is used depends upon the cause of the problem. Reduced fertility may have its origins in the male or the female partner or may be due to a combination of factors from both.[1-6]

The most obvious cause is a failure of ovulation in the female or spermatogenesis in the male. This may have various causes, including damage or abnormal formation of the gonads, a failure of hypothalamic/pituitary stimulation, abnormal feedback as in the polycystic ovary syndrome, or suppression of gonadal function as in hyperprolactinaemia. These conditions and their management are briefly discussed under Hypogonadism (above), Ovarian Dysfunction (below), Polycystic Ovary Syndrome (below), and Hyperprolactinaemia (above).

The first-line treatment for anovulatory infertility in women (the primary problem in about 25 to 30% of infertile couples[1]) is clomiphene. This has been reported to produce ovulation in up to 70% of anovulatory women,[1,2] although amenorrhoeic women are claimed to respond less well than those with oligomenorrhoea.[2] Because of concerns about a possibly increased risk of ovarian cancer (see p.1439) it has been suggested that no more than 6 cycles of therapy should be given: 3 cycles of treatment at increasing doses are generally enough to tell if the patient will respond.[1,2] Combination of clomiphene with a mid-cycle injection of chorionic gonadotrophin has also been tried,[2] with variable results.[7,8] Tamoxifen is a possible alternative in those who cannot tolerate clomiphene,[9,10] and may be useful where abnormalities of cervical mucus contribute to infertility.

In anovulatory women who fail to respond to clomiphene there is a choice of second-line therapy. Direct administration of gonadotrophins with follicle-stimulating activity, such as human menopausal gonadotrophins or recombinant human follicle-stimulating hormone,[11,12] may be appropriate in hypogonadotrophic women with low oestrogen levels, and can be effective even in others.

The risks of ovarian hyperstimulation and multiple pregnancies are considerable however, and close monitoring is mandatory, using ovarian ultrasound to assess follicle development.[1,2] Once one to three follicles are sufficiently mature, chorionic gonadotrophin is given to induce ovulation, and thereafter for luteal support. Aggregate pregnancy rates of about 10 to 25% per cycle have been reported with such treatment.[1] Women with polycystic ovary syndrome (see below) respond less well than hypogonadotrophic patients,[1,2] and are at greater risk of the ovarian hyperstimulation syndrome.[2]

The other alternative is pulsatile administration of gonadorelin (gonadotrophin releasing hormone) or its analogues. It is primarily indicated in women with hypothalamic causes of anovulation, in whom pregnancy rates approaching 30% per cycle have been stated to occur,[1,2] and again is less effective in women with polycystic ovary syndrome than in hypogonadotrophic patients. However, the risks of ovarian hyperstimulation and multiple pregnancy are lower than with direct administration of gonadotrophins, and gonadorelin therapy is considered by commentators to be the preferred therapy in anovulatory women with hypergonadotrophic amenorrhoea.[1]

Where anovulation is secondary to hyperprolactinaemia treatment with bromocriptine can restore fertility (see above). The use of bromocriptine in infertility of unknown cause does not seem to be justified.[1]

Producing a response in men with impaired sperm production can be difficult.[3-6,13] In men with hypogonadotrophic hypogonadism replacement therapy with a substance with luteinising hormone activity such as chorionic gonadotrophin is given to stimulate spermatogenesis and followed if necessary by an agent such as menopausal gonadotrophins which have follicle-stimulating and luteinising activity.[5,14] Treatment must often be continued for 12 months or more to permit development and maturation of spermatozoa, but 70% of these men show some degree of spermatogenesis with this therapy.[4] Once initiated, spermatogenesis may be maintained with chorionic gonadotrophin therapy alone. Pulsatile administration of gonadorelin may restore gonadotrophin secretion and correct infertility in men with hypogonadotrophic hypogonadism in whom the pituitary-gonadal axis is intact, such as those with Kallmann's syndrome.[15,16] Again, 12 months' therapy or more may be required.[4]

In idiopathic oligospermia, however, results of drug therapy have been disappointing, including trials with gonadorelin, and with testolactone and mesterolone; testosterone rebound therapy (in which high doses are given to suppress endogenous pituitary function, and then abruptly stopped, in the hope of provoking a rebound) is not recommended.[5] The antioestrogens, clomiphene and tamoxifen have both been used in subfertile men,[5,6] but with little convincing evidence of benefit.

Where infertility is due to obstruction or inflammation of the fallopian tubes in the woman or the ductal system in the man treatment may be difficult, and the return of normal fertility unlikely: microsurgical techniques may offer hope for a return of patency, but many patients will require *in-vitro* fertilisation in order to conceive. Where infection is the cause, appropriate anti-infective agents may be useful.[3,4] (See also under Pelvic Inflammatory Disease, p.135.) Autoantibodies to spermatozoa in some men may interfere with sperm motility; immunosuppression with corticosteroids (prednisolone[17] or methylprednisolone[18]) has been associated with successful pregnancy in such cases, but the usual risks of corticosteroid therapy apply and must be balanced against the equivocal evidence of benefit.[4,6]

Endometriosis (p.1442) is another important cause of infertility in women, although the reason for the association is not fully understood. It is not clear that treatment improves fertility even where there is symptomatic improvement, although conservative surgery may do so in severe disease.

A variety of other agents has been employed, on a more or less empirical basis, in the management of infertility. Such agents include nonsteroidal anti-inflammatory drugs, guaiphenesin to improve cervical mucus quality, kallidinogenase because of its supposed role in male genital-tract function, and oxpentifylline to increase sperm count and motility. Growth hormone or one of its analogues has been used as an adjunct to ovarian stimulation with gonadotrophins.

Where other methods fail, assisted reproduction may be considered, including *in vitro* fertilisation or gamete or zygote intrafallopian transfer.[1,2,4,6] In particular, intracytoplasmic sperm injection has reportedly revolutionised the treatment of male factor infertility.[13] Gonadotrophins with or without clomiphene, together with a gonadorelin analogue to desensitise the pituitary, are used to stimulate follicular maturation and ovulation so that the ova can be collected. So called 'long protocols' in which gonadorelin agonists are started in the midluteal phase of the menstrual cycle or earlier and are maintained until chorionic gonadotrophin is given, appear to give better results than short ('flare-up') or ultrashort regimens, in which gonadorelin agonists are given for less time.[19-21] One study has suggested that better results may be given if nafarelin is used rather than leuprorelin.[22]

1. Collins JA, Hughes EG. Pharmacological interventions for the induction of ovulation. *Drugs* 1995; **50:** 480–94.
2. Hamilton M. Treatment of infertility: anovulatory infertility in women. *Prescribers' J* 1996; **36:** 46–54.
3. Skakkebaek NE, *et al.* Pathogenesis and management of male infertility. *Lancet* 1994; **343:** 1473–9.
4. Wu FC-W. Treatment of infertility: infertility in men. *Prescribers' J* 1996; **36:** 55–61.
5. Howards SS. Treatment of male infertility. *N Engl J Med* 1995; **332:** 312–17.
6. Wardle PG. Treatment of male infertility. *Prescribers' J* 1990; **30:** 124–30.
7. Nash LD. The treatment of luteal phase dysfunction with clomiphene citrate and human chorionic gonadotrophin (HCG). *Infertility* 1982; **5:** 87–104.
8. Fisch P, *et al.* Unexplained infertility: evaluation of treatment with clomiphene citrate and human chorionic gonadotropin. *Fertil Steril* 1989; **51:** 828–33.
9. Messinis IE, Nillius SJ. Comparison between tamoxifen and clomiphene for induction of ovulation. *Acta Obstet Gynecol Scand* 1982; **61:** 377–9.
10. Roumen FJME, *et al.* Treatment of infertile women with a deficient postcoital test with two antiestrogens: clomiphene and tamoxifen. *Fertil Steril* 1984; **41:** 237–43.
11. Chuong CJ, *et al.* Successful pregnancy after treatment with recombinant human follicle stimulating hormone. *Lancet* 1993; **341:** 1101.
12. Hornnes P, *et al.* Recombinant human follicle-stimulating hormone treatment leads to normal follicular growth, estradiol secretion, and pregnancy in a World Health Organization group II anovulatory woman. *Fertil Steril* 1993; **60:** 724–6.
13. Lewis-Jones DI, Gazvani MR. Male infertility: modern management and prognosis. *Br J Hosp Med* 1997; **58:** 271–6.

14. Finkel DM, *et al.* Stimulation of spermatogenesis by gonadotropins in men with hypogonadotropic hypogonadism. *N Engl J Med* 1985; **313:** 651–5.
15. Shargil AA. Treatment of idiopathic hypogonadotropic hypogonadism in men with luteinizing hormone-releasing hormone: a comparison of treatment with daily injections and with the pulsatile infusion pump. *Fertil Steril* 1987; **47:** 492–501.
16. Crowley WF, Whitcomb RW. Gonadotropin-releasing hormone deficiency in men: diagnosis and treatment with exogenous gonadotropin-releasing hormone. *Am J Obstet Gynecol* 1990; **163:** 1752–8.
17. Hendry WF, *et al.* Comparison of prednisolone and placebo in subfertile men with antibodies to spermatozoa. *Lancet* 1990; **335:** 85–8.
18. Shulman JF, Shulman S. Methylprednisolone treatment of immunologic infertility in the male. *Fertil Steril* 1982; **38:** 591–9.
19. Urbancsek J, Witthaus E. Midluteal buserelin is superior to early follicular phase buserelin in combined gonadotropin-releasing hormone analog and gonadotropin stimulation in in vitro fertilization. *Fertil Steril* 1996; **65:** 966–71.
20. Tan S-L, *et al.* Cumulative conception and live-birth rates after in vitro fertilization with and without the use of long, short, and ultrashort regimens of the gonadotropin-releasing hormone agonist buserelin. *Am J Obstet Gynecol* 1994; **171:** 513–20.
21. Filicori M, *et al.* Different gonadotropin and leuprorelin ovulation induction regimens markedly affect follicular fluid hormone levels and folliculogenesis. *Fertil Steril* 1996; **65:** 387–93.
22. Martin MC, *et al.* The choice of a gonadotropin-releasing hormone analog influences outcome of in vitro fertilization treatment. *Am J Obstet Gynecol* 1994; **170:** 1629–34.

Lactation inhibition and induction

Lactation is the physiological secretion of milk post partum. Milk production by the breast is induced by prolactin while oxytocin promotes milk ejection into the milk ducts; both prolactin and oxytocin secretion are stimulated by suckling.

Lactation inhibition. The breast engorgement with consequent discomfort and galactorrhoea triggered by prolactin secretion post partum can be problematic in women who choose not to breast feed or are unable to do so. Oestrogens were formerly employed to suppress lactation in such women, but this use is now considered inappropriate because of an increased risk of thromboembolism. Bromocriptine is a potent inhibitor of prolactin secretion: it has been given post partum in short treatment courses (about 14 days) to suppress lactation[1,2] and is more effective than an oestrogen for this purpose.[2] However, bromocriptine is a potent agent which has also been associated with severe adverse effects in some women receiving it, and its use for lactation suppression is no longer advocated in a number of countries. Other dopaminergic agents with similar actions such as cabergoline, lysuride, metergoline, and quinagolide have also been used to suppress lactation. Although one commentator has suggested that cabergoline, which is generally better tolerated than bromocriptine, may be a better choice for lactation inhibition,[3] the same general objections as for bromocriptine apply to all these drugs. Non-pharmacological methods, such as the avoidance of nipple stimulation, and if necessary the use of mild analgesics, are generally to be preferred.

Lactation induction. Drug therapy has also been used occasionally to stimulate lactation, although mechanical stimulation of the nipple remains the primary method.[4] Dopamine antagonists, of which metoclopramide has been the most widely used, can produce modest increases in breast milk production; it has been suggested that therapy should be limited to one or two weeks, and there has been some concern about the presence of these drugs in breast milk.[4,5] Protirelin has been given intranasally to stimulate lactation by increasing serum prolactin concentrations, but is expensive, and a suitable commercial preparation is unavailable.[4] The use of oxytocin nasal spray to promote milk ejection is not recommended, as mothers may become dependent upon its action.[4]

1. Duchesne C, Leke R. Bromocriptine mesylate for prevention of postpartum lactation. *Obstet Gynecol* 1981; **57:** 464–7.
2. Walker S, *et al.* Controlled trial of bromocriptine, quinoestrol, and placebo in suppression of puerperal lactation. *Lancet* 1975; **ii:** 842–5.
3. Webster J. A comparative review of the tolerability profiles of dopamine agonists in the treatment of hyperprolactinaemia and inhibition of lactation. *Drug Safety* 1996; **14:** 228–38. Correction. *ibid*; 342.
4. Anderson PO, Valdés V. Increasing breast milk supply. *Clin Pharm* 1993; **12:** 479–80.
5. Kauppila A, *et al.* Metoclopramide and breast feeding: transfer into milk and the newborn. *Eur J Clin Pharmacol* 1983; **25:** 819–23.

Ovarian dysfunction

Primary ovarian dysfunction may be due to failure of the ovaries to form normally, as in Turner's syndrome (see below), or their degeneration before puberty; there may be premature failure, effectively an early menopause, due to low initial follicle numbers or to destruction of follicles by autoantibodies, chemotherapy, radiotherapy, infection, or trauma; or there may be some other condition such as the polycystic ovary syndrome (see below). Alternatively, ovarian dysfunction can be secondary to decreased gonadotrophic stimulation which may occur with weight loss or due to a defect in the hypothalamic/pituitary axis (see also under Hypogonadism, above).

Primary dysfunction is often associated with high concentrations of circulating gonadotrophins, whereas in hypothalamic or pituitary dysfunction the gonadotrophin concentrations are of course low.

Women with primary ovarian dysfunction generally require sex hormone replacement therapy. Conception is rarely possible in such women. In women with chronic anovulation secondary to gonadotrophin deficiency due to hypothalamic or pituitary dysfunction, ovulation may be induced with clomiphene citrate, gonadotrophins, or the pulsatile administration of gonadorelin (see under Infertility, above).

Polycystic ovary syndrome. The polycystic ovary syndrome (PCOS) comprises enlargement of the ovaries with multiple follicular cysts and a thickened, whitish, capsule; there is persistent elevation of serum luteinising hormone concentrations, with a tendency to increased androgen and oestrogen concentrations. Women typically present with erratic menstruation, hirsutism, and obesity, although not all these features may be present; fertility is also often impaired. In severely affected women there may be associated hyperinsulinaemia with insulin resistance.

Management is essentially symptomatic. Patients should be encouraged to lose weight if obese; weight loss alone may be sufficient to improve menstrual regularity, hirsutism, and fertility. Clinical commentators suggest that symptoms of hyperandrogenism can be treated with an anti-androgen such as cyproterone acetate or spironolactone together with an oestrogen or a combined contraceptive pill;[1-3] flutamide has also been employed as an anti-androgen in these patients (see also the discussion of the management of hirsutism, p.1441). In women who do not desire pregnancy, a low-dose oral contraceptive is also the recommended means of treating amenorrhoea or oligomenorrhoea.[2,3] An alternative is the cyclic administration of a progestogen which lacks androgenic properties, in order to induce withdrawal bleeding (anovular women who do not receive hormonal treatment may be at increased risk of endometrial cancer).[2,3]

In patients who wish to conceive clomiphene citrate is the initial treatment of choice to induce ovulation, but although ovulation may be induced in up to 80% of cases, pregnancy rates are only about half this figure.[3] In patients who do not respond to clomiphene, a human menopausal gonadotrophin with follicle-stimulating activity may be tried followed by chorionic gonadotrophin (see also under Infertility, above). Human gonadotrophins such as urofollitrophin or the recently developed recombinant follicle-stimulating hormone, which lack luteinising hormone activity, may be preferable[4] as patients with polycystic ovary syndrome already have raised luteinising hormone concentrations. The use of pulsatile gonadorelin and its analogues in patients with polycystic ovary syndrome appears to be less effective than in hypogonadotrophic hypogonadism (see Infertility, above) and is held to be contra-indicated by some manufacturers. However, pretreatment with a gonadorelin analogue administered continuously for 8 weeks, to suppress gonadotrophin production, before the pulsatile administration of gonadorelin, has produced improved ovulation and pregnancy rates.[5] Patients must be monitored carefully during any therapy to induce ovulation, as women with polycystic ovaries are more prone to multiple follicle development and ovarian hyperstimulation:[1] a low-dose regimen of follicle stimulating hormone has been reported to reduce this risk.[4,6] An alternative to drug therapy is the use of laparoscopic ovarian diathermy, which appears to be as effective as gonadotrophin therapy in inducing ovulation in women resistant to clomiphene.[7]

Occasional reports suggest some benefit from octreotide[8] and bromocriptine[9] in normalising the hormonal environment. (The latter is most likely to be useful in women with associated hyperprolactinaemia—see above.)

It has been suggested that hyperinsulinism may play a pathogenetic role in stimulating ovarian androgen production in polycystic ovary syndrome;[10] some small studies have reported an improvement in hyperandrogenism[11,12] and in subsequent fertility[11] associated with metformin treatment although others have reported negligible benefit.[13] Treatment with metformin has also been reported to improve the ovulatory response to clomiphene, as well as increasing the rate of spontaneous ovulation.[14]

1. White MC, Turner EI. Polycystic ovary syndrome 2: diagnosis and management. *Br J Hosp Med* 1994; **51:** 349–52. Correction. *ibid.*; **52:** 122.
2. Franks S. Polycystic ovary syndrome. *N Engl J Med* 1995; **333:** 853–61. Correction. *ibid*; 1435.
3. Harrington DJ, Balen AH. Polycystic ovary syndrome: aetiology and management. *Br J Hosp Med* 1996; **56:** 17–20.
4. Shoham Z, *et al.* Polycystic ovarian syndrome: safety and effectiveness of stepwise and low-dose administration of purified follicle-stimulating hormone. *Fertil Steril* 1991; **55:** 1051–6.
5. Filicori M, *et al.* Polycystic ovary syndrome: abnormalities and management with pulsatile gonadotropin-releasing hormone and gonadotropin-releasing hormone analogs. *Am J Obstet Gynecol* 1990; **163:** 1737–42.
6. White DM, *et al.* Induction of ovulation with low-dose gonadotropins in polycystic ovary syndrome: an analysis of 109 pregnancies in 225 women. *J Clin Endocrinol Metab* 1996; **81:** 3821–4.
7. Gadir AA, *et al.* Ovarian electrocautery versus human menopausal gonadotrophins and pure follicle stimulating hormone therapy in the treatment of patients with polycystic ovarian disease. *Clin Endocrinol (Oxf)* 1990; **33:** 585–92.
8. Prelević GM, *et al.* Inhibitory effect of Sandostatin on secretion of luteinising hormone and ovarian steroids in polycystic ovary syndrome. *Lancet* 1990; **336:** 900–3.
9. Pehrson JJ, *et al.* Bromocriptine, sex steroid metabolism, and menstrual patterns in the polycystic ovary syndrome. *Ann Intern Med* 1986; **105:** 129–30.
10. Utiger RD. Insulin and the polycystic ovary syndrome. *N Engl J Med* 1996; **335:** 657–8.
11. Velazquez EM, *et al.* Metformin therapy in polycystic ovary syndrome reduces hyperinsulinemia, insulin resistance, hyperandrogenemia, and systolic blood pressure, while facilitating normal menses and pregnancy. *Metabolism* 1994; **43:** 647–54.
12. Nestler JE, Jakubowicz DJ. Decreases in ovarian cytochrome P450c17α activity and serum free testosterone after reduction of insulin secretion in polycystic ovary syndrome. *N Engl J Med* 1996; **335:** 617–23.
13. Ehrmann DA, *et al.* Effects of metformin on insulin secretion, insulin action, and ovarian steroidogenesis in women with polycystic ovary syndrome. *J Clin Endocrinol Metab* 1997; **82:** 524–30.
14. Nestler JE, *et al.* Effects of metformin on spontaneous and clomiphene-induced ovulation in the polycystic ovary syndrome. *N Engl J Med* 1998; **338:** 1876–80.

Turner's syndrome. Turner's syndrome is a congenital disorder associated with the absence of an X or Y chromosome, resulting in an individual with only a single X chromosome who is female in phenotype but in whom the ovaries do not develop. In addition to this gonadal dysgenesis, which results in infertility and primary amenorrhoea, various physical abnormalities may be present including short stature, a short webbed neck and characteristic facial appearance, shield-like chest, multiple naevi, and certain renal and cardiovascular abnormalities. Hypothyroidism and glucose intolerance may occur.

As with other forms of ovarian failure hormone replacement therapy with oestrogen and intermittent progestogen is indicated in women with Turner's syndrome, in order to produce sexual maturation and the development of secondary sexual characteristics as well as to avoid complications such as osteoporosis. Clinical opinion has generally been that therapy should begin with low doses of oestrogen in girls of prepubertal age, gradually increasing the dose to promote slow development of secondary sexual characteristics and eventual breakthrough bleeding, at which point a cyclic progestogen should be added to oestrogen maintenance.[1,2] In the UK ethinyloestradiol has been widely used in girls with Turner's syndrome, but commentators in both the UK and the US suggest that this is inappropriate,[1,2] and that replacement should be with a natural oestrogen such as oestradiol, in suitably modest doses. (Good comparative studies of these options are lacking.[3]) Application of a transdermal oestradiol patch may be a convenient way to achieve oestrogen replacement in these women, although during adolescence oestrogen requirements are greater than those in normal menopausal women, for whom most transdermal formulations have been developed.[2] Oral contraceptives have been used for maintenance in adult women with

Turner's syndrome (again often containing ethinyloestradiol)[1] but it has been suggested that these supply too high a dose of oestrogen.[2]

A minority of patients with Turner's syndrome have some residual ovarian function, and there are a few reports of pregnancy in such patients.[2] In women without ovaries it may be possible to maintain pregnancy by appropriate endocrine replacement following implantation of a fertilised donor egg.

Short stature is the most common clinical manifestation of Turner's syndrome. Therapy with growth hormone has been widely tried, but despite a number of studies which reported benefit,[4-7] particularly when combined with an anabolic steroid such as stanozolol or oxandrolone, other results have suggested that the increase in final height is not likely to be great.[8,9] There is also some concern about the possible adverse effect on height of beginning oestrogen therapy too soon.[2]

1. Masters KW. Treatment of Turner's syndrome—a concern. *Lancet* 1996; **348:** 681–2.
2. Saenger P. Turner's syndrome. *N Engl J Med* 1996; **335:** 1749–54.
3. Conway GS, *et al.* Treatment of Turner's syndrome. *Lancet* 1996; **348:** 1590–1.
4. Buchanan CR, *et al.* Growth hormone in short, slowly growing children and those with Turner's syndrome. *Arch Dis Child* 1987; **62:** 912–16.
5. Rongen-Westerlaken C, *et al.* Methionyl human growth hormone in Turner's syndrome. *Arch Dis Child* 1988; **63:** 1211–17.
6. Takano K, *et al.* Turner's syndrome: treatment of 203 patients with recombinant human growth hormone for one year: a multicentre study. *Acta Endocrinol (Copenh)* 1989; **120:** 559–68.
7. Rosenfeld RG, *et al.* Growth hormone therapy of Turner's syndrome: beneficial effect on adult height. *J Pediatr* 1998; **132:** 319–24.
8. Van den Broeck J, *et al.* Final height after long-term growth hormone treatment in Turner syndrome. *J Pediatr* 1995; **127:** 729–35.
9. Taback SP, *et al.* Does growth-hormone supplementation affect adult height in Turner's syndrome? *Lancet* 1996; **348:** 25–7.

Precocious puberty

Precocious puberty is commonly understood to mean the development of secondary sexual characteristics before the age of 8 years in girls or 9 years in boys; it is four to five times more common in girls. It is either central, due to premature activation of the hypothalamic-pituitary-gonadal axis, or peripheral, due to secretion of extrapituitary gonadotrophins or gonadal steroids independent of gonadorelin secretion from the hypothalamus or pituitary gonadotrophins. In many cases the cause is not apparent, and they are classified as idiopathic. A small proportion of cases are due to tumours. Central precocious puberty may be caused by CNS lesions secondary to diseases such as encephalitis, meningitis, or granuloma, or due to head trauma. Peripheral precocious puberty can be associated with congenital or familial syndromes such as McCune-Albright syndrome or familial testotoxicosis (familial male precocious puberty). Congenital adrenal hyperplasia (see p.1020) can also produce premature sexual development in boys and virilisation in girls.

Apart from early sexual maturation and the associated emotional distress, the chief clinical consequence of precocious puberty is short stature as an adult, due to premature closure of the epiphyses under the influence of sex steroids.[1-3]

Gonadorelin analogues have replaced agents such as medroxyprogesterone acetate (which suppressed secondary sexual characteristics but were often ineffective in preventing epiphyseal fusion) as the treatment of choice in central precocious puberty.[2,3] The continuous rather than pulsatile administration of gonadorelin can paradoxically suppress gonadotrophin secretion by desensitisation and down regulation of pituitary receptors. Although originally given daily, by subcutaneous injection or nasal insufflation, intramuscular depot preparations are more convenient,[4] and probably now more widely used.[3] Treatment with gonadorelin analogues suppresses sexual development and also skeletal maturation; most studies have reported an improvement in final height,[2,5] although children with concomitant growth hormone deficiency (for example after cranial irradiation) may need additional therapy with somatropin or its analogues for maximum benefit.[6] Discontinuation of treatment should be individualised on the basis of final height potential and the patient and family's wishes.[3]

In the peripheral forms of precocious puberty the gonadorelin analogues are ineffective.[2] Any underlying condition such as a gonadal or adrenal neoplasm should be sought and treated appropriately. Otherwise, therapy is aimed at suppressing premature sexual maturation. Medroxyprogesterone acetate retains some usefulness in these conditions,[2] while the aromatase inhibitor testolactone has been used with some success to block oestrogen biosynthesis in girls with the McCune-Albright syndrome to treat the associated precocious puberty.[7,8] Although ineffective when given alone, testolactone was reported to be of benefit when combined with the anti-androgen, spironolactone, in boys with testotoxicosis;[9] a reduction in the rate of bone maturation was reported. Response diminished with long-term treatment, but could be restored by the addition of a gonadorelin analogue, deslorelin, to therapy.[11]

Other agents with anti-androgenic properties such as cyproterone acetate[3] or ketoconazole[10] have also been tried in boys with precocious puberty, but the use of the former is no longer considered appropriate.

1. Anonymous. Precocious puberty. *Lancet* 1991; **337:** 1194–5.
2. Wheeler MD, Styne DM. Drug treatment in precocious puberty. *Drugs* 1991; **41:** 717–28.
3. Merke DP, Cutler GB. Evaluation and management of precocious puberty. *Arch Dis Child* 1996; **75:** 269–71.
4. Neely EK, *et al.* Two-year results of treatment with depot leuprolide acetate for central precocious puberty. *J Pediatr* 1992; **121:** 634–40.
5. Paul D, *et al.* Long term effect of gonadotropin-releasing hormone agonist therapy on final and near-final height in 26 children with true precocious puberty treated at a median age of less than 5 years. *J Clin Endocrinol Metab* 1995; **80:** 546–51.
6. Cara JF, *et al.* Height prognosis of children with true precocious puberty and growth hormone deficiency: effect of combination therapy with gonadotropin releasing hormone agonist and growth hormone. *J Pediatr* 1992; **120:** 709–15.
7. Feuillan PP, *et al.* Treatment of precocious puberty in the McCune-Albright syndrome with the aromatase inhibitor testolactone. *N Engl J Med* 1986; **315:** 1115–19.
8. Feuillan PP, *et al.* Long term testolactone therapy for precocious puberty in girls with the McCune-Albright syndrome. *J Clin Endocrinol Metab* 1993; **77:** 647–51.
9. Laue L, *et al.* Treatment of familial male precocious puberty with spironolactone and testolactone. *N Engl J Med* 1989; **320:** 496–502.
10. Holland FJ, *et al.* Ketoconazole in the management of precocious puberty not responsive to LHRH-analogue therapy. *N Engl J Med* 1985; **312:** 1023–8. Correction. *ibid.*; 1652.
11. Laue L, *et al.* Treatment of familial male precocious puberty with spironolactone, testolactone, and deslorelin. *J Clin Endocrinol Metab* 1993; **76:** 151–5.

Premenstrual syndrome

The gonadorelin analogues have been used to treat patients with severe symptoms attributable to the premenstrual syndrome (p.1456), together with 'add-back' therapy with oestrogen plus progestogen to prevent the symptoms of oestrogen deficiency.

Syndrome of inappropriate ADH secretion

Antidiuretic hormone (ADH; vasopressin) is secreted from the posterior pituitary gland in response to a rise in plasma osmolality resulting from total body water deficit, thus maintaining water homoeostasis. In some patients, however, secretion of ADH occurs despite hypotonicity of the extracellular fluid and normal or raised fluid volume, and such patients are said to have the syndrome of inappropriate ADH secretion (SIADH). With severe water excess, the resultant hyponatraemia may result in symptoms ranging from lassitude or headache to profound neurological symptoms such as confusion, convulsions, or coma. Some patients may experience inappropriate thirst as well as ADH secretion, thus exacerbating their condition. For a discussion of sodium homoeostasis and dilutional hyponatraemia, see p.1150.

The causes of SIADH are manifold. ADH may be secreted inappropriately either from the pituitary gland itself or ectopically from a variety of malignancies, most commonly from small-cell bronchial carcinoma. Other conditions which may precipitate SIADH include CNS disorders, infections such as encephalitis and meningitis, head trauma, acute porphyria, or pulmonary diseases such as tuberculosis and pneumonia. Alternatively, SIADH may be drug-induced; drugs associated with the condition include carbamazepine, chlorpropamide, cytotoxic agents such as cyclophosphamide and the vinca alkaloids, oxytocin, some antipsychotics, and tricyclic antidepressants.

Diagnosis of SIADH is initially prompted by the presence of hyponatraemia and corresponding plasma hypo-osmolality with or without neurological symptoms. Hypervolaemia, persistent excess sodium excretion, lack of oedema, and normality of both renal and adrenal function are confirmatory.

The treatment of SIADH differs depending on the severity and duration of the hyponatraemia, but is based on raising the plasma-sodium concentration cautiously in conjunction with reduction of hypervolaemia. Mild degrees of water excess are frequently asymptomatic and may not require specific therapy, but patients with SIADH often have a more severe disorder and initially treatment is best aimed at the underlying cause of the SIADH, such as treatment of the offending infection, malignancy or otherwise, or removal of a causative drug. If such treatment is not possible or if symptoms persist, water restriction may be considered. However, fluid restriction is an unpleasant form of treatment, particularly for patients who retain inappropriate thirst, and may not be tolerable. In these patients demeclocycline may be given to antagonise the effect of ADH on the renal tubules. Lithium has been given as an alternative, and phenytoin has been used occasionally to inhibit pituitary ADH secretion. Diuretics such as frusemide (in conjunction with oral sodium chloride) have also been tried in an attempt to optimise diuresis while retaining sodium. In severe acute water intoxication treatment is initially best undertaken to correct the profound hyponatraemia with intravenous infusion of hypertonic (up to 5%) or isotonic sodium chloride often with concurrent frusemide or other loop diuretic to avoid volume expansion. Dexamethasone has been used to treat associated cerebral oedema but its degree of efficacy is unclear.

Some references to SIADH and its management are given below.

1. Miyagawa CI. The pharmacologic management of the syndrome of inappropriate secretion of antidiuretic hormone. *Drug Intell Clin Pharm* 1986; **20:** 527–31.
2. Kinzie BJ. Management of the syndrome of inappropriate secretion of antidiuretic hormone. *Clin Pharm* 1987; **6:** 625–33.
3. Kovacs L, Robertson GL. Syndrome of inappropriate antidiuresis. *Endocrinol Metab Clin North Am* 1992; **21:** 859–75.

Atosiban (9359-h)

Atosiban *(USAN, rINN)*.

ORF-22164; RWJ-22164. 1-(3-Mercaptopropionic acid)-2-[3-(*p*-ethoxyphenyl)-D-alanine]-4-L-threonine-8-L-ornithineoxytocin.

$C_{43}H_{67}N_{11}O_{12}S_2$ = 994.2.

CAS — 90779-69-4.

Atosiban is a peptide analogue of oxytocin (p.1257) but with oxytocin antagonist properties. It has been investigated by intravenous infusion as a tocolytic in the management of premature labour, but there is some concern about adverse effects on the fetus.

References.

1. Shubert PJ. Atosiban. *Clin Obstet Gynecol* 1995; **38:** 722–4.
2. Valenzuela GJ, *et al.* Placental passage of the oxytocin antagonist atosiban. *Am J Obstet Gynecol* 1995; **172:** 1304–6.
3. Goodwin TM, *et al.* Dose ranging study of the oxytocin antagonist atosiban in the treatment of preterm labor. *Obstet Gynecol* 1996; **88:** 331–6.

Buserelin Acetate (14039-p)

Buserelin Acetate *(BANM, USAN, rINNM)*.

HOE-766; S74-6766 (buserelin); D-Ser (Bu^t)^6 Pro^9 NEt LHRH acetate. (6-*O*-*tert*-Butyl-D-serine)-des-10-glycinamidegonadorelin ethylamide acetate; 5-Oxo-L-prolyl-L-histidyl-L-tryptophyl-L-seryl-L-tyrosyl-*O*-*tert*-butyl-D-seryl-L-leucyl-L-arginyl-*N*-ethyl-L-prolinamide acetate.

$C_{60}H_{86}N_{16}O_{13},C_2H_4O_2$ = 1299.5.

CAS — 57982-77-1 (buserelin); 68630-75-1 (buserelin acetate).

Pharmacopoeias. Eur. (see p.viii) includes Buserelin.

1.05 g of buserelin acetate is approximately equivalent to 1 g of buserelin.

Buserelin (Ph. Eur.) (Buserelinum) is described as a white or slightly yellowish hygroscopic powder. Sparingly **soluble** in water and in dilute mineral acids. **Store** in airtight containers at 2° to 8°. Protect from light.

Stability. A reminder that the expiry date of buserelin nasal spray is only 5 weeks after opening the container.[1]

1. Cowan DB. Buserelin nasal spray expires five weeks after bottle opened. *Br Med J* 1993; **306:** 1478.

Adverse Effects and Precautions

As for Gonadorelin, p.1247.

Effects on the bones. In a study[1] involving 46 patients with symptomatic locally advanced or metastatic prostate cancer, various doses of buserelin or triptorelin were used and produced objective improvement in 26 of 35 given buserelin and 8 of 11 given triptorelin. However 17 of 32 patients who had bone pain at the start of treatment had an increase in bone pain which resolved after the first week; one patient who had no initial bone pain developed such pain on receiving the gonadorelin analogue. Additional symptoms to increased bone pain included lymphoedema in 4, increased serum-creatinine concentration in 1, and one patient who developed signs of compression of the spinal cord with complete sphincter dysfunction and weakness in the legs.

To prevent adverse effects arising from the initial increase in circulating testosterone, cyproterone acetate has been given for three days before and for one week after initiation of gonadorelin analogue therapy.[2] Another anti-androgen, nilutamide, has been given concomitantly with buserelin for a similar purpose.[3]

Bone loss has been reported in premenopausal women given buserelin for endometriosis;[4,5] formation of ovarian cysts was reported in women receiving buserelin as part of an *in-vitro* fertilisation and embryo transfer programme.[6]

1. Waxman J, *et al.* Importance of early tumour exacerbation in patients treated with long acting analogues of gonadotrophin releasing hormone for advanced prostatic cancer. *Br Med J* 1985; **291:** 1387–8.
2. Waxman J. Early tumour exacerbation in patients treated with long acting analogues of gonadotrophin releasing hormones. *Br Med J* 1986; **292:** 58.
3. Kuhn J-M, *et al.* Prevention of the transient adverse effects of a gonadotropin-releasing hormone analogue (buserelin) in metastatic prostatic carcinoma by administration of an antiandrogen (nilutamide). *N Engl J Med* 1989; **321:** 413–18.
4. Matta WH, *et al.* Hypogonadism induced by luteinising hormone releasing hormone agonist analogues: effects on bone density in premenopausal women. *Br Med J* 1987; **294:** 1523–4.
5. Devogelaer J-P, *et al.* LHRH analogues and bone loss. *Lancet* 1987; **i:** 1498.
6. Feldberg D, *et al.* Ovarian cyst formation: a complication of gonadotropin-releasing hormone agonist therapy. *Fertil Steril* 1989; **51:** 42–5.

Effects on the cardiovascular system. Hypertension in one patient associated with buserelin acetate.[1]

1. Barrett JFR, Dalton ME. Hypertension in association with buserelin. *Br Med J* 1987; **294:** 1101.

Pharmacokinetics

Buserelin is completely absorbed following subcutaneous injection, with peak plasma concentrations occurring about 1 hour after a dose. It accumulates in liver and kidneys as well as in the anterior pituitary. It is metabolised by tissue peptidases and is excreted in urine and bile as unchanged drug and metabolites. The half-life after injection is stated to be about 80 minutes.

Uses and Administration

Buserelin acetate is an analogue of gonadorelin (see p.1248) with similar properties. It is used for the suppression of testosterone in the treatment of malignant neoplasms of the prostate; it is also used in the treatment of endometriosis and as an adjunct to ovulation induction with gonadotrophins in the treatment of infertility. It has also been used in precocious puberty and has been tried as a contraceptive and in the treatment of fibroids (see below).

In advanced prostatic carcinoma treatment is started with the equivalent of 500 μg of buserelin being injected subcutaneously every 8 hours for 7 days. On the eighth day treatment is changed to the nasal route with 100 μg of buserelin being sprayed into each nostril 6 times daily (usually before and after meals). An acceptable response should be achieved within 4 to 6 weeks. Since there is initial increase in circulating testosterone, an anti-androgen such as cyproterone acetate may be given for at least 3 days before beginning buserelin therapy, and continued for at least 3 weeks, to avoid the risk of a disease flare.

In endometriosis the equivalent of 150 μg of buserelin is sprayed into each nostril three times daily. The usual duration of therapy is 6 months which should not be exceeded.

For pituitary desensitisation before ovulation induction with gonadotrophins the equivalent of 150 μg buserelin is given intranasally four times daily, beginning either in the early follicular phase (day 1) or midluteal phase (day 21) of the menstrual cycle. Alternatively, the equivalent of 200 to 500 μg of buserelin may be given daily as a subcutaneous injection. Therapy should be continued until pituitary down-regulation occurs, which normally takes 2 to 3 weeks; if necessary 300 μg four times daily intranasally, or 500 μg twice daily subcutaneously may be given. Gonadotrophin treatment is then added to buserelin therapy until an appropriate stage of follicular development, when both are withdrawn and chorionic gonadotrophin is given to induce ovulation.

General reviews of buserelin.

1. Brogden RN, *et al.* Buserelin: a review of its pharmacodynamic and pharmacokinetic properties, and clinical profile. *Drugs* 1990; **39:** 399–437.

Contraception. There have been reports of buserelin given intranasally providing effective contraception (p.1434) in women.[1-4] It also been tried as a postcoital contraceptive.[5] However, such methods remain investigational.

1. Bergquist C, *et al.* Peptide contraception in women: inhibition of ovulation by chronic intranasal LRH agonist therapy. *Ups J Med Sci* 1984; **89:** 99–106.
2. Lemay A, *et al.* Inhibition of ovulation during discontinuous intranasal luteinizing hormone-releasing hormone agonist dosing in combination with gestagen-induced bleeding. *Fertil Steril* 1985; **43:** 868–77.
3. Lemay A, *et al.* Endometrial histology during intermittent intranasal luteinizing hormone-releasing hormone (LH-RH) agonist sequentially combined with an oral progestogen as an antiovulatory contraceptive approach. *Fertil Steril* 1987; **48:** 775–82.
4. Fraser HM, *et al.* Luteinizing hormone releasing hormone agonist for contraception in breast feeding women. *J Clin Endocrinol Metab* 1989; **69:** 996–1002.
5. Lemay A, *et al.* Gonadotroph and corpus luteum responses to two successive intranasal doses of a luteinizing hormone-releasing hormone agonist at different days after the midcycle luteinizing hormone surge. *Fertil Steril* 1983; **39:** 661–7.

Endometriosis. Gonadorelin analogues such as buserelin have a role in the management of endometriosis (p.1442), but the need for long-term therapy limits their value because of the risk of osteoporosis; 'add-back' therapy with concomitant hormone replacement is being investigated.

Among 400 patients given up to 1.2 mg of buserelin daily intranasally for 6 months, improvement in endometriosis was noted in 79 of 101 evaluable patients.[1] Other studies have confirmed the effectiveness of intranasal buserelin in the treatment of endometriosis.[2,3] However, incomplete suppression of endometrial foci has been reported following intranasal buserelin therapy.[4] Buserelin administered subcutaneously, by injection[3] or infusion,[5] has been found to be effective. In comparing different routes of administration, intranasal and subcutaneous buserelin were found to be equally effective in one study[3] but in another,[6] a subcutaneous implant (6.6 mg injected at 6-weekly intervals on 3 occasions) was superior to intranasal buserelin (300 μg three times daily).

1. Anonymous. LHRH analogues in endometriosis. *Lancet* 1986; **ii:** 1016–18.
2. Franssen AMHW, *et al.* Endometriosis: treatment with gonadotropin-releasing hormone agonist buserelin. *Fertil Steril* 1989; **51:** 401–8.
3. Lemay A, *et al.* Efficacy of intranasal or subcutaneous luteinizing hormone-releasing hormone agonist inhibition of ovarian function in the treatment of endometriosis. *Am J Obstet Gynecol* 1988; **158:** 233–6.
4. Nisolle-Pochet M, *et al.* Histologic study of ovarian endometriosis after hormonal therapy. *Fertil Steril* 1988; **49:** 423–6.
5. Lemay A, *et al.* Prevention of follicular maturation in endometriosis by subcutaneous infusion of luteinizing hormone-releasing hormone agonist started in the luteal phase. *Fertil Steril* 1988; **49:** 410–17.
6. Donnez J, *et al.* Administration of nasal buserelin as compared with subcutaneous buserelin implant for endometriosis. *Fertil Steril* 1989; **52:** 27–30.

Fibroids. Like other gonadorelin analogues (see also p.1248) buserelin has been used to reduce the volume of uterine fibroids.[1-4] It has been given by various routes and in various regimens including subcutaneous injection of approximately 6 μg in pulses every 45 minutes,[1,2] intranasal administration of 100 μg 12 times daily[2] or 300 μg three times daily,[3] and the combination of subcutaneous administration of buserelin 200 μg every 8 hours for 14 days followed by 400 μg intranasally 3 times daily thereafter.[4] Treatment periods of up to 6 months resulted in significant shrinkage of fibroids although they tended to return to pretreatment size within 12 months of stopping buserelin.

1. Healy DL, *et al.* Shrinkage of a uterine fibroid after subcutaneous infusion of a LHRH agonist. *Br Med J* 1984; **289:** 1267–8.
2. Healy DL. The use of LHRH analogues in the treatment of uterine fibroids. *Gynecol Endocrinol* 1989; **3** (suppl 2): 33–49.
3. Matta WHM, *et al.* Long-term follow-up of patients with uterine fibroids after treatment with the LHRH agonist buserelin. *Br J Obstet Gynaecol* 1989; **96:** 200–6.
4. Maheux R, *et al.* Use of intranasal luteinizing hormone-releasing hormone agonist in uterine leiomyomas. *Fertil Steril* 1987; **47:** 229–33.

Infertility. Pregnancies have been successfully achieved following the use of buserelin combined with gonadotrophic hormone therapy for induction of ovulation.[1-4] This treatment has also been successful as an aid to improving *in-vitro* fertilisation procedures.[5-10] Buserelin with gonadotrophic hormones has been found to result in pregnancies in women previously unresponsive to clomiphene citrate,[2,8] although there may be a greater risk of multiple births.[7]

The regimens used in *in-vitro* fertilisation may be characterised as long, in which the gonadorelin analogue is given for 2 weeks or more, short, in which it is given for about 8 to 10 days of the menstrual cycle, and ultrashort, where it is given for 3 days only. A comparative study of such regimens found that the best results in all age groups were consistently associated with the long buserelin protocol.[11] The timing of buserelin administration may also be important. Starting buserelin in the midluteal phase of the cycle has been reported to produce more rapid pituitary down regulation and higher pregnancy rates from *in-vitro* fertilisation than when buserelin was begun in the early follicular phase.[10]

For a general discussion of the management of infertility, see p.1239.

1. Fleming R, *et al.* Pregnancy after ovulation induction in a patient with menopausal gonadotropin levels after chemotherapy. *Lancet* 1984; **i:** 399.
2. Armitage M, *et al.* Successful treatment of infertility due to polycystic ovary disease using a combination of luteinising hormone releasing hormone agonist and low dosage menotrophin. *Br Med J* 1987; **295:** 96.
3. Fleming R, *et al.* Combined gonadotropin-releasing hormone analog and exogenous gonadotropins for ovulation induction in infertile women: efficacy related to ovarian function assessment. *Am J Obstet Gynecol* 1988; **159:** 376–81.
4. Remorgida V, *et al.* Administration of pure follicle-stimulating hormone during gonadotropin-releasing hormone agonist therapy in patients with clomiphene-resistant polycystic ovarian disease: hormonal evaluations and clinical perspectives. *Am J Obstet Gynecol* 1989; **160:** 108–13.
5. Porter RN, *et al.* Induction of ovulation for in-vitro fertilisation using buserelin and gonadotropins. *Lancet* 1984; **ii:** 1284.
6. Shaw RW, *et al.* Twin pregnancy after pituitary desensitisation with LHRH agonist and pure FSH. *Lancet* 1985; **ii:** 506–7.
7. Rutherford AJ, *et al.* Improvement of in vitro fertilisation after treatment with buserelin, an agonist of luteinising hormone releasing hormone. *Br Med J* 1988; **296:** 1765–8.
8. Owen EJ, *et al.* The use of a short regimen of buserelin, a gonadotrophin-releasing hormone agonist, and human menopausal gonadotrophin in assisted conception cycles. *Hum Reprod* 1989; **4:** 749–53.
9. MacLachlan V, *et al.* A controlled study of luteinizing hormone-releasing hormone agonist (buserelin) for the induction of folliculogenesis before in vitro fertilization. *N Engl J Med* 1989; **320:** 1233–7.
10. Urbancsek J, Witthaus E. Midluteal buserelin is superior to early follicular phase buserelin in combined gonadotropin-releasing hormone analog and gonadotropin stimulation in in vitro fertilization. *Fertil Steril* 1996; **65:** 966–71.
11. Tan S-L, *et al.* Cumulative conception and live-birth rates after in vitro fertilization with and without the use of long, short, and ultrashort regimens of the gonadotrophin-releasing hormone agonist buserelin. *Am J Obstet Gynecol* 1994; **171:** 513–20.

Malignant neoplasms. The long-term use of buserelin in men decreases the testicular concentration of testosterone. For this reason it is used in the treatment of prostatic cancer (p.491), which is androgen-dependent.[1-6] Gonadorelin analogues are an effective alternative to orchidectomy, sometimes combined with an anti-androgen for enhanced effect, and play a major role in the management of advanced, incurable disease.

Other reports of malignant neoplasms treated with buserelin include its use in metastatic breast cancer[7,8] and meningioma.[9] For further discussion of these malignant neoplasms and their management, see p.485 and p.485, respectively.

1. Waxman JH, *et al.* Treatment with gonadotrophin releasing hormone analogue in advanced prostatic cancer. *Br Med J* 1983; **286:** 1309–12.
2. Lock MTWT, *et al.* Long-term effects of buserelin on plasma testosterone and luteinizing hormone concentrations. *Lancet* 1985; **ii:** 1236–7.
3. Waxman J, *et al.* A pharmacological evaluation of a new 3-month depot preparation of buserelin for prostatic cancer. *Cancer Chemother Pharmacol* 1989; **25:** 219–20.
4. Volmer MC, *et al.* Lung metastases of prostate carcinoma cleared by intranasal GRH analogue. *Lancet* 1985; **i:** 1507.
5. Klign JGM, *et al.* Combined treatment with buserelin and cyproterone acetate in metastatic prostatic carcinoma. *Lancet* 1985; **ii:** 493.
6. Labrie F, *et al.* Combined treatment with flutamide and surgical or medical (LHRH agonist) castration in metastatic prostatic cancer. *Lancet* 1986; **i:** 48–9.
7. Klijn JGM, de Jong FH. Treatment with a luteinising-hormone-releasing-hormone analogue (buserelin) in premenopausal patients with metastatic breast cancer. *Lancet* 1982; **i:** 1213–16.
8. Falkson G, Falkson HC. CAF and nasal buserelin in the treatment of premenopausal women with metastatic breast cancer. *Eur J Cancer Clin Oncol* 1989; **25:** 737–41.
9. van Şeters AP, *et al.* Symptomatic relief of meningioma by buserelin maintenance therapy. *Lancet* 1989; **i:** 564–5.

Porphyria. Buserelin in combination with medroxyprogesterone acetate suppressed cyclic and premenstrual exacerbations of acute porphyria (p.983) in 2 patients. Doses used were 300 μg buserelin intranasally in the evenings of days 1 to 21 of the menstrual cycle and 10 mg medroxyprogesterone acetate daily by mouth from day 12 to 21. Both patients were free from porphyric attacks during the reported 11 months of treatment.[1]

1. Bargetzi MJ, *et al.* Premenstrual exacerbations in hepatic porphyria: prevention by intermittent administration of an LH-RH agonist in combination with a gestagen. *JAMA* 1989; **261:** 864.

Precocious puberty. The gonadorelin analogues have largely replaced other treatments in the management of central precocious puberty (p.1241). For some references to the use of buserelin in precocious puberty, see below.

1. Ward PS, *et al.* Reversible inhibition of central precocious puberty with a long acting GnRH analogue. *Arch Dis Child* 1985; **60:** 872–4.
2. Stanhope R, *et al.* Reversible inhibition of central precocious puberty with a long acting GnRH analogue. *Arch Dis Child* 1986; **61:** 95–9.
3. Drop SLS, *et al.* The effect of treatment with an LH-RH agonist (buserelin) on gonadal activity growth and bone maturation in children with central precocious puberty. *Eur J Pediatr* 1987; **146:** 272–8.
4. Cacciari E, *et al.* Long-term follow-up and final height in girls with central precocious puberty treated with luteinizing hormone-releasing hormone analogue nasal spray. *Arch Pediatr Adolesc Med* 1994; **148:** 1194–9.

Premenstrual syndrome. Like other gonadorelin analogues, buserelin,[1] usually with hormone replacement therapy to prevent menopausal symptoms, may be considered in women for whom other drug treatments for premenstrual syndrome (p.1456) are ineffective.

1. Hussain SY, *et al.* Buserelin in premenstrual syndrome. *Gynecol Endocrinol* 1992; **6:** 57–64.

Preparations

Proprietary Preparations (details are given in Part 3)
Aust.: Suprecur; Suprefact; ***Belg.:*** Suprefact; ***Canad.:*** Suprefact; ***Fr.:*** Bigonist; Suprefact; ***Ger.:*** Profact; Suprecur; Suprefact†; ***Irl.:*** Suprecur; Suprefact; ***Ital.:*** Suprefact; ***Neth.:*** Suprecur; Suprefact; ***Norw.:*** Suprecur; Suprefact; ***S.Afr.:*** Suprecur†; Suprefact; ***Spain:*** Suprecur; Suprefact; ***Swed.:*** Suprecur; Suprefact; ***Switz.:*** Suprefact; ***UK:*** Suprecur; Suprefact.

Carbetocin (4825-a)

Carbetocin *(BAN, rINN).*

2,1-Desamino-4,1-desthio-$O^{4,2}$-methyl[1-homocysteine]oxytocin; 1-Butyric acid-2-[3-(*p*-methoxyphenyl)-L-alanine]oxytocin.

$C_{45}H_{69}N_{11}O_{12}S$ = 988.2.

CAS — 37025-55-1.

Carbetocin is a synthetic analogue of oxytocin (p.1257) reported to have a longer duration of action.

References.

1. Sweeney G, *et al.* Pharmacokinetics of carbetocin, a long-acting oxytocin analogue, in nonpregnant women. *Curr Ther Res* 1990; **47:** 528–40.
2. Hunter DJS, *et al.* Effect of carbetocin, a long-acting oxytocin analog on the postpartum uterus. *Clin Pharmacol Ther* 1992; **52:** 60–7.
3. Silcox J, *et al.* Transfer of carbetocin into human breast milk. *Obstet Gynecol* 1993; **82:** 456–9.
4. Dansereau J, *et al.* Double-blind comparison of carbetocin versus oxytocin in preventing uterine atony post cesarean section. *Eur J Obstet Gynecol Reprod Biol* 1996; **69;** 37.

Chorionic Gonadotrophin (5927-s)

Chorionic Gonadotrophin *(BAN, rINN).*

CG; Choriogonadotrophin; Chorionic Gonadotropin; Gonadotrophinum Chorionicum; HCG; hCG; Human Chorionic Gonadotrophin; Pregnancy-urine Hormone; PU.

CAS — 9002-61-3.

Pharmacopoeias. In *Chin., Eur.* (see p.viii), *Jpn,* and *US.*

A preparation of a glycoprotein substance secreted by the placenta and obtained from the urine of pregnant women. It is a white or almost white amorphous powder. The Ph. Eur. specifies a preparation containing not less than 2500 units per mg. The USP specifies a potency of not less than 1500 USP units per mg.

Soluble in water. **Store** at 2° to 8° in airtight containers; protect from light.

Units

650 units of human chorionic gonadotrophin are contained in one ampoule of the third International Standard (1986).

70 units of the alpha subunit of human chorionic gonadotrophin for immunoassay are contained in one ampoule of the first International Reference Preparation (1975).

70 units of the beta subunit of human chorionic gonadotrophin for immunoassay are contained in one ampoule of the first International Reference Preparation (1975).

Adverse Effects and Precautions

Side-effects that have been reported include headache, tiredness, changes in mood, depression, restlessness, oedema, (especially in males), and pain on injection. Treatment for cryptorchidism may produce precocious puberty. Gynaecomastia has been reported. Ovarian hyperstimulation may occur, with marked ovarian enlargement or cyst formation, acute abdominal pain, ascites, pleural effusion, hypovolaemia, shock, and thrombo-embolic disorders in severe cases.

Chorionic gonadotrophin should be given with care to patients in whom androgen-induced fluid retention might be a hazard as in asthma, epilepsy, migraine, or cardiovascular disorders, including hypertension, or renal disorders. Hypersensitivity reactions may occur and it is recommended that patients suspected to be susceptible should be given skin tests before treatment. It should not be given to patients with disorders that might be exacerbated by androgen release such as carcinoma of the prostate or precocious puberty.

Pharmacokinetics

Following intramuscular administration peak concentrations of chorionic gonadotrophin occur about 6 hours after a dose. It is distributed primarily to the gonads. Blood concentrations decline in a biphasic manner, with half-lives of between about 6 and 11 hours, and 23 to 38 hours respectively. About 10 to 12% of an intramuscular dose is excreted in urine within 24 hours.

Uses and Administration

Chorionic gonadotrophin is a hormone produced by the placenta and obtained from the urine of pregnant women. Its effects are predominantly those of the gonadotrophin, luteinising hormone (p.1254), which is responsible for triggering ovulation and formation of the corpus luteum in women, and stimulates the production of testosterone by the testes in men.

Chorionic gonadotrophin is given to women to induce ovulation after follicular development has been stimulated with follicle-stimulating hormone or human menopausal gonadotrophins in the treatment of anovulatory infertility due to absent or low concentrations of gonadotrophins. A single dose of 5000 to 10 000 units is given by intramuscular injection to mimic the midcycle peak of luteinising hormone which normally stimulates ovulation. Up to 3 repeat injections of up to 5000 units each may be given within the following 9 days to prevent insufficiency of the corpus luteum. Chorionic gonadotrophin is also given in conjunction with menotrophin and sometimes also clomiphene citrate as an adjunct to *in vitro* fertilisation procedures and other assisted conception techniques involving superovulation and oocyte collection.

In males it has been used in the treatment of prepubertal cryptorchidism. Regimens vary widely, but doses usually range from 500 to 4000 units three times weekly by intramuscular injection.

It is also given for male infertility associated with hypogonadotrophic hypogonadism. Again, there is considerable variation in the dosage regimen, and doses have varied from 500 to 4000 units two to three times weekly. An agent with follicle-stimulating activity such as menotrophin is often added to enable normal spermatogenesis.

In the treatment of delayed puberty associated with hypogonadism in males, an initial dose of 500 to 1500 units is given twice weekly; the dose should be titrated against plasma-testosterone concentration.

Chorionic gonadotrophin has been used in the treatment of obesity but there is no evidence to support its value.

Cryptorchidism. Although surgery remains the treatment with the best success rate in cryptorchidism it is often reserved for boys who do not respond to a trial of hormonal therapy (see p.1236). Gonadorelin or chorionic gonadotrophin appear to be of some benefit, although only a minority of cases will respond;[1] they may be given in combination.[2] Chorionic gonadotrophin is also used as an adjuvant to surgery, to render the testis palpable.[3] Some further references to use of chorionic gonadotrophin for cryptorchidism are given below.[4-6]

1. Pyörälä S, *et al.* A review and meta-analysis of hormonal treatment of cryptorchidism. *J Clin Endocrinol Metab* 1995; **80:** 2795–9.
2. Nane I, *et al.* Primary gonadotropin releasing hormone and adjunctive human chorionic gonadotropin treatment in cryptorchidism: a clinical trial. *Urology* 1997; **49:** 108–11.
3. Polascik TJ, *et al.* Reappraisal of the role of human chorionic gonadotropin in the diagnosis and treatment of the nonpalpable testis: a 10-year experience. *J Urol (Baltimore)* 1996; **156:** 804–6.
4. Garagorri JM, *et al.* Results of early treatment of cryptorchidism with human chorionic gonadotropin. *J Pediatr* 1982; **101:** 923–7.
5. Rajfer J, *et al.* Hormonal therapy of cryptorchidism: a randomized, double-blind study comparing human chorionic gonadotropin and gonadotropin-releasing hormone. *N Engl J Med* 1986; **314:** 466–70.
6. Urban MD, *et al.* HCG stimulation in children with cryptorchidism. *Clin Pediatr (Phila)* 1987; **26:** 512–14.

Delayed puberty. Use of chorionic gonadotrophin may be appropriate in boys with delayed puberty due to hypogonadotrophic hypogonadism (p.1237).

Infertility. In women with anovulatory infertility chorionic gonadotrophin can be used to provoke ovulation and provide luteal support once maturation of a suitable number of follicles has been stimulated by other means. It is used similarly in the various protocols for assisted reproduction. In men with hypogonadotrophic hypogonadism it is employed to stimulate and maintain spermatogenesis. The management of male and female infertility, including the role of chorionic gonadotrophin, is discussed on p.1239.

Malignant neoplasms. Control of Kaposi's sarcoma (p.496) has been reported in a few patients given high-dose intramuscular chorionic gonadotrophin, but regrowth occurred when dosage was reduced or withdrawn.[1] Another study, using lower doses, was discontinued due to toxicity and lack of benefit,[2] but others have confirmed benefit following intralesional injection.[3] There is some suggestion that preparations vary in their activity against the tumour, and that it is not chorionic gonadotrophin itself, but some impurity, (perhaps a ribonuclease[4]) which is the active principle.[3,5,6]

Chorionic gonadotrophin (LDI-200) is also reported to be under investigation in the treatment of acute leukaemia. For the more conventional management of these diseases see p.478.

1. Harris PJ. Treatment of Kaposi's sarcoma and other manifestations of AIDS with human chorionic gonadotropin. *Lancet* 1995; **346:** 118–19.
2. Bower M, *et al.* Human chorionic gonadotropin for AIDS-related Kaposi's sarcoma. *Lancet* 1995; **346:** 642.
3. Gill PS, *et al.* The effects of preparations of human chorionic gonadotropin on AIDS-related Kaposi's sarcoma. *N Engl J Med* 1996; **335:** 1261–9. Correction. *ibid.* 1997; **336:** 1115.
4. Griffiths SJ, *et al.* Ribonuclease inhibits Kaposi's sarcoma. *Nature* 1997; **390:** 568.
5. Gill PS, *et al.* Intralesional human chorionic gonadotropin for Kaposi's sarcoma. *N Engl J Med* 1997; **336:** 1188.
6. von Overbeck J, *et al.* Human chorionic gonadotropin for AIDS-related Kaposi's sarcoma. *Lancet* 1995; **346:** 642–3.

Obesity. A meta-analysis[1] involving 24 trials concluded that there was no evidence that chorionic gonadotrophin was effective in the treatment of obesity (p.1476).

1. Lijesen GKS, *et al.* The effect of human chorionic gonadotropin (HCG) in the treatment of obesity by means of the Simeons therapy: a criteria-based meta-analysis. *Br J Clin Pharmacol* 1995; **40:** 237–43.

Preparations

BP 1998: Chorionic Gonadotrophin Injection;
USP 23: Chorionic Gonadotropin for Injection.

Proprietary Preparations (details are given in Part 3)
Aust.: Pregnyl; Profasi; ***Austral.:*** APL; Pregnyl; Profasi; ***Belg.:*** Pregnyl; Profasi†; ***Canad.:*** APL; Pregnyl; Profasi HP; ***Ger.:*** Choragon; Predalon; Pregnesin; Primogonyl; ***Irl.:*** Gonadotraphon LH; Pregnyl; Profasi; ***Ital.:*** Gonasi HP; Neogonadil†; Pregnyl†; Profasi HP; ***Neth.:*** Pregnyl; Profasi; ***Norw.:*** Physex†; Pregnyl; Profasi; ***S.Afr.:*** APL; Pregnyl; Profasi; ***Spain:*** Physex; Pregnyl; Profasi HP; ***Swed.:*** Pregnyl; Profasi; ***Switz.:*** Pregnyl; Primogonyl†; Profasi; ***UK:*** Choragon; Gonadotraphon LH†; Pregnyl; Profasi; ***USA:*** APL; Chorex; Chorigon†; Choron; Follutein†; Glukor†; Gonic; Pregnyl; Profasi.

Corticorelin (16592-m)

Corticorelin *(rINN)*.

Corticoliberin; Corticotrophin-releasing Hormone; Corticotropin-releasing Factor; CRF; CRH.

$C_{208}H_{344}N_{60}O_{63}S_2$ (human) = 4757.5 (human).

A polypeptide isolated from the hypothalamus.

Adverse Effects

Flushing of the face and mild dyspnoea may follow injection of corticorelin; hypotension has been reported, especially following large doses.

Loss of consciousness, lasting for 10 seconds to 5 minutes, occurred in 3 patients, two of whom had Cushing's disease and one who had secondary adrenal insufficiency, following intravenous injection of corticorelin 200 µg.[1] The 2 patients with Cushing's disease had a slight accompanying fall in blood pressure. In a fourth patient, receiving corticosteroid and thyroid hormone replacement therapy, injection of corticorelin was associated with a sharp fall in systolic blood pressure and subsequent asystole. These serious side-effects were not noted by others[2,3] and were variously attributed to impurities,[2] high dosage,[2] vasovagal syncope,[3] or to the fact that the corticorelin used in the study was of ovine rather than human origin.[3] The authors of the original study[1] have since stated[4] that lowering of the dose from 200 µg administered intravenously over 10 seconds to 100 µg over 60 seconds has stopped serious adverse effects but that ovine corticorelin was still preferred because of its longer duration of action and lower incidence of hypotensive adverse effects. There has, however, been a further report of chest pain accompanied by a fall in blood pressure in a patient receiving corticorelin at a dose of 100 µg.[5]

1. Hermus A, *et al.* Serious reactions to corticotropin-releasing factor. *Lancet* 1983; **i:** 776.
2. Schulte HM, *et al.* Safety of corticotropin-releasing factor. *Lancet* 1983; **i:** 1222.
3. Oppermann D. Safety of human and ovine corticotropin-releasing hormone. *Lancet* 1986; **ii:** 1031–2.
4. Hermus ARMM, *et al.* Safety of human and ovine corticotropin-releasing hormone. *Lancet* 1986; **ii:** 1032–3.
5. Paloma VC, *et al.* Chest pain after intravenous corticotropin-releasing hormone. *Lancet* 1989; **i:** 222.

Uses and Administration

Corticorelin is a hypothalamic releasing hormone that stimulates the release of corticotrophin (p.1244) from the anterior pituitary. It is used in the differential diagnosis of Cushing's syndrome (p.1236) and other adrenal disorders. Doses of 100 µg, or of 1 µg per kg body-weight, as the triflutate derivative, have been given by intravenous injection; higher doses have been given but may be associated with an increased risk of adverse effects (see above).

It is also under investigation in other disorders including shock, respiratory distress syndrome and asthma, rheumatoid arthritis, and cerebral and pulmonary oedema.

Diagnosis and testing. The role of corticorelin as a diagnostic agent has been reviewed.[1-5] It is considered effective in the differential diagnosis of adrenal disorders including Cushing's syndrome: patients with pituitary Cushing's syndrome have an exaggerated increase in plasma-corticotrophin and plasma-cortisol concentrations in response to corticorelin, whereas those with adrenal or ectopic syndrome have no response.[6-8] Other methods used to diagnose Cushing's syndrome include measurement of plasma-corticotrophin by radio-immunoassay, a low-dose or overnight high-dose dexamethasone suppression test, radiographic techniques including computed tomography, and bilateral simultaneous inferior petrosal sinus sampling (BSIPSS).[3] The corticorelin stimulation test is of comparable diagnostic efficacy to the dexamethasone suppression test,[9,10] although false results have been obtained with both tests.[9] The corticorelin stimulation test is considered somewhat unreliable if the disease is due to low-grade ectopic secretion of corticotrophin by small tumours.[4,7,8] A combination of the dexamethasone and corticorelin tests is reportedly more accurate than either alone.[1,10,11]

1. Chrousos GP, *et al.* Clinical applications of corticotropin-releasing factor. *Ann Intern Med* 1985; **102:** 344–58.
2. Taylor AL, Fishman LM. Corticotropin-releasing hormone. *N Engl J Med* 1988; **319:** 213–22.
3. Kaye TB, Crapo L. The Cushing syndrome: an update on diagnostic tests. *Ann Intern Med* 1990; **112:** 434–44.
4. Daughaday WH. Clinical applications of corticotropin releasing hormone. *Mayo Clin Proc* 1990; **65:** 1026–8.
5. Anonymous. CRH test in the 1990s. *Lancet* 1990; **336:** 1416.
6. Chrousos GP, *et al.* The corticotropin-releasing factor stimulation test: an aid in the evaluation of patients with Cushing's syndrome. *N Engl J Med* 1984; **310:** 622–6.
7. Sebastian JP, *et al.* CRH test. *Lancet* 1991; **337:** 233.
8. McCarthy MI, *et al.* CRH test. *Lancet* 1991; **337:** 233–4.
9. Hermus AR, *et al.* The corticotropin-releasing-hormone test versus the high-dose dexamethasone test in the differential diagnosis of Cushing's syndrome. *Lancet* 1986; **ii:** 540–4.
10. Nieman LK, *et al.* The ovine corticotropin-releasing hormone stimulation test and the dexamethasone suppression test in the differential diagnosis of Cushing's syndrome. *Ann Intern Med* 1986; **105:** 862–7.
11. Yanovski JA, *et al.* Corticotropin-releasing hormone stimulation following low-dose dexamethasone administration: a new test to distinguish Cushing's syndrome from pseudo-Cushing's states. *JAMA* 1993; **269:** 2232–8.

Preparations

Proprietary Preparations (details are given in Part 3)
Ger.: CRH; ***Neth.:*** Corticobiss†; CRH; ***USA:*** Acthrel.

Corticotrophin (1461-v)

Corticotrophin *(BAN)*.

Corticotropin *(rINN)*; ACTH; Adrenocorticotrophic Hormone; Adrenocorticotrophin; Corticotropinum.

CAS — 9002-60-2 (corticotrophin); 9050-75-3 (corticotrophin zinc hydroxide); 8049-55-6 (corticotropin zinc hydroxide).

Pharmacopoeias. In *Eur.* (see p.viii). *US* includes only as a preparation in the form of an injection.

Corticotrophin is a substance obtained from the anterior lobe of the pituitary gland of mammals used by man for food (the Ph. Eur. specifies *pigs*) and contains the polypeptide corticotrophic principle that increases the rate at which corticoid hormones are secreted by the adrenal gland. It contains not less than 70 units per mg. A white or almost white hygroscopic powder or flakes. The Ph. Eur. specifies that a 1% solution has a pH of 3.0 to 5.0; Corticotrophin for Injection USP 23 has a pH of 2.5 to 6.0 when reconstituted. **Store** at a temperature not exceeding 25°. Protect from light.

Units

5 units of porcine corticotrophin for bioassay are contained in approximately 50 µg (with lactose 5 mg) in one ampoule of the third International Standard (1962).

Adverse Effects

Corticotrophin stimulates the adrenals to produce cortisol (hydrocortisone) and mineralocorticoids; it therefore has the potential to produce similar adverse glucocorticoid and mineralocorticoid effects to those of the corticosteroids (see p.1010). In particular, its mineralocorticoid properties may produce marked sodium and water retention; considerable potassium loss may also occur.

Corticotrophin can induce sensitisation, and severe hypersensitivity reactions, including anaphylaxis, may occur.

Whereas corticosteroids replace endogenous cortisol (hydrocortisone) and thereby induce adrenal atrophy, corticotrophin's stimulant effect induces hypertrophy. Withdrawal of corticotrophin may therefore be easier than withdrawal of corticosteroids; nevertheless, the ability of the hypothalamic-pituitary-adrenal axis to respond to stress is still reduced, and abrupt withdrawal of corticotrophin may result in symptoms of hypopituitarism (see Withdrawal, below).

Reports of the adverse effects observed in children given corticotrophin for infantile spasms.

1. Riikonen R, Donner M. ACTH therapy in infantile spasms: side effects. *Arch Dis Child* 1980; **55:** 664–72.
2. Hanefeld F, *et al.* Renal and pancreatic calcification during treatment of infantile spasms with ACTH. *Lancet* 1984; **i:** 901.
3. Riikonen R, *et al.* Disturbed calcium and phosphate homeostasis during treatment with ACTH of infantile spasms. *Arch Dis Child* 1986; **61:** 671–6.
4. Perheentupa J, *et al.* Adrenocortical hyporesponsiveness after treatment with ACTH of infantile spasms. *Arch Dis Child* 1986; **61:** 750–3.

Effects on blood pressure. A hypertensive crisis following intravenous administration of tetracosactrin resulted in the discovery of an adrenaline-secreting phaeochromocytoma in a patient.[1] It was suggested that caution should be observed when using corticotrophin in patients with postural hypotension in whom the diagnosis of phaeochromocytoma has not been excluded.

1. Jan T, *et al.* Epinephrine-producing pheochromocytoma with hypertensive crisis after corticotropin injection. *Am J Med* 1990; **89:** 824–5.

Withdrawal

Corticotrophin administration may depress the pituitary adrenal axis. Abrupt withdrawal of corticotrophin may therefore produce adrenocortical and pituitary unresponsiveness, and therapy should be stopped gradually. See also Withdrawal under Corticosteroids, p.1012.

Precautions

As for Corticosteroids, p.1013.

Phaeochromocytoma. See under Effects on Blood Pressure, in Adverse Effects above.

Interactions

Interactions seen with corticotrophin are liable to be similar to those with corticosteroids (p.1014).

Uses and Administration

Corticotrophin is a naturally occurring hormone of the anterior lobe of the pituitary gland which induces hyperplasia and increase in weight of the adrenal gland and the secretion of adrenocortical hormones, especially cortisol (hydrocortisone), some mineralocorticoids, such as corticosterone, and, to a lesser extent, androgens. It has little effect on aldosterone secretion which proceeds independently.

Secretion of corticotrophin by the functioning pituitary gland is controlled by the release of corticorelin from the hypothalamus and is also regulated by a negative feedback mechanism involving concentrations of circulating glucocorticoids. Conditions of stress may also stimulate secretion.

Corticotrophin may be used diagnostically to investigate adrenocortical insufficiency. It has also been used therapeutically in most of the conditions (with the exception of the adrenal deficiency states and adrenocortical overactivity) for which systemic corticosteroid therapy is indicated (p.1015). Such use is now fairly limited. However, corticotrophin is used in certain neurological disorders such as infantile spasms and multiple sclerosis. The synthetic polypeptide tetracosactrin (p.1261), which has the same amino-acid sequence as the first 24 residues of human corticotrophin, may be preferred as less antigenic.

Corticotrophin has been available for injection in two forms. One form is a plain injection that may be administered by the subcutaneous, intramuscular, or intravenous routes. The other form includes the long-acting depot preparations in which the viscosity is increased by the addition of gelatin or in which corticotrophin is combined with zinc hydroxide. The gelatin-containing depot preparation is administered subcutaneously or intramuscularly, the zinc hydroxide-containing depot preparation is administered intramuscularly; neither should be given intravenously. Individual responses to therapeutic corticotrophin vary considerably and doses must be adjusted accordingly.

For diagnostic purposes the corticotrophin test is based on the measurement of plasma-cortisol concentrations before and after injection. The plain preparation is used in doses of 10 to 25 units in 500 mL of glucose 5% infused intravenously over 8 hours.

For therapeutic purposes typical initial doses for the plain type of injection have been up to 20 units four times daily by the subcutaneous or intramuscular routes, and for the depot preparations about 20 to 80 units every 24 to 72 hours by the subcutaneous route (for the gelatin-containing preparation) or the intramuscular route (for both types of depot preparation). As soon as possible the dosage should be reduced gradually to the minimum necessary to control symptoms.

Octacosactrin is another polypeptide analogue of corticotrophin; it has the same sequence as the first 28 residues.

Epilepsy. The use of corticotrophin in the management of infantile spasms is referred to under Corticosteroids, p.1020.

References.

1. Hrachovy RA, *et al.* High-dose, long-duration versus low-dose, short-duration corticotropin therapy for infantile spasms. *J Pediatr* 1994; **124:** 803–6.
2. Baram TZ, *et al.* High-dose corticotropin (ACTH) versus prednisone for infantile spasms: a prospective, randomized, blinded study. *Pediatrics* 1996; **97:** 375–9.

Multiple sclerosis. Short-term courses of corticotrophin have been used to speed recovery from acute exacerbations of multiple sclerosis (p.620). Such treatment does not affect the degree of recovery or the overall course of the disease. Doses vary, but one schedule is 80 units daily intramuscularly or intravenously for 5 days followed by 40 units for another 5 days.[1] Successive treatments may be less beneficial.[2,3]

1. Giesser B. Multiple sclerosis: current concepts in management. *Drugs* 1985; **29:** 88–95.
2. Weiner HL, Hafler DA. Immunotherapy of multiple sclerosis. *Ann Neurol* 1988; **23:** 211–22.
3. Carter JL, Rodriguez M. Immunosuppressive treatment of multiple sclerosis. *Mayo Clin Proc* 1989; **64:** 664–9.

Post-dural puncture headache. There are anecdotal reports of the relief of headache associated with dural puncture by corticotrophin (or tetracosactrin),[1,2] although, as discussed on p.1282, in many cases patients respond simply to bed rest and hydration, with analgesics as needed.

1. Collier BB. Treatment for postdural puncture headache. *Br J Anaesth* 1994; **72:** 366–7.
2. Foster P. ACTH treatment for post-lumbar puncture headache. *Br J Anaesth* 1994; **73:** 429.

Preparations

USP 23: Corticotropin for Injection; Corticotropin Injection; Corticotropin Zinc Hydroxide Injectable Suspension; Repository Corticotropin Injection.

Proprietary Preparations (details are given in Part 3)
Austral.: Acthar†; ***Canad.:*** Actharn†; ***Ger.:*** Acethropan†; ***Irl.:*** Acthar; ***S.Afr.:*** Acthar; ***Swed.:*** Acton prolongatum†; ***UK:*** Acthar; ***USA:*** Acthar.

Demoxytocin (12630-q)

Demoxytocin *(rINN).*

Deamino-oxytocin; Desamino-oxytocin; ODA-914. 1-(3-Mercaptopropionic acid)-oxytocin.

$C_{43}H_{65}N_{11}O_{12}S_2$ = 992.2.

CAS — 113-78-0.

Demoxytocin is a synthetic analogue of oxytocin (p.1257) and has similar properties. It is given as buccal tablets, for the induction of labour (p.1411), in doses of 50 units every half-hour until a normal contraction rhythm is established, when the dose should be reduced to 25 units every half hour. Dosage should not exceed a maximum of 500 units. For the augmentation of labour, 25 units or 50 units if necessary every half-hour has been recommended. Twenty-five or 50 units may be given 5 to 10 minutes before nursing to stimulate milk ejection, although it is suggested that oxytocics should not be used for this purpose, see p.1240.

Preparations

Proprietary Preparations (details are given in Part 3)
Ital.: Sandopart; ***S.Afr.:*** Sandopart†; ***Switz.:*** Sandopart†.

Deslorelin (10811-t)

Deslorelin *(BAN, USAN, rINN).*

D-Trp LHRH-PEA. 5-Oxo-L-prolyl-L-histidyl-L-tryptophyl-L-seryl-L-tyrosyl-D-tryptophyl-L-leucyl-L-arginyl-N-ethyl-L-prolinamide.

$C_{64}H_{83}N_{17}O_{12}$ = 1282.5.

CAS — 57773-65-6.

Deslorelin is an analogue of gonadorelin (p.1247) investigated in the treatment of precocious puberty and for prostate cancer; it has also been tried in endometriosis.

References.

1. Labrie F, *et al.* Long term treatment with luteinising hormone releasing hormone agonists and maintenance of serum testosterone to castration concentrations. *Br Med J* 1985; **291:** 369–70.
2. Pescovitz OH, *et al.* NIH experience with precocious puberty: diagnostic subgroups and response to short term luteinizing hormone releasing hormone analog therapy. *J Pediatr* 1986; **108:** 47–54.
3. Comite F, *et al.* Luteinizing hormone releasing hormone analogue therapy for central precocious puberty: long-term effect on somatic growth, bone maturation, and predicted height. *JAMA* 1986; **255:** 2613–16.
4. Manasco PK, *et al.* Six-year results of luteinizing hormone releasing hormone (LHRH) agonist treatment in children with LHRH-dependent precocious puberty. *J Pediatr* 1989; **115:** 105–8.

Desmopressin (5922-b)

Desmopressin *(BAN, rINN).*

DDAVP; Desmopressinum. 1-(3-Mercaptopropionic acid)-8-D-arginine-vasopressin; [1-Deamino,8-D-arginine]vasopressin.

$C_{46}H_{64}N_{14}O_{12}S_2$ = 1069.2.

CAS — 16679-58-6.

Pharmacopoeias. In *Eur.* (see p.viii).

A white fluffy powder. **Soluble** in water, in glacial acetic acid, and in alcohol. **Store** at 2° to 8°. Protect from light and moisture.

Desmopressin Acetate (5923-v)

Desmopressin Acetate *(BANM, USAN, rINNM).*

$C_{46}H_{64}N_{14}O_{12}S_2,C_2H_4O_2,3H_2O$ = 1183.3.

CAS — 62288-83-9 (anhydrous desmopressin acetate); 62357-86-2 (desmopressin acetate trihydrate).

Units

27 units of desmopressin are contained in approximately 27 μg of desmopressin (with 5 mg of human albumin and citric acid) in one ampoule of the first International Standard (1980).

Adverse Effects and Precautions

Rare adverse effects with desmopressin include headache, nausea, and mild abdominal cramps; there may be pain and swelling at the site of injection. With large intravenous doses hypotension, with tachycardia and facial flushing, may occur; some patients may experience an increase in blood pressure. Occasionally there may be cerebral or coronary thrombosis. Hypersensitivity reactions have also occurred. The antidiuretic action of desmopressin may produce water intoxication and hyponatraemia, occasionally leading to convulsions. Nasal administration may cause local irritation, congestion and epistaxis.

Precautions to be observed during the administration of desmopressin are similar to those for vasopressin (see p.1263). It should not be used in patients with type IIB von Willebrand's disease, in whom the release of clotting factors may lead to platelet aggregation and thrombocytopenia. When desmopressin is used diagnostically, or for the treatment of enuresis, the fluid intake should be limited to a minimum and only to satisfy thirst for 8 hours following administration (see also below).

Effects on the cardiovascular system. Facial flushing and warmth following intravenous desmopressin reflect a vasodilator action[1] or may be due to an opioid mechanism in the CNS.[2] A drop in diastolic blood pressure of about 14 mmHg and an increase in heart rate of 20 beats per minute are the rule during intravenous infusion of desmopressin in doses of 400 ng per kg body-weight or more.[1] The hypotensive effects of desmopressin were responsible for a serious reaction, involving cyanosis and dyspnoea, in a 21-month-old child with cyanotic heart disease.[3] Thrombosis (including myocardial infarction)[4-6] and cerebral infarction[7] have been associated rarely with the use of intravenous desmopressin.

Manufacturers also warn of the possibility of an increase in blood pressure.

1. Brommer EJP, *et al.* Desmopressin and hypotension. *Ann Intern Med* 1985; **103:** 962.
2. Pigache RM. Facial flushing induced by vasopressin-like peptides lacking pressor activity. *J Clin Pharmacol* 1984; **17:** 369–71.
3. Israels SJ, Kobrinsky NL. Serious reaction to desmopressin in a child with cyanotic heart disease. *N Engl J Med* 1989; **320:** 1563–4.
4. Anonymous. Desmopressin and arterial thrombosis. *Lancet* 1989; **i:** 938–9.
5. Mannucci PM, Lusher JM. Desmopressin and thrombosis. *Lancet* 1989; **ii:** 675–6.
6. Hartmann S, Reinhart W. Fatal complication of desmopressin. *Lancet* 1995; **345:** 1302–3. Correction. *ibid.;* 1648.
7. Grunwald Z, Sather SDC. Intraoperative cerebral infarction after desmopressin administration in infant with end-stage renal disease. *Lancet* 1995; **345:** 1364–5.

Effects on electrolytes. There have been a number of reports of seizures due to hyponatraemia and water intoxication following intranasal[1-6] or intravenous[7] desmopressin. In the UK, the Committee on Safety of Medicines noted in March 1996 that it had received reports of hyponatraemic convulsions in 21 children and 3 adults receiving desmopressin (which it somewhat inaccurately described as vasopressin).[8] It was recommended that when this drug was used to treat primary nocturnal enuresis the risks of concomitant hyponatraemia should be minimised by avoiding concomitant use of drugs, such as tricyclic antidepressants, that increase endogenous ADH secretion; by keeping to the recommended starting dose; by avoiding excessive fluid intake, including during swimming; and by stopping treatment temporarily if vomiting or diarrhoea occurred, to allow recovery of normal fluid and electrolyte balance.

1. Simmonds EJ, *et al.* Convulsions and coma after intranasal desmopressin in cystic fibrosis. *Br Med J* 1988; **297:** 1614.
2. Salvatoni A, *et al.* Hyponatremia and seizures during desmopressin acetate treatment in hypothyroidism. *J Pediatr* 1990; **116:** 835–6.
3. Davis RC, *et al.* Nocturnal enuresis. *Lancet* 1992; **340:** 1550.
4. Hamed M, *et al.* Hyponatraemic convulsion associated with desmopressin and imipramine treatment. *Br Med J* 1993; **306:** 1169.
5. Hourihane J, Salisbury AJ. Use caution in prescribing desmopressin for nocturnal enuresis. *Br Med J* 1993; **306:** 1545.
6. Robson WLM, Leung AKC. Hyponatraemia following desmopressin. *Br Med J* 1993; **307:** 64–5.
7. Shepherd LL, *et al.* Hyponatremia and seizures after intravenous administration of desmopressin acetate for surgical hemostasis. *J Pediatr* 1989; **114:** 470–2.
8. Committe on Safety of Medicines/Medicines Control Agency. Hyponatraemic convulsions in patients with enuresis treated with vasopressin. *Current Problems* 1996; **22:** 4.

Effects on mental function. Paranoid psychosis occurred after desmopressin therapy in a patient with Alzheimer's dementia.[1]

1. Collins GB, *et al.* Paranoid psychosis after DDAVP therapy for Alzheimer's dementia. *Lancet* 1981; **ii:** 808.

Tolerance. In 3 uraemic patients desmopressin infusion produced an initial shortening of the bleeding time but following repeated infusions this response was reduced and there was even some increase in base-line bleeding times.[1] Two infusions of desmopressin 300 ng per kg body-weight in one day appear to induce a near maximum response; different treatment is required subsequently.

1. Canavese C, *et al.* Reduced response of uraemic bleeding time to repeated doses of desmopressin. *Lancet* 1985; **i:** 867–8.

Interactions

As for Vasopressin, p.1264.

Pharmacokinetics

Desmopressin is absorbed from the nasal mucosa with a bioavailability of 10 to 20%. Following oral administration it is largely destroyed in the gastrointestinal tract but sufficient is absorbed following high doses to produce therapeutic effects. When given intravenously desmopressin exhibits biphasic pharmacokinetics, with half-lives of about 8 minutes and 75 minutes for the 2 phases respectively.

References.

1. Fjellestad-Paulsen A, *et al.* Pharmacokinetics of 1-deamino-8-D-arginine vasopressin after various routes of administration in healthy volunteers. *Clin Endocrinol (Oxf)* 1993; **38:** 177–82.
2. Lam KSL, *et al.* Pharmacokinetics, pharmacodynamics, long-term efficacy and safety of oral 1-deamino-8-D-arginine vasopressin in adult patients with central diabetes insipidus. *Br J Clin Pharmacol* 1996; **42:** 379–85.

Uses and Administration

Desmopressin is a synthetic analogue of vasopressin (see p.1263). It has greater antidiuretic activity and a more prolonged action than vasopressin or lypressin. It also stimulates factor VIII and plasminogen activator activity in the blood, but has little pressor activity.

Desmopressin is used similarly to vasopressin in the diagnosis and treatment of cranial diabetes insipidus, and in the treatment of nocturnal enuresis and tests of renal function. It is also used in the management of mild or moderate haemophilia and type I von Willebrand's disease, and in tests of fibrinolytic response. Desmopressin may also relieve headache due to lumbar puncture.

It is given as the acetate, by mouth, as a solution intranasally, and by injection. The intranasal dose is approximately ten times that required intravenously and the oral dose about ten times greater than the intranasal dose.

In the control of cranial diabetes insipidus, desmopressin acetate is given by mouth in usual initial doses of 100 μg three times daily. Doses may be adjusted according to response, with maintenance doses usually between 100 and 200 μg three times daily though total doses of between 100 μg and 1200 μg daily have been used. It may also be used intranasally in usual doses of 10 to 40 μg of desmopressin acetate daily as a single dose or in divided doses; children aged 3 months to 12 years may be given 5 to 30 μg intranasally daily. It may also be administered subcutaneously, intramuscularly, or intravenously in a dose of 1 to 4 μg daily; a dose from 0.4 μg has been suggested in children and infants. A single intranasal dose of 20 μg or 2 μg subcutaneously or intramuscularly has been given in the diagnosis of diabetes insipidus. Doses of 10 to 40 μg intranasally or 2 μg by injection have been used to test renal function.

In the management of primary nocturnal enuresis desmopressin acetate is given in usual doses of 200 to 400 μg by mouth or 20 to 40 μg intranasally at bedtime. The need for continued treatment should be reassessed after 3 months by withdrawing desmopressin for at least 1 week. For the control of nocturia in patients with multiple sclerosis 10 to 20 μg intranasally at bedtime is recommended (but see Urinary Incontinence, below)

Desmopressin acetate is given by intravenous infusion to boost concentrations of factor VIII before surgical procedures in patients with mild to moderate haemophilia or type I von Willebrand's disease. The usual dose is 0.3 or 0.4 μg (300 or 400 ng) per kg body-weight by slow intravenous infusion over 15 to 30 minutes just before surgery. It may be used similarly to treat spontaneous or trauma-induced bleeding episodes in these patients.

For diagnosis of fibrinolytic response desmopressin acetate may be given by intravenous infusion in doses of 0.4 μg per kg over 20 minutes; a sample of venous blood is taken 20 minutes after completing the infusion and tested for fibrinolytic activity on fibrin plates.

Desmopressin acetate has also been given in a dose of 4 μg subcutaneously or intramuscularly for the treatment or prophylaxis of headache due to lumbar puncture, repeated if necessary after 24 hours.

Diabetes insipidus. Desmopressin is the usual treatment for cranial diabetes insipidus (p.1237).

Haemorrhagic disorders. Desmopressin is used in the management of patients with mild haemophilia A, carriers of haemophilia with low factor VIII concentrations, and patients with von Willebrand's disease, as discussed on p.707. Intravenous injection of desmopressin is immediately followed by tranexamic acid to inhibit the enhanced fibrinolytic activity.[1] The resultant three- to fivefold increase in all factor VIII activities should be sufficient to allow minor surgery, providing the basal concentration of the most deficient factor VIII activity is 7% or more. With higher basal factor VIII concentrations, more major surgery such as cholecystectomy or thoracotomy may be possible. Desmopressin can also be given intranasally but the factor VIII response is less predictable than with injection. The use of desmopressin as an alternative to blood products has been recommended whenever possible in the treatment of these disorders, as a precaution against infection with HIV.[2] The references listed below give further information on the use of desmopressin in haemophilia and/or von Willebrand's disease.[3-8]

Bleeding due to liver disease has been controlled by desmopressin,[9,10] as has that associated with uraemia[11-14] (but for a report of tolerance to the effects of repeated doses of desmopressin in uraemic patients, see under Adverse Effects and Precautions, above), and there are reports of bleeding being controlled in other disorders such as telangiectasia,[15] and platelet storage deficiency,[16] and in patients with acquired antibodies to factor VIII.[17] See also p.1264 and p.1261 for references to the use of vasopressin and another of its synthetic analogues, terlipressin, respectively, in the treatment of haemorrhagic disorders.

Desmopressin has been tried in surgical procedures with conflicting results.[18-21] It has been suggested that it may only be useful in patients with inadequate haemostatic mechanisms undergoing cardiac surgery[22] and that its usefulness in noncardiac surgery needs further study.[23] A possible role for desmopressin has been proposed in the control of surgical bleeding in patients whose religious beliefs preclude the use of blood products.[24] It has been reported to be effective in postoperative aspirin-related bleeding that was previously unresponsive to administration of clotting factors,[25] and may be helpful for the prevention of excessive blood loss in patients who have received aspirin within 7 days of cardiac bypass surgery.[26]

1. Anonymous. DDAVP in haemophilia and von Willebrand's disease. *Lancet* 1983; **ii:** 774–5.
2. Jones P. HIV infection and haemophilia. *Arch Dis Child* 1991; **66:** 364–8.
3. Anonymous. Desmopressin for hemophilia and other coagulation disorders. *Med Lett Drugs Ther* 1984; **26:** 82.
4. Kobrinsky NL, *et al.* Shortening of bleeding time by 1-deamino-8-D-arginine vasopressin in various bleeding disorders. *Lancet* 1984; **i:** 1145–8.
5. de la Fuente B, *et al.* Response of patients with mild and moderate hemophilia A and von Willebrand's disease to treatment with desmopressin. *Ann Intern Med* 1985; **103:** 6–14.
6. Vicente V, *et al.* Intranasal desmopressin in mild hemophilia A. *Ann Intern Med* 1985; **103:** 807–8.
7. Prince S. An alternative to blood product therapy for dental extractions in the mild to moderate haemophiliac patient. *Br Dent J* 1987; **162:** 256–7.
8. Rose EH, Aledort LM. Nasal spray desmopressin (DDAVP) for mild hemophilia A and von Willebrand disease. *Ann Intern Med* 1991; **114:** 563–8.
9. Burroughs AK, *et al.* Desmopressin and bleeding time in patients with cirrhosis. *Br Med J* 1985; **291:** 1377–81.
10. Rak K, *et al.* Desmopressin and bleeding time in patients with cirrhosis. *Br Med J* 1986; **292:** 138.
11. Mannucci PM, *et al.* Deamino-8-D-arginine vasopressin shortens the bleeding time in uremia. *N Engl J Med* 1983; **308:** 8–12.
12. Shapiro MD, Kelleher SP. Intranasal deamino-8-D-arginine vasopressin shortens the bleeding time in uremia. *Am J Nephrol* 1984; **4:** 260–1.
13. Viganò GL, *et al.* Subcutaneous desmopressin (DDAVP) shortens the bleeding time in uremia. *Am J Hematol* 1989; **31:** 32–5.
14. Jacquot C, *et al.* Addition of desmopressin to recombinant human erythropoietin in treatment of haemostatic defect of uraemia. *Lancet* 1988; **i:** 420.
15. Quitt M, *et al.* The effect of desmopressin on massive gastrointestinal bleeding in hereditary telangiectasia unresponsive to treatment with cryoprecipitate. *Arch Intern Med* 1990; **150:** 1744–6.
16. Nieuwenhuis HK, Sixma JJ. 1-Desamino-8-D-arginine vasopressin (desmopressin) shortens the bleeding time in storage pool deficiency. *Ann Intern Med* 1988; **108:** 65–7.
17. Naorose-Abidi SM, *et al.* Desmopressin therapy in patients with acquired factor VIII inhibitors. *Lancet* 1988; **i:** 366.
18. Salzman EW, *et al.* Treatment with desmopressin acetate to reduce blood loss after cardiac surgery: a double-blind randomized trial. *N Engl J Med* 1986; **314:** 1402–6.
19. Kobrinsky NL, *et al.* 1-Desamino-8-D-arginine vasopressin (desmopressin) decreases operative blood loss in patients having Harrington rod spinal fusion surgery: a randomized, double-blinded, controlled trial. *Ann Intern Med* 1987; **107:** 446–50. Correction. *ibid.* 1988; **108:** 496.
20. Hackmann T, *et al.* A trial of desmopressin (1-desamino-8-D-arginine vasopressin) to reduce blood loss in uncomplicated cardiac surgery. *N Engl J Med* 1989; **321:** 1437–43.
21. Cattaneo M, Mannucci PM. Desmopressin and blood loss after cardiac surgery. *Lancet* 1993; **342:** 812.
22. Salzman EW. Desmopressin and surgical hemostasis. *N Engl J Med* 1990; **322:** 1085.
23. Anonymous. Can drugs reduce surgical blood loss? *Lancet* 1988; **i:** 155–6.
24. Martens PR. Desmopressin and Jehovah's witness. *Lancet* 1989; **i:** 1322.
25. Chard RB, *et al.* Use of desmopressin in the management of aspirin-related and intractable haemorrhage after cardiopulmonary bypass. *Aust N Z J Surg* 1990; **60:** 125–8.
26. Sheridan DP, *et al.* Use of desmopressin acetate to reduce blood transfusion requirements during cardiac surgery in patients with acetylsalicylic-acid-induced platelet dysfunction. *Can J Surg* 1994; **37:** 33–6.

Memory disorders. Desmopressin 4 μg daily by intramuscular injection for 6 weeks failed to have any beneficial effect on the impairment of memory arising from severe head injuries in 6 men, aged 24 to 36 years, injured in road traffic accidents 3 to 8 years previously, none of whom had diabetes insipidus.[1] A subsequent course of lypressin also failed to have any beneficial effect. In a more recent study,[2] intranasal desmopressin 20 μg daily administered for a mean of 4.3 days from 16 to 40 hours after closed-head injury significantly improved information processing and short-term verbal logical memory.

1. Jenkins JS, *et al.* Desmopressin in post-traumatic amnesia. *Lancet* 1979; **ii:** 1245–6.
2. Filipová M, *et al.* Clinical efficacy of 1-desamino-8-D-arginine-vasopressin (DDAVP) in short-term recovery from minor head injury. *Hum Psychopharmacol Clin Exp* 1989; **4:** 47–50.

Nocturnal enuresis. Desmopressin is one of the main drugs used as an alternative or adjunct to nonpharmacological methods for the treatment of nocturnal enuresis in children (p.453). Secretion of vasopressin during the night in normal individuals reduces urine output and it has been suggested that nocturnal enuresis in some children might be due to impaired nocturnal secretion of vasopressin. However, a recent study[1] found no difference in nocturnal vasopressin levels or urine production in enuretic and non-enuretic children, but did find that children with nocturnal enuresis required a greater output of vasopressin to regulate plasma osmolality; other evidence has suggested that developmental delay in 2 separate areas of the CNS is involved.[2] Nonetheless, it has been shown that administration of the synthetic vasopressin analogue, desmopressin, at night can be effective in the short-term control of nocturnal enuresis[3] and many now consider it to be the drug of choice in terms of safety. It should not be given when enuresis is due to polydipsia as desmopressin may provoke water intoxication and convulsions due to hyponatraemia. For precautions to be observed when desmopressin is used to treat enuresis see under Effects on Electrolytes, above.

1. Eggert P, Kühn B. Antidiuretic hormone regulation in patients with primary nocturnal enuresis. *Arch Dis Child* 1995; **73:** 508–11.
2. Koff SA. Cure of nocturnal enuresis: why isn't desmopressin very effective? *Pediatr Nephrol* 1996; **10:** 667–70.
3. Moffat MEK, *et al.* Desmopressin acetate and nocturnal enuresis: how much do we know? *Pediatrics* 1993; **92:** 420–5.

Orthostatic hypotension. The first drug tried in patients with orthostatic hypotension (p.1040) who cannot be managed by non pharmacological methods is usually fludrocortisone, but desmopressin is sometimes useful in patients with central neurological abnormalities.[1]

1. Mathias CJ, *et al.* The effect of desmopressin on nocturnal polyuria, overnight weight loss, and morning postural hypotension in patients with autonomic failure. *Br Med J* 1986; **293:** 353–4.

Post dural puncture headache. References to the use of desmopressin in lumbar-puncture headache;[1-4] results have generally been disappointing. As mentioned on p.1282 in many cases patients respond to conservative treatment with bed rest, hydration, and analgesics.

1. Durward WF, Harrington H. Headache after lumbar puncture. *Lancet* 1976; **ii:** 1403–4.
2. Widerlöv E, Lindström L. DDAVP and headache after lumbar puncture. *Lancet* 1979; **i:** 548.
3. Hansen PE, Hansen JH. DDAVP, a synthetic analogue of vasopressin, in prevention of headache after lumbar puncture and lumbar pneumoencephalography. *Acta Neurol Scand* 1979; **60:** 183–8.
4. Cowan JMA, *et al.* DDAVP in the prevention of headache after lumbar puncture. *Br Med J* 1980; **280:** 224.

Renal function testing. Desmopressin was equally effective by the intranasal and intramuscular routes in assessment of the urine-concentrating capacity of the kidneys in a dose of 40 μg and 2 μg respectively.[1] It was noted that urine-concentrating ability decreased with advancing age.[2] Experience in 32 adults suggested that desmopressin was as effective as vasopressin tannate for assessing renal function and that a suitable dose was 40 μg intranasally at 8 a.m. after overnight water deprivation.[3] It was also suggested that desmopressin be used routinely by the intranasal route and that it be administered by the intramuscular route to check results if technical difficulties arose.[4] Intramuscular desmopressin 4 μg was found suitable for assessing renal function in sedentary subjects or hospital inpatients[5] and intranasal desmopressin 40 μg was useful in early diagnosis of renal dysfunction caused by chronic abuse of analgesics.[6] In lithium-treated patients a test of urine osmolality using desmopressin before and after 14 hours of total fluid deprivation was a safe, convenient, and reliable means of estimating renal concentrating capacity.[7]

1. Monson JP, Richards P. Desmopressin urine concentration test. *Br Med J* 1978; **1:** 24.
2. Monson JP, Richards P. Age and urine concentration after desmopressin. *Br Med J* 1978; **1:** 1054–5.
3. Delin K, *et al.* Urinary concentration test with desmopressin. *Br Med J* 1978; **1:** 757–8.
4. Delin K, *et al.* Assessment of renal concentrating ability. *Br Med J* 1979; **1:** 888–9.
5. Curtis JR, Donovan BA. Assessment of renal concentrating ability. *Br Med J* 1979; **1:** 304–5.
6. Wambach G, *et al.* Detection of renal impairment in cases of chronic abuse of analgesics by administration of desamino-D-arginine vasopressin. *Arzneimittelforschung* 1989; **39:** 387–90.
7. Asplund K, *et al.* DDAVP test in assessment of renal function during lithium therapy. *Lancet* 1979; **i:** 491.

Urinary incontinence. Desmopressin given intranasally appeared to be effective in reducing voiding frequency/incontinence when studied in 26 patients with multiple sclerosis whose bladder dysfunction had previously been unresponsive to antimuscarinic therapy.[1] However a review of studies using desmopressin to treat nocturia in patients with multiple sclerosis cast doubt on the clinical relevance of the limited reductions achieved in voiding frequency.[2]

1. Fredrikson S. Nasal spray desmopressin treatment of bladder dysfunction in patients with multiple sclerosis. *Acta Neurol Scand* 1996; **94:** 31–4.
2. Ferreira E, Letwin SR. Desmopressin for nocturia and enuresis associated with multiple sclerosis. *Ann Pharmacother* 1998; **32:** 114–16.

Preparations

BP 1998: Desmopressin Injection; Desmopressin Intranasal Solution.

Proprietary Preparations (details are given in Part 3)

Aust.: Minirin; ***Austral.:*** Minirin; Octostim; ***Belg.:*** Minirin; ***Canad.:*** DDAVP; Octostim; ***Fr.:*** Minirin; ***Ger.:*** DDAVP; Minirin; ***Irl.:*** Desmospray; Desmotabs; ***Ital.:*** Emosint; Minirin/DDAVP; ***Neth.:*** Minrin; Octostim; ***Norw.:*** Minirin; Octostim; ***S.Afr.:*** DDAVP†; ***Spain:*** Minurin; ***Swed.:*** Minirin; Octostim; ***Switz.:*** Minirin; Octostim; ***UK:*** DDAVP; Desmospray; Desmotabs; ***USA:*** Concentraid†; DDAVP; Stimate.

Felypressin (5924-g)

Felypressin *(BAN, USAN, rINN).*

Phelypressine; PLV2. [2-Phenylalanine,8-lysine]vasopressin; Cys-Phe-Phe-Gln-Asn-Cys-Pro-Lys-Gly-NH_2.

$C_{46}H_{65}N_{13}O_{11}S_2$ = 1040.2.

CAS — 56-59-7.

Felypressin is a synthetic analogue of vasopressin (p.1263) with similar actions. Its antidiuretic effects are less than those of vasopressin. It is used as a vasoconstrictor in local anaesthetic injections for dental use when sympathomimetics should be avoided. It is also an ingredient of preparations used in the treatment of pain and inflammation of the mouth.

Preparations

Proprietary Preparations (details are given in Part 3)

Multi-ingredient: ***Belg.:*** Trigat†; ***Fr.:*** Collupressine.

Used as an adjunct in: ***Austral.:*** Citanest Dental; ***Ger.:*** Xylonest; ***Irl.:*** Citanest with Octapressin; ***Ital.:*** Citanest con Octapressin; ***Neth.:*** Citanest Octapressine; ***Norw.:*** Citanest Octapressin; ***S.Afr.:*** Citanest Octopressin†; ***Spain:*** Citanest Octapressin; ***Swed.:*** Citanest Octapressin; ***Switz.:*** Xylonest-Octapressin; ***UK:*** Citanest with Octapressin.

Follicle-stimulating Hormone

(15579-r)

FSH.

Follitropin Alfa (17626-v)

Follitropin Alfa *(BAN, rINN).*

$C_{437}H_{682}N_{122}O_{134}S_{13}$ (α-subunit); $C_{538}H_{833}N_{145}O_{171}S_{13}$ (β-subunit) = 10206 (α-subunit); 12485 (β-subunit).

CAS — 9002-68-0 (follitropin alfa); 56832-30-5 (α- subunit); 110909-60-9 (β-subunit); 146479-72-3 (follitropin alfa).

Follitropin Beta (5037-r)

Follitropin Beta *(BAN, rINN).*

Org-32489.

$C_{437}H_{682}N_{122}O_{134}S_{13}$ (α-subunit); $C_{538}H_{833}N_{145}O_{171}S_{13}$ (β-subunit) = 10206 (α-subunit); 12485 (β-subunit).

CAS — 169108-34-3 (follitropin beta); 150490-84-9 (follitropin beta); 56832-30-5 (α-subunit); 110909-60-9 (β-subunit).

Units

80 units of human pituitary follicle-stimulating hormone are contained in approximately 4.17 µg (with 5 mg of mannitol and 1 mg human serum albumin) in one ampoule of the first International Standard (1986).

Adverse Effects and Precautions

As for Human Menopausal Gonadotrophins, p.1252.

In a few countries, gonadotrophins derived from cadaver pituitary glands have been used in the treatment of infertility, and a small number of patients are reported to have acquired Creutzfeldt-Jakob disease from such preparations.[1] However, most countries have preferred to use gonadotrophins derived from urine,[1] and these in their turn are being replaced with recombinant products;[2] such preparations do not carry the risk of transmitting the disease.

1. Healy DL, Evans J. Creutzfeldt-Jakob disease after pituitary gonadotrophins. *Br Med J* 1993; **307:** 517–18.
2. Eshkol A, Page ML. Human gonadotrophin preparations. *Br Med J* 1994; **308:** 789.

Pharmacokinetics

Follitropins alfa and beta are slowly absorbed following subcutaneous or intramuscular injection, with an absolute bioavailability of about 70 to 80%. Peak plasma concentrations of follitropin beta have been stated to occur about 12 hours after subcutaneous or intramuscular injection. Accumulation occurs with repeated doses, reaching a steady state within 3 to 4 days. Follitropins are slowly eliminated from the body, with terminal half-life ranging from 12 to 70 hours. About one-eighth of a dose of follitropin alfa is reported to be excreted in the urine.

References.

1. Karlsson MO, *et al.* The population pharmacokinetics of recombinant- and urinary-human follicle stimulating hormone in women. *Br J Clin Pharmacol* 1998; **45:** 13–20.

Uses and Administration

Follicle-stimulating hormone is a gonadotrophic hormone secreted by the anterior lobe of the pituitary gland, together with another gonadotrophin, luteinising hormone (see p.1254).

These gonadotrophins stimulate the normal functioning of the gonads and the secretion of sex hormones in both men and women. In women, follicle-stimulating hormone stimulates the development and maturation of the follicles and ova; in men it has a role in spermatogenesis.

Recombinant human follicle-stimulating hormones (follitropins alfa or beta) are used in the treatment of female infertility due to anovulation, in women who have not responded to treatment with clomiphene (see p.1239).

The dosage and schedule of treatment must be determined according to the needs of each patient; it is usual to monitor response by studying the patient's urinary oestrogen excretion or by ultrasonic visualisation of follicles or both. Treatment is usually begun with 75 to 150 units daily by subcutaneous injection for 7 or 14 days; if there is no response, dosage is increased at 7 or 14 day intervals until an adequate but not excessive response is achieved. Treatment is then stopped and followed after 1 or 2 days by a single dose of chorionic gonadotrophin 5000 to 10 000 units to induce ovulation. In menstruating patients treatment should be started within the first 7 days of the menstrual cycle. It has been suggested by the UK manufacturers of follitropin alfa that a daily dose of 225 units is the usual maximum, and that if a patient fails to respond adequately after 4 weeks of treatment that cycle should be abandoned and the patient should subsequently begin the next cycle at a higher starting dose.

Follitropins are also employed as part of *in-vitro* fertilisation or other assisted reproductive technologies. For this purpose doses of 150 to 225 units daily are generally given, for at least 4 days, commencing on the 2nd or 3rd day of the cycle. Thereafter the dose may be adjusted individually based on ovarian response; adequate follicular development generally occurs within about 5 to 10 days of treatment. Pituitary downregulation with a gonadorelin analogue may be employed in conjunction with follitropin therapy, in which case the gonadorelin analogue is generally begun about 2 weeks before follitropin, and the 2 are then continued concomitantly until follicular development is adequate. A single dose of up to 10 000 units of chorionic gonadotrophin is then given to induce final follicular maturation and oocyte retrieval performed about 35 hours later.

Other substances with follicle-stimulating activity are used similarly: these include human menopausal gonadotrophins (p.1252), which have both luteinising and follicle-stimulating activity, and urofollitrophin (p.1263).

Preparations

Proprietary Preparations (details are given in Part 3)

Aust.: Gonal-F; ***Austral.:*** Puregon; ***Fr.:*** Gonal-F; ***Ger.:*** Gonal-F; Puregon; ***Irl.:*** Gonal-F; Puregon; ***Ital.:*** Gonal-F; Puregon; ***Neth.:*** Gonal-F; Puregon; ***Norw.:*** Gonal-F; Puregon; ***Swed.:*** Gonal-F; Puregon; ***Switz.:*** Gonal-F; ***UK:*** Gonal-F; Puregon; ***USA:*** Follistim; Gonal-F.

Gonadorelin (5925-q)

Gonadorelin *(BAN, rINN).*

Abbott-41070 (gonadorelin acetate); AY-24031 (gonadorelin hydrochloride); Follicle Stimulating Hormone-releasing Factor; GnRH; Gonadoliberin; Gonadorelinum; Gonadotrophin-releasing Hormone; Hoe-471; LH/FSH-RF; LH/FSH-RH; LH-RF; LH-RH; Luliberin; Luteinising Hormone-releasing Factor.

5-Oxo-L-prolyl-L-histidyl-L-tryptophyl-L-seryl-L-tyrosylglycyl-L-leucyl-L-arginyl-L-prolylglycinamide.

$C_{55}H_{75}N_{17}O_{13}$ = 1182.3.

CAS — 33515-09-2 (gonadorelin or gonadorelin monohydrochloride); 34973-08-5 (gonadorelin diacetate, anhydrous); 52699-48-6 (gonadorelin diacetate, tetrahydrate); 51952-41-1 (gonadorelin xHCl).

NOTE. Gonadorelin Acetate and Gonadorelin Hydrochloride are *USAN*.

Pharmacopoeias. In *Fr., Ger., Neth.,* and *Swiss.*

Eur. (see p.viii) includes a monograph for Gonadorelin Acetate. *Br.* also includes a monograph for Gonadorelin Hydrochloride.

A decapeptide obtained by synthesis. The acetate or hydrochloride is described as a white or faintly yellowish-white powder. **Soluble** in water and in 1% v/v glacial acetic acid; sparingly soluble in methyl alcohol. **Store** in airtight containers at a temperature of 2° to 8°. Protect from light.

Units

31 units of gonadorelin for bioassay are contained in approximately 50 µg of gonadorelin acetate (with lactose 2.5 mg and human plasma albumin 0.5 mg) in one ampoule of the first International Reference Preparation (1980).

Adverse Effects

Gonadorelin and its analogues are generally well tolerated but may cause gastro-intestinal adverse effects, usually nausea and abdominal pain or discomfort. There may be headache or lightheadedness, and an increase in menstrual bleeding. Continued therapy with gonadorelin analogues results in paradoxical suppression of the pituitary gonadal axis: in premenopausal women this may produce menopausal symptoms, including vaginal dryness, hot flushes, and loss of libido. If sufficiently prolonged the suppression of circulating oestrogens may lead to a decrease in trabecular bone density. In men, hot flushes and sexual dysfunction have occurred. Breast swelling and tenderness in men have been reported infrequently with gonadorelin analogues. Other adverse effects reportedly associated with gonadorelin analogue therapy, and presumably related to changes in the hormonal milieu, include mood changes, nervousness, palpitations, acne and dry skin, alterations in liver function tests and blood lipids, decreased glucose tolerance, and changes in scalp and body hair. Ovarian hyperstimulation (as seen with chorionic gonadotrophin, p.1243), although rare, has occurred in women given gonadorelin.

Reactions or pain may occur at the site of injection with rash (local or generalised), thrombophlebitis, swelling, or pruritus. Hypersensitivity reactions, including bronchospasm and anaphylaxis, have been reported.

Other effects may be a consequence of the particular use of gonadorelin or its analogues. Tumour flare, due to an initial surge in testosterone concentrations, has been reported in the initial stages of treatment for cancer of the prostate and concomitant anti-androgen therapy may be given prophylactically. Flare may manifest as an increase in bone pain; occasionally there has been a worsening of urinary-tract symptoms with haematuria and urinary obstruction. An initial increase in signs and symptoms has also been reported in women with breast cancer receiving gonadorelin analogues; hypercalcaemia has occurred in those with metastatic disease.

Hypersensitivity. Acquired hypersensitivity led to an anaphylactic reaction following intravenous administration of gonadorelin to a man who had been receiving pulsatile subcutaneous gonadorelin therapy for 10 weeks.[1]

1. Potashnik G, *et al.* Anaphylactic reaction to gonadotropin-releasing hormone. *N Engl J Med* 1993; **328:** 815.

Precautions

Gonadorelin should not generally be used in patients with pituitary adenoma. It is also recommended that patients with weight-related amenorrhoea should not receive gonadorelin until their weight is corrected. While it has been recommended by at least one manufacturer that gonadorelin should not be used in women with polycystic ovary disease or with endometriotic cysts, gonadorelin and its analogues have produced improvement in polycystic disease, in uterine fibroids, and gonadorelin analogues have been used with benefit in endometriosis. Gonadorelin should be discontinued if the patient becomes pregnant. Contraceptive measures should be taken to protect against unwanted ovulation.

Interactions

Drugs affecting pituitary secretion of gonadotrophins may alter the response to gonadorelin; other hormonal therapy and corticosteroids can affect the response. Spironolactone and levodopa can stimulate gonadotrophins while phenothiazines, dopamine antagonists, digoxin, and sex hormones can inhibit gonadotrophin secretion.

Pharmacokinetics

Gonadorelin is poorly absorbed from the gastro-intestinal tract. It has a terminal plasma half-life of only 10 to 40 minutes after intravenous injection. It is hydrolysed in the plasma and excreted in the urine as inactive metabolites.

Gonadorelin analogues are absorbed following oral, intramuscular, intranasal, or rectal administration and have a longer half-life.

Uses and Administration

Gonadorelin is a synthetic form of hypothalamic gonadotrophin-releasing hormone. It stimulates the synthesis and release of follicle-stimulating hormone and, in particular, luteinising hormone in the anterior lobe of the pituitary. The secretion of endogenous gonadotrophin-releasing hormone is pulsatile and is controlled by several factors including circulating sex hormones. Gonadotrophic hormones, released from the pituitary gland in response to gonadorelin, stimulate secretion of sex hormones from the gonads. A single dose of gonadorelin or one of its analogues has the effect of increasing circulating sex hormones; continued administration leads to down-regulation of gonadorelin-receptor synthesis in the pituitary and results in a paradoxical reduction in sex-hormone secretion. It is sometimes used as the hydrochloride or acetate.

Gonadorelin is used in the diagnosis of hypothalamic-pituitary-gonadal dysfunction. Assessment is usually based on the response to a dose of gonadorelin of 100 μg by intravenous or subcutaneous injection. In females, where possible, it should be given early in the follicular stage of the menstrual cycle.

Gonadorelin is also used in the treatment of amenorrhoea and infertility associated with hypogonadotrophic hypogonadism and multifollicular ovaries. Weight-related amenorrhoea should have been corrected by diet. Treatment in such conditions is based on an intermittent pulse pump providing 5 to 20 μg over one minute every 90 minutes for up to 6 months or until conception.

Gonadorelin, or more usually its analogues such as buserelin, goserelin, leuprorelin, nafarelin, and triptorelin (which are more potent and have a longer duration of action) are used in contraception, cryptorchidism, malignant neoplasms (especially of the prostate), and in delayed and precocious puberty.

Reviews of gonadorelin and its analogues.

1. Fraser HM, Waxman J. Gonadotrophin releasing hormone analogues for gynaecological disorders and infertility. *Br Med J* 1989; **298:** 475–6.
2. Conn PM, Crowley WF. Gonadotropin-releasing hormone and its analogues. *N Engl J Med* 1991; **324:** 93–103.

Benign prostatic hyperplasia. The gonadorelin analogues have been tried in the management of benign prostatic hyperplasia (p.1446) but are considered unsatisfactory for indefinite use. See also under Leuprorelin Acetate, p.1253, and Nafarelin Acetate, p.1254.

Contraception. The gonadorelin analogues have been investigated as contraceptives,[1] but contraceptives based on oestrogens and progestogens remain the standard for hormonal contraceptive therapy (p.1434). For references to the use of buserelin and nafarelin in contraception see p.1242 and p.1254 respectively.

1. Anonymous. LHRH analogues for contraception. *Lancet* 1987; **i:** 1179–81.

Cryptorchidism. Whether gonadorelin or its analogues have a role in the management of cryptorchidism is a matter of debate; surgery remains the treatment with the best success rate, but hormonal therapy, with gonadorelin or chorionic gonadotrophin or both, is widely employed (see p.1236). Some references to the use of gonadorelin in cryptorchidism, with variable results, are listed below.[1-5] Meta-analysis has suggested a success rate of about 20% overall, although this may be reduced when care is taken to exclude retractile testes.[6]

1. Illig R, *et al.* Treatment of cryptorchidism by intranasal synthetic luteinising-hormone releasing hormone: results of a collaborative double-blind study. *Lancet* 1977; **ii:** 518–20.
2. Klidjian AM, *et al.* Luteinising hormone releasing hormone for incomplete descent of the testis. *Arch Dis Child* 1985; **60:** 568–71.
3. Witjes JA, *et al.* Use of luteinizing-hormone-releasing hormone nasal spray in the treatment of cryptorchidism: is there still an indication: a clinical study in 78 boys with 103 undescended testicles. *Eur Urol* 1990; **17:** 226–8.
4. Rajfer J, *et al.* Hormonal therapy of cryptorchidism: a randomized, double-blind study comparing human chorionic gonadotropin and gonadotropin-releasing hormone. *N Engl J Med* 1986; **314:** 466–70.
5. de Muinck Keizer-Schrama SMPF, *et al.* Double-blind, placebo-controlled study of luteinising-hormone-releasing-hormone nasal spray in treatment of undescended testes. *Lancet* 1986; **i:** 876–80.
6. Pyörälä S, *et al.* A review and meta-analysis of hormonal treatment of cryptorchidism. *J Clin Endocrinol Metab* 1995; **80:** 2795–9.

Delayed and precocious puberty. For mention of the use of gonadorelin or its analogues in delayed and precocious puberty, see p.1237 and p.1241 respectively. Benefit in delayed puberty is most likely in those cases where it is secondary to hypogonadism (see p.1239).

Diagnosis of hypothalamic and pituitary dysfunction. References to gonadorelin in the diagnosis of hypothalamic-pituitary-gonadal dysfunction[1-6] including one[5] suggesting its abandonment on the grounds that it offered no help in classifying patients with amenorrhoea or determining the therapeutic potential of treatment with gonadorelin.

1. Mortimer CH, *et al.* Luteinizing hormone and follicle stimulating hormone-releasing hormone test in patients with hypothalamic-pituitary-gonadal dysfunction. *Br Med J* 1973; **4:** 73–7.
2. Yoshimoto Y, *et al.* Restoration of normal pituitary gonadotropin reserve by administration of luteinizing-hormone-releasing hormone in patients with hypogonadotropic hypogonadism. *N Engl J Med* 1975; **292:** 242–5.
3. Sagel J, *et al.* The role of luteinizing hormone-releasing hormone in the diagnosis of constitutional delayed puberty. *Postgrad Med J* 1975; **51:** 611–14.
4. Ginsburg J, *et al.* Use of clomiphene and luteinizing hormone/follicle stimulating hormone-releasing hormone in investigation of ovulatory failure. *Br Med J* 1975; **3:** 130–3.
5. Adulwahid NA, *et al.* Diagnostic tests with luteinising hormone releasing hormone should be abandoned. *Br Med J* 1985; **291:** 1471–2.
6. Eckert KL, *et al.* A single-sample, subcutaneous gonadotropin-releasing hormone test for central precocious puberty. *Pediatrics* 1996; **97:** 517–19.

Disturbed behaviour. For mention of the use of triptorelin in men with paraphilias, see p.1262.

Endometriosis. Gonadorelin analogues are effective in the management of endometriosis (p.1442), but the need for long-term therapy to prevent recurrence limits their value, because of the risk of osteoporosis; 'add-back' therapy with concomitant hormone replacement is being investigated. Some references to gonadorelin analogues producing improvements in endometriosis are listed below.

For further references, see Buserelin Acetate, p.1242, Leuprorelin Acetate, p.1253, and Nafarelin Acetate, p.1254.

1. Meldrum DR, *et al.* "Medical oophorectomy" using a long-acting GNRH agonist—a possible new approach to the treatment of endometriosis. *J Clin Endocrinol Metab* 1982; **54:** 1081–3.
2. Cedars MI, *et al.* Treatment of endometriosis with a long-acting gonadotropin-releasing hormone agonist plus medroxyprogesterone acetate. *Obstet Gynecol* 1990; **75:** 641–5.
3. Barbieri RL. Gonadotropin-releasing hormone agonists and estrogen-progestogen replacement therapy. *Am J Obstet Gynecol* 1990; **162:** 593–5.
4. Shaw RW. LHRH analogues in the treatment of endometriosis—comparative results with other treatments. *Baillieres Clin Obstet Gynaecol* 1988; **2:** 659–75.
5. Henzl MR. Gonadotropin-releasing hormone (GnRH) agonists in the management of endometriosis: a review. *Clin Obstet Gynecol* 1988; **31:** 840–56.

Fibroids. Uterine fibroids (leiomyomas) are benign tumours of uterine smooth muscle found in about 20% of women older than 30 years. They may given rise to menstrual problems, pelvic discomfort, infertility, and miscarriage. Although small fibroids may not require treatment, the management of symptomatic fibroids has traditionally been surgical. However, because they are oestrogen responsive the use of gonadorelin and its analogues in the treatment of uterine fibroids has been discussed.[1-3] Results have been encouraging but it is uncertain whether such treatment will provide an alternative to surgery since when treatment stops uterine and fibroid volume tend to return to pretreatment values. Hot flushes and vaginal dryness are a common problem with gonadorelin therapy and bone loss may occur. The administration of oestrogens, once the uterine fibroid size has significantly reduced, has been tried in order to counteract these side-effects. Subcutaneous injection of long-acting depot preparations of gonadorelin or its analogues appear to be the preferred method of administration and it is considered that this treatment is a valuable pre-operative adjunct to surgery, simplifying the procedure by reducing the size and vascularity of the fibroid. However, concern has been expressed that the use of gonadorelin analogues for treating fibroids may complicate the differentiation of benign and malignant growths.[4]

For further references to gonadorelin analogues being used in the treatment of fibroids, see Buserelin Acetate, p.1242, Goserelin Acetate, p.1249, Leuprorelin Acetate, p.1253, Nafarelin Acetate, p.1254, and Triptorelin, p.1262.

1. Anonymous. Uterine fibroids: medical treatment or surgery? *Lancet* 1986; **ii:** 1197.
2. Baird DT, West CP. Medical management of fibroids. *Br Med J* 1988; **296:** 1684–5.
3. Friedman AJ, *et al.* Efficacy and safety considerations in women with uterine leiomyomas treated with gonadotropin-releasing hormone agonists: the estrogen threshold hypothesis. *Am J Obstet Gynecol* 1990; **163:** 1114–19.
4. Meyer WR, *et al.* Unsuspected leiomyosarcoma: treatment with a gonadotropin-releasing hormone analogue. *Obstet Gynecol* 1990; **75** (suppl): 529–32.

Growth retardation. The use of gonadorelin analogue to delay precocious puberty may improve the final height of children with the disorder. However, the use of a gonadorelin analogue with growth hormone in short but otherwise normal children is controversial—see under Triptorelin, p.1262.

Hirsutism. For reference to the use of gonadorelin analogues such as leuprorelin in the treatment of hirsutism, see p.1253.

Infertility. Gonadorelin and its analogues are used in the management of infertility related to hypogonadotrophic hypogonadism in both women and men (p.1239). Some further references are given below. See also under Buserelin Acetate, p.1242, Leuprorelin Acetate, p.1253, and Triptorelin, p.1262.

1. Lingle L, Hart LL. Gonadotropin-releasing hormone in infertility. *DICP Ann Pharmacother* 1989; **23:** 246–8.
2. Thomas AK, *et al.* Induction of ovulation with subcutaneous pulsatile gonadotropin-releasing hormone: correlation with body weight and other parameters. *Fertil Steril* 1989; **51:** 786–90.
3. Homburg R, *et al.* One hundred pregnancies after treatment with pulsatile luteinising hormone releasing hormone to induce ovulation. *Br Med J* 1989; **298:** 809–12.
4. Kovacs GT, *et al.* Induction of ovulation with gonadotrophin-releasing hormone—life-table analysis of 50 courses of treatment. *Med J Aust* 1989; **151:** 21–6.
5. Santoro N. Efficacy and safety of intravenous pulsatile gonadotropin-releasing hormone: Lutrepulse for injection. *Am J Obstet Gynecol* 1990; **163:** 1759–64.
6. Nachtigall LB, *et al.* Adult-onset idiopathic hypogonadotropic hypogonadism–a treatable form of male infertility. *N Engl J Med* 1997; **336:** 410–15.

Malignant neoplasms. Gonadorelin analogues are used, sometimes with anti-androgens such as cyproterone acetate or flutamide, in the treatment of prostatic cancer (p.491) where they provide an alternative to orchidectomy in the management of advanced disease. They have also been tried in neoplasms of the breast, endometrium, ovary, and pancreas where their use is much less well established. For discussion of these malignancies and their management, see under Choice of Antineoplastic, p.476.

Analogues used include buserelin acetate (see p.1242), goserelin acetate (see p.1249), leuprorelin acetate (see p.1253), and triptorelin (see p.1262).

Mastalgia. Gonadorelin analogues such as goserelin may be effective in severe refractory mastalgia (see p.1443).

Polycystic ovary syndrome. Gonadorelin analogues have been tried in polycystic ovary syndrome (p.1240) even though it is contra-indicated in this condition by some manufacturers. Pulsatile gonadorelin achieves a higher ovulatory rate in women with multifollicular ovaries than in those with large polycystic ovaries and the incidences of early miscarriage and abortion are higher in those with polycystic ovaries. Ovulation rate can be improved by pretreatment with a gonadorelin analogue for 8 weeks before using gonadorelin; Filicori *et al.*[1] employed this technique and 38% of patients achieved pregnancy. The rate of spontaneous abortion was also decreased from 50 to 38% after administration.

Further references to polycystic ovary syndrome including its treatment with gonadorelin analogues are listed below.[2-5]

1. Filicori M, *et al.* Polycystic ovary syndrome: abnormalities and management with pulsatile gonadotropin-releasing hormone and gonadotropin-releasing hormone analogs. *Am J Obstet Gynecol* 1990; **163:** 1737–42.
2. Stuckey BGA, *et al.* Continuous gonadotropin-releasing hormone for ovulation induction in polycystic ovarian disease. *Fertil Steril* 1987; **48:** 1055–7.
3. Eshel A, *et al.* Pulsatile luteinizing hormone-releasing hormone therapy in women with polycystic ovary syndrome. *Fertil Steril* 1988; **49:** 956–60.
4. Burger CW, *et al.* Ovulation induction with pulsatile luteinizing hormone-releasing hormone in women with clomiphene citrate-resistant polycystic ovary-like disease: endocrine results. *Fertil Steril* 1989; **51:** 20–9.
5. Homburg R, *et al.* Combined luteinizing hormone releasing hormone analogue and exogenous gonadotrophins for the treatment of infertility associated with polycystic ovaries. *Hum Reprod* 1990; **5:** 32–5.

Porphyria. For mention of the use of buserelin in a regimen to suppress cyclic premenstrual exacerbations of acute porphyria, see p.1243.

Premenstrual syndrome. In women in whom other drug treatments for premenstrual syndrome (p.1456) are ineffective, use of a gonadorelin analogue, usually with hormone replacement therapy to prevent menopausal symptoms, may be considered. Short-term use (3 months) has been used to confirm the diagnosis of premenstrual syndrome, or to predict the response to bilateral oophorectomy when this is being considered. Some references to the use of gonadorelin analogues in premenstrual syndrome are given below.[1-4]

1. Mortola JF, *et al.* Successful treatment of severe premenstrual syndrome by combined use of gonadotropin-releasing hormone agonist and estrogen/progestin. *J Clin Endocrinol Metab* 1991; **72:** 252A–F.
2. Hussain SY, *et al.* Buserelin in premenstrual syndrome. *Gynecol Endocrinol* 1992; **6:** 57–64.
3. Mortola JF. Applications of gonadotropin-releasing hormone analogues in the treatment of premenstrual syndrome. *Clin Obstet Gynecol* 1993; **36:** 753–63.
4. Mezrow G, *et al.* Depot leuprolide acetate with estrogen and progestin add-back for long-term treatment of premenstrual syndrome. *Fertil Steril* 1994; **62:** 932–7.

Preparations

BP 1998: Gonadorelin Injection.

Proprietary Preparations (details are given in Part 3)
Aust.: Kryptocur; Lutrelef; Relefact LH-RH; ***Austral.:*** HRF; Relefact LH-RH†; ***Belg.:*** HRF; Kryptocur; Lutrelef†; ***Canad.:*** Factrel; Lutrepulse; Relisorm; ***Fr.:*** Lutrelef; Pulstit†; Stimu-LH; ***Ger.:*** GnRH†; Kryptocur; Lutrelef; Relefact LH-RH; ***Irl.:*** Cryptocur†; Fertiral†; HRF; Relefact LH-RH; ***Ital.:*** HRF†; Kryptocur; Lutrelef; Relisorm L†; ***Neth.:*** Cryptocur; HRF; Lutrelef; Relefact LH-RH; ***Norw.:*** Lutrefact†; Lutrelef†; ***S.Afr.:*** HRF; ***Spain:*** Luforan; ***Swed.:*** Lutrelef; ***Switz.:*** Kryptocur; Lutrelef; Relisorm L; ***UK:*** Fertiral; HRF; Relefact LH-RH; ***USA:*** Factrel; Lutrepulse.
Multi-ingredient: ***UK:*** Relefact LH-RH/TRH†.

Goserelin Acetate (16845-p)

Goserelin Acetate *(BANM, rINNM)*.

ICI-118630 (goserelin); D-Ser $(Bu^t)^6$ $Azgly^{10}$-LHRH Acetate.

3-[5-Oxo-L-prolyl-L-histidyl-L-tryptophyl-L-seryl-L-tyrosyl-(3-*O-tert*-butyl)-D-seryl-L-leucyl-L-arginyl-L-prolyl]carbazamide acetate.

$C_{59}H_{84}N_{18}O_{14},C_2H_4O_2$ = 1329.5.

CAS — 65807-02-5 (goserelin).

NOTE. Goserelin is *USAN*.

1.05 g of goserelin acetate is approximately equivalent to 1 g of goserelin.

Adverse Effects and Precautions

As for Gonadorelin, p.1247. Some women may experience vaginal bleeding during initial therapy, which normally resolves spontaneously.

Pituitary apoplexy. A report of pituitary apoplexy (a clinical syndrome caused by haemorrhage and infarction of a pituitary adenoma) in an elderly patient with a symptomless pituitary adenoma who was given goserelin for advanced prostate cancer.[1] The patient developed headache, vomiting, visual disturbances, gradual impairment of consciousness, intermittent fever, and progressive hyponatraemia. Symptoms responded to prednisolone replacement therapy.

1. Ando S, *et al.* Pituitary apoplexy after goserelin. *Lancet* 1995; **345:** 458.

Pharmacokinetics

Goserelin is almost completely absorbed following subcutaneous injection, and has a serum elimination half-life of 2 to 4 hours, which may be increased in patients with impaired renal function. More than 90% of a dose is excreted in urine, as unchanged drug and metabolites.

Uses and Administration

Goserelin acetate is an analogue of gonadorelin (see p.1248) with similar properties. It is used for the suppression of gonadal sex hormone production in the treatment of malignant neoplasms of the prostate, in advanced breast cancer in pre- and peri-menopausal women, and in the management of endometriosis and uterine fibroids. It is also given before surgery for endometrial reduction and as an adjunct to ovulation induction with gonadotrophins in the treatment of infertility.

Goserelin acetate is available as depot preparations; with one such preparation a dose equivalent to 3.6 mg of goserelin injected subcutaneously into the anterior abdominal wall provides effective suppression of oestradiol or testosterone for 28 days. A full response should be achieved by the end of this period and treatment is continued with repeated doses at 28-day intervals; in endometriosis, therapy is given for up to 6 months while in women with anaemia as a result of uterine fibroids it is continued, with concomitant iron supplementation, for up to 3 months before surgery. In men with prostate cancer preparations supplying the equivalent of 10.8 mg of goserelin, given every 12 weeks, may also be employed.

In the treatment of prostatic cancer an anti-androgen such as cyproterone acetate may be given for several days before beginning goserelin therapy and continued for at least 3 weeks, to avoid the risk of a disease flare.

Regimens for oocyte collection for *in-vitro* fertilisation employ gonadorelin analogues for pituitary desensitisation before ovulation induction with gonadotrophins. The equivalent of 3.6 mg of goserelin is given as a subcutaneous depot injection and serum-oestradiol concentrations monitored until they decline to levels similar to those in the early follicular phase, a process which usually takes 7 to 21 days. Once downregulation occurs gonadotrophin therapy is begun until an appropriate stage of follicular development, when it is withdrawn and chorionic gonadotrophin is given to induce ovulation.

Goserelin has also been given in other sex-hormone-related conditions.

Reviews of goserelin.

1. Chrisp P, Goa KL. Goserelin: a review of its pharmacodynamic and pharmacokinetic properties, and clinical use in sex hormone-related conditions. *Drugs* 1991; **41:** 254–88.
2. Perry CM, Brogden RN. Goserelin: a review of its pharmacodynamic and pharmacokinetic properties, and therapeutic use in benign gynaecological disorders. *Drugs* 1996; **51:** 319–46.

Endometriosis. Gonadorelin analogues such as goserelin are effective in the management of endometriosis (p.1442), but the need for long-term therapy to prevent recurrence limits their value because of the risk of osteoporosis; 'add-back' therapy, with concomitant hormone replacement, is being investigated.

References.

1. Shaw RW, *et al.* An open randomized comparative study of the effect of goserelin depot and danazol in the treatment of endometriosis. *Fertil Steril* 1992; **58:** 265–72.

Fibroids. Gonadorelin analogues such as goserelin have been tried as an adjunct or an alternative to surgery in the treatment of uterine fibroids (p.1248), although there has been some concern that this might complicate the diagnosis of malignancy. Some further references are listed below.

1. Lumsden MA, *et al.* Goserelin therapy before surgery for uterine fibroids. *Lancet* 1987; **i:** 36–7.
2. Lumsden MA, *et al.* Treatment with the gonadotrophin releasing hormone-agonist goserelin before hysterectomy for uterine fibroids. *Br J Obstet Gynaecol* 1994; **101:** 438–42.
3. Benagiano G, *et al.* Zoladex (goserelin acetate) and the anemic patient: results of a multicenter fibroid study. *Fertil Steril* 1996; **66:** 223–9.

Malignant neoplasms. Goserelin 3.6 mg injected subcutaneously as a depot preparation every 28 days is effective[1,2] in the treatment of prostate cancer (p.491). It has produced a response comparable with that of orchidectomy (surgical removal of the testes) in patients with metastatic prostate cancer.[3-5] Goserelin combined with the anti-androgen flutamide also produced an overall survival similar to that of orchidectomy.[6] There is some evidence that adjuvant therapy with goserelin may improve survival in patients with locally advanced prostate cancer when combined with radiotherapy.[7]

Goserelin may also be used as hormonal therapy in premenopausal women with advanced breast cancer, either alone[8,9] or combined with tamoxifen,[10] and is said to be as effective as oophorectomy.[9]

There are reports of goserelin producing a response in pancreatic cancer,[11] and in adenocarcinoma of the salivary glands.[12] However, its role in the management of these malignancies is less well established. For discussions of the conventional management of malignancies of the breast and pancreas see p.485 and p.491 respectively.

1. Williams G, *et al.* Biodegradable polymer luteinising hormone releasing hormone analogue for prostatic cancer: use of a new peptide delivery system. *Br Med J* 1984; **289:** 1580–1.
2. Ahmed SR, *et al.* Preliminary report on use of depot formulation of LHRH analogue ICI-118630 (Zoladex) in patients with prostatic cancer. *Br Med J* 1985; **290:** 185–7.
3. Ryan PG, Peeling WB. UK trials of treatment for M1 prostatic cancer: the LH-RH analogue Zoladex vs orchidectomy. *Am J Clin Oncol* 1988; **11** (suppl 2): S169–72.
4. Peeling WB, *et al.* Phase III studies to compare goserelin (Zoladex) with orchiectomy and with diethylstilbestrol in treatment of prostatic carcinoma. *Urology* 1989; **33** (suppl): 45–52.
5. Soloway M, *et al.* A phase III, multicenter comparison of depot Zoladex and orchiectomy in patients with previously-untreated, stage D_2 prostrate cancer. *Gynecol Endocrinol* 1988; **2** (suppl 1): 60.
6. Iversen P, *et al.* Zoladex and flutamide versus orchiectomy in the treatment of advanced prostatic cancer: a combined analysis of two European studies, EORTC 30853 and DAPROCA 86. *Cancer* 1990; **66** (suppl): 1067–73.
7. Bolla M, *et al.* Improved survival in patients with locally advanced prostrate cancer treated with radiotherapy and goserelin. *N Engl J Med* 1997; **337:** 295–300.
8. Dixon AR, *et al.* Goserelin (Zoladex) in premenopausal advanced breast cancer: duration of response and survival. *Br J Cancer* 1990; **62:** 868–70.
9. Bajetta E, *et al.* Goserelin in premenopausal advanced breast cancer: clinical and endocrine evaluation of responsive patients. *Oncology* 1994; **51:** 262–9.
10. Jonat W, *et al.* A randomised study to compare the effect of the luteinising hormone releasing hormone (LHRH) analogue goserelin with or without tamoxifen in pre- and perimenopausal patients with advanced breast cancer. *Eur J Cancer* 1995; **31A:** 137–42.
11. Andrén-Sandberg Å. Treatment with an LHRH analogue in patients with advanced pancreatic cancer: a preliminary report. *Acta Chir Scand* 1990; **156:** 549–51.
12. van der Hulst RWM, *et al.* Partial remission of parotid gland carcinoma after goserelin. *Lancet* 1994; **344:** 817.

Mastalgia. For reference to the use of goserelin in mastalgia, see under Danazol, p.1443.

Preparations

Proprietary Preparations (details are given in Part 3)
Aust.: Zoladex; ***Austral.:*** Zoladex; ***Belg.:*** Zoladex; ***Canad.:*** Zoladex; ***Fr.:*** Zoladex; ***Ger.:*** Zoladex; ***Irl.:*** Zoladex; ***Ital.:*** Zoladex; ***Neth.:*** Zoladex; ***Norw.:*** Zoladex; ***S.Afr.:*** Zoladex; ***Spain:*** Zoladex; ***Swed.:*** Zoladex; ***Switz.:*** Zoladex; ***UK:*** Zoladex; ***USA:*** Zoladex.

Growth Hormone (3882-t)

Growth Hormone *(BAN)*.

GH; Phyone; Somatotrophin; Somatotropin; STH.

CAS — 9002-72-6.

Somatrem (12012-b)

Somatrem *(BAN, USAN, pINN)*.

Met-HGH; Methionyl Human Growth Hormone.

$C_{995}H_{1537}N_{263}O_{301}S_8$ = 22 256.

CAS — 82030-87-3.

Somatrem is an analogue of somatropin containing an additional (methionyl) amino-acid residue. It may be produced in bacteria from recombinant DNA. Sometribove (*BAN*) is methionyl bovine growth hormone, sometripor (*BAN*) is methionyl porcine growth hormone, and somidobove (*BAN*) is synthetic bovine growth hormone.

Somatropin (5933-q)

Somatropin *(BAN, USAN, rINN)*.

CB-311; HGH; Human Growth Hormone; LY-137998.

$C_{990}H_{1528}N_{262}O_{300}S_7$ = 22 125.

CAS — 12629-01-5.

Pharmacopoeias. In *Eur.* (see p.viii), which also includes Somatropin Bulk Solution.

Somatropin is synthetic human growth hormone having the normal structure of the major (22K) component of natural human pituitary growth hormone. It consists of a single polypeptide chain of 191 amino acids with disulphide linkages between positions 53 and 165 and between 182 and 189. For labelling purposes, the name may carry in parentheses an approved code in lower case letters indicative of the method of production: (epr) indicates production by enzymatic conversion of a precursor produced by a bacterium genetically modified by recombinant DNA technology; (rbe) indicates production from bacteria genetically modified by recombinant DNA technology; (rmc) indicates production from genetically engineered and transformed mammalian (mouse) cells.

A white or almost white powder, containing not less than 2.5 units per mg. **Store** at 2° to 8° in airtight containers. The bulk solution should be stored at −20° in airtight containers.

Units

4.4 units of human growth hormone (somatropin) are contained in 1.75 mg of freeze-dried purified human growth hormone, with 20 mg of glycine, 2 mg of mannitol, 2 mg of lactose, and 2 mg of sodium bicarbonate, in one ampoule of the first International Standard (1987).

The first International Standard for Somatropin (1994) has a defined content of 2 mg of protein per ampoule, with a specific activity of 3 units per mg of protein. Commercial preparations vary somewhat in the number of units per mg.

References.

1. WHO. WHO Expert Committee on biological standardization: forty-fourth report. *WHO Tech Rep Ser 848* 1994.
2. WHO. WHO Expert Committee on biological standardization: forty-fifty report *WHO Tech Rep Ser 858* 1995.

Adverse Effects and Precautions

Antibodies to growth hormone have been formed in some patients but these rarely seem to affect growth. There may be redness, itching, lumps, or lipoatrophy at the site of injection. Transient dose-related fluid retention with peripheral oedema has occurred; headache, muscle and joint pain, and cases of benign intracranial hypertension have been reported. Although growth hormone has diabetogenic effects, high acute dosage has been associated with hypoglycaemia.

Therapy is contra-indicated in patients with active neoplasms or intracranial lesions and should be discontinued if evidence of tumour growth develops. Growth hormones should not be used for growth promotion in patients with closed epiphyses. Because of the diabetogenic effect of growth hormone it should be given with care to patients with diabetes mellitus; adjustment of antidiabetic therapy may be necessary. Hypothyroidism may develop during treatment, and may result in suboptimal response. For the suggestion that growth hormone should not be used to treat acute catabolic states, as in patients with severe burns or who are otherwise critically ill, see Burns, under Uses and Administration, below.

Benign intracranial hypertension. Benign intracranial hypertension (pseudotumor cerebri) had occurred in 22 children and 1 adult given growth hormone treatment between 1986 and 1993.[1] Eight further cases were identified in a subsequent report in 1995.[2] Three patients treated with mecasermin also developed benign intracranial hypertension. Symptoms such as headache and papilloedema resolved when treatment was stopped. In a report of another case[3] it was pointed out that diagnosis may be complicated by the not infrequent occurrence of headache in patients receiving growth hormone; these normally resolved spontaneously.

1. Malozowski S, *et al.* Growth hormone, insulin-like growth factor I, and benign intracranial hypertension. *N Engl J Med* 1993; **329:** 665–6.
2. Malozowski S, *et al.* Benign intracranial hypertension in children with growth hormone deficiency treated with growth hormone. *J Pediatr* 1995; **126:** 996–9.
3. Price DA, *et al.* Benign intracranial hypertension induced by growth hormone treatment. *Lancet* 1995; **345:** 458–9.

Carcinogenicity. Despite fears to the contrary studies in children given growth hormone after cranial irradiation for brain tumours or CNS leukaemia have found no evidence that therapy with growth hormone increased the relapse rate.[1,2] Nevertheless, 5 cases of acute leukaemia have been reported among patients in Japan treated with growth hormones, a 9.4-fold increase over the expected incidence,[3] and other cases have been reported subsequently.[4,5] An international workshop convened in 1988 to review known leukaemia cases in patients treated with growth hormones in Europe, North America, Japan, and Australia since 1959 found the observed incidence of leukaemia in growth-hormone-treated patients to represent a 2-fold increase over the expected rate.[6] After a careful review of the data it was concluded that there may be a small increase in leukaemia incidence associated with growth hormone treatment of growth hormone-deficient patients, but that it was not clear that this was actually attributable to growth hormone. A later study involving 6284 patients treated with growth hormone between 1963 and 1985 in the USA confirmed an increase of about 2.5-fold in the incidence of leukaemia in this population, but noted that many of the patients had other risk factors for leukaemia.[7] It has been suggested that growth hormone deficiency is itself a risk factor for leukaemia and that perhaps this, rather than growth hormone treatment is related to the increased incidence of leukaemia in these patients.[8] If there is any risk it is relatively small, and in view of the essential nature of growth hormone therapy in growth hormone-deficient children it would be inappropriate and unwise to withhold it.[6]

Further reports of malignancies associated with growth hormone therapy include two children with Bloom's syndrome (a rare chromosomal disorder affecting DNA replication), one of whom developed B-cell non-Hodgkin's lymphoma and the other stem-cell leukaemia.[9]

1. Clayton PE, *et al.* Does growth hormone cause relapse of brain tumours? *Lancet* 1987; **i:** 711–13.
2. Ogilvy-Stuart AL, *et al.* Growth hormone and tumour recurrence. *Br Med J* 1992; **304:** 1601–5.
3. Watanabe S, *et al.* Leukaemia in patients treated with growth hormone. *Lancet* 1988; **i:** 1159.
4. Delemarre-Van de Waal HA, *et al.* Leukaemia in patients treated with growth hormone. *Lancet* 1988; **i:** 1159.
5. Watanabe S, *et al.* Leukemia and other malignancies among GH users. *J Pediatr Endocrinol* 1993; **6:** 99–108.
6. Fisher DA, *et al.* Leukaemia in patients treated with growth hormone. *Lancet* 1988; **i:** 1159–60.
7. Fradkin JE, *et al.* Risk of leukemia after treatment with pituitary growth hormone. *JAMA* 1993; **270:** 2829–32.
8. Rapaport R, *et al.* Relationship of growth hormone deficiency and leukemia. *J Pediatr* 1995; **126:** 759–61.
9. Brock PR, *et al.* Malignant disease in Bloom's syndrome children treated with growth hormone. *Lancet* 1991; **337:** 1345–6.

Creutzfeldt-Jakob disease. Reports in 1985 of a small number of deaths from Creutzfeldt-Jakob disease in patients under 40 years of age who had received growth hormone extracted from human pituitary glands resulted in the suspension of the distribution of pituitary-derived growth hormone by the licensing authorities in a number of countries, including Australia, Canada, the Netherlands, the UK, and the USA.[1-5] Preparations of non-pituitary-derived growth hormone are now available that are free from contamination with Creutzfeldt-Jakob virus. However, because of the long incubation period of this virus, cases of infection are still being reported in patients who had received pituitary-derived growth hormone years previously.[6-9]

1. Brown P, *et al.* Potential epidemic of Creutzfeldt-Jakob disease from human growth hormone therapy. *N Engl J Med* 1985; **313:** 728–33. Correction. *ibid.*; 967.
2. Powell-Jackson J, *et al.* Creutzfeldt-Jakob disease after administration of human growth hormone. *Lancet* 1985; **ii:** 244–6.
3. Anonymous. Human growth hormone distribution discontinued. *FDA Drug Bull* 1985; **15:** 17–18.
4. Lazarus L. Suspension of the Australian human pituitary hormone programme. *Med J Aust* 1985; **143:** 57–9.
5. Bannister BA, McCormick A. Creutzfeldt-Jakob disease with reference to the safety of pituitary growth hormone. *J Infect* 1987; **14:** 7–12.
6. Fradkin JE, *et al.* Creutzfeldt-Jakob disease in pituitary growth hormone recipients in the United States. *JAMA* 1991; **265:** 880–4.
7. Buchanan CR, *et al.* Mortality, neoplasia, and Creutzfeldt-Jakob disease in patients treated with human pituitary growth hormone in the United Kingdom. *Br Med J* 1991; **302:** 824–8.
8. Billette de Villemeur T, *et al.* Creutzfeldt-Jakob disease in children treated with growth hormone. *Lancet* 1991; **337:** 864–5.
9. Macario ME, *et al.* Pituitary growth hormone and Creutzfeldt-Jakob disease. *Br Med J* 1991; **302:** 1149.

Effects on carbohydrate metabolism. Symptomatic diabetes mellitus developed in a child given somatropin for familial short stature.[1] In another case[2] nonketotic hyperglycaemia developed within weeks of beginning growth hormone therapy in a 22-month-old child, leading to convulsions and metabolic acidosis; the patient died despite correction of the hyperglycaemia.

1. Botero D, *et al.* Symptomatic non-insulin-dependent diabetes mellitus during therapy with recombinant human growth hormone. *J Pediatr* 1993; **123:** 590–2.
2. Garg AK, Hyperglycemia during replacement growth hormone therapy. *J Pediatr* 1994; **125:** 329.

Effects on immune function. Growth hormone is generally considered to interact with the immune system although there is a lack of evidence that this is clinically significant.[1,2] There has been a report of acute renal transplant rejection in 2 children receiving treatment for growth retardation with somatropin.[3] In both children renal function of the transplant was stable for several years before somatropin was started, and growth hormone therapy had continued for some months before rejection occurred. It was suggested that during the first months of growth hormone therapy in transplant recipients, immunosuppressive therapy should be increased and transplant function carefully monitored.

1. Church JA, *et al.* Immune functions in children treated with biosynthetic growth hormone. *J Pediatr* 1989; **115:** 420–3.
2. Rapaport R, Oleske J. Immune function during growth hormone therapy. *J Pediatr* 1990; **116:** 669–70.
3. Tydén G, *et al.* Acute renal graft rejection after treatment with human growth hormone. *Lancet* 1990; **336:** 1455–6.

Effects on skeletal muscle. A report of mild inflammatory myositis, with myalgia and muscle weakness, in 2 patients receiving growth hormone therapy.[1] It was suggested that the effect might be due to *m*-cresol used as a preservative in the preparation.

1. Yordam N. Myositis associated with growth hormone therapy. *J Pediatr* 1994; **125:** 671.

Gynaecomastia. A report of 22 cases of prepubertal gynaecomastia diagnosed during growth hormone treatment.[1]

1. Malozowski S, Stadel BV. Prepubertal gynecomastia during growth hormone therapy. *J Pediatr* 1995; **126:** 659–61.

Hypersensitivity. Generalised urticaria in a patient given somatropin was overcome by a desensitisation regimen.[1] The patient was subsequently maintained uneventfully on daily injections of somatropin.

1. Walker SB, *et al.* Systemic reaction to human growth hormone treated with acute desensitization. *Pediatrics* 1992; **90:** 108–9.

Iron supplementation. The view has been expressed[1] that given the increased production of haemoglobin and the prevalence of iron deficiency in patients treated with growth hormone, supplementation with iron should be considered in patients receiving growth hormone treatment.

1. Vihervuori E, *et al.* Increases in hemoglobin concentration and iron needs in response to growth hormone treatment. *J Pediatr* 1994; **125:** 242–5.

Pancreatitis. A report of acute pancreatitis in a patient with pseudohypoparathyroidism and growth hormone deficiency following the institution of growth hormone treatment.[1] Ten further cases of acute pancreatitis associated with growth hormone treatment had been reported to the FDA at the time of writing.

1. Malozowski S, *et al.* Acute pancreatitis associated with growth hormone therapy for short stature. *N Engl J Med* 1995; **332:** 401–2.

Interactions

High doses of corticosteroids may inhibit the growth promoting effects of growth hormone.

Pharmacokinetics

Somatropin is well absorbed after subcutaneous or intramuscular injection with a bioavailability varying from about 60 to 80%; peak serum concentrations may not be achieved for several hours. After intravenous injection it has a half-life of about 20 to 30 minutes but after subcutaneous or intramuscular administration serum concentrations decline with a half-life of 3 to 5 hours, due to more prolonged release from the injection site. It is metabolised in the liver and kidneys and excreted in bile.

A study of the pharmacokinetics of somatropin following transdermal jet injection in healthy subjects suggested that absorption was more rapid and peak serum concentration higher than after conventional subcutaneous injection of the same dose.[1] However this did not seem to result in any difference in the total amount absorbed, nor in the biological effect of the drug.

1. Verhagen A, *et al.* Pharmacokinetics and pharmacodynamics of a single dose of recombinant human growth hormone after subcutaneous administration by jet-injection: comparison with conventional needle-injection. *Eur J Clin Pharmacol* 1995; **49:** 69–72.

Uses and Administration

Somatropin is synthetic human growth hormone and somatrem its methionyl analogue. Growth hormone is an anabolic hormone secreted by the anterior lobe of the pituitary, varying in size and amino-acid sequence between animal species. It promotes growth of skeletal, muscular, and other tissues, stimulates protein anabolism, and affects fat and mineral metabolism. The hormone has a diabetogenic action on carbohydrate metabolism.

Secretion is pulsatile and dependent on neural and hormonal influences including a hypothalamic release-inhibiting hormone (see Somatostatin, p.1261), and a hypothalamic releasing hormone (see Somatorelin, p.1260). Sleep, hypoglycaemia, and physical or emotional stress result in increased secretion of growth hormone. The effects of growth hormone on skeletal growth are mediated by the somatomedins (see p.1260).

Somatropin or somatrem is given to children with open epiphyses for the treatment of short stature due to growth hormone deficiency (pituitary dwarfism) following assessment of pituitary function. Somatropin is also used in children with some other forms of growth retardation, for example in Turner's syndrome or that due to chronic renal insufficiency. In adults, somatropin is given for confirmed growth hormone deficiency. It is also used in the management of wasting or cachexia associated with AIDS.

Doses should be individualised for each patient. Manufacturers vary somewhat in their estimates of the number of units per mg for somatropin and although some countries specify labelling in mg, others require labelling in units or both. Somatrem may be given in doses similar to those of somatropin.

In children with growth hormone deficiency, the usual dose in the UK is 0.5 to 0.7 units per kg body-weight, or 12 to 20 units per m^2 body-surface, weekly. (This corresponds to about 0.18 to 0.26 mg per kg weekly.) This weekly dose may be given by intramuscular injection in 3 divided doses or by subcutaneous injection, usually in 6 or 7 divided doses. Similar dosage regimens are employed in other countries. In Turner's syndrome (gonadal dysgenesis) higher doses are suggested of up to about 1 unit per kg or 28 units per m^2 weekly in 6 or 7 divided doses by subcutaneous injection. Similar doses may be employed in children with growth retardation due to chronic renal insufficiency.

In adults with growth hormone deficiency lower doses are recommended. A suggested initial dose is 0.125 units per kg weekly, divided into daily subcutaneous injections, and increased according to requirements up to a maximum of 0.25 units per kg per week. Dosage requirements may decline with increasing age.

In the treatment of wasting or cachexia in patients with AIDS somatropin is given is doses of 0.1 mg per kg daily by subcutaneous injection at bedtime.

Administration in adults. Growth hormone continues to be secreted in adult life, although secretion and activity gradually decline with increasing age, and it appears to play a role in maintaining skeletal and lean body-mass amongst other things. In adults with growth hormone deficiency (usually secondary to pituitary adenoma or its treatment) replacement therapy with growth hormone improves bone mineral density, decreases fat mass and increases lean body-mass, resting metabolic rate, and in some cases improves feelings of well being.[1-7] Doses need to be lower than in children:[1,2] an initial dose of 0.0125 units per kg body-weight daily, increased if necessary at 2- to 3-week intervals, has been suggested.[1]

Less well established is the use of growth hormone in otherwise healthy elderly patients.[8-11] Considerable controversy has attended suggestions that growth hormone therapy may retard or reverse some of the metabolic effects of ageing, and there is some concern that these patients may be at increased risk of adverse effects: in one small study 6 of 12 healthy elderly subjects given growth hormone therapy withdrew due to symptoms of carpal tunnel syndrome, fluid retention, or arthralgia.[10]

Other uses for growth hormone in adult patients are discussed below.

1. Powrie J, *et al.* Growth hormone replacement therapy for growth hormone-deficient adults. *Drugs* 1995; **49:** 656–63.
2. Shalet SM. Growth hormone deficiency and replacement in adults. *Br Med J* 1996; **313:** 314.
3. Salomon F, *et al.* The effects of treatment with recombinant human growth hormone on body composition and metabolism in adults with growth hormone deficiency. *N Engl J Med* 1989; **321:** 1797–1803.
4. Jørgensen JOL, *et al.* Beneficial effects of growth hormone treatment in GH-deficient adults. *Lancet* 1989; **i:** 1221–5.
5. Whitehead HM, *et al.* Growth hormone treatment of adults with growth hormone deficiency: effect on fat and carbohydrate metabolism. *Diabetes* 1990; **39** (suppl 1): 298.
6. Baum HBA, *et al.* Effects of physiologic growth hormone therapy on bone density and body composition in patients with adult-onset growth hormone deficiency: a randomized, placebo-controlled trial. *Ann Intern Med* 1996; **125:** 883–90.
7. Cuneo RC, *et al.* The Australian multicenter trial of growth hormone (GH) treatment in GH-deficient adults. *J Clin Endocrinol Metab* 1998; **83:** 107–116.
8. Rudman D, *et al.* Effects of human growth hormone in men over 60 years old. *N Engl J Med* 1990; **323:** 1–6.
9. Marcus R, *et al.* Effects of short term administration of recombinant human growth hormone to elderly people. *J Clin Endocrinol Metab* 1990; **70:** 519–27.
10. Yarasheski KE, Zachwieja JJ. Growth hormone therapy for the elderly: the fountain of youth proves toxic. *JAMA* 1993; **270:** 1694.
11. Papadakis MA, *et al.* Growth hormone replacement in healthy older men improves body composition but not functional ability. *Ann Intern Med* 1996; **124:** 708–16.

Burns. In children with severe burns requiring skin grafts, somatropin 0.2 mg per kg body-weight daily by intramuscular injection reduced donor-site healing times and hospitalisation times; subcutaneous somatropin 0.1 mg per kg daily was ineffective.[1] However, the manufacturers have recommended that somatropin should not be used to treat acute catabolic states in critically ill and burn patients, as there is some evidence that mortality may be increased. The management of burns is described on p.1073.

1. Herndon DN, *et al.* Effects of recombinant human growth hormone on donor-site healing in severely burned children. *Ann Surg* 1990; **212:** 424–9.

Cachexia. Treatment with subcutaneous growth hormone has been reported to reverse weight loss and improve body wasting in subjects with HIV disease,[1-3] and somatropin is licensed for this indication in the USA. Dosage may be important: most studies have used doses of around 0.1 mg per kg body-weight, but a study using lower doses, alone or combined with mecasermin, reported only modest improvement.[4] Mecasermin alone was of uncertain value.

Growth hormone therapy has also been reported to improve metabolic indicators of malnutrition when given together with parenteral nutrition to patients undergoing haemodialysis.[5]

1. Krentz AJ, *et al.* Anthropometric, metabolic, and immunological effects of recombinant human growth hormone in AIDS and AIDS-related complex. *J Acquir Immune Defic Syndr* 1993; **6:** 245–51.
2. Mulligan K, *et al.* Anabolic effects of recombinant human growth hormone in patients with wasting associated with human immunodeficiency virus infection. *J Clin Endocrinol Metab* 1993; **77:** 956–62.
3. Schambelan M, *et al.* Recombinant human growth hormone in patients with HIV-associated wasting: a randomized, placebo-controlled trial. *Ann Intern Med* 1996; **125:** 873–82.
4. Waters D, *et al.* Recombinant human growth hormone, insulin-like growth factor 1, and combination therapy in AIDS-associated wasting: a randomized, double-blind, placebo-controlled trial. *Ann Intern Med* 1996; **125:** 865–72.
5. Schulman G, *et al.* The effects of recombinant human growth hormone and intradialytic parenteral nutrition in malnourished haemodialysis patients. *Am J Kidney Dis* 1993; **21:** 527–34.

Cardiomyopathies. Administration of growth hormone for 12 weeks to patients with heart failure secondary to dilated cardiomyopathy (p.785) produced an increase in left-ventricular mass but no improvement in clinical status.[1]

1. Osterziel KJ, *et al.* Randomised, double-blind, placebo-controlled trial of human recombinant growth hormone in patients with chronic heart failure due to dilated cardiomyopathy. *Lancet* 1998; **351:** 1233–7.

Fibromyalgia. Symptomatic improvement was reported after several months in a study of daily subcutaneous growth hormone injection in women with fibromyalgia,[1] a painful form of soft-tissue rheumatism (p.4), and low levels of insulin-like growth factor 1 (IGF-1).

1. Bennett RM, *et al.* A randomized, double-blind, placebo-controlled study of growth hormone in the treatment of fibromyalgia. *Am J Med* 1998; **104:** 227–31.

Growth retardation. For a discussion of the management of growth retardation, including the role of growth hormone, see p.1237. Where growth retardation is associated with growth hormone deficiency, growth hormone replacement therapy is an appropriate treatment, and significantly improves growth velocity, although there are some doubts about the extent of the benefit in terms of final height. The use of growth hormone in children with short stature but without clinical growth hormone deficiency is, however, controversial and of unproven efficacy.

Guidelines[1] have been issued in the USA for the appropriate use of growth hormone in children with short stature. These consider the use of growth hormone unproven other than in growth hormone deficiency and probably Turner's syndrome (but see p.1240) and chronic renal insufficiency.

1. Drug and Therapeutics Committee, Lawson Wilkins Pediatric Endocrine Society. Guidelines for the use of growth hormone in children with short stature. *J Pediatr* 1995; **127:** 857–67.

Infertility. Studies[1,2] have found that somatropin sensitises the ovary to stimulation by gonadotrophins and it has been suggested that it may have a role in the management of female infertility in patients resistant to conventional ovarian stimulation.[1] However, some workers have found it of little value.[3] Growth hormone has also been tried similarly to enhance spermatogenesis in infertile men unresponsive to conventional therapy.[4,5]

For a discussion of infertility and the more usual drugs used in its management, see p.1239.

1. Homburg R, *et al.* Cotreatment with human growth hormone and gonadotropins for induction of ovulation: a controlled clinical trial. *Fertil Steril* 1990; **53:** 254–60.
2. Yoshimura Y, *et al.* Effects of growth hormone on follicle growth, oocyte maturation, and ovarian steroidogenesis. *Fertil Steril* 1993; **59:** 917–23.
3. Levron J, *et al.* No beneficial effects of human growth hormone therapy in normal ovulatory patients with a poor ovarian response to gonadotropins. *Gynecol Obstet Invest* 1993; **35:** 65–8.
4. Shoham Z, *et al.* Cotreatment with growth hormone for induction of spermatogenesis in patients with hypogonadotropic hypogonadism. *Fertil Steril* 1992; **57:** 1044–51.
5. Ovesen PG. *et al.* Vaeksthormonbehandling af maend med nedsat saedkvalitet. *Ugeskr Laeger* 1998; **160:** 176–80.

Osteogenesis imperfecta. For reference to possible benefit from growth hormone therapy in patients with osteogenesis imperfecta, see p.730.

Osteomalacia. As mentioned on p.730, there has been some interest in the use of growth hormone in children with hypophosphataemic rickets.

Ulcers. Severe necrotic ulceration of the heel, sufficiently deep to expose the calcaneum, in a diabetic patient, responded to an extemporaneous preparation containing 4 units of somatropin in 50 mL of an ointment vehicle based on cod-liver oil and soft white paraffin. On doubling the concentration of somatropin the rate of healing appeared to accelerate.[1]

For a discussion of diabetic foot disease and other diabetic complications see p.315. The management of wounds and ulcers is discussed on p.1076.

1. Waagø H. Local treatment of ulcers in diabetic foot with human growth hormone. *Lancet* 1987; **i:** 1485.

Veterinary and agricultural use. Bovine growth hormone or bovine somatotrophin (bovine somatotropin; BST) can increase milk yield. Some references to the debate on the safety of this practice follow.

1. Anonymous. Bovine somatotropin and human health. *Lancet* 1988; **ii:** 376.
2. Davis C. Safety of bovine somatotropin. *Lancet* 1988; **ii:** 629.
3. Brunner E. Safety of bovine somatotropin. *Lancet* 1988; **ii:** 629.
4. Daughaday WH, Barbano DM. Bovine somatotropin supplementation of dairy cows: is the milk safe? *JAMA* 1990; **264:** 1003–5. Correction. *ibid.* 1991; **265:** 1393.
5. Mepham TB. Bovine somatotrophin and public health. *Br Med J* 1991; **302:** 483–4.
6. Kronfeld DS. Bovine somatotropin. *JAMA* 1991; **265:** 1389.
7. Daughaday WH, Barbano DM. Bovine somatotropin. *JAMA* 1991; **265:** 1389–90.

Preparations

BP 1998: Somatropin Injection.

Proprietary Preparations (details are given in Part 3)

Aust.: Genotropin; Humatrope; Norditropin; Saizen; ***Austral.:*** Genotropin; Humatro-Pen; Humatrope; Norditropin; Saizen; Somatonorm†; ***Belg.:*** Genotonorm; Humatrope; Norditropin; Saizen†; Zomacton; ***Canad.:*** Humatrope; Protropin; Saizen; ***Fr.:*** Genotonorm; Maxomat; Norditropine; Saizen; Umatrope; ***Ger.:*** Genotropin; Grorm†; Humatrope; Norditropin; Saizen; Zomacton; ***Irl.:*** Genotropin; Norditropin; Saizen; Somatonorm†; Zomacton; ***Ital.:*** Genotropin; Grorm†; Humatrope; Norditropin; Saizen; Somatonorm†; Zomacton; ***Neth.:*** Genotropin; Humatrope; Norditropin; Zomacton; ***Norw.:*** Genotropin; Humatrope; Norditropin; Saizen; ***S.Afr.:*** Genotropin; Humatrope; Norditropin; Saizen; ***Spain:*** Genotonorm; Humatrope; Norditropin; Saizen; Somatonorm†; Zomacton; ***Swed.:*** Genotropin; Humatrope; Norditropin; Saizen; Somatonorm†; Zomacton; ***Switz.:*** Genotropin; Humatrope; Norditropine; Saizen; ***UK:*** Genotropin; Humatrope; Norditropin; Saizen; Zomacton; ***USA:*** Genotropin; Humatrope; Norditropin; Nutropin; Protropin; Serostim.

Histrelin Acetate (15849-b)

Histrelin Acetate *(rINNM)*.

ORF-17070 (histrelin); RWJ-17070 (histrelin). 5-Oxo-L-prolyl-L-histidyl-L-tryptophyl-L-seryl-L-tyrosyl-N^{τ}-benzyl-D-histidyl-L-luecyl-L-arginyl-*N*-ethyl-L-prolinamide acetate.

CAS — 76712-82-8 (histrelin).

Adverse Effects and Precautions

As for Gonadorelin, p.1247.

Uses and Administration

Histrelin is an analogue of gonadorelin (p.1248) with similar properties. It is used for the suppression of gonadal sex hormone production in children with central precocious puberty (p.1241). It is given by subcutaneous injection as the acetate, in usual doses equivalent to 10 µg of histrelin per kg body-weight daily.

It has been investigated in various other disorders, including malignant neoplasms of the prostate (p.491) and disorders related to the menstrual cycle. It is also under investigation in the treatment of acute intermittent porphyria.

References.

1. Anderson KE, *et al.* A gonadotropin releasing hormone analogue prevents cyclical attacks of porphyria. *Arch Intern Med* 1990; **150:** 1469–74.
2. Mortola JF, *et al.* Successful treatment of severe premenstrual syndrome by combined use of gonadotropin-releasing hormone agonist and estrogen/progestin. *J Clin Endocrinol Metab* 1991; **72:** 252A–F.
3. Barradell LB, McTavish D. Histrelin: a review of its pharmacological properties and therapeutic role in central precocious puberty. *Drugs* 1993; **45:** 570–88.

Preparations

Proprietary Preparations (details are given in Part 3)

USA: Supprelin.

Human Menopausal Gonadotrophins (17585-l)

Human Menopausal Gonadotrophins *(BAN)*.
HMG; Org-31338; Urogonadotrophin.

A purified extract of human postmenopausal urine containing follicle-stimulating hormone (FSH) and luteinising hormone (LH); the relative *in-vivo* activity is expressed as a ratio. Human menopausal gonadotrophins with a ratio of FSH:LH of 1:1 are known as menotrophin (see below).

Menotrophin (5930-b)

Menotrophin *(BAN)*.
Menotropins *(USAN)*; Menotropinum.
CAS — 9002-68-0.
Pharmacopoeias. In *Aust., Belg., Br., It., Neth., Port.,* and *US.*

Human menopausal gonadotrophins, containing follicle-stimulating hormone and luteinising hormone activity in a ratio of approximately 1:1. Chorionic gonadotrophin obtained from the urine of pregnant women may be added to achieve such a ratio.

Menotrophin is an off-white or slightly yellow powder containing not less than 40 units of follicle-stimulating hormone activity per mg and not less than 40 units of luteinising hormone activity per mg.

Soluble in water. **Store** at 2° to 8° in airtight containers. Protect from light.

Units

54 units of follicle-stimulating hormone and 46 units of luteinising hormone are contained in one ampoule of the third International Standard (1993).

Adverse Effects

Human menopausal gonadotrophins may cause dose-related ovarian hyperstimulation varying from mild ovarian enlargement and abdominal discomfort to severe hyperstimulation with marked ovarian enlargement or cyst formation, acute abdominal pain, ascites, pleural effusion, hypovolaemia, shock and thrombo-embolic disorders. Rupture of ovarian cysts and intraperitoneal haemorrhage has occurred, usually after pelvic examination. Fatalities have been reported.

There is a risk of multiple births. Hypersensitivity reactions and local reactions at the injection site may occur.

Ovarian hyperstimulation syndrome occurring with human menopausal gonadotrophins treatment in 4 women progressed to acute adnexal torsion[1] and in another became severe and was accompanied by deep venous thrombosis.[2]

1. Kemmann E, *et al.* Adnexal torsion in menotropin-induced pregnancies. *Obstet Gynecol* 1990; **76:** 403–6.
2. Kaaja R, *et al.* Severe ovarian hyperstimulation syndrome and deep venous thrombosis. *Lancet* 1989; **ii:** 1043.

Precautions

Human menopausal gonadotrophins should not be given to pregnant patients. Use should be avoided in patients with abnormal genital bleeding, hormone sensitive malignancies such as those of the breast, uterus, prostate, ovaries or testes, or ovarian cysts or enlargement not caused by the polycystic ovary syndrome. Pituitary or hypothalamic lesions, adrenal or thyroid disorders, and hyperprolactinaemia should be appropriately treated to exclude them as causes of infertility before attempting therapy with human menopausal gonadotrophins. Patients who experience ovarian enlargement are at risk of rupture; pelvic examinations should be avoided or carried out with care and the recommendation has been made that sexual intercourse should be avoided while there is such a risk.

Interactions

In women who show evidence of excessive ovarian stimulation while receiving human menopausal gonadotrophins the administration of drugs with luteinising-hormone (LH) activity increases the risk of ovarian hyperstimulation syndrome.

Uses and Administration

Human menopausal gonadotrophins possess both follicle-stimulating hormone (FSH) activity (see p.1247) and luteinising hormone (LH) activity (see p.1254).

Human menopausal gonadotrophins are used in the treatment of male and female infertility due to hypogonadism. In anovulatory infertility unresponsive to clomiphene human menopausal gonadotrophins are administered to induce follicular maturation and are followed by treatment with chorionic gonadotrophin to stimulate ovulation and corpus luteum formation, a topic discussed further on p.1239. In women with polycystic ovary syndrome a gonadorelin analogue may be given beforehand to suppress pituitary gonadotrophin production (see p.1240).

The dosage and schedule of treatment must be determined according to the needs of each patient; it is usual to monitor response by studying the patient's urinary oestrogen excretion or by ultrasonic visualisation of follicles, or both. Human menopausal gonadotrophins may be given daily by intramuscular injection to provide a dose of 75 to 150 units of FSH and gradually adjusted if necessary until an adequate response is achieved. Treatment is then stopped and followed after 1 or 2 days by single doses of chorionic gonadotrophin 5000 to 10 000 units (see p.1243). In menstruating patients treatment should be started within the first 7 days of the menstrual cycle. In the UK it has been suggested that the treatment course should be abandoned if no response is seen in 3 weeks although in the US the manufacturers recommend that an individual course of menotrophin should not exceed 12 days. This course may be repeated at least twice more if necessary.

An alternative schedule is to give three equal doses of menotrophin, each providing 225 to 375 units of FSH on alternate days followed by chorionic gonadotrophin one week after the first dose.

In *in-vitro* fertilisation procedures or other assisted conception techniques human menopausal gonadotrophins are used in conjunction with chorionic gonadotrophin and sometimes also clomiphene citrate or a gonadorelin analogue. Stimulation of follicular growth is produced by human menopausal gonadotrophins in a dose providing 75 to 300 units of FSH daily, usually beginning on the 2nd or 3rd day of the cycle. An example of a combined regimen involves clomiphene citrate 100 mg on days 2 to 6, with human menopausal gonadotrophins beginning on day 5 in a dose providing 150 to 225 units of FSH daily. Treatment is continued until an adequate response is obtained and the final injection of human menopausal gonadotrophins is followed 1 to 2 days later with up to 10 000 units of chorionic gonadotrophin. Oocyte retrieval is carried out about 32 to 36 hours later.

In men with hypogonadotrophic hypogonadism (p.1239), spermatogenesis is stimulated with chorionic gonadotrophin and then human menopausal gonadotrophins are added in a dose of 75 or 150 units of FSH two or three times weekly. Treatment should be continued for at least 3 or 4 months.

Infertility. References to the use of human menopausal gonadotrophins in the management of female infertility[1-12] often with other agents including buserelin,[2,3] chorionic gonadotrophin,[4] clomiphene citrate,[5,6] leuprorelin,[7] ethinyloestradiol,[8] and triptorelin.[9] Anecdotal report suggests that human menopausal gonadotrophins may be more effective than urofollitrophin in treating anovulatory infertility,[10] perhaps because the luteinising hormone content plays some role in follicular development. However, in contrast, others have found the use of a pure recombinant follicle-stimulating hormone to be associated with higher pregnancy rates than human menopausal gonadotrophins when employed in regimens for in-vitro fertilisation.[12]

For a discussion of infertility and its management, including the role of human menopausal gonadotrophins, see p.1239.

1. Serhal PF, *et al.* Unexplained infertility—the value of Pergonal superovulation combined with intrauterine insemination. *Fertil Steril* 1988; **49:** 602–6.
2. Fleming R, *et al.* Combined gonadotropin-releasing hormone analog and exogenous gonadotropins for ovulation induction in infertile women: efficacy related to ovarian function assessment. *Am J Obstet Gynecol* 1988; **159:** 376–81.
3. MacLachlan V, *et al.* A controlled study of luteinizing hormone-releasing hormone agonist (buserelin) for the induction of folliculogenesis before in vitro fertilization. *N Engl J Med* 1989; **320:** 1233–7.
4. Yuen BH, *et al.* Comparison of the outcome of ovulation induction therapy in an in vitro fertilization program employing a low-dose and an individually adjusted high-dose schedule of human menopausal gonadotropins. *Am J Obstet Gynecol* 1985; **151:** 172–5.
5. Kemmann E, Jones JR. Sequential clomiphene citrate-menotropin therapy for induction or enhancement of ovulation. *Fertil Steril* 1983; **39:** 772–9.
6. Afnan AMM, *et al.* Pulsatile gonadotropin administration in in-vitro fertilisation. *Lancet* 1984; **i:** 1239.
7. Lewinthal D, *et al.* Induction of ovulation with luprolide acetate and human menopausal gonadotropin. *Fertil Steril* 1988; **49:** 585–8.
8. Check JH, *et al.* Ovulation induction and pregnancy with an estrogen-gonadotropin stimulation technique in a menopausal woman with marked hypoplastic ovaries. *Am J Obstet Gynecol* 1989; **160:** 405–6.
9. Zorn JR, *et al.* Never on a Sunday: programming for IVF-ET and GIFT. *Lancet* 1987; **i:** 385–6.
10. Vine S, *et al.* Human gonadotrophin preparations. *Br Med J* 1994; **308:** 1509–10.
11. White DM, *et al.* Induction of ovulation with low-dose gonadotropins in polycystic ovary syndrome: an analysis of 109 pregnancies in 225 women. *J Clin Endocrinol Metab* 1996; **81:** 3821–4.
12. Out HJ, *et al.* Recombinant follicle-stimulating hormone (follitropin beta, Puregon) yields higher pregnancy rates in in vitro fertilization than urinary gonadotropins. *Fertil Steril* 1997; **68:** 138–42.

Preparations

BP 1998: Menotrophin Injection;
USP 23: Menotropins for Injection.

Proprietary Preparations (details are given in Part 3)
Aust.: Humegon; Pergonal; ***Austral.:*** Humegon; Pergonal†; ***Belg.:*** Humegon; Pergonal†; ***Canad.:*** Humegon; Pergonal; ***Fr.:*** Humegon; Inductor†; Neo-Pergonal; ***Ger.:*** Humegon; Menogon; Pergonal; ***Irl.:*** Humegon; Pergonal; ***Ital.:*** Pergogreen; Pergonal†; ***Jpn:*** Gonadoryl†; ***Neth.:*** Humegon; Pergonal; ***Norw.:*** Humegon; Pergonal†; ***S.Afr.:*** Humegon; Pergonal; ***Spain:*** HMG; Pergonal; ***Swed.:*** Humegon†; Pergogreen†; Pergonal†; ***Switz.:*** Humegon; Pergogreen; Pergonal; ***UK:*** Humegon; Menogon; Normegon; Pergonal; ***USA:*** Humegon; Pergonal; Repronex.

Lanreotide Acetate (17187-r)

Lanreotide Acetate *(BANM, USAN, rINNM)*.
BIM-23014C. 3-(2-Naphthyl)-D-alanyl-L-cysteinyl-L-tyrosyl-D-tryptophyl-L-lysyl-L-valyl-L-cysteinyl-L-threoninamide cyclic (2→7)-disulfide acetate.
$C_{54}H_{69}N_{11}O_{10}S_2,x(C_2H_4O_2)$.
CAS — 108736-35-2 (lanreotide); 127984-74-1 (lanreotide acetate).

Adverse Effects and Precautions

As for Octreotide Acetate, p.1255.

Interactions

As for Octreotide Acetate, p.1255.

Pharmacokinetics

Following intramuscular administration of sustained-release lanreotide an initial rapid liberation of the drug is followed by more prolonged release with an apparent half-life of about 5 days. The absolute bioavailability is stated to be about 50%.

Uses and Administration

Lanreotide is a somatostatin analogue with similar general properties to those of octreotide (see p.1255). It is given, as a long-acting intramuscular depot injection, in the treatment of acromegaly (see p.1235), as well as in the management of carcinoid tumours (see p.477).

Lanreotide is administered as the acetate. The usual dose, in both acromegaly and the carcinoid syndrome, is the equivalent of 30 mg of lanreotide by intramuscular depot injection every 14 days, increased if necessary to 30 mg every 10 days.

Lanreotide has been tried for the prevention of restenosis in coronary blood vessels following angioplasty.

References.

1. Parmar H, *et al.* Therapeutic response to somatostatin analogue, BIM-23014, in metastatic prostatic cancer. *Clin Exp Metastasis* 1992; **10:** 3–11.
2. Heron I, *et al.* Pharmacokinetics and efficacy of a long-acting formulation of the new somatostatin analog BIM 23014 in patients with acromegaly. *J Clin Endocrinol Metab* 1993; **76:** 721–7.
3. Emanuelsson H, *et al.* Long-term effects of angiopeptin treatment in coronary angioplasty: reduction in clinical events but not angiographic restenosis. *Circulation* 1995; **91:** 1689–96.
4. Eriksson B, *et al.* The use of new somatostatin analogues, lanreotide and octastatin, in neuroendocrine gastro-intestinal tumours. *Digestion* 1996; **57** (suppl 1): 77–80.

Preparations

Proprietary Preparations (details are given in Part 3)
Fr.: Somatuline; ***Ital.:*** Ipstyl; ***Spain:*** Somatulina; ***UK:*** Somatuline.

Leuprorelin Acetate (12895-s)

Leuprorelin Acetate *(BANM, rINNM)*.

Abbott-43818; Leuprolide Acetate *(USAN)*; TAP-144. 5-Oxo-L-prolyl-L-histidyl-L-tryptophyl-L-seryl-L-tyrosyl-D-leucyl-L-leucyl-L-arginyl-*N*-ethyl-L-prolinamide acetate.

$C_{59}H_{84}N_{16}O_{12},C_2H_4O_2 = 1269.5.$

CAS — 53714-56-0 (leuprorelin); 74381-53-6 (leuprorelin acetate).

Adverse Effects and Precautions

As for Gonadorelin, p.1247.

Benign intracranial hypertension. A report of increased intracranial pressure associated with leuprorelin treatment in one patient.[1]

1. Arber N, *et al.* Pseudotumor cerebri associated with leuprorelin acetate. *Lancet* 1990; **335:** 668.

Effects on the eyes. Therapy with leuprorelin may be associated with blurred vision, usually lasting 1 to 2 hours after injection, but in rare instances more prolonged.[1] Haemorrhage or occlusion of intra-ocular blood vessels, ocular pain, and lid oedema have also been reported but the association is less well established.

1. Fraunfelder FT, Edwards R. Possible ocular adverse effects associated with leuprolide injections. *JAMA* 1995; **273:** 773–4.

Hypersensitivity. A report of recurrent anaphylaxis in a patient given a depot injection of leuprorelin acetate, requiring both acute and chronic management.[1]

1. Letterie GS, *et al.* Recurrent anaphylaxis to a depot form of GnRH analogue. *Obstet Gynecol* 1991; **78:** 943–6.

Local reactions. Local reactions, including erythema, pain, induration, and sterile abscess are particularly associated with depot injections of gonadorelin analogues such as leuprorelin and triptorelin;[1-4] they may also occur with subcutaneous daily injection.[1] It has been suggested that the depot vehicle, a lactic acid-glycolic acid copolymer, may be responsible for many, although not all, such reactions.[1-4] Reactions are claimed to be more prevalent in children than in adults:[4] an incidence of about 5% of patients has been suggested. Reactions are apparently idiosyncratic, and may occur at any time during therapy, may be intermittent, or may never recur.[4]

1. Manasco PK, *et al.* Local reactions to depot leuprolide therapy for central precocious puberty. *J Pediatr* 1993; **123:** 334–5.
2. Neely EK, *et al.* Local reactions to depot leuprolide therapy for central precocious puberty. *J Pediatr* 1993; **123:** 335.
3. Tonini G, *et al.* Local reactions to luteinizing hormone releasing hormone analog therapy. *J Pediatr* 1995; **126:** 159.
4. Neely EK, *et al.* Local reactions to luteinizing hormone releasing hormone analog therapy. *J Pediatr* 1995; **126:** 159–60.

Pharmacokinetics

Leuprorelin acetate is not active when given orally but is well absorbed following subcutaneous or intramuscular injection. Following parenteral administration it has an elimination half-life of about 3 hours.

References.

1. Sennello LT, *et al.* Single-dose pharmacokinetics of leuprolide in humans following intravenous and subcutaneous administration. *J Pharm Sci* 1986; **75:** 158–60.

Uses and Administration

Leuprorelin acetate is an analogue of gonadorelin (see p.1248) with similar properties. Continuous administration is used for the suppression of gonadal sex hormone production in the treatment of malignant neoplasms of the prostate, in central precocious puberty and in the management of endometriosis and uterine fibroids. It is also given before uterine surgery for endometrial reduction, and may be used in the treatment of breast cancer in premenopausal women.

In the management of advanced prostate cancer, leuprorelin acetate may be given by subcutaneous injection in a usual single daily dose of 1 mg. It is also given subcutaneously or intramuscularly as depot preparations but the dosage and route of administration of these may differ between countries. In the UK, 3.75 mg may be given once a month, by subcutaneous or intramuscular injection, or 11.25 mg may be given subcutaneously every 3 months. In the USA, however, the dose administered is 7.5 mg monthly, 22.5 mg every 3 months, or 30 mg every 4 months, and the preparation is given intramuscularly. An anti-androgen such as cyproterone acetate may be given for several days before beginning leuprorelin therapy and continued for about 3 weeks, to avoid the risk of a disease flare.

For the management of endometriosis and uterine fibroids, leuprorelin acetate 3.75 mg monthly may be given as a single depot injection, intramuscularly or subcutaneously. Alternatively, 11.25 mg may be given as an intramuscular depot every 3 months. Treatment should be initiated during the first 5 days of the menstrual cycle, and may be continued for up to 6 months for endometriosis, while in women with anaemia due to uterine fibroids it is continued, with concomitant iron supplementation, for up to 3 months. As preparation for uterine surgery a single 3.75 mg depot injection may be given 5 to 6 weeks before the procedure.

In the management of central precocious puberty leuprorelin acetate has been given by intramuscular depot injection in a dose of 0.3 mg per kg bodyweight every 4 weeks, adjusted according to response. Doses of 50 μg per kg daily by subcutaneous injection, adjusted according to response, have also been used.

Leuprorelin acetate has also been given in other sex-hormone-related disorders and has been tried in some gastro-intestinal disorders such as irritable bowel syndrome.

General references.

1. Plosker GL, Brogden RN. Leuprorelin: a review of its pharmacology and therapeutic use in prostatic cancer, endometriosis and other sex hormone-related disorders. *Drugs* 1994; **48:** 930–67.

Administration. Favourable luteinising hormone response in healthy subjects to leuprorelin administered transdermally via electrically powered patches.[1]

1. Meyer BR, *et al.* Transdermal versus subcutaneous leuprolide: a comparison of acute pharmacodynamic effect. *Clin Pharmacol Ther* 1990; **48:** 340–5.

Benign prostatic hyperplasia. For a discussion of the management of benign prostatic hyperplasia, including mention of the use of gonadorelin analogues and the view that they are unsatisfactory for indefinite therapy, see p.1446. References to the use of leuprorelin are cited below.[1]

1. Gabrilove JL, *et al.* Effect of long-acting gonadotropin-releasing hormone analog (leuprolide) therapy on prostatic size and symptoms in 15 men with benign prostatic hypertrophy. *J Clin Endocrinol Metab* 1989; **69:** 629–32.

Endometriosis. Gonadorelin analogues such as leuprorelin are effective in the management of endometriosis (p.1442) but the need for long-term therapy to prevent recurrence limits their value because of the risk of osteoporosis; 'add-back' therapy, with concomitant hormone replacement, is being investigated. Some references to the use of leuprorelin in endometriosis are given below.

1. Rivlin ME, *et al.* Leuprolide acetate in the management of ureteral obstruction caused by endometriosis. *Obstet Gynecol* 1990; **75:** 532–6.
2. Seltzer VL, Benjamin F. Treatment of pulmonary endometriosis with a long-acting GnRH agonist. *Obstet Gynecol* 1990; **76:** 929–31.

Fibroids. Gonadorelin analogues may be of some benefit as an adjunct or alternative to surgery in women with uterine fibroids—see p.1248, although there has been some concern that this might complicate the diagnosis of malignancy. Some further references are listed below.

1. Friedman AJ, *et al.* Treatment of leiomyomata with intranasal or subcutaneous leuprolide, a gonadotropin-releasing hormone agonist. *Fertil Steril* 1987; **48:** 560–4.
2. Schlaff WD, *et al.* A placebo-controlled trial of a depot gonadotropin-releasing hormone analogue (leuprolide) in the treatment of uterine leiomyomata. *Obstet Gynecol* 1989; **74:** 856–62.
3. Friedman AJ, *et al.* Treatment of leiomyomata uteri with leuprolide acetate depot: a double-blind, placebo-controlled, multicenter study. *Obstet Gynecol* 1991; **77:** 720–5.
4. Meyer WR, *et al.* Unsuspected leiomyosarcoma: treatment with a gonadotropin-releasing hormone analogue. *Obstet Gynecol* 1990; **75:** 529–32.

Hirsutism. The mainstay of drug treatment for hirsutism (p.1441) has been an anti-androgen, usually cyproterone acetate or spironolactone. Although gonadorelin analogues such as leuprorelin have been used, and are effective, they must be given parenterally or nasally and may produce menopausal effects, notably osteoporosis.

References.

1. Rittmaster RS, Thompson DL. Effect of leuprolide and dexamethasone on hair growth and hormone levels in hirsute women: the relative importance of the ovary and the adrenal in the pathogenesis of hirsutism. *J Clin Endocrinol Metab* 1990; **70:** 1096–1102.
2. Elkind-Hirsch KE, *et al.* Combination gonadotropin-releasing hormone agonist and oral contraceptive therapy improves treatment of hirsute women with ovarian hyperandrogenism. *Fertil Steril* 1995; **63:** 970–8.

Infertility. Gonadorelin analogues are used in the treatment of infertility—see p.1239. Some references to the use of leuprorelin in female infertility are given below.

1. Stone BA, *et al.* Gonadotrophin and estradiol levels during ovarian stimulation in women treated with leuprolide acetate. *Obstet Gynecol* 1989; **73:** 990–5.
2. Sathanandan M, *et al.* Adjuvant leuprolide in normal, abnormal, and poor responders to controlled ovarian hyperstimulation for in vitro fertilization/gamete intrafallopian transfer. *Fertil Steril* 1989; **51:** 998–1006.
3. Filicori M, *et al.* Different gonadotropin and leuprorelin ovulation induction regimens markedly affect follicular fluid hormone levels and folliculogenesis. *Fertil Steril* 1996; **65:** 387–93.

Malignant neoplasms. Gonadorelin analogues are used as an alternative to orchidectomy in the management of malignant neoplasms of the prostate (p.491). Studies indicating benefit from leuprorelin therapy, alone or with an anti-androgen, are listed below.[1-6] Leuprorelin also suppresses oestrogen concentrations to values within the postmenopausal range[7] in premenopausal women with breast cancer (p.485). There are also reports of endometrial cancer,[8] and ovarian cancer[9] responding to leuprorelin, but the role of the gonadorelin analogues in these conditions is much less well established (see p.487 and p.491, respectively).

1. The Leuprolide Study Group. Leuprolide versus diethylstilbestrol for metastatic prostate cancer. *N Engl J Med* 1984; **311:** 1281–6.
2. Giraud B. Interim report of a large French multicentre study of efficacy and safety of 3.75 mg leuprorelin depot in metastatic prostatic cancer. *J Int Med Res* 1990; **18** (suppl 1): 84–9.
3. Rizzo M, *et al.* Leuprorelin acetate depot in advanced prostatic cancer: a phase II multicentre trial. *J Int Med Res* 1990; **18** (suppl 1): 114–25.
4. Crawford ED, *et al.* A controlled trial of leuprolide with and without flutamide in prostatic carcinoma. *N Engl J Med* 1989; **321:** 419–24.
5. Nabors W, Crawford ED. Luteinizing hormone releasing hormone agonists: the US experience. *J Int Med Res* 1990; **18** (suppl 1): 31–4.
6. Schellhammer PF, *et al.* A controlled trial of bicalutamide versus flutamide, each in combination with luteinizing hormone-releasing hormone analogue therapy, in patients with advanced prostate carcinoma: analysis of time to progression. *Cancer* 1996; **78:** 2164–9.
7. Dowsett M, *et al.* A dose-comparative endocrine-clinical study of leuprorelin in premenopausal breast cancer patients. *Br J Cancer* 1990; **62:** 834–7.
8. Gallagher CJ, *et al.* A new treatment for endometrial cancer with gonadotrophin releasing-hormone analogue. *Br J Obstet Gynaecol* 1991; **98:** 1037–41.
9. Bruckner HW, Motwani BT. Treatment of advanced refractory ovarian carcinoma with a gonadotropin-releasing hormone analogue. *Am J Obstet Gynecol* 1989; **161:** 1216–18.

Precocious puberty. The gonadorelin analogues have replaced other agents as the drugs of choice for the treatment of central precocious puberty (p.1241). Daily subcutaneous injections of leuprorelin acetate 4 to 50 μg per kg body-weight for up to about 25 months have resulted in a reduction in linear growth rate and rate of bone age advancement in children with central precocious puberty.[1] Monthly intramuscular administration of a depot preparation was also suitable.[2,3]

1. Lee PA, *et al.* Effects of leuprolide in the treatment of central precocious puberty. *J Pediatr* 1989; **114:** 321–4.
2. Kappy M, *et al.* Suppression of gonadotropin secretion by a long-acting gonadotropin-releasing hormone analog (leuprolide acetate, Lupron depot) in children with precocious puberty. *J Clin Endocrinol Metab* 1989; **69:** 1087–9.
3. Neely EK, *et al.* Two-year results of treatment with depot leuprolide acetate for central precocious puberty. *J Pediatr* 1992; **121:** 634–40.

Premenstrual syndrome. In women in whom other drug treatments for premenstrual syndrome (p.1456) are ineffective, use of a gonadorelin analogue, usually with hormone replacement therapy to prevent menopausal symptoms, may be considered.

References to the use of leuprorelin in premenstrual syndrome are given below.

1. Mezrow G, *et al.* Depot leuprolide acetate with estrogen and progestin add-back for long-term treatment of premenstrual syndrome. *Fertil Steril* 1994; **62:** 932–7.

Preparations

Proprietary Preparations (details are given in Part 3)
Aust.: Enantone; ***Austral.:*** Lucrin; ***Belg.:*** Lucrin; ***Canad.:*** Lupron; ***Fr.:*** Enantone; Lucrin; ***Ger.:*** Carcinil; Enantone; Enantone-Gyn; Trenantone; Uno-Enantone; ***Irl.:*** Prostap; ***Ital.:*** Enantone; ***Jpn:*** Leuplin; ***Neth.:*** Lucrin; ***Norw.:*** Enanton; Procren; ***S.Afr.:*** Lucrin; ***Spain:*** Ginecrin; Procrin; ***Swed.:*** Enanton; Procren; ***Switz.:*** Lucrin; ***UK:*** Prostap; ***USA:*** Lupron.

Luteinising Hormone (5931-v)

Human Interstitial-cell-stimulating Hormone; ICSH; LH; Lutropin.

CAS — 9002-67-9; 39341-83-8 (human).

Units

35 units of human pituitary luteinising hormone are contained in approximately 5.8 μg (with 1 mg of human albumin, 5 mg of mannitol, and 1 mg of sodium chloride) in one ampoule of the second International Standard (1988).

10 units of the alpha subunit of human pituitary luteinising hormone are contained in approximately 10 μg (with 0.5 mg of human albumin, 2.5 mg of lactose, and 45 μg of sodium chloride) in one ampoule of the first International Standard (1984).

10 units of the beta subunit of human pituitary luteinising hormone are contained in 10 μg (with 0.5 mg of human albumin, 2.5 mg of lactose, and 45 μg of sodium chloride) in one ampoule of the first International Standard (1984).

Uses and Administration

Luteinising hormone (LH; interstitial-cell-stimulating hormone; ICSH) is a gonadotrophin secreted by the anterior lobe of the pituitary together with another gonadotrophin, follicle-stimulating hormone (FSH) (p.1247).

These gonadotrophins stimulate the normal functioning of the gonads and the secretion of sex hormones in both men and women. In women, follicle-stimulating hormone stimulates the development and maturation of the follicles and ova. As the follicle develops it produces oestrogen in increasing amounts which at mid-cycle stimulates the release of LH. This causes rupture of the follicle with ovulation and converts the follicle into the corpus luteum which secretes progesterone. In men, luteinising hormone stimulates the interstitial cells of the testis to secrete testosterone, which in turn has a direct effect on the seminiferous tubules.

Gonadotrophic substances with luteinising or follicle-stimulating activity or both are used in the treatment of fertility disorders (see p.1239), chiefly in females but also in males. Such substances include chorionic gonadotrophin which possesses LH activity (see p.1243) and human menopausal gonadotrophins which possess both LH and FSH activity (see p.1252). A recombinant DNA-derived human luteinising hormone (rechLH) is being investigated as an alternative to chorionic gonadotrophin or for administration in conjunction with FSH.

References.

1. DeCherney AH, Naftolin F. Recombinant DNA-derived human luteinizing hormone: basic science rapidly applied to clinical medicine. *JAMA* 1988; **259:** 3313–14.
2. Simon JA, *et al.* Characterization of recombinant DNA derived-human luteinizing hormone in vitro and in vivo: efficacy in ovulation induction and corpus luteum support. *JAMA* 1988; **259:** 3290–5.
3. Hull M, *et al.* Recombinant human luteinising hormone: an effective new gonadotropin preparation. *Lancet* 1994; **344:** 334–5.
4. Imthurn B, *et al.* Recombinant human luteinising hormone to mimic mid-cycle LH surge. *Lancet* 1996; **348:** 332–3.
5. Agrawal R, *et al.* Pregnancy after treatment with three recombinant gonadotropins. *Lancet* 1997; **349:** 29–30.

Melanocyte-stimulating Hormone (5936-w)

B Hormone; Chromatophore Hormone; Intermedin; Melanotropin; MSH; Pigment Hormone.

CAS — 9002-79-3.

Melanocyte-stimulating hormone is a polypeptide isolated from the pars intermedia of the pituitary of fish and amphibia which causes dispersal of melanin granules in the skin of fish and amphibia and allows adaptation to the environment.

In adult humans, the pituitary gland lacks a distinct intermediate lobe, and the pituitary is not thought to secrete melanocyte-stimulating hormone (MSH) directly. However, the precursor molecule, pro-opiomelanocortin, is cleaved in the pituitary into corticotrophin (p.1244), the glycoprotein β-lipotrophin (β-LPH), and an amino-terminal peptide. Subsequent processing in other tissues, such as the brain and gastro-intestinal tract, may yield three forms of MSH, α-MSH (via corticotrophin cleavage), β-MSH, and γ-MSH. The presence and function of these melanocyte-stimulating hormones in man are uncertain. A receptor analogous to that in amphibians is apparently lacking in humans; effects on skin pigmentation emanating from the pituitary are primarily mediated by corticotrophin.

Release of melanocyte-stimulating hormone is inhibited in animals by melanostatin; there is also evidence for a hypothalamic releasing factor (MRF).

Melanocyte-stimulating hormone is under investigation, as α-MSH, in the prevention and treatment of ischaemic intrinsic acute renal failure.

Alpha melanocyte-stimulating hormone (α-MSH) has neurotrophic actions during development and has been investigated for its potential in promoting recovery of nerve function after injury.[1]

1. Choo V. Healing with recovery of function. *Lancet* 1993; **342:** 673.

Preparations

Proprietary Preparations (details are given in Part 3)

Multi-ingredient: *Ital.:* Retinovix†.

Melanostatin (5937-e)

Intermedin-inhibiting Factor; Melanocyte-stimulating-hormone-release-inhibiting Factor; Melanotropin Release-inhibiting Factor; MIF. Pro-Leu-Gly-NH_2.

CAS — 9083-38-9.

Melanostatin is a tripeptide obtained from the hypothalamus which inhibits the release of melanocyte-stimulating hormone (see above) in animals. However, there is little evidence of its activity in man. It has been tried in the treatment of depression and parkinsonism but with little benefit.

Nafarelin Acetate (16907-g)

Nafarelin Acetate *(BANM, USAN, rINNM).*

D-Nal(2)[6]-LHRH acetate hydrate; RS-94991298. 5-Oxo-L-prolyl-L-histidyl-L-tryptophyl-L-seryl-L-tyrosyl-3-(2-naphthyl)-D-alanyl-L-leucyl-L-arginyl-L-prolylglycinamide acetate hydrate.

$C_{66}H_{83}N_{17}O_{13},xC_2H_4O_2,yH_2O$.

CAS — 76932-56-4 (nafarelin); 86220-42-0 (nafarelin acetate).

Adverse Effects and Precautions

As for Gonadorelin, p.1247.

Effects on electrolytes. A report of severe hyperkalaemia in a woman receiving nafarelin therapy for uterine fibroids.[1] Despite serum potassium greater than 10 mmol per litre she had no symptoms and the electrocardiogram was normal. Hyperkalaemia resolved without treatment following discontinuation of nafarelin.

1. Hata T, *et al.* Severe hyperkalaemia with nafarelin. *Lancet* 1996; **347:** 333.

Pharmacokinetics

Nafarelin is rapidly absorbed following intranasal administration with peak plasma concentrations achieved within 20 minutes of a dose, although bioavailability is only about 3%. The plasma half-life is about 3 to 4 hours. Nafarelin is metabolised by peptidases in the body; following subcutaneous administration it is excreted in urine, as metabolites and a small amount of unchanged drug, and in the faeces.

Uses and Administration

Nafarelin acetate is an analogue of gonadorelin (see p.1248) with similar properties. It is used for the treatment of endometriosis in usual doses equivalent to 200 μg of nafarelin twice daily intranasally, doubled after 2 months if amenorrhoea has not occurred. Treatment should begin on days 2 to 4 of the menstrual cycle, and may be continued for up to 6 months.

Nafarelin acetate is also used in the treatment of central precocious puberty, and as an adjunct to ovulation induction with gonadotrophins in the treatment of infertility.

For central precocious puberty the usual dose is the equivalent of nafarelin 800 μg intranasally (400 μg in each nostril) twice daily. If adequate suppression is not achieved at this dose it may be increased to 600 μg three times daily in alternate nostrils.

Regimens for oocyte collection for *in vitro* fertilisation employ gonadorelin analogues for pituitary desensitisation before ovulation induction with gonadotrophins; the equivalent of 400 μg of nafarelin is given intranasally twice daily, beginning either in the early follicular phase (day 2) or midluteal phase (day 21) of the menstrual cycle. Therapy should be continued until downregulation is achieved; if this does not occur within 12 weeks therapy should be withdrawn. Once downregulation occurs gonadotrophin treatment is added to nafarelin therapy until an appropriate stage of follicular development, when both are withdrawn and chorionic gonadotrophin is given to induce ovulation.

Nafarelin has also been given in other sex hormone-related conditions.

Benign prostatic hyperplasia. Prostate size decreased by a mean of 24.2% in 9 men treated for benign prostatic hyperplasia for 6 months with nafarelin acetate 400 μg daily subcutaneously.[1] Six months after the end of treatment, prostate size approached that of pretreatment values.

For a discussion of benign prostatic hyperplasia and its management, including the view that gonadorelin analogues are unsuitable for indefinite therapy, see p.1446.

1. Peters CA, Walsh PC. The effect of nafarelin acetate, a luteinizing-hormone-releasing hormone agonist, on benign prostatic hyperplasia. *N Engl J Med* 1987; **317:** 599–604.

Contraception. Nafarelin 125 or 250 μg daily intranasally as the sole means of contraception (p.1434) inhibited ovulation; no pregnancies occurred during 59 treatment months in 30 women,[1] or during 222 months in 47 women.[2] However, such methods remain investigational.

1. Gudmundsson JA, *et al.* Inhibition of ovulation by intranasal nafarelin, a new superactive agonist of GnRH. *Contraception* 1984; **30:** 107–14.
2. Gudmundsson JA, *et al.* Intranasal peptide contraception by inhibition of ovulation with the gonadotropin-releasing hormone superagonist nafarelin: six months' clinical results. *Fertil Steril* 1986; **45:** 617–23.

Endometriosis. Gonadorelin analogues are effective in the management of endometriosis (p.1442), but the need for long-term therapy to prevent recurrence limits their value because of the risk of osteoporosis; 'add-back' therapy, with concomitant hormone replacement, is under investigation. Some references to the use of nafarelin in endometriosis are listed below.

1. Schriock E, *et al.* Treatment of endometriosis with a potent agonist of gonadotropin-releasing hormone (nafarelin). *Fertil Steril* 1985; **44:** 583–8.
2. Henzl MR, *et al.* Administration of nasal nafarelin as compared with oral danazol for endometriosis: a multicenter double-blind comparative clinical trial. *N Engl J Med* 1988; **318:** 485–9.
3. Burry KA. Nafarelin in the management of endometriosis: quality of life assessment. *Am J Obstet Gynecol* 1992; **166:** 735–9.
4. Hornstein MD, *et al.* Retreatment with nafarelin for recurrent endometriosis symptoms: efficacy, safety, and bone mineral density. *Fertil Steril* 1997; **67:** 1013–18.

Fibroids. Gonadorelin analogues such as nafarelin have been tried as an adjunct or alternative to surgery in the treatment of uterine fibroids (see p.1248), although there has been some concern that this might complicate the diagnosis of malignancy. Some further references are listed below.

1. Andreyko JL, *et al.* Use of an agonistic analog of gonadotropin-releasing hormone (nafarelin) to treat leiomyomas: assessment by magnetic resonance imaging. *Am J Obstet Gynecol* 1988; **158:** 903–10.

Infertility. Gonadorelin analogues are used in the treatment of infertility (p.1239). As well as being used directly they are employed in regimens to induce superovulation to enable ova collection and *in vitro* fertilisation, and use of nafarelin has been reported to produce a higher rate of successful pregnancies than leuprorelin in one *in vitro* fertilisation programme.[1]

1. Martin MC, *et al.* The choice of a gonadotropin-releasing hormone analog influences outcome of in vitro fertilization treatment. *Am J Obstet Gynecol* 1994; **170:** 1629–34.

Precocious puberty. Nafarelin preserved adult height potential in girls with idiopathic precocious puberty (p.1241) having a poor initial height prognosis.[1] However, reviewers have noted that results from earlier studies into other features of precocious puberty have been equivocal.[2]

1. Kreiter M, *et al.* Preserving adult height potential in girls with idiopathic true precocious puberty. *J Pediatr* 1990; **117:** 364–70.
2. Chrisp P, Goa KL. Nafarelin: a review of its pharmacodynamic and pharmacokinetic properties, and clinical potential in sex hormone-related conditions. *Drugs* 1990; **39:** 523–51.

Preparations

Proprietary Preparations (details are given in Part 3)

Austral.: Synarel; *Belg.:* Synarel; *Canad.:* Synarel; *Fr.:* Synarel; *Ger.:* Synarela; *Irl.:* Synarel; *Neth.:* Synarel; *Norw.:* Synarela; *S.Afr.:* Synarel; *Swed.:* Synarela; *Switz.:* Synrelina; *UK:* Synarel; *USA:* Synarel.

Octreotide Acetate (16932-q)

Octreotide Acetate (BANM, USAN, rINNM).

SMS-201-995 (octreotide). 2-(D-Phenylalanyl-L-cystyl-L-phenylalanyl-D-tryptophyl-L-lysyl-L-threonyl-L-cystyl)-(2R,3R)-butane-1,3-diol acetate; D-Phenylalanyl-L-cysteinyl-L-phenylalanyl-D-tryptophyl-L-lysyl-L-threonyl-N-[(1R,2R)-2-hydroxy-1-(hydroxymethyl)propyl]-L-cysteinamide cyclic (2→7) disulphide acetate.

$C_{49}H_{66}N_{10}O_{10}S_2,xC_2H_4O_2$ = 1019.3 (octreotide).

CAS — 83150-76-9 (octreotide); 79517-01-4 (octreotide acetate).

Incompatibility. Apparent loss of insulin has been reported from a total parenteral nutrient solution containing octreotide; there may be an incompatibility.[1] Also the manufacturers had suggested that octreotide might be adsorbed onto plastics. However, a solution containing octreotide 200 µg per mL as the acetate was reported to be stable at 5° or −20° for up to 60 days when stored in polypropylene syringes.[2]

1. Rosen GH. Potential incompatibility of insulin and octreotide in total parenteral nutrient solutions. *Am J Hosp Pharm* 1989; **46:** 1128.
2. Ripley RG, *et al.* Stability of octreotide acetate in polypropylene syringes at 5 and −20°C. *Am J Health-Syst Pharm* 1995; **52:** 1910–11.

Adverse Effects and Precautions

There may be a transient local reaction at the site of injection of octreotide. Systemic side-effects are mainly gastro-intestinal and may include anorexia, nausea, vomiting, diarrhoea and steatorrhoea, abdominal discomfort, and flatulence. Administration between meals or at bedtime may reduce these gastro-intestinal effects.

Gallstones may develop on long-term therapy; there have been isolated reports of hepatic dysfunction and of biliary colic associated with drug withdrawal. Hypoglycaemia may occur, especially in patients with insulinomas, but there is also a risk of hyperglycaemia or impaired glucose tolerance. Thyroid function should be monitored during octreotide therapy because of the possibility of hypothyroidism. Checks should be made for gallstones before prolonged therapy and at 6- to 12-month intervals during treatment. Cardiac rhythm should be monitored during intravenous administration of octreotide. Doses may need to be adjusted in patients with end-stage renal failure, in whom the clearance of octreotide is reduced.

Effects on the biliary tract. Octreotide has an inhibitory effect on gallbladder motility accounting for the development of gallstones and biliary colic.[1-6]

1. McKnight JA, *et al.* Changes in glucose tolerance and development of gall stones during high dose treatment with octreotide for acromegaly. *Br Med J* 1989; **299:** 604–5.
2. Buscail L, *et al.* Gall stones and treatment with octreotide for acromegaly. *Br Med J* 1989; **299:** 1162.
3. Wass JAH, *et al.* Gall stones and treatment with octreotide for acromegaly. *Br Med J* 1989; **299:** 1162–3.
4. Ho KY, *et al.* Therapeutic efficacy of the somatostatin analog SMS 201-995 (octreotide) in acromegaly: effects of dose and frequency and long-term safety. *Ann Intern Med* 1990; **112:** 173–81.
5. James RA, *et al.* Biliary colic on abrupt withdrawal of octreotide. *Lancet* 1991; **338:** 1527.
6. Bigg-Wither GW, *et al.* Effects of long term octreotide on gall stone formation and gall bladder function. *Br Med J* 1992; **304:** 1611–12.

Effects on carbohydrate metabolism. Changes in glucose tolerance were observed over 12 months in patients treated with octreotide 600 to 1500 µg daily subcutaneously for acromegaly.[1] Of 3 patients with normal glucose tolerance initially, one remained normal, one developed impaired glucose tolerance, and one became diabetic. Of 4 with impaired glucose tolerance initially, 2 remained unchanged, one became diabetic, and the other returned to normal. There has been a report of deterioration in glucose tolerance leading to death from diabetic ketoacidosis occurring after cessation of octreotide treatment in a patient with acromegaly and insulin-resistant diabetes mellitus.[2]

See also Diabetes Mellitus and Hyperinsulinism under Uses and Administration, below.

1. McKnight JA, *et al.* Changes in glucose tolerance and development of gall stones during high dose treatment with octreotide for acromegaly. *Br Med J* 1989; **299:** 604–5.
2. Abrahamson MJ. Death from diabetic ketoacidosis after cessation of octreotide in acromegaly. *Lancet* 1990; **336:** 318–19.

Effects on the liver. A report of hepatitis occurring during treatment of an acromegalic patient with octreotide 300 µg daily subcutaneously.[1] Liver enzyme values returned to normal within 2 months of withdrawing octreotide.

1. Arosio M, *et al.* Acute hepatitis after treatment of acromegaly with octreotide. *Lancet* 1988; **ii:** 1498.

Effects on the pancreas. Reports of pancreatitis associated with octreotide.[1-3] It has been suggested that octreotide-induced pancreatitis may result from spasm of the sphincter of Oddi, resulting in retention of activated pancreatic enzymes due to outflow obstruction.[3]

1. Fredenrich A, *et al.* Acute pancreatitis after short-term octreotide. *Lancet* 1991; **338:** 52–3.
2. Sadoul J-L, *et al.* Acute pancreatitis following octreotide withdrawal. *Am J Med* 1991; **90:** 763–4.
3. Bodemar G, Hjortswang H. Octreotide-induced pancreatitis: an effect of increased contractility of Oddi sphincter. *Lancet* 1996; **348:** 1668–9.

Effects on the skin. Diffuse loss of scalp hair has been reported in 4 of 7 women who received octreotide; after withdrawal of octreotide in 3 of the women there was a complete recovery of scalp hair.[1]

1. Jönsson A, Manhem P. Octreotide and loss of scalp hair. *Ann Intern Med* 1991; **115:** 913.

Interactions

Octreotide has been associated with alterations in nutrient absorption: there is a theoretical possibility that it may affect the absorption of orally administered drugs. Patients receiving insulin or oral hypoglycaemic drugs may require dose adjustments of these agents if octreotide is given concomitantly, and the bioavailability of bromocriptine is increased by concomitant octreotide administration. It has been suggested that dosage of beta blockers, calcium-channel blockers, or agents to control fluid and electrolyte balance may also need to be adjusted.

Cyclosporin. For a reference to octreotide reducing serum concentrations of cyclosporin, see p.522.

Pharmacokinetics

Octreotide is rapidly absorbed following subcutaneous injection, with peak plasma concentrations reached about 25 to 30 minutes after a dose, and is distributed to body tissues. It is said to exhibit non-linear pharmacokinetics, with reduced clearance at high doses. Octreotide is removed from the body with a plasma elimination half-life of approximately 1.5 hours; half-life is prolonged in elderly patients and in renal failure. About a third of a dose is excreted unchanged in the urine.

Uses and Administration

Octreotide is an octapeptide analogue of somatostatin (see p.1261) with similar properties but a longer duration of action.

It is used as the acetate in the symptomatic management of carcinoid tumours and other secretory neoplasms such as VIPomas. Octreotide acetate is also used in the short-term treatment of acromegaly and the prevention of complications following pancreatic surgery, and has been investigated in the treatment of a variety of other disorders including variceal haemorrhage, diarrhoea associated with AIDS, and the dumping syndrome.

In the management of **secretory neoplasms** octreotide acetate is given subcutaneously in an initial dose equivalent to 50 µg of octreotide once or twice daily gradually increased, according to response, to up to 600 µg daily in 2 to 4 divided doses. Higher doses have been used.

Where a rapid response is required, the initial dose may be given by the intravenous route. In the UK the manufacturers state that it should be diluted not less than 1 in 1 or not more than 1 in 9 in sodium chloride 0.9%, but in the USA the manufacturers permit the use of the undiluted solution as an intravenous bolus in emergencies; alternatively the dose may be given by intermittent infusion over 15 to 30 minutes, diluted in 50 to 200 mL of sodium chloride 0.9% or glucose 5%.

Once control has been established maintenance therapy with a depot preparation may be possible; initially 20 mg by intramuscular injection every 4 weeks is suggested. Subcutaneous injection with a rapid-acting preparation should be continued for 2 weeks after the first depot injection to provide symptomatic cover, and may be added to therapy when necessary thereafter. Maintenance doses of the depot preparation may be adjusted after 3 months to between 10 and 30 mg every 4 weeks, as necessary.

In **acromegaly**, the usual dose is the equivalent of 100 to 200 µg of octreotide three times daily by subcutaneous injection. In the USA it is suggested that dosage begin with 50 µg three times daily in order to minimise gastro-intestinal disturbance. Once control has been established maintenance therapy with a depot preparation is possible; an initial dose equivalent to 20 mg of octreotide given intramuscularly once a month has been recommended for patients with acromegaly, adjusted after 3 months to between 10 and 30 mg monthly.

For the prevention of complications following **pancreatic surgery** the equivalent of 0.1 mg of octreotide may be given 3 times daily by subcutaneous injection of a rapid-acting preparation; treatment is given for 7 consecutive days, beginning at least 1 hour before laparotomy on the day of operation.

General reviews of octreotide.

1. Mosdell KW, Visconti JA. Emerging indications for octreotide therapy, part 1. *Am J Hosp Pharm* 1994; **51:** 1184–92.
2. Mosdell KW, Visconti JA. Emerging indications for octreotide therapy, part 2. *Am J Hosp Pharm* 1994; **51:** 1317–30.
3. Bloom SR, O'Shea D. Octreotide. *Prescribers' J* 1996; **36:** 120–4.
4. Lamberts SWJ, *et al.* Octreotide. *N Engl J Med* 1996; **334:** 246–54.

Acromegaly. Although surgery remains the most important method of treatment, octreotide may be useful in the management of acromegaly (p.1235) particularly in the frail and elderly patient, since it can reduce growth hormone concentrations and tumour size, and may improve cardiovascular parameters.[1-6] Continuous subcutaneous infusion may be more effective than intermittent injection.[7] Sustained-release octreotide also appears to be of value.[8]

1. Chanson P, *et al.* Cardiovascular effects of the somatostatin analog octreotide in acromegaly. *Ann Intern Med* 1990; **113:** 921–5.
2. Ho KY, *et al.* Therapeutic efficacy of the somatostatin analog SMS 201-995 (octreotide) in acromegaly: effects of dose and frequency and long-term safety. *Ann Intern Med* 1990; **112:** 173–81.
3. Vance ML, Harris AG. Long-term treatment of 189 acromegalic patients with the somatostatin analog octreotide: results of the International Multicenter Acromegaly Study Group. *Arch Intern Med* 1991; **151:** 1573–8.
4. Ezzat S, *et al.* Octreotide treatment of acromegaly: a randomized, multicenter study. *Ann Intern Med* 1992; **117:** 711–18.
5. Acromegaly Therapy Consensus Development Panel. Consensus statement: benefits versus risks of medical therapy for acromegaly. *Am J Med* 1994; **97:** 468–73.
6. van der Lely AJ, *et al.* A risk-benefit assessment of octreotide in the treatment of acromegaly. *Drug Safety* 1997; **17:** 317–24.
7. Harris AG, *et al.* Continuous versus intermittent subcutaneous infusion of octreotide in the treatment of acromegaly. *J Clin Pharmacol* 1995; **35:** 59–71.
8. Gillis JC, *et al.* Octreotide long-acting release (LAR): a review of its pharmacological properties and therapeutic use in the management of acromegaly. *Drugs* 1997; **53:** 681–99.

Carcinoid syndrome and other secretory neoplasms. For a discussion of carcinoid tumours and other secretory neoplasms, including reference to the important role of octreotide, see p.477.

Cardiovascular disorders. There have been reports of benefit from octreotide in patients with postprandial hypotension and orthostatic hypotension associated with autonomic neuropathy.[1-3] It is one of many drugs that have been tried in orthostatic hypotension (see p.1040). Octreotide has also produced rapid and sustained cardiac improvement in patients with acromegaly.[4] (See also above.) Promising results have also been seen in 3 patients with primary hypertrophic cardiomyopathy.[5]

1. Hoeldtke RD, *et al.* Treatment of autonomic neuropathy with a somatostatin analogue SMS-201-995. *Lancet* 1986; **ii:** 602–5.
2. Hoeldtke RD, Israel BC. Treatment of orthostatic hypotension with octreotide. *J Clin Endocrinol Metab* 1989; **68:** 1051–9.
3. Woo J, *et al.* Treatment of severe orthostatic hypotension with the somatostatin analogue octreotide. *Aust N Z J Med* 1990; **20:** 822–3.
4. Chanson P, *et al.* Cardiovascular effects of the somatostatin analog octreotide in acromegaly. *Ann Intern Med* 1990; **113:** 921–5.
5. Günal AI, *et al.* Short term reduction of left ventricular mass in primary hypertrophic cardiomyopathy by octreotide injections. *Heart* 1996; **76:** 418–21.

Cushing's syndrome. It has been suggested[1] that octreotide may be useful in the diagnosis, and possibly the treatment, of Cushing's syndrome (p.1236).

1. Woodhouse NJY, *et al.* Acute and long-term effects of octreotide in patients with ACTH-dependent Cushing's syndrome. *Am J Med* 1993; **95:** 305–8.

Diabetes mellitus. Although octreotide has been reported to impair glucose tolerance, and even precipitate frank diabetes (see Effects on Carbohydrate Metabolism, under Adverse Effects, above), its variable effects on blood glucose and insulin have led to investigations[1-3] of its possible benefits in diabetes mellitus (p.313). There is also some suggestion that it may be of benefit in the treatment or prevention of diabetic nephropathy.[4] Benefit has been reported from the use of octreotide in patients with diabetic diarrhoea—see Gastro-intestinal Disorders, below.

1. Rios MS, *et al.* Somatostatin analog SMS 201-995 and insulin needs in insulin-dependent diabetic patients studied by means of an artificial pancreas. *J Clin Endocrinol Metab* 1986; **63:** 1071–4.
2. Hadjidakis DJ, *et al.* The effects of the somatostatin analogue SMS 201-995 on carbohydrate homeostasis of insulin-dependent diabetics as assessed by the artificial endocrine pancreas. *Diabetes Res Clin Pract* 1988; **5:** 91–8.
3. Candrina R, Giustina G. Effect of a new long-acting somatostatin analogue (SMS 201-995) on glycemic and hormonal profiles in insulin-treated type II diabetic patients. *J Endocrinol Invest* 1988; **11:** 501–7.
4. Serri O, *et al.* Somatostatin analogue, octreotide, reduces increased glomerular filtration rate and kidney size in insulin-dependent diabetes. *JAMA* 1991; **265:** 888–92.

Diagnosis and testing. Radiolabelled octreotide or derivatives such as pentetreotide may be used successfully to visualise various malignant neoplasms which express somatostatin receptors.[1-6] Somatostatin receptor scintigraphy is the most sensitive method for imaging lesions in patients with Zollinger-Ellison syndrome.[6]

Octreotide may also have a role in the diagnosis of Cushing's syndrome, a topic discussed in more detail on p.1236.

1. Krenning EP, *et al.* Localisation of endocrine-related tumours with radioiodinated analogue of somatostatin. *Lancet* 1989; **i:** 242–4.
2. Lamberts SWJ, *et al.* Somatostatin-receptor imaging in the localization of endocrine tumors. *N Engl J Med* 1990; **323:** 1246–9.
3. van Eijck CHJ, *et al.* Somatostatin-receptor scintigraphy in primary breast cancer. *Lancet* 1994; **343:** 640–3.
4. McCready VR, Hickish TF. Somatostatin imaging function. *Lancet* 1994; **343:** 617.
5. Dominioni L, *et al.* Localisation of carcinoid tumour with radiolabelled octreotide and intraoperative gamma detection. *Lancet* 1994; **344:** 1783.
6. Gibril F, *et al.* Somatostatin receptor scintigraphy: its sensitivity compared with that of other imaging methods in detecting primary and metastatic gastrinomas: a prospective study. *Ann Intern Med* 1996; **125:** 26–34.

Eye disorders. A report of response to octreotide in a patient with bilateral cystoid macular oedema, a refractory form of retinal oedema.[1] The problem recurred when octreotide was twice discontinued and each time responded to resumption of octreotide injections.

1. Kuijpers RWAM, *et al.* Treatment of cystoid macular edema with octreotide. *N Engl J Med* 1998; **338:** 624–6.

Gastro-intestinal disorders. Somatostatin inhibits gastric and intestinal secretion and the production of various active substances in the gastro-intestinal tract. It also reduces splanchnic arterial blood flow and portal and gastric mucosal blood flow. These properties are made use of, usually in the form of octreotide, in the management of a number of gastro-intestinal disorders. Octreotide has been used particularly in the treatment of **endocrine tumours** of the gastro-intestinal tract (see Carcinoid Syndrome, p.477).

The antisecretory properties of octreotide have also been of benefit in patients with **diarrhoea** associated with a variety of conditions including AIDS,[1-4] amyloidosis,[5] diabetes mellitus,[6-8] microvillous atrophy,[9] bone-marrow transplantation,[10] and enterocolitis induced by gold therapy.[11] Octreotide has also been used to reduce the output from postoperative small-bowel fistulae[12] and may also be useful in decreasing faecal mass or jejunal efflux in patients with the short-bowel syndrome and jejunostomies or ileostomies.[13,14] Octreotide therapy resulted in closure of small bowel fistulae in almost 80% of patients in one study[12] and in accelerated healing of pancreatic cutaneous fistulae.[15,16] The management of more conventional forms of diarrhoea is discussed on p.1168.

There have been mixed results with octreotide in the treatment of **gastro-intestinal bleeding**. Although a large multicentre study[17] showed that octreotide had no benefit compared with placebo in the management of bleeding upper gastro-intestinal ulcers, a later meta-analysis suggested there might be some benefit.[18] Octreotide appears to be at least as effective as vasopressin or terlipressin in controlling **variceal haemorrhage**. It also appears to be as effective as balloon tamponade,[19] and there is some evidence that it is as effective as sclerotherapy.[20] Two large controlled studies have suggested that combination of octreotide with endoscopic ligation[21] or sclerotherapy[22] reduces the risk of rebleeding. Octreotide has also produced some benefit (combined with regular sclerotherapy), in the long-term management of patients with cirrhotic portal hypertension.[23] For further discussion of the management of variceal haemorrhage, see p.1576.

Other gastro-intestinal disorders in which octreotide might be useful include **dumping syndrome**[24,25] (further discussed on p.1169), reactive (or postprandial) **hypoglycaemia**,[26,27] **protein-losing enteropathy** associated with intestinal lymphangiectasia,[28] prevention of **NSAID-induced gastric injury**,[29] and **vomiting** secondary to bowel obstruction in patients terminally ill with cancer.[30,31]

1. Cook DJ, *et al.* Somatostatin treatment for cryptosporidial diarrhea in a patient with the acquired immunodeficiency syndrome (AIDS). *Ann Intern Med* 1988; **108:** 708–9.
2. Robinson EN, Fogel R. SMS 201-995, a somatostatin analogue and diarrhea in the acquired immunodeficiency syndrome (AIDS). *Ann Intern Med* 1988; **109:** 680–1.
3. Clotet B, *et al.* Efficacy of the somatostatin analogue (SMS-201-995), Sandostatin, for cryptosporidial diarrhoea in patients with AIDS. *AIDS* 1989; **3:** 857–8.
4. Kim-Sing A, *et al.* Palliative high-dose octreotide in a case of severe AIDS-related diarrhea. *Ann Pharmacother* 1994; **28:** 806–7.
5. O'Connor CR, O'Dorisio TM. Amyloidosis, diarrhea, and a somatostatin analogue. *Ann Intern Med* 1989; **110:** 665–6.
6. Tsai S-T, *et al.* Diabetic diarrhea and somatostatin. *Ann Intern Med* 1986; **104:** 894.
7. Michaels PE, Cameron RB. Octreotide is cost-effective therapy in diabetic diarrhea. *Arch Intern Med* 1991; **151:** 2469.
8. Mourad FH, *et al.* Effective treatment of diabetic diarrhoea with somatostatin analogue, octreotide. *Gut* 1992; **33:** 1578–80.
9. Couper RTL, *et al.* Clinical response to the long acting somatostatin analogue SMS 201-995 in a child with congenital microvillus atrophy. *Gut* 1989; **30:** 1020–4.
10. Crouch MA, *et al.* Octreotide acetate in refractory bone marrow transplant-associated diarrhea. *Ann Pharmacother* 1996; **30:** 331–6.
11. Dorta G, *et al.* Treatment of gold-induced enteritis with octreotide. *Lancet* 1993; **342:** 179.
12. Nubiola-Calonge P, *et al.* Blind evaluation of the effect of octreotide (SMS 201-995), a somatostatin analogue, on small-bowel fistula output. *Lancet* 1987; **ii:** 672–4.
13. Ladefoged K, *et al.* Effect of a long acting somatostatin analogue SMS 201-995 on jejunostomy effluents in patients with severe short bowel syndrome. *Gut* 1989; **30:** 943–9.
14. Nightingale JMD, *et al.* Jejunal efflux in short bowel syndrome. *Lancet* 1990; **336:** 765–8.
15. Prinz RA, *et al.* Treatment of pancreatic cutaneous fistulas with a somatostatin analog. *Am J Surg* 1988; **155:** 36–42.
16. Heij HA, *et al.* A comparison of the effects of two somatostatin analogues in a patient with an external pancreatic fistula. *Pancreas* 1986; **1:** 188–90.
17. Christiansen J, *et al.* Placebo-controlled trial with the somatostatin analogue SMS 201-995 in peptic ulcer bleeding. *Gastroenterology* 1989; **97:** 568–74.
18. Imperiale TF, Birgisson S. Somatostatin or octreotide compared with H_2 antagonists and placebo in the management of acute nonvariceal upper gastrointestinal hemorrhage: a meta-analysis. *Ann Intern Med* 1997; **127:** 1062–71. Correction. *ibid.* 1998; **128:** 245.
19. O'Donnell LJD, Farthing MJG. Octreotide and bleeding oesophageal varices. *Lancet* 1989; **ii:** 1276.
20. Jenkins SA, *et al.* A multicentre randomised trial comparing octreotide and injection sclerotherapy in the management and outcome of acute variceal haemorrhage. *Gut* 1997; **41:** 526–33.
21. Sung JJY, *et al.* Prospective randomised study of effect of octreotide on rebleeding from oesophageal varices after endoscopic ligation. *Lancet* 1995; **346:** 1666–9.
22. Besson I, *et al.* Sclerotherapy with or without octreotide for acute variceal bleeding. *N Engl J Med* 1995; **333:** 555–60.
23. Jenkins SA, *et al.* Randomised trial of octreotide for long term management of cirrhosis after variceal haemorrhage. *Br Med J* 1997; **315:** 1338–41.
24. Hopman WPM, *et al.* Treatment of the dumping syndrome with the somatostatin analogue SMS 201-995. *Ann Surg* 1988; **207:** 155–9.
25. Farthing MJA. Octreotide in dumping and short bowel syndromes. *Digestion* 1993; **54** (suppl 1): 47–52.
26. D'Cruz DP, *et al.* Long-term symptomatic relief of postprandial hypoglycaemia following gastric surgery with a somatostatin analogue. *Postgrad Med J* 1989; **65:** 116–17.
27. Lehnert H, *et al.* Treatment of severe reactive hypoglycemia with a somatostatin analogue (SMS 201-995). *Arch Intern Med* 1990; **150:** 2401–2.
28. Bac DJ, *et al.* Octreotide for protein-losing enteropathy with intestinal lymphangiectasia. *Lancet* 1995; **345:** 1639.
29. Scheiman JM, *et al.* Reduction of non-steroidal anti-inflammatory drug induced gastric injury and leucocyte endothelial adhesion by octreotide. *Gut* 1997; **40:** 720–5.
30. Khoo D, *et al.* control of emesis in bowel obstruction in terminally ill patients. *Lancet* 1992; **339:** 375–6.
31. Crawford R, Quigley C. Octreotide. *Prescribers' J* 1996; **36:** 231–2.

Hypercalcaemia. There have been individual reports of hypercalcaemia associated with raised plasma concentrations of parathyroid hormone-related protein (humoral hypercalcaemia) being successfully controlled with octreotide in patients with malignant pancreatic endocrine tumours[1,2] and adrenal phaeochromocytoma.[3] In two of these patients,[2,3] hypercalcaemia had previously been resistant to treatment with bisphosphonates. Octreotide also resolved hypercalcaemia occurring in a patient with VIPoma and vasoactive intestinal peptide concentrations declined.[4]

For a discussion on hypercalcaemia of malignancy and its management, including the role of octreotide, see p.1148.

1. Wynick D, *et al.* Treatment of a malignant pancreatic endocrine tumour secreting parathyroid hormone related protein. *Br Med J* 1990; **300:** 1314–15.
2. Dodwell D, *et al.* Treatment of a pancreatic tumour secreting parathyroid hormone related protein. *Br Med J* 1990; **300:** 1653.
3. Harrison M, *et al.* Somatostatin analogue treatment for malignant hypercalcaemia. *Br Med J* 1990; **300:** 1313–14. Correction. *ibid.*; **301:** 97 [dosage error].
4. Venkatesh S, *et al.* Somatostatin analogue: use in the treatment of vipoma with hypercalcaemia. *Am J Med* 1989; **87:** 356–7.

Hyperinsulinism. As well as reactive hypoglycaemia (see Gastro-intestinal Disorders, above), octreotide has been used to control inappropriate insulin secretion, both in the short-term and long-term, in children with hypoglycaemia of infancy,[1-3] or nesidioblastosis.[4-6] It has also been used to treat a patient with hyperinsulinaemia induced by quinine.[7] For mention of investigations of octreotide for the reverse effect, see Diabetes Mellitus, above.

1. Kirk JMW, *et al.* Somatostatin analogue in short term management of hyperinsulinism. *Arch Dis Child* 1988; **63:** 1493–4.
2. DeClue TJ, *et al.* Linear growth during long-term treatment with somatostatin analog (SMS 201-995) for persistent hyperinsulinemic hypoglycemia of infancy. *J Pediatr* 1990; **116:** 747–50.
3. Thornton PS, *et al.* Short- and long-term use of octreotide in the treatment of congenital hyperinsulinism. *J Pediatr* 1993; **123:** 637–43.
4. Hindmarsh P, Brook CGD. Short-term management of nesidioblastosis using the somatostatin analogue SMS 201-995. *N Engl J Med* 1987; **316:** 221–2.
5. Delemarre-van de Waal HA, *et al.* Long-term treatment of an infant with nesidioblastosis using a somatostatin analogue. *N Engl J Med* 1987; **316:** 222–3.
6. Behrens R, *et al.* Unusual course of neonatal hyperinsulinaemic hypoglycaemia (nesidioblastosis). *Arch Dis Child* 1998; **78:** F156.
7. Phillips RE, *et al.* Effectiveness of SMS 201-995, a synthetic, long-acting somatostatin analogue, in treatment of quinine-induced hyperinsulinaemia. *Lancet* 1986; **i:** 713–16.

Infertility. Octreotide reduced circulating insulin and luteinising hormone concentrations and lowered androgen production in women with polycystic ovary syndrome.[1] This should assist in the development of ovulatory cycles. (For a discussion of the polycystic ovary syndrome and its management, see p.1240).

There has been a report of a pregnancy occurring in a previously infertile woman, resistant to clomiphene, who was treated with octreotide for acromegaly.[2] The neonate had no malformations and developed normally.

For a discussion of infertility and the more usual drugs used in its management, see p.1239.

1. Prelević GM, *et al.* Inhibitory effect of Sandostatin on secretion of luteinising hormone and ovarian steroids in polycystic ovary syndrome. *Lancet* 1990; **336:** 900–3.
2. Landolt AM, *et al.* Successful pregnancy in a previously infertile woman treated with SMS-201-995 for acromegaly. *N Engl J Med* 1989; **320:** 671–2.

Malignant neoplasms. See under Carcinoid Syndrome, above. For mention of the use of octreotide to treat vomiting associated with malignant gastro-intestinal obstruction see Gastro-intestinal Disorders, above. Octreotide has also proved of benefit in bone pain due to metastatic gastrinoma (see Pain, below).

MENINGIOMA. Octreotide suppressed severe headaches associated with meningioma in a patient;[1] doses were increased to 500 μg three times daily subcutaneously because of tolerance. The patient was able to discontinue octreotide following subsequent surgical removal of the tumour. It was also thought that octreotide had had a beneficial effect on the meningioma size.

1. Rünzi MW, *et al.* Successful treatment of meningioma with octreotide. *Lancet* 1989; **i:** 1074.

THYMOMA. A patient with thymoma and pure red-cell aplasia, in whom corticosteroids alone failed to control anaemia, experienced complete remission following treatment with octreotide and prednisone, and subsequently remained well on long-term maintenance therapy with octreotide 500 μg twice daily and prednisone 200 μg per kg body-weight daily.[1]

1. Palmieri G, *et al.* Successful treatment of a patient with a thymoma and pure red-cell aplasia with octreotide and prednisone. *N Engl J Med* 1997; **336:** 263–5.

Nesidioblastosis. For reference to the use of octreotide in nesidioblastosis, see Hyperinsulinism, above.

Pain. Octreotide 120 to 480 μg daily was administered by continuous intrathecal infusion to 5 patients with cancer pain that had been poorly controlled by opioid analgesics.[1] All patients obtained good pain relief, 3 reporting pain to be totally absent. Sustained decrease in incapacitating bone pain has also been reported in a patient with skeletal metastasis of a gastrinoma who was given subcutaneous octreotide 100 μg three times daily.[2] The pain of hypertrophic pulmonary osteoarthropathy (a paraneoplastic syndrome of periostitis, arthropathy, and gynaecomastia seen particularly with squamous cell lung cancer) has also been reported to respond to octreotide.[3] However, a controlled study of octreotide in cancer pain found that it was no better than placebo in most patients.[4] (General guidelines for the management of cancer pain are discussed on p.8.) Octreotide has also been reported to ease headache associated with meningioma (above), and pituitary adenoma (see below).

1. Penn RD, *et al.* Intrathecal octreotide for cancer pain. *Lancet* 1990; **335:** 738.
2. Burgess JR, *et al.* Effective control of bone pain by octreotide in a patient with metastatic gastrinoma. *Med J Aust* 1996; **164:** 725–7.
3. Johnson SA, *et al.* Treatment of resistant pain in hypertrophic pulmonary osteoarthropathy with subcutaneous octreotide. *Thorax* 1997; **52:** 298–9.
4. De Conno F, *et al.* Subcutaneous octreotide in the treatment of pain in advanced cancer patients. *J Pain Symptom Manage* 1994; **9:** 34–8.

Pancreatic disorders. For reference to the use of octreotide in the treatment of pancreatic endocrine tumours and pancreatic fistulae, see under Carcinoid Syndrome (p.477) and also Gastro-intestinal Disorders, above.

Pituitary adenoma. Pituitary adenomas, which may be responsible for conditions such as acromegaly (p.1235), or hyperprolactinaemia (p.1238), may respond to therapy with octreotide by shrinkage of the tumour and an improvement in symptoms such as headaches and visual disturbances or reduction in the secretion of active hormones, or both. Some references are listed below.

1. Williams G, *et al.* Analgesic effect of somatostatin analogue (octreotide) in headache associated with pituitary tumours. *Br Med J* 1987; **295:** 247–8.
2. Orme SM, *et al.* Shrinkage of thyrotrophin secreting pituitary adenoma treated with octreotide. *Postgrad Med J* 1991; **67:** 466–8.
3. Donckier J, *et al.* Shrinkage of inoperable adenomas in cavernous sinus with high-dose octreotide. *Lancet* 1993; **342:** 301.
4. Chanson P, *et al.* Octreotide therapy for thyroid-stimulating hormone-secreting pituitary adenomas: a follow-up of 52 patients. *Ann Intern Med* 1993; **119:** 236–40.
5. Thapar K, *et al.* Antiproliferative effect of the somatostatin analogue octreotide on growth hormone-producing pituitary tumors: results of a multicenter randomized trial. *Mayo Clin Proc* 1997; **72:** 893–900.

Pretibial myxoedema. A patient receiving thyroxine replacement after subtotal thyroidectomy who developed severe pretibial myxoedema (deposition of glycosaminoglycans in the subcutaneous tissue of the shins) was treated by surgical removal of the myxoedematous tissue and subsequent maintenance with octreotide.[1] Prolonged control of the myxoedema, which tends to recur after surgery, was considered possibly to be due to the drug.

1. Derrick EK, *et al.* Successful surgical treatment of severe pretibial myxoedema. *Br J Dermatol* 1995; **133:** 317–18.

Raised intracranial pressure. For a reference to octreotide being tried in benign intracranial hypertension, see p.796.

Sleep apnoea. A report of improvement in the severity of sleep apnoea in acromegalic patients treated with octreotide.[1]

1. Grunstein RR, *et al.* Effect of octreotide, a somatostatin analog, on sleep apnea in patients with acromegaly. *Ann Intern Med* 1994; **121:** 478–83.

Preparations

Proprietary Preparations (details are given in Part 3)
Aust.: Sandostatin; ***Austral.:*** Sandostatin; ***Belg.:*** Sandostatine; ***Canad.:*** Sandostatin; ***Fr.:*** Sandostatine; ***Ger.:*** Sandostatin; ***Irl.:*** Sandostatin; ***Ital.:*** Longastatina; Samilstin; Sandostatina; ***Neth.:*** Sandostatine; ***Norw.:*** Sandostatin; ***S.Afr.:*** Sandostatin; ***Spain:*** Sandostatin; ***Swed.:*** Sandostatin; ***Switz.:*** Sandostatine; ***UK:*** Sandostatin; ***USA:*** Sandostatin.

Ornipressin (5938-l)

Ornipressin (*rINN*).

[8-Ornithine]-vasopressin.

$C_{45}H_{63}N_{13}O_{12}S_2$ = 1042.2.

CAS — 3397-23-7.

Ornipressin is a synthetic derivative of vasopressin (see p.1263) with similar actions. It is reported to be a strong vasoconstrictor with only weak antidiuretic properties and is used to reduce bleeding during surgery. A solution containing up to 5 units in 20 to 60 mL of sodium chloride injection (0.9%) is infiltrated into the area involved. Ornipressin is also used for bleeding oesophageal varices, the management of which is discussed on p.1576. For this purpose it has been given by intravenous infusion: a dose of 20 units over 20 minutes, diluted in 100 mL of 0.9% sodium chloride injection has been suggested. Continuous infusion over 24 or 48 hours has also been advocated.

Adverse effects. Acute pulmonary oedema occurred in a patient following infiltration of ornipressin (12 units in 40 mL isotonic saline) as a local vasoconstrictor during surgery.[1] It was suggested that no more than 0.1 unit per kg body-weight should be administered in this manner.

1. Borgeat A, *et al.* Acute pulmonary oedema following administration of ornithine-8-vasopressin. *Br J Anaesth* 1990; **65:** 548–51.

Liver disorders. Following beneficial results in one patient,[1] ornipressin was given by intravenous infusion at a dose of 6 units per hour over a period of 4 hours to 9 patients with cirrhosis of the liver.[2] All patients responded; renal function improved during infusion and there was reversal of the hyperdynamic state of the circulation. No major adverse effects were reported. Previous experience[1] indicated that treatment could be maintained for several days by continuous infusion of 1.5 units per hour.

1. Lenz K, *et al.* Enhancement of renal function with ornipressin in a patient with decompensated cirrhosis. *Gut* 1985; **26:** 1385–6.
2. Lenz K, *et al.* Beneficial effect of 8-ornithin vasopressin on renal dysfunction in decompensated cirrhosis. *Gut* 1989; **30:** 90–6.

Preparations

Proprietary Preparations (details are given in Part 3)
Aust.: POR 8; ***Austral.:*** POR 8; ***Ger.:*** POR 8; ***S.Afr.:*** POR 8†; ***Switz.:*** POR 8.

Oxytocin (5940-g)

Oxytocin (*BAN, rINN*).

Alpha-hypophamine; Oxytocinum. Cys-Tyr-Ile-Gln-Asn-Cys-Pro-Leu-Gly-NH_2 cyclic (1→6) disulphide; [2-Leucine,7-isoleucine]vasopressin.

$C_{43}H_{66}N_{12}O_{12}S_2$ = 1007.2.

CAS — 50-56-6.

Pharmacopoeias. In *Chin., Eur.* (see p.viii), *Jpn,* and *US,* as oxytocin or a concentrated solution or injection, or more than one of these.

A cyclic nonapeptide having the structure of the hormone produced by the posterior lobe of the pituitary that stimulates contraction of the uterus and milk ejection in receptive mammals. It may be obtained from the gland of domestic animals used for food by man, or prepared by synthesis; the Ph. Eur. definition requires the latter.

A white or almost white powder, or a clear colourless solution. As a solid, it contains not less than 560 units per mg, calculated with reference to the peptide content; as a liquid it contains not less than 150 units per mL. **Store** at 2° to 8° in airtight containers.

Units

12.5 units of oxytocin for bioassay are contained in approximately 21.4 μg of synthetic peptide (with human albumin 5 mg) in one ampoule of the fourth International Standard (1978).

Adverse Effects

Administration of oxytocin in high doses or to those hypersensitive to it may cause violent uterine contractions leading to uterine rupture and extensive laceration of the soft tissues, fetal bradycardia, fetal arrhythmias, and fetal asphyxiation, and perhaps fetal or maternal death.

Maternal deaths from severe hypertension and subarachnoid haemorrhage have occurred. Postpartum haemorrhage and fatal afibrinogenaemia have been reported but may be due to obstetric complications. Water retention leading to hyponatraemia and intoxication, with pulmonary oedema, convulsions, coma, and even death may occur, especially when oxytocin is given intravenously over prolonged periods. Vasopressin-like activity (see p.1263) is more likely with oxytocin of natural origin but may occur even with the synthetic peptide.

Anaphylactic and other hypersensitivity reactions, cardiac arrhythmias, pelvic haematomas, and nausea and vomiting may occur. Rapid intravenous injection has produced acute transient hypotension, together with flushing and reflex tachycardia.

There are reports of neonatal jaundice and retinal haemorrhage associated with the use of oxytocin in the management of labour. Adverse effects following the intranasal administration of oxytocin have included nasal irritation, rhinorrhoea, lachrymation, uterine bleeding, and violent uterine contractions.

Commenting on the misuse of oxytocin in labour,[1] Taylor and Taylor observed that statements on the management of labour were often misinterpreted as meaning that all labouring women who fail to make adequate progress in terms of cervical dilatation should be given oxytocin. They pointed out that this would only be true if poor progress was due to poor uterine action, and would be dangerous where there was disproportion and that the decision to use oxytocin required careful assessment by an experienced obstetrician. In the previous 2 years the authors had seen one case of fractured pelvis, 2 of ruptured uterus, and 7 of cerebral palsy from fetal hypoxia, all of which were thought to be due to the ill-advised use of oxytocin to augment labour.

For reference to haemorrhage and to neonatal hyperbilirubinaemia occurring after an oxytocin challenge test, see under Uses and Administration, below.

1. Taylor RW, Taylor M. Misuse of oxytocin in labour. *Lancet* 1988; **i:** 352.

Jaundice. Analysis of neonatal jaundice in 12 461 single births confirmed a higher incidence in offspring of mothers given oxytocin, independent of gestational age at birth, sex, race, epidural analgesia, method of delivery, and birthweight, each of which was also associated with jaundice.[1] In a total of 90 infants born to mothers after oxytocin-induced labour in 2 studies,[2,3] haematological disturbances were noted. These included erythrocyte fragility or reduction in erythrocyte deformability, hyponatraemia, hypo-osmolality, and an increase in serum-bilirubin concentration. Glucose injection, used as a vehicle for oxytocin may have further aggravated these changes.[3]

1. Friedman L, *et al.* Factors influencing the incidence of neonatal jaundice. *Br Med J* 1978; **1:** 1235–7.
2. Buchan PC. Pathogenesis of neonatal hyperbilirubinaemia after induction of labour with oxytocin. *Br Med J* 1979; **2:** 1255–7.
3. Singhi S, Singh M. Pathogenesis of oxytocin-induced neonatal hyperbilirubinaemia. *Arch Dis Child* 1979; **54:** 400–2.

Neonatal administration. No adverse effects had been reported in 2 infants who had inadvertently been injected with oxytocin.[1]

1. Donatini B, *et al.* Inadvertent administration of uterotonics to neonates. *Lancet* 1993; **341:** 839–40.

Water intoxication. Oxytocin-induced water intoxication is most likely to arise as a result of prolonged attempts to empty the uterus in missed abortion or mid-trimester termination of pregnancy, but it has also been described after oxytocin infusion in other conditions including induction of labour.[1] Irrespective of the oxytocin concentration, patients in virtually all the reported cases have received more than 3.5 litres of infused fluid. Convulsions and somnolence associated with hyponatraemia have also been reported in a patient who was drinking more than 5 litres of herbal tea daily while using intranasal oxytocin 8 times a day or more.[2]

Another factor contributing to hyponatraemia is the antidiuretic effect of the pethidine and morphine commonly used for analgesia with oxytocin infusions. Water intoxication usually presents with fits and loss of consciousness but in some cases there may be preceding signs such as raised venous pressure, bounding pulse, and tachycardia. Diagnosis is confirmed by profound hyponatraemia; the mechanism appears to be more complex than simply haemodilution by the infused water. Treatment consists of controlling convulsions and maintaining an airway; oxytocin infusion must be stopped and isotonic, or even hypertonic, saline may be infused. Diuresis may then be assisted with frusemide. The prime objective, however, should be prevention; no patient should receive more than 3 litres of fluid containing oxytocin, and a careful fluid balance record is essential.

1. Feeney JG. Water intoxication and oxytocin. *Br Med J* 1982; **285:** 243.
2. Mayer-Hubner B. Pseudotumour cerebri from intranasal oxytocin and excessive fluid intake. *Lancet* 1996; **347:** 623.

Precautions

Oxytocin should not be given where spontaneous labour or vaginal delivery are liable to harm either the mother or the fetus. This includes significant cephalopelvic disproportion or unfavourable presentation of the fetus, placenta praevia or vasa praevia, cord presentation or prolapse, mechanical obstruction to delivery, fetal distress or hypertonic uterine contractions. It should not be used where there is a predisposition to uterine rupture, as in multiple pregnancy or high parity, polyhydramnios, or the presence of a uterine scar from previous caesarean section. Oxytocin should not be employed for prolonged periods in resistant uterine inertia, severe pre-eclampsia, or severe cardiovascular disorders.

When given for induction or enhancement of labour particular care is needed in borderline cephalopelvic disproportion, less severe degrees of cardiovascular disease, and in patients over 35 years of age or with other risk factors. Careful monitoring of fetal heart rate and uterine motility is essential so that dosage of oxytocin can be adjusted to individual response; the drug should be given by intravenous infusion, preferably by means of a syringe pump. Infusion should be discontinued immediately if fetal distress or uterine hyperactivity occur.

Over-vigorous labour should be avoided in cases of fetal death in utero, or where there is meconium-stained amniotic fluid, because there is a risk of amniotic fluid embolism.

The risk of water intoxication should be borne in mind, particularly when high doses of oxytocin are administered over a long time. Infusion volumes should be kept low, and in such circumstances an electrolyte-based infusion fluid should be used rather than glucose solution. Fluid intake by mouth should be restricted and a fluid balance chart maintained; serum electrolytes should be measured if electrolyte imbalance is suspected.

For the suggestion that oxytocin challenge testing should be employed with caution in women whose offspring might be at risk of hyperbilirubinaemia, see under Uses and Administration, below.

Interactions

Oxytocin may enhance the vasopressor effects of sympathomimetics.

Pharmacokinetics

Oxytocin undergoes enzymatic destruction in the gastro-intestinal tract but it is rapidly absorbed from the mucous membranes when administered buccally or intranasally. It is metabolised by the liver and kidneys with a plasma half-life of only a few minutes. Only small amounts are excreted unchanged in the urine.

References.

1. Seitchik J, *et al.* Oxytocin augmentation of dysfunctional labor IV: oxytocin pharmacokinetics. *Am J Obstet Gynecol* 1984; **150:** 225–8.

Uses and Administration

Oxytocin is a cyclic nonapeptide secreted by the hypothalamus and stored in the posterior lobe of the pituitary gland. It may be prepared from the gland of mammals or by synthesis.

Oxytocin causes contraction of the uterus, the effect increasing with the duration of pregnancy due to proliferation of oxytocin receptors. Small doses increase the tone and amplitude of the uterine contractions; large or repeated doses result in tetany. Oxytocin also stimulates the smooth muscle associated with the secretory epithelium of the lactating breast causing the ejection of milk but having no direct effect on milk secretion. It has a weak antidiuretic action.

Oxytocin is used for the induction and augmentation of labour, to control postpartum bleeding and uterine hypotonicity in the third stage of labour, and to promote lactation in cases of faulty milk ejection. It is also used in missed abortions, but other measures may be preferred.

For the induction or augmentation of labour oxytocin may be given by slow intravenous infusion preferably by means of an infusion pump. A solution containing 5 units in 500 mL of a physiological electrolyte solution such as 0.9% sodium chloride is generally recommended but more concentrated solutions may be given via infusion pump. Infusion is begun at an initial rate of 0.5 to 4 milliunits per minute (US sources suggest no more than 2 milliunits per minute) and then gradually increased by increments of 1 to 2 milliunits per minute, at intervals of at least 20 minutes, until a contraction pattern similar to that of normal labour is achieved. A rate of up to 6 milliunits per minute is reported to produce plasma oxytocin concentrations comparable to those in natural labour but doses of up to 20 milliunits or more per minute may be required. Once labour is progressing, oxytocin infusion may be gradually withdrawn. Fetal heart rate and uterine contractions should be monitored continuously.

For the treatment and prevention of postpartum haemorrhage oxytocin may be given by slow intravenous injection in a dose of 5 units; this may be followed in severe cases by intravenous infusion of 5 to 20 units in 500 mL of a suitable non-hydrating diluent. An alternative for the prophylaxis of postpartum haemorrhage in the routine management of the third stage of labour is the intramuscular injection of oxytocin 5 units with ergometrine 500 µg with or after delivery of the baby's shoulders. In the USA a dose of 10 units of oxytocin, by intravenous infusion at a rate of 20 to 40 milliunits per minute, or as an intramuscular injection, has been recommended for treatment of postpartum haemorrhage.

In missed abortion a suggested dose in the UK is 5 units by slow intravenous injection, followed if necessary by intravenous infusion at a rate of 20 to 40 milliunits per minute or higher.

Oxytocin nasal spray is used to facilitate lactation; the usual dose is one spray into one or both nostrils 2 to 3 minutes before suckling. However, there is a danger that the mother may become dependent upon its action and such usage is not generally recommended (see p.1240).

Oxytocin has also been given, as the citrate, in the form of a buccal tablet to induce labour; however, absorption is irregular following buccal administration and this route has been superseded by intravenous infusion.

An oxytocin challenge test has been used to evaluate fetal distress in pregnant patients at high-risk.

Synthetic derivatives of oxytocin such as demoxytocin (see p.1245) have been used similarly.

Labour induction and augmentation. Oxytocin infusions have proved to be one of the most successful agents for induction and augmentation of labour, as discussed on p.1411. There have been numerous studies on the dosage of oxytocin required to induce or augment labour,[1-8] which increasingly favour low-dose regimens, starting at infusion rates of 1 milliunit per minute or less. However, it has been pointed out that no one regimen has been clearly proved superior.[9]

1. Seitchik J, Castillo M. Oxytocin augmentation of dysfunctional labor I: clinical data. *Am J Obstet Gynecol* 1982; **144:** 899–905.
2. Seitchik J, Castillo M. Oxytocin augmentation of dysfunctional labor III: multiparous patients. *Am J Obstet Gynecol* 1983; **145:** 777–80.
3. Seitchik J, *et al.* Oxytocin augmentation of dysfunctional labor V: an alternative oxytocin regimen. *Am J Obstet Gynecol* 1985; **151:** 757–61.
4. Wein P. Efficacy of different starting doses of oxytocin for induction of labor. *Obstet Gynecol* 1989; **74:** 863–8.
5. Blakemore KJ, *et al.* A prospective comparison of hourly and quarter-hourly oxytocin dose increase intervals for the induction of labor at term. *Obstet Gynecol* 1990; **75:** 757–61.
6. Mercer B, *et al.* Labor induction with continuous low-dose oxytocin infusion: a randomized trial. *Obstet Gynecol* 1991; **77:** 659–63.
7. Akoury HA, *et al.* Oxytocin augmentation of labour and perinatal outcome in nulliparas. *Obstet Gynecol* 1991; **78:** 227–30.
8. Satin AJ, *et al.* High versus low-dose oxytocin for labor stimulation. *Obstet Gynecol* 1992; **80:** 111–16.
9. Xenakis EM-J, Piper JM. Chemotherapeutic induction of labour: a rational approach. *Drugs* 1997; **54:** 61–8.

Oxytocin challenge test. The oxytocin challenge test (OCT) is designed to detect placental insufficiency, and identify fetuses at risk of still-birth or complications during labour. In a study, it was performed on 399 occasions in 305 women with pregnancies at risk and a gestational age of 36 weeks or more.[1] Oxytocin 1 milliunit per minute was given by infusion pump and increased every 5 to 10 minutes until a contraction rate of 3 per 10 minutes was achieved. Less than 10% of late or variable decelerations of fetal heart rate (FHR) was judged negative; 10 to 29% was judged equivocal; and 30% or more was judged positive. The finding of a positive or equivocal response to the OCT was considered a prediction of decelerations of the FHR during parturition, though the type of risk might vary. Following the performance of 100 OCT's in 90 pregnant women considered at risk[2] it was concluded that a negative result is a reliable test of fetal well-being which should encourage obstetricians to await spontaneous onset of labour in preference to intervention. However, there have been reports of fetal death occurring despite a negative response to the OCT.[3-5] Adverse effects associated with the OCT have included haemorrhage occurring in a patient after the second of two tests (the patient was found to have a major placenta praevia)[6] and neonatal hyperbilirubinaemia.[7] The latter effect led to the suggestion that the OCT should be used with caution in women whose babies might be at risk from hyperbilirubinaemia.

1. Schulman H, *et al.* Quantitative analysis in the oxytocin challenge test. *Am J Obstet Gynecol* 1977; **129:** 239–44.
2. Sellappah S, Wagman H. Oxytocin challenge test as an out patient procedure. *Br J Clin Pract* 1984; **38:** 255–8.
3. Marcum RG. False negative oxytocin challenge test. *Am J Obstet Gynecol* 1977; **127:** 894.
4. Lorenz RP, Pagano JS. A case of intrauterine fetal death after a negative oxytocin challenge test. *Am J Obstet Gynecol* 1978; **130:** 232.
5. Dittman R, Belcher J. False-negative oxytocin challenge test. *N Engl J Med* 1978; **298:** 56.
6. Ng KH, Wong WP. Risk of haemorrhage in oxytocin stress test. *Br Med J* 1976; **2:** 698–9.
7. Peleg D, Goldman JA. Oxytocin challenge test and neonatal hyperbilirubinaemia. *Lancet* 1976; **ii:** 1026.

Postpartum haemorrhage. Oxytocin is used for the prophylaxis and treatment of postpartum haemorrhage. It may be combined with ergometrine, but comparative studies of the combination versus oxytocin alone have produced contradictory results, as discussed under Ergometrine Maleate, p.1575.

Retained placenta. Oxytocin 100 units injected into the vein of the umbilical cord removed retained placentas within a shorter time than did placebo.[1] The removal of the placenta is important to allow contraction of the myometrium and prevention of excessive blood loss, and is one reason for the use of oxytocin in the active management of the third stage of labour, as discussed under Postpartum Haemorrhage—see above and on p.1575.

1. Wilken-Jensen C, *et al.* Removing a retained placenta by oxytocin—a controlled study. *Am J Obstet Gynecol* 1989; **161:** 155–6.

Preparations

BP 1998: Ergometrine and Oxytocin Injection; Oxytocin Injection;
USP 23: Oxytocin Injection; Oxytocin Nasal Solution.

Proprietary Preparations (details are given in Part 3)
Aust.: Pitocin; Syntocinon; ***Austral.:*** Syntocinon; ***Belg.:*** Syntocinon; ***Canad.:*** Syntocinon†; Toesen†; ***Fr.:*** Syntocinon; ***Ger.:*** Orasthin; Pitocin†; Syntocinon; ***Irl.:*** Syntocinon; ***Ital.:*** Syntocinon; ***Neth.:*** Piton-S†; Syntocinon; ***Norw.:*** Pitocin; Syntocinon; ***S.Afr.:*** Syntocinon; ***Spain:*** Syntocinon; ***Swed.:*** Partocon; Syntocinon; ***Switz.:*** Syntocinon; ***UK:*** Syntocinon; ***USA:*** Pitocin; Syntocinon†.

Multi-ingredient: ***Austral.:*** Syntometrine; ***Ger.:*** Syntometrin; ***Irl.:*** Syntometrine; ***S.Afr.:*** Syntometrine; ***UK:*** Syntometrine.

Posatirelin (10389-r)

Posatirelin (*rINN*).

(2*S*)-*N*-[(1*S*)-1-[[(2*S*)-2-Carbamoyl-1-pyrrolidinyl]carbonyl]-3-methylbutyl]-6-oxopipecolamide.

$C_{17}H_{28}N_4O_4$ = 352.4.

CAS — 78664-73-0.

Posatirelin is an analogue of protirelin (see p.1259). It is claimed to have beneficial effects on CNS function, and is under investigation in the management of dementia of various causes.

References.

1. Parnetti L, *et al.* Posatirelin for the treatment of late-onset Alzheimer's disease: a double-blind multicentre study vs citicoline and ascorbic acid. *Acta Neurol Scand* 1995; **92:** 135–40.
2. Parnetti L, *et al.* Posatirelin in the treatment of vascular dementia: a double-blind multicentre study vs placebo. *Acta Neurol Scand* 1996; **93:** 456–63.
3. Reboldi G, *et al.* Pharmacokinetic profile and endocrine effects of posatirelin treatment in healthy elderly subjects. *J Clin Pharmacol* 1996; **36:** 823–31.

Powdered Pituitary (Posterior Lobe) (5943-s)

Hypophysis Cerebri Pars Posterior; Hypophysis Sicca; Ipofisi Posteriore; Pituitarium Posterius Pulveratum; Pituitary; Posterior Pituitary.

NOTE. Pituitary Extract (Posterior) is *BAN*.

Pharmacopoeias. In *Aust.* which specifies not less than 1 unit of oxytocic activity per mg. *US* includes Posterior Pituitary Injection.

A preparation from the posterior lobes of mammalian pituitary bodies.

Adverse Effects, Treatment, and Precautions

Similar to those for oxytocin (see p.1257) and for vasopressin (see p.1263). Allergic symptoms, including anaphylaxis, have occasionally been reported.

Uses and Administration

Powdered pituitary (posterior lobe) has oxytocic, pressor, antidiuretic, and hyperglycaemic actions and has generally been replaced by compounds or preparations with more specific actions such as oxytocin (p.1258) and desmopressin (p.1245).

It is an ingredient of a number of preparations of combined tissue extracts promoted as tonics or for a variety of non-endocrine disorders.

Preparations

USP 23: Posterior Pituitary Injection.

Proprietary Preparations (details are given in Part 3)
Spain: Acetuber.

Prolactin (5944-w)

Galactin; Lactogen; Lactogenic Hormone; Lactotropin; LMTH; LTH; Luteomammotropic Hormone; Luteotrophic Hormone; Luteotropin; Mammotropin.

CAS — 9002-62-4; 12585-34-1 (sheep); 56832-36-1 (ox); 9046-05-3 (pig).

Prolactin is a water-soluble protein from the anterior pituitary; it is structurally related to growth hormone (p.1249). In *animals,* prolactin has a wide variety of actions and is involved in reproduction, parental care, feeding of the young, electrolyte balance, and growth and development. In humans it has a definite role in inducing milk production; oxytocin (see p.1258) stimulates milk ejection. Relatively high concentrations of prolactin have been found in amniotic fluid. Placental lactogen has been shown to have prolactin-like activity. Prolactin secretion is stimulated by suckling and, for a few months after delivery, it has an inhibitory effect on the ovaries, acting as a natural contraceptive.

The hypothalamus can both stimulate and inhibit prolactin secretion by the anterior pituitary; the inhibitory influence is predominant and is mediated through a dopaminergic system. Dopamine binds to the lactotrope D_2 receptor to inhibit prolactin synthesis and release. Noradrenaline and gamma-aminobutyric acid are also inhibitory as are dopaminergic drugs such as bromocriptine. Although protirelin (see p.1259) has prolactin-releasing activity, there is evidence for the existence of a separate hypothalamic releasing factor (PRF). Prolactin secretion may also be stimulated by methyldopa, metoclopramide, reserpine, opioid analgesics, and neuroleptics of the phenothiazine or butyrophenone type.

Hyperprolactinaemia, which is associated with a variety of other endocrine disorders, is discussed on p.1238.

Prolactin has been given by intramuscular injection in the management of lactation disorders and some forms of menstrual disturbance.

Preparations

Proprietary Preparations (details are given in Part 3)
Ital.: Ferolactan†.

Protirelin (5945-e)

Protirelin *(BAN, USAN, rINN).*

Abbott-38579; Lopremone; Protirelinum; Synthetic TRH; Thyrotrophin-releasing Hormone; Thyrotropin-releasing Hormone; TRF; TRH. L-Pyroglutamyl-L-histidyl-L-prolinamide; 1-[*N*-(5-Oxo-L-prolyl)-L-histidyl]-L-prolinamide; Glu-His-Pro-NH_2.

$C_{16}H_{22}N_6O_4$ = 362.4.

CAS — 24305-27-9.

Pharmacopoeias. In *Eur.* (see p.viii) and *Jpn,* which also includes the tartrate.

A synthetic tripeptide with the same sequence of amino acids as the natural hormone. A white or yellowish-white hygroscopic powder. Very **soluble** in water; freely soluble in methyl alcohol. **Store** in airtight containers at a temperature of 2° to 8°. Protect from light.

Adverse Effects

Protirelin given by intravenous injection may cause headache, nausea, a desire to micturate, flushing, dizziness, and a strange taste. These effects have been attributed to contraction of smooth muscles by the bolus injection. Hypertension and an increased pulse rate, or hypotension, have occasionally been reported as have a few cases of amaurosis and convulsions.

Amaurosis. Of 4 patients with pituitary tumours who developed severe headache after protirelin injection, one also developed amaurosis, apparently associated with pituitary apoplexy.[1] Visual acuity improved after surgery.

1. Drury PL, *et al.* Transient amaurosis and headache after thyrotropin releasing hormone. *Lancet* 1982; **i:** 218–19.

Effects on the cardiovascular system. Increased blood pressure has been reported in women given protirelin antenatally,[1,2] and the view has been expressed that although the magnitude of the change is unlikely to be clinically significant in normotensive women, a much greater rise seen in pre-eclamptic women was severe enough to increase the risk of cerebral haemorrhage.[2]

1. ACTOBAT Study Group. Australian collaborative trial of antenatal thyrotropin-releasing hormone (ACTOBAT) for prevention of neonatal respiratory disease. *Lancet* 1995; **345:** 877–82.
2. Peek MJ, *et al.* Hypertensive effect of antenatal thyrotropin-releasing hormone in pre-eclampsia. *Lancet* 1995; **345:** 793. Correction. *ibid.*; 1124.

Effects on the CNS. Adverse effects reported following injection of 400 µg of protirelin included unconsciousness, hypotension, and convulsions.[1] In another patient with a history of convulsions, injection of 500 µg of protirelin induced epileptic seizures.[2]

1. Dolva LØ, *et al.* Side effects of thyrotrophin releasing hormone. *Br Med J* 1983; **287:** 532.
2. Maeda K, Tanimoto K. Epileptic seizures induced by thyrotropin releasing hormone. *Lancet* 1981; **i:** 1058–9.

Effects on the respiratory system. A report of bronchospasm in an asthmatic boy given protirelin intravenously.[1]

For the suggestion that protirelin may provoke bronchospasm in patients with motor neurone disease, see under Precautions, below.

1. McFadden RG, *et al.* TRH and bronchospasm. *Lancet* 1981; **ii:** 758–9.

Effect on sexual function. On questioning, 7 of 16 women reported a sensation of mild vaginal sexual arousal occurring 1 to 3 minutes after intravenous injection of protirelin.[1] Four women also experienced urinary sensations, and 3 described an urge to urinate with no sexual component.

1. Blum M, Pulini M. Vaginal sensations after injection of thyrotropin releasing hormone. *Lancet* 1980; **ii:** 43.

Precautions

Protirelin should be given with care to patients with ischaemic heart disease, obstructive airways disease, or severe hypopituitarism. Administration of protirelin while the patient is lying down may reduce the incidence of hypotension.

A report of pituitary apoplexy following combined testing of anterior pituitary function in a patient with a pituitary tumour.[1] Of the drugs given, protirelin was thought most likely to have an aetiological role.

See also Amaurosis, under Adverse Effects, above.

1. Chapman AJ, *et al.* Pituitary apoplexy after combined test of anterior pituitary function. *Br Med J* 1985; **291:** 26.

Eclampsia. For the suggestion that the hypertensive effects of protirelin increase the risk of cerebral haemorrhage in pre-eclamptic women, see Effects on the Cardiovascular System under Adverse Effects, above.

Motor neurone disease. Preliminary results suggest that in some patients with amyotrophic lateral sclerosis intravenous injection of protirelin may result in acute bronchospasm.[1] Five of 25 patients experienced falls in FEV_1 of more than 20%; in 2, a 15% decrease in arterial-oxygen pressure occurred. Patients with sclerosis and weakened respiratory muscles should be warned of this potential side-effect.

1. Braun SR, *et al.* Pulmonary effects of thyrotropin-releasing hormone in amyotrophic lateral sclerosis. *Lancet* 1984; **ii** 529–30.

Interactions

Lamberg and Gordin have reviewed the drugs influencing the response to protirelin.[1] The secretion of thyrotrophin appears to be modulated by dopaminergic and noradrenergic pathways at both the hypothalamic and pituitary level. Dopamine and bromocriptine have depressed the response to protirelin; levodopa is a powerful depressant. Partial depression has been reported after the administration of chlorpromazine, thioridazine, and phentolamine, all of which have alpha-receptor blocking properties. Beta-receptors do not appear to be involved in the thyrotrophin response to protirelin whereas the antiserotonin agent, cyproheptadine, has an inhibitory effect. Aspirin and corticosteroids with predominantly glucocorticoid activity have also depressed the response. An enhanced response to protirelin has been seen after the administration of theophylline. Oestrogens may also increase the response in men but not usually in women; when combined with a progestogen a slightly depressed response has been reported.

Other drugs reported to depress the response to protirelin include lithium[2] and ranitidine.[3]

1. Lamberg B-A, Gordin A. Abnormalities of thyrotrophin secretion and clinical implications of the thyrotrophin releasing hormone stimulation test. *Ann Clin Res* 1978; **10:** 171–83.
2. Lauridsen UB, *et al.* Lithium and the pituitary-thyroid axis in normal subjects. *J Clin Endocrinol Metab* 1974; **39:** 383–5.
3. Tarditi E, *et al.* Impaired TSH response to TRH after intravenous ranitidine in man. *Experientia* 1983; **39:** 109–10.

Uses and Administration

Protirelin is a hypothalamic releasing hormone which stimulates the release of thyrotrophin (see p.1262) from the anterior lobe of the pituitary. It also has prolactin-releasing activity. It may be obtained by synthesis.

Protirelin may be used in the assessment of the hypothalamic-pituitary-thyroid axis in the diagnosis of mild hyperthyroidism (p.1489) or hypothyroidism (p.1490), and ophthalmic Graves' disease, although in many cases immunoassays for thyroid-stimulating hormone are now preferred. The response to protirelin may be used for differentiating between primary and secondary hypothyroidism but care is required in interpreting the results of the test and it should not be used alone in establishing the diagnosis. Protirelin is given with gonadorelin (see p.1248) in the assessment of anterior pituitary function.

Protirelin is given intravenously usually in doses of 200 to 500 µg. A suggested intravenous dose in children is 1 µg per kg body-weight in the UK, but in the USA a dose of 7 µg per kg has been recommended.

Protirelin is under investigation in the treatment of motor neurone disease, and in the prevention of neonatal respiratory distress syndrome, but results have been variable.

Protirelin tartrate has been given in the treatment of neurological disorders.

Neonatal respiratory distress syndrome. The regulation of fetal lung development is under multihormonal control and thyroid hormones appear to stimulate pulmonary maturation. However, the thyroid hormones and thyrotrophin do not cross the placenta sufficiently for them to be employed for prenatal treatment in premature labours where neonatal respiratory distress syndrome (p.1025) may develop, and therefore therapy with protirelin has been investigated.[1] Protirelin has been given with corticosteroids to the mother and some beneficial effects have been noted.[1] One study using protirelin 400 µg every 8 hours for 4 doses has indicated that antenatal protirelin reduced the incidence of chronic lung disease when given with corticosteroids but did not affect the incidence of respiratory distress syndrome.[2] However, a large multicentre study involving 1234 women found that in those assigned to treatment with protirelin 200 µg every 12 hours, up to a maximum of 4 doses, in addition to corticosteroid therapy, there were no beneficial effects on outcome compared with those women given corticosteroids only;[3] in fact, respiratory distress syndrome and need for ventilation were greater in the offspring of mothers given protirelin. Subsequent follow-up appeared to confirm the disadvantages of protirelin in this cohort;[4] however the unexpected conclusions of this study have aroused some controversy.[5-7]

1. de Zegher F, *et al.* Prenatal treatment with thyrotrophin releasing hormone to prevent neonatal respiratory distress. *Arch Dis Child* 1992; **67:** 450–4.
2. Ballard RA, *et al.* Respiratory disease in very-low-birthweight infants after prenatal thyrotropin-releasing hormone and glucocorticoid. *Lancet* 1992; **339:** 510–5.
3. ACTOBAT Study Group. Australian collaborative trial of antenatal thyrotropin-releasing hormone (ACTOBAT) for prevention of neonatal respiratory disease. *Lancet* 1995; **345:** 877–82.
4. Crowther CA, *et al.* Australian collaborative trial of antenatal thyrotropin-releasing hormone: adverse effects at 12-month follow-up. *Pediatrics* 1997; **99:** 311–17.
5. Ballard RA, *et al.* Thyrotropin-releasing hormone for prevention of neonatal respiratory disease. *Lancet* 1995; **345:** 1572.
6. Moya FR, Maturana A. Thyrotropin-releasing hormone for prevention of neonatal respiratory disease. *Lancet* 1995; **345:** 1572–3.
7. McCormick MC. The credibility of the ACTOBAT follow-up study. *Pediatrics* 1997; **99:** 476–8.

Neurological disorders. Intravenous infusion of very high doses of protirelin at rates of 2 to 19 mg per minute produced moderate to excellent improvement in neurological deficits in studies involving 17 patients with amyotrophic lateral sclerosis, a form of motor neurone disease (p.1625) and slight to moderate benefit in a further patient with chronic juvenile proximal spinal muscular atrophy.[1] Benefit was evident within 30 seconds of the start of infusion but was sustained for only half to one hour afterwards. However, the subsequent consensus of opinion was that protirelin could not be recommended for patients with motor neurone disease, although some of its analogues may be of value.[2]

Other neurological disorders in which there are reports of protirelin having some beneficial effects include ataxia of spinocerebellar degeneration.[3,4] In general the management of cerebellar ataxia is mainly supportive.

1. Engel WK, *et al.* Effect on weakness and spasticity in amyotrophic lateral sclerosis of thyrotropin-releasing hormone. *Lancet* 1983; **ii:** 73–5.
2. Goonetilleke A. Current therapies in motor neurone disease. *Br J Hosp Med* 1995; **53:** 314–17.
3. Bonuccelli U, *et al.* Oral thyrotropin-releasing hormone treatment in inherited ataxias. *Clin Neuropharmacol* 1988; **11:** 520–8.
4. Filla A, *et al.* Sperimentazione cronica del TRH per via intramuscolare nelle degenerazioni spino-cerebellari: studio in doppio cieco cross-over su 30 soggetti. *Riv Neurol* 1989; **59:** 83–8.

Preparations

Proprietary Preparations (details are given in Part 3)
Aust.: Antepan; Relefact TRH; Thyroliberin TRH†; ***Belg.:*** TRH UCB; ***Canad.:*** Relefact TRH; ***Fr.:*** Stimu-TSH; ***Ger.:*** Antepan; Relefact TRH; Thyroliberin; ***Ital.:*** Irtonin; Xantium; ***Jpn:*** Hirtonin; ***Neth.:*** Relefact TRH; ***Spain:*** TRH Prem†; ***Swed.:*** Thyrefact; ***Switz.:*** Relefact TRH; ***UK:*** TRH-Cambridge; ***USA:*** Thypinone; Thyrel-TRH.

Multi-ingredient: ***UK:*** Relefact LH-RH/TRH†.

Somatomedins (16990-k)

IGFs; Insulin-like Growth Factors; Sulphation Factors.

A group of polypeptide hormones related to insulin and usually known individually as insulin-like growth factors (IGFs), with molecular weights of about 7000 to 8000. They are synthesised in the liver, kidney, muscle, and other tissues.

Mecasermin (15906-x)

Mecasermin *(BAN, rINN).*

IGF-I; Insulin-like growth factor I (human); Somatomedin C.

$C_{331}H_{512}N_{94}O_{101}S_7$ = 7648.6.

CAS — 68562-41-4; 67763-96-6.

Units

150 000 units of insulin-like growth factor I are contained in one ampoule of the first International Standard (1994). For practical purposes 1 international unit can be assumed to be equivalent to 1 μg of insulin-like growth factor I.

Adverse Effects

Since the somatomedins are considered to be responsible for many of the actions of growth hormone similar adverse effects (see p.1250) might be expected.

Syncope in the absence of hypoglycaemia has been reported in patients receiving mecasermin by intravenous bolus, accompanied in some cases by convulsions, asystole, bradycardia, hypotension, or dizziness.[1] Reports appear to have ceased since recommendations that mecasermin not be given intravenously at rates greater than 24 μg per kg body-weight per hour. In addition, mid- and long-term effects of treatment have resulted in adverse effects similar to those associated with growth hormone therapy, including benign intracranial hypertension, gynaecomastia, and acromegalic changes of the features.[1] Arthralgia, nerve palsies, and hypophosphataemia and dyspnoea have been associated with high-dose intravenous bolus therapy.[2]

For a reference to benign intracranial hypertension associated with mecasermin therapy, see under Growth Hormone, p.1250. For concerns about an increased risk of retinopathy in diabetic patients receiving mecasermin, see under Diabetes Mellitus, below.

1. Malozowski S, Stadel B. Risks and benefits of insulin-like growth factor. *Ann Intern Med* 1994; **121:** 549.
2. Usala A-L. Risks and benefits of insulin-like growth factor. *Ann Intern Med* 1994; **121:** 550.

Uses and Administration

The somatomedins are a group of polypeptide hormones, some of which are involved in mediating the effects of growth hormone in the body. IGF-I (mecasermin) is believed to be responsible for many of the anabolic effects of growth hormone. It is secreted primarily by the liver, regulated principally by growth hormone and insulin secretion; IGF-I may also be secreted in other tissues, where it may exert local hormonal (paracrine) effects. In the circulation, IGF-I is almost completely protein bound; 6 binding proteins have been identified, production of some of which is also under the control of growth hormone. In addition to its anabolic effects IGF-I, which is structurally related to insulin, also has potent hypoglycaemic properties.

IGF-I is available as mecasermin, a product of recombinant DNA technology. It has been used in the treatment of children with Laron-type dwarfism, in whom an abnormality of the growth hormone receptor results in an inability to secrete endogenous IGF-I. Long-term administration (several months) with a dose of 150 μg per kg body-weight daily by subcutaneous injection has been reported to produce significant improvement in linear growth in children with this condition. It has also been given to children with growth-attenuating antibodies to growth hormone.

Mecasermin is also being investigated in the management of diabetes mellitus and insulin resistance and is being tried in various other disorders including motor neurone disease, osteoporosis, cachexia, and some peripheral neuropathies.

IGF-II is thought to play an important role in fetal growth, although its function in adults is uncertain. It is closely related in structure to IGF-I, but is not under the control of growth hormone.

General reviews.

1. Laron Z. Somatomedin-1 (insulin-like growth factor-I) in clinical use: facts and potential. *Drugs* 1993; **45:** 1–8.
2. Bondy CA, *et al.* Clinical uses of insulin-like growth factor I. *Ann Intern Med* 1994; **124:** 593–601.
3. Le Roith D. Insulin-like growth factors. *N Engl J Med* 1997; **336:** 633–40.

Diabetes mellitus. There has been considerable interest in the therapeutic potential of mecasermin in diabetes mellitus;[1,2] in particular, several reports and small studies have suggested it can improve insulin sensitivity in patients with insulin resistance.[3-6] A small randomised study[7] has found that mecasermin 40 μg per kg body-weight daily by subcutaneous injection improved metabolic control when added to insulin therapy in patients with type 1 diabetes. However although there was no evidence of an increase in diabetic complications in this study the known proliferative effects of mecasermin have raised concern about a possibly increased risk of diabetic retinopathy;[8] some studies have been halted because of this possibility.

For a general discussion of diabetes mellitus and its management, see p.313.

1. Kolaczynski JW, Caro JF. Insulin-like growth factor-1 therapy in diabetes: physiologic basis, clinical benefits, and risks. *Ann Intern Med* 1994; **120:** 47–55.
2. Dunger DB. Insulin and insulin-like growth factors in diabetes mellitus. *Arch Dis Child* 1995; **72:** 469–71.
3. Hussain MA, Froesch ER. Treatment of type A insulin resistance with insulin-like growth factor-I. *Lancet* 1993; **341:** 1536–7.
4. Ishihama H, *et al.* Long term follow up in type A insulin resistant syndrome treated by insulin-like growth factor I. *Arch Dis Child* 1994; **71:** 144–6.
5. Moses AC, *et al.* Insulin-like growth factor I (rhIGF-I) as a therapeutic agent for hyperinsulinemic insulin-resistant diabetes mellitus. *Diabetes Res Clin Pract* 1995; **28** (suppl): 185–94.
6. Hirano T, Adachi M. Insulin-like growth factor 1 therapy for type B insulin resistance. *Ann Intern Med* 1997; **127:** 245–6.
7. Acerini CL, *et al.* Randomised placebo-controlled trial of human recombinant insulin-like growth factor I plus intensive insulin therapy in adolescents with insulin-dependent diabetes mellitus. *Lancet* 1997; **350:** 1199–1204.
8. Møller N, Ørskov H. Does IGF-I therapy in insulin-dependent diabetes mellitus limit complications? *Lancet* 1997; **350:** 1188–9.

Growth retardation. References[1,2] to the use of mecasermin in patients with Laron-type dwarfism (growth hormone resistance). For a discussion of growth retardation and its management see p.1237.

1. Laron Z, *et al.* Effect of acute administration of insulin-like growth factor I in patients with Laron-type dwarfism. *Lancet* 1988; **ii:** 1170–72.
2. Laron Z, *et al.* Effects of insulin-like growth factor on linear growth, head circumference, and body fat in patients with Laron-type dwarfism. *Lancet* 1992; **339:** 1258–61.

Motor neurone disease. Mecasermin is under investigation for the management of amyotrophic lateral sclerosis,[1] a form of motor neurone disease (p.1625).

1. Lai EC, *et al.* Effect of recombinant human insulin-like growth factor-1 on progression of ALS: a placebo-controlled study. *Neurology* 1997; **49:** 1621–30.

Osteoporosis. Mecasermin has been investigated as a stimulant of bone formation in osteoporosis (p.731). Some references are given below.

1. Ebeling PR, *et al.* Short-term effects of recombinant human insulin-like growth factor I on bone turnover in normal women. *J Clin Endocrinol Metab* 1993; **77:** 1384–7.
2. Rubin CG, *et al.* Treating a patient with the Werner syndrome and osteoporosis using recombinant human insulin-like growth factor. *Ann Intern Med* 1994; **121:** 655–8.

Somatorelin (3765-j)

Somatorelin *(rINN).*

GHRF; GHRH; GRF; GRF-44; Growth Hormone-releasing Factor (Human); Growth Hormone-releasing Hormone; Somatoliberin.

$C_{215}H_{358}N_{72}O_{66}S$ = 5039.7.

CAS — 83930-13-6.

Sermorelin Acetate (2499-b)

Sermorelin Acetate *(BANM, USAN, rINNM).*

GRF(1-29)NH_2; Growth hormone-releasing factor (human)-(1-29)-peptide amide. Tyr-Ala-Asp-Ala-Ile-Phe-Thr-Asn-Ser-Tyr-Arg-Lys-Val-Leu-Gly-Gln-Leu-Ser-Ala-Arg-Lys-Leu-Leu-Gln-Asp-Ile-Met-Ser-Arg-NH_2 acetate hydrate.

$C_{149}H_{246}N_{44}O_{42}S.xC_2H_4O_2.yH_2O$ = 3357.9 (sermorelin).

CAS — 86168-78-7 (sermorelin); 114466-38-5 (sermorelin acetate).

Adverse Effects and Precautions

Facial flushing and pain at the injection site may occur after injection of sermorelin acetate. Headache, nausea and vomiting, dysgeusia, and tightness in the chest have also been reported. Antibodies to somatorelin may develop on repeated administration.

Sermorelin should be used with care in patients with epilepsy or diabetes mellitus. Sermorelin should not be used to treat growth retardation in children in whom the growth hormone response to stimulation tests is inadequate. Treatment should cease once the epiphyses have closed. Uncontrolled hypothyroidism may impair response to sermorelin.

Uses and Administration

Somatorelin is a peptide secreted by the hypothalamus which promotes the release of growth hormone from the anterior pituitary. It exists as 44-, 40-, and 37-amino-acid peptides; the 44-amino acid form may possibly be converted to the smaller forms but all are reported to be active, the activity residing in the first 29 amino-acid residues. Sermorelin is a synthetic peptide corresponding to the 1–29 amino acid sequence of somatorelin.

Sermorelin is used in the form of the acetate for the diagnosis of growth hormone deficiency. The usual dose is the equivalent of sermorelin 1 μg per kg body-weight by intravenous injection in the morning following an overnight fast. A normal response to sermorelin indicates that the somatotrophs are functional, but does not exclude growth hormone deficiency due to hypothalamic dysfunction; it must be used in conjunction with other tests in establishing a diagnosis.

Sermorelin is also used for the treatment of growth hormone deficiency in children; doses of the equivalent of 30 μg per kg, as the acetate, may be given once daily at bedtime by subcutaneous injection. Sermorelin has also been tried as an adjunct to gonadotrophin therapy in the induction of ovulation and has been investigated in the treatment of HIV-associated wasting.

Somatorelin (in its 40- or 44-amino-acid forms) has been used in the assessment of growth hormone deficiency.[1-3] It has usually been given as a single intravenous injection in doses of 1 μg per kg body-weight or total doses of up to 200 μg. Subsequent normal or exaggerated increases in serum-growth hormone concentrations have occurred in healthy subjects,[1,2] and in patients with hypothalamic tumours[3] or acromegaly,[2] but not in patients with hypopituitarism.[2] A synthetic 29-amino-acid sequence of somatorelin, sermorelin acetate is now available for the diagnosis of growth hormone deficiency. However, it has been suggested that the test is not useful for screening as it does not test the hypothalamic-pituitary axis, and that it should not be used in routine clinical practice.[4]

The 44- and 40-amino-acid forms of somatorelin, known as GRF(1-44) and GRF(1-40) (hpGRF-40), as well as sermorelin, have been investigated for the treatment of growth hormone deficiency.[5-8] Generally an increase in growth-hormone secretion occurred accompanied by an increase in growth rate. Various treatment regimens have been tried. Patients have received somatorelin or sermorelin subcutaneously. Somatorelin has been given in 3-hourly pulses day and night,[5] in 4 nocturnal pulses,[6] or once daily.[8] Sermorelin has been given twice daily.[6,7] For a discussion of growth retardation and its management, including mention of the use of growth hormone releasing hormone as an alternative to growth hormone treatment, see p.1237.

Sermorelin has also been investigated for intranasal administration.[9]

1. Thorner MO, *et al.* Human pancreatic growth-hormone-releasing factor selectively stimulates growth-hormone secretion in man. *Lancet* 1983; **i:** 24–8. Correction. *ibid.*; 256.
2. Wood SM, *et al.* Abnormalities of growth hormone release in response to human pancreatic growth hormone releasing factor (GRF (1-44)) in acromegaly and hypopituitarism. *Br Med J* 1983; **286:** 1687–91.
3. Grossman A, *et al.* Growth-hormone-releasing factor in growth hormone deficiency: demonstration of a hypothalamic defect in growth hormone release. *Lancet* 1983; **ii:** 137–8.
4. Hindmarsh PC, Swift PGF. An assessment of growth hormone provocation tests. *Arch Dis Child* 1995; **72:** 362–8.
5. Thorner MO, *et al.* Acceleration of growth in two children treated with human growth hormone-releasing factor. *N Engl J Med* 1985; **312:** 4–9.
6. Smith PJ, Brook CGD. Growth hormone releasing hormone or growth hormone treatment in growth hormone insufficiency? *Arch Dis Child* 1988; **63:** 629–34.
7. Ross RJM, *et al.* Treatment of growth-hormone deficiency with growth-hormone-releasing hormone. *Lancet* 1987; **i:** 5–8.
8. Wit JM, *et al.* Short-term effect on growth of two doses of GRF 1-44 in children with growth hormone deficiency: comparison with growth induced by methionyl-GH administration. *Horm Res* 1987; **27:** 181–9.
9. Vance ML, *et al.* The effect of intravenous, subcutaneous, and intranasal GH-RH analog, [Nle^{27}]GHRH(1-29)-NH_2, on growth hormone secretion in normal men: dose-response relationships. *Clin Pharmacol Ther* 1986; **40:** 627–33.

Preparations

Proprietary Preparations (details are given in Part 3)
Aust.: Geref; ***Belg.:*** Geref†; ***Canad.:*** Geref; ***Fr.:*** Gerel†; ***Ger.:*** Geref†; ***Irl.:*** Geref; ***Ital.:*** Geref; Relsyne†; ***Neth.:*** GHRH; Somatobiss†; ***Norw.:*** Geref; ***S.Afr.:*** Geref; ***Spain:*** Geref; ***Swed.:*** Geref; Groliberin†; ***Switz.:*** Geref; Somatobiss†; ***UK:*** Geref; ***USA:*** Geref.

Somatostatin (5946-l)

Somatostatin *(BAN, rINN)*.

GH-RIF; GHRIH; Growth-hormone-release-inhibiting Hormone; Somatostatinum; Somatotrophin-release-inhibiting Factor. Ala-Gly-Cys-Lys-Asn-Phe-Phe-Trp-Lys-Thr-Phe-Thr-Ser-Cys cyclic (3→14) disulphide.

$C_{76}H_{104}N_{18}O_{19}S_2$ = 1637.9.

CAS — 38916-34-6.

Pharmacopoeias. In *Eur.* (see p.viii).

A cyclic tetradecapeptide having the structure of the hypothalamic hormone that inhibits the release of growth hormone, produced by chemical synthesis and containing not more than 15% w/w of acetic acid.

A white amorphous powder. Freely **soluble** in water and in acetic acid; practically insoluble in dichloromethane. **Store** in airtight containers at a temperature of 2° to 8°. Protect from light.

Adverse Effects and Precautions

Abdominal discomfort, flushing, nausea, and bradycardia have been associated with overly rapid administration. Because of the short half-life of somatostatin adverse effects are generally transitory on stopping or reducing the infusion. Concomitant parenteral nutrition has been suggested because of the inhibitory effects of somatostatin on intestinal absorption; blood sugar should be monitored since somatostatin may interfere with carbohydrate metabolism.

Effects on the kidneys. Somatostatin has been reported to have an inhibitory effect on renal function[1,2] and severe water retention and hyponatraemia have been reported.[3]

1. Walker BJ, *et al.* Somatostatin and water excretion. *Lancet* 1983; **i:** 1101–2.
2. Vora JP, *et al.* Effect of somatostatin on renal function. *Br Med J* 1986; **292:** 1701–2.
3. Halma C, *et al.* Life-threatening water intoxication during somatostatin therapy. *Ann Intern Med* 1987; **107:** 518–20.

Uses and Administration

Somatostatin is a polypeptide obtained from the hypothalamus or by synthesis. The naturally occurring form has a cyclic structure. Although somatostatin derived from the hypothalamus is a 14-amino-acid peptide, a longer, 28-amino-acid form also exists in some tissues. It inhibits the release of growth hormone (see p.1249) from the anterior pituitary. It also inhibits the release of thyrotrophin (see p.1262) and corticotrophin (see p.1244) from the pituitary, glucagon and insulin from the pancreas, and appears to have a role in the regulation of duodenal and gastric secretions. In the CNS it appears to play a role in the perception of pain.

It has been tried in a variety of disorders including upper gastro-intestinal haemorrhage (p.1576), insulin resistance, and the management of hormone-secreting tumours and other hypersecretory disorders, but it has a very short duration of action and several analogues of somatostatin have been produced in an attempt to prolong its activity as well as making its inhibitory effects more specific: octreotide (see p.1255) is such an analogue.

Somatostatin is usually given as the acetate. In the treatment of gastro-intestinal haemorrhage, somatostatin acetate equivalent to somatostatin 3.5 μg per kg body-weight per hour has been given by intravenous infusion.

Preparations

Proprietary Preparations (details are given in Part 3)
Aust.: Curastatin; Somatin; Somatolan; Stilamin; ***Belg.:*** Modustatine; Stilamin†; ***Canad.:*** Stilamin; ***Fr.:*** Modustatine; ***Ger.:*** Aminopan; Stilamin†; ***Ital.:*** Etaxene; Ikestatina; Modustatina; Nastoren; Resurmide; Somacur†; Stilamin; Zecnil; ***Neth.:*** Somatofalk; ***Spain:*** Somiaton; Somonal; ***Switz.:*** Stilamin.

Terlipressin (12796-g)

Terlipressin *(BAN, rINN)*.

Triglycyl-lysine-vasopressin. *N*-[*N*-(*N*-Glycylglycyl)glycyl]lypressin; Gly-Gly-Gly-Cys-Tyr-Phe-Gln-Asn-Cys-Pro-Lys-Gly-NH_2 cyclic (4→9) disulphide.

$C_{52}H_{74}N_{16}O_{15}S_2$ = 1227.4.

CAS — 14636-12-5.

Adverse Effects, Treatment, and Precautions

As for Vasopressin, p.1263.

The pressor and antidiuretic effects of terlipressin are reported to be less marked than those of vasopressin.

Effects on electrolytes. A report of hypokalaemia in a patient receiving terlipressin.[1]

1. Stéphan F, Paillard F. Terlipressin-exacerbated hypokalaemia. *Lancet* 1998; **351:** 1249–50.

Uses and Administration

Terlipressin is an inactive prodrug which is slowly converted in the body to lypressin, and has the general physiological actions of vasopressin (see p.1264).

It is used in the control of bleeding oesophageal varices, in doses of 2 mg by intravenous injection, followed by 1 or 2 mg every 4 to 6 hours if necessary, until bleeding is controlled, for up to 72 hours.

The acetate has been used similarly.

Variceal haemorrhage. In a study in patients with bleeding oesophageal varices (p.1576), patients responded better to terlipressin given by intravenous bolus injection than to vasopressin given by intravenous infusion.[1] There was no significant difference in mortality between the two drugs. A placebo-controlled study in patients with confirmed or suspected cirrhosis of the liver[2] showed that terlipressin was effective in controlling variceal bleeding and that significantly fewer patients receiving terlipressin died from bleeding or secondary hepatic failure than those receiving placebo. Early administration of terlipressin and glyceryl trinitrate (before endoscopy) has also been shown to reduce bleeding and mortality rates in cirrhotic patients with active upper gastro-intestinal bleeding.[3] Comparison of a regimen of terlipressin given by intravenous bolus injection, plus glyceryl trinitrate given sublingually, with balloon tamponade in variceal bleeding suggested similar efficacy.[4] However, tamponade was successful in all patients that were previously unresponsive to terlipressin plus glyceryl trinitrate whereas this drug combination failed in all patients previously unresponsive to tamponade.

1. Freeman JG, *et al.* Controlled trial of terlipressin ('Glypressin') versus vasopressin in the early treatment of oesophageal varices. *Lancet* 1982; **ii:** 66–8.
2. Söderlund C, *et al.* Terlipressin (triglycyl-lysine vasopressin) controls acute bleeding oesophageal varices: a double-blind, randomized, placebo-controlled trial. *Scand J Gastroenterol* 1990; **25:** 622–30.
3. Levacher S, *et al.* Early administration of terlipressin plus glyceryl trinitrate to control active upper gastrointestinal bleeding in cirrhotic patients. *Lancet* 1995; **346:** 865–8.
4. Fort E, *et al.* A randomized trial of terlipressin plus nitroglycerin vs balloon tamponade in the control of acute variceal hemorrhage. *Hepatology* 1990; **11:** 678–81.

Preparations

Proprietary Preparations (details are given in Part 3)
Aust.: Glycylpressin; ***Belg.:*** Glypressin; ***Fr.:*** Glypressine; ***Ger.:*** Glycylpressin; ***Irl.:*** Glypressin; ***Ital.:*** Glipressina; ***Neth.:*** Glypressin; ***Switz.:*** Glypressine; ***UK:*** Glypressin.

Tetracosactrin (1465-s)

Tetracosactrin *(BAN)*.

Tetracosactide *(rINN)*; α^{1-24}-Corticotrophin; β^{1-24}-Corticotrophin; Cosyntropin *(USAN)*; Tetracosactido; Tetracosactidum. Corticotrophin-(1–24)-tetracosapeptide; Ser-Tyr-Ser-Met-Glu-His-Phe-Arg-Trp-Gly-Lys-Pro-Val-Gly-Lys-Lys-Arg-Arg-Pro-Val-Lys-Val-Tyr-Pro.

$C_{136}H_{210}N_{40}O_{31}S$ = 2933.4.

CAS — 16960-16-0.

Pharmacopoeias. In *Eur.* (see p.viii).

Tetracosactrin is a synthetic tetracosapeptide that increases the rate at which corticoid hormones are secreted by the adrenal gland. Its amino acid sequence is the same as that of the first 24 residues of human corticotrophin. The Ph. Eur. specifies not less than 800 units per mg.

Tetracosactrin is a white to yellow amorphous powder. Sparingly **soluble** in water. **Store** at 2° to 8° under an atmosphere of nitrogen. Protect from light.

Units

490 units of tetracosactrin for bioassay are contained in approximately 490 μg of synthetic tetracosactrin with mannitol 20 mg in one ampoule of the first International Reference Preparation (1981).

Adverse Effects

As for Corticotrophin, p.1244. Severe or fatal hypersensitivity reactions have occurred.

Withdrawal

As for Corticotrophin, p.1244.

Precautions

As for Corticosteroids, p.1013. Tetracosactrin is contra-indicated in patients with a history of allergic disorders such as asthma.

Since hypersensitivity reactions may not occur for up to 1 hour after injection sufficient time should be allowed for recovery after administration at the hospital or surgery. Self-administration is not recommended.

Interactions

As for Corticosteroids, p.1014.

Pharmacokinetics

Following intravenous injection tetracosactrin exhibits triphasic pharmacokinetics. It is rapidly eliminated from plasma, mostly by distribution to the adrenal glands and kidneys. It is metabolised by serum endopeptidases into inactive oligopeptides, and then by aminopeptidases into free amino acids. Most of a dose is excreted in urine within 24 hours. The terminal half-life of tetracosactrin is about 3 hours.

Uses and Administration

Tetracosactrin is a synthetic polypeptide with general properties similar to those of corticotrophin (see p.1244). Tetracosactrin is used diagnostically to investigate adrenocortical insufficiency (p.1017).

Although tetracosactrin, like corticotrophin, has also been used therapeutically for most of the conditions in which systemic corticosteroid therapy is indicated, it is now rarely used for such indications.

Tetracosactrin is usually employed in the form of the acetate although doses are often expressed in terms of tetracosactrin itself.

For diagnostic purposes tetracosactrin acetate is used intramuscularly or intravenously as a plain injection in the first instance then, if results are inconclusive, intramuscularly as a long-acting depot injection. The initial test using the plain injection is based on the measurement of plasma-cortisol concentrations immediately before and exactly 30 minutes after an intramuscular or intravenous injection equivalent to 250 μg of tetracosactrin; adrenocortical function may be regarded as normal if there is a rise in the cortisol concentration of at least 200 nmol per litre (70 μg per litre). A suggested intravenous dose in children has been 250 μg per 1.73 m^2 body-surface.

If the results of this test are equivocal the long-acting depot preparation may be used, the adult dose being 1 mg of tetracosactrin acetate given intramuscularly with adrenocortical function being regarded as normal if plasma-cortisol concentrations have steadily increased to 1000 to 1800 nmol per litre 5 hours after the injection. A three day test, for example with 1 mg of the depot preparation given each morning, is also used to differentiate between primary and secondary adrenocortical insufficiency; this is preceded on the first day and followed on the fourth day by the test using the plain injection. A marked improvement in the second assessment suggests secondary adrenocortical insufficiency.

For therapeutic purposes tetracosactrin acetate has been given by intramuscular injection as the long-acting depot preparation. The usual initial adult dose of tetracosactrin acetate is 1 mg daily (or 1 mg every 12 hours in acute cases), reduced after the acute symptoms have been controlled to 0.5 to 1 mg every 2 or 3 days or 1 mg weekly.

Preparations

BP 1998: Tetracosactide Injection; Tetracosactide Zinc Injection.

Proprietary Preparations (details are given in Part 3)
Aust.: Synacthen; *Belg.:* Cortrosyn†; Synacthen; *Canad.:* Cortrosyn; Synacthen Depot; *Fr.:* Synacthene; *Ger.:* Synacthen; Synacthen Depot; *Irl.:* Synacthen; Synacthen Depot†; *Ital.:* Cortrosyn; Synacthen; *Neth.:* Cortrosyn†; Synacthen; *Norw.:* Synacthen; *S.Afr.:* Synacthen Depot; *Spain:* Nuvacthen Depot; *Swed.:* Synacthen; *Switz.:* Synacthen; Synacthen Retard; *UK:* Synacthen; Synacthen Depot; *USA:* Cortrosyn.

Thyrotrophin (5947-y)

Thyrotrophin *(BAN, rINN)*.

Thyroid-stimulating Hormone; Thyrotrophic Hormone; Thyrotropin; TSH.

CAS — 9002-71-5.

A glycoprotein from the anterior pituitary with a molecular weight in man of about 30 000.

Units

0.037 units of human pituitary thyrotrophin for immunoassay and bioassay are contained in approximately 7.5 μg of thyrotrophin, with albumin 1 mg and lactose 5 mg, in one ampoule of the second International Reference Preparation (1983).

Adverse Effects

Infrequent side-effects of thyrotrophin include nausea, vomiting, headache, a desire to micturate, and flushing. High doses may produce excessive thyroid stimulation, with angina, tachycardia or arrhythmias, dyspnoea, sweating, nervousness and irritability. Hypersensitivity reactions, including skin rash and urticaria, erythema and swelling at the injection site, and anaphylaxis have occurred, particularly on repeated administration.

Precautions

Thyrotrophin should not be given to patients with recent myocardial infarction or uncorrected adrenocortical insufficiency, including adrenocortical insufficiency secondary to hypopituitarism. Care is also required in patients with cardiovascular disease.

Uses and Administration

Thyrotrophin is a glycoprotein secreted by the anterior lobe of the pituitary and with an alpha subunit essentially the same as that of the gonadotrophins. Its main actions are to increase the iodine uptake by the thyroid and the formation and secretion of the thyroid hormones. It may produce hyperplasia of thyroid tissue. Thyrotrophin secretion is controlled by a hypothalamic releasing hormone (Protirelin, see p.1259) and by circulating thyroid hormones; somatostatin (see p.1261) may inhibit the release of thyrotrophin.

Thyrotrophin has been used in conjunction with radio-iodine in the diagnosis of hypothyroidism (p.1490) and to differentiate between primary and secondary hypothyroidism, but direct radio-immunoassay of circulating endogenous thyroid-stimulating hormone may be preferred. Thyrotrophin increases the uptake of radio-iodine by the thyroid and has been used as a diagnostic tool and as an adjunct in the treatment of certain types of thyroid cancer.

The usual dose is 10 units daily by intramuscular or subcutaneous injection; depending upon the indication this dose may be given for between 1 and 8 days.

Malignant neoplasms of the thyroid. Patients with thyroid carcinoma (p.494) may undergo surgery or radio-iodine treatment or both and subsequently receive thyroid hormone therapy. Continuous monitoring for tumour recurrence in subsequent years requires interruption of thyroid hormone treatment, with consequent hypothyroidism. A study[1] comparing administration of thyrotrophin with withdrawal of thyroid hormones as a prelude to radio-iodine scanning found that the former did stimulate radio-iodine uptake but that the sensitivity of scanning was less than after thyroid hormone withdrawal. Withdrawal was still the best option in these patients, but thyrotrophin might be considered an alternative where this was refused.[1,2]

1. Ladenson PW, *et al.* Comparison of administration of recombinant human thyrotropin with withdrawal of thyroid hormone for radioactive iodine scanning in patients with thyroid carcinoma. *N Engl J Med* 1997; **337:** 888–96.
2. Utiger RD. Follow-up of patients with thyroid carcinoma. *N Engl J Med* 1997; **337:** 928–30.

Preparations

Proprietary Preparations (details are given in Part 3)
Canad.: Thytropar†; *USA:* Thytropar.

Triptorelin (16834-v)

Triptorelin *(BAN, USAN, rINN)*.

AY-25650; BIM-21003; BN-52014; CL-118532; Triptoreline; D-Trp⁶-LHRH; [6-D-Tryptophan] luteinising hormone-releasing factor. 5-Oxo-L-prolyl-L-histidyl-L-tryptophyl-L-seryl-L-tyrosyl-D-tryptophyl-L-leucyl-L-arginyl-L-prolylglycinamide.

$C_{64}H_{82}N_{18}O_{13}$ = 1311.4.

CAS — 57773-63-4.

Adverse Effects and Precautions

As for Gonadorelin, p.1247.

For a report of disease flare in patients given triptorelin for prostatic cancer, see Buserelin Acetate, p.1242.

Local reactions. For reference to local reactions occurring following injection of gonadorelin analogues, including triptorelin, see p.1253.

Sepsis. A report of 2 patients in whom triptorelin therapy led to sepsis caused by expulsion of necrotic fibroids through the cervix.[1]

1. Ellenbogen A, *et al.* Complication of triptorelin treatment for uterine myomas. *Lancet* 1989; **ii:** 167–8.

Pharmacokinetics

Triptorelin is rapidly absorbed following subcutaneous injection, with peak plasma concentrations achieved about 40 minutes after a dose. The biological half-life has been stated to be about 7.5 hours, although longer half-lives have been reported in patients with prostate cancer, and shorter half-lives in some groups of healthy subjects.

References.

1. Müller FO, *et al.* Pharmacokinetics of triptorelin after intravenous bolus administration in healthy males and in males with renal or hepatic insufficiency. *Br J Clin Pharmacol* 1997; **44:** 335–41.

Uses and Administration

Triptorelin is an analogue of gonadorelin (see p.1248) with similar properties, used for the suppression of gonadal sex hormone production in the treatment of malignant neoplasms of the prostate, in precocious puberty, and in the management of endometriosis, female infertility, and uterine fibroids. It is used either as the base or as the acetate or embonate; doses are given in terms of the base. It is given as a daily subcutaneous injection or monthly as an intramuscular depot preparation.

In the treatment of prostate cancer 3.0 or 3.75 mg of the depot preparation is given intramuscularly every 4 weeks; the first dose may be preceded by 0.1 mg daily for 7 days by subcutaneous injection. An anti-androgen such as cyproterone acetate may be given for several days before beginning therapy with gonadorelin analogues and continued for about 3 weeks to avoid the risk of a disease flare.

Similar doses of the depot preparation may be given for up to 6 months in the management of endometriosis or uterine fibroids, with treatment begun during the first 5 days of the menstrual cycle. In the management of female infertility doses of 0.1 mg subcutaneously daily, in conjunction with gonadotrophins, have been recommended from the second day of the menstrual cycle for about 10 to 12 days. In children with precocious puberty a dose of 50 μg of depot triptorelin per kg body-weight may be given intramuscularly every 4 weeks.

Delayed and precocious puberty. Gonadorelin analogues such as triptorelin[1,2] are used in the management of central precocious puberty (see p.1241). They may also be effective in delayed puberty (p.1237) although they are most likely to be helpful where this is due to hypogonadism. A reference to the use of triptorelin to differentiate gonadotrophin deficiency from constitutional delayed puberty is given below.[3]

1. Roger M, *et al.* Long term treatment of male and female precocious puberty by periodic administration of a long-acting preparation of D-trp⁶-luteinizing hormone-releasing hormone microcapsules. *J Clin Endocrinol Metab* 1986; **62:** 670–7.
2. Oostdijk W, *et al.* Final height in central precocious puberty after long term treatment with a slow release GnRH agonist. *Arch Dis Child* 1996; **75:** 292–7.
3. Zamboni G, *et al.* Use of the gonadotropin-releasing hormone agonist triptorelin in the diagnosis of delayed puberty in boys. *J Pediatr* 1995; **126:** 756–8.

Disturbed behaviour. Combined therapy with triptorelin, which suppressed testosterone secretion by inhibiting the pituitary gonadal axis, and supportive psychotherapy, has been tried in the treatment of men with paraphilias (see p.636): a reduction in abnormal sexual thoughts and behaviours has been reported, although the study was uncontrolled.[1]

1. Rösler A, Witztum E. Treatment of men with paraphilia with a long-acting analogue of gonadotropin-releasing hormone. *N Engl J Med* 1998; **338:** 416–22.

Endometriosis. Gonadorelin analogues are effective in the management of endometriosis (p.1442), but the need for long-term therapy to prevent recurrence limits their value because of the risk of osteoporosis; 'add-back' therapy, with concomitant hormone replacement, is being investigated.

Fibroids. Gonadorelin analogues have been tried as an alternative to surgery in the treatment of uterine fibroids (see p.1248), despite some concern that this may complicate the diagnosis of malignancy. Some further references to the use of triptorelin are listed below.

1. van Leusden HAIM. Rapid reduction of uterine myomas after short-term treatment with microencapsulated D-Trp⁶-LHRH. *Lancet* 1986; **ii:** 1213.
2. Schneider D, *et al.* GnRH analogue-induced uterine shrinkage enabling a vaginal hysterectomy and repair in large leiomyomatous uteri. *Obstet Gynecol* 1991; **78:** 540–1.

Growth retardation. As discussed on p.1237 gonadorelin analogues have been given in combination with growth hormone to short girls without growth hormone deficiency, in an attempt to delay puberty and bone maturation and thus maximise the final height achieved. However, there is some doubt about the extent of benefit, and in any case the concept of such treatment in children who are not clinically deficient in growth hormone is controversial, and some authorities do not consider it appropriate.

For a reference to such combination treatment employing triptorelin, see below.

1. Saggese G, *et al.* Combination treatment with growth hormone and gonadotropin-releasing hormone analogs in short normal girls. *J Pediatr* 1995; **126:** 468–73.

Infertility. Gonadorelin analogues are used in the management of infertility related to hypogonadotrophic hypogonadism in both men and women. For a discussion of infertility and its management, including the role of gonadorelin analogues, see p.1239. Triptorelin 1.8 mg intramuscularly was added to a schedule of norethisterone and human menopausal gonadotrophin[1] to prevent spontaneous surges of luteinising hormone as part of a carefully timed programme of ovarian stimulation which enabled follicular aspiration for *in-vitro* fertilisation to be carried out usually on a weekday and avoided the need for clinical and laboratory staff to be on duty 7 days a week.

1. Zorn JR, *et al.* Never on a Sunday: programming for IVF-ET and GIFT. *Lancet* 1987; **i:** 385–6.

Malignant neoplasms. Lung and bone metastases cleared in a patient with prostatic carcinoma (p.491) given triptorelin daily by subcutaneous injection.[1] The initial dose was 500 μg daily for the first 7 days after which it was reduced to 100 μg daily. Two multicentre studies[2,3] found slow-release triptorelin (in the form of microcapsules releasing 100 μg daily, given intramuscularly once a month) to be as effective as orchidectomy in the initial treatment of advanced prostatic cancer. There are reports of responses to triptorelin in advanced adenocarcinoma of the pancreas,[4] advanced ovarian cancer[5] (although others have been unable to show any benefit in a randomised study[6]), and lung metastases of breast cancer.[7] However, the role of gonadorelin analogues in the management of these malignancies, which are discussed on p.491, p.491, and p.485, remains to be determined.

1. Comaru-Schally AM, *et al.* Clearance of lung metastases of prostate carcinoma after treatment with LH-RH agonist. *Lancet* 1984; **ii:** 281–2.
2. Parmar H, *et al.* Randomised controlled study of orchidectomy vs long-acting D-TRP-6-LHRH microcapsules in advanced prostatic carcinoma. *Lancet* 1985; **ii:** 1201–5.
3. Boccardo F, *et al.* D-TRP-6-LH-RH treatment of advanced prostatic cancer. *Lancet* 1986; **i:** 621.
4. Gonzalez-Barcena D, *et al.* Response to D-TRP-6-LH-RH in advanced adenocarcinoma of pancreas. *Lancet* 1986; **ii:** 154.
5. Parmar H, *et al.* Response to D-Trp-6-luteinising hormone releasing hormone (Decapeptyl) microcapsules in advanced ovarian cancer. *Br Med J* 1988; **296:** 1229.
6. Emons G, *et al.* Luteinizing hormone-releasing hormone agonist triptorelin in combination with cytotoxic chemotherapy in patients with advanced ovarian carcinoma: a prospective double-blind randomized trial. *Cancer* 1996; **78:** 1452–60.
7. Sanchez-Garrido F, *et al.* Clearance of lung metastases of breast carcinoma after treatment with triptorelin in postmenopausal woman. *Lancet* 1995; **345:** 868.

Preparations

Proprietary Preparations (details are given in Part 3)
Aust.: Decapeptyl; ***Belg.:*** Decapeptyl; ***Fr.:*** Decapeptyl; ***Ger.:*** Decapeptyl; ***Irl.:*** Decapeptyl; ***Ital.:*** Decapeptyl; ***Neth.:*** Decapeptyl; ***S.Afr.:*** Decapeptyl; ***Spain:*** Decapeptyl; ***Swed.:*** Decapeptyl; ***Switz.:*** Decapeptyl; ***UK:*** Decapeptyl.

Urofollitrophin (12013-v)

Urofollitrophin *(BAN).*
Urofollitropin *(USAN, rINN)*; Urofollitropinum.
CAS — 97048-13-0.
Pharmacopoeias. In *Eur.* (see p.viii).

A dry preparation containing menopausal gonadotrophin obtained from the urine of postmenopausal women. It contains not less than 90 units of follicle-stimulating hormone per mg; the ratio of units of luteinising hormone to units of follicle-stimulating hormone is not more than 1:60.

A practically white or slightly yellow powder. **Soluble** in water. **Store** in airtight containers at a temperature of 2° to 8°. Protect from light.

Urofollitrophin is a gonadotrophin, obtained from the urine of postmenopausal women, possessing follicle-stimulating hormone (FSH) activity but virtually no luteinising activity. For details of the actions of FSH, see p.1247.

Urofollitrophin is used similarly to human menopausal gonadotrophins (see p.1252) in the treatment of female infertility with the exception that being without luteinising hormone activity, it can be used in patients where any increase in luteinising hormone activity is not required, as in polycystic ovarian disease. Urofollitrophin is given subcutaneously or intramuscularly in a dosage adjusted according to the patient's response. Usually a dose providing 75 to 150 units of FSH daily is given initially. When an adequate response is achieved, as determined by oestrogen monitoring or ultrasonic visualisation of follicles, treatment is stopped and chorionic gonadotrophin is administered to induce ovulation. Treatment with urofollitrophin should be discontinued if there is no response after 4 weeks although treatment may again be attempted in future cycles.

Urofollitrophin is also used in conjunction with other agents as part of *in vitro* fertilisation procedures. Urofollitrophin in a dose providing 75 to 300 units of FSH is given daily, usually beginning from day 2 or 3 of the menstrual cycle. Alternatively, therapy has been initiated with clomiphene citrate and continued with urofollitrophin, or urofollitrophin may be given after suppression of gonadotrophin release with a gonadorelin analogue. Treatment is continued until an adequate response is obtained and the final injection of urofollitrophin is followed 1 to 2 days later with 5000 to 10 000 units of chorionic gonadotrophin. Oocyte retrieval is performed 34 to 35 hours later.

Urofollitrophin is also used in conjunction with chorionic gonadotrophin to stimulate spermatogenesis in the treatment of male infertility, although a preparation with combined luteinising activity, such as human menopausal gonadotrophins, may be preferred. The usual dose provides 75 units of FSH daily, or 75 to 150 units 2 to 3 times a week, together with a simultaneous dose of chorionic gonadotrophin 1000 to 2000 units. Treatment should be continued for at least 3 or 4 months. For a brief discussion of hypogonadism see p.1239.

Infertility. For reference to the use of preparations with follicle-stimulating hormone activity in infertility, see p.1239. The management of women with polycystic ovary syndrome is discussed in more detail on p.1240. Some further references are listed below.

1. Remorgida V, *et al.* Administration of pure follicle-stimulating hormone during gonadotropin-releasing hormone agonist therapy in patients with clomiphene-resistant polycystic ovarian disease: hormonal evaluations and clinical perspectives. *Am J Obstet Gynecol* 1989; **160:** 108–13.
2. Buvat J, *et al.* Purified follicle-stimulating hormone in polycystic ovary syndrome: slow administration is safer and more effective. *Fertil Steril* 1989; **52:** 553–9.
3. McFaul PB, *et al.* Treatment of clomiphene citrate-resistant polycystic ovarian syndrome with pure follicle-stimulating hormone or human menopausal gonadotropin. *Fertil Steril* 1990; **53:** 792–7.

Preparations

BP 1998: Urofollitropin Injection.

Proprietary Preparations (details are given in Part 3)
Aust.: Fertinorm; ***Austral.:*** Metrodin; ***Belg.:*** Metrodin†; ***Canad.:*** Fertinorm; Metrodin; ***Fr.:*** Fertiline; Metrodine; ***Ger.:*** Fertinorm; ***Irl.:*** Metrodin; ***Ital.:*** Metrodin; ***Neth.:*** Follegon; Metrodin; ***Norw.:*** Fertinorm†; ***S.Afr.:*** Metrodin; ***Spain:*** Fertinorm†; Neo Fertinorm; ***Swed.:*** Fertinorm†; ***Switz.:*** Metrodin; ***UK:*** Metrodin; Orgafol; ***USA:*** Fertinex; Metrodin.

Vapreotide (13864-w)

Vapreotide *(USAN, rINN).*
BMY-41606; RC-160. D-Phenylalanyl-L-cysteinyl-L-tyrosyl-D-tryptophyl-L-lysyl-L-valyl-L-cysteinyl-L-tryptophanamide cyclic (2→7)-disulfide.
$C_{57}H_{70}N_{12}O_9S_2$ = 1131.4.
CAS — 103222-11-3.

Vapreotide is a somatostatin analogue similar to octreotide (p.1255). It is under investigation in the management of various gastro-intestinal and neoplastic disorders.

References.

1. Stiefel F, Morant R. Vapreotide, a new somatostatin analogue in the palliative management of obstructive ileus in advanced cancer. *Support Care Cancer* 1993; **1:** 57–8.
2. Eriksson B, *et al.* The use of new somatostatin analogues, lanreotide and octastatin, in neuroendocrine gastro-intestinal tumours. *Digestion* 1996; **57** (suppl 1): 77–80.

Vasopressin (5948-j)

ADH; Antidiuretic Hormone; Beta-Hypophamine.
CAS — 11000-17-2 (vasopressin injection).

NOTE. Vasopressin Injection is *rINN.*
Pharmacopoeias. In *US*, which includes both argipressin and lypressin in this title.
Vasopressin Injection is included in *Jpn.*

The pressor and antidiuretic principle of the posterior lobe of the pituitary gland. It may be prepared by synthesis or by extraction from the glands of healthy, domestic animals used for food in man. The USP states that its vasopressor activity is not less than 300 USP units per mg. **Store** in airtight containers at 2° to 8°.

Argipressin (5949-z)

Argipressin *(BAN, rINN).*
[8-Arginine]vasopressin; AVP; CI-107 (argipressin tannate).
Cys-Tyr-Phe-Gln-Asn-Cys-Pro-Arg-Gly-NH_2 cyclic (1→6) disulphide.
$C_{46}H_{65}N_{15}O_{12}S_2$ = 1084.2.
CAS — 113-79-1.

NOTE. Argipressin Tannate is *USAN.*

Argipressin is a form of vasopressin obtained from most mammals including man but excluding pig. It is usually prepared synthetically. Lypressin (see below) is vasopressin from pig.

Units

8.2 units of argipressin for bioassay are contained in approximately 20 µg of synthetic peptide acetate (with human albumin 5 mg and citric acid) in one ampoule of the first International Standard (1978).

Lypressin (5934-p)

Lypressin *(BAN, USAN, rINN).*
L-8; Lipressina; LVP. [8-Lysine]vasopressin; Cys-Tyr-Phe-Gln-Asn-Cys-Pro-Lys-Gly-NH_2 cyclic (1→6) disulphide.
$C_{46}H_{65}N_{13}O_{12}S_2$ = 1056.2.
CAS — 50-57-7.
Pharmacopoeias. Lypressin Injection is included in *Eur.* (see p.viii).

A form of vasopressin which is usually prepared synthetically, or may be extracted from the posterior pituitary of pigs. The Ph. Eur. injection has a pH of 3.7 to 4.3. **Store** at a temperature of 2° to 15° and avoid freezing.

Units

7.7 units of lypressin are contained in approximately 23.4 µg of synthetic peptide (with albumin 5 mg and citric acid) in one ampoule of the first International Standard (1978).

Vasopressin Tannate (5950-p)

The water-insoluble tannate of the pressor principle of the posterior lobe of the pituitary.

Adverse Effects

Large parenteral doses of vasopressin may give rise to marked pallor, pounding headache, sweating, tremor, nausea, vomiting, diarrhoea, eructation, cramp, and a desire to defaecate; some of these effects may also be noted following large intranasal doses of lypressin. In women, vasopressin may cause uterine cramps of a menstrual character. Hyponatraemia with water retention and signs of water intoxication can occur.

Hypersensitivity reactions have occurred and include urticaria and bronchial constriction. Anaphylactic shock and cardiac arrest have been reported.

Vasopressin may constrict coronary arteries. Chest pain, myocardial ischaemia, and infarction have occurred following injection, and fatalities have been reported. Other cardiovascular effects include occasional reports of arrhythmias and bradycardia, as well as hypertension. Peripheral vasoconstriction has resulted in gangrene, and thrombosis as well as local irritation at the injection site may occur.

Following intranasal use (usually as lypressin) nasal congestion, irritation, and ulceration have been reported occasionally; systemic effects at usual intranasal doses are mostly reported to be mild.

Effects on the heart. Arrhythmias, including ventricular tachycardia and fibrillation,[1] torsade de pointes,[2-4] and asystole[5] are among the adverse effects of vasopressin administration. Paradoxical bradycardia and hypotension has also been reported.[6]

1. Kelly KJ, *et al.* Vasopressin provocation of ventricular dysrhythmia. *Ann Intern Med* 1980; **92:** 205–6.
2. Eden E, *et al.* Ventricular arrhythmia induced by vasopressin: torsade de pointes related to vasopressin-induced bradycardia. *Mt Sinai J Med* 1983; **50:** 49–51.
3. Stein LB, *et al.* Fatal torsade de pointes occurring in a patient receiving intravenous vasopressin and nitroglycerin. *J Clin Gastroenterol* 1992; **15:** 171–4.
4. Faigel DO, *et al.* Torsade de pointes complicating the treatment of bleeding esophageal varices: association with neuroleptics, vasopressin, and electrolyte imbalance. *Am J Gastroenterol* 1995; **90:** 822–4.
5. Fitz JD. Vasopressin induction of ventricular ectopy. *Arch Intern Med* 1982; **142:** 644.
6. Kraft W, *et al.* Paradoxical hypotension and bradycardia after intravenous arginine vasopressin. *J Clin Pharmacol* 1998; **38:** 283–6.

Ischaemia. Reports of ischaemia and infarction associated with vasopressin.

1. Greenwald RA, *et al.* Local gangrene: a complication of peripheral Pitressin therapy for bleeding esophageal varices. *Gastroenterology* 1978; **74:** 744–6.
2. Colombani P. Upper extremity gangrene secondary to superior mesenteric artery infusion of vasopressin. *Dig Dis Sci* 1982; **27:** 367–9.
3. Lambert M, *et al.* Reversible ischemic colitis after intravenous vasopressin therapy. *JAMA* 1982; **247:** 666–7.
4. Anderson JR, Johnston GW. Development of cutaneous gangrene during continuous peripheral infusion of vasopressin. *Br Med J* 1983; **287:** 1657–8.
5. Reddy KR, *et al.* Bilateral nipple necrosis after intravenous vasopressin therapy. *Arch Intern Med* 1984; **144:** 835–6.
6. Brearly S, *et al.* A lethal complication of peripheral vein vasopressin infusion. *Hepatogastroenterology* 1985; **32:** 224–5.
7. Sweren BS, Bohlman ME. Gastric and splenic infarction: a complication of intraarterial vasopressin infusion. *Cardiovasc Intervent Radiol* 1989; **12:** 207–9.
8. Maceyko RF, *et al.* Vasopressin-associated cutaneous infarcts, alopecia, and neuropathy. *J Am Acad Dermatol* 1994; **31:** 111–13.

Treatment of Adverse Effects

The antidiuretic effects on water retention and sodium imbalance may be treated by water restriction and a temporary withdrawal of vasopressin. Severe cases may require osmotic diuresis alone or with frusemide.

A report of the localised intravenous and intra-arterial administration of guanethidine in the treatment of a patient with extravasation of vasopressin.[1] The intra-arterial administration of guanethidine was considered to have helped to avoid necrotic changes.

1. Crocker MC. Intravascular guanethidine in the treatment of extravasated vasopressin. *N Engl J Med* 1981; **304:** 1430.

Precautions

Vasopressin should not be used in patients with chronic nephritis with nitrogen retention, and should be avoided or given only with extreme care, and in small doses, to patients with vascular disease, especially of the coronary arteries.

It should be given with care to patients with asthma, epilepsy, migraine, heart failure, or other conditions which might be aggravated by water retention. Fluid intake should be adjusted to avoid hyponatraemia and water intoxication. Care is also required in hypertension or other conditions that may be exacerbated by a rise in blood pressure. Nasal absorption of vasopressin may be impaired in patients with rhinitis.

Abuse. Vasopressin or its analogues have been abused as so-called 'smart drugs' for their supposed effect on memory recall and cognition.

Resistance. Antibodies to vasopressin were detected in 6 of 28 patients being treated for diabetes insipidus, all of whom experienced a decrease in antidiuretic effect with previously effective argipressin or lypressin therapy;[1] desmopressin and chlorpropamide remained effective in these patients. There have been reports of patients with diabetes insipidus of pregnancy unresponsive to argipressin but responsive to desmopressin.[2] This was probably due to excessive placental production of vasopressinase, an enzyme which degrades argipressin.

1. Vokes TJ, *et al.* Antibodies to vasopressin in patients with diabetes insipidus: implications for diagnosis and therapy. *Ann Intern Med* 1988; **108:** 190–5.
2. Shah SV, Thakur V. Vasopressinase and diabetes insipidus of pregnancy. *Ann Intern Med* 1988; **109:** 435–6.

Interactions

The antidiuretic effects of vasopressins might be expected to be enhanced in some patients receiving chlorpropamide, clofibrate, carbamazepine, fludrocortisone, urea, or tricyclic antidepressants; lithium, heparin, demeclocycline, noradrenaline, and alcohol may decrease the antidiuretic effect. Ganglion-blocking agents may increase sensitivity to the pressor effects of vasopressins.

Cimetidine. A report of severe bradycardia and heart block leading to asystole in a patient given combined vasopressin and cimetidine therapy.[1]

1. Nikolic G, Singh JB. Cimetidine, vasopressin and chronotropic incompetence. *Med J Aust* 1982; **2:** 435–6.

Uses and Administration

Vasopressin is secreted by the hypothalamus and stored in the posterior lobe of the pituitary gland. It may be prepared from the gland of mammals or by synthesis. Vasopressin has a direct antidiuretic action on the kidney, increasing tubular reabsorption of water. It also constricts peripheral blood vessels and causes contraction of the smooth muscle of the intestine, gallbladder, and urinary bladder. It has practically no oxytocic activity.

Vasopressin, which is usually administered parenterally or intranasally in the synthetic forms of argipressin or lypressin, is used in the treatment of diabetes insipidus due to a deficiency in antidiuretic hormone. It is ineffective in nephrogenic diabetes insipidus. It should not be used to raise the blood pressure. Argipressin has also been used in the prevention and treatment of postoperative abdominal distension, and was formerly given to remove gas in abdominal visualisation procedures. Argipressin or lypressin are used in the treatment of bleeding oesophageal varices.

In the treatment of cranial diabetes insipidus to control polyuria, argipressin may be administered subcutaneously or intramuscularly; a suggested dose in the UK is 5 to 20 units every 4 hours. In the USA, 5 to 10 units given 2 or 3 times daily or more has been suggested. Alternatively, lypressin may be given as a nasal spray, the usual dose for diabetes insipidus being 4 to 10 units 3 or 4 times daily; an extra dose may be given at bedtime to eliminate nocturia. Dosage should be adjusted as required; more frequent administration may be needed. Argipressin has also been given intranasally. A long-acting oily suspension of vasopressin tannate was formerly used by intramuscular injection in diabetes insipidus.

In the management of variceal bleeding argipressin may be given by intravenous infusion. For intravenous use an initial dose of 20 units in 100 mL of glucose (5%) injection, infused over 15 minutes has been suggested. Lypressin is also sometimes administered intravenously for bleeding oesophageal varices.

Administration. Results[1] suggesting that although intravenous administration of argipressin produced much higher plasma concentrations than intranasal administration, the latter evoked a greater CNS response.

1. Pietrowsky R, *et al.* Brain potential changes after intranasal vs intravenous administration of vasopressin: evidence for a direct nose-brain pathway for peptide effects in humans. *Biol Psychiatry* 1996; **39:** 332–40.

Administration in children. Vasopressin administered by continuous intravenous infusion in an average dose of 9 milliunits per kg body-weight per hour was safe and effective in five children who had diabetes insipidus as a manifestation of severe brain injury.[1] It has also been used safely in two children aged 3 years and under with postoperative diabetes insipidus; the dose used was 1.5 to 3 milliunits per kg per hour.[2]

1. Ralston C, Butt W. Continuous vasopressin replacement in diabetes insipidus. *Arch Dis Child* 1990; **65:** 896–7.
2. McDonald JA, *et al.* Treatment of the young child with postoperative central diabetes insipidus. *Am J Dis Child* 1989; **143:** 201–4.

Advanced cardiac life support. In a preliminary study argipressin 40 units by intravenous injection appeared to be of value in the treatment of cardiac arrest due to ventricular fibrillation.[1] Spontaneous circulation returned in 16 of 20 patients so treated; 14 were successfully resuscitated on arrival in hospital and 8 survived to be discharged. In comparison, of 20 patients treated with 1 mg of adrenaline intravenously only 7 were resuscitated and 3 survived till discharge. Vasopressin is not part of the standard management in cardiopulmonary resuscitation, although adrenaline is (see p.779); these results suggest that further comparative study is warranted.

1. Lindner KH, *et al.* Randomised comparison of epinephrine and vasopressin in patients with out-of-hospital ventricular fibrillation. *Lancet* 1997; **349:** 535–7.

Diabetes insipidus. For a discussion of diabetes insipidus and its management, including reference to the use of vasopressin analogues (particularly desmopressin), see p.1237.

Nocturnal enuresis. For references to the use of the vasopressin analogue, desmopressin, in nocturnal enuresis, see p.1246.

Variceal haemorrhage. Vasopressin has been widely used to control bleeding from oesophageal varices, as discussed on p.1576. However, terlipressin, and more recently octreotide, have been found to have some advantages over vasopressin, and octreotide is increasingly preferred for this purpose. Reviews of the treatment of variceal haemorrhage[1-10] do, however, generally cite vasopressin as a well-known treatment. Glyceryl trinitrate has been given with the aim of counteracting the adverse cardiac effects of vasopressin while potentiating its beneficial effects on portal pressure.[3-7]

References listed below also give information on the use of vasopressin in the management of some other haemorrhagic disorders, including cyclophosphamide-induced haemorrhagic cystitis, massive haemorrhage in Crohn's disease, blood loss in abortion or caesarean section, and haemoptysis.[11-15]

1. Hussey KP. Vasopressin therapy for upper gastrointestinal tract hemorrhage: has its efficacy been proven? *Arch Intern Med* 1985; **145:** 1263–7.
2. Anonymous. Management of acute variceal bleeding. *Lancet* 1988; **ii:** 999–1000.
3. Terblanche J, *et al.* Controversies in the management of bleeding esophageal varices. *N Engl J Med* 1989; **320:** 1393–8.
4. Schaffner JA. Acute upper gastrointestinal bleeding. *Drugs* 1989; **37:** 97–104.
5. Stump DL, Hardin TC. The use of vasopressin in the treatment of upper gastrointestinal haemorrhage. *Drugs* 1990; **39:** 38–53.
6. Gimson AE, Westaby D. The management of an episode of variceal bleeding. *Postgrad Med J* 1991; **67:** 140–6.
7. MacDougall BRD, *et al.* Portal hypertension—25 years of progress. *Gut* 1991; **32** (suppl): S18–S24.
8. Bornman PC, *et al.* Management of oesophageal varices. *Lancet* 1994; **343:** 1079–84.
9. Williams SGJ, Westaby D. Management of variceal haemorrhage. *Br Med J* 1994; **308:** 1213–17.
10. Sung JJY. Non-surgical treatment of variceal haemorrhage. *Br J Hosp Med* 1997; **57:** 162–6.
11. Pyeritz RE, *et al.* An approach to the control of massive hemorrhage in cyclophosphamide-induced cystitis by intravenous vasopressin: a case report. *J Urol (Baltimore)* 1978; **120:** 253–4.
12. Mellor JA, *et al.* Massive gastrointestinal bleeding in Crohn's disease: successful control by intra-arterial vasopressin infusion. *Gut* 1982; **23:** 872–4.
13. Schulz KF, *et al.* Vasopressin reduces blood loss from second-trimester dilatation and evacuation abortion. *Lancet* 1985; **ii:** 353–6.
14. Noseworthy TW, Anderson BJ. Massive hemoptysis. *Can Med Assoc J* 1986; **135:** 1097–9.
15. Lurie S, *et al.* Subendometrial vasopressin to control intractable placental bleeding. *Lancet* 1997; **349:** 698.

Preparations

Ph. Eur.: Lypressin Injection;
USP 23: Lypressin Nasal Solution; Vasopressin Injection.

Proprietary Preparations (details are given in Part 3)
Austral.: Pitressin; ***Canad.:*** Pitressin†; Pressyn; ***Fr.:*** Diapid; ***Ger.:*** Pitressin; Vasopressin; ***Irl.:*** Pitressin; Syntopressin; ***Neth.:*** Vasopressine†; ***S.Afr.:*** Vasopressin†; ***Spain:*** Vasopressina; ***Swed.:*** Postacton†; Vasopressin†; ***Switz.:*** Vasopressine†; ***UK:*** Pitressin; Syntopressin; ***USA:*** Diapid; Pitressin.

Used as an adjunct in: ***Ger.:*** Neo-Lidocaton; ***Ital.:*** Neo-Lidocaton†; ***Switz.:*** Neo-Lidocaton†.

Lipid Regulating Drugs

This chapter describes hyperlipidaemias and the role of lipid regulating drugs in their management. The principal groups of lipid regulating drugs described are the statins [3-hydroxy-3-methylglutaryl-coenzyme A (HMG-CoA) reductase inhibitors], fibric acid derivatives and related compounds (the fibrates), the bile-acid binding resins, derivatives of nicotinic acid, and the omega-3 marine triglycerides.

Hyperlipidaemias

Hyperlipidaemia, the elevation of lipid concentrations in plasma, is the manifestation of a disorder in the synthesis and degradation of plasma lipoproteins and may reflect a high-fat diet. A major concern in patients with hyperlipidaemia is their increased risk of ischaemic heart disease.

The **lipids** that are of relevance in hyperlipidaemias are cholesterol, an essential component of cell membranes and a precursor of steroid hormone synthesis, and triglyceride, an important energy source. They are transported in the blood as lipoproteins.

Lipoproteins are complex particles comprising a hydrophilic coat of phospholipids, free cholesterol, and specific polypeptides termed apolipoproteins (apoproteins) around a core of varying proportions of triglyceride and of cholesterol which is present as cholesteryl ester. The lipoproteins are characterised by their density which in general increases as they are metabolised and the proportion of cholesteryl ester to triglyceride increases. Table 1, below, lists the principal lipoproteins and their associated lipids.

Table 1. Principal lipoproteins and associated lipids.

Lipoprotein	Lipid
Chylomicron	Triglyceride
VLDL	Triglyceride
IDL	Cholesterol and triglyceride
LDL	Cholesterol
HDL	Cholesterol

The lowest density lipoproteins are the **chylomicrons** which transport triglyceride derived from dietary fat, and the **VLDL** (very low-density lipoproteins; pre-β lipoproteins) which transport endogenous triglyceride mainly synthesised in the liver, to peripheral tissues. The triglyceride is hydrolysed in the peripheral tissues by lipoprotein lipase, which is activated by apolipoprotein CII present in the lipoproteins. Both chylomicrons and VLDL are progressively depleted of triglyceride yielding increasingly dense lipoprotein particles termed 'remnant' particles. Chylomicron remnants are cleared rapidly from plasma by the liver where they are metabolised, releasing free cholesterol. VLDL remnants which include **IDL** (intermediate-density lipoproteins; broad β-lipoproteins) may also be cleared by the liver or converted to **LDL** (low-density lipoprotein; β-lipoprotein). **HDL** (high-density lipoproteins; α-lipoproteins) are synthesised in the liver and small intestine and have a role in the transport of cholesterol from the peripheral tissues to the liver. Cholesterol not utilised in the liver is secreted in the bile as bile acids and unesterified cholesterol. The majority is reabsorbed from the intestines and a small proportion is excreted in the faeces.

Hyperlipidaemias, sometimes referred to as dyslipidaemias, have been classified in various ways.[1] They may be described in terms of which lipid is elevated in the plasma, that is, as **hypercholesterolaemia**, **hypertriglyceridaemia**, or **'mixed' hyperlipidaemia** (where plasma concentrations of both cholesterol and triglyceride are raised). Alternatively, they may be described according to the lipoprotein abnormality and termed **hyperlipoproteinaemias**. This latter method, devised by Fredrickson, was adapted by the WHO and is still in common use. The WHO classification defines six types of hyperlipoproteinaemia, types I, IIa, IIb, III, IV, and V (see Table 2, below). Neither of these classification systems offers any information on the aetiology of the hyperlipidaemia, for instance, whether primary or secondary.

Primary hyperlipidaemias are those where the raised plasma-lipid concentration is the result of a genetic defect. The major primary hyperlipidaemias are given in Table 3, p.1266. They include **monogenic hyperlipidaemias**, that is those which are the result of a single genetic defect and **polygenic** or **multifactorial hyperlipidaemias**, those where the raised plasma-lipid concentrations are the result of an interaction between genetic, dietary, and other environmental factors. The majority of people with hypercholesterolaemia fall into this latter group; the disorder is termed **common, polygenic**, or **multifactorial hypercholesterolaemia** and is generally associated with only mild or moderate elevation of plasma-cholesterol concentrations. Hyperlipidaemias caused by single genetic defects generally produce higher plasma-lipid concentrations.

Secondary hyperlipidaemias are those where the raised plasma-lipid concentration is caused by another disease state or by drug therapy. Diseases producing hypertriglyceridaemia include diabetes mellitus, chronic renal failure, and bulimia. Hypercholesterolaemia can occur in hypothyroidism, nephrotic syndrome, biliary obstruction, and anorexia nervosa. Drugs that may produce hypertriglyceridaemia and/or hypercholesterolaemia include thiazide diuretics (in high doses) and corticosteroids. Excessive alcohol intake may produce elevated plasma-triglyceride concentrations. Primary and secondary causes of hyperlipidaemia can co-exist in any individual.

The degree of hyperlipidaemia seen in patients with primary or secondary hyperlipidaemia is influenced by various factors, including, importantly, diet. A diet rich in saturated fat and cholesterol and poor in fibre can produce hypercholesterolaemia. Obesity further predisposes to hyperlipidaemia. Other factors that may influence lipid concentrations include acute trauma (such as myocardial infarction), pregnancy, lack of exercise, smoking, and environmental factors (such as climate and water hardness).

The majority of people with hyperlipidaemia have plasma-lipid concentrations that are only mildly or moderately elevated, and they exhibit no **clinical symptoms**. At the other end of the spectrum, severe hypercholesterolaemia can cause tendon, tuberous, or planar xanthomas, xanthelasma, and arcus corneae; it is also associated with an increased risk of ischaemic stroke. Severe hypertriglyceridaemia can cause acute severe abdominal pain due to pancreatitis, hepatic and splenic enlargement, eruptive xanthomas, and lipaemia retinalis. Of particular significance though is the relationship between some hyperlipidaemias and premature ischaemic heart disease (before the age of 65) (see Table 3, p.1266). In patients with very severe hypercholesterolaemia, such as familial hypercholesterolaemia, ischaemic heart disease may be very premature; in those with the heterozygous form onset of heart disease during their 20s or 30s is not unusual, and in the rarer homozygous form ischaemic heart disease may develop by the age of 10.

Table 2. Classification of hyperlipoproteinaemias.

WHO classification	Lipoproteins elevated	Plasma lipids affected: Cholesterol	Plasma lipids affected: Triglyceride
I	Chylomicrons	Normal or elevated	Elevated
IIa	LDL	Elevated	Normal
IIb	LDL and VLDL	Elevated	Elevated
III	VLDL with abnormally high cholesterol content	Elevated	Elevated
IV	VLDL	Normal or elevated	Elevated
V	Chylomicrons and VLDL	Elevated	Elevated

Lipids and ischaemic heart disease. It is now well-established that hypercholesterolaemia is associated with an increased risk of atherosclerosis (see p.782) and consequently ischaemic heart disease. Epidemiological data show a progressive and continuous relationship between plasma-cholesterol concentrations and mortality from ischaemic heart disease. The 30-year follow-up of 4374 men and women from the Framingham Study[2] confirmed this continuous relationship which appeared strongest in subjects under 50 years of age, with a 9% increase in death from cardiovascular disease for each 10 mg per dL (0.26 mmol per litre) rise in total plasma-cholesterol concentration. Plasma-cholesterol concentrations of 5.2 mmol per litre (200 mg per dL) or less are associated with a low risk of ischaemic heart disease. The increased total plasma-cholesterol concentration associated with ischaemic heart disease is due mainly to raised LDL-cholesterol. In contrast, HDL-cholesterol is inversely associated with ischaemic heart disease. Low plasma concentrations of HDL-cholesterol (below 0.9 mmol per litre or 35 mg per dL) are generally associated with increased risk of ischaemic heart disease, whereas high concentrations are protective. An association between plasma-triglyceride concentrations and risk of ischaemic heart disease is less certain.[3] Some triglyceride-rich lipoproteins such as chylomicron remnant particles and IDL are atherogenic and the risk of heart disease increases as triglyceride concentrations increase in patients with high total cholesterol and low HDL-cholesterol concentrations, but hypertriglyceridaemia alone (greater than 2.3 mmol per litre or 200 mg per dL) is not an independent risk factor for ischaemic heart disease.

Since the association between plasma-cholesterol concentrations and ischaemic heart disease is continuous there has been much debate over what should be considered a 'desirable' lipid concentration, at what point lipid-lowering treatment with diet and/or lipid regulating drugs is required, and how people with hyperlipidaemia should be identified (screening). Guidelines[4-8] have attempted to clarify who should be treated. Bearing in mind that hypercholesterolaemia is only one of several risk factors for ischaemic heart disease and should never be treated in isolation, British[5] and European guidelines[7] have advised that, in general, if total plasma cholesterol remains above 5 mmol per litre and LDL-cholesterol above 3 mmol per litre despite dietary therapy then drug therapy should be added to dietary therapy. US guidelines[8] have suggested that drug treatment should be considered for an adult who, despite dietary therapy, has a LDL cholesterol level of 190 mg or more per dL without two other risk factors or 160 mg or more per dL with two other risk factors. Risk and treatment tables have been designed to aid decisions about cholesterol lowering and primary prevention of ischaemic heart disease[5,7,39] (in patients with no established ischaemic heart disease). They cover variables such as sex and age, and presence or absence of the risk factors of hypertension, smoking, diabetes mellitus, and left ventricular hypertrophy. They are not intended to be used for decision making regarding secondary prevention (patients with established ischaemic heart disease).

Studies of cholesterol-lowering therapy have shown a reduction in coronary events, and angiography has demonstrated favourable effects on coronary artery lesions. The reduction in coronary events is seen in both dietary and drug studies and has been most evident in patients at high risk, that is, those with established ischaemic heart disease (secondary prevention). There is also evidence of benefit for primary prevention.

Table 3. Primary hyperlipidaemias.

	WHO type	Prevalence	Typical lipid concentrations (mmol/L) Cholesterol	Triglyceride	Risk of IHD	Pancreatitis
Common (polygenic) hypercholesterolaemia	IIa, IIb	Very common	6.5 to 9.0	< 2.3	+	–
Familial hypercholesterolaemia	IIa, IIb	Moderately common	7.5 to 16.0	< 2.3	+++	–
Familial hypertriglyceridaemia	IV, V	Common	6.5 to 12.0	10 to 30	?	++
Familial combined hyperlipidaemia	IIa, IIb, IV, and V	Common	6.5 to 10.0	2.3 to 12.0	++	–
Familial dysbetalipoproteinaemia or remnant hyperlipoproteinaemia	III	Uncommon	9.0 to 14.0	9.0 to 14.0	++	+
Abnormal lipoprotein lipase function	I	Rare	< 6.5	10.0 to 30.0	–	+++

+ = elevated risk; – = no risk; ? = uncertain risk; IHD = ischaemic heart disease

One concern has been that there might be an association between low cholesterol concentrations and increased morbidity and mortality from non-cardiac causes including haemorrhagic stroke, cancer, accidents and suicide, and chronic respiratory, liver, and bowel disease.[9-14] However, some consider that, with the possible exception of haemorrhagic stroke, the association may not be causal,[10,15-17] and confounding factors may explain the relationship.[9] Also, diseases such as cancer may produce low cholesterol concentrations rather than be a result of them.[9,10] The increased non-cardiac mortality has generally been restricted to studies of lipid regulating drugs,[18,19] although it has also been seen with dietary therapy alone.[20]

Some studies[21-25] (those using drugs other than the statins) suggested that the maximum beneficial response to intervention may be delayed for several years after the start of therapy. Analysis of results of observational and randomised studies[24] indicated that little reduction in risk of ischaemic heart disease occurs in the first two years of treatment and that the full reduction is achieved within five years. Also cholesterol concentrations had been reduced by only about 10 to 15% on average, which may not be adequate to produce significant reductions in ischaemic heart disease mortality.

The statins have a more marked cholesterol-lowering effect than the older lipid regulating drugs such as cholestyramine and clofibrate and in, for example, the large Scandinavian Simvastatin Survival Study (4S),[26,42,43] simvastatin was effective for the **secondary prevention** of ischaemic heart disease in patients with elevated cholesterol concentrations without increasing non-cardiac mortality. Reviews[27-29] of this and other studies have concluded that there is now clear evidence of benefit from reducing raised cholesterol concentrations in patients with pre-existing ischaemic heart disease. Another statin, pravastatin, has been found in the Cholesterol and Recurrent Events (CARE) Trial[30,40] to be of benefit for secondary prevention in patients who have average, rather than elevated, cholesterol concentrations and such use has been advocated.[31] Data from the WOSCOPS trials[33,41] and others[32] also indicate that pravastatin is effective for **primary prevention** in moderate hypercholesterolaemia. Similar findings have been published for lovastatin.[44]

The primary and secondary prevention studies have been predominantly in middle-aged men and more studies are needed in women and the elderly to determine appropriate lipid-lowering strategies in these groups. In the 4S trial[43] with simvastatin the risk for major coronary events was reduced for women as well as for men although the number of women studied was too few to assess effects on mortality. It has been suggested[34] that dietary manipulation aimed at reducing plasma-cholesterol concentrations may have a detrimental effect on the lipid profile in women at low risk of ischaemic heart disease. This assertion is based on findings that, in women, low HDL is a more consistent risk factor for cardiovascular disease than high LDL, and diets designed to reduce LDL concentrations would also reduce HDL concentrations.

Screening programmes have been introduced to identify people with hyperlipidaemia; in the USA it has been recommended that all adults should have their blood-lipid concentrations measured.[6] However, since the value of treatment in the vast proportion of those tested is questioned, many consider that routine cholesterol measurements in healthy people are not warranted.[19,35,36] Screening is recommended for patients with symptomatic ischaemic heart disease or peripheral vascular disease, in those with clinical signs of hyperlipidaemia, with a family history of ischaemic heart disease or hyperlipidaemia, and with other risk factors for ischaemic heart disease.[4,5,7,35,36] It should always be carried out as part of an assessment of overall risk status for heart disease.

A full lipoprotein analysis will identify those patients whose mild hypercholesterolaemia is due to very high plasma concentrations of HDL-cholesterol and thus avoid them undergoing inappropriate dietary or drug therapy. The triglyceride and HDL-cholesterol measurement may also influence the choice of drug as lipid regulating drugs differ in their effects on LDL- and HDL-cholesterol and triglycerides. Once a significant hyperlipidaemia has been identified then further investigations may determine whether the hyperlipidaemia is secondary to another condition or is a primary abnormality. Some secondary hyperlipidaemias respond to treatment of the underlying disease, for example hypothyroidism, whereas others may require lipid regulating therapy in addition to treatment of the primary condition, for example in diabetes mellitus and renal disease.

Lipids and stroke. Some of the studies already mentioned above, as well as investigating the coronary effects of lipid lowering in patients with established ischaemic heart disease, also looked at the effect on non-cardiac atherosclerosis. Two studies with pravastatin[20,30] and one with simvastatin[42] have indicated a reduction in the risk of stroke.

Treatment of hyperlipidaemias. The main aim of treatment in patients with hypercholesterolaemia is to reduce the risk of developing ischaemic heart disease or the occurrence of further cardiovascular or cerebrovascular events in those with clinical evidence of ischaemic heart disease or peripheral vascular disease. In patients with severe hypertriglyceridaemia treatment is indicated to prevent attacks of acute pancreatitis. Treatment may also be indicated to promote the regression or non-progression of disfiguring xanthomas. The main methods of treating hyperlipidaemias are dietary and lifestyle changes and the administration of lipid regulating drugs. Some surgical and other procedures may also be used in familial hypercholesterolaemia (see below).

The basis of **dietary therapy** is weight reduction in the obese and a reduction in total fat intake. UK dietary recommendations include a reduction in saturated fatty acids, restriction of *trans* fatty acids, and increased consumption of long-chain n-3 polyunsaturated fatty acids; earlier restrictions on dietary intake of cholesterol and n-6 polyunsaturated fatty acids still stand.[37]

Dietary changes should be combined with other lifestyle changes such as cessation of smoking, increasing physical exercise, and reducing alcohol intake. A reduced alcohol intake is especially advised in those with hypertriglyceridaemia. A more rigorous diet than that often recommended may be necessary for diet alone to be of much value.[38] Drug therapy is frequently necessary.

The principal groups of **lipid regulating drugs** (hypolipidaemic drugs) are the statins, fibric acid derivatives and related compounds, bile-acid binding resins, nicotinic acid and its derivatives, and the omega-3 marine triglycerides. Their main effects on lipids are shown in Table 4.

Table 4. Lipid regulating drugs and their activities.

Drug group	Typical drugs	Principal lipids affected
Bile-acid binding resins	Cholestyramine Colestipol	LDL-cholesterol ↓
Fibric acid derivatives and related compounds	Bezafibrate Clofibrate Fenofibrate Gemfibrozil	VLDL-triglycerides ↓ HDL-cholesterol ↑ LDL-cholesterol ↑ or ↓
Nicotinic acid and derivatives	Acipimox Nicofuranose Nicotinic acid	VLDL-triglycerides ↓ HDL-cholesterol ↑ LDL-cholesterol ↓ (modest)
Statins	Atorvastatin Cerivastatin Fluvastatin Lovastatin Pravastatin Simvastatin	LDL-cholesterol ↓ Triglycerides ↓ (modest)
Miscellaneous drugs	Omega-3 marine triglycerides	VLDL-triglycerides ↓

In general, **drug therapy** should only be initiated after an adequate trial of dietary modification has failed to reduce plasma-lipid concentrations sufficiently and should always be an adjunct to dietary modification and not a substitute for it. Patients who are likely to require drug therapy include those with severe hyperlipidaemia (familial hypercholesterolaemia, familial combined hyperlipidaemia, and familial dysbetalipoproteinaemia), those with clinical manifestations of ischaemic heart disease or peripheral vascular disease or who have undergone coronary artery bypass surgery, and those with major risk factors.

The major primary hyperlipidaemias may be treated as follows.

- COMMON (POLYGENIC) HYPERCHOLESTEROLAEMIA. In this condition drug therapy may be considered if a sufficient trial of dietary modification fails to produce an adequate reduction in plasma-cholesterol concentrations. The decision to begin drug therapy will depend on the degree of hypercholesterolaemia, together with other risk factors, and the presence of ischaemic heart disease or peripheral vascular disease. Treatment with one lipid regulating drug is usually sufficient. First-line drugs are now the statins; bile-acid binding resins or, if not tolerated, fibric acid derivatives, were previously used. Dextrothyroxine and neomycin have been used in patients with hypercholesterolaemia but have generally been abandoned in favour of more effective or safer drugs.
- FAMILIAL HYPERCHOLESTEROLAEMIA. Patients with familial hypercholesterolaemia usually have very high plasma-cholesterol concentrations which rarely respond adequately to diet alone and drug therapy is therefore often necessary in this high-risk group. The first-line drugs are the statins. In severe cases combination therapy is usually required. A statin together with a bile-acid binding resin may be used. A low dose of the bile-acid binding resin may be sufficient. In the homozygous form of familial hypercholesterolaemia, in which there is a lack of functional LDL-receptors, bile-acid binding resins are not effective. In some forms of familial hypercholesterolaemia, and where plasma-cholesterol concentrations are very high, plasma-triglyceride concentrations may also be raised. In these cases a fibric acid derivative or nicotinic acid may be effective, and in more severe cases the combination of a bile-acid binding resin together with a fibric acid derivative or a statin may be used. In patients with the homozygous form liver transplantation is the most definitive treatment. Plasma exchange (weekly or fortnightly) or more selective procedures such as LDL apheresis, including the use of heparin to precipitate LDL (the HELP system—Heparin Extracorporeal LDL Precipitation) may also be used in combination with lipid regulating drugs. Gene therapy is under investigation as a treatment for familial hypercholesterolaemia.
- FAMILIAL HYPERTRIGLYCERIDAEMIA. In patients with familial hypertriglyceridaemia dietary therapy is generally adequate, but drugs may be required if there is a high risk of acute pancreatitis or if there is a family history of atherosclerosis. The risk of acute pancreatitis is high when plasma-triglyceride concentrations are above 20 mmol per litre. Nicotinic acid or the fibric acid derivatives, particularly gemfibrozil, are generally recommended and may be used in combination in severe cases. Omega-3 marine triglycerides may also be of value. In severe intractable hypertriglyceridaemia, particularly type V hyperlipoproteinaemia, norethisterone has been suggested for women or oxandrolone for men.
- FAMILIAL COMBINED HYPERLIPIDAEMIA.Drug therapy may be used in patients who do not respond to dietary therapy alone. The choice will depend on the predominant lipid abnormality. A fibric acid derivative is the first choice in cases where hypertriglyceridaemia is predominant. A statin is first choice when hypercholesterolaemia predominates, and nicotinic acid is useful where plasma concentrations of triglyceride and cholesterol are elevated to a similar degree. Bile-acid binding resins should not be used alone since they can aggravate hypertriglyceridaemia, but they may be useful in combination with a triglyceride-lowering drug in some patients. Treatment with a combination of drugs that lowers both cholesterol and triglyceride concentrations may be required in some patients especially in those with markedly raised plasma concentrations of triglyceride or cholesterol, as treatment of these patients with drugs effective against only the predominant lipid may produce a rise in the plasma-concentrations of the other lipid. Many different combinations of lipid regulating drugs have been used, including combinations of statins and fibric acid derivatives; this combination is not recommended for routine use because of the possibility of increased adverse effects, but may be useful in selected patients. The choice of treatment in these cases is largely empirical as responses are not always predictable in individual patients.
- FAMILIAL DYSBETALIPOPROTEINAEMIA. (remnant hyperlipoproteinaemia; remnant particle disease). In this lipid disorder the degree of hyperlipidaemia is usually severe and, although it may respond remarkably to dietary therapy, drug treatment is usually necessary. Fibric acid derivatives are the first-choice drugs. Statins or nicotinic acid may also be used.
- ABNORMAL LIPOPROTEIN LIPASE FUNCTION. (chylomicronaemia). No drugs currently available are useful in this disorder. The condition is treated with severe restriction of dietary fat, and the diet may be supplemented by medium chain triglycerides to improve tolerability.

1. Beaumont JL, *et al.* Classification of hyperlipidaemias and hyperlipoproteinaemias. *Bull WHO* 1970; **43:** 891–915.
2. Anderson KM, *et al.* Cholesterol and mortality: 30 years of follow-up from the Framingham Study. *JAMA* 1987; **257:** 2176–80.
3. NIH Consensus Development Panel on Triglyceride, High-Density Lipoprotein, and Coronary Heart Disease. Triglyceride, high-density lipoprotein, and coronary heart disease. *JAMA* 1993; **269:** 505–10.
4. Betteridge DJ, *et al.* Management of hyperlipidaemia: guidelines of the British Hyperlipidaemia Association. *Postgrad Med J* 1993; **69:** 359–69.
5. Wood D, *et al.* Joint British recommendations on prevention of coronary heart disease in clinical practice. *Heart* 1998; **80** (suppl 2): S1-S29.
6. Expert Panel on Detection, Evaluation, and Treatment of High Blood Cholesterol in Adults. Summary of the second report of the National Cholesterol Education Program (NCEP) expert panel on detection, evaluation, and treatment of high blood cholesterol in adults (Adult Treatment Panel II). *JAMA* 1993; **269:** 3015–23.
7. Wood D, *et al.* Prevention of coronary heart disease in clinical practice: recommendations of the second joint task force of European and other societies on coronary prevention. *Eur Heart J* 1998; **19:** 1434–1503.
8. National Cholesterol Education Program. Second report of the expert panel on detection, evaluation, and treatment of high blood cholesterol in adults (adult treatment panel II). *Circulation* 1994; **89:** 1329–1445.
9. Jacobs D, *et al.* Report of the conference on low blood cholesterol: mortality associations. *Circulation* 1992; **86:** 1046–60.
10. Law MR, *et al.* Assessing possible hazards of reducing serum cholesterol. *Br Med J* 1994; **308:** 373–9.
11. Davey Smith G, *et al.* Plasma cholesterol concentration and mortality: the Whitehall Study. *JAMA* 1992; **267:** 70–6.
12. Newman TB, Hulley SB. Carcinogenicity of lipid-lowering drugs. *JAMA* 1996; **275:** 55–60.
13. Zureik M, *et al.* Serum cholesterol concentration and death from suicide in men: Paris prospective study I. *Br Med J* 1996; **313:** 649–51.
14. Golomb BA. Cholesterol and violence: is there a connection? *Ann Intern Med* 1998; **128:** 478–87.
15. Marmot M. The cholesterol papers. *Br Med J* 1994; **308:** 351–2.
16. Dalen JE, Dalton WS. Does lowering cholesterol cause cancer? *JAMA* 1996; **275:** 67–8.
17. Brown SL. Lowered serum cholesterol and low mood. *Br Med J* 1996; **313:** 637–8.
18. Davey Smith G, Pekkanen J. Should there be a moratorium on the use of cholesterol lowering drugs? *Br Med J* 1992; **304:** 431–4.
19. Davey Smith G, *et al.* Cholesterol lowering and mortality: the importance of considering initial level of risk. *Br Med J* 1993; **306:** 1367–73. Correction. *ibid.*; 1648.
20. The Long-Term Intervention with Pravastatin in Ischaemic Disease (LIPID) Study Group. Prevention of cardiovascular events and death with pravastatin in patients with coronary heart disease and a broad range of initial cholesterol levels. *N Engl J Med* 1998; **339:** 1349–57.
21. Lipid Research Clinics Program. The Lipid Research Clinics Coronary Primary Prevention Trial results I: reduction in incidence of coronary heart disease. *JAMA* 1984; **251:** 351–64.
22. Frick MH, *et al.* Helsinki Heart Study: primary-prevention trial with gemfibrozil in middle-aged men with dyslipidemia. *N Engl J Med* 1987; **317:** 1237–45.
23. Manninen V, *et al.* Lipid alterations and decline in the incidence of coronary heart disease in the Helsinki Heart Study. *JAMA* 1988; **260:** 641–51.
24. Law MR, *et al.* By how much and how quickly does reduction in serum cholesterol concentration lower risk of ischaemic heart disease? *Br Med J* 1994; **308:** 367–73.
25. Oliver MF, *et al.* A co-operative trial in the primary prevention of ischaemic heart disease using clofibrate: report from the Committee of Principal Investigators. *Br Heart J* 1978; **40:** 1069–1118.
26. Scandinavian Simvastatin Survival Study Group. Randomised trial of cholesterol lowering in 4444 patients with coronary heart disease: the Scandinavian Simvastatin Survival Study (4S). *Lancet* 1994; **344:** 1383–9.
27. Oliver M, *et al.* Lower patients' cholesterol now. *Br Med J* 1995; **310:** 1280–1.
28. van Boven AJ, *et al.* The 4S study: implications for prescribing. *Drugs* 1996; **51:** 507–14.
29. Pedersen TR, Tobert JA. Benefits and risks of HMG-CoA reductase inhibitors in the prevention of coronary heart disease: a reappraisal. *Drug Safety* 1996; **14:** 11–24.
30. Sacks FM, *et al.* The effect of pravastatin on coronary events after myocardial infarction in patients with average cholesterol levels. *N Engl J Med* 1996; **335:** 1001–9.
31. Byrne CD, Wild SH. Lipids and secondary prevention of ischaemic heart disease. *Br Med J* 1996; **313:** 1273–4.
32. Shepherd J, *et al.* Prevention of coronary heart disease with pravastatin in men with hypercholesterolemia. *N Engl J Med* 1995; **333:** 1301–7.
33. West of Scotland Coronary Prevention Group. West of Scotland Coronary Prevention Study: identification of high-risk groups and comparison with other cardiovascular intervention trials. *Lancet* 1996; **348:** 1339–42.
34. Crouse JR. Gender, lipoproteins, diet, and cardiovascular risk: sauce for the goose may not be sauce for the gander. *Lancet* 1989; **i:** 318–20.
35. American College of Physicians. Guidelines for using serum cholesterol, high-density lipoprotein cholesterol, and triglyceride levels as screening tests for preventing coronary heart disease in adults. *Ann Intern Med* 1996; **124:** 515–17.
36. Garber AM, *et al.* Cholesterol screening in asymptomatic adults, revisited. *Ann Intern Med* 1996; **124:** 518–31.
37. DoH. Nutritional aspects of cardiovascular disease. *Report on health and social subjects 46*. London: HMSO, 1994.
38. Ramsay LE, *et al.* Dietary reduction of serum cholesterol concentration: time to think again. *Br Med J* 1991; **303:** 953–7.
39. Ramsay LE, *et al.* The Sheffield table for primary prevention of coronary heart disease: corrected. *Lancet* 1996; **348:** 1251–2.
40. Sacks FM, *et al.* Relationship between plasma LDL concentrations during treatment with pravastatin and recurrent coronary events in the Cholesterol and Recurrent Events Trial. *Circulation* 1998; **97:** 1446–52.
41. West of Scotland Coronary Prevention Study Group. Influence of pravastatin and plasma lipids on clinical events in the West of Scotland Coronary Prevention Study (WOSCOPS). *Circulation* 1998; **97:** 1440–5.
42. Pedersen TR, *et al.* Effect of simvastatin on ischemic signs and symptoms in the Scandinavian Simvastatin Survival Study (4S). *Am J Cardiol* 1998; **81:** 333–5.
43. Miettinen TA, *et al.* Cholesterol-lowering therapy in women and elderly patients with myocardial infarction or angina pectoris: findings from the Scandinavian Simvastatin Survival Study (4S). *Circulation* 1997; **96:** 211–18.
44. Downs JR, *et al.* Primary prevention of acute coronary events with lovastatin in men and women with average cholesterol levels: results of AFCAPS/TexCAPS. *JAMA* 1998; **279:** 1615–22.

Acipimox (12316-x)

Acipimox *(BAN, rINN).*

K-9321. 5-Methylpyrazine-2-carboxylic acid 4-oxide.

$C_6H_6N_2O_3$ = 154.1.

CAS — 51037-30-0.

Adverse Effects and Precautions

Acipimox may cause peripheral vasodilatation resulting in flushing, itching, and a sensation of heat. Rash and erythema may occur. Gastro-intestinal disturbances including heartburn, epigastric pain, nausea, and diarrhoea have been reported, as well as headache and malaise. Urticaria, angioedema, and bronchospasm may occur rarely.

Acipimox is contra-indicated in patients with peptic ulceration. It should not be given to patients with renal impairment if the creatinine clearance is less than 30 mL per minute; extended dose intervals should be employed if the creatinine clearance is 30 to 60 mL per minute.

In a study involving 3009 hyperlipidaemic patients with type 2 diabetes,[1] adverse effects to acipimox occurred in 8.8% resulting in withdrawal in 5.5% of patients. The most frequent adverse effects involved the skin (57.6%), gastro-intestinal tract (25.8%), and CNS (9.7%). Labial oedema occurred in 3 cases and an urticarial eruption, collapse, and dyspnoea in one. The incidence of adverse effects was almost twice as high in females as in males, the difference being mainly due to a greater incidence of flushing, pruritus, and skin rashes. The incidence was not affected by age. There was a mean 15.3% reduction in fasting blood glucose concentrations and an 8.5% reduction in glycosylated haemoglobin during treatment with acipimox.

1. Lavezzari M, *et al.* Results of a phase IV study carried out with acipimox in type II diabetic patients with concomitant hyperlipoproteinaemia. *J Int Med Res* 1989; **17:** 373–80.

Pharmacokinetics

Acipimox is rapidly and completely absorbed from the gastro-intestinal tract and peak plasma concentrations occur within 2 hours. It does not bind to plasma proteins and the plasma half-life is about 2 hours. It is not significantly metabolised and is excreted in the urine, largely unchanged.

Uses and Administration

Acipimox is a lipid regulating drug related to nicotinic acid (p.1351). It is used in the treatment of type IIa, IIb, or IV hyperlipoproteinaemias.

It is given by mouth in usual doses of 500 to 750 mg daily in divided doses, taken with meals. Doses of up to 1200 mg daily have been used.

Hyperlipidaemias. Acipimox is used in the management of hyperlipidaemias (p.1265) and produces effects on plasma lipoproteins similar to those of nicotinic acid although it may not be as potent in its lipid modifying effect. Acipimox was developed to overcome the problems of compliance resulting from nicotinic acid's adverse effects. Its primary action is thought to be the inhibition of lipolysis thus reducing the availability of free fatty acids for the hepatic production of very-low-density lipoprotein (VLDL) and this in turn leads to a decrease in low-density lipoprotein (LDL) production. Increases in high-density lipoprotein (HDL) may also occur. The overall effect is a reduction in VLDL-triglyceride and total triglyceride concentrations and an increase in HDL-cholesterol concentrations, but only a modest reduction in LDL-cholesterol or total-cholesterol concentrations.[1-6]

Acipimox has been shown to be effective in the treatment of hyperlipidaemias in diabetic patients, and has generally produced a reduction in blood-glucose concentrations.[5,6] A patient with type A insulin-resistance syndrome, who had diabetes and severe hypertriglyceridaemia with very high fasting insulin and non-esterified fatty acids, responded to treatment with acipimox 500 mg twice daily in a modified-release form.[7]

1. Sommariva D, *et al.* Changes in lipoprotein cholesterol and triglycerides induced by acipimox in type IV and type II hyperlipoproteinemic patients. *Curr Ther Res* 1985; **37:** 363–8.
2. Ball MJ, *et al.* Acipimox in the treatment of patients with hyperlipidaemia: a double blind trial. *Eur J Clin Pharmacol* 1986; **31:** 201–4.
3. Taskinen M-R, Nikkilä EA. Effects of acipimox on serum lipids, lipoproteins and lipolytic enzymes in hypertriglyceridemia. *Atherosclerosis* 1988; **69:** 249–55.
4. Crepaldi G, *et al.* Plasma lipid lowering activity of acipimox in patients with type II and type IV hyperlipoproteinaemia. *Atherosclerosis* 1988; **70:** 115–21.
5. Dulbecco A, *et al.* Effect of acipimox on plasma glucose levels in patients with non-insulin-dependent diabetes mellitus. *Curr Ther Res* 1989; **46:** 478–83.
6. Lavezzari M, *et al.* Results of a phase IV study carried out with acipimox in type II diabetic patients with concomitant hyperlipoproteinaemia. *J Int Med Res* 1989; **17:** 373–80.
7. Kumar S, *et al.* Suppression of non-esterified fatty acids to treat type A insulin resistance syndrome. *Lancet* 1994; **343:** 1073–4.

Preparations

Proprietary Preparations (details are given in Part 3)
Aust.: Olbetam; ***Belg.:*** Olbetam; ***Ger.:*** Olbemox; ***Irl.:*** Olbetam; ***Ital.:*** Olbetam; ***Neth.:*** Nedios; ***S.Afr.:*** Olbetam; ***Switz.:*** Olbetam; ***UK:*** Olbetam.

Atorvastatin Calcium (14543-n)

Atorvastatin Calcium *(BANM, USAN, rINNM).*

CI-981. Calcium (βR,δR)-2-(p-fluorophenyl)-β,δ-dihydroxy-5-isopropyl-3-phenyl-4-(phenylcarbamoyl)pyrrole-1-heptanoic acid (1:2) trihydrate.

$C_{66}H_{68}CaF_2N_4O_{10},3H_2O$ = 1209.4.

CAS — 134523-00-5 (atorvastatin); 134523-03-8 (atorvastatin calcium).

Adverse Effects and Precautions

As for Simvastatin, p.1278.

General references.

1. Black DM, *et al.* An overview of the clinical safety profile of atorvastatin (Lipitor), a new HMG-CoA reductase inhibitor. *Arch Intern Med* 1998; **158:** 577–84.

Effects on the blood. An immune thrombocytopenia attributed to atorvastatin has been reported in 1 patient.[1] Adverse haematological reactions had not been noted when the patient previously received simvastatin.

1. González-Ponte ML, *et al.* Atorvastatin-induced severe thrombocytopenia. *Lancet* 1998; **352:** 1284.

Effects on the skin. Toxic epidermal necrolysis apparently caused by atorvastatin has been reported.[1] The authors were not aware of this adverse effect previously having been associated with any of the statin lipid regulating drugs.

1. Pfeiffer CM, *et al.* Toxic epidermal necrolysis from atorvastatin. *JAMA* 1998; **279:** 1613–14.

Interactions

As for Simvastatin, p.1279.

Pharmacokinetics

Atorvastatin is rapidly absorbed from the gastro-intestinal tract. It has low absolute bioavailability of about 12% due to presystemic clearance in the gastro-intestinal mucosa and/or first-pass metabolism in the liver, its primary site of action. Atorvastatin is metabolised by cytochrome P450 3A4 to a number of compounds which are also active inhibitors of HMG-CoA reductase. The mean plasma elimination half-life of atorvastatin is about 14 hours although the half-life of inhibitory activity for HMG-CoA reductase is approximately 20 to 30 hours due to the contribution of the active metabolites. It is 98% bound to plasma proteins. Atorvastatin is excreted as metabolites, primarily in the bile.

Uses and Administration

Atorvastatin, a 3-hydroxy-3-methylglutaryl coenzyme A (HMG-CoA) reductase inhibitor (a statin), is a lipid regulating drug with actions on plasma lipids similar to those of simvastatin (p.1279). It is used in the treatment of hypercholesterolaemias and combined (mixed) hyperlipidaemia (p.1265).

Atorvastatin is given by mouth as the calcium salt although doses are expressed in terms of the base. The initial dose is 10 mg daily which may be adjusted at intervals of 4 weeks up to a maximum of 80 mg daily.

General reviews.

1. Lea AP, McTavish D. Atorvastatin: a review of its pharmacology and therapeutic potential in the management of hyperlipidaemias. *Drugs* 1997; **53:** 828–47.

Preparations

Proprietary Preparations (details are given in Part 3)
Austral.: Lipitor; ***Ital.:*** Lipitor; Torvast; Totalip; Xarator; ***Neth.:*** Lipitor; ***S.Afr.:*** Lipitor; ***Swed.:*** Lipitor; ***UK:*** Lipitor; ***USA:*** Lipitor.

Beclobrate (12421-r)

Beclobrate *(BAN, rINN).*

Sgd-24774. Ethyl (±)-2-(4-p-chlorobenzylphenoxy)-2-methylbutyrate.

$C_{20}H_{23}ClO_3$ = 346.8.

CAS — 55937-99-0.

Beclobrate, a fibric acid derivative (see Bezafibrate, below), was used as a lipid regulating drug, but liver toxicity led to its withdrawal.

Benfluorex Hydrochloride (12424-n)

Benfluorex Hydrochloride *(pINNM).*

JP-992; SE-780. 2-[α-Methyl-3-(trifluoromethyl)phenethylamino]ethyl benzoate hydrochloride.

$C_{19}H_{20}F_3NO_2,HCl$ = 387.8.

CAS — 23602-78-0 (benfluorex); 35976-51-3 (benfluorex, ±); 23642-66-2 (benfluorex hydrochloride).

Benfluorex hydrochloride is a lipid regulating drug used in the treatment of hyperlipidaemias (p.1265). It has also been used as an adjunct in the management of type 2 diabetes mellitus (p.313).

It is given in usual doses of 150 mg three times daily by mouth with meals.

Preparations

Proprietary Preparations (details are given in Part 3)
Fr.: Mediator; ***Ital.:*** Balans†; Mediaxal; Minolip†; ***Spain:*** Modulator; ***Switz.:*** Mediaxal.

Bezafibrate (12441-h)

Bezafibrate *(BAN, USAN, rINN).*

BM-15075; LO-44. 2-[4-(2-p-Chlorobenzamidoethyl)phenoxy]-2-methylpropionic acid.

$C_{19}H_{20}ClNO_4$ = 361.8.

CAS — 41859-67-0.

Pharmacopoeias. In It.

Adverse Effects

The commonest side-effects of bezafibrate therapy are gastro-intestinal upsets including anorexia, nausea, and gastric discomfort. Other adverse effects reported to occur less frequently include headache, dizziness, vertigo, fatigue, skin rashes, pruritus, alopecia, impotence, and anaemia and leucopenia. Raised serum-aminotransferase concentrations have occasionally been reported. Elevated creatine phosphokinase concentrations during bezafibrate therapy may be associated with a syndrome of myositis, myopathy, and rarely rhabdomyolysis; patients with hypoalbuminaemia resulting from the nephrotic syndrome or other renal impairment may be at increased risk. Bezafibrate may increase the lithogenic index, but although there have been isolated reports of gallstones there is no evidence that the administration of bezafibrate is associated with an increased frequency of this adverse effect.

Effects on hypoglycaemic control. Reductions in fasting blood-glucose concentrations of between 4 and 10% occurred during long-term therapy with bezafibrate in hyperlipidaemic diabetic patients.[1,2] Jones *et al.*[3] suggested that bezafibrate could be considered as additional or alternative therapy in patients with type 2 diabetes mellitus.

1. Rüth E, Vollmar J. Verbesserung der diabeteseinstellung unter der therapie mit bezafibrat. *Dtsch Med Wochenschr* 1982; **107:** 1470–3.
2. Bruneder H, Klein HJ. Hyperlipoproteinämie und diabetes mellitus: langzeitbehandlung mit bezafibrat bei 115 patienten. *Med Welt* 1984; **35:** 357–60.
3. Jones IR, *et al.* Lowering of plasma glucose concentrations with bezafibrate in patients with moderately controlled NIDDM. *Diabetes Care* 1990; **13:** 855–63.

Effects on the kidneys. A report of renal failure associated with bezafibrate.[1] See also Effects on Skeletal Muscle, below.

1. Lipkin GW, Tomson CRV. Severe reversible renal failure with bezafibrate. *Lancet* 1993; **341:** 371.

Effects on the nervous system. Peripheral neuropathy occurred in a patient given bezafibrate and was substantiated by nerve conduction studies.[1]

1. Ellis CJ, *et al.* Peripheral neuropathy with bezafibrate. *Br Med J* 1994; **309:** 929.

Effects on skeletal muscle. The UK Committee on Safety of Medicines has noted that myositis and myopathy are well known to occur with lipid regulating drugs such as fibrates and statins.[1] Rhabdomyolysis, presenting as muscle pain with elevated creatine phosphokinase and myoglobinuria leading to renal failure, has also been reported but appears to be rare. Worldwide reporting did not indicate marked differences in the risk of the reactions with individual drugs. Patients with renal impairment, and possibly with hypothyroidism, may be at increased risk of muscle toxicity.

1. Committee on Safety of Medicines/Medicines Control Agency. Rhabdomyolysis associated with lipid-lowering drugs. *Current Problems* 1995; **21:** 3.

Headache. Severe recurrent headaches were associated with bezafibrate administration in one patient.[1] The headaches started about 24 hours after therapy with bezafibrate began, and recurred about 1 hour after each dose.

1. Hodgetts TJ, Tunnicliffe C. Bezafibrate-induced headache. *Lancet* 1989; **i:** 163.

Precautions

Bezafibrate should not be given to patients with severe liver or kidney impairment, primary biliary cirrhosis, gallstones or gallbladder disorders, or hypoalbuminaemic states such as the nephrotic syndrome.

Patients with renal impairment and possibly with hypothyroidism may be at increased risk of the muscle toxicity associated with fibrates and statins (see Adverse Effects, above). Combined treatment with a fibrate and a statin may increase the risk of serious muscle toxicity. The UK Committee on Safety of Medicines[1] has advised that patients treated with these drugs should consult their doctor if they develop muscle pain, tenderness, or weakness and treatment should be stopped if muscle toxicity is suspected clinically or if creatine phosphokinase is markedly raised or progressively rising.

1. Committee on Safety of Medicines/Medicines Control Agency. Rhabdomyolysis associated with lipid-lowering drugs. *Current Problems* 1995; **21:** 3.

Diabetes mellitus. See Effects on Hypoglycaemic Control, under Adverse Effects, above.

Renal impairment. See under Uses and Administration, below.

Interactions

Bezafibrate and other fibrates may enhance the effects of oral anticoagulants; the dose of anticoagulant should be reduced when treatment with a fibrate is started, and then adjusted gradually if necessary. Recommendations concerning the amount that the anticoagulant dose should be reduced by vary between the manufacturers of the differing fibrates and are sometimes not even specified; the manufacturers of bezafibrate suggest a reduction of up to 50% in the dosage of anticoagulant. The mechanism of the interaction has not yet been determined. Fibrates have been reported to displace warfarin from protein binding sites but other mechanisms are probably also involved.

A number of other drugs may be displaced from plasma proteins by fibrates including tolbutamide and other sulphonylurea antidiabetics, phenytoin, and, in patients with hypoalbuminaemia, frusemide. The interaction with antidiabetics is complex since bezafibrate has been shown to alter glucose tolerance in both diabetic and non-diabetic patients. The dosage of antidiabetics may need adjusting during concomitant bezafibrate therapy.

There is an increased risk of myopathy if fibrates are given concurrently with statins.

Increased cyclosporin concentrations and associated nephrotoxicity have been reported when the drug was administered concomitantly with bezafibrate.

Pharmacokinetics

Bezafibrate is readily absorbed from the gastro-intestinal tract. Plasma protein binding is about 95%. The plasma elimination half-life is about 2 hours. Most of a dose is excreted in the urine, about half as unchanged drug, the remainder as metabolites including the glucuronide conjugate. A small proportion of the dose appears in the faeces.

References.

1. Abshagen U, *et al.* Disposition pharmacokinetics of bezafibrate in man. *Eur J Clin Pharmacol* 1979; **16:** 31–8.
2. Abshagen U, *et al.* Steady-state kinetics of bezafibrate and clofibrate in healthy female volunteers. *Eur J Clin Pharmacol* 1980; **17:** 305–8.

Old age. In a study comparing the pharmacokinetics of bezafibrate in 19 elderly patients with younger healthy subjects,[1] maximum plasma concentrations were 1.6 times higher in the elderly group (median 12.1 mg per litre against 7.7 mg per litre) and half-life was increased by 3.8 times (median 6.6 hours against 1.7 hours). The differences could not be attributed solely to diminished renal function in elderly patients. Dosage adjustments in elderly patients should not therefore be based on renal function alone.

1. Neugebauer G, *et al.* Steady-state kinetics of bezafibrate retard in hyperlipidemic geriatric patients. *Klin Wochenschr* 1988; **66:** 250–6.

Renal impairment. For a report of the half-life of bezafibrate in patients with impaired renal function, see under Uses and Administration, below.

Uses and Administration

Bezafibrate, a fibric acid derivative, is a lipid regulating drug. It is used in the treatment of type IIa, type IIb, type III, type IV, and type V hyperlipoproteinaemias. It reduces elevated plasma concentrations of triglycerides by reducing the concentration of very-low-density lipoproteins (VLDL). It reduces elevated plasma concentrations of cholesterol to a lesser extent, but the effect is variable.

Bezafibrate is given in a usual dose of 200 mg three times daily by mouth taken with or after food; 200 mg twice daily may occasionally be adequate for maintenance particularly in the treatment of hypertriglyceridaemia. A 400-mg modified-release tablet is also available and is given as a single daily dose of 400 mg.

General reviews.

1. Goa KL, *et al.* Bezafibrate: an update of its pharmacology and use in the management of dyslipidaemia. *Drugs* 1996; **52:** 725–53.

Administration in renal impairment. Bezafibrate is generally contra-indicated in severe renal dysfunction but the manufacturer has stated that it may be given to patients with renal impairment depending on creatinine clearance. Suggested doses are: creatinine clearance 40 to 60 mL per minute, 400 mg daily; 15 to 40 mL per minute, 200 mg daily or on alternate days; less than 15 mL per minute and dialysis patients, 200 mg on every third day.

In a study in patients with impaired renal function[1] the half-life of bezafibrate was reported to be prolonged to 4.6 hours in 3 patients with creatinine clearance greater than 40 mL per minute, 7.8 hours in 8 patients with creatinine clearance of 20 to 40 mL per minute, and 20.1 hours in a patient with creatinine clearance of 13 mL per minute. Williams *et al.*[2] reported an accelerated decline in renal function in 2 patients with advanced chronic renal failure during bezafibrate therapy, and suggested that further dosage reductions would be necessary to avoid excessive plasma-bezafibrate concentrations in uraemic patients.

1. Anderson P, Norbeck H-E. Clinical pharmacokinetics of bezafibrate in patients with impaired renal function. *Eur J Clin Pharmacol* 1981; **21:** 209–14.
2. Williams AJ, *et al.* The short term effects of bezafibrate on the hypertriglyceridaemia of moderate to severe uraemia. *Br J Clin Pharmacol* 1984; **18:** 361–7.

Hyperlipidaemias. Bezafibrate is a typical member of the fibric acid derivative group of drugs (the fibrates) used in the treatment of hyperlipidaemias (p.1265). One of the primary actions of the fibrates is to promote the catabolism of triglyceride-rich lipoproteins, in particular very-low-density lipoproteins (VLDL), apparently mediated by an enhanced activity of lipoprotein lipase.[1] They may also interfere with the synthesis of VLDL, possibly by inhibiting hepatic acetyl coenzyme A carboxylase. The effect of fibrates on low-density lipoprotein-cholesterol (LDL-cholesterol) depends on the overall lipoprotein status of the patient. In hypertriglyceridaemic patients the response depends on underlying LDL-cholesterol concentrations and the type of lipoprotein abnormality, while in normotriglyceridaemic patients with type IIa hyperlipoproteinaemia the LDL-cholesterol tends to decrease. In these patients bezafibrate and fenofibrate may reduce LDL-cholesterol concentrations more effectively than clofibrate or gemfibrozil. High-density lipoprotein-cholesterol (HDL-cholesterol) concentrations are increased by fibrate therapy in both hypertriglyceridaemic and normotriglyceridaemic patients, although there have been a few reports of unexpected falls in HDL-cholesterol with bezafibrate[2,3] and ciprofibrate (see p.1271).

Fibrates have three actions on sterol metabolism:[1] they inhibit the synthesis of cholesterol, they inhibit the synthesis of bile acids, and they enhance the secretion of cholesterol in bile. It is these latter two effects which are responsible for the raised cholesterol saturation of bile, which may lead to the formation of gallstones in some patients. However, other factors appear to be necessary since gallstones only develop in relatively few patients.

Bezafibrate has been shown to reduce cholesterol and triglyceride concentrations in patients with type IIa, IIb, and IV hyperlipoproteinaemias and in diabetic patients with lipid abnormalities.[4] Comparative studies have shown it to be at least as effective as clofibrate and fenofibrate, and to be more so than gemfibrozil in the short, but possibly not long, term.[4] It is less effective than ciprofibrate (except for effects on HDL-cholesterol).[4]

The influence of long-term bezafibrate administration on mortality from **ischaemic heart disease** has been investigated. In the Bezafibrate Coronary Atherosclerosis Intervention Trial (BECAIT)[5,6] treatment for 5 years in young men (less than 45 years of age) following myocardial infarction resulted in fewer coronary events and slowed the progression of focal coronary atherosclerosis when compared with placebo.

1. Grundy SM, Vega GL. Fibric acids: effects on lipids and lipoprotein metabolism. *Am J Med* 1987; **83** (suppl 5B): 9–20.
2. Capps NE. Lipid profiles on fibric-acid derivatives. *Lancet* 1994; **344:** 684–5.
3. McLeod AJ, *et al.* Abnormal lipid profiles on fibrate derivatives. *Lancet* 1996; **347:** 261.
4. Goa KL, *et al.* Bezafibrate: an update of its pharmacology and use in the management of dyslipidaemia. *Drugs* 1996; **52:** 725–53.
5. Ericsson C-G, *et al.* Angiographic assessment of effects of bezafibrate on progression of coronary artery disease in young male postinfarction patients. *Lancet* 1996; **347:** 849–53.
6. Ericsson C-G, *et al.* Effect of bezafibrate treatment over five years on coronary plaques causing 20% to 50% diameter narrowing (The Bezafibrate Coronary Atherosclerosis Intervention Trial (BECAIT)). *Am J Cardiol* 1997; **80:** 1125–9.

Preparations

Proprietary Preparations (details are given in Part 3)
Aust.: Bezalip; ***Belg.:*** Cedur; Eulitop; ***Canad.:*** Bezalip; ***Fr.:*** Befizal; ***Ger.:*** Azufibrat; Befibrat; Beza; Beza Lande; Beza Puren; Bezacur; Bezamerck; Cedur; Durabezur; Lipox; Regadrin B; Sklerofibrat; ***Ital.:*** Bezalip; Hadiel; ***Jpn:*** Bezalip; ***Neth.:*** Bezalip; ***S.Afr.:*** Bezalip; ***Spain:*** Difaterol; Eulitop; Reducterol; ***Swed.:*** Bezalip; ***Switz.:*** Cedur; ***UK:*** Bezalip; Bezalip Mono.

Binifibrate (18698-g)

Binifibrate *(rINN).*

2-(4-Chlorophenoxy)-2-methylpropionic acid ester with 1,3-dinicotinoyloxypropan-2-ol.

$C_{25}H_{23}ClN_2O_7$ = 498.9.

CAS — 69047-39-8.

Binifibrate, a derivative of clofibrate (p.1271) and nicotinic acid (p.1351), is a lipid regulating drug used in the treatment of hyperlipidaemias (p.1265). The usual dose is 600 mg three times daily by mouth.

Preparations

Proprietary Preparations (details are given in Part 3)
Spain: Antopal; Aterozot†; Biniwas; Clearon.

Cerivastatin Sodium (656-p)

Cerivastatin Sodium *(BANM, USAN, rINNM).*

Bay-W-6228. Sodium {S-[R*,S*-(E)]}-7-[4-(4-fluorophenyl)-5-(methoxymethyl)-2,6-bis(1-methylethyl)-3-pyridinyl]-3,5-dihydroxy-6-heptenoate.

$C_{26}H_{33}FNNaO_5$ = 481.5.

CAS — 143201-11-0.

Adverse Effects and Precautions

As for Simvastatin, p.1278.

Interactions

As for Simvastatin, p.1279.

Pharmacokinetics

Cerivastatin is readily and almost completely absorbed from the gastro-intestinal tract. The absolute bioavailability is reported to be about 60%. Cerivastatin undergoes metabolism in the liver, its primary site of action. The three major metabolites are also active inhibitors of HMG-CoA reductase. Cerivastatin is about 99% bound to plasma proteins. The plasma elimination half-life of cerivastatin has been reported to be approximately 2 to 3 hours. It is excreted as metabolites, about 30% in the urine and 70% in the faeces.

Uses and Administration

Cerivastatin, a 3-hydroxy-3-methylglutaryl coenzyme A (HMG-CoA) reductase inhibitor (a statin), is a lipid regulating drug with actions on plasma lipids similar to those of simvastatin (p.1279).

It is used in the treatment of hypercholesterolaemias, particularly in type IIa and type IIb hyperlipoproteinaemias (p.1265).

Cerivastatin is given by mouth as the sodium salt. The initial dose is 100 µg once daily in the evening. The dose may be adjusted in increments of 100 µg at intervals of at least 4 weeks up to a maximum of 300 µg once daily. A maximum dose of 200 µg once daily has been recommended in patients with moderate to severe renal impairment.

General reviews.

1. McClellan KJ, *et al.* Cerivastatin. *Drugs* 1998; **55:** 415–20.

Preparations

Proprietary Preparations (details are given in Part 3)
Neth.: Lipobay; ***Swed.:*** Lipobay; ***UK:*** Lipobay; ***USA:*** Baycol.

Cholestyramine (1344-d)

Cholestyramine *(BAN).*

Colestyramine *(rINN)*; Cholestyramine Resin; MK-135.

CAS — 11041-12-6.

Pharmacopoeias. In US.

Cholestyramine is a strongly basic anion-exchange resin containing quaternary ammonium functional groups which are attached to a styrene-divinylbenzene copolymer (about 2% divinylbenzene). It is used in the chloride form.

A white to buff-coloured, hygroscopic, fine powder, odourless or with a slight amine-like odour. It loses not more than 12% of its weight on drying.

Practically **insoluble** in water, in alcohol, in chloroform, and in ether. A 1% aqueous slurry has a pH of 4 to 6. **Store** in airtight containers.

Adverse Effects

The most common side-effect of cholestyramine is constipation; faecal impaction may develop and haemorrhoids may be aggravated. Other gastro-intestinal side-effects include abdominal discomfort or pain, heartburn, flatulence, nausea, vomiting, and diarrhoea.

Cholestyramine in high doses may cause steatorrhoea by interfering with the absorption of fats from the gastro-intestinal tract and therefore decreased absorption of fat-soluble vitamins, such as vitamins A, D, and K, may occur. Chronic administration of cholestyramine may thus result in an increased bleeding tendency due to hypoprothrombinaemia associated with vitamin K deficiency; it also has a potential to cause osteoporosis due to impaired calcium and vitamin D absorption.

Due to the fact that cholestyramine is the chloride form of an anion-exchange resin, prolonged use may produce hyperchloraemic acidosis, particularly in children.

Skin rashes and pruritus of the tongue, skin, and perianal region have occasionally occurred.

Results of the Lipid Research Clinics Coronary Primary Prevention Trial[1] involving 3806 men given cholestyramine or placebo for an average of 7.4 years. Gastro-intestinal side-effects occurred frequently in both groups but especially in the cholestyramine group. In the first year 68% of the cholestyramine group experienced at least one gastro-intestinal side-effect compared with 43% of the placebo group; by the seventh year the incidence had diminished so that approximately equal percentages of patients were affected (29% and 26% respectively). Constipation and heartburn, especially, were more frequent in the cholestyramine group which also reported more abdominal pain, belching or bloating, gas, and nausea. These side-effects were usually not severe and could be dealt with by standard clinical means.

The incidence of malignant neoplasms was similar in the two groups although there were differences in incidence at some sites. In particular, there were 21 cases of malignancy in the gastro-intestinal tract (8 fatal) in the cholestyramine group compared with 11 cases (1 fatal) in the placebo group. The number of colon cancers was identical in both groups. However, Oliver commented that 6 rare cancers of the buccal cavity or pharynx in the cholestyramine group should not pass unnoticed.[2]

1. Lipid Research Clinics Program. The Lipid Research Clinics Coronary Primary Prevention Trial results. *JAMA* 1984; **251:** 351–64.
2. Oliver MF. Hypercholesterolaemia and coronary heart disease: an answer. *Br Med J* 1984; **288:** 423–4.

Precautions

Cholestyramine powder should be administered as a suspension in water or a flavoured vehicle to minimise the risk of oesophageal obstruction.

Cholestyramine should not be used in patients with complete biliary obstruction as it is unlikely to be effective.

Because of the risk of vitamin deficiencies, supplements of vitamins A, D, E, and K should be considered during prolonged therapy with cholestyramine; if given by mouth they need to be in a water-miscible form. Parenteral administration, particularly of vitamin K for hypoprothrombinaemia, may be necessary if a deficiency becomes established. Reduced serum-folate concentrations have also been reported in children with familial hypercholesterolaemia and it has been suggested that supplementation with folic acid should be considered in such circumstances.

Interactions

Cholestyramine may delay or reduce the absorption of other drugs, particularly acidic drugs, administered concomitantly. Enterohepatic circulation may be reduced. Delayed or reduced absorption of thiazide diuretics, propranolol, digoxin and related alkaloids, loperamide, phenylbutazone, barbiturates, oestrogens, progestogens, thyroid hormones, warfarin, and some antibacterials, has either been reported or may be expected. It is therefore recommended that other drugs should be taken at least 1 hour before, or 4 to 6 hours after, the administration of cholestyramine.

Uses and Administration

Cholestyramine is a bile-acid binding resin and lipid regulating drug. It is used in the treatment of hypercholesterolaemias, particularly type IIa hyperlipoproteinaemia, and for the primary prevention of ischaemic heart disease in middle-aged men with primary hypercholesterolaemia. Cholestyramine is also used for the relief of diarrhoea associated with ileal resection, Crohn's disease, vagotomy, diabetic vagal neuropathy, and radiation, and to relieve the pruritus associated with the deposition in dermal tissue of excess bile acids in patients with partial biliary obstruction or primary biliary cirrhosis.

Cholestyramine is not absorbed from the gastro-intestinal tract but it adsorbs, and combines with, the bile acids in the intestine to form an insoluble complex that is excreted in the faeces. The normal reabsorption of bile acids is thus prevented and this leads to an increased oxidation of cholesterol to bile acids to replace those partially removed from the enterohepatic circulation. The overall effect is a reduction of total plasma-cholesterol concentration, mainly by lowering low-density lipoprotein (LDL)-cholesterol; this may be accompanied by moderate increases in plasma triglyceride and high-density lipoprotein (HDL)-cholesterol concentrations. Since the uses of cholestyramine are based upon the removal of intestinal bile acids it is unlikely that a response will be achieved in patients with complete biliary obstruction.

Cholestyramine may be introduced gradually over 3 to 4 weeks to minimise gastro-intestinal effects.

In hyperlipidaemias and diarrhoea the usual dose by mouth is 12 to 24 g daily, administered either as a single dose or in up to 4 divided doses. Dosage should be adjusted according to the patient's response and may be increased to 36 g daily if necessary. Lower doses may be adequate in some forms of hyperlipidaemia.

In pruritus doses of 4 to 8 g daily are usually sufficient.

A suggested dose of cholestyramine for children over 6 years of age is 240 mg per kg body-weight daily in divided doses.

Cholestyramine should be administered as a suspension in water or a flavoured vehicle.

Administration in children. Plasma-cholesterol concentrations were lowered in children given cholestyramine alone[1] or with dietary restrictions[2,3] for periods ranging from 1 to 8 years. Long-term treatment with cholestyramine had no adverse effects on physical growth[2,3] and development or sexual maturation.[2] However, West and Lloyd[1] found compliance to be a problem with only 48% of patients complying with treatment after 8 years.

1. West RJ, Lloyd JK. Long-term follow-up of children with familial hypercholesterolaemia treated with cholestyramine. *Lancet* 1980; **ii:** 873–5.
2. Glueck CJ, *et al.* Safety and efficacy of long-term diet and diet plus bile acid-binding resin cholesterol-lowering therapy in 73 children heterozygous for familial hypercholesterolemia. *Pediatrics* 1986; **78:** 338–48.
3. Tonstad S, *et al.* Efficacy and safety of cholestyramine therapy in peripubertal and prepubertal children with familial hypercholesterolemia. *J Pediatr* 1996; **129:** 42–9.

Antibiotic-associated colitis. Cholestyramine binds *Clostridium difficile* toxins and has been tried as an alternative to vancomycin or metronidazole in patients with diarrhoea associated with *C. difficile* toxins following antibiotic therapy (p.123). In general cholestyramine is given following a course of vancomycin or metronidazole in patients suffering multiple relapses.[1-3]

1. Bartlett JG. Treatment of Clostridium difficile colitis. *Gastroenterology* 1985; **89:** 1192–5.
2. Pruksananonda P, Powell KR. Multiple relapses of Clostridium difficile-associated diarrhea responding to an extended course of cholestyramine. *Pediatr Infect Dis J* 1989; **8:** 175–8.
3. Satin AJ, *et al.* Relapsing Clostridium difficile toxin-associated colitis in ovarian cancer patients treated with chemotherapy. *Obstet Gynecol* 1989; **74:** 487–9.

Biliary disorders. Beneficial responses were reported with cholestyramine in the management of congenital nonobstructive nonhaemolytic hyperbilirubinaemia (Crigler-Najjar disease) in 2 infants.[1,2] It has also produced a beneficial effect in 1 patient with sclerosing cholangitis.[3]

1. Arrowsmith WA, *et al.* Comparison of treatments for congenital nonobstructive nonhaemolytic hyperbilirubinaemia. *Arch Dis Child* 1975; **50:** 197–201.
2. Odièvre M, *et al.* Case of congenital nonobstructive, nonhaemolytic jaundice: successful long-term phototherapy at home. *Arch Dis Child* 1978; **53:** 81–2.
3. Polter DE, *et al.* Beneficial effect of cholestyramine in sclerosing cholangitis. *Gastroenterology* 1980; **79:** 326–33.

Hyperlipidaemias. Cholestyramine and other bile-acid binding resins, sometimes called bile-acid sequestrants,[1-3] are used in conjunction with dietary modification in the treatment of hyperlipidaemias (p.1265) in patients with raised low-density lipoprotein (LDL)-cholesterol concentrations such as those with heterozygous familial hypercholesterolaemia. Their action is mediated through an increase in the synthesis of LDL-receptors on hepatocytes. Thus they are ineffective in patients with homozygous familial hypercholesterolaemia who lack functional LDL-receptors. They may stimulate very-low-density lipoprotein (VLDL) production and thereby increase triglyceride concentrations. If they are to be used in patients with raised triglyceride concentrations, combination with nicotinic acid or a fibric acid derivative will be necessary. These combinations also produce enhanced cholesterol-lowering effects.[4,5]

Results of the Lipid Research Clinics Coronary Primary Prevention Trial[6] in 3806 middle-aged men with primary hypercholesterolaemia (type II hyperlipoproteinaemia) demonstrated that treatment with cholestyramine reduced the incidence of **ischaemic heart disease** in patients at high risk when compared with placebo, chiefly by reduction of total plasma-cholesterol and LDL-cholesterol concentrations.[7] However, there was a larger number of violent and accidental deaths in the treatment group. In the National Heart, Lung and Blood Institute (NHLBI) Type II Coronary Intervention Study in 116 patients with type II hyperlipoproteinaemia and ischaemic heart disease,[8,9] the progression of ischaemic heart disease, assessed angiographically after 5 years, was moderately reduced by cholestyramine.

The side-effects of cholestyramine may be reduced by using a low-dosage regimen. The dose-response curve for cholestyramine is non-linear and 8 g daily can often achieve a 10 to 20% reduction in LDL cholesterol.[10]

1. LaRosa J. Review of clinical studies of bile acid sequestrants for lowering plasma lipid levels. *Cardiology* 1989; **76** (suppl 1): 55–64.
2. Shepherd J. Mechanism of action of bile acid sequestrants and other lipid-lowering drugs. *Cardiology* 1989; **76** (suppl 1): 65–74.
3. Ast M, Frishman WH. Bile acid sequestrants. *J Clin Pharmacol* 1990; **30:** 99–106.
4. Curtis LD, *et al.* Combination treatment with cholestyramine and bezafibrate for heterozygous familial hypercholesterolaemia. *Br Med J* 1988; **297:** 173–5.
5. Jones AF, *et al.* Gemfibrozil plus cholestyramine in familial hypercholesterolaemia. *Lancet* 1988; **i:** 776.
6. Lipid Research Clinics Program. The Lipid Research Clinics Coronary Primary Prevention trial results 1: reduction in incidence of coronary heart disease. *JAMA* 1984; **251:** 351–64.
7. Lipid Research Clinics Program. The Lipid Research Clinics Coronary Primary Prevention trial results 2: the relationship of reduction in incidence of coronary heart disease in cholesterol lowering. *JAMA* 1984; **251:** 365–74.
8. Brensike JF, *et al.* Effects of therapy with cholestyramine on progression of coronary arteriosclerosis: results of the NHLBI Type II Coronary Intervention Study. *Circulation* 1984; **69:** 313–24.
9. Levy RI, *et al.* The influence of changes in lipid values induced by cholestyramine and diet on progression of coronary artery disease: results of the NHLBI Type II Coronary Intervention Study. *Circulation* 1984; **69:** 325–37.
10. Illingworth DR. Treatment of hyperlipidaemia. *Br Med Bull* 1990; **46:** 1025–58.

Preparations

USP 23: Cholestyramine for Oral Suspension.

Proprietary Preparations (details are given in Part 3)
Aust.: Quantalan; ***Austral.:*** Questran; ***Belg.:*** Questran; ***Canad.:*** Novo-Cholamine; Questran; ***Fr.:*** Questran; ***Ger.:*** Colestyr; Lipocol; Quantalan; Vasosan; ***Irl.:*** Questran; ***Ital.:*** Colestrol; Questran; ***Neth.:*** Questran; ***Norw.:*** Questran; ***S.Afr.:*** Questran; ***Spain:*** Lismol; Questran; Resincolestiramina; ***Swed.:*** Questran; ***Switz.:*** Quantalan; ***UK:*** Cholemin; Questran; ***USA:*** Prevalite; Questran.

Ciprofibrate (15316-r)

Ciprofibrate *(BAN, USAN, rINN).*

Win-35833. 2-[4-(2,2-Dichlorocyclopropyl)phenoxy]-2-methylpropionic acid.

$C_{13}H_{14}Cl_2O_3$ = 289.2.

CAS — 52214-84-3.

Adverse Effects and Precautions

As for Bezafibrate, p.1268.

Interactions

As for Bezafibrate, p.1268.

NSAIDs. Acute renal failure due to rhabdomyolysis in one patient has been attributed to an interaction between ciprofibrate and ibuprofen.[1] Ibuprofen was believed to have displaced ciprofibrate from protein binding sites. The use of radiological contrast media may also have been a contributory factor.

1. Ramachandran S, *et al.* Acute renal failure due to rhabdomyolysis in presence of concurrent ciprofibrate and ibuprofen treatment. *Br Med J* 1997; **314:** 1593.

Pharmacokinetics

Ciprofibrate is readily absorbed from the gastro-intestinal tract; peak plasma concentrations occur within 1 to 4 hours. Ciprofibrate is highly protein bound. It is excreted in the urine as unchanged drug and as glucuronide conjugates. The elimination half-life varies from about 38 to 86 hours in patients on long-term therapy.

Uses and Administration

Ciprofibrate, a fibric acid derivative, is a lipid regulating drug with actions on plasma lipids similar to those of bezafibrate (p.1269).

It is used in the treatment of type IIa, type IIb, type III, and type IV hyperlipoproteinaemias (p.1265). The usual dose is 100 mg daily by mouth.

Administration in renal impairment. Ciprofibrate is contra-indicated in patients with severe renal dysfunction. The manufacturer has suggested reducing the dose to 100 mg every other day for patients with moderate renal impairment.

Renal clearance of ciprofibrate was reduced and elimination half-life approximately doubled in patients with severe renal impairment.[1] Mild renal insufficiency slowed the urinary excretion of ciprofibrate but not its extent. The clearance of ciprofibrate was unaffected by haemodialysis.

1. Ferry N, *et al.* The influence of renal insufficiency and haemodialysis on the kinetics of ciprofibrate. *Br J Clin Pharmacol* 1989; **28:** 675–81.

Hyperlipidaemias. Similarly to other fibric acid derivatives (see under Bezafibrate, p.1269) ciprofibrate is stated to reduce elevated low-density lipoprotein (LDL)-cholesterol and very-low-density lipoprotein (VLDL)-triglyceride concentrations and to increase high-density lipoprotein (HDL)-cholesterol concentrations. There have, however, been reports of an abnormal response to ciprofibrate, namely a fall in HDL-cholesterol rather than the expected rise. In one patient the effect was seen when the dose of ciprofibrate was increased from 100 to 200 mg daily;[1] in another it occurred with 100 mg daily.[2]

1. Chandler HA, Batchelor AJ. Ciprofibrate and lipid profile. *Lancet* 1994; **344:** 128–9.
2. McLeod AJ, *et al.* Ciprofibrate and lipid profile. *Lancet* 1994; **344:** 955.

Preparations

Proprietary Preparations (details are given in Part 3)
Belg.: Hyperlipen; ***Fr.:*** Bi-Lipanor†; Lipanor; ***Neth.:*** Modalim; ***Switz.:*** Hyperlipen; ***UK:*** Modalim.

Clinofibrate (16584-m)

Clinofibrate *(rINN).*

S-8527. 2,2′-[Cyclohexylidenebis(4-phenyleneoxy)]bis[2-methylbutyric acid].

$C_{28}H_{36}O_6$ = 468.6.

CAS — 30299-08-2.

Pharmacopoeias. In *Jpn.*

Clinofibrate, a fibric acid derivative (see Bezafibrate, p.1268), is a lipid regulating drug used in the treatment of hyperlipidaemias (p.1265). The usual dose is 200 mg two or three times daily by mouth.

Preparations

Proprietary Preparations (details are given in Part 3)
Aust.: Lipoclin; ***Jpn:*** Lipoclin.

Clofibrate (1341-x)

Clofibrate *(BAN, USAN, rINN).*

AY-61123; Clofibratum; Ethyl *p*-Chlorophenoxyisobutyrate; Ethyl Clofibrate; ICI-28257; NSC-79389. Ethyl 2-(4-chlorophenoxy)-2-methylpropionate.

$C_{12}H_{15}ClO_3$ = 242.7.

CAS — 637-07-0 (clofibrate); 882-09-7 (clofibric acid).

Pharmacopoeias. In *Chin., Eur.* (see p.viii), *Jpn,* and *US.*

A clear colourless to pale yellow liquid with a characteristic odour. Ph. Eur. **solubilities** are: very slightly soluble in water; miscible with alcohol and ether. USP solubilities are: insoluble in water; soluble in acetone, alcohol, and chloroform. **Store** in airtight containers. Protect from light.

Aluminium Clofibrate (1342-r)

Aluminium Clofibrate *(BAN, rINN).*

Alufibrate; Aluminum Clofibrate. Bis[2-(4-chlorophenoxy)-2-methylpropionato]hydroxyaluminium.

$C_{20}H_{21}AlCl_2O_7$ = 471.3.

CAS — 24818-79-9; 14613-01-5.

Calcium Clofibrate (16291-y)

Calcium Clofibrate *(rINN).*

$C_{20}H_{20}CaCl_2O_6$ = 467.4.

CAS — 39087-48-4.

Magnesium Clofibrate (8041-a)

Magnesium Clofibrate *(rINN).*

Clomag; UR-112.

$C_{20}H_{20}Cl_2MgO_6$ = 451.6.

CAS — 14613-30-0.

Adverse Effects and Precautions

As for Bezafibrate, p.1268.

Additional side-effects occasionally reported with clofibrate include vomiting, diarrhoea, dyspepsia, flatulence, weight gain, drowsiness, and hepatomegaly.

Large-scale long-term studies have demonstrated an increased incidence of cholecystitis, gallstones, and sometimes pancreatitis in patients receiving clofibrate, and some studies, but not all, have indicated an increased incidence of certain cardiovascular disorders, including cardiac arrhythmias. The unexpected finding of an increased mortality rate in patients taking clofibrate in the WHO study (see below) produced serious concern over the long-term safety of clofibrate.

Doubts over the safety of clofibrate for long-term prophylaxis were raised following 2 large-scale studies; the Coronary Drug Project[1] and the WHO Co-operative Trial.[2] The Coronary Drug Project showed that while clofibrate was generally well tolerated, there was an increased incidence of serious effects over the 5-year study period. These included cholelithiasis (3.0% against 1.3% with placebo), pulmonary embolism or thrombophlebitis (5.2% against 3.3%), arrhythmias other than atrial fibrillation, new cases of intermittent claudication, and new angina pectoris. Other findings included an increased incidence of palpable spleen, and enlarged, firm, or tender liver. Anticoagulant therapy was required in 37% more patients taking clofibrate than placebo. Further analysis of the results[3] showed that the incidence of cholelithiasis or cholecystitis over the first 6 years was 4.0% in the clofibrate group compared with 2.6% in the placebo group.

In the WHO study[2] there was a higher incidence of cholelithiasis and a slight excess of thrombo-embolism, but no evidence of an increased incidence of intermittent claudication. More importantly, the long-term safety of clofibrate was thrown into doubt by the finding that, although clofibrate reduced the incidence of non-fatal myocardial infarction, the overall death rate was higher in the clofibrate group than in the control groups. The excess deaths were related to a range of disorders with no single disorder predominating. Follow-up after 9.6 years[4] and 13.2 years[5] indicated that the excess of deaths from causes other than ischaemic heart disease was almost entirely confined to the period of exposure to clofibrate; the excess during the treatment period was 47% from all causes compared with 5% after treatment ended. The causes of death were spread over a range of malignant and non-malignant disorders.

1. The Coronary Drug Project Research Group. Clofibrate and niacin in coronary heart disease. *JAMA* 1975; **231:** 360–80.
2. Oliver MF, *et al.* A co-operative trial in the primary prevention of ischaemic heart disease using clofibrate. *Br Heart J* 1978; **40:** 1069–1118.
3. The Coronary Drug Project Research Group. Gall bladder disease as a side effect of drugs influencing lipid metabolism. *N Engl J Med* 1977; **296:** 1185–90.
4. Oliver MF, *et al.* WHO cooperative trail on primary prevention of ischaemic heart disease using clofibrate to lower serum cholesterol: mortality follow-up. *Lancet* 1980; **ii:** 379–85. Correction. *ibid.*; 490.
5. Oliver MF, *et al.* WHO cooperative trial on primary prevention of ischaemic heart disease using clofibrate to lower serum cholesterol: final mortality follow-up. *Lancet* 1984; **ii:** 600–604.

Effects on the kidneys. Renal failure has been reported[1,2] in patients taking clofibrate. See also Effects on Skeletal Muscle, under Adverse Effects of Bezafibrate, p.1268.

1. Dosa S, *et al.* Acute-on-chronic renal failure precipitated by clofibrate. *Lancet* 1976; **i:** 250.
2. Cumming A. Acute renal failure and interstitial nephritis after clofibrate treatment. *Br Med J* 1980; **281:** 1529–30.

Effects on the nervous system. Peripheral neuropathy developed in a patient given clofibrate.[1] Symptoms resolved when clofibrate was withdrawn.

1. Gabriel R, Pearce JMS. Clofibrate-induced myopathy and neuropathy. *Lancet* 1976; **ii:** 906.

Effects on the respiratory system. Eosinophilic pneumonia in 1 patient associated with the use of clofibrate.[1]

1. Hendrickson RM, Simpson F. Clofibrate and eosinophilic pneumonia. *JAMA* 1982; **247:** 3082.

Interactions

As for Bezafibrate, p.1268.

The manufacturers of clofibrate have suggested that, in patients taking oral anticoagulants, the dose of anticoagulant should be reduced to about a half when treatment with clofibrate is started, and then adjusted gradually if necessary.

Pharmacokinetics

Clofibrate is readily absorbed from the gastro-intestinal tract and is rapidly hydrolysed to its active metabolite, chlorophenoxyisobutyric acid (clofibric acid), which is extensively bound to plasma proteins. The plasma half-life is about 17 hours. It is excreted in the urine, predominantly in the form of a glucuronide conjugate.

References.

1. Cailleux A, *et al.* Etude pharmacocinétique des hypolipémiants dérivés de l'acide clofibrique chez l'homme après administration unique et répétée. *Therapie* 1976; **31:** 637–45.
2. Gugler R. Clinical pharmacokinetics of hypolipidaemic drugs. *Clin Pharmacokinet* 1978; **3:** 425–39.

Uses and Administration

Clofibrate, a fibric acid derivative, is a lipid regulating drug with actions on plasma lipids similar to those of bezafibrate (p.1269). It is used in the treatment of type III hyperlipoproteinaemia; it may also be helpful in some patients with severe hypertriglyceridaemia due to type IIb, type IV, or type V hyperlipoproteinaemias.

The usual dose, by mouth, is 20 to 30 mg per kg body-weight daily in 2 or 3 divided doses after food. In adults, doses are commonly in the range 1.5 to 2 g daily.

The aluminium, calcium, and magnesium salts of clofibrate have also been used in the treatment of hyperlipidaemias.

Clofibrate has been used for the prophylaxis of ischaemic heart disease but is no longer recommended for this purpose because of the incidence of adverse effects during long-term treatment. For further details see under Adverse Effects, above.

Administration in renal impairment. Clofibrate should generally be avoided in patients with renal impairment.

The plasma half-life of total clofibric acid has been reported[1] to be extended from about 17 hours in healthy subjects to a mean of about 130 hours in 5 patients with renal failure undergoing haemodialysis. Goldberg *et al.*[2] found that a dose of 1.0 to 1.5 g of clofibrate per week effectively lowered plasma-triglyceride concentrations without causing toxicity in 11 hypertriglyceridaemic patients undergoing haemodialysis.

1. Faed EM, McQueen EG. Plasma half-life of clofibric acid in renal failure. *Br J Clin Pharmacol* 1979; **7:** 407–10.
2. Goldberg AP, *et al.* Control of clofibrate toxicity in uraemic hypertriglyceridemia. *Clin Pharmacol Ther* 1977; **21:** 317–25.

Hyperlipidaemias. Like other fibric acid derivatives clofibrate is used in the treatment of hyperlipidaemias (p.1265). It reduces elevated plasma-triglyceride concentrations probably mainly by an effect on lipoprotein lipase (see Bezafibrate, p.1269).

Several studies involving clofibrate investigated whether reduction of elevated serum-lipids would reduce the incidence of **ischaemic heart disease**. The two largest long-term studies were the Coronary Drug Project[1] which involved over 8000 subjects with confirmed previous myocardial infarctions, and the WHO Co-operative Trial[2] in over 15 000 healthy men. The Coronary Drug Project found no reduction in total mortality, nor in fatal or non-fatal major ischaemic heart disease. The overall incidence of major ischaemic heart disease was reduced in the clofibrate group compared with hyperlipidaemic controls in the WHO Co-operative Trial, the difference being confined to non-fatal myocardial infarctions. The increased incidence in both cardiovascular and non-cardiovascular diseases in subjects taking clofibrate, in particular the incidence of cholelithiasis and, in the WHO study, the excess mortality in the clofibrate group[3,4] (see also under Adverse Effects, above) has meant that clofibrate is no longer used for the prophylaxis of ischaemic heart disease. Other fibric acid derivatives, for example gemfibrozil (p.1274), are, however, used prophylactically.

1. The Coronary Drug Project Research Group. Clofibrate and niacin in coronary heart disease. *JAMA* 1975; **231:** 360–80.
2. Oliver MF, *et al.* A co-operative trial in the primary prevention of ischaemic heart disease using clofibrate. *Br Heart J* 1978; **40:** 1069–1118.
3. Oliver MF, *et al.* WHO cooperative trial on primary prevention of ischaemic heart disease using clofibrate to lower serum cholesterol: mortality follow-up. *Lancet* 1980; **ii:** 379–85. Correction. *ibid.*; 490.
4. Oliver MF, *et al.* WHO cooperative trial on primary prevention of ischaemic heart disease using clofibrate to lower serum cholesterol: final mortality follow-up. *Lancet* 1984; **ii:** 600–604.

Neonatal jaundice. Clofibrate has been found to be effective both in the treatment of jaundice in term infants and for prophylaxis in premature infants.[1] In a study involving 93 term infants with jaundice, clofibrate 50 mg per kg bodyweight as a single oral dose reduced the intensity and duration of jaundice compared with placebo. As a prophylactic measure, clofibrate was shown to reduce the degree of jaundice in premature infants when the plasma concentration of clofibric acid reached 140 μg per mL within 24 hours of clofibrate administration. The dose required to achieve this was estimated to be 100 to 150 mg per kg.

1. Gabilan JC, *et al.* Clofibrate treatment of neonatal jaundice. *Pediatrics* 1990; **86:** 647–8.

Preparations

BP 1998: Clofibrate Capsules;
USP 23: Clofibrate Capsules.

Proprietary Preparations (details are given in Part 3)
Aust.: Arterioflexin; Regelan; ***Austral.:*** Arterioflexin†; Atromid-S; Col†; ***Belg.:*** Atromidin; ***Canad.:*** Atromid-S; Novo-Fibrate; ***Fr.:*** Lipavlon; ***Ger.:*** atherolipin†; Regelan N; Skleromexe†; ***Irl.:*** Atromid-S; ***Ital.:*** Atromidin†; Clofinit†; Geromid†; Lipavil†; Sepik†; ***Neth.:*** Clofi†; ***S.Afr.:*** Atromid-S; ***Spain:*** Neo Atromid; ***Swed.:*** Atromidin; ***Switz.:*** Regelan; ***UK:*** Atromid-S; ***USA:*** Atromid-S.

Multi-ingredient: ***Ger.:*** Anti-Lipide-ratiopharm†; Lipofacton†; vasoatherolip†; ***Ital.:*** Clopir†; Ellemger†; S.trat.os†; Sinteroid†; ***S.Afr.:*** Lipaten; ***Spain:*** Arteriobrate; ***Switz.:*** Liaptene†.

Clofibride (1345-n)

Clofibride *(rINN).*

MG-46. 3-Dimethylcarbamoylpropyl 2-(4-chlorophenoxy)-2-methylpropionate.

$C_{16}H_{22}ClNO_4$ = 327.8.

CAS — 26717-47-5.

Clofibride, a fibric acid derivative (see Bezafibrate, p.1268), is a lipid regulating drug that has been used in the treatment of hypercholesterolaemia and hypertriglyceridaemia.

The active metabolite of clofibride is clofibric acid (chlorophenoxyisobutyric acid). Hydroxy-4-*N*-dimethylbutyramide is an additional metabolite.

Preparations

Proprietary Preparations (details are given in Part 3)
Fr.: Lipenan†.

Colestipol Hydrochloride (1346-h)

Colestipol Hydrochloride *(BANM, USAN, rINNM).*

U-26597A.

CAS — 26658-42-4 (colestipol); 50925-79-6 (colestipol); 37296-80-3 (colestipol hydrochloride).

Pharmacopoeias. In Br. and US.

Colestipol is a basic anion-exchange resin. It is the hydrochloride of a copolymer of diethylenetriamine and epichlorohydrin (1-chloro-2,3-epoxypropane).

Yellow to orange hygroscopic beads. Each g binds not less than 1.1 mEq and not more than 1.7 mEq of sodium cholate, calculated as the cholate binding capacity.

Swells but does not dissolve in water or dilute aqueous solutions of acid or alkali. Practically **insoluble** in alcohol and dichloromethane. The supernatant of a 10% w/w suspension in water has a pH of 6.0 to 7.5. **Store** in airtight containers.

Adverse Effects and Precautions

As for Cholestyramine, p.1269.

Reductions in total serum-thyroxine and thyroxine-binding globulin concentrations were found during routine monitoring of thyroid function in patients receiving colestipol and nicotinic acid, but were considered to be benign.[1]

1. Cashin-Hemphill L, *et al.* Alterations in serum thyroid hormonal indices with colestipol-niacin therapy. *Ann Intern Med* 1987; **107:** 324–9.

Interactions

As for Cholestyramine, p.1270.

Uses and Administration

Colestipol hydrochloride is a bile-acid binding resin. It is not absorbed from the gastro-intestinal tract but binds bile acids in the intestines and has actions similar to those of cholestyramine (p.1270).

It is a lipid regulating drug and is used in the treatment of hypercholesterolaemias, particularly type IIa hyperlipoproteinaemia.

Colestipol hydrochloride is available as granules and is administered as a suspension in water or a flavoured vehicle. The recommended initial dose is 5 g daily or twice daily, increasing gradually at intervals of 1 to 2 months to up to 30 g daily in single or two divided doses as necessary.

In the USA, colestipol hydrochloride is also available as tablets; doses range from 2 to 16 g daily.

Hyperlipidaemias. Colestipol is a bile-acid binding resin used similarly to cholestyramine (p.1270) in the treatment of hyperlipidaemias (p.1265).

Colestipol on its own[1] or with nicotinic acid[2,3] has been reported to be effective in the prophylaxis of **ischaemic heart disease**. The Cholesterol-Lowering Atherosclerosis Study (CLAS)[2] in middle-aged men with progressive atherosclerosis who had undergone coronary bypass surgery showed that colestipol plus nicotinic acid reduced blood concentrations of total cholesterol, triglycerides, and low-density lipoprotein (LDL)-cholesterol, and increased those of high-density lipoprotein (HDL)-cholesterol. Drug treatment also reduced progression of atherosclerosis, development of new lesions in native coronary arteries, and changes in venous bypass grafts. Benefits were maintained after 4 years.[3]

The side-effects of colestipol may be reduced by using a low-dose regimen. The dose-response curve for colestipol is non-linear and 10 g daily can often achieve a 10 to 20% reduction in LDL cholesterol.[4] In a study of patients with moderate hypercholesterolaemia,[5] colestipol 10 g daily (as granules in suspension), either as a single dose in the morning or evening or in two divided doses was effective and well-tolerated. In another study[6] in patients with moderate primary hypercholesterolaemia lower doses of colestipol (2.5 g three times daily) taken together with psyllium (also 2.5 g three times daily) were as effective and better tolerated than higher doses of colestipol alone (5 g three times daily).

1. Dorr AE, *et al.* Colestipol hydrochloride in hypercholesterolemic patients—effect on serum cholesterol and mortality. *J Chron Dis* 1978; **31:** 5–14.
2. Blankenhorn DH, *et al.* Beneficial effects of combined colestipol-niacin therapy on coronary atherosclerosis and coronary venous bypass grafts. *JAMA* 1987; **257:** 3233–40.
3. Cashin-Hemphill L, *et al.* Beneficial effects of colestipol-niacin on coronary atherosclerosis: a 4-year follow-up. *JAMA* 1990; **264:** 3013–17.
4. Illingworth DR. Treatment of hyperlipidaemia. *Br Med Bull* 1990; **46:** 1025–58.
5. Lyons D, *et al.* Colestipol at varying dosage intervals in the treatment of moderate hypercholesterolaemia. *Br J Clin Pharmacol* 1994; **37:** 59–62.
6. Spence JD, *et al.* Combination therapy with colestipol and psyllium mucilloid in patients with hyperlipidemia. *Ann Intern Med* 1995; **123:** 493–9.

Preparations

BP 1998: Colestipol Granules;
USP 23: Colestipol Hydrochloride for Oral Suspension.

Proprietary Preparations (details are given in Part 3)
Austral.: Colestid; ***Belg.:*** Colestid; ***Canad.:*** Colestid; ***Ger.:*** Cholestabyl; Colestid; ***Irl.:*** Colestid; ***Neth.:*** Colestid; ***Norw.:*** Lestid; ***S.Afr.:*** Colestid†; ***Spain:*** Colestid; ***Swed.:*** Lestid; ***Switz.:*** Colestid; ***UK:*** Colestid; ***USA:*** Colestid.

Colextran Hydrochloride (12634-e)

Colextran Hydrochloride *(rINNM).*

DEAE-dextran Hydrochloride; Detaxtran Hydrochloride; Diethylaminoethyl-dextran Hydrochloride. Dextran 2-(diethylamino)ethyl ether hydrochloride.

CAS — 9064-91-9 (colextran hydrochloride); 9015-73-0 (colextran).

Colextran hydrochloride, an anion-exchange resin, is a lipid regulating drug used in the treatment of hyperlipidaemias (p.1265). It is given in a usual dose of 2 to 3 g daily by mouth in divided doses.

Preparations

Proprietary Preparations (details are given in Part 3)
Ital.: Dexide; Nolipid; Pulsar; Rationale; ***Spain:*** Dexide.

Dextrothyroxine Sodium (9004-r)

Dextrothyroxine Sodium *(BANM, USAN, rINN).*

Sodium Dextrothyroxine; 3,5,3′,5′-Tetraiodo-D-thyronine Sodium; D-Thyroxine Sodium. Sodium 4-*O*-(4-hydroxy-3,5-di-iodophenyl)-3,5-di-iodo-D-tyrosinate hydrate.

$C_{15}H_{10}I_4NNaO_4(+xH_2O)$ = 798.9 (anhydrous).

CAS — 51-49-0 (dextrothyroxine); 137-53-1 (dextrothyroxine sodium, anhydrous); 7054-08-2 (dextrothyroxine sodium, hydrate).

Adverse Effects

Most adverse effects of dextrothyroxine are due to the drug's metabolic activity. Cardiac changes include angina pectoris, extrasystoles, ectopic beats, supraventricular tachycardia, and ECG evidence of ischaemic heart disease.

Other adverse effects include insomnia, nervousness, tremor, diuresis, loss of weight, sweating, flushing, fever, alopecia, menstrual irregularities, nausea, vomiting, decreased appetite, diarrhoea, constipation, skin rashes, and pruritus. The development of gallstones has also occasionally been reported. The general adverse effects of thyroid hormones are described on p.1497.

Effects on the heart. In the Coronary Drug Project, treatment with dextrothyroxine sodium was stopped after 36 months when it was found that the mortality in the 1083 patients receiving it was 18.4% higher than in those receiving placebo.[1] The excess mortality was mainly due to deaths from coronary and other cardiovascular causes, and was concentrated in a subgroup of patients with pre-existing cardiovascular disease or hypertension: the incidence of recurrent non-fatal myocardial infarction was also higher.

Adverse effects included, in addition to cardiovascular disorders, decreased glucose tolerance, possible abnormalities of hepatic function, and hypermetabolism attributable to hyperthyroid activity. Dextrothyroxine used in the study was shown to contain less than 0.5% of levothyroxine, equivalent to less than 30 μg of levothyroxine from the daily dose of 6 mg of dextrothyroxine. However, samples of commercially available dextrothyroxine were found to contain 0.8 to 1.0% of levothyroxine.[2]

1. The Coronary Drug Project Research Group. The Coronary Drug Project: findings leading to further modifications of its protocol with respect to dextrothyroxine. *JAMA* 1972; **220:** 996–1008.
2. Scheiffele E, Schultze KW. The Coronary Drug Project. *JAMA* 1972; **221:** 918.

Hyperthyroidism. Hyperthyroidism occurred in a patient during treatment with dextrothyroxine 4 mg daily.[1] The patient became euthyroid when dextrothyroxine was discontinued and symptoms recurred when dextrothyroxine was reintroduced.

1. Hazenburg HJA, *et al.* Dextrothyroxine induced hyperthyroidism in a patient with heterozygous familial hypercholesterolaemia. *Neth J Med* 1987; **31:** 117–21.

Precautions

Dextrothyroxine is contra-indicated in patients with hypertension or heart disease including angina pectoris, myocardial infarction, cardiac arrhythmias, and heart failure. It is also contra-indicated in patients with advanced liver or kidney disease. The precautions to be taken with thyroid hormones in general are described on p.1497.

Interactions

Dextrothyroxine may enhance the effects of anticoagulants. It may increase the requirements of insulin or oral hypoglycaemics. The interactions of thyroid hormones in general are described on p.1498.

Uses and Administration

Dextrothyroxine is the D-isomer of thyroxine but has only weak thyroid hormone activity. It is a lipid regulating drug that reduces elevated plasma-cholesterol concentrations, particularly the low-density lipoprotein (LDL) fraction.

Dextrothyroxine is used as the sodium salt in the treatment of hypercholesterolaemia in type II hyperlipoproteinaemia (p.1265) but this use is severely limited by cardiotoxicity. The initial dose is 1 to 2 mg daily, increased by 1 to 2 mg at monthly intervals until a satisfactory response is achieved, up to a maximum of 4 to 8 mg daily by mouth.

Dextrothyroxine was formerly used to treat hypothyroidism.

Preparations

Proprietary Preparations (details are given in Part 3)
Canad.: Choloxin; ***Ger.:*** Dynothel; Eulipos†; ***Ital.:*** Lisolipin†; ***USA:*** Choloxin.

Divistyramine (16609-t)

Divistyramine, a bile-acid binding resin, is a lipid regulating drug that has been used similarly to cholestyramine (p.1269) in the treatment of hyperlipidaemias (p.1265). It has also been used for the relief of pruritus in patients with partial biliary obstruction. It has been given by mouth in usual doses of 6 to 9 g daily as a suspension in a suitable vehicle.

Preparations

Proprietary Preparations (details are given in Part 3)
Switz.: Ipocol†.

Etofibrate (12719-c)

Etofibrate *(rINN).*

2-Nicotinoyloxyethyl 2-(4-chlorophenoxy)-2-methylpropionate.

$C_{18}H_{18}ClNO_5$ = 363.8.

CAS — 31637-97-5.

Etofibrate, a derivative of clofibrate (p.1271) and nicotinic acid (p.1351), is a lipid regulating drug used in the treatment of hyperlipidaemias (p.1265). The usual dose is 300 mg three times daily by mouth.

Preparations

Proprietary Preparations (details are given in Part 3)
Aust.: Lipo-Merz; ***Ger.:*** Lipo-Merz; ***Spain:*** Afloyan; ***Switz.:*** Lipo-Merz.

Fenofibrate (1348-b)

Fenofibrate *(BAN, rINN).*

LF-178; Procetofene. Isopropyl 2-[4-(4-chlorobenzoyl)phenoxy]-2-methylpropionate.

$C_{20}H_{21}ClO_4$ = 360.8.

CAS — 49562-28-9.

Pharmacopoeias. In *Chin.* and *Eur.* (see p.viii).

A white or almost white, crystalline powder. Practically **insoluble** in water; slightly soluble in alcohol; very soluble in dichloromethane. **Protect** from light.

Adverse Effects and Precautions

As for Bezafibrate, p.1268.

The most common adverse effects in both long- and short-term studies of fenofibrate have been gastro-intestinal disturbances, occurring in about 3 to 5% of patients.[1] Other adverse effects include dermatological, musculoskeletal, and neurological disorders. There has been no evidence yet of an increased incidence of gallstones, although some increases in the indices of bile lithogenicity have been reported.[1-3]

For a report of the half-life being prolonged in patients with renal impairment, see Administration in Renal Impairment, under Uses and Administration, below.

1. Brown WV. Treatment of hypercholesterolaemia with fenofibrate: a review. *Curr Med Res Opin* 1989; **11:** 321–30.
2. Blane GF. Comparative toxicity and safety profile of fenofibrate and other fibric acid derivatives. *Am J Med* 1987; **83** (suppl 5B): 26–36.
3. Palmer RH. Effects of fibric acid derivatives on biliary lipid composition. *Am J Med* 1987; **83** (suppl 5B): 37–43.

Interactions

As for Bezafibrate, p.1268.

The manufacturers of fenofibrate suggest that in patients taking oral anticoagulants, the dose of anticoagulant should be reduced by about one-third when treatment with fenofibrate is started, and then adjusted gradually if necessary.

Pharmacokinetics

Fenofibrate is readily absorbed from the gastro-intestinal tract when taken with food; absorption is substantially reduced if fenofibrate is administered after an overnight fast. It is rapidly hydrolysed to its active metabolite fenofibric acid which is extensively bound to plasma albumin. The plasma elimination half-life is about 20 hours. Fenofibric acid is excreted predominantly in the urine, mainly as the glucuronide conjugate, but also as a reduced form of fenofibric acid and its glucuronide.

References.

1. Chapman MJ. Pharmacology of fenofibrate. *Am J Med* 1987; **83** (suppl 5B): 21–5.

Uses and Administration

Fenofibrate, a fibric acid derivative, is a lipid regulating drug with actions on plasma lipids similar to those of bezafibrate (p.1269).

It is used in the treatment of type IIa, type IIb, type III, type IV, and type V hyperlipoproteinaemias.

The usual initial dose, by mouth, is 300 mg daily in divided doses with food. Doses may be adjusted according to response to between 200 and 400 mg daily. Children may be given 5 mg per kg bodyweight daily.

Preparations containing micronised fenofibrate are available that have improved bioavailability and thus may allow a lower total daily dose. The recommended initial dose is about 200 mg daily depending upon the formulation used.

General references.

1. *Am J Med* 1987; **83** (suppl 5B).
2. *Cardiology* 1989; **76** (suppl 1): 1–54.
3. Adkins JC, Faulds D. Micronised fenofibrate: a review of its pharmacodynamic properties and clinical efficacy in the management of dyslipidaemia. *Drugs* 1997; **54:** 615–33.

Administration in renal impairment. Fenofibrate is generally contra-indicated in patients with severe renal dysfunction, but the UK manufacturers have stated that fenofibrate may be given in mild or moderate renal impairment in reduced doses. They have suggested doses of 200 or 100 mg daily for creatinine clearances of 60 or 20 mL per minute, respectively.

The plasma half-life of fenofibric acid has been shown to be prolonged to up to about 360 hours in patients with renal disease following a single dose of fenofibrate.[1] No correlation was found between the elimination half-life and serum creatinine concentrations or creatinine clearance. Fenofibrate metabolites were not removed by haemodialysis. Significant accumulation of fenofibric acid occurs on repeated daily dosing in renal insufficiency.

1. Desager JP, *et al.* Effect of hemodialysis on plasma kinetics of fenofibrate in chronic renal failure. *Nephron* 1982; **31:** 51–4.

Hyperlipidaemias. Like other fibric acid derivatives, fenofibrate is used in the treatment of hyperlipidaemias (p.1265). It reduces elevated plasma-triglyceride concentrations probably mainly by an effect on lipoprotein lipase[1] (see Bezafibrate, p.1269). Substantial reductions in plasma-cholesterol concentrations have been reported in healthy subjects[1] and in patients with type IIa and IIb hyperlipoproteinaemias.[2-4] Low-density lipoprotein (LDL)-cholesterol concentrations were increased in patients with type IV or V hyperlipoproteinaemias with low base-line LDL-cholesterol concentrations.[5] In addition, high-density lipoprotein (HDL)-cholesterol concentrations are generally increased.[1,3,4] A uricosuric effect has also been reported.[1]

Although patient numbers have generally been small,[1] comparative studies have suggested that fenofibrate reduces cholesterol concentrations to a greater extent than clofibrate. Overall, the effect of fenofibrate was comparable with bezafibrate and ciprofibrate although the effects on individual lipoproteins differed somewhat. Fenofibrate was less effective than simvastatin[6] at reducing elevated cholesterol concentrations but more effective at reducing elevated triglyceride concentrations.

1. Balfour JA, *et al.* Fenofibrate: a review of its pharmacodynamic and pharmacokinetic properties and therapeutic use in dyslipidaemia. *Drugs* 1990; **40:** 260–90.
2. Brown WV, *et al.* Effects of fenofibrate on plasma lipids: double-blind, multicenter study in patients with type IIA or IIB hyperlipidemia. *Arteriosclerosis* 1986; **6:** 670–8.
3. Brown WV. Treatment of hypercholesterolaemia with fenofibrate: a review. *Curr Med Res Opin* 1989; **11:** 321–30.
4. Superko HR. A review of combined hyperlipidaemia and its treatment with fenofibrate. *J Int Med Res* 1989; **17:** 99–112.
5. Seidehamel RJ. Fenofibrate in type IV and type V hyperlipoproteinemia. *Cardiology* 1989; **76** (suppl 1): 23–32.
6. Stohler R, *et al.* Effects of simvastatin and fenofibrate on serum lipoproteins and apolipoproteins in primary hypocholesterolaemia. *Eur J Clin Pharmacol* 1989; **37:** 199–203.

Preparations

Proprietary Preparations (details are given in Part 3)
Aust.: Fenolip; Lipcor†; Lipsin; ***Belg.:*** Lipanthyl; ***Canad.:*** Lipidil; ***Fr.:*** Lipanthyl; Secalip; ***Ger.:*** durafenat; Lipanthyl; Lipidil; Normalip; ***Ital.:*** Fulcro; Lipanthyl; Lipidax†; Lipil†; Lipoclar; Lipofene; Liposit†; Nolipax; Scleril; Tilene; Volutine; ***S.Afr.:*** Lipsin; ***Spain:*** Liparison; Lipovas†; Secalip; ***Switz.:*** Lipanthyl; ***UK:*** Lipantil; ***USA:*** Tricor.

Fluvastatin Sodium (5928-w)

Fluvastatin Sodium *(BANM, USAN, rINNM).*

XU-62-320. Sodium (±)-(3R*,5S*,6E)-7-[3-(p-Fluorophenyl)-1-isopropylindol-2-yl]-3,5-dihydroxy-6-heptenoate.

$C_{24}H_{25}FNNaO_4$ = 433.4.

CAS — 93957-54-1 (fluvastatin); 93957-55-2 (fluvastatin sodium).

Adverse Effects and Precautions

As for Simvastatin, p.1278.

Interactions

The interactions of statins with other drugs are described under simvastatin (p.1279). However, similar interactions appear not to have been reported with fluvastatin although caution is advised when using such combinations.

General reviews.

1. Garnett WR. Interactions with hydroxymethylglutaryl-coenzyme A reductase inhibitors. *Am J Health-Syst Pharm* 1995; **52:** 1639–45.

Pharmacokinetics

Fluvastatin, unlike simvastatin or lovastatin, is active without the need for hydrolysis. It is rapidly and completely absorbed from the gastro-intestinal tract and undergoes extensive first-pass metabolism in the liver, its primary site of action. An absolute bioavailability of 24% has been reported. It is more than 98% bound to plasma proteins. It is excreted mainly in the faeces (about 90%) with only about 6% being excreted in the urine.

General reviews.

1. Desager J-P, Horsmans Y. Clinical pharmacokinetics of 3-hydroxy-3-methylglutaryl-coenzyme A reductase inhibitors. *Clin Pharmacokinet* 1996; **31:** 348–71.
2. Lennernäs H, Fager G. Pharmacodynamics and pharmacokinetics of the HMG-CoA reductase inhibitors: similarities and differences. *Clin Pharmacokinet* 1997; **32:** 403–25.

Uses and Administration

Fluvastatin, a 3-hydroxy-3-methylglutaryl coenzyme A (HMG-CoA) reductase inhibitor (a statin), is a lipid regulating drug with actions on plasma lipids similar to those of simvastatin (p.1279).

It is used in the treatment of hypercholesterolaemias particularly in type IIa and type IIb hyperlipoproteinaemias. It is also given prophylactically in hypercholesterolaemic patients with ischaemic heart disease.

Fluvastatin is given by mouth as the sodium salt, but doses are expressed in terms of the base. The initial dose is 20 to 40 mg once daily in the evening, increased if necessary at intervals of 4 weeks up to 40 mg twice daily.

General reviews.

1. Deslypere JP. The role of HMG-CoA reductase inhibitors in the treatment of hyperlipidemia: a review of fluvastatin. *Curr Ther Res* 1995; **56:** 111–28.
2. Plosker GL, Wagstaff AJ. Fluvastatin: a review of its pharmacology and use in the management of hypercholesterolaemia. *Drugs* 1996; **51:** 433–59.
3. Schectman G, Hiatt J. Dose–response characteristics of cholesterol-lowering drug therapies: implications for treatment. *Ann Intern Med* 1996; **125:** 990–1000.

Hyperlipidaemias. Fluvastatin, like other statins, is used in the treatment of hyperlipidaemias (p.1265) and a general discussion of the lipid regulating effects of statins can be found in simvastatin (p.1279).

Studies[1,2] have confirmed the ability of fluvastatin to reduce low-density lipoprotein (LDL)-cholesterol in patients with primary[1,2] or combined[2] hypercholesterolaemia; it was also well-tolerated.

1. Davidson MH. Fluvastatin long-term Extension Trial (FLUENT): summary of efficacy and safety. *Am J Med* 1994; **96** (suppl 6A): 41S–44S.
2. Beil S, *et al.* Fluvastatin lipid-lowering effect in routine practice conditions (FLIRT): results of a drug surveillance study. *Clin Drug Invest* 1997; **14:** 146–53.

Preparations

Proprietary Preparations (details are given in Part 3)
Aust.: Lescol; ***Austral.:*** Lescol; Vastin; ***Belg.:*** Lescol; ***Canad.:*** Lescol; ***Fr.:*** Fractal; Lescol; ***Ger.:*** Cranoc; LOCOL; ***Irl.:*** Lescol; ***Ital.:*** Lescol; Lipaxan; Primesin; ***Neth.:*** Canef; Lescol; ***Norw.:*** Canef; Lescol; ***S.Afr.:*** Lescol; ***Spain:*** Lescol; Lymetel; ***Swed.:*** Canef; Lescol; ***Switz.:*** Lescol; ***UK:*** Lescol; ***USA:*** Lescol.

Gemfibrozil (1349-v)

Gemfibrozil *(BAN, USAN, rINN).*

CI-719. 2,2-Dimethyl-5-(2,5-xylyloxy)valeric acid.

$C_{15}H_{22}O_3$ = 250.3.

CAS — 25812-30-0.

Pharmacopoeias. In *Br.* and *US.*

A white or almost white waxy crystalline solid. M.p. 58° to 61°. Practically **insoluble** in water; soluble in alcohol and in chloroform; soluble to freely soluble in methyl alcohol. **Store** in airtight containers. Protect from light.

Adverse Effects and Precautions

As for Bezafibrate, p.1268.

In the Helsinki Heart Study,[1] 11.3% of 2051 patients taking gemfibrozil reported various moderate to severe upper gastro-intestinal tract symptoms during the first year of treatment compared with 7% of 2030 patients taking placebo. No differences were seen between gemfibrozil and placebo groups in haemoglobin concentrations, urinary-protein, or urinary-sugar concentrations.

There was no significant difference in the total number of cancers between the gemfibrozil and placebo groups nor in the number of operations for gallstones or for cataract surgery. A higher number of deaths in the gemfibrozil group was mainly due to accident or violence and intracranial haemorrhage.

A follow-up study[2] reported that gastro-intestinal symptoms remained more common in patients taking gemfibrozil. Although there was no significant difference between the gemfibrozil and placebo groups cholecystectomies were consistently more common in those receiving gemfibrozil during the entire 8.5-year observation period. Cancer occurred equally in both groups, but there was increased mortality attributable to cancer in the gemfibrozil group, mainly during the last 1.5 years of follow-up.

1. Frick MH, *et al.* Helsinki Heart Study: primary-prevention trial with gemfibrozil in middle-aged men with dyslipidemia: safety of treatment, changes in risk factors, and incidence of coronary heart disease. *N Engl J Med* 1987; **317:** 1237–45.
2. Huttunen JK, *et al.* The Helsinki Heart Study: an 8.5-year safety and mortality follow-up. *J Intern Med* 1994; **235:** 31–9.

Effects on hypoglycaemic control. There have been conflicting reports of the effects of gemfibrozil on glucose metabolism in hyperlipidaemic diabetic patients. In a study of 14 diabetic patients[1] treated with gemfibrozil for 9 to 23 weeks control of diabetes was not generally impaired and appeared in some cases to be slightly improved. Konttinen *et al.*[2] reported a slight increase in antidiabetic therapy requirements in 9 of 20 patients and a decrease in 1. Testori *et al.*[3] reported a decrease in fasting and oral glucose tolerance test-stimulated glucose concentrations in patients with impaired glucose tolerance but not in those with normal glucose tolerance. No reduction in insulin secretion was noted. Two other studies[4,5] found no clinically significant changes in glucose metabolism in stable diabetics taking gemfibrozil. In another,[6] gemfibrozil was associated with decreased hyperglycaemia in diabetics whose blood-glucose concentrations were not well controlled.

1. de Salcedo I, *et al.* Gemfibrozil in a group of diabetics. *Proc R Soc Med* 1976; **69** (suppl 2): 64–70.
2. Konttinen A, *et al.* The effect of gemfibrozil on serum lipids in diabetic patients. *Ann Clin Res* 1979; **11:** 240–5.
3. Testori GP, *et al.* Effect of gemfibrozil treatment on glucose tolerance in hypertriglyceridemic patients with normal or impaired glucose tolerance. *Curr Ther Res* 1990; **47:** 390–5.
4. Leaf DA, *et al.* The hypolipidemic effects of gemfibrozil in type V hyperlipidemia. *JAMA* 1989; **262:** 3154–60.
5. Pagani A, *et al.* Effect of short-term gemfibrozil administration on glucose metabolism and insulin secretion in non-insulin-dependent diabetics. *Curr Ther Res* 1989; **45:** 14–20.
6. Notarbartolo A, *et al.* Effects of gemfibrozil in hyperlipidemic patients with or without diabetes. *Curr Ther Res* 1993; **53:** 381–93.

Effects on the nervous system. The Adverse Drug Reactions Advisory Committee in Australia has received reports of paraesthesia occurring in 6 patients in association with gemfibrozil treatment.[1]

1. Anonymous. Paraesthesia and neuropathy with hypolipidaemic agents. *Aust Adverse Drug React Bull* 1993; **12:** 6.

Effects on sexual function. Impotence and loss of libido has been reported in 3 patients[1-3] during gemfibrozil treatment. In 2 of the men[1,2] bezafibrate did not produce this adverse effect. The UK Committee on Safety of Medicines was reported to be aware of a further 6 cases.[2] Of a further 3 cases reported from Spain of impotence associated with gemfibrozil, one patient had previously reacted similarly to clofibrate.[4]

1. Pizarro S, *et al.* Gemfibrozil-induced impotence. *Lancet* 1990; **336:** 1135.
2. Bain SC, *et al.* Gemfibrozil-induced impotence. *Lancet* 1990; **336:** 1389.
3. Bharani A. Sexual dysfunction after gemfibrozil *Br Med J* 1992; **305:** 693.
4. Figueras A, *et al.* Gemfibrozil-induced impotence. *Ann Pharmacother* 1993; **27:** 982.

Effects on skeletal muscle. For reports of rhabdomyolysis in patients taking gemfibrozil with lovastatin, see p.1275.

Effects on the skin. Psoriasis was exacerbated in a patient within 2 weeks of starting gemfibrozil therapy and recurred when gemfibrozil was subsequently reintroduced.[1]

1. Fisher DA, *et al.* Exacerbation of psoriasis by the hypolipidemic agent, gemfibrozil. *Arch Dermatol* 1988; **124:** 854–5.

Gallstones. Gemfibrozil increased the concentration of cholesterol in bile and decreased the output of bile acids in 8 normolipaemic male subjects.[1] This resulted in an increase in the lithogenic index in both gallbladder and hepatic bile, although no cholesterol crystals were detected in gallbladder bile. In the Helsinki Heart Study[2] no significant increase in gallstone operations was reported among 2051 patients taking gemfibrozil compared with 2030 taking placebo. However, a follow-up study[3] reported that cholecystectomies were consistently more common in those receiving gemfibrozil during the entire 8.5-year observation period, suggesting that gemfibrozil is lithogenic like other fibric acid derivatives.

1. Leiss O, *et al.* Effect of gemfibrozil on biliary lipid metabolism in normolipemic subjects. *Metabolism* 1985; **34:** 74–82.
2. Frick MH, *et al.* Helsinki Heart Study: primary-prevention trial with gemfibrozil in middle-aged men with dyslipidemia: safety of treatment, changes in risk factors, and incidence of coronary heart disease. *N Engl J Med* 1987; **317:** 1237–45.
3. Huttunen JK, *et al.* The Helsinki Heart Study: an 8.5-year safety and mortality follow-up. *J Intern Med* 1994; **235:** 31–9.

Headache. Headaches occurred 30 to 90 minutes after each dose of gemfibrozil in 2 patients.[1,2] In both patients, the headaches were accompanied by dry mouth, and in 1 also by blurred vision. The headaches stopped when gemfibrozil was withdrawn and recurred one week after re-exposure.

1. Arellano F, *et al.* Gemfibrozil-induced headache. *Lancet* 1988; **i:** 705.
2. Alvarez-Sabin J, *et al.* Gemfibrozil-induced headache. *Lancet* 1988; **ii:** 1246.

Interactions

As for Bezafibrate, p.1268.

Antidiabetics. For mention of the effect, in some patients, of gemfibrozil on antidiabetic therapy requirement, see Effects on Hypoglycaemic Control, above.

Lipid regulating drugs. The bioavailability of gemfibrozil was reduced by the concomitant administration of *colestipol*, but was unaffected when gemfibrozil was taken either 2 hours before or 2 hours after colestipol.[1]

For reports of rhabdomyolysis in patients taking gemfibrozil with *lovastatin*, see Effects on Skeletal Muscle, under Adverse Effects of Lovastatin, p.1275.

1. Forland SC, *et al.* Apparent reduced absorption of gemfibrozil when given with colestipol. *J Clin Pharmacol* 1990; **30:** 29–32.

Pharmacokinetics

Gemfibrozil is readily absorbed from the gastro-intestinal tract; peak concentrations in plasma occur within 1 to 2 hours; the half-life is about 1.5 hours. Plasma protein binding of gemfibrozil is about 98%. About 70% of a dose is excreted in the urine mainly as glucuronide conjugates of gemfibrozil and its metabolites; little is excreted in the faeces.

Uses and Administration

Gemfibrozil, a fibric acid derivative, is a lipid regulating drug with actions on plasma lipids similar to those of bezafibrate (p.1269).

It is used in the treatment of type IIa, type IIb, type III, type IV, and type V hyperlipoproteinaemias. It is also indicated for the primary prevention of ischaemic heart disease in hyperlipidaemic middle-aged men who have not responded to dietary and other measures: in the USA this use is restricted to type IIb patients who also have low HDL-cholesterol concentrations. The usual dose, by mouth, is 1.2 g daily in 2 divided doses given 30 minutes before the morning and evening meals. The dosage range may vary between 0.9 and 1.5 g daily.

Reviews.

1. Todd PA, Ward A. Gemfibrozil: a review of its pharmacodynamic and pharmacokinetic properties, and therapeutic use in dyslipidaemia. *Drugs* 1988; **36:** 314–39.
2. Spencer CM, Barradell LB. Gemfibrozil: a reappraisal of its pharmacological properties and place in the management of dyslipidaemia. *Drugs* 1996; **51:** 982–1018.

Administration in renal impairment. Although in the USA gemfibrozil is not recommended in patients with severe renal impairment, the UK manufacturer suggests that patients with renal impairment could be given a starting dose of 900 mg daily, adjusted according to response.

In a study[1] of the pharmacokinetics of gemfibrozil in 17 patients with stable chronic renal failure the mean plasma half-life was 1.8 and 1.9 hours after multiple and single doses respectively, which was comparable with that reported in patients with normal renal function. Gemfibrozil clearance was independent of renal function, but the kinetics of gemfibrozil metabolites were not evaluated.

Beneficial responses[2] were seen in lipid and lipoprotein concentrations in 5 of 6 uraemic patients treated with gemfibrozil 1200 mg daily for six months and in 6 nephrotic patients given gemfibrozil 800 mg daily for 4 months. No significant adverse effects or signs of organ toxicity were seen.

1. Evans JR, *et al.* The effect of renal function on the pharmacokinetics of gemfibrozil. *J Clin Pharmacol* 1987; **27:** 994–1000.
2. Manninen V, *et al.* Gemfibrozil treatment of dyslipidaemias in renal failure with uraemia or in the nephrotic syndrome. *Res Clin Forums* 1982; **4:** 113–18.

Hyperlipidaemias. Gemfibrozil is classified as a fibric acid derivative and is used in the treatment of hyperlipidaemias (p.1265). It has effects on plasma-lipid concentrations similar to those described under bezafibrate (p.1269). The major effects of gemfibrozil have been a reduction in plasma-triglyceride concentrations and an increase in high-density lipoprotein (HDL)-cholesterol concentrations. A reduction in very-low-density lipoprotein (VLDL)-triglyceride appears to be largely responsible for the fall in plasma triglyceride, although reductions in HDL- and low-density lipoprotein (LDL)-triglycerides have also been reported.[1-3] The effect of gemfibrozil on total cholesterol has been more variable. In general LDL-cholesterol may be decreased in patients with pre-existing high concentrations and raised in those with low concentrations.[1,2,4] The increase in HDL-cholesterol concentrations has resulted in favourable changes to the ratios of HDL-cholesterol to LDL-cholesterol and to total cholesterol.[4,5] Gemfibrozil has successfully raised HDL-cholesterol concentrations in patients with isolated low levels of HDL-cholesterol, but otherwise normal cholesterol concentrations.[6]

The Helsinki Heart Study[7] assessed gemfibrozil for the primary prevention of **ischaemic heart disease** in middle-aged men with hyperlipidaemia. In this study 4081 middle-aged men with raised serum concentrations of non-HDL cholesterol (Fredrickson type IIa, type IIb, and type IV hyperlipoproteinaemias) but with no coronary symptoms were randomly assigned to gemfibrozil 600 mg or placebo twice daily for 5 years; 2859 subjects completed the study, but all subjects initially randomised were followed for 5 years and included in the analysis. There was an overall reduction of 34% in the incidence of fatal and non-fatal myocardial infarctions and cardiac deaths in the gemfibrozil group compared with the placebo group, with the greatest reduction seen during years 3 to 5. On conclusion of this 5-year controlled study all participants were offered gemfibrozil with follow-up for a further 3.5 years.[8] Direct comparison with a placebo group was thus not possible, but long-term treatment with gemfibrozil seemed to postpone coronary events for about 5 years. Effects on safety and mortality were reported separately (see under Adverse Effects and Precautions, above).

1. Olsson AG, *et al.* Effect of gemfibrozil on lipoprotein concentrations in different types of hyperlipoproteinaemia. *Proc R Soc Med* 1976; **69** (suppl 2): 28–31.
2. Nikkilä EA, *et al.* Gemfibrozil: effect on serum lipids, lipoproteins, postheparin plasma lipase activities and glucose tolerance in primary hypertriglyceridaemia. *Proc R Soc Med* 1976; **69** (suppl 2): 58–63.
3. Kesäniemi YA, Grundy SM. Influence of gemfibrozil and clofibrate on metabolism of cholesterol and plasma triglycerides in man. *JAMA* 1984; **251:** 2241–6.
4. Manninen V, *et al.* Lipid alterations and decline in the incidence of coronary heart disease in the Helsinki Heart Study. *JAMA* 1988; **260:** 641–51.
5. Lewis JE, Multicenter Collaborative Study Group. Clinical use of gemfibrozil: a controlled multicenter trial. *Pract Cardiol* 1983; **9:** 99–118.
6. Miller M, *et al.* Effect of gemfibrozil in men with primary isolated low high-density lipoprotein cholesterol: a randomised, double-blind, placebo-controlled, crossover study. *Am J Med* 1993; **94:** 7–12.
7. Frick MH, *et al.* Helsinki Heart Study: primary-prevention trial with gemfibrozil in middle-aged men with dyslipidemia: safety of treatment, changes in risk factors, and incidence of coronary heart disease. *N Engl J Med* 1987; **317:** 1237–45.
8. Heinonen OP, *et al.* The Helsinki Heart Study: coronary heart disease incidence during an extended follow-up. *J Intern Med* 1994; **235:** 41–9.

Preparations

BP 1998: Gemfibrozil Capsules; Gemfibrozil Tablets;
USP 23: Gemfibrozil Capsules; Gemfibrozil Tablets.

Proprietary Preparations (details are given in Part 3)
Aust.: Gevilon; ***Austral.:*** Ausgem; Gemfibromax; Jezil; Lipazil; Lopid; ***Belg.:*** Lopid; ***Canad.:*** Lopid; ***Fr.:*** Lipur; ***Ger.:*** Gevilon; ***Irl.:*** Lopid; ***Ital.:*** Fibrocit; Gemlipid; Genlip; Lipozid; Lopid; ***Neth.:*** Lopid; ***S.Afr.:*** Lopid; ***Spain:*** Bolutol; Decrelip; Litarek; Lopid; Pilder; Taborcil; Tentroc†; Trialmin; ***Swed.:*** Lopid; ***Switz.:*** Gevilon; ***UK:*** Emfib; Lopid; ***USA:*** Gemcor; Lopid†.

Homonicotinic Acid (12827-x)

3-Pyridylacetic acid.

$C_7H_7NO_2$ = 137.1.

CAS — 501-81-5.

Homonicotinic acid is a lipid regulating drug.

Preparations

Proprietary Preparations (details are given in Part 3)
Ital.: Minedil†.

Multi-ingredient: ***Ital.:*** Geriavit†.

Lifibrol (13818-b)

Lifibrol *(USAN, rINN)*.

K-12148. (±)-*p*-[4-(*p*-*tert*-Butylphenyl)-2-hydroxybutoxy]benzoic acid.

$C_{21}H_{26}O_4$ = 342.4.

CAS — 96609-16-4.

Lifibrol is under investigation as a lipid regulating drug for the treatment of hypercholesterolaemia.

References.

1. Schwandt P, *et al.* Safety and efficacy of lifibrol upon four-week administration to patients with primary hypercholesterolaemia. *Eur J Clin Pharmacol* 1994; **47:** 133–8.
2. Locker PK, *et al.* Lifibrol: a novel lipid-lowering drug for the therapy of hypercholesterolemia. *Clin Pharmacol Ther* 1995; **57:** 73–88.

Lovastatin (16894-k)

Lovastatin (*BAN, USAN, rINN*).

L-154803; MB-530B; 6α-Methylcompactin; Mevinolin; MK-803; Monacolin K; MSD-803. (3R,5R)-7-{(1S,2S,6R,8S,8aR)-1,2,6,7,8,8a-Hexahydro-2,6-dimethyl-8-[(S)-2-methylbutyryloxy]-1-naphthyl}-3-hydroxyheptan-5-olide.

$C_{24}H_{36}O_5$ = 404.5.

CAS — 75330-75-5.

Pharmacopoeias. In US.

A white to off-white crystalline powder. Practically **insoluble** in water and in petroleum spirit; freely soluble in chloroform; soluble in acetone, in acetonitrile, and in methyl alcohol; sparingly soluble in alcohol. **Store** at 8° or below in airtight containers under nitrogen.

Adverse Effects and Precautions

As for Simvastatin, p.1278.

Adverse effects led to withdrawal of lovastatin in 21 of 745 patients receiving the drug for about 5 years.[1] They included asymptomatic elevation of hepatic aminotransferases in 10 patients, gastro-intestinal symptoms in 3, rash in 2, myopathy in 2, myalgia in 1, arthralgia in 1, insomnia in 1, and weight gain in 1.

1. Lovastatin Study Groups. Lovastatin 5-year safety and efficacy study: Lovastatin Study Groups I through IV. *Arch Intern Med* 1993; **153:** 1079–87.

Effects on the blood. Haemolytic anaemia in one patient has been attributed to lovastatin;[1] no adverse effect was seen in the patient when given simvastatin.

1. Robbins MJ, *et al.* Lovastatin-induced hemolytic anemia; not a class-specific reaction. *Am J Med* 1995; **99:** 328–9.

Effects on the eyes. Lens opacities were found in 13 of 101 patients taking lovastatin following an 18-week study.[1] However, no further deterioration was seen in 11 of these patients who continued to take lovastatin at follow-up after an average of 26 months from the start of treatment.

No differences were found in the development of lens opacities or in changes in visual acuity between patients treated with lovastatin for 48 weeks and patients taking placebo in a study of 8245 patients.[2]

1. Hunninghake DB, *et al.* Lovastatin: follow-up ophthalmologic data. *JAMA* 1988; **259:** 354–5.
2. Laties AM, *et al.* The human lens after 48 weeks of treatment with lovastatin. *N Engl J Med* 1990; **323:** 683–4.

Effects on the nervous system. Paraesthesias developed in a 47-year-old woman about two years after starting treatment with lovastatin.[1] Symptoms disappeared a few weeks after treatment was discontinued, but reappeared two weeks after starting treatment with pravastatin. Symptoms again abated a few weeks after pravastatin was discontinued.

1. Jacobs MB. HMG-CoA reductase inhibitor therapy and peripheral neuropathy. *Ann Intern Med* 1994; **120:** 970.

Effects on sexual function. Low sperm count associated with lovastatin therapy was reported in one patient.[1]

1. Hildebrand RD, Hepperlen TW. Lovastatin and hypospermia. *Ann Intern Med* 1990; **112:** 549–50.

Effects on skeletal muscle. Muscle disorders are well-recognised adverse effects of lipid regulating drugs such as the fibrates and statins (see Simvastatin, p.1278).

There have been reports of myopathy and rhabdomyolysis in patients receiving lovastatin in combination with azithromycin,[1] clarithromycin,[1] danazol,[2] erythromycin,[3] gemfibrozil,[4-6] itraconazole,[7] and nicotinic acid,[8] and in patients receiving immunosuppressive therapy (often including cyclosporin) following transplant surgery.[9-11] There has also been a report of rhabdomyolysis in a patient taking lovastatin on its own.[12] Muscle weakness and soreness associated with lovastatin was relieved in one patient by the administration of ubidecarenone.[13]

1. Grunden JW, Fisher KA. Lovastatin-induced rhabdomyolysis possibly associated with clarithromycin and azithromycin. *Ann Pharmacother* 1997; **31:** 859–63.
2. Dallaire M, Chamberland M. Rhabdomyolyse sévère chez un patient recevant lovastatine, danazol et doxycycline. *Can Med Assoc J* 1994; **150:** 1991–4.
3. Ayanian JZ, *et al.* Lovastatin and rhabdomyolysis. *Ann Intern Med* 1988; **109:** 682–3.
4. Kogan AD, Orenstein S. Lovastatin-induced acute rhabdomyolysis. *Postgrad Med J* 1990; **66:** 294–6.
5. Marais GE, Larson KK. Rhabdomyolysis and acute renal failure induced by combination lovastatin and gemfibrozil therapy. *Ann Intern Med* 1990; **112:** 228–30.
6. Pierce LR, *et al.* Myopathy and rhabdomyolysis associated with lovastatin-gemfibrozil combination therapy. *JAMA* 1990; **264:** 71–5.
7. Lees RS, Lees AM. Rhabdomyolysis from the coadministration of lovastatin and the antifungal agent itraconazole. *N Engl J Med* 1995; **333:** 664–5.
8. Reaven P, Witztum JL. Lovastatin, nicotinic acid, and rhabdomyolysis. *Ann Intern Med* 1988; **109:** 597–8.
9. Norman DJ, *et al.* Myolysis and acute renal failure in a heart-transplant recipient receiving lovastatin. *N Engl J Med* 1988; **318:** 46–7.
10. East C, *et al.* Rhabdomyolysis in patients receiving lovastatin after cardiac transplantation. *N Engl J Med* 1988; **318:** 47–8.
11. Corpier CL, *et al.* Rhabdomyolysis and renal injury with lovastatin use: report of two cases in cardiac transplant recipients. *JAMA* 1988; **260:** 239–41.
12. Wallace CS, Mueller BA. Lovastatin-induced rhabdomyolysis in the absence of concomitant drugs. *Ann Pharmacother* 1992; **26:** 190–2.
13. Walravens PA, *et al.* Lovastatin, isoprenes, and myopathy. *Lancet* 1989; **ii:** 1097–8.

Effects on sleep patterns. For reports of the effects of statins, including lovastatin, on sleep patterns, see Simvastatin, p.1278.

Pregnancy. For a report suggesting that exposure to lovastatin during pregnancy has no adverse outcome, see Simvastatin, p.1279.

Interactions

As for Simvastatin, p.1279.

General reviews.

1. Garnett WR. Interactions with hydroxymethylglutaryl-coenzyme A reductase inhibitors. *Am J Health-Syst Pharm* 1995; **52:** 1639–45.

Raised concentrations of lovastatin have occurred in patients also given *mibefradil*. Lovastatin has been associated with both hyperthyroidism[1] and hypothyroidism[2] in patients taking *thyroxine*. Bleeding and increases in prothrombin time have been reported in patients taking lovastatin with coumarin *anticoagulants* (see under Warfarin, p.969).

For reports of interactions of lovastatin with *azithromycin, clarithromycin, danazol, erythromycin, gemfibrozil, immunosuppressants, itraconazole,* and *nicotinic acid*, see Effects on Skeletal Muscle, above.

1. Lustgarten BP. Catabolic response to lovastatin therapy. *Ann Intern Med* 1988; **109:** 171–2.
2. Demke DM. Drug interaction between thyroxine and lovastatin. *N Engl J Med* 1989; **321:** 1341–2.

Pharmacokinetics

Lovastatin is absorbed from the gastro-intestinal tract and is hydrolysed in the liver to its active β-hydroxyacid form. Three other metabolites have also been isolated. Lovastatin undergoes extensive first-pass metabolism in the liver, its primary site of action, and less than 5% of the oral dose has been reported to reach the circulation. Peak plasma concentrations occur within 2 to 4 hours, and steady-state concentrations are achieved after 2 to 3 days with daily administration. Both lovastatin and its β-hydroxyacid metabolite are extensively bound (more than 95%) to plasma proteins. It is mainly excreted in the bile; about 85% of the administered dose has been recovered from the faeces and about 10% from the urine. The half-life of the active metabolite is 1 to 2 hours.

General reviews.

1. Desager J-P, Horsmans Y. Clinical pharmacokinetics of 3-hydroxy-3-methylglutaryl-coenzyme A reductase inhibitors. *Clin Pharmacokinet* 1996; **31:** 348–71.
2. Lennernäs H, Fager G. Pharmacodynamics and pharmacokinetics of the HMG-CoA reductase inhibitors: similarities and differences. *Clin Pharmacokinet* 1997; **32:** 403–25.

Uses and Administration

Lovastatin, a 3-hydroxy-3-methylglutaryl coenzyme A (HMG-CoA) reductase inhibitor (a statin), is a lipid regulating drug with actions on plasma lipids similar to those of simvastatin (p.1279).

Lovastatin is used in the treatment of hypercholesterolaemias, particularly in type IIa and IIb hyperlipoproteinaemias. It is also given prophylactically in hypercholesterolaemic patients with ischaemic heart disease.

Lovastatin is given in an initial dose of 10 to 20 mg daily in the evening with food, increased, if necessary, at intervals of 4 weeks or more to 80 mg daily in single or divided doses. In patients taking immunosuppressants an initial dose of 10 mg daily is recommended; the daily dose should not exceed 20 mg.

General reviews.

1. McKenney JM. Lovastatin: a new cholesterol-lowering agent. *Clin Pharm* 1988; **7:** 21–36.
2. Henwood JM, Heel RC. Lovastatin: a preliminary review of its pharmacodynamic properties and therapeutic use in hyperlipidaemia. *Drugs* 1988; **36:** 429–54.
3. Frishman WH, *et al.* Lovastatin and other HMG-CoA reductase inhibitors. *J Clin Pharmacol* 1989; **29:** 975–82.
4. Schectman G, Hiatt J. Dose–response characteristics of cholesterol-lowering drug therapies: implications for treatment. *Ann Intern Med* 1996; **125:** 990–1000.

Hyperlipidaemias. Lovastatin, like other statins, is used in the treatment of hyperlipidaemias (p.1265) and a general discussion of the lipid regulating effects of statins can be found in simvastatin (p.1279).

Lovastatin is effective in the treatment of primary hypercholesterolaemia. In the Expanded Clinical Evaluation of Lovastatin (EXCEL) study[1,2] involving more than 8000 patients with moderate hypercholesterolaemia, lovastatin lowered low-density lipoprotein (LDL)-cholesterol, total cholesterol, and triglyceride concentrations and increased high-density lipoprotein (HDL)-cholesterol concentrations in both men and women; benefit was maintained in those followed up for 2 years.[3] Lovastatin appeared to be more effective than nicotinic acid at reducing LDL-cholesterol in patients with primary hypercholesterolaemia, but less effective at increasing HDL-cholesterol; lovastatin was better tolerated.[4] Hypercholesterolaemia is a risk factor for **ischaemic heart disease** and lovastatin may be given for the secondary prevention of atherosclerotic heart disease. In the Asymptomatic Carotid Artery Progression Study (ACAPS)[5] lovastatin appeared to be of benefit in patients with early carotid artery atherosclerosis, although in another study it failed to prevent restenosis after coronary angioplasty.[6] Benefit has also been demonstrated[7] with lovastatin in primary prevention of coronary disease in men and women and even in those with only average cholesterol levels.

1. Bradford RH, *et al.* Expanded clinical evaluation of lovastatin (EXCEL) study results: I. efficacy in modifying plasma lipoproteins and adverse event profile in 8245 patients with moderate hypercholesterolemia. *Arch Intern Med* 1991; **151:** 43–9.
2. Bradford RH, *et al.* Efficacy and tolerability of lovastatin in 3390 women with moderate hypercholesterolemia. *Ann Intern Med* 1993; **118:** 850–5.
3. Bradford RH, *et al.* Expanded clinical evaluation of lovastatin (EXCEL) study results: two-year efficacy and safety follow-up. *Am J Cardiol* 1994; **74:** 667–73.
4. Illingworth DR, *et al.* Comparative effects of lovastatin and niacin in primary hypercholesterolemia. *Arch Intern Med* 1994; **154:** 1586–95.
5. Furberg CD, *et al.* Effect of lovastatin on early carotid atherosclerosis and cardiovascular events. *Circulation* 1994; **90:** 1679–87.
6. Weintraub WS, *et al.* Lack of effect of lovastatin on restenosis after coronary angioplasty. *N Engl J Med* 1994; **331:** 1331–7.
7. Downs JR, *et al.* Primary prevention of acute coronary events with lovastatin in men and women with average cholesterol levels: results of AFCAPS/TexCAPS. *JAMA* 1998; **279:** 1615–22.

Preparations

USP 23: Lovastatin Tablets.

Proprietary Preparations (details are given in Part 3)
Aust.: Mevacor; ***Canad.:*** Mevacor; ***Ger.:*** Mevinacor; ***Norw.:*** Mevacor; ***Spain:*** Lipofren; Mevacor; Nergadan; Taucor; ***USA:*** Mevacor.

Meglutol (18802-y)

Meglutol (*USAN, rINN*).

CB-337. 3-Hydroxy-3-methylglutaric acid.

$C_6H_{10}O_5$ = 162.1.

CAS — 503-49-1.

Meglutol is a lipid regulating drug used in the treatment of hyperlipidaemias (p.1265). The usual dose is 1.5 to 3 g daily in divided doses by mouth.

Preparations

Proprietary Preparations (details are given in Part 3)
Ital.: Lipoglutaren†; Mevalon.

Melinamide (16885-c)

Melinamide (*rINN*).

AC-223. N-(α-Methylbenzyl)linoleamide.

$C_{26}H_{41}NO$ = 383.6.

CAS — 14417-88-0.

Melinamide is a lipid regulating drug that has been used in the treatment of hyperlipidaemias (p.1265).

Preparations

Proprietary Preparations (details are given in Part 3)
Jpn: Artes†.

Mevastatin (16591-h)

Mevastatin (*rINN*).

Compactin; CS-500; ML-236B. (1S,7S,8S,8aR)-1,2,3,7,8,8a-Hexahydro-7-methyl-8-{2-[(2R,4R)-tetrahydro-4-hydroxy-6-oxo-2H-pyran-2-yl]ethyl}-1-naphthyl (S)-2-methylbutyrate.

$C_{23}H_{34}O_5$ = 390.5.

CAS — 73573-88-3.

Mevastatin, which has been isolated from *Penicillium citrinum*, is a lipid regulating drug. It is a 3-hydroxy-3-methylglutaryl coenzyme A (HMG-CoA) reductase inhibitor (a statin) (see Simvastatin, p.1278) but is no longer used in clinical practice because of reports of toxicity in *animals*.

Nicofibrate Hydrochloride (1353-n)

Nicofibrate Hydrochloride (*rINNM*).

Clofenpyride Hydrochloride. 3-Pyridylmethyl 2-(4-chlorophenoxy)-2-methylpropionate hydrochloride.

$C_{16}H_{16}ClNO_3,HCl = 342.2.$

CAS — 31980-29-7 (nicofibrate); 17413-51-3 (nicofibrate hydrochloride).

Nicofibrate hydrochloride, a derivative of clofibrate (p.1271) and nicotinic acid (p.1351), is a lipid regulating drug used in the treatment of hyperlipidaemias (p.1265). The usual dose is 400 mg two or three times daily by mouth.

Preparations

Proprietary Preparations (details are given in Part 3)
Ital.: Arterium V†; ***Spain:*** Arterium; Atepium†.

Omega-3 Triglycerides (3897-m)

Docosahexaenoic Acid (16610-l)

DHA. Docosahexa-4,7,10,13,16,19-enoic acid.

$C_{22}H_{32}O_2 = 328.5.$

NOTE. DHA is also used as a synonym for dihydroxyacetone.

Eicosapentaenoic Acid (12685-f)

EPA. Eicosapenta-5,8,11,14,17-enoic acid.

$C_{20}H_{30}O_2 = 302.5.$

CAS — 25378-27-2.

NOTE. EPA is also used as a synonym for pheneturide.

Omega-3 Marine Triglycerides (3899-v)

Omega-3 Marine Triglycerides (*BAN*).

Pharmacopoeias. In *Eur.* (see p.viii).

A mixture of mono-, di-, and triglycerides of omega-3 acids but containing mainly triglycerides. The omega-3 acids are from the body oil of fatty fish species from the Engraulidae, Carangidae, Clupeidae, Osmeridae, Salmonidae, and Scrombroidae families. The acids consist of alpha-linolenic acid, moroctic acid, eicosatetraenoic acid, eicosapentaenoic acid (timnodonic acid), heneicosapentaenoic acid, clupanodonic acid, and docosahexaenoic acid (cervonic acid). The total amount of omega-3 acids expressed as triglycerides is not less than 60% and that of both eicosapentaenoic acid and docosahexaenoic acid together, expressed as triglycerides, is not less than 45%. Tocopherol may be added as an antoxidant.

A pale yellow liquid. Practically **insoluble** in water; slightly soluble in dehydrated alcohol; very soluble in acetone. **Store** in airtight containers under inert gas. Protect from light.

Adverse Effects and Precautions

Omega-3 marine triglycerides and similar preparations may cause nausea and eructation, particularly at higher doses. Some preparations may also contain significant amounts of vitamins A and D and long-term use can cause toxicity. There is also a theoretical possibility of vitamin E deficiency with long-term use. Some concern has been expressed over the high calorific value and cholesterol content of some preparations.

Omega-3 triglycerides have antithrombotic activity and should be given with caution to patients with haemorrhagic disorders or to those receiving anticoagulants or other drugs affecting coagulation. They should also be used with caution in asthmatic patients sensitive to aspirin.

Fever, myalgia, sore throat, and tender lymphadenopathy lasting for 3 weeks were associated with omega-3 triglycerides in a 68-year-old woman.[1] Symptoms recurred within 48 hours of restarting administration.

1. Ogden P, *et al.* Reactive lymphoid hyperplasia after omega-3 fatty acid supplementation. *Ann Intern Med* 1988; **109:** 843–4.

Effects on the blood. Epistaxis was associated with omega-3 marine triglyceride treatment in 8 of 11 patients.[1] Prolonged bleeding time was noted in 3 patients.

1. Clarke JTR, *et al.* Increased incidence of epistaxis in adolescents with familial hypercholesterolemia treated with fish oil. *J Pediatr* 1990; **116:** 139–41.

Effects on the gastro-intestinal tract. High-dose purified eicosapentaenoic acid ethyl ester produced loose motions with passage of unabsorbed oil in the stool.[1]

1. Hawthorne AB, *et al.* Fish oil revisited. *Lancet* 1989; **ii:** 811.

Effects on hypoglycaemic control. A deterioration in glycaemic control has been reported in both type 1 and type 2 diabetic patients taking omega-3 marine triglycerides and fish oil preparations.[1-6] However, improved insulin sensitivity has also been reported.[7]

1. Glauber H, *et al.* Adverse metabolic effect of omega-3 fatty acids in non-insulin-dependent diabetes mellitus. *Ann Intern Med* 1988; **108:** 663–8.
2. Kasim SE, *et al.* Effects of omega-3 fish oils on lipid metabolism, glycemic control, and blood pressure in type II diabetic patients. *J Clin Endocrinol Metab* 1988; **67:** 1–5.
3. Schectman G, *et al.* Effect of fish oil concentrate on lipoprotein composition in NIDDM. *Diabetes* 1988; **37:** 1567–73.
4. Hendra TJ, *et al.* Effects of fish oil supplements in NIDDM subjects: controlled study. *Diabetes Care* 1990; **13:** 821–9.
5. Vessby B, Boberg M. Dietary supplementation with n-3 fatty acids may impair glucose homeostasis in patients with non-insulin-dependent diabetes mellitus. *J Intern Med* 1990; **228:** 165–71.
6. Stacpoole PW, *et al.* Dose-response effects of dietary marine oil on carbohydrate and lipid metabolism in normal subjects and patients with hypertriglyceridemia. *Metabolism* 1989; **38:** 946–56.
7. Popp-Snijders C, *et al.* Dietary supplementation of omega-3 polyunsaturated fatty acids improves insulin sensitivity in non-insulin-dependent diabetics. *Diabetes Res* 1987; **4:** 141–7.

Uses and Administration

The omega-3 marine triglycerides contain triglycerides of the omega-3 fatty acids, particularly eicosapentaenoic acid and docosahexaenoic acid. These long-chain n-3 polyunsaturated fatty acids are precursors of eicosanoids in *fish* and when taken by man they compete with the precursor arachidonic acid. Their actions in man include a hypolipidaemic action, especially a reduction in plasma triglycerides; an anti-inflammatory action; and an antiplatelet effect.

Fish oils are a source of omega-3 triglycerides and preparations such as omega-3 marine triglycerides are thus used in patients with severe hypertriglyceridaemia. They are also marketed as dietary supplements.

A wide range of doses have been employed. The usual dose by mouth is 5 g twice daily with food.

Fish oils and other omega-3 fatty acid preparations have been widely promoted as dietary supplements and a wide range of preparations of varying composition and potency is available. The interest in marine fish oils arose following observations that populations with a diet rich in marine fish oils generally have a low incidence of cardiovascular disease. In addition the incidence of asthma, psoriasis, and auto-immune diseases have been reported to be lower among Eskimos than in populations consuming a typical western diet, although the incidence of haemorrhagic stroke and epilepsy may be higher.

The omega-3 fatty acids eicosapentaenoic acid and docosahexaenoic acid are long-chain n-3 polyunsaturated fatty acids. They compete with arachidonic acid for inclusion in cyclo-oxygenase and lipoxygenase pathways: their antithrombotic activity is attributed to effects on prostanoid synthesis, promoting vasodilatation, a reduction in platelet aggregation, increased bleeding time and decreased platelet counts. Their anti-inflammatory activity is attributed to effects on leukotriene synthesis. Omega-3 fatty acids also have hypolipidaemic activity (below). Other effects reported include an increase in erythrocyte deformability, a decrease in blood viscosity, and a reduction in blood pressure.[1-4] Beneficial effects have been reported with omega-3 fatty acids in some inflammatory and auto-immune disorders including rheumatoid arthritis (p.2)[5,17,18] and psoriasis (p.1075),[6,7] but in later studies neither administration by the oral[8] nor the topical[9] route was effective in psoriasis. Other conditions in which some response has been noted include Behçet's syndrome (p.1018),[10] Raynaud's syndrome (p.794),[11] Crohn's disease[12] and ulcerative colitis (p.1171),[13] renal transplantation (p.499),[14] cystic fibrosis (p.119),[15] and glomerular kidney disease (p.1021).[16]

Overall, it would appear that an increase in seafood in the diet could have a beneficial effect in many people, but it is not clear if healthy people gain any benefit from going a stage further by taking supplements of fish oil or omega-3 triglycerides.

1. Knapp HR, FitzGerald GA. The antihypertensive effects of fish oils: a controlled study of polyunsaturated fatty acid supplements in essential hypertension. *N Engl J Med* 1989; **320:** 1037–43.
2. Bønaa KH, *et al.* Effect of eicosapentaenoic and docosahexaenoic acids on blood pressure in hypertension: a population-based intervention trial from the Tromsø study. *N Engl J Med* 1990; **322:** 795–801.
3. Appel LJ, *et al.* Does supplementation of diet with 'fish oil' reduce blood pressure? A meta-analysis of controlled clinical trials. *Arch Intern Med* 1993; **153:** 1429–38.
4. Morris MC, *et al.* Does fish oil lower blood pressure? A meta-analysis of controlled trials. *Circulation* 1993; **88:** 523–33.
5. Kremer JM, *et al.* Fish-oil fatty acid supplementation in active rheumatoid arthritis: a double-blinded, controlled, crossover study. *Ann Intern Med* 1987; **106:** 497–503.
6. Gupta AK, *et al.* Double-blind, placebo-controlled study to evaluate the efficacy of fish oil and low-dose UVB in the treatment of psoriasis. *Br J Dermatol* 1989; **120:** 801–7.
7. Lassus A, *et al.* Effects of dietary supplementation with polyunsaturated ethyl ester lipids (Angiosen) in patients with psoriasis and psoriatic arthritis. *J Int Med Res* 1990; **18:** 68–73.
8. Søyland E, *et al.* Effect of dietary supplementation with very-long-chain n-3 fatty acids in patients with psoriasis. *N Engl J Med* 1993; **328:** 1812–16.
9. Henneicke-von Zepelin H-H, *et al.* Highly purified omega-3-polyunsaturated fatty acids for topical treatment of psoriasis: results of a double-blind, placebo-controlled multicentre study. *Br J Dermatol* 1993; **129:** 713–17.
10. Kürkçüoğlu N, Tandoğdu R. The effect of "MaxEPA" in the treatment of patients with Behcet's disease. *Br J Dermatol* 1989; **121:** 667–8.
11. DiGiacomo RA, *et al.* Fish-oil dietary supplementation in patients with Raynaud's phenomenon: a double-blind, controlled, prospective study. *Am J Med* 1989; **86:** 158–64.
12. Belluzzi A, *et al.* Effect of an enteric-coated fish-oil preparation on relapses in Crohn's disease. *N Engl J Med* 1996; **334:** 1557–60.
13. Salomon P, *et al.* Treatment of ulcerative colitis with fish oil n-3-ω-fatty acid: an open trial. *J Clin Gastroenterol* 1990; **12:** 157–61.
14. Homan van der Heide JJ, *et al.* Effect of dietary fish oil on renal function and rejection in cyclosporine-treated recipients of renal transplants. *N Engl J Med* 1993; **329:** 769–73.
15. Lawrence R, Sorrell T. Eicosapentaenoic acid in cystic fibrosis: evidence of a pathogenetic role for leukotriene B_4. *Lancet* 1993; **342:** 465–9.
16. Donadio JV, *et al.* A controlled trial of fish oil in IgA nephropathy. *N Engl J Med* 1994; **331:** 1194–9.
17. Lau CS, *et al.* Effects of fish oil supplementation on non-steroidal anti-inflammatory drug requirement in patients with mild rheumatoid arthritis—a double-blind placebo controlled study. *Br J Rheumatol* 1993; **32:** 982–9.
18. Geusens P, *et al.* Long-term effect of omega-3 fatty acid supplementation in active rheumatoid arthritis: a 12-month, double-blind, controlled study. *Arthritis Rheum* 1994; **37:** 824–9.

Hyperlipidaemias. The omega-3 fatty acids eicosapentaenoic acid and docosahexaenoic acid have hypolipidaemic activity. The most consistent effect is a dose-dependent reduction in triglyceride concentrations due to a reduction in very-low-density lipoproteins (VLDL). Variable responses have been seen in cholesterol, low-density lipoprotein (LDL)-cholesterol, and high-density lipoprotein (HDL)-cholesterol concentrations. However, the results of early studies may have been confounded by the cholesterol content of fish oils used. The hypolipidaemic effects from studies using omega-3 fatty acid preparations have been more consistent. There is some doubt as to whether the hypotriglyceridaemic effect is sustained during long-term therapy.

Omega-3 fatty acids are used in the treatment of hypertriglyceridaemia (p.1265) but there is insufficient evidence of any effect on the incidence of **ischaemic heart disease** in the long-term. In a large long-term study increased dietary intake of omega-3 fatty acids did not substantially reduce the risk of ischaemic heart disease in men who had initially been free of known cardiovascular disease.[1] Some,[2,3] but not other[4] studies have shown a decrease in coronary vessel restenosis after angioplasty.

1. Ascherio A, *et al.* Dietary intake of marine n-3 fatty acids, fish intake, and the risk of coronary disease among men. *N Engl J Med* 1995; **332:** 977–82.
2. Dehmer GJ, *et al.* Reduction in the rate of early restenosis after coronary angioplasty by a diet supplemented with n-3 fatty acids. *N Engl J Med* 1988; **319:** 733–40.
3. Gapinski JP, *et al.* Preventing restenosis with fish oils following coronary angioplasty: a meta-analysis. *Arch Intern Med* 1993; **153:** 1595–1601.
4. Reis GJ, *et al.* Randomised trial of fish oil for prevention of restenosis after coronary angioplasty. *Lancet* 1989; **ii:** 177–81.

Preparations

Proprietary Preparations (details are given in Part 3)
Aust.: Eicosapen; ***Austral.:*** EPA†; Fishaphos; Maxepa; ***Fr.:*** Maxepa; Mega 65; ***Ger.:*** Bilatin Fischol; Eicosapen; Lipiscor; ***Ital.:*** Esapent; Eskim; Fish Factor; Maxepa; Seacor; ***Norw.:*** Omacor; ***Switz.:*** Ameu; Eicosapen; Epacaps; Omega-3; ***UK:*** Best EPA; Flowmega; Gamma EPA; Marinepa; Maxepa; Pure Omega; Triomar; ***USA:*** Cardi-Omega 3; EFA Plus†; Maxepa; Mega-MaxEPA†; Promega; Tricol Softgels.

Multi-ingredient: ***Austral.:*** Bioglan E-Plus; Bioglan Maxepa; Efamol Marine Capsules†; Epo + Maxepa + Vitamin E Herbal Plus Formula 8; Himega; Lifesystem Herbal Plus Formula 9 Fatty Acids And Vitamin E; Macro Maxepa; Maxepa & EPO; Maxepa Plus; Naudicelle Marine; Naudicelle plus Epanoil†; Naudicelle Plus†; ***Fr.:*** Bionagrol Plus; Elteans; Liparmonyl†; Omegacoeur; Synerbiol; ***Ital.:*** Agedin Plus; Dermana; Ictom 3; Trofinerv; ***UK:*** Efacal; Efalex; Efamarine; Efanatal; Efatime; EPOC Marine; Epopa; Galmarin; Gamma Marine; Naudicelle Forte; Naudicelle Plus; Naudicelle SL; Super GammaOil Marine; ***USA:*** Efamol PMS†; Marine Lipid Concentrate; Sea-Omega; SuperEPA.

Pantethine (13075-b)

(*R*)-*NN'*-[Dithiobis(ethyleneiminocarbonylethylene)]bis(2,4-dihydroxy-3,3-dimethylbutyramide).

$C_{22}H_{42}N_4O_8S_2 = 554.7.$

CAS — 16816-67-4.

Pharmacopoeias. In *Jpn.*

Pantethine is a component of coenzyme A. It is a lipid regulating drug used in the treatment of hyperlipidaemias (p.1265). The usual dose is 600 to 1200 mg daily by mouth in divided doses.

Preparations

Proprietary Preparations (details are given in Part 3)
Ital.: Analip; Lipodel; Pantetina; ***Jpn:*** Pantosin; ***Spain:*** Atarone; Liponet; Obliterol.

Multi-ingredient: ***Ital.:*** Analip†; Carpantin; Fosfolip†; Glutestere B-Complesso†.

Pirifibrate (13134-f)

Pirifibrate *(rINN)*.

EL-466. 6-Hydroxymethyl-2-pyridylmethyl 2-(4-chlorophenoxy)-2-methylpropionate.

$C_{17}H_{18}ClNO_4$ = 335.8.

CAS — 55285-45-5.

Pirifibrate, a fibric acid derivative (see Bezafibrate, p.1268), is a lipid regulating drug used in the treatment of hyperlipidaemias (p.1265). The usual dose is 750 mg twice daily by mouth.

Preparations

Proprietary Preparations (details are given in Part 3)
Spain: Bratenol.

Pirozadil (3912-s)

Pirozadil *(rINN)*.

722-D. 2,6-Pyridinediyldimethylene bis(3,4,5-trimethoxybenzoate).

$C_{27}H_{29}NO_{10}$ = 527.5.

CAS — 54110-25-7.

Pirozadil, a nicotinic acid derivative, is a lipid regulating drug used in the treatment of hyperlipidaemias (p.1265). Usual doses are 1.5 to 3 g daily in divided doses by mouth.

Pirozadil has been shown to reduce total and low-density lipoprotein-cholesterol concentrations in patients with hypercholesterolaemias.[1,2] Adverse effects in 2 of 15 patients[1] included oedema, palpitations, and numbness of the extremities. This latter effect was sufficiently severe to necessitate withdrawal of treatment in one patient.

1. Shinomiya M, *et al.* Effect of pirozadil on lipids, lipoproteins and apolipoproteins in Japanese with type IIa hyperlipoproteinaemia. *Arzneimittelforschung* 1987; **37:** 1069–71.
2. Masana L, *et al.* Treatment of diet-resistant polygenic hypercholesterolaemic patients with a new nicotinate derivative: in vivo and in vitro low density lipoprotein metabolic studies. *J Clin Pharmacol* 1989; **29:** 201–6.

Preparations

Proprietary Preparations (details are given in Part 3)
Spain: Pemix.

Plafibride (13139-b)

Plafibride *(rINN)*.

ITA-104. 1-[2-(4-Chlorophenoxy)-2-methylpropionyl]-3-morpholinomethylurea.

$C_{16}H_{22}ClN_3O_4$ = 355.8.

CAS — 63394-05-8.

Plafibride, a fibric acid derivative (see Bezafibrate, p.1268), is a lipid regulating drug that has been used in the treatment of hyperlipidaemias.

Preparations

Proprietary Preparations (details are given in Part 3)
Spain: Idonor†.

Pravastatin Sodium (3758-z)

Pravastatin Sodium *(BANM, USAN, rINNM)*.

CS-514; Eptastatin Sodium; 3β-Hydroxycompactin Sodium; SQ-31000. Sodium (3*R*,5*R*)-7-{(1*S*,2*S*,6*S*,8*S*,8a*R*)-1,2,6,7,8,8a-hexahydro-6-hydroxy-2-methyl-8-[(*S*)-2-methylbutyryloxy]-1-naphthyl}-3,5-dihydroxyheptanoate.

$C_{23}H_{35}O_7Na$ = 446.5.

CAS — 81093-37-0 (pravastatin); 81131-70-6 (pravastatin sodium).

Adverse Effects and Precautions

As for Simvastatin, p.1278.

Effects on mental function. For comments on the depressive symptoms reported in patients receiving statins, including pravastatin, see under Simvastatin, p.1278.

Effects on the nervous system. For a report of paraesthesias associated with pravastatin therapy, see under Lovastatin, p.1275.

Effects on skeletal muscle. Muscle disorders are well-recognised adverse effects of lipid regulating drugs such as the fibrates and statins (see Simvastatin, p.1278).

An inflammatory myopathy resembling dermatomyositis developed in a woman treated for 5 months with pravastatin.[1]

1. Schalke BB, *et al.* Pravastatin-associated inflammatory myopathy. *N Engl J Med* 1992; **327:** 649–50.

Interactions

The interactions of statins with other drugs are described under simvastatin (p.1279). However, similar interactions appear not to have been reported with pravastatin although caution is advised when using such combinations.

General reviews.

1. Garnett WR. Interactions with hydroxymethylglutaryl-coenzyme A reductase inhibitors. *Am J Health-Syst Pharm* 1995; **52:** 1639–45.

Pharmacokinetics

Pravastatin, unlike simvastatin or lovastatin, is active without the need for hydrolysis. Following absorption from the gastro-intestinal tract it undergoes extensive first-pass metabolism in the liver, its primary site of action. The absolute bioavailability of pravastatin is 17%. Approximately 50% of the circulating drug is bound to plasma proteins. The plasma elimination half-life of pravastatin is 1.5 to 2 hours. Pravastatin is excreted mainly in faeces (about 70%) via the bile with a smaller proportion excreted in the urine (about 20%).

General reviews.

1. Quion JAV, Jones PH. Clinical pharmacokinetics of pravastatin. *Clin Pharmacokinet* 1994; **27:** 94–103.
2. Desager J-P, Horsmans Y. Clinical pharmacokinetics of 3-hydroxy-3-methylglutaryl-coenzyme A reductase inhibitors. *Clin Pharmacokinet* 1996; **31:** 348–71.
3. Lennernäs H, Fager G. Pharmacodynamics and pharmacokinetics of the HMG-CoA reductase inhibitors: similarities and differences. *Clin Pharmacokinet* 1997; **32:** 403–25.

Uses and Administration

Pravastatin, a 3-hydroxy-3-methylglutaryl coenzyme A (HMG-CoA) reductase inhibitor (a statin), is a lipid regulating drug with actions on plasma lipids similar to those of simvastatin (p.1279).

Pravastatin is used in the treatment of hypercholesterolaemias, particularly in type IIa and IIb hyperlipoproteinaemias. It is also given prophylactically in hypercholesterolaemic patients for both primary and secondary prevention of ischaemic heart disease. It is also used in patients with a previous myocardial infarction to reduce the risk of stroke.

Pravastatin is given by mouth as the sodium salt in usual doses of 10 to 40 mg once daily at bedtime. The dose may be adjusted at intervals of not less than 4 weeks.

General reviews.

1. Raasch RH. Pravastatin sodium, a new HMG-CoA reductase inhibitor. *DICP Ann Pharmacother* 1991; **25:** 388–94.
2. McTavish D, Sorkin EM. Pravastatin: a review of its pharmacological properties and therapeutic potential in hypercholesterolaemia. *Drugs* 1991; **42:** 65–89.
3. Jungnickel PW, *et al.* Pravastatin: a new drug for the treatment of hypercholesterolemia. *Clin Pharm* 1992; **11:** 677–89.
4. Schectman G, Hiatt J. Dose-response characteristics of cholesterol-lowering drug therapies: implications for treatment. *Ann Intern Med* 1996; **125:** 990–1000.
5. Haria M, McTavish D. Pravastatin: a reappraisal of its pharmacological properties and clinical effectiveness in the management of coronary heart disease. *Drugs* 1997; **53:** 299–336.

Hyperlipidaemias. Pravastatin, like other statins, is used in the treatment of hyperlipidaemias (p.1265) and a general discussion of the effects of statins can be found in simvastatin (p.1279).

Pravastatin is effective for the treatment of primary hypercholesterolaemia; it lowers low-density lipoprotein (LDL)-cholesterol concentrations and also increases high-density (HDL)-cholesterol.[1] Hypercholesterolaemia is a risk factor for **ischaemic heart disease** and pravastatin has been shown to have a protective effect in men with moderate hypercholesterolaemia and no history of myocardial infarction.[2,3,5] Benefit has also been demonstrated in both men and women with a previous infarction.[4,6] Lowering lipid concentrations in patients with previous myocardial infarction has also reduced the frequency of **stroke**.[4,7]

1. Rubenfire M, *et al.* The effect of pravastatin on plasma lipoprotein and apolipoprotein levels in primary hypercholesterolemia. *Arch Intern Med* 1991; **151:** 2234–40.
2. Shepherd J, *et al.* Prevention of coronary heart disease with pravastatin in men with hypercholesterolemia. *N Engl J Med* 1995; **333:** 1301–7.
3. West of Scotland Coronary Prevention Group. West of Scotland Coronary Prevention Study: identification of high-risk groups and comparison with other cardiovascular intervention trials. *Lancet* 1996; **348:** 1339–42.
4. Sacks FM, *et al.* The effect of pravastatin on coronary events after myocardial infarction in patients with average cholesterol levels. *N Engl J Med* 1996; **335:** 1001–9.
5. West of Scotland Coronary Prevention Study Group. Influence of pravastatin and plasma lipids on clinical events in the West of Scotland Coronary Prevention Study (WOSCOPS). *Circulation* 1998; **97:** 1440–5.
6. Sacks FM, *et al.* Relationship between plasma LDL concentrations during treatment with pravastatin and recurrent coronary events in the Cholesterol and Recurrent Events Trial. *Circulation* 1998; **97:** 1446–52.
7. The Long-Term Intervention with Pravastatin in Ischaemic Disease (LIPID) Study Group. Prevention of cardiovascular events and death with pravastatin in patients with coronary heart disease and a broad range of initial cholesterol levels. *N Engl J Med* 1998; **339:** 1349–57.

Preparations

Proprietary Preparations (details are given in Part 3)
Aust.: Pravachol; Selipran; ***Austral.:*** Pravachol; ***Belg.:*** Pravasine; ***Canad.:*** Pravachol; ***Fr.:*** Elisor; Vasten; ***Ger.:*** Liprevil; Mevalotin; Pravasin; ***Irl.:*** Lipostat; ***Ital.:*** Aplactin; Prasterol; Pravaselect; Sanaprav; Selectin; ***Jpn:*** Mevalotin; ***Neth.:*** Selektine; ***Norw.:*** Pravachol; ***S.Afr.:*** Prava; ***Spain:*** Bristacol; Lipemol; Liplat; Prareduct; ***Swed.:*** Pravachol; ***Switz.:*** Mevalotin; Selipran; ***UK:*** Lipostat; ***USA:*** Pravachol.

Probucol (1356-b)

Probucol *(BAN, USAN, rINN)*.

DH-581. 4,4′-(Isopropylidenedithio)bis(2,6-di-*tert*-butylphenol).

$C_{31}H_{48}O_2S_2$ = 516.8.

CAS — 23288-49-5.

Pharmacopoeias. In US.

A white to off-white crystalline powder. Practically **insoluble** in water; soluble in alcohol and petroleum spirit; freely soluble in chloroform and propyl alcohol. **Protect** from light.

Adverse Effects and Precautions

The commonest side-effects of probucol therapy are gastro-intestinal upsets with diarrhoea occurring in about 10% of patients; flatulence, abdominal pain, nausea, and vomiting may also occur. Hypersensitivity reactions including angioedema have been reported.

Fatal cardiac arrhythmias have been reported in *animals* and prolonged QT intervals in man. Probucol should be given with caution to patients with recent myocardial damage, severe ventricular arrhythmias, cardiovascular-associated syncope, or prolonged QT interval. The risk of arrhythmias may be increased in patients taking tricyclic antidepressants, class I or III antiarrhythmics, or phenothiazines.

Side-effects reported during a 1-year study involving 88 patients given probucol decreased after the first 3 months of therapy.[1] The most common was loose stools or diarrhoea; constipation was reported much less frequently. Other side-effects which occurred were flatulence, vertigo, dizziness, a different odour of the skin, and pruritus. No patient withdrew from the study because of side-effects.

1. McCaughan D. Nine years of treatment with probucol. *Artery* 1982; **10:** 56–70.

Effects on the heart. Prolongation of the QT interval in *animal* studies was first reported by Troendle *et al.*[1] of the FDA. Four of eight *monkeys* given probucol and an atherogenic diet died, apparently of ventricular arrhythmias. Evaluation of 198 patients who had received probucol for 5 years or more, revealed that changes in the QT interval had occurred with increases predominating. In 42 patients studied[2] for up to 2 years, no correlation was found between blood concentrations of probucol and lengthening of the QT interval; although nearly half the patients showed a lengthening of the QT interval on probucol the overall change was not statistically significant. There was no clinical or electrocardiographic evidence of arrhythmias in any patient. In an analysis of 48 men who had taken probucol as part of a multifactorial primary prevention study,[3] probucol was found to increase QT interval compared with controls. However, prolongations were modest. Correlation was seen between QT changes and serum triglyceride concentrations. Although serious cardiac arrhythmias were not noted in these studies, there have been individual reports of potentially fatal polymorphic ventricular tachycardia (torsade de pointes) in patients with probucol-associated prolongation of the QT interval.[4,5]

1. Troendle G, *et al.* Probucol and the QT interval. *Lancet* 1982; **i:** 1179.
2. Dujovne CA, *et al.* Electrocardiographic effects of probucol: a controlled prospective clinical trial. *Eur J Clin Pharmacol* 1984; **26:** 735–9.
3. Naukkarinen V, *et al.* Probucol-induced electrocardiographic changes in a five-year primary prevention of vascular diseases. *Curr Ther Res* 1989; **45:** 232–7.
4. Gohn DC, Simmons TW. Polymorphic ventricular tachycardia (torsade de pointes) associated with the use of probucol. *N Engl J Med* 1992; **326:** 1435–6.
5. Kajinami K, *et al.* Propranolol for probucol-induced QT prolongation with polymorphic ventricular tachycardia. *Lancet* 1993; **341:** 124–5.

Interactions

The risk of arrhythmias in patients receiving probucol may be increased in those taking arrhythmogenic drugs concurrently (see Adverse Effects and Precautions, above).

For reference to the effect of probucol on cyclosporin concentrations, see p.522.

Pharmacokinetics

The absorption of probucol from the gastro-intestinal tract is limited and variable, and is stated to be at a maximum if taken with food. Concentrations in blood rise slowly and reach steady-state after 3 to 4 months of continuous treatment. Probucol accumulates in adipose tissue and concentrations fall only slowly, over several months, when treatment is withdrawn. Excretion is considered to be chiefly by the biliary system into the faeces.

Uses and Administration

Probucol is a lipid regulating drug that has been used in the treatment of hypercholesterolaemia, particularly type IIa hyperlipoproteinaemia. It lowers total plasma-cholesterol concentrations, mainly by reducing low-density lipoprotein (LDL)-cholesterol and high-density lipoprotein (HDL)-cholesterol concentrations. It has little effect on triglyceride or very-low-density lipoprotein (VLDL)-cholesterol concentrations. It may cause regression of xanthomas.

The usual dose by mouth is 500 mg twice daily, given with the morning and evening meals.

Administration in the elderly. Probucol reduced total cholesterol and LDL-cholesterol concentrations more markedly in patients over 65 years of age than in younger patients.[1]

1. Morisaki N, *et al.* Effects of long-term treatment with probucol on serum lipoproteins in cases of familial hypercholesterolemia in the elderly. *J Am Geriatr Soc* 1990; **38:** 15–18.

Hyperlipidaemias. Probucol has been used in the treatment of hyperlipidaemias (p.1265). It lowers plasma concentrations of low-density lipoprotein (LDL) cholesterol by about 10 to 20% and high-density lipoprotein (HDL) cholesterol by about 30% in hyperlipidaemic subjects.[1] The reduction in LDL-cholesterol appears to be mainly due to an increase in the fractional catabolic rate of LDL. An independent antioxidant effect may also contribute to the clinical action of probucol.[1,2]

Hypercholesterolaemia is a known risk factor for atherosclerosis and reduction of raised LDL-cholesterol concentrations is of benefit in the secondary prevention of **ischaemic heart disease**. The antoxidant effect of probucol could be of additional benefit. The significance of the reduction in HDL-cholesterol is not yet known: such a reduction could be expected to increase the risk, although this has not been observed in clinical studies.[1,2]

1. Buckley MM-T, *et al.* Probucol: a reappraisal of its pharmacological properties and therapeutic use in hypercholesterolaemia. *Drugs* 1989; **37:** 761–800.
2. Zimetbaum P, *et al.* Probucol: pharmacology and clinical application. *J Clin Pharmacol* 1990; **30:** 3–9.

Preparations

USP 23: Probucol Tablets.

Proprietary Preparations (details are given in Part 3)
Aust.: Lurselle†; ***Austral.:*** Lurselle; ***Canad.:*** Lorelco†; ***Fr.:*** Lurselle†; ***Ger.:*** Lurselle; ***Ital.:*** Lurselle†; ***S.Afr.:*** Lurselle; ***Spain:*** Bifenabid; Panesclerina†; Superlipid; ***Switz.:*** Lurselle†; ***UK:*** Lurselle†; ***USA:*** Lorelco†.

Ronifibrate (2922-m)

Ronifibrate (*rINN*).

I-612. 3-Hydroxypropyl nicotinate, 2-(4-chlorophenoxy)-2-methylpropionate (ester).

$C_{19}H_{20}ClNO_5$ = 377.8.

CAS — 42597-57-9.

Ronifibrate, a derivative of clofibrate (p.1271) and nicotinic acid (p.1351), is a lipid regulating drug used in the treatment of hyperlipidaemias (p.1265). The usual dose is 500 mg by mouth up to three times daily.

Preparations

Proprietary Preparations (details are given in Part 3)
Ital.: Cloprane.

Simfibrate (1358-g)

Simfibrate (*rINN*).

CLY-503; Diclofibrate. Trimethylene bis[2-(4-chlorophenoxy)-2-methylpropionate].

$C_{23}H_{26}Cl_2O_6$ = 469.4.

CAS — 14929-11-4.

Pharmacopoeias. In *Jpn.*

Simfibrate, a fibric acid derivative (see Bezafibrate, p.1268), is a lipid regulating drug used in the treatment of hyperlipidaemias (p.1265). The usual dose is 0.75 to 1.5 g daily by mouth in divided doses.

Preparations

Proprietary Preparations (details are given in Part 3)
Ital.: Cholesolvin; Sinfibrex†; ***Jpn:*** Cholesolvin.

Simvastatin (2452-l)

Simvastatin (*BAN, USAN, rINN*).

L-644128-000U; MK-733; Synvinolin; Velastatin. (1*S*,3*R*,7*S*,8*S*,8a*R*)-1,2,3,7,8,8a-Hexahydro-3,7-dimethyl-8-{2-[(2*R*,4*R*)-tetrahydro-4-hydroxy-6-oxo-2*H*-pyran-2-yl]ethyl}-1-naphthyl 2,2-dimethylbutyrate.

$C_{25}H_{38}O_5$ = 418.6.

CAS — 79902-63-9.

Pharmacopoeias. In *US.*

A white to off-white powder. Practically **insoluble** in water; freely soluble in alcohol, in chloroform, and in methyl alcohol; sparingly soluble in propylene glycol; very slightly soluble in petroleum spirit. **Store** under nitrogen.

Adverse Effects and Precautions

The commonest adverse effects of therapy with simvastatin and other statins are gastro-intestinal disturbances. Other adverse effects reported include headache, skin rashes, dizziness, blurred vision, insomnia, and dysgeusia. Reversible increases in serum-aminotransferase concentrations may occur and liver function should be monitored. Hepatitis and pancreatitis have been reported. A hypersensitivity syndrome whose features have included angioedema has been reported. Myopathy, characterised by myalgia and muscle weakness and associated with increased creatine phosphokinase concentrations, has been reported, especially in patients taking simvastatin concurrently with immunosuppressants, fibric acid derivatives, or nicotinic acid. Rarely, rhabdomyolysis with acute renal failure may develop.

Simvastatin should not be given to patients with acute liver disease or unexplained persistent raised serum-aminotransferase concentrations or to those with porphyria. It should be avoided during pregnancy since there is a possibility that it could interfere with fetal sterol synthesis; there have been a few reports of congenital abnormalities associated with statins (but see below). It should be discontinued if marked or persistent increases in serum-aminotransferase or creatine-phosphokinase concentrations occur. It should be used with caution in patients with severe renal impairment.

In February 1992 the UK CSM briefly reviewed the adverse effects that had been reported to it since simvastatin was made available in the UK in May 1989.[1] There had been 257 000 prescriptions and 738 reports to the CSM. Abnormal hepatic function (36 reports) and myalgia (48) were 2 of the most frequently reported reactions and included 5 reports of hepatitis and 2 of jaundice. Other muscle effects included myositis (3), myopathy (10), and asymptomatic increases in serum creatinine kinase concentrations(7). Gastro-intestinal side-effects accounted for 20% of the reports; skin, neurological and musculoskeletal effects for 15% each; psychiatric effects for 10%; liver effects for 7%; and visual effects for 4%.

1. Committee on Safety of Medicines. Simvastatin. *Current Problems 33* 1992.

Effects on the blood. Thrombotic thrombocytopenic purpura has been described in a patient within 24 hours of taking the second dose of newly-initiated simvastatin therapy.[1] No other precipitating factor was apparent.

1. McCarthy LJ, *et al.* Thrombotic thrombocytopenic purpura and simvastatin. *Lancet* 1998; **352:** 1284–5.

Effects on the hair. Since its introduction in Australia 16 cases of alopecia in association with the use of simvastatin had been reported to the Adverse Drug Reactions Advisory Committee.[1] Most cases involved either excessive hair loss or hair thinning, although two cases of hair loss in patches and one resembling alopecia areata were reported. Onset occurred between 3 days and 15 months of starting therapy.

1. Anonymous. Simvastatin and alopecia. *Aust Adverse Drug React Bull* 1993; **12:** 7.

Effects on the kidneys. Proteinuria was reported in 10 patients taking simvastatin 40 mg daily.[1] The protein loss was of a pattern typical for increased glomerular permeability. In 2 patients proteinuria disappeared when simvastatin was withdrawn and recurred on its subsequent reintroduction.

Renal failure due to rhabdomyolysis has been reported rarely (see under Effects on Skeletal Muscle, below).

1. Deslypere JP, *et al.* Proteinuria as complication of simvastatin treatment. *Lancet* 1990; **336:** 1453.

Effects on mental function. A few cases have been reported of depressive symptoms developing in patients treated with pravastatin[1] or simvastatin.[2] The symptoms appeared during the first few weeks or months of treatment. However, a randomised placebo-controlled study[3] involving over 600 patients did not find that simvastatin treatment was associated with mood disturbances.

1. Lechleitner M, *et al.* Depressive symptoms in hypercholesterolaemic patients treated with pravastatin. *Lancet* 1992; **340:** 910.
2. Duits N, Bos FM. Depressive symptoms and cholesterol-lowering drugs. *Lancet* 1993; **341:** 114.
3. Wardle J, *et al.* Randomised placebo controlled trial of effect on mood of lowering cholesterol concentration. *Br Med J* 1996; **313:** 75–8.

Effects on the nervous system. Since its introduction in Australia 22 cases of paraesthesia associated with simvastatin had been reported to the Adverse Drug Reactions Advisory Committee.[1] Symptoms most frequently involved the face, scalp, tongue, and limbs and ranged from hypoaesthetic to hyperaesthetic sensations. In a few cases symptoms occurred immediately on starting treatment while in others they appeared up to one year after initiating therapy. Symptoms disappeared shortly after treatment was withdrawn; in 5 cases symptoms recurred on rechallenge. Four cases of more serious neurological damage had also been reported.

1. Anonymous. Paraesthesia and neuropathy with hypolipidaemic agents. *Aust Adverse Drug React Bull* 1993; **12:** 6.

Effects on sexual function. Impotence has been reported[1] in 5 men receiving simvastatin. No sexual difficulties were noted when fluvastatin was substituted in 4 of them.

1. Jackson G. Simvastatin and impotence. *Br Med J* 1997; **315:** 31.

Effects on skeletal muscle. The UK Committee on Safety of Medicines has noted that myositis and myopathy are well known to occur with lipid regulating drugs such as fibrates and statins.[1] Rhabdomyolysis, presenting as muscle pain with elevated creatine phosphokinase and myoglobinuria leading to renal failure, has also been reported but appears to be rare. Worldwide reporting did not indicate marked differences in the risk of the reactions with individual drugs. Patients with renal impairment and possibly with hypothyroidism may be at increased risk of muscle toxicity, as may those given *cyclosporin* and a statin concomitantly. Combined treatment with a *fibrate* and a statin may also increase the risk of serious muscle toxicity. The Committee advised that patients treated with fibrates or statins should consult their doctor if they develop muscle pain, tenderness, or weakness and treatment should be stopped if muscle toxicity is suspected clinically or if creatine phosphokinase is markedly raised or progressively rising. Rhabdomyolysis has occurred in 2 patients receiving simvastatin and *itraconazole*[2,3] and in 1 patient given *nefazodone*.[4]

The problem of muscle disorders, as a class effect, associated with statins (namely fluvastatin, pravastatin, and simvastatin) has also been noted by the Adverse Drug Reactions Advisory Committee in Australia.[5]

1. Committee on Safety of Medicines/Medicines Control Agency. Rhabdomyolysis associated with lipid-lowering drugs. *Current Problems* 1995; **21:** 3.
2. Segaert MF, *et al.* Drug-interaction-induced rhabdomyolysis. *Nephrol Dial Transplant* 1996; **11:** 1846–7.
3. Horn M. Coadministration of itraconazole with hypolipidemic agents may induce rhabdomyolysis in healthy individuals. *Arch Dermatol* 1996; **132:** 1254.
4. Jacobson RH, *et al.* Myositis and rhabdomyolysis associated with concurrent use of simvastatin and nefazodone. *JAMA* 1997; **277:** 296.
5. Adverse Drug Reactions Advisory Committee (ADRAC). Fluvastatin and muscle disorders—a class effect. *Aust Adverse Drug React Bull* 1997; **16:** 3.

Effects on sleep patterns. Patients taking lovastatin have been reported to experience a reduction in the length of continuous sleep while no such effect was observed with pravastatin.[1] A similar sleep disturbance has been reported with simvastatin.[2] It was suggested that pravastatin might be less likely to affect sleep since it is hydrophilic and does not penetrate the brain easily. However, there have been conflicting reports: in other studies neither lovastatin,[3] pravastatin,[4] nor simvastatin,[3-5] had any adverse effect on sleep, but there have been further individual reports of sleep disturbances with lovastatin.[6,7]

1. Schaefer EJ. HMG-CoA reductase inhibitors for hypercholesterolemia. *N Engl J Med* 1988; **319:** 1222.
2. Barth JD, *et al.* Inhibitors of hydroxymethylglutaryl coenzyme A reductase for treating hypercholesterolaemia. *Br Med J* 1990; **301:** 669.
3. Black DM, *et al.* Sleep disturbances and HMG CoA reductase inhibitors. *JAMA* 1990; **264:** 1105.
4. Eckernäs S-Å, *et al.* The effects of simvastatin and pravastatin on objective and subjective measures of nocturnal sleep: a comparison of two structurally different HMG CoA reductase inhibitors in patients with primary moderate hypercholesterolaemia. *Br J Clin Pharmacol* 1993; **35:** 284–9.
5. Keech AC, *et al.* Absence of effects of prolonged simvastatin therapy on nocturnal sleep in a large randomized placebo-controlled study. *Br J Clin Pharmacol* 1996; **42:** 483–90.
6. Rosenson RS, Goranson NL. Lovastatin-associated sleep and mood disturbances. *Am J Med* 1993; **95:** 548–9.
7. Sinzinger H, *et al.* Sleep disturbance and appetite loss after lovastatin. *Lancet* 1994; **343:** 973.

Pregnancy. Postmarketing surveillance identified 134 cases of unintentional exposure to lovastatin or simvastatin during pregnancy in which the outcome was known.[1] Although there were 9 reports of congenital anomalies these consisted of a spectrum of unrelated malformations and the frequency did not exceed that expected in the general population. It was therefore considered that these drugs did not adversely affect outcome of pregnancy.

1. Manson JM, *et al.* Postmarketing surveillance of lovastatin and simvastatin exposure during pregnancy. *Reprod Toxicol* 1996; **10:** 439–46.

Interactions

There is an increased risk of myopathy if certain drugs such as immunosuppressants (notably cyclosporin), fibric acid derivatives, or nicotinic acid are given concurrently with statins; for further details see Effects on Skeletal Muscle, under Adverse Effects, above. Bleeding and increases in prothrombin time have been reported in patients taking simvastatin with coumarin anticoagulants. Raised concentrations of simvastatin have occurred in patients also given mibefradil.

General reviews.

1. Garnett WR. Interactions with hydroxymethylglutaryl-coenzyme A reductase inhibitors. *Am J Health-Syst Pharm* 1995; **52:** 1639–45.

Pharmacokinetics

Simvastatin is absorbed from the gastro-intestinal tract and is hydrolysed to its active β-hydroxyacid form. Other active metabolites have been detected and a number of inactive metabolites are also formed. Simvastatin undergoes extensive first-pass metabolism in the liver, its primary site of action. Less than 5% of the oral dose has been reported to reach the circulation as active metabolites. Both simvastatin and its β-hydroxyacid metabolite are about 95% bound to plasma proteins. It is mainly excreted in the faeces via the bile as metabolites. About 10 to 15% is recovered in the urine, mainly in inactive forms. The half-life of the active metabolite is 1.9 hours.

General reviews.

1. Mauro VF. Clinical pharmacokinetics and practical applications of simvastatin. *Clin Pharmacokinet* 1993; **24:** 195–202.
2. Desager J-P, Horsmans Y. Clinical pharmacokinetics of 3-hydroxy-3-methylglutaryl-coenzyme A reductase inhibitors. *Clin Pharmacokinet* 1996; **31:** 348–71.
3. Lennernäs H, Fager G. Pharmacodynamics and pharmacokinetics of the HMG-CoA reductase inhibitors: similarities and differences. *Clin Pharmacokinet* 1997; **32:** 403–25.

Uses and Administration

Simvastatin is a lipid regulating drug; it is a competitive inhibitor of 3-hydroxy-3-methylglutaryl coenzyme A reductase (HMG-CoA reductase), the rate-determining enzyme for cholesterol synthesis. HMG-CoA reductase inhibitors (also called statins) reduce total cholesterol, low-density lipoprotein (LDL)-cholesterol, and very-low-density lipoprotein (VLDL)-cholesterol concentrations in plasma. They also tend to reduce triglycerides and to increase high-density lipoprotein (HDL)-cholesterol concentrations. They are considered to exert their hypocholesterolaemic action by stimulating an increase in LDL-receptors on hepatocyte membranes thereby increasing the clearance of LDL from the circulation.

Simvastatin is used in the treatment of hypercholesterolaemias, particularly in type IIa and IIb hyperlipoproteinaemias. Statins may not be effective in patients with homozygous familial hypercholesterolaemia who lack functional LDL-receptors. Simvastatin is also given prophylactically in hypercholesterolaemic patients with ischaemic heart disease.

Simvastatin is given by mouth in an initial dose of 5 to 10 mg in the evening; an initial dose of 20 mg may be used in patients with ischaemic heart disease. The dose may be adjusted at intervals of not less than 4 weeks up to a maximum of 40 mg once daily in the evening. A maximum of 10 mg daily is recommended in those taking immunosuppressants.

General reviews.

1. Todd PA, Goa KL. Simvastatin: a review of its pharmacological properties and therapeutic potential in hypercholesterolaemia. *Drugs* 1990; **40:** 583–607.
2. Mauro VF, MacDonald JL. Simvastatin: a review of its pharmacology and clinical use. *DICP Ann Pharmacother* 1991; **25:** 257–64.
3. Plosker GL, McTavish D. Simvastatin: a reappraisal of its pharmacology and therapeutic efficacy in hypercholesterolaemia. *Drugs* 1995; **50:** 334–63.
4. Vaughan CJ, *et al.* Statins do more than just lower cholesterol. *Lancet* 1996; **348:** 1079–82. Correction. *ibid.* 1997; **349:** 214.
5. Schectman G, Hiatt J. Dose–response characteristics of cholesterol-lowering drug therapies: implications for treatment. *Ann Intern Med* 1996; **125:** 990–1000.

Hyperlipidaemias. Statins, including simvastatin, are used in the treatment of hyperlipidaemias (p.1265) and are effective in reducing total cholesterol and low-density lipoprotein (LDL)-cholesterol concentrations in patients with hypercholesterolaemia.[1-4] They are also of value in the secondary prevention of ischaemic heart disease.

Statins have been shown to be more effective in reducing LDL-cholesterol concentrations than bile-acid binding resins or fibric acid derivatives, typically achieving reductions of 20 to 40%. Concentrations of high-density lipoprotein (HDL)-cholesterol are increased, or unchanged, resulting in an improvement of the LDL:HDL-cholesterol ratio. Combination of statins with bile-acid binding resins has been shown to produce additional reductions in LDL-cholesterol concentrations of up to about 60%. However, there is concern over enhanced adverse effects with combinations of statins and nicotinic acid or fibric acid derivatives.

STUDIES WITH SIMVASTATIN. An interim report of the 5-year Oxford Cholesterol Study in over 600 patients at increased risk of ischaemic heart disease confirmed the efficacy and safety of simvastatin as a lipid regulating drug at follow-up after 3 years.[5] Total cholesterol, LDL-cholesterol, and triglyceride concentrations were all substantially reduced and there were small increases in HDL-cholesterol. Since hypercholesterolaemia is a known risk factor for atherosclerosis, there is much interest in the value of this lipid regulating effect in the prophylaxis of **ischaemic heart disease**. Large placebo-controlled studies with simvastatin for the secondary prevention of ischaemic heart disease, the Multicentre Anti-Atheroma Study (MAAS)[6] and the Scandinavian Simvastatin Survival Study (4S)[7,8,9] have indicated a beneficial effect when cholesterol levels are reduced in patients with ischaemic heart disease. In MAAS, reduction of atherogenic lipoproteins was claimed to slow the coronary atherosclerotic process in patients with moderate hypercholesterolaemia and known ischaemic heart disease. Overall, in 4S, simvastatin was associated with improved survival and no apparent increase in non-cardiac mortality in patients with angina pectoris or previous myocardial infarction. The risk for major coronary events in this trial was reduced for women as well as for men although there were too few women studied to assess effects on mortality. Additionally, there was some evidence[8] that simvastatin retarded progression of **non-cardiac atherosclerosis** as the risk of peripheral vascular disease (such as intermittent claudication) and cerebrovascular disease (stroke and transient ischaemic attacks) was reduced.

1. Hoeg JM, Brewer HB. 3-Hydroxy-3-methylglutaryl-coenzyme A reductase inhibitors in the treatment of hypercholesterolemia. *JAMA* 1987; **258:** 3532–6.
2. Illingworth DR, Bacon S. Hypolipidemic effects of HMG-CoA reductase inhibitors in patients with hypercholesterolemia. *Am J Cardiol* 1987; **60:** 33G–42G.
3. Grundy SM. HMG-CoA reductase inhibitors for treatment of hypercholesterolemia. *N Engl J Med* 1988; **319:** 24–33.
4. Slater EE, MacDonald JS. Mechanism of action and biological profile of HMG CoA reductase inhibitors. *Drugs* 1988; **36** (suppl 3): 72–82.
5. Keech A, *et al.* Three-year follow-up of the Oxford Cholesterol Study: assessment of the efficacy and safety of simvastatin in preparation for a large mortality study. *Eur Heart J* 1994; **15:** 255–69.
6. MAAS Investigators. Effect of simvastatin on coronary atheroma: the Multicentre Anti-Atheroma Study (MAAS). *Lancet* 1994; **344:** 633–8. Correction. *ibid.*: 762.
7. Scandinavian Simvastatin Survival Study Group. Randomised trial of cholesterol lowering in 4444 patients with coronary heart disease: the Scandinavian Simvastatin Survival Study (4S). *Lancet* 1994; **344:** 1383–9.
8. Pedersen TR, *et al.* Effect of simvastatin on ischemic signs and symptoms in the Scandinavian Simvastatin Survival Study (4S). *Am J Cardiol* 1998; **81:** 333–5.
9. Miettinen TA, *et al.* Cholesterol-lowering therapy in women and elderly patients with myocardial infarction or angina pectoris: findings from the Scandinavian Simvastatin Survival Study (4S). *Circulation* 1997; **96:** 4211–18.

Preparations

USP 23: Simvastatin Tablets.

Proprietary Preparations (details are given in Part 3)
Aust.: Zocord; ***Austral.:*** Lipex; Zocor; ***Belg.:*** Zocor; ***Canad.:*** Zocor; ***Fr.:*** Lodales; Zocor; ***Ger.:*** Denan; Zocor; ***Irl.:*** Zocor; ***Ital.:*** Liponorm; Medipo; Sinvacor; Sivastin; Zocor; ***Neth.:*** Zocor; ***Norw.:*** Zocor; ***S.Afr.:*** Zocor; ***Spain:*** Colemin; Pantok; Zocor; ***Swed.:*** Zocord; ***Switz.:*** Zocor; ***UK:*** Zocor; ***USA:*** Zocor.

Sitosterol (1359-q)

β-Sitosterin; β-Sitosterol. Stigmast-5-en-3β-ol.
$C_{29}H_{50}O = 414.7$.
CAS — 83-46-5.

Sitosterol is a naturally occurring phytosterol that is used as a lipid regulating drug in the treatment of hyperlipidaemias (p.1265). The usual dose is 3 to 6 g daily in divided doses by mouth.

It is also used in benign prostatic hyperplasia (p.1446) in usual initial doses of 20 mg three times daily by mouth reducing to 10 mg three times daily for long-term therapy.

References.

1. Berges RR, *et al.* Randomised, placebo-controlled, double-blind clinical trial of β-sitosterol in patients with benign prostatic hyperplasia. *Lancet* 1995; **345:** 1529–32.
2. Klippel KF, *et al.* A multicentric, placebo-controlled, double-blind clinical trial of β-sitosterol (phytosterol) for the treatment of benign prostatic hyperplasia. *Br J Urol* 1997; **80:** 427–32.

Preparations

Proprietary Preparations (details are given in Part 3)
Ger.: Azuprostat M; Flemun; Harzol; Liposit; LP-Truw mono; Prostasal; Sito-Lande; Triastonal.

Multi-ingredient: ***UK:*** Cholasitrol; Sitosterol-B†.

Sorbinicate (13262-q)

Sorbinicate *(rINN).*
D-Glucitol hexanicotinate.
$C_{42}H_{32}N_6O_{12} = 812.7$.
CAS — 6184-06-1.

Sorbinicate, a derivative of nicotinic acid, is a lipid regulating drug that has been used in the treatment of hyperlipidaemias.

Preparations

Proprietary Preparations (details are given in Part 3)
Ital.: Nicosterolo†.

Theofibrate (12720-s)

Theofibrate *(USAN).*
Etofylline Clofibrate *(rINN)*; ML-1024. 2-(Theophyllin-7-yl)ethyl 2-(4-chlorophenoxy)-2-methylpropionate.
$C_{19}H_{21}ClN_4O_5 = 420.8$.
CAS — 54504-70-0.

Theofibrate, a fibric acid derivative (see Bezafibrate, p.1268), is a lipid regulating drug used in the treatment of hyperlipidaemias (p.1265). The usual dose is 250 mg two or three times daily by mouth.

Preparations

Proprietary Preparations (details are given in Part 3)
Aust.: Duolip; ***Ger.:*** Duolip; ***Switz.:*** Duolip.

Tiadenol (1360-d)

Tiadenol *(rINN).*
LL-1558. 2,2′-(Decamethylenedithio)diethanol.
$C_{14}H_{30}O_2S_2 = 294.5$.
CAS — 6964-20-1.

Tiadenol is a lipid regulating drug used in the treatment of hyperlipidaemias (p.1265). The usual dose is 1.2 to 2.4 g daily by mouth in divided doses.

Preparations

Proprietary Preparations (details are given in Part 3)
Fr.: Fonlipol; ***Ital.:*** Delipid†; Eulip; Fonlipol†; Tiabrenolo; Tiaclar†; Tiaden; Tiaterol†; ***Spain:*** Endol; Millaterol†; Norlipol†.

Tocofibrate (3916-y)

Tocofibrate *(rINN)*.
2,5,7,8-Tetramethyl-2-(4,8,12-trimethyltridecyl)-6-chromanyl 2-(4-chlorophenoxy)-2-methylpropionate.
$C_{39}H_{59}ClO_4$ = 627.3.
CAS — 50465-39-9.

Tocofibrate, a fibric acid derivative (see Bezafibrate, p.1268), is a lipid regulating drug used in the treatment of hyperlipidaemias (p.1265). The usual dose is 800 mg by mouth three times daily.

Preparations

Proprietary Preparations (details are given in Part 3)
Spain: Transferal.

Tocopheryl Nicotinate (7899-j)

Vitamin E Nicotinate. (±)-α-Tocopherol nicotinate.
$C_{35}H_{53}NO_3$ = 535.8.
CAS — 51898-34-1; 16676-75-8.

Tocopheryl nicotinate is a lipid regulating drug and a vasodilator. It is used in the treatment of hyperlipidaemias (p.1265). The usual dose is 100 to 200 mg three times daily by mouth.

Preparations

Proprietary Preparations (details are given in Part 3)
Ger.: Renascin†; ***Ital.:*** Renascin†; ***Jpn:*** Juvela; ***Spain:*** Disclar; Vitaber PP + E.

Multi-ingredient: ***Ital.:*** Evitex; ***Spain:*** Esclerobion†; Evitex A E Fuerte.

Local Anaesthetics

Local anaesthetics are compounds that produce reversible loss of sensation by preventing or diminishing the conduction of sensory nerve impulses near to the site of their application or injection. Also, because their mode of action is to decrease permeability of the nerve cell membrane to sodium ions, they are considered to have a membrane stabilising effect.

Clinically useful local anaesthetics have the same general chemical configuration of an amine portion joined to an aromatic residue by an ester or amide link. The type of linkage is important in determining the properties of the drug.

For a classification of local anaesthetics, see Table 1, below.

Table 1. Classification of local anaesthetics.

Amide type	Ester type
Bupivacaine	*Esters of benzoic acid*
Butanilicaine	Amylocaine
Carticaine	Cocaine
Cinchocaine	Propanocaine
Clibucaine	*Esters of meta-aminobenzoic acid*
Ethyl parapiperidino-acetylaminobenzoate	Clormecaine
Etidocaine	Proxymetacaine
Lignocaine	*Esters of para-aminobenzoic acid*
Mepivacaine	Amethocaine
Oxethazaine	Benzocaine
Prilocaine	Butacaine
Ropivacaine	Butoxycaine
Tolycaine	Butyl aminobenzoate
Trimecaine	Chloroprocaine
Vadocaine	Oxybuprocaine
Miscellaneous	Parethoxycaine
Bucricaine	Procaine
Dimethisoquin	Propoxycaine
Diperodon	Tricaine
Dyclocaine	
Ethyl chloride	
Ketocaine	
Myrtecaine	
Octacaine	
Pramoxine	
Propipocaine	

Adverse Effects

Adverse effects apparent after local anaesthesia may be caused by the anaesthetic or errors in technique, or may be the result of blockade of the sympathetic nervous system. Local anaesthetics may produce systemic adverse effects as a result of raised plasma concentrations that arise when the rate of uptake into the circulation exceeds the rate of breakdown, for example, following

- excessive dosage or rate of administration
- accidental intravascular injection
- absorption of large amounts through mucous membranes or damaged skin
- absorption of large amounts from inflamed or highly vascular areas.

Adverse effects may also be caused by concomitantly administered vasoconstrictors.

Hypersensitivity reactions are rare and generally limited to local anaesthetics of the ester type. There appears to be no cross-sensitivity between ester- and amide-type local anaesthetics. Idiosyncrasy to local anaesthetics has been reported. Hypersensitivity reactions to preservatives in local anaesthetic preparations have been reported.

The systemic toxicity of local anaesthetics mainly involves the CNS and the cardiovascular system. Excitation of the CNS may be manifested by restlessness, excitement, nervousness, paraesthesias, dizziness, tinnitus, blurred vision, nausea and vomiting, muscle twitching and tremors, and convulsions. Numbness of the tongue and perioral region, and lightheadedness followed by sedation may appear as early signs of systemic toxicity. Excitation when it occurs may be transient and followed by depression with drowsiness, respiratory failure, and coma. There may be effects on the cardiovascular system with myocardial depression and peripheral vasodilatation resulting in hypotension and bradycardia; arrhythmias and cardiac arrest may occur. Hypotension often accompanies spinal and epidural anaesthesia; inappropriate positioning of the patient may be a contributory factor for women in labour.

Some local anaesthetics cause methaemoglobinaemia (see under Effects on the Blood, below).

Fetal intoxication has occurred following the use of local anaesthetics in labour, either as a result of the transplacental diffusion or after accidental injection of the fetus.

Prolonged use of topical anaesthetics in the eye causes corneal damage.

Reviews.

1. Reynolds F. Adverse effects of local anaesthetics. *Br J Anaesth* 1987; **59:** 78–95.
2. McCaughey W. Adverse effects of local anaesthetics. *Drug Safety* 1992; **7:** 178–189.
3. Berde CB. Toxicity of local anesthetics in infants and children. *J Pediatr* 1993; **122** (suppl): S14–S20.
4. Naguib M, *et al.* Adverse effects and drug interactions associated with local and regional anaesthesia. *Drug Safety* 1998; **18:** 221–50.

Adverse effects of central block. The most prominent adverse effects associated with spinal or epidural anaesthesia (i.e. central nerve block—see below) involve the cardiovascular system.[1] Sympathetic block results in venodilatation, reduced venous return, decreased cardiac output, and hypotension. Higher levels of neural block may result in the added effects of vagus nerve block. Other cardiovascular complications may include bradycardia or heart block.[1] Unexpected cardiac arrest has also been reported after spinal anaesthesia.[1,2] Cardiovascular effects may also arise from systemic absorption (see below).

Total spinal anaesthesia from extreme spread of a block produces unconsciousness, hypotension, and respiratory arrest. Less extensive spread to the cervical region is usually associated with nausea, agitation, and hypotension.[1]

Systemic toxicity is primarily a complication of epidural block as larger doses are required than for spinal block, although serum concentrations attained with epidural block are usually lower than those required to produce CNS effects (unless there is inadvertent injection into an epidural vein). As concentrations increase symptoms progress from numbness of the tongue, lightheadedness, visual disturbances, and muscular twitching through to unconsciousness, convulsions, coma, respiratory arrest, and cardiovascular depression. Arrhythmias, heart block, and cardiovascular collapse appear to be more common with the lipid-soluble long-acting drugs such as bupivacaine, and special care should be taken to avoid fast bolus injections.[1]

Post-dural puncture headache is probably the most common neurological complication related to these procedures and may be accompanied by tinnitus or photophobia. It is considered to be caused by leakage of CSF following puncture of the dura mater.[1] It has been pointed out that headache following spinal block may rarely be caused by meningitis.[3] Cranial nerve lesions have also occurred after spinal anaesthesia.[1,2] Reversible loss of hearing in the low frequency range, usually affecting both ears, has been reported rarely following spinal anaesthesia but has not been found in patients who received epidural block,[4,5] although transient effects on the auditory system of the neonate may occur after maternal epidural anaesthesia.[6] Puncture of the dura with leakage of CSF appears to be an important feature of hearing loss following spinal anaesthesia, although the precise mechanism is not known.[7] Neurological complications associated with these blocks may also rarely include paraplegia caused by arachnoiditis, or trauma or compression of the spinal cord following development of a haematoma or abscess.[1,2] Cauda equina syndrome, the symptoms of which include urinary retention, loss of perineal sensation, loss of sexual function, and faecal incontinence, is also a rare complication which can present many months after spinal anaesthesia.[8]

Perioperative shivering has been associated with epidural anaesthesia.[9]

Patients receiving epidural analgesia during labour appear to have an increased risk of developing pyrexia and this may result in fetal compromise.[10]

Hypotension is a problem with spinal or epidural anaesthesia and may be particularly exaggerated during pregnancy (see under Overdosage, below, for the management of such hypotension). A study[11] to compare the haemodynamic effects of spinal with epidural anaesthesia showed that spinal anaesthesia was associated with greater haemodynamic changes than epidural anaesthesia. The results of a further study[12] using hyperbaric bupivacaine suggest that greater haemodynamic stability is achieved with continuous spinal anaesthesia than with a single bolus spinal injection, although there is a possible risk of neurotoxicity if excessive doses of local anaesthetic are required. Studies using epidural bupivacaine with[13] or without[14] adrenaline showed no alteration in uteroplacental or fetal haemodynamics.

Backache is a frequent postoperative complication following epidural, spinal, or general anaesthesia; there is debate about whether it occurs more frequently with epidural or spinal block.[1,15-17]

1. Parnass SM, Schmidt KJ. Adverse effects of spinal and epidural anaesthesia. *Drug Safety* 1990; **5:** 179–94.
2. Wildsmith JAW, Lee JA. Neurological sequelae of spinal anaesthesia. *Br J Anaesth* 1989; **63:** 505–7.
3. Harding SA, *et al.* Meningitis after combined spinal-extradural anaesthesia in obstetrics. *Br J Anaesth* 1994; **73:** 545–7.
4. Panning B, *et al.* Transient low-frequency hypoacousia after spinal anaesthesia. *Lancet* 1983; **ii:** 582.
5. Wang LP, *et al.* Transient hearing loss following spinal anaesthesia. *Anaesthesia* 1987; **42:** 1258–63.
6. Bozynski MEA, *et al.* Effect of prenatal lignocaine on auditory brain stem evoked response. *Arch Dis Child* 1989; **64:** 934–8.
7. Broome IJ. Hearing loss and dural puncture. *Lancet* 1993; **341:** 667–8.
8. Kalmanovitch DVA, Simmons P. Post-anaesthetic complications in the home. *Prescribers' J* 1988; **28:** 124–31.
9. Anonymous. Perioperative shivering. *Lancet* 1991; **338:** 547–8.
10. Fusi L, *et al.* Maternal pyrexia associated with the use of epidural analgesia in labour. *Lancet* 1989; **i:** 1250–2.
11. Robson SC, *et al.* Maternal and fetal haemodynamic effects of spinal and extradural anaesthesia for elective caesarean section. *Br J Anaesth* 1992; **68:** 54–9.
12. Robson SC, *et al.* Incremental spinal anaesthesia for elective caesarean section: maternal and fetal haemodynamic effects. *Br J Anaesth* 1993; **70:** 634–8.
13. Alahuhta S, *et al.* Effects of extradural bupivacaine with adrenaline for caesarean section on uteroplacental and fetal circulation. *Br J Anaesth* 1991; **67:** 678–82.
14. Alahuhta S, *et al.* Uteroplacental and fetal haemodynamics during extradural anaesthesia for caesarean section. *Br J Anaesth* 1991; **66:** 319–23.
15. MacArthur C, *et al.* Epidural anaesthesia and long term backache after childbirth. *Br Med J* 1990; **301:** 9–12.
16. Murphy JD. Epidural anaesthesia and long term backache after childbirth. *Br Med J* 1990; **301:** 385.
17. Russell R, *et al.* Assessing long term backache after childbirth. *Br Med J* 1993; **306:** 1299–1303.

Effects on the blood. METHAEMOGLOBINAEMIA. Methaemoglobinaemia has been reported following the use of several local anaesthetics including amethocaine,[1] benzocaine,[1-3] and lignocaine[1] but is more commonly associated with the use of prilocaine.[4-6] It may occur following local injection or topical administration. It has been suggested that the effect is due to the presence of an aniline group in the structure or, in the case of lignocaine and prilocaine, metabolism to an aniline-like structure. Methaemoglobinaemia may result from the use of usual doses or may occur in patients exposed to toxic concentrations of local anaesthetic.[1,6] The effect for prilocaine may be dose-related with 8 mg per kg body-weight usually being needed to produce symptoms.[7] However, methaemoglobinaemia has occurred in a 12-week infant following the topical application of a eutectic preparation of prilocaine and lignocaine.[5] Although increases in methaemoglobin concentrations are small following the use of this mixture in infants[8] and children[9] it appears that infants are particularly susceptible to induced methaemoglobinaemia during the first 3 months of life probably due to their limited enzyme capacity.[8] The UK manufacturers of one eutectic prilocaine/lignocaine preparation do not recommend using it in infants under 1 year of age. Concomitant administration of other drugs such as sulphonamides[5] or antimalarials[7] may predispose to methaemoglobinaemia. Patients with haemoglobinopathies or glucose-6-phosphate dehydrogenase deficiency may also be at greater risk.[1]

1. Olson ML, McEvoy GK. Methemoglobinemia induced by local anesthetics. *Am J Hosp Pharm* 1981; **38:** 89–93.
2. Rodriguez LF, *et al.* Benzocaine-induced methemoglobinemia: report of a severe reaction and review of the literature. *Ann Pharmacother* 1994; **28:** 643–9.
3. Tush GM, Kuhn RJ. Methemoglobinemia induced by an over-the-counter medication. *Ann Pharmacother* 1996; **30:** 1251–4.
4. Mandel S. Methemoglobinemia following neonatal circumcision. *JAMA* 1989; **261:** 702.
5. Jakobson B, Nilsson A. Methemoglobinemia associated with a prilocaine-lidocaine cream and trimetoprim-sulphamethoxazole: a case report. *Acta Anaesthesiol Scand* 1985; **29:** 453–5.
6. Knobeloch L, *et al.* Prilocaine-induced methemoglobinemia—Wisconsin, 1993. *JAMA* 1994; **272:** 1403–4.

7. Reynolds F. Adverse effects of local anaesthetics. *Br J Anaesth* 1987; **59:** 78–95.
8. Nilsson A, *et al.* Inverse relationship between age-dependent erythrocyte activity of methaemoglobin reductase and prilocaine-induced methaemoglobinaemia during infancy. *Br J Anaesth* 1990; **64:** 72–6.
9. Frayling IM, *et al.* Methaemoglobinaemia in children treated with prilocaine-lignocaine cream. *Br Med J* 1990; **301:** 153–4.

Effects on the ears. Symptoms such as vertigo, nausea, and nystagmus, which have been reported following the use of local anaesthetics in the external[1] or middle ear,[2] may result from penetration of the local anaesthetic into the inner ear. For reference to hearing loss associated with spinal block, see under Adverse Effects of Central Block, above.

1. Raine NMN, Whittet HB. Emla cream and induced vertigo. *Br J Hosp Med* 1994; **51:** 614–15.
2. Blair Simmons F, *et al.* Lidocaine in the middle ear: a unique cause of vertigo. *Arch Otolaryngol* 1973; **98:** 42–3.

Hypersensitivity. Local anaesthetics may provoke types I and IV hypersensitivity reactions.[1,2] Type I reactions (e.g. anaphylaxis) to local anaesthetics are generally rare and occur more frequently with the ester-type than with the amide-type drugs.[2-5] Nevertheless, severe or fatal reactions have been associated not only with ester-type local anaesthetics such as amethocaine[6] and procaine[7] but also with the amide-type local anaesthetics lignocaine[8-11] and prilocaine.[8] Intolerance may also have been the cause of death in one patient who received mepivacaine for paracervical anaesthesia.[12] Hypotension encountered during dental anaesthesia is usually a vasovagal response unrelated to the type of local anaesthetic used and may be prevented by the use of diazepam.[4,5] Some patients diagnosed as being hypersensitive to local anaesthetics may have reacted to preservatives in the preparations.[5] Skin testing has been proposed to detect allergies but if it is undertaken drugs should be tested individually as patients may react to some but not all drugs of one type.[8] Although the reliability of skin testing has been questioned,[5] it may be of benefit in patients who will require future local anaesthesia and when a patient's history does not rule out a possible allergic reaction.[2] However, testing itself can cause severe or anaphylactic reactions.[13,14] Patients sensitised by topical application may subsequently develop anaphylactic reactions when treated systemically.[13] The use of sensitisers such as benzocaine or amethocaine in lozenges or throat sprays may also sensitise patients.[15] Topical use of related compounds such as para-aminobenzoic acid in sunscreens can produce cross-hypersensitivity reactions with some ester-type local anaesthetics.[5]

For reports of the incidence of allergy to local anaesthetics determined by patch testing, see under individual monographs.

1. Canfield DW, Gage TW. A guideline to local anesthetic allergy testing. *Anesth Prog* 1987; **34:** 157–63.
2. Eggleston ST, Lush LW. Understanding allergic reactions to local anaesthetics. *Ann Pharmacother* 1996; **30:** 851–7.
3. Adriani J, *et al.* The allergenicity of lidocaine and other amide and related local anesthetics. *Anesthesiol Rev* 1986; **13:** 30–6.
4. Anonymous. *Br Med J* 1980; **280:** 1360. Correction. *ibid.*; **281:** 211.
5. Parnass SM, Schmidt KJ. Adverse effects of spinal and epidural anesthesia. *Drug Safety* 1990; **5:** 179–94.
6. Moriwaki K, *et al.* A case report of anaphylactic shock induced by tetracaine used for spinal anesthesia. *Masui* 1986; **35:** 1279–84.
7. MacLachlan D, Forrest AL. Procaine and malignant hyperthermia. *Lancet* 1974; **i:** 355.
8. Fisher MM, Pennington JC. Allergy to local anaesthesia. *Br J Anaesth* 1982; **54:** 893–4.
9. Howard JJ, *et al.* Adult respiratory distress syndrome following administration of lidocaine. *Chest* 1982; **81:** 644–5.
10. Promisloff RA, DuPont DC. Death from ARDS and cardiovascular collapse following lidocaine administration. *Chest* 1983; **83:** 585.
11. Ruffles SP, Ayres JG. Fatal bronchospasm after topical lignocaine before bronchoscopy. *Br Med J* 1987; **294:** 1658–9.
12. Grimes DA, Cates W. Deaths from paracervical anesthesia used for first-trimester abortion, 1972–1975. *N Engl J Med* 1976; **295:** 1397–9.
13. Mulvey PM. Allergy to local anaesthetics. *Med J Aust* 1980; **1:** 386.
14. Brown DT, *et al.* Allergic reaction to an amide local anaesthetic. *Br J Anaesth* 1981; **53:** 435–7.
15. Verbov J. Drug eruptions. *Practitioner* 1979; **222:** 400–9.

Pregnancy. For discussions covering the adverse effects associated with the use of epidural or spinal blocks during labour, see under Adverse Effects of Central Block, above and under Labour Pain on p.9.

For adverse effects on the fetus associated with paracervical block, see Peripheral Nerve Block under Local Anaesthetic Techniques, below.

Treatment of Adverse Effects

Absorption of local anaesthetics from the site of injection may be reduced, if necessary, by applying a tourniquet. When systemic reactions to local anaesthetics occur steps should be taken to maintain the circulation and respiration and to control convulsions. A patent airway must be established and oxygen given, together with assisted ventilation if necessary. The circulation should be maintained with infusions of intravenous fluids. Vasopressors have been suggested in the treatment of marked hypotension although their use is accompanied by a risk of CNS excitation. Vasopressors should not be given to patients receiving oxytocic drugs. Convulsions may be controlled by the intravenous administration of diazepam or thiopentone sodium but these drugs may also depress respiration and the circulation. A short-acting neuromuscular blocker, together with endotracheal intubation and artificial respiration, has been used when convulsions persist. Methaemoglobinaemia may be treated by the intravenous administration of methylene blue.

Overdosage. Activated charcoal has been suggested for use in the treatment of oral overdosage with drugs such as lignocaine.[1]

Treatment of CNS toxicity following intravenous injection of local anaesthetics is dependent upon the duration of the reaction.[2] Most seizures associated with intravenous injection abate rapidly and treatment is mainly dependent upon maintaining adequate oxygenation. If seizures continue for 1 or 2 minutes the use of thiopentone or diazepam is indicated. Suxamethonium may also be needed for skeletal muscle relaxation and to aid intubation. It has been suggested that since diazepam or barbiturates could seriously exacerbate circulatory and respiratory depression, suxamethonium with ventilation might be preferable as it rapidly and consistently stops convulsions and does not depress the myocardium.[3] However, suxamethonium might also cause hyperkalaemia and thus exacerbate lignocaine cardiotoxicity.

For the treatment of bradycardia insertion of a temporary pacemaker should be considered.[1,4]

Hypotension should be managed by the use of intravenous fluids but vasopressors may be necessary for continuing hypotension. Isoprenaline may be useful in the presence of myocardial depression.[1,4] Some consider the response to intravenous fluids to be too slow to be of use in the treatment of hypotension associated with *spinal* or *epidural block* and recommend the use of vasopressors first.[5] It is preferable to use a drug that constricts veins to a greater degree than arteries as the fall in blood pressure is largely due to decreased venous return and there is only minimal arteriolar dilatation.[2] In cases of high spinal or epidural blockade use of a drug such as ephedrine that can produce tachycardia may be beneficial to offset induced bradycardia. For patients who could be at risk from an increase in heart rate phenylephrine may be preferable. Ephedrine is the drug of choice during pregnancy as phenylephrine can decrease uteroplacental perfusion. Ephedrine has also been recommended for prophylactic use before spinal or epidural block in patients at high risk of hypotension. It has been administered as a single intramuscular injection[6] as well as by the more usual intravenous route. One group[7] found that another alpha-adrenergic drug, metaraminol, was marginally more effective than ephedrine in preventing hypotension during spinal block but, in contrast to ephedrine, metaraminol caused a decrease in heart rate. The same group[8] observed that fluid loading with a colloid enhanced the limited ability of ephedrine as a peripheral vasoconstrictor.

1. Denaro CP, *et al.* Poisoning due to class 1B antiarrhythmic drugs: lignocaine, mexiletine and tocainide. *Med Toxicol Adverse Drug Exp* 1989; **4:** 412–28.
2. Parnass SM, Schmidt KJ. Adverse effects of spinal and epidural anaesthesia. *Drug Safety* 1990; **5:** 179–94.
3. Zaccara G, *et al.* Clinical features, pathogenesis and management of drug-induced seizures. *Drug Safety* 1990; **5:** 109–51.
4. Henry J, Volans G. ABC of poisoning: cardiac drugs. *Br Med J* 1984; **289:** 1062–4.
5. Anonymous. Epidural block for caesarean section and circulatory changes. *Lancet* 1989; **ii:** 1076–8.
6. Sternlo J-E, *et al.* Prophylactic im ephedrine in bupivacaine spinal anaesthesia. *Br J Anaesth* 1995; **74:** 517–20.
7. Critchley LAH, *et al.* Hypotension during subarachnoid anaesthesia: haemodynamic analysis of three treatments. *Br J Anaesth* 1994; **72:** 151–5.
8. Critchley LAH, *et al.* Hypotension during subarachnoid anaesthesia: haemodynamic effects of ephedrine. *Br J Anaesth* 1995; **74:** 373–8.

Post-dural puncture headache. Headache following puncture of the dura mater (post-dural puncture headache) during procedures such as lumbar puncture or central nerve blocks for spinal anaesthesia is thought to be caused by subsequent leakage of CSF.[1] With conservative therapy such as bed rest, analgesics, and hydration symptoms in the majority of patients with mild post-dural headache will be relieved within 1 to 2 days.[1] The value of bed rest has, however, been questioned as evidence of its effectiveness is weak.[2] If the headache persists for a further 24 hours measures such as epidural saline[1] or dextran[3] or the use of intravenous caffeine and sodium benzoate[1,4] may be effective; oral caffeine has also been shown to be of benefit.[3] If this is unsuccessful then the epidural injection of autologous blood to form a blood patch over the dural puncture can be employed.[1] Desmopressin is also used for the treatment of post-dural puncture headache but results have generally been disappointing.[5-8] There have been anecdotal reports of success using corticotrophin or tetracosactrin.[9,10] The type of needle used for lumbar puncture may have a bearing on the incidence of post-dural puncture headache.[2]

1. Parnass SM, Schmidt KJ. Adverse effects of spinal and epidural anaesthesia. *Drug Safety* 1990; **5:** 179–94.
2. Broadley SA, Fuller GN. Lumbar puncture needn't be a headache. *Br Med J* 1997; **315:** 1324–5.
3. Choi A, *et al.* Pharmacologic management of postdural puncture headache. *Ann Pharmacother* 1996; **30:** 831–9.
4. Jarvis AP, *et al.* Intravenous caffeine for postdural puncture headache. *Anesth Analg* 1986; **65:** 316–17.
5. Durward WF, Harrington H. Headache after lumbar puncture. *Lancet* 1976; **ii:** 1403–4.
6. Widerlöv E, Lindström L. DDAVP and headache after lumbar puncture. *Lancet* 1979; **i:** 548.
7. Hansen PE, Hansen JH. DDAVP, a synthetic analogue of vasopressin, in prevention of headache after lumbar puncture and lumbar pneumoencephalography. *Acta Neurol Scand* 1979; **60:** 183–8.
8. Cowan JMA, *et al.* DDAVP in the prevention of headache after lumbar puncture. *Br Med J* 1980; **280:** 224.
9. Collier BB. Treatment for post dural puncture headache. *Br J Anaesth* 1994; **72:** 366–7.
10. Foster P. ACTH treatment for post-lumbar puncture headache. *Br J Anaesth* 1994; **73:** 429.

Precautions

As with any drug local anaesthetics are contra-indicated in patients with known hypersensitivity. However, it might be possible to avoid reactions by using a local anaesthetic of the alternative chemical type. Cross sensitivity can occur between ester-type local anaesthetics based on para-aminobenzoic acid and para-aminobenzoic acid and hydroxybenzoate preservatives. Facilities for resuscitation should be available when local anaesthetics are administered parenterally.

Local anaesthetics should be given cautiously to the elderly, to the debilitated, to children, and to patients with epilepsy, impaired cardiac conduction or respiratory function, shock, or liver damage; patients with myasthenia gravis are particularly susceptible to the effects of local anaesthetics. The ester type of local anaesthetic is contra-indicated in patients with low plasma-cholinesterase concentrations. Techniques such as epidural or spinal anaesthesia should not be employed in patients with cerebrospinal diseases, cardiogenic or hypovolaemic shock, or altered coagulation status nor in those with pyogenic infection of the skin at or adjacent to the injection site.

Because of the risk of systemic adverse effects when local anaesthetics are absorbed too rapidly, they should not be injected into or applied to inflamed or infected tissues or to damaged skin or mucosa. For similar reasons, the rate of injection should not be too rapid and great care must be taken to avoid inadvertent intravascular injection. The risk of adverse effects from the uptake of local anaesthetics into the circulation may be reduced by the inclusion of adrenaline to produce vasoconstriction, but the lowest effective concentration of adrenaline should be used. Solutions containing adrenaline should not, however, be used for producing anaesthesia in appendages such as digits, because the profound ischaemia that follows may lead to gangrene. Mepivacaine and prilocaine produce less vasodilatation at low concentrations than other local anaesthetics; they may therefore be useful in cases where the addition of vasoconstrictors is contra-indicated. However, moderate to high concentrations of all local anaesthetics, with the exception of cocaine, produce vasodilatation.

When used in the mouth or throat, local anaesthetics may impair swallowing and increase the risk of aspiration. Patients who have received local anaesthetics for procedures such as laryngoscopy or tracheoscopy should be cautioned not to eat or drink for at least 3 to 4 hours after the anaesthetic.

The cornea may be damaged by prolonged topical application of local anaesthetics, particularly cocaine. Patients should be warned not to rub or touch the eye while anaesthesia persists and the anaesthetised eye should be protected from dust and bacterial contamination.

Local anaesthetics may be ototoxic and should not be instilled into the middle ear.

The application of local anaesthetics to the skin for prolonged periods or to extensive areas should be avoided.

Precautions for central block. Epidural or spinal block may rarely result in paraplegia caused by an induced haematoma or abscess producing arachnoiditis, trauma, or compression of the spinal cord.[1] These blocks have therefore in general been considered to be unsuitable for use in patients with pre-existing neurological disease, infection at the puncture site, or blood disorders or in those receiving aspirin or full-dose anticoagulant therapy.[1] Epidural or spinal block in patients receiving low-dose anticoagulant therapy to prevent post-operative deep-vein thrombosis is still controversial.[1,2]

Thrombelastography has been used as a predictor of bleeding in patients on anticoagulant therapy before regional anaesthesia.[3] It identifies patients with an unusually sensitive response to subcutaneous heparin but it does not seem to be useful in evaluating the extent of platelet dysfunction after aspirin. A study in the USA[4] involving 891 patients found that low-dose aspirin during pregnancy did not increase the risk of bleeding complications during epidural anaesthesia compared with placebo; it was considered that the recommendation to stop aspirin 7 to 10 days before delivery was unjustified.

The risks of regional anaesthesia involving epidural or spinal blocks in patients with cardiovascular disease have been discussed by Reilly.[5] Studies have used various parameters of outcome such as mortality, postoperative cardiac events, or development of myocardial ischaemia to assess the benefits of regional anaesthesia and general anaesthesia. Regional anaesthesia may reduce early postoperative mortality but with little difference in the long-term outcome. There appears to be little evidence of a difference in re-infarction rate but a lower incidence of postoperative cardiac failure has been associated with regional analgesia as compared with general anaesthesia.

1. Parnass SM, Schmidt KJ. Adverse effects of spinal and epidural anaesthesia. *Drug Safety* 1990; **5:** 179–94.
2. Stow PJ, Burrows FA. Anticoagulants in anaesthesia. *Can J Anaesth* 1987; **34:** 632–49.
3. Mallett SV, Platt M. Role of thrombelastography in bleeding diatheses and regional anaesthesia. *Lancet* 1991; **338:** 765–6.
4. Sibai BM, *et al.* Low-dose aspirin in nulliparous women: safety of continuous epidural block and correlation between bleeding time and maternal-neonatal bleeding complications. *Am J Obstet Gynecol* 1995; **172:** 1553–7.
5. Reilly CS. Regional analgesia and myocardial ischaemia. *Br J Anaesth* 1993; **71:** 467–8.

Epilepsy. In a retrospective study[1] of labour in patients with a history of epilepsy, convulsions occurred in 5 of 18 patients who received epidural analgesia and in 3 of 33 patients who did not. Although the trend for epileptic women to be at greater risk of epidural-induced convulsions was not significant in this study, excess use of local anaesthetics in these patients should be avoided.

1. Anderson S. Management of epilepsy. *Lancet* 1990; **336:** 1127.

Malignant hyperthermia. Despite the long-held view that amide-type local anaesthetics should be avoided in patients with or susceptible to malignant hyperthermia an extensive search of the literature revealed no specific reference to malignant hyperthermia being caused solely by the use of these agents.[1] The Malignant Hyperthermia Association of the United States has been reported as stating that all local anaesthetics appear to be safe for people susceptible to malignant hyperthermia.[2]

1. Adragna MG. Medical protocol by habit—the avoidance of amide local anesthetics in malignant hyperthermia susceptible patients. *Anesthesiology* 1985; **62:** 99–100.
2. Brownell AKW, Paasuke RT. Use of local anesthetics in malignant hyperthermia. *Can Med Assoc J* 1986; **134:** 993–4.

Pregnancy. For discussions covering the precautions associated with the use of epidural or spinal blocks during labour, see under Precautions for Central Block, above, and under Labour Pain, p.9.

Tachyphylaxis. The effect of successive epidural injections of 2% solutions of lignocaine, mepivacaine, or prilocaine was reduced by 25 to 30% with each injection when the interval between the disappearance of analgesia and re-injection was more than 10 minutes but anaesthesia was augmented if this interval was less than 10 minutes.[1] Such tachyphylaxis, associated with the prolonged epidural administration of all local anaesthetics, has been reviewed more recently.[2]

1. Bromage PR, *et al.* Tachyphylaxis in epidural analgesia 1: augmentation and decay of local anesthesia. *J Clin Pharmacol* 1969; **9:** 30–8.
2. Mogensen T. Tachyphylaxis to epidural local anaesthetics. *Dan Med Bull* 1995; **42:** 141–6.

Test dose. A test dose is recommended in epidural block to check for accidental intravenous or intrathecal injection but negative results should be treated with caution.[1] Accidental intravenous placement of the needle is notoriously more difficult to detect than inadvertent subarachnoid placement. Adrenaline has been added to the test solution to aid detection of intravenous injection but is considered by some to be of little value.[2,3] For reference to the questionable value of skin testing to detect hypersensitivity to local anaesthetics, see under Hypersensitivity in Adverse Effects, above.

1. Scott DB. Test doses in extradural block. *Br J Anaesth* 1988; **61:** 129–30.
2. Thornburn J. Limitations of adrenaline test doses in obstetric patients undergoing extradural anaesthesia. *Br J Anaesth* 1989; **62:** 578–81.
3. Narchi P, *et al.* Heart rate response to an iv test dose of adrenaline and lignocaine with and without atropine pretreatment. *Br J Anaesth* 1991; **66:** 583–6.

Interactions

The metabolism of local anaesthetics derived from esters may be inhibited by anticholinesterases thus increasing the risk of systemic toxicity.

Ester derivatives such as amethocaine, benzocaine, or procaine that are hydrolysed to para-aminobenzoic acid may antagonise the activity of aminosalicylic acid or sulphonamides. Ester-type local anaesthetics such as procaine and cocaine that are hydrolysed by plasma cholinesterase may competitively enhance the neuromuscular blocking activity of suxamethonium.

There is an increased risk of myocardial depression when amide-type local anaesthetics such as bupivacaine, lignocaine, or ropivacaine are administered concomitantly with antiarrhythmics.

If local anaesthetics containing adrenaline are given for epidural or paracervical block during labour the use of an oxytocic drug post partum may lead to severe hypertension. There is no clinical evidence of dangerous interactions between adrenaline-containing local anaesthetics and MAOIs or tricyclic antidepressants. Great care should however be taken to avoid inadvertent intravenous administration of the local anaesthetic preparation.

For further details of interactions between local anaesthetics and other drugs, see under individual monographs.

Pharmacokinetics

Most local anaesthetics are readily absorbed through mucous membranes, and through damaged skin. Local anaesthetics are weak bases and at tissue pH can diffuse through connective tissue and cellular membranes to reach the nerve fibre where ionisation can occur. While some local anaesthetics are active in the cationic form, others are active in the non-ionised form.

Anaesthetics of the ester type are hydrolysed by esterases in the plasma and, to a lesser extent, in the liver. The effect of spinal anaesthetics lasts until the drug is taken up into the blood circulation since there is little esterase in the spinal fluid.

Amide-type anaesthetics are metabolised in the liver and, in some cases, the kidneys. While there is little protein binding with most ester-type anaesthetics, the amide types are considerably bound.

References.
1. Wildsmith JAW, *et al.* Plasma concentrations of local anaesthetics after interscalene brachial plexus block. *Br J Anaesth* 1977; **49:** 461–6.
2. Nau H. Clinical pharmacokinetics in pregnancy and perinatology I: placental transfer and fetal side effects of local anaesthetic agents. *Dev Pharmacol Ther* 1985; **8:** 149–81.
3. Kanto J. Obstetric analgesia: clinical pharmacokinetic considerations. *Clin Pharmacokinet* 1986; **11:** 283–98.
4. Tucker GT. Pharmacokinetics of local anaesthetics. *Br J Anaesth* 1986; **58:** 717–31.
5. Burm AGL. Clinical pharmacokinetics of epidural and spinal anaesthesia. *Clin Pharmacokinet* 1989; **16:** 283–311.
6. Smith C. Pharmacology of local anaesthetic agents. *Br J Hosp Med* 1994; **52:** 455–60.

Uses and Administration

Local anaesthetics act by preventing the generation and transmission of impulses along nerve fibres and at nerve endings; depolarisation and ion-exchange are inhibited. The effects are reversible. The anaesthetic base must penetrate the lipoprotein nerve sheath before it can act and therefore drugs with high lipid-solubility tend to have a greater potency and duration of action and a faster onset than drugs with low lipid-solubility. Also as only unionised base can penetrate nerve membranes, the lower the pK_a of the local anaesthetic the better. In general, loss of pain (analgesia) occurs before loss of sensory and autonomic function (anaesthesia) and loss of motor function (paralysis), but this may depend on the drug used and the site of administration. The effectiveness of an anaesthetic depends on the concentration attained at the nerve fibre. The latent period before the onset of action may also vary according to the concentration used and the method of administration.

Local anaesthetics are generally administered as acidic solutions of the water-soluble hydrochloride salts; alkalinisation of these solutions may increase the speed of onset and reduce the pain associated with injection (see below). Formulations employing the carbonated base rather than the hydrochloride have also been used to increase the speed of onset (see below). When adrenaline is added, a solution of about pH 3 to 5 is necessary to ensure stability.

Local anaesthetics may be administered in many different ways (see under Local Anaesthetic Techniques, below), some compounds being more suitable than others for a particular route of administration. They vary in their anaesthetic potency and speed of onset and duration of action.

The potency of local anaesthetics is traditionally compared against procaine, which, having a low potency, is given the relative anaesthetic potency value of 1. Other relative anaesthetic potency values are amethocaine 8-10, bupivacaine 8, chloroprocaine 1-2, etidocaine 4-6, lignocaine 2, mepivacaine 2, and prilocaine 2.

Speed of onset and duration of action depend on the anaesthetic technique employed, the type of block, and the site of administration. The most protein bound drugs tend to have the longest duration of action.

The dosage of individual local anaesthetics depends on the injection site and the procedure used. The smallest effective dose and the lowest effective concentration should be used. Smaller doses are usually needed in the elderly, in children, in debilitated patients, and in cardiac disease. Doses should also be reduced in the presence of hepatic disease. Meticulous attention to technique is essential particularly in nerve block and spinal procedures. Injections for central nerve blocks, such as epidural (including caudal block) and spinal block should not contain preservatives.

The speed of onset and duration of action of local anaesthetics are increased by the addition of a vasoconstrictor, which has the effect of reducing the uptake of the local anaesthetic into the circulation from the injection site. Solutions containing adrenaline 1 in 200 000 are generally advocated, although higher concentrations such as 1 in 80 000 may be used in dentistry where the total dose is small. The total amount of adrenaline injected should not exceed 500 µg although the amount of adrenaline absorbed varies considerably with the site of administration; some consider that the maximum dose should be 200 µg. Other vasoconstrictors including noradrenaline are also used, but authorities in the UK consider that noradrenaline should not be used since it presents no advantages and when administered at relatively high concentrations has occasionally been associated with severe hypertensive episodes. Vasoconstrictors should not be used when producing a nerve block in an appendage, as gangrene may occur. Vasoconstrictors have been added to injections for spinal block, but their use is not recommended because of the danger of reducing the blood supply to the spinal cord.

Action. The intrinsic vasoactivity of a local anaesthetic can influence its rate of removal from the site of action and therefore its duration of action. Ester-type local anaesthetics such as amethocaine and procaine are more likely to produce vasodilatation than amide-type local anaesthetics such as cinchocaine, lignocaine, mepivacaine, and prilocaine following intradermal administration.[1] However, cocaine differs from other ester-type local anaesthetics in that it produces vasoconstriction. The amide-type local anaesthetics can produce vasoconstriction but, apart from prilocaine, their vasoconstrictor activity has generally been found to decline with increasing concentration,[1,2] and, in one study, lignocaine and bupivacaine produced more vasodilatation than vasoconstriction at the higher concentrations tested.[2] Mepivacaine has produced greater and more consistent vasoconstriction than lignocaine, cinchocaine, or prilocaine following intradermal injection[1] but this greater vasoactivity is not always evident.[3]

1. Willatts DG, Reynolds F. Comparison of the vasoactivity of amide and ester local anaesthetics: an intradermal study. *Br J Anaesth* 1985; **57:** 1006–11.
2. Aps C, Reynolds F. The effect of concentration on vasoactivity of bupivacaine and lignocaine. *Br J Anaesth* 1976; **48:** 1171–4.
3. Goebel WM, *et al.* Comparative circulatory levels of 2 per cent mepivacaine and 2 per cent lignocaine. *Br Dent J* 1980; **148:** 261–4.

CARBONATED SOLUTIONS. The use of carbonated solutions of local anaesthetics (prepared by treatment of the base with carbon dioxide) instead of the usual hydrochloride salts has been discussed in several reviews.[1-3] Although some early studies indicated that carbonated solutions of bupivacaine, lignocaine, or prilocaine produced earlier onset of anaesthesia and improved the quality of epidural or brachial plexus blocks not all subsequent studies have confirmed these results. A method for preparing carbonated solutions has been given by Bromage[4] but proprietary preparations of such solutions of bupivacaine or lignocaine may be available in some countries.

1. Covino BG. Pharmacology of local anaesthetic agents. *Br J Anaesth* 1986; **58:** 701–16.
2. Burm AGL. Clinical pharmacokinetics of epidural and spinal anaesthesia. *Clin Pharmacokinet* 1989; **16:** 283–311.
3. Carrie LES. Extradural, spinal or combined block for obstetric surgical anaesthesia. *Br J Anaesth* 1990; **65:** 225–33.
4. Bromage PR. Improved conduction blockade in surgery and obstetrics: carbonated local anesthetics. *Can Med Assoc J* 1967; **97:** 1377–84.

PH OF SOLUTIONS. The pain associated with infiltration of local anaesthetics can be reduced by buffering the solution to physiological pH with sodium bicarbonate.[1,2] Although buffering itself does not appear to compromise the efficacy of anaesthesia,[2] alkalinisation of the solution may reduce the solubility of the local anaesthetic and cause precipitation.[2-4] To enhance stability local anaesthetic solutions are usually prepared to have an acidic pH and it is therefore recommended that if solutions are buffered they should be used immediately.[2]

Similar pH adjustments for solutions for intravenous regional anaesthesia have been reported to reduce the amount of local venous irritation and thrombophlebitis[5] and to increase the speed of onset and the duration of the block.[6] Alkalinisation of a solution used for epidural block for caesarean section has been reported to result in a more rapid onset of action and denser block.[7]

Alkalinisation has also been used to hasten the onset of peripheral nerve block[8] by increasing the proportion of the lipid-soluble nonionised free base but the effect in epidural block has been inconsistent.[9,10]

1. McKay W, *et al.* Sodium bicarbonate attenuates pain on skin infiltration with lidocaine, with or without epinephrine. *Anesth Analg* 1987; **66:** 572–4.
2. Cristoph RA, *et al.* Pain reduction in local anesthetic administration through pH buffering. *Ann Emerg Med* 1988; **17:** 117–20.
3. Bourget P, *et al.* Factors influencing precipitation of pH-adjusted bupivacaine solutions. *J Clin Pharm Ther* 1990; **15:** 197–204.
4. Nakano NI. Temperature-dependent aqueous solubilities of lidocaine, mepivacaine, and bupivacaine. *J Pharm Sci* 1979; **68:** 667–8.
5. Yudenfreund SM, *et al.* pH-Buffered 2-chloroprocaine for intravenous regional anesthesia. *DICP Ann Pharmacother* 1989; **23:** 614–15.
6. Armstrong P, *et al.* Effect of alkalinization of prilocaine on IV regional anaesthesia. *Br J Anaesth* 1989; **63:** 625P–626P.
7. Fernando R, Jones HM. Comparison of plain and alkalinized local anaesthetic mixtures of lignocaine and bupivacaine for elective extradural caesarean section. *Br J Anaesth* 1991; **67:** 699–703.
8. Coventry DM, Todd JG. Alkalinization of bupivacaine for sciatic nerve blockade. *Br J Anaesth* 1989; **62:** 227P.
9. Burm AGL. Clinical pharmacokinetics of epidural and spinal anaesthesia. *Clin Pharmacokinet* 1989; **16:** 283–311.
10. Carrie LES. Extradural, spinal or combined block for obstetric surgical anaesthesia. *Br J Anaesth* 1990; **65:** 225–33.

Anorectal disorders. See under Surface Anaesthesia, below.

Cancer pain. For the role of local anaesthetics in the management of cancer pain, see p.8.

Cough. Drugs such as lignocaine or bupivacaine have been administered by inhalation in severe intractable cough,[1-4] including cough caused by malignant neoplasms. Cough suppression is produced by an indirect peripheral action on sensory receptors, but as all protective pulmonary reflexes may be lost and bronchospasm may be induced, nebulised local anaesthetics should be used in controlled circumstances only; there may also be temporary loss of the swallowing reflex. The management of cough in general is discussed on p.1052.

1. Howard P, *et al.* Lignocaine aerosol and persistent cough. *Br J Dis Chest* 1977; **71:** 19–24.
2. Stewart CJ, Coady TJ. Suppression of intractable cough. *Br Med J* 1977; **i:** 1660–1.
3. Sanders RV, Kirkpatrick MB. Prolonged suppression of cough after inhalation of lidocaine in a patient with sarcoid. *JAMA* 1984; **252:** 2456–7.
4. Brown RC, Turton CWG. Cough and angiotensin converting enzyme inhibition. *Br Med J* 1988; **296:** 1741.

Endoscopy. Local anaesthetics such as lignocaine are sometimes used before endoscopy to improve patient comfort and facilitate passage of the endoscope. As mentioned in the discussion on drugs used in endoscopy (see p.638) some consider that the use of local anaesthetics for procedures such as gastro-intestinal endoscopy should probably be reserved for those patients who prefer to undergo endoscopy without sedation as their use in addition to premedication with opioids or benzodiazepines appears to serve little purpose. Some references to the use of lignocaine in endoscopic procedures are given below.

1. Chuah SY, *et al.* Topical anaesthesia in upper gastrointestinal endoscopy. *Br Med J* 1991; **303:** 695.
2. Jameson JS, *et al.* Topical anaesthesia improves toleration for upper gastrointestinal endoscopy. *Gut* 1992; **33** (suppl): S51.
3. Randell T, *et al.* Topical anaesthesia of the nasal mucosa for fibreoptic airway endoscopy. *Br J Anaesth* 1992; **68:** 164–7.

Intraoperative and postoperative pain. For details of the use of local anaesthetics in the management of surgical and postoperative pain, see p.11 and also under Pain in Infants and Children, p.7.

OPHTHALMIC SURGERY. Techniques used to achieve local anaesthesia for ophthalmic surgery include administering a portion of the local anaesthetic by *retrobulbar injection*; some is used for block of the facial nerve, and the rest is used to induce paralysis of the eyelids. A mixture of equal parts of bupivacaine 0.5% and lignocaine 2% solutions may be useful.[1] Addition of hyaluronidase to the local anaesthetic may increase the success rate for obtaining complete ocular akinesia and anaesthesia.[2]

Adrenaline, usually in a concentration of 1 in 200 000, is commonly included to prolong the duration and increase the extent of the block unless contra-indicated by the presence of orbital vascular pathology.[3]

Because of the complications associated with retrobulbar injection, other methods of local anaesthesia have been tried including *peribulbar injection* and *injection into sub-Tenon's space*;[3,4] some prefer to induce anaesthesia by *subconjunctival injection* of bupivacaine 0.5%[5] or lignocaine 2%[6,7] sometimes in conjunction with eye drops such as amethocaine 1% but the degree of akinesia achieved may be inferior[7] to that from retrobulbar injection.

Injections of local anaesthetics in or around the eye can themselves be painful and topical application of a cream containing a eutectic mixture of lignocaine and prilocaine has been used to alleviate any pain associated with these procedures.[8]

The use of local anaesthetics appears to prevent the endocrine and metabolic response to the stress of ophthalmic surgery when the surgery is carried out under local anaesthesia alone[9,10] but an increase in serum-cortisol concentration has been observed in the postoperative period in patients whose ophthalmic surgery had been carried out under a combination of general and local anaesthesia.[10] The efficacy of local anaesthetics in reducing increases in intra-ocular pressure induced by intubation is unclear (see under Anaesthesia on p.1302).

1. Oji E, Oji A. Bupivacaine and lignocaine for ophthalmic surgery. *Br J Ophthalmol* 1987; **71:** 66–8.
2. Thomson I. Addition of hyaluronidase to lignocaine with adrenaline for retrobulbar anaesthesia in the surgery of senile cataract. *Br J Ophthalmol* 1988; **72:** 700–2.
3. Hamilton RC. Techniques of orbital regional anaesthesia. *Br J Anaesth* 1995; **75:** 88–92.
4. Berry CB, Murphy PM. Regional anaesthesia for cataract surgery. *Br J Hosp Med* 1993; **49:** 689–701.
5. Redmond RM, Dallas NL. Extracapsular cataract extraction under local anaesthesia without retrobulbar injection. *Br J Ophthalmol* 1990; **74:** 203–4.
6. Smith R. Cataract extraction without retrobulbar anaesthetic injection. *Br J Ophthalmol* 1990; **74:** 205–7.
7. Khoo CY. Local anaesthesia without retrobulbar injection. *Br J Ophthalmol* 1990; **74:** 639.
8. Sunderraj P, *et al.* A double-masked evaluation of lignocaine-prilocaine cream (EMLA) used to alleviate the pain of retrobulbar injection. *Br J Ophthalmol* 1991; **75:** 130–2.
9. Barker JP, *et al.* Local analgesia prevents the cortisol and glycaemic responses to cataract surgery. *Br J Anaesth* 1990; **64:** 442–5.
10. Barker JP, *et al.* Retrobulbar block fails to prevent an increase in serum cortisol concentration on emergence from anaesthesia after cataract surgery. *Br J Anaesth* 1994; **72:** 119–21.

ORTHOPAEDIC SURGERY. The use of central or peripheral nerve blocks for orthopaedic surgery has been reviewed by McKenzie and Loach.[1] McKenzie has also discussed the topic of thrombo-embolism associated with anaesthesia.[2] The incidence of postoperative deep vein thrombosis and possibly pulmonary thrombo-embolism following orthopaedic surgery appears to be lower in patients who receive spinal or epidural anaesthesia compared with those who undergo general anaesthesia. Local anaesthetics may have an important role to play in mediating a prophylactic effect. A large study would be needed to determine if regional anaesthesia reduces overall mortality, but in studies that showed a reduction in early postoperative mortality associated with spinal block, the long-term outcome was unaffected.

Intravenous regional anaesthesia has been used for manipulation of fractures and minor surgical procedures of the limbs and, when properly conducted, is considered to be a simple and safe method of anaesthesia.[3] Complications can develop when this technique is employed by those without adequate knowledge and training.[3,4] Fatalities have occurred with bupivacaine.[5] As all local anaesthetics have the potential to produce convulsions and cardiotoxicity it is recommended that an anaesthetist be present with resuscitation facilities; patients should also be fasted.[3,4]

Local infiltration of a local anaesthetic compared favourably with intravenous regional anaesthesia for manipulation of Colles' fractures in terms of satisfactory anaesthesia, ease and speed of performance, and lack of complications.[6] However, pain scores were higher in those patients receiving local infiltration.

1. McKenzie PJ, Loach AB. Local anaesthesia for orthopaedic surgery. *Br J Anaesth* 1986; **58:** 779–89.
2. McKenzie PJ. Deep venous thrombosis and anaesthesia. *Br J Anaesth* 1991; **66:** 4–7.
3. Armstrong P, *et al.* Anaesthesia and Colles' fractures. *Br Med J* 1990; **300:** 261.
4. Goold JE. Intravenous regional anaesthesia. *Br J Hosp Med* 1985; **33:** 335–40.
5. Heath ML. Deaths after intravenous regional anaesthesia. *Br Med J* 1982; **285:** 913–14.
6. Cobb AG, Houghton GR. Local anaesthetic infiltration versus Bier's block for Colles' fractures. *Br Med J* 1985; **291:** 1683–4.

Labour pain. For the role of epidural analgesia with local anaesthetics in the relief of labour pain, see p.9.

Low back pain. For the role of local anaesthetics in the management of low back pain, see p.10.

Mouth ulceration. For the role of local anaesthetics in the management of mouth ulceration, see p.1172.

Pain. The general management of pain is discussed on p.4. Local anaesthetics are used in a variety of situations for the management of pain. They are usually given by local injection or applied topically but are sometimes used intravenously in techniques such as intravenous regional anaesthesia, which involves the continuous infusion of local anaesthetics such as lignocaine to produce general analgesia. However, the technique is potentially dangerous and seldom employed.

Postherpetic neuralgia. For the role of local anaesthetics in the management of postherpetic neuralgia, see p.10.

Soft-tissue rheumatism. For the role of local anaesthetics in the management of soft-tissue rheumatism, see p.4.

Spasticity. The management of spasticity (p.1303) involves physiotherapy together with the use of antispastic drugs. Other approaches to treatment include nerve blocks with local anaesthetics; these can improve spasticity but should generally only be used when further muscle relaxation would not increase disability.

Local Anaesthetic Techniques

Local anaesthetics are employed in several techniques. In order of increasing level of anaesthesia they are: surface or topical anaesthesia; infiltration anaesthesia; and regional nerve block, including peripheral nerve block, sympathetic nerve block, and central nerve block which includes epidural and spinal (intrathecal or subarachnoid) block. Local anaesthetics may also be given intravenously for regional anaesthesia.

Surface anaesthesia. Surface or topical anaesthesia blocks the sensory nerve endings in the skin or mucous membranes. Penetration of intact skin by local anaesthetics is generally poor whereas absorption through mucous membranes may be rapid. However percutaneous anaesthesia can be achieved by application of a eutectic mixture of lignocaine and prilocaine to intact skin (see Eutectic Mixtures under Lignocaine, p.1296). Other methods of improving dermal delivery of local anaesthetics include a transdermal patch of lignocaine, and an iontophoretic drug delivery system incorporating lignocaine and adrenaline. Anaesthesia of the skin and subcutaneous tissues is also discussed under Infiltration Anaesthesia, below.

Many local anaesthetics are effective surface anaesthetics, a notable exception being procaine. There are a number of special uses of topical anaesthesia including anaesthetising the cornea during ophthalmological procedures and the throat and larynx before intubation and bronchoscopy. Great care is necessary when employing local anaesthetics to anaesthetise the urethra; if trauma has occurred, rapid absorption of the drug may occur and give rise to serious adverse effects. Absorption from the respiratory tract is also rapid and care is essential to avoid administering a toxic dose. Eutectic mixtures may be of value in providing surface anaesthesia for a number of minor medical or surgical procedures.

Local anaesthetics have been included in topical preparations to relieve the pain of haemorrhoids (p.1170) but good evidence of their efficacy is lacking. Similar uses include pain relief in pruritus ani and anal fissure. Excessive application of local anaesthetics to the rectal mucosa should be avoided as absorption can occur; use for periods of no longer than a few days is recommended to prevent sensitisation of the anal skin. Local anaesthetics are sometimes included in topical preparations for the relief of pruritus (p.1075). However, they are only marginally effective and can very occasionally cause sensitisation. The use of local anaesthetics in rubefacient and topical analgesic preparations is discussed on p.7.

Infiltration anaesthesia. Infiltration anaesthesia is produced by injection of a local anaesthetic directly into and around the field of operation without attempting to identify individual nerves. The drug used should not be absorbed too rapidly otherwise the anaesthesia will wear off too quickly for practical use; some local anaesthetics require the addition of a vasoconstrictor in low concentrations, which can increase the duration of infiltration anaesthesia and reduce peak plasma concentrations of the local anaesthetic. Infiltration anaesthesia is extensively used in dentistry.

Anaesthesia of small areas by infiltration techniques requires a relatively large amount of local anaesthetic, which is not a problem for minor surgery but would be for more extensive areas that required anaesthesia. The amount of local anaesthetic used can be reduced and the duration of anaesthesia increased by blocking specific nerves that innervate the area. This may be carried out at several levels. In *field block* anaesthesia subcutaneous injection of a local anaesthetic close to the nerves around the area to be anaesthetised blocks sensory nerve paths. This is a form of infiltration anaesthesia, but the technique requires less drug for a given area to be anaesthetised.

Regional nerve block. Regional nerve block anaesthesia involves specific blocks at the levels of major nerves or spinal roots, and may include peripheral nerve block, sympathetic nerve block, and central nerve block including epidural and spinal block. For a discussion of the use of nerve blocks in the management of pain, see p.6.

PERIPHERAL NERVE BLOCK. Peripheral nerve block anaesthesia involves injection into or around a peripheral nerve or plexus supplying the part to be anaesthetised; motor fibres may be blocked as well as sensory fibres. Examples of this type of block include brachial plexus block, intercostal nerve block, paracervical block, and pudendal block. Adrenaline is often added as a vasoconstrictor.

As mentioned under Labour Pain on p.9, the technique of *paracervical local anaesthetic block* has largely fallen out of favour because of the high incidence of fetal arrhythmias, acidosis, and asphyxia and isolated reports of fetal death.

SYMPATHETIC NERVE BLOCK. Sympathetic nerve block such as stellate ganglion blockade and lumbar sympathectomy is used in the management of a range of painful conditions and vascular diseases (see under Sympathetic Pain Syndromes on p.11). Temporary block is obtained using local anaesthetics such as lignocaine or bupivacaine but permanent block may be produced with use of neurolytic agents such as phenol (see Pain, p.1122) or alcohol (see Pain, p.1100).

CENTRAL NERVE BLOCK. Central nerve block includes epidural and spinal block.

Epidural block (also referred to as *extradural* or *peridural block*) is used to provide analgesia or anaesthesia in surgical and obstetric procedures by injecting the local anaesthetic alone or with a small dose of an opioid analgesic into the epidural space. Introduction of a cannula into the epidural space enables prolonged analgesia or anaesthesia to be provided through the use of 'top-up' doses or continuous infusion of the drugs. In obstetrics the injection is made in the lumbar region in order to block the roots of sensory nerves supplying the uterus and lower birth canal. In *caudal block* an epidural injection is made through the sacral hiatus. A test dose at the intended injection site is recommended before starting epidural anaesthesia to ensure that the main dose is not injected intravascularly or into the subarachnoid space.

For the adverse effects of and precautions for central block, see above.

Spinal block (also referred to as *subarachnoid* or *intrathecal block*) is produced by injecting a solution of a suitable drug within the spinal subarachnoid space, causing temporary paralysis of the nerves with which it comes into contact. Vasoconstrictors have been added to prolong the duration of the block but the effect was not always clinically useful and there was a danger of restricting the blood supply to the spinal cord; therefore this practice is not recommended. The somatic level at which anaesthesia occurs depends on many factors including the specific gravity or baricity of the anaesthetic solution used and the positioning of the patient.

References.

1. Commission on the provision of surgical services. *Report of the working party on pain after surgery.* London: Royal College of Surgeons of England and College of Anaesthetists, 1990.
2. Schulte-Steinberg O, Rahlfs VW. Spread of extradural analgesia following caudal injection in children: a statistical study. *Br J Anaesth* 1977; **49:** 1027–34.
3. Wolf AR, *et al.* Postoperative analgesia after paediatric orchidopexy: evaluation of a bupivacaine-morphine mixture. *Br J Anaesth* 1990; **64:** 430–5.
4. Naguib M, *et al.* Ketamine for caudal analgesia in children: comparison with caudal bupivacaine. *Br J Anaesth* 1991; **67:** 559–64.
5. Gallagher TM. Regional anaesthesia for surgical treatment of inguinal hernia in preterm babies. *Arch Dis Child* 1993; **69:** 623–4.
6. Tobias JD, *et al.* Use of continuous caudal block to relieve lower-extremity ischemia caused by vasculitis in a child with meningococcemia. *J Pediatr* 1989; **115:** 1019–21.
7. Casey WF. Which spinal anaesthetic? *Br J Hosp Med* 1988; **40:** 425.
8. Wildsmith JAW. Intrathecal or extradural: which approach for surgery? *Br J Anaesth* 1987; **59:** 397–8.
9. Carrie LES. Extradural, spinal or combined block for obstetric surgical anaesthesia. *Br J Anaesth* 1990; **65:** 225–33.
10. Kestin IG. Spinal anaesthesia in obstetrics. *Br J Anaesth* 1991; **66:** 596–607.
11. Sullivan JM, Ramanathan KB. Management of medical problems in pregnancy—severe cardiac disease. *N Engl J Med* 1985; **313:** 304–9.
12. Ward RM, Hutton P. Factors modifying the use of anaesthetic drugs in the elderly. *Br Med Bull* 1990; **46:** 156–68.
13. Stone PA, *et al.* Complications of spinal anaesthesia following extradural block for caesarean section. *Br J Anaesth* 1989; **62:** 335–7.
14. Benedetti C, Tiengo M. Continuous subarachnoid analgesia in labour. *Lancet* 1990; **335:** 225.
15. Bonnet F, *et al.* Prevention of tourniquet pain by spinal isobaric bupivacaine with clonidine. *Br J Anaesth* 1989; **63:** 93–6.

Intravenous regional anaesthesia. Intravenous regional anaesthesia (Bier's block) involves injection of a dilute solution of local anaesthetic into a suitable limb vein after exsanguination and application of a tourniquet, in order to produce anaesthesia distal to it. Arterial flow must remain occluded for at least 20 minutes after injection and adrenaline should not be used.

For references to the use of intravenous regional anaesthesia for manipulation of fractures and minor surgical procedures of the limbs, see under Orthopaedic Surgery, above.

Amethocaine (7603-v)

Amethocaine *(BAN)*.

Tetracaine *(rINN)*. 2-Dimethylaminoethyl 4-butylaminobenzoate.

$C_{15}H_{24}N_2O_2$ = 264.4.

CAS — 94-24-6.

Pharmacopoeias. In *Chin.* and *US.*

A white or light yellow waxy solid. M.p. 41° to 46°. Very slightly **soluble** in water; soluble 1 in 5 of alcohol and 1 in 2 of chloroform or of ether. **Store** in airtight containers. Protect from light.

Amethocaine Hydrochloride (7604-g)

Amethocaine Hydrochloride *(BANM)*.

Tetracaine Hydrochloride *(rINNM)*; Dicainum; Tetracaini Hydrochloridum; Tetracainii Chloridum.

$C_{15}H_{24}N_2O_2,HCl$ = 300.8.

CAS — 136-47-0.

NOTE. AME and TET are codes approved by the BP for use on single unit doses of eye drops containing amethocaine hydrochloride where the individual container may be too small to bear all the appropriate labelling information.

Pharmacopoeias. In *Chin., Eur.* (see p.viii), *Int., Jpn, Pol.,* and *US.*

A white, odourless, slightly hygroscopic, polymorphic, crystalline powder. Freely to very **soluble** in water; soluble in alcohol; practically insoluble in ether. The Ph. Eur. specifies that a 1% solution in water has a pH of 4.5 to 6.5; the USP specifies a pH of 5.0 to 6.0 for a 1% solution of Sterile Tetracaine Hydrochloride. **Incompatible** with alkalis. **Store** in airtight containers. Protect from light. Aqueous solutions should be discarded if they contain crystals or are discoloured or cloudy.

Adverse Effects and Treatment

As for Local Anaesthetics in general, p.1281.

Amethocaine has high systemic toxicity. Absorption of amethocaine from mucous membranes is rapid and adverse reactions can occur abruptly without the appearance of prodromal signs or convulsions; fatalities have occurred.

A stinging sensation may occur when amethocaine is used in the eye. Mild erythema at the site of application is frequently seen with topical administration; slight oedema or pruritus occur less commonly.

Urethral stricture. There has been a report[1] of a sudden increase in the incidence of urethral stricture following transurethral surgery, which may have been due to an increase in the concentration of amethocaine hydrochloride in the lubricant gel from 0.1 to 3%.

1. Pansadoro V. Role of local anaesthetics in urethral strictures after transurethral surgery. *Lancet* 1990; **336:** 64.

Precautions

As for Local Anaesthetics in general, p.1282.

Amethocaine should not be applied to inflamed, traumatised, or highly vascular surfaces. It should not be used to provide anaesthesia for bronchoscopy or cystoscopy, as lignocaine is a safer alternative.

Interactions

For interactions associated with local anaesthetics, see p.1283.

Pharmacokinetics

See under Local Anaesthetics, p.1283.

Uses and Administration

Amethocaine, a para-aminobenzoic acid ester, is a potent local anaesthetic with actions and uses similar to those described on p.1283. It is used for surface anaesthesia and spinal anaesthesia; its use in other local anaesthetic techniques is restricted by its systemic toxicity.

Amethocaine is generally used as the hydrochloride in solutions and creams, and as the base in gels or ointments.

For *anaesthesia of the eye*, solutions containing 0.5 to 1.0% amethocaine hydrochloride and ointments containing 0.5% amethocaine have been used. Instillation of a 0.5% solution produces anaesthesia within 25 seconds that lasts for 15 minutes or longer and is suitable for use before minor surgical procedures.

For *topical anaesthesia*, a 1% cream or a 0.5% ointment has been used. These preparations have been used for painful conditions of the *anus or rectum*. A 4% gel is used as a *percutaneous local anaesthetic* before *venepuncture or venous cannulation*. The gel is applied to the centre of the area to be anaesthetised and covered with an occlusive dressing. Gel and dressing are removed after 30 minutes for venepuncture and after 45 minutes for venous cannulation. A single application generally provides anaesthesia for 4 to 6 hours. This method is not suitable for premature infants or those less than 1 month of age.

Amethocaine hydrochloride has also been used in the *mouth* in sprays and lozenges.

Amethocaine has also been used for *spinal anaesthesia* usually as a 0.5% solution.

Action. For a comparison of the vasoactivity of amethocaine with some other local anaesthetics, see p.1284.

Spinal block. A study[1] in 40 patients indicated that for patients undergoing caesarean section with spinal anaesthesia (see Central Nerve Block, p.1285) doses of 12 or 14 mg of amethocaine provided better intraoperative analgesia than doses of 8 or 10 mg without leading to excessive spread of the block.

1. Hirabayashi Y, *et al.* Visceral pain during Caesarean section: effect of varying dose of spinal amethocaine. *Br J Anaesth* 1995; **75:** 266–8.

Surface anaesthesia. A topical gel formulation of amethocaine 4% in Carbomer 1.5% appears to provide more rapid and prolonged surface anaesthesia (see p.1284) than a eutectic mixture of lignocaine and prilocaine.[1] In a double-blind placebo-controlled study[2] the amethocaine gel formulation was significantly better than the eutectic mixture in reducing pain caused by laser treatment of portwine stains. Application of about 500 mg of the amethocaine gel under an occlusive dressing for 30 minutes has been found to be adequate for reliable anaesthesia in children undergoing venepuncture;[3] 1 g applied for 40 minutes has produced acceptable anaesthesia for venous cannulation both in children[4] and in adults.[5] The same formulation appears to be equally effective when incorporated into a transdermal patch.[6]

There have been reports of seizures and death in children following the use of a mixture of amethocaine, adrenaline, and cocaine on mucosal surfaces.[7] Amethocaine should not be applied to traumatised, inflamed, or highly vascular surfaces. A gel containing a mixture of lignocaine, adrenaline, and amethocaine has been found to be an effective alternative to the cocaine-containing preparation.[8]

Amethocaine has also been incorporated into a mucosa-adhesive polymer film to relieve the pain of oral lesions resulting from radiation and antineoplastic therapy.[9]

1. McCafferty DF, *et al.* In vivo assessment of percutaneous local anaesthetic preparations. *Br J Anaesth* 1989; **62:** 17–21.
2. McCafferty DF, *et al.* Effect of percutaneous local anaesthetics on pain reduction during pulse dye laser treatment of portwine stains. *Br J Anaesth* 1997; **78:** 286–9.
3. Woolfson AD, *et al.* Clinical experiences with a novel percutaneous amethocaine preparation: prevention of pain due to venepuncture in children. *Br J Clin Pharmacol* 1990; **30:** 273–9.
4. Lawson RA, *et al.* Evaluation of an amethocaine gel preparation for percutaneous analgesia before venous cannulation in children. *Br J Anaesth* 1995; **75:** 282–5.
5. O'Connor B, Tomlinson AA. Evaluation of the efficacy and safety of amethocaine gel applied topically before venous cannulation in adults. *Br J Anaesth* 1995; **74:** 706–8.
6. McCafferty DF, Woolfson AD. New patch delivery system for percutaneous local anaesthesia. *Br J Anaesth* 1993; **71:** 370–4.
7. Wong S, Hart LL. Tetracaine/adrenaline/cocaine for local anesthesia. *DICP Ann Pharmacother* 1990; **24:** 1181–3.
8. Ernst AA, *et al.* Lidocaine adrenaline tetracaine gel versus tetracaine adrenaline cocaine gel for topical anesthesia in linear scalp and facial lacerations in children aged 5 to 17 years. *Pediatrics* 1995; **95:** 255–8.
9. Yotsuyanagi T, *et al.* Mucosa-adhesive film containing local analgesic. *Lancet* 1985; **ii:** 613.

Preparations

BP 1998: Tetracaine Eye Drops;
USP 23: Benzocaine, Butamben, and Tetracaine Hydrochloride Gel; Benzocaine, Butamben, and Tetracaine Hydrochloride Ointment; Benzocaine, Butamben, and Tetracaine Hydrochloride Topical Aerosol; Benzocaine, Butamben, and Tetracaine Hydrochloride Topical Solution; Cocaine and Tetracaine Hydrochlorides and Epinephrine Topical Solution; Procaine and Tetracaine Hydrochlorides and Levonordefrin Injection; Tetracaine and Menthol Ointment; Tetracaine Hydrochloride Cream; Tetracaine Hydrochloride for Injection; Tetracaine Hydrochloride in Dextrose Injection; Tetracaine Hydrochloride Injection; Tetracaine Hydrochloride Ophthalmic Solution; Tetracaine Hydrochloride Topical Solution; Tetracaine Ointment; Tetracaine Ophthalmic Ointment.

Proprietary Preparations (details are given in Part 3)
Canad.: Pontocaine; Supracaine; ***Ger.:*** Oto-Flexiole N; ***S.Afr.:*** Anethaine†; Covostet; ***Spain:*** Anest Compuesto; Anestesia Topi Braun C/A; Anestesia Topica And Far†; Anestesico; Lubricante Urol†; ***UK:*** Ametop; Anethaine; ***USA:*** Ak-T-Caine; Pontocaine; Viractin.

Multi-ingredient: ***Aust.:*** Dynexan; Herviros; Neocones; Tonexol; ***Belg.:*** Anesthesique Double; ***Canad.:*** Panocaine; ZAP†; ***Fr.:*** Amygdospray; Broncorinol maux de gorge; Cantalene; Codetricine vitamine C; Collucalmyl†; Colluspir†; Drill; Eludril; Eufosyl†; Hexomedine; Lysofon; Oromedine; Oroseptol; Oroseptol Lysozyme; Otylol; Pharyngine a la Vitamine C†; Solutricine Tetracaine; Tyrcine; ***Ger.:*** Acoin; Biofenicol-N†; Bronchovydrin†; Brox-Aerosol N†; Dexa-Biofenicol-N†; Dynexan†; Furacin-Otalgicum†; Gingicaine D; Herviros; Incut†; Ophtocain; Para Muc†; Sprucaine Spray†; Targophagin†; ***Irl.:*** Norgotin†; ***Ital.:*** Corizzina; Donalg; Lasoproct; Recto-Reparil; Ruscoroid; Uretral†; ***S.Afr.:*** Dynexan; Pernicream†; ***Spain:*** Anesti Doble; Anestina Braun; Angicola†; Blastoestimulina; Carbocaina; Cortison Chemicetina†; Dentikrisos; Neocones; Otocusi Enzimatico†; Otogen Calmante; Resorborina; Topicaina; Topicaina Miro†; Vinciseptil Otico; ***Switz.:*** Adrectal; Angidine; Collunosol†; Diabetosan†; Dynexan; Eludril; Mucosan†; Neocones; Stomaqualine†; Tonex; Tonexol†; Tyrothricine + Gramicidine; ***UK:*** Eludril; ***USA:*** Cetacaine; Stypto-Caine.

Amylocaine Hydrochloride (7605-q)

Amylocaine Hydrochloride *(BANM)*.

Amyleinii Chloridum; Amylocain. Hydrochlor.; Chlorhydrate d'Amyléine. 1-(Dimethylaminomethyl)-1-methylpropyl benzoate hydrochloride.

$C_{14}H_{21}NO_2,HCl = 271.8.$

CAS — 644-26-8 (amylocaine hydrochloride); 532-59-2 (amylocaine hydrochloride).

Pharmacopoeias. In Belg.

Amylocaine, a benzoic acid ester, is a local anaesthetic (p.1281) used mainly as the hydrochloride in a range of preparations for application to the skin or mucous membranes. It has also been used in preparations for the relief of painful anorectal conditions and has been included in oral mixtures for the relief of coughs.

Preparations

Proprietary Preparations (details are given in Part 3)

Multi-ingredient: ***Belg.:*** Babygencal; Dentophar; Dequalinium; Glottyl†; Rectovasol; Tablettes pour la Gorge Medica†; ***Canad.:*** Pommade Midy; Rhino-Mex; ***Fr.:*** Anolan†; Arpha†; Artralgon; Avenoc; Biphedrine Aqueuse†; Bronchodermine; Buccawalter; Campho-Pneumine; Chloridia†; Collustan; Dolodent; Elenol; Frazoline; Glottyl; Humex†; Hyalurectal†; Migralgine; Parkipan; Pastilles M.B.C†; Pholcones; Pommade Midy†; Pulmoll; Suppositoires Midy†; ***Ital.:*** Dentinale; Proctosedyl; Rinoleina Adulti†; ***Spain:*** Eucalyptospirine; Eucalyptospirine Lact; Hemodren Compuesto; Sanovox†; ***Switz.:*** Stix†.

Benzocaine (7608-w)

Benzocaine *(BAN, rINN)*.

Anaesthesinum; Anesthamine; Benzocainum; Ethoform; Éthoforme; Ethyl Aminobenzoate; Ethylis Aminobenzoas. Ethyl 4-aminobenzoate.

$C_9H_{11}NO_2 = 165.2.$

CAS — 94-09-7.

Pharmacopoeias. In *Chin., Eur.* (see p.viii), *Int., Jpn, Pol.,* and *US.*

Colourless or white crystals or a white odourless crystalline powder. M.p. 88° to 92°. **Soluble** 1 in 2500 of water, 1 in 5 of alcohol, 1 in 2 of chloroform, and 1 in 4 of ether; dissolves in dilute acids; soluble 1 in 30 to 50 of almond oil or olive oil. **Protect** from light.

Adverse Effects and Treatment

As for Local Anaesthetics in general, p.1281.

Hypersensitivity. The incidence of positive reactions in patients patch tested with benzocaine has ranged from 3.3 to 5.9%.[1,2] Patch testing with benzocaine has been recommended by The International Contact Dermatitis Research Group as an indicator of contact hypersensitivity to local anaesthetics. However, Beck and Holden[3] found that of 40 patients who had had positive reactions to benzocaine with amethocaine and cinchocaine 21 were not allergic to benzocaine alone.

1. Rudzki E, Kleniewska D. The epidemiology of contact dermatitis in Poland. *Br J Dermatol* 1970; **83:** 543–5.
2. Bandmann H-J, *et al.* Dermatitis from applied medicaments. *Arch Dermatol* 1972; **106:** 335–7.
3. Beck MH, Holden A. Benzocaine—an unsatisfactory indicator of topical local anaesthetic sensitization for the UK. *Br J Dermatol* 1988; **118:** 91–4.

Precautions

As for Local Anaesthetics in general, p.1282.

Interactions

For interactions associated with local anaesthetics, see p.1283.

Pharmacokinetics

See under Local Anaesthetics, p.1283.

Uses and Administration

Benzocaine, a para-aminobenzoic acid ester, is a local anaesthetic used for surface anaesthesia (p.1284); it has low potency and systemic toxicity. It is used, often in combination with other drugs such as analgesics, antiseptics, antibacterials, antifungals, and antipruritics, for the temporary local relief of pain associated with dental conditions, oropharyngeal disorders, haemorrhoids, anal pruritus, and ear pain.

Lozenges containing benzocaine in usual doses of up to 10 mg are used for the relief of sore throat. Gels, pastes, solutions, and sprays containing benzocaine in concentrations of up to 20% have been used for surface anaesthesia of the mouth and throat.

Benzocaine is used in ear drops, creams, ointments, lotions, solutions, sprays, gels, and suppositories in concentrations up to 20% for topical analgesia and anaesthesia.

Benzocaine has also been used as the hydrochloride.

Obesity. It has been reported[1] that despite the inclusion of benzocaine in some over-the-counter appetite suppressants there is no good evidence of its value in obesity. The usual strategies for the treatment of obesity are discussed on p.1476.

1. Anonymous. A nasal decongestant and a local anesthetic for weight control? *Med Lett Drugs Ther* 1979; **21:** 65–6.

Preparations

USP 23: Antipyrine and Benzocaine Otic Solution; Antipyrine, Benzocaine, and Phenylephrine Hydrochloride Otic Solution; Benzocaine and Menthol Topical Aerosol; Benzocaine Cream; Benzocaine Gel; Benzocaine Lozenges; Benzocaine Ointment; Benzocaine Otic Solution; Benzocaine Topical Aerosol; Benzocaine Topical Solution; Benzocaine, Butamben, and Tetracaine Hydrochloride Gel; Benzocaine, Butamben, and Tetracaine Hydrochloride Ointment; Benzocaine, Butamben, and Tetracaine Hydrochloride Topical Aerosol; Benzocaine, Butamben, and Tetracaine Hydrochloride Topical Solution.

Proprietary Preparations (details are given in Part 3)
Aust.: Anaestherit; ***Austral.:*** Applicaine; Topicaine; ***Canad.:*** Anbesol Baby; Baby Orajel; Orajel; Sirop Dentition; Teething Syrup†; Topicaine; ***Ger.:*** Anaesthesierende Salbe†; Anaesthesin; Flavamed Halstabletten; Subcutin N; Zahnerol N; ***Ital.:*** Gengivarium; ***Spain:*** Dentispray; Hurricaine; Lanacane; ***Switz.:*** Orajel; ***UK:*** Burneze; Lanacane; Vicks Ultra Chloraseptic; ***USA:*** 3 in 1 Toothache Relief; Americaine Anesthetic; Americaine Anesthetic Lubricant; Baby Anbesol; Baby Orajel; BanSmoke; Benzocol†; Benzodent; Chigger-Tox; Dent's Extra Strength Toothache Gum; Dent's Lotion-Jel; Dent's Maximum Strength Toothache Drops; Dermoplast; Detane; Diet Ayds; Hurricaine; Lanacane; Medamint†; Mycinettes; Numzident; Orabase Baby; Orabase Gel; Orabase-B; Orajel; Oratect†; Otocain; Red Cross Canker Sore Medication; SensoGARD; Slim Mint; Spec-T; Trocaine; Unguentine†; Vicks Children's Chloraseptic; Zilabrace†; Zilactin-B Medicated; ZilaDent†.

Multi-ingredient: numerous preparations are listed in Part 3.

Bucricaine Hydrochloride (3391-d)

Bucricaine Hydrochloride *(rINNM)*.

Centbucridine (base or hydrochloride). 9-(Butylamino)-1,2,3,4-tetrahydroacridine monohydrochloride.

$C_{17}H_{22}N_2,HCl = 290.8.$

CAS — 316-15-4 (bucricaine); 76958-83-3 (bucricaine hydrochloride); 82636-28-0 (bucricaine hydrochloride).

Bucricaine is a local anaesthetic that has been applied topically for surface anaesthesia of the eye and given by injection for infiltration anaesthesia, peripheral nerve blocks, and spinal block.

References.

1. Vacharajani GN, *et al.* A comparative study of centbucridine and lidocaine in dental extraction. *Int J Clin Pharmacol Res* 1983; **3:** 251–5.
2. Dasgupta D, *et al.* Randomised double-blind study of centbucridine and lignocaine for subarachnoid block. *Indian J Med Res* 1983; **77:** 512–16.

Bupivacaine Hydrochloride (7609-e)

Bupivacaine Hydrochloride *(BANM, USAN, rINNM)*.

AH-2250; Bupivcaini Hydrochloridum; LAC-43; Win-11318. (±)-(1-Butyl-2-piperidyl)formo-2',6'-xylidide hydrochloride monohydrate.

$C_{18}H_{28}N_2O,HCl,H_2O = 342.9.$

CAS — 2180-92-9 (bupivacaine); 18010-40-7 (bupivacaine hydrochloride, anhydrous); 14252-80-3 (bupivacaine hydrochloride, monohydrate).

Pharmacopoeias. In *Chin., Eur.* (see p.viii), *Int., Pol.,* and *US.*

A white odourless crystalline powder or colourless crystals. Freely **soluble** to soluble in water; freely soluble in alcohol; slightly soluble in acetone and in chloroform. A 1% solution in water has a pH of 4.5 to 6.0. **Protect** from light.

Stability of solutions. For a discussion of the effect that pH has on the stability of local anaesthetic solutions and the pain associated with their injection, see p.1284.

For reference to the stability of admixtures of bupivacaine and fentanyl in solution, with or without adrenaline, see under Fentanyl Citrate, p.38.

Adverse Effects and Treatment

As for Local Anaesthetics in general, p.1281.

Bupivacaine appears to be more cardiotoxic than other local anaesthetics. Cardiac arrest due to bupivacaine can be resistant to electrical defibrillation and a successful outcome may require prolonged resuscitative efforts.

For reference to the toxic threshold for bupivacaine plasma concentrations, see Absorption under Pharmacokinetics, below.

Effects on the cardiovascular system. Bupivacaine[1,2] and etidocaine[2] appear to be more cardiotoxic than most other commonly used local anaesthetics and marked cardiovascular depression may occur at plasma concentrations only slightly above those for CNS toxicity.[2] Fatalities have occurred. Simultaneous seizures and cardiovascular collapse may develop rapidly following inadvertent intravascular injection and even prompt oxygenation and blood pressure support might not prevent cardiac arrest.[2] Ventricular fibrillation which is very resistant to normal methods of defibrillation may develop. Since lignocaine and the other local anaesthetics have additive effects on the CNS bretylium may be preferable to lignocaine for the treatment of induced arrhythmias.[1] Fatal cardiotoxicity has occurred following the use of bupivacaine in intravenous regional anaesthesia, possibly due to leakage past the tourniquet, and the use of bupivacaine in this technique should be avoided.[1] Fatalities have also been associated with the use of 0.75% solutions for epidural anaesthesia in obstetric patients and this strength is no longer recommended for obstetric anaesthesia. See also Labour Pain under Uses and Administration, below.

1. Anonymous. Cardiotoxicity of local anaesthetic drugs. *Lancet* 1986; **ii:** 1192–4.
2. Albright GA. Cardiac arrest following regional anesthesia with etidocaine or bupivacaine. *Anesthesiology* 1979; **51:** 285–7.

Effects on the eyes. Bilateral retinal haemorrhages developed in a 47-year-old woman[1] after receiving a caudal block with bupivacaine 0.5%. The haemorrhages cleared and her usual vision returned by 3 months.

1. Ling C, *et al.* Bilateral retinal haemorrhages following epidural injection. *Br J Ophthalmol* 1993; **77:** 316—17.

Prolonged block. Reports of prolonged block following the use of bupivacaine in regional anaesthesia.[1,2]

1. Pathy GV, Rosen M. Prolonged block with recovery after extradural analgesia for labour. *Br J Anaesth* 1975; **47:** 520–2.
2. Brockway MS, *et al.* Prolonged brachial plexus block with 0.42% bupivacaine. *Br J Anaesth* 1989; **63:** 604–5.

Precautions

As for Local Anaesthetics in general, p.1282.

Bupivacaine is contra-indicated for use in intravenous regional anaesthesia (Bier's block) and for paracervical block in obstetrics. The 0.75% solution is contra-indicated for epidural block in obstetrics.

Porphyria. Bupivacaine is thought to be safe for use in patients with acute porphyrias.[1] The course of anaesthesia was uneventful in one patient with acute intermittent porphyria who was given spinal bupivacaine for caesarean section.[2]

1. Moore MR, McColl KEL. *Porphyria: drug lists.* Glasgow Porphyria Research Unit, University of Glasgow, 1991.
2. McNeill MJ, Bennet A. Use of regional anaesthesia in a patient with acute porphyria. *Br J Anaesth* 1990; **64:** 371–3.

Renal impairment. Spinal block after the administration of 3 mL bupivacaine 0.75% was reported to be more rapid in onset and of shorter duration in patients with chronic renal failure when compared with control patients.[1]

1. Orko R, *et al.* Subarachnoid anaesthesia with 0.75% bupivacaine in patients with chronic renal failure. *Br J Anaesth* 1986; **58:** 605–9.

Interactions

For interactions associated with local anaesthetics, see p.1283.

Antiarrhythmics. There is an increased risk of myocardial depression when bupivacaine and antiarrhythmics are administered concomitantly.

Beta blockers. *Propranolol* reduced the clearance of bupivacaine by 35% in 6 healthy subjects.[1] There is therefore the risk of increased bupivacaine toxicity if these 2 drugs are administered concomitantly.

1. Bowdle TA, *et al.* Propranolol reduces bupivacaine clearance. *Anesthesiology* 1987; **66:** 36–8.

Histamine H_2-receptor antagonists. Studies of the effect of H_2-receptor antagonists on the pharmacokinetics of bupivacaine have yielded variable results. While one group of workers[1] found that pretreatment with *cimetidine* decreased the clearance of bupivacaine others have failed to find any significant pharmacokinetic effects.[2,3] Similarly pretreatment with *ranitidine* has either increased plasma concentrations of bupivacaine[4] or had no significant effect.[3]

1. Noble DW, *et al.* Effects of H-2 antagonists on the elimination of bupivacaine. *Br J Anaesth* 1987; **59:** 735–7.
2. Pihlajamäki KK. Lack of effect of cimetidine on the pharmacokinetics of bupivacaine in healthy subjects. *Br J Clin Pharmacol* 1988; **26:** 403–6.
3. Flynn RJ, *et al.* Does pretreatment with cimetidine and ranitidine affect the disposition of bupivacaine? *Br J Anaesth* 1989; **62:** 87–91.
4. Wilson CM. Plasma bupivacaine concentrations associated with extradural anaesthesia for caesarean section: influence of pretreatment with ranitidine. *Br J Anaesth* 1986; **58:** 1330P–1331P.

Local anaesthetics. For reference to the effect of bupivacaine on the protein binding of lignocaine and mepivacaine respectively, see under Lignocaine, p.1294 and Mepivacaine, p.1297.

Pharmacokinetics

Bupivacaine is about 95% bound to plasma proteins. Reported half-lives are from 1.5 to 5.5 hours in adults and about 8 hours in neonates. It is metabolised in the liver and is excreted in the urine principally as metabolites with only 5 to 6% as unchanged drug.

Bupivacaine is distributed into breast milk in small quantities. It crosses the placenta but the ratio of fetal concentrations to maternal concentrations is relatively low. Bupivacaine also diffuses into the cerebrospinal fluid.

See also under Local Anaesthetics, p.1283.

Absorption. The toxic threshold for bupivacaine plasma concentrations is considered by some to lie in the range of 2 to 4 µg per mL[1] and in the UK the maximum single recommended dose for bupivacaine is 150 mg (equivalent to approximately 2 mg per kg body-weight). Administration of bupivacaine for regional anaesthesia of the head and neck in a mean total dose of 3.4 mg per kg body-weight has produced mean peak plasma concentrations of 3.56 and 4.95 µg per mL when administered with or without adrenaline respectively, without producing toxicity.[2] Similarly, intrapleural administration of bupivacaine 0.5% in a dose of 2.5 mg per kg has produced mean peak plasma concentrations of 2.57 and 3.22 µg per mL when given with or without adrenaline respectively without producing toxicity.[3] A further study[4] in which a 72-hour interpleural infusion of bupivacaine hydrochloride with adrenaline was administered to cholecystectomy patients showed appreciable interpatient variability in steady-state plasma drug concentrations (range 1.3 to 3.2 µg per mL; mean 2.1 µg per mL); no patient suffered any adverse effects. Bilateral intercostal nerve blocks using bupivacaine 2 mg per kg have also produced concentrations within the presumed toxic range without adverse effects but the use of adrenaline with this block did not reliably reduce peak plasma-bupivacaine concentrations.[5]

Stellate ganglion block with bupivacaine 0.25% has produced a mean peak plasma concentration of 0.34 and 0.47 µg per mL after doses of 10 or 20 mL respectively.[6] Administration of bupivacaine 0.5% in a dose of 3 mg per kg with or without adrenaline for sciatic and femoral nerve block produced mean peak plasma concentrations below 0.8 µg per mL.[7]

Bupivacaine is rapidly absorbed from the synovial membrane of the knee during arthroscopy but plasma concentrations did not exceed 350 ng per mL after controlled pressure-irrigation with isotonic solutions containing up to 200 mg.[8] Although one group of workers found that the maximum plasma concentrations of bupivacaine after intra-articular injection of 30 mL of a 0.5% solution for arthroscopy was 875 ng per mL they suggested that adrenaline should probably be added to minimise absorption.[9]

1. Tucker GT. Pharmacokinetics of local anaesthetics. *Br J Anaesth* 1986; **58:** 717–31.
2. Neill RS, Watson R. Plasma bupivacaine concentrations during combined regional and general anaesthesia for resection and reconstruction of head and neck carcinomata. *Br J Anaesth* 1984; **56:** 485–92.
3. Gin T, *et al.* Effect of adrenaline on venous plasma concentrations of bupivacaine after interpleural administration. *Br J Anaesth* 1990; **64:** 662–6.
4. Kastrissios H, *et al.* The disposition of bupivacaine following a 72h interpleural infusion in cholecystectomy patients. *Br J Clin Pharmacol* 1991; **32:** 251–4.
5. Bodenham A, Park GR. Plasma concentrations of bupivacaine after intercostal nerve block in patients after orthotopic liver transplantation. *Br J Anaesth* 1990; **64:** 436–41.
6. Hardy PAJ, Williams NE. Plasma concentrations of bupivacaine after stellate ganglion block using two volumes of 0.25% bupivacaine plain solution. *Br J Anaesth* 1990; **65:** 243–4.
7. Misra U, *et al.* Plasma concentrations of bupivacaine following combined sciatic and femoral 3 in 1 nerve blocks in open knee surgery. *Br J Anaesth* 1991; **66:** 310–13.
8. Debruyne D, *et al.* Monitoring serum bupivacaïne levels during arthroscopy. *Eur J Clin Pharmacol* 1985; **27:** 733–5.
9. Butterworth JF, *et al.* Effect of adrenaline on plasma concentrations of bupivacaine following intra-articular injection of bupivacaine for knee arthroscopy. *Br J Anaesth* 1990; **65:** 537–9.

SURFACE ANAESTHESIA. Studies of the absorption of bupivacaine following surface application.

1. McBurney A, *et al.* Absorption of lignocaine and bupivacaine from the respiratory tract during fibreoptic bronchoscopy. *Br J Clin Pharmacol* 1984; **17:** 61–6.

Pregnancy. Bupivacaine crosses the placenta to a lesser degree than lignocaine or mepivacaine following maternal injection. Values of 0.2 to 0.4 have been reported[1,2] for the ratio of fetal to maternal concentrations for bupivacaine compared with values of 0.5 to 0.7 quoted[2,3] for lignocaine and mepivacaine. The greater degree of protein-binding of bupivacaine compared with these other drugs not only limits the amount of bupivacaine available to cross the placenta but also reduces the relative amount of free drug in the fetal circulation[2] (see also under Protein Binding, below). Addition of adrenaline to the injection does not appear to affect the placental transfer rate of bupivacaine.[4] Measurement of a beta-phase half-life of 25 hours in the neonate compared with 1.25 hours in mothers suggests that the neonate is less able to metabolise bupivacaine.[5]

1. Denson DD, *et al.* Serum bupivacaine concentrations in term parturients following continuous epidural analgesia for labor and delivery. *Ther Drug Monit* 1984; **6:** 393–8.
2. Blogg CE, Simpson BR. Obstetric analgesia and the newborn baby. *Lancet* 1974; **i:** 1283.
3. Poppers PJ. Evaluation of local anaesthetic agents for regional anaesthesia in obstetrics. *Br J Anaesth* 1975; **47:** 322–7.
4. Reynolds F, *et al.* Effect of time and adrenaline on the feto-maternal distribution of bupivacaine. *Br J Anaesth* 1989; **62:** 509–14.
5. Caldwell J, *et al.* Pharmacokinetics of bupivacaine administered epidurally during childbirth. *Br J Clin Pharmacol* 1976; **3:** 956P–957P.

Protein binding. The two major binding proteins for bupivacaine in serum are α-1-acid glycoprotein, the influence of which is predominant at low concentrations, and albumin, which plays the major role at high concentrations. Reduction in pH from 7.4 to 7.0 decreases the affinity of the α_1-acid glycoprotein for bupivacaine but has no effect on albumin affinity.[1] Serum-protein binding of bupivacaine is reduced during pregnancy but it is considered that the increase in free bupivacaine concentrations is unlikely to cause a clinically significant increase in the risk of CNS or cardiovascular toxicity.[2] As fetal plasma contains little α_1-acid glycoprotein the binding capacity for bupivacaine is reduced and this may contribute to the difference between maternal and fetal plasma concentration at delivery[3] (see also under Pregnancy, above).

Ageing, uncomplicated by disease, does not affect the serum-protein binding of bupivacaine.[4]

1. Denson D, *et al.* Alpha$_1$-acid glycoprotein and albumin in human serum bupivacaine binding. *Clin Pharmacol Ther* 1984; **35:** 409–15.
2. Denson DD, *et al.* Bupivacaine protein binding in the term parturient: effects of lactic acidosis. *Clin Pharmacol Ther* 1984; **35:** 702–9.
3. Petersen MC, *et al.* Relationship between the transplacental gradients of bupivacaine and α_1-acid glycoprotein. *Br J Clin Pharmacol* 1981; **12:** 859–62.
4. Veering BT, *et al.* Age does not influence the serum protein binding of bupivacaine. *Br J Clin Pharmacol* 1991; **32:** 501–3.

Uses and Administration

Bupivacaine hydrochloride is a local anaesthetic of the amide type with actions and uses similar to those described on p.1283. It has a slow onset and a long duration of action. The speed of onset and duration of action are increased by the addition of a vasoconstrictor and absorption into the circulation from the site of injection is reduced. Doses of bupivacaine are expressed in terms of the anhydrous hydrochloride. Slow accumulation occurs with repeated doses. It is used mainly for infiltration and regional nerve blocks, particularly epidural block, but is contra-indicated for obstetric paracervical block and for use in intravenous regional anaesthesia (Bier's block). The 0.75% solution is contra-indicated for epidural block in obstetrics. (Local anaesthetic techniques are discussed on p.1284.) The carbonated solution of bupivacaine is also available in some countries for injection (see p.1284).

The concentration of bupivacaine solution used affects the extent of motor blockade achieved. A 0.25% solution generally produces incomplete motor block, a 0.5% solution will usually produce motor block and some muscle relaxation, and complete motor block and muscle relaxation can be achieved with a 0.75% solution. The dosage of bupivacaine used depends on the site of injection and the procedure used.

The manufacturers state that the maximum dose of bupivacaine hydrochloride is determined by the status of the patient and the site of injection. In the UK the suggested general maximum single dose is 150 mg followed if necessary by doses of up to 50 mg every 2 hours.

In the USA the recommended single maximum dose is 175 mg of plain bupivacaine hydrochloride or 225 mg when given with adrenaline; doses may be repeated at intervals of not less than 3 hours but the total daily dose should not exceed 400 mg.

The dose should be reduced in the elderly, in children, and in debilitated patients, and in cardiac or hepatic disease. A test dose of bupivacaine, preferably with adrenaline, should be given before commencing epidural block to detect inadvertent intravascular administration. Subsequent doses should be given in small increments.

For *infiltration anaesthesia* bupivacaine is used as a 0.25% solution in doses up to the recommended maximum (see above). When a longer duration of anaesthesia is required, as in dental or surgical procedures of the maxillary and mandibular area, a 0.5% solution with adrenaline 1 in 200 000 may be used in a dose of 9 mg (1.8 mL) per injection site. This dose may be repeated once after 2 to 10 minutes if needed, but a total dose of 90 mg (18 mL) should not be exceeded over a single dental sitting. For *peripheral nerve blocks* the usual dose is 12.5 mg (5 mL) as a 0.25% solution or 25 mg (5 mL) as a 0.5% solution. The usual recommended maximum single dose is 150 mg in the UK and 175 mg in the USA. For *sympathetic nerve block* 50 to 125 mg (20 to 50 mL) as a 0.25% solution is recommended. A 0.75% solution has been used for *ret-*

robulbar block in ophthalmic surgery in a dose of 15 to 30 mg (2 to 4 mL).

For *lumbar epidural block* in surgery a 0.25% solution may be used in a dose of 25 to 50 mg (10 to 20 mL) or as a 0.5% solution in a dose of 50 to 100 mg (10 to 20 mL). Lower doses of 15 to 30 mg (6 to 12 mL) as the 0.25% solution or 30 to 60 mg (6 to 12 mL) as the 0.5% solution have been recommended for analgesia during labour. A 0.75% solution is also used for induction of lumbar epidural block in non-obstetric surgery in a single dose of 75 to 150 mg (10 to 20 mL). For *caudal block* in surgery 37.5 to 75 mg (15 to 30 mL) as a 0.25% solution or 75 to 150 mg (15 to 30 mL) as a 0.5% solution may be used. For analgesia during labour a dose of 25 to 50 mg (10 to 20 mL) as a 0.25% solution or 50 to 100 mg (10 to 20 mL) as a 0.5% solution has been recommended. Solutions with or without adrenaline may be used for these procedures apart from dental infiltration, when adrenaline is added to the solution (see above).

Hyperbaric solutions of bupivacaine without adrenaline may be used for *spinal anaesthesia*. Preparations containing 0.5% are available and are given in doses of 10 to 20 mg (2 to 4 mL).

Bupivacaine is usually administered as a racemic mixture but the S(−)-isomer (levobupivacaine) is under investigation.

Reviews.

1. McClellan KJ, Spencer CM. Levobupivacaine. *Drugs* 1998; **56:** 355–62.

Action. Addition of potassium chloride 0.2 mmol to 40 mL of bupivacaine 0.25% solution resulted in a more rapid onset of sensory loss than the same dose of plain bupivacaine in patients undergoing brachial plexus block for forearm or hand surgery.[1]

Hyaluronidase did not increase the speed of onset of brachial plexus block produced by bupivacaine 0.5%, with or without adrenaline, but did reduce the duration of anaesthesia.[2]

Administration of bupivacaine encapsulated in liposomes can prolong postsurgical analgesic action without motor block.[3,4]

For a comparison of the vasoactivity of bupivacaine and some other local anaesthetics, see p.1284.

1. Parris MR, Chambers WA. Effects of the addition of potassium to prilocaine or bupivacaine: studies on brachial plexus blockade. *Br J Anaesth* 1986; **58:** 297–300.
2. Keeler JF, *et al.* Effect of addition of hyaluronidase to bupivacaine during axillary brachial plexus block. *Br J Anaesth* 1992; **68:** 68–71.
3. Boogaerts S, *et al.* Epidural administration of liposomal bupivacaine for the management of postsurgical pain. *Br J Anaesth* 1993; **70:** (suppl 1): 104.
4. Boogaerts JG, *et al.* Pharmacokinetic-pharmacodynamic specific behaviour of liposome-associated bupivacaine in humans. *Br J Anaesth* 1995; **74** (suppl 1): 74.

Administration in children. See under Intraoperative and Postoperative Pain, below.

Administration in renal impairment. For a report that the onset and duration of spinal anaesthesia with bupivacaine is altered in renal impairment, see under Precautions, above.

Intraoperative and postoperative pain. A 0.5% solution of bupivacaine has been instilled through an indwelling catheter in doses of 50 mg into surgical wounds to provide postoperative analgesia after splenectomy or cholecystectomy.[1] Injection of bupivacaine 0.5% in a dose of 100 mg with or without adrenaline has been used to produce paravertebral block for pain relief after cholecystectomy.[2-4] Bupivacaine administered intraperitoneally, however, appears to be ineffective in the management of post-cholecystectomy pain.[5,6]

Administration of bupivacaine 0.25% as a continuous infusion through a paravertebral catheter for pain relief after thoracotomy produced significantly less hypotension and urinary retention than epidural administration.[7] Continuous intercostal infusion of bupivacaine for pain relief after thoracotomy was also associated with a low incidence of complications, and provided an effective adjunct to systemic opioids.[8]

Bupivacaine has also been administered by continuous infusion in other peripheral nerve blocks to provide postoperative analgesia including intercostal nerve block[9,10] and brachial plexus block.[11,12] Solutions containing 0.5% have been administered intrapleurally in doses up to 2.5 mg per kg body-weight with adrenaline for operations on the trunk including cholecystectomy;[13,14] a 0.25% solution has also been tried similarly in doses of 25 mg for thoracotomy.[15]

Intra-abdominal instillation of bupivacaine 2 mg per kg body-weight has been found to shorten postoperative colonic adynamic ileus after abdominal surgery.[16] A 0.5% solution of bupivacaine administered in a dose of 5 mg into the vas deferens was effective in the prevention of acute pain and chronic discomfort following vasectomy.[17]

Use of bilateral local infiltration with bupivacaine 0.25% significantly reduced the incidence of wide complex extrasystoles associated with stimulation of the trigeminal nerve in patients undergoing third molar extraction under general anaesthesia.[18] Epidural administration of bupivacaine with an opioid analgesic has been tried for use in patient-controlled analgesia.[19] Addition of bupivacaine reduced the dose of fentanyl required for equivalent analgesia, but there was no demonstrable clinical benefit from using this combination compared with epidural fentanyl alone.[20]

The management of postoperative pain is discussed on p.11.

For details of the use of bupivacaine in ophthalmic surgery, see under Uses and Administration of Local Anaesthetics, p.1284.

1. Levack ID, *et al.* Abdominal wound perfusion for the relief of postoperative pain. *Br J Anaesth* 1986; **58:** 615–19.
2. Giesecke K, *et al.* Paravertebral block during cholecystectomy: effect on circulatory and hormonal responses. *Br J Anaesth* 1988; **61:** 652–6.
3. Kumar CM. Paravertebral block for post-cholecystectomy pain relief. *Br J Anaesth* 1989; **63:** 129.
4. Giesecke K. Paravertebral block for post-cholecystectomy pain relief. *Br J Anaesth* 1989; **63:** 129.
5. Thiry E, *et al.* Intraperitoneal bupivacaine does not reduce postoperative pain after laparoscopic cholecystectomy. *Br J Anaesth* 1994; **72** (suppl 1): 120.
6. Fuhrer Y, *et al.* Effects on postoperative pain and pharmacokinetics of intraperitoneal bupivacaine after laparoscopic cholecystectomy. *Br J Anaesth* 1995; **74** (suppl 1): 141.
7. Matthews PJ, Govenden V. Comparison of continuous paravertebral and extradural infusions of bupivacaine for pain relief after thoracotomy. *Br J Anaesth* 1989; **62:** 204–5.
8. Dryden CM, *et al.* Efficacy of continuous intercostal bupivacaine for pain relief after thoracotomy. *Br J Anaesth* 1993; **70:** 508–10.
9. Hashimi H, Stewart AL. Perceptions of pain relief after surgery. *Br Med J* 1990; **301:** 338.
10. Broka S, *et al.* Continuous intercostal analgesia and thoracic surgery. *Br J Anaesth* 1995; **74** (suppl 1): 141–2.
11. Rosenberg PH, *et al.* Plasma concentrations of bupivacaine and two of its metabolites during continuous interscalene brachial plexus block. *Br J Anaesth* 1991; **66:** 25–30.
12. Parikh RK, *et al.* Prolonged postoperative analgesia for arthrolysis of the elbow joint. *Br J Anaesth* 1995; **74:** 469–71.
13. Mogg GA, *et al.* Pharmacokinetics of interpleural bupivacaine in patients undergoing cholecystectomy. *Br J Anaesth* 1990; **64:** 657–61.
14. Gin T, *et al.* Effect of adrenaline on venous plasma concentrations of bupivacaine after interpleural administration. *Br J Anaesth* 1990; **64:** 662–6.
15. Debruyne D, *et al.* Clinical pharmacokinetics after repeated intrapleural bupivacaine administration. *Clin Pharmacokinet* 1990; **18:** 240–4.
16. Rimbäck G, et al. Effect of intra-abdominal bupivacaine instillation on postoperative colonic motility. *Gut* 1986; **27:** 170–5.
17. Paxton LD, *et al.* Intra-vas deferens bupivacaine for prevention of acute pain and chronic discomfort after vasectomy. *Br J Anaesth* 1995; **74:** 612–13.
18. Wilson IH, *et al.* Regional analgesia with bupivacaine in dental anaesthesia. *Br J Anaesth* 1986; **58:** 401–5.
19. Cooper DW, Turner G. Patient-controlled extradural analgesia to compare bupivacaine, fentanyl and bupivacaine with fentanyl in the treatment of postoperative pain. *Br J Anaesth* 1993; **70:** 503–7.
20. Cooper DW, *et al.* Patient-controlled extradural analgesia with bupivacaine, fentanyl, or a mixture of both, after Caesarean section. *Br J Anaesth* 1996; **76:** 611–15.

IN CHILDREN. Bupivacaine 0.25% injected intra-operatively up to a maximum dose of 1.5 mg per kg body-weight with adrenaline has been used in infants for the control of postoperative pain due to pyloromyotomy and appears to attenuate some of the cardiac and respiratory effects associated with the use of general anaesthesia alone.[1] Doses of 2.5 mg of bupivacaine per year of age administered as a 0.5% solution have been used for ilio-inguinal nerve block for analgesia in children undergoing herniotomy.[2] A study[3] in infants undergoing abdominal surgery found that an epidural infusion of bupivacaine produced comparable analgesia to an intravenous infusion of morphine. It was considered that bupivacaine might be preferable to morphine in neonates and young infants who are particularly prone to respiratory depression, but older children might require additional sedation or analgesia to prevent restlessness in the postoperative period.

1. McNicol LR, *et al.* Peroperative bupivacaine for pyloromyotomy pain. *Lancet* 1990; **335:** 54–5.
2. Smith BAC, Jones SEF. Analgesia after herniotomy in a paediatric day unit. Br Med J 1982; 285; 1466.
3. Wolf AR, Hughes D. Pain relief for infants undergoing abdominal surgery: comparison of infusions of IV morphine and extradural bupivacaine. *Br J Anaesth* 1993; **70:** 10–16.

Labour pain. For a discussion of the management of labour pain, including mention of the use of local anaesthetics, see p.9.

Crawford[1] found from experience in nearly 1000 patients that 8 mL of a 0.5% solution of bupivacaine with adrenaline was the optimum dose for epidural block during labour; pain relief lasted for about 2 hours. Decreasing the concentration of the final dose to 0.25% reduced the persistence of sensory and motor nerve block after delivery. Other workers[2] found that bupivacaine 0.375% was the most suitable concentration for epidural analgesia when using a regimen of regular 'top-up' doses of 0.5 mg per kg body-weight about every 90 minutes. However, the use of low doses of bupivacaine 0.25% for epidural analgesia in primiparous women was associated with a lower incidence of forceps delivery and oxytocin augmentation.[3] Although an even lower concentration of bupivacaine (0.0625%) used in combination with sufentanil[4] produced analgesia similar to that with 0.125% bupivacaine used alone, the duration of the second stage of labour and the incidence of instrumental and surgical delivery were not reduced. Similar results were obtained using bupivacaine 0.0625% with diamorphine 0.005%; in addition pruritus and drowsiness produced by diamorphine were considered to be troublesome in many patients.[5]

Intrathecal injections of bupivacaine with or without an opioid are sometimes used[6,7] with epidural injections to achieve a faster onset of analgesia and a reduced degree of motor block in the management of labour pain. Intrathecal injections containing bupivacaine have also been given alone[8,9] for the management of labour pain but the use of this route alone is usually associated with anaesthesia and management of postoperative pain in caesarean section. Bupivacaine has also been tried with lignocaine for epidural anaesthesia in caesarean section in order to reduce the dose of bupivacaine and minimise cardiotoxicity.[10]

1. Crawford JS. Lumbar epidural block in labour: a clinical analysis. *Br J Anaesth* 1972; **44:** 66–74.
2. Purdy G, *et al.* Continuous extradural analgesia in labour: comparison between "on demand" and regular "top-up" injections. *Br J Anaesth* 1987; **59:** 319–24.
3. Turner MJ, *et al.* Primiparous women using epidural analgesia. *Br Med J* 1990; **300:** 123.
4. Auroy Y, Benhamou D. Extradural analgesia for labour: 0.125% bupivacaine vs 0.0625% bupivacaine with 0.2 μg mL^{-1} sufentanil. *Br J Anaesth* 1995; **74** (suppl 1): 105–6.
5. Bailey CR, *et al.* diamorphine-bupivacaine mixture compared with plain bupivacaine for analgesia. *Br J Anaesth* 1994; **72:** 58–61.
6. Stacey RGW, *et al.* Single space combined spinal-extradural technique for analgesia in labour. *Br J Anaesth* 1993; **71:** 499–502.
7. Collis RE, *et al.* Randomised comparison of combined spinal-epidural and standard epidural analgesia in labour. *Lancet* 1995; **345:** 1413–16.
8. Kestin IG, *et al.* Analgesia for labour and delivery using incremental diamorphine and bupivacaine via a 32-gauge intrathecal catheter. *Br J Anaesth* 1992; **68:** 244–7.
9. McHale S, *et al.* Continuous subarachnoid infusion of 0.125% bupivacaine for analgesia during labour. *Br J Anaesth* 1992; **69:** 634–6.
10. Howell P, *et al.* Comparison of four local extradural anaesthetic solutions for elective Caesarean section. *Br J Anaesth* 1990; **65:** 648–53.

Preparations

BP 1998: Bupivacaine and Adrenaline Injection; Bupivacaine Injection;
USP 23: Bupivacaine Hydrochloride and Epinephrine Injection; Bupivacaine Hydrochloride in Dextrose Injection; Bupivacaine Hydrochloride Injection.

Proprietary Preparations (details are given in Part 3)
Aust.: Carboneural; Carbostesin; ***Austral.:*** Marcain; Marcain Spinal Heavy; ***Belg.:*** Marcaine; ***Canad.:*** Marcaine; Sensorcaine; ***Fr.:*** Marcaine; ***Ger.:*** Bucain; Carbostesin; ***Irl.:*** Marcain; ***Ital.:*** Bupiforan; Marcaina; ***Neth.:*** Marcaine; Marcaine glucose; ***Norw.:*** Marcain; ***S.Afr.:*** Macaine; Regibloc; ***Spain:*** Svedocain Sin Vasoconstr; ***Swed.:*** Marcain; ***Switz.:*** Carbostesin; ***UK:*** Marcain; ***USA:*** Marcaine; Sensorcaine.

Multi-ingredient: ***Austral.:*** Marcain plus Fentanyl; Marcain plus Pethidine.

Butacaine Sulphate (7610-b)

Butacaine Sulphate *(BANM, rINNM)*.

Butacain. Sulph.; Butacaine Sulfate. 3-Dibutylaminopropyl 4-aminobenzoate sulphate.

$(C_{18}H_{30}N_2O_2)_2,H_2SO_4 = 711.0.$

CAS — 149-16-6 (butacaine); 149-15-5 (butacaine sulphate).

Butacaine, a para-aminobenzoic acid ester, is a local anaesthetic (p.1281) used for surface anaesthesia. It has been used topically, as the sulphate, in solutions for dental pain and in ear and nasal drops.

Preparations

Proprietary Preparations (details are given in Part 3)

Multi-ingredient: ***Fr.:*** Relaxoddi; Rhinamide; ***Spain:*** Topicaina; Topicaina Mirot†.

Butanilicaine Hydrochloride (9855-a)

Butanilicaine Hydrochloride *(BANM, rINNM)*.

$C_{13}H_{19}ClN_2O,HCl = 291.2.$

CAS — 6027-28-7.

Butanilicaine Phosphate (7611-v)

Butanilicaine Phosphate *(BANM, rINNM)*.

$C_{13}H_{19}ClN_2O,H_3PO_4 = 352.8.$

CAS — 2081-65-4.

Butanilicaine is an amide local anaesthetic (p.1281) that has been used for infiltration or nerve block anaesthesia.

Preparations

Proprietary Preparations (details are given in Part 3)
Ger.: Hostacain†.

Butoxycaine Hydrochloride (11333-y)

Butoxycaini Hydrochloridum. 2-Diethylaminoethyl-(*p*-butoxybenzoate) hydrochloride.

$C_{17}H_{27}NO_3,HCl = 329.9.$

CAS — 3772-43-8 (butoxycaine); 2350-32-5 (butoxycaine hydrochloride).

Butoxycaine, a para-aminobenzoic acid ester, is a local anaesthetic (p.1281) that has been used as the base or hydrochloride for surface anaesthesia.

Preparations

Proprietary Preparations (details are given in Part 3)
Ger.: Stadacain†.

Multi-ingredient: ***Ger.:*** Bismolan; Branolind L†; Hamo-ratiopharm; Mastu NH†; Stas Halstabletten†.

Butyl Aminobenzoate (7613-q)

Butamben *(USAN)*; Butoforme. Butyl 4-aminobenzoate.

$C_{11}H_{15}NO_2 = 193.2.$

CAS — 94-25-7.

Pharmacopoeias. In *Fr.* and *US.*

A white, odourless, crystalline powder. M.p. 57° to 59°. **Soluble** 1 in 7000 of water; soluble in alcohol, in ether, in chloroform, in fixed oils, and in dilute acids. It slowly hydrolyses when boiled with water.

Butyl Aminobenzoate Picrate (9857-x)

Abbott-34842; Butamben Picrate *(USAN)*.

$(C_{11}H_{15}NO_2)_2.C_6H_3N_3O_7 = 615.6.$

CAS — 577-48-0.

Butyl aminobenzoate, a para-aminobenzoic acid ester, is a local anaesthetic (p.1281) that has been used for surface anaesthesia of the skin and mucous membranes. It has also been used for relief of pain and pruritus associated with anorectal disorders.

Butyl aminobenzoate picrate is applied to the skin as a 1% ointment.

Preparations

USP 23: Benzocaine, Butamben, and Tetracaine Hydrochloride Gel; Benzocaine, Butamben, and Tetracaine Hydrochloride Ointment; Benzocaine, Butamben, and Tetracaine Hydrochloride Topical Aerosol; Benzocaine, Butamben, and Tetracaine Hydrochloride Topical Solution; Erythromycin Ethylsuccinate Injection.

Proprietary Preparations (details are given in Part 3)
USA: Butesin Picrate.

Multi-ingredient: ***Austral.:*** Butesin Picrate; ***Belg.:*** Nestosyl; ***Fr.:*** Ginkor Procto; Nestosyl; Preparation H; Rhino-Sulforgan†; Tyrothricine Lafran; ***Spain:*** Alvogil; Topicaina; ***Switz.:*** Alvogyl; ***USA:*** Cetacaine.

Carticaine Hydrochloride (7614-p)

Carticaine Hydrochloride *(BANM)*.

Articaine Hydrochloride *(rINNM)*; 40 045; Hoe-045. Methyl 4-methyl-3-(2-propylaminopropionamido)thiophene-2-carboxylate hydrochloride.

$C_{13}H_{20}N_2O_3S,HCl = 320.8.$

CAS — 23964-58-1 (carticaine); 23964-57-0 (carticaine hydrochloride).

Carticaine hydrochloride is an amide local anaesthetic (p.1281). It has been used as a 1 or 2% solution with or without adrenaline for infiltration and regional anaesthesia. A 4% solution of carticaine hydrochloride with adrenaline is used similarly in dentistry. A 5% hyperbaric solution of carticaine hydrochloride with glucose has been used for spinal anaesthesia.

Preparations

Proprietary Preparations (details are given in Part 3)
Aust.: Ubistesin; Ultracain Dental; ***Canad.:*** Ultracaine D-S; ***Fr.:*** Alphacaine; ***Ger.:*** Ubistesin; Ultracain; Ultracain D-S; Ultracain Hyperbar; Ultracain-Suprarenin; ***Ital.:*** Citocartin; Septanest; Ultracain D-S; ***Neth.:*** Ultracain D-S; Ultracain Hyperbaar; ***Switz.:*** Rudocaine; Septanest; Ubistesin; Ultracaine D-S.

Chloroprocaine Hydrochloride (7615-s)

Chloroprocaine Hydrochloride *(rINNM)*.

2-Diethylaminoethyl 4-amino-2-chlorobenzoate hydrochloride.

$C_{13}H_{19}ClN_2O_2,HCl = 307.2.$

CAS — 133-16-4 (chloroprocaine); 3858-89-7 (chloroprocaine hydrochloride).

Pharmacopoeias. In *US.*

A white odourless crystalline powder. **Soluble** 1 in 20 of water and 1 in 100 of alcohol; very slightly soluble in chloroform; practically insoluble in ether. Solutions in water are acid to litmus. Discoloured solutions should not be used.

pH of solutions. For a discussion of the effect that pH has on the stability of local anaesthetic solutions and the pain associated with their injection, see p.1284.

Adverse Effects, Treatment, and Precautions

As for Local Anaesthetics in general, p.1281.

Interactions

For interactions associated with local anaesthetics, see p.1283.

Pharmacokinetics

Chloroprocaine is hydrolysed rapidly in the circulation by plasma cholinesterase. It has a half-life of 19 to 26 seconds in adults. It is excreted in the urine mainly as metabolites.

See also under Local Anaesthetics, p.1283.

Uses and Administration

Chloroprocaine, a para-aminobenzoic acid ester, is a local anaesthetic with actions and uses similar to those described on p.1283. It has properties similar to those of procaine (p.1299). It has a rapid onset (6 to 12 minutes) and short duration (one hour) of action.

Chloroprocaine is used as the hydrochloride with or without preservative for infiltration and peripheral nerve block. Solutions without preservative may also be used for central nerve block including lumbar and caudal epidural blocks. It may be given, if necessary, with adrenaline 1 in 200 000 to delay absorption and reduce toxicity. Chloroprocaine is not an effective surface anaesthetic. It should not be used for spinal anaesthesia. (Local anaesthetic techniques are discussed on p.1284.)

The dosage of chloroprocaine used depends on the site of injection and the procedure used. For *mandibular nerve block* a 2% solution is used in a dose of 40 to 60 mg (2 to 3 mL) and for *infra-orbital nerve block* a dose of 10 to 20 mg (0.5 to 1.0 mL) as a 2% solution is used. A 2% solution is also used for *brachial plexus block* in a dose of 600 to 800 mg (30 to 40 mL). For *digital nerve block* a 1% solution without adrenaline is used in a dose of 30 to 40 mg (3 to 4 mL). In obstetrics a dose of 200 mg (10 mL) per side as a 2% solution is suggested for *pudendal block*, and for a *paracervical block* a 1% solution in a dose of 30 mg (3 mL) at each of 4 sites. For *lumbar epidural block* 40 to 50 mg (2.0 to 2.5 mL) as a 2% solution or 60 to 75 mg (2.0 to 2.5 mL) as a 3% solution is used for each segment to be anaesthetised, the usual total dose being 300 to 750 mg with smaller repeat doses being given at intervals of 40 to 50 minutes. For *caudal block* a dose of 300 to 500 mg (15 to 25 mL) of a 2% solution or 450 to 750 mg (15 to 25 mL) of a 3% solution may be given and repeated at intervals of 40 to 60 minutes.

In adults single doses of chloroprocaine hydrochloride without adrenaline should not exceed 800 mg and single doses with adrenaline 1 in 200 000 should not exceed 1 g.

Dosages should be reduced for children, elderly, and debilitated patients and those with cardiac disease. For children concentrations of 0.5 to 1.0% are suggested for infiltration and 1.0 to 1.5% for nerve block procedures.

Preparations

USP 23: Chloroprocaine Hydrochloride Injection.

Proprietary Preparations (details are given in Part 3)
Canad.: Nesacaine; ***Switz.:*** Ivracain; Nesacain; ***USA:*** Nesacaine.

Cinchocaine (7616-w)

Cinchocaine *(BAN, rINN)*.

Cincainum; Dibucaine. 2-Butoxy-*N*-(2-diethylaminoethyl)cinchoninamide; 2-Butoxy-*N*-(2-diethylaminoethyl)quinoline-4-carboxamide.

$C_{20}H_{29}N_3O_2 = 343.5.$

CAS — 85-79-0.

Pharmacopoeias. In *US.*

A white to off-white powder, with a slight characteristic odour. M.p. 62° to 66°. **Soluble** 1 in 4600 of water, 1 in 0.7 of alcohol, 1 in 0.5 of chloroform, and 1 in 1.4 of ether. It darkens on exposure to light. **Store** in airtight containers. Protect from light.

Cinchocaine Hydrochloride (7617-e)

Cinchocaine Hydrochloride *(BANM, rINNM)*.

Cincaini Chloridum; Cinchocaini Hydrochloridum; Dibucaine Hydrochloride; Dibucainium Chloride; Percainum; Sovcainum.

$C_{20}H_{29}N_3O_2,HCl = 379.9.$

CAS — 61-12-1.

NOTE. This compound was originally marketed under the name Percaine, but accidents occurred owing to the confusion of this name with procaine.

Pharmacopoeias. In *Eur.* (see p.viii), *Jpn*, and *US.*

Fine, colourless or white to off-white, odourless, crystals or white to off-white crystalline powder; it is hygroscopic. M.p. 96° to 100°. It agglomerates very easily. Very to freely **soluble** in water; freely soluble in alcohol, in acetone, in chloroform, and in dichloromethane. A 2% solution in water has a pH of 5.0 to 6.0. Cinchocaine hydrochloride darkens on exposure to light. **Store** in airtight containers. Protect from light.

Cinchocaine is an amide local anaesthetic (p.1281) that is now generally used for surface anaesthesia. It is one of the most potent and toxic of the long-acting local anaesthetics and its parenteral use was restricted to spinal anaesthesia.

For surface anaesthesia cinchocaine has been used, as the base or hydrochloride, in creams and ointments containing up to 1.0% and in suppositories for the temporary relief of pain and itching associated with skin and anorectal conditions. Cinchocaine benzoate has also been used topically.

Action. For a comparison of the vasoactivity of cinchocaine and some other local anaesthetics, see p.1284.

Determination of plasma cholinesterase activity. For mention of the use of cinchocaine in the determination of plasma cholinesterase activity, see under Precautions of Suxamethonium Chloride, p.1321.

Preparations

USP 23: Dibucaine Cream; Dibucaine Hydrochloride Injection; Dibucaine Ointment.

Proprietary Preparations (details are given in Part 3)

Aust.: Nupercainal†; ***Austral.:*** Nupercaine Heavy; ***Canad.:*** Nupercainal; ***Ger.:*** DoloPosterine N; ***Swed.:*** Cincain; ***Switz.:*** Nupercainal; ***UK:*** Nupercainal; ***USA:*** Nupercainal.

Multi-ingredient: ***Aust.:*** Ciloprin cum Anaesthetico; Scheriproct; Ultraproct; ***Austral.:*** Proctocort†; Proctosedyl; Scheriproct; Ultraproct; ***Belg.:*** Hemosedan; Scheriproct; Tri-histalex; Ultraproct; ***Canad.:*** Nupercainal; Proctosedyl; Proctosone; ***Fr.:*** Anti-Hemorroidaires; Deliproct; Ultraproct; ***Ger.:*** Anumedin; Faktu; Otobacid N; Procto-Kaban; Proctospre; Scheriproct; Ultraproct; ***Irl.:*** Proctosedyl; Scheriproct; Ultraproct; ***Ital.:*** Algolisina; Ultraproct; ***Neth.:*** Proctosedyl; Ultraproct†; ***Norw.:*** Proctosedyl; Scheriproct; ***S.Afr.:*** Cepacaine; Proctosedyl; Scheriproct; ***Spain:*** Anestesia Loc Braun S/A; Ruscus; Scheriproct; Ultraproct†; ***Swed.:*** Proctosedyl; Scheriproct N; ***Switz.:*** Ciloprine ca; Decatylene Neo; Faktu; Locaseptil-Neo; Locaseptil†; Proctosedyl†; Proctospre; Scheriproct; Ultraproct; ***UK:*** Proctosedyl; Scheriproct; Ultraproct; Uniroid; Uniroid-HC; ***USA:*** Corticaine.

Used as an adjunct in: ***Aust.:*** Butazolidin; Delta-Tomanol; ***Ger.:*** Butazolidin; ***Switz.:*** Butazolidine.

Clibucaine Hydrochloride (11598-z)

Clibucaine Hydrochloride *(rINNM)*.

2',4'-Dichloro-β-piperidinobutyranilide hydrochloride.

$C_{15}H_{20}Cl_2N_2O,HCl = 351.7.$

CAS — 15302-10-0 (clibucaine).

Clibucaine hydrochloride is an amide local anaesthetic (p.1281). It has been included in lozenges used for the treatment of mouth and throat disorders.

Preparations

Proprietary Preparations (details are given in Part 3)

Multi-ingredient: ***Switz.:*** Batramycine†.

Clormecaine Hydrochloride (14175-c)

Clormecaine Hydrochloride *(rINNM)*.

2-(Dimethylamino)-ethyl 3-amino-4-chlorobenzoate hydrochloride.

$C_{11}H_{15}ClN_2O_2,HCl = 279.2.$

CAS — 13930-34-2 (clormecaine).

Clormecaine hydrochloride, a meta-aminobenzoic acid ester, is a local anaesthetic (p.1281) that has been administered by mouth in conjunction with antacids for the symptomatic relief of peptic ulcer and gastric hyperacidity.

Preparations

Proprietary Preparations (details are given in Part 3)

Multi-ingredient: ***Ital.:*** Placacid†.

Coca (7618-l)

Coca Leaves; Hoja de Coca.

The dried leaves of *Erythroxylum coca* (Bolivian or Huanuco leaf) or of *E. truxillense* (Peruvian or Truxillo leaf) (Erythroxylaceae), indigenous to Bolivia and Peru and cultivated in Colombia and Indonesia.

Coca leaves contain about 0.7 to 1.5% of total alkaloids, of which cocaine, cinnamyl-cocaine, and α-truxilline are the most important.

Coca was formerly used for its stimulant action and for the relief of gastric pain, nausea, and vomiting, but it has no place in modern medicine. The practice of coca leaf chewing still continues in South America.

Cocaine (7619-y)

Cocaine *(BAN)*.

Cocaína; Methyl Benzoylecgonine. (*1R,2R,3s,5S*)-2-Methoxycarbonyltropan-3-yl benzoate.

$C_{17}H_{21}NO_4$ = 303.4.

CAS — 50-36-2.

NOTE. The following names have also been used to describe various forms of cocaine: basuco, bazooka, bernice, blow, C, charlie, coke, crack, flake, freebase, girl, gold dust, her, lady, leaf, nose candy, pasta, rock, she, snow, space dust, toot, white girl, white lady.

Pharmacopoeias. In Br., It., and US.

Colourless to white crystals or white crystalline powder obtained from the leaves of *Erythroxylum coca* and other spp. of *Erythroxylum*, or by synthesis. M.p. 96° to 98°. It is slightly volatile. BP **solubilities** are: practically insoluble in water; freely soluble in alcohol and in ether; very soluble in chloroform; soluble in arachis oil; slightly soluble in liquid paraffin. USP solubilities are: soluble 1 in 600 of water, 1 in 7 of alcohol, 1 in 1 of chloroform, 1 in 3.5 of ether, 1 in 12 of olive oil, 1 in 80 to 100 of liquid paraffin. A saturated solution in water is alkaline to phenolphthalein or litmus. **Protect** from light.

Cocaine Hydrochloride (7620-g)

Cocaine Hydrochloride *(BANM)*.

Chloridrato de Cocaína; Cocaine Hydrochlor.; Cocaini Hydrochloridum; Cocainium Chloratum.

$C_{17}H_{21}NO_4$,HCl = 339.8.

CAS — 53-21-4.

NOTE. CCN is a code approved by the BP for use on single unit doses of eye drops containing cocaine hydrochloride where the individual containers may be too small to bear all the appropriate labelling information.

Pharmacopoeias. In Chin., Eur. (see p.viii), Jpn, Pol., and US.

Odourless hygroscopic colourless crystals or white crystalline powder. M.p. about 197° with decomposition. Cocaine hydrochloride 1.12 g is approximately equivalent to 1 g of cocaine. **Soluble** 1 in 0.5 of water, 1 in 3.5 of alcohol, and 1 in 15 of chloroform; soluble in glycerol; practically insoluble in ether. Solutions are adversely affected by alkalis. **Protect** from moisture and light.

Stability of solutions. A stability study[1] was conducted in response to queries over conflicting data on the incompatibility of cocaine hydrochloride solutions and phenol. Some pharmacists had reported that cocaine hydrochloride eye drops preserved with phenol had shown no sign of physical incompatibility. The BPC 1973 states that cocaine hydrochloride is incompatible with phenol but suggests that cocaine hydrochloride solutions may be preserved with chlorocresol. The study found that there was no sign of physical incompatibility in aqueous solutions containing cocaine hydrochloride 5% and phenol 0.5% stored for a year at temperatures of 0° to 37° but there was a fall in pH, greatest at the higher temperatures, which was suggestive of chemical change. It was recommended that such solutions should be stored in a cool place.

1. *PSGB Lab Report P/75/14* 1975.

Adverse Effects

As for Local Anaesthetics in general, p.1281, but cocaine differs from other local anaesthetics in that it acts as a potent indirect-acting sympathomimetic. It stimulates the CNS causing agitation, dilated pupils, tachycardia, hypertension, hallucinations, hypertonia, and hyperreflexia. Convulsions, coma, and metabolic acidosis may develop. Symptoms of CNS stimulation and sympathetic overactivity are very marked in overdosage with cocaine. A single dose of 1.2 g may be fatal, but some persons have a cocaine idiosyncrasy and severe toxicity may occur after doses of only 20 mg. Systemic absorption of small doses may slow the heart, but with increasing doses tachycardia, hypertension, and ventricular fibrillation occur.

Topical application of cocaine to the cornea can cause corneal damage with clouding, pitting, sloughing, and occasionally ulceration. Topical application to the nose or mouth has been reported to cause loss of smell and taste respectively.

Prolonged use of cocaine by nasal inhalation may cause mucosal damage or perforation of the nasal septum.

Excessive concentrations of cocaine should not be used topically as, in addition to risks of systemic toxicity following absorption, lasting local damage may occur.

Abuse. Cocaine abuse and its effects have been discussed in a number of reviews.[1-5]

Cocaine abuse was once only in the form of chewing of Coca leaves containing small amounts of cocaine but processing of the leaves has led to abuse with a variety of more dangerous preparations containing higher concentrations of cocaine.[6] Coca paste, produced by maceration of the leaves with petrol and sulphuric acid, contains about 40 to 90% of cocaine sulphate and is smoked with tobacco or cannabis. Treatment of coca paste with hydrochloric acid produces cocaine hydrochloride, which is abused by intravenous injection, either alone or with diamorphine, or by sniffing to achieve nasal absorption. Alkaloidal cocaine (cocaine base; 'freebase'), which is abused by smoking, is produced by treating cocaine hydrochloride with alkali, followed either by heating (to form 'crack' cocaine) or by extracting the base from ether or another organic solvent. The route of administration of cocaine determines the rate and extent of its absorption, although once absorbed, the pharmacokinetics are independent of route. The route of administration rather than the form of cocaine used is important in determining the abuse potential; intravenous cocaine hydrochloride and smoked cocaine base have a greater potential for abuse than intranasal cocaine hydrochloride because of their greater rapidity and intensity of effects. The psychological effects of cocaine abuse may be described by a cycle of initial euphoria followed by dysphoria and finally schizophreniform psychosis.[6,7] Euphoria may be accompanied by other symptoms of stimulation such as sexual arousal, anorexia, insomnia, hyperexcitability, loquacity, and grandiosity and users may appear manic. After a short time these feelings are replaced by symptoms of dysphoria including considerable anxiety, fear, depression, apathy, irritability, suspiciousness. Dysphoria may be ameliorated by repeated administration, so the user develops the need to take the drug continuously to feel relatively well, but repeated administration appears to diminish the intensity of the effects.[6] During euphoria and dysphoria users may experience a wide range of physical symptoms including palpitations, headache, dizziness, gastro-intestinal effects, hyperhidrosis, tremors, tachycardia, hypertension, fever, and myoclonic jerks. Seizures can also occur following repeated use. In chronic abusers psychological deterioration may eventually occur, resulting in loss of mental function, compulsive disorders, suicidal ideation, psychopathic disorders, and ultimately a psychosis resembling acute paranoid schizophrenia similar to that seen with amphetamines.[6,7] Symptoms may include paranoia, stereotyped behaviour, delusions, loss of impulse control, violence, and visual, olfactory, auditory, gustatory, and tactile hallucinations. Overdosage can result in death due to status epilepticus, hyperthermia, ventricular tachycardia, and cardiac or respiratory arrest.[6]

For further details of the adverse effects of cocaine abuse, including effects due to use during pregnancy, see below.

1. Johanson C-E, Fischman MW. The pharmacology of cocaine related to its abuse. *Pharmacol Rev* 1989; **41:** 3–52.
2. Warner EA. Cocaine abuse. *Ann Intern Med* 1993: **119:** 226–35.
3. Strang J, *et al.* Cocaine in the UK—1991. *Br J Psychiatry* 1993; **162:** 1–13.
4. Das G. Cocaine abuse in North America: a milestone in history. *J Clin Pharmacol* 1993; **33:** 296–310.
5. Hatsukami DK, Fischman MW. Crack cocaine and cocaine hydrochloride: are the differences myth or reality? *JAMA* 1996; **276:** 1580–8.
6. Arif A, ed. *Adverse health consequences of cocaine abuse.* Geneva: WHO, 1987.
7. Leikin JB, *et al.* Clinical features and management of intoxication due to hallucinogenic drugs. *Med Toxicol Adverse Drug Exp* 1989; **4:** 324–50.

EFFECTS ON THE BLOOD. References.

1. Leissinger CA. Severe thrombocytopenia associated with cocaine use. *Ann Intern Med* 1990; **112:** 708–10.

EFFECTS ON THE CARDIOVASCULAR SYSTEM. There appears to be no relationship between underlying heart disease and the risk of cocaine-induced cardiac effects and cardiac events can occur regardless of the route of abuse.[1] Cardiovascular toxicity due to cocaine may be related to individual sensitivity and therefore may not be predictable or dose dependent.[2] Patients with plasma cholinesterase deficiency are particularly at risk for sudden death.[3] Other risk factors for cardiovascular disease, such as cigarette smoking may exacerbate the cardiac toxicity of cocaine.[4,5] Cocaine blocks reuptake of catecholamines at adrenergic nerve endings and thus produces sympathetic stimulation of the cardiovascular system. Accumulation of catecholamines predisposes the myocardium to arrhythmias,[6] and sinus tachycardia, supraventricular or ventricular tachyarrhythmias, myocarditis, and sudden arrhythmic death may occur.[6-8] Severe hypertension can lead to cerebrovascular accidents and stroke has occurred even in young adults without other predisposing conditions.[9,10] Aortic dissection[11,12] and rupture of the aorta have also occurred.[3] Myocardial infarction and ischaemia have been associated with cocaine abuse[1,3,6] but self-limiting chest pain without signs of myocardial infarction also commonly occurs;[7] asymptomatic myocardial ischaemia manifesting as episodes of ST segment elevation has also been reported during withdrawal of cocaine.[13] The mechanism for these changes remains to be resolved but coronary vasospasm,[13] vasoconstriction,[14] coronary thrombosis,[15,16] and direct myocardiotoxicity[17] are among the suggested causes. Some workers[18] have found that the timing of the coronary vasoconstriction correlated with blood concentration of cocaine's active metabolites, benzoylecgonine and ethyl methyl ecgonine.

Vasoconstriction due to cocaine may also produce ischaemia in the fingers, toes, spinal cord,[7] kidneys,[19] spleen,[20] and intestines.[21] Other reported cardiovascular effects include dilated cardiomyopathy.[22]

1. VanDette JM, Cornish LA. Medical complications of illicit cocaine use. *Clin Pharm* 1989; **8:** 401–11.
2. Thadani PV. Cardiovascular toxicity of cocaine: underlying mechanisms. *J Appl Cardiol* 1990; **5:** 317–20.
3. Cregler LL, Mark H. Medical complications of cocaine abuse. *N Engl J Med* 1986; **315:** 1495–1500.
4. Moliterno DJ, *et al.* Coronary-artery vasoconstriction induced by cocaine, cigarette smoking, or both. *N Engl J Med* 1994; **330:** 454–9.
5. Higgins ST, *et al.* Influence of cocaine use on cigarette smoking. *JAMA* 1994; **272:** 1724.
6. Loper KA. Clinical toxicology of cocaine. *Med Toxicol Adverse Drug Exp* 1989; **4:** 174–85.
7. Anonymous. Acute reactions to drugs of abuse. *Med Lett Drugs Ther* 1990; **32:** 92–4.
8. Bauman JL, *et al.* Cocaine-related sudden cardiac death: a hypothesis correlating basic science and clinical observations. *J Clin Pharmacol* 1994; **34:** 902–11.
9. Kaku DA, Lowenstein DH. Emergence of recreational drug abuse as a major risk factor for stroke in young adults. *Ann Intern Med* 1990; **113:** 821–7.
10. Levine SR, *et al.* Cerebrovascular complications of the use of the "crack" form of alkaloidal cocaine. *N Engl J Med* 1990; **323:** 699–704.
11. Edwards J, Rubin RN. Aortic dissection and cocaine abuse. *Ann Intern Med* 1987; **107:** 779–80.
12. Jaffe BD, *et al.* Cocaine-induced coronary-artery dissection. *N Engl J Med* 1994; **330:** 510–11.
13. Nademanee K, *et al.* Myocardial ischemia during cocaine withdrawal. *Ann Intern Med* 1989; **111:** 876–80.
14. Lange RA, *et al.* Cocaine-induced coronary-artery vasoconstriction. *N Engl J Med* 1989; **321:** 1557–62.
15. Minor RL, *et al.* Cocaine-induced myocardial infarction in patients with normal coronary arteries. *Ann Intern Med* 1991; **115:** 797–806.
16. Kugelmass AD, Ware JA. Cocaine and coronary artery thrombosis. *Ann Intern Med* 1992; **116:** 776–7.
17. Peng S-K, *et al.* Direct cocaine cardiotoxicity demonstrated by endomyocardial biopsy. *Arch Pathol Lab Med* 1989; **113:** 842–5.
18. Brogan WC, *et al.* Recurrent coronary vasoconstriction caused by intranasal cocaine: possible role for metabolites. *Ann Intern Med* 1992; **116:** 556–61.
19. Sharff JA. Renal infarction associated with intravenous cocaine use. *Ann Emerg Med* 1984; **13:** 1145–7.
20. Novielli KD, Chambers CV. Splenic infarction after cocaine use. *Ann Intern Med* 1991; **114:** 251–2.
21. Freudenberger RS, *et al.* Intestinal infarction after intravenous cocaine administration. *Ann Intern Med* 1990; **113:** 715–16.
22. Chokshi SK, *et al.* Reversible cardiomyopathy associated with cocaine intoxication. *Ann Intern Med* 1989; **111:** 1039–40.

EFFECTS ON THE KIDNEYS. For reference to renal failure following rhabdomyolysis associated with cocaine abuse, see under Effects on the Muscles, below. There has been a report[1] of acute renal failure occurring in a 16-year-old girl secondary to cocaine abuse but without evidence of rhabdomyolysis.

For reference to renal infarction due to cocaine abuse, see under Effects on the Cardiovascular System, above.

1. Leblanc M, *et al.* Cocaine-induced acute renal failure without rhabdomyolysis. *Ann Intern Med* 1994; **121:** 721–2.

EFFECTS ON THE LUNGS. The abuse of cocaine by smoking the free base has resulted in a range of pulmonary complications not previously encountered with other methods of abuse for cocaine. Associated adverse effects have included pulmonary oedema, hypersensitivity pneumonitis, pulmonary haemorrhage, obliterative bronchiolitis, abnormalities of pulmonary function, pneumomediastinum, and pneumothorax.[1] Severe or life-threatening exacerbations of asthma have also been reported.[2]

1. Ettinger NA, *et al.* A review of the respiratory effects of smoking cocaine. *Am J Med* 1989; **87:** 664–8.
2. Rubin RB, Neugarten J. Cocaine-associated asthma. *Am J Med* 1990; **88:** 438–9.

EFFECTS ON THE MOUTH. Gingival necrosis following local application of cocaine to the gingivae has been reported in 2 patients.[1]

1. Parry J, *et al.* Mucosal lesions due to oral cocaine use. *Br Dent J* 1996; **180:** 462–4.

EFFECTS ON THE MUSCLES. Rhabdomyolysis, sometimes progressing to renal failure, has been associated with free-base smoking or injection of cocaine hydrochloride.[1-3]

1. Roth D, *et al.* Acute rhabdomyolysis associated with cocaine intoxication. *N Engl J Med* 1988; **319:** 673–7.
2. Herzlich BC, *et al.* Rhabdomyolysis related to cocaine abuse. *Ann Intern Med* 1988; **109:** 335–6.
3. Pogue VA, Nurse HM. Cocaine-associated acute myoglobinuric renal failure. *Am J Med* 1989; **86:** 183–6.

EFFECTS ON SEXUAL FUNCTION. While the initial euphoria of cocaine abuse may be accompanied by sexual arousal, sexual dysfunction can occur[1] and male infertility has been reported.[2]

1. Cregler LL, Mark H. Medical complications of cocaine abuse. *N Engl J Med* 1986; **315:** 1495–1500.
2. Bracken MB, *et al.* Association of cocaine use with sperm concentration, motility, and morphology. *Fertil Steril* 1990; **53:** 315–22.

OVERDOSAGE. References to fatal overdosage from cocaine abuse.

1. Mittleman RE, Wetli CV. Death caused by recreational cocaine use. *JAMA* 1984; **252:** 1889–93.
2. Cowart V. National concern about drug abuse brings athletes under unusual scrutiny. *JAMA* 1986; **256:** 2457–65.
3. Greenland VC, *et al.* Vaginally administered cocaine overdose in a pregnant woman. *Obstet Gynecol* 1989; **74:** 476–7.

PREGNANCY AND BREAST FEEDING. The effects of cocaine abuse during pregnancy have been reviewed.[1-3] Women who abuse cocaine during pregnancy appear to have an increased risk of spontaneous abortion,[4] abruptio placentae[5,6] and associated still-births,[7] premature labour,[8-10] and other birth complications.[8-10] These effects may be due to vasoconstriction by cocaine increasing maternal blood pressure and reducing placental blood flow.[11] Uterine rupture[12] during pregnancy and rupture of ectopic pregnancies[13] have also been associated with cocaine. Neonates born to mothers abusing cocaine have an increased risk of intra-uterine growth retardation and may have lower birth-weight, smaller head size, and shorter length.[5,7-9,14-16] Cocaine is possibly teratogenic and congenital abnormalities associated with abuse include cardiovascular abnormalities,[9,17,18] limb reduction defects,[19] intestinal atresia or infarction,[19] skull defects,[7] and genito-urinary tract anomalies.[20] Neurobehavioural impairment[21] and signs of transient CNS irritability[22] may also occur. Some workers[23,24] have found effects on cognition and motor delays while others have found effects on arousal and attention regulation rather than cognitive processes.[25] Cocaine can increase neonatal cerebral blood flow[26] and cerebral infarction and associated seizures have occurred in neonates whose mothers took cocaine near to the onset of labour.[27] Evidence on the risk of intraventricular haemorrhage is conflicting.[6,23]

Acute intoxication has been reported in a breast-fed child whose mother was using cocaine intranasally.[28]

1. Slutsker L. Risks associated with cocaine use during pregnancy. *Obstet Gynecol* 1992; **79:** 778–89.
2. Volpe JJ. Effects of cocaine use on the fetus. *N Engl J Med* 1992; **327:** 399–407. Correction. *ibid.*; 1039.
3. Wiggins RC. Pharmacokinetics of cocaine in pregnancy and effects on fetal maturation. *Clin Pharmacokinet* 1992; **22:** 85–93.
4. Chasnoff IJ, *et al.* Cocaine use in pregnancy. *N Engl J Med* 1985; **315:** 666–9.
5. Dombrowski MP, *et al.* Cocaine abuse is associated with abruptio placentae and decreased birth weight, but not shorter labor. *Obstet Gynecol* 1991; **77:** 139–41.
6. Dusick AM, *et al.* Risk of intracranial hemorrhage and other adverse outcomes after cocaine exposure in a cohort of 323 very low birth weight infants. *J Pediatr* 1993; **122:** 438–45.
7. Bingol N, *et al.* Teratogenicity of cocaine in humans. *J Pediatr* 1987; **110:** 93–6.
8. Mastrogiannis DS, *et al.* Perinatal outcome after recent cocaine usage. *Obstet Gynecol* 1990; **76:** 8–11.
9. Little BB, *et al.* Cocaine abuse during pregnancy: maternal and fetal implications. *Obstet Gynecol* 1989; **73:** 157–60.
10. Spence MR, *et al.* The relationship between recent cocaine use and pregnancy outcome. *Obstet Gynecol* 1991; **78:** 326–9.
11. Farrar HC, Kearns GL. Cocaine: clinical pharmacology and toxicology. *J Pediatr* 1989; **115:** 665–75.
12. Gonsoulin W, *et al.* Rupture of unscarred uterus in primigravid woman in association with cocaine abuse. *Am J Obstet Gynecol* 1990; **163:** 526–7.
13. Thatcher SS, *et al.* Cocaine use and acute rupture of ectopic pregnancies. *Obstet Gynecol* 1989; **74:** 478–9.
14. Zuckerman B, *et al.* Effects of maternal marijuana and cocaine use on fetal growth. *N Engl J Med* 1989; **320:** 762–8.
15. Chasnoff IJ, *et al.* Temporal patterns of cocaine use in pregnancy: perinatal outcome. *JAMA* 1989; **261:** 1741–4.
16. Little BB, Snell LM. Brain growth among fetuses exposed to cocaine in utero: asymmetrical growth retardation. *Obstet Gynecol* 1991; **77:** 361–4.
17. Lipshultz SE, *et al.* Cardiovascular abnormalities in infants prenatally exposed to cocaine. *J Pediatr* 1991; **118:** 44–51.
18. Shaw GM, *et al.* Maternal use of cocaine during pregnancy and congenital cardiac anomalies. *J Pediatr* 1991; **118:** 167–8.
19. Hoyme HE, *et al.* Prenatal cocaine exposure and fetal vascular disruption. *Pediatrics* 1990; **85:** 743–7.
20. Chávez GF, *et al.* Maternal cocaine use during early pregnancy as a risk factor for congenital urogenital anomalies. *JAMA* 1989; **262:** 795–8.
21. Singer LT, *et al.* Neurobehavioural sequelae of fetal cocaine exposure. *J Pediatr* 1991; **119:** 667–72.
22. Doberczak TM, *et al.* Neonatal neurologic and electroencephalographic effects of intrauterine cocaine exposure. *J Pediatr* 1988; **113:** 354–8.
23. Singer LT, *et al.* Increased incidence of intraventricular hemorrhage and developmental delay in cocaine-exposed, very low birth weight infants. *J Pediatr* 1994; **124:** 765–71.
24. Azuma SD, Chasnoff IJ. Outcome of children prenatally exposed to cocaine and other drugs: a path analysis of three-year data. *Pediatrics* 1993; **92:** 396–402.
25. Mayes LC, *et al.* Information processing and developmental assessments in 3-month-old infants exposed prenatally to cocaine. *Pediatrics* 1995; **95:** 539–45.
26. van der Bor M, *et al.* Increased cerebral blood flow velocity in infants of mothers who abuse cocaine. *Pediatrics* 1990; **85:** 733–6.
27. Chasnoff IJ, *et al.* Perinatal cerebral infarction and maternal cocaine use. *J Pediatr* 1986; **108:** 456–9.
28. Chasnoff IJ, *et al.* Cocaine intoxication in a breast-fed infant. *Pediatrics* 1987; **80:** 836–8.

Treatment of Adverse Effects

As for Local Anaesthetics in general, p.1282.

Cocaine overdosage. In the emergency management of overdosage with cocaine the general aims are to establish adequate ventilation and support the circulation. If oral ingestion of a large amount is suspected the stomach should be emptied and activated charcoal administered.[1] A tourniquet may be applied to limit absorption if the drug was injected. Patients who have swallowed packages containing cocaine for the purpose of smuggling, may be given laxatives but surgical intervention may be required if signs of toxicity appear.[2] Sedation with intravenous diazepam may be sufficient to manage the symptoms of cocaine overdose. Sedation with benzodiazepines may also be appropriate initial therapy for hypertension or tachyarrhythmias since the excessive sympathetic tone is largely centrally mediated.[3] Severe arrhythmias may require treatment with intravenous propranolol although, following a report of paradoxical hypertension presumably due to unopposed α-adrenergic stimulation, a beta blocker with both α- and β-adrenergic effects such as labetalol is preferred by some if hypertension is also present;[2,4] sodium nitroprusside[3,4] or phentolamine[3,5] may also be used. Although labetalol can reduce the hypertension it does not alleviate cocaine-induced coronary vasoconstriction;[6] it has therefore been suggested that glyceryl trinitrate would be preferable for patients with cocaine-induced chest pain.[5,6] There is concern about the use of lignocaine for the treatment of cocaine-induced arrhythmias as lignocaine may enhance toxicity.[5] Calcium-channel blockers such as verapamil may also be of use as an antagonist for coronary artery vasoconstriction induced by cocaine.[5] Diazepam should be used to manage seizures[1,4] but if they cannot be controlled phenytoin can be used as an adjunct.[1] Hyperthermia should be treated with physical cooling but the use of dantrolene may also be necessary.[1] Control of anxiety and agitation with benzodiazepines when combined with rapid cooling may also have the effect of decreasing heat production in hyperthermic patients.[3] Metabolic acidosis should be monitored and treated where necessary.[1,4] Short-acting barbiturates or benzodiazepines may be used for dysphoric agitation but drugs that lower the seizure threshold such as phenothiazines or haloperidol should be avoided.[1]

1. Loper KA. Clinical toxicology of cocaine. *Med Toxicol Adverse Drug Exp* 1989; **4:** 174–85.
2. Ramrakha P, Barton I. Drug smuggler's delirium. *Br Med J* 1993; **306:** 470–1.
3. Anonymous. Acute reactions to drugs of abuse. *Med Lett Drugs Ther* 1996; **38:** 43–6.
4. Farrar HC, Kearns GL. Cocaine: clinical pharmacology and toxicology. *J Pediatr* 1989; **115:** 665–75.
5. Hollander JE. The management of cocaine-associated myocardial ischemia. *N Engl J Med* 1995; **333:** 1267–72.
6. Boehrer JD, *et al.* Influence of labetalol on cocaine-induced coronary vasoconstriction in humans. *Am J Med* 1993; **94:** 608–10.

Withdrawal. Cocaine can produce psychological dependence but does not produce a major physical withdrawal syndrome. The management of cocaine abuse and dependence has been reviewed.[1-3] There is no advantage to gradual withdrawal and it is best for the patient to discontinue the drug abruptly.[1,4] The three major psychiatric complications associated with cocaine withdrawal are dysphoric agitation, severe depression, and psychotic symptoms.[1] Dysphoric agitation is best treated with diazepam; propranolol may also be used in more persistent cases. Depressive symptoms during the acute post-cocaine phase are usually transient and require no treatment other than close observation. Desipramine has been used with equivocal results; it appears to be of most benefit in patients who have antecedent or consequent symptoms of severe depression.[2] Trazodone and imipramine have also been tried but had more adverse effects than desipramine.[2] Antipsychotics such as chlorpromazine, haloperidol, and promazine have been used successfully to manage patients with psychotic symptoms associated with cocaine dependence.[1]

Several drugs have been tried in the maintenance of abstinence from cocaine.[1] Lithium may be useful in patients with bipolar disorder or cyclothymic personality. Methylphenidate may be helpful in patients with attention deficit disorders but has potential for abuse itself. Phenothiazine derivatives have been tried in the control of impulsive behaviour and to decrease cocaine craving, although adverse effects may limit their acceptability. Carbamazepine has been reported to suppress the craving for cocaine although this has not been supported by subsequent trials.[2] Buprenorphine is under investigation to suppress cocaine and opioid use in patients dependent on both drugs.[2] Anxiolytics or antidepressants are considered unlikely to be of benefit in maintaining abstinence.[2] MAOIs such as phenelzine have been used in a manner analogous to the use of disulfiram in alcohol abuse to provoke unpleasant reactions if patients relapse.[5]

There is evidence to suggest that cocaine use affects the dopaminergic modulation of CNS function, and several drugs that interact with the dopamine system have been tried in the treatment of cocaine abuse and dependence, but with mixed results.[2]

1. Arif A, ed. *Adverse health consequences of cocaine abuse.* Geneva: WHO, 1987.
2. Mendelson JH, Mello NK. Management of cocaine abuse and dependence. *N Engl J Med* 1996; **334:** 965–72.
3. Kleber HD. Pharmacotherapy, current and potential, for the treatment of cocaine dependence. *Clin Neuropharmacol* 1995; **18** (suppl 1): S96–S109.
4. DoH. *Drug misuse and dependence: guidelines on clinical management.* London: HMSO, 1991.
5. Brewer C. Cocaine and crack. *Br Med J* 1989; **299:** 792.

Precautions

As for Local Anaesthetics in general, p.1282.

Since some patients have a marked sensitivity to cocaine the administration of a test dose before use on mucous membranes has been suggested. Cocaine should not be applied to damaged mucosa because of the risk of systemic toxicity from enhanced absorption. Ophthalmic preparations of cocaine should not be applied to the eyes for prolonged periods as damage to the cornea may occur not only from the local action of cocaine, but also from loss of the protective eyelid reflexes. As with other mydriatics, there is also a risk of cocaine precipitating angle-closure glaucoma in patients predisposed to the condition. Patients receiving cocaine for surface anaesthesia should be monitored for possible cardiovascular effects. Cocaine should be used with great caution in patients with hypertension, cardiovascular disease, or thyrotoxicosis. It is not recommended for use during pregnancy or breast feeding.

Abuse. Cocaine is subject to abuse. See under Adverse Effects, above.

Gilles de la Tourette's syndrome. Gilles de la Tourette's syndrome, which had been well controlled for 10 years by haloperidol, was precipitated in a 27-year-old man following intranasal use of cocaine on one occasion.[1]

1. Mesulam M-M. Cocaine and Tourette's syndrome. *N Engl J Med* 1986; **315:** 398.

Myasthenia gravis. Report of a patient in whom cocaine abuse first unmasked and then exacerbated myasthenia gravis.[1]

1. Berciano J, *et al.* Myasthenia gravis unmasked by cocaine abuse. *N Engl J Med* 1991; **325:** 892.

Porphyria. Cocaine has been associated with clinical exacerbations of porphyria and is considered unsafe in porphyric patients.[1]

1. Moore MR, McColl KEL. *Porphyria: drug lists.* Glasgow: Porphyria Research Unit, University of Glasgow, 1991.

Interactions

For interactions associated with local anaesthetics, see p.1283.

Cocaine and adrenaline enhance each other's sympathomimetic effects and should preferably not be used in association. Caution is needed if cocaine is used with other drugs that may also potentiate the action of catecholamines such as guanethidine or MAOIs.

Adrenaline. There has recently been a report[1] of 3 cases of arrhythmias associated with the use of a paste containing cocaine 25% and adrenaline 0.18% for local anaesthesia of the nasal mucosa. The amount of cocaine applied to the nasal mucosa in the above 3 cases ranged from about 2.5 to 4.5 mg per kg body-weight; the maximum recommended dose of cocaine alone in healthy adults is 1.5 mg per kg.

1. Nicholson KEA, Rogers JEG. Cocaine and adrenaline paste: a fatal combination? *Br Med J* 1995; **311:** 250–1.

Alcohol. In the presence of alcohol, cocaine is metabolised to its ethyl homologue cocaethylene.[1] Cocaethylene appears to have the same stimulant effects as cocaine but it has a longer half-life and *animal* studies suggest that it is more toxic than the parent drug.

1. Randall T. Cocaine, alcohol mix in body to form even longer lasting, more lethal drug. *JAMA* 1992; **267:** 1043–4.

Beta blockers. *Propranolol* potentiated cocaine-induced coronary vasoconstriction following intranasal administration of cocaine in a placebo-controlled study.[1]

1. Lange RA, *et al.* Potentiation of cocaine-induced coronary vasoconstriction by beta-adrenergic blockade. *Ann Intern Med* 1990; **112:** 897–903.

Haloperidol. For the effect of cocaine on haloperidol, see under Chlorpromazine, p.653.

Pharmacokinetics

Cocaine may be slowly absorbed from some sites because of the vasoconstriction it produces, but absorption occurs from all sites of application, including mucous membranes and the gastro-intestinal tract, and may be enhanced when there is inflammation. Cocaine is rapidly absorbed when smoked.

Cocaine is rapidly metabolised by plasma esterases and hepatic esterases to ecgonine methyl ester. Benzoylecgonine, another major metabolite of cocaine, may be produced by spontaneous hydrolysis. Cocaine is also demethylated to the active metabolite norcocaine which is not excreted but undergoes further metabolism. There is considerable interindividual variation in the plasma half-life of cocaine possibly due to differences in esterase activity.

Cocaine and its metabolites are excreted in the urine, approximately 10% appearing as unchanged drug. Cocaine and its metabolites may be detectable in urine for several days or even weeks after administration. Cocaine crosses the blood-brain barrier and accumulates within the CNS. It does not appear to undergo rapid metabolism within the brain and concentrations in the CNS following acute intoxication may greatly exceed those in plasma.

Cocaine crosses the placenta and the presence of its metabolites in neonatal hair has been used to indicate intra-uterine exposure. Cocaine is distributed into breast milk.

See also under Local Anaesthetics, p.1283.

References.

1. Busto U, *et al.* Clinical pharmacokinetics of non-opiate abused drugs. *Clin Pharmacokinet* 1989; **16:** 1–26.
2. Graham K, *et al.* Determination of gestational cocaine exposure by hair analysis. *JAMA* 1989; **262:** 3328–30.
3. Burke WM, Ravi NV. Urinary excretion of cocaine. *Ann Intern Med* 1990; **112:** 548–9.
4. Ravi NV, Burke WM. Cocaine and traffic accident fatalities in New York City. *JAMA* 1990; **263:** 2887.
5. Schenker S, *et al.* The transfer of cocaine and its metabolites across the term human placenta. *Clin Pharmacol Ther* 1993; **53:** 329–39.

Absorption. Cocaine is rapidly absorbed from the pulmonary vasculature when smoked and the speed of onset of its effects is similar to that obtained after intravenous injection.[1] Absorption from mucous membranes is delayed by vasoconstriction and peak plasma concentrations of up to 474 ng per mL have been obtained 15 to 120 minutes after application of doses of 1.5 to 2 mg per kg body-weight to the nasal mucosa as a 10% cocaine hydrochloride solution;[2,3] cocaine may still be detectable in the nose several hours later and this may result in prolonged systemic absorption.[2] In one study it was estimated that only 5% of the total dose of cocaine hydrochloride used prior to nasal surgery was absorbed from the nasal mucosa following application of 500 mg of cocaine hydrochloride as a 25% paste with adrenaline or 200 mg as a 10% solution with adrenaline (Moffett's solution) and blood concentrations were well below those associated with toxicity[4] (but see also Adrenaline, under Interactions, above). Peak serum concentrations of cocaine have been obtained after 50 to 90 minutes following oral administration and are similar to those obtained after nasal application.[3]

1. Farrar HC, Kearns GL. Cocaine: clinical pharmacology and toxicology. *J Pediatr* 1989; **115:** 665–75.
2. Van Dyke C, *et al.* Cocaine: plasma concentrations after intranasal application in man. *Science* 1976; **191:** 859–61.
3. Van Dyke C, *et al.* Oral cocaine: plasma concentrations and central effects. *Science* 1978; **200:** 211–13.
4. Quiney RE. Intranasal topical cocaine: Moffett's method or topical cocaine paste? *J Laryngol Otol* 1986; **100:** 279–83.

Uses and Administration

Cocaine, a benzoic acid ester, is a local anaesthetic with actions and uses similar to those described on p.1283. It is used as a surface anaesthetic but, because of systemic adverse effects and its abuse potential, its use is now almost entirely restricted to surgery of the ear, nose, and throat. It has been largely replaced by other drugs in ophthalmology because of its corneal toxicity, although it may still be useful in removal or debridement of the corneal epithelium. Cocaine also blocks the uptake of catecholamines at adrenergic nerve endings and potentiates the action of catecholamines. Its sympathomimetic actions cause tachycardia, peripheral vasoconstriction, a rise in blood pressure, and mydriasis. The use of cocaine in association with drugs such as adrenaline increases the risk of cardiac arrhythmias. Despite this hazard some use this combination in otolaryngology to improve the operative field and reduce absorption.

When applied to mucous membranes, surface anaesthesia develops rapidly and persists for 30 minutes or longer depending on the concentration of cocaine used, the dose, and on the vascularity of the tissue.

Cocaine hydrochloride is used for the administration of cocaine in aqueous solutions. Solutions containing up to 4% have been used in ophthalmology (but see Precautions, above).

Solutions containing up to 10% of cocaine are applied to the nasal mucosa in otolaryngological procedures. Pastes containing up to 25% of cocaine have also been applied.

In order to avoid systemic effects, the usual maximum total dose recommended for application to the nasal mucosa in healthy adults is 1.5 mg per kg body-weight. It should be used only by those skilled in the precautions needed to minimise absorption and the consequent risk of arrhythmias.

Cocaine has been used in conjunction with diamorphine or morphine for the relief of severe pain, especially in terminal illness, but this use is now obsolete.

Cocaine solutions should never be administered by injection; other local anaesthetics are equally effective and much safer.

A review of cocaine and its uses.

1. Middleton RM, Kirkpatrick MB. Clinical use of cocaine: a review of the risks and benefits. *Drug Safety* 1993; **9:** 212–17.

Preparations

USP 23: Cocaine and Tetracaine Hydrochlorides and Epinephrine Topical Solution; Cocaine Hydrochloride Tablets for Topical Solution.

Dimethisoquin Hydrochloride (7622-p)

Dimethisoquin Hydrochloride *(BANM, USAN)*.

Quinisocaine Hydrochloride *(rINNM)*; Chinisocainum Hydrochloride; Dimethisoquinium Chloride. 2-(3-Butyl-1-isoquinolyloxy)-*NN*-dimethylethylamine hydrochloride.

$C_{17}H_{24}N_2O,HCl = 308.8$.

CAS — 86-80-6 (dimethisoquin); 2773-92-4 (dimethisoquin hydrochloride).

Dimethisoquin hydrochloride is a local anaesthetic (p.1281) available in some countries for use as a surface anaesthetic in the form of an ointment or cream in a concentration of 0.5% or as suppositories. It is used for the relief of pruritus, anogenital or anorectal irritation, and minor skin conditions.

Preparations

Proprietary Preparations (details are given in Part 3)

Belg.: Quotane†; ***Fr.:*** Quotane; ***Ger.:*** Haenal; Isochinol; ***Switz.:*** Isochinol.

Multi-ingredient: ***Fr.:*** Rectoquotane.

Diperodon Hydrochloride (7624-w)

Diperodon Hydrochloride *(BANM, rINNM)*.

Diperocaine Hydrochloride. 3-Piperidinopropylene bis(phenylcarbamate) hydrochloride.

$C_{22}H_{27}N_3O_4,HCl = 433.9$.

CAS — 101-08-6 (anhydrous diperodon); 51552-99-9 (diperodon monohydrate); 537-12-2 (diperodon hydrochloride).

Diperodon is a local anaesthetic (p.1281) that has been used as the base or the hydrochloride for surface anaesthesia.

Preparations

Proprietary Preparations (details are given in Part 3)

Multi-ingredient: ***UK:*** Cold Sore Ointment†; ***USA:*** A-Caine; Bactine First Aid Antibiotic Plus Anesthetic; Hemet†; Hemocaine†.

Dyclocaine Hydrochloride (7625-e)

Dyclocaine Hydrochloride *(BANM)*.

Dyclonine Hydrochloride *(rINNM)*; Dyclocaini Chloridum. 4′-Butoxy-3-piperidinopropiophenone hydrochloride.

$C_{18}H_{27}NO_2,HCl = 325.9$.

CAS — 586-60-7 (dyclocaine); 536-43-6 (dyclocaine hydrochloride).

Pharmacopoeias. In US.

White crystals or white crystalline powder, with a slight odour. **Soluble** 1 in 60 of water, 1 in 24 of alcohol, and 1 in 2.3 of chloroform; soluble in acetone; practically insoluble in ether and in hexane. A 1% solution in water has a pH of 4.0 to 7.0. **Store** in airtight containers. Protect from light.

Dyclocaine hydrochloride is a local anaesthetic (p.1281) used for topical anaesthesia of the skin and mucous membranes in concentrations of 0.5 or 1.0%. Single doses in excess of 200 mg should generally not be used. Lozenges containing up to 3 mg have been used for the temporary relief of pain associated with sore throats or mouth irritation. It may cause irritation at the site of application and should not be given by injection or used in the eyes.

Preparations

USP 23: Dyclonine Hydrochloride Gel; Dyclonine Hydrochloride Topical Solution.

Proprietary Preparations (details are given in Part 3)

Canad.: Sucrets for Kids; ***USA:*** Dyclone; Oradex-C†; Sucrets.

Multi-ingredient: ***Canad.:*** Skin Shield; Tanac; ***USA:*** Cepacol Maximum Strength Sore Throat; Skin Shield; Tanac.

Ethyl Chloride (3108-b)

Aethylium Chloratum; Chlorethyl; Cloruro de Etilo; Ethylis Chloridum; Hydrochloric Ether; Monochlorethane. Chloroethane.

$C_2H_5Cl = 64.51$.

CAS — 75-00-3.

Pharmacopoeias. In Aust., Belg., Br., Pol., and US.

At ambient temperatures and pressures ethyl chloride is gaseous but condenses, when slightly compressed, into a colourless, mobile, flammable, very volatile liquid with an ethereal odour. If prepared from Industrial Methylated Spirit it may contain a small variable proportion of methyl chloride. B.p. 12° to 13°.

Slightly **soluble** in water; miscible with alcohol and with ether. It is neutral to litmus. **Store** in airtight containers preferably hermetically sealed at a temperature not exceeding 15°. Protect from light.

CAUTION. Ethyl chloride is highly flammable and mixtures of the gas with 5 to 15% of air are explosive.

Adverse Effects and Precautions

As for Chloroform, p.1221.

Cutaneous sensitisation can occur rarely. Thawing of frozen tissue following surgery may be painful and prolonged spraying onto the skin can cause chemical frostbite. Freezing may also distort the histological structure of biopsy specimens. Ethyl chloride should not be applied to broken skin or mucous membranes.

Uses and Administration

Owing to its low boiling-point and the intense cold produced by evaporation, ethyl chloride has been used as a local anaesthetic in minor surgery but this procedure is not generally recommended. It has also been used topically for the relief of pain. Ethyl chloride was formerly used as an inhalational anaesthetic but has no place in modern anaesthetic practice.

Preparations

Proprietary Preparations (details are given in Part 3)
Ger.: Chloraethyl "Dr Henning"; Cloraethyl "Dr. Henning"†; Holsten aktiv; WariActiv; ***Spain:*** Cloretilo Chemirosa; ***Switz.:*** Chlorethyl.

Multi-ingredient: ***Austral.:*** Frezan†; ***Spain:*** Talgo Odontalgico; ***USA:*** Fluro-Ethyl.

Ethyl *p*-Piperidinoacetylaminobenzoate

(8638-n)

EPAB; SA-7. 4-[(1-Piperidinylacetyl)amino]benzoic acid ethyl ester.

$C_{16}H_{22}N_2O_3$ = 290.4.

CAS — 41653-21-8.

Ethyl *p*-piperidinoacetylaminobenzoate is an amide local anaesthetic (p.1281) that has been given by mouth for the symptomatic relief of gastritis.

Preparations

Proprietary Preparations (details are given in Part 3)
Jpn: Sulcain.

Etidocaine Hydrochloride (7626-l)

Etidocaine Hydrochloride *(BANM, rINNM).*

W-19053. (±)-2-(*N*-Ethylpropylamino)butyro-2′,6′-xylidide hydrochloride.

$C_{17}H_{28}N_2O,HCl$ = 312.9.

CAS — 36637-18-0 (etidocaine); 36637-19-1 (etidocaine hydrochloride).

NOTE. Etidocaine is *USAN*.

Adverse Effects, Treatment, and Precautions

As for Local Anaesthetics in general, p.1281.

Effects on the cardiovascular system. For a discussion of the cardiotoxicity of etidocaine, see under the Adverse Effects of Bupivacaine Hydrochloride, p.1286.

Interactions

For interactions associated with local anaesthetics, see p.1283.

Pharmacokinetics

Etidocaine is rapidly absorbed into the circulation after parenteral injection and is about 95% bound to plasma proteins. It crosses the placenta but the ratio of fetal to maternal concentrations is relatively low. It also diffuses across the blood-brain barrier. Etidocaine is metabolised in the liver and its numerous metabolites are excreted in the urine; about 1% of the drug is excreted unchanged. The plasma elimination half-life of etidocaine is 2 to 3 hours in adults.

See also under Local Anaesthetics, p.1283.

Pregnancy. Following maternal injection etidocaine rapidly crosses the placenta[1] but the degree of transfer is less than for other local anaesthetics including bupivacaine.[2] The ratio of fetal to maternal concentrations of etidocaine varies but values up to about 0.35 are usual.[1,2] Some metabolites appear to be transferred to a greater degree than the parent compound[1]. Etidocaine is highly protein bound but the fraction of unbound drug in plasma increases in pregnant women during delivery.[1] Protein binding of etidocaine is also reduced in fetal plasma.[3] Although neonates are able to metabolise etidocaine it appears that they are less able to do so than adults; a mean elimination half-life of 6.42 hours has been reported in neonates.[3]

1. Morgan DJ, *et al.* Disposition and placental transfer of etidocaine in pregnancy. *Eur J Clin Pharmacol* 1977; **12:** 359–65.
2. Poppers PJ. Evaluation of local anaesthetic agents for regional anaesthesia in obstetrics. *Br J Anaesth* 1975; **47:** 322–7.
3. Morgan D, *et al.* Pharmacokinetics and metabolism of the anilide local anaesthetics in neonates: 11: etidocaine. *Eur J Clin Pharmacol* 1978; **13:** 365–71.

Uses and Administration

Etidocaine hydrochloride is a local anaesthetic of the amide type with actions and uses similar to those described on p.1283. It has a rapid onset and a long duration of action. Etidocaine is used for infiltration anaesthesia, peripheral nerve block, and epidural anaesthesia, usually with adrenaline 1 in 200 000. (Local anaesthetic techniques are discussed on p.1284.)

The dosage of etidocaine used depends on the site of injection and the procedure used. The maximum dose should not generally exceed 300 mg when given without adrenaline, or 400 mg when given with adrenaline. Generally, additional incremental doses may be administered every 2 to 3 hours.

For *infiltration anaesthesia* a 0.5% solution may be used in a dose of 5 to 400 mg (1 to 80 mL). For dentistry a dose of 15 to 75 mg (1 to 5 mL) may be given as a 1.5% solution with adrenaline. For *peripheral nerve blocks* a 0.5% solution may be used in a dose of 25 to 400 mg (5 to 80 mL) or a 1.0% solution in a dose of 50 to 400 mg (5 to 40 mL). For *retrobulbar block* a 1% solution may be used in a dose of 20 to 40 mg (2 to 4 mL) or a 1.5% solution in a dose of 30 to 60 mg (2 to 4 mL).

When given by *epidural injection* etidocaine hydrochloride produces a profound degree of motor blockade and although the degree of abdominal muscle relaxation produced may be desirable in some obstetrical procedures it makes this drug unsuitable for use in vaginal deliveries. A dose of 100 to 300 mg (10 to 30 mL) may be injected as a 1% solution or 150 to 300 mg (10 to 20 mL) as a 1.5% solution for lumbar epidural block prior to surgery, including caesarean section. Lower doses of 50 to 150 mg (10 to 30 mL) as a 0.5% solution or 50 to 200 mg (5 to 20 mL) as a 1% solution are suggested for gynaecological procedures. For caudal anaesthesia 50 to 150 mg (10 to 30 mL) as a 0.5% solution or 100 to 300 mg (10 to 30 mL) as a 1% solution may be given.

Preparations

Proprietary Preparations (details are given in Part 3)
Aust.: Duranest; ***Austral.:*** Duranest†; ***Fr.:*** Duranest; ***Ger.:*** Duranest; ***Swed.:*** Duranest†; ***USA:*** Duranest.

Ketocaine Hydrochloride (12882-b)

Ketocaine Hydrochloride *(rINNM).*

Chetocaina Cloridrata. 2′-(2-Di-isopropylaminoethoxy)butyrophenone hydrochloride.

$C_{18}H_{29}NO_2,HCl$ = 327.9.

CAS — 1092-46-2 (ketocaine); 1092-47-3 (ketocaine hydrochloride).

Ketocaine hydrochloride is a local anaesthetic (p.1281) that has been used as a surface anaesthetic in suppositories or ointments for anorectal disorders.

Preparations

Proprietary Preparations (details are given in Part 3)

Multi-ingredient: ***Ital.:*** Proctolyn; Proctonide†.

Lignocaine (7602-b)

Lignocaine *(BAN).*

Lidocaine *(rINN)*; Lidocainum. 2-Diethylaminoaceto-2′,6′-xylidide.

$C_{14}H_{22}N_2O$ = 234.3.

CAS — 137-58-6.

Pharmacopoeias. In *Eur.* (see p.viii), *Int., Jpn,* and *US.*

A white to slightly yellow crystalline powder with a characteristic odour. M.p. 66° to 70°. Practically **insoluble** in water; very soluble in alcohol, in chloroform, or in dichloromethane; freely soluble in ether; dissolves in oils.

Lignocaine forms a mixture with prilocaine that has a melting-point lower than that of either ingredient. This **eutectic** mixture is used in the preparation of topical dosage forms.

Lignocaine Hydrochloride (7601-m)

Lignocaine Hydrochloride *(BANM).*

Lidocaine Hydrochloride *(rINNM)*; Lidocaini Hydrochloridum; Lignoc. Hydrochlor.

$C_{14}H_{22}N_2O,HCl,H_2O$ = 288.8.

CAS — 73-78-9 (lignocaine hydrochloride, anhydrous); 6108-05-0 (lignocaine hydrochloride, monohydrate).

NOTE. LIDFLN is a code approved by the BP for use on single unit doses of eye drops containing lignocaine hydrochloride and fluorescein sodium where the individual container may be too small to bear all the appropriate labelling information.

Pharmacopoeias. In *Chin., Eur.* (see p.viii), *Int., Pol.,* and *US.*

A white odourless crystalline powder. M.p. 74° to 79°. Lignocaine hydrochloride monohydrate 1.23 g or anhydrous lignocaine hydrochloride 1.16 g is approximately equivalent to 1 g of lignocaine. Ph. Eur. **solubilities** are: very soluble in water; freely soluble in alcohol; practically insoluble in ether. USP solubilities are: very soluble in water and in alcohol; soluble in chloroform; insoluble in ether. A 0.5% solution in water has a pH of 4.0 to 5.5. **Protect** from light.

Incompatibility. Lignocaine hydrochloride has been reported to be incompatible in solution with amphotericin,[1] sulphadiazine sodium,[2] methohexitone sodium,[2] cephazolin sodium,[3] or phenytoin sodium.[4] See also under Stability, below.

The lignocaine content of buffered cardioplegic solutions has been reported[5] to decrease when stored in polyvinyl chloride containers at ambient temperature, but not when stored at 4°. This loss appeared to result from pH-dependent sorption of lignocaine onto the plastic and did not occur when lignocaine solutions were stored in glass bottles.

1. Whiting DA. Treatment of chromoblastomycosis with high local concentrations of amphotericin B. *Br J Dermatol* 1967; **79:** 345–51.
2. Riley BB. Incompatibilities in intravenous solutions. *J Hosp Pharm* 1970; **28:** 228–40.
3. Kleinberg ML, *et al.* Stability of antibiotics frozen and stored in disposable hypodermic syringes. *Am J Hosp Pharm* 1980; **37:** 1087–8.
4. Kirschenbaum HL, *et al.* Stability and compatibility of lidocaine hydrochloride with selected large-volume parenterals and drug additives. *Am J Hosp Pharm* 1982; **39:** 1013–15.
5. Lackner TE, *et al.* Lidocaine stability in cardioplegic solution stored in glass bottles and polyvinyl chloride bags. *Am J Hosp Pharm* 1983; **40:** 97–101.

pH of solutions. For the effect pH has on the surface tension and administration of lignocaine solutions by infusion, see under Administration in Uses and Administration, below.

For a discussion of the effect that pH has on the stability of local anaesthetic solutions and the pain associated with their injection, see p.1284.

Stability. Although there was no decrease in the lignocaine content of lignocaine hydrochloride and adrenaline injection during transport and storage under tropical conditions, the content of adrenaline fell to almost zero in some samples after several months; supply of the injection as a dry powder and separate solvent should be considered for the tropics.[1]

Acid stable drugs such as adrenaline hydrochloride, noradrenaline acid tartrate, or isoprenaline may begin to deteriorate within several hours of admixture with lignocaine hydrochloride as lignocaine solutions may raise the pH of the final solution above the maximum pH for their stability. Such extemporaneous mixtures should be used promptly after preparation.[2]

1. Abu-Reid IO, *et al.* Stability of drugs in the tropics: a study in Sudan. *Int Pharm J* 1990; **4:** 6–10.
2. Parker EA. Xylocaine hydrochloride 2% injection. *Am J Hosp Pharm* 1971; **28:** 805.

Adverse Effects and Treatment

As for Local Anaesthetics in general, p.1281.

Effects on the CNS. A report[1] of suspected psychotic reactions associated with the use of lignocaine in 6 patients given intravenous lignocaine for the treatment of cardiac disorders.

1. Turner WM. Lidocaine and psychotic reactions. *Ann Intern Med* 1982; **97:** 149–50.

Effects on the skin. Erythema and pigmentation of the upper lip in a child following local dental infiltration of lignocaine was attributed to a type of fixed drug eruption.[1]

1. Curley RK, *et al.* An unusual cutaneous reaction to lignocaine. *Br Dent J* 1987; **162:** 113–14.

Overdosage. The most serious effects of lignocaine intoxication are on the CNS and cardiovascular system and overdosage can result in severe hypotension, asystole, bradycardia, apnoea, seizures, coma, cardiac arrest, respiratory arrest, and death. Intoxication with lignocaine is relatively common and can occur as a result of acute overdosage following poor control of intravenous maintenance infusions or after accidental injection of concentrated solutions. However, it more commonly results from inadvertent intravascular administration during regional anaesthesia or from too rapid injection of therapeutic doses particularly in patients with circulatory insufficiency or when clearance is reduced due to heart failure, liver disease, old age, or through interaction with other drugs.[1] Seizures have also been reported after excessive doses administered subcutaneously.[2] Although the bioavailability of lignocaine is low it may be sufficient to result in significant toxicity when swallowed[1] and there have been reports of CNS toxicity, seizures, and death in children[3-7] and adults[8-10] following the ingestion of topical solutions and after the use of viscous preparations in the mouth. Lignocaine is absorbed from mucous membranes and serious toxicity has been reported after urethral[11] or rectal[12] instillation of lignocaine preparations.

The treatment of overdosage from local anaesthetics is discussed on p.1282.

1. Denaro CP, Benowitz NL. Poisoning due to class 1B antiarrhythmic drugs: lignocaine, mexiletine and tocainide. *Med Toxicol Adverse Drug Exp* 1989; **4:** 412–28.
2. Pelter MA, *et al.* Seizure-like reaction associated with subcutaneous lidocaine injection. *Clin Pharm* 1989; **8:** 767–8.
3. Sakai RI, Lattin JE. Lidocaine ingestion. *Am J Dis Child* 1980; **134:** 323.
4. Rothstein P, *et al.* Prolonged seizures associated with the use of viscous lidocaine. *J Pediatr* 1982; **101:** 461–3.
5. Mofenson HC, *et al.* Lidocaine toxicity from topical mucosal application. *Clin Pediatr (Phila)* 1983; **22:** 190–2.
6. Giard MJ, *et al.* Seizures induced by oral viscous lidocaine. *Clin Pharm* 1983; **2:** 110.
7. Amitai Y, *et al.* Death following accidental lidocaine overdose in a child. *N Engl J Med* 1986; **314:** 182–3.
8. Parish RC, *et al.* Seizures following oral lidocaine for esophageal anesthesia. *Drug Intell Clin Pharm* 1985; **19:** 199–201.
9. Fruncillo RJ, *et al.* CNS toxicity after ingestion of topical lidocaine. *N Engl J Med* 1982; **306:** 426–7.
10. Geraets DR, *et al.* Toxicity potential of oral lidocaine in a patient receiving mexiletine. *Ann Pharmacother* 1992; **26:** 1380–1.
11. Dix VW, Tresidder GC. Collapse after use of lignocaine jelly for urethral anaesthesia. *Lancet* 1963; **i:** 890.
12. Pottage A, Scott DB. Safety of "topical" lignocaine. *Lancet* 1988; **i:** 1003.

Pregnancy. The overall effect of maternal epidural anaesthesia appears to be beneficial for the fetus (see under Labour Pain, p.9) but the use of lignocaine may produce transient effects in the auditory system of the neonate.[1]

1. Bozynski MEA, *et al.* Effect of prenatal lignocaine on auditory brain stem evoked response. *Arch Dis Child* 1989; **64:** 934–8.

Precautions

As for Local Anaesthetics in general, p.1282.

In general lignocaine should not be given to patients with hypovolaemia, heart block or other conduction disturbances, and should be used with caution in patients with congestive heart failure, bradycardia, or respiratory depression. Lignocaine is metabolised in the liver and must be given with caution to patients with hepatic insufficiency. The plasma half-life of lignocaine may be prolonged in conditions that reduce hepatic blood flow such as cardiac and circulatory failure. Metabolites of lignocaine may accumulate in patients with renal impairment.

The intramuscular injection of lignocaine may increase creatine phosphokinase concentrations that can interfere with the diagnosis of acute myocardial infarction.

Cerebrovascular disorders. Administration of lignocaine 5 mg per kg body-weight by intravenous infusion over 30 minutes was associated with a 12% reduction in cerebral blood flow in healthy subjects although it returned to normal within 60 minutes.[1] Cerebral blood flow in patients with diabetes was lower than in healthy subjects, but was unaffected by lignocaine infusion, indicating reduced cerebrovascular reactivity.

1. Kastrup J, *et al.* Intravenous lidocaine and cerebral blood flow: impaired microvascular reactivity in diabetic patients. *J Clin Pharmacol* 1990; **30:** 318–23.

Renal impairment. See under Uses and Administration, below.

Interactions

For interactions associated with local anaesthetics, see p.1283.

The clearance of lignocaine may be reduced by propranolol and cimetidine (see below). The cardiac depressant effects of lignocaine are additive with those of beta blockers and of other antiarrhythmics including intravenous phenytoin; long-term administration of enzyme-inducers such as phenytoin may increase dosage requirements of lignocaine (see below). Hypokalaemia produced by acetazolamide, loop diuretics, and thiazides antagonises the effect of lignocaine.

Antiarrhythmics. Lignocaine toxicity, arising from the use of an oral preparation containing lignocaine, has been reported[1] in a patient who was receiving *mexiletine*.

1. Geraets DR, *et al.* Toxicity potential of oral lidocaine in a patient receiving mexiletine. *Ann Pharmacother* 1992; **26:** 1380–1.

Antiepileptics. Studies in healthy subjects and patients with epilepsy[1,2] suggest that long-term administration of drugs such as *phenytoin* or *barbiturates* may increase dosage requirements for lignocaine due to induction of drug-metabolising microsomal enzymes. Administration of phenytoin can also increase plasma concentrations of α_1-acid glycoprotein and thereby reduce the free fraction of lignocaine in plasma.[3]

1. Heinonen J, *et al.* Plasma lidocaine levels in patients treated with potential inducers of microsomal enzymes. *Acta Anaesthesiol Scand* 1970; **14:** 89–95.
2. Perucca E, Richens A. Reduction of oral bioavailability of lignocaine by induction of first pass metabolism in epileptic patients. *Br J Clin Pharmacol* 1979; **8:** 21–31.
3. Routledge PA, *et al.* Lignocaine disposition in blood in epilepsy. *Br J Clin Pharmacol* 1981; **12:** 663–6.

Beta blockers. Significant increases in plasma-lignocaine concentrations have occurred during concomitant therapy with *propranolol*[1-4] owing to a reduction in the clearance of lignocaine from plasma. A similar interaction has been observed with *nadolol*[3] and *metoprolol*,[2] although in another study[5] metoprolol did not alter the pharmacokinetics of lignocaine. The hepatic metabolism of lignocaine may be reduced as a result of a fall in hepatic blood flow associated with reduced cardiac output or it may be caused by direct inhibition of hepatic microsomal enzymes.[6] Significant impairment of lignocaine clearance would therefore be most likely to occur with those drugs that lack intrinsic sympathomimetic activity and have a greater effect on cardiac output or with the more lipid-soluble drugs that have greater effects on microsomal oxygenases. Results of one study[4] suggest that the reduction in clearance produced by propranolol is mainly by direct inhibition of metabolism rather than by lowering of hepatic blood flow.

1. Ochs HR, *et al.* Reduction in lidocaine clearance during continuous infusion and by coadministration of propranolol. *N Engl J Med* 1980; **303:** 373–7.
2. Conrad KA, *et al.* Lidocaine elimination: effects of metoprolol and of propranolol. *Clin Pharmacol Ther* 1983; **33:** 133–8.
3. Schneck DW, *et al.* Effects of nadolol and propranolol on plasma lidocaine clearance. *Clin Pharmacol Ther* 1984; **36:** 584–7.
4. Bax NDS, *et al.* The impairment of lignocaine clearance by propranolol—major contribution from enzyme inhibition. *Br J Clin Pharmacol* 1985; **19:** 597–603.
5. Miners JO, *et al.* Failure of 'therapeutic' doses of β-adrenoceptor antagonists to alter the disposition of tolbutamide and lignocaine. *Br J Clin Pharmacol* 1984; **18:** 853–60.
6. Tucker GT, *et al.* Effects of β-adrenoceptor antagonists on the pharmacokinetics of lignocaine. *Br J Clin Pharmacol* 1984; **17:** 21S–28S.

H_2-receptor antagonists. There have been numerous studies[1-4] of the interaction between *cimetidine* and lignocaine but differences between the studies makes interpretation of the overall clinical significance of the results difficult. Cimetidine appears to reduce the hepatic metabolism of lignocaine; it may also reduce its clearance by decreasing hepatic blood flow. Significant increases in plasma-lignocaine concentrations have been reported. Changes in protein binding are not generally important but patients with myocardial infarction who have increased levels of α_1-acid glycoprotein may be partially protected from increases in concentrations of free lignocaine.[5] Since it is not possible to identify those patients at risk all patients receiving these drugs concurrently should be closely monitored for signs of toxicity. The use of other H_2-receptor antagonists may be preferable. In studies in healthy subjects *ranitidine* either had no effect on lignocaine kinetics[6] or produced changes consistent with small reductions in hepatic blood flow.[7]

1. Feely J, *et al.* Increased toxicity and reduced clearance of lidocaine by cimetidine. *Ann Intern Med* 1982; **96:** 592–4.
2. Knapp AB, *et al.* The cimetidine-lidocaine interaction. *Ann Intern Med* 1983; **98:** 174–7.
3. Patterson JH, *et al.* Influence of a continuous cimetidine infusion on lidocaine plasma concentrations in patients. *J Clin Pharmacol* 1985; **25:** 607–9.
4. Bauer LA, *et al.* Cimetidine-induced decrease in lidocaine metabolism. *Am Heart J* 1984; **108:** 413–15.
5. Berk SI, *et al.* The effect of oral cimetidine on total and unbound serum lidocaine concentrations in patients with suspected myocardial infarction. *Int J Cardiol* 1987; **14:** 91–4.
6. Feely J, Guy E. Lack of effect of ranitidine on the disposition of lignocaine. *Br J Clin Pharmacol* 1983; **15:** 378–9.
7. Robson RA, *et al.* The effect of ranitidine on the disposition of lignocaine. *Br J Clin Pharmacol* 1985; **20:** 170–3.

Local anaesthetics. Although a number of drugs were shown to reduce the amount of lignocaine bound to α_1-acid glycoprotein only the displacement produced by *bupivacaine* was considered to be of possible clinical significance.[1]

There is concern about the use of lignocaine to treat *cocaine*-induced arrhythmias as lignocaine may enhance toxicity.[2]

1. Goolkasian DL, *et al.* Displacement of lidocaine from serum α_1-acid glycoprotein binding sites by basic drugs. *Eur J Clin Pharmacol* 1983; **25:** 413–17.
2. Hollander JE. The management of cocaine-associated myocardial ischemia. *N Engl J Med* 1995; **333:** 1267–72.

Neuromuscular blockers. The possible interaction between neuromuscular blockers and antiarrhythmics including lignocaine is discussed under the Interactions of Atracurium, p.1306.

Oral contraceptives. For mention of the effect of oral contraceptives on the protein binding of lignocaine, see under Protein Binding in Pharmacokinetics, below.

Smoking. The effects of smoking on lignocaine therapy are unclear. Studies in a limited number of patients have found reduced systemic bioavailability suggestive of induction of drug-metabolising activity[1] and an inconsistent effect on protein binding.[2,3]

1. Huet P-M, Lelorier J. Effects of smoking and chronic hepatitis B on lidocaine and indocyanine green kinetics. *Clin Pharmacol Ther* 1980; **28:** 208–15.
2. McNamara PJ, *et al.* Effect of smoking on binding of lidocaine to human serum proteins. *J Pharm Sci* 1980; **69:** 749–51.
3. Davis D, *et al.* The effects of age and smoking on the plasma protein binding of lignocaine and diazepam. *Br J Clin Pharmacol* 1985; **19:** 261–5.

Pharmacokinetics

Lignocaine is readily absorbed from the gastro-intestinal tract, from mucous membranes, and through damaged skin. Absorption through intact skin is poor. It is rapidly absorbed from injection sites including muscle.

After an intravenous dose lignocaine is rapidly and widely distributed into highly perfused tissues followed by redistribution into skeletal muscle and adipose tissue. Lignocaine is bound to plasma proteins, including α_1-acid glycoprotein (AAG). The extent of binding is variable but is approximately 66%. Plasma protein binding of lignocaine depends in part on the concentrations of both lignocaine and AAG. Any alteration in the concentration of AAG can greatly affect plasma concentrations of lignocaine (see under Protein Binding, below).

Plasma concentrations decline rapidly after an intravenous dose with an initial half-life of less than 30 minutes; the elimination half-life is 1 to 2 hours but may be prolonged if infusions are given for longer than 24 hours or if hepatic blood flow is reduced.

Lignocaine is largely metabolised in the liver and any alteration in liver function or hepatic blood flow can have a significant effect on its pharmacokinetics and dosage requirements. First-pass metabolism is extensive and bioavailability is about 35% after oral administration. Metabolism in the liver is rapid and approximately 90% of a given dose is dealkylated to form monoethylglycinexylidide (MEGX) and glycinexylidide (GX). Both of these metabolites may contribute to the therapeutic and toxic effects of lignocaine and since their half-lives are longer than that of lignocaine, accumulation, particularly of glycinexylidide, may occur during prolonged infusions. Further metabolism occurs and metabolites are excreted in the urine with less than 10% of unchanged lignocaine. Reduced clearance of lignocaine has been found in patients with heart failure, alcoholic liver disease, or chronic or viral hepatitis. Concomitant therapy with drugs that alter hepatic blood flow or induce drug-metabolising microsomal enzymes can also affect the clearance of lignocaine (see under Interactions, above). Renal impairment does not affect the clearance of lignocaine but accumulation of its active metabolites can occur and may lead to toxicity.

Lignocaine crosses the placenta and blood-brain barrier; it is distributed into breast milk.

See also under Local Anaesthetics, p.1283.

References.

1. Nattel S, *et al.* The pharmacokinetics of lignocaine and β-adrenoceptor antagonists in patients with acute myocardial infarction. *Clin Pharmacokinet* 1987; **13:** 293–316.
2. Bodenham A, *et al.* The altered pharmacokinetics and pharmacodynamics of drugs commonly used in critically ill patients. *Clin Pharmacokinet* 1988; **14:** 347–73.
3. Shammas FV, Dickstein K. Clinical pharmacokinetics in heart failure: an updated review. *Clin Pharmacokinet* 1988; **15:** 94–113.

Absorption. SURFACE APPLICATION. Serum-lignocaine concentrations were usually so low as to be unmeasurable in patients who gargled and expectorated 15 mL (300 mg) of a 2% viscous solution before endoscopy[1] and mean peak serum concentrations of lignocaine were below those associated with toxicity following endotracheal application of 100 mg of lignocaine by spray.[2] The relative bioavailability of lignocaine has been found to be higher when applied to the upper respiratory tract than after administration to the lower respiratory tract.[3] Acceptably low plasma-lignocaine concentrations were noted with the following regimen used before bronchoscopy: a 4% lignocaine solution gargled for 30 seconds, a 2% solution sprayed onto the oropharynx, a 2% jelly applied to the oropharynx and nasal passages, and a 1% solution injected through a bronchoscope.[4] However, the absorption of lignocaine applied intranasally can be highly variable.[5] One study indicated that, for bronchoscopy, administration of lignocaine by inhalation from a nebuliser rather than by direct spray results in lower peak serum concentrations.[6]

1. Fazio A, *et al.* Lidocaine serum concentrations following endoscopy. *Drug Intell Clin Pharm* 1987; **21:** 752–3.
2. Scott DB, *et al.* Plasma lignocaine concentrations following endotracheal spraying with an aerosol. *Br J Anaesth* 1976; **48:** 899–902.
3. McBurney A, *et al.* Absorption of lignocaine and bupivacaine from the respiratory tract during fibreoptic bronchoscopy. *Br J Clin Pharmacol* 1984; **17:** 61–6.
4. Ameer B, *et al.* Systemic absorption of topical lidocaine in elderly and young adults undergoing bronchoscopy. *Pharmacotherapy* 1989; **9:** 74–81.
5. Scavone JM, *et al.* The bioavailability of intranasal lignocaine. *Br J Clin Pharmacol* 1989; **28:** 722–4.
6. Labedzki L, *et al.* Reduced systemic absorption of intrabronchial lidocaine by high-frequency nebulization. *J Clin Pharmacol* 1990; **30:** 795–7.

Protein binding. Lignocaine is markedly bound to α_1-acid glycoprotein (AAG), an acute phase protein which is increased after trauma, surgery, burns, myocardial infarction, in chronic inflammatory disorders such as Crohn's disease, and in cancer. Protein binding may therefore be greatly increased in these conditions and reduced in neonates, the nephrotic syndrome, and in liver disease when AAG concentrations are lower than normal. This may result in an eightfold variation in the free fraction of lignocaine between these conditions.[1] Measurement of free drug concentrations may be a better guide to dosage requirements than measurement of total plasma concentrations.[2] AAG concentrations may also be reduced by oestrogens[3] leading to a higher free fraction of lignocaine in women than in men and the free fraction is further increased during pregnancy and in women taking oral contraceptives.[3,4] Protein binding may also be affected by other concomitant drug therapy or smoking (for further details, see under Interactions, above).

1. Routledge PA. Pharmacological terms: protein binding. *Prescribers' J* 1988; **28:** 34–5.
2. Shand DG. α_1-Acid glycoprotein and plasma lidocaine binding. *Clin Pharmacokinet* 1984; **9** (suppl 1): 27–31.
3. Routledge PA, *et al.* Sex-related differences in the plasma protein binding of lignocaine and diazepam. *Br J Clin Pharmacol* 1981; **11:** 245–50.
4. Wood M, Wood AJJ. Changes in plasma drug binding and α_1-acid glycoprotein in mother and newborn infant. *Clin Pharmacol Ther* 1981; **29:** 522–6.

Uses and Administration

Lignocaine is a local anaesthetic of the amide type with actions and uses similar to those described on p.1283. It is used for infiltration and regional nerve blocks. It has a rapid onset of action and anaesthesia is obtained within a few minutes depending on the site of administration; it has an intermediate duration of action. The speed of onset and duration of action of lignocaine are increased by the addition of a vasoconstrictor and absorption into the circulation from the site of injection is reduced. The carbonated solution of lignocaine is also available in some countries for injection (see p.1284). Lignocaine is also a useful surface anaesthetic but it should be remembered that it may be rapidly and extensively absorbed following topical application to mucous membranes and systemic effects may occur. Hyaluronidase (p.1588) has been added to preparations of lignocaine used for surface and infiltration anaesthesia but it may also enhance systemic absorption. (Local anaesthetic techniques are discussed on p.1284.)

Lignocaine is a class Ib antiarrhythmic used in the treatment of ventricular arrhythmias, especially after myocardial infarction. It has been given by intravenous infusion in the treatment of refractory status epilepticus.

Lignocaine is included in some injections, such as depot corticosteroids, to prevent pain, itching, and other local irritation. Lignocaine sodium is included in intramuscular injections of some antibacterials to reduce the pain on injection produced by the antibacterial.

The dose of lignocaine hydrochloride used for **local anaesthesia** depends on the site of injection and the procedure used. When given with adrenaline, the suggested general maximum dose of lignocaine hydrochloride is 500 mg; without adrenaline, the maximum recommended single dose in the UK is 200 mg and in the USA, 300 mg, except for spinal anaesthesia (see below). Lignocaine hydrochloride solutions containing adrenaline 1 in 200 000 are used for infiltration anaesthesia and nerve blocks; higher concentrations of adrenaline are seldom necessary, except in dentistry, in which case, solutions of lignocaine hydrochloride with adrenaline 1 in 80 000 may be used. Doses of lignocaine should be reduced in children, the elderly, and in debilitated patients. A test dose of lignocaine, preferably with adrenaline, should be given before commencing epidural block to detect inadvertent intravenous administration.

- For percutaneous *infiltration anaesthesia* recommended doses in the USA using 0.5% or 1.0% solutions are 5 to 300 mg (1 to 60 mL of a 0.5% solution, or 0.5 to 30 mL of a 1.0% solution).
- The dosage of lignocaine hydrochloride in *peripheral nerve block* depends on the route of administration. The manufacturer in the USA suggests that for brachial plexus block 225 to 300 mg (15 to 20 mL) as a 1.5% solution may be given; for intercostal nerve block 30 mg (3 mL) is given as a 1% solution; for paracervical block a 1% solution is used in a dose of 100 mg (10 mL) on each side, repeated not more frequently than every 90 minutes; for paravertebral block a 1% solution may be used in doses of 30 to 50 mg (3 to 5 mL); a 1% solution is recommended for pudendal block in doses of 100 mg (10 mL) on each side; for retrobulbar block a 4% solution may be used in doses of 120 to 200 mg (3 to 5 mL).
- Lignocaine hydrochloride is also used for *sympathetic nerve block* as a 1% solution; suggested doses are 50 mg (5 mL) for cervical block and 50 to 100 mg (5 to 10 mL) for lumbar block.
- For *epidural anaesthesia* 2 to 3 mL of solution is needed for each dermatome to be anaesthetised but usual total doses in the USA and recommended concentrations are: lumbar epidural 250 to 300 mg (25 to 30 mL) of a 1% solution for analgesia and 225 to 300 mg (15 to 20 mL) as a 1.5% solution or 200 to 300 mg (10 to 15 mL) as a 2% solution for anaesthesia, and for thoracic epidural a 1% solution may be used at doses of 200 to 300 mg (20 to 30 mL). In obstetric caudal analgesia 200 to 300 mg (20 to 30 mL) is used as a 1% solution and in surgical caudal anaesthesia a 1.5% solution may be used in doses of 225 to 300 mg (15 to 20 mL). For continuous epidural anaesthesia, the maximum doses should not be repeated more frequently than every 90 minutes.
- A hyperbaric solution of 1.5% or 5% lignocaine hydrochloride in glucose 7.5% solution is available for *spinal anaesthesia*; adrenaline should not be used. Doses of up to 50 mg (1.0 mL) of a 5% solution and 9 to 15 mg (0.6 to 1.0 mL) of a 1.5% solution have been used during labour for a normal vaginal delivery. Up to 75 mg (1.5 mL) of the 5% solution has been used for caesarean section and 75 to 100 mg (1.5 to 2 mL) for other surgical procedures.
- For *intravenous regional anaesthesia* a 0.5% solution without adrenaline has been used in doses of 50 to 300 mg (10 to 60 mL). In the USA, a maximum dose of 4 mg per kg body-weight has been recommended for adults, and 3 mg per kg as a 0.25 or 0.5% solution has been recommended for children.
- Lignocaine may be used in a variety of formulations for *surface anaesthesia*.

  Lignocaine ointment is used for *anaesthesia of skin and mucous membranes* with a maximum recommended total dose of 35 g of 5% ointment (equivalent to 1.75 g of lignocaine base) in 24 hours.

  Gels are used for *anaesthesia of the urinary tract* and the dose used varies in different countries. The manufacturers in the UK have suggested the following doses given as a 2% gel: in females 100 to 200 mg of lignocaine hydrochloride is inserted into the urethra several minutes before examination; in males 400 mg is instilled in 2 portions, or 600 to 800 mg in 3 to 4 portions. The doses used in the USA are lower: in females 60 to 100 mg of lignocaine hydrochloride is inserted into the urethra several minutes before examination; in males 100 to 200 mg is used before catheterisation and 600 mg before sounding or cystoscopy; the US manufacturers suggest that not more than 600 mg should be given in this form in any 12-hour period. A dose of 200 to 400 mg of a 2% gel is also recommended in the UK for endoscopy. A quantity of the gel containing about 100 mg of lignocaine hydrochloride is used to lubricate tubing for endotracheal insertion.

  Topical solutions are used for *surface anaesthesia of mucous membranes of the mouth, throat, and upper gastro-intestinal tract*. For painful conditions of the mouth and throat a 2% solution may be used: 300 mg (15 mL) may be rinsed and ejected or, for pharyngeal pain, the solution is gargled and swallowed if necessary; it should not be used more frequently than every 3 hours. The recommended maximum daily dose in the USA for topical oral solutions is 2.4 g. Doses of 40 to 300 mg of a 4% solution (1 to 7.5 mL) are used before bronchoscopy, bronchography, laryngoscopy, oesophagoscopy, endotracheal intubation, and biopsy in the mouth and throat. Lignocaine in a strength of 10% has also been used as a spray for application to mucous membranes for the prevention of pain during various procedures including use in otorhinolaryngology, dentistry, introduction of instruments into the respiratory and gastro-intestinal tracts, and in obstetrics. The dose depends on the extent of the site to be anaesthetised; 10 to 50 mg is generally sufficient for dentistry and otorhinolaryngology; for other procedures, the maximum dose in a 24-hour period is 200 mg. For laryngotracheal anaesthesia 160 mg of lignocaine hydrochloride as a 4% spray is instilled as a single dose into the lumen of the larynx and trachea.

  Lignocaine is used *rectally* as suppositories, ointments, and creams in the treatment of haemorrhoids and other painful perianal conditions.

  Eye drops containing lignocaine hydrochloride 4% with fluorescein are used in tonometry.

  A *eutectic mixture* containing lignocaine base 2.5% and prilocaine base 2.5% is applied as a cream under an occlusive dressing to produce *surface anaesthesia of the skin* before procedures requiring needle puncture, surgical treatment of localised lesions, and split skin grafting; it has been used similarly, but without an occlusive dressing, before removal of genital warts (see also under Eutectic Mixtures, below). Other methods of improving dermal delivery include a *transdermal patch* of lignocaine, and an *iontophoretic drug delivery system* incorporating lignocaine and adrenaline.

For the treatment of **ventricular arrhythmias** lignocaine is given intravenously as the hydrochloride. It may be used in advanced cardiac life support for cardiac arrest due to ventricular fibrillation and pulseless ventricular tachycardia when direct current shocks (together with adrenaline) have failed to restore a normal rhythm. For adults, a dose of 100 mg (or 1.5 mg per kg if based on body-weight) can be given and repeated after 3 to 5 minutes to a total dose of 3 mg per kg if necessary. The endotracheal route has been employed when intravenous access cannot be obtained, although doses should probably be increased from those employed intravenously; the precise endotracheal dose has not yet been established, however. Lignocaine is also used in other ventricular arrhythmias in which the patient is in a more stable condition. In these circumstances lignocaine is usually given as a loading dose followed by an infusion. Usual doses are 50 to 100 mg or 1.0 to 1.5 mg per kg body-weight as a direct intravenous injection at a rate of 25 to 50 mg per minute. If no effect is seen within 5 to 10 minutes of this loading dose, it may be repeated once or twice to a maximum dose of 200 to 300 mg in 1 hour. A continuous intravenous infusion is usually commenced after loading, at a dose of 1 to 4 mg per minute. It is rarely necessary to continue this infusion for longer than 24 hours, but in the event that a longer infusion is required, the dose may need to be reduced to avoid potential toxicity resulting from an increase in the half-life. Dosage may need to be reduced in patients with heart failure or liver disorders.

In emergency situations, lignocaine hydrochloride has also been given for arrhythmias by intramuscular injection into the deltoid muscle in a dose of 300 mg, repeated if necessary after 60 to 90 minutes.

Action. For a comparison of the vasoactivity of lignocaine and some other local anaesthetics, see p.1284.

Administration. Doubts over the value of recommended maximum doses for local anaesthetics have been raised by Scott.[1,2] Systemic toxic effects of local anaesthetics are related to blood concentrations and, as absorption varies considerably according to the site of injection, recommendation of a single maximum dose without regard to the site of the procedure is meaningless. If one assumes that a plasma-lignocaine concentration of 5 μg per mL is required for toxicity then this would be achieved by injection of 300 mg in the intercostal area, 500 mg epidurally, 600 mg in the region of the brachial plexus, or 1000 mg subcutaneously. The reduction of peak concentrations obtained by the addition of adrenaline is also dependent on the site of injection. Furthermore, most cases of severe toxicity do not result from overdosage but from inadvertent intravascular injection or too rapid injection.

The pH of lignocaine solutions can affect intravenous administration and should be kept low. Such solutions should be infused using a volume pump rather than a drop counting device for at alkaline pH lignocaine can lower surface tension and thereby alter the drop size.[3] For references to the use of buffered solutions of local anaesthetics such as lignocaine to reduce the pain associated with infiltration of the anaesthetic, see pH of solutions, p.1284.

1. Scott DB. "Maximum recommended doses" of local anaesthetic drugs. *Br J Anaesth* 1989; **63:** 373–4.
2. Scott DB. Safe use of lignocaine. *Br Med J* 1989; **299:** 56.
3. Leor R, *et al.* The influence of pH on the intravenous delivery of lidocaine solutions. *Eur J Clin Pharmacol* 1990; **39:** 521–3.

Administration in renal impairment. The pharmacokinetics of lignocaine and its metabolite monoethylglycinexylidide appear to be unaffected in patients with renal failure except that accumulation of the metabolite glycinexylidide may occur during infusions of 12 hours or more.[1] Data to predict the amount of lignocaine and glycinexylidide removed during haemodialysis have been provided by several workers.[2,3] Lignocaine does not appear to be removed during haemofiltration.[4]

1. Collinsworth KA, *et al.* Pharmacokinetics and metabolism of lidocaine in patients with renal failure. *Clin Pharmacol Ther* 1975; **18:** 59–64.
2. Gibson TP, Nelson HA. Drug kinetics and artificial kidneys. *Clin Pharmacokinet* 1977; **2:** 403–26.
3. Lee CC, Marbury TC. Drug therapy in patients undergoing haemodialysis: clinical pharmacokinetic considerations. *Clin Pharmacokinet* 1984; **9:** 42–66.
4. Saima S, *et al.* Negligible removal of lidocaine during arteriovenous hemofiltration. *Ther Drug Monit* 1990; **12:** 154–6.

Burns. Lignocaine given intravenously has been reported to have produced pain relief in a few patients with second-degree burns.[1]

1. Jönsson A, *et al.* Inhibition of burn pain by intravenous lignocaine infusion. *Lancet* 1991; **338:** 151–2.

Cardiac arrhythmias. Lignocaine is classified as a class Ib antiarrhythmic drug (p.776) and may be used in the treatment of ventricular arrhythmias, including those associated with cardiac arrest and myocardial infarction. It is usually administered intravenously. Dosage details are given in Uses and Administration, above. Some forms of ventricular tachycardia may be terminated by the use of lignocaine; the overall treatment options are described under Cardiac Arrhythmias, p.782. Guidelines for cardiopulmonary resuscitation, including the use of lignocaine, are described under Advanced Cardiac Life Support, p.779.

Lignocaine has been considered for the *prophylaxis* of ventricular fibrillation in patients with proven or suspected myocardial infarction. However, while some studies have identified a protective effect,[1,2] in others this has not been shown to be accompanied by a reduction in mortality and might even have increased it.[3,4] Nevertheless, one review of the available evidence[5] concluded that lignocaine prophylaxis was a reasonable policy for patients at highest risk of ventricular fibrillation such as those with acute transmural infarction, under 65 years of age, and within 6 hours of the onset of infarction symptoms.

It has been suggested that increased mortality sometimes seen with lignocaine might be associated with the duration of administration; a recent study[6] found that patients who received a bolus dose of lignocaine followed by a 40-hour continuous infusion for prophylaxis of ventricular arrhythmias experienced more episodes of heart failure than patients who received the bolus dose followed by an 8-hour infusion.

1. Horwitz RI, Feinstein AR. Improved observational method for studying therapeutic efficacy: suggestive evidence that lidocaine prophylaxis prevents death in acute myocardial infarction. *JAMA* 1981; **246:** 2455–9.
2. Koster RW, Dunning AJ. Intramuscular lidocaine for prevention of lethal arrhythmias in the prehospitalization phase of acute myocardial infarction. *N Engl J Med* 1985; **313:** 1105–10.
3. MacMahon S, *et al.* Effects of prophylactic lidocaine in suspected acute myocardial infarction: an overview of results from the randomized, controlled trials. *JAMA* 1988; **260:** 1910–16.
4. Hine LK, *et al.* Meta-analytic evidence against prophylactic use of lidocaine in acute myocardial infarction. *Ann Intern Med* 1989; **149:** 2694–8.
5. Nattel S, Arenal A. Antiarrhythmic prophylaxis after acute myocardial infarction: is lidocaine still useful? *Drugs* 1993; **45:** 9–14.
6. Pharand C, *et al.* Lidocaine prophylaxis for fatal ventricular arrhythmias after acute myocardial infarction. *Clin Pharmacol Ther* 1995; **57:** 471–8.

Diabetic neuropathy. Lignocaine may be one of the drugs worth trying in patients with diabetic neuropathy (p.9) who do not respond to the usual therapy. In a double-blind crossover study[1] involving 15 patients with moderate or severe painful diabetic neuropathy, lignocaine 5 mg per kg body-weight by intravenous infusion improved symptoms more effectively than placebo. In the 11 patients who responded to lignocaine, relief of symptoms lasted from 3 to 21 days.

1. Kastrup J, *et al.* Treatment of chronic painful diabetic neuropathy with intravenous lidocaine infusion. *Br Med J* 1986; **292:** 173.

Hiccup. A protocol for the management of intractable hiccups may be found under Chlorpromazine, p.655. Lignocaine is one of a large number of drugs that has been tried in the treatment of hiccups without strong evidence of their efficacy. It has been given in the form of a 2% viscous solution taken by mouth. Nebulised lignocaine has also been tried.[1]

1. Neeno TA, Rosenow EC. Intractable hiccups: consider nebulized lidocaine. *Chest* 1996; **110:** 1129–30.

Intubation. Lignocaine has produced conflicting results when used to attenuate the pressor response and rise in intraocular pressure induced by procedures such as tracheal intubation.[1-5] For an overall discussion of this problem, see under Anaesthesia, p.1302.

1. Tam S, *et al.* Attenuation of circulatory responses to endotracheal intubation using intravenous lidocaine: a determination of the optimal time of injection. *Can Anaesth Soc J* 1985; **32:** S65.
2. Miller CD, Warren SJ. IV lignocaine fails to attenuate the cardiovascular response to laryngoscopy and tracheal intubation. *Br J Anaesth* 1990; **65:** 216–19.
3. Murphy DF, *et al.* Intravenous lignocaine pretreatment to prevent intraocular pressure rise following suxamethonium and tracheal intubation. *Br J Ophthalmol* 1986; **70:** 596–8.
4. Drenger B, Pe'er J. Attenuation of ocular and systemic responses to tracheal intubation by intravenous lignocaine. *Br J Ophthalmol* 1987; **71:** 546–8.
5. Mostafa SM, *et al.* Effects of nebulized lignocaine on the intraocular pressure responses to tracheal intubation. *Br J Anaesth* 1990; **64:** 515–17.

Migraine and cluster headache. Despite periodic renewed interest, lignocaine has so far failed to find an accepted role in the management of migraine (p.443) or cluster headache (p.443). Intravenous lignocaine has been tried for the emergency parenteral treatment of migraine, but in a comparative study with dihydroergotamine or chlorpromazine it was found to be less effective than either.[1] More recently, intranasal instillation of lignocaine has produced rapid relief of headache in some patients with acute migraine but early relapse of headache was common.[2]

Intranasal instillation of lignocaine has also been reported to be effective in aborting individual attacks of headache during cluster periods in patients with cluster headache.[3,4]

1. Bell R, *et al.* A comparative trial of three agents in the treatment of acute migraine headache. *Ann Emerg Med* 1990; **19:** 1070–82.
2. Maizels M, *et al.* Intranasal lidocaine for treatment of migraine: a randomized, double-blind, controlled trial. *JAMA* 1996; **276:** 319–21.
3. Kittrelle JP, *et al.* Cluster headache: local anesthetic abortive agents. *Arch Neurol* 1985; **42:** 496–8.
4. Robbins L. Intranasal lidocaine for cluster headache. *Headache* 1995; **35:** 83–4.

Pleurodesis. Lignocaine has been instilled intrapleurally as a 1% solution in doses of up to 300 mg to relieve the severe chest pain associated with the use of tetracycline for pleurodesis.[1-3] While the larger doses were significantly more effective[2] toxic plasma concentrations were less likely to occur if a dose of 3 mg per kg body-weight or less was used.[3]

1. Harbecke RG. Intrapleurally given tetracycline with lidocaine. *JAMA* 1980; **244:** 1899–1900.
2. Sherman S, *et al.* Optimum anesthesia with intrapleural lidocaine during chemical pleurodesis with tetracycline. *Chest* 1988; **93:** 533–6.
3. Wooten SA, *et al.* Systemic absorption of tetracycline and lidocaine following intrapleural instillation. *Chest* 1988; **94:** 960–3.

Status epilepticus. Lignocaine hydrochloride may be used to control status epilepticus resistant to more conventional treatment (see p.337). It has a rapid onset of action but its effect is short-lived and continuous infusion may be necessary.[1] However, despite its efficacy in treating status epilepticus it has been noted that doses producing high plasma concentrations can result in CNS toxicity including seizures.[1] Recurrence of seizures associated with the withdrawal of prolonged lignocaine therapy may be due to accumulated lignocaine metabolites exerting an excitatory effect on the nervous system when the inhibitory effect of lignocaine is being reduced.[2]

Lignocaine was used instead of diazepam for 42 episodes of status epilepticus in 36 patients who either had limited pulmonary reserve or who had not responded to intravenous diazepam.[3] Lignocaine 1.5 to 2 mg per kg body-weight (usually a dose of 100 mg) was administered as a single intravenous dose over 2 minutes. This dose was repeated once if there was no positive response to the first dose (11 episodes) or the seizures recurred (19 episodes). Subsequently a continuous infusion of lignocaine at a rate of 3 to 4 mg per kg per hour was given in the 7 episodes that recurred after the second dose; 5 of these showed a positive response. The 11 episodes not responding to the first dose did not respond to the second dose or to a continuous infusion.

1. Bauer J, Elger CE. Management of status epilepticus in adults. *CNS Drugs* 1994; **1:** 26–44.
2. Wallin A, *et al.* Lidocaine treatment of neonatal convulsions, a therapeutic dilemma. *Eur J Clin Pharmacol* 1989; **36:** 583–6.
3. Pascual J, *et al.* Role of lidocaine (lignocaine) in managing status epilepticus. *J Neurol Neurosurg Psychiatry* 1992; **55:** 49–51.

Surface anaesthesia. EUTECTIC MIXTURES. A cream, containing lignocaine 2.5% and prilocaine 2.5% in a eutectic mixture, can produce local anaesthesia when applied topically to intact skin and appears to be of value in a number of minor medical or surgical procedures both in adults and in children.[1-3] Applications that have been tried include venepuncture for blood sampling, intravenous or arterial cannulation, retrobulbar injections, lumbar puncture, curettage of molluscum contagiosum lesions, genital wart removal, split skin grafting, laser treatment, extracorporeal shock wave therapy, separation of preputial adhesions, and circumcision. It has also been tried as an anaesthetic for the ear drum in preparation for otological procedures such as myringotomy and grommet insertion but is potentially ototoxic and should not be used in the presence of a perforation. Postherpetic neuralgia (p.10) has also been treated with some success.[4,5]

The eutectic cream is usually applied to skin under an occlusive dressing for at least 60 minutes although it has been suggested that for children aged 1 to 5 years 30 minutes may be sufficient.[6] The manufacturers suggest a maximum application time of 5 hours. The onset and duration of the effect may be affected by the site of application.[2] When used for the removal of genital warts an occlusive dressing is not necessary and the application time recommended by the manufacturer is 5 to 10 minutes. The level of anaesthesia begins to decline after 10 to 15 minutes when applied to the genital mucosa and any procedure should be started immediately. Systemic absorption of lignocaine and prilocaine appears to be minimal when applied to intact skin[6] even after treating large areas or leaving the cream in place for many hours.[7] However, the UK manufacturers recommend that it should not be used for children under 1 year of age as excessive absorption can lead to methaemoglobinaemia, owing to the presence of prilocaine (see under Effects on the Blood, p.1281). However, eutectic mixtures of lignocaine and prilocaine have been used to reduce the pain of puncture procedures[8] and for circumcision[9] in neonates, and appear to be safe and efficacious.

The eutectic cream should not be used on wounds or mucous membranes (except for genital warts in adults) and should not be used for atopic dermatitis. It should not be applied to or near the eyes because it causes corneal irritation, and it should not be instilled in the middle ear. It should be used with caution in patients with anaemia or congenital or acquired methaemoglobinaemia. Transient paleness, redness, and oedema may occur following application.

Some studies suggested that a topical gel formulation of amethocaine 4% can produce longer and more rapid anaesthesia than the above lignocaine with prilocaine cream (see p.1285). It has also been suggested[10] that topical amethocaine may have practical advantages over the eutectic mixture of lignocaine and prilocaine, which has to be applied for at least one hour and is therefore of no value for emergency procedures; it also causes vasoconstriction at the site of application, which can make venepuncture difficult.

1. Lee JJ, Rubin AP. Emla cream and its current uses. *Br J Hosp Med* 1993; **50:** 463–6.
2. Buckley MM, Benfield P. Eutectic lidocaine/prilocaine cream: a review of the topical anaesthetic/analgesic efficacy of a eutectic mixture of local anaesthetics (EMLA). *Drugs* 1993; **46:** 126–51.
3. Koren G. Use of the eutectic mixture of local anesthetics in young children for procedure-related pain. *J Pediatr* 1993; **122** (suppl): S30–S35.
4. Litman SJ, *et al.* Use of EMLA cream in the treatment of post-herpetic neuralgia. *J Clin Anesth* 1996; **8:** 54–7.
5. Kost RG, Straus SE. Postherpetic neuralgia—pathogenesis, treatment, and prevention. *N Engl J Med* 1996; **335:** 32–42.
6. Hanks GW, White I. Local anaesthetic creams. *Br Med J* 1988; **297:** 1215–16.
7. Scott DB. Topical anaesthesia of intact skin. *Br J Parenter Ther* 1986; **7:** 134–5.
8. Gourrier E, *et al.* Use of EMLA® cream in a department of neonatology. *Pain* 1996; **68:** 431–4.
9. Taddio A, *et al.* Efficacy and safety of lidocaine-prilocaine cream for pain during circumcision. *N Engl J Med* 1997; **336:** 1197–1201.
10. Russell SCS, Doyle E. Paediatric anaesthesia. *Br Med J* 1997; **314:** 201–3.

Tinnitus. Tinnitus is the perception of a noise that arises or appears to arise within the head.

Objective tinnitus may be audible to others and arises from lesions outside the auditory system. Subjective tinnitus (tinnitus aurium) originates from sites within the auditory system and is perceived only by the patient. A simple and remediable cause of tinnitus can be impacted ear wax. Tinnitus is often associated with head injury, vertigo, and hearing loss, including age-related and noise-induced hearing loss. It may also be a symptom of an underlying disorder such as Ménière's disease, may be associated with anxiety or depressive disorders, or may be a manifestation of drug toxicity (for example with aspirin or quinine). In such cases, treatment of the underlying disorder or removal of the offending drug can resolve the tinnitus.

Treatment of tinnitus is difficult although reassurance and counselling are often effective in helping patients to tolerate their condition. Maskers or, if the tinnitus is associated with hearing loss, hearing aids are also used; surgery is rarely indicated. Treatment with a wide variety of drugs has been tried. Intravenous lignocaine has proven to be effective in reducing or eliminating tinnitus but the effect only lasts for a few hours and is, therefore, impractical for most patients. Efforts to find an effective oral analogue of lignocaine have not, so far, been successful. Other drugs that have been tried include the antiepileptics carbamazepine and phenytoin, and the loop diuretic frusemide, but unacceptable adverse effects limit their use.

References.

1. Luxon LM. Tinnitus: its causes, diagnosis, and treatment. *Br Med J* 1993; **306:** 1490–1.
2. Robson AK, Birchall JP. Management of tinnitus. *Prescribers' J* 1994; **34:** 1–7.
3. Coles RRA. Drug treatment of tinnitus in Britain. In: Reich GE, Vernon JA, eds. *Proceedings of the fifth international tinnitus seminar.* Portland: American Tinnitus Association, 1995.
4. Vesterager V. Tinnitus—investigation and management. *Br Med J* 1997; **314:** 728–31.

Preparations

BP 1998: Lidocaine and Adrenaline Injection; Lidocaine and Chlorhexidine Gel; Lidocaine Gel; Lidocaine Injection; Sterile Lidocaine Solution;
USP 23: Lidocaine Hydrochloride and Dextrose Injection; Lidocaine Hydrochloride and Epinephrine Injection; Lidocaine Hydrochloride Injection; Lidocaine Hydrochloride Jelly; Lidocaine Hydrochloride Oral Topical Solution; Lidocaine Hydrochloride Topical Solution; Lidocaine Ointment; Lidocaine Oral Topical Solution; Lidocaine Topical Aerosol; Neomycin and Polymyxin B Sulfates and Lidocaine Cream; Neomycin and Polymyxin B Sulfates, Bacitracin Zinc, and Lidocaine Ointment; Neomycin and Polymyxin B Sulfates, Bacitracin, and Lidocaine Ointment.

Proprietary Preparations (details are given in Part 3)
Aust.: Lidocorit; Neo-Xylestesin; Neo-Xylestesin forte; Neurolid; Xylanaest; Xylocain; Xylocard; Xyloneural; ***Austral.:*** Fargo†; Nurocain; Nurocain with Sympathin†; Ora-Sed Lotion†; Seda-Gel; Stud 100; Xylocaine; Xylocaine Heavy; Xylocaine Special Adhesive; Xylocard; ***Belg.:*** Otoralgyl; Xylocaine; Xylocaine Visqueuse; Xylocard; ***Canad.:*** Family Medicated Sunburn Relief; Lidodan; Solarcaine Lidocaine; Xylocaine; Xylocard; ***Fr.:*** Mesocaine; Otoralgyl; Xylocaine; Xylocard; ***Ger.:*** Anaesthol; Corafusin†; Heweneural; Licain; Lidesthesin; Lidocaton; Lidoject; LidoPosterine; Neo-Lidocaton; neo-Novutox†; Nor-Anaesthol; Sagittaproct; Xylestesin; Xylestesin-A; Xylestesin-S; Xylocain; Xylocain f.d. Kardiologie; Xylocitin; Xyloneural; ***Irl.:*** Xylocaine; Xylocard; ***Ital.:*** Ecocain; Lident Adrenalina; Lident Andrenor; Lidrian; Luan; Odontalg; Ortodermina; Resina Carbolica Dentilin; Xilo-Mynol; Xylocaina; Xylonor; ***Jpn:*** Penles; ***Neth.:*** Dentiform†; Dentinox; Otalgan; Xylocaine; Xylocard; ***Norw.:*** Xylocain; Xylocard; ***S.Afr.:*** Lidocaton†; Peterkaien; Pharmacaine†; Remicaine; Remicard; Xylocaine; Xylocaine Heavy; Xylotox; ***Spain:*** Aeroderm; Anestecidan Noradrenalin†; Anestecidan Simple†; Cidancaina†; Curadent; Llorentecaina Noradrenal; Xilonibsa; Xylocaina; Xylonor 2% Sin Vasoconst; Xylonor Especial; ***Swed.:*** Xylocain; Xylocain tung; Xylocard; ***Switz.:*** Kenergon; Lidocaton; Lignospan; Lubogliss; Neo-Lidocaton†; Rapidocaine; Sedagul; Solarcaine; Xylesine; Xylestesin-F; Xylestesin-S "special"; Xylocain; Xylocard; Xyloneural; Xylonor; ***UK:*** Laryng-O-Jet; Lignostab-A; Lignostab-N†; Mouth Gel†; Pensacaine with Adrenaline†; Rinstead; Strepsils Direct Action Spray; Vagisil; Woodwards Teething Gel; Xylocaine; Xylocaine 2% Plain; Xylocaine Accordion; Xylocard; Xylotox; ***USA:*** Anestacon; Dentipatch; Dermaflex; Dilocaine; Dr Scholl's Cracked Heel Relief; Duo-Trach Kit; L-Caine†; Lidoject; LidoPen; Nervocaine; no more burn†; no more ouchies†; Nulicaine; Octocaine; Xylocaine; Zilactin-L.

Multi-ingredient: numerous preparations are listed in Part 3.

Mepivacaine Hydrochloride (7633-e)

Mepivacaine Hydrochloride *(BANM, rINNM).*

Mepivacaini Chloridum; Mepivicaini Hydrochloridum. (1-Methyl-2-piperidyl)formo-2′,6′-xylidide hydrochloride.

$C_{15}H_{22}N_2O,HCl = 282.8.$

CAS — 96-88-8 (mepivacaine); 22801-44-1 ((±)-mepivacaine); 1722-62-9 (mepivacaine hydrochloride).

Pharmacopoeias. In *Eur.* (see p.viii), *Jpn,* and *US.*

A white odourless crystalline powder. Freely **soluble** in water, in alcohol, and in methyl alcohol; very slightly soluble in chloroform and in dichloromethane; practically insoluble in ether. A 2% solution in water has a pH of 4.0 to 5.0.

pH of solutions. For a discussion of the effect that pH has on the stability of local anaesthetic solutions and the pain associated with their injection, see p.1284.

Adverse Effects, Treatment, and Precautions

As for Local Anaesthetics in general, p.1281.

Interactions

For interactions associated with local anaesthetics, see p.1283.

Studies *in vitro* showed that bupivacaine dramatically reduced the binding of mepivacaine to α-1-acid glycoprotein.[1]

1. Hartrick CT, *et al.* Influence of bupivacaine on mepivacaine protein binding. *Clin Pharmacol Ther* 1984; **36:** 546–50.

Pharmacokinetics

Mepivacaine is highly bound to plasma proteins (about 78%). The plasma half-life has been reported to be about 2 to 3 hours in the adult and about 9 hours in the neonate. It is rapidly metabolised in the liver and less than 10% of a dose is reported to be excreted unchanged in the urine. Several metabolites are also excreted via the kidneys and include glucuronide conjugates of hydroxy compounds and an *N*-demethylated compound, 2′,6′-pipecoloxylidide (PPX). Over 50% of a dose is excreted as metabolites into the bile but these probably undergo enterohepatic circulation as only small amounts are excreted in the faeces. Mepivacaine crosses the placenta.

See also under Local Anaesthetics, p.1283.

Pregnancy. There is considerable transfer of mepivacaine across the placenta following maternal administration and the ratio of fetal to maternal concentrations is in the order of 0.7.[1] Although neonates have a very limited capacity to metabolise mepivacaine it appears they are able to eliminate the drug.[2]

1. Lurie AO, Weiss JB. Blood concentration of mepivacaine and lidocaine in mother and baby after epidural anesthesia. *Am J Obstet Gynecol* 1970; **106:** 850–6.
2. Meffin P, *et al.* Clearance and metabolism of mepivacaine in the human neonate. *Clin Pharmacol Ther* 1973; **14:** 218–25.

Uses and Administration

Mepivacaine hydrochloride is a local anaesthetic of the amide type with actions and uses similar to those described on p.1283. It is used for infiltration, peripheral nerve block, and epidural anaesthesia. (Local anaesthetic techniques are discussed on p.1284.) Mepivacaine has a rapid onset and an intermediate duration of action. The speed of onset and duration of action are increased by the addition of a vasoconstrictor and absorption into the circulation from the site of injection is reduced.

The dosage of mepivacaine used depends on the site of injection and the procedure used. An adult dose of mepivacaine hydrochloride should not generally exceed 400 mg and the total dose in 24 hours should not exceed 1 g. Doses should be reduced in the elderly, in debilitated patients, and in those with cardiac or hepatic impairment. A suggested maximum dose for children, especially less than 3 years of age, is 5 to 6 mg per kg body-weight. Concentrations of less than 2% should also be used for children less than 3 years of age.

For *infiltration anaesthesia* up to 400 mg of a 1% (40 mL) or 0.5% (80 mL) solution is used. For *dental infiltration and nerve block* a 2% solution with a vasoconstrictor or a 3% plain solution is used. For anaesthesia at a single site in the jaw a dose of 36 mg (1.8 mL) of the 2% solution or 54 mg (1.8 mL) of the 3% solution is used. For anaesthesia of the entire oral cavity 180 mg (9 mL) of the 2% solution or 270 mg (9 mL) of the 3% solution is used. Some recommend that no more than 300 mg should be administered at a single dental sitting.

For *peripheral nerve blocks,* namely *cervical, brachial plexus, intercostal,* and *pudendal blocks,* 1 or 2% solutions may be used in doses of 50 to 400 mg (5 to 40 mL) as a 1% solution, or 100 to 400 mg (5 to 20 mL) as a 2% solution. For pudendal block half of the dose is injected on each side. For *paracervical block* a dose of up to 100 mg (10 mL) of a 1% solution on each side has been suggested allowing an interval of 5 minutes between sides. This may be repeated at an interval of not less than 90 minutes, and for a combined paracervical and pudendal block up to 150 mg (15 mL) of a 1% solution is injected on each side. For therapeutic nerve block in the management of pain 10 to 50 mg (1 to 5 mL) of a 1% solution or 20 to 100 mg (1 to 5 mL) of a 2% solution may be given.

For *epidural anaesthesia* usual doses are: 150 to 300 mg (15 to 30 mL) of a 1% solution, 150 to 375 mg (10 to 25 mL) of a 1.5% solution, or 200 to 400 mg (10 to 20 mL) of a 2% solution. Hyperbaric solutions of mepivacaine hydrochloride without adrenaline have also been used for spinal anaesthesia.

Mepivacaine has been included in the intramuscular injections of other drugs to minimise the pain produced at the injection site.

Mepivacaine has also been used as a surface anaesthetic but other local anaesthetics such as lignocaine are more effective.

Action. For a comparison of the vasoactivity of mepivacaine and some other local anaesthetics, see p.1284.

Preparations

USP 23: Mepivacaine Hydrochloride and Levonordefrin Injection; Mepivacaine Hydrochloride Injection.

Proprietary Preparations (details are given in Part 3)
Aust.: Scandicain; Scandonest; ***Austral.:*** Carbocaine; ***Belg.:*** Scandicaine; ***Canad.:*** Carbocaine; Polocaine; ***Ger.:*** Meaverin; Meaverin "A" mit Adrenalin; Meaverin "N" mit Noradrenaline; Meaverin hyperbar; Mecain; Mepicaton; Mepihexal; Mepivastesin; Mepivastesin forte†; Scandicain; Scandicain "N3"†; ***Ital.:*** Carbocaina; Mepi-Mynol; Mepicain; Mepident; Mepiforan; Optocain; ***Neth.:*** Scandicaine; ***Norw.:*** Carbocain; ***S.Afr.:*** Carbocaine; Scandonest; ***Spain:*** Isogaine; Scandinibsa; ***Swed.:*** Carbocain; ***Switz.:*** Mepicaton; Scandicain; Scandonest; ***USA:*** Carbocaine; Carbocaine with Neo-Cobefrin; Isocaine; Polocaine.

Multi-ingredient: ***Ger.:*** Meaverin; Scandicain†; Thesit.

Used as an adjunct in: ***Aust.:*** Estradurin; Triodurin; ***Ger.:*** Estradurin; ***Ital.:*** Estradurin†; ***Jpn:*** Amasulin; Bestcall; Lilacillin; Pansporin; Takesulin; ***Neth.:*** Estradurin; ***Norw.:*** Estradurin; ***Swed.:*** Estradurin; Triodurin†; ***Switz.:*** Estradurin; ***UK:*** Estradurin†.

Myrtecaine (12986-l)

Myrtecaine *(rINN).*

Nopoxamine. 2-[2-(10-Norpin-2-en-2-yl)ethoxy]triethylamine.

$C_{17}H_{31}NO = 265.4.$

CAS — 7712-50-7.

Myrtecaine is a local anaesthetic (p.1281) used topically as the base or lauryl sulphate in rubefacient preparations for the treatment of muscle and joint pain. Myrtecaine lauryl sulphate is also used in preparations with antacids for the symptomatic relief of gastro-intestinal disorders.

Preparations

Proprietary Preparations (details are given in Part 3)

Multi-ingredient: ***Aust.:*** Acidrine; Kalisyl; Latesyl; Rheugesal; ***Belg.:*** Acidrine; Algesal; ***Fr.:*** Acidrine; Algesal Suractive; ***Ger.:*** Acidrine; Algesal; Algesalona; ***Ital.:*** Acidrine; ***Neth.:*** Algesal Forte; ***S.Afr.:*** Analgen†; ***Spain:*** Algesal; ***Switz.:*** Algesal; Algesalona.

Octacaine Hydrochloride (13036-x)

Octacaine Hydrochloride *(pINNM)*.

3-Diethylaminobutyranilide hydrochloride.

$C_{14}H_{22}N_2O,HCl = 270.8$.

CAS — 13912-77-1 (octacaine); 59727-70-7 (octacaine hydrochloride).

Octacaine hydrochloride is a local anaesthetic (p.1281) that has been used for surface anaesthesia.

Preparations

Proprietary Preparations (details are given in Part 3)

Multi-ingredient: ***Ger.:*** Batrax; ***Switz.:*** Batramycine.

Oxethazaine (7638-c)

Oxethazaine *(BAN, USAN)*.

Oxetacaine *(rINN)*; Wy-806. 2,2'-(2-Hydroxyethylimino)bis[*N*-(αα-dimethylphenethyl)-*N*-methylacetamide].

$C_{28}H_{41}N_3O_3 = 467.6$.

CAS — 126-27-2 (oxethazaine); 13930-31-9 (oxethazaine hydrochloride).

Pharmacopoeias. In Br. and Jpn.

A white or almost white powder. Practically **insoluble** in water; freely soluble in methyl alcohol; very soluble in chloroform; soluble in ethyl acetate.

Oxethazaine is an amide anaesthetic (p.1281) that is stated to have a prolonged action. It is administered by mouth in conjunction with antacids for the symptomatic relief of gastro-oesophageal reflux disease (p.1170). It has also been used as the hydrochloride in ointments and suppositories for the relief of pain associated with haemorrhoids.

Preparations

Proprietary Preparations (details are given in Part 3)

Ital.: Emoren; ***Jpn:*** Strocain.

Multi-ingredient: ***Aust.:*** Tepilta; ***Austral.:*** Mucaine; ***Belg.:*** Muthesa; ***Canad.:*** Mucaine; ***Fr.:*** Mutesa; ***Ger.:*** Tepilta; ***Irl.:*** Mucaine; ***Ital.:*** Mucoxin; ***S.Afr.:*** Mucaine; ***Spain:*** Natrocitral; Roberfarin; Tepilta; ***Switz.:*** Muthesa; ***UK:*** Mucaine.

Oxybuprocaine Hydrochloride

(7639-k)

Oxybuprocaine Hydrochloride *(BANM, rINNM)*.

Benoxinate Hydrochloride; Oxybuprocaini Hydrochloridum. 2-Diethylaminoethyl 4-amino-3-butoxybenzoate hydrochloride.

$C_{17}H_{28}N_2O_3,HCl = 344.9$.

CAS — 99-43-4 (oxybuprocaine); 5987-82-6 (oxybuprocaine hydrochloride).

NOTE. BNX is a code approved by the BP for use on single unit doses of eye drops containing oxybuprocaine hydrochloride where the individual container may be too small to bear all the appropriate labelling information.

Pharmacopoeias. In Eur. (see p.viii), Jpn, and US.

White or slightly off-white or colourless crystals or crystalline powder, odourless or with a slight characteristic odour. It is polymorphic. **Soluble** 1 in 0.8 of water, 1 in 2.6 of alcohol, and 1 in 2.5 of chloroform; practically insoluble in ether. Aqueous solutions have a pH of 4.5 to 6.0. **Protect** from light.

Adverse Effects, Treatment, and Precautions

As for Local Anaesthetics in general, p.1281.

Effects on the eyes. Fibrinous iritis and moderate corneal swelling occurred in 2 patients following the use of a 0.4% or 1.0% solution of oxybuprocaine hydrochloride for topical anaesthesia of the eye for minor surgery.[1] The effects may have been due to inadvertent entry of the drug into the anterior chamber of the eye.

1. Haddad R. Fibrinous iritis due to oxybuprocaine. *Br J Ophthalmol* 1989; **73:** 76–7.

Interactions

For interactions associated with local anaesthetics, see p.1283.

Uses and Administration

Oxybuprocaine, a para-aminobenzoic acid ester, is a local anaesthetic with actions and uses similar to those described on p.1283. It is used for surface anaesthesia (p.1284) and is reported to be less irritant than amethocaine when applied to the conjunctiva in therapeutic concentrations.

Oxybuprocaine is used as the hydrochloride in a 0.4% solution in short ophthalmological procedures. One drop instilled into the conjunctival sac anaesthetises the surface of the eye sufficiently to allow tonometry after 60 seconds and a further drop after 90 seconds provides adequate anaesthesia for the fitting of contact lenses. Three drops at 90-second intervals produces sufficient anaesthesia after 5 minutes for removal of a foreign body from the corneal epithelium, or for incision of a Meibomian cyst through the conjunctiva. The sensitivity of the cornea is normal again after about 1 hour.

A 1% solution of oxybuprocaine hydrochloride is also available for surface anaesthesia of the nose and throat.

Preparations

USP 23: Benoxinate Hydrochloride Ophthalmic Solution; Fluorescein Sodium and Benoxinate Hydrochloride Ophthalmic Solution.

Proprietary Preparations (details are given in Part 3)

Aust.: Flurekain; Fortasept; Novain; ***Belg.:*** Novesine; Unicaine; ***Fr.:*** Cebesine; Novesine; ***Ger.:*** Benoxinat SE; Conjuncain-EDO; Novesine; Novesine 1%; Oxbarukain; Vesiform S†; ***Ital.:*** Novesina; ***Neth.:*** Novesine 1% KNO†; ***S.Afr.:*** Novesin; ***Spain:*** Benoxinato; Prescaina; ***Switz.:*** Novesin; Novesine†.

Multi-ingredient: ***Austral.:*** Fluress; ***Belg.:*** Anesthesique Double; ***Canad.:*** Fluress; ***Fr.:*** Collu-Blache†; ***Ger.:*** duraultra forte†; Thilorbin; ***Spain:*** Anesti Doble; Fluotest; ***Swed.:*** Fluress; ***Switz.:*** Collu-Blache; Mebucaine; ***USA:*** Flu-Oxinate; Flurate; Fluress; Flurox.

Parethoxycaine Hydrochloride (13082-m)

Parethoxycaine Hydrochloride *(rINNM)*.

2-Diethylaminoethyl 4-ethoxybenzoate hydrochloride.

$C_{15}H_{23}NO_3,HCl = 301.8$.

CAS — 94-23-5 (parethoxycaine); 136-46-9 (parethoxycaine hydrochloride).

Parethoxycaine hydrochloride, a para-aminobenzoic acid ester, is a local anaesthetic (p.1281) used in pastilles for painful conditions of the mouth and throat, and in a cream for insect bites.

Preparations

Proprietary Preparations (details are given in Part 3)

Fr.: Maxicaine.

Multi-ingredient: ***Fr.:*** Maxi-Tyro†; Mousticreme†.

Pramoxine Hydrochloride (7642-l)

Pramoxine Hydrochloride *(BANM)*.

Pramocaine Hydrochloride *(rINNM)*; Pramoxinium Chloride. 4-[3-(4-Butoxyphenoxy)propyl]morpholine hydrochloride.

$C_{17}H_{27}NO_3,HCl = 329.9$.

CAS — 140-65-8 (pramoxine); 637-58-1 (pramoxine hydrochloride).

Pharmacopoeias. In US.

A white or almost white crystalline powder; it may have a faint aromatic odour. Freely **soluble** in water and alcohol; soluble 1 in 35 of chloroform; very slightly soluble in ether. A 1% solution in water has a pH of about 4.5. **Store** in airtight containers.

Pramoxine hydrochloride is a local anaesthetic (p.1281) used for surface anaesthesia. It is used alone or with corticosteroids and other drugs, usually in a concentration of 1%, in a wide range of formulations for the relief of pain and itching associated with minor skin conditions and anorectal disorders. Initial burning or stinging may occur following topical application. It should not be used for the nose or eyes. The base has been used in suppositories.

A review[1] of an aerosol foam containing pramoxine 1% with hydrocortisone 1% for the relief of puerperal perineal pain concluded that it did not offer any advantages over traditional remedies and its routine use could not be recommended.

1. Anonymous. Epifoam after childbirth for perineal pain. *Drug Ther Bull* 1987; **25:** 39–40.

Preparations

USP 23: Pramoxine Hydrochloride Cream; Pramoxine Hydrochloride Jelly.

Proprietary Preparations (details are given in Part 3)

Canad.: Tronothane†; ***Fr.:*** Tronothane; ***Ital.:*** Tronotene; ***S.Afr.:*** Anugesic; ***USA:*** Anti Itch; Fleet Pain Relief; Fleet Relief†; Prax; Proctofoam; Tronothane.

Multi-ingredient: ***Canad.:*** Anugesic-HC; Anusol Plus; Aveeno Anti-Itch; PrameGel; Pramox HC; Proctofoam-HC; Sarna-P; ***Ger.:*** Proctofoam-HC†; ***Irl.:*** Anugesic-HC; Proctofoam-HC; ***Ital.:*** Proctocort†; ***Neth.:*** Creme bij Wondjes†; Nestosyl†; Proctofoam-HC†; ***S.Afr.:*** Anugesic; Proctofoam; ***UK:*** Anugesic-HC; Epifoam†; Proctocream HC; Proctofoam-HC; ***USA:*** 1 + 1-F; Analpram-HC; Anusol; Aveeno Anti-Itch; Betadine Plus First Aid Antibiotics & Pain Reliever; Caladryl; Caladryl Clear; Cortic; Enzone; Epifoam; Gentz†; Hemorid For Women; Itch-X; Oti-Med; Otomar-HC; Phicon; Phicon-F; PrameGel; Pramosone; Proctocream HC; Proctofoam-HC; Tri-Otic; Tronolane; Zone-A†; Zoto-HC.

Prilocaine Hydrochloride (7643-y)

Prilocaine Hydrochloride *(BANM, USAN, rINNM)*.

Astra-1512; L-67; Propitocaine Hydrochloride. 2-Propylaminopropiono-o-toluidide hydrochloride.

$C_{13}H_{20}N_2O,HCl = 256.8$.

CAS — 721-50-6 (prilocaine); 1786-81-8 (prilocaine hydrochloride).

Pharmacopoeias. In Eur. (see p.viii) and US.

A white odourless crystalline powder or colourless crystals. M.p. 166° to 171°. **Soluble** 1 in 3.5 of water, 1 in 4.2 of alcohol, and 1 in 175 of chloroform; very slightly soluble in acetone; practically insoluble in ether.

Prilocaine forms a mixture with lignocaine that has a melting-point lower than that of either ingredient. This **eutectic** mixture is used in the preparation of topical dosage forms.

pH of solutions. For a discussion of the effect that pH has on the stability of local anaesthetic solutions and the pain associated with their injection, see p.1284.

Adverse Effects, Treatment, and Precautions

As for Local Anaesthetics in general, p.1281.

Methaemoglobinaemia apart, prilocaine is considered to be the least toxic of the amide-type local anaesthetics.

Methaemoglobinaemia and cyanosis, attributed to the metabolite *o*-toluidine, appear to occur more frequently with prilocaine than with other local anaesthetics (see p.1281). Symptoms usually occur when doses of prilocaine hydrochloride exceed about 8 mg per kg body-weight but the very young may be more susceptible. Methaemoglobinaemia has been observed in neonates whose mothers received prilocaine shortly before delivery and it has also been reported following prolonged topical application of a prilocaine/lignocaine eutectic mixture in children. The UK manufacturers of such a eutectic mixture have contra-indicated its use in infants under 1 year of age. Methaemoglobinaemia may be treated by administering oxygen followed, if necessary, by an injection of methylene blue.

Prilocaine should be avoided in patients with anaemia, congenital or acquired methaemoglobinaemia, cardiac or ventilatory failure, or hypoxia.

Effects on the CNS. For reference to the prilocaine serum concentrations associated with CNS toxicity, see under Absorption in Pharmacokinetics, below.

Interactions

For interactions associated with local anaesthetics, see p.1283.

Methaemoglobinaemia may occur at lower doses of prilocaine in patients receiving concomitant therapy with other drugs known to cause such conditions (e.g. sulphonamides such as sulphamethoxazole in co-trimoxazole).

Neuromuscular blockers. For a possible interaction between *mivacurium* and prilocaine, see under Atracurium, p.1307.

Pharmacokinetics

Prilocaine hydrochloride is reported to be 55% bound to plasma proteins. It is rapidly metabolised mainly in the liver and also in the kidneys and is excreted in the urine mainly as metabolites. One of the principal metabolites excreted in the urine is *o*-toluidine, which is believed to cause the methaemoglobinaemia observed after large doses. Prilocaine crosses the placenta and during prolonged epidural anaesthesia may produce methaemoglobinaemia in the fetus. It is distributed into breast milk.

See also under Local Anaesthetics, p.1283.

Absorption. Peak serum concentrations of prilocaine hydrochloride attained after the use of 8.5 mL of a 1% solution for retrobulbar and facial nerve block were well below the concentration of 20 μg per mL associated with CNS toxicity due to prilocaine.[1]

1. Goggin M, *et al.* Serum concentrations of prilocaine following retrobulbar block. *Br J Anaesth* 1990; **64:** 107–9.

Uses and Administration

Prilocaine hydrochloride is a local anaesthetic of the amide type with actions and uses similar to those described on p.1283. It has a similar anaesthetic potency to lignocaine. However, it has a slower onset of action, less vasodilator activity, and a slightly longer duration of action; it is also less toxic. Prilocaine is used for infiltration anaesthesia and nerve blocks in solutions of 0.5%, 1%, and 2%. For intravenous regional anaesthesia 0.5% and 1% solutions are used, and for epidural block and for analgesia, a 2% solution is used. A 3% solution with the vasoconstrictor felypressin (p.1246) or a 4% solution without are used for dental procedures. (Local anaesthetic techniques are discussed on p.1284.) Carbonated solutions of prilocaine have also been tried in some countries in epidural and brachial plexus nerve blocks (see p.1284). Prilocaine is used for surface anaesthesia in a eutectic mixture with lignocaine.

The dosage of prilocaine used depends on the site of injection and the procedure used. The maximum recommended dose in adults for prilocaine is 400 mg if used alone, or 300 mg if used with felypressin. Doses should be reduced for elderly or debilitated patients. The dose for children over 6 months of age is up to 5 mg per kg body-weight. For dental infiltration or nerve blocks, the usual adult dose of prilocaine hydrochloride without felypressin is 40 to 80 mg; children under 10 years of age generally require about 40 mg. The usual adult dose of prilocaine hydrochloride with felypressin 0.03 units per mL is 30 to 150 mg; children under 10 years of age generally require 30 to 60 mg.

A eutectic mixture of prilocaine base 2.5% and lignocaine base 2.5% is applied as a cream under an occlusive dressing to produce surface anaesthesia of the skin before procedures requiring needle puncture, surgical treatment of localised lesions, and split skin grafting; it has been used similarly, but without an occlusive dressing, before removal of genital warts.

Action. For a comparison of the vasoactivity of prilocaine and some other local anaesthetics, see p.1284.

Infiltration anaesthesia. Addition of felypressin at a concentration of 0.03 units per mL to prilocaine 3% injection did not reduce plasma concentrations of prilocaine after infiltration of a 60-mg dose into the upper premolar region.[1]

1. Cannell H, Whelpton R. Systemic uptake of prilocaine after injection of various formulations of the drug. *Br Dent J* 1986; **160:** 47–9.

Surface anaesthesia. For references to the use of prilocaine and lignocaine as a eutectic mixture for topical anaesthesia of intact skin and removal of genital warts, see Eutectic Mixtures under Lignocaine Hydrochloride, p.1296.

Preparations

BP 1998: Prilocaine Injection;
USP 23: Prilocaine and Epinephrine Injection; Prilocaine Hydrochloride Injection.

Proprietary Preparations (details are given in Part 3)
Austral.: Citanest; Citanest Dental; Citanest Plain; ***Belg.:*** Citanest; ***Canad.:*** Citanest; ***Ger.:*** Xylonest; ***Irl.:*** Citanest; Citanest with Octapressin; ***Ital.:*** Citanest con Octapressin; ***Neth.:*** Citanest; Citanest Octapressine; ***Norw.:*** Citanest Octapressin; ***S.Afr.:*** Citanest Octopressin†; ***Spain:*** Citanest; Citanest Octapressin; ***Swed.:*** Citanest; Citanest Octapressin; ***Switz.:*** Xylonest; Xylonest-Octapressin; ***UK:*** Citanest; Citanest with Octapressin; ***USA:*** Citanest.

Multi-ingredient: ***Aust.:*** Emla; ***Austral.:*** Emla; ***Belg.:*** Emla; ***Canad.:*** Emla; ***Fr.:*** Emla; ***Ger.:*** Emla; ***Irl.:*** Emla; ***Ital.:*** Emla; ***Neth.:*** Emla; ***Norw.:*** Citanest; Emla; ***S.Afr.:*** Emla; ***Swed.:*** Emla; ***Switz.:*** Emla; ***UK:*** Emla; ***USA:*** Emla.

Procaine Hydrochloride (7644-j)

Procaine Hydrochloride *(BANM, rINNM).*

Allocaine; Ethocaine Hydrochloride; Novocainum; Procaini Hydrochloridum; Procainii Chloridum; Procainium Chloride; Syncaine. 2-Diethylaminoethyl 4-aminobenzoate hydrochloride.

$C_{13}H_{20}N_2O_2,HCl = 272.8.$

CAS — 59-46-1 (procaine); 51-05-8 (procaine hydrochloride).

Pharmacopoeias. In *Chin., Eur.* (see p.viii), *Int., Jpn, Pol.,* and *US.*

Small colourless or white odourless crystals or a white crystalline powder. **Soluble** 1 in 1 of water and 1 in 15 of alcohol; slightly soluble in chloroform; practically insoluble in ether. A 2% solution in water has a pH of 5.0 to 6.5. **Incompatibility** has been reported with aminophylline, barbiturates, magnesium sulphate, phenytoin sodium, sodium bicarbonate, and amphotericin. **Protect** from light.

Stability of solutions. Degradation of procaine in a cardioplegic solution containing magnesium, sodium, potassium, and calcium salts was found to be temperature dependent.[1] At a storage temperature of 6° the shelf-life of the solution was 5 weeks and this was increased to 9 weeks when the storage temperature was −10°. Using carbon dioxide instead of nitrogen in the head space did not affect stability of procaine.

1. Synave R, *et al.* Stability of procaine hydrochloride in a cardioplegic solution containing bicarbonate. *J Clin Hosp Pharm* 1985; **10:** 385–8.

Adverse Effects and Treatment

As for Local Anaesthetics in general, p.1281.

Severe hypotension leading to cardiac arrest and death developed in 1 patient following the infusion of 600 mg of procaine for malignant hyperthermia.[1]

1. MacLachlan D, Forrest AL. Procaine and malignant hyperthermia. *Lancet* 1974; **i:** 355.

Hypersensitivity. Of 600 persons with dermatitis or eczema submitted to patch testing with 2% aqueous solution of procaine hydrochloride, 4.8% gave a positive reaction.[1]

For reports of hypersensitivity including anaphylactic reactions associated with procaine and other local anaesthetics, see under Adverse Effects of Local Anaesthetics, p.1282.

1. Rudzki E, Kleniewska D. The epidemiology of contact dermatitis in Poland. *Br J Dermatol* 1970; **83:** 543–5.

Precautions

As for Local Anaesthetics in general, p.1282.

Systemic lupus erythematosus. The limited theoretical risk from using procaine for local anaesthesia in patients who have had procainamide-induced systemic lupus erythematosus was aired some years ago.[1-3]

1. Dubois EL. Procaine anesthesia after procainamide-induced systemic erythematosus. *JAMA* 1977; **238:** 2201.
2. Alarcón-Segovia D. Procaine anesthesia after procainamide-induced systemic erythematosus. *JAMA* 1977; **238:** 2201.
3. Lee SL. Procaine anesthesia after procainamide-induced systemic erythematosus. *JAMA* 1977; **238:** 2201.

Interactions

For interactions associated with local anaesthetics, see p.1283.

Diuretics. Concomitant administration of *acetazolamide* extends the plasma half-life of procaine.[1]

1. Calvo R, *et al.* Effects of disease and acetazolamide on procaine hydrolysis by red blood cell enzymes. *Clin Pharmacol Ther* 1980; **27:** 179–83.

Pharmacokinetics

Procaine is poorly absorbed from mucous membranes but is readily absorbed following parenteral administration and rapidly hydrolysed by plasma cholinesterase to para-aminobenzoic acid and diethylaminoethanol; some may also be metabolised in the liver. Only about 6% is bound to plasma proteins. About 80% of the para-aminobenzoic acid is excreted unchanged or conjugated in the urine. About 30% of the diethylaminoethanol is excreted in the urine, the remainder being metabolised in the liver.

See also under Local Anaesthetics, p.1283.

Uses and Administration

Procaine hydrochloride, a para-aminobenzoic acid ester, is a local anaesthetic with actions and uses similar to those described on p.1283. Because of its poor penetration of intact mucous membranes, procaine is ineffective for surface application and has been chiefly used by injection, although in general it has been replaced by lignocaine and other local anaesthetics. It has a slow onset of action and a short duration of action. It has vasodilator activity and therefore a vasoconstrictor may be added to delay absorption and increase the duration of action. Procaine has mainly been used for infiltration anaesthesia, peripheral nerve blocks, and spinal anaesthesia. (Local anaesthetic techniques are discussed on p.1284.) It has also been used in cardioplegic solutions to protect the myocardium during cardiac surgery.

For *infiltration anaesthesia* 0.25 to 0.5% solutions of procaine hydrochloride have been used in doses of 350 to 600 mg.

For *peripheral nerve block* a usual dose of 500 mg of procaine hydrochloride has been given as a 0.5% (100 mL), 1.0% (50 mL), or 2.0% (25 mL) solution. Doses up to 1 g have been used. For infiltration and peripheral nerve block adrenaline has been added to solutions in general to give a final concentration of 1 in 200 000 to 1 in 100 000.

Procaine hydrochloride has been used with propoxycaine in dentistry.

Procaine forms poorly soluble salts or conjugates with some drugs, for example penicillin, and is used to prolong their action after injection. It may also reduce the pain of injection.

Procaine-*N*-glucoside hydrochloride is included in a preparation for gastro-intestinal disorders, and procaine ascorbate is included in a multivitamin preparation.

Action. For a comparison of the vasoactivity of procaine and some other local anaesthetics, see p.1284.

Preparations

USP 23: Procaine and Phenylephrine Hydrochlorides Injection; Procaine and Tetracaine Hydrochlorides and Levonordefrin Injection; Procaine Hydrochloride and Epinephrine Injection; Procaine Hydrochloride Injection; Propoxycaine and Procaine Hydrochlorides and Levonordefrin Injection; Propoxycaine and Procaine Hydrochlorides and Norepinephrine Bitartrate Injection.

Proprietary Preparations (details are given in Part 3)

Aust.: Geroaslan H3; Gerovital H3; Novanaest; ***Canad.:*** Novocain; ***Fr.:*** Gero†; ***Ger.:*** Hewedolor Procain; Lophakomp-Procain N; Novocain; Pasconeural-Injektopas 1%; Procaneural; ***Ital.:*** Lenident; ***Spain:*** Anestesia Loc Braun C/A; Venocaina; ***Switz.:*** Syntocaine; ***USA:*** Novocain.

Multi-ingredient: ***Aust.:*** Aslavital†; Biolecit H3; Causat; DH 112†; Gerontin; KH3; Regenerin; ***Austral.:*** Cardioplegia Solution; Cellaforte†; ***Belg.:*** Otocalmine; Rhinofluine†; Tympalgine; ***Fr.:*** Antiseptique-Calmante; Arpha†; Novitan; Otylol; Pastilles M.B.C†; Peridil-Heparine†; Rectophedrol; Stom-Antiba†; X-Adene; ***Ger.:*** B_1-Neurischian†; Bellaravil-retard†; Bellaravil†; Cardioplegin N; Causat B12 N; Causat N; Claudemor†; Dodecatol N; Echtrovit-K; Glutisal†; Hewedolor plus Coffein; Impletol; KH3; Melcain†; Myo-Melcain†; Neurotropan-Hy†; Neurotropan-M†; NeyChondrin "N" (Revitorgan-Dilutionen "N" Nr. 68); Ney-Pulpin "N" (Revitorgan-Dilutionen "N" Nr. 10); Otalgan; Otodolor; Pasconeural-Injektopas; Rectoparin†; Revicain; Revicain Comp; Revicain Comp Plus; Rutibal†; Ulcumel†; Veno-Kattwiga N; Zettaviran†; ***Ital.:*** Citroftalmina; Citroftalmina VC; Dentosedina; Gastrosanol†; Mios; Neo-Ustiol; Oftalzina; Otalgan; Otomidone; Otopax; Rinantipiol; Spasmodil Complex†; Zincoimidazyl†; ***S.Afr.:*** Universal Earache Drops; ***Spain:*** Anestesia Loc Braun S/A; Anestina Braun; Co Bucal; Coliriocilina Adren Astr; Dentol Topico; Eupnol; Hepadigest; Higado Potenciado Medic; Kanafosal; Kanafosal Predni; KH3 Powel; Neocolan; Nulacin Fermentos; Oftalmol Dexa; Oftalmol Ocular; Otalgan; Otonasal; Otosedol; Otosmo†; Pomada Oftalm Antisep†; Tangenol; ***Switz.:*** Anaestalgin; Ginvapast; Nasello; Otalgan; Otosan; ***UK:*** KH3; ***USA:*** Ravocaine and Novocain.

Used as an adjunct in: ***Ger.:*** Eukalisan N; Redox-Injektopas; ***Ital.:*** Neuroftal; ***Spain:*** Sulmetin; Sulmetin Papaverina; ***Switz.:*** Dolo-Neurobion†; ***UK:*** Achromycin†; ***USA:*** Hemocyte; Hytinic; Licoplex DS.

Propanocaine Hydrochloride (7645-z)

Propanocaine Hydrochloride *(rINNM).*

467D_3. 3-Diethylamino-1-phenylpropyl benzoate hydrochloride.

$C_{20}H_{25}NO_2,HCl = 347.9.$

CAS — 493-76-5 (propanocaine); 1679-79-4 (propanocaine hydrochloride).

Propanocaine hydrochloride, a benzoic acid ester, is a local anaesthetic (p.1281) that has been used topically for surface anaesthesia.

Preparations

Proprietary Preparations (details are given in Part 3)

Multi-ingredient: ***Fr.:*** Lelong Irritations; ***Spain:*** Detraine.

Propipocaine (19750-h)

Propipocaine *(rINN)*.

Propoxypiperocaine. 3-Piperidino-4'-propoxypropiophenone.

$C_{17}H_{25}NO_2$ = 275.4.

CAS — 3670-68-6.

Propipocaine is a local anaesthetic (p.1281) that has been used for surface anaesthesia.

Preparations

Proprietary Preparations (details are given in Part 3)
Ger.: Anaesthesie†.

Multi-ingredient: ***Ger.:*** Nifucin.

Propoxycaine Hydrochloride (7646-c)

Propoxycaine Hydrochloride *(rINNM)*.

Propoxycainium Chloride. 2-Diethylaminoethyl 4-amino-2-propoxybenzoate hydrochloride.

$C_{16}H_{26}N_2O_3$,HCl = 330.8.

CAS — 86-43-1 (propoxycaine); 550-83-4 (propoxycaine hydrochloride).

Pharmacopoeias. In *US.*

A white odourless crystalline solid. It discolours on prolonged exposure to light and air. **Soluble** 1 in 2 of water, 1 in 10 of alcohol, and 1 in 80 of ether; practically insoluble in acetone and in chloroform. A 2% solution in water has a pH of about 5.4. **Protect** from light.

Propoxycaine hydrochloride, a para-aminobenzoic acid ester, is a local anaesthetic (p.1281). It has been used in a concentration of 0.4% in combination with procaine hydrochloride 2% solution with a vasoconstrictor for infiltration anaesthesia and nerve block in dental procedures. Propoxycaine has a more rapid onset and a longer duration of action than that of procaine. Usual doses of propoxycaine hydrochloride are 7.2 mg for anaesthesia at a single site and 36 mg for anaesthesia of the entire oral cavity.

Preparations

USP 23: Propoxycaine and Procaine Hydrochlorides and Levonordefrin Injection; Propoxycaine and Procaine Hydrochlorides and Norepinephrine Bitartrate Injection.

Proprietary Preparations (details are given in Part 3)

Multi-ingredient: ***USA:*** Ravocaine and Novocain.

Proxymetacaine Hydrochloride

(7647-k)

Proxymetacaine Hydrochloride *(BANM, rINNM)*.

Proparacaine Hydrochloride. 2-Diethylaminoethyl 3-amino-4-propoxybenzoate hydrochloride.

$C_{16}H_{26}N_2O_3$,HCl = 330.8.

CAS — 499-67-2 (proxymetacaine); 5875-06-9 (proxymetacaine hydrochloride).

NOTE. PROX is a code approved by the BP for use on single unit doses of eye drops containing proxymetacaine hydrochloride where the individual container may be too small to bear all the appropriate labelling information. PROXFLN is a similar code approved for eye drops containing proxymetacaine hydrochloride and fluorescein sodium.

Pharmacopoeias. In *Br.* and *US.*

A white to off-white or faintly buff-coloured, odourless or almost odourless, crystalline powder. **Soluble** in water, in warm alcohol, in chloroform, or in methyl alcohol; very soluble in dehydrated alcohol; practically insoluble in ether. A 1% solution in water has a pH of 5.7 to 6.4. **Protect** from light.

Adverse Effects, Treatment, and Precautions

As for Local Anaesthetics in general, p.1281.

A severe immediate-type corneal reaction may rarely occur. Allergic contact dermatitis has also been reported.

Exacerbation of Stevens-Johnson syndrome has been reported[1] in one woman after ophthalmic anaesthesia with proxymetacaine hydrochloride.

1. Ward B, *et al.* Dermatologic reaction in Stevens-Johnson syndrome after ophthalmic anesthesia with proparacaine hydrochloride. *Am J Ophthalmol* 1978; **86:** 133–5.

Interactions

For interactions associated with local anaesthetics, see p.1283.

Pharmacokinetics

See under Local Anaesthetics, p.1283.

Uses and Administration

Proxymetacaine hydrochloride, a meta-aminobenzoic acid ester, is a local anaesthetic with actions and uses similar to those described on p.1283. It is used for surface anaesthesia (p.1284) in ophthalmology in a concentration of 0.5%. Proxymetacaine is of similar potency to amethocaine in equal concentrations and induces anaesthesia within about 20 seconds. The duration of action may be 15 minutes or longer. Instillation of 1 or 2 drops permits tonometry after 30 seconds. For removal of foreign bodies or sutures from the cornea 1 or 2 drops are instilled every 5 to 10 minutes for 1 to 3 doses or 1 or 2 drops are instilled 2 to 3 minutes before the procedure. For deeper anaesthesia such as needed for cataract extraction 1 drop is instilled every 5 to 10 minutes to a total of 5 to 7 applications.

Trigeminal neuralgia. There have been anecdotal reports that proxymetacaine eye drops relieved trigeminal neuralgia (p.12) refractory to carbamazepine.[1,2]

1. Zavon MR, Fichte CM. Trigeminal neuralgia relieved by ophthalmic anesthetic. *JAMA* 1991; **265:** 2807.
2. Zavon MR, Fichte CM. Trigeminal neuralgia relieved by optical anesthesia. *JAMA* 1991; **266:** 1649.

Preparations

BP 1998: Proxymetacaine Eye Drops;
USP 23: Fluorescein Sodium and Proparacaine Hydrochloride Ophthalmic Solution; Proparacaine Hydrochloride Ophthalmic Solution.

Proprietary Preparations (details are given in Part 3)
Austral.: Alcaine; Ophthaine†; Ophthetic; ***Belg.:*** Alcaine†; ***Canad.:*** Ak-Taine; Alcaine; Diocaine; Ophthetic; RO-Parcaine†; ***Ger.:*** Chibro-Kerakain; Ophthetic†; Proparakain-POS; ***Irl.:*** Ophthaine; ***Norw.:*** Alcaine; ***S.Afr.:*** Ophthetic; ***Switz.:*** Alcaine; ***UK:*** Ophthaine; ***USA:*** Ak-Taine; Alcaine; Kainair†; Ocu-caine; Ophthaine†; Ophthetic; Parcaine.

Multi-ingredient: ***Canad.:*** Dioflur-P†; Fluoracaine; ***USA:*** Fluoracaine.

Ropivacaine Hydrochloride (7300-y)

Ropivacaine Hydrochloride *(BANM, rINNM)*.

AL-281. (*S*)-2',6'-Dimethyl-1-propylpiperidine-2-carboxanilide hydrochloride monohydrate.

$C_{17}H_{26}N_2O$,HCl,H_2O = 328.9.

CAS — 84057-95-4 (ropivacaine); 98717-15-8 (anhydrous ropivacaine hydrochloride); 132112-35-7 (ropivacaine hydrochloride monohydrate).

Adverse Effects and Treatment

As for Local Anaesthetics in general, p.1281.

Effects on the cardiovascular system. Ropivacaine is structurally related to bupivacaine, but data from extensive *animal* studies suggest that ropivacaine may be less cardiotoxic than bupivacaine.[1] Results from a study[2] in 12 healthy male volunteers support these data; at doses producing CNS symptoms cardiovascular changes, such as depression of conduction and diastolic function, were less pronounced with ropivacaine than with bupivacaine.

1. Cederholm I. Preliminary risk-benefit analysis of ropivacaine in labour and following surgery. *Drug Safety* 1997; **16:** 391–402.
2. Knudsen K, *et al.* Central nervous and cardiovascular effects of i.v. infusions of ropivacaine, bupivacaine and placebo in volunteers. *Br J Anaesth* 1997; **78:** 507–14.

Precautions

As for Local Anaesthetics in general, p.1282.

Interactions

For interactions associated with local anaesthetics, see p.1283.

Concomitant administration of ropivacaine with general anaesthetics, opioid analgesics, or drugs structurally related to amide-type local anaesthetics (e.g. certain antiarrhythmics) may result in potentiation of adverse effects.

Drugs such as fluvoxamine or verapamil that inhibit CYP1A isoenzymes have the potential to produce increased plasma concentrations of ropivacaine.

Pharmacokinetics

Ropivacaine is about 94% bound to plasma proteins. The terminal elimination half-life has been reported to be 1.8 hours. It is extensively metabolised in the liver, predominantly by aromatic hydroxylation which is mediated by the cytochrome P450 isoenzyme CYP1A. The metabolites are excreted mainly in the urine; about 1% of a dose is excreted as unchanged drug. Some metabolites also have a local anaesthetic effect but less than that of ropivacaine. Ropivacaine crosses the placenta.

See also under Local Anaesthetics, p.1283.

Uses and Administration

Ropivacaine hydrochloride is a local anaesthetic of the amide type with actions and uses similar to those described on p.1283. It is a long-acting local anaesthetic, although onset and duration of action are dependent upon the administration site; the presence of a vasoconstrictor such as adrenaline has no effect. Like bupivacaine (p.1286) ropivacaine has a differential blocking effect on nerve fibres and, at the lowest concentration used, there is good differentiation between sensory and motor block. The onset and duration of sensory block produced by ropivacaine is generally similar to that obtained with bupivacaine but the motor block is often slower in onset, shorter in duration, and less intense. Ropivacaine is used for epidural blocks, peripheral nerve blocks, and infiltration anaesthesia and field blocks. At high doses it produces surgical anaesthesia, whereas at lower doses it is used for the management of acute pain such as labour pain (p.9) and postoperative pain (p.11).

Ropivacaine hydrochloride is administered in concentrations of 0.2 to 1.0%. The dosage depends on the site of injection and the procedure used. (Local anaesthetic techniques are discussed on p.1284.) The dose of ropivacaine should be reduced in the elderly, in children, and in acutely ill or debilitated patients. A test dose of lignocaine with adrenaline should be given before commencing epidural block with ropivacaine to detect inadvertent intravascular administration.

For **surgical anaesthesia**, doses of ropivacaine hydrochloride for *lumbar epidural block* are 75 to 150 mg (15 to 30 mL) as a 0.5% solution, or 112.5 to 187.5 mg (15 to 25 mL) as a 0.75% solution, or 150 to 200 mg (15 to 20 mL) as a 1.0% solution; for caesarean section, doses are 100 to 150 mg (20 to 30 mL) as a 0.5% solution or 112.5 to 150 mg (15 to 20 mL) as a 0.75% solution. Doses for *thoracic epidural block* to establish a block for post-operative pain relief are 25 to 75 mg (5 to 15 mL) as a 0.5% solution or 37.5 to 112.5 mg (5 to 15 mL) as a 0.75% solution; the actual dose used depends on the level of the injection. For *peripheral nerve blocks* of major nerves such as the brachial plexus nerve, doses are 175 to 250 mg (35 to 50 mL) as a 0.5% solution. For *infiltration anaesthesia* and *field block* up to 200 mg (40 mL) as a 0.5% solution or up to 225 mg (30 mL) as a 0.75% solution may be used.

In the management of **acute pain** ropivacaine hydrochloride is used as a 0.2% solution; 0.5% solutions may be used for infiltration. Doses for *lumbar epidural block* are 20 to 40 mg (10 to 20 mL) as an initial bolus followed by 20 to 30 mg (10 to 15 mL) at intervals of not less than 30 minutes. Alternatively, 12 to 20 mg (6 to 10 mL) per hour may be given as a continuous epidural infusion although, in the management of labour pain, doses of up to 28 mg (14 mL) per hour may be required. Doses for *thoracic epidural block* are 8 to 16 mg (4 to 8 mL) per hour as a continuous infusion. For *infiltration anaesthesia* doses are 2 to 200 mg (1 to 100 mL) of a 0.2% solution or 5 to 200 mg (1 to 40 mL) as a 0.5% solution.

References.

1. Markham A, Faulds D. Ropivacaine: a review of its pharmacology and therapeutic use in regional anaesthesia. *Drugs* 1996; **52:** 429–49.
2. McClure JH. Ropivacaine. *Br J Anaesth* 1996; **76:** 300–307
3. Morton C. Ropivacaine. *Br J Hosp Med* 1997; **58:** 97–100.

Preparations

Proprietary Preparations (details are given in Part 3)
Aust.: Naropin; ***Austral.:*** Naropin; ***Ger.:*** Naropin; ***Irl.:*** Naropin; ***Ital.:*** Naropina; ***Neth.:*** Naropin; ***Swed.:*** Narop; ***UK:*** Naropin; ***USA:*** Naropin.

Tolycaine Hydrochloride (7649-t)

Tolycaine Hydrochloride *(BANM, rINNM).*

Methyl 2-(2-diethylaminoacetamido)-*m*-toluate hydrochloride.

$C_{15}H_{22}N_2O_3,HCl = 314.8.$
CAS — 3686-58-6 (tolycaine); 7210-92-6 (tolycaine hydrochloride).

Tolycaine hydrochloride is an amide local anaesthetic (p.1281).

Preparations

Proprietary Preparations (details are given in Part 3)
Used as an adjunct in: ***Ger.:*** Tardocillin.

Tricaine Mesylate (11077-y)

Metacaine Mesylate. Ethyl 3-aminobenzoate methanesulphonate.

$C_{10}H_{15}NO_5S = 261.3.$
CAS — 886-86-2.

Tricaine mesylate is a derivative of an isomer of benzocaine (see p.1286) and although it has been used as a local anaesthetic in human medicine it is now mainly used as an anaesthetic and tranquilliser for fish and other cold-blooded animals.

Trimecaine Hydrochloride (7650-l)

Trimecaine Hydrochloride *(pINNM).*

Trimecainium Chloratum. 2-Diethylamino-2′,4′,6′-trimethylacetanilide hydrochloride.

$C_{15}H_{24}N_2O,HCl = 284.8.$
CAS — 616-68-2 (trimecaine); 1027-14-1 (trimecaine hydrochloride).

Trimecaine hydrochloride is an amide local anaesthetic (p.1281).

Preparations

Proprietary Preparations (details are given in Part 3)
Used as an adjunct in: ***Aust.:*** Ketazon; ***Ger.:*** Ketazon.

Vadocaine (3771-l)

Vadocaine *(rINN).*

ORK-242. (±)-6′-Methoxy-2-methyl-1-piperidinepropiono-2′,4′-xylidide.

$C_{18}H_{28}N_2O_2 = 304.4.$
CAS — 72005-58-4.

Vadocaine is an amide local anaesthetic (p.1281) that has been studied as the hydrochloride for its antitussive action.

References.

1. Silvasti M, *et al.* Steady state pharmacokinetics of the new antitussive compound vadocaine hydrochloride. *Arzneimittelforschung* 1990; **40:** 453–6.

Muscle Relaxants

The muscle relaxants included in this chapter are of 3 main types and are listed in Table 1, below.

Table 1. Classification of muscle relaxants.

Centrally acting relaxants	Neuromuscular blockers
Afloqualone	Competitive blockers
Baclofen	*Aminosteroidal*
Carisprodol	Pancuronium
Chlorphenesin carbamate	Pipecuronium
Chlorzoxazone	Rapacuronium
Cyclobenzaprine	Rocuronium
Eperisone	Vecuronium
Idrocilamide	*Benzylisoquinolinium*
Mephenesin	Alcuronium
Metaxalone	Atracurium
Methocarbamol	Cisatracurium
Pridinol	Doxacurium
Thiocolchicoside	Gallamine
Tizanidine	Metocurine
Tolperisone	Mivacurium
	Tubocurarine
Directly acting relaxants	Depolarising blockers
Dantrolene	Decamethonium
	Suxamethonium

Centrally acting relaxants. These generally have a selective action on the CNS and are principally used for relieving painful muscle spasms or spasticity occurring in musculoskeletal and neuromuscular disorders. Their mechanism of action may be due to their CNS-depressant activity.

Directly acting relaxants. Dantrolene is a drug which has a direct action on skeletal muscle and is used for the relief of spasticity associated with a variety of conditions.

Neuromuscular blockers (myoneuronal blockers). These drugs affect transmission at the neuromuscular junction and are used as adjuncts to general anaesthesia, particularly to enable adequate muscle relaxation to be achieved with light anaesthesia. There are 2 main types of neuromuscular blockers: competitive (or non-depolarising neuromuscular blockers) and depolarising neuromuscular blockers.

- *Competitive neuromuscular blockers* act by competing with acetylcholine for receptors on the motor end-plate. Their action can be opposed by increasing the local concentration of acetylcholine, for example by giving an anticholinesterase such as neostigmine (p.1393). Tubocurarine (p.1322) was formerly the standard reference drug of this type but its use has declined, therefore details of the actions and uses of competitive neuromuscular blockers are discussed under Atracurium, p.1304.
- *Depolarising neuromuscular blockers* act by depolarising the motor end-plate to prevent the normal response to acetylcholine; their action is not reversed by anticholinesterases. Suxamethonium (p.1319) is the standard reference drug of this type.

Also included in this chapter are miscellaneous blocking drugs, such as botulinum A toxin, which inhibits the release of acetylcholine at the motor nerve terminals.

For details of drugs used to relax *smooth muscle* see the chapters on Antimuscarinics, p.453 and Gastro-intestinal Drugs, p.1167.

General references.

1. Agoston S, *et al.* Clinical pharmacokinetics of neuromuscular blocking drugs. *Clin Pharmacokinet* 1992; **22:** 94–115.
2. Book WJ, *et al.* Adverse effects of depolarising neuromuscular blocking agents: incidence, prevention and management. *Drug Safety* 1994; **10:** 331–49.
3. Abel M, *et al.* Adverse effects of nondepolarising neuromuscular blocking agents: incidence, prevention and management. *Drug Safety* 1994; **10:** 420–38.
4. Hunter JM. New neuromuscular blocking drugs. *N Engl J Med* 1995; **332:** 1691–9.
5. Naguib M, Magboul MMA. Adverse effects of neuromuscular blockers and their antagonists. *Drug Safety* 1998; **18:** 99–116.
6. Guay J, *et al.* Clinical pharmacokinetics of neuromuscular relaxants in pregnancy. *Clin Pharmacokinet* 1998; **34:** 483–96.

Anaesthesia

Generally, *competitive neuromuscular blockers*, having a slower onset and a longer duration of action, are used in major operations, while the *depolarising neuromuscular blockers* (usually suxamethonium), with a much faster onset and shorter duration, are used for minor operations or manipulations and particularly for intubation. Following administration of suxamethonium to aid intubation, a longer-acting competitive drug may then be given to maintain muscle relaxation throughout the operation. Neuromuscular blockers can be classified by their onset and duration of action (see Table 2, below) but it should be borne in mind that onset and duration of action are dose-dependent and can therefore vary. Competitive neuromuscular blockers with a short to intermediate duration of action, such as atracurium and vecuronium, are more widely employed than those with a longer duration of action such as pancuronium. Because of the adverse effects such as myalgia associated with suxamethonium, alternative neuromuscular blockers have been investigated for intubation and some now question the use of suxamethonium for elective procedures,[1] especially in day-case patients.[2] Some competitive blockers such as vecuronium have a relatively rapid onset of action but are considered to act too slowly to enable rapid intubation in an emergency[3] when suxamethonium remains the drug of choice. The newer competitive blocker rocuronium has an onset of action only slightly slower than that of suxamethonium and may be suitable for use in emergencies when suxamethonium is contra-indicated;[4] unfortunately it has a long duration of action. Competitive blockers with more rapid onset are being evaluated. One study found that it was necessary to use an opioid such as alfentanil as part of the induction regimen in order to obtain intubating conditions with rocuronium similar to those with suxamethonium.[32]

Competitive neuromuscular blockers have also been administered in divided doses in an attempt to shorten the onset to paralysis and thus provide an alternative to suxamethonium for intubation.[5] This so-called *priming principle* involves administration of a small initial dose, termed the priming dose, followed by a large paralysing dose. Priming may be with 2 doses of the same competitive relaxant or a combination of 2 different relaxants which may then exhibit synergism. However, some consider[5] that this technique is associated with an unacceptable incidence of adverse effects and that it has no role in clinical anaesthesia.

Table 2. Relative speed of onset and duration of action of neuromuscular blockers.

Neuromuscular blocker	Onset*	Duration†
Alcuronium	Intermediate	Intermediate
Atracurium	Intermediate	Short/Intermediate
Cisatracurium	Intermediate	Short/Intermediate
Doxacurium	Slow	Long
Gallamine	Rapid	Intermediate
Metocurine	Rapid/Intermediate	Intermediate/Long
Mivacurium	Intermediate	Short
Pancuronium	Rapid	Long
Pipercuronium	Intermediate	Intermediate/Long
Rocuronium	Rapid	Intermediate
Suxamethonium	Ultra-rapid	Ultra-short
Tubocurarine	Intermediate/Slow	Intermediate
Vecuronium	Rapid	Intermediate

*Onset:	†Duration:
Ultra-rapid, less than 1 minute	Ultra-short, less than 8 minutes
Rapid, 1 to 2 minutes	Short, 8 to 20 minutes
Intermediate, 2 to 4 minutes	Intermediate, 20 to 50 minutes
Slow, more than 4 minutes	Long, more than 50 minutes

Onset and duration of action are dose-dependent

The use of anaesthetic regimens that avoid the need for a neuromuscular blocker during intubation has also been investigated. Although the general anaesthetic propofol has been tried alone[6] some consider it to be inadequate[7,8] due to undesirable haemodynamic responses and intolerance of the tracheal tube. Propofol with alfentanil was considered to produce suitable conditions for intubation in studies in adults[9-11] and in children.[12,13] In one study[12] coughing and limb movements were more common with propofol and alfentanil than with propofol and suxamethonium but it appears that the coughing may be reduced by concomitant administration of lignocaine.[11]

One group of workers[14] found that using a very low dose of suxamethonium after alfentanil and propofol produced good conditions for nasal intubation without the incidence of myalgia associated with full-dose suxamethonium. Low doses of rocuronium have also been found to improve conditions for tracheal intubation after induction with propofol and alfentanil.[15] Induction with propofol and alfentanil has enabled standard doses of vecuronium to produce conditions for rapid tracheal intubation comparable to those achieved with suxamethonium.[16]

Procedures such as intubation can cause an undesirable pressor response resulting in increased heart rate and arterial blood pressure. They can also cause an increase in intracranial pressure and intra-ocular pressure. Furthermore, the use of suxamethonium to facilitate intubation, is itself associated with a transient increase in intra-ocular pressure. Small doses of a competitive neuromuscular blocker have been given before suxamethonium to prevent this rise in intra-ocular pressure, but such a measure is not considered to be effective.[17] Opioids such as alfentanil and fentanyl appear to be effective in attenuating both the pressor response[18-20] and the rise in intra-ocular pressure[21,22] associated with intubation but the use of lignocaine has produced conflicting results.[23-27] Many anaesthetics, with the exception of ketamine, reduce intra-ocular pressure to some extent and prior administration of thiopentone may help to counteract the effect of suxamethonium.[28]

Other drugs that have been used or tried in the prevention of the haemodynamic response to intubation include magnesium sulphate[29] and propofol.[30,31]

1. Steyn M, Morton NS. Tracheal intubation without neuromuscular block. *Br J Anaesth* 1994; **73:** 862–7.
2. Cartwright DP. Suxamethonium in day-case anaesthesia. *Br J Anaesth* 1993; **71:** 918–19.
3. Williams A, *et al.* Clinical experience with Org NC45 (Norcuron) as the sole muscle relaxant. *Can Anaesth Soc J* 1982; **29:** 567–72.
4. Hunter JM. Rocuronium: the newest aminosteroid neuromuscular blocking drug. *Br J Anaesth* 1996; **76:** 481–3
5. Jones RM. The priming principle: how does it work and should we be using it? *Br J Anaesth* 1989; **63:** 1–3.
6. Keaveny JP, Knell PJ. Intubation under induction doses of propofol. *Anaesthesia* 1988; **43S:** 80–1.
7. Saarnivaara L, Klemola U-M. Injection pain, intubating conditions and cardiovascular changes following induction of anaesthesia with propofol alone or in combination with alfentanil. *Acta Anaesthesiol Scand* 1991; **35:** 19–23.
8. Rodney GE, *et al.* Propofol or propofol/alfentanil compared to thiopentone/succinylcholine for intubation of healthy children. *Can J Anaesth* 1992; **39:** A129.
9. Alcock R, *et al.* Comparison of alfentanil with suxamethonium in facilitating nasotracheal intubation in day-case anaesthesia. *Br J Anaesth* 1993; **70:** 34–7.
10. Coghlan SFE, *et al.* Use of alfentanil with propofol for nasotracheal intubation without neuromuscular block. *Br J Anaesth* 1993; **70:** 89–91.
11. Davidson JAH, Gillespie JA. Tracheal intubation after induction of anaesthesia with propofol, alfentanil and i.v. lignocaine. *Br J Anaesth* 1993; **70:** 163–6.
12. Steyn MP, *et al.* Tracheal intubation without neuromuscular block in children. *Br J Anaesth* 1994; **72:** 403–6.
13. McConaghy P, Bunting HE. Assessment of intubating conditions in children after induction with propofol and varying doses of alfentanil. *Br J Anaesth* 1994; **73:** 596–9.
14. Nimmo SM, *et al.* Effectiveness and sequelae of very low-dose suxamethonium for nasal intubation. *Br J Anaesth* 1995; **74:** 31–4.
15. Barclay K, *et al.* Low-dose rocuronium improves conditions for tracheal intubation after induction of anaesthesia with propofol and alfentanil. *Br J Anaesth* 1997; **78:** 92–4.
16. Groener R, Moyes DG. Rapid tracheal intubation with propofol, alfentanil and a standard dose of vecuronium. *Br J Anaesth* 1997; **79:** 384–5.
17. Book WJ, *et al.* Adverse effects of depolarising neuromuscular blocking agents: incidence, prevention and management. *Drug Safety* 1994; **10:** 331–49.
18. Crawford DC, *et al.* Effects of alfentanil on the pressor and catecholamine responses to tracheal intubation. *Br J Anaesth* 1987; **59:** 707–12.

19. Scheinin B, *et al.* Alfentanil obtunds the cardiovascular and sympathoadrenal responses to suxamethonium-facilitated laryngoscopy and intubation. *Br J Anaesth* 1989; **62:** 385–92.
20. Chung F, Evans D. Low-dose fentanyl: haemodynamic response during induction and intubation in geriatric patients. *Can Anaesth Soc J* 1985; **32:** 622–8.
21. Mostafa SM, *et al.* Comparison of effects of fentanyl and alfentanil on intra-ocular pressure. *Anaesthesia* 1986; **41:** 493–8.
22. Sweeney J, *et al.* Modification by fentanyl and alfentanil of the intraocular pressure response to suxamethonium and tracheal intubation. *Br J Anaesth* 1989; **63:** 688–91.
23. Tam S, *et al.* Attenuation of circulatory responses to endotracheal intubation using intravenous lidocaine: a determination of the optimal time of injection. *Can Anaesth Soc J* 1985; **32:** S65.
24. Miller CD, Warren SJ. I.V. lignocaine fails to attenuate the cardiovascular response to laryngoscopy and tracheal intubation. *Br J Anaesth* 1990; **65:** 216–19.
25. Murphy DF, *et al.* Intravenous lignocaine pretreatment to prevent intraocular pressure rise following suxamethonium and tracheal intubation. *Br J Ophthalmol* 1986; **70:** 596–8.
26. Drenger B, Pe'er J. Attenuation of ocular and systemic responses to tracheal intubation by intravenous lignocaine. *Br J Ophthalmol* 1987; **71:** 546–8.
27. Mostafa SM, *et al.* Effects of nebulized lignocaine on the intraocular pressure responses to tracheal intubation. *Br J Anaesth* 1990; **64:** 515–17.
28. Holloway KB. Control of the eye during general anaesthesia for intraocular surgery. *Br J Anaesth* 1980; **52:** 671–9.
29. Ashton WB, *et al.* Attenuation of the pressor response to tracheal intubation by magnesium sulphate with and without alfentanil in hypertensive proteinuric patients undergoing caesarean section. *Br J Anaesth* 1991; **67:** 741–7.
30. Brossy MJ, *et al.* Haemodynamic and catecholamine changes after induction of anaesthesia with either thiopentone or propofol with suxamethonium. *Br J Anaesth* 1994; **72:** 596–8.
31. Gin T, *et al.* Plasma catecholamines and neonatal condition after induction of anaesthesia with propofol or thiopentone at caesarean section. *Br J Anaesth* 1993; **70:** 311–116.
32. Sparr HJ, *et al.* Influence of induction technique on intubating conditions after rocuronium in adults: comparison with rapid-sequence induction using thiopentone and suxamethonium. *Br J Anaesth* 1996; **77:** 339–42.

Intensive care

The use of neuromuscular blockers in patients requiring mechanical ventilation as part of intensive care has been discussed in a number of reviews.[1,2] Neuromuscular blockers are used to provide additional relaxation and facilitate ventilatory support in patients who fail to respond to sedation alone. It is important to ensure that such patients are adequately sedated before these drugs are administered. Patients who are considered most likely to benefit are those with spontaneous respiration that is counterproductive to mechanical ventilation. Patients with little inherent respiratory muscle activity are less likely to obtain an improvement in oxygenation. Neuromuscular blockers may also improve control of intracranial pressure in patients with intracranial hypertension including prevention of rises in intracranial pressure associated with routine tracheobronchial suction.

Pancuronium has been widely used as a neuromuscular blocker in intensive care because of its tendency to increase arterial pressure but it can also produce tachycardia. Vecuronium and atracurium have relatively few cardiovascular effects but there has been some concern over the ability of a metabolite of atracurium to cross the blood-brain barrier and accumulate in the CNS (see under Pharmacokinetics, p.1307). Tachyphylaxis may occur and dosage requirements may be increased in patients with burns or in those receiving prolonged therapy. Dose modification may also be necessary in patients with renal or hepatic impairment.

When rapid reversal of paralysis is necessary an anticholinesterase such as neostigmine may be used but relatively little is known about the efficacy of anticholinesterases in reversing prolonged paralysis.[3] Prolonged neuromuscular blockade may be related to dosage and since the pharmacodynamics and pharmacokinetics of neuromuscular blockers may be altered in patients in intensive care close monitoring of neuromuscular blockade is advised.[1,2] Other factors which may potentiate neuromuscular blockade include drug interactions, electrolyte imbalance, hypothermia, or changes in acid-base balance.[1] An acute myopathy has followed prolonged use, most commonly with aminosteroid neuromuscular blockers.

Neonatal intensive care. Neuromuscular blockers such as pancuronium bromide are used in neonatal intensive care to obtain muscle relaxation during mechanical ventilation in infants with severe pulmonary disease, especially in those whose respiratory efforts are out of phase with the ventilator.[4] They are only used in infants at high risk of complications such as *pneumothorax* or *intraventricular haemorrhage*.

Abolition of spontaneous respiration during mechanical ventilation has had variable effects on the incidence of *pneumothorax* in infants with respiratory distress syndrome. Although a reduced incidence was found in one study[5] involving infants of less than 33 weeks' gestation, in another study[6] the incidence was reduced only in infants with a gestational age of 27 to 32 weeks; no reduction was obtained in those below 26 weeks' gestation. Paralysis also failed to reduce the incidence of pneumothorax or interstitial emphysema in a study[7] of infants with hyaline membrane disease but did appear to speed recovery of lung function.

The aetiology of *intraventricular haemorrhage* remains obscure but there is a well recognised association with gestational age;[8] less mature neonates are more susceptible and the incidence decreases sharply after 30 weeks' gestation. There appears to be an association between fluctuating cerebral blood-flow velocity in the first day of life and subsequent development of intraventricular haemorrhage.[9] Respiratory paralysis from the first day of life until 72 hours of age has been reported[10] to stabilise both cerebral and arterial blood-flow velocity and to produce a decrease in the incidence and severity of intraventricular haemorrhage in infants with respiratory distress syndrome. However, respiratory paralysis has also been reported to have no effect on the development of intraventricular haemorrhage.[5,6]

The use of neuromuscular blockers in the newborn is not without complications. Multiple joint contractures, possibly potentiated by concomitant use of aminoglycosides or phenobarbitone, have been reported[11,12] in infants given pancuronium and regular passive limb movements should be performed during paralysis. Marked oedema, severe disturbances of fluid balance, and renal failure followed by death have been reported in 2 neonates.[13] Hypoxaemia may develop following induction of paralysis unless a significant increase in ventilator support is made;[5,9,14] hypotension may also occur.[15] Drugs such as pancuronium which are metabolised in the liver and excreted in the urine have a prolonged action in premature infants.[4] As with adults (see above), continuous use of neuromuscular blockers in neonates has been associated with prolonged neuromuscular block on discontinuation.[16]

1. Coursin DB, *et al.* Muscle relaxants in critical care. *Curr Opin Anaesthesiol* 1993; **6:** 341–6.
2. Elliot JM, Bion JF. The use of neuromuscular blocking drugs in intensive care practice. *Acta Anaesthesiol Scand* 1995; **39** (suppl 106): 70–82.
3. Watling SM, Dasta JF. Prolonged paralysis in intensive care unit patients after the use of neuromuscular blocking agents: a review of the literature. *Crit Care Med* 1994; **22:** 884–93.
4. Levene MI, Quinn MW. Use of sedatives and muscle relaxants in newborn babies receiving mechanical ventilation. *Arch Dis Child* 1992; **67:** 870–3.
5. Greenough A, *et al.* Pancuronium prevents pneumothoraces in ventilated premature babies who actively expire against positive pressure inflation. *Lancet* 1984; **i:** 1–3.
6. Cooke RWI, Rennie JM. Pancuronium and pneumothorax. *Lancet* 1984; **i:** 286–7.
7. Pollitzer MJ, *et al.* Pancuronium during mechanical ventilation speeds recovery of lungs of infants with hyaline membrane disease. *Lancet* 1981; **i:** 346–8.
8. Miall-Allen VM, *et al.* Blood pressure fluctuation and intraventricular hemorrhage in the preterm infant of less than 31 weeks' gestation. *Pediatrics* 1989; **83:** 657–61.
9. Perlman JM, *et al.* Fluctuating cerebral blood-flow velocity in respiratory distress syndrome. *N Engl J Med* 1983; **309:** 204–9.
10. Perlman JM, *et al.* Reduction in intraventricular hemorrhage by elimination of fluctuating cerebral blood-flow velocity in preterm infants with respiratory distress syndrome. *N Engl J Med* 1985; **312:** 1353–7.
11. Sinha SK, Levene MI. Pancuronium bromide induced joint contractures in the newborn. *Arch Dis Child* 1984; **59:** 73–5.
12. Fanconi S, *et al.* Effects of paralysis with pancuronium bromide on joint mobility in premature infants. *J Pediatr* 1995; **127:** 134–6.
13. Reynolds EOR, *et al.* Muscle relaxation and periventricular hemorrhage. *N Engl J Med* 1985; **313:** 955–6.
14. Philips JB, *et al.* Hypoxaemia in ventilated neonates after pancuronium paralysis. *Lancet* 1979, **i:** 877.
15. McIntosh N. Hypotension associated with pancuronium use in the newborn. *Lancet* 1985; **ii:** 279.
16. Björklund LJ. Use of sedatives and muscle relaxants in newborn babies receiving mechanical ventilation. *Arch Dis Child* 1993; **69:** 544.

Muscle spasm

Spasm is a painful involuntary contraction of muscle which can cause involuntary movement, interfere with function, and cause distortion. It is a symptom of many muscular and other types of disorders and treatment should primarily be aimed at the underlying cause. Centrally acting muscle relaxants and benzodiazepines are used to treat muscle spasms such as *splinting* that occur in response to local trauma or musculoskeletal and joint disorders. Splinting is a reflex muscular spasm that produces muscular rigidity and acts as a protective mechanism to prevent movement and further damage of the affected part. Short courses of muscle relaxants may be considered in the management of acute low back pain (p.10).

Cramps are muscle spasms of abrupt onset that occur at rest and usually last for a few seconds or minutes. They are often precipitated by dehydration and hyponatraemia produced by vigorous exercise, excessive sweating, diarrhoea, and vomiting or may be associated with drug therapy or haemodialysis. Pregnant women, the elderly, and those with peripheral vascular disease, appear to be particularly susceptible to *night cramps* of the feet or legs, the cause of which is not well understood.

The management of muscle cramps has been reviewed.[1] Quinine has traditionally been the standard treatment for nocturnal cramps but there has been concern over its efficacy and potential for adverse effects, especially in the elderly. In the USA, for example, the FDA ruled that quinine products should no longer be used for the management of nocturnal cramps.[2,3] A meta-analysis[4] concluded that although quinine was effective in the treatment of nocturnal cramps in ambulatory patients the risk of serious adverse effects should be borne in mind. It was recommended that patients should be closely monitored while the efficacy of quinine is assessed over a period of at least 4 weeks. Some authorities recommend that treatment be stopped every 3 months to see whether it is still needed.[5] A number of other drugs have been tried for nocturnal cramps but there is little convincing evidence to support their use.[1,2]

Haemodialysis-induced cramp (p.1151) is a common complication occurring during or after dialysis.[1,6] Its aetiology is not clear but response to blood volume expansion with hypertonic solutions such as glucose, mannitol, or saline suggests that hypovolaemia may be involved. Haemodialysis-induced cramp has also been reported to respond to quinine.

1. McGee SR. Muscle cramps. *Arch Intern Med* 1990; **150:** 511–18.
2. FDA. Drug products for the treatment and/or prevention of nocturnal leg muscle cramps for over-the-counter human use. *Fed Regist* 1994; **59:** 43234–52.
3. Nightingale SL. Quinine for nocturnal leg cramps. *ACP J Club* 1995; **123:** 86.
4. Man-Son-Hing M, Wells G. Meta-analysis of efficacy of quinine for treatment of nocturnal leg cramps in elderly people. *Br Med J* 1995; **310:** 13–17.
5. Anonymous. Quinine for nocturnal leg cramps? *Drug Ther Bull* 1996; **34:** 7–8.
6. Mujais SK. Muscle cramps during hemodialysis. *Int J Artif Organs* 1994; **17:** 570–2.

Spasticity

The term, spasticity, has been loosely applied to various disorders of motor control resulting from CNS disease. The concept of spasticity generally includes symptoms such as increased muscle tone, exaggerated stretch reflexes, impaired voluntary movement, weakness, loss of dexterity, abnormal posture, and often disturbed gait. In some patients muscle spasm and pain may be more distressing than impaired movement. Other complications may include contractures, pressure sores, and infection. Spasticity is a feature of many neurological conditions, particularly spinal lesions, such as in multiple sclerosis, cerebral palsy, head injury, and stroke.

Spasticity is disabling and difficult to treat when severe, but mild or moderate forms may be effectively managed by conservative treatment. Some patients may even use spasticity to provide a means of posture control and care should be taken that treatment does not lead to increased disability.

Various discussions on the management of spasticity have been published.[1,2] The mainstay of management is physiotherapy together with antispastic drugs. Baclofen, dantrolene, and diazepam are the drugs most often used. These 3 drugs act via different mechanisms which are not fully understood.

Baclofen is thought to act at the spinal cord level but may also have supraspinal sites of action. It is a powerful neuronal depressant and may exert its inhibitory effects by acting as an agonist at GABA (gamma aminobutyric acid) receptors. *Diazepam* is also thought to act centrally by enhancing the response to GABA. In contrast, *dantrolene* acts directly on muscles possibly by interfering with release of calcium from muscular sarcoplasmic reticulum thus interfering with contraction. All these are usually given by mouth but baclofen may also be given intrathecally in severe chronic spasticity.[3,4] Administration directly into the spinal subarachnoid space allows immediate delivery to the site of action in the spinal cord and hence allows considerably lower doses to be used than those given orally. It has been reported,[5] that some patients receiving long-term intrathecal baclofen treatment, have been able to stop their therapy without symptoms of spasticity re-appearing, and that others have been able to reduce the dosage required.

Tizanidine, a recently introduced centrally acting relaxant and α-adrenergic agonist, may also be of value for spasticity. It can produce additive effects with baclofen thereby allowing a reduction in the dosage of both drugs; use with benzodiazepines is not recommended because of the potential for interactions.

Other drugs which may produce some benefit or are being studied in spasticity include *other benzodiazepines*, *clonidine*, and *memantine*.

Other approaches to treatment include nerve blocks using *local anaesthetics*; they should generally only be used when further muscle relaxation would not increase disability. *Chemical neurolysis* using alcohol or phenol is only considered when there is intractable continuous pain. Local injections of *botulinum A toxin* have produced some encouraging results in the management of limb spasticity in post-stroke patients and in children with cerebral palsy; its temporary effect may be an advantage over chemical neurolysis but some consider that the need for regular injections is unlikely to be acceptable to children.[6]

Nondrug treatments have included electrical stimulation techniques such as transcutaneous nerve stimulation and dorsal column stimulation; vibration applied to agonist spastic muscles to improve voluntary movement; cooling to decrease afferent inputs from peripheral receptors; and orthopaedic surgery or neurosurgery.

1. Young RR. Spasticity: a review. *Neurology* 1994; **44** (suppl 9): S12–S20.
2. Ko Ko C, Ward AB. Management of spasticity. *Br J Hosp Med* 1997; **58:** 400–5.
3. McLean BN. Intrathecal baclofen in severe spasticity. *Br J Hosp Med* 1993; **49:** 262–7.
4. Anonymous. Intrathecal baclofen for spasticity. *Med Lett Drugs Ther* 1994; **36:** 21–2.
5. Dressnandt J, Conrad B. Lasting reduction of severe spasticity after ending chronic treatment with intrathecal baclofen. *J Neurol Neurosurg Psychiatry* 1996; **60:** 168–73.
6. Neville B. Botulinum toxin in the cerebral palsies. *Br Med J* 1994; **309:** 1526–7.

Tetanus

The clinical manifestations of tetanus following infection with *Clostridium tetani* are caused by the highly potent neurotoxin tetanospasmin produced by its germinating spores. For the antibacterial treatment and prevention of tetanus and neutralisation of tetanospasmin, see p.145.

The muscular symptoms of generalised tetanus include trismus (lockjaw), glottal spasm, generalised muscle spasm, opisthotonus (spasm of the back muscles resulting in backward arching of the body), respiratory spasm, and paralysis. Other complications include electrolyte disturbances and autonomic dysfunction leading to cardiovascular effects such as hypertension, tachycardia, and peripheral vasoconstriction. Patients may have a milder form in which the twitching and muscle spasms are limited to the area near the site of the injury but this localised tetanus is rare and can progress to the generalised form.

Benzodiazepines such as diazepam are useful for controlling the neuromuscular manifestations and can also reduce patient anxiety and produce sedation. *Opioid analgesics* can be added to treatment to provide analgesia and additional sedation. *Chlorpromazine* is sometimes used in combination with benzodiazepines to minimise rigidity and muscle spasms. Centrally acting muscle relaxants have also been used to control muscle spasms. *Baclofen* has been given by the intrathecal route but its therapeutic range in severe tetanus may be very narrow and deep coma and loss of spontaneous respiration has been reported. When muscle spasms are severe or interfere with respiration, *competitive neuromuscular blockers* have been used, in addition to benzodiazepine sedation, to control spasms and to induce therapeutic paralysis so mechanical ventilation can be initiated. Various drugs have been tried to control autonomic overactivity including *beta blockers* and *morphine*. Electrolyte disturbance is corrected with calcium and magnesium salts.

References.

1. Attygalle D, Karalliedde L. Unforgettable tetanus. *Eur J Anaesthesiol* 1997; **14:** 122–33.
2. Ernst ME, *et al.* Tetanus: pathophysiology and management. *Ann Pharmacother* 1997; **31:** 1507–13.

Afloqualone (12331-t)

Afloqualone *(rINN)*.

HQ-495. 6-Amino-2-fluoromethyl-3-*o*-tolylquinazolin-4(3*H*)-one.

$C_{16}H_{14}FN_3O$ = 283.3.

CAS — 56287-74-2.

Afloqualone is a centrally acting skeletal muscle relaxant that has been given by mouth for the treatment of muscle spasm associated with musculoskeletal conditions. Photosensitivity reactions have been reported.

References.

1. Ishikawa T, *et al.* Photoleukomelanodermatitis (Kobori) induced by afloqualone. *J Dermatol* 1994; **21:** 430–3.

Preparations

Proprietary Preparations (details are given in Part 3)
Jpn: Arofuto†.

Alcuronium Chloride (5701-j)

Alcuronium Chloride *(BAN, USAN, rINN)*.

Alcuronii Chloridum; Allnortoxiferin Chloride; Diallylnortoxiferine Dichloride; Diallyltoxiferine Chloride; Ro-4-3816. *NN'*-Diallylbisnortoxiferinium dichloride.

$C_{44}H_{50}Cl_2N_4O_2$ = 737.8.

CAS — 23214-96-2 (alcuronium); 15180-03-7 (alcuronium chloride).

Pharmacopoeias. In *Eur.* (see p.viii).

A white or slightly greyish-white, crystalline powder. Freely **soluble** in water and in methyl alcohol; soluble in alcohol; practically insoluble in cyclohexane. **Store** in an airtight container under nitrogen. Protect from light.

Adverse Effects, Treatment, and Precautions

As for competitive neuromuscular blockers in general (see Atracurium, p.1304).

Alcuronium chloride can induce histamine release to some degree. Anaphylactoid reactions have been associated with the use of alcuronium. It has some vagolytic action and may produce tachycardia; hypotension may also occur.

Hypersensitivity. Reports of anaphylactoid reactions to alcuronium.

See also under Suxamethonium Chloride, p.1320.

1. Fisher M, Baldo B. Adverse reactions to alcuronium: an Australian disease? *Med J Aust* 1983; **i:** 630–2.
2. Fisher MM, Munro I. Life-threatening anaphylactoid reactions to muscle relaxants. *Anesth Analg* 1983; **62:** 559–64.

Porphyria. Alcuronium was considered to be unsafe in patients with acute porphyria because it has been shown to be porphyrinogenic in *animals* or *in-vitro* systems.[1]

1. Moore MR, McColl KEL. *Porphyria: drug lists.* Glasgow: Porphyria Research Unit, University of Glasgow, 1991

Pregnancy. Alcuronium crosses the placenta. No evidence of neuromuscular block was seen in any of the neonates born to 12 women who received alcuronium 15 to 30 mg by intravenous injection, 5.0 to 10.5 minutes before delivery[1] but caution is advised if alcuronium is given in obstetrics in high doses or for a prolonged period.

1. Ho PC, *et al.* Caesarean section and placental transfer of alcuronium. *Anaesth Intensive Care* 1981; **9:** 113–18.

Renal impairment. Alcuronium is excreted mainly by the kidneys and accumulation, with prolonged paralysis, may therefore be expected in patients with renal impairment given large or repeated doses. A prolonged elimination half-life has been reported in anuria.[1] However, doses of 160 μg per kg body-weight have been used without any problems in patients with chronic renal failure undergoing renal transplantation.[2] The average duration of action of this dose was 37 minutes and any residual neuromuscular blockade at the end of surgery was successfully reversed using atropine and neostigmine.

1. Raaflaub J, Frey P. Zur pharmakokinetik von diallylnortoxiferin beim menschen. *Arzneimittelforschung* 1972; **22:** 73–8.
2. Kaushik S, *et al.* Use of alcuronium in patients undergoing renal transplantation. *Br J Anaesth* 1984; **56:** 1229–33.

Interactions

For interactions associated with competitive neuromuscular blockers, see Atracurium, p.1306.

Pharmacokinetics

When given intravenously, alcuronium is widely distributed throughout the body tissues and crosses the placenta. It is excreted unchanged, mainly in urine. Small amounts are also excreted in bile. The elimination half-life is about 3 hours.

References.

1. Raaflaub J, Frey P. Zur pharmakokinetik von diallylnortoxiferin beim menschen. *Arzneimittelforschung* 1972; **22:** 73–8.
2. Walker J, *et al.* Clinical pharmacokinetics of alcuronium chloride in man. *Eur J Clin Pharmacol* 1980; **17:** 449–57.

Uses and Administration

Alcuronium chloride is a benzylisoquinolinium competitive neuromuscular blocker (see Atracurium, p.1308) that is used for endotracheal intubation and to provide muscle relaxation in general anaesthesia for surgical procedures (see Anaesthesia, p.1302). An initial dose of 200 to 250 μg per kg bodyweight has been given intravenously. Supplementary doses of one-sixth to one-quarter the initial dose are reported to provide relaxation for additional periods of similar duration to the first. The above doses produce muscle relaxation within about 2 minutes and the effect lasts for about 20 to 30 minutes.

Preparations

Proprietary Preparations (details are given in Part 3)
Aust.: Alloferin; ***Austral.:*** Alloferin†; ***Ger.:*** Alloferin; ***Neth.:*** Alloferin†; ***S.Afr.:*** Alloferin; ***Switz.:*** Alloferine†; ***UK:*** Alloferin†.

Atracurium Besylate (12405-r)

Atracurium Besylate *(BAN, USAN)*.

Atracurium Besilate *(rINN)*; 33A74; BW-33A. 2,2'-(3,11-Dioxo-4,10-dioxatridecamethylene)bis(1,2,3,4-tetrahydro-6,7-dimethoxy-2-methyl-1-veratrylisoquinolinium) di(benzenesulphonate).

$C_{53}H_{72}N_2O_{12},2C_6H_5O_3S$ = 1243.5.

CAS — 64228-81-5.

Pharmacopoeias. In *It.*

The commercial preparation of atracurium is a mixture of 10 stereoisomers of which cisatracurium constitutes about 15%.

Cisatracurium Besylate (17507-r)

Cisatracurium Besylate *(BAN)*.

Cisatracurium Besilate *(rINN)*; Bésilate de Cisatracurium; Besilato de Cisatracurio; BW-51W (cisatracurium); BW-51W89 (cisatracurium); 51W89 (cisatracurium). (1*R*,1'*R*,2*R*,2'*R*)-2,2'-(3,11-Dioxo-4,10-dioxatridecamethylene)bis(1,2,3,4-tetrahydro-6,7-dimethoxy-2-methyl-1-veratrylisoquinolinium) dibenzenesulfonate.

CAS — 96946-42-8.

Incompatibility. Neuromuscular blockers are generally incompatible with alkaline solutions, for example barbiturates such as thiopentone sodium. It is good practice not to administer neuromuscular blockers in the same syringe, or simultaneously through the same needle, as other drugs.

Adverse Effects

The adverse effects of competitive neuromuscular blockers are generally similar although they differ in their propensity to cause histamine release and cardiovascular effects. Histamine release and associated cardiovascular effects appear to be rare with the aminosteroidal blockers. Competitive neuromuscular blockers with vagolytic activity may produce tachycardia and a rise in blood pressure. The use of blockers which lack an effect on the vagus may result in bradycardia during anaesthesia due to the effects of other drugs employed or as a result of vagal stimulation. Reduction in blood pressure with compensatory tachycardia may occur with some competitive neuromuscular blockers due in part to sympathetic ganglion blockade or the release of histamine. Reduction in gastro-intestinal motility and tone may occur as a result of ganglionic blockade.

Histamine release may also lead to wheal-and-flare effects at the site of injection, flushing, occasionally bronchospasm, and rarely anaphylactoid reactions.

Malignant hyperthermia has been associated rarely with competitive neuromuscular blockers.

In overdosage there is prolonged apnoea due to paralysis of the intercostal muscles and diaphragm, with cardiovascular collapse and the effects of histamine release.

Atracurium and its isomer cisatracurium have no significant vagal or ganglionic blocking activity at recommended doses. Unlike atracurium, cisatracurium does not induce histamine release and is therefore associated with greater cardiovascular stability.

For possible risks from their major metabolite laudanosine, see under Pharmacokinetics, below.

In 3 large-scale surveillance studies involving a total of 6106 patients, 3346 of whom were given atracurium, the overall incidence of adverse events in the atracurium groups was 10%,[1] 13%,[2] and 29%.[3] This compared with an incidence of 18% in patients given alcuronium, 13% in patients given a neuromuscular blocker other than atracurium, and 40% in patients given vecuronium, respectively. Severe reactions with atracurium were infrequent. No patient experienced cardiac arrest or anaphylaxis and there were no reports of difficulty in antagonism of neuromuscular blockade. Adverse effects possibly related to histamine release in the atracurium groups were hypotension (in 3.4, 1.8, and 15% of patients), bronchospasm or wheezing (0.2, 1.5, and 0.4%), tachycardia (1.9, 0.1, and 0.4%), and rash (2.5, 0.3, and 1.0%). Other cardiovascular events reported included hypertension (1.1, 1.4, and 0.6%) and bradycardia (0.6, 0.8, and 12%). Hypotension and tachycardia occurred significantly less often in patients given atracurium compared with those given alcuronium but cutaneous reactions occurred more often. No other significant differences were observed in the incidence of adverse events in patients given atracurium compared with those receiving another neuromuscular blocker.

1. Beemer GH, *et al.* Adverse reactions to atracurium and alcuronium: a prospective surveillance study. *Br J Anaesth* 1988; **61:** 680–4.
2. Jick H, *et al.* Atracurium—a post-marketing surveillance study: methods and US experience. *Br J Anaesth* 1989; **62:** 590–5.
3. Lawson DH, *et al.* Atracurium—a post-marketing surveillance study: UK study and discussion. *Br J Anaesth* 1989; **62:** 596–600.

Effects on body temperature. Malignant hyperthermia has been associated with competitive neuromuscular blockers on rare occasions. Two cases of mild malignant hyperthermia have been reported[1] where tubocurarine was probably the triggering drug. Each episode developed in a member of a known malignant hyperthermia family and developed despite preventive measures such as prophylactic cooling, and avoidance of potent inhalation anaesthetics and depolarising muscle relaxants. Another case[2] was associated with the use of pancuronium.

1. Britt BA, *et al.* Malignant hyperthermia induced by curare. *Can Anaesth Soc J* 1974; **21:** 371–5.
2. Waterman PM, *et al.* Malignant hyperthermia: a case report. *Anesth Analg* 1980; **59:** 220–1.

Effects on the muscles. For reference to acute myopathy and prolonged muscle weakness after withdrawal of long-term continuous infusions of competitive neuromuscular blockers, see under Intensive Care, p.1303.

Hypersensitivity. Reports[1,2] of severe anaphylactoid reactions following administration of atracurium. For a discussion of hypersensitivity reactions associated with neuromuscular blockers, see under Suxamethonium Chloride, p.1320.

1. Stirton-Hopkins C. Life-threatening reaction to atracurium. *Br J Anaesth* 1988; **60:** 597–8.
2. Oh TE, Horton JM. Adverse reactions to atracurium. *Br J Anaesth* 1989; **62:** 467–8.

Treatment of Adverse Effects

It is essential to maintain assisted respiration in patients who have received a competitive neuromuscular blocker until spontaneous breathing is fully restored; in addition a cholinesterase inhibitor such as neostigmine is usually given intravenously, in association with atropine or glycopyrronium, to hasten reversal of the neuromuscular block. Patients need to be closely monitored after reversal of block to ensure that muscle relaxation does not return.

Severe hypotension may require intravenous fluid replacement and cautious administration of a pressor agent; the patient should be positioned to facilitate venous return from the muscles.

Administration of an antihistamine before induction of neuromuscular blockade may be of value in preventing histamine-induced adverse effects in patients with asthma or those susceptible to bronchospasm.

Reversal of neuromuscular blockade. For a discussion of the use of anticholinesterases for reversal of residual neuromuscular block produced by intermediate- or short-acting blockers after surgical or similar procedures, see under Neostigmine, p.1395.

Precautions

Doses of neuromuscular blockers need to be carefully titrated for individual patients according to response; monitoring of the degree of block is recommended in order to reduce the risk of overdosage. Patients who have received a neuromuscular blocker should always have their respiration assisted or controlled until the drug has been inactivated or antagonised.

Atracurium and other competitive neuromuscular blockers should be used with great care, if at all, in respiratory insufficiency or pulmonary disease and in the dehydrated or severely ill patient. The response to neuromuscular blockers is often unpredictable in patients with neuromuscular disorders and they should be used with great caution in these patients (see below). Caution is also needed in patients with a history of conditions such as asthma where release of histamine would be a hazard. Care is also required in patients with a history of hypersensitivity to any neuromuscular blocker.

Resistance to the effects of competitive neuromuscular blockers may occur in patients with burns (see below). The effect of competitive neuromuscular blockers may vary in patients with hepatic impairment. Resistance appears to occur to the actions of some blockers such as doxacurium, metocurine, pancuronium, and tubocurarine while for some other blockers, including mivacurium and rocuronium, a prolonged action in patients with hepatic impairment may necessitate a reduction in the usual dosage.

Competitive neuromuscular blockers excreted mainly in the urine should be used with caution in renal impairment; a reduction in dosage may be necessary. Dosage reductions are also required in obese patients, to take account of ideal body weight. Doses may need to be reduced in infants and neonates due to increased sensitivity to competitive muscle relaxants.

The effects of competitive neuromuscular blockers are increased by metabolic or respiratory acidosis and hypokalaemia, hypermagnesaemia, hypocalcaemia, and hypophosphataemia. Competitive neuromuscular blockade may also be enhanced by raised body temperature and reduced in hypothermia.

In contrast to other competitive neuromuscular blockers, reduction in body temperature may necessitate a dosage reduction for *atracurium and its isomer cisatracurium* since cooling reduces the rate of inactivation of atracurium and cisatracurium, but physiological variations in body temperature and pH will not significantly affect their action.

Burns. The dose requirements of competitive neuromuscular blockers are increased in patients with burns,[1-3] the dose correlating with both the extent of the burn and time after injury. This resistance is usually not seen in patients with less than 10% body-surface burns but if more than 40% of the body-surface is affected the dose of competitive blocker may need to be up to five times higher than in patients without burns. Resistance peaks about 2 weeks after injury, persists for many months in patients with major burns, and decreases gradually with healing of the burn. The mechanism of resistance is multifactorial but may be partly explained by increased protein binding, increased volume of distribution, and increased numbers of acetylcholine receptors at the motor end-plate requiring more muscle relaxant to produce a given effect. Despite the high doses of competitive relaxants that are required, recovery from neuromuscular blockade is not seriously impaired and their effects can be reversed with usual doses of an anticholinesterase.

1. Martyn J, *et al.* Clinical pharmacology of muscle relaxants in patients with burns. *J Clin Pharmacol* 1986; **26:** 680–5.
2. Anonymous. Neuromuscular blockers in patients with burns. *Lancet* 1988; **ii:** 1003–4.
3. Tschida SJ, *et al.* Resistance to nondepolarizing neuromuscular blocking agents. *Pharmacotherapy* 1996; **16:** 409–18.

Cardiopulmonary bypass. The effect of cardiopulmonary bypass on the pharmacokinetics and pharmacodynamics of competitive neuromuscular blockers can be complex but generally their dosage may need to be reduced. Although the intensity of neuromuscular blockade of most competitive neuromuscular blockers is reduced by hypothermia[1] used during cardiopulmonary bypass, their administration during this procedure is associated with rises in plasma concentrations, reduced clearance, and prolongation of the elimination half-life.[2-5] Various mechanisms, including reduced distribution to highly perfused tissues such as the lungs, have been proposed to explain this effect.[2] For atracurium, it appears that it is a reduction in the temperature-dependent inactivation by Hofmann elimination during hypothermia which enables lower doses to be used.[6]

1. Buzello W, *et al.* Unequal effects of cardiopulmonary bypass-induced hypothermia on neuromuscular blockade from constant infusion of alcuronium, d-tubocurarine, pancuronium, and vecuronium. *Anesthesiology* 1987; **66:** 842–6.
2. Walker JS, *et al.* Alcuronium kinetics in patients undergoing cardiopulmonary bypass surgery. *Br J Clin Pharmacol* 1983; **15:** 237–44.
3. Walker JS, *et al.* Altered d-tubocurarine disposition during cardiopulmonary bypass surgery. *Clin Pharmacol Ther* 1984; **35:** 686–94.
4. Wierda JMKH, Agoston S. Pharmacokinetics of vecuronium during hypothermic bypass. *Br J Anaesth* 1989; **63:** 627P–628P.
5. Smeulers NJ, *et al.* Hypothermic cardiopulmonary bypass influences the concentration-response relationship and the biodisposition of rocuronium. *Eur J Anaesthesiol* 1995; **12** (suppl 11): 91–4.
6. Flynn PJ, *et al.* Use of atracurium in cardiac surgery involving cardiopulmonary bypass with induced hypothermia. *Br J Anaesth* 1984; **56:** 967–72.

Hepatic impairment. Alterations in the pharmacokinetics of atracurium and cisatracurium in patients with hepatic impairment (see under Pharmacokinetics, below) do not appear to be clinically significant and a reduction in dosage is not generally recommended.

Neuromuscular disorders. Caution is needed if competitive neuromuscular blockers are given to patients with neuromuscular disease since severe complications have been reported.[1] Increased response may be seen in patients with paraplegia or quadriplegia, but resistance has been reported in patients with hemiplegia. Increased response also may occur in patients with amyotrophic lateral sclerosis, neurofibromatosis, and poliomyelitis; this is of little concern unless the respiratory muscles are involved when prolonged apnoea may occur. Patients with myasthenia gravis usually show increased sensitivity to competitive relaxants although small doses have been given without complications. During remission of myasthenia gravis a normal response is usual but since remission is often incomplete, small intermittent doses are advised. A significantly greater exaggeration of response is seen in patients with the myasthenic syndrome. Both normal and increased responses have been reported in patients with myotonias or muscular dystrophies but exquisite sensitivity occurs in patients with ocular muscular dystrophy. A normal response to competitive relaxants may be expected in patients with multiple sclerosis, muscular denervation, Parkinson's disease, and tetanus.

1. Azar I. The response of patients with neuromuscular disorders to muscle relaxants: a review. *Anesthesiology* 1984; **61:** 173–87.

Pregnancy. Results of a controlled study[1] have indicated that the pharmacokinetics of atracurium are unaltered during pregnancy; it is concluded that atracurium could be given in usual doses during pregnancy or in the postpartum period. Atracurium 300 μg per kg body-weight given to 26 women undergoing caesarean section, with subsequent incremental doses of 100 or 200 μg per kg if necessary, produced good surgical relaxation in all patients without any complications.[2] Of the 26 neonates delivered, respiration was established within 90 seconds in 21, with an Apgar score of 10 at 5 minutes. The remaining 5 neonates were delivered by caesarean section because of fetal distress and were slower to start breathing.

1. Guay J, *et al.* Pharmacokinetics of atracurium in pregnant women. *Clin Drug Invest* 1996; **11:** 167–73.
2. Frank M, *et al.* Atracurium in obstetric anaesthesia: a preliminary report. *Br J Anaesth* 1983; **55:** 113S-114S.

Renal impairment. Although some differences in the pharmacokinetics of atracurium and cisatracurium have been reported in patients with renal impairment (see under Pharmacokinetics, below) duration of their neuromuscular blocking action is not significantly dependent on renal function and usual doses may be given to patients with renal impairment.[1,2] Atracurium has been given by infusion to patients with end-stage renal failure[3] when the initial dose required for induction of neuromuscular block was 37% higher than that required by patients without renal impairment; an increase that could be explained by the larger extracellular fluid volume in patients with chronic renal failure.

Although the pharmacokinetics of atracurium and cisatracurium are not appreciably different in renal impairment, those of their metabolites may be (see under Pharmacokinetics, below) and therefore it has been suggested that neuromuscular function should be monitored during use of atracurium.[4]

1. Hunter JM, *et al.* Use of the muscle relaxant atracurium in anephric patients: preliminary communication. *J R Soc Med* 1982; **75:** 336–340.

2. Boyd AH, *et al.* Pharmacodynamics of the 1R cis-1'R cis isomer of atracurium (51W89) in health and chronic renal failure. *Br J Anaesth* 1995; **74:** 400–404.
3. Gramstad L. Atracurium, vecuronium and pancuronium in end-stage renal failure: dose-response properties and interactions with azathioprine. *Br J Anaesth* 1987; **59:** 995–1003.
4. Vandenbrom RHG, *et al.* Pharmacokinetics and neuromuscular blocking effects of atracurium besylate and two of its metabolites in patients with normal and impaired renal function. *Clin Pharmacokinet* 1990; **19:** 230–40.

Resistance. The aetiology of resistance to competitive blockers is not clear but might be due to pharmacodynamic or pharmacokinetic alterations associated with disease states such as burn injuries (see above) or concomitant drug therapy (see under Interactions, below). One review[1] noted that there had been numerous case reports of resistance to competitive neuromuscular blockers; most had been associated with single dose administration or short-term intermittent therapy but more recent reports had documented resistance in 9 patients during continuous infusions of whom 7 had received atracurium and 2 rocuronium. Resistance to atracurium had followed 2 different patterns. Patients had required either usual or raised doses for initial control but both groups had subsequently required progressive increases. Most patients with resistance to atracurium were successfully managed by transfer to pancuronium or doxacurium.

1. Tschida SJ, *et al.* Resistance to nondepolarizing neuromuscular blocking agents. *Pharmacotherapy* 1996; **16:** 409–18.

Tourniquets. Atracurium might be unsuitable for neuromuscular blockade of a limb which has been isolated with a tourniquet in order to provide a bloodless field for surgery.[1] Atracurium undergoes non-enzymatic degradation in plasma and would therefore continue to degrade locally leading to a loss of blockade in the limb and this could not be corrected by further doses unless the tourniquet was deflated.

1. Shannon PF. Neuromuscular block and tourniquets. *Br J Anaesth* 1994; **73:** 726.

Interactions

A number of drugs may influence neuromuscular transmission and thus interfere with the action of both competitive and depolarising neuromuscular blockers, resulting in potentiation or antagonism of neuromuscular block. Some interactions may be advantageous such as the reversal of competitive neuromuscular block by anticholinesterases. In general, adverse interactions are potentially more serious in patients with impaired neuromuscular function (see Neuromuscular Disorders, above, and under Suxamethonium Chloride, p.1320).

Drug interactions affecting neuromuscular blockers of either type (competitive and depolarising) as well as those specific for competitive neuromuscular blockers are discussed below; well-established interactions are covered as are interactions that have only been the subject of anecdotal reports. For drug interactions specific to depolarising neuromuscular blockers see under Interactions in Suxamethonium Chloride, p.1321.

Reviews.

1. Feldman S, Karalliedde L. Drug interactions with neuromuscular blockers. *Drug Safety* 1996; **15:** 261–73.

Antiarrhythmics. Lignocaine, procainamide, quinidine, and verapamil all have some neuromuscular blocking activity and may enhance the block produced by neuromuscular blockers. Large doses of *lignocaine* may reduce the release of acetylcholine and act directly on the muscle membrane. *Quinidine* has a curare-like action at the neuromuscular junction and depresses the muscle action potential. If administered during recovery from neuromuscular block it can result in muscle weakness and apnoea and it should be avoided, if possible, in the immediate postoperative period. Calcium-channel blockers such as *verapamil* may interfere with the release of acetylcholine and prolonged administration may lead to a reduction in intracellular calcium concentration. Potentiation of neuromuscular blockade has been reported[1] and the block may be resistant to reversal with neostigmine; edrophonium may be required.

1. van Poorten JF, *et al.* Verapamil and reversal of vecuronium neuromuscular blockade. *Anesth Analg* 1984; **63:** 155–7.

Antibacterials. Some antibacterials in very high concentration can produce a muscle paralysis which may be additive to or synergistic with that produced by neuromuscular blockers. The neuromuscular block produced by antibacterials may be enhanced in patients with intracellular potassium deficiency, low plasma-calcium concentration, neuromuscular disease, or a tendency to a high plasma-antibacterial concentration, for example following large doses or in renal impairment. The interaction appears to be more important for competitive muscle relaxants. The antibacterials most commonly implicated are aminoglycosides, lincosamides, polymyxins, and, more rarely, tetracyclines.

The *aminoglycosides* diminish release of and sensitivity to acetylcholine and their effect can be reversed, at least in part, by calcium, fampridine, or an anticholinesterase. The interaction can occur with most routes of aminoglycoside administration. There are reports of potentiation of neuromuscular blockade occurring with many different aminoglycoside-neuromuscular blocker combinations[1-6] and all aminoglycosides should be used with extreme caution during surgery and in the postoperative period.

The *lincosamides* (*clindamycin* and *lincomycin*) can prolong the action of muscle relaxants producing a neuromuscular block that may be difficult to reverse with calcium or anticholinesterases.[7,8] Patients should be monitored for prolonged paralysis.

There have been reports of prolonged apnoea[2,5,8] following the use of *polymyxins* (*colistin, polymyxin B*) with a neuromuscular blocker. The block is difficult to reverse; calcium may be partially successful, but neostigmine may increase the block.

Tetracyclines have weak neuromuscular blocking properties; potentiation of neuromuscular block has been reported in patients with myasthenia gravis.[2] Reversal of the block may be partly achieved with calcium, but the value of anticholinesterases is questionable.

The *ureidopenicillins* (*azlocillin* and *mezlocillin*), and the closely related *piperacillin* and *apalcillin*, are reported to prolong the block produced by vecuronium.[9,10]

Vancomycin has been reported to increase neuromuscular blockade by vecuronium.[11] Prolonged paralysis and apnoea has occurred in a patient recovering from suxamethonium-induced blockade after being given vancomycin.[12]

1. Hall DR, *et al.* Gentamicin, tubocurarine, lignocaine and neuromuscular blockade. *Br J Anaesth* 1972; **44:** 1329–32.
2. Pittinger CB, *et al.* Antibiotic-induced paralysis. *Anesth Analg Curr Res* 1970; **49:** 487–501.
3. Waterman PM, Smith RB. Tobramycin-curare interaction. *Anesth Analg Curr Res* 1977; **56:** 587–8.
4. Regan AG, Perumbetti PPV. Pancuronium and gentamicin interaction in patients with renal failure. *Anesth Analg* 1980; **59:** 393.
5. Giala MM, Paradelis AG. Two cases of prolonged respiratory depression due to interaction of pancuronium with colistin and streptomycin. *J Antimicrob Chemother* 1979; **5:** 234–5.
6. Jedeikin R, *et al.* Prolongation of neuromuscular blocking effect of vecuronium by antibiotics. *Anaesthesia* 1987; **42:** 858–60.
7. Booij LHD, *et al.* Neostigmine and 4-aminopyridine antagonism of lincomycin-pancuronium neuromuscular blockade in man. *Anesth Analg* 1978; **57:** 316–21.
8. de Gouw NE, *et al.* Interaction of antibiotics on pipecuronium-induced neuromuscular blockade. *J Clin Anesth* 1993; **5:** 212–15.
9. Tryba M. Wirkungsverstäkung nicht-depolarisierender muskelrelaxantien durch acylaminopenicilline: untersuchungen am beispiel von vecuronium. *Anaesthesist* 1985; **34:** 651–5.
10. Tryba M, Klemm D. Wechselwirkungen zwischen acylaminopenicillinen und nicht depolarisierenden muskelrelaxantien. *Fortschr Antimikrob Antineoplast Chemother* 1985; **4–7:** 1827–33.
11. Huang KC, *et al.* Vancomycin enhances the neuromuscular blockade of vecuronium. *Anesth Analg* 1990; **70:** 194–6.
12. Albrecht RF, Lanier WL. Potentiation of succinylcholine-induced phase II block by vancomycin. *Anesth Analg* 1993; **77:** 1300–2.

Anticholinesterases. *Neostigmine* and *edrophonium* inhibit both acetylcholinesterase and plasma cholinesterase and are used clinically to antagonise competitive neuromuscular blockade. Conversely they enhance the action of depolarising muscle relaxants thus prolonging neuromuscular block, although suxamethonium-induced phase II block can be reversed with an anticholinesterase. See also Interactions in Suxamethonium Chloride, p.1321.

Antiepileptics. Resistance to competitive neuromuscular blockers has been reported in patients receiving chronic treatment with *carbamazepine*[1,2] or *phenytoin*[3] and rapid recovery from neuromuscular block may occur. However, atracurium[1] and mivacurium[4] appear to be unaffected by chronic carbamazepine therapy and the effect of chronic phenytoin treatment on atracurium has usually been minimal[3] although one study[5] has reported quicker recovery. A report of sensitivity to vecuronium in one patient[6] suggests that acute administration of phenytoin may increase rather than decrease the effect of competitive neuromuscular blockers.

1. Ebrahim Z, *et al.* Carbamazepine therapy and neuromuscular blockade with atracurium and vecuronium. *Anesth Analg* 1988; **67:** S55.
2. Whalley DG, Ebrahim Z. Influence of carbamazepine on the dose-response relationship of vecuronium. *Br J Anaesth* 1994; **72:** 125–6.
3. Ornstein E, *et al.* The effect of phenytoin on the magnitude and duration of neuromuscular block following atracurium or vecuronium. *Anesthesiology* 1987; **67:** 191–6.
4. Spacek A, *et al.* Chronic carbamazepine therapy does not influence mivacurium-induced neuromuscular block. *Br J Anaesth* 1996; **77:** 500–502.
5. Tempelhoff R, *et al.* Resistance to atracurium-induced neuromuscular blockade in patients with intractable seizure disorders treated with anticonvulsants. *Anesth Analg* 1990; **71:** 665–9.
6. Baumgardner JE, Bagshaw R. Acute versus chronic phenytoin therapy and neuromuscular blockade. *Anaesthesia* 1990; **45:** 493–4.

Antineoplastics. It has been recommended that atracurium should be used with care in patients receiving anti-oestrogenic drugs,[1] following a case of prolonged neuromuscular blockade with atracurium in a patient receiving *tamoxifen*. See also under Interactions in Suxamethonium Chloride, p.1321.

1. Naguib M, Gyasi HK. Antiestrogenic drugs and atracurium—a possible interaction? *Can Anaesth Soc J* 1986; **33:** 682–3.

Aprotinin. Caution has been advised when aprotinin and neuromuscular blockers are used concomitantly following reports of apnoea.[1,2]

1. Chasapakis G, Dimas C. Possible interaction between muscle relaxants and the kallikrein-trypsin inactivator "Trasylol". *Br J Anaesth* 1966; **38:** 838–9.
2. Marcello B, Porati U. Trasylol e blocco neuromuscolare: nota preventiva. *Minerva Anestesiol* 1967; **33:** 814–5.

Benzodiazepines. There are conflicting reports of the effect of *diazepam* on neuromuscular blockers; potentiation,[1] or antagonism[1] of neuromuscular block, and a lack of interaction[2-4] have all been reported.

1. Feldman SA, Crawley BE. Interaction of diazepam with the muscle-relaxant drugs. *Br Med J* 1970; **2:** 336–8.
2. Driessen JJ, *et al.* Benzodiazepines and neuromuscular blocking drugs in patients. *Acta Anaesthesiol Scand* 1986; **30:** 642–6.
3. Bradshaw EG, Maddison S. Effect of diazepam at the neuromuscular junction. *Br J Anaesth* 1979; **51:** 955–60.
4. Asbury AJ, *et al.* Effect of diazepam on pancuronium-induced neuromuscular blockade maintained by a feedback system. *Br J Anaesth* 1981; **53:** 859–63.

Beta blockers. There is conflicting evidence for the effect of beta blockers on the activity of neuromuscular blockers. Lack of effect on depolarising neuromuscular block[1] and antagonism[2,3] or enhancement[4,5] of both competitive and depolarising block have been reported. The exact mechanism of interaction is not clear. There have also been reports of some neuromuscular blockers such as atracurium[6,7] and alcuronium[8] increasing the hypotension and bradycardia associated with the use of anaesthesia in patients receiving beta blockers; these include reports in patients using beta blockers in eye drops for glaucoma.

1. McCammon RL, *et al.* The effect of esmolol on the onset and duration of succinylcholine-induced neuromuscular blockade. *Anesthesiology* 1985; **63:** A317.
2. Varma YS, *et al.* Effect of propranolol hydrochloride on the neuromuscular blocking action of d-tubocurarine and succinylcholine in man. *Indian J Med Res* 1972; **60:** 266–72.
3. Varma YS, *et al.* Comparative effect of propranolol, oxprenolol and pindolol on neuromuscular blocking action of d-tubocurarine in man. *Indian J Med Res* 1973; **61:** 1382–6.
4. Rozen MS, Whan FM. Prolonged curarization associated with propranolol. *Med J Aust* 1972; **1:** 467–8.
5. Murthy VS, *et al.* Cardiovascular and neuromuscular effects of esmolol during induction of anesthesia. *J Clin Pharmacol* 1986; **26:** 351–7.
6. Glynne GL. Drug Interaction? *Anaesthesia* 1984; **39:** 293.
7. Rowlands DE. Drug Interaction? *Anaesthesia* 1984; **39:** 1252.
8. Yate B, Mostafa SM. Drug Interaction? *Anaesthesia* 1984; **39:** 728.

Botulinum A toxin. The neuromuscular block induced by botulinum A toxin (p.1310) is enhanced by competitive neuromuscular blockers.

Calcium-channel blockers. Both *nifedipine* and *verapamil* enhance the effect of competitive neuromuscular blockers. See also under Antiarrhythmics, above.

Cardiac inotropes. Pancuronium or suxamethonium may interact with cardiac glycosides[1] resulting in an increased incidence of arrhythmias; the interaction is more likely with pancuronium.

1. Bartolone RS, Rao TLK. Dysrhythmias following muscle relaxant administration in patients receiving digitalis. *Anesthesiology* 1983; **58:** 567–9.

Corticosteroids. Antagonism of the neuromuscular blocking effects of pancuronium[1] and vecuronium[2] has been reported in patients taking corticosteroids. This interaction may occur only with long-term corticosteroid treatment and may be expected with all competitive neuromuscular blockers.

1. Azar I, *et al.* Resistance to pancuronium in an asthmatic patient treated with aminophylline and steroids. *Can Anaesth Soc J* 1982; **29:** 280–2.
2. Parr SM, *et al.* Betamethasone-induced resistance to vecuronium: a potential problem in neurosurgery? *Anaesth Intensive Care* 1991; **19:** 103–5.

Diuretics. *Frusemide*, and possibly *mannitol*, have been reported to enhance tubocurarine neuromuscular block in patients with renal failure,[1] but antagonism of tubocurarine by frusemide has also occurred.[2] Small doses of frusemide (less than 100 μg per kg) may inhibit protein kinase which inhibits muscle contraction and potentiates neuromuscular blockade, whereas high doses inhibit phosphodiesterase increasing cAMP activity and resulting in antagonism of neuromuscular blockade. The potassium-depleting effect of diuretics may enhance the effect of competitive neuromuscular blockers.

1. Miller RD, *et al.* Enhancement of d-tubocurarine neuromuscular blockade by diuretics in man. *Anesthesiology* 1976; **45:** 442–5.
2. Azar I, *et al.* Furosemide facilitates recovery of evoked twitch response after pancuronium. *Anesth Analg* 1980; **59:** 55–7.

Ganglion blockers. Prolonged neuromuscular blockade has been reported[1,2] in patients receiving neuromuscular blockers and *trimetaphan*. Trimetaphan may have direct neuromuscular blocking activity and some activity against plasma cholinesterase.

1. Wilson SL, *et al.* Prolonged neuromuscular blockade associated with trimethaphan: a case report. *Anesth Analg Curr Res* 1976; **55:** 353–6.
2. Poulton TH, *et al.* Prolonged apnea following trimethaphan and succinylcholine. *Anesthesiology* 1979; **50:** 54–6.

General anaesthetics. Neuromuscular blockers are potentiated in a dose-dependent manner by inhalation anaesthetics.[1-4] The dose of neuromuscular blocker may need to be reduced by up to 70%[1] depending on the anaesthetic used and its concentration, and on the choice of blocker; the interaction is of greater clinical importance with competitive blockers. *Isoflurane, enflurane, desflurane*, and *sevoflurane* produce the greater potentiation, followed by *halothane* and *cyclopropane*. Reversal of competitive block with an anticholinesterase has been reported to be reduced.[5,6] See also under Interactions in Suxamethonium Chloride, p.1321.

Potentiation of the neuromuscular blocking effects of tubocurarine[7] and atracurium[8] has been reported following the intravenous administration of *ketamine*. Results from studies *in vitro* suggest that ketamine decreases sensitivity to acetylcholine and it would therefore be expected to potentiate all neuromuscular blockers, but no interaction was reported for pancuronium.[7] Early data[9] suggesting that ketamine potentiates suxamethonium-induced blockade have not been confirmed by later studies.[7,10] For incompatibility between neuromuscular blockers and alkaline solutions such as thiopentone sodium, see under Incompatibility, above.

1. Cannon JE, *et al.* Continuous infusion of vecuronium: the effect of anesthetic agents. *Anesthesiology* 1987; **67:** 503–6.
2. Swen J, *et al.* Interaction between nondepolarizing neuromuscular blocking agents and inhalation anesthetics. *Anesth Analg* 1989; **69:** 752–5.
3. Ghourin AF, White PF. Comparative effects of desflurane and isoflurane on vecuronium-induced neuromuscular blockade. *J Clin Anesth* 1992; **4:** 34–8.
4. Vanlinthout LEM, *et al.* Effect of isoflurane and sevoflurane on the magnitude and time course of neuromuscular block produced by vecuronium, pancuronium and atracurium. *Br J Anaesth* 1996; **76:** 389–95.
5. Delisle S, Bevan DR. Impaired neostigmine antagonism of pancuronium during enflurane anaesthesia in man. *Br J Anaesth* 1982; **54:** 441–5.
6. Gill SS, *et al.* Edrophonium antagonism of atracurium during enflurane anaesthesia. *Br J Anaesth* 1990; **64:** 300–5.
7. Johnston RR, *et al.* The interaction of ketamine with d-tubocurarine, pancuronium, and succinylcholine in man. *Anesth Analg Curr Res* 1974; **53:** 496–501.
8. Toft P, Helbo-Hansen S. Interaction of ketamine with atracurium. *Br J Anaesth* 1989; **62:** 319–20.
9. Bovill JG, *et al.* Current status of ketamine anaesthesia. *Lancet* 1971; **i:** 1285–8.
10. Helbo-Hansen HS, *et al.* Ketamine does not affect suxamethonium-induced neuromuscular blockade in man. *Eur J Anaesthesiol* 1989; **6:** 419–23.

Histamine H_2 antagonists. There are conflicting reports of the effects of histamine H_2 antagonists on neuromuscular blockade. *Cimetidine* has been variously reported to prolong suxamethonium-induced paralysis[1] or to have no effect.[2] *Famotidine* and *ranitidine* have been reported[2] not to interact with suxamethonium. Cimetidine, but not ranitidine, has been reported[3] to delay recovery from vecuronium-induced neuromuscular block. Neither drug appeared to affect recovery after the use of atracurium.

1. Kambam JR, *et al.* Effect of cimetidine on duration of action of succinylcholine. *Anesth Analg* 1987; **66:** 191–2.
2. Turner DR, *et al.* Neuromuscular block by suxamethonium following treatment with histamine type 2 antagonists or metoclopramide. *Br J Anaesth* 1989; **63:** 348–50.
3. McCarthy G, *et al.* Effect of H2-receptor antagonist pretreatment on vecuronium- and atracurium-induced neuromuscular blockade. *Br J Anaesth* 1991; **66:** 713–15.

Immunosuppressants. Antagonism of the neuromuscular blocking effects of competitive neuromuscular blockers has been reported with *azathioprine*,[1] although the effect may not be clinically important. Azathioprine probably inhibits phosphodiesterase activity at the motor nerve terminal resulting in increased release of acetylcholine. There have been reports of prolonged neuromuscular blockade with atracurium, pancuronium, and vecuronium in some patients receiving *cyclosporin* intravenously.[2,3] This effect has been attributed to interaction with polyethoxylated castor oil used as the solvent for cyclosporin but a similar reaction has been reported in a patient receiving cyclosporin by mouth.[4]

1. Gramstad L. Atracurium, vecuronium and pancuronium in end-stage renal failure: dose-response properties and interaction with azathioprine. *Br J Anaesth* 1987; **59:** 995–1003.
2. Crosby E, Robblee JA. Cyclosporine-pancuronium interaction in a patient with a renal allograft. *Can J Anaesth* 1988; **35:** 300–2.
3. Sidi A, *et al.* Prolonged neuromuscular blockade and ventilatory failure after renal transplantation and cyclosporine. *Can J Anaesth* 1990; **37:** 543–8.
4. Ganjoo P, Tewari P. Oral cyclosporine-vecuronium interaction. *Can J Anaesth* 1994; **41:** 1017.

Lithium. There have been isolated reports of prolonged neuromuscular blockade following the use of neuromuscular blockers in patients receiving lithium.[1,2]

1. Borden H, *et al.* The use of pancuronium bromide in patients receiving lithium carbonate. *Can Anaesth Soc J* 1974; **21:** 79–82.
2. Hill GE, *et al.* Potentiation of succinylcholine neuromuscular blockade by lithium carbonate. *Anesthesiology* 1976; **44:** 439–42.

Local anaesthetics. Healthy subjects who had undergone regional anaesthesia of the forearm experienced symptoms suggestive of local anaesthetic toxicity on deflation of the tourniquet cuff when mivacurium and prilocaine had been used together for anaesthesia;[1] administration of prilocaine or mivacurium alone did not produce such an effect. It was considered unlikely that the effect was due entirely to prilocaine inhibition of metabolism of mivacurium by plasma cholinesterase.[2]

The interaction between neuromuscular blockers and lignocaine is discussed under Antiarrhythmics above.

1. Torrance JM, *et al.* Low-dose mivacurium supplementation of prilocaine i.v. regional anaesthesia. *Br J Anaesth* 1997; **78:** 222–3.
2. Torrance JM, *et al.* Interactions between mivacurium and prilocaine. *Br J Anaesth* 1997; **78:** 262.

Magnesium salts. Parenteral magnesium salts may potentiate the effects of neuromuscular blockers;[1] the neuromuscular block is deepened and prolonged and a reduction in the dose of the blocker may be needed. Magnesium salts should be used with caution in the postoperative period since administration shortly after recovery from neuromuscular block can lead to recurarisation.[2] Magnesium salts reduce release of and sensitivity to acetylcholine, thus contributing to neuromuscular blockade.

1. Ghoneim MM, Long JP. The interaction between magnesium and other neuromuscular blocking agents. *Anesthesiology* 1970; **32:** 23–7.
2. Fuchs-Buder T, Tassonyi E. Magnesium sulphate enhances residual neuromuscular block induced by vecuronium. *Br J Anaesth* 1996; **76:** 565–6.

MAOIs. There appears to be a theoretical hazard with pancuronium in patients receiving MAOIs since it releases stored adrenaline, but alcuronium, atracurium, or vecuronium appear to be suitable alternatives.

Neuromuscular blockers. A competitive neuromuscular blocker given shortly before a depolarising blocker antagonises the depolarising neuromuscular block. This interaction has been used clinically to reduce muscle fasciculations caused by suxamethonium (see Anaesthesia, p.1302 and Effects on the Muscles, p.1319) and tried for other adverse effects associated with suxamethonium (see Effects on Plasma-potassium Concentration, p.1320). To achieve this antagonism a small non-paralysing dose of a competitive blocker is administered before suxamethonium. If a paralysing dose of a competitive blocker is followed some time later with a dose of suxamethonium, for example to facilitate abdominal closure, the resulting neuromuscular block is influenced by the competitive blocker used, the depth of residual block, the dose of suxamethonium, and whether an anticholinesterase is given; antagonism, enhancement, and a combination of the two have been observed.[1,2]

A competitive blocker is often given following the short-acting suxamethonium to maintain neuromuscular blockade during long procedures. The action of the competitive blocker has been reported to be considerably potentiated and prolonged in these circumstances.[3,4]

Combination of competitive blockers may have additive or synergistic effects and the interaction may differ depending on which blocker is given first. Caution is needed if a small dose of a shorter-acting blocker is given near the end of an operation in which a long-acting blocker has been given previously, since the resulting block may be greater than expected and much longer than desired.[5-7]

1. Scott RPF, Norman J. Effect of suxamethonium given during recovery from atracurium. *Br J Anaesth* 1988; **61:** 292–6.
2. Black AMS. Effect of suxamethonium given during recovery from atracurium. *Br J Anaesth* 1989; **62:** 348–9.
3. d'Hollander AA, *et al.* Clinical and pharmacological actions of a bolus injection of suxamethonium: two phenomena of distinct duration. *Br J Anaesth* 1983; **55:** 131–4.
4. Ono K, *et al.* Influence of suxamethonium on the action of subsequently administered vecuronium or pancuronium. *Br J Anaesth* 1989; **62:** 324–6.
5. Rashkovsky OM, *et al.* Interaction between pancuronium bromide and vecuronium bromide. *Br J Anaesth* 1985; **57:** 1063–6.
6. Middleton CM, *et al.* Use of atracurium or vecuronium to prolong the action of tubocurarine. *Br J Anaesth* 1989; **62:** 659–63.
7. Kim KS, *et al.*Interactions between mivacurium and pancuronium. *Br J Anaesth* 1997; **79:** 19–23.

Sex hormones. Resistance to the neuromuscular blocking effects of suxamethonium and vecuronium in one patient was attributed to prior long-term therapy with *testosterone*,[1] although the exact mechanism could not be explained. See also under Interactions in Suxamethonium Chloride, p.1321.

1. Reddy P, *et al.* Resistance to muscle relaxants in a patient receiving prolonged testosterone therapy. *Anesthesiology* 1989; **70:** 871–3.

Smoking. Preliminary work suggests that smoking might affect the dose requirements for neuromuscular blockers. One group of workers[1] found that smokers needed more vecuronium than non-smokers; it was considered that the effect might be explained at the receptor level although possible increased metabolism of vecuronium could not be excluded. This was in contrast to an earlier study[2] in which the amount of atracurium required was reduced in smokers.

1. Teiriä H, *et al.* Effect of smoking on dose requirements for vecuronium. *Br J Anaesth* 1996; **76:** 154–5.
2. Kroeker KA, *et al.* Neuromuscular blockade in the setting of chronic nicotine exposure. *Anesthesiology* 1994; **81:** A1120.

Sympathomimetics. Intravenous *salbutamol* has been reported to enhance the blockade obtained with pancuronium and vecuronium.[1] See also under Interactions in Suxamethonium Chloride, p.1321.

1. Salib Y, Donati F. Potentiation of pancuronium and vecuronium neuromuscular blockade by intravenous salbutamol. *Can J Anaesth* 1993; **40:** 50–3.

Xanthines. Resistance to neuromuscular block with pancuronium, requiring an increase in dosage or transfer to vecuronium, has been reported in patients receiving *aminophylline* with[1] or without[2] corticosteroid therapy. It was suggested that this effect might be due to inhibition of phosphodiesterase by aminophylline resulting in increased release of acetylcholine at the nerve terminal.

1. Azar I, *et al.* Resistance to pancuronium in an asthmatic patient treated with aminophylline and steroids. *Can Anaesth Soc J* 1982; **29:** 280–2.
2. Daller JA, *et al.* Aminophylline antagonizes the neuromuscular blockade of pancuronium but not vecuronium. *Crit Care Med* 1991; **19:** 983–5.

Pharmacokinetics

Following intravenous injection both atracurium besylate and cisatracurium besylate undergo spontaneous degradation via Hofmann elimination (a non-enzymatic breakdown process occurring at physiological pH and temperature) to produce laudanosine and other metabolites. There is also ester hydrolysis by non-specific plasma esterases. The metabolites have no neuromuscular blocking activity.

About 80% of atracurium besylate is bound to plasma proteins. Atracurium besylate and its metabolites cross the placenta in clinically insignificant amounts. Excretion of atracurium and cisatracurium is in urine and bile, mostly as metabolites. The elimination half-life has been reported to be approximately 20 minutes for atracurium and 22 to 29 minutes for cisatracurium but laudanosine has an elimination half-life of about 3 hours.

Atracurium and cisatracurium are degraded by Hofmann elimination and metabolised by non-specific plasma esterases. Hofmann elimination is generally believed to be the main route of degradation but *in-vitro* work suggests ester hydrolysis is more important.[1] Both routes are independent of renal and hepatic function and no dosage reduction is recommended for elderly patients or those with impaired renal or hepatic function. However, the elimination half-life of atracurium has been found to be slightly longer in elderly patients[2] and in those with hepatic cirrhosis[3] compared with young and healthy patients, although others[4] have found no change in the pharmacokinetics of atracurium in the elderly. Renal and hepatic involvement in the metabolism of atracurium[2] may help to explain any tendency to reduced elimination but this does not appear to be clinically significant. Although clearance of cisatracurium has been reported to be reduced in patients with renal failure[5] this appears to have little significant effect on its pharmacodynamics.[6] Differences in the pharmacokinetics of cisatracurium in patients with hepatic impairment have been reported to be minor.[7]

The major biotransformation product of atracurium and cisatracurium is *laudanosine* which has no clinical neuromuscular blocking activity. It is more lipid soluble than atracurium and cisatracurium and has a half-life of around 3 hours compared with one of approximately 20 minutes for atracurium. Higher plasma-laudanosine concentrations have been reported in patients with renal failure[5,8,9] than in patients with normal renal function. The elimination half-life of laudanosine was found to be significantly greater in patients with hepatic cirrhosis[3] and in elderly patients[2] compared with healthy and young patients respectively. Laudanosine crosses the blood-brain barrier in man. The concentration of laudanosine in the CSF increases during an infusion of atracurium and the CSF-to-plasma ratio gradually increases. A ratio of 0.14 was found at 125 to 140 minutes[10] during an infusion of atracurium at a mean rate of 510 μg per kg per hour. No evidence of CNS stimulation has been reported in man although patients given atracurium[11] had a 20% higher mean arterial-thiopentone concentration at awakening compared with patients given vecuronium, suggesting that laudanosine may have had a minor stimulatory effect on the CNS. The blood-brain barrier appears to be effective in preventing a very high concentration of laudanosine from reaching the CNS and it is considered unlikely[12] that concentrations great enough to provoke seizures will be reached. Cisatracurium may be associated with the production of less laudanosine than atracurium.[13]

1. Stiller RL, *et al.* In vitro degradation of atracurium in human plasma. *Br J Anaesth* 1985; **57:** 1085–8.
2. Kent AP, *et al.* Pharmacokinetics of atracurium and laudanosine in the elderly. *Br J Anaesth* 1989; **63:** 661–6.
3. Parker CJR, Hunter JM. Pharmacokinetics of atracurium and laudanosine in patients with hepatic cirrhosis. *Br J Anaesth* 1989; **62:** 177–83.
4. d'Hollander AA, *et al.* Clinical evaluation of atracurium besylate requirement for a stable muscle relaxation during surgery: lack of age-related effects. *Anesthesiology* 1983; **59:** 237–40.
5. Eastwood NB, *et al.* Pharmacokinetics of 1R-cis 1'R-cis atracurium besylate (51W89) and plasma laudanosine concentrations in health and chronic renal failure. *Br J Anaesth* 1995; **75:** 431–5
6. Boyd AH, *et al.* Pharmacodynamics of the 1R cis-1'R cis isomer of atracurium (51W89) in health and chronic renal failure. *Br J Anaesth* 1995; **74:** 400–404.
7. De Wolf AM, *et al.* Pharmacokinetics and pharmacodynamics of cisatracurium in patients with end-stage liver disease undergoing liver transplantation. *Br J Anaesth* 1996; **76:** 624–8.
8. Fahey MR, *et al.* Effect of renal failure on laudanosine excretion in man. *Br J Anaesth* 1985; **57:** 1049–51.
9. Vandenbrom RHG, *et al.* Pharmacokinetics and neuromuscular blocking effects of atracurium besylate and two of its metabolites in patients with normal and impaired renal function. *Clin Pharmacokinet* 1990; **19:** 230–40.
10. Eddleston JM, *et al.* Concentrations of atracurium and laudanosine in cerebrospinal fluid and plasma during intracranial surgery. *Br J Anaesth* 1989; **63:** 525–30.
11. Beemer GH, *et al.* Production of laudanosine following infusion of atracurium in man and its effects on awakening. *Br J Anaesth* 1989; **63:** 76–80.
12. Yate PM, *et al.* Clinical experience and plasma laudanosine concentrations during the infusion of atracurium in the intensive therapy unit. *Br J Anaesth* 1987; **59:** 211–17.
13. Boyd AH, *et al.* Comparison of the pharmacokinetics and pharmacodynamics of an infusion of cis-atracurium (51W89) or atracurium in critically ill patients undergoing mechanical ventilation in an intensive therapy unit. *Br J Anaesth* 1996; **76:** 382–8.

Uses and Administration

Competitive neuromuscular blockers act by competing with acetylcholine for receptors on the motor end-plate of the neuromuscular junction to produce blockade. The muscles that produce fine rapid movements such as those of the face are the first to be affected followed by those of the limbs and torso; the last to be affected are those of the diaphragm. The paralysis is reversible with recovery occurring in reverse order. Restoration of normal neuromuscular function can be hastened by increasing the concentration of acetylcholine at the motor end-plate by giving an anticholinesterase such as neostigmine.

Atracurium besylate and cisatracurium besylate are competitive benzylisoquinolinium neuromuscular blockers. Cisatracurium besylate, the *Rcis,1'Rcis*-isomer of atracurium besylate, is approximately three times more potent than the mixture of isomers that constitute atracurium besylate. Following an intravenous dose of atracurium muscle relaxation begins in about 2 minutes and lasts for 15 to 35 minutes; onset may be slightly longer for cisatracurium.

Atracurium besylate and cisatracurium besylate are used for endotracheal intubation and to provide muscle relaxation in general anaesthesia for surgical procedures (see Anaesthesia, p.1302) and to aid controlled ventilation (see Intensive Care, p.1303).

For **atracurium besylate**, the usual initial dose for adults and children over 1 month of age is 300 to 600 μg per kg body-weight by intravenous injection. Subsequent doses of 80 to 200 μg per kg may be given as necessary. It is recommended that in patients with cardiovascular disease the initial dose should be administered over a period of 60 seconds.

Atracurium besylate may also be given by continuous intravenous infusion at a rate of 5 to 10 μg per kg per minute to maintain neuromuscular block during prolonged procedures.

For **cisatracurium besylate**, a usual initial dose for adults is 150 μg per kg body-weight. The neuromuscular block may be extended with a maintenance dose of 30 μg per kg approximately every 20 minutes. The usual initial dose for children over 2 years is 100 μg per kg body-weight. The neuromuscular block may be extended with a maintenance dose of 20 μg per kg approximately every 9 minutes.

Cisatracurium besylate may also be given by continuous intravenous infusion at an initial rate of 3 μg per kg per minute followed by a rate of 1 to 2 μg per kg per minute after stabilisation.

Reviews.

1. Hughes R. Atracurium—the first years. *Clin Anaesthesiol* 1985; **3:** 331–45.
2. Reilly CS, Nimmo WS. New intravenous anaesthetics and neuromuscular blocking drugs: a review of their properties and clinical use. *Drugs* 1987; **34:** 98–135.
3. Bryson HM, Faulds D. Cisatracurium besilate: a review of its pharmacology and clinical potential in anaesthetic practice. *Drugs* 1997; **53:** 848–66.

Administration in infants and children. Children generally require larger doses of competitive neuromuscular blockers on a weight basis than adolescents or adults to achieve similar degrees of neuromuscular blockade and may recover more quickly. However, neonates and infants under 1 year of age are more sensitive and usual doses may produce prolonged neuromuscular blockade.

Electroconvulsive therapy. Competitive neuromuscular blockers have been used to reduce the intensity of muscle contractions and minimise trauma in patients receiving electroconvulsive therapy but suxamethonium (p.1319) is generally preferred because of its short duration of action.

Intravenous regional anaesthesia. Competitive neuromuscular blockers and/or opioid analgesics have been added to the local anaesthetic used in intravenous regional anaesthesia (p.1285) to improve the quality of anaesthesia. However atracurium (see Tourniquets under Precautions, above) and mivacurium (see Tourniquets, p.1317) might be unsuitable for such use.

Shivering. Various drugs have been tried in the treatment of postoperative shivering (p.1219). There are reports of neuromuscular blockers being used to treat shivering after cardiac surgery in order to reduce cardiovascular stress;[1] one study[2] has suggested that vecuronium might be preferable to pancuronium as it does not increase myocardial work and may be associated with fewer complications.

1. Cruise C, *et al.* Comparison of meperidine and pancuronium for the treatment of shivering after cardiac surgery. *Can J Anaesth* 1992; **39:** 563–8.
2. Dupuis J-Y, *et al.* Pancuronium or vecuronium for the treatment of shivering after cardiac surgery. *Anesth Analg* 1994; **79:** 472–81.

Tetanus. For a comment on the role of competitive neuromuscular blockers in the management of muscle spasms caused by tetanus, see p.1304.

Preparations

Proprietary Preparations (details are given in Part 3)
Aust.: Nimbex; Tracrium; ***Austral.:*** Nimbex; Tracrium; ***Belg.:*** Tracrium; ***Canad.:*** Tracrium; ***Fr.:*** Nimbex; Tracrium; ***Ger.:*** Nimbex; Tracrium; ***Irl.:*** Nimbex; Tracrium; ***Ital.:*** Nimbex; Tracrium; ***Neth.:*** Nimbex; Tracrium; ***Norw.:*** Nimbex; Tracrium; ***S.Afr.:*** Nimbex; Tracrium; ***Spain:*** Nimbex; Tracrium; ***Swed.:*** Nimbex; Tracrium; ***Switz.:*** Tracrium; ***UK:*** Nimbex; Tracrium; ***USA:*** Nimbex; Tracrium.

Baclofen (5702-z)

Baclofen *(BAN, USAN, rINN)*.

Aminomethyl Chlorohydrocinnamic Acid; Ba-34647; Baclofenum. β-Aminomethyl-*p*-chlorohydrocinnamic acid; (*RS*)-Amino-3-(4-chlorophenyl)butyric acid.

$C_{10}H_{12}ClNO_2$ = 213.7.

CAS — 1134-47-0.

Pharmacopoeias. In *Eur.* (see p.viii), *Jpn, Pol.,* and *US.*

A white or almost white, odourless or practically odourless, crystalline powder. It exhibits polymorphism. Slightly **soluble** in water; very slightly soluble in alcohol and methyl alcohol; practically insoluble in acetone, chloroform, and ether; dissolves in dilute mineral acids and alkali hydroxides. **Store** in airtight containers.

Adverse Effects

Adverse effects associated with baclofen are often transient and dose-related. They may be minimised by increasing doses gradually or controlled by a reduction in dosage.

The most common side-effects include drowsiness, nausea, dizziness, confusion, fatigue, muscular pain and weakness, and hypotension. Other side-effects include euphoria, hallucinations, mental depression, headache, tinnitus, paraesthesias, slurred speech, dry mouth, taste alterations, vomiting, diarrhoea or constipation, ataxia, nystagmus, tremors, insomnia, visual disturbances, skin rashes, pruritus, increased sweating, urinary disturbances, respiratory or cardiovascular depression, blood sugar changes, alterations in liver function values, and a paradoxical increase in spasticity.

Overdosage may lead to muscular hypotonia, drowsiness, respiratory depression, coma, and convulsions (see also below).

Abrupt withdrawal of baclofen may result in a withdrawal syndrome (see under Precautions, below).

Effects on the nervous system. Epilepsy, progressing to status epilepticus, has been associated with the use of baclofen in a patient who had had no previous history of seizures.[1] Baclofen had been given in a dose of 80 mg daily and symptoms had resolved following gradual withdrawal and the use of antiepileptics.

1. Rush JM, Gibberd FB. Baclofen-induced epilepsy. *J R Soc Med* 1990; **83:** 115–16.

Treatment of Adverse Effects

Treatment of overdosage is symptomatic. Following ingestion of baclofen the stomach should be emptied by emesis or lavage. Activated charcoal may be given. For the use of physostigmine salicylate in the treatment of intrathecal baclofen overdosage, see below.

Overdosage. Atropine sulphate 600 μg intravenously[1] successfully treated baclofen overdosage in one patient who had ingested 420 mg and had failed to improve after gastric lavage and induced diuresis. Bradycardia, hypotension, hypothermia, and respiratory depression all improved and no further treatment was needed.

Baclofen may be administered intrathecally and accidental overdosage has caused respiratory depression, decreased alertness, coma, muscle weakness, and vomiting.[2] Mild intrathecal bolus overdoses of baclofen in patients without cardiac compromise can be treated using physostigmine, but physostigmine proved to be ineffective in a patient who accidentally received 10 mg of baclofen intrathecally[3] and in such severe overdosage respiratory support and time to recover is needed.[4] A lumbar tap to remove about 30 to 50 mL of cerebrospinal fluid may help to reduce the intrathecal concentration of baclofen if implemented soon after the overdose. Physostigmine salicylate is given intravenously in a dose of 1 to 2 mg over 5 minutes and may be repeated at intervals of 30 to 60 minutes.[2,4]

1. Ferner RE. Atropine treatment for baclofen overdose. *Postgrad Med J* 1981; **57:** 580–1.
2. Müller-Schwefe G, Penn RD. Physostigmine in the treatment of intrathecal baclofen overdose. *J Neurosurg* 1989; **71:** 273–5.
3. Saltuari L, *et al.* Failure of physostigmine in treatment of acute severe intrathecal baclofen intoxication. *N Engl J Med* 1990; **322:** 1533.
4. Penn RD, Kroin JS. Failure of physostigmine in treatment of acute severe intrathecal baclofen intoxication. *N Engl J Med* 1990; **322:** 1533–4.

Precautions

Baclofen is contra-indicated in patients with peptic ulcer and should be used with caution in those with a history of peptic ulcer. It should also be used with caution in patients with severe psychiatric disorders or epilepsy or convulsive disorders since these disorders may be exacerbated by baclofen. Liver function should be monitored in patients with liver disease; patients with renal impairment need a reduced dose. Baclofen should be used with caution in patients with respiratory impairment. Observations of increased blood sugar concentrations suggest caution in patients with diabetes mellitus. Care is also required in the elderly in whom adverse effects may be more common and in patients with cerebrovascular disease who tolerate baclofen poorly. It should be used with caution in patients who use their spasticity to maintain posture or to increase function. Urine retention may be exacerbated in patients with hypertonic bladder sphincters. Baclofen may cause drowsiness; patients affected should not drive or operate machinery.

Abrupt withdrawal of baclofen may result in a withdrawal syndrome and exacerbation of spasticity; dosage should be reduced gradually over at least 1 to 2 weeks, or longer if symptoms occur.

Anaesthesia. Acute bradycardia and hypotension occurred following rib retraction in 3 patients given baclofen 30 mg by mouth 90 minutes before thoracic surgery under general anaesthesia, but not in a further 3 patients given placebo.[1] Administration of atropine and ephedrine relieved bradycardia and hypotension in 2 patients, but a brief cardiac arrest occurred in 1. Administration of baclofen may disturb autonomic control of the circulation during general anaesthesia and surgery.

1. Sill JC, *et al.* Bradycardia and hypotension associated with baclofen used during general anaesthesia. *Anesthesiology* 1986; **64:** 255–8.

Peptic ulcer. Results of a study of baclofen-stimulated gastric acid secretion in 10 healthy subjects given 600 μg per kg body-weight intravenously suggested that patients on baclofen might be at risk from baclofen-induced hyperacidity.[1]

1. Pugh S, *et al.* Clinical and experimental significance of the newly discovered activity of baclofen (PCP-GABA) as a stimulant of gastric acid secretion. *Gut* 1985; **26:** A545.

Porphyria. Baclofen was considered to be unsafe in patients with acute porphyria because it has been shown to be porphyrinogenic in *in-vitro* systems.[1]

1. Moore MR, McColl KEL. *Porphyria: drug lists.* Glasgow: Porphyria Research Unit, University of Glasgow, 1991.

Renal impairment. Reports of baclofen toxicity in patients with severely impaired renal function.[1] Most patients had received 15 mg or more of baclofen daily although one patient who had received the manufacturer's suggested dose of 5 mg daily still developed toxic symptoms after only 4 days of treatment.

1. Chen K-S, *et al.* Baclofen toxicity in patients with severely impaired renal function. *Ann Pharmacother* 1997; **31:** 1315–20.

Respiratory disorders. Baclofen might precipitate bronchoconstriction in susceptible individuals. A patient with asthma developed symptomatic bronchoconstriction after taking baclofen on two separate occasions.[1] Another patient who had a history of exercise-induced dyspnoea and wheezing was found to have bronchial hyperresponsiveness to methacholine only after taking baclofen.

1. Dicpinigaitis PV, *et al.* Baclofen-induced bronchoconstriction. *Ann Pharmacother* 1993; **27:** 883–4.

Withdrawal. Psychiatric reactions including hallucinations, paranoia, delusions, psychosis, anxiety, confusion, and agitation have been reported[1-4] following abrupt withdrawal of baclofen; symptoms have generally resolved on restarting. Convulsions have also been reported.[5] Except for serious adverse reactions, the dose of baclofen should be gradually reduced. In the UK the Committee on Safety of Medicines recommends reduction over at least 1 to 2 weeks or longer if symptoms occur.

1. Lees AJ, *et al.* Hallucinations after withdrawal of baclofen. *Lancet* 1977; **i:** 858.
2. Stein R. Hallucinations after sudden withdrawal of baclofen. *Lancet* 1977; **ii:** 44–5.
3. Harrison SA, Wood CA. Hallucinations after preoperative baclofen discontinuation in spinal cord injury patients. *Drug Intell Clin Pharm* 1985; **19:** 747–9.
4. Committee on Safety of Medicines/Medicines Control Agency. Severe withdrawal reactions with baclofen. *Current Problems* 1997; **23:** 3.
5. Barker I, Grant IS. Convulsions after abrupt withdrawal of baclofen. *Lancet* 1982; **ii:** 556–7.

Interactions

Alcohol and other CNS depressants may exacerbate the CNS effects of baclofen and should be avoided; severe aggravation of hyperkinetic symptoms may possibly occur in patients taking lithium. There may be increased weakness if baclofen is given to patients taking a tricyclic antidepressant and there may be an increased hypotensive effect if it is given to patients receiving antihypertensive therapy.

Dopaminergics. For reports of patients with Parkinson's disease taking levodopa who have experienced adverse effects when given baclofen, see under Levodopa, on p.1139.

NSAIDs. Report of an elderly patient who developed baclofen toxicity after concomitant ibuprofen therapy was started.[1] It appeared that acute renal insufficiency caused by ibuprofen had impaired baclofen excretion.

1. Dahlin PA, George J. Baclofen toxicity associated with declining renal clearance after ibuprofen. *Drug Intell Clin Pharm* 1984; **18:** 805–8.

Pharmacokinetics

Baclofen is rapidly and almost completely absorbed from the gastro-intestinal tract following an oral dose. The peak plasma concentration occurs about 1 to 3 hours following ingestion, but the rate and extent of absorption vary between patients, and vary inversely with the dose. Following oral administration some baclofen crosses the blood-brain barrier with concentrations in CSF corresponding to about 12% of those in the plasma. Approximately 30% of baclofen is bound to plasma proteins. About 70 to 80% of a dose is excreted in the urine mainly as unchanged drug; about 15% is metabolised in the liver. The elimination half-life of baclofen is about 3 to 4 hours in plasma and about 5 hours in the CSF.

Absorption. A crossover study in 5 healthy subjects given baclofen 20 mg by mouth after an overnight fast or a standardised breakfast showed that baclofen was rapidly absorbed in both cases, and the rate and extent of absorption were not significantly altered by the presence of food.[1] There is no need to modify the current practice of giving baclofen with food to minimise gastro-intestinal side-effects.

1. Peterson GM, *et al.* Food does not affect the bioavailability of baclofen. *Med J Aust* 1985; **142:** 689–90.

Uses and Administration

Baclofen, an analogue of gamma-aminobutyric acid (p.1582), is a centrally acting skeletal muscle relaxant. It interferes with the release of excitatory neurotransmitters and inhibits monosynaptic and polysynaptic transmission at the spinal cord level. It may also act at supraspinal sites producing CNS depression. Baclofen is one of the drugs commonly used for the symptomatic relief of spasticity associated with a variety of conditions.

The initial dose of baclofen is 5 mg three times daily by mouth preferably with or after food or milk. The total daily dose is increased by 15 mg every fourth day (i.e. the dosage regimen is 5 mg three times a day for 3 days, 10 mg three times a day for 3 days, then 15 mg three times a day for 3 days) until either a dose of 20 mg three times a day is reached or until the desired therapeutic effect is obtained. Higher doses have been used. Doses of more than 80 to 100 mg daily are not generally recommended although doses of up to 150 mg daily have been given to carefully supervised patients.

In the UK a dosage range of 0.75 to 2 mg per kg body-weight daily has been used for children; in children over 10 years a maximum daily dosage of 2.5 mg per kg may be given. The usual starting dose is 2.5 mg given four times daily increased cautiously about every 3 days until the desired therapeutic effect is obtained. The recommended daily maintenance doses are: 12 months to 2 years of age, 10 to 20 mg; 2 to 6 years, 20 to 30 mg; 6 to 10 years, 30 to 60 mg.

Doses should be reduced in renal impairment; 5 mg daily has been suggested (but see also under Precautions, above).

If no benefit is apparent within 6 to 8 weeks of achieving the maximum dosage, therapy should probably be gradually withdrawn.

Baclofen is also given by continuous intrathecal infusion in the treatment of spasticity in patients not tolerating or not adequately responding to baclofen by mouth. Before beginning the intrathecal regimen any existing antispastic therapy should be gradually withdrawn to avoid overdosage or drug interactions. Intrathecal test doses are given initially to determine if there is going to be any benefit before implanting a controlled infusion pump. Test doses start at 25 or 50 μg and are increased by 25 μg every 24 hours until a dose of 100 μg is reached or a positive response of about 4 to 8 hours is obtained. Patients who fail to respond to a test dose of up to 100 μg are considered to be unsuitable for intrathecal treatment. For patients showing a positive response lasting for longer than 8 to 12 hours, the test dose that was required to produce the response can then be given as a 24-hour infusion; if the response to the test dose lasted 8 to 12 hours or less, then a dose equivalent to twice the test dose is given. Daily dosage can then be adjusted as required. A usual maintenance dose is within the range of 300 to 800 μg daily.

Dystonias. There have been isolated reports of improvement in patients with various forms of dystonia (p.1141) treated with baclofen[1,2] although there has also been a report[3] of a patient whose condition deteriorated during baclofen therapy.

1. Narayan RK, *et al.* Intrathecal baclofen for intractable axial dystonia. *Neurology* 1991; **41:** 1141–2.
2. Greene PE, Fahn S. Baclofen in the treatment of idiopathic dystonia in children. *Mov Disord* 1992; **7:** 48–52.
3. Silbert PL, Stewart-Wynne EG. Increased dystonia after intrathecal baclofen. *Neurology* 1992; **42:** 1639–40.

Hiccup. Baclofen has been given by mouth in daily divided doses ranging from 10 to 80 mg for the management of intractable hiccup (p.655) poorly controlled by other drugs.

References.

1. Burke AM, *et al.* Baclofen for intractable hiccups. *N Engl J Med* 1988; **319:** 1354.
2. Lance JW, Bassil GT. Familial intractable hiccup relieved by baclofen. *Lancet* 1989; **ii:** 276–7.
3. Yaqoob M, *et al.* Baclofen for intractable hiccups. *Lancet* 1989; **ii:** 562–3.
4. Ramirez FC, Graham DY. Treatment of intractable hiccup with baclofen: results of a double-blind randomized, controlled, cross-over study. *Am J Gastroenterol* 1992; **87:** 1789–91.
5. Ramirez FC, Graham DY. Hiccups, compulsive water drinking, and hyponatremia. *Ann Intern Med* 1993; **118:** 649.

Pain. Like some other muscle relaxants baclofen is used in the management of painful conditions associated with muscle spasm or spasticity (see below). The use of muscle relaxants for conditions such as low back pain is referred to on p.10. Baclofen does not appear to possess conventional analgesic activity[1] but may potentiate the analgesia produced by opioid analgesics.[2] However, it appears to be of use in the management of trigeminal neuralgia (p.12) and is sometimes added to treatment when response to first-line drugs alone is inadequate.[3]

1. Terrence CF, *et al.* Is baclofen an analgesic? *Clin Neuropharmacol* 1983; **6:** 241–5.
2. Panerai AE, *et al.* Baclofen prolongs the analgesic effect of fentanyl in man. *Br J Anaesth* 1985; **57:** 954–5.
3. Fromm GH, *et al.* Baclofen in the treatment of trigeminal neuralgia: double-blind study and long-term follow-up. *Ann Neurol* 1984; **15:** 240–4.

Spasticity. Baclofen is one of the main drugs used in the management of spasticity (see p.1303). It is used in spasticity to reduce muscle spasm and pain especially in spinal cord lesions in conditions such as multiple sclerosis or paraplegia.

Patients with severe spasticity often require high doses of baclofen by mouth before a response occurs. Some may fail to respond because adverse effects limit increases in dosage. Intrathecal administration is therefore sometimes tried as this produces much higher concentrations in the CNS than oral administration.[1,2] Intrathecal administration may be by bolus injection or by continuous infusion; infusion is probably preferred[3] to minimise the risk of overdosage. There is a large interindividual variation in the dose required to produce improvement in spasticity; doses of 12 to 1500 μg per day by continuous infusion[2,4-9] have produced improvement in some adults and children with spinal cord injuries, multiple sclerosis, and cerebral spasticity. An increased dose of baclofen may be given at night to prevent spasms that interfere with sleep. Although reports of tolerance to the effect of intrathecal baclofen have raised doubt[10] over whether long-term benefit can be maintained, a number of workers have achieved long-term efficacy.[6,11] It has been reported[12] that some patients receiving long-term intrathecal baclofen treatment have been able to stop their therapy without symptoms of spasticity re-appearing and others have been able to reduce the dosage required.

1. McLean BN. Intrathecal baclofen in severe spasticity. *Br J Hosp Med* 1993; **49:** 262–7.
2. Anonymous. Intrathecal baclofen for spasticity. *Med Lett Drugs Ther* 1994; **36:** 21–2.
3. Penn RD, Kroin JS. Intrathecal baclofen. *N Engl J Med* 1989; **321:** 1414–15.
4. Penn RD, Kroin JS. Continuous intrathecal baclofen for severe spasticity. *Lancet* 1985; **ii:** 125–7.
5. Dralle D, *et al.* Intrathecal baclofen for spasticity. *Lancet* 1985; **ii:** 1003.
6. Penn RD, *et al.* Intrathecal baclofen for severe spinal spasticity. *N Engl J Med* 1989; **320:** 1517–21.
7. Dralle D, *et al.* Intrathecal baclofen for cerebral spasticity. *Lancet* 1989; **ii:** 916.
8. Albright AL, *et al.* Intrathecal baclofen for spasticity in cerebral palsy. *JAMA* 1991; **265:** 1418–22.
9. Albright AL, *et al.* Continuous intrathecal baclofen infusion for spasticity of cerebral origin. *JAMA* 1993; **270:** 2475–7.
10. Lewis KS, Mueller WM. Intrathecal baclofen for severe spasticity secondary to spinal cord injury. *Ann Pharmacother* 1993; **27:** 767–74.
11. Azouvi P, *et al.* Intrathecal baclofen administration for control of severe spinal spasticity: functional improvement and long-term follow-up. *Arch Phys Med Rehabil* 1996; **77:** 35–9.
12. Dressnandt J, Conrad B. Lasting reduction of severe spasticity after ending chronic treatment with intrathecal baclofen. *J Neurol Neurosurg Psychiatry* 1996; **60:** 168–73.

Stiff-man syndrome. There has been an anecdotal report[1] of benefit with intrathecal baclofen in a patient with stiff-man syndrome (p.667) inadequately controlled with other drugs or oral baclofen. However, in a double-blind placebo-controlled study[2] in 3 patients clinical improvement was evident in only one patient when receiving intrathecal baclofen.

1. Seitz RJ, *et al.* Stiff-person syndrome with anti-glutamic acid decarboxylase autoantibodies: complete remission of symptoms after intrathecal baclofen administration. *J Neurol* 1995; **242:** 618–22.
2. Silbert PL, *et al.* Intrathecal baclofen therapy in stiff-man syndrome: a double-blind, placebo-controlled trial. *Neurology* 1995; **45:** 1893–7.

Tardive dyskinesia. Baclofen is one of many drugs that have been tried in antipsychotic-induced tardive dyskinesia (p.650) but its efficacy is unclear. While patients in some double-blind studies[1] have obtained improvement with baclofen other double-blind studies[2] suggest that it is unlikely to be more effective than placebo.

1. Ananth J, *et al.* Baclofen in the treatment of tardive dyskinesia. *Curr Ther Res* 1987; **42:** 111–14.
2. Glazer WM, *et al.* The treatment of tardive dyskinesia with baclofen. *Psychopharmacology (Berl)* 1985; **87:** 480–3.

Tetanus. The management of tetanus is described on p.1304 and p.145. There are case reports of beneficial responses with baclofen 1 or 2 mg daily by continuous intrathecal infusion.[1] However, the therapeutic range of intrathecal baclofen in severe tetanus may be very narrow and deep coma with loss of spontaneous respiration and reflexes has been reported[2] following an increase in dosage from 1.2 mg to 2 mg daily. This adverse effect could be fatal in the absence of ventilatory support. In an attempt to avoid the risk of secondary infection from an indwelling intraspinal catheter intermittent intrathecal administration of baclofen has also been employed.[3]

1. Müller H, *et al.* Intrathecal baclofen in tetanus. *Lancet* 1986; **i:** 317–18.
2. Romijn JA, *et al.* Reversible coma due to intrathecal baclofen. *Lancet* 1986; **ii:** 696.
3. Demaziere J, *et al.* Intermittent intrathecal baclofen for severe tetanus. *Lancet* 1991; **337:** 427.

Urinary incontinence. Baclofen has been used with some benefit in the management of urinary incontinence and retention (p.454) secondary to lesions of the spinal cord.

References.

1. Hachen HJ, Krucker V. Clinical and laboratory assessment of the efficacy of baclofen (Lioresal®) on urethral sphincter spasticity in patients with traumatic paraplegia. *Eur Urol* 1977; **3:** 237–40.
2. Leyson JFJ, *et al.* Baclofen in the treatment of detrusor-sphincter dyssynergia in spinal cord injury patients. *J Urol (Baltimore)* 1980; **124:** 82–4.
3. Kums JJM, Delhaas EM. Intrathecal baclofen infusion in patients with spasticity and neurogenic bladder disease. *World J Urol* 1991; **9:** 153–6.

Preparations

BP 1998: Baclofen Oral Solution; Baclofen Tablets;
USP 23: Baclofen Tablets.

Proprietary Preparations (details are given in Part 3)

Aust.: Lioresal; ***Austral.:*** Clofen; Lioresal; ***Belg.:*** Lioresal; ***Canad.:*** Lioresal; Nu-Baclo; ***Fr.:*** Lioresal; ***Ger.:*** Lebic; Lioresal; ***Irl.:*** Lioresal; ***Ital.:*** Lioresal; ***Neth.:*** Lioresal; ***Norw.:*** Lioresal; ***S.Afr.:*** Clinispas†; Lioresal; Neurospas†; ***Spain:*** Lioresal; ***Swed.:*** Lioresal; ***Switz.:*** Lioresal; ***UK:*** Baclospas; Balgifen; Lioresal; ***USA:*** Lioresal.

Botulinum A Toxin (18860-d)

Botulinum A toxin is a neurotoxin produced by *Clostridium botulinum*.

Residual botulinum A toxin or spillages should be inactivated by autoclaving or use of a dilute hypochlorite solution (1% available chlorine).

Units

The dose of botulinum A toxin preparations is expressed in terms of units. The manufacturers state that one unit corresponds to the median lethal dose (LD_{50}) injected intraperitoneally into mice under defined conditions. However, the available preparations are employed at different doses for the same indications, and the units of one preparation cannot be considered to apply to another.

It has been suggested that the difference between botulinum A toxin preparations may not only be confined to just a numerical dosage adjustment.[1] Reviews of the literature have suggested that there may also be a difference in the incidence of adverse effects. The reported frequency of dysphagia for Dysport (28% and 44%) in patients with spasmodic torticollis was greater than that for Botox (9.5 to 17%). This variation might relate to differences in bioactivity not recognised by the mouse lethality bioassay.

1. Borodic G. Therapeutic botulinum toxin. *Lancet* 1994; **344:** 1370.

Adverse Effects

Injections of botulinum A toxin have been associated with a transient burning sensation, bruising at the injection site, and local weakness. Deep or misplaced injections may paralyse nearby muscle groups and excessive doses may paralyse distant muscles.

The most common adverse effects following the injection of botulinum A toxin into muscles surrounding the eye, such as in the management of blepharospasm, hemifacial spasm, or strabismus are ptosis, lachrymation, photophobia, and ocular irritation. Some patients may be unable to close the eyelid completely. Other adverse effects that have been reported include ectropion and entropion, and diplopia. Patients experience a reduction in blinking and this can lead to dry eye, keratitis, and corneal damage. Angle-closure glaucoma has been reported. Vertical deviation has also occurred in patients treated for horizontal strabismus. Needle penetrations of the eye during treatment of strabismus have resulted in vitreous and retrobulbar haemorrhages.

Dysphagia is the most common adverse effect following injection of botulinum A toxin into neck muscles in the treatment of spasmodic torticollis and there may be pooling of saliva with risk of aspiration in severely affected patients (*important*, see also under Precautions, below). Dry mouth, paralysis of the vocal cords, and weakness of the neck muscles may also occur. Generalised weakness, malaise, nausea, and visual disturbances have occasionally been reported. Other effects which have occurred rarely include drowsiness, stiffness, ptosis, and headache. Respiratory difficulties, associated with the use of large doses, have occurred on rare occasions.

Overdosage can produce a widespread paralysis.

There have been occasional reports of hypersensitivity reactions such as skin rashes and influenza-like symptoms.

Adverse effects most frequently associated with injection of botulinum A toxin into the lower limb include falling, leg pain, and general weakness; lethargy and leg cramps have also been reported.

Antibody formation. Neutralising antibodies that reduce or abolish the beneficial effects of treatment have been found in a small proportion of patients who have received prolonged treatment with botulinum A toxin.[1] In a review[2] of the use of botulinum A toxin it was stated that there was growing concern over the development of antibodies after repeated injections as many of the conditions for which botulinum toxin is indicated are chronic and require indefinite treatment. Antibody formation was reported to be more common with high-dose indications such as spasmodic torticollis than in low-dose indications such as blepharospasm. The occurrence of antibodies appeared to correlate with the dose per injection, the quantity of botulinum protein given per injection, the number of injections given, and the frequency of injections.

1. Hambleton P, *et al.* Antitoxins and botulinum toxin treatment. *Br Med J* 1992; **304:** 959–60.
2. Borodic GE, Pearce LB. New concepts in botulinum toxin therapy. *Drug Safety* 1994; **11:** 145–52.

Biliary colic. A 43-year-old woman with no previous history of gallbladder disease experienced single episodes of biliary colic after each of 3 sessions of treatment with botulinum A toxin for blepharospasm.[1] Botulinum A toxin might have exerted a systemic effect to block acetylcholine release leading to gallbladder hypomotility with delayed emptying and stasis.

1. Schnider P, *et al.* Gallbladder dysfunction induced by botulinum A toxin. *Lancet* 1993; **342:** 811–12.

Dysphagia. By November 1993, the UK Committee on Safety of Medicines had received 4 reports of severe dysphagia with choking in patients who had received injections of botulinum A toxin into the neck muscles as a treatment for torticollis.[1] The dysphagia developed 5 to 7 days after the injection and in one patient it was persisting 6 weeks after the injection. The dysphagia led to aspiration of the stomach contents into the lungs and one patient with a history of poor lung function died from bronchopneumonia.

See also under Units, above for further reference to dysphagia as an adverse effect.

1. Committee on Safety of Medicines/Medicines Control Agency. Reminder: botulinum type A toxin (Dysport)—severe dysphagia with unlicensed route of administration. *Current Problems* 1993; **19:** 11.

Glaucoma. Acute angle-closure glaucoma has been reported[1] in an 83-year-old woman after a series of injections of botulinum A toxin for the treatment of blepharospasm.

1. Corridan P, *et al.* Acute angle-closure glaucoma following botulinum toxin injection for blepharospasm. *Br J Ophthalmol* 1990; **74:** 309–10.

Treatment of Adverse Effects

The use of artificial tears may relieve keratitis and dry eye (see p.1470). In the event of overdosage general supportive care is required. The patient should be monitored for several days for signs of paralysis and artificial respiration may be necessary. It is doubtful that specific botulinum antitoxin (p.1506) will be of value although some consider that it might help if given within 30 minutes of overdosage.

Precautions

Botulinum A toxin is contra-indicated in generalised disorders of muscle activity such as myasthenia gravis. Injections, especially those into the neck, should be made with great care to avoid unintended paralysis (see also below). It is also contra-indicated in pregnancy and breast feeding. As with other biological products, the potential for botulinum A toxin to cause anaphylaxis should be considered. Deep or misplaced injections should be avoided; the relevant anatomy, and any alterations due to previous surgery, must be understood before injecting.

SPECIFIC CAUTIONS WHEN TREATING BLEPHAROSPASM, HEMIFACIAL SPASM, OR STRABISMUS. Reduced blinking can lead to corneal exposure, persistent epithelial defect, and corneal ulceration, especially in patients with VIIth cranial nerve disorders; corneal sensation should be carefully tested in previously treated eyes, injection into the lower eye-lid area avoided, and any resulting epithelial defect vigorously treated.

SPECIFIC CAUTIONS WHEN TREATING LOWER LIMB SPASTICITY IN CHILDREN WITH CEREBRAL PALSY OR SPASMODIC TORTICOLLIS. Botulinum A toxin should only be used by specialists experienced in the diagnosis and management of these disorders and who have received training.

Interactions

Botulinum A toxin should not be given with (or before) aminoglycosides or spectinomycin. Interactions may also occur with other drugs that have neuromuscular blocking activity, including lincosamides, polymyxins, tetracyclines, and muscle relaxants.

Uses and Administration

Botulinum A toxin causes neuromuscular blockade by inhibiting the calcium-ion mediated release of acetylcholine at the motor nerve terminals, resulting in a diminished endplate potential and subsequent flaccid paralysis of the affected muscles. The paralysis persists until new nerve terminals form, usually within 2 to 3 months. Botulinum A toxin is given as a complex with haemagglutinin by local injection in the treatment of hemifacial spasm, blepharospasm, spasmodic torticollis, and lower limb spasticity in children with cerebral palsy. Botulinum A toxin has also been used for the management of strabismus and is being investigated for use in the management of several other disorders.

Doses of botulinum A toxin are expressed in terms of units, which have not been standardised between preparations (see under Units, above). Doses are therefore specific to each individual preparation; further details are given below.

Botulinum B toxin and *botulinum F toxin* are under investigation for the treatment of similar neuromuscular disorders; being antigenically distinct they have the potential for use in patients who develop resistance to botulinum toxin treatment due to the development of antibodies to type A toxin.

Reviews.

1. Elston JS. The clinical use of botulinum toxin. *Semin Ophthalmol* 1988; **III:** 249–60.
2. Jankovic J, Brin MF. Therapeutic uses of botulinum toxin. *N Engl J Med* 1991; **324:** 1186–94.
3. Moore A. Botulinum toxin. *Prescribers' J* 1991; **31:** 197–202.
4. Borodic GE, Pearce LB. New concepts in botulinum toxin therapy. *Drug Safety* 1994; **11:** 145–52.
5. Hughes AJ. Botulinum toxin in clinical practice. *Drugs* 1994; **48:** 888–93.

Achalasia. The treatment of choice for achalasia (see Oesophageal Motility Disorders, p.1174) is mechanical dilatation of the lower oesophageal sphincter, or if necessary surgery, but more recently injection of botulinum A toxin[1,2] has been found to be effective. Such an approach has been recommended in patients thought to be at risk from mechanical dilation or surgery.[3] However, there has been a call[4] for more data on long-term efficacy as well as for a comparative study against mechanical dilation.

1. Pasricha PJ, *et al.* Intrasphincteric botulinum toxin for the treatment of achalasia. *N Engl J Med* 1995; **332:** 774–8. Correction. *ibid.*; **333:** 75.
2. Cuillière C, *et al.* Achalasia: outcome of patients treated with intrasphincteric injection of botulinum toxin. *Gut* 1997; **41:** 87–92.
3. Cohen S, Parkman HP. Treatment of achalasia—from whalebone to botulinum toxin. *N Engl J Med* 1995; **332:** 815–6.
4. Vantrappen G. Being toxic to the oesophagus. *Gut* 1997; **41:** 131–2.

Anal fissure. Anal fissure is a superficial tear in the mucosa of the distal anal canal characterized by pain on defaecation, rectal bleeding, and spasm of the anal sphincter. Healing, which is usually uneventful, may be helped by conservative management with bran and bulk laxatives and topical local anaesthetics for pain relief. Surgical treatment has been used for patients who develop a chronic condition but since this has been associated with high rates of long-term incontinence and recurrence alternative treatments are being investigated. As hypertonicity of the internal anal sphincter may be involved in the pathophysiology of chronic anal fissure, local injections of botulinum A toxin have been used to produce paresis of this sphincter.[1,2] The duration of the effect appears to be long enough to allow complete healing of the fissure in most patients although some may relapse; temporary incontinence had been the only adverse effect reported. Topical application of nitrates can relax the anal sphincter and there have been reports[3,4] of encouraging results in the treatment of anal fissure using glyceryl trinitrate or isosorbide dinitrate ointments. Follow-up[5] of patients treated with glyceryl trinitrate indicated that after 24 to 38 months most had not experienced further problems or had had occasional recurrences which in the majority of cases had responded to further topical treatment.

1. Jost WH, Schimrigk K. Botulinum toxin in therapy of anal fissure. *Lancet* 1995; **345:** 188–9.
2. Maria G, *et al.* A comparison of botulinum toxin and saline for the treatment of chronic anal fissure. *N Engl J Med* 1998; **338:** 217–20.
3. Banerjee AK. Treating anal fissure: glyceryl trinitrate ointment may remove the need for surgery. *Br Med J* 1997; **314:** 1638–9.
4. Lund JN, Scholefield JH. A randomised, prospective, double-blind, placebo-controlled trial of glyceryl trinitrate ointment in treatment of anal fissure. *Lancet* 1997; **349:** 11–14. Correction. *ibid.*: 656.
5. Lund JN, Scholefield JH. Follow-up of patients with chronic anal fissure treated with topical glyceryl trinitrate. *Lancet* 1998; **352:** 1681.

Anismus. Anismus is a condition in which inappropriate contraction of the anal sphincters occurs when bowel evacuation is attempted; it seems to be a form of dystonia.

Treatment with botulinum A toxin was investigated in 7 patients with intractable constipation due mainly to anismus.[1] The toxin was injected bilaterally into the puborectalis muscle using an electromyographically guided needle; patients were allowed to continue with their laxatives throughout the study if required. Symptoms improved in all but one of the patients, although two patients could not be regarded as treatment successes because they developed faecal incontinence; four patients had an excellent clinical outcome.

1. Hallan RI, *et al.* Treatment of anismus in intractable constipation with botulinum A toxin. *Lancet* 1988; **ii:** 714–17.

Blepharospasm. Blepharospasm is a focal dystonia characterised by repeated involuntary blinking caused by spasms of the orbicularis oculi muscle of the eye and in some cases this may lead to functional blindness. Blepharospasm is often associated with other dystonias of the head and neck such as in Meige syndrome where patients also suffer from involuntary contractures of the muscles around the mouth. Oral drug treatment as used for dystonias in general (see p.1141) is usually ineffective and surgery (facial nerve avulsion) is often followed by recurrent spasm.[1] Local injections of botulinum A toxin into the orbicularis oculi muscle mimic the effect of surgical denervation of the muscle and are reported[2-4] to have been effective in over 70% of patients, although there appear to be few controlled studies.[5] Symptomatic improvement has been reported to last from about 9 to 15 weeks and there appears to be no increase in duration of effect following multiple injections. In one retrospective study in patients with blepharospasm and Meige syndrome treatment with botulinum A toxin was still effective in most patients 11 years after the start of therapy.[4]

Doses of botulinum A toxin are expressed in terms of units, which have not been standardised between preparations. Doses are therefore *specific to each individual preparation.* For blepharospasm botulinum A toxin is injected into the orbicularis oculi of the upper and lower lids; injection into additional sites in the brow area and upper facial area may be indicated if the spasms interfere with vision. In the UK *the preparation Botox* is injected intramuscularly in an initial dose of 1.25 to 2.50 units at each site to a total of up to 25 units per eye. An effect is usually obtained within 3 days and reaches a peak after 1 to 2 weeks; each treatment lasts for about 3 months. If the response lasts less than 2 months the dose may be increased to 5 units at each site but the total dose administered in a 12-week period should not exceed 100 units. Administration more frequently than every 3 months confers no additional benefit. For *the preparation Dysport* the initial dose is a total of 120 units per eye given as subcutaneous injections of 20 or 40 units per site. Subsequently the total dose may need to be reduced to 60 to 80 units per eye. With this preparation the relief of symptoms may begin within 2 to 4 days with a maximum effect being obtained within 2 weeks. Injections of Dysport may need to be repeated every 8 weeks.

1. Kennedy RH, *et al.* Treatment of blepharospasm with botulinum toxin. *Mayo Clin Proc* 1989; **64:** 1085–90.
2. Grandas F. Blepharospasm: a review of 264 patients. *J Neurol Neurosurg Psychiatry* 1988; **51:** 767–72.
3. Elston JS. The management of blepharospasm and hemifacial spasm. *J Neurol* 1992; **239:** 5–8.
4. Mauriello JA, *et al.* Treatment selections of 239 patients with blepharospasm and Meige syndrome over 11 years. *Br J Ophthalmol* 1996; **80:** 1073–6.
5. Jankovic J, Orman J. Botulinum A toxin for cranial-cervical dystonia: a double blind, placebo-controlled study. *Neurology* 1987; **37:** 616–23.

Hand dystonia. Hand dystonia, or hand cramp, is a type of focal dystonia (see p.1141). It is more commonly reported in people who perform repetitive movements with their hands, such as writers, keyboard operators, and musicians. Treatment has usually been with antimuscarinics, although with limited success. A double-blind study reported that 8 out of 10 patients had greater subjective improvement in focal hand dystonia, compared with placebo, after treatment with botulinum A toxin given by the intramuscular route; objective improvement in muscle strength was seen in 6 patients.[1] However, pain and severe weakness in the shoulder region resembling neuralgic amyotrophy has been reported[2] in 2 patients injected with botulinum A toxin for writer's cramp. It was considered that if unexplained pain occurred in the shoulder or upper arm after a first injection of botulinum A toxin further injections were contra-indicated.

1. Cole R, *et al.* Double-blind trial of botulinum toxin for treatment of focal hand dystonia. *Mov Disord* 1995; **10:** 466–71.
2. Sheean GL, *et al.* Pain and remote weakness in limbs injected with botulinum toxin A for writer's cramp. *Lancet* 1995; **346:** 154–6.

Hemifacial spasm. Hemifacial spasm is characterised by involuntary unilateral synchronous contractions of muscles innervated by the facial nerve. The spasms usually begin with twitching of muscles around the eye or mouth but as the disease progresses their frequency increases and they spread to involve the rest of the facial muscles. Hemifacial spasm may be improved by surgery but there is a risk of irreversible paralysis. Few drugs are effective for hemifacial spasm but carbamazepine has been reported to have been of help on occasions. Reports suggest that injections of botulinum A toxin may be effective in relieving symptoms in about 75% of patients but there do not appear to be any studies comparing it against other treatments. Repeat injections are required by most patients every 3 to 4 months but long-term efficacy appears to be maintained. Dosage regimens of botulinum A toxin used in hemifacial spasm are similar to those used for blepharospasm (see above) although an electromyographically guided needle may be required to identify small muscles around the mouth.

References.

1. Elston JS. The management of blepharospasm and hemifacial spasm. *J Neurol* 1992; **239:** 5–8.
2. Chen R-S, *et al.* Botulinum toxin A injection in the treatment of hemifacial spasm. *Acta Neurol Scand* 1996; **94:** 207–11.

Hyperhidrosis. A number of drugs and surgical techniques have been used in the treatment of hyperhidrosis (p.1074). Botulinum A toxin has been tried in the management of focal hyperhidrosis because of its ability to block cholinergic transmission at nerve terminals innervating the sweat glands. Encouraging results have been obtained in patients with severe resistant focal hyperhidrosis using intradermal[1] or subcutaneous[2,3] injections but evidence of efficacy at present comes mainly from anecdotal reports and small controlled studies. Some workers[4] prefer to use intradermal injections for palmar hyperhidrosis in order to minimise the risk of reversible weakness of the small muscles of the hand reported with subcutaneous injection.

1. Naumann M, *et al.* Focal hyperhidrosis: effective treatment with intracutaneous botulinum toxin. *Arch Dermatol* 1998; **134:** 301–4.
2. Schnider P, *et al.* Double-blind trial of botulinum A toxin for the treatment of focal hyperhidrosis of the palms. *Br J Dermatol* 1997; **136:** 548–52.
3. Schnider P, *et al.* Uses of botulinum toxin. *Lancet* 1997; **349:** 953.
4. Heckmann M, *et al.* Optimizing botulinum toxin therapy for hyperhidrosis. *Br J Dermatol* 1998; **138:** 553–4.

Laryngeal dystonias. Botulinum A toxin has been tried in the treatment of spasmodic dysphonia,[1,2] focal laryngeal dystonia,[3] and dysfunctional spasm following total laryngectomy.[4]

1. Ludlow CL. Treatment of speech and voice disorders with botulinum toxin. *JAMA* 1990; **264:** 2671–5.
2. Liu TC, *et al.* Prospective study of patients' subjective responses to botulinum toxin injection for spasmodic dysphonia. *J Otolaryngol* 1996; **25:** 66–74.
3. Marion M-H, *et al.* Stridor and focal laryngeal dystonia. *Lancet* 1992; **339:** 457–8.
4. Crary MA, *et al.* Using botulinum toxin A to improve speech and swallowing function following total laryngectomy. *Arch Otolaryngol Head Neck Surg* 1996; **122:** 760–3.

Nystagmus. Nystagmus is characterised by an involuntary, rapid, rhythmic movement of the eyeball. Various treatments including surgery, corrective spectacles, and drug therapy have all been tried but none appear to be ideal. Retrobulbar injection of botulinum A toxin was associated with an improvement in visual acuity when tried in 6 patients with acquired nystagmus and debilitating symptoms such as oscillopsia (oscillating vision).[1] The amplitude of the nystagmus was reduced but the frequency was generally unchanged. However, the need for repeated injections and adverse effects such as diplopia limited patient acceptability.

1. Repka MX, *et al.* Treatment of acquired nystagmus with botulinum neurotoxin A. *Arch Ophthalmol* 1994; **112:** 1320–4.

Ocular surgery. Ptosis is a common adverse effect of botulinum A toxin (see Adverse Effects, above). Therapeutic ptosis induced with botulinum toxin may be a useful adjunct in the management of patients undergoing epikeratoplasty since it promotes stabilisation of the epithelium on the graft.[1]

1. Freegard T, *et al.* Therapeutic ptosis with botulinum toxin in epikeratoplasty. *Br J Ophthalmol* 1993; **77:** 820–2.

Pain. There have been anecdotal reports of the use of botulinum A toxin in the treatment of painful disorders such as postcholecystectomy pain associated with sphincter of Oddi dysfunction,[1] and relief of orofacial pain associated with temporomandibular joint dysfunction[2] and facial arthromyalgia.[3] Promising results have been obtained from an open study[4] investigating botulinum toxin as a treatment for chronic refractory tennis elbow in 14 patients. The general management of pain is discussed on p.4 with separate sections on colic pain on p.8, orofacial pain on p.10, postoperative pain on p.11, and soft-tissue rheumatism, p.4.

1. Pasricha PJ, *et al.* Intrasphincteric injection of botulinum toxin for suspected sphincter of Oddi dysfunction. *Gut* 1994; **35:** 1319–21.
2. Girdler NM. Use of botulinum toxin to alleviate facial pain. *Br J Hosp Med* 1994; **52:** 363.
3. Girdler NM. Uses of botulinum toxin. *Lancet* 1997; **349:** 953.
4. Morré HHE, *et al.* Treatment of chronic tennis elbow with botulinum toxin. *Lancet* 1997; **349:** 1746.

Spasmodic torticollis. Spasmodic torticollis (cervical dystonia) is a focal dystonia (p.1141) characterised by spasmodic rotation of the head as a result of dystonic spasm of the neck muscles. The head may turn to one side (torticollis), extend (retrocollis), or flex (antecollis). Spasms may be repetitive or sustained. Response of spasmodic torticollis to drug therapy is usually poor and surgery has been associated with potentially serious complications. Intramuscular injections of botulinum A toxin have been shown to be effective but dysphagia, which can have severe consequences (see under Adverse Effects, above) occurs in a significant number of patients. Other side-effects have included lethargy, local weakness, vertigo, and dysphonia.

When injecting botulinum A toxin localisation of the involved muscles with electromyographic guidance may be useful. Multiple injection sites allow more uniform contact with the innervation areas of the dystonic muscle and are especially useful in larger muscles. Bilateral injection of the sternocleidomastoid muscle is not recommended as there is an increased risk of adverse effects, especially dysphagia. Reduced doses may be required for elderly or underweight patients or others with reduced muscle mass. Doses of botulinum A toxin are expressed in terms of units which have not been standardised between preparations. Doses are therefore *specific to each individual preparation.*

In the UK the usual initial dose of botulinum A toxin *as the preparation Dysport* is 500 units injected in divided doses into the two or three most active neck muscles.

- For *rotational torticollis*, 350 units is given initially into the splenius capitis muscle (ipsilateral to the direction of the chin/head rotation) and 150 units into the sternocleidomastoid muscle (contralateral to rotation).
- For *laterocollis*, 350 units is given initially into the ipsilateral splenius capitis muscle and 150 units into the ipsilateral sternocleidomastoid muscle; if associated with *shoulder elevation*, ipsilateral trapezoid or levator scapulae muscles may also require treatment; if 3 muscles need treatment, 300 units are injected into the splenius capitis muscle, 100 units into the sternocleidomastoid muscle, and 100 units into the third muscle.
- For *retrocollis*, 250 units is given into each of the splenius capitis muscles which may be followed after 6 weeks by bilateral trapezius injections in a dose of up to 250 units per muscle; bilateral splenii injections may increase the risk of neck muscle weakness.

Subsequent doses may range from 250 to 1000 units, although higher doses may be accompanied by an increase in adverse effects such as dysphagia; doses above 1000 units are not recommended. An initial effect is usually observed within 1 week; injections usually need to be repeated every 8 to 12 weeks.

Recommended doses in the UK for botulinum A toxin *as the preparation Botox* are listed below but the manufacturer has stated that in practice the maximum total dose is not usually more than 200 units. No more than 50 units should be given at any one injection site; limiting the dose injected into the sternocleidomastoid muscle to less than 100 units may reduce the risk of dysphagia.

- *Type I* (head rotated toward side of shoulder elevation)—sternocleidomastoid muscle: total dosage of 50 to 100 units divided amongst at least 2 sites; levator scapulae: total of 50 units amongst 1 to 2 sites; scalene: total of 25 to 50 units amongst 1 to 2 sites; splenius capitis: total of 25 to 75 units amongst 1 to 3 sites; trapezius: total of 25 to 100 units amongst 1 to 8 sites.
- *Type II* (head rotation only)—sternocleidomastoid muscle: total dosage of 25 to 100 units divided amongst at least 2 sites if more than 25 units is given.
- *Type III* (head tilted toward side of shoulder elevation)—sternocleidomastoid muscle: total dosage of 25 to 100 units at posterior border divided amongst at least 2 sites if more than 25 units is given; levator scapulae: total of 25 to 100 units amongst at least 2 sites; scalene: total of 25 to 75 units amongst at least 2 sites; trapezius: total of 25 to 100 units amongst 1 to 8 sites.
- *Type IV* (bilateral posterior cervical muscle spasm with elevation of the face)—splenius capitis and splenius cervicis: a total dosage of 50 to 200 units divided amongst 2 to 8 sites and which include both sides of the neck.

References.

1. Blackie JD, Lees AJ. Botulinum toxin treatment in spasmodic torticollis. *J Neurol Neurosurg Psychiatry* 1990; **53:** 640–3.
2. Greene P, *et al.* Double-blind, placebo-controlled trial of botulinum toxin injections for the treatment of spasmodic torticollis. *Neurology* 1990; **40:** 1213–18.
3. Anderson TJ, *et al.* Botulinum toxin treatment of spasmodic torticollis. *J R Soc Med* 1992; **85:** 524–9.
4. Brans JWM, *et al.* Botulinum toxin versus trihexyphenidyl in cervical dystonia: a prospective, randomized, double-blind controlled trial. *Neurology* 1996; **46:** 1066–72.

Spasticity. The mainstay of management of spasticity, as discussed on p.1303, is physiotherapy together with antispastic drugs. Chemical neurolysis should only be considered when there is intractable continuous pain. Local injections of botulinum A toxin, as an alternative to chemical neurolysis, have been of benefit in the management of limb spasticity in post-stroke patients[1-3] and children with cerebral palsy.[4-6] However, children may find the need for repeated injections unacceptable.[4]

In the UK, botulinum A toxin as the preparation Botox is used in the management of dynamic equinus foot deformity associated with spasticity in children with cerebral palsy. For children over 2 years of age the recommended total dose is 4 units per kg body-weight injected into each of 2 sites in the medial and lateral heads of the gastrocnemius muscle. When both lower limbs are to be injected on the same occasion this total dose should be divided between the 2 limbs. Clinical improvement generally occurs within the first 2 weeks. Repeat doses should not be given more frequently than every 2 months.

1. Simpson DM, *et al.* Botulinum toxin type A in the treatment of upper extremity spasticity: a randomized, double-blind, placebo-controlled trial. *Neurology* 1996; **46:** 1306–10.
2. Bhakta BB, *et al.* Use of botulinum toxin in stroke patients with severe upper limb spasticity. *J Neurol Neurosurg Psychiatry* 1996; **61:** 30–5.
3. Burbaud P, *et al.* A randomised, double blind, placebo controlled trial of botulinum toxin in the treatment of spastic foot in hemiparetic patients. *J Neurol Neurosurg Psychiatry* 1996; **61:** 265–9.
4. Neville B. Botulinum toxin in the cerebral palsies. *Br Med J* 1994; **309:** 1526–7.
5. Zelnik N, *et al.* The role of botulinum toxin in the treatment of lower limb spasticity in children with cerebral palsy—a pilot study. *Isr J Med Sci* 1997; **33:** 129–33.
6. Carr LJ, *et al.* Position paper on the use of botulinum toxin in cerebral palsy. *Arch Dis Child* 1998; **79:** 271–3.

Stiff-man syndrome. Report[1] of a patient with stiff-man syndrome (p.667) who had marked improvement of ambulation and cessation of pain following injection of botulinum A toxin into affected paraspinal muscles.

1. Davis D, Jabbari B. Significant improvement of stiff-person syndrome after paraspinal injection of botulinum toxin A. *Mov Disord* 1993; **8:** 371–3.

Strabismus. Botulinum A toxin has been used to weaken overactive extra-ocular muscles as an alternative or adjunct to surgery in the correction of strabismus (p.1389). Not all patients respond to botulinum A toxin and many patients who do respond require more than one injection to maintain improvement. Botulinum A toxin does not appear to offer a better degree of correction than traditional surgery and it has been suggested that it should be reserved for use in patients unresponsive to or unsuitable for surgery. In the USA botulinum A toxin as the preparation Botox is indicated for the treatment of strabismus in patients 12 years of age or older. Depending on the direction and degree of deviation to be corrected the recommended initial dose of Botox to be injected into any one extra-ocular muscle ranges from 1.25 to 5.0 units. Paralysis is usually seen within the first 2 days and increases in intensity during the first week. The paralysis lasts for 2 to 6 weeks and gradually resolves over a further 2 to 6 weeks. It is recommended that patients are re-examined 7 to 14 days after injection to assess the effect of the dose given. If treatment is required for residual or recurrent strabismus, patients are either given treatment at the previous dosage if response was judged to have been adequate or up to twice the previous dose if paralysis had been incomplete. Repeat injections should not be administered until the effects of the previous dose have dissipated. No more than 25 units should be injected into any one muscle; the US manufacturer recommends that the cumulative dose in a 30-day period should not exceed 200 units. Injections should be diluted with 0.9% sodium chloride solution so that the volume administered is between 0.05 mL and 0.15 mL. Injections should also be made using an electromyographically guided needle to aid location of the target muscle.

References.

1. Biglan AW, *et al.* Management of strabismus with botulinum A toxin. *Ophthalmology* 1989; **96:** 935–43.
2. Carruthers JDA, *et al.* Botulinum vs adjustable suture surgery in the treatment of horizontal misalignment in adult patients lacking fusion. *Arch Ophthalmol* 1990; **108:** 1432–5.
3. Lyons CJ, *et al.* Botulinum toxin therapy in dysthyroid strabismus. *Eye* 1990; **4:** 538–42.
4. McNeer KW. An investigation of the clinical use of botulinum toxin A as a postoperative adjustment procedure in the therapy of strabismus. *J Pediatr Ophthalmol Strabismus* 1990; **27:** 3–9.
5. Scott AB, *et al.* Botulinum treatment of childhood strabismus. *Ophthalmology* 1990; **97:** 1434–8.
6. Petitto VB, Buckley EG. Use of botulinum toxin in strabismus after retinal detachment surgery. *Ophthalmology* 1991; **98:** 509–13.
7. Elston J. Is botulinum toxin helpful in squint management? *Br J Ophthalmol* 1998; **82:** 105.
8. Tejedor J, Rodríguez JM. Retreatment of children after surgery for acquired esotropia: reoperation versus botulinum injection. *Br J Ophthalmol* 1998; **82:** 110–14.

Tremor. Local injection of botulinum A toxin[1,2] has been tried in patients with essential tremor (p.831) that fails to respond to conventional treatment.

1. Henderson JM, *et al.* Botulinum toxin A in non-dystonic tremors. *Eur Neurol* 1996; **36:** 29–35.
2. Jankovic J, *et al.* A randomized, double-blind, placebo-controlled study to evaluate botulinum toxin type A in essential hand tremor. *Mov Disord* 1996; **11:** 250–6.

Vaginismus. Report[1] of one patient who had relief of vaginismus (painful involuntary spasm of the vaginal or perianal muscles severe enough to prevent intercourse) for more than 24 months after injection of botulinum toxin into the vaginal wall muscles.

1. Brin MF, Vapnek JM. Treatment of vaginismus with botulinum toxin injections. *Lancet* 1997; **349:** 252–3.

Preparations

Proprietary Preparations (details are given in Part 3)
Austral.: Botox; ***Canad.:*** Botox; ***Fr.:*** Botox; Dysport; ***Ger.:*** Botox; ***Irl.:*** Botox; Dysport; ***Ital.:*** Botox; Dysport; ***Norw.:*** Botox; ***Swed.:*** Botox; ***Switz.:*** Botox; ***UK:*** Botox; Dysport; ***USA:*** Botox; Oculinum†.

Carbolonium Bromide (5703-c)

Carbolonium Bromide (BAN).

Hexcarbacholine Bromide *(rINN)*; Choline Bromide Hexamethylenedicarbamate; Hexacarbacholine Bromide. NN'-Hexamethylenebis[(2-carbamoyloxyethyl)trimethylammonium] dibromide.

$C_{18}H_{40}Br_2N_4O_4$ = 536.3.

CAS — 13309-41-6 (carbolonium); 306-41-2 (carbolonium bromide).

Carbolonium bromide is a neuromuscular blocker which produces an initial depolarising neuromuscular block that is rapidly converted to a phase II (competitive type) blockade. Its actions are more prolonged than those of other depolarising neuromuscular blockers such as suxamethonium (p.1321).

Preparations

Proprietary Preparations (details are given in Part 3)
Ger.: Imbretil†.

Carisoprodol (5704-k)

Carisoprodol (BAN, rINN).

Isopropylmeprobamate. 2-Methyl-2-propyltrimethylene carbamate isopropylcarbamate.

$C_{12}H_{24}N_2O_4$ = 260.3.

CAS — 78-44-4.

Pharmacopoeias. In US.

A white crystalline powder with a slight characteristic odour. M.p. 91° to 94°. **Soluble** 1 in 2083 of water, 1 in 2.5 of alcohol and of acetone, and 1 in 2.3 of chloroform. **Store** in airtight containers.

Adverse Effects, Treatment, and Precautions

As for Meprobamate, p.678.

An idiosyncratic reaction may occur within minutes of a dose in patients who have not previously received carisoprodol. The symptoms, which include severe weakness and central disturbances, usually subside over several hours. There may be a short-lived quadriplegia. Cross reactivity can occur with its metabolite meprobamate.

Overdosage may result in stupor, coma, shock, respiratory depression, and rarely death.

It should be used with caution in patients with impaired hepatic or renal function. As carisoprodol is concentrated in breast milk, it is perhaps best avoided during breast feeding.

Carisoprodol may cause drowsiness therefore patients affected should not drive or operate machinery.

Dependence. There has been a case report of carisoprodol dependence probably due to its metabolism to meprobamate.[1] The patient experienced symptoms of meprobamate withdrawal which resolved with a reducing dose schedule of meprobamate.

1. Luehr JG, *et al.* Mail-order (veterinary) drug dependence. *JAMA* 1990; **263:** 657.

Porphyria. Carisoprodol has been associated with acute attacks of porphyria and is considered unsafe in patients with acute porphyria.[1]

1. Moore MR, McColl KEL. *Porphyria: drug lists.* Glasgow: Porphyria Research Unit, University of Glasgow, 1991.

Interactions

The CNS effects of carisoprodol may be potentiated by alcohol or other CNS depressants.

Pharmacokinetics

Carisoprodol is absorbed from the gastro-intestinal tract. It is metabolised in the liver and excreted in urine as metabolites, including meprobamate. It is distributed in substantial amounts into breast milk.

References.

1. Olsen H, *et al.* Carisoprodol elimination in humans. *Ther Drug Monit* 1994; **16:** 337–40.

Uses and Administration

Carisoprodol is a centrally acting skeletal muscle relaxant whose mechanism of action is not completely understood but may be related to its sedative actions. Following administration by mouth its effects begin within about 30 minutes and last for 4 to 6 hours. It is used as an adjunct in the short-term symptomatic treatment of painful muscle spasm (p.1303) associated with musculoskeletal conditions. A usual dose is 350 mg given three to four times daily by mouth. Half the usual dose or less is recommended in elderly patients. It is also given with analgesics in compound preparations.

Headache. Carisoprodol is available in some countries in compound analgesic preparations for the treatment of tension-type headache (muscle-contraction headache), but results for muscle relaxants in general are disappointing and they appear to have little place in the management of tension-type headache (p.444).

Preparations

USP 23: Carisoprodol and Aspirin Tablets; Carisoprodol Tablets; Carisoprodol, Aspirin, and Codeine Phosphate Tablets.

Proprietary Preparations (details are given in Part 3)
Canad.: Soma; ***Ger.:*** Sanoma; ***Norw.:*** Somadril; ***Spain:*** Somalgit; ***Swed.:*** Somadril; ***UK:*** Carisoma; ***USA:*** Rela†; Soma.

Multi-ingredient: ***Ital.:*** Flectomas†; Flexidone; Soma Complex; Teknadone†; ***Norw.:*** Somadril Comp†; ***Spain:*** Flexagil; Relaxibys; ***Swed.:*** Somadril Comp; ***Switz.:*** Lagaflex†; ***USA:*** Sodol Compound; Soma Compound; Soma Compound with Codeine.

Chlorphenesin Carbamate (5705-a)

Chlorphenesin Carbamate *(BANM, USAN, pINNM)*.

U-19646. 3-(4-Chlorophenoxy)propane-1,2-diol 1-carbamate.

$C_{10}H_{12}ClNO_4$ = 245.7.

CAS — 104-29-0 (chlorphenesin); 886-74-8 (chlorphenesin carbamate).

Pharmacopoeias. In *Jpn.*

Adverse Effects and Precautions

Chlorphenesin carbamate produces drowsiness and dizziness. There may also be nausea, headache, weakness, confusion, agitation, and insomnia. Hypersensitivity reactions have been reported. There are rare reports of blood disorders.

It should be used with caution in patients with hepatic impairment. Patients affected by drowsiness should not drive or operate machinery.

Interactions

The CNS effects of chlorphenesin carbamate may be potentiated by alcohol or other CNS depressants.

Pharmacokinetics

Chlorphenesin carbamate is readily and completely absorbed from the gastro-intestinal tract and partly metabolised in the liver. It is excreted in the urine, mainly as the glucuronide.

Uses and Administration

Chlorphenesin carbamate is a centrally acting skeletal muscle relaxant related to mephenesin (p.1315). Its mode of action may be related to general depressant effects on the CNS. It is used as an adjunct in the symptomatic treatment of painful muscle spasm (p.1303) associated with musculoskeletal conditions. The usual initial dose is 800 mg three times daily given by mouth reduced to 400 mg four times daily or less once a response has been achieved. It has been recommended that chlorphenesin carbamate should not be administered for longer than 8 weeks.

Chlorphenesin base (p.376) is used as an antifungal.

Preparations

Proprietary Preparations (details are given in Part 3)
USA: Maolate.

Chlorzoxazone (5706-t)

Chlorzoxazone *(BAN, rINN)*.

Chlorobenzoxazolinone. 5-Chlorobenzoxazol-2(3*H*)-one.

$C_7H_4ClNO_2$ = 169.6.

CAS — 95-25-0.

Pharmacopoeias. In *US.*

A white or almost white, practically odourless crystalline powder. Slightly **soluble** in water; sparingly soluble in alcohol, in isopropyl alcohol, and in methyl alcohol; soluble in solutions of alkali hydroxides and ammonia. **Store** in airtight containers.

Adverse Effects and Treatment

The most common side-effects of chlorzoxazone are drowsiness and dizziness. There may occasionally also be gastro-intestinal irritation and gastro-intestinal bleeding has been reported. Other effects that have occurred are headache, overstimulation, and rarely sensitivity reactions including skin rashes, petechiae, ecchymoses, urticaria and pruritus; very rarely, angioedema or anaphylactoid reactions may occur. Some patients taking chlorzoxazone have developed jaundice and liver damage suspected to be caused by the drug.

Following overdosage there may be gastro-intestinal disturbances, drowsiness, dizziness, headache, malaise, and sluggishness followed by marked loss of muscle tone, hypotension, and respiratory depression. Treatment consists of emptying the stomach by lavage or emesis, followed by administration of activated charcoal and supportive therapy.

Effects on the liver. Hepatotoxicity, sometimes fatal, has been associated with chlorzoxazone treatment.[1]

1. Powers BJ, *et al.* Chlorzoxazone hepatotoxic reactions: an analysis of 21 identified or presumed cases. *Arch Intern Med* 1986; **146:** 1183–6.

Torticollis. There has been a report of a patient with a spasmodic torticollis-like syndrome, consisting of tonic deviation of the head to the right, clenching of the teeth, and dysarthria, which developed repeatedly within 2 hours of ingesting chlorzoxazone for low back pain.[1] Intravenous injection of benztropine mesylate 1 mg gave rapid relief of symptoms.

1. Rosin MA. Chlorzoxazone-induced spasmodic torticollis. *JAMA* 1981; **246:** 2575.

Precautions

Chlorzoxazone should not be given to patients with impaired liver function and should be discontinued if signs of liver toxicity appear. Patients should be advised to report to their doctor any signs or symptoms of possible liver toxicity such as fever, rash, jaundice, dark urine, anorexia, nausea, vomiting, or right upper quadrant pain. Chlorzoxazone may cause drowsiness; patients affected should not drive or operate machinery.

The urine of patients taking chlorzoxazone may be coloured orange or reddish-purple by a phenolic metabolite.

Porphyria. Chlorzoxazone has been associated with clinical exacerbations of porphyria and is considered unsafe in porphyric patients.[1]

1. Moore MR, McColl KEL. *Porphyria: drug lists.* Glasgow: Porphyria Research Unit, University of Glasgow, 1991.

Interactions

The CNS effects of chlorzoxazone may be enhanced by alcohol and other CNS depressants.

Disulfiram. A study[1] of the efficacy of disulfiram as an inhibitor of the cytochrome P450 isozyme 2E1 (an enzyme involved in the metabolism of chlorzoxazone) found that a single 500-mg dose of disulfiram reduced plasma clearance of chlorzoxazone by 85% resulting in a doubling of peak plasma concentrations and prolongation of chlorzoxazone's elimination half-life from a mean of 0.92 to 5.1 hours.

1. Kharasch ED, *et al.* Single-dose disulfiram inhibition of chlorzoxazone metabolism: a clinical probe for P450 2E1. *Clin Pharmacol Ther* 1993; **53:** 643–50.

Isoniazid. Isoniazid inhibited the clearance of chlorzoxazone by 56% when given to 10 slow acetylator subjects resulting in an increase in sedation, headache, and nausea.[1] Two days after discontinuation of isoniazid there had been a rebound increase in the clearance of chlorzoxazone by 56% over the pre-isoniazid clearance value. Similar but less pronounced effects have also been reported[2] in rapid acetylators with chlorzoxazone's pharmacokinetic parameters returning to base-line values in 2 days.

1. Zand R, *et al.* Inhibition and induction of cytochrome P4502E1-catalyzed oxidation by isoniazid in humans. *Clin Pharmacol Ther* 1993; **54:** 142–9.
2. O'Shea D, *et al.* Modulation of CYP2E1 activity by isoniazid in rapid and slow N-acetylators. *Br J Clin Pharmacol* 1997; **43:** 99–103.

Pharmacokinetics

Chlorzoxazone is reported to be completely absorbed after oral administration and peak plasma concentrations are achieved after 1 to 2 hours. It is rapidly metabolised in the liver, mainly to 6-hydroxychlorzoxazone, and excreted in the urine primarily as the glucuronide. The elimination half-life of chlorzoxazone is about 1 hour.

Uses and Administration

Chlorzoxazone is a centrally acting skeletal muscle relaxant with sedative properties. It is claimed to inhibit muscle spasm by exerting an effect primarily at the level of the spinal cord and subcortical areas of the brain. Following oral administration its effects begin within an hour and last for 3 to 4 hours.

It is used as an adjunct in the symptomatic treatment of painful muscle spasm (p.1303) associated with musculoskeletal conditions. The usual initial dose is 500 mg three or four times daily by mouth; the dose can often be reduced subsequently to 250 mg three or four times daily, although doses of up to 750 mg three or four times daily may be given if necessary. Chlorzoxazone is also given with analgesics in compound preparations.

Preparations

USP 23: Chlorzoxazone Tablets.

Proprietary Preparations (details are given in Part 3)
Ital.: Biomioran†; ***S.Afr.:*** Paraflex†; ***Swed.:*** Paraflex; ***Switz.:*** Escoflex†; ***USA:*** Paraflex; Parafon Forte DSC; Remular-S.

Multi-ingredient: ***Aust.:*** Parafon; ***Canad.:*** Acetazone Forte; Acetazone Forte C8; Back-Aid; Parafon Forte; Parafon Forte C8; Tylenol Aches & Strains; ***Ger.:*** Paraflex spezial†; ***S.Afr.:*** Parafon†; ***Swed.:*** Paraflex comp.; ***Switz.:*** Escoflex Compositum†; Parafon; Zafor; ***USA:*** Algisin†; Flexaphen; Mus-Lax†; Spasgesic†.

Cyclobenzaprine Hydrochloride (5708-r)

Cyclobenzaprine Hydrochloride *(USAN, rINNM)*.

MK-130 (cyclobenzaprine); Proheptatriene Hydrochloride; Ro-4-1557 (cyclobenzaprine); RP-9715 (cyclobenzaprine). 3-(5*H*-Dibenzo[*a,d*]cyclohepten-5-ylidene)-*NN*-dimethylpropylamine hydrochloride.

$C_{20}H_{21}N,HCl$ = 311.8.

CAS — 303-53-7 (cyclobenzaprine); 6202-23-9 (cyclobenzaprine hydrochloride).

Pharmacopoeias. In *US.*

A white or off-white odourless crystalline powder. Freely **soluble** in water, in alcohol, and in methyl alcohol; sparingly soluble in isopropyl alcohol; slightly soluble in chloroform and in dichloromethane; practically insoluble in hydrocarbons.

Adverse Effects, Treatment, and Precautions

Cyclobenzaprine hydrochloride is structurally related to the tricyclic antidepressants and shares their adverse effects and precautions (see Amitriptyline, p.273).

It may cause drowsiness; patients affected should not drive or operate machinery.

Neuroleptic malignant syndrome. Report of a neuroleptic malignant-like syndrome associated with cyclobenzaprine in a 36-year-old man.[1] It was not clear whether the syndrome was due to an idiosyncratic reaction or to an overdose.

1. Theoharides TC, *et al.* Neuroleptic malignant-like syndrome due to cyclobenzaprine. *J Clin Psychopharmacol* 1995; **15:** 79–81.

Interactions

Cyclobenzaprine is structurally related to the tricyclic antidepressants and may be subject to similar interactions (see Amitriptyline, p.276). The CNS effects of cyclobenzaprine may be enhanced by alcohol or other CNS depressants.

Pharmacokinetics

Cyclobenzaprine hydrochloride is readily and almost completely absorbed from the gastro-intestinal tract although plasma concentrations vary considerably among individuals given the same dose. About 93% is bound to plasma proteins and has a reported elimination half-life of 1 to 3 days. It is extensively metabolised, principally to glucuronide conjugates, and excreted in the urine. Some unchanged drug appears in the bile and is excreted in the faeces.

Uses and Administration

Cyclobenzaprine hydrochloride is a centrally acting skeletal muscle relaxant, related to the tricyclic antidepressants. It acts mainly at the brain stem to decrease tonic somatic motor activity influencing both alpha and gamma motor systems. Additional activity at spinal cord sites may be involved. Following oral administration its effects begin within 1 hour; the effects of a single dose have been reported to last as long as 12 to 24 hours.

It is used as an adjunct in the symptomatic treatment of painful muscle spasm (p.1303) associated with musculoskeletal conditions. The usual dose is 10 mg three times daily given by mouth; the daily dose should not exceed 60 mg. Treatment for more than 2 or 3 weeks is not recommended.

References.

1. Katz WA, Dube J. Cyclobenzaprine in the treatment of acute muscle spasm: review of a decade of clinical experience. *Clin Ther* 1988; **10:** 216–28.

Fibromyalgia. Studies of the efficacy of cyclobenzaprine in the management of fibromyalgia, a painful musculoskeletal disorder which usually responds poorly to analgesics have produced conflicting results[1,2] but a small percentage of patients may obtain some relief.[2] In one study[2] involving 208 patients with fibromyalgia improvement 1 month after starting treatment was shown in 21% of patients receiving amitriptyline, 12% of those receiving cyclobenzaprine, and in none of those given placebo. Although the percentage of patients with improvement had increased at the 3 and 6 month assessments there was no longer a significant difference between the groups. Cyclobenzaprine had been given in an initial dosage of 10 mg at night and increased to 30 mg daily. An earlier study[3] found that 30 mg daily was not more effective than 10 mg at night but resulted in a higher incidence of adverse effects.

1. Reynolds WJ, *et al.* The effects of cyclobenzaprine on sleep physiology and symptoms in patients with fibromyalgia. *J Rheumatol* 1991; **18:** 452–4.
2. Carette S, *et al.* Comparison of amitriptyline, cyclobenzaprine, and placebo in the treatment of fibromyalgia: a randomized, double-blind clinical trial. *Arthritis Rheum* 1994; **37:** 32–40.
3. Santandrea S, *et al.* A double-blind crossover study of two cyclobenzaprine regimens in primary fibromyalgia syndrome. *J Int Med Res* 1993; **21:** 74–80.

Preparations

USP 23: Cyclobenzaprine Hydrochloride Tablets.

Proprietary Preparations (details are given in Part 3)
Canad.: Flexeril; Novo-Cycloprine; ***Ital.:*** Flexiban; ***Spain:*** Yurelax; ***USA:*** Flexeril.

Dantrolene Sodium (5709-f)

Dantrolene Sodium *(BANM, USAN, rINNM)*.

F-440; F-368 (dantrolene). The hemiheptahydrate of the sodium salt of 1-[5-(4-nitrophenyl)furfurylideneamino]imidazolidine-2,4-dione.

$C_{14}H_9N_4NaO_5,3\frac{1}{2}H_2O$ = 399.3.

CAS — 7261-97-4 (dantrolene); 14663-23-1 (anhydrous dantrolene sodium); 24868-20-0 (dantrolene sodium, hemiheptahydrate).

Pharmacopoeias. In *Jpn.*

Adverse Effects

Adverse effects associated with dantrolene sodium tend to occur at the start of treatment, but are often short lived and can be controlled by adjusting the dose. The most common side-effects are drowsiness, dizziness, fatigue, muscle weakness, and malaise. Diarrhoea may be severe enough to necessitate withdrawal. If diarrhoea recurs following reintroduction of dantrolene, then treatment should probably be stopped permanently. Other side-effects reported include nausea and vomiting, anorexia, constipation, abdominal cramps, gastro-intestinal bleeding, tachycardia, unstable blood pressure, dyspnoea, rashes (often acneform), pruritus, chills and fever, headache, myalgia, nervousness, insomnia, confusion, visual disturbances, mental depression, dysphagia and speech disturbances, and seizures. Haematuria, crystalluria, urinary frequency and retention, and incontinence may occur. Rare but serious adverse effects include hepatotoxicity which may be fatal (see below) and pleural effusion with pericarditis.

Serious side-effects do not appear to be a problem with the short-term use of intravenous dantrolene sodium in the treatment of malignant hyperthermia.

Effects on the liver. Dantrolene has caused hepatotoxicity with raised liver enzyme values, jaundice, and hepatitis;[1,2] fatalities have been reported.[1] Not all patients experienced symptoms such as anorexia, nausea, or abdominal discomfort before the onset of disease and the severity of hepatic injury was unrelated to clinical presentation. In the first report[1] the 14 fatalities occurred with doses in excess of 200 mg daily. The onset of hepatic injury was usually between 1 and 6 months after starting treatment and fatalities were not reported in the first 2 months. Only rarely did injury develop before 45 days of treatment. Females appeared to be at greater risk of serious liver injury and the severity of reaction appeared to be age-related with all fatalities occurring in patients over 30 years of age. The liver injury was usually hepatocellular and might include ascending cholangitis; there was no evidence of hypersensitivity.

1. Utili R, *et al.* Dantrolene-associated hepatic injury: incidence and character. *Gastroenterology* 1977; **72:** 610–16.
2. Wilkinson SP, *et al.* Hepatitis from dantrolene sodium. *Gut* 1979; **20:** 33–6.

Lymphomas. Fatal lymphocytic lymphoma in one patient was associated with prolonged dantrolene therapy 600 mg daily for progressive spastic paraplegia.[1]

1. Wan HH, Tucker JS. Dantrolene and lymphocytic lymphoma. *Postgrad Med J* 1980; **56:** 261–2.

Precautions

It is recommended that dantrolene sodium should not be given to patients with active liver disease. Liver-function tests should be performed in all patients before and during treatment; if abnormal values are found, treatment should generally be discontinued. The risk of liver injury may be increased in patients over 30 years of age, in females (especially those taking oestrogens), and with doses above 400 mg per day (see under Effects on the Liver, above). Dantrolene sodium should be used with caution in patients with cardiac or pulmonary disorders. It should not be given to patients who use their spasticity to maintain posture or function or to patients with acute muscle spasm.

Dantrolene sodium may cause drowsiness; patients affected should not drive or operate machinery.

Interactions

The CNS effects of dantrolene sodium may be enhanced by alcohol or other CNS depressants. Concomitant administration with oestrogens may possibly increase the risk of liver damage.

Calcium-channel blockers. Severe hyperkalaemia and myocardial depression occurred following administration of dantrolene intravenously for prophylaxis of malignant hyperthermia in a patient also taking verapamil for angina.[1] The peak serum-potassium concentration was 7.1 mmol per litre 2.5 hours after the dantrolene infusion. Nifedipine was substituted for verapamil in a subsequent operation and only a small increase in serum potassium occurred following administration of dantrolene. Ventricular fibrillation and cardiovascular collapse associated with hyperkalaemia have been seen with this combination in *animal* studies and the manufacturers recommend that calcium-channel blockers and intravenous dantrolene should not be used together.

1. Rubin AS, Zablocki AD. Hyperkalaemia, verapamil, and dantrolene. *Anesthesiology* 1987; **66:** 246–9.

Pharmacokinetics

Dantrolene sodium is slowly and incompletely absorbed from the gastro-intestinal tract. It is metabolised in the liver mainly to the hydroxylated and acetamide metabolites which have weak muscle relaxant activity. It is excreted in the urine, mainly as metabolites with a small amount of unchanged dantrolene; some is excreted in the bile. Dantrolene is bound extensively to plasma proteins. The elimination half-life following oral administration is about 9 hours.

Uses and Administration

Dantrolene sodium is a muscle relaxant with a direct action on skeletal muscle. It uncouples muscular contraction from excitation, probably by interfering with the release of calcium from the sarcoplasmic reticulum.

It is given by mouth for the symptomatic relief of chronic, severe spasticity (p.1303) due to a variety of conditions and is one of the main drugs used. It is also given, usually by intravenous injection, for the treatment of malignant hyperthermia.

For spasticity, the initial dose is 25 mg daily by mouth increased gradually as necessary, at 7-day intervals, over about 7 weeks to a maximum dose of 100 mg four times daily. If no response is achieved within 45 days treatment should be discontinued. In the UK dantrolene is not recommended for use in children, but in the USA a suggested dose for children is 0.5 mg per kg body-weight once daily, increased gradually if necessary to 2 mg per kg three times daily; administration four times daily may be necessary for some children but a dose of 100 mg 4 times daily should not be exceeded.

In the treatment of malignant hyperthermia, dantrolene sodium is given, together with supportive measures, in an initial dose of 1 mg per kg body-weight by rapid intravenous injection, repeated, if necessary, to a total dose of 10 mg per kg. In the USA, doses of 1 to 2 mg per kg by mouth 4 times daily have been recommended for up to 3 days after the crisis to prevent recurrence, and similar doses have been given for 1 to 2 days before surgery in individuals thought to be at risk of developing the syndrome. Prophylactic doses may also be given intravenously; 2.5 mg per kg has been recommended, infused over about 60 minutes, starting about 75 minutes before anticipated anaesthesia, with further administration during anaesthesia and surgery if signs of malignant hyperthermia develop.

Hyperthermia. Dantrolene is used in the treatment of hyperthermia associated with muscle rigidity and fulminant hypermetabolism of skeletal muscle which occurs in the neuroleptic malignant syndrome (see below and p.651) and in malignant hyperthermia (see below). There is also anecdotal evidence that dantrolene may produce beneficial effects for the treatment of similar symptoms resulting from poisoning with various agents such as carbon monoxide,[1] MAOIs,[2] and methylenedioxyethamphetamine.[3] However, following suggestions that it may also be of use in cocaine intoxication, the manufacturers[4] warned physicians that they should not regard dantrolene as an effective treatment for all types of hyperthermia and rigidity accompanying poisoning.

Dantrolene may hasten cooling when used as part of treatment for heat stroke (see under Fever and Hyperthermia, p.1) but does not appear to affect outcome.[5]

1. Ten Holter JBM, Schellens RLLAM. Dantrolene sodium for treatment of carbon monoxide poisoning. *Br Med J* 1988; **296:** 1772–3.
2. Kaplan RF, *et al.* Phenelzine overdose treatment with dantrolene sodium. *JAMA* 1986; **255:** 642–4.
3. Tehan B. Ecstasy and dantrolene. *Br Med J* 1993; **306:** 146.
4. Fox AW. More on rhabdomyolysis associated with cocaine intoxication. *N Engl J Med* 1989; **321:** 1271.
5. Channa AB, *et al.* Is dantrolene effective in heat stroke patients? *Crit Care Med* 1990; **18:** 290–2.

MALIGNANT HYPERTHERMIA. Malignant hyperthermia (malignant hyperpyrexia) is a rare but potentially fatal syndrome associated with general anaesthesia. The aetiology is not completely understood but appears to be a disorder of muscle fibres in which a sudden increase in the concentration of calcium in muscle cytoplasm initiates a series of metabolic disturbances. The disorder appears to be genetically determined and is more common in males. In susceptible individuals a reaction may be induced by inhalation anaesthetics (mainly halogenated hydrocarbons), suxamethonium, prolonged anaesthesia, pre-operative exercise, muscle trauma, fever, or anxiety. However, many reactions occur in individuals who have had uneventful general anaesthesia previously. Early signs and symptoms of the syndrome include tachycardia, unstable blood pressure, hypercapnia, rising temperature, and hyperventilation followed by metabolic acidosis and hyperkalaemia. Muscle rigidity develops in many patients and later there may be evidence of muscle damage including raised serum concentrations of creatine phosphokinase and other enzymes, myoglobinaemia, and myoglobinuria. Hyperthermia develops relatively late. Other late complications may include renal failure, intravascular coagulopathy, and pulmonary oedema.

Treatment should be started as soon as possible after symptoms appear. Dantrolene may be given in a dose of 1 mg per kg body-weight by rapid intravenous injection; injections may be repeated at this dosage until symptoms subside or a total dose of 10 mg per kg has been given in a 15-minute period.[1] An average dose of about 2.5 mg per kg is usually effective. This use of dantrolene has been discussed in several reviews.[1,2] If symptoms reappear the regimen may be repeated. Supportive treatment must also be started including immediate withdrawal of anaesthesia, administration of oxygen, correction of acidosis with sodium bicarbonate, control of hyperkalaemia with insulin, and cooling procedures (see p.1). The incidence of reactions in susceptible individuals can be reduced by avoiding triggering agents. Prophylactic administration of dantrolene has also been used but one group of workers[3] who reported a high incidence of adverse effects in a small study of susceptible patients given dantrolene did not recommend its routine use. Susceptibility to malignant hyperthermia can be detected by histological examination of muscle fibres obtained by biopsy and study of their response to caffeine and/or halothane *in vitro*.

Dantrolene has been suggested[4] for use as a secondary drug in the treatment of a related and potentially fatal syndrome that has developed in some children following induction of anaesthesia with halothane and suxamethonium (see also p.1320).

1. Britt BA. Dantrolene. *Can Anaesth Soc J* 1984; **31:** 61–75.
2. Ward A, *et al.* Dantrolene: a review of its pharmacodynamic and pharmacokinetic properties and therapeutic use in malignant hyperthermia, the neuroleptic malignant syndrome and an update of its use in muscle spasticity. *Drugs* 1986; **32:** 130–68.
3. Wedel DJ, *et al.* Clinical effects of intravenously administered dantrolene. *Mayo Clin Proc* 1995; **70:** 241–6.
4. Rosenberg H, Gronert GA. Intractable cardiac arrest in children given succinylcholine. *Anesthesiology* 1992; **77:** 1054.

Neuroleptic malignant syndrome. Dantrolene has been used, usually alone or with bromocriptine, in the treatment of neuroleptic malignant syndrome (p.651) although some workers have not found it to be of use.[1] Doses reported for dantrolene have varied greatly.[2,3] For those patients unable to swallow and when rapid control of symptoms is required, doses of 1 mg or more per kg body-weight have been given initially by intravenous injection. Up to 600 mg has been given daily by mouth in divided doses.

1. Rosebush PI, *et al.* The treatment of neuroleptic malignant syndrome: are dantrolene and bromocriptine useful adjuncts to supportive care? *Br J Psychiatry* 1991; **159:** 709–12.
2. Ward A, *et al.* Dantrolene: a review of its pharmacodynamic and pharmacokinetic properties and therapeutic use in malignant hyperthermia, the neuroleptic malignant syndrome and an update of its use in muscle spasticity. *Drugs* 1986; **32:** 130–68.
3. Harpe C, Stoudemire A. Aetiology and treatment of neuroleptic malignant syndrome. *Med Toxicol* 1987; **2:** 166–76.

Preparations

Proprietary Preparations (details are given in Part 3)

Aust.: Dantamacrin; ***Austral.:*** Dantrium; ***Belg.:*** Dantrium; ***Canad.:*** Dantrium; ***Fr.:*** Dantrium; ***Ger.:*** Dantamacrin; ***Irl.:*** Dantrium; ***Ital.:*** Danlene†; Dantrium; ***Neth.:*** Dantrium; ***S.Afr.:*** Dantrium; ***Switz.:*** Dantamacrin; ***UK:*** Dantrium; ***USA:*** Dantrium.

Decamethonium Iodide (5711-c)

Decamethonium Iodide *(BAN)*.

Decamethonium Biiodatum; Decametonium Iodidum. *NN'*-Decamethylenebis(trimethylammonium) di-iodide.

$C_{16}H_{38}I_2N_2$ = 512.3.

CAS — 156-74-1 (decamethonium); 541-22-0 (decamethonium bromide); 1420-40-2 (decamethonium iodide).

NOTE. Decamethonium Bromide is *rINN*.

Decamethonium is a depolarising neuromuscular blocker with actions and uses similar to those of suxamethonium chloride (p.1319). The effect of a single intravenous injection lasts for 15 to 20 minutes, but onset of action is slower than with suxamethonium. It is excreted mainly in the urine as unchanged drug. It is now used mainly as the iodide salt although the bromide was also formerly employed.

Doxacurium Chloride (4961-m)

Doxacurium Chloride *(BAN, USAN, rINN).*

BW-A938U. A mixture of the (1*R*,1′*S*,2*S*,2′*R*), (1*R*,1′*R*,2*S*,2′*S*), and (1*S*,1′*S*,2*R*,2′*R*) stereoisomers (a *meso* isomer and two enantiomers respectively) of 1,1′,2,2′,3,3′,4,4′-octahydro-6,6′,7,7′,8,8′-hexamethoxy-2,2′-dimethyl-1,1′-bis(3,4,5-trimethoxybenzyl)-2,2′-[butanedioylbis(oxytrimethylene)]di-isoquinolinium dichloride, all of which are in a *trans* configuration at the 1 and 2 positions of the isoquinolinium rings.

$C_{56}H_{78}Cl_2N_2O_{16}$ = 1106.1.

CAS — 106819-53-8 (doxacurium chloride, meso isomer); 83348-52-1 (doxacurium chloride, total racemate).

Adverse Effects, Treatment, and Precautions

As for competitive neuromuscular blockers in general (see Atracurium, p.1304). Doxacurium has little histamine-releasing activity and causes negligible vagal or sympathetic blockade so that significant cardiovascular side-effects are not a problem.

Renal impairment. Although the duration of neuromuscular block and speed of recovery following the use of doxacurium were found to be prolonged in patients with renal failure when compared with patients with normal renal function, the differences were considered not to be significant.[1]

1. Cashman JN, *et al.* Neuromuscular block with doxacurium (BW A938U) in patients with normal or absent renal function. *Br J Anaesth* 1990; **64:** 186–92.

Interactions

For interactions associated with competitive neuromuscular blockers, see Atracurium, p.1306.

Pharmacokinetics

Following intravenous administration, doxacurium chloride is excreted mainly unchanged in the urine and bile. The elimination half-life is reported to be about 2 hours.

Uses and Administration

Doxacurium chloride is a benzylisoquinolinium competitive neuromuscular blocker (see Atracurium, p.1308). It is used for endotracheal intubation and to provide muscle relaxation in general anaesthesia for surgical procedures (see Anaesthesia, p.1302) and to aid controlled ventilation (see below).

Dosages are expressed in terms of the equivalent amount of doxacurium base. The usual initial dose is 50 µg per kg body-weight intravenously; maintenance doses of 5 to 10 µg per kg are employed. At the above dose muscle relaxation occurs within about 5 minutes and the effect lasts for about 100 minutes. For more prolonged procedures an initial dose of 80 µg per kg may be used, which produces muscle relaxation in about 4 minutes and the effects last for about 2½ hours.

Reviews.

1. Mirakhur RK. Newer neuromuscular blocking drugs: an overview of their clinical pharmacology and therapeutic use. *Drugs* 1992; **44:** 182–99.

Administration in the elderly. There are several studies that have shown that the duration of action of doxacurium is prolonged in the elderly, although the precise mechanism for this prolongation is subject to debate.[1-3] Since both the onset of action and recovery are delayed some consider[4] that doxacurium may not be suitable for use in the elderly for surgical procedures of less than one hour.

1. Levy G. Effect of advanced age on the pharmacodynamics of doxacurium. *Clin Pharmacol Ther* 1994; **55:** 359.
2. Varin F, *et al.* Effect of advanced age on the pharmacodynamics of doxacurium. *Clin Pharmacol Ther* 1994; **55:** 359–60.
3. Schmith VD, *et al.* Effect of advanced age on the pharmacodynamics of doxacurium. *Clin Pharmacol Ther* 1994; **55:** 360–2.
4. Martlew RA, Harper NJN. The clinical pharmacology of doxacurium in young adults and in elderly patients. *Anaesthesia* 1995; **50:** 779–82.

Administration in infants and children. As for some other neuromuscular blockers, children over 2 years of age have been found to require more doxacurium per kg body-weight than adults to achieve a similar degree of neuromuscular blockade,[1] and the dosage requirement may be almost twice as great as that for adults.[2] Children may also recover more quickly.[1] However, the sensitivity of infants under one year of age appears to be increased.[2]

1. Goudsouzian NG, *et al.* Neuromuscular and cardiovascular effects of doxacurium in children anaesthetized with halothane. *Br J Anaesth* 1989; **62:** 263–8.
2. Taivainen T, Meretoja OA. Doxacurium in infants, children and adolescents during balanced anaesthesia. *Br J Anaesth* 1995; **74** (suppl 1): 98–9.

Intensive care. Experience of the use of doxacurium to facilitate mechanical ventilation in patients in intensive care (see p.1303) is relatively limited. It appears to offer prolonged neuromuscular block without the tachycardia associated with pancuronium; recovery after prolonged administration may also be faster than with pancuronium.[1] There has been an anecdotal report of the successful management with doxacurium of 4 patients who had developed tachyphylaxis to long-term administration to atracurium.[2]

1. Murray MJ, *et al.* Double-blind, randomized multicenter study of doxacurium vs. pancuronium in intensive care unit patients who require neuromuscular-blocking agents. *Crit Care Med* 1995; **23:** 450–8.
2. Coursin DB, *et al.* Doxacurium infusion in critically ill patients with atracurium tachyphylaxis. *Am J Health-Syst Pharm* 1995; **52:** 635–9.

Preparations

Proprietary Preparations (details are given in Part 3)
Canad.: Nuromax; ***USA:*** Nuromax.

Eperisone Hydrochloride (16629-d)

Eperisone Hydrochloride *(rINNM).*

4′-Ethyl-2-methyl-3-piperidinopropiophenone hydrochloride.

$C_{17}H_{25}NO,HCl$ = 295.8.

CAS — 64840-90-0 (eperisone).

Eperisone hydrochloride is a centrally acting skeletal muscle relaxant that is used in the symptomatic treatment of muscle spasm (p.1303) and spasticity (p.1303). It may also have a vasodilatory action. The usual initial dose is 50 mg three times daily by mouth, after food.

Preparations

Proprietary Preparations (details are given in Part 3)
Jpn: Myonal.

Fazadinium Bromide (5714-t)

Fazadinium Bromide *(BAN, rINN).*

AH-8165D. 1,1′-Azobis(3-methyl-2-phenyl-1*H*-imidazo[1,2-*a*]pyridinium) dibromide.

$C_{28}H_{24}Br_2N_6$ = 604.3.

CAS — 36653-54-0 (fazadinium); 49564-56-9 (fazadinium bromide).

Fazadinium bromide is a competitive neuromuscular blocker (see Atracurium, p.1304) but its use has been limited by a high incidence of adverse cardiovascular effects.

Preparations

Proprietary Preparations (details are given in Part 3)
Ital.: Fazadon†.

Gallamine Triethiodide (5720-k)

Gallamine Triethiodide *(BANM, rINN).*

Benzcurine Iodide; Gallamini Triethiodidum; Gallamone Triethiodide. 2,2′,2″-(Benzene-1,2,3-triyltrioxy)tris(tetraethylammonium) tri-iodide.

$C_{30}H_{60}I_3N_3O_3$ = 891.5.

CAS — 153-76-4 (gallamine); 65-29-2 (gallamine triethiodide).

Pharmacopoeias. In *Eur.* (see p.viii), *Int.*, and *US.*

A white, or almost white, hygroscopic odourless amorphous powder. Very **soluble** in water; slightly to sparingly soluble in alcohol; very slightly soluble in chloroform; practically insoluble in dichloromethane and in ether. A 2% solution in water has a pH of 5.3 to 7.0. **Store** in airtight containers. Protect from light.

Adverse Effects, Treatment, and Precautions

As for competitive neuromuscular blockers in general (see Atracurium, p.1304). Tachycardia often develops due to the vagolytic action of gallamine triethiodide and blood pressure may occasionally be raised. It has a small histamine-releasing effect; occasional anaphylactoid reactions have been reported. It should be avoided in patients hypersensitive to iodine. Although competitive muscle relaxants have been given with great care to patients with myasthenia gravis (see Neuromuscular Disorders, p.1305), the manufacturer of gallamine triethiodide recommends that it should not be used in such patients.

Cardiopulmonary bypass. Alterations in the pharmacokinetics of competitive neuromuscular blockers in patients undergoing surgery involving cardiopulmonary bypass usually necessitate the use of reduced doses (see p.1305). However, the pharmacokinetics of gallamine in patients undergoing cardiopulmonary bypass appear not to differ significantly from those in control patients.[1]

1. Shanks CA, *et al.* Gallamine disposition in open-heart surgery involving cardiopulmonary bypass. *Clin Pharmacol Ther* 1983; **33:** 792–9.

Renal impairment. Gallamine triethiodide is excreted unchanged in the urine and some consider that it should be avoided in severe renal impairment since prolonged paralysis may occur. Significantly prolonged elimination half-life and reduced clearance have been reported[1] in patients with chronic renal failure given gallamine triethiodide in initial doses of 2 mg per kg body-weight intravenously.

1. Ramzan MI, *et al.* Gallamine disposition in surgical patients with chronic renal failure. *Br J Clin Pharmacol* 1981; **12:** 141–7.

Interactions

For interactions associated with competitive neuromuscular blockers, see Atracurium, p.1306.

Pharmacokinetics

Following intravenous administration gallamine triethiodide is distributed throughout body tissues. It is not metabolised, and is excreted in the urine as unchanged drug.

Uses and Administration

Gallamine triethiodide is a benzylisoquinolinium competitive neuromuscular blocker (see Atracurium, p.1308). Muscle relaxation occurs within about 1 to 2 minutes following intravenous injection and lasts for about 20 to 30 minutes. It is used to provide muscle relaxation in general anaesthesia for surgical procedures (see Anaesthesia, p.1302) and to aid mechanical ventilation (see Intensive Care, p.1303).

An initial test dose of 20 mg may be given intravenously to the patient before anaesthesia to determine undue sensitivity. In the UK, initial doses of 80 to 120 mg by intravenous injection have been recommended, with further doses of 20 to 40 mg as required. In children, a dose of 1.5 mg per kg body-weight has been recommended, reduced to 600 µg per kg for neonates.

In the USA and some other countries lower doses have generally been employed; an initial dose of 1 mg per kg intravenously, up to a maximum of 100 mg, with additional doses of 0.5 to 1 mg per kg after about 30 to 40 minutes or longer if required.

Where intravenous administration is not feasible, gallamine triethiodide may be given intramuscularly, with or without hyaluronidase.

Preparations

BP 1998: Gallamine Injection;
USP 23: Gallamine Triethiodide Injection.

Proprietary Preparations (details are given in Part 3)
Austral.: Flaxedil; ***Belg.:*** Flaxedil†; ***Canad.:*** Flaxedil; ***Fr.:*** Flaxedil†; ***Neth.:*** Flaxedil; ***S.Afr.:*** Flaxedil†; ***Spain:*** Miowas G; ***UK:*** Flaxedil; ***USA:*** Flaxedil†.

Idrocilamide (12842-t)

Idrocilamide *(rINN).*

LCB-29. *N*-(2-Hydroxyethyl)cinnamamide.

$C_{11}H_{13}NO_2$ = 191.2.

CAS — 6961-46-2.

Adverse Effects

When given by mouth idrocilamide was reported to produce abdominal pain, nausea, and drowsiness. Excitement, euphoria and hallucinations, and mental depression may occur.

Uses and Administration

Idrocilamide is a centrally acting muscle relaxant that has been given by mouth or intramuscular injection for the symptomatic treatment of painful muscle spasm associated with musculoskeletal conditions. It is reported to have local muscle relaxant and anti-inflammatory effects and is now mainly used topically.

Preparations

Proprietary Preparations (details are given in Part 3)
Belg.: Srilane; ***Fr.:*** Srilane; ***Switz.:*** Talval.

Mephenesin (5722-t)

Mephenesin *(BAN, rINN).*

Cresoxydiol; Glykresin. 3-(*o*-Tolyloxy)propane-1,2-diol.

$C_{10}H_{14}O_3$ = 182.2.

CAS — 59-47-2.

Pharmacopoeias. In *It.*

Adverse Effects

Given by mouth, mephenesin may produce lassitude, drowsiness, weakness, loss of appetite, nausea, and vomiting. Allergic reactions may rarely occur. Overdosage may produce visual disturbances, motor incoordination, hypotonia, a fall in blood pressure, and respiratory paralysis.

Precautions

Mephenesin may cause drowsiness; patients affected should not drive or operate machinery.

Porphyria. Mephenesin was considered to be unsafe in patients with acute porphyria because it has been shown to be porphyrinogenic in *animals* or *in-vitro* systems.[1]

1. Moore MR, McColl KEL. *Porphyria: drug lists.* Glasgow: Porphyria Research Unit, University of Glasgow, 1991.

Interactions

The CNS effects of mephenesin may be enhanced by alcohol or other CNS depressants.

Pharmacokinetics

Mephenesin is readily absorbed from the gastro-intestinal tract and distributed throughout most tissues of the body. It is metabolised mainly in the liver and excreted in urine as metabolites and a small amount of unchanged drug.

Uses and Administration

Mephenesin is a centrally acting skeletal muscle relaxant used for the symptomatic treatment of painful muscle spasm (p.1303) associated with musculoskeletal conditions. Its clinical usefulness is considered to be limited by its brief duration of action. It is given by mouth in doses of 1.5 to 3 g daily in divided doses. It is also applied topically, usually with rubefacients.

Preparations

Proprietary Preparations (details are given in Part 3)
Belg.: Decontractyl†; ***Fr.:*** Decontractyl; ***Ger.:*** DoloVisano M; Rexoxyl†; ***Ital.:*** Relaxar†.

Multi-ingredient: ***Belg.:*** Algipan; Decontractyl; ***Canad.:*** Decontractyl; ***Fr.:*** Algipan†; Decontractyl; Traumalgyl; ***Ital.:*** Relaxar; ***S.Afr.:*** Spasmend.

Metaxalone (5724-r)

Metaxalone *(BAN, USAN, rINN).*

AHR-438. 5-(3,5-Xylyloxymethyl)oxazolidin-2-one.

$C_{12}H_{15}NO_3$ = 221.3.

CAS — 1665-48-1.

Adverse Effects, Treatment, and Precautions

As for Chlorzoxazone, p.1313.

Metaxalone may cause drowsiness; patients affected should not drive or operate machinery.

Patients taking metaxalone excrete in the urine a metabolite which gives a false positive reaction to copper sulphate-based tests for glycosuria.

Interactions

The CNS effects of metaxalone may be enhanced by alcohol and other CNS depressants.

Pharmacokinetics

Metaxalone is absorbed from the gastro-intestinal tract, metabolised in the liver, and excreted in urine as metabolites. The plasma elimination half-life is about 2 to 3 hours.

Uses and Administration

Metaxalone is a centrally acting skeletal muscle relaxant. Its mode of action may be related to its sedative properties.

It is used as an adjunct in the symptomatic treatment of painful muscle spasm (p.1303) associated with musculoskeletal conditions. The usual dose is 800 mg three or four times daily by mouth.

Preparations

Proprietary Preparations (details are given in Part 3)
USA: Skelaxin.

Methocarbamol (5725-f)

Methocarbamol *(BAN, rINN).*

Guaiphenesin Carbamate. 2-Hydroxy-3-(2-methoxyphenoxy)propyl carbamate.

$C_{11}H_{15}NO_5$ = 241.2.

CAS — 532-03-6.

Pharmacopoeias. In US.

A white powder, odourless or with a slight characteristic odour. M.p. about 94° or, if previously ground to a fine powder, about 90°. **Soluble** 1 in 40 of water at 20°; sparingly soluble in chloroform; soluble in alcohol only with heating; practically insoluble in *n*-hexane. **Store** in airtight containers.

Adverse Effects

Side-effects reported with methocarbamol include nausea, anorexia, lightheadedness, dizziness, lassitude, drowsiness, restlessness, anxiety, confusion, blurred vision, fever, headache, convulsions, and hypersensitivity reactions including rashes, pruritus, urticaria, angioedema, and conjunctivitis with nasal congestion.

After injection patients may experience flushing and a metallic taste; incoordination, diplopia, nystagmus, vertigo, syncope, hypotension, bradycardia, and anaphylaxis have been reported. There may be sloughing and thrombophlebitis at the site of injection.

Precautions

Methocarbamol is contra-indicated in coma or pre-coma states, brain damage, myasthenia gravis, or in patients with a history of epilepsy. Caution is advisable in renal or hepatic impairment. Methocarbamol may cause drowsiness; patients affected should not drive or operate machinery.

Preparations for injection may contain, as a solvent, a macrogol which could increase existing acidosis and urea retention in patients with renal impairment; such preparations should not be used in patients with known or suspected renal disease.

Methocarbamol could cause discoloration of the urine, which became brown to black or green on standing.[1]

1. Baran RB, Rowles B. Factors affecting coloration of urine and feces. *J Am Pharm Assoc* 1973; **NS13:** 139–42.

Interactions

The CNS effects of methocarbamol may be potentiated by alcohol or other CNS depressants. Methocarbamol has also been reported to potentiate the effects of anorectics and antimuscarinics.

Pharmacokinetics

Methocarbamol is rapidly and almost completely absorbed from the gastro-intestinal tract following oral administration. Its plasma half-life is reported to be about 1 to 2 hours. It is metabolised by dealkylation and hydroxylation and is excreted in urine primarily as the glucuronide and sulphate conjugates of its metabolites. A small amount is excreted in faeces.

Uses and Administration

Methocarbamol is a centrally acting skeletal muscle relaxant whose action may be due to general depressant effects on the CNS.

Methocarbamol is used as an adjunct in the symptomatic treatment of painful muscle spasm (p.1303) associated with musculoskeletal conditions. It is sometimes given with analgesics in compound preparations for the treatment of musculoskeletal pain.

The usual initial dose by mouth for muscle spasm is 1.5 g four times daily, reduced to a maintenance dose of about 4 g daily after 2 to 3 days. A dose of 750 mg three times daily may be sufficient for a therapeutic effect. Methocarbamol has been given by intramuscular injection in a dose of up to 500 mg into each gluteal region at intervals of 8 hours. It has also been given intravenously at a rate of not more than 300 mg per minute, by slow injection or by infusion in sodium chloride or glucose injection. The parenteral route should not be used for more than 3 consecutive days and the dose should not exceed 3 g daily. The patient should remain lying down during, and for 10 to 15 minutes after, intravenous administration. The injection is hypertonic and extravasation should be avoided.

Half the maximum daily dose or less may be sufficient for elderly patients.

Preparations

USP 23: Methocarbamol Injection; Methocarbamol Tablets.

Proprietary Preparations (details are given in Part 3)
Austral.: Robaxin†; ***Canad.:*** Robaxin; ***Fr.:*** Lumirelax; ***Ger.:*** Ortoton; Traumacut†; ***Ital.:*** Miowas†; ***S.Afr.:*** Robaxin; ***Spain:*** Miowas†; Robaxin; ***Swed.:*** Robaxin; ***UK:*** Robaxin; ***USA:*** Robaxin.

Multi-ingredient: ***Canad.:*** Aspirin Backache; Robaxacet; Robaxacet-8; Robaxisal; Robaxisal-C; ***Fr.:*** Lumirelax†; ***Ger.:*** Ortoton Plus; ***Irl.:*** Robaxisal; ***S.Afr.:*** Robaxisal; ***Spain:*** Robaxisal; Robaxisal Compuesto; ***Swed.:*** Robaxisal Forte; ***UK:*** Robaxisal Forte†; ***USA:*** Robaxisal.

Metocurine Iodide (5726-d)

Metocurine Iodide *(USAN).*

Dimethyl Tubocurarine Iodide; (+)-*O,O'*-Dimethylchondrocurarine Di-iodide; Dimethyltubocurarine Iodide; Trimethyltubocurarine Iodide. (+)-6,6',7',12'-Tetramethoxy-2,2,2',2'-tetramethyltubocuraranium di-iodide.

$C_{40}H_{48}I_2N_2O_6$ = 906.6.

CAS — 5152-30-7 (metocurine); 7601-55-0 (metocurine iodide).

NOTE. The name dimethyltubocurarine iodide was based on the old empirical formula for tubocurarine (p.1322).

Pharmacopoeias. In US.

A white to pale yellow crystalline powder. **Soluble** 1 in 400 of water and 1 in 10 000 of alcohol, chloroform, and of ether; slightly soluble in 3N hydrochloric acid and dilute solutions of sodium hydroxide. **Store** in airtight containers.

Adverse Effects, Treatment, and Precautions

As for competitive neuromuscular blockers in general (see Atracurium, p.1304).

Metocurine iodide has a moderate risk of inducing histamine release. Allergic reactions may occur in patients sensitive to iodine. Metocurine has some ganglion blocking activity and cardiovascular side-effects may occur.

Renal impairment. A study involving 5 patients with renal failure undergoing transplantation showed that the mean elimination half-life of metocurine was 11.4 hours, compared with 6.0 hours in 5 healthy subjects and plasma clearance was significantly reduced.[1] However, the serum concentration required to produce 90% blockade was significantly elevated in patients with renal failure. There was considerable variation in the duration of neuromuscular blockade in patients with renal failure, one remaining well relaxed for 6 hours while one was well relaxed for only 10 minutes. If patients with renal failure are given metocurine, monitoring is imperative to ensure adequate relaxation without overdosage.

1. Brotherton WP, Matteo RS. Pharmacokinetics and pharmacodynamics of metocurine in humans with and without renal failure. *Anesthesiology* 1981; **55:** 273–6.

Interactions

For interactions associated with competitive neuromuscular blockers, see Atracurium, p.1306.

Pharmacokinetics

Following intravenous administration metocurine iodide is rapidly distributed. About 50% is excreted unchanged in urine in 48 hours and 2% is excreted in bile. The elimination half-life is reported to be around 3.6 hours.

Pregnancy. Metocurine crossed the placenta in small but detectable amounts in 18 women undergoing caesarean section.[1] The concentration of metocurine in the umbilical vein was 4, 7, 12, and 12% of that in the maternal vein when the drug was given 2, 4, 6, and 10 minutes before delivery. All infants were in good condition at delivery with a mean Apgar score of 10 at 5 minutes.

1. Kivalo I, Saarikoski S. Placental transfer of ^{14}C-dimethyltubocurarine during caesarean section. *Br J Anaesth* 1976; **48:** 239–42.

Uses and Administration

Metocurine iodide is a benzylisoquinolinium competitive neuromuscular blocker (see Atracurium, p.1308). Following a single intravenous dose muscle relaxation occurs in 1 to 4 minutes and is maintained for about 25 to 90 minutes. It is used for endotracheal intubation and to provide muscle relaxation in general anaesthesia for surgical procedures (see Anaesthesia, p.1302) and electroconvulsive therapy and to aid controlled ventilation (see Intensive Care, p.1303).

The initial dose of metocurine iodide for intubation is usually 200 to 400 µg per kg body-weight by intravenous injection over 30 to 60 seconds and further doses of 0.5 to 1 mg may be given as required for muscle relaxation. For muscle relaxation during electroconvulsive therapy average doses totalling 2 to 3 mg have been employed.

Preparations

USP 23: Metocurine Iodide Injection.

Proprietary Preparations (details are given in Part 3)
Canad.: Metubine; ***USA:*** Metubine.

Mivacurium Chloride (5500-v)

Mivacurium Chloride *(BAN, USAN, rINN).*

BW-B1090U. A mixture of the stereoisomers of (*E*)-1,1',2,2',3,3',4,4'-octahydro-6,6',7,7'-tetramethoxy-2,2'-dimethyl-1,1'-bis(3,4,5-trimethoxybenzyl)-2,2'-[oct-4-enedioylbis(oxytrimethylene)]di-isoquinolinium dichloride.

$C_{58}H_{80}Cl_2N_2O_4$ = 940.2.

CAS — 106861-44-3 (mivacurium chloride, total racemate).

Adverse Effects, Treatment, and Precautions

As for competitive neuromuscular blockers in general (see Atracurium, p.1304). Mivacurium chloride has no significant vagal or ganglion blocking activity at recommended doses. It may induce histamine release especially when given in large doses rapidly.

Mivacurium should be used with caution, if at all, in patients with plasma cholinesterase deficiency, since its duration of action will be prolonged in such patients.

Burns. In common with other competitive muscle relaxants patients with burns may develop resistance to mivacurium and require increased doses (see under Atracurium, p.1305). However, as these patients may also have reduced plasma cholinesterase activity dosage requirements could also be reduced. The manufacturer recommends that such patients should be given a test dose of 150 to 200 µg per kg body-weight with subsequent dosage adjustments being guided by monitoring of the block.

Hepatic and renal impairment. The pharmacokinetics of mivacurium have been studied in patients with kidney[1-3] or liver impairment.[1,4,5] Compared with healthy subjects, the duration of relaxation produced by mivacurium was approximately 1.5 times greater than normal in patients with kidney disease and up to about 3 times greater than normal in patients with liver impairment. The reduced plasma-cholinesterase activity in the patients with liver impairment may have played an important part in this effect. Although an anticholinesterase such as neostigmine hastens recovery by only a few minutes in healthy subjects its use may be indicated in patients in whom recovery is delayed.[2]

1. Cook DR, *et al.* Pharmacokinetics of mivacurium in normal patients and in those with hepatic or renal failure. *Br J Anaesth* 1992; **69:** 580–5.
2. Phillips BJ, Hunter JM. Use of mivacurium chloride by constant infusion in the anephric patient. *Br J Anaesth* 1992: **68:** 492–8.
3. Head-Rapson AG, *et al.* Pharmacokinetics and pharmacodynamics of the three isomers of mivacurium in health, in end-stage renal failure and in patients with impaired renal function. *Br J Anaesth* 1995; **75:** 31–6.

4. Devlin JC, *et al.* Pharmacodynamics of mivacurium chloride in patients with hepatic cirrhosis. *Br J Anaesth* 1993; **71:** 227–31.
5. Head-Rapson AG, *et al.* Pharmacokinetics of the three isomers of mivacurium and pharmacodynamics of the chiral mixture in hepatic cirrhosis. *Br J Anaesth* 1994; **73:** 613–18.

Neuromuscular disorders. Neuromuscular blockade was successfully achieved with mivacurium in an obese elderly patient with myasthenia gravis requiring surgery.[1] Only about half the usual dose was required and even then recovery was delayed. See Atracurium, p.1305 for a discussion of the use of competitive neuromuscular blockers in patients with neuromuscular disorders.

1. Seigne RD, Scott RPF. Mivacurium chloride and myasthenia gravis. *Br J Anaesth* 1994; **72:** 468–9.

Plasma cholinesterase deficiency. There have been reports of prolonged neuromuscular block produced by mivacurium in patients with plasma cholinesterase deficiency.[1-4] Time to full recovery had varied; one patient required up to 8 hours.

1. Goudsouzian NG, *et al.* Prolonged neuromuscular block from mivacurium in two patients with cholinesterase deficiency. *Anesth Analg* 1993; **77:** 183–5.
2. Sockalingam I, Green DW. Mivacurium-induced prolonged neuromuscular block. *Br J Anaesth* 1995; **74:** 234–6.
3. Fox MH, Hunt PCW. Prolonged neuromuscular block associated with mivacurium. *Br J Anaesth* 1995; **74:** 237–8.
4. Zimmer S. Mivacurium and prolonged neuromuscular block. *Br J Anaesth* 1995; **75:** 823.

Tourniquets. It has been suggested that mivacurium might be unsuitable for neuromuscular blockade of a limb which has been isolated with a tourniquet in order to provide a bloodless field for surgery.[1] Mivacurium is largely inactivated by the enzymatic action of plasma cholinesterase and would therefore continue to degrade locally leading to a loss of blockade in the limb and this could not be corrected by further doses unless the tourniquet was deflated. However, Torrance *et al.*[2] found that, as for other competitive neuromuscular blockers, the use of mivacurium to supplement regional anaesthesia produced prolonged muscle weakness well beyond cuff deflation. This suggests that mivacurium is not broken down in the ischaemic limb and that recovery is not dependent on plasma concentrations of mivacurium.

See also Local Anaesthetics, under Interactions in Atracurium, p.1307, for a report of symptoms suggestive of local anaesthetic toxicity when prilocaine and mivacurium were used together.

1. Shannon PF. Neuromuscular block and tourniquets. *Br J Anaesth* 1994; **73:** 726.
2. Torrance JM, *et al.* Low-dose mivacurium supplementation of prilocaine i.v. regional anaesthesia. *Br J Anaesth* 1997; **78:** 222–3.

Interactions

For interactions associated with competitive neuromuscular blockers, see Atracurium, p.1306.

Pharmacokinetics

Mivacurium is administered as a mixture of 3 stereoisomers, 2 of which (*cis-trans* and *trans-trans*) are considered to account for most of the neuromuscular blocking effect. All 3 isomers are inactivated by plasma cholinesterase. Renal and hepatic mechanisms are involved in their elimination with excretion in urine and bile.

Uses and Administration

Mivacurium chloride is a benzylisoquinolinium competitive neuromuscular blocker (see Atracurium, p.1308).

Following intravenous injection muscle relaxation occurs within 2 to 2.5 minutes with a duration of action of about 10 to 20 minutes. It is used for endotracheal intubation and to provide muscle relaxation in general anaesthesia for surgical procedures (see Anaesthesia, p.1302) and to aid controlled ventilation (see Intensive Care, p.1303).

Doses are expressed in terms of mivacurium base. The initial dose by intravenous injection is 70 to 250 μg per kg body-weight. Doses up to 150 μg per kg may be administered over 5 to 15 seconds but higher doses should be given over 30 seconds. In patients with asthma or cardiovascular disease, or those who are sensitive to falls in arterial blood pressure, administration should be over 60 seconds. A suggested method for administration of a dose of 250 μg per kg for tracheal intubation is to give one injection of 150 μg per kg followed 30 seconds later by an injection of 100 μg per kg. Maintenance doses of 100 μg per kg may be given at intervals of 15 minutes. In children aged 2 to 6 months an initial dose of 150 μg per kg has been given; in children aged 7 months to 12 years, an initial dose of 200 μg per kg has been given. A maintenance dose of 100 μg per kg may be given every 6 to 9 minutes for children aged 2 months to 12 years. Reduced doses may be required in elderly patients. For obese patients weighing more than 30% over their ideal body-weight the manufacturer recommends that the initial dose should be based upon their ideal body-weight and not actual body-weight. Mivacurium chloride may also be administered by continuous intravenous infusion for maintenance of block. For adults the initial rate is 8 to 10 μg per kg per minute adjusted every 3 minutes if necessary by increments of 1 μg per kg per minute to a usual dose of 6 to 7 μg per kg per minute; in children aged 2 months to 12 years the usual dose is 11 to 14 μg per kg per minute.

Reviews.

1. Mirakhur RK. Newer neuromuscular blocking drugs: an overview of their clinical pharmacology and therapeutic use. *Drugs* 1992; **44:** 182–99.
2. Frampton JE, McTavish D. Mivacurium: a review of its pharmacology and therapeutic potential in general anaesthesia. *Drugs* 1993; **45:** 1066–89.
3. Feldman S. Mivacurium. *Br J Hosp Med* 1997; **57:** 199–201.

Action. Mivacurium has a shorter duration of action than most other competitive neuromuscular blockers. Studies[1-3] suggest that it is a useful alternative to suxamethonium for the production of neuromuscular block of short duration and has the advantage that its block can be reversed with an anticholinesterase. For a discussion of the choice of anticholinesterase for reversal of neuromuscular block produced by short-acting blockers such as mivacurium, see under Neostigmine, p.1395. Although its onset of action may be accelerated by giving a priming dose,[4] mivacurium has a slower onset than suxamethonium and so may not be a suitable alternative[5] when rapid intubation is required. For a general review of neuromuscular blockers, see Anaesthesia, p.1302.

1. Brandom BW, *et al.* Comparison of mivacurium and suxamethonium administered by bolus and infusion. *Br J Anaesth* 1989; **62:** 488–93.
2. Caldwell JE, *et al.* Comparison of the neuromuscular block induced by mivacurium, suxamethonium or atracurium during nitrous oxide-fentanyl anaesthesia. *Br J Anaesth* 1989; **63:** 393–9.
3. Goldberg ME, *et al.* Comparison of tracheal intubating conditions and neuromuscular blocking profiles after intubating doses of mivacurium chloride or succinylcholine in surgical outpatients. *Anesth Analg* 1989; **69:** 93–9.
4. Haxby EJ, *et al.* Mivacurium priming intervals. *Br J Anaesth* 1994; **72:** 485P.
5. Anonymous. Mivacurium—a new neuromuscular blocker. *Med Lett Drugs Ther* 1992; **34:** 82.

Administration in the elderly. In a study[1] comparing the effects of mivacurium in elderly and young adults the duration of neuromuscular effects was prolonged in elderly patients by about 30%. The mean infusion requirement in elderly patients was 3.67 μg per kg body-weight per minute compared with 5.5 μg per kg per minute in young adults.

1. Maddineni VR, *et al.* Neuromuscular and haemodynamic effects of mivacurium in elderly and young adult patients. *Br J Anaesth* 1994; **73:** 608–12.

Preparations

Proprietary Preparations (details are given in Part 3)
Aust.: Mivacron; ***Austral.:*** Mivacron; ***Belg.:*** Mivacron; ***Canad.:*** Mivacron; ***Fr.:*** Mivacron; ***Ger.:*** Mivacron; ***Irl.:*** Mivacron; ***Ital.:*** Mivacron; ***Neth.:*** Mivacron; ***Norw.:*** Mivacron; ***S.Afr.:*** Mivacron; ***Spain:*** Mivacron; ***Swed.:*** Mivacron; ***Switz.:*** Mivacron; ***UK:*** Mivacron; ***USA:*** Mivacron.

Pancuronium Bromide (5727-n)

Pancuronium Bromide *(BAN, USAN, rINN)*.

NA-97; Org-NA-97; Pancuronii Bromidum. 1,1′-(3α,17β-Diacetoxy-5α-androstan-2β,16β-ylene)bis(1-methylpiperidinium) dibromide.

$C_{35}H_{60}Br_2N_2O_4$ = 732.7.

CAS — 15500-66-0.

Pharmacopoeias. In *Eur.* (see p.viii).

White or almost white, hygroscopic crystalline powder. Freely or very **soluble** in water; freely soluble in alcohol; practically insoluble in ether. **Store** in airtight containers. Protect from light.

Adverse Effects, Treatment, and Precautions

As for competitive neuromuscular blockers in general (see Atracurium, p.1304).

Pancuronium has a vagolytic action but does not produce ganglionic blockade. It has a small histamine-releasing effect. Hypersensitivity reactions are relatively rare but bradycardia, bronchospasm, hypotension, and cardiovascular collapse have been reported. Pancuronium has been associated with excessive salivation is some patients.

Pancuronium should be used with caution in patients with raised catecholamine concentrations, or who are receiving drugs with sympathomimetic effects, as cardiovascular side-effects are more likely in these patients.

Hepatic impairment. Prolonged neuromuscular blockade may occur in patients with liver disease given pancuronium bromide since increased elimination half-life with increased volume of distribution and reduced clearance has been reported.[1] However, the expanded distribution volume may necessitate an increase in the dose of pancuronium in these patients[1,2] and may be interpreted as resistance to the neuromuscular blocking effects of pancuronium.

1. Duvaldestin P, *et al.* Pancuronium pharmacokinetics in patients with liver cirrhosis. *Br J Anaesth* 1978; **50:** 1131–6.
2. Ward ME, *et al.* Althesin and pancuronium in chronic liver disease. *Br J Anaesth* 1975; **47:** 1199–1204.

Hypersensitivity. Reports of anaphylactoid or anaphylactic reactions associated with pancuronium bromide.

1. Brauer FS, Ananthanarayan CR. Histamine release by pancuronium. *Anesthesiology* 1978; **49:** 434–5.
2. Patriarca G, *et al.* Pancuronium allergy: a case report. *Br J Anaesth* 1989; **62:** 210–12.
3. Moneret-Vautrin DA, *et al.* Simultaneous anaphylaxis to thiopentone and a neuromuscular blocker: a study of two cases. *Br J Anaesth* 1990; **64:** 743–5.

Renal impairment. Prolonged neuromuscular blockade may occur following administration of pancuronium to patients with severe renal impairment. Pancuronium distributes rapidly into extracellular fluid following intravenous injection and the initial neuromuscular blockade produced will depend upon the peak drug concentration in this fluid. Since extracellular fluid volume is increased in chronic renal failure such patients may require a larger initial dose of pancuronium and a 45% increase in dose requirement has been reported[1] in patients with end-stage renal failure. Renal excretion is the main route of elimination and prolonged elimination half-life with reduced clearance may be expected in renal failure; total dose requirements may be reduced. The main infusion rate of pancuronium to maintain 90% blockade in patients with end-stage renal failure was reported to be 61.5% less than for patients with normal renal function.

1. Gramstad L. Atracurium, vecuronium and pancuronium in end-stage renal failure. *Br J Anaesth* 1987; **59:** 995–1003.

Interactions

For interactions associated with competitive neuromuscular blockers, see Atracurium, p.1306.

Pharmacokinetics

Following intravenous injection pancuronium bromide is rapidly distributed into body tissues; about 80% may be bound to plasma proteins. A small proportion is metabolised in the liver to metabolites with weak neuromuscular blocking activity. It is largely excreted in urine as unchanged drug and metabolites; a small amount is excreted in bile. The plasma elimination half-life is about 2 hours.

Pregnancy. In 15 patients undergoing caesarean section[1] given pancuronium bromide 100 μg per kg body-weight intravenously with other agents, mean maternal arterial and umbilical venous serum concentrations of pancuronium bromide and metabolites were 520 and 120 ng per mL respectively at delivery (mean of 13 minutes after injection), giving a fetal to maternal ratio of 0.23.

1. Wingard LB, *et al.* Modified fluorometric quantitation of pancuronium bromide and metabolites in human maternal and umbilical serums. *J Pharm Sci* 1979; **68:** 914–15.

Uses and Administration

Pancuronium bromide is an aminosteroidal competitive neuromuscular blocker (see Atracurium, p.1308). Muscle relaxation occurs within about 1.5 to 2 minutes of intravenous administration and lasts for about 45 to 60 minutes.

Pancuronium bromide is used for endotracheal intubation and to provide muscle relaxation in general anaesthesia for surgical procedures (see Anaesthesia, p.1302) and in the management of patients on assisted ventilation (see Intensive Care, p.1303).

The initial dose for intubation is usually 40 to 100 μg per kg body-weight by intravenous injection, with maintenance doses of 10 to 20 μg per kg. Children may be given similar doses. Doses of 30 to 40 μg per kg initially have been suggested in neonates, with maintenance doses of 10 to 20 μg per kg as necessary; in the USA, dosage based on an initial test dose of 20 μg per kg has been advocated for the neonate. Adult patients under intensive care who require assisted ventilation for conditions such as intractable status asthmaticus or tetanus may be given 60 μg per kg intravenously every 1 to 1½ hours or less frequently.

Fetal paralysis. Pancuronium bromide 100 μg per kg estimated fetal-weight administered into the umbilical vein produced fetal paralysis for about 40 minutes during intravascular exchange transfusion.[1] A dose of 200 to 300 μg per kg produced fetal paralysis for about 1 to 8 hours for more complicated transfusion procedures.[2] No adverse effects were reported.

1. Copel JA, *et al.* The use of intravenous pancuronium bromide to produce fetal paralysis during intravascular transfusion. *Am J Obstet Gynecol* 1988; **158:** 170–1.
2. Moise KJ, *et al.* Intravenous pancuronium bromide for fetal neuromuscular blockade during intrauterine transfusion for red-cell alloimmunization. *Obstet Gynecol* 1989; **74:** 905–8.

Neuroleptic malignant syndrome. Pancuronium is one of several drugs for which there have been isolated reports[1] of success in the management of neuroleptic malignant syndrome (p.651).

1. Sangal R, Dimitrijevic R. Neuroleptic malignant syndrome: successful treatment with pancuronium. *JAMA* 1985; **254:** 2795–6.

Preparations

BP 1998: Pancuronium Injection.

Proprietary Preparations (details are given in Part 3)
Aust.: Pavulon; ***Austral.:*** Pavulon; ***Canad.:*** Pavulon; ***Irl.:*** Pavulon; ***Ital.:*** Pavulon; ***Neth.:*** Pavulon; ***Norw.:*** Pavulon; ***S.Afr.:*** Curon-B; Pavulon; ***Spain:*** Pavulon; ***Swed.:*** Pavulon; ***Switz.:*** Pavulon; ***UK:*** Pavulon; ***USA:*** Pavulon.

Pipecuronium Bromide (19664-b)

Pipecuronium Bromide *(BAN, USAN, rINN)*.

Pipecurium Bromide; RGH-1106. 1,1,1′,1′-Tetramethyl-4,4′-(3α,17β-diacetoxy-5α-androstan-2β,16β-diyl)dipiperazinium dibromide.

$C_{35}H_{62}Br_2N_4O_4$ = 762.7.

CAS — 52212-02-9 (anhydrous pipecuronium bromide); 68399-57-5 (pipecuronium bromide dihydrate).

Adverse Effects, Treatment, and Precautions

As for competitive neuromuscular blockers in general (see Atracurium, p.1304). Pipecuronium is reported to have no significant cardiovascular adverse effects or histamine-related effects.

Interactions

For interactions associated with competitive neuromuscular blockers, see Atracurium, p.1306.

Pharmacokinetics

Following intravenous administration, pipecuronium is excreted in the urine mainly unchanged and as the less active 3-desacetyl metabolite. Values of about 1.7 and 2.3 hours have been reported for the mean elimination half-life.

Uses and Administration

Pipecuronium bromide is an aminosteroidal competitive neuromuscular blocker (see Atracurium, p.1308). Following intravenous injection muscle relaxation occurs within 2.5 to 3 minutes with a duration of action of about 30 minutes to 2 hours, depending on the dose.

Pipecuronium bromide is used for endotracheal intubation and to provide muscle relaxation in general anaesthesia for surgical procedures (see Anaesthesia, p.1302) and to aid mechanical ventilation (see Intensive Care, p.1303). Doses of 50 to 85 μg per kg body-weight intravenously have been recommended with subsequent doses of 10 to 15 μg per kg. Doses may need to be reduced in the presence of renal impairment; a dose of 50 μg per kg has been recommended for patients with a creatinine clearance of less than 40 mL per minute.

Reviews.

1. Mirakhur RK. Newer neuromuscular blocking drugs: an overview of their clinical pharmacology and therapeutic use. *Drugs* 1992; **44:** 182–99.

Preparations

Proprietary Preparations (details are given in Part 3)
Aust.: Arpilon; ***Ger.:*** Arpilon†; ***Ital.:*** Arduan; ***Neth.:*** Arpilon†; ***Switz.:*** Arpilon†; ***USA:*** Arduan.

Pridinol Mesylate (5729-m)

Pridinol Mesilate *(rINNM)*; C-238 (pridinol). 1,1-Diphenyl-3-piperidinopropan-1-ol methanesulphonate.

$C_{20}H_{25}NO,CH_3SO_3H$ = 391.5.

CAS — 511-45-5 (pridinol); 968-58-1 (pridinol hydrochloride); 6856-31-1 (pridinol mesylate).

Pridinol mesylate is a centrally acting muscle relaxant used in the symptomatic treatment of muscle spasm (p.1303). The usual initial dose by mouth is 2 to 8 mg three times daily, reduced to 4 to 8 mg daily for maintenance treatment. It is also given by intramuscular injection, and has been applied in compound topical preparations.

Pridinol is used as the hydrochloride for its antimuscarinic properties in the management of parkinsonism (p.1128).

Preparations

Proprietary Preparations (details are given in Part 3)
Ger.: Lyseen; Parks; ***Ital.:*** Lyseen.

Multi-ingredient: ***Ger.:*** Parks-Plus†; ***Ital.:*** Algolisina.

Rapacuronium Bromide (17374-n)

Rapacuronium Bromide *(BAN, rINN)*.

Org-9487. 1-(3α-Acetoxy-2β-piperidino-17β-propionyloxy-5α-androstan-16β-yl)-1-allylpiperidinium bromide.

$C_{37}H_{61}BrN_2O_4$ = 677.8.

CAS — 156137-99-4.

Rapacuronium bromide is an aminosteroidal competitive neuromuscular blocker (see Atracurium, p.1304). It is an analogue of vecuronium (p.1323) with a more rapid onset of muscle relaxation. It is being studied as a potential alternative to suxamethonium.

References

1. Wierda JMKH, *et al.* Time course of action and endotracheal intubating conditions of Org 9487, a new short-acting steroidal muscle relaxant; a comparison with succinylcholine. *Anesth Analg* 1993; **77:** 579–84.
2. van den Broek L, *et al.* Pharmacodynamics and pharmacokinetics of an infusion of Org 9487, a new short-acting steroidal neuromuscular blocking agent. *Br J Anaesth* 1994; **73:** 331–5.
3. Connolly FM, *et al.* Time course of action of Org 9487 with or without reversal: comparison with suxamethonium. *Br J Anaesth* 1995; **74:** 473P.
4. Meretoja OA, *et al.* A fast-onset short acting non-depolarizing neuromuscular blocker, ORG 9487, in infants and children. *Br J Anaesth* 1996; **76** (suppl 2): 95.
5. Mills KG, *et al.* Pharmacodynamics of Org 9487: onset and recovery characteristics of single and three incremental bolus doses. *Br J Anaesth* 1996; **77:** 684P–685P.

Rocuronium Bromide (13930-b)

Rocuronium Bromide *(BAN, USAN, rINN)*.

Org-9426. 1-Allyl-1-(3α,17β-dihydroxy-2β-morpholino-5α-androstan-16β-yl)pyrrolidinium bromide 17-acetate; 1-(17β-Acetoxy-3α-hydroxy-2β-morpholino-5α-androstan-16β-yl)-1-allylpyrrolidinium bromide.

$C_{32}H_{53}BrN_2O_4$ = 609.7.

CAS — 119302-91-9.

Adverse Effects, Treatment, and Precautions

As for competitive neuromuscular blockers in general (see Atracurium, p.1304). Rocuronium is reported to have minimal cardiovascular and histamine-releasing effects. High doses have mild vagolytic activity. It should be used with caution in patients with hepatic or renal impairment.

Severe transient burning pain associated with injection of rocuronium was considered[1] to be responsible for the spontaneous movement sometimes seen in the arm or wrist into which rocuronium is administered. It is recommended that rocuronium should be administered only when a deep stage of unconsciousness has been achieved.

1. Borgeat A, Kwiatkowski D. Spontaneous movements associated with rocuronium: is pain on injection the cause? *Br J Anaesth* 1997; **79:** 382–3.

Hepatic impairment. There have been conflicting reports of the pharmacokinetics and pharmacodynamics of rocuronium in patients with hepatic impairment. In contrast to earlier studies[1,2] van Miert *et al.*[3] found a significant reduction in the plasma clearance of rocuronium in patients with cirrhosis. The elimination half-life has been variously reported to be unchanged[1] or prolonged[2,3] with delayed recovery.[3] Some studies[2,3] found that the onset of action was not affected while one group of workers[1] reported a delay.

1. Khalil M, *et al.* Pharmacokinetics and pharmacodynamics of rocuronium in patients with cirrhosis. *Anesthesiology* 1994; **80:** 1241–7.
2. Magorian T, *et al.* The pharmacokinetics and neuromuscular effects of rocuronium bromide in patients with liver disease. *Anesth Analg* 1995; **80:** 754–9.
3. van Miert MM, *et al.* The pharmacokinetics and pharmacodynamics of rocuronium in patients with hepatic cirrhosis. *Br J Clin Pharmacol* 1997; **44:** 139–44.

Renal impairment. In a study[1] of the pharmacokinetics and neuromuscular effects of rocuronium the clearance of rocuronium was reduced in patients with renal failure when compared with healthy patients but the accompanying increase in duration of clinical relaxation did not reach statistical significance. However, it was recommended that rocuronium should be used with caution in the presence of renal failure as there were large interpatient variations in both clinical response and pharmacokinetic parameters in patients with renal failure.

1. Cooper RA, *et al.* Time course of neuromuscular effects and pharmacokinetics of rocuronium bromide (ORG 9426) during isoflurane anaesthesia in patients with and without renal failure. *Br J Anaesth* 1993; **71:** 222–6.

Interactions

For interactions associated with competitive neuromuscular blockers, see Atracurium, p.1306.

Pharmacokinetics

Following intravenous administration plasma concentrations of rocuronium follow a three compartment open model. There is an initial distribution phase with a half-life of 1 to 2 minutes followed by a slower distribution phase with a half-life of 14 to 18 minutes. It is reported to be about 30% bound to plasma proteins. The elimination half-life is about 1.4 to 1.6 hours. Up to 30% of a dose may be excreted in the urine within 24 hours. There is some evidence that rocuronium may also be excreted in the bile. The main metabolite of rocuronium, 17-desacetylrocuronium, is reported to have a weak neuromuscular blocking effect.

References.

1. Khuenl-Brady KS, Sparr H. Clinical pharmacokinetics of rocuronium bromide. *Clin Pharmacokinet* 1996; **31:** 174–83.
2. McCoy EP, *et al.* Pharmacokinetics of rocuronium after bolus and continuous infusion during halothane anaesthesia. *Br J Anaesth* 1996; **76:** 29–33.
3. Wierda JMKH, *et al.* Pharmacokinetics and pharmacokinetic-dynamic modelling of rocuronium in infants and children. *Br J Anaesth* 1997; **78:** 690–5.

Intensive care. The pharmacokinetics of rocuronium appear to differ between intensive care patients receiving prolonged administration and surgical patients.[1] The volume of distribution at steady state may be increased, the plasma clearance decreased, and the terminal half-life prolonged. Recovery time on discontinuation may also be longer.

1. Sparr HJ, *et al.* Pharmacodynamics and pharmacokinetics of rocuronium in intensive care patients. *Br J Anaesth* 1997; **78:** 267–73.

Pregnancy. The mean concentration of rocuronium in venous plasma of 32 patients given a dose of 600 μg per kg body-weight before undergoing caesarean section was 2412 ng per mL at delivery;[1] the ratio of mean concentrations of rocuronium in umbilical venous plasma to maternal venous plasma at this time was 0.16. In 12 of these patients the mean concentration of rocuronium in umbilical arterial plasma was 271 ng per mL giving a ratio of 0.62 for the mean concentration of rocuronium in arterial to venous umbilical plasma. The concentration of 17-desacetylrocuronium in maternal venous plasma was 178 ng per mL and was less than 25 ng per mL in umbilical plasma.

1. Abouleish E, *et al.* Rocuronium (Org 9426) for Caesarean section. *Br J Anaesth* 1994; **73:** 336–41.

Uses and Administration

Rocuronium bromide is an aminosteroidal competitive neuromuscular blocker (see Atracurium, p.1308). Following intravenous injection it produces muscle relaxation within 1 to 2 minutes with a duration of about 30 to 50 minutes. Rocuronium bromide is used for endotracheal intubation and to provide muscle relaxation in general anaesthesia for surgical procedures (see Anaesthesia, p.1302) and to aid controlled ventilation (see Intensive Care, p.1303).

A usual initial dose is 600 μg per kg body-weight by intravenous injection with maintenance doses of 150 μg per kg by injection; maintenance may also be by infusion at a rate of 300 to 600 μg per kg per hour although higher rates have been used. Similar doses to those used in adults have been used in infants and children older than one month but maintenance doses may be required more frequently.

For obese patients weighing more than 30% over their ideal body-weight the UK manufacturer recommends that doses should be reduced by taking into account lean body-mass; in the USA the manufacturer recommends that dosage should be based on actual body-weight.

Reviews and discussions.

1. Mirakhur RK. Newer neuromuscular blocking drugs: an overview of their clinical pharmacology and therapeutic use. *Drugs* 1992; **44:** 182–9.
2. Hunter JM. Rocuronium: the newest aminosteroid neuromuscular blocking drug. *Br J Anaesth* 1996; **76:** 481–3.

Administration in children. Conditions for intubation in a study involving 70 children were judged to be good to excellent within one minute of intravenous administration of rocuronium 600 or 900 μg per kg body-weight with a trend to better conditions with the higher dose.[1]

1. Fuchs-Buder T, Tassonyi E. Intubating conditions and time course of rocuronium-induced neuromuscular block in children. *Br J Anaesth* 1996; **77:** 335–8.

INTRAMUSCULAR ROUTE. Intramuscular injection of rocuronium 1 mg per kg body-weight into the deltoid muscle permitted tracheal intubation to be carried out in lightly anaesthetised infants after 2.5 minutes.[1] In children a dose of 1.8 mg per kg enabled tracheal intubation after 3 minutes. However, the mean time to initial recovery after these doses was 57 minutes in infants and 70 minutes in children.

1. Reynolds LM, *et al.* Intramuscular rocuronium in infants and children: dose-ranging and tracheal intubating conditions. *Anesthesiology* 1996; **85:** 231–9.

Preparations

Proprietary Preparations (details are given in Part 3)
Belg.: Esmeron; ***Canad.:*** Zemuron; ***Fr.:*** Esmeron; ***Ger.:*** Esmeron; ***Irl.:*** Esmeron; ***Ital.:*** Esmeron; ***Neth.:*** Esmeron; ***Norw.:*** Esmeron; ***S.Afr.:*** Esmeron; ***Spain:*** Esmeron; ***Swed.:*** Esmeron; ***Switz.:*** Esmeron; ***UK:*** Esmeron; ***USA:*** Zemuron.

Styramate (5730-t)

Styramate *(BAN, rINN).*

β-Hydroxyphenethyl carbamate.

$C_9H_{11}NO_3$ = 181.2.

CAS — 94-35-9.

Styramate is a centrally acting skeletal muscle relaxant that was formerly used in the symptomatic treatment of painful muscle spasm associated with musculoskeletal conditions.

Preparations

Proprietary Preparations (details are given in Part 3)
Multi-ingredient: *S.Afr.:* Sinaxamol†.

Suxamethonium Chloride (5732-r)

Suxamethonium Chloride *(BAN, pINN).*

Choline Chloride Succinate; Succicurarium Chloride; Succinylcholine Chloride; Suxamethonii Chloridum; Suxametonklorid.

2,2′-Succinyldioxybis(ethyltrimethylammonium) dichloride dihydrate.

$C_{14}H_{30}Cl_2N_2O_4,2H_2O$ = 397.3.

CAS — 306-40-1 (suxamethonium); 55-94-7 (suxamethonium bromide); 71-27-2 (anhydrous suxamethonium chloride); 6101-15-1 (suxamethonium chloride dihydrate); 541-19-5 (suxamethonium iodide).

Pharmacopoeias. In *Chin., Eur.* (see p.viii), *Int., Jpn, Pol.,* and *US.*

A white or almost white, odourless, hygroscopic, crystalline powder. Suxamethonium 1 mg is equivalent to 1.37 mg of suxamethonium chloride dihydrate and to 1.24 mg of anhydrous suxamethonium chloride. **Soluble** 1 in 1 of water and 1 in 350 of alcohol; slightly soluble in chloroform; practically insoluble in ether. A 0.5% solution in water has a pH of 4.0 to 5.0. **Store** in airtight containers. Protect from light.

Incompatibility. Incompatibilities of neuromuscular blockers are discussed under Atracurium, p.1304.

Stability. A study of the loss of potency of suxamethonium chloride 20 mg per mL in water indicated that decomposition occurred at a considerably higher rate at 40° than at 25° and that the pH range of maximum stability was 3.75 to 4.50 for unbuffered solutions.[1] Assuming the usual conditions of manufacturing, transit, and storage the total loss of potency was estimated to be 7% and 9% respectively for injections kept at room temperature for 4 and 6 weeks. If unbuffered suxamethonium chloride injection complying with USP pH limits (3.0 to 4.5) must be stored at room temperature, it should not be kept for longer than 4 weeks.

1. Boehm JJ, *et al.* Shelf life of unrefrigerated succinylcholine chloride injection. *Am J Hosp Pharm* 1984; **41:** 300–2.

Adverse Effects

The neuromuscular blocking action of suxamethonium chloride is terminated by the enzyme plasma cholinesterase and prolonged apnoea may occur in patients with an atypical enzyme or with low enzyme activity. Apnoea may also occur following development of phase II block (see Uses and Administration, below) after high or repeated doses of suxamethonium chloride, although tachyphylaxis may also occur with repeated doses.

Administration of suxamethonium chloride results in transient fasciculations during the onset of depolarising block. Rhabdomyolysis, myoglobinaemia, and myoglobinuria have been reported and may be associated with muscle damage following fasciculations. Postoperative muscle pain occurs in some patients but is not directly related to the degree of fasciculation. A transient rise in intra-gastric pressure may occur secondary to fasciculation of abdominal muscles. A transient increase in intra-ocular pressure often occurs. Depolarisation of skeletal muscle produces an immediate increase in plasma-potassium concentration and this can have serious consequences in some patients (see below).

Stimulation of the vagus nerve and parasympathetic ganglia by suxamethonium chloride may be followed by bradycardia, other arrhythmias, and hypotension and may be exacerbated by the raised plasma-potassium concentration; cardiac arrest has been reported. Tachycardia and an increase in blood pressure due to stimulation of sympathetic ganglia have also been reported.

Suxamethonium chloride may cause an increase in salivary, bronchial, and gastric secretion and other muscarinic effects. Salivary gland enlargement has occurred.

Direct release of histamine from mast cells occurs but this is not the main mechanism of hypersensitivity reactions (see Hypersensitivity, below). Flushing, skin rash, bronchospasm, and shock have been reported.

Other reported effects include prolonged respiratory depression and apnoea.

Administration of suxamethonium chloride is implicated in the development of malignant hyperthermia in those patients with a genetic predisposition to the syndrome (see Dantrolene Sodium, p.1314).

Reviews of the adverse effects of suxamethonium.

1. Book WJ, *et al.* Adverse effects of depolarising neuromuscular blocking agents: incidence, prevention and management. *Drug Safety* 1994; **10:** 331–49.

Effects on intra-ocular pressure. Administration of suxamethonium is often followed 20 to 30 seconds later by a transient increase in intra-ocular pressure which may be due in part to contracture of extra-ocular muscles. If suxamethonium is administered during eye surgery after incision of the eyeball or to patients with penetrating eye injury there is a theoretical risk that any increase in intra-ocular pressure may result in extrusion of ocular contents and loss of sight. However, there appear to be few reports of vitreous extrusion associated with suxamethonium[1] and a large retrospective study[2] has failed to find any evidence that suxamethonium caused additional eye damage in patients with penetrating eye injuries. Furthermore the procedure of intubation is associated with a greater increase in intra-ocular pressure than that seen with suxamethonium. Nonetheless, opinion on the safety of suxamethonium in eye surgery varies. While some suggest that a rapid competitive neuromuscular blocker would be preferable to aid intubation in patients with penetrating eye injuries, after incision of the eyeball, and in glaucoma others advocate that the risk of a transient rise of intra-ocular pressure in these situations should be weighed against the need for rapid intubation.[1,3] For a discussion on the use of various agents to counteract the rise in intra-ocular pressure associated with suxamethonium and intubation in general, see under Anaesthesia, p.1302.

1. Book WJ, *et al.* Adverse effects of depolarising neuromuscular blocking agents: incidence, prevention and management. *Drug Safety* 1994; **5:** 331–49.
2. Libonati MM, *et al.* The use of succinylcholine in open eye surgery. *Anesthesiology* 1985; **62:** 637–40.
3. Edmondson L. Intraocular pressure and suxamethonium. *Br J Anaesth* 1997; **79:** 146.

Effects on the muscles. Muscle fasciculations and postoperative muscle pain commonly follow administration of suxamethonium. Fasciculations (generalised and desynchronised contractions of skeletal muscle fibres) occur during the onset of depolarising block in almost all patients given suxamethonium and may cause muscle damage. They are seen especially in the 'fine' muscles of the hands and face and can be useful as an indication that suxamethonium is working. Attempts have been made to prevent their development with the aim of reducing postoperative muscle pain. However, there appears to be no direct correlation between the extent of visible fasciculations and muscle pain.[1] Slow infusion of suxamethonium[2] or administration in divided doses[3] reduces fasciculations but not muscle pain.

Postoperative muscle pain is one of the most common side-effects of suxamethonium and has been noted in about 50% of patients, although the reported incidence varies widely from near zero to almost 100%.[4] It usually occurs on the first postoperative day and most commonly affects muscles of the neck, shoulders, and upper abdomen. The incidence and severity of muscle pain is increased in patients who are mobile soon after surgery and in females, but it occurs less often in children and pregnant women.[4-6] The mechanism of suxamethonium-induced muscle pain is not fully understood; there have been many attempts to prevent it. Most commonly, pretreatment with a small dose of a competitive neuromuscular blocker has reduced both visible fasciculations and the incidence and severity of muscle pain,[1,7-10] but has the disadvantage that it may delay the onset and reduce the intensity of subsequent suxamethonium block[11] and impair conditions for intubation[1,11] (see under Interactions in Atracurium, p.1307). Pretreatment with a small dose (10 mg) of suxamethonium in a 'self-taming' technique appears to offer no protection against muscle pain.[1] There have been reports that thiopentone can reduce the incidence of myalgia and muscle fasciculations[12] and prevent increases in serum concentrations of myoglobin and creatinine kinase induced by suxamethonium.[13] Treatment with benzodiazepines[14-17] has produced conflicting results. Pretreatment with the prostaglandin synthetase inhibitors aspirin,[18] lysine aspirin,[19] or diclofenac,[20] but not ketorolac,[21] has been reported to reduce postoperative muscle pain without abolishing visible fasciculations or diminishing the intensity of neuromuscular block. Not all methods have concentrated on drug treatment. A simple regimen of stretching exercises before premedication has reduced the incidence of both fasciculations and postoperative muscle pain.[5]

Suxamethonium may also produce an increase in jaw tension (masseter spasm or trismus)[22] in both adults[23] and children[24,25] during the onset of neuromuscular blockade. Tracheal intubation is greatly hindered in affected patients. It is not possible to predict which patients will show this response and the mechanism is unknown, although in about 50% of patients it may indicate the onset of malignant hyperthermia. Pretreatment with a paralysing dose of a competitive neuromuscular blocker prevents the response[25] but it is not known whether this is clinically useful.

1. O'Sullivan EP, *et al.* Differential effects of neuromuscular blocking agents on suxamethonium-induced fasciculations and myalgia. *Br J Anaesth* 1988; **60:** 367–71.
2. Feingold A, Velazquez JL. Suxamethonium infusion rate and observed fasciculations: a dose-response study. *Br J Anaesth* 1979; **51:** 241–5.
3. Wilson DB, Dundee JW. Failure of divided doses of succinylcholine to reduce the incidence of muscle pains. *Anesthesiology* 1980; **52:** 273–5.
4. Riding JE. Minor complications of general anaesthesia. *Br J Anaesth* 1975; **47:** 91–101.
5. Magee DA, Robinson RJS. Effect of stretch exercises on suxamethonium induced fasciculations and myalgia. *Br J Anaesth* 1987; **59:** 596–601.
6. Anonymous. Suxamethonium myalgia. *Lancet* 1988; **ii:** 944–5.
7. Bennetts FE, Khalil KI. Reduction of post-suxamethonium pains by pretreatment with four non-depolarising agents. *Br J Anaesth* 1981; **53:** 531–6.
8. Erkola O, *et al.* Five non-depolarizing muscle relaxants in precurarization. *Acta Anaesthesiol Scand* 1983; **27:** 427–32.
9. Sosis M, *et al.* Comparison of atracurium and d-tubocurarine for prevention of succinylcholine myalgia. *Anesth Analg* 1987; **66:** 657–9.
10. Findlay GP, Spittal MJ. Rocuronium pretreatment reduces suxamethonium-induced myalgia: comparison with vecuronium. *Br J Anaesth* 1996; **76:** 526–9.
11. Pauca AL, *et al.* Inhibition of suxamethonium relaxation by tubocurarine and gallamine pretreatment during induction of anaesthesia in man. *Br J Anaesth* 1975; **47:** 1067–73.
12. Manani G, *et al.* The influence of thiopentone and alfathesin on succinylcholine-induced fasciculations and myalgias. *Can Anaesth Soc J* 1981; **28:** 253–8.
13. Noguchi I, *et al.* Effects of different doses of thiopentone on the increase in serum myoglobin induced by suxamethonium in children. *Br J Anaesth* 1993; **71:** 291–3.
14. Chestnutt WN, *et al.* A comparison of the efficacy of benzodiazepines with tubocurarine in prevention of suxamethonium-induced muscle pain *Br J Clin Pharmacol* 1984; **17:** 222P.
15. Fahmy NR, *et al.* Diazepam prevents some adverse effects of succinylcholine. *Clin Pharmacol Ther* 1979; **26:** 395–8.
16. Davies AO. Oral diazepam pre-medication reduces the incidence of post-succinylcholine muscle pains. *Can Anaesth Soc J* 1983; **30:** 603–6.
17. Verma RS, *et al.* Diazepam and succinylcholine-induced muscle pains. *Anesth Analg* 1978; **57:** 295–7.
18. McLoughlin C, *et al.* Suxamethonium induced myalgia and the effect of pre-operative administration of oral aspirin: a comparison with a standard treatment and an untreated group. *Anaesthesia* 1988; **43:** 565–7.
19. Naguib M, *et al.* Effect of pre-treatment with lysine acetyl salicylate on suxamethonium-induced myalgia. *Br J Anaesth* 1987; **59:** 606–10.

20. Kahraman S, *et al.* Effect of preoperative i.m. administration of diclofenac on suxamethonium-induced myalgia. *Br J Anaesth* 1993; **71:** 238–41.
21. Leeson-Payne CG, *et al.* Use of ketorolac in the prevention of suxamethonium myalgia. *Br J Anaesth* 1994; **73:** 788–90.
22. Saddler JM. Jaw stiffness—an ill understood condition. *Br J Anaesth* 1991; **67**: 515–16.
23. Leary NP, Ellis FR. Masseteric muscle spasm as a normal response to suxamethonium. *Br J Anaesth* 1990; **64:** 488–92.
24. Van Der Spek AFL, *et al.* Changes in resistance to mouth opening induced by depolarizing and non-depolarizing neuromuscular relaxants. *Br J Anaesth* 1990; **64:** 21–7.
25. Smith CE, *et al.* Pretreatment with non-depolarizing neuromuscular blocking agents and suxamethonium-induced increases in resting jaw tension in children. *Br J Anaesth* 1990; **64:** 577–81.

Effects on plasma-potassium concentration. Suxamethonium administration is followed by depolarisation of motor end-plates in skeletal muscle resulting in an immediate increase in plasma-potassium concentration. The rise is usually small, being about 0.5 mmol or less per litre, but suxamethonium is best avoided in patients whose plasma-potassium concentration is already high, such as those with renal impairment. An exaggerated response, with severe hyperkalaemia resulting in ventricular fibrillation and cardiac arrest, has been reported in patients with burns,[1,2] massive trauma, neuromuscular disease (see under Neuromuscular Disorders in Precautions, below), and severe long-lasting sepsis.[3] See also Children in Precautions, below for reference to fatal cardiac arrest associated with hyperkalaemia in children. With burns or trauma the period of greatest risk is from about 10 to 90 days after the injury, but may be further prolonged if there is delayed healing or persistent infection. These patients may still react abnormally to suxamethonium 2 years after the injury. In neuromuscular disease the greatest risk period is usually from 3 weeks to 6 months after onset, but severe hyperkalaemia may occur after 24 to 48 hours or later than 6 months. Patients with severe sepsis for more than a week should be considered at risk of hyperkalaemia and no suxamethonium should be given until the infection has cleared. The mechanism of this hyperkalaemic response appears to be a supersensitivity of acetylcholine receptors in which the entire muscle fibre membrane, rather than discrete motor end-plate sites, becomes directly excitable by depolarising drugs. Depolarisation by suxamethonium thus results in release of potassium over the entire muscle fibre membrane and hyperkalaemia results.

Various methods have been tried to attenuate the hyperkalaemia, including pretreatment with a small dose of a competitive neuromuscular blocker[3,4] or with suxamethonium itself.[5,6] No method is sufficiently reliable to be used clinically.

Anaesthetics such as thiopentone and halothane can increase the hyperkalaemic response.[4]

1. Martyn J, *et al.* Clinical pharmacology of muscle relaxants in patients with burns. *J Clin Pharmacol* 1986; **26:** 680–5.
2. Anonymous. Neuromuscular blockers in patients with burns. *Lancet* 1988; **ii:** 1003–4.
3. Kohlschütter B, *et al.* Suxamethonium-induced hyperkalaemia in patients with severe intra-abdominal infections. *Br J Anaesth* 1976; **48:** 557–62.
4. Dhanaraj VJ, *et al.* A study of the changes in serum potassium concentration with suxamethonium using different anaesthetic agents. *Br J Anaesth* 1975; **47:** 516–19.
5. Magee DA, Gallagher EG. "Self-taming" of suxamethonium and serum potassium concentration. *Br J Anaesth* 1984; **56:** 977–9.
6. Plötz J, Schreiber W. Side effects induced by suxamethonium on the skeletal muscle and their prevention. *Br J Anaesth* 1985; **57:** 1044–5.

Hypersensitivity. Hypersensitivity reactions to neuromuscular blockers occur more commonly in women than in men,[1,2] in atopic patients and those who have a history of asthma or allergy,[2] and in patients who have had a previous reaction to anaesthetic drugs.[2] Circulatory collapse, flushing, skin rash, urticaria, and bronchospasm have occurred in hypersensitivity reactions associated with suxamethonium;[1,3,4] deaths have been reported.[3,5] The exact mechanism by which neuromuscular blockers produce hypersensitivity reactions is still uncertain; they all have a direct effect on mast cells, releasing histamine without immunological involvement, and could cause anaphylactoid reactions. Histamine release associated with use of aminosteroidal blockers is rare compared with the benzylisoquinolinium blockers.[6] Tubocurarine is considered to be the most potent releaser of histamine, with pancuronium and vecuronium having only very weak activity. Suxamethonium is considered to have only 1% of the histamine-releasing activity of tubocurarine but is more likely to produce serious hypersensitivity reactions. A type I immediate hypersensitivity reaction involving IgE antibodies is considered to be the mechanism of most hypersensitivity reactions associated with neuromuscular blockers.[2,5,7,8] Antibodies reacting with neuromuscular blockers, including suxamethonium, have been demonstrated.[5,8] The antibodies appear to be directed against quaternary or tertiary ammonium-ion groups which are present in neuromuscular blockers; such groups are also found in other drugs, cosmetics, disinfectants, and foods. This may help explain the cross-reactivity reported between different neuromuscular blockers[1,2,5,8,9] and how sensitisation occurs without prior exposure to any neuromuscular blocker.[2,5] At least 50% of patients sensitive to one neuromuscular blocker will react to one or more others[10] with some patients sensitive to most.[1] Intradermal skin tests are used to investigate and predict sensitivity to neuromuscular blockers, but their interpretation is controversial and it cannot be concluded that all patients with positive skin tests will have clinical sensitivity.[1,10] Although radioallergosorbent tests can detect antibodies to suxamethonium, alcuronium, and thiopentone[3,11] some consider that their routine use is not justified as reactions could be avoided by taking an adequate patient history.[12]

1. Youngmen PR, *et al.* Anaphylactoid reactions to neuromuscular blocking agents: a commonly undiagnosed condition? *Lancet* 1983; **ii:** 597–9.
2. Fisher MM, Munro I. Life-threatening anaphylactoid reactions to muscle relaxants. *Anesth Analg* 1983; **62:** 559–64.
3. Brahams D. Fatal reaction to suxamethonium: case for screening by radioallergosorbent test? *Lancet* 1989; **i:** 1400–1.
4. Moneret-Vautrin DA, *et al.* Simultaneous anaphylaxis to thiopentone and a neuromuscular blocker: a study of two cases. *Br J Anaesth* 1990; **64:** 743–5.
5. Fisher M, Baldo B. Adverse reactions to alcuronium: an Australian disease? *Med J Aust* 1983; **1:** 630–2.
6. Naguib M, *et al.* Histamine-release haemodynamic changes produced by rocuronium, vecuronium, mivacurium, atracurium and tubocurarine. *Br J Anaesth* 1995; **75:** 588–92.
7. Vervloet D. Anaphylactoid reactions to suxamethonium. *Lancet* 1983; **ii:** 1197.
8. Harle DG, *et al.* Detection of IgE antibodies to suxamethonium after anaphylactoid reactions during anaesthesia. *Lancet* 1984; **I:** 930–2.
9. Harle DG, *et al.* Cross-reactivity of metocurine, atracurium, vecuronium and fazadinium with IgE antibodies from patients unexposed to these drugs but allergic to other myoneural blocking drugs. *Br J Anaesth* 1985; **57:** 1073–6.
10. Withington DE. Relevance of histamine to the anaesthetist. *Br J Hosp Med* 1988; **40:** 264–70.
11. Assem ESK. Anaphylactic anaesthetic reactions: the value of paper radioallergosorbent tests for IgE antibodies to muscle relaxants and thiopentone. *Anaesthesia* 1990; **45:** 1032–8.
12. Noble DW, Yap PL. Screening for antibodies to anaesthetics. *Br Med J* 1989; **299:** 2.

Treatment of Adverse Effects

Following administration of suxamethonium chloride assisted respiration should be maintained until spontaneous respiration has been fully restored. Transfusion of fresh whole blood, frozen plasma, or other source of plasma cholinesterase will help the destruction of the suxamethonium when prolonged paralysis is a result of atypical or low serum concentrations of plasma cholinesterase. Anticholinesterases should not usually be used since they potentiate the usual phase I block (see under Uses and Administration, below). If the neuromuscular block ceases to be depolarising in type and acquires some features of a competitive block (phase II block) the cautious use of an anticholinesterase may be considered. A short-acting anticholinesterase such as edrophonium may be given intravenously and if an obvious improvement is maintained for several minutes, neostigmine may be given with atropine.

Severe hypersensitivity reactions should be treated promptly with supportive and symptomatic measures.

If malignant hyperthermia develops, it may be treated as described under Dantrolene Sodium, p.1314.

The muscarinic effects of suxamethonium chloride, such as bradycardia and excessive salivary secretion, may be reduced by giving an antimuscarinic such as atropine before suxamethonium. A small dose of a competitive neuromuscular blocker given before suxamethonium has been used to reduce some of the adverse effects of suxamethonium on the muscles (see Effects on the Muscles, above).

Precautions

Doses of neuromuscular blockers need to be carefully titrated for individual patients according to response; monitoring of the degree of block is recommended in order to reduce the risk of overdosage. Patients who have received a neuromuscular blocker should always have their respiration assisted or controlled until the drug has been inactivated or antagonised.

Suxamethonium chloride is contra-indicated in patients with atypical plasma cholinesterase and should be used with caution in patients with reduced plasma cholinesterase activity (see below) which may occur in certain disease states and following exposure to certain drugs. Plasma cholinesterase concentrations fall during pregnancy and the puerperium and therefore maternal paralysis may be mildly prolonged. Suxamethonium is contra-indicated in patients with burns, massive trauma, renal impairment with a raised plasma-potassium concentration, severe long-lasting sepsis, and severe hyperkalaemia since suxamethonium-induced rises in plasma-potassium concentration can have serious consequences in such patients. It is contra-indicated in patients with a history of hypersensitivity to the drug and, because of the possibility of cross-sensitivity (see above), should be used with caution when hypersensitivity to any neuromuscular blocker has previously occurred. Suxamethonium should be avoided in patients with a penetrating eye injury or glaucoma or those about to undergo incision of the eyeball in eye surgery because of the risks from increased intra-ocular pressure. Suxamethonium chloride produces muscle contractions before relaxation and should therefore be used with caution in patients with bone fractures. It is contra-indicated in patients with a family history of malignant hyperthermia.

The response to suxamethonium chloride is often unpredictable in patients with neuromuscular disorders and it should be used with great caution in these patients (see below). Caution is also needed if it is given to a patient with cardiac or respiratory disease. Children may be at special risk from cardiac arrest associated with hyperkalaemia, see below.

Hypothermia may enhance the neuromuscular blocking effects of suxamethonium chloride and an increase in body temperature may reduce them.

Children. Reports of fatal cardiac arrests[1,2] in apparently healthy children and adolescents, who were subsequently found to have had undiagnosed myopathies, led in the USA to restrictions on the use of suxamethonium in this age group contra-indicating it except for emergency tracheal intubation or where an immediate securing of an airway is essential. Many anaesthetists disagreed[2] with this contra-indication and an FDA Committee advised[3] that the contra-indication should be replaced by a warning about the possibility of cardiac arrest associated with hyperkalaemia with special attention being paid to male children who are considered to be at the highest risk. One British anaesthetist who questioned the rationale behind restricting the elective use of suxamethonium pointed out that alternatives to suxamethonium had not been demonstrated to be as safe or effective for airway management.[4] The rare occurrence of cardiac arrest in children might be further reduced by taking a careful family history to exclude undiagnosed myopathies and by using an intravenous as opposed to inhalation induction when suxamethonium is to be used. A survey had found that most cases of cardiac arrest in children in the UK associated with the use of suxamethonium had been caused by vagal overactivity in non-atropinised patients.

1. Rosenberg H, Gronert GA. Intractable cardiac arrest in children given succinylcholine. *Anesthesiology* 1992; **77:** 1054.
2. Book WJ, *et al.* Adverse effects of depolarising neuromuscular blocking agents: incidence, prevention and management. *Drug Safety* 1994; **10:** 331–49.
3. *FDC Reports Pink Sheet* 1994; June 13: 16.
4. Hopkins PM. Use of suxamethonium in children. *Br J Anaesth* 1995; **75:** 675–7.

Neuromuscular disorders. Caution is needed if suxamethonium is to be given to patients with neuromuscular disease since severe complications have been reported.[1] Hyperkalaemia and cardiac arrhythmias or cardiac arrest have been reported following administration of suxamethonium to patients with hemiplegia, diffuse intracranial lesions (head injury, encephalitis, ruptured cerebral aneurysm), tetanus, paraplegia, acute anterior horn cell disease, and muscular dystrophies. An exaggerated response to suxamethonium has been reported in the myasthenic syndrome but resistance may occur in patients with neurofibromatosis. Resistance may also occur in patients with myasthenia gravis, but uneventful administration has also been reported although early onset of phase II block is possible in these patients. Muscle contractures and hyperkalaemia may be expected in amyotrophic lateral sclerosis and muscular denervation. The response to suxamethonium is unpredictable in patients with myotonias and it should be avoided in those patients. It is recommended that suxamethonium is also avoided in hemiplegia, paraplegia, muscular denervation, and muscular dystrophies.

1. Azar I. The response of patients with neuromuscular disorders to muscle relaxants: a review. *Anesthesiology* 1984; **61:** 173–87.

Plasma cholinesterase deficiency. Suxamethonium is normally rapidly hydrolysed by plasma cholinesterase and the clinical effects usually last for only several minutes. Activity of the enzyme varies between individuals and prolonged paralysis following suxamethonium is commonly due to a hereditary or acquired reduction in plasma cholinesterase activity. The genes involved in the control of plasma cholinesterase production are termed usual, atypical (dibucaine-resistant), fluoride-resistant, and silent. About 96% of the population are homozygous for the normal gene. The commonest variant in western populations is the atypical form with about 3 to 4% of the population being heterozygous for this variant. They exhibit a slightly prolonged response to suxamethonium. Homozygotes for the atypical variant have a frequency of about 0.04%. They exhibit markedly prolonged apnoea following a standard dose of suxamethonium but can be readily identified by biochemical tests. The fluoride-resistant and silent variants occur very rarely. A measure of plasma cholinesterase activity can be obtained from the percentage inhibition of the enzyme by the local anaesthetic cinchocaine (commonly known in this context by its American name, dibucaine) to give the dibucaine number. Most normal people have a dibucaine number of about 80.

Acquired plasma cholinesterase deficiency is clinically less important than genetically determined deficiency. The enzyme is synthesised in the liver and **severe liver impairment** or malnutrition may cause abnormally low enzyme levels with some prolongation of suxamethonium activity. Reduced enzyme activity may also be found in severe anaemia, burns, cancer, collagen diseases, severe dehydration, severe infections, malnutrition, myocardial infarction, myxoedema, and renal impairment; plasmapheresis or plasma exchange removes significant amounts of plasma cholinesterase.

During **pregnancy** there is a rapid fall in plasma cholinesterase concentration which persists throughout pregnancy and for up to several weeks into the puerperium. The concentration of atypical plasma cholinesterase is also reduced in pregnancy and the puerperium. A number of **drugs** reduce plasma cholinesterase synthesis or activity and may prolong suxamethonium paralysis as discussed under Interactions, below.

References.

1. Wood GJ, Hall GM. Plasmapheresis and plasma cholinesterase. *Br J Anaesth* 1978; **50:** 945–9.
2. Evans RT, Wroe JM. Plasma cholinesterase changes during pregnancy: their interpretation as a cause of suxamethonium-induced apnoea. *Anaesthesia* 1980; **35:** 651–4.
3. Lumley J. Prolongation of suxamethonium following plasma exchange. *Br J Anaesth* 1980; **52:** 1149–50.
4. Williams FM. Clinical significance of esterases in man. *Clin Pharmacokinet* 1985; **10:** 392–403.
5. Robson N, *et al.* Plasma cholinesterase changes during the puerperium. *Anaesthesia* 1986; **41:** 243–9.
6. Cherala SR, *et al.* Placental transfer of succinylcholine causing transient respiratory depression in the newborn. *Anaesth Intensive Care* 1989; **17:** 202–4.

Renal impairment. Suxamethonium chloride may be given in usual doses to patients with renal failure[1] but should be avoided if hyperkalaemia is also present (see Effects on Plasma-potassium Concentration above).

1. Ryan DW. Preoperative serum cholinesterase concentration in chronic renal failure. *Br J Anaesth* 1977; **49:** 945–9.

Interactions

A number of drugs may interact with depolarising neuromuscular blockers such as suxamethonium. The mechanisms of interaction may include a direct effect on neuromuscular transmission or an alteration of enzyme activity and may result in potentiation or antagonism of neuromuscular block. In general, interactions with suxamethonium are potentially more serious in patients with impaired neuromuscular function (see Neuromuscular Disorders, above) and in patients with reduced activity of plasma cholinesterase enzyme (see above).

Interactions common to competitive and depolarising neuromuscular blockers are covered under Atracurium, p.1306 whereas those specific for depolarising blockers are discussed below; well established interactions are covered as are interactions that have only been the subject of anecdotal reports.

Antiarrhythmics. See under Atracurium, p.1306.

Antibacterials. See under Atracurium, p.1306.

Anticholinesterases. The action of suxamethonium can be markedly prolonged in patients using eye drops containing *ecothiopate*, a long-acting anticholinesterase which inhibits both acetylcholinesterase and plasma cholinesterase. Following systemic absorption of ecothiopate, plasma cholinesterase activity may rapidly be reduced to 5% or less of normal and prolonged apnoea after administration of suxamethonium has occurred. On discontinuing ecothiopate, enzyme activity remains depressed for 1 to 2 months. If a patient has used ecothiopate eye drops in the previous 2 months, suxamethonium should not be given unless normal plasma cholinesterase activity can be demonstrated; a competitive neuromuscular blocker is preferable. Exposure to *organophosphorus insecticides* may also reduce plasma cholinesterase activity resulting in prolonged paralysis following administration of suxamethonium; enzyme activity may be totally abolished. Anticholinesterase such as *neostigmine* enhance the action of suxamethonium although suxamethonium-induced phase II block can be reversed with an anticholinesterase. Care should be taken if there is a need to use suxamethonium for urgent short procedures after a competitive-neuromuscular-induced block has been antagonised with an anticholinesterase as the resulting block may be greatly prolonged.[1] Inhibition of plasma cholinesterase with *tacrine* has been used clinically to potentiate and prolong the action of suxamethonium, although this is no longer widely practised.

1. Fleming NW, *et al.* Neuromuscular blocking action of suxamethonium after antagonism of vecuronium by edrophonium, pyridostigmine or neostigmine. *Br J Anaesth* 1996; **77:** 492–5.

Antiepileptics. The mean time to recovery from suxamethonium-induced neuromuscular block was 14.3 minutes in 9 patients receiving chronic treatment with phenytoin and/or carbamazepine compared with 10.0 minutes in 9 patients not receiving antiepileptics.[1]

1. Melton AT, *et al.* Prolonged duration of succinylcholine in patients receiving anticonvulsants: evidence for mild upregulation of acetylcholine receptors? *Can J Anaesth* 1993; **40:** 939–42.

Antineoplastics. *Cyclophosphamide* has been reported to prolong the neuromuscular block produced by suxamethonium through reduction of plasma cholinesterase activity, possibly by alkylation of the enzyme.[1] Since enzyme activity may be reduced by up to 70% for several days to several weeks, it was suggested[2] that suxamethonium should be avoided if possible in patients receiving cyclophosphamide. Other alkylating agents also reported to reduce plasma cholinesterase activity include *mustine, thiotepa*, and *tretamine*.[2]

1. Walker IR, *et al.* Cyclophosphamide, cholinesterase and anaesthesia. *Aust N Z J Med* 1972; **3:** 247–51.
2. Zsigmond EK, Robins G. The effect of a series of anti-cancer drugs on plasma cholinesterase activity. *Can Anaesth Soc J* 1972; **19:** 75–82.

Aprotinin. See under Atracurium, p.1306.

Benzodiazepines. See under Atracurium, p.1306.

Beta blockers. See under Atracurium, p.1306.

Cardiac inotropes. See under Atracurium, p.1306.

Ganglion blockers. See under Atracurium, p.1307.

General anaesthetics. Tachyphylaxis and phase II block (see below) develop earlier, and after smaller total doses of suxamethonium, when inhalation anaesthetics are used. Halothane may increase the incidence of arrhythmias associated with suxamethonium and may potentiate suxamethonium-induced muscle damage.[1] Suxamethonium should be used with caution with other drugs that might produce additive cardiovascular effects. Severe bradycardia and asystole have occurred when used in anaesthetic regimens with propofol and opioids such as fentanyl.

See also under Interactions in Atracurium, p.1307.

1. Laurence AS, Henderson P. Serum myoglobin after suxamethonium administration to children: effect of pretreatment before iv and inhalation induction. *Br J Anaesth* 1986; **58:** 126P.

Histamine H_2 antagonists. See under Atracurium, p.1307.

Lithium. See under Atracurium, p.1307.

Local anaesthetics. *Procaine, cocaine*, and *chloroprocaine* are ester-type local anaesthetics which are hydrolysed by plasma cholinesterase and may competitively enhance the neuromuscular blocking activity of suxamethonium. See also Antiarrhythmics under Atracurium, p.1306.

Magnesium salts. See under Atracurium, p.1307.

MAOIs. Reduction of plasma cholinesterase activity by *phenelzine* has been reported[1] to cause significant prolongation of suxamethonium paralysis. Enzyme activity may be reduced to 10% of normal and recovery may take up to a month. The dosage of suxamethonium may need to be substantially reduced or a competitive neuromuscular blocker used.

1. Bodley PO, *et al.* Low serum pseudocholinesterase levels complicating treatment with phenelzine. *Br Med J* 1969; **3:** 510–12.

Metoclopramide. Dose-dependent prolongation of suxamethonium-induced neuromuscular blockade has been reported in patients given metoclopramide.[1,2] The potent inhibitory effect of metoclopramide on plasma cholinesterase may account for this interaction.

1. Turner DR, *et al.* Neuromuscular block by suxamethonium following treatment with histamine type 2 antagonists or metoclopramide. *Br J Anaesth* 1989; **63:** 348–50.
2. Kao YJ, *et al.* Dose-dependent effect of metoclopramide on cholinesterases and suxamethonium metabolism. *Br J Anaesth* 1990; **65:** 220–4.

Neuromuscular blockers. See under Atracurium, p.1307.

Sex hormones. *Oestrogens* and oestrogen-containing *oral contraceptives* reduce plasma cholinesterase activity[1] possibly due to suppression of hepatic synthesis of the enzyme, but little prolongation of suxamethonium paralysis may be expected since activity is reduced by only about 20%. See also under Atracurium, p.1307.

1. Robertson GS, Aberd MB. Serum protein and cholinesterase changes in association with contraceptive pills. *Lancet* 1967; **i:** 232–5.

Sympathomimetics. *Bambuterol* can inhibit plasma cholinesterase activity and so prolong the activity of suxamethonium.[1] Phase II block has been reported in some patients with abnormal plasma cholinesterase.[2]

1. Staun P, *et al.* The influence of 10 mg and 20 mg bambuterol on the duration of succinylcholine-induced neuromuscular blockade. *Acta Anaesthesiol Scand* 1990; **34:** 498–500.
2. Bang U, *et al.* The effect of bambuterol on plasma cholinesterase activity and suxamethonium-induced neuromuscular blockade in subjects heterozygous for abnormal plasma cholinesterase. *Acta Anaesthesiol Scand* 1990; **34:** 600–4.

Pharmacokinetics

After injection, suxamethonium is rapidly hydrolysed by plasma cholinesterase in plasma. One molecule of choline is split off rapidly to form succinylmonocholine which is then slowly hydrolysed to succinic acid and choline. Only a small proportion of suxamethonium is excreted unchanged in the urine. Succinylmonocholine has weak muscle-relaxant properties mainly of a competitive nature.

The gene responsible for the expression of plasma cholinesterase exhibits polymorphism and enzyme activity varies between individuals (see under Precautions, above).

Small amounts of suxamethonium do cross the placenta but clinical experience indicates that the neonate is not adversely affected when it has been used for caesarean section.

Uses and Administration

Suxamethonium is a depolarising neuromuscular blocker used to produce muscle relaxation. It acts as an acetylcholine agonist at the neuromuscular junction, combining with cholinergic receptors of the motor end-plate to produce depolarisation which may produce transient fasciculations. Suxamethonium is resistant to breakdown by acetylcholinesterase, the depolarisation is prolonged, and the refractory period of the motor end-plate extended. This prevents repolarisation and subsequent depolarisation and a flaccid muscle paralysis occurs. This initial depolarisation block is commonly known as a **phase I block.** The muscles that produce fine rapid movements such as those of the face are the first to be affected followed by those of the limbs, abdomen, and chest; the diaphragm is affected last. Recovery occurs in reverse order. When excessive amounts of suxamethonium accumulate at the neuromuscular junction, for example following high or prolonged dosage, the nature of the block may change to one with characteristics similar to competitive block. This is commonly termed **phase II block** or **dual block** and may be associated with prolonged neuromuscular blockade and apnoea.

Following intravenous injection suxamethonium chloride acts in about 30 to 60 seconds and has a duration of action of about 2 to 6 minutes. Following intramuscular injection it acts in 2 to 3 minutes and has a duration of action of about 10 to 30 minutes. It is used in surgical and other procedures in which a rapid onset and brief duration of muscle relaxation is needed (see Anaesthesia, p.1302), including intubation, endoscopies, and electroconvulsive therapy. It is normally given by intravenous injection, usually as the chloride (but the bromide and iodide have also been used). Suxamethonium has to be given after induction of general anaesthesia because paralysis is usually preceded by painful muscle fasciculations. A competitive neuromuscular blocker may sometimes be given before suxamethonium to try to reduce some of the adverse effects on the muscles (see under Effects on the Muscles, above). Premedication with an antimuscarinic may be of value in reducing bradycardia and excessive salivation. Assisted respiration is necessary.

An initial test dose of 0.1 mg per kg of suxamethonium chloride may be given intravenously if increased sensitivity is suspected. The response to suxamethonium varies considerably and the usual single dose of suxamethonium chloride for an adult is 0.3 to 1.1 mg per kg body-weight by intravenous injection with a usual range of 20 mg to a maximum total of 100 mg. Supplementary doses of 50 to 100% of the initial dose may be administered at 5 to 10 minute intervals if required but the total dose given by repeated intravenous injection or continuous infusion (see below) should not exceed 500 mg per hour. Infants and children are more resistant to suxamethonium than adults. A recommended intravenous dose for infants under one year of age is 2 mg per kg; a dose of 1 mg per kg is recommended for children 1 to 12 years old.

When a suitable vein is inaccessible suxamethonium chloride has been given by intramuscular injection, a suggested dose being 2.5 to 4 mg per kg body-weight to a maximum total of 150 mg. The intramuscular dose for infants is up to 4 to 5 mg per kg and for older children up to 4 mg per kg to a maximum total of 150 mg.

For prolonged procedures in adults sustained relaxation may be obtained by continuous intravenous infusion of a 0.1 to 0.2% solution. A rate of 2 to 5 mg per minute is usually adequate but may be adjusted as necessary. The total dose given by repeated intravenous injection (see above) or continuous infusion should not exceed 500 mg per hour.

Preparations

BP 1998: Suxamethonium Chloride Injection;
USP 23: Succinylcholine Chloride for Injection; Succinylcholine Chloride Injection.

Proprietary Preparations (details are given in Part 3)
Aust.: Lysthenon; ***Austral.:*** Scoline; ***Belg.:*** Myoplegine; ***Canad.:*** Anectine; Quelicin; ***Fr.:*** Celocurine; ***Ger.:*** Lysthenon; Pantolax; Succicuran; Succinyl†; ***Irl.:*** Anectine; ***Ital.:*** Midarine; Myotenlis; ***Neth.:*** Succinyl†; ***Norw.:*** Curacit; ***S.Afr.:*** Scoline; ***Spain:*** Anectine; Mioflex; ***Swed.:*** Celocurin; ***Switz.:*** Lysthenon; Midarine; Succinolin; Succinyl†; ***UK:*** Anectine; Scoline†; ***USA:*** Anectine; Quelicin; Sucostrin†.

Thiocolchicoside (13324-v)

Thiocolchicoside *(rINN)*.

3,10-Di(demethoxy)-3-glucopyranosyloxy-10-methylthiocolchicine.

$C_{27}H_{33}NO_{10}S$ = 563.6.
CAS — 602-41-5.

Pharmacopoeias. In Fr.

Thiocolchicoside is a muscle relaxant which has been claimed to possess GABA-mimetic and glycinergic actions. It is used in the symptomatic treatment of painful muscle spasm (p.1303). The usual initial dose is 16 mg daily by mouth. It has also been given intramuscularly, in doses up to 8 mg daily, or applied as cream or ointment. Photosensitivity reactions may occur.

Preparations

Proprietary Preparations (details are given in Part 3)
Fr.: Coltramyl; Miorel; ***Ital.:*** Muscoril.

Multi-ingredient: ***Ital.:*** Tioscina; ***Spain:*** Adalgur; Liviane Compuesto; Neurosido†.

Tizanidine Hydrochloride (13357-j)

Tizanidine Hydrochloride *(BANM, USAN, rINNM)*.

AN-021; DS-103-282; DS-103-282-ch. 5-Chloro-*N*-(2-imidazolin-2-yl)-2,1,3-benzothiadiazol-4-ylamine hydrochloride.

$C_9H_8ClN_5S,HCl$ = 290.2.
CAS — 51322-75-9 (tizanidine); 64461-82-1 (tizanidine hydrochloride).

Tizanidine hydrochloride 1.14 mg is approximately equivalent to 1 mg of tizanidine.

Adverse Effects and Precautions

Tizanidine hydrochloride may cause drowsiness; patients affected should not drive or operate machinery. Other adverse effects include dry mouth, fatigue, dizziness or vertigo, muscle pain and weakness, insomnia, anxiety, headache, bradycardia, nausea, and gastro-intestinal disturbances. Hallucinations have occurred on rare occasions. Many adverse effects have been found to be dose related and slow titration of doses appears to reduce the frequency of occurrence. Hypotension may occur. Increases in liver enzymes and rarely acute hepatitis have been associated with tizanidine and it is contra-indicated in patients with severe hepatic dysfunction. In the UK it is recommended that liver function should be monitored in all patients for the first 4 months and in those who develop symptoms suggestive of hepatic dysfunction. Treatment should be discontinued if liver enzymes are persistently raised. Caution is required in the elderly and in patients with renal insufficiency.

Interactions

The CNS effects of tizanidine may be enhanced by alcohol or other CNS depressants. There may be an additive hypotensive effect when tizanidine is used in patients receiving antihypertensive therapy; bradycardia may also be enhanced if given with beta blockers or digoxin. The clearance of tizanidine has been reported to be lower in women receiving hormonal contraceptives.

Antiepileptics. For reference to an interaction between tizanidine and phenytoin, see p.356.

Pharmacokinetics

Tizanidine is absorbed from the gastro-intestinal tract and peak plasma concentrations have occurred 1 to 2 hours after administration by mouth. Tizanidine undergoes extensive first-pass metabolism in the liver and is excreted mainly in the urine as inactive metabolites. Elimination half-lives of 2.1 to 4.2 hours have been reported.

Uses and Administration

Tizanidine hydrochloride is a centrally acting skeletal muscle relaxant. It is an α_2-adrenergic agonist structurally related to clonidine (p.841) and acts mainly at the level of the spinal cord.

It is used as an adjunct in the management of spasticity associated with multiple sclerosis or spinal cord disorders, and in the symptomatic treatment of painful muscle spasm (p.1303) associated with musculoskeletal conditions. Tizanidine hydrochloride is usually given in divided doses by mouth. The usual initial daily dose is the equivalent of 2 mg of the base given as a single dose. The daily dose may be increased thereafter according to response in steps of 2 mg at intervals of at least 3 to 4 days, usually up to 24 mg daily given in 3 to 4 divided doses. The maximum recommended dose is 36 mg daily. For patients with renal insufficiency, treatment is also started with 2 mg once daily, but thereafter it is advised to slowly increase the once-daily dose before increasing the frequency of administration. Maintenance doses have been given in some countries in the form of modified-release preparations.

References.

1. Hutchinson DR. Modified release tizanidine: a review. *J Int Med Res* 1989; **17:** 565–73.

Premedication. The value of tizanidine as a premedicant is being studied.[1] A dose of tizanidine 12 mg appears to have sedative and sympatholytic effects comparable with clonidine 150 μg.

1. Meittinen TJ, *et al.* The sedative and sympatholytic effects of oral tizanidine in healthy volunteers. *Anesth Analg* 1996; **82:** 817–20.

Spasticity. The use of tizanidine in the management of spasticity (p.1303) associated with cerebral and spinal disorders has been discussed.[1,2] Its antispastic efficacy had been demonstrated in several placebo-controlled studies and in comparative studies it had produced similar improvements in muscle tone to baclofen or diazepam. Carefully titrated doses of tizanidine and baclofen used together may have additive beneficial effects[1,2] but use with benzodiazepines is not recommended because of potential interactions.[1] It was considered that tizanidine might have the advantage of being better tolerated than baclofen.

1. Wagstaff AJ, Bryson HM. Tizanidine: a review of its pharmacology, clinical efficacy and tolerability in the management of spasticity associated with cerebral and spinal disorders. *Drugs* 1997; **53:** 435–52.
2. Anonymous. Tizanidine for spasticity. *Med Lett Drugs Ther* 1997; **39:** 62–3.

Preparations

Proprietary Preparations (details are given in Part 3)
Aust.: Sirdalud; ***Belg.:*** Sirdalud; ***Ger.:*** Sirdalud; ***Ital.:*** Sirdalud; ***Jpn:*** Ternelin; ***Neth.:*** Sirdalud; ***Spain:*** Sirdalud; ***Switz.:*** Sirdalud; ***UK:*** Zanaflex; ***USA:*** Zanaflex.

Tolperisone Hydrochloride (5735-n)

Tolperisone Hydrochloride *(BANM, rINNM)*.

N-553. 2,4′-Dimethyl-3-piperidinopropiophenone hydrochloride.

$C_{16}H_{23}NO,HCl$ = 281.8.
CAS — 728-88-1 (tolperisone); 3644-61-9 (tolperisone hydrochloride).

Pharmacopoeias. In Jpn.

Tolperisone hydrochloride is a centrally acting muscle relaxant that has been used for the symptomatic treatment of spasticity (p.1303) and muscle spasm (p.1303), in usual doses of 50 to 150 mg three times daily by mouth.

Preparations

Proprietary Preparations (details are given in Part 3)
Aust.: Mydocalm; ***Ger.:*** Mydocalm; ***Jpn:*** Muscalm†; ***Switz.:*** Mydocalm.

Tubocurarine Chloride (5736-h)

Tubocurarine Chloride *(BAN, rINN)*.

d-Tubocurarine Chloride; (+)-Tubocurarine Chloride Hydrochloride Pentahydrate; Tubocurarini Chloridum. (+)-7′,12′-Dihydroxy-6,6′-dimethoxy-2,2′,2′-trimethyltubocuraranium dichloride pentahydrate.

$C_{37}H_{42}Cl_2N_2O_6,5H_2O$ = 771.7 (The empirical formula of tubocurarine chloride was formerly considered to be $C_{38}H_{44}Cl_2N_2O_6,5H_2O$).
CAS — 57-95-4 (tubocurarine); 57-94-3 (anhydrous tubocurarine chloride); 6989-98-6 (tubocurarine chloride, pentahydrate).

Pharmacopoeias. In *Eur.* (see p.viii), *Int.*, *Jpn*, and *US.*

The chloride of (+)-tubocurarine. It may be obtained from extracts of the stems of *Chondodendron tomentosum* (Menispermaceae) and is one of the active principles of curare, by which name it is sometimes referred to in anaesthetic literature. It is a white or slightly yellowish-white or greyish-white, crystalline powder.

Ph. Eur. **solubilities** are: soluble in water and in alcohol; practically insoluble in acetone and in ether; dissolves in solutions of alkali hydroxides. USP solubilities are: soluble 1 in 20 of water and 1 in 45 of alcohol. A 1% solution in water has a pH of 4.0 to 6.0. **Store** in airtight containers.

Adverse Effects, Treatment, and Precautions

As for competitive neuromuscular blockers in general (see Atracurium, p.1304). A transient fall in blood pressure commonly occurs, due in part to ganglionic blockade and the release of histamine; there may be an increase in heart rate. Tubocurarine has a greater propensity to cause histamine release than other competitive neuromuscular blockers in clinical use. Tubocurarine should be used with caution in patients with renal impairment. Resistance to the effect of tubocurarine may occur in patients with hepatic impairment.

Interactions

For interactions associated with competitive neuromuscular blockers, see Atracurium, p.1306.

Pharmacokinetics

Tubocurarine chloride is a quaternary ammonium compound and absorption from the gastro-intestinal tract following oral administration is extremely poor. Absorption is slow and irregular when given intramuscularly. Following intravenous injection tubocurarine is widely distributed throughout body tissues; less than 50% is bound to plasma proteins. Following a single dose extensive redistribution to tissues is responsible for the termination of activity, but after a large single dose or repeated small doses tissue saturation occurs and renal excretion becomes the main determinant of duration. When given in usual doses it does not pass the blood-brain barrier, and does not appear to cross the placenta in significant amounts. Up to 75% of a dose is excreted unchanged in the urine in 24 hours, and up to 12% in bile. Biliary excretion is increased in renal impairment. A small proportion of a dose is metabolised in the liver.

Uses and Administration

Tubocurarine is a benzylisoquinolinium competitive neuromuscular blocker (see Atracurium, p.1308). Following intravenous injection of tubocurarine chloride neuromuscular block appears within one minute and lasts for about 30 minutes; the maximum effect is attained within 2 to 5 minutes. Tubocurarine chloride has been used similarly to other competitive neuromuscular blockers to produce muscle relaxation in various procedures but has largely been replaced by other drugs with fewer cardiovascular effects and a lower potential for histamine release.

Doses used have varied according to the degree of muscle relaxation required. In the UK initial doses of 15 to 30 mg have been given intravenously to adults with additional doses of 5 to 10 mg given at intervals of 25 to 60 minutes if required to maintain muscle relaxation. In the USA lower doses have generally been used. An initial dose of 6 to 9 mg intravenously has been suggested followed by 3 to 4.5 mg after 3 to 5 minutes if necessary; additional doses of 3 mg may be given as required for prolonged procedures. Tubocurarine should be given with caution in reduced doses to patients with renal impairment; if large or repeated doses are given neuromuscular block may be prolonged. Tubocurarine chloride has also been used to control the muscle spasms of tetanus (p.1304).

Preparations

USP 23: Tubocurarine Chloride Injection.

Proprietary Preparations (details are given in Part 3)
Canad.: Tubarine†; ***Ital.:*** Tubarine†; ***Spain:*** Curarina Miro; ***UK:*** Jexin†; Tubarine†.

Vecuronium Bromide (14012-x)

Vecuronium Bromide *(BAN, USAN, rINN).*

Org-NC-45. 1-(3α,17β-Diacetoxy-2β-piperidino-5α-androstan-16β-yl)-1-methylpiperidinium bromide.

$C_{34}H_{57}BrN_2O_4$ = 637.7.

CAS — 50700-72-6.

Incompatibility. A solution containing vecuronium bromide 1 mg per mL was found to be visually incompatible with frusemide.[1] For incompatibilities of competitive neuromuscular blockers in general, see under Atracurium on p.1304.

1. Chiu MF, Schwartz ML. Visual compatibility of injectable drugs used in the intensive care unit. *Am J Health-Syst Pharm* 1997; **54:** 64–5.

Adverse Effects, Treatment, and Precautions

As for competitive neuromuscular blockers in general (see Atracurium, p.1304).

Vecuronium bromide has little histamine-releasing activity although a local reaction at the site of injection has been reported. Bronchospasm and anaphylactoid reactions have been rarely reported. Also it has little vagolytic or ganglion-blocking activity and at usual doses vecuronium bromide produces no significant adverse cardiovascular effects.

Caution may be needed in patients with hepatic or renal impairment; dosage adjustments may be required in renal failure.

Elderly. It has been recommended that neuromuscular function should be monitored in elderly patients receiving vecuronium since there may be a risk of prolonged block.[1]

1. Slavov V, *et al.* Comparison of duration of neuromuscular blocking effect of atracurium and vecuronium in young and elderly patients. *Br J Anaesth* 1995; **74:** 709–11.

Hepatic impairment. The duration of action of vecuronium is reported to be significantly prolonged in patients with cholestasis[1] or cirrhosis with oesophageal varices[2] given a dose of 200 μg per kg body-weight intravenously. Plasma clearance was significantly reduced and the elimination half-life significantly increased from a mean of 58 to 98 minutes.[1] A dose of 150 μg per kg was found to have a similar onset and duration of action in patients with hepatic impairment and healthy controls,[2] but a dose of 100 μg per kg had a slower onset and slightly shorter duration of action in those with liver disturbance.[3] Following a dose of vecuronium, rapid and extensive hepatic uptake occurs which largely determines its short duration of action. However, as the dose increases this mechanism becomes saturated and hepatic elimination becomes more important in terminating activity. This would help to explain the variation in results seen with the different doses. Caution is needed if large single doses or repeated doses are given to patients with hepatic impairment.

1. Lebrault C, *et al.* Pharmacokinetics and pharmacodynamics of vecuronium in patients with cholestasis. *Br J Anaesth* 1986; **58:** 983–7.
2. Hunter JM, *et al.* The use of different doses of vecuronium in patients with liver dysfunction. *Br J Anaesth* 1985; **57:** 758–64.
3. Bell CF, *et al.* Use of atracurium and vecuronium in patients with oesophageal varices. *Br J Anaesth* 1985; **57:** 160–8.

Renal impairment. A small proportion of vecuronium bromide is excreted in urine and it may be given in usual doses to patients with renal failure.[1,2] No clinically significant difference in elimination half-life, clearance, or duration of action were reported[1] between patients with renal failure and those with normal renal function. The onset of neuromuscular block may be slightly slower in renal failure[2] and these patients may require an increase of around 20% in the initial dose of vecuronium.[3] However, the dosage requirement for maintenance of neuromuscular block may be reduced by about 20%[3] and slight prolongation of block may occur if dosage is not adjusted, but reversal of residual block with neostigmine is prompt and effective.[2]

Resistance to vecuronium has been reported[2] in 2 anephric patients. Total doses of 620 and 660 μg per kg body-weight produced maximum neuromuscular block of 77% and 36% but despite the high doses used there were no adverse effects or residual curarisation.

1. Fahey MR, *et al.* Pharmacokinetics of Org NC 45 (Norcuron) in patients with and without renal failure. *Br J Anaesth* 1981; **53:** 1049–53.
2. Hunter JM, *et al.* Comparison of vecuronium, atracurium and tubocurarine in normal patients and in patients with no renal function. *Br J Anaesth* 1984; **56:** 941–51.
3. Gramstad L. Atracurium, vecuronium and pancuronium in end-stage renal failure: dose-response properties and interactions with azathioprine. *Br J Anaesth* 1987; **59:** 995–1003.

Interactions

For interactions associated with competitive neuromuscular blockers, see Atracurium, p.1306.

Pharmacokinetics

Following intravenous administration vecuronium is rapidly distributed. It is taken up by the liver and partly metabolised; the metabolites have some neuromuscular blocking activity. It is excreted mainly in bile as unchanged drug and metabolites; some is also excreted in urine. The plasma elimination half-life is reported to range from about 30 to 80 minutes.

Pregnancy. The proportion of vecuronium crossing the placenta following doses of 60 to 80 μg per kg body-weight was considered clinically insignificant and its use during obstetric anaesthesia was considered safe for the newborn.[1]

1. Demetriou M, *et al.* Placental transfer of Org NC 45 in women undergoing caesarean section. *Br J Anaesth* 1982; **54:** 643–5.

Uses and Administration

Vecuronium bromide is an aminosteroidal competitive neuromuscular blocker (see Atracurium, p.1308).

Following intravenous injection muscle relaxation occurs within about 1.5 to 2 minutes and lasts for about 20 to 30 minutes.

Vecuronium bromide is used for endotracheal intubation and to provide muscle relaxation in general anaesthesia for surgical procedures (see Anaesthesia, p.1302) and to aid controlled ventilation (see Intensive Care, p.1303). The usual initial dose for intubation is 80 to 100 μg per kg body-weight by intravenous injection. Higher initial doses ranging from 150 to 300 μg per kg have sometimes been used for other procedures. However, it is recommended that the dose should not exceed 100 μg per kg in caesarean section or neonatal surgery. Maintenance doses of 20 to 30 μg per kg may be given as required during prolonged procedures; in the USA a lower maintenance dose of 10 to 15 μg per kg is recommended. Neuromuscular blockade may also be maintained with an intravenous infusion given at a rate of 0.8 to 1.4 μg per kg per minute but should be preceeded by an initial bolus injection of 40 to 100 μg per kg. The manufacturers recommend that in obese patients the dosage of vecuronium should be reduced taking into account lean body-mass.

Children older than 5 months can be given adult doses but children up to 1 year may have a more rapid response and the high initial dose for intubation may not be necessary. Neonates and infants below 5 months of age may be more sensitive to vecuronium and it is recommended that they should be given an initial test dose of 10 to 20 μg per kg, followed by increments according to response. The duration of action and recovery is longer in neonates and infants than in children and adults and they may require smaller maintenance doses administered less frequently.

Reviews of vecuronium.

1. Miller RD, *et al.* Clinical pharmacology of vecuronium and atracurium. *Anesthesiology* 1984; **61:** 444–53.
2. Reilly CS, Nimmo WS. New intravenous anaesthetics and neuromuscular blocking drugs: a review of their properties and clinical use. *Drugs* 1987; **34:** 98–135.

Preparations

Proprietary Preparations (details are given in Part 3)
Aust.: Norcuron; ***Austral.:*** Norcuron; ***Belg.:*** Norcuron; ***Canad.:*** Norcuron; ***Ger.:*** Norcuron; ***Irl.:*** Norcuron; ***Ital.:*** Norcuron; ***Neth.:*** Norcuron; ***Norw.:*** Norcuron; ***S.Afr.:*** Norcuron; ***Spain:*** Norcuron; ***Swed.:*** Norcuron; ***Switz.:*** Norcuron; ***UK:*** Norcuron; ***USA:*** Norcuron.

Nonionic Surfactants

A surfactant is a compound that can reduce the interfacial tension between 2 immiscible phases. This is due to the molecule containing 2 localised regions, one being hydrophilic in nature and the other hydrophobic.

The properties of nonionic surfactants are largely dependent on the proportions of these 2 groups in the molecule. Hydrophilic groups include the oxyethylene group ($-O.CH_2.CH_2-$) and the hydroxyl group ($-OH$). By varying the number of these groups in a hydrophobic molecule, such as a fatty acid, substances are obtained which range from strongly hydrophobic and water-insoluble compounds, such as glyceryl monostearate, to strongly hydrophilic and water-soluble compounds, such as the macrogols. These 2 extreme types are not satisfactory as emulsifying agents, though they are useful stabilisers in the presence of efficient emulsifying agents. Between these extremes are the nonionic emulsifying agents in which the proportions of hydrophilic and hydrophobic groups are more evenly balanced; these include some of the macrogol esters and ethers and sorbitan derivatives. By virtue of the processes used in their manufacture, nonionic surfactants are usually mixtures of related compounds; the properties of a particular material may vary from one manufacturer to another and there may be variation in batches from an individual source.

Nonionic surfactants differ from anionic surfactants (p.1468) by the absence of charge on, or ionisation of, the molecule; they are generally less irritant than anionic or cationic surfactants.

In addition to their use as emulsifiers some nonionic surfactants are also used in pharmacy as solubilising and wetting agents. Nonionic surfactants have applications in the food, cosmetic, paint, pesticide, and textile industries as well as being used as oil slick dispersants. Some macrogol ethers such as nonoxinol 9 are used as spermicides.

Since nonionic surfactants do not ionise to any great extent in solution, they are generally compatible with both anionic and cationic substances, but they reduce the antimicrobial action of many preservatives.

Nonionic surfactants may be classified according to their hydrophilic-lipophilic balance (HLB). This is an arbitrary scale of values denoting the relative affinity of the surfactant for oil and water. Lipophilic surfactants have low HLB values (less than 10) and are generally used as antifoaming agents, water-in-oil emulsifying agents, and as wetting agents; hydrophilic surfactants have higher HLB values (greater than 10) and are generally used as oil-in-water emulsifying agents and solubilising agents.

The range of nonionic surfactants used in pharmaceutical practice is large and their classification can be varied and complex. The principal groups of nonionic surfactants are outlined below.

Glycol and glycerol esters are a group of nonionic surfactants consisting of fatty acid esters of glycols and glycerol. Hydrophobic properties predominate and these compounds are poor emulsifying agents if used alone, though they are useful stabilisers for both oil-in-water and water-in-oil emulsions. If a small amount of soap, sulphated fatty alcohol, or other surfactant is added to the esters, a 'self-emulsifying' product is formed which is capable of producing satisfactory oil-in-water emulsions. **Acetoglycerides** are mixed glyceryl esters in which the glycerol is esterified partly with a fatty acid and partly with acetic acid.

Macrogol esters are polyoxyethylene esters of fatty acids, mainly stearates. The hydrophilic properties of the oxyethylene group are weaker than those of the hydroxyl group but by introducing a sufficient number into a fatty acid molecule, substances are produced in which the hydrophilic and hydrophobic properties are sufficiently well balanced for the esters to act as efficient oil-in-water emulsifying agents. They may also be used as wetting and solubilising agents. Since the ester linkage is prone to hydrolysis, these compounds are less resistant to acids and alkalis than the macrogol ethers.

Macrogol ethers are condensation products prepared by reaction between fatty alcohols or alkylphenols and ethylene oxide. The ether linkage confers good stability to acids and alkalis. Macrogol ethers are widely used in the preparation of oil-in-water emulsions and as wetting and solubilising agents.

Sorbitan derivatives are derivatives of the cyclic mono- or di-anhydrides of sorbitol. They consist of *sorbitan esters* which are prepared by esterification of one or more of the hydroxyl groups in the anhydrides with a fatty acid such as stearic, palmitic, oleic, or lauric acid, and *polysorbates* which are polyoxyethylene derivatives of the sorbitan esters. Sorbitan esters are oil-soluble, water-dispersible, nonionic surfactants which are effective water-in-oil emulsifiers. Polysorbates are more hydrophilic, water-soluble compounds and are used as oil-in-water emulsifying agents. By varying the number of oxyethylene groups in the molecule, and the type of fatty acid in the sorbitan ester, surfactants with a wide range of properties may be obtained.

Poloxamers are copolymers of polyoxyethylene and polyoxypropylene. They are used as oil-in-water emulsifiers and as solubilising and wetting agents in a variety of pharmaceutical preparations intended for internal use.

Other nonionic compounds with surface activity such as the higher fatty alcohols are covered in the chapter on Paraffins and Similar Bases (p.1382).

Acetoglycerides (9971-f)

Acetoglycerides are mixed glyceryl esters in which the glycerol is esterified partly with a fatty acid and partly with acetic acid.

Diacetylated Monoglycerides (486-g)

Pharmacopoeias. In *USNF.*

Consists of glycerol esterified with edible fat-forming fatty acids and acetic acid.

A clear liquid. Very **soluble** in alcohol 80%, vegetable oils, and mineral oils; sparingly soluble in alcohol 70%. **Store** in airtight containers. Protect from light.

Mono- and Di-acetylated Monoglycerides

(13601-w)

Pharmacopoeias. In *USNF.*

Consists of glycerol esterified with edible fat-forming fatty acids and acetic acid.

A white to pale yellow waxy solid. M.p. about 45°. Practically **insoluble** in water; soluble in chloroform and ether; slightly soluble in carbon disulphide. **Store** in airtight containers. Protect from light.

Diacetylated monoglycerides and mono- and di-acetylated monoglycerides have been used as plasticisers.

---

p-Di-isobutyl-phenoxypolyethoxyethanol

(9985-v)

p-Di-isobutyl-phenoxypolyethoxyethanol is used as a spermicide.

Preparations

Proprietary Preparations (details are given in Part 3)
Canad.: Ortho-Gynol; ***Ger.:*** Ortho-Gynol†; ***Neth.:*** Ortho-Gynol†; ***UK:*** Ortho-Gynol†.

Ethylene Glycol Monostearate (433-c)

Ethylene Glycol Stearate; Éthylène Glycol (Stéarate d'); Ethylenglycoli Monostearas; Ethyleni Glycoli Stearas.

CAS — 111-60-4 (ethylene glycol monostearate); 4219-49-2 (ethylene glycol monopalmitate).

Pharmacopoeias. In *Eur.* (see p.viii).

A white or almost white, waxy solid consisting of a mixture of the palmitic and stearic acid esters of ethylene glycol and containing not less than 50% of monoesters from stearic acid and not more than 5% of free ethylene glycol. M.p. 54° to 60°. Practically **insoluble** in water; soluble in hot alcohol and in acetone. **Protect** from light.

Ethylene glycol monostearate has the properties of and is used for the same purposes as glyceryl monostearate or self-emulsifying glyceryl monostearate (below). Ethylene glycol monolaurate and mono-oleate, and diethylene glycol monostearate, monolaurate, and mono-oleate, have also been used.

Glyceryl Behenate (3270-j)

Pharmacopoeias. In *USNF.*

A mixture of glycerides of fatty acids, mainly behenic acid.

A fine powder with a faint odour. M.p. about 70°. Practically **insoluble** in water and in alcohol; soluble in chloroform. **Store** in airtight containers at a temperature not exceeding 35°.

Glyceryl behenate is used as a lubricant and binder in tablet-making.

Glyceryl Mono-oleate (434-k)

Monolein.

CAS — 25496-72-4 (glyceryl mono-oleate).

A mixture of the glycerides of oleic acid and other fatty acids, consisting mainly of the mono-oleate.

Glyceryl mono-oleate has similar properties to glyceryl monostearate or self-emulsifying glyceryl monostearate (below).

Glyceryl Monostearate (435-a)

Glycérol (Monostéarate de); Glyceroli Monostearas; GMS; Monostearin.

CAS — 31566-31-1 (glyceryl monostearate); 26657-96-5 (glyceryl monopalmitate).

Pharmacopoeias. In *Eur.* (see p.viii), *Int.*, *Jpn*, and *Pol.* Also in *USNF.*

Glyceryl Monostearate 40–50 (Ph. Eur.) is a mixture of monoacylglycerols, mostly stearoyl- and palmitoylglycerol, together with variable quantities of di- and tri-acylglycerols. It contains between 40 and 50% of 1-monoacylglycerols, calculated as 2,3-dihydroxypropyl stearate ($C_{21}H_{42}O_4$ = 358.6), and not more than 6% of free glycerol.

A white or almost white hard waxy mass or unctuous powder or flakes. M.p. 54° to 64°. Practically **insoluble** in water; soluble in ether and at 60° in alcohol. **Store** in airtight containers. Protect from light.

Glyceryl Monostearate (USNF) contains not less than 90% of monoglycerides of saturated fatty acids, chiefly glyceryl monostearate ($C_{21}H_{42}O_4$ = 358.6) and glyceryl monopalmitate ($C_{19}H_{38}O_4$ = 330.5). It may contain a suitable antioxidant.

A white wax-like solid, beads, or flakes with a slight fatty odour. M.p. not below 55°. **Insoluble** in water but may be dispersed in hot water with the aid of a small amount of soap or other suitable surfactant; soluble 1 in 10 of chloroform, 1 in 100 of ether and methyl alcohol, 1 in 33 of isopropyl alcohol; dissolves in hot organic solvents. **Store** in airtight containers. Protect from light.

Self-emulsifying Glyceryl Monostearate

(436-t)

Monostearin Emulsificans; Self-emulsifying Mono- and Diglycerides of Food Fatty Acids; Self-emulsifying Monostearin.

Pharmacopoeias. In *Br.*

A mixture consisting principally of mono-, di-, and triglycerides of stearic and palmitic acids, and of minor proportions of other fatty acids; it may also contain free fatty acids, free glycerol, and soap. The BP specifies that it contains not less than 30% of monoglycerides, not more than 7% of free glycerol, and not more than 6% of soap, calculated as sodium oleate, all calculated with reference to the anhydrous substance.

A white to cream-coloured, hard, waxy solid with a faint fatty odour. **Dispersible** in hot water; soluble in hot dehydrated alcohol and hot liquid paraffin; soluble in hot vegetable oils, but may give turbid solutions at concentrations below 20%.

Because of the presence of soap, it is **incompatible** with acids and high concentrations of ionisable salts, hard water, calcium compounds, zinc oxide, and oxides of heavy metals.

Uses

Glyceryl monostearate is a poor water-in-oil emulsifying agent but it is a useful stabiliser of water-in-oil and oil-in-water emulsions in preparations for internal and external use. It has emollient properties. Glyceryl monostearate is also used in the food and cosmetic industries.

It is usual to add a small amount of soap, sulphated fatty alcohol, or other surfactant, to glyceryl monostearate, which has the effect of making the product self-emulsifying and capable of producing satisfactory oil-in-water emulsions. Self-emulsifying glyceryl monostearate is used as an emulsifying agent for oils, fats, solvents, and waxes in the preparation of bases of the non-emulsified, emulsified, and vanishing-cream types. It is not intended for inclusion in preparations for internal use.

Aqueous preparations containing self-emulsifying glyceryl monostearate should contain a preservative to prevent fungal or bacterial growth.

Macrogol Cetostearyl Ethers

(10485-r)

Macrogoli Aetherum Cetostearylicum.

Pharmacopoeias. In *Eur.* (see p.viii), which gives standards for compounds containing from 2 to 33 units of ethylene oxide per molecule (nominal value).

Mixtures of ethers of mixed macrogols with linear fatty alcohols, mainly cetostearyl alcohol. They may contain some free macrogols and various amounts of free cetostearyl alcohol.

White or yellowish-white waxy, unctuous masses, pellets, microbeads, or flakes.

Macrogol cetostearyl ethers with low numbers of ethylene oxide units per molecule are practically **insoluble** in water; soluble in alcohol and in dichloromethane. Macrogol cetostearyl ethers with higher numbers of ethylene oxide units per molecule are dispersible or soluble in water; soluble in alcohol and in dichloromethane.

Macrogol cetostearyl ethers solidify at 32° to 52°. **Store** in airtight containers.

Cetomacrogol 1000

(445-x)

Cetomacrogol 1000 *(BAN, rINN).*

Polyethylene Glycol 1000 Monocetyl Ether; Polyoxyethylene Glycol 1000 Monocetyl Ether.

CAS — 9004-95-9; 68439-49-6.

Pharmacopoeias. In *Br.* and *Int.*

A macrogol ether containing 20 to 24 oxyethylene groups in the polyoxyethylene chain. It is represented by the formula $CH_3.[CH_2]_m.[O.CH_2.CH_2]_n.OH$, where *m* may be 15 or 17 and *n* may be 20 to 24.

An odourless or almost odourless cream-coloured waxy unctuous mass, pellets, or flakes, melting when heated, to a clear brownish-yellow liquid. M.p. not lower than 38°.

Soluble in water, alcohol, and acetone; practically insoluble in petroleum spirit. It has been reported to be **incompatible** with phenols and to reduce the antibacterial activity of quaternary ammonium compounds. Cetomacrogol may separate from solutions in the presence of a high concentration of electrolytes.

Macrogol cetostearyl ethers are used as surfactants and emulsifiers. Cetomacrogol 1000 is used with cetostearyl alcohol (for example, in the form of Cetomacrogol Emulsifying Wax BP 1998) as an emulsifying agent for making oil-in-water emulsions that are unaffected by moderate concentrations of electrolytes and that are stable over a wide pH range. It is also used to disperse volatile oils in water to form transparent sols.

Preparations

BP 1998: Cetomacrogol Emulsifying Wax *(Emulsifying Wax, Non-ionic).*

Proprietary Preparations (details are given in Part 3)

Multi-ingredient: ***UK:*** Lipobase.

Polyoxyl 20 Cetostearyl Ether

(459-m)

Pharmacopoeias. In *USNF.*

A mixture of the monocetostearyl (mixed hexadecyl and octadecyl) ethers of mixed macrogols, the average polymer length being equivalent to 17.2 to 25.0 oxyethylene units.

A cream-coloured waxy unctuous mass melting, when heated, to a clear brownish-yellow liquid. **Soluble** in water, alcohol, and acetone; practically insoluble in petroleum spirit. A 10% solution in water has a pH of 4.5 to 7.5. **Store** in a cool place in airtight containers.

Macrogol Lauryl Ethers

(13605-j)

α-Dodecyl-ω-hydroxypoly(oxyethylene); Laureth Compounds; Lauromacrogols; Macrogoli Aetherum Laurilicum; Polyoxyl Lauryl Ethers.

CAS — 9002-92-0.

Pharmacopoeias. In *Eur.* (see p.viii), which gives standards for compounds containing from 3 to 23 units of ethylene oxide per molecule (nominal value).

Mixtures of ethers of mixed macrogols with linear fatty alcohols, mainly lauryl alcohol, represented by the formula $C_{12}H_{25}(OCH_2CH_2)_nOH$. They may contain some free macrogols and various amounts of free lauryl alcohol.

Macrogol lauryl ethers with 3 to 5 units of ethylene oxide per molecule are colourless liquids. Practically **insoluble** in water and in petroleum spirit; soluble or dispersible in alcohol.

Macrogol lauryl ethers with 9 to 23 units of ethylene oxide per molecule are white, waxy masses. **Soluble** or dispersible in water; soluble in alcohol; practically insoluble in petroleum spirit.

Macrogol lauryl ethers should be **stored** in airtight containers.

Laureth 2

(11352-c)

A mixture of monolauryl ethers of macrogols where the average value of *n* in the formula given above is 2.

Laureth 4

(447-f)

Laureth 4 *(USAN).*

CAS — 9002-92-0.

A mixture of monolauryl ethers of macrogols where the average value of *n* in the formula given above is 4.

Laureth 9

(448-d)

Laureth 9 *(USAN).*

Lauromacrogol 400 *(rINN)*; Polidocanol.

CAS — 9002-92-0; 3055-99-0.

NOTE. Lauromacrogol 400 has sometimes been erroneously described as containing 8, rather than 9, oxyethylene groups.

Pharmacopoeias. In *Jpn.*

A mixture of monolauryl ethers of macrogols where the average value of *n* in the formula given above is 9.

Adverse Effects

There have been occasional reports of allergic skin reactions following the topical application of preparations containing laureth compounds.

A 63-year-old man developed pulmonary oedema, a dramatic fall in heart rate, transient left pyramidal syndrome and died following sclerotherapy with laureth 9 to control gastric variceal bleeding;[1] the fatality was attributed to the action of the drug that had passed into the systemic circulation. Another patient has been described[2] who suffered a reversible ischaemic neurological deficit after sclerotherapy with laureth 9 for varicose veins of the leg.

1. Paterlini A, *et al.* Heart failure and endoscopic sclerotherapy of variceal bleeding. *Lancet* 1984; **i:** 1241.

2. Van der Plas JPL, *et al.* Reversible ischaemic neurological deficit after sclerotherapy of varicose veins. *Lancet* 1994; **343:** 428.

Uses and Administration

Macrogol lauryl ethers (laureth compounds) have been used as surfactants and spermicides. Laureth 9 is used as a sclerosant (see under Ethanolamine Oleate, p.1576) in the treatment of oesophageal and gastric varices and has been used as a local anaesthetic and antipruritic in combination topical preparations.

Preparations

Proprietary Preparations (details are given in Part 3)

Aust.: Aethoxysklerol; ***Belg.:*** Aethoxysklerol; ***Fr.:*** Aetoxisclerol; Veinosclerol; ***Ger.:*** Aethoxysklerol; Hamo-Europuran N; Recessan; ***Ital.:*** Atossisclerol Kreussler; ***Neth.:*** Aethoxysklerol; ***Spain:*** Etoxisclerol; ***Swed.:*** Aethoxysklerol; ***Switz.:*** Aethoxysklerol.

Multi-ingredient: ***Aust.:*** Balneum Hermal Plus; Dentinox; Paididont; Prurimix; Recessan; Solcoseryl comp; Vonum; ***Austral.:*** Alcos-Anal†; Collomack†; ***Belg.:*** Neo-Alcos-Anal; ***Canad.:*** Fostex CM†; ***Ger.:*** Acoin; Alcos-Anal; Anaesthesulf P; Azulon liquidum Homburg†; Balneum Plus; Brand- u. Wundgel-Medice N; Collomack; Corti-Dynexan; Dentinox N; Dermaethyl-H†; Dermaethyl†; Dexamed†; Dynexan MHP†; HAEMO-Exhirud; Hamoagil†; Hepathrombin-Procto†; Hexamon N; Inflam; Meaverin; Medigel; Mediphon†; Optiderm; Pruriderm ultra†; Rectosellan H; Rectosellan N†; Sagittaproct S; Scandicain†; Siozwo†; Solcoseryl Dental; Tamposit N; Tamposit†; Thesit; Thesit P; Thrombimed†; Transpulmin†; Varitan N; Vaxicum N; Vehiculan NF†; Vivisun; Vonum cutan†; ***Irl.:*** Balneum Plus; ***Ital.:*** Optiderm; ***Norw.:*** Alcos-Anal; ***S.Afr.:*** Tyrogel†; ***Switz.:*** Alcos-Anal†; Balneum Plus; Baume†; Decasept; Dentinox; Eludril; Optiderm; Oxydermine; Pruri-med; Ralur; Solcoseryl Dental; Sportusal; Sportusal Spray sine heparino; ***UK:*** Anacal; Balneum Plus; ***USA:*** Lubrin.

Macrogol Monomethyl Ethers

(15825-t)

Polyethylene Glycol Monomethyl Ethers. α-Methyl-ω-hydroxypoly(oxyethylene).

CAS — 9004-74-4.

Pharmacopoeias. In *USNF* which gives standards for compounds having nominal average molecular weights in the range of 350 to 10 000.

A series of monomethyl ethers of macrogols of differing chain lengths, represented by the formula $CH_3(OCH_2CH_2)_nOH$. The name is usually designated by a number that corresponds approximately to its average molecular weight.

As the average molecular weight increases the water solubility and solubility in organic solvents decreases while viscosity increases. Liquid grades occur as clear to slightly hazy, colourless or practically colourless, slightly hygroscopic, viscous liquids with a slight characteristic odour. Solid grades occur as practically odourless, white, waxy, plastic material or as creamy white flakes, beads, or powders. **Store** in airtight containers.

Macrogol monomethyl ethers may be used as ointment bases, solvents, and plasticisers.

Macrogol Oleyl Ethers

(10492-x)

Macrogoli Aetherum Oleicum.

Pharmacopoeias. In *Eur.* (see p.viii), which gives standards for compounds containing from 2 to 20 units of ethylene oxide per molecule (nominal value).

Mixtures of ethers of mixed macrogols with linear fatty alcohols, mainly oleyl alcohol. They may contain some free macrogols and various amounts of free oleyl alcohol.

Macrogol oleyl ethers with 2 to 5 units of ethylene oxide per molecule are yellow liquids. Practically **insoluble** in water and in petroleum spirit; soluble in alcohol.

Macrogol oleyl ethers with 10 to 20 units of ethylene oxide per molecule are yellowish-white, waxy masses. **Dispersible** or soluble in water; soluble in alcohol; practically insoluble in petroleum spirit.

Macrogol oleyl ethers should be **stored** in airtight containers. Protect from light.

Polyoxyl 10 Oleyl Ether

(460-t)

Polyethylene Glycol Mono-oleyl Ether.

CAS — 9004-98-2.

Pharmacopoeias. In *USNF.*

A mixture of the mono-oleyl ethers of mixed macrogols, the average polymer length being equivalent to 8.6 to 10.4 oxyethylene units. It may contain suitable stabilisers.

A soft white semisolid or pale yellow liquid with a bland odour. **Soluble** in water and alcohol; dispersible in liquid paraffin and propylene glycol with possible separation on standing. **Store** in a cool place in airtight containers.

Macrogol oleyl ethers such as polyoxyl 10 oleyl ether are used as surfactants.

Menfegol

(748-l)

Menfegol *(rINN).*

Menphegol. α-[*p*-(*p*-Menthyl)phenyl]-ω-hydroxypoly(oxyethylene).

CAS — 57821-32-6.

Menthylphenyl ethers of macrogols represented by the formula $C_{16}H_{23}(OCH_2CH_2)_nOH$.

Menfegol is a nonionic surfactant used as a spermicide.

Mono- and Di-glycerides (487-q)

E471 (mono- and di-glycerides of fatty acids).

Pharmacopoeias. In *USNF.*

A mixture of glycerol mono- and di-esters, with minor amounts of tri-esters, of fatty acids from edible oils. It contains not less than 40% of monoglycerides. It may contain suitable stabilisers.

It varies in consistency from yellow liquids through ivory-coloured plastics to hard, ivory-coloured solids having a bland odour. Practically **insoluble** in water; soluble in alcohol, chloroform, other chlorinated hydrocarbons, and ethyl acetate. **Store** in airtight containers. Protect from light.

Mono- and di-glycerides is used as an emulsifying agent.

Nonoxinols (450-k)

Macrogol Nonylphenyl Ethers; Nonoxynols. α-(4-Nonylphenyl)-ω-hydroxypoly(oxyethylene).

CAS — 26027-38-3.

NOTE. Nonoxinol is *BAN* and *rINN*. The name may be followed by a figure indicating the approximate number of oxyethylene groups in the polyoxyethylene chain.
USAN specifies Nonoxynol 4, Nonoxynol 9, Nonoxynol 15, and Nonoxynol 30.

A series of nonylphenyl ethers of macrogols of differing chain lengths, represented by the formula $C_{15}H_{23}.[O.CH_2.CH_2]_n.OH$.

Nonoxinol 9 (452-t)

Nonoxinol 9 *(BAN, rINN).*

Nonoxynol 9 *(USAN).* α-(4-Nonylphenyl)-ω-hydroxynona(oxyethylene).

$C_{33}H_{60}O_{10}$ (nominal) = 616.8.

Pharmacopoeias. In *US.*

A colourless to light yellow, clear viscous liquid. **Soluble** in water, alcohol, and maize oil. **Store** in airtight containers.

Nonoxinol 10 (453-x)

Nonoxinol 10 *(BAN, rINN).*

Nonoxynol 10. α-(4-Nonylphenyl)-ω-hydroxydeca(oxyethylene).

$C_{35}H_{64}O_{11}$ (nominal) = 660.9.

Pharmacopoeias. In *USNF.*

A colourless to light amber viscous liquid with an aromatic odour. **Soluble** in water and in polar organic solvents. **Store** in airtight containers.

Nonoxinol 11 (9983-m)

Nonoxinol 11 *(BAN, rINN).*

Nonoxynol 11. α-(4-Nonylphenyl)-ω-hydroxyundeca(oxyethylene).

$C_{37}H_{68}O_{12}$ (nominal) = 704.9.

Adverse Effects and Precautions

Nonoxinols used as vaginal spermicides may cause local irritation.

Pregnancy. Although maternal use of spermicidal contraceptives has been linked to an increased frequency of congenital abnormalities, including trisomy, the comment has been made that such studies are probably flawed by recall bias.[1] Meta-analysis of nine studies also supported the view that peri- and postconceptual maternal use of spermicides was not associated with adverse fetal outcome.[2]

1. Mishell DR. Contraception. *N Engl J Med* 1989; **320:** 777–87.
2. Einarson TR, *et al.* Maternal spermicide use and adverse reproductive outcome: a meta-analysis. *Am J Obstet Gynecol* 1990; **162:** 655–60.

Toxic shock syndrome. Thirteen cases of the toxic shock syndrome associated with the use of a vaginal contraceptive sponge impregnated with nonoxinol 9 were reviewed.[1] These had been reported in the USA up to November 1984. In 4 of the cases, there were other predisposing conditions; postpartum use, use during menstruation, and prolonged retention.

1. Faich G, *et al.* Toxic shock syndrome and the vaginal contraceptive sponge. *JAMA* 1986; **255:** 216–18.

Urinary-tract infection. Use of spermicidal foam or jelly containing nonoxinol 9 may disturb the normal vaginal flora and predispose to colonisation with *Escherichia coli* and the development of bacteriuria.[1] An increased risk of acute *E. coli* urinary-tract infection has been reported[2] associated with the use of condoms coated with nonoxinol 9.

1. Hooton TM, *et al.* Escherichia coli bacteriuria and contraceptive method. *JAMA* 1991; **265:** 64–9.
2. Fihn SD, *et al.* Association between use of spermicide-coated condoms and Escherichia coli urinary tract infection in young women. *Am J Epidemiol* 1996; **144:** 512–20.

Uses

Nonoxinols have surface active properties and may be used as solubilising agents. Nonoxinol 9 is used as a spermicide for contraception (p.1434).

Antimicrobial activity. It has been suggested that nonoxinol 9, when used as a spermicidal contraceptive, may also provide some protection against sexually transmitted diseases, including chlamydial and gonococcal infections.[1,2] It has also been tried in herpes simplex infections (p.597) and in the prophylaxis of human immunodeficiency virus (HIV) infection, but it is not clear whether it is of clinical benefit.[2] Indeed, a double-blind placebo-controlled study[3] involving 1292 HIV-negative female sex workers found that it did not reduce the rate of new HIV, gonorrhoea, or chlamydia infection.

1. North BB. Vaginal contraceptives: effective protection from sexually transmitted diseases for women? *J Reprod Med* 1988; **33:** 307–311.
2. Anonymous. Multipurpose spermicides. *Lancet* 1992; **340:** 211–13.
3. Roddy RE, *et al.* A controlled trial of nonoxynol 9 film to reduce male-to-female transmission of sexually transmitted diseases. *N Engl J Med* 1998; **339:** 504–10.

Preparations

Proprietary Preparations (details are given in Part 3)
Aust.: Contraceptivum†; Delfen; Patentex; ***Austral.:*** Delfen; Lubarol; Ortho-Creme; ***Belg.:*** Delfen†; Gynintim Film; Patentex; ***Canad.:*** Advantage 24; Delfen; Emko†; Encare; K-Y Personal Lubricant; Lifestyles; Ortho-Gynol II; Ramses; Sheik; Titan; Today†; Trojan; ***Fr.:*** Patentex; Semicid; ***Ger.:*** Ortho-Gel; Patentex Oval N; Patentex†; ***Irl.:*** Delfen; Gynol II; Ortho-Creme; Orthoforms; ***Ital.:*** C-Film; Patentex Ovuli†; ***Neth.:*** Delfen†; ***S.Afr.:*** Delfen; Emko†; Patentex†; ***Spain:*** C-Film†; Lineafarm; Nacha; Nobliten; Yadalan; ***Switz.:*** C-Film; Delfen; Patentex Oval N; Syn-A-Gen; ***UK:*** C-Film; Delfen; Double Check; Duracreme; Duragel; Gynol II; Ortho-Creme; Orthoforms; Staycept Pessaries†; Today; Two's Company†; ***USA:*** Advantage 24; Because; Delfen; Emko; Encare; Excita; Gynol; Koromex; Ortho-Creme†; Ramses; Semicid; Sheik Elite; Shur-Seal; Today; VCF.

Multi-ingredient: ***Canad.:*** Protectaid; ***Ger.:*** A-gen 53; ***Ital.:*** Agena; Betaform Habitat; Florigien; Vironox; ***Spain:*** Lavolen.

Octoxinols (456-d)

Macrogol Tetramethylbutylphenyl Ethers; Octoxynols; Octylphenoxy Polyethoxyethanol. α-[4-(1,1,3,3-Tetramethylbutyl)phenyl]-ω-hydroxypoly(oxyethylene).

CAS — 9002-93-1.

NOTE. Octoxinol is *BAN* and *rINN*. The name may be followed by a figure indicating the approximate number of oxyethylene groups in the polyoxyethylene chain.
USAN specifies Octoxynol 9.

A series of tetramethylbutylphenyl ethers of macrogols of differing chain lengths, represented by the formula $C_{14}H_{21}.[O.CH_2.CH_2]_n.OH$.

Octoxinol 9 (457-n)

Octoxinol 9 *(BAN, rINN).*

Octoxynol 9 *(USAN).*

$C_{32}H_{58}O_{10}$ (nominal) = 602.8.

Pharmacopoeias. In *USNF.*

A clear, pale yellow, viscous liquid with a faint odour. **Miscible** with water, alcohol, and acetone; soluble in toluene; practically insoluble in petroleum spirit. **Store** in airtight containers.

Uses

Octoxinols have surface active properties and may be used as solubilising agents. They are also used as spermicides.

Preparations

Proprietary Preparations (details are given in Part 3)
Austral.: Ortho-Gynol; Summer's Eve Disposable; ***Switz.:*** Ortho-Gynol†; ***UK:*** Staycept Jelly†; ***USA:*** Koromex; Ortho-Gynol.

Multi-ingredient: ***Austral.:*** Summer's Eve Feminine; ***USA:*** Feminique; Massengill; Massengill Disposable; New Freshness†; Summer's Eve Disposable.

Poloxamers (463-f)

Polyethylene-polypropylene glycol. α-Hydro-ω-hydroxypoly(oxyethylene)poly(oxypropylene)poly(oxyethylene) block copolymer.

CAS — 9003-11-6.

NOTE. Poloxamer is *BAN* and *rINN*. The name is followed by a figure, the first 2 digits of which, when multiplied by 100, correspond to the approximate average molecular weight of the polyoxypropylene portion and the third digit, when multiplied by 10, corresponds to the percentage by weight of the polyoxyethylene portion.
USAN specifies Poloxamer 182D, Poloxamer 182LF, Poloxamer 188, Poloxamer 188LF, and Poloxamer 331.
Poloxalene (*BAN, USAN, rINN*) is also a poloxamer.

Pharmacopoeias. In *USNF* under the title Poloxamer where specifications are given for Poloxamer 124, Poloxamer 188, Poloxamer 237, Poloxamer 338, and Poloxamer 407.

A series of nonionic polyoxyethylene-polyoxypropylene copolymers with the general formula $HO(C_2H_4O)_a(C_3H_6O)_b(C_2H_4O)_aH$.

The available grades vary from liquids to solids. A 2.5% solution in water has a pH of 5.0 to 7.5. Poloxamers have been reported to be **incompatible** with phenols. **Store** in airtight containers.

Poloxalene (464-d)

Poloxalene *(BAN, USAN, rINN).*

SKF-18667.

Pharmacopoeias. In *US* for veterinary use only.

A liquid poloxamer in which *a* in the general formula given above averages 12 and *b* averages 34; it has a molecular weight of about 3000. A colourless or pale yellow liquid. **Soluble** in water, in chloroform, and in ethylene dichloride. **Store** in airtight containers.

Poloxamer 188 (465-n)

Poloxamer 188 *(BAN, USAN, rINN).*

Poloxalkol.

NOTE. Compounded preparations of danthron and poloxamer 188 have the British Approved Name Co-danthramer; the proportions are expressed in the form *x/y*, where *x* and *y* are the strengths in milligrams of danthron and poloxamer respectively.

Pharmacopoeias. In *Br.* Also in *USNF* under the group title Poloxamer.

The BP specifies a poloxamer in which *a* in the general formula given above is about 75 and *b* about 30; it has an average molecular weight of 8350. The USNF specifies a poloxamer in which *a* averages 80 and *b* averages 27; it has an average molecular weight of 7680 to 9510.

White or almost white waxy flakes or powder, odourless or with a very mild odour. M.p. 52° to 55°. Freely **soluble** in water, alcohol, and methyl alcohol; practically insoluble in ether. **Store** in airtight containers.

Poloxamer 407 (9988-p)

Poloxamer 407 *(BAN, rINN).*

Pharmacopoeias. In *USNF* under the group title Poloxamer.

A poloxamer in which *a* in the general formula given above averages 101 and *b* averages 56; it has an average molecular weight of 9840 to 14 600.

A white solid, odourless or with a very mild odour. M.p. about 56°. Freely **soluble** in water, alcohol, and isopropyl alcohol. **Store** in airtight containers.

Precautions

Poloxamers may increase the absorption of liquid paraffin and other fat-soluble substances.

Uses and Administration

Poloxamers are used as emulsifying agents for intravenous fat emulsions, as solubilising agents to maintain clarity in elixirs and syrups, and as wetting agents for antibiotics. They may also be used in ointment or suppository bases and as tablet binders or coaters.

Poloxamer 188 is used as a wetting agent in the treatment of constipation. It is usually administered in combination with a laxative such as danthron. Poloxamer 188 has also been used as an emulsifying agent in fluorocarbon blood substitutes. Poloxamer 188 has been investigated for its ability to improve blood flow in sickle-cell crisis; it has also been tried in myocardial infarction. Other investigational uses include the treatment of burns.

Poloxamer 407 is used in solutions for contact lens care as is poloxamer 338.

Poloxalene is used as a defoaming agent in the treatment of bloat in ruminants.

Preparations

Proprietary Preparations (details are given in Part 3)
Austral.: Clerz; Coloxyl; Pliagel; ***Fr.:*** Alkenide; Idrocol.

Multi-ingredient: ***Aust.:*** Actizyme; ***Austral.:*** Comfortcare GP Dual Action; ***Irl.:*** Codalax; ***Ital.:*** Ultimex†; ***UK:*** Ailax; Codalax; ***USA:*** Baby Orajel Tooth and Gum Cleanser.

Polyoxyl Castor Oils (9982-h)

Macrogolglyceroli Ricinoleas; Polyethoxylated Castor Oils.

Pharmacopoeias. In *Eur.* (see p.viii), which gives standards for compounds containing ricinoleyl glycerol ethoxylated with 30 to 50 molecules of ethylene oxide per molecule (nominal value).

Mixtures containing mainly ethoxylated ricinoleyl glycerol, with small amounts of macrogol ricinoleate and the corresponding free glycols.

Clear, yellow, viscous liquids. Relative density about 1.05; viscosity, at 25°, 500 to 800 mPa s.

Freely **soluble** in water and in alcohol; very soluble in dichloromethane. **Protect** from light.

Polyoxyl 35 Castor Oil (18355-g)

Pharmacopoeias. In *USNF.*

A mixture of the triricinoleate ester of ethoxylated glycerol with smaller amounts of macrogol ricinoleate and the corresponding free glycols. It is produced by reacting 1 mole of glycerol ricinoleate with about 35 moles of ethylene oxide.

A yellow oily liquid with a faint characteristic odour. Sp. gr. 1.05 to 1.06; viscosity at 25°, 650 to 850 mPa s. Very **soluble** in water; soluble in alcohol and ethyl acetate; practically insoluble in mineral oils. **Store** in airtight containers.

Polyethoxylated castor oils are reported to affect polyvinyl chloride containers and apparatus adversely.

Adverse Effects

Polyoxyl castor oils (such as Cremophor EL), used as vehicles in various intravenous injections, have been associated with severe anaphylactoid reactions, hyperlipidaemias, alterations in blood viscosity, and erythrocyte aggregation.

References.

1. Bagnarello AG, *et al.* Unusual serum lipoprotein abnormality induced by the vehicle of miconazole. *N Engl J Med* 1977; **296:** 497–9.
2. Forrest ARW, *et al.* Long-term Althesin infusion and hyperlipidaemia. *Br Med J* 1977; **2:** 1357–8.
3. Dye D, Watkins J. Suspected anaphylactic reaction to Cremophor EL. *Br Med J* 1980; **280:** 1353.
4. Howrie DL, *et al.* Anaphylactoid reactions associated with parenteral cyclosporine use: possible role of Cremophor EL. *Drug Intell Clin Pharm* 1985; **19:** 425–7.
5. Chapuis B, *et al.* Anaphylactic reaction to intravenous cyclosporine. *N Engl J Med* 1985; **312:** 1259.
6. Siddall SJ, *et al.* Anaphylactic reactions to teniposide. *Lancet* 1989; **i:** 394.

Uses

Polyoxyl castor oils are macrogol esters used as emulsifying and solubilising agents. Polyoxyl 35 castor oil has been used as a solvent in vehicles for various intravenous injections.

Polyoxyl Hydrogenated Castor Oils

(19834-g)

Macrogolglyceroli Hydroxystearas.

Pharmacopoeias. In *Eur.* (see p.viii), which gives standards for compounds containing trihydroxystearyl glycerol ethoxylated with 7 to 60 molecules of ethylene oxide per molecule (nominal value).

Mixtures of mainly ethoxylated trihydroxystearyl glycerol with small amounts of macrogol hydroxystearate and the corresponding free glycols.

Polyoxyl hydrogenated castor oils with less than 10 units of ethylene oxide per molecule are yellowish, turbid, viscous liquids. Practically **insoluble** in water; dispersible in alcohol; soluble in acetone.

Polyoxyl hydrogenated castor oils with more than 20 units of ethylene oxide per molecule are white or yellowish, semi-liquid or pasty masses. Freely **soluble** in water, in alcohol, and in acetone; practically insoluble in petroleum spirit.

Polyoxyl 40 Hydrogenated Castor Oil

(18356-q)

Pharmacopoeias. In *USNF.*

A mixture of the trihydroxystearate ester of ethoxylated glycerol, with smaller amounts of macrogol trihydroxystearate and the corresponding free glycols. It is produced by reacting 1 mole of glycerol trihydroxystearate with about 40 to 45 moles of ethylene oxide.

A white to yellowish paste or pasty liquid with a faint odour. Congealing range 20° to 30°. Very **soluble** in water; soluble in alcohol and ethyl acetate; practically insoluble in mineral oils. **Store** in airtight containers.

Polyoxyl hydrogenated castor oils are used as surfactants.

Polyoxyl Stearates (13602-e)

Macrogol Stearates; Macrogoli Stearas; Polyoxyethylene Glycol Stearates; Polyoxyethylene Stearates.

CAS — 9004-99-3.

NOTE. Two systems of nomenclature are used for these compounds, which have the general formula $C_{17}H_{35}COO.[O.CH_2CH_2]_n.H$. The number '8' in the names 'Polyoxyl 8 Stearate' or 'Polyoxyethylene 8 Stearate' refers to the approximate polymer length in oxyethylene units. The number '400' in the names 'Macrogol Stearate 400' or 'Polyoxyethylene Glycol 400 Stearate' refers to the average molecular weight of the polymer chain.

Pharmacopoeias. In *Eur.* (see p.viii), which gives standards for compounds with average polymer lengths equivalent to 6 to 100 ethylene oxide units per molecule (nominal value).

Mixtures of the mono- and di-esters of mainly stearic acid and macrogols. They may contain some free macrogols.

White or slightly yellowish waxy masses. **Soluble** in alcohol and in isopropyl alcohol. Polyoxyl stearates containing 6 to 9 units of ethylene oxide per molecule are practically insoluble but freely dispersible in water; miscible with fatty oils and with waxes. Polyoxyl stearates containing 20 to 100 units of ethylene oxide per molecule are soluble in water; practically insoluble in fatty oils and in waxes.

Polyoxyl stearates should be **stored** in airtight containers.

Incompatibilities. Polyoxyl stearates have been reported to be generally stable with electrolytes and weak acids or bases although strong acids or bases may cause hydrolysis and saponification. Discoloration or precipitation may occur with phenolic substances and complexation with preservatives. Decrease in the antimicrobial activity of bacitracin, chloramphenicol, phenoxymethylpenicillin, and tetracycline has been stated to occur with concentrations of polyoxyl stearates exceeding 5%.

Polyoxyl 8 Stearate (440-z)

Polyoxyl 8 Stearate *(BAN, USAN).*

Macrogol Stearate 400 *(rINN)*; Macrogol Ester 400; Polyoxyethylene 8 Stearate; Polyoxyethylene Glycol 400 Stearate.

NOTE. The serial number 430 was used in the UK to identify polyoxyl 8 stearate when it was a permitted emulsifier and stabiliser in food.

A mixture of the monostearate and distearate esters of mixed macrogols and the corresponding free glycols, the average polymer length being equivalent to about 8 oxyethylene units.

Polyoxyl 40 Stearate (441-c)

Polyoxyl 40 Stearate *(BAN, USAN).*

Macrogol Stearate 2000 *(rINN)*; Estearato de Polioxila 40; Macrogol Ester 2000; Polyoxyethylene 40 Stearate; Stearethate 40.

NOTE. The serial number 431 was used in the UK to identify polyoxyl 40 stearate when it was a permitted emulsifier and stabiliser in food.

Pharmacopoeias. In *Jpn.* Also in *USNF.*

A mixture of the monostearate and distearate esters of mixed macrogols, the average polymer length being equivalent to about 40 oxyethylene units.

A waxy solid which is white to light tan in colour and is odourless or has a faint fatty odour. Congealing range 37° to 47°.

Soluble in water, alcohol, acetone, and ether; practically insoluble in liquid paraffin and vegetable oils. **Store** in airtight containers.

Polyoxyl 50 Stearate (442-k)

Polyoxyethylene 50 Stearate.

Pharmacopoeias. In *USNF.*

A mixture of the monostearate and distearate esters of mixed macrogols and the corresponding free glycols, the average polymer length being equivalent to about 50 oxyethylene units.

A cream-coloured soft waxy solid with a faint fatty odour. M.p. about 45°. **Soluble** 1 in 0.7 of water, 1 in 13 000 of dehydrated alcohol, 1 in 0.45 of chloroform, and 1 in 14 000 of ether. Soluble in isopropyl alcohol. **Store** in airtight containers.

Polyoxyl stearates are macrogol esters which are used as emulsifying and solubilising agents. Polyoxyl 8 monolaurate, and the mono-oleate and di-oleate esters have also been used.

Preparations

Proprietary Preparations (details are given in Part 3)

Multi-ingredient: ***Austral.:*** Blink-N-Clean†; ***Ger.:*** Lens Fresh.

Polysorbates (13603-l)

A series of mixtures of fatty acid esters of sorbitol and its anhydrides copolymerised with approximately 20 moles of ethylene oxide for each mole of sorbitol and its anhydrides.

Incompatibilities. Polysorbates have been reported to be stable with electrolytes and weak acids and bases although saponification may occur in the presence of strong acids and bases. Discoloration or precipitation may occur with phenolic substances. The oleic acid esters are sensitive to oxidation. For reference to the possible incompatibility of polysorbate 80 with hydroxybenzoates, see p.1117.

Polysorbate 20 (472-d)

Polysorbate 20 *(BAN, USAN, rINN).*

432; Polyoxyethylene 20 Sorbitan Monolaurate; Polysorbatum 20; Sorbimacrogol Laurate 300; Sorboxaethenum Laurinicum.

$C_{58}H_{114}O_{26}$ (approximate).

CAS — 9005-64-5.

Pharmacopoeias. In *Eur.* (see p.viii) and *Int.* Also in *USNF.*

A mixture of partial lauric esters of sorbitol and its anhydrides copolymerised with approximately 20 moles of ethylene oxide for each mole of sorbitol and its anhydrides. The lauric acid used for esterification may contain variable amounts of other fatty acids.

A clear or slightly opalescent yellowish or brownish-yellow oily liquid with a faint characteristic odour. Relative density about 1.1. **Miscible** with water, with alcohol, with methyl alcohol, with dioxan, and with ethyl acetate; practically insoluble in liquid paraffin. **Store** in airtight containers. Protect from light.

Polysorbate 40 (427-a)

Polysorbate 40 *(BAN, USAN, rINN).*

434; Polyoxyethylene 20 Sorbitan Monopalmitate; Sorbimacrogol Palmitate 300.

$C_{62}H_{122}O_{26}$ (approximate).

CAS — 9005-66-7.

Pharmacopoeias. In *USNF.*

A mixture of palmitic esters of sorbitol and its anhydrides copolymerised with approximately 20 moles of ethylene oxide for each mole of sorbitol and its anhydrides.

A yellow liquid with a faint characteristic odour. **Miscible** with water and alcohol; practically insoluble in liquid paraffin and in fixed oils. **Store** in airtight containers. Protect from light.

Polysorbate 60 (474-h)

Polysorbate 60 *(BAN, USAN, rINN).*

435; Polyoxyethylene 20 Sorbitan Monostearate; Polysorbatum 60; Sorbimacrogol Stearate 300; Sorboxaethenum Stearinicum.

$C_{64}H_{126}O_{26}$ (approximate).

CAS — 9005-67-8.

Pharmacopoeias. In *Eur.* (see p.viii), *Int.*, and *Pol.* Also in *USNF.*

A mixture of partial stearic esters of sorbitol and its anhydrides copolymerised with approximately 20 moles of ethylene oxide for each mole of sorbitol and its anhydrides. The stearic acid used for esterification may contain variable amounts of other fatty acids, especially palmitic acid.

A lemon to orange-coloured oily liquid or semi-gel or yellowish-brown gelatinous mass which becomes a clear liquid above 25°; it has a faint characteristic odour. Relative density about 1.1. **Miscible** with water, with alcohol, with methyl alcohol, with ethyl acetate, and with toluene; practically insoluble in liquid paraffin and in fixed oils. **Store** in airtight containers. Protect from light.

Polysorbate 65 (475-m)

Polysorbate 65 *(BAN, USAN, rINN).*

436; Polyoxyethylene 20 Sorbitan Tristearate; Sorbimacrogol Tristearate 300.

$C_{100}H_{194}O_{28}$ (approximate).

CAS — 9005-71-4.

A mixture of mainly tristearate esters of sorbitol and its anhydrides copolymerised with approximately 20 moles of ethylene oxide for each mole of sorbitol and its anhydrides.

A tan-coloured waxy solid with a faint characteristic odour. **Dispersible** in water; soluble in alcohol, liquid paraffin, and fixed oils. **Store** in airtight containers. Protect from light.

Polysorbate 80 (476-b)

Polysorbate 80 *(BAN, USAN, rINN).*

433; Olethytan 20; Polyäthylenglykol-Sorbitanoleat; Polyoxyethylene 20 Sorbitan Mono-oleate; Polysorbatum 80; Polysorbitanum 80 Oleinatum; Sorbimacrogol Oleate 300; Sorboxaethenum Oleinicum; Sorethytan 20 Mono-oleate.

$C_{64}H_{124}O_{26}$ (approximate).

CAS — 9005-65-6.

Pharmacopoeias. In *Chin.*, *Eur.* (see p.viii), *Int.*, *Jpn*, and *Pol.* Also in *USNF.*

A mixture of partial oleic esters of sorbitol and its anhydrides copolymerised with approximately 20 moles of ethylene oxide for each mole of sorbitol and its anhydrides.

A clear yellowish or brownish-yellow oily liquid with a faint characteristic odour. Relative density about 1.08; viscosity, at 25°, about 400 mPa s. **Miscible** with water, with alcohol, with ethyl acetate, and with methyl alcohol; practically insoluble in liquid paraffin and in fixed oils. **Store** in airtight containers. Protect from light.

Polysorbate 85 (477-v)

Polysorbate 85 *(BAN, USAN, rINN).*

Polyoxyethylene 20 Sorbitan Trioleate; Sorbimacrogol Trioleate 300.

$C_{100}H_{188}O_{28}$ (approximate).

CAS — 9005-70-3.

A mixture of mainly trioleate esters of sorbitol and its anhydrides copolymerised with approximately 20 moles of ethylene oxide for each mole of sorbitol and its anhydrides.

An amber-coloured oily liquid with a faint characteristic odour. **Dispersible** in water; soluble in alcohol. **Store** in airtight containers. Protect from light.

Adverse Effects and Precautions

Polysorbates may increase the absorption of fat-soluble substances.

There have been occasional reports of hypersensitivity following topical application of preparations containing polysorbates.

Fatalities in low birth-weight infants associated with the injection of a polysorbate-containing preparation are discussed below.

Effects in infants. Following the introduction in the USA of an intravenous preparation of vitamin E (E-Ferol) there were a number of reports of unusual liver and kidney disorders with 38 deaths being reported among treated low birth-weight infants. Affected infants had unexplained hypotension, thrombocytopenia, renal dysfunction, hepatomegaly, cholestasis, ascites, and metabolic acidosis;[1-3] the preparation was subsequently withdrawn from the market in April 1984 about 5 months after it was introduced. *In-vitro* evidence was produced demonstrating that E-Ferol suppressed the response of human lymphocytes to phytohaemagglutinin. However, it was the mixture of polysorbates, polysorbate 20 and in particular polysorbate 80, that was shown to be responsible for this suppression rather than the α-tocopherol acetate component. Despite this *in-vitro* data, overwhelming infection was not a feature in the affected infants.[2] Large doses of polysorbates were unavoidably injected when E-Ferol was used and it was suggested that polysorbates may accumulate as a result of an alteration in the metabolism by low birth-weight infants; polysorbate-induced alteration of membrane fluidity in cells of vessel walls may have led to changes in structure and function.[2]

1. Alade SL, *et al.* Polysorbate 80 and E-Ferol toxicity. *Pediatrics* 1986; **77:** 593–7.
2. Balistreri WF, *et al.* Lessons from the E-Ferol tragedy. *Pediatrics* 1986; **78:** 503–6.
3. Golightly LK, *et al.* Pharmaceutical excipients: adverse effects associated with inactive ingredients in drug products. *Med Toxicol* 1988; **3:** 128–65 and 209–240.

Hypersensitivity. Local inflammatory reactions following intramuscular injection of a vitamin A preparation were considered[1] to be due to a hypersensitivity reaction to polysorbate 80, included as an excipient.

1. Shelley WB, *et al.* Polysorbate 80 hypersensitivity. *Lancet* 1995; **345:** 1312–13.

Uses

Polysorbates are hydrophilic nonionic surfactants which are used as emulsifying agents for the preparation of stable oil-in-water emulsions in pharmaceutical products; they are frequently used with a sorbitan ester in varying proportions to produce products with a range of texture and consistency. Polysorbates have also been used in the formulation of insecticide and herbicide sprays, industrial detergents, and cosmetic products. They are also used as emulsifiers in the food industry.

Polysorbates are used as solubilising agents for a variety of substances including essential oils and oil-soluble vitamins such as vitamins A, D, and E, and as wetting agents in the formulation of oral and parenteral suspensions. However, see Adverse Effects and Precautions, above.

Polysorbates may also be used for their surfactant properties in preparations for the removal of ear wax, and for the management of dry eyes and upper respiratory-tract disorders.

Preparations

Proprietary Preparations (details are given in Part 3)

Belg.: Oleosorbate; ***Canad.:*** Tears Encore; ***Fr.:*** Cerumenol; Oleosorbate†.

Multi-ingredient: ***Aust.:*** Expigen; Nasimild†; ***Fr.:*** Fluisedal; Fluisedal sans promethazine; Prorhinel; ***Ger.:*** Broncho Sanol†; Prorhinel; ***Neth.:*** Prorhinel†; ***Norw.:*** Expigen; ***S.Afr.:*** Dilinct; Expigen; Panadoc†; ***Switz.:*** Prorhinel; Rhinocure; Rhinocure Simplex; ***USA:*** Viva-Drops.

Propylene Glycol Diacetate (18363-g)

Propanediol diacetate.

$C_7H_{12}O_4$ = 160.2.

CAS — 623-84-7 (1,2-isomer); 628-66-0 (1,3-isomer).

Pharmacopoeias. In *USNF.*

A clear, colourless liquid with a mild, fruity odour. **Soluble** in water. A 5% solution has a pH of 4 to 6. Sp. gr. 1.04 to 1.06. **Store** in airtight containers and avoid contact with metals.

Propylene glycol diacetate is an emulsifying and/or solubilising agent, and a solvent. It is included in some external preparations for ear infection.

Preparations

Proprietary Preparations (details are given in Part 3)

Austral.: VoSoL.

Multi-ingredient: ***Canad.:*** VoSoL; VoSoL HC; ***USA:*** AA-HC Otic; Acetasol; Acetasol HC; VoSoL; VoSoL HC.

Propylene Glycol Monostearate (437-x)

Propylene Glycol Stearate; Propylèneglycol (Stéarate de); Propylenglycoli Monostearas; Prostearin.

CAS — 1323-39-3 (propylene glycol monostearate); 29013-28-3 (propylene glycol monopalmitate).

Pharmacopoeias. In *Eur.* (see p.viii). Also in *USNF.*

A mixture of the propylene glycol mono- and di-esters of stearic and palmitic acids. Ph. Eur. specifies not less than 50% of mono-esters produced from the condensation of propylene glycol and stearic acid. USNF specifies not less than 90% of mono-esters, chiefly propylene glycol monostearate and propylene glycol monopalmitate.

White or almost white, wax-like solid, beads, or flakes, with a slight agreeable fatty odour. Congealing temperature not less than 45°; m.p. 33° to 40°. Practically **insoluble** in water but it may be dispersed in hot water with the aid of a small amount of soap or other suitable surfactant; soluble in alcohol, in acetone, in ether, and in fixed and mineral oils. **Protect** from light.

Propylene glycol monostearate is obtainable commercially in the pure, non-dispersible form, or in the self-emulsifying form containing a small proportion of soap or other primary emulsifying agent.

Propylene glycol monostearate is used as a stabiliser or emulsifier similarly to glyceryl monostearate or self-emulsifying glyceryl monostearate (p.1325). Propylene glycol monolaurate and mono-oleate have also been used.

Quillaia (469-v)

Panama Wood; Quillaia Bark; Quillaiae Cortex; Seifenrinde; Soap Bark.

CAS — 631-01-6 (quillaic acid).

Pharmacopoeias. In *Aust., Br., Fr.,* and *Swiss.*

The dried inner part of the bark of *Quillaja saponaria* and other species of *Quillaja* (Rosaceae), containing not less than 22% of alcohol (45%)-soluble extractive. It is odourless or almost odourless, but the dust or powder is strongly sternutatory.

It contains 2 amorphous saponin glycosides, quillaic acid and quillaiasapotoxin.

Adverse Effects

Quillaia taken by mouth has been reported to produce gastro-intestinal irritation. It has been suggested that the ingestion of large amounts may produce liver damage, respiratory failure, convulsions, and coma.

Uses

Quillaia is used as an emulsifying agent and frothing agent; it is often used in combination with tragacanth mucilage or another thickening agent. Quillaia is also used for its surfactant properties in preparations for skin and respiratory-tract disorders.

Preparations

BP 1998: Quillaia Liquid Extract; Quillaia Tincture.

Proprietary Preparations (details are given in Part 3)

Fr.: Sebocalm†.

Multi-ingredient: ***Fr.:*** Coaltar Saponine le Beuf; ***Ital.:*** Soluzione Composta Alcoolica Saponosa di Coaltar; ***Spain:*** Mercufila Coaltar†; ***Swed.:*** Quilla simplex; ***Switz.:*** Expectoran avec codeine†; Expectoran Codein; Expectoran†.

Sorbitan Esters (13604-y)

A series of mixtures of the partial esters of sorbitol and its mono- and di-anhydrides with fatty acids.

Sorbitan Monolaurate (478-g)

Sorbitan Monolaurate *(BAN, USAN).*

Sorbitan Laurate *(rINN)*; 493; Sorbitani Lauras.

$C_{18}H_{34}O_6$ (approximate).

CAS — 1338-39-2.

Pharmacopoeias. In *Eur.* (see p.viii). Also in *USNF.*

A mixture of the partial esters of sorbitol and its mono- and di-anhydrides with lauric acid.

A yellow to brownish-yellow or amber-coloured viscous oily liquid with a bland characteristic odour. Relative density about 0.98. Practically **insoluble** but dispersible in water; miscible with alcohol; soluble in liquid paraffin; slightly soluble in cottonseed oil and ethyl acetate. **Store** in airtight containers. Protect from light.

Sorbitan Mono-oleate (479-q)

Sorbitan Mono-oleate *(BAN).*

Sorbitan Oleate *(rINN)*; 494; NSC-406239; Sorbitan Mono-oleate *(USAN)*; Sorbitani Oleas.

$C_{24}H_{44}O_6$ (approximate).

CAS — 1338-43-8.

Pharmacopoeias. In *Eur.* (see p.viii). Also in *USNF.*

A mixture of the partial esters of sorbitol and its mono- and di-anhydrides with oleic acid.

A yellow to brownish-yellow or amber-coloured viscous oily liquid with a bland characteristic odour. Practically **insoluble** but dispersible in water; practically insoluble in propylene glycol; slightly soluble in ether; soluble in fatty oils producing a hazy solution; miscible with alcohol. Relative density about 0.99. **Store** in airtight containers. Protect from light.

Sorbitan Monopalmitate (480-d)

Sorbitan Monopalmitate *(BAN, USAN).*

Sorbitan Palmitate *(rINN)*; 495; Sorbitani Palmitas.

$C_{22}H_{42}O_6$ (approximate).

CAS — 26266-57-9.

Pharmacopoeias. In *Eur.* (see p.viii). Also in *USNF.*

A mixture of the partial esters of sorbitol and its mono- and di-anhydrides with palmitic acid.

A cream-coloured or yellowish or yellow powder, waxy flakes, or hard masses with a faint fatty odour. Practically **insoluble** in water; slightly soluble in alcohol; soluble in warm dehydrated alcohol; soluble in fatty oils; soluble with haze in warm liquid paraffin and arachis oil. M.p. 44° to 51°. **Protect** from light.

Sorbitan Monostearate (481-n)

Sorbitan Monostearate *(BAN, USAN).*

Sorbitan Stearate *(rINN)*; 491; Sorbitani Stearas.

$C_{24}H_{46}O_6$ (approximate).

CAS — 1338-41-6.

Pharmacopoeias. In *Eur.* (see p.viii). Also in *USNF.*

A mixture of the partial esters of sorbitol and its mono- and di-anhydrides with stearic acid.

A cream-coloured to pale yellow to tan waxy solid. M.p. 50° to 55°. Practically **insoluble** but dispersible in water; slightly soluble in alcohol; practically insoluble in acetone; soluble, with haze, above 50° in ethyl acetate and liquid paraffin. **Protect** from light.

Sorbitan Sesquioleate (482-h)

Sorbitan Sesquioleate *(BAN, USAN, rINN).*

$C_{33}H_{60}O_{6.5}$ (approximate).

CAS — 8007-43-0.

Pharmacopoeias. In *Jpn* and *Swiss.* Also in *USNF.*

A mixture of the partial esters of sorbitol and its mono- and di-anhydrides with oleic acid.

A yellow to amber-coloured, oily viscous liquid. Practically **insoluble** in water and in propylene glycol; soluble in alcohol, in isopropyl alcohol, in cottonseed oil, and in liquid paraffin. **Store** in airtight containers.

Sorbitan Trioleate (483-m)

Sorbitan Trioleate *(BAN, USAN, rINN).*

Sorbitani Trioleas.

$C_{60}H_{108}O_8$ (approximate).

CAS — 26266-58-0.

Pharmacopoeias. In *Eur.* (see p.viii). Also in *USNF.*

A mixture of the partial tri-esters of sorbitol and its mono- and di-anhydrides with oleic acid.

A yellow to brownish yellow or amber-coloured viscous oily liquid which becomes a pale yellow, light yellowish, or brown solid below 25°. Practically **insoluble**, but dispersible, in water; freely soluble in ether; soluble in isopropyl alcohol, in methyl alcohol, in corn oil, in cottonseed oil, and in liquid paraffin; slightly soluble to soluble in alcohol; practically insoluble in ethylene glycol and in propylene glycol. Relative density about 0.98. **Store** in airtight containers. Protect from light.

Sorbitan Tristearate (484-b)

Sorbitan Tristearate *(BAN, USAN, rINN)*.

492.

$C_{60}H_{114}O_8$ (approximate).

CAS — 26658-19-5.

A mixture of the partial tri-esters of sorbitol and its mono- and di-anhydrides with stearic acid.

Adverse Effects

There have been occasional reports of hypersensitive skin reactions following the topical application of creams containing sorbitan esters.

References.

1. Finn OA, Forsyth A. Contact dermatitis due to sorbitan monolaurate. *Contact Dermatitis* 1975; **1:** 318.
2. Hannuksela M, *et al.* Allergy to ingredients of vehicles. *Contact Dermatitis* 1976; **2:** 105–10.
3. Austad J. Allergic contact dermatitis to sorbitan monooleate (Span 80). *Contact Dermatitis* 1982; **8:** 426–7.
4. Boyle J, Kennedy CTC. Contact urticaria and dermatitis to Alphaderm. *Contact Dermatitis* 1984; **10:** 178.

Uses

Sorbitan esters are lipophilic nonionic surfactants which are used as emulsifying agents in the preparation of emulsions, creams, and ointments for pharmaceutical and cosmetic use. When used alone they produce stable water-in-oil emulsions but they are frequently used in combination with a polysorbate in varying proportions to produce water-in-oil or oil-in-water emulsions or creams with a variety of different textures and consistencies. Sorbitan esters are also used as emulsifiers and stabilisers in food.

Sucrose Esters (485-v)

E473 (sucrose esters of fatty acids).

Esterification of 1 or more hydroxyl groups in sucrose with a fatty acid such as stearic or palmitic acid produces nonionic compounds which possess surface-active properties. Commercial sucrose esters are mixtures of the mono-, di-, and tri-esters of palmitic and stearic acids with sucrose; various grades are available.

The sucrose esters are used as dispersing and emulsifying agents in food and cosmetic preparations.

Tyloxapol (461-x)

Tyloxapol *(BAN, USAN, rINN)*.

Superinone.

CAS — 25301-02-4.

Pharmacopoeias. In US.

A polymer of 4-(1,1,3,3-tetramethylbutyl)phenol with ethylene oxide and formaldehyde.

A viscous amber liquid, sometimes slightly turbid, with a slight aromatic odour. Slowly but freely **miscible** with water; soluble in chloroform, glacial acetic acid, carbon disulphide, carbon tetrachloride, and toluene. A 5% solution in water has a pH of 4.0 to 7.0. Tyloxapol should not be allowed to come into contact with metals. **Store** in airtight containers.

Adverse Effects

Slight inflammation of the eyelids has been reported after prolonged use of aqueous inhalations. It has been reported that occasional febrile reactions may occur.

Uses and Administration

Tyloxapol is a nonionic surfactant of the alkyl aryl polyether alcohol type. Solutions have been used as an aqueous inhalation as a mucolytic agent for tenacious bronchopulmonary secretions. It is also employed in solutions used to cleanse contact lenses. It has also been used as a vehicle for aerosol medication and for antibacterial agents administered in irrigation solutions for pyogenic bone or joint infections.

Preparations

Proprietary Preparations (details are given in Part 3)

Aust.: Tacholiquin; ***Belg.:*** Alevaire†; ***Canad.:*** Enuclene; ***Fr.:*** Translight; ***Ger.:*** Enuclen N; Tacholiquin; ***Spain:*** Lacermucin; ***Switz.:*** Tacholiquin†; ***USA:*** Enuclene.

Multi-ingredient: *Ger.:* Complete.

Nutritional Agents and Vitamins

Nutrition in Health (3839-c)

The principal constituents of food are carbohydrates, fats, minerals, proteins, vitamins, indigestible fibre, and water. Energy is provided by the metabolism of carbohydrates, fats, surplus protein, and alcohol.

Carbohydrates found in foods may be classified according to their degree of polymerisation into three main groups, namely sugars, oligosaccharides, and polysaccharides; all of these are made up only of carbon, hydrogen, and oxygen. Sugars can be further subdivided into *monosaccharides* (single-molecule sugars), such as fructose and glucose, *disaccharides* (whose molecules consist of two monosaccharides joined together), such as lactose and sucrose, and *sugar alcohols* (polyols) such as sorbitol and mannitol. *Oligosaccharides* typically consist of 3 to 9 monosaccharides joined together, and include malto-oligosaccharides such as maltodextrins. *Polysaccharides* consist of many monosaccharides joined together and include starches and non-starch polysaccharides such as cellulose. Non-starch polysaccharides are the major fraction of dietary fibre, and many authorities now consider this term is preferable to dietary fibre.

Fats have the same elemental composition as carbohydrates, but with a lower proportion of oxygen. Dietary fat is usually in the form of triglycerides, esters of glycerol with three fatty acid molecules. Essential fatty acids are ones which cannot be made in the body and which must be supplied by the food.

Proteins are made up of carbon, hydrogen, oxygen, and nitrogen; most proteins also contain sulphur and some contain phosphorus. They are required for the regulation of body processes such as growth and tissue maintenance, and excess protein can be converted into carbohydrate and used to provide energy.

Proteins consist of chains of **amino acids** of which there are *essential* and *non-essential* types. Essential amino acids cannot be synthesised in sufficient amounts in the body and must therefore be present in food; non-essential amino acids can be synthesised in the body. Essential amino acids are also known as indispensable amino acids. There are eight essential amino acids: isoleucine, leucine, lysine, methionine, phenylalanine, threonine, tryptophan, and valine. Arginine and histidine are also essential for infant growth while synthesis of cysteine, taurine, and tyrosine may be inadequate in premature infants.

Several inorganic elements, or minerals, are essential dietary constituents; those which are required in relatively small amounts are known as **trace elements** (see p.1332). Their main function is to act as essential cofactors in various enzyme systems.

Vitamins and their role in health are described on p.1332.

Human requirements. Guidance on intakes of energy and protein has been made available by various bodies or authorities.[1-3] For an explanation of the relevant nomenclature and terms used in the UK and USA, see under Vitamins, p.1332.

1. Subcommittee on the tenth edition of the RDAs, Food and Nutrition Board, Commission on Life Sciences, National Research Council. *Recommended dietary allowances.* 10th ed. Washington, DC: National Academy Press, 1989.
2. WHO. Diet, nutrition, and the prevention of chronic diseases: report of a WHO study group. *WHO Tech Rep Ser 797* 1990.
3. DoH. Dietary reference values for food energy and nutrients for the United Kingdom: report of the panel on dietary reference values of the committee on medical aspects of food policy. *Report on health and social subjects 41.* London: HMSO, 1991.

Dietary Modification (3840-s)

Infants, children, elderly people, and pregnant or lactating women have particular nutritional requirements, but in most cases, provided that they are is in good general health, adjustment to intake is all that is required rather than extensive modification or supplementation.

Dietary modification is important in the management of a variety of disorders. Calorie restriction is fundamental to the management of obesity, although it may be difficult to motivate patients to accept long-term changes to their eating patterns, and some fashionable diets are at best of little value.

The role of diet in the aetiology of cardiovascular disorders (such as salt intake in hypertension and fat intake in ischaemic heart disease) is recognised to be of importance and is leading to public health campaigns for healthier eating patterns.

Dietary modification is also an accepted part of the management of diabetes mellitus, while protein restriction is important in the management of uraemia or hepatic encephalopathy.

There are also various metabolic disorders such as phenylketonuria, or forms of intolerance to dietary components, such as coeliac disease, in which the diet must be modified to exclude or drastically reduce certain food components.

Amino acid metabolic disorders. Various inborn errors of amino-acid metabolism are known. They are not common but their consequences are often serious or fatal. Although in some cases there is no effective treatment, early diagnosis is important as some conditions can be managed by dietary modification and/or the use of vitamins. Two of the better known syndromes, homocystinuria and phenylketonuria, are discussed briefly below. Cystinosis, another autosomal recessive disorder of amino acid metabolism, is discussed on p.1569.

Homocystinuria. Homocystinuria in its classical form is an autosomal recessive disorder due to a genetic deficiency of the enzyme cystathionine synthetase, resulting in accumulation of homocysteine (oxidised extracellularly to homocystine).[1] Manifestations may include mental retardation, atherosclerosis, thrombo-embolism, osteoporosis, and ocular symptoms including lens dislocation, glaucoma, cataract, and retinal detachment. Dietary restriction of methionine together with cystine supplements has been used for treatment; some patients may respond to treatment with B vitamins (pyridoxine, cobalamins, and folic acid),[1,2] or to betaine.[3-6]

Phenylketonuria. Phenylketonuria is an autosomal recessive disorder which is usually due to a defect in the enzyme phenylalanine hydroxylase. This results in raised blood concentrations of phenylalanine in the neonate, and if untreated produces a syndrome of skin rash, depigmentation, hypertonia, seizures, and severe mental retardation. The disease is controlled by use of a synthetic diet very low in phenylalanine,[7-11] and if started early this can permit relatively normal intellectual development. High-dose tyrosine does not appear to be an effective alternative to a diet low in phenylalanine.[12,13]

1. Isherwood DM. Homocystinuria. *Br Med J* 1996; **313:** 1025–6.
2. Schuh S, *et al.* Homocystinuria and megaloblastic anemia responsive to vitamin B_{12} therapy. *N Engl J Med* 1984; **310:** 686–90.
3. Smolin LA, *et al.* The use of betaine for the treatment of homocystinuria. *J Pediatr* 1981; **99:** 467–72.
4. Wilcken DEL, *et al.* Homocystinuria—the effects of betaine in the treatment of patients not responsive to pyridoxine. *N Engl J Med* 1983; **309:** 448–53.
5. Holme E, *et al.* Betaine for treatment of homocystinuria caused by methylenetetrahydrofolate reductase deficiency. *Arch Dis Child* 1989; **64:** 1061–4.
6. Anonymous. Betaine for homocystinuria. *Med Lett Drugs Ther* 1997; **39:** 12.
7. Rylance G. Outcome of early detected and early treated phenylketonuria patients. *Postgrad Med J* 1989; **65** (suppl 2): S7–9.
8. Link R. Phenylketonuria diet in adolescents— energy and nutrient intake—is it adequate? *Postgrad Med J* 1989; **65** (suppl 2): S21–4.
9. American Academy of Pediatrics Committee on Genetics. Maternal phenylketonuria. *Pediatrics* 1991; **88:** 1284–5.
10. Thompson GN, *et al.* Pregnancy in phenylketonuria: dietary treatment aimed at normalising maternal plasma phenylalanine concentration. *Arch Dis Child* 1991; **66:** 1346–9.
11. Medical Research Council. Report of the Medical Research Council Working Party on Phenylketonuria. Recommendations on the dietary management of phenylketonuria. *Arch Dis Child* 1993; **68:** 426–7.
12. Pietz J, *et al.* Effect of high-dose tyrosine supplementation on brain function in adults with phenylketonuria. *J Pediatr* 1995; **127:** 936–43.
13. Smith ML, *et al.* Randomised controlled trial of tyrosine supplementation on neuropsychological performance in phenylketonuria. *Arch Dis Child* 1998; **78:** 116–21.

Cardiovascular disease. Modification of the diet may be helpful in patients with, or at risk of, cardiovascular disease. In patients with hypertension (p.788), reduction in salt intake forms one of the non-pharmacological measures that may be tried before commencing drug therapy or used as an adjunct to such therapy.

Dietary changes may also be helpful in reducing the risk of ischaemic heart disease, although the evidence is less clear. For both the general population, and that proportion of it considered at high risk, the basis of dietary management is a reduction in the total intake of dietary fat, and in particular of saturated fatty acids. An increased intake of long chain n-3 polyunsaturated fatty acids has been recommended and also a restriction on *trans* fatty acids. Dietary cholesterol should be restricted although it may make less of a contribution to plasma cholesterol levels than dietary saturates.[1] For a discussion on the control of blood lipid levels to modify the risk of ischaemic heart disease, see Hyperlipidaemias, p.1265.

For discussion of the possibility that antioxidant vitamins may reduce the risk of ischaemic heart disease see under Vitamins, p.1333. The link between folic acid, homocysteine, and ischaemic heart disease is discussed on p.1341.

1. DoH. Nutritional aspects of cardiovascular disease. *Report on health and social subjects 46.* London: HMSO, 1994. [COMA report.]

Coeliac disease. Coeliac disease (gluten-sensitive enteropathy) is an inflammatory disorder of the small intestine that results from an immunological reaction to the gliadin fraction of gluten (p.1585). The inflammation leads to mucosal atrophy with subsequent malabsorption, although the extent and severity of mucosal inflammation varies widely, and some patients are asymptomatic. In adults, anaemia and mild gastro-intestinal symptoms that may be confused with irritable bowel syndrome are the usual symptoms. In infants and children there may be growth retardation or failure to thrive, and gastro-intestinal symptoms may be more marked. Other nutritional deficiencies, including calcium malabsorption leading to osteopenia, may also occur, and mouth ulcers are also common.

Treatment of coeliac disease involves a strict, life-long, gluten-free diet. Nutritional supplements may be necessary at the start of treatment but can usually be stopped once mucosal recovery has occurred. Diagnosis is confirmed by normalisation of the mucosa on repeat biopsy after 3 to 4 months. Dermatitis herpetiformis (p.1073) is a non-gastro-intestinal manifestation of coeliac disease. Patients may have no gastro-intestinal symptoms, although mucosal abnormalities are generally apparent on biopsy. These patients also respond to a gluten-free diet. Patients with coeliac disease have an increased incidence of small-bowel lymphoma and a slight increase in the incidence of some other gastro-intestinal cancers. There is some evidence that this incidence is reduced in patients maintaining a strict diet.

Reviews.

1. Duggan JM. Recent developments in our understanding of adult coeliac disease. *Med J Aust* 1997; **166:** 312–15.
2. Ferguson A. Coeliac disease. *Prescribers' J* 1997; **37:** 206–12.
3. Mäki M, Collin P. Coeliac disease. *Lancet* 1997; **349:** 1755–9.
4. Barr GD, Grehan MJ. Coeliac disease. *Med J Aust* 1998; **169:** 109–14.

Diabetes mellitus. Dietary control is important in both type 1 and type 2 diabetes mellitus (p.313); in the latter condition such control, combined possibly with increased exercise, may be all that is required to correct the condition. In addition to reduction in the intake of sugar, and an increase in fibre intake (which may also lower blood sugar concentrations), the correction of obesity removes one of the factors associated with insulin resistance.

Hepatic encephalopathy. Dietary modification forms an important part of the treatment of hepatic encephalopathy (see p.1170).

Inflammatory bowel disease. In inflammatory bowel diseases (p.1171) dietary modification or supplementation may often be necessary to maintain the nutritional status of the patient. Such supplementation may be oral, nasogastric, or parenteral.

Elemental diets have been shown to be effective in the management of Crohn's disease,[1] although they are apparently of less importance in ulcerative colitis. The terminology surrounding the use of these diets has been elucidated by Payne-James and Silk.[2] They have stated that the term elemental diet was originally coined to describe diets containing free amino acids and glucose and was often prefixed by the phrase 'chemically defined'. However, in recent years the term had come to embrace diets whose nitrogen sources included peptides and were often also called predigested diets. They believed that the term elemental diet could be used for either type but that for those with an amino acid nitrogen source the term chemically defined elemental diet should be used whereas for those with a peptide nitrogen source predigested elemental diet was suitable. The term polymeric diet should be used for those diets with a whole protein nitrogen source.

1. Teahon K, *et al.* Ten years' experience with an elemental diet in the management of Crohn's disease. *Gut* 1990; **31:** 1133–7.
2. Payne-James JJ, Silk DBA. Use of elemental diets in the treatment of Crohn's disease by gastroenterologists. *Gut* 1990; **31:** 1424.

Malignant neoplasms. For a brief discussion of the idea that an increased intake of antoxidant vitamins might reduce the risk of developing malignancies, see under Vitamins, p.1333.

Obesity. Obesity is relatively common in the developed world, and is accompanied by an increased risk of cardiovascular disease, diabetes, and other disorders. Methods such as dietary modification, behaviour therapy, and exercise with adjunctive drug therapy, where indicated (see p.1476) can produce weight loss, but the essence of treatment is a reduction in calorific intake, usually to around 1000 kcal (4200 kJ) daily for a woman or 1500 kcal (6300 kJ) for a man. Very low calorie diets (less than 600 to 800 kcal per day) may also be tried. For weight loss to be achieved and sustained, eating behaviour must be permanently modified, which may pose difficulties. The intake of foods such as fats, alcohol, and sugars, particularly the former, should be reduced but it is obviously important to maintain an adequate intake of essential nutrients.

Artificial sweeteners or other non-sucrose sweeteners are often used as part of weight-reducing diets as well as being widely used in the food industry. Intense and bulk sweeteners are included in this chapter, although some such as mannitol (p.900) have additional uses and are described in other chapters.

Renal failure. A resurgence of interest in possible interventions that may be of value in preventing or slowing the progression of chronic renal failure (p.1152) has led again to evaluation of low-protein diets. Patients with renal failure who adopt a protein-restricted diet have fewer symptoms of uraemia than those on a normal diet.[1] Some results have also suggested that protein restriction can slow the progression of renal failure,[2] but the value of low protein diets in delaying the onset of end-stage renal disease has been the subject of much controversy. Two large multicentre studies provided little evidence of a substantial benefit,[3,4] but meta-analyses have consistently provided support for dietary protein restriction.[5,6] It has been suggested that the benefit of other interventions such as the use of ACE inhibitors,[7] as well as the difficulties in obtaining patient compliance with such a restrictive diet,[8] may have limited the benefits to be obtained from protein restriction, but there is also evidence that response and outcome vary depending on the cause of renal failure.[4,9]

1. Klahr S. Chronic renal failure: management. *Lancet* 1991; **338:** 423–7.
2. Mallick NP. Dietary protein and progression of chronic renal disease. *Br Med J* 1994; **309:** 1101–2.
3. Locatelli F, *et al.* Prospective, randomised, multicentre trial of effect of protein restriction on progression of chronic renal insufficiency. *Lancet* 1991; **337:** 1299–1304.
4. Klahr S, *et al.* The effects of dietary protein restriction and blood-pressure control on the progression of chronic renal disease. *N Engl J Med* 1994; **330:** 877–84.
5. Fouque D, *et al.* Controlled low protein diets in chronic renal insufficiency: meta-analysis. *Br Med J* 1992; **304:** 216–20.
6. Pedrini MT, *et al.* The effect of dietary protein restriction on the progression of diabetic and nondiabetic renal diseases: a meta-analysis. *Ann Intern Med* 1996; **124:** 627–32.
7. Shiigai T, *et al.* Dietary protein restriction and blood-pressure control in chronic renal insufficiency. *N Engl J Med* 1994; **331:** 405.
8. Barsotti G, Giovannetti S. Low-protein diet and chronic renal failure. *Lancet* 1991; **338:** 442.
9. Locatelli F, *et al.* Low-protein diet and chronic renal failure. *Lancet* 1991; **338:** 442–3.

Enteral and Parenteral Nutrition

(3841-w)

Malnutrition of varying degrees is not uncommon in hospitalised patients, and some form of nutritional support is important in patients who cannot eat an adequate normal diet. Such support should provide for the patient's requirements for energy, in the form of carbohydrate and fat, nitrogen as amino acids or protein, water and electrolytes; where appropriate, vitamins and trace elements should also be supplied. The decision to initiate nutritional support depends on the patient's clinical condition: indications may include unconsciousness, obstruction or inability to swallow, inflammatory bowel disease, fistula, short bowel syndrome, and weakness and malnutrition associated with trauma, surgery, or malignant disease. If possible, nutritional support should be by the enteral route; it is easier, more physiological, and somewhat less prone to complications than the parenteral route.

Enteral nutrition includes feeding by mouth, by nasogastric or nasoenteric tube, or directly into a gastrostomy or other enterostomy. It may be supplemental, if normal food intake is possible but inadequate, or total. Individual patients vary in their requirements according to age, size, and metabolic state, but a diet supplying 2000 to 3000 kcal of energy and 10 to 15 g of nitrogen (as 60 to 90 g of protein) in 2 to 3 litres of fluid is fairly typical; because absorption from the gastro-intestinal tract is incomplete requirements are higher than by the parenteral route. Preparations containing whole protein are generally preferred; elemental diets, in which nitrogen is supplied as amino acids or oligopeptides, are less well tolerated and less palatable, although they may have a role in impaired digestion or when a zero-residue diet is desired.

Although considered safer than parenteral nutrition, enteral feeding is not without complications. Patients may be at risk of oesophagitis, aspiration, and regurgitation as a result of the tube insertion; other potential problems include diarrhoea, nausea and vomiting, gastric retention, hyperglycaemia, fluid and electrolyte disturbances, and infection of the feed regimen.

Parenteral nutrition is reserved for situations in which it is impossible to meet nutritional requirements by the enteral route. Like enteral nutrition it may be given supplementally or as the sole source of body requirements (total parenteral nutrition or TPN). Although parenteral nutrition may be given short-term via a peripheral vein, the thrombophlebitis produced by invariably hyperosmolar nutrition solutions means that a central venous catheter, usually into the subclavian vein, is the normal route of administration.

The formulation of the nutritional solution must be adjusted according to the patient's requirements. The solution should supply sufficient energy to allow for the resting energy expenditure (around 25 kcal per kg body-weight in the average adult) but must also take into account any increased energy expenditure of illness. Conversely, starvation can reduce resting metabolism and energy requirements. Various formulae exist for the calculation of energy expenditure in patients. Energy is best supplied in the form of carbohydrate (at least 30%, and preferably 60% of energy requirements should be in this form) with some fat. Glucose is the optimal carbohydrate energy source, while fat is supplied as a lipid emulsion, often of soya oil. Nitrogen is supplied as amino acids, but to ensure that these are used for protein synthesis rather than as sources of energy it is important to control the ratio of non-protein energy to nitrogen in the solution. A ratio of 150 to 200 kcal per g of nitrogen is usually considered optimal but in hypercatabolic patients (e.g. in sepsis) lower ratios of 120 kcal per g or less may be appropriate. All essential amino acids are supplied although there is some variation between solutions as to which non-essential amino acids are present.

Parenteral nutrition must also supply the patient's requirements for fluid, essential electrolytes such as sodium, potassium, and calcium (as well as phosphate, since glucose infusion may provoke hypophosphataemia), and, particularly if treatment is prolonged, vitamins and trace elements. If glucose loading produces signs of hyperglycaemia insulin may be added to correct it.

The major complication of parenteral nutrition is infection of the catheter, which can lead to septicaemia. Other problems may include venous thrombosis or air embolism, extravasation due to misplacement of the catheter tip, and metabolic disturbances. Adverse effects of overfeeding include respiratory and hepatic dysfunction. Complications of long-term total parenteral nutrition include gallbladder sludging, gallstones, cholestasis, and abnormal liver function tests.

Stability and compatibility. The complex nature of solutions for parenteral nutrition renders them susceptible to compatibility problems.[1-12] Stability is dependent upon several factors including pH and relative concentrations of the components. Amino acids exert a buffering effect on the overall pH of mixed solutions containing amino acids, glucose, and fat emulsions but amino acids with glucose undergo the Maillard reaction (browning) and the life of combined solutions is therefore limited. Solutions containing electrolytes, particularly divalent cations, are not stable, and aggregation will eventually occur. Additives should be added only if there is known compatibility, and any additions performed aseptically before the start of the infusion. In general mixed parenteral nutrition solutions should be used immediately after preparation and administered to the patient within 24 hours.

1. Allwood MC. Compatibility and stability of TPN mixtures in big bags. *J Clin Hosp Pharm* 1984; **9:** 181–98.
2. Niemiec PW, Vanderveen TW. Compatibility considerations in parenteral nutrient solutions. *Am J Hosp Pharm* 1984; **41:** 893–911.
3. Parry VA, *et al.* Effect of various nutrient ratios on the emulsion stability of total nutrient admixtures. *Am J Hosp Pharm* 1986; **43:** 3017–22.
4. Hardy G. Ten years of TPN with 3 litre bags. *Pharm J* 1987; **239:** HS26–HS28.
5. Johnson OL, *et al.* The destabilization of parenteral feeding emulsions by heparin. *Int J Pharmaceutics* 1989; **53:** 237–40.
6. Takagi J, *et al.* Sterility of total parenteral nutrient solutions stored at room temperature for seven days. *Am J Hosp Pharm* 1989; **46:** 973–7.
7. Tripp MG, *et al.* Stability of total nutrient admixtures in a dual-chamber flexible container. *Am J Hosp Pharm* 1990; **47:** 2496–503.
8. Vaughan LM, *et al.* Incompatibility of iron dextran and a total nutrient admixture. *Am J Hosp Pharm* 1990; **47:** 1745–6.
9. Washington C. The stability of intravenous fat emulsions in total parenteral nutrition mixtures. *Int J Pharmaceutics* 1990; **66:** 1–21.
10. Manning RJ, Washington C. Chemical stability of total parenteral nutrition mixtures. *Int J Pharmaceutics* 1992; **81:** 1–20.
11. Neuzil J, *et al.* Oxidation of parenteral lipid emulsion by ambient and phototherapy lights: potential toxicity of routine parenteral feeding. *J Pediatr* 1995; **126:** 785–90.
12. Trissel LA, *et al.* Compatibility of parenteral nutrient solutions with selected drugs during simulated Y-site administration. *Am J Health-Syst Pharm* 1997; **54:** 1295–1300.

Adverse effects and precautions. ENTERAL NUTRITION. Reviewing the complications of enteral nutrition Bastow has noted[1] that many of the problems encountered can be avoided by using a fine bore tube, administering the feed by continuous infusion, and by careful monitoring of the patient for metabolic abnormalities.

Complexation of the nutrients with aluminium-containing antacids, also given via the tube, may occur and this deposition of solid masses may cause oesophageal obstruction.[2]

Although diarrhoea has been widely believed to be a common occurrence in patients receiving enteral nutrition it may not necessarily be caused by the tube feeding itself;[3,4] concomitant drug therapy can often be implicated. However, enteral feeding has been shown to be associated with increased colonic secretion, which can be reversed by infusion of short-chain fatty acids.[5]

1. Bastow MD. Complications of enteral nutrition. *Gut* 1986; **21** (suppl 1): 51–5.
2. Valli C, *et al.* Interaction of nutrients with antacids: a complication during enteral tube feeding. *Lancet* 1986; **i:** 747–8.
3. Edes TE, *et al.* Diarrhea in tube-fed patients: feeding formula not necessarily the cause. *Am J Med* 1990; **88:** 91–3.
4. Heimburger DC. Diarrhea with enteral feeding: will the real cause please stand up? *Am J Med* 1990; **88:** 89–90.
5. Bowling TE, *et al.* Reversal by short-chain fatty acids of colonic fluid secretion induced by enteral feeding. *Lancet* 1993; **342:** 1266–8.

PARENTERAL NUTRITION. A common complication of parenteral nutrition is infection of the intravenous feeding catheter site which can lead to septicaemia. de Cicco and co-workers[1] suggested that infection and colonisation of central venous catheters could be reduced if the catheter was tunnelled through subcutaneous tissue before emerging through the skin. Strict aseptic techniques should be used for changing the dressing or bags containing the nutrient fluids.

Thrombophlebitis can occur following the use of both peripheral and central veins. Although it has been suggested that infusion of hyperosmolar solutions via a central line is less likely to produce thrombophlebitis, because the feed is immediately diluted by a large volume of blood, Dollery and colleagues[2,3] found that major thrombotic complications such as pulmonary embolism and right atrial thrombosis were more common than hitherto recognised in children and adolescents receiving long term parenteral nutrition via central catheters. Kohlhardt and Smith[4] have reported that the use of a fine-bore silicone catheter peripherally may avoid the need for central vein cannulation and Madan and others[5] have confirmed a lower incidence of thrombophlebitis when fine-bore silicone catheters rather than teflon ones were used for peripheral administration of parenteral nutrition. The addition of heparin to the feed, and the use of local hydrocortisone and glyceryl trinitrate, has also been reported to prolong the survival of peripheral infusion sites.[6] Extravasation may also be a problem, particularly with hyperosmolar solutions, and has led to severe tissue damage; hyaluronidase or thiomucase may be used in the treatment of such extravasation.[7]

Parenteral nutrition may be associated with atrophic changes in the mucosal structure and enzymic activity of the intestine, leading to increased permeability with a possible increased risk of bacteraemia and endotoxaemia. These changes, which have been attributed to lack of glutamine (which is unstable in solution), can reportedly be prevented by addition of glutamine-releasing dipeptides to solutions for total parenteral nutrition.[8] Addition of glutamine has also been reported to improve nitrogen balance—see p.1345. For discussion of the possible benefits associated with addition of branched-chain amino acids see below.

1. de Cicco M, *et al.* Source and route of microbial colonisation of parenteral nutrition catheters. *Lancet* 1989; **ii:** 1258–61.
2. Dollery CM, *et al.* Thrombosis and embolism in long-term central venous access for parenteral nutrition. *Lancet* 1994; **344:** 1043–5.
3. Dollery CM. Pulmonary embolism in parenteral nutrition. *Arch Dis Child* 1996; **74:** 95–8.
4. Kohlhardt SR, Smith RC. Fine bore silicone catheters for peripheral intravenous nutrition in adults. *Br Med J* 1989; **299:** 1380–1.
5. Madan M, *et al.* Influence of catheter type on occurrence of thrombophlebitis during peripheral intravenous nutrition. *Lancet* 1992; **339:** 101–103.
6. Moclair AE, *et al.* Total parenteral nutrition via a peripheral vein: a comparison of heparinised and non-heparinised regimens. *Int J Pharm Pract* 1991; **1:** 38–40.
7. Gil M-E, Mateu J. Treatment of extravasation from parenteral nutrition solution. *Ann Pharmacother* 1998; **32:** 51–5.
8. van der Hulst RRWJ, *et al.* Glutamine and the preservation of gut identity. *Lancet* 1993; **341:** 1363–5.

Uses. Parenteral and enteral nutrition now have an established place either for supplemental use or for providing total nutritional requirements in many conditions. General reviews as well as those pertaining to special groups of patients or disorders have been published.[1-12]

1. Cochran EB, *et al.* Parenteral nutrition in pediatric patients. *Clin Pharm* 1988; **7:** 351–66.
2. Anonymous. Nutrition and the metabolic response to injury. *Lancet* 1989; **i:** 995–7.
3. Cochran EB, *et al.* Parenteral nutrition in the critically ill patient. *Clin Pharm* 1989; **8:** 783–99.
4. American College of Physicians. Parenteral nutrition in patients receiving cancer chemotherapy. *Ann Intern Med* 1989; **110:** 734–6.
5. Driscoll DF, Blackburn GL. Total parenteral nutrition 1990: a review of its current status in hospitalised patients, and the need for patient-specific feeding. *Drugs* 1990; **40:** 346–63.
6. Pennington C. Parenteral nutrition at home. *Prescribers' J* 1990; **30:** 271–8.
7. The Veterans Affairs Total Parenteral Nutrition Cooperative Study Group. Perioperative total parenteral nutrition in surgical patients. *N Engl J Med* 1991; **325:** 525–32.
8. Matuchansky C, *et al.* Cyclical parenteral nutrition. *Lancet* 1992; **340:** 588–92.
9. Golden MHN, Briend A. Treatment of malnutrition in refugee camps. *Lancet* 1993; **342:** 360.
10. Elia M. Changing concepts of nutrient requirements in disease: implications for artificial nutritional support. *Lancet* 1995; **345:** 1279–84.
11. Mattox TW, *et al.* Recent advances: parenteral nutrition support. *Ann Pharmacother* 1995; **29:** 174–80.
12. Souba WW. Nutritional support. *N Engl J Med* 1997; **336:** 41–8.

BRANCHED-CHAIN AMINO ACIDS. In the stressed hypercatabolic patient, as seen in sepsis, trauma, or major surgery, standard forms of nutritional support sometimes fail to produce a positive nitrogen balance. Recognition of altered protein metabolism in these patients, and specifically that of the branched-chain amino acids leucine, isoleucine, and valine, has led to the theory that increasing the exogenous supply of these branched-chain amino acids will be beneficial and result in an improvement of protein synthesis. In a review and discussion on this topic Teasley and Buss[1] concluded that the numerous clinical studies that have been performed so far have yielded variable results and that the use of branched-chain amino acid-enriched solutions in nutritional support thus remains controversial. This conclusion was also supported by Oki and Cuddy[2] who published a review at the same time.

In some metabolic disorders such as maple syrup urine disease, reduction or elimination of the intake of branched-chain amino acids, rather than supplementation, is a necessary part of management.[3]

1. Teasley KM, Buss RL. Do parenteral nutrition solutions with high concentrations of branched-chain amino acids offer significant benefits to stressed patients? *DICP Ann Pharmacother* 1989; **23:** 411–16.
2. Oki JC, Cuddy PG. Branched-chain amino acid support of stressed patients. *DICP Ann Pharmacother* 1989; **23:** 399–410.
3. Berry GT, *et al.* Branched-chain amino acid-free parenteral nutrition in the treatment of acute metabolic decompensation in patients with maple syrup urine disease. *N Engl J Med* 1991; **324:** 175–9.

Trace Elements (17190-c)

Trace elements are inorganic substances found in small amounts in the tissues and required for various metabolic processes; together with the vitamins (see below) they are sometimes referred to as micronutrients. The elements considered essential are chromium, copper, fluorine, iodine, iron, manganese, molybdenum, selenium, and zinc. Iron, in the form of haem, plays an essential role in oxygen transport while iodine is required by the thyroid for the formation of thyroid hormones; most of the other essential trace elements are cofactors for various enzymes. Trace elements probably essential include boron, nickel, silicon, and vanadium; it has been suggested on the basis of *animal* studies that there might be a requirement for tin.

Well-defined deficiency syndromes exist for copper, iodine, iron, selenium, and zinc; although deficiency of other trace elements is possible, their deficiency syndromes are not well defined because of their ubiquity in the diet. Guidance concerning the intake of various trace elements has been published—see also Human Requirements under Vitamins, below.

References.

1. WHO. *Trace elements in human nutrition and health.* Geneva: WHO, 1996.

Vitamins (7820-j)

Vitamins are organic substances required by the body in small amounts for various metabolic processes. They are not synthesised in the body, or are synthesised in small or insufficient quantities. Vitamins are sometimes classified as fat soluble or water soluble. Substances in the vitamin A, D, E, and K groups are generally fat soluble, and biotin, folic acid, niacin, pantothenic acid, vitamins B_1, B_2, B_6, and B_{12}, and vitamin C substances are generally water soluble.

Vitamin deficiency may result from an inadequate diet, perhaps due to increased requirements such as during pregnancy, or may be induced by disease or drugs. Vitamins may be used clinically for the prevention and treatment of specific vitamin deficiency states and details of these uses are provided under the individual drug monographs.

Large doses of vitamins (megavitamin therapy) have been proposed for a variety of disorders, but adequate evidence of their value is lacking. Excessive intakes of most water-soluble vitamins have little effect due to their rapid excretion in urine, but excessive intakes of fat-soluble vitamins accumulate in the body and are potentially dangerous.

Water-soluble vitamins are liable to degrade in solution especially if exposed to light. Addition of vitamin mixtures to infusion solutions for parenteral nutrition should therefore be carried out as soon as possible before infusion. Solutions should be used within 24 hours of preparation and be protected from light.

Human requirements. Vitamins and trace elements are essential nutrients and in many countries guidance has been published concerning their intake.

In the UK various terms are used to define intake:[1]

- estimated average requirement (EAR) is used for the requirements of energy, proteins, vitamins, or minerals of a group of people and usually about half will need more and half less than the specified figure
- lower reference nutrient intake (LRNI) is applied to proteins, vitamins, or minerals and is that amount that is enough for only a few people who have low needs
- reference nutrient intake (RNI) is also applied to proteins, vitamins, or minerals and is an amount that is enough, or more than enough, for about 97% of people in a group
- a safe intake is used to indicate an intake or range of intakes where there is not enough information to estimate EAR, LRNI, or RNI, but rather it is an amount enough for almost everyone but is not so large as to cause undesirable effects
- dietary reference value (DRV) is used to cover EAR, LRNI, RNI, and safe intake.

It is emphasised in the report that these intakes are not meant to be recommendations for any individual or group; they do not reflect either a recommendation that such an amount should be taken daily in the diet or as a supplement. They are intended rather as yardsticks for the assessment of dietary surveys and food supply statistics; to provide guidance on appropriate dietary composition and meal provision; or for food labelling purposes in which case it is envisaged that an EAR will be used.

In the USA the National Academy of Sciences has traditionally set recommended dietary allowances (RDAs),[2] defined as the levels of intake of essential nutrients that, on the basis of scientific knowledge, are judged to be adequate to meet the known nutrient needs of practically all healthy persons. The allowances are amounts that are intended to be consumed as part of a normal diet. However, new dietary reference intakes (DRIs) are being developed, which will include 3 reference values in addition to the traditional RDA as follows:

- the estimated average requirement is the intake that meets the needs of half the individuals in a group
- the adequate intake is the mean intake level that appears to sustain a desired marker of health, and will be set when there is insufficient evidence to establish an RDA
- the tolerable upper intake level is the maximum intake that is not likely to adversely affect health.

Information pertaining to the requirements of specific vitamins and minerals is provided under the individual monographs.

1. DoH. Dietary reference values for food energy and nutrients for the United Kingdom: report of the panel on dietary reference values of the committee on medical aspects of food policy. *Report on health and social subjects 41.* London: HMSO, 1991.
2. Subcommittee on the tenth edition of the RDAs, Food and Nutrition Board, Commission on Life Sciences, National Research Council. *Recommended dietary allowances.* 10th ed. Washington, DC: National Academy Press, 1989.

Supplementation. An adequate dietary intake of vitamins is necessary for good health but whether vitamin supplementation in the absence of any demonstrable deficiency is beneficial or even worthwhile remains debatable.

It is generally considered that healthy persons eating a normal balanced diet should have no need for vitamin supplementation. A review of the topic[1] pointed out that the vitamins that people chose for self medication are often not the ones that are actually present in inadequate amounts in their diets and the commercial preparations available often do not make it clear whether the amounts they contain are near the physiological requirements or many times greater. Supplementation should concentrate on groups of people at risk of deficiency such as neonates, who need vitamin K; pregnant and lactating women, who need calcium, folic acid, and iron; and certain groups who need vitamin D; vegans and their infants may require vitamin B_{12} supplements. A multivitamin supplement might be considered for some groups such as the elderly and those with reduced calorie intake. However, one might have difficulty in finding a good multivitamin preparation containing all 13 vitamins but no non-vitamins. Also with many of the multivitamin preparations the doses and ratios vary inexplicably.

In a review of supplementation specifically in children Kendall concluded that, provided schoolchildren and adolescents eat a wide variety of foods, there was no need for vitamin supplementation.[2] However, it was recommended that supplementation with vitamins A, C, and D should be given to those between the ages of 6 months and 2 years and preferably up to the age of 5 years.

A subsequent study supports the suggestion that supplementation may be of some benefit in the elderly. Chandra[3] reported evidence that supplementation with modest, physiological doses of vitamins and trace elements resulted in an improvement in immune response and a decreased frequency of infection in elderly subjects. It was suggested that dosage might be crucial and that excessive doses of micronutrients could impair rather than improve immune response.

1. Truswell S. Who should take vitamin supplements? *Br Med J* 1990; **301:** 135–6. Correction. *ibid.*; 354.
2. Kendall HE. Vitamin and mineral supplements for children. *Pharm J* 1990; **245:** 460–2.
3. Chandra RK. Effect of vitamin and trace-element supplementation on immune responses and infection in elderly subjects. *Lancet* 1992; **340:** 1124–7.

MENTAL FUNCTION. Administration of vitamin and mineral supplements to children was reported in 1988 to increase non-verbal intelligence[1] and the topic has remained highly controversial since. In the following two years more studies were published but these failed to substantiate the earlier possible effect and concluded that vitamin supplementation did not improve mental functioning or reasoning in children.[2,3] Suggestions were made shortly after these publications that there may be a subset of children with poor nutritional status who may, in fact, receive some benefit[4] but this again was disputed.[5]

In 1991 another study was published,[6] this time coinciding with the launch of the proprietary product used in the study, with the publication of a book on the subject, and with the showing on British television of a documentary concerning the study. This study purported to demonstrate that supplementation with exactly the recommended dietary allowances of vitamins improved the IQ of children, a finding that was said not to occur significantly with other quantities of vitamin supplementation. This view attracted extremely harsh criticism[7-9] from physicians, nutritionists, psychologists, and epidemiologists.

1. Benton D, Roberts G. Effect of vitamin and mineral supplementation on intelligence of a sample of schoolchildren. *Lancet* 1988; **i:** 140–3.
2. Naismith DJ, *et al.* Can children's intelligence be increased by vitamin and mineral supplements? *Lancet* 1988; **ii:** 335.
3. Crombie IK, *et al.* Effect of vitamin and mineral supplementation on verbal and non-verbal reasoning of schoolchildren. *Lancet* 1990; **335:** 744–7.
4. Benton D, Buts J-P. Vitamin/mineral supplementation and intelligence. *Lancet* 1990; **335:** 1158–60.
5. Crombie IK, *et al.* Vitamin/mineral supplementation and intelligence. *Lancet* 1990; **336:** 175.
6. Schoenthaler SJ, *et al.* Controlled trial of vitamin-mineral supplementation: effects on intelligence and performance. *Personality Indiv Diff* 1991; **12:** 351–62.
7. Whitehead RG. Vitamins, minerals, schoolchildren, and IQ. *Br Med J* 1991; **302:** 548.
8. Peto R. Vitamins and IQ. *Br Med J* 1991; **302:** 906.
9. Anonymous. Brains and vitamins. *Lancet* 1991; **337:** 587–8.

PROPHYLAXIS OF ISCHAEMIC HEART DISEASE. As discussed on p.782, hypercholesterolaemia is a major risk factor for the development of atherosclerosis and consequently ischaemic heart disease (including angina and myocardial infarction). Treatment of hypercholesterolaemia with lipid regulating drugs is discussed under Hyperlipidaemias (p.1265). Since oxidation of lipids, particularly low-density-lipoprotein (LDL) cholesterol,[1] has been proposed as a factor in atherogenesis, another approach has been to try and prevent atherosclerosis by the use of dietary antioxidants such as vitamins E and C and betacarotene. Prospective epidemiological studies have revealed a reduced risk of ischaemic heart disease in individuals taking vitamin E supplements,[2,3] and those with a high carotene intake (particularly smokers).[2] In a further prospective cohort study,[4] dietary vitamin E consumption, but not vitamin E supplementation, was associated with decreased risk of death from ischaemic heart disease. Conversely, in these studies,[2-4] intake of vitamin C did not appear to be associated with a decreased risk of ischaemic heart disease. Data from some studies assessing serum or fat concentrations also provide evidence that high betacarotene concentrations are associated with decreased cardiovascular disease.[5-7]

However, despite these promising epidemiological data, results from randomised placebo-controlled trials have generally failed to find any benefit for vitamin E or betacarotene supplements in the primary or secondary prevention of ischaemic heart disease. In the Alpha Tocopherol, Beta Carotene Cancer Prevention (ATBC) study, which monitored cardiovascular disease as a secondary end-point, vitamin E was not associated with a decreased incidence of ischaemic heart disease, and betacarotene was associated with a small increased risk.[8] In further analyses, neither supplement appreciably altered the incidence of angina pectoris,[9] nor showed any beneficial effect on cardiovascular deaths in the subset of men with previous myocardial infarction.[10] Similarly, neither the Betacarotene and Retinol Efficacy Trial (CARET)[11] nor the Skin Cancer Prevention Study[7] found an effect for betacarotene supplementation on the risk of death from cardiovascular disease. In studies specifically on cardiovascular end-points, no benefit from betacarotene supplements was seen in a large, randomised, placebo-controlled study[12] in healthy men and an initial study[13] of supplementation with high-dose vitamin E in patients with evidence of ischaemic heart disease failed to show any beneficial effect on cardiovascular deaths. It has been suggested that the lack of effect of vitamin E in some of these studies may be due to an insufficiently high dose of tocopherol, since the effect seems chiefly to be seen in those receiving 100 units or more daily.[2,3] Further large-scale studies are underway; the Heart Outcomes Prevention Evaluation (HOPE) trial and the Heart Protection Study are assessing the effect of vitamin E and a 'cocktail' of vitamin E, vitamin C, and betacarotene, respectively, on the development of ischaemic heart disease in high risk subjects.[14] For a discussion of the possibility that folic acid may reduce ischaemic heart disease through its homocysteine-lowering effect, see p.1341.

1. Jha P, *et al.* The antioxidant vitamins and cardiovascular disease: a critical review of epidemiologic and clinical trial data. *Ann Intern Med* 1995; **123:** 860–72. Correction. *ibid.* 1996; **124:** 934.
2. Rimm EB, *et al.* Vitamin E consumption and the risk of coronary heart disease in men. *N Engl J Med* 1993; **328:** 1450–6.
3. Stampfer MJ, *et al.* Vitamin E consumption and the risk of coronary disease in women. *N Engl J Med* 1993; **328:** 1444–9.
4. Kushi LH, *et al.* Dietary antioxidant vitamins and death from coronary heart disease in postmenopausal women. *N Engl J Med* 1996; **334:** 1156–62.
5. Morris DL, *et al.* Serum carotenoids and coronary heart disease: the Lipid Research Clinics Coronary Primary Prevention Trial and Follow-up Study. *JAMA* 1994; **272:** 1439–41.
6. Kardinaal AFM, *et al.* Antioxidants in adipose tissue and risk of myocardial infarction: the EURAMIC study. *Lancet* 1993; **342:** 1379–84.
7. Greenberg ER, *et al.* Mortality associated with low plasma concentration of beta carotene and the effect of oral supplementation. *JAMA* 1996; **275:** 699–703.
8. The Alpha-Tocopherol, Beta-Carotene Cancer Prevention Study Group. The effect of vitamin E and beta carotene on the incidence of lung cancer and other cancers in male smokers. *N Engl J Med* 1994; **330:** 1029–35.
9. Rapola JM, *et al.* Effect of vitamin E and beta carotene on the incidence of angina pectoris. *JAMA* 1996; **275:** 693–8. Correction. *ibid.* 1998; **279:** 1528.
10. Rapola JM, *et al.* Randomised trial of α-tocopherol and β-carotene supplements on incidence of major coronary events in men with previous myocardial infarction. *Lancet* 1997; **349:** 1715–20.
11. Omenn GS, *et al.* Effects of a combination of beta carotene and vitamin A on lung cancer and cardiovascular disease. *N Engl J Med* 1996; **334:** 1150–5.
12. Hennekens CH, *et al.* Lack of effect of long-term supplementation with beta carotene on the incidence of malignant neoplasms and cardiovascular disease. *N Engl J Med* 1996; **334:** 1145–9.
13. Stephens NG, *et al.* Randomised controlled trial of vitamin E in patients with coronary disease: Cambridge Heart Antioxidant Study (CHAOS). *Lancet* 1996; **347:** 781–6.
14. Lonn EM, Yusuf S. Is there a role for antioxidant vitamins in the prevention of cardiovascular diseases? An update of epidemiological and clinical trials data. *Can J Cardiol* 1997; **13:** 957–65.

PROPHYLAXIS OF MALIGNANT NEOPLASMS. Diet has long been hypothesised to play a role in the development of cancer. There is evidence that a diet rich in fruit and vegetables is associated with a lower incidence of malignant disease, particularly of the respiratory and digestive tracts.[1] It has been hypothesised that some of the benefits of such a diet derive from the role of antioxidant vitamins such as the carotenoids and vitamins C and E in scavenging free radicals.[2,3] However, it is by no means certain that these are the only, or necessarily the most important, dietary components responsible for benefit, since components such as dietary fibre may also play a role. In addition, different antioxidants may vary in their properties and efficacy,[3,4] and the appropriate dosage remains largely conjectural, and perhaps as a result the evidence of benefit is often conflicting.

Several clinical trials of the use of **vitamin A** or **betacarotene** in the secondary or primary prevention of malignancy have been reported. Prolongation of disease-free interval in patients with various malignant neoplasms was reported in 1 study of betacarotene,[5] and another reported remission of oral leukoplakia in patients treated with betacarotene and vitamin A.[6] Vitamin A alone was reported to reduce the incidence of primary tobacco-related neoplasms in a study of patients treated surgically for lung cancer.[7] However, other results have largely failed to substantiate any benefit for secondary prevention. No reduction in the incidence of new skin cancers,[8] or in malignant transformation of cervical dysplasia,[9] or in new colorectal adenomas[10] was reported in 3 other studies. In a primary prevention study, a combination of betacarotene, vitamin E, and selenium was associated with a reduction in stomach and oesophageal cancers in a population at high risk of these cancers and with a diet low in micronutrients in China.[11] In contrast, other primary prevention studies have failed to show any benefit, and possibly some harm, from betacarotene supplements in well-nourished populations. A study in smokers[12,13] showed an increase in lung cancer and associated mortality in those receiving betacarotene (20 mg daily), but not those receiving vitamin E (50 mg daily). Similarly, an increased risk of lung cancer was noted in recipients of betacarotene (30 mg daily) with vitamin A (25 000 units daily) in another study in individuals at high risk of lung cancer, and this study was stopped early as a result.[14,15] A third study in healthy men found no benefit or harm for betacarotene supplements (50 mg on alternate days) in terms of incidence of malignant neoplasms, including those of the lung.[16]

Vitamin C has also been proposed for this purpose but there is no real evidence to justify it. It certainly appears to be ineffective as adjuvant therapy in the treatment of advanced malignancy,[17] and combination with betacarotene and vitamin E failed to show any effect in preventing colorectal adenoma.[10] At physiological concentrations vitamin C is an important antioxidant,[3] but supplementation is unlikely to be justified in anyone eating a balanced diet.[1]

Vitamin E substances are also known to play an important antioxidant role in the body. Animal studies have suggested that they should inhibit tumour production, and the Chinese study mentioned above found combined antioxidant therapy including vitamin E to be of benefit in the primary prevention of stomach and oesophageal cancers.[11] Other studies in western populations have generally been disappointing; vitamin E had no effect on lung cancer incidence in those at risk,[12,13] and did not prevent the development of new colorectal adenomas.[10] However, further analysis of the lung-cancer study[18] suggests that vitamin E may have protected against prostate cancer.

Results from the Nurses' Health Study have indicated that prolonged use of multivitamins was associated with reduced risk of developing cancer of the colon.[19] This effect was thought to be due to the **folate** component and could be demonstrated after 15 years of use, but not after shorter-term ingestion. Dietary folate was also associated with a modest reduction in risk for colon cancer.

At present, therefore, the only conclusion that appears uncontroversial is that a diet involving frequent consumption of fruit and vegetables is likely to be beneficial.[1] However, given the present difficulties in treating many malignancies once they develop (p.476), interest in the topic seems likely to continue.

1. Austoker J. Diet and cancer. *Br Med J* 1994; **308:** 1610–14.
2. Hennekens CH. Antioxidant vitamins and cancer. *Am J Med* 1994; **97** (suppl 3A): 2S–4S.
3. Halliwell B. Free radicals, antioxidants, and human disease: curiosity, cause, or consequence? *Lancet* 1994; **344:** 721–4.
4. Hankinson SE, Stampfer MJ. All that glitters is not beta carotene. *JAMA* 1994; **272:** 1455–6.
5. Santamaria L, *et al.* First clinical report (1980-1988) of cancer chemoprevention with betacarotene plus canthaxanthin supplemented to patients after radical treatment. *Boll Chim Farm* 1988; **127:** 57S–60S.
6. Stich HF, *et al.* Remission of oral leukoplakias and micronuclei in tobacco/betel quid chewers treated with beta-carotene and with beta-carotene plus vitamin A. *Int J Cancer* 1988; **42:** 195–9.
7. Pastorino U, *et al.* Adjuvant treatment of stage I lung cancer with high-dose vitamin A. *J Clin Oncol* 1993; **11:** 1216–22.
8. Greenberg ER, *et al.* A clinical trial of beta carotene to prevent basal-cell and squamous-cell cancers of the skin. *N Engl J Med* 1990 **323:** 789–95.
9. de Vet HCW, *et al.* The effect of beta-carotene on the regression and progression of cervical dysplasia: a clinical experiment. *J Clin Epidemiol* 1991; **44:** 273–83.
10. Greenberg ER, *et al.* A clinical trial of antioxidant vitamins to prevent colorectal adenoma. *N Engl J Med* 1994; **331:** 141–7.
11. Blot WJ, *et al.* Nutrition intervention trials in Linxian, China: supplementation with specific vitamin/mineral combinations, cancer incidence, and disease-specific mortality in the general population. *J Natl Cancer Inst* 1993; **85:** 1483–92.
12. The Alpha-Tocopherol, Beta-Carotene Cancer Prevention Study Group. The effect of vitamin E and beta carotene on the incidence of lung cancer and other cancers in male smokers. *N Engl J Med* 1994; **330:** 1029–35.
13. Albanes D, *et al.* α-Tocopherol and β-carotene supplements and lung cancer incidence in the alpha-tocopherol, beta-carotene cancer prevention study: effects of base-line characteristics and study compliance. *J Natl Cancer Inst* 1996; **88:** 1560–70.
14. Omenn GS, *et al.* Effects of a combination of beta carotene and vitamin A on lung cancer and cardiovascular disease. *N Engl J Med* 1996; **334:** 1150–5.
15. Omenn GS, *et al.* Risk factors for lung cancer and for intervention effects in CARET, the Beta-Carotene and Retinol Efficacy Trial. *J Natl Cancer Inst* 1996; **88:** 1550–9.
16. Hennekens CH, *et al.* Lack of effect of long-term supplementation with beta carotene on the incidence of malignant neoplasms and cardiovascular disease. *N Engl J Med* 1996; **334:** 1145–9.
17. Moertel CG, *et al.* High-dose vitamin C versus placebo in the treatment of patients with advanced cancer who have had no prior chemotherapy: a randomized double-blind comparison. *N Engl J Med* 1985; **312:** 137–41.
18. Heinonen OP, *et al.* Prostate cancer and supplementation with α-tocopherol and β-carotene: incidence and mortality in a controlled trial. *J Natl Cancer Inst* 1998; **90:** 440–6.
19. Giovannucci E, *et al.* Multivitamin use, folate, and colon cancer in women in the Nurses' Health Study. *Ann Intern Med* 1998; **129:** 517–24.

Acesulfame Potassium (14035-b)

Acesulfame Potassium *(BANM, rINNM).*

Acesulfame K; Acesulfamum Kalicum; E950; H73-3293; HOE-095K. The potassium salt of 6-methyl-1,2,3-oxathiazin-4(3*H*)-one 2,2-dioxide.

$C_4H_4KNO_4S = 201.2.$

CAS — 55589-62-3.

Pharmacopoeias. In *Eur.* (see p.viii).

A white, crystalline powder or colourless crystals. **Soluble** in water, very slightly soluble in alcohol and in acetone.

Acesulfame potassium is an intense sweetener about 200 times as sweet as sucrose. It is used in foods and does not appear to be affected by cooking.

Preparations

Proprietary Preparations (details are given in Part 3)

Multi-ingredient: ***Ital.:*** Dulcex†.

Alanine (572-b)

Alanine *(USAN, rINN).*

A; Ala; L-Alanine; Alaninum. L-2-Aminopropionic acid.

$C_3H_7NO_2 = 89.09.$

CAS — 56-41-7.

Pharmacopoeias. In *Eur.* (see p.viii) and *US.*

Colourless or white or almost white odourless crystals or crystalline powder. Freely **soluble** in water; very slightly soluble in alcohol and slightly soluble in 80% alcohol; practically insoluble in ether. A 5% solution in water has a pH of 5.5 to 7.0. **Protect** from light.

Alanine is an aliphatic amino acid. It is used as a dietary supplement.

Hypoglycaemia. References to the investigational use of alanine in the management of insulin-induced hypoglycaemia.[1-3]

1. Wiethop BV, Cryer PE. Glycemic actions of alanine and terbutaline in IDDM. *Diabetes Care* 1993; **16:** 1124–30.
2. Wiethop BV, Cryer PE. Alanine and terbutaline in treatment of hypoglycemia in IDDM. *Diabetes Care* 1993; **16:** 1131–6.
3. Saleh TY, Cryer PE. Alanine and terbutaline in the prevention of nocturnal hypoglycemia in IDDM. *Diabetes Care* 1997; **20:** 1231–6.

Preparations

Proprietary Preparations (details are given in Part 3)
Multi-ingredient: *UK:* Amino MS.

Arginine (573-v)

Arginine (*rINN*).

Arg; L-Arginine; Argininum; R. L-2-Amino-5-guanidinovaleric acid.

$C_6H_{14}N_4O_2$ = 174.2.

CAS — 74-79-3.

Pharmacopoeias. In *Eur.* (see p.viii) and *US.*

White or almost white crystalline powder, or white or colourless, practically odourless crystals. Freely **soluble** in water; sparingly or very slightly soluble in alcohol; practically insoluble in ether. **Protect** from light.

Arginine Glutamate (574-g)

Arginine Glutamate (*BAN, USAN, rINNM*).

L-Arginine L-glutamate.

$C_6H_{14}N_4O_2,C_5H_9NO_4$ = 321.3.

CAS — 4320-30-3.

Arginine Hydrochloride (575-q)

Arginine Hydrochloride (*USAN, rINNM*).

L-Arginine Monohydrochloride; Arginini Hydrochloridum.

$C_6H_{14}N_4O_2,HCl$ = 210.7.

CAS — 1119-34-2.

Pharmacopoeias. In *Chin., Eur.* (see p.viii), *Jpn,* and *US.*
Fr. also includes Arginine Aspartate.

Practically odourless white or colourless crystals or white or almost white powder. Freely **soluble** in water; very slightly soluble in alcohol; practically insoluble in ether. **Protect** from light.

Adverse Effects and Precautions

Nausea, vomiting, flushing, headache, numbness, and local venous irritation may occur if arginine solutions are infused too rapidly. Elevated plasma-potassium concentrations have been reported in uraemic patients and arginine should therefore be administered with caution to patients with renal disease or anuria. Arginine hydrochloride should be administered cautiously to patients with electrolyte disturbances as its high chloride content could lead to the development of hyperchloraemic acidosis.

Extravasation. A report[1] of necrosis following extravasation of a 10% solution of arginine hydrochloride. Both osmotic and local hyperkalaemic effects had been proposed as a mechanism for the injury.

1. Bowlby HA, Elanjian SI. Necrosis caused by extravasation of arginine hydrochloride. *Ann Pharmacother* 1992; **26:** 263–4.

Hyperkalaemia. Two alcoholic patients with severe liver disease and moderate renal insufficiency developed severe hyperkalaemia following administration of arginine hydrochloride and one died.[1] Both patients had received a total dose of 300 mg of spironolactone some time before arginine hydrochloride administration, but the contribution of spironolactone to the hyperkalaemia was not known.

1. Bushinsky DA, Gennari FJ. Life-threatening hyperkalemia induced by arginine. *Ann Intern Med* 1978; **89:** 632–4.

Hypersensitivity. A 10-year-old boy experienced an anaphylactic reaction 5 minutes after the start of an infusion of a 5% arginine hydrochloride solution in a test for growth-hormone output.[1] This was considered to be a very rare event and only one other apparent allergic reaction had been reported to the manufacturers.

1. Tiwary CM, *et al.* Anaphylactic reaction to arginine infusion. *N Engl J Med* 1973; **288:** 218.

Uses and Administration

Arginine is an aliphatic amino acid which is essential for infant growth. It is used as a dietary supplement.

Arginine stimulates the release of growth hormone by the pituitary gland and may be used instead of, or in addition to, other tests such as insulin-induced hypoglycaemia, for the evaluation of growth disorders; false-positive and false-negative results are relatively common and evaluation therefore should not be made on the basis of a single arginine test. It is used as a 10% solution of the hydrochloride in usual doses of 30 g by intravenous infusion given over 30 minutes; children should be given 500 mg per kg body-weight.

Arginine is used in certain conditions accompanied by hyperammonaemia; for further details see below.

Arginine hydrochloride has also been used as an acidifying agent. In severe metabolic alkalosis intravenous doses (in grams) have been calculated by multiplying the desired decrease in plasma-bicarbonate concentration (mEq or mmol per litre) by the patient's body-weight (in kg) and then dividing by 9.6. In forced acid diuresis to hasten drug elimination after overdose a suggested dose has been 10 g intravenously over 30 minutes.

Arginine may also be employed in the form of the acetylasparaginate, aspartate, citrate, glutamate, oxoglurate, tidiacicate (thiazolidine-2,4-dicarboxylate), and timonacicate (thiazolidine-4-carboxylate). Formulation as an arginine salt is used to improve the solubility of a number of drugs, notably analgesics and antibiotics.

Hyperammonaemia. Hyperammonaemia is a characteristic feature of inborn errors of the urea cycle and is particularly severe in ornithine carbamoyl transferase (OCT) deficiency and carbamoyl phosphate synthetase (CPS) deficiency. During the urea cycle, waste ammonia, in the form of the ammonium ion, is normally condensed with bicarbonate and ATP to form carbamoyl phosphate which undergoes several more reactions, including one leading to the synthesis of arginine, and ultimate transformation to urea for excretion. Thus, in defects of this cycle ammonia accumulates and arginine synthesis is deficient. Hyperammonaemia is often associated with respiratory alkalosis in patients with urea cycle disorders.

The basis of treatment is dietary protein restriction, to decrease the requirement for waste nitrogen synthesis, and the administration of drugs to stimulate alternative pathways of waste nitrogen excretion. These include arginine, citrulline, sodium benzoate, sodium phenylacetate, and sodium phenylbutyrate. In the initial management of severe hyperammonaemia, haemodialysis is required.

Arginine supplements are given except in hyperargininaemia,[1] although citrulline may be used in some cases instead.[2] Walter and Leonard[1] have quoted oral doses of arginine 0.5 to 2 g daily for long-term management of OCT and CPS deficiency, and up to 700 mg per kg daily for argininosuccinate synthetase (AS) or argininosuccinate lysase (AL) deficiencies. Intravenous doses quoted for the treatment of severe hyperammonaemia or encephalopathy were arginine 200 to 800 mg per kg body-weight given as a loading dose over 4 hours, followed by a constant infusion of 200 to 800 mg per kg daily, the dose range varying with the specific defect in the cycle.

Patients also receive concomitant treatment with sodium benzoate and sodium phenylacetate[2-5] or sodium phenylbutyrate[5-7] unless suffering from AL deficiency, which can usually be managed with protein restriction and arginine alone.[4] When sodium benzoate is conjugated with glycine and excreted as hippuric acid it provides an alternative pathway of nitrogen excretion, while sodium phenylacetate and sodium phenylbutyrate provide a second and even more effective pathway by conjugation with glutamine.

The usual initial doses of sodium benzoate and sodium phenylacetate in affected infants are 250 mg of each per kg body-weight daily by intravenous infusion, followed by 250 to 500 mg of each per kg daily by constant infusion.[4,5] Infusion is continued until the drugs can be taken orally; although earlier protocols were based on oral sodium benzoate, oral sodium phenylbutyrate is now preferred at a dosage of 450 to 600 mg per kg daily.[5-7] It has been suggested that carnitine supplementation should be added to minimise the adverse effects in patients treated with benzoate.[8]

Hyperammonaemia and hepatic encephalopathy can also arise from a variety of other causes and although arginine has been advocated many authorities do not consider such use beneficial; however, intravenous sodium benzoate and sodium phenylacetate have successfully been used to manage transient severe hyperammonaemia in patients being treated for acute leukaemia.[9]

For the management of hepatic encephalopathy, see p.1170.

Hyperargininaemia, resulting from arginase deficiency, is associated with vomiting, convulsions, physical and mental retardation, and sometimes hyperammonaemia. It has been successfully managed in one patient by dietary supplementation with lysine and ornithine,[10] although the long-term effects of the raised arginine concentrations were unknown.

1. Walter JH, Leonard JV. Inborn errors of the urea cycle. *Br J Hosp Med* 1987; **38:** 176–83.
2. Msall M, *et al.* Neurologic outcome in children with inborn errors of urea synthesis: outcome of urea-cycle enzymopathies. *N Engl J Med* 1984; **310:** 1500–5.
3. Brusilow SW, *et al.* New pathways of nitrogen excretion in inborn errors of urea synthesis. *Lancet* 1979; **ii:** 452–4.
4. Brusilow SW, *et al.* Treatment of episodic hyperammonemia in children with inborn errors of urea synthesis. *N Engl J Med* 1984; **310:** 1630–4.
5. Maestri NE, *et al.* Prospective treatment of urea cycle disorders. *J Pediatr* 1991; **119:** 923–8.
6. Maestri NE, *et al.* Long-term survival of patients with argininosuccinate synthetase deficiency. *J Pediatr* 1995; **127:** 929–35.
7. Maestri NE, *et al.* Long-term treatment of girls with ornithine transcarbamylase deficiency. *N Engl J Med* 1996; **335:** 855–9.
8. Sakuma T. Alteration of urinary carnitine profile induced by benzoate administration. *Arch Dis Child* 1991; **66:** 873–5.
9. Watson AJ, *et al.* Transient idiopathic hyperammonaemia in adults. *Lancet* 1985; **ii:** 1271–4.
10. Kang SS, *et al.* Hyperargininemia: effect of ornithine and lysine supplementation. *J Pediatr* 1983; **103:** 763–5.

Hypotensive action. Arginine is the physiological precursor of nitric oxide (endothelium-derived relaxing factor; EDRF) and this has been suggested as an explanation for the hypotensive effect that has been reported in healthy subjects[1-3] and hypertensive patients[1,4] given infusions of arginine, although effects of arginine unrelated to nitric oxide generation cannot be excluded.[4] Decrease in plasma-cholesterol concentrations has also been reported in 2 hypercholesterolaemic patients given arginine infusions.[5] It has even been suggested that arginine might be suitable for the short-term control of hypertension,[3] although in the absence of controlled studies of its effect this must be considered speculative.

For a discussion of hypertension and its conventional management, see p.788.

1. Nakaki T, *et al.* L-arginine-induced hypotension. *Lancet* 1990; **336:** 696.
2. Hishikawa K, *et al.* L-arginine-induced hypotension. *Lancet* 1991; **337:** 683–4.
3. Petros AJ, *et al.* L-arginine-induced hypotension. *Lancet* 1991; **337:** 1044–5.
4. Pedrinelli R, *et al.* Pressor, renal and endocrine effects of L-arginine in essential hypertensives. *Eur J Clin Pharmacol* 1995; **48:** 195–201.
5. Korbut R, *et al.* Effect of L-arginine on plasminogen-activator inhibitor in hypertensive patients with hypercholesterolemia. *N Engl J Med* 1993; **328:** 287–8.

Malignant neoplasms. Dietary supplementation with arginine for 3 days before each cycle of chemotherapy for breast cancer (p.485) was associated with high response rates in a pilot study,[1] a finding which was considered to justify further evaluation.

1. Brittenden J, *et al.* Dietary supplementation with L-arginine in patients with breast cancer (>4cm) receiving multimodality treatment: report of a feasibility study. *Br J Cancer* 1994; **69:** 918–21.

Preparations

USP 23: Arginine Hydrochloride Injection.

Proprietary Preparations (details are given in Part 3)
Aust.: Sangenor; ***Belg.:*** Dynamisan; ***Fr.:*** Acdril†; Dynamisan; Energitum; Eucol†; Hepagrume; Sargenor; Tiadilon; ***Ger.:*** Eubiol; Leberam†; ***Ital.:*** Bioarginina; Dynamisan; Sargenor; Spermargin†; Sulfile; ***Spain:*** Hepacitol; Livercrom; Potenciator; Sargenor; Sorbenor; ***Switz.:*** Dynamisan; ***USA:*** R-Gene.

Multi-ingredient: ***Aust.:*** Leberinfusion; Rocmaline; ***Austral.:*** Anti-Flab†; ***Fr.:*** Activarol; Arginotri-B; Arnilose; Citrarginine; Epuram; Hepargitol; Liporex†; Rocmaline; Viridex†; ***Ger.:*** Glutarsin E; Hepasteril A†; Hepasteril†; Rocmalat†; Sterofundin CH compositum†; Sterofundin CH†; ***Ital.:*** Calciofix; Citruplexina†; Glutargin; Ipoazotal; Ipoazotal Complex; Isoram; Polilevo; Somatron; Tonoplus; Vitasprint Complex; ***Spain:*** Dynamogen; Sanieb; ***Switz.:*** Activital; Arginotri-B; Vitasprint Complex.

Arrowroot (12393-w)

Amylum Marantae; Araruta; Maranta.

The starch granules of the rhizomes of *Maranta arundinacea* (Marantaceae).

Arrowroot has the general properties of starch (p.1356). It has been used as a suspending agent in the preparation of barium meals and has sometimes been used in place of starch in tablet manufacture.

Aspartame (2374-j)

Aspartame *(BAN, USAN, rINN)*.

APM; Aspartamum; E951; SC-18862. Methyl *N*-L-α-aspartyl-L-phenylalaninate; 3-Amino-*N*-(α-methoxycarbonylphenethyl)succinamic acid; *N*-L-α-aspartyl-L-phenylalanine, 1-methyl ester.

$C_{14}H_{18}N_2O_5$ = 294.3.

CAS — 22839-47-0.

Pharmacopoeias. In *Eur.* (see p.viii). Also in *USNF.*

A white odourless slightly hygroscopic crystalline powder with an intensely sweet taste.

Sparingly or slightly **soluble** in water and in alcohol; practically insoluble in dichloromethane and in hexane. A 0.8% solution in water has a pH of 4.0 to 6.5.

Store in airtight containers.

In the presence of moisture it hydrolyses to form aspartylphenylalanine and a diketopiperazine derivative, with a resulting loss of sweetness.

Adverse Effects and Precautions

Excessive use of aspartame should be avoided by patients with phenylketonuria since one of its metabolic products is phenylalanine. Aspartame's sweetness is lost during prolonged cooking.

The safety and side-effects of aspartame as a pharmaceutical excipient have been reviewed.[1,2]

Aspartame is hydrolysed in the gastro-intestinal tract to its 3 primary constituents, methanol, aspartic acid, and phenylalanine. However, even with extraordinary consumption, methanol toxicity stemming from aspartame use is extremely unlikely. Aspartate concentrations in blood do not rise significantly following a very large dose (50 to 100 mg per kg body-weight) and therefore toxicity related to aspartate is also not expected to occur. Despite the similarity of aspartate to glutamate studies in glutamate-sensitive persons have shown that they are not affected by aspartame consumption. Plasma concentrations of phenylalanine are also unlikely to be markedly elevated following modest consumption of aspartame by healthy persons but persons with phenylketonuria should avoid or limit their use of aspartame.

A number of adverse effects have been reported[1,2] following the use of aspartame, either as spontaneously recorded complaints from consumers or as published case reports in the medical literature. Most frequently reported problems have been headache, neuropsychiatric or behavioural symptoms, seizures, gastro-intestinal symptoms, and hypersensitivity or dermatological symptoms. Available data do not provide evidence for serious widespread health consequences attendant upon the use of aspartame but it would appear that certain individuals may have an unusual sensitivity to the product.

Studies have confirmed aspartame's lack of effect on children's behaviour or cognitive function.[3,4]

An increased incidence of brain cancer was postulated to be related to aspartame use in a recent report;[5] however, the USA Food and Drug Administration maintain that the available evidence does not support an association.[6]

1. Golightly LK, *et al.* Pharmaceutical excipients: adverse effects associated with 'inactive' ingredients in drug products (part II). *Med Toxicol* 1988; **3:** 209–40.
2. American Academy of Pediatrics. "Inactive" ingredients in pharmaceutical products: update. *Pediatrics* 1997; **99:** 268–78.
3. Shaywitz BA, *et al.* Aspartame, behavior, and cognitive function in children with attention deficit disorder. *Pediatrics* 1994; **93:** 70–5.
4. Wolraich ML, *et al.* Effects of diets high in sucrose or aspartame on the behavior and cognitive performance of children. *N Engl J Med* 1994; **330:** 301–7.
5. Olney JW, *et al.* Increasing brain tumor rates: is there a link to aspartame? *J Neuropathol Exp Neurol* 1996; **55:** 1115–23.
6. Anonymous. Aspartame: no apparent link with brain tumours. *WHO Drug Inf* 1997; **11:** 18–19.

Uses

Aspartame is an intense sweetening agent about 180 to 200 times as sweet as sucrose. It is used in foods, beverages, and pharmaceuticals. Each g provides approximately 17 kJ (4 kcal).

Preparations

Proprietary Preparations (details are given in Part 3)

Fr.: D Sucril; ***Ital.:*** Aspartina; Dietason†; Dolcor; Futura; Le Sucrine†; Microcal†; Suaviter; Vantaggio; Weight Watchers Punto.

Multi-ingredient: ***Ital.:*** Doldieta; Dulcex†; Weight Watchers Punto.

Aspartic Acid (576-p)

Aspartic Acid *(USAN, pINN)*.

Acidum Asparticum; Asp; L-Aspartic Acid; D. L-Aminosuccinic acid.

$C_4H_7NO_4$ = 133.1.

CAS — 56-84-8.

Pharmacopoeias. In *Eur.* (see p.viii).

A white or almost white crystalline powder, or colourless crystals. Slightly **soluble** in water; practically insoluble in alcohol and in ether. It dissolves in dilute solutions of alkali hydroxides and in dilute mineral acids. **Protect** from light.

Aspartic acid is an aliphatic amino acid. It is used as a dietary supplement.

Betacarotene (7824-a)

Betacarotene *(rINN)*.

all-*trans*-β-Carotene; Beta Carotene *(USAN)*; Betacarotenum; E160(a); Provitamin A. β,β-Carotene; *(all-E)*-1,1′-(3,7,12,16-Tetramethyl-1,3,5,7,9,11,13,15,17-octadecanonaene-1,18-diyl)bis[2,6,6-trimethylcyclohexene].

$C_{40}H_{56}$ = 536.9.

CAS — 7235-40-7.

Pharmacopoeias. In *Eur.* (see p.viii) and *US.*

Red or reddish brown to violet-brown crystals or crystalline powder. Practically **insoluble** in water and in alcohol; soluble in chloroform and in carbon disulphide; sparingly soluble in ether, in petroleum spirit, and in vegetable oils; slightly soluble in cyclohexane; practically insoluble in methyl alcohol, in acids, and in alkalis. **Store** in airtight containers at a temperature not exceeding 25°. Protect from light.

Carotene exists in 3 isomeric forms, all of which are converted to some extent into vitamin A in the livers of man and animals. Of the 3 isomers of carotene, the *beta* compound is more active than the *alpha-* or *gamma-*isomers. The vitamin A activity of plants is due to the presence of *alpha-*, *beta-*, and *gamma-*carotenes and to kryptoxanthine; that of animal tissues is due to both vitamin A and carotene, while fish-liver oils contain vitamin A but no carotene.

Units

Vitamin A activity in foods is currently expressed in terms of retinol equivalents: 6 μg of betacarotene represents 1 retinol equivalent (or 10 of the former International units for provitamin A—see p.1358).

Adverse Effects and Precautions

Loose stools may occasionally occur during treatment with betacarotene and the skin may assume a slightly yellow discoloration. Bruising and arthralgia have been reported rarely.

Excessive intake of betacarotene does not result in hypervitaminosis A (see Pharmacokinetics, below).

Carcinogenicity. For reference to the finding of an increased incidence of lung cancers in individuals receiving betacarotene supplements, compared with those receiving placebo, in studies investigating the ability of betacarotene to protect against malignancy, see under Prophylaxis of Malignant Neoplasms, p.1333.

Effects on the skin. Yellow pigmentation of the skin may result from an unusually high consumption of carrots or other source of carotene,[1] or from a defect in the enzyme that normally metabolises betacarotene to vitamin A.[2] Hypercarotenaemia can be distinguished from jaundice by the fact that the sclerae retain their normal white colour. Pigmentation occurs first on the palms and soles and may extend to the nasolabial folds. Although it has been stated that the condition is harmless as the body converts carotene to retinol only in amounts as required,[1] others consider that long-standing hypercarotenaemia can have clinical sequelae:[2] neutropenia[3] and amenorrhoea[4] have been reported to be associated with the condition.

1. Sharman IM. Hypercarotenaemia. *Br Med J* 1985; **290:** 95.
2. Vaughan Jones SA, Black MM. Metabolic carotenaemia. *Br J Dermatol* 1994; **131:** 145.
3. Shoenfeld Y, *et al.* Neutropenia induced by hypercarotenaemia. *Lancet* 1982; **i:** 1245.
4. Kemmann E, *et al.* Amenorrhoea associated with carotenemia. *JAMA* 1983; **249:** 926–9.

Pharmacokinetics

Gastro-intestinal absorption of betacarotene depends on the presence of bile and is increased by dietary fat. About 20 to 60% of betacarotene is metabolised to retinol in the intestinal wall, and a small amount is converted to vitamin A in the liver. The proportion of betacarotene converted to vitamin A decreases as the intake of betacarotene increases, and high doses of betacarotene do not lead to abnormally high serum concentrations of vitamin A. Unchanged betacarotene is distributed to various tissues including fat, the adrenal glands, and ovaries.

References.

1. Wang X-D. Review: absorption and metabolism of β-carotene. *J Am Coll Nutr* 1994; **13:** 314–25.

Human requirements

Carotenes, of which betacarotene has the highest activity, are major dietary sources of vitamin A—see p.1359.

Uses and Administration

Betacarotene is a carotenoid precursor of vitamin A (p.1358). It is used for the prevention of vitamin A deficiency at a dose of 6 to 15 mg daily. In the treatment of vitamin A deficiency, vitamin A is preferred to betacarotene.

Betacarotene may be given by mouth to reduce the severity of photosensitivity reactions in patients with erythropoietic protoporphyria (see also below). Doses are in the range of 30 to 300 mg daily for adults and 30 to 150 mg daily for children depending upon severity; they may be taken as either single daily doses or divided doses but should preferably be taken with meals. The protection offered by betacarotene is not total and generally 2 to 6 weeks of treatment resulting in a yellow coloration of palms and soles is necessary before patients should attempt to increase their exposure to sunlight.

Betacarotene and other carotenoids (alphacarotene and gammacarotene) are used as colouring agents for foods.

Betacarotene has antoxidant activity and has been studied for its possible protective benefit in a number of disorders.

Age-related macular degeneration. A study in patients with age-related macular degeneration (p.618) indicated that the risk of developing this disorder (a leading cause of irreversible blindness among elderly persons) was markedly decreased amongst those with the highest carotenoid intake;[1] in particular, lutein and zeaxanthin, or green leafy vegetables (which contain high concentrations of these carotenoids) were associated with a lower risk. Increasing the intake of these carotenoids may be of benefit in reducing the development of this disorder.

1. Seddon JM, *et al.* Dietary carotenoids, vitamins A, C, and E, and advanced age-related macular degeneration. *JAMA* 1994; **272:** 1413–20.

Deficiency states. A study in Senegalese children suffering from vitamin A deficiency as defined by abnormal results on eye cytology found that supplementation with betacarotene (in a single dose equivalent to 200 000 units of vitamin A) was as effective as a single 200 000 unit dose of vitamin A palmitate in reversing the ocular changes.[1] Since betacarotene is less toxic than vitamin A itself it would have some advantages for vitamin A supplementation, either as an oral supplement or by encouraging the consumption of carotenoid-rich fruit and vegetables. A study in Indonesian women found that a betacarotene supplement improved vitamin A status, whereas an additional daily portion of dark-green leafy vegetables containing a similar amount of betacarotene did not.[2] However, others contend that consumption of food sources of carotenoids are effective in improving vitamin A status in deficiency states,[3,4] and that it may not be appropriate to extrapolate these findings to vitamin A deficient children.[3,5] WHO policy is still to promote dietary adjustment wherever vitamin A deficiency is endemic.[5]

For further discussion of vitamin A deficiency and the value of supplementation in various disease states, see under Vitamin A Substances, p.1359.

1. Carlier C, *et al.* A randomised controlled trial to test equivalence between retinyl palmitate and β carotene for vitamin A deficiency. *Br Med J* 1993; **307:** 1106–10.
2. de Pee S, *et al.* Lack of improvement in vitamin A status with increased consumption of dark-green leafy vegetables. *Lancet* 1995; **346:** 75–81.
3. Reddy V. Vitamin A status and dark green leafy vegetables. *Lancet* 1995; **346:** 1634–5.
4. Underwood BA. Vitamin A status and dark green leafy vegetables. *Lancet* 1995; **346:** 1635.
5. WHO. Vitamin A status: is dietary replacement practicable. *WHO Drug Inf* 1995; **9:** 141.

Ischaemic heart disease. There are results from epidemiological studies suggesting the potential benefits of dietary betacarotene in preventing ischaemic heart disease, particularly in smokers; however, randomised placebo-controlled studies of betacarotene supplements have returned negative results, as discussed on p.1333.

Malignant neoplasms. Epidemiologists have often expressed interest in whether diet and nutrition are important factors in the development of cancer and particular attention has been given to carotenoids and especially betacarotene. Because some evidence from epidemiological studies did indeed appear to show that higher dietary intakes had a protective effect several randomised placebo-controlled trials examining the use of betacarotene supplements in the primary or secondary prevention of malignancy were instigated. However, the results of studies so far published have generally been disappointing. Moreover, some results suggest that supplementation with betacarotene may actually be harmful: an increase in lung cancer was seen in those at risk for this malignancy (see p.1333).

Porphyria. Betacarotene is the most widely used systemic agent for the management of erythropoietic protoporphyria,[1] a non-acute porphyria characterised by cutaneous photosensitivity (p.983). It is often administered with canthaxanthin to reduce the skin discoloration caused by betacarotene alone.

1. Todd DJ. Erythropoietic protoporphyria. *Br J Dermatol* 1994; **131:** 751–66.

Preparations

USP 23: Beta Carotene Capsules; Oil- and Water-soluble Vitamins Capsules; Oil- and Water-soluble Vitamins Tablets; Oil-soluble Vitamins Capsules; Oil-soluble Vitamins Tablets.

Proprietary Preparations (details are given in Part 3)
Aust.: Carotaben; ***Austral.:*** B-Tene; Solatene†; ***Ger.:*** BellaCarotin mono; Carotaben; ***Ital.:*** Tannisol; ***Neth.:*** Carotaben; ***S.Afr.:*** Vitaforce Carotene A†; ***Swed.:*** Karotena ACO†; ***Switz.:*** Carotaben; ***UK:*** Arocin; Biocarotine; Pervita; ***USA:*** Max-Caro†; Provatene†; Solatene†.

Multi-ingredient: ***Aust.:*** Oleovit A; Oleovit A + D; ***Austral.:*** Antioxidant Tablets; Beta A-C; Cold Sore Tablets; Eye Health Herbal Plus Formula 4; Ginkgo ACE†; Lifesystem Herbal Plus Formula 5 Eye Relief; Lifesystem Herbal Plus Formula 8 Echinacea; Odourless Garlic; Sinus and Hayfever; ***Fr.:*** Difrarel; Phenoro; ***Ger.:*** Carotin; Sonnenbraun; ***Ital.:*** Aclon Lievit; Agedin Plus; Angstrom Viso/Labbra Alta Protezione; Ecamannan; Eccarvit; Fotoretin†; Levudin; Mirtilene; Solecin; Tannidin Plus; ***Spain:*** Aceite Acalorico; Mirtilus; ***Switz.:*** Apotrin; Difrarel†; Linola gras; Phenoro†; Visaline; ***USA:*** Antiox.

Biotin (7859-g)

Biotin *(pINN)*.

Biotinum; Coenzyme R; Vitamin H. *cis*-5-(Hexahydro-2-oxo-1*H*-thieno[3,4-*d*]imidazol-4-yl)valeric acid.

$C_{10}H_{16}N_2O_3S$ = 244.3.

CAS — 58-85-5.

Pharmacopoeias. In *Eur.* (see p.viii) and *US.*

A white crystalline powder or colourless crystals. Very slightly **soluble** in water and in alcohol; practically insoluble in other common organic solvents. It dissolves in dilute solutions of alkali hydroxides. **Store** in airtight containers. Protect from light.

Biotin is traditionally considered to be a vitamin B substance. It is an essential coenzyme in fat metabolism and in other carboxylation reactions. Biotin deficiency may result in the urinary excretion of organic acids and changes in skin and hair. Deficiency of biotin is very unlikely in man because of its widespread distribution in food. Egg-yolk and offal are especially good sources. Biotin deficiency has been reported however during long-term parenteral nutrition and in patients with biotinidase deficiency, an inherited metabolic disorder.

Biotin combines with avidin, a glycoprotein present in raw egg-white, to form an inactive compound.

Deficiency states. References to the successful use of biotin to treat deficiency of biotinidase, the enzyme responsible for the recycling and functioning of biotin.

1. Wolf B, *et al.* Clinical findings in four children with biotinidase deficiency detected through a statewide neonatal screening program. *N Engl J Med* 1985; **313:** 16–19.
2. Hurvitz H, *et al.* Biotinidase deficiency associated with severe combined immunodeficiency. *Lancet* 1989; **ii:** 228–9.
3. McVoy JRS, *et al.* Partial biotinidase deficiency: clinical and biochemical features. *J Pediatr* 1990; **116:** 78–83.
4. Lara EB, *et al.* Biotinidase deficiency in black children. *J Pediatr* 1990; **116:** 750–2.

Human requirements. In the United Kingdom neither a reference nutrient intake (RNI) nor an estimated average requirement (EAR) (see p.1332) has been set for biotin although it was considered that an intake of between 10 and 200 μg daily was both safe and adequate.[1] Similarly in the United States an adequate intake of 30 μg daily has been set for adults.[2]

1. DoH. Dietary reference values for food energy and nutrients for the United Kingdom: report of the panel on dietary reference values of the committee on medical aspects of food policy. *Report on health and social subjects 41.* London: HMSO, 1991.
2. Standing Committee on the Scientific Evaluation of Dietary Reference Intakes of the Food and Nutrition Board. *Dietary Reference Intakes for thiamin, riboflavin, niacin, vitamin B_6, folate, vitamin B_{12}, pantothenic acid, biotin, and choline.* Washington, DC: National Academy Press, 1998.

Preparations

USP 23: Oil- and Water-soluble Vitamins Capsules; Oil- and Water-soluble Vitamins Tablets; Water-soluble Vitamins Capsules; Water-soluble Vitamins Tablets.

Proprietary Preparations (details are given in Part 3)
Aust.: Medobiotin; ***Austral.:*** Biotinas†; ***Ger.:*** BIO-H-TIN; Deacura; Gabunat; Medobiotin; Priorin Biotin; Rombellin; ***Ital.:*** Biodermatin; Diathynil†.

Multi-ingredient: ***Fr.:*** Arbum; Forcapil; ***Ger.:*** Carotin; Sonnenbraun; ***Ital.:*** Herbavit; ***Spain:*** Lacerdermol.

Carnitine (12528-s)

Levocarnitine *(BAN, USAN, rINN)*; L-Carnitine. (*R*)-(3-Carboxy-2-hydroxypropyl)trimethylammonium hydroxide, inner salt; (*R*)-3-Hydroxy-4-trimethylammoniobutyrate.

$C_7H_{15}NO_3$ = 161.2.

CAS — 541-15-1.

NOTE. The configuration for Carnitine *(rINN)* is not specified.
Pharmacopoeias. In *Eur.* (see p.viii) and *US.*

White odourless, hygroscopic crystals or crystalline powder. Freely **soluble** in water and hot alcohol; practically insoluble in acetone and in ether. A 5% solution in water has a pH of 6.5 to 8.5. **Store** in airtight containers.

Adverse Effects

Gastro-intestinal disturbances such as nausea, vomiting, diarrhoea, and abdominal cramps have been reported following the administration of L-carnitine. Body odour has also been noticed in some patients.

Of 30 patients given DL-carnitine intravenously after dialysis sessions 3 developed myasthenia-like symptoms but following administration of only L-carnitine to these 3 the symptoms did not occur.[1] It was considered that in anuric uraemic patients the D-isomer was not excreted adequately and that accumulation had blocked neuromuscular transmission. It was therefore suggested that L-carnitine, rather than the DL-form, should be employed.

1. Bazzato G, *et al.* Myasthenia-like syndrome after D,L but not L-carnitine. *Lancet* 1981; **i:** 1209.

Uses and Administration

L-Carnitine is an amino acid derivative which is an essential cofactor of fatty acid metabolism.

Carnitine is used in the treatment of primary carnitine deficiency and has also been tried in carnitine deficiency secondary to a variety of defects of intermediary metabolism or other conditions such as haemodialysis. Both the L- and the DL-isomers have been used, but it is believed that only L-carnitine is effective and in addition, that DL-carnitine supplementation can lead to carnitine deficiency.

In primary carnitine deficiency, up to 200 mg per kg body-weight daily by mouth may be required, administered in 2 to 4 divided doses. Rarely, higher doses of up to 400 mg per kg daily may be needed. When administered intravenously, up to 100 mg per kg daily is given in 3 to 4 divided doses by slow intravenous injection over 2 to 3 minutes.

In patients with carnitine deficiency secondary to haemodialysis, the recommended dose is 20 mg per kg intravenously after each dialysis session, adjusted according to plasma-carnitine concentrations. A maintenance dose of 1 g daily by mouth may be considered.

Carnitine is under investigation for the treatment of zidovudine-induced mitochondrial myopathy.

Carnitine hydrochloride, carnitine orotate, and bicarnitine chloride have also been used.

Carnitine, which has been the subject of several reviews,[1-4] occurs as distinct L- and D-isomers although naturally-occurring carnitine is almost exclusively the L-isomer. In higher animals carnitine is an essential co-factor of fatty acid metabolism in the heart, liver, and skeletal muscle. It is normally synthesised in the liver, brain, and kidneys in sufficient quantities to meet human requirements but dietary sources such as meat and dairy products also provide carnitine. In plasma and tissues carnitine is present in the free form and as acylcarnitine esters of which acetylcarnitine (see p.1542) is the most abundant.

It has been pointed out that L-carnitine should be used in therapeutics in preference to DL-carnitine, which is the form often present in over-the-counter preparations and dietary supplements. This is because the biochemical and pharmacological profiles of the two isomers are very different with L-carnitine acting as a substrate for carnitine acetyltransferase while D-carnitine acts as a competitive inhibitor; also, L-carnitine-induced stimulation of palmitate oxidation is competitively inhibited by D-palmitoylcarnitine. Such differences in the activities of the isomers are thus believed to account for findings of benefit only with the L-isomer or unwanted effects when D-carnitine or DL-carnitine was administered.[1,3]

Primary carnitine deficiency is a disorder of the membrane transport of carnitine and patients have presented with hypoglycaemia and encephalopathy, skeletal myopathy, and cardiomyopathy. Therapy with carnitine in these primary deficiency states is considered to have a rational basis.[1,2] Secondary carnitine deficiency occurs in many inherited metabolic disorders and especially in the organic acidurias and disorders of beta-oxidation. Some authors have said that the benefit of therapy with carnitine is limited in organic acidurias[2] and unproven or doubtful in disorders of beta-oxidation[2,5,6] while others have disagreed with this view believing treatment may be worthwhile.[7,8]

Carnitine deficiency may also arise during the long-term administration of drugs such as valproic acid,[1] pivampicillin,[9,10] or pivmecillinam,[9] which are conjugated with carnitine. Investigations are in progress to assess whether carnitine supplementation can prevent or reverse this type of carnitine deficiency but treatment with carnitine, although it raised plasma-carnitine concentrations, had no more effect than placebo on the well-being of children receiving valproic acid therapy in one such study.[11]

Since carnitine supplementation has been associated with a reduction[18] in the incidence of haemodialysis-induced cramps (p.1303) it has been suggested that these cramps might be due in part to carnitine deficiency.

There is also some evidence[1,12] that carnitine supplements may be of benefit to low birth-weight preterm infants, but a double-blind study[13] failed to confirm this effect. However, premature infants at particular risk of carnitine deficiency, such as those on long-term parenteral nutrition, may benefit.[4,14] Some workers consider that carnitine supplements may be advisable in full-term infants receiving formula feeds.[15]

Low concentrations of carnitine have also been reported to occur in a variety of other conditions and there is some evidence that carnitine supplementation may exert a cardioprotective role. Benefit in patients with cardiomyopathies,[1] reduction of infarct size and prevention of arrhythmias in patients with myocardial infarction,[1,2] increased exercise tolerance in patients with angina[1,2] or intermittent claudication,[2] and protection from the cardiotoxicity of the anthracycline antineoplastics[1] have all been described in patients given carnitine supplementation. However, the use of carnitine in healthy subjects in an attempt to improve athletic performance is controversial.[16]

One case report has described a dramatic response of long-standing leg ulcers to carnitine therapy in a patient with sickle-cell disease.[17]

1. Goa KL, Brogden RN. L-Carnitine: a preliminary review of its pharmacokinetics, and its therapeutic use in ischaemic cardiac disease and primary and secondary carnitine deficiencies in relationship to its role in fatty acid metabolism. *Drugs* 1987; **34:** 1–24.
2. Anonymous. Carnitine deficiency. *Lancet* 1990; **335:** 631–3.
3. Li Wan Po A. Carnitine: a scientifically exciting molecule. *Pharm J* 1990; **245:** 388–9.
4. Walter JH. L-carnitine. *Arch Dis Child* 1996; **74:** 475–8.
5. Anonymous. Medium chain acyl CoA dehydrogenase deficiency. *Lancet* 1991; **338:** 544–5.
6. Rinaldo P, *et al.* Effect of treatment with glycine and L-carnitine in medium-chain acyl-coenzyme A dehydrogenase deficiency. *J Pediatr* 1993; **122:** 580–4.
7. Winter SC, *et al.* Carnitine deficiency. *Lancet* 1990; **335:** 981–2.
8. Chalmers RA, *et al.* Carnitine deficiency. *Lancet* 1990; **335:** 982.
9. Holme E, *et al.* Carnitine deficiency induced by pivampicillin and pivmecillinam therapy. *Lancet* 1989; **ii:** 469–73.
10. Melegh B. Carnitine supplementation in pivampicillin treatment. *Lancet* 1989; **ii:** 1096.
11. Freeman JM, *et al.* Does carnitine administration improve the symptoms attributed to anticonvulsant medications?: a double-blinded, crossover study. *Pediatrics* 1994; **93:** 893–5.
12. Shortland GJ, Walter JH. L-carnitine. *Lancet* 1990; **335:** 1215.
13. Shortland GJ, *et al.* Randomised controlled trial of L-carnitine as a nutritional supplement in preterm infants. *Arch Dis Child Fetal Neonatal Ed* 1998; **78:** F185–F188.
14. Sulkers EJ, *et al.* L-carnitine. *Lancet* 1990; **335:** 1215.
15. Giovannini M, *et al.* Is carnitine essential in children? *J Int Med Res* 1991; **19:** 88–102.
16. Tonda ME, Hart LL. N,N-dimethylglycine and L-carnitine as performance enhancers in athletes. *Ann Pharmacother* 1992; **26:** 935–7.
17. Harrell HL. L-Carnitine for leg ulcers. *Ann Intern Med* 1990; **113:** 412.
18. Ahmad S, *et al.* Multicenter trial of L-carnitine in maintenance hemodialysis patients II: clinical and biochemical effects. *Kidney Int* 1990; **38:** 912–8.

Preparations

USP 23: Levocarnitine Injection; Levocarnitine Oral Solution; Levocarnitine Tablets.

Proprietary Preparations (details are given in Part 3)
Canad.: Carnitor; ***Fr.:*** Levocarnil; ***Ger.:*** Biocarn; L-Carn; Nefrocarnit; ***Ital.:*** Anetin; Briocor; Cardimet; Cardiogen; Carnicor; Carnidex†; Carnitolo; Carnitop; Carnovis; Carnum; Carrier;

Carvis; Carvit; Elleci; Eucar; Eucarnil; Farnitin; Framil; Karrer; Kernit; Lefcar; Levocarvit; Medocarnitin; Metina; Miocardin; Miocor; Miotonal; Neo Cardiol; Transfert; ***Spain:*** Carnicor; Secabiol; ***Switz.:*** Elcarnitol†; ***UK:*** Carnitor; Elcarn; ***USA:*** Carnitor; VitaCarn.

Multi-ingredient: ***Fr.:*** Arkotonic; ***Ital.:*** Biocarnil; Carpantin; Cerebrix†; Co-Carnetina B12; Normo-Calcium†; ***Spain:*** Hepadif; Histiotone†; Malandil; ***UK:*** Slimswift Day Trim†.

Choline Chloride (7875-g)

Choline Chloride *(rINN)*.

Cholinii Chloridum. 2-Hydroxyethyltrimethylammonium chloride.

$C_5H_{14}ClNO$ = 139.6.

CAS — 62-49-7 (choline); 67-48-1 (choline chloride).

Pharmacopoeias. In *Aust.* and *Fr.*

Choline is an acetylcholine precursor. It is involved in lipid metabolism and acts as a methyl donor in various other metabolic processes. Choline has traditionally been considered to be a vitamin B substance although its functions do not justify its classification as a vitamin. Choline can be synthesised in the body. However, its absence in total parenteral nutrition causes hepatic steatosis, and it is also thought to be a requirement in the diet of neonates. Sources of choline, which occurs mostly as lecithin, include egg-yolk and vegetable and animal fat.

Choline is used as a dietary supplement and has been used to treat liver disorders such as fatty liver and cirrhosis. It has been tried in the management of Alzheimer's disease (p.1386) but without success. Choline is used as the bitartrate, dihydrogen citrate, and orotate salts as well as the chloride.

Human requirements. In the USA, an adequate intake of 550 mg daily in men and 425 mg daily in women has been determined for choline.[1]

1. Standing Committee on the Scientific Evaluation of Dietary Reference Intakes of the Food and Nutrition Board. *Dietary Reference Intakes for thiamin, riboflavin, niacin, vitamin B_6, folate, vitamin B_{12}, pantothenic acid, biotin, and choline.* Washington, DC: National Academy Press, 1998.

Preparations

Proprietary Preparations (details are given in Part 3)
Austral.: Becholine D†; ***Fr.:*** Hepagrume; ***Ger.:*** Neurotropan.

Multi-ingredient: ***Aust.:*** Orocholin; ***Austral.:*** Gingo A; Ginkgo ACE†; Liv-Detox; ***Belg.:*** Sulfarlem Choline; ***Fr.:*** Citrocholine; Citrocholine vit. C 250†; Cystichol; Desintex-Choline; Hepacholine Sorbitol; Kalicitrine; Liporex†; Phosphocholine†; Romarinex-Choline; ***Ger.:*** Enterotropin†; Hepabionta comp†; Hepalipon N; Hepalixier†; Hepatofalk; Hepatofalk Neu; Hepavis†; Hepsan†; Neurotropan-Hy†; Neurotropan-M†; Orotofalk†; Sterofundin CH compositum†; Tutofusin LC†; ***Ital.:*** Citrosorbina B6†; Emofol†; Epa-Treis; Glutestere B-Complesso†; Itahepar†; Litrison; ***S.Afr.:*** Hepavite; ***Spain:*** Antibiofilus; Hepato Fardi; ***Switz.:*** Sebo Lotion†; ***UK:*** Fat-Solv; Lipotropic Factors; ***USA:*** Ak-Biocholine; Ilopan-Choline.

Chondroitin Sulphate–Iron Complex (14169-a)

Ferropolichondrum.

CAS — 54391-57-0.

Chondroitin sulphate-iron complex is employed as a source of iron (p.1346) for iron-deficiency anaemia (p.702). It is given by mouth in doses containing the equivalent of up to 90 mg of iron daily.

Preparations

Proprietary Preparations (details are given in Part 3)
Ital.: Condrofer; Ferrol; Isairon; ***Jpn:*** Blutal.

Chromium (18958-w)

Cr = 51.9961.

Chromium Trichloride (12560-s)

Chromic Chloride.

$CrCl_3$ = 158.4.

CAS — 10025-73-7 (anhydrous chromium trichloride); 10060-12-5 (chromium trichloride hexahydrate).

Pharmacopoeias. US has a monograph for chromium trichloride hexahydrate.

Chromium Trichloride Hexahydrate (USP 23) occurs as dark green, odourless, slightly deliquescent crystals. **Soluble** in water and in alcohol; slightly soluble in acetone; practically insoluble in ether. **Store** in airtight containers.

Adverse Effects

Trivalent salts of chromium, such as chromium trichloride, are generally considered to produce few adverse effects. However, hexavalent forms of chromium are notably toxic (see under Chromium Trioxide, p.1562).

Effects on the kidneys. Two cases of renal failure were attributed to ingestion of excessive doses of chromium picolinate (a trivalent chromium salt) in women with no previous history of renal dysfunction.[1,2] For mention of decreases in glomerular filtration rate in children receiving chromium-supplemented total parenteral nutrition, see below.

1. Wasser WG, *et al.* Chronic renal failure after ingestion of over-the-counter chromium picolinate. *Ann Intern Med* 1997; **126:** 410.
2. Cerulli J, *et al.* Chromium picolinate toxicity. *Ann Pharmacother* 1998; **32:** 428–31.

Uses and Administration

Chromium is an essential trace element that potentiates insulin action thus influencing carbohydrate, lipid, and protein metabolism. Dietary sources rich in chromium include brewers' yeast, meat, whole grains, and nuts. Chromium trichloride has been given as a chromium supplement in total parenteral nutrition. Chromium picolinate is used as a chromium supplement, and is being investigated for improving glycaemic control in patients with diabetes mellitus.

Human requirements. In the United Kingdom neither a reference nutrient intake (RNI) nor an estimated average requirement (EAR) (see p.1332) has been set for chromium although a safe and adequate intake was believed to be above 25 μg daily for adults.[1] Similarly, in the United States a recommended dietary allowance has not been published and the safe and adequate intake for adults was believed to be 50 to 200 μg daily.[2] WHO considers that the minimum population mean intake likely to meet normal needs for chromium might be approximately 33 μg daily, and that supplementation of this element should not exceed 250 μg daily until more is known.[3]

1. DoH. Dietary reference values for food energy and nutrients for the United Kingdom: report of the panel on dietary reference values of the committee on medical aspects of food policy. *Report on health and social subjects 41.* London: HMSO, 1991.
2. Subcommittee on the tenth edition of the RDAs, food and Nutrition Board, Commission on Life Sciences, National Research Council. *Recommended dietary allowances.* 10th ed. Washington, DC: National Academy Press, 1989.
3. WHO. Chromium. In: *Trace elements in human nutrition and health.* Geneva: WHO, 1996: 155–60.

Supplementation. Although a daily chromium intake of 0.2 μg per kg body-weight has been suggested in children receiving total parenteral nutrition (TPN), a study in 15 children[1] receiving long-term parenteral nutrition found that supplementation at about this level was associated with serum-chromium concentrations 4 to 42 times higher than the mean value in 15 children not receiving TPN. Raised serum-chromium concentrations were associated with a decrease in glomerular filtration rate; one year after discontinuing chromium supplementation, which reduced intake to 0.05 μg per kg daily (as contaminants of water and TPN solutions), chromium concentrations, although lower, were still higher than controls and renal function had not altered. The authors have subsequently discontinued chromium supplementation in both children and adults, since chromium contamination of TPN solutions appears adequate to prevent deficiency, although it is acknowledged that signs of chromium deficiency may take some years to appear. Chromium contamination in various preparations used in paediatric parenteral nutrition has been studied.[2]

1. Moukarzel AA, *et al.* Excessive chromium intake in children receiving total parenteral nutrition. *Lancet* 1992; **339:** 385–8.
2. Hak EB, *et al.* Chromium and zinc contamination of parenteral nutrient solution components commonly used in infants and children. *Am J Health-Syst Pharm* 1998; **55:** 150–4.

Preparations

USP 23: Chromic Chloride Injection.

Proprietary Preparations (details are given in Part 3)
Austral.: Chrometrace†; ***Canad.:*** Micro Cr; ***USA:*** Chroma-Pak.

Multi-ingredient: ***Austral.:*** Digestaid; ***Canad.:*** Formula CI; ***Fr.:*** Bio-Chrome.

Citrulline (16582-n)

N^5-(Aminocarbonyl)-L-ornithine; N^δ-Carbamylornithine. α-Amino-δ-ureidovaleric acid.

$C_6H_{13}N_3O_3$ = 175.2.

CAS — 372-75-8.

Citrulline is an amino acid which is involved in the urea cycle. Citrulline and citrulline malate are used as dietary supplements.

Citrulline has been given as an alternative to arginine in the management of hyperammonaemia due to urea cycle disorders (p.1334).

Lysinuric protein intolerance is another condition associated with hyperammonaemia and similar neurological sequelae. In this condition there is no deficiency of urea-cycle enzymes but a deficiency of urea-cycle substrate, such as ornithine, which results in reduced synthesis of citrulline. Supplements of citrulline given with meals have been reported to have resulted in a substantial increase in protein tolerance, striking acceleration in linear growth, and an increase in bone mass in a child with this disorder who presented with osteoporosis.[1]

1. Carpenter TO, *et al.* Lysinuric protein intolerance presenting as childhood osteoporosis: clinical and skeletal response to citrulline therapy. *N Engl J Med* 1985; **312:** 290–4.

Preparations

Proprietary Preparations (details are given in Part 3)
Fr.: Stimol; ***Switz.:*** Stimufor†.

Multi-ingredient: ***Fr.:*** Epuram; ***Ital.:*** Citruplexina†; Energon Rende†; Ideolider; Ipoazotal; Ipoazotal Complex; Polilevo.

Cod-liver Oil (7890-v)

Cod-liver Oil *(BAN)*.

Aceite de Hígado de Bacalao; Cod Liver Oil; Huile de Foie de Morue; Iecoris Aselli Oleum; Lebertran; Ol. Morrh.; Óleo de Bacalhau; Oleum Jecoris Aselli; Oleum Morrhuae; Olio di Fegato di Merluzzo.

CAS — 8001-69-2.

Pharmacopoeias. In *Eur.* (see p.viii), *Jpn, Pol.,* and *US.*

The fatty oil obtained from the fresh liver of the cod, *Gadus morrhua* and other species of Gadidae, solid substances being removed by cooling and filtering. Ph. Eur. includes Cod-liver Oil (Type A) and Cod-liver Oil (Type B). For both types, Ph. Eur. specifies not less than 600 units (180 μg) and not more than 2500 units (750 μg) of vitamin A per g and not less than 60 units (1.5 μg) and not more than 250 units (6.25 μg) of vitamin D (cholecalciferol) per g. The USP specifies not less than 850 units (225 μg) of vitamin A and not less than 85 units (2.125 μg) of vitamin D per g, and permits up to 1% of a suitable flavour or flavours.

A clear yellowish viscous liquid with a slightly fishy but not rancid odour. Practically **insoluble** in water; slightly soluble in alcohol; freely soluble in ether, in chloroform, in carbon disulphide, and in ethyl acetate; miscible with petroleum spirit. **Store** in well-filled airtight containers preferably under an inert gas. Protect from light.

Uses and Administration

Cod-liver oil is a rich source of vitamin D (p.1366) and a good source of vitamin A (p.1358). It also contains several essential fatty acids.

Cod-liver oil dressings or ointment have been advocated to accelerate healing in burns, ulcers, pressure sores, and superficial wounds, but controlled observations have failed to substantiate claims of their value.

Preparations

Proprietary Preparations (details are given in Part 3)
Aust.: Adecaps; ***Austral.:*** Hypol; ***Belg.:*** Surmoruine; ***Ger.:*** Unguentolan; ***Ital.:*** Dermovitamina; Merluzzina†; ***Spain:*** Aceite Geve Concentrado; ***Switz.:*** Morrhulan.

Multi-ingredient: ***Aust.:*** Dermilon†; Dermowund; Desitin; Leukichtan; Mirfulan; Pudan-Lebertran-Zinksalbe; Vitapan; Vulpuran; ***Austral.:*** Covitol†; Hypol; Mac†; Rashaway†; ***Belg.:*** Mitosyl; Newderm; Peneytol†; Polyseptol; Pyal; Vitamorrhuine; ***Canad.:*** Caldesene; Desitin; ***Fr.:*** Eryteal; Fletagex†; Halivite; ***Ger.:*** Adebilan†; Chlortesin-N†; Dermilon; Desitin; Elbozon†; Gelovitall†; Jacosulfon†; Kremulsion†; Leukona-Wundsalbe; Mirfulan; Mirfulan Spray N; Mitosyl; Rectosellan N†; Swansol-Wundsalbe†; ***Irl.:*** Caldease; Morhulin; ***Ital.:*** Dermosteril†; Fosfarsile Yunior; Idustatin; Neo-Ustiol; Steril Zeta; Trofo 5; Viocidina; ***Norw.:*** Aselli; Jecoderm†; ***S.Afr.:*** Achromide; Daromide†; Ung Vernleigh; ***Spain:*** Avril; Recto Menaderm; Siete Mares Higado Bacal; ***Switz.:*** Keroderm; Mitosyl†; Perles d'huile de foie de morue du Dr Geistlich; Phlogidermil; Vita-Hexin; Vita-Merfen†; ***UK:*** Hofels Cod Liver Oil and Garlic†; M & M; Morhulin; Scott's Emulsion; Woodwards Nappy Rash Ointment; ***USA:*** A and D Medicated; Caldesene; Clocream; Desitin; Diaparene Peri-Anal†; Diaper Rash; Dyprotex; Medicone Dressing; Primaderm-B.

Copper (5284-y)

Cu = 63.546.

CAS — 7440-50-8.

Calcium Copperedetate (12505-h)

Calcium [ethylenediaminetetra-acetato(4—)-*N,N′,O,O′*]copper (II) dihydrate.

$C_{10}H_{12}CaCuN_2O_8,2H_2O$ = 427.9.

CAS — 66317-91-7 (anhydrous calcium copperedetate).

Pharmacopoeias. In *BP(Vet).*

A blue, odourless or almost odourless, crystalline powder. It contains 9.1 to 9.7% of Ca and 14.4 to 15.3% of Cu. Freely **soluble** in water, the solution gradually precipitating the insoluble tetrahydrate; practically insoluble in alcohol.

Copper Chloride (5288-k)

Cupric Chloride.

$CuCl_2,2H_2O$ = 170.5.

CAS — 7447-39-4 (anhydrous copper chloride); 10125-13-0 (copper chloride dihydrate).

Pharmacopoeias. In *US.*

Bluish-green deliquescent crystals. Freely **soluble** in water; soluble in alcohol; slightly soluble in ether. **Store** in airtight containers.

Copper Gluconate (18507-g)

Copper D-gluconate (1:2); Bis(D-gluconato-O^1,O^2) copper.

$C_{12}H_{22}CuO_{14}$ = 453.8.

CAS — 527-09-3.

Pharmacopoeias. In *US.*

Copper Sulphate (5285-j)

Copper Sulph.; Cuivre (Sulfate de); Cupr. Sulph.; Cupri Sulfas; Cupri Sulphas; Cupric Sulfate; Kupfersulfat; Sulfato de Cobre.

Copper (II) sulphate pentahydrate.

$CuSO_4,5H_2O$ = 249.7.

CAS — 7758-98-7 (anhydrous copper sulphate); 7758-99-8 (copper sulphate pentahydrate).

NOTE. Crude copper sulphate is sometimes known as 'blue copperas', 'blue stone', and 'blue vitriol'.

Pharmacopoeias. In *Eur.* (see p.viii) and *US. Eur.* also includes Anhydrous Copper Sulphate.

Blue crystals or crystalline powder. It slowly effloresces in air. The exsiccated salt is nearly white.

Soluble 1 in 3 of water, 1 in 0.5 of boiling water, 1 in 500 of alcohol, and 1 in 3 of glycerol; soluble in methyl alcohol. **Store** in airtight containers.

Anhydrous Copper Sulphate (Ph. Eur.) is a greenish grey, very hygroscopic, powder. Freely **soluble** in water; slightly soluble in methyl alcohol; practically insoluble in alcohol. **Store** in airtight containers.

Adverse Effects

Adverse effects from copper have tended to arise following absorption of the metal from cooking utensils and during dialysis. Ingestion of copper from cooking utensils is associated mainly with hepatotoxicity. Dialysis procedures may supply copper through the water supply or from parts of the equipment and when this happens patients may suffer haemolysis and other haematological reactions with kidney involvement as well as hepatotoxicity; the toxicity is generally a result of poor equipment maintenance.

Adverse effects attributed to copper have been reported in women with copper-containing intra-uterine devices. There have been isolated case reports of various effects such as allergy and endometrial changes. However, with these devices it is difficult to separate those adverse effects that are due to the device from those due solely to the copper.

The symptoms of Wilson's disease (hepatolenticular degeneration) (see p.992) are due to an accumulation of copper in various parts of the body.

Copper salts if ingested can produce severe gastro-intestinal effects and there may be systemic absorption of copper leading to the effects discussed above. The use of sprays of copper salts in agriculture has been associated with lung changes. Treatment of copper poisoning is symptomatic and may involve the use of a chelating agent to remove any absorbed metal. Dialysis has been tried.

Effects on the liver. A report of cirrhosis and acute liver failure attributable to chronic excessive copper supplement ingestion.[1]

1. O'Donohue J, *et al.* Micronodular cirrhosis and acute liver failure due to chronic copper self-intoxication. *Eur J Gastroenterol Hepatol* 1993; **5:** 561–2.

Interactions

Large doses of zinc supplements may inhibit the gastro-intestinal absorption of copper.

Uses and Administration

Copper is an essential trace element although severe copper deficiency, which is associated with anaemia, neutropenia, and bone demineralisation, is rare in humans. Copper sulphate is added to parenteral feeds as a source of copper in the prophylaxis and treatment of deficiency states. Doses that have been employed for prophylaxis range from 0.5 to 1.5 mg (7.9 to 23.6 μmol) of copper daily although up to 3 mg daily has been suggested in established deficiency; infants have received 20 μg (0.3 μmol) of copper per kg body-weight daily. The dose should be governed by the serum-copper concentration which in healthy adults ranges between 0.7 and 1.6 μg per mL (0.01 to 0.025 μmol per mL).

Copper sulphate and other soluble salts of copper have an astringent action on mucous surfaces and in strong solutions they are corrosive.

Copper has a contraceptive effect when present in the uterus and is added to some intra-uterine contraceptive devices; for further details, see below. It is also reported to have an antimicrobial action.

Copper sulphate has been used to prevent the growth of algae in reservoirs, ponds, and swimming pools and as a molluscicide in the control of fresh-water snails that act as intermediate hosts in the life-cycle of the parasites causing schistosomiasis.

Reagents containing copper sulphate are used in tests for reducing sugars.

In veterinary medicine calcium copperedetate, copper methionate, and cuproxoline are used for the prevention and treatment of copper deficiency.

Copper bracelets are worn as a folk remedy for rheumatic disorders: there is no good evidence to justify such a practice.

Copper (Cuprum Metallicum; Cuprum Met.) is used in homoeopathic medicine.

Contraception. In a statement from the Medical Advisory Committee of the Family Planning Association and the National Association of Family Planning Doctors in Great Britain the following points were made.[1] Intra-uterine devices (IUDs) are believed to exert their contraceptive effect (p.1434) by interfering with the reproductive process before the ovum reaches the intra-uterine cavity and the copper released from copper-bearing IUDs probably potentiates this effect. Like all devices which are placed in the uterus, copper IUDs are subject to deposition of cellular debris and of calcium and magnesium salts. The calcium and magnesium salts were once thought to reduce the effectiveness of IUDs, but this is not so as the copper ions are still able to diffuse. Copper IUDs first became available in the 1970s and in the early models the thin copper wire wound around the stem of the device sometimes fragmented or disappeared completely. Subsequent development led to devices that are both more effective and have a longer life. This has been achieved by increasing the wire thickness, by the preparation of a silver-core copper wire, and by the use of solid copper collars or sleeves on the device. The modern copper IUDs in use today should be regarded as being clinically effective and safe for at least five years. Copper IUDs are the most effective available method for postcoital contraception (p.1434). Traditional copper IUDs are T-shaped and rigid or semi-rigid. Newer forms include an implantable frameless device, which may be more suitable for nulliparous women.

1. Newton J, Tacchi D. Long-term use of copper intrauterine devices. *Lancet* 1990; **335:** 1322–3.

Deficiency states. Acquired copper deficiency is very rare and the small number of cases have usually involved patients on total parenteral nutrition or in one case[1] enteral nutrition.

In the United Kingdom dietary reference values (see p.1332) have been published for copper.[2] Although an estimated average requirement (EAR) could not be derived a reference nutrient intake (RNI) of 1.2 mg (19 μmol) daily was set for adults; RNIs of lower values were also specified for infants and children.[2]

In the United States a recommended dietary allowance has not been set for copper because of the uncertainty concerning the quantitative human requirements. Rather, a safe and adequate range has been specified of 1.5 to 3 mg daily for adults; lower values were also given for infants and children of various age groups.[3]

WHO has estimated a minimum population mean intake of 1.2 mg daily for women and 1.3 mg daily for men, and safe upper limits of population mean intakes of 10 mg daily for women and 12 mg daily for men;[4] values are also estimated for infants and children.

Menkes' disease is an X-linked genetic disorder associated with a defect in copper transport, which almost invariably results in death due to progressive cerebral degeneration by the age of 3 years. Early initiation of treatment with copper-histidine complex may be of benefit in such children.[5]

1. Masugi J, *et al.* Copper deficiency anemia and prolonged enteral feeding. *Ann Intern Med* 1994; **121:** 386.
2. DoH. Dietary reference values for food energy and nutrients for the United Kingdom: report of the panel on dietary reference values of the committee on medical aspects of food policy. *Report on health and social subjects 41.* London: HMSO, 1991.
3. Subcommittee on the tenth edition of the RDAs, Food and Nutrition Board, Commission on Life Sciences, National Research Council. *Recommended dietary allowances.* 10th ed. Washington, DC: National Academy Press, 1989.
4. WHO. Copper. In: *Trace elements in human nutrition and health.* Geneva: WHO, 1996: 123–43.
5. Sarkar B, *et al.* Copper-histidine therapy for Menkes' disease. *J Pediatr* 1993; **123:** 828–30.

Schistosomiasis. Although most control programmes for schistosomiasis (p.95) use niclosamide as a molluscicide, and copper salts have largely been abandoned for snail control, copper sulphate is still used for this purpose in Egypt.[1]

1. WHO. The control of schistosomiasis: second report of the WHO expert committee. *WHO Tech Rep Ser 830* 1993.

Preparations

BPC 1973: Compound Ferrous Sulphate Tablets;
USP 23: Cupric Chloride Injection; Cupric Sulfate Injection.

Proprietary Preparations (details are given in Part 3)
Austral.: Coppertrace†; Multiload; ***Canad.:*** Gyne-T; Micro Cu; ***Fr.:*** Gyne-T; Metacuprol; ML Cu 250; ML Cu 375; Remoplexe; Sterilet T au Cuivre†; ***Ger.:*** Cuprenase†; Gyne-T; Multiload; ***Irl.:*** Multiload; Ortho Gyne-T; ***Ital.:*** Copper T†; Gravigard; Mini-Gravigard; ML Cu 250†; No-Gravid; Ortho-Neo-T†; Telo Cypro; ***Neth.:*** Gyne-T; Multiload; ***S.Afr.:*** Cuprocept CCL; Dalcept; Fincoid†; Multiload; Tricept; ***Switz.:*** Fincoid; Multiload; SOF-T; ***UK:*** Gynefix; Multiload; Novagard†; Ortho Gyne-T; ***USA:*** Cu-7†; Paragard T380A; Tatum-T†.

Multi-ingredient: ***Austral.:*** Alcusal; Alcusal Sport; Ascoxal; ***Canad.:*** Nova-T; ***Fr.:*** Bioceanat; Dermalibour; Dermo-Sulfuryl; Dermocreme; Dermocuivre; Dexaderme Kefranet†; Femiplexe; Laccoderme Dalibour†; Nova-T; Oligoderm; Ramet Dalibour; Ramet Pain; Sanoformine; Septalibour; Tot'hema; Vitacuivre†; ***Ger.:*** Nova-T; Silvapin Sauerstoffbad mit Fichtennadelol†; Silvapin Sauerstoffbad†; Sulfolitruw†; ***Irl.:*** Ferrotab; ***Ital.:*** Nova-T; Silver-Nova T†; ***Neth.:*** Nova-T; ***Norw.:*** Ascoxal; ***S.Afr.:*** Nova-T; ***Spain:*** Acnosan; Ferroce†; ***Swed.:*** Ascoxal; ***Switz.:*** Nova-T; ***UK:*** Folicin†; Foresight Iron Formula; Nova-T; ***USA:*** ORA5.

Cyclamic Acid (2389-r)

Cyclamic Acid *(BAN, USAN).*

Cyclam. Acid; E952; Hexamic Acid. *N*-Cyclohexylsulphamic acid.

$C_6H_{13}NO_3S$ = 179.2.

CAS — 100-88-9.

Calcium Cyclamate (2379-t)

Calc. Cyclam.; Calcium Cyclohexanesulfamate; Cyclamate Calcium; E952. Calcium *N*-cyclohexylsulphamate dihydrate.

$C_{12}H_{24}CaN_2O_6S_2,2H_2O$ = 432.6.

CAS — 139-06-0 (anhydrous calcium cyclamate); 5897-16-5 (calcium cyclamate dihydrate).

Sodium Cyclamate (2409-s)

Sodium Cyclamate *(BAN, rINN).*

Cyclamate Sodium; E952; Natrii cyclamas; Sod. Cyclam.; Sodium Cyclohexanesulphamate. Sodium *N*-cyclohexylsulphamate.

$C_6H_{12}NNaO_3S$ = 201.2.

CAS — 139-05-9.

Pharmacopoeias. In *Eur.* (see p.viii).

White crystalline powder or colourless crystals. Freely **soluble** in water; slightly soluble in alcohol; very slightly soluble in ether. A 10% solution in water has a pH of 5.5 to 7.5.

Cyclamic acid and its calcium and sodium salts are intense sweetening agents. In dilute solutions (up to about 0.17%) sodium cyclamate is about 30 times as sweet as sucrose but this factor decreases at higher concentrations. When the concentration approaches 0.5%, a bitter taste becomes noticeable. It is stable to heat.

The use of cyclamates as artificial sweeteners in food, soft drinks, and artificial sweetening tablets was at one time prohibited in Great Britain and some other countries because of concern about the metabolite cyclohexylamine, but has since been reappraised to allow their use.

Preparations

Proprietary Preparations (details are given in Part 3)
Canad.: Sucaryl.

Multi-ingredient: ***Austral.:*** Sucaryl; ***Fr.:*** Humex†; Sucaryl; ***Ital.:*** Diet Sucaryl.

Cysteine (16183-s)

Cysteine *(rINN).*

C; Cys; L-Cysteine. L-2-Amino-3-mercaptopropionic acid.

$C_3H_7NO_2S$ = 121.2.

CAS — 52-90-4.

Pharmacopoeias. In *Ger.*

Cysteine Hydrochloride (579-e)

Cysteine Hydrochloride *(rINNM).*

920; Cys Hydrochloride; L-Cysteine Hydrochloride Monohydrate; Cysteini Hydrochloridum Monohydricum. L-2-Amino-3-mercaptopropionic acid hydrochloride monohydrate.

$C_3H_7NO_2S,HCl,H_2O$ = 175.6.

CAS — 52-89-1 (anhydrous L-cysteine hydrochloride); 7048-04-6 (L-cysteine hydrochloride monohydrate).

Pharmacopoeias. In *Eur.* (see p.viii) and *US.*

White or colourless crystals or crystalline powder. Ph. Eur. **solubilities** are: freely soluble in water; slightly soluble in alcohol; practically insoluble in ether. USP solubilities are: soluble in water, in alcohol, and in acetone.

Cysteine is an aliphatic amino acid. Cysteine and cysteine hydrochloride are used as dietary supplements.

Cysteine and cysteine hydrochloride are included in preparations used in ophthalmology; eye drops have been used to prevent corneal ulceration after chemical burns.

Cysteine, like other sulfhydryl-containing drugs, could produce a false-positive result in the nitroprusside test for ketone bodies used in diabetes and suspected hepatocellular injury.[1]

1. Csako G, Elin RJ. Unrecognized false-positive ketones from drugs containing free-sulfhydryl group(s). *JAMA* 1993; **269:** 1634.

Preparations

USP 23: Cysteine Hydrochloride Injection.

Proprietary Preparations (details are given in Part 3)

Multi-ingredient: ***Austral.:*** Ginkgo ACE†; ***Fr.:*** Co-A†; Lobamine-Cysteine; Phakan; Vita-Iodurol; Vita-Iodurol ATP; ***Ger.:*** Cheihepar†; Choldestal†; Hepalixier†; Hepaticum "Mletzko"†; Hepatofalk Neu; Prohepar†; Reducdyn†; *Switz.:* Lobamine-Cysteine; Phakolen.

Cystine (580-b)

Cystine *(USAN)*.

L-Cystine; Cystinum; Di(α-aminopropionic)-β-disulphide; β,β′-Dithiodialanine. L-3,3′-Dithiobis(2-aminopropionic acid).

$C_6H_{12}N_2O_4S_2$ = 240.3.

CAS — 56-89-3.

Pharmacopoeias. In *Eur.* (see p.viii).

A white crystalline powder. Practically **insoluble** in water and in alcohol. It dissolves in dilute solutions of alkali hydroxides. **Protect** from light.

Cystine is an aliphatic amino acid. It is used as a dietary supplement.

Low-methionine diets in conjunction with cystine supplementation have been used in the treatment of congenital homocystinuria (see Amino Acid Metabolic Disorders, p.1330).

Preparations

Proprietary Preparations (details are given in Part 3)
Fr.: Gelucystine; Hexaphane; ***Ital.:*** Cistidil; Mavigen Sebo; ***Spain:*** Vitacrecil.

Multi-ingredient: ***Aust.:*** Gelacet; Pantogar; ***Canad.:*** Amino-Cerv; ***Fr.:*** Arbum; Cystichol; Forcapil; Solacy; Totephan; ***Ger.:*** Gelacet N; Gerontamin; Pantovigar; ***Switz.:*** Gelacet; Pantogar; Solacy†; ***USA:*** Amino-Cerv.

Dextrin (581-v)

Dextrin *(BAN)*.

British Gum; Dextrinum Album; Starch Gum.

CAS — 9004-53-9.

Pharmacopoeias. In *Aust., Br., Chin., Fr., Ger.,* and *Jpn.* Also in *US-NF.*

Starch partially hydrolysed by heating with or without the aid of suitable acids and buffers. The BP specifies maize or potato starch.

A white, pale yellow, or brown powder with a slight characteristic odour. BP **solubilities** are: very soluble in boiling water forming a mucilaginous solution; slowly soluble in cold water; practically insoluble in alcohol and ether. The USNF states that the solubility of dextrin in water varies; that it is usually very soluble, but often contains an insoluble portion.

Dextrin, a glucose polymer, is a source of carbohydrate sometimes used in oral dietary supplements and tube feeding. Glucose is rapidly released in the gastro-intestinal tract but because of the high average molecular weight of dextrin, solutions have a lower osmolarity than isocaloric solutions of glucose. Additionally, preparations based on dextrin and intended for dietary supplementation usually have a low electrolyte content and are free of lactose and sucrose. These properties make such preparations suitable for dietary supplementation in a variety of diseases including certain gastro-intestinal disorders where malabsorption is a problem, in disaccharide intolerance (without isomaltose intolerance), and in acute and chronic hepatic and renal diseases where protein, mineral, and fluid restriction are often necessary.

Dextrin is also used as a tablet and capsule diluent, and as a binding, suspending, and viscosity-increasing agent. It has also been used as an adhesive and stiffening agent for surgical dressings.

Icodextrin (*BAN*), which is a (1→4)-α-D-glucan with a weight-average molecular weight of about 20 000 and more than 85% of its molecules with molecular weights between 1640 and 45 000, is used in dialysis fluids as an alternative to glucose-based solutions (see also below).

Commenting on the disadvantages of glucose in dialysis fluids, Stein and others reported results in 11 patients[1] receiving continuous ambulatory peritoneal dialysis (CAPD) who had suffered repeated fluid overload from glucose-based dialysis solutions, suggesting that replacement of glucose with dextrin as the osmotic agent could reverse fluid overload and possibly reduce the frequency of exchange. However, Martis and colleagues[2] considered that the proposed frequency of exchange would not provide adequate removal of urea, and suggested that in addition to underdialysis there would be an accumulation of poorly-metabolisable glucose polymers in the blood. Icodextrin may not be associated with these disadvantages.

1. Stein A, *et al.* Glucose polymer for ultrafiltration failure in CAPD. *Lancet* 1993; **341:** 1159.
2. Martis L, *et al.* CAPD with dialysis solution containing glucose polymer. *Lancet* 1993; **342:** 176–7.

Preparations

USNF 18: Liquid Glucose.

Proprietary Preparations (details are given in Part 3)
Austral.: Poly-Joule; ***Canad.:*** Caloreen†; ***Fr.:*** Caloreen; ***Irl.:*** Caloreen; ***S.Afr.:*** Caloreen; ***UK:*** Caloreen.

Multi-ingredient: ***Fr.:*** Picot.

Ferric Ammonium Citrate (5034-a)

381; Ferricum Citricum Ammoniatum; Iron and Ammonium Citrate.

CAS — 1185-57-5.

Pharmacopoeias. In *Chin.*

A complex of ammonium ferric citrate containing about 21.5% of iron.

Ferric ammonium citrate is given by mouth as a source of iron (see p.1346) for iron-deficiency anaemia (p.702).

It is also used as a food additive to fortify bread.

Preparations

Proprietary Preparations (details are given in Part 3)
Ital.: Sciroppo Fenoglio.

Multi-ingredient: ***Aust.:*** Ferrovin-Chinaeisenwein; ***Belg.:*** Ferrifol B12; Rubraton†; ***Canad.:*** Heparos; Maltlevol; ***Ger.:*** Praefeminon plus; ***Ital.:*** Emopon; Ferriseltz; Neo-Cromaton Bicomplesso Ferro†; ***Neth.:*** Pleegzuster†; ***UK:*** Ironorm; Lexpec with Iron; Lexpec with Iron-M; ***USA:*** Geritol; Geritonic.

Ferric Pyrophosphate (11422-j)

Iron Pyrophosphate.

$Fe_4(P_2O_7)_3$ = 745.2.

CAS — 10058-44-3.

Ferric pyrophosphate is given by mouth as a source of iron (see p.1346) for iron-deficiency anaemia (p.702).

Preparations

Proprietary Preparations (details are given in Part 3)
Ital.: Ferro Angelini†.

Multi-ingredient: ***Austral.:*** Incremin Iron; ***Canad.:*** Incremin with Iron†; ***USA:*** Incremin with Iron; Kovitonic; Troph-Iron†; Vitafol; Vitalize.

Ferrocholinate (5042-a)

Ferrocholinate *(rINN)*.

$C_{11}H_{20}FeNO_9,2H_2O$ = 402.2.

CAS — 1336-80-7.

A chelate prepared by reacting equimolar quantities of freshly precipitated ferric hydroxide with choline dihydrogen tartrate.

Ferrocholinate is given by mouth as a source of iron (see p.1346) for iron-deficiency anaemia (p.702).

Preparations

Proprietary Preparations (details are given in Part 3)
Ital.: Emofer†; ***Spain:*** Podertonic.

Multi-ingredient: ***Ital.:*** Redinon Cortex†; ***Spain:*** Cromatonbic 5000 Ferro†.

Ferrous Ascorbate (12749-f)

$C_{12}H_{14}FeO_{12}$ = 406.1.

CAS — 24808-52-4.

Ferrous ascorbate is used as a source of iron (see p.1346) for iron-deficiency anaemia (p.702). It is given by mouth as the anhydrous form in usual dose units of 245 mg and as a hydrated form in usual dose units of 275 mg; both forms provide about 33 mg of iron per dose unit; the total dose is usually up to the equivalent of 200 mg of iron daily.

Preparations

Proprietary Preparations (details are given in Part 3)
Canad.: Ascofer; ***Fr.:*** Ascofer; ***Spain:*** Ferro Semar; ***Switz.:*** Ascofer†.

Multi-ingredient: ***Aust.:*** China-Eisenwein.

Ferrous Aspartate (5044-x)

$C_8H_{12}FeN_2O_8,4H_2O$ = 392.1.

Ferrous aspartate is used as a source of iron (see p.1346) for iron-deficiency anaemia (p.702). It has been given by mouth in doses of up to 1.4 g daily (equivalent to about 200 mg of iron daily).

Preparations

Proprietary Preparations (details are given in Part 3)
Belg.: Spartocine; ***Ger.:*** Grandelat eisen†; Spartocine N; ***Ital.:*** Spartocina†.

Ferrous Chloride (18204-j)

Iron (II) chloride tetrahydrate.

$FeCl_2,4H_2O$ = 198.8.

CAS — 7758-94-3 (anhydrous ferrous chloride); 13478-10-9 (ferrous chloride tetrahydrate).

Ferrous chloride is used as a source of iron (see p.1346) for iron-deficiency anaemia (p.702). It is given by mouth in usual doses of about 350 to 700 mg daily in divided doses (equivalent to about 100 to 200 mg of iron daily).

Preparations

Proprietary Preparations (details are given in Part 3)
Fr.: Fer UCB; ***Ger.:*** Ferro 66; ***Ital.:*** Cotone Emostatico; ***Switz.:*** Ferrascorbin.

Multi-ingredient: ***Switz.:*** Ferrascorbin.

Ferrous Fumarate (5054-f)

Ferrosi Fumaras.

$C_4H_2FeO_4$ = 169.9.

CAS — 141-01-5.

Pharmacopoeias. In *Chin., Eur.* (see p.viii), *Int.,* and *US.*

A fine reddish-orange to reddish-brown powder, odourless or with a slight odour; 200 mg contains about 65 mg of iron. Slightly **soluble** in water; very slightly soluble in alcohol. **Store** in airtight containers. Protect from light.

Ferrous fumarate is used as a source of iron (see p.1346) for iron-deficiency anaemia (p.702). It is given by mouth in usual doses of up to 600 mg daily (equivalent to about 200 mg of iron daily); doses of up to 1.2 g daily (equivalent to about 400 mg of iron daily) may be used if necessary.

Preparations

BP 1998: Ferrous Fumarate and Folic Acid Tablets; Ferrous Fumarate Oral Suspension; Ferrous Fumarate Tablets;
USP 23: Ferrous Fumarate and Docusate Sodium Extended-release Tablets; Ferrous Fumarate Tablets.

Proprietary Preparations (details are given in Part 3)
Aust.: Ferretab; Ferrobet; ***Belg.:*** Ferrum Hausmann; Ferumat; ***Canad.:*** Neo-Fer; Novo-Fumar; Palafer; ***Fr.:*** Fumafer; ***Ger.:*** Ferrokapsul; Ferrolande†; Ferrum Hausmann; Ferrum Klinge†; Rulofer N; ***Irl.:*** Fersaday†; Galfer; ***Ital.:*** Ferro-12; ***Neth.:*** Ferumat†; ***Norw.:*** Neo-Fer; ***S.Afr.:*** Fersamal†; ***Swed.:*** Erco-Fer; ***Switz.:*** Ferrum Hausmann; ***UK:*** Ferrocap†; Fersaday; Fersamal; Galfer; ***USA:*** Femiron; Feostat; Ferancee; Ferocyl; Ferretts†; Ferro-Sequels; Ferromar; Fumasorb†; Fumerin†; Hemaspan; Hemocyte; Ircon; Nephro-Fer; Span-FF†; Vitron-C†.

Multi-ingredient: ***Aust.:*** Ferretab comp; Trinsicon; ***Austral.:*** Children's Calcium With Minerals; Medinat PMT-Eze; ***Belg.:*** Gestiferrol; ***Canad.:*** Appedrine; Caltrate + Iron & Vitamin D; Dexatrim; Fortiplex; Palafer CF; Prevencal & D & Fer; Trinsicon†; ***Ger.:*** Blutquick Forte S; Hemoxier†; ***Irl.:*** BC 500 with Iron; Ferrocap F; Folex; Galfer FA; Givitol; Multivite Plus†; ***S.Afr.:*** Pregamal; Trinsicon; ***Spain:*** Anemotron†; Foliferron; ***Swed.:*** Erco-Fer vitamin; ***Switz.:*** Blastoifer†; Duofer; Duofer Fol; Farnolith†; Ferrum Fol B Hausmann†; ***UK:*** Ferrocap F 350†; Folex-350; Galfer FA; Galfer-Vit†; Givitol; Iron Jelloids; Meterfolic†; Pregaday; ***USA:*** ABC to Z; Berocca Plus; Berplex; Caltrate + Iron & Vitamin D; Certagen; Cevi-Fer; Chromagen; Chromagen FA; Chromagen Forte; Contrin; Estrostep Fe; Fergon Iron Plus Calcium†; Ferotrinsic; Ferro-Dok; Fetrin; Formula B Plus; Fumatinic; Geriot; Gevral T; Hem Fe†; Hemocyte-F; Ircon-FA; Livitamin with Intrinsic Factor†; Livitamin†; Livitrinsic-f; Loestrin Fe; Nestabs FA; Parvlex; Perihemin†; Polytinic; Pronemia Hematinic; Stuartinic; Tabron†; Thera Hematinic; Theragenerix-H; Tolfrinic; TriHEMIC; Trinsicon; Trinsicon M†; Vitafol; Yelets; Zodeac.

Ferrous Gluceptate (13440-s)

Ferrous Glucoheptonate.

$Fe(C_7H_{13}O_8)_2$ = 506.2.

CAS — 25126-38-9.

Ferrous gluceptate is given by mouth as a source of iron (see p.1346) for iron-deficiency anaemia (p.702).

Preparations

Proprietary Preparations (details are given in Part 3)

Multi-ingredient: ***Spain:*** Clamarvit; Normovite Antianem Iny; Normovite Antianemico.

Ferrous Gluconate (5058-m)

Eisen(II)-Gluconat; Ferrosi Gluconas. Iron(II) di(D-gluconate).

$C_{12}H_{22}FeO_{14},xH_2O$.

CAS — 299-29-6 (anhydrous ferrous gluconate); 12389-15-0 (ferrous gluconate dihydrate).

Pharmacopoeias. In Eur. (see p.viii).

Pol. and *US.* specify the dihydrate.

Greenish-yellow to grey powder or granules. It may have a slight odour resembling that of burnt sugar. It contains not less than 11.8% and not more than 12.5% of ferrous iron calculated on the dried material; 600 mg of the dihydrate contains about 70 mg of iron. Freely but slowly **soluble** in water producing a greenish-brown solution, more readily soluble in hot water; practically insoluble in alcohol. A 10% solution in water has a pH of 4.0 to 5.5 three to four hours after preparation.

Store in airtight containers. Protect from light.

Ferrous gluconate is used as a source of iron (see p.1346) for iron-deficiency anaemia (p.702). It is given by mouth in doses of up to 1.8 g daily (equivalent to up to 210 mg of iron daily). A ferric iron compound, ferric sodium gluconate has been employed similarly.

Preparations

BP 1998: Ferrous Gluconate Tablets;
USP 23: Ferrous Gluconate Capsules; Ferrous Gluconate Elixir; Ferrous Gluconate Tablets.

Proprietary Preparations (details are given in Part 3)
Aust.: Ferro-Agepha; Losferron; ***Austral.:*** Fergon; ***Belg.:*** Losferron; ***Canad.:*** Fertinic; Novo-Ferrogluc; ***Fr.:*** Losferon; ***Ger.:*** Ferrlecit; Ferrominerase†; Ferrum Verla; Losan Fe; Losferron; Rulofer G; ***Irl.:*** Fergon; ***Ital.:*** Actiferro; Cromatonferro; Emoferrina; Epaplex 40; Extrafer; Ferlixit; Ferrematos; Ferri-Emina; Ferritin Oti; Ferrosprint; Fevital Simplex; Fisiofer; Gibifer; Glucoferro; Hemocromo; Inferil; Ipocromo; Ironax; Lisiofer; Losferron; Rossepar; Rubroferrina; Sustemial; ***Neth.:*** Losferron; ***Spain:*** Glutaferro; ***Switz.:*** Loesfer; ***UK:*** Fergon†; ***USA:*** Fergon; Ferralet†; Simron†.

Multi-ingredient: ***Aust.:*** Ferro-Kobalt†; Losferron-Fol; ***Fr.:*** Tot'hema; Triogene; ***Ger.:*** Athensa-ferro-Saft†; Biovital Forte N; Blutquick Forte; Blutquick Forte S; Ferro-B 12 Ehrl†; Ferro-C-Calcium; Folsana; Hemoxier†; ***Irl.:*** Cyfol†; ***Ital.:*** Ferritin Complex; Sideritrina†; ***S.Afr.:*** Ferlucon†; Kiddie Vite; ***Spain:*** Clamarvit; ***Switz.:*** Duofer; Duofer Fol; Ferrascorbin; Loesfer + acide folique; ***UK:*** Feravol-F†; Feravol-G†; Ferfolic SV; Foresight Iron Formula; ***USA:*** Compete; Fergon Plus†; Ferralet Plus; Hemocyte; Hemocyte-V; Hytinic; Iromin-G; Licoplex DS; Mission Surgical Supplement.

Ferrous Glycine Sulphate (5059-b)

Ferrous Aminoacetosulphate.

CAS — 14729-84-1.

A chelate of ferrous sulphate and glycine.

Ferrous glycine sulphate is used as a source of iron (see p.1346) for iron-deficiency anaemia (p.702). It is given by mouth in doses containing the equivalent of up to 150 mg of iron daily.

Preparations

Proprietary Preparations (details are given in Part 3)
Austral.: Plesmet†; ***Ger.:*** Ferro sanol; Ferro sanol duodenal; ***Irl.:*** Ferrocontin Continus†; Plesmet; ***Spain:*** Glutaferro; ***Switz.:*** Ferro-sanol duodenal; ***UK:*** Ferrocontin Continus†; Plesmet.

Multi-ingredient: ***Irl.:*** Ferrocontin Folic Continus†; ***Ital.:*** Epaglifer†; ***UK:*** Ferrocontin Folic Continus†.

Ferrous Lactate (5060-x)

Iron Lactate.

$C_6H_{10}FeO_6,3H_2O$ = 288.0.

CAS — 5905-52-2 (anhydrous ferrous lactate); 6047-24-1 (ferrous lactate trihydrate).

Ferrous lactate is used as a source of iron (see p.1346) for iron-deficiency anaemia (p.702).

Preparations

Proprietary Preparations (details are given in Part 3)
S.Afr.: Ferro Drops L; ***Spain:*** Cromatonbic Ferro.

Multi-ingredient: ***Aust.:*** Anthozym.

Ferrous Oxalate (5061-r)

Ferrum Oxalicum Oxydulatum; Iron Protoxalate.

$C_2FeO_4,2H_2O$ = 179.9.

CAS — 516-03-0 (anhydrous ferrous oxalate); 6047-25-2 (ferrous oxalate dihydrate).

Pharmacopoeias. In Belg.

Ferrous oxalate is used as a source of iron (see p.1346) for iron-deficiency anaemia (p.702). It has been given by mouth in doses of up to 300 mg daily (equivalent to up to 90 mg of iron daily).

Preparations

Proprietary Preparations (details are given in Part 3)
Multi-ingredient: ***Fr.:*** Disulone; Ducase.

Ferrous Succinate (5062-f)

$C_4H_4FeO_4$ = 171.9.

CAS — 10030-90-7.

Ferrous succinate is used as a source of iron (see p.1346) for iron-deficiency anaemia (p.702). It is given by mouth in doses of up to about 300 mg daily (equivalent to up to about 100 mg of iron daily).

Preparations

Proprietary Preparations (details are given in Part 3)
Canad.: Cerevon; ***Fr.:*** Inofer; ***Ger.:*** Ferrlecit 2; ***Irl.:*** Ferromyn†; ***Swed.:*** Ferromyn S; ***UK:*** Ferromyn†.

Multi-ingredient: ***Ger.:*** Multibionta-Eisen†.

Ferrous Sulphate (5063-d)

Eisen(II)-Sulfat; Ferreux (Sulfate); Ferrosi Sulfas; Ferrous Sulfate; Ferrum Sulfuricum Oxydulatum; Iron Sulphate; Iron(II) Sulphate Heptahydrate.

$FeSO_4,7H_2O$ = 278.0.

CAS — 7720-78-7 (anhydrous ferrous sulphate); 7782-63-0 (ferrous sulphate heptahydrate).

NOTE. Crude ferrous sulphate is known as Green Vitriol or Green Copperas.

Pharmacopoeias. In Chin., Eur. (see p.viii), *Int.*, *Jpn*, and *US.*

Swiss also includes ferrous sulphate sesquihydrate.

Odourless bluish-green crystals or granules or a pale green crystalline powder, containing about 60 mg of iron in 300 mg. It is efflorescent in dry air; on exposure to moist air it is oxidised and becomes brown in colour due to the formation of basic ferric sulphate.

Soluble 1 in 1.5 of water and 1 in 0.5 of boiling water; practically insoluble in alcohol. A 5% solution in water has a pH of 3.0 to 4.0. **Store** in airtight containers.

Dried Ferrous Sulphate (5064-n)

Dried Ferrous Sulfate (*USAN*); Exsiccated Ferrous Sulphate; Ferrosi Sulfas Exsiccatus.

CAS — 13463-43-9.

Pharmacopoeias. In *Aust.*, *Br.*, *Int.*, and *US.*

Ferrous sulphate deprived of part of its water of crystallisation by drying at 40°. The USP specifies that it consists primarily of the monohydrate with varying amounts of the tetrahydrate. A greyish-white to buff-coloured powder. The BP specifies 86 to 90% of $FeSO_4$; the USP specifies 86 to 89% of $FeSO_4$.

Slowly but almost completely **soluble** in freshly boiled and cooled water; practically insoluble in alcohol.

Ferrous sulphate is used as a source of iron (see p.1346) for iron-deficiency anaemia (p.702). It is given by mouth and the dried form is frequently used in solid dosage forms and the heptahydrate in liquid dosage forms. Usual doses of dried ferrous sulphate are up to 600 mg daily (equivalent to 180 to 195 mg of iron daily, this figure being somewhat variable depending on the purity and water content of the salt).

Ferrous sulphate oxidised with nitric and sulphuric acids yields ferric subsulphate solution, also known as Monsel's solution, which has been used as a haemostatic.

Preparations

BP 1998: Ferrous Sulphate Tablets; Paediatric Ferrous Sulphate Oral Solution;
BPC 1973: Compound Ferrous Sulphate Tablets;
USP 23: Ferrous Sulfate Oral Solution; Ferrous Sulfate Syrup; Ferrous Sulfate Tablets.

Proprietary Preparations (details are given in Part 3)
Aust.: Ferro-Gradumet; Ferrograd C; Infa-Tardyferon; Tardyferon; ***Austral.:*** Ferro-Gradumet; Fespan†; ***Belg.:*** Fer-In-Sol†; Fero-Grad; Fero-Gradumet; Resoferon; ***Canad.:*** Fer-In-Sol; Fero-Grad; Ferodan; Novo-Ferrosulfate; Slow-Fe; ***Fr.:*** Fero-Grad vitamine C; ***Ger.:*** Aktiferrin N; Ceferro; Dreisafer; Eisen-Diasporal; Eisendragees-ratiopharm; Eryfer; Ferro 66 DL†; Haemoprotect; Kendural C; Plastufer; Resoferix†; Tardyferon; Vitaferro; ***Irl.:*** Feospan; Fer-In-Sol; Ferrograd; Ferrograd C; Slow-Fe†; ***Ital.:*** Eryfer†; Fer-In-Sol; Ferro-Grad; Ferro-Grad C; ***Neth.:*** Eryfer†; Ferro-Gradumet; Liquifer; ***Norw.:*** Duroferon; Ferro-Retard; Ferromax; ***S.Afr.:*** Fero-Grad; Fesofor†; ***Spain:*** Fero-Gradumet; ***Swed.:*** Duroferon; ***Switz.:*** Ferro-Gradumet; Resoferon; ***UK:*** Feospan; Ferrograd; Ferrograd C; Ironorm; Slow-Fe; ***USA:*** Fe^{50}; Feosol; Fergen-sol; Fer-In-Sol; Fer-Iron; Feratab; Fero-Grad; Fero-Gradumet; Ferospace; Ferra-TD†; Ferralyn†; Irospan; Mol-Iron; Slow-Fe.

Multi-ingredient: ***Aust.:*** Aktiferrin; Aktiferrin compositum; Ferrograd-Fol; Ferrum-Quarz; Kephalodoron; Tardyferon-Fol; ***Austral.:*** Fefol; FGF Tabs; Irontona; ***Canad.:*** Iberet; Slow-Fe Folic; ***Fr.:*** Ionarthrol; Tardyferon; Tardyferon B_9; ***Ger.:*** Aktiferrin E F†; Biovital N; Eryfer comp.; Ferro Cytofol†; Ferro sanol comp; Ferro-Folgamma; Ferro-Folsan; Ferro-Folsan plus†; Ferro-Folsaure-Vicotrat†; Ferrophor†; Hamatopan; Hamatopan F; Kendural-Fol-500; Kendural-Plus; Plastulen N; Tardyferon-Fol; ***Irl.:*** Fefol; Fefol-Vit†; Ferrograd Folic; Ferrotab; Fesovit; Folferite†; Pregnavite Forte F†; Slow-Fe Folic†; ***Ital.:*** Cura; Ferro-Grad Folic; Vitamucin con Ferro†; ***Norw.:*** Pregnifer; ***S.Afr.:*** Effee; Fefol; Fefol-Vit†; Fero-Folic; Foliglobin; Iberet; Laxicaps†; ***Spain:*** Ferriwas B12 Fuerte†; Ferroce†; Iberet; Pildoras Ferrug Sanatori; Tardyferon; Vitagama Fluor Complex; ***Switz.:*** Actiferrine; Actiferrine-F Nouvelle formule; Fero-Folic; Gyno-Tardyferon; Infa-Tardyferon†; Kendural; Resoferon fol B†; Tardyferon; ***UK:*** Bidor; Dencyl; Ditemic; Fefol; Fefol Z†; Fefol-Vit†; Feospan Z†; Feravol†; Ferrograd Folic; Fesovit Z; Fesovit†; Folicin†; Fortespan; Ironorm; Pregnavite Forte F; Slow-Fe Folic; ***USA:*** Aqua Ban Plus; Fero-Folic; Generet; Gerivites; Iberet; Iberet-Folic-500; Multibret Hematinic†; Multibret-Folic†; Reticulex†.

Ferrous Tartrate (5065-h)

Ferrosi Tartras.

$C_4H_4FeO_6,2\frac{1}{2}H_2O$ = 249.0.

CAS — 2944-65-2 (anhydrous ferrous tartrate).

Ferrous tartrate is used as a source of iron (see p.1346) for iron-deficiency anaemia (p.702). It is given by mouth in doses of up to 1 g daily (equivalent to up to 224 mg of iron daily).

Folic Acid (7860-f)

Folic Acid (*BAN, rINN*).

Acidum Folicum; Folacin; Folinsyre; PGA; Pteroylglutamic Acid; Pteroylmonoglutamic Acid; Vitamin B_9; Vitamin B_{11}. *N*-[4-(2-Amino-4-hydroxypteridin-6-ylmethylamino)benzoyl]-L(+)-glutamic acid.

$C_{19}H_{19}N_7O_6$ = 441.4.

CAS — 59-30-3 (folic acid); 6484-89-5 (sodium folate).

Pharmacopoeias. In *Chin.*, *Eur.* (see p.viii), *Int.*, *Jpn*, *Pol.*, and *US.*

A yellow to orange brown, odourless crystalline powder.

Very slightly **soluble** or practically insoluble in water; practically insoluble in most organic solvents such as alcohol, acetone, chloroform, and ether. It readily dissolves in dilute solutions of alkali hydroxides and carbonates; soluble in hydrochloric acid and in sulphuric acid. **Protect** from light.

Stability in solution. Folic acid has been reported to precipitate in some proprietary amino acid solutions and in the presence of high concentrations of calcium ions, but it appears to be stable and remain in solution provided the pH remains above 5. There have also been reports of folic acid being absorbed by the polyvinyl chloride container and administration set; however other studies have not substantiated such observations.[1]

1. Allwood MC. Compatibility and stability of TPN mixtures in big bags. *J Clin Hosp Pharm* 1984; **9:** 181–98.

Adverse Effects

Folic acid is generally well tolerated. Gastro-intestinal disturbances and hypersensitivity reactions have been reported rarely.

Precautions

Folic acid should never be given alone or in conjunction with inadequate amounts of vitamin B_{12} for the treatment of undiagnosed megaloblastic anaemia, since folic acid may produce a haematopoietic response in patients with a megaloblastic anaemia due to vitamin B_{12} deficiency without preventing aggravation of neurological symptoms. This masking of the true deficiency state can lead to serious neurological damage, such as subacute combined degeneration of the cord (see also below).

Caution is advised in patients who may have folate-dependent tumours.

The issue of fortification of food with folic acid to reduce the number of infants born with neural tube defects (see below) has created debate on the risks of masking vitamin B_{12} deficiency, particularly in the elderly. As mentioned in Precautions, above, it is accepted that folic acid should not be used in megaloblastic anaemia due to vitamin B_{12} deficiency, because it will not prevent the neurological manifestations of this deficiency, and may delay the diagnosis. Masking of vitamin B_{12} deficiency has been noted with daily doses of folic acid of 5 mg, and it is generally considered that very low doses do not have this effect. It has also been stated that folic acid may precipitate the neurological manifestations of vitamin B_{12} deficiency; however, a review of the evidence suggests this is unlikely.[1]

Nevertheless, concerns regarding neurological effects of vitamin B_{12} deficiency in the elderly have led to adoption of a level of folic acid fortification in the USA that is accepted will not provide optimum protection against neural tube defects, but that is hoped will minimise any risks.[2] It has been suggested that concomitant fortification with vitamin B_{12} might also be a solution.

1. Dickinson CJ. Does folic acid harm people with vitamin B_{12} deficiency? *Q J Med* 1995; **88:** 357–64.
2. Tucker KL, *et al.* Folic acid fortification of the food supply: potential benefits and risks for the elderly population. *JAMA* 1996; **276:** 1879–85. Correction. *ibid.* 1997; **277:** 714.

Interactions

Folate deficiency states may be produced by a number of drugs including antiepileptics, oral contraceptives, antituberculous drugs, alcohol, and folic acid antagonists such as aminopterin, methotrexate, pyrimethamine, trimethoprim, and sulphonamides. In some instances, such as during methotrexate or antiepileptic therapy, replacement therapy with folinic acid or folic acid may become necessary in order to prevent megaloblastic anaemia developing; folate supplementation has reportedly decreased serum-phenytoin concentrations in a few cases (see p.357).

Antiepileptic-associated folate deficiency is discussed further under phenytoin, p.353.

References.

1. Lambie DG, Johnson RH. Drugs and folate metabolism. *Drugs* 1985; **30:** 145–55.

Pharmacokinetics

Folic acid is rapidly absorbed from the gastro-intestinal tract, mainly from the duodenum and jejunum. Dietary folates are stated to be less well absorbed than crystalline folic acid. The naturally occurring folate polyglutamates are largely deconjugated and reduced by dihydrofolate reductase in the intestines to form 5-methyltetrahydrofolate, which appears in the portal circulation, where it is extensively bound to plasma proteins. Folic acid administered therapeutically enters the portal circulation largely unchanged since it is a poor substrate for reduction by dihydrofolate reductase. It is converted to the metabolically active form 5-methyltetrahydrofolate in the plasma and liver.

The principal storage site of folate is the liver; it is also actively concentrated in the CSF.

Folate undergoes enterohepatic circulation. Folate metabolites are eliminated in the urine and folate in excess of body requirements is excreted unchanged in the urine. Folate is distributed into breast milk. Folic acid is removed by haemodialysis.

Human Requirements

Body stores of folate in healthy persons have been reported as being between 5 to 10 mg, but may be much higher. About 150 to 200 µg of folate a day is considered a suitable average intake for all healthy persons except women of child-bearing potential and pregnant women who require additional folic acid to protect against neural tube defects in their offspring (see below). Folate is present, chiefly combined with several L(+)-glutamic acid moieties, in many foods, particularly liver, kidney, yeast, nuts, and leafy green vegetables. The vitamin is readily oxidised to unavailable forms and is easily destroyed during cooking.

In the United Kingdom dietary reference values (see p.1332) have been published for folate.[1] In the United States recommended dietary allowances (RDAs) had been set, and have recently been reviewed[2] under the programme to set Dietary Reference Intakes (see p.1332). Differing amounts are recommended for infants and children of varying ages, for adult males and females, and for pregnant and lactating women. In the UK the Reference Nutrient Intake (RNI) for adult males and females is 200 µg daily and the Estimated Average Requirement (EAR) is 150 µg daily. In the USA an RDA of 400 µg daily for adult men and women has recently been set; the EAR is 320 µg of folate daily.

Folate requirements are increased during pregnancy; an RNI of 300 µg daily has been suggested for pregnant women in the UK and an RDA of 600 µg daily in the USA. In the light of recent confirmation of the value of folate in preventing neural tube defects, it is now recommended that women planning a pregnancy receive supplemental folic acid before conception and during the first trimester (see below). To increase the intake in women of childbearing age, folic acid fortification of grain-based foods has been adopted in the USA, and advocated in other countries including the UK. However, there remains some debate over the appropriate level of fortification to optimise prevention of neural tube defects and to minimise the risks of masking underlying vitamin B_{12} deficiency in the elderly.

1. DoH. Dietary reference values for food energy and nutrients for the United Kingdom: report of the panel on dietary reference values of the committee on medical aspects of food policy. *Report on health and social subjects 41*. London: HMSO, 1991.
2. Standing Committee on the Scientific Evaluation of Dietary Reference Intakes of the Food and Nutrition Board. *Dietary Reference Intakes for thiamin, riboflavin, niacin, vitamin B_6, folate, vitamin B_{12}, pantothenic acid, biotin, and choline.* Washington, DC: National Academy Press, 1998.

Uses and Administration

Folic acid is a member of the vitamin B group. Folic acid is reduced in the body to tetrahydrofolate, which is a coenzyme for various metabolic processes including the synthesis of purine and pyrimidine nucleotides, and hence in the synthesis of DNA; it is also involved in some amino-acid conversions, and in the formation and utilisation of formate. Deficiency, which can result in megaloblastic anaemia (p.703), develops when the dietary intake is inadequate (as in malnutrition) when there is malabsorption (as in sprue), increased utilisation (as in pregnancy or conditions such as haemolytic anaemia), increased loss (as in haemodialysis), or as a result of the administration of folate antagonists and other drugs that interfere with normal folate metabolism (see under Interactions, above).

Folic acid is used in the treatment and prevention of the folate deficiency state. It does not correct folate deficiency due to dihydrofolate reductase inhibitors; calcium folinate (p.1342) is used for this purpose. Folic acid is also used in women of child-bearing potential and pregnant women to protect against neural tube defects in their offspring. This is discussed in more detail in Neural Tube Defects, below.

For the treatment of folate-deficient megaloblastic anaemia it is recommended in the UK that folic acid is given by mouth in doses of 5 mg daily for 4 months; up to 15 mg daily may be necessary in malabsorption states. Continued administration of folic acid 5 mg every 1 to 7 days by mouth may be necessary in chronic haemolytic states such as thalassaemia major or sickle-cell anaemia, depending on the diet and rate of haemolysis; similar doses may be necessary in some patients receiving renal dialysis in order to prevent deficiency.

In the USA the usual recommended therapeutic dose for folate deficiency is lower; folic acid 0.25 to 1.0 mg daily by mouth is suggested until a haematopoietic response has been obtained, although some patients require higher doses, especially in malabsorption states. The usual maintenance dose is 0.4 mg daily.

In the prophylaxis of megaloblastic anaemia of pregnancy, the usual dose is 200 to 500 µg daily in the UK, and up to 1 mg daily in the USA.

For women of child-bearing potential at high risk of having a pregnancy affected by neural tube defect, the dose of folic acid is 4 or 5 mg daily starting before pregnancy (in the USA the recommendation is 4 weeks before) and continued through the first trimester. For other women of child-bearing potential the dose in the UK is 400 µg daily.

Folic acid may also be administered by intramuscular, intravenous, or subcutaneous injection as the sodium salt.

Deficiency states. Reviews of the use of folic acid in conditions associated with folate deficiency.

1. Davis RE. Clinical chemistry of folic acid. *Clin Chem* 1986; **25:** 233–94.
2. Crellin R, *et al.* Folates and psychiatric disorders: clinical potential. *Drugs* 1993; **45:** 623–36.
3. Wickramasinghe SN. Folate and vitamin B_{12} deficiency and supplementation. *Prescribers' J* 1997; **37:** 88–95.

Ischaemic heart disease. Elevated blood-homocysteine concentrations appear to be an independent risk factor for atherosclerosis and ischaemic heart disease (p.782),[1] and there is evidence that they are inversely related to blood-folate concentrations.[2] Epidemiological studies[3,4] indicate that individuals with a high intake of folate or vitamin B_6 from vitamin supplements or food are at lower risk of ischaemic heart disease. Furthermore, meta-analyses suggest that administration of folic acid reduces blood-homocysteine levels,[2,5] and that vitamin B_{12}, but not B_6, may have an additional effect.[5] Thus, there is growing interest in conducting prospective randomised trials to assess the effect of folic acid in the primary or secondary prevention of ischaemic heart disease. In a small study[6] in renal transplant recipients with hyperhomocysteinaemia, vitamin B_6 was effective in reducing post-methionine-loading plasma homocysteine concentrations, and folic acid plus vitamin B_{12} was effective in lowering fasting plasma homocysteine concentrations. The authors concluded that all three of these B-group vitamins may have a role in reducing atherosclerotic outcomes in this patient group.[6]

1. Welch GN, Loscalzo J. Homocysteine and atherosclerosis. *N Engl J Med* 1998; **338:** 1042–50.
2. Boushey CJ, *et al.* A quantitative assessment of plasma homocysteine as a risk factor for vascular disease: probable benefits of increasing folic acid intakes. *JAMA* 1995; **274:** 1049–57.
3. Morrison HI, *et al.* Serum folate and risk of fatal coronary heart disease. *JAMA* 1996; **275:** 1893–6.
4. Rimm EB, *et al.* Folate and vitamin B_6 from diet and supplements in relation to risk of coronary heart disease among women. *JAMA* 1998; **279:** 359–64.
5. Homocysteine Lowering Trialists' Collaboration. Lowering blood homocysteine with folic acid based supplements: meta-analysis of randomised trials. *Br Med J* 1998; **316:** 894–8.
6. Bostmon AG, *et al.* Treatment of hyperhomocysteinemia in renal transplant recipients. *Ann Intern Med* 1997; **127:** 1089–92.

Neural tube defects. Failure of the fetal neural tube to fuse normally during the first 4 weeks of pregnancy may result in one of several congenital defects. These include anencephaly (absence of the brain and cranial vault) and spina bifida (failure of the vertebrae to fuse). The latter ranges from spina bifida occulta, where neurological abnormalities are rare, to meningocoele or meningomyelocoele, where the meninges, or meninges and spinal cord, herniate outwards through the vertebral defect and which may be associated with hydrocephalus and paralysis of the lower limbs and sphincters.

The reasons for this failure in normal development are not well understood and appear to include both environmental and genetic factors. The risk is increased in certain geographical areas, and in the offspring of parents with previous children who had neural tube defects, or of parents who themselves suffer from the condition.

A defect in the methylenetetrahydrofolate reductase gene has been identified, which is estimated to occur in about 5 to 15% of white populations, and appears to result in an increased requirement for folates, and an increased risk of recurrent early pregnancy loss and neural tube defects.[1,2] Since the 1960s there has been some evidence that the mother's folate status was significant, and in the early 1980s two groups published evidence for claims that the oral administration of folic acid, with or without other vitamins, in the period around conception, reduced the incidence of neural tube defect in the offspring of mothers who had previously borne children with the defect.[3,4]

Although criticised on several grounds, the conclusions of these studies were borne out by a large multicentre study initiated by the Medical Research Council (MRC) of the UK.[5] This study was terminated early because of overwhelming evidence that folic acid 4 mg daily taken from before conception until the twelfth week of gestation by women with a history of a previous pregnancy affected by a neural tube defect reduced the incidence of such defect by about two-thirds. Multivitamins alone (A, D, B_1, B_2, nicotinamide, B_6, and C) did not demonstrate a similar benefit.

Prevention of recurrence. In the light of the MRC study, it is recommended in the UK that in couples with spina bifida or a history of previous offspring with neural tube defect, all those women who may become pregnant should receive folic acid 5 mg daily (in the absence of a commercially-available 4 mg dosage form) until the twelfth week of pregnancy.[6] In the USA, recommendations are 4 mg of folic acid daily from at least four weeks before conception through the first 3 months of pregnancy.[7] It must be borne in mind that only about 60 to 70% of neural tube defects appear to be folate-sensitive, and parents should be counselled appropriately.

The investigators in the MRC trial acknowledged that a 4 mg dose may not be optimal, and both early[3,4] and later[8] studies imply that much lower doses of folic acid may reduce the risk of recurrence, but this has yet to be clearly demonstrated. Furthermore, the optimum length of time that supplements should be given to these women before conception is unknown.

Prevention of occurrence. First occurrences of neural tube defects account for about 95% of cases, and there are obvious public health implications if the benefits of folate in mothers known to be at risk can be extended to the general population. A study in Hungary[9] indicated that folic acid 0.8 mg daily with multivitamins, taken for at least one month before conception and until the third month of gestation decreased the incidence of first occurrence of neural tube defects. A case control study in the USA[10] (where the normal incidence of neural tube defect is much lower than Hungary) suggested that a periconceptional folic acid intake of as little as 0.4 mg daily reduced the occurrence of the disorder by 60%.

With such results in mind the US Public Health Service has recommended that all women of childbearing age who are capable of pregnancy should receive folic acid 0.4 mg daily although care should be taken to keep folate consumption below 1 mg daily except under medical supervision.[11] Such universal coverage would allow for the problem of unplanned pregnancies but would be difficult to achieve, other than by fortification of dietary staples with folate. Food fortification has therefore been adopted in the USA, at a level of 140 μg of folic acid per 100 g of cereal-grain product. While this amount will probably be insufficient to provide maximum reduction in the incidence of neural tube defects,[12,13] it was chosen to minimise the risk of masking vitamin B_{12} deficiency in the elderly.[14] Efforts to increase the use of folic acid supplements in women of childbearing potential are still advocated.

In the UK, the current recommendation is that all women planning a pregnancy should take an extra 0.4 mg of folic acid daily before conception and during the first twelve weeks of pregnancy, bringing the average folate intake to about 0.6 mg daily.[6] In unplanned pregnancies, supplementation should begin as soon as pregnancy is suspected. As in the USA food fortification is being considered and some food is already fortified on a voluntary basis; however, the current emphasis is on education. Patients receiving antiepileptic drugs are at increased risk of neural tube defect and it has been suggested that folic acid supplementation for such patients should be at the level used for prevention of recurrence,[15] i.e. 4 or 5 mg daily.

The mechanism by which folic acid protects against neural tube defects is unknown, but various theories have been postulated including a positive effect in promoting neural tube closure,[16] or a selective abortifacient effect on affected fetuses (terathanasia),[17] although the latter has been disputed.[18] There is some evidence that low maternal vitamin B_{12} concentrations are an independent risk factor for neural tube defects,[19,20] perhaps indicating a role for methionine synthase in their aetiology, and suggesting that additional supplementation with cobalamins be warranted, or that methionine supplements could be investigated as an alternative to folic acid.[21] Interestingly, the results from the Hungarian programme[22,23] and from other studies[24,25] suggest that multivitamin supplements (including folic acid) may also reduce the occurrence of other congenital abnormalities.

1. Molly AM, *et al.* Thermolabile variant of 5,10-methylenetetrahydrofolate reductase associated with low red-cell folates: implications for folate intake recommendations. *Lancet* 1997; **349:** 1591–3.
2. Nelen WLDM, *et al.* Recurrent early pregnancy loss and genetic-related disturbances in folate and homocysteine metabolism. *Br J Hosp Med* 1997; **58:** 511–13.
3. Smithells RW, *et al.* Apparent prevention of neural tube defects by periconceptional vitamin supplementation. *Arch Dis Child* 1981; **56:** 911–18.
4. Laurence KM, *et al.* Double-blind randomised controlled trial of folate treatment before conception to prevent recurrence of neural tube defects. *Br Med J* 1981; **282:** 1509–11.
5. MRC Vitamin Study Research Group. Prevention of neural tube defects: results of the Medical Research Council vitamin study. *Lancet* 1991; **338:** 131–7.
6. DoH. *Folic acid and the prevention of neural tube defects: report from an expert advisory group.* London: Department of Health, 1992.
7. Centers for Disease Control. Use of folic acid for prevention of spina bifida and other neural tube defects—1983-1991 *MMWR* 1991; **40:** 513–16.
8. Kirke PN, *et al.* A randomised trial of low dose folic acid to prevent neural tube defects. *Arch Dis Child* 1992; **67:** 1442–6.
9. Czeizel AE, Dudás I. Prevention of the first occurrence of neural-tube defects by periconceptional vitamin supplementation. *N Engl J Med* 1992; **327:** 1832–5.
10. Werler MM, *et al.* Periconceptional folic acid exposure and risk of occurrent neural tube defects. *JAMA* 1993; **269:** 1257–61.
11. Centers for Disease Control. Recommendations for use of folic acid to reduce number of spina bifida cases and other neural tube defects. *JAMA* 1993; **269:** 1233–8.
12. Daly S, *et al.* Minimum effective dose of folic acid for food fortification to prevent neural-tube defects. *Lancet* 1997; **350:** 1666–9.
13. Brown JE, *et al.* Predictors of red cell folate level in women attempting pregnancy. *JAMA* 1997; **277:** 548–52.
14. Tucker KL, *et al.* Folic acid fortification of the food supply: potential benefits and risks for the elderly population. *JAMA* 1996; **276:** 1879–85. Correction. *ibid.* 1997; **277:** 714.
15. Girling JC, Shennan AH. Epilepsy and pregnancy. *Br Med J* 1993; **307:** 937.
16. Zhao Q, *et al.* Prenatal folic acid treatment suppresses acrania and meroanencephaly in mice mutant for the Cart1 homeobox gene. *Nat Genet* 1996; **13:** 275–83.
17. Hook EB, Czeizel AE. Can terathanasia explain the protective effect of folic-acid supplementation on birth defects? *Lancet* 1997; **350:** 513–15.
18. Burn J, Fisk NM. Terathanasia, folic acid, and birth defects. *Lancet* 1997; **350:** 1322–3.
19. Kirke PN, *et al.* Maternal plasma folate and vitamin B_{12} are independent risk factors for neural tube defects. *Q J Med* 1993; **86:** 703–8.
20. Mills JL, *et al.* Homocysteine metabolism in pregnancies complicated by neural-tube defects. *Lancet* 1995; **345:** 149–51.
21. Klein NW. Folic acid and prevention of spina bifida. *JAMA* 1996; **275:** 1636.
22. Czeizel AE. Prevention of congenital abnormalities by periconceptional multivitamin supplementation. *Br Med J* 1993; **306:** 1645–8.
23. Czeizel AE. Reduction of urinary tract and cardiovascular defects by periconceptional multivitamin supplementation. *Am J Med Genet* 1996; **62:** 179–83.
24. Shaw GM, *et al.* Risks of orofacial clefts in children born to women using multivitamins containing folic acid periconceptionally. *Lancet* 1995; **346:** 393–6.
25. Botto LD, *et al.* Periconceptional multivitamin use and the occurrent of conotruncal heart defects: results from a population-based, case-control study. *Pediatrics* 1996; **98:** 911–17.

Preparations

BP 1998: Ferrous Fumarate and Folic Acid Tablets; Folic Acid Tablets;
USP 23: Folic Acid Injection; Folic Acid Tablets; Oil- and Water-soluble Vitamins Capsules; Oil- and Water-soluble Vitamins Tablets; Water-soluble Vitamins Capsules; Water-soluble Vitamins Tablets.

Proprietary Preparations (details are given in Part 3)
Aust.: Folamin†; Folsan; ***Austral.:*** Folasic†; Folicid†; Megafol; ***Belg.:*** Folavit†; ***Canad.:*** Folvite; Novo-Folacid; ***Fr.:*** Speciafoldine; ***Ger.:*** Folarell; Folsan; Lafol; ***Irl.:*** Clonfolic; ***Ital.:*** Folico†; Folina; ***Spain:*** Acfol; ***Swed.:*** Folacin; ***Switz.:*** Foli-Rivo; Folvite; ***UK:*** Folatine; Folicare; Lexpec; Preconceive; ***USA:*** Folvite.

Multi-ingredient: ***Aust.:*** Aktiferrin compositum; Beneuran compositum; Ferretab comp; Ferrograd-Fol; Losferron-Fol; Tardyferon-Fol; Trinsicon; ***Austral.:*** Children's Calcium With Minerals; Fefol; FGF Tabs; ***Belg.:*** Ferrifol B12; Gestiferrol; Neo Genyl†; Rubraton†; ***Canad.:*** Folacin 12; Palafer CF; Slow-Fe Folic; Trinsicon†; ***Fr.:*** Tardyferon B_9; ***Ger.:*** Aktiferrin E F†; B 12 compositum N†; B_{12}-Fol-Vicotrat; Eryfer comp.; Ferro Cytofol†; Ferro sanol comp; Ferro-B 12 Ehrl†; Ferro-Folgamma; Ferro-Folsan; Ferro-Folsan plus†; Ferro-Folsaure-Vicotrat†; Folgamma; Folicombin; Folsana; Hamatopan F; Hepagrisevit Forte-N; Hepagrisevit-Depot†; Hepasteril†; Kendural-Fol-500; Medivitan N; Medyn; Mersol; mono-Hepagrisevit†; Plastulen N; Rulofer†; Selectafer N; Tardyferon-Fol; ***Irl.:*** Cyfol†; Fefol; Fefol-Vit†; Ferrocap F; Ferrocontin Folic Continus†; Ferrograd Folic; Folex; Folferite†; Galfer FA; Givitol; Multivite Plus†; Pregnavite Forte F†; Slow-Fe Folic†; ***Ital.:*** Efargen; Emofol†; Epargriseovit; Ferro-Grad Folic; Ferro-Tre; Folepar B12; Liverest†; Oro B12; Oromag B12†; Protidepar 100†; Protidepar†; Trivitepar B12†; Vitamucin con Ferro†; ***Norw.:*** Pregnifer; ***S.Afr.:*** Effee; Fefol; Fefol-Vit†; Fero-Folic; Ferrimed; Foliglobin; Hepabionta; Pregamal; Trinsicon; ***Spain:*** Ferriwas B12 Fuerte†; Foliferron; Hepa Factor; Normovite Antianem Iny; Normovite Antianemico; Yectofer Compuesto†; ***Switz.:*** Actiferrine-F Nouvelle formule; Duofer Fol; Fero-Folic; Ferrum Fol B Hausmann†; Gyno-Tardyferon; Loesfer + acide folique; Maltofer Fol; Resoferon fol B†; ***UK:*** Dencyl; Fefol; Fefol Z†; Fefol-Vit†; Feravol-F†; Ferfolic SV; Ferrocap F 350†; Ferrocontin Folic Continus†; Ferrograd Folic; Folex-350; Folic Plus; Folicin†; Fortespan; Galfer FA; Givitol; Hematinic; Ironorm; Lexpec with Iron; Lexpec with Iron-M; Meterfolic†; Pregaday; Pregnavite Forte F; Slow-Fe Folic; ***USA:*** ABC to Z; Berocca Plus; Berplex; Centurion A–Z; Certagen; Cevi-Fer; Chromagen FA; Chromagen Forte; Compete; Contrin; Feocyte; Fero-Folic; Ferotrinsic; Ferralet Plus; Formula B Plus; Fumatinic; Geriot; Geritol Complete; Gevral T; Hemocyte-F; Iberet-Folic-500; Ircon-FA; Iromin-G; Kovitonic; Livitrinsic-f; Multibret-Folic†; Nephro-Fer Rx; Nestabs FA; Niferex Forte†; Nu-Iron Plus; Nu-Iron V; Parvlex; Perihemin†; Polytinic; Pronemia Hematinic; Reticulex†; Tabron†; Thera Hematinic; Theragenerix-H; Theravee Hematinic; TriHEMIC; Trinsicon; Vita-Feron; Vitafol; Yelets; Zodeac.

Folinic Acid (7862-n)

Citrovorum Factor; Formyl Tetrahydropteroylglutamic Acid; Leucovorin. 5-Formyltetrahydropteroylglutamate; *N*-[4-(2-Amino-5-formyl-5,6,7,8-tetrahydro-4-hydroxypteridin-6-ylmethylamino)benzoyl]-L(+)-glutamic acid.

$C_{20}H_{23}N_7O_7$ = 473.4.

CAS — 58-05-9.

Calcium Folinate (7863-h)

Calcium Folinate *(BAN, rINN).*

Calcium Folinate-SF; Calcium Leucovorin; Leucovorin Calcium; NSC-3590. Calcium 5-formyltetrahydropteroylglutamate; Calcium *N*-[4-(2-amino-5-formyl-5,6,7,8-tetrahydro-4-hydroxypteridin-6-ylmethylamino)benzoyl]-L(+)glutamate.

$C_{20}H_{21}CaN_7O_7$ = 511.5.

CAS — 1492-18-8 (anhydrous calcium folinate); 41927-89-3 (calcium folinate pentahydrate); 6035-45-6 (calcium folinate pentahydrate).

Pharmacopoeias. In *Eur.* (see p.viii), *Int., Jpn,* and *US.*

A white, yellowish-white, or yellow, odourless, amorphous or crystalline powder. Practically **insoluble** in alcohol and in acetone. A 2.5% solution has a pH of 6.8 to 8.0. **Store** in airtight containers. Protect from light.

Calcium folinate and fluorouracil, with or without 5% glucose, were incompatible when mixed in various ratios and stored in polyvinyl chloride containers at various temperatures.[1]

1. Trissel LA, *et al.* Incompatibility of fluorouracil with leucovorin calcium or levoleucovorin calcium. *Am J Health-Syst Pharm* 1995; **52:** 710–15.

Adverse Effects

Occasional hypersensitivity reactions have been reported; pyrexia has occurred rarely after injections.

Precautions

As for Folic Acid, p.1340.

Interactions

As for Folic Acid, p.1341.

Folinic acid should not be administered simultaneously with a folic acid antagonist such as methotrexate as this may nullify the effect of the antagonist. Folinic acid enhances the toxicity, as well as the antineoplastic action, of fluorouracil, especially on the gastro-intestinal tract.

Pharmacokinetics

Calcium folinate is well absorbed after oral and intramuscular administration and, unlike folic acid (p.1341), is rapidly converted to biologically active folates. Folate is concentrated in the liver and CSF although distribution occurs to all body tissues. Folates are mainly excreted in the urine, with small amounts in the faeces.

References.

1. McGuire BW, *et al.* Pharmacokinetics of leucovorin calcium after intravenous, intramuscular, and oral administration. *Clin Pharm* 1988; **7:** 52–8.
2. Wolfrom C, *et al.* Pharmacokinetic study of methotrexate, folinic acid and their serum metabolites in children treated with high-dose methotrexate and leucovorin rescue. *Eur J Clin Pharmacol* 1990; **39:** 377–83.
3. Zittoun J, *et al.* Pharmacokinetic comparison of leucovorin and levoleucovorin. *Eur J Clin Pharmacol* 1993; **44:** 569–73.
4. Mader RM, *et al.* Pharmacokinetics of rac-leucovorin vs [S]-leucovorin in patients with advanced gastrointestinal cancer. *Br J Clin Pharmacol* 1994; **37:** 243–8.
5. Schmitz JC, *et al.* Disposition of folic acid and its metabolites: a comparison with leucovorin. *Clin Pharmacol Ther* 1994; **55:** 501–8.

Uses and Administration

Folinic acid is the 5-formyl derivative of tetrahydrofolic acid, the active form of folic acid. Folinic acid is used principally as an antidote to folic acid antagonists, such as methotrexate (p.548), which block the conversion of folic acid to tetrahydrofolate by binding the enzyme dihydrofolate reductase. It does not block the antimicrobial action of folate antagonists such as trimethoprim or pyrimethamine, but may reduce their haematological toxicities.

Folinic acid, as calcium folinate, can be administered by mouth, by intramuscular injection, or by intravenous injection or infusion. Doses of calcium folinate are given in terms of folinic acid.

In cases of inadvertent overdosage of a folic acid antagonist, folinic acid should be administered as soon as possible and preferably within the first hour. Doses equal to or greater than the dose of methotrexate have been recommended. Alternatively it has been stated that where large overdoses of methotrexate have been given, calcium folinate may be given by intravenous infusion in a dose equivalent to 75 mg of folinic acid within 12 hours, followed by 12 mg intramuscularly every 6 hours for 4 doses. In less severe overdosage 6 to 12 mg of folinic acid intramuscularly every 6 hours for 4 doses may be adequate. Although vincristine is not a folic acid antagonist, folinic acid has also been proposed for some manifestations of vincristine toxicity overdosage—see p.570.

Folinic acid is used in conjunction with high-dose methotrexate antineoplastic therapy to reduce the toxicity of the methotrexate ('folinic acid rescue';

'calcium leucovorin rescue'). Folinic acid is given after an appropriate interval, usually of up to 24 hours, has elapsed for methotrexate to exert its antineoplastic effect and the objective is to maintain plasma concentrations of reduced folates at a level equivalent to or greater than the plasma-methotrexate concentration. Dosage must therefore be adapted according to the methotrexate regimen, and the patient's ability to clear the antineoplastic. In general, doses of up to 120 mg have been given over 12 to 24 hours, by intramuscular injection or intravenous injection or infusion, followed by 12 to 15 mg intramuscularly, or 15 mg by mouth, every 6 hours for the next 48 hours. With doses of methotrexate below 100 mg, folinic acid 15 mg by mouth every 6 hours for 48 to 72 hours may suffice.

Folinic acid is also used to enhance the cytotoxic effect of fluorouracil in advanced colorectal cancer (see p.536) although conclusive survival benefits have not yet been shown. One suggested regimen is folinic acid 200 mg per m^2 body-surface by slow intravenous injection over at least 3 to 5 minutes followed by fluorouracil at an initial dose of 370 mg per m^2 intravenously; the treatment is given daily for 5 consecutive days and may be repeated at intervals of 21 to 28 days. Lower doses of folinic acid (20 mg per m^2 by intravenous injection followed by fluorouracil 425 mg per m^2) have also been used.

Folinic acid, like folic acid, is effective in the treatment of folate-deficient megaloblastic anaemia (see p.703). Doses of 15 mg daily by mouth have been suggested. If given intramuscularly a dose of up to 1 mg daily has been recommended on the grounds that higher doses have not been proven to be any more effective. It is unsuitable for megaloblastic anaemia secondary to vitamin-B_{12} deficiencies.

Calcium levofolinate, the active laevo-isomer, is used similarly to calcium folinate, in doses half those recommended for the racemic form. Calcium mefolinate is also used.

HIV infection and AIDS. Calcium folinate has been used to reduce the toxicity of pyrimethamine and trimethoprim in patients with HIV infection. However, adjunctive administration of oral calcium folinate to patients with AIDS receiving co-trimoxazole for the treatment of *Pneumocystis carinii* pneumonia (PCP), was associated with a higher rate of therapeutic failure and a decrease in survival and did not reduce the frequency of dose-limiting co-trimoxazole toxicity.[1] Calcium folinate did not reduce the toxicity of co-trimoxazole being used for the primary prophylaxis of PCP.[2]

1. Safrin S, *et al.* Adjunctive folinic acid with trimethoprim-sulfamethoxazole for Pneumocystis carinii pneumonia in AIDS patients is associated with an increased risk of therapeutic failure and death. *J Infect Dis* 1994; **170:** 912–17.
2. Bozzette SA, *et al.* The tolerance for zidovudine plus thrice weekly or daily trimethoprim-sulfamethoxazole with and without leucovorin for primary prophylaxis in advanced HIV disease. *Am J Med* 1995; **98:** 177–82.

Preparations

USP 23: Leucovorin Calcium Injection; Leucovorin Calcium Tablets.

Proprietary Preparations (details are given in Part 3)
Aust.: Cehafolin; Isovorin; Levorin; Ribofolin; ***Belg.:*** Elvorine; Ledervorin; ***Fr.:*** Elvorine; Folinoral; Lederfoline; Osfolate; Perfolate; ***Ger.:*** FOLI-cell; Imofolin†; Lederfolat; Rescuvolin; Ribofolin; ***Ital.:*** Biofolic; Calcifolin; Calfolex; Calinat; Citofolin; Disintox†; Ecofol; Emovis; Folaren; Foliben; Folidar; Folinac; Folinvit; Foliplus; Folix; Furoic; Lederfolin; Levofolene; Osfolato; Perfolin; Prefolic; Resfolin; Sanifolin; Tonofolin; ***Neth.:*** Isovorin; Ledervorin; ***Norw.:*** Rescuvolin; ***S.Afr.:*** Refolinon; Rescuvolin; ***Spain:*** Cromatonbic Folinico; Folaxin; Folidan; Isovorin; Lederfolin; ***Swed.:*** Citrec; Isovorin; Rescuvolin; ***Switz.:*** Isovorin; Osfolate; ***UK:*** Isovorin; Lederfolin; Refolinon; ***USA:*** Wellcovorin.

Multi-ingredient: ***Ital.:*** Adinepar†; Bio-Rex†; Disintox Cortex†; Divical; Dopatox†; Emazian B12; Emazian Cortex†; Emoantitossina; Emonucleosina Cortex†; Emopon; Eparmefolin; Epartonno†; Exepin Cortex†; Ferplex Fol†; Ferritin Complex; Ferrofolin; Ferrofolin Venti†; Folinemic Cortex†; Folinemic†; For Liver; Fruttidasi†; Globuleno†; Hepa-Factor; Hepa-Factor Complex†; Idropan B; Ipavit; Legofer Folinico†; Liverasten†; NE 300†; Neo-Cromaton Cortex†; Nepatim†; Siderofolin†; Sulton; Tonoliver 10000†; Tonoliver Ferro†; ***Spain:*** Cromatonbic 5000 Ferro†; Cromatonbic 5000†.

Fructose (595-e)

D-Fructose; Fructosum; Fruit Sugar; Laevulose; Laevulosum; Levulose. D-(−)-Fructopyranose.
$C_6H_{12}O_6$ = 180.2.
CAS — 57-48-7.

Pharmacopoeias. In *Eur.* (see p.viii), *Jpn*, and *US.*

Odourless colourless crystals or a white crystalline powder with a sweet taste. Very or freely **soluble** in water; soluble 1 in 15 of alcohol, and 1 in 14 of methyl alcohol.

Adverse Effects

Large doses of fructose given by mouth may cause flatulence, abdominal pain, and diarrhoea. Lactic acidosis and hyperuricaemia may follow intravenous infusions; fatalities have occurred.

Urticaria in one patient associated with the ingestion of certain foods was found to be caused by D-psicose, a minor constituent of high-fructose syrup, which is used as a sweetening agent.[1]

1. Nishioka K, *et al.* Urticaria induced by D-psicose. *Lancet* 1983; **ii:** 1417–18.

Precautions

Fructose should not be given to patients with hereditary fructose intolerance.

It should be given with caution to patients with impaired kidney function or severe liver damage.

Pharmacokinetics

Fructose is absorbed from the gastro-intestinal tract but more slowly than glucose. It is metabolised more rapidly than glucose, mainly in the liver where it is phosphorylated and a part is converted to glucose; other metabolites include lactic acid and pyruvic acid. Although it has often been considered that the metabolism of fructose is not dependent on insulin and that insulin is not necessary for its conversion to glycogen, glucose is a metabolic product of fructose and requires the presence of insulin for its further metabolism.

Uses and Administration

Fructose is sweeter than sucrose or sorbitol. It is used as a sweetener in foods for diabetics; in the UK it has been advised that the intake of fructose be limited to 25 g daily in persons with diabetes mellitus.

Fructose has been employed as an alternative to glucose in parenteral nutrition but its use is not recommended because of the risk of lactic acidosis. Use by intravenous infusion in the treatment of severe alcohol poisoning is also no longer recommended.

Solutions of fructose with glucose have been used in the treatment of nausea and vomiting (p.1172) including vomiting of pregnancy.

A reiteration of the view that the use of intravenous infusions containing fructose and sorbitol, which remain popular in some countries, should be abandoned.[1] Not only can they lead to life-threatening build-up of lactic acid, they have led to fatalities in patients with undiagnosed hereditary fructose intolerance.

1. Collins J. Time for fructose solutions to go. *Lancet* 1993; **341:** 600.

Preparations

BP 1998: Fructose Intravenous Infusion;
USP 23: Fructose and Sodium Chloride Injection; Fructose Injection.

Proprietary Preparations (details are given in Part 3)
Aust.: Laevoral; Laevosan; ***Fr.:*** Fruxucre; ***Ital.:*** Fructal; Fructan; Fructopiran; Fructosil; Laevosan; ***Switz.:*** Laevoral†; ***UK:*** Levugen.

Multi-ingredient: ***Austral.:*** Anvatrol†; Emetrol; ***Fr.:*** Arnilose; ***Ger.:*** Alinda†; Gallexier; Reducdyn†; ***Ital.:*** Eparema-Levul; Liozim; Retinosio Vitaminico†; Sucrinburck†; Vitalmix; Weight Watchers Punto; ***Norw.:*** Invertos; ***Spain:*** Levulosalino Isot; Levupotasico; Levusalino; ***USA:*** Emecheck†; Emetrol; Naus-A-Way†.

Gleptoferron (16821-d)

Gleptoferron (*BAN, USAN, rINN*).
$C_7H_{14}O_8.(C_6H_{10}O_5)_n.FeOOH$.
CAS — 57680-55-4.

A macromolecular complex of ferric hydroxide and dextranglucoheptonic acid.

Gleptoferron has been employed for iron-deficiency anaemia in veterinary medicine. It was given by intramuscular injection.

Glucose (17536-m)

Anhydrous Glucose (582-g)

Anhydrous Dextrose; Dextrosum Anhydricum; D-Glucose; Glucosum Anhydricum. D-(+)-Glucopyranose.
$C_6H_{12}O_6$ = 180.2.
CAS — 50-99-7.

Pharmacopoeias. In *Eur.* (see p.viii), *Int.*, *Jpn*, *Pol.*, and *US.*
Some pharmacopoeias include anhydrous glucose and/or glucose monohydrate as separate monographs whereas others permit the anhydrous and/or monohydrate under a single monograph.

Anhydrous Glucose (Ph. Eur.) is a white crystalline powder with a sweet taste. Freely **soluble** in water; sparingly soluble in alcohol.

Dextrose (USP 23), which is either anhydrous or the monohydrate, is a white odourless crystalline or granular powder or colourless crystals with a sweet taste. **Soluble** 1 in 1 of water and 1 in 100 of alcohol; very soluble in boiling water; soluble in boiling alcohol.

Anhydrous glucose 0.9 g is approximately equivalent to glucose monohydrate 1 g.

A 5.05% solution of anhydrous glucose in water is iso-osmotic with serum.

Both Glucose Intravenous Infusion (BP 1998) and Dextrose Injection (USP 23) may be prepared from either anhydrous glucose or glucose monohydrate. However, the potency of the BP preparation is expressed in terms of anhydrous glucose whereas that of the USP is expressed in terms of glucose monohydrate. The BP directs that when glucose is required as a diluent for official injections or intravenous infusions, Glucose Intravenous Infusion 5% should be used.

Glucose Monohydrate (584-p)

Dextrosum Monohydridicum; D-Glucose Monohydrate; Glucosum Monohydridicum; Glycosum; Grape Sugar. D-(+)-Glucopyranose monohydrate.
$C_6H_{12}O_6,H_2O$ = 198.2.
CAS — 5996-10-1.

Pharmacopoeias. In *Chin.*, *Eur.* (see p.viii), *Int.*, and *US.*
Some pharmacopoeias include anhydrous glucose and/or glucose monohydrate as separate monographs whereas others permit the anhydrous and/or monohydrate under a single monograph.
Eur. includes Liquid Glucose. *USNF* includes Dextrose Excipient and Liquid Glucose.

Glucose (Ph. Eur.) is a white crystalline powder with a sweet taste. **Solubilities** are as for Anhydrous Glucose (above).

Dextrose (USP 23) is either anhydrous or the monohydrate. For further details see Anhydrous Glucose (above).

Glucose monohydrate 1.1 g is approximately equivalent to anhydrous glucose 1 g.

A 5.51% solution of glucose monohydrate in water is iso-osmotic with serum.

Liquid Glucose (Ph. Eur.) is a clear colourless or brown viscous liquid containing a mixture of glucose, di- and polysaccharides obtained by hydrolysis of starch, in aqueous solution. It contains not less than 70.0 and not more than 99.5% of dry matter. **Miscible** with water. It may partly or totally solidify at room temperature, liquefying again on heating to 50°. Liquid Glucose (USNF) is a similar product, described as containing chiefly glucose, dextrins, maltose, and water. It should be **stored** in airtight containers.

Adverse Effects and Precautions

Intravenous administration of glucose solutions (particularly hyperosmotic solutions, which also have a low pH) may cause local pain, vein irritation, and thrombophlebitis, and tissue necrosis if extravasation occurs. Some of these reactions may be due to degradation products present after autoclaving or to poor administration technique. Intravenous infusion can lead to the development of fluid and electrolyte disturbances including hypokalaemia, hypomagnesaemia, and hypophosphataemia. Prolonged administration or rapid infusion of large volumes of iso-osmotic solutions may cause oedema or water intoxication; conversely, prolonged or rapid administration of hyperosmotic solutions may result in dehydration as a consequence of the induced hyperglycaemia.

The use of hyperosmotic glucose solutions is contra-indicated in patients with anuria, intracranial or in-traspinal haemorrhage, and in delirium tremens where there is dehydration.

It has been suggested that glucose solutions should not be used after acute ischaemic strokes as hyper-glycaemia has been implicated in increasing cerebral ischaemic brain damage and in impairing recovery.

Glucose solutions should not be administered through the same infusion equipment as whole blood as haemolysis and clumping can occur.

Pregnancy. Glucose solutions are commonly employed as hydrating fluids and as vehicles for the administration of other drugs. It has been suggested that if used during labour the glucose load on the mother may lead to fetal hyperglycaemia, hyperinsulinaemia, and acidosis, with subsequent neonatal hypoglycaemia and jaundice.[1,2] Others[3] have found no evidence of such an effect, and note that the number of patients included in such reports is often small and the selection criteria not homogeneous.

1. Kenepp NB, *et al.* Fetal and neonatal hazards of maternal hydration with 5% dextrose before caesarean section. *Lancet* 1982; **i:** 1150–2.
2. Singhi S, *et al.* Hazards of maternal hydration with 5% dextrose. *Lancet* 1982; **ii:** 335–6.
3. Piquard F, *et al.* Does fetal acidosis develop with maternal glucose infusion during normal labor? *Obstet Gynecol* 1989; **74:** 909–14.

Stroke. It has been stated that glucose infusion should be avoided after ischaemic stroke.[1,2] Experimental and clinical studies have purported to show that increased blood-glucose concentrations worsen cerebral ischaemic brain damage and impair recovery. The mechanism responsible is believed to be the increase in ischaemic tissue of lactate with resultant acidosis; the precise manner in which the lactate damages or impairs recovery of tissue is not, however, known.

1. Scheinberg P. Controversies in the management of cerebral vascular disease. *Neurology* 1988; **38:** 1609–16.
2. WHO. Stroke—1989: recommendations on stroke prevention, diagnosis, and therapy: report of the WHO task force on stroke and other cerebrovascular disorders. *Stroke* 1989; **20:** 1407–31.

Pharmacokinetics

Glucose is rapidly absorbed from the gastro-intestinal tract. Peak plasma concentrations of glucose occur about 40 minutes after oral administration of glucose to hypoglycaemic patients. It is metabolised via pyruvic or lactic acid to carbon dioxide and water with the release of energy. All body cells are capable of oxidising glucose and it forms the principal source of energy in cellular metabolism.

Uses and Administration

Glucose, a monosaccharide, is administered by mouth or by intravenous infusion in the treatment of carbohydrate and fluid depletion. It is the preferred source of carbohydrate in parenteral nutrition regimens (p.1331) and is used in oral rehydration solutions (p.1152) for the prevention and treatment of dehydration due to acute diarrhoeal diseases (p.1168).

Glucose is also used in the treatment of hypoglycaemia (see below) and is administered orally in the glucose tolerance test as a diagnostic aid for diabetes mellitus (see p.313).

The way in which the strengths of glucose solutions for intravenous use are expressed varies in different countries. Although the BP requires that the strength be expressed in terms of anhydrous glucose, the USP states that strengths are expressed in terms of glucose monohydrate. Thus, the term glucose 5% may represent, depending on origin, either 50 g per litre of anhydrous glucose (equivalent to about 55 g per litre of glucose monohydrate) or 50 g per litre of glucose monohydrate (equivalent to about 45 g per litre of anhydrous glucose). As the manner in which such preparations are referred to in the medical literature is sometimes ambiguous, it has not always been possible to state clearly in *Martindale* whether the strengths of glucose solutions mentioned relate to the anhydrous or hydrated form; however, in *Martindale*, unless otherwise specified, glucose injection is a 5% solution to distinguish it from more concentrated forms. For many practical purposes it is probably less important to know the exact way in which the strength of a given concentration is expressed than to avoid confusion between completely different strengths such as 5, 10, and 50% as the more concentrated forms are associated with special side-effects and precautions.

Glucose solution 5% (5.05% anhydrous, 5.51% monohydrate) is iso-osmotic with blood and is the strength often employed for fluid depletion; it may be administered via a peripheral vein. Glucose solutions with a concentration greater than 5% are hyperosmotic and are generally used as a carbohydrate source; a 50% solution is often employed in the treatment of severe hypoglycaemia (but see also Hypoglycaemia, below). Hyperosmotic solutions should generally be administered via a central vein although some authorities have considered that concentrations up to 10% may be administered via a peripheral vein for short periods provided the site is alternated regularly. In the emergency treatment of hypoglycaemia it may be necessary to use a peripheral vein but the solution should be given slowly; a suggested rate for glucose 50% in such circumstances is 3 mL per minute.

The dose of glucose is variable and is dependent on individual patient requirements; serum-glucose concentrations may need to be carefully monitored. The maximum rate of glucose utilisation has been estimated to be about 500 to 800 mg per kg body-weight per hour.

Strongly hyperosmotic glucose solutions (25 to 50%) have also been used to reduce cerebrospinal pressure (p.796) and cerebral oedema caused by delirium tremens or acute alcohol intoxication (p.1099) although they do not appear to be widely employed. Glucose solution 50% has also been used as a sclerosing agent in the treatment of varicose veins and as an irritant to produce adhesive pleuritis.

Ectopic pregnancy. Ectopic pregnancy (implantation of the fertilised ovum outside the womb) is now recognised at earlier stages as a result of improved diagnostic techniques. Surgery remains the mainstay of treatment, but although conservative surgical techniques may be employed in an attempt to preserve fertility, nonsurgical methods have been increasingly investigated. The best established therapy is with methotrexate (p.550), but prostaglandins or hyperosmolar glucose solutions have also been employed.

The local instillation of 10 to 20 mL of glucose 50% into unruptured tubes has been found by Lang and associates to be a safe and satisfactory alternative to combined therapy consisting of dinoprost injected into the gestational sac, sulprostone intramuscularly, and oestrogens to effect luteolysis.[1] No side-effects were reported by 16 women who received glucose in this manner whereas 9 of 15 who received the prostaglandins and oestrogens reported abdominal cramps which ceased only after discontinuation of sulprostone, 6 were subfebrile, and 2 had signs of imminent tubal rupture. It was believed that the mechanism of action of hyperosmolar glucose in destroying the developing ectopic pregnancy was probably due to necrobiosis by dehydrating the cells.

Thompson subsequently queried whether methotrexate was likely to cause any more local damage to the fallopian tubes than glucose.[2] In reply Lang and Hönigl[3] still believed that damage to the tubal wall with glucose was unlikely and additionally pointed out corrections to the urinary concentrations of chorionic gonadotrophin as published in the original article.

1. Lang PF, *et al.* Conservative treatment of ectopic pregnancy with local injection of hyperosmolar glucose solution or prostaglandin-$F_{2\alpha}$: a prospective randomised study. *Lancet* 1990; **336:** 78–81.
2. Thompson GR. Hyperosmolar glucose solution or prostaglandin-$F_{2\alpha}$ for ectopic pregnancy. *Lancet* 1990; **336:** 685.
3. Lang PF, Hönigl W. Hyperosmolar glucose solution or prostaglandin-$F_{2\alpha}$ for ectopic pregnancy. *Lancet* 1990; **336:** 685.

Glycogen storage disease. Starch may be a more acceptable alternative to glucose in the control of the hypoglycaemia of type I glycogen storage disease, see p.1356.

Haemodialysis-induced cramp. Suggestions that haemodialysis-induced cramps (p.1151) are due to hypovolaemia (see p.1303) are supported by the efficacy of volume expansion with hypertonic solutions in the management of such cramps. Intravenous infusion of 50 mL of glucose 50% solution has been used as an effective alternative to infusion of sodium chloride or mannitol.[1,2]

1. Milutinovich J, *et al.* Effect of hypertonic glucose on the muscular cramps of hemodialysis. *Ann Intern Med* 1979; **90:** 926–8.
2. Canzanello VJ, *et al.* Comparison of 50% dextrose water, 25% mannitol, and 23.5% saline for the treatment of hemodialysis-associated muscle cramps. *Trans Am Soc Artif Intern Organs* 1991; **37:** 649–52.

Hyperkalaemia. Insulin, together with glucose to prevent hypoglycaemia, is given to stimulate the cellular uptake of potassium in the emergency treatment of moderate to severe hyperkalaemia (p.1149). Usually, 50 mL of glucose 50% is administered.

Hypoglycaemia. Glucose is used to correct insulin-induced hypoglycaemia, as discussed on p.323, either by mouth or by infusion of a hypertonic solution. For intravenous infusion up to 50 mL of a 50% solution is given. Glucose 10 or 20% may be used but larger volumes are required. Although 50% glucose solution has been generally used to correct hypoglycaemia in children, some workers consider that so concentrated a solution is associated with unacceptable morbidity and possible mortality, and that it should be replaced by the 10% solution for this purpose.[1] A 5 or 10% solution is used to prevent the hypoglycaemia associated with insulin infusion for the treatment of diabetic ketoacidosis, once blood-glucose concentration has fallen below 10 mmol per litre (see p.316).

1. Winrow AP, *et al.* Paediatric resuscitation: don't use 50% dextrose. *Br Med J* 1993; **306:** 1612.

Myocardial infarction. Some results in diabetic and nondiabetic patients have suggested that the value of a glucose, insulin, and potassium combination in patients with myocardial infarction should perhaps be reconsidered, despite earlier failures (see p.791).

Preparations

BP 1998: Glucose Intravenous Infusion; Glucose Irrigation Solution; Potassium Chloride and Glucose Intravenous Infusion; Potassium Chloride, Sodium Chloride and Glucose Intravenous Infusion; Sodium Chloride and Glucose Intravenous Infusion;
Ph. Eur.: Anticoagulant Acid-Citrate-Glucose Solutions (ACD); Anticoagulant Citrate-Phosphate-Glucose Solution (CPD);
USNF 18: Dextrose Excipient; Liquid Glucose;
USP 23: Alcohol in Dextrose Injection; Anticoagulant Citrate Dextrose Solution; Anticoagulant Citrate Phosphate Dextrose Adenine Solution; Anticoagulant Citrate Phosphate Dextrose Solution; Dextrose and Sodium Chloride Injection; Dextrose Injection; Half-strength Lactated Ringer's and Dextrose Injection; Lactated Ringer's and Dextrose Injection; Modified Lactated Ringer's and Dextrose Injection; Multiple Electrolytes and Dextrose Injection Type 1; Multiple Electrolytes and Dextrose Injection Type 2; Multiple Electrolytes and Dextrose Injection Type 3; Multiple Electrolytes and Dextrose Injection Type 4; Potassium Chloride in Dextrose and Sodium Chloride Injection; Potassium Chloride in Dextrose Injection; Potassium Chloride in Lactated Ringer's and Dextrose Injection; Ringer's and Dextrose Injection; Sodium Chloride and Dextrose Tablets.

Proprietary Preparations (details are given in Part 3)
Aust.: Glucosan; ***Canad.:*** Glucodex; ***Ger.:*** Dextro med†; Dextromon†; Glucosteril; ***Irl.:*** Hycal; ***Ital.:*** Energen; ***Spain:*** Apir Glucoibys; Apir Glucosado; Apiroflex Glucosada; Glucosmon; ***UK:*** Glucodin; ***USA:*** Dex4 Glucose; Glutose; Insulin Reaction.

Multi-ingredient: numerous preparations are listed in Part 3.

Glutamic Acid (586-w)

Glutamic Acid *(USAN, rINN).*

620; Acidum Glutamicum; E; Glu; L-Glutamic Acid; Glutaminic Acid. L-(+)-2-Aminoglutaric acid.

$C_5H_9NO_4$ = 147.1.

CAS — 56-86-0.

Pharmacopoeias. In *Chin.* and *Eur.* (see p.viii).

A white crystalline powder or colourless crystals. Freely **soluble** in boiling water; slightly soluble in cold water; practically insoluble in alcohol, in acetic acid, in acetone, and in ether. **Protect** from light.

Glutamic Acid Hydrochloride (587-e)

Glutamic Acid Hydrochloride *(rINNM).*

Aciglumin; Glu Hydrochloride. L-(+)-2-Aminoglutaric acid hydrochloride.

$C_5H_9NO_4,HCl$ = 183.6.

CAS — 138-15-8.

Pharmacopoeias. In *Ger.*

Levoglutamide (598-j)

Levoglutamide *(pINN).*

Gln; L-Glutamine; Q. L-Glutamic acid 5-amide; L-(+)-2-Aminoglutaramic acid.

$C_5H_{10}N_2O_3$ = 146.1.

CAS — 56-85-9.

Pharmacopoeias. In *Ger.*

Glutamic acid is an aliphatic amino acid which is degraded readily in the body to form levoglutamide (glutamine). Glutamic acid and levoglutamide are used as dietary supplements.

Glutamic acid hydrochloride, which releases hydrochloric acid in the stomach, has been used in the symptomatic treatment of achlorhydria or hypochlorhydria in usual doses by mouth of 0.5 to 1 g with meals.

Parenteral nutrition. Profound depletion of glutamine in skeletal muscle is characteristic of injury, and suggestions that glutamine is involved in the regulation of muscle protein synthesis have led to studies[1-5] of supplementation with levoglutamide or more stable peptide derivatives in parenteral nutrition regimens for patients with injury and infection.

Supplementation of parenteral nutrition regimens with levoglutamide has been shown to reduce clinical infection in patients who have undergone bone-marrow transplantation[2] or who have suffered multiple trauma.[5] A further study has shown improved mortality among intensive-care patients given parenteral feeds supplemented with glutamine.[4]

The use of levoglutamide coupled with alanine (L-alanyl-L-glutamine; Ala-Gln) has been described.[1] In patients undergoing major uncomplicated surgery on the lower gastro-intestinal tract, a significantly better postoperative nitrogen balance was achieved in those whose total parenteral nutrition regimen had been supplemented with about 20 g daily of this dipeptide (equivalent to about 12 g daily of glutamine) when compared with a control group. Others[3] have shown that supplementation of total parenteral nutrition solutions with a glutamine dipeptide (glycyl-L-glutamine), in quantities equivalent to 0.23 g of glutamine per kg body-weight daily, prevented the increased intestinal permeability and atrophic changes in the intestinal mucosa associated with unsupplemented solutions. Such changes may be associated with decreased immunity and bacteraemia, which may explain the reduction in clinical infection mentioned above.

It has also been postulated that muscle protein catabolism after trauma may be due to a shortage of α-ketoglutarate rather than glutamine; glutamine is formed from α-ketoglutarate, which has the same carbon skeleton. Wernerman and co-workers[6] have shown that supplementation of total parenteral nutrition with α-ketoglutarate or a dipeptide, ornithine-α-ketoglutarate, reduces muscle protein depletion and suggested this may be a more physiological way of providing glutamine.

1. Stehle P, *et al.* Effect of parenteral glutamine peptide supplements on muscle glutamine loss and nitrogen balance after major surgery. *Lancet* 1989; **i:** 231–3.
2. Ziegler TR, *et al.* Clinical and metabolic efficacy of glutamine-supplemented parenteral nutrition after bone marrow transplantation: a randomized, double-blind, controlled study. *Ann Intern Med* 1992; **116:** 821–8.
3. van der Hulst RRWJ, *et al.* Glutamine and the preservation of gut integrity. *Lancet* 1993; **334:** 1363–5.
4. Griffiths RD, *et al.* Six-month outcome of critically ill patients given glutamine-supplemented parenteral nutrition. *Nutrition* 1997; **13:** 295–302.
5. Houdijk APJ, *et al.* Randomised trial of glutamine-enriched enteral nutrition on infectious morbidity in patients with multiple trauma. *Lancet* 1998; **352:** 772–6.
6. Wernerman J, *et al.* α-Ketoglutarate and postoperative muscle catabolism. *Lancet* 1990; **335:** 701–3.

Vincristine neurotoxicity. Neurotoxicity is a relatively common adverse reaction experienced with vincristine (see p.570). A double-blind placebo-controlled randomised study involving 84 patients found that the administration of glutamic acid 1.5 g daily by mouth in divided doses during a 6-week induction chemotherapy course decreased vincristine-induced neurotoxicity.[1] The mechanism by which glutamic acid may inhibit vincristine toxicity was not known although various proposals were discussed and further trials were considered warranted.

Inadvertent intrathecal administration of vincristine has resulted in paralysis and death although there has been one case where this was prevented. One of the manufacturers of vincristine (*Lilly*) has stated[2] that details of this case will be included in data sheets and package inserts, adding though that the role of glutamic acid cannot be determined. Successful treatment included removal of cerebrospinal fluid and flushing the subarachnoid space with lactated Ringer's solution together with the administration of glutamic acid 10 g intravenously over 24 hours followed by 500 mg three times daily by mouth until neurological dysfunction stabilised.

1. Jackson DV, *et al.* Amelioration of vincristine neurotoxicity by glutamic acid. *Am J Med* 1988; **84:** 1016–22.
2. Dyke RW. Treatment of inadvertent intrathecal injection of vincristine. *N Engl J Med* 1989; **321:** 1270–1.

Preparations

Proprietary Preparations (details are given in Part 3)
Aust.: Dipeptiven; Neuroglutamin; ***Austral.:*** Muripsin†; ***Ger.:*** Dipeptamin; Glutamin-Verla; Gluti-Agil; Pepsaletten N; ***Ital.:*** Dipeptiven; Glutacerebro; Glutaven; Memoril; ***Norw.:*** Glutacid; ***Spain:*** Glutaneurina B6 Fte†; ***Swed.:*** Dipeptiven; Hypochylin; ***UK:*** Dipeptiven; Muripsin†; ***USA:*** Acidulin†.

Multi-ingredient: ***Aust.:*** Aslavital†; Pansan; ***Austral.:*** Aspartatol; Bioglan Digestive Zyme†; Liv-Detox; Prozyme; ***Fr.:*** Catarstat; Glutaminol B_6†; Phakan; Viridex†; Vita-Dermacide; YSE Glutamique; ***Ger.:*** Glutarsin E; Pansan†; Pepsaldra†; Vitasprint B_{12}; ***Ital.:*** Briogen; Canulase†; Cerebrix†; Dalivit†; Deadyn†; Energon Rende†; Esaglut; Fosfo Plus; Fosfoglutil†; Fosglutamina B6†; Glivitom†; Gluserin B12†; Glutamin Fosforo; Memoserina S; Memovit B12; Mnemina Fosforo†; Vitasprint; Vitasprint Complex; ***S.Afr.:*** Lentogesic; Spasmo-Canulase; ***Spain:*** Agudil; Cerebrmente†; Espasmo Canulasa; Gammamida Complex; Gastro Gobens; Gastroglutal; Jorkil; Mederebro Compuesto; Nucleserina; Tebetane Compuesto; ***Switz.:*** Ginkovit†; Phakolen; Spasmo-Canulase; Vitasprint Complex; ***UK:*** Amino MS; Fat-Solv; Slimswift Day Trim†; ***USA:*** Prevenzyme†.

Glycine (589-y)

Glycine *(rINN).*

Aminoacetic Acid; G; Gly; Glycinum; Glycocoll; Sucre de Gélatine.

$C_2H_5NO_2$ = 75.07.

CAS — 56-40-6.

Pharmacopoeias. In *Eur.* (see p.viii), *Jpn,* and *US.*

A white odourless crystalline powder. **Soluble** 1 in 4 of water at 25°, 1 in 2.6 at 50°, 1 in 1.9 at 75°, and 1 in 1.5 at 100°; soluble 1 in 1254 of alcohol; very slightly soluble or practically insoluble in ether. A 5% solution in water has a pH of 5.9 to 6.4.

Adverse Effects and Precautions

Systemic absorption of glycine irrigation solutions can lead to disturbances of fluid and electrolyte balance and cardiovascular and pulmonary disorders.

Glycine irrigation should be used cautiously in patients with hepatic impairment since any absorption and consequent metabolism may cause hyperammonaemia. The possible effects on fluid and electrolyte balance warrant cautious use in patients with cardiopulmonary or renal dysfunction; glycine irrigation is contra-indicated in anuric patients.

Reports and discussions concerning adverse effects, including disturbances of fluid and electrolyte balance, after the use of glycine irrigation solutions and precautions to be observed.

1. Ovassapian A, *et al.* Visual disturbances: an unusual symptom of transurethral prostatic resection reaction. *Anesthesiology* 1982; **57:** 332–4.
2. Sinclair JF, *et al.* Absorption of 1.5% glycine after percutaneous ultrasonic lithotripsy for renal stone disease. *Br Med J* 1985; **291:** 691–2.
3. Goble NM, *et al.* Absorption of 1.5% glycine after percutaneous ultrasonic lithotripsy for renal stone disease. *Br Med J* 1985; **291:** 966–7.
4. Miller RA, Whitfield HN. Absorption of 1.5% glycine after percutaneous ultrasonic lithotripsy for renal stone disease. *Br Med J* 1985; **291:** 967.
5. Hahn RG, Rundgren M. Vasopressin and amino acid concentrations in serum following absorption of irrigating fluid containing glycine and ethanol. *Br J Anaesth* 1989; **63:** 337–9.
6. Baumann R, *et al.* Absorption of glycine irrigating solution during transcervical resection of endometrium. *Br Med J* 1990; **300:** 304–5.
7. Boto TCA, *et al.* Absorption of irrigating fluid during transcervical resection of endometrium. *Br Med J* 1990; **300:** 748.
8. Rao PN. Absorption of irrigating fluid during transcervical resection of endometrium. *Br Med J* 1990; **300:** 748–9.
9. Wiener J, Gregory L. Absorption of irrigating fluid during transcervical resection of endometrium. *Br Med J* 1990; **300:** 749.
10. Magos AL, *et al.* Absorption of irrigating fluid during transcervical resection of endometrium. *Br Med J* 1990; **300:** 1079.
11. Istre O, *et al.* Postoperative cerebral oedema after transcervical endometrial resection and uterine irrigation with 1.5% glycine. *Lancet* 1994; **344:** 1187–9.
12. Beutler JJ, Koomans HA. Safety and transcervical endometrial resection. *Lancet* 1995; **345:** 55.
13. Hahn RG, Persson P-G. Acute myocardial infarction after prostatectomy. *Lancet* 1996; **347:** 355.

Uses and Administration

Glycine is the simplest of the amino acids. It is used as a dietary supplement.

Glycine is sometimes used in conjunction with antacids in the treatment of gastric hyperacidity. It is also used as an ingredient of some aspirin preparations with the object of reducing gastric irritation.

Sterile solutions of glycine 1.5% in water, which are hypotonic and non-conductive, are used as urogenital irrigation solutions during certain surgical procedures, particularly transurethral resection of the prostate.

Glycine hydrochloride has also been used.

Preparations

BP 1998: Glycine Irrigation Solution;
USP 23: Glycine Irrigation.

Proprietary Preparations (details are given in Part 3)
Fr.: Gyn-Hydralin; Uro 3000.

Multi-ingredient: ***Aust.:*** Centramin; ***Austral.:*** Cal-Alkyline; Digest-eze†; Proacid; ***Fr.:*** Activarol; Cristopal; Magnesium Glycocolle Lafarge; Phakan; ***Ger.:*** Pansan†; Panzynorm forte†; Robusanon†; ***Ital.:*** Detoxicon; Digestivo Antonetto; Exepin Cortex†; Nevrostenina B12†; ***Spain:*** Actilevol C†; Sanieb; Tebetane Compuesto; ***Switz.:*** Phakolen; Regla pH; ***UK:*** Slimswift Night Trim†; ***USA:*** Calglycine Antacid.

Used as an adjunct in: ***Austral.:*** Disprin Direct; ***Fr.:*** Juvepirine; Sargepirine; ***Ger.:*** Godamed; ***Ital.:*** Aspiglicina; Geyfritz; ***Spain:*** Dulcipirina†; Okal.

Halibut-liver Oil (7825-t)

Aceite de Higado de Hipogloso; Heilbuttleberöl; Ol. Hippogloss.; Oleum Hippoglossi; Oleum Jecoris Hippoglossi.

CAS — 8001-46-5.

Pharmacopoeias. In *Aust.* and *Br.*

The fixed oil extracted from the fresh or suitably preserved liver of the halibut species belonging to the genus *Hippoglossus* (Pleuronectidae). It contains not less than 30 000 units of vitamin A activity per g. Halibut-liver oil may contain up to about 3000 units of vitamin D activity per g. Halibut-liver oil containing 30 000 units of vitamin A in 1 g contains approximately 4000 units in 0.15 mL.

A pale to golden-yellow liquid with a fishy but not rancid odour and taste. Practically **insoluble** in alcohol; miscible with chloroform, ether, and petroleum spirit. **Store** in well-filled containers. Protect from light.

Halibut-liver oil is used as a means of administering vitamins A (p.1358) and D (p.1366); the proportion of vitamin A to vitamin D is usually greater in halibut-liver oil than in cod-liver oil (p.1337). It is usually given in capsules.

Preparations

BP 1998: Halibut-liver Oil Capsules.

Proprietary Preparations (details are given in Part 3)
Ger.: Viton†; ***Switz.:*** Halibut.

Multi-ingredient: ***Aust.:*** Vitawund; ***Fr.:*** Eryteal; Preparation H; ***Ger.:*** Vita-Merfen N†; ***Switz.:*** A Vogel Capsules polyvitaminees; Perles d'huile de foie de morue du Dr Geistlich.

Histidine (591-q)

Histidine *(USAN, rINN).*

H; His; L-Histidine; Histidinum. L-2-Amino-3-(1*H*-imidazol-4-yl)propionic acid.

$C_6H_9N_3O_2$ = 155.2.

CAS — 71-00-1 (L-histidine); 645-35-2 (anhydrous L-histidine hydrochloride).

Pharmacopoeias. In *Eur.* (see p.viii) and *US.*

Eur. also includes Histidine Hydrochloride Monohydrate.

Colourless or white odourless crystals or crystalline powder. **Soluble** in water; very slightly soluble in alcohol; practically insoluble in ether. A 2% solution in water has a pH of 7.0 to 8.5. **Protect** from light.

Histidine Hydrochloride Monohydrate (Ph. Eur.) is a white crystalline powder or colourless crystals. Freely **soluble** in water; slightly soluble in alcohol; practically insoluble in ether. A 5% solution has a pH of 3 to 5. **Protect** from light.

Histidine is a heterocyclic amino acid which is essential for infant growth and which may be essential for some other groups, such as patients with uraemia. Histidine and histidine hydrochloride are used as dietary supplements.

Histidine, like glycine, is sometimes used in conjunction with antacids in the treatment of gastric hyperacidity.

Preparations

Proprietary Preparations (details are given in Part 3)
Ger.: Histinorm†; Histiplus†.

Purified Honey (592-p)

Clarified Honey; Gereinigter Honig; Mel Depuratum; Mel Despumatum; Miel Blanc; Strained Honey.

Pharmacopoeias. In *Chin., Fr., Ger.,* and *Jpn.*

Purified honey is obtained by purification of the honey from the comb of the bee, *Apis mellifera* and other species of *Apis* (Apidae).

Honey, which contains about 70 to 80% of glucose and fructose, is used as a demulcent and sweetening agent, especially in linctuses and cough mixtures (p.1052).

Honey has been identified as a source of *Clostridium botulinum* spores and thus recommendations have been made that honey should not be given to infants because of the risk of causing infant botulism.[1]

1. Arnon SS, *et al.* Honey and other environmental risk factors for infant botulism. *J Pediatr* 1979; **94:** 331–6.

Anecdotal reports and traditional usage dating back to Ancient Egypt suggest that honey may be of some value as a wound dressing. Its antibacterial properties are attributed both to high osmolality and the liberation of hydrogen peroxide, but may vary with the source:[1,2] in Europe, some of the best activity has been seen with lime-flower honey.[2] A group from India[3] has reported that these properties offer a potentially simple and cheap means of preserving skin grafts in developing countries, with 100% uptake of reconstituted grafts stored for up to 6 weeks and 80% uptake of those stored for 7 to 12 weeks. However, concern has been expressed since honey may contain not only chemical contaminants but clostridial spores (see also above), and it has been suggested[2] that to be medically acceptable honey must be sterile, residue-free, and of measured antibacterial activity.

Sugar (p.1357) has been used similarly to honey in treating wounds. The management of wounds and ulcers is described on p.1076.

1. Greenwood D. Honey for superficial wounds and ulcers. *Lancet* 1993; **341:** 90–1.
2. Postmes T, *et al.* Honey for wounds, ulcers, and skin graft preservation. *Lancet* 1993; **341:** 756–7.
3. Subrahmanyam M. Storage of skin grafts in honey. *Lancet* 1993; **341:** 63–4.

Preparations

Proprietary Preparations (details are given in Part 3)
Ger.: M2 Woelm†; ***Ital.:*** Oramil.

Multi-ingredient: ***Aust.:*** Thierry; ***Canad.:*** Herbal Cough Expectorant; Mielocol; ***Ger.:*** Adebilan†; Kneipp Brustkaramellen†; Melrosum Codein Hustensirup; ***Ital.:*** Apiserum con Telergon 1; Bebimix; Bioton; Biovigor; Biovigor Polline†; Camegel; Cocktail Reale; Fon Wan Eleuthero; Fon Wan Ginsenergy; Fon Wan Pocket Energy; Fon Wan Pollen; Liozim; Miegel; Neo Trefogel†; Nerex; Nutrigel; Vitalmix; ***Neth.:*** Melrosum; ***Switz.:*** Neo-Angin au miel et citron; ***UK:*** Buttercup Syrup (Honey and Lemon flavour); Fisherman's Friend Honey Cough Syrup†; Herb and Honey Cough Elixir; Honey & Molasses; Jackson's Children's Cough Pastilles; Lemsip Dry Tickly Cough; Lemsip Linctus†; M & M; Meltus Honey & Lemon; Regina Royal Five; Sanderson's Throat Specific; Throaties Catarrh Pastilles; Throaties Family Cough Linctus; Venos Honey & Lemon.

Iron (5031-z)

Ferrum.

Fe = 55.845.

CAS — 7439-89-6.

Pharmacopoeias. Aust. and It. include a monograph for reduced iron.

Practically **insoluble** in water and alcohol; almost completely soluble in dilute mineral acids.

Adverse Effects

The astringent action of iron preparations sometimes produces gastro-intestinal irritation and abdominal pain with nausea and vomiting when administered orally. These irritant side-effects are usually related to the amount of elemental iron taken rather than the type of preparation. Other gastro-intestinal effects may include either diarrhoea or constipation. Side-effects may be reduced by administration with or after food (rather than on an empty stomach) or by beginning therapy with a small dose and increasing gradually. Modified-release products are claimed to produce fewer side-effects but this may only reflect the lower availability of iron from these preparations. Oral liquid preparations containing iron salts may blacken the teeth and should be drunk through a straw. The faeces of patients taking iron salts may be coloured black.

The adverse effects associated with iron given parenterally are described under iron dextran (see p.1348).

Since absorbed iron is conserved by the body, iron overload, with increased storage of iron in various tissues (haemosiderosis), may occur as a result of excessive oral or, in particular, parenteral therapy. Patients mistakenly given iron therapy when not suffering from iron-deficiency anaemia are also at risk as are those with pre-existing iron storage or absorption diseases.

Acute iron overdosage can be divided into four stages. In the first phase, which occurs up to 6 hours after oral ingestion, gastro-intestinal toxicity, notably vomiting and diarrhoea, predominates. Other effects may include cardiovascular disorders such as hypotension and tachycardia, metabolic changes including acidosis and hyperglycaemia, and CNS depression ranging from lethargy to coma. Patients with only mild to moderate poisoning do not generally progress past this first phase. The second phase may occur at 6 to 24 hours after ingestion and is characterised by a temporary remission or clinical stabilisation. In the third phase gastro-intestinal toxicity recurs together with shock, metabolic acidosis, convulsions, coma, hepatic necrosis and jaundice, hypoglycaemia, coagulation disorders, oliguria or renal failure, and pulmonary oedema. The fourth phase may occur several weeks after ingestion and is characterised by gastro-intestinal obstruction and possibly late hepatic damage.

Relatively small amounts of iron may produce symptoms of toxicity. It has been stated that more than the equivalent of 30 mg of iron per kg body-weight could lead to some symptoms of toxicity and that in a young child the equivalent of about 75 mg of iron per kg should be regarded as extremely dangerous. Estimates of acute lethal dosages have ranged from the equivalent of 180 mg of iron per kg upwards. Serum-iron concentrations have also been employed as an indication of the severity of overdosage: a peak concentration of 5 μg or more per mL is reportedly associated with moderate to severe poisoning in many patients.

Effects on the cardiovascular system. For a suggestion that iron overload may contribute to ischaemic heart disease, see under Precautions, below.

Effects on growth. Iron supplementation in iron-replete children has been reported to adversely affect their growth—see below, under Precautions.

Iron overload. Because the body lacks a mechanism for the excretion of excess iron, abnormally high absorption or repeated blood transfusion will result in iron overload, leading eventually to haemochromatosis. The consequences of haemochromatosis include pigment deposition in skin and other organs, mild liver dysfunction, endocrine dysfunction (failure of the adolescent growth spurt, hypogonadism, sometimes diabetes and hypothyroidism), and heart disease (pericarditis, heart failure, and arrhythmias). If unchecked, the iron build-up can lead to death, mainly through heart failure or arrhythmia. Where the increased iron intake cannot be avoided (as in patients receiving regular transfusions for β-thalassaemia—see p.704) treatment with the iron chelating agent desferrioxamine is used to retard accumulation.

Treatment of Adverse Effects

In treating acute iron poisoning, speed is essential to reduce absorption of iron from the alimentary tract. Emesis or lavage should be considered and serum-iron concentrations may be an aid to estimating the severity of poisoning. Chelation therapy with desferrioxamine may be necessary and the procedure described under desferrioxamine mesylate (see p.976) should be followed.

Other measures include the symptomatic management and therapy of metabolic and cardiovascular disorders.

General references.

1. Proudfoot AT, *et al.* Management of acute iron poisoning. *Med Toxicol* 1986; **1:** 83–100.
2. Mann KV, *et al.* Management of acute iron overdose. *Clin Pharm* 1989; **8:** 428–40.

Overdosage. References highlighting the specific problem of iron overdose in children.[1,2] Child-resistant packaging and warning labels may be helpful in reducing the problem.

1. Anonymous. Iron-containing drugs and supplements: accidental poisoning. *WHO Drug Inf* 1995; **9:** 159–60.
2. Fitzpatrick R, Murray V. Iron toxicity: dietary supplements. *Pharm J* 1996; **256:** 666.

Pregnancy. Limited data on the treatment of iron overdose in pregnancy from the UK National Teratology Information Service, suggested that treatment with desferrioxamine should not be withheld if clinically indicated.[1-3] Most pregnancies had a normal outcome.

1. McElhatton PR, *et al.* The consequences of iron overdose and its treatment with desferrioxamine in pregnancy. *Hum Exp Toxicol* 1991; **10:** 251–9.
2. McElhatton PR, *et al.* Outcome of pregnancy following deliberate iron overdose by the mother. *Hum Exp Toxicol* 1993; **12:** 579.
3. McElhatton PR, *et al.* The outcome of pregnancy following iron overdose by the mother. *Br J Clin Pharmacol* 1998; **45:** 212P–213P.

Precautions

Iron compounds should not be given to patients receiving repeated blood transfusions or to patients with anaemias not produced by iron deficiency unless iron deficiency is also present. Oral iron therapy should not be administered concomitantly with parenteral iron. Care should be taken in patients with iron-storage or iron-absorption diseases such as haemochromatosis, haemoglobinopathies, or existing gastro-intestinal diseases such as inflammatory bowel disease, intestinal strictures and diverticulae.

Liquid preparations containing iron salts should be well diluted with water and swallowed through a straw to prevent discoloration of the teeth.

There has been concern, for a number of reasons, about the potential consequences of iron supplementation in individuals and groups who are not actually iron-deficient. Apart from the suggestion that certain populations may be at somewhat increased risk of microbial infection following supplementation (see Infections, below), there is some evidence that supplementation in non-iron-deficient children may retard their growth.[1] It has also been proposed that iron may be associated with ischaemic heart disease, by modifying low density lipoprotein in ways which increase its atherogenic potential and by sensitising the myocardium to ischaemic injury.[2,3] Although the role of iron in the pathogenesis of coronary heart disease is at present undecided, the use of iron should, it has been suggested, be restricted to patients with proven iron deficiency or to pregnancy.[2]

1. Idjradinata P, *et al.* Adverse effect of iron supplementation on weight gain of iron-replete young children. *Lancet* 1994; **343:** 1252–4.
2. Burt MJ, *et al.* Iron and coronary heart disease. *Br Med J* 1993; **307:** 575–6.
3. Sullivan JL. Iron and coronary heart disease: iron makes myocardium vulnerable to ischaemia. *Br Med J* 1993; **307:** 1066–7.

Infections. Iron is not only an essential element for humans but is also essential for many micro-organisms. Thus, it has been suggested that persons with either adequate iron stores or iron overload may provide optimum conditions for microbial growth and therefore be susceptible to an increased incidence and severity of infection; conversely, iron-deficiency anaemia may offer some protection against infections. The topic has been reviewed[1] and although there is no evidence that small amounts of iron supplements or iron-fortified food in normal people will render them more prone to infection[2] there is some evidence that in populations with a high prevalence of endemic infectious disease such as malaria, iron therapy may be followed by a higher incidence of infectious complications or by a flare-up of existing low-grade disease. Therefore, the routine use of iron supplements in such communities has been questioned;[3,4] however, an increasing number of studies have failed to demonstrate a detrimental effect.[5-8]

1. Hershko C, *et al.* Iron and infection. *Br Med J* 1988; **296:** 660–4.
2. Bullen JJ, Ward CG. Iron and infection. *Br Med J* 1988; **296:** 1539.
3. Oppenheimer SJ, *et al.* Iron supplementation increases prevalence and effects of malaria: report on clinical studies in Papua New Guinea. *Trans R Soc Trop Med Hyg* 1986; **80:** 603–12.
4. Smith AW, *et al.* The effects on malaria of treatment of iron-deficiency anaemia with oral iron in Gambian children. *Ann Trop Paediatr* 1989; **9:** 17–23.
5. Harvey PWJ, *et al.* The effect of iron therapy on malarial infection in Papua New Guinean schoolchildren. *Am J Trop Med Hyg* 1989; **40:** 12–18.
6. Boele van Hensbroek M, *et al.* Iron, but not folic acid, combined with effective antimalarial therapy promotes haematological recovery in African children after acute falciparum malaria. *Trans R Soc Trop Med Hyg* 1995; **89:** 672–6.
7. van den Hombergh J, *et al.* Does iron therapy benefit children with severe malaria-associated anaemia? A clinical trial with 12 weeks supplementation of oral iron in young children from the Turiani Division, Tanzania. *J Trop Pediatr* 1996; **42:** 220–7.
8. Menendez C, *et al.* Randomised placebo-controlled trial of iron supplementation and malaria chemoprophylaxis for prevention of severe anaemia and malaria in Tanzanian infants. *Lancet* 1997; **350:** 844–50.

Interference with diagnostic tests. Although studies *in vitro* have demonstrated that iron (ferrous sulphate) will cause a false-positive result in the Hemoccult test for blood in faeces, this does not occur *in vivo* in persons receiving oral iron therapy.[1,2] An explanation for the difference in these findings is that hydrogen peroxide in the Hemoccult developer converts ferrous ions in solution to ferric ions, which cause oxidation in the test, whereas *in vivo* the iron is probably eliminated in the faeces in the form of non-reactive insoluble iron precipitates.[2]

1. Kulbaski MJ, *et al.* Oral iron and the Hemoccult test: a controversy on the teaching wards. *N Engl J Med* 1989; **320:** 1500.
2. McDonnell M, Elta G. More on oral iron and the Hemoccult test. *N Engl J Med* 1989; **321:** 1684.

Porphyria. Erythropoietic protoporphyria was exacerbated by oral iron therapy in four patients;[1] a further patient had a variable reaction to iron, being able to tolerate it on some occasions but suffering from exacerbation of porphyria on others.[2]

1. Milligan A, *et al.* Erythropoietic protoporphyria exacerbated by oral iron therapy. *Br J Dermatol* 1988; **119:** 63–6.
2. McClements BM, *et al.* Erythropoietic protoporphyria and iron therapy. *Br J Dermatol* 1990; **122:** 423–6.

Interactions

Iron salts are not well absorbed by mouth, and administration with food may further impair their absorption.

Compounds containing calcium and magnesium, including antacids and mineral supplements, and bicarbonates, carbonates, oxalates, or phosphates, may also impair the absorption of iron by the formation of insoluble complexes. Similarly the absorption of both iron salts and tetracyclines is diminished when they are taken concomitantly by mouth. If treatment with both drugs is required, a time interval of about 2 to 3 hours should be allowed between them. A suitable interval is also advised if an iron supplement is required in patients receiving trientine. Zinc salts may decrease the absorption of iron.

Some agents, such as ascorbic acid and citric acid, may actually increase the absorption of iron.

The response to iron may be delayed in patients receiving concomitant parenteral chloramphenicol therapy.

Iron salts can also decrease the absorption of other drugs and thus reduce their bioavailability and clinical effect. Drugs so affected included bisphosphonates, fluoroquinolones, levodopa, methyldopa, penicillamine, and tetracycline. Iron salts may reduce the efficacy of thyroxine (p.1498).

Interactions with parenteral iron are mentioned under Iron Dextran, p.1348.

Reviews.

1. Campbell NRC, Hasinoff BB. Iron supplements: a common cause of drug interactions. *Br J Clin Pharmacol* 1991; **31:** 251–5.

Pharmacokinetics

Iron is irregularly and incompletely absorbed from the gastro-intestinal tract, the main sites of absorption being the duodenum and jejunum. Absorption is aided by the acid secretion of the stomach and by some dietary acids (such as ascorbic acid) and is more readily affected when the iron is in the ferrous state or is part of the haem complex (haem-iron). Absorption is also increased in conditions of iron deficiency or in the fasting state but is decreased if the body stores are overloaded. Only about 5 to 15% of the iron ingested in food is normally absorbed.

Following absorption the majority of iron is bound to transferrin and transported to the bone marrow where it is incorporated into haemoglobin; the remainder is contained within the storage forms, ferritin or haemosiderin, or as myoglobin, with smaller amounts occurring in haem-containing enzymes or in plasma bound to transferrin.

Only very small amounts of iron are excreted as the majority released after the destruction of the haemoglobin molecule is re-used. This conservation of body iron, and lack of an excretory mechanism for excess iron, is the reason for the development of iron overload with excessive iron therapy or repeated transfusions.

General references.

1. Harju E. Clinical pharmacokinetics of iron preparations. *Clin Pharmacokinet* 1989; **17:** 69–89.

Human Requirements

The body contains about 4 g of iron most of which is present as haemoglobin.

Apart from haemorrhage, iron is mainly lost from the body in the faeces, urine, from skin, and sweat, but the total loss is very small. Iron is also lost in small amounts in breast milk and in menstrual blood. In healthy men and postmenopausal women the loss is replaced by the absorption of about 1 mg of iron daily; about 1.5 to 2 mg needs to be absorbed daily by premenopausal women. In childhood and adolescence, the need is proportionately greater because of growth. Iron absorption is variable but is usually between 5 and 15% and therefore a dietary allowance containing the equivalent of about 10 mg of iron daily is usually sufficient for men and postmenopausal women; up to 15 mg daily may be necessary for premenopausal women with normal menstrual blood losses; some authorities recommend higher amounts or supplements during pregnancy. For further details concerning dietary requirements, see below and for a discussion of prophylactic iron given during pregnancy, see Iron-deficiency Anaemia, under Uses and Administration, below.

Good dietary sources of haem-iron are animal products such as meat and fish; non-haem-iron is also found in animal products and in vegetable products such as legumes and some leafy vegetables, but some vegetable products with a high iron content also contain phosphates or phytates which inhibit absorption by the formation of unabsorbable complexes.

In the United Kingdom, dietary reference values (DRV)[1] and in the United States, recommended dietary allowances (RDA)[2] have been published for iron.

In the UK the estimated average requirement (EAR) for adult males and postmenopausal females is 6.7 mg daily and the reference nutrient intake (RNI) is 8.7 mg daily; for premenopausal females, but without heavy menstrual blood losses, the EAR and RNI are 11.4 and 14.8 mg daily respectively. Amounts for infants, children, and adolescents, which are proportionately higher than those for adults, are also given. No increase is considered necessary during pregnancy or lactation.[1]

In the USA the RDA for adult males and postmenopausal females is 10 mg daily and that for premenopausal women is 15 mg. Amounts for infants, children, and adolescents, again proportionately higher than for adults, are also provided. No increase is considered necessary during lactation although an increase to 30 mg during pregnancy is considered warranted.[2]

The Food and Agriculture Organization of the United Nations together with the World Health Organization has also published guidelines concerning iron requirements and these take into account many factors including bioavailability of iron in the diet.[3]

For an explanation of the definitions, DRV, EAR, RNI, and RDA, see under Vitamins, p.1332.

1. DoH. Dietary reference values for food energy and nutrients for the United Kingdom: report of the panel on dietary reference values of the committee on medical aspects of food policy. *Report on health and social subjects 41*. London: HMSO, 1991.
2. Subcommittee on the tenth edition of the RDAs, Food and Nutrition Board, Commission on Life Sciences, National Research Council. *Recommended dietary allowances*. 10th ed. Washington, DC: National Academy Press, 1989.
3. FAO/WHO. *Requirements of vitamin A, iron, folate and vitamin B_{12}: report of a joint FAO/WHO expert consultation*. Rome: Food and Agriculture Organization of the United Nations, 1988.

Uses and Administration

Iron is an essential constituent of the body, being necessary for haemoglobin formation and for the oxidative processes of living tissues. Iron deficiency results in defective erythropoiesis and anaemia. Iron and iron salts should only be given for the treatment or prophylaxis of iron-deficiency anaemias (see below). They should not be given for the treatment of other types of anaemia except where iron deficiency is also present. Iron-deficiency anaemias respond readily to iron therapy but the underlying cause of the anaemia should be determined and treated.

The preferred route for the administration of iron is by mouth, usually as soluble ferrous salts, which are better absorbed than ferric salts. The usual adult dose for the treatment of iron-deficiency anaemia is 100 to 200 mg of iron daily in divided doses. The usual adult prophylactic dose is 60 to 120 mg of iron daily. There are various recommendations for children's doses and up to 2 mg of iron per kg bodyweight three times daily for treatment and 1 mg per kg daily for prophylaxis of iron-deficiency anaemia has been employed. Therapy is generally continued until haemoglobin concentrations reach normal values, which may take some weeks, and then for a further 3 months or more to restore body-iron stores.

Further information concerning the dosage of iron salts and compounds used is provided in the individual monographs; this information, however, tends to reflect the amounts of iron contained in different salts or available commercial preparations and therefore, in some instances, may not be within the general range of iron dosages as quoted above.

The iron content of various iron salts is tabulated in Table 1, below.

Table 1. Approximate amounts of different iron salts that supply 60mg of elemental iron.

Iron salt	Amount
Ferrous ascorbate (anhydrous)	437 mg
Ferrous aspartate (tetrahydrate)	422 mg
Ferrous carbonate (anhydrous)	125 mg
Ferrous chloride (tetrahydrate)	214 mg
Ferrous fumarate (anhydrous)	183 mg
Ferrous gluceptate (anhydrous)	544 mg
Ferrous gluconate (dihydrate)	518 mg
Ferrous lactate (trihydrate)	310 mg
Ferrous oxalate (dihydrate)	193 mg
Ferrous succinate (anhydrous)	185 mg
Ferrous sulphate (dried)	186 mg
Ferrous sulphate (heptahydrate)	300 mg
Ferrous tartrate (hemipentahydrate)	268 mg

Some oral preparations of iron are presented in modified-release dosage forms and these preparations are claimed to result in reduced gastro-intestinal side-effects and have the advantage of once-daily dosing. The preparations are designed to release the iron gradually along the gut but in some instances the iron may not have been released until the preparation reaches a part of the gut where absorption is poor thus resulting in sub-optimal dosing.

Iron can also be given parenterally in circumstances where oral therapy cannot be undertaken and such use is typified by iron dextran (see p.1348).

Anoxic seizures. Recent findings[1] of a reduction in the frequency of breath-holding episodes in children treated with iron suggest that there might be a relationship between anoxic seizures (p.456) and iron deficiency.[2]

1. Daoud AS, *et al.* Effectiveness of iron therapy on breath-holding spells. *J Pediatr* 1997; **130:** 547–50.
2. Hannon DW. Breath-holding spells: waiting to inhale, waiting for systole, or waiting for iron therapy? *J Pediatr* 1997; **130:** 510–12.

Iron-deficiency anaemia. Iron deficiency eventually results in anaemia (p.702), usually of a microcytic, hypochromic type, and because iron requirements are increased during infancy, puberty, pregnancy, and menstruation, such anaemias are most common in women and children.[1] Although any underlying cause for the iron deficiency should be sought and treated, most iron-deficiency anaemias respond well to treatment with oral iron.[2] The usual dose is sufficient of a ferrous salt to supply about 100 to 200 mg of elemental iron daily, with the aim of increasing haemoglobin concentrations by 0.1 to 0.2 g per 100 mL per day or 2 g per 100 mL over 3 to 4 weeks.[2] Treatment is continued for about 3 months once haemoglobin concentrations have returned to the normal range, in order to aid replenishment of iron stores. Parenteral iron therapy is rarely indicated. Prophylactic administration may be justifiable in certain groups, such as in pregnancy and in pre-school children, but there is some debate as to its value, and its use in the former has declined.[3-7] (For the possible problems associated with iron supplementation in those who are not deficient, see under Precautions, above.) Usual prophylactic doses provide about 60 to 120 mg of elemental iron daily. Intermittent iron supplementation is under study.[8]

1. De Maayer EM, *et al. Preventing and controlling iron deficiency anaemia through primary health care: a guide for health administrators and programme managers*. Geneva: WHO, 1989.
2. Smith AG. Prescribing iron. *Prescribers' J* 1997; **37:** 82–7.
3. Hibbard BM. Iron and folate supplements during pregnancy: supplementation is valuable only in selected patients. *Br Med J* 1988; **297:** 1324 and 1326.
4. Horn E. Iron and folate supplements during pregnancy: supplementing everyone treats those at risk and is cost effective. *Br Med J* 1988; **297:** 1325 and 1327.
5. US Preventive Services Task Force. Routine iron supplementation during pregnancy: policy statement. *JAMA* 1993; **270:** 2846–8.
6. US Preventive Services Task Force. Routine iron supplementation during pregnancy: review article. *JAMA* 1993; **270:** 2848–54.

7. Anonymous. Routine iron supplements in pregnancy are unnecessary. *Drug Ther Bull* 1994; **32:** 30–1.
8. Cook JD. Iron supplementation: is less better? *Lancet* 1995; **346:** 587.

Iron Dextran (5066-m)

Iron-Dextran Complex.

CAS — 9004-66-4.

Pharmacopoeias. Br., Chin., and *US* include Iron Dextran Injection.

A complex of ferric hydroxide with dextrans. The BP injection specifies dextrans of weight average molecular weight between 5000 and 7500, and the USP injection specifies partially hydrolysed dextran of low molecular weight.

Adverse Effects and Treatment

Severe anaphylactoid reactions may occur after administration of iron dextran and fatalities have been reported. It is therefore recommended that administration takes place where there are facilities for the emergency treatment of such reactions, that certain precautions be observed, and that test doses be employed (see Precautions, below).

Intravenous administration may be associated with peripheral vascular flushing, tachycardia, and hypotension and syncope; thrombophlebitis may also occur at the site of injection, although the incidence may be reduced by administering iron dextran in sodium chloride 0.9% rather than glucose 5%. Intramuscular injection is associated with local reactions, pain, and staining at the site of injection; leakage along the injection track may occur unless the proper administration technique is employed (see under Uses and Administration, below). Other immediate reactions with either route include nausea, vomiting, and taste disturbance.

Patients may also experience delayed reactions 1 to 2 days after administration of iron dextran, such as arthralgia, myalgia, regional lymphadenopathy, chills, fever, paraesthesia, dizziness, malaise, headache, nausea, vomiting, and haematuria.

Overdose of parenteral iron is unlikely to be associated with any acute manifestations. Unwarranted parenteral iron therapy will result in iron overload and excess storage of iron (haemochromatosis) in the long term. The consequences of this include liver and endocrine dysfunction and heart disease (see Iron Overload, p.1346), and possibly an increased risk of infection (see Infections, under Precautions for Iron, p.1346). Iron overload may require chelation therapy with desferrioxamine (p.976).

Intramuscular injection of iron complexes such as iron dextran has resulted in sarcomas at the injection site in *animals*. There is some evidence that this may occur in humans.

Effects on the blood. A 1-year-old girl with Down's syndrome and iron-deficiency anaemia was given three intramuscular injections of iron dextran over 6 days (to a total of 30 mg per kg body-weight). Pancytopenia developed subsequently, which reappeared when challenged with iron dextran. Tests indicated an allergic pathogenesis for the pancytopenia.[1]

For further discussion of hypersensitivity reactions to iron dextran, see under Hypersensitivity, below.

1. Hurvitz H, *et al.* Pancytopenia caused by iron-dextran. *Arch Dis Child* 1986; **61:** 194–6.

Hypersensitivity. The Boston Collaborative Drug Surveillance Program monitored consecutively 32 812 medical inpatients. Drug-induced anaphylaxis occurred in 1 of 169 patients given iron dextran; the route of administration was not stated in this report.[1]

Hamstra and colleagues investigated 481 persons who received a total of 2099 intravenous injections of iron dextran and found 3 life-threatening immediate anaphylactoid reactions; 8 severe delayed reactions were also observed as were many other reactions of a less serious nature.[2] In a more recent series,[3] 10 of 573 patients experienced anaphylactoid reactions after intravenous administration of iron dextran. Other serious reactions included 1 case of cardiac arrest, and 3 cases of dyspnoea, hypertension, or chest pain.

There has been a report of a lupus-like disorder associated with administration of iron dextran;[4] the illness resolved with appropriate treatment but recurred on rechallenge.

For discussion of pancytopenia believed to have an underlying allergic pathogenesis, see under Effects on the Blood, above.

1. Porter J, Jick H. Drug-induced anaphylaxis, convulsions, deafness, and extrapyramidal symptoms. *Lancet* 1977; **i:** 587–8.
2. Hamstra RD, *et al.* Intravenous iron dextran in clinical medicine. *JAMA* 1980; **243:** 1726–31.
3. Fishbane S, *et al.* The safety of intravenous iron dextran in hemodialysis patients. *Am J Kidney Dis* 1996; **28:** 529–34.
4. Oh VMS. Iron dextran and systemic lupus erythematosus. *Br Med J* 1992; **305:** 1000.

Overdosage. A 29-year-old woman was given 32 mL iron dextran (Imferon) intravenously. Twenty-four hours later she developed muscle cramps, bilateral frontal headaches, with subsequent neck stiffness, and marked opisthotonia with photophobia.[1] The haemoglobin concentration did not rise following the infusion of iron which indicated there had been no iron deficiency. Thus, abnormally high concentrations of free iron had followed the iron therapy and this free iron was able to cross into the cerebrospinal fluid and was responsible for the meningitic symptoms.

1. Shuttleworth D, *et al.* Meningism due to intravenous iron dextran. *Lancet* 1983; **ii:** 453.

Precautions

Iron dextran is contra-indicated in patients with severe liver damage or acute kidney infection. It is also contra-indicated in persons with a history of hypersensitivity to the preparation. Teratogenicity has been demonstrated in non-anaemic *animals* given the equivalent of about three times the maximum human dose and its use should be avoided in pregnancy if possible.

Additionally, iron dextran should be employed with caution in patients with a history of allergic disorders or asthma and in these patients the intramuscular, and not the intravenous, route should be employed. Patients with rheumatoid arthritis may experience a worsening of symptoms when given iron dextran intravenously. Patients with other inflammatory disorders such as lupus erythematosus may be at increased risk of delayed reactions. Large doses of iron dextran by infusion may lead to serum discoloration; this should not be mistaken as evidence of haemolysis. Oral iron salts should be discontinued before administration of parenteral iron.

A test dose should be given before administration of a full therapeutic dose (see Uses and Administration, below) and emergency measures for the treatment of allergic reactions should be available (see Anaphylactic Shock, p.816). Patients should be kept under observation for at least 1 hour after administration of a test dose or following intravenous administration.

Iron dextran formulated with phenol as a preservative is intended for administration by the intramuscular route only.

Interactions

There is some evidence that enalapril may potentiate the adverse systemic reactions seen with intravenous iron therapy.[1]

Parenterally administered chloramphenicol may delay the response to iron therapy in anaemia.

1. Rolla G, *et al.* Systemic reactions to intravenous iron therapy in patients receiving angiotensin-converting enzyme inhibitor. *J Allergy Clin Immunol* 1994; **93:** 1074–5.

Pharmacokinetics

After intramuscular injection iron dextran is absorbed primarily through the lymphatic system: about 60% is absorbed after 3 days and up to 90% after 1 to 3 weeks. The reticuloendothelial cells gradually separate iron from the iron-dextran complex; the distribution and elimination of iron is described on p.1347. Absorption of drug inadvertently deposited in subcutaneous tissue may take months or even years.

References.

1. Spruill WJ. Timing iron dextran doses when plasmapheresis is required. *Clin Pharm* 1990; **9:** 419–20.

Uses and Administration

Iron dextran should be used only in the treatment of proven iron-deficiency anaemia (p.702) where oral therapy, as described on p.1347, is ineffective or impracticable.

It is given by deep intramuscular injection into the upper outer quadrant of the buttock; to prevent leakage along the injection track, the subcutaneous tissue is drawn to one side before the needle is inserted. It may also be given intravenously at a rate not exceeding the equivalent of 50 mg iron (1 mL) per minute.

Prior to commencing therapy, all patients should receive a test dose of 0.5 mL administered via the intended route, and should be observed for adverse reactions (see Precautions, above).

For iron-deficiency anaemia, total dosage is calculated according to the haemoglobin concentration and body-weight of the patient; allowance is also made for additional iron to replenish iron stores. Iron dextran injection is usually supplied with a table from which the recommended dose can be obtained for patients of different weights and haemoglobin (Hb) status. There may be variations between countries in the doses obtained from such tables. Doses can also be calculated from various formulae. Typical formulae used for a preparation containing the equivalent of 50 mg of iron per mL are as follows:

Dose in mL =

$$\{0.0476 \times \text{body-weight (kg)} \times [14.8 - \text{Hb level (g/100 mL)}]\}$$
$$+$$
$$\text{1 mL per 5 kg body-weight, to a maximum of 14 mL}$$

Dose in mL for children up to 15 kg =

$$\{0.0476 \times \text{body-weight (kg)} \times [12 - \text{Hb level (g/100 mL)}]\}$$
$$+$$
$$\text{1 mL per 5 kg body-weight.}$$

Using these formulae a 70-kg man with a haemoglobin value of 5.9 g per 100 mL would be given a total of 2.2 g of iron (44 mL of the iron dextran preparation). An alternative formula is:

$$\{0.0442 \times \text{body-weight (kg)} \times [\text{desired Hb level (g/100 mL)} - \text{measured Hb level}]\}$$
$$+$$
$$(0.26 \times \text{body-weight})$$

In adults, the calculated lean body-weight should normally be used in this formula rather than the actual body-weight. Note that doses obtained from tables or the above formulae are for iron-deficiency anaemia, and are not suitable for iron replacement for simple blood loss.

The total dose requirement may be administered as a series of intramuscular injections daily or once or twice weekly in inactive patients. A suggested dosage per intramuscular injection for children is: less than 5 kg body-weight, up to 0.5 mL (25 mg); 5 to 9 kg, up to 1 mL (50 mg). Adults and larger children normally receive 2 mL (100 mg).

Iron dextran is also administered intravenously either by total-dose infusion (TDI) or as an undiluted injection. In total-dose infusion, the total dose calculated according to the haemoglobin concentration (as outlined above) is given by slow intravenous infusion in about 500 mL of sodium chloride 0.9% or glucose 5%; sodium chloride may be preferable due to the reduced incidence of thrombophlebitis. The initial rate for the 0.5 mL test dose should not exceed 5 drops per minute but provided that this is well tolerated the rate of infusion may be increased progressively to 45 to 60 drops per minute.

For undiluted administration the total dose is also calculated according to the haemoglobin concentration. A test dose of 0.5 mL of the iron dextran preparation should be given by slow intravenous injection. If, after an observation period of about 1 hour, this test dose has been well tolerated, the therapeutic dose may be given either as a single dose, or divided and given as a series of injections. Patients given iron dextran intravenously should be observed closely for at least one hour after administration.

Anaemia of chronic renal failure. US guidelines for the treatment of anaemia of chronic renal failure[1] recommend the regular use of small intravenous doses of iron dextran to prevent iron deficiency and promote improved erythropoiesis; oral iron is usually insufficient to maintain adequate iron stores in these patients, particularly when also treated with erythropoietin.

1. National Kidney Foundation. NKF-DOQI clinical practice guidelines for the treatment of anemia of chronic renal failure. *Am J Kidney Dis* 1997; **30** (suppl 3): S192–S240.

Preparations

BP 1998: Iron Dextran Injection;
USP 23: Iron Dextran Injection.

Proprietary Preparations (details are given in Part 3)
Austral.: Imferon†; ***Belg.:*** Imferon†; ***Neth.:*** Imferon†; ***S.Afr.:*** Imferon†; ***Spain:*** Imferon; ***Switz.:*** Imferdex†; ***UK:*** Imferon†; ***USA:*** DexFerrum; INFeD.

Multi-ingredient: ***Spain:*** Imferon B12†.

Iron Polymaltose (12864-h)

Ferromaltose; Ferrum Polyisomaltose.

A complex of ferric hydroxide and isomaltose.

Iron polymaltose is used as a source of iron (p.1346) for iron-deficiency anaemia (p.702). It is given by mouth in doses containing the equivalent of up to 240 mg of iron daily. It is also given parenterally, the total dose being calculated and given by intravenous infusion or, preferably, as a series of intramuscular injections containing the equivalent of up to 200 mg of iron in a single day; injections are usually given only every few days. For further information relating to the parenteral use of iron, see Iron Dextran, p.1348.

Preparations

Proprietary Preparations (details are given in Part 3)
Aust.: Ferrum Hausmann; ***Austral.:*** Ferrum H; ***Belg.:*** Ferrum Hausmann; ***Fr.:*** Maltofer; ***Ger.:*** Ferrum Hausmann; ***Irl.:*** Ferrum; ***Ital.:*** Intrafer; ***S.Afr.:*** Ferrimed; Ferrimed DS; ***Switz.:*** Ferrum Hausmann; Maltofer.

Multi-ingredient: ***S.Afr.:*** Ferrimed; ***Switz.:*** Maltofer Fol.

Iron Sorbitol (5070-f)

Astra-1572; Iron Sorbitex *(USAN)*; Iron-Sorbitol-Citric Acid Complex.
CAS — 1338-16-5.

Pharmacopoeias. Br. and *US* include injections of iron sorbitol.

A complex of ferric iron, sorbitol, and citric acid, stabilised with dextrin and sorbitol.

Adverse Effects, Treatment, and Precautions

As for Iron Dextran, p.1348.

There may be severe systemic reactions with cardiac complications which may be fatal, such as complete atrioventricular block, ventricular tachycardia, or ventricular fibrillation. A transient metallic taste or loss of taste may occur.

The urine of patients treated with iron sorbitol may become dark on standing.

Iron sorbitol should not be administered intravenously.

A description of adverse events in three patients with the malabsorption syndrome treated with intramuscular injections of iron sorbitol.[1] Two patients died; in one, findings were consistent with anaphylaxis and in the other cardiac toxicity was considered to be due to a direct effect. In the third patient direct cardiac toxicity was also implicated.

1. Karhunen P, *et al.* Reaction to iron sorbitol injection in three cases of malabsorption. *Br Med J* 1970; **2:** 521–2.

Interactions

As for Iron Dextran, p.1348.

Pharmacokinetics

About 66% of iron sorbitol is absorbed within 3 hours of intramuscular injection, most of it directly into the blood circulation, and some via the lymphatic system. Almost all is absorbed within about 10 days. Clearance of iron sorbitol from the plasma is rapid, and is mainly via the reticuloendothelial system, as described for Iron Dextran, p.1348.

Uses and Administration

Iron sorbitol should be used only in the treatment of proven iron-deficiency anaemia (p.702) where oral therapy, as described on p.1347, is ineffective or impracticable.

It is given by deep intramuscular injection into the upper outer quadrant of the buttock; to prevent leakage along the injection track, the subcutaneous tissue is drawn to one side before the needle is inserted.

Total dosage is calculated according to body-weight and the haemoglobin concentration of the blood, and tables are usually provided with iron sorbitol injections for this purpose. The recommended single dose is the equivalent of 1.5 mg of iron per kg body-weight up to a maximum of 100 mg per injection; these doses are then given daily until the total dosage has been achieved. Iron sorbitol is not recommended in children under 3 kg in body-weight.

Iron sorbitol should not be administered intravenously.

Preparations

BP 1998: Iron Sorbitol Injection;
USP 23: Iron Sorbitex Injection.

Proprietary Preparations (details are given in Part 3)
Aust.: Jectofer; ***Canad.:*** Jectofer; ***Ger.:*** Jectofer; ***Irl.:*** Jectofer; ***Neth.:*** Jectofer; ***Norw.:*** Jectofer; ***Spain:*** Yectofer; ***Swed.:*** Jectofer; ***UK:*** Jectofer.

Multi-ingredient: ***Spain:*** Yectofer Compuesto†.

Iron Succinyl-Protein Complex (19370-y)

Iron Proteinsuccinylate; ITF-282.
CAS — 93615-44-2.

Iron succinyl-protein complex is a source of iron (p.1346) used for iron-deficiency anaemia (p.702). It is given by mouth in doses of up to 1.6 g daily (equivalent to up to 80 mg of iron daily).

References.

1. Köpeke W, Sauerland MC. Meta-analysis of efficacy and tolerability data on iron proteinsuccinylate in patients with iron deficiency anemia of different severity. *Arzneimittelforschung* 1995; **45:** 1211–16.

Preparations

Proprietary Preparations (details are given in Part 3)
Ital.: Ferlatum; Ferplex; Ferremon; Ferrofolin Simplex; Folinemic Ferro; Legofer; Pernexin; Proteoferrina; Rekord Ferro; ***Spain:*** Ferplex; Ferrocur; Lactoferrina.

Multi-ingredient: ***Ital.:*** Ferplex Fol†; Ferrofolin; Legofer Folinico†; Siderofolin†.

Isoleucine (593-s)

Isoleucine *(USAN, rINN)*.

I; Ile; L-Isoleucine; Isoleucinum. L-2-Amino-3-methylvaleric acid.

$C_6H_{13}NO_2$ = 131.2.
CAS — 73-32-5.

Pharmacopoeias. In *Eur.* (see p.viii), *Jpn*, and *US*.

White, or almost white, practically odourless crystalline powder or flakes. Ph. Eur. states sparingly **soluble** in water whereas the USP states soluble in water; slightly soluble in alcohol; practically insoluble in ether. It dissolves in dilute mineral acids and in dilute solutions of alkali hydroxides. A 1% solution in water has a pH of 5.5 to 7.0. **Protect** from light.

Isoleucine is a branched-chain amino acid which is an essential constituent of the diet. It is used as a dietary supplement. It is also an ingredient of several preparations that have been promoted for disorders of the liver.

Preparations

Proprietary Preparations (details are given in Part 3)

Multi-ingredient: ***Ger.:*** Bramin-hepa; Falkamin; Lactostrict†; ***Ital.:*** Falkamin; Isobranch; Isoram.

Isomalt (14038-q)

Isomalt *(BAN)*.

BAY-i-3930; E953; Isomaltitol.

An approximately equimolar mixture of 6-*O*-(α-D-glucopyranosyl)-D-glucitol ($C_{12}H_{24}O_{11}$ = 344.3) and 1-*O*-(α-D-glucopyranosyl)-D-mannitol dihydrate ($C_{12}H_{24}O_{11}$,$2H_2O$ = 380.3).

A white, odourless, crystalline, slightly hygroscopic solid with a sweet taste.

Isomalt is a sugar alcohol (polyol) used as a bulk sweetener in foods. The ingestion of large quantities may produce flatulence and have a laxative effect.

A WHO Expert Committee reported[1] that isomalt is partly metabolised in the small intestine to glucose, mannitol, and sorbitol and the remaining isomalt is completely metabolised by the flora of the large intestine. The Australian manufacturers have commented that the hydrolysis and absorption is minimal and does not significantly affect blood-sugar or insulin concentrations; they consider isomalt to be suitable for use by diabetic patients.[2]

1. FAO/WHO. Evaluation of certain food additives and contaminants: twenty-ninth report of the joint FAO/WHO expert committee on food additives. *WHO Tech Rep Ser 733* 1986.
2. Barnes JA. Martindale and isomalt. *Aust J Pharm* 1994; **75:** 183.

Lactose (594-w)

Lactosum; Lattosio; Milk Sugar; Saccharum Lactis. 4-*O*-β-D-Galactopyranosyl-(1→4)-α-D-glucopyranose monohydrate.

$C_{12}H_{22}O_{11}$,H_2O = 360.3.
CAS — 63-42-3 (anhydrous lactose); 5989-81-1 (lactose monohydrate); 10039-26-6 (lactose monohydrate, cyclic); 64044-51-5 (lactose monohydrate, open form).

Pharmacopoeias. In *Chin., Eur.* (see p.viii), *Int., Jpn*, and *Pol.* Also in *USNF.* Some pharmacopoeias include separate monographs for Anhydrous Lactose and Lactose Monohydrate.

A disaccharide obtained from the whey of milk. White or almost white odourless crystalline powder with a slightly sweet taste.

Lactose may exist in a number of distinct forms depending upon the crystallisation and drying processes employed. The forms can vary in the contents of crystalline and amorphous lactose, the amounts of α- and β-lactose, and in their hydration states. The α-form of lactose exists in either the anhydrous or monohydrate state whereas the β-form exists only in the anhydrous state. Lactose (Ph. Eur.) and Lactose Monohydrate (USNF) are the α-form. Anhydrous Lactose (Ph. Eur., USNF) specifies the β-form or a mixture of the α- and β-forms. Commercial lactose is mainly the α-monohydrate.

Slowly **soluble** 1 in 5 of water and soluble 1 in 2.6 of boiling water; practically insoluble in alcohol. **Store** in airtight containers.

A 9.75% solution in water is iso-osmotic with blood.

Adverse Effects and Precautions

Lactose intolerance occurs due to a deficiency of the intestinal enzyme lactase. Ingestion of lactose by patients with lactase deficiency leads to a clinical syndrome of abdominal pain, diarrhoea, distension, and flatulence; symptoms may also occur in persons without such a deficiency who have ingested excessive amounts of lactose.

Lactose is contra-indicated in patients with galactosaemia, the glucose-galactose malabsorption syndrome, or lactase deficiency.

Lactose intolerance. A review of lactose intolerance.[1] The capacity of the infant intestine to produce lactase, the enzyme responsible for digesting lactose, is retained into adulthood only by a minority of the world's population, mostly of north European descent; in Africa and Asia more than 90% of the population are lactase deficient. Because of the ubiquity of lactose in the diet and the consequent frequency of abdominal symptoms, attempts have been made to treat lactose intolerance by dietary exclusion (which need not be complete since lactase deficiency is rarely absolute). An alternative is enzyme replacement therapy with β-galactosidase from micro-organisms (see Tilactase, p.1637), but the role of such therapy has yet to be fully determined. The findings of one study[2] suggested that, in adults with lactose intolerance, the use of lactose-digestive aids is unnecessary if lactose intake is limited to the equivalent of 240 mL of milk or less a day.

For the use of soya in infants intolerant to cows' milk, see p.1356.

1. Anonymous. Lactose intolerance. *Lancet* 1991; **338:** 663–4.
2. Suarez FL, *et al.* A comparison of symptoms after the consumption of milk or lactose-hydrolysed milk by people with self-reported severe lactose intolerance. *N Engl J Med* 1995; **333:** 1–4.

Pharmacokinetics

Lactose is hydrolysed by lactase in the small intestine to glucose and galactose, which are then absorbed.

Uses and Administration

Lactose, the carbohydrate component of milk, is less sweet than sucrose.

Lactose is widely used in pharmaceutical manufacturing. In the production of capsules or tablets it may be employed as a diluent, bulking agent, filler, or excipient and in powders as a bulking agent. Lactose is also used as a carrier for drugs in dry powder inhalers. Characteristics such as particle size make different grades of lactose suitable for different applications.

Preparations

Proprietary Preparations (details are given in Part 3)
Aust.: Sorbifen Baby; ***Canad.:*** Novo-Plus; ***Ger.:*** Medilet.

Multi-ingredient: ***Aust.:*** Ichth-Oestren; Joghurt Milkitten; ***Ger.:*** Eugalan Topfer forte; Eugalan Topfer forte LC; ***Spain:*** Vacuosa Ultra Adsorb†; ***Switz.:*** Spuman a la camomille†; Spuman†.

Leucine (597-y)

Leucine *(USAN, rINN)*.

α-Aminoisocaproic Acid; L; Leu; L-Leucine; Leucinum. L-2-Amino-4-methylvaleric acid.

$C_6H_{13}NO_2$ = 131.2.

CAS — 61-90-5.

Pharmacopoeias. In *Eur.* (see p.viii), *Jpn*, and *US*.

Shiny flakes or a white or almost white, practically odourless crystalline powder. Sparingly **soluble** in water; practically insoluble in alcohol and in ether. It dissolves in dilute solutions of mineral acids and of alkali hydroxides. A 1% solution in water has a pH of 5.5 to 7.0. **Protect** from light.

Leucine is a branched-chain amino acid which is an essential constituent of the diet. It is used as a dietary supplement. It is also an ingredient of several preparations that have been promoted for disorders of the liver.

Preparations

Proprietary Preparations (details are given in Part 3)

Multi-ingredient: ***Fr.:*** Revitalose; ***Ger.:*** Bramin-hepa; Falkamin; Lactostrict†; ***Ital.:*** Falkamin; Isobranch; Isoram.

Lysine (12141-y)

Lysine *(USAN, rINN)*.

K; Lys; L-Lysine. L-2,6-Diaminohexanoic acid.

$C_6H_{14}N_2O_2$ = 146.2.

CAS — 56-87-1.

Pharmacopoeias. In *Ger.* as the monohydrate.

Lysine Acetate (669-y)

Lysine Acetate *(rINNM)*.

Lys Acetate; L-Lysine Monoacetate. L-2,6-Diaminohexanoic acid acetate.

$C_6H_{14}N_2O_2,C_2H_4O_2$ = 206.2.

CAS — 57282-49-2.

Pharmacopoeias. In *US*.

White odourless crystals or crystalline powder. Freely **soluble** in water.

Lysine Hydrochloride (599-z)

Lysine Hydrochloride *(USAN, rINNM)*.

Lys Hydrochloride; L-Lysine Monohydrochloride; Lysini Hydrochloridum. L-2,6-Diaminohexanoic acid hydrochloride.

$C_6H_{14}N_2O_2,HCl$ = 182.6.

CAS — 657-27-2.

Pharmacopoeias. In *Eur.* (see p.viii), *Jpn*, and *US*.

A white odourless crystalline powder or colourless crystals. Freely **soluble** in water; slightly soluble in alcohol; practically insoluble in ether. **Protect** from light.

Lysine is an aliphatic amino acid which is an essential constituent of the diet. Lysine and lysine hydrochloride are used as dietary supplements.

Hyperargininaemia. Lysine has been used with ornithine to manage symptoms in a patient with hyperargininaemia—see under Hyperammonaemia, p.1334.

Preparations

Proprietary Preparations (details are given in Part 3)

Switz.: Ambifon†; ***USA:*** Enisyl†.

Multi-ingredient: ***Austral.:*** Cold Sore Relief; Cold Sore Tablets; Incremin Iron; Vitaline; ***Canad.:*** Coba-12†; ***Fr.:*** Acti 5; Curasten; Revitalose; ***Ital.:*** Biocarnil; Calciofix; Cerebrix†; Combivit†; Gliviton†; Incremin; Oroticon Lisina†; ***Spain:*** Acticinco; Calcioretard; Euzymina Lisina; Malandil; ***UK:*** Amino MS; Labophylline†; ***USA:*** Klorvess.

Malt Extract (601-c)

Extractum Bynes.

It contains 50% or more of maltose, together with dextrin, glucose, and small amounts of other carbohydrates, and protein. It is prepared from malted grain of barley (*Hordeum distichon* or *H. vulgare*) or a mixture of this with not more than 33% of malted grain of wheat (*Triticum aestivum* or *T. turgidum*).

Malt extract has nutritive properties. It is chiefly used as a vehicle in preparations containing cod-liver oil (p.1337) and halibut-liver oil (p.1345). It is a useful flavouring agent for masking bitter tastes.

A product known as malt soup extract, obtained from barley grains, and containing 73% maltose together with 12% other polymeric carbohydrates as well as small amounts of proteins, electrolytes, and vitamins, is sometimes used as a laxative. For discussion of constipation and its management, see p.1168.

Preparations

Proprietary Preparations (details are given in Part 3)

USA: Maltsupex.

Multi-ingredient: ***Austral.:*** Waterbury's Compound†; ***Fr.:*** Elixir Contre La Toux Weleda; Galactogil; ***Ital.:*** Syllamalt†; ***Switz.:*** Optilax; ***USA:*** Syllamalt.

Maltitol (13690-b)

E965; Hydrogenated Maltose; D-Maltitol; Maltitolum. α-D-Glucopyranosyl-1,4-D-glucitol.

$C_{12}H_{24}O_{11}$ = 344.3.

CAS — 585-88-6.

Pharmacopoeias. In *Eur.* (see p.viii).

A white crystalline powder. Very **soluble** in water; practically insoluble in alcohol.

Maltitol Syrup (10169-s)

E965; Hydrogenated Glucose Syrup; Hydrogenated High Maltose-glucose Syrup; Liquid Maltitol; Maltitolum Liquidum.

Pharmacopoeias. In *Eur.* (see p.viii).

A clear, colourless, syrupy liquid. It is an aqueous solution of a hydrogenated, part hydrolysed starch, containing not less than 70% w/w of solid matter composed of a mixture of mainly maltitol with sorbitol and hydrogenated oligo- and polysaccharides. On the dried basis, it contains not less than 50% of maltitol and not more than 8% of sorbitol. **Miscible** with water and with glycerol.

Hydrogenated glucose syrup is a generic term encompassing products of widely varying composition and it was concluded that such products containing up to 90% of maltitol should more properly be called maltitol syrup.[1] This was subsequently amended to include products containing up to 98% maltitol.[2] Preparations containing a minimum of 98% of maltitol were designated the title maltitol.

1. FAO/WHO. Evaluation of certain food additives and contaminants: thirty-third report of the joint FAO/WHO expert committee on food additives. *WHO Tech Rep Ser 776* 1989.
2. FAO/WHO. Evaluation of certain food additives and contaminants: forty-first report of the joint FAO/WHO expert committee on food additives. *WHO Tech Rep Ser 837* 1993.

Maltitol and maltitol syrup are bulk sweeteners used in foods; they are considered to be less cariogenic than sucrose. The ingestion of large quantities may produce flatulence and diarrhoea.

Preparations

USNF 18: Maltitol Solution.

Maltodextrin (602-k)

Pharmacopoeias. In *Swiss.* Also in *USNF*.

A glucose polymer prepared by the partial hydrolysis of starch.

White hygroscopic powder or granules. Freely **soluble** or readily dispersible in water; slightly soluble to practically insoluble in dehydrated alcohol. A 20% solution has a pH of between 4 and 7. **Store** in airtight containers at a temperature not exceeding 30° and a relative humidity not exceeding 50%.

Maltodextrin, a malto-oligosaccharide, is a source of carbohydrate often used in oral dietary supplements and tube feeding. Glucose is rapidly released in the gastro-intestinal tract but because of the high average molecular weight of maltodextrin, solutions have a lower osmolarity than isocaloric solutions of glucose. Additionally, preparations based on maltodextrin and intended for dietary supplementation usually have a low electrolyte content and are free of other sugars such as fructose, galactose, lactose, and sucrose. These properties make such preparations suitable for dietary supplementation in a variety of diseases including certain gastro-intestinal disorders where malabsorption is a problem, in disaccharide intolerance (without isomaltose intolerance), and in acute and chronic hepatic and renal diseases where protein, mineral, and fluid restriction are often necessary.

Maltodextrin is also employed as a pharmaceutical excipient.

Preparations

Proprietary Preparations (details are given in Part 3)

Austral.: Maxijul; ***Canad.:*** Moducal†; ***Irl.:*** Fibrosine; ***Ital.:*** Fantomalt; Maltovis.

Multi-ingredient: ***Fr.:*** Gumilk; ***Ital.:*** Doldieta.

Maltose (603-a)

4-*O*-α-D-Glucopyranosyl-β-D-glucopyranose.

$C_{12}H_{22}O_{11}$ = 342.3.

CAS — 69-79-4 (anhydrous maltose); 6363-53-7 (maltose monohydrate).

Pharmacopoeias. In *Jpn*.

It is obtained from starch by hydrolysis with amylase. The hydration of maltose depends on the solvent from which it is crystallised.

Maltose, a disaccharide composed of two glucose molecules, is less sweet than sucrose. It is often present with other sugars in mixtures used as carbohydrate sources.

Adverse effects. Hyponatraemia developed in a patient with acute renal failure after liver transplantation following intravenous infusion of normal immunoglobulin in 10% maltose.[1] The effect which recurred on each of four successive infusions resembled that of hyperglycaemia and was thought to be due to accumulation of maltose and other osmotically active metabolites in the extracellular fluid.

1. Palevsky PM, *et al.* Maltose-induced hyponatremia. *Ann Intern Med* 1993; **118:** 526–8.

Preparations

USNF 18: Liquid Glucose.

Proprietary Preparations (details are given in Part 3)

Jpn: Martos-10.

Multi-ingredient: ***Fr.:*** Picot.

Manganese (5303-d)

Mn = 54.938049.

CAS — 7439-96-5.

Manganese Chloride (18463-w)

$MnCl_2.4H_2O$ = 197.9.

CAS — 7773-01-5 (anhydrous manganese chloride); 13446-34-9 (manganese chloride tetrahydrate).

Pharmacopoeias. In *US*.

Large, irregular, pink, odourless, translucent crystals. **Soluble** in water and alcohol; practically insoluble in ether. **Store** in airtight containers. A 5% solution has a pH between 3.5 and 6.0.

Manganese Gluconate (18506-v)

Bis(D-gluconato-O^1,O^2) manganese; Manganese D-gluconate.

$C_{12}H_{22}MnO_{14}$ = 445.2.

Pharmacopoeias. In *US* which allows either the anhydrous or dihydrate form.

Manganese Sulphate (5304-n)

Manganese Sulfate. Manganese (II) sulphate tetrahydrate.

$MnSO_4.4H_2O$ = 223.1.

CAS — 7785-87-7 (anhydrous manganese sulphate); 10034-96-5 (manganese sulphate monohydrate); 10101-68-5 (manganese sulphate tetrahydrate).

Pharmacopoeias. In *Br.* and *Fr. Br.*, *Fr.*, and *US* include the monohydrate.

Manganese Sulphate (BP 1998) (the tetrahydrate form) is described as pale pink odourless or almost odourless crystals or crystalline powder. Freely **soluble** in water; practically insoluble in alcohol.

Manganese Sulphate Monohydrate (BP 1998) is described as pale red hygroscopic crystals. Freely **soluble** in water; practically insoluble in alcohol. **Store** in airtight containers.

Manganese Sulfate (USP 23) (the monohydrate form) is described as pale red, slightly efflorescent crystals, or purple, odourless powder. **Soluble** in water; insoluble in alcohol. **Store** in airtight containers.

Adverse Effects

Acute poisoning due to ingestion of manganese or manganese salts is rare. The main symptoms of chronic poisoning, either from injection or usually inhalation of manganese dust or fumes in air, include extrapyramidal symptoms that can lead to progressive deterioration in the central nervous system.

Cholestatic liver disease, and possibly changes in the basal ganglia, have been reported to be associated with hypermanganesaemia in children receiving long-term parenteral nutrition;[1,2] manganese accumulation may be secondary to impaired biliary excretion.[3] Manganese supplementation in such patients requires re-appraisal and whole blood manganese concentrations should be monitored regularly. A low-dose regimen of not more than 1 μg (0.018 μmol) per kg body-weight daily has been suggested,[2,3] which is the dose recommended by the American Society of Clinical Nutrition.[4] Manganese accumulation in the basal ganglia has been observed in patients with liver cirrhosis.[5]

1. Reynolds AP, *et al.* Manganese in long term paediatric parenteral nutrition. *Arch Dis Child* 1994; **71:** 527–8.
2. Fell JME, *et al.* Manganese toxicity in children receiving long-term parenteral nutrition. *Lancet* 1996; **347:** 1218–21.
3. Beath SV, *et al.* Manganese toxicity and parenteral nutrition. *Lancet* 1996; **347:** 1773–4. Correction. *ibid.* **348:** 416.
4. Greene HL, *et al.* Guidelines for the use of vitamins, trace elements, calcium, magnesium, and phosphorus in infants and children receiving total parenteral nutrition: report of the Subcommittee on Pediatric Parenteral Nutrient Requirements from the Committee on Clinical Practice Issues of The American Society for Clinical Nutrition. *Am J Clin Nutr* 1988; **48:** 1324–42.

5. Krieger D, *et al.* Manganese and chronic hepatic encephalopathy. *Lancet* 1995; **346:** 270–4.

Pharmacokinetics

Absorption of manganese from the gastro-intestinal tract is variable, ranging from 3 to 50%. There is some evidence that the amount absorbed decreases as intake increases, suggesting a homoeostatic response. In the circulation, manganese is bound to transmanganin, a beta-1-globulin. Manganese is stored in the brain, kidneys, pancreas, and liver. It is excreted in bile, and undergoes enterohepatic circulation.

Uses and Administration

Manganese is an essential trace element and small amounts of a salt such as the chloride or sulphate are sometimes added to solutions for total parenteral nutrition. Suggested doses are 275 μg (5 μmol) elemental manganese daily for adults and children over 40 kg body-weight, and 1 μg (0.0182 μmol) per kg body-weight for infants and children to a maximum of 15 μg (see also under Adverse Effects, above).

Manganese compounds or salts that have been used in therapeutics in addition to those mentioned above include manganese amino acid chelate, manganese dioxide, manganese gluconate, and manganese hydrogen citrate.

Human requirements. In the United Kingdom neither a reference nutrient intake (RNI) nor an estimated average requirement (EAR) (see p.1332) has been set for manganese although a safe intake for adults was believed to lie above 1.4 mg (26 μmol) daily.[1] Similarly, in the United States a recommended dietary allowance has not been published but the safe and adequate range for adults was considered to be 2 to 5 mg daily.[2] WHO has not proposed a safe range of mean population intakes for manganese since neither intakes resulting in deficiency nor threshold toxicity levels have been established.[3] Diets high in unrefined cereals, nuts, leafy vegetables, and tea will be high in manganese.

1. DoH. Dietary reference values for food energy and nutrients for the United Kingdom: report of the panel on dietary reference values of the committee on medical aspects of food policy. *Report on health and social subjects 41*. London: HMSO, 1991.
2. Subcommittee on the tenth edition of the RDAs, Food and Nutrition Board, Commission on Life Sciences, National Research Council. *Recommended dietary allowances*. 10th ed. Washington, DC: National Academy Press, 1989.
3. WHO. Manganese. In: *Trace elements in human nutrition and health*. Geneva: WHO, 1996; 163–7.

Preparations

BPC 1973: Compound Ferrous Sulphate Tablets;
USP 23: Manganese Chloride Injection; Manganese Sulfate Injection.

Proprietary Preparations (details are given in Part 3)
Austral.: Mangatrace†; ***Canad.:*** Micro Mn; ***Fr.:*** Mangaplexe.

Multi-ingredient: ***Fr.:*** Dienol†; Ionarthrol; Megasthenyl; Oligoderm; Tot'hema; ***Ger.:*** Aksekapseln†; diabetoSome (Revitorgan)†; Sulfolitruw†; ***Irl.:*** Ferrotab; ***Ital.:*** Ferrlecit†; ***UK:*** Folicin†.

Molybdenum (16901-d)

Mo = 95.94.

Ammonium Molybdate (18365-p)

Hexaammonium molybdate tetrahydrate.

$(NH_4)_6Mo_7O_{24},4H_2O$ = 1235.9.

CAS — 12054-85-2.

Pharmacopoeias. In *US.*

Colourless or slightly green or yellow crystals. **Soluble** in water; practically insoluble in alcohol. **Store** in airtight containers.

Sodium Molybdate (18511-h)

Na_2MoO_4 = 205.9.

Pharmacopoeias. In *Ger.*, which also includes a monograph for the dihydrate.

Adverse Effects

Very high intakes of molybdenum, and associated increases in xanthine oxidase activity, may result in hyperuricaemia, and possibly gout. Molybdenum intoxication may impair the utilisation of copper.

Uses and Administration

Molybdenum is an essential trace element and small amounts, in the form of ammonium molybdate or sodium molybdate, are sometimes added to solutions for total parenteral nutrition. A suggested dose is about 20 to 120 μg (0.2 to 1.2 μmol) elemental molybdenum daily.

Ammonium molybdate is used in veterinary medicine to treat copper poisoning in sheep.

Human requirements. In the United Kingdom neither a reference nutrient intake (RNI) nor an estimated average requirement (EAR) (see p.1332) has been set for molybdenum although a safe intake was believed to be between 50 and 400 μg (0.5 and 4 μmol) daily for adults.[1] Similarly, in the United States a recommended dietary allowance has not been published but a safe and adequate range was considered to be 75 to 250 μg daily for adults.[2] WHO make the suggestion that the adult basal requirement for molybdenum could be about 25 μg daily, corresponding to approximately 0.4 μg per kg body-weight.[3]

Foods contributing to dietary molybdenum include milk, beans, breads, and cereals; however, extreme regional variations occur in molybdenum contents of food crops due to soil differences.

1. DoH. Dietary reference values for food energy and nutrients for the United Kingdom: report of the panel on dietary reference values of the committee on medical aspects of food policy. *Report on health and social subjects 41*. London: HMSO, 1991.
2. Subcommittee on the tenth edition of the RDAs, Food and Nutrition Board, Commission on Life Sciences, National Research Council. *Recommended dietary allowances*. 10th ed. Washington, DC: National Academy Press, 1989.
3. WHO. Molybdenum. In: *Trace elements in human nutrition and health*. Geneva: WHO, 1996; 144–54.

Preparations

USP 23: Ammonium Molybdate Injection.

Proprietary Preparations (details are given in Part 3)
Fr.: Molybdene Injectable; ***USA:*** Molypen.

Multi-ingredient: ***Ger.:*** Sulfolitruw†.

Monosodium Glutamate (617-n)

621; Chinese Seasoning; MSG; Natrii Glutamas; Sodium Glutamate. Sodium hydrogen L-(+)-2-aminoglutarate monohydrate.

$C_5H_8NNaO_4,H_2O$ = 187.1.

CAS — 142-47-2 (anhydrous).

Pharmacopoeias. In *USNF. Chin.* includes the injection.

White, practically odourless, free-flowing crystals or crystalline powder. It may have either a slightly sweet or slightly salty taste. Monosodium glutamate 32 g is approximately equivalent to anhydrous monosodium glutamate 29 g or glutamic acid 25 g. Freely **soluble** in water; sparingly soluble in alcohol. A 5% solution in water has a pH of 6.7 to 7.2. **Store** in airtight containers.

Monosodium glutamate is widely used as a flavour enhancer and imparts a meaty flavour.

In susceptible individuals, ingestion of foods containing monosodium glutamate may result in flushing, facial pressure, chest pain, headache, and nausea. The symptoms tend to occur within an hour of eating 3 g or more of monosodium glutamate on an empty stomach.

Nicotinic Acid (7865-b)

Nicotinic Acid *(rINN).*

375; Acidum Nicotinicum; Niacin; Nikotinsäure. Pyridine-3-carboxylic acid.

$C_6H_5NO_2$ = 123.1.

CAS — 59-67-6.

NOTE. Some published sources use the term niacin as a generic term to include both nicotinic acid and nicotinamide; in the USP the title niacin is applied specifically to nicotinic acid.

Pharmacopoeias. In *Chin., Eur.* (see p.viii), *Int., Jpn,* and *US.*

White, odourless or almost odourless, crystals or crystalline powder.

Soluble 1 in 60 of water; soluble or freely soluble in boiling water and in boiling alcohol; practically insoluble in ether; dissolves in dilute solutions of alkali hydroxides and carbonates. **Protect** from light.

Nicotinamide (7864-m)

Nicotinamide *(rINN).*

Niacinamide; Nicotinamidum; Nicotinic Acid Amide; Nicotylamide; Vitamin B_3; Vitamin PP. Pyridine-3-carboxamide.

$C_6H_6N_2O$ = 122.1.

CAS — 98-92-0.

Pharmacopoeias. In *Chin., Eur.* (see p.viii), *Int., Jpn, Pol.,* and *US.*

A white crystalline powder or colourless crystals, odourless or with a faint characteristic odour. **Soluble** 1 in 1.5 of water, 1 in 10 of boiling water, and 1 in 5.5 of alcohol; slightly soluble in ether; soluble in glycerol. A 5% solution in water has a pH of 6.0 to 7.5. **Store** in airtight containers.

Adverse Effects and Treatment

Nicotinic acid has a vasodilator action and when given by mouth or by injection in therapeutic doses it may cause flushing, a sensation of heat, faintness, and a pounding in the head. These symptoms are transient and various strategies have been proposed to reduce them (see below). Nicotinamide does not have a vasodilator action.

Other adverse effects which have been reported, especially following high doses of nicotinic acid, include dryness of the skin, pruritus, hyperpigmentation, abdominal cramps, diarrhoea, nausea and vomiting, anorexia, activation of peptic ulcer, amblyopia, jaundice and impairment of liver function, decrease in glucose tolerance, hyperglycaemia, and hyperuricaemia. Most of these effects subside on withdrawal of the drug.

Topical nicotinamide may cause dryness of the skin and, less frequently, pruritus, erythema, burning sensation, and irritation.

Nicotinic acid produces frequent adverse effects, but they are not usually serious, tend to decrease with time, and some can be minimised by following appropriate instructions for use.[1,2] Dermal and gastro-intestinal reactions are most common. Truncal and facial flushing are reported in 90 to 100% of treated patients in large clinical trials; they appear to be prostaglandin-mediated and can be reduced with aspirin 75 mg or 325 mg given shortly before nicotinic acid administration, or simply by giving the nicotinic acid with food, and by starting therapy with a low dose and gradually increasing this. Flushing may be less common with modified-release formulations.[2] Significant elevations of liver enzymes are occasionally seen with nicotinic acid therapy. They are more common in patients given large dosage increases over short periods of time, and in patients treated with modified-release formulations. Palumbo[3] has suggested that since effects on liver function may in some instances lead to hepatic failure and are more common with modified-release dosage forms the use of crystalline immediate-release preparations should be preferred, a view shared by other commentators.[4] However, although studies appear to confirm a more frequent association of hepatotoxicity with modified-release dosage forms[5-7] it should be borne in mind that these effects can also occur with the immediate-release preparations, especially at high doses. There is also a suggestion that not all modified-release preparations are alike in their effects.[8] (For further references to hepatotoxicity, see below.)

Nicotinic acid can reduce glucose tolerance, and this may be problematic in patients with diabetes mellitus,[2,4] although nicotinamide has been investigated in the prevention of diabetes mellitus (see below). Nicotinic acid also decreases urinary excretion of uric acid, which may result in elevation of serum uric acid and exacerbation of pre-existing gout.[2]

1. Knodel LC, Talbert RL. Adverse effects of hypolipidaemic drugs. *Med Toxicol* 1987; **2:** 10–32.
2. American Society of Health-System Pharmacists. ASHP therapeutic position statement on the safe use of niacin in the management of dyslipidemias. *Am J Health-Syst Pharm* 1997; **54:** 2815–19.
3. Palumbo PJ. Rediscovery of crystalline niacin. *Mayo Clin Proc* 1991; **66:** 112–13.
4. Kreisberg RA. Niacin: a therapeutic dilemma—"one man's drink is another's poison". *Am J Med* 1994; **97:** 313–16.
5. McKenney JM, *et al.* A comparison of the efficacy and toxic effects of sustained- vs immediate-release niacin in hypercholesterolemic patients. *JAMA* 1994; **271:** 672–7.
6. Rader JI, *et al.* Hepatic toxicity of unmodified and time-release preparations of niacin. *Am J Med* 1992; **92:** 77–81.
7. Gray DR, *et al.* Efficacy and safety of controlled-release niacin in dyslipoproteinemic veterans. *Ann Intern Med* 1994; **121:** 252–8.
8. Lavie CJ, Milani RV. Safety and side-effects of sustained-release niacin. *JAMA* 1994; **272:** 513–14.

Effects on the eyes. Retrospective survey of hyperlipidaemic patients suggested that dry eyes (sicca syndromes), blurred vision, and swollen eyelids might be associated with nicotinic acid therapy in some patients.[1] The effects appeared to be dose-related and reversible. In 2 patients treatment was discontinued because of symptoms suggestive of cystoid macular oedema. Three other cases of nicotinic acid maculopathy have been reported.[2]

1. Fraunfelder FW, *et al.* Adverse ocular effects associated with niacin therapy. *Br J Ophthalmol* 1995; **79:** 54–6.
2. Callanan D, *et al.* Macular edema associated with nicotinic acid (niacin). *JAMA* 1998; **279:** 1702.

Effects on the liver. As mentioned above hepatotoxicity may occur with nicotinic acid, particularly at high doses or with modified-release dosage forms, but toxicity at low doses and with immediate-release preparations has also been seen.

Further references.

1. Mullin GE, *et al.* Fulminant hepatic failure after ingestion of sustained-release nicotinic acid. *Ann Intern Med* 1989; **iii:** 253–5.
2. Knopp RH. Niacin and hepatic failure. *Ann Intern Med* 1989; **iii:** 769.
3. Henkin Y, *et al.* Rechallenge with crystalline niacin after drug-induced hepatitis from sustained-release niacin. *JAMA* 1990; **264:** 241–3.
4. Hodis HN. Acute hepatic failure associated with the use of low-dose sustained-release niacin. *JAMA* 1990; **264:** 181.
5. Etchason JA, *et al.* Niacin-induced hepatitis: a potential side effect with low-dose time-release niacin. *Mayo Clin Proc* 1991; **66:** 23–8.
6. Rader JI, *et al.* Hepatic toxicity of unmodified and time-release preparations of niacin. *Am J Med* 1992; **92:** 77–81.

Effects on the muscles. Myopathy has been noted with nicotinic acid.[1] Rhabdomyolysis has occurred when nicotinic acid was given with lovastatin (see p.1275).

1. Litin SC, Anderson CF. Nicotinic-acid associated myopathy: a report of three cases. *Am J Med* 1989; **86:** 481–3.

Precautions

Nicotinic acid should be given cautiously to patients with a history of peptic ulcer disease, and to patients with diabetes mellitus, gout, or impaired liver function.

Interactions

There may be an increased risk of myopathy or rhabdomyolysis when nicotinic acid is used concurrently with statins (p.1275). Nicotinic acid may increase the requirements for insulin or oral hypoglycaemics.

Antiepileptics. For the effect of nicotinamide on carbamazepine, see p.342.

Nicotine. In a patient receiving nicotinic acid as part of her regular medication addition of therapy with transdermal nicotine patches was followed by flushing and dizziness after usual doses of nicotinic acid.[1] The patient had experienced such reactions 3 years previously on commencing nicotinic acid therapy, but not subsequently, and it was suggested that an interaction might be responsible.

1. Rockwell KA. Potential interaction between niacin and transdermal nicotine. *Ann Pharmacother* 1993; **27:** 1283–4.

Pharmacokinetics

Nicotinic acid and nicotinamide are readily absorbed from the gastro-intestinal tract following oral administration and widely distributed in the body tissues. Nicotinic acid appears in breast milk. The main route of metabolism is their conversion to *N*-methylnicotinamide and the 2-pyridone and 4-pyridone derivatives; nicotinuric acid is also formed. Small amounts of nicotinic acid and nicotinamide are excreted unchanged in urine following therapeutic doses; however the amount excreted unchanged is increased with larger doses.

References.

1. Gugler R. Clinical pharmacokinetics of hypolipidaemic drugs. *Clin Pharmacokinet* 1978; **3:** 425–39.
2. Weiner M. Clinical pharmacology and pharmacokinetics of nicotinic acid. *Drug Metab Rev* 1979; **9:** 99–106.

Human Requirements

The daily human requirement of nicotinic acid, though not definitely known, is probably about 15 to 20 mg. Yeast, meat, fish, potatoes, green vegetables, and wholemeal cereals are good sources of nicotinic acid and nicotinamide. However they may be present in a bound, unabsorbable form in cereals, especially maize. Nicotinic acid can also be obtained from the conversion of tryptophan in the body, 60 mg of dietary tryptophan being considered equivalent to 1 mg of dietary nicotinic acid, so requirements are influenced by dietary protein intake and if protein intake is adequate there is little need for any preformed vitamin in the diet. There is generally little loss of nicotinic acid from foods during cooking.

In the United Kingdom dietary reference values (see p.1332) have been published for nicotinic acid[1] and in the United States recommended dietary allowances (RDAs) have been set.[2] In the UK the reference nutrient intake (RNI) is 6.6 mg niacin equivalent per 1000 kcal daily and the estimated average requirement (EAR) is 5.5 mg niacin equivalent per 1000 kcal daily for adult males and females. One niacin equivalent is equal to 1 mg of dietary nicotinic acid or 60 mg of dietary tryptophan. In the US the RDAs are also expressed in niacin equivalents and are 16 mg daily for adult males and 14 mg daily for adult females; the EAR is 12 mg daily in males and 11 mg daily in females.

1. DoH. Dietary reference values for food energy and nutrients for the United Kingdom: report of the panel on dietary reference values of the committee on medical aspects of food policy. *Report on health and social subjects 41.* London: HMSO, 1991.
2. Standing Committee on the Scientific Evaluation of Dietary Reference Intakes of the Food and Nutrition Board. *Dietary Reference Intakes for thiamin, riboflavin, niacin, vitamin B_6, folate, vitamin B_{12}, pantothenic acid, biotin, and choline.* Washington, DC: National Academy Press, 1998.

Uses and Administration

Nicotinic acid and nicotinamide, the form which occurs naturally in the body, are water-soluble vitamin B substances which are converted to nicotinamide adenine dinucleotide (Nadide, p.1606) and nicotinamide adenine dinucleotide phosphate (NADP). These coenzymes are involved in electron transfer reactions in the respiratory chain.

Nicotinic acid deficiency develops when the dietary intake is inadequate. Deficiency leads to the development of a syndrome known as pellagra, characterised by skin lesions, especially on areas exposed to sunlight, with hyperpigmentation and hyperkeratinisation. Other symptoms include diarrhoea, abdominal pain, glossitis, stomatitis, loss of appetite, headache, lethargy, and mental and neurological disturbances. Nicotinic acid deficiency may occur in association with other vitamin B-complex deficiency states, for example in alcoholism.

Nicotinic acid and nicotinamide are used in the treatment and prevention of nicotinic acid deficiency. Nicotinamide is preferred as it does not cause vasodilatation. They are usually given by mouth, the preferred route, but may also be administered by the intramuscular route or by slow intravenous administration. Doses of up to 500 mg daily (of either compound) in divided doses have been recommended.

Nicotinic acid has been employed for its vasodilator action in the treatment of a variety of disorders; its value is not considered to be established.

In high doses, nicotinic acid has beneficial effects on blood lipid profiles, and has been used, in conjunction with dietary modification and often in association with other lipid regulating drugs, in hyperlipidaemias (see below). Initial doses of up to 600 mg daily by mouth in divided doses, gradually increased over 2 to 4 weeks to doses of up to 6 g daily have been given; side-effects may be a limiting factor.

Topical nicotinamide is used in the treatment of mild to moderate inflammatory acne (see below), typically as a 4% gel.

Nicotinamide has been shown to inhibit the destruction of pancreatic beta cells *in vitro* and is therefore being investigated in the prevention and treatment of type 1 diabetes mellitus (see below).

Acne. Topical nicotinamide may be used in the treatment of inflammatory acne (p.1072); nicotinamide 4% was as effective as clindamycin 1% when applied topically twice a day for 8 weeks.[1]

1. Shalita AR, *et al.* Topical nicotinamide compared with clindamycin gel in the treatment of inflammatory acne vulgaris. *Int J Dermatol* 1995; **34:** 434–7.

Diabetes mellitus. Nicotinamide has been reported to induce remission in patients with newly diagnosed type 1 diabetes mellitus (p.313), and may delay the onset of disease.[1,2] However, nicotinic acid can affect glucose tolerance and should be used with care in established diabetes (see under Adverse Effects and Precautions, above).

1. Elliott RB, Chase HP. Prevention or delay of type 1 (insulin-dependent) diabetes mellitus in children using nicotinamide. *Diabetologia* 1991; **34:** 362–5.
2. Pozilli P, *et al.* Meta-analysis of nicotinamide treatment in patients with recent onset insulin dependent diabetes. *Diabetes Care* 1996; **19:** 1357–63.

Hyperlipidaemias. Nicotinic acid is reported to have a favourable effect on blood-lipid profiles, raising high-density lipoprotein (HDL)-cholesterol and lowering low-density lipoprotein (LDL)-cholesterol. Immediate-release preparations exhibit this effect to a greater degree than modified-release preparations (although modified-release preparations may be better at lowering LDL-cholesterol).[1] Nicotinic acid was less effective than lovastatin at reducing LDL-cholesterol in patients with primary hypercholesterolaemia, but more effective at increasing HDL-cholesterol; lovastatin was better tolerated.[2] The first-line treatment for hyperlipidaemias remains dietary and lifestyle modification; where this fails, drug therapy may be considered (p.1265). Nicotinic acid is used particularly in familial hypertriglyceridaemia, or in familial combined hyperlipidaemia when both triglyceride and cholesterol concentrations are similarly elevated.

1. McKenney JM, *et al.* A comparison of the efficacy and toxic effects of sustained- vs immediate-release niacin in hypercholesterolemic patients. *JAMA* 1994; **271:** 672–7.
2. Illingworth DR, *et al.* Comparative effects of lovastatin and niacin in primary hypercholesterolemia: a prospective trial. *Arch Intern Med* 1994; **154:** 1586–95.

Pemphigus. Oral treatment with nicotinamide and a tetracycline[1,2] has controlled lesions in pemphigus and pemphigoid (p.1075).

1. Sawai T, *et al.* Pemphigus vegetans with oesophageal involvement: successful treatment with minocycline and nicotinamide. *Br J Dermatol* 1995; **132:** 668–70.
2. Kolbach DN, *et al.* Bullous pemphigoid successfully controlled by tetracycline and nicotinamide. *Br J Dermatol* 1995; **133:** 88–90.

Preparations

BP 1998: Nicotinamide Tablets; Nicotinic Acid Tablets; Vitamins B and C Injection;
BPC 1973: Compound Vitamin B Tablets; Strong Compound Vitamin B Tablets; Vitamins Capsules;
USP 23: Niacin Injection; Niacin Tablets; Niacinamide Injection; Niacinamide Tablets; Oil- and Water-soluble Vitamins Capsules; Oil- and Water-soluble Vitamins Oral Solution; Oil- and Water-soluble Vitamins Tablets; Water-soluble Vitamins Capsules; Water-soluble Vitamins Tablets.

Proprietary Preparations (details are given in Part 3)
Aust.: Nicovitol; ***Austral.:*** Bioglan Tri-B3†; Nikacid†; Papulex; Tri-B3†; ***Belg.:*** Ucemine PP; ***Canad.:*** Papulex; ***Fr.:*** Nicobion; ***Ger.:*** Nicobion; Niconacid†; ***Irl.:*** Papulex; ***Swed.:*** Nicangin; ***UK:*** Papulex; ***USA:*** Endur-acin†; Nia-Bid; Niacels†; Niacor; Niaplus†; Niaspan; Nico-400; Nicobid Tempules; Nicolar; Nicotinex; Slo-Niacin.

Multi-ingredient: numerous preparations are listed in Part 3.

Ornithine (608-d)

Ornithine *(rINN)*.

α,δ-Diaminovaleric Acid; L-Ornithine. L-2,5-Diaminovaleric acid.

$C_5H_{12}N_2O_2$ = 132.2.

CAS — 70-26-8.

Pharmacopoeias. Ger. includes Ornithine Aspartate and Ornithine Hydrochloride.

Ornithine is an aliphatic amino acid. It is used as a dietary supplement.

The aspartate, hydrochloride, and oxoglurate have been used in the treatment of hyperammonaemia (p.1334) and liver disorders.

Preparations

Proprietary Preparations (details are given in Part 3)
Aust.: Cere; Hepa; Ornicetil; ***Fr.:*** Cetornan; Ornicetil; ***Ger.:*** Hepa-Merz; Hepa-Merz KT; Hepa-Vibolex†; Ornicetil†; ***Ital.:*** Ornicetil; Ornicetil S; Ornil; Ornil KG; ***Spain:*** Ornicetil; ***Switz.:*** Ornicetil.

Multi-ingredient: ***Austral.:*** Anti-Flab†; ***Fr.:*** Arnilose; Epuram; Ornitaine; ***Ger.:*** Hepa-Merz†; ***Ital.:*** Citruplexina†; Ipoazotal; Ipoazotal Complex; Polilevo; Somatron; ***Spain:*** Sedionbel†; ***UK:*** Slimswift Night Trim†.

Pantothenic Acid (7866-v)

Pantothenic Acid *(BAN)*.

Vitamin B_5. (+)-(*R*)-3-(2,4-Dihydroxy-3,3-dimethylbutyramido)propionic acid.

$C_9H_{17}NO_5$ = 219.2.

CAS — 79-83-4.

Calcium Pantothenate (7867-g)

Calcium Pantothenate *(BANM, rINN)*.

Calcii Pantothenas; Dextro Calcium Pantothenate.

$(C_9H_{16}NO_5)_2Ca$ = 476.5.

CAS — 137-08-6 (calcium D-pantothenate); 6381-63-1 (calcium DL-pantothenate); 599-54-2 (DL-pantothenic acid).

Pharmacopoeias. In *Chin., Eur.* (see p.viii), *Jpn, Pol.* and *US.*
US also has a monograph for Racemic Calcium Pantothenate.
Ger. also includes Sodium Pantothenate.

A white, odourless, slightly hygroscopic powder. Ph. Eur. **solubilities** are: freely soluble in water; slightly soluble in alcohol; practically insoluble in ether. The USP has: soluble 1 in 3 of water; soluble in glycerol; practically insoluble in alcohol, in chloroform, and in ether. A 5% solution has a pH of 6.8 to 8.0. The USP specifies that the physiological activity of racemic calcium pantothenate is approximately one-half that of calcium pantothenate. **Store** in airtight containers.

Adverse Effects

Pantothenic acid is reported to be generally non-toxic.

Pharmacokinetics

Pantothenic acid is readily absorbed from the gastro-intestinal tract following oral administration. It is widely distributed in the body tissues and appears in breast milk. About 70% of pantothenic acid is excreted unchanged in the urine and about 30% in the faeces.

Human Requirements

Pantothenic acid is widely distributed in foods. Meat, legumes, and whole grain cereals are particularly rich sources; other good sources include eggs, milk, vegetables, and fruits.

In the United Kingdom neither a reference nutrient intake (RNI) nor an estimated average requirement (EAR) has been set (see p.1332) for pantothenic acid although an intake of 3 to 7 mg daily for adults was believed to be adequate.[1] Similarly, in the United States a recommended dietary allowance has not been published but an adequate intake for adults was believed to be 5 mg daily, increased to 6 mg in pregnancy and 7 mg during lactation.[2]

1. DoH. Dietary reference values for food energy and nutrients for the United Kingdom: report of the panel on dietary reference values of the committee on medical aspects of food policy. *Report on health and social subjects 41.* London: HMSO, 1991.
2. Standing Committee on the Scientific Evaluation of Dietary Reference Intakes of the Food and Nutrition Board. *Dietary Reference Intakes for thiamin, riboflavin, niacin, vitamin B_6, folate, vitamin B_{12}, pantothenic acid, biotin, and choline.* Washington, DC: National Academy Press, 1998.

Uses and Administration

Pantothenic acid is traditionally considered to be a vitamin B substance. It is a component of coenzyme A which is essential in the metabolism of carbohydrate, fat, and protein.

Deficiency of pantothenic acid is unlikely in man because of its widespread distribution in food.

Pantothenic acid has no accepted therapeutic uses in human medicine, though it has been administered by mouth as a nutritional supplement, often as the calcium salt and usually in conjunction with other vitamins of the B group.

Preparations

USP 23: Calcium Pantothenate Tablets; Oil- and Water-soluble Vitamins Capsules; Oil- and Water-soluble Vitamins Oral Solution; Oil- and Water-soluble Vitamins Tablets; Water-soluble Vitamins Capsules; Water-soluble Vitamins Tablets.

Proprietary Preparations (details are given in Part 3)
Austral.: Pantonate; ***Canad.:*** Calpan; ***Ger.:*** Kerato Biciron N; ***Spain:*** Pantenil†; ***Switz.:*** Pantothen; ***UK:*** Cantopal; ***USA:*** Dexol TD†.

Multi-ingredient: ***Aust.:*** Lemuval; Pantogar; Salbei-Halspastillen; ***Austral.:*** Bioglan Zn-A-C; Hair and Skin Formula; Septacene†; Slimrite†; ***Belg.:*** Prurivax†; Sili-Met-San; Vitapantol; ***Fr.:*** Calced†; Dossifil; Forcapil; Modane; Sulfo-Thiorine Pantothenique†; Thiopheol†; Thiopon Pantothenique; ***Ger.:*** Aksekapseln†; Ansudoral†; Azupanthenol; Carotin; Crinocedin†; Pantovigar; Potsilo; Sonnenbraun; Spersantovit†; Vidirakt N†; ***Ital.:*** Esaglut; Fevital†; Fisiolax†; Fruttidasi†; Gliviton†; Lasonil H; Lasoproct; Nuleron; P-Cortin†; Silisan; Vitecaf; ***Spain:*** Calcio 20 Complex; Hubergrip; Lacerdermol; Lucil†; Lupidon; Modane; Pantenil; Pulmofasa; Pulmofasa Antihist; Resorpil†; Tasumicina†; Tri Hachemina; ***Switz.:*** Cortifluid N; Decasept; Osa; Pantogar; Sili-Met-San.

Phenylalanine (610-k)

Phenylalanine *(USAN, rINN).*

α-Aminohydrocinnamic Acid; F; Phe; L-Phenylalanine; Phenylalaninum. L-2-Amino-3-phenylpropionic acid.

$C_9H_{11}NO_2$ = 165.2.

CAS — 63-91-2.

Pharmacopoeias. In *Eur.* (see p.viii), *Jpn,* and *US.*

White odourless crystals, flakes, or crystalline powder. Sparingly **soluble** in water; very slightly soluble in alcohol and in methyl alcohol; practically insoluble in ether; dissolves in dilute solutions of alkali hydroxides and in dilute mineral acids. A 1% solution in water has a pH of 5.4 to 6.0. **Protect** from light.

Phenylalanine is an aromatic amino acid which is an essential constituent of the diet. It is used as a dietary supplement.

Phenylalanine intake should be restricted in patients with phenylketonuria (see Amino Acid Metabolic Disorders, p.1330).

Vitiligo. There is no totally effective treatment for vitiligo (localised hypopigmentation, p.1075). Oral or topical photochemotherapy with psoralens is generally considered to be the best available treatment, but experimental therapy includes UVA phototherapy with either khellin or phenylalanine. Administration of phenylalanine in doses of up to 100 mg per kg body-weight by mouth in conjunction with UVA/sunlight led to beneficial results in more than 90% of 200 patients with vitiligo.[1] Optimal repigmentation of the vitiliginous macules was noted in early disease, but prolonged treatment still induced repigmentation in long-standing cases. Repigmentation occurred mainly in areas rich in follicles. Such treatment is contra-indicated in phenylketonuria and in pregnancy.

1. Cormane RH, *et al.* Treatment of vitiligo with L-phenylalanine and light. *Br J Dermatol* 1986; **115:** 587.

The symbol † denotes a preparation no longer actively marketed

Preparations

Proprietary Preparations (details are given in Part 3)
USA: Endorphenyl.

Multi-ingredient: ***Fr.:*** Revitalose.

Polysaccharide-Iron Complex (11509-r)

Polysaccharide-iron complex is used as a source of iron (p.1346) for iron-deficiency anaemia (p.702). It is given by mouth in doses containing the equivalent of up to 300 mg of iron daily.

Preparations

Proprietary Preparations (details are given in Part 3)
Belg.: Ferricure; ***Canad.:*** Niferex; ***Irl.:*** Niferex†; ***Spain:*** Niferex†; ***UK:*** Niferex; ***USA:*** Hytinic; Niferex; Niferex with Vitamin C†; Nu-Iron.

Multi-ingredient: ***USA:*** Niferex Forte†; Nu-Iron Plus; Nu-Iron V.

Proline (613-x)

Proline *(USAN, rINN).*

P; Pro; L-Proline; Prolinum. L-Pyrrolidine-2-carboxylic acid.

$C_5H_9NO_2$ = 115.1.

CAS — 147-85-3.

Pharmacopoeias. In *Eur.* (see p.viii) and *US.*

White or almost white odourless crystals or crystalline powder. Very **soluble** or freely soluble in water; freely soluble in alcohol; practically insoluble in butyl alcohol, in ether, and in isopropyl alcohol. **Protect** from light.

Proline is a heterocyclic amino acid. It is used as a dietary supplement.

Saccharated Iron Oxide (5067-b)

Eisenzucker; Ferric Oxide, Saccharated; Ferrum Oxydatum Saccharatum; Oxyde de Fer Sucré.

CAS — 8047-67-4.

Pharmacopoeias. In *Aust.* and *Swiss.*

A form of saccharated iron oxide is used as a source of iron (p.1346) for iron-deficiency anaemia (p.702). It is given by mouth in doses of up to 300 mg daily (equivalent to up to 120 mg of iron daily). It is also given intravenously.

Preparations

Proprietary Preparations (details are given in Part 3)
Aust.: Ferrivenin; ***Ital.:*** Ferroven; Ferrum Hausmann; Unifer; ***Switz.:*** Venofer.

Multi-ingredient: ***Aust.:*** Ferrovin-Eisenelixier; ***Ger.:*** Hicoton; Rulofer†; Selectafer N; ***Switz.:*** B_{12}N-Compositum.

Saccharin (2404-b)

Benzoic Acid Sulphimide; Benzoic Sulfimide; Benzosulphimide; E954; Gluside; Sacarina; Saccarina; Saccharinum; o-Sulfobenzimide; Zaharina. 1,2-Benzisothiazolin-3-one 1,1-dioxide.

$C_7H_5NO_3S$ = 183.2.

CAS — 81-07-2.

Pharmacopoeias. In *Eur.* (see p.viii). Also in *USNF.*

White odourless or faintly aromatic crystals or crystalline powder with an intensely sweet taste.

Soluble 1 in 290 of water, 1 in 25 of boiling water, and 1 in about 30 of alcohol; slightly soluble in chloroform and in ether; readily dissolves in dilute ammonia solution and in solutions of alkali hydroxides and, with the evolution of carbon dioxide, in solutions of alkali carbonates. A saturated solution in water is acid to litmus.

Saccharin Ammonium (13556-r)

Ammonium Saccharin.

$C_7H_8N_2O_3S$ = 200.2.

CAS — 6381-61-9.

Saccharin Calcium (2405-v)

Calcium Benzosulphimide; Calcium Saccharin; E954.

$C_{14}H_8CaN_2O_6S_2,3\frac{1}{2}H_2O$ = 467.5.

CAS — 6485-34-3 (anhydrous saccharin calcium); 6381-91-5 (hydrated saccharin calcium).

Pharmacopoeias. In *US.*

White odourless or faintly aromatic crystals or crystalline powder with an intensely sweet taste. **Soluble** 1 in 2.6 of water and 1 in 4.7 of alcohol.

Saccharin Sodium (2406-g)

E954; Saccharin Sod.; Saccharinnatrium; Saccharinum Natricum; Saccharoidum Natricum; Sodium Benzosulphimide; Sodium Saccharin; Soluble Gluside; Soluble Saccharin.

$C_7H_4NNaO_3S$ = 205.2.

CAS — 128-44-9 (anhydrous saccharin sodium); 6155-57-3 (saccharin sodium dihydrate).

Pharmacopoeias. In *Chin., Eur.* (see p.viii), *Int., Jpn,* and *US.*

Colourless or white crystals or a white crystalline powder, odourless or faintly aromatic with an intensely sweet taste. When in powdered form it usually contains about one-third the theoretical amount of water of hydration as a result of efflorescence. **Soluble** 1 in 1.5 of water and 1 in 50 of alcohol; practically insoluble in ether. **Store** in airtight containers.

Adverse Effects

There have been rare reports of hypersensitivity and photosensitivity reactions with saccharin.

Saccharin-associated bladder tumours in *rats* given high doses have been the cause of much concern and investigation. However, it is now generally accepted that these are not applicable to saccharin use as a sweetener by man.

Effects on the liver. Elevated liver enzyme values in an elderly woman followed administration of two different medications sweetened with saccharin sodium.[1] Findings resolved on discontinuation of all preparations containing saccharin, and were subsequently found to recur on rechallenge with a small amount of saccharin sodium.

1. Negro F, *et al.* Hepatotoxicity of saccharin. *N Engl J Med* 1994; **331:** 134–5.

Pharmacokinetics

Saccharin is readily absorbed from the gastro-intestinal tract. It is almost all excreted unchanged in the urine within 24 to 48 hours.

Uses and Administration

Saccharin and its salts are intense sweeteners, a dilute solution having about 300 times the sweetening power of sucrose. They are used in pharmaceuticals and in foods and beverages and are heat stable. They have no food value. The salts are more often used than saccharin itself as they are considered to be more palatable.

Preparations

USP 23: Saccharin Sodium Oral Solution; Saccharin Sodium Tablets.

Proprietary Preparations (details are given in Part 3)
Fr.: Gaosucryl†; Sucredulcor.

Multi-ingredient: ***Austral.:*** Sucaryl; ***Fr.:*** Sucaryl; ***Ital.:*** Diet Sucaryl; Sucrinburck†.

Safflower Oil (7367-s)

Pharmacopoeias. In *US.*

Jpn includes Safflower, the flower of *Carthamus tinctorius.*

The refined fixed oil obtained from the seeds of the safflower, or false (bastard) saffron, *Carthamus tinctorius* (Compositae). It contains about 75% of linoleic acid as well as various saturated fatty acids.

It thickens and becomes rancid on prolonged exposure to air. **Store** in airtight containers. Protect from light.

Safflower oil has similar actions and uses to those of soya oil, p.1355. Emulsions containing a mixture of safflower oil 5% and soya oil 5%, or 10% and 10% respectively, are given as part of total parenteral nutrition regimens.

For reference to the association of lipid emulsion administration, as part of a parenteral nutrition regimen, with the development of sinus bradycardia, see under Soya Oil, p.1355.

Preparations

Proprietary Preparations (details are given in Part 3)

Multi-ingredient: ***Canad.:*** Liposyn†; ***Ger.:*** Abbolipid; LP-Truw†; ***Ital.:*** Liposyn; ***Swed.:*** Liposyn; ***Switz.:*** A Vogel Capsules polyvitaminees; ***UK:*** Efamol Safflower & Linseed; Epopa; Exzem Oil; ***USA:*** Liposyn II; Microlipid.

Selenium (16982-k)

Se = 78.96.

Potassium Selenate (13159-p)

K_2SeO_4 = 221.2.

CAS — 7790-59-2.

Pharmacopoeias. In *BP(Vet).*

Colourless, odourless or almost odourless crystals or a white crystalline powder. Freely **soluble** in water.

Selenious Acid (3941-j)

Monohydrated selenium dioxide.

H_2SeO_3 = 129.0.

CAS — 7783-00-8.

Pharmacopoeias. In *US.*

Store in airtight containers.

Sodium Selenite (16987-f)

Na_2SeO_3 = 172.9.

CAS — 10102-18-8.

Pharmacopoeias. In *BP(Vet).*

White to slightly greyish pink granular powder. Freely **soluble** in water; practically insoluble in alcohol and in ether.

Adverse Effects

Overdosage of selenium has been associated with loss of hair, nail changes, diarrhoea, dermatitis, garlic odour of breath, fatigue, and peripheral neuropathy.

References.

1. Clark RF, *et al.* Selenium poisoning from a nutritional supplement. *JAMA* 1996; **275:** 1087–8.

Pharmacokinetics

Selenium compounds are generally readily absorbed from the gastro-intestinal tract. Selenium is stored in red blood cells, the liver, spleen, heart, and nails. It is converted in tissues to its metabolically active forms. Selenium is excreted in the urine, and to a lesser extent in the faeces.

Uses and Administration

Selenium is an essential trace element and is an integral part of the enzyme system glutathione peroxidase; this enzyme protects intracellular structures against oxidative damage. Deficiency of selenium has been associated with an endemic form of cardiomyopathy, Keshan disease, seen in one part of China. Selenium is present in foods mainly as the amino acids selenomethionine and selenocysteine and derivatives.

Selenious acid and its sodium salt, sodium selenite, are used as a source of selenium, especially for patients with deficiency states following prolonged parenteral nutrition. Suggested doses for addition to total parenteral nutrition are 31.5 µg elemental selenium daily for adults and children greater than 40 kg body-weight, and 2 µg per kg body-weight daily for infants and children to a maximum of 30 µg daily.

Selenate and selenite salts are used for selenium deficiency states in veterinary medicine.

Human requirements. In the United Kingdom dietary reference values (DRV)[1] and in the United States recommended dietary allowances (RDA)[2] have been published for selenium. In the UK the reference nutrient intake for adult males and females is 75 and 60 µg daily respectively; values are also given for infants and children of varying ages and for lactating women. The UK report also noted that there was no convincing evidence that high intakes protected against cancer or cardiovascular disease; indeed, there was even some evidence that high intakes disturbed selenium homoeostasis and it was recommended that the maximum safe intake from all sources should be set at 450 µg daily for adult males. In the US, the RDA for adult males and females is set at 70 and 55 µg daily, respectively, and again values are also given for infants and children as well as pregnant and lactating women. WHO have recommended a lower limit of the safe range of population mean intakes of dietary selenium of 40 µg daily for adult males and 30 µg daily for adult females.[3] A maximum daily safe dietary selenium intake of 400 µg was suggested for adults.

1. DoH. Dietary reference values for food energy and nutrients for the United Kingdom: report of the panel on dietary reference values of the committee on medical aspects of food policy. *Report on health and social subjects 41.* London: HMSO, 1991.
2. Subcommittee on the tenth edition of the RDAs, Food and Nutrition Board, Commission on Life Sciences, National Research Council. *Recommended dietary allowances.* 10th ed. Washington, DC: National academy press, 1989.
3. WHO. Selenium. In: *Trace elements in human nutrition and health.* Geneva: WHO, 1996; 105–22.

Prophylaxis of malignant neoplasms. Selenium supplementation did not protect against the development of new basal or squamous cell carcinomas, of the skin in a study of patients with a history of these cancers.[1] However, analysis of secondary end-points indicated a reduced incidence of various other cancers in this study group.[1] Subsequent study has suggested, in particular, an association between low selenium intake and the risk of prostate cancer; incidence was reduced by 63% in patients receiving the supplement.[2] Another group has also reported an inverse correlation between surrogate measurements of long-term selenium intake and the risk of advanced prostate cancer.[3]

1. Clark LC, *et al.* Effects of selenium supplementation for cancer prevention in patients with carcinoma of the skin: a randomized controlled trial. *JAMA* 1996; **276:** 1957–63. Correction. *ibid.* 1997; **277:** 1520.
2. Clark LC, *et al.* Decreased incidence of prostate cancer with selenium supplementation: results of a double-blind cancer prevention trial. *Br J Urol* 1998; **81:** 730–4.
3. Yoshizawa K, *et al.* Study of prediagnostic selenium level in toenails and the risk of advanced prostate cancer. *J Natl Cancer Inst* 1998; **90:** 1219–24.

Preparations

USP 23: Selenious Acid Injection.

Proprietary Preparations (details are given in Part 3)
Aust.: Selen; ***Canad.:*** Micro Se; ***Fr.:*** Celnium; Plexium; Selenion; ***Ger.:*** Cefasel; selenase; Selit; Seltrans; ***Swed.:*** Selen†; ***USA:*** Sele-Pak; Selepen.

Multi-ingredient: ***Austral.:*** Vitaglow Selemite B Tablets; ***Canad.:*** Vita-E Plus Selenium; ***Fr.:*** Bio-Selenium; Selenium-ACE; ***Ital.:*** Fosfarsile Forte; Neomyrt Plus; Tannidin Plus; ***S.Afr.:*** Selenium-ACE†; ***Swed.:*** Selen + E†; ***UK:*** Lipase-Se Enzyme†; Se-Power; Selenium-ACE.

Serine (616-d)

Serine *(USAN, rINN).*

β-Hydroxyalanine; S; Ser; L-Serine; Serinum. L-2-Amino-3-hydroxypropionic acid.

$C_3H_7NO_3$ = 105.1.

CAS — 56-45-1.

Pharmacopoeias. In *Eur.* (see p.viii) and *US.*

White, or almost white, odourless crystalline powder or colourless crystals. **Soluble** or freely soluble in water; practically insoluble in alcohol and in ether.

Serine is an aliphatic amino acid. It is used as a dietary supplement.

Preparations

Proprietary Preparations (details are given in Part 3)

Multi-ingredient: ***Ger.:*** Sulfolitruw†.

Sodium Ironedetate (5071-d)

Sodium Ironedetate *(BAN).*

Sodium Feredetate *(rINN).* The monohydrated iron chelate of the monosodium salt of ethylenediamine-*NNN′N′*-tetra-acetic acid; Iron (III) sodium ethylenediaminetetra-acetate monohydrate.

$C_{10}H_{12}FeN_2NaO_8,H_2O$ = 385.1.

CAS — 15708-41-5 (anhydrous sodium ironedetate).

Sodium ironedetate is used as a source of iron (p.1346) for iron-deficiency anaemia (p.702). It is given by mouth in doses of up to 1.42 g daily (equivalent to up to about 205 mg of iron daily).

Preparations

Proprietary Preparations (details are given in Part 3)
Fr.: Ferrostrane; ***Ital.:*** Ferro Complex; ***Switz.:*** Ferrostrene†; ***UK:*** Sytron.

Sorbitol (619-m)

E420; D-Sorbitol; Sorbitolum. D-Glucitol.

$C_6H_{14}O_6$ = 182.2.

CAS — 50-70-4.

Pharmacopoeias. In *Chin., Eur.* (see p.viii), *Jpn,* and *Pol.* Also in *USNF.*

US includes only Sorbitol Solution.

Ph. Eur. specifies a white crystalline powder. The USNF specifies a white hygroscopic powder, granules, or flakes with a sweet taste; it permits small amounts of other polyhydric alcohols. **Soluble** 1 in 0.45 of water; sparingly or slightly soluble in alcohol; slightly soluble in acetic acid and in methyl alcohol; practically insoluble in ether.

A 5.48% solution of sorbitol hemihydrate is iso-osmotic with serum. **Store** in airtight containers.

Incompatibility. For reference to the incompatibility of sorbitol with hydroxybenzoates, see p.1117.

Adverse Effects and Precautions

As for Fructose, p.1343.

Effects on electrolyte balance. Sorbitol is employed as a vehicle in some proprietary preparations of activated charcoal intended to reduce drug absorption after poisoning; the sorbitol increases the palatability of the preparation and also produces an osmotic diarrhoea that facilitates elimination of the activated charcoal and adsorbed drug. Repeated doses of such preparations are often advocated but a case report has described a patient with end-stage renal failure in whom profuse watery diarrhoea and subsequent hypernatraemia was induced by the sorbitol.[1]

1. Gazda-Smith E, Synhavsky A. Hypernatraemia following treatment of theophylline toxicity with activated charcoal and sorbitol. *Arch Intern Med* 1990; **150:** 689 and 692.

Effects on the gastro-intestinal tract. Sorbitol is often used as a sweetener in sugar-free liquid preparations and the risk of sorbitol-induced diarrhoea associated with such products has been highlighted.[1-3] Chronic sorbitol-induced diarrhoea with associated pneumatosis intestinalis has been reported in a child receiving 21.7 g sorbitol daily in liquid medications.[4]

Colonic necrosis in a renal transplant recipient who received sodium polystyrene sulphonate suspension in sorbitol enemas for hyperkalaemia has been attributed to the sorbitol component.[5] It was subsequently pointed out that the manufacturers' instructions to give a cleansing enema both before and after the resin enema had not been followed and that this complication had never been reported when the product was administered properly.[6] It has also been suggested that sorbitol contributed to the morbidity in a patient who developed septicaemia as a complication of intestinal pseudo-obstruction, following the use of charcoal with sorbitol to treat self-poisoning with theophylline.[7] It was suggested that gaseous distension following bacterial metabolism of sorbitol had rendered the bowel wall ischaemic, facilitating passage of bacteria or of endotoxin into the systemic circulation.

1. Brown AM, Masson E. 'Hidden' sorbitol in proprietary medicines - a cause for concern? *Pharm J* 1990; **245:** 211.
2. Edes TE, *et al.* Diarrhea in tube-fed patients: feeding formula not necessarily the cause. *Am J Med* 1990; **88:** 91–3.
3. Johnston KR, *et al.* Gastrointestinal effects of sorbitol as an additive in liquid medications. *Am J Med* 1994; **97:** 185–91.
4. Duncan B, *et al.* Medication-induced pneumatosis intestinalis. *Pediatrics* 1997; **99:** 633–6.
5. Wootton FT, *et al.* Colonic necrosis with Kayexalate-Sorbitol enemas after renal transplantation. *Ann Intern Med* 1989; **111:** 947–9.
6. Shepard KV. Cleansing enemas after sodium polystyrene sulfonate enemas. *Ann Intern Med* 1990; **112:** 711.
7. Longdon P, Henderson A. Intestinal pseudo-obstruction following the use of enteral charcoal and sorbitol and mechanical ventilation with papaveretum sedation for theophylline poisoning. *Drug Safety* 1992; **7:** 74–7.

Pharmacokinetics

Sorbitol is poorly absorbed from the gastro-intestinal tract following oral or rectal administration. It is metabolised mainly in the liver, to fructose (see p.1343), a reaction catalysed by the enzyme sorbitol dehydrogenase. Some sorbitol may be converted directly to glucose by the enzyme aldose reductase.

Uses and Administration

Sorbitol is a polyhydric sugar alcohol (polyol) with half the sweetening power of sucrose. It occurs naturally in many fruits and vegetables and is prepared commercially by the reduction of glucose.

It has been employed as a 30% solution as an alternative to glucose in parenteral nutrition (p.1331) but its use is not recommended because of the risk of lactic acidosis.

Sorbitol may be administered by mouth or rectally as an osmotic laxative in the management of constipation (p.1168); doses of 20 to 50 g have been suggested.

Solutions containing about 3% of sorbitol are used as irrigating fluids in transurethral surgical procedures.

Sorbitol was formerly given intravenously as a 50% solution as an osmotic diuretic.

Sorbitol also acts as a bulk sweetening agent. It is used in limited quantities as a sweetener in energy-reduced diabetic food products. It is also used as an alternative to sucrose in many sugar-free oral liquid preparations and in sugar-free foods as it is less likely to cause dental caries.

Sorbitol also has humectant and stabilising properties and is used in various pharmaceutical and cosmetic products including toothpaste.

Preparations

BP 1998: Sorbitol Intravenous Infusion;
Ph. Eur.: Sorbitol Solution (70 per cent) (Crystallising); Sorbitol Solution (70 per cent) (Non-crystallising);
USNF 18: Noncrystallizing Sorbitol Solution;
USP 23: Sorbitol Solution.

Proprietary Preparations (details are given in Part 3)
Austral.: Sorbilax; ***Belg.:*** Syn MD; ***Fr.:*** Hepagrume; Sorbostyl†; ***Ital.:*** Sorbilande†; ***Swed.:*** Cystosol; Resulax; Sorbitur; ***Switz.:*** Syn MD.

Multi-ingredient: ***Aust.:*** Glandosane; Lemazol; Microklist; Resectal; Tromgallol; Yal; ***Austral.:*** Aquae; Carbosorb S; Emtobil†; Medevac; Microlax; ***Belg.:*** Bilagol; Microlax; Spagulax S†; ***Canad.:*** Charcodote; Microlax; Moi-Stir; Salivart; ***Fr.:*** Arnilose; Artisial; Hepacholine Sorbitol; Hepargitol; Liporex†; Megabyl; Microlax; Modulite; Nivabetol; Norbiline; Ornitaine; Schoum; Sorbocitryl†; Spagulax au Sorbitol; Syaline-spray†; Vitaphakol; ***Ger.:*** Artisial; Bilibyk/KM-Suspension†; Cholebrine-Reizmahlzeit†; Dr. Hotz Vollbad; Flacar; Glandosane; Klysma Sorbit; Lemazol†; Microklist; Osmofundin 20%†; Sorbosan†; Sterofundin

OH⁻†; Tirgon†; Tutofusin S; Yal; *Irl.:* Luborant; *Ital.:* Bilarvis†; Citroepatina; Citrosorbina B6†; Liverchin†; Macrolax; Magisbile; Malto Mannite Magnesiaca†; Norbiline; Novilax; Prontoclisma†; Si-Cliss; Sorbiclis; Tamarmanna†; Weight Watchers Punto; *Neth.:* Microlax; *Norw.:* Klyx; Microlax; *S.Afr.:* Agofell; Microlax; *Spain:* Gastroalgine; Hepadif; Levaliver; Meneparol Sol†; Norbiline†; Polisilan Gel; Primperan Complex; Sualyn; Sugarbil; Sugarceton; Sulmetin†; Vitaphakol; *Swed.:* Klyx; Microlax; Somanol; Vi-Siblin S; *Switz.:* Cital; Glandosane; Microklist; Purisole; Vitaphakol; Yal; *UK:* Glandosane; Luborant; Relaxit; *USA:* Actidose with Sorbitol; Glandosane; Moi-Stir; Salivart.

Soya Oil (7369-e)

Soja Bean Oil; Sojae Oleum; Soyabean Oil; Soya-bean Oil; Soybean Oil.

Pharmacopoeias. In *Chin., Eur.* (see p.viii), *Jpn*, and *US*.
Eur. also includes Hydrogenated Soya-bean Oil. *Ger.* also includes Partially Hydrogenated Soya Oil.

Ph. Eur. specifies: the refined fatty oil obtained from the seeds of *Glycine soja* and *Glycine max (G. hispida)* (Leguminosae). A clear pale yellow liquid. Practically **insoluble** in alcohol; miscible with ether and with petroleum spirit. **Store** in well-filled containers. Protect from light.

The USP specifies: the refined fixed oil obtained from the seeds of the soya plant *Glycine soja*. A clear pale yellow oily liquid with a characteristic odour. **Insoluble** in water; miscible with chloroform and with ether. **Store** in airtight containers. Protect from light.

Hydrogenated Soya-bean Oil (Ph. Eur.) is obtained by refining, bleaching, hydrogenation, and deodorisation of soya oil. It consists mainly of triglycerides of palmitic and stearic acids. A white mass or powder which melts to a clear, pale yellow liquid when heated. Practically **insoluble** in water; very slightly soluble in alcohol; freely soluble in dichloromethane, in light petroleum after heating, and in toluene. **Protect** from light.

Incompatibility. For mention of the compatibility and stability of solutions and emulsions for parenteral nutrition see under Enteral and Parenteral Nutrition, p.1331.

Adverse Effects

Hypersensitivity reactions including fever and chills have been reported following the infusion of soya oil emulsion although they are considered to be fairly rare. Other rare immediate reactions include dyspnoea, cyanosis, nausea, vomiting, headache, and chest and back pain.

Too rapid infusion of soya oil emulsion or prolonged infusion or its administration to patients with impaired fat metabolism has been associated with the 'overload syndrome'. This is manifested by blood disorders such as bone-marrow depression, anaemia, thrombocytopenia, and spontaneous bleeding, hepatosplenomegaly, raised liver enzyme values, hyperlipidaemia, seizures, and shock. Pigmentation of tissues after prolonged therapy with lipid emulsion infusions has also been reported.

Soya protein-based infant feeds can be antigenic and cause gastro-intestinal adverse effects in sensitive individuals.

Bacteraemia. Although coagulase-negative staphylococci are constituents of the normal microflora of the skin they are also the most common blood-culture isolates and cause of sepsis in neonatal intensive care units. A strong association has been demonstrated between the administration of lipids through peripheral venous catheters made of Teflon and development of coagulase-negative staphylococcal bacteraemia in neonates.[1] However, the benefits of parenteral lipids in providing nutritional support for premature infants clearly outweighed the risks; investigation of catheters made of other materials, or other delivery systems, might reduce the opportunity for coagulase-negative staphylococci to adhere and come into contact with nutrient-rich growth media in the form of lipid emulsions. Others also took the view that this work should not lead to the abandonment of parenteral lipids in such infants;[2] vancomycin should be considered for the initial management of coagulase-negative staphylococcal bacteraemia should it occur.

1. Freeman J, *et al.* Association of intravenous lipid emulsion and coagulase-negative staphylococcal bacteremia in neonatal intensive care units. *N Engl J Med* 1990; **323:** 301–8.
2. Klein JO. From harmless commensal to invasive pathogen: coagulase-negative staphylococci. *N Engl J Med* 1990; **323:** 339–40.

Effects on the cardiovascular system. Development of sinus bradycardia has been reported in a patient receiving total parenteral nutrition which included the administration of a soya oil-based emulsion.[1] The authors suggested that it might be wise to administer fat emulsion only through a peripheral vein. However, sinus bradycardia has been reported following the administration of a safflower oil-based emulsion via a peripheral vein as part of a TPN regimen.[2]

1. Sternberg A, *et al.* Intralipid-induced transient sinus bradycardia. *N Engl J Med* 1981; **304:** 422–3.
2. Traub SL, *et al.* Sinus bradycardia associated with peripheral lipids and total parenteral nutrition. *J Parenter Enteral Nutr* 1985; **9:** 358–60.

Effects on the endocrine system. Soya is a rich source of phyto-oestrogens including isoflavones, and it has recently been demonstrated that infants fed soya-based formula have high serum concentrations of these substances.[1] It has been suggested that these may be sufficient to exert biological effects, bringing the safety of soya-based formulae into question. As yet, effects have not been observed clinically, but further studies are needed to assess the short- and long-term effects of soya-based products.[2]

1. Setchell KDR, *et al.* Exposure of infants to phyto-oestrogens from soy-based infant formula. *Lancet* 1997; **350:** 23–7.
2. Essex C. Phytoestrogens and soy based infant formula. *Br Med J* 1996; **313:** 507–8.

Effects on the nervous system. Jellinek reported CNS disorders in 2 patients receiving infusions of fractionated soya emulsion including convulsions, coma, and cortical blindness in one young woman.[1] A similar case was attributed to fat embolism,[2] but occurring after what the manufacturers pointed out was a faster than recommended infusion[3] may perhaps have represented a fat-overload syndrome.

1. Jellinek EH. Dangers of intravenous fat infusions. *Lancet* 1976; **ii:** 967.
2. Estbe JP, Malledant Y. Fat embolism after lipid emulsion infusion. *Lancet* 1991; **337:** 673.
3. McCracken M. Fat embolism after lipid emulsion infusion. *Lancet* 1991; **337:** 983.

Hypersensitivity. Urticaria has been reported in two patients following the administration intravenously of soya oil emulsions.[1,2] In one case the patient had previously received the emulsion for 19 days without ill-effect.[1]

Anaphylactic reactions have been documented after the ingestion of several foods or foodstuffs containing, or prepared from, soya beans, although the exact allergen remains unknown. In one patient who suffered anaphylactic attacks after eating such products a specific IgE-antibody response to the allergen Kunitz soybean trypsin inhibitor was demonstrated.[3] This was not, however, the only allergen present in soya beans as other patients who had a negative response to this allergen had positive responses in whole soya bean tests.

IgE antibodies to soya bean antigens have also been found in workers who suffered from asthma after handling soya beans[4,5] leading to the suggestion that an allergic mechanism had been responsible; the asthma was believed to have been due to the dust released during the handling of the beans.

1. Kamath KR, *et al.* Acute hypersensitivity reaction to Intralipid. *N Engl J Med* 1981; **304:** 360.
2. Hiyama DT, *et al.* Hypersensitivity following lipid emulsion infusion in an adult patient. *J Parenter Enteral Nutr* 1989; **13:** 318–20.
3. Moroz LA, Yang WH. Kunitz soybean trypsin inhibitor: a specific allergen in food anaphylaxis. *N Engl J Med* 1980; **302:** 1126–8.
4. Sunyer J, *et al.* Case-control study of serum immunoglobulin-E antibodies reactive with soybean in epidemic asthma. *Lancet* 1989; **i:** 179–82.
5. Hernando L, *et al.* Asthma epidemics and soybean in Cartagena (Spain). *Lancet* 1989; **i:** 502.

Pulmonary fat emboli. Pulmonary fat emboli or microemboli, sometimes fatal, have occurred in several infants who received infusions of fat emulsions based on soya oil.[1-3]

In one case[3] the patient's serum, which contained a high concentration of C-reactive protein, agglutinated the fat emulsion and this finding was considered to support the hypothesis that microemboli are formed by agglutination of fat emulsion in the bloodstream by C-reactive protein. The authors of this report did not consider the precise pathogenesis to be clear, nor did they know whether the condition was preventable, but did suggest that it may be prudent either to ensure that the C-reactive protein concentration was normal (less than 10 mg per litre) or to perform a creaming test to determine which babies may embolise the infused fat emulsion. However, other studies,[4] while not excluding a role of C-reactive protein in agglutination, have failed to find any correlation between raised concentrations of this protein and the rate of agglutination.

1. Barson AJ, *et al.* Fat embolism in infancy after intravenous fat infusions. *Arch Dis Child* 1978; **53:** 218–23.
2. Levene MI, *et al.* Pulmonary fat accumulation after Intralipid infusion in the preterm infant. *Lancet* 1980; **ii:** 815–8.
3. Hulman G, Levene M. Intralipid microemboli. *Arch Dis Child* 1986; **61:** 702–3.
4. Zagara G, *et al.* C-reactive protein and serum agglutination in vivo of intravenous fat emulsions. *Lancet* 1989; **i:** 733.

Precautions

Intravenous soya oil emulsion should not be given to patients with severe liver disease, acute shock, or severe or pathological hyperlipidaemia, or when the ability to metabolise fat may otherwise be impaired. Caution has also been advised in patients with pulmonary disease, renal insufficiency, uncompensated diabetes mellitus, hyperthyroidism, sepsis, and some disorders of blood coagulation. However, if administration is considered in such patients, the elimination of fat should be monitored daily.

Egg-yolk phospholipids may be used as emulsifiers in some preparations and therefore such fat emulsions should not be given to patients with severe egg allergy.

Fat emulsions may extract phthalate plasticisers from administration bags and sets and therefore non-phthalate containing equipment should be used wherever possible. Soya-based infant feeds should be avoided in infants with documented cows' milk protein-induced enteropathy or enterocolitis, as these infants are frequently also sensitive to soya protein.

Neonatal hyperbilirubinaemia. The use of intravenous lipid emulsions in hyperbilirubinaemic neonates and the relationship between the resulting increase in plasma free fatty acids and bilirubin has been subject to debate.

In a review of neonatal bilirubin toxicity[1] early work was discussed in which it had been suggested that because fat particles can bind free bilirubin, intravenous fat may help decrease the risk of kernicterus. However, because intravenous fat is metabolised to free fatty acids, and long chain fatty acids are tightly bound to albumin, mention was also made of the converse proposal that bilirubin displacement may occur during fat therapy, increasing the infant's risk for bilirubin encephalopathy. *In vitro* studies were also reviewed which had indicated that bilirubin was not displaced from albumin until free fatty acids in plasma approached a 4 or 5:1 ratio with albumin as well as evidence suggesting that fatty acids may alter bilirubin binding by causing significant conformational changes in the albumin molecule.

A study in 20 preterm infants[2] showed that in those of less than 30 weeks gestation fat emulsion 1 g per kg body-weight infused over a 15-hour period had minimal risk of significantly decreasing bilirubin binding to albumin since the free fatty acid to albumin ratio remained at approximately 2:1; however, at higher doses of 2 or 3 g per kg over the same time period there did appear to be some risk of decreased binding. Infants older than 30 weeks were always at less risk irrespective of the dose used. A later study[3] involving 38 neonates of 27 to 34 weeks gestation, demonstrated that varying the administration regimen with different infusion rates and intermittent and constant dosing (maximum dose and rate being 4 g per kg over 16 hours) appeared to have little effect on serum concentrations of total and apparent unbound bilirubin, although there was a trend towards greater variability in apparent unbound concentrations with the intermittent regimen. Serum concentrations of apparent unbound bilirubin as high as 45 nmol per litre were observed without any detectable clinical signs of encephalopathy.

1. Walker PC. Neonatal bilirubin toxicity: a review of kernicterus and the implications of drug-induced bilirubin displacement. *Clin Pharmacokinet* 1987; **13:** 26–50.
2. Spear ML, *et al.* The effect of 15-hour fat infusions of varying dosage on bilirubin binding to albumin. *J Parenter Enteral Nutr* 1985; **9:** 144–7.
3. Brans YW, *et al.* Influence of intravenous fat emulsion on serum bilirubin in very low birthweight neonates. *Arch Dis Child* 1987; **62:** 156–60.

Uses and Administration

Emulsions of fractionated soya oil containing 10, 20, or 30% are given by slow intravenous infusion as part of total parenteral nutrition regimens (p.1331), usually in conjunction with amino acid and carbohydrate solutions. The solutions and emulsions may be administered at separate sites, administered at the same site through a Y-connector, or combined in one admixture. Fat emulsions provide a high energy intake in a relatively small volume. They may also be used to prevent or correct essential fatty acid deficiency. When used as a calorie source the dose of the emulsion is determined by the energy requirements and clinical status of the patient; the amount, generally, should not comprise more than 60% of patients' total calorie intake. For the prevention and correction of fatty acid deficiency about 5 to 10% of total calorific intake should be as an intravenous fat emulsion.

The composition and dosage recommendations of commercial preparations do differ slightly but they should be started slowly. Suggested initial rates for the 10% and 20% products are 1 mL per minute and 0.5 mL per minute respectively for 15 to 30 minutes. The rate may then be increased and up to about 500 mL (or 10 mL per kg body-weight) of 10% or 250 mL (or 5 mL per kg) of 20% emulsion may be given on the first day. The total daily dosage may then be increased gradually on subsequent days; suggested daily dose ranges are 500 to 1500 mL of a 10% or 500 to 1000 mL of a 20% emulsion and suggested rates of administration are 500 mL of a 10% emulsion over a period of not less than 3 hours, and 500 mL of a 20% emulsion over not less than 5 hours. Where a 30% emulsion is used, a dose of 333 mL or about 4.75 mL per kg body-weight has been recommended, given over 5 hours or more; the first dose should not exceed 3 mL per kg.

Soya oil also has emollient properties and is used as a bath additive in the treatment of dry skin conditions.

Preparations made from whole soya beans, utilising soya oil and soya protein are used as the basis of lactose-free vegetable milks for infants and patients with lactose or similar disaccharide intolerance or with an allergy to cows' milk protein (see also below).

Administration. Haumont and colleagues[1] have suggested that it is the concentration of phospholipid solubilisers, and particularly the excess present as free phospholipid liposomes, that determines the effect of lipid emulsions on plasma-lipid concentrations. In 20 premature infants requiring parenteral nutrition, infusion of up to 4 g of fat per kg body-weight daily as a 20% emulsion (twice the usual maximum dose) had less effect on plasma lipid concentrations than 2 g per kg daily as a 10% emulsion; the difference was thought to be due to the fact that the 20% emulsion was relatively liposome-poor, with a ratio of phospholipids to triglycerides of 0.06, whereas the liposome-rich 10% emulsion had a ratio of 0.12. The authors suggested that the 10% emulsion should not be used in preterm infants.

For discussion of the potential risks of kernicterus if lipid infusions are given to hyperbilirubinaemic neonates, see under Precautions, above.

1. Haumont D, *et al.* Effect of liposomal content of lipid emulsions on plasma lipid concentrations in low birth weight infants receiving parenteral nutrition. *J Pediatr* 1992; **121:** 759–63.

Food intolerance. The American Academy of Pediatrics currently recommends[1] that soya-based infant feeds are appropriate for use in galactosaemia and hereditary lactase deficiency, and documented allergy to cows' milk protein. However, infants with documented cows' milk protein enteropathy or enterocolitis should receive hydrolysed protein formula, as they are likely to be sensitive to soya protein. They conclude that soya-based infant feeds have no proven role in the prevention of atopic disease or in the management of infantile colic.

The FDA has warned against the use of soya-based drinks intended for adults as the sole source for nutrition for infants.[2] It was stated that soya drinks can lead to severe protein and calorie malnutrition, multiple vitamin and mineral deficiency, and death in infants who receive no other source of nourishment, and should not be confused with soya-based infant formulas, which are specially formulated to meet the nutritional needs of infants.

For reference to the use of soya-based foods themselves causing allergic reactions, see under Hypersensitivity, above. Lactose intolerance in adults is briefly discussed on p.1349.

1. American Academy of Pediatrics. Soy protein-based formulas: recommendations for use in infant feeding. *Pediatrics* 1998; **101:** 148–53.
2. Nightingale S. Warnings issued about practices, products: soy drink warning. *JAMA* 1985; **254:** 1428.

Preparations

Proprietary Preparations (details are given in Part 3)
Aust.: Balneum Hermal; Elolipid; Intralipid; Lipofundin; Lipovenos; Olbad Cordes; Solipid; ***Austral.:*** Intralipid; Soypliment†; ***Belg.:*** Intralipid; Lipovenoes; ***Canad.:*** Intralipid; ***Fr.:*** Balneum normal†; Endolipide; Intralipide; Ivelip; Lipoven; ***Ger.:*** Balneum; Deltalipid; Hoecutin Olbad; Intralipid; Kneipp Neurodermatitis-Bad; Lipofundin; Olbad Cordes; Salvilipid; ***Irl.:*** Balneum; Intralipid; Lipofundin S; ***Ital.:*** Intralipid; Ivelip; Lipofundin S; Lipovenos; Soyacal†; ***Jpn:*** Intrafat; ***Neth.:*** Intralipid; ***Norw.:*** Intralipid; Lipovenos; ***S.Afr.:*** Intralipid; ***Spain:*** Ivelip; Lipofundina MCT/LCT; Lipovenos; ***Swed.:*** Emulsan†; Intralipid; Lipovenos; ***Switz.:*** Balneum; Intralipid; Lipidem; Lipovenos; Olbad Cordes (Bain huileux Cordes)†; ***UK:*** Balneum; Intralipid; Ivelip; Lipofundin; Lipovenos; Soyacal; ***USA:*** Intralipid; Liposyn III.

Multi-ingredient: ***Aust.:*** Badeol; Balneum Hermal mit Teer; Balneum Hermal Plus; Kabi Mix E; Lipofundin mit MCT; Olbad Cordes comp; Oleosint; PE-Mix; TriMix E; ***Austral.:*** Hypol; ***Belg.:*** Medialipide; ***Canad.:*** Liposyn†; ***Fr.:*** Clinoleic; Ivemix; KabiMix; Medialipide; Piascledine; Trive; Vitrimix KV; ***Ger.:*** Abbolipid; Balneoconzen; Balneovit O†; Balneum mit Schwefel†; Balneum mit Teer†; Balneum Plus; Derma Bad†; Lipovenos; Nutrifundin†; Oleobal; Sulfo-Olbad Cordes; Windol Basisbad; ***Irl.:*** Balneum Plus; Balneum with Tar; Vitrimix KV; ***Ital.:*** KabiMix; Lipofundin MCT; Liposyn; Piascledine; ***Neth.:*** KabiMix; Vitrimix KV; ***Norw.:*** Ivamix; KabiMix; Vasolipid; Vitrimix; ***S.Afr.:*** Lipofundin MCT/LCT; Lipovenous; ***Spain:*** KabiMix; Trive; ***Swed.:*** KabiMix; Liposyn; Structolipid; Vasolipid; Vitrimix; ***Switz.:*** Antidry; Balneum Plus; Demosvelte N; Lipofundin MCT; Melisol; Sulfo-Olbad Cordes†; Vitrimix; ***UK:*** Balneum Plus; Balneum with Tar†; Clinomel; KabiMix; Lipofundin MCT/LCT; Phytolife Plus; Vitrimix KV; ***USA:*** Anusol; Liposyn II.

Starch (1641-s)

Almidón; Amido; Amidon; Amilo; Amylum; Stärke.

CAS — 9005-25-8 (starch); 9005-82-7 (α-amylose); 9004-34-6 (β-amylose); 9037-22-3 (amylopectin).

NOTE. Starch (BP) may be maize starch, rice starch, potato starch, wheat starch, or tapioca starch (cassava starch). Starch (USNF) is maize starch, wheat starch, tapioca starch, or potato starch.

Pharmacopoeias. Some or all of the starches described are included in *Chin., Eur.* (see p.viii), *Int., Jpn,* and *Pol.* Also in *USNF. Eur.* also includes Pregelatinised Starch, *Br.* also includes Sterilisable Maize Starch, *USNF* also includes Pregelatinized Starch, and *US* includes Absorbable Dusting Powder and Topical Starch.

Polysaccharide granules obtained from the caryopsis of maize, *Zea mays*, rice, *Oryza sativa*, wheat, *Triticum aestivum (T. vulgare)*, from the tubers of potato, *Solanum tuberosum* or from the rhizomes of cassava, *Manihot utilissima*. Maize starch is also known as corn starch. Starch contains amylose and amylopectin, both polysaccharides based on α-glucose.

A very fine, white, odourless, powder which creaks when pressed between the fingers, or irregular angular masses. Maize starch may be slightly yellowish.

Practically **insoluble** in cold water and in alcohol. **Store** in airtight containers.

Adverse Effects

The use of starch glove powders by surgeons[1] has resulted in contamination of the patients' surgical wound by starch and in the development of complications such as inflammation, adhesions, and granulomatous lesions. In addition, glove starch powder may be a risk factor in the development of latex allergy, and may act as a vector for bacterial pathogens.

1. Haglaund U, Junghanns K, eds. Glove powder—the hazards which demand a ban. *Eur J Surg* 1997; **163** (suppl 579): 1–55.

Effects of cassava. In 1985 the World Health Organization added malnutrition-related diabetes (which included the type previously known as Tropical diabetes) to its classification of diabetes mellitus.[1] Epidemiological evidence had suggested an association between fibrocalculous pancreatic diabetes (a subclass of malnutrition-related diabetes) and the consumption of cassava root (tapioca, manioc), which for many people living in tropical developing countries, where protein intake was low, was the main source of food energy. Cassava root contains several cyanogenic substances and although food preparation and processing could reduce the cyanide content, there was the possibility that in persons with an inadequate protein intake, particularly if deficient in sulphur-containing amino acids which are involved in detoxification pathways, accumulation of cyanides might occur. The WHO, however, did consider that further research was necessary to firmly establish any relation between this type of diabetes and high levels of cassava consumption. In a review which appeared in the following year[2] the cassava/malnutrition hypothesis was thought to be attractive, but unproven; also there was strong evidence against it being the only cause. Many studies and reports have since been published but still no definitive answer appears to have emerged.

Neurotoxicity including spastic paraparesis[3] and optic neuropathy[4] caused by exposure to cyanide after ingestion of cassava root has been reported.

1. WHO. Diabetes mellitus: report of a WHO study group. *WHO Tech Rep Ser 727* 1985.
2. Abu-Bakare A, *et al.* Tropical or malnutrition-related diabetes: a real syndrome? *Lancet* 1986; **i:** 1135–8.
3. Cliff J, *et al.* Association of high cyanide and low sulphur intake in cassava-induced spastic paraparesis. *Lancet* 1985; **ii:** 1211–3.
4. Freeman AG. Optic neuropathy and chronic cyanide toxicity. *Lancet* 1986; **i:** 441–2.

Uses and Administration

Starch is absorbent and is widely used in dusting-powders, either alone or mixed with zinc oxide or other similar substances. Starch is used as a surgical glove powder; because adverse effects have occurred care should be taken to minimise contamination of the wound. It is incorporated in many tablets as a disintegrating agent.

A starch mucilage is given by mouth in the treatment of iodine poisoning.

Rice-based solutions have been tried in the prevention and treatment of dehydration due to acute diarrhoeal diseases (p.1168) and may have advantages under certain circumstances over conventional oral rehydration solutions.

Glycogen storage diseases. Type I glycogen storage disease, in which hypoglycaemia is a predominant symptom, has been successfully managed by continuous nocturnal nasogastric infusion of glucose and frequent daytime feedings. However, such a regimen requires good patient compliance and monitoring of the night-time infusions. As an alternative, a more standard diet together with uncooked corn starch suspensions prepared with tap water at room temperature and taken every 6 hours in doses of 1.75 to 2.5 g per kg body-weight have been reported[1] to be very satisfactory in maintaining normoglycaemia. In one infant, in whom starch was not satisfactory, the lack of response was considered to be due to inadequate pancreatic amylase activity and although it was subsequently reported[2] that addition of a pancreatic enzyme concentrate had produced some improvement, the response was still inadequate to maintain normoglycaemia for more than 2 hours. It was considered that other amylase preparations should be identified for possible use in such patients.

Renal complications can also arise in type I glycogen storage disease as a consequence of a range of metabolic abnormalities. Corn starch therapy has been reported to have caused the amelioration of proximal renal tubular dysfunction in 3 patients who had previously only received frequent daytime feeding as therapy. In 16 other patients who had previously received treatment with corn starch or glucose infusions such renal dysfunction was not identified and it was considered that the rapid response to therapy may explain why renal tubular dysfunction is not found more frequently in these patients.[3]

1. Chen Y-T, *et al.* Cornstarch therapy in type 1 glycogen-storage disease. *N Engl J Med* 1984; **310:** 171–5.
2. Chen Y-T, Sidbury JB. Cornstarch therapy in type 1 glycogen-storage disease. *N Engl J Med* 1984; **311:** 128–9.
3. Chen Y-T, *et al.* Amelioration of proximal renal tubular dysfunction in type I glycogen storage disease with dietary therapy. *N Engl J Med* 1990; **323:** 590–3.

Preparations

BP 1998: Compound Zinc Paste; Dithranol Paste; Sterilisable Maize Starch; Talc Dusting Powder;
Ph. Eur.: Pregelatinised Starch;
USNF 18: Pregelatinized Starch;
USP 23: Absorbable Dusting Powder; Topical Starch.

Stevioside (16994-r)

Eupatorin; Rebaudin; Stevin; Steviosin.

$C_{38}H_{60}O_{18}$ = 804.9.

CAS — 57817-89-7.

A glycoside extracted from the leaves of yerba dulce, *Stevia rebaudiana* (Compositae).

Stevioside has about 300 times the sweetness of sucrose and has been used as a sweetening agent in foods. An extract of the leaves of *Stevia rebaudiana* which contains stevioside as well as other glycosides including rebaudioside A, has been used similarly.

References.

1. Crammer B, Ikan R. Sweet glycosides from the stevia plant. *Chem Br* 1986; **22:** 915–16 and 918.

Sucralose (5781-q)

Sucralose *(BAN)*.

TGS; Trichlorogalactosucrose. 1,6-Dichloro-1,6-dideoxy-β-D-fructofuranosyl 4-chloro-4-deoxy-α-D-galactopyranoside.

$C_{12}H_{19}Cl_3O_8$ = 397.6.

CAS — 56038-13-2.

Sucralose is used as a sweetening agent. It is reported to have between about 300 and 1000 times the sweetening power of sucrose.

References.

1. Anonymous. Sucralose—a new artificial sweetener. *Med Lett Drugs Ther* 1998; **40:** 67–8.

Sucrose (660-b)

Azúcar; Cane Sugar; Refined Sugar; Sacarosa; Saccharose; Saccharum; Sucre; Sucrosum; Zucker. β-D-Fructofuranosyl-α-D-glucopyranoside.

$C_{12}H_{22}O_{11}$ = 342.3.

CAS — 57-50-1.

Pharmacopoeias. In *Chin., Eur.* (see p.viii), *Jpn*, and *Pol.* Also in *USNF.*

USNF also includes Compressible Sugar, Confectioner's Sugar, and Sugar Spheres.

Colourless or white, odourless, lustrous, dry crystals, crystalline masses, or white crystalline powder, with a sweet taste, obtained from sugar-cane, *Saccharum officinarum* (Gramineae), sugar-beet, *Beta vulgaris* (Chenopodiaceae), and other sources.

Soluble 1 in 0.5 of water, 1 in 0.2 of boiling water, and 1 in 170 of alcohol; practically insoluble in dehydrated alcohol. A solution in water is neutral to litmus.

Sucrose may be contaminated by traces of heavy metals or sulphites and this may lead to **incompatibility** with active ingredients when sucrose is used as a pharmaceutical excipient. Syrup preserved with hydroxybenzoates has been reported to be incompatible with a range of compounds.

Adverse Effects and Precautions

Sucrose consumption increases the incidence of dental caries.

Sucrose should be administered with care to patients with diabetes mellitus. It is contra-indicated in patients with the glucose-galactose malabsorption syndrome, fructose intolerance, or sucrase-isomaltase deficiency.

Conclusions and recommendations of the Panel on Dietary Sugars after reviewing the evidence relating to sugars in the diet and the health of the population in the UK.[1]

No evidence was found that the consumption of most sugars naturally incorporated into the cellular structure of foods (intrinsic sugars) represented a threat to health and consideration was therefore mainly directed towards the dietary use of sugars not so incorporated (extrinsic sugars), of which sucrose was the principal non-milk extrinsic sugar.

There was extensive evidence suggesting that sugars were the most important dietary factor in the cause of dental caries and it was recommended that consumption of non-milk extrinsic sugars should be decreased.

It was considered that dietary sugars may contribute to the development of obesity, a condition which plays an important part in the aetiology of a number of diseases. For the majority of the population, who had normal plasma lipids and normal glucose tolerance, the consumption of sugars within the present range carried no special metabolic risks but those persons consuming more than about 200 g daily should replace the excess with starch. It was, however, recommended that those with special medical problems such as diabetes or hypertriglyceridaemia should restrict non-milk extrinsic sugar to less than about 20 to 50 g daily unless otherwise instructed by their own physician or dietitian. It was also concluded that current consumption of sugars, particularly sucrose, played no direct causal role in the development of cardiovascular (atherosclerotic coronary, peripheral, or cerebral vascular) disease, essential hypertension, or diabetes mellitus, and also had no significant specific effects on behaviour or psychological function. Although links between sucrose intake and certain other diseases (such as colorectal cancer, renal and biliary calculi, and Crohn's disease) had been proposed it was not felt that the evidence was adequate to justify any general dietary recommendations.

The conclusions of a joint FAO/WHO consultation on carbohydrates in human nutrition[2] were broadly in agreement with the above. However, they note that the terms intrinsic and extrinsic sugars have not gained wide acceptance, either in the UK or other countries in the world, and they recommended against the use of these terms.

1. DoH. Dietary sugars and human disease: report of the panel on dietary sugars of the committee on medical aspects of food policy. *Report on health and social subjects 37.* London: HMSO, 1989.
2. FAO/WHO. *Carbohydrates in human nutrition: report of a joint FAO/WHO expert consultation. FAO Food and Nutrition 66.* Rome: Food and Agriculture Organization of the United Nations, 1998.

Effects on the kidneys. Acute renal failure with severe hyponatraemia has been reported in one patient following the use of granulated sugar to treat an infected pneumonectomy wound cavity.[1] The authors noted that intravenous sucrose had long been known to be nephrotoxic in both animal models and man and considered that mild renal insufficiency before sucrose intoxication may have contributed to the nephrosis. A follow-up comment was, however, made that the nephrotoxicity may have been caused by gentamicin, a solution of which had been used to irrigate the cavity prior to packing the wound.[2]

1. Debure A, *et al.* Acute renal failure after use of granulated sugar in deep infected wound. *Lancet* 1987; **i:** 1034–5.
2. Archer H, *et al.* Toxicity of topical sugar. *Lancet* 1987; **i:** 1485–6.

Pharmacokinetics

Sucrose is hydrolysed in the small intestine by the enzyme sucrase to glucose and fructose, which are then absorbed. Sucrose is excreted unchanged in the urine when given intravenously.

Uses and Administration

Sucrose, a disaccharide, is used as a sweetening agent. It is commonly used as household sugar. If the sweetness of sucrose is taken as 100, fructose has a value of about 173, glucose 74, maltose 32, galactose 32, and lactose 16.

Sucrose is used as a tablet excipient and lozenge basis, and as a suspending and viscosity-increasing agent. Syrups prepared from concentrated solutions of sucrose form the basis of many linctuses.

Cough. Sucrose syrups are used as demulcents in linctuses used for treating cough (p.1052).

Diagnostic test for gastro-intestinal damage. Sucrose is not absorbed from the healthy gastro-intestinal tract. It has been proposed[1] that the absorption of sucrose could be used as a diagnostic test of gastro-intestinal damage.

1. Sutherland LR, *et al.* A simple non-invasive marker of gastric damage: sucrose permeability. *Lancet* 1994; **343:** 998–1000.

Gastro-intestinal spasm. For mention of a beneficial effect of sucrose solution in infantile colic, see p.1170.

Hiccup. Administration of a teaspoon of dry granulated sugar resulted in the immediate cessation of hiccup in 19 of 20 patients;[1] 12 of the patients had suffered from hiccup for less than 6 hours but in the remaining 8 persistent hiccup had been present for 24 hours to 6 weeks. The effect may be due to stimulation of the pharynx. A protocol for the treatment of intractable hiccup (p.655) suggests that swallowing dry granulated sugar is one of the first treatments that should be tried.

1. Engleman EG, *et al.* Granulated sugar as treatment for hiccups in conscious patients. *N Engl J Med* 1971; **285:** 1489.

Pain. A systematic review[1] concluded that sucrose solutions could reduce physiological and behavioural indicators of stress and pain in neonates undergoing painful procedures although there had been some doubt expressed[2] over whether this indicated effective analgesia. The review[1] was unable to determine an optimal dose, but 1 mL of a 25% solution or 2 mL of a 50% solution has been reported to reduce crying time in premature[3] and full-term[4] infants, respectively, when administered 2 minutes before heel prick sampling. Similarly, 2 mL of a 75% sucrose solution by mouth reduced crying time in infants receiving intramuscular vaccines.[5] For management of pain in infants and children, see p.7.

1. Stevens B, Ohlsson A. Sucrose in Neonates Undergoing Painful Procedures (updated 18 February 1998). Available in the Cochrane Library; Issue 3. Oxford: Update Software; 1998.
2. Anonymous. Pacifiers, passive behaviour, and pain. *Lancet* 1992; **339:** 275–6.
3. Ramenghi LA, *et al.* Reduction of pain response in premature infants using intraoral sucrose. *Arch Dis Child* 1996; **74:** F126–F128.
4. Haouari N, *et al.* The analgesic effect of sucrose in full term infants: a randomised controlled trial. *Br Med J* 1995; **310:** 1498–1500.
5. Lewindon PJ, *et al.* Randomised controlled trial of sucrose by mouth for the relief of infant crying after immunisation. *Arch Dis Child* 1998; **78:** 453–6.

Wound healing. Sugar, either in the form of granulated sugar[1,2] or pastes composed of caster sugar and icing sugar,[3,4] has been used successfully in the treatment of a variety of wounds (p.1076) including open mediastinitis after cardiac surgery,[1] large abscesses and bed sores,[3,4] and diabetic ulcers.[2] Debridement of the wound is believed to be due partly to the osmotic effect of sugar and partly to the mechanical cleansing action but it is not known how sugar stimulates granulation tissue to form.[3,4] Once granulation tissue is well established and the wound is shrinking, an alternative wound preparation, such as an alginate, hydrocolloid, or hydrogel, should be used as sugar pastes cause bleeding.[5] Sugar is also effective at deodorising malodorous wounds. The use of the combined caster and icing sugar pastes, of which details of the formulas used are provided in the original publications,[3,4] has been advocated as a way to overcome the problems of possible non-sterility and contamination of commercial granulated sugar.[3,4]

Honey (p.1345) has been used similarly.

1. Trouillet JL, *et al.* Use of granulated sugar in treatment of open mediastinitis after cardiac surgery. *Lancet* 1985; **ii:** 180–4.
2. Quatraro A, *et al.* Sugar and wound healing. *Lancet* 1985; **ii:** 664.
3. Gordon H, *et al.* Sugar and wound healing. *Lancet* 1985; **ii:** 663–4.
4. Middleton KR, Seal D. Sugar as an aid to wound healing. *Pharm J* 1985; **235:** 757–8.
5. Seal DV, Middleton K. Healing of cavity wounds with sugar. *Lancet* 1991; **338:** 571–2.

Preparations

BP 1998: Syrup *(Simple Syrup)*;
USNF 18: Compressible Sugar; Confectioner's Sugar; Sugar Spheres; Syrup.

Invert Sugar (661-v)

CAS — 8013-17-0.

Pharmacopoeias. Br. and *US* include preparations of invert sugar.

An equimolecular mixture of glucose and fructose which may be prepared by the hydrolysis of sucrose with a suitable mineral acid such as hydrochloric acid.

Invert sugar has similar actions and uses to those of glucose (p.1343) and fructose (p.1343). It has been used as a 5 and 10% solution as an alternative to glucose in parenteral nutrition but, as with fructose, such use cannot be recommended.

A syrup of invert sugar is used as a stabilising agent; when mixed with suitable proportions of sucrose-based syrup it will help to prevent crystallisation of the sucrose.

Preparations

BP 1998: Invert Syrup;
USP 23: Invert Sugar Injection; Multiple Electrolytes and Invert Sugar Injection Type 1; Multiple Electrolytes and Invert Sugar Injection Type 2; Multiple Electrolytes and Invert Sugar Injection Type 3.

Proprietary Preparations (details are given in Part 3)

Multi-ingredient: ***Norw.:*** Travert; ***S.Afr.:*** Emex; ***USA:*** Travert.

Thaumatin (12877-q)

Thaumatin *(BAN).*

E957; Katemfe.

CAS — 53850-34-3.

A mixture in the ratio of 2:1 of two polypeptides thaumatin I and thaumatin II, each consisting of 207 amino acid residues and having a molecular weight of about 22 000, derived from the fruit of *Thaumatococcus daniellii* (Scitamineae).

An odourless, cream-coloured, proteinaceous powder with an intensely sweet taste.

Thaumatin is a protein whose amino-acid range excludes histidine. It is an intense sweetener whose sweetness builds up gradually but persists for up to an hour, and is considered to be by far the sweetest of such compounds in use. It is used as a sweetener and flavour modifier in foods and drinks but is unstable to heat.

Threonine (662-g)

Threonine *(USAN, rINN).*

β-Methylserine; T; Thr; L-Threonine; Threoninum. L-2-Amino-3-hydroxybutyric acid.

$C_4H_9NO_3$ = 119.1.

CAS — 72-19-5.

Pharmacopoeias. In *Eur.* (see p.viii), *Jpn*, and *US.*

White crystalline powder or colourless to white odourless crystals. Freely **soluble** or soluble in water; practically insoluble in alcohol, in dehydrated alcohol, in chloroform, and in ether. A 2.5 or 5% solution in water has a pH of 5.0 to 6.5.

Threonine is an aliphatic amino acid which is an essential constituent of the diet. It is used as a dietary supplement.

Threonine has been investigated for the treatment of various spastic disorders.

Motor neurone disease. Threonine was shown to be ineffective[1] in motor neurone disease (p.1625).

1. Blin O, *et al.* A double-blind, placebo-controlled trial of L-threonine in amyotrophic lateral sclerosis. *J Neurol* 1992; **239:** 79–81.

Tyrosine (665-s)

Tyrosine *(USAN, rINN).*

Tyr; L-Tyrosine; Tyrosinum; Y. L-2-Amino-3-(4-hydroxyphenyl)propionic acid.

$C_9H_{11}NO_3$ = 181.2.

CAS — 60-18-4.

Pharmacopoeias. In *Eur.* (see p.viii) and *US.*

Colourless or white odourless crystals or crystalline powder. Very slightly **soluble** in water; practically insoluble in alcohol and in ether. It dissolves in dilute mineral acids and in dilute solutions of alkali hydroxides. **Protect** from light.

Tyrosine is an aromatic amino acid. It is used as a dietary supplement.

Phenylketonuria. Tyrosine was not an effective alternative to a diet low in phenylalanine in patients with phenylketonuria, see under Amino Acid Metabolic Disorders, p.1330.

Preparations

Proprietary Preparations (details are given in Part 3)

Multi-ingredient: ***Austral.:*** Aussie Tan Pre-Tan; ***Ger.:*** K_5 "spezial"†; ***UK:*** Amino MS; ***USA:*** Catemine.

Valine (666-w)

Valine *(USAN, rINN).*

α-Aminoisovaleric Acid; V; Val; L-Valine; Valinum. (S)-2-Amino-3-methylbutanoic acid.

$C_5H_{11}NO_2$ = 117.1.

CAS — 72-18-4.

Pharmacopoeias. In *Eur.* (see p.viii), *Jpn,* and *US.*

White or almost white, odourless crystalline powder or colourless crystals. **Soluble** in water; very slightly soluble or practically insoluble in alcohol; practically insoluble in acetone, and in ether. A 5% solution in water has a pH of 5.5 to 7.0. **Protect** from light.

Valine is a branched-chain amino acid which is an essential constituent of the diet. It is used as a dietary supplement. It is also an ingredient of several preparations that have been promoted for disorders of the liver.

Preparations

Proprietary Preparations (details are given in Part 3)

Ger.: Horm-Valin†.

Multi-ingredient: ***Fr.:*** Revitalose; ***Ger.:*** Bramin-hepa; Falkamin; Lactostrict†; ***Ital.:*** Falkamin; Isobranch; Isoram.

Vitamin A Substances (7823-k)

Antixerophthalmic Vitamin; Axerophtholum; Vitaminum A.

Pharmacopoeias. In *Eur.* (see p.viii) and *US.*

Chin. includes a monograph for the acetate. *Jpn* and *Pol.* include monographs for the acetate and the palmitate. *Br.* also includes a monograph for Natural Vitamin A Ester Concentrate. *Eur.* also includes monographs for Synthetic Vitamin A Concentrate (Oily Form) (Synthetic Retinol Concentrate (Oily Form)), Synthetic Vitamin A Concentrate (Powder Form) (Synthetic Retinol Concentrate (Powder Form)), and Synthetic Vitamin A Concentrate (Water-dispersible Form) (Synthetic Retinol Concentrate (Water-dispersible Form)).

Vitamin A (USP 23) may consist of retinol (vitamin A alcohol; $C_{20}H_{30}O$ = 286.5; *CAS*—68-26-8) or its esters formed from edible fatty acids, principally acetic and palmitic acids. It is a light yellow to red oil which may solidify upon refrigeration; practically odourless or with a mild fishy odour but no rancid odour or taste. In liquid form, it is **insoluble** in water and in glycerol; very soluble in chloroform and in ether; soluble in dehydrated alcohol and in vegetable oils. In solid form, may be dispersible in water. It may be diluted with edible oils or be incorporated in solid edible carriers or excipients, and may contain suitable antoxidants, dispersants, and antimicrobial agents. It should be **stored** in airtight containers, preferably under an atmosphere of inert gas. Protect from light.

Natural Vitamin A Ester Concentrate (BP 1998) consists of a natural ester or a mixture of natural esters of retinol or of a solution of the ester or mixture of esters in arachis oil or other suitable vegetable oil. It contains not less than 485 000 units of vitamin A per g. It is a yellow oil or mixture of oil and crystalline material with a faint odour. Practically **insoluble** in water; soluble or partly soluble in alcohol; miscible with chloroform, ether, or petroleum spirit. **Store** in airtight containers at 8° to 15°. Protect from light.

Synthetic Vitamin A Concentrate (Oily Form) (Ph. Eur.) (Synthetic Retinol Concentrate (Oily Form) (BP 1998)) consists of an ester or a mixture of esters of retinol (the acetate, propionate, or palmitate) prepared by synthesis. It may be diluted with a suitable vegetable oil. It contains not less than 500 000 units of vitamin A per g. It is a yellow to brownish yellow oily liquid; practically **insoluble** in water; soluble or partly soluble in dehydrated alcohol; miscible with organic solvents. **Store** at 8° to 15°. Protect from light.

Synthetic Vitamin A Concentrate (Powder Form) (Ph. Eur.) (Synthetic Retinol Concentrate (Powder Form) (BP 1998)) is again an ester or mixture of esters of retinol (the acetate, propionate, or palmitate) prepared by synthesis and dispersed in a matrix of gelatin or acacia or other suitable material. It contains not less than 250 000 units of vitamin A per g. It is a yellowish powder. Practically **insoluble** in water or may swell or form an emulsion, depending on formulation. **Store** in airtight containers at 8° to 15°. Protect from light.

Synthetic Vitamin A Concentrate (Water-dispersible Form) (Ph. Eur.) (Synthetic Retinol Concentrate (Water-dispersible Form) (BP 1998)) consists of an ester or a mixture of esters of retinol (the acetate, propionate, or palmitate) prepared by synthesis to which suitable solubilisers have been added. It contains not less than 100 000 units of vitamin A per g. It is a yellow or yellowish liquid of variable opalescence and viscosity. **Store** in airtight containers. Protect from light.

Stability. The compatibility and stability of components of total parenteral nutrition solutions have been reviewed.[1,2] Retinol is known to be rapidly broken down by exposure to ultraviolet light, and daylight causes rapid degradation. Covering the bag reduces or prevents degradation, depending on the effectiveness of the cover although simple shading on the side of the bag nearest to the daylight can be beneficial. However, up to 50% of the vitamin can be degraded during passage through the administration set. It has been shown that the presence of amino acids offers some protection and the presence of a fat emulsion affords considerable protection.

A number of studies have shown that vitamin A binds to plastics, especially polyvinyl chloride. It is now clear that sorption to bags and administration sets depends on the ester used. While the acetate ester is strongly bound, the palmitate shows little or no tendency to adsorb to polyvinyl chloride. It must be concluded that vitamin A losses will occur during parenteral nutrition, although not during storage in the refrigerator if light-protected.

A study of essential drugs shipped by Unicef to the tropics[3] found that the elevated temperatures in transit reduced the activity of retinol capsules by 1.5%, but this was considered of no medical or practical significance.

1. Allwood MC. Compatibility and stability of TPN mixtures in big bags. *J Clin Hosp Pharm* 1984; **9:** 181–98.
2. Niemiec PW, Vanderveen TW. Compatibility considerations in parenteral nutrient solutions. *Am J Hosp Pharm* 1984; **41:** 893–911.
3. Hogerzeil HV, *et al.* Stability of essential drugs during shipment to the tropics. *Br Med J* 1992; **304:** 210–14.

Units

The International Standards for vitamin A and for provitamin A were discontinued in 1954 and 1956 respectively but the International units for these substances have continued to be widely used. In 1960–1, the WHO Expert Committee on Biological Standardization stated that the International unit for vitamin A is equivalent to the activity of 0.000344 mg of pure all-*trans* vitamin A acetate and the International unit for provitamin A is equivalent to the activity of 0.0006 mg of pure all-*trans* β-carotene.

The activity of one International unit is contained in 0.0003 mg of all-*trans* retinol, in 0.00055 mg of all-*trans* retinol palmitate, and in 0.000359 mg of all-*trans* retinol propionate.

The USP unit is defined as the specific biologic activity of 0.0003 mg of the all-*trans* isomer of retinol, and is equivalent to the International unit.

Vitamin A activity in foods is currently expressed in terms of retinol equivalents: 1 retinol equivalent is defined as 1 μg of all-*trans* retinol, 6 μg of all-*trans* beta carotene, or 12 μg of other provitamin A carotenoids.

Adverse Effects and Precautions

The administration of excessive amounts of vitamin A substances over long periods can lead to toxicity, known as hypervitaminosis A. This is characterised by fatigue, irritability, anorexia and loss of weight, vomiting and other gastro-intestinal disturbances, low-grade fever, hepatosplenomegaly, skin changes (yellowing, dryness, sensitivity to sunlight), alopecia, dry hair, cracking and bleeding lips, anaemia, headache, hypercalcaemia, subcutaneous swelling, nocturia, and pains in bones and joints. Symptoms of chronic toxicity may also include raised intracranial pressure and papilloedema mimicking brain tumours, tinnitus, visual disturbances which may be severe, and painful swelling over the long bones. Symptoms usually clear on withdrawal of vitamin A, but in children premature closure of the epiphyses of the long bones may result in arrested bone growth.

Acute vitamin A intoxication may occur with very high doses and is characterised by sedation, dizziness, nausea and vomiting, erythema, pruritus, desquamation, and increased intracranial pressure (resulting in bulging fontanelle in infants).

Hypervitaminosis A does not appear to be a problem with large doses of carotenoids (see Pharmacokinetics under Betacarotene, p.1335).

Enhanced susceptibility to the effects of vitamin A may be seen in children and in patients with liver disease.

Excessive doses of vitamin A should be avoided in pregnancy because of potential teratogenic effects; for further details see Pregnancy, below.

Gastro-intestinal absorption of vitamin A may be impaired in cholestatic jaundice and fat-malabsorption conditions.

Benign intracranial hypertension. High doses of vitamin A cause increased intracranial pressure, and, in infants, this is manifested as bulging of the fontanelle. In one study,[1] 11.5% of infants receiving 3 doses of 50 000 units of vitamin A at monthly intervals had bulging fontanelle, compared with 1% of infants receiving placebo. The bulging lasted between 24 and 72 hours and subsided without treatment,[1] and did not appear to be associated with any physical or developmental abnormalities on long-term follow-up.[2] In another study in neonates, bulging fontanelle occurred in 4.6% of recipients of vitamin A 50 000 units and 2.7% of placebo recipients 24 hours after administration.[3]

1. de Francisco A, *et al.* Acute toxicity of vitamin A given with vaccines in infancy. *Lancet* 1993; **342:** 526–7.
2. van Dillen J, *et al.* Long-term effect of vitamin A with vaccines. *Lancet* 1996; **347:** 107.
3. Agoestina T, *et al.* Safety of one 52 μmol (50 000 IU) oral dose of vitamin A administered to neonates. *Bull WHO* 1994; **72:** 859–68.

Carcinogenicity. For mention of the *increased* risk of lung cancer in high-risk individuals receiving betacarotene and vitamin A, when compared with placebo, in a study investigating vitamins in lung cancer prevention, see Prophylaxis of Malignant Neoplasms, p.1333.

Effects on the blood. Normochromic macrocytic anaemia developed in a patient who had been receiving vitamin A 150 000 IU daily by mouth for several months.[1] The patient's haemoglobin returned to normal when vitamin A was discontinued, and the accompanying symptoms of perioral dermatitis and glossitis also disappeared.

1. White JM. Vitamin-A-induced anaemia. *Lancet* 1984; **ii:** 573.

Effects on the immune system. Vitamin A deficiency is generally associated with impaired immunity, and treatment of deficiency results in reductions in morbidity and mortality from a number of infectious diseases (see below). However, a few studies have shown increased prevalence of diarrhoea and/or respiratory tract infections with high doses of vitamin A. There is a possibility that high single doses of vitamin A may temporarily attenuate the immune response in non-deficient children.[1] For mention that high-dose vitamin A supplements have been associated with a reduced response to measles vaccine in some studies, see p.1518.

1. Anonymous. Childhood morbidity, immunity and micronutrients. *WHO Drug Inf* 1996; **10:** 12–16.

Effects on the liver. Vitamin A is stored in the Dissë space of liver cells and excess administration can lead to fibrosis and obstruction of sinusoidal blood flow, causing non-cirrhotic portal hypertension and hepatocellular dysfunction.[1] Although hepatotoxicity has typically been reported with habitual ingestion of doses of vitamin A greater than 50 000 units daily, a case of severe hepatic fibrosis, with jaundice and hepatomegaly, has been reported in a patient who had been taking 25 000 units daily for at least 6 years in a multivitamin supplement.[2]

1. Sherlock S. The spectrum of hepatotoxicity due to drugs. *Lancet* 1986; **ii:** 440–4.
2. Kowalski TE, *et al.* Vitamin A hepatotoxicity: a cautionary note regarding 25,000 IU supplements. *Am J Med* 1994; **97:** 523–8.

Hypersensitivity. Local inflammatory reactions and severe anaphylactoid reactions have occurred in patients receiving vitamin A injections, and are usually attributed to solubilisers such as polyoxyl castor oils (p.1327), and, less commonly, polysorbates (p.1328).

A case of cutaneous hypersensitivity to retinol palmitate, and not other injection ingredients, has been described.[1]

1. Shelley WB, *et al.* Hypersensitivity to retinol palmitate injection. *Br Med J* 1995; **311:** 232.

Pregnancy. The fact that synthetic vitamin A derivatives such as isotretinoin are teratogenic (p.1085) has prompted concern about the potential teratogenicity of high doses of vitamin A.

A prospective cohort study found that a total daily intake of vitamin A from all sources of greater than 15 000 units during early pregnancy was associated with a significantly increased risk of birth defects of structures arising from the cranial neural crest.[1] When vitamin A intake from supplements was analysed separately, an apparent vitamin A threshold dose for the development of birth defects of 10 000 units daily was suggested. However, this study has been criticised[2,3] and some suggest the data allows for a higher threshold dose.[3] A further study found no significant difference in birth defect rates between women consuming greater than 8000 or 10 000 units of vitamin A daily in the period around conception (as supplements and fortified cereals) and those consuming less than 5000 units daily.[4]

Following earlier case reports in the USA suggesting that large doses of vitamin A (equivalent to about ten times the daily recommended dietary allowance of 2250 units) taken in early pregnancy may cause birth defects, the UK Chief Medical Officer cautioned women against the use of vitamin A supplements except under medical supervision.[5] Additionally, advice was given that liver or liver products should not be eaten because high concentrations of vitamin A had been detected in some samples of animal liver. Concern has been expressed that the avoidance of liver or liver products may result in inadequate nutrition in some and that a less alarmist view may have been to suggest a limitation on intake rather than total prohibition.[6,7]

The American College of Obstetricians and Gynecologists has recommended that women who are pregnant or planning pregnancy should ensure that any vitamin supplements they take contain a daily dose of vitamin A of no more than 5000 units.[8] The Australian Adverse Drug Reactions Advisory Committee has advised women in this category to avoid vitamin A supplements and to not exceed the recommended daily allowance of 2500 units from all sources.[9]

1. Rothman KJ, *et al.* Teratogenicity of high vitamin A intake. *N Engl J Med* 1995; **333:** 1369–73.
2. Werler MM, *et al.* Teratogenicity of high vitamin A intake. *N Engl J Med* 1996; **334:** 1195–6.
3. Watkins M, *et al.* Teratogenicity of high vitamin A intake. *N Engl J Med* 1996; **334:** 1196.
4. Mills JL, *et al.* Vitamin A and birth defects. *Am J Obstet Gynecol* 1997; **177:** 31–6.
5. Department of Health. *Women cautioned: watch your vitamin A intake.* London: Department of Health, 1990 (18 October).
6. Nelson M. Vitamin A, liver consumption, and risk of birth defects. *Br Med J* 1990; **301:** 1176.
7. Sanders TAB. Vitamin A and pregnancy. *Lancet* 1990; **336:** 1375.
8. American College of Obstetricians and Gynecologists. Vitamin A supplementation during pregnancy. *Int J Gynecol Obstet* 1993; **40:** 175.
9. Adverse Drug Reactions Advisory Committee. Vitamin A and birth defects. *Aust Adverse Drug React Bull* 1996; **15:** 14–15.

Interactions

Absorption of vitamin A from the gastro-intestinal tract may be reduced by the presence of neomycin, cholestyramine, or liquid paraffin.

There is an increased risk of hypervitaminosis A if vitamin A is coadministered with synthetic retinoids such as acitretin, isotretinoin, and tretinoin.

There is conflicting evidence regarding the effect of vitamin A on the response to measles vaccine (see p.1518).

Pharmacokinetics

Vitamin A substances are readily absorbed from the gastro-intestinal tract but absorption may be reduced in the presence of fat malabsorption, low protein intake, or impaired liver or pancreatic function. Vitamin A esters are hydrolysed by pancreatic enzymes to retinol, which is then absorbed and re-esterified. Some retinol is stored in the liver. It is released from the liver bound to a specific α_1-globulin (retinol-binding protein) in the blood. The retinol not stored in the liver undergoes glucuronide conjugation and subsequent oxidation to retinal and retinoic acid; these and other metabolites are excreted in urine and faeces. Vitamin A does not readily diffuse across the placenta (but see Pregnancy, above), but is present in breast milk.

References.

1. Hartmann D, *et al.* Pharmacokinetic modelling of the plasma concentration-time profile of the vitamin retinyl palmitate following intramuscular administration. *Biopharm Drug Dispos* 1990; **11:** 689–700.

Human Requirements

Dietary vitamin A is derived from 2 sources, *preformed retinoids* from animal sources such as liver, kidney, dairy produce, and eggs (fish-liver oils are the most concentrated natural source), and *provitamin carotenoids* which can be obtained from many plants; these are converted to retinol in the body but are less effectively utilised. Carotenes (α, β, and γ) are major sources and of these, β-carotene (beta-carotene—see p.1335) has the highest vitamin A activity and is the most plentiful in food. Variable amounts of β-carotenes are found in carrots and dark green or yellow vegetables. Red palm oil is a good source of α- and β-carotenes.

In the United Kingdom dietary reference values (see p.1332) have been published[1] for vitamin A and similarly in the United States recommended daily allowances have been set.[2] Differing amounts are recommended for infants and children of varying ages, for adult males and females, and for pregnant and lactating women (but see Pregnancy, above). In the UK the reference nutrient intake (RNI) for adult males and females is 700 and 600 μg retinol equivalents (approximately 2330 and 2000 units) daily, respectively and the estimated average requirement (EAR) is 500 and 400 μg retinol equivalents (approximately 1660 and 1330 units) daily, respectively. This UK report[1] also highlighted the toxicity associated with large doses of vitamin A and recommended that regular intakes should not exceed 9000 μg (30 000 units) daily in adult men and 7500 μg (25 000 units) daily in adult women. Figures were also given for infants and children who were said to be more sensitive to the effects of vitamin A. These limits did not apply to therapeutic doses of vitamin A used under medical supervision.[1] In pregnancy the RNI is 700 μg retinol equivalents (2330 units) daily and in nursing mothers 950 μg (3160 units) daily. In the USA the allowances for adult males and females are 1000 and 800 μg retinol equivalents (approximately 3330 and 2660 units) daily, respectively.[2]

1. DoH. Dietary reference values for food energy and nutrients for the United Kingdom: report of the panel on dietary reference values of the committee on medical aspects of food policy. *Report on health and social subjects 41.* London: HMSO, 1991.
2. Subcommittee on the tenth edition of the RDAs, Food and Nutrition Board, Commission on Life Sciences, National Research Council. *Recommended dietary allowances.* 10th ed. Washington, DC: National Academy Press, 1989.

Uses and Administration

Vitamin A, a fat-soluble vitamin, is essential for growth, for the development and maintenance of epithelial tissue, and for vision, particularly in dim light. Vitamin A deficiency develops when the dietary intake is inadequate and is seen more frequently in young children than in adults. It is rare in developed countries but remains a major problem in many developing countries. Prolonged deficiency leads to xerophthalmia or "dry eye", the initial symptom of which is night blindness which may progress to severe eye lesions and blindness. Other symptoms include changes in the skin and mucous membranes.

Vitamin A is used in the treatment and prevention of vitamin A deficiency. It may be administered by mouth in an oil- or water-based form, the oil-based generally being the preferred type. It can also be administered by intramuscular injection of a water-miscible form; oil-miscible preparations of vitamin A are poorly absorbed from injection sites following intramuscular injection and are not usually used for administration by this route. For further details concerning vitamin A supplementation, including doses for the treatment and prophylaxis of xerophthalmia, see under Deficiency States, below.

Vitamin A supplements are often given to patients with primary biliary cirrhosis or chronic cholestatic liver disease as deficiencies are common in these disorders. An intramuscular dose of 10 000 units every 2 to 4 months has been suggested.

Vitamins A and D have been used together as cream or ointment in the treatment of minor skin disorders including abrasions. Vitamin A has also been used alone to treat various skin disorders including acne and psoriasis. It has been tried in patients with retinitis pigmentosa to retard the decline in retinal function.

Deficiency states. Vitamin A deficiency is relatively rare in developed countries and is usually only seen in certain medical conditions such as biliary cirrhosis or cholestatic jaundice. However, it is a continuing problem in many developing countries and children appear to be particularly vulnerable.

In the developing countries where dietary intake may often be less than desirable, infections such as measles, acute respiratory diseases, and diarrhoea can be major precipitating factors of vitamin A deficiency. Thus WHO have targeted elimination of vitamin A deficiency as an important strategy in child health,[1,2] and as part of the Expanded Programme on Immunization. They recommend the use of vitamin A supplements in the treatment of vitamin A deficiency (see Xerophthalmia, below) and to prevent vitamin A deficiency where the periodic administration of supplements is determined to be the most feasible and effective method of improving vitamin A status. In universal distribution programmes,[2] supplemental doses are given to all preschool-age children at a dose of 200 000 units every 4 to 6 months, with infants between the ages of 6 and 12 months receiving half this dose. Infants aged less than 6 months may receive 50 000 units if they are not breast fed or if they are breast fed and their mothers have not received supplemental vitamin A. Mothers in high-risk regions should receive 200 000 units within 8 weeks of delivery of a child. Targeted distribution programmes involve vitamin A supplementation to children and pregnant women in specific high-risk areas.[2] Doses used in children are similar to those used in universal programmes, but doses used in pregnant women should not exceed 10 000 units daily, or 25 000 units weekly.

A number of studies have indicated that general supplementation with vitamin A decreases both mortality rates and morbidity among children in developing countries with a high prevalence of vitamin A deficiency.[3-6] Although not all studies have confirmed these findings,[7,8] two meta-analyses concur that the effect is likely to be genuine especially as regards measles infection,[9,10] and researchers and commentators have agreed that overall improvement of vitamin A status is worthwhile and necessary.[7,11] Some studies have evaluated mortality specifically in infants less than 6 months of age. In one study there was no overall benefit on early infant mortality with a tendency for the relative risk of mortality to increase with improved nutritional status,[12] whereas another reported a decrease in mortality in the first year of life.[13] A study in vitamin-A-deficient children has demonstrated abnormalities in T-cell subsets which are corrected by vitamin A supplementation,[14] and it has been proposed that the apparent effects of vitamin A on morbidity and mortality may be due to modulation of immune function (see also above). In countries in which vitamin A deficiency is not widespread some form of supplementation may still be considered. In the UK, the Department of Health has recommended routine supplementation with 700 units of vitamin A daily, together with ascorbic acid and vitamin D, in children aged 6 months to 2 years, or preferably up to 5 years of age, particularly in winter and early spring; some infants from 1 month of age may also benefit.

Anaemia. There has been a study among pregnant Indonesian women with nutritional anaemia that demonstrated a beneficial effect for vitamin A on haemoglobin when given with iron supplementation.[15]

Diarrhoea. Several of the large mortality trials already mentioned reported that vitamin A supplementation was associated with reduced mortality attributed to diarrhoea,[4-6] but one did not.[7] The effect on morbidity from diarrhoea is even less clear. A reduction in the severity, but not the incidence, of diarrhoea has been noted in two studies.[16,17] However, in one study in children with subclinical vitamin A deficiency, there was an increased prevalence of diarrhoea for 2 weeks after vitamin A supplementation,[18] and in another study, vitamin A increased the incidence of diarrhoea in children aged less than 30 months.[19]

Measles. Vitamin A supplementation has an important role in the prevention of complications from measles.[9,10] Two studies specifically addressing vitamin A status and measles have found that complications such as pneumonia and diarrhoea were less common in children who had received supplements at the time of diagnosis than in those given a placebo.[20,21] There is thus now a body of opinion supporting the view that vitamin A supplements in doses of 200 000[22] or 400 000[23] units should be given to children in developing countries with clinical measles. Studies in the USA have indicated that even among well-nourished children from a developed country, vitamin A deficiency in measles patients is not uncommon,[24,25] and vitamin A supplementation needs to be considered in children at risk.[26]

Respiratory-tract infections. The mortality trials mentioned did not show a consistent impact for vitamin A supplementation on death from non-measles-related respiratory infections.[4-6] Similarly, other studies have found no benefit of vitamin A on subsequent respiratory morbidity.[16,17,27] A meta-analysis of trials reporting pneumonia morbidity and mortality found no overall benefit or harm from vitamin A supplementation.[28] However, an increased prevalence of symptoms of respiratory infections associated with vitamin A supplementation has been noted in two studies,[18,19] particularly in children with adequate nutritional status.

Vitamin A was not effective for the treatment of childhood non-measles-related lower respiratory-tract infections[29] or pneumonia.[30] Similarly, there was no benefit from vitamin A in the treatment of respiratory syncytial virus infection in children in two studies.[31,32] In one of these studies there was a tendency for vitamin A to improve outcomes in the subgroup of severely ill children,[31] and in the other there was a slight increase in duration of hospitalisation in low-risk children receiving vitamin A.[32]

Shigellosis. A single high-dose vitamin A supplement reduced the severity of acute shigellosis in children in Bangladesh.[33]

Xerophthalmia. Vitamin A deficiency is responsible in many developing countries for visual problems which may culminate in xerophthalmia and blindness. Supplementation with vitamin A as recommended by WHO and discussed above will raise the vitamin A status of the individual and act prophylactically against the development of xerophthalmia. For the treatment of xerophthalmia (which includes night blindness, conjunctival xerosis with Bitot's spots, corneal xerosis, corneal ulceration, and keratomalacia) WHO have stated that oral doses of vitamin A, preferably in an oil-based preparation, are the treatment of choice and should be given immediately the disorder is recognised.[2] All patients over 1 year of age (with the exception of women of reproductive age, see below) should receive 200 000 units by mouth immediately on diagnosis; infants aged 6 to 12 months should receive 100 000 units, and those aged less than 6 months, 50 000 units. The dose should be repeated the next day, and again at least 2 weeks later. In women of reproductive age there is a need to balance the possible teratogenic effects of vitamin A should they be pregnant (see above) with the serious consequences of xerophthalmia. WHO recommend that when there are severe signs of active xerophthalmia (i.e. acute corneal lesions) high dose vitamin A treatment should be given as described above for those aged over 1 year. When only less severe signs are present (night blindness, Bitot's spots), women of reproductive age should receive a daily oral dose of 5000 to 10 000 units for at least 4 weeks. Alternatively, a weekly dose of not more than 25 000 units may be substituted.

Although xerophthalmia is far less common in developed countries, vitamin A deficiency should be considered in all patients with recurrent conjunctival or corneal disorders associated with gastro-intestinal or liver disease.[34]

1. Potter AR. Reducing vitamin A deficiency. *Br Med J* 1997; **314:** 317–18.
2. WHO/UNICEF/IVACG Task Force. *Vitamin A supplements: a guide to their use in the treatment and prevention of vitamin A deficiency and xerophthalmia*. 2nd ed. Geneva: WHO, 1997.
3. Rahmathullah L, *et al*. Reduced mortality among children in southern India receiving a small weekly dose of vitamin A. *N Engl J Med* 1990; **323:** 929–35.
4. West KP, *et al*. Efficacy of vitamin A in reducing preschool child mortality in Nepal. *Lancet* 1991; **338:** 67–71.
5. Daulaire NMP, *et al*. Childhood mortality after a high dose of vitamin A in a high risk population. *Br Med J* 1992; **304:** 207–10.
6. Ghana VAST Study Team. Vitamin A supplementation in northern Ghana: effects on clinic attendances, hospital admissions, and child mortality. *Lancet* 1993; **342:** 7–12.
7. Vijayaraghavan K, *et al*. Effect of massive dose of vitamin A on morbidity and mortality in Indian children. *Lancet* 1990; **336:** 1342–5.
8. Herrera MG, *et al*. Vitamin A supplementation and child survival. *Lancet* 1992; **340:** 267–71.
9. Glasziou PP, Mackerras DEM. Vitamin A supplementation in infectious diseases: a meta-analysis. *Br Med J* 1993; **306:** 366–70.
10. Fawzi WW, *et al*. Vitamin A supplementation and child mortality: a meta-analysis. *JAMA* 1993; **269:** 898–903.
11. Anonymous. Vitamin A and malnutrition/infection complex in developing countries. *Lancet* 1990; **336:** 1349–51.
12. West KP, *et al*. Mortality of infants <6 mo of age supplemented with vitamin A: a randomized double-masked trial in Nepal. *Am J Clin Nutr* 1995; **62:** 143–8.
13. Humphrey JH, *et al*. Impact of neonatal vitamin A supplementation on infant morbidity and mortality. *J Pediatr* 1996; **128:** 489–96.
14. Semba RD, *et al*. Abnormal T-cell subset proportions in vitamin-A-deficient children. *Lancet* 1993; **341:** 5–8.
15. Suharno D, *et al*. Supplementation with vitamin A and iron for nutritional anaemia in pregnant women in West Java, Indonesia. *Lancet* 1993; **342:** 1325–8.
16. Barreto ML, *et al*. Effect of vitamin A supplementation on diarrhoea and acute lower-respiratory-tract infections in young children in Brazil. *Lancet* 1994; **344:** 228–31.
17. Bhandari N, *et al*. Impact of massive dose of vitamin A given to preschool children with acute diarrhoea on subsequent respiratory and diarrhoeal morbidity. *Br Med J* 1994; **309:** 1404–7.
18. Stansfield SK, *et al*. Vitamin A supplementation and increased prevalence of childhood diarrhoea and acute respiratory infections. *Lancet* 1993; **342:** 578–82.
19. Dibley MJ, *et al*. Vitamin A supplementation fails to reduce incidence of acute respiratory illness and diarrhea in preschool-age Indonesian children. *J Nutr* 1996; **126:** 434–42.
20. Barclay AJG, *et al*. Vitamin A supplements and mortality related to measles: a randomised clinical trial. *Br Med J* 1987; **294:** 294–6.
21. Hussey GD, Klein M. A randomized, controlled trial of vitamin A in children with severe measles. *N Engl J Med* 1990; **323:** 160–4.
22. Toole MJ, *et al*. Measles prevention and control in emergency settings. *Bull WHO* 1989; **67:** 381–8.
23. Chan M. Vitamin A and measles in third world children. *Br Med J* 1990; **301:** 1230–1.
24. Arrieta AC, *et al*. Vitamin A levels in children with measles in Long Beach, California. *J Pediatr* 1992; **121:** 75–8.
25. Butler JC, *et al*. Measles severity and serum retinol (vitamin A) concentration among children in the United States. *Pediatrics* 1993; **91:** 1176–81.
26. Committee on Infectious Diseases of the American Academy of Pediatrics. Vitamin A treatment of measles. *Pediatrics* 1993; **91:** 1014–15.
27. Kartasasmita CB, *et al*. Plasma retinol level, vitamin A supplementation and acute respiratory infections in children of 1-5 years old in a developing country. *Tubercle Lung Dis* 1995; **76:** 563–9.
28. The Vitamin A and Pneumonia Working Group. Potential interventions for the prevention of childhood pneumonia in developing countries: a meta-analysis of data from field trials to assess the impact of vitamin A supplementation on pneumonia morbidity and mortality. *Bull WHO* 1995; **73:** 609–19.
29. Kjolhede CL, *et al*. Clinical trial of vitamin A as adjuvant treatment for lower respiratory tract infections. *J Pediatr* 1995; **126:** 807–12.
30. Nacul LC, *et al*. Randomised, double blind, placebo controlled clinical trial of efficacy of vitamin A treatment in non-measles childhood pneumonia. *Br Med J* 1997; **315:** 505–10.
31. Dowell SF, *et al*. Treatment of respiratory syncytial virus infection with vitamin A: a randomized placebo-controlled trial in Santiago, Chile. *Pediatr Infect Dis J* 1996; **15:** 782–6.
32. Bresee JS, *et al*. Vitamin A therapy for children with respiratory syncytial virus infection: a multicenter trial in the United States. *Pediatr Infect Dis J* 1996; **15:** 777–82.
33. Hossain S, *et al*. Single dose vitamin A treatment in acute shigellosis in Bangladeshi children: randomised double blind controlled trial. *Br Med J* 1998; **316:** 422–6.
34. Watson NJ, *et al*. Vitamin A deficiency and xerophthalmia in the United Kingdom. *Br Med J* 1995; **310:** 1050–1. Correction. *ibid.*: 1320.

HIV infection and AIDS. A study in Malawi found that the rates of vertical transmission of HIV infection (birth of seropositive infants to seropositive mothers) were inversely related to maternal vitamin A status;[1] vitamin A deficiency during pregnancy was associated with a threefold to fourfold increased risk of mother-to-child transmission of HIV. This was not incompatible with the role of vitamin A in immunity and maintenance of mucosal surfaces, and since both HIV infection and pregnancy are risk factors for vitamin A deficiency, it was suggested that nutritional intervention to reduce vitamin A deficiency might help combat mother-to-child transmission. However, another study[2] in Tanzania, for which vertical transmission data are not yet available, found no evidence of an effect of vitamin A on birth outcomes in HIV-infected women and the authors pointed out that serum concentrations of vitamin A might be a marker of the stage of HIV disease rather than being causally related to outcome. The study did however find that multivitamin supplements reduced the risk of low birthweight and size for age, and of premature birth, in the offspring of these women.[2] Means of reducing the risk of HIV infection in neonates (see HIV Infection Prophylaxis, p.601) are of considerable interest.

1. Semba RD, *et al*. Maternal vitamin A deficiency and mother-to-child transmission of HIV-1. *Lancet* 1994; **343:** 1593–7.
2. Fawzi WW, *et al*. Randomised trial of effects of vitamin supplements on pregnancy outcomes and T-cell counts in HIV-1-infected women in Tanzania. *Lancet* 1998; **351:** 1477–82.

Malignant neoplasms. Epidemiological studies suggest that antoxidant vitamins such as the vitamin A substances may play a role in preventing the development of malignancy but there is currently little evidence from prospective studies to support this (see p.1333). Conversely, synthetic retinoids such as tretinoin (all-*trans*-retinoic acid) have an established role in treating some cancers (see p.1094).

Retinitis pigmentosa. Retinitis pigmentosa is the name applied to a group of slowly progressive hereditary degenerative diseases of the retina that often results in blindness in adulthood. The rod and cone photoreceptors in the retina are primarily affected and initial symptoms include night blindness and intolerance to light. Later signs include infiltration of pigment from the retinal pigmentary epithelium into the retinal layers. Various treatments have been tried but none appear to have any proven benefit. Results of one large double-blind study[1] suggest that whereas treatment with vitamin A might slow the decline in visual acuity treatment with vitamin E appears to have a deleterious effect on the rate of decline. In 3 patients with retinitis pigmentosa and a defect in α-tocopherol-transfer protein associated with vitamin E deficiency, vitamin E administration did appear to delay the rate of vision decline.[2] Transplantation of the retina is being investigated as a treatment for retinitis pigmentosa.[3]

1. Berson EL, *et al*. A randomized trial of vitamin A and vitamin E supplementation for retinitis pigmentosa. *Arch Ophthalmol* 1993; **111:** 761–2.
2. Yokota T, *et al*. Retinitis pigmentosa and ataxia caused by a mutation in the gene for the α-tocopherol-transfer protein. *N Engl J Med* 1996; **335:** 1770–1.
3. Anonymous. Transplantation as a therapy for retinitis pigmentosa? *Br J Ophthalmol* 1997; **81:** 430.

Preparations

BPC 1973: Vitamins A and D Capsules; Vitamins Capsules; ***USP 23:*** Oil- and Water-soluble Vitamins Capsules; Oil- and Water-soluble Vitamins Oral Solution; Oil- and Water-soluble Vitamins Tablets; Oil-soluble Vitamins Capsules; Oil-soluble Vitamins Tablets; Oleovitamin A and D; Oleovitamin A and D Capsules; Vitamin A Capsules.

Proprietary Preparations (details are given in Part 3)
Aust.: Arcavit A; Avitol; Oleovit A; ***Austral.:*** Dermalife; Micelle A†; ***Belg.:*** Acaren†; Arovit†; Dagravit A; ***Canad.:*** A-Mulsion; Aquasol A†; Arovit; ***Fr.:*** A 313; Arovit; Avibon; ***Ger.:*** A-Mulsin; A-Vicotrat; Oculotect; Ophtol-A; Ophtosan; Solan-M; Vitadral; ***Ital.:*** Akeral†; Amirale†; Arovit; Avitina†; Euvitol; Idrurto A†; Primavit†; Repervit; Vit-A-N; ***Neth.:*** Dagravit A Forte; ***S.Afr.:*** Arovit; ***Spain:*** Arovit†; Auxina A Masiva; Biominol A; Dif Vitamin A Masivo; Ido A 50†; Ledovit A†; Mulsal A Megadosis; Rinocusi Vitaminico; ***Swed.:*** Arovit; ***Switz.:*** Arovit; Axerol†; Oculotect; ***UK:*** Biovit-A; Ro-A-Vit; ***USA:*** Aquasol A; Del-Vi-A; Palmitate-A 5000; Pedi-Vit-A; Retinol-A; Vit-A-Drops.

Multi-ingredient: numerous preparations are listed in Part 3.

Vitamin B Substances (17537-b)

The B vitamin group includes the B_1 substances (thiamine and its derivatives), B_2 (riboflavine), B_6 (pyridoxine and derivatives), and B_{12} (the cobalamins). In addition, nicotinic acid and its derivatives (p.1351) and folic acid (p.1340) are held to be part of the group, as is pantothenic acid (p.1352), but these latter substances are not generally referred to by their traditional B nomenclature.

Vitamin B_1 Substances (14738-l)

Acetiamine Hydrochloride (12309-r)

Acetiamine Hydrochloride (*rINNM*).

Acethiamine Hydrochloride; Diacethiamine Hydrochloride. *N*-(5-Acetoxy-3-acetylthiopent-2-en-2-yl)-*N*-(4-amino-2-methylpyrimidin-5-ylmethyl)formamide hydrochloride monohydrate.

$C_{16}H_{22}N_4O_4S,HCl,H_2O$ = 420.9.
CAS — 299-89-8 (acetiamine).

Benfotiamine (7831-k)

Benfotiamine (*rINN*).

S-Benzoylthiamine *O*-Monophosphate. *N*-(4-Amino-2-methylpyrimidin-5-ylmethyl)-*N*-(2-benzoylthio-4-dihydroxyphosphinyloxy-1-methylbut-1-enyl)formamide.

$C_{19}H_{23}N_4O_6PS$ = 466.4.
CAS — 22457-89-2.

Bisbentiamine (7832-a)

Bisbentiamine (*rINN*).

O-Benzoylthiamine Disulphide. *NN'*-{Dithiobis[2-(2-benzoyloxyethyl)-1-methylvinylene]}bis[*N*-(4-amino-2-methylpyrimidin-5-ylmethyl)formamide].

$C_{38}H_{42}N_8O_6S_2$ = 770.9.
CAS — 2667-89-2.

Cycotiamine (7837-d)

Cycotiamine (*rINN*).

CCT; Cyclocarbothiamine. *N*-(4-Amino-2-methylpyrimidin-5-ylmethyl)-*N*-[1-(2-oxo-1,3-oxathian-4-ylidene)ethyl]formamide.

$C_{13}H_{16}N_4O_3S$ = 308.4.
CAS — 6092-18-8.

Fursultiamine (7838-n)

Fursultiamine (*rINN*).

Thiamine Tetrahydrofurfuryl Disulphide; TTFD. *N*-(4-Amino-2-methylpyrimidin-5-ylmethyl)-*N*-[4-hydroxy-1-methyl-2-(tetrahydrofurfuryldithio)but-1-enyl]formamide.

$C_{17}H_{26}N_4O_3S_2$ = 398.5.
CAS — 804-30-8.

Octotiamine (7839-h)

Octotiamine (*rINN*).

TATD; Thioctothiamine. *N*-[2-(3-Acetylthio-7-methoxycarbonylheptyldithio)-4-hydroxy-1-methylbut-1-enyl]-*N*-(4-amino-2-methylpyrimidin-5-ylmethyl)formamide.

$C_{23}H_{36}N_4O_5S_3$ = 544.8.
CAS — 137-86-0.

Prosultiamine (13182-q)

Prosultiamine (*rINN*).

DTPT; Thiamine Propyl Disulphide. *N*-(4-Amino-2-methylpyrimidin-5-ylmethyl)-*N*-(4-hydroxy-1-methyl-2-propyldithiobut-1-enyl)formamide.

$C_{15}H_{24}N_4O_2S_2$ = 356.5.
CAS — 59-58-5.

Sulbutiamine (7834-x)

Sulbutiamine (*rINN*).

Bisibutiamine; *O*-Isobutyrylthiamine Disulphide. *NN'*-{Dithiobis[2-(2-isobutyryloxyethyl)-1-methylvinylene]}bis[*N*-(4-amino-2-methylpyrimidin-5-ylmethyl)formamide].

$C_{32}H_{46}N_8O_6S_2$ = 702.9.
CAS — 3286-46-2.

Thiamine Hydrochloride (7829-d)

Thiamine Hydrochloride *(BANM, rINNM).*

Aneurine Hydrochloride; Thiamin Hydrochloride; Thiamine Chloride; Thiamini Hydrochloridum; Thiaminii Chloridum; Vitamin B_1. 3-(4-Amino-2-methylpyrimidin-5-ylmethyl)-5-(2-hydroxyethyl)-4-methylthiazolium chloride hydrochloride.

$C_{12}H_{17}ClN_4OS,HCl$ = 337.3.

CAS — 59-43-8 (thiamine); 67-03-8 (thiamine hydrochloride).

Pharmacopoeias. In *Chin., Eur.* (see p.viii), *Int., Jpn, Pol.,* and *US.* Thiamine hydrobromide is included in *Int.*

Colourless or white crystals or white or almost white crystalline powder with a faint characteristic odour.

Soluble 1 in 1 of water and 1 in 170 of alcohol; soluble in glycerol; practically insoluble in ether. A 2.5% solution in water has a pH of 2.7 to 3.3. **Store** in airtight nonmetallic containers. Protect from light.

Sterile solutions of pH 4 or less lose activity only very slowly but neutral or alkaline solutions deteriorate rapidly, especially in contact with air. When exposed to air, the anhydrous material rapidly absorbs about 4% of water.

Thiamine Nitrate (7830-c)

Thiamine Nitrate *(BANM, rINNM).*

Aneurine Mononitrate; Thiamine Mononitrate; Thiamini Nitras; Vitamin B_1 Mononitrate. 3-(4-Amino-2-methylpyrimidin-5-ylmethyl)-5-(2-hydroxyethyl)-4-methylthiazolium nitrate.

$C_{12}H_{17}N_5O_4S$ = 327.4.

CAS — 532-43-4.

Pharmacopoeias. In *Eur.* (see p.viii), *Int., Jpn, Pol.,* and *US.*

Small white or colourless crystals or a white or almost white crystalline powder with a slight characteristic odour. **Soluble** 1 in 44 of water; freely soluble in boiling water; slightly soluble in alcohol and in methyl alcohol; very slightly soluble in chloroform. The Ph. Eur. states that a 2% solution in water has a pH of 6.8 to 7.6 and the USP that it has a pH between 6.0 and 7.5. **Store** in airtight nonmetallic containers. Protect from light.

Stability. A review of the compatibility and stability of components of total parenteral nutrition solutions when mixed in 1- or 3-litre flexible containers.[1] Thiamine is incompatible with reducing agents such as sulphites. The thiamine molecule is cleaved into pyrimidine and thiazole moieties. The rate of hydrolytic cleavage increases with increasing pH, and may be rapid at pH 6. Some studies have shown that thiamine degrades rapidly in amino acid infusion solutions containing thiosulphite, especially above pH 6.5. More recent studies have suggested that the degradation effect of thiosulphite is concentration-dependent. Negligible losses were reported after storage of 3-litre containers in the refrigerator for 7 days, especially in the absence of trace elements. Thiamine has been found to be more stable if the sulphite concentration does not exceed 0.05%. It can be concluded that thiamine losses will be insignificant under normal conditions of the preparation, storage, and administration of 3-litre parenteral nutrition solutions.

1. Allwood MC. Compatibility and stability of TPN mixtures in big bags. *J Clin Hosp Pharm* 1984; **9:** 181–98.

Adverse Effects and Precautions

Adverse effects seldom occur following administration of thiamine, but hypersensitivity reactions have occurred, mainly after parenteral administration. These reactions have ranged in severity from very mild to, very rarely, fatal anaphylactic shock (see below).

Hypersensitivity. The UK Committee on Safety of Medicines had received, between 1970 and July 1988, 90 reports of adverse reactions associated with the use of an injection containing high doses of vitamins B and C. The most frequent reactions were 41 cases of anaphylaxis, 13 cases of dyspnoea or bronchospasm, and 22 cases of rash or flushing; 78 of the reactions occurred during, or shortly after, intravenous injection and the other 12 after intramuscular injection.[1] They recommended that parenteral treatment be used only when essential, and that, when used, facilities for treating anaphylaxis should be available. They also recommended that, when the intravenous route was used, the injection be administered slowly (over 10 minutes). Various authors[2,3] have noted that parenteral treatment is *essential* for the prophylaxis and treatment of Wernicke's encephalopathy (see below).

1. Committee on Safety of Medicines. Parentrovite & allergic reactions. *Current Problems 24* 1989.
2. Wrenn KD, Slovis CM. Is intravenous thiamine safe? *Am J Emerg Med* 1992; **10:** 165.
3. Thomson AD, Cook CCH. Parenteral thiamine and Wernicke's encephalopathy: the balance of risks and concerns. *Alcohol Alcohol* 1997; **32:** 207–9.

The symbol † denotes a preparation no longer actively marketed

Pharmacokinetics

Small amounts of thiamine are well absorbed from the gastro-intestinal tract following oral administration, but the absorption of doses larger than about 5 mg is limited. It is also rapidly absorbed following intramuscular administration. It is widely distributed to most body tissues, and appears in breast milk. Within the cell thiamine is mostly present as the diphosphate. Thiamine is not stored to any appreciable extent in the body and amounts in excess of the body's requirements are excreted in the urine as unchanged thiamine or as metabolites.

References.

1. Weber W, *et al.* Nonlinear kinetics of the thiamine cation in humans: saturation of nonrenal clearance and tubular reabsorption. *J Pharmacokinet Biopharm* 1990; **18:** 501–23.
2. Tallaksen CME, *et al.* Kinetics of thiamin and thiamin phosphate esters in human blood, plasma and urine after 50 mg intravenously or orally. *Eur J Clin Pharmacol* 1993; **44:** 73–8.

Human Requirements

Thiamine requirements are directly related to the carbohydrate intake and the metabolic rate. A daily dietary intake of about 0.9 to 1.5 mg of thiamine is recommended for healthy men and about 0.8 to 1.1 mg for healthy women. Cereals, nuts, peas, beans, and yeast are rich sources of thiamine. Pork and some other meats especially liver, heart, or kidneys, and also fish, contain significant amounts. Flour and bakery products are often enriched with thiamine. Considerable losses of thiamine may result from cooking processes.

In the United Kingdom dietary reference values (see p.1332) have been published for thiamine[1] and similarly in the United States recommended dietary allowances (RDAs) have been set.[2] In the UK for adult males and females the reference nutrient intake (RNI) is 0.4 mg per 1000 kcal daily and the estimated average requirement (EAR) is 0.3 mg per 1000 kcal daily. In the USA an RDA of 1.2 mg daily in adult males and 1.1 mg daily in females is recommended.

1. DoH. Dietary reference values for food energy and nutrients for the United Kingdom: report of the panel on dietary reference values of the committee on medical aspects of food policy. *Report on health and social subjects 41.* London: HMSO, 1991.
2. Standing Committee on the Scientific Evaluation of Dietary Reference Intakes of the Food and Nutrition Board. *Dietary Reference Intakes for thiamin, riboflavin, niacin, vitamin B_6, folate, vitamin B_{12}, pantothenic acid, biotin, and choline.* Washington, DC: National Academy Press, 1998.

Uses and Administration

Thiamine is a water-soluble vitamin, although some of its derivatives have greater lipophilicity. It is an essential coenzyme for carbohydrate metabolism in the form of the diphosphate (thiamine pyrophosphate, cocarboxylase). Thiamine deficiency develops when the dietary intake is inadequate; severe deficiency leads to the development of a syndrome known as beri-beri. Chronic 'dry' beri-beri is characterised by peripheral neuropathy, muscle wasting and muscle weakness, and paralysis. Acute 'wet' beri-beri is characterised by cardiac failure and oedema. Wernicke-Korsakoff syndrome (demyelination of the central nervous system) may develop in severe cases of thiamine deficiency. Severe thiamine deficiency, characterised by lactic acidosis and neurological deterioration, has been reported within a relatively short time of the initiation of thiamine-free total parenteral nutrition; some deaths have occurred.

Thiamine is used in the treatment and prevention of thiamine deficiency. It is usually given by mouth, the preferred route, but may if necessary be administered by the intramuscular or intravenous routes (but see Hypersensitivity, above); intravenous injections should be given slowly over 10 minutes. In the treatment of mild chronic thiamine deficiency usual doses of 10 to 25 mg daily by mouth, in single or divided doses have been recommended. In severe thiamine deficiency doses of up to 300 mg daily are given, and even higher daily doses may be employed in Wernicke-Korsakoff syndrome by the intravenous route.

Thiamine is usually given as either the hydrochloride or nitrate salts although other salts such as the dicamsylate, disulphide, monophosphate (monophosphothiamine) or pyrophosphate may be employed.

Other compounds that possess vitamin B_1 activity and may be used as alternatives to thiamine include acetiamine, benfotiamine, bisbentiamine, fursultiamine, octotiamine, prosultiamine, and sulbutiamine.

Wernicke-Korsakoff syndrome. The Wernicke-Korsakoff syndrome is a manifestation of thiamine deficiency seen particularly in alcoholics, but which may accompany other conditions including starvation or prolonged fasting, or persistent vomiting. It was originally classified as two separate disorders, Wernicke's encephalopathy and Korsakoff's syndrome, but these are now thought to represent aspects of a single pathological process.

Classical Wernicke's symptoms comprise confusion, ataxia, ophthalmoplegia, and nystagmus. Ophthalmoplegia and ataxia may precede the mental symptoms by some days. Hypothermia may be seen, and collapse and sudden death may occur in some patients. The manifestations of Korsakoff's syndrome are short-term memory loss, learning deficits, and confabulation. The conditions are associated with demyelination and glial proliferation, as well as haemorrhagic lesions, mainly in the periventricular regions of the brain; characteristic biochemical abnormalities include raised serum-pyruvate concentration, which has been postulated as a cause of encephalopathy.[1]

Early recognition and treatment is important, both because of the risk of collapse and sudden death,[2] and to pre-empt irreversible damage to the CNS. Korsakoff symptoms respond less well to treatment than those associated with Wernicke's encephalopathy,[3] and may indeed only become evident on treatment.

Treatment is with parenteral thiamine, preferably intravenously, to ensure adequate absorption; any risks of parenteral treatment are considered justifiable.[4] Although as little as 2 or 3 mg may be enough to reverse the ocular symptoms, which generally begin to improve in 1 to 6 hours, doses of at least 100 mg should be given initially. (In practice a typical dose is 500 mg given intravenously with other vitamins every 8 hours, for 2 days if symptoms persist, and followed by 100 mg twice daily by mouth, or 250 mg daily intravenously until the patient can take oral thiamine.[4,5]) The ataxia and acute confusional state may also resolve dramatically although improvement may not be noted for days or months. The effects of the syndrome on memory are much harder to reverse. Some 25% of patients make a full, and 50% a partial, recovery.[3]

1. Petrie WM, Ban TA. Vitamins in psychiatry: do they have a role? *Drugs* 1985; **30:** 58–65.
2. Reuler JB, *et al.* Wernicke's encephalopathy. *N Engl J Med* 1985; **312:** 1035–9.
3. Anonymous. Korsakoff's syndrome. *Lancet* 1990; **336:** 912–13.
4. Cook CCH, Thomson AD. B-complex vitamins in the prophylaxis and treatment of Wernicke-Korsakoff syndrome. *Br J Hosp Med* 1997; **57:** 461–5.
5. Chataway J, Hardman E. Thiamine doses for alcohol withdrawal. *Br J Hosp Med* 1994; **51:** 615.

Preparations

BP 1998: Thiamine Injection; Thiamine Tablets; Vitamins B and C Injection;
BPC 1973: Compound Vitamin B Tablets; Strong Compound Vitamin B Tablets; Vitamins Capsules;
USP 23: Oil- and Water-soluble Vitamins Capsules; Oil- and Water-soluble Vitamins Oral Solution; Oil- and Water-soluble Vitamins Tablets; Thiamine Hydrochloride Elixir; Thiamine Hydrochloride Injection; Thiamine Hydrochloride Tablets; Thiamine Mononitrate Elixir; Water-soluble Vitamins Capsules; Water-soluble Vitamins Tablets.

Proprietary Preparations (details are given in Part 3)

Aust.: Beneuran; Bevitol; Judolor†; ***Austral.:*** Beta-Sol; Betamin; Invite B_1†; ***Belg.:*** Aneurol; Benerva; Beneurol; Beston†; Betamine; Tabiomyl†; ***Canad.:*** Betaxin; Bewon; ***Fr.:*** Arcalion; Benerva; Bevitine; Vitanevril Fort†; ***Ger.:*** Aneurin; B_1-Vicotrat; Benfogamma; Betabion; Judolor†; Lophakomp-B1; ***Irl.:*** Benerva; ***Ital.:*** Benerva; Betabion; Bisolvit†; Bivitasi; CO-B1†; Cocarvit†; Pirofosfasi†; Trifosfaneurina†; ***Jpn:*** Biotamin; Cometamin; Neuvita; ***Spain:*** Arcalion; Benerva; Glutaneurina B6 Fte†; Neurostop; Surmenalit; Vitantial†; ***Swed.:*** Benerva; Betabion; ***Switz.:*** Arcalion; Benerva; ***UK:*** Benerva; ***USA:*** Thiamilate.

Multi-ingredient: numerous preparations are listed in Part 3.

Vitamin B_2 Substances (14733-q)

Riboflavine (7843-r)

Riboflavine *(BAN)*.

Riboflavin *(rINN)*; E101; Lactoflavin; Riboflavinum; Vitamin B_2; Vitamin G. 7,8-Dimethyl-10-(1′-D-ribityl)isoalloxazine; 3,10-Dihydro-7,8-dimethyl-10-(D-*ribo*-2,3,4,5-tetrahydroxypentyl)benzopteridine-2,4-dione.

$C_{17}H_{20}N_4O_6$ = 376.4.

CAS — 83-88-5.

Pharmacopoeias. In *Chin., Eur.* (see p.viii), *Int., Jpn, Pol.,* and *US.*

A yellow to orange-yellow crystalline powder with a slight odour.

Very slightly **soluble** in water; more soluble in 0.9% sodium chloride solution than in water; practically insoluble in alcohol, in chloroform, and in ether; soluble in dilute alkali solutions. **Store** in airtight containers. Protect from light. When dry it is not appreciably affected by light, but in solution light induces rapid deterioration, especially in the presence of alkali.

Riboflavine Sodium Phosphate (7842-x)

Riboflavine Sodium Phosphate *(BANM)*.

Riboflavin Sodium Phosphate *(rINNM)*; Riboflavin 5′-Phosphate Sodium; Riboflavine Phosphate (Sodium Salt); Riboflavini Natrii Phosphas; Vitamin B_2 Phosphate. The sodium salt of riboflavine 5′-phosphate.

$C_{17}H_{20}N_4NaO_9P$ = 478.3.

CAS — 130-40-5.

Pharmacopoeias. In *Eur.* (see p.viii) and *Jpn.*

US specifies the dihydrate salt.

A fine yellow to orange-yellow, odourless or almost odourless, crystalline hygroscopic powder. Riboflavine sodium phosphate 1.27 g is approximately equivalent to 1 g of riboflavine. Ph. Eur. states that it is **soluble** and the USP sparingly soluble in water; very slightly soluble in alcohol; practically insoluble in ether. A 1% solution in water has a pH of 5.0 to 6.5. **Store** in airtight containers. Protect from light. When dry, it is not affected by diffused light, but when in solution light induces rapid deterioration.

Stability. A review of the compatibility and stability of components of total parenteral nutrition solutions when mixed in 1- or 3-litre flexible containers.[1] Unpublished studies have indicated that light-induced losses of riboflavine can amount to 40% after 8 hours, and 55% after a typical 24-hour administration period. Losses during passage through the administration set can lead to a further 2% loss. It is important, therefore, to include an adequate overage in a parenteral nutrition regimen to allow for these losses. As with other losses caused by exposure to daylight, commencing infusion in the evening ensures that the patient receives greater amounts of this vitamin.

1. Allwood MC. Compatibility and stability of TPN mixtures in big bags. *J Clin Hosp Pharm* 1984; **9:** 181–98.

Adverse Effects and Precautions

No adverse effects have been reported with the use of riboflavine. Large doses of riboflavine result in a bright yellow discoloration of the urine which may interfere with certain laboratory tests.

Pharmacokinetics

Riboflavine is absorbed from the gastro-intestinal tract. Although riboflavine is widely distributed to body tissues little is stored in the body.

Riboflavine is converted in the body to the coenzyme flavine mononucleotide (FMN; riboflavine 5′-phosphate) and then to another coenzyme flavine adenine dinucleotide (FAD). About 60% of FMN and FAD are bound to plasma proteins. Riboflavine is excreted in urine, partly as metabolites. As the dose increases, larger amounts are excreted unchanged. Riboflavine crosses the placenta and is distributed into breast milk.

Human Requirements

The riboflavine requirement is often related to the energy intake but it appears to be more closely related to resting metabolic requirements. A daily dietary intake of about 1.1 to 1.7 mg of riboflavine is recommended. Liver, kidney, fish, eggs, milk, cheese, yeast, and some green vegetables such as broccoli and spinach are the richest sources of riboflavine. In general, little loss of riboflavine occurs during cooking, but considerable losses may occur if foods, especially milk, are exposed to sunlight.

In the United Kingdom dietary reference values (see p.1332) have been published for riboflavine[1] and similarly in the United States recommended dietary allowances (RDAs) have been set.[2] Differing amounts are recommended for infants and children of varying ages, for adult males and females of varying ages, and for pregnant and lactating women; in the USA the differing amounts recommended for the differing age groups have been said to reflect the changes in caloric intakes at these ages. In the UK the reference nutrient intake (RNI) is 1.3 mg daily and 1.1 mg daily for adult males and females respectively; the estimated average requirement (EAR) is 1.0 mg daily and 0.9 mg daily respectively. In the USA the RDAs for adult males and females are 1.3 and 1.1 mg daily respectively.

1. DoH. Dietary reference values for food energy and nutrients for the United Kingdom: report of the panel on dietary reference values of the committee on medical aspects of food policy. *Report on health and social subjects 41.* London: HMSO, 1991.

2. Standing Committee on the Scientific Evaluation of Dietary Reference Intakes of the Food and Nutrition Board. *Dietary Reference Intakes for thiamin, riboflavin, niacin, vitamin B_6, folate, vitamin B_{12}, pantothenic acid, biotin, and choline.* Washington, DC: National Academy Press, 1998.

Uses and Administration

Riboflavine, a water-soluble vitamin, is essential for the utilisation of energy from food. The active, phosphorylated forms, flavine mononucleotide (FMN) and flavine adenine dinucleotide (FAD), are involved as coenzymes in oxidative/reductive metabolic reactions. Riboflavine is also necessary for the functioning of pyridoxine and nicotinic acid.

Riboflavine deficiency develops when the dietary intake is inadequate. Deficiency leads to the development of a well-defined syndrome known as ariboflavinosis, characterised by cheilosis, angular stomatitis, glossitis, keratitis, surface lesions of the genitalia, and seborrhoeic dermatitis. There may also be normocytic anaemia and ocular symptoms including itching and burning of the eyes, photophobia, and corneal vascularisation. Some of these symptoms may, in fact, represent deficiencies of other vitamins such as pyridoxine or nicotinic acid which do not function correctly in the absence of riboflavine. Riboflavine deficiency may also occur in association with other vitamin B-complex deficiency states such as pellagra.

Riboflavine is used in the treatment and prevention of riboflavine deficiency. It is usually given in doses of 1 or 2 mg by mouth, the preferred route. Doses of up to 30 mg daily in single or divided doses have been used. Riboflavine is also a component of intramuscular or intravenous multivitamin injections.

Riboflavine tetrabutyrate has also been used.

Riboflavine is also used as a colouring agent for food.

Migraine. Results from an open pilot study[1] and a placebo-controlled trial[2] have suggested that riboflavine in high doses (400 mg daily) might be of some benefit in the prophylaxis of migraine attacks (p.443).

1. Schoenen J, *et al.* High-dose riboflavin as a prophylactic treatment of migraine: results of an open pilot study. *Cephalalgia* 1994; **14:** 328–9.

2. Schoenen J, *et al.* Effectiveness of high-dose riboflavin in migraine prophylaxis: a randomized controlled trial. *Neurology* 1998; **50:** 466–70.

Preparations

BP 1998: Vitamins B and C Injection;
BPC 1973: Compound Vitamin B Tablets; Strong Compound Vitamin B Tablets; Vitamins Capsules;
USP 23: Oil- and Water-soluble Vitamins Capsules; Oil- and Water-soluble Vitamins Oral Solution; Oil- and Water-soluble Vitamins Tablets; Riboflavin Injection; Riboflavin Tablets; Water-soluble Vitamins Capsules; Water-soluble Vitamins Tablets.

Proprietary Preparations (details are given in Part 3)

Belg.: Berivine; Ribon; ***Fr.:*** Beflavine; ***Ger.:*** Werdo†; ***Ital.:*** Beflavina†.

Multi-ingredient: some preparations are listed in Part 3.

Vitamin B_6 Substances (14734-p)

Pyridoxine is only one of 3 similar compounds that may be referred to as vitamin B_6; the other two are pyridoxal and pyridoxamine.

Pyridoxine Hydrochloride (7847-h)

Pyridoxine Hydrochloride *(BANM, rINNM)*.

Adermine Hydrochloride; Piridossina Cloridrato; Pyridoxini Hydrochloridum; Pyridoxinii Chloridum; Pyridoxinium Chloride; Pyridoxol Hydrochloride; Vitamin B_6. 3-Hydroxy-4,5-bis(hydroxymethyl)-2-picoline hydrochloride.

$C_8H_{11}NO_3,HCl$ = 205.6.

CAS — 65-23-6 (pyridoxine); 58-56-0 (pyridoxine hydrochloride).

Pharmacopoeias. In *Chin., Eur.* (see p.viii), *Int., Jpn, Pol.,* and *US.*

A white or almost white crystalline powder, or crystals.

Soluble 1 in 5 of water and 1 in 115 of alcohol; practically insoluble in chloroform and in ether. A 5% solution in water has a pH of 2.4 to 3.0. **Store** in airtight containers. Protect from light.

Stability. A review of the compatibility and stability of components of total parenteral nutrition solutions when mixed in 1- or 3-litre flexible containers.[1] Pyridoxine is light sensitive although degradation is far less than is observed with vitamin A or riboflavine. No losses have been reported unless the solution was exposed to direct sunlight when destruction of more than 80% of the added pyridoxine occurred in 8 hours. Under normal conditions therefore, pyridoxine losses would be small.

1. Allwood MC. Compatibility and stability of TPN mixtures in big bags. *J Clin Hosp Pharm* 1984; **9:** 181–98.

Adverse Effects and Precautions

Long-term administration of large doses of pyridoxine is associated with the development of severe peripheral neuropathies; the dose below which these do not occur is controversial (see below).

Effects on the nervous system. Severe sensory neuropathy has been described in patients receiving large doses of pyridoxine (2 to 6 g daily) for periods of 2 to 40 months.[1] It has, however, been debated as to whether smaller doses may produce such effects. Some contend that amounts of pyridoxine below this level are unlikely to produce toxic effects[2,3] although there have been some case reports[4,5] with amounts up to about 500 mg daily. Following a review of the possible toxicity associated with lower doses of pyridoxine, proposals were put forward in the UK to limit the dose freely available in dietary supplements to 10 mg daily; products supplying up to 50 mg daily would continue to be available from pharmacies and higher doses would only be available on prescription.[6] These proposals have been heavily contested.[6,7] An upper limit of 100 mg daily has been suggested in the USA.[7]

1. Schaumburg H, *et al.* Sensory neuropathy from pyridoxine abuse: a new megavitamin syndrome. *N Engl J Med* 1983; **309:** 445–8.
2. Pauling L. Sensory neuropathy from pyridoxine abuse. *N Engl J Med* 1984; **310:** 197.
3. Baker H, Frank O. Sensory neuropathy from pyridoxine abuse. *N Engl J Med* 1984; **310:** 197.
4. Berger A, Schaumburg HH. More on neuropathy from pyridoxine abuse. *N Engl J Med* 1984; **311:** 986.
5. Waterston JA, Gilligan BS. Pyridoxine neuropathy. *Med J Aust* 1987; **146:** 640–2.
6. Collier J. Vitamin B-6: food or medicine? *Br Med J* 1998; **317:** 92–3.
7. Anonymous. Still time for rational debate about vitamin B_6. *Lancet* 1998; **351:** 1523.

Interactions

Pyridoxine reduces the effects of levodopa (see p.1140), but this does not occur if a dopa decarboxylase inhibitor is also given. It has also been reported to decrease serum concentrations of phenobarbitone (p.351). Many drugs may increase the requirements for pyridoxine; such drugs include isoniazid, penicillamine, and oral contraceptives.

Pharmacokinetics

Pyridoxine, pyridoxal, and pyridoxamine are readily absorbed from the gastro-intestinal tract following oral administration and are converted to the active forms pyridoxal phosphate and pyridoxamine phosphate. They are stored mainly in the liver where there is oxidation to 4-pyridoxic acid and other inactive metabolites which are excreted in the urine. As the dose increases, proportionally greater amounts are excreted unchanged in the urine. Pyridoxal crosses the placenta and also appears in breast milk.

Human Requirements

For adults, the daily requirement of pyridoxine is probably about 1.5 to 2 mg and this amount is present in most normal diets. The requirement tends to increase as protein intake increases due to the role of the vitamin in amino acid metabolism. Meats, especially chicken, kidney, and liver, cereals, eggs, fish, and certain vegetables and fruits are good sources of pyridoxine.

In the United Kingdom[1] dietary reference values (see p.1332) have been published for vitamin B_6 and similarly in the United States recommended dietary allowances (RDAs) have been set.[2] Differing amounts are recommended for infants and children of varying ages, for adult males and females, and during pregnancy and lactation. In the UK the reference nutrient intake (RNI) is 15 µg per g of protein daily for adult males and females and the estimated average requirement (EAR) is 13 µg per g of protein daily for the same group. In the USA the RDA for adult men ranges from 1.3 to 1.7 mg daily and that for adult women ranges from 1.3 to 1.5 mg daily.[2]

1. DoH. Dietary reference values for food energy and nutrients for the United Kingdom: report of the panel on dietary reference values of the committee on medical aspects of food policy. *Report on health and social subjects 41*. London: HMSO, 1991.
2. Standing Committee on the Scientific Evaluation of Dietary Reference Intakes of the Food and Nutrition Board. *Dietary Reference Intakes for thiamin, riboflavin, niacin, vitamin B_6, folate, vitamin B_{12}, pantothenic acid, biotin, and choline.* Washington, DC: National Academy Press, 1998.

Uses and Administration

Pyridoxine, a water-soluble vitamin, is involved principally in amino acid metabolism, but is also involved in carbohydrate and fat metabolism. It is also required for the formation of haemoglobin.

Deficiency of pyridoxine is rare in humans because of its widespread distribution in foods. Pyridoxine deficiency may however be drug-induced and can occur, for instance, during isoniazid therapy. Inadequate utilisation of pyridoxine may result from certain inborn errors of metabolism. Pyridoxine deficiency may lead to sideroblastic anaemia, dermatitis, cheilosis, and neurological symptoms such as peripheral neuritis, and convulsions.

Pyridoxine is used in the treatment and prevention of pyridoxine deficiency states. It is usually given by mouth, the preferred route, but may also be administered by the subcutaneous, intramuscular, or intravenous routes. Doses of up to 150 mg daily have been used in general deficiency states; higher doses of up to 400 mg daily have been used in the treatment of sideroblastic anaemias (see below); and similar doses have been used to treat certain metabolic disorders such as homocystinuria (see Amino Acid Metabolic Disorders, below) or primary hyperoxaluria (below). Pyridoxine has also been used to treat seizures due to hereditary syndromes of pyridoxine deficiency or dependency in infants.

Pyridoxine has also been tried in a wide variety of other disorders, including the treatment of depression and other symptoms associated with the premenstrual syndrome (see below) and the use of oral contraceptives, although it is only one of many agents advocated, and its efficacy has been questioned.

Pyridoxine is usually administered as the hydrochloride although other salts such as the citrate, oxoglurate, phosphate, and phosphoserinate, have also been employed. The pidolate (metadoxine) has been investigated in alcoholism (see below).

For the use of pyridoxine in the prophylaxis of isoniazid-induced peripheral neuritis and for the treatment of acute isoniazid toxicity, see under Isoniazid, p.219.

Pyridoxal phosphate may be used to treat vitamin B_6 deficiency.

Alcoholism. Pyridoxine and its pidolate, known as metadoxine, have been tried in the treatment of alcohol poisoning and alcoholism. One study showed pyridoxine to be ineffective in acute alcohol poisoning[1] but another[2] suggested that the pidolate might be of benefit as an adjunct in the management of alcohol withdrawal (p.1099).

1. Mardel S, *et al.* Intravenous pyridoxine in acute ethanol intoxication. *Hum Exp Toxicol* 1994; **13:** 321–3.
2. Rizzo A, *et al.* Uso terapeutico della metadoxina nell'alcolismo cronico: studio clinico in doppio cieco su pazienti ricoverati in un reparto di medicina generale. *Clin Ter* 1993; **142:** 243–50.

Amino acid metabolic disorders. Reports of the use of pyridoxine in various inborn errors of amino acid metabolism.[1,2] Some patients with homocystinuria respond to pyridoxine with or without cobalamins and folate. Dietary methionine restriction and betaine or choline may also be required (see p.1330). For the use of pyridoxine in primary hyperoxaluria, another inherited metabolic disorder, see below.

1. Boers GHJ, *et al.* Heterozygosity for homocystinuria in premature peripheral and cerebral occlusive arterial disease. *N Engl J Med* 1985; **313:** 709–15.
2. Hayasaka S, *et al.* Clinical trials of vitamin B_6 and proline supplementation for gyrate atrophy of the choroid and retina. *Br J Ophthalmol* 1985; **69:** 283–90.

Anaemias. Some patients with acquired or hereditary sideroblastic anaemia (p.704) that is severe enough to require treatment will respond to high doses (up to 400 mg daily) of pyridoxine, and a trial is considered worthwhile in all patients.

Carpal tunnel syndrome. Pyridoxine has been advocated by some[1] for patients with carpal tunnel syndrome (see Soft-tissue Rheumatism, p.4), but there is controversy surrounding its efficacy,[2] and a study found pyridoxine to be no more effective than placebo.[3]

1. Lewis PJ. Pyridoxine supplements may help patients with carpal tunnel syndrome. *Br Med J* 1995; **310:** 1534.
2. Copeland DA, Stoukides CA. Pyridoxine in carpal tunnel syndrome. *Ann Pharmacother* 1994; **28:** 1042–4.
3. Spooner GR, *et al.* Using pyridoxine to treat carpal tunnel syndrome. *Can Fam Physician* 1993; **39:** 2122–7.

Epilepsy. Pyridoxine-dependent epilepsy is an autosomal recessive disorder associated with decreased central γ-aminobutyric acid (GABA) concentrations and elevated cerebral glutamate concentrations. Untreated patients suffer from progressive encephalopathy, mental retardation, and intractable epilepsy; lifelong supplementation with pyridoxine can control epileptic symptoms but mental retardation may still develop. Test doses of pyridoxine intravenously, repeated at intervals of 10 minutes up to a total of 500 mg if necessary, have been suggested in the diagnosis of pyridoxine-dependent epilepsy; if the patient responds then a daily oral dose of 5 mg per kg body-weight is suggested although there is no real consensus on the appropriate dosage.[1] A study in one patient[2] found that although pyridoxine 5 mg per kg body-weight reduced glutamate concentrations in cerebrospinal fluid from their untreated value of 200 times normal limits, it did so only to 10 times the normal value, despite remission of symptoms. Doses of 10 mg per kg daily were required to normalise CSF glutamate, and it was suggested that this was a more appropriate target for therapy.

1. Gospe SM. Current perspectives on pyridoxine-dependent seizures. *J Pediatr* 1998; **132:** 919–23.
2. Baumeister FAM, *et al.* Glutamate in pyridoxine-dependent epilepsy: neurotoxic glutamate concentration in the cerebrospinal fluid and its normalization by pyridoxine. *Pediatrics* 1994; **94:** 318–21.

Ischaemic heart disease. For mention of the possible link between vitamin B_6, hyperhomocysteinaemia, and atherosclerosis and ischaemic heart disease, see under Folic Acid p.1341.

Premenstrual syndrome. Pyridoxine has been widely used in the premenstrual syndrome (p.1456) despite controversy over its effectiveness. West has said that, in theory, depressive symptoms may be provoked by pyridoxine deficiency because of its role as a coenzyme in the production of certain neurotransmitters, but that it is difficult to attribute any of the other symptoms of the premenstrual syndrome to pyridoxine deficiency and doses of 50 mg are no more effective than a placebo.[1] Reviewing published studies of the use of pyridoxine in the premenstrual syndrome Kleijnen and co-workers also concluded that there was no evidence that such treatment was efficacious.[2] If pyridoxine is used, the dosage should be restricted (50 mg daily) because of concerns (see above) about neurotoxicity.[3]

1. West CP. The premenstrual syndrome. *Prescribers' J* 1987; **27** (2): 9–15.
2. Kleijnen J, *et al.* Vitamin B_6 in the treatment of the premenstrual syndrome—a review. *Br J Obstet Gynaecol* 1990; **97:** 847–52.
3. Severino SK, Moline ML. Premenstrual syndrome: identification and management. *Drugs* 1995; **49:** 71–82.

Primary hyperoxaluria. Primary hyperoxaluria (as distinct from the various forms secondary to other disorders) is a genetic disorder characterised by excessive synthesis and urinary excretion of oxalic acid. Two forms are known, type I (glycolic aciduria) and type II (L-glyceric aciduria), associated with different enzyme defects. They are marked by recurrent calcium oxalate kidney stones, or nephrocalcinosis, leading to renal failure, together with extrarenal deposition of calcium oxalate and frequently severe peripheral vascular insufficiency. Treatment with high doses of pyridoxine may help decrease oxalate excretion particularly in type I disease.[1,2] A few patients may respond to lower (physiological) doses.[3] Such treatment can be combined with an oral orthophosphate supplement, which helps reduce renal deposition of calcium oxalate, and the combination appears to preserve renal function.[4] Therapy with magnesium salts, citrate, and thiazide diuretics has also been suggested. In patients in whom renal failure develops, the results of kidney transplantation have been disappointing, due to deposition of calcium oxalate in the new kidney, although concomitant liver transplantation can correct the enzyme defect.[5]

1. Alinei P, *et al.* Pyridoxine treatment of type 1 hyperoxaluria. *N Engl J Med* 1984; **311:** 798.
2. de Zegher F, *et al.* Successful treatment of infantile type I primary hyperoxaluria complicated by pyridoxine toxicity. *Lancet* 1985; **ii:** 392–3.
3. Yendt ER, Cohanim M. Response to a physiologic dose of pyridoxine in type I primary hyperoxaluria. *N Engl J Med* 1985; **312:** 953–7.
4. Milliner DS, *et al.* Results of long-term treatment with orthophosphate and pyridoxine in patients with primary hyperoxaluria. *N Engl J Med* 1994; **331:** 1553–8.
5. Watts RWE, *et al.* Combined hepatic and renal transplantation in primary hyperoxaluria type I: clinical report of nine cases. *Am J Med* 1991; **90:** 179–88.

Preparations

BP 1998: Pyridoxine Tablets; Vitamins B and C Injection;
BPC 1973: Strong Compound Vitamin B Tablets;
USP 23: Oil- and Water-soluble Vitamins Capsules; Oil- and Water-soluble Vitamins Oral Solution; Oil- and Water-soluble Vitamins Tablets; Pyridoxine Hydrochloride Injection; Pyridoxine Hydrochloride Tablets; Water-soluble Vitamins Capsules; Water-soluble Vitamins Tablets.

Proprietary Preparations (details are given in Part 3)
Aust.: Benadon; ***Austral.:*** Invite B_6†; Pyroxin; ***Belg.:*** Bedoxine; ***Canad.:*** Carthamex; Hexa-Betalin†; ***Fr.:*** Becilan; Dermo 6; ***Ger.:*** B_6-Vicotrat; Benadon†; Bonasanit; Hexobion; Lophakomp-B6; Pyragamma†; ***Irl.:*** Benadon; Complement Continus; ***Ital.:*** Benadon; Glutarase†; Memosprint; Metadoxil; Vivox†; Xanturenasi; ***Norw.:*** AFI-B_6; ***S.Afr.:*** Beesix†; Lactosec; ***Spain:*** Beglunina; Benadon; Conductasa; Dermo Chabre B6†; Duplicalcio 150; Glutaneurina B6 Fte†; Godabion B6; Serfoxide; Sibevit†; ***Swed.:*** Benadon; ***Switz.:*** Benadon; Complement Continus; ***UK:*** Benadon; Complement Continus; Orovite Complement B_6; Woman Kind; ***USA:*** Aminoxin; Hexa-Betalin†; Nestrex; Rodex TD†; Rodex†.

Multi-ingredient: numerous preparations are listed in Part 3.

Vitamin B_{12} Substances (14752-w)

Vitamin B_{12} is the name generally used for a group of related cobalt-containing compounds, also known as cobalamins, of which cyanocobalamin and hydroxocobalamin are the principal forms in clinical use.

Cyanocobalamin (7853-d)

Cyanocobalamin *(BAN, rINN).*

Cobamin; Cyanocobalaminum; Cycobemin. *Coα*-[α-(5,6-Dimethylbenzimidazolyl)]-*Coβ*-cyanocobamide.

$C_{63}H_{88}CoN_{14}O_{14}P$ = 1355.4.

CAS — 68-19-9.

Pharmacopoeias. In *Chin., Eur.* (see p.viii), *Int., Jpn, Pol.,* and *US.*

Dark red crystals or crystalline or amorphous powder. In the anhydrous form it is very hygroscopic and when exposed to air it may absorb about 12% of water.

Soluble 1 in 80 of water; the Ph. Eur. states that it is sparingly soluble, and the USP that it is soluble, in alcohol; practically insoluble in acetone, in chloroform, and in ether. **Store** in airtight containers. Protect from light.

Hydroxocobalamin (7854-n)

Hydroxocobalamin *(BAN, USAN, rINN).*

Hydroxocobalaminum; Idrossocobalamina. *Coα*-[α-(5,6-Dimethylbenzimidazolyl)]-*Coβ*-hydroxocobamide.

$C_{62}H_{89}CoN_{13}O_{15}P$ = 1346.4.

CAS — 13422-51-0.

Pharmacopoeias. In *Int., It.,* and *US.*

Int. also includes Hydroxocobalamin Chloride and Hydroxocobalamin Sulphate. *Jpn* has Hydroxocobalamin Acetate. *Eur.* (see p.viii) includes the acetate, chloride, and sulphate.

Hydroxocobalamin occurs either as the acetate ($C_{64}H_{93}CoN_{13}O_{17}P$), the chloride ($C_{62}H_{90}ClCoN_{13}O_{15}P$) or the sulphate ($C_{124}H_{180}Co_2N_{26}O_{34}P_2S$). The hydrated form of hydroxocobalamin has been referred to as aquocobalamin.

Dark red, odourless or almost odourless crystals or crystalline powder. Some decomposition may occur on drying. The anhydrous form is very hygroscopic.

Soluble 1 in 50 of water and 1 in 100 of alcohol; sparingly soluble in methyl alcohol; practically insoluble in acetone, in chloroform, and in ether. A 2% solution in water has a pH of 8 to 10. The USP has **store** at a temperature not exceeding 15° and the Ph. Eur. between 2° and 8°. Store in airtight containers. Protect from light.

Adverse Effects and Precautions

Allergic hypersensitivity reactions have occurred rarely following the parenteral administration of the vitamin B_{12} compounds cyanocobalamin and hydroxocobalamin.

Arrhythmias secondary to hypokalaemia have occurred at the beginning of parenteral treatment with hydroxocobalamin.

Cyanocobalamin or hydroxocobalamin should, if possible, not be given to patients with suspected vitamin B_{12} deficiency without first confirming the diagnosis, and should not be used to treat megaloblastic anaemia of pregnancy. Regular monitoring of the blood is advisable. Administration of doses greater than 10 μg daily may produce a haematological response in patients with folate deficiency; indiscriminate use may mask the precise diagnosis. Conversely, folate may mask vitamin B_{12} deficiency (see p.1340).

Cyanocobalamin should not be used for Leber's disease or tobacco amblyopia since these optic neuropathies may degenerate further.

Antibodies to hydroxocobalamin-transcobalamin II complex have developed during hydroxocobalamin therapy.

Analysis, by the Boston Collaborative Drug Surveillance Program, of data on 15 438 patients hospitalised between 1975 and 1982 detected 3 allergic skin reactions attributed to cyanocobalamin among 168 recipients of the drug.[1] For the purposes of the study, reactions were defined as being generalised morbilliform exanthems, urticaria, or generalised pruritus only.

1. Bigby M, *et al.* Drug-induced cutaneous reactions: a report from the Boston Collaborative Drug Surveillance Program on 15 438 consecutive inpatients, 1975 to 1982. *JAMA* 1986; **256:** 3358–63.

Interactions

Absorption of vitamin B_{12} from the gastro-intestinal tract may be reduced by neomycin, aminosalicylic acid, histamine H_2-receptor antagonists, and colchicine. Serum concentrations may be decreased by concurrent administration of oral contraceptives. Many of these interactions are unlikely to be of clinical significance but should be taken into account when performing assays for blood concentrations. Parenteral chloramphenicol may attenuate the effect of vitamin B_{12} in anaemia.

Pharmacokinetics

Vitamin B_{12} substances bind to intrinsic factor, a glycoprotein secreted by the gastric mucosa, and are then actively absorbed from the gastro-intestinal tract. Absorption is impaired in patients with an absence of intrinsic factor, with a malabsorption syndrome or with disease or abnormality of the gut, or after gastrectomy. Absorption from the gastro-intestinal tract can also occur by passive diffusion; little of the vitamin present in diets is absorbed in this manner although the process becomes increasingly important with larger amounts such as those used therapeutically. Vitamin B_{12} is extensively bound to specific plasma proteins called transcobalamins; transcobalamin II appears to be involved in the rapid transport of the cobalamins to tissues. Vitamin B_{12} is stored in the liver, excreted in the bile, and undergoes extensive enterohepatic recycling; part of an administered dose is excreted in the urine, most of it in the first 8 hours; urinary excretion, however, accounts for only a small fraction in the reduction of total body stores acquired by dietary means. Vitamin B_{12} diffuses across the placenta and also appears in breast milk.

After injection of cyanocobalamin a large proportion is excreted in the urine within 24 hours; the body retains only 55% of a 100-μg dose and 15% of a 1000-μg dose. Body stores of vitamin B_{12} amount to 2000 to 3000 μg which is believed to be enough for 3 to 4 years. If 1000 μg is injected monthly, the 150 μg retained lasts for about 1 month. Hydroxocobalamin is better retained than cyanocobalamin; 90% of a 100-μg dose and 30% of a 1000-μg dose are retained and that range is believed to be enough for 2 to 10 months.[1]

1. Anonymous. Time to drop cyanocobalamin? *Drug Ther Bull* 1984; **22:** 43.

Intranasal absorption. For references to the intranasal absorption of cyanocobalamin and hydroxocobalamin, see Administration, below.

Human Requirements

For adults, the daily requirement of vitamin B_{12} is probably about 1 to 2 μg and this amount is present in most normal diets. Vitamin B_{12} occurs only in animal products; it does not occur in vegetables, therefore strict vegetarian (vegan) diets that exclude dairy products may provide an inadequate amount although it has been said that many years of vegetarianism are necessary before a deficiency is produced, if at all. Meats, especially liver and kidney, milk, eggs, and other dairy products, and fish are good sources of vitamin B_{12}.

In the United Kingdom[1] dietary reference values (see p.1332) have been published for vitamin B_{12} and similarly in the United States recommended dietary allowances (RDAs) have been set.[2] Differing amounts are recommended for infants and children of varying ages, adults and pregnant and lactating women. In the UK the reference nutrient intake (RNI) is 1.5 μg daily for adult males and females and the estimated average requirement (EAR) is 1.25 μg daily. In the USA the RDA for adults is 2.4 μg daily.

1. DoH. Dietary reference values for food energy and nutrients for the United Kingdom: report of the panel on dietary reference values of the committee on medical aspects of food policy. *Report on health and social subjects 41*. London: HMSO, 1991.
2. Standing Committee on the Scientific Evaluation of Dietary Reference Intakes of the Food and Nutrition Board. *Dietary Reference Intakes for thiamin, riboflavin, niacin, vitamin B_6, folate, vitamin B_{12}, pantothenic acid, biotin, and choline*. Washington, DC: National Academy Press, 1998.

Uses and Administration

Vitamin B_{12}, a water-soluble vitamin, occurs in the body mainly as methylcobalamin (mecobalamin) and as adenosylcobalamin (cobamamide) and hydroxocobalamin. Mecobalamin and cobamamide act as coenzymes in nucleic acid synthesis. Mecobalamin is also closely involved with folic acid in several important metabolic pathways.

Vitamin B_{12} deficiency may occur in strict vegetarians with an inadequate dietary intake, although it has been said that it may take many years of an inadequate intake before a deficiency is produced. Deficiency is more likely in patients with malabsorption syndromes or metabolic disorders, nitrous oxide-induced megaloblastosis, or following gastrectomy or extensive ileal resection. Deficiency leads to the development of megaloblastic anaemias and demyelination and other neurological damage. A specific anaemia known as pernicious anaemia develops in patients with an absence of the intrinsic factor necessary for good absorption of the vitamin from dietary sources.

Vitamin B_{12} preparations are used in the treatment and prevention of vitamin B_{12} deficiency. It is desirable to identify the exact cause of deficiency before commencing therapy. Hydroxocobalamin is generally preferred to cyanocobalamin; it binds more firmly to plasma proteins and is retained in the body longer (see under Pharmacokinetics, above). Cyanocobalamin and hydroxocobalamin are generally administered by the intramuscular route, although cyanocobalamin may be given by mouth and intranasal formulations are being developed (see under Administration, below). Oral cyanocobalamin may be used in treating or preventing vitamin B_{12} deficiency of dietary origin.

In pernicious anaemia and other macrocytic anaemias without neurological involvement, cyanocobalamin and hydroxocobalamin may be administered in doses of 250 to 1000 μg intramuscularly on alternate days for 1 to 2 weeks, then 250 μg weekly until the blood count returns to normal. Maintenance doses of 1000 μg are administered monthly (for cyanocobalamin) or every 2 to 3 months (for hydroxocobalamin). If there is neurological involvement, cyanocobalamin or hydroxocobalamin may be given in doses of 1000 μg on alternate days and continued for as long as improvement occurs. For the prophylaxis of anaemia associated with vitamin B_{12} deficiency resulting from gastrectomy or malabsorption syndromes cyanocobalamin may be given in doses of 250 to 1000 μg intramuscularly each month and hydroxocobalamin in doses of 1000 μg intramuscularly every 2 or 3 months. For vitamin B_{12} deficiency of dietary origin, cyanocobalamin 50 to 150 μg may be taken daily by mouth between meals. Lower doses for the administration of both cyanocobalamin and hydroxocobalamin are recommended in the USA.

Treatment usually results in rapid haematological improvement and a striking clinical response. However, neurological symptoms respond more slowly and in some cases remission may not be complete.

Hydroxocobalamin may also be given in the treatment of tobacco amblyopia and Leber's optic atrophy; initial doses are 1000 μg daily for 2 weeks intramuscularly followed by 1000 μg twice weekly for as long as improvement occurs. Thereafter, 1000 μg is administered every 1 to 3 months.

Cyanocobalamin and hydroxocobalamin are also used in the Schilling test to investigate vitamin B_{12} absorption and deficiency states. They are administered in a non-radioactive form together with cyanocobalamin radioactively-labelled with cobalt-57 or cobalt-58 and the amount of radioactivity excreted in the urine can be used to assess absorption status. A differential Schilling test, in which the forms of cyanocobalamin are given under different conditions can provide information concerning the cause of the malabsorption. Cobamamide and mecobalamin may also be used for vitamin B_{12} deficiency.

Administration. The small amounts of vitamin B_{12} present in the diet are absorbed from the gastro-intestinal tract by an active process which involves binding with intrinsic factor. As intrinsic factor is absent in patients who have developed pernicious anaemia it has often been assumed that oral treatment with vitamin B_{12} preparations will therefore be ineffective. This, however, is not necessarily so, as larger amounts of vitamin B_{12} may be absorbed by passive diffusion although a considerable amount does still remain totally unabsorbed. Thus recent attention has been given again to the use of oral cobalamins for the treatment of pernicious anaemia.[1,2] It is now considered that oral doses of 1000 μg daily will provide an adequate amount and will be a suitable alternative to injections given at monthly or so intervals. It has been stated that cyanocobalamin is also effective when given intranasally,[3] with peak plasma concentrations greater than those achievable orally, and that this may offer another alternative to injection. The intranasal absorption of hydroxocobalamin has also been studied.[4]

1. Lederle FA. Oral cobalamin for pernicious anemia: medicine's best kept secret? *JAMA* 1991; **265:** 94–5.
2. Hathcock JN, Troendle GJ. Oral cobalamin for treatment of pernicious anemia? *JAMA* 1991; **265:** 96–7.
3. Romeo VD, *et al.* Intranasal cyanocobalamin. *JAMA* 1992; **268:** 1268–9.
4. van Asselt DZB, *et al.* Nasal absorption of hydroxocobalamin in healthy elderly adults. *Br J Clin Pharmacol* 1998; **45:** 83–6.

Amino acid metabolic disorders. References to the use of hydroxocobalamin in the treatment of inborn errors of vitamin B_{12} metabolism.[1-6] Some patients with homocystinuria (p.1330) or methylmalonic aciduria have responded to cobalamins.

1. Schuh S, *et al.* Homocystinuria and megaloblastic anemia responsive to vitamin B_{12} therapy. *N Engl J Med* 1984; **310:** 686–90.
2. Hoffbrand AV, *et al.* Hereditary abnormal transcobalamin II previously diagnosed as congenital dihydrofolate reductase deficiency. *N Engl J Med* 1984; **310:** 789–90.
3. Shinnar S, Singer HS. Cobalamin C mutation (methylmalonic aciduria and homocystinuria) in adolescence. *N Engl J Med* 1984; **311:** 451–4.
4. Bhatt HR, *et al.* Treatment of hydroxocobalamin-resistant methylmalonic acidaemia with adenosylcobalamin. *Lancet* 1986; **ii:** 465.
5. van der Meer SB, *et al.* Prenatal treatment of a patient with vitamin B_{12}-responsive methylmalonic acidemia. *J Pediatr* 1990; **117:** 923–6.
6. Andersson HC, Shapira E. Biochemical and clinical response to hydroxocobalamin versus cyanocobalamin treatment in patients with methylmalonic acidemia and homocystinuria (cblC). *J Pediatr* 1998; **132:** 121–4.

Cyanide toxicity. Hydroxocobalamin combines with cyanide to form cyanocobalamin, and thus may be used as an antidote to cyanide toxicity (p.1407). Hydroxocobalamin is reported to be effective in controlling cyanide toxicity due to nitroprusside infusion,[1] and after exposure to inhaled combustion products in residential fires.[2]

1. Zerbe NF, Wagner BKJ. Use of vitamin B12 in the treatment and prevention of nitroprusside-induced cyanide toxicity. *Crit Care Med* 1993; **21:** 465–7.

2. Houeto P, *et al.* Relation of blood cyanide to plasma cyanocobalamin concentration after a fixed dose of hydroxocobalamin in cyanide poisoning. *Lancet* 1995; **346:** 605–8.

Deficiency states. The emergence of new metabolic assays for homocysteine and methylmalonic acid has led to the identification of subtle vitamin B_{12} deficiency[1,2] without the overt manifestations of megaloblastic anaemia (p.703) or neurological disease; this condition appears to be particularly common in the elderly.[1] At present, there is no clear clinical rationale for treating subtle deficiency.[1] However, preliminary findings from a recent study suggest it may be linked to some immunological impairment, identified as impaired antibody responses to pneumococcal vaccine.[3] Moreover, hyperhomocysteinaemia has been identified as a risk factor for atherosclerosis and ischaemic heart disease, and there is increasing interest in the potential of B vitamins, including B_{12}, to reduce homocysteine concentrations and therefore atherosclerotic outcomes, as discussed under Folic Acid, p.1341.

Dietary vitamin B_{12} deficiency in infants may lead to developmental abnormalities.[4,5]

1. Carmel R. Subtle cobalamin deficiency. *Ann Intern Med* 1996; **124:** 338–40.

2. Green R. Screening for vitamin B_{12} deficiency: caveat emptor. *Ann Intern Med* 1996; **124:** 509–11.

3. Fata FT, *et al.* Impaired antibody responses to pneumococcal polysaccharide in elderly patients with low serum vitamin B_{12} levels. *Ann Intern Med* 1996; **124:** 299–304.

4. Emery ES, *et al.* Vitamin B12 deficiency: a cause of abnormal movements in infants. *Pediatrics* 1997; **99:** 255–6.

5. von Schenck U, *et al.* Persistence of neurological damage induced by dietary vitamin B-12 deficiency in infancy. *Arch Dis Child* 1997; **77:** 137–9.

Neural tube defects. It has been found that an abnormality in homocysteine metabolism is present in many women who give birth to children with neural tube defects (p.1341); the enzyme methionine synthase, which converts homocysteine to methionine, requires both folate and vitamin B_{12} as cofactors, and low maternal vitamin B_{12} concentrations may be an independent risk factor for neural tube defects.[1] If confirmed, this would suggest that additional supplementation with cobalamins may be warranted.

1. Mills JL, *et al.* Homocysteine metabolism in pregnancies complicated by neural-tube defects. *Lancet* 1995; **345:** 149–51.

Preparations

BP 1998: Cyanocobalamin Injection; Cyanocobalamin Tablets; Hydroxocobalamin Injection;
USP 23: Cyanocobalamin Injection; Hydroxocobalamin Injection; Oil- and Water-soluble Vitamins Capsules; Oil- and Water-soluble Vitamins Oral Solution; Oil- and Water-soluble Vitamins Tablets; Water-soluble Vitamins Capsules; Water-soluble Vitamins Tablets.

Proprietary Preparations (details are given in Part 3)

Aust.: Erycytol; Hepavit; ***Austral.:*** Cytamen; Neo-Cytamen; ***Belg.:*** Forta B; Hydroxo; Novobedouze; ***Canad.:*** Rubramin; ***Fr.:*** Cobanzyme; Cyanokit; Dibencozan†; Dodecavit; Dolonevran†; Hydroxo†; Indusil T; Novobedouze†; Paxom†; ***Ger.:*** Ambe 12; Aquo-Cytobion; B 12-L 90; B12-Depot-Hevert; B12-Ehrl; B12-Horfervit; B12-Rotexmedica; B12-Steigerwald; B_{12} Ankermann; B_{12}-AS; B_{12}-Depot-Vicotrat; B_{12}-Vicotrat; Berubi-long†; Berubi†; Chibro B12†; Cytobion; Depogamma†; Hamo-Vibolex; Lophakomp-B 12; Lophakomp-B 12 Depot; Millevit†; Novidroxin; Vicapan N; Vit-Alboform†; Vita-Brachont; Vitamin B12 forte; ***Irl.:*** Cytacon; Cytamen; Neo-Cytamen; ***Ital.:*** Anabasi†; Cobaforte; Cobamide†; Cobergon†; Dobetin; Eritrovit B12; Fravit B12†; Idrobamina†; Idrossamina†; Indusil; Maximal†; Natur B12†; Neo-Cytamen; OH B12; Reticulogen; Zidovit†; ***Jpn:*** Calomide-S; Methycobal; ***Neth.:*** Betolvex†; Hydrocobamine; ***Norw.:*** Betolvex; ***S.Afr.:*** Betolvex; Cobalatec; Cytacon†; Cytamen†; Noritive-12; Nubee 12†; ***Spain:*** Ambritan; Asimil B12; B12 Latino Depot†; Cobaldocemetil†; Cromatonbic B12; Indusil†; Isopto B 12; Lifaton B12; Megamilbedoce; Optovite B12; Reticulogen Fortific; Zimadoce; ***Swed.:*** Behepan; Betolvex; ***Switz.:*** Arcored†; Betolvex; Cobazymase†; Hydroxo†; Novobedouze†; Vitarubin; ***UK:*** Cemac B12; Cobalin-H; Cytacon; Cytamen; Neo-Cytamen; ***USA:*** Cobolin-M†; Crystamine; Crysti 1000; Cyanoject; Cyomin; Ener-B; Hydro Cobex; Hydro-Crysti-12; Hydrobexan†; LA-12; Nascobal; Rubesol-1000†; Rubramin PC.

Multi-ingredient: numerous preparations are listed in Part 3.

Vitamin C Substances (14732-g)

Several substances have vitamin C activity, notably ascorbic acid and its calcium and sodium salts. Natural products with a high vitamin C content are black currant and rose fruit.

Ascorbic Acid (7881-b)

Ascorbic Acid *(BAN, rINN).*

Acidum Ascorbicum; L-Ascorbic Acid; Cevitamic Acid; E300; Vitamin C. The enolic form of 3-oxo-L-gulofuranolactone; 2,3-Didehydro-L-*threo*-hexono-1,4-lactone.

$C_6H_8O_6$ = 176.1.
CAS — 50-81-7.

Pharmacopoeias. In *Chin., Eur.* (see p.viii), *Int., Jpn, Pol.,* and *US.*

Odourless or almost odourless, colourless crystals or white or slightly yellow crystalline powder. It discolours on exposure to air and moisture. **Soluble** 1 in 3 of water; soluble or sparingly soluble in alcohol; practically insoluble in chloroform and in ether. **Store** in airtight nonmetallic containers. Protect from light. A 5% solution in water has a pH of 2.1 to 2.6. Solutions of ascorbic acid deteriorate rapidly in air.

Black Currant (7882-v)

Cassis; Rib. Nig.; Ribes Nigrum.

Pharmacopoeias. In *Br.*

The fresh ripe fruit of *Ribes nigrum* (Grossulariaceae) together with their pedicels and rachides. It has a strong, characteristic odour and a pleasantly acidic taste.

Calcium Ascorbate (16560-a)

Calcium Ascorbate *(BANM, rINNM).*

Calcii Ascorbas; E302.

$(C_6H_7O_6)_2Ca,2H_2O$ = 426.3.
CAS — 5743-27-1.

Pharmacopoeias. In *Eur.* (see p.viii) and *US.*

A white to slightly yellow crystalline powder; practically odourless. Freely **soluble** in water; the USP has slightly soluble, and the Ph. Eur. practically insoluble, in alcohol; practically insoluble in ether. A 10% solution has a pH between 6.8 and 7.4. **Store** in airtight nonmetallic containers. Protect from light.

Rose Fruit (7883-g)

Brier Fruit; Cynosbati Fructus; Cynosbati Pseudofructus; Dog Rose Fruits; Églantier; Hips; Hypanthium Rosae; Rosae Fructus; Rose Hips.

Pharmacopoeias. In *Fr., Ger., Jpn,* and *Swiss.*

The fruits of *Rosa canina* (Rosaceae) or other species of *Rosa.*

Sodium Ascorbate (7880-m)

Sodium Ascorbate *(BANM, rINN).*

E301; Monosodium L-Ascorbate. 3-Oxo-L-gulofuranolactone sodium enolate.

$C_6H_7NaO_6$ = 198.1.
CAS — 134-03-2.

Pharmacopoeias. In *Fr.* and *US.*

White or very faintly yellow, odourless or practically odourless, crystals or crystalline powder. It gradually darkens on exposure to light.

Soluble 1 in 1.3 of water; very slightly soluble in alcohol; practically insoluble in chloroform and ether. A 10% solution in water has a pH of 7 to 8. **Store** in airtight containers. Protect from light.

Stability. A review of the compatibility and stability of components of total parenteral nutrition solutions when mixed in 1- or 3-litre flexible containers.[1] Ascorbic acid is likely to be one of the least stable additives, although its degradation depends on a number of inter-related factors. It is oxidised in aqueous solutions by reaction with dissolved oxygen. The most important factors with respect to the rate and extent of degradation are dissolved oxygen and the presence of catalysts, especially copper ions. A second stage of ascorbic acid degradation occurs due to the permeation of oxygen through plastic which can lead to the degradation of 2.0 to 2.5 mg ascorbic acid per hour at room temperature. Another factor that influences degradation is the observation that cysteine and cystine inhibit the catalytic effect of copper. Therefore, if the infusion includes these amino acids, degradation rates can be lower. Ascorbic acid losses in TPN mixtures have been estimated from various studies. Following the addition of 500 mg ascorbic acid to the 3-litre bag, approximately 10% loss has been recorded in 24 hours at ambient temperature with exclusion of copper; with addition of trace elements to the 3-litre bag, up to 40% of the vitamin may be degraded within 2 to 3 hours. If less than 200 mg ascorbic acid is added to each bag, the patient may receive negligible amounts. Either a large excess of ascorbic acid must be added to ensure adequate daily requirements are met, or vitamins and trace elements are administered on alternate days. It should also be noted that one degradation product of ascorbic acid is oxalic acid which may be present in clinically significant quantities if considerable amounts of ascorbic acid have degraded.

1. Allwood MC. Compatibility and stability of TPN mixtures in big bags. *J Clin Hosp Pharm* 1984; **9:** 181–98.

Adverse Effects and Precautions

Ascorbic acid is usually well tolerated. Large doses are reported to cause diarrhoea and other gastro-intestinal disturbances. It has also been stated that large doses may result in hyperoxaluria and the formation of renal calcium oxalate calculi and ascorbic acid should therefore be given with care to patients with hyperoxaluria (see Effects on the Kidneys, below). Tolerance may be induced with prolonged use of large doses, resulting in symptoms of deficiency when intake is reduced to normal.

Large doses of ascorbic acid have resulted in haemolysis in patients with glucose-6-phosphate dehydrogenase (G6PD) deficiency (see below).

Effects on the blood. There are reports of haemolysis in patients with glucose-6-phosphate dehydrogenase deficiency following large doses of ascorbic acid either intravenously[1,2] or in soft drinks.[3] There has also been a report[4] of a patient with paroxysmal nocturnal haemoglobinuria suffering haemolysis following the ingestion of large amounts of ascorbic acid in a soft drink. There is concern that the large quantities of vitamin C in feeds for premature neonates may have a pro-oxidant effect, and lead to haemolysis. However, a double-blind study found no increase in erythrocyte destruction or hyperbilirubinaemia in premature neonates receiving vitamin C.[5]

1. Campbell GD, *et al.* Ascorbic acid-induced hemolysis in G-6-PD deficiency. *Ann Intern Med* 1975; **82:** 810.
2. Rees DC, *et al.* Acute haemolysis induced by high dose ascorbic acid in glucose-6-phosphate dehydrogenase deficiency. *Br Med J* 1993; **306:** 841–2.
3. Mehta JB, *et al.* Ascorbic-acid-induced haemolysis in G-6-PD deficiency. *Lancet* 1990; **336:** 944.
4. Iwamoto N, *et al.* Haemolysis induced by ascorbic acid in paroxysmal nocturnal haemoglobinuria. *Lancet* 1994; **343:** 357.
5. Doyle J, *et al.* Does vitamin C cause hemolysis in premature newborn infants? Results of a multicenter double-blind, randomized, controlled trial. *J Pediatr* 1997; **130:** 103–9.

Effects on the kidneys. Although renal impairment associated with excessive oxalate excretion has been reported following the administration of large doses of ascorbic acid[1-3] it has been considered that healthy persons can ingest large amounts of ascorbic acid with relatively small increases in oxalate excretion[4,5] and without an increased risk of oxalate stone formation.

1. Reznik VM, *et al.* Does high-dose ascorbic acid accelerate renal failure? *N Engl J Med* 1980; **302:** 1418–19.
2. Swartz RD, *et al.* Hyperoxaluria and renal insufficiency due to ascorbic acid administration during total parenteral nutrition. *Ann Intern Med* 1984; **100:** 530–1.
3. Balcke P, *et al.* Ascorbic acid aggravates secondary hyperoxalemia in patients on chronic hemodialysis. *Ann Intern Med*1984; **101:** 344–5.
4. Tsao CS. Ascorbic acid administration and urinary oxalate. *Ann Intern Med* 1984; **101:** 405–6.
5. Wandzilak TR, *et al.* Effect of high dose vitamin C on urinary oxalate levels. *J Urol (Baltimore)* 1994; **151:** 834–7.

Effects on the teeth. A report of dental enamel erosion which was attributed to the daily ingestion of chewable ascorbic acid tablets over a period of 3 years.[1] The tablets lowered the pH of the saliva to a level at which calcium was lost from the tooth enamel.

1. Giunta JL. Dental erosion resulting from chewable vitamin C tablets. *J Am Dent Assoc* 1983; **107:** 253–6.

Interference with laboratory tests. Ascorbic acid, a strong reducing agent, interferes with laboratory tests involving oxidation and reduction reactions. Falsely-elevated or false-negative test results may be obtained from plasma, faeces, or urine samples depending on such factors as the dose of ascorbic acid and specific method employed.

Interactions

For the effect of ascorbic acid on various drugs see under desferrioxamine (p.976), hormonal contraceptives (p.1433), fluphenazine (p.654), and warfarin (p.969). Ascorbic acid may increase the absorption of iron in iron-deficiency states.

Pharmacokinetics

Ascorbic acid is readily absorbed from the gastro-intestinal tract and is widely distributed in the body tissues. Plasma concentrations of ascorbic acid rise as the dose ingested is increased until a plateau is reached with doses of about 90 to 150 mg daily. Body stores of ascorbic acid in health are about 1.5 g although larger stores may occur with intakes higher than 200 mg daily. The concentration is higher in leucocytes and platelets than in erythrocytes and plasma. In deficiency states the concentration in leucocytes declines later and at a slower rate, and has been considered to be a better criterion for the evaluation of deficiency than the concentration in plasma.

Ascorbic acid is reversibly oxidised to dehydroascorbic acid; some is metabolised to ascorbate-2-sulphate, which is inactive, and oxalic acid which are excreted in the urine. Ascorbic acid in excess of the body's needs is also rapidly eliminated unchanged in the urine; this generally occurs with intakes exceeding 200 mg daily. Ascorbic acid crosses the placenta and is distributed into breast milk. It is removed by haemodialysis.

Human Requirements

A daily dietary intake of about 30 to 60 mg of vitamin C has been recommended for adults. There is, however, wide variation in individual requirements. Humans are unable to form their own ascorbic acid and so a dietary source is necessary. Most dietary ascorbic acid is obtained from fruit and vegetable sources; only small amounts are present in milk and animal tissues. Relatively rich sources include rose hips (rose fruit), black currant, citrus fruits, leafy vegetables, tomatoes, potatoes, and green and red peppers.

Ascorbic acid is readily destroyed during cooking processes. Considerable losses may also occur during storage.

In the United Kingdom[1] dietary reference values (see p.1332) have been published for vitamin C and similarly in the United States recommended dietary allowances have been set.[2] Differing amounts are recommended for infants and children of varying ages, for adult males and females, and for pregnant and lactating women. In the UK the reference nutrient intake (RNI) is 40 mg daily for adult males and females and the estimated average requirement (EAR) is 30 mg daily. In the USA the recommended amount for adults is 60 mg daily; in general the amount recommended in the USA for all ages and groups is higher than that set in the UK. Because smokers are known to have low vitamin C concentrations it is recommended by the US authorities that such persons should have an intake of at least 100 mg daily.

1. DoH. Dietary reference values for food energy and nutrients for the United Kingdom: report of the panel on dietary reference values of the committee on medical aspects of food policy. *Report on health and social subjects 41*. London: HMSO, 1991.
2. Subcommittee on the tenth edition of the RDAs, Food and Nutrition Board, Commission on Life Sciences, National Research Council. *Recommended dietary allowances* 10th ed. Washington, DC: National Academy Press, 1989.

Uses and Administration

Vitamin C, a water-soluble vitamin, is essential for the synthesis of collagen and intercellular material. Vitamin C deficiency develops when the dietary intake is inadequate. It is rare in adults, but may occur in infants, alcoholics, or the elderly. Deficiency leads to the development of a well-defined syndrome known as scurvy. This is characterised by capillary fragility, bleeding (especially from small blood vessels and the gums), normocytic or macrocytic anaemia, cartilage and bone lesions, and slow healing of wounds.

Vitamin C is used in the treatment and prevention of deficiency. It completely reverses symptoms of deficiency. It is usually given by mouth, the preferred route, as ascorbic acid, and is often given to infants in the form of a suitable fruit juice such as orange juice or as black currant or rose hip syrups. Ascorbic acid may be administered, as sodium ascorbate, by the intramuscular route, and also by the intravenous or subcutaneous routes. Doses of 25 to 75 mg daily in the prevention of deficiency, and 250 mg or more daily in divided doses for the treatment of deficiency, have been recommended.

Ascorbic acid may be given with desferrioxamine in the treatment of patients with thalassaemia, to improve the chelating action of desferrioxamine, thereby increasing the excretion of iron (see p.704). In iron deficiency states ascorbic acid may increase gastro-intestinal iron absorption and ascorbic acid or ascorbate salts are therefore included in some oral iron preparations. Ascorbic acid or sodium ascorbate have been used in treating methaemoglobinaemia. Ascorbic acid has been used to acidify urine. It has also been tried in the treatment of many other disorders, as discussed in the review below, but there is little evidence of beneficial effect.

Eye drops containing potassium ascorbate have been used for the treatment of chemical burns. Potassium ascorbate 10% is used alternately with sodium citrate 10%; it is believed that the ascorbate works by mopping up free oxygen radicals thus aiding in the prevention of corneal epithelial damage.

Ascorbic acid and calcium and sodium ascorbates are used as antoxidants in pharmaceutical manufacturing and in the food industry.

A beneficial effect of 'megadose' ascorbic acid therapy has been claimed for an extraordinary number of conditions and the subject has been reviewed by Ovesen.[1] These conditions include the common cold, asthma, atherosclerosis, cancer, psychiatric disorders, increased susceptibility to infections due to abnormal leucocyte function, infertility, and osteogenesis imperfecta; it has also been tried in treatment of wound healing, pain in Paget's disease, and opioid withdrawal. Ovesen concluded that generally there are only few properly controlled studies which substantiate these claims, and confirmation by controlled studies is required. This is certainly true of the proposed use of vitamin C to prevent cancer. Data from the few studies that have been conducted have failed to show any benefit from vitamin C (see p.1333).

As for the common cold (p.595), published findings suggest that ascorbic acid might produce a reduction in the severity of a cold but not in its incidence,[2] except perhaps in men with a low vitamin C intake.[3]

Another field in which it has been proposed that vitamin C might produce benefit is in the prevention of ischaemic heart disease, in which oxidation by free radicals is thought to play a role. However, in general, data from prospective epidemiological studies have not revealed a link between vitamin C intake and ischaemic heart disease (see p.1333). Ascorbic acid is also one of a number of agents for which reports of benefit exist in idiopathic thrombocytopenic purpura (see p.1023).

1. Ovesen L. Vitamin therapy in the absence of obvious deficiency: what is the evidence? *Drugs* 1984; **27:** 148–70.
2. Hemilä H. Does vitamin C alleviate the symptoms of the common cold?—a review of current evidence. *Scand J Infect Dis* 1994; **26:** 1–6.
3. Hemilä H. Vitamin C intake and susceptibility to the common cold. *Br J Nutr* 1997; **77:** 59–72.

Preparations

BP 1998: Ascorbic Acid Injection; Ascorbic Acid Tablets; Black Currant Syrup; Vitamins B and C Injection;
BPC 1973: Vitamins Capsules;
USP 23: Ascorbic Acid Injection; Ascorbic Acid Oral Solution; Ascorbic Acid Tablets; Oil- and Water-soluble Vitamins Capsules; Oil- and Water-soluble Vitamins Oral Solution; Oil- and Water-soluble Vitamins Tablets; Water-soluble Vitamins Capsules; Water-soluble Vitamins Tablets.

Proprietary Preparations (details are given in Part 3)
Aust.: Ascorbin; Bioagil; C-Vit; Calcascorbin; Ce-Limo; Cebion; Cevitol; Irocovit C; Mel-C; Redoxon; Tetesept Vitamin C; Vicedent; ***Austral.:*** Ascorbt†; Bioglan Cal C; Cecon; Flavettes†; Invite C†; Megavit C 1000†; Potent C†; Pro-C; Redoxon; Sugarless C; Supa C; Supervite C†; ***Belg.:*** C-Dose; C-Will; Cenol; Cetamine; Cevi-drops†; Cevitan†; Redoxon; ***Canad.:*** Action; Apo-C; Ascorbex; Balanced C Complex; C Forte; C-1000; C-3000; Ce-Vi-Sol†; Ester-C; Kamu Jay; Kyolic 103; Ortic C; Redoxon; Revitalose C; Timed Release C; Vita-C; ***Fr.:*** Arkovital C; Laroscorbine; Midy Vitamine C; Tempodia; Vitacemil†; Vitascorbol; ***Ger.:*** Ascorell; Ascorvit; ASS OPT; ASS-Kreuz; Cebion; Cebion N; Cedoxon†; Ceglycon†; Cetebe; Hermes Cevitt; ***Irl.:*** Redoxon; Rubex; ***Ital.:*** Acidylina; Agrumina; Aran C†; Ascomed; Ascorbin†; Ascorgil†; Aster C†; Bio-Ci; C Monovit; C-Lisa; C-Tard; Cantan†; Cebion; Cecon; Cevigen†; Cevit†; Ciergin†; Duo-C; Dynaphos-C; Ergofit; Idro-C; Lemonvit; Redoxon; Vici; Vicitina; Vigovit C†; Vincit†; Zig C; ***Neth.:*** C-Will; Dagravit C†; Davitamon C†; Redoxon; ***Norw.:*** AFI-C; ***S.Afr.:*** Cebion†; Redoxon; Scorbex; ***Spain:*** Biocatines C Fuerte†; Caramelos Vit C; Cebion; Cecrisina†; Citrolider; Citrovit; Junce; Ledovit C; Redoxon; Top Fit-C†; Upsa C; Yoguis C†; ***Swed.:*** C-vimin; Ido-C; ***Switz.:*** C-Naryl; Cegrovit; Redoxon; Vicemex; Vita-Ce; ***UK:*** Buffered C; Buffered C 500; Redoxon; ***USA:*** Alba CE; Ascorbicap; Ce-Vi-Sol; Cebid; Cecon; Cee-1000 TD†; Cee-500†; Cenolate; Cevalin; Cevi-Bid; Dull-C; Flavorcee; N'ice Vitamin C; Sunkist; Vita-C.

Multi-ingredient: numerous preparations are listed in Part 3.

Vitamin D Substances (7892-q)

The term vitamin D is used for a range of closely related sterol compounds including alfacalcidol, calcifediol, calcitriol, cholecalciferol, dihydrotachysterol, and ergocalciferol.

Alfacalcidol (7885-p)

Alfacalcidol *(BAN, rINN).*

EB-644; 1α-Hydroxycholecalciferol; 1α-Hydroxyvitamin D_3; 1α-OHD_3. (5*Z*,7*E*)-9,10-Secocholesta-5,7,10(19)-triene-1α,3β-diol.

$C_{27}H_{44}O_2$ = 400.6.

CAS — 41294-56-8.

Pharmacopoeias. In *Eur.* (see p.viii).

White or almost white crystals which are sensitive to air, heat, and light. Practically **insoluble** in water; freely soluble in alcohol; soluble in fatty oils. Reversible isomerisation to pre-alfacalcidol may take place in solution. **Store** at 2° to 8° in airtight containers under an atmosphere of nitrogen. The contents of an opened container should be used immediately. Protect from light.

Calcifediol (7886-s)

Calcifediol *(USAN, rINN).*

25-Hydroxycholecalciferol; 25-Hydroxyvitamin D_3; 25-$(OH)D_3$; U-32070E. (5*Z*,7*E*)-9,10-Secocholesta-5,7,10-(19)-triene-3β,25-diol monohydrate.

$C_{27}H_{44}O_2,H_2O$ = 418.7.

CAS — 19356-17-3 (anhydrous calcifediol); 63283-36-3 (calcifediol monohydrate).

Pharmacopoeias. In *Eur.* (see p.viii) and *US.*

White or almost white crystals which are sensitive to air, heat, and light. Practically **insoluble** in water; freely soluble in alcohol; soluble in fatty oils. Reversible isomerisation to pre-calcifediol may take place in solution. **Store** at 2° to 8° in airtight containers under an atmosphere of nitrogen. The contents of an opened container should be used immediately. Protect from light.

Calcitriol (7887-w)

Calcitriol *(BAN, USAN, rINN).*

Calcitriolum; 1,25-Dihydroxycholecalciferol; 1α,25-Dihydroxycholecalciferol; 1α,25-Dihydroxyvitamin D_3; 1α,25$(OH)_2D_3$; Ro-21-5535. (5*Z*,7*E*)-9,10-Secocholesta-5,7,10(19)-triene-1α,3β,25-triol.

$C_{27}H_{44}O_3$ = 416.6.

CAS — 32222-06-3.

Pharmacopoeias. In *Eur.* (see p.viii).

White or almost white crystals. Practically **insoluble** in water; freely soluble in alcohol; soluble in ether and in fatty oils. It is sensitive to air, heat, and light. **Store** at 2 to 8° in airtight containers, under an atmosphere of nitrogen. The contents of an opened container should be used immediately. Protect from light.

Cholecalciferol (7888-e)

Cholecalciferol *(BAN).*

Colecalciferol *(rINN)*; Activated 7-Dehydrocholesterol; Cholecalciferolum; Vitamin D_3. (5*Z*,7*E*)-9,10-Secocholesta-5,7,10(19)-trien-3β-ol.

$C_{27}H_{44}O$ = 384.6.

CAS — 67-97-0.

Pharmacopoeias. In *Chin., Eur.* (see p.viii), *Int., Jpn, Pol.,* and *US.*
Eur. also includes monographs for Cholecalciferol Concentrate (Oily Form), Cholecalciferol Concentrate (Powder Form), and Cholecalciferol Concentrate (Water-dispersible Form). *US* also includes Cholecalciferol Solution.

The naturally occurring form of vitamin D. It is produced from 7-dehydrocholesterol, a sterol present in mammalian skin, by ultraviolet irradiation. White or almost white, odourless crystals which are sensitive to air, heat, and light. Practically **insoluble** in water; freely soluble or soluble in alcohol; freely soluble in ether; soluble in chloroform and in fatty oils. Solutions in volatile solvents are unstable and should be used immediately. **Store** at a temperature of 2 to 8° in hermetically sealed containers in which the air has been replaced by nitrogen. The contents of an opened container should be used immediately. Protect from light.

Dihydrotachysterol (7891-g)

Dihydrotachysterol *(BAN, rINN).*

Dichysterol. (5*E*,7*E*,22*E*)-10α-9,10-Secoergosta-5,7,22-trien-3β-ol.

$C_{28}H_{46}O$ = 398.7.

CAS — 67-96-9.

Pharmacopoeias. In *Br.* and *US.*

Odourless or almost odourless colourless or white crystals or white crystalline powder. Practically **insoluble** in water; soluble in alcohol; freely or very soluble in chloroform; freely soluble in ether; sparingly soluble in arachis oil. **Store** at a temperature not exceeding 15° in hermetically sealed glass containers in which the air has been replaced by nitrogen. Protect from light.

Ergocalciferol (7884-q)

Ergocalciferol *(BAN, rINN).*

Calciferol; Ergocalciferolum; Irradiated Ergosterol; Viosterol; Vitamin D_2. (5Z,7E,22E)-9,10-Secoergosta-5,7,10(19),22-tetraen-3β-ol.

$C_{28}H_{44}O$ = 396.6.

CAS — 50-14-6.

Pharmacopoeias. In *Chin., Eur.* (see p.viii), *Int., Jpn,* and *US.*

An antirachitic substance obtained from ergosterol, a sterol present in fungi and yeasts, by ultraviolet irradiation. White or almost white, odourless, crystals or white or slightly yellow crystalline powder. It is sensitive to air, heat, and light.

Practically **insoluble** in water; freely soluble or soluble in alcohol and in ether; soluble in chloroform and in fatty oils. Solutions in volatile solvents are unstable and should be used immediately. **Store** at a temperature of 2 to 8° in hermetically sealed containers in which the air has been replaced by nitrogen. The contents of an opened container should be used immediately. Protect from light.

Stability. A review of the compatibility and stability of components of total parenteral solutions when mixed in 1- or 3-litre flexible containers.[1] Vitamin D may bind strongly to plastic which can lead to significant losses to the bag and administration set. Vitamin D losses from paediatric TPN mixtures have been estimated to be about 30 to 36% over a 24-hour administration period. The quantity of vitamin D delivered depends on infusion rate, type of administration set, composition of mixture, and total volume infused.

1. Allwood MC. Compatibility and stability of TPN mixtures in big bags. *J Clin Hosp Pharm* 1984; **9:** 181–98.

Units

The Second International Standard Preparation (1949) of vitamin D consisted of bottles containing approximately 6 g of a solution of cholecalciferol in vegetable oil (1000 units per g). This standard has now been discontinued.

NOTE. One unit of vitamin D is contained in 25 ng of cholecalciferol or ergocalciferol (i.e. 1 mg of cholecalciferol or ergocalciferol is equivalent to 40 000 units of vitamin D).

Adverse Effects and Treatment

Excessive intake of vitamin D leads to the development of hypercalcaemia and its associated effects including hypercalciuria, ectopic calcification, and renal and cardiovascular damage (for a discussion of vitamin-D mediated hypercalcaemia and its treatment, see p.1148). Symptoms of overdosage include anorexia, lassitude, nausea and vomiting, diarrhoea, polyuria, sweating, headache, thirst, and vertigo. Interindividual tolerance to vitamin D varies considerably; infants and children are generally more susceptible to its toxic effects. The vitamin should be withdrawn if toxicity occurs. It has been stated that vitamin D dietary supplementation may be detrimental in persons already receiving an adequate intake through their diet and exposure to sunlight since the difference between therapeutic and toxic concentrations is relatively small.

Calcitriol, which is more potent than the other forms of vitamin D, might reasonably be expected to pose a greater risk of toxicity; however, its effects are reported to be reversed more rapidly on withdrawal than when other derivatives are used.

Hypersensitivity reactions have occurred.

Vitamin D is the most likely of all vitamins to cause overt toxicity. Doses of 60 000 units per day can cause hypercalcaemia, with muscle weakness, apathy, headache, anorexia, nausea and vomiting, bone pain, ectopic calcification, proteinuria, hypertension, and cardiac arrhythmias. Chronic hypercalcaemia can lead to generalised vascular calcification, nephrocalcinosis, and rapid deterioration of renal function.[1]

Hypercalcaemia has been reported in one person following brief industrial exposure to cholecalciferol.[2]

A study in children treated for renal osteodystrophy has provided some evidence that hypercalcaemia may occur more frequently with calcitriol than with ergocalciferol.[3] Another such study has suggested that vitamin D has nephrotoxic properties independent of the degree of induced hypercalcaemia, and that the decline in renal function may be more marked with calcitriol.[4]

Topical calcitriol may affect calcium homoeostasis, and hypercalcaemia has been reported in some studies.[5] For mention of the effect of other vitamin D analogues used in psoriasis on calcium homoeostasis, see p.1080.

1. Anonymous. *Med Lett Drugs Ther* 1984; **26:** 73.
2. Jibani M, Hodges NH. Prolonged hypercalcaemia after industrial exposure to vitamin D_3. *Br Med J* 1985; **290:** 748–9.
3. Hodson EM, *et al.* Treatment of childhood renal osteodystrophy with calcitriol or ergocalciferol. *Clin Nephrol* 1985; **24:** 192–200.
4. Chan JCM, *et al.* A prospective, double-blind study of growth failure in children with chronic renal insufficiency and the effectiveness of treatment with calcitriol versus dihydrotachysterol. *J Pediatr* 1994; **124:** 520–8.
5. Bourke JF, *et al.* Vitamin D analogues in psoriasis: effects on systemic calcium homeostasis. *Br J Dermatol* 1996; **135:** 347–54.

Precautions

Vitamin D should not be administered to patients with hypercalcaemia. It should be administered with caution to infants as they may have increased sensitivity to its effects and should be used with care in patients with renal impairment or calculi, or heart disease, who might be at increased risk of organ damage if hypercalcaemia occurred. Plasma phosphate concentrations should be controlled during vitamin D therapy to reduce the risk of ectopic calcification.

It is advised that patients receiving pharmacological doses of vitamin D should have their plasma-calcium concentration monitored at regular intervals, especially initially and if symptoms suggest toxicity (see above). Similar monitoring is recommended in infants if they are breast fed by mothers receiving vitamin D.

Pregnancy. Hypercalcaemia during pregnancy may produce congenital disorders in the offspring, and neonatal hypoparathyroidism. However, the risks to the fetus of untreated maternal hypoparathyroidism are considered greater than the risks of hypercalcaemia due to vitamin D therapy. Indeed, one report noted increased requirements for vitamin D preparations during pregnancy for the treatment of hypoparathyroidism;[1] the doses tended to need increasing during the second half of pregnancy. In one woman in whom the dose of calcitriol was kept at the increased level after delivery (in an attempt to allow for the calcium loss involved in breast feeding) hypercalcaemia developed; this did not occur in 2 women who did not breast feed and in whom the dose of the vitamin D preparations was reduced soon after delivery.[1]

1. Caplan RH, Beguin EA. Hypercalcaemia in a calcitriol-treated hypoparathyroid woman during lactation. *Obstet Gynecol* 1990; **76:** 485–9.

Interactions

There is an increased risk of hypercalcaemia if vitamin D is coadministered with thiazide diuretics and calcium. Plasma-calcium concentrations should be monitored in patients receiving the drugs concurrently. Some antiepileptics may increase vitamin D requirements (e.g. carbamazepine, phenobarbitone, phenytoin, and primidone).

Danazol. A report of hypercalcaemia associated with danazol in a patient maintained on alfacalcidol therapy for hypoparathyroidism.[1] Introduction of danazol appeared to reduce the maintenance requirement for alfacalcidol.

1. Hepburn NC, *et al.* Danazol-induced hypercalcaemia in alphacalcidol-treated hypoparathyroidism. *Postgrad Med J* 1989; **65:** 849–50.

Thyroxine. Three patients receiving dihydrotachysterol and calcium for postoperative hypoparathyroidism, following thyroidectomy, developed hypercalcaemia when their concomitant thyroxine therapy was discontinued before a radioiodine scan.[1] The dose of dihydrotachysterol should be reduced and serum-calcium concentrations should be monitored when thyroid treatment is interrupted, since elimination of dihydrotachysterol may be delayed in hypothyroidism.

1. Lamberg B-A, Tikkanen MJ. Hypercalcaemia due to dihydrotachysterol treatment in patients with hypothyroidism after thyroidectomy. *Br Med J* 1981; **283:** 461–2.

Pharmacokinetics

Vitamin D substances are well absorbed from the gastro-intestinal tract. The presence of bile is essential for adequate intestinal absorption; absorption may be decreased in patients with decreased fat absorption.

Vitamin D and its metabolites circulate in the blood bound to a specific α-globulin. Vitamin D can be stored in adipose and muscle tissue for long periods of time. It is slowly released from such storage sites and from the skin where it is formed in the presence of sunlight or ultraviolet light. Ergocalciferol and cholecalciferol have a slow onset and a long duration of action; calcitriol and its analogue alfacalcidol, however, have a more rapid action and shorter half-lives.

Cholecalciferol and ergocalciferol are hydroxylated in the liver by the enzyme vitamin D 25-hydroxylase to form 25-hydroxycholecalciferol (calcifediol) and 25-hydroxyergocalciferol respectively. These compounds undergo further hydroxylation in the kidneys by the enzyme vitamin D 1-hydroxylase to form the active metabolites 1,25-dihydroxycholecalciferol (calcitriol) and 1,25-dihydroxyergocalciferol respectively. Further metabolism also occurs in the kidneys, including the formation of the 1,24,25-trihydroxy derivatives. Of the synthetic analogues, alfacalcidol is converted rapidly in the liver to calcitriol, and dihydrotachysterol is hydroxylated, also in the liver, to its active form 25-hydroxydihydrotachysterol.

Vitamin D compounds and their metabolites are excreted mainly in the bile and faeces with only small amounts appearing in urine; there is some enterohepatic recycling but it is considered to have a negligible contribution to vitamin D status. Certain vitamin D substances may be distributed into breast milk.

Human Requirements

The daily requirements of vitamin D in adults are small and may be met mainly by exposure to sunlight and/or obtained from the diet. A daily dietary intake of about 200 to 400 units (5 to 10 μg of cholecalciferol or ergocalciferol) of vitamin D is generally considered adequate for healthy adults. In comparison with older adults in the age range of 25 years upwards the requirements per kg body-weight are greater in infants, children, and young adults and during pregnancy and lactation. Requirements may also be higher in people who are not exposed to adequate sunlight such as the elderly or housebound.

Vitamin D is present in few foods. Fish-liver oils, especially cod-liver oil, are good sources of vitamin D. Other sources, which contain much smaller amounts, include butter, eggs, and liver. Some foods are often fortified with vitamin D and milk and margarine will therefore also provide a supply of vitamin D. Cooking processes do not appear to affect the activity of vitamin D.

In the United Kingdom dietary reference values (see p.1332) for vitamin D have only been published for selected groups of the population.[1] In the US Recommended Dietary Allowances had been set,[2] and have recently been replaced by Dietary Reference Intakes (see p.1332). Differing amounts are recommended for infants and children of varying ages, for adults, and for pregnant and lactating women. In the UK a dietary intake was considered unnecessary for adults living a normal lifestyle who were being exposed to solar radiation; for those confined indoors a Reference Nutrient Intake (RNI) of 10 μg [as cholecalciferol or ergocalciferol] daily was set. This RNI of 10 μg daily was also considered to be applicable to all persons aged 65 years or more and to pregnant and lactating women. RNIs were set for children up to the age of 3 years; dietary intake was considered unnecessary for older children. Mention was made that in order to achieve the above reference nutrient intakes, supplementation of the diet may actually be required and supplementation was also recommended for Asian women and children in the UK. In the USA the traditional Recommended Dietary Allowances were: 7.5 μg during the first 6 months of life but if infants were breast fed and not exposed to sunlight it was recommended that a supplement of 5 to 7.5 μg daily should be given; 10 μg for all persons up to the age of 24 years; 5 μg for all persons over the age of 24 years; and 10 μg for all pregnant or lactating women. Under the new Dietary Reference Intakes, Adequate Intakes have been set for vitamin D.[3] These are: 5 μg per day (as cholecalciferol) for all persons from birth through to age 50 years, including pregnant or lactating women; 10 μg per day for adults aged 51 to 70 years; and 15 μg per day for those aged greater than 70 years.

1. DoH. Dietary reference values for food energy and nutrients for the United Kingdom: report of the panel on dietary reference values of the committee on medical aspects of food policy. *Report on health and social subjects 41*. London: HMSO, 1991.
2. Subcommittee on the tenth edition of the RDAs, Food and Nutrition Board, Commission on Life Sciences, National Research Council. *Recommended dietary allowances*. 10th ed. Washington, DC: National Academy Press, 1989.
3. Standing Committee on the Scientific Evaluation of Dietary Reference Intakes of the Food and Nutrition Board. *Dietary Reference Intakes for calcium, phosphorus, magnesium, vitamin D, and fluoride*. Washington, DC: National Academy Press, 1997.

Uses and Administration

Vitamin D compounds are fat-soluble sterols, sometimes considered to be hormones or hormone precursors, which are essential for the proper regulation of calcium and phosphate homoeostasis and bone mineralisation.

Vitamin D deficiency develops when there is inadequate exposure to sunlight or a lack of the vitamin in the diet. Deficiency generally takes a prolonged period of time to develop due to slow release of the vitamin from body stores. Deficiency may occur in some infants who are breast fed without supplemental vitamin D or exposure to sunlight, in the elderly whose mobility and thus exposure to light may be impaired, and in persons with fat malabsorption syndromes; certain disease states such as renal failure may also affect the metabolism of vitamin D substances to metabolically active forms and thus result in deficiency. Deficiency leads to the development of a syndrome characterised by hypocalcaemia, hypophosphataemia, undermineralisation or demineralisation of bone, bone pain, bone fractures, and muscle weakness, known in adults as osteomalacia (see below). In children, in whom there may be growth retardation and skeletal deformity, especially of the long bones, it is known as rickets.

Vitamin D compounds are used in the treatment and prevention of vitamin D deficiency states and hypocalcaemia associated with disorders such as hypoparathyroidism, and renal osteodystrophy, as indicated by the cross-references given below.

A variety of forms and analogues of vitamin D are available, and the choice of agent depends on the cause of the condition to be treated and the relative properties of the available agents. Cholecalciferol and ergocalciferol are equal in potency, and have a slow onset and relatively prolonged duration of action. Dihydrotachysterol has relatively weak antirachitic activity, but its actions are faster in onset and less persistent than those of the calciferols and it does not require renal hydroxylation. Calcifediol, an intermediate metabolite, has some action of its own but is also converted to the more potent 1,25-dihydroxycholecalciferol (calcitriol); calcitriol and its analogue alfacalcidol are the most potent and rapidly acting of the vitamin D substances.

- For the treatment of simple nutritional deficiencies **cholecalciferol** or **ergocalciferol** are generally preferred. They are usually given by mouth, but may also be administered by intramuscular injection. A dose of 10 μg (400 units) daily is generally sufficient in adults for the prevention of simple deficiency states. Deficiency due to malabsorption states or liver disease often requires higher doses for treatment, of up to 1 mg (40 000 units) daily. Doses of up to 2.5 mg (100 000 units) daily may be used in the treatment of hypocalcaemia due to hypoparathyroidism.
- Where large doses are required it may be preferable to use one of the more potent derivatives. In particular, when renal function is impaired as in renal osteodystrophy, with consequent reduction in the conversion of calciferols to their active metabolites, then alfacalcidol or calcitriol, which do not require renal hydroxylation, should be given. **Calcitriol** is given by mouth or by intravenous injection. Usual initial adult doses of 0.25 μg daily or on alternate days are given by mouth, increased if necessary, in steps of 0.25 μg at intervals of 2 to 4 weeks, to a usual dose of 0.5 to 1 μg daily. Initial doses intravenously are usually 0.5 μg three times a week increased if necessary in steps of 0.25 to 0.5 μg at intervals of 2 to 4 weeks, to a usual dose of 0.5 to 3 μg three times a week. Alternatively, **alfacalcidol** is given in initial doses of 1 μg daily by mouth, or 0.5 μg for elderly patients. Doses of 0.25 to 1 μg daily may be given for maintenance. Suggested doses for children under 20 kg are 0.05 μg (50 ng) per kg body-weight daily and for premature infants and neonates a dose of 0.05 to 0.1 μg (50 to 100 ng) per kg daily. Doses of alfacalcidol may also be given by intravenous injection over 30 seconds.
- Of the other available forms, **calcifediol**, the 25-hydroxylated metabolite of cholecalciferol, is given in usual adult doses of 50 to 100 μg daily or 100 to 200 μg on alternate days by mouth. For hypocalcaemic tetany due to hypoparathyroidism, **dihydrotachysterol** is given in initial adult doses of 0.25 to 2.5 mg daily by mouth, depending on severity. Maintenance doses have ranged from 0.25 mg per week to 1 mg daily. **Paricalcitol** is another vitamin D analogue which is used to treat the secondary hyperparathyroidism associated with chronic renal failure.

When vitamin D substances are given in pharmacological doses, dosage must be individualised for each patient, and should be based on regular monitoring of plasma-calcium concentrations (initially weekly, and then every 2 to 4 weeks), to optimise clinical response and avoid hypercalcaemia.

Vitamin D, usually in the form of calcitriol, may be used in the treatment of osteoporosis (see below). In established postmenopausal osteoporosis, calcitriol 0.25 μg twice daily is recommended. Vitamin D and calcium supplements are often given as adjuncts to other therapies in osteoporosis.

Calcitriol has been used in the management of psoriasis (see below).

Calciferol derivatives are used as a rodenticide.

General references.

1. Fraser DR. Vitamin D. *Lancet* 1995; **345:** 104–7.
2. van der Wielen RPJ, *et al.* Serum vitamin D concentrations among elderly people in Europe. *Lancet* 1995; **346:** 207–10.
3. Gloth FM, *et al.* Vitamin D deficiency in homebound elderly persons. *JAMA* 1995; **274:** 1683–6.
4. Nellen JFJB, *et al.* Hypovitaminosis D in immigrant women: slow to be diagnosed. *Br Med J* 1996; **312:** 570–2.
5. Thomas MK, *et al.* Hypovitaminosis D in medical inpatients. *N Engl J Med* 1998; **338:** 777–83.

Hyperparathyroidism. Vitamin D has been employed for certain forms of hyperparathyroidism. The secondary hyperparathyroidism of renal osteodystrophy (p.732) may respond to oral or intravenous treatment with calcitriol, or its analogue alfacalcidol,[1-3] which do not require renal hydroxylation for activation. However, doses capable of suppressing parathyroid hormone secretion may lead to hypercalcaemia[3] and a decline in renal function[4] (see also under Adverse Effects, above), which may limit their value.

1. Andress DL, *et al.* Intravenous calcitriol in the treatment of refractory osteitis fibrosa of chronic renal failure. *N Engl J Med* 1989; **321:** 274–9.
2. Argilés À, *et al.* High-dose alfacalcidol for anaemia in dialysis. *Lancet* 1993; **342:** 378–9.
3. Quarles LD, *et al.* Prospective trial of pulse oral versus intravenous calcitriol treatment of hyperparathyroidism in ESRD. *Kidney Int* 1994; **45:** 1710–21.
4. Chan JCM, *et al.* A prospective, double-blind study of growth failure in children with chronic renal insufficiency and the effectiveness of treatment with calcitriol versus dihydrotachysterol. *J Pediatr* 1994; **124:** 520–8.

Hypoparathyroidism. Although parenteral calcium salts may be given acutely for hypocalcaemic tetany, long-term treatment of hypoparathyroidism (p.733) usually aims at correction of associated hypocalcaemia with oral vitamin D compounds, which increase the intestinal absorption of calcium. If dietary calcium is inadequate these may be combined with calcium supplementation.

Hypoparathyroidism in *pregnancy* poses severe risks of fetal hyperparathyroidism with neonatal hypocalcaemic rickets, which may be fatal. Treatment with calcium and either cholecalciferol or ergocalciferol in doses of 1.25 to 2.5 mg daily, or dihydrotachysterol 0.25 to 1.0 mg daily is essential.[1]

1. Hague WM. Treatment of endocrine diseases. *Br Med J* 1987; **294:** 297–300.

Malignant neoplasms. The active form of vitamin D, calcitriol (1,25-dihydroxycholecalciferol) has been found to promote tissue differentiation and to inhibit cellular proliferation *in vitro*. These findings have prompted workers to investigate the potential role and efficacy of vitamin D metabolites or analogues (sometimes referred to as deltanoids) in malignant neoplasms and in other disorders of cell growth such as psoriasis (see below).

Animal and *in vitro* studies with alfacalcidol have led to the suggestion that evaluation should be undertaken in malignant disease of the human breast.[1] A study in humans has been performed with the calcitriol derivative calcipotriol (p.1080); in this trial calcipotriol used topically in advanced or cutaneous metastatic breast cancer was considered to exert some positive effects and further investigation was considered warranted.[2] Regression of T-cell lymphoma of the skin (mycosis fungoides, p.482) has been reported following application of calcipotriol,[3] and following systemic treatment with calcitriol and a retinoid in a patient who failed to respond to topical calcipotriol.[4] However, 3 other patients with cutaneous T-cell lymphoma failed to respond to calcitriol and isotretinoin,[5] which may have been because of the phenotype or stage of the disease.[6] Systemic treatment, again with calcitriol and a retinoid, has also been reported to produce regression of actinic keratoses and non-melanoma skin cancers in 4 patients (p.492).[7]

1. Colston KW, *et al.* Possible role for vitamin D in controlling breast cancer cell proliferation. *Lancet* 1989; **i:** 188–91.
2. Bower M, *et al.* Topical calcipotriol treatment in advanced breast cancer. *Lancet* 1991; **337:** 701–2. Correction. *ibid.*; 1618.
3. Scott-Mackie P, *et al.* Calcipotriol and regression in T-cell lymphoma of skin. *Lancet* 1993; **342:** 172.
4. French LE, *et al.* Remission of cutaneous T-cell lymphoma with combined calcitriol and acitretin. *Lancet* 1994; **344:** 686–7.
5. Thomsen K. Cutaneous T-cell lymphoma and calcitriol and isotretinoin treatment. *Lancet* 1995; **345:** 1583.
6. French LE, Saurat J-H. Treatment of cutaneous T-cell lymphoma by retinoids and calcitriol. *Lancet* 1995; **346:** 376–7.
7. Majewski S, *et al.* Combination of isotretinoin and calcitriol for precancerous and cancerous skin lesions. *Lancet* 1994; **344:** 1510–11.

Osteomalacia. Treatment of osteomalacia (p.730) primarily aims at correcting any underlying deficiency states, and vitamin D substances, calcium, or phosphate supplements may be given by mouth as necessary. Where rickets is due to impaired synthesis of calcitriol (type I pseudodeficiency) or receptor resistance (type II pseudodeficiency) replacement therapy with calcitriol may be indicated (in the latter case with very high dose calcium),[1] while X-linked hypophosphataemic rickets is generally treated with phosphate supplementation and calcitriol, although vitamin D alone is also effective.[2] The use of single large doses of a vitamin D substance (stosstherapie), for the prophylaxis of rickets, is highly controversial because of problems with toxicity, although it may be effective in patients with rickets due to proven vitamin D deficiency.[3]

1. Hochberg Z, *et al.* Calcium therapy for calcitriol-resistant rickets. *J Pediatr* 1992; **121:** 803–8.
2. Seikaly MG, *et al.* The effect of phosphate supplementation on linear growth in children with X-linked hypophosphatemia. *Pediatrics* 1994; **94:** 478–81.
3. Shah BR, Finberg L. Single-day therapy for nutritional vitamin D-deficiency rickets: a preferred method. *J Pediatr* 1994; **125:** 487–90.

PREGNANCY AND THE NEONATE. Most infants receive adequate calcium and vitamin D during pregnancy and during breast feeding or bottle feeding to prevent the development of rickets. However, it is considered that there are certain groups of women whose infants may be at special risk of neonatal rickets and these include those suffering economic deprivation, those living at high latitudes, and Asian immigrants in northern Europe, especially in winter. It is therefore suggested that pregnant women in such circumstances should receive supplements as the diet and sunshine exposure may not be providing adequate calcium (1 to 1.2 g daily) or vitamin D (400 units daily).[1]

Rickets may be more problematical in the premature infant as vitamin D requirements may be increased. Although there is no evidence that routine administration is necessary or desirable, healing of illness as a result of rickets may be achieved rapidly by the use of alfacalcidol 100 to 200 ng per kg body-weight daily.[2]

1. Misra R, Anderson DC. Providing the fetus with calcium. *Br Med J* 1990; **300:** 1220–1.
2. Brooke OG. Supplementary vitamin D in infancy and childhood. *Arch Dis Child* 1983; **58:** 573–4.

Osteopetrosis. For mention of the use of high-dose calcitriol in the management of juvenile osteopetrosis, see under Corticosteroids, p.1024.

Osteoporosis. Studies using vitamin D for the treatment of osteoporosis (p.731) have produced conflicting results.[1-6] However, in patients over 75 years of age, in whom dietary deficiencies are common, calcium and vitamin D supplements are recommended.

Vitamin D may be used in the prevention of corticosteroid-induced osteoporosis, see p.1011.

1. Ott SM, Chesnut CH. Calcitriol treatment is not effective in postmenopausal osteoporosis. *Ann Intern Med* 1989; **110:** 267–74.
2. Gallagher JC, Goldgar D. Treatment of postmenopausal osteoporosis with high doses of synthetic calcitriol: a randomized controlled study. *Ann Intern Med* 1990; **113:** 649–55.
3. Tilyard MW, *et al.* Treatment of postmenopausal osteoporosis with calcitriol or calcium. *N Engl J Med* 1992; **326:** 357–62.
4. Chapuy MC, *et al.* Effect of calcium and cholecalciferol treatment for three years on hip fractures in elderly women. *Br Med J* 1994; **308:** 1081–2.

Phytomenadione (7903-k)

Phytomenadione (*BAN, rINN*).

Methylphytylnaphthochinonum; Phylloquinone; Phytomenad.; Phytomenadionum; Phytonadione; Vitamin K_1. 2-Methyl-3-[3,7,11,15-tetramethylhexadec-2-enyl] naphthalene-1,4-dione.

$C_{31}H_{46}O_2$ = 450.7.

CAS — 84-80-0.

Pharmacopoeias. In *Chin., Eur.* (see p.viii), *Int., Jpn,* and *US.*

Phytomenadione is a mixture of the *trans* (*E*) and *cis* (*Z*) isomers. Ph. Eur. specifies that it contains not less than 75% of *trans*-phytomenadione, and also allows not more than 4% of *trans*-epoxyphytomenadione. The USP specifies a content of not more than 21% of *cis*-phytomenadione. A clear, intense yellow to amber, very viscous, odourless or almost odourless, oily liquid, which is stable in air but decomposes on exposure to sunlight. Practically **insoluble** in water; sparingly or slightly soluble in alcohol; miscible with ether and with fatty oils; soluble in dehydrated alcohol and in chloroform. **Store** in airtight containers. Protect from light. Aqueous dispersions of phytomenadione for injection should not be allowed to freeze.

Incompatibility. A review of the compatibilities of nutritional agents and drugs in parenteral nutrition solutions.[1] Phytomenadione is reported to be visually compatible for 24 hours in parenteral nutrition solutions containing typical additives. Although concern has been expressed about the instability of phytomenadione to light, only 10 to 15% loss of potency occurs over 24 hours on exposure to sunlight or fluorescent light. Phytomenadione passes through an inline filter with negligible loss.

1. Niemiec PW, Vanderveen TW. Compatibility considerations in parenteral nutrient solutions. *Am J Hosp Pharm* 1984; **41:** 893–911.

Stability. A polyethoxylated castor oil formulation of phytomenadione was stable for at least 30 days at room temperature when repackaged in amber glass dropper bottles.[1] When refrigerated at 4 to 8°, it was stable in both plastic and amber glass bottles.

1. Wong VK, Ho PC. Stability of Konakion repackaged in dropper bottles for oral administration. *Aust J Hosp Pharm* 1996; **26:** 641–4.

Adverse Effects and Precautions

Intravenous administration of phytomenadione has caused severe reactions resembling hypersensitivity or anaphylaxis; symptoms have included facial flushing, sweating, chest constriction and chest pain, dyspnoea, cyanosis, and cardiovascular collapse; fatalities have been reported. It is not clear if these reactions were caused by phytomenadione itself or by polyethoxylated castor oil which is present as a surfactant in some parenteral formulations; reports of possible reactions with formulations that do not contain polyethoxylated castor oil are unconfirmed. Such reactions have generally been associated with a too rapid rate of infusion but have also been reported even when the solution was diluted and infused slowly. Pain and swelling may occur at the injection site following administration of phytomenadione. Localised skin reactions have been reported following intramuscular or subcutaneous injection of phytomenadione.

Administration of menadione and menadiol sodium phosphate to neonates, especially premature infants, has been associated with the development of haemolytic anaemia, hyperbilirubinaemia, and kernicterus, and such use is not recommended. Phytomenadione has a lower risk of haemolysis. Menadione and menadiol sodium phosphate have also been reported to cause haemolysis in patients with glucose-6-phosphate dehydrogenase deficiency or vitamin E deficiency.

Phytomenadione in its colloidal formulation is solubilised with lecithin and a bile salt, thus should be given with caution to patients with severely impaired liver function and to premature neonates weighing less than 2.5 kg, since the bile salt may displace bilirubin.

Carcinogenicity. A case-control study from the UK[1] suggested an increased risk of cancer in children who had received vitamin K at birth for the prevention of haemorrhagic disease of the newborn (see below). A further study[2] by the same authors indicated that this risk was associated with intramuscular, but not oral, administration, and was strongest for childhood leukaemia. In response to these data, the British Paediatric Association recommended that the oral route of administration be preferred for prophylaxis,[3] whereas the American Academy of Pediatrics continued to advocate the intramuscular route.[4]

Subsequent studies from the USA,[5] Sweden,[6] Denmark,[6,7] Germany,[8] and England[9] did not confirm an increased risk of childhood cancer, including leukaemias, after the use of intramuscular vitamin K. More recently, 4 further studies were published.[10-13] Two of the reports, a case-control study in Scotland[10] and an ecological study in Britain,[11] showed no increased risk of any cancers with the use of intramuscular vitamin K. A third case-control study in England and Wales[12] found a borderline association between intramuscular vitamin K and cancers, particularly leukaemia. In the fourth study, a case-control study in northern England,[13] there was an increased risk (odds ratio 1.79) of acute lymphoblastic leukaemia developing 1 to 6 years after birth in children who had received intramuscular vitamin K. In 1998 an expert working group formed by the UK Medicines Control Agency and the Committee on Safety of Medicines reviewed all the available studies.[14] They concluded that there was no increased risk of solid tumours with vitamin K, and that, although an increased risk of leukaemia could not be excluded, observed results were compatible with chance. Moreover, they could not identify a plausible mechanism for a carcinogenic effect of vitamin K. The UK Department of Health[15] now advocates either oral or intramuscular prophylaxis, and recommends that the parents should be involved in the decision on which route of administration is used.

1. Golding J, *et al.* Factors associated with childhood cancer in a national cohort study. *Br J Cancer* 1990; **62:** 304–8.
2. Golding J, *et al.* Childhood cancer, intramuscular vitamin K, and pethidine given during labour. *Br Med J* 1992; **305:** 341–6.
3. British Paediatric Association. *Vitamin K prophylaxis in infancy.* London, 1992: British Paediatric Association.
4. American Academy of Pediatrics Vitamin K Ad Hoc Task Force. Controversies concerning vitamin K and the newborn. *Pediatrics* 1993; **91:** 1001–3.
5. Klebanoff MA, *et al.* The risk of childhood cancer after neonatal exposure to vitamin K. *N Engl J Med* 1993; **329:** 905–8.
6. Ekelund H, *et al.* Administration of vitamin K to newborn infants and childhood cancer. *Br Med J* 1993; **307:** 89–91.
7. Olsen JH, *et al.* Vitamin K regimens and incidence of childhood cancer in Denmark. *Br Med J* 1994; **308:** 895–6.
8. von Kries R, *et al.* Vitamin K and childhood cancer: a population based case-control study in Lower Saxony, Germany. *Br Med J* 1996; **313:** 199–203.
9. Ansell P, *et al.* Childhood leukaemia and intramuscular vitamin K: findings from a case-control study. *Br Med J* 1996; **313:** 204–5.
10. McKinney PA, *et al.* Case-control study of childhood leukaemia and cancer in Scotland: findings for neonatal intramuscular vitamin K. *Br Med J* 1998; **316:** 173–7.
11. Passmore SJ, *et al.* Ecological studies of relation between hospital policies on neonatal vitamin K administration and subsequent occurrence of childhood cancer. *Br Med J* 1998; **316:** 184–9.
12. Passmore SJ, *et al.* Case-control studies of relation between childhood cancer and neonatal vitamin K administration. *Br Med J* 1998; **316:** 178–184.
13. Parker L, *et al.* Neonatal vitamin K administration and childhood cancer in the north of England: retrospective case-control study. *Br Med J* 1998; **316:** 189–93.
14. Committee on Safety of Medicines/Medicines Control Agency. Safety of intramuscular vitamin K (Konakion). *Current Problems* 1998; **24:** 3–4.
15. Department of Health. *Vitamin K for newborn babies.* London, 1998: Department of Health.

Effects on the blood. Cerebral arterial thrombosis developed in 2 patients with malabsorption syndromes due to coeliac disease during treatment with vitamin K for severe deficiency of vitamin-K-dependent coagulation factors. An increased tendency to thrombotic events had previously been reported to be present in patients with intestinal inflammatory disorders. It was suggested that if bleeding did occur in such patients treatment should be with plasma infusions or small doses of vitamin K but that vitamin K deficiency should not be specifically treated since a gluten-free diet or corticosteroids given for the gastro-intestinal disorder will result in a gradual correction.[1]

1. Florholmen J, *et al.* Cerebral thrombosis in two patients with malabsorption syndrome treated with vitamin K. *Br Med J* 1980; **281:** 541.

Hypersensitivity. References to hypersensitivity reactions to intravenous phytomenadione preparations containing polyethoxylated castor oil.[1-3]

1. Hopkins CS. Adverse reaction to a Cremophor-containing preparation of intravenous vitamin K. *Intensive Therapy Clin Monit* 1988; **9:** 254–5.
2. de la Rubia J, *et al.* Anaphylactic shock and vitamin K_1. *Ann Intern Med* 1989; **110:** 943.
3. Martinez-Abad M, *et al.* Vitamin K_1 and anaphylactic shock. *DICP Ann Pharmacother* 1991; **25:** 871–2.

Interactions

Vitamin K decreases the effects of oral anticoagulants (see p.969), and is used to counteract excessive effects of these drugs, see below. Vitamin K may reduce the response to resumed therapy with anticoagulants for a week or more.

Pharmacokinetics

The fat-soluble vitamin K compounds phytomenadione and menadione require the presence of bile for their absorption from the gastro-intestinal tract; the water-soluble derivatives of menadione can be absorbed in the absence of bile. Vitamin K accumulates mainly in the liver but is stored in the body only for short periods of time. Vitamin K does not appear to cross the placenta readily and it is poorly distributed into breast milk. Phytomenadione is rapidly metabolised to more polar metabolites and is excreted in bile and urine as glucuronide and sulphate conjugates.

Absorption. Absorption of phytomenadione from the colloidal (micellar) preparation was more irregular and unpredictable after intramuscular than intravenous administration in healthy adults;[1] when used as an antidote to anticoagulant drugs, this formulation should be given intravenously. In neonates, plasma phytomenadione concentrations were within or above the adult fasting plasma range 24 days after receiving a single dose of the colloidal preparation either orally (3 mg) or intramuscularly (1.5 mg).[2]

1. Soedirman JR, *et al.* Pharmacokinetics and tolerance of intravenous and intramuscular phylloquinone (vitamin K_1) mixed micelles formulation. *Br J Clin Pharmacol* 1996; **41:** 517–23.
2. Schubiger G, *et al.* Vitamin K_1 concentration in breast-fed neonates after oral or intramuscular administration of a single dose of a new mixed-micellar preparation of phylloquinone. *J Pediatr Gastroenterol Nutr* 1993; **16:** 435–9.

Human Requirements

The minimum daily requirements of vitamin K are not clearly defined but an intake of about 1 μg per kg body-weight daily appears to be adequate. Vitamin K requirements in normal adults can be met from the average diet and from the synthesis of menaquinones (also known as vitamin K_2) by bacterial action in the intestine. Vitamin K occurs naturally as phytomenadione (vitamin K_1) which is present in many foods, especially leafy green vegetables such as cabbage and spinach, and is also present in liver, cows' milk, egg-yolk, and some cereals.

In the United Kingdom neither a reference nutrient intake (RNI) nor an estimated average requirement (EAR) (see p.1332) has been set for vitamin K although an intake of 1 μg per kg body-weight daily was considered to be both safe and adequate for adults; a higher intake based on body-weight of about 2 μg per kg body-weight daily (10 μg daily) was believed to be justified in infants due to the absence of hepatic menaquinones in early life and reliance on dietary vitamin K alone. It was stated that all babies should receive prophylactic vitamin K at birth[1] and for further details concerning neonatal use, see Haemorrhagic Disease of the Newborn below.

In the United States, recommended dietary allowances have been published for vitamin K. Differing amounts are recommended for infants, children, and adult males and females of varying ages but in general the amount is approximately equivalent to 1 μg per kg body-weight daily.[2]

1. DoH. Dietary reference values for food energy and nutrients for the United Kingdom: report of the panel on dietary reference values of the committee on medical aspects of food policy. *Report on health and social subjects 41.* London: HMSO, 1991.
2. Subcommittee on the tenth edition of the RDAs, Food and Nutrition Board, Commission on Life Sciences, National Research Council. *Recommended dietary allowances.* 10th ed. Washington, DC: National Academy Press, 1989.

Uses and Administration

Vitamin K is an essential cofactor in the hepatic synthesis of prothrombin (factor II) and other blood clotting factors (factors VII, IX, and X, and proteins C and S) and in the function of proteins such as osteocalcin important for bone development.

Vitamin K deficiency may develop in neonates, and can lead to haemorrhagic disease of the newborn. Vitamin K deficiency is uncommon in adults, but may occur in patients with malabsorption syndromes, obstructive jaundice or hepatic disease. Deficiency leads to the development of hypoprothrombinaemia, in which the clotting time of the blood is prolonged and spontaneous bleeding can occur. Coumarin anticoagulants interfere with vitamin K metabolism, and their effects can be antagonised by giving vitamin K.

Vitamin K compounds are used in the treatment and prevention of haemorrhage associated with vitamin

K deficiency. The dose of vitamin K should be carefully controlled by prothrombin-time estimations.

Phytomenadione is a naturally occurring vitamin K substance. It is the only vitamin K compound used to reverse hypoprothrombinaemia and haemorrhage caused by anticoagulant therapy. It is not effective as a heparin antidote. For over-anticoagulation, the dose depends on the international normalised ratio (INR) and the degree of haemorrhage, as discussed under the Treatment of Adverse Effects of Warfarin, p.965. Typical doses of phytomenadine are 0.5 to 5 mg by slow intravenous injection or up to 5 mg orally. Other suggested doses, e.g. in manufacturers' literature, include the following: subcutaneous, intramuscular, or intravenous phytomenadione for severe haemorrhage in initial doses of 2.5 to 10 mg up to 20 or 25 mg, and very rarely up to 50 mg; oral phytomenadione for less severe haemorrhage in initial doses of 10 to 20 mg; and oral phytomenadione 5 to 10 mg for raised INR with no haemorrhage. Similar doses have been used in hypoprothrombinaemia due to certain cephalosporins (p.180). Depending on the solubilising agents used, some formulations of phytomenadione are more suitable for intravenous use than others, and administration details vary.

In the treatment of haemorrhagic disease of the newborn phytomenadione may be given in a dose of 1 mg intravenously or intramuscularly and, if necessary, further doses may be given 8-hourly. As a prophylactic measure, a single dose of 0.5 to 1 mg may be given intramuscularly to the newborn infant, or 2 mg orally followed by a second dose of 2 mg after 4 to 7 days; for further details see below.

Menadiol sodium phosphate is a water-soluble derivative of menadione, a synthetic lipid-soluble vitamin K analogue. It may be used for the prevention of vitamin K deficiency in patients with malabsorption syndromes in whom oral phytomenadione may be inefficiently absorbed. It is given in usual doses equivalent to 10 to 40 mg of menadiol phosphate daily by mouth.

Menadiol dibutyrate and menatetrenone have also been used and the latter has been investigated in the management of osteoporosis. Acetomenaphthone has been used in preparations promoted for the relief of chilblains.

Action. References to the action of vitamin K and the role of vitamin K-dependent coagulation proteins and carboxyglutamate-containing proteins such as osteocalcin.

1. Friedman PA. Vitamin K-dependent proteins. *N Engl J Med* 1984; **310:** 1458–60.
2. Rick ME. Protein C and protein S: vitamin K-dependent inhibitors of blood coagulation. *JAMA* 1990; **263:** 701–3.
3. Shearer MJ. Vitamin K. *Lancet* 1995; **345:** 229–34.

Haemorrhagic disease of the newborn. Haemorrhagic disease of the newborn (HDN; vitamin K deficiency bleeding; VKDB) of which 3 types have been recognised, is associated with a clotting defect due to vitamin K deficiency. In early HDN bleeding occurs at the time of delivery or during the first 24 hours of life and is typically seen in infants whose mothers have taken drugs that affect vitamin K metabolism such as warfarin, some antiepileptics, rifampicin, or isoniazid. Classic HDN, the most common type, usually occurs at 2 to 5 days of age and breast feeding is an important factor as human breast milk has a much lower content of vitamin K than either cow's milk or infant formulas. Late HDN presents frequently as intracranial haemorrhage in infants over one month of age. The vitamin-K deficiency in these cases can be either idiopathic (usually in breast-fed infants who did not receive vitamin K at birth) and/or can be a secondary manifestation of other disorders such as chronic diarrhoea, cystic fibrosis or other malabsorption syndromes, biliary atresia, or α_1-antitrypsin deficiency.[1]

Treatment of HDN involves use of parenteral phytomenadione, usually 1 mg initially with further doses depending on response. More immediate treatment, in the form of blood transfusion or blood clotting factors, may be needed to compensate for severe blood loss and delayed response to vitamin K. HDN, particularly the late type, carries a high risk of morbidity or death; therefore, the emphasis has been on prevention. It has long been known that administration of vitamin K to the neonate soon after birth can reduce the incidence of HDN. Menadiol sodium phosphate was formerly used, but reports in the 1950s of jaundice and kernicterus in infants given this vitamin K analogue caused concern, and led to the preferential use of phytomenadione either intramuscularly or orally. Administration of phytomenadione, usually as a single intramuscular injection, has been standard practice for neonates considered at high risk of HDN, such as those who had a complicated delivery, those born prematurely, and those whose mothers were receiving antiepileptic therapy. Since it is not possible to selectively identify all neonates that are at risk for HDN, the routine administration of phytomenadione to all neonates has been advocated. However, such practice has been controversial, particularly as regards the route of administration.[2,3] Some have considered that oral administration is less invasive and more acceptable to parents.[3] However, there has also been concern about the adequacy of absorption of orally administered phytomenadione, and the lack of a suitable oral formulation. In addition, there was some evidence[4-6] to suggest that a single intramuscular dose was more effective than a single oral dose in preventing late HDN, and that repeated oral doses might be required, which may be less convenient and carry the risk of poor compliance. More recently, a possible increased risk of childhood cancer in neonates treated with intramuscular, but not oral, phytomenadione has been reported (see above). Although the association remains controversial, it led to recommendations for the preferential use of oral vitamin K in neonates at low-risk of HDN in some countries, including the UK[7] and Germany,[8] whereas other countries, including the USA,[9] still preferred the intramuscular route for all neonates.

There is still no agreement on the most effective oral dose and its frequency of administration, and study of this has been complicated by the lack of a suitable oral preparation of phytomenadione.[10,11] Options currently available for oral administration include the polyethoxylated castor oil and polysorbate-80 containing preparations (unlicensed for oral use) and the colloidal, micelle formulation (licensed for oral use in some countries). These preparations are packaged in glass ampoules, therefore are unsuitable for parents to administer at home. The colloidal preparation may be absorbed more reliably (see above).

The 1992 recommendations of the British Paediatric Society[7] for oral use of the polyethoxylated castor oil formulation suggested a single dose of 0.5 mg on the day of birth. For breast-fed babies, additional doses of 0.5 mg at 7 to 10 days and at 4 to 6 weeks, or 0.2 mg at weekly intervals for 26 weeks, or 0.05 mg daily for 26 weeks, were recommended. Current UK doses[12] for the colloidal preparation in healthy term neonates are 2 mg soon after birth, then 2 mg at 4 to 7 days. Exclusively breast-fed infants should be given a third oral dose of 2 mg one month after birth. Further monthly doses of 2 mg have been recommended while the infant remains exclusively breast-fed. A report[13] of the failure of prophylaxis in 3 breast-fed babies (2 of whom had unidentified cholestatic liver disease) who received 2 doses of this formulation, as recommended in Switzerland, emphasises the importance of the third, and possibly, other, follow-up doses. The most recent advice from the UK Department of Health[12] advocates that all newborn infants should receive vitamin K prophylaxis, both oral and intramuscular administration should be available, and that parents should be involved in the decision on which route of administration is used.

Various other oral regimens have been investigated or are in use. In the Netherlands a regimen of 1 mg orally or intramuscularly at birth, followed by 25 μg daily or 1 mg weekly by mouth from 1 week to 3 months of age has been found satisfactory.[14,15] In Germany[8,15] and Australia[15] the suggested oral regimen for the polyethoxylated castor oil formulation was 1 mg at birth, at 3 to 10 days and at weeks 3 to 6, although some failures have been reported in babies receiving this regimen,[8] and the Australian data confirm it is less effective than a single intramuscular dose.[15] One hospital in the USA has satisfactorily used, for many years, a single 2-mg dose administered via nasogastric tube to neonates after birth.[16] In Denmark, a 2-mg dose at birth followed by a weekly dose of 1 mg during the first 3 months of life has effectively prevented any late HDN in healthy breast-fed babies.[17]

Although phytomenadione crosses the placenta slowly and to a limited extent, it is nevertheless recommended that pregnant women receiving drugs that are vitamin K antagonists (particularly antiepileptics) should receive vitamin K 10 to 20 mg daily from 36 weeks gestation.[18] This is in addition to the requirement that their neonates, who are at high risk of HDN, receive intramuscular phytomenadione soon after birth. Maternal phytomenadione administration has been investigated as a means of improving vitamin K status in breast-fed neonates. In 1 study,[19] 5 mg daily for 12 weeks was effective for this purpose.

1. Hathaway WE. Haemostatic disorders in the newborn. In: Bloom AL, Thomas DP, eds. *Haemostasis and thrombosis.* 2nd ed. Edinburgh: Churchill Livingstone, 1987: 554–69.
2. Tripp JH, McNinch AW. Haemorrhagic disease and vitamin K. *Arch Dis Child* 1987; **62:** 436–7.
3. Brown SG, *et al.* Should intramuscular vitamin K prophylaxis for haemorrhagic disease of the newborn be continued? A decision analysis. *N Z Med J* 1989; **102:** 3–5.
4. Clarkson PM, James AG. Parenteral vitamin K_1: the effective prophylaxis against haemorrhagic disease for all newborn infants. *N Z Med J* 1990; **103:** 95–6.
5. McNinch AW, Tripp JH. Haemorrhagic disease of the newborn in the British Isles: two year prospective study. *Br Med J* 1991; **303:** 1105–9.
6. Von Kries R. Neonatal vitamin K. *Br Med J* 1991; **303:** 1083–4.
7. British Paediatric Association. *Vitamin K prophylaxis in infancy.* London, 1992: British Paediatric Association.
8. von Kries R, *et al.* Repeated oral vitamin K prophylaxis in West Germany: acceptance and efficacy. *Br Med J* 1995; **310:** 1097–8.
9. American Academy of Pediatrics Vitamin K Ad Hoc Task Force. Controversies concerning vitamin K and the newborn. *Pediatrics* 1993; **91:** 1001–3.
10. Barton JS, *et al.* Neonatal vitamin K prophylaxis in the British Isles: current practice and trends. *Br Med J* 1995; **310:** 632–3.
11. Rennie JM, Kelsall AWR. Vitamin K prophylaxis in the newborn—again. *Arch Dis Child* 1994; **70:** 248–51.
12. Department of Health. *Vitamin K for newborn babies.* London, 1998: Department of Health.
13. Baenziger O, *et al.* Oral vitamin K prophylaxis for newborn infants: safe enough? *Lancet* 1996; **348:** 1456.
14. Cornelissen M, Hirasing R. Vitamin K for neonates. *Br Med J* 1994; **309:** 484–5.
15. Cornelissen M, *et al.* Prevention of vitamin K deficiency bleeding: efficacy of different multiple oral dose schedules of vitamin K. *Eur J Pediatr* 1997; **156:** 126–30.
16. Clark FI, James EJP. Twenty-seven years of experience with oral vitamin K_1 therapy in neonates. *J Pediatr* 1995; **127:** 301–4.
17. Nørgaard Hansen K, Ebbesen F. Neonatal vitamin K prophylaxis in Denmark: three years' experience with oral administration during the first three months of life compared with one oral administration at birth. *Acta Paediatr Scand* 1996; **85:** 1137–9.
18. Delgado-Escueta AV, Janz D. Consensus guidelines: preconception counseling, management, and care of the pregnant woman with epilepsy. *Neurology* 1992; **42** (suppl 5): 149–60.
19. Greer FR, *et al.* Improving the vitamin K status of breastfeeding infants with maternal vitamin K supplements. *Pediatrics* 1997; **99:** 88–92.

Neonatal intraventricular haemorrhage. Vitamin K crosses the placenta slowly and to a limited extent,[1,2] but sufficiently to warrant studies to assess whether antenatal administration of phytomenadione to the mother may reduce the incidence or severity of intraventricular haemorrhage (p.709) in the preterm neonate. Two studies did find that such antenatal administration had a beneficial outcome[3,4] but this finding was not confirmed by a subsequent study.[5] Moreover, a larger randomised controlled study failed to find any benefit from vitamin K prophylaxis.[6]

1. Yang Y-M, *et al.* Maternal-fetal transport of vitamin K_1 and its effects on coagulation in premature infants. *J Pediatr* 1989; **115:** 1009–13.
2. Kazzi NJ, *et al.* Placental transfer of vitamin K_1 in preterm pregnancy. *Obstet Gynecol* 1990; **75:** 334–7.
3. Pomerance JJ, *et al.* Maternally administered antenatal vitamin K_1: effect on neonatal prothrombin activity, partial thromboplastin time, and intraventricular hemorrhage. *Obstet Gynecol* 1987; **70:** 235–41.
4. Morales WJ, *et al.* The use of antenatal vitamin K in the prevention of early neonatal intraventricular hemorrhage. *Am J Obstet Gynecol* 1988; **159:** 774–9.
5. Kazzi NJ, *et al.* Maternal administration of vitamin K does not improve the coagulation profile of preterm infants. *Pediatrics* 1989; **84:** 1045–50.
6. Thorp JA, Antepartum vitamin K and phenobarbital for preventing intraventricular hemorrhage in the premature newborn: a randomized, double-blind, placebo-controlled trial. *Obstet Gynecol* 1994; **83:** 70–6.

Preparations

BP 1998: Menadiol Phosphate Injection; Menadiol Phosphate Tablets; Phytomenadione Injection; Phytomenadione Tablets; ***USP 23:*** Menadiol Sodium Diphosphate Injection; Menadiol Sodium Diphosphate Tablets; Menadione Injection; Oil- and Water-soluble Vitamins Capsules; Oil- and Water-soluble Vitamins Tablets; Oil-soluble Vitamins Capsules; Oil-soluble Vitamins Tablets; Phytonadione Injection; Phytonadione Tablets.

Proprietary Preparations (details are given in Part 3)
Aust.: Kavitol†; Konakion; Vikaman; ***Austral.:*** K Thrombin; Konakion; ***Belg.:*** Konakion; ***Canad.:*** Konakion†; ***Ger.:*** Kanavit; Konakion; ***Irl.:*** Konakion; Synkavit†; ***Ital.:*** Konakion; ***Jpn:*** Glakay; Kaytwo; Kaywan†; ***Neth.:*** Konakion; ***Norw.:*** Konakion; ***S.Afr.:*** Konakion; ***Spain:*** Kaergona Hidrosoluble; Konakion; ***Swed.:*** Konakion; ***Switz.:*** Konakion; ***UK:*** Konakion; Synkavit; ***USA:*** Aquamephyton; Konakion; Mephyton.

Multi-ingredient: ***Austral.:*** Chilblain Formula; ***Belg.:*** Hemocoavit†; ***Canad.:*** Duo-CVP with Vitamin K†; ***Fr.:*** Bilkaby; ***Ger.:*** Styptobion†; ***Irl.:*** Bio-Calcium + D_3 + K; ***Ital.:*** Askarutina†; Streptan†; ***S.Afr.:*** Pernivit†; ***Spain:*** Caprofides Hemostatico; Citroflavona Solu†; Cromoxin K; Quercetol K; Vitaendil C K P.

Xylitol (667-e)

E967; Xylit; *meso*-Xylitol.

$C_5H_{12}O_5$ = 152.1.

CAS — 87-99-0 (xylitol); 16277-71-7 (D-xylitol).

Pharmacopoeias. In *Eur.* (see p.viii) and *Jpn.* Also in *USNF.*

A polyhydric alcohol (polyol) related to the pentose sugar, xylose (p.1645).

White odourless crystals or crystalline powder. It has a sweet taste and produces a cooling sensation in the mouth. **Soluble** 1 in about 0.65 of water; sparingly soluble in alcohol.

Adverse Effects

Large amounts taken by mouth may cause diarrhoea and flatulence. Ingestion of xylitol is not likely to lead to hyperoxaluria which can occur with intravenous infusion. Hyperuricaemia, changes in liver-function tests, and acidosis (including lactic acidosis) have occurred after intravenous infusion.

Uses and Administration

Xylitol is used as a bulk sweetener in foods. It is also used as a sweetening agent in sugar-free preparations as it is non-cariogenic and is less likely to cause dental caries than sucrose. It was formerly considered as a substitute for glucose in intravenous nutrition but such use has generally been abandoned due to adverse effects.

Mouth and ear infections. Chewing-gum containing xylitol appears to have a useful role in the prevention of dental caries (p.132).[1] The findings of one trial[2] also suggest that xylitol chewing gum may have a preventative effect against acute otitis media (p.134).

1. Edgar WM. Sugar substitutes, chewing gum and dental caries—a review. *Br Dent J* 1998; **184:** 29–32.
2. Uhari M, *et al.* Xylitol chewing gum in prevention of acute otitis media: double blind randomised trial. *Br Med J* 1996; **313:** 1180–4.

Preparations

Proprietary Preparations (details are given in Part 3)
Irl.: Oralbalance.

Multi-ingredient: ***Austral.:*** Saliva Orthana†; ***Ger.:*** Cardioplegin N; Duocal†; Kalium-Magnesium-Asparaginat; Kaloplasmal; Salvi Cal GX; ***Ital.:*** Dentosan "Pagni" Collutorio†; Dentosan Ortodontico Collutorio; Neo-Stomygen; ***Swed.:*** Salivin†; ***UK:*** Saliva Orthana; Salivace; ***USA:*** Optimoist.

Dried Yeast (7840-a)

Brewers' Yeast; Cerevisiae Fermentum Siccatum; Faex Siccata; Fermento de Cerveja; Levedura Sêca; Levure de Bière; Saccharomyces Siccum; Trockenhefe.

Pharmacopoeias. In *Aust., Chin.,* and *Jpn.*

Unicellular fungi belonging to the family Saccharomycetaceae, dried by a process which avoids decomposition of the vitamins present. The chief species are *Saccharomyces cerevisiae, S. carlsbergensis,* and *S. monacensis.* Dried yeast contains thiamine, nicotinic acid, riboflavine, pyridoxine, pantothenic acid, biotin, folic acid, cyanocobalamin, aminobenzoic acid, inositol, and chromium.

Dried yeast is a rich source of vitamins of the B group. It has been used for the prevention and treatment of vitamin B deficiency in doses of 1 to 8 g daily by mouth. Yeast is an ingredient of some preparations for treating haemorrhoids, and some preparations intended to restore normal gastro-intestinal flora. Yeast is widely used in brewing.

Preparations

Proprietary Preparations (details are given in Part 3)
Belg.: Preparation H Sperti; ***Fr.:*** Microlev; ***Ger.:*** Faexojodan; Furunkulosin; Levurinetten N; ***Ital.:*** Lievitovit 300; Preparazione H; Zimocel.

Multi-ingredient: ***Aust.:*** Levurinetten; Sperti Praparation H; ***Austral.:*** ML 20; Plantiodine Plus; Preparation H; Vitaglow Selemite B Tablets; ***Canad.:*** Preparation H; ***Fr.:*** Actisoufre; Calciforte; Carbolevure; Carbophagix; Fluorocalciforte; Phytophanere; Preparation H; Solacy; Spasmag; ***Ger.:*** Adebilan†; Diabetylin N†; Etmocard†; Haut-Vital; Hepsan†; Imbak; Katulcin†; Mederma†; Menstrualin†; Pantovigar; Sperti Praparation H; Worishofener Nervenpflege Dr. Kleinschrod†; ***Irl.:*** Preparation H; ***Ital.:*** Aclon Lievit; Alvear Complex; Bio Ritz†; Bio-Real; Complesso B Antitossico Jamco; Enzygaster†; Eurogel; Florelax; Lactisporin; Lactivis; Lactolife; Lactovit; Levudin; Lievigran†; Lievistar; Lievital†; Lievitosohn; Lievitovit; Sillix; Vigogel; ***Neth.:*** Sperti Preparation H; ***S.Afr.:*** Revaton; Vitaforce 21-Plus†; ***Spain:*** Actilevol C†; Osspulvit Vitaminado†; Preparacion H; ***Switz.:*** A Vogel Capsules polyvitaminees; Carbolevure; Ginkovit†; Pantogar; Solacy†; Sperti Preparation H; ***UK:*** B Complex; Brewers Yeast; Brewers Yeast with Garlic; Phillips P.T.Y. Yeast Tablets; Preparation H; Yeast Vite; ***USA:*** Medicone; Preparation H; Rectagene Medicated Balm; Wyanoids Relief Factor.

Zinc (5327-p)

Zn = 65.39.
CAS — 7440-66-6.

Zinc Chloride (5329-w)

Zinci Chloridum; Zincum Chloratum.
$ZnCl_2$ = 136.3.
CAS — 7646-85-7.
Pharmacopoeias. In *Eur.* (see p.viii), *Jpn, Pol.,* and *US.*

A white or almost white, odourless, deliquescent, crystalline powder or granules or opaque white masses or sticks.

Soluble 1 in 0.5 of water, 1 in 1.5 of alcohol, and 1 in 2 of glycerol. An approximately 10% solution in water has a pH of 4.6 to 5.5. **Store** in airtight non-metallic containers.

Zinc chloride almost always contains some oxychloride which produces a slightly turbid aqueous solution. Turbid solutions, except when intended for ophthalmic use, may be cleared by adding gradually a small amount of dilute hydrochloric acid. Solutions of zinc chloride should be filtered through asbestos or sintered glass, since they dissolve paper and cotton wool.

Zinc Gluconate (17035-v)

$C_{12}H_{22}O_{14}Zn$ = 455.7.
CAS — 4468-02-4.
Pharmacopoeias. In *US.*

White or almost white powder or granules. Zinc gluconate 350 mg is approximately equivalent to 50 mg of zinc. **Soluble** in water; very slightly soluble in alcohol. A 1% solution has a pH of 5.5 to 7.5.

Zinc Sulphate (5330-m)

Zinc Sulfate; Zinci Sulfas; Zincum Sulfuricum.
$ZnSO_4,7H_2O$ = 287.6.
CAS — 7733-02-0 (anhydrous zinc sulphate); 7446-20-0 (zinc sulphate heptahydrate).

NOTE. 'White vitriol' or 'white copperas' is crude zinc sulphate.
ZSU is a code approved by the BP for use on single unit doses of eye drops containing zinc sulphate where the individual container may be too small to bear all the appropriate labelling information.

Pharmacopoeias. In *Chin., Eur.* (see p.viii), *Jpn,* and *Pol.*
US includes the monohydrate and the heptahydrate.

Odourless, colourless, transparent, efflorescent crystals or white crystalline powder. Each g of zinc sulphate represents 3.5 mmol of zinc. Zinc sulphate 220 mg is approximately equivalent to 50 mg of zinc.

Soluble 1 in 0.6 of water and 1 in 2.5 of glycerol; practically insoluble in alcohol. A 5% solution in water has a pH of 4.4 to 5.6.

Store in airtight non-metallic containers.

Adverse Effects, Treatment, and Precautions

The most frequent adverse effects of zinc salts (the gluconate and sulphate) administered by mouth are gastro-intestinal and include abdominal pain, dyspepsia, nausea, vomiting, diarrhoea, gastric irritation, and gastritis. These are particularly common if zinc salts are taken on an empty stomach, and may be reduced by administration with meals.

In acute overdosage zinc salts are corrosive, due to the formation of zinc chloride by stomach acid; treatment consists of administration of milk or alkali carbonates and activated charcoal. The use of emetics or gastric lavage should be avoided.

Prolonged administration of high doses of zinc supplements by mouth or parenterally leads to copper deficiency with associated sideroblastic anaemia and neutropenia. Zinc toxicity has occurred after the use of contaminated water in haemodialysis solutions. High serum zinc concentrations may be reduced by using a chelating drug such as sodium calciumedetate (p.994).

Metal fume fever is an occupational disease associated with inhalation of freshly-oxidised metal fumes, most commonly from zinc, iron or copper. It is characterised by fever, nausea, dyspnoea, and chest pain, and is generally self-limiting and does not appear to be associated with long-term sequelae.

Parenteral nutrition. Zinc was found to be a common contaminant of various components used for total parenteral nutrition (TPN), and rubber stoppers or glass may have been the source.[1] Levels of zinc found may exceed daily requirements even before the addition of supplementary zinc. The authors suggested it may be important to routinely monitor zinc status in patients receiving long-term TPN, particularly infants and children.

1. Hak EB, *et al.* Chromium and zinc contamination of parenteral nutrient solution components commonly used in infants and children. *Am J Health-Syst Pharm* 1998; **55:** 150–4.

Interactions

The absorption of zinc may be reduced by iron supplements, penicillamine, phosphorus-containing preparations, and tetracyclines. Zinc supplements reduce the absorption of copper, ciprofloxacin (p.187), iron, norfloxacin, penicillamine, and tetracyclines (p.260).

Pharmacokinetics

Zinc is incompletely absorbed from the gastro-intestinal tract, and absorption is reduced in the presence of some dietary constituents such as phytates. Bioavailability of dietary zinc varies widely between different sources, but is approximately 20 to 30%. Zinc is distributed throughout the body with the highest concentrations found in muscle, bone, skin, and prostatic fluids. It is primarily excreted in the faeces, and regulation of faecal losses is important in zinc homoeostasis. Small amounts are lost in urine and perspiration.

Human Requirements

In the United Kingdom dietary reference values (DRV)[1] and in the United States recommended dietary allowances (RDA)[2] have been published for zinc. In the UK the reference nutrient intake (RNI) for adult males and females is 9.5 and 7.0 mg daily respectively; values are also given for infants and children of varying ages and for lactating women. In the USA the RDA for adult males and females is set at 15 and 12 mg daily respectively, again with values for infants, children, pregnant and lactating women also being given. The US report also recommends that because of possible toxicity chronic ingestion of zinc supplements exceeding 15 mg daily should only be under medical supervision. WHO recommend lower limits of the safe ranges of population mean intakes of dietary zinc for 3 categories of diets based on high, moderate, and low zinc bioavailability: values are 4.0, 6.5, and 13.1 mg dietary zinc daily for women, and 5.6, 9.4, and 18.7 mg dietary zinc daily for men, respectively.[3] They recommend an upper limit of the safe range of population mean intakes of zinc of 35 mg per day for women, and 45 mg per day for men.

1. DoH. Dietary reference values for food energy and nutrients for the United Kingdom: report of the panel on dietary reference values of the committee on medical aspects of food policy. *Report on health and social subjects 41.* London: HMSO, 1991.
2. Subcommittee on the tenth edition of the RDAs, Food and Nutrition Board, Commission on Life Sciences, National Research Council. *Recommended dietary allowances.* 10th ed. Washington, DC: National Academy Press, 1989.
3. WHO. Zinc. In: *Trace elements in human nutrition and health.* Geneva: WHO, 1996: 72–104.

Uses and Administration

Zinc is an essential element of nutrition and traces are present in a wide range of foods. It is a constituent of many enzyme systems and is present in all tissues. Features of zinc deficiency include growth retardation and defects of rapidly-dividing tissues such as the skin, the immune system, and the intestinal mucosa. Water-soluble zinc salts are used as supplements to correct zinc deficiency; for example, in malabsorption syndromes, during parenteral feeding, in conditions with increased body losses (trauma, burns, and protein-losing states), and in acrodermatitis enteropathica (a rare genetic disorder characterised by severe zinc deficiency). They have been tried in the treatment of a large number of conditions that may be related to zinc deficiency. In deficiency states, zinc is usually given by mouth as the sulphate, the sulphate monohydrate, or the gluconate, in doses of up to 50 mg of elemental zinc three times daily. When intravenous supplements are required, zinc chloride or zinc sulphate may be given; a suggested dose for parenteral nutrition is 6.5 mg of elemental zinc (100 µmol) daily.

Oral zinc salts, commonly the acetate (p.1646), may be used as copper absorption inhibitors in Wilson's disease (p.992).

Zinc sulphate is used topically in a variety of skin conditions mainly for its astringent properties. The insoluble zinc salts, commonly the oxide (p.1096), are used similarly. Zinc sulphate is also used as an astringent in eye drops. Zinc chloride has been employed for its powerful caustic and astringent properties, usually in very dilute solution, in, for example, mouthwashes.

Common cold. Zinc salts, in the form of lozenges, have been tried in the treatment of the common cold (p.595) with variable results.[1-5]

1. Al-Nakib W, *et al.* Prophylaxis and treatment of rhinovirus colds with zinc gluconate lozenges. *J Antimicrob Chemother* 1987; **20:** 893–901.
2. Douglas RM, *et al.* Failure of effervescent zinc acetate lozenges to alter the course of upper respiratory tract infections in Australian adults. *Antimicrob Agents Chemother* 1987; **31:** 1263–5.
3. Smith DS, *et al.* Failure of zinc gluconate in treatment of acute upper respiratory tract infections. *Antimicrob Agents Chemother* 1989; **33:** 646–8.
4. Mossad SB, *et al.* Zinc gluconate lozenges for treating the common cold: a randomized, double-blind, placebo-controlled study. *Ann Intern Med* 1996; **125:** 81–8.
5. Macknin ML, *et al.* Zinc gluconate lozenges for treating the common cold in children: a randomized controlled trial. *JAMA* 1998; **279:** 1962–7.

Deficiency states. General references.

1. Bryce-Smith D. Zinc deficiency—the neglected factor. *Chem Br* 1989; **25:** 783–6.

DIARRHOEA. Chronic diarrhoea can be a sign of zinc deficiency, and diarrhoea can lead to excessive zinc losses and zinc deficiency when dietary zinc is inadequate. Zinc supplements have been shown to reduce the intensity and duration of acute diarrhoea (p.1168) in malnourished children in India[1] and Bangladesh.[2] In a further study in Guatemala,[3] zinc supplements reduced the incidence of diarrhoeal episodes.

1. Sazawal S, *et al.* Zinc supplementation in young children with acute diarrhea in India. *N Engl J Med* 1995; **333:** 839–44.
2. Roy SK, *et al.* Randomised controlled trial of zinc supplementation in malnourished Bangladeshi children with acute diarrhoea. *Arch Dis Child* 1997; **77:** 196–200.
3. Ruel MT, *et al.* Impact of zinc supplementation on morbidity from diarrhea and respiratory infections among rural Guatemalan children. *Pediatrics* 1997; **99:** 808–13.

GROWTH RETARDATION. Growth retardation (p.1237) in a group of short Japanese children without endocrine abnormalities was found to be associated with mild to moderate zinc deficiency; supplementation with zinc sulphate 5 mg per kg body-weight daily by mouth over 6 months resulted in an improvement in growth velocity despite unchanged growth hormone production.[1]

1. Nakamura T, *et al.* Mild to moderate zinc deficiency in short children: effect of zinc supplementation on linear growth velocity. *J Pediatr* 1993; **123:** 65–9.

TASTE DISORDERS. Zinc appears to be effective for the treatment of taste disturbances (p.656) associated with zinc deficiency but there is insufficient evidence to determine its efficacy for taste dysfunction secondary to conditions that do not involve low serum zinc concentrations.[1]

1. Heyneman CA. Zinc deficiency and taste disorders. *Ann Pharmacother* 1996; **30:** 186–7.

Preparations

BP 1998: Zinc Sulphate Eye Drops; Zinc Sulphate Lotion *(Lotio Rubra)*;
USP 23: White Lotion; Zinc Chloride Injection; Zinc Sulfate Injection; Zinc Sulfate Ophthalmic Solution.

Proprietary Preparations (details are given in Part 3)
Aust.: Solvezink; Virudermin†; ***Austral.:*** Bioglan Zinc Chelate; Zincaps; Zinctrace†; ***Canad.:*** Anusol; Anuzinc; Micro Zn; PMS-Egozinc; ***Fr.:*** Hexaphane; Rubozinc; Vitazinc; Zymizinc; ***Ger.:*** Solvezink; Virudermin; Zink-D; Zinkamin; Zinkit; Zinkorot; ***Norw.:*** Solvezink; ***S.Afr.:*** ZN 220; ***Swed.:*** Solvezink; ***Switz.:*** Collazin; Virudermin; ***UK:*** Solvazinc; Sootheye†; Z Span; Zincomed†; Zincosol; ***USA:*** Eye-Sed; Orazinc; Verazinc; Zinca-Pak; Zincate.

Multi-ingredient: numerous preparations are listed in Part 3.

Organic Solvents

Most of the solvents described in this chapter have no specific therapeutic use. Additional solvents used in pharmacy and described in other chapters include alcohols, chlorinated hydrocarbons such as chloroform and trichloroethylene, fixed oils, glycols, paraffins, and water.

Organic solvents are widely used in industry and toxicity may follow acute or chronic exposure. Adverse effects may occur due to inhalation, ingestion, or absorption through the skin. Organic solvents are irritant to the skin and mucous membranes, and also commonly affect the CNS. They may sensitise the myocardium to catecholamines and cardiac arrhythmias may occur. Chronic exposure may lead to central and peripheral neurotoxicity, as well as to renal toxicity and hepatotoxicity.

References.

1. White RF, Proctor SP. Solvents and neurotoxicity. *Lancet* 1997; **349:** 1239–43.

Abuse. Since they are volatile liquids and have CNS effects many organic solvents are implicated in volatile substance abuse. Clinical features of intoxication are similar to those of alcohol intoxication, with initial CNS stimulation followed by CNS depression, which may progress to delirium, convulsions, coma, and death. Sudden death due to cardiac arrhythmias has also been reported.

1. Proceedings of a meeting on substance abuse. *Hum Toxicol* 1989; **8:** 253–334.
2. Ashton CH. Solvent abuse. *Br Med J* 1990; **300:** 135–6.

Acetone (6501-j)

Dimethyl Ketone; 2-Propanone.

$CH_3.CO.CH_3$ = 58.08.

CAS — 67-64-1.

Pharmacopoeias. In *Eur.* (see p.viii). Also in *USNF.*

A clear, colourless, volatile, mobile, flammable liquid with a characteristic odour. Relative density 0.790 to 0.793; sp. gr. not more than 0.789.

Miscible with water, alcohol, chloroform, ether, and most volatile oils. A 50% solution in water is neutral to litmus. **Store** in airtight containers. Protect from light.

Adverse Effects and Treatment

Inhalation of acetone vapour causes excitement followed by CNS depression with headache, restlessness, and fatigue, leading to coma and respiratory depression in severe cases. Vomiting and haematemesis may occur. There may be a latent period before the onset of symptoms of acetone poisoning. Similar symptoms may be observed after ingestion of acetone although hyperglycaemia has also been reported. The vapour is irritant to mucous membranes in high concentrations.

Acetone is commonly implicated in volatile substance abuse (p.1375).

Treatment of adverse effects consists of removal from exposure and general supportive and symptomatic measures. Gastric lavage may be worthwhile if acetone has been recently ingested; activated charcoal may be administered.

For the possible effect of acetone on the metabolism of acetonitrile, see under Acetonitrile, below.

Pharmacokinetics

Acetone is absorbed through the lungs following inhalation. Some absorption occurs from the gastro-intestinal tract. It is mostly excreted unchanged, predominantly through the lungs and also in the urine.

Uses

Acetone is widely used as an industrial, pharmaceutical, and domestic solvent; it is also used as an extraction solvent in food processing.

A suggestion that topical application of acetone might be useful in the dissolution of sea urchin spines.[1]

1. Millar JS. Clinical curio: treatment of sea urchin stings. *Br Med J* 1984; **288:** 390.

Acetonitrile (6502-z)

Ethanenitrile; Methyl Cyanide.

$CH_3.CN$ = 41.05.

CAS — 75-05-8.

A colourless liquid with an aromatic odour. Wt per mL about 0.79 g. B.p. about 81°.

Acetonitrile emits highly toxic fumes of hydrogen cyanide when heated to decomposition or when reacted with acids or oxidising agents. **Store** in airtight containers.

Adverse Effects and Treatment

As for cyanides (see Hydrocyanic Acid, p.1407).

There have been several reports, including one fatality, of cyanide poisoning in infants following ingestion of artificial nail removers containing acetonitrile.[1,2] As acetonitrile is slowly metabolised to cyanide, serious toxic effects may not occur until several hours after ingestion and there is the danger that these products may be confused with acetone-based nail polish removers which are less toxic. In a report of an adult who died after ingestion of acetonitrile, the onset of symptoms was delayed for 24 hours. It was considered that concomitant ingestion of acetone had slowed the metabolism of acetonitrile.[3]

1. Caravati EM, Litovitz TL. Pediatric cyanide intoxication and death from an acetonitrile-containing cosmetic. *JAMA* 1988; **260:** 3470–3.
2. Losek JD, *et al.* Cyanide poisoning from a cosmetic nail remover. *Pediatrics* 1991; **88:** 337–40.
3. Boggild MD, *et al.* Acetonitrile ingestion: delayed onset of cyanide poisoning due to concurrent ingestion of acetone. *Postgrad Med J* 1990; **66:** 40–1.

Pharmacokinetics

Acetonitrile undergoes metabolism to cyanide. Cyanide is responsible for the toxicity of acetonitrile.

Uses

Acetonitrile is used as an industrial solvent. It may also be present in artificial nail removers.

Amyl Acetate (6503-c)

$C_7H_{14}O_2$ = 130.2.

CAS — 123-92-2 (iso-amyl acetate); 53496-15-4 (sec-amyl acetate); 628-63-7 (n-amyl acetate).

A mixture of isomers, principally *iso-*, *sec-*, and *n*-amyl acetate. *iso*-Amyl acetate is a clear colourless liquid with a sharp, fruity odour. Wt per mL about 0.87 g. B.p. about 140°. Slightly **soluble** in water; miscible with alcohol and ether. **Store** in airtight containers.

Adverse Effects

Prolonged exposure to amyl acetate may produce headache, fatigue, and depression of the CNS. Irritation of mucous membranes may also occur.

Effects on the heart. A 27-year-old man developed headache, nausea, and vomiting after using a paint containing amyl acetate as the solvent in an unventilated room.[1] Some days later chest pain and dyspnoea developed; he was admitted to hospital 2 weeks after exposure with heart failure which slowly responded to treatment.

1. Weissberg PL, Green ID. Methyl-cellulose paint possibly causing heart failure. *Br Med J* 1979; **ii:** 1113–14.

Uses

Amyl acetate is used as a pharmaceutical and industrial solvent.

Amylene Hydrate (4004-b)

Aethyldimethylmethanolum; Dimethylethyl Carbinol; Tertiary Amyl Alcohol. 2-Methylbutan-2-ol.

$C_5H_{12}O$ = 88.15.

CAS — 75-85-4.

Pharmacopoeias. In *Aust.* Also in *USNF.*

A clear, colourless, volatile liquid with a camphoraceous odour. Sp. gr. 0.803 to 0.807. B.p. 97° to 103°.

Freely **soluble** in water; miscible with alcohol, chloroform, ether, and glycerol. Solutions of amylene hydrate in water are neutral to litmus. **Store** in airtight containers.

Adverse Effects

Amylene hydrate is irritant and has a depressant effect on the CNS.

Uses

Amylene hydrate is used as a pharmaceutical solvent. It was formerly used as a hypnotic.

Aniline (6504-k)

Phenylamine.

$C_6H_5.NH_2$ = 93.13.

CAS — 62-53-3.

A colourless or pale yellow oily liquid with a characteristic odour, readily darkening to brown on exposure to air and light. Wt per mL about 1.02 g. B.p. about 183°. **Store** in airtight containers. Protect from light.

CAUTION. *Suitable precautions should be taken to avoid skin contact with aniline as it can penetrate skin and produce systemic toxicity.*

Adverse Effects and Treatment

Inhalation, ingestion, or cutaneous absorption of aniline results in methaemoglobinaemia, with cyanosis, headache, weakness, stupor, and coma. Irritation, nausea and vomiting, and cardiac arrhythmias may occur. Haemolysis has been reported and may give rise to kidney damage or jaundice. Death is usually a result of cardiovascular collapse.

Treatment may involve methylene blue (p.985), transfusions, or haemodialysis. Gastric lavage may be performed after ingestion; activated charcoal may be administered.

Bladder papillomas have been reported in workers previously exposed to aniline. Commercial aniline may be contaminated with β-naphthylamine, a potential carcinogen.

Uses

Aniline is a solvent with wide industrial applications.

Benzene (6505-a)

Phenyl Hydride.

C_6H_6 = 78.11.

CAS — 71-43-2.

NOTE. Benzene may be known as 'benzina', 'benzol', 'benzole', or 'benzolum'. However, 'benzol' is also used to describe a mixture of hydrocarbons and 'benzin' or 'benzine' is used as a name for a petroleum distillate (see also Petroleum Spirit, p.1380).

Pharmacopoeias. In *Aust.*

A clear colourless flammable liquid with a characteristic aromatic odour. Wt per mL about 0.88 g. B.p. about 80°. **Store** in airtight containers.

Adverse Effects, Treatment, and Precautions

Symptoms of acute poisoning following inhalation or ingestion of benzene include initial excitement or euphoria followed by CNS depression with headache, dizziness, blurred vision, and ataxia, which in severe cases may progress to coma (accompanied by hyperactive reflexes), convulsions, and death from respiratory failure. Other symptoms include nausea and irritation of the mucous membranes; ventricular arrhythmias may occur. Direct skin contact with liquid benzene may result in marked irritation, and dermatitis may develop on prolonged or repeated exposure.

Prolonged industrial exposure to benzene vapour has been associated with adverse effects on the gastro-intestinal tract and the CNS but in particular with marked effects on the bone marrow and blood. Decreases in the numbers of red or white blood cells or of platelets may occur, producing symptoms of headache, fatigue, anorexia, pallor, and petechiae. In severe cases pancytopenia or aplastic anaemia may develop. Leukaemia, particularly acute non-lymphoblastic leukaemia has also developed, often many years after exposure to benzene has ceased. These effects have been reported in workers exposed to relatively high concentrations of the vapour (around 200 ppm or more) but reduced red blood cell counts and anaemia have also been reported at lower concentrations. Chromosome abnormalities have been observed after prolonged exposure to benzene, particularly at the higher concentrations associated with blood dyscrasias; however, the significance of these abnormalities in the development of leukaemia is unclear.

Treatment of poisoning consists of symptomatic and supportive measures. Gastric lavage may be performed for acute intoxication if the patient presents soon after ingestion but care must be taken to avoid aspiration. Activated charcoal may be administered. In chronic poisoning, repeated blood transfusions may be necessary. Adrenaline and other sympathomimetics should be avoided because of the risk of precipitating cardiac arrhythmias.

Reviews.

1. Health and Safety Executive. Benzene. *Toxicity Review 4.* London: HMSO, 1982.

Malignant neoplasms. Epidemiological data have supported an association between benzene exposure and acute non-lymphoblastic leukaemia, but the risk following low levels of exposure (1 to 10 ppm) was not clear.[1] A large cohort study[2] has suggested that there is an increased risk of acute non-lymphoblastic leukaemia and of non-Hodgkins lymphoma with benzene exposure at levels below 10 ppm.

1. Austin H, *et al.* Benzene and leukemia: a review of the literature and a risk assessment. *Am J Epidemiol* 1988; **127:** 419–39.
2. Hayes RB, *et al.* Benzene and the dose-related incidence of hematologic neoplasms in China. *J Natl Cancer Inst* 1997; **89:** 1065–71.

Pregnancy. An evaluation of the USA National Natality and Fetal Mortality Survey noted that maternal or paternal occupational exposure to agents such as benzene was associated with an increased risk of still-birth and that paternal exposure to benzene increased the risk of low-birth-weight infants.[1]

1. Savitz DA, *et al.* Effect of parents' occupational exposures on risk of stillbirth, preterm delivery, and small-for-gestational-age infants. *Am J Epidemiol* 1989; **129:** 1201–18.

Pharmacokinetics

Benzene is absorbed by inhalation, and ingestion, but is not significantly absorbed through the skin. Some is excreted unchanged from the lungs. Oxidation to phenol and related quinol compounds occurs, the metabolites being excreted in the urine as conjugates of sulphuric or glucuronic acid.

Uses

Benzene was formerly applied as a pediculicide. Its use as an industrial solvent is decreasing.

Butyl Acetate (12482-e)

n-Butyl acetate.

$C_6H_{12}O_2$ = 116.2.

CAS — 123-86-4.

A clear, colourless flammable liquid with a strong fruity odour. Wt per mL about 0.88 g. B.p. 123° to 126°. Slightly **soluble** in water; miscible with alcohol. **Store** in airtight containers.

Adverse Effects

Butyl acetate is irritant. High concentrations may cause depression of the CNS.

Uses

Butyl acetate is used as an industrial solvent and as an extraction solvent in food processing.

Butyl Alcohol (16556-f)

n-Butanol; *n*-Butyl Alcohol. Butan-1-ol.

$C_4H_{10}O$ = 74.12.

CAS — 71-36-3.

Pharmacopoeias. In *USNF.*

A clear, colourless, mobile liquid with a vinous odour. Sp. gr. 0.807 to 0.809. B.p. about 118°. **Soluble** in water; miscible with alcohol, ether, and many other organic solvents. **Store** in airtight containers at a temperature not exceeding 40°.

CAUTION. *Suitable precautions should be taken to avoid skin contact with butyl alcohol as it can penetrate skin and produce systemic toxicity.*

Adverse Effects

Butyl alcohol may be irritant and may cause mild CNS depression with headache, dizziness, and drowsiness.

References to the toxicity of butyl alcohol.

1. Butanols—four isomers: 1-butanol, 2-butanol, tert-butanol, isobutanol. *Environmental Health Criteria 65.* Geneva: WHO, 1987.
2. 1-Butanol. *Health and Safety Guide.* Geneva: WHO, 1987.

Uses

Butyl alcohol is used as an industrial and pharmaceutical solvent and as an extraction solvent in food processing.

Butylamine (12484-y)

n-Butylamine.

$C_4H_{11}N$ = 73.14.

CAS — 109-73-9.

A colourless to pale yellow flammable liquid with an ammoniacal odour. Wt per mL about 0.744 g. B.p. about 78°. **Miscible** with water, alcohol, and ether. **Store** in airtight containers.

CAUTION. *Suitable precautions should be taken to avoid skin contact with butylamine as it can penetrate skin and produce systemic toxicity.*

Adverse Effects

Butylamine is irritant. Symptoms of CNS depression may be observed after exposure to high concentrations of the vapour.

Uses

Butylamine is used as a solvent.

Carbon Disulphide (6506-t)

Carbon Bisulphide; Carbonei Sulfidum; Carboneum Bisulfuratum; Carboneum Sulfuratum; Schwefelkohlenstoff.

CS_2 = 76.14.

CAS — 75-15-0.

Pharmacopoeias. In *Aust.*

A clear, colourless, volatile, flammable liquid with a chloroform-like odour. Commercial grades have an unpleasant odour described by some as being reminiscent of decaying radishes. Wt per mL about 1.26 g. B.p. about 46°. **Store** in airtight containers.

The vapour mixed with air in the proportions of 1 to 50% is highly explosive.

CAUTION. *Suitable precautions should be taken to avoid skin contact with carbon disulphide as it can penetrate skin and produce systemic toxicity.*

Adverse Effects and Treatment

Carbon disulphide is irritant. Toxic effects may occur as a result of inhalation, ingestion, or absorption through the skin.

Acute poisoning may result in gastro-intestinal disturbances and euphoria, followed by depression of the CNS. Symptoms include headache, dizziness, mood changes, and in severe cases, manic psychoses, delirium, hallucinations, coma, convulsions, and death due to respiratory failure.

Chronic poisoning has been associated with occupational exposure to carbon disulphide vapour for prolonged periods. It is characterised by peripheral neuropathies; CNS effects such as headache, fatigue, insomnia, tremor, emotional lability, extrapyramidal disorders, manic-depressive psychoses and encephalopathy; gastro-intestinal effects including anorexia, dyspepsia, and ulcerative changes; and effects on the eye. Occupational exposure to carbon disulphide has been shown to be associated with an increased incidence of mortality from coronary heart disease. The action of carbon disulphide on endocrine function has resulted in menstrual irregularities, an increased incidence of spontaneous abortions and premature births, loss of libido, sperm abnormalities, and decreased serum-thyroxine concentrations; there is limited evidence of impaired glucose tolerance.

Treatment consists of removal from exposure and general supportive and symptomatic measures. Gastric lavage may be performed after ingestion; activated charcoal may be administered. Adrenaline and other sympathomimetics should be avoided because of the risk of precipitating cardiac arrhythmias. Peripheral neuropathies may be only slowly reversible.

Reviews of the toxicity of carbon disulphide.

1. Carbon Disulfide. *Environmental Health Criteria 10.* Geneva: WHO, 1979.
2. WHO. Recommended health-based limits in occupational exposure to selected organic solvents. *WHO Tech Rep Ser 664* 1981.
3. Health and Safety Executive. Carbon disulphide. *Toxicity Review 3.* London: HMSO, 1981.

Effects on endocrine function. A retrospective study of 265 female workers in the rayon industry exposed for at least one year to carbon disulphide, and 291 non-exposed female workers.[1] Levels of exposure to carbon disulphide varied over the study period from 0.7 to 30.6 mg per m^3. Women exposed to carbon disulphide had a higher risk of menstrual disturbances than non-exposed women. However, there was no difference between the 2 groups in incidence of toxaemia, emesis gravidarum, spontaneous abortion, premature or overdue delivery, or congenital malformation.

1. Zhou SY, *et al.* Effects of occupational exposure to low-level carbon disulfide (CS_2) on menstruation and pregnancy. *Ind Health* 1988; **26:** 203–14.

Effects on the heart. Studies demonstrating an increased incidence of mortality from cardiovascular disease in workers occupationally exposed to carbon disulphide.[1-3] The evidence suggests that the risk decreases after cessation of exposure.

1. Nurminen M, Hernberg S. Effects of intervention on the cardiovascular mortality of workers exposed to carbon disulphide: a 15 year follow up. *Br J Ind Med* 1985; **42:** 32–5.
2. Sweetnam PM, *et al.* Exposure to carbon disulphide and ischaemic heart disease in a viscose rayon factory. *Br J Ind Med* 1987; **44:** 220–7.
3. MacMahon B, Monson RR. Mortality in the US rayon industry. *J Occup Med* 1988; **30:** 698–705.

Pharmacokinetics

Carbon disulphide is rapidly absorbed after inhalation and ingestion, and is also absorbed through intact skin. It is excreted unchanged through the lungs and in the urine predominantly as metabolites.

Uses

Carbon disulphide is used as an industrial solvent and has been used, in the vapour form, as an insecticide.

Carbon Tetrachloride (767-z)

Tetrachloromethane.

CCl_4 = 153.8.

CAS — 56-23-5.

Pharmacopoeias. In *Belg.*

A clear, colourless, mobile, liquid with a chloroform-like odour. Sp. gr. 1.588 to 1.590. B.p. 76° to 78°. Practically **insoluble** in water; miscible with alcohol, chloroform, ether, petroleum spirit, and fixed and volatile oils. **Store** in airtight containers at a temperature not exceeding 30°. Protect from light.

CAUTION. *Avoid contact with carbon tetrachloride; the vapour and liquid are poisonous. Care should be taken not to vaporise carbon tetrachloride in the presence of a flame because of the production of harmful gases, mainly phosgene.*

Adverse Effects

Individual response to carbon tetrachloride varies widely; a few millilitres of carbon tetrachloride inhaled or given by mouth have proved fatal and its toxicity appears to be increased by alcohol. Symptoms of poisoning follow ingestion, inhalation, or application but develop more rapidly after inhalation.

Carbon tetrachloride is irritant; repeated application of carbon tetrachloride to the skin may result in dermatitis. Aspiration may result in pulmonary oedema.

Adverse effects after acute exposure from any route include gastro-intestinal disturbances such as nausea, vomiting, and abdominal pain, and CNS disturbances such as headache, dizziness, and drowsiness, with progression to convulsions, coma, and death from respiratory depression or circulatory collapse. Death may also occur as a result of ventricular arrhythmia. Hepatic and renal cellular necrosis can occur and are associated with free radical production; symptoms usually begin a few days or up to 2 weeks after acute exposure to carbon tetrachloride. Kidney damage may present as oliguria, progressing to proteinuria, anuria, weight gain, and oedema. Symptoms of liver damage include anorexia, jaundice, and hepatomegaly. If hepatorenal necrosis is not fatal recovery is eventually complete.

Symptoms of chronic poisoning are similar to those of acute poisoning; in addition, paraesthesias, visual disturbances, anaemia, and aplastic anaemia have occurred. Carcinogenicity has been demonstrated in *animals.*

References.

1. Melamed E, Lavy S. Parkinsonism associated with chronic inhalation of carbon tetrachloride. *Lancet* 1977; **i:** 1015.
2. Johnson BP, *et al.* Cerebellar dysfunction after acute carbon tetrachloride poisoning. *Lancet* 1983; **ii:** 968.
3. Perez AJ, *et al.* Acute renal failure after topical application of carbon tetrachloride. *Lancet* 1987; **i:** 515–6.
4. Health and Safety Executive. Carbon tetrachloride, chloroform. *Toxicity Review 23.* London: HMSO, 1992.
5. Manno M, Rezzadore M. Critical role of ethanol abuse in carbon tetrachloride poisoning. *Lancet* 1994; **343:** 232.

Treatment of Adverse Effects

If carbon tetrachloride vapour has been inhaled remove the patient to the fresh air. Remove clothing contaminated by liquid and wash the skin. If carbon tetrachloride has been recently ingested gastric lavage may be performed and activated charcoal may be administered.

The usual symptomatic and supportive measures should be instituted. Hepatic and renal function should be monitored closely. Haemodialysis or peritoneal dialysis may be needed if renal function is impaired. Adrenaline or other sympathomimetics should be avoided because of the risk of precipitating cardiac arrhythmias.

Acetylcysteine (p.1054) may be administered to patients recently exposed to carbon tetrachloride in an attempt to prevent or modify liver and kidney damage.

Experimental studies and anecdotal reports suggest that hyperbaric oxygen therapy is of potential benefit in the treatment of carbon tetrachloride poisoning.[1]

1. Burkhart KK, *et al.* Hyperbaric oxygen treatment for carbon tetrachloride poisoning. *Drug Safety* 1991; **6:** 332–8.

Pharmacokinetics

Carbon tetrachloride is readily absorbed after inhalation and from the gastro-intestinal tract. It is also absorbed through the skin. Metabolism to reactive free radicals is thought to account for the hepatorenal toxicity of carbon tetrachloride.

Carbon tetrachloride is slowly excreted from the body via the lungs and the urine.

Uses

Carbon tetrachloride is employed in industry as a solvent and degreaser. It was formerly used in certain types of fire extinguisher and as an industrial and domestic dry cleaner but has been largely replaced for this purpose by less toxic substances. Carbon tetrachloride has also been used for the fumigation of cereals.

Carbon tetrachloride was formerly given by mouth as an anthelmintic but it has been superseded by equally effective and less toxic drugs.

Cyclohexane (6507-x)

Hexahydrobenzene; Hexamethylene.

C_6H_{12} = 84.16.

CAS — 110-82-7.

A colourless, flammable liquid. Wt per mL about 0.78 g. B.p. about 81°. **Store** in airtight containers.

Adverse Effects

Cyclohexane is irritant, and may also have central nervous system effects.

Reviews of the toxicity of cyclohexane.

1. Health and Safety Executive. Cyclohexane, cumene, para-dichlorobenzene (p-DCB), chlorodifluoromethane (CFC 22). *Toxicity Review 25.* London: HMSO, 1991.

Uses

Cyclohexane is used as an industrial solvent.

Dichloromethane (6521-a)

Methylene Chloride; Methyleni Chloridum.

CH_2Cl_2 = 84.93.

CAS — 75-09-2.

Pharmacopoeias. In *Eur.* (see p.viii). Also in *USNF.*

A clear, colourless, mobile, volatile liquid with a chloroform-like odour. Non-flammable. Relative density 1.320 to 1.332; sp. gr. 1.318 to 1.322. Distilling range 39.5° to 40.5°. Its vapour is not explosive when mixed with air. Phosgene is produced on heating of dichloromethane.

Sparingly **soluble** in water; miscible with alcohol, ether, and with fixed and volatile oils. **Store** in airtight containers. Protect from light.

Adverse Effects and Treatment

Acute exposure to dichloromethane vapour may depress the CNS; symptoms progress from headache and dizziness to coma and death in severe cases. Pulmonary oedema has been reported. Significant exposure may result in raised blood concentrations of carboxyhaemoglobin and symptoms of carbon monoxide poisoning. Cardiovascular effects have been attributed to hypoxia secondary to carboxyhaemoglobinaemia. There has been a report of haemolysis following acute ingestion of dichloromethane.

Chronic occupational exposure to dichloromethane vapour has produced gastro-intestinal disturbances in addition to symptoms observed after acute poisoning. Dichloromethane is a common constituent of paint strippers and may be implicated in volatile substance abuse (p.1375).

The liquid is irritant and high concentrations of the vapour are irritant to the eyes.

Treatment of acute poisoning consists of removal from exposure and supportive and symptomatic measures. Carboxyhaemoglobinaemia should be managed as for carbon monoxide poisoning (p.1164) by administration of 100% oxygen; hyperbaric oxygen may be indicated. Activated charcoal may be administered following ingestion. Adrenaline and other sympathomimetics should be avoided because of the risk of precipitating cardiac arrhythmias.

References.

1. Methylene Chloride. *Environmental Health Criteria 32.* Geneva: WHO, 1984.
2. Health and Safety Executive. Dichloromethane (methylene chloride). *Toxicity Review 12.* London: HMSO, 1985.
3. Methylene chloride. *Health and Safety Guide 6.* Geneva: WHO, 1987.
4. Rioux JP, Myers RAM. Methylene chloride poisoning: a paradigmatic review. *J Emerg Med* 1988; **6:** 227–38.
5. Manno M, *et al.* Double fatal inhalation of dichloromethane. *Hum Exp Toxicol* 1992; **11:** 540–5.

Pharmacokinetics

Dichloromethane is rapidly absorbed following inhalation and is also absorbed after ingestion and slowly through intact skin. It appears to be partially metabolised to carbon dioxide and carbon monoxide which are exhaled, although significant blood-carboxyhaemoglobin concentrations may be attained. Some unchanged dichloromethane is exhaled and small amounts are excreted in the urine.

Uses

Dichloromethane is used as a pharmaceutical and industrial solvent. It is also employed as an extraction solvent in food processing.

Dichloromethane is widely used in paint strippers.

Dichloropropane (19073-b)

Propylene Dichloride. 1,2-Dichloropropane.

$C_3H_6Cl_2$ = 113.0.

CAS — 78-87-5.

A colourless, mobile, flammable liquid. Wt per mL about 1.16 g. B.p. about 96°. **Store** in airtight containers.

Adverse Effects

Dichloropropane is irritant; high concentrations may result in CNS depression.

A report of acute renal failure, haemolytic anaemia, acute liver disease, and disseminated intravascular coagulation following intentional inhalation of a stain remover containing dichloropropane; the patient recovered following blood transfusions and haemodialysis.[1]

1. Locatelli F, Pozzi C. Relapsing haemolytic-uraemic syndrome after organic solvent sniffing. *Lancet* 1983; **ii:** 220.

Uses

Dichloropropane is used as an industrial solvent, dry cleaning agent, and agricultural defumigant.

Diethyl Phthalate (6508-r)

Diethylis Phthalas; Ethyl Phthalate. The diethyl ester of benzene-1,2-dicarboxylic acid.

$C_{12}H_{14}O_4$ = 222.2.

CAS — 84-66-2.

Pharmacopoeias. In *Eur.* (see p.viii). Also in *USNF.*

A clear, colourless or very slightly yellow, practically odourless oily liquid. Relative density 1.117 to 1.121; sp. gr. 1.118 to 1.122 at 20°.

Practically **insoluble** in water; miscible with alcohol, ether, and usual organic solvents. **Store** in airtight containers.

Adverse Effects

Diethyl phthalate is irritant and, in high concentrations, causes CNS depression.

References.

1. Health and Safety Executive. Review of the toxicity of the esters of o-phthalic acid (phthalate esters). *Toxicity Review 14.* London: HMSO, 1986.
2. Kamrin MA, Mayor GH. Diethyl phthalate: a perspective. *J Clin Pharmacol* 1991; **31:** 484–9.

Uses

Diethyl phthalate is used as a denaturant of alcohol, for example in surgical spirit, and as a solvent and plasticiser.

Preparations

BP 1998: Surgical Spirit.

Dimethyl Sulphoxide (6509-f)

Dimethyl Sulphoxide *(BAN).*

Dimethyl Sulfoxide *(USAN, rINN);* Dimethylis Sulfoxidum; DMSO; Methyl Sulphoxide; NSC-763; SQ-9453; Sulphinylbismethane.

C_2H_6OS = 78.13.

CAS — 67-68-5.

Pharmacopoeias. In *Eur.* (see p.viii) and *US.*

A colourless hygroscopic odourless liquid or crystals. F.p. not lower than 18.3°. Relative density 1.100 to 1.104; sp. gr. 1.095 to 1.097.

Miscible with water, alcohol, and ether; practically insoluble in acetone, in alcohol, in chloroform, and in ether. **Store** in airtight glass containers. Protect from light.

Adverse Effects and Treatment

High concentrations of dimethyl sulphoxide applied to the skin may cause burning discomfort, itching, erythema, vesiculation, and urticaria. Continued use may result in scaling.

Systemic effects may occur after administration by any route and include gastro-intestinal disturbances, drowsiness, headache, and hypersensitivity reactions. A garlic-like odour on the breath and skin is attributed to the formation of dimethyl sulphide (see Pharmacokinetics, below). Intravascular haemolysis has been reported following intravenous administration. Local discomfort and spasm may occur when given by bladder instillation.

Treatment of adverse effects consists of symptomatic and supportive measures. Gastric lavage may be helpful after acute ingestion, although it should be remembered that absorption is rapid.

Reviews.

1. Brobyn RD. The human toxicology of dimethyl sulfoxide. *Ann N Y Acad Sci* 1975; **243:** 497–506.
2. Willhite CC, Katz PI. Toxicology updates: dimethyl sulfoxide. *J Appl Toxicol* 1984; **4:** 155–60.

Dimethyl sulphoxide administered by intravenous infusion for spinal cord injury to 14 patients has caused transient haemolysis and haemoglobinuria.[1] Infusion strengths greater than 10% were associated with grossly discoloured urine but there was no evidence of kidney damage. In two patients, raised liver and muscle enzyme concentrations, mild jaundice, and evidence of haemolysis developed after receiving dimethyl sulphoxide intravenously for arthritis.[2] One also developed acute renal tubular necrosis, deterioration in level of consciousness, and evidence of cerebral infarction. Acute, reversible neurological deterioration in one patient has been associated with intravenous dimethyl sulphoxide.[3]

Serum hyperosmolality[4] has been reported in a patient who had pre-existing diabetes insipidus after receiving haematopoietic stem cells cryopreserved in dimethyl sulphoxide following chemotherapy for a malignant germ-cell tumour; symptoms included severe headache, confusion, and abdominal pain.

1. Muther RS, Bennett WM. Effects of dimethyl sulfoxide on renal function in man. *JAMA* 1980; **244:** 2081–3.
2. Yellowlees P, *et al.* Dimethylsulphoxide-induced toxicity. *Lancet* 1980; **ii:** 1004–6.
3. Bond GR, *et al.* Dimethylsulphoxide-induced encephalopathy. *Lancet* 1989; **i:** 1134–5.
4. Thomé S, *et al.* Dimethylsulphoxide-induced serum hyperosmolality after cryopreserved stem-cell graft. *Lancet* 1994; **344:** 1431–2.

Precautions

When used as a penetrating basis for other drugs applied topically, dimethyl sulphoxide may enhance their toxic effects.

Since dimethyl sulphoxide has been associated with lens changes in *animals*, the manufacturers recommend assessment of ophthalmic function every 6 months during long-term treatment of cystitis with intravesical instillation of dimethyl sulphoxide. Liver and renal function should also be assessed at intervals of 6 months. Bladder instillation may be harmful in patients with urinary-tract malignancy because of vasodilatation.

Interactions

For mention of an interaction between dimethyl sulphoxide and sulindac, see p.87.

Pharmacokinetics

Dimethyl sulphoxide is readily absorbed after administration by all routes. It is metabolised by oxidation to dimethyl sulphone and by reduction to dimethyl sulphide. Dimethyl sulphoxide and the sulphone metabolite are excreted in the urine and faeces. Dimethyl sulphide is excreted through the lungs and skin and is responsible for the characteristic odour from patients.

Uses and Administration

Dimethyl sulphoxide is a highly polar substance which has exceptional solvent properties for both organic and inorganic chemicals, and is widely used as an industrial solvent.

It has been reported to have a wide spectrum of pharmacological activity including membrane penetration, anti-inflammatory effects, local analgesia, weak bacteriostasis, diuresis, vasodilatation, dissolution of collagen, and free-radical scavenging.

The principal use of dimethyl sulphoxide is as a vehicle for drugs such as idoxuridine (p.613); it aids penetration of the drug into the skin, and so may enhance the drug's effect. It is also used as a 50% aqueous solution for bladder instillation for the symptomatic relief of interstitial cystitis; doses of 50 mL are instilled and allowed to remain for 15 minutes. Treatment is repeated every 2 weeks initially.

Dimethyl sulphoxide has been administered orally, intravenously, or topically for a wide range of indications including cutaneous and musculoskeletal disorders, but evidence of beneficial effects is limited.

Dimethyl sulphoxide is used as a cryoprotectant for various human tissues.

Reviews.

1. Trice JM, Pinals RS. Dimethyl sulfoxide: a review of its use in the rheumatic disorders. *Semin Arthritis Rheum* 1985; **15:** 45–60.
2. Swanson BN. Medical use of dimethyl sulfoxide (DMSO). *Rev Clin Basic Pharm* 1985; **5:** 1–33.

Cryopreservation. Dimethyl sulphoxide is used as a cryoprotectant in various assisted conception techniques.[1] Adverse effects have been reported in patients receiving haematopoietic stem cells cryopreserved in dimethyl sulphoxide (see under Adverse Effects, above).

1. Trounson AO. Cryopreservation. *Br Med Bull* 1990; **46:** 695–708.

Extravasation of antineoplastics. Several reports have suggested a role for topical dimethyl sulphoxide in the treatment of anthracycline extravasation.[1-4] The problem of antineoplastic extravasation and its management is discussed further on p.474.

1. Lawrence HJ, Goodnight SH. Dimethyl sulfoxide and extravasation of anthracycline agents. *Ann Intern Med* 1983; **98:** 1025.
2. Olver IN, *et al.* A prospective study of topical dimethyl sulfoxide for treating anthracycline extravasation. *J Clin Oncol* 1988; **6:** 1732–5.
3. Rospond RM, Engel LM. Dimethyl sulfoxide for treating anthracycline extravasation. *Clin Pharm* 1993; **12:** 560–1.
4. Bertelli G, *et al.* Dimethylsulphoxide and cooling after extravasation of antitumour agents. *Lancet* 1993; **341:** 1098.

Gallstones. For mention of the use of dimethyl sulphoxide to dissolve gallstones, see Methyl *tert*-Butyl Ether, p.1379.

Interstitial cystitis. Interstitial cystitis is an inflammatory condition of the bladder of unknown aetiology. Symptoms include pain, urinary frequency, urinary urgency, and nocturia. Many treatments have been tried, including local and systemic drug therapy and surgery.

Bladder instillations of a 50% aqueous solution of dimethyl sulphoxide appear to alleviate symptoms.[1,2] It has been suggested that the chief effect of dimethyl sulphoxide may be on sensory nerves since there appears to be no significant alteration in the endoscopic or morphological appearance of the bladder after treatment.[3] Treatment has successfully been repeated at relapse.[3]

Oral administration of pentosan polysulphate sodium (p.928) may also provide some relief of symptoms.

1. Fowler JE. Prospective study of intravesical dimethyl sulfoxide in treatment of suspected early interstitial cystitis. *Urology* 1981; **18:** 21–6.
2. Perez-Marrero R, *et al.* A controlled study of dimethyl sulfoxide in interstitial cystitis. *J Urol (Baltimore)* 1988; **140:** 36–9.
3. Ryan PG, Wallace DMA. Are we making progress in the drug treatment of disorders of the bladder, prostate, and penis? *J Clin Pharm Ther* 1990; **15:** 1–12.

Raised intracranial pressure. Intravenous osmotic diuretics, particularly mannitol, are used to lower raised intracranial pressure (p.796). Small preliminary studies[1,2] indicate that intravenous administration of dimethyl sulphoxide can control raised intracranial pressure refractory to other treatments but some workers[1] have encountered problems with fluid overload and difficulties with administration.

1. Marshall LF, *et al.* Dimethyl sulfoxide for the treatment of intracranial hypertension: a preliminary trial. *Neurosurgery* 1984; **14:** 659–63.
2. Karaca M, *et al.* Dimethyl sulphoxide lowers ICP after closed head trauma. *Eur J Clin Pharmacol* 1991; **40:** 113–14.

Preparations

USP 23: Dimethyl Sulfoxide Irrigation.

Proprietary Preparations (details are given in Part 3)
Canad.: Kemsol; Rimso; ***Ger.:*** Rheumabene; ***UK:*** Rimso; ***USA:*** Rimso.

Multi-ingredient: ***Ger.:*** Dolobene; Verrumal; ***Spain:*** Artrodesmol Extra; ***Switz.:*** Dolo Demotherm; Dolobene; Histalgane; Histalgane mite; Neo-Liniment†; Roll-bene; Sportusal; Sportusal Spray sine heparino; Verra-med; Verrumal.

Dimethylacetamide (6510-z)

Acetyldimethylamine; DMAC. *NN*-Dimethylacetamide.
$C_4H_9NO = 87.12$.
CAS — 127-19-5.

A clear, colourless liquid. Wt per mL about 0.94 g. B.p. about 165°. **Miscible** with water and most organic solvents.

CAUTION. *Suitable precautions should be taken to avoid skin contact with dimethylacetamide as it can penetrate skin and produce systemic toxicity.*

Adverse Effects

As for Dimethylformamide (below), although a disulfiram-like reaction with alcohol has not been reported.

A review[1] of the toxicology of dimethylacetamide in *animals* and in man with reference to its use as a vehicle for antineoplastic agents.

1. Kim S-N. Preclinical toxicology and pharmacology of dimethylacetamide, with clinical notes. *Drug Metab Rev* 1988; **19:** 345–68.

Uses

Dimethylacetamide is used as an industrial and pharmaceutical solvent.

Dimethylformamide (6511-c)

DMF. *NN*-Dimethylformamide.
$C_3H_7NO = 73.09$.
CAS — 68-12-2.

A colourless liquid. Wt per mL about 0.95 g. B.p. about 153°.

CAUTION. *Suitable precautions should be taken to avoid skin contact with dimethylformamide as it can penetrate skin and produce systemic toxicity.*

Adverse Effects and Precautions

Dimethylformamide is irritant. Gastro-intestinal effects including nausea, vomiting, loss of appetite, and abdominal pain, CNS effects such as headache, dizziness, and weakness, and liver damage have been reported in workers occupationally exposed to the liquid or vapour. Some workers exposed to dimethylformamide have experienced a disulfiram-like effect after consumption of alcohol.

Reviews of the adverse effects of dimethylformamide.

1. Dimethylformamide. *Environmental Health Criteria 114.* Geneva: WHO, 1991.

Effects on the liver. Elevated liver enzyme values were found in 36 of 58 (62%) workers in a fabric coating factory.[1] Exposure to the solvent, dimethylformamide, was considered to be the most likely cause. Symptoms reported by workers were generally mild and included anorexia, abdominal pain, nausea, headache, dizziness, and a disulfiram-type reaction to alcohol.

Hepatotoxicity has occurred following acute poisoning with a veterinary drug formulated in dimethylformamide. There were only minor increases in liver enzyme values in one such patient who was treated early with acetylcysteine.[2]

1. Redlich CA, *et al.* Liver disease associated with occupational exposure to the solvent dimethylformamide. *Ann Intern Med* 1988; **108:** 680–6.
2. Buylaert W, *et al.* Hepatotoxicity of N,N-dimethylformamide (DMF) in acute poisoning with the veterinary euthanasia drug T-61. *Hum Exp Toxicol* 1996; **15:** 607–11.

Malignant neoplasms. There have been reports of testicular cancer in men occupationally exposed to dimethylformamide.[1] Such an association could not, however, be substantiated by epidemiological data on 3859 male employees exposed to dimethylformamide between 1950 and 1970 and followed up to 1984.[2] It has been suggested that although dimethylformamide may not itself be carcinogenic, it may increase absorption through the skin of heavy metal carcinogens, possibly including chromates.[3]

1. Levin SL, *et al.* Testicular cancer in leather tanners exposed to dimethylformamide. *Lancet* 1987; **ii:** 1153.
2. Chen JL, Kennedy GL. Dimethylformamide and testicular cancer. *Lancet* 1988; **i:** 55.
3. Ducatman AM. Dimethylformamide, metal dyes, and testicular cancer. *Lancet* 1989; **i:** 911.

Pharmacokinetics

Dimethylformamide is absorbed after inhalation and through intact skin. It is excreted mainly in the urine as metabolites.

Uses

Dimethylformamide is used as an industrial solvent.

Dioxan (6512-k)

Diethylene Dioxide; Diethylene Ether; Dioxane. 1,4-Dioxane.
$C_4H_8O_2 = 88.11$.
CAS — 123-91-1.

NOTE. Do not confuse dioxan and dioxin (p.1572).

A colourless flammable liquid with an ethereal odour. Wt per mL about 1.03 g. B.p. about 101°. **Store** in airtight containers.

CAUTION. *It is dangerous to distil or evaporate dioxan unless precautions have been taken to remove explosive peroxides. Suitable precautions should be taken to avoid skin contact with dioxan as it can penetrate skin and produce systemic toxicity.*

Adverse Effects and Treatment

Dioxan vapour is irritant to mucous membranes. High concentrations may cause nausea and vomiting, and depression of the CNS with headache, dizziness, drowsiness, and in severe cases unconsciousness. On repeated exposure, severe liver and kidney damage, including necrotic changes, can occur and may be fatal. Direct contact with liquid dioxan can result in dermatitis. Dioxan has been shown to be carcinogenic in *animals.*

Treatment consists of removal from exposure and general supportive and symptomatic measures.

Pharmacokinetics

Dioxan is absorbed after inhalation and through the skin. It is metabolised by oxidation to β-hydroxyethoxy-acetic acid.

Uses

Dioxan is used as an industrial solvent.

Epichlorohydrin (16293-z)

1-Chloro-2,3-epoxypropane.
$C_3H_5ClO = 92.52$.
CAS — 106-89-8.

A colourless, flammable liquid. Wt per mL about 1.18 g. B.p. 115° to 118°. The vapour forms explosive mixtures with air. Harmful gases including phosgene are liberated on heating of epichlorohydrin. **Store** in airtight containers.

CAUTION. *Suitable precautions should be taken to avoid skin contact with epichlorohydrin as it can penetrate skin and produce systemic toxicity.*

Adverse Effects

Epichlorohydrin is irritant. It has been shown to be carcinogenic to *animals*.

References to the toxicity of epichlorohydrin.

1. Epichlorohydrin. *Environmental Health Criteria 33.* Geneva: WHO, 1984.
2. Epichlorohydrin. *Health and Safety Guide 8.* Geneva: WHO, 1987.
3. Health and Safety Executive. Ammonia, 1-chloro-2,3-epoxypropane (epichlorohydrin), carcinogenicity of cadmium and its compounds. *Toxicity Review 24.* London: HMSO, 1991.

Uses

Epichlorohydrin is used as an industrial solvent.

Solvent Ether (6513-a)

Aether; Aether Aethylicus; Aether Solvens; Diethyl Ether; Eter; Ether; Éther rectifié; Ethyl Ether; Ethyl Oxide.
$(C_2H_5)_2O = 74.12$.
CAS — 60-29-7.

NOTE. Solvent ether is not intended for anaesthesia; only ether of a suitable quality (see p.1223) should be so used.

Pharmacopoeias. In *Eur.* (see p.viii), *Jpn, Pol.,* and *US* .

A colourless, clear, very volatile, flammable, very mobile liquid with a characteristic sweet, pungent odour. It volatilises very quickly and by so doing reduces temperature. Though ether is one of the lightest of liquids, its vapour is very heavy, being 2½ times heavier than air. Relative density 0.714 to 0.716; sp. gr. 0.713 to 0.716. B.p. about 35°. **Soluble** in water and hydrochloric acid; miscible with alcohol, chloroform, dichloromethane, petroleum spirit, and fixed and volatile oils. **Store** at 8° to 15° in airtight containers. Protect from light.

CAUTION. *Ether is very volatile and flammable and mixtures of its vapour with oxygen, nitrous oxide, or air at certain concentrations are explosive. It should not be used in the presence of an open flame or any electrical apparatus liable to produce a spark; precautions should be taken against the production of static electrical discharge. Explosive peroxides are generated by the atmospheric oxidation of solvent ether and it is dangerous to distil a sample which contains peroxides.*

Adverse Effects

As for Anaesthetic Ether, p.1223. Ingestion of 30 to 60 mL may be fatal.

A report of interstitial cystitis following attempted dissolution of a Foley catheter balloon with ether.[1]

1. Nellans RE, *et al.* Ether cystitis. *JAMA* 1985; **254:** 530.

Uses

Solvent ether is widely used as a pharmaceutical and industrial solvent, and is used as an extraction solvent in food processing.

For reference to the use of ether ear drops to remove maggots in the ear, see under Turpentine Oil, p.1641.

Ethyl Acetate (6514-t)

Acetic Ether; Aethylis Acetas; Aethylium Aceticum; Ethyl Ethanoate; Ethylis Acetas.
$C_4H_8O_2 = 88.11$.
CAS — 141-78-6.

Pharmacopoeias. In *Eur.* (see p.viii)and *Pol.* Also in *USNF.*

A colourless, clear, volatile, flammable liquid with a fragrant, refreshing, slightly acetous fruity odour. Relative density 0.898 to 0.902; sp. gr. 0.894 to 0.898. B.p. 76° to 78°. **Soluble** in water; miscible with alcohol, acetone, dichloromethane, ether, and with fixed and volatile oils. **Store** in airtight containers at a temperature not exceeding 30°. Protect from light.

Adverse Effects

Ethyl acetate is irritant to mucous membranes. High concentrations may cause depression of the CNS. Ethyl acetate may be implicated in volatile substance abuse (p.1375).

For discussion of neurotoxicity after occupational exposure to solvents and the absence of such an effect with ethyl acetate, see under Toluene, p.1381.

Uses

Ethyl acetate is used as a flavour and solvent in pharmaceutical preparations. It is also employed in industry as a solvent and is used as an extraction solvent in food processing.

Formamide (6516-r)

Carbamaldehyde; Methanamide.
$CH_3NO = 45.04$.
CAS — 75-12-7.

A colourless, oily liquid. B.p. 210°. Wt per mL, about 1.13 g.

Adverse Effects

Formamide is reported to be irritant.

Uses

Formamide is used as an industrial solvent.

Glycofurol (9935-a)

Glycofurol 75; Tetraglycol; Tetrahydrofurfuryl Alcohol Polyethylene Glycol Ether. α-(Tetrahydrofuranyl)-ω-hydroxypoly(oxyethylene).
CAS — 9004-76-6.

A clear, colourless, almost odourless liquid. Wt per mL about 1.08 g. B.p. 80° to 100°. **Incompatible** with oxidising agents. **Store** under nitrogen in airtight containers. Protect from light.

Uses

Glycofurol is used as a pharmaceutical solvent for injections.

Hexachloroethane (780-l)

$C_2Cl_6 = 236.7$.
CAS — 67-72-1.

Pharmacopoeias. In *Aust.*

Hexachloroethane is a chlorinated hydrocarbon used in industry as a solvent. Eye irritation and photophobia have resulted from industrial exposure to the vapour. It was formerly used in veterinary medicine as an anthelmintic, but has been superseded by less toxic drugs.

n-Hexane (9931-j)

C_6H_{14} = 86.18.
CAS — 110-54-3.

A colourless, flammable, volatile liquid with a faint odour. Wt per mL about 0.66 g. B.p. about 69°. **Store** in airtight containers.

Adverse Effects

n-Hexane is irritant. Acute exposure to the vapour may result in CNS depression with headache, drowsiness, dizziness, and in severe cases unconsciousness. Chronic occupational exposure and abuse of *n*-hexane have been associated with the development of peripheral neuropathies. *n*-Hexane is a constituent of some adhesives and may be implicated in volatile substance abuse (p.1375). Some adverse effects of petrol have been attributed to its content of *n*-hexane.

References.

1. Health and Safety Executive. *n*-Hexane. *Toxicity Review 18.* London: HMSO, 1987.
2. *n*-Hexane. *Environmental Health Criteria 122.* Geneva: WHO, 1991.
3. *n*-Hexane. *Health and Safety Guide 59.* Geneva: WHO, 1991.

Effects on the nervous system. There have been many reports of peripheral neuropathy attributed to the abuse of and occupational exposure to *n*-hexane, although symptoms tend to be milder in the latter.[1] Tetraplegia has occurred in severe cases. There is typically a clinical deterioration several weeks after exposure followed by a slow recovery which, in severe cases, may not be complete. It has been suggested that methyl ethyl ketone potentiates the peripheral neuropathy induced by *n*-hexane. Occupational exposure to *n*-hexane has also been associated with cranial nerve neuropathy.

Parkinsonism in a leather worker, possibly associated with exposure to solvents, predominantly *n*-hexane has been noted.[2]

For further discussion of neurotoxicity after occupational exposure to solvents including *n*-hexane, see under Toluene, p.1381.

1. Lolin Y. Chronic neurological toxicity associated with exposure to volatile substances. *Hum Toxicol* 1989; **8:** 293–300.
2. Pezzoli G, *et al.* Parkinsonism due to n-hexane exposure. *Lancet* 1989; **ii:** 874.

Pharmacokinetics

n-Hexane is absorbed by inhalation and to a limited extent through the skin. Oxidative metabolites, including 2,5-hexanedione are excreted in the urine largely as conjugates. Some unchanged *n*-hexane is excreted via the lungs.

Uses

n-Hexane is widely used as an industrial solvent, as a solvent in glues, and as an extraction solvent in food processing.

Preparations

Proprietary Preparations (details are given in Part 3)
Multi-ingredient: ***Austral.:*** Sacsol.

Kerosene (6517-f)

Kerosine; 'Paraffin'.
CAS — 8008-20-6.

Kerosene is a mixture of hydrocarbons, chiefly members of the alkane series, distilled from petroleum. It is a clear, colourless liquid with a characteristic odour. Sp. gr. about 0.8 g. B.p. 180° to 300°. An odourless grade is available. **Store** in airtight containers.

Adverse Effects

The chief danger from ingestion of kerosene is pneumonitis and attendant pulmonary complications resulting from aspiration. Spontaneous or induced vomiting increases the risk of aspiration. Ingestion of kerosene results in a burning sensation in the mouth and throat, gastro-intestinal disturbances, and possibly cough, dyspnoea, and transient cyanosis. There may be excitation followed by depression of the central nervous system, with weakness, dizziness, drowsiness, confusion, incoordination, and restlessness progressing to convulsions, coma, and respiratory depression in severe cases. Cardiac arrhythmias have been reported.

The course of poisoning from inhalation is similar to that following ingestion although CNS and cardiac effects are more likely. Kerosene is irritant.

Abuse. A case of volatile substance abuse (seep.1375) involving kerosene by inhalation and ingestion has been reported.[1]

1. Sarathi P, *et al.* Kerosene abuse by inhalation and ingestion. *Am J Psychiatry* 1992; **149:** 710.

Treatment of Adverse Effects

Treatment of kerosene poisoning is supportive and symptomatic. Every precaution should be taken to avoid aspiration of kerosene into the lungs. Most authorities agree that emesis and gastric lavage should generally be avoided unless an additional toxin such as a pesticide has been ingested. Activated charcoal may be administered. Adrenaline and other sympathomimetics should be avoided because of the risk of precipitating cardiac arrhythmias.

Uses

Kerosene is used as a degreaser and cleaner and as an illuminating and fuel oil in kerosene ('paraffin') lamps and stoves. The odourless grade has been used as a solvent in the preparation of some insecticide sprays.

2-Methoxyethanol (12943-n)

Ethylene Glycol Monomethyl Ether.
$C_3H_8O_2$ = 76.09.
CAS — 109-86-4.

A clear, colourless to slightly yellow liquid. Wt per mL about 0.96 g. B.p. about 125°. **Miscible** with water, acetone, alcohol, ether, dimethylformamide, and glycerol. **Store** in airtight containers.

CAUTION. *Suitable precautions should be taken to avoid skin contact with 2-methoxyethanol as it can penetrate skin and produce systemic toxicity.*

Adverse Effects

2-Methoxyethanol is irritant to mucous membranes. Ingestion may result in CNS depression with confusion, weakness, and in severe cases coma and death from respiratory depression. Nausea, metabolic acidosis, and kidney damage may also occur. Prolonged industrial exposure to the vapour has been associated with severe effects on the CNS characterised by headache, dizziness, lethargy, weakness, ataxia, tremor, disorientation, mental changes, weight loss, and visual disturbances. Anaemia has also been reported.

References to the toxicity of 2-methoxyethanol and other glycol ethers.

1. Health and Safety Executive. Glycol ethers. *Toxicity Review 10.* London: HMSO, 1985.
2. 2-Methoxyethanol, 2-ethoxyethanol, and their acetates. *Environmental Health Criteria 115.* Geneva: WHO, 1990.
3. Browning RG, Curry SC. Clinical toxicology of ethylene glycol monoalkyl ethers. *Hum Exp Toxicol* 1994; **13:** 325–35.

Uses

2-Methoxyethanol is used as an industrial solvent.

Methyl Alcohol (556-b)

Methanol.
CH_3OH = 32.04.
CAS — 67-56-1.
Pharmacopoeias. In *Ger.* Also in *USNF.*

A clear, colourless, flammable liquid with a characteristic odour. Wt per mL about 0.79 g. B.p. about 65°. **Miscible** with water, alcohol, ether, and most other organic solvents. **Store** in airtight containers.

CAUTION. *Suitable precautions should be taken to avoid skin contact with methyl alcohol as it can penetrate skin and produce systemic toxicity.*

Adverse Effects

Immediate signs of acute poisoning following ingestion of methyl alcohol resemble those of alcohol intoxication (see p.1099), but are milder. Characteristic symptoms of methyl alcohol poisoning are caused by toxic metabolites and develop after a latent period of about 12 to 24 hours or longer with concomitant alcohol consumption. The outstanding features of poisoning are metabolic acidosis with rapid, shallow breathing, visual disturbances which often proceed to irreversible blindness, and severe abdominal pain. Other symptoms include headache, gastro-intestinal disturbances, pain in the back and extremities, and coma which in severe cases may terminate in death due to respiratory failure or, rarely, to circulatory collapse. Mania and convulsions occasionally occur. Individual response to methyl alcohol varies widely. Ingestion of 30 mL is considered to be potentially fatal.

Absorption of methyl alcohol through the skin or inhalation of the vapour may also lead to toxic systemic effects.

References to the adverse effects of methyl alcohol.

1. Jacobsen D, McMartin KE. Methanol and ethylene glycol poisonings: mechanism of toxicity, clinical course, diagnosis and treatment. *Med Toxicol* 1986; **1:** 309–34.
2. Anderson TJ, *et al.* Neurologic sequelae of methanol poisoning. *Can Med Assoc J* 1987; **136:** 1177–9.
3. Cavalli A, *et al.* Severe reversible cardiac failure associated with methanol intoxication. *Postgrad Med J* 1987; **63:** 867–8.
4. Shapiro L, *et al.* Unusual case of methanol poisoning. *Lancet* 1993; **341:** 112.

Treatment of Adverse Effects

Recent ingestion of methyl alcohol should be treated by gastric lavage; activated charcoal may be administered. Metabolic acidosis should be corrected immediately with intravenous sodium bicarbonate. Treatment with alcohol, which delays the oxidation of methyl alcohol to its toxic metabolites, should also be initiated, the dosage being adjusted to achieve and maintain a blood-alcohol concentration of 1 to 2 mg per mL. An oral dose of about 50 g (equivalent to 150 mL of 40% v/v alcohol) for an adult of around 70 kg body-weight has been suggested; the alcohol should be well diluted before administration. If required, an alcohol infusion may then be given for which the following doses have been used: 120 mL of 10% alcohol or 250 mL of 5% alcohol per hour. For alcoholic patients or those with induced liver enzymes, the dose of alcohol should be increased accordingly. Suggested doses are 145 mL of 10% alcohol or 300 mL of 5% alcohol per hour.

Haemodialysis may be indicated to increase the removal of methyl alcohol and its toxic metabolites. Peritoneal dialysis has been used but is less efficient. Some authorities recommend initiation of haemodialysis if the amount of methyl alcohol ingested exceeds 30 g (equivalent to about 40 mL), if the blood-methyl alcohol concentration is greater than 500 μg per mL, or if severe metabolic acidosis or visual complications develop. If haemodialysis is used, a constant blood-alcohol concentration may be ensured either by increasing the alcohol infusion rate or by addition of alcohol to the dialysate fluid. Treatment should not be discontinued prematurely since oxidation and excretion of methyl alcohol may continue for several days; patients should, therefore, be closely observed and monitored. Suitable supportive treatment should be carried out as required.

References indicating blood-formate concentrations to be a better predictor of the severity of methyl alcohol poisoning than concentrations of methyl alcohol.

1. Osterloh JD, *et al.* Serum formate concentrations in methanol intoxication as a criterion for hemodialysis. *Ann Intern Med* 1986; **104:** 200–3.
2. Mahieu P, *et al.* Predictors of methanol intoxication with unfavourable outcome. *Hum Toxicol* 1989; **8:** 135–7.

Pharmacokinetics

Methyl alcohol is readily absorbed from the gastro-intestinal tract and distributed throughout the body fluids. It may also be absorbed by inhalation or through large areas of skin. Oxidation by alcohol dehydrogenase with formation of formaldehyde and formic acid takes place mainly in the liver and also in the kidneys. These metabolites are thought to be largely responsible for the characteristic symptoms of methyl alcohol poisoning. Metabolism is much slower than for ethyl alcohol, which competitively inhibits the metabolism of methyl alcohol. Oxidation and excretion may continue for several days after ingestion. Elimination of unchanged methyl alcohol via the lungs and in the urine is a minor route of excretion.

Uses

Methyl alcohol is used as a pharmaceutical and industrial solvent. It is also used as 'wood naphtha' to denature alcohol in the preparation of industrial methylated spirits. Methyl alcohol is also used as an extraction solvent in food processing.

Methyl *tert*-Butyl Ether (19482-r)

Methyl Terbutyl Ether; Methyl Tertiary Butyl Ether; MTBE. 2-Methoxy-2-methylpropane.
$C_5H_{12}O$ = 88.15.
CAS — 1634-04-4.

A volatile, flammable liquid. Wt per mL about 0.74 g. B.p. about 55°. **Store** in airtight containers.

CAUTION. *Explosive peroxides may be generated by the atmospheric oxidation of methyl tert-butyl ether, but the risk is lower than with solvent ether.*

Adverse Effects

Methyl *tert*-butyl ether is irritant and may cause CNS depression. See under Uses and Administration below for adverse effects that have been reported after use as a gallstone solvent.

Uses and Administration

Methyl *tert*-butyl ether is a solvent which is used for the rapid dissolution of cholesterol gallstones.

Gallstones. An alternative to bile acid therapy in patients with gallstones (p.1642) who are not considered suitable for surgery is direct instillation of a solvent into the gallbladder.

Methyl *tert*-butyl ether has been used to dissolve cholesterol gallstones; stones rich in calcium or pigments are not dissolved.[1] Unfortunately incomplete dissolution and residual debris can lead to recurrence of stone formation.[2] The solvent is most commonly instilled via a percutaneous transhepatic catheter,[1,3] although other routes have been used.[4] Thistle *et al.*[3] treated 75 patients with gallbladder stones with continuous infusion and aspiration of methyl *tert*-butyl ether 4 to 6 times a minute for an average of 5 hours a day for one to 3 days. At least 95% of the stone mass was dissolved in 72 patients. Gallbladder stones recurred in 4 patients between 6 and 16 months after the procedure; seven of 51 patients with residual stone fragments had an episode of biliary colic during 6 to 42 months of follow-up. Nausea, sometimes with emesis, occurred in about one-third of patients. Overflow of solvent from the gallbladder can result in absorption from the gastro-intestinal tract; methyl *tert*-butyl ether is detected on the breath and sedation can occur. One patient in whom overflow occurred developed ulcerative duodenitis and intravascular haemolysis. Coma and acute renal failure have also complicated treatment and have been attributed to leakage alongside the catheter rather than overflow of solvent.[5] Other workers[6,7] have obtained similar results for the dissolution of gallstones. One group[6] found that nausea and vomiting could be reduced if the treatment time was kept short and the perfusion volume was kept as low as possible; they also managed to prevent bile leakage and haemorrhage using a tissue adhesive or subcutaneous administration of ceruletide to contract the gallbladder. Dissolution of gallbladder stones with methyl *tert*-butyl ether is likely to remain confined to specialist centres for use in patients unsuitable for surgical treatment.[1] A combination of litholytic modalities such as dissolution with solvents or bile acids, or lithotripsy may overcome some of the disadvantages of individual treatments.[8]

Methyl *tert*-butyl ether has been instilled via a nasobiliary catheter to dissolve stones in the common bile duct. Although effective in some cases,[9] further study has indicated disappointing overall results.[1,10]

Various combinations of drugs have been investigated to dissolve pigment-rich or mixed stones. For common bile-duct stones these include a cocktail of dimethyl sulphoxide 60%, methyl *tert*-butyl ether 20%, and sodium bicarbonate 20%, and a regimen of alternating infusions of pentyl ether and edetic acid-urea 10%.[11] A similar regimen of methyl hexyl ether and edetic acid-urea has been used successfully in 2 patients with calcified gallbladder stones.[12]

1. Bouchier IAD. Gall stones. *Br Med J* 1990; **300:** 592–7.
2. Maudgal DP, Northfield TC. A practical guide to the nonsurgical treatment of gallstones. *Drugs* 1991; **41:** 185–92.
3. Thistle JL, *et al.* Dissolution of cholesterol gallbladder stones by methyl *tert*-butyl ether administered by percutaneous transhepatic catheter. *N Engl J Med* 1989; **320:** 633–9.
4. Foerster E-Ch, *et al.* Direct dissolution of gallbladder stones. *Lancet* 1989; **i:** 954.
5. Ponchon T, *et al.* Renal failure during dissolution of gallstones by methyl-*tert*-butyl ether. *Lancet* 1988; **ii:** 276–7.
6. Hellstern A, *et al.* Gall stone dissolution with methyl tert-butyl ether: how to avoid complications. *Gut* 1990; **31:** 922–5.
7. McNulty J, *et al.* Dissolution of cholesterol gall stones using methyltertbutyl ether: a safe effective treatment. *Gut* 1991; **32:** 1550–3.
8. Salen G, Tint GS. Nonsurgical treatment of gallstones. *N Engl J Med* 1989; **320:** 665–6.
9. Murray WR, *et al.* Choledocholithiasis—in vivo stone dissolution using methyl tertiary butyl ether (MTBE). *Gut* 1988; **29:** 143–5.
10. Neoptolemos JP, *et al.* How good is methyl tert-butyl (MTBE) for common bile duct (CBD) stone dissolution? *Gut* 1989; **30:** A736–7.
11. Anonymous. Gallstones, bile acids, and the liver. *Lancet* 1989; **ii:** 249–51.
12. Swobodnik W, *et al.* Dissolution of calcified gallbladder stones by treatment with methyl-hexyl ether and urea-EDTA. *Lancet* 1988; **ii:** 216.

Methyl Butyl Ketone (10649-h)

2-Hexanone; Methyl *n*-Butyl Ketone. Hexan-2-one.

$C_6H_{12}O$ = 100.2.

CAS — 591-78-6.

A colourless, volatile liquid. Wt per mL about 0.82 g. B.p. about 127°. **Store** in airtight containers.

CAUTION. *Suitable precautions should be taken to avoid skin contact with methyl butyl ketone as it can penetrate skin and produce systemic toxicity.*

Methyl Isobutyl Ketone (6520-k)

Hexone; Isopropylacetone; MIBK. 4-Methylpentan-2-one.

$C_6H_{12}O$ = 100.2.

CAS — 108-10-1.

Pharmacopoeias. In *USNF.*

A transparent, colourless, mobile, volatile liquid with a faint ketonic and camphoraceous odour. Sp. gr. not more than 0.799. Distilling range 114° to 117°. Slightly **soluble** in water; miscible with alcohol and ether. **Store** in airtight containers.

CAUTION. *Suitable precautions should be taken to avoid skin contact with methyl isobutyl ketone as it can penetrate skin and produce systemic toxicity.*

Adverse Effects

Methyl butyl ketone and methyl isobutyl ketone may depress the CNS in high concentrations. Their vapours are irritating to mucous membranes. Methyl isobutyl ketone may be implicated in volatile substance abuse (p.1375).

References.

1. Methyl isobutyl ketone. *Environmental Health Criteria 117.* Geneva: WHO, 1990.
2. Methyl isobutyl ketone. *Health and Safety Guide 58.* Geneva: WHO, 1991.

Effects on the nervous system. Peripheral neuropathy[1] has occurred following occupational exposure to methyl butyl ketone, particularly an outbreak of neuropathy in a printing plant after the replacement of methyl isobutyl ketone by methyl butyl ketone in a solvent mixture with methyl ethyl ketone. Methyl ethyl ketone may have potentiated the neurotoxicity induced by methyl butyl ketone.

For further discussion of neurotoxicity after occupational exposure to solvents including methyl butyl ketone, see under Toluene, p.1381.

1. Lolin Y. Chronic neurological toxicity associated with exposure to volatile substances. *Hum Toxicol* 1989; **8:** 293–300.

Uses

Methyl isobutyl ketone is used as an industrial and pharmaceutical solvent and also as an alcohol denaturant. Methyl butyl ketone is used as an industrial solvent.

Methyl Chloride (6519-n)

Monochloromethane. Chloromethane.

CH_3Cl = 50.49.

CAS — 74-87-3.

A colourless gas compressed to a colourless liquid with an ethereal odour. B.p. about −24°. **Store** in airtight containers.

Adverse Effects and Treatment

Symptoms of methyl chloride intoxication often appear after a latent period of several hours and are similar after acute or chronic exposure to the vapour. Symptoms include gastro-intestinal disturbances such as nausea, vomiting, and abdominal pain, and signs of CNS depression including headache, weakness, drowsiness, confusion, visual disturbances, and incoordination progressing to convulsions, coma, and death from respiratory depression in severe cases. There have been a few reports of liver and kidney damage.

Treatment consists of removal from exposure and supportive and symptomatic measures. Neurological effects may persist for many months.

References to the toxicity of methyl chloride.

1. Repko JD, Lasley SM. Behavioral, neurological, and toxic effects of methyl chloride: a review of the literature. *CRC Crit Rev Toxicol* 1979; **6:** 283–302.

Uses

Methyl chloride is used as an industrial solvent. It has been used as an aerosol propellant and refrigerant and was formerly used as a local anaesthetic.

Methyl Ethyl Ketone (16890-y)

Ethyl Methyl Ketone; MEK. Butan-2-one.

C_4H_8O = 72.11.

CAS — 78-93-3.

A colourless flammable liquid with an acetone-like odour. Wt per mL about 0.81 g. B.p. 79° to 81°. **Soluble** in water; miscible with alcohol and ether. **Store** in airtight containers.

Adverse Effects

Methyl ethyl ketone is irritant. Inhalation may result in mild CNS effects including headache and dizziness; nausea and vomiting may also occur.

Methyl ethyl ketone may be implicated in volatile substance abuse (p.1375).

Effects on the nervous system. There are isolated reports of neurotoxicity produced by methyl ethyl ketone alone.[1] These include one of retrobulbar neuritis and one of peripheral neuropathy. It has been suggested, however, that methyl ethyl ketone potentiates the peripheral neuropathy induced by methyl butyl ketone and *n*-hexane.

For further discussion of neurotoxicity after occupational exposure to solvents including methyl ethyl ketone, see under Toluene, p.1381.

1. Lolin Y. Chronic neurological toxicity associated with exposure to volatile substances. *Hum Toxicol* 1989; **8:** 293–300.

Uses

Methyl ethyl ketone is used as an industrial solvent and as an extraction solvent in food processing.

Octyldodecanol (6347-x)

Octyldodecanolum.

$C_{20}H_{42}O$ = 298.5.

Pharmacopoeias. In *Eur.* (see p.viii). Also in *USNF.*

Consists chiefly of 2-octyldodecanol with small amounts of related alcohols.

Clear, water-white or colourless to yellowish, free-flowing oily liquid. Relative density 0.830 to 0.850. Practically **insoluble** in water; soluble in alcohol and in ether. **Store** in airtight containers. Protect from light.

Octyldodecanol is used as a pharmaceutical solvent.

Petroleum Spirit (6518-d)

Light Petroleum; Petroleum Benzin; Petroleum Ether; Solvent Hexane.

Pharmacopoeias. In *Aust., Ger., Jpn.,* and *Pol.* Various boiling ranges are specified.

Swiss describes Benzinum Medicinale, consisting mainly of hexane and heptane.

A purified distillate of petroleum, consisting of a mixture of the lower members of the paraffin series of hydrocarbons. It is a colourless, transparent, very volatile, highly flammable liquid with a characteristic odour. It is available in a variety of boiling ranges.

NOTE. The motor fuel termed 'petrol' in the UK and 'gasoline' in the USA is a mixture of volatile hydrocarbons of variable composition containing paraffins (alkanes), olefins (alkenes), cycloparaffins, and aromatic compounds.

Adverse Effects and Treatment

As for Kerosene, p.1379. Petroleum spirit and petrol, being more volatile and of lower viscosity than kerosene, are more likely to be inhaled and to cause aspiration pneumonitis. The toxicity of petrol varies with its composition; some adverse effects have been attributed to lead additives or to the content of *n*-hexane or benzene. Petrol may be implicated in volatile solvent abuse (p.1375).

References to the toxicity of petroleum spirit.[1-3]

For discussion of neurotoxicity after occupational exposure to solvents including petrol, see under Toluene, p.1381.

1. Selected petroleum products. *Environmental Health Criteria 20.* Geneva: WHO, 1982.
2. Daniels AM, Latcham RW. Petrol sniffing and schizophrenia in a Pacific island paradise. *Lancet* 1984; **i:** 389.
3. Eastwell HD. Elevated lead levels in petrol "sniffers". *Med J Aust* 1985; **143** (suppl): S63–4.

Uses

Petroleum spirit and other petroleum distillates are used as pharmaceutical solvents.

Propylene Carbonate (5451-l)

4-Methyl-1,3-dioxolan-2-one.

$C_4H_6O_3$ = 102.1.

CAS — 108-32-7.

Pharmacopoeias. In *USNF.*

A clear colourless mobile liquid. Freely **soluble** in water; miscible with alcohol and with chloroform; practically insoluble in petroleum spirit. **Store** in airtight containers.

Uses

Propylene carbonate is used as a solvent in oral and topical pharmaceuticals and for cellulose-based polymers and plasticisers. It has been used as a nonvolatile, stabilising liquid carrier in hard gelatin capsules.

Tetrachloroethane (6522-t)

Acetylene Tetrachloride; Perchloroethylene. 1,1,2,2-Tetrachloroethane.

$C_2H_2Cl_4$ = 167.8.

CAS — 79-34-5.

A colourless liquid with a chloroform-like odour. B.p. about 146°. Wt per mL about 1.59 g. **Store** in airtight containers.

CAUTION. *Suitable precautions should be taken to avoid skin contact with tetrachloroethane as it can penetrate skin and produce systemic toxicity.*

Adverse Effects and Treatment

As for Carbon Tetrachloride, p.1376. Tetrachloroethane is probably the most toxic of the chlorinated hydrocarbons. Poisoning can occur through percutaneous absorption as well as ingestion or inhalation.

Uses

Tetrachloroethane is used as an industrial solvent.

Tetrachloroethylene (813-v)

Perchloroethylene; Tetrachloroethylenum.

C_2Cl_4 = 165.8.

CAS — 127-18-4.

Adverse Effects and Treatment

As for Carbon Tetrachloride, p.1376. Symptoms, especially following administration by mouth when used therapeutically, are less severe.

The vapour or liquid may be irritating to skin or mucous membranes.

Tetrachloroethylene may be implicated in volatile substance abuse (p.1375). Dependence may follow habitual inhalation of small quantities of tetrachloroethylene vapour.

References to adverse effects of tetrachloroethylene.

1. Tetrachloroethylene. *Environmental Health Criteria 31.* Geneva: WHO, 1984.
2. Tetrachloroethylene. *Health and Safety Guide.* Geneva: WHO, 1987.

3. Health and Safety Executive. Tetrachloroethylene (tetrachloroethene, perchloroethylene). *Toxicity Review 17*. London: HMSO, 1987.
4. Bagnell PC, Ellenberger HA. Obstructive jaundice due to a chlorinated hydrocarbon in breast milk. *Can Med Assoc J* 1977; **117:** 1047–8.
5. Mutti A, *et al.* Nephropathies and exposure to perchloroethylene in dry-cleaners. *Lancet* 1992; **340:** 189–93.

Pharmacokinetics

Tetrachloroethylene is slightly absorbed from the gastro-intestinal tract; absorption is increased in the presence of alcohol and fats or oils. It is absorbed following inhalation and after direct contact with the skin. It is excreted unchanged in expired air; initial elimination is rapid but a proportion may be retained and excreted slowly.

Metabolites of tetrachloroethylene, mainly trichloroacetic acid, have been found in the urine.

Uses and Administration

Tetrachloroethylene is a chlorinated hydrocarbon widely used as a solvent in industry. It was formerly given by mouth as an anthelmintic, but has been superseded by equally effective and less toxic drugs.

Toluene (6523-x)

Methylbenzene; Phenylmethane; Toluol; Toluole.

C_7H_8 = 92.14.

CAS — 108-88-3.

A colourless, volatile, flammable liquid with a characteristic odour. Wt per mL about 0.87 g. B.p. about 111°. **Store** in airtight containers.

CAUTION. *Suitable precautions should be taken to avoid skin contact with toluene as it can penetrate skin and produce systemic toxicity.*

Adverse Effects, Treatment, and Precautions

Toluene has similar acute toxicity to benzene (p.1375) but is a less serious industrial hazard. Adverse effects are treated similarly to benzene. It is a common constituent of adhesives and is frequently implicated in volatile substance abuse (p.1375). Commercial toluene may contain benzene, and this may perhaps influence the pattern of adverse effects. In addition to acute toxic effects, toluene abuse has been associated with damage to the nervous system, kidneys, liver, heart, and lungs (see below). Chronic poisoning caused by occupational exposure to toluene has resulted mainly in nervous system disorders.

Reviews.

1. WHO. Recommended health-based limits in occupational exposure to selected organic solvents. *WHO Tech Rep Ser 664* 1981.
2. Toluene. *Environmental Health Criteria 52*. Geneva: WHO, 1985.
3. Health and Safety Executive. Toluene. *Toxicity Review 20*. London: HMSO, 1989.

The non-neurological toxicity following volatile substance abuse has been reviewed.[1] Chronic toluene abuse may result in damage to the *kidneys*; renal tubular acidosis and glomerulonephritis have been described, although evidence for the latter is only circumstantial. Renal tubular acidosis has been regarded as reversible; however, there are reports suggesting that damage to renal tubules is permanent.

The few reports linking chronic toluene abuse with *liver* damage cover hepatomegaly and hepatorenal failure. Effects on the *heart* are usually acute; sudden death has resulted from ventricular dysrhythmias. Chronic myocarditis with fibrosis has been reported. Chronic toluene inhalation can cause damage to the *lungs*. Autopsies in a few patients have shown changes indicative of emphysema.

Nervous system toxicity has also been reviewed.[2] Cerebellar dysfunction has occurred after toluene abuse; an acute intoxication phase, which usually subsides within weeks of abstinence, is followed by a chronic phase which may be permanent. Diffuse CNS disease such as encephalopathy, dementia, and multifocal brain injury may also develop. An association between toluene abuse and peripheral neuropathy has not been confirmed; muscle weakness may be a result of electrolyte and fluid disturbances. The review cites individual reports of choreoathetosis, epilepsy, and optic atrophy with anosmia and deafness after toluene abuse. Some of these neurological effects, particularly cerebellar effects and diffuse CNS disease have also occurred after occupational exposure to toluene.

Some studies have noted an excess mortality from motor neurone disease among leather workers,[3] although this has not been confirmed by others.[4] Occupational exposure to solvents has been postulated as the cause.[3] Of the many agents currently used in leather work, those with known or probable neurotoxic effects are *n*-hexane, methyl butyl ketone, toluene, and methyl ethyl ketone. Ethyl acetate is commonly used but has no recognised neurological side-effects.[3] A Swedish study of workers in a range of occupations has found some support for an increased risk of amyotrophic lateral sclerosis after occupational exposure to solvents, probably toluene and petrol.[5] Another Swedish study found an association between multiple sclerosis and occupational exposure to solvents, especially white spirit and petrol.[5]

1. Marjot R, McLeod AA. Chronic non-neurological toxicity from volatile substance abuse. *Hum Toxicol* 1989; **8:** 301–6.
2. Lolin Y. Chronic neurological toxicity associated with exposure to volatile substances. *Hum Toxicol* 1989; **8:** 293–300.
3. Hawkes CH, *et al.* Motoneuron disease: a disorder secondary to solvent exposure? *Lancet* 1989; **i:** 73–6.
4. Martyn CN. Motoneuron disease and exposure to solvents. *Lancet* 1989; **i:** 394.
5. Gunnarsson L-G, Lindberg G. Amyotrophic lateral sclerosis in Sweden 1970-83 and solvent exposure. *Lancet* 1989; **i:** 958.

Pregnancy. Retrospective surveys of pregnancies in mothers with a history of solvent abuse suggested that toluene abuse during pregnancy can cause preterm delivery and perinatal death. It was suggested that toluene may be teratogenic as intra-uterine exposure was associated with prenatal and postnatal growth retardation, microcephaly, impairment of mental development, and facial dysmorphia.[1-3] It is uncertain if these results can be extrapolated to cover occupational exposure. Although some studies of occupational exposure to solvents during pregnancy have suggested an association,[4] there is little consistent evidence to link exposure to any particular solvent with spontaneous abortion, retarded fetal development, still-birth, or congenital malformation.[5]

1. Wilkins-Haug L, Gabow PA. Toluene abuse during pregnancy: obstetric complications and perinatal outcomes. *Obstet Gynecol* 1991; **77:** 504–9.
2. Arnold GL, *et al.* Toluene embryopathy: clinical delineation and developmental follow-up. *Pediatrics* 1994; **93:** 216–20.
3. Pearson MA, *et al.* Toluene embryopathy: delineation of the phenotype and comparison with fetal alcohol syndrome. *Pediatrics* 1994; **93:** 211–15.
4. McDonald JC, *et al.* Chemical exposures at work in early pregnancy and congenital defect: a case-referent study. *Br J Ind Med* 1987; **44:** 527–33.
5. Scott A. *Br Med J* 1992; **304:** 369.

Pharmacokinetics

Toluene is absorbed by inhalation, ingestion, and to some extent through the skin. It is rapidly metabolised mainly by oxidation to benzoic acid which is excreted in the urine largely as the glycine conjugate hippuric acid; *o*-, *m*-, and *p*-cresol are minor urinary metabolites. Some unchanged toluene is excreted through the lungs.

Uses

Toluene is widely used as an industrial solvent.

Trichloroethane (6524-r)

Methylchloroform; α-Trichloroethane. 1,1,1-Trichloroethane.

$C_2H_3Cl_3$ = 133.4.

CAS — 71-55-6.

A colourless, slightly hygroscopic liquid. Sp. gr. about 1.31. B.p. about 74°. Practically **insoluble** in water; miscible with alcohol, chloroform, and ether. Non-flammable. **Store** in airtight containers.

Adverse Effects and Treatment

Acute intoxication with trichloroethane may result in initial excitement followed by depression of the CNS with dizziness, drowsiness, headache, lightheadedness, and ataxia, progressing to coma and death from respiratory depression in severe cases. Death may also occur from ventricular arrhythmias. Fatalities have occurred following accidental exposure to high concentrations of trichloroethane in confined spaces. Trichloroethane is commonly used in dry cleaning, typewriter correction fluids, and as a solvent for plaster removal and is frequently implicated in volatile substance abuse (p.1375).

Nausea, vomiting, and diarrhoea have been reported following ingestion. Trichloroethane is a mild irritant.

Treatment of adverse effects consists of removal from exposure and general supportive and symptomatic measures. Activated charcoal may be administered. Adrenaline and other sympathomimetics should be avoided because of the risk of precipitating cardiac arrhythmias.

Reviews.

1. Health and Safety Executive. 1,1,1-Trichloroethane. *Toxicity Review 9*. London: HMSO, 1984.

According to a brief review of non-neurological toxicity from volatile substance abuse,[1] there were no reports of damage to the *liver* after the abuse of trichloroethane. There was a report of hepatotoxicity following acute occupational exposure, but this might have been a hypersensitivity reaction. There was another report[2] of fatty liver disease in 4 patients with a history of occupational exposure to trichloroethane although there has been some debate over the validity of the association for 2 of these cases.[3,4]

Effects on the *heart* were considered usually to be acute and sudden death from ventricular arrhythmias had occurred in abusers. There have, however, been a few cases of chronic cardiac toxicity after both abuse and occupational exposure.[1]

1. Marjot R, McLeod AA. Chronic non-neurological toxicity from volatile substance abuse. *Hum Toxicol* 1989; **8:** 301–6.
2. Hodgson MJ, *et al.* Liver disease associated with exposure to 1,1,1-trichloroethane. *Arch Intern Med* 1989; **149:** 1793–8.
3. Guzelian PS. 1,1,1-Trichloroethane and the liver. *Arch Intern Med* 1991; **151:** 2321–2.
4. Hodgson MJ, Vanthiel DH. 1,1,1-Trichloroethane and the liver. *Arch Intern Med* 1991; **151:** 2322 and 2325–6.

Effects on the skin. A report of scleroderma in 3 patients occupationally exposed to trichloroethylene and, in 2 cases, also to trichloroethane.[1]

1. Flindt-Hansen H, Isager H. Scleroderma after occupational exposure to trichlorethylene and trichlorethane. *Acta Derm Venereol (Stockh)* 1987; **67:** 263–4.

Pharmacokinetics

Trichloroethane is absorbed after inhalation, ingestion, and through intact skin. Small amounts are metabolised to trichloroethanol and trichloroacetic acid and excreted in the urine, but it is largely excreted unchanged through the lungs over a period of days.

Uses

Trichloroethane has wide applications as an industrial solvent. It is commonly used in dry cleaning, typewriter correction fluids, and as a solvent for plaster removal.

Preparations

Proprietary Preparations (details are given in Part 3)
UK: Zoff.

Multi-ingredient: ***Austral.:*** Sacsol NF.

White Spirit (6525-f)

A mixture of hydrocarbons available as a colourless liquid. **Store** in airtight containers.

Adverse Effects and Treatment

As for Kerosene, p.1379.

References to the toxicity of white spirit.[1]

For discussion of neurotoxicity after occupational exposure to solvents including white spirit, see under Toluene, p.1381.

1. Selected petroleum products. *Environmental Health Criteria 20*. Geneva: WHO, 1982.

Uses

White spirit is used as an industrial solvent.

Xylene (6526-d)

Xylol; Xylole.

C_8H_{10} = 106.2.

CAS — 1330-20-7; 108-38-3 (m-xylene); 95-47-6 (o-xylene); 106-42-3 (p-xylene).

Pharmacopoeias. In Aust.

A mixture of *o*-, *m*-, and *p*-dimethylbenzene in which the *m*-isomer predominates.

A colourless, volatile, flammable liquid. Wt per mL about 0.86 g. B.p. about 138° to 142°. **Store** in airtight containers.

CAUTION. *Suitable precautions should be taken to avoid skin contact with xylene as it can penetrate skin and produce systemic toxicity.*

Adverse Effects, Treatment, and Precautions

The acute toxicity of xylene is similar to that of benzene (p.1375) but is less marked. Adverse effects are treated similarly to benzene.

Xylene has been implicated in volatile substance abuse (p.1375). Commercial xylene may contain benzene, and this may perhaps influence the pattern of adverse effects.

Xylene should not be used to dissolve ear wax if the tympanic membrane is perforated.

References.

1. WHO. Recommended health-based limits in occupational exposure to selected organic solvents. *WHO Tech Rep Ser 664* 1981.
2. Health and Safety Executive. Xylenes. *Toxicity Review 26*. London: HMSO, 1992.

Effects on the eyes. Eye injuries due to accidental contact with paints containing xylene have been reported.[1] The injuries resembled alkali burns and were treated in a similar manner.

1. Ansari EA. Ocular injury with xylene - a report of two cases. *Hum Exp Toxicol* 1997; **16:** 273–5.

Effects on the nervous system. References to the adverse effects of xylene on the nervous system.

1. Arthur LJH, Curnock DA. Xylene-induced epilepsy following innocent glue sniffing. *Br Med J* 1982; **284:** 1787.
2. Roberts FP, *et al.* Near-pure xylene causing reversible neuropsychiatric disturbance. *Lancet* 1988; **ii:** 273.

Pharmacokinetics

Xylene is absorbed after inhalation, ingestion, and to some extent through the skin. It is rapidly metabolised by oxidation to the corresponding *o*-, *m*-, or *p*-methylbenzoic(toluic) acids and excreted in the urine largely as the glycine conjugate, methylhippuric acid (toluric acid). Xylenols are minor metabolites and are excreted in the urine as the glucuronide and sulphate conjugates. Some unchanged xylene is excreted through the lungs.

Uses

Xylene is used as an industrial and pharmaceutical solvent and in preparations to dissolve ear wax.

Preparations

Proprietary Preparations (details are given in Part 3)
Fr.: Cerulyse; ***Ital.:*** Cerulisina; ***Switz.:*** Novo-Cerusol.

Paraffins and Similar Bases

This chapter includes a number of substances used mainly as bases for the preparation of creams, ointments, other topical preparations, and suppositories. They are used either as inert carriers for drugs or for their various emulsifying and emollient properties. Some are also used to improve the texture, stability, or water repellent properties of the final preparation. The bases discussed include petroleum hydrocarbons, animal fats and waxes, vegetable oils, and silicones. Other substances used in the preparation of bases can be found in Soaps and other Anionic Surfactants (p.1468) and in Nonionic Surfactants (p.1324).

Hard Paraffin (6401-w)

905 (mineral hydrocarbons); Hartparaffin; Paraff. Dur.; Paraffin; Paraffin Wax; Paraffinum Durum; Paraffinum Solidum.

CAS — 8002-74-2.

Pharmacopoeias. In *Chin., Eur.* (see p.viii), *Int., Jpn,* and *Pol.* Also in *USNF.*

USNF includes additionally Synthetic Paraffin.

A mixture of solid saturated hydrocarbons obtained from petroleum.

It is a colourless or white, odourless, translucent solid, showing a crystalline structure, and is slightly greasy to the touch. The melted substance is free from fluorescence in daylight. It has a congealing range of 47° to 65°.

Practically **insoluble** in water and in alcohol; freely soluble in chloroform, in dichloromethane, in ether, in volatile oils, and in most warm fixed oils; slightly soluble in dehydrated alcohol. An alcoholic extract is neutral to litmus. **Protect** from light.

Synthetic Paraffin (USNF) is a very hard odourless white wax containing mostly long-chain, unbranched, saturated hydrocarbons, with a small amount of branched hydrocarbons. The average molecular weight may range from 400 to 1400.

Hard paraffin is employed principally as a stiffening ingredient in ointment bases. It is also used in creams, and as a coating for capsules and tablets.

A variety of hard paraffin (m.p. 43° to 46°) is employed in physiotherapy in the form of paraffin-wax baths for the relief of pain in inflamed joints and sprains.

The injection of paraffins may produce granulomatous reactions.

Preparations

BP 1998: Paraffin Ointment *(Unguentum Paraffini)*; Simple Ointment *(Ung. Simp.; Unguentum Simplex)*; Wool Alcohols Ointment *(Ung. Alcoh. Lan.)*.

Proprietary Preparations (details are given in Part 3)

Multi-ingredient: ***UK:*** Melrose.

Liquid Paraffin (6402-e)

905 (mineral hydrocarbons); Dickflüssiges Paraffin; Heavy Liquid Petrolatum; Huile de Vaseline Épaisse; Liquid Petrolatum; Mineral Oil; Oleum Petrolei; Oleum Vaselini; Paraffinum Liquidum; Paraffinum Subliquidum; Vaselinöl; Vaselinum Liquidum; White Mineral Oil.

CAS — 8012-95-1.

Pharmacopoeias. In *Chin., Eur.* (see p.viii), *Jpn, Pol.,* and *US.*

Liquid paraffin is a mixture of liquid saturated hydrocarbons obtained from petroleum. The USP permits a suitable stabiliser.

It is a transparent, colourless, odourless, or almost odourless, oily liquid, free, or practically free, from fluorescence by daylight. Practically **insoluble** in water, in ether, and in hydrocarbons; practically insoluble to slightly soluble in alcohol; miscible with fixed oils (except castor oil) and soluble in volatile oils. **Store** in airtight containers. Protect from light.

Light Liquid Paraffin (6403-l)

Dünnflüssiges Paraffin; Huile de Vaseline Fluide; Light Liquid Petrolatum; Light Mineral Oil; Light White Mineral Oil; Paraff. Liq. Lev.; Paraffinum Liquidum Leve; Paraffinum Liquidum Tenue; Paraffinum Perliquidum; Spray Paraffin; Vaselina Liquida.

Pharmacopoeias. In *Eur.* (see p.viii) and *Jpn.* Also in *USNF. US* also includes Topical Light Mineral Oil.

Light liquid paraffin is a mixture of liquid saturated hydrocarbons obtained from petroleum. The USNF permits a suitable stabiliser. It has similar characteristics to Liquid Paraffin, but a lower kinematic viscosity.

Adverse Effects and Precautions

Excessive dosage by mouth, or rectum, may result in anal seepage and irritation. Liquid paraffin is absorbed to a slight extent and may give rise to foreign-body granulomatous reactions. Similar reactions have followed the injection of liquid paraffin and may be considerably delayed in onset. Injection may also cause vasospasm and prompt surgical removal may be required to prevent severe damage. Lipoid pneumonia has been reported following the aspiration of liquid paraffin.

Chronic ingestion of liquid paraffin may rarely be associated with impaired absorption of fat-soluble vitamins and possibly other compounds. It should not be used when abdominal pain, nausea, or vomiting is present. Prolonged use should be avoided. Also it should not be used in children under 3 years of age.

Haematological changes and deposition of food grade liquid paraffins in the liver, spleen, and lymph nodes has occurred during feeding studies in *rats.*[1]

1. FAO/WHO. Evaluation of certain food additives and contaminants: forty-fourth report of the joint FAO/WHO expert committee on food additives. *WHO Tech Rep Ser 859* 1995.

Granuloma. References.

1. Bloem JJ, van der Waal I. Paraffinoma of the face: a diagnostic and therapeutic problem. *Oral Surg* 1974; **38:** 675–80.
2. Albers DD, *et al.* Oil granuloma of the ureter. *J Urol (Baltimore)* 1984; **132:** 114.

Lipoid pneumonia. References.

1. Varkey B, Kutty AVP. Lipoid pneumonia with lipoid granulomata in scalene node. *Ann Intern Med* 1976; **84:** 176–7.
2. Anonymous. Case records of the Massachusetts general hospital. *N Engl J Med* 1977; **296:** 1105–11.
3. Becton DL, *et al.* Lipoid pneumonia in an adolescent girl secondary to use of lip gloss. *J Pediatr* 1984; **105:** 421–3.
4. Beermann B, *et al.* Lipoid pneumonia: an occupational hazard of fire eaters. *Br Med J* 1984; **289:** 1728–9.

Uses and Administration

Taken internally, liquid paraffin acts as a lubricant and, since it keeps the stools soft, it has been used in the symptomatic treatment of constipation (p.1168), although its use is generally not recommended. Up to 45 mL has been given daily by mouth, usually in the evening but should not be taken immediately before going to bed. Liquid paraffin is an ingredient of several preparations that contain other laxatives such as cascara, magnesium hydroxide, or phenolphthalein. It has also been given as an enema in a usual dose of 120 mL.

Externally, liquid paraffin may be used as an ingredient of ointment bases, as an emollient and cleanser in certain skin conditions, and as an ophthalmic lubricant in the management of dry eye (p.1470).

Light liquid paraffin has similar uses to liquid paraffin.

Preparations

BP 1998: Cetomacrogol Emulsifying Ointment; Cetrimide Emulsifying Ointment; Emulsifying Ointment; Liquid Paraffin and Magnesium Hydroxide Oral Emulsion *(Emuls. Paraff. Liq. et Mag. Hydrox.; Mist. Mag. Hydrox. et Paraff. Liq.)*; Liquid Paraffin Oral Emulsion *(Emuls. Paraff. Liq.; Emulsio Paraffini Liquidi)*; Simple Eye Ointment *(Eye Ointment Basis)*; Wool Alcohols Ointment *(Ung. Alcoh. Lan.)*;

USP 23: Bland Lubricating Ophthalmic Ointment; Mineral Oil Emulsion; Mineral Oil Enema; Topical Light Mineral Oil.

Proprietary Preparations (details are given in Part 3)

Austral.: Derma-Oil†; Hamilton Bath Oil; Hamilton Shower Oil†; ***Belg.:*** Lansoyl; ***Canad.:*** Bebia†; Fleet Enema Mineral Oil; Lansoyl; Nujol; Skin Conditioner & Bath Oil; Therapeutic Bath Oil; ***Fr.:*** Lansoyl; Laxamalt; Lubentyl; Nujol; Nutra Nutraderme; Parlax†; Restrical; ***Ger.:*** Granugenol†; Obstinol mild; Oleatum; Salus-Ol†; Sanato-Lax†; ***Irl.:*** Alcoderm; Lansoyl†; Oilatum Gel; ***Ital.:*** Agarol Rosa†; Duratirs; Laxil†; ***Spain:*** Emuliquen Simple; Hodernal; ***Switz.:*** Lansoyl; Laxamalt; Lubentyl†; Oleatum fett†; ***UK:*** Cetraben Bath Oil; Keri; Oilatum Fragrance Free; Oilatum Gel; Oilatum Skin Therapy; Oilatum Soap; ***USA:*** Agoral Plain†; Kondremul; Liqui-Doss; Milkinol; Neo-Cultol.

Multi-ingredient: ***Aust.:*** Balneum Hermal F; ***Austral.:*** Agarol; Alpha Keri; Alpha Keri Tar; Cleansing Lotion; DermaVeen Shower and Bath; Duratears; E45; Ego Prickly Heat Powder†; Egozite Baby Cream; Granugen; Hamilton Skin Lotion; Lacri-Lube; Oilatum Emollient; Oilatum Plus; Parachoc; QV Tar†; Rikoderm; Soov Prickly Heat; ***Belg.:*** Agarol; Duratears; Lacrytube; ***Canad.:*** Agarol; Agarol Plain; Akwa Tears; Alpha Keri; Duolube; Duratears; Episec; Huile de Bain Therapeutique; Hypotears; Lacri-Lube; Laxarol; Lubriderm; Lubriderm Daily UV Defense; Magnolax; Oculube; Optilube; Penederm; Stancare; Therapeutic Bath Oil; Therapeutic Skin Lotion; Ti-Lub; ***Fr.:*** Balmex; Balneum surgras; Cerat Inalterable; Colarine†; Cold Cream Naturel; Lubentyl a la Magnesie; Molagar†; Parapsyllium; Parlax Compose†; Transitol; Transulose; ***Ger.:*** Agarol; Balneovit O†; Balneum F; Befelka-Oel; Coliquifilm; Derma Bad†; Gleitgelen; Granugen†; Hoecutin Olbad F; Obstinol; Oleobal; Parfenac Basisbad; Sanato-Lax-forte†; Windol Basisbad; ***Irl.:*** Agarol; Balmandol†; Diprobath; Emulsiderm; Hydromol; Lacri-Lube; Milpar; Oilatum Emollient; Petrolagar No. 1†; Petrolagar No. 2; Petrolagar with Phenolphthalein; Polytar Emollient; ***Ital.:*** Agarol†; Dacriosol†; Emulsione Lassativa†; Lacrilube; ***Neth.:*** Agarol†; Duratears Z†; Siccatears†; ***Norw.:*** Simplex; ***S.Afr.:*** Agarol; Lacrilube; Millypar; Oilatum Emollient†; ***Spain:*** Aceite Acalorico; Agarol; Emuliquen Antiespasmodic†; Emuliquen Laxante; Lubrifilm; ***Switz.:*** Agarol; Antidry; Balmandol; Balneum F; Ceralba†; Coliquifilm; Duratears; Falqui; Lubentyl a la Magnesie†; Melisol; Paragar; Paragol; Woloderma†; ***UK:*** Agarol; Alpha Keri; Balmandol†; BMS†; Cetraben; Dermol; Diprobath; Emmolate; Emulsiderm; Epaderm; Hydromol Cream; Hydromol Emollient; Imuderm; Infaderm; Lacri-Lube; Lipobase; Lubri-Tears; Lubrifilm†; Mil-Par; Oilatum Emollient; Oilatum Plus; Petrolagar†; Polytar Emollient; Refresh Night Time; Savlon Bath Oil†; ***USA:*** Agoral; Akwa Tears; Alpha Keri; Desitin Creamy; Dry Eyes; Duratears Naturale; Haley's M-O; Hemorid For Women; Hypotears; Kondremul with Cascara†; Kondremul with Phenolphthalein; Lacri-Lube; LubriTears; Puralube; Refresh PM; Tears Again; Tears Renewed; Throat Discs; Vagisil; ZBT.

White Soft Paraffin (6404-y)

905 (mineral hydrocarbons); Paraff. Moll. Alb.; Paraffinum Molle Album; Vaselina Branca; Vaseline Officinale; White Petrolatum; White Petroleum Jelly.

Pharmacopoeias. In *Aust., Br., Chin., Fr., Ger., Int., It., Jpn, Pol., Port., Swiss,* and *US.* Many pharmacopoeias use the title Vaselinum Album; in Great Britain the name 'Vaseline' is a trade-mark.

White soft paraffin is bleached yellow soft paraffin. The USP permits a suitable stabiliser.

Yellow Soft Paraffin (6405-j)

Paraff. Moll. Flav.; Paraffinum Molle Flavum; Petrolatum; Petroleum Jelly; Vaselina Amarela; Yellow Petrolatum; Yellow Petroleum Jelly.

CAS — 8009-03-8.

Pharmacopoeias. In *Aust., Br., Chin., Jpn, Pol., Port., Swiss,* and *US.* Many pharmacopoeias use the title Vaselinum Flavum; in Great Britain the name 'Vaseline' is a trade-mark.

A purified semi-solid mixture of hydrocarbons obtained from petroleum. It is a pale yellow to yellow or light amber-coloured, translucent, soft, unctuous mass, not more than slightly fluorescent by daylight even when melted, and odourless when rubbed on the skin. The USP permits a suitable stabiliser. The BP has a drop point of 42° to 60°. The USP has a m.p. of 38° to 60°.

Practically **insoluble** in water and in alcohol; soluble in carbon disulphide, chloroform, ether, petroleum spirit, and most fixed and volatile oils, the solutions sometimes showing a slight opalescence. **Protect** from light.

Adverse Effects

Adverse effects of white soft paraffin or yellow soft paraffin are rare when used in topical preparations, but sensitivity reactions and acne have been reported following topical use. Granulomatous reactions following absorption or injection and lipoid pneumonia following aspiration have occurred.

A report of burns to the scalp, face, and hands in 5 patients who accidentally ignited their hair following the application of paraffin-based hair grease.[1] Four patients suffered inhalation injury, 2 of whom required intubation.

1. Bascom R, *et al.* Inhalation injury related to use of petrolatum-based hair grease. *J Burn Care Rehabil* 1984; **5:** 327–30.

Hypersensitivity. Studies on the allergenicity of white soft paraffin and yellow soft paraffin products.[1-3] Considering their widespread use there are very few reports of sensitivity; white soft paraffin is generally less sensitising than yellow soft paraffin, although allergenicity differs from product to product. The allergenic components are probably polycyclic aromatic hydrocarbons present as impurities and quantities found in a particular paraffin depend on the source and purification method. Only the purest forms should be used in pharmaceuticals, cosmetics, and for patch testing, and highly purified white soft paraffin is preferred to yellow soft paraffin.

1. Dooms-Goossens A, Degreef H. Contact allergy to petrolatums (I). Sensitising capacity of different brands of yellow and white petrolatums. *Contact Dermatitis* 1983; **9:** 175–85.
2. Dooms-Goossens A, Degreef H. Contact allergy to petrolatums (II). Attempts to identify the nature of the allergens. *Contact Dermatitis* 1983; **9:** 247–56.
3. Dooms-Goossens A, Dooms M. Contact allergy to petrolatums (III). Allergenicity prediction and pharmacopoeial requirements. *Contact Dermatitis* 1983; **9:** 352–9.

Uses and Administration

Soft paraffin is used as an ointment basis and as an emollient in the management of skin disorders. It is not readily absorbed by the skin. Sterile dressings containing soft paraffin are used for wound dressing and as a packing material. Soft paraffin is also included in ointments used as ophthalmic lubricants in the management of dry eye (see p.1470). Application of soft paraffin has also been used for the eradication of pubic lice from the eyelashes (see p.1401).

Preparations

BP 1998: Cetomacrogol Emulsifying Ointment; Cetrimide Emulsifying Ointment; Emulsifying Ointment; Paraffin Ointment *(Unguentum Paraffini)*; Simple Eye Ointment *(Eye Ointment Basis)*; Simple Ointment *(Ung. Simp.; Unguentum Simplex)*; Wool Alcohols Ointment *(Ung. Alcoh. Lan.)*;
USP 23: Bland Lubricating Ophthalmic Ointment; Hydrophilic Ointment; Hydrophilic Petrolatum; Petrolatum Gauze; White Ointment; Yellow Ointment.

Proprietary Preparations (details are given in Part 3)

Austral.: Jelonet; Uni Salve; Unitulle; ***Canad.:*** Aquaphor; Vaseline; ***Fr.:*** Jelonet; Unitulle; ***Ital.:*** Jelonet; Lomatuell H; ***S.Afr.:*** Jelonet; ***Spain:*** Lacrilube; ***UK:*** Dermamist; Jelonet; Paratulle; Vaseline; ***USA:*** Uni Salve†.

Multi-ingredient: ***Aust.:*** Tiroler Steinol; ***Austral.:*** Blistex Medicated Lip Conditioner; DermaVeen Moisturising; Duratears; E45; Lacri-Lube; ***Belg.:*** Duratears; Lacrytube; ***Canad.:*** Akwa Tears; Chapstick Medicated Lip Balm; Diaper Guard; Duolube; Duratears; Hydrophil; Hypotears; Lacri-Lube; Moisturel; Oculube; Optilube; Prevex; ***Fr.:*** Oxythyol; Transitol; Transulose; ***Ger.:*** Coliquifilm; ***Irl.:*** Lacri-Lube; ***Ital.:*** Dacriosol†; Lacrilube; ***Neth.:*** Duratears Z†; Siccatears†; ***Norw.:*** Simplex; ***S.Afr.:*** Lacrilube; ***Spain:*** Lubrifilm; Tears Lubricante; Vaselina Boricada; Vaselina Mentolada; ***Switz.:*** Coliquifilm; ***UK:*** Cetraben; Epaderm; Hewletts; Imuderm; Lacri-Lube; Lipobase; Lubri-Tears; Lubrifilm†; Melrose; Refresh Night Time; ***USA:*** Akwa Tears; Bottom Better; Chapstick Medicated Lip Balm; Desitin Creamy; Diaper Guard; Dry Eyes; Duratears Naturale; Hemorid For Women; Hypotears; Lacri-Lube; LubriTears; Puralube; Refresh PM; Tears Again; Tears Renewed; Triple Care Extra Protective Cream.

Alkyl Benzoate (19787-z)

Alkyl (C12-15) Benzoate.

Pharmacopoeias. In *USNF.*

Alkyl benzoate consists of esters of a mixture of C12 to C15 primary and branched alcohols and benzoic acid. It is a clear, practically colourless, oily liquid. Practically **insoluble** in water, in glycerol, and in propylene glycol. Soluble in alcohol, in isopropyl alcohol, in acetone, in ethyl acetate, in isopropyl myristate, in isopropyl palmitate, in liquid paraffin, in vegetable oils, in volatile silicones, and in wool fat. **Store** in airtight containers. Protect from light.

Alkyl benzoate has emollient properties. It may be used as an oily vehicle.

White Beeswax (6407-c)

901 (beeswax); Cera Alba; Cera Blanca; Cêra Branca; Cire Blanche; Gebleichtes Wachs; White Wax.

CAS — 8012-89-3.

Pharmacopoeias. In *Eur.* (see p.viii), *Jpn,* and *Pol.* Also in *USNF.*

White beeswax is bleached yellow beeswax.

Yellow Beeswax (6408-k)

901 (beeswax); Cêra Amarela; Cera Amarilla; Cera Flava; Cire Jaune; Gelbes Wachs; Yellow Wax.

CAS — 8012-89-3.

Pharmacopoeias. In *Chin., Eur.* (see p.viii), and *Jpn.* Also in *USNF.*

The wax obtained by melting with hot water the walls of the honeycomb of the bee, *Apis mellifera* (Apidae), and removing the foreign matter. It occurs as yellow or light brown pieces or plates with a faint and characteristic honey-like odour, brittle when cold, soft and malleable when warmed in the hand. Ph. Eur. has a drop point of 61° to 65°; USNF has a melting range of 62° to 65°.

Ph. Eur. **solubilities** are: practically insoluble in water; partially soluble in hot alcohol and in ether; completely soluble in fatty and essential oils. USP solubilities are: insoluble in water; sparingly soluble in alcohol; completely soluble in chloroform, in ether, in fixed and volatile oils, and in warm carbon disulphide.

Yellow beeswax is used as a stiffening agent in ointments and creams, and enables water to be incorporated to produce water-in-oil emulsions. White beeswax is similarly employed; it is occasionally used to adjust the melting-point of suppositories.

A sterile preparation of white beeswax, hard paraffin, and isopropyl palmitate (Sterile Surgical Bone Wax) has been used to control bleeding from damaged bone in orthopaedic surgery. It should not be confused with Aseptic Surgical Wax (BPC 1949), also known as Horsley's Wax, which contained yellow beeswax, olive oil, and phenol in a mercuric chloride solution and was used to control haemorrhage in bone or cranial surgery.

Hypersensitivity to beeswax has been reported.

Preparations

BP 1998: Paraffin Ointment *(Unguentum Paraffini)*;
USP 23: Rose Water Ointment; White Ointment; Yellow Ointment.

Proprietary Preparations (details are given in Part 3)

Multi-ingredient: ***Aust.:*** Tiroler Steinol; ***Fr.:*** Balmex; Cerat Inalterable; Cold Cream Naturel; ***Ger.:*** Paradiol†; ***Switz.:*** Ceralba†.

Cetostearyl Alcohol (6410-e)

Alcohol Cetylicus et Stearylicus; Alcool Cetostearilico; Cetearyl Alcohol; Cetostearyl Alc.; Cetylstearylalkohol.

CAS — 8005-44-5; 67762-27-0.

Pharmacopoeias. In *Eur.* (see p.viii), *Int.,* and *Pol.* Also in *USNF.*

A mixture of solid aliphatic alcohols, mainly stearyl and cetyl alcohols. It contains not less than 90% of stearyl plus cetyl alcohols and not less than 40% of stearyl alcohol.

A white or pale yellow wax-like mass, plates, flakes, or granules, with a faint characteristic odour. M.p. 48° to 56°.

Practically **insoluble** in water; freely soluble in ether; soluble in alcohol and petroleum spirit. When melted, it is miscible with fatty oils, with liquid paraffin, and with melted wool fat.

Emulsifying Cetostearyl Alcohol (Type A) (Ph. Eur.) is a mixture containing not less than 80% cetostearyl alcohol and not less than 7% sodium cetostearyl sulphate. **Emulsifying Cetostearyl Alcohol (Type B)** (Ph. Eur.) is a mixture containing not less than 80% cetostearyl alcohol and not less than 7% sodium lauryl sulphate. Both are a white or pale yellow, wax-like mass, plates, flakes, or granules. **Soluble** in hot water giving an opalescent solution; practically insoluble in cold water; slightly soluble in alcohol.

Cetostearyl alcohol is used in creams, ointments, and other topical preparations as a stiffening agent and emulsion stabiliser. In conjunction with suitable hydrophilic substances as in Emulsifying Wax, it produces oil-in-water emulsions which are stable over a wide pH range. It is also used to improve the emollient properties of paraffin ointments.

Cetostearyl alcohol can cause hypersensitivity.

Preparations

BP 1998: Cetomacrogol Emulsifying Wax *(Emulsifying Wax, Non-ionic)*; Cetrimide Emulsifying Ointment; Emulsifying Wax;
USNF 18: Emulsifying Wax.

Proprietary Preparations (details are given in Part 3)

Multi-ingredient: ***UK:*** Lipobase; Neutrogena Dermatological Cream.

Cetyl Alcohol (6411-l)

Alcohol Cetylicus; Álcool Cetílico; Cetanol; 1-Hexadecanol; Hexadecyl Alcohol.

CAS — 36653-82-4; 124-29-8.

Pharmacopoeias. In *Eur.* (see p.viii), *Int., Jpn,* and *Pol.* Also in *USNF.*

A mixture of solid aliphatic alcohols consisting chiefly of cetyl alcohol, $C_{16}H_{33}OH$. USNF specifies not less than 90% of cetyl alcohol, the remainder consisting chiefly of related alcohols.

It occurs as white unctuous mass, powder, flakes, cubes, or granules, with a faint characteristic odour. M.p. 45° to 52°. Practically **insoluble** in water; freely to sparingly soluble in alcohol; freely soluble in ether; miscible when melted with animal and vegetable oils, liquid paraffin, and melted wool fat.

Cetyl alcohol is used in topical preparations for its emollient, water absorptive, stiffening, and weak emulsifying properties. It may be incorporated into suppositories to raise the melting-point and may be used in the coating of delayed release solid dose forms.

Cetyl alcohol can cause hypersensitivity.

Cetyl Esters Wax (6430-z)

Synthetic Spermaceti.

Pharmacopoeias. In *Int.* Also in *USNF.*

A mixture consisting primarily of esters of saturated fatty alcohols (C_{14} to C_{18}) and saturated fatty acids (C_{14} to C_{18}). White to off-white translucent flakes with a crystalline structure and a pearly lustre when caked; it has a faint odour. M.p. 43° to 47°.

Practically **insoluble** in water and cold alcohol; soluble in chloroform, ether, fixed and volatile oils, and boiling alcohol; slightly soluble in petroleum spirit. **Store** in a dry place.

Cetyl esters wax is used as a stiffening agent and emollient in creams and ointments as a replacement for natural spermaceti obtained from the sperm whale and the bottle-nosed whale.

Preparations

USP 23: Rose Water Ointment.

Cholesterol (6412-y)

Cholesterin; Cholesterolum. Cholest-5-en-3β-ol.

$C_{27}H_{46}O$ = 386.7.

CAS — 57-88-5.

Pharmacopoeias. In *Eur.* (see p.viii), *Jpn,* and *Pol.* Also in *USNF.*

White or faintly yellow, almost odourless, pearly leaflets, needles, powder, or granules. It acquires a yellow to pale tan colour on prolonged exposure to light. M.p. 147° to 150°.

Practically **insoluble** in water; slowly soluble 1 in 100 of alcohol and 1 in 50 of dehydrated alcohol; soluble to sparingly soluble in acetone; soluble in chloroform, dioxan, ether, ethyl acetate, petroleum spirit, and vegetable oils. **Protect** from light.

Cholesterol imparts water-absorbing power to ointments and is used as an emulsifying agent. It has emollient activity.

Cholesteryl benzoate is used as an ingredient in dermatological preparations.

Coconut Oil (6413-j)

Aceite de Coco; Coconut Butter; Oleum Cocois; Oleum Cocos Raffinatum; Oleum Cocosis.

CAS — 8001-31-8.

Pharmacopoeias. In *Br.* and *Jpn.*

A white or pearl-white unctuous mass, odourless or with an odour of coconut, obtained by expression from the dried solid part of the endosperm of the coconut, the fruit of *Cocos nucifera* (Palmae). M.p. 23° to 26°.

Freely **soluble** in alcohol (at 60°), in chloroform, and in ether. It readily becomes rancid on exposure to air. **Store** at a temperature not exceeding 25° in well-filled containers. Protect from light.

NOTE. Fractionated coconut oil (thin vegetable oil) is used as a source of medium-chain triglycerides (p.1599).

Coconut oil forms a readily absorbable ointment basis. It is also used in food manufacturing.

Emulsifying Wax (6021-r)

Anionic Emulsifying Wax; Cera Emulsificans; Cetylanum; Emulsif. Wax.

CAS — 8014-38-8.

Pharmacopoeias. In *Br. and Ger.*

Emulsifying Wax (*USNF*) is prepared from cetostearyl alcohol containing a polysorbate.

It is prepared from 9 parts of cetostearyl alcohol and 1 part of sodium lauryl sulphate or sodium salts of similar sulphated higher primary aliphatic alcohols.

It is an almost white or pale yellow waxy solid or flakes, becoming plastic when warm, with a faint characteristic odour. Practically **insoluble** in water, forming an emulsion; partly soluble in alcohol.

Emulsifying wax added to fatty or paraffin bases facilitates the preparation of oil-in-water emulsions which are absorbed and are non-greasy when rubbed into the skin. It is a constituent of many hydrophilic ointment bases for so-called 'washable' ointments.

Emulsifying ointment which contains emulsifying wax with white soft paraffin and liquid paraffin was found to have major sunscreen activity in clinically normal skin.[1] It should not be used before phototherapy or in phototesting procedures.

1. Cox NH, Sharpe G. Emollients, salicylic acid, and ultraviolet erythema. *Lancet* 1990; **335:** 53–4.

Preparations

BP 1998: Aqueous Cream *(Hydrous Emulsifying Ointment; Simple Cream)*; Emulsifying Ointment.

Proprietary Preparations (details are given in Part 3)

Multi-ingredient: ***UK:*** Epaderm.

Hard Fat (6415-c)

Adeps Neutralis; Adeps Solidus; Glycérides Semi-synthétiques Solides; Hartfett; Massa Estearínica; Neutralfett.

Pharmacopoeias. In *Eur.* (see p.viii), *Int.,* and *Pol.* Also in *USNF.*

A mixture of triglycerides, diglycerides, and monoglycerides obtained either by esterification of fatty acids of natural origin with glycerol or by trans esterification of natural fats.

A white to almost white, waxy, brittle mass, almost odourless and free from rancid odour. The Ph. Eur. has a melting-point of 30° to 45° but specifies that it does not differ by more than 2° from the nominal value; the USNF has a range not greater than 4° between 27° to 44°. The melted substance is colourless or slightly yellowish and forms a stable white emulsion when shaken with an equal amount of hot water.

Practically **insoluble** in water; slightly soluble in alcohol; freely soluble in ether. **Store** in airtight containers at a temperature 5° or more below the melting-point. Protect from light.

The name Hard Fat is applied to a range of bases with varying degrees of hardness and differing melting ranges used for the preparation of suppositories.

Isopropyl Myristate (6416-k)

Isopropylis Myristas.

$(CH_3)_2CH.O.CO.(CH_2)_{12}.CH_3$ = 270.5.

CAS — 110-27-0.

Pharmacopoeias. In *Eur.* (see p.viii). Also in *USNF.*

A clear colourless or almost colourless, almost odourless, mobile oily liquid; congeals at about 5°.

Immiscible with water; miscible with alcohol, dichloromethane, ether, fatty oils, and with liquid paraffin; practically insoluble in glycerol and in propylene glycol. **Store** in airtight containers. Protect from light. **Incompatible** with hard paraffin.

Isopropyl myristate is resistant to oxidation and hydrolysis and does not become rancid. It is absorbed fairly readily by the skin and is used as a basis for relatively nongreasy emollient ointments and creams. It is also used as a solvent for many substances applied externally.

Other isopropyl fatty acid esters, including di-isopropyl adipate, isopropyl laurate, isopropyl linoleate, and isopropyl palmitate (below) have similar properties and are used for similar purposes to those of isopropyl myristate.

Preparations

Proprietary Preparations (details are given in Part 3)
Spain: Nucoa.

Multi-ingredient: ***Canad.:*** Domol†; ***Irl.:*** Diprobath; Emulsiderm; Hydromol; ***UK:*** Dermol; Diprobath; Emulsiderm; Hydromol Cream; Hydromol Emollient.

Isopropyl Palmitate (6417-a)

Isopropylis Palmitas.

$(CH_3)_2CH.O.CO.(CH_2)_{14}.CH_3$ = 298.5.

CAS — 142-91-6.

Pharmacopoeias. In *Eur.* (see p.viii). Also in *USNF.*

A clear, colourless, mobile, oily liquid with a slight odour. **Immiscible** with water; miscible with alcohol, dichloromethane, ether, fatty oils, and liquid paraffin; soluble in acetone, castor oil, chloroform, cottonseed oil, and ethyl acetate; practically insoluble in glycerol and propylene glycol. **Store** in airtight containers. Protect from light.

Isopropyl palmitate has properties and uses similar to those of isopropyl myristate (above).

Laurocapram (16870-s)

Laurocapram *(USAN, rINN).*

N-0252. 1-Dodecylazacycloheptan-2-one; 1-Dodecylhexahydro-2*H*-azepin-2-one.

$C_{18}H_{35}NO$ = 281.5.

CAS — 59227-89-3.

Laurocapram (Azone) has been investigated for enhancing the penetration of drugs through the skin.

Microcrystalline Wax (6422-z)

907 (refined microcrystalline wax).

Pharmacopoeias. In *USNF.*

A mixture of straight-chain, branched-chain, and cyclic hydrocarbons, obtained by solvent fractionation of the still bottom fraction of petroleum by suitable dewaxing or de-oiling means.

A white or cream-coloured odourless waxy solid. Melting range 54° to 102°. Practically **insoluble** in water; sparingly soluble in dehydrated alcohol; soluble in chloroform, ether, volatile oils, and in most warm fixed oils. **Store** in airtight containers.

Microcrystalline wax is used as a stiffening agent in creams and ointments and as a tablet and capsule coating agent.

Oleic Acid (1319-f)

Acidum Oleicum; Ölsäure.

CAS — 112-80-1 ($C_{18}H_{34}O_2$).

Pharmacopoeias. In *Eur.* (see p.viii). Also in *USNF.*

Oleic acid is obtained by hydrolysis of fats or fixed oils. It is a clear, yellowish or brownish oily liquid with a characteristic lard-like odour. On exposure to air it darkens in colour and the odour becomes more pronounced.

It consists chiefly of (*Z*)-octadec-9-enoic acid [$CH_3.(CH_2)_7.CH:CH.(CH_2)_7.CO_2H$ = 282.5] and varying amounts of saturated and other unsaturated fatty acids. Congealing point not above 10°.

Practically **insoluble** in water; miscible with alcohol, chloroform, dichloromethane, ether, and fixed and volatile oils. **Store** at 8° to 15° in airtight containers. Protect from light.

Oleic acid forms soaps with alkaline substances and is used as an emulsifying or solubilising agent. It occurs in edible fats and oils which are used as foods or food components.

Preparations

BP 1998: Chloroxylenol Solution *(Roxenol)*; White Liniment *(White Embrocation).*

Oleyl Alcohol (6423-c)

CAS — 143-28-2.

Pharmacopoeias. In *USNF.*

A mixture of unsaturated and saturated high molecular weight fatty alcohols consisting chiefly of oleyl alcohol, $C_{18}H_{36}O$ = 268.5.

A clear colourless to light yellow oily liquid with a faint characteristic odour. Practically **insoluble** in water; soluble in alcohol, ether, isopropyl alcohol, and light liquid paraffin. **Store** in well-filled airtight containers.

Oleyl alcohol is used as an emollient and as an emulsifying and solubilising agent. The acetate has also been used.

Fractionated Palm Kernel Oil (6425-a)

Pharmacopoeias. In *Br.*

A white, solid, odourless or almost odourless, brittle fat, obtained by selective solvent fractionation and hydrogenation of the natural oil from the kernels of *Elaeis guineensis* (Palmae). M.p. 31° to 36°.

Practically **insoluble** in water and alcohol; miscible with chloroform, ether, and petroleum spirit. **Store** at a temperature not exceeding 25°.

Fractionated palm kernel oil is used as a basis for suppositories. It has also been used in food manufacturing. The unfractionated oil has been used as an emollient and as an ointment basis.

Preparations

Proprietary Preparations (details are given in Part 3)

Multi-ingredient: ***Ger.:*** Demozem†.

Shea Butter (13235-b)

A natural fat obtained from the kernel of the fruit of *Butyrospermum parkii* (Sapotaceae) indigenous to W. Africa.

Shea butter is used as an ointment and cream basis.

Silicones (13600-s)

Silicones are polymers with a structure consisting of alternate atoms of silicon and oxygen, with organic groups attached to the silicon atoms. As the degree of polymerisation increases, the products become more viscous and the various grades are distinguished by a number, approximately corresponding to the viscosity of the particular grade. Silicones may be fluids (or oils), greases, waxes, resins, or rubbers depending on the degree of polymerisation.

Dimethicones (6428-r)

Dimethicones *(BAN).*

Dimeticone *(rINN)*; 900; Dimethicone *(USAN)*; Dimethyl Silicone Fluid; Dimethylpolysiloxane; Dimethylsiloxane; Dimeticonum; Huile de Silicone; Methyl Polysiloxane; Permethylpolysiloxane; Silicone Oil; Siliconum Liquidum. Poly(dimethylsiloxane).

$CH_3.[Si(CH_3)_2.O]_nSi(CH_3)_3$.

CAS — 9006-65-9.

Pharmacopoeias. In *Chin.* and *Eur.* (see p.viii). Also in *USNF. USNF* also includes Cyclomethicone, a fully methylated cyclic siloxane.

Dimethicones are fluid silicones in which the organic group is a methyl radical. The Ph. Eur. describes dimethicones with a kinematic viscosity between 20 and 1300 mm^2 per second, those with a nominal viscosity of 50 mm^2 per second or less being intended for external use. The USNF allows a range of nominal viscosities between 20 and 30 000 centistokes.

Dimethicones are clear colourless, odourless liquids. Practically **insoluble** in water, acetone, and methyl alcohol; very slightly soluble to practically insoluble in dehydrated alcohol; miscible with ethyl acetate, methyl ethyl ketone, and toluene; very slightly soluble in isopropyl alcohol; soluble in amyl acetate, chlorinated hydrocarbons, ether, *n*-hexane, petroleum spirit, and xylene. **Store** in airtight containers.

Simethicone (activated dimethicone), a mixture of liquid dimethicones with silicon dioxide, is described on p.1213.

Adverse Effects

Adverse effects from the clinical use of silicones appear to be rare. Foreign-body reactions have been reported following their use as joint implants. Other implants, notably breast implants, usually for reconstruction following mastectomy or for cosmetic purposes, carry the risk of migration of silicone with cyst formation and other complications; accidental intravascular injection has been fatal. Late adverse ocular effects can follow the intravitreal injection of liquid silicone in the management of retinal detachment.

Connective-tissue disorders. Since the introduction of silicone breast implants in the early 1960s there have been numerous anecdotal reports of various connective-tissue disorders occurring in women who have undergone breast reconstruction or augmentation with these implants. Scleroderma has been the most frequently reported disorder; others have included systemic lupus erythematosus, rheumatoid arthritis, and inflammatory myopathies. A syndrome of vague musculoskeletal symptoms, fever, and fatigue has also been reported. These cases led the FDA to call for a moratorium in the US on the use of silicone breast implants in January 1992. However, with the exception of one study of self-reported symptoms which showed only a small increase in risk,[1] large epidemiological studies[2-5] and a review by the Medical Devices Agency in the UK have so far failed to show any association between silicone breast implants and connective-tissue disorders.

1. Hennekens CH, *et al.* Self-reported breast implants and connective-tissue diseases in female health professionals: a retrospective cohort study. *JAMA* 1996; **275:** 616–21.
2. Gabriel SE, *et al.* Risk of connective-tissue diseases and other disorders after breast implantation. *N Engl J Med* 1994; **330:** 1697–1702.
3. Sánchez-Guerrero J, *et al.* Silicone breast implants and the risk of connective-tissue diseases and symptoms. *N Engl J Med* 1995; **332:** 1666–70.
4. Silverman BG, *et al.* Reported complications of silicone gel breast implants: an epidemiologic review. *Ann Intern Med* 1996; **124:** 744–56.
5. Nyrén O, *et al.* Risk of connective tissue disease and related disorders among women with breast implants: a nation-wide retrospective cohort study in Sweden. *Br Med J* 1998; **316:** 417–22.

Uses and Administration

Dimethicones and other silicones are water-repellent and have a low surface tension. They are used in topical barrier preparations for protecting the skin against water-soluble irritants. Creams, lotions, and ointments containing a dimethicone are employed for the prevention of bedsores and napkin rash and to protect the skin against trauma due to incontinence or stoma discharge. Silicone preparations should not be applied where free drainage is necessary or to inflamed or abraded skin. Silicones, usually a dimethicone, are also used topically as wound dressings.

Silicones have also been used for arthroplasty in rheumatic disorders, by intravitreal injection for retinal detachment, and by subcutaneous injection or implantation in reconstructive or cosmetic surgery.

Dimethicones, in particular simethicone (activated dimethicone) (p.1213), are used in the treatment of flatulence.

Retinal detachment. Retinal detachment is separation of the retina from the underlying retinal pigmentary epithelium and usually requires surgical repair. Intravitreal injection of liquid silicone may be used for retinal tamponade following or in conjunction with surgery in complicated or persistent detachment of the retina.[1,2] Late complications following its use may include cataract, glaucoma, and keratopathy.

1. Chan C, Okun E. The question of ocular tolerance to intravitreal liquid silicone: a long-term analysis. *Ophthalmology* 1986; **93:** 651–60.
2. Gray RH, *et al.* Fluorescein angiographic findings in three patients with long-term intravitreal liquid silicone. *Br J Ophthalmol* 1989; **73:** 991–5.

Preparations

Proprietary Preparations (details are given in Part 3)

Austral.: Dermafilm†; Egozite Protective Baby Lotion; Instru-Safe; Rosken Skin Repair; Silic 15; ***Canad.:*** Barrier Cream; Barriere; Protecto-Derm; ***Fr.:*** Cica-Care; Ophtasiloxane; ***Ger.:*** Jaikin N; Symadal; ***Ital.:*** Radioced; ***UK:*** Cica-Care.

Multi-ingredient: ***Aust.:*** Ceolat Compositum; Evalgan; Riker Silicone-Spray; ***Austral.:*** Derma Care†; Dermalife Plus; Dimethicream; Eczema Cream; Egozite Baby Cream; Formicare Skin Relief†; Hamilton Skin Repair Cream; Nappy-Mate; Ungvita; ***Belg.:*** Rikosol Silicone†; ***Canad.:*** Blistex Lip Balm; Blistex Lip Tone; Blistex Sunblock†; Blistex Ultra Lip Balm; Complex 15; Diaper Guard; Dyprotex†; Moisturel; Silon†; Soft Lips; ***Fr.:*** Balmex; ***Ger.:*** Evalgan†; ***Irl.:*** Conotrane; Siopel; Sprilon; Vasogen; ***Ital.:*** Angstrom Viso/Labbra Alta Protezione; Rikospray; Silicogamma†; ***S.Afr.:*** Arola Rosebalm; Rikerspray†; Siopel; ***Spain:*** Dermo H Infantil; Nevasona†; Proskin; S 13†; Silidermil; Tegunal; ***Swed.:*** Silon; ***UK:*** Bioglan Effervescent Granules; Cal-A-Cool†; Cobadex; Conotrane; Cymex; Savlon Nappy Rash Cream†; Silastic; Siopel; Sprilon; Vasogen; ***USA:*** Blistex Lip Balm; Dermasil; Diaper Guard; Dyprotex; Maxilube; Medacote; Mentholatum Cherry Ice; Mentholatum Natural Ice; Mentholatum Softlips; Mentholatum Softlips Lipbalm; Mentholatum Softlips Lipbalm (UV); Unicare†.

Squalane (6431-c)

Cosbiol; Dodecahydrosqualene; Perhydrosqualène; Spinacane. 2,6,10,15,19,23-Hexamethyltetracosane.

$C_{30}H_{62}$ = 422.8.

CAS — 111-01-3.

Pharmacopoeias. In *USNF.*

A saturated hydrocarbon obtained by hydrogenation of squalene, an aliphatic triterpene occurring in some fish oils.

It is a colourless, almost odourless, transparent oil. Practically **insoluble** in water; very slightly soluble in dehydrated alcohol; miscible with chloroform and with ether; slightly soluble in acetone. **Store** in airtight containers.

Squalane is a saturated derivative of squalene, a constituent of human sebum. It is miscible with human sebum and is included in topical preparations to increase skin permeability. It is also used as an emollient.

Stearyl Alcohol (6432-k)

Alcohol Stearylicus; Alcool Stéarylique; 1-Octadecanol; Octadecyl Alcohol.

CAS — 112-92-5.

Pharmacopoeias. In *Eur.* (see p.viii), *Jpn,* and *Pol.* Also in *USNF.*

A mixture of solid alcohols being mainly (90 to 95%) stearyl alcohol ($C_{18}H_{37}OH$).

White unctuous flakes, granules, or mass with a faint characteristic odour. M.p. 55° to 60°. Practically **insoluble** in water; soluble in alcohol; freely soluble in ether; miscible when melted with fatty oils, liquid paraffin, and melted wool fat.

Stearyl alcohol is used to thicken ointments and creams and to increase their water-holding capacity; it has emollient and weak emulsifying properties. It is also used in controlled release solid dose formulations.

Stearyl alcohol can cause hypersensitivity.

Theobroma Oil (6435-x)

Beurre de Cacao; Burro di Cacao; Butyrum Cacao; Cacao Butter; Cocoa Butter; Kakaobutter; Manteca de Cacao; Manteiga de Cacau; Ol. Theobrom.; Oleum Cacao; Oleum Theobromatis.

CAS — 8002-31-1.

Pharmacopoeias. In *Aust., Br., Fr., Ger., It., Jpn, Neth.,* and *Pol.* Also in *USNF.*

A solid fat expressed from the roasted seeds of *Theobroma cacao* (Sterculiaceae). It is a yellowish-white, somewhat brittle solid with a slight odour of cocoa. M.p. 31° to 34°.

Slightly **soluble** in alcohol; freely soluble in chloroform, ether, and petroleum spirit; soluble in boiling dehydrated alcohol. **Store** at a temperature not exceeding 25°.

Theobroma oil is employed as a basis for suppositories. If it is heated to more than 36° during preparation the solidification point will be appreciably lowered due to the formation of metastable states, leading to subsequent difficulty in setting. It is a major ingredient of chocolate.

Wool Alcohols (6436-r)

Alcoholes Adipis Lanae; Alcoholia Lanae; Alcolanum; Lanalcolum; Lanolin Alcohols; Wollwachsalkohole; Wool Wax Alcohols.

CAS — 8027-33-6.

Pharmacopoeias. In *Eur.* (see p.viii). Also in *USNF.*

A mixture of sterols and higher aliphatic alcohols obtained from wool fat and containing not less than 30% of sterols calculated as cholesterol.

It is a pale yellow to brownish-yellow solid, somewhat brittle when cold but plastic when warm, with a faint characteristic odour. M.p. not below 56° to 58°. It may contain a suitable antoxidant.

Practically **insoluble** in water; slightly soluble in alcohol; soluble in boiling dehydrated alcohol and dichloromethane; freely soluble in chloroform and petroleum spirit; soluble or freely soluble in ether. **Store** at a temperature not exceeding 25°. Protect from light. **Incompatible** with coal tar, ichthammol, resorcinol, and phenol.

Wool alcohols is an emulsifying agent and emulsion stabiliser used in the preparation of water-in-oil creams and ointments. It increases the water absorbing capacity of hydrocarbon mixtures; the addition of 5% of wool alcohols permits a threefold increase in the amount of water which can be incorporated in soft paraffin and such emulsions are not 'cracked' by the addition of weak acids.

It has an emollient action on the skin and is used in preparations for dry skin and dry eyes.

Derivatives of wool alcohols with similar uses include acetylated wool alcohols and ethoxylated wool alcohols.

Wool alcohols may cause hypersensitivity.

Preparations

BP 1998: Wool Alcohols Ointment *(Ung. Alcoh. Lan.).*

Proprietary Preparations (details are given in Part 3)

Austral.: Eucerin (Anhydrous).

Multi-ingredient: ***Austral.:*** Oilatum Emollient; ***Canad.:*** Lacri-Lube; ***Ger.:*** Coliquifilm; ***Irl.:*** Oilatum Emollient; ***Ital.:*** Lacrilube; ***S.Afr.:*** Oilatum Emollient†; ***Switz.:*** Ceralba†; Coliquifilm; ***UK:*** BMS†; Emmolate; Oilatum Emollient; Refresh Night Time; Savlon Bath Oil†; ***USA:*** Refresh PM.

Wool Fat (6437-f)

Adeps Lanae; Anhydrous Lanolin; Cera Lanae; Graisse de Suint Purifiée; Lanoléine; Lanolin; Lanolina; Purified Lanolin; Refined Wool Fat; Suarda; Wollfett; Wollwachs.

CAS — 8006-54-0.

Pharmacopoeias. In *Chin., Eur.* (see p.viii), *Int., Jpn, Pol.,* and *US.* Some pharmacopoeias include Hydrous Wool Fat which is prepared by the addition of water to wool fat.

US also includes under the title Modified Lanolin a grade that has been processed to reduce the contents of free lanolin alcohols and detergent and pesticide residues.

A purified anhydrous waxy substance obtained from the wool of the sheep, *Ovis aries* (Bovidae). It is a pale yellow unctuous substance with a characteristic odour; melted wool fat is a clear or almost clear, yellow liquid. Drop point and melting range 38° to 44°. It may contain a suitable antoxidant. 10 g absorbs not less than 20 mL of water.

Practically **insoluble** in water; sparingly soluble in cold alcohol; slightly soluble in boiling alcohol; soluble to freely soluble in ether; freely soluble in chloroform; it forms an opalescent solution in petroleum spirit. **Store** at temperature not exceeding 25°.

Wool fat is used in the formulation of water-in-oil creams and ointments. When mixed with a suitable vegetable oil or with soft paraffin it gives emollient creams which penetrate the skin. It can absorb about 30% of water.

Derivatives and modifications of wool fat include poloxyl lanolin (ethoxylated lanolin), isopropyl lanolate, lanolin oil, and lanolin wax. Hydrogenated wool fat (hydrogenated lanolin) is a mixture of higher aliphatic alcohols and sterols obtained from the hydrogenation of wool fat.

Hydrous wool fat (hydrous lanolin) is an ointment basis prepared by the addition of water to wool fat. The Ph. Eur. specifies wool fat 75% and water 25%.

Wool fat can cause sensitivity reactions.

General reviews.

1. Barnett G. Lanolin and derivatives. *Cosmet Toilet* 1986; **101** (Mar): 23–44.

Reports of pesticide residues in wool fat and comments on risks.

1. Copeland CA, *et al.* Pesticide residue in lanolin. *JAMA* 1989; **261:** 242.
2. Cade PH. Pesticide in lanolin. *JAMA* 1989; **262:** 613.
3. Copeland CA, Wagner SL. Pesticide in lanolin. *JAMA* 1989; **262:** 613.

Lanolin treated to remove both detergent and natural free fatty alcohols reduced the incidence of hypersensitivity in lanolin-sensitive patients to almost zero.[1]

1. Clark EW, *et al.* Lanolin with reduced sensitizing potential. *Contact Dermatitis* 1977; **3:** 69–74.

Preparations

BP 1998: Simple Eye Ointment *(Eye Ointment Basis)*; Simple Ointment *(Ung. Simp.; Unguentum Simplex)*;
USP 23: Modified Lanolin.

Proprietary Preparations (details are given in Part 3)

Canad.: Lanolelle; Masse†; ***Ital.:*** Vitlan†; ***S.Afr.:*** Duratears; ***UK:*** Medilan; ***USA:*** Uni Derm†.

Multi-ingredient: ***Aust.:*** Tiroler Steinol; ***Austral.:*** Alpha Keri; Alpha Keri Tar; Duratears; E45; Lacri-Lube; Rikoderm; Soothe'n Heal; ***Belg.:*** Duratears; Lacrytube; ***Canad.:*** Akwa Tears; Alpha Keri; Dermolan†; Duratears; Huile de Bain Therapeutique; Lubriderm; Lubriderm Daily UV Defense; Optilube; Stancare; Therapeutic Bath Oil; Therapeutic Skin Lotion; ***Fr.:*** Oxythyol; ***Irl.:*** Lacri-Lube; ***Ital.:*** Dacriosol†; ***Neth.:*** Duratears Z†; ***S.Afr.:*** Lacrilube; ***Spain:*** Lubrifilm; Tears Lubricante; ***Switz.:*** Duratears; ***UK:*** Alpha Keri; Hewletts; Lacri-Lube; Lubri-Tears; Lubrifilm†; Melrose; ***USA:*** Akwa Tears; Alpha Keri; Bottom Better; Dry Eyes; Duratears Naturale; Lacri-Lube; LubriTears.

Parasympathomimetics

Parasympathomimetics may be classified into 2 distinct pharmacological groups:

- cholinergic agonists, such as bethanechol, carbachol, methacholine, and pilocarpine which act directly on effector cells to mimic the effects of acetylcholine. They are sometimes referred to as cholinomimetics or true parasympathomimetics; some such as bethanechol, carbachol, and methacholine are choline esters
- anticholinesterases (cholinesterase inhibitors) which inhibit the enzymic hydrolysis of acetylcholine by acetylcholinesterase and other cholinesterases, thereby prolonging and enhancing its actions in the body. They may be classified by the length of time taken to restore active enzyme following binding of enzyme to drug. The 'reversible' anticholinesterases such as ambenonium, neostigmine, physostigmine, and pyridostigmine generally produce enzyme inhibition for a few hours, whereas 'irreversible' anticholinesterases such as dyflos and ecothiopate produce extremely prolonged inhibition, and return of cholinesterase activity depends on synthesis of new enzyme. Centrally acting reversible anticholinesterases include donepezil, rivastigmine, and tacrine.

Parasympathomimetics have a variety of uses, which are discussed in the following sections. Some are administered topically for their miotic action in the treatment of glaucoma and strabismus. Those that are anticholinesterases are given systemically to reverse the neuromuscular blockade of neuromuscular blockers; they are also used in myasthenia gravis and for dementia of the Alzheimer's type. Other uses of parasympathomimetics, which are discussed elsewhere, have included decreased gastro-intestinal motility (p.1168) such as paralytic ileus and postoperative urinary retention (p.454).

A number of drugs, such as fampridine and guanidine, which enhance the release of acetylcholine from nerve terminals are also discussed in this chapter.

References.

1. Goyal RK. Muscarinic receptor subtypes: physiology and clinical implications. *N Engl J Med* 1989; **321:** 1022–9.

Dementia

Dementia is a syndrome in which impairment of cortical or subcortical function leads to deterioration of cognitive processes or intellectual abilities including memory, judgement, language, communication, and abstract thinking. Unlike delirium there is no gross clouding of consciousness. There may be changes in personality and behaviour disturbances. Dementia is usually progressive, though not always irreversible, and loss of social and other skills often leads to complete dependence on others.

Although dementia is more prevalent in the elderly it is not an inevitable consequence of ageing. Dementia can result from a large number of conditions including:

- *neurodegenerative diseases*: Alzheimer's disease, Pick's disease, Huntington's chorea, Parkinson's disease, Lewy-body disease, multiple sclerosis, progressive supranuclear palsy
- *vascular diseases*: multiple cerebral infarcts, occlusion of carotid artery, cranial arteritis
- *trauma*: subdural haematoma
- *neoplasms*
- *CNS infections*: encephalitis, syphilis, toxoplasmosis, AIDS, Creutzfeldt-Jakob disease
- *endocrine/metabolic disorders*: hypothyroidism, uraemia, hepatic failure, cardiac failure, respiratory failure, hypoxia
- *toxic insults*: alcohol, solvents, heavy metals, drug therapy
- *hydrocephalus*
- *nutritional deficiency*: vitamin B_{12}, folic acid, thiamine
- *depression*

Of the above, Alzheimer's disease is the most common cause of dementia and accounts for over half of all patients; about one-third of dementia cases are due to vascular disease.

Treatment employed in dementia can be broadly divided into that which controls disturbed behaviour (p.636) and that which tries to improve or preserve cognitive function (see below). Although many drugs have been tried in the management of cognitive impairment most have produced little or no benefit.

ALZHEIMER'S DISEASE. Alzheimer's disease is a progressive degenerative condition affecting mainly patients over 60 years of age. Death usually occurs within 10 years of onset. The rare early-onset form of Alzheimer's disease (familial Alzheimer's disease) is sometimes referred to as pre-senile dementia. Apart from age other risk factors include Down's syndrome and a family history. Presence of the ε4 allele of apolipoprotein E is another risk factor; it correlates with prevalence and age of onset in some forms of Alzheimer's disease but use for routine clinical or predictive testing is controversial. Pathological features include general atrophy of the brain with loss of neurones and reduced synaptic density in the cerebral cortex. There also appears to be damage to cholinergic neurones in the forebrain resulting in acetylcholine deficiency in the cortex. The main histological features of Alzheimer's disease are the presence of senile plaques consisting of a central core of β-amyloid protein and neurofibrillary tangles associated with a modified form of the endogenous protein tau.

Dialysis dementia, an irreversible condition which has occurred in dialysis patients, has been associated with excess aluminium in the dialysing fluid but the role of aluminium in Alzheimer's disease, if any, is unclear. High concentrations of aluminium silicates have been found in the core of senile plaques and aluminium appears to accumulate in neurofibrillary tangles.

Deficiencies in numerous neurotransmitters have been found in patients with Alzheimer's disease but reduced choline acetyltransferase activity leading to reduced synthesis of acetylcholine remains the most consistent defect correlating with the severity of the condition. A number of methods have been tried in an attempt to increase acetylcholine concentrations in the brain including administration of *acetylcholine precursors*, *cholinesterase inhibitors*, *enhancers of acetylcholine release*, and *cholinergic agonists*. However, none replace lost cholinergic neurones and therefore none affect overall progression of the disease.

Treatments using *precursors of acetylcholine* such as lecithin or choline alone are not considered to produce useful improvements.

Tacrine and donepezil are the main *cholinesterase inhibitors* used. Tacrine may delay cognitive decline in some patients with mild or moderate Alzheimer's disease but many patients cannot tolerate the doses required and have to stop therapy because of gastro-intestinal effects or signs of hepatotoxicity. Some consider that it is difficult to interpret the effectiveness of tacrine from the available data and there appears to be a lack of long-term studies. Donepezil may also produce modest improvements; it appears to be better tolerated than tacrine and hepatotoxicity has not been reported. Rivastigmine is another recently introduced cholinesterase inhibitor. Other cholinesterase inhibitors which have been tried or are under study for use in Alzheimer's disease include physostigmine, eptastigmine, galantamine, and metriphonate.

Fampridine and linopirdine, which *enhance acetylcholine release from nerve terminals* have also been tried in Alzheimer's disease but there is little evidence of clinical benefit.

Limited improvement has been reported with some *cholinergic agonists* but pilocarpine may exacerbate the dementia. Muscarinic M_1 agonists such as xanomeline are being investigated on the basis that muscarinic M_1 receptors appear to be preserved throughout the course of Alzheimer's disease.

An alternative line of investigation is the *stimulation of nicotinic receptors* using nicotine. A hypothesis that free radicals may initiate and maintain mechanisms responsible for neurodegeneration in Alzheimer's disease has prompted the investigation of drugs such as α-tocopherol and selegiline for antoxidant therapy but their value remains to be confirmed.

Neurotropic or nootropic drugs such as piracetam have also been tried in Alzheimer's disease and other dementias but there is little convincing evidence of clinical usefulness.

Many drugs with *vasodilator activity* were originally tried in dementia when it was believed that the condition was due to 'cerebrovascular insufficiency' (p.785), but overall there is little convincing evidence of benefit. Ergot derivatives such as co-dergocrine mesylate and nicergoline have been the most commonly used; however, any effectiveness is now attributed to their action as metabolic enhancers or nootropic drugs and their place in therapy has still to be established.

Observations in women receiving *hormone replacement therapy* (HRT) have suggested that oestrogens can reduce the risk and delay the onset of Alzheimer's disease in elderly women and a long-term study on the value of HRT for prevention of Alzheimer's disease is in progress. The effect of oestrogens on cognitive function in postmenopausal women who already have mild or moderate Alzheimer's disease is also being studied. Some retrospective studies also indicate an inverse association between the use of *anti-inflammatory drugs* such as NSAIDs and the risk of developing Alzheimer's disease.

VASCULAR DEMENTIA. Vascular dementia is a syndrome produced by ischaemic, hypoxic, or haemorrhagic brain lesions. Vessel occlusion is the most common cause of vascular dementia and produces a variety of cognitive deficits depending on the site of ischaemia. Among the major forms of dementia recognised are those due to multiple infarcts, single strategic infarcts, and subcortical white matter ischaemia (Binswanger's disease). It has a more acute onset than dementia due to Alzheimer's disease and in contrast to the continuous progression of Alzheimer's disease has a stepwise progression. Risk factors for this type of dementia appear to be as for stroke (p.799) in general and similar methods for prevention and treatment may be of use.

LEWY-BODY DEMENTIA. Dementia of the Lewy-body type is distinguished from other types of dementia by a state of fluctuating cognitive impairment and confusion; hallucinations, paranoid delusions, a tendency to fall for no apparent reason, and transient clouding or loss of consciousness are also characteristic symptoms. In addition, mild extrapyramidal symptoms may be present and there is increased susceptibility to the extrapyramidal adverse effects of antipsychotics (see the Elderly, under Precautions of Chlorpromazine on p.652).

1. Cummings JL. Dementia: the failing brain. *Lancet* 1995; **345:** 1481–4. Correction. *ibid.*; 1551.
2. Fleming KC, *et al.* Dementia: diagnosis and evaluation. *Mayo Clin Proc* 1995; **70:** 1093–1107.
3. Gooch MD, Stennett DJ. Molecular basis of Alzheimer's disease. *Am J Health-Syst Pharm* 1996; **53:** 1545–57.
4. Amar K, Wilcock G. Vascular dementia. *Br Med J* 1996; **312:** 227–31.
5. Konno S, *et al.* Classification, diagnosis and treatment of vascular dementia. *Drugs Aging* 1997; **11:** 361–73.
6. Parnetti L, *et al.* Cognitive enhancement therapy for Alzheimer's disease: the way forward. *Drugs* 1997; **53:** 752–68.
7. American Psychiatric Association. Practice guideline for the treatment of patients with Alzheimer's disease and other dementias of late life. *Am J Psychiatry* 1997; **154** (suppl): 1–39.
8. Benzi G, Moretti A. Is there a rationale for the use of acetylcholinesterase inhibitors in the therapy of Alzheimer's disease? *Eur J Pharmacol* 1998; **346:** 1–13.
9. Small GW. Treatment of Alzheimer's disease: current approaches and promising developments. *Am J Med* 1998; **104** (suppl 4A): 32S–38S.
10. Eccles M, *et al.* North of England evidence based guidelines development project: guideline for the primary care management of dementia. *Br Med J* 1998; **317:** 802–8.

Eaton-Lambert myasthenic syndrome

Eaton-Lambert myasthenic syndrome is a rare disorder that like myasthenia gravis (see below) is an auto-immune disease of the neuromuscular junction. However, unlike myasthenia gravis, in which auto-antibodies affect acetylcholine receptors, patients with Eaton-Lambert syndrome have auto-antibodies that act presynaptically to reduce release of acetylcholine. The muscle weakness of this syndrome mostly affects the proximal muscles, particularly those of the limbs, and respiratory and ocular muscles are usually spared. Autonomic symptoms including dry mouth, constipation, and impotence are also common. Over half of patients also develop small cell carcinoma of the lung. Response to treatment with anticholinesterases alone is poor; treatment with 3,4-diaminopyridine, which increases acetylcholine release, appears to be more effective. The use of similar drugs such as guanidine and fampridine is limited by severe adverse effects. Some patients may obtain additional benefit when anticholinesterases are used in addition to 3,4-diaminopyridine. Because of the auto-immune basis of Eaton-Lambert syndrome immunosuppressive treatment and plasma exchange similar to that employed in myasthenia gravis are also used. Treatment with corticosteroids does not appear to induce the initial exacerbation of symptoms that can occur in myasthenia gravis.

1. Newsom-Davis J. Myasthenia gravis and the Lambert-Eaton myasthenic syndrome. *Prescribers' J* 1993; **33:** 205–12.

Glaucoma and ocular hypertension

Intra-ocular pressure rises when there is an imbalance between production and drainage of aqueous humour in the eye. Aqueous humour is secreted by the ciliary body and flows into the posterior chamber of the eye. It then passes through the pupil into the anterior chamber from where about 75% drains from the eye through the trabecular meshwork into Schlemm's canal and then into the episcleral veins. The remainder is removed by the uveoscleral route, passing through the ciliary muscle and finally into the episcleral tissues.

The term **ocular hypertension** is used to describe intra-ocular pressure above an upper normal value of 21 mmHg when there are no signs of optic nerve damage. The term **glaucoma** is used to describe a group of conditions characterised by cupping of the optic disc and damage of the optic nerve and is associated with visual loss. Although it was once thought that raised intra-ocular pressure was an essential feature of glaucoma, it is now recognised that glaucoma can occur and progress in patients with an intra-ocular pressure within the normal range. Also, some patients may have raised intra-ocular pressure for many years without evidence of glaucoma. Whether these patients would receive long-term benefit from a reduction in intra-ocular pressure is under study but many ophthalmologists consider that therapy is indicated if the intra-ocular pressure is higher than 30 mmHg. Raised intra-ocular pressure is now considered to be only one of several risk factors for glaucoma, but as it is the only one that can be altered, current therapy for glaucoma is directed at lowering it. The aim is not just to reduce intra-ocular pressure to a normal value but to a level at which damage to the optic nerve ceases.[1-4]

Raised intra-ocular pressure associated with glaucoma is usually due to reduced outflow of aqueous humour from the eye. Glaucoma is described as open-angle or angle-closure depending on the mechanism of the obstruction of drainage and may be acute or chronic. Glaucoma may also be referred to as primary or secondary. Primary glaucoma is usually associated with a direct disturbance of aqueous outflow whereas secondary glaucoma develops as a consequence of a number of diseases or of trauma.

The most common form of glaucoma is **chronic open-angle glaucoma** (simple glaucoma; wide-angle glaucoma) which is due to blockage in drainage through the trabecular meshwork. Intra-ocular pressure increases gradually, and the condition is usually asymptomatic until well advanced and severe damage has occurred. Usually, both eyes are affected. Risk factors include old age, diabetes, Afro-Caribbean race, a family history, and myopia. A 'steroid glaucoma' may be produced, after a few weeks of treatment with eye drops containing corticosteroids, in patients predisposed to open-angle glaucoma; the risk with systemic corticosteroids appears to be less.

In contrast, **angle-closure glaucoma** (closed-angle glaucoma; narrow-angle glaucoma) usually occurs as an acute emergency. Patients present with a painful red eye, sweating, and nausea and vomiting as a result of a rapid rise in intra-ocular pressure. This can result from blockage of the flow of aqueous humour into the anterior chamber. The resulting rise in intra-ocular pressure bows the iris against the trabecular meshwork restricting aqueous outflow and thereby further raising intra-ocular pressure. It usually occurs in patients with hypermetropia who have a shallow anterior chamber and a narrow filtration angle. The use of mydriatics in such patients is contra-indicated as dilatation of the pupil can precipitate an acute attack of angle-closure glaucoma.

ANTIGLAUCOMA DRUGS. Although many drugs are effective in reducing intra-ocular pressure there is little data on their long-term effect on visual field changes in glaucoma.[3,5] Drugs used in the treatment of glaucoma lower intra-ocular pressure by a variety of mechanisms and their effects are often additive. Their use has been discussed in a number of reviews.[1,2,4,6]

Beta blockers inhibit beta receptors in the ciliary epithelium and thereby reduce the secretion of aqueous humour. They are often the drugs of first choice for initial and maintenance treatment of open-angle and other chronic glaucomas and of ocular hypertension; other drugs are used with them when further reductions in intra-ocular pressure are required. They are better tolerated than miotics but can produce systemic effects, and their safety, particularly in the elderly, has been questioned.[7,8] Studies suggest that individual topical beta blockers are probably equally effective in reducing intra-ocular pressure but if a nonselective beta blocker is used an additional reduction in pressure may not be obtained with adrenaline.[9]

Parasympathomimetic miotics facilitate trabecular drainage by constricting the pupil and pulling open the trabecular meshwork. However, this can cause blurred vision and browache, especially in younger patients, and the small pupil may cause problems if central vision is already limited. Parasympathomimetic miotics also reduce uveoscleral outflow and this can cause a paradoxical increase in intra-ocular pressure in patients with a recessed anterior angle. They should not be used in the presence of inflammation as adhesions may form between the pupil and the lens (posterior synechiae). Pilocarpine is the miotic most frequently employed and is indicated in the treatment of open-angle glaucoma and other chronic glaucomas. It is often added to treatment with other drugs when further reductions in intra-ocular pressure are required. It requires frequent instillation and this may lead to problems with compliance. Carbachol is sometimes used when resistance or intolerance to pilocarpine develops. Physostigmine is more potent than pilocarpine but is poorly tolerated and is rarely used now; it was used with pilocarpine but rarely alone. Stronger or longer-acting anticholinesterase miotics such as demecarium and ecothiopate can cause pupillary block and induce angle-closure glaucoma. They are usually only used in patients refractory to other antiglaucoma treatment or in those in whom the lens of the eye has been removed (aphakic patients). Pilocarpine is also used in the emergency treatment of angle-closure glaucoma before surgery or laser therapy.

Sympathomimetics such as adrenaline or dipivefrine increase outflow of aqueous humour through the trabecular meshwork and the uveoscleral route and may also reduce its rate of production. They are used in open-angle glaucoma and other chronic glaucomas usually when further reductions in intra-ocular pressure are required in patients receiving beta blockers (but may not produce an additive effect if used with a nonselective beta blocker).[9] As they produce pupillary dilatation they can induce an acute attack if used in angle-closure glaucoma. Adrenaline can cause eye irritation and produce systemic effects. Dipivefrine is converted into adrenaline by corneal esterases and ocular adverse effects are usually less than with adrenaline itself.

Carbonic anhydrase inhibitors such as acetazolamide, reduce production of aqueous humour by a mechanism independent of their diuretic action. They are used as part of the emergency treatment of angle-closure glaucoma to produce a rapid reduction in intra-ocular pressure before surgery or laser therapy. They are also added to treatment in open-angle glaucoma and other chronic glaucomas in patients refractory to treatment with beta blockers, sympathomimetics, and short-acting miotics, but many patients are unable to tolerate prolonged therapy when they are given systemically. More recently introduced topical carbonic anhydrase inhibitors, such as dorzolamide, have a lower potential to produce adverse effects. Dorzolamide is used similarly to other topical drugs either alone or as an adjunct in patients resistant to or intolerant of beta blockers.

Osmotic diuretics reduce vitreous volume and can produce a marked reduction in intra-ocular pressure. They are used in the short-term management of glaucoma when a rapid reduction in intra-ocular pressure is required before surgery. Mannitol and urea are both given intravenously and have a faster onset than glycerol or isosorbide given orally.

Several other drugs are used topically in glaucoma and ocular hypertension. Guanethidine reduces aqueous secretion and is used either alone or in combination to enhance and prolong the effect of adrenaline; prolonged use can cause fibrosis and corneal changes. More recent introductions include apraclonidine, brimonidine, and latanoprost. Apraclonidine is an alpha$_2$-adrenoceptor agonist derivative of clonidine which lowers intra-ocular pressure by reducing production of aqueous humour. It is used alone or as an adjunct to other drugs in the control of intra-ocular pressure associated with ocular surgery or in the short-term to delay laser treatment or surgery for patients with glaucoma not adequately controlled with other drugs; tachyphylaxis and ocular irritation limit its long-term use. Brimonidine is another alpha$_2$-adrenoceptor agonist used similarly. Latanoprost is a prostaglandin $F_{2\alpha}$ analogue which is effective when used topically once a day and is currently indicated for use in patients intolerant of or not adequately controlled by other drugs. It lowers intra-ocular pressure by increasing uveoscleral outflow. It appears to be well-tolerated but may cause a potentially irreversible increase in brown pigmentation of the iris; the long-term significance of this effect is unknown. Similar drugs used in some countries include the alpha-adrenergic agonist clonidine, the alpha-adrenergic antagonist dapiprazole, and the prostaglandin $F_{2\alpha}$ analogue unoprostone.

DIAGNOSIS OF GLAUCOMA. *Open-angle glaucoma* is asymptomatic in its early stages and the use of screening methods for detecting early disease is of great importance. Measurement of intra-ocular pressure alone is a poor diagnostic tool and a combination of direct examination of the optic nerve together with visual field examination and intra-ocular pressure tonometry is considered to be more reliable.[4] Provocative tests such as placing the patient prone in a dark room are sometimes used to identify eyes suffering from or at risk of angle-closure glaucoma. Short-acting mydriatics have also been used but are not without risk. Long-term follow-up of patients whose treatment had been determined by the use of a provocative test using phenylephrine with pilocarpine has suggested that this test is neither sensitive nor specific.[10]

TREATMENT OF GLAUCOMA. *Open-angle glaucoma* is frequently treated first with a topical beta blocker. Adrenaline and a miotic such as pilocarpine are then added as necessary to control intra-ocular pressure. Other drugs such as a topical carbonic anhydrase inhibitor may also be required. It has been suggested that each type of drug should be tried alone first before resorting to combination therapy. If further reduction of intra-ocular pressure is required a systemic carbonic anhydrase inhibitor may be used but long-term treatment is poorly tolerated. If this is unsuccessful, surgery (trabeculectomy) or laser treatment (trabeculoplasty) is usually indicated. Laser treatment appears to be as effective as topical drug therapy[11] although its effects may be short-lived.[12] It has been suggested that it might be of use in the initial treatment of older patients who cannot use eye drops or when surgery needs to be postponed or is contra-indicated.[4] However, the early use of surgery is now often advocated in Europe, especially for younger patients, although this is still a subject of debate in the USA. Some consider that there is an unnecessary risk of continuing visual loss while drug treatment is being evaluated, and they advocate surgery as the primary treatment.[13] The earlier use of surgical intervention is supported by evidence that long-term drug therapy[14] or laser treatment[4] may have a deleterious effect on the outcome of subsequent surgery and by evidence that surgery is more effective than drug or laser treatment in producing long-term intra-ocular pressure control.[12]

It is essential to start treatment for an *acute attack of angle-closure glaucoma* within 24 to 48 hours. If treatment is delayed adhesions may form between the iris and the cornea (peripheral anterior synechiae) and the trabecular meshwork may be damaged. *Chronic angle-closure glaucoma* may then develop with permanently raised intra-ocular pressure which ultimately leads to total loss of vision (absolute glaucoma). The initial treatment aims to produce a rapid reduction in intra-ocular pressure. A miotic such as pilocarpine is used topically to constrict the pupil while a carbonic anhydrase inhibitor such as acetazolamide is given by mouth or by intravenous injection. Osmotic diuretics such as mannitol or urea given intravenously or glycerol or isosorbide given orally may also be used. When intra-ocular pressure has been reduced sufficiently, laser therapy or surgery is performed on both eyes to increase drainage of aqueous humour. If further topical treatment is required after surgery, treatment is usually as for open-angle glaucoma. Beta blockers, with or without adrenaline, are preferred to pilocarpine as there is a risk of posterior synechiae forming when pilocarpine is used.

Glaucoma filtering surgery such as trabeculectomy can be highly effective in reducing intra-ocular pressure, but in some groups of patients, such as children, Afro-Caribbeans, or those who have had previous ocular surgery, there is a high failure rate, usually due to formation of scar tissue.[15] The scar formation is associated with proliferation of fibroblasts and the subconjunctival injection of antiproliferative drugs such as fluorouracil has been shown to reduce the failure rate of surgery but at a cost of increased epithelial toxicity and conjunctival wound leaks.[15] A study group[16] reporting on the long-term follow-up of patients treated with fluorouracil recommended that fluorouracil should still be used in the surgical management of glaucoma in patients with a history of ocular surgery, but in view of the increased incidence of late-onset conjunctival wound leaks, suggested caution in its use in eyes with good prognoses at the dosage they employed. The use of a single intraoperative topical application of mitomycin has been investigated as an alternative to the regimen of multiple injections required with fluorouracil. Rates of success comparable with those for fluorouracil have been achieved but a plea for caution has been made[17] over the risk of adverse effects that could affect vision and the need to determine long-term safety of antiproliferative drugs. Other drugs are also being studied as antiproliferative agents. Whether the use of antiproliferative drugs is of benefit to all patients undergoing glaucoma surgery is under study.[7]

Postoperative ocular hypertension may occur following surgery on the anterior chamber of the eye or procedures such as trabeculoplasty. Acetylcholine or carbachol instilled directly into the anterior chamber of the eye (intracameral instillation) are used intra-operatively to reduce early postoperative rises in intra-ocular pressure in procedures such as cataract extraction. The short action of acetylcholine can be an advantage as prolonged miosis is associated with severe postoperative pain. However, some consider carbachol to be the more effective drug;[18,19] standard antiglaucoma drugs including beta blockers, pilocarpine, apraclonidine, and carbonic anhydrase inhibitors have also been used for prophylaxis of postoperative ocular hypertension.

1. Hurvitz LM, *et al.* New developments in the drug treatment of glaucoma. *Drugs* 1991; **41:** 514–32.
2. Quigley HA. Open-angle glaucoma. *N Engl J Med* 1993; **328:** 1097–1106.
3. Liesegang TJ. Glaucoma: changing concepts and future directions. *Mayo Clin Proc* 1996; **71:** 689–94.
4. Anonymous. The management of primary open angle glaucoma. *Drug Ther Bull* 1997; **35:** 4–6.
5. Rossetti L, *et al.* Randomized clinical trials on medical treatment of glaucoma: are they appropriate to guide clinical practice? *Arch Ophthalmol* 1993; **111:** 96–103.
6. Taniguchi T, Kitazawa Y. A risk-benefit assessment of drugs used in the management of glaucoma. *Drug Safety* 1994; **11:** 68–74.
7. Diggory P, Franks W. Medical treatment of glaucoma—a reappraisal of the risks. *Br J Ophthalmol* 1996; **80:** 85–9.
8. O'Donoghue E. β Blockers and the elderly with glaucoma: are we adding insult to injury? *Br J Ophthalmol* 1995; **79:** 794–6.
9. Sorensen SJ, Abel SR. Comparison of the ocular beta-blockers. *Ann Pharmacother* 1996; **30:** 43–54.
10. Wishart PK. Does the pilocarpine phenylephrine provocative test help in the management of acute and subacute angle closure glaucoma? *Br J Ophthalmol* 1991; **75:** 284–7.
11. Glaucoma Laser Trial Research Group. The glaucoma laser trial (GLT) and glaucoma laser trial follow-up study: 7. results. *Am J Ophthalmol* 1995; **120:** 718–31.
12. Migdal C, *et al.* Long-term functional outcome after early surgery compared with laser and medicine in open-angle glaucoma. *Ophthalmology* 1994; **101:** 1651–7.
13. Hitchings RA. Primary surgery for primary open angle glaucoma—justified or not? *Br J Ophthalmol* 1993; **77:** 445–8.
14. Broadway D, *et al.* Adverse effects of topical antiglaucomatous medications on the conjunctiva. *Br J Ophthalmol* 1993; **77:** 590–6.
15. Khaw PT, *et al.* 5-Fluorouracil and beyond. *Br J Ophthalmol* 1991; **75:** 577–8.
16. The Fluorouracil Filtering Surgery Study Group. Five-year follow-up of the Fluorouracil Filtering Surgery Study. *Am J Ophthalmol* 1996; **121:** 349–66.
17. Khaw PT. Antiproliferative agents and the prevention of scarring after surgery: friend or foe? *Br J Ophthalmol* 1995; **79:** 627.
18. Ruiz RS, *et al.* Effects of carbachol and acetylcholine on intraocular pressure after cataract extraction. *Am J Ophthalmol* 1989; **107:** 7–10.
19. Hollands RH, *et al.* Control of intraocular pressure after cataract extraction. *Can J Ophthalmol* 1990; **25:** 128–32.

Myasthenia gravis

The pathogenesis of myasthenia gravis and its management have been reviewed.[1-5] The disorder is characterised by defective neuromuscular transmission and consequent muscular weakness due to formation of auto-antibodies to acetylcholine receptors. The thymus appears to be involved in many patients and some have a thymoma. There appear to be several types of myasthenia and a number of classifications have been proposed. Classifications based on the distribution and severity of symptoms include ocular myasthenia, where the disease is clinically confined to the extra-ocular muscles and mild or moderate generalised myasthenia, also affecting muscles other than the extra-ocular muscles; acute fulminating myasthenia; and late severe myasthenia. Another classification, based on the age of onset and the presence, or absence of thymoma, divides patients into those with thymoma; those without thymoma and onset before age of 40; and those without thymoma and onset after 40 years of age. Other types of myasthenia include transient neonatal myasthenia, which may persist for 1 to 6 weeks in the infants of myasthenic mothers due to transplacental passage of receptor antibodies, penicillamine-induced myasthenia, and congenital myasthenia (see under 3,4-Diaminopyridine, p.1390).

DIAGNOSIS OF MYASTHENIA GRAVIS. Although all patients have circulating antibodies to acetylcholine receptors they are undetectable by radioimmunoassay in about 15% of patients who are described as having seronegative myasthenia. Patients may often be tested first for their reaction to an anticholinesterase. Intravenous edrophonium preceded by atropine (Tensilon test) is the most commonly used anticholinesterase test because of its rapid onset and short duration of action. However severe adverse effects can occasionally occur so testing should only be undertaken when facilities for endotracheal intubation and controlled ventilation are immediately available. A positive result is considered to be a rapid but temporary increase in muscle strength. Repetitive nerve stimulation is also used as a diagnostic test but, like the anticholinesterase test, is not specific for myasthenia gravis.

TREATMENT OF MYASTHENIA GRAVIS. Symptomatic treatment is with an anticholinesterase; pyridostigmine and neostigmine are those most commonly used. Most patients prefer pyridostigmine as it produces less muscarinic adverse effects and has a longer duration of action, although the quicker onset of action of neostigmine may offer an advantage at the beginning of the day. The dose must be adjusted to give the optimum therapeutic response but muscle strength may not be restored to normal and some patients must live with a degree of disability. The effect may vary for different muscles and the dosage should be adjusted so that the bulbar and respiratory muscles receive optimum treatment. Edrophonium may be employed to establish whether the patient is underdosed or overdosed.

Corticosteroids are the main immunosuppressive drugs used and are indicated for patients who are seriously ill prior to thymectomy, for those unsuitable for thymectomy (see below), and for those who are insufficiently improved postoperatively. They are also useful in patients with ocular myasthenia, who as a group respond poorly to anticholinesterases and to thymectomy, provided that their disability is severe enough to warrant long-term corticosteroid treatment with its attendant side-effects. Various dosage regimens appear to be in use. Some start with low doses such as 5 to 20 mg of prednisolone daily (or on alternate days to reduce the risk of steroid-induced exacerbations of weakness) and increase the dose slowly thereafter according to response; an improvement is usually seen after a few weeks. Others use more aggressive regimens to obtain a more rapid response and start with large doses such as 60 to 100 mg of prednisolone daily. Whichever method is used, once clinical benefit has been obtained the regimen should be modified to administration on alternate days with the dose being slowly tapered when the patient is in remission. It should be remembered that patients receiving corticosteroids require less anticholinesterase therapy and, if the dosage of the anticholinesterase is not reduced, an initial deterioration in the myasthenia may occur in the first few weeks of treatment (see also under Interactions of Neostigmine, p.1394). In the majority of patients it is not usually possible to withdraw corticosteroids completely but some patients may be maintained satisfactorily on as little as 10 mg on alternate days. If remission cannot be maintained on low-dose prednisolone, addition of azathioprine at a dosage of 2 to 3 mg per kg body-weight daily may be considered. Addition of azathioprine to treatment may allow a reduction in the dose of both corticosteroids and anticholinesterases. Azathioprine may also be of use when corticosteroids are contra-indicated or when response to corticosteroids alone is insufficient, but since it has a much slower onset of action than corticosteroids it is not usually used alone. Cyclosporin has been effective in some patients unresponsive to anticholinesterases and corticosteroids but serious adverse effects including nephrotoxicity may limit its use; the time to response is similar to that with corticosteroids. Other drugs such as cyclophosphamide and methotrexate have also been tried.

Plasma exchange provides a dramatic but short-lived improvement and is useful as a short-term measure in myasthenic crisis to improve ill patients while other therapies take effect, but there is no evidence that repeated plasma exchange combined with immunosuppression is superior to immunosuppression alone.

Thymectomy may be offered to all patients sufficiently fit to undergo surgery unless they have minimal symptoms, purely ocular disease, or late onset or seronegative disease. Thymectomy is usually avoided in prepubertal children because of concern over the effect on growth and the development of the immune system and it has been suggested that symptomatic treatment with anticholinesterases should be continued until adolescence, when the disease often improves spontaneously. Following thymectomy, remission or improvement may be expected in about 80% of patients without thymomas, although this may take some years; the response is poorer in those with thymomas.

Other forms of treatment, such as high-dose intravenous normal immunoglobulins are mostly nonspecific and have generally been used only in patients refractory to all other treatment.

1. Havard CWH, Fonseca V. New treatment approaches to myasthenia gravis. *Drugs* 1990; **39:** 66–73.
2. Keys PA, Blume RP. Therapeutic strategies for myasthenia gravis. *DICP Ann Pharmacother* 1991; **25:** 1101–8.
3. Newsom-Davis J. Myasthenia gravis and the Lambert-Eaton myasthenic syndrome. *Prescribers' J* 1993; **33:** 205–12.
4. Drachman DB. Myasthenia gravis. *N Engl J Med* 1994; **330:** 1797–1810.
5. Evoli A, *et al.* A practical guide to the recognition and management of myasthenia gravis. *Drugs* 1996; **52:** 662–70.

Reversal of mydriasis

Topical miotics (mydriolytics) are sometimes used to reverse the effects of mydriatics following surgery or ophthalmoscopic examination but do not appear to be in routine clinical use. Pilocarpine can counteract the mydriatic effect of topical sympathomimetics, such as phenylephrine and hydroxyamphetamine, but is ineffective against mydriasis produced by antimuscarinics, such as homatropine, and may impair vision further when used with tropicamide. Furthermore, there is also the risk that pilocarpine might precipitate angle-closure glaucoma in susceptible patents. Dapiprazole appears to be safer than pilocarpine when used to reverse sympathomimetic-induced mydriasis and is effective to some degree against tropicamide-induced mydriasis. It also appears to enhance recovery of accommodation after the use of cycloplegics.

The rate of reversal of mydriasis is generally slower in patients with dark irides than in those with lighter irides.

Strabismus

Strabismus, sometimes referred to as a squint or cast, is a lack of coordination of the visual axes of the eyes so that the eyes are usually either turned towards (convergent strabismus) or away (divergent strabismus) from each other. It can arise from a physical defect of the attachment of the extra-ocular muscles to the eye or from paralysis, spasms, or overactivity affecting the extra-ocular muscles of one of the eyes. In young children strabismus or other conditions which prevent a clear image being formed on the retina can result in visual impairment (amblyopia) in the affected eye if not treated.

Treatment for strabismus often consists of eye exercises, and methods to force preferential use of the affected eye by restricting vision through the healthy eye. This is accomplished either by using an eye patch or by penalisation with glasses or the cycloplegic drug atropine. However, as prolonged use of atropine eye drops may be required there is a risk of systemic toxicity. Surgery may sometimes be necessary. Extra-ocular injection of botulinum A toxin has been used to weaken an overactive extra-ocular eye muscle as an aid to eye realignment; repeated injections may be required. Long-acting parasympathomimetic miotics such as demecarium, dyflos, and ecothiopate have been used in the diagnosis and management of convergent strabismus (esotropia) due to excessive accommodation. With any form of treatment care has to be taken not to induce amblyopia in the healthy eye.

Aceclidine Hydrochloride (4503-d)

Aceclidine Hydrochloride *(rINNM)*.

3-Acetoxyquinuclidine hydrochloride; 3-Quinuclidinyl acetate hydrochloride.

$C_9H_{15}NO_2,HCl$ = 205.7.

CAS — 827-61-2 (aceclidine); 6109-70-2 (aceclidine hydrochloride).

NOTE. Aceclidine is *USAN*.

Adverse Effects, Treatment, and Precautions

As for Neostigmine, p.1394. For adverse effects and precautions of miotics, see also Pilocarpine, p.1397.

Uses and Administration

Aceclidine hydrochloride is a parasympathomimetic miotic which is a cholinergic agonist. It is used in eye drops to lower intra-ocular pressure in patients with glaucoma (p.1387).

Preparations

Proprietary Preparations (details are given in Part 3)
Belg.: Glaucocare; ***Fr.:*** Glaucostat; ***Ger.:*** Glaucotat; ***Ital.:*** Glaunorm; ***Neth.:*** Glaucocare; ***Spain:*** Glaucostat; ***Switz.:*** Glaucostat.

Multi-ingredient: ***Belg.:*** Glaucofrin; ***Fr.:*** Glaucadrine; ***Ger.:*** Glaucadrin†; ***Neth.:*** Glaucofrin; ***Switz.:*** Glaucadrine.

Acetylcholine Chloride (4506-m)

Acetylcholine Chloride *(BAN, rINN)*.

Acetylcholini Chloridum. (2-Acetoxyethyl)trimethylammonium chloride.

$C_7H_{16}ClNO_2$ = 181.7.

CAS — 51-84-3 (acetylcholine); 60-31-1 (acetylcholine chloride).

Pharmacopoeias. In *Aust., Belg., Swiss,* and *US.*

Jpn includes Acetylcholine Chloride for Injection.

White or off-white crystals or crystalline powder. Very **soluble** in water; freely soluble in alcohol; practically insoluble in ether. Aqueous solutions of acetylcholine chloride are unstable and should be prepared immediately before use. **Incompatible** with alkalis. **Store** in airtight containers.

Adverse Effects

Because it is rapidly hydrolysed in the body by cholinesterases the toxicity of acetylcholine is normally relatively low.

Adverse effects of the choline esters include nausea and vomiting, abdominal pain, flushing, sweating, salivation, lachrymation, rhinorrhoea, eructation, diarrhoea, urinary frequency, headache, difficulty in visual accommodation, bradycardia, peripheral vasodilatation leading to hypotension, and bronchoconstriction.

Treatment of Adverse Effects

Atropine sulphate may be given intravenously, intramuscularly, or subcutaneously to control the muscarinic effects of the choline esters. Supportive treatment may be required.

Precautions

Choline esters are contra-indicated in intestinal or urinary obstruction or where increased muscular activity of the urinary or gastro-intestinal tract is liable to be harmful. They are also contra-indicated in asthma and obstructive airways disease, in cardiovascular disorders including bradycardia or heart block and recent myocardial infarction, and in hypotension, vagotonia, epilepsy, parkinsonism, hyperthyroidism, peptic ulceration, and pregnancy.

Interactions

As for Neostigmine, p.1394. Acetylcholine is hydrolysed in the body by cholinesterase and its effects are markedly prolonged and enhanced by prior administration of anticholinesterases.

Beta blockers. A report[1] of severe bronchospasm with subsequent pulmonary oedema following intra-ocular injection of acetylcholine chloride in a patient also receiving metoprolol by mouth.

1. Rasch D, *et al.* Bronchospasm following intraocular injection of acetylcholine in a patient taking metoprolol. *Anesthesiology* 1983; **59:** 583–5.

NSAIDs. According to a manufacturer of acetylcholine chloride ophthalmic preparations there have been reports of acetylcholine and carbachol being ineffective when used in patients treated with topical (ophthalmic) NSAIDs.

Uses and Administration

Acetylcholine is an endogenous chemical transmitter with a very wide range of actions in the body; it is a powerful quaternary ammonium parasympathomimetic but its action is transient as it is rapidly destroyed by cholinesterase. It is released from postganglionic parasympathetic nerves and also from some postganglionic sympathetic nerves to produce peripheral actions which correspond to those of muscarine. It is accordingly a vasodilator and cardiac depressant, a stimulant of the vagus and the parasympathetic nervous system, and it has a tonic action on smooth muscle. It also increases lachrymal, salivary, and other secretions. All the muscarinic actions of acetylcholine are abolished by atropine.

Acetylcholine also has actions which correspond to those of nicotine and is accordingly a stimulant of skeletal muscle, the autonomic ganglia, and the adrenal medulla. The nicotinic actions of acetylcholine on skeletal muscle are blocked by competitive neuromuscular blockers; they are also inhibited by massive administration or discharge of acetylcholine itself which has clinical application in relation to the mode of action of suxamethonium (p.1321).

Acetylcholine chloride is used as a miotic to reduce postoperative rises in intra-ocular pressure associated with cataract surgery, penetrating keratoplasty, iridectomy, and other anterior segment surgery (see p.1387) but is ineffective when applied topically as it is hydrolysed more rapidly than it can penetrate the cornea. Doses of 0.5 to 2 mL of a freshly prepared 1% solution of acetylcholine chloride are therefore instilled directly into the anterior chamber of the eye (intracameral instillation). Miosis occurs within seconds and lasts for about 20 minutes.

Diagnosis and testing. AUTONOMIC FAILURE. Acetylcholine has been used in a sweat-spot test for autonomic neuropathy in diabetic patients.[1] An area on the dorsum of the foot is painted with iodine and starch, followed by intradermal injection of acetylcholine into the centre of the area. Sweat produced in response to acetylcholine reacts with the iodine and starch to produce fine black dots corresponding to the pores of the sweat glands; a normal response is indicated by a uniform distribution of dark spots whereas in diabetic autonomic neuropathy this pattern is lost to a varying degree. A similar test has been carried out[2] to assess sympathetic nerve function and therefore predict the success of lumbar sympathectomy in patients with critical limb ischaemia.

1. Ryder REJ, *et al.* Acetylcholine sweatspot test for autonomic denervation. *Lancet* 1988; **i:** 1303–1305.
2. Altomare DF. Acetylcholine sweat test: an effective way to select patients for lumbar sympathectomy. *Lancet* 1994; **344:** 976–8.

Preparations

USP 23: Acetylcholine Chloride for Ophthalmic Solution.

Proprietary Preparations (details are given in Part 3)
Austral.: Miochol; ***Belg.:*** Miochol; ***Canad.:*** Miochol; ***Ger.:*** Miochol-E; ***Ital.:*** Miochol-E; Miovisin; ***Neth.:*** Miochol†; ***S.Afr.:*** Covochol; Miochol-3; ***Swed.:*** Miochol; ***UK:*** Miochol; ***USA:*** Miochol.

Ambenonium Chloride (4507-b)

Ambenonium Chloride *(BAN, rINN)*.

Ambestigmini Chloridum; Win-8077. *N,N'*-Oxalylbis(*N*-2-aminoethyl-*N*-2-chlorobenzyldiethylammonium) dichloride.

$C_{28}H_{42}Cl_4N_4O_2$ = 608.5.

CAS — 7648-98-8 (ambenonium); 115-79-7 (anhydrous ambenonium chloride); 52022-31-8 (ambenonium chloride tetrahydrate).

Pharmacopoeias. In *Jpn.*

Adverse Effects, Treatment, and Precautions

As for Neostigmine, p.1394.

It produces fewer muscarinic side-effects than neostigmine. As there is only slight warning of overdosage, routine administration of atropine with ambenonium is contra-indicated because the muscarinic symptoms of overdosage may be suppressed leaving only the more serious nicotinic effects (fasciculation and paralysis of voluntary muscle).

Pharmacokinetics

Ambenonium chloride is poorly absorbed from the gastro-intestinal tract. It does not appear to be hydrolysed by cholinesterases.

Uses and Administration

Ambenonium is a quaternary ammonium compound which is a reversible inhibitor of cholinesterase activity with actions similar to those of neostigmine (p.1394), but of longer duration. Ambenonium chloride is given by mouth in the treatment of myasthenia gravis (p.1388) and may be of value in patients who cannot tolerate neostigmine or pyridostigmine. It is administered 3 or 4 times daily, usually in doses of 5 to 25 mg, adjusted according to individual response.

Preparations

Proprietary Preparations (details are given in Part 3)
Fr.: Mytelase; ***Swed.:*** Mytelase; ***USA:*** Mytelase.

Bethanechol Chloride (4509-g)

Bethanechol Chloride *(BAN)*.

Carbamylmethylcholine Chloride. (2-Carbamoyloxypropyl)trimethylammonium chloride.

$C_7H_{17}ClN_2O_2$ = 196.7.

CAS — 674-38-4 (bethanechol); 590-63-6 (bethanechol chloride).

Pharmacopoeias. In *Jpn* and *US.*

Colourless or white hygroscopic crystals or white crystalline powder usually having a slight amine-like odour. There are two crystalline forms.

Freely **soluble** in water and in alcohol; practically insoluble in chloroform and in ether. A 1% solution in water has a pH of 5.5 to 6.5. The manufacturers state that solutions of bethanechol chloride may be autoclaved at 120° for 20 minutes without discoloration or loss of potency. **Store** in airtight containers.

Stability. References to the stability of oral liquid preparations of bethanechol chloride prepared extemporaneously from tablets.

1. Schlatter JL, Saulnier J-L. Bethanechol chloride oral solutions: stability and use in infants. *Ann Pharmacother* 1997; **31:** 294–6.
2. Allen LV, Erickson MA. Stability of bethanechol chloride, pyrazinamide, quinidine sulfate, rifampin, and tetracycline hydrochloride in extemporaneously compounded oral liquids. *Am J Health-Syst Pharm* 1998; **55:** 1804–9.

Adverse Effects and Treatment

As described for choline esters under Acetylcholine Chloride, p.1389.

Precautions

As described for choline esters under Acetylcholine Chloride, p.1389.

Bethanechol should not be given by the intravenous or intramuscular routes as very severe muscarinic adverse effects are liable to occur, calling for emergency administration of atropine.

Autonomic neuropathy. Patients with autonomic neuropathy might be more susceptible to the adverse effects of bethanechol and they should be started on low-dosage regimens and observed closely for signs of toxicity.[1]

1. Caraco Y, *et al.* Bethanechol-induced cholinergic toxicity in diabetic neuropathy. *DICP Ann Pharmacother* 1990; **24:** 327–8.

Interactions

As for Neostigmine, p.1394.

Pharmacokinetics

Bethanechol chloride is poorly absorbed from the gastro-intestinal tract. It is not hydrolysed by cholinesterases. The UK manufacturer has stated that at standard doses bethanechol does not cross the blood-brain barrier.

Uses and Administration

Bethanechol chloride, a choline ester, is a quaternary ammonium parasympathomimetic which has predominantly the muscarinic actions of acetylcholine (p.1389). It is not inactivated by cholinesterases so that its actions are more prolonged than those of acetylcholine. Bethanechol chloride has little if any nicotinic activity and is used for its actions on the bladder and gastro-intestinal tract. It is used as an alternative to catheterisation in the treatment of urinary retention and has also been used for gastric atony and retention, abdominal distension following surgery, congenital megacolon, and gastro-oesophageal reflux disease.

It is given, usually in doses of 5 mg subcutaneously or 10 to 50 mg by mouth, both up to 4 times daily, but dosage must be adjusted individually. Oral doses should be taken on an empty stomach. The effects usually occur within 5 to 15 minutes of a subcutaneous dose, or 30 to 90 minutes of an oral dose, and disappear within about 1 to 2 hours depending on the dose and route of administration used. For a warning to avoid intravenous or intramuscular administration, see under Precautions, above.

Decreased gastro-intestinal motility. Parasympathomimetics such as bethanechol enhance gastric contractions and increase intestinal motility and form just one of many treatments that have been used in conditions associated with decreased gastro-intestinal motility (p.1168).

References.

1. Malagelada J-R, *et al.* Gastric motor abnormalities in diabetic and postvagotomy gastroparesis: effect of metoclopramide and bethanechol. *Gastroenterology* 1980; **78:** 286–93.

Gastro-oesophageal reflux disease. The management of gastro-oesophageal reflux disease is discussed on p.1170. Prokinetic drugs such as bethanechol have been tried but their value is not clear; treatment is more usually with a proton pump inhibitor or histamine H_2-receptor antagonist.

References.

1. Saco LS, *et al.* Double-blind controlled trial of bethanechol and antacid versus placebo and antacid in the treatment of erosive esophagitis. *Gastroenterology* 1982; **82:** 1369–73.
2. Thanick KD, *et al.* Reflux esophagitis: effect of oral bethanechol on symptoms and endoscopic findings. *Ann Intern Med* 1980; **93:** 805–8.
3. Thanick K, *et al.* Bethanechol or cimetidine in the treatment of symptomatic reflux esophagitis: a double-blind control study. *Arch Intern Med* 1982; **142:** 1479–81.
4. Strickland AD, Chang JHT. Results of treatment of gastroesophageal reflux with bethanechol. *J Pediatr* 1983; **103:** 311–15.

Reversal of antimuscarinic effects. Bethanechol chloride has been given by mouth to alleviate antimuscarinic side-effects of tricyclic antidepressants, including dry mouth due to salivary gland inhibition, bladder inhibition, and constipation.[1,2]

1. Everett HC. The use of bethanechol chloride with tricyclic antidepressants. *Am J Psychiatry* 1975; **132:** 1202–4.
2. Everett HC. Dry mouth and delayed dissolution of nitroglycerin. *N Engl J Med* 1984; **310:** 1122.

Stuttering. A double-blind placebo-controlled study[1] in 10 patients with stuttering (p.674) on the whole failed to confirm an earlier report[2] of benefit using bethanechol although 2 patients who did respond elected to continue treatment after the study.

1. Kampman K, Brady JP. Bethanechol in the treatment of stuttering. *J Clin Psychopharmacol* 1993; **13:** 284–5.
2. Hays P. Bethanechol chloride in treatment of stuttering. *Lancet* 1987; **i:** 271.

Urinary incontinence and retention. Patients with overflow incontinence may suffer from a continuous dribbling of urine as a consequence of an overdistended bladder produced by urinary retention. This may result from reduced detrusor contraction. Bethanechol is one of the parasympathomimetics that have been given to increase detrusor activity, but there have been doubts about the effectiveness of such treatment (see p.454). Bethanechol was also one of the parasympathomimetics used in the management of postoperative urinary retention but they have generally been superseded by catheterisation.

References.

1. Finkbeiner AE. Is bethanechol chloride clinically effective in promoting bladder emptying: a literature review. *J Urol (Baltimore)* 1985; **134:** 443–9.

Preparations

USP 23: Bethanechol Chloride Injection; Bethanechol Chloride Tablets.

Proprietary Preparations (details are given in Part 3)
Aust.: Myocholine; ***Austral.:*** Urecholine; Urocarb; ***Belg.:*** Muscaran; ***Canad.:*** Duvoid; Myotonachol; Urecholine; ***Ger.:*** Myocholine; ***Ital.:*** Urecholine; ***S.Afr.:*** Urecholine; ***Spain:*** Myo Hermes; ***Switz.:*** Myocholine; ***UK:*** Myotonine; ***USA:*** Duvoid; Myotonachol; Urecholine.

Carbachol (4511-d)

Carbachol *(BAN, rINN)*.

Carbach.; Carbacholine; Carbacholum; Carbacholum Chloratum; Choline Chloride Carbamate. *O*-Carbamoylcholine chloride; (2-Carbamoyloxyethyl)trimethylammonium chloride.

$C_6H_{15}ClN_2O_2$ = 182.6.

CAS — 51-83-2.

NOTE. CAR is a code approved by the BP for use on single unit doses of eye drops containing carbachol where the individual container may be too small to bear all the appropriate labelling information.

Pharmacopoeias. In *Aust., It., Pol., Swiss,* and *US.*

Store in airtight containers.

Incompatibility. Chlorocresol (0.025 to 0.1%) and chlorbutol (0.5%) were both found to be incompatible with a solution of carbachol (0.8%) and sodium chloride (0.69%), very slight precipitates forming on heating and increasing on standing.[1]

1. *PSGB Lab Report No.911* 1962.

Adverse Effects and Treatment

As described for choline esters under Acetylcholine Chloride, p.1389. Carbachol has substantial nicotinic activity which may be unmasked by the use of atropine to counteract muscarinic effects. Carbachol also produces adverse effects similar to those of other miotics such as pilocarpine (p.1397) when used in the eye but may produce more ciliary spasm than pilocarpine.

Effects on the gastro-intestinal tract. A report[1] of fatal oesophageal rupture following subcutaneous injection of carbachol to relieve urinary retention.

1. Cochrane P. Spontaneous oesophageal rupture after carbachol therapy. *Br Med J* 1973; **1:** 463–4.

Overdosage. A report[1] of life-threatening attacks of profuse sweating, intestinal cramps, explosive defaecation, hypothermia, hypotension, and bradycardia in a 36-year-old man following deliberate poisoning with 30 to 40 mg of carbachol. The patient's 10-year-old son had died after poisoning with a similar dose of carbachol.

1. Sangster B, *et al.* Two cases of carbachol intoxication. *Neth J Med* 1979; **22:** 27–8.

Precautions

As described for choline esters under Acetylcholine Chloride, p.1389. For precautions when used as a miotic see under Pilocarpine, p.1397. Carbachol should not be given by the intravenous or intramuscular routes as very severe muscarinic adverse effects are liable to occur, calling for emergency treatment with atropine.

Interactions

NSAIDs. According to a manufacturer of acetylcholine chloride ophthalmic preparations there have been reports of acetylcholine and carbachol being ineffective when used in patients treated with topical (ophthalmic) NSAIDs.

Uses and Administration

Carbachol, a choline ester, is a quaternary ammonium parasympathomimetic with the muscarinic and nicotinic actions of acetylcholine (p.1389). It is not inactivated by cholinesterases so that its actions are more prolonged than those of acetylcholine.

Carbachol has a miotic action and eye drops containing 0.75 to 3% are sometimes used up to four times daily to lower intra-ocular pressure in glaucoma usually in conjunction with other miotics. Miosis occurs within 10 to 20 minutes of instillation of carbachol eye drops and lasts for 4 to 8 hours; reduction in intra-ocular pressure lasts for 8 hours.

Carbachol is also administered intra-ocularly, up to 0.5 mL of a 0.01% solution being instilled into the anterior chamber of the eye (intracameral instillation), to produce miosis in ocular surgery, and reduce postoperative rises in intra-ocular pressure. The maximum degree of miosis is usually obtained within 2 to 5 minutes of intra-ocular instillation and miosis lasts for 24 to 48 hours.

Carbachol has been used as an alternative to catheterisation in the treatment of urinary retention (p.454) in a dose of 2 mg given three times daily by mouth on a empty stomach, although catheterisation is generally preferred. For the acute symptoms of postoperative urinary retention doses of 250 μg have been given subcutaneously repeated twice if necessary at 30-minute intervals. For a warning to avoid intravenous or intramuscular administration, see under Precautions, above. Carbachol has also been used in some countries for the treatment of decreased gastro-intestinal motility (p.1168).

Dry mouth. Carbachol has been used as an alternative to pilocarpine in the treatment of radiation-induced xerostomia.[1] The overall treatment of dry mouth is discussed on p.1470.

1. Joensuu H. Treatment for post-irradiation xerostomia. *N Engl J Med* 1994; **330:** 141–2.

Glaucoma and ocular hypertension. Carbachol is sometimes used as an alternative to pilocarpine in the management of glaucoma (p.1387) when resistance or intolerance to pilocarpine develops. It is also instilled into the anterior chamber of the eye (intracameral instillation) to minimise postoperative rises in intra-ocular pressure associated with ocular surgery, and is considered by some[1,2] to be more effective than acetylcholine.

1. Ruiz RS, *et al.* Effects of carbachol and acetylcholine on intramuscular pressure after cataract extraction. *Am J Ophthalmol* 1989; **107:** 7–10.
2. Hollands RH, *et al.* Control of intraocular pressure after cataract extraction. *Can J Ophthalmol* 1990; **25:** 128–32.

Preparations

USP 23: Carbachol Intraocular Solution; Carbachol Ophthalmic Solution.

Proprietary Preparations (details are given in Part 3)
Austral.: Miostat; ***Belg.:*** Miostat; ***Canad.:*** Miostat; ***Ger.:*** Carbamann; Doryl; Jestryl; ***Neth.:*** Miostat†; ***Swed.:*** Isopto Karbakolin; ***Switz.:*** Doryl; Miostat; Spersacarbachol; ***USA:*** Carbastat; Miostat.

Multi-ingredient: ***Ital.:*** Mios; ***Spain:*** Risunal A†; Risunal B†.

Choline Alfoscerate (4848-h)

Choline Alfoscerate *(rINN)*.

Choline Glycerophosphate; L-α-Glycerylphosphorylcholine. Choline hydroxide, (*R*)-2,3-dihydroxypropyl hydrogen phosphate, inner salt.

$C_8H_{20}NO_6P$ = 257.2.

CAS — 28319-77-9.

Choline alfoscerate is reported to be a precursor of acetylcholine and has been tried in the treatment of Alzheimer's disease and other dementias (p.1386), although this type of treatment is not considered to produce useful improvement.

References.

1. Di Perri R, *et al.* A multicentre trial to evaluate the efficacy and tolerability of α-glycerylphosphorylcholine versus cytosine diphosphocholine in patients with vascular dementia. *J Int Med Res* 1991; **19:** 330–41.
2. Parnetti L *et al.* Multicentre study of l-α-glyceryl-phosphorylcholine vs ST200 among patients with probable senile dementia of Alzheimer's type. *Drugs Aging* 1993; **3:** 159–64.

Preparations

Proprietary Preparations (details are given in Part 3)
Ital.: Brezal; Delecit; Gliatilin.

Demecarium Bromide (4512-n)

Demecarium Bromide *(BAN, rINN)*.

BC-48. *N,N'*-Decamethylenebis(*N,N,N*-trimethyl-3-methylcarbamoyloxyanilinium) dibromide.

$C_{32}H_{52}Br_2N_4O_4$ = 716.6.

CAS — 56-94-0.

Pharmacopoeias. In *US.*

A white or slightly yellow, slightly hygroscopic, crystalline powder. Freely **soluble** in water and in alcohol; soluble in ether; sparingly soluble in acetone. A 1% solution in water has a pH of 5 to 7. **Store** in airtight containers. Protect from light.

Adverse Effects

As for Neostigmine, p.1394 and Ecothiopate Iodide, p.1392. For adverse effects of miotics, see also Pilocarpine, p.1397.

Treatment of Adverse Effects

As for Ecothiopate Iodide, p.1392.

Pralidoxime has been reported to be more active in counteracting the effects of dyflos and ecothiopate than of demecarium.

Precautions

As for Neostigmine, p.1394 and Ecothiopate Iodide, p.1392. For precautions of miotics, see also Pilocarpine, p.1397.

Interactions

As for Ecothiopate Iodide, p.1392.

Uses and Administration

Demecarium is a quaternary ammonium compound which is a reversible inhibitor of cholinesterase with a long duration of action similar to that of ecothiopate iodide (p.1392). Its miotic action begins within about 15 to 60 minutes of its application and may persist for a week or more. It causes a reduction in intra-ocular pressure that is maximal in 24 hours and may persist for 9 days or more.

Demecarium bromide has been used in the treatment of open-angle glaucoma (p.1387), particularly in aphakic patients and when other drugs have proved inadequate. The dosage varies, 1 or 2 drops of a 0.125% or 0.25% solution being instilled from twice weekly, preferably at bedtime, to twice daily. Demecarium bromide has also been used in the diagnosis and management of accommodative convergent strabismus (p.1389).

Preparations

USP 23: Demecarium Bromide Ophthalmic Solution.

Proprietary Preparations (details are given in Part 3)
UK: Tosmilen†; ***USA:*** Humorsol.

3,4-Diaminopyridine (19064-m)

3,4-Diaminopyridine has similar actions and uses to fampridine (p.1393) but is reported to be more potent in enhancing the release of acetylcholine from nerve terminals. It is used in the Eaton-Lambert myasthenic syndrome and other myasthenic conditions. It has been tried in multiple sclerosis and in botulism. There have been isolated reports of seizures and 3,4-diaminopyridine is therefore contra-indicated in patients with epilepsy.

Congenital myasthenia. Congenital or hereditary myasthenia is a heterogeneous group of rare disorders associated with various defects in neuromuscular transmission including presynaptic impairment of acetylcholinesterase release, postsynaptic abnormality of acetylcholine receptors, or a deficiency of acetylcholinesterase.[1] Symptoms may be similar to those of myasthenia gravis (p.1388) but there are no immunological abnormalities. Although some forms may respond to anticholinesterases, therapy is usually unsatisfactory. Experience in 16 patients[2] has suggested that 3,4-diaminopyridine used alone or with anticholinesterases may be of benefit.

1. Engel AG. Congenital myasthenic syndromes. *Neurol Clin North Am* 1994; **12:** 401–37.
2. Palace J, *et al.* 3,4-Diaminopyridine in the treatment of congenital (hereditary) myasthenia. *J Neurol Neurosurg Psychiatry* 1991; **54:** 1069–72.

Eaton-Lambert myasthenic syndrome. Administration of 3,4-diaminopyridine by mouth in daily doses of up to 100 mg has been found[1] to be effective in the treatment of both the motor and autonomic deficits of patients with Eaton-Lambert syndrome (p.1386). A usual starting dose of 10 mg given three or four times daily increasing if necessary to a maximum of 20 mg given five times daily has been used.[2] Adverse effects appear to be mainly mild and dose related.[1] Most patients experience some form of paraesthesia up to 60 minutes after administration.[1,2] 3,4-Diaminopyridine can produce mild excitatory effects and some patients may experience difficulty in sleeping.

1. McEvoy KM, *et al.* 3,4-Diaminopyridine in the treatment of Lambert-Eaton myasthenic syndrome. *N Engl J Med* 1989; **321:** 1567–71.
2. Newsom-Davis J. Myasthenia gravis and the Lambert-Eaton myasthenic syndrome. *Prescribers' J* 1993; **33:** 205–212.

Multiple sclerosis. 3,4-Diaminopyridine has been tried in the management of multiple sclerosis (p.620). In a crossover study[1] involving 36 patients with multiple sclerosis, 3,4-diaminopyridine given in a dosage of up to 100 mg daily improved symptoms of leg weakness to a greater extent than placebo but paraesthesia and abdominal pain which occurred in most patients were dose-limiting in some.

1. Bever CT, *et al.* Treatment with oral 3,4-diaminopyridine improves leg strength in multiple sclerosis patients: results of a randomized, double-blind, placebo-controlled, crossover trial. *Neurology* 1996; **47:** 1457–62.

Distigmine Bromide (4513-h)

Distigmine Bromide *(BAN, rINN).*

BC-51; Bispyridostigmine Bromide; Hexamarium Bromide. 3,3′-[N,N′-Hexamethylenebis(methylcarbamoyloxy)]bis(1-methylpyridinium bromide).

$C_{22}H_{32}Br_2N_4O_4$ = 576.3.

CAS — 15876-67-2.

Pharmacopoeias. In *Jpn.*

Adverse Effects, Treatment, and Precautions

As for Neostigmine, p.1394. The anticholinesterase action of distigmine, and hence its adverse effects, may be prolonged, and if treatment with atropine is required it should be maintained for at least 24 hours. The UK manufacturer has advised that it should be avoided in pregnancy.

Interactions

As for Neostigmine, p.1394.

Pharmacokinetics

Distigmine is poorly absorbed from the gastro-intestinal tract.

Uses and Administration

Distigmine is a quaternary ammonium compound which is a reversible inhibitor of cholinesterase activity with actions similar to those of neostigmine (p.1394) but more prolonged. Maximum inhibition of plasma cholinesterase occurs 9 hours after a single intramuscular dose, and persists for about 24 hours.

Distigmine bromide has been administered by intramuscular injection or by mouth on an empty stomach. It is one of several drugs that have been used in the prevention and treatment of postoperative gastro-intestinal atony (p.1168). It has also been used in postoperative urinary retention (p.454), although it has been superseded by catheterisation. A dose of 500 µg of distigmine bromide was injected intramuscularly about 24 to 72 hours after surgery and repeated at intervals of 1 to 3 days until normal function was restored. Alternatively it was given by mouth in a dose of 5 mg daily thirty minutes before breakfast. A similar dose by mouth, given daily or on alternate days, has been employed in the management of neurogenic bladder.

Distigmine bromide in conjunction with short-acting parasympathomimetics may also be given by mouth for the treatment of myasthenia gravis (p.1388), but patients being treated with parasympathomimetics tend to prefer pyridostigmine. The initial dose is 5 mg daily before breakfast, increased at intervals of 3 to 4 days if necessary to a maximum of 20 mg daily; children may be given up to 10 mg daily according to age.

Preparations

Proprietary Preparations (details are given in Part 3)
Aust.: Ubretid; ***Austral.:*** Ubretid†; ***Ger.:*** Ubretid; ***Irl.:*** Ubretid; ***Neth.:*** Ubretid; ***S.Afr.:*** Ubretid; ***Switz.:*** Ubretid; ***UK:*** Ubretid.

Donepezil Hydrochloride (3627-b)

Donepezil Hydrochloride *(BANM, rINNM).*

E-2020; ER-4111 (donepezil). (±)-2-[(1-Benzyl-4-piperidyl)methyl]-5,6-dimethoxy-1-indanone hydrochloride.

$C_{24}H_{29}NO_3,HCl$ = 416.0.

CAS — 120014-06-4 (donepezil); 120011-70-3 (donepezil hydrochloride).

Adverse Effects, Treatment, and Precautions

Generally as for Neostigmine, p.1394. Adverse effects of donepezil notably include nausea, vomiting, diarrhoea, fatigue, insomnia, and muscle cramps. Less frequent adverse effects reported include headache and dizziness; syncope, bradycardia, and sinoatrial and atrioventricular block have occurred rarely. Psychiatric disturbances, including hallucinations, agitation, and aggressive behaviour, have been reported. Minor increases in plasma-creatine kinase have occurred and there is potential for bladder outflow obstruction and for convulsions.

Effects of the skin. A report[1] of purpuric rash associated with donepezil.

1. Bryant CA, *et al.* Purpuric rash with donepezil treatment. *Br Med J* 1998; **317:** 787.

Interactions

As for Neostigmine, p.1394. Hepatic metabolism of donepezil via the cytochrome P450 system has been demonstrated and plasma concentrations of donepezil may be raised by drugs such as ketoconazole, itraconazole, and erythromycin that inhibit the isoenzyme CYP3A4 and by fluoxetine and quinidine which inhibit the isoenzyme CYP2D6; plasma concentrations may be reduced by enzyme inducers such as rifampicin, phenytoin, carbamazepine, and alcohol.

Pharmacokinetics

Donepezil hydrochloride is well absorbed from the gastro-intestinal tract, maximum plasma concentrations being achieved within 3 to 4 hours. It is about 95% bound to plasma proteins. Donepezil undergoes partial metabolism via the cytochrome P450 system to 4 major metabolites. About 11% of a dose is present in plasma as 6-*O*-desmethyl donepezil which has similar activity to the parent compound. Over 10 days, about 57% of a dose is recovered from the urine as unchanged drug and metabolites, and 14.5% from the faeces; 28% remains unrecovered suggesting accumulation. The elimination half-life is about 70 hours. Steady-state concentrations are achieved within 3 weeks of the start of therapy.

Uses and Administration

Donepezil hydrochloride, a piperidine derivative, is a reversible and specific inhibitor of acetylcholinesterase with actions similar to those of neostigmine (p.1394). It is highly selective for the CNS and is used for the symptomatic treatment of mild to moderately severe dementia in Alzheimer's disease. Donepezil hydrochloride is given in an initial dose of 5 mg by mouth once daily in the evening and increased if necessary after 4 to 6 weeks to a maximum of 10 mg once daily. Clinical benefit should be reassessed on a regular basis.

Alzheimer's disease. Donepezil hydrochloride is used in the symptomatic treatment of mild to moderately severe dementia in Alzheimer's disease (p.1386). It appears to produce modest benefits in some patients.[1,2] Although there are no comparative studies of donepezil and tacrine it has been suggested[3-5] that donepezil may prove preferable as it appears to be better tolerated and hepatotoxicity has not been reported to be a problem. Longer term randomised trials of donepezil were considered necessary to evaluate benefits and costs.[6] An advisory committee in the UK recommended that treatment with donepezil should be under specialist supervision, that benefit should be assessed at 12 weeks, and treatment only continued if there was evidence of benefit.[7]

1. Rogers SL, Friedhoff LT. Donepezil Study Group. The efficacy and safety of donepezil in patients with Alzheimer's disease: results of a multicentre, randomized, double-blind, placebo-controlled trial. *Dementia* 1996; **7:** 293–303.
2. Rogers SL, *et al.* A 24-week, double-blind, placebo-controlled trial of donepezil in patients with Alzheimer's disease. *Neurology* 1998; **50:** 136–45.
3. American Psychiatric Association. Practice guideline for the treatment of patients with Alzheimer's disease and other dementias of late life. *Am J Psychiatry* 1997; **154** (suppl): 1–39.
4. Shintani EY, Uchida KM. Donepezil: an anticholinesterase inhibitor for Alzheimer's disease. *Am J Health-Syst Pharm* 1997; **54:** 2805–10.
5. Barner EL, Gray SL. Donepezil use in Alzheimer disease. *Ann Pharmacother* 1998; **32:** 70–7.
6. Eccles M, *et al.* North of England evidence based guidelines development project: guideline for the primary care management of dementia. *Br Med J* 1998; **317:** 802–8.
7. Standing Medical Advisory Committee (SMAC). *The use of donepezil for Alzheimer's disease.* UK: Department of Health, May 1998.

Preparations

Proprietary Preparations (details are given in Part 3)
Irl.: Aricept; ***Ital.:*** Memac; ***Swed.:*** Aricept; ***UK:*** Aricept; ***USA:*** Aricept.

Dyflos (4514-m)

Dyflos *(BAN).*

DFP; Difluorophate; Di-isopropyl Fluorophosphate; Di-isopropylfluorophosphonate; Fluostigmine; Isoflurophate. Di-isopropyl phosphorofluoridate.

$C_6H_{14}FO_3P$ = 184.1.

CAS — 55-91-4.

Pharmacopoeias. In *US.*

A clear, colourless, or faintly yellow liquid. Specific gravity about 1.05. Sparingly **soluble** in water; soluble in alcohol and in vegetable oils. It is decomposed by moisture with the evolution of hydrogen fluoride. **Store** at 8° to 15° in sealed containers.

CAUTION. *The vapour of dyflos is very toxic. The eyes, nose, and mouth should be protected when handling dyflos, and contact with the skin should be avoided. Dyflos can be removed from the skin by washing with soap and water. Contaminated material should be immersed in a 2% aqueous solution of sodium hydroxide for several hours.*

Adverse Effects

As for Neostigmine, p.1394 and Ecothiopate Iodide, p.1392. For adverse effects of miotics, see also Pilocarpine, p.1397.

The anticholinesterase action of dyflos, and hence its adverse effects, may be prolonged. Its vapour is extremely irritating to the eye and mucous membranes.

Systemic toxicity also occurs after inhalation of the vapour. Prolonged use of dyflos in the eye may cause slowly reversible depigmentation of the lid margins in dark-skinned patients.

Treatment of Adverse Effects

As for Ecothiopate Iodide, p.1392.

Precautions

As for Neostigmine, p.1394 and Ecothiopate Iodide, p.1392. For precautions of miotics, see also Pilocarpine, p.1397.

Interactions

As for Ecothiopate Iodide, p.1392.

Pharmacokinetics

Dyflos is readily absorbed from the gastro-intestinal tract, from skin and mucous membranes, and from the lungs. Dyflos interacts with cholinesterases producing stable phosphonylated and phosphorylated derivatives which are then hydrolysed by phosphorylphosphatases. These products of hydrolysis are excreted mainly in the urine.

Uses and Administration

Dyflos is an irreversible inhibitor of cholinesterases with actions similar to those of ecothiopate iodide (p.1392). Dyflos has a powerful miotic action which begins within 5 to 10 minutes and may persist for up to 4 weeks; it causes a reduction in intra-ocular pressure which is maximal in 24 hours and may persist for a week.

Dyflos has been used mainly in the treatment of open-angle glaucoma (p.1387), particularly in aphakic patients and when other drugs have proved inadequate. It was also employed in the diagnosis and management of accommodative convergent strabismus (p.1389).

Dyflos is administered locally usually as a 0.025% ophthalmic ointment preferably at night before retiring.

Preparations

USP 23: Isoflurophate Ophthalmic Ointment.

Proprietary Preparations (details are given in Part 3)
USA: Floropryl.

Ecothiopate Iodide (4515-b)

Ecothiopate Iodide *(BAN, rINN)*.

Echothiophate Iodide; Ecostigmine Iodide; MI-217. (2-Diethoxyphosphinylthioethyl)trimethylammonium iodide.

$C_9H_{23}INO_3PS$ = 383.2.

CAS — 6736-03-4 (ecothiopate); 513-10-0 (ecothiopate iodide).

Pharmacopoeias. In *Jpn* and *US*.

A white crystalline hygroscopic powder with an alliaceous odour. **Soluble** 1 in 1 of water, 1 in 25 of dehydrated alcohol, and 1 in 3 of methyl alcohol; practically insoluble in other organic solvents. A solution in water has a pH of about 4. **Store** in airtight containers preferably at a temperature below 0°. Protect from light.

Adverse Effects

As for Neostigmine, p.1394. For adverse effects of miotics, see also Pilocarpine, p.1397.

Ecothiopate is an irreversible cholinesterase inhibitor; its action, and hence its adverse effects, may be prolonged.

Plasma and erythrocyte cholinesterases may be diminished by treatment with eye drops of ecothiopate, or other long-acting anticholinesterases and systemic toxicity occurs more frequently than with shorter-acting miotics. Acute iritis, retinal detachment, or precipitation of acute glaucoma may occasionally follow treatment with ecothiopate and iris cysts (especially in children) or lens opacities may develop following prolonged treatment.

Treatment of Adverse Effects

In systemic poisoning, atropine sulphate may be given parenterally with pralidoxime chloride as for intoxication with organophosphorus insecticides (see p.992); subconjunctival injection of pralidoxime has been employed to reverse severe ocular adverse effects. Supportive treatment, including assisted ventilation, should be given as necessary.

To prevent or reduce development of iris cysts in patients receiving ecothiopate eye drops, phenylephrine eye drops may be given simultaneously.

Precautions

As for Neostigmine, p.1394. For precautions of miotics, see also under Pilocarpine, p.1397. In general ecothiopate, in common with other long-acting anticholinesterases, should be used only where therapy with other drugs has proved ineffective. Ecothiopate iodide should not be used in patients with iodine hypersensitivity.

Interactions

As for Neostigmine, p.1394. Plasma and erythrocyte cholinesterases may be depressed for a considerable time after discontinuation of long-acting anticholinesterases such as ecothiopate.

Uses and Administration

Ecothiopate is an irreversible inhibitor of cholinesterase with actions similar to those of neostigmine (p.1394), but much more prolonged. Its miotic action begins within 10 to 30 minutes of its application and may persist for 1 to 4 weeks; it causes a reduction in intra-ocular pressure which is maximal after 24 hours and may persist for days or weeks.

Ecothiopate iodide is used mainly in the treatment of open-angle glaucoma (p.1387), particularly in aphakic patients and when other drugs have proved inadequate. It is administered as drops of a 0.03 to 0.25% solution. The manufacturers recommend twice daily administration to allow for diurnal variations in intra-ocular pressure, although a single dose has also been used once daily or on alternate days. It is advisable to give the single dose or one of the two daily doses at bedtime.

Ecothiopate iodide eye drops are also used in the diagnosis and management of accommodative convergent strabismus (p.1389).

Preparations

USP 23: Echothiophate Iodide for Ophthalmic Solution.

Proprietary Preparations (details are given in Part 3)
Austral.: Phospholine Iodide; ***Belg.:*** Phospholine Iodide; ***Canad.:*** Phospholine Iodide; ***Fr.:*** Phospholine Iodide; ***Ger.:*** Phospholinjodid†; ***Ital.:*** Phospholine Iodide†; ***Neth.:*** Phospholine Iodide; ***Switz.:*** Phospholine†; ***UK:*** Phospholine Iodide; ***USA:*** Phospholine Iodide.

Edrophonium Chloride (4516-v)

Edrophonium Chloride *(BAN, rINN)*.

Edrophonii Chloridum. Ethyl(3-hydroxyphenyl)dimethylammonium chloride.

$C_{10}H_{16}ClNO$ = 201.7.

CAS — 312-48-1 (edrophonium); 116-38-1 (edrophonium chloride).

Pharmacopoeias. In *Br., Int., Jpn,* and *US*.

A white odourless crystalline powder. **Soluble** 1 in 0.5 of water and 1 in 5 of alcohol; practically insoluble in chloroform and in ether. A 10% solution in water has a pH of 4 to 5. **Protect** from light.

Adverse Effects, Treatment, and Precautions

As for Neostigmine, p.1394.

Interactions

As for Neostigmine, p.1394.

Uses and Administration

Edrophonium is a quaternary ammonium compound which is a reversible inhibitor of cholinesterase activity. It has actions similar to those of neostigmine (p.1394) but its effect on skeletal muscle is claimed to be particularly prominent. Its action is rapid in onset and of short duration. In patients with myasthenia gravis, there is immediate subjective improvement and muscle strength increases. This effect usually lasts only for about 5 to 15 minutes, after which time the typical signs and symptoms return; because of its brief action the drug is not suitable for the routine treatment of myasthenia gravis.

Edrophonium chloride is used in **myasthenia gravis** (p.1388) both diagnostically and to distinguish between its under- or over-treatment with other anticholinesterases. The usual *diagnostic procedure* is to inject 2 mg intravenously and, if no adverse reaction occurs within 30 to 45 seconds, to continue with the injection of a further 8 mg. In the UK the recommended total dose for children is 100 μg per kg body-weight, one-fifth of the dose being given initially, followed 30 seconds later by the remainder if no adverse effect develops. In the USA the manufacturers suggest a total dose of 5 mg for children weighing less than 34 kg and 10 mg for heavier children with one-fifth of the dose being given initially followed by increments of 1 mg every 30 to 45 seconds; the suggested total dose for infants is 0.5 mg. When intravenous injection is difficult edrophonium may be given by intramuscular injection; the usual dose in adults is 10 mg while children below 34 kg in weight may be given 2 mg and heavier children 5 mg; infants may be given 0.5 to 1 mg intramuscularly or subcutaneously. Atropine should always be available when the test is carried out in order to treat any severe muscarinic reactions that may occur.

To *detect under- or over-treatment*, test doses of 1 to 2 mg of edrophonium chloride are given intravenously to distinguish severe symptoms of myasthenia gravis due to inadequate therapy, from the effects of overdosage with anticholinesterase drugs. If treatment has been inadequate, edrophonium chloride will produce an immediate amelioration of symptoms, whereas in cholinergic crises due to over-treatment the symptoms will be temporarily aggravated. The manufacturers suggest administration one hour after the last dose of treatment but other authorities recommend administration just before the next dose is due. It is advised that testing should only be undertaken when facilities for endotracheal intubation and controlled ventilation are immediately available.

Edrophonium chloride was originally introduced for the **reversal of neuromuscular blockade** in anaesthesia. In the UK the recommended dose for the reversal of the effects of competitive neuromuscular blockers is 500 to 700 μg per kg body-weight given by intravenous injection over several minutes either with or after atropine sulphate 0.6 mg; in the USA a dose of 10 mg of edrophonium chloride is given over 30 to 45 seconds and repeated as required up to a maximum of 40 mg. The brevity of its action limits its value. Where prolonged apnoea occurs in a patient treated with a depolarising neuromuscular blocker, such as suxamethonium, edrophonium 10 mg may be given intravenously with atropine to determine the presence of phase II block (see p.1321).

Edrophonium bromide has been used similarly to edrophonium chloride.

Reversal of neuromuscular blockade. For a discussion of whether edrophonium might be more suitable than neostigmine for reversal of residual block after the use of the shorter-acting competitive neuromuscular blockers, see under Uses and Administration of Neostigmine, p.1395.

Snake bite. For the use of anticholinesterases in the treatment of snake-bite, see under Uses and Administration of Neostigmine, p.1395.

Tetrodotoxin poisoning. Management of poisoning due to tetrodotoxin, a heat stable neuromuscular blocking toxin found in various marine animals, such as puffer fish, is mainly symptomatic and supportive. Reports[1,2] on the effectiveness of intravenous anticholinesterases such as edrophonium or neostigmine in reversing muscle weakness in tetrodotoxin poisoning have been conflicting. Although it appears that anticholinesterases may only be effective during partial block produced by tetrodotoxin some consider[3] that, as there is no specific antidote, any measure that brings about improvement may be tried.

1. Chew SK, *et al.* Anticholinesterase drugs in the treatment of tetrodotoxin poisoning. *Lancet* 1984; **ii:** 108.
2. Tibballs J. Severe tetrodotoxic fish poisoning. *Anaesth Intensive Care* 1988; **16:** 215–17.
3. Karalliedde L. Management of puffer fish poisoning. *Br J Anaesth* 1995; **75:** 500.

Preparations

BP 1998: Edrophonium Injection;
USP 23: Edrophonium Chloride Injection.

Proprietary Preparations (details are given in Part 3)
Canad.: Enlon; Tensilon; ***Irl.:*** Tensilon†; ***S.Afr.:*** Tensilon; ***Spain:*** Anticude; ***UK:*** Camsilon; ***USA:*** Enlon; Enlon-Plus; Reversol; Tensilon.

Eptastigmine (13786-l)

Eptastigmine *(rINN)*.

N-Demethyl-*N*-heptylphysostigmine. (3a*S*,8a*R*)-1,2,3,3a,8,8a-Hexahydro-1,3a,8-trimethylpyrrolo[2,3-*b*]indol-5-yl heptylcarbamate.

$C_{21}H_{33}N_3O_2$ = 359.5.

CAS — 101246-68-8.

Eptastigmine is a long-acting inhibitor of cholinesterase activity; it is a lipophilic derivative of physostigmine (p.1395). It is being studied in the oral treatment of Alzheimer's disease (p.1386) but has been reported to produce adverse haematological effects.

References.

1. Unni LK, *et al.* Kinetics of cholinesterase inhibition by eptastigmine in man. *Eur J Clin Pharmacol* 1991; **41:** 83–4.
2. Auteri A, *et al.* Pharmacodynamics and pharmacokinetics of eptastigmine in elderly subjects. *Eur J Clin Pharmacol* 1993; **45:** 373–6.
3. Imbimbo BP, *et al.* Relationship between pharmacokinetics and pharmacodynamics of eptastigmine in young healthy volunteers. *J Clin Pharmacol* 1995; **35:** 285–90.
4. Canal N, Imbimbo BP. Eptastigmine Study Group. Relationship between pharmacodynamic activity and cognitive effects of eptastigmine in patients with Alzheimer's disease. *Clin Pharmacol Ther* 1996; **60:** 218–28.
5. Canal N, *et al.* Eptastigmine Study Group. A 25-week, double-blind, randomized, placebo-controlled, trial of eptastigmine in patients with diagnosis of probable Alzheimer's disease. *Eur J Neurol* 1996; **3** (suppl 5): 238.

Eseridine Salicylate (4522-m)

Eseridine Salicylate (*rINNM*).

Eserine Aminoxide Salicylate; Eserine Oxide Salicylate; Physostigmine Aminoxide Salicylate; Physostigmine *N*-Oxide Salicylate. (4a*S*,9a*S*)-2,3,4,4a,9,9a-Hexahydro-2,4a,9-trimethyl-1,2-oxazino[6,5-*b*]indol-6-ylmethylcarbamate salicylate.

$C_{15}H_{21}N_3O_3,C_7H_6O_3$ = 429.5.

CAS — 25573-43-7 (eseridine); 5995-96-0 (eseridine salicylate).

Eseridine salicylate, a derivative of physostigmine, is an inhibitor of cholinesterase activity that has been given by mouth in preparations for dyspepsia and other gastric disorders.

References.

1. Astier A, Petitjean O. Pharmacokinetics of an anticholinesterasic agent (eserin N-oxyde) in humans after administration of two galenic forms. *J Pharmacol Clin* 1985; **4:** 521–7.

Preparations

Proprietary Preparations (details are given in Part 3)
Fr.: Geneserine.

Fampridine (12364-v)

Fampridine (*USAN, rINN*).

EL-970. 4-Aminopyridine; 4-Pyridinamine.

$C_5H_6N_2$ = 94.11.

CAS — 504-24-5.

Fampridine enhances the release of acetylcholine from nerve terminals and has been used intravenously to reverse the effects of competitive neuromuscular blockers. It has also been tried by mouth and intravenously in the management of a number of neurological disorders including Eaton-Lambert myasthenic syndrome (p.1386), multiple sclerosis (p.620), spinal cord injury, and Alzheimer's disease (p.1386), and for the reversal of neuromuscular blockade in patients with botulism (p.1506).

Fampridine has also been considered as a specific antidote in poisoning with calcium-channel blockers such as verapamil (p.961).

Adverse effects, especially seizures, may limit its use.

References.

1. Evenhuis J, *et al.* Pharmacokinetics of 4-aminopyridine in human volunteers. *Br J Anaesth* 1981; **53:** 567–9.
2. Wesseling H, *et al.* Effects of 4-aminopyridine in elderly patients with Alzheimer's disease. *N Engl J Med* 1984; **310:** 988–9.
3. Ter Wee PM, *et al.* 4-Aminopyridine and haemodialysis in the treatment of verapamil intoxication. *Hum Toxicol* 1985; **4:** 327–9.
4. Davidson M, *et al.* 4-Aminopyridine in the treatment of Alzheimer's disease. *Biol Psychiatry* 1988; **23:** 485–90.
5. Hansebout RR, *et al.* 4-Aminopyridine in chronic spinal cord injury: a controlled, double-blind, crossover study in eight patients. *J Neurotrauma* 1993; **10:** 1–18.

Multiple sclerosis. Fampridine has potassium-channel blocking activity and has been tried in the treatment of multiple sclerosis (p.620) to improve conduction in demyelinated fibres; improvements have been reported in walking, dexterity, and vision, but only small numbers of patients have been studied.

References.

1. Davis FA, *et al.* Orally administered 4-aminopyridine improves clinical signs in multiple sclerosis. *Ann Neurol* 1990; **27:** 186–92.
2. Van Diemen HAM, *et al.* 4-Aminopyridine in patients with multiple sclerosis: dosage and serum level related to efficacy and safety. *Clin Neuropharmacol* 1993; **16:** 195–204.
3. Bever CT, *et al.* The effects of 4-aminopyridine in multiple sclerosis patients: results of a randomized, placebo-controlled, double-blind, concentration-controlled, crossover trial. *Neurology* 1994; **44:** 1054–9.
4. Schwid SR, *et al.* Quantitative assessment of sustained-release 4-aminopyridine for symptomatic treatment of multiple sclerosis. *Neurology* 1997; **48:** 817–21.

Galantamine Hydrobromide (4517-g)

Galantamine Hydrobromide (*rINNM*).

Galanthamine Hydrobromide; Galanthamini Hydrobromidum. 1,2,3,4,6,7,7a,11c-Octahydro-9-methoxy-2-methylbenzofuro[4,3,2-*efg*][2]benzazocin-6-ol hydrobromide.

$C_{17}H_{21}NO_3,HBr$ = 368.3.

CAS — 357-70-0 (galantamine); 1953-04-4 (galantamine hydrobromide).

Pharmacopoeias. In *Chin.*

The hydrobromide of galantamine, an alkaloid which has been obtained from the Caucasian snowdrop (Voronov's snowdrop), *Galanthus woronowii* (Amaryllidaceae), and related species.

Galantamine hydrobromide is a reversible inhibitor of cholinesterase activity, with actions similar to those of neostigmine (p.1394). It has been used in Alzheimer's disease (p.1386), in various neuromuscular disorders, and to curtail the muscle relaxation produced by competitive neuromuscular blockers.

References.

1. Weinstock M, *et al.* Effect of physostigmine on morphine-induced postoperative pain and somnolence. *Br J Anaesth* 1982; **54:** 429–34.
2. Westra P, *et al.* Pharmacokinetics of galanthamine (a long-acting anticholinesterase drug) in anaesthetized patients. *Br J Anaesth* 1986; **58:** 1303–7.
3. Bickel U, *et al.* Pharmacokinetics of galanthamine in humans and corresponding cholinesterase inhibition. *Clin Pharmacol Ther* 1991; **50:** 420–8.
4. Kweitz H, *et al.* Galanthamine, a selective nontoxic acetylcholinesterase inhibitor is significantly superior over placebo in the treatment of SDAT. *Neuropsychopharmacology* 1994; **10** (suppl): 130S.
5. Fulton B, Benfield P. Galanthamine. *Drugs Aging* 1996; **9:** 60–5.

Preparations

Proprietary Preparations (details are given in Part 3)
Aust.: Nivalin; ***Ital.:*** Nivalina†.

Guanidine Hydrochloride (12807-c)

Carbamidine Hydrochloride; Iminourea Hydrochloride.

CH_5N_3,HCl = 95.53.

CAS — 113-00-8 (guanidine); 50-01-1 (guanidine hydrochloride).

Guanidine hydrochloride enhances the release of acetylcholine from nerve terminals. It has been given by mouth to reverse neuromuscular blockade in patients with botulism (p.1506), but its efficacy has not been established. Guanidine hydrochloride has also been tried in Eaton-Lambert myasthenic syndrome (p.1386) and other neurological disorders, but its use has been associated with bone-marrow suppression in some patients.

References.

1. Kaplan JE, *et al.* Botulism, type A, and treatment with guanidine. *Ann Neurol* 1979; **6:** 69–71.
2. Critchley EMR, *et al.* Outbreak of botulism in North West England and Wales. *Lancet* 1989; **ii:** 849–53.
3. Neal KR, Dunbar EM. Improvement in bulbar weakness with guanoxan in type B botulism. *Lancet* 1990; **335:** 1286–7.

Linopirdine (10977-a)

Linopirdine (*USAN, rINN*).

DuP-996. 1-Phenyl-3,3-bis(4-pyridylmethyl)-2-indolinone; 1,3-Dihydro-1-phenyl-3,3-bis(4-pyridinylmethyl)-2*H*-indol-2-one.

$C_{26}H_{21}N_3O$ = 391.5.

CAS — 105431-72-9.

Linopirdine is reported to enhance the release of acetylcholine, and possibly other neurotransmitters, from nerve terminals. It has been given by mouth in studies of the treatment of Alzheimer's disease (p.1386) but there is little evidence of clinical benefit.

References.

1. Pieniaszek HJ, *et al.* Single-dose pharmacokinetics, safety, and tolerance of linopirdine (DUP 996) in healthy young adults and elderly volunteers. *J Clin Pharmacol* 1995; **35:** 22–30.
2. Rockwood K, *et al.* A randomized, controlled trial of linopirdine in the treatment of Alzheimer's disease. *Can J Neurol Sci* 1997; **24:** 140–5.

Methacholine Chloride (4520-n)

Methacholine Chloride (*BAN, rINN*).

Acetyl-β-methylcholine Chloride; Amechol Chloride; Methacholinium Chloratum. (2-Acetoxypropyl)trimethylammonium chloride.

$C_8H_{18}ClNO_2$ = 195.7.

CAS — 55-92-5 (methacholine); 62-51-1 (methacholine chloride).

Pharmacopoeias. In *Fr., It., Swiss,* and *US.*

Colourless, or white, very hygroscopic crystals, or a white crystalline powder, odourless or with a slight odour. **Soluble** 1 in 1.2 of water, 1 in 1.7 of alcohol, and 1 in 2.1 of chloroform. Solutions in water are neutral to litmus. **Store** in airtight containers.

Adverse Effects and Treatment

As for Acetylcholine Chloride, p.1389. Severe adverse cholinergic effects have followed the oral and parenteral administration of methacholine and these routes are no longer used.

Precautions

As for Neostigmine, p.1394.

Methacholine has the potential to produce severe bronchoconstriction and it should not be used for inhalation challenge tests in patients with clinically apparent asthma, wheezing, or poor pulmonary function.

Methacholine should not be given orally or parenterally.

Interactions

As for Neostigmine, p.1394. Methacholine is slowly hydrolysed by acetylcholinesterase, and its effects are markedly enhanced by prior administration of anticholinesterases.

Uses and Administration

Methacholine is a quaternary ammonium parasympathomimetic with the muscarinic actions of acetylcholine (p.1389). It is hydrolysed by acetylcholinesterase at a considerably slower rate than acetylcholine and is more resistant to hydrolysis by nonspecific cholinesterases so that its actions are more prolonged.

Inhalation of nebulised solutions of methacholine chloride are used to provoke bronchoconstriction in the diagnosis of bronchial airway hypersensitivity (but see also below and Precautions, above).

Methacholine chloride has been used in eye drops as a miotic.

Diagnosis and testing. ASTHMA. Inhalation of methacholine chloride is used as a challenge test in the diagnosis of bronchial airway hypersensitivity.[1-5] While some clinicians consider that methacholine is too dangerous for routine use in the diagnosis of asthma and that its use should rarely be necessary,[6] others report that it is of use in carefully selected patients and rarely dangerous if used according to the directions.[7] A modification of the conventional test for use in children has been described.[8]

1. Clifford RD, *et al.* Prevalence of atopy and range of bronchial response to methacholine in 7 and 11 year old school children. *Arch Dis Child* 1989; **64:** 1126–32.
2. Clifford RD, *et al.* Associations between respiratory symptoms, bronchial response to methacholine, and atopy in two age groups of school children. *Arch Dis Child* 1989; **64:** 1133–9.
3. Cabanes LR, *et al.* Bronchial hyperresponsiveness to methacholine in patients with impaired left ventricular function. *N Engl J Med* 1989; **320:** 1317–22.
4. Scanlon PD, Beck KC. Methacholine inhalation challenge. *Mayo Clin Proc* 1994; **69:** 1118–19.
5. Siersted HC, *et al.* Interrelationships between diagnosed asthma, asthma-like symptoms, and abnormal airway behaviour in adolescence: the Odense Schoolchild Study. *Thorax* 1996; **51:** 503–9.
6. Anonymous. Methacholine for diagnosis of asthma. *Med Lett Drugs Ther* 1987; **29:** 60.
7. Anonymous. Methacholine for diagnosis of asthma: an additional note. *Med Lett Drugs Ther* 1987; **29:** 74.
8. Noviski N, *et al.* Bronchial provocation determined by breath sounds compared with lung function. *Arch Dis Child* 1991; **66:** 952–5.

Preparations

Proprietary Preparations (details are given in Part 3)
USA: Provocholine.

Milameline (3156-l)

Milameline (*rINN*).

CI-979 (milameline hydrochloride); Milamelina; Milaméline; RU-35926 (milameline hydrochloride). 1,2,5,6-Tetrahydro-1-methylnicotinaldehyde (*E*)-*O*-methyloxime.

$C_8H_{14}N_2O$ = 154.2.

CAS — 139886-32-1 (milameline); 139886-04-7 (milameline hydrochloride).

NOTE. Milameline Hydrochloride is *USAN*.

Milameline is reported to be a selective muscarinic M_1 agonist; it is under investigation for the management of Alzheimer's disease.

Neostigmine (15576-a)

Neostigmine (*BAN*).

3-(Dimethylcarbamoyloxy)trimethylanilinium ion.

$C_{12}H_{19}N_2O_2$ = 223.3.

CAS — 59-99-4.

Neostigmine Bromide (4501-r)

Neostigmine Bromide (*BANM, pINN*).

Neostig. Brom.; Neostigmini Bromidum; Neostigminii Bromidum; Neostigminum Bromatum; Synstigminium Bromatum.

$C_{12}H_{19}BrN_2O_2$ = 303.2.

CAS — 114-80-7.

Pharmacopoeias. In *Chin., Eur.* (see p.viii), *Int.,* and *US.*

Hygroscopic, colourless crystals or a white crystalline powder. Very **soluble** in water; freely soluble in alcohol. **Store** in airtight containers. Protect from light.

References.

1. Porst H, Kny L. Kinetics of the degradation of neostigmine bromide in aqueous solution. *Pharmazie* 1985; **40:** 713–17.

Neostigmine Methylsulphate (4502-f)

Neostigmine Methylsulphate *(BANM)*.

Neostig. Methylsulph.; Neostigmine Methylsulfate; Neostigmine Metilsulfate; Neostigmini Metilsulfas; Proserinum.

$C_{13}H_{22}N_2O_6S$ = 334.4.

CAS — 51-60-5.

Pharmacopoeias. In *Chin., Eur.* (see p.viii), *Int., Jpn, Pol.*, and *US.*

Hygroscopic, colourless crystals or a white crystalline powder. Very **soluble** in water; freely soluble in alcohol; practically insoluble in ether. **Store** in airtight containers. Protect from light.

Adverse Effects

The side-effects of neostigmine are chiefly due to excessive cholinergic stimulation and most commonly include increased salivation, nausea and vomiting, abdominal cramps, and diarrhoea. Allergic reactions have been reported; rashes have been associated with the use of the bromide salt. Neostigmine penetrates the blood-brain barrier poorly and CNS effects are usually only seen with high doses.

Overdosage may lead to a 'cholinergic crisis', characterised by both muscarinic and nicotinic effects. These effects may include excessive sweating, lachrymation, increased peristalsis, involuntary defaecation and urination or desire to urinate, miosis, ciliary spasm, nystagmus, bradycardia and other arrhythmias, hypotension, muscle cramps, fasciculations, weakness and paralysis, tight chest, wheezing, and increased bronchial secretion combined with bronchoconstriction. CNS effects include ataxia, convulsions, coma, slurred speech, restlessness, agitation, and fear. Death may result from respiratory failure, due to a combination of the muscarinic, nicotinic and central effects, or cardiac arrest.

It has been reported that a paradoxical increase in blood pressure and heart rate may result from nicotinic stimulation of sympathetic ganglia, especially where atropine has been given to reverse the muscarinic effects (see under Treatment of Adverse Effects, below).

In patients with myasthenia gravis, in whom other symptoms of overdosage may be mild or absent, the major symptom of cholinergic crisis is increased muscular weakness, which must be differentiated from the muscular weakness caused by an exacerbation of the disease itself (myasthenic crisis).

The adverse effects of parasympathomimetics applied topically for their miotic action are discussed under Pilocarpine on p.1397.

Treatment of Adverse Effects

If neostigmine has been taken by mouth the stomach should be emptied by lavage. When necessary maintenance of respiration should take priority. Atropine sulphate should be given in usual doses of 1 to 2 mg, preferably intravenously, or else intramuscularly and repeated as necessary to control the muscarinic effects; some authorities suggest doses of up to 4 mg. Nicotinic effects, including muscle weakness and paralysis, are not antagonised by atropine; the use of small doses of a competitive neuromuscular blocker has been suggested for the control of muscle twitching. Use of the cholinesterase inhibitor pralidoxime as an adjunct to atropine has also been suggested (see p.992). Further supportive treatment should be given as required.

Precautions

Neostigmine is contra-indicated in patients with mechanical intestinal or urinary-tract obstruction, or peritonitis. It should be used with extreme caution in patients who have undergone recent intestinal or bladder surgery and in patients with bronchial asthma. It should be used with caution in patients with cardiovascular disorders including arrhythmias, bradycardia, recent myocardial infarction, and hypotension, as well as in patients with vagotonia, epilepsy, hyperthyroidism, parkinsonism, renal impairment, or peptic ulcer. When neostigmine is given by injection, atropine should always be available to counteract any excessive reactions; atropine may also be given before, or with, neostigmine to prevent or minimise muscarinic side-effects but this may mask the initial symptoms of overdosage and lead to cholinergic crisis.

The UK manufacturer has advised that as the severity of myasthenia gravis often fluctuates considerably during pregnancy, particular care is needed to avoid cholinergic crisis caused by overdosage; it has also been reported that neonatal myasthenia may follow administration of large doses during pregnancy. The amount of neostigmine distributed into breast milk is very small but breast-fed infants need to be monitored.

Large doses of neostigmine by mouth should be avoided in conditions where there may be increased absorption from the gastro-intestinal tract. It should be avoided in patients known to be hypersensitive to neostigmine; the bromide ion from neostigmine bromide may contribute to the allergic reaction.

The precautions of parasympathomimetics applied topically for their miotic action are discussed under Pilocarpine on p.1397.

Neuromuscular disorders. Treatment of residual non-depolarising neuromuscular block by administration of neostigmine in association with atropine to a patient with dystrophia myotonica was only partly effective, and following a second dose of both drugs complete neuromuscular block developed.[1] In a second patient, with a history of progressive muscle dystrophy, the administration of neostigmine to reverse residual non-depolarising blockade gave rise to a tonic response in the indirectly stimulated muscle. The type and degree of the response to neostigmine, and probably other anticholinesterases, cannot be predicted in patients with neuromuscular disease.

A patient with sero-negative ocular myasthenia gravis had exaggerated responses to both vecuronium and neostigmine.[2] The dose of neuromuscular blockers and their antagonists used in patients with myasthenia gravis should be titrated carefully regardless of the severity of the condition.

1. Buzello W, *et al.* Hazards of neostigmine in patients with neuromuscular disorders: report of two cases. *Br J Anaesth* 1982; **54:** 529–34.
2. Kim J-M, Mangold J. Sensitivity to both vecuronium and neostigmine in a sero-negative myasthenic patient. *Br J Anaesth* 1989; **63:** 497–500.

Renal impairment. The dosage of neostigmine may need to be adjusted in patients with renal impairment. Cronnelly *et al.*[1] found that a mean serum elimination half-life of 79.8 minutes obtained in patients with normal renal function was prolonged to 181.1 minutes in anephric patients.

1. Cronnelly R, *et al.* Renal function and the pharmacokinetics of neostigmine in anesthetized man. *Anesthesiology* 1979; **51:** 222–6.

Interactions

Drugs that possess neuromuscular blocking activity, such as the aminoglycosides, clindamycin, colistin, cyclopropane, and the halogenated inhalational anaesthetics, may antagonise the effects of neostigmine. A number of drugs, including quinine, chloroquine, hydroxychloroquine, quinidine, procainamide, propafenone, lithium, and the beta blockers, that have the potential to aggravate myasthenia gravis may reduce the effectiveness of treatment with parasympathomimetics. Prolonged bradycardia has also occurred in patients receiving beta blockers following administration of neostigmine. Anticholinesterases, such as neostigmine, can inhibit the metabolism of suxamethonium and enhance and prolong its action.

Concomitant ophthalmic use of anticholinesterases, such as ecothiopate, should be undertaken with care in patients receiving neostigmine systemically for myasthenia gravis, because of possible additive toxicity.

Antimuscarinics such as atropine antagonise the muscarinic effects of neostigmine.

Beta blockers. There have been several reports of bradycardia and hypotension following administration of neostigmine or physostigmine to patients receiving beta blockers[1-4] but no significant changes in heart rate were noted in a study of pyridostigmine given to 8 patients taking beta blockers.[5] Beta blockers have the potential to aggravate the symptoms of myasthenia gravis and may therefore reduce the effectiveness of parasympathomimetic treatment.

1. Sprague DH. Severe bradycardia after neostigmine in a patient taking propranolol to control paroxysmal atrial tachycardia. *Anesthesiology* 1975; **42:** 208–10.
2. Seidl DC, Martin DE. Prolonged bradycardia after neostigmine administration in a patient taking nadolol. *Anesth Analg* 1984; **63:** 365–7.
3. Baraka A, Dajani A. Severe bradycardia following physostigmine in the presence of beta-adrenergic blockade: a case report. *Middle East J Anesthesiol* 1984; **7:** 291–3.
4. Eldor J, *et al.* Prolonged bradycardia and hypotension after neostigmine administration in a patient receiving atenolol. *Anaesthesia* 1987; **42:** 1294–7.
5. Arad M, *et al.* Safety of pyridostigmine in hypertensive patients receiving beta blockers. *Am J Cardiol* 1992; **69:** 518–22.

Calcium-channel blockers. Concomitant use of calcium-channel blockers such as verapamil and neuromuscular blockers may produce an enhanced muscle block which is resistant to reversal with neostigmine[1] but which may be reversed by edrophonium.[2]

1. van Poorten JF, *et al.* Verapamil and reversal of vecuronium neuromuscular blockade. *Anesth Analg* 1984; **63:** 155–7.
2. Jones RM, *et al.* Verapamil potentiation of neuromuscular blockade: failure of reversal with neostigmine but prompt reversal with edrophonium. *Anesth Analg* 1985; **64:** 1021–5.

Corticosteroids. Although use of glucocorticoids alone may improve strength in myasthenic patients, administration of methylprednisolone to patients receiving neostigmine or pyridostigmine has exacerbated symptoms and produced profound weakness often necessitating assisted ventilation.[1] Since the adverse effects of concomitant therapy usually occur before any expected benefits it has been suggested that the glucocorticoid should be given on alternate days in small doses which are increased gradually until the optimal effect is achieved.[2]

1. Brunner NG, *et al.* Corticosteroids in management of severe, generalized myasthenia gravis: effectiveness and comparison with corticotrophin therapy. *Neurology* 1972; **22:** 603–10.
2. Jubiz W, Meikle AW. Alterations of glucocorticoid actions by other drugs and disease states. *Drugs* 1979; **18:** 113–21.

Pharmacokinetics

Neostigmine is a quaternary ammonium compound and as the bromide is poorly absorbed from the gastro-intestinal tract. Following parenteral administration as the methylsulphate, neostigmine is rapidly eliminated and is excreted in the urine both as unchanged drug and metabolites. Neostigmine undergoes hydrolysis by cholinesterases and is also metabolised in the liver. Protein binding to human serum albumin is reported to range from 15 to 25%. Penetration into the CNS is poor. Neostigmine crosses the placenta and very small amounts are distributed into breast milk.

Neostigmine appears to be poorly and variably absorbed when administered by mouth. In 3 myasthenic patients peak plasma concentrations were obtained 1 to 2 hours after a single 30-mg dose by mouth and the mean plasma half-life was 0.87 hours; bioavailability was estimated to be 1 to 2%.[1] Mean plasma half-lives of 0.89 and 1.20 hours have been obtained following intravenous[1] and intramuscular[2] injections of neostigmine methylsulphate respectively, although again only a few patients were studied. Metabolism and biliary excretion may play significant roles in the elimination of neostigmine.[2] About 80% of a dose may be excreted in the urine within 24 hours; about 50% of a dose as unchanged drug and 15% as 3-hydroxyphenyltrimethylammonium.[2] Mean plasma elimination half-lives for neostigmine have been found to be shorter in infants (0.65 hours) and children (0.80 hours) compared with adults (1.12 hours) but this does not appear to be related to its duration of effect in antagonising neuromuscular blockade.[3] The half-life is prolonged in renal failure.

1. Aquilonius S-M, *et al.* A pharmacokinetic study of neostigmine in man using gas chromatography–mass spectrometry. *Eur J Clin Pharmacol* 1979; **15:** 367–71.
2. Somani SM, *et al.* Kinetics and metabolism of intramuscular neostigmine in myasthenia gravis. *Clin Pharmacol Ther* 1980; **28:** 64–8.
3. Fisher DM, *et al.* The neuromuscular pharmacology of neostigmine in infants and children. *Anesthesiology* 1983; **59:** 220–5.

Uses and Administration

Neostigmine is a quaternary ammonium compound which inhibits cholinesterase activity and thus prolongs and intensifies the physiological actions of acetylcholine (p.1389). It probably also has direct effects on skeletal muscle fibres. The anticholinesterase actions of neostigmine are reversible.

Neostigmine is used in the treatment of myasthenia gravis, and has been used as an alternative to edrophonium in the diagnosis of myasthenia gravis (p.1388). It is used in anaesthesia to reverse the neuromuscular blockade produced by competitive neuromuscular blockers (see below). It is also used in the management of paralytic ileus. Neostigmine has been used in the management of postoperative urinary retention (p.454) but has generally been superseded by catheterisation. It is sometimes used to lower intra-ocular pressure in the management of glaucoma (p.1387) and to reduce rises in intra-ocular pressure associated with ophthalmic surgery although other parasympathomimetics are usually used when such miotics are required.

Neostigmine is given as the bromide and as the methylsulphate. Neostigmine bromide is given by mouth and has been used topically as eye drops; the methylsulphate is administered by intramuscular, intravenous, or subcutaneous injection.

The manufacturers state that 0.5 mg of neostigmine methylsulphate by intravenous injection is approximately equivalent in effect to 1 to 1.5 mg of neostigmine methylsulphate by intramuscular or subcutaneous injection, or 15 mg of neostigmine bromide by mouth.

In the treatment of **myasthenia gravis**, neostigmine is given by mouth as the bromide in a total daily dose usually between 75 and 300 mg, divided throughout the day, and if necessary the night, according to individual response; larger portions of the total dose may be given at times of greater fatigue. The maximum daily dose that most patients can tolerate is 180 mg. A usual total daily dose in children is 15 to 90 mg by mouth. In patients in whom oral therapy is impractical neostigmine methylsulphate may be given in doses of 0.5 to 2.5 mg by intramuscular or subcutaneous injection at intervals, giving a total daily dose usually in the range 5 to 20 mg. Single doses in children have ranged from 200 to 500 µg.

In the treatment of neonatal myasthenia gravis doses in the range 50 to 250 µg of the methylsulphate by intramuscular or subcutaneous injection, or 1 to 5 mg of the bromide by mouth, have been given usually every 4 hours; treatment is rarely needed beyond 8 weeks of age.

To **reverse neuromuscular blockade** produced by competitive neuromuscular blockers, the usual adult dose used in the UK is 50 to 70 µg per kg body-weight given by intravenous injection over a period of 60 seconds; in the USA lower doses of 0.5 to 2 mg are used. Additional neostigmine may be given until the muscle power is normal but a total of 5 mg should not be exceeded. The patient should be well ventilated until complete recovery of normal respiration is assured. To counteract any muscarinic effects 0.6 to 1.2 mg of atropine sulphate is administered by intravenous injection with or before the dose of neostigmine; it has been suggested that in the presence of bradycardia atropine sulphate should be administered several minutes before neostigmine. Glycopyrronium bromide has been used as an alternative to atropine sulphate.

In the treatment of paralytic ileus and postoperative urinary retention, doses of 15 to 30 mg of the bromide by mouth, or more usually 0.5 mg of the methylsulphate by subcutaneous or intramuscular injection, have been used.

Neostigmine bromide has been administered as eye drops to lower intra-ocular pressure in the treatment of glaucoma.

Decreased gastro-intestinal motility. Parasympathomimetics enhance gastric contractions and increase intestinal motility and have been used in a variety of conditions associated with decreased gastro-intestinal motility (p.1168). Some workers[1,2] have reported good results using intravenous neostigmine in the treatment of acute colonic pseudo-obstruction, a condition that appears to be due to parasympathomimetic dysfunction. It has therefore been suggested that parasympathomimetics might be tried as an alternative to colonic decompression or surgery when conservative management has failed or a rapid resolution is required. Neostigmine has also been used in the treatment of severe constipation due to disrupted intestinal motility.[3,4]

1. Hutchinson R, Griffiths C. Acute colonic pseudo-obstruction: a pharmacological approach. *Ann R Coll Surg Engl* 1992; **74:** 364–7.
2. Stephenson BM, *et al.* Parasympathomimetic decompression of acute colonic pseudo-obstruction. *Lancet* 1993; **342:** 1181–2.
3. Miller LS. Neostigmine for severe constipation with spinal cord lesions. *Ann Intern Med* 1984; **101:** 279.
4. Thurtle OA, *et al.* Intractable constipation in malignant phaeochromocytoma: combined treatment with adrenergic blockade and cholinergic drugs. *J R Soc Med* 1984; **77:** 327–8.

Growth hormone deficiency. For reference to the potential value of intranasal administration of neostigmine with somatorelin in the treatment of short stature in children, see under Uses and Administration of Pyridostigmine, p.1398.

Reversal of neuromuscular blockade. Anticholinesterases have commonly been used after surgery to antagonise residual neuromuscular block induced by the long-acting competitive neuromuscular blockers. However, since the introduction of intermediate-acting blockers such as atracurium and vecuronium and shorter-acting blockers such as mivacurium there has been continuing debate[1,2] on whether anticholinesterases can be used in reduced doses or even omitted for these blockers. Decreasing the dosage of the anticholinesterase may reduce its adverse effects. Nausea and vomiting may be less common in patients not given neostigmine after the use of a competitive blocker,[3,4] and omission of neostigmine also avoids any adverse effects it may have on gut anastomoses. One commentator[1] considered that the wide variation in recovery time with aminosteroid blockers such as rocuronium was an indication for always using at least a small dose of anticholinesterase when these drugs were used. However, it was suggested that if the block was being carefully monitored and recovery was established a reduced dose of 1.25 mg of neostigmine might be preferable following a benzylisoquinolinium blocker such as atracurium or mivacurium. In children, smaller doses of an anticholinesterase could be used, even after an aminosteroid blocker, and after a blocker such as mivacurium, they may not be needed at all.

It has been suggested that because of its shorter duration of action edrophonium might be more suitable than neostigmine to antagonise residual block for blockers with shorter actions. Edrophonium also has lesser effects on the vagus, a more rapid onset of action, and may be associated with a lower incidence of nausea and vomiting than neostigmine.[5] Neostigmine can cause clinically significant neuromuscular blockade if it is given to a patient who has already recovered a large degree of neuromuscular function[6,7] but edrophonium appears not to re-induce blockade on repeat administration.[8] However, the antagonism produced by edrophonium is not adequately and reliably sustained especially following profound block.[9,10] It has also been suggested that edrophonium might be more appropriate than neostigmine for use with mivacurium. Neostigmine inhibits plasma cholinesterase responsible for the metabolism of mivacurium and its use can in theory delay rather than speed recovery although in practice there is considered to be little evidence for such an effect.[1]

1. Hunter JM. Is it always necessary to antagonize residual neuromuscular block? Do children differ from adults? *Br J Anaesth* 1996; **77:** 707–9.
2. Fawcett WJ. Neuromuscular block in children. *Br J Anaesth* 1997; **78:** 627.
3. King MJ, *et al.* Influence of neostigmine on postoperative vomiting. *Br J Anaesth* 1988; **61:** 403–6.
4. Ding Y, *et al.* Use of mivacurium during laparoscopic surgery: effect of reversal drugs on postoperative recovery. *Anesth Analg* 1994; **78:** 450–4.
5. Watcha MF, *et al.* Effect of antagonism of mivacurium-induced neuromuscular block on postoperative emesis in children. *Anesth Analg* 1995; **80:** 713–17.
6. Hughes R, *et al.* Neuromuscular blockade by neostigmine. *Br J Anaesth* 1979; **51:** 568P.
7. Payne JP, *et al.* Neuromuscular blockade by neostigmine in anaesthetized man. *Br J Anaesth* 1980; **52:** 69–75.
8. Astley BA, *et al.* Electrical and mechanical responses after neuromuscular blockade with vecuronium, and subsequent antagonism with neostigmine or edrophonium. *Br J Anaesth* 1987; **59:** 983–8.
9. Caldwell JE, *et al.* Antagonism of profound neuromuscular blockade induced by vecuronium or atracurium: comparison of neostigmine with edrophonium. *Br J Anaesth* 1986; **58:** 1285–9.
10. Mirakhur RK, *et al.* Antagonism of vecuronium-induced neuromuscular blockade with edrophonium or neostigmine. *Br J Anaesth* 1987; **59:** 473–7.

Snake bite. The general management of snake bites is discussed on p.1534. Numerous reports from India have claimed benefit for anticholinesterases in the treatment of neurotoxic envenoming from snake bites but failure to distinguish between cobra and krait bites, lack of controls, and inadequate information about other therapy vitiate the claims.[1] However, anticholinesterases have been shown in 2 double-blind studies to be more effective than placebo[2] and antivenom[3] in the treatment of snake bite due to the Philippine cobra (*Naja naja philippinensis*). Neostigmine has recently been reported[4] to have been effective in reversing paralysis in 2 patients bitten by *Micrurus frontalis* (a coral snake). Anticholinesterases would be expected to be of little value for bites from snakes whose venom contains neurotoxins which act presynaptically, including the Asian krait, the Australian tiger snake, and the taipan[5] and although beneficial results have been reported in individual patients,[6] overall results are considered to be inconsistent.[2,7] However, it is recommended that a test dose of edrophonium preceded by atropine should be given to patients with neurological signs who have been bitten by a snake of any species and if improvement occurs, a longer acting anticholinesterase such as neostigmine can be administered.[2]

1. Reid HA. Venoms and antivenoms. *Trop Dis Bull* 1983; **80:** 23.
2. Watt G, *et al.* Positive response to edrophonium in patients with neurotoxic envenoming by cobras (Naja naja philippinensis). *N Engl J Med* 1986; **315:** 1444–8.
3. Watt G, *et al.* Comparison of Tensilon® and antivenom for the treatment of cobra-bite paralysis. *Trans R Soc Trop Med Hyg* 1989; **83:** 570–3.
4. Vital Brazil O, Vieira RJ. Neostigmine in the treatment of snake accidents caused by Micrurus frontalis: report of two cases. *Rev Inst Med Trop S Paulo* 1996; **38:** 61–7.
5. Brophy T, Sutherland SK. Use of neostigmine after snake bite. *Br J Anaesth* 1979; **51:** 264–5.
6. Warrell DA, *et al.* Severe neurotoxic envenoming by the Malayan krait Bungarus candidus (Linnaeus): response to antivenom and anticholinesterase. *Br Med J* 1983 **286:** 678–80.
7. Trevett AJ, *et al.* Failure of 3,4-diaminopyridine and edrophonium to produce significant clinical benefit in neurotoxicity following the bite of Papuan taipan *(Oxyuranus scutellatus canni). Trans R Soc Trop Med Hyg* 1995; **89:** 444–6.

Tetrodotoxin poisoning. For reference to the use of neostigmine in the treatment of tetrodotoxin poisoning caused by eating puffer fish, see under Uses and Administration of Edrophonium Chloride, p.1392.

Preparations

BP 1998: Neostigmine Injection; Neostigmine Tablets;
USP 23: Neostigmine Bromide Tablets; Neostigmine Methylsulfate Injection.

Proprietary Preparations (details are given in Part 3)
Aust.: Normastigmin; Prostigmin; ***Austral.:*** Prostigmin†; ***Belg.:*** Prostigmine; Robinul-Neostigmine; ***Canad.:*** Prostigmin; ***Fr.:*** Prostigmine; ***Ger.:*** Neoeserin†; Prostigmin†; ***Irl.:*** Prostigmin; ***Ital.:*** Intrastigmina; Prostigmina; ***Neth.:*** Prostigmin; ***Norw.:*** Prostigmin; Robinul-Neostigmin; ***S.Afr.:*** Prostigmin†; ***Spain:*** Prostigmine; ***Swed.:*** Robinul-Neostigmin; ***Switz.:*** Prostigmine; Robinul-Neostigmine; ***UK:*** Prostigmin†; Robinul-Neostigmine; ***USA:*** Neostigmine Min-I-Mix; Prostigmin.

Multi-ingredient: ***Aust.:*** Normastigmin mit Pilocarpin; Pilostigmin Puroptal; ***Ger.:*** Syncarpin; ***Spain:*** Risunal A†; Risunal B†.

Paraoxon (14240-s)

E-600. Diethyl *p*-nitrophenyl phosphate.

$C_{10}H_{14}NO_6P$ = 275.2.

CAS — 311-45-5.

Paraoxon is a potent inhibitor of cholinesterase activity which has been used with other miotics in the treatment of glaucoma. It is the active metabolite of the organophosphorus insecticide parathion (p.1409) and therefore produces similar toxicity but with a faster onset.

Preparations

Proprietary Preparations (details are given in Part 3)

Multi-ingredient: ***Ital.:*** Mios.

Physostigmine (4521-h)

Physostigmine *(BAN)*.

Eserine. (3a*S*,8a*R*)-1,2,3,3a,8,8a-Hexahydro-1,3a,8-trimethylpyrrolo[2,3-*b*]indol-5-yl methylcarbamate.

$C_{15}H_{21}N_3O_2$ = 275.3.

CAS — 57-47-6.

Pharmacopoeias. In US.

An alkaloid obtained from the calabar bean (ordeal bean; chopnut), the seed of *Physostigma venenosum* (Leguminosae). It occurs as a white, odourless, microcrystalline powder which acquires a red tint on exposure to heat, light, air, or contact with traces of metals. M.p. not lower than 103°.

Slightly **soluble** in water; very soluble in chloroform and in dichloromethane; freely soluble in alcohol; soluble in fixed oils. **Store** in airtight containers. Protect from light.

Physostigmine Salicylate (4523-b)

Physostigmine Salicylate *(BANM)*.

Eserine Salicylate; Eserini Salicylas; Physostig. Sal.; Physostigmine Monosalicylate; Physostigmini Salicylas; Physostigminii Salicylas.

$C_{15}H_{21}N_3O_2,C_7H_6O_3$ = 413.5.

CAS — 57-64-7.

Pharmacopoeias. In *Eur.* (see p.viii), *Int., Jpn, Pol.,* and *US.*

Colourless or white odourless crystals or white powder. It becomes red on exposure to heat, light, air, and contact with traces of metals; the colour develops more quickly in the presence of moisture.

Ph. Eur. **solubilities** are: sparingly soluble in water; soluble in alcohol; very slightly soluble in ether. USP solubilities are: 1 in 75 of water, 1 in 16 of alcohol, 1 in 6 of chloroform, and 1 in 250 of ether. A 0.9% solution in water has a pH of 5.1 to 5.9. **Store** in airtight containers. Protect from light.

Aqueous solutions are unstable. Solutions for injection should not be used if more than slightly discoloured.

Physostigmine Sulphate (4524-v)

Physostigmine Sulphate *(BANM)*.

Ésérine (Sulfate D'); Eserine Sulphate; Eserini Sulfas; Physostig. Sulph.; Physostigmine Sulfate; Physostigmini Sulfas.

$(C_{15}H_{21}N_3O_2)_2,H_2SO_4 = 648.8.$

CAS — 64-47-1.

Pharmacopoeias. In *Eur.* (see p.viii) and *US.*

A white or almost white, odourless, hygroscopic crystalline powder. It becomes red on exposure to heat, light, air, and on contact with traces of metals; the colour develops more quickly in the presence of moisture.

Ph. Eur. **solubilities** are: very soluble in water; freely soluble in alcohol; practically insoluble in ether. USP solubilities are: 1 in 4 of water, 1 in 0.4 of alcohol, and 1 in 1200 of ether. A 1% solution in water has a pH of 3.5 to 5.5. **Store** in well-filled airtight glass containers. Protect from light. Aqueous solutions are unstable.

Adverse Effects, Treatment, and Precautions

Systemic effects as for Neostigmine, p.1394. For adverse effects and precautions for topical miotics see also under Pilocarpine, p.1397.

Systemic toxic effects of physostigmine are usually more severe than those occurring with neostigmine. Physostigmine crosses the blood-brain barrier and may therefore produce CNS effects. Physostigmine is not well tolerated when used in the eyes for long periods and may produce follicles in the conjunctiva; hypersensitivity reactions are also common. Prolonged use of ophthalmic ointments containing physostigmine may cause depigmentation of the lid margins in dark-skinned patients.

Overdosage. The use of atropine in the management of a patient who had taken 1 g of physostigmine had to be abandoned after it produced tachycardia and multifocal ventricular ectopic beats.[1] However, in a similar case of severe poisoning a slow intravenous injection of propranolol 5 mg reduced the high pulse rate and controlled pulse irregularities despite frequent intravenous administration of atropine.[2]

1. Cumming G, *et al.* Treatment and recovery after massive overdosage of physostigmine. *Lancet* 1968; **ii:** 147–9.
2. Valero A. Treatment of severe physostigmine poisoning. *Lancet* 1968; **ii:** 459–60.

Interactions

As for Neostigmine, p.1394.

Pharmacokinetics

Physostigmine is readily absorbed from the gastro-intestinal tract, subcutaneous tissues, and mucous membranes. It is largely destroyed in the body by hydrolysis of the ester linkage by cholinesterases; a 1-mg dose injected subcutaneously has been claimed to be destroyed in 2 hours. It crosses the blood-brain barrier. Little is excreted in the urine.

From studies in 5 subjects there appear to be marked interindividual differences in the absorption and metabolism of physostigmine salicylate after administration of doses of up to 4 mg by mouth and it has been suggested that physostigmine may undergo a saturable presystemic metabolism.[1-3] Oral bioavailability has ranged from 5.2 to 11.7% in 3 of the subjects.[3]

In a study[4] of a single application of a physostigmine (base) transdermal system in 6 subjects, the mean absolute bioavailability was 36% (range 12.6 to 53.2%); the interindividual variability in absolute bioavailability was decreased by about 30% in comparison with administration of an oral solution of physostigmine salicylate. There was continued absorption of physostigmine following removal of the transdermal system, indicating a drug reservoir in the skin.

In a study[5] of 9 patients with Alzheimer's disease, a mean elimination half-life for physostigmine of 16.4 minutes was reported following intravenous administration of physostigmine salicylate. Cholinesterase inhibition was more prolonged than that suggested by its elimination half-life.

1. Gibson M, *et al.* Physostigmine concentrations after oral doses. *Lancet* 1985; **i:** 695–6.
2. Sharpless NS, Thal LJ. Plasma physostigmine concentrations after oral administration. *Lancet* 1985; **i:** 1397–8.
3. Whelpton R, Hurst P. Bioavailability of oral physostigmine. *N Engl J Med* 1985; **313:** 1293–4.
4. Walker K, *et al.* Pharmacokinetics of physostigmine in man following a single application of a transdermal system. *Br J Clin Pharmacol* 1995; **39:** 59–63.
5. Asthana S, *et al.* Clinical pharmacokinetics of physostigmine in patients with Alzheimer's disease. *Clin Pharmacol Ther* 1995; **58:** 299–309.

Uses and Administration

Physostigmine is a reversible tertiary amine inhibitor of cholinesterase activity with actions similar to those of neostigmine (p.1394). Physostigmine has been used, alone or more usually in combination with other miotics such as pilocarpine, to decrease intra-ocular pressure in glaucoma (p.1387). It is a more potent miotic than pilocarpine but is rarely tolerated for prolonged periods. When it is used in glaucoma physostigmine has usually been administered as eye drops containing 0.25 or 0.5% of the salicylate or as an ophthalmic ointment containing 0.25% of the sulphate.

Physostigmine crosses the blood-brain barrier and has been used to reverse the central as well as the peripheral effects of agents with antimuscarinic actions in postoperative patients and following overdosage but such treatment is not usually recommended. Physostigmine is under investigation in the management of Alzheimer's disease.

Alzheimer's disease. Physostigmine is being studied in the symptomatic management of Alzheimer's disease (p.1386). However, published studies have involved small numbers of patients and have been of limited duration. Results[1-4] using oral physostigmine have been conflicting but it appears that it might produce small improvements in memory impairment. Modified-release preparations, including transdermal patches,[5] are also being studied to overcome the problems associated with physostigmine's short half-life.

1. Stern Y, *et al.* Long-term administration of oral physostigmine in Alzheimer's disease. *Neurology* 1988; **38:** 1837–41.
2. Thal LJ, *et al.* Chronic oral physostigmine without lecithin improves memory in Alzheimer's disease. *J Am Geriatr Soc* 1989; **37:** 42–48.
3. Jenike MA, *et al.* Oral physostigmine treatment for patients with presenile and senile dementia of the Alzheimer's type: a double-blind placebo-controlled trial. *J Clin Psychiatry* 1990; **51:** 3–7.
4. Sano M, *et al.* Safety and efficacy of oral physostigmine in the treatment of Alzheimer disease. *Clin Neuropharmacol* 1993; **16:** 61–9.
5. Levy A, *et al.* Transdermal physostigmine in the treatment of Alzheimer's disease. *Alzheimer Dis Assoc Disord* 1994; **8:** 15–21.

Anaesthesia. Physostigmine has been given postoperatively to reverse CNS effects and reduce arousal time[1] in patients who have received antimuscarinics, antihistamines, benzodiazepines, or other drugs such as droperidol but its routine use is not recommended. It has also been tried in patients who have received ketamine[2] or morphine[3] and appears to reverse sedation without adversely affecting analgesia.

1. Brebner J, Hadley L. Experiences with physostigmine in the reversal of adverse post-anaesthetic effects. *Can Anaesth Soc J* 1976; **23:** 574–81.
2. Balmer HGR, Wyte SR. Antagonism of ketamine by physostigmine. *Br J Anaesth* 1977; **49:** 510.
3. Weinstock M, *et al.* Effect of physostigmine on morphine-induced postoperative pain and somnolence. *Br J Anaesth* 1982; **54:** 429–33.

Antimuscarinic poisoning. As physostigmine penetrates the blood-brain barrier it has been used to reverse the central effects of poisoning with agents having antimuscarinic actions including tricyclic antidepressants, antihistamines, some antiemetics, some antiparkinsonian drugs, and phenothiazines. However, reviewers agree that in general such a use is inappropriate and hazardous. Physostigmine does not appear to affect the mortality rate in tricyclic antidepressant poisoning[1] and its use can lead to severe cardiac[2,3] and respiratory effects[2,3] and to convulsions.[3,4] In uncomplicated cases of overdosage the safest treatment could be to await the spontaneous remission of toxicity.[2] If used at all, physostigmine should be reserved for treatment of life-threatening symptoms such as uncontrollable convulsions, coma with respiratory depression, or severe hypertension.[5] Physostigmine has a shorter duration of action than most antimuscarinics and a considerably shorter duration of action than most tricyclics, therefore reports of the successful use of physostigmine have highlighted the need for repeated doses or continuous administration over periods of hours or days.[6,7]

1. Aquilonius S-M, Hedstrand U. The use of physostigmine as an antidote in tricyclic anti-depressant intoxication. *Acta Anaesthesiol Scand* 1978; **22:** 40–5.
2. Caine ED. Anticholinergic toxicity. *N Engl J Med* 1979; **300:** 1278.
3. Newton RW. Physostigmine salicylate in the treatment of tricyclic antidepressant overdosage. *JAMA* 1975; **231:** 941–3.
4. Knudsen K, Heath A. Effects of self poisoning with maprotiline. *Br Med J* 1984; **288:** 601–3.
5. Anonymous. Treatment of acute drug abuse reactions. *Med Lett Drugs Ther* 1987; **29:** 83–5.
6. Pall H, *et al.* Experiences with physostigminesalicylate in tricyclic antidepressant poisoning. *Acta Pharmacol Toxicol* 1977; **41** (suppl 2): 171–8.
7. Brier RH. Physostigmine dose for tricyclic drug overdose. *Ann Intern Med* 1978; **89:** 579.

Baclofen overdosage. For references to the use of physostigmine in the treatment of baclofen overdosage, see p.1308.

Cerebellar ataxias. Double-blind controlled studies indicate that physostigmine[1,2] can produce symptomatic improvement in some patients with cerebellar ataxia including those with hereditary forms of spinocerebellar degeneration such as Friedreich's ataxia.

1. Rodriguez-Budelli MM, *et al.* Action of physostigmine on inherited ataxias. *Adv Neurol* 1978; **21:** 195–202.
2. Aschoff JC, *et al.* Physostigmin in der behandlung von kleinhirnataxien. *Nervenarzt* 1996; **67:** 311–18.

Withdrawal syndromes. Physostigmine has been reported[1,2] to have produced beneficial results when tried in the management of the symptoms of alcohol withdrawal (p.1099).

1. Powers JS, *et al.* Physostigmine for treatment of delirium tremens. *J Clin Pharmacol* 1981; **21:** 57–60.
2. Stojek A, *et al.* Local physostigmine in the management of early alcohol withdrawal. *Br J Addict* 1987; **82:** 927–30.

Preparations

USP 23: Physostigmine Salicylate Injection; Physostigmine Salicylate Ophthalmic Solution; Physostigmine Sulfate Ophthalmic Ointment.

Proprietary Preparations (details are given in Part 3)
Aust.: Anticholium; ***Ger.:*** Anticholium; ***USA:*** Antilirium†.

Multi-ingredient: ***Belg.:*** Miotic Double; ***Ger.:*** Isopto Pilomin; Miopos-POS stark†; Pilo-Eserin.

Pilocarpine (4525-g)

Pilocarpine *(BAN)*.

(3*S*,4*R*)-3-Ethyldihydro-4-[(1-methyl-1*H*-imidazol-5-yl)methyl]furan-2(3*H*)-one.

$C_{11}H_{16}N_2O_2 = 208.3.$

CAS — 92-13-7.

Pharmacopoeias. In *US.*

An alkaloid obtained from the leaves of jaborandi, *Pilocarpus microphyllus* (Rutaceae) and other species of *Pilocarpus*. A viscous, hygroscopic, oily liquid or crystals. M.p. about 34°. **Soluble** in water, in alcohol, and in chloroform; sparingly soluble in ether; practically insoluble in petroleum spirit. **Store** at a temperature not exceeding 8° in airtight containers. Protect from light.

Pilocarpine Borate (16189-z)

$C_{11}H_{16}N_2O_2,xBH_3O_3.$

CAS — 16509-56-1.

Pilocarpine Hydrochloride (4526-q)

Pilocarpine Hydrochloride *(BANM)*.

Pilocarp. Hydrochlor.; Pilocarpine Monohydrochloride; Pilocarpini Chloridum; Pilocarpini Hydrochloridum; Pilocarpinium Chloratum.

$C_{11}H_{16}N_2O_2,HCl = 244.7.$

CAS — 54-71-7.

NOTE. PIL is a code approved by the BP for use on single unit doses of eye drops containing pilocarpine hydrochloride where the individual container may be too small to bear all the appropriate labelling information.

Pharmacopoeias. In *Eur.* (see p.viii), *Int.*, *Jpn*, *Pol.*, and *US.*

Odourless hygroscopic colourless white crystals or a white or almost white crystalline powder.

Ph. Eur. **solubilities** are: very soluble in water and in alcohol. USP solubilities are: soluble 1 in 0.3 of water, 1 in 3 of alcohol, and 1 in 360 of chloroform; insoluble in ether. A 5% solution in water has a pH of 3.5 to 4.5. **Store** in airtight containers. Protect from light.

Stability. Pilocarpine hydrochloride oral solution, prepared from powder or eye drops and buffered at pH 5.5, was found[1] to be stable for 60 days at 25° and for 90 days at 4°.

1. Fawcett JP, *et al.* Formulation and stability of pilocarpine oral solution. *Int J Pharm Pract* 1994; **3:** 14–18.

Pilocarpine Nitrate (4527-p)

Pilocarpine Nitrate *(BANM)*.

Pilocarp. Nit.; Pilocarpine Mononitrate; Pilocarpini Nitras; Pilocarpinii Nitras; Pilocarpinium Nitricum.

$C_{11}H_{16}N_2O_2,HNO_3 = 271.3.$

CAS — 148-72-1.

NOTE. PIL is a code approved by the BP for use on single unit doses of eye drops containing pilocarpine nitrate where the individual container may be too small to bear all the appropriate labelling information.

Pharmacopoeias. In *Chin.*, *Eur.* (see p.viii), *Int.*, and *US.*

Colourless or white crystals, or white or almost white crystalline powder. **Soluble** 1 in 4 of water and 1 in 75 of alcohol; practically insoluble in chloroform and in ether. A 5% solution in water has a pH of 3.5 to 4.5. **Store** in airtight containers. Protect from light.

Adverse Effects, Treatment, and Precautions

Systemic effects and cautions are as for Neostigmine, p.1394.

In relation to the *oral* use of pilocarpine as a sialogogue sweating is noted as a common problem; caution is needed to avoid dehydration in patients who may sweat excessively and who cannot maintain an adequate fluid intake. Paradoxical hypertension and constipation, confusion, and increased urinary frequency are also specifically included among the adverse effects reported. Additionally contra-indications include pregnancy. The manufacturer recommends that it should not be given when miosis is undesirable such as in patients with acute iritis or angle-closure glaucoma. An eye examination should be carried out before starting treatment. In addition pilocarpine should be given with care to those with cognitive or psychiatric disturbances, with renal calculi or renal impairment, or with biliary-tract disorders. Dosage should be reduced in patients with hepatic impairment.

Following *ocular* administration pilocarpine is usually better tolerated than the anticholinesterases, but in common with other miotics may produce ciliary spasm, ocular pain and irritation, blurred vision, lachrymation, myopia, and browache. Conjunctival vascular congestion, superficial keratitis, vitreous haemorrhage, and increased pupillary block have been reported. Lens opacities have occurred following prolonged use. Treatment with miotics should be stopped if symptoms of systemic toxicity develop.

Miotics are contra-indicated in conditions where pupillary constriction is undesirable such as acute iritis, acute uveitis, anterior uveitis, and some forms of secondary glaucoma. They should be avoided in acute inflammatory disease of the anterior segment of the eye. If possible, treatment with long-acting miotics should be discontinued before surgery on the eye as there is an increased risk of hyphaema. Miotics should be used with extreme caution in patients with a history of retinal detachment and in young patients with myopia. Miosis may cause blurred vision and difficulty with dark adaptation and caution is necessary with night driving or when hazardous tasks are undertaken in poor illumination. Miotics should not be used by patients wearing soft contact lenses.

Systemic adverse effects after the ophthalmic use of pilocarpine are thought to be rare and reports of toxicity appear to involve elderly patients treated for acute angle-closure glaucoma prior to surgery and who received 2 to 5 times the usual daily dose of pilocarpine in a few hours.[1]

1. Everitt DE, Avorn J. Systemic effects of medications used to treat glaucoma. *Ann Intern Med* 1990; **112:** 120–5.

Alzheimer's disease. In patients with dementia of Alzheimer type, CNS symptoms may be induced or exacerbated by the use of pilocarpine eye drops.[1,2]

1. Reyes PF, *et al.* Mental status changes induced by eye drops in dementia of the Alzheimer type. *J Neurol Neurosurg Psychiatry* 1987; **50:** 113–15.
2. Fraunfelder FT, Morgan R. The aggravation of dementia by pilocarpine. *JAMA* 1994; **271:** 1742–3.

Asthma. A reminder that topical miotics can precipitate bronchospasm in susceptible patients.[1] However, the severity of bronchospasm induced by carbachol has been reported to be less than that produced by timolol. Bronchospastic complications are much less likely to occur with pilocarpine but have nevertheless been reported. As inhalations of methacholine are used to induce bronchospasm in the diagnosis of latent asthma, the risk of exacerbating asthma should be considered before methacholine is used in the eye.

1. Prakash UBS, *et al.* Pulmonary complications from ophthalmic preparations. *Mayo Clin Proc* 1990; **65:** 521–9.

Glaucoma. Miotics usually lower intra-ocular pressure by decreasing the resistance to outflow of aqueous humour from the anterior chamber through the trabecular network. However, they appear to reduce uveoscleral outflow and this may cause a paradoxical rise in intra-ocular pressure in patients with severely compromised trabecular outflow as was reported in a patient with post-traumatic angle-recession glaucoma.[1] It has been recommended that the use of pilocarpine should be avoided after drainage operations for glaucoma because its miotic effect can increase the occurrence of posterior pupillary synechiae; a topical beta blocker is usually adequate if control of intra-ocular pressure is required.[2] Pilocarpine-induced miosis was shown to cause a significant deterioration in visual field in patients with chronic open-angle glaucoma in one study.[3] It was suggested that this factor should be an important consideration when choosing therapy for glaucoma, particularly in cases where field loss approaches the permitted legal minimum for driving. Of 53 patients receiving long-term therapy with pilocarpine gel, 15 developed a corneal haze which persisted for at least 2 years in 13; although the patients remained asymptomatic the long-term effects were unknown.[4] Many patients using the gel also developed superficial punctate keratitis which usually cleared spontaneously during treatment.

1. Bleiman BS, Schwartz AL. Paradoxical intraocular pressure response to pilocarpine: a proposed mechanism and treatment. *Arch Ophthalmol* 1979; **97:** 1305–6.
2. Phillips CI, *et al.* Posterior synechiae after glaucoma operations: aggravation by shallow anterior chamber and pilocarpine. *Br J Ophthalmol* 1987; **71:** 428–32.
3. Webster AR, *et al.* The effect of pilocarpine on the glaucomatous visual field. *Br J Ophthalmol* 1993; **77:** 721–5.
4. Johnson DH, *et al.* Corneal changes during pilocarpine gel therapy. *Am J Ophthalmol* 1986; **101:** 13–15.

Hypersensitivity. Contact urticaria involving the eyelids has been reported[1] in a patient following treatment with pilocarpine eye drops for glaucoma.

1. O'Donnell BF, Foulds IS. Contact allergic dermatitis and contact urticaria due to topical ophthalmic preparations. *Br J Ophthalmol* 1993; **77:** 740–1.

Retinal detachment. The use of miotics has been implicated in numerous reports as a cause of retinal detachment but reviews of the subject have concluded that there is little factual evidence to support the association.[1,2] However, there is circumstantial evidence that retinal detachment is more likely to occur with strong miotics. Furthermore, patients with myopia or pre-existing retinal damage appear to be at greater risk and there is the possibility that even low concentrations of relatively mild miotics such as 1% pilocarpine might precipitate retinal detachment.

1. Alpar JJ. Miotics and retinal detachment: a survey and case report. *Ann Ophthalmol* 1979; **11:** 395–401.
2. Beasley H, Fraunfelder FT. Retinal detachments and topical ocular miotics. *Ophthalmology* 1979; **86:** 95–8.

Interactions

As for Neostigmine, p.1394.

Pharmacokinetics

Mean elimination half-lives for pilocarpine have been reported to be 0.76 and 1.35 hours following oral administration of 5 and 10 mg doses of the hydrochloride respectively. Inactivation of pilocarpine is thought to occur at neuronal synapses and probably in plasma. Pilocarpine and its inactive metabolites, including pilocarpic acid are excreted in the urine.

Uses and Administration

Pilocarpine is a tertiary amine direct-acting parasympathomimetic with primarily the muscarinic effects of acetylcholine (p.1389). It is used mainly in the treatment of glaucoma and dry mouth, and has also been used as a diaphoretic in diagnostic tests for cystic fibrosis and leprosy. Topical application of pilocarpine to the eye produces miosis (pupil constriction) by contraction of the iris sphincter muscle; contraction of the ciliary muscle results in increased accommodation. Constriction of the pupil also pulls open the trabecular meshwork in the eye and this in turn facilitates drainage of aqueous humour and reduction of intra-ocular pressure. Following the use of eye drops, miosis occurs in about 10 to 30 minutes and lasts 4 to 8 hours while peak reduction in intra-ocular pressure occurs within 75 minutes and the reduction usually persists for 4 to 14 hours.

Pilocarpine is used in the treatment of open-angle **glaucoma** (p.1387) and is commonly administered with topical beta blockers or sympathomimetic drugs. It is used as the hydrochloride or the nitrate, usually as 0.5 to 4% eye drops administered 4 times daily, the dose being adjusted individually. Solutions containing 0.25 to 10% of the hydrochloride are also available and the higher strengths may sometimes be required in patients with heavily pigmented irides. A modified-release system inserted into the conjunctival sac and releasing 20 or 40 μg of pilocarpine per hour for 7 days and a 4% ophthalmic gel have also been used. Pilocarpine may also be used as part of the emergency treatment of acute attacks of angle-closure glaucoma prior to surgery.

The miotic action of pilocarpine has been used to antagonise the effects of sympathomimetic mydriatics on the eye and in surgical procedures on the eye. Pilocarpine borate has been used similarly in ophthalmology to the hydrochloride and nitrate.

Pilocarpine hydrochloride is used in the treatment of **dry mouth** following radiotherapy for malignant neoplasms of the head and neck. It increases salivary flow only in patients with residual salivary gland function. The initial dose is 5 mg by mouth three times a day with or immediately after meals, increased gradually if necessary after 4 to 8 weeks until an adequate response is obtained, up to a maximum of 10 mg three times a day. Treatment should be discontinued if no improvement is obtained after 3 months of use.

Diagnosis and testing. CYSTIC FIBROSIS. The fact that individuals with cystic fibrosis have abnormally high concentrations of sodium and chloride in their sweat has been used in the diagnosis of this condition and pilocarpine iontophoresis has been used to promote sweating as part of that test.[1]

1. Gibson LE, Cooke RE. A test for concentration of electrolytes in sweat in cystic fibrosis of the pancreas utilizing pilocarpine by iontophoresis. *Pediatrics* 1959; **23:** 545–9.

LEPROSY. The induction of sweat secretion by intradermal injection of pilocarpine nitrate has been used to assess the functional status of dermal nerves in patients with leprotic skin lesions.[1]

1. Joshi PB. Pilocarpine test in assesment of therapeutic efficacy in maculoanaesthetic leprosy. *Lepr India* 1976; **48:** 55–60.

Dry mouth. Pilocarpine is used as a sialogogue in the treatment of dry mouth (p.1470) following radiotherapy for head and neck cancer. It is also being investigated as a treatment for dry mouth in the auto-immune disease, Sjögren's syndrome.[1]

1. Wiseman LR, Faulds D. Oral pilocarpine: a review of its pharmacological properties and clinical potential in xerostomia. *Drugs* 1995; **49:** 143–55.

Reversal of mydriasis. Pilocarpine has been used to reverse the effects of mydriatics following surgery or ophthalmoscopic examination but other miotics may be preferred (see p.1388). It counteracts the mydriatic effects of sympathomimetics, such as phenylephrine and hydroxyamphetamine[1] but is ineffective against mydriasis produced by antimuscarinics, such as homatropine,[1] and may impair vision further when used with tropicamide.[2] Furthermore, there is also the risk of pilocarpine precipitating angle-closure glaucoma in susceptible patients (see under Glaucoma, above).

1. Anastasi LM, *et al.* Effect of pilocarpine in counteracting mydriasis. *Arch Ophthalmol* 1968; **79:** 710–15.
2. Nelson ME, Orton HP. Counteracting the effects of mydriatics: does it benefit the patient? *Arch Ophthalmol* 1987; **105:** 486–9.

Preparations

BP 1998: Pilocarpine Hydrochloride Eye Drops; Pilocarpine Nitrate Eye Drops;
USP 23: Pilocarpine Hydrochloride Ophthalmic Solution; Pilocarpine Nitrate Ophthalmic Solution; Pilocarpine Ocular System.

Proprietary Preparations (details are given in Part 3)

Aust.: Pilocarpol†; Piloftal; Pilogel; ***Austral.:*** Isopto Carpine; Ocusert; Pilopt; PV Carpine; ***Belg.:*** Isopto Carpine; Pilo; ***Canad.:*** Diocarpine; Isopto Carpine; Miocarpine; Pilopine HS; RO-Carpine†; Spersacarpine†; ***Fr.:*** Chibro-Pilocarpine; Pilo; Vitacarpine†; ***Ger.:*** Asthenopin; Borocarpin-S; Chibro-Pilocarpin†; Pilo-Stulln; Pilocarpol; Pilogel; Pilomann; Pilomann-Ol; Pilopos; Spersacarpin; Vistacarpin; ***Irl.:*** Isopto Carpine; Pilogel; PV Carpine†; Salagen; Sno Pilo†; ***Ital.:*** Dropilton; Liocarpina; Pilogel; Pilotonina; ***Neth.:*** Isopto Carpine†; Pilogel†; Salagen; ***Norw.:*** Isopto Carpine; Pilo; ***S.Afr.:*** Isopto Carpine; Pilogel; PV Carpine; ***Spain:*** Antodrel†; Carpinplast†; Isopto Carpina; ***Swed.:*** Licarpin; Spersacarpine†; ***Switz.:*** Isopto Carpine; Pilo; Pilogel HS; PV Carpine†; Spersacarpine; ***UK:*** Isopto Carpine; Ocusert; Pilogel; Salagen; Sno Pilo; ***USA:*** Adsorbocarpine; Akarpine; Isopto Carpine; Ocu-Carpine; Ocusert; Pilagan; Pilocar; Pilopine HS; Piloptic; Pilopto-Carpine; Pilostat; Salagen; Storzine.

Multi-ingredient: ***Aust.:*** Betacarpin; Normastigmine mit Pilocarpin; Pilostigmin Puroptal; Thiloadren; Timpilo; ***Austral.:*** Timpilo; ***Belg.:*** Miotic Double; Normoglaucon; Rhinofluine†; Timpilo†; ***Canad.:*** E-Pilo; Timpilo; ***Fr.:*** Carpilo; Montavon; Neosyncarpine†; Timpilo; ***Ger.:*** Augentropfen Thilo†; Borocarpin-N†; Borocarpin†; Glauko Biciron; Isopto Pilomin; Miopos-POS stark†; Normoglaucon; Piladren†; Pilo-Eserin; Syncarpin; Thiloadren N; Timpilo; ***Ital.:*** Equiton; Mios; Pilodren; Ripix; Timicon; ***Neth.:*** Normoglaucon; Timpilo-2; ***Norw.:*** Fotil; Timpilo; ***Spain:*** Frikton†; Lucil†; Resorpil†; ***Swed.:*** Fotil; Timpilo; ***Switz.:*** Pilofrine†; Ripix; Timpilo; ***USA:*** E-Pilo; PE.

Pyridostigmine Bromide (4528-s)

Pyridostigmine Bromide *(BAN, rINN)*.

Pyridostig. Brom.; Pyridostigmine (Bromure De); Pyridostigmini Bromidum. 3-Dimethylcarbamoyloxy-1-methylpyridinium bromide.

$C_9H_{13}BrN_2O_2$ = 261.1.

CAS — 155-97-5 (pyridostigmine); 101-26-8 (pyridostigmine bromide).

Pharmacopoeias. In *Chin., Eur.* (see p.viii), *Int., Jpn,* and *US.*

A white or almost white deliquescent crystalline powder with an agreeable characteristic odour. Very **soluble** or freely soluble in water and in alcohol; freely soluble in chloroform; slightly soluble in petroleum spirit; practically insoluble in ether. **Store** in airtight containers. Protect from light.

Adverse Effects, Treatment, and Precautions

As for Neostigmine, p.1394. It has been stated that muscarinic adverse effects occur less frequently with pyridostigmine treatment than with neostigmine.

Psychosis. Postoperative psychosis which developed in a patient with myasthenia gravis who received large doses of pyridostigmine bromide has been attributed to bromide intoxication[1] but this diagnosis has been challenged.[2]

1. Rothenberg DM, *et al.* Bromide intoxication secondary to pyridostigmine bromide therapy. *JAMA* 1990; **263:** 1121–2.
2. Senecal P-E, Osterloh J. Confusion from pyridostigmine bromide: was there bromide intoxication? *JAMA* 1990; **264:** 454–5.

Renal impairment. In patients receiving pyridostigmine for the reversal of non-depolarising muscular blockade following anaesthesia pyridostigmine kinetics were not significantly different in 5 following renal transplantation from those in 5 with normal renal function but in 4 anephric patients the elimination half-life was significantly increased and the plasma clearance significantly decreased.[1] It appeared that approximately 75% of the plasma clearance of pyridostigmine depended on renal function.

1. Cronnelly R, *et al.* Pyridostigmine kinetics with and without renal function. *Clin Pharmacol Ther* 1980; **28:** 78–81.

Interactions

As for Neostigmine, p.1394.

Pharmacokinetics

Pyridostigmine bromide is poorly absorbed from the gastro-intestinal tract. It undergoes hydrolysis by cholinesterases and is also metabolised in the liver. Pyridostigmine is excreted mainly in the urine as unchanged drug and metabolites. Pyridostigmine crosses the placenta and very small amounts are distributed into breast milk. Penetration into the CNS is poor.

One group of workers[1] suggest that data from previous pharmacokinetic studies of pyridostigmine may be at variance due to the analytical methods used or inappropriate storage conditions of plasma samples and recommended that samples should be acidified and stored at −75°. They measured a mean terminal elimination half-life of 200 minutes in 11 healthy subjects given 60 mg of pyridostigmine by mouth; maximum plasma concentrations were obtained 1 to 5 hours after dosing. The mean terminal elimination half-life following a 4-mg intravenous infusion in 10 of these subjects was 97 minutes. Oral bioavailability was calculated to vary from 11.5 to 18.9%. In an earlier study administration of food did not appear to affect bioavailability but did delay the time taken to achieve peak plasma concentrations.[2] It appears that 75% of the plasma clearance of pyridostigmine depends on renal function.[3] 3-Hydroxy-*N*-methylpyridinium has been identified as one of the 3 metabolites isolated from the urine of patients taking pyridostigmine.[4]

1. Breyer-Pfaff U, *et al.* Pyridostigmine kinetics in healthy subjects and patients with myasthenia gravis. *Clin Pharmacol Ther* 1985; **37:** 495–501.
2. Aquilonius S-M, *et al.* Pharmacokinetics and oral bioavailability of pyridostigmine in man. *Eur J Clin Pharmacol* 1980; **18:** 423–8.
3. Cronnelly R, *et al.* Pyridostigmine kinetics with and without renal function. *Clin Pharmacol Ther* 1980; **28:** 78–81.
4. Somani SM, *et al.* Pyridostigmine in man. *Clin Pharmacol Ther* 1972; **13:** 393–9.

Distribution into breast milk. Pyridostigmine was present in breast milk from 2 nursing mothers receiving maintenance therapy for myasthenia gravis in a concentration between 36 and 113% of that in maternal plasma,[1] but in both cases the dose ingested per kg body-weight by the nursing infant was 0.1% or less of that ingested by the mother. Maternal medication with pyridostigmine should be no obstacle to breast feeding, at least with doses in the range of 180 to 300 mg daily.

1. Hardell L-I, *et al.* Pyridostigmine in human breast milk. *Br J Clin Pharmacol* 1982; **14:** 565–7.

Uses and Administration

Pyridostigmine is a quaternary ammonium compound which is a reversible inhibitor of cholinesterase activity with actions similar to those of neostigmine (p.1394), but is slower in onset and of longer duration. It is administered as the bromide.

Pyridostigmine is mainly used in the treatment of myasthenia gravis (p.1388). It has also been used in the treatment of paralytic ileus. Pyridostigmine is sometimes used to reverse the neuromuscular blockade produced by competitive neuromuscular blockers but is generally considered less satisfactory than neostigmine. Pyridostigmine has been used in the management of postoperative urinary retention (p.454) but has generally been superseded by catheterisation.

In **myasthenia gravis**, total daily doses may range from 0.3 to 1.2 g by mouth; some authorities advise that the daily dose should not exceed 720 mg. The dose should be divided throughout the day and, if necessary, the night according to the response of the patient and larger portions of the total daily dose may be given at times of greater fatigue. A suggested dose for children is 7 mg per kg body-weight daily in 5 or 6 divided doses. An alternative regimen is an initial dose of 30 mg for children under 6 years or 60 mg for those aged 6 to 12 years. This is increased gradually by increments of 15 to 30 mg daily until a satisfactory response is obtained, which is usually within the dosage range of 30 to 360 mg daily. It has been given as modified-release tablets, usually once or twice daily but these offer less flexibility of dosage. If necessary it has also been given by intramuscular injection or in severe cases by very slow intravenous injection. However, administration by the intravenous route is hazardous and, if used, atropine must be available to counteract any severe muscarinic reactions.

In the treatment of neonatal myasthenia doses in the range 50 to 150 μg per kg by intramuscular injection or 5 to 10 mg by mouth have been given every 4 to 6 hours; however, neostigmine has generally been preferred. Treatment is rarely needed beyond 8 weeks of age.

To **reverse neuromuscular blockade** produced by competitive neuromuscular blockers, doses of 10 to 20 mg have been given intravenously, preceded by atropine sulphate 0.6 to 1.2 mg to counteract any muscarinic effects. Glycopyrronium bromide has been used as an alternative to atropine.

In the treatment of paralytic ileus and postoperative urinary retention pyridostigmine bromide has been given by mouth in doses of 60 to 240 mg.

Decreased gastro-intestinal motility. Parasympathomimetics such as pyridostigmine enhance gastric contractions and increase intestinal motility and form one of many treatments that have been used in a variety of conditions associated with decreased gastro-intestinal motility (p.1168).

Pyridostigmine, generally in doses of 60 mg up to 3 times daily, has been used to relieve severe constipation in patients with impaired intestinal motility due to Parkinson's disease.[1]

1. Sadjadpour K. Pyridostigmine bromide and constipation in Parkinson's disease. *JAMA* 1983; **249:** 1148.

Growth hormone deficiency. The hypothalamic cholinergic system plays an important role in mechanisms for releasing growth hormone.[1] Activation of muscarinic receptors induces growth hormone release probably through inhibition of somatostatin release. The cholinesterase inhibitor pyridostigmine greatly potentiates rises in growth hormone induced by somatorelin but unexpectedly, direct muscarinic agonists apparently fail to induce growth hormone release. Studies in children indicate that intravenous administration of somatorelin preceded by pyridostigmine given by mouth is the most powerful single test of the secretory integrity of somatotrophs. The test differentiates growth hormone deficiency due to pituitary secretory inability from that due to a hypothalamic defect and permits a rational approach to replacement therapy. However, pyridostigmine given alone or with somatorelin does not appear to be useful for the treatment of short stature in children but administration of neostigmine and somatorelin by the intranasal route appears to be potentially useful.

The management of growth retardation is discussed on p.1237, and includes a comment that there is some dispute over whether stimulated growth hormone secretion tests are superior to measurements of circulating somatomedins in detecting growth hormone deficiency.

1. Müller EE, *et al.* Involvement of brain catecholamines and acetylcholine in growth hormone deficiency states: pathophysiological, diagnostic and therapeutic implications. *Drugs* 1991; **41:** 161–77.

Nerve gas poisoning. Pyridostigmine has been administered prophylactically to protect soldiers against attack with nerve gas agents (p.1606) which inhibit acetylcholinesterase.[1] Pyridostigmine binds reversibly to acetylcholinesterase and provides a protected store from which acetylcholinesterase is later released.[1,2] Prophylaxis with pyridostigmine greatly enhances the efficacy of treatment with atropine and pralidoxime against exposure to soman but it is not effective alone and may not be uniformly effective against other nerve agents.[1] Administration of 30 mg of pyridostigmine every 8 hours provides the optimum level of protection[2] and although adverse effects are common at this dosage the performance of military duties is not impaired.[3] However, neurological symptoms in veterans suffering the so-called Gulf War Syndrome appear to be more common in those who reported exposure to a range of potentially toxic substances which include pyridostigmine.[4] It has been suggested that these symptoms may be evidence of organophosphate-induced polyneuropathy resulting from exposure to a combination of organophosphorus compounds and other cholinesterase inhibitors such as pyridostigmine.[5] A study in *hens*[6] (a species susceptible to anticholinesterases) has also found symptoms of enhanced neurotoxicity when pyridostigmine, the insect repellent diethyltoluamide, and the pyrethroid insecticide permethrin were used together.

1. Dunn MA, Sidell FR. Progress in medical defense against nerve agents. *JAMA* 1989; **262:** 649–52.
2. Ministry of Defence. *Medical manual of defence against chemical agents.* London: HMSO, 1987. (JSP312).
3. Keeler JR, *et al.* Pyridostigmine used as a nerve agent pretreatment under wartime conditions. *JAMA* 1991; **266:** 693–5.
4. The Iowa Persian Gulf Study Group. Self-reported illness and health status among gulf war veterans: a population-based study. *JAMA* 1997; **277:** 238–45.
5. Haley RW, Kurt TL. Self-reported exposure to neurotoxic chemical combinations in the gulf war: a cross-sectional epidemiologic study. *JAMA* 1997; **277:** 231–7.
6. Abou-Donia MB, *et al.* Neurotoxicity resulting from coexposure to pyridostigmine bromide, DEET, and permethrin: implications of gulf war chemical exposure. *J Toxicol Environ Health* 1996; **48:** 35–56.

Post-poliomyelitis syndrome. Pyridostigmine has been reported to be of benefit in reducing fatigue associated with post-poliomyelitis syndrome.[1] A suggested[2] dose is 30 mg daily increased gradually to about 60 mg three times daily but side effects are common.

1. Trojan DA, Cashman NR. Anticholinesterases in post-poliomyelitis syndrome. *Ann N Y Acad Sci* 1995; **753:** 285–95.
2. Thorsteinsson G. Management of postpolio syndrome. *Mayo Clin Proc* 1997; **72:** 627–38.

Preparations

BP 1998: Pyridostigmine Injection; Pyridostigmine Tablets;
USP 23: Pyridostigmine Bromide Injection; Pyridostigmine Bromide Syrup; Pyridostigmine Bromide Tablets.

Proprietary Preparations (details are given in Part 3)
Aust.: Mestinon; ***Austral.:*** Mestinon†; ***Belg.:*** Mestinon; ***Canad.:*** Mestinon; Regonol; ***Fr.:*** Mestinon; ***Ger.:*** Kalymin; Mestinon; ***Irl.:*** Mestinon; ***Ital.:*** Mestinon; ***Neth.:*** Mestinon; ***Norw.:*** Mestinon; ***S.Afr.:*** Mestinon; ***Spain:*** Mestinon; ***Swed.:*** Mestinon; ***Switz.:*** Mestinon; ***UK:*** Mestinon; ***USA:*** Mestinon; Regonol.

Rivastigmine (17993-v)

Rivastigmine *(rINN)*.

ENA-713; SDZ-ENA-713. (−)-*m*[(*S*)-l-(Dimethylamino)ethyl] phenyl ethylmethylcarbamate.

$C_{14}H_{22}N_2O_2$ = 250.3.

CAS — 123441-03-2.

Adverse Effects, Treatment, and Precautions

Generally as for Neostigmine, p.1394. Adverse effects with rivastigmine notably include nausea, vomiting, anorexia, dizziness, somnolence, and asthenia. Other common adverse effects include abdominal pain, diarrhoea, dyspepsia, agitation, confusion, depression, headache, insomnia, sweating, tremor, malaise, and upper-respiratory-tract and urinary-tract infections. Rare cases of angina, gastro-intestinal haemorrhage, and syncope have been observed. There is a potential for bladder outflow obstruction and seizures. Use of rivastigmine has been associated with weight loss and monitoring of patients' weight during treatment is recommended. Female patients have been found to be more susceptible to nausea, vomiting, anorexia, and weight loss.

Interactions

As for Neostigmine, p.1394.

Pharmacokinetics

Rivastigmine is readily absorbed from the gastro-intestinal tract and peak plasma concentrations are reached in about one hour. Administration with food delays absorption by about 1.5 hours and reduces maximum plasma concentrations. Rivastigmine is about 40% bound to plasma proteins and readily crosses the blood-brain barrier. It is rapidly and extensively metabolised, primarily by cholinesterase-mediated hydrolysis to the weakly active decarbamylated metabolite. The plasma half-life of rivastigmine is reported to be about one hour and more than 90% of a dose is excreted in the urine within 24 hours. Less than 1% of a dose appears in the faeces.

Uses and Administration

Rivastigmine is a carbamate type reversible acetylcholinesterase inhibitor. It is selective for the CNS and is used for the symptomatic treatment of mild to moderately severe Alzheimer's disease (p.1386). It is given as the hydrogen tartrate but doses are expressed in terms of the equivalent amount of base. An initial dose is 1.5 mg given twice daily with food. Thereafter, the dose may be increased according to response by increments of 1.5 mg twice daily at intervals of at least 2 weeks to a maximum dose of 6 mg twice daily. Clinical benefit should be reassessed on a regular basis.

References.

1. Anand R, *et al.* Efficacy and safety results of the early phase studies with Excelon™ (ENA-713) in Alzheimer's disease: an overview. *J Drug Dev Clin Pract* 1996; **8:** 109–116.

Preparations

Proprietary Preparations (details are given in Part 3)
UK: Exelon.

Tacrine Hydrochloride (1447-q)

Tacrine Hydrochloride *(BANM, USAN, rINNM).*

CI-970; Tetrahydroaminoacridine Hydrochloride; THA.
1,2,3,4-Tetrahydroacridin-9-ylamine hydrochloride.
$C_{13}H_{14}N_2$,HCl = 234.7.
CAS — 321-64-2 (tacrine); 1684-40-8 (tacrine hydrochloride).

Adverse Effects and Treatment

As for Neostigmine, p.1394.

A major adverse effect of tacrine involves the liver.

Effects on the CNS. A report of tonic or tonic-clonic seizures in 6 of 78 patients given tacrine for mild or moderate dementia of the Alzheimer's type.[1]

1. Lebert F, *et al.* Convulsive effects of tacrine *Lancet* 1996; **347:** 1339–40.

Effects on the liver. A major adverse effect of tacrine therapy is hepatotoxicity. Examination of data from 2446 patients aged at least 50 years who received tacrine for Alzheimer's disease suggested that raised serum-alanine aminotransferase (ALT) levels are likely to occur in about 50% of patients; most cases developed within the first 12 weeks of therapy.[1] The increase is usually asymptomatic and mild, and resolves upon dosage reduction or discontinuation of treatment. However, a small percentage of patients may develop life-threatening hepatotoxicity, which cannot be predicted before treatment starts. No significant correlation has been found between plasma-tacrine concentrations and hepatotoxicity,[2] although frequent monitoring of serum-ALT concentrations during the first 12 weeks of therapy can identify these highly susceptible individuals. However, hepatotoxicity may occur after this time, and an asymptomatic increase in serum-ALT concentrations has been reported in one patient after more than 80 weeks of therapy.[3]

For guidelines on the monitoring of serum-alanine aminotransferase concentrations during tacrine therapy, see Precautions, below.

1. Watkins PB, *et al.* Hepatotoxic effects of tacrine administration in patients with Alzheimer's disease. *JAMA* 1994; **271:** 992–8.
2. Ford JM, *et al.* Serum concentrations of tacrine hydrochloride predict its adverse effects in Alzheimer's disease. *Clin Pharmacol Ther* 1993; **53:** 691–5.
3. Terrell PS, *et al.* Late-onset alanine aminotransferase increase with tacrine. *Ann Pharmacother* 1996; **30:** 301.

Precautions

As for Neostigmine, p.1394. Tacrine should be used with care in patients with impaired liver function or who have a history of such impairment.

Serum-alanine aminotransferase concentrations should be monitored in patients receiving continuous treatment with tacrine. Monitoring should be carried out every other week for at least the first 16 weeks of therapy, followed by monthly for 2 months and then every 3 months thereafter. Weekly monitoring is recommended in patients with elevated aminotransferase levels that are greater than twice the upper limit of the normal range.

If signs of liver involvement worsen, the dose should be reduced or withdrawn. It has been recommended that a threefold to fivefold increase of alanine aminotransferase concentrations calls for a reduction in the dose by 40 mg daily. If increases are above that tacrine should be withdrawn. Withdrawal is also imperative should jaundice develop, confirmed by elevated total bilirubin levels. Treatment with tacrine may be reconsidered once signs of liver dysfunction return to normal. Patients who develop jaundice should not be treated again with tacrine.

Abrupt discontinuation of tacrine therapy or a large reduction in the dose may be associated with behavioural disturbances and a decline in cognitive function.

Interactions

As for Neostigmine, p.1394. Since tacrine is metabolised in the liver by the cytochrome P450 enzyme system (principally CYP1A2), drugs that either inhibit or induce the same isoenzymes may raise or lower plasma concentrations of tacrine.

Cimetidine, a nonspecific inhibitor of the cytochrome P450 enzyme system, has been shown to inhibit the metabolism of tacrine resulting in reduced oral clearance and an increase in plasma concentrations.[1,2] A similar effect has been reported[3] with *fluvoxamine* which inhibits the cytochrome P450 isoenzyme CYP1A2, but *quinidine*, an inhibitor of CYP2D6, appears to have no effect on tacrine metabolism.[1] *Cigarette smoking* has been reported to markedly reduce plasma-tacrine concentrations.[4] Tacrine may inhibit the metabolism of other drugs, such as *theophylline* (see p.770), which are metabolised by the same cytochrome P450 isoenzyme.

1. de Vries TM. Effect of cimetidine and low-dose quinidine on tacrine pharmacokinetics in humans. *Pharm Res* 1993; **10:** S337.
2. Forgue ST, *et al.* Inhibition of tacrine oral clearance by cimetidine. *Clin Pharmacol Ther* 1996; **59:** 444–9.
3. Becquemont L, *et al.* Influence of the CYP1A2 inhibitor fluvoxamine on tacrine pharmacokinetics in humans. *Clin Pharmacol Ther* 1997; **61:** 619–27.
4. Welty D, *et al.* The effect of smoking on the pharmacokinetics and metabolism of Cognex® in healthy volunteers. *Pharm Res* 1993; **10:** S334.

Pharmacokinetics

Tacrine is rapidly absorbed from the gastro-intestinal tract but large interindividual variations in oral bioavailability and the time to achieve peak plasma concentrations have been reported. The presence of food in the stomach reduces the absorption of tacrine by about 30 to 40%. Tacrine is subject to an extensive first-pass effect in the liver, and is metabolised by the cytochrome P450 system (principally CYP1A2) to several metabolites, the main one of which is the 1-hydroxy metabolite velnacrine (p.1400). Tacrine is 55% bound to plasma proteins. Little unchanged drug is excreted in urine.

In 3 studies in a total of 21 patients peak plasma concentrations of tacrine hydrochloride have been achieved 0.5 to 3 hours after oral administration of doses of 25 or 50 mg and oral bioavailability has ranged from less than 5% to up to 36%.[1-3] Mean elimination half-lives were 1.37 and 1.59 hours after the 25 mg dose and 2.14 and 3.2 hours after the 50 mg dose. Tacrine's elimination appears to be mainly by metabolism in the liver and less than 3% of a dose was recovered unchanged in the urine of one patient.[1] Plasma concentrations of tacrine's main metabolite 1-hydroxy-9-aminotetrahydroacridine (velnacrine) rapidly exceed those of the parent compound and elimination half-lives of 43 and 81 minutes were found for this metabolite in 2 patients studied.[2] Further information is provided in the review by Madden *et al.*[4]

1. Forsyth DR, *et al.* Pharmacokinetics of tacrine hydrochloride in Alzheimer's disease. *Clin Pharmacol Ther* 1989; **46:** 634–41.
2. Hartvig P, *et al.* Clinical pharmacokinetics of intravenous and oral 9-amino-1,2,3,4-tetrahydroacridine, tacrine. *Eur J Clin Pharmacol* 1990; **38:** 259–63.
3. Sitar DS, *et al.* Bioavailability and pharmacokinetic disposition of tacrine HCl in elderly patients with Alzheimer's disease. *Clin Pharmacol Ther* 1995; **57:** 198.
4. Madden S, *et al.* Clinical pharmacokinetics of tacrine. *Clin Pharmacokinet* 1995; **28:** 449–57.

Uses and Administration

Tacrine hydrochloride is a centrally acting reversible cholinesterase inhibitor used in the treatment of mild to moderate dementia of the Alzheimer's type (p.1386).

The initial dose of tacrine hydrochloride expressed in terms of tacrine is 10 mg four times a day for a minimum of 6 weeks. Dosage should not be increased during this period because the potential exists for a delay in onset of increased liver enzyme concentrations. Serum-alanine aminotransferase concentrations should be monitored regularly (see Precautions, above) and, if there is no significant increase, doses may be increased by 40 mg daily at six-week intervals until a satisfactory response is obtained, up to a maximum of 160 mg daily in four divided doses. Tacrine should be taken on an empty stomach to improve absorption, although it can be taken with food by patients in whom gastro-intestinal adverse effects may be a problem.

Tacrine has been used to prolong the action of suxamethonium and to antagonise competitive neuromuscular blockers. It has also been used as a respiratory stimulant and has been used as an adjunct to morphine therapy to reduce opioid-induced respiratory depression.

Alzheimer's disease. Tacrine is used in the symptomatic management of Alzheimer's disease (p.1386). It may delay cognitive decline in some patients with mild or moderate Alzheimer's disease but many cannot tolerate the dosage required and have to stop treatment because of gastro-intestinal effects or signs of hepatotoxicity. Although there have been numerous studies of the use of tacrine in Alzheimer's disease a review[1] of double-blind randomised controlled trials found few methodologically suitable for analysis and no convincing evidence of clinical effectiveness. It was also noted that there were no data from controlled studies of longer than 6 months. However, some consider[2-6] that a cautious trial of tacrine might be warranted in patients with mild to moderate Alzheimer's disease and various guidelines on its use have been issued.[5,6]

1. Qizilbash N, *et al.* The efficacy of tacrine in Alzheimer's disease. Dementia & Cognitive Impairment Module of The Cochrane Database of Systematic Reviews (updated 1 September 1997). Available in The Cochrane Library; Issue 4. Oxford: Update Software; 1997.
2. Crimson ML. Tacrine: first drug approved for Alzheimer's disease. *Ann Pharmacother* 1994; **28:** 744–51.
3. Davis KL, Powchik P. Tacrine. *Lancet* 1995; **345:** 625–30.
4. Samuels SC, Davis KL. A risk-benefit assessment of tacrine in the treatment of Alzheimer's disease. *Drug Safety* 1997; **16:** 66–77.
5. Lyketsos CG, *et al.* Guidelines for the use of tacrine in Alzheimer's disease: clinical application and effectiveness. *J Neuropsychiatr Clin Neurosci* 1996; **8:** 67–73.
6. American Psychiatric Association. Practice guideline for the treatment of patients with Alzheimer's disease and other dementias of late life. *Am J Psychiatry* 1997; **154** (suppl): 1–39.

Preparations

Proprietary Preparations (details are given in Part 3)
Aust.: Cognex; *Austral.:* Cognex; THA; *Belg.:* Cognex; *Fr.:* Cognex; *Ger.:* Cognex; *Spain:* Cognex; *Swed.:* Cognex; *Switz.:* Cognex; *USA:* Cognex.

Multi-ingredient: *Austral.:* Mortha†.

Velnacrine Maleate (5350-q)

Velnacrine Maleate *(BANM, USAN, rINNM).*

HP-029; P-83-6029A. (±)-9-Amino-1,2,3,4,-tetrahydro-1-acridinol maleate (1:1).

$C_{13}H_{14}N_2O,C_4H_4O_4$ = 330.3.

CAS — 104675-29-8 (velnacrine); 112964-98-4 (velnacrine); 118909-22-1 (velnacrine maleate); 112964-99-5 (velnacrine maleate).

Velnacrine inhibits cholinesterase activity and has actions similar to those of tacrine (above) of which it is a metabolite. Velnacrine maleate given by mouth has been studied in the treatment of Alzheimer's disease but the manufacturer stopped development in 1994.

References.

1. Clipp EC, Moore MJ. Caregiver time use: an outcome measure in clinical trial research of Alzheimer's disease. *Clin Pharmacol Ther* 1995; **58:** 228–36.
2. Zemlan FP, *et al.* Velnacrine for the treatment of Alzheimer's disease: a double-blind, placebo-controlled trial. *J Neural Transm* 1996; **103:** 1105–16.

Xanomeline (17456-m)

Xanomeline *(USAN, rINN).*

LY-246708. 3-[4-(Hexyloxy)-1,2,5-thiadiazol-3-yl]-1,2,5,6-tetrahydro-1-methylpyridine.

$C_{14}H_{23}N_3OS$ = 281.4.

CAS — 131986-45-3.

Xanomeline is reported to be a selective muscarinic M_1 agonist. The tartrate is being studied in the management of Alzheimer's disease.

References.

1. Sramek JJ, *et al.* The safety and tolerance of xanomeline tartrate in patients with Alzheimer's disease. *J Clin Pharmacol* 1995; **35:** 800–806.
2. Bodick NC, *et al.* Effects of xanomeline, a selective muscarinic receptor agonist, on cognitive function and behavioral symptoms in Alzheimer disease. *Arch Neurol* 1997; **54:** 465–73.

Zifrosilone (17651-g)

Zifrosilone *(USAN, rINN).*

MDL-73745. 2,2,2-Trifluoro-3′-(trimethylsilyl)acetophenone.

$C_{11}H_{13}F_3OSi$ = 246.3.

CAS — 132236-18-1.

Zifrosilone is an inhibitor of cholinesterase activity under investigation for the management of Alzheimer's disease.

References.

1. Cutler NR, *et al.* Acetylcholinesterase inhibition by zifrosilone: pharmacokinetics and pharmacodynamics. *Clin Pharmacol Ther* 1995; **58:** 54–61.

Pesticides and Repellents

This chapter describes compounds used as pesticides and as insect repellents. The term pesticide covers fungicides, herbicides, insecticides (including acaricides), molluscicides, and rodenticides, among others. Most of the pesticides included here are used in clinical or veterinary medicine or in vector control against human or animal disease. Some are used primarily in an agricultural or horticultural setting and are included because of their potential toxicity.

Pesticides can be absorbed during application, by consumption of treated or contaminated products, or by accidental contamination and they may be stored or retained in the tissues. International regulations and controls operate to reduce the risk to both public and user. Values for acceptable daily intakes of pesticides are provided by the Food and Agriculture Organization of the United Nations and the World Health Organization (WHO) through the WHO Technical Report series of publications or, more recently, through *Pesticides Residues in Food: yearly evaluations*, FAO Plant Production and Protection Papers, Rome.

Classification of the main pesticides included in this chapter is given in Table 1 (below).

The **fungicides** included in this chapter are some of those used in the management of plant disease.

Herbicides are used for weed control both in the domestic setting and professionally in agriculture and horticulture. Those here have been included primarily because they are toxic and have been associated with many cases of poisoning.

Many biting insects can cause unpleasant reactions and the use of **insect repellents** can help to overcome this. Perhaps more importantly, the correct use of insect repellents plays a major role in personal protection against a number of communicable diseases transmitted by insect vectors. Examples are babesiosis (ticks), Lyme disease (ticks), malaria (mosquitoes), relapsing fevers (lice and ticks), spotted fevers (ticks), and typhus fever (fleas, lice, and mites). Some compounds such as diethyltoluamide and dimethyl phthalate are effective as repellents while others such as benzyl benzoate and some of the pyrethroids are effective both as repellents and insecticides.

Insecticides have numerous applications. They are used in the treatment of ectoparasitic infections such as pediculosis (lice infections) (below) and in the vector control (below) of a number of communicable diseases that are spread by insects. Acaricides are used to treat scabies (mite infections) (below) and are included within the broad classification of insecticides although acari (mites) are not, technically, insects. Insecticides are also widely used in veterinary practice and in agriculture and horticulture.

The insecticides used in veterinary practice are often classified as topical or systemic ectoparasiticides. Topical ectoparasiticides, as the name implies, are applied topically to the host animal (such as dogs or cats) to kill its ectoparasites (such as fleas). In the case of systemic ectoparasiticides the term 'systemic' refers to the ingestion of the insecticide by the ectoparasite from the host's blood; the insecticide may be present in the host's blood either as a result of absorption through the skin after topical application or after systemic administration.

Molluscicides are used in agriculture or horticulture or in the domestic garden to control snail and slug pests. Additionally, molluscicides such as niclosamide (described in the Anthelmintics chapter on p.105) are used against the freshwater snail vector *Bulinus* in the control of schistosomiasis.

Table 1. Classification of pesticides.

Fungicides	Benomyl, cycloheximide, hexachlorobenzene
Herbicides	Dichlorophenoxyacetic acid, dinitro-*o*-cresol, dinitrophenol, diquat, glyphosate, paraquat, trichlorophenoxyacetic acid
Insect repellents	Butopyronoxyl, dibutyl phthalate, diethyltoluamide, dimethyl phthalate, dioctyl adipate, ethohexadiol, piperonal
Insecticides	
Carbamate	Bendiocarb, carbaryl, carbosulfan, methomyl, propoxur
Chlorinated	Chlordane, dicophane, dieldrin, endosulfan, endrin, heptachlor, lindane
Organophosphorus	Azamethiphos, bromophos, chlorfenvinphos, chlorpyrifos, coumaphos, cythioate, diazinon, dichlorvos, dimethoate, dioxathion, fenitrothion, fenthion, heptenophos, iodofenphos, malathion, parathion, phosmet, phoxim, pirimiphos-methyl, propetamphos, pyraclofos, temefos
Pyrethroid	Bioallethrin, cyfluthrin, cyhalothrin, cypermethrin, deltamethrin, esdepallethrine, fenvalerate, flumethrin, permethrin, phenothrin, pyrethrum flower, resmethrin, tetramethrin
Miscellaneous	Amitraz, benzyl benzoate, chloropicrin, copper oleate, cymiazole, cyromazine, diflubenzuron, ethylene dibromide, ethylene dichloride, fipronil, fluvalinate, lufenuron, methoprene, methyl bromide, monosulfiram, rotenone
Molluscicides	Endod, metaldehyde
Rodenticides	Aluminium phosphide, antu, brodifacoum, bromadiolone, chlorophacinone, coumatetralyl, difenacoum, diphenadione, flocoumafen, fluoroacetamide, norbormide, red squill, sodium fluoroacetate

Rodenticides may be used to exterminate rats and mice when they are likely to be vectors for diseases such as leptospirosis, plague, rat-bite fever, and some haemorrhagic fevers. Many of them are anticoagulants. Warfarin is a commonly used rodenticide but is described elsewhere (p.964).

Clinical Uses of Pesticides and Repellents

Pediculosis

Two species of louse cause pediculosis in man; these are *Pediculus humanus* with its two varieties, *Pediculus humanus capitis* (the head louse) and *Pediculus humanus humanus* (the body louse), and *Pthirus pubis* (*Phthirus pubis*) (the pubic or crab louse). Unlike the head louse, the body louse is an important vector for a number of infections including epidemic typhus (p.149), trench fever (p.146), and relapsing fever (p.140).

Insecticides used in the treatment of pediculosis include malathion, and some pyrethroids such as bioallethrin, permethrin, phenothrin, and tetramethrin. Carbaryl is also effective, although there has been some concern over a theoretical risk of carcinogenicity. Lindane has been used for pubic lice, but many strains of head lice are resistant.

In the UK it has been common for the recommended drugs for the treatment of head lice to be rotated periodically to reduce the emergence of resistance, a problem observed with the newer pyrethroids as well as older insecticides such as lindane. Lotions are preferred to shampoo for head lice since contact time with the insecticide is longer and treatment is thus more effective. Treatment is usually repeated after 7 days. Egg cases ('nits') can be removed by combing the wet hair with a fine tooth comb. A head louse repellent containing piperonal is available.

Malathion has also been suggested for treatment of infections of the eye lashes and brows with pubic lice (pthiriasis or phthiriasis palpebrarum). Other treatments have included the application of a thick layer of yellow soft paraffin or application of yellow mercuric oxide 1% eye ointment twice daily for about 7 or 8 days or a single application of fluorescein eye drops.

Clothing and bed linen of persons with body lice should be washed in hot water or dry cleaned and ironed.

Topical or systemic antimicrobials should be given as necessary for secondary infections.

References.

1. Burgess IF. Human lice and their management. *Adv Parasitol* 1995; **36:** 271–342.

Scabies

Scabies is a parasitic infection of the skin by the mite *Sarcoptes scabiei*. The predominant symptom is pruritus which is caused by an allergic reaction to the parasite and may not occur until several weeks after infection for the first time. Subsequent infections usually result in pruritus after a few days. Pruritus may persist for some months after effective treatment with an acaricide but is not necessarily an indication for further acaricidal treatment; rather, antipruritics should be used. A severe crusted form (Norwegian scabies) may occur rarely, particularly in immunocompromised or incapacitated patients.

Treatment is with the acaricides permethrin or malathion applied, preferably as aqueous lotions, to clean, cool, dry skin over the entire body and left on for 8 to 24 hours, depending upon the preparation. The preparation should be reapplied to the hands whenever they are washed during this period. In adults, it is not usually necessary to treat the face and scalp, but these areas should be treated in young children or patients with atypical or crusted scabies. A single treatment is usually effective, but treatment may be repeated after 7 to 10 days if necessary. Close family and personal contacts should be treated at the same time. Other drugs used topically in the treatment of scabies include benzyl benzoate, crotamiton, lindane, and sulphur; monosulfiram is used in combination with benzyl benzoate. A single oral dose of ivermectin may be effective.

In addition to treatment with an acaricide, symptomatic treatment of the itching with crotamiton, calamine lotion, or systemic antihistamines or corticosteroids may be required.

References.

1. Elgart ML. A risk-benefit assessment of agents used in the treatment of scabies. *Drug Safety* 1996; **14:** 386–93.

Vector control

Many pests are involved in the transmission of communicable diseases and vector control[1,2] is an important part of the fight against such diseases. Insecticides are employed in the control of filariasis (p.95) (*Aedes, Anopheles, Culex,* and *Mansonia* mosquitoes);[3] leishmaniasis (p.575) (*Phlebotomus* or *Lutzomyia* sandflies);[4] malaria (p.422) (*Anopheles* mosquitoes);[5-8] onchocerciasis (p.95) (*Simulium* blackflies);[9] African trypanosomiasis (p.577) (*Glossina* tsetse flies);[10] and South American trypanosomiasis (p.578) (*Triatoma* bugs).[11] The insecticide temefos has proved useful in dracunculiasis (p.93) (crustacean host to the guinea worm larvae). In some cases, as in filariasis or onchocerciasis, the insecticides employed act primarily against the larval stage of the insect vector, whereas in other situations, as in malaria, activity is against the adult insect; in trypanosomiasis, activity is directed against both adult and immature stages. The majority of the experience gained in insecticidal vector control has probably been in malaria, and, for instance, a positive effect seen in the control of leishmaniasis has been considered to be mainly a byproduct of the concomitant malaria control programmes.

Insect repellents can provide personal protection against many insect vectors. For example, in malaria, insect repellents as well as the use of insecticides are important in preventing mosquito bites.

Molluscicides are employed in the control of schistosomiasis (p.95) (*Bulinus* snails).[12]

Rodenticides are also extremely valuable in the vector control of some diseases such as leptospirosis (p.129), plague (p.138), rat-bite fever (p.117), and some haemorrhagic fevers (p.595).

1. Chavasse DC, Yap HH, eds. *Chemical methods for the control of vectors and pests of public health importance.* Geneva: WHO, 1997.
2. Rozendaal JA. *Vector control: methods for use by individuals and communities.* Geneva: WHO, 1997.
3. WHO. Lymphatic filariasis: the disease and its control. *WHO Tech Rep Ser 821* 1992.
4. WHO. Control of the leishmaniases. *WHO Tech Rep Ser 793* 1990.
5. Rozendaal JA. Impregnated mosquito nets and curtains for self-protection and vector control. *Trop Dis Bull* 1989; **86:** R1–R41.
6. WHO. Practical chemotherapy of malaria: report of a WHO scientific group. *WHO Tech Rep Ser 805* 1990.
7. WHO. *International travel and health: vaccination requirements and health advice.* Geneva: WHO, 1996.
8. WHO. Vector control for malaria and other mosquito-borne diseases. *WHO Tech Rep Ser 857* 1995.
9. WHO. Report of a WHO expert committee on onchocerciasis control. *WHO Tech Rep Ser 852* 1995.
10. WHO. Epidemiology and control of African trypanosomiasis: report of a WHO expert committee. *WHO Tech Rep Ser 739* 1986.
11. WHO. Control of Chagas disease: report of a WHO expert committee. *WHO Tech Rep Ser 811* 1991.
12. WHO. The control of schistosomiasis: second report of the WHO expert committee. *WHO Tech Rep Ser 830* 1993.

Aluminium Phosphide (16410-b)

Aluminum Phosphide.

AlP = 57.96.

CAS — 20859-73-8 (aluminium phosphide); 7803-51-2 (phosphine); 1314-84-7 (zinc phosphide).

Aluminium phosphide is used for the fumigation of grain and as a rodenticide. It releases phosphine (PH_3) in the presence of moisture and this accounts for its pesticidal activity. Phosphine gas has a garlic-like odour repulsive to man and domestic animals but apparently not to *rats*. Zinc phosphide is used similarly.

References to poisoning associated with aluminium phosphide.

1. Wilson R, *et al.* Acute phosphine poisoning aboard a grain freighter. *JAMA* 1980; **244:** 148–50.
2. Singh S, *et al.* Aluminium phosphide ingestion. *Br Med J* 1985; **290:** 1110–11.

Amitraz (18372-q)

Amitraz (*BAN, USAN, pINN*).

U-36059. N,N'[(Methylimino)dimethylidyne]di-2,4-xylidine.

$C_{19}H_{23}N_3$ = 293.4.

CAS — 33089-61-1.

Pharmacopoeias. In *BP(Vet)*. Also in *US*, for veterinary use only.

A white to buff-coloured powder. Practically **insoluble** in water; decomposes slowly in alcohol; freely soluble in acetone.

Amitraz is used as a topical ectoparasiticide in veterinary practice; it is effective against various lice, mites, and ticks.

References to poisoning with amitraz.

1. Jorens PG, *et al.* An unusual poisoning with the unusual pesticide amitraz. *Hum Exp Toxicol* 1997; **16:** 600–1.
2. Aydin K, *et al.* Amitraz poisoning in children: clinical and laboratory findings of eight cases. *Hum Exp Toxicol* 1997; **16:** 680–2.

Antu (16411-v)

1-(1-Naphthyl)-2-thiourea.

$C_{11}H_{10}N_2S$ = 202.3.

CAS — 86-88-4.

Antu was formerly used as a rodenticide. The carcinogenic risk from naphthylamine impurities restricted its use.

Azamethiphos (15581-z)

Azamethiphos (*BAN*).

CGA-18809; OMS-1825. *S*-[(6-Chloro-2,3-dihydro-2-oxo-1,3-oxazolo[4,5-*b*]pyridin-3-yl)methyl] *O,O*-dimethyl phosphorothioate.

$C_9H_{10}ClN_2O_5PS$ = 324.7.

CAS — 35575-96-3.

Azamethiphos is an organophosphorus insecticide (p.1408) used in veterinary practice for the control of ectoparasites in the environment.

Bendiocarb (18020-g)

2,3-Isopropylidenedioxyphenyl methylcarbamate.

$C_{11}H_{13}NO_4$ = 223.2.

CAS — 22781-23-3.

Bendiocarb is a carbamate insecticide (p.1403) for agricultural and household use.

Benomyl (18837-n)

Methyl 1-(butylcarbamoyl)benzimidazol-2-ylcarbamate.

$C_{14}H_{18}N_4O_3$ = 290.3.

CAS — 17804-35-2.

Benomyl is a fungicide used for the treatment and control of fungal plant diseases.

Although experimental evidence in *animals* has suggested a possible link between benomyl and congenital eye defects (anophthalmia) the association could not be substantiated in humans.[1-4]

1. Gilbert R. "Clusters" of anophthalmia in Britain. *Br Med J* 1993; **307:** 340–1.
2. Bianchi F, *et al.* Clusters of anophthalmia. *Br Med J* 1994; **308:** 205.
3. Kristensen P, Irgens LM. Clusters of anophthalmia. *Br Med J* 1994; **308:** 205–6.
4. Castilla EE. Clusters of anophthalmia. *Br Med J* 1994; **308:** 206.

Benzyl Benzoate (3569-w)

Benzoato de Bencilo; Benzoato de Benzilo; Benzoesäurebenzylester; Benzyl Benz.; Benzylis Benzoas.

$C_6H_5.CO.O.CH_2.C_6H_5$ = 212.2.

CAS — 120-51-4.

Pharmacopoeias. In *Eur.* (see p.viii), *Int.*, *Jpn*, and *US.*

Colourless or almost colourless crystals or a clear colourless or almost colourless oily liquid with a faintly aromatic odour. F.p. is not below 17° or 18°. Practically **insoluble** in water and in glycerol; miscible with alcohol, with chloroform, with dichloromethane, with ether, and with fatty and essential oils. **Store** at a temperature not exceeding 40° in well-filled airtight containers. Protect from light.

Adverse Effects and Treatment

Benzyl benzoate is irritant to the eyes and mucous membranes and it may be irritant to the skin. Hypersensitivity reactions have been reported. If ingested, benzyl benzoate may cause stimulation of the CNS and convulsions. Systemic symptoms have been reported following excessive topical use. Treatment of poisoning involves gastric lavage if accidentally ingested or washing of the skin following topical use; appropriate symptomatic measures should also be instituted.

Uses and Administration

Benzyl benzoate is an acaricide used in the treatment of scabies (p.1401) although other treatments are generally preferred. It is customary to apply benzyl benzoate as a 25% application to the whole body, usually from the neck down; the application is repeated, without bathing, on the next day and washed off 24 hours later; a third application may sometimes be necessary. Benzyl benzoate is not generally recommended for infants and children, but if used the application should be diluted to minimise the risk of irritation, although this also reduces efficacy.

Benzyl benzoate has also been used as a pediculicide.

Benzyl benzoate is also used as a solubilising agent.

Preparations

BP 1998: Benzyl Benzoate Application;
USP 23: Benzyl Benzoate Lotion.

Proprietary Preparations (details are given in Part 3)
Austral.: Ascabiol; Benzemul; ***Ger.:*** Acarosan; Antiscabiosum; ***Irl.:*** Ascabiol; ***Ital.:*** Mom Lozione Preventiva; ***S.Afr.:*** Ascabiol; ***UK:*** Ascabiol.

Multi-ingredient: ***Austral.:*** Anusol; Anusol-HC†; ***Belg.:*** Pulmex; Pulmex Baby; ***Fr.:*** Allerbiocid S; Ascabiol; ***Ger.:*** Kontakto Derm Lotio; Labocane; ***Irl.:*** Anugesic-HC; Anusol-HC; Sudocrem; ***Ital.:*** Antiscabbia Candioli al DDT Terapeutico; Balsamico F. di M.†; Mom Zanzara; Tioderma†; ***S.Afr.:*** Anugesic; Anusol-HC; ***Spain:*** Tulgrasum Cicatrizante; Yacutin; ***Swed.:*** Tenutex; ***Switz.:*** Anusol; ***UK:*** Anugesic-HC; Anusol-HC; Sudocrem; ***USA:*** Anumed; Anumed HC; Anuprep Hemorrhoidal†; Anusol; Hemril; Rectagene II†.

Bioallethrin (16537-t)

Bioallethrin (*BAN*).

Allethrin I; Depallethrin. (*RS*)-3-Allyl-2-methyl-4-oxocyclopent-2-enyl (1*R*,3*R*)-2,2-dimethyl-3-(2-methylprop-1-enyl)cyclopropanecarboxylate.

$C_{19}H_{26}O_3$ = 302.4.

CAS — 584-79-2 (RS-bioallethrin); 28434-00-6 (S-bioallethrin).

Bioallethrin is a pyrethroid insecticide (p.1410). It is used topically, in conjunction with the synergist piperonyl butoxide (p.1409), in the treatment of pediculosis (p.1401). It is also used in anti-mosquito devices and for the control of household insect pests.

Preparations

Proprietary Preparations (details are given in Part 3)
Ital.: Zanzevia†; ***UK:*** Actomite.

Multi-ingredient: ***Austral.:*** Paralice; ***Belg.:*** Para; ***Canad.:*** Para; ***Fr.:*** Para Special Poux; Parasidose†; ***Ger.:*** Jacutin N; Spregal; ***Ital.:*** Zanzevia†; ***Neth.:*** Para-Speciaal; ***UK:*** Fortefog.

Brodifacoum (16545-t)

WBA-8119. 3-[3-(4'-Bromobiphenyl-4-yl)-1,2,3,4-tetrahydro-1-naphthyl]-4-hydroxycoumarin.

$C_{31}H_{23}BrO_3$ = 523.4.

CAS — 56073-10-0.

Brodifacoum is an anticoagulant rodenticide. It is reported to be effective in warfarin-resistant strains of rodents.

Brodifacoum, a second-generation anticoagulant rodenticide, inhibits prothrombin synthesis to cause bleeding that may be occult.[1] It is absorbed from the gastro-intestinal tract; dermal absorption is possible. Poisons containing 100 mg per kg of bait are not hazardous to man; more concentrated forms are particularly hazardous and their availability should be restricted. Baits, which should be prepared only by trained personnel, should contain a suitable marker-dye.

There have been reports of poisoning with brodifacoum.[2,3]

1. WHO. Safe use of pesticides: ninth report of the WHO expert committee on vector biology and control. *WHO Tech Rep Ser 720* 1985.
2. Watts RG, *et al.* Accidental poisoning with a superwarfarin compound (brodifacoum) in a child. *Pediatrics* 1990; **86:** 883–7.
3. Ross GS, *et al.* An acquired hemorrhagic disorder from long-acting rodenticide ingestion. *Arch Intern Med* 1992; **152:** 410–12.

Bromadiolone (3862-z)

3-[3-(4'-Bromobiphenyl-4-yl)-3-hydroxy-1-phenylpropyl]-4-hydroxycoumarin.

$C_{30}H_{23}BrO_4$ = 527.4.

CAS — 28772-56-7.

Bromadiolone is an anticoagulant rodenticide.

Bromadiolone, a second-generation anticoagulant rodenticide, inhibits prothrombin synthesis to cause bleeding that may be occult.[1] It is absorbed from the gastro-intestinal tract; dermal absorption is possible. Poisons containing 100 mg per kg of bait are not hazardous to man; more concentrated forms are particularly hazardous and their availability should be restricted. Baits, which should be prepared only by trained personnel, should contain a suitable marker-dye.

There have been reports of poisoning with bromadiolone.[2]

1. WHO. Safe use of pesticides: ninth report of the WHO expert committee on vector biology and control. *WHO Tech Rep Ser 720* 1985.
2. Greeff MC, *et al*. "Superwarfarin" (bromodialone) poisoning in two children resulting in prolonged anticoagulation. *Lancet* 1987; **ii:** 1269.

Bromophos (18104-w)

OMS-658. *O*-4-Bromo-2,5-dichlorophenyl *O,O*-dimethyl phosphorothioate.

$C_8H_8BrCl_2O_3PS$ = 366.0.

CAS — 2104-96-3.

Bromophos is an organophosphorus insecticide (p.1408) used in veterinary practice for the control of ectoparasites in the environment. It is also used as an agricultural insecticide.

Butopyronoxyl (2551-z)

Indalone. Butyl 3,4-dihydro-2,2-dimethyl-4-oxo-2*H*-pyran-6-carboxylate.

$C_{12}H_{18}O_4$ = 226.3.

CAS — 532-34-3.

Butopyronoxyl has been used as an insect repellent.

Carbamate Insecticides (3561-h)

The carbamate insecticides are *N*-substituted esters of carbamic acid. Those described in this chapter are listed in Table 1 (p.1401).

References.

1. WHO. Carbamate pesticides: a general introduction. *Environmental Health Criteria 64*. Geneva: WHO, 1986.

Adverse Effects

As for Organophosphorus Insecticides, p.1408.

The carbamates are cholinesterase inhibitors, differing from the organophosphorus insecticides in that the inhibition they produce is generally less intense and more rapidly reversible. Also they do not appear to enter the CNS as readily so that severe central effects are uncommon.

Treatment of Adverse Effects

If carbamate insecticides have been ingested the stomach should be emptied by lavage. Contaminated clothing should be removed and the skin washed with soap and water. Treatment is largely symptomatic and supportive and includes atropine but this may not always be necessary due to the rapidly reversible nature of the cholinesterase inhibition produced. Pralidoxime or other oximes should *not* be given.

References.

1. WHO. Safe use of pesticides: fourteenth report of the WHO expert committee on vector biology and control. *WHO Tech Rep Ser 813* 1991.
2. Proudfoot A, ed. *Pesticide poisoning: notes for the guidance of medical practitioners*. 2nd ed. London: DoH, The Stationery Office, 1996.

Carbaryl (3570-m)

Carbaryl *(BAN)*.

Carbaril *(pINN)*; OMS-29. 1-Naphthyl methylcarbamate.

$C_{12}H_{11}NO_2$ = 201.2.

CAS — 63-25-2.

Pharmacopoeias. In *Br.*

A white to off-white or light grey powder which darkens on exposure to light. Very slightly **soluble** in water; soluble in alcohol and in acetone. **Store** at a temperature not exceeding 25°. Protect from light.

Adverse Effects and Treatment

As for Carbamate Insecticides, p.1403. Carbaryl may be absorbed following ingestion, inhalation, or skin contamination.

Carbaryl has been reported to produce neoplasms in *mice* and *rats* and in late 1995 the UK Department of Health advised that it would be prudent to consider carbaryl as a potential human carcinogen; its medicinal use was limited to prescription only. However, the Department of Health emphasised that the risk was a theoretical one and that any risk from the intermittent use of head lice preparations was likely to be very small.

Uses and Administration

Carbaryl is a carbamate insecticide (p.1403). It is used as a 0.5 or 1.0% lotion or shampoo in the treatment of head and pubic pediculosis (p.1401). Lotions are generally preferred to shampoos as the contact time is longer. Aqueous lotions are preferred to treat pubic lice because alcoholic lotions are irritant to excoriated skin and the genitalia; aqueous lotions may also be preferable in asthmatic subjects or children to avoid alcoholic fumes. Skin or hair treated with an alcohol-based preparation should be allowed to dry naturally.

Carbaryl is also used as a topical ectoparasiticide in veterinary practice and as an agricultural, horticultural, and household insecticide.

Preparations

BP 1998: Carbaryl Lotion.

Proprietary Preparations (details are given in Part 3)
Irl.: Carylderm; Defesto C†; Derbac-C; ***Ital.:*** Ikecrin†; ***UK:*** Carylderm; Clinicide†; Mitchell Expel Anti Lice Spray; Suleo-C.

Carbosulfan (5368-k)

2,3-Dihydro-2,2-dimethylbenzofuran-7-yl (dibutylaminothio)methylcarbamate.

$C_{20}H_{32}N_2O_3S$ = 380.5.

Carbosulfan is a carbamate insecticide (p.1403) used for the larvicidal treatment of rivers in the control of onchocerciasis (p.95).

Chlordane (18055-k)

1,2,4,5,6,7,8,8-Octachloro-2,3,3a,4,7,7a-hexahydro-4,7-methanoindene.

$C_{10}H_6Cl_8$ = 409.8.

CAS — 57-74-9.

Chlordane is a chlorinated insecticide (p.1403). Its use is limited, or even prohibited, in some countries because of toxicity due to its persistent nature.

References.

1. Chlordane. *Environmental Health Criteria 34*. Geneva: WHO, 1984.
2. Kutz FW, *et al*. A fatal chlordane poisoning. *J Toxicol Clin Toxicol* 1983; **20:** 167–74.

Chlorfenvinphos (18108-j)

Chlorfenvinphos *(BAN)*.

Clofenvinfos *(rINN)*. 2-Chloro-1-(2,4-dichlorophenyl)vinyl diethyl phosphate.

$C_{12}H_{14}Cl_3O_4P$ = 359.6.

CAS — 470-90-6.

Chlorfenvinphos is an organophosphorus insecticide (p.1408) used in agriculture.

Chlorinated Insecticides (3562-m)

The chlorinated or organochlorine insecticides were widely used, but because of persistence in man many have been banned or restricted. Those described in this chapter are listed in Table 1 (p.1401).

References.

1. WHO. Polychlorinated biphenyls and terphenyls. *Environmental Health Criteria 2*. Geneva: WHO, 1976.

Adverse Effects

Chlorinated or organochlorine insecticides form a very wide group and the toxicity of individual members varies considerably. In general these insecticides produce symptoms consistent with CNS stimulation. They may be absorbed through the respiratory and gastro-intestinal tracts and through the skin.

Symptoms of acute poisoning include nausea and vomiting, paraesthesia, giddiness, tremors, convulsions, coma, and respiratory failure. Liver, kidney, and myocardial toxicity have been reported. Effects on the blood include agranulocytosis and aplastic anaemia. Symptoms may be complicated by the effects of the solvent.

Chlorinated insecticides have been reported to enhance microsomal hepatic enzyme activity. Skin reactions can follow contact with insecticides.

Polychlorinated biphenyl (PCB) and terphenyl compounds were formerly used as insecticides in many countries. They are stored in body fat and are not readily excreted except in breast milk, although they possibly cross the placenta; because of this and because of accidental contamination they remain a cause for concern. The related polybrominated biphenyl compounds (PBB) which have no insecticidal uses have also been absorbed by the public following accidental contamination of the food chain.

Some chlorinated insecticides have weak oestrogenic effects; it has been proposed that exposure may increase the risk of breast cancer.

Treatment of Adverse Effects

If chlorinated insecticides have been ingested the stomach should be emptied by lavage. Contaminated clothing should be removed and the skin washed with soap and water. Treatment is largely symptomatic and supportive with treatment of CNS stimulation such as hyperactivity and convulsions.

References.

1. WHO. Safe use of pesticides: fourteenth report of the WHO expert committee on vector biology and control. *WHO Tech Rep Ser 813* 1991.
2. Proudfoot A, ed. Pesticide poisoning: notes for the guidance of medical practitioners. 2nd ed. London: DoH, The Stationery Office, 1996.

Chlorophacinone (18199-w)

LM-91. 2-[2-(4-Chlorophenyl)-2-phenylacetyl]indane-1,3-dione.

$C_{23}H_{15}ClO_3$ = 374.8.

CAS — 3691-35-8.

Chlorophacinone is an indanedione derivative used as an anticoagulant rodenticide. It is also reported to uncouple oxidative phosphorylation with consequent stimulation of cellular metabolism which may contribute to its toxicity.

References to poisoning with chlorophacinone.

1. Burucoa C, *et al*. Chlorophacinone intoxication: biological and toxicological study. *J Toxicol Clin Toxicol* 1989; **27:** 79–89.

Chloropicrin (12554-e)

Nitrochloroform. Trichloronitromethane.

CCl_3NO_2 = 164.4.

CAS — 76-06-2.

A slightly oily liquid with an intense odour.

Chloropicrin is a lachrymatory agent and is intensely irritating to the skin and mucous membranes. It is an insecticide and is used for fumigating stored grain and soil. Chloropicrin is also added to other fumigants as a warning gas.

Chlorpyrifos (18112-w)

Chlorpyrifos *(BAN)*.

O,O-Diethyl *O*-3,5,6-trichloro-2-pyridyl phosphorothioate.

$C_9H_{11}Cl_3NO_3PS$ = 350.6.

CAS — 2921-88-2.

Chlorpyrifos is an organophosphorus insecticide (p.1408) used in agriculture.

Copper Oleate (12608-s)

$Cu(C_{18}H_{33}O_2)_2$ = 626.5.

CAS — 1120-44-1.

Copper oleate has been used topically as an insecticide for the treatment of pediculosis (p.1401).

Preparations

Proprietary Preparations (details are given in Part 3)
Ger.: Cuprex†.

Coumaphos (18115-y)

Coumaphos *(BAN)*.

Coumafos *(rINN)*; Bayer-21199. *O*-3-Chloro-4-methyl-7-coumarinyl *O,O*-diethyl phosphorothioate.

$C_{14}H_{16}ClO_5PS$ = 362.8.

CAS — 56-72-4.

Coumaphos is an organophosphorus insecticide (p.1408) used as a topical ectoparasiticide in veterinary practice.

Coumatetralyl (16406-p)

4-Hydroxy-3-(1,2,3,4-tetrahydro-1-naphthyl)coumarin.

$C_{19}H_{16}O_3$ = 292.3.

CAS — 5836-29-3.

Coumatetralyl is an anticoagulant rodenticide.

Cycloheximide (12620-v)

Cycloheximide *(USAN)*.

Cicloheximide *(rINN)*; U-4527. 3-{(2*R*)-2-[(1*S*,3*S*,5*S*)-3,5-Dimethyl-2-oxocyclohexyl]-2-hydroxyethyl}glutarimide.

$C_{15}H_{23}NO_4$ = 281.3.

CAS — 66-81-9.

Cycloheximide is an antimicrobial substance produced by strains of *Streptomyces griseus*. It has antifungal properties and has been used for the treatment and control of certain mycotic plant diseases.

Cyfluthrin (3855-c)

Cyfluthrin *(BAN)*.

Bay-VI-1704; Cyfluthin. (*RS*)-α-Cyano-4-fluoro-3-phenoxybenzyl (1*RS*,3*RS*; 1*RS*,3*SR*)-3-(2,2-dichlorovinyl)-2,2-dimethylcyclopropanecarboxylate.

$C_{22}H_{18}Cl_2FNO_3$ = 434.3.

CAS — 68359-37-5.

Cyfluthrin is a pyrethroid insecticide (p.1410) used in agriculture.

Cyhalothrin (15318-d)

Cyhalothrin *(BAN)*.

PP-563. (*RS*)-α-Cyano-3-phenoxybenzyl (*Z*)-(1*RS*,3*RS*)-3-(2-chloro-3,3,3-trifluoropropenyl)-2,2-dimethylcyclopropanecarboxylate.

$C_{23}H_{19}ClF_3NO_3$ = 449.8.

CAS — 68085-85-8.

Cyhalothrin is a pyrethroid insecticide (p.1410) that is used, particularly as a mixture of the (*Z*)-(1*R*,3*R*) *S* ester and the (*Z*)-(1*S*,3*S*) *R* ester (known as lambda-cyhalothrin), for the control of insect pests in public health. It has also been used in agriculture.

References.

1. Cyhalothrin. *Environmental Health Criteria 99*. Geneva: WHO, 1990.

Cymiazole (3886-d)

CGA-50439; CGA-192357 (cymiazole hydrochloride); Xymiazole. 2,4-Dimethyl-*N*-(3-methyl-2(3*H*)-thiazolylidene)benzenamine.

$C_{12}H_{14}N_2S$ = 218.3.

CAS — 61676-87-7 (cymiazole); 121034-85-3 (cymiazole hydrochloride).

Cymiazole is a pesticide used in beekeeping.

Cypermethrin (19015-k)

Cypermethrin *(BAN)*.

(*RS*)-α-Cyano-3-phenoxybenzyl (1*RS*,3*RS*)-(1*RS*,3*RS*)-3-(2,2-dichlorovinyl)-2,2-dimethylcyclopropanecarboxylate.

$C_{22}H_{19}Cl_2NO_3$ = 416.3.

CAS — 52315-07-8.

Cypermethrin, an isomeric mixture containing alpha-cypermethrin, is a pyrethroid insecticide (p.1410) used as a topical ectoparasiticide in veterinary practice. It is also used in agriculture. Zeta-cypermethrin is also used.

References.

1. Cypermethrin. *Environmental Health Criteria 82*. Geneva: WHO, 1989.
2. Alpha-cypermethrin. *Environmental Health Criteria 142*. Geneva: WHO, 1992.

Preparations

Proprietary Preparations (details are given in Part 3)

Multi-ingredient: *UK:* Fortefog.

Cyromazine (4874-b)

Cyromazine *(BAN, rINN)*.

CGA-72662. *N*-Cyclopropyl-1,3,5-triazine-2,4,6-triamine.

$C_6H_{10}N_6$ = 166.2.

CAS — 66215-27-8.

Cyromazine is used as a topical ectoparasiticide in veterinary practice and as an agricultural insecticide.

Cythioate (3573-g)

Cythioate *(BAN)*.

O,O-Dimethyl *O*-(4-sulphamoylphenyl) phosphorothioate.

$C_8H_{12}NO_5PS_2$ = 297.3.

CAS — 115-93-5.

Cythioate is an organophosphorus insecticide (p.1408) used as a systemic ectoparasiticide in veterinary practice; it is administered by mouth to the host animal.

Daminozide (10683-b)

N-Dimethylaminosuccinamic acid.

$C_6H_{12}N_2O_3$ = 160.2.

CAS — 1596-84-5.

Daminozide is a plant growth regulator that has been used in pesticides to improve fruit crops. There have been concerns about residues of the chemical in the fruit.

Deltamethrin (16614-c)

Deltamethrin *(BAN)*.

Decamethrin; NRDC-161. (*S*)-α-Cyano-3-phenoxybenzyl (1*R*,3*R*)-3-(2,2-dibromovinyl)-2,2-dimethylcyclopropanecarboxylate.

$C_{22}H_{19}Br_2NO_3$ = 505.2.

CAS — 52918-63-5.

Deltamethrin is a pyrethroid insecticide (p.1410) used in the vector control of malaria (p.422). It is also used as a topical ectoparasiticide in veterinary practice and as an agricultural and household insecticide.

References.

1. Deltamethrin health and safety guide. *IPCS Health and Safety Guide 30*. Geneva: WHO, 1989.
2. Deltamethrin. *Environmental Health Criteria 97*. Geneva: WHO, 1990.

Diazinon (18132-j)

Diazinon *(BAN)*.

Dimpylate *(rINN)*. *O,O*-Diethyl *O*-(2-isopropyl-6-methylpyrimidin-4-yl) phosphorothioate.

$C_{12}H_{21}N_2O_3PS$ = 304.3.

CAS — 333-41-5.

Diazinon is an organophosphorus insecticide (p.1408) used as a systemic ectoparasiticide in veterinary practice; it is applied topically to the host animal. It is also employed as an insecticide in agriculture and horticulture.

References.

1. Wagner SL, Orwick DL. Chronic organophosphate exposure associated with transient hypertonia in an infant. *Pediatrics* 1994; **94:** 94–7.

Dibromochloropropane (12642-e)

1,2-Dibromo-3-chloropropane.

$C_3H_5Br_2Cl$ = 236.3.

CAS — 96-12-8.

Dibromochloropropane has been used as a pesticide. Low sperm counts and evidence of testicular damage have occurred in workers exposed to dibromochloropropane.

Dibutyl Phthalate (2553-k)

Butyl Phthalate; DBP. Dibutyl benzene-1,2-dicarboxylate.

$C_{16}H_{22}O_4$ = 278.3.

CAS — 84-74-2.

Pharmacopoeias. In *Eur.* (see p.viii).

A clear, oily, colourless or very slightly yellow liquid. Practically **insoluble** in water; miscible with alcohol and with ether. **Store** in airtight containers.

Adverse Effects and Precautions

Dibutyl phthalate has occasionally caused hypersensitivity reactions. As with other phthalates contact with plastics should be avoided.

Uses and Administration

Dibutyl phthalate has been used as an insect repellent although it is slightly less effective than dimethyl phthalate (p.1405). It is less volatile and less easily removed by washing than dimethyl phthalate, and its chief use therefore has been for the impregnation of clothing.

Dibutyl phthalate has also been employed as a plasticiser.

Preparations

Proprietary Preparations (details are given in Part 3)

Multi-ingredient: *S.Afr.:* Mylol.

Dichlorophenoxyacetic Acid (3576-s)

2,4-D. 2,4-Dichlorophenoxyacetic acid.

$C_8H_6Cl_2O_3$ = 221.0.

CAS — 94-75-7.

Adverse Effects, Treatment, and Precautions

Most cases of poisoning with dichlorophenoxyacetic acid have involved its ingestion with other herbicides; the solvent may also play a part in any toxicity. There is little pattern to the range of adverse effects which may occur following ingestion, inhalation, or topical exposure.

Observed adverse effects have involved the central and peripheral nervous system, muscles, and the cardiovascular system. Gastro-intestinal effects are common with poisoning. Hepatotoxicity, nephrotoxicity, and pulmonary disorders have been observed but it is not clear that dichlorophenoxyacetic acid contributed to the toxicity. The role of phenoxyacetic acids in cancer is discussed under trichlorophenoxyacetic acid (p.1410).

Ingested material should be removed by lavage. Contaminated clothing should be removed and the skin washed with soap and water. Forced alkaline diuresis has been reported to be effective in removing dichlorophenoxyacetic acid. Further treatment is symptomatic.

References.

1. 2,4-Dichlorophenoxyacetic acid (2,4-D). *Environmental Health Criteria 29*. Geneva: WHO, 1984.
2. 2,4-Dichlorophenoxyacetic acid (2,4-D)—environmental aspects. *Environmental Health Criteria 84*. Geneva: WHO, 1989.
3. Friesen EG, *et al.* Clinical presentation and management of acute 2,4-D oral ingestion. *Drug Safety* 1990; **5:** 155–9.
4. Flanagan RJ, *et al.* Alkaline diuresis for acute poisoning with chlorophenoxy herbicides and ioxynil. *Lancet* 1990; **335:** 454–8.

Uses

Dichlorophenoxyacetic acid is a herbicide widely used for weed control in cereals and other crops. It is usually used as its salts or esters in combination with other herbicides.

Dichlorvos (3577-w)

Dichlorvos *(BAN, USAN, rINN)*.

DDVP; NSC-6738; OMS-14; SD-1750. 2,2-Dichlorovinyl dimethyl phosphate.

$C_4H_7Cl_2O_4P$ = 221.0.

CAS — 62-73-7.

Pharmacopoeias. In *Fr.* for veterinary use.

Dichlorvos is an organophosphorus insecticide (p.1408) of short persistence, effective against a wide range of insects. It is sometimes used as a fumigant. It is also used as a topical ectoparasiticide in veterinary practice. It has also been used for the extermination of insects in aircraft (disinsection).

References.

1. Dichlorvos health and safety guide. *IPCS Health and Safety Guide 18*. Geneva: WHO, 1988.
2. Dichlorvos. *Environmental Health Criteria 79*. Geneva: WHO, 1989.

Dicophane (3578-e)

Clofenotane *(rINN)*; Chlorofenotano; Chlorophenothane; Chlorphenothanum; DDT; Dichlorodiphenyltrichloroethane; Dichophanum. 1,1,1-Trichloro-2,2-bis(4-chlorophenyl)ethane.

$C_{14}H_9Cl_5$ = 354.5.

CAS — 50-29-3.

Pharmacopoeias. In *Aust.* and *It.*

Adverse Effects and Treatment

As for Chlorinated Insecticides, p.1403.

References.

1. DDT and its derivatives. *Environmental Health Criteria 9*. Geneva: WHO, 1979.
2. DDT and its derivatives—environmental aspects. *Environmental Health Criteria 83*. Geneva: WHO, 1989.

Carcinogenicity. Some small epidemiological studies have suggested that certain organochlorines, namely 1,1-dichloro-2,2-bis(*p*-chlorophenyl)ethylene (DDE), a metabolite of dicophane, and polychlorinated biphenyls (PCBs), might increase the risk of breast cancer in women. However, reanalysis[1] of the available data indicated that an association with breast cancer was unlikely for dicophane; there was no evidence for an association with the polychlorinated biphenyls. Any link between exposure to dicophane and the development of testicular cancer in men was also refuted[2] following long-term monitoring of populations in Scandinavia.

1. Key T, Reeves G. Organochlorines in the environment and breast cancer. *Br Med J* 1994; **308:** 1520–1.
2. Ekbom A, *et al.* DDT and testicular cancer. *Lancet* 1996; **347:** 553–4.

Effects on fertility. A metabolite of dicophane, 1,1-dichloro-2,2-bis-(*p*-chlorophenyl)ethylene (DDE), was reported[1] to have anti-androgenic properties in *rats* and exposure to dicophane might account for a previously reported decline in male fertility and an increase in male reproductive abnormalities.

1. Keke WR, *et al.* Persistent DDT metabolite p,p'-DDE is a potent androgen receptor antagonist. *Nature* 1995; **375:** 581–5.

Pharmacokinetics

Dicophane may be absorbed after ingestion or inhalation or through the skin. Dicophane is stored in the body, particularly in body fat, and is very slowly eliminated. It crosses the placenta and appears in breast milk. It is metabolised in the body to the ethylene derivative, 1,1-dichloro-2,2-bis(*p*-chlorophenyl)ethylene (DDE); the acetic acid derivative (DDA) also appears in the urine.

Uses

Dicophane is a chlorinated insecticide (p.1403). It is a stomach and contact poison and retains its activity for long periods under a variety of conditions. It is effective against disease vectors such as fleas, lice, and mosquitoes and has been applied topically for pediculosis (p.1401) and scabies (p.1401), although more suitable alternatives exist.

Because of the extreme persistence of dicophane, concern in respect of its effect in the environment, and the problem of resistance, the widespread use of dicophane is now generally discouraged. It is no longer used in some countries while in others its use is limited.

Despite reservations regarding the use of dicophane for vector control, many endemic countries have relied on it for the control of both malaria and visceral leishmaniasis. A WHO study group[1] reviewed the current situation and concluded that dicophane might be used provided that all the following conditions were met. Namely that: it was used only for indoor spraying; it was known to be effective; it was manufactured to WHO's specifications; and the necessary safety precautions were taken in its use and disposal. However, they recommended further investigation of the effects of dicophane in breast milk and of suspected carcinogenicity, as well as clarification of the significance of the reduced density of muscarinic receptors caused by dicophane.

1. WHO. Vector control for malaria and other mosquito-borne diseases. *WHO Tech Rep Ser 857* 1995.

Preparations

Proprietary Preparations (details are given in Part 3)
Fr.: Benzochloryl†; *Ital.:* Polvere Cruz Verde†.

Multi-ingredient: *Ital.:* Antiscabbia Candioli al DDT Terapeutico; Pyr†.

Dieldrin (3579-l)

Dieldrin *(BAN, pINN).*
CAS — 60-57-1 (HEOD).

Dieldrin contains about 85% of (1*R*,4*S*,5*S*,8*R*)-1,2,3,4,10,10-hexachloro-6,7-epoxy-1,4,4a,5,6,7,8,8a-octahydro-1,4:5,8-dimethanonaphthalene (HEOD), $C_{12}H_8Cl_6O$ = 380.9. The remaining 15% is mainly chlorinated organic compounds related to HEOD.

Adverse Effects and Treatment

As for Chlorinated Insecticides, p.1403.

Dieldrin is more toxic than dicophane (above) and is readily absorbed through the skin.

References.

1. Aldrin and dieldrin. *Environmental Health Criteria 91.* Geneva: WHO, 1989.
2. Aldrin and dieldrin health and safety guide. *IPCS Health and Safety Guide 21.* Geneva: WHO, 1989.
3. Høyer AP, *et al.* Organochlorine exposure and risk of breast cancer. *Lancet* 1998; **352:** 1816–20.

Uses

Dieldrin is a chlorinated insecticide (p.1403) formerly used as a sheep dip. Its use is now limited to a few specified purposes such as termite control.

Diethyltoluamide (2554-a)

Diethyltoluamide *(BAN, rINN).*
DEET. *NN*-Diethyl-*m*-toluamide.
$C_{12}H_{17}NO$ = 191.3.
CAS — 134-62-3.
Pharmacopoeias. In *US.*

A colourless liquid with a faint pleasant odour. Practically **insoluble** in water and glycerol; miscible with alcohol, carbon disulphide, chloroform, ether, and isopropyl alcohol. **Store** in airtight containers.

Adverse Effects and Precautions

Occasional hypersensitivity to diethyltoluamide has been reported. Diethyltoluamide should not be applied near the eyes, to mucous membranes, to broken skin, or to areas of skin flexion as irritation or blistering may occur. Systemic toxicity has been reported following application of large topical doses, particularly in children.

Hypersensitivity and anaphylaxis has been described in one patient after exposure to diethyltoluamide.[1] Toxic encephalopathy has been noted in children who received liberal applications of this compound;[2] seizures have also been reported,[3] and there have been cases of manic psychosis[4] and cardiovascular toxicity (sinus bradycardia and orthostatic hypotension)[5] associated with topical application. Toxic reactions, including death, have been reported following the ingestion of large amounts of diethyltoluamide-containing insect repellents.[6]

1. Miller JD. Anaphylaxis associated with insect repellent. *N Engl J Med* 1982; **307:** 1341–2.
2. Roland EH, *et al.* Toxic encephalopathy in a child after brief exposure to insect repellents. *Can Med Assoc J* 1985; **132:** 155–6.
3. Anonymous. Seizures temporally associated with use of DEET insect repellent—New York and Connecticut. *Arch Dermatol* 1989; **125:** 1619–20.
4. Snyder JW, *et al.* Acute manic psychosis following the dermal application of N,N-diethyl-m-toluamide (DEET) in an adult. *J Toxicol Clin Toxicol* 1986; **24:** 429–39.
5. Clem JR, *et al.* Insect repellent (N,N-diethyl-m-toluamide) cardiovascular toxicity in an adult. *Ann Pharmacother* 1993; **27:** 289–93.
6. Tenenbein M. Severe toxic reactions and death following the ingestion of diethyltoluamide-containing insect repellents. *JAMA* 1987; **258:** 1509–11.

Uses

Diethyltoluamide is an insect repellent which is effective against mosquitoes as well as blackflies, harvest-bugs or chiggers, midges, ticks, and fleas. It is considered to be of value for personal protection against malaria (p.422). It has also been used as a repellent against leeches. It may be applied to skin and clothing.

Preparations

USP 23: Diethyltoluamide Topical Solution.

Proprietary Preparations (details are given in Part 3)
Fr.: Item Repulsif Antipoux; *Ger.:* Autan; *Ital.:* Lozione Cruz Verde Zanzara†; Sinezan†; Zanzipik; *S.Afr.:* Mylol; *UK:* Bug Guards; Dusk; Jungle Formula Insect Repellent; Mijex; Ultrathon.

Multi-ingredient: *Canad.:* Muskol; *Ital.:* Cruzzy; Entom; Lozione Cruz Verde con Erogatore†; *S.Afr.:* Mylol; *Switz.:* Pellit†; *UK:* Jungle Formula Insect Repellent Plus U.V. Sunscreens; Mijex.

Difenacoum (3864-k)

3-(3-Biphenyl-4-yl-1,2,3,4-tetrahydro-1-naphthyl)-4-hydroxycoumarin.
$C_{31}H_{24}O_3$ = 444.5.
CAS — 56073-07-5.

Difenacoum is an anticoagulant rodenticide.

Difenacoum, a second-generation anticoagulant rodenticide inhibits prothrombin synthesis to cause bleeding that may be occult.[1] It is absorbed from the gastro-intestinal tract; dermal absorption is possible. Poisons containing 100 mg per kg of bait are not hazardous to man; more concentrated forms are particularly hazardous and their availability should be restricted. Baits, which should be prepared only by trained personnel, should contain a suitable marker-dye.

There have been reports of poisoning with difenacoum.[2,3]

1. WHO. Safe use of pesticides: ninth report of the WHO expert committee on vector biology and control. *WHO Tech Rep Ser 720* 1985.
2. Barlow AM, *et al.* Difenacoum (Neosorexa) poisoning. *Br Med J* 1982; **285:** 541.
3. Butcher GP, *et al.* Difenacoum poisoning as a cause of haematuria. *Hum Exp Toxicol* 1992; **11:** 553–4.

Diflubenzuron (18066-x)

1-(4-Chlorophenyl)-3-(2,6-difluorobenzoyl)urea.
$C_{14}H_9ClF_2N_2O_2$ = 310.7.
CAS — 35367-38-5.

Diflubenzuron is an insecticide and larvicide that acts as a growth regulator by interfering with the formation of cuticle. It is used in agriculture and for the control of disease vectors.

Diflubenzuron possesses residual activity against mosquito larvae.

Dimethoate (11646-q)

Fosfamid. *O,O*-Dimethyl *S*-methylcarbamoylmethyl phosphorodithioate.
$C_5H_{12}NO_3PS_2$ = 229.3.
CAS — 60-51-5.

Dimethoate is an organophosphorus insecticide (p.1408) used in agriculture.

References.

1. Dimethoate health and safety guide. *IPCS Health and Safety Guide 20.* Geneva: WHO, 1988.
2. Dimethoate. *Environmental Health Criteria 90.* Geneva: WHO, 1989.
3. Jovanović D, *et al.* A case of unusual suicidal poisoning by the organophosphorus insecticide dimethoate. *Hum Exp Toxicol* 1990; **9:** 49–51.

Dimethyl Phthalate (2555-t)

DMP; Methyl Phthalate. Dimethyl benzene-1,2-dicarboxylate.
$C_{10}H_{10}O_4$ = 194.2.
CAS — 131-11-3.
Pharmacopoeias. In *Br.* and *Fr.*

A colourless or faintly coloured liquid, odourless or almost odourless.

Slightly **soluble** in water; miscible with alcohol, ether, and most organic solvents.

Adverse Effects and Precautions

Dimethyl phthalate may cause temporary smarting and should not be applied near the eyes or to mucous membranes. As with other phthalates contact with plastics should be avoided.

Uses

Dimethyl phthalate is an insect repellent.

Preparations

Proprietary Preparations (details are given in Part 3)

Multi-ingredient: *Fr.:* Mousticreme†; *Ger.:* Kulan†; *S.Afr.:* Mylol; *Switz.:* Pellit†.

Dinitro-o-cresol (18085-d)

DNOC. 4,6-Dinitro-*o*-cresol.
$C_7H_6N_2O_5$ = 198.1.
CAS — 534-52-1.

Dinitro-*o*-cresol is a dinitrophenol formerly used as an insecticide and herbicide. It increases metabolism by uncoupling oxidative phosphorylation and was also formerly used in obesity. Fatal poisoning has occurred.

Dinitrophenol (3580-v)

2,4-Dinitrophenol.
$C_6H_4N_2O_5$ = 184.1.
CAS — 51-28-5.

Dinitrophenol is used as a herbicide. Since dinitrophenol increases metabolism by uncoupling oxidative phosphorylation it was formerly used in the treatment of obesity. Fatal poisoning has occurred.

Dioctyl Adipate (19235-g)

DEHA; Di-(2-ethylhexyl)adipate.
$C_{22}H_{42}O_4$ = 370.6.

Dioctyl adipate is used as an insect repellent. It is also used as a plasticiser by the plastics industry: concern about the migration of this and other plasticisers into foodstuffs from polythene films used to wrap them ('cling film') have led to its use at lower concentrations.

Preparations

Proprietary Preparations (details are given in Part 3)
UK: Protec.

Dioxathion (3581-g)

Dioxathion *(BAN).*
Dioxation *(rINN).* It consists mainly of *cis* and *trans* isomers of *S,S'*-1,4-dioxan-2,3-diyl bis(*O,O*-diethyl phosphorodithioate).
$C_{12}H_{26}O_6P_2S_4$ = 456.5.
CAS — 78-34-2.

Dioxathion is an organophosphorus insecticide (p.1408) that has been used in agriculture and as a topical ectoparasiticide in veterinary practice.

Diphenadione (4812-y)

Diphenadione *(BAN, pINN).*
Diphacinone. 2-(Diphenylacetyl)indan-1,3-dione.
$C_{23}H_{16}O_3$ = 340.4.
CAS — 82-66-6.

Diphenadione is used as an anticoagulant rodenticide.

Diquat Dibromide (3584-s)

9,10-Dihydro-8a,10a-diazoniaphenanthrene dibromide; 1,1′-Ethylene-2,2′-bipyridyldiylium dibromide.

$C_{12}H_{12}Br_2N_2$ = 344.0.

CAS — 2764-72-9 (diquat); 85-00-7 (diquat dibromide).

Diquat dibromide is a contact herbicide used in agriculture and horticulture. It has similar adverse effects to those of paraquat (p.1409).

References.

1. Paraquat and diquat. *Environmental Health Criteria 39.* Geneva: WHO, 1984.

Endod (19131-r)

Endod is obtained from the dried fruits of *Phytolacca dodecandra* (Phytolaccaceae) and has molluscicidal properties. It has been investigated for the control of the snail vector of schistosomiasis.

References.

1. Goldsmith MF. Out of Africa comes the fruit of long research: possible self-reliant control of schistosomiasis. *JAMA* 1991; **265:** 2650–1.

Endosulfan (18067-r)

1,4,5,6,7,7-Hexachloro-8,9,10-trinorborn-5-en-2,3-ylenebismethylene sulphite.

$C_9H_6Cl_6O_3S$ = 406.9.

CAS — 115-29-7.

Endosulfan is a chlorinated insecticide (p.1403) used in agriculture.

References.

1. Endosulfan. *Environmental Health Criteria 40.* Geneva: WHO, 1984.
2. Endosulfan health and safety guide. *IPCS Health and Safety Guide 17.* Geneva: WHO, 1988.

Endrin (18068-f)

(1*R*,4*S*,4a*S*,5*S*,6*S*,7*R*,8*R*,8a*R*)-1,2,3,4,10,10-Hexachloro-1,4,4a,5,6,7,8,8a-octahydro-6,7-epoxy-1,4:5,8-dimethanonaphthalene.

$C_{12}H_8Cl_6O$ = 380.9.

CAS — 72-20-8.

Endrin is a chlorinated insecticide (p.1403), but its use was prohibited, at least in some countries, because of toxicity and persistence in the environment.

General references to endrin,[1-4] including reports of poisoning.[2,3]

1. Endrin health and safety guide. *IPCS Health and Safety Guide 60.* Geneva: WHO, 1991.
2. Anonymous. Acute convulsions associated with endrin poisoning—Pakistan. *JAMA* 1985; **253:** 334–5.
3. Runhaar EA, *et al.* A case of fatal endrin poisoning. *Hum Toxicol* 1985; **4:** 241–7.
4. Endrin. *Environmental Health Criteria 130.* Geneva: WHO, 1992.

Esdepallethrine (13425-w)

(*S*)-3-Allyl-2-methyl-4-oxocyclopent-2-enyl (1*R*,3*R*)-2,2-dimethyl-3-(2-methylprop-1-enyl)-cyclopropanecarboxylate.

$C_{19}H_{26}O_3$ = 302.4.

CAS — 28434-00-6.

Esdepallethrine is a pyrethroid insecticide (p.1410). It is employed as an acaricide in combination with piperonyl butoxide (p.1409) in the topical treatment of scabies (p.1401).

Esdepallethrine is also used in devices and sprays to control insects, including mosquitoes.

Preparations

Proprietary Preparations (details are given in Part 3)

Multi-ingredient: ***Canad.:*** Scabene; ***Fr.:*** A-Par; Acardust; Spregal; ***Ital.:*** Acardust; ***Switz.:*** Acardust.

Ethohexadiol (2556-x)

Ethylhexanediol. 2-Ethylhexane-1,3-diol.

$C_8H_{18}O_2$ = 146.2.

CAS — 94-96-2.

Ethohexadiol is an insect repellent. It may be applied topically to the skin and to clothing. It has been used in conjunction with dimethyl phthalate.

Preparations

Proprietary Preparations (details are given in Part 3)

UK: Z.Stop†.

Multi-ingredient: ***Ger.:*** Kulan†.

Ethylene Dibromide (12710-q)

EDB. 1,2-Dibromoethane.

$C_2H_4Br_2$ = 187.9.

CAS — 106-93-4.

Ethylene dibromide is an insecticidal fumigant and a lead scavenger used in the petroleum industry. Its use has been restricted in certain areas because of carcinogenicity in experimental *animals* and because of evidence of persistence in fruit and cereals that have undergone fumigation.

Ethylene dibromide is more toxic than carbon tetrachloride or ethylene dichloride. It is irritant to the eyes, skin, and mucous membranes. Inhalation leads to drowsiness, CNS depression, and possibly pulmonary oedema. Contact with the skin causes blistering and it is readily absorbed. Kidney and liver damage may occur.

Reports of poisoning due to ethylene dibromide.

1. Letz GA, *et al.* Two fatalities after acute occupational exposure to ethylene dibromide. *JAMA* 1984; **252:** 2428–31.

Ethylene Dichloride (12711-p)

Brocide; Dutch Liquid. 1,2-Dichloroethane.

$C_2H_4Cl_2$ = 98.96.

CAS — 107-06-2.

Ethylene dichloride is an insecticidal fumigant. It is also used in the petroleum industry and as an industrial solvent. Exposure to the vapour may cause lachrymation and corneal clouding, nasal irritation, and vertigo due to the depressant effect on the CNS. Contact with the skin may cause dermatitis. Kidney and liver damage, hypotension and cardiac impairment, gastro-intestinal disturbances, haemorrhage, coma, and pulmonary oedema may follow absorption after inhalation, topical application, or ingestion.

Ethylene dichloride has been reported to be carcinogenic in experimental *animals.*

References.

1. 1,2 Dichloroethane. *Environmental Health Criteria 62.* Geneva: WHO, 1987.
2. 1,2-Dichloroethane health and safety guide. *IPCS Health and Safety Guide 55.* Geneva: WHO, 1991.

Fenitrothion (18142-c)

Fenitrothion *(BAN).*

O,O-Dimethyl *O*-4-nitro-*m*-tolyl phosphorothioate.

$C_9H_{12}NO_5PS$ = 277.2.

CAS — 122-14-5.

Fenitrothion is an organophosphorus insecticide (p.1408) used as a topical ectoparasiticide in veterinary medicine. It is also used as an agricultural insecticide.

References.

1. Fenitrothion. *Environmental Health Criteria 133.* Geneva: WHO, 1992.
2. Bouma MJ, Nesbit R. Fenitrothion intoxication during spraying operations in the malaria programme for Afghan refugees in North West Frontier Province of Pakistan. *Trop Geogr Med* 1995; **47:** 12–14.

Fenthion (3586-e)

Fenthion *(BAN).*

Bayer-29493; S-752. *O,O*-Dimethyl *O*-4-methylthio-*m*-tolyl phosphorothioate.

$C_{10}H_{15}O_3PS_2$ = 278.3.

CAS — 55-38-9.

Pharmacopoeias. In *BP(Vet).*

A yellowish-brown oily substance. Practically **immiscible** with water; miscible with alcohol and with chloroform.

Fenthion is an organophosphorus insecticide (p.1408) used as a systemic ectoparasiticide in veterinary practice; it is applied topically to the host animal. Fenthion has also been used in agriculture.

Macular changes have been detected in the eyes of workers regularly exposed to fenthion.[1] It was considered that there was a need for long-term studies on subjects exposed to different organophosphorus compounds to assess their role in producing macular changes.

1. Misra UK, *et al.* Some observations on the macula of pesticide workers. *Hum Toxicol* 1985; **4:** 135–45.

Fenvalerate (11799-n)

Fenvalerate *(BAN).*

(*RS*)-α-Cyano-3-phenoxybenzyl (*RS*)-2-(4-chlorophenyl)-3-methylbutyrate.

$C_{25}H_{22}ClNO_3$ = 419.9.

CAS — 51630-58-1.

Fenvalerate is a pyrethroid insecticide (p.1410) used as a topical ectoparasiticide in veterinary practice. It has also been used as an insecticide in agriculture and horticulture.

Esfenvalerate, one of the stereoisomers of fenvalerate, is also used as an agricultural insecticide.

Fipronil (672-p)

Fipronil *(BAN).*

MB-46030; RM-1601. (*RS*)-5-Amino-1-(2,6-dichloro-4-trifluoromethylphenyl)-4-(trifluoromethylsulfinyl)pyrazole-3-carbonitrile.

$C_{12}H_4Cl_2F_6N_4OS$ = 437.1.

CAS — 120068-37-3.

Fipronil is used as a topical ectoparasiticide in veterinary practice.

Flocoumafen (3073-s)

Flocoumafene; OMS-3047. 4-Hydroxy-3-[1,2,3,4-tetrahydro-3-[4-(4-trifluoromethylbenzyloxy)phenyl]-1-naphthyl]coumarin.

$C_{33}H_{25}F_3O_4$ = 542.5.

CAS — 90035-08-8.

Flocoumafen is a coumarin derivative used as an anticoagulant rodenticide. It is said to be effective in rodents resistant to other anticoagulant rodenticides.

Flumethrin (15321-a)

Flumethrin *(BAN).*

α-Cyano-4-fluoro-3-phenoxybenzyl 3-(β,4-dichlorostyryl)-2,2-dimethylcyclopropanecarboxylate.

$C_{28}H_{22}Cl_2FNO_3$ = 510.4.

CAS — 69770-45-2.

Flumethrin is a pyrethroid insecticide (p.1410) used as a topical ectoparasiticide in veterinary practice.

Reports of poisoning with flumethrin.

1. Box SA, Lee MR. A systemic reaction following exposure to a pyrethroid insecticide. *Hum Exp Toxicol* 1996; **15:** 389–90.

Fluoroacetamide (7731-y)

Compound 1081.

$FCH_2.CONH_2$ = 77.06.

CAS — 640-19-7.

Fluoroacetamide is a rodenticide and produces adverse effects similar to those of sodium fluoroacetate (p.1410).

Fluvalinate (3885-f)

ZR-3210. Cyano(3-phenoxyphenyl)methyl ester of *N*-[2-chloro-4-(trifluoromethyl)phenyl]-DL-valine.

$C_{26}H_{22}ClF_3N_2O_3$ = 502.9.

CAS — 69409-94-5.

Fluvalinate is a pesticide used in beekeeping.

Glyphosate (11805-g)

N-(Phosphonomethyl)glycine.

$C_3H_8NO_5P$ = 169.1.

CAS — 1071-83-6.

Glyphosate is used as a herbicide.

Reports of poisoning with glyphosate products[1-3] and guidelines for treatment[4] have been published. The toxicity has been believed to be largely due to the inclusion in the herbicide (Roundup) formulation of a surfactant, polyoxyethyleneamine.

1. Sawada Y, *et al.* Probable toxicity of surface-active agent in commercial herbicide containing glyphosate. *Lancet* 1988; **i:** 299.
2. Talbot AR, *et al.* Acute poisoning with a glyphosate-surfactant herbicide ('Roundup'): a review of 93 cases. *Hum Exp Toxicol* 1991; **10:** 1–8.
3. Menkes DB, *et al.* Intentional self-poisoning with glyphosate-containing herbicides. *Hum Exp Toxicol* 1991; **10:** 103–7.
4. Proudfoot A, ed. *Pesticide poisoning: notes for the guidance of medical practitioners.* 2nd ed. London: DoH, The Stationery Office, 1996.

Heptachlor (18074-x)

1,4,5,6,7,8,8-Heptachloro-3a,4,7,7a-tetrahydro-4,7-methanoindene.

$C_{10}H_5Cl_7$ = 373.3.
CAS — 76-44-8.

Heptachlor is a chlorinated insecticide (p.1403), but its use was prohibited, at least in some countries, because of its persistent nature.

References.

1. Heptachlor. *Environmental Health Criteria 38.* Geneva: WHO, 1984.
2. Heptachlor health and safety guide. *IPCS Health and Safety Guide 14.* Geneva: WHO, 1988.

Heptenophos (18147-r)

Hoe-02982. 7-Chlorobicyclo[3.2.0]hepta-2,6-dien-6-yl dimethyl phosphate.

$C_9H_{12}ClO_4P$ = 250.6.
CAS — 23560-59-0.

Heptenophos is an organophosphorus insecticide (p.1408) that has been used in veterinary care for the control of ectoparasites. It is also used in agriculture.

Hexachlorobenzene (12823-c)

HCB.

C_6Cl_6 = 284.8.
CAS — 118-74-1.

NOTE. Hexachlorobenzene should not be confused with gamma benzene hexachloride (lindane).

Hexachlorobenzene has been used as an agricultural fungicide. It is not biodegradable to any significant extent and hexachlorobenzene residues in food have arisen as a result of its occurrence in industrial wastes as well as its use as a fungicide; its use is banned in some countries.

Hexachlorobenzene is reported to be distributed into breast milk.

Porphyria cutanea tarda[1] and parkinsonism[2] have both been reported in subjects who had ingested seed crops treated with hexachlorobenzene. In a further report the symptoms of porphyria in some patients have been said to persist for many years.[3]

1. Cam C, Nigogosyan G. Acquired toxic porphyria cutanea tarda due to hexachlorobenzene. *JAMA* 1963; **183:** 88–91.
2. Chapman LJ, *et al.* Parkinsonism and industrial chemicals. *Lancet* 1987; **i:** 332–3.
3. Cripps DJ, *et al.* Porphyria turcica due to hexachlorobenzene: a 20 to 30 year follow-up study on 204 patients. *Br J Dermatol* 1984; **111:** 413–22.

Hydrocyanic Acid (7751-k)

Prussic Acid.
CAS — 74-90-8.

An aqueous solution containing hydrogen cyanide, HCN = 27.03. A colourless liquid with a characteristic almond odour.

CAUTION. *Hydrocyanic acid and its vapour are intensely poisonous.*

Adverse Effects and Precautions

Cyanides interfere with the oxygen uptake of cells by inhibition of cytochrome oxidase, an enzyme necessary for cellular oxygen transport.

Poisoning by cyanides may occur from inhalation of the vapour, ingestion, or absorption through the skin. Poisoning may arise from cyanide pesticides, industrial accidental exposure, or the inhalation of fumes from some burning plastics. Poisoning may also occur from cyanide-containing plants or fruits.

When large doses of hydrocyanic acid are taken, unconsciousness occurs within a few seconds and death within a few minutes. With smaller toxic doses the symptoms, which occur within a few minutes, may include constriction of the throat, nausea, vomiting, giddiness, headache, palpitation, hyperpnoea then dyspnoea, bradycardia, (initially there may be tachycardia), unconsciousness, and violent convulsions, followed by death. The characteristic smell of bitter almonds may not be obvious and not all individuals can detect it. Cyanosis is not prominent. Similar but usually slower effects occur with cyanide salts.

The fatal dose of hydrocyanic acid (HCN) for man is considered to be about 50 mg and of the cyanides about 250 mg.

Treatment of Adverse Effects

Treatment must be given rapidly but should not involve the use of antidotes unless it is certain that cyanide has been absorbed and poisoning is severe.

Cyanide is absorbed very rapidly on inhalation and the poisoned patient should be removed from the area and given oxygen. Steps should be taken to ensure that the airway is adequate. Contaminated clothing should be removed and skin washed. If the patient is conscious, amyl nitrite inhalations may be given for up to 30 seconds every minute but the value of this practice is questionable. Should the patient be unconscious or nearly so, then in the UK and some other countries it is the practice to give dicobalt edetate (p.979) by injection since it forms a stable complex with the cyanide ion. However, cyanide poisoning should be confirmed as absence of cyanide puts the patient at risk from the adverse effects of dicobalt edetate. The recommended dose of dicobalt edetate is 300 mg given intravenously over about 1 to 5 minutes depending on the severity of the poisoning and repeated once or twice depending on the response. It is customary to give 50 mL of glucose 50% intravenously after each injection, although the value of this has been questioned. An alternative treatment is to inject, as soon as possible, 10 mL of sodium nitrite injection (3%) intravenously over 3 to 5 minutes; using the same needle and vein continue with an injection of 12.5 g of sodium thiosulphate (50 mL of a 25% solution or 25 mL of a 50% solution) administered over a period of about 10 minutes. Sodium nitrite converts haemoglobin to methaemoglobin, which competes with cytochrome oxidase for cyanide with the formation of cyanmethaemoglobin; sodium thiosulphate aids the conversion or inactivation of cyanide from cyanmethaemoglobin to thiocyanate. If toxic symptoms recur, the injections of nitrite and thiosulphate may be repeated at half the initial doses. Appropriate measures should be instituted to correct hypotension and acidosis. Hydroxocobalamin has also been investigated in the management of cyanide toxicity.

If cyanide has been ingested, one of the above procedures should be instituted and the stomach then rapidly emptied by lavage.

Some references concerning the management of cyanide poisoning.[1-3] The use of solutions A and B (15.8% ferrous sulphate in 0.3% citric acid, and 6% sodium carbonate respectively) as so-called oral antidotes in persons exposed to cyanide has been condemned as ineffective and lacking scientific evidence.[2]

1. Langford RM, Armstrong RF. Algorithm for managing injury from smoke inhalation. *Br Med J* 1989; **299:** 902–5.
2. Koizumi A. Fighting myths. *Lancet* 1994; **344:** 559–60.
3. Proudfoot A, ed. *Pesticide poisoning: notes for the guidance of medical practitioners.* 2nd ed. London: DoH, The Stationery Office, 1996.

Uses

Cyanides have various industrial applications. Hydrocyanic acid and cyanide salts produce hydrogen cyanide which has been used as a gas for the eradication of rabbits, rodents, and some other pests. Cyanide salts that might be encountered include calcium cyanide, mercuric cyanide, potassium cyanide, potassium ferricyanide, potassium sodium cyanide, and sodium cyanide.

Imidacloprid (8311-n)

Bay-NTN-33893. 1-[(6-Chloro-3-pyridinyl)methyl]-4,5-dihydro-*N*-nitro-1*H*-imidazol-2-amine.

$C_9H_{10}ClN_5O_2$ = 255.7.
CAS — 105827-78-9; 138261-41-3.

Imidacloprid is used as a topical ectoparasiticide in veterinary practice.

Iodofenphos (3863-c)

Iodofenphos *(BAN).*

Jodfenphos. *O*-2,5-Dichloro-4-iodophenyl *O,O*-dimethyl phosphorothioate.

$C_8H_8Cl_2IO_3PS$ = 413.0.
CAS — 18181-70-9.

Iodofenphos is an organophosphorus insecticide (p.1408) used in veterinary practice for the control of ectoparasites in the environment. It is also used as an agricultural insecticide. It is an effective mosquito larvicide.

Lindane (3587-l)

Lindane *(BAN, USAN, rINN).*

666; Benhexachlor; Gamma Benzene Hexachloride; Gamma-BHC; Gamma-HCH; HCH; Hexicide. 1α,2α,3β,4α,5α,6β-Hexachlorocyclohexane.

$C_6H_6Cl_6$ = 290.8.
CAS — 58-89-9.

Pharmacopoeias. In *Eur.* (see p.viii), *Int.*, and *US.*

A white or almost white crystalline powder with a slight musty odour. Practically **insoluble** in water; freely soluble in acetone and in chloroform; soluble in dehydrated alcohol; slightly soluble in ethylene glycol. **Protect** from light.

Adverse Effects and Treatment

As for Chlorinated Insecticides, p.1403.

There has been some concern over the application of higher than normal concentrations of lindane to the skin in the treatment of scabies and pediculosis; children are considered to be particularly at risk. Resistance has limited its use in pediculosis, so children with that infection tend not to be exposed to it anyway. However, use has continued in scabies and here treatment should be avoided in young children and in women who are breast feeding or are pregnant. Lindane should also be avoided in patients with a history of epilepsy or who have a low body-weight.

Seizures have been reported following the topical use of lindane.[1] In reply, one of the manufacturers stated that up to the end of 1983 they were aware of 21 cases of convulsive disorders apparently associated with the use of their product; it had been used by over 40 million people. Of the 21 cases the seizures were definitely or probably caused by the product in 11 but in 9 of them the seizures were associated with ingestion or excessive use.[2]

Isolated reports of adverse effects associated with lindane include disseminated intravascular coagulation and subsequent death after oral ingestion[3] and aplastic anaemia after prolonged topical exposure (twice daily application for three weeks).[4]

1. Etherington JD. Major epileptic seizures and topical gamma-benzene hexachloride. *Br Med J* 1984; **289:** 228.
2. Kelly VT. Major epileptic seizures and topical gammabenzene hexachloride. *Br Med J* 1984; **289:** 837.
3. Rao CVSR, *et al.* Disseminated intravascular coagulation in a case of fatal lindane poisoning. *Vet Hum Toxicol* 1988; **30:** 132–4.
4. Rauch AE, *et al.* Lindane (Kwell)-induced aplastic anemia. *Arch Intern Med* 1990; **150:** 2393–5.

Uses and Administration

Lindane is a chlorinated insecticide (p.1403). It has been used topically in a concentration of 1% for scabies (p.1401) in selected patients and has also been used in pediculosis (p.1401) but use for head lice is restricted by resistance.

Lindane has been used for the control of disease vectors including mosquitoes, lice, and fleas but resistance has developed. It has also been used as an agricultural and a horticultural insecticide, but its use is prohibited or restricted in many countries.

Preparations

USP 23: Lindane Cream; Lindane Lotion; Lindane Shampoo.

Proprietary Preparations (details are given in Part 3)
Aust.: Jacutin; ***Belg.:*** Lencid†; Quellada; ***Canad.:*** GBH†; Hexit; Kwellada; ***Fr.:*** Aphtiria; Elentol; Scabecid; ***Ger.:*** Jacutin; Quellada H; ***Irl.:*** Lorexane†; Quellada; ***Neth.:*** Jacutin†; ***S.Afr.:*** Gambex; Quellada; ***Switz.:*** Jacutin; ***UK:*** Quellada†; ***USA:*** G-well; Kwell†.

Multi-ingredient: ***Fr.:*** Elenol; ***Spain:*** Sudosin; Yacutin.

Lufenuron (15417-m)

Lufenuron *(BAN, rINN).*

CGA-184699. 1-[2,5-Dichloro-4-(1,1,2,3,3,3-hexafluoropropoxy)phenyl]-3-(2,6-difluorobenzoyl)urea; (*RS*)-*N*-[2,5-Dichloro-4-(1,1,2,3,3,3-hexafluoropropoxy)phenylcarbamoyl]-2,6-difluorobenzamide.

$C_{17}H_8Cl_2F_8N_2O_3$ = 511.1.
CAS — 103055-07-8.

Lufenuron is used as a systemic ectoparasiticide in veterinary practice; it is given by mouth to the host animal.

Malathion (3590-q)

Malathion *(BAN).*

Carbofos; Compound 4047; OMS-1. Diethyl 2-(dimethoxyphosphinothioylthio)succinate.

$C_{10}H_{19}O_6PS_2$ = 330.4.
CAS — 121-75-5.

Pharmacopoeias. In *Eur.* (see p.viii) and *US.*

A clear, colourless or yellow to deep brown liquid with a characteristic odour. Congeals at about 2.9°. Slightly **soluble** in water; miscible with alcohols, ethers, esters, ketones, aromatic and alkylated aromatic hydrocarbons, and vegetable oils. **Store** in airtight containers. Protect from light.

The manufacturers have reported that malathion is sensitive to heat and is degraded at temperatures above 30°.

Adverse Effects and Treatment

As for Organophosphorus Insecticides, p.1408.

Malathion is one of the safer organophosphorus insecticides but its toxicity may be increased by the presence of impurities.

Acute renal insufficiency has been described in one patient associated with excessive exposure to a malathion spray.[1] The condition resolved without specific treatment. Renal toxicity had not previously been associated with organophosphorus pesticides. Mild transient renal insufficiency and proteinuria, together with several other late complications including cardiac arrhythmias, pulmonary oedema and diffuse interstitial fibrosis, and muscle weakness due to peripheral neuropathy, were seen subsequent to recovery from the initial cholinergic toxicity in a second case of acute poisoning, due to ingestion of malathion.[2]

1. Albright RK, *et al.* Malathion exposure associated with acute renal failure. *JAMA* 1983; **250:** 2469.
2. Dive A, *et al.* Unusual manifestations after malathion poisoning. *Hum Exp Toxicol* 1994; **13:** 271–4.

Uses and Administration

Malathion is an organophosphorus insecticide (p.1408). It is used in the treatment of head and pubic pediculosis (p.1401) and in scabies (p.1401); lotions of 0.5% and shampoos of 1% are commonly available. Lotions are generally preferred to shampoos as the contact time is longer. Aqueous lotions are preferred to treat pubic lice and scabies because alcoholic lotions are irritant to excoriated skin and the genitalia; aqueous lotions may also be preferable in asthmatic subjects or children to avoid alcoholic fumes. Skin or hair treated with an alcohol-based preparation should be allowed to dry naturally.

Malathion is also used in veterinary care, agriculture, and horticulture. It is widely used for adult and larval mosquito control although resistance occurs.

Preparations

USP 23: Malathion Lotion.

Proprietary Preparations (details are given in Part 3)
Austral.: Cleensheen; KP 24†; Lice Rid; ***Belg.:*** Prioderm; Radikal; ***Fr.:*** Prioderm; ***Ger.:*** Organoderm†; ***Irl.:*** Derbac-M; Malfesto†; Prioderm; ***Ital.:*** Aftir Gel; ***Neth.:*** Noury Hoofdlotion†; Prioderm; ***Norw.:*** Prioderm; ***Swed.:*** Prioderm; ***Switz.:*** Lusap; Prioderm; ***UK:*** Derbac-M; Prioderm; Quellada-M; Suleo-M; ***USA:*** Ovide.

Multi-ingredient: ***Fr.:*** Para Plus.

Metaldehyde (3591-p)

$(C_2H_4O)_x$.
CAS — 9002-91-9.

A cyclic polymer of acetaldehyde.

Adverse Effects and Treatment

Symptoms of poisoning by metaldehyde may be delayed and include vomiting and diarrhoea, fever, drowsiness, convulsions, and coma. Death from respiratory failure may occur within 48 hours. Kidney and liver damage may occur.

Treatment is symptomatic.

References.

1. Longstreth WT, Pierson DJ. Metaldehyde poisoning from slug bait ingestion. *West J Med* 1982; **137:** 134–7.
2. Proudfoot A, ed. *Pesticide poisoning: notes for the guidance of medical practitioners.* 2nd ed. London: DoH, The Stationery Office, 1996.

Uses

Metaldehyde is a molluscicide used in pellets against slugs and snails. It is also reported to be an ingredient of some firelighters.

'Meta' is compressed metaldehyde which has been used as a solid fuel burning with a non-luminous carbon-free flame.

Methomyl (18035-y)

S-Methyl *N*-(methylcarbamoyloxy)thioacetimidate.
$C_5H_{10}N_2O_2S$ = 162.2.
CAS — 16752-77-5.

Methomyl is a carbamate insecticide (p.1403) that has been used in agriculture.

Reports of poisoning with methomyl and its management.

1. Martinez-Chuecos J, *et al.* Management of methomyl poisoning. *Hum Exp Toxicol* 1990; **9:** 251–4.

Methoprene (3592-s)

Methoprene *(rINN).*

ZR-515. Isopropyl 11-methoxy-3,7,11-trimethyldodeca-2(*E*),4(*E*)-dienoate.
$C_{19}H_{34}O_3$ = 310.5.
CAS — 40596-69-8.

Methoprene is an insect growth regulator which mimics the action of insect juvenile hormones and, if it is applied at the appropriate period of sensitivity, it causes death by preventing the transformation of larva to pupa. It is used against a variety of insects including fleas and mosquitoes. It is used in veterinary practice for the control of ectoparasites in the environment, rather than being applied to the animals themselves.

Methyl Bromide (2257-s)

Bromomethane; Monobromomethane.
CH_3Br = 94.94.
CAS — 74-83-9.

Adverse Effects, Treatment, and Precautions

Methyl bromide is a vesicant. Toxic effects after inhalation or percutaneous absorption are mainly due to neurotoxicity and include dizziness, headache, vomiting, blurred vision, weakness, ataxia, confusion, mania, hallucinations, mental depression, convulsions, pulmonary oedema, and coma. Renal and hepatic toxicity may also occur and death may be due to circulatory collapse or respiratory failure. Onset of symptoms may be preceded by a latent period. Concentrations of 1% or more are irritant to the eyes. Treatment is symptomatic although dimercaprol or acetylcysteine therapy has been tried. Rubber absorbs and retains methyl bromide and should not therefore be used in protective clothing.

A report of optic atrophy from occupational exposure to methyl bromide and a discussion of its neurotoxicity.[1]

1. Chavez CT, *et al.* Methyl bromide optic atrophy. *Am J Ophthalmol* 1985; **99:** 715–19.

Uses

Methyl bromide has been used as an insecticidal fumigant for soil and some foodstuffs.

When supplied for fumigation it usually contains chloropicrin as a lachrymatory warning agent.

Methyl bromide has been used as a gaseous disinfectant; it has low antimicrobial activity but good penetrating power.

Methyl bromide was formerly used with carbon tetrachloride in some fire extinguishers. It has also been used as a refrigerant.

Monosulfiram (3595-l)

Monosulfiram *(BAN).*

Sulfiram *(rINN)*; Sulfiramum. Tetraethylthiuram monosulphide.
$C_{10}H_{20}N_2S_3$ = 264.5.
CAS — 95-05-6.
Pharmacopoeias. In *Aust.* .

Adverse Effects and Precautions

An erythematous rash has occasionally been reported. Monosulfiram produces effects similar to those of disulfiram (p.1573) if ingested with alcohol. As there may be a risk of absorption following the application of monosulfiram to the whole body, patients are advised to abstain from alcohol for at least 48 hours.

The reactions to alcohol occasionally reported in patients who have applied monosulfiram solution[1,2] resemble those seen with disulfiram. Analysis has shown that monosulfiram solutions exposed to room light undergo photochemical conversion to disulfiram, and that the concentration of disulfiram, and the ability of the solution to inhibit aldehyde dehydrogenase and hence the metabolism of alcohol, increases with the duration of such storage.[3,4] Whether patients who have applied monosulfiram solution should avoid direct light immediately afterwards remains to be elucidated.[4]

1. Blanc D, Deprez P. Unusual adverse reaction to an acaricide. *Lancet* 1990; **335:** 1291–2.
2. Burgess I. Adverse reactions to monosulfiram. *Lancet* 1990; **336:** 873.
3. Mays DC, *et al.* Photolysis of monosulfiram: a mechanism for its disulfiram-like reaction. *Clin Pharmacol Ther* 1994; **55:** 191.
4. Lipsky JJ, *et al.* Monosulfiram, disulfiram, and light. *Lancet* 1994; **343:** 304.

Uses and Administration

Monosulfiram is a pesticide that has been used as an acaricide, either alone or in conjunction with benzyl benzoate, in the treatment of scabies (p.1401), although other treatments are now preferred.

Monosulfiram has also been used as a pesticide in veterinary practice.

Preparations

Proprietary Preparations (details are given in Part 3)
Irl.: Tetmosol†; ***S.Afr.:*** Tetmosol; ***UK:*** Tetmosol†.

Multi-ingredient: ***Fr.:*** Ascabiol.

Naphthalene (3596-y)

Naphthalin.
$C_{10}H_8$ = 128.2.
CAS — 91-20-3.

Adverse Effects, Treatment, and Precautions

Ingestion of naphthalene can produce headache, nausea and vomiting, diarrhoea, profuse perspiration, dysuria, haematuria, acute haemolytic anaemia, coma, and convulsions. Doses as low as 2 g have proved fatal to the small child. Treatment is symptomatic and includes emptying the stomach by lavage. Blood transfusions may be required. The vapour is irritating to the eyes; chronic exposure has led to cataract formation. Haemolysis may occur in persons with glucose-6-phosphate dehydrogenase deficiency.

A report[1] of haemolytic anaemia in a neonate, attributed to inhalation of naphthalene by the mother during the twenty-eighth week of gestation.

1. Athanasion M, *et al.* Hemolytic anemia in a female newborn infant whose mother inhaled naphthalene before delivery. *J Pediatr* 1997; **130:** 680–1.

Uses

Naphthalene has been used in lavatory deodorant discs and in mothballs. It has also been used as a soil fumigant.

Norbormide (3597-j)

McN-1025. 5-[α-Hydroxy-α-(2-pyridyl)benzyl]-7-[α-(2-pyridyl)benzylidene]-8,9,10-trinorborn-5-ene-2,3-dicarboximide.
$C_{33}H_{25}N_3O_3$ = 511.6.
CAS — 991-42-4.

Norbormide is a selective rodenticide effective against most species of rats, in which it produces extreme irreversible peripheral vasoconstriction. It is not very toxic to other rodents.

Organophosphorus Insecticides (3564-v)

The organophosphorus or organophosphate insecticides may be esters, amides, or thiol derivatives of phosphoric, phosphonic, phosphorothioic, or phosphonothioic acids.

Those described in this chapter are listed in Table 1 (p.1401).

References.

1. WHO. Organophosphorus insecticides: a general introduction. *Environmental Health Criteria 63.* Geneva: WHO, 1986.

Adverse Effects

Organophosphorus insecticides are potent cholinesterase inhibitors and can be very toxic. This inhibition results in both muscarinic and nicotinic effects with some central involvement.

Toxic effects may include abdominal cramps, nausea, vomiting, diarrhoea, pancreatitis, urinary incontinence, miosis or mydriasis, weakness, respiratory disturbances, lachrymation, increased salivation and sweating, bradycardia or tachycardia, hypotension or hypertension, cyanosis, muscular twitching, and convulsions. Some organophosphorus compounds cause delayed neuropathy. CNS symptoms include restlessness, anxiety, dizziness, confusion, coma, and depression of the respiratory or cardiovascular system. Patients may experience mental disturbances. Inhalation or external contact can cause local as well as systemic effects.

Repeated exposure may have a cumulative effect though the organophosphorus insecticides are, in contrast to the chlorinated insecticides, rapidly metabolised and excreted and are not appreciably stored in body tissues.

References to the adverse effects and poisoning encountered with organophosphorus compounds such as insecticides (including sheep dips).

1. WHO. Safe use of pesticides: fourteenth report of the WHO expert committee on vector biology and control. *WHO Tech Rep Ser 813* 1991.
2. Proudfoot A, ed. *Pesticide poisoning: notes for the guidance of medical practitioners.* 2nd ed. London: DoH, The Stationery Office, 1996.
3. Minton NA, Murray VSG. A review of organophosphate poisoning. *Med Toxicol* 1988; **3:** 350–75.
4. Dunn MA, Sidell FR. Progress in medical defense against nerve agents. *JAMA* 1989; **262:** 649–52.
5. Karalliedde L, Senanayake N. Organophosphorus insecticide poisoning. *Br J Anaesth* 1989; **63:** 736–50.
6. Öztürk MA, *et al.* Anticholinesterase poisoning in Turkey—clinical, laboratory and radiologic evaluation of 269 cases. *Hum Exp Toxicol* 1990; **9:** 273–9.
7. Murray VSG, Volans GN. Management of injuries due to chemical weapons. *Br Med J* 1991; **302:** 129–30.
8. Lotti M. Treatment of acute organophosphate poisoning. *Med J Aust* 1991; **154:** 51–5.
9. Casey P, Vale JA. Deaths from pesticide poisoning in England and Wales: 1945–1989. *Hum Exp Toxicol* 1994; **13:** 95–101.
10. Eyer P. Neuropsychopathological changes by organophosphorus compounds—a review. *Hum Exp Toxicol* 1995; **14:** 857–64.
11. Steenland K. Chronic neurological effects of organophosphate pesticides. *Br Med J* 1996; **312:** 1312–13.

Treatment of Adverse Effects

Rapid treatment is essential. If organophosphorus insecticides have been ingested the stomach should be emptied by lavage. Contaminated clothing should be removed and the skin, including any areas contaminated by vomiting or hypersecretion, should receive copious and prolonged washing with soap and water. Contamination of the eye is treated by washing of the conjunctiva. The patient should be treated with atropine (p.456) and either pralidoxime (p.992) or obidoxime (p.988) and symptomatic treatment should be instituted. Diazepam is sometimes given; it may be necessary to give it parenterally in moderate to severe poisoning to control muscle fasciculations and convulsions; oral administration in mild poisoning may be helpful in relieving anxiety. The patient should be observed for signs of deterioration due to delayed absorption.

Paraquat (3600-c)

1,1′-Dimethyl-4,4′-bipyridyldiylium ion.

$C_{12}H_{14}N_2$ = 186.3.

CAS — 4685-14-7.

Paraquat Dichloride (3601-k)

$C_{12}H_{14}Cl_2N_2$ = 257.2.

CAS — 1910-42-5.

Adverse Effects

Concentrated solutions of paraquat may cause irritation of the skin, inflammation, and possibly blistering; cracking and shedding of the nails; and delayed healing of cuts and wounds. It is not significantly absorbed from undamaged skin. A few fatalities have occurred following skin contact but these appear to have been associated with prolonged contact and concentrated solutions.

Splashes in the eye cause severe inflammation, which may be delayed for 12 to 24 hours, corneal oedema, reduced visual acuity, and extensive superficial stripping of the corneal and conjunctival epithelium, which usually slowly heals. Inhalation of dust or spray may cause nasal bleeding.

Paraquat weedkillers available for use in domestic gardens contain 2.5% w/v paraquat sometimes in association with other herbicides such as diquat. While this strength of paraquat can cause nausea and vomiting as well as some respiratory changes when ingested, it is not considered to be a lethal form.

Most of the cases of severe poisoning follow the ingestion or sometimes injection of the concentrated forms of paraquat herbicide (20% w/v), the distribution of which is restricted to agriculturalists and horticulturalists. In many cases this ingestion is intentional. It is considered that patients who ingest 20 to 40 mg per kg body-weight suffer moderate to severe poisoning; most but not all die up to about 2 or 3 weeks after ingestion. Severe acute poisoning occurs with ingestion of higher doses. The irritant effects of paraquat are reflected in oesophageal ulceration and gastro-intestinal effects. There is widespread organ damage, most notably involving the kidneys and lungs. In such poisoning death is virtually certain and occurs rapidly.

Preparations of paraquat may contain an emetic or a laxative and some contain a malodorous agent to deter ingestion.

General references concerning paraquat toxicity and its treatment.

1. Paraquat and diquat. *Environmental Health Criteria 39*. Geneva: WHO, 1984.
2. Bismuth C, *et al.* Paraquat poisoning. *Drug Safety* 1990; **5:** 243–51.
3. Pond SM. Manifestations and management of paraquat poisoning. *Med J Aust* 1990; **152:** 256–9.
4. Paraquat Health and Safety Guide. *Health and Safety Guide 51*. Geneva: WHO, 1991.
5. WHO. Safe use of pesticides: fourteenth report of the WHO expert committee on vector biology and control. *WHO Tech Rep Ser 813* 1991.
6. Proudfoot A, ed. *Pesticide poisoning: notes for the guidance of medical practitioners*. 2nd ed. London: DoH, The Stationery Office, 1996.

Treatment of Adverse Effects

Following contact with paraquat, contaminated clothing should be removed and the skin washed with soap and water. The eyes, if splashed, should be irrigated; later topical therapy may involve the symptomatic use of antibacterials or corticosteroids.

There is no specific treatment for paraquat poisoning and the immediate aim is to remove or inactivate the paraquat. Initial management involves the oral administration of an adsorbent, preferably activated charcoal given in a dose of 100 g together with a laxative and followed by 50 g of charcoal every 4 hours until the charcoal is seen in the stool. Gastric lavage is considered to be of doubtful value. Fuller's earth and bentonite are alternative oral adsorbents. When none of these adsorbents is available a suspension of clay or of uncontaminated soil should be considered if medical attention is likely to be delayed. A 30% suspension of Fuller's earth has been used in a dose of 200 to 500 mL every 2 hours for three doses. Alternatively a suspension of 7% bentonite may be employed. Magnesium sulphate or mannitol are used with Fuller's earth or bentonite in order to hasten bowel evacuation and prevent obstruction due to the adsorbent. Patients may require intensive supportive therapy, but oxygen should not be given initially as it appears to enhance the pulmonary toxicity of paraquat; however, it may be needed in later stages as part of palliative care.

Methods aimed at hastening elimination such as forced diuresis, peritoneal dialysis, haemodialysis, and haemoperfusion have been tried but the former two appear to be ineffective and results with the latter two methods have varied; no method is of proven value.

For some general references concerning the treatment of paraquat toxicity, see under Adverse Effects, above.

Once paraquat has been absorbed moderate to severe poisoning may result in acute renal failure, hepatitis, and pulmonary fibrosis; death may occur after 2 to 3 weeks. Pulse therapy with cyclophosphamide and methyl prednisolone might be of benefit in such patients.[1]

1. Lin J-L, *et al.* Pulse therapy with cyclophosphamide and methylprednisolone in patients with moderate to severe paraquat poisoning: a preliminary report. *Thorax* 1996; **51:** 661–3.

Uses

Paraquat is a contact herbicide widely used as the dichloride in agriculture and horticulture. Liquid concentrates are supplied in the UK only to approved users.

Parathion (18168-m)

O,O-Diethyl *O*-4-nitrophenyl phosphorothioate.

$C_{10}H_{14}NO_5PS$ = 291.3.

CAS — 56-38-2.

Parathion is an organophosphorus insecticide (p.1408) that has been used in agriculture and horticulture. Its metabolite diethyl nitrophenyl phosphate (paraoxon, p.1395) contributes to its toxicity.

Reports of poisoning with parathion.

1. Anastassiades CJ, Ioannides M. Organophosphate poisoning and auricular fibrillation. *Br Med J* 1984; **289:** 290.
2. Golsousidis H, Kokkas V. Use of 19 590 mg of atropine during 24 days of treatment, after a case of unusually severe parathion poisoning. *Hum Toxicol* 1985; **4:** 339–40.
3. Clifford NJ, Nies AS. Organophosphate poisoning from wearing a laundered uniform previously contaminated with parathion. *JAMA* 1989; **262:** 3035–6.

Permethrin (13097-w)

Permethrin *(BAN, USAN, rINN)*.

3-Phenoxybenzyl (1*RS*,3*RS*)-(1*RS*,3*SR*)-3-(2,2-dichlorovinyl)-2,2-dimethylcyclopropanecarboxylate.

$C_{21}H_{20}Cl_2O_3$ = 391.3.

CAS — 52645-53-1.

Permethrin is a pyrethroid insecticide (p.1410). It is used in the treatment of head pediculosis (p.1401) as a 1% application; there have been signs of resistance. It is also employed as an acaricide in the treatment of scabies (p.1401) as a 5% cream.

Permethrin is also used as a topical ectoparasiticide in veterinary practice and as an agricultural, horticultural, and household insecticide.

Permethrin is active against mosquitoes and is widely used for the impregnation of bednets and curtains in the control of malaria (p.422). It is also active against blackflies in the adult and larval stages and is used for the larvicidal treatment of rivers in the control of onchocerciasis (p.95). It is also active against tsetse flies.

Permethrin is suitable for aircraft disinsection.

References.

1. Permethrin. *Environmental Health Criteria 94*. Geneva: WHO, 1990.

Preparations

Proprietary Preparations (details are given in Part 3)
Austral.: Lyclear; Nix; Pyrifoam; Quellada; ***Belg.:*** Nix; Zalvor; ***Canad.:*** Nix; ***Fr.:*** Nix; ***Irl.:*** Lyclear; ***Ital.:*** Nix; ***Neth.:*** Loxazol; ***Norw.:*** Nix; ***S.Afr.:*** Lyclear; ***Swed.:*** Nix; ***Switz.:*** Loxazol; ***UK:*** Lyclear; Residex P55; ***USA:*** Acticin; Elimite; Nix.

Multi-ingredient: ***Belg.:*** Shampoux; ***Fr.:*** Anti-Ac; Charlieu Anti-Poux; Heldis†; Para Plus; Pyreflor; Sanytol.

Phenothrin (3602-a)

Phenothrin *(BAN, rINN)*.

3-Phenoxybenzyl (1*RS*,3*RS*)-(1*RS*,3*SR*)-2,2-dimethyl-3-(2-methylprop-1-enyl)cyclopropanecarboxylate.

$C_{23}H_{26}O_3$ = 350.5.

CAS — 26002-80-2.

Phenothrin is a pyrethroid insecticide (p.1410). It is used for the treatment of head and pubic pediculosis (p.1401) as a 0.2% alcoholic or a 0.5% aqueous lotion; as with permethrin there have been signs of resistance.

Phenothrin is also used as a household insecticide and for the disinsection of public areas and aircraft.

General references.

1. d-Phenothrin. *Environmental Health Criteria 96*. Geneva: WHO, 1990.
2. d-Phenothrin health and safety guide. *IPCS Health and Safety Guide 32*. Geneva: WHO, 1989.

References to the use of phenothrin for aircraft disinsection.

1. Russell RC, Paton R. In-flight disinsection as an efficacious procedure for preventing international transport of insects of public health importance. *Bull WHO* 1989; **67:** 543–7.

Preparations

Proprietary Preparations (details are given in Part 3)
Belg.: Hegor†; ***Fr.:*** Hegor Antipoux†; Itax Antipoux; Item Antipoux; Parasidose; ***Irl.:*** Headmaster; ***Ital.:*** Cruzzy; Mom Shampoo Schiuma; ***Jpn:*** Sumithrin†; ***UK:*** Full Marks; ***USA:*** Pronto.

Multi-ingredient: ***Fr.:*** Itax Antipoux; ***Ital.:*** Mom Shampoo Antiparassitario; Neo Mom.

Phosmet (18175-h)

Phosmet *(BAN)*.

O,O-Dimethyl phthalimidomethyl phosphorodithioate.

$C_{11}H_{12}NO_4PS_2$ = 317.3.

CAS — 732-11-6.

Phosmet is an organophosphorus insecticide (p.1408) used as a systemic ectoparasiticide in veterinary practice; it is applied topically to the host animal. It has also been used in agriculture and horticulture.

Phoxim (18178-v)

Phoxim *(BAN)*.

Bayer-9053. 2-(Diethoxyphosphinothioyloxyimino)-2-phenylacetonitrile.

$C_{12}H_{15}N_2O_3PS$ = 298.3.

CAS — 14816-18-3.

Phoxim is an organophosphorus insecticide (p.1408) used for the larvicidal treatment of rivers in the control of onchocerciasis (p.95).

Piperonal (17600-a)

Heliotropin; Piperonylaldehyde. 1,3-Benzodioxole-5-carboxaldehyde.

$C_8H_6O_3$ = 150.1.

CAS — 120-57-0.

Piperonal is used as an insect repellent against head lice (see Pediculosis, p.1401).

Preparations

Proprietary Preparations (details are given in Part 3)
Fr.: Para Repulsif; ***UK:*** Rappell.

Piperonyl Butoxide (3603-t)

Piperonyl Butoxide *(BAN)*.

5-[2-(2-Butoxyethoxy)ethoxymethyl]-6-propyl-1,3-benzodioxole.

$C_{19}H_{30}O_5$ = 338.4.

CAS — 51-03-6.

Pharmacopoeias. In *BP(Vet)*.

A yellow or pale brown oily liquid with a faint characteristic odour.

Very slightly **soluble** in water; miscible with alcohol, chloroform, ether, and petroleum oils.

Piperonyl butoxide is used as a synergist for pyrethrin and pyrethroid insecticides. Mixtures of piperonyl butoxide and pyrethrins or pyrethroids are used in the treatment of pediculosis (p.1401).

Piperonyl butoxide is considered to cause a variety of gastro-intestinal effects as well as mild CNS depression.

Preparations

Proprietary Preparations (details are given in Part 3)

Multi-ingredient: ***Austral.:*** Banlice; Lyban; Meditox†; Paralice; Sundown with Insect Repellant; ***Belg.:*** Para; Pyriderm; Shampoux; ***Canad.:*** Lice Enz†; Para; Pronto; R & C; Scabene; ***Fr.:*** A-Par; Acardust; Anti-Ac; Charlieu Anti-Poux; Heldis†; Itax Antipoux; Marie Rose†; Para Plus; Para Special Poux; Parasidose†; Pyreflor; Spray-Pax; Spregal; ***Ger.:*** Goldgeist; Jacutin N; Quellada P; Spregal; ***Ital.:*** Acardust; Baygon N; Cruzzy; Cruzzy Antiparassitario; Entom; Lozione Cruz Verde con Erogatore†; Mafu; Mom Piretro Emulsione; Pyr†; Shampoo Antiparassitario al Piretro Cruz Verde†; Zanzevia†; ***Neth.:*** Crinopex-N; Para-Speciaal; ***Norw.:*** Rinsoderm; ***S.Afr.:*** Quell P†; ***Swed.:*** Crinopex; ***Switz.:*** A-Par; Acardust; ***UK:*** Buzpel; Fortefog; Patriot; Prevent; ***USA:*** A-200; Barc; Blue; Clear Total Lice Elimination System; Control-L†; End Lice; InnoGel Plus; Lice Enz†; Pronto; Pyrinex; Pyrinyl II; Pyrinyl Plus; R & C; RID; Tegrin-LT; Tisit; Triple X.

Pirimiphos-Methyl (18181-d)

O-2-Diethylamino-6-methylpyrimidin-4-yl *O,O*-dimethyl phosphorothioate.

$C_{11}H_{20}N_3O_3PS$ = 305.3.

CAS — 29232-93-7.

Pirimiphos-methyl is an organophosphorus insecticide (p.1408). It is used in agriculture and domestically.

Propetamphos (18182-n)

Propetamphos *(BAN)*.

Isopropyl (*E*)-3-[(ethylamino)(methoxy)phosphinothio-oxy]but-2-enoate.

$C_{10}H_{20}NO_4PS$ = 281.3.

CAS — 31218-83-4.

Propetamphos is an organophosphorus insecticide (p.1408) used as a topical ectoparasiticide in veterinary practice.

Propoxur (18039-k)

Propoxur *(BAN)*.

2-Isopropoxyphenyl methylcarbamate.

$C_{11}H_{15}NO_3$ = 209.2.

CAS — 114-26-1.

Propoxur is a carbamate insecticide (p.1403) used as a topical ectoparasiticide in veterinary practice.

Preparations

Proprietary Preparations (details are given in Part 3)
Ital.: Pulvis-3.

Pyraclofos (5372-y)

(*RS*)-[*O*-1-(4-Chlorophenyl)pyrazol-4-yl *O*-ethyl *S*-propyl phosphorothioate].

$C_{14}H_{18}ClN_2O_3PS$ = 360.8.

CAS — 77458-01-6.

Pyraclofos is an organophosphorus insecticide (p.1408) used for the larvicidal treatment of rivers in the control of onchocerciasis (p.95).

Pyrethrum Flower (3604-x)

Chrysanthème Insecticide; Dalmatian Insect Flowers; Insect Flowers; Insektenblüten; Piretro; Pyrethri Flos.

CAS — 8003-34-7 (pyrethrum); 121-21-1 (pyrethrin I); 121-29-9 (pyrethrin II); 25402-06-6 (cinerin I); 121-20-0 (cinerin II).

Pharmacopoeias. In *Aust.* Also in *BP(Vet). US* includes Pyrethrum Extract.

Pyrethrum Flower (BP(Vet)) is the dried flowerheads of *Chrysanthemum cinerariaefolium* (Compositae), containing not less than 1% of pyrethrins of which not less than one-half consists of pyrethrin I.

Pyrethrum Extract (USP 23) is a mixture of three naturally occurring esters of Chrysanthemic acid (pyrethrins I: pyrethrin 1, cinerin 1, and jasmolin 1) and three esters of pyrethric acid (pyrethrins II: pyrethrin 2, cinerin 2, and jasmolin 2). It is a pale yellow liquid having a bland, flowery odour. Practically insoluble in water; soluble in liquid paraffin and in most organic solvents. **Store** in airtight containers. Protect from light.

Adverse Effects and Precautions

Pyrethrum is irritant to the eyes and mucosa. Hypersensitivity reactions have been reported.

Uses

Pyrethrum flower is mainly used for the preparation of pyrethrum extracts containing a mixture of chrysanthemic acid and pyrethric acid esters (pyrethrins I and II).

Pyrethrins in the form of pyrethrum extract have a long history of use as insecticides. Pyrethrum is rapidly toxic to many insects. It has a much quicker knock-down effect than dicophane or lindane, but it is less persistent and less stable. Its action can be enhanced by certain substances such as piperonyl butoxide (p.1409) and pyrethrins with piperonyl butoxide are used clinically in the treatment of pediculosis (p.1401). Pyrethroid insecticides (synthetic analogues of pyrethrins) such as permethrin and phenothrin are also used clinically; deltamethrin and permethrin are among those used for the vector control of malaria.

Pyrethrum, pyrethrins, and pyrethroids are also used as topical ectoparasiticides in veterinary practice and as agricultural, horticultural, and household insecticides.

Preparations

Proprietary Preparations (details are given in Part 3)
Ital.: Moskill†.

Multi-ingredient: ***Belg.:*** Pyriderm; ***Fr.:*** Marie Rose†; Spray-Pax; ***Ger.:*** Goldgeist; Quellada P; ***Ital.:*** Cruzzy; Cruzzy Antiparassitario; Entom; Lozione Cruz Verde con Erogatore†; Pyr†; Shampoo Antiparassitario al Piretro Cruz Verde†; ***Neth.:*** Crinopex-N; ***Norw.:*** Rinsoderm; ***Swed.:*** Crinopex; ***Switz.:*** A-Par; ***USA:*** Clear Total Lice Elimination System.

Red Squill (2028-t)

CAS — 507-60-8 (scilliroside).

A red variety of *Urginea maritima*, which contains, in addition to cardiac glycosides, an active principle, scilliroside.

Red squill is very toxic to rats and has been incorporated in rat poisons; it has neurotoxic and cardiotoxic properties.

Resmethrin (11863-c)

5-Benzyl-3-furylmethyl (1*RS*,3*RS*)-(1*RS*,3*SR*)-2,2-dimethyl-3-(2-methylprop-1-enyl)cyclopropanecarboxylate.

$C_{22}H_{26}O_3$ = 338.4.

CAS — 10453-86-8.

Resmethrin is a pyrethroid insecticide (p.1410) used in veterinary practice for the control of ectoparasites in the environment. Resmethrin is also used as an agricultural, horticultural, and household insecticide, but is not synergised by pyrethrum synergists such as piperonyl butoxide (p.1409).

Rotenone (3606-f)

Rotenonum. (2*R*,6a*S*,12a*S*)-1,2,6,6a,12,12a-Hexahydro-2-isopropenyl-8,9-dimethoxychromeno[3,4-*b*]furo[2,3-*h*]chromen-6-one.

$C_{23}H_{22}O_6$ = 394.4.

CAS — 83-79-4.

Rotenone is a non-systemic insecticide used in agriculture and in horticulture.

Rotenone is the active ingredient of derris (the dried rhizome and roots of *Derris elliptica*; also known as tuba root or akertuba) and of lonchocarpus (the dried root of *Lonchocarpus utilis*; also known as cube root, timbo, or barbusco). Powdered forms of derris and of lonchocarpus have been used as insecticides and fish poisons.

Sodium Fluoroacetate (7734-c)

Compound 1080; Sodium Monofluoroacetate.

$FCH_2.CO_2Na$ = 100.0.

CAS — 62-74-8.

Adverse Effects, Treatment, and Precautions

Sodium fluoroacetate is highly toxic, the lethal dose if ingested being about 2 to 10 mg per kg body-weight. Toxic effects may be delayed for several hours after absorption by mouth or inhalation, and include nausea and vomiting, apprehension, muscle twitching, cardiac irregularities, convulsions, respiratory failure, coma, and death usually due to ventricular fibrillation.

Treatment is generally supportive and symptomatic.

Uses

Sodium fluoroacetate is a highly effective rodenticide but must be used with great caution because of its toxicity to other animals and to man.

Temefos (3609-h)

Temefos *(USAN, rINN)*.

27165; Temephos. *O,O'*-(Thiodi-*p*-phenylene) *O,O,O',O'*-tetramethyl bis(phosphorothioate).

$C_{16}H_{20}O_6P_2S_3$ = 466.5.

CAS — 3383-96-8.

Temefos is an organophosphorus insecticide (p.1408). It is effective against the larvae of mosquitoes, blackflies, and other insects, and is used for the larvicidal treatment of rivers in the control of onchocerciasis (p.95). It is also effective against the crustacean host to the larvae of the guinea worm and is used in the control of dracunculiasis (p.93); treatment of drinking water is both effective and acceptable.

Tetrachlorvinphos (18193-b)

ENT-25841; SD-8447. 2-Chloro-1-(2,4,5-trichlorophenyl)vinyl dimethyl phosphate.

$C_{10}H_9Cl_4O_4P$ = 366.0.

CAS — 961-11-5; 22248-79-9 (Z-tetrachlorvinphos); 22350-76-1 (E-tetrachlorvinphos).

Tetrachlorvinphos is an organophosphorus insecticide (p.1408) used as an ectoparasiticide in veterinary practice.

Tetramethrin (3610-a)

Tetramethrin *(rINN)*.

Cyclohex-1-ene-1,2-dicarboximidomethyl (1*RS*,3*RS*)-(1*RS*,3*SR*)-2,2-dimethyl-3-(2-methylprop-1-enyl)cyclopropanecarboxylate.

$C_{19}H_{25}NO_4$ = 331.4.

CAS — 7696-12-0.

Tetramethrin is a pyrethroid insecticide (p.1410) used in the treatment of pediculosis (p.1401). It is also used in veterinary practice for the control of ectoparasites in the environment and as a household insecticide.

Preparations

Proprietary Preparations (details are given in Part 3)

Multi-ingredient: ***Fr.:*** Itax Antipoux; ***Ital.:*** Baygon N; Mafu; Mom Piretro Emulsione; Mom Shampoo Antiparassitario; Neo Mom.

Trichlorophenoxyacetic Acid (3611-t)

2,4,5-T. 2,4,5-Trichlorophenoxyacetic acid.

$C_8H_5Cl_3O_3$ = 255.5.

CAS — 35915-18-5.

Trichlorophenoxyacetic acid is a selective herbicide with similar actions to dichlorophenoxyacetic acid (p.1404). It is usually used in ester formulations. It was used as a defoliating agent in the Vietnam war in conjunction with dichlorophenoxyacetic acid.

Swedish studies initially indicated that there was an increased incidence of soft tissue sarcoma, Hodgkin's disease, and non-Hodgkin's lymphoma with phenoxy herbicides. Other studies have failed to demonstrate such a connection with the exception of non-Hodgkin's lymphoma.[1-4]

These herbicides were used for defoliation in Vietnam as Agent Orange, which consisted of a mixture of dichlorophenoxyacetic acid, trichlorophenoxyacetic acid, and the impurity TCDD (dioxin), and concern has been expressed that they may have contributed to an increased incidence of cancer among exposed subjects as well as an adverse effect on the offspring of those subjects. This has been a matter of considerable debate,[5] prompting a series of biennial reassessments of the health effects of Agent Orange by the US National Academy of Sciences' Institute of Medicine.[6]

1. Anonymous. Phenoxy herbicides, trichlorophenols, and soft-tissue sarcomas. *Lancet* 1982; **i:** 1051–2.
2. Coggon D, Acheson ED. Do phenoxy herbicides cause cancer in man? *Lancet* 1982; **i:** 1057–9.
3. Hoar SK, *et al.* Agricultural herbicide use and risk of lymphoma and soft-tissue sarcoma. *JAMA* 1986; **256:** 1141–7.
4. The Selected Cancers Cooperative Study Group. The association of selected cancers with service in the US military in Vietnam. *Arch Intern Med* 1990; **150:** 2473–83, 2485–92, and 2495–2505.
5. McCarthy M. Agent Orange. *Lancet* 1993; **342:** 362.
6. Stephenson J. New IOM report links Agent Orange exposure to risk of birth defect in Vietnam vets' children. *JAMA* 1996; **275:** 1066–7.

Prostaglandins

'Prostaglandin' was the name given by von Euler to a substance found in extracts and secretions from the human prostate gland and seminal vesicles which greatly lowered the blood pressure after injection into animals and stimulated the isolated intestine and uterus. There is now known to be an extensive family of prostaglandins and related compounds which are involved in many different biological functions. The prostaglandins, along with thromboxanes and leukotrienes are all derived from 20-carbon polyunsaturated fatty acids and are collectively termed eicosanoids. In man, the most common precursor is arachidonic acid (eicosatetraenoic acid) whereas eicosapentaenoic acid is a predominant precursor in fish and marine animals.

Arachidonic acid is released from cell-membrane phospholipids by the enzyme phospholipase A_2 and is then rapidly metabolised by several enzymes, the major ones being cyclo-oxygenase (prostaglandin synthetase) and lipoxygenase. The prostaglandins, thromboxanes, and prostacyclin (sometimes collectively termed prostanoids) all contain ring structures and are products of arachidonic-acid oxidation by cyclo-oxygenase, an enzyme widely distributed in cell membranes. The leukotrienes are products of the lipoxygenase pathway. The initial step in the cyclo-oxygenase pathway is the formation of cyclic endoperoxide prostaglandin G_2 (PGG_2) which is then reduced to the endoperoxide prostaglandin H_2 (PGH_2). Prostaglandin H_2 is then converted to the primary prostaglandins prostaglandin D_2, prostaglandin E_2, and prostaglandin $F_{2\alpha}$, to thromboxane A_2 (TXA_2) via the enzyme thromboxane synthetase, or to prostacyclin (PGI_2) via the enzyme prostacyclin synthetase. These products are further metabolised and rapidly inactivated in the body. The secondary prostaglandins, prostaglandin A_2 (PGA_2), prostaglandin B_2 (PGB_2), and prostaglandin C_2 (PGC_2) are derived from prostaglandin E_2, but are formed during extraction and probably do not occur biologically.

The prostaglandins are all derivatives of the carbon skeleton 7-(2-octylcyclopentyl)heptanoic acid (also known as prostanoic acid). All natural prostaglandins have a double bond at position 1,2 and a hydroxyl group at position 3 of the octyl side-chain. Depending on the substitutions on the cyclopentane ring, the main series of prostaglandins are distinguished by the letters A, B, C, D, E, and F; the members of each series are further subdivided by subscript numbers which indicate the degree of unsaturation in the side-chains—hence, those derived from eicosatrienoic acid (dihomo-γ-linolenic acid) have the subscript 1, those derived from arachidonic acid have the subscript 2, and those derived from eicosapentaenoic acid have the subscript 3. In man, only prostaglandins of the '2' series appear to be of physiological importance. Thromboxane A_2 has an oxane rather than a cyclopentane ring; it is chemically unstable and breaks down to thromboxane B_2. Prostacyclin has a double-ring structure and breaks down to 6-keto-prostaglandin $F_{1\alpha}$.

Endogenous prostaglandins are autacoids; they can be formed by virtually all tissues and cells in response to a variety of stimuli, produce a wide range of effects, and are involved in the regulation of virtually all biological functions. Prostaglandins appear to act through various receptor-mediated mechanisms. Some of their effects are mediated within cells by activation or inhibition of adenylate cyclase and the regulation of cyclic adenosine monophosphate production. At one time prostaglandin E_2 and prostaglandin $F_{2\alpha}$ were thought to be of paramount importance, but with the discovery of thromboxane A_2, prostacyclin, and the leukotrienes it was realised that these primary prostaglandins belong to a large family of physiologically active eicosanoids. Thromboxane A_2 induces platelet aggregation and constricts arterial smooth muscle whereas prostacyclin causes vasodilatation and prevents platelet aggregation; the balance between these opposing actions has an important role in the regulation of intravascular platelet aggregation and thrombus formation. The leukotrienes are important mediators of inflammation.

The pharmacological properties of prostaglandins are wide-ranging and include contraction or relaxation of smooth muscle in the blood vessels, bronchi, uterus, and gastro-intestinal tract; inhibition of gastric acid secretion; and effects on platelet aggregation, the endocrine system, and metabolic processes. Individual prostaglandins vary greatly in their activities and potencies; their actions also depend on the animal species, on the tissues in which they are acting, and on the concentration present, and entirely opposite actions may be elicited with very small structural changes in the molecule.

The diverse **clinical applications** of prostaglandins reflect their wide-ranging physiological and pharmacological properties. Synthetic analogues have been developed with the aim of obtaining compounds which are more stable, have a longer duration of action, and a more specific effect.

- prostaglandins used to soften and dilate the cervix and as uterine stimulants in obstetrics and gynaecology include: dinoprost (prostaglandin $F_{2\alpha}$) (p.1414) and its analogue carboprost (p.1414); dinoprostone (prostaglandin E_2) (p.1414) and its analogue sulprostone (p.1420); and gemeprost (p.1418) and misoprostol (p.1419), analogues of prostaglandin E_1
- prostaglandins used as vasodilators and inhibitors of platelet aggregation include: alprostadil (prostaglandin E_1) (p.1412) and its analogue limaprost (p.1419); and epoprostenol (prostacyclin) (p.1417) and its analogue iloprost (p.1419)
- prostaglandins used as inhibitors of gastric acid secretion and to protect the gastro-intestinal mucosa include misoprostol (p.1419)
- prostaglandin analogues such as latanoprost (p.1419) are used in glaucoma
- synthetic analogues of prostaglandin F_1 and $F_{2\alpha}$ are used as luteolytics (causing regression of the corpus luteum in the ovary) in veterinary medicine.

References.

1. Moncada S, Vane JR. Arachidonic acid metabolites and the interactions between platelets and blood-vessel walls. *N Engl J Med* 1979; **300:** 1142–7.
2. Crawford MA. Background to essential fatty acids and their prostanoid derivatives. *Br Med Bull* 1983; **39:** 210–13.
3. Bakhle YS. Synthesis and catabolism of cyclo-oxygenase products. *Br Med Bull* 1983; **39:** 214–18.
4. Blackwell GJ, Flower RJ. Inhibition of phospholipase. *Br Med Bull* 1983; **39:** 260–4.
5. Higgs GA, Vane JR. Inhibition of cyclo-oxygenase and lipoxygenase. *Br Med Bull* 1983; **39:** 265–70.
6. Wardle EN. Guide to the prostaglandins. *Br J Hosp Med* 1985; **34:** 229–32.
7. Hawkey CJ, Rampton DS. Prostaglandins and the gastrointestinal mucosa: are they important in its function, disease, or treatment? *Gastroenterology* 1985; **89:** 1162–88.
8. Nies AS. Prostaglandins and the control of the circulation. *Clin Pharmacol Ther* 1986; **39:** 481–8.
9. Halushka PV, *et al.* Thromboxane, prostaglandin and leukotriene receptors. *Annu Rev Pharmacol Toxicol* 1989; **29:** 213–39.

Labour induction and augmentation

During the final 4 to 5 weeks of pregnancy the cervix normally undergoes a 'ripening' process so that at parturition it is not a barrier to delivery from the uterus. Since endogenous prostaglandins, particularly prostaglandin E_2, play an important role in this process exogenous prostaglandins have been given to women in whom the cervix is insufficiently ripe at term.[1-3] The oral antiprogestogen mifepristone has also been tried.[4]

Dinoprostone (prostaglandin E_2) is the most widely used prostaglandin; dinoprost (prostaglandin $F_{2\alpha}$) has sometimes been used (as have other prostaglandins) but is associated with a higher incidence of adverse effects. Various routes of administration have been employed. The intravenous and oral routes have been associated with frequent adverse, particularly gastro-intestinal, effects and intravaginal administration as pessaries or gel is now preferred. The intracervical and extra-amniotic routes are sometimes employed, and while these routes are probably more effective than the intravaginal route, they are more invasive and are generally used only when the cervix is particularly unripe or when the intravaginal route has produced a poor response. One study[5] found that intravenous infusion of low-dose oxytocin was as effective as intracervical dinoprostone for achieving subsequent vaginal delivery in women with an unripe cervix, although dinoprostone recipients were more likely to have spontaneous onset of labour during ripening.

If labour does not start when the cervix is ripe then **labour induction** may be considered. The most widely used induction technique is amniotomy (deliberate rupture of the fetal membranes), often followed by slow intravenous infusion of oxytocin to stimulate uterine contractions. Alternatively prostaglandins, particularly dinoprostone, may be used to induce contractions and mifepristone has been tried.[4]

Oxytocin is administered by slow intravenous infusion at a usual initial rate of 0.5 to 4 milliunits per minute gradually increased by increments of 1 to 2 milliunits per minute at intervals of about 20 to 60 minutes. However, there have been conflicting findings about the dose. Some have used low doses effectively[6-8] (e.g. starting at 0.5 or 0.7 milliunits per minute) and found them to be as effective as higher dose regimens with a reduced incidence of uterine hyperstimulation.[7] Others report that the failure of induction was less frequent with higher doses (starting at 6 milliunits per minute), although there was a higher rate of caesarean section for fetal distress.[9]

When dinoprostone is used for labour induction it is usually given intravaginally as gel which has been found to be more effective than pessaries.[10] Dinoprostone given this way produces similar results to oxytocin infusions[11] with the advantage of lower rates of neonatal jaundice and postpartum haemorrhage. It is also less invasive and as its effects are more akin to spontaneous labour, it is more popular with the mother than oxytocin. Intracervical dinoprostone gel, originally developed as a method of combining cervical ripening and then labour induction, is more invasive and appears to offer no advantage over the intravaginal route. Misoprostol intravaginally has also been studied and has compared favourably with intracervical dinoprostone.[12,13] However, the use of amniotomy followed by intravenous infusion of oxytocin remains widely employed for labour induction, although some workers[14] do not recommend its routine use. In pregnancies at term, premature rupture of the fetal membranes (i.e. before labour begins) might increase the risk of both maternal and fetal infection.[15] The usual practice in such situations has often been to induce labour immediately, either with oxytocin intravenously or dinoprostone vaginally. Some have suggested expectant management as an alternative to immediate induction,[16] but this has been criticised.[15]

Oxytocin or a prostaglandin may also be used for **labour augmentation**. Doses of oxytocin are similar to those used for induction. Low-dose regimens starting at 1 milliunit per minute intravenously, have proved successful[17,18] and are increasingly used, although higher doses starting at 6 milliunits per minute[9] have been given. Comparison of the two approaches[9] found that high doses led to shorter labour, fewer forceps deliveries, and a lower incidence of caesarean section for dystocia, but more commonly resulted in uterine hyperstimulation.

Dinoprostone is the prostaglandin most often used for augmentation of labour. As with its use for induction, dinoprostone results in lower incidences of neonatal jaundice and of postpartum haemorrhage, and is more popular with mothers than oxytocin. It is usually given intravaginally as a gel or pessaries. A gel may be given intracervically, but this is a more invasive route. Oral dinoprostone tablets have been used despite their gastro-intestinal side-effects, and are considered to be more useful for augmentation than for induction.

Once delivery has successfully been initiated, management of the third stage of labour may be considered to reduce the risks of postpartum haemorrhage. Ergometrine or oxytocin or both are usually employed for this purpose, as discussed on p.1575.

1. Embrey MP. Prostaglandins in human reproduction. *Br Med J* 1981; **283:** 1563–6.
2. Zanini A, *et al.* Pre-induction cervical ripening with prostaglandin E_2 gel: intracervical versus intravaginal route. *Obstet Gynecol* 1990; **76:** 681–3.
3. Rayburn WF. Prostaglandin E_2 gel for cervical ripening and induction of labor: a critical analysis. *Am J Obstet Gynecol* 1989; **160:** 529–34.
4. Frydman R, *et al.* Labor induction in women at term with mifepristone (RU 486): a double-blind, randomized, placebo-controlled study. *Obstet Gynecol* 1992; **80:** 972–5.
5. Jackson GM, *et al.* Cervical ripening before induction of labor: a randomized trial of prostaglandin E_2 gel versus low-dose oxytocin. *Am J Obstet Gynecol* 1994; **171:** 1092–6.
6. Blakemore KJ, *et al.* A prospective comparison of hourly and quarter-hourly oxytocin dose increase intervals for the induction of labor at term. *Obstet Gynecol* 1990; **75:** 757–61.
7. Mercer B, *et al.* Labor induction with continuous low-dose oxytocin infusion: a randomized trial. *Obstet Gynecol* 1991; **77:** 659–63.
8. Wein P. Efficacy of different starting doses of oxytocin for induction of labor. *Obstet Gynecol* 1989; **74:** 863–8.
9. Satin AJ, *et al.* High- versus low-dose oxytocin for labor stimulation. *Obstet Gynecol* 1992; **80:** 111–16.
10. Mahmood TA. A prospective comparative study on the use of prostaglandin E_2 gel (2 mg) and prostaglandin E_2 tablet (3 mg) for the induction of labour in primigravid women with unfavourable cervices. *Eur J Obstet Gynecol Reprod Biol* 1989; **33:** 169–75.
11. Silva-Cruz A, *et al.* Prostaglandin E_2 gel compared to oxytocin for medically-indicated labour induction at term: a controlled clinical trial. *Pharmatherapeutica* 1988; **5:** 228–32.
12. Chuck FJ, *et al.* Labor induction with intravaginal misoprostol versus intracervical prostaglandin E_2 gel (Prepidil gel): randomized comparison. *Am J Obstet Gynecol* 1995; **173:** 1137–42.
13. Varaklis K, *et al.* Randomised controlled trial of vaginal misoprostol and intracervical prostaglandin E_2 gel for induction of labor at term. *Obstet Gynecol* 1995; **86:** 541–4.
14. Thornton JG, Lilford RJ. Active management of labour: current knowledge and research issues. *Br Med J* 1994; **309:** 366–9.
15. Duff P. Premature rupture of the membranes at term. *N Engl J Med* 1996; **334:** 1053–4.
16. Hannah ME, *et al.* Induction of labor compared with expectant management for prelabor rupture of the membranes at term. *N Engl J Med* 1996; **334:** 1005–10.
17. Seitchik J, Castillo M. Oxytocin augmentation of dysfunctional labor I: clinical data. *Am J Obstet Gynecol* 1982; **144:** 899–905.
18. Seitchik J, Castillo M. Oxytocin augmentation of dysfunctional labor III: multiparous patients. *Am J Obstet Gynecol* 1983; **145:** 777–80.
19. Akoury HA, *et al.* Oxytocin augmentation of labor and perinatal outcome in nulliparas. *Obstet Gynecol* 1991; **78:** 227–30.

Termination of pregnancy

One of the main factors influencing the choice of method for termination of pregnancy is the stage of gestation.[1]

Menstrual extraction, which involves aspiration of the uterine cavity and induction of uterine bleeding is sometimes used when menstruation is no more than **14 days** overdue. Dilatation and vacuum aspiration is a common method for termination of pregnancy at up to **63 days** of amenorrhoea. Termination may also be achieved medically with the oral antiprogestogenic drug mifepristone followed by a prostaglandin. Withdrawal of the progesterone influence on the uterus through the action of mifepristone may result in uterine contractions; mifepristone may also increase the myometrial sensitivity to prostaglandins. Prostaglandins soften and dilate the cervix and stimulate uterine contractions. Mifepristone is probably not sufficiently effective when given alone and is therefore usually followed 36 to 48 hours later by a low dose of a prostaglandin analogue, usually gemeprost administered intravaginally, although sulprostone has been used. Mifepristone may also be combined effectively with prostaglandin E analogues, notably misoprostol given orally or vaginally. Prostaglandins have been used alone but are now usually combined with mifepristone.

Methotrexate has also been investigated. Intramuscular methotrexate followed 3 days later by intravaginal misoprostol was more effective than misoprostol alone for termination at 56 days or less;[2] the combination was re- [illegible] to be less successful after 57 to 63 days' gesta- [illegible]ter studies[4,5] however found the combination to be safe and effective in terminating pregnancies up to 63 days' gestation; in these the misoprostol was administered up to 7 days after the methotrexate.

Intravaginal administration of isosorbide mononitrate is being investigated for cervical ripening.[6]

Termination at later stages of pregnancy is generally associated with higher morbidity and mortality.

Standard methods at **9 to 14 weeks** of gestation are surgical (dilatation and vacuum aspiration). There has been very little clinical study of medical methods although preparation of the cervix with prostaglandins intravaginally is common.

At **more than 14 weeks** cervical preparation and medical induction is usually performed, again with mifepristone followed by a prostaglandin. Prostaglandins administered intravaginally include gemeprost and misoprostol, but usually in repeated doses. Parenteral administration can involve carboprost intramuscularly or sulprostone intravenously. Intra-amniotic dinoprost or extra-amniotic dinoprostone have been used when none of the above prostaglandins were available but such methods of administration carry additional risks. The frequency of side-effects with prostaglandins is reported to be generally higher with intra-amniotic than with extra-amniotic administration. Other methods have included the intra-amniotic administration of hypertonic sodium chloride and the intra-amniotic administration of hyperosmolar urea augmented with dinoprost.

1. WHO. Medical methods for termination of pregnancy: report of a WHO scientific group. *WHO Tech Rep Ser 871* 1997.
2. Creinin MD, Vittinghoff E. Methotrexate and misoprostol vs misoprostol alone for early abortion: a randomized controlled trial. *JAMA* 1994; **272:** 1190–5.
3. Creinin MD. Methotrexate and misoprostol for abortion at 57–63 days gestation. *Contraception* 1994; **50:** 511–15.
4. Hausknecht RU. Methotrexate and misoprostol to terminate early pregnancy. *N Engl J Med* 1995; **333:** 537–40.
5. Creinin MD, *et al.* A randomized trial comparing misoprostol three and seven days after methotrexate for early abortion. *Am J Obstet Gynecol* 1995; **173:** 1578–84.
6. Thomson AJ, *et al.* Randomised trial of nitric oxide donor versus prostaglandin for cervical ripening before first-trimester termination of pregnancy. *Lancet* 1998; **352:** 1093–6.

Alfaprostol (18611-g)

Alfaprostol *(BAN, USAN, rINN).*

K-11941; Ro-22-9000. Methyl (*Z*)-7-{(1*R*,2*S*,3*R*,5*S*)-2-[(3*S*)-5-cyclohexyl-3-hydroxypent-1-ynyl]-3,5-dihydroxycyclopentyl}hept-5-enoate.

$C_{24}H_{38}O_5$ = 406.6.

CAS — 74176-31-1.

Alfaprostol is a synthetic analogue of dinoprost (prostaglandin $F_{2\alpha}$). It is used as a luteolytic in veterinary medicine.

Alprostadil (8071-n)

Alprostadil *(BAN, USAN, rINN).*

PGE_1; Prostaglandin E_1; U-10136. (*E*)-(8*R*,11*R*,12*R*,15*S*)-11,15-Dihydroxy-9-oxoprost-13-enoic acid; 7-{(1*R*,2*R*,3*R*)-3-Hydroxy-2-[(*E*)-(3*S*)-3-hydroxyoct-1-enyl]-5-oxocyclopentyl}heptanoic acid.

$C_{20}H_{34}O_5$ = 354.5.

CAS — 745-65-3.

NOTE. In *Martindale* the term alprostadil is used for the exogenous form and prostaglandin E_1 for the endogenous form.

Pharmacopoeias. In US.

Jpn includes Alprostadil Alfadex.

A white to off-white crystalline powder. M.p. about 110°. Freely **soluble** in alcohol; soluble in acetone; very slightly soluble in chloroform and ether; slightly soluble in ethyl acetate. **Store** between 2° and 8° in airtight containers.

Adverse Effects, Treatment, and Precautions

The adverse effects reported most commonly in infants with congenital heart disease treated with alprostadil are apnoea, fever, flushing, hypotension, bradycardia, tachycardia, diarrhoea, and convulsions. Other adverse effects reported include oedema, cardiac arrest, hypokalaemia, disseminated intravascular coagulation, and cortical proliferation of the long bones. Weakening of the wall of the ductus arteriosus and pulmonary artery may occur following prolonged infusion. Alprostadil should be avoided in neonates with respiratory distress syndrome and should be used with caution in those with bleeding tendencies; blood pressure and respiratory status should be monitored during infusion.

Adverse effects reported in adults given alprostadil have included headache, flushing, hypotension, diarrhoea, and pain and inflammation at the infusion site.

Following intracavernosal injection of alprostadil for the treatment of impotence, the most frequently reported adverse effect is pain during erection. Penile fibrosis, fibrotic nodules, and Peyronie's disease have been reported. Priapism may occur (see below). Intracavernosal injection of alprostadil should be avoided in patients with sickle-cell disease, myeloma, leukaemias, complicating penile deformities, or other conditions predisposing to prolonged erection.

A review[1] of the incidence of side-effects in 492 infants with critical congenital heart disease treated with alprostadil at 56 centres in the USA over a 3-year period. At least one intercurrent medical event was reported in 213 infants (43%) during therapy, but only 49% of these reactions were believed to be related to or probably related to alprostadil administration. *Cardiovascular events* (cutaneous vasodilatation or oedema, rhythm or conduction disturbances, and hypotension) occurred in 90 infants (18%) and were thought to be related to alprostadil in 54% of occurrences. Intra-aortic infusion of alprostadil, used more commonly in cyanotic infants, was associated with a significantly greater incidence of cutaneous dilatation than the intravenous route; although reversed by repositioning the catheter, intravenous infusion was considered preferable. Cardiovascular effects were more likely in infants of less than 2 kg birth-weight or when the duration of infusion exceeded 48 hours. *Central nervous system events* (seizure-like activity, temperature elevation, irritability, or lethargy) occurred in 81 infants (16%) and were more frequent when the duration of infusion exceeded 48 hours. *Respiratory depression* (apnoea or hypoventilation), the most worrying side-effect, occurred in 58 infants (12%) and was thought to be related to alprostadil in 68% of occurrences. It was significantly more common in cyanotic infants and those weighing less than 2 kg at birth and was the most common reason for discontinuing infusion of alprostadil. Assisted ventilation should be readily available before initiating therapy with alprostadil. *Metabolic abnormalities* (hypoglycaemia or hypocalcaemia) occurred in 12 infants. *Gastro-intestinal disturbances* also occurred in 12. Diarrhoea was the most common disturbance; necrotising enterocolitis and hyperbilirubinaemia were isolated occurrences. *Infections* (sepsis or wound infections) in 12 infants, *haematological abnormalities* (haemorrhage, disseminated intravascular coagulation, and thrombocytopenia) in 9, and *renal failure* or *insufficiency* in 9 were generally not considered to be related to alprostadil infusion. There was insufficient data to confirm earlier reports of histological changes in the ductus arteriosus wall[2] and in the small pulmonary arteries.[3]

1. Lewis AB, *et al.* Side effects of therapy with prostaglandin E_1 in infants with critical congenital heart disease. *Circulation* 1981; **64:** 893–8.
2. Gittenberger-de Groot AC, *et al.* Histopathology of the ductus arteriosus after prostaglandin E_1 administration in ductus dependent cardiac anomalies. *Br Heart J* 1978; **40:** 215–20.
3. Haworth SG, *et al.* Effect of prostaglandin E_1 on pulmonary circulation in pulmonary atresia: a quantitative morphometric study. *Br Heart J* 1980 **43:** 306–14.

Effects on the bones. Periosteal or cortical hyperostosis has been reported in infants following long-term therapy with alprostadil for cyanotic congenital heart disease.[1-3] A retrospective review of 30 infants[2] treated with alprostadil revealed radiographic signs of periosteal reactions in 5. Changes could be detected after even short courses of therapy; 3 developed relatively mild periosteal changes in the ribs after infusions ranging from 9 to 205 hours and one had involvement of the left femur after infusion for 71 hours. Resolution of lesions had occurred in most bones 6 to 12 months later. In a further study,[4] radiological evidence of cortical hyperostosis was found in 53 of 86 infant heart transplant recipients who had received alprostadil infusion pre-operatively. Of 53 of the infants who had received alprostadil for less than 30 days, 21 were affected (2 severely). Correspondingly, of those treated for 30 to 60 days, 18 of 22 were affected (13 severely). All 14 infants treated for more than 60 days were affected (7 severely). Since the associated bone changes may persist for months after discontinuation of alprostadil, caution should be exercised to avoid misdiagnosis.

1. Ueda K, *et al.* Cortical hyperostosis following long-term administration of prostaglandin E_1 in infants with cyanotic congenital heart disease. *J Pediatr* 1980; **97:** 834–6.
2. Ringel RE, *et al.* Periosteal changes secondary to prostaglandin administration. *J Pediatr* 1983; **103:** 251–3.

3. Williams JL. Periosteal hyperostosis resulting from prostaglandin therapy. *Eur J Radiol* 1986; **6:** 231–2.
4. Woo K, *et al.* Cortical hyperostosis: a complication of prolonged prostaglandin infusion in infants awaiting cardiac transplantation. *Pediatrics* 1994; **93:** 417–20.

Effects on the gastro-intestinal tract. Hyperplasia of the antral mucosa, resulting in gastric outlet obstruction, has been reported in several neonates receiving alprostadil infusion.[1,2] It was suggested that this effect was dose-dependent.[1] Regression of the obstruction usually occurred following cessation of therapy.

1. Peled N, *et al.* Gastric-outlet obstruction induced by prostaglandin therapy in neonates. *N Engl J Med* 1992; **327:** 505–10.
2. Merkus PJFM, *et al.* Prostaglandin E1 and gastric outlet obstruction in infants. *Lancet* 1993; **342:** 747.

Effects on the metabolism. Severe hyperglycaemia with apparent ketoacidosis occurred during infusion with alprostadil postoperatively in the infant of a diabetic mother.[1] The manufacturers had received reports of hyperglycaemia associated with alprostadil in 5 infants, one of whom had a diabetic mother.

1. Cohen MH, Nihill MR. Postoperative ketotic hyperglycaemia during prostaglandin E_1 infusion in infancy. *Pediatrics* 1983; **71:** 842–4.

Priapism. If priapism occurs following the use of alprostadil for erectile dysfunction, its treatment should not be delayed more than 6 hours. Initial therapy is by penile aspiration. If aspiration is unsuccessful a sympathomimetic with action on alpha adrenergic receptors is given by cautious intracavernosal injection, with continuous monitoring of blood pressure and pulse. Extreme caution is necessary in patients with coronary heart disease, hypertension, cerebral ischaemia, or if taking an antidepressant. Low doses and dilute solutions are recommended as follows:

- intracavernosal injection of phenylephrine 100 to 200 micrograms (0.5 to 1 mL of a 200 microgram per mL solution) every 5 to 10 minutes; maximum total dose 1 mg (if a suitable strength of phenylephrine injection is not available one may be specially prepared by diluting 0.1 mL of the phenylephrine 1% (10 mg per mL) injection to 5 mL with sodium chloride 0.9%)

alternatively

- intracavernosal injection of adrenaline 10 to 20 micrograms (0.5 to 1 mL of a 20 microgram per mL solution) every 5 to 10 minutes; maximum total dose 100 micrograms (if a suitable strength of adrenaline is not available one may be specially prepared by diluting 0.1 mL of the adrenaline 1 in 1000 (1 mg per mL) injection to 5 mL with sodium chloride 0.9%)

alternatively

- intracavernosal injection of metaraminol may be used, but it should be noted that fatal hypertensive crises have been reported; a maximum total dose of up to 1 mg has been suggested (prepared by diluting 0.1 mL of metaraminol 1% (10 mg per mL) injection to 5 mL with sodium chloride 0.9%), given by careful slow injection.

If necessary the sympathomimetic injections can be followed by further penile aspiration. If sympathomimetics are unsuccessful, urgent surgical referral is required.

Pharmacokinetics

Following infusion alprostadil is rapidly metabolised by oxidation during passage through the pulmonary circulation. It is excreted in the urine as metabolites within about 24 hours.

References.

1. Cox JW, *et al.* Pulmonary extraction and pharmacokinetics of prostaglandin E_1 during continuous intravenous infusion in patients with adult respiratory distress syndrome. *Am Rev Respir Dis* 1988; **137:** 5–12.
2. Cawello W, *et al.* Dose proportional pharmacokinetics of alprostadil (prostaglandin E_1) in healthy volunteers following intravenous infusion. *Br J Clin Pharmacol* 1995; **40:** 273–6.

Uses and Administration

Alprostadil is a prostaglandin which causes vasodilatation and prevents platelet aggregation. The endogenous substance is termed prostaglandin E_1. It is used mainly in congenital heart disease and in impotence (below).

Alprostadil is given to maintain the patency of the ductus arteriosus in neonates with congenital heart disease until surgery is possible. It is administered by continuous intravenous infusion beginning with doses of 50 to 100 nanograms per kg body-weight per minute; doses should be reduced as soon as possible to the lowest dosage necessary to maintain response. Some workers recommend a lower starting dose. It may also be administered by continuous infusion through an umbilical artery catheter placed at the ductal opening.

Intracavernosal injections of alprostadil are used in the treatment of impotence due to erectile dysfunction. Alprostadil is used in an initial dose of 2.5 μg and increased incrementally until an optimal dose is established. The second dose should be 5 μg if some response to the first dose is observed or 7.5 μg if there is no response; subsequent increments should be of 5 to 10 μg until the optimum dose is found. In cases of erectile dysfunction of neurogenic origin secondary to spinal cord injury a suggested initial dose is 1.25 μg, with a second dose of 2.5 μg, and third dose and subsequent increments of 5 μg. While ascertaining optimum dose, the interval between doses should be at least 1 day if there has been a partial response; in the case of no response to an administered dose the next higher one may be given within one hour. Subsequently the optimal dose should be administered not more than once daily and not more than three times per week. The usual dose range is 5 to 20 μg and the maximum recommended dose is 60 μg.

Alprostadil may also be injected intracavernosally in the diagnosis of erectile dysfunction in doses ranging from 5 to 20 μg.

Alprostadil alfadex (a combination of alprostadil with α-cyclodextrin) is available in some countries for intracavernosal injection in the treatment of erectile dysfunction. Urethral suppositories containing alprostadil are also used in doses of 125 μg to 1000 μg.

Erectile dysfunction. Alprostadil has been given by intracavernosal injection as an aid to the diagnosis and treatment of erectile dysfunction (p.1614). The dose of alprostadil most commonly used in treatment is between 5 and 20 μg; doses of 2.5 to 100 μg have been reported, although it is recommended that doses should not exceed 60 μg. A dose-related response has been demonstrated[1-3] and dose-related local pain may occur.[1,4,5] In comparative studies alprostadil was at least as effective as papaverine either alone or in combination with phentolamine in producing erections,[4,5] and may be effective in patients who do not respond to papaverine;[6] it may also be safer.[7] Alprostadil has also been given in conjunction with papaverine and phentolamine.[8]

Alprostadil has also been used as a pellet (or micro-suppository) which is inserted into the urethra and delivers the drug across the urethral membrane.[9]

1. Schramek P, Waldhauser M. Dose-dependent effect and side-effect of prostaglandin E_1 in erectile dysfunction. *Br J Clin Pharmacol* 1989; **28:** 567–71.
2. Linet OI, Ogrinc FG. Efficacy and safety of intracavernosal alprostadil in men with erectile dysfunction. *N Engl J Med* 1996; **334:** 873–7.
3. Garceau RJ, *et al.* Dose-response studies of intracavernous injection therapy with alprostadil in Asian and Australian men with erectile dysfunction. *Curr Ther Res* 1996; **57:** 50–61.
4. Waldhauser M, Schramek P. Efficiency and side effects of prostaglandin E_1 in the treatment of erectile dysfunction. *J Urol (Baltimore)* 1988; **140:** 525–7.
5. Lee LM, *et al.* Prostaglandin E_1 versus phentolamine/papaverine for the treatment of erectile impotence: a double-blind comparison. *J Urol (Baltimore)* 1989; **141:** 549–55.
6. Sarosdy MF, *et al.* A prospective double-blind trial of intracorporeal papaverine versus prostaglandin E_1 in the treatment of impotence. *J Urol (Baltimore)* 1989; **141:** 551–3.
7. Anonymous. Alprostadil for erectile impotence. *Drug Ther Bull* 1995; **33:** 61–2.
8. Govier FE, *et al.* Experience with triple-drug therapy in a pharmacological erection program. *J Urol (Baltimore)* 1993; **150:** 1822–4.
9. Padma-Nathan H, *et al.* Treatment of men with erectile dysfunction with transurethral alprostadil. *N Engl J Med* 1997; **336:** 1–7.

Ergotamine poisoning. Alprostadil[1,2] has been used to treat the circulatory disturbances in ergotamine poisoning (p.446) and is one of many drugs that have been employed.

1. Levy JM, *et al.* Prostaglandin E_1 for alleviating symptoms of ergot intoxication: a case report. *Cardiovasc Intervent Radiol* 1984; **7:** 28–30.
2. Horstmann R, *et al.* Kritische extremitätenischämie durch ergotismus. *Dtsch Med Wochenschr* 1993; **118:** 1067–71.

Haemorrhagic cystitis. Bladder irrigation with alprostadil produced resolution of severe haemorrhagic cystitis in 5 of 6 children who had undergone bone-marrow transplantation.[1] Alprostadil was administered via a catheter and retained for 1 hour each day for at least 7 consecutive days.

1. Trigg ME, *et al.* Prostaglandin E_1 bladder instillations to control severe hemorrhagic cystitis. *J Urol (Baltimore)* 1990; **143:** 92–4.

Hepatic disorders. Encouraging results were reported in 17 patients with fulminant or subfulminant *viral hepatitis* (p.595) following administration of alprostadil in doses of up to 600 nanograms per kg body-weight per hour [10 nanograms per kg per minute] for up to 28 days.[1] Twelve patients responded with clinical, biochemical, and histological improvement. Oral administration of dinoprostone was necessary to maintain remission in 5 patients with non-A non-B hepatitis although prostaglandin therapy was subsequently successfully withdrawn from 2 of these patients. The 5 patients who did not respond had advanced disease with stage 4 encephalopathy at the start of treatment. In another study,[2] 11 of 12 liver transplant recipients who had developed recurrent hepatitis B infection responded to intravenous alprostadil followed by oral dinoprostone or misoprostol or in one case to oral therapy alone. Eight of the patients responded for a sustained period. Prostaglandins were studied because they had previously been shown to have a cytoprotective effect in experimentally induced hepatitis or in isolated hepatocytes, but the mechanism by which they exerted a beneficial effect was uncertain.

Combined intravenous therapy with glucagon, insulin, and alprostadil formulated in lipid microspheres has also been found effective in preventing *acute fulminant liver failure* after hepatic arterial infusion of antineoplastic chemotherapy.[3]

1. Sinclair SB, *et al.* Biochemical and clinical response of fulminant viral hepatitis to administration of prostaglandin E: a preliminary report. *J Clin Invest* 1989; **84:** 1063–9.
2. Flowers M, *et al.* Prostaglandin E in the treatment of recurrent hepatitis B infection after orthotopic liver transplantation. *Transplantation* 1994; **58:** 183–92.
3. Ikegami T, *et al.* Randomized control trial of lipo-prostaglandin E_1 in patients with acute liver injury induced by Lipiodol-targeted chemotherapy. *Clin Pharmacol Ther* 1995; **57:** 582–9.

Peripheral vascular disease. Various prostaglandins including alprostadil[1-8] have been used in the treatment of peripheral vascular disease (p.794), particularly in severe Raynaud's syndrome, but do not constitute mainline therapy.

1. Anonymous. Prostaglandins and peripheral vascular disease. *Lancet* 1983; **i:** 1199.
2. Kyle V, Hazleman B. Prostaglandin E_1 and peripheral vascular disease. *Lancet* 1983; **ii:** 282.
3. Clifford PC, *et al.* Treatment of vasospastic disease with prostaglandin E_1. *Br Med J* 1980; **281:** 1031–4.
4. Martin MFR, Tooke JE. Effects of prostaglandin E_1 on microvascular haemodynamics in progressive systemic sclerosis. *Br Med J* 1982; **285:** 1688–90.
5. Langevitz P, *et al.* Treatment of refractory ischemic skin ulcers in patients with Raynaud's phenomenon with PGE_1 infusions. *J Rheumatol* 1989; **16:** 1433–5.
6. Sethi GK, *et al.* Intravenous infusion of prostaglandin E_1 (PGE_1) in management of limb ischemia. *Am Surg* 1986; **52:** 474–8.
7. Telles GS, *et al.* Prostaglandin E_1 in severe lower limb ischaemia: a double-blind controlled trial. *Br J Surg* 1984; **71:** 506–8.
8. Mohrland JS, *et al.* A multiclinic, placebo-controlled, double-blind study of prostaglandin E_1 in Raynaud's syndrome. *Ann Rheum Dis* 1985; **44:** 754–60.

Preparations

USP 23: Alprostadil Injection.

Proprietary Preparations (details are given in Part 3)
Aust.: Caverject; Minprog; Prostavasin; ***Austral.:*** Caverject; Prostin VR; ***Belg.:*** Caverject; Prostin VR; ***Canad.:*** Caverject; Prostin VR; ***Fr.:*** Caverject; Edex; Prostine VR; ***Ger.:*** Minprog; Prostavasin; ***Irl.:*** Caverject; Viridal; ***Ital.:*** Alprostar; Caverject; Prostavasin; Prostin VR; ***Jpn:*** Liple; Prostandin; ***Neth.:*** Caverject; Prostin VR; ***Norw.:*** Caverject; Prostivas; ***S.Afr.:*** Caverject; Prostin VR; ***Spain:*** Caverject; Sugiran; ***Swed.:*** Caverject; Prostivas; ***Switz.:*** Caverject; Prostin VR; ***UK:*** Caverject; Muse; Prostin VR; Viridal; ***USA:*** Edex; Muse; Prostin VR.

Beraprost (6462-d)

Beraprost *(USAN, rINN)*.

ML-1229; ML-1129 (beraprost sodium); TRK-100 (beraprost sodium). (±)-(1*R*,2*R*,3a*S*,8b*S*)-2,3,3a,8b-Tetrahydro-2-hydroxy-1-[(*E*)-(3*S*,-4*RS*)-3-hydroxy-4-methyl-1-octen-6-ynyl]-1*H*-cyclopenta[*b*]benzofuran-5-butyric acid.

$C_{24}H_{30}O_5$ = 398.5.

CAS — 88430-50-6 (beraprost); 88475-69-8 (beraprost sodium).

NOTE. Beraprost Sodium is also *USAN*.

Beraprost is a synthetic analogue of epoprostenol (prostacyclin) which causes vasodilatation and prevents platelet aggregation. It is being studied in several disorders including peripheral vascular disease, pulmonary hypertension, and thrombotic thrombocytopenic purpura and is given by mouth as the sodium salt.

Preparations

Proprietary Preparations (details are given in Part 3)
Jpn: Dorner.

Carboprost (8074-b)

Carboprost *(BAN, USAN, rINN).*

15-Me-PGF$_{2\alpha}$; Methyldinoprost; (15*S*)-15-Methylprostaglandin F$_{2\alpha}$; U-32921. (5*Z*,13*E*)-(8*R*,9*S*,11*R*,12*R*,15*S*)-9,11,15-Trihydroxy-15-methylprosta-5,13-dienoic acid; (*Z*)-7-{(1*R*,2*R*,3*R*,5*S*)-3,5-Dihydroxy-2-[(*E*)-(3*S*)-3-hydroxy-3-methyloct-1-enyl]cyclopentyl}hept-5-enoic acid.

$C_{21}H_{36}O_5$ = 368.5.

CAS — 35700-23-3.

Carboprost Methyl (8075-v)

Carboprost Methyl *(BANM, USAN, rINNM).*

U-36384. The methyl ester of carboprost.

$C_{22}H_{38}O_5$ = 382.5.

CAS — 35700-21-1.

Carboprost Trometamol (8076-g)

Carboprost Trometamol *(BANM, rINNM).*

Carboprost Tromethamine *(USAN)*; U-32921E.

$C_{21}H_{36}O_5,C_4H_{11}NO_3$ = 489.6.

CAS — 58551-69-2.

Pharmacopoeias. In *US.*

A compound of carboprost with trometamol in a ratio of 1:1. Carboprost trometamol 1.3 µg is approximately equivalent to 1 µg of carboprost. **Store** at −25° to −10°.

Adverse Effects and Precautions

As for Dinoprostone, p.1415.

Carboprost may cause bronchospasm and, less frequently, dyspnoea and pulmonary oedema. Patients with cardiopulmonary disorders should be monitored for reductions in arterial-oxygen content.

Once a prostaglandin has been given to terminate pregnancy it is essential that termination take place; if the prostaglandin is unsuccessful other measures should be used.

Uses and Administration

Carboprost is a synthetic 15-methyl analogue of dinoprost (prostaglandin F$_{2\alpha}$). It is a uterine stimulant with a more prolonged action than dinoprost; the presence of the methyl group delays inactivation by enzymic dehydrogenation.

Carboprost is used for the termination of pregnancy (p.1412) and for the treatment of refractory postpartum haemorrhage due to uterine atony (p.1575). It is usually administered intramuscularly as the trometamol salt.

For the termination of second trimester pregnancy (between the 13th and 20th weeks of gestation) the equivalent of 250 µg of carboprost is given by deep intramuscular injection and repeated every 1½ to 3½ hours depending on the uterine response; if necessary the dose may be increased to 500 µg, but the total dose given should not exceed 12 mg of carboprost. If preferred a test dose of 100 µg may be given initially. Alternatively carboprost trometamol has been administered intra-amniotically in a dose equivalent to 2.5 mg of the base over five minutes; this dose may be repeated after 24 hours if termination has not occurred and the membranes are intact.

Carboprost methyl given as vaginal pessaries has been tried for termination of pregnancy in the second trimester.

For the treatment of postpartum haemorrhage the equivalent of 250 µg of carboprost is given by deep intramuscular injection as the trometamol salt at intervals of about 90 minutes; the interval may be reduced if necessary, but should not be less than 15 minutes. A total dose of 2 mg should not be exceeded.

Haemorrhagic cystitis. Carboprost trometamol instilled into the bladder successfully controlled cyclophosphamide-induced haemorrhagic cystitis (p.516) in 15 of 24 bone-marrow transplant patients.[1] The dose consisted of 50 mL of solutions containing 2 to 10 µg per mL instilled four times daily for 7 days.

1. [illegible], *et al.* Intravesicular carboprost for the treatment of [illegible]gic cystitis after marrow transplantation. *Urology* [illegible]11–15.

Preparations

USP 23: Carboprost Tromethamine Injection.

Proprietary Preparations (details are given in Part 3)
Neth.: Prostin/15M; ***Swed.:*** Prostinfenem; ***UK:*** Hemabate; ***USA:*** Hemabate.

Cicaprost (2842-m)

Cicaprost *(rINN).*

ZK-96480. {2-[(2*E*,3a*S*,4*S*,5*R*,6a*S*)-Hexahydro-5-hydroxy-4-[(3*S*,4*S*)-3-hydroxy-4-methyl-1,6-nonadiynyl]-2-(1*H*)-pentalenylidene]ethoxy}acetic acid.

$C_{22}H_{30}O_5$ = 374.5.

CAS — 95722-07-9.

Cicaprost is a synthetic analogue of epoprostenol (prostacyclin) that has been studied for the oral treatment of peripheral vascular disease. It has also been given as cicaprost betadex.

References.

1. Lau CS, *et al.* A randomised, double-blind study of cicaprost, an oral prostacyclin analogue, in the treatment of Raynaud's phenomenon secondary to systemic sclerosis. *Clin Exp Rheumatol* 1993; **11:** 35–40.

Ciprostene Calcium (18972-p)

Ciprostene Calcium *(USAN, pINNM).*

9β-Methyl Carbacyclin Calcium; 9β-Methylcarbacyclin Calcium; U-61431F. Calcium (*Z*)-(3a*S*,5*R*,6*R*,6a*R*)-hexahydro-5-hydroxy-6-[(*E*)-(3*S*)-3-hydroxy-1-octenyl]-3a-methyl-$\Delta^{2(1H),\delta}$pentalenevalerate.

$(C_{22}H_{35}O_4)_2Ca$ = 767.1.

CAS — 81845-44-5 (ciprostene); 81703-55-1 (ciprostene calcium).

Ciprostene, a vasodilator and platelet aggregation inhibitor, is a stable analogue of epoprostenol (prostacyclin). It has been studied in peripheral vascular disease and has been given as the calcium salt by intravenous infusion.

References.

1. The Ciprostene Study Group. The effect of ciprostene in patients with peripheral vascular disease (PVD) characterized by ischemic ulcers. *J Clin Pharmacol* 1991; **31:** 81–7.

Cloprostenol Sodium (8077-q)

Cloprostenol Sodium *(BANM, USAN, rINNM).*

ICI-80996. Sodium (±)-(*Z*)-7-{(1*R*,2*R*,3*R*,5*S*)-2-[(*E*)-(3*R*)-4-(3-chlorophenoxy)-3-hydroxybut-1-enyl]-3,5-dihydroxycyclopentyl}hept-5-enoate.

$C_{22}H_{28}ClNaO_6$ = 446.9.

CAS — 40665-92-7 (cloprostenol); 55028-72-3 (cloprostenol sodium).

Pharmacopoeias. In *BP(Vet).*

A white or almost white amorphous hygroscopic powder. Freely **soluble** in water, in alcohol, and in methyl alcohol; practically insoluble in acetone. **Store** in airtight containers. Protect from light.

Cloprostenol sodium is a synthetic analogue of dinoprost (prostaglandin F$_{2\alpha}$). It is used as a luteolytic in veterinary medicine.

Dinoprost (2931-b)

Dinoprost *(BAN, USAN, rINN).*

PGF$_{2\alpha}$; Prostaglandin F$_{2\alpha}$; U-14583. (5*Z*,13*E*)-(8*R*,9*S*,11*R*,12*R*,15*S*)-9,11,15-Trihydroxyprosta-5,13-dienoic acid; (*Z*)-7-{(1*R*,2*R*,3*R*,5*S*)-3,5-Dihydroxy-2-[(*E*)-(3*S*)-3-hydroxyoct-1-enyl]cyclopentyl}hept-5-enoic acid.

$C_{20}H_{34}O_5$ = 354.5.

CAS — 551-11-1.

NOTE. In *Martindale* the term dinoprost is used for the exogenous form and prostaglandin F$_{2\alpha}$ for the endogenous form.

Pharmacopoeias. In *Jpn.*

Dinoprost Trometamol (8081-m)

Dinoprost Trometamol *(BANM, rINNM).*

Dinoprost Tromethamine *(USAN)*; Dinoprostum Trometamoli; PGF$_{2\alpha}$ THAM; Prostaglandin F$_{2\alpha}$ Trometamol; U-14583E.

$C_{20}H_{34}O_5,C_4H_{11}NO_3$ = 475.6.

CAS — 38562-01-5.

Pharmacopoeias. In *Eur.* (see p.viii) and *US.*

A compound of dinoprost with trometamol in a ratio of 1:1. A white or almost white powder. Dinoprost trometamol 1.3 µg is approximately equivalent to 1 µg of dinoprost. Very **soluble** in water; freely soluble in alcohol and dimethylformamide; slightly soluble in chloroform; soluble in methyl alcohol; practically insoluble in acetonitrile. **Store** in airtight containers.

Adverse Effects and Precautions

As for Dinoprostone, p.1415.

Dinoprost can cause bronchoconstriction and bronchospasm with wheezing and dyspnoea has occurred, especially in asthmatic patients.

Once a prostaglandin has been given to terminate pregnancy it is essential that termination take place; if the prostaglandin is unsuccessful other measures should be used.

Uses and Administration

Dinoprost is a prostaglandin of the F series (p.1411) with actions on smooth muscle; the endogenous substance is termed prostaglandin F$_{2\alpha}$ and is rapidly metabolised in the body. It induces contraction of uterine muscle at any stage of pregnancy and is reported to act predominantly as a vasoconstrictor on blood vessels and as a bronchoconstrictor on bronchial muscle.

Dinoprost is used principally for the termination of pregnancy (p.1412). It may also be used for missed abortion, hydatidiform mole, and fetal death *in utero*. Dinoprost has also been given for the induction of labour but, because it has a higher incidence of adverse effects than dinoprostone, is no longer recommended for routine use by most authorities; more appropriate treatment is discussed on p.1411.

Dinoprost is usually administered intra-amniotically for termination of pregnancy. It may be given intravenously, but this route has been associated with a high incidence of adverse effects and is generally only used for missed abortion or hydatidiform mole. The extra-amniotic route has also been used. Dinoprost is given as the trometamol salt, doses being expressed in terms of the equivalent amount of dinoprost. It should not be administered continuously for more than two days.

For the termination of pregnancy during the second trimester 40 mg of dinoprost is administered intra-amniotically by slowly injecting 8 mL of a solution containing 5 mg per mL into the amniotic sac. In the USA a further dose of 10 to 40 mg after 24 hours has been suggested if the membranes are still intact.

Dinoprost has also been given by intravenous infusion for the termination of pregnancy, missed abortion, or hydatidiform mole, a solution containing 50 µg per mL of dinoprost being infused at a rate of 25 µg per minute for at least 30 minutes, then maintained or increased to 50 µg per minute according to response and maintained at this rate for at least 4 hours before increasing further.

For the induction of labour dinoprost has been given intravenously. A suggested dosage regimen has been 2.5 µg per minute infused as a solution containing 15 µg per mL for at least 30 minutes and then maintained or increased according to the patient's response; in the USA the suggested dose has been 2.5 µg per minute infused as a solution containing 50 µg per mL, the dose being doubled every hour if necessary to a maximum of 20 µg per minute. In fetal death *in utero* higher doses may be required and an initial rate of 5 µg per minute has been used with increases at intervals of not less than 1 hour.

Ileus. Ileus induced by administration of vinca alkaloids to 3 patients with carcinoma of the lung was successfully relieved by the intravenous infusion of dinoprost 0.3 to 0.5 µg per kg body-weight per minute for 2 hours twice daily.[1] For a brief discussion of ileus and its usual treatment, see under Decreased Gastro-intestinal Motility, p.1168.

1. Saito H, *et al.* Prostaglandin F$_{2\alpha}$ in the treatment of vinca alkaloid-induced ileus. *Am J Med* 1993; **95:** 549–51.

Preparations

BP 1998: Dinoprost Injection;
USP 23: Dinoprost Tromethamine Injection.

Proprietary Preparations (details are given in Part 3)
Austral.: Prostin F2 Alpha; ***Fr.:*** Prostine F$_2$ Alpha; ***Ger.:*** Minprostin F$_{2\alpha}$; ***Irl.:*** Prostin F2 Alpha; ***Ital.:*** Prostin F2 Alpha†; ***Jpn:*** Prostarmon.F†; ***S.Afr.:*** Prostin F2 Alpha; ***Swed.:*** Prostin†; ***UK:*** Prostin F2 Alpha.

Dinoprostone (8082-b)

Dinoprostone *(BAN, USAN, rINN).*

Dinoprostonum; PGE$_2$; Prostaglandin E$_2$; U-12062. (5*Z*,13*E*)-(8*R*,11*R*,12*R*,15*S*)-11,15-Dihydroxy-9-oxoprosta-5,13-dienoic acid; (*Z*)-7-{(1*R*,2*R*,3*R*)-3-Hydroxy-2-[(*E*)-(3*S*)-3-hydroxyoct-1-enyl]-5-oxocyclopentyl}hept-5-enoic acid.

$C_{20}H_{32}O_5$ = 352.5.

CAS — 363-24-6.

NOTE. In *Martindale* the term dinoprostone is used for the exogenous form and prostaglandin E$_2$ for the endogenous form.

Pharmacopoeias. In *Eur.* (see p.viii).

A white or almost white, crystalline powder or colourless crystals. Practically *insoluble* in water; freely soluble in alcohol; very soluble in methyl alcohol. Store below −15°.

Adverse Effects

The incidence and severity of adverse reactions to dinoprostone are dose-related and also depend to some extent on the route of administration; the intravenous route has been associated with a high incidence of adverse effects. Nausea, vomiting, diarrhoea, and abdominal pain are common. Transient cardiovascular symptoms have included flushing, shivering, headache, dizziness, and hypotension; there have been rare reports of sudden cardiovascular collapse. Hypertension has also been reported. Convulsions and EEG changes have occurred rarely. Local tissue irritation and erythema may follow intravenous administration; the erythema disappears 2 to 5 hours after infusion. Temporary pyrexia and a raised white cell count may occur but generally revert to normal after termination of the infusion. Local infection may follow intra- or extra-amniotic therapy. Excessive uterine activity may occur and there have been occasional reports of uterine rupture following the use of prostaglandins to terminate pregnancy or induce labour; fetal distress and, rarely, fetal death have occurred during the induction of labour.

Dinoprostone, although generally acting as a bronchodilator, may cause bronchoconstriction in some individuals.

Side-effects were evaluated in 626 patients[1] undergoing abortion (usually in the second trimester), using extra-amniotic or intra-amniotic dinoprost or dinoprostone, often with oxytocin. Vomiting occurred in 291, diarrhoea in 28, pyrexia in 34, transient hypotension (fall in systolic blood pressure of at least 20 mmHg) in 25, transient bronchospasm in 2 patients given extra-amniotic dinoprost, and blood loss exceeding 250 mL in 68 (38 lost more than 500 mL). There were no convulsions even though 8 patients were epileptics receiving antiepileptic therapy. Three patients sustained lacerations to the cervix. Five patients complained of breast soreness or lactation; these symptoms may have been under-reported. Overall 14 patients were re-admitted; 13 because of excessive vaginal bleeding and 1 because of pelvic infection.

A later report describes the cumulative experience in 3313 pregnancies[2] in which dinoprostone gel was used for induction of term labour or cervical ripening. Adverse effects were rare. Vomiting, fever, and diarrhoea occurred in approximately 0.2% of mothers and were difficult to distinguish from the effects of concurrent drug therapy. Detectable myometrial activity was dose related and more common after intravaginal than after intracervical administration. Myometrial activity was reported in 0.6 to 6% of patients following intravaginal application and hyperstimulation was virtually non-existent at an intracervical dose of 0.5 mg. Fetal effects were negligible in the absence of uterine hyperstimulation.

1. MacKenzie IZ, *et al.* Prostaglandin-induced abortion: assessment of operative complications and early morbidity. *Br Med J* 1974; **4:** 683–6.
2. Rayburn WF. Prostaglandin E_2 gel for cervical ripening and induction of labor: a critical analysis. *Am J Obstet Gynecol* 1989; **160:** 529–34.

A modified-release pessary formulation of dinoprostone (Propess) was withdrawn from the UK market in 1990 following several reports of problems with its use. Khouzam and Ledward[1] reported adverse effects including vaginismus, severe pain, and gastro-intestinal disturbances in 2 patients and an unduly short labour in a third. They attributed this to "dose dumping". This suggestion was refuted by Graham,[2] and it was suggested by MacKenzie and Taylor[3] that a more likely explanation was increased sensitivity to prostaglandins in some patients, particularly in multiparae and those in whom the cervix is ripe. A further problem arose from the necessity to remove the pessary to terminate its action. Vaginismus prevented removal in the case reported by Khouzam and Ledward;[1] Bex *et al.*[4] reported difficulty in retrieving pessaries in 3 patients due to adherence to the vaginal mucosa and difficulties were also experienced by Baravilala *et al.*[5] and MacKenzie and Taylor.[3] Concern was also expressed that in some instances pessaries were never recovered despite thorough searches.[4,5] A retrievable pessary (Propess-RS) was made available in 1995 to overcome some of the above problems; each pessary is supplied in a knitted polyester pouch to which is attached a drawstring to aid removal.

1. Khouzam MN, Ledward RS. Difficulties with controlled release prostaglandin E_2 pessaries. *Lancet* 1990; **336:** 119.
2. Graham NB. Controlled-release prostaglandin E_2 pessary and cervical ripening. *Lancet* 1990; **336:** 562.
3. MacKenzie IZ, Taylor AVG. Controlled-release prostaglandin E_2 pessary and cervical ripening. *Lancet* 1990; **336:** 562.
4. Bex P, *et al.* Difficulties with controlled release prostaglandin E_2 pessaries. *Lancet* 1990; **336:** 119.
5. Baravilala WR, *et al.* Controlled release prostaglandin E_2 pessaries. *Lancet* 1990; **336:** 437.

Effects on the bones. Reversible widening of cranial sutures occurred in 2 newborn infants given dinoprostone intravenously for 95 and 97 days in addition to the reversible periosteal reactions of the long bones and bone thickening previously described in infants given prostaglandins of the E series long-term.[1]

1. Hoevels-Guerich H, *et al.* Widening of cranial sutures after long-term prostaglandin E_2 therapy in two newborn infants. *J Pediatr* 1984; **105:** 72–4.

Effects on the cardiovascular system. Severe cardiovascular disorders reported with the intra-amniotic or intravaginal administration of dinoprost or dinoprostone have included cardiac arrhythmias in 3 patients,[1,2] fatal in 2 of them;[2] hypotension, tachypnoea, and tachycardia in 3 patients[3,4] with associated pyrexias in 2 patients;[3] fatal myocardial infarction in a patient who had several high-risk factors for ischaemic heart disease;[5] and severe hypertension in 1 patient.[6]

1. Burt RL, *et al.* Hypokalemia and cardiac arrhythmia associated with prostaglandin-induced abortion. *Obstet Gynecol* 1977; **50:** 45S–46S.
2. Cates W, Jordaan HVF. Sudden collapse and death of women obtaining abortions induced with prostaglandin $F_{2\alpha}$. *Am J Obstet Gynecol* 1979; **133:** 398–400.
3. Phelan JP, *et al.* Dramatic pyrexic and cardiovascular response to intravaginal prostaglandin E_2. *Am J Obstet Gynecol* 1978; **132:** 28–32.
4. Cameron IT, Baird DT. Sudden collapse after intra-amniotic prostaglandin E_2 injection. *Lancet* 1984; **ii:** 1046.
5. Patterson SP, *et al.* A maternal death associated with prostaglandin E_2. *Obstet Gynecol* 1979; **54:** 123–4.
6. Veber B, *et al.* Severe hypertension during postpartum haemorrhage after i.v. administration of prostaglandin E2. *Br J Anaesth* 1992; **68:** 623–4.

Effects on fertility. Of 105 women who wished to conceive following second-trimester abortion with prostaglandins, 104 did so.[1] Conception occurred within 24 months in 99 women and after a longer delay in 5.

1. MacKenzie IZ, Fry A. A prospective self-controlled study of fertility after second-trimester prostaglandin-induced abortion. *Am J Obstet Gynecol* 1988; **158:** 1137–40.

Effects on the fetus. A woman who failed to abort despite receiving carboprost intravaginally 7 weeks after conception gave birth at 34 weeks' gestation to an infant with hydrocephalus and abnormal digits.[1]

For reports of adverse effects on the fetus due to hyperstimulation of the uterus during labour, see under Effects on the Uterus, below.

1. Collins FS, Mahoney MJ. Hydrocephalus and abnormal digits after failed first-trimester prostaglandin abortion attempt. *J Pediatr* 1983; **102:** 620–1.

Effects on the gastro-intestinal system. Hypotension and apnoea induced by dinoprostone infusions have been suggested by some[1] as a cause of necrotising enterocolitis in infants with symptomatic congenital heart disease although others[2] do not support this view.

1. Leung MP, *et al.* Necrotizing enterocolitis in neonates with symptomatic congenital heart disease. *J Pediatr* 1988; **113:** 1044–6.
2. Miller MJS, Clark DA. Congenital heart disease and necrotizing enterocolitis. *J Pediatr* 1989; **115:** 335–6.

Effects on the neonate. Aspiration of the undissolved remnants of a dinoprostone vaginal tablet caused neonatal respiratory distress due to mechanical obstruction of the airways: there was no evidence to suggest absorption of dinoprostone from the tablet matrix.[1]

For other neonatal effects see under Effects on the Bones, above.

1. Andersson S, *et al.* Neonatal respiratory distress caused by aspiration of a vaginal tablet containing prostaglandin. *Br Med J* 1987; **295:** 25–6.

Effects on the nervous system. Convulsions and EEG changes have been occasionally reported during the administration of prostaglandins for termination of pregnancy. Lyneham[1] reported convulsions in 5 of 320 women following intra-amniotic dinoprost administration, but other authors[2-4] have not encountered problems in other large series of patients given dinoprost or dinoprostone by various routes despite the inclusion of patients with a history of epilepsy. However Brandenburg *et al.*[5] reported convulsions in 3 of 4 epileptic patients following intramuscular administration of sulprostone.

1. Lyneham RC, *et al.* Convulsions and electroencephalogram abnormalities after intra-amniotic prostaglandin $F_{2\alpha}$. *Lancet* 1973; **ii:** 1003–5.
2. MacKenzie IZ, *et al.* Convulsions and prostaglandin-induced abortion. *Lancet* 1973; **ii:** 1323.
3. Thiery M, *et al.* Prostaglandins and convulsions. *Lancet* 1974; **i:** 218.
4. Fraser IS, Gray C. Electroencephalogram changes after prostaglandin. *Lancet* 1974; **i:** 360.
5. Brandenburg H, *et al.* Convulsions in epileptic women after administration of prostaglandin E_2 derivative. *Lancet* 1990; **336:** 1138.

Effects on the uterus. Fatal amniotic fluid embolism occurred following induction of labour with dinoprostone pessaries in a 37-year-old woman.[1] Although administration of dinoprostone was not considered to be solely responsible, the high pressure gradient produced in the uterus could have been a predisposing factor. Amniotic fluid embolism was also found post mortem in a patient who died of intracerebral haemorrhage[2] following a precipitate labour induced by a dinoprostone pessary. The infant also died from intracranial haemorrhage following the spontaneous vaginal delivery. Again, hyperstimulation of the uterus could have been implicated.

Hypertonic uterine contractions also followed application of dinoprostone 5 mg as a gel.[3] The intensity of the contractions was eventually decreased with terbutaline.

Uterine hyperstimulation may also lead to fetal distress. Intrauterine fetal death occurred in 2 high-risk pregnancies[4] following insertion into the extra-amniotic space of dinoprost 10 mg in Tylose gel. Placental abruption and neonatal death following the administration of a 3-mg dinoprostone vaginal pessary was also reported in a woman with a retained IUD but an otherwise uncomplicated pregnancy.[5]

Uterine or cervical rupture has been reported following the termination of pregnancy with dinoprost given intra-amniotically;[6] dinoprostone given intra-amniotically,[7,8] intravenously,[9] or extra-amniotically;[10] and carboprost given intramuscularly.[11] Vergote *et al.*[11] noted that uterine rupture was not always suspected, but should be considered if established uterine contractions disappear or there is vaginal blood loss without concomitant progressive dilatation. Rupture has also followed the use of dinoprostone pessaries for the induction of labour;[12,13] rupture of a uterine scar occurred in 2 patients.[14] Larsen *et al.*[15] have also reported complications following the use of dinoprostone to induce labour in grand multiparae; one patient given dinoprostone by mouth developed severe postpartum haemorrhage due to uterine rupture and died and another given dinoprostone vaginally was found to have a ruptured uterus following delivery of a stillborn infant. They considered that induction of labour with dinoprostone was not safer than carefully controlled oxytocin infusion with amniotomy. They recommended restricting the vaginal dose of dinoprostone in grand multiparae to 3 mg if the cervix is unripe, to 2 mg if the cervix is ripe, and advised that administration should not be repeated for at least 24 hours.

1. Less A, *et al.* Vaginal prostaglandin E_2 and fatal amniotic fluid embolus. *JAMA* 1990; **263:** 3259–60.
2. Stronge J, *et al.* A neonatal and maternal death following the administration of intravaginal prostaglandin. *J Obstet Gynaecol* 1987; **7:** 271–2.
3. Chamberlin RO, *et al.* Uterine hyperstimulation resulting from intravaginal prostaglandin E_2: a case report. *J Reprod Med* 1987; **32:** 233–5.
4. Quinn MA, Murphy AJ. Fetal death following extra-amniotic prostaglandin gel: report of two cases. *Br J Obstet Gynaecol* 1981; **88:** 650–1.
5. Simmons K, Savage W. Neonatal death associated with induction of labour with intravaginal prostaglandin E_2: case report. *Br J Obstet Gynaecol* 1984; **91:** 598–9.
6. Karim SMM, Ratnam SS. Mid-trimester termination. *Br Med J* 1974; **4:** 161–2.
7. Fraser IS. Complications of prostaglandin-induced abortion. *Br Med J* 1974; **4:** 404.
8. Emery S, *et al.* Uterine rupture after intra-amniotic injection of prostaglandin E_2. *Br Med J* 1979; **2:** 51.
9. Smith AM. Rupture of uterus during prostaglandin-induced abortion. *Br Med J* 1975; **i:** 205.
10. Traub AI, Ritchie JWK. Rupture of the uterus during prostaglandin-induced abortion. *Br Med J* 1979; **2:** 496.
11. Vergote I, *et al.* Uterine rupture due to 15-methyl prostaglandin $F_{2\alpha}$. *Lancet* 1982; **ii:** 1402.
12. Claman P, *et al.* Uterine rupture with the use of vaginal prostaglandin E_2 for induction of labor. *Am J Obstet Gynecol* 1984; **150:** 889–90.
13. Keller F, Joyce TH. Uterine rupture associated with the use of vaginal prostaglandin E_2 suppositories. *Can Anaesth Soc J* 1984; **31:** 80–2.
14. Bromham DR, Anderson RS. Uterine scar rupture in labour induced with vaginal prostaglandin E_2. *Lancet* 1980; **ii:** 485–6.
15. Larsen JV, *et al.* Uterine hyperstimulation and rupture after induction of labour with prostaglandin E_2. *S Afr Med J* 1984; **65:** 615–16.

Overdosage. Severe adverse effects have been attributed to inappropriate systemic absorption of prostaglandins. Ross and Whitehouse[1] reported rigors, vomiting, severe abdominal pain, and an intense desire to urinate and defaecate in 3 patients given dinoprostone intra-amniotically, together with urea in 2, for mid-trimester abortion; one patient had peripheral vasoconstriction and a rapid low-volume pulse, with hypotension, and another had peripheral cyanosis. Craft and Bowen-Simpkins[2] attributed these symptoms to a relatively large dose of prostaglandin rapidly reaching the systemic circulation, possibly as a result of displacement of the needle or cannula and Karim[3] suggested that prior administration of urea would increase the rate of absorption of prostaglandins from the amniotic cavity. In a further report[4] flushing, severe headache, and nausea immediately after a test dose of dinoprost 2.5 mg was also thought to be due to incorrect positioning of the needle in the amniotic cavity with consequent injection into the systemic circulation; Karim[3] suggested that at least part of the dose had been injected into the peritoneal cavity.

Severe reactions have also been reported with prostaglandins given to abort hydatidiform moles. A 20-year-old woman given 20 mg of dinoprostone by injection into the uterine cavity developed profound hypotension, bradycardia, and rigors, followed by nausea, vomiting, suprapubic pain, an increased pulse rate, pyrexia, and generalised flushing.[5] Karim[3] pointed out that because of the absence of fetal membranes in a molar pregnancy, intra-uterine administration was similar to extra-amniotic administration and the dose used had been 100 times higher than the usual extra-amniotic dose. However, in a similar patient[6] 'extra-amniotic' instillation of dinoprostone 200 μg was followed immediately by nausea, retching, severe abdominal pain, dizziness, difficulty in breathing and the production of frothy blood-stained sputum, an imperceptible pulse, and hypotension; since there is no extra-amniotic space in a hydatidiform mole the dinoprostone had probably been injected directly into the maternal circulation.

1. Ross AH, Whitehouse WL. Adverse reactions to intra-amniotic urea and prostaglandin. *Br Med J* 1974; **1:** 642.
2. Craft I, Bowen-Simpkins P. Adverse reactions to intra-amniotic urea and prostaglandin. *Br Med J* 1974; **2:** 446.
3. Karim SMM. Adverse reactions to intra-amniotic prostaglandin. *Br Med J* 1974; **3:** 347.
4. Brown R. Adverse reactions to intra-amniotic prostaglandin. *Br Med J* 1974; **2:** 382.
5. Smith AM. Adverse reactions to intra-amniotic prostaglandin. *Br Med J* 1974; **2:** 382–3.
6. McNicol E, Gray H. Adverse reaction to extra-amniotic prostaglandin E_2. *Br J Obstet Gynaecol* 1977; **84:** 229–30.

Precautions

Dinoprostone should not be given to patients in whom oxytocic drugs are generally contra-indicated (see Oxytocin, p.1257), or where there is hypertonic uterine inertia, where prolonged contractions of the uterus are considered inappropriate, as, for example, in patients with a history of caesarean section or major uterine surgery, where major degrees of cephalopelvic disproportion may be present, where fetal malpresentation is present, where there is suspicion of fetal distress, where there is a history of difficult labour or traumatic delivery, in grand multiparae with 6 or more previous term pregnancies, or in those with a history of pelvic inflammatory disease. Since prostaglandins enhance the effects of oxytocin use of the 2 drugs together or in sequence should be carefully monitored.

Dinoprostone is contra-indicated in active cardiac, pulmonary, renal, or hepatic disease. Dinoprostone should be used with caution in patients with glaucoma or raised intra-ocular pressure, asthma or a history of asthma, epilepsy or a history of epilepsy, hepatic or renal dysfunction, or cardiovascular disease.

In the induction of labour cephalopelvic relationships should be carefully evaluated before use. During use uterine activity, fetal status, and the progress of cervical dilatation should be carefully monitored to detect adverse responses, such as hypertonus, sustained uterine contractions, or fetal distress. In patients with a history of hypertonic uterine contractility or tetanic uterine contractions, uterine activity and the state of the fetus should be continuously monitored throughout labour. Where high-tone myometrial contractions are sustained the possibility of uterine rupture should be considered.

Dinoprostone should not be administered by the myometrial route, since there is a possible association with cardiac arrest in severely ill patients. The extra-amniotic route should not be used in patients with cervicitis or vaginal infections. Vaginal preparations of dinoprostone should not be used in the induction of labour once the membranes are ruptured.

In the therapeutic termination of pregnancy, fetal damage has been observed in cases of incomplete termination and the appropriate treatment for complete evacuation of the uterus should therefore be instituted whenever termination is unsuccessful or incomplete. Dinoprostone should not be used for termination in patients with pelvic infection, unless adequate treatment has already been started.

Administration. For the hazards of unintentional systemic absorption of prostaglandins following their intra-uterine administration for the termination of pregnancy and abortion of hydatidiform moles, see Overdosage in Adverse Effects, above.

Interactions

Dinoprostone enhances the effects of oxytocin on the uterus.

Marked hypertension, vomiting, and severe dyspnoea occurred following the sequential administration of oxytocin, methylergometrine, and dinoprost within the space of 10 minutes to a woman with postpartum haemorrhage.[1]

1. Cohen S, *et al.* Severe systemic reactions following administration of different ureotonic [uterotonic] drugs. *N Y State J Med* 1983; **83:** 1060–1.

Uses and Administration

Dinoprostone is a prostaglandin of the E series (p.1411) with actions on smooth muscle; the endogenous substance is termed prostaglandin E_2 and is rapidly metabolised in the body. It induces contraction of uterine muscle at any stage of pregnancy and is reported to act predominantly as a vasodilator on blood vessels and as a bronchodilator on bronchial muscle. Dinoprostone is used in the UK principally in the induction of labour (p.1411); it may also be used for the termination of pregnancy (p.1412), missed abortion, hydatidiform mole, and fetal death *in utero*.

Dinoprostone is usually administered vaginally. It may also be given intravenously, extra-amniotically, or by mouth, but the intravenous route has been associated with a high incidence of adverse effects and is generally only used for missed abortion or hydatidiform mole; continuous administration for more than two days is not recommended.

For the **induction of labour** dinoprostone is administered to ripen (soften and dilate) the cervix before the membranes are ruptured and to induce labour at term. The cervical gel used for the former purpose contains 500 μg in 2.5 mL, whereas the vaginal gel used for induction of labour contains 1 or 2 mg per 2.5 mL; the more concentrated vaginal gel should not be administered into the cervical canal. Pessaries containing 3 mg are also available for labour induction. These are not bioequivalent to the vaginal gel and their dosage is different.

To soften and dilate the cervix before induction of labour dinoprostone 500 μg is administered as cervical gel. For induction of labour the dose as vaginal gel is 1 mg (or 2 mg in primigravida patients with unfavourable induction features) followed, if necessary, by a further 1 or 2 mg after 6 hours; a total dose of 3 mg (or 4 mg in unfavourable primigravida patients) should not be exceeded. Alternatively a vaginal pessary containing 3 mg may be used and this may be followed, if necessary, by a further 3 mg after 6 to 8 hours; a total dose of 6 mg should not be exceeded. A modified-release pessary delivering 5 mg over 12 hours can be employed instead. If this does not produce satisfactory cervical ripening within 8 to 12 hours then it should be removed and a second and final modified-release pessary administered to be retained for not more than 12 hours.

Dinoprostone may be given by mouth for the induction of labour in an initial dose of 0.5 mg, repeated hourly, and increased if necessary to 1 mg hourly until an adequate response is achieved; single doses of 1.5 mg should not be exceeded. Oral administration has, however, generally been replaced by intravaginal administration since the latter is associated with fewer gastro-intestinal side-effects.

Dinoprostone has been given intravenously for the induction of labour but is no longer recommended for routine use by most authorities. A suggested intravenous dosage regimen has been 250 nanograms of dinoprostone per minute infused as a solution containing 1.5 μg per mL for 30 minutes, the dose being subsequently maintained or increased according to the patient's response; in fetal death *in utero* higher doses may be required and an initial rate of 500 nanograms per minute has been used with increases at intervals of not less than 1 hour.

For the **termination of pregnancy** in the second trimester 1 mL of a solution containing 100 μg of dinoprostone per mL may be instilled extra-amniotically through a suitable Foley catheter, with subsequent doses of 1 or 2 mL given at intervals usually of 2 hours, according to response. Dinoprostone has also been given intravenously for the termination of pregnancy and for missed abortion or hydatidiform mole. A suggested dosage regimen is the intravenous infusion of a solution containing 5 μg per mL at a rate of 2.5 μg per minute for 30 minutes, then maintained or increased to 5 μg per minute; this rate should be maintained for at least 4 hours before making further increases.

In the USA dinoprostone pessaries are used for the termination of second trimester pregnancy, a dose of 20 mg being administered intravaginally and repeated every 3 to 5 hours according to response; a total dose of 240 mg should not be exceeded. Pessaries are also used in the USA in missed abortion, fetal death *in utero*, and benign hydatidiform mole.

Dinoprostone is used in some centres to maintain the patency of ductus arteriosus (see below).

Haemorrhagic cystitis. Dinoprostone instilled into the bladder for 4 hours and repeated for 4 days successfully improved severe cyclophosphamide-induced haemorrhagic cystitis (p.516) in a bone marrow transplant recipient.[1]

1. Mohiuddin J, *et al.* Treatment of cyclophosphamide-induced cystitis with prostaglandin E_2. *Ann Intern Med* 1984; **101:** 142.

Hepatic disorders. See under Alprostadil, p.1413, for reference to the use of prostaglandins, including dinoprostone, in the treatment of viral hepatitis.

Patent ductus arteriosus. The short-term use of prostaglandins, particularly alprostadil and dinoprostone, to maintain the patency of ductus arteriosus until surgery can be performed to correct the malformation is well-established. Treatment for a longer period, especially with oral dinoprostone, may facilitate later surgery by allowing growth of the infants and their pulmonary arteries.

Beneficial responses to long-term administration of dinoprostone have been reported by Silove *et al.*[1] in 60 of 62 infants and by Thanopoulos *et al.*[2] in 22 infants. Thanopoulos *et al.* encountered severe adverse effects in 4 of 11 infants given dinoprostone by intravenous infusion at an initial dose of 0.05 μg per kg body-weight per minute. Silove *et al.* recommended a dose regimen consisting of oral administration of dinoprostone in an initial dose of 20 to 25 μg per kg body-weight hourly, decreasing the frequency of doses after the first week. Treatment is continued for up to 4 weeks initially and a decision then made whether to proceed with surgery or to plan a longer course of treatment to encourage further growth. When gastro-intestinal absorption is expected to be poor or when oral treatment is ineffective low doses of dinoprostone may be given intravenously, beginning with the infusion of 0.003 μg per kg per minute; it is rarely necessary to increase the dose for more than a few hours and doses as high as 0.01 to 0.02 μg per kg per minute are exceptional.

1. Silove ED, *et al.* Evaluation of oral and low dose intravenous prostaglandin E_2 in management of ductus dependent congenital heart disease. *Arch Dis Child* 1985; **60:** 1025–30.
2. Thanopoulos BD, *et al.* Prostaglandin E_2 administration in infants with ductus-dependent cyanotic congenital heart disease. *Eur J Pediatr* 1987; **146:** 279–82.

Pemphigus. Erosive oral lesions in 3 patients[1] with pemphigus vulgaris (p.1075) that had previously been refractory to standard corticosteroid therapy resolved on sucking oral dinoprostone tablets 1.5 to 3 mg daily. Symptoms recurred within weeks of ceasing dinoprostone therapy but could be controlled by courses of 0.5 to 1 mg daily for 1 to 2 weeks, when required.

1. Morita H, *et al.* Clinical trial of prostaglandin E_2 on the oral lesions of pemphigus vulgaris. *Br J Dermatol* 1995; **132:** 165–6.

Peripheral vascular disease. Various prostaglandins including dinoprostone have been used in the treatment of peripheral vascular disease (p.794), particularly in severe Raynaud's syndrome, but do not constitute mainline therapy.

References.

1. Eriksson G, *et al.* Topical prostaglandin E_2 for chronic leg ulcers. *Lancet* 1986; **i:** 905.
2. Eriksson G, *et al.* Topical prostaglandin E_2 in the treatment of chronic leg ulcers—a pilot study. *Br J Dermatol* 1988; **118:** 531–6.

Postpartum haemorrhage. Dinoprostone and other prostaglandins have been used to control severe postpartum haemorrhage (p.1575) unresponsive to ergometrine and oxytocin. Beneficial response to continuous intra-uterine irrigation with dinoprostone solution 1.5 μg per mL was seen in 22 patients with postpartum haemorrhage unresponsive to other treatment.[1] Postpartum haemorrhage was controlled in another patient using a dinoprostone 3-mg vaginal suppository held against the uterine wall.[2]

1. Peyser MR, Kupfermine MJ. Management of severe postpartum hemorrhage by intrauterine irrigation with prostaglandin E_2. *Am J Obstet Gynecol* 1990; **162:** 694–6.
2. Markos AR. Prostaglandin E_2 intrauterine suppositories in the treatment of secondary postpartum hemorrhage. *J R Soc Med* 1989; **82:** 504–5.

Preparations

Proprietary Preparations (details are given in Part 3)
Aust.: Cerviprost; Prepidil; Prostin E2; ***Austral.:*** Prostin E2; ***Belg.:*** Prepidil; Prostin E2; ***Canad.:*** Prepidil; Prostin E2; ***Fr.:*** Prepidil; Prostine E_2; ***Ger.:*** Cerviprost; Minprostin E_2; Prepidil; ***Irl.:*** Prepidil; Prostin E2; ***Ital.:*** Prepidil; Prostin E2; ***Jpn:*** Prostarmon.E†; ***Neth.:*** Cerviprost†; Prepidil; Prostin E2; ***Norw.:*** Cerviprost†; Minprostin; ***S.Afr.:*** Prandin E_2; Prepidil; Prostin E2; ***Spain:*** Gravidex; Prepidil; ***Swed.:*** Cerviprost†; Minprostin; Propess; ***Switz.:*** Cerviprost; Prepidil; Prostin E2; ***UK:*** Prepidil; Propess; Prostin E2; ***USA:*** Cervidil; Prepidil; Prostin E2.

Enisoprost (16621-z)

Enisoprost *(USAN, rINN)*.

SC-34301. (±)-Methyl (*Z*)-7-{(1*R*,2*R*,3*R*)-3-hydroxy-2-[(*E*)-(4*RS*)-4-hydroxy-4-methyl-1-octenyl]-5-oxocyclopentyl}-4-heptenoate.

$C_{22}H_{36}O_5$ = 380.5.
CAS — 81026-63-3.

Enisoprost is a synthetic analogue of alprostadil (prostaglandin E_1) that has been investigated as an adjunct to cyclosporin therapy in organ transplant recipients to reduce acute transplant rejection and to diminish the nephrotoxic effects of cyclosporin; however, results have generally been disappointing.

References.

1. Adams MB and The Enisoprost Renal Transplant Study Group. Enisoprost in renal transplantation. *Transplantation* 1992; **53:** 338–45.
2. Pollak R, *et al.* A trial of the prostaglandin El analogue, enisoprost, to reverse chronic cyclosporine-associated renal dysfunction. *Am J Kidney Dis* 1992; **20:** 336–41.
3. Ismail T, *et al.* Enisoprost in liver transplantation. *Transplantation* 1995; **59:** 1298–1301.

Enprostil (16628-f)

Enprostil *(BAN, USAN, rINN)*.

RS-84135. Methyl (*E*)-(11*R*,15*R*)-11,15-dihydroxy-9-oxo-16-phenoxy-17,18,19,20-tetranorprosta-4,5,13-trienoate; Methyl 7-{(*E*)-(3*R**)-3-hydroxy-2-[(1*R**,2*R**,3*R**)-3-hydroxy-4-phenoxybut-1-enyl]-5-oxocyclopentyl}hepta-4,5-dienoate.

$C_{23}H_{28}O_6$ = 400.5.
CAS — 73121-56-9.

Enprostil, a synthetic analogue of dinoprostone (prostaglandin E_2), inhibits gastric acid secretion. It has been given by mouth in the treatment of peptic ulcer disease.

References.

1. Goa KL, Monk JP. Enprostil: a preliminary review of its pharmacodynamic and pharmacokinetic properties, and therapeutic efficacy in the treatment of peptic ulcer disease. *Drugs* 1987; **34:** 539–59.

Epoprostenol (8084-g)

Epoprostenol *(USAN, rINN)*.

PGI_2; PGX; Prostacyclin; Prostaglandin I_2; Prostaglandin X; U-53217. (5*Z*,13*E*)-(8*R*,9*S*,11*R*,12*R*,15*S*)-6,9-Epoxy-11,15-dihydroxyprosta-5,13-dienoic acid; (*Z*)-5-{(3a*R*,4*R*,5*R*,6a*S*)-5-Hydroxy-4-[(*E*)-(3*S*)-3-hydroxyoct-1-enyl]perhydrocyclopenta[*b*]furan-2-ylidene}valeric acid.

$C_{20}H_{32}O_5$ = 352.5.
CAS — 35121-78-9.

NOTE. In *Martindale* the term epoprostenol is used for the exogenous form and prostacyclin for the endogenous form.

Epoprostenol Sodium (8085-q)

Epoprostenol Sodium *(BAN, USAN, rINNM)*.

U-53217A.

$C_{20}H_{31}NaO_5$ = 374.4.
CAS — 61849-14-7.

Stability in solution. Epoprostenol is unstable at physiological pH and solutions for infusion are prepared in an alkaline glycine buffer at pH 10.5. The half-life in aqueous solution of pH 7.4 has been reported to be less than 3 minutes at 37°,[1] but increased stability has been reported in plasma, albumin, or whole blood.[1,2]

1. El Tahir KEH, *et al.* Stability of prostacyclin in human plasma. *Clin Sci* 1980; **59:** 28P–29P.
2. Mikhailidis DP, *et al.* Infusion of prostacyclin (epoprostenol). *Lancet* 1982; **ii:** 767.

Adverse Effects and Precautions

The incidence of adverse reactions to epoprostenol is dose-related. Side-effects during intravenous infusion commonly include hypotension, increased heart rate, flushing, and headache. Dosage should be reduced or the epoprostenol infusion stopped if excessive hypotension occurs. Bradycardia together with pallor, sweating, nausea, and abdominal discomfort may occur. Erythema over the intravenous infusion site has been noted. Other side-effects reported have included nausea and vomiting, diarrhoea, jaw pain or nonspecific musculoskeletal pain, anxiety, nervousness, or tremor, flu-like symptoms, hyperglycaemia, drowsiness, and chest pain.

A study in 24 healthy subjects investigated the incidence of adverse effects with intravenous infusions of epoprostenol of up to 10 ng per kg body-weight per minute for up to 100 minutes.[1] Subjects varied in their susceptibility to epoprostenol but the same sequence of events was usually present. A change in pre-ejection period and facial flushing was often apparent at an infusion rate of 2 to 2.5 ng per kg per minute. A rise in heart rate and change in other cardiovascular variables was present when the infusion rate had increased to 4 to 5 ng per kg per minute; headache, generally the dose-limiting factor, was usually present at this dose and increased as the dose was raised, as did the other effects. Erythema over the vein and 'vagal reflex' only appeared after at least 1 hour of infusion; 'vagal reflex' took only a few seconds to develop.

Early studies showing that high doses were well tolerated had been conducted using a form of epoprostenol probably only half as potent as the commercially available product. It was proposed that 4 ng per kg per minute should in general be the maximum infusion rate for prolonged infusions, although higher rates could be tolerated in anaesthetised patients. Careful attention to infusion technique is necessary and monitoring of the heart rate is advisable in view of the suddenness with which the 'vagal reflex' can occur. Most of the adverse effects reported here have responded to a reduction in dosage.

1. Pickles H, O'Grady J. Side effects occurring during administration of epoprostenol (prostacyclin, PGI_2), in man. *Br J Clin Pharmacol* 1982; **14:** 177–85.

Effects on the blood. Reports of rebound platelet activation during continuous epoprostenol infusion.[1,2]

1. Yardumian DA, Machin SJ. Altered platelet function in patients on continuous infusion of epoprostenol. *Lancet* 1984; **i:** 1357.
2. Sinzinger H, *et al.* Rebound platelet activation during continuous epoprostenol infusion. *Lancet* 1984; **ii:** 759.

Effects on the cardiovascular system. Evidence that epoprostenol and its analogue iloprost can induce myocardial ischaemia in patients with coronary artery disease.[1]

1. Bugiardini R, *et al.* Myocardial ischemia induced by prostacyclin and iloprost. *Clin Pharmacol Ther* 1985; **38:** 101–8.

Effects on mental state. Symptoms of depression were associated with intravenous epoprostenol therapy in 4 patients.[1]

1. Ansell D, *et al.* Depression and prostacyclin infusion. *Lancet* 1986; **ii:** 509.

Interactions

Since epoprostenol is a potent vasodilator and inhibitor of platelet aggregation, care should be taken in patients receiving other vasodilators or anticoagulants concomitantly. The hypotensive effects of epoprostenol may be exacerbated by using acetate in dialysis fluids.

Pharmacokinetics

Endogenous prostacyclin is a product of arachidonic acid metabolism with a very short half-life. Following intravenous infusion epoprostenol is hydrolysed rapidly to the more stable but much less active 6-keto-prostaglandin $F_{1\alpha}$ (6-oxo-prostaglandin $F_{1\alpha}$). Unlike many other prostaglandins, epoprostenol is not inactivated in the pulmonary circulation.

Uses and Administration

Epoprostenol is a prostaglandin (p.1411) which causes vasodilatation and prevents platelet aggregation. The endogenous substance is termed prostacyclin. It is used mainly in extracorporeal procedures and in pulmonary hypertension.

Epoprostenol is given as the sodium salt and doses are expressed in terms of the base. It is unstable in solution at physiological pH and also has a very short duration of action because of its rapid hydrolysis *in vivo*. It must therefore be administered by continuous infusion. Great care must be taken in preparing a suitably diluted solution for infusion and only diluent as supplied by the manufacturer, should be used to reconstitute epoprostenol.

Epoprostenol is used to **prevent platelet aggregation** when blood is brought into contact with nonbiological surfaces such as in extracorporeal circulation, especially in renal dialysis patients. It is administered by continuous intravenous infusion or into the blood supplying the extracorporeal circulation. The usual dose for renal dialysis is 5 nanograms per kg body-weight per minute intravenously before dialysis, then 5 nanograms per kg per minute into the arterial inlet of the dialyser during dialysis.

In the long-term treatment of primary **pulmonary hypertension** a dose-ranging procedure is performed first in order to establish the maximum infusion rate that can be tolerated. Epoprostenol should then be administered by continuous infusion through a central venous catheter the initial rate being 4 nanograms per kg body-weight per minute *less than* the maximum-tolerated infusion rate; if the maximum-tolerated infusion rate is less than 5 nanograms per kg per minute, then the initial rate should be one-half of this maximum rate. Dosage is then adjusted according to the patient's response. Increases or decreases of 1 to 2 nanograms per kg per minute may be made at intervals of at least 15 minutes.

The discovery, properties, and clinical applications of prostacyclin have been reviewed by Vane.[1] Prostaglandin endoperoxides, isolated in the early 1970s by Samuelsson and others were found to be transformed by thromboxane synthetase in platelets to thromboxane A_2, which caused platelet aggregation and vascular contraction. In contrast, prostaglandin endoperoxides were transformed by blood vessel microsomes to prostacyclin, which had potent anti-aggregatory properties and relaxed vascular strips. It was suggested that a balance between the amounts of thromboxane A_2 formed by platelets and prostacyclin formed by blood vessel walls might be critical for thrombus formation and this concept is now well established. Prostacyclin is the main product of arachidonic acid in vascular tissues, endothelial cells from vessel walls being the most active producers. It is a strong hypotensive agent through vasodilatation of vascular beds, including the pulmonary and cerebral circulations, and is also a potent endogenous inhibitor of platelet aggregation. Inhibition of aggregation is achieved by stimulation of adenylate cyclase, leading to an increase in cyclic adenosine monophosphate (cAMP) levels in the platelets. By inhibiting several steps in the activation of the arachidonic acid metabolic cascade, prostacyclin exerts an overall control of platelet aggregability. Prostacyclin also increases cAMP levels in cells other than platelets and thus the prostacyclin/thromboxane A_2 system may have wider biological significance in cell regulation.

Discussing the pharmacological interactions between prostacyclin and thromboxanes Whittle and Moncada[2] expressed the opinion that endogenous prostacyclin and thromboxane A_2 now appear to be of more physiological and pathological importance than the more classical prostanoids prostaglandin E_2 and prostaglandin $F_{2\alpha}$. They have directly opposing pharmacological actions in many systems, such as on platelet function, vascular smooth muscle, bronchopulmonary function, and gastro-intestinal integrity. Thus prostanoid-mediated control of cellular and tissue function may reflect an interactive modulation between prostacyclin and thromboxane A_2 with imbalance resulting in dysfunction, for example in platelet and vascular disorders. Thromboxane A_2 has both bronchoconstrictor and pulmonary irritant actions and has brought about marked changes in respiratory function in experimental models; prostacyclin may oppose these effects on both the pulmonary vasculature and bronchial smooth muscle. Thromboxane A_2 has induced marked renal vasoconstriction *in vitro* whereas renal vasodilatation and stimulation of the release of renin has followed the administration of epoprostenol [exogenous prostacyclin] in *animals*. In contrast to the pro-ulcerogenic actions of thromboxane A_2, epoprostenol and its analogues, like other prostaglandins, have potent gastro-intestinal anti-ulcer properties which can be disassociated from their gastric antisecretory properties. The term 'cytoprotection' has been used to describe this ability of exogenous prostaglandins to prevent gastro-intestinal damage; endogenous prostaglandins might have a similar protective role. Epoprostenol also has a cytoprotective effect against experimental damage in the gastric mucosa, myocardium, and liver whereas thromboxane A_2 has a cytolytic effect.

1. Vane JR. Adventures and excursions in bioassay—the stepping stones to prostacyclin. *Postgrad Med J* 1983; **59:** 743–58.
2. Whittle BJR, Moncada S. Pharmacological interactions between prostacyclin and thromboxanes. *Br Med Bull* 1983; **39:** 232–8.

Acute respiratory distress syndrome. Encouraging results[1,2] have been seen with inhaled epoprostenol in the treatment of acute respiratory distress syndrome (p.1017).

1. Walmrath D, *et al.* Aerosolised prostacyclin in adult respiratory distress syndrome. *Lancet* 1993; **342:** 961–2.
2. Walmrath D, *et al.* Direct comparison of inhaled nitric oxide and aerosolized prostacyclin in acute respiratory distress syndrome. *Am J Respir Crit Care Med* 1996; **153:** 991–6.

Extracorporeal circulation. Epoprostenol has been used to inhibit the platelet aggregation which results from blood in extracorporeal circulations, such as those used in haemodialysis, cardiopulmonary bypass, and haemoperfusion, coming into contact with artificial surfaces. This platelet aggregation can lead to thrombocytopenia and bleeding and the aggregates may block filters in the circuits; embolisation of aggregates may cause cerebral dysfunction after cardiopulmonary bypass.

Epoprostenol has been used with heparin[1] or as the sole antithrombotic[2-4] in patients with renal failure undergoing haemodialysis; it is considered to have a role in patients at risk of bleeding with routine heparin anticoagulation. Zusman *et al.*[2] found it necessary to reduce the infusion rate of epoprostenol from 4 nanograms per kg per minute to as little as 0.25 nanograms per kg per minute in some patients because of a fall in blood pressure, but Turney *et al.*[3,5] did not encounter clinically significant hypotension. Clotting in the extracorporeal circuit has been reported in patients given epoprostenol as sole antithrombotic treatment.[6,7] Although their experience indicates that many patients will dialyse successfully with epoprostenol alone, Rylance *et al.*[7] suggest that an infusion of epoprostenol 5 nanograms per kg per minute, together with a small bolus dose of heparin (500 to 1000 units) at the start of dialysis and further bolus doses to maintain a small prolongation of activated whole-blood clotting-time, will permit safe haemodialysis, especially in the patient who is bleeding, by protecting platelets and preventing fibrin generation.

1. Turney JH, *et al.* Platelet protection and heparin sparing with prostacyclin during regular dialysis therapy. *Lancet* 1980; **ii:** 219–22.
2. Zusman RM, *et al.* Hemodialysis using prostacyclin instead of heparin as the sole antithrombotic agent. *N Engl J Med* 1981; **304:** 934–9.
3. Turney JH, *et al.* Prostacyclin in extracorporeal circulations. *Lancet* 1981; **i:** 1101.
4. Swartz RD, *et al.* Epoprostenol (PGI_2, prostacyclin) during high-risk hemodialysis: preventing further bleeding complications. *J Clin Pharmacol* 1988; **28:** 818–25.
5. Turney JH, Weston MJ. Dialysis without anticoagulants. *Lancet* 1981; **ii:** 693.
6. Knudsen F, *et al.* Epoprostenol as sole antithrombotic treatment during haemodialysis. *Lancet* 1984; **ii:** 235–6.
7. Rylance PB, *et al.* Epoprostenol during haemodialysis. *Lancet* 1984; **ii:** 744–5.

Heart failure. Epoprostenol has been investigated for the treatment of heart failure (p.785) but development was abandoned due to an increase in mortality associated with long-term use of the drug.[1]

1. Phillips BB, Gandhi AJ. Epoprostenol in the treatment of congestive heart failure. *Am J Health-Syst Pharm* 1997; **54:** 2613–15.

Peripheral vascular disease. Various prostaglandins including epoprostenol have been used for their vasodilating effect in the treatment of peripheral vascular disease (p.794), particularly in severe Raynaud's syndrome, but do not constitute mainline therapy.

References.

1. Szczeklik A, *et al.* Successful therapy of advanced arteriosclerosis obliterans with prostacyclin. *Lancet* 1979; **i:** 1111–14.
2. Dowd PM, *et al.* Treatment of Raynaud's phenomenon by intravenous infusion of prostacyclin (PGI_2). *Br J Dermatol* 1982; **160:** 81–9.
3. Belch JJF, *et al.* Intermittent epoprostenol (prostacyclin) infusion in patients with Raynaud's syndrome: a double-blind controlled trial. *Lancet* 1983; **i:** 313–15.
4. Belch JJF, *et al.* Epoprostenol (prostacyclin) and severe arterial disease: a double-blind trial. *Lancet* 1983; **i:** 315–17.
5. Burns EC, *et al.* Raynaud's disease. *Arch Dis Child* 1985; **60:** 537–41.
6. De San Lazaro C, *et al.* Prostacyclin in severe peripheral vascular disease. *Arch Dis Child* 1985; **60:** 370–84.
7. Denning DW, *et al.* Peripheral symmetrical gangrene successfully treated with epoprostenol and tissue plasminogen activator. *Lancet* 1986; **ii:** 1401–2.
8. Willis AL, *et al.* Effects of prostacyclin and orally active stable mimetic agent RS-93427-007 on basic mechanisms of atherogenesis. *Lancet* 1986; **ii:** 682–3.
9. Leaker B, *et al.* Treatment of acute renal failure, symmetrical peripheral gangrene, and septicaemia with plasma exchange and epoprostenol. *Lancet* 1987; **i:** 156.
10. Negus D, *et al.* Intra-arterial prostacyclin compared to Praxilene in the management of severe lower limb ischaemia: a double-blind trial. *J Cardiovasc Surg* 1987; **28:** 196–9.

Pulmonary hypertension. Epoprostenol was originally introduced into the management of primary pulmonary hypertension (p.796) to sustain patients long enough for them to have heart-lung transplantation. Recently, encouraging results (sustained clinical improvement and probable improved survival) have been reported in some patients given long-term[1-4,8] intravenous therapy by portable infusion pumps. Inhaled epoprostenol, a method of administration that may overcome some of the adverse effects associated with the parenteral route, has been used with some success in adults[5,6] with primary or secondary pulmonary hypertension and in neonates[7] with persistent pulmonary hypertension of the newborn.

1. Barst RJ, *et al.* Survival in primary pulmonary hypertension with long-term continuous intravenous prostacyclin. *Ann Intern Med* 1994; **121:** 409–15. Correction. *ibid.* 1995; **122:** 238.
2. Barst RJ, *et al.* A comparison of continuous intravenous epoprostenol (prostacyclin) with conventional therapy for primary pulmonary hypertension. *N Engl J Med* 1996; **334:** 296–301.
3. Shapiro SM, *et al.* Primary pulmonary hypertension: improved long-term effects and survival with continuous intravenous epoprostenol infusion. *J Am Coll Cardiol* 1997; **30:** 343–9.
4. McLaughlin VV, *et al.* Reduction in pulmonary vascular resistance with long-term epoprostenol (prostacyclin) therapy in primary pulmonary hypertension. *N Engl J Med* 1998; **338:** 273–7.
5. Olschewski H, *et al.* Aerosolized prostacyclin and iloprost in severe pulmonary hypertension. *Ann Intern Med* 1996; **124:** 820–4.
6. Mikhail G, *et al.* An evaluation of nebulized prostacyclin in patients with primary and secondary pulmonary hypertension. *Eur Heart J* 1997; **18:** 1499–1504.
7. Bindl L, *et al.* Aerosolised prostacyclin for pulmonary hypertension in neonates. *Arch Dis Child* 1994; **71:** F214–F216.
8. Higenbottam T, *et al.* Long term intravenous prostaglandin (epoprostenol or iloprost) for treatment of severe pulmonary hypertension. *Heart* 1998; **80:** 151–5.

Stroke. The role of prostaglandins in ischaemic brain damage is controversial[1] and results with epoprostenol in patients with ischaemic stroke (p.799) have been inconclusive. There was no evidence of improved mortality or morbidity in patients with acute cerebral infarction given epoprostenol 5 nanograms per kg body-weight per minute by intravenous infusion, when compared with placebo,[2] and although some benefit was seen in a further study in patients with completed ischaemic stroke[3] the improvement was not sustained. Also a randomised controlled study in 80 patients with ischaemic stroke showed no benefit.[4]

1. Dearden NM. Ischaemic brain. *Lancet* 1985; **ii:** 255–9.
2. Martin JF, *et al.* Prostacyclin in cerebral infarction. *N Engl J Med* 1985; **312:** 1642.
3. Huczynski J, *et al.* Double-blind controlled trial of the therapeutic effects of prostacyclin in patients with completed ischaemic stroke. *Stroke* 1985; **16:** 810–14.
4. Yatsu FM, *et al.* Prostacyclin infusion in acute ischaemic strokes. In: Rose FC, ed. *Stroke: epidemiological, therapeutic and socio-economic aspects*. London: Royal Society of Medicine, 1986: 73–9.

Thrombotic microangiopathies. Platelet aggregation has a major role in the pathogenesis of thrombotic thrombocytopenic purpura and the related disorder, haemolytic-uraemic syndrome (p.726). Prostacyclin deficiency has been demonstrated in both conditions, but results with epoprostenol have been variable. Intravenous infusion of epoprostenol was ineffective in 2 patients with thrombotic thrombocytopenic purpura refractory to standard therapy,[1,2] but was associated with complete remission in 2 further patients.[3,4] The patient treated successfully by Payton *et al.*[4] responded dramatically to the intravenous infusion of epoprostenol gradually increased to 8 nanograms per kg body-weight per minute, continued for 7 days, and then given for a further 12 days at a dose of 4 nanograms per kg per minute for 8 hours a day; they suggested that epoprostenol should be started early, used in the maximum tolerable dose, and continued for as long as circulating platelet aggregates can be detected. A further patient with intractable thrombotic thrombocytopenic purpura responded to treatment with epoprostenol in association with nafazatrom, a stimulant of prostacyclin synthesis.[5]

Prolonged epoprostenol infusion may have contributed to the recovery of a patient with postpartum haemolytic-uraemic syndrome and evidence of prostacyclin deficiency[6] and 3 children with haemolytic-uraemic syndrome also responded to treatment with epoprostenol.[7]

1. Budd GT, *et al.* Prostacyclin therapy of thrombotic thrombocytopenic purpura. *Lancet* 1980; **ii:** 915.
2. Johnson JE, *et al.* Ineffective epoprostenol therapy for thrombotic thrombocytopenic purpura. *JAMA* 1983; **250:** 3089–91.
3. Fitzgerald GA, *et al.* Intravenous prostacyclin in thrombotic thrombocytopenic purpura. *Ann Intern Med* 1981; **95:** 319–22.
4. Payton CD, *et al.* Successful treatment of thrombotic thrombocytopenic purpura by epoprostenol infusion. *Lancet* 1985; **i:** 927–8.
5. Durrant STS, *et al.* Nafazatrom in treatment of thrombotic thrombocytopenic purpura. *Lancet* 1985; **ii:** 842.
6. Webster J, *et al.* Prostacyclin deficiency in haemolytic-uraemic syndrome. *Br Med J* 1980; **281:** 271.
7. Beattie TJ, *et al.* Prostacyclin infusion in haemolytic-uraemic syndrome of children. *Br Med J* 1981; **283:** 470.

Preparations

Proprietary Preparations (details are given in Part 3)
Aust.: Flolan; ***Irl.:*** Flolan; ***Ital.:*** Flolan; ***Neth.:*** Flolan; ***Spain:*** Flolan; ***UK:*** Flolan.

Etiproston Trometamol (10706-a)

Etiproston Trometamol *(rINNM)*.

Etiproston Tromethamine. Trometamol salt of (*Z*)-7-[(1*R*,2*R*,3*R*,5*S*)-3,5-dihydroxy-2-[(*E*)-2-[2-(phenoxymethyl)-1,3-dioxolan-2-yl]vinyl] cyclopentyl]-5-heptenoic acid.

$C_{24}H_{32}O_7,C_4H_{11}NO_3$ = 553.6.

CAS — 59619-81-7 (etiproston).

Etiproston trometamol is a synthetic analogue of dinoprost (prostaglandin $F_{2\alpha}$). It is used as a luteolytic in veterinary medicine.

Gemeprost (8088-w)

Gemeprost *(BAN, USAN, rINN)*.

16,16-Dimethyl-*trans*-Δ^2-prostaglandin E_1 methyl ester; ONO-802; SC-37681. Methyl (2*E*,13*E*)-(8*R*,11*R*,12*R*,15*R*)-11,15-dihydroxy-16,16-dimethyl-9-oxoprosta-2,13-dienoate; Methyl (*E*)-7-{(1*R*,2*R*,3*R*)-3-hydroxy-2-[(*E*)-(3*R*)-3-hydroxy-4,4-dimethyloct-1-enyl]-5-oxocyclopentyl}hept-2-enoate.

$C_{23}H_{38}O_5$ = 394.5.

CAS — 64318-79-2.

Adverse Effects and Precautions

Gemeprost is given vaginally as pessaries and systemic adverse effects such as nausea, vomiting, and diarrhoea are relatively mild. Other reported side-effects have included headache, muscle weakness, dizziness, flushing, chills, backache, dyspnoea, chest pain, palpitations, and mild pyrexia. Vaginal bleeding and mild uterine pain may occur.

Uterine rupture has been reported rarely, most commonly in multiparous women and in those with a history of uterine surgery.

The effects of gemeprost on the fetus are not known. Once a prostaglandin has been given to terminate pregnancy it is essential that termination take place; if the prostaglandin is unsuccessful other measures should be used.

Gemeprost should be used with caution in patients with obstructive airways disease, cardiovascular disease, raised intra-ocular pressure, cervicitis, or vaginitis.

The incidence of vomiting (19 or 35%) and diarrhoea (12 or 19%) in 2 studies of patients treated with gemeprost pessaries was similar to that seen with other prostaglandins, but gemeprost was reported to cause less uterine pain.[1,2]

1. Cameron IT, Baird DT. The use of 16,16-dimethyl-trans-Δ^2 prostaglandin E_1 methyl ester (gemeprost) vaginal pessaries for the termination of pregnancy in the early second trimester: a comparison with extra-amniotic prostaglandin E_2. *Br J Obstet Gynaecol* 1984; **91:** 1136–40.
2. Andersen LF, *et al.* Termination of second trimester pregnancy with gemeprost vaginal pessaries and intra-amniotic $PGF_{2\alpha}$: a comparative study. *Eur J Obstet Gynecol Reprod Biol* 1989; **31:** 1–7.

Effects on the cardiovascular system. Periods of ventricular standstill of up to 6 seconds were observed in a patient during treatment with gemeprost vaginal pessaries.[1] The patient required temporary cardiac pacing, but no persistent cardiac rhythm disturbances were detected on follow-up.

1. Kalra PA, *et al.* Cardiac standstill induced by prostaglandin pessaries. *Lancet* 1989; **i:** 1460–1.

Uses and Administration

Gemeprost is a synthetic analogue of alprostadil (prostaglandin E_1). It is used to soften and dilate the cervix and as a uterine stimulant in the termination of pregnancy (p.1412). In the first trimester, a pessary containing gemeprost 1 mg is inserted into the vagina 3 hours before surgery to ripen the cervix. Gemeprost may also be used for termination of pregnancy in the second trimester when a 1-mg pessary is inserted every 3 hours to a maximum of 5 pessaries. Should this course be ineffective one further course may be given after an interval of 24 hours. In the case of intra-uterine fetal death only one course of five pessaries should be given. Vaginal gemeprost is also used following the administration of oral mifepristone (p.1451) in the termination of pregnancy.

Preparations

Proprietary Preparations (details are given in Part 3)
Austral.: Cervagem; ***Fr.:*** Cervageme; ***Ger.:*** Cergem; ***Ital.:*** Cervidil; ***Jpn:*** Preglandin; ***Neth.:*** Cervagem†; ***Norw.:*** Cervagem; ***Swed.:*** Cervagem; ***UK:*** Cervagem†.

Iloprost (16847-w)

Iloprost *(BAN, rINN)*.

Ciloprost; ZK-36374. *(E)*-(3a*S*,4*R*,5*R*,6a*S*)-Hexahydro-5-hydroxy-4-[(*E*)-(3*S*,4*RS*)-3-hydroxy-4-methyl-1-octen-6-ynyl]-$\Delta^{2(1H),\delta}$-pentalenevaleric acid.

$C_{22}H_{32}O_4$ = 360.5.

CAS — 73873-87-7.

Iloprost Trometamol (17902-s)

Iloprost Trometamol *(BANM, rINNM)*.

Ciloprost Tromethamine; Iloprost Tromethamine.

Adverse Effects and Precautions

As for Epoprostenol, p.1417.

Effects on the cardiovascular system. Hypotension was observed[1] in 2 of 6 patients during administration of iloprost. Both patients recovered rapidly when iloprost was discontinued, although one required intravenous atropine to correct sinus bradycardia.

Evidence of myocardial ischaemia was reported in 4 of 33 patients with coronary artery disease during iloprost infusion.[2] The same authors[3] noted a similar effect in 4 of 28 patients with stable angina in a subsequent study. According to one study,[4] there might be an increased risk of thromboembolism in some patients given iloprost, due to platelet activation and enhanced coagulation.

1. Upward JW, *et al.* Hypotension in response to iloprost, a prostacyclin analogue. *Br J Clin Pharmacol* 1986; **21:** 241–3.
2. Bugiardini R, *et al.* Myocardial ischemia induced by prostacyclin and iloprost. *Clin Pharmacol Ther* 1985; **38:** 101–8.
3. Bugiardini R, *et al.* Effects of iloprost, a stable prostacyclin analog, on exercise capacity and platelet aggregation in stable angina pectoris. *Am J Cardiol* 1986; **58:** 453–9.
4. Kovacs IB, *et al.* Infusion of a stable prostacyclin analogue, iloprost, to patients with peripheral vascular disease: lack of antiplatelet effect but risk of thromboembolism. *Am J Med* 1991; **90:** 41–6.

Uses and Administration

Iloprost, a vasodilator and platelet aggregation inhibitor, is a stable analogue of the prostaglandin epoprostenol (prostacyclin). It is given by intravenous infusion as the trometamol salt in the treatment of peripheral vascular disease. The usual dose is the equivalent of 0.5 to 2 nanograms of iloprost per kg body-weight per minute for 6 hours each day.

Administration of iloprost by mouth is under investigation.

Reviews.

1. Grant SM, Goa KL. Iloprost: a review of its pharmacodynamic and pharmacokinetic properties, and therapeutic potential in peripheral vascular disease, myocardial ischaemia and extracorporeal circulation procedures. *Drugs* 1992; **43:** 889–924.

Peripheral vascular disease. Various prostaglandins including iloprost have been used in the treatment of peripheral vascular disease (p.794), particularly in severe Raynaud's syndrome, but do not constitute mainline therapy.

References.

1. Kaukinen S, *et al.* Hemodynamic effects of iloprost, a prostacyclin analog. *Clin Pharmacol Ther* 1984; **36:** 464–9.
2. Chiesa R, *et al.* Use of stable prostacyclin analogue ZK 36374 to treat severe lower limb ischaemia. *Lancet* 1985; **ii:** 95–6.
3. Waller PC, *et al.* Placebo controlled trial of iloprost in patients with stable intermittent claudication. *Br J Clin Pharmacol* 1986; **21:** 562P–563P.
4. Rademaker M, *et al.* Prolonged increase in digital blood flow following iloprost infusion in patients with systemic sclerosis. *Postgrad Med J* 1987; **63:** 617–20.
5. McHugh NJ, *et al.* Infusion of iloprost, a prostacyclin analogue, for treatment of Raynaud's phenomenon in systemic sclerosis. *Ann Rheum Dis* 1988; **47:** 43–7.
6. Yardumian DA, *et al.* Successful treatment of Raynaud's syndrome with iloprost, a chemically stable prostacyclin analogue. *Br J Rheumatol* 1988; **27:** 220–6.
7. Rademaker M, *et al.* Comparison of intravenous infusions of iloprost and oral nifedipine in treatment of Raynaud's phenomenon in patients with systemic sclerosis: a double blind randomised study. *Br Med J* 1989; **298:** 561–4.
8. Stafford PJ, *et al.* Multiple microemboli after disintegration of clot during thrombolysis for acute myocardial infarction. *Br Med J* 1989; **299:** 1310–12.
9. Visona A, *et al.* Clinical and hemodynamic effects of iloprost in patients with peripheral vascular disease. *Curr Ther Res* 1989; **45:** 794–803.
10. Fiessinger JN, Schäfer M. Trial of iloprost versus aspirin treatment for critical limb ischaemia of thromboangiitis obliterans. *Lancet* 1990; **335:** 555–7.
11. Zahavi J, *et al.* Ischaemic necrotic toes associated with antiphospholipid syndrome and treated with iloprost. *Lancet* 1993; **342:** 862.
12. Tait IS, *et al.* Management of intra-arterial injection injury with iloprost. *Lancet* 1994; **343:** 419.
13. Belch JJF, *et al.* Oral iloprost as a treatment for Raynaud's syndrome: a double blind multicentre placebo controlled study. *Ann Rheum Dis* 1995; **54:** 197–200.
14. Motz E, *et al.* Intra-arterial iloprost for limb ischaemia. *Lancet* 1995; **346:** 1295.

Pulmonary hypertension. Epoprostenol is an accepted part of the management of pulmonary hypertension (p.796) and iloprost, a stable analogue, has been studied. Both aerosolised[1] administration and continuous intravenous infusion[2] have been employed with beneficial results.

1. Olschewski H, *et al.* Aerosolized prostacyclin and iloprost in severe pulmonary hypertension. *Ann Intern Med* 1996; **124:** 820–4.
2. Higenbottam TW, *et al.* Treatment of pulmonary hypertension with the continuous infusion of a prostacyclin analogue, iloprost. *Heart* 1998; **79:** 175–9.

Preparations

Proprietary Preparations (details are given in Part 3)
Aust.: Ilomedin; ***Fr.:*** Ilomedine; ***Ger.:*** Ilomedin; ***Ital.:*** Endoprost; Ilomedin; ***Neth.:*** Ilomedine; ***Norw.:*** Ilomedin; ***Swed.:*** Ilomedin; ***Switz.:*** Ilomedin.

Latanoprost (16780-q)

Latanoprost *(BAN, USAN, rINN)*.

PhXA-41; XA-41. Isopropyl *(Z)*-7-{(1*R*,2*R*,3*R*,5*S*)-3,5-dihydroxy-2-[(3*R*)-3-hydroxy-5-phenylpentyl]cyclopentyl}-5-heptenoate.

$C_{26}H_{40}O_5$ = 432.6.

CAS — 130209-82-4.

Adverse Effects and Precautions

Latanoprost eye drops may produce a gradual increase in the amount of brown pigment in the iris, due to increased melanin content of melanocytes. This change in eye colour is most evident in patients with mixed colour irises. Darkening, thickening, and lengthening of eye lashes may occur and darkening of the palpebral skin has been reported rarely. Iritis and/or uveitis has also been reported rarely.

The use of latanoprost eye drops has been associated with systemic adverse reactions. In a case report[1] of 2 patients with latanoprost-associated hypertension the authors mentioned that other events including peripheral and facial oedema, dyspnoea, exacerbation of asthma, tachycardia, and chest pain or angina pectoris had been reported.

1. Peak AS, Sutton BM. Systemic adverse effects associated with topically applied latanoprost. *Ann Pharmacother* 1998; **32:** 504–5.

Uses and Administration

Latanoprost is a synthetic analogue of dinoprost (prostaglandin $F_{2\alpha}$) that is used topically to reduce intra-ocular pressure in patients with open-angle glaucoma and ocular hypertension (p.1387). One drop of a 0.005% solution is instilled once daily in the evening.

Preparations

Proprietary Preparations (details are given in Part 3)
Austral.: Xalatan; ***Ital.:*** Xalatan; ***Neth.:*** Xalatan; ***Swed.:*** Xalatan; ***UK:*** Xalatan; ***USA:*** Xalatan.

Limaprost (2957-j)

Limaprost *(rINN)*.

ONO-1206; OP-1206. *(E)*-7-{(1*R*,2*R*,3*R*)-3-Hydroxy-2-[(*E*)-(3*S*,5*S*)-3-hydroxy-5-methyl-1-nonenyl]-5-oxocyclopentyl}-2-heptenoic acid.

$C_{22}H_{36}O_5$ = 380.5.

CAS — 88852-12-4.

Limaprost is a synthetic analogue of alprostadil (prostaglandin E_1). It is given by mouth for the treatment of peripheral vascular disease.

References.

1. Shono T, Ikeda K. Rapid effect of oral limaprost in Raynaud's disease in childhood. *Lancet* 1989; **i:** 908.
2. Murai C, *et al.* Oral limaprost for Raynaud's phenomenon. *Lancet* 1989; **ii:** 1218.

Preparations

Proprietary Preparations (details are given in Part 3)
Jpn: Opalmon.

Luprostiol (8089-e)

Luprostiol *(BAN, rINN)*.

(±)-*(Z)*-7-{(1*S*,2*R*,3*R*,5*S*)-2-[(2*S*)-3-(3-Chlorophenoxy)-2-hydroxypropylthio]-3,5-dihydroxycyclopentyl}hept-5-enoic acid.

$C_{21}H_{29}ClO_6S$ = 445.0.

CAS — 67110-79-6.

Luprostiol is a synthetic analogue of dinoprost (prostaglandin $F_{2\alpha}$). It is used as a luteolytic in veterinary medicine.

Meteneprost (8090-b)

Meteneprost *(USAN, rINN)*.

9-Deoxo-16,16-dimethyl-9-methylene-prostaglandin E_2; U-46785. (5*Z*,13*E*)-(8*R*,11*R*,12*R*,15*R*)-11,15-Dihydroxy-16,16-dimethyl-9-methyleneprosta-5,13-dienoic acid; *(Z)*-7-{(1*R*,2*R*,3*R*)-3-Hydroxy-2-[(*E*)-(3*R*)-3-hydroxy-4,4-dimethyloct-1-enyl]-5-methylenecyclopentyl}hept-5-enoic acid.

$C_{23}H_{38}O_4$ = 378.5.

CAS — 61263-35-2.

Meteneprost is a synthetic derivative of dinoprostone (prostaglandin E_2). It is a uterine stimulant and has been studied for the termination of pregnancy.

Misoprostol (16898-r)

Misoprostol *(BAN, USAN, rINN)*.

SC-29333. (±)-Methyl 7-{(1*R*,2*R*,3*R*)-3-hydroxy-2-[(*E*)-(4*RS*)-4-hydroxy-4-methyloct-1-enyl]-5-oxocyclopentyl}heptanoate; (±)-Methyl (13*E*)-11,16-dihydroxy-16-methyl-9-oxoprost-13-enoate.

$C_{22}H_{38}O_5$ = 382.5.

CAS — 59122-46-2.

Adverse Effects

The commonest side-effect occurring with misoprostol is diarrhoea. Other gastro-intestinal effects include abdominal pain, dyspepsia, flatulence, and nausea and vomiting. Increased uterine contractility and abnormal vaginal bleeding (including menorrhagia and intermenstrual bleeding) have been reported with misoprostol. Other adverse effects include skin rashes, headache, and dizziness. Hypotension is rarely seen at recommended doses.

A summary of data on misoprostol presented to the FDA.[1] During controlled studies the most common adverse effect was diarrhoea (8.2% compared with 3.1% for placebo); it was dose-related but usually mild, only 8 of 2003 subjects receiving misoprostol having withdrawn because of incapacitating diarrhoea. Headaches and abdominal discomfort were also reported. The effects of misoprostol on the uterus and the potential risks of uterine bleeding or abortion in pregnant women were of more concern. In nonpregnant women taking part in the controlled studies there were menstrual complaints in 15 of 410 (3.7%) receiving misoprostol compared with 2 of 115 (1.7%) given placebo. In a study in pregnant women who had elected to undergo first trimester abortion, all 6 who had a spontaneous expulsion of the uterine contents had received 1 or 2 doses of misoprostol 400 μg the previous evening, while none of those given placebo aborted spontaneously; overall 25 of the 56 women receiving misoprostol experienced uterine bleeding compared with only 2 of 55 on placebo.

1. Lewis JH. Summary of the 29th meeting of the Gastrointestinal Drugs Advisory Committee, Food and Drug Administration—June 10, 1985. *Am J Gastroenterol* 1985; **80:** 743–5.

Effects on the fetus. For reports of congenital malformations possibly associated with the misuse of misoprostol, see under Termination of Pregnancy in Uses and Administration, below.

Precautions

Misoprostol should not be given to patients who are pregnant or who may become pregnant because it can cause uterine contraction.

Inflammatory bowel disease. Life-threatening diarrhoea was reported in a patient with unrecognised Crohn's disease following six doses of misoprostol.[1]

1. Kornbluth A, *et al.* Life-threatening diarrhea after short-term misoprostol use in a patient with Crohn ileocolitis. *Ann Intern Med* 1990; **113:** 474–5.

Pharmacokinetics

Misoprostol is reported to be rapidly absorbed and metabolised to its active form (misoprostol acid, SC-30695) following administration by mouth. Administration with food reduces the rate but not the extent of absorption. Misoprostol acid is further metabolised by oxidation in a number of body organs and is excreted mainly in the urine. The plasma elimination half-life is reported to be between 20 and 40 minutes.

References.

1. Schoenhard G, *et al.* Metabolism and pharmacokinetic studies of misoprostol. *Dig Dis Sci* 1985; **30** (suppl): 126S–128S.
2. Karim A, *et al.* Effects of food and antacid on oral absorption of misoprostol, a synthetic prostaglandin E_1 analog. *J Clin Pharmacol* 1989; **29:** 439–43.

Uses and Administration

Misoprostol is a synthetic analogue of alprostadil (prostaglandin E_1).

It is used in the treatment of benign gastric and duodenal ulceration including that associated with NSAIDs. The usual dose by mouth is 800 μg daily in two to four divided doses with food.

Misoprostol is also used in conjunction with NSAIDs to prevent NSAID-induced ulcers. The usual prophylactic dose is 200 μg two to four times daily. A dose of 100 μg four times daily has been suggested for patients not tolerating the higher dose. Some preparations of NSAIDs contain misoprostol in an attempt to limit their adverse effects on the gastro-intestinal mucosa.

General reviews.

1. Walley TJ. Misoprostol. *Prescribers' J* 1993; **33:** 78–82.

Labour induction and augmentation. Prostaglandins are well established for the induction of labour (p.1411) and several studies have investigated the use of misoprostol. Given vaginally misoprostol was as effective as intravenous oxytocin[1] and more effective than intracervical dinoprostone gel.[2-5] Using misoprostol tablets, doses employed have been 50 μg vaginally increased every 2 hours[1] or every 4 hours[2,4,5] or 25 μg vaginally increased every 2 hours[3] according to the patient's response. Misoprostol has also been given orally in doses of 50 μg every 4 hours.[6]

Misoprostol has also been tried for active management of the third stage of labour (see Postpartum Haemorrhage under Ergometrine, p.1575).

1. Margulies M, *et al.* Misoprostol to induce labour. *Lancet* 1992; **339:** 64.
2. Chuck FJ, Huffacker BJ. Labor induction with intravaginal misoprostol versus intracervical prostaglandin E_2 gel (Prepidil gel): randomized comparison. *Am J Obstet Gynecol* 1995; **173:** 1137–42.
3. Varaklis K, *et al.* Randomized controlled trial of vaginal misoprostol and intracervical prostaglandin E_2 gel for induction of labor at term. *Obstet Gynecol* 1995; **86:** 541–4.
4. Mundle WR, Young DC. Vaginal misoprostol for induction of labor: a randomized controlled trial. *Obstet Gynecol* 1996; **88:** 521–5.
5. Buser D, *et al.* A randomized comparison between misoprostol and dinoprostone for cervical ripening and labor induction in patients with unfavorable cervices. *Obstet Gynecol* 1997; **89:** 581–5.
6. Windrim R, *et al.* Oral administration of misoprostol for labor induction: a randomized controlled trial. *Obstet Gynecol* 1997: **89:** 392–7.

Organ and tissue transplantation. Misoprostol 200 μg four times daily improved renal function in cyclosporin-treated recipients of renal transplants.[1] The number of patients who had acute graft rejection was lower in the misoprostol group than in the placebo group.

Improvement of renal function in transplant recipients by misoprostol or other prostaglandin E_1 analogues could be the result of an immunosuppressant effect[1,2] or the inhibition of renal thromboxane.[3] Prolonged therapy would be necessary to prevent chronic nephrotoxicity.[3]

However, misoprostol does not appear to have gained a role in the usual management of renal transplantation (p.499).

1. Moran M, *et al.* Prevention of acute graft rejection by the prostaglandin E_1 analogue misoprostol in renal-transplant recipients treated with cyclosporine and prednisone. *N Engl J Med* 1990; **322:** 1183–8.
2. Perl A. Role of a prostaglandin E_1 analogue in the prevention of acute graft rejection by cyclosporine. *N Engl J Med* 1990; **323:** 831–2.
3. Di Palo FQ, *et al.* Role of a prostaglandin E_1 analogue in the prevention of acute graft rejection by cyclosporine. *N Engl J Med* 1990; **323:** 832–3.

Peptic ulcer disease. Although misoprostol can produce benefit in duodenal[1,2] and gastric[3,4] ulcers, prostaglandins are generally considered to have no advantages over other forms of therapy for peptic ulceration (p.1174), and their adverse effects can be troublesome. One area in which they may have a role, however, is in the prophylaxis and treatment of peptic ulceration in patients taking NSAIDs. There is good evidence that misoprostol can reduce the risk of gastric and duodenal ulcer formation in patients on long-term NSAID treatment,[5-10] and it appears more effective in this respect than histamine H_2-receptor antagonists,[7] for which evidence of benefit against gastric injury is less persuasive. However, misoprostol's abdominal adverse effects, particularly diarrhoea and abdominal cramps, may limit its usefulness and patient acceptability and omeprazole, which is equally effective in preventing NSAID-induced ulceration, is better tolerated.[9] Improved formulations, in which the active isomer of misoprostol is bound to a polymer, may reduce adverse effects;[11] reducing the dose might increase patient acceptability without reducing effectiveness.[10]

1. Brand DL, *et al.* Misoprostol, a synthetic PGE_1 analog, in the treatment of duodenal ulcers: a multicenter double-blind study. *Dig Dis Sci* 1985; **30** (suppl): 147S–158S.
2. Bright-Asare P, *et al.* Efficacy of misoprostol (twice daily dosage) in acute healing of duodenal ulcer: a multicenter double-blind controlled trial. *Dig Dis Sci* 1986; **31** (suppl): 63S–67S.
3. Agrawal NM, *et al.* Healing of benign gastric ulcer: a placebo-controlled comparison of two dosage regimens of misoprostol, a synthetic analog of prostaglandin E_1. *Dig Dis Sci* 1985; **30** (suppl): 164S–170S.
4. Rachmilewitz D, *et al.* A multicenter international controlled comparison of two dosage regimens of misoprostol with cimetidine in treatment of gastric ulcer in outpatients. *Dig Dis Sci* 1986; **31** (suppl): 75S–80S.
5. Graham DY, *et al.* Duodenal and gastric ulcer prevention with misoprostol in arthritis patients taking NSAIDs. *Ann Intern Med* 1993; **119:** 257–62.
6. Silverstein FE, *et al.* Misoprostol reduces serious gastrointestinal complications in patients with rheumatoid arthritis receiving nonsteroidal anti-inflammatory drugs. *Ann Intern Med* 1995; **123:** 241–9.
7. Koch M, *et al.* Prevention of nonsteroidal anti-inflammatory drug-induced gastrointestinal mucosal injury: a meta-analysis of randomized controlled clinical trials. *Arch Intern Med* 1996; **156:** 2321–32.
8. Champion GD, *et al.* NSAID-induced gastrointestinal damage: epidemiology, risk and prevention, with an evaluation of the role of misoprostol: an Asia-Pacific perspective and consensus. *Drugs* 1997; **53:** 6–19.
9. Hawkey CJ, *et al.* Omeprazole compared with misoprostol for ulcers associated with nonsteroidal antiinflammatory drugs. *N Engl J Med* 1998; **338:** 727–34.
10. Raskin JB, *et al.* Misoprostol dosage in the prevention of nonsteroidal anti-inflammatory drug-induced gastric and duodenal ulcers: a comparison of three regimens. *Ann Intern Med* 1995; **123:** 344–50.
11. Perkins WE, *et al.* Polymer delivery of the active isomer of misoprostol: a solution to the intestinal side effect problem. *J Pharmacol Exp Ther* 1994; **269:** 151–6.

Postpartum haemorrhage. Prostaglandins are used in the treatment of established postpartum haemorrhage (p.1575) and one study[1] has indicated that misoprostol, given orally immediately after delivery, is effective in preventing bleeding although further comparative trials are needed.

1. El-Refaey H, *et al.* Use of oral misoprostol in the prevention of postpartum haemorrhage. *Br J Obstet Gynaecol* 1997; **104:** 336–9.

Termination of pregnancy. Prostaglandins are widely employed for the termination of pregnancy (p.1412) and misoprostol has been studied both for cervical preparation and for inducing uterine contractions.

Vaginal administration of misoprostol is effective for cervical ripening prior to surgical termination in the first trimester.[1] Oral administration of misoprostol following the administration of mifepristone orally is effective in terminating early pregnancy of up to 63 days and especially so at up to 49 days.[2,3] Misoprostol can also be given vaginally.[4,15] In addition, vaginal misoprostol in combination with intramuscular methotrexate has been studied.[5-7]

Misoprostol on its own is only a weak abortifacient and is often ineffective when used alone for the termination of pregnancy, although it has been widely misused for this purpose in some countries, notably Brazil.[8-10] Anecdotal reports[10-12] and one small controlled study[16] have associated such misuse during the first trimester of pregnancy with congenital malformations, particularly of the neonates' skull, though the manufacturers had found no evidence of teratogenicity in *animals.*[13]

Intravaginal misoprostol has been reported to be as effective as dinoprostone for termination of pregnancy during the second trimester.[14]

1. El-Refaey H, *et al.* Cervical priming with prostaglandin E1 analogues, misoprostol and gemeprost. *Lancet* 1994; **343:** 1207–9. Correction. *ibid.*; 1650.
2. Peyron R, *et al.* Early termination of pregnancy with mifepristone (RU 486) and the orally active prostaglandin misoprostol. *N Engl J Med* 1993; **328:** 1509–13.
3. Spitz IM, *et al.* Early pregnancy termination with mifepristone and misoprostol in the United States. *N Engl J Med* 1998; **338:** 1241–7.
4. El-Refaey H, *et al.* Induction of abortion with mifepristone (RU 486) and oral or vaginal misoprostol. *N Engl J Med* 1995; **332:** 983–7.
5. Creinin MD, Vittinghoff E. Methotrexate and misoprostol vs misoprostol alone for early abortion: a randomized controlled trial. *JAMA* 1994; **272:** 1190–5.
6. Hausknecht RU. Methotrexate and misoprostol to terminate early pregnancy. *N Engl J Med* 1995; **333:** 537–40.
7. Creinin MD, *et al.* A randomized trial comparing misoprostol three and seven days after methotrexate for early abortion. *Am J Obstet Gynecol* 1995; **173:** 1578–84.
8. Costa SH, Vessey MP. Misoprostol and illegal abortion in Rio de Janeiro, Brazil. *Lancet* 1993; **341:** 1258–61.
9. Coêlho HLL, *et al.* Misoprostol and illegal abortion in Fortaleza, Brazil. *Lancet* 1993; **341:** 1261–3. Correction. *ibid.*; 1486.
10. Fonseca W, *et al.* Misoprostol and congenital malformations. *Lancet* 1991; **338:** 56.
11. Shepard TH. Möbius syndrome after misoprostol: a possible teratogenic mechanism. *Lancet* 1995; **346:** 780.
12. Gonzalez CH, *et al.* Congenital abnormalities in Brazilian children associated with misoprostol misuse in first trimester of pregnancy. *Lancet* 1998; **351:** 1624–7.
13. Downie WW. Misuse of misoprostol. *Lancet* 1991; **338:** 247.
14. Jain JK, Mishell DR. A comparison of intravaginal misoprostol with prostaglandin E_2 for termination of second-trimester pregnancy. *N Engl J Med* 1994; **331:** 290–3.
15. Ashok PW, *et al.* Termination of pregnancy at 9-13 weeks' amenorrhoea with mifepristone and misoprostol. *Lancet* 1998; **52:** 542–3.
16. Pastuszak AL, *et al.* Use of misoprostol during pregnancy and Möbius' syndrome in infants. *N Engl J Med* 1998; **338:** 1881–5.

Preparations

Proprietary Preparations (details are given in Part 3)
Aust.: Cyprostol; ***Austral.:*** Cytotec; ***Belg.:*** Cytotec; ***Canad.:*** Cytotec; ***Fr.:*** Cytotec; ***Ger.:*** Cytotec; ***Irl.:*** Cytotec; ***Ital.:*** Cytotec; Misodex; Symbol†; ***Neth.:*** Cytotec; ***Norw.:*** Cytotec; ***S.Afr.:*** Cytotec; ***Spain:*** Cytotec; Menpros; ***Swed.:*** Cytotec; ***Switz.:*** Cytotec; ***UK:*** Cytotec; ***USA:*** Cytotec.

Used as an adjunct in: ***Austral.:*** Arthrotec; ***Canad.:*** Arthrotec; ***Ger.:*** Arthotec; ***Irl.:*** Arthrotec; ***Ital.:*** Artrotec; Misofenac; ***Neth.:*** Arthrotec; ***Norw.:*** Arthrotec; ***S.Afr.:*** Arthrotec; ***Swed.:*** Arthrotec; ***Switz.:*** Arthrotec; ***UK:*** Arthrotec; Condrotec; Napratec; ***USA:*** Arthrotec.

Nocloprost (3146-w)

Nocloprost *(rINN).*

(*Z*)-7-[(1*R*,2*R*,3*R*,5*R*)-5-Chloro-3-hydroxy-2-[(*E*)-(3*R*)-3-hydroxy-4,4-dimethyl-1-octenyl]cyclopentyl]-5-heptenoic acid.

$C_{22}H_{37}ClO_4$ = 401.0.

CAS — 79360-43-3.

Nocloprost is a synthetic analogue of dinoprostone (prostaglandin E_2) that has been investigated in the treatment of peptic ulcer disease.

References.

1. Täuber U, *et al.* Pharmacokinetics of nocloprost in human volunteers and its relation to dose. *Eur J Clin Pharmacol* 1993; **44:** 497–500.

Ornoprostil (2971-l)

Ornoprostil *(rINN).*

OU-1308. Methyl (−)-(1*R*,2*R*,3*R*)-3-hydroxy-2-[(*E*)-(3*S*,5*S*)-3-hydroxy-5-methyl-1-nonenyl]-ε,5-dioxocyclopentaneheptanoate.

$C_{23}H_{38}O_6$ = 410.5.

CAS — 70667-26-4.

Ornoprostil is a synthetic prostaglandin analogue that has been used in the treatment of peptic ulcer disease.

Preparations

Proprietary Preparations (details are given in Part 3)
Jpn: Alloca†; Rowok†.

Rosaprostol (16980-z)

Rosaprostol *(rINN).*

9-Hydroxy-19,20-bis-nor-prostanoic Acid; IBI-C83. 2-Hexyl-5-hydroxycyclopentaneheptanoic acid, mixture of (1*RS*,2*SR*,5*RS*) and (1*RS*,2*SR*,5*SR*) isomers.

$C_{18}H_{34}O_3$ = 298.5.

CAS — 56695-65-9.

Rosaprostol is a synthetic prostaglandin derivative that inhibits gastric acid secretion. It has been given by mouth in the treatment of peptic ulcer disease.

Preparations

Proprietary Preparations (details are given in Part 3)
Ital.: Rosal†.

Sulprostone (8096-w)

Sulprostone *(USAN, rINN).*

CP-34089; 16-Phenoxy-ω-17,18,19,20-tetranor-prostaglandin E_2-methylsulfonylamide; SHB-286; ZK-57671. (*Z*)-7-{(1*R*,2*R*,3*R*)-3-Hydroxy-2-[(*E*)-(3*R*)-3-hydroxy-4-phenoxybut-1-enyl]-5-oxocyclopentyl}-*N*-(methylsulphonyl)hept-5-enamide.

$C_{23}H_{31}NO_7S$ = 465.6.

CAS — 60325-46-4.

Adverse Effects and Precautions

As for Dinoprostone, p.1415.

Once a prostaglandin has been given to terminate pregnancy it is essential that termination take place; if the prostaglandin is unsuccessful other measures should be used.

Effects on the cardiovascular system. A 31-year-old woman died from cardiovascular shock during an abortion induced by mifepristone followed by sulprostone. She had 12 children, one previous abortion, and was a heavy cigarette smoker.[1] Four other deaths with sulprostone had not been associated with abortion.

1. Anonymous. A death associated with mifepristone/sulprostone. *Lancet* 1991; **337:** 969–70.

Effects on the nervous system. Convulsions occurred in 3 of 4 epileptic patients following administration of sulprostone.[1]

1. Brandenburg H, *et al.* Convulsions in epileptic women after administration of prostaglandin E_2 derivative. *Lancet* 1990; **336:** 1138.

Uses and Administration

Sulprostone is a synthetic derivative of dinoprostone (prostaglandin E_2). It is a uterine stimulant and is used for dilatation of the cervix prior to surgical termination of pregnancy in the first trimester and for the termination of pregnancy in the second trimester (p.1412). It is also used to control postpartum haemorrhage (p.1575). Sulprostone is administered by intravenous infusion. A dose of 500 μg over 3 to 6 hours has been suggested for cervical dilatation in the first trimester and a similar dose over about 2 hours is given for postpartum haemorrhage. For termination of pregnancy in the second trimester an infusion at a rate of 100 μg per hour for up to 10 hours is recommended; if necessary the infusion rate may be increased to up to 500 μg per hour, to a maximum total dose of 1.5 mg. If unsuccessful the course may be repeated once 12 to 24 hours later. Sulprostone has also been administered extra-amniotically and locally into the cervix. It has also been administered by the intramuscular route, but this is no longer recommended.

Preparations

Proprietary Preparations (details are given in Part 3)
Aust.: Nalador; ***Fr.:*** Nalador; ***Ger.:*** Nalador; ***Ital.:*** Nalador; ***Neth.:*** Nalador; ***Switz.:*** Nalador.

Tiaprost Trometamol (8097-e)

Tiaprost Trometamol *(BANM, rINNM).*

Trometamol salt of (±)-(*Z*)-7-{(1*R*,2*R*,3*R*,5*S*)-3,5-dihydroxy-2-[(*E*)-(3*RS*)-3-hydroxy-4-(3-thienyloxy)but-1-enyl]cyclopentyl}hept-5-enoic acid.

$C_{20}H_{28}O_6S,C_4H_{11}NO_3$ = 517.6.

CAS — 71116-82-0 (tiaprost).

Tiaprost trometamol is a synthetic analogue of dinoprost (prostaglandin $F_{2\alpha}$). It is used as a luteolytic in veterinary medicine.

Unoprostone (15932-f)

Unoprostone *(rINN).*

UF-021 (unoprostone isopropyl). (+)-(*Z*)-7-[(1*R*,2*R*,3*R*,5*S*)-3,5-Dihydroxy-2-(3-oxodecyl)cyclopentyl]-5-heptenoic acid.

$C_{22}H_{38}O_5$ = 382.5.

CAS — 120373-36-6 (unoprostone); 120373-24-2 (unoprostone isopropyl).

Unoprostone is a synthetic analogue of dinoprost (prostaglandin $F_{2\alpha}$) that is used topically as the isopropyl ester for the treatment of glaucoma and ocular hypertension.

References.

1. Yamamoto T, *et al.* Clinical evaluation of UF-021 (Rescula; isopropyl unoprostone). *Surv Ophthalmol* 1997; **41** (suppl 2): S99–S103.

Preparations

Proprietary Preparations (details are given in Part 3)

Jpn: Rescula.

Radiopharmaceuticals

Radioactive compounds are used in medicine as sources of radiation for radiotherapy and for diagnostic purposes. They have numerous uses in research and industry.

Sealed radioactive sources are bonded or encapsulated to prevent the escape of the radioactive material and are used as supplied. Unsealed sources, on the other hand, are radioactive materials usually in liquid, particulate, or gaseous form that are removed from their containers for application. Radiopharmaceuticals come within this category.

The aim of this chapter is to provide background information on the radionuclides that are used as radiopharmaceuticals. Care is required in the preparation, handling, use, and disposal of these compounds; they are thus best dealt with by those with suitable experience and training.

Atomic Structure

An atom is composed of a central positively charged nucleus around which, and at relatively great distances away, negatively charged electrons revolve in orbits. The electrons are arranged round the atomic nucleus in a series of 'shells' in each of which is a limited number of orbits.

The nucleus consists of 2 main kinds of particles known as protons, each of unit positive charge, and neutrons, which are uncharged; the total number of these particles in the nucleus is known as the *mass number.*

Each electron carries a negative charge which is of the same size as the positive charge of the proton, so that in the neutral atom the number of electrons is equal to the number of protons in the nucleus.

The number of protons in the nucleus is known as the *atomic number*, which determines the number of electrons in the extranuclear structure. Thus all the atoms of a particular chemical element have the same atomic number. But while the number of protons (atomic number) in a given element is constant, the number of neutrons in the atoms, and thus their masses (mass numbers), may vary. These different forms of the same element are known as isotopes of the element and these isotopes differ in some of their physical properties.

Some isotopes may be stable, the differences between them arising solely from their difference in mass; others may be radioactive (*radioisotopes*), their nuclei changing spontaneously and emitting particles or electromagnetic waves, or both.

Most of the naturally occurring isotopes are stable, though there are a number which are unstable and therefore radioactive, for example, uranium-235. In addition, artificial radionuclides are prepared by converting stable nuclei into unstable forms and even naturally occurring radionuclides may be prepared by artificial means.

The symbol used for a nuclide is a development of the chemical symbol for the atom, with the mass number as a superscript and the atomic number as a subscript; thus the symbols for the 3 hydrogen isotopes—common hydrogen, deuterium, and tritium—are ${}^{1}_{1}H$, ${}^{2}_{1}H$, and ${}^{3}_{1}H$, and the symbols for the 3 naturally occurring uranium isotopes are ${}^{234}_{92}U$, ${}^{235}_{92}U$, and ${}^{238}_{92}U$; as the atomic number can be inferred from the chemical symbol it is the usual practice to omit the subscript. It is also common practice to write out the full name of the element followed by the mass number e.g. chromium-51 for ${}^{51}Cr$.

Emissions from Radioisotopes

The 3 main types of emission from radioactive substances are *alpha particles, beta particles,* and *gamma-rays.* Most sources emit more than one type of radiation.

Alpha particles are positively charged particles (helium nuclei), each consisting of 2 protons and 2 neutrons.

Beta particles (β^- or β^+) are identical with electrons or positrons but arise from the nucleus. They are emitted with great velocity and their energies are spread over a spectrum. Positrons are similar to electrons, having a similar mass but a positive charge.

Gamma-rays are electromagnetic radiations or *photons* with a wavelength much shorter than those of light.

In certain cases, e.g. chromium-51, *electron capture* (EC) occurs, an electron from an inner shell being absorbed by the nucleus with the production of an *X-ray* characteristic of the daughter atom or emission of an *Auger electron.*

The type of emission from a radionuclide largely determines its usefulness in medicine. Those emitting alpha particles are very little used partly because detection and measurement are difficult. Positron-emitters, such as carbon-11, fluorine-18, nitrogen-13, and oxygen-15, have become more popular in recent years and are used in positron-emission tomography where the radiation is measured from within the body as opposed to computed tomography where the energy is supplied from an external source. Single photon emission tomography is another technique like position-emission tomography that provides views of slices through the body and this technique employs gamma-ray emitting radionuclides which are the most accessible and the most common radiation source in radiopharmaceuticals.

The radiation data given under the radionuclides described in the following pages show the half-life, the energy of the radiation of particles in million electronvolts (MeV), and the percentage of total number of transformations which gives rise to the emission of the particular radiation. Since one transformation may give rise to more than one gamma-ray the percentages do not necessarily add up to 100%. X-rays, together with minor emissions, have been omitted unless they are a significant part of the total emission.

Decay of Radionuclides

A radionuclide will consist of unstable atoms which will at some time undergo an energy change with the emission of ionising radiation, those which are actually undergoing this change, and those which have undergone the change. In quantitative terms this transition occurs at a rate which is characteristic of the radionuclide and it is expressed as its half-life—the time required for the activity to fall by one-half. Many radionuclides have complex decay characteristics with several possible energies of emitted particles and radiation. Some radionuclides may be in an excited or metastable state denoted by the suffix m attached to the mass number (e.g. Technetium-99m) and undergo *isomeric transition* (IT) with the release of γ-rays.

The activity of radionuclides is measured in terms of the rate of transformation or disintegration. The unit is the becquerel (Bq)=1 transformation per second; the curie (Ci) was formerly used as the unit of activity; 1 Ci=3.7×10^{10} Bq.

Supply, Preparation, and Control

A wide range of radionuclides and specially formulated radiopharmaceuticals is available from specialised manufacturers. However, there are national controls on the use, transport, storage, and disposal of such compounds. Authority and guidance should be sought from the relevant bodies and authorities before using such compounds.

Generators are special features in the supply of radionuclides. They are receptacles containing a parent and daughter nuclide in equilibrium and from which the daughter nuclide, which usually has a short half-life, may be eluted. Generators are available for the production of indium-113m and technetium-99m. Generators are also available for some positron-emitters.

Storage conditions for radiopharmaceuticals should be such as to prevent the inadvertent emission of radioactivity as well as to meet the storage requirements for the pharmaceutical that has been labelled. Thus due account still has to be paid, for instance, to the effects of temperature and light. Radiopharmaceuticals are liable to decomposition by self-irradiation effects which may cause degradation of solvent, preservative, or other compounds. There can also be a continuous formation of oxidising and reducing chemical species arising from the effect of the radioactivity on any chemical substances present in the radiopharmaceutical, even in minute amounts.

Adverse Effects

The internal irradiation of tissues following the administration of radionuclides carries similar dangers to exposure to ionising radiation from an external source, and local high irradiation doses may arise if these nuclides are specifically localised in a tissue. The most serious danger is genetic damage prior to and during the reproductive period. Tissues whose cells are in a continuous state of multiplication are particularly sensitive to the effects of radiation.

Untoward effects of exposure to the larger doses of irradiation include leucopenia, anaemia, inflammation of the skin, radiation sickness, and neoplasms.

In considering the effect of a given radionuclide it is usual to calculate the dose to the organ most critically affected, and also the dose to the whole body.

In considering the adverse effects of radiopharmaceuticals one should not forget the effects that might arise from the carrier or from contaminants.

General Uses

Radiopharmaceuticals are used widely in many branches of medicine and surgery, mainly for the diagnosis and sometimes for the treatment of disease. They can provide information not available using other diagnostic techniques such as contrast media, ultrasound, and computed tomography or other external irradiation. Interesting developments have followed the tagging of monoclonal antibodies with radionuclides.

Many investigations involve the oral or parenteral administration of radionuclides or labelled compounds followed usually by an imaging procedure. Some investigations involve the measurement of radioactive concentrations in organs, tissues, blood, urine, or faeces. The quantities used are always the smallest which will give the desired accuracy of image or of measurement.

Radiological Terms

Alpha particles. Nuclei of helium atoms emitted by radioactive atomic nuclei.

Annihilation. The interaction and disappearance of a positive and a negative electron with the conversion of their energy into electromagnetic radiation.

Atomic number (Z). The number of protons in the atomic nucleus.

Auger effect. The emission of an electron from an atom due to the filling of a vacancy in an inner electron shell.

Becquerel (Bq). The SI unit of activity, defined as 1 transformation per second. The curie was formerly used as the unit of activity. 1 Bq=2.7×10^{-11} Ci.

Beta particles. Electrons or positrons emitted by radioactive atomic nuclei.

Carrier-free. A preparation in which substantially all the atoms of the activated element present are radioactive. Material of high specific activity is often loosely referred to as 'carrier-free'.

Curie (Ci). Now superseded as a unit of activity by the becquerel. A curie (Ci) represented 3.7×10^{10} transformations per second. 1 Ci=3.7×10^{10} Bq.

Daughter. Of a given nuclide, any nuclide that originates from it by radioactive decay.

Electron capture (EC). A mode of radioactivity decay involving the capture of an orbital electron by its nucleus.

Gamma-radiation. Electromagnetic radiation emitted in the process of a change in configuration of a nucleus or particle annihilation and having wavelengths shorter than those of X-rays.

Gray (Gy). The SI unit of absorbed dose, defined as 1 J per kg. The rad was formerly used as the unit of absorbed dose. 1 Gy=100 rads.

Isomeric transition (IT). The decay of one isomer to another having a lower energy state. The transition is accompanied by the emission of gamma-radiation.

Isomers. Nuclides with the same mass number and atomic number but with nuclei having different energy states.

Isotopes. Nuclides with the same atomic number but different mass numbers.

Nuclide. A species of atom having a specific mass number, atomic number, and nuclear energy state.

Photon. A quantum of electromagnetic radiation.

Positron. A positive beta particle.

Rad (radiation absorbed dose).

Now superseded as a unit of absorbed dose by the gray. A rad is equal to 10^{-2} J per kg. The röntgen and the rad in soft tissue are approximately equivalent in magnitude for moderate energies. 1 rad=10^{-2} Gy.

Radioactive decay. The spontaneous change of a nucleus resulting in the emission of a particle or a photon.

Radioactivity. The property of certain nuclides of spontaneously emitting particles or photons or of undergoing spontaneous fission.

Radioisotope. An isotope that is radioactive.

Radionuclide. A nuclide that is radioactive.

Rem (röntgen-equivalent-man).

Now superseded as a unit of dose equivalent by the sievert (Sv). A rem is numerically equal to the absorbed dose in rads multiplied by the appropriate quality factor defining the biological effect and by any other modifying factors. The sievert is the joule per kg (J kg^{-1}) equal to 100 rem.

Röntgen (R). A unit of exposure of X- or gamma-radiation, equal to 2.58×10^{-4} coulombs per kg in air superseded by the SI unit of exposure, the coulomb per kg (C kg^{-1}). 1 C kg^{-1}=3.876×10^{3} R.

Sievert (Sv). The SI unit of dose equivalent numerically equal to the absorbed dose in grays multiplied by the appropriate quality factor defining the biological effect and by any other modifying factors expressed in J per kg.

Specific activity. The activity per unit mass of a material containing a radioactive substance.

X-rays. Electromagnetic radiation other than annihilation radiation originating in the extranuclear part of the atom and having wavelengths much shorter than those of visible light.

Carbon-11 (9907-j)

CAS — 14333-33-6.

HALF-LIFE. 20.4 minutes.

Carbon-11 is a positron-emitter which is used in positron-emission tomography (p.1422). Compounds which have been labelled with carbon-11 include L-methionine for the detection of malignant neoplasms, acetic acid and palmitic acids for the study of myocardial metabolism, and raclopride for the study of CNS dopaminergic D_2 receptors. Labelled carbon monoxide may be used to assess blood volume.

Preparations

USP 23: Methionine C 11 Injection; Raclopride C 11 Injection; Sodium Acetate C 11 Injection.

Carbon-14 (5853-q)

CAS — 14762-75-5.

HALF-LIFE. 5730 years.

Carbon-14 has been used to label many organic compounds that may be employed in breath tests.

Chromium-51 (5854-p)

CAS — 14392-02-0.

HALF-LIFE. 27.7 days.

Chromium-51, as sodium chromate (^{51}Cr), is used to label red blood cells so that red-cell survival and red-cell volume can be measured. Chromium-51 activity in the faeces can be used to estimate gastro-intestinal blood losses. Red blood cells labelled with chromium-51 and damaged by heat before re-injection have been used for spleen scanning.

As chromium edetate (^{51}Cr) given intravenously, chromium-51 is used in the determination of the glomerular filtration rate.

As chromic chloride (^{51}Cr), chromium-51 has been administered intravenously for the determination of loss of serum protein into the gastro-intestinal tract.

Preparations

Ph. Eur.: Chromium(^{51}Cr) Edetate Injection; Sodium Chromate(^{51}Cr) Sterile Solution;
USP 23: Sodium Chromate Cr 51 Injection.

Proprietary Preparations (details are given in Part 3)
USA: Chromitope.

Cobalt-57 (5855-s)

CAS — 13981-50-5.

HALF-LIFE. 271 days.

Cobalt-57, in the form of an aqueous solution or capsules of cyanocobalamin (^{57}Co), is given by mouth for the measurement of absorption of vitamin B_{12} in the diagnosis of pernicious anaemia and other malabsorption syndromes. It is also used with cyanocobalamin (^{58}Co), see below.

Preparations

Ph. Eur.: Cyanocobalamin(^{57}Co) Capsules; Cyanocobalamin(^{57}Co) Solution;
USP 23: Cyanocobalamin Co 57 Capsules; Cyanocobalamin Co 57 Oral Solution.

Proprietary Preparations (details are given in Part 3)
USA: Cobratope.

Multi-ingredient: ***UK:*** Dicopac.

Cobalt-58 (5856-w)

CAS — 13981-38-9.

HALF-LIFE. 70.8 days.

Cobalt-58, in the form of an aqueous solution of cyanocobalamin (^{58}Co) is given by mouth for the measurement of absorption of vitamin B_{12} in the diagnosis of pernicious anaemia and other malabsorption syndromes.

The different energies of cobalt-57 and cobalt-58 facilitate separation of the isotopes in a mixture. Advantage is taken of this to differentiate between failure of absorption due to lack of intrinsic factor (pernicious anaemia) and that due to ileal malabsorption by the simultaneous administration of free cyanocobalamin (^{58}Co) and cyanocobalamin (^{57}Co) bound to intrinsic factor. A dual isotope kit has been used for this purpose.

Preparations

Ph. Eur.: Cyanocobalamin(^{58}Co) Solution.

Proprietary Preparations (details are given in Part 3)
USA: Rubratope.

Multi-ingredient: ***UK:*** Dicopac.

Fluorine-18 (19185-l)

CAS — 13981-56-1.

HALF-LIFE. 110 minutes.

Fluorine-18 is a positron-emitting radionuclide which is used in positron-emission tomography (p.1422).

Fludeoxyglucose (^{18}F) (2-deoxy-2-fluoro-^{18}F-α-D-glucopyranose; ^{18}F-fluorodeoxyglucose) is given by intravenous injection for the assessment of cerebral and myocardial glucose metabolism in various physiological or pathological states including stroke and myocardial ischaemia. It is also employed for the detection of malignant tumours including those of the brain, liver, lung, and thyroid gland. Fluorodopa (^{18}F) is also used in cerebral imaging.

Preparations

Ph. Eur.: Fludeoxyglucose (^{18}F) Injection;
USP 23: Fludeoxyglucose F 18 Injection; Fluorodopa F 18 Injection; Sodium Fluoride F 18 Injection.

Gallium-67 (5858-l)

CAS — 14119-09-6.

HALF-LIFE. 3.26 days.

Gallium-67 is used in the form of an intravenous injection of gallium citrate (^{67}Ga).

Gallium citrate (^{67}Ga) is concentrated in some malignant tumours of the lymphatic system, as well as in some other tissues, and is used for tumour visualisation. Concentration also occurs in inflammatory lesions and the injection is therefore employed for the localisation of focal inflammatory sites, such as may occur in abscesses, osteomyelitis, or sarcoidosis. Gallium scans have proved useful for the detection of the various infections and malignancies that may be encountered in patients with AIDS.

Preparations

Ph. Eur.: Gallium(^{67}Ga) Citrate Injection;
USP 23: Gallium Citrate Ga 67 Injection.

Gold-198 (5859-y)

CAS — 10043-49-9.

HALF-LIFE. 65 hours (2.7 days).

Gold-198, as colloidal gold (^{198}Au) with most of the activity associated with particles of diameter 5 to 20 nm, has been used by intrapleural or intraperitoneal injection in the treatment of malignant ascites and malignant pleural effusion.

The above injection has also been given intravenously for the measurement of liver blood flow, in liver scanning, and for general investigations of the reticuloendothelial system. Since the gamma-ray energies are not particularly good for scanning and the radiation dose to the patient is relatively high, it has generally been superseded by more suitable agents such as technetium-99m-labelled compounds.

Indium-111 (5860-g)

CAS — 15750-15-9.

HALF-LIFE. 67 hours (2.8 days).

Indium-111 as indium (^{111}In) complexed with pentetic acid (pentetate) is used diagnostically in cerebrospinal fluid studies.

Leucocytes labelled with indium (^{111}In) hydroxyquinoline are used for the location of inflammatory lesions; applications have been the detection or localisation of abscesses, infections including those occurring in patients with AIDS, inflammatory bowel diseases such as Crohn's disease or ulcerative colitis, and transplant rejection. Platelets have been similarly labelled and used for the detection of thrombi and for the investigation of thrombocytopenia.

Colloids have been prepared using indium chloride (^{111}In) and have been used for investigation of the lymphatic system. Indium (^{111}In) bleomycin has been given by intravenous injection used for the detection of tumours. Indium (^{111}In) pentetreotide is used for the detection and localisation of tumours originating from neuroendocrine cells.

Several different monoclonal antibodies, such as altumomab pentetate, capromab pendetide, imciromab pentetate, and satumomab pendetide, have been labelled with indium-111. Applications include the detection, diagnosis, and evaluation of malignant neoplasms of the colon, rectum, prostate, and ovaries as well as the detection and localisation of myocardial infarction.

Preparations

Ph. Eur.: Indium(^{111}In) Chloride Solution; Indium(^{111}In) Oxine Solution; Indium(^{111}In) Pentetate Injection;
USP 23: Indium In 111 Chloride Solution; Indium In 111 Oxyquinoline Solution; Indium In 111 Pentetate Injection; Indium In 111 Pentetreotide Injection; Indium In 111 Satumomab Pendetide Injection.

Proprietary Preparations (details are given in Part 3)
Ital.: Myoscint; Octreoscan; OncoScint CR 103; Scintifor C†; ***Spain:*** OncoScint CR 103; ***UK:*** OncoScint CR 103†; ***USA:*** OncoScint CR/OV.

Indium-113m (5861-q)

CAS — 14885-78-0 (indium-113).

HALF-LIFE. 99.5 minutes.

Indium-113m is a daughter of tin-113 ($^{113}_{50}$Sn, half-life 115 days, γ- and X-radiation) and because of its short half-life is normally prepared just before use by elution from a sterile generator consisting of tin-113 adsorbed on an ion-exchange material contained in a column.

Indium-113m may be used for labelling a variety of materials with differing physical properties including particles and colloids suited to scanning procedures for various organs and tissues. Chelates with pentetic acid have also been used. The short half-life of indium-113m and its lack of β-emission have allowed large doses to be given with a small radiation dose to the patient. High count rates for scanning are therefore achieved.

Iodine-123 (5862-p)

CAS — 15715-08-9.

HALF-LIFE. 13.2 hours.

Iodine-123 has similar adverse effects and precautions to those of iodine-131 (see below).

Its principal use is in thyroid uptake tests and thyroid imaging when it is given by mouth or intravenous injection as sodium iodide (^{123}I).

Sodium iodohippurate (^{123}I) is employed intravenously in tests of renal function and in renal imaging.

Iobenguane (^{123}I) (*m*-iodobenzylguanidine (^{123}I))is given intravenously for the localisation of certain tumours, for example phaeochromocytomas, and for the evaluation of neuroblastoma. It is also used for functional studies of the adrenal medulla and myocardium.

Various monoclonal antibodies have been labelled with iodine-123; potential applications include the detection of malignant neoplasms.

Preparations

Ph. Eur.: Iobenguane(^{123}I) Injection; Sodium Iodide(^{123}I) Solution; Sodium Iodohippurate(^{123}I) Injection;
USP 23: Iobenguane I 123 Injection; Iodohippurate Sodium I 123 Injection; Sodium Iodide I 123 Capsules; Sodium Iodide I 123 Solution.

Iodine-125 (5863-s)

CAS — 14158-31-7.

HALF-LIFE. 60.1 days.

Iodine-125 has similar adverse effects and precautions to those of iodine-131 (see below).

Iodine-125 is not very suitable for the external counting of radioactivity in the thyroid gland because its γ-energy is weak and tissue absorption is high. However, it is very suitable for radioimmunoassays *in vitro* and because it has a long half-life it is preferred as a label for many compounds to detect and estimate drugs and hormones in body fluids.

Iodine-125 may be used orally as sodium iodide (^{125}I), in the diagnosis of thyroid disorders.

Sodium iothalamate (^{125}I) has been used intravenously in the determination of glomerular filtration rate and sodium iodohippurate (^{125}I), intravenously for the measurement of effective renal plasma flow.

Iodine-125, as iodinated (^{125}I) human fibrinogen, has been used intravenously to demonstrate and locate deep vein thrombosis of the leg. Iodinated (^{125}I) fibrinogen has also been used in the measurement of fibrinogen metabolism in certain disturbances of blood coagulation.

Iodinated (^{125}I) albumin has been used for the determination of blood or plasma volume.

Preparations

BP 1998: Iodinated(^{125}I) Albumin Injection;
Ph. Eur.: Dried Human Iodinated(^{125}I) Fibrinogen; Sodium Iodide(^{125}I) Solution;
USP 23: Iodinated I 125 Albumin Injection; Iothalamate Sodium I 125 Injection.

Iodine-131 (5864-w)

CAS — 10043-66-0.

HALF-LIFE. 8.04 days.

Adverse Effects

A small percentage of patients treated with iodine-131 for thyrotoxicosis become hypothyroid each year and eventually most patients will require thyroid replacement therapy. Hypoparathyroidism has also been reported. Radiation thyroiditis with soreness may develop shortly after treatment. There may be severe and potentially dangerous swelling of the thyroid especially in patients with large goitres and this has on rare occasions produced asphyxiation. Leukaemia and carcinoma of the thyroid have occasionally been reported, particularly in young patients. However retrospective studies have shown no increased incidence in adults after iodine-131 treatment for thyrotoxicosis.

In the treatment of thyroid carcinoma, the larger doses of radioactive iodine sometimes cause nausea and vomiting a few days after ingestion, which may be due to gastritis as iodine-131 is also concentrated in gastric mucosa. Large doses depress the bone marrow.

Precautions

The use of sodium iodide (^{131}I) is contra-indicated, even in diagnostic doses, during pregnancy and lactation. Sodium iodide (^{131}I) should not be given to patients with large toxic nodular goitres or to patients with severe thyrotoxic heart disease. There is some controversy as to whether radio-iodine therapy exacerbates Graves' ophthalmopathy (see p.1489).

Many drugs have been reported to interfere with thyroid- or other organ-function studies and checks should be made on any treatment the patient might be receiving before any estimations are carried out.

Uses and Administration

Iodine radioisotopes are mainly used in studies of thyroid function and in the treatment of hyperthyroidism (p.1489) and some forms of thyroid carcinoma (p.494).

Iodine radioisotopes can be incorporated into many compounds including liothyronine and thyroxine, triglycerides and fatty acids, such as triolein and oleic acid, and proteins, such as iodinated human albumin, with varying degrees of stability and with little or no change in the biological activity of the labelled molecule. It is common practice to saturate the thyroid with non-radioactive iodine when uptake of radiation by the gland is not desired (see Radiation Protection, p.1494).

Sodium iodide (^{131}I) is given by mouth and by intravenous injection in studies of thyroid function, particularly in measurements of the uptake of iodine by the thyroid, and in thyroid scanning. It is also used in the treatment of hyperthyroidism and in the treatment of malignant neoplasm of the thyroid.

Injections containing iobenguane (^{131}I) (*m*-iodobenzylguanidine (^{131}I)) may be employed for the localisation and treatment of phaeochromocytoma (p.795) and neuroblastoma (p.494).

Human albumin iodinated with iodine-131 is employed in the determination of the blood or plasma volume.

Sodium iodohippurate (^{131}I) is used intravenously for renal function tests and for renal imaging.

Rose bengal sodium (^{131}I) has been given intravenously in tests of liver function.

Iodinated (^{131}I) norcholesterol (6β-iodomethyl-19-norcholest-5(10)-en-3β-ol (^{131}I)) has been used for adrenal scintigraphy by slow intravenous injection.

Various monoclonal antibodies labelled with iodine-131 are used for the detection of malignant neoplasms and some are being investigated for therapeutic purposes.

Preparations

Ph. Eur.: Iobenguane(^{131}I) Injection for Diagnostic Use; Iobenguane(^{131}I) Injection for Therapeutic Use; Iodinated(^{131}I) Norcholesterol Injection; Sodium Iodide(^{131}I) Capsules for Diagnostic Use; Sodium Iodide(^{131}I) Solution; Sodium Iodohippurate(^{131}I) Injection;
USP 23: Iodinated I 131 Albumin Aggregated Injection; Iodinated I 131 Albumin Injection; Iodohippurate Sodium I 131 Injection; Rose Bengal Sodium I 131 Injection; Sodium Iodide I 131 Capsules; Sodium Iodide I 131 Solution.

Proprietary Preparations (details are given in Part 3)
USA: Hipputope; Iodotope.

Iron-59 (5866-l)

CAS — 14596-12-4.

HALF-LIFE. 44.6 days.

Iron-59, in the form of ferrous citrate (^{59}Fe) or ferric citrate (^{59}Fe) is used by intravenous injection in the measurement of iron absorption and utilisation. Ferric chloride (^{59}Fe) has been given for the same purpose.

Preparations

BP 1998: Ferric Citrate(^{59}Fe) Injection.

Krypton-81m (18354-v)

CAS — 15678-91-8.

HALF-LIFE. 13.1 seconds.

Krypton-81m is a daughter of rubidium-81 ($^{81}_{37}$Rb; half-life 4.58 hours), and is prepared immediately before use by elution from a generator containing rubidium-81 adsorbed on a suitable ion-exchange column using humidified air or oxygen as the eluent. Krypton-81m is used as a gas in lung ventilation studies.

Preparations

USP 23: Krypton Kr 81m.

Nitrogen-13 (16918-s)

CAS — 13981-22-1.

HALF-LIFE. 9.96 minutes.

Nitrogen-13 is a positron-emitting radionuclide which is used in positron-emission tomography (p.1422). In the form of ammonia (^{13}N) it is given intravenously for imaging blood flow in organs such as the heart, brain, and liver. Nitrogen gas (^{13}N) may be used for pulmonary ventilation studies.

Preparations

USP 23: Ammonia N 13 Injection.

Oxygen-15 (17602-x)

HALF-LIFE. 2 minutes.

Oxygen-15 is a positron-emitting radionuclide used in positron-emission tomography (p.1422). It is employed in the form of water (^{15}O) and is given intravenously to study cerebral and myocardial perfusion.

Oxygen gas, carbon dioxide, and carbon monoxide have also been labelled with oxygen-15.

Preparations

USP 23: Water O 15 Injection.

Phosphorus-32 (5869-z)

CAS — 14596-37-3.

HALF-LIFE. 14.3 days.

Phosphorus-32, given as sodium phosphate (^{32}P), is used intravenously in the treatment of polycythaemia vera (p.495). Phosphorus-32 is taken up by the rapidly proliferating haematopoietic cells sufficiently to reduce their reproduction. Sodium phosphate (^{32}P) is also employed intravenously in the treatment of chronic myeloid (p.480) and chronic lymphocytic leukaemia (p.480) and in the palliative treatment of bone metastases.

Chromic phosphate (^{32}P) is administered intraperitoneally or intrapleurally in the treatment of malignant effusions (p.484); it may also be given by interstitial injection for the treatment of ovarian (p.491) or prostatic carcinoma (p.491).

Preparations

Ph. Eur.: Sodium Phosphate(^{32}P) Injection;
USP 23: Chromic Phosphate P 32 Suspension; Sodium Phosphate P 32 Solution.

Proprietary Preparations (details are given in Part 3)
USA: Phosphocol.

Rhenium-186 (3879-n)

CAS — 14998-63-1.

HALF-LIFE. 90.6 hours.

Rhenium-186 has been used in colloidal form for the treatment of arthritic joint conditions. Rhenium-186 etidronate has been investigated for the treatment of painful bone metastases. Monoclonal antibodies labelled with rhenium-186 have been investigated for the treatment of various malignant neoplasms.

Rubidium-82 (11869-f)

CAS — 14391-63-0.

HALF-LIFE. 75 seconds.

Rubidium-82 is a positron-emitting radionuclide which is used in positron-emission tomography (p.1422). Rubidium chloride (^{82}Rb) is administered intravenously for cardiac imaging.

Preparations

USP 23: Rubidium Chloride Rb 82 Injection.

Proprietary Preparations (details are given in Part 3)
USA: CardioGen 82.

Samarium-153 (12226-a)

HALF-LIFE. 47 hours.

Samarium-153, in the form of samarium lexidronam (samarium-EDTMP) (^{153}Sm), is used for the palliative treatment of painful bone metastases (p.484). It is given by intravenous injection.

Preparations

Proprietary Preparations (details are given in Part 3)
USA: Quadramet.

Selenium-75 (5872-w)

CAS — 14265-71-5.

HALF-LIFE. 118.5 days.

Selenium-75 in the form of 6β-[(methyl[^{75}Se]seleno)methyl]-19-norcholest-5(10)-en-3β-ol [selenonorcholestenol (^{75}Se)] is used in adrenal scintigraphy.

Selenium-75 in the form of tauroselcholic acid (^{75}Se) (^{75}SeHCAT) is used in the measurement of bile acid absorption for the assessment of ileal function.

Preparations

Proprietary Preparations (details are given in Part 3)
UK: Scintadren.

Strontium-89 (3881-a)

CAS — 14158-27-1.

HALF-LIFE. 50.5 days.

Strontium-89, in the form of strontium chloride (^{89}Sr), is used for the palliation of pain in patients with bone metastases (p.484); it is given intravenously.

References.

1. Robinson RG, *et al.* Strontium 89 therapy for the palliation of pain due to osseous metastases. *JAMA* 1995; **274:** 420–4.

Preparations

USP 23: Strontium Chloride Sr 89 Injection.

Proprietary Preparations (details are given in Part 3)
Canad.: Metastron; ***Fr.:*** Metastron; ***Ital.:*** Metastron; ***Spain:*** Metastron; ***UK:*** Metastron; ***USA:*** Metastron.

Technetium-99m (5878-c)

CAS — 14133-76-7 (technetium-99).

HALF-LIFE. 6.02 hours.

Adverse Effects

Hypersensitivity reactions have been reported with technetium-99m preparations.

Uses and Administration

Technetium-99m is a daughter of molybdenum-99 ($^{99}{}_{42}$Mo, half-life 66.2 hours) and because of its short half-life is normally prepared just before use by elution from a sterile generator consisting of molybdenum-99 adsorbed on to alumina in a glass column. Technetium-99m as pertechnetate ($^{99m}TcO_4^-$) is obtained by elution with a sterile solution of sodium chloride 0.9%. Radiopharmaceuticals of technetium-99m are prepared shortly after elution to reduce loss by decay.

Because it has a short half-life and can be administered in relatively large doses, and because the energy of its γ-emission is readily detected, technetium-99m is very widely used, either as the pertechnetate or in the form of various labelled compounds, particles, and colloids for scanning bone and organs such as the brain, heart, kidney, liver, lung, spleen, and thyroid.

Sodium pertechnetate (^{99m}Tc) is used intravenously for angiography and for imaging blood pools, brain, salivary glands, and thyroid gland; the oral route may also be employed for brain and thyroid imaging. Topical application to the eye is used for studying nasolachrymal drainage and the intraurethral route for imaging the urinary tract. Potassium perchlorate may be given before administration of the pertechnetate to prevent uptake in the thyroid or choroid plexus and thus enhance visualisation in other organs.

Macroaggregates of human albumin labelled with technetium-99m [macrosalb (^{99m}Tc)] are used in lung scanning for the detection of abnormal lung perfusion patterns; following the intravenous injection of a suspension of suitable particle size, usually 10 to 100 μm, the particles become trapped in the lung capillaries enabling ischaemic areas to be defined. Labelled albumin microspheres of particle size 10 to 50 μm are used similarly.

When technetium-99m bound to human serum albumin is administered intravenously it becomes evenly distributed in the circulation and highly vascular organs or pools of blood may be readily located. Such a preparation is used in the examination of the heart.

Technetium-99m in the form of a colloid, such as albumin, sulphur, antimony sulphide, or tin, is used intravenously for the examination of the liver, spleen, and bone marrow. Sulphur colloid (^{99m}Tc) may be given orally for oesophageal and gastro-intestinal imaging.

Technetium-99m complexes of iminodiacetic acid derivatives, such as disofenin, etifenin, lidofenin, and mebrofenin are employed intravenously in the investigation of hepatic function and in the imaging of the hepatobiliary system.

Agents used intravenously in both brain and renal imaging are technetium-99m-labelled gluconate, gluceptate, and pentetate. Other technetium-99m-labelled compounds are used in brain and kidney scanning; for instance, labelled bicisate and exametazime have been employed in brain imaging and mertiatide and succimer have been used in kidney studies.

For bone scanning various labelled phosphate compounds may be used and include medronate, oxidronate, and pyrophosphate, all given intravenously. Technetium-99m as the pyrophosphate is also used in cardiac scintigraphy. Technetium-99m medronate and pyrophosphate are also used to label red blood cells for use in blood pool scintigraphy, cardiac scintigraphy, detection of gastro-intestinal bleeding, and testicular scintigraphy.

Compounds employed intravenously in cardiac imaging include technetium-99m-labelled sestamibi, teboroxime, and tetrofosmin.

Technetium-99m-labelled leucocytes (prepared using exametazime) are employed for localisation of sites of inflammation or infection.

Monoclonal antibodies, such as arcitumomab, labelled with technetium-99m are used for the detection and localisation of malignant neoplasms.

Many other technetium-99m-labelled compounds have been prepared and used in different clinical studies for the examination of different organs or systems. Like radio-iodine, technetium-99m in various forms has been used to detect deep-vein thrombosis of the legs. Use with other radionuclides includes subtraction scanning with thallium-201 to detect parathyroid tumours.

Preparations

Ph. Eur.: Sodium Pertechnetate(^{99m}Tc) Injection (Fission); Sodium Pertechnetate(^{99m}Tc) Injection (Non-fission); Technetium (^{99m}Tc) Mertiatide Injection; Technetium(^{99m}Tc) Colloidal Rhenium Sulphide Injection; Technetium(^{99m}Tc) Colloidal Sulphur Injection; Technetium(^{99m}Tc) Colloidal Tin Injection; Technetium(^{99m}Tc) Etifenin Injection; Technetium(^{99m}Tc) Gluconate Injection; Technetium(^{99m}Tc) Human Albumin Injection; Technetium(^{99m}Tc) Macrosalb Injection; Technetium(^{99m}Tc) Medronate Injection; Technetium(^{99m}Tc) Microspheres Injection; Technetium(^{99m}Tc) Pentetate Injection; Technetium(^{99m}Tc) Succimer Injection; Technetium(^{99m}Tc) Tin Pyrophosphate Injection;
USP 23: Sodium Pertechnetate Tc 99m Injection; Technetium Tc 99m (Pyro- and trimeta-) Phosphates Injection; Technetium Tc 99m Albumin Aggregated Injection; Technetium Tc 99m Albumin Colloid Injection; Technetium Tc 99m Albumin Injection; Technetium Tc 99m Disofenin Injection; Technetium Tc 99m Etidronate Injection; Technetium Tc 99m Exametazime Injection; Technetium Tc 99m Gluceptate Injection; Technetium Tc 99m Lidofenin Injection; Technetium Tc 99m Mebrofenin Injection; Technetium Tc 99m Medronate Injection; Technetium Tc 99m Mertiatide Injection; Technetium Tc 99m Oxidronate Injection; Technetium Tc 99m Pentetate Injection; Technetium Tc 99m Pyrophosphate Injection; Technetium Tc 99m Red Blood Cells Injection; Technetium Tc 99m Sestamibi Injection; Technetium Tc 99m Succimer Injection; Technetium Tc 99m Sulfur Colloid Injection; Technetium Tc 99m Tetrofosmin Injection.

Proprietary Preparations (details are given in Part 3)

Aust.: Cardiolite; ***Canad.:*** Choletec; ***Fr.:*** Cardiolite; Ceretec; Myoview; Neurolite; ***Ital.:*** CEA-Scan; Ceretec; Myoview; TechneScan MAG3; ***Spain:*** Myoview; Neurolite; ***UK:*** Ceretec; Myoview; ***USA:*** CardioTec; CEA-Scan; Choletec; Macrotec; MDP-Squibb; OsteoScan; Phosphotec; Techneplex; Tesuloid.

Thallium-201 (5879-k)

CAS — 15064-65-0.

HALF-LIFE. 73.1 hours.

Thallium-201, in the form of thallous chloride (^{201}Tl), is administered by intravenous injection for scanning the myocardium in the investigation of acute myocardial infarction. It is also used for myocardial perfusion imaging in cardiac stress testing of patients with ischaemic heart disease. Adenosine (p.813), dipyridamole (p.857), or dobutamine (p.860) may be used to induce pharmacological stress in those patients unable to tolerate exercise.

Other uses include the localisation of parathyroid adenomas and hyperplasia by thallium-201 and technetium-99m subtraction scanning.

Preparations

Ph. Eur.: Thallous(^{201}Tl) Chloride Injection;
USP 23: Thallous Chloride Tl 201 Injection.

Tritium (5881-e)

Hydrogen-3.

CAS — 10028-17-8.

HALF-LIFE. 12.3 years.

Tritium, in the form of tritiated water, has been used to determine the total body water by a dilution technique.

Preparations

Ph. Eur.: Tritiated(^{3}H) Water Injection.

Xenon-127 (9910-s)

CAS — 13994-19-9.

HALF-LIFE. 36.41 days.

Xenon-127 has similar physical properties to those of xenon-133 (see below) and is also used by inhalation for pulmonary function studies and lung imaging.

Preparations

USP 23: Xenon Xe 127.

Xenon-133 (5882-l)

CAS — 14932-42-4.

HALF-LIFE. 5.25 days.

Xenon-133 is an inert gas with relatively low solubility in plasma. In the gaseous form, it is mixed with air or oxygen in a bag or in a closed or open circuit spirometer. When the administration of gas is stopped, xenon-133 is excreted promptly and completely through the lungs. It is used by inhalation in pulmonary function studies and lung imaging as well as in cerebral blood flow studies. It has also been employed for these purposes in the form of an injection in sodium chloride 0.9%.

Preparations

Ph. Eur.: Xenon(^{133}Xe) Injection;
USP 23: Xenon Xe 133; Xenon Xe 133 Injection.

Yttrium-90 (5883-y)

CAS — 10098-91-6.

HALF-LIFE. 64.1 hours.

Yttrium-90, in the form of a colloidal suspension of yttrium silicate (^{90}Y) is suitable for instillation into pleural or peritoneal cavities in the treatment of malignant pleural effusion (p.484) or malignant ascites (p.781).

Yttrium-90, as either yttrium citrate (^{90}Y) or yttrium silicate (^{90}Y), is also used in the treatment of arthritic conditions of joints.

Yttrium-90 conjugated to various monoclonal antibodies is being investigated for the treatment of malignant neoplasms.

Sex Hormones

The male and female sex organs, the adrenal cortex, and the placenta produce steroidal hormones which influence the development and maintenance of structures directly and indirectly associated with reproduction. The secretion of these sex hormones is controlled by gonadotrophic hormones of the anterior lobe of the pituitary gland; the secretion of these gonadotrophic hormones is in turn influenced by the hypothalamus and also by the concentration of circulating sex hormones. There are 3 groups of endogenous sex hormones, androgens, oestrogens, and progestogens, all of which are derived from the same steroidal precursors. The progestogenic hormone, progesterone is formed from pregnenolone, and both of these compounds may be converted to androgen precursors such as androstenedione. Androstenedione is converted to the androgenic hormone testosterone by hydroxysteroid dehydrogenases. Oestrogenic hormones are synthesised from androstenedione (and also from testosterone) by the action of aromatase.

Testosterone is the main androgenic hormone formed in the interstitial (Leydig) cells of the testes. A small proportion of circulating testosterone is also derived from the metabolism of less potent androgens secreted by the adrenal cortex and ovaries. In many target tissues testosterone is then converted to the more active dihydrotestosterone by 5α-reductase. Some testosterone also undergoes peripheral conversion to oestradiol.

Testosterone controls the development and maintenance of the male sex organs and the male secondary sex characteristics. It also produces systemic anabolic effects, such as increased retention of nitrogen, calcium, sodium, potassium, chloride, and phosphate. This leads to an increase in water retention and bone growth. The skin becomes more vascular and less fatty and erythropoiesis is increased.

Numerous derivatives of testosterone have been developed. Alkylation at the 17α position results in derivatives that are orally active (e.g. methyltestosterone, stanozolol) and esterification of the 17β-hydroxyl group increases lipid solubility and is used to prepare long-acting intramuscular preparations (e.g. testosterone enanthate). Removal of the 19-methyl group is reported to improve the anabolic to androgenic ratio (e.g. nandrolone). The derivatives also vary in their plasma protein binding affinity, and degree of conversion to dihydrotestosterone and aromatic conversion to oestrogen. Numerous other structural modifications have been made.

Oestradiol is the most active of the naturally occurring oestrogens formed from androgen precursors in the ovarian follicles of premenopausal women. In men and postmenopausal women (and to an insignificant extent in premenopausal women) oestrogens are also formed in adipose tissue from adrenal androgens.

Oestrogens control the development and maintenance of the female sex organs, secondary sex characteristics, and mammary glands as well as certain functions of the uterus and its accessory organs (particularly the proliferation of the endometrium, the development of the decidua, and the cyclic changes in the cervix and vagina). Large amounts of oestradiol are also formed in the placenta; in late pregnancy, this increases the spontaneous activity of the uterine muscle and its response to oxytocic drugs. The additional activity of progesterone is essential for the complete biological function of the female sex organs.

A number of oestrogens are used therapeutically. Ethinyl substitution at the C17 position has led to the development of synthetic oestrogens such as ethinyloestradiol and mestranol, which have greatly improved potency and oral activity. Oral activity of natural oestrogens is improved by esterification (e.g. oestradiol valerate) or by conjugation (e.g. oestrone sulphate). Esterification also increases solubility in lipid vehicles and is used to prepare long-acting intramuscular preparations.

A number of nonsteroidal oestrogens, including broparestrol, chlorotrianisene, dienoestrol, hexestrol, and stilboestrol, have also been used.

Progesterone is the main hormone secreted by the corpus luteum. It acts on the endometrium by converting the proliferative phase induced by oestrogen to a secretory phase thereby preparing the uterus to receive the fertilised ovum. Progesterone has a catabolic action and causes a slight rise in basal body temperature during the secretory phase of menstruation. Large quantities of progesterone are also produced by the placenta during pregnancy. During pregnancy it suppresses uterine motility and is responsible for the further development of the breasts.

Progestogens (gestagens, progestagens, progestins) are synthetic compounds with actions similar to those of progesterone. They are administered either as progesterone derivatives or as 19-nortestosterone analogues. The 19-nortestosterone analogues (such as norethisterone and norgestrel) possess some androgenic activity, but some newer norgestrel derivatives (desogestrel, gestodene, and norgestimate) have little androgenic activity. The progesterone derivatives dydrogesterone, hydroxyprogesterone, and medroxyprogesterone are less androgenic than the 19-nortestosterone analogues. The progesterone derivatives chlormadinone, and particularly cyproterone, have anti-androgenic activity.

The principal natural and synthetic sex hormones covered in this chapter are thus:

- **androgens and anabolic steroids**, typified by testosterone (p.1464)
- **oestrogens**, typified by oestradiol (p.1455)
- **progestogens**, typified by progesterone (p.1459).

Other related substances also described in this chapter are:

- drugs with predominantly **weak androgenic** properties such as danazol (p.1441) and gestrinone (p.1447)
- drugs which combine **oestrogenic and progestogenic** properties such as tibolone (p.1466)
- drugs with predominantly **anti-androgenic** properties. These include the progesterone derivative cyproterone acetate, the nonsteroidal 5α-reductase inhibitor finasteride, and the plant extract saw palmetto. Those anti-androgens that are used principally in the hormonal treatment of prostate cancer are covered in the Antineoplastics chapter. These include the nonsteroidal drugs bicalutamide (p.507), flutamide (p.537), and nilutamide (p.556)
- drugs with predominantly **anti-oestrogenic** properties. These include the nonsteroidal anti-oestrogens clomiphene, cyclofenil, and the more selective nonsteroidal anti-oestrogens ormeloxifene and raloxifene. Those anti-oestrogens used in the hormonal treatment of breast cancer are covered in the Antineoplastics chapter. These include the oestrogen receptor antagonists tamoxifen (p.563) and toremifene (p.567), and various nonsteroidal aromatase inhibitors such as formestane (p.537) and anastrozole (p.504)
- drugs with predominantly **antiprogestogenic** properties such as the progestogen derivative mifepristone.

The activity of endogenous sex hormones can be modulated by gonadotrophins, and gonadorelin and its analogues, and these are discussed in the Hypothalamic and Pituitary Hormones chapter, beginning on p.1235.

The therapeutic application of sex hormones and related substances is broad and covers many circumstances where hormonal manipulation is desirable. Major applications are the use of oestrogens and progestogens for **contraception** (see Hormonal Contraceptives, p.1434) and for the alleviation of **menopausal symptoms** (see Hormone Replacement Therapy, p.1437). A physiological application is the use of an androgen or an oestrogen in the management of **delayed puberty** and **hypogonadism**, (see Testosterone, p.1465 or Oestradiol, p.1456). Other clinical applications include the management of **benign prostatic hyperplasia** (p.1446), **endometriosis** (p.1442), **gynaecomastia** (p.1442), **hirsutism** (p.1441), **infertility** (p.1239), **mastalgia** (p.1443), **menorrhagia** (p.1461), and **premenstrual syndrome** (p.1456). Hormonal manipulation also has an important role in the treatment of **malignant neoplasms** of the breast (p.485), prostate (p.491), and endometrium (p.487).

Hormonal Contraceptives (9021-f)

Hormonal contraceptives are currently only available for women although preparations for men are being evaluated. Oral hormonal contraceptives for women are divided into 2 main types: 'combined' (containing an oestrogen and a progestogen) and 'progestogen-only'. Parenteral progestogen-only preparations have also been developed and include subcutaneous implants and depot intramuscular injections. Progesterone-containing intra-uterine devices are also available.

Progestogens inhibit ovulation by suppressing the necessary mid-cycle surge of luteinising hormone. However, the low doses in progestogen-only oral contraceptives do not suppress it reliably in all cycles. Contraceptive efficacy is instead achieved by thickening the cervical mucus so that it is not readily penetrated by sperm, and by preventing proliferation of the endometrium so that it remains unfavourable for implantation of any fertilised ova. Intra-uterine progestogen-only devices act similarly; the physical presence of the system in the uterus may also contribute to overall contraceptive efficacy. Parenteral progestogen-only contraceptives on the other hand provide reliable suppression of ovulation.

Oestrogens inhibit ovulation by suppressing the mid-cycle release of follicle-stimulating hormone. They act synergistically with progestogens in combined oral contraceptives to provide regular and consistent suppression of ovulation.

Combined oral preparations are also available for *emergency contraception* after unprotected coitus; they prevent implantation of any fertilised ova.

Adverse Effects

Many reports have been published of adverse effects associated with the use of **combined oral contraceptives**. The data has mostly been gained retrospectively and often involves older preparations containing higher doses of oestrogen and progestogen than are used currently.

There may be gastro-intestinal side-effects such as nausea or vomiting, chloasma (melasma), and other skin or hair changes, headache, water retention, weight gain, breast tenderness, and changes in libido.

Menstrual irregularities such as spotting, breakthrough bleeding, or amenorrhoea can occur during treatment. These effects may result from the relative balance of oestrogenic and progestogenic effects of particular products and their incidence may be reduced by changing to a different product. For example, early or mid-cycle spotting or absence of withdrawal bleeding may require a preparation with a greater oestrogen to progestogen ratio, or less progestogen as in multiphasic preparations, or temporary supplementation with an oestrogen.

Intolerance to contact lenses has been reported and vision may deteriorate in myopic patients. Some patients may experience depression and other mental changes. Preparations containing a progestogen with androgenic properties such as levonorgestrel and norgestrel may be associated with increased oiliness of the skin and acne. Conversely, acne may be improved with progestogens such as norgestimate or desogestrel.

There is an increased risk of cardiovascular disease and associated mortality related, at least in part, to the oestrogen content of combined oral contraceptives. The incidence of cardiovascular side-effects is probably less with the newer lower-dose preparations than with the older higher-dose preparations. Increased mortality from myocardial infarction is much greater with increased age and in cigarette smokers, although some evidence suggests that healthy women aged over 35 years who do not smoke are not at increased risk. Other risk factors include a family history of arterial disease, diabetes mellitus, hypertension, obesity, and migraine. Thrombosis may be more common when factor V Leiden is present or in patients with blood groups A, B, or AB. Specific risk factors for venous thrombo-embolism include a family history of venous thrombo-embolism, varicose veins and, again obesity. Recent evidence has also indicated that the risk of venous thrombo-embolism varies according to the progestogen component of combined oral contraceptives; a higher incidence has been associated with desogestrel and gestodene than with levonorgestrel, norethisterone, and ethynodiol. For further discussion see Venous Thrombo-embolism, below.

Combined oral contraceptives may cause hypertension and there may be reduced glucose tolerance and changes in lipid metabolism. Liver function can be impaired, although jaundice is rare. There appears to be a marked increase (though the incidence is still very low) in the relative risk of benign liver tumours. Malignant liver tumours have also been reported.

Combined oral contraceptives are reported to slightly increase the risk of cervical cancer (although other factors may be involved) and breast cancer, but to protect against ovarian cancer and endometrial cancer. For further discussion, see Carcinogenicity, below.

As with combined oral contraceptives, **progestogen-only contraceptives** may cause nausea, vomiting, headache, breast discomfort, depression, skin disorders, and weight gain. Menstrual irregularities such as amenorrhoea, breakthrough bleeding, spotting, and menorrhagia are more common with progestogen-only contraceptives, and are particularly common with parenteral preparations. Available progestogen-only contraceptives carry less risk of thrombo-embolic and cardiovascular disease than combined oral contraceptives.

Carcinogenicity. Concern has often been expressed as to whether the use of hormonal contraceptives by normally healthy women may either cause or increase the risk of developing malignant neoplasms. To investigate any possible link between such use and cancer, two main types of study have been employed by epidemiologists, namely the prospective study and the case-control study. Many factors have made direct comparison of results difficult and such factors include the type and composition of oral contraceptive used (which has changed over the years), the age of the patient, the age at which the contraceptives were first used, and the sexual and obstetric history of the patient. Overall, however, the evidence indicates that combined oral contraceptives in fact exert a protective effect against the development of endometrial and ovarian carcinoma. However, there is a small increase in risk of breast cancer during use and for 10 years after discontinuation. In addition, there does appear to be a slight risk of cervical cancer with the prolonged use of combined oral contraceptives and a negligible risk of liver cancer. For further details concerning the effects on individual organs, see the following sections. It should be noted that even where the relative risk has been shown to be substantially increased this will not translate into many new cases of a rare cancer, and this contributes to the difficulties of assessing clinical relevance. It is also worthy of note that two large prospective cohort studies (the Nurses' Health Study and the Royal College of General Practitioners' study) found no evidence of a difference in overall mortality between women who had used oral contraceptives and those who had not.[1,4] Some general reviews on hormonal contraceptives and cancer are cited below.[2,3]

1. Colditz GA, *et al.* Oral contraceptive use and mortality during 12 years of follow-up: the Nurses' Health Study. *Ann Intern Med* 1994; **120:** 821–6.
2. WHO. Oral contraceptives and neoplasia: report of a WHO scientific group. *WHO Tech Rep Ser 817* 1992.
3. La Vecchia C, *et al.* Oral contraceptives and cancer: a review of the evidence. *Drug Safety* 1996; **14:** 260–72.
4. Beral V, *et al.* Mortality associated with oral contraceptive use: 25 year follow up of cohort of 46 000 women from Royal College of General Practitioners' oral contraception study. *Br Med J* 1999; **318:** 96–100.

BREAST. Numerous epidemiological studies have been published on the potential link between hormonal contraceptives and breast cancer. Most of these data relate to **combined oral contraceptives**, which are the most widely used form. The breast cancer risk from use of these contraceptives will require monitoring for some time to come as the first users of oral contraceptives continue to age, and because of the changing patterns of use.

Early studies from the 1980s variously failed to show any significant increase in risk of breast cancer in women who had ever used hormonal contraceptives compared with those who had never done so,[1-4] or showed an increase in risk,[5] or identified a risk in specific sub-groups of users.[6-12] Potential identified risk factors, for which much of the evidence is conflicting, included current use,[10] duration of use,[7,11] age at first use,[6] duration of use before a first full-term pregnancy,[7,8] nulliparity,[9] high-dose preparations,[11] and family history of breast cancer.[12] It was also reported that use of oral contraceptives might lead to an accelerated presentation of breast cancer,[13] or an increased risk of invasive cancer.[4]

In response to these studies, the Committee on Safety of Medicines in the UK,[14] the Food and Drug Administration in the USA,[15] and the International Committee for Research in Reproduction[16] issued advice that the available evidence did not require a change in prescribing practice. This advice has not been subsequently changed, although patients should be informed of the possible small increase in risk of breast cancer, which has to be weighed against established benefits of therapy.[23]

From 1990 to 1995, over 20 major studies have been published on the oral contraceptive-breast cancer issue, and have been reviewed by La Vecchia *et al.*[17] In general, these studies have shown some excess breast cancer risk in current or recent users of oral contraceptives, but no excess risk for use more than 5 years previously. In contrast to some earlier studies, duration of use tended not to affect risk, neither did any of the major recognised risk factors for breast cancer.

More recently, a Collaborative Group on Hormonal Factors in Breast Cancer was set up to re-analyse all the worldwide epidemiological evidence on breast cancer risk and hormonal contraceptives. The group identified individual data on 53 297 women with breast cancer, and 100 239 controls (women without breast cancer) from 54 studies, and have published a summary of their findings,[18] and a further detailed review.[19] They reported that women currently using oral contraceptives have a slight increase in the relative risk of breast cancer (1.24; 95% confidence intervals 1.15 to 1.33), and that this risk decreases after stopping use, and is no longer significant after 10 or more years. There was a weak trend towards an increase in risk with increasing duration of use. Thus, it appears that the risk of breast cancer increases soon after first exposure, does not increase with duration of exposure, and returns to normal 10 years after cessation of exposure.[18]

Cancers diagnosed in those who had ever used hormonal contraceptives were clinically less advanced than in those who had never done so.[18] Further information is required on whether this is related to earlier diagnosis or a biological effect of the hormones. In addition, data on breast cancer mortality are required.

When analysed by age at first use, the risk was largest in those women who started use as teenagers. Because of the trend towards earlier use, further review of long-term data is required.[18] The most important risk factor is, however, the age at which women discontinue the contraceptive; the greater the age at stopping, the more breast cancers are diagnosed.[23]

There was no difference in risk between nulliparous women, parous women who began use of oral contraceptives before their first child, and parous women who began use of oral contraceptives after the birth of their first child.[18]

Low-dose oral contraceptives were not associated with a decreased risk of breast cancer.[18] When preparations were grouped according to oestrogen dose (less than 50 μg, 50 μg, and greater than 50 μg), there was, if anything, a decrease in breast cancer risk with increasing dose among women who had stopped use 10 or more years before, largely due to a reduction in breast cancer risk in those who had used the highest dose preparations.

There are far fewer data on risk of breast cancer with **progestogen-only contraceptives**, which are less frequently used than combined preparations.

A WHO study published in 1991 indicated that, overall, depot medroxyprogesterone acetate did not increase the risk of breast cancer (relative risk compared with never users 1.21; 95% confidence intervals 0.96 to 1.53) and that risk did not increase with duration of use.[20] However, there appeared to be a slight increase in risk within the first 4 years of use, especially in women under 35 years of age. These findings agreed with those of a smaller study by Paul *et al.*[21] in which women who had used depot medroxyprogesterone acetate for 2 years or longer before the age of 25 had a relative risk of 4.6. Pooled analysis of these 2 studies indicated that current or recent use was the key factor.[22] The relative risk of breast cancer in women who had used medroxyprogesterone acetate in the last 5 years was 2.0, and there was no increased risk in women who had ceased use more than 5 years previously, regardless of their duration of use.

The Collaborative Group on Hormonal Factors in Breast Cancer reported that there was some evidence of an increased risk of breast cancer for use of oral or injectable progestogens in the previous 5 years (relative risk 1.17), and no risk 10 or more years after stopping use.[18] These findings were broadly similar to those for combined preparations. As for combined preparations, the most important factor is the age at discontinuation. For women who stop by age 30 after 5 years use of a progestogen-only preparation there would be an estimated increase from 44 to 46 or 47 cases per 10 000 compared with those who have never used a hormonal contraceptive. For 5 years use stopping by age 40 there would be an estimated increase from 160 to 170 cases diagnosed in the following 10 years.[23]

1. Ellery C, *et al.* A case-control study of breast cancer in relation to the use of steroid contraceptive agents. *Med J Aust* 1986; **144:** 173–6.
2. Paul C, *et al.* Oral contraceptives and breast cancer: a national study. *Br Med J* 1986; **293:** 723–6.
3. The Cancer and Steroid Hormone Study of the Centers for Disease Control and the National Institute of Child Health and Human Development. Oral-contraceptive use and the risk of breast cancer. *N Engl J Med* 1986; **315:** 405–11.
4. Stanford JL, *et al.* Oral contraceptives and breast cancer: results from an expanded case-control study. *Br J Cancer* 1989; **60:** 375–81.
5. Miller DR, *et al.* Breast cancer before age 45 and oral contraceptive use: new findings. *Am J Epidemiol* 1989; **129:** 269–80.
6. Pike MC, *et al.* Breast cancer in young women and use of oral contraceptives: possible modifying effect of formulation and age at use. *Lancet* 1983; **ii:** 926–30.
7. Meirik O, *et al.* Oral contraceptive use and breast cancer in young women: a joint national case-control study in Sweden and Norway. *Lancet* 1986; **ii:** 650–4.
8. McPherson K, *et al.* Early oral contraceptive use and breast cancer: results of another case-control study. *Br J Cancer* 1987; **56:** 653–60.
9. Meirik O, *et al.* Breast cancer and oral contraceptives: patterns of risk among parous and nulliparous women—further analysis of the Swedish-Norwegian material. *Contraception* 1989; **39:** 471–5.
10. Romieu I, *et al.* Prospective study of oral contraceptive use and risk of breast cancer in women. *J Natl Cancer Inst* 1989; **81:** 1313–21.
11. UK National Case-Control Study Group. Oral contraceptive use and breast cancer risk in young women. *Lancet* 1989; **i:** 973–82.
12. UK National Case-Control Study Group. Oral contraceptive use and breast cancer risk in young women: subgroup analyses. *Lancet* 1990; **335:** 1507–9.
13. Kay CR, Hannaford PC. Breast cancer and the pill—a further report from the Royal College of General Practitioners' oral contraception study. *Br J Cancer* 1988; **58:** 675–80.
14. Committee on Safety of Medicines. Oral contraceptives and carcinoma of the breast. *Current Problems 26* 1989.
15. Anonymous. Cancer risks of oral contraception. *Lancet* 1989; **i:** 84.
16. International Committee for Research in Reproduction. Oral contraceptives and breast cancer. *JAMA* 1989; **262:** 206–7.
17. La Vecchia C, *et al.* Oral contraceptives and cancer: a review of the evidence. *Drug Safety* 1996; **14:** 260–72.
18. Collaborative Group on Hormonal Factors in Breast Cancer. Breast cancer and hormonal contraceptives: collaborative reanalysis of individual data on 53 297 women with breast cancer and 100 239 women without breast cancer from 54 epidemiological studies. *Lancet* 1996; **347:** 1713–27.
19. Collaborative Group on Hormonal Factors in Breast Cancer. Breast cancer and hormonal contraceptives: further results. *Contraception* 1996; **54** (suppl): 1S–106S.
20. WHO Collaborative Study of Neoplasia and Steroid Contraceptives. Breast cancer and depot-medroxyprogesterone acetate: a multinational study. *Lancet* 1991; **338:** 833–8.

21. Paul C, *et al.* Depot medroxyprogesterone (Depo-Provera) and risk of breast cancer. *Br Med J* 1989; **299:** 759–62.
22. Skegg DCG, *et al.* Depot medroxyprogesterone acetate and breast cancer: a pooled analysis of the World Health Organization and New Zealand studies. *JAMA* 1995; **273:** 799–804.
23. Committee on Safety of Medicines/Medicines Control Agency. Oral contraceptives and breast cancer. *Current Problems* 1998; **24:** 2–3.

CERVIX. It is often considered difficult to carry out satisfactory epidemiological studies on the relationship between hormonal contraceptives and cervical cancer because of the many known variables and factors which may influence the development of this type of neoplasm. For example, sexual activity *per se,* and multiple sexual partners (both of the woman and her partner) increase the risk, while the use of other non-hormonal barrier methods of contraception may offer some protection against cervical neoplasia. Nevertheless, there have been some suggestions that the use of oral contraceptives may be associated with an increased risk.

Two UK cohort studies from the 1980s revealed an increased risk of cervical cancer in women receiving oral contraceptives that was shown to increase with increasing duration of use.[1,2]

In 1992, WHO reviewed these cohort data, and data from 18 case-controlled studies carried out up to 1990.[3] They concluded that use of oral contraceptives for more than 5 years was associated with a modest increase in the relative risk of cervical squamous cell carcinoma (in the order of 1.3 to 1.8). Additional potential risk factors included recent or current use and high oestrogen dose. Of known risk factors for cervical cancer, women with multiple sexual partners, genital infection, or high parity had higher risks associated with oral contraceptives.[3].

Most cervical cancers are squamous cell carcinomas, but it has been proposed that oral contraceptive use might be a particular risk factor for the rarer adenocarcinoma of the cervix, the incidence of which has risen in younger women. Reviewing studies up to 1990, WHO concluded that data were insufficient to draw firm conclusions on links between oral contraceptives and the risk of cervical adenocarcinoma.[3] A case-controlled study from 1994 found an increased risk of adenocarcinoma of the cervix in users of oral contraceptives.[4] Any use of oral contraceptives was associated with an approximate doubling of risk, and use for more than 12 years was associated with a relative risk 4.4 times greater than that in women who never used an oral contraceptive. More recently, a WHO study reported that the strength of the observed relationship for cervical adenocarcinomas and adenosquamous carcinomas and oral contraceptives was about the same as that for invasive squamous cell cervical carcinomas.[5]

Human papilloma virus (HPV) has a role in the aetiology of cervical cancer and women who are HPV positive using oral contraceptives may be at increased risk of cervical neoplasm.[6]

Data on the risk of cervical cancer with **progestogen-only contraceptives** are limited. WHO have investigated any possible link between the use of medroxyprogesterone acetate as a long-acting injectable contraceptive and cervical neoplasia. Analysis showed a small non-significant elevated risk (1.11; 95% confidence interval 0.9 to 1.29), and no clear association with duration of use.[7]

1. Vessey MP, *et al.* Neoplasia of the cervix uteri and contraception: a possible adverse effect of the pill. *Lancet* 1983; **ii:** 930–4.
2. Beral V, *et al.* Oral contraceptive use, and malignancies of the genital tract: results from the Royal College of General Practitioners' oral contraception study. *Lancet* 1988; **ii:** 1331–5.
3. WHO. Oral contraceptives and neoplasia: report of a WHO scientific group. *WHO Tech Rep Ser 817* 1992.
4. Ursin G, *et al.* Oral contraceptive use and adenocarcinoma of cervix. *Lancet* 1994; **344:** 1390–4.
5. Thomas DB, Ray RM. Oral contraceptives and invasive adenocarcinomas and adenosquamous carcinomas of the uterine cervix. *Am J Epidemiol* 1996; **144:** 281–9.
6. La Vecchia C, *et al.* Oral contraceptives and cancer: a review of the evidence. *Drug Safety* 1996; **14:** 260–72.
7. WHO Collaborative Study of Neoplasia and Steroid Contraceptives. Depot-medroxyprogesterone acetate (DMPA) and risk of invasive squamous cell cervical cancer. *Contraception* 1992; **45:** 299–312.

ENDOMETRIUM. It has been reliably demonstrated that **combined oral contraceptives** decrease the risk of endometrial cancer. WHO analysed data from case-control and cohort studies published up to 1990,[1] including data from the large Cancer and Steroid Hormone Study (CASH) in the USA,[2] and reported that there was a highly significant trend of decreasing risk of endometrial cancer with increasing duration of use of combined oral contraceptives. The reduction in risk was estimated to be 20% after 1 year and 50% after 4 years' use.[1] The protective effect was observed for endometrial cancer with and without squamous elements,[1,2] and was found to persist for at least 15 years after cessation of use.[2] A more recent study with longer term follow-up indicated that the protection persists for at least 20 years.[3] Thus, further follow-up is required to determine the true duration of protection.

The results of the WHO Collaborative Study on Neoplasia and Steroid Contraceptives suggested that protection may be greater with preparations containing high-dose progestogen.[4] However, a more recent study found that risk of endometrial cancer was unrelated to progestogen potency of the oral contraceptive, although this study also reported no protective effect for less than 5 years' use.[5]

Unopposed menopausal oestrogen replacement therapy is known to increase the risk of endometrial cancer (see p.1435), and it has been suggested that the protective effect of oral contraceptives may be reduced in women who subsequently use this. There is some evidence that this may be the case.[3,5]

There are limited data on the effect of **progestogen-only contraceptives** on the risk of endometrial cancer, although they would be expected to be protective. Results from the WHO Collaborative Study[6] suggest that depot medroxyprogesterone acetate reduced the risk of endometrial cancer; the estimated relative risk in those who had used this parenteral contraceptive was 0.21. However, many of the women in this study received supplemental oestrogen to control menstrual irregularity, and were therefore technically taking a form of combined therapy.[7] There was some evidence that the protective effect of medroxyprogesterone acetate was greater in women who had not received oestrogen,[7] and this requires further study.

1. WHO. Oral contraceptives and neoplasia: report of a WHO scientific group. *WHO Tech Rep Ser 817* 1992.
2. The Cancer and Steroid Hormone Study of the Centers for Disease Control and the National Institute of Child Health and Human Development. Combination oral contraceptive use and the risk of endometrial cancer. *JAMA* 1987; **257:** 796–800.
3. Stanford JL, *et al.* Oral contraceptives and endometrial cancer: do other risk factors modify the association? *Int J Cancer* 1993; **54:** 243–8.
4. Rosenblatt KA, *et al.* Hormonal content of combined oral contraceptives in relation to the reduced risk of endometrial carcinoma. *Int J Cancer* 1991; **49:** 870–4.
5. Voigt LF, *et al.* Recency, duration, and progestin content of oral contraceptives in relation to the incidence of endometrial cancer. *Cancer Causes Control* 1994; **5:** 227–33.
6. WHO Collaborative Study of Neoplasia and Steroid Contraceptives. Depot-medroxyprogesterone acetate (DMPA) and risk of endometrial cancer. *Int J Cancer* 1991; **49:** 186–90.
7. Szarewski A, Guillebaud J. Safety of DMPA. *Lancet* 1991; **338:** 1157–8.

LIVER. The use of **combined oral contraceptives** has been rarely associated with liver tumours, both benign (hepatic adenomas and focal nodular hyperplasia)[1] and malignant (hepatocellular carcinoma).[1,2]

Hepatocellular carcinomas are associated with hepatitis B, and are relatively common in countries where this is endemic but rare elsewhere. Case-control studies in populations at high risk for hepatocellular carcinoma suggest that the use or oral contraceptives does not appear to significantly affect the risk, although long-term data are scanty.[3,4] In contrast, case-control studies in countries where the prevalence of hepatitis B is low have shown an increased risk of hepatocellular carcinoma among users of oral contraceptives, particularly after long-term use (reviewed by WHO[1] and La Vecchia[2]). However, because the malignancy is so rare, this increased risk may be negligible.[2] For example, there has been no increase in mortality from liver cancer in young women in the UK since the introduction and use of oral contraceptives.[5] Similar findings have been reported for the USA and Sweden.[6]

There are limited data specifically on **progestogen-only contraceptives**. Results from a WHO study[7] provided no evidence that use of medroxyprogesterone acetate as a long-acting injectable contraceptive altered the risk of developing liver cancer but the power of the study to detect any small alterations in risk was low.

1. WHO. Oral contraceptives and neoplasia: report of a WHO scientific group. *WHO Tech Rep Ser 817* 1992.
2. La Vecchia C, *et al.* Oral contraceptives and cancer: a review of the evidence. *Drug Safety* 1996; **14:** 260–72.
3. The WHO Collaborative Study of Neoplasia and Steroid Contraceptives. Combined oral contraceptives and liver cancer. *Int J Cancer* 1989; **43:** 254–9.
4. Kew MC, *et al.* Contraceptive steroids as a risk factor for hepatocellular carcinoma: a case/control study in South African black women. *Hepatology* 1990; **11:** 298–302.
5. Mant JWF, Vessey MP. Trends in mortality from primary liver cancer in England and Wales 1975-1992: influence of oral contraceptives. *Br J Cancer* 1995; **72:** 800–3.
6. Waetjen LE, Grimes DA. Oral contraceptives and primary liver cancer: temporal trends in three countries. *Obstet Gynecol* 1996; **88:** 945–9.
7. Anonymous. Depot-medroxyprogesterone acetate (DMPA) and cancer: memorandum from a WHO meeting. *Bull WHO* 1986; **64:** 375–82.

OVARY. There is convincing evidence that **combined oral contraceptives** reduce the risk of ovarian cancer,[1,2] possibly as a function of their inhibition of ovulation. Relative risks for ovarian cancer have variously been reported as 0.4 to 0.8 in those who have ever used oral contraceptives, and decrease with increasing duration of use. There is evidence that there may be a delay of several years before the protective effect becomes apparent, but that it persists for as long as 20 years after cessation of use.[3] The protective effect has been noted for both malignant and borderline malignant tumours, and for each of the major histological subtypes of epithelial ovarian cancer.

Recently it has been suggested that newer lower-dose oestrogen preparations may be slightly less protective than higher-dose preparations.[4] The relative risk for use of high-dose preparations was 0.68, and for low-dose preparations was 0.81.

It has been suggested that the protective effect against ovarian cancer has significant implications for public health. For example, it was estimated that oral contraceptive use may have prevented nearly one-quarter of deaths expected to occur due to ovarian cancer in 1986 in women aged 54 years or less in England and Wales.[5]

There are few data on the effects of **progestogen-only contraceptives** on the risk of ovarian cancer. WHO have investigated the effect of depot medroxyprogesterone acetate on ovarian cancer, and found that it was not associated with either a decrease or increase in risk (relative risk 1.07; 95% confidence interval 0.6 to 1.8).[6] This is perhaps surprising since the preparation, like combined oral contraceptives, inhibits ovulation.

1. Franceschi S, *et al.* Pooled analysis of 3 European case-control studies of epithelial ovarian cancer III: oral contraceptive use. *Int J Cancer* 1991; **49:** 61–5.
2. Whittemore AS, *et al.* Characteristics relating to ovarian cancer risk: collaborative analysis of 12 US case-control studies II: invasive epithelial ovarian cancers in white women. *Am J Epidemiol* 1992; **136:** 1184–1203.
3. Rosenberg L, *et al.* A case-control study of oral contraceptive use and invasive epithelial ovarian cancer. *Am J Epidemiol* 1994; **139:** 654–61.
4. Rosenblatt KA, *et al.* High-dose and low-dose combined oral contraceptives: protection against epithelial ovarian cancer and the length of the protective effect. *Eur J Cancer* 1992; **28A:** 1872–6.
5. Villard-Mackintosh L, *et al.* The effects of oral contraceptives and parity on ovarian cancer trends in women under 55 years of age. *Br J Obstet Gynaecol* 1989; **96:** 783–8.
6. WHO Collaborative Study of Neoplasia and Steroid Contraceptives. Depot-medroxyprogesterone acetate (DMPA) and risk of epithelial ovarian cancer. *Int J Cancer* 1991; **49:** 191–5.

SKIN. Although there have been some suggestions of a possible association between the use of oral contraceptives and the development of malignant melanoma[1-3] most studies, including recent analyses of relatively large numbers of women suffering from malignant melanoma, found no such association with either current or prior use of oral contraceptive preparations.[4-9] A meta-analysis of 18 case-control studies confirmed the lack of association.[10]

1. Beral V, *et al.* Malignant melanoma and oral contraceptive use among women in California. *Br J Cancer* 1977; **36:** 804–9.
2. Lerner AB, *et al.* Effects of oral contraceptives and pregnancy on melanomas. *N Engl J Med* 1979; **301:** 47.
3. Beral V, *et al.* Oral contraceptive use and malignant melanoma in Australia. *Br J Cancer* 1984; **50:** 681–5.
4. Bain C, *et al.* Oral contraceptive use and malignant melanoma. *J Natl Cancer Inst* 1982; **68:** 537–9.
5. Helmrich SP, *et al.* Lack of an elevated risk of malignant melanoma in relation to oral contraceptive use. *J Natl Cancer Inst* 1984; **72:** 617–20.
6. Green A, Bain C. Hormonal factors and melanoma in women. *Med J Aust* 1985; **142:** 446–8.
7. Østerlind A, *et al.* The Danish case-control study of cutaneous malignant melanoma III: hormonal and reproductive factors in women. *Int J Cancer* 1988; **42:** 821–4.
8. Palmer JR, *et al.* Oral contraceptive use and risk of cutaneous malignant melanoma. *Cancer Causes Control* 1992; **3:** 547–54.
9. Holly EA, *et al.* Cutaneous melanoma in women III: reproductive factors and oral contraceptive use. *Am J Epidemiol* 1995; **141:** 943–50.
10. Gefeller O, *et al.* Cutaneous malignant melanoma in women and the role of oral contraceptives. *Br J Dermatol* 1998; **138:** 122–4.

Ectopic pregnancy. Pregnancies in users of oral (but not parenteral) progestogen-only contraceptives are more likely to be ectopic than are pregnancies occurring in the general population. Oral progestogen-only contraceptives do not reliably inhibit ovulation and therefore offer less protection against ectopic pregnancy than against intra-uterine pregnancy. Early references to this effect are cited below.[1-5] Since parenteral progestogen-only contraceptives provide reliable suppression of ovulation, like combined oral contraceptives, they protect against both ectopic pregnancies and functional ovarian cysts. In the case of the levonorgestrel-releasing progestogen-only implant the risk of ectopic pregnancy is believed to be reduced overall, but the proportion of ectopic to intra-uterine pregnancies is increased among the very few pregnancies that do occur.

1. Bonnar J. Progestagen-only contraception and tubal pregnancies. *Lancet* 1974; **i:** 170–1.
2. Bonnar J. Progestogen-only contraceptive and tubal pregnancies. *Br Med J* 1974; **1:** 287.
3. Huntington KM. Progestagen-only contraception and tubal pregnancies. *Lancet* 1974; **i:** 360.
4. Liukko P, Erkkola R. Low-dose progestogens and ectopic pregnancy. *Br Med J* 1976; **2:** 1257.
5. Corcoran R, Howard R. Low-dose progestagens and ectopic pregnancy. *Lancet* 1977; **i:** 98–9.

Effects on carbohydrate metabolism. The potential effects of oral contraceptives on glucose tolerance are of particular concern because of the risk that impaired glucose tolerance will exacerbate their cardiovascular effects.[1] Early studies suggested that the prevalence of abnormal glucose tolerance in oral contraceptive users was increased from about 4 to 35% but subsequent studies produced conflicting results. Possible reasons for these discrepancies may include failure to discriminate between differing doses of oestrogen and between the differing types and doses of progestogen used in the preparation. It has been shown that the decrease in glucose tolerance is related not only to oestrogen doses greater than 75 μg daily but also to the type of progestogen. As most oral contraceptives used currently contain lower doses of oestrogen the important question is whether such low-dose preparations have deleterious effects. Levonorgestrel has been reported to be the most potent progestogen in decreasing glucose tolerance[2] whereas preliminary results of another study have suggested that a combined oral contraceptive containing norethisterone does not result in a deterioration of glucose tolerance.[3] It is therefore considered[1] that preparations containing high doses of levonorgestrel should be prescribed for long-term use only after the most careful consideration, especially in patients with a past history of gestational diabetes or with impaired glucose tolerance.

However, a subsequent study has suggested that glucose tolerance testing may not be the best way of assessing the effects of oral contraceptives on carbohydrate metabolism.[4] In this study, in which insulin and C-peptide production was also measured, it was found that although levonorgestrel-containing combined preparations had a greater effect on glucose tolerance, desogestrel- or norethindrone-containing preparations produced a similar degree of insulin resistance, suggesting that this depends on the oestrogenic component, and is modified by the progestogen.

Despite these effects, data from the Nurses' Health Study indicate that oral contraceptives do not appear to increase the risk of developing type 2 diabetes mellitus.[5,6] However a study in the USA, in breast-feeding women of Hispanic origin who had experienced recent gestational diabetes, suggested that the use of progestogen-only, but not combined, contraceptives was associated with an increased risk of developing type 2 diabetes mellitus in this group.[7]

1. Taylor R. Drugs and glucose tolerance. *Adverse Drug React Bull* 1986; (Dec.): 452–5.
2. Perlman JA, *et al.* Oral glucose tolerance and the potency of contraceptive progestins. *J Chron Dis* 1985; **38:** 857–64.
3. Wynn V. Effect of duration of low-dose oral contraceptive administration on carbohydrate metabolism. *Am J Obstet Gynecol* 1982; **142:** 739–46.
4. Godsland IF, *et al.* Insulin resistance, secretion, and metabolism in users of oral contraceptives. *J Clin Endocrinol Metab* 1991; **74:** 64–70.
5. Rimm EB, *et al.* Oral contraceptive use and the risk of type 2 (non-insulin-dependent) diabetes mellitus in a large prospective study of women. *Diabetologia* 1992; **35:** 967–72.
6. Chasan-Taber L, *et al.* A prospective study of oral contraceptives and NIDDM among US women. *Diabetes Care* 1997; **20:** 330–5.
7. Kjos SL, *et al.* Contraception and the risk of type 2 diabetes mellitus in Latina women with prior gestational diabetes mellitus. *JAMA* 1998; **280:** 533–8.

Effects on the cardiovascular system. Soon after their introduction in the 1960s it became apparent that **combined oral contraceptives** were associated with an increased risk of cardiovascular effects including *hypertension, venous thrombo-embolism, myocardial infarction*, and *stroke*. Consequently, there are a number of contra-indications and precautions relating to their use in women with risk factors for cardiovascular disease (see under Precautions, below).

Changing patterns of use, and a progressive reduction in doses, have meant a continued need to evaluate the risks associated with oral contraceptives.

Current use of lower-dose combined oral contraceptives (less than 50 μg oestrogen) increases blood pressure in many women, and also results in a small but significant increased risk of venous thrombo-embolism. Any increased risk of myocardial infarction and stroke is low in women aged less than 35 years who do not smoke and who do not have pre-existing hypertension. Further details of these adverse effects are covered in the following sections.

The effect of progestogens on the cardiovascular risk profile of oral contraceptives has not been established. Some of the newer progestogens have been reported to have more favourable effects on plasma lipids (see below) and there is some suggestion that they may have a lower risk of myocardial infarction, but there are insufficient data to confirm or refute this. Recently, however, it has been reported that desogestrel and gestodene are associated with 1.5 to 2 times the risk of venous thrombo-embolism than older progestogens.

The Nurses' Health Study found no association between ever having used oral contraceptives and death from cardiovascular disease.[1] The Royal College of General Practitioners' study reported an increase in death from cerebrovascular disease with current or recent (within 10 years) use of oral contraceptives, but not for past use (greater than 10 years).[4]

Some general reviews are cited below.[2,3]

1. Colditz GA, *et al.* Oral contraceptive use and mortality during 12 years of follow-up: the Nurses' Health Study. *Ann Intern Med* 1994; **120:** 821–6.
2. WHO. WHO Scientific Group Meeting on Cardiovascular Disease and Steroid Hormone Contraceptive: summary of conclusions. *Wkly Epidem Rec* 1997; **72:** 361–3.
3. Chasan-Taber L, Stampfer MJ. Epidemiology of oral contraceptives and cardiovascular disease. *Ann Intern Med* 1998; **128:** 467–77.
4. Beral V, *et al.* Mortality associated with oral contraceptive use: 25 year follow up of cohort of 46 000 women from Royal College of General Practitioners' oral contraception study. *Br Med J* 1999; **318:** 96–100.

HYPERTENSION. In a one-year prospective multicentre study[1] involving 704 women under the age of 35 using a combined oral contraceptive containing levonorgestrel 250 μg and ethinyloestradiol 50 μg and 703 women using a non-hormonal intra-uterine contraceptive device, those using the oral contraceptive developed higher systolic and diastolic blood pressures (systolic pressures were 3.6 to 5.0 mmHg higher, diastolic pressures were 1.9 to 2.7 mmHg higher). Only 4 women receiving oral contraceptives developed hypertension. A similar increase in blood pressure was noted in a study[2] involving 222 users of combined oral contraceptives containing 30 μg ethinyloestradiol. There was a greater increase in blood pressure for those preparations containing 250 μg levonorgestrel than those containing 150 μg levonorgestrel.

More recently, data from the Nurses' Health Study[3] showed an increased risk (relative risk 1.8) for the development of hypertension in women taking lower-dose combined oral contraceptives. Increasing doses of progestogen were positively associated with hypertension, and the lowest risk occurred in women receiving triphasic preparations, which have the lowest total dose of progestogen. A recent UK study[4] found a small increase in blood pressure of 2.3/1.6 mmHg associated with the use of combined oral contraceptives. In this study, progestogen-only oral contraceptives were not associated with an increase in blood pressure.

In a study of malignant hypertension in 34 women of childbearing age (defined as 15 to 44 years of age), 11 of the women were taking oral contraceptives at presentation and, of these, 6 were known to have had normal blood pressure immediately before starting to take oral contraceptives.[5]

1. WHO Task Force on Oral Contraceptives. The WHO multicentre trial of the vasopressor effects of combined oral contraceptives 1: comparisons with IUD. *Contraception* 1989; **40:** 129–45.
2. Khaw K-T, Peart WS. Blood pressure and contraceptive use. *Br Med J* 1982; **285:** 403–7.
3. Chasan-Taber L, *et al.* Prospective study of oral contraceptives and hypertension among women in the United States. *Circulation* 1996; **94:** 483–9.
4. Dong W, *et al.* Blood pressure in women using oral contraceptives: results from the Health Survey for England 1994. *J Hypertens* 1997; **15:** 1063–8.
5. Lim KG, *et al.* Malignant hypertension in women of childbearing age and its relation to the contraceptive pill. *Br Med J* 1987; **294:** 1057–9.

MYOCARDIAL INFARCTION. Case-control studies from the 1970s and early 1980s revealed an increased risk of acute myocardial infarction in users of oral contraceptives (generally of the high-dose type) relative to those never having used them.[1,2] Several large cohort studies have provided similar findings.[3-6] Among current users the reported relative risk of myocardial infarction has varied between about 1.8 and 6.4,[1-3,5,6] whereas in women having used oral contraceptives in the past the reported relative risk has varied between about 0.8 and 2.5.[2-5] Women who smoke while using oral contraceptives are at a greatly increased risk,[1,5,7] those smoking more than 15 to 25 cigarettes per day having at least a twentyfold increased risk of myocardial infarction compared with non-smoking non-oral contraceptive users.[1,5]

More recently, data on combined oral contraceptives that have lower oestrogen doses have revealed at most small and non-significant increases in risk of acute myocardial infarction associated with oral contraceptive use.[8,9]

These studies have principally been from the USA or the UK. Most recently, the WHO Collaborative Study of Cardiovascular Disease and Steroid Hormone Contraception have reported the findings of an international multicentre case-control study.[10] The overall odds ratio for acute myocardial infarction in current users of combined oral contraceptives was 5.01 in Europe and 4.78 in Africa, Asia, and Latin America. This increase in risk reflected use in women who had coexistent risk factors such as smoking, and who had not had their blood pressure checked before use. Thus, when the background incidence of acute myocardial infarction is taken into account, use of combined oral contraceptives in non-smoking women aged less than 35 years is associated with an excess of 3 per million women-years, and this is likely to be lower in those women who have their blood pressure screened before and during use. However, in older women who smoke, the excess risk associated with the use of combined oral contraceptives is substantial (400 per million women-years). There was no increase in risk associated with past use of oral contraceptives irrespective of duration of use.

There has been interest in the effect of different progestogen components on the risk of myocardial infarction. Limited data from the WHO study[10] and from the USA[11] suggest no difference in risk between desogestrel or gestodene compared with levonorgestrel. Analysis of European data[12] suggest a reduction in risk with gestodene- and desogestrel-containing products compared with other progestogens (0.28; 95% confidence intervals 0.09 to 0.86). A recent WHO Scientific Group meeting concluded that available data do not allow the conclusion that risk of myocardial infarction is related to progestogen type.[13] Moreover, there is probably a small increased risk of venous thrombo-embolism associated with desogestrel or gestodene (see below).

1. Shapiro S, *et al.* Oral-contraceptive use in relation to myocardial infarction. *Lancet* 1979; **i:** 743–7.
2. Slone D, *et al.* Risk of myocardial infarction in relation to current and discontinued use of oral contraceptives. *N Engl J Med* 1981; **305:** 420–4.
3. Royal College of General Practitioners' Oral Contraception Study. Further analyses of mortality in oral contraceptive users. *Lancet* 1981; **i:** 541–6.
4. Stampfer MJ, *et al.* A prospective study of past use of oral contraceptive agents and risk of cardiovascular diseases. *N Engl J Med* 1988; **319:** 1313–17.
5. Croft P, Hannaford PC. Risk factors for acute myocardial infarction in women: evidence from the Royal College of General Practitioners' oral contraception study. *Br Med J* 1989; **298:** 165–8.
6. Vessey MP, *et al.* Mortality among oral contraceptive users: 20 year follow up of women in a cohort study. *Br Med J* 1989; **299:** 1487–91.
7. Goldbaum GM, *et al.* The relative impact of smoking and oral contraceptive use on women in the United States. *JAMA* 1987; **258:** 1339–42.
8. Thorogood M, *et al.* Is oral contraceptive use still associated with an increased risk of fatal myocardial infarction? Report of a case-control study. *Br J Obstet Gynaecol* 1991; **98:** 1245–53.
9. Sidney S, *et al.* Myocardial infarction and use of low-dose oral contraceptives: a pooled analysis of 2 US studies. *Circulation* 1998; **98:** 1058–63.
10. WHO Collaborative Study of Cardiovascular Disease and Steroid Hormone Contraception. Acute myocardial infarction and combined oral contraceptives: results of an international multicentre case-control study. *Lancet* 1997; **349:** 1202–9.
11. Jick H, *et al.* Risk of acute myocardial infarction and low-dose combined oral contraceptives. *Lancet* 1996; **347:** 627–8.
12. Lewis MA, *et al.* The use of oral contraceptives and the occurrence of acute myocardial infarction in young women: results from the transnational study on oral contraceptives and the health of young women. *Contraception* 1997; **56:** 129–40.
13. WHO. WHO Scientific Group Meeting on Cardiovascular Disease and Steroid Hormone Contraceptives: summary of conclusions. *Wkly Epidem Rec* 1997; **72:** 361–3.

STROKE. Current use of **combined oral contraceptives** has been associated with an increased risk of stroke, with most data relating to older high-dose oestrogen preparations. In general this association has been strongest for ischaemic stroke, and relatively weak for haemorrhagic stroke.[1] A subsequent Danish study found that low-dose oral contraceptives (30 to 40 μg of oestrogen) were associated with a lower risk of cerebral thrombo-embolism than preparations containing 50 μg oestrogen.[2]

Data on 2198 cases of stroke (haemorrhagic, ischaemic, and unclassified) and 6086 controls have recently been reported from the WHO Collaborative Study of Cardiovascular Disease and Steroid Hormone Contraception.[3,4] For all strokes combined, odds ratios for the current use of lower-dose (less than 50 μg oestrogen) and higher dose preparations were 1.41 (95% confidence intervals 0.90 to 2.20) and 2.71 (1.70 to 4.32), respectively, in Europe, and 1.86 (1.49 to 2.33) and 1.92 (1.48 to 2.50), respectively, in Africa, Asia, and Latin America. In Europe, it was estimated that the incidence rate of stroke in women aged 20 to 44 years was 4.8 per 100 000 women-years, and that this was increased to 6.7 per 100 000 in users of lower-dose preparations and 12.9 per 100 000 in users of higher-dose preparations.[3]

The risk of haemorrhagic stroke was significant only in women aged greater than 35 years, those who had a history of hypertension, and those who were current smokers.[3]

The overall odds ratio for ischaemic stroke was 2.99 (1.65 to 5.40) in Europe and 2.93 (2.15 to 4.00) in Africa, Asia, and Latin America.[4] Odds ratios were lower in women aged less than 35 years, those who did not smoke, those with no history of hypertension, and those who reported that their blood pressure had been checked before use. Duration of current use and past use were unrelated to risk.[4] A further small European case-control study[5] reported that there was no significant difference in risk of ischaemic stroke between low-dose oral contraceptives containing second generation progestogens and those containing desogestrel, gestodene, or norgestimate.

Similar findings to those of the WHO study have also been published from the USA.[6] Low-dose preparations (less than 50 μg oestrogen) were associated with a nonsignificant increase in ischaemic stroke; the odds ratio was 1.18 (0.54 to 2.59).

Data for **progestogen-only contraceptives** are limited. The Danish study reported no increase in cerebral thrombo-embolic attacks in users of oral progestogen-only contraceptives; the odds ratio was 0.9 (0.4 to 2.4).[2]

1. Vessey MP, *et al.* Oral contraceptives and stroke: findings in a large prospective study. *Br Med J* 1984; **289:** 530–1.
2. Lidegaard Ø. Oral contraception and risk of a cerebral thromboembolic attack: results of a case-control study. *Br Med J* 1993; **306:** 956–63.
3. WHO Collaborative Study of Cardiovascular Disease and Steroid Hormone Contraception. Haemorrhagic stroke, overall stroke risk, and combined oral contraceptives: results of an international, multicentre, case-control study. *Lancet* 1996; **348:** 505–10.

4. WHO Collaborative Study of Cardiovascular Disease and Steroid Hormone Contraception. Ischaemic stroke and combined oral contraceptives: results of an international, multicentre, case-control study. *Lancet* 1996; **348:** 498–505.
5. Heinemann LAJ, *et al.* Case-control study of oral contraceptives and risk of thromboembolic stroke: results from international study on oral contraceptives and health of young women. *Br Med J* 1997; **315:** 1502–4.
6. Petitti DB, *et al.* Stroke in users of low-dose oral contraceptives. *N Engl J Med* 1996; **335:** 8–15.

VENOUS THROMBO-EMBOLISM. Use of **combined oral contraceptives** has long been known to be associated with an increased risk of venous thrombo-embolic events including deep-vein thrombosis and pulmonary embolism. This increased risk applies both to idiopathic events and events associated with surgery or trauma, and is limited to current users and is not associated with duration of use. Most early data relate to high-dose combined preparations, and it has been suggested by some studies,[1] but not others,[2,3] that preparations containing lower doses of oestrogen may be associated with a decreased risk.

The WHO Collaborative Study of Cardiovascular Disease and Steroid Hormone Contraception reported data from over 10 times more cases than any previous study.[4] The increased risk of idiopathic deep-vein thrombosis and/or pulmonary embolism associated with current use of combined oral contraceptives was 4.15 (95% confidence intervals 3.09 to 5.57) in Europe and 3.25 (2.59 to 4.08) in Africa, Asia, and Latin America. The increased risk was apparent within 4 months of starting use, was unaffected by duration of use, and had disappeared within 3 months of stopping use. Risk was unaffected by age, hypertension, or smoking (in contrast to myocardial infarction, see above), but was increased in those with a body-mass index greater than 25 kg per m^2 and in those with a history of hypertension of pregnancy. Of preparations containing progestogens of the norethisterone or norgestrel type, risk was nonsignificantly less with lower-dose oestrogen than with high-dose oestrogen.

The progestogen component has generally been considered to be unrelated to thrombo-embolic events; therefore, it came as a surprise when WHO found a higher risk in combined oral contraceptives containing *desogestrel* or *gestodene* than in those containing older progestogens.[4] These risk data were the subject of a separate report,[5] and were subsequently confirmed by 3 further case-control studies.[6-8] The increased risk varied from 4.8 to 9.1 compared with non-users, and was found to be 1.5 to 2.6 times higher than for preparations containing levonorgestrel or other progestogens. One study estimated that the probability of death from venous thromboembolism was 20 per million users per year for desogestrel- and gestodene-containing products and 14 per million users per year for products containing low-dose oestrogen with other progestogens, compared with 5 per million per year for non-users.[8] The risk was especially high in women with the factor V Leiden mutation,[7] who are at increased risk of thrombosis, but screening to exclude these women from using oral contraceptives was not considered necessary.[9]

Regulatory agencies have reacted in different ways to these data. The UK Committee on Safety of Medicines (CSM) has advised restriction in prescribing of these products (see Cardiovascular Disease under Precautions, below), as have some other European authorities, and ongoing studies are being monitored. The most recent study also showed an increased risk of 1.68 for desogestrel and gestodene versus older progestogens; however, further logistic regression rendered the risk nonsignificant.[10]

The findings of these studies, and the regulatory action, have been the subject of numerous published letters and articles. It has been suggested that the effect could be due to preferential prescribing of gestodene or desogestrel products in individuals at possible increased risk of cardiovascular events, since the products have been marketed as being better in this regard.[11] Additionally, it has been suggested that attrition of susceptible users occurs with preparations used for longer periods (the 'healthy user' effect), and that this may favour older products.[11] Both of these hypotheses have been disputed.[12] However, considering all the data, a WHO scientific group meeting concluded that preparations containing desogestrel or gestodene probably carry a small excess risk of venous thrombo-embolism beyond that attributable to levonorgestrel-containing preparations.[13]

The mechanism behind differences in thrombotic potential is not known, but there are some *in-vitro* data suggesting that oral contraceptives may induce a resistance to the blood's natural anticoagulation system, and that this resistance is greater with products containing desogestrel and gestodene compared with older progestogens.[14]

More recently, reports have identified an increased risk of cerebral-vein thrombosis with oral contraceptives.[15,16]

1. Vessey M, *et al.* Oral contraceptives and venous thromboembolism: findings in a large prospective study. *Br Med J* 1986; **292:** 526.
2. Kierkegaard A. Deep vein thrombosis and the oestrogen content in oral contraceptives—an epidemiological analysis. *Contraception* 1985; **31:** 29–41.
3. Helmrich SP, *et al.* Venous thromboembolism in relation to oral contraceptive use. *Obstet Gynecol* 1987; **69:** 91–5.
4. WHO Collaborative Study Group. Venous thromboembolic disease and combined oral contraceptives: results of international multicentre case-control study. *Lancet* 1995; **346:** 1575–82.
5. WHO Collaborative Study Group. Effect of different progestagens in low oestrogen oral contraceptives on venous thromboembolic disease. *Lancet* 1995; **346:** 1582–8.
6. Jick H, *et al.* Risk of idiopathic cardiovascular death and nonfatal venous thromboembolism in women using oral contraceptives with differing progestagen components. *Lancet* 1995; **346:** 1589–93.
7. Bloemenkamp KWM, *et al.* Enhancement by factor V Leiden mutation of risk of deep-vein thrombosis associated with oral contraceptives containing a third-generation progestagen. *Lancet* 1995; **346:** 1593–6.
8. Spitzer WO, *et al.* Third generation oral contraceptives and risk of venous thromboembolic disorders: an international case-control study. *Br Med J* 1996; **312:** 83–8.
9. Vandenbroucke JP, *et al.* Factor V Leiden: should we screen oral contraceptive users and pregnant women? *Br Med J* 1996; **313:** 1127–30.
10. Farmer RDT, *et al.* Population-based study of risk of venous thromboembolism associated with various oral contraceptives. *Lancet* 1997; **349:** 83–8.
11. Lewis MA, *et al.* The increased risk of venous thromboembolism and the use of third generation progestagens: role of bias in observational research. *Contraception* 1996; **54:** 5–13.
12. Farley TMM, *et al.* Oral contraceptives and thrombotic diseases: impact of new epidemiologic studies. *Contraception* 1996; **54:** 193–5.
13. WHO. WHO Scientific Group Meeting on Cardiovascular Disease and Steroid Hormone Contraceptives: summary of conclusions. *Wkly Epidem Rec* 1997; **72:** 361–3.
14. Rosing J, *et al.* Oral contraceptives and venous thrombosis: different sensitivities to activated protein C in women using second- and third-generation oral contraceptives. *Br J Haematol* 1997; **97:** 233–8.
15. de Bruijn SFTM, *et al.* Case-control study of risk of cerebral sinus thrombosis in oral contraceptive users who are carriers of hereditary prothrombotic conditions. *Br Med J* 1998; **316:** 589–92.
16. Martinelli I, *et al.* High risk of cerebral-vein thrombosis in carriers of a prothrombin-gene mutation and in users of oral contraceptives. *N Engl J Med* 1998; **338:** 1793–7.

Effects on the ears. In the Royal College of General Practitioners' study of oral contraception in the UK,[1] by 1981 there had been 13 cases of newly occurring otosclerosis in each of the groups of oral contraceptive users (101 985 woman-years) and controls (146 534 woman-years); this showed a non-significant relative risk of 1.29. Although, by analogy with pregnancy, it may be prudent to suppose that oral contraceptives could exacerbate pre-existing otosclerosis, the data do not support the view that the condition is associated with their use.

1. Kay CR, Wingrave SJ. Oral contraceptives and otosclerosis. *Br Med J* 1984; **288:** 1164.

Effects on the eyes. Analysis of data from 2 large UK cohort studies suggested that oral contraceptive use does not increase the risk of eye disease, with the possible exception of retinal vascular lesions.[1]

1. Vessey MP, *et al.* Oral contraception and eye disease: findings in two large cohort studies. *Br J Ophthalmol* 1998; **82:** 538–42.

Effects on fertility. Following the discontinuation of hormonal contraceptives some patients may experience amenorrhoea, anovulation, and infertility. This infertility, however, has been shown by most studies to be only temporary.

Data from the Oxford Family Planning Association study[1] have indicated that impairment of fertility after oral contraceptives was only very slight and short-lived in women who had previously had a baby. In nulliparous women aged 25 to 29 years impairment of fertility was more severe but the effect had almost entirely disappeared after 48 months. In the older, aged 30 to 34 years, nulliparous women there was even more impairment of fertility but this was not permanent as by 72 months after stopping oral contraceptive use the numbers of women who had not conceived were similar to a group who had previously used non-hormonal methods of contraception.

After injectable progestogen-only contraceptives, smaller studies have again indicated that there are no long-lasting effects on fertility;[2] but it has also been suggested that a return to ovulation occurs significantly earlier in prior norethisterone enanthate users than in medroxyprogesterone users.[3]

Infertility may also be related to the presence of pelvic inflammatory disease; for further details concerning the role of oral contraceptives in this disorder, see below.

1. Anonymous. "Pill" use appears to impair fertility in a certain group of women. *Pharm J* 1986; **236:** 227.
2. Fotherby K, *et al.* Return of ovulation and fertility in women using norethisterone enanthate. *Contraception* 1984; **29:** 447–55.
3. Garza-Flores J, *et al.* Return to ovulation following the use of long-acting injectable contraceptives: a comparative study. *Contraception* 1985; **31:** 361–6.

Effects on the gallbladder. Data from the Royal College of General Practitioners' (RCGP) oral contraception study accumulated up to December 1979 revealed no overall increased risk of gallbladder disease in the long-term, despite the indications of earlier data and other studies relating to short-term use.[1] Further studies have identified an increased risk of gallbladder disease in oral contraceptive users under the age of 30[2] or 20.[3] The latest data from the RCGP study show an increase in risk of mild hepatitis during the first 4 years of oral contraceptive use, possibly reflecting gallstone-associated cholestasis.[4] This risk then decreased to less than that seen in women who had never used oral contraceptives.

1. Wingrave SJ, Kay CR. Oral contraceptives and gallbladder disease: Royal College of General Practitioners' oral contraception study. *Lancet* 1982; **ii:** 957–9.
2. Scragg RKR, *et al.* Oral contraceptives, pregnancy, and endogenous oestrogen in gall stone disease—a case-control study. *Br Med J* 1984; **288:** 1795–9.
3. Strom BL, *et al.* Oral contraceptives and other risk factors for gallbladder disease. *Clin Pharmacol Ther* 1986; **39:** 335–41.
4. Hannaford PC, *et al.* Combined oral contraceptives and liver disease. *Contraception* 1997; **55:** 145–51.

Effects on the gastro-intestinal tract. The prevalence of recent oral contraceptive use in women with colonic Crohn's disease was significantly higher than in those with small-bowel Crohn's disease or ulcerative colitis.[1] In 399 patients with Crohn's disease the colon was involved more than twice as often in women as in men. It was suggested that oral contraceptive usage may predispose to a colitis that resembles colonic Crohn's disease.

An examination of the data on chronic inflammatory bowel disease obtained in the Oxford Family Planning Association contraceptive study revealed the following incidences of disease per 1000 woman-years of observation: ulcerative colitis, 0.26 in oral contraceptive users and 0.11 in non-users; Crohn's disease, 0.13 in users and 0.07 in non-users.[2] The use of oral contraceptives was therefore more strongly associated with ulcerative colitis than with Crohn's disease although even that association fell short of conventional levels of significance. The suggestion that oral contraceptives have an aetiological role in chronic inflammatory bowel disease cannot yet be regarded as established. This was borne out by the contrary findings of a further study[3] which showed a stronger association between oral contraceptive use and Crohn's disease than between oral contraceptive use and ulcerative colitis.

1. Rhodes JM, *et al.* Colonic Crohn's disease and use of oral contraception. *Br Med J* 1984; **288:** 595–6.
2. Vessey M, *et al.* Chronic inflammatory bowel disease, cigarette smoking, and use of oral contraceptives: findings in a large cohort study of women of childbearing age. *Br Med J* 1986; **292:** 1101–3.
3. Entrican JH, Sircus W. Chronic inflammatory bowel disease, cigarette smoking, and use of oral contraceptives. *Br Med J* 1986; **292:** 1464.

Effects on lipids. Because combined oral contraceptives have been reported to be associated with an excess risk of various adverse cardiovascular events (see above) and because other epidemiological evidence suggests that the composition of blood lipids may be one of several factors involved in the aetiology of some of these disorders, many workers have investigated the biochemical profiles of women taking various formulations of oral contraceptives. Results have often been contradictory and conflicting as the net effect is the result of opposing actions of the oestrogen and the progestogen components, and depends on the ratio between these. In general, the oestrogen component increases triglycerides, but decreases low-density lipoproteins, whereas the progestogen component tends to decrease high-density lipoproteins and increase low-density lipoproteins, particularly if it is androgenic (19-nortestosterone-derived progestogens). Newer non-androgenic progestogens such as desogestrel and gestodene appear to have a less detrimental effect on serum lipids. However, the contribution of these lipid changes to the incidence of cardiovascular disease in oral contraceptive users is uncertain. In particular, contrary to expectations, desogestrel and gestodene appear to be associated with a higher risk of venous thrombo-embolism than older progestogens (see above).

Some references to the effects of various oral contraceptives on serum lipid profiles are given below.[1-10]

For further details concerning the proposed role of the various serum lipids and subfractions in the aetiology of cardiovascular disease, see under Hyperlipidaemias, p.1265.

1. Smith RP, Sizto R. Metabolic effects of two triphasic formulations containing ethinyl estradiol and dl-norgestrel. *Contraception* 1983; **28:** 189–99.
2. Wahl P, *et al.* Effect of estrogen/progestin potency on lipid/lipoprotein cholesterol. *N Engl J Med* 1983; **308:** 862–7.
3. Deslypere JP, *et al.* Effect of long term hormonal contraception on plasma lipids. *Contraception* 1985; **31:** 633–42.
4. WHO Task Force on Oral Contraceptives. A randomized double-blind study of the effects of two low-dose combined oral contraceptives on biochemical aspects: report from a seven-centred study. *Contraception* 1985; **32:** 223–6.
5. Luoma PV, *et al.* One year study of effects of an oestrogen-dominant oral contraceptive on serum high-density lipoprotein cholesterol, apolipoproteins A-I and A-II and hepatic microsomal function. *Eur J Clin Pharmacol* 1987; **31:** 563–8.
6. Bertolini S, *et al.* Effects of three low-dose oral contraceptive formulations on lipid metabolism. *Acta Obstet Gynecol Scand* 1987; **66:** 327–32.
7. Burkman RT, *et al.* Lipid and lipoprotein changes associated with oral contraceptive use: a randomized clinical trial. *Obstet Gynecol* 1988; **71:** 33–8.
8. Notelovitz M, *et al.* Lipid and lipoprotein changes in women taking low-dose, triphasic oral contraceptives: a controlled, comparative, 12-month clinical trial. *Am J Obstet Gynecol* 1989; **160:** 1269–80.
9. Patsch W, *et al.* The effect of triphasic oral contraceptives on plasma lipids and lipoproteins. *Am J Obstet Gynecol* 1989; **161:** 1396–1401.
10. Godsland IF, *et al.* The effects of different formulations of oral contraceptive agents on lipid and carbohydrate metabolism. *N Engl J Med* 1990; **323:** 1375–81.

Effects on mental state. A review of drug-induced mental depression concluded that since mood disturbance is common during the menstrual cycle and particularly in the premenstrual phase it is difficult to evaluate the possible association of depression with oral contraceptives.[1] The evidence, however, suggests that the incidence is a little greater than with control subjects but it is still only 4 to 6%. A later review[2] came to a similar conclusion that in a number of surveys in which oral contraceptives have been compared with either placebo or an intra-uterine device no increase in depression or other nervous symptoms has been found.

1. Tyrer PJ. Drug-induced depression. *Prescribers' J* 1981; **21:** 237–42.
2. King DJ. Drug-induced psychiatric syndromes. *Prescribers' J* 1986; **26:** 50–8.

Effects on the musculoskeletal system. BONE DENSITY. Postmenopausal women who have previously used combined oral contraceptives appear to have improved bone mineral density compared with those who have not.[1] In contrast, users of the progestogen-only contraceptive medroxyprogesterone acetate may have reductions in bone mineral density, although these appear to be reversible on discontinuation of the drug.[2] A small study has prospectively analysed the effect of combined oral contraceptives and parenteral progestogen-only contraceptives on bone mass in adolescents.[3] After 1 year of use, bone mineral density decreased by 1.5% in users of depot medroxyprogesterone acetate, but increased in users of combined oral contraceptives or levonorgestrel implants, and in control subjects. A later study in women who had used depot medroxyprogesterone acetate for between 1 and 16 years found that although there was a slight reduction in bone density compared with age-specific population means this was not sufficient to be of clinical importance.[4]

1. Kritz-Silverstein D, Barrett-Connor E. Bone mineral density in postmenopausal women as determined by prior oral contraceptive use. *Am J Public Health* 1993; **83:** 100–2.
2. Cundy T, *et al.* Recovering of bone density in women who stop using medroxyprogesterone acetate. *Br Med J* 1994; **308:** 247–8.
3. Cromer BA, *et al.* A prospective comparison of bone density in adolescent girls receiving depot medroxyprogesterone acetate (Depo-Provera), levonorgestrel (Norplant), or oral contraceptives. *J Pediatr* 1996; **129:** 671–6.
4. Gbolade B, *et al.* Bone density in long term users of depot medroxyprogesterone acetate. *Br J Obstet Gynaecol* 1998; **105:** 790–4.

RHEUMATOID ARTHRITIS. While reviews[1] have commented on the rare reports of arthritis or arthropathies attributed to oral contraceptives some large studies have investigated the incidence of rheumatoid arthritis in oral contraceptive users. A negative association between the use of oral contraceptives and the development of rheumatoid arthritis has been reported in four studies[2-5] thus giving rise to the suggestion that oral contraceptive use may, in fact, have some sort of protective role. These findings were not, however, substantiated by other workers[6-8] who found no association, either beneficial or detrimental, between the use of oral contraceptives and the later development of rheumatoid arthritis. A recent meta-analysis found no conclusive evidence of a protective effect of oral contraceptives on rheumatoid arthritis risk.[9]

1. Hart FD. Drug-induced arthritis and arthralgia. *Drugs* 1984; **28:** 347–54.
2. Wingrave SJ, Kay CR. Reduction in incidence of rheumatoid arthritis associated with oral contraceptives: Royal College of General Practitioners' oral contraception study. *Lancet* 1978; **i:** 569–71.
3. Vandenbroucke JP, *et al.* Oral contraceptives and rheumatoid arthritis: further evidence for a preventive effect. *Lancet* 1982; **ii:** 839–42.
4. Hazes JMW, *et al.* Reduction of the risk of rheumatoid arthritis among women who take oral contraceptives. *Arthritis Rheum* 1990; **33:** 173–9.
5. Spector TD, *et al.* The pill, parity, and rheumatoid arthritis. *Arthritis Rheum* 1990; **33:** 782–9.
6. Linos A, *et al.* Case-control study of rheumatoid arthritis and prior use of oral contraceptives. *Lancet* 1983; **i:** 1299–1300.
7. del Junco DJ, *et al.* Do oral contraceptives prevent rheumatoid arthritis? *JAMA* 1985; **254:** 1938–41.
8. Hannaford PC, *et al.* Oral contraceptives and rheumatoid arthritis: new data from the Royal College of General Practitioners' oral contraception study. *Ann Rheum Dis* 1990; **49:** 744–6.
9. Pladevall-Vila M, *et al.* Controversy of oral contraceptives and risk of rheumatoid arthritis: meta-analysis of conflicting studies and review of conflicting meta-analyses with special emphasis on analysis of heterogeneity. *Am J Epidemiol* 1996; **144:** 1–14.

Effects on the nervous system. Chorea has been reported following administration of oral contraceptives;[1,2] the choreic movements stopped within 2 to 8 weeks of discontinuing therapy.

1. Lane RJM, Routledge PA. Drug-induced neurological disorders. *Drugs* 1983; **26:** 124–47.
2. Wadlington WB, *et al.* Chorea associated with the use of oral contraceptives: report of a case and review of the literature. *Clin Pediatr (Phila)* 1981; **20:** 804–6.

Effects on the pancreas. Reports of pancreatitis secondary to hyperlipidaemia associated with the use of combined oral contraceptives.[1,2]

1. Parker WA. Estrogen-induced pancreatitis. *Clin Pharm* 1983; **2:** 75–9.
2. Stuyt PMJ, *et al.* Pancreatitis induced by oestrogen in a patient with type I hyperlipoproteinaemia. *Br Med J* 1986; **293:** 734.

Effects on the skin. Oral contraceptives may cause chloasma, and those containing androgenic progestogens may cause or aggravate acne and hirsutism. More rarely, oral contraceptives have been implicated in photosensitivity associated with drug-induced lupus erythematosus.[1] A survey of people using UV-A sunbeds at commercial premises in the UK revealed that the prevalence of pruritus, nausea, and skin rashes as side-effects to the sunbeds was higher in women taking oral contraceptives than in women receiving no medication.[2] There has been a report of hidradenitis suppurativa, a condition resulting in the recurrence of boils at the axillary apocrine sweat glands, anogenital region, and breasts, occurring in 7 women using oral contraceptives.[3]

For mention of the refuted association between oral contraceptives and malignant melanoma, see Skin under Carcinogenicity above.

1. Smith AG. Drug-induced photosensitivity. *Adverse Drug React Bull* 1989; (Jun.): 508–11.
2. Diffey BL. Use of UV-A sunbeds for cosmetic tanning. *Br J Dermatol* 1986; **115:** 67–76.
3. Stellon AJ, Wakeling M. Hidradenitis suppurativa associated with use of oral contraceptives. *Br Med J* 1989; **298:** 28–9.

Effects on the uterus. The Oxford Family Planning Association study found that the risk of developing uterine leiomyomas (uterine fibroids) was reduced by the use of oral contraceptives.[1] The observed reduction in risk was approximately 17% with each five years of oral contraceptive use, and was not thought to be due to selective prescribing.[2,3] The authors hypothesised that unopposed oestrogen may be a risk factor for uterine fibroids, and that the reduced risk with oral contraceptives might be analogous to the reduction in endometrial carcinoma seen with these drugs (see above).[1] However, another case-control study involving 390 women with leiomyomas failed to find a protective (or detrimental) effect with oral contraceptive use.[4]

1. Ross RK, *et al.* Risk factors for uterine fibroids: reduced risk associated with oral contraceptives. *Br Med J* 1986; **293:** 359–62.
2. Ratner H. Risk factors for uterine fibroids: reduced risk associated with oral contraceptives. *Br Med J* 1986; **293:** 1027.
3. Ross RK, *et al.* Risk factors for uterine fibroids: reduced risk associated with oral contraceptives. *Br Med J* 1986; **293:** 1027.
4. Parazzini F, *et al.* Oral contraceptive use and risk of uterine fibroids. *Obstet Gynecol* 1992; **79:** 430–3.

Pelvic inflammatory disease. Concern over the generalisation that oral contraceptives protect against all forms of pelvic inflammatory disease led to an evaluation of the validity of this association by analysing published epidemiological evidence and reviewing relevant information from other disciplines.[1] Most studies have been limited to hospitalised women who represent less than 25% of all cases of pelvic inflammatory disease and are likely to have relatively severe forms of the disease. These studies have also failed to distinguish between gonococcal and non-gonococcal disease. While oral contraceptives may provide some protection against gonococcal pelvic inflammatory disease, epidemiological and biological evidence suggests that infection with *Chlamydia trachomatis*, the leading cause of non-gonococcal disease, is enhanced by oral contraceptives; in 12 of the 14 epidemiological studies a two- to threefold increase in the prevalence of cervical *C. trachomatis* infection was demonstrated in oral contraceptive users. It was concluded that the suggestion that oral contraceptives protect against all forms of pelvic inflammatory disease was premature. It was also considered that any protection against clinically apparent pelvic inflammatory disease does not guarantee protection against tubal factor infertility.

Others[2] have expressed the view that a more critical examination of past studies was warranted since none of the data cited by Washington *et al.*[1] were corrected for factors which may possibly affect risk such as age, marital status, sexual behaviour, obstetric history, or history of urethritis in sexual partner. However, Washington *et al.*[3] pointed out that one of the studies originally cited plus one later study controlled for these variables and that these studies found a statistically significant association between oral contraceptive use and *C. trachomatis* infection. Another subsequent study[4] confirmed this association and in addition noted a positive relationship between oral contraceptive use and *Neisseria gonorrhoeae* infection. Interestingly, rates of gonococcal infection appeared higher for preparations containing more androgenic progestogens. A recent case-control study involving 141 women with pelvic inflammatory disease and 739 controls suggested that oral contraceptive use protected against symptomatic disease in women already infected with *C. trachomatis* but not in those infected with *N. gonorrhoeae*.[5]

In a study on the relationship of tubal infertility to oral contraceptive use, past contraceptive use was studied in 283 nulliparous infertile women and in 3833 women at delivery.[6] No association between past oral contraceptive use and tubal infertility was observed in cases with or without a history of pelvic inflammatory disease. It may, however, be misleading to group all oral contraceptive users into a single category since a considerable variation in risk by type of formulation was observed. Users of oestrogen-dominant oral contraceptives (containing 75 μg or more of oestrogen together with a progestogen with enhanced oestrogenic activity such as ethynodiol diacetate or norethisterone acetate) had an elevated risk for tubal infertility while users of low-oestrogen preparations (containing 50 μg or less of oestrogen together with norgestrel or norethisterone) had no increased risk. Age at first use of oral contraceptives also appeared to be a variable factor. Women who had first used a low-oestrogen preparation between the ages of 20 and 24 years had a decreased risk of tubal infertility, while women who had first used other types of formulations before the age of 20 years had a significantly elevated risk. Two experimental observations may be relevant to the apparent difference in risk with regard to the oestrogenic activity. Cervical mucus under the influence of oestrogens tends to be thin and clear with sperm penetration favoured and this may also favour bacterial ascent. Also, although progesterone appears to be necessary for the initiation of chlamydial infection, oestrogen may be more important in its spread. It was concluded that this study offers more reason for women to avoid oral contraceptives with a high oestrogenic content.

1. Washington AE, *et al.* Oral contraceptives, Chlamydia trachomatis infection, and pelvic inflammatory disease: a word of caution about protection. *JAMA* 1985; **253:** 2246–50.
2. Gall SA. Oral contraceptives and Chlamydia infections. *JAMA* 1986; **255:** 38.
3. Washington AE, *et al.* Oral contraceptives and Chlamydia infections. *JAMA* 1986; **255:** 38–9.
4. Louv WC, *et al.* Oral contraceptive use and the risk of chlamydial and gonococcal infections. *Am J Obstet Gynecol* 1989; **160:** 396–402.
5. Wølner-Hanssen P, *et al.* Decreased risk of symptomatic chlamydial pelvic inflammatory disease associated with oral contraceptive use. *JAMA* 1990; **263:** 54–9.
6. Cramer DW, *et al.* The relationship of tubal infertility to barrier method and oral contraceptive use. *JAMA* 1987; **257:** 2446–50.

Precautions

Before hormonal contraceptives are given the woman should undergo an appropriate medical examination and her medical history should be carefully evaluated. Regular examination is recommended during use. The contraceptive effectiveness of combined and progestogen-only preparations may be reduced during episodes of vomiting or diarrhoea and extra contraceptive measures may be necessary. For precautions to be observed if a 'pill' is missed, see under Uses and Administration, below.

Combined oral contraceptives are *contra-indicated* in women with markedly impaired liver function or cholestasis, the Dubin-Johnson or Rotor syndromes, hepatic adenoma, porphyria, oestrogen-dependent neoplasms such as breast or endometrial cancer, cardiovascular disease (see also below) including previous or current thrombo-embolic disorders, or high risk of them, and arterial disease or multiple risk factors for it, thrombophlebitis, disorders of lipid metabolism, undiagnosed vaginal bleeding, possible pregnancy, or a history during pregnancy of pruritus, chorea, herpes, deteriorating otosclerosis, or cholestatic jaundice. They are also contra-indicated in severe or focal migraine (or where there are other risk factors for cardiovascular disease) and should be used with caution in other forms of migraine (for further details, see below). They should be *administered with caution* to women with a history of diabetes mellitus, mental depression, asthma, epilepsy, gallbladder disease, sickle-cell disease, or conditions influenced by fluid retention. They should also be used with caution in those with varicose veins (and should be avoided in thrombo-phlebitis or where the restrictions outlined under Venous Thrombo-embolism apply, see below). Where not actually contra-indicated, they should also be used with caution in those with a risk factor for cardiovascular disease such as cigarette smoking, obesity, hypertension, or a family history of cardiovascular disorders (see also below). Current opinion is that low-dose combined oral contraceptives may be used in women over the age of 35 years provided they do not smoke and have no other risk factors for cardiovascular disease, but that they should be avoided over the age of 50 years. Administration to those undergoing surgery or prolonged bed rest may increase the risk of thrombo-embolic episodes and it is generally recommended that use of combined oral contraceptives should be discontinued 4 to 6 weeks before major elective surgery (see also below). Combined oral contraceptives should not be used after recent evacuation of a hydatidiform mole until urine and plasma gonadotrophin concentrations have returned to normal. They should be avoided in nursing mothers as lactation may be reduced (see also below). Increased concentrations of thyroxine-binding globulin, reflected in increased levels of protein-bound iodine, occur and while the thyroid state is generally unaffected, some tests of thyroid function give abnormal results. Cortisol-binding globulin may also be increased and some other laboratory test values may be affected. Contact lenses may irritate.

Progestogen-only contraceptives, whether oral or injectable, may be used when oestrogenic-containing preparations are contra-indicated but certain contra-indications and precautions must still be observed. They are contra-indicated in women with undiagnosed vaginal bleeding, possible pregnancy, severe arterial disease, hormone-dependent neoplasms, porphyria, and severe liver disease such as hepatic adenoma.

Like combined oral contraceptives they should not be used after recent evacuation of a hydatidiform mole. Progestogen-only contraceptives should be used with care in women with heart disease, malabsorption syndromes, liver dysfunction including recurrent cholestatic jaundice, or a history of jaundice in pregnancy. Oral progestogen-only contraceptives should also be used with care in past ectopic pregnancy (see above) or functional ovarian cysts. Despite unsatisfactory evidence of hazard, other suggested cautions for progestogen-only contraceptives include diabetes mellitus, hypertension, migraine, and thrombo-embolic disorders.

Cardiovascular disease. Combined oral contraceptives are associated with a number of arterial and venous risk factors. Progestogen-only contraceptives are associated with fewer risk factors, although they still need to be avoided when arterial disease is severe.

ARTERIAL DISEASE. UK sources have recommended that combined oral contraceptives may be used with **caution** if any **one** of the following factors are present, but should be **avoided** if **two or more** factors are present: *family history of arterial disease* in first-degree relative aged under 45 years (avoiding if atherogenic lipid profile as well as family history of arterial disease); *diabetes mellitus* (avoiding if diabetic complications present); *hypertension* (avoiding if severe); *smoking* (avoiding if 40 or more cigarettes daily); *age over 35 years* (avoiding if over 50 years); *obesity* (avoiding if body-mass index exceeds 39 kg per m^2—and avoiding gestodene or desogestrel if it exceeds 30 kg per m^2, see under Venous Thrombo-embolism, below); *migraine,* see under Migraine, below.

VENOUS THROMBO-EMBOLISM. Combined oral contraceptives increase the risk of venous thrombo-embolism and should not be used in women at special risk for thrombosis such as those with known thrombotic coagulation abnormalities or a personal history of venous or arterial thrombosis.

In the light of evidence indicating an increased risk of venous thrombo-embolism with combined oral contraceptives containing *desogestrel* or *gestodene* (see above), the UK Committee on Safety of Medicines has advised additional precautions for these products. As well as the usual precautions, it is advised they should not be used by obese women (body-mass index greater than 30 kg per m^2), those with varicose veins, or those with a history of thrombosis of any cause. Moreover, it is recommended that they should be used only in women who are intolerant of other combined oral contraceptives and who are prepared to accept an increased risk of venous thrombo-embolism. Some other regulatory bodies have also made recommendations regarding the use of these products, but the European Committee on Proprietary Medicinal Products has not.

Lupus erythematosus. A short comment that despite there being occasional reports of lupus being exacerbated by oral contraceptives, the vast majority of patients with systemic lupus erythematosus experience no adverse effects, especially from low oestrogen preparations.[1]

1. Hughes GRV. The management of systemic lupus erythematosus. *Prescribers' J* 1987; **27:** 1.

Migraine. UK sources have recommended that combined oral contraceptives be **contra-indicated** in: migraine with typical focal aura; severe migraine regularly lasting longer than 72 hours despite treatment; and migraine treated with an ergot derivative. They also recommend **caution** in migraine without focal aura and migraine controlled with a 5-HT$_1$ agonist. A woman receiving a combined oral contraceptive should report any increase in headache frequency or the onset of focal symptoms. If focal neurological symptoms not typical of aura persist for longer than one hour the combined oral contraceptive should be discontinued and the woman referred urgently to a neurologist.

Porphyria. Oral contraceptives have been associated with acute attacks of porphyria and are considered unsafe in patients with acute porphyria.[1] The progestogen content is considered more hazardous than the oestrogen content.

1. Moore MR, McColl KEL. *Porphyria: drug lists.* Glasgow: Porphyria Research Unit, University of Glasgow, 1991.

Pregnancy and breast feeding. In contrast to the numerous cases of congenital malformations reported after the use of high doses of sex hormones for hormonal pregnancy tests, there have been only a few suggestions that continued administration of oral contraceptives during early pregnancy may result in congenital limb reduction deformities,[1-3] and one case of neonatal choreoathetosis following prenatal exposure to oral contraceptives.[4]

Many studies, conversely, have shown no evidence that the use of oral contraceptives is associated with congenital malformations or teratogenic effects, whether past use (discontinued before conception), use after the last menstrual period, or known use in early pregnancy.[5-10] A meta-analysis[11] of some of these, plus other studies, confirmed this. The relative risk for all malformations with use of oral contraceptives was estimated to be 0.99 (95% confidence intervals 0.83 to 1.19). The use of oral contraceptives in early pregnancy also appears unlikely to increase the risk of hypospadia in male fetuses (see also p.1455).[12] For a discussion of the ectopic pregnancy risk in users of hormonal contraceptives, see above.

1. Janerich DT, *et al.* Oral contraceptives and congenital limb reduction defects. *N Engl J Med* 1974; **291:** 697–700.
2. McCredie J, *et al.* Congenital limb defects and the pill. *Lancet* 1983; **ii:** 623.
3. Kricker A, *et al.* Congenital limb reduction deformities and use of oral contraceptives. *Am J Obstet Gynecol* 1986; **155:** 1072–8.
4. Profumo R, *et al.* Neonatal choreoathetosis following prenatal exposure to oral contraceptives. *Pediatrics* 1990; **86:** 648–9.
5. Robinson SC. Pregnancy outcome following oral contraceptives. *Am J Obstet Gynecol* 1971; **109:** 354–8.
6. Royal College of General Practitioners' Oral Contraception Study. The outcome of pregnancy in former oral contraceptive users. *Br J Obstet Gynaecol* 1976; **83:** 608–16.
7. Rothman KJ, Louik C. Oral contraceptives and birth defects. *N Engl J Med* 1978; **299:** 522–4.
8. Vessey M, *et al.* Outcome of pregnancy in women using different methods of contraception. *Br J Obstet Gynaecol* 1979; **86:** 548–56.
9. Linn S, *et al.* Lack of association between contraceptive usage and congenital malformations in offspring. *Am J Obstet Gynecol* 1983; **147:** 923–8.
10. Källén B. Maternal use of oral contraceptives and Down syndrome. *Contraception* 1989; **39:** 503–6.
11. Bracken MB. Oral contraception and congenital malformations in offspring: a review and meta-analysis of the prospective studies. *Obstet Gynecol* 1990; **76:** 552–7.
12. Raman-Wilms L, *et al.* Fetal genital effects of first trimester sex hormone exposure: a meta-analysis. *Obstet Gynecol* 1995; **85:** 141–9.

BREAST FEEDING. Combined oral contraceptives may diminish the volume of breast milk and should be avoided until weaning (or for at least 6 months after birth). Progestogen-only oral contraceptives do not affect lactation, but should not be given until 3 weeks after birth to avoid an increased risk of breakthrough bleeding. Similarly, progestogen-only parenteral contraceptives should not be given until 5 or 6 weeks after birth if a woman is breast feeding; they may be started within 5 days if she is not breast feeding, provided she is warned that heavy or prolonged bleeding may occur. Very small amounts of both oestrogens and progestogens are distributed into the breast milk.

Sickle-cell disease. In *sickle-cell disease* there is an increased risk of thrombosis; oral contraceptive use also carries an increased risk of thrombosis but it is by no means certain that the two risks are additive. Some manufacturers have specifically warned against the use of combined oral contraceptives in sickle-cell disease but it has also been considered that there is no contra-indication to the use of low-dose combined preparations[1,2] or that a progestogen-only pill[3] or depot injection of medroxyprogesterone acetate,[4] be used.

For *sickle-cell trait* there is no increased risk of thrombosis and no contra-indication to the use of a combined preparation, as well as none to the use of a progestogen-only preparation. Many women with sickle-cell trait have, unnecessarily, been denied the use of oral contraceptives in the mistaken belief that what may have an adverse effect in sickle-cell disease may have a similar adverse outcome in the trait.[3]

1. Freie HMP. Sickle cell diseases and hormonal contraception. *Acta Obstet Gynecol Scand* 1983; **62:** 211–17.
2. Howard RJ, *et al.* Contraceptives, counselling, and pregnancy in women with sickle cell disease. *Br Med J* 1993; **306:** 1735–7.
3. Evans DIK. Should patients who say that they have "sickle cells" be prescribed the contraceptive pill? *Br Med J* 1984; **289:** 425.
4. Guillebaud J. Sickle cell disease and contraception. *Br Med J* 1993; **307:** 506–7.

Surgery. Case reports and epidemiological studies showing an increased risk of idiopathic deep-vein thrombosis and pulmonary embolism in young women taking **combined oral contraceptives** (see above) led to the widespread belief that oral contraceptives may predispose to deep-vein thrombosis postoperatively. A report by Vessey *et al.*[1] showed that the incidence of deep-vein thrombosis postoperatively in young women taking combined oral contraceptives was about twice that of women not taking contraceptives but the difference was not statistically significant. For studies in which iodine-125 fibrinogen scans were used to diagnose thrombosis postoperatively, the incidences were 4.6% in patients undergoing gynaecological operations,[2] 0% in patients undergoing abdominal operations,[3] and 20% in patients undergoing emergency appendectomies.[4] Some have considered[5] that the risk to young women of becoming pregnant from discontinuing oral contraceptives or of developing side-effects from prophylaxis may be greater than the risk of developing postoperative deep-vein thrombosis. They have suggested that, until further data are available, combined oral contraceptives should not be withheld from young women who require abdominal operations and that the routine use of prophylaxis in women on these drugs is probably unnecessary, particularly if they have no other risk factors. This advice is also broadly similar to that proposed later in the UK by the Thromboembolic Risk Factors (THRIFT) Consensus Group.[6] They suggested that unless there were other risk factors there was insufficient evidence to support a policy of routinely stopping combined oral contraceptives before major surgery. Additionally, there was insufficient evidence to support routine specific thrombo-embolic prophylaxis in women without additional risk factors.

Nevertheless, in general the advice given in an earlier review[7] still stands, that, if possible, combined oral contraceptives should be discontinued 4 weeks before major elective surgery and all surgery of the legs, and that prophylactic heparin should be considered where this was not possible. They can normally be recommended at the first menses occurring at least 2 weeks after full mobilisation. It has also been pointed out[8,9] that for patients awaiting surgery who require contraception, a progestogen-only oral contraceptive or an injection of medroxyprogesterone acetate may be suitable since neither preparation increases the risk of thrombosis.

1. Vessey M, *et al.* Oral contraceptives and venous thromboembolism: findings in a large prospective study. *Br Med J* 1986; **292:** 526.
2. Tso SC, *et al.* Deep vein thrombosis and changes in coagulation and fibrinolysis after gynaecological operations in Chinese: the effect of oral contraceptives and malignant disease. *Br J Haematol* 1980; **46:** 603–12.
3. Gallus AS, *et al.* Oral contraceptives and surgery: reduced antithrombin and antifactor XA levels without postoperative venous thrombosis in low-risk patients. *Thromb Res* 1984; **35:** 513–26.
4. Sagar S, *et al.* Oral contraceptives, antithrombin III activity, and postoperative deep-vein thrombosis. *Lancet* 1976; **i:** 509–11.
5. Sue-Ling H, Hughes LE. Should the pill be stopped preoperatively? *Br Med J* 1988; **296:** 447–8.
6. Thromboembolic Risk Factors (THRIFT) Consensus Group. Risk of and prophylaxis for venous thromboembolism in hospital patients. *Br Med J* 1992; **305:** 567–74.
7. Guillebaud J. Surgery and the pill. *Br Med J* 1985; **291:** 498–9.
8. Guillebaud J. Should the pill be stopped preoperatively? *Br Med J* 1988; **296:** 786–7.
9. Guillebaud J, Robinson GE. Stopping the pill. *Br Med J* 1991; **302:** 789.

Interactions

Enzyme-inducing drugs may cause failure of **combined oral contraceptives** by increasing their metabolism and clearance. This effect is well established for a number of *antiepileptics, griseofulvin*, and *rifamycin antibacterials*, and has also been suggested for some *antivirals* and for *modafinil*. Although less well documented, these interactions would also be expected to apply to **progestogen-only contraceptives**. Orally administered *tretinoin* may cause failure of low-dose progestogen-only contraceptives, and may possibly affect combined oral contraceptives. Rarely, *broad-spectrum antibacterials* have been associated with combined oral contraceptive failure, possibly by reducing enterohepatic recycling of the oestrogen component. As the doses of oestrogen and progestogens in oral contraceptives have decreased, reports of menstrual irregularities and unintended pregnancies attributed to these drug interactions have increased. Further details of drugs affecting hormonal contraceptives are given below under specific headings.

Oral contraceptives may, as well as being affected themselves by drug interactions, *affect other drugs*. Compounds undergoing oxidative metabolism may have their plasma concentration raised by oral contraceptives through an inhibitory action. Conversely, oral contraceptives appear to induce glucuronidation of some drugs thus reducing their plasma concentration. Oral contraceptives may also antagonise the actions of a number of drugs. Drugs affected include the following:

- some analgesics (increased clearance of paracetamol and morphine)
- anticoagulants (increased and decreased effects reported; see p.969)
- some antidepressants (reduced effectiveness, but also increased toxicity; see p.277)
- antidiabetics (antagonism of effect)
- antihypertensives (antagonism of effect)
- benzodiazepines (increased or decreased clearance; see p.665)
- clofibrate (increased clearance and antagonism of effect)
- corticosteroids (reduced clearance and enhanced effect; see p.1014)
- cyclosporin (increased toxicity; see p.522)
- lignocaine (increased free fraction due to altered protein binding; see p.1295)
- xanthines (decreased clearance; see p.770).

Reviews of drug interactions with oral contraceptives.

1. Brodie MJ. Oral contraceptives. *Prescribers' J* 1983; **23:** 140–3.
2. D'Arcy PF. Drug interactions with oral contraceptives. *Drug Intell Clin Pharm* 1986; **20:** 353–62.
3. Back DJ, Orme ML'E. Pharmacokinetic drug interactions with oral contraceptives. *Clin Pharmacokinet* 1990; **18:** 472–84.
4. Shenfield GM. Oral contraceptives: are drug interactions of clinical significance? *Drug Safety* 1993; **9:** 21–37.

Antibacterials. An interaction between the *rifamycins (rifampicin* and *rifabutin)* and oral contraceptives is well established (see Rifamycins, below) and alternative contraceptive measures are necessary. A variety of *broad-spectrum antibacterials* have been reported to decrease oral contraceptive efficacy. Some studies have pointed to interference with intestinal flora involved in enterohepatic circulation of oestrogens as being a likely mechanism for this interaction. Although up until 1985 there had been 32 reports[1] of unintended pregnancies in women receiving *penicillins* (25 of them with *ampicillin)* the ability of antibacterials to inhibit oral contraceptive efficacy remains unproven. The data are consistent, however, with the supposition that efficacy is occasionally impaired. Several cases of unintended pregnancies have been reported following the use of *tetracyclines*. It is recommended that additional contraceptive precautions should be used while taking, and for 7 days after stopping, a short course of any broad-spectrum antibacterial. If the course of antibacterial exceeds 2 weeks resistance to impairment of intestinal flora develops and additional precautions become unnecessary.

With regard to other antibacterials, in theory any one with significant effects on intestinal flora could affect contraceptive efficacy. Isolated cases of pregnancy have been reported following the use of *cephalosporins, chloramphenicol, dapsone, isoniazid, nitrofurantoin, sulphonamides,* and *co-trimoxazole* but it is impossible to determine which, if any, of these interactions is real.

1. Back DJ, *et al.* Evaluation of Committee on Safety of Medicines yellow card reports on oral contraceptive-drug interactions with anticonvulsants and antibiotics. *Br J Clin Pharmacol* 1988; **25:** 527–32.

RIFAMYCINS. *Rifampicin* regularly results in menstrual irregularities and occasionally in unintended pregnancies in women receiving oral contraceptives. It is a potent enzyme inducer and considerably enhances the metabolism of oral contraceptives. Because of its potent effect, a non-hormonal method of contraception such as an intra-uterine device is recommended during, and for 4 to 8 weeks after stopping, rifampicin therapy. Similarly, other forms of contraception are recommended during *rifabutin* therapy.

TRIACETYLOLEANDOMYCIN. Severe pruritus and jaundice may occur if oral contraceptives and triacetyloleandomycin are administered concurrently.[1] It has been suggested that their hepatic effects may be additive or synergistic, and that concurrent use should be avoided.

1. Miguet J-P, *et al.* Jaundice from troleandomycin and oral contraceptives. *Ann Intern Med* 1980; **92:** 434.

Antiepileptics. Oral contraceptive failure and breakthrough bleeding have been reported in numerous cases during periods of concurrent antiepileptic therapy.[1-4] *Phenytoin,* barbiturates such as *phenobarbitone* and *primidone*, and *carbamazepine* have been most frequently implicated, and *oxcarbazepine*, *ethosuximide,* and *topiramate* may interact similarly. These drugs increase clearance of oral contraceptives by enzyme induction, so diminishing their effect. In women receiving such antiepileptics use of non-hormonal contraceptives such as the intra-uterine device should be considered. If these are unsuitable, an oral contraceptive with an increased oestrogen content of 50 to 100 µg is generally adequate. Alternatively, a standard monophasic preparation may be given for 3 cycles without a break followed by a tablet-free interval of 4 days (tricycling). Switching to a non-interacting antiepileptic such as valproate could be considered.

1. Kenyon IE. Unplanned pregnancy in an epileptic. *Br Med J* 1972; **1:** 686–7.
2. Hempel E, Klinger W. Drug stimulated biotransformation of hormonal steroid contraceptives: clinical implications. *Drugs* 1976; **12:** 442–8.
3. Mattson RH, Cramer JA. Epilepsy, sex hormones, and antiepileptic drugs. *Epilepsia* 1985; **26** (suppl 1): S40–S51.
4. Back DJ, *et al.* Evaluation of Committee on Safety of Medicines yellow card reports on oral contraceptive-drug interactions with anticonvulsants and antibiotics. *Br J Clin Pharmacol* 1988; **25:** 527–32.

Antifungals. Menstrual irregularities and pregnancies have been reported in women receiving oral contraceptives and *griseofulvin* concurrently[1,2] and more studies are needed to confirm the existence of the interaction and the mechanism of action involved. Additional contraceptive measures should be considered in women using the two drugs concurrently (and for at least 7 days after stopping griseofulvin). There have also been anecdotal reports[3,4] of menstrual irregularities and contraceptive failure with *fluconazole, itraconazole,* and *ketoconazole*, and similar advice applies to these if pregnancy is to be avoided with certainty.

1. van Dijke CPH, Weber JCP. Interaction between oral contraceptives and griseofulvin. *Br Med J* 1984; **288:** 1125–6.
2. Back DJ, *et al.* Evaluation of Committee on Safety of Medicines yellow card reports on oral contraceptive-drug interactions with anticonvulsants and antibiotics. *Br J Clin Pharmacol* 1988; **25:** 527–32.
3. Pillans PI, Sparrow MJ. Pregnancy associated with a combined oral contraceptive and itraconazole. *N Z Med J* 1993; **106:** 436.
4. Meyboom RHB, *et al.* Disturbance of withdrawal bleeding during concomitant use of itraconazole and oral contraceptives. *N Z Med J* 1997; **110:** 300.

Antivirals. A number of antivirals are likely to accelerate the metabolism of oestrogens and progestogens; theoretically therefore, they may decrease the efficacy of hormonal contraceptives. This has been suggested for *HIV-protease inhibitors* (see Indinavir, p.614) such as *nelfinavir* and *ritonavir,*[1] and for *nevirapine*. An alternative form of contraception should be considered.

1. Ouellet D, *et al.* Effect of ritonavir on the pharmacokinetics of ethinyl oestradiol in healthy female volunteers. *Br J Clin Pharmacol* 1998; **46:** 111–16.

Stimulants. *Modafinil* induces hepatic enzymes and may reduce the efficacy of oral contraceptives. It has been suggested that when oral contraceptives are used concurrently, a preparation containing at least 50 µg of ethinyloestradiol should be used.

Vitamins. Large supplements of vitamin C have been reported to increase serum ethinyloestradiol concentrations in women taking oral contraceptives,[1] but a further study showed no effect.[2]

1. Back DJ, *et al.* Interaction of ethinyloestradiol with ascorbic acid in man. *Br Med J* 1981; **282:** 1516.
2. Zamag NM, *et al.* Absence of an effect of high vitamin C dosage on the systemic availability of ethinyl estradiol in women using a combination oral contraceptive. *Contraception* 1993; **48:** 377–91.

Pharmacokinetics

For a discussion of the pharmacokinetics of oestrogens and progestogens, see Oestradiol, p.1455 and Progesterone, p.1460, respectively. The extent of binding of progestogens to serum sex-hormone binding globulin may be altered when they are administered with an oestrogen. Oestrogens increase serum concentrations of sex-hormone binding globulin, and progestogens differ in their ability to suppress this effect.

Reference to the effects of hormonal contraceptives on binding proteins.[1]

1. Fotherby K. Interactions of contraceptive steroids with binding proteins and the clinical implications. *Ann N Y Acad Sci* 1988; **538:** 313–20.

Uses and Administration

The main use of hormonal contraceptives is for contraception, but combined oral contraceptives are also commonly used in menstrual disorders such as dysmenorrhoea (p.9), premenstrual syndrome (p.1456), and menorrhagia (p.1461), particularly where contraception is also required. Combined oral contraceptives are also used in polycystic ovary syndrome (p.1240) and Turner's syndrome (p.1240), and may be used in endometriosis (p.1442); those containing non-androgenic progestogens may be used in acne (p.1072) and hirsutism (p.1441).

Combined oral contraceptives containing both an oestrogen and a progestogen, are the most effective type of oral contraceptive for general use. The synthetic ethinyl derivatives ethinyloestradiol and mestranol are the oestrogens typically used in such preparations. The progestogenic component is a 19-nortestosterone derivative such as desogestrel, ethynodiol diacetate, gestodene, levonorgestrel, lynoestrenol, norethisterone, norethisterone acetate, norgestimate, or norgestrel. Preparations may be *monophasic* (containing a fixed dose of oestrogen and progestogen), or *biphasic* or *triphasic* (when the dose of progestogen, or both the progestogen and oestrogen, are varied through the cycle). Phased preparations are designed to mimic more closely the pattern of endogenous hormone secretion and may provide better cycle control than monophasic preparations. More rarely, *sequential* preparations are used, which contain an oestrogen alone for part of the cycle. Combined oral contraceptives are taken for 21 days (or occasionally 22 days) followed by an interval of 7 days (or 6 days) when menstrual bleeding will occur. Some preparations include 21 (or 22) active tablets plus 7 (or 6) inert tablets to remove the need for counting days ('every day' preparations). The oestrogen content of most preparations is currently in the range of 20 to 50 µg daily although higher doses were often formerly used. A formulation containing the lowest dose of oestrogen compatible with good cycle control should be chosen, considering the following:

- *low-strength* preparations (ethinyloestradiol 20 µg) are most appropriate for obese or older women, provided a combined oral contraceptive is considered otherwise suitable
- *standard strength* preparations (ethinyloestradiol 30 or 35 µg in monophasic, or 30 to 40 µg in phased) are appropriate for most other women
- *high-strength* preparations (ethinyloestradiol 50 µg or mestranol 50 µg) are generally used only in circumstances where bioavailability of the oestrogen is reduced, such as concomitant use of some enzyme-inducing drugs (see Interactions, above).

When first **starting** combined oral contraceptives, if first tablet is taken on the first day of the menstrual cycle (the first day of bleeding) additional contraceptive precautions are unnecessary. If the first tablet is taken on the fourth day of the cycle or later, additional contraceptive precautions should be undertaken for 7 days (or 14 days for 'every day' preparations in case the inert tablets are inadvertently taken first). If amenorrhoea is present and pregnancy has been excluded, combined oral contraceptives may be started on any day, but additional precautions should be used for the first 7 days. Combined oral contraceptives should be started on the same day after abortion or miscarriage. In women not breast feeding, they may be started 3 weeks postpartum; progestogen-only contraceptives are preferred in breast-feeding women (see under Precautions above). When **changing** to a combined preparation containing a different progestogen, the new preparation should be started on the day following the last active tablet of the old preparation. If a tablet-free interval is taken then extra contraceptive precautions are necessary for the first 7 days of the new preparation. In the case of 'every day' preparations, to allow for the fact that the inert tablets may inadvertently be taken first, extra contraceptive precautions are necessary during the first 14 days. Meticulous regularity of dosage is essential and contraceptive protection may be lost if a dose is not taken at the proper time or is missed. If a **missed tablet** is not taken within 12 hours, then the missed tablet or tablets should be discarded and the remaining tablets of that month's course should be taken as usual, but with extra contraceptive measures for the next 7 days. If these 7 days run into the last 7 days of the cycle, then the tablet-free interval (or the 7 inert tablets) should be omitted and the next cycle of tablets started immediately. Similarly, extra contraceptive measures are advised during, and for 7 days after recovery from, vomiting and diarrhoea.

Progestogen-only oral contraceptives are suitable for women when an oestrogen component is contra-indicated. They are taken continuously, usually **starting** on day one of the menstrual cycle, with no interval during menstrual bleeding. They may be associated with a higher failure rate than the combined preparations. Regularity in taking the doses is even more important with this type of preparation; contraceptive efficacy is reduced if a dose is delayed by more than 3 hours. Commonly used progestogens include the 19-nortestosterone derivatives ethynodiol diacetate, levonorgestrel, and norethisterone. When **changing** from a combined oral contraceptive preparation to a progestogen-only contraceptive, the new tablets should be started immediately with no tablet-free interval (or inert tablets taken). If there is a gap in administration of active ingredients, then extra contraceptive precautions are required for 7 days. If a **missed tablet** is delayed by more than 3 hours, it should be taken as soon as possible and the next tablet taken at the correct time. Additional contraceptive methods should be used for the next 7 days. Additional contraceptive methods are also required during, and for 7 days after recovery from, vomiting and diarrhoea.

Progestogens are also used alone as **parenteral contraceptives** and provide a very high level of contraceptive efficacy. They are usually given within the first 5 days of the menstrual cycle. Medroxyprogesterone acetate is given by intramuscular injection as a long-acting depot preparation in a dose of 150 mg to provide contraception for up to a 3-month period. Norethisterone enanthate is used similarly in a dose of 200 mg to provide protection for up to 2 months. Injectable contraceptives are usually used to provide short-term protection or are used in women unable to use other methods. Long-acting injections containing both an oestrogen and a progestogen have been investigated. Levonorgestrel is used in the form of a subcutaneous implant providing contraception for 5 years.

Progestogen-releasing intra-uterine devices are also available. One such device releases 20 μg of levonorgestrel every 24 hours and provides contraception for 5 years. It is usually inserted within 7 days of the onset of menstruation.

Postcoital hormonal contraceptives (the Yuzpe method) have to be taken within 72 hours after an act of unprotected intercourse to be effective. They should be used only in **emergencies** and not as a routine method of contraception. A preparation available for such use consists of tablets each containing ethinyloestradiol 50 μg and norgestrel 500 μg or levonorgestrel 250 μg. Two tablets should be taken within 72 hours and a further 2 tablets exactly 12 hours later. Alternatively, levonorgestrel 750 μg may be given alone and repeated after 12 hours (for details see below).

Choice of contraceptive method. Contraception is used for fertility control, and some methods have additional non-contraceptive health benefits. There are a wide variety of regular methods including periodic abstinence (natural family planning), male and female barrier methods, intra-uterine devices (IUDs), female hormonal contraceptives, and female or male sterilisation. In addition, female hormonal contraceptives and copper IUDs are available for emergency (postcoital) contraception. The methods employed for contraceptive purposes can be grouped into three categories: those that prevent ovulation, those that prevent fertilisation of the ovum, and those that prevent implantation of the fertilised ovum. None of the available contraceptive methods are effective once implantation of a fertilised ovum has occurred, i.e. they are not abortifacients.

A large number of factors will influence the choice of contraceptive method. Those relating to the woman include age (and therefore likely fertility), parity, medical disorders, risk of sexually transmitted diseases, smoking status, breast feeding, and cultural and religious considerations. Those relating to the method include its failure rate, reversibility, ease of use, mechanism of action, adverse effects, and non-contraceptive benefits.

The most reliable reversible methods for contraception are those for which there can be no 'user' failure such as *progestogen injections* and *implants*, and progestogen or copper *intra-uterine devices* (IUDs). These methods have reported failure rates of between 0.09 and 2% during the first year of use. The duration of action of the various progestogen injections is up to 2 or 3 months, whereas progestogen implants and progestogen IUDs are effective for up to 3 or 5 years. These long-acting progestogen preparations thicken cervical mucus, so preventing sperm penetration, and suppress the endometrium, so preventing implantation. In addition, they suppress ovulation; the degree of suppression is complete for injectable preparations, about 50% for implants, and low for the progestogen IUDs. Copper IUDs were traditionally thought to act by preventing implantation, but it is now thought that the biochemical changes which they produce in the uterus also prevent fertilisation. They are effective and have a prolonged action (up to 5 or 10 years), but they have been associated with an increased rate of pelvic inflammatory disease and ectopic pregnancy. IUDs are generally unsuitable for nulliparous women and those at increased risk of sexually transmitted diseases.

Of methods subject to 'user' failure, *combined oral contraceptives* are the most effective. They have a reported failure rate during the first year of 0.1% if used perfectly, but 3% in typical practice. Their principal mechanism of action is to prevent ovulation, and they also decrease the chances of fertilisation and implantation. Combined oral contraceptives offer the non-contraceptive advantages of avoidance of dysmenorrhoea, pre-menstrual tension, and iron-deficiency anaemia, and in the long-term they protect against endometrial and ovarian cancer. However, they do not protect against sexually transmitted diseases, they are unsuitable for older women who smoke, and long-term use carries a slight increased risk of breast cancer.

Progestogen-only oral contraceptives have a 0.5% failure rate during the first year of use if taken correctly, which is slightly higher than that for combined preparations; in practice, failure rates of from 1 to 10% have been reported. Regularity in taking them is essential; a dose should not be delayed for more than 3 hours. They act primarily to decrease the chance of fertilisation and implantation since they prevent ovulation in only 14 to 40% of cycles. They are useful for women who are breast feeding, for those who smoke and are more than 35 years of age, and if medical conditions contra-indicate the use of oestrogens.

Barrier methods, including both male and female condoms, vaginal sponges containing spermicide, and diaphragms and cervical caps used in conjunction with spermicide, act as a mechanical barrier to prevent fertilisation, and inactivate sperm. Barrier methods decrease the risk of sexually transmitted diseases and a shift towards their use has occurred since the emergence of HIV infection in particular. However, barrier methods are not as effective in preventing conception as hormonal contraception and copper IUDs. Even when used correctly, failure rates in the first year of use vary from 3% for the male condom to 11.5% with the cervical cap plus spermicide. Spermicides, such as nonoxinol 9, may be used alone as foam or as dissolvable vaginal tablets or pessaries, or as a spermicide-containing polyvinyl alcohol film placed over the cervix. However, they are generally considered relatively ineffective when used as the sole method of contraception, and such use is not recommended.

Natural family planning methods such as periodic abstinence using the calendar, temperature, cervical mucus ('Billings') or sympto-thermal methods require high motivation to learn and practice effectively. However, they may be the only acceptable method to some people. More recently, measurement of urine concentrations of oestrone glucuronide and luteinising hormone has been used as a predictor of the timing of ovulation and hence the risk of becoming pregnant. Traditional methods such as withdrawal (coitus interruptus) are widely used in some areas, but are considered relatively ineffective.

Various other methods of contraception are under investigation including injectable, transdermal, and vaginal forms of combined hormonal contraceptives, and the use of gonadorelin analogues to prevent ovulation. Contraceptive vaccines are also being investigated. Although there has been some investigation of **male contraception**, and weekly intramuscular injection of high-dose testosterone or nandrolone to produce azoospermia has been investigated with some success, development of an oral contraceptive dosage form for males has been slow. Use of a progestogen pill, with 'add-back' testosterone, is being studied.

The available irreversible methods of contraception are surgical male or female *sterilisation*. The use of mepacrine for non-surgical sterilisation has been attempted but has proved extremely controversial.

References.

1. WHO. Facts about once-a-month injectable contraceptives: memorandum from a WHO meeting. *Bull WHO* 1993; **71:** 677–89.
2. Matlin SA. Prospects for pharmacological male contraception. *Drugs* 1994; **48:** 851–63.
3. Baird DT, Glasier AF. Hormonal contraception. *N Engl J Med* 1993; **328:** 1543–9.
4. Flemming CF. Oral contraception. *Prescribers' J* 1994; **34:** 227–34.
5. Weisberg E. Prescribing oral contraceptives. *Drugs* 1995; **49:** 224–31.
6. Anonymous. Long-acting progestogen-only contraception. *Drug Ther Bull* 1996; **34:** 93–6.
7. Anonymous. Choice of contraceptives. *Med Lett Drugs Ther* 1995; **37:** 9–12. Additional note. *ibid.*: 36.
8. WHO. *Contraceptive Method Mix: guidelines for policy and service delivery.* Geneva: World Health Organization, 1994.
9. Belfield T, ed. *FPA Contraceptive Handbook: a guide for family planning and other health professionals.* 2nd ed. London: Family Planning Association, 1997.

EMERGENCY CONTRACEPTION. Emergency contraception[1-3] can be used after unprotected intercourse but before a fertilised ovum has been implanted. Methods that act after implantation are considered abortifacients. The two most commonly used emergency contraceptives are *oral contraceptives* and *copper IUDs*.

The oral contraceptive used has typically been a preparation containing high-dose oestrogen together with a progestogen, taken within 72 hours of intercourse, and repeated 12 hours later (the Yuzpe regimen or so-called 'morning after pill'). This preparation is thought to act by a variety of mechanisms, which may depend on when in the menstrual cycle it is used. It may prevent implantation, prevent or delay ovulation, disrupt ovum transport, and alter corpus luteum function. Reported efficacy rates vary between 75 and 80%. Levonorgestrel alone (without an oestrogen) is also used as an emergency contraceptive. A large WHO multicentre study recently found that levonorgestrel 750 μg alone within 72 hours of intercourse and repeated after 12 hours was more effective than the Yuzpe regimen and better tolerated.[4] Both regimens were most effective when given within 24 hours of intercourse.

Copper, but not progestogen, IUDs can be inserted up to 120 hours after unprotected intercourse for postcoital contraception. They have a failure rate of less than 1% when used for emergency contraception. Thus, when efficacy is a priority the IUD is the emergency contraceptive method of choice.

Drugs under investigation for use as emergency contraceptives include *mifepristone*. When taken as a single dose within 72 hours of unprotected intercourse this has been reported to be 100% effective. It appears to act by inhibiting ovulation or, if ovulation has occurred, by preventing implantation. Although mifepristone is also effective after implantation, it cannot be considered to interrupt pregnancy if used before implantation (5 to 7 days after fertilisation).

References.

1. Anonymous. Hormonal emergency contraception. *Drug Ther Bull* 1993; **31:** 27–8.
2. Glasier A. Emergency postcoital contraception. *N Engl J Med* 1997; **337:** 1058–64.
3. Kubba A, Wilkinson C. Emergency contraception update. *Br J Fam Plann* 1998; **23:** 135–7.
4. Task Force on Postovulatory Methods of Fertility Regulation. Randomised controlled trial of levonorgestrel versus the Yuzpe regimen of combined oral contraceptives for emergency contraception. *Lancet* 1998; **352:** 428–33.

Hormone Replacement Therapy

(19996-n)

The menopause is defined as the permanent cessation of cyclical menstruation due to loss of ovarian follicular activity. It is therefore determined in retrospect, conventionally after a period of 1 year without menstruation. In the few years prior to the menopause (the menopausal transition), ovarian oestradiol secretion declines, sometimes in a fluctuating manner, and there is a resultant increase in pituitary follicle-stimulating hormone (FSH) secretion. The menopausal transition may be characterised by irregular menstrual cycles and dysfunctional uterine bleeding, and fertility is much reduced compared with the early reproductive years. The term perimenopause is used to cover the menopausal transition and the first year after the menopause, and may last 3 to 5 years. It has sometimes been referred to as the climacteric. Oestrogen concentrations reach their minimum and FSH concentrations their maximum about 4 years after the menopause. After the menopause the ovaries may continue to produce some androgens, which together with adrenal androgens are converted to oestrogens (predominantly oestrone) in the periphery, but oestrogen concentrations are much lower than in premenopausal women. The median age for the natural menopause is about 51 years. If the menopause occurs in women aged 40 years or less, it is considered premature. The menopause may be induced by surgical removal of both ovaries, or sometimes by antineoplastic drugs or radiotherapy.

The decline in oestrogen concentrations during the perimenopause may be associated with both acute and long-term effects. However, some of these may be difficult to differentiate from the effects of ageing, and the incidence varies geographically. Established *acute symptoms* can include vasomotor instability, manifesting as hot flushes and night sweats, and vaginal atrophy and dyspareunia. Nonspecific symptoms include palpitations, headache, backache, and psychological symptoms such as tiredness, lack of concentration, loss of libido, irritability, insomnia, and depression. Insomnia may occur secondary to night sweats. There is little evidence that depressive illness is disproportionally increased at the menopause. Urinary problems are common in ageing women, and may occur in the perimenopause, but the extent that these are due to lack of oestrogens has not been determined. An established *long-term consequence* of the decline in oestrogen concentrations is an increased risk of bone fractures resulting from an increase in the rate of bone resorption. In addition, decline in oestrogen concentrations is associated with adverse effects on blood lipoproteins, and this may be a risk factor for cardiovascular disease.

Acute and longer term effects of the menopause may be managed by using hormone replacement therapy (HRT) with oestrogens, with or without progestogens.

Adverse Effects

When oestrogens are used for menopausal hormone replacement therapy (HRT), adverse effects include nausea and vomiting, weight changes, breast enlargement and tenderness, premenstrual-like syndrome, fluid retention, changes in liver function, cholestatic jaundice, rashes and chloasma (melasma), depression, headache, and decreased tolerance of contact lenses. Transdermal delivery systems may cause contact sensitisation (possibly severe hypersensitivity reactions on continued exposure), and headache has been reported on vigorous exercise. Use of oestrogen without a progestogen results in endometrial hyperplasia and an increased risk of endometrial carcinoma (see below). The addition of a progestogen for 10 to 14 days of a 28-day cycle reduces this risk but results in regular withdrawal bleeding towards the end of the progestogen. Use of continuous progestogen and oestrogen avoids withdrawal bleeding, but may result in irregular breakthrough bleeding, particularly in the early stages of therapy, or if used within 12 months of the last menstrual period. Current use of menopausal HRT is associated with an increased risk of venous thromboembolism (see below). Long-term use of menopausal HRT therapy may be associated with an increased risk of breast cancer (see below).

Reviews.

1. Winship KA. Unopposed oestrogens. *Adverse Drug React Acute Poisoning Rev* 1987; **1:** 37–66.
2. Evans MP, *et al.* Hormone replacement therapy: management of common problems. *Mayo Clin Proc* 1995; **70:** 800–5.

Carcinogenicity. Use of unopposed oestrogen as menopausal hormone replacement therapy (HRT) in women with a uterus increases the risk of endometrial cancer, irrespective of the route of administration. This risk is reduced, although possibly not eliminated completely, by the use of a progestogen. Although less well established, there is mounting evidence that long-term use of oestrogens as HRT is associated with an increased risk of breast cancer, and that the addition of a progestogen does not decrease or increase this risk. The exact extent of the risk and its implications for prescribing practice remain controversial.

Because of continuing modifications in regimens for HRT there is a continuing need to monitor the incidence of various cancers in users of this therapy.

BREAST. Early age at menarche and late age at menopause increase the risk of breast cancer, and surgical oophorectomy at an early age decreases the risk of breast cancer. In addition, higher concentrations of unbound endogenous oestrogens in postmenopausal women appear to increase the risk of developing breast cancer.[1] Such risk factors have prompted concerns that menopausal hormone replacement therapy (HRT) might be associated with an increased risk of breast cancer.

Reviews and analyses of studies published during the 1970s and/or 1980s on the use of unopposed oestrogen replacement therapy in postmenopausal women have generally shown that there is an associated moderate increase in the risk of breast cancer; figures for overall relative risk compared with non-oestrogen users ranged from under 1 to up to 2.[2-4] One of these, a meta-analysis of studies from 1976 to 1989, by Steinberg *et al.*[3] further showed that although the relative risk of breast cancer rose to 1.3 after 15 years of oestrogen use, it did not appear to rise at all until after 5 years' use. A similar meta-analysis by Dupont and Page[4] differentiated between low-dose oestrogens and high-dose oestrogens; those taking 0.625 mg daily of conjugated oestrogens had a risk of breast cancer 1.08 times higher than non-oestrogen users, whereas the relative risk in those taking 1.25 mg daily or more was up to 2.0. A more recent meta-analysis[5] differentiated between current use of HRT, duration of use, and use at any time. The highest relative risk of breast cancer was associated with current use (1.4); use for 10 years or more was associated with a relative risk of about 1.2, and having ever used HRT was not associated with an increased risk. The most robust data to date have been provided by the Collaborative Group on Hormonal Factors in Breast Cancer, who reanalysed about 90% of the worldwide evidence on breast cancer and the use of HRT.[6] They reported that the relative risk of having breast cancer diagnosed was increased by a factor of 1.023 for each year of use, being 1.35 for 5 or more years of use. However, this effect was reduced on cessation of use, and had largely disappeared after about 5 years. In women who started therapy at age 50, the cumulative excess number of breast cancers diagnosed per 1000 women between age 50 and 70 were estimated to be 2, 6, and 12 for 5, 10, and 15 years use, respectively, from a base-line of 45 per 1000 in never-users.[6]

Most data relate to the use of unopposed oestrogen. There has been speculation both that the concomitant use of progestogen in HRT could reduce the risk of breast cancer and that it may increase it. An early indication from the study by Bergkvist *et al.*[7] suggested an increased relative risk of 4.4 in the small subgroup using long-term combined therapy, but because of the large confidence intervals they considered these results were inconclusive. Analysis of the Nurses Health Study cohort has provided evidence that current use of oestrogen and progestogen is associated with a similar increased relative risk of breast cancer to that of unopposed oestrogen (1.4 versus 1.3).[8] However, a case-control study[9] found no increased risk of breast cancer either for oestrogen plus a progestogen, unopposed oestrogen, or for long duration of use. The Collaborative Group on Hormonal Factors in Breast Cancer[6] found no evidence of marked differences between preparations containing oestrogens alone and those containing oestrogens and progestogens.

The public health perspective of any increased risk of breast cancer will depend on the background risk. This is high in Western countries, so a small increased relative risk would equate to a large absolute increase in number of cases.[10]

If menopausal oestrogen therapy increases the risk of breast cancer, there is a need to ascertain whether these cancers can be detected early, how aggressive they are, and what the mortality rate from them is. Currently, there are limited data on these points. A recent study[11] indicated that the use of HRT decreases the sensitivity and specificity of screening mammography (resulting in more false positives and more false negatives), apparently because it increases radiographic breast density, so decreasing the ability to interpret the mammogram. This is of concern for the success of screening programmes, and has been suggested as a factor in the increased detection of interval cancers (those detected between screening appointments).[12] However, there are also data suggesting that breast cancers in women on HRT may be of better prognostic grade.[13] The Collaborative Group on Hormonal Factors in Breast Cancer reported that breast cancers were more likely to be localised in current or recent users of HRT, but that there was evidence of an increased risk of metastasis with increasing duration of use.[6] Follow-up of most studies is currently insufficient to give a clear indication of mortality risk with long-term use. Early data from a UK cohort study[14] suggested a decreased risk of breast cancer mortality, but after further follow-up the risk was no longer reduced.[15] Recent data[8] from the Nurses Health Study cohort suggest an increase in risk of death from breast cancer in the subset of women currently using HRT with 5 years or more of use (1.45). Similarly, although mortality was lower overall, a trend towards an increased risk of death from breast cancer (1.9; 95% confidence interval 0.4 to 8.4) was seen in a study of long-term use (mean of 17 years).[16]

The risk of breast cancer may be increased further by the use of HRT in women who are already at an increased risk. Although a recent study found a modest increase in risk in these women, it was not significantly higher, and there was a reduced total mortality rate.[17] It is unclear whether use of HRT in breast cancer survivors increases the risk of subsequent recurrence and associated mortality (see also under Precautions, below).

1. Toniolo PG, *et al.* A prospective study of endogenous estrogens and breast cancer in postmenopausal women. *J Natl Cancer Inst* 1995; **87:** 190–7.
2. Henderson BE. The cancer question: an overview of recent epidemiologic and retrospective data. *Am J Obstet Gynecol* 1989; **161:** 1859–64.
3. Steinberg KK, *et al.* A meta-analysis of the effect of estrogen replacement therapy on the risk of breast cancer. *JAMA* 1991; **265:** 1985–90.
4. Dupont WD, Page DL. Menopausal estrogen replacement therapy and breast cancer. *Arch Intern Med* 1991; **151:** 67–72.
5. Colditz GA, *et al.* Hormone replacement therapy and risk of breast cancer: results from epidemiologic studies. *Am J Obstet Gynecol* 1993; **168:** 1473–80.
6. Collaborative Group on Hormonal Factors in Breast Cancer. Breast cancer and hormone replacement therapy: collaborative reanalysis of data from 51 epidemiological studies of 52 705 women with breast cancer and 108 411 women without breast cancer. *Lancet* 1997; **350:** 1047–59. Correction. *ibid.*; 1484.
7. Bergkvist L, *et al.* The risk of breast cancer after estrogen and estrogen—progestin replacement. *N Engl J Med* 1989; **321:** 293–7.
8. Colditz GA, *et al.* The use of estrogens and progestins and the risk of breast cancer in postmenopausal women. *N Engl J Med* 1995; **332:** 1589–93.
9. Stanford JL, *et al.* Combined estrogen and progestin hormone replacement therapy in relation to risk of breast cancer in middle-aged women. *JAMA* 1995; **274:** 137–42.
10. WHO. Research on the menopause in the 1990s: report of a WHO scientific group. *WHO Tech Rep Ser 866* 1996.
11. Laya MB, *et al.* Effect of estrogen replacement therapy on the specificity and sensitivity of screening mammography. *J Natl Cancer Inst* 1996; **88:** 643–9.
12. Cohen EL. Effect of hormone replacement therapy on cancer detection by mammography. *Lancet* 1997; **349:** 1624.
13. Harding C, *et al.* Hormone replacement therapy and tumour grade in breast cancer: prospective study in screening unit. *Br Med J* 1996; **312:** 1646–7. Correction. *ibid.*; **313:** 198.
14. Hunt K, *et al.* Long-term surveillance of mortality and cancer incidence in women receiving hormone replacement therapy. *Br J Obstet Gynaecol* 1987; **94:** 620–35.
15. Hunt K, *et al.* Mortality in a cohort of long-term users of hormone replacement therapy: an updated analysis. *Br J Obstet Gynaecol* 1990; **97:** 1080–6.
16. Ettinger B, *et al.* Reduced mortality associated with long-term postmenopausal estrogen therapy. *Obstet Gynecol* 1996; **87:** 6–12.
17. Sellers TA, *et al.* The role of hormone replacement therapy in the risk for breast cancer and total mortality in women with a family history of breast cancer. *Ann Intern Med* 1997; **127:** 973–80.

CERVIX. Studies of the effect of hormone replacement therapy on cervical cancer risk are likely to be subject to the potential confounding of other risk factors such as sexual activity. There are few data on this risk, but one recent study suggests oestrogens do not increase, and may decrease, the risk of cervical cancer.[1]

1. Parazzini, F, *et al.* Case-control study of oestrogen replacement therapy and risk of cervical cancer. *Br Med J* 1997; **315:** 85–8.

ENDOMETRIUM. The increased incidence of endometrial hyperplasia and risk of cancer in women receiving unopposed oestrogen replacement therapy is well established. An analysis of case control studies published during the 1970s and 1980s revealed a relative risk of developing endometrial cancer of 1.4 to 7.6 in women who had ever used oestrogen, and a relative risk of 3.1 to 15 in long-term users, compared with nonusers.[1] Risk was also increased with higher doses of oestrogens. In general, endometrial cancer in oestrogen users was of a better prognostic stage, and survival rates were better, than in nonusers.[1] An elevated risk of endometrial cancer persists for a number of years after discontinuation of unopposed oestrogen therapy.[2]

Addition of a progestogen to oestrogen replacement therapy reduces the incidence of endometrial hyperplasia and cancer. However, the extent to which the addition of a progestogen alters the risks and benefits of oestrogen replacement therapy, and the optimum progestogen type, and dose and duration, have not been fully elucidated.

As regards risk of endometrial cancer, preliminary data from a cohort study revealed that the addition of cyclical progestogen to oestrogen therapy reduced this risk compared with oestrogen therapy alone.[3] A further case-control study confirmed that progestogens decreased the relative risk, and that the reduction in risk was greater when progestogens were used for 10 or more days per month than when they were used for less than 10 days per month.[4] Two much larger case-control studies have confirmed these findings.[5,6] However, 1 of these studies[5] reported that in long-term users the addition of a progestogen did not reduce the risk of endometrial cancer to that seen in nonusers—after 5 years of use, the relative risk of endometrial cancer with hormone replacement therapy containing 10 or more days of progestogen per month was 2.5 (95% confidence intervals 1.1 to 5.5). This finding remains to be confirmed.

Use of progestogens for 10 days of an 84 day cycle (long cycle) has been suggested to improve acceptability of combined hormone replacement therapy. However one study of a long-cycle regimen was discontinued because of an increased risk of endometrial hyperplasia and atypia compared with a conventional monthly cycle regimen.[7]

Some newer regimens of hormone replacement therapy employ continuous low-doses of progestogen with oestrogen, which avoid withdrawal bleeding. Data on the incidence of endometrial hyperplasia from randomised trials of these regimens have been reassuring.[8,9] Continuous norethisterone plus ethinyloestradiol,[8] and continuous medroxyprogesterone plus conjugated oestrogens,[9] protected the endometrium against the hyperplasia seen with the oestrogen alone. Continuous therapy was as effective as cyclical therapy containing 12 days' progestogen.[9] The first data on endometrial cancer risk from continuous combined hormone replacement therapy suggests that it is as protective as sequential therapy with the progestogen administered for 10 or more days per month (odds ratio 1.07 per 5 years of use for both regimens).[6]

1. Henderson BE. The cancer question: an overview of recent epidemiologic and retrospective data. *Am J Obstet Gynecol* 1989; **161:** 1859–64.
2. Rubin GL, *et al.* Estrogen replacement therapy and the risk of endometrial cancer: remaining controversies. *Am J Obstet Gynecol* 1990; **162:** 148–54.
3. Persson I, *et al.* Risk of endometrial cancer after treatment with oestrogens alone or in conjunction with progestogens: results of a prospective study. *Br Med J* 1989; **298:** 147–51.
4. Voigt LF, *et al.* Progestagen supplementation of exogenous oestrogens and risk of endometrial cancer. *Lancet* 1991; **338:** 274–7.
5. Beresford S, *et al.* Risk of endometrial cancer in relation to use of oestrogen combined with cyclic progestagen therapy in postmenopausal women. *Lancet* 1997; **349:** 458–61.
6. Pike MC, *et al.* Estrogen-progestin replacement therapy and endometrial cancer. *J Natl Cancer Inst* 1997; **89:** 1110–16.
7. Cerin A, *et al.* Adverse endometrial effects of long-cycle estrogen and progestogen replacement therapy. *N Engl J Med* 1996; **334:** 668–9.
8. Speroff L, *et al.* The comparative effect on bone density, endometrium, and lipids of continuous hormones as replacement therapy (CHART Study). *JAMA* 1996; **276:** 1397–1403.
9. The Writing Group for the PEPI trial. Effects of hormone replacement therapy on endometrial histology in postmenopausal women. *JAMA* 1996; **275:** 370–5.

GASTRO-INTESTINAL TRACT. Evidence of an effect of oestrogen replacement therapy on colorectal cancer is ambiguous, since studies have reported both an increased and a decreased incidence; meta-analysis has suggested no overall effect.[1] However, subsequent cohort studies did suggest a lower incidence of colon cancer in those who had received oestrogens.[2,3] This was most pronounced in current users in whom the relative risk was about one third to one half of that for women who had never taken oestrogen. Similarly, a large case-control study also reported a significant reduction in colon cancer, but not rectal cancer.[4]

1. MacLennan SC, *et al.* Colorectal cancer and oestrogen replacement therapy: a meta-analysis of epidemiological studies. *Med J Aust* 1995; **162:** 491–3.
2. Calle EE, *et al.* Estrogen replacement therapy and risk of fatal colon cancer in a prospective cohort of postmenopausal women. *J Natl Cancer Inst* 1995; **87:** 517–23.
3. Grodstein F, *et al.* Postmenopausal hormone use and risk for colorectal cancer and adenoma. *Ann Intern Med* 1998; **128:** 705–12.
4. Newcomb PA, Storer BE. Postmenopausal hormone use and risk of large-bowel cancer. *J Natl Cancer Inst* 1995; **87:** 1067–71.

OVARY. There was no clear evidence that the use of oestrogen replacement therapy altered the risk of invasive ovarian cancer in various case-control studies reviewed by the Collaborative Ovarian Cancer Group.[1] However, a more recent cohort study has suggested that long-term oestrogen replacement therapy may increase the risk of fatal ovarian cancer.[2]

1. Whittemore AS, *et al.* Characteristics relating to ovarian cancer risk: collaborative analysis of 12 US case-control studies. *Am J Epidemiol* 1992; **136:** 1184–1203.
2. Rodriguez C, *et al.* Estrogen replacement therapy and fatal ovarian cancer. *Am J Epidemiol* 1995; **141:** 828–35.

Effects on the cardiovascular system. Various facts support the theory that oestrogens may be cardioprotective. For example, mortality rates for cardiovascular disease in women are lower than those in men at all ages. In addition, women who have a surgically induced menopause at a young age are at increased risk of coronary heart disease compared with women who have a natural menopause.

Conversely, use of high doses of oestrogens for malignant disease is associated with an increased risk of cardiovascular events. Similarly, use of oestrogens in combined oral contraceptives carries a small increased risk of cardiovascular disease (see p.1429). Moreover, an early study in men surviving a myocardial infarction found that high doses of conjugated oestrogens (5 mg daily) were associated with a higher incidence of subsequent coronary events than placebo (see p.1457).

However, the majority of large observational studies have revealed a decreased risk of coronary heart disease and mortality in women receiving menopausal hormone replacement therapy (HRT) compared with those who have never received this therapy (see below). Although progestogens may reduce the beneficial effects of oestrogens on some lipids, available data suggest that use of combined HRT is still cardioprotective. The reduction in risk has been estimated as 30 to 50%, although biases such as the healthy user effect are likely to play a part in this estimate and some results from controlled studies have cast doubt on the extent of any reduction in risk. Whether HRT reduces the risk of stroke is even less clear (see below) and it appears to be associated with an *increased* risk of venous thrombo-embolism (see below).

The mechanisms by which oestrogen exerts its cardiovascular effects are not fully understood. Oestrogen has beneficial effects of lipoproteins, but adverse effects on triglycerides (see below). Similarly, it has beneficial effects on some, and adverse effects on other, mediators of thrombosis. Oestrogen may also have a direct beneficial effect on the coronary vasculature.

CORONARY HEART DISEASE. In 1991, Stampfer and Colditz reviewed 31 case-control and cohort studies on the risk of coronary heart disease in women using menopausal hormone replacement therapy (HRT).[1] Four studies showed an adverse trend, 2 showed no effect on risk, and 25 showed a trend to reduction in risk or a significant reduction in risk. The summary relative risk was 0.56, with estimated 95% confidence intervals of 0.50 to 0.61. Other reviews have reported similar reductions in risk.[2,3] Much of the data relates to the use of unopposed oestrogen, which is no longer recommended in women with a uterus because of the risk of endometrial cancer (see above).

There has been concern that the addition of progestogen might negate or reduce the cardiovascular benefits of oestrogens by reducing the oestrogen-induced rise in serum high-density-lipoprotein cholesterol concentrations. It has been postulated that this may be particularly true for progestogens derived from nortestosterone rather than progesterone. Results from the Postmenopausal Estrogen/Progestin Interventions Trial (PEPI) indicated that the beneficial effects on blood lipoproteins and fibrinogen, although greatest with unopposed oestrogen, were still present when combined with medroxyprogesterone or micronised progesterone (micronised progesterone was preferable to medroxyprogesterone).[4] Moreover, the UK Medical Research Council Study reported a fairly even balance between possibly beneficial and adverse effects on lipid concentrations and coagulability when conjugated oestrogens alone were compared with conjugated oestrogens plus norgestrel (a nortestosterone derivative).[5] Similar results were reported in the CHART study for ethinyloestradiol with or without norethisterone.[6] Although reassuring, these 3 studies provide information only on surrogate end-points.

The most recent data from the Nurses' Health Study cohort[7] show a greater reduction in the risk of major coronary heart disease among women receiving an oestrogen plus a progestogen (relative risk 0.4) than those receiving an oestrogen alone (0.6), as compared with the risk in women not using hormones. Recent *in vitro* data suggest that progestogens may actually protect against atherosclerosis via inhibition of smooth muscle cell proliferation.[8]

As regards duration of HRT use, it appears that current use is the most important factor for cardiovascular risk reduction. Users with coronary risk factors appear to derive greater benefit from HRT than those at low risk of coronary artery disease.[9] Of concern, the Nurses' Health Study reported that the apparent benefit from HRT decreased with increasing duration of use beyond 10 years because of an increase in mortality from breast cancer.[9]

In contrast to previous findings, a recent retrospective case-control study[10] did not find a decreased risk of myocardial infarction in women currently using combined HRT or oestrogens alone. The authors of this study suggest that the benefit of HRT may not be as large as has been estimated in some qualitative overviews, and emphasise the need for data from randomised trials.[10] This has been confirmed by results[11] of the Heart and Estrogen/progestin Replacement Study, a randomised placebo-controlled trial in women with established coronary heart disease. Combined HRT with conjugated oestrogens plus medroxyprogesterone produced no overall benefit in reducing the occurrence of myocardial infarction or death due to ischaemic heart disease in these women. This overall lack of effect was due to an initial increase in cardiac events during the first year, with a later beneficial effect. These worrying results have suggested that HRT should not be used for secondary prevention in women with heart disease, in contrast to some earlier suggestions (see also under Uses and Administration, below), but the extent to which they can be extrapolated to women without pre-existing heart disease is unclear. It is hoped that the results of other ongoing randomised studies such as the Womens Health Initiative will provide a more definitive answer.

1. Stampfer MJ, Colditz GA. Estrogen replacement therapy and coronary heart disease: a quantitative assessment of the epidemiologic evidence. *Prev Med* 1991; **20:** 47–63.
2. Grady D, *et al.* Hormone therapy to prevent disease and prolong life in postmenopausal women. *Ann Intern Med* 1992; **117:** 1016–37.
3. Barrett-Connor E, Bush TL. Estrogen and coronary heart disease in women. *JAMA* 1991; **265:** 1861–7.
4. The Writing Group for the PEPI Trial. Effects of estrogen or estrogen/progestin regimens on heart disease risk factors in postmenopausal women: the Postmenopausal Estrogen/Progestin Interventions (PEPI) Trial. *JAMA* 1995; **273:** 199–208. Correction. *ibid.*; **274:** 1676.
5. Medical Research Council's General Practice Research Framework. Randomised comparison of oestrogen versus oestrogen plus progestogen hormone replacement therapy in women with hysterectomy. *Br Med J* 1996; **312:** 473–8.
6. Speroff L, *et al.* The comparative effect on bone density, endometrium, and lipids of continuous hormones as replacement therapy (CHART Study): a randomized controlled trial. *JAMA* 1996; **276:** 1397–1403.
7. Grodstein F, *et al.* Postmenopausal estrogen and progestin use and the risk of cardiovascular disease. *N Engl J Med* 1996; **335:** 453–61. Correction. *ibid.*; 1046.
8. Lee W-S, *et al.* Progesterone inhibits arterial smooth muscle cell proliferation. *Nature Med* 1997; **3:** 1005–1008.
9. Grodstein F, *et al.* Postmenopausal hormone therapy and mortality. *N Engl J Med* 1997; **336:** 1769–75.
10. Sidney S, *et al.* Myocardial infarction and the use of estrogen and estrogen-progestogen in postmenopausal women. *Ann Intern Med* 1997; **127:** 501–8.
11. Hulley S, *et al.* Randomized trial of estrogen plus progestin for secondary prevention of coronary heart disease in postmenopausal women. *JAMA* 1998; **280:** 605–13.

HYPERTENSION. Although high doses of oestrogens have been associated with increased blood pressure, in normotensive women, use of menopausal hormone replacement therapy (HRT) has little effect on blood pressure or may be associated with a small decrease. Similarly, there is some evidence that HRT does not alter blood pressure in hypertensive women.[1]

1. Lip GYH, *et al.* Hormone replacement therapy and blood pressure in hypertensive women. *J Hum Hypertens* 1994; **8:** 491–4.

STROKE. The Framingham Study suggested a more than two-fold increased risk of stroke in women using menopausal hormone replacement therapy.[1] However, subsequent studies reporting risk of stroke separately from other cardiovascular events have shown either no effect on risk[2] or a decreased risk in the order of 30 to 50%.[3,4]

Recent data from the Nurses' Health Study cohort[5] revealed little association between the risk of stroke of any type and current use of unopposed oestrogens or oestrogen plus progestogen. However, they reported a trend towards an increased risk of stroke in current users of high-dose oestrogen therapy (1.25 mg or higher). Similarly, a large Danish case-control study found that unopposed oestrogens or oestrogen plus progestogen had no effect on the risk of non-fatal haemorrhagic or thrombo-embolic stroke.[6]

1. Wilson PWF, *et al.* Postmenopausal estrogen use, cigarette smoking, and cardiovascular morbidity in women over 50: the Framingham study. *N Engl J Med* 1985; **313:** 1038–43.
2. Stampfer MJ, *et al.* Postmenopausal estrogen therapy and cardiovascular disease: ten-year follow-up from the Nurses' Health Study. *N Engl J Med* 1991; **325:** 756–62.
3. Paganini-Hill A, *et al.* Postmenopausal oestrogen treatment and stroke: a prospective study. *Br Med J* 1988; **297:** 519–22.
4. Finucane FF, *et al.* Decreased risk of stroke among postmenopausal hormone users: results from a national cohort. *Arch Intern Med* 1993; **153:** 73–9.
5. Grodstein F, *et al.* Postmenopausal estrogen and progestin use and the risk of cardiovascular disease. *N Engl J Med* 1996; **335:** 453–61. Correction. *ibid.*; 1406.
6. Tønnes Pedersen A, *et al.* Hormone replacement therapy and risk of non-fatal stroke. *Lancet* 1997; **350:** 1277–83.

VENOUS THROMBO-EMBOLISM. Traditionally it has been assumed that, unlike combined oral contraceptives, menopausal hormone replacement therapy (HRT) is not associated with an increased risk of venous thrombo-embolism.

However, 4 recent observational studies have provided substantial evidence that there is an increased risk of deep vein thrombosis and/or pulmonary embolism in women receiving HRT.[1-4] The relative risk of venous thrombo-embolism was found to be 2.1 to 3.6 in current users compared with past-users or those who had never received HRT. This equates to an excess of 16 to 23 cases per 100 000 women per year. One study found that the increase in risk was restricted to the first year of use.[4] Another reported an increased risk with increasing oestrogen dose.[2]

The UK Committee on Safety of Medicines considers that these data do not affect the risk-benefit ratio of therapy in women without predisposing factors for venous thrombo-embolism.[5] However, in some women with predisposing factors, such as a personal or family history of venous thrombo-embolism, severe varicose veins, obesity, surgery, trauma or prolonged bed-rest, the risk of venous thrombo-embolism may exceed the benefits.

Preliminary evidence from a randomised placebo-controlled trial[6] supports the findings of the observational studies above.

1. Daly E, *et al.* Risk of venous thromboembolism in users of hormone replacement therapy. *Lancet* 1996; **348:** 977–80.
2. Jick H, *et al.* Risk of hospital admission for idiopathic venous thromboembolism among users of postmenopausal oestrogens. *Lancet* 1996; **348:** 981–83.
3. Grodstein F, *et al.* Prospective study of exogenous hormones and risk of pulmonary embolism in women. *Lancet* 1996; **348:** 983–7.
4. Pérez Gutthann S, *et al.* Hormone replacement therapy and risk of venous thromboembolism: population based case-control study. *Br Med J* 1997; **314:** 796–800.
5. Committee on Safety of Medicines/Medicines Control Agency. Risk of venous thromboembolism with hormone replacement therapy. *Current Problems* 1996; **22:** 9–10.
6. Grady D, Furberg C. Venous thromboembolic events associated with hormone replacement therapy. *JAMA* 1997; **278:** 477.

Effects on lipids. Oestrogens increase serum high-density-lipoprotein cholesterol and decrease low-density-lipoprotein cholesterol concentrations, effects that are considered favourable and may be a mechanism behind their reduction in coronary heart disease in postmenopausal women (see above). However, they may also increase serum triglyceride concentrations, which is undesirable. Severe hypertriglyceridaemia and pancreatitis have occurred in women with hypertriglyceridaemia treated with oestrogens.[1,2] Use of concomitant progestogen reduces oestrogen-induced hypertriglyceridaemia.[2]

1. Glueck CJ, *et al.* Severe hypertriglyceridemia and pancreatitis when estrogen replacement therapy is given to hypertriglyceridemic women. *J Lab Clin Med* 1994; **123:** 59–64.
2. Isley WL, Oki J. Estrogen-induced pancreatitis after discontinuation of concomitant medroxyprogesterone therapy. *Am J Med* 1997; **102:** 416–17.

Pancreatitis. Unopposed oestrogen has been associated with pancreatitis in women with hypertriglyceridaemia (see above).

Precautions

Before menopausal hormone replacement therapy (HRT) is given the woman should undergo an appropriate medical examination and her medical history should be carefully evaluated. Regular examination is recommended during use.

HRT should be avoided in women with active thrombophlebitis or thrombo-embolic disease or undiagnosed abnormal vaginal bleeding, and abnormal vaginal bleeding during therapy should be investigated (see below). HRT is also contra-indicated in women with oestrogen-dependent neoplasms such as those of the breast or endometrium, and is usually considered contra-indicated in women with a history of these conditions although this has been debated (see below). Active liver disease and porphyria are also generally considered to be contra-indications.

Prolonged exposure to unopposed oestrogens increases the risk of endometrial cancer whatever the route of administration (see above). HRT should be used with caution in women with predisposing factors to thrombo-embolism (see also above), migraine, a history of breast nodules or fibrocystic disease, uterine fibroids, or a history of endometriosis. Consideration should be given to temporarily stopping HRT 4 weeks prior to elective surgery.

Cautions for HRT for which the evidence is less well established include diabetes, asthma, epilepsy, hypertension, cardiac or renal disease, melanoma, otosclerosis, multiple sclerosis, and systemic lupus erythematosus.

Doses of oestrogen in HRT are insufficient to provide contraception. Therapy is contra-indicated in known or suspected pregnancy, and in women who are breast feeding.

Endometriosis. Endometriosis may be reactivated by unopposed oestrogen use in postmenopausal women. This has occurred, even in women who have previously undergone hysterectomy and bilateral oophorectomy for endometriosis.[1,2] Reactivation of endometriosis can result in ureteric obstruction and consequent renal damage.[1,2] Use of combined hormone replacement therapy rather than unopposed oestrogen has been advocated for women who have radical surgery for endometriosis.[1]

1. Manyonda IT, *et al.* Obstructive uropathy from endometriosis after hysterectomy and oophorectomy; two case reports. *Eur J Obstet Gynecol Reprod Biol* 1989; **31:** 195–8.
2. Brough RJ, O'Flynn K. Recurrent pelvic endometriosis and bilateral ureteric obstruction associated with hormone replacement therapy. *Br Med J* 1996; **312:** 1221–2.

Malignant neoplasms. A discussion on the use of hormone replacement therapy (HRT) with oestrogen in patients previously treated for endometrial or breast cancer.[1] Experience suggested that it may be used safely in patients who had been previously treated for endometrial cancer and, although there was little or no experience of its use in women previously treated for breast cancer, that it was not contra-indicated in all such women; the benefit-risk ratio should be considered for each individual.

Several workers have highlighted the lack of information about the risks of HRT in patients with a history of breast cancer, and have agreed that such therapy should not necessarily be withheld in these patients provided that the risks are understood.[2-5] Short-term continuous combined HRT in selected women with severe menopausal symptoms has been suggested.[6] Others suggest that HRT should be combined with tamoxifen in such patients.[3,7]

1. Creasman WT. Estrogen replacement therapy: is previously treated cancer a contraindication? *Obstet Gynecol* 1991; **77:** 308–12.
2. Lobo RA. Hormone replacement therapy: oestrogen replacement after treatment for breast cancer? *Lancet* 1993; **341:** 1313–14.
3. Powles TJ, *et al.* Hormone replacement after breast cancer. *Lancet* 1993; **342:** 60–1.
4. DiSaia PJ, *et al.* Hormone replacement therapy in breast cancer. *Lancet* 1993; **342:** 1232.
5. Cobleigh MA, *et al.* Estrogen replacement therapy in breast cancer survivors: a time for change. *JAMA* 1994; **272:** 540–5.
6. Eden JA. Estrogen replacement therapy in survivors of breast cancer: a risk-benefit assessment. *Drugs Aging* 1996; **8:** 127–33.
7. Powles TJ, Hickish T. Breast cancer response to hormone replacement therapy withdrawal. *Lancet* 1995; **345:** 1442.

Vaginal bleeding. Menopausal hormone replacement therapy (HRT) is contra-indicated in patients with undiagnosed abnormal vaginal bleeding, which may be a symptom of endometrial carcinoma. The causes of abnormal vaginal bleeding in women receiving HRT and guidelines on their investigation and treatment have been reviewed.[1,2]

1. Good AE. Diagnostic options for assessment of postmenopausal bleeding. *Mayo Clin Proc* 1997; **72:** 345–9.
2. Spencer CP, *et al.* Management of abnormal bleeding in women receiving hormone replacement therapy. *Br Med J* 1997; **315:** 37–42.

Interactions

Drugs that increase the hepatic metabolism of oestrogens and progestogens have been associated with failure of the combined oral contraceptive (see p.1432). Important examples include rifamycins, some antiepileptics, and griseofulvin. It is not unreasonable to assume that these drugs would also be associated with decreased effectiveness of hormone replacement therapy (HRT), but there appears to be little information on this (see below).

Although oral contraceptives may antagonise or reduce the effects of a number of drugs (see p.1432), the lower doses of oestrogens used in HRT are considered less likely to induce interactions, although the possibility remains.

Alcohol. Acute ingestion of an alcoholic beverage led to a threefold increase in circulating oestradiol in women on menopausal hormone replacement therapy (HRT).[1] The authors suggest that drinking habits may need to be considered when deciding on an appropriate dose of HRT.

1. Ginsburg ES, *et al.* Effects of alcohol ingestion on estrogens in postmenopausal women. *JAMA* 1996; **276:** 1747–51.

Antiepileptics. A report of phenytoin diminishing the effect of conjugated oestrogens in a menopausal woman.[1]

1. Notelovitz M, *et al.* Interaction between estrogen and Dilantin in a menopausal woman. *N Engl J Med* 1981; **304:** 788–9.

Pharmacokinetics

For a discussion of the pharmacokinetics of oestrogens and progestogens, see Oestradiol, p.1455 and Progesterone, p.1460, respectively. The extent of binding of progestogens to serum sex-hormone binding globulin may be altered when they are administered with an oestrogen. Oestrogens increase serum concentrations of sex-hormone binding globulin, and progestogens differ in their ability to suppress this effect.

Uses and Administration

The most commonly used oestrogens in menopausal hormone replacement therapy (HRT) are natural oestrogens such as oestradiol and conjugated oestrogens. Dosages of oestrogens used in HRT are generally lower than those used in combined oral contraceptives, and do not therefore provide contraception.

Various routes of administration for the different oestrogenic compounds used for HRT are available, including the oral route, subcutaneous implants, topical applications for vulvovaginal use, and transdermal skin patches and gels. Generally, if prolonged therapy (for more than 2 to 4 weeks) with an oestrogen by any route is envisaged in a woman with an intact uterus, a progestogen is required to prevent endometrial proliferation. This may be administered by mouth cyclically for 10 to 14 days per cycle or continuously; transdermal preparations are now also available. Both progesterone derivatives such as medroxyprogesterone and dydrogesterone, and 19-nortestosterone analogues such as norethisterone and norgestrel are used. Doses of progestogens for HRT are similar to those used in combined oral contraceptives.

Administration. In a discussion of the relative merits of oral and transdermal oestrogen therapy[1] it was suggested that there was circumstantial and theoretical evidence to suppose that transdermal therapy might be preferable in women who smoke, who suffer from migraine, hepatobiliary disease, or hypertriglyceridaemia, or who have a history of thrombo-embolism. In contrast, oral administration might be preferable in patients with hypercholesterolaemia. However, studies to examine these suppositions were needed. Various alternatives to oral oestrogen therapy have been reviewed.[2,3]

For reviews of oestradiol administration as implants or given transdermally, see p.1456.

1. Lufkin EG, Ory SJ. Relative value of transdermal and oral estrogen therapy in various clinical situations. *Mayo Clin Proc* 1994; **69:** 131–5.
2. Baker VL. Alternatives to oral estrogen replacement: transdermal patches, percutaneous gels, vaginal creams and rings, implants, and other methods of delivery. *Obstet Gynecol Clin North Am* 1994; **21:** 271–97.
3. Jewelewicz R. New developments in topical estrogen therapy. *Fertil Steril* 1997; **67:** 1–12.

Benefits and risks of HRT. ACUTE MENOPAUSAL SYMPTOMS. Where symptoms are severe enough to warrant treatment, hormone replacement therapy (HRT) with oestrogens is the mainstay of treatment for *vasomotor symptoms and atrophic vaginitis*. Commentators[1,2] have suggested that there are few contra-indications to the treatment of women with acute symptoms, although undiagnosed vaginal bleeding, before or during therapy, should always be investigated, as it can be a sign of endometrial cancer.

In addition, women with active thrombophlebitis or thrombo-embolic disorders should not receive HRT, and the risk-benefit should be considered carefully in women with predisposing risk factors for venous thrombo-embolism. HRT should also not be used in women with oestrogen-dependent cancer, although some have suggested that short-term HRT need not necessarily be withheld in women who have survived breast cancer if menopausal symptoms are severe and unresponsive to other measures (see also Malignant Neoplasms under Precautions, above).

If the woman is in the perimenopause she is potentially fertile, and HRT does not provide contraception. It is now considered that, in women under 50 years of age and free of all risk factors for venous and arterial disease, a low-oestrogen dose combined oral contraceptive (p.1433) can be used to provide both relief of menopausal symptoms and contraception. If HRT is used in perimenopausal women, then non-hormonal contraceptive measures should be used if required (see p.1434).

Perimenopausal women with a uterus should also receive a cyclical progestogen, which will cause regular withdrawal bleeding. An alternative is the levonorgestrel intra-uterine device with concomitant oral or transdermal oestrogen.[3] In women with a uterus who are postmenopausal (greater than 12 months) continuous combined HRT may be used, which induces an atrophic endometrium. An alternative is the hormonal agent tibolone, which does not require concomitant progestogen. Women without a uterus, and who have not had endometriosis, may receive continuous oestrogen alone. For a discussion of the risks of endometrial cancer with HRT, see under Adverse Effects, above.

In women experiencing solely *vaginal symptoms*, HRT administered just for a few weeks may be sufficient. This may be administered vaginally. In women experiencing vasomotor symptoms, oral or transdermal HRT is required. Most women do not require exogenous oestrogens to control hot flushes for more than 3 to 5 years; the lowest dose that controls symptoms is given, and therapy is tapered over a few years and withdrawn if prophylactic cover of long-term effects is not required.[2]

Nonspecific symptoms may also improve in women administered HRT. For example, oestrogens have reduced the incidence of urinary-tract infections,[4] and dysuria and incontinence (see below), although good evidence is somewhat scanty. Similarly, many women report improved mood and well-being when given oestrogens,[1,2] although it is unclear to what extent this is due to relief of other symptoms. True depression does not respond to HRT, and needs to be identified and treated appropriately. Moreover, the addition of progestogens carries some risk of adverse effects on mood such as depression, anxiety, and irritability. Nonpharmacological measures that may benefit some women with vasomotor symptoms include regular physical activity and stress management. Alternative medical therapies that may be tried include the progestogens megestrol and medroxyprogesterone, clonidine or veralipride.[5,6] However, the evidence for the efficacy of these alternative therapies is less conclusive than that for HRT. Evening primrose oil is not effective.[7] Women in cultures with diets high in plant oestrogens have low incidences of menopausal vasomotor symptoms suggesting a potential benefit from such diets.[8]

LONG-TERM EFFECTS. Reliable estimates of the true benefits and risks for long-term HRT in postmenopausal women are not available, and hence for many women the balance of these risks remains controversial.[9,10] There are extensive data[8] from observational studies on the beneficial effects on fracture rates and cardiovascular disease, and the risks for development of breast cancer and endometrial cancer, and the possible effects on overall mortality. However, the women receiving HRT in these studies may differ from women not receiving HRT, and the extent of any bias resulting from this is unclear. Randomised prospective studies are underway, but the first results will not be reported for a number of years. In the meantime, various authors have used the available data to suggest clinical guidelines.[1-3,11,12]

It is generally agreed that all women who have had a *premature natural or induced menopause* should receive HRT until the age of 50 years, unless there are specific contra-indications to therapy (mentioned in the discussion of acute symptoms above). Considerations as to how long they need to continue HRT after the usual age for the menopause are probably the same as for other women.

Women who have, or who are at risk of developing *osteoporosis* should generally receive long-term HRT (see also below). Risk factors for osteoporosis include familial predisposition, sedentary lifestyle, cigarette smoking, low body-weight, corticosteroid therapy, and a subnormal peak bone mass, for example, due to a calcium-deficient diet in childhood and adolescence. Where possible, treatment should be combined with adequate dietary calcium, weight-bearing exercise, and cessation of smoking.

Women who have, or are at risk of developing, *coronary heart disease* have also been considered likely to benefit from HRT (but see also below).

Women who are at high risk of *breast cancer* should probably not receive long-term HRT (see also Malignant Neoplasms under Precautions, above). Those with a family history of breast cancer may be at particular risk.

Most authors agree that a woman should make an informed choice regarding HRT based on how she values each potential effect. In general, studies that have modelled the various risks have estimated that the overall benefits of long-term HRT starting at about age 50 are likely to outweigh the risks except in women who are at high risk of breast cancer.[12,13] An important consideration in these analyses is that the data on incidence of each of the diseases are specific to the USA. Incidence rates of hip fracture, cardiovascular disease, and breast cancer vary widely between countries,[8] which may affect the choice. For example, a preliminary analysis using data from Italy suggested that use of HRT for 10 years was likely to result in an overall reduction in life expectancy in Italian women, who are at a low risk of ischaemic heart disease.[14]

The appropriate duration of HRT is also debated. For optimal benefits on bone and vasculature it is anticipated that HRT should be continued for 10 to 20 years or more.[11] However, the breast cancer risk increases with increasing duration of use. Moreover, the incidence of breast cancer may exceed that of cardiovascular disease in women aged less than 60 years. Therefore, some have suggested that the best age to start HRT in asymptomatic women for prevention of osteoporosis and heart disease may be at age 65.[15]

Long-term HRT for the treatment and prevention of osteoporosis and cardiovascular disease is administered orally or transdermally. As mentioned above, oestrogens alone are suitable for women without a uterus who have not had endometriosis. In other women, a progestogen is also required to reduce the risk of endometrial hyperplasia and carcinoma (see also Carcinogenicity under Adverse Effects, above) or recurrence of endometriosis. This may be administered cyclically in perimenopausal women, but continuous administration is likely to be preferred in women who have been postmenopausal for more than 1 year since it avoids withdrawal bleeding. Tibolone is an alternative in women who have been postmenopausal for more than 1 year. Non-hormonal options for osteoporosis prophylaxis or treatment include bisphosphonates, as discussed on p.731. The selective oestrogen-receptor modulator raloxifene is also available.

1. Jacobs HS, Loeffler FE. Postmenopausal hormone replacement therapy. *Br Med J* 1992; **305:** 1403–8.
2. Notelovitz M. Estrogen replacement therapy: indications, contraindications, and agent selection. *Am J Obstet Gynecol* 1989; **161:** 1832–41.
3. Anonymous. Hormone replacement therapy. *Drug Ther Bull* 1996; **34:** 81–4.
4. Raz R, Stamm WE. A controlled trial of intravaginal estriol in postmenopausal women with recurrent urinary tract infections. *N Engl J Med* 1993; **329:** 753–6.
5. Young RL, *et al.* Management of menopause when estrogen cannot be used. *Drugs* 1990; **40:** 220–30.
6. Luchero MA, McCloskey WW. Alternatives to estrogen for the treatment of hot flushes. *Ann Pharmacother* 1997; **31:** 915–17.
7. Chenoy R, *et al.* Effect of oral gamolenic acid from evening primrose oil on menopausal flushing. *Br Med J* 1994; **308:** 501–3.
8. WHO. Research on the menopause in the 1990s. *WHO Tech Rep Ser 866* 1996.
9. Toozs-Hobson P, Cardoz L. Hormone replacement therapy for all? Universal prescription is desirable. *Br Med J* 1996; **313:** 350–1.
10. Jacobs HS. Hormone replacement therapy for all? Not for everybody. *Br Med J* 1996; **313:** 351–2.
11. American College of Physicians. Guidelines for counselling postmenopausal women about preventive hormone therapy. *Ann Intern Med* 1992; **117:** 1038–41.
12. Grady D, *et al.* Hormone therapy to prevent disease and prolong life in postmenopausal women. *Ann Intern Med* 1992; **117:** 1016–37.
13. Col NF, *et al.* Patient-specific decisions about hormone replacement therapy in postmenopausal women. *JAMA* 1997; **277:** 1140–7.
14. Panico S, *et al.* Hormone replacement therapy may not always be right choice to prevent cardiovascular disease. *Br Med J* 1996; **313:** 687.
15. Prince RL, Geelhoed EA. When should postmenopausal women start taking oestrogen replacement therapy? *Med J Aust* 1995; **162:** 173–4.

Cardiovascular disorders. Observational studies have shown a decreased risk of coronary heart disease and consequent mortality in women receiving menopausal hormone replacement therapy (HRT), see under Adverse Effects, above, and oestrogens are known to have some beneficial effects on the plasma lipid profile (see above). Therefore, some have advocated the use of HRT as a possible alternative, or adjunct, to lipid regulating drugs in postmenopausal women with hypercholesterolaemia.[1] Hyperlipidaemias and their more usual treatments are discussed on p.1265.

However, results from a randomised study[2] in women with established coronary heart disease have shown an initial increase in adverse cardiac events when HRT was given, and although some benefit was seen after 4 or 5 years there was no overall decrease in myocardial infarction or cardiac death.

Data from a recent randomised crossover study[3] showed that both simvastatin and continuous conjugated oestrogens plus medroxyprogesterone had beneficial effects on plasma lipoprotein concentrations, but that simvastatin was more effective than the hormones. In addition, the hormones increased, whereas simvastatin decreased, triglyceride concentrations.

Some observational studies have reported that women receiving HRT have better survival rates after revascularisation procedures (p.797) than women not receiving this therapy.[4,5]

1. Expert Panel on Detection, Evaluation, and Treatment of High Blood Cholesterol in Adults. Summary of the second Report of the National Cholesterol Education Program (NCEP) Expert Panel on Detection, Evaluation, and Treatment of High Blood Cholesterol in Adults (Adult Treatment Panel II). *JAMA* 1993; **269:** 3015–23.
2. Hulley S, *et al.* Randomized trial of estrogen plus progestin for secondary prevention of coronary heart disease in postmenopausal women. *JAMA* 1998; **280:** 650–13.
3. Darling GM, *et al.* Estrogen and progestin compared with simvastatin for hypercholesterolemia in postmenopausal women. *N Engl J Med* 1997; **337:** 595–601.
4. O'Keefe JH, *et al.* Estrogen replacement therapy after coronary angioplasty in women. *J Am Coll Cardiol* 1997; **29:** 1–5.
5. Sullivan JM, *et al.* Effect on survival of estrogen replacement therapy after coronary artery bypass grafting. *Am J Cardiol* 1997; **79:** 847–50.

Dementia. Several observational studies[1-3] in women receiving hormone replacement therapy have suggested that oestrogens can reduce the risk and delay the onset of Alzheimer's disease (p.1386) in postmenopausal women. However, a recent meta-analysis[6] concluded that studies conducted so far had had substantial methodological problems and that results had been conflicting. A long-term study of the value of hormone replacement therapy in Alzheimer's disease (Womens Health Initiative Clinical Trial) is in progress. Preliminary reports[4,5] suggest that treatment with oestrogens may also be of benefit in women who already have Alzheimer's disease; results of further studies are awaited.

1. Tang M-X,*et al.* Effect of oestrogen during menopause on risk and age at onset of Alzheimer's disease. *Lancet* 1996; **348:** 429–32.
2. Paganini-Hill A, Henderson VW. Estrogen replacement therapy and risk of Alzheimer disease. *Arch Intern Med* 1996; **156:** 2213–17.
3. Kawas C, *et al.* A prospective study of estrogen replacement therapy and the risk of developing Alzheimer's disease: the Baltimore Longitudinal Study of Aging. *Neurology* 1997; **48:** 1517–21.
4. Ohkura T, *et al.* Long-term estrogen replacement therapy in female patients with dementia of the Alzheimer type: 7 case reports. *Dementia* 1995; **6:** 99–107.
5. Schneider LS, *et al.* Potential role for estrogen replacement in the treatment of Alzheimer's dementia. *Am J Med* 1997; **103** (suppl 3A): 46S–50S.
6. Yaffe K, *et al.* Estrogen therapy in postmenopausal women: effects on cognitive function and dementia. *JAMA* 1998; **279:** 688–95.

Hyperparathyroidism. Oestrogens may ameliorate some consequences of hyperparathyroidism in postmenopausal women as well as mitigate osteoporosis,[1-4] but any long-term benefits are, as mentioned on p.733, uncertain.

1. Anonymous. Medical management of primary hyperparathyroidism. *Lancet* 1984; **ii:** 727–8.
2. Marcus R, *et al.* Conjugated estrogens in the treatment of postmenopausal women with hyperparathyroidism. *Ann Intern Med* 1984; **100:** 633–40.
3. Selby PL, Peacock M. Ethinyl estradiol and norethindrone in the treatment of primary hyperparathyroidism in postmenopausal women. *N Engl J Med* 1986; **314:** 1481–5.
4. Coe FL, *et al.* Is estrogen preferable to surgery for postmenopausal women with primary hyperparathyroidism? *N Engl J Med* 1986; **314:** 1508–9.

Osteoporosis. Oestrogens have a direct antiresorptive effect on bone, and will increase bone mass density (BMD). Suggested minimum daily doses are 0.625 mg of conjugated oestrogens, 2 mg of oestradiol by mouth or 50 μg transdermally, and 15 μg of ethinyloestradiol.[1] Addition of a progestogen (required to prevent endometrial hyperplasia in women with a uterus) does not impair the beneficial effect of oestrogens on BMD, whether administered cyclically or continuously.[2,3] Oestrogens are currently the preferred method of treating and preventing postmenopausal osteoporosis, as discussed on p.731. Unresolved issues are the duration of therapy required to prevent fractures in old age,[4] and the ideal age to start therapy to obtain the maximum benefits to the bone with the minimum risk of breast cancer.

Oestrogens are also used in women to reduce the risk of corticosteroid-induced osteoporosis (see p.1011).

1. Jacobs HS, Loeffler FE. Postmenopausal hormone replacement therapy. *Br Med J* 1992; **305:** 1403–8.
2. The Writing Group for the PEPI trial. Effects of hormone therapy on bone mineral density: results from the Postmenopausal Estrogen/Progestin Interventions (PEPI) trial. *JAMA* 1996; **276:** 1389–96.
3. Speroff L, *et al.* The comparative effect on bone density, endometrium, and lipids of continuous hormones as replacement therapy (CHART Study): a randomized controlled trial. *JAMA* 1996; **276:** 1397–1403.
4. Schneider DL, *et al.* Timing of postmenopausal estrogen for optimal bone mineral density: the Rancho Bernardo study. *JAMA* 1997; **277:** 543–7.

Urinary incontinence. Urinary incontinence (p.454) may be one of a number of acute symptoms associated with a decline in oestrogen levels (see above). Studies[1,2] suggest that oestrogens used with alpha-adrenoceptor agonists are effective in the management of female stress incontinence and this combination has been advocated for use in postmenopausal patients with mild symptoms. Unfortunately addition of a progestogen to treatment to reduce the risk of endometrial carcinoma in women with an intact uterus might exacerbate the incontinence.[3] The value of oestrogens used without an alpha-adrenoceptor agonist in urinary incontinence is less clear. Some workers[4] consider that oestrogens may be of use for symptoms of urgency, frequency, and nocturia in postmenopausal patients with urge incontinence; it has been suggested that hypoestrogenism may reduce the sensory threshold of the bladder.[5] A meta-analysis of 23 studies concluded that oestrogen therapy subjectively improved urinary incontinence in postmenopausal women but many of the studies examined were considered to be deficient in some respect.[6] A later well-designed study[7] found that hormone replacement therapy did not improve measures of incontinence in such patients although there was the possibility that concomitant progestogen therapy might have affected efficacy.

1. Walter S, *et al.* Stress urinary incontinence in postmenopausal women treated with oral estrogen (estriol) and an alpha-adrenoceptor-stimulating agent (phenylpropanolamine): a randomized double-blind placebo-controlled study. *Int Urogynecol J* 1990; **1:** 74–9.
2. Hilton P, *et al.* Oral and intravaginal estrogens alone and in combination with alpha-adrenergic stimulation in genuine stress incontinence. *Int Urogynecol J* 1990; **1:** 80–6.
3. Benness C, *et al.* Do progestogens exacerbate urinary incontinence in women on HRT? *Neurourol Urodyn* 1991; **10:** 316–17.
4. Cardozo L. Role of estrogens in the treatment of female urinary incontinence. *J Am Geriatr Soc* 1990; **38:** 326–8.
5. Fantl JA, *et al.* Postmenopausal urinary incontinence: comparison between non-estrogen-supplemented and estrogen-supplemented women. *Obstet Gynecol* 1988; **71:** 823–8.
6. Fantl JA *et al.* Estrogen therapy in the management of urinary incontinence in postmenopausal women: a meta-analysis: first report of the hormones and urogenital therapy committee. *Obstet Gynecol* 1994; **83:** 12–18.
7. Fantl JA, *et al.* Efficacy of estrogen supplementation in the treatment of urinary incontinence. *Obstet Gynecol* 1996; **88:** 745–9.

Algestone Acetophenide (9022-d)

Algestone Acetophenide *(USAN, rINNM).*

Alphasone Acetophenide; Dihydroxyprogesterone Acetophenide; SQ-15101. 16α,17α-(1-Phenylethylidenedioxy)pregn-4-ene-3,20-dione; 16α,17α-Isopropylidenedioxypregn-4-ene-3,20-dione.

$C_{29}H_{36}O_4$ = 448.6.

CAS — 595-77-7 (algestone); 24356-94-3 (algestone acetophenide).

Algestone acetophenide is a progestogen (see Progesterone, p.1459) that has been given by intramuscular injection in monthly doses of 150 mg in conjunction with oestradiol enanthate as a hormonal contraceptive (see p.1426). It has also been applied topically in the treatment of acne.

Preparations

Proprietary Preparations (details are given in Part 3)
Ital.: Neolutin Depositum†.

Multi-ingredient: ***Spain:*** Topasel.

Allyloestrenol (9023-n)

Allyloestrenol *(BAN).*

Allylestrenol *(rINN).* 17α-Allylestr-4-en-17β-ol.

$C_{21}H_{32}O$ = 300.5.

CAS — 432-60-0.

Allyloestrenol is a progestogen (see Progesterone, p.1459) structurally related to progesterone that has been given in threatened and habitual abortion, and to prevent premature labour. However, with the exception of proven progesterone deficiency, such use is no longer recommended. In threatened abortion in progesterone-deficient women a suggested dose is 5 mg three times daily by mouth for 5 to 7 days.

A case-control study of allyloestrenol use in pregnancy during 1980 to 1984 in Hungary indicated that it was not teratogenic.[1]

1. Czeizel A, Huiskes N. A case-control study to evaluate the risk of congenital anomalies as a result of allylestrenol therapy during pregnancy. *Clin Ther* 1988; **10:** 725–39.

Preparations

Proprietary Preparations (details are given in Part 3)
Aust.: Gestanon; ***Belg.:*** Gestanon†; ***Ger.:*** Gestanon†; ***Ital.:*** Gestanon†; ***S.Afr.:*** Gestanin†; ***Spain:*** Gestanon†; ***Switz.:*** Gestanon†; ***UK:*** Gestanin†.

Altrenogest (12346-m)

Altrenogest *(BAN, USAN, rINN).*

A-35957; A-41300; RH-2267; RU-2267. 17α-Allyl-17β-hydroxy-19-norandrosta-4,9,11-trien-3-one; 17β-Hydroxy-19,21,24-trinorchola-4,9,11,22-tetraen-3-one.

$C_{21}H_{26}O_2$ = 310.4.

CAS — 850-52-2.

Altrenogest is a progestogen (see Progesterone, p.1459) used in veterinary medicine.

Broparestrol (12456-s)

Broparestrol *(rINN).*

α-Bromo-β-(4-ethylphenyl)stilbene.

$C_{22}H_{19}Br$ = 363.3.

CAS — 479-68-5.

Broparestrol is a synthetic nonsteroidal oestrogen (see Stilboestrol, p.1462) that is an ingredient of preparations promoted for topical use in acne and similar skin disorders. It has been given in neoplastic disease.

Preparations

Proprietary Preparations (details are given in Part 3)

Multi-ingredient: ***Fr.:*** Acnestrol.

Chlormadinone Acetate (9027-v)

Chlormadinone Acetate *(BANM, USAN, rINNM).*

NSC-92338. 6-Chloro-17-hydroxypregna-4,6-diene-3,20-dione acetate.

$C_{23}H_{29}ClO_4$ = 404.9.

CAS — 1961-77-9 (chlormadinone); 302-22-7 (chlormadinone acetate).

Pharmacopoeias. In *Fr., Jpn.,* and *Pol.*

Adverse Effects and Precautions

As for progestogens in general (see Progesterone, p.1459).

Effects on the skin. A report of autoimmune dermatitis in one patient associated with chlormadinone acetate.[1]

1. Katayama I, Nishioka K. Autoimmune progesterone dermatitis with persistent amenorrhoea. *Br J Dermatol* 1985; **112:** 487–91.

Interactions

As for progestogens in general (see Progesterone, p.1460).

Uses and Administration

Chlormadinone acetate is a progestogen structurally related to progesterone (p.1460) that may have some anti-androgenic activity. It is given by mouth either alone or in combination with ethinyloestradiol or mestranol in the treatment of menstrual disorders such as menorrhagia (p.1461) and endometriosis (p.1442) at doses of 2 to 10 mg daily. It may also be used as the progestogen component of combined oral contraceptives (see p.1433) at a dose of 1 to 2 mg daily, particularly in women with androgen-dependent conditions such as acne and hirsutism.

Preparations

Proprietary Preparations (details are given in Part 3)
Fr.: Luteran; ***Ger.:*** Gestafortin; ***Jpn:*** Prostal.

Multi-ingredient: ***Fr.:*** Lutestral; ***Ger.:*** Eunomin†; Gestamestrol N; Menova†; Neo-Eunomin; Ovosiston; ***Switz.:*** Neo-Eunomine.

Chlorotrianisene (9029-q)

Chlorotrianisene *(BAN, rINN).*

NSC-10108; Tri-*p*-anisylchloroethylene. Chlorotris(4-methoxyphenyl)ethylene.

$C_{23}H_{21}ClO_3$ = 380.9.

CAS — 569-57-3.

Pharmacopoeias. In *Chin.,* and *US.*

Store in airtight containers.

Chlorotrianisene is a synthetic nonsteroidal oestrogen structurally related to stilboestrol (p.1462). It has a prolonged action.

Chlorotrianisene has been given by mouth for the treatment of menopausal symptoms in usual doses of 12 to 25 mg daily cyclically or continuously. A similar regimen has been used in the treatment of female hypogonadism.

Chlorotrianisene has also been given in similar doses for prostatic carcinoma.

Preparations

USP 23: Chlorotrianisene Capsules.

Proprietary Preparations (details are given in Part 3)
Belg.: Tace†; ***Ger.:*** Merbentul†; ***Spain:*** Tace; ***Switz.:*** Tace†; ***USA:*** Tace.

Clomiphene Citrate (9031-n)

Clomiphene Citrate *(BANM, USAN).*

Clomifene Citrate *(rINNM)*; Chloramiphene Citrate; Clomifeni Citras; MER-41; MRL-41; NSC-35770. A mixture of the *E* and *Z* isomers of 2-[4-(2-chloro-1,2-diphenylvinyl)phenoxy]triethylamine dihydrogen citrate.

$C_{26}H_{28}ClNO,C_6H_8O_7$ = 598.1.

CAS — 911-45-5 (clomiphene); 15690-57-0 ((E)-clomiphene); 15690-55-8 ((Z)-clomiphene); 50-41-9 (clomiphene citrate); 7599-79-3 ((E)-clomiphene citrate); 7619-53-6 ((Z)-clomiphene citrate).

NOTE. Clomiphene may be separated into its *Z* and *E* isomers, zuclomiphene and enclomiphene.

Pharmacopoeias. In *Chin., Eur.* (see p.viii), *Int., Jpn,* and *US.*

A white to pale yellow, odourless or almost odourless, crystalline powder. It contains 30 to 50% of the *Z* isomer. Slightly **soluble** in water; sparingly soluble in alcohol; freely soluble in methyl alcohol; slightly soluble in chloroform; practically insoluble in ether. **Protect** from light.

Adverse Effects

The incidence and severity of adverse effects of clomiphene citrate tend to be related to the dose employed. The most commonly reported adverse effects are reversible ovarian enlargement and cyst formation, vasomotor flushes resembling menopausal symptoms, and abdominal or pelvic discomfort or pain, sometimes with nausea or vomiting. Ovarian hyperstimulation syndrome has occurred. Breast tenderness, abnormal uterine bleeding, weight gain, headache, and endometriosis have also been reported. Transient visual disturbances such as after-images and blurring of vision may occur, and there have been rare reports of cataracts. Skin reactions such as allergic rashes and urticaria have occasionally been reported and reversible hair loss has been reported rarely. CNS disturbances have included convulsions, dizziness, lightheadedness, nervous tension, fatigue, vertigo, insomnia, and depression. Abnormalities in liver function tests and jaundice have sometimes been reported.

Following therapy with clomiphene citrate there is an increased risk of multiple births, but rarely more than twins. Although there have been reports of congenital disorders such as neural tube defects or Down's syndrome in infants born to women treated with clomiphene the role of the drug in the causation of these defects has not been established and the incidence is reported to be similar to that in women with other types of infertility problems. There is an increased risk of ectopic pregnancy.

Carcinogenicity. There have been a number of reports suggesting an association between drug therapy to treat infertility by stimulating ovulation and the subsequent development of ovarian cancer.[1-5] Concern has focussed in particular on the use of clomiphene citrate and gonadotrophins, and a study has reported an increased risk of ovarian cancer in women who had prolonged clomiphene therapy (for one year or more) although not in those who received the drug for a shorter period.[6] No association between gonadotrophin therapy and ovarian cancer was noted in this study. The conclusions of this study are only tentative, since the numbers who developed ovarian cancer were small, and it has been pointed out that a successfully achieved pregnancy may reduce the risk of some other cancers, and that the risks and benefits of the procedure are not easy to balance.[7] However, as a matter of prudence the UK Committee on Safety of Medicines has recommended that clomiphene should not normally be used for more than 6 cycles.[8]

1. Fishel S, Jackson P. Follicular stimulation for high tech pregnancies: are we playing it safe? *Br Med J* 1989; **299:** 309–11.
2. Kulkarni R, McGarry JM. Follicular stimulation and ovarian cancer. *Br Med J* 1989; **299:** 740.
3. Dietl J. Ovulation and ovarian cancer. *Lancet* 1991; **338:** 445.
4. Willemsen W, *et al.* Ovarian stimulation and granulosa-cell tumour. *Lancet* 1993; **341:** 986–8.
5. Tewari K, *et al.* Fertility drugs and malignant germ-cell tumour of ovary in pregnancy. *Lancet* 1998; **351:** 957–8.
6. Rossing MA, *et al.* Ovarian tumors in a cohort of infertile women. *N Engl J Med* 1994; **331:** 77–6.
7. Whittemore AS. The risk of ovarian cancer after treatment for infertility. *N Engl J Med* 1994; **331:** 805–6.
8. Committee on Safety of Medicines/Medicines Control Agency. Clomiphene (Clomid, Serophene): possible association with ovarian cancer. *Current Problems* 1995; **21:** 7.

Effects on the CNS. A report of convulsions following administration of clomiphene citrate to an infertile woman;[1] only five other cases had been reported since 1963.

1. Rimmington MR, *et al.* Convulsions after clomiphene citrate. *Br Med J* 1994; **309:** 512.

Effects on the eyes. As mentioned above, clomiphene may cause visual disturbances, which resolve on cessation of treatment. However, visual symptoms have persisted in a few cases.[1]

1. Purvin VA. Visual disturbance secondary to clomiphene citrate. *Arch Ophthalmol* 1995; **113:** 482–4.

Effects on the fetus. Discussions and individual reports of congenital disorders after treatment of the mother with clomiphene,[1-10] plus evidence that the incidence of fetal disorders is not increased following infertility treatment.[11-13]

1. Dyson JL, Kohler HG. Anencephaly and ovulation stimulation. *Lancet* 1973; **i:** 1256–7.
2. Field B, Kerr C. Ovulation stimulation and defects of neural-tube closure. *Lancet* 1974; **ii:** 1511.
3. Singh M, Singhi S. Possible relationship between clomiphene and neural tube defects. *J Pediatr* 1978; **93:** 152.
4. Halal F, *et al.* Méga-urètre, hypospadias et anus imperforé chez un nouveau-né: rôle possible du clomiphène pris par la mère. *Can Med Assoc J* 1980; **122:** 1159–60.
5. Cornel MC, *et al.* Ovulation induction and neural tube defects. *Lancet* 1989; **i:** 1386.
6. Czeizel A. Ovulation induction and neural tube defects. *Lancet* 1989; **ii:** 167.
7. Cuckle H, Wald N. Ovulation induction and neural tube defects. *Lancet* 1989; **ii:** 1281.
8. Cornel MC, *et al.* Ovulation induction, in-vitro fertilisation, and neural tube defects. *Lancet* 1989; **ii:** 1530.
9. Vollset SE. Ovulation induction and neural tube defects. *Lancet* 1990; **337:** 178.
10. White L, *et al.* Neuroectodermal tumours in children born after assisted conception. *Lancet* 1990; **336:** 1577.
11. Mills JL, *et al.* Risk of neural tube defects in relation to maternal fertility and fertility drug use. *Lancet* 1990; **336:** 103–4.
12. Rosa F. Ovulation induction and neural tube defects. *Lancet* 1990; **336:** 1327.
13. Werler MM, *et al.* Ovulation induction and risk of neural tube defects. *Lancet* 1994; **344:** 445–6.

Precautions

Clomiphene is contra-indicated in patients with liver disease and the potential for toxicity should be considered in patients with a history of liver dysfunction. It should not be used in pregnancy, or in patients with undiagnosed abnormal uterine bleeding; some sources suggest it should also be avoided in patients with hormone-dependent tumours, and in those with pre-existing mental depression or thrombophlebitis because of the risk of exacerbation. The cause of infertility should be investigated. The patient should be warned of the possibility of multiple births, particularly if higher doses are used.

Patients undergoing therapy with clomiphene, particularly those with polycystic ovaries, should receive the lowest doses possible to minimise ovarian enlargement or cyst formation. The patient should be instructed to report any abdominal or pelvic pain as this may indicate the presence or enlargement of ovarian cysts. They should also be evaluated for the presence of ovarian cyst before each cycle of treatment. If abnormal enlargement occurs, clomiphene should not be given until the ovaries have returned to pre-treatment size, and subsequent doses should be reduced. Treatment should be discontinued if visual disturbances develop and the patient warned that this might affect their ability to drive or operate machinery. Long-term cyclic therapy is not recommended, because of the uncertainty regarding increased risk of ovarian cancer (see above): in the UK a maximum of 6 cycles of treatment is advised.

Pharmacokinetics

Clomiphene citrate is absorbed from the gastro-intestinal tract. It is metabolised in the liver and slowly excreted via the bile. Unchanged drug and metabolites are excreted in the faeces. The biological half-life is reported to be 5 days although traces are found in the faeces for up to 6 weeks. Enterohepatic recirculation takes place. The *E*-isomer is reported to be less well absorbed and more rapidly eliminated than the *Z*-isomer.

References.

1. Szutu M, *et al.* Pharmacokinetics of intravenous clomiphene isomers. *Br J Clin Pharmacol* 1989; **27:** 639–40.

Uses and Administration

Clomiphene is chemically related to chlorotrianisene and has both oestrogenic and anti-oestrogenic properties, the latter residing principally in the *E*-isomer. Its action in stimulating ovulation is believed to be related to its anti-oestrogenic properties. It stimulates the secretion of pituitary gonadotrophic hormones, probably by blocking the negative feedback effect of oestrogens at receptor sites in the hypothalamus and pituitary.

Clomiphene is the most widely-used drug in the treatment of anovulatory infertility (p.1239). Therapy with clomiphene will not be successful unless the woman, though anovulatory, is capable of ovulation and her partner is fertile. It is ineffective in primary pituitary or primary ovarian failure. The usual dose by mouth is 50 mg of the citrate daily for 5 days, starting on or about the 5th day of the menstrual cycle or at any time if there is amenorrhoea. If ovulation does not occur, a course of 100 mg daily for 5 days may be given starting as early as 30 days after the previous one. Women should be examined for pregnancy and ovarian enlargement or cysts between cycles. In general, 3 courses of therapy are adequate to assess whether ovulation is obtainable. If ovulation has not occurred, the diagnosis should be re-evaluated. Once ovulation is established, each cycle of clomiphene should be started on or about the 5th day of the cycle. If pregnancy has not occurred after a total of about 6 cycles, further clomiphene therapy is not recommended.

Clomiphene has also been used in conjunction with gonadotrophins and in *in-vitro* fertilisation programmes.

Clomiphene has also been used in the treatment of male infertility due to oligospermia to stimulate gonadotrophin release and enhance spermatogenesis.

Preparations

BP 1998: Clomifene Tablets;
USP 23: Clomiphene Citrate Tablets.

Proprietary Preparations (details are given in Part 3)
Aust.: Clomid; Serophene; ***Austral.:*** Clomid; Serophene; ***Belg.:*** Clomid; Pergotime†; ***Canad.:*** Clomid; Serophene; ***Fr.:*** Clomid; Pergotime; ***Ger.:*** Clomhexal; Clostilbegyt; Dyneric; Pergotime; ***Irl.:*** Clomid; Serophene; ***Ital.:*** Clomid; Prolifen; Serofene; ***Neth.:*** Clomid; Serophene; ***Norw.:*** Clomivid; Pergotime; ***S.Afr.:*** Clomid; Serophene; ***Spain:*** Clomifen; Omifin; ***Swed.:*** Clomivid; Pergotime; ***Switz.:*** Clomid; Serophene; ***UK:*** Clomid; Serophene; ***USA:*** Clomid; Milophene†; Serophene.

Clostebol Acetate (9032-h)

Clostebol Acetate *(BAN, rINNM).*

4-Chlorotestosterone Acetate; Chlortestosterone Acetate. 4-Chloro-3-oxoandrost-4-en-17β-yl acetate; 4-Chloro-17β-hydroxyandrost-4-en-3-one acetate.

$C_{21}H_{29}ClO_3$ = 364.9.

CAS — 1093-58-9 (clostebol); 855-19-6 (clostebol acetate).

Clostebol acetate has anabolic properties (see Testosterone, p.1464) and is given in doses of 30 mg weekly by intramuscular injection, or 15 mg 2 or 3 times daily by mouth, for 3 weeks followed by a 3-week pause. It may also be applied topically to wounds and ulcers, and has been used as an ophthalmological preparation.

Preparations

Proprietary Preparations (details are given in Part 3)
Ger.: Megagrisevit mono; Steranabol†; ***Ital.:*** Alfa-Trofodermin†; Clostene†.

Multi-ingredient: ***Fr.:*** Trofoseptine†; ***Ital.:*** Trofodermin.

Cyclofenil (9033-m)

Cyclofenil *(BAN, rINN).*

F-6066; H-3452; ICI-48213. 4,4′-(Cyclohexylidenemethylene)bis(phenyl acetate).

$C_{23}H_{24}O_4$ = 364.4.

CAS — 2624-43-3.

Cyclofenil is a nonsteroidal anti-oestrogen that has been used in the treatment of anovulatory infertility due to hypothalamic-pituitary dysfunction.

It has been given by mouth in doses of 200 mg three times daily for 5 days, in a cyclical regimen for 3 to 4 cycles. It has also been given for menstrual disorders and in the management of menopausal symptoms.

Preparations

Proprietary Preparations (details are given in Part 3)
Ger.: Fertodur†; ***Ital.:*** Fertodur†; Neoclym; ***Switz.:*** Fertodur†; ***UK:*** Rehibin†.

Cyproterone Acetate (9034-b)

Cyproterone Acetate *(BANM, USAN, rINNM).*

Cyproteroni Acetas; NSC-81430; SH-714; SH-881 (cyproterone). 6-Chloro-1β,2β-dihydro-17α-hydroxy-3′*H*-cyclopropa[1,2]pregna-1,4,6-triene-3,20-dione acetate.

$C_{24}H_{29}ClO_4$ = 416.9.

CAS — 2098-66-0 (cyproterone); 427-51-0 (cyproterone acetate).

Pharmacopoeias. In *Eur.* (see p.viii).

A white or almost white, crystalline powder. Practically **insoluble** in water; sparingly soluble in dehydrated alcohol; freely soluble in acetone; soluble in methyl alcohol; very soluble in dichloromethane. **Protect** from light.

Adverse Effects

When given to men cyproterone inhibits spermatogenesis, reduces the volume of ejaculate, and causes infertility; these effects are slowly reversible. Abnormal spermatozoa may be produced. Gynaecomastia is common and permanent enlargement of the mammary glands may occur; galactorrhoea and benign nodules have been reported rarely. There may be initial sedation and depressive mood changes. Patients may experience alterations in hair pattern, skin reactions, weight changes, and anaemia. Osteoporosis may occur rarely. Altered liver function and breathlessness may occur. There have also been reports of hepatitis, jaundice, and hepatic failure, sometimes fatal, developing usually after several months of high-dose cyproterone therapy, but its association with liver cancer is uncertain.

When low-dose cyproterone is given with ethinyloestradiol to women, adverse effects associated with combined oral contraceptives (see p.1426) may occur.

Carcinogenicity. See Effects on the Liver, below.

Effects on the cardiovascular system. Combined oral contraceptives are associated with a small increased risk of cardiovascular disease (see p.1429). Deep-vein thrombosis associated with antibodies to cyproterone acetate in women using oral contraceptives containing cyproterone acetate and ethinyloestradiol has been reported.[1,2]

1. Leroy O, *et al.* Deep venous thrombosis and antibodies to cyproterone acetate. *Lancet* 1990; **336:** 509.
2. Beaumont V, Beaumont J-L. Thrombosis and antibodies to cyproterone acetate. *Lancet* 1991; **337:** 113.

Effects on the eyes. Bilateral optic atrophy in one elderly male patient was thought to be associated with cyproterone.[1] No other cases were known either from the published literature or from the manufacturers' records.

1. Markus H, Polkey M. Visual loss and optic atrophy associated with cyproterone acetate. *Br Med J* 1992; **305:** 159.

Effects on the liver. There have been numerous reports of hepatic reactions associated with cyproterone acetate. In February 1995, the UK Committee on Safety of Medicines noted that it had received 96 reports of reactions including hepatitis, cholestatic jaundice, and hepatic failure, following cyproterone treatment;[1] 33 cases had led to fatalities. Nearly all (91) of the cases were in elderly men typically receiving high doses (300 mg) for prostatic cancer, and toxicity usually developed after several months of treatment. In view of this it was recommended that the use of cyproterone acetate in prostatic cancer be restricted to short courses for the testosterone flare associated with the commencement of gonadorelin analogue therapy, or for hot flushes after surgical or chemical castration, or for patients unresponsive to, or intolerant of, other treatments.

Although there is little doubt of the risk of hepatotoxicity, suggestions of an association between cyproterone therapy and the development of liver cancer remain contentious. There are individual reports of hepatocellular carcinoma developing in patients receiving cyproterone,[2,3] and some evidence *in vitro* of the formation of DNA adducts in exposed hepatocytes,[4] but there does not seem to be clinical evidence to support any association between use of cyproterone acetate and the development of liver tumours.[4,5]

1. Committee on Safety of Medicines/Medicines Control Agency. Hepatic reactions with cyproterone acetate (Cyprostat, Androcur). *Current Problems* 1995; **21:** 1.
2. Watanabe S, *et al.* Three cases of hepatocellular carcinoma among cyproterone users. *Lancet* 1994; **344:** 1567–8.
3. Rüdiger T, *et al.* Hepatocellular carcinoma after treatment with cyproterone acetate combined with ethinyloestradiol. *Lancet* 1995; **345:** 452–3.
4. Lewis S. Warning on cyproterone. *Lancet* 1995; **345:** 247.
5. Rabe T, *et al.* Liver tumours in women on oral contraceptives. *Lancet* 1994; **344:** 1568–9.

Precautions

When used for hypersexuality, cyproterone is contra-indicated in men with liver diseases or malignant or wasting diseases. In addition, it should not be given to men with severe chronic depression, severe diabetes with vascular changes, sickle-cell anaemia, or to those with a history of thrombo-embolic disorders. It may delay bone maturation and testicular development and so should not be given to immature youths. When used for prostate cancer, there are no absolute contra-indications to the use of cyproterone, but the above conditions should prompt cautious consideration of the risks and benefits.

In men treated with cyproterone, liver function should be monitored before treatment, and whenever any symptoms or signs suggestive of hepatotoxicity occur. If cyproterone-induced hepatotoxicity occurs, treatment should be withdrawn. In men with prostate cancer, it may be advisable to limit the duration of treatment (see Effects on the Liver, above). Men with diabetes require careful monitoring of diabetic control. Since anaemia has been observed, regular blood counts are recommended during treatment. Adrenocortical suppression has been reported and function should be monitored regularly during treatment. Patients should be advised that the initial sedative effects may interfere with driving and the operation of machinery.

When cyproterone is given in conjunction with ethinyloestradiol to women the precautions for combined oral contraceptives (see p.1431) should be observed.

Pregnancy. Administration of cyproterone during pregnancy might carry a risk of feminisation of a male fetus. However, there are a few case reports of healthy male infants born to mothers who had inadvertently taken a combination of cyproterone acetate and ethinyloestradiol during the early stages of pregnancy,[1,2] and of a male fetus that was found to have no malformations after abortion was induced.[3] For further information on oral contraceptive use in pregnancy, see p.1432.

1. Statham BN, *et al.* Conception during 'Diane' therapy—a successful outcome. *Br J Dermatol* 1985; **113:** 374.
2. Bye P. Comments on 'conception during "Diane" therapy—a successful outcome'. *Br J Dermatol* 1986; **114:** 516.
3. Bergh T, Bakos O. Exposure to antiandrogen during pregnancy: case report. *Br Med J* 1987; **294:** 677–8.

Interactions

The manufacturers state that alcohol may reduce the effectiveness of cyproterone acetate.

When given in conjunction with ethinyloestradiol to women, interactions similar to those for combined oral contraceptives (see p.1432) might be anticipated.

Pharmacokinetics

Cyproterone acetate is slowly absorbed from the gastro-intestinal tract with peak plasma concentrations being achieved in 3 to 4 hours. The terminal elimination half-life is about 38 hours. Cyproterone is metabolised in the liver; about 35% of a dose is excreted in urine as free and conjugated metabolites, the remainder being excreted in the faeces. The principal metabolite, 15β-hydroxycyproterone, has antiandrogenic activity.

Uses and Administration

Cyproterone acetate is a progestogen with antiandrogenic properties.

It is used for the control of libido in severe hypersexuality or sexual deviation in adult males (p.636). The usual dose by mouth is 50 mg twice daily after meals.

It is also used in males for the palliative treatment of prostatic carcinoma (p.491) where other drugs are ineffective or not tolerated, to control disease flare or hot flushes associated with gonadorelin analogue therapy, and to control hot flushes associated with orchidectomy. The usual initial dose for disease flare or palliation is 300 mg daily in 2 to 3 divided doses after meals and maintenance treatment is continued with doses of 200 to 300 mg daily, but there is a risk of hepatotoxicity with long-term therapy. For the treatment of hot flushes, doses of 50 to 150 mg daily in 1 to 3 divided doses are given.

Cyproterone acetate may be used in conjunction with ethinyloestradiol in females for the control of acne (see below) and idiopathic hirsutism (see below), and also provides contraception in these women. The usual doses are 2 mg of cyproterone acetate with 35 µg of ethinyloestradiol given daily for 21 days of each menstrual cycle; the first treatment course should start on the first day of the menstrual cycle and each subsequent course started after 7 tablet-free days have followed the preceding course.

Cyproterone acetate has also been given by depot intramuscular injection.

Acne. Comparisons of cyproterone acetate 2 mg with either 35 or 50 µg of ethinyloestradiol in the treatment of refractory acne (p.1072) in women[1-3] have shown that, in general, both combinations were effective but that the lower dose of oestrogen was considered more acceptable for long-term therapy.

1. Colver GB, *et al.* Cyproterone acetate and two doses of oestrogen in female acne; a double-blind comparison. *Br J Dermatol* 1988; **118:** 95–9.
2. Fugère P, *et al.* Cyproterone acetate/ethinyl estradiol in the treatment of acne: a comparative dose-response study of the estrogen component. *Contraception* 1990; **42:** 225–34.
3. Anonymous. Dianette for women with acne. *Drug Ther Bull* 1990; **28:** 15–16.

Hidradenitis suppurativa. Some reports of a beneficial response of female hidradenitis suppurativa, an androgen-dependent disorder of the skin and hair in the pubic and axillary regions, to cyproterone acetate with ethinyloestradiol.[1-3]

1. Mortimer PS, *et al.* A double-blind controlled cross-over trial of cyproterone acetate in females with hidradenitis suppurativa. *Br J Dermatol* 1986; **115:** 263–8.
2. Sawers RS, *et al.* Control of hidradenitis suppurativa in women using combined antiandrogen (cyproterone acetate) and oestrogen therapy. *Br J Dermatol* 1986; **115:** 269–74.
3. Mortimer PS, *et al.* Mediation of hidradenitis suppurativa by androgens. *Br Med J* 1986; **292:** 961.

Hirsutism. Hirsutism is an abnormal growth in females of coarse pigmented terminal hair in an adult male pattern, and is one of the clinical expressions of hyperandrogenism. Most women with hirsutism have increased concentrations of circulating androgens from the ovaries associated with polycystic ovary syndrome (p.1240).[1] In rare cases, the adrenal gland is the primary source of increased androgens, for example, in congenital adrenal hyperplasia (p.1020). In a few cases, severe hirsutism is associated with frank virilisation due to massively increased circulating androgen concentrations from an androgen-secreting tumour.[2] Hirsutism is an adverse effect of androgenic progestogens, such as norgestrel, used in hormonal contraceptives and hormone replacement therapy. Androgens and anabolic steroids may also cause hirsutism in females.

Treatment for hirsutism employs topical cosmetic treatments such as bleaching, shaving, plucking, and electrolysis, and in the mildest cases this may be all that is required. However, such mechanical means of treatment are more usually combined with drug therapy to prevent further conversion of vellus to terminal hair, and to slow the regrowth of terminal hair, which may become lighter and softer. Because the growth cycle of hair is long, a response to therapy may not be seen for 6 to 12 months.

The mainstay of drug therapy for hirsutism is an anti-androgen, the most commonly used being the steroidal anti-androgens *cyproterone acetate* and *spironolactone*. To increase efficacy (by suppressing ovarian androgen production) and minimise the chance of conception (because of the risk of feminisation of a male fetus), cyclical *ethinyloestradiol* is commonly used with cyproterone acetate, while combined (nonandrogenic) *hormonal contraceptives* are commonly used with spironolactone, which has no progestogenic activity. Cyproterone acetate may be used in a low-dose combined preparation containing cyproterone acetate 2 mg with ethinyloestradiol 35 µg.[1,2] In more severe hirsutism, the two drugs may be prescribed separately in a 'reversed sequential regimen', with cyproterone acetate 50 to 150 mg given on days 5 to 15 of the menstrual cycle and ethinyloestradiol 30 to 50 µg on days 5 to 26.[1-3] When a satisfactory response has been achieved, the cyproterone dosage is gradually reduced, and eventually the low-dose combination preparation may be sufficient.

In some countries spironolactone is the drug of choice for the treatment of hirsutism, particularly if there is associated obesity and hypertension; doses of up to 300 mg daily have been given initially, with the aim of reducing the dose when hair growth has been controlled.[3] *Flutamide, finasteride,* and *leuprorelin* have also been shown to be effective. The condition has also been reported to respond to *ketoconazole*.

Although non-androgenic oral contraceptives have a role in reducing hyperandrogenism in polycystic ovary syndrome and corticosteroids have a role in congenital adrenal hyperplasia, neither is generally considered sufficient to reduce the hirsutism associated with these diseases, and an anti-androgen is usually added to the therapy.[2]

1. Conway GS, Jacobs HS. Hirsutism. *Br Med J* 1990; **301:** 619–20.
2. Rittmaster RS. Hirsutism. *Lancet* 1997; **349:** 191–5.
3. Delahunt JW. Hirsutism: practical therapeutic guidelines. *Drugs* 1993; **45:** 223–31.

Preparations

Proprietary Preparations (details are given in Part 3)

Aust.: Andro-Diane; Androcur; ***Austral.:*** Androcur; Cyprone; ***Belg.:*** Androcur; ***Canad.:*** Androcur; ***Fr.:*** Androcur; ***Ger.:*** Androcur; ***Irl.:*** Androcur; ***Ital.:*** Androcur; ***Neth.:*** Androcur; ***Norw.:*** Androcur; ***S.Afr.:*** Androcur; ***Spain:*** Androcur; ***Swed.:*** Androcur; ***Switz.:*** Androcur; ***UK:*** Androcur; Cyprostat.

Multi-ingredient: ***Aust.:*** Climen; Diane; ***Austral.:*** Brenda-35 ED; Climen; Diane ED; ***Belg.:*** Climen; Diane; ***Fr.:*** Climene; Diane; ***Ger.:*** Climen; Diane; ***Irl.:*** Dianette; ***Ital.:*** Climen; Diane; ***Neth.:*** Climene; Diane; ***Norw.:*** Diane; ***S.Afr.:*** Climen; Diane; ***Spain:*** Diane; ***Switz.:*** Climen†; Diane; ***UK:*** Dianette.

Danazol (9035-v)

Danazol *(BAN, USAN, pINN).*

Win-17757. 17α-Pregna-2,4-dien-20-yno[2,3-*d*]isoxazol-17β-ol.

$C_{22}H_{27}NO_2$ = 337.5.

CAS — 17230-88-5.

Pharmacopoeias. In *Chin.,* and *US.*

A white or pale yellow crystalline powder. Practically **insoluble** in water and petroleum spirit; sparingly soluble in alcohol; freely soluble in chloroform, slightly soluble in ether; soluble in acetone. **Store** in airtight containers. Protect from light.

Adverse Effects

Side-effects of danazol that reflect inhibition of the pituitary-ovarian axis include amenorrhoea (occasionally persistent), hot flushes, sweating, reduction in breast size, changes in libido, vaginitis, emotional lability, and nervousness.

Side-effects attributable to androgenic activity include acne, oily skin or hair, mild hirsutism, oedema, gain in weight, deepening of the voice, androgenic alopecia, and rarely clitoral hypertrophy. Testicular atrophy and a reduction in spermatogenesis may occur.

Other side-effects include gastro-intestinal disturbances, increased or decreased blood cell counts, headache, backache, dizziness, tremor, depression, fatigue, sleep disorders, muscle spasm or cramp, skin rash, hyperglucagonaemia, abnormal glucose tolerance, decreased serum high-density-lipoprotein cholesterol, increased serum low-density-lipoprotein cholesterol, and elevation of liver-function test values and rarely cholestatic jaundice. Some patients may experience tachycardia and hypertension. Benign intracranial hypertension and visual disturbances have occurred.

Effects on carbohydrate metabolism. Diabetes mellitus developed in a patient receiving danazol 400 mg twice daily for endometriosis.[1] The diabetes developed 8 weeks after initiation of danazol therapy and resolved completely after the drug was discontinued.

1. Seifer DB, *et al.* Insulin-dependent diabetes mellitus associated with danazol. *Am J Obstet Gynecol* 1990; **162:** 474–5.

Effects on the liver. As with other 17α-alkylated steroids (see p.1464), cholestatis, peliosis hepatis, and hepatic adenomas have been associated with danazol. Some references to these effects are cited below.[1-5]

1. Ohsawa T, Iwashita S. Hepatitis associated with danazol. *Drug Intell Clin Pharm* 1986; **20:** 889.
2. Boue F, *et al.* Danazol and cholestatic hepatitis. *Ann Intern Med* 1986; **105:** 139–40.
3. Fermand JP, *et al.* Danazol-induced hepatocellular adenoma. *Am J Med* 1990; **88:** 529–30.
4. Bray GP, *et al.* Resolution of danazol-induced cholestatis with S-adenosylmethionine. *Postgrad Med J* 1993; **69:** 237–9.
5. Makdisi WJ, *et al.* Fatal peliosis of the liver and spleen in a patient with agnogenic myeloid metaplasia treated with danazol. *Am J Gastroenterol* 1995; **90:** 317–8.

Effects on the skin. Erythema multiforme developed in two patients receiving danazol for profuse bleeding.[1]

1. Gately LE, Andes WA. Danazol and erythema multiforme. *Ann Intern Med* 1988; **109:** 85.

Precautions

Danazol should be used with caution in conditions which may be adversely affected by fluid retention, such as in cardiac, hepatic, and renal disorders, migraine, and epilepsy. It should also be used with care in patients with a history of thrombosis, and should not be used in patients with a thrombo-embolic disorder. Also, it should not be given to patients with marked hepatic, cardiac or kidney dysfunction, undiagnosed genital bleeding, androgen-dependent tumours, or to patients with porphyria as it may enhance porphyrin metabolism. As with other 17α-alkylated compounds, there is an increased risk of liver disorders and liver function should be monitored during therapy.

Danazol should not be given during pregnancy because of a possible androgenic effect on the female fetus (see below), and non-hormonal contraception is recommended during treatment. Danazol should also not be given to breast-feeding mothers. Caution is required in children and adolescents since precocious sexual development may occur in boys and virilisation in girls, and premature epiphyseal closure may occur in both sexes.

Porphyria. Danazol has been associated with clinical exacerbations of porphyria and is considered unsafe in porphyric patients.[1]

1. Moore MR, McColl KEL. *Porphyria: drug lists.* Glasgow: Porphyria Research Unit, University of Glasgow, 1991.

Pregnancy. Reports of masculinisation of female infants born to mothers who had received danazol during pregnancy.[1-3]

1. Shaw RW, Farquhar JW. Female pseudohermaphroditism associated with danazol exposure in utero: case report. *Br J Obstet Gynaecol* 1984; **91:** 386–9.
2. Kingsbury AC. Danazol and fetal masculinization: a warning. *Med J Aust* 1985; **143:** 410–11.
3. Brunskill PJ. The effects of fetal exposure to danazol. *Br J Obstet Gynaecol* 1992; **99:** 212–15.

Interactions

Therapy with danazol may inhibit the hepatic metabolism of a number of drugs including carbamazepine (see p.342), cyclosporin (see p.522), warfarin (see p.969), and possibly tacrolimus (see p.563). Introduction of danazol appeared to reduce the maintenance requirement for alfacalcidol (see p.1367).

Pharmacokinetics

Danazol is absorbed from the gastro-intestinal tract and metabolised in the liver; absorption is said to be markedly increased if it is taken with food. A half-life of about 4.5 hours has been reported. 2-Hydroxymethylethisterone is said to be the major metabolite.

Uses and Administration

Danazol suppresses the pituitary-ovarian axis by inhibiting pituitary output of gonadotrophins. It has weak androgenic activity.

Danazol has been given by mouth in the treatment of a variety of conditions including endometriosis, some benign breast disorders such as mastalgia and fibrocystic breast disease, gynaecomastia, menorrhagia associated with dysfunctional uterine bleeding, and prevention of hereditary angioedema. It may also be employed for the pre-operative thinning of the endometrium prior to hysteroscopic endometrial ablation, and has been tried in a variety of other conditions including pubertal or pre-pubertal breast hypertrophy and various blood disorders.

When given to women, treatment with danazol should be started on day 1 of the menstrual cycle or after pregnancy has been otherwise excluded.

In **endometriosis** the usual dose is 200 to 800 mg daily in 2 to 4 divided doses, adjusted according to the response. Therapy is given for 3 to 6 months or continued for up to 9 months if necessary.

In the treatment of **benign breast disorders** the usual initial dose is 100 to 400 mg daily in 2 divided doses, subsequently adjusted according to response, and continued for 3 to 6 months. For **gynaecomastia** 200 mg daily has been given to male adolescents, increased after 2 months to 400 mg daily if no response occurs; adult men may be given 400 mg daily initially. Therapy is usually tried for 6 months.

In dysfunctional uterine bleeding manifesting as **menorrhagia** doses of 200 mg daily have been employed and treatment is reviewed after 3 months.

In the management of **hereditary angioedema** doses of 200 mg two or three times daily are given, adjusted according to the patient's response.

For **pre-operative thinning** of the endometrium the usual dose is 400 to 800 mg daily for 3 to 6 weeks.

Blood disorders. While danazol may produce thrombocytopenia and leucopenia it may also have a beneficial effect in some blood disorders. It has been reported that danazol increases plasma concentrations of factor VIII and factor IX and may therefore be beneficial in the treatment of the haemorrhagic disorders (p.707) **haemophilia A or haemophilia B** (Christmas disease).[1,2] However, other workers have failed to substantiate these results and indeed have sometimes suggested that danazol may even increase the frequency of bleeding in such patients.[3-6]

In one report, danazol was found to increase plasma concentrations of protein C and protein S (inhibitors of blood coagulation) in a patient with end-stage renal disease.[7] This led to the suggestion that it and stanozolol may be useful in end-stage renal disease with hypercoagulability after dialysis.

Treatment with danazol has been reported to be beneficial in the treatment of **idiopathic thrombocytopenic purpura** (p.1023) resulting in increased platelet counts,[8-12] although in one study[10] 7 of 10 patients derived no benefit. A study investigating the possible mode of action in this disorder[13] indicated that danazol may mediate an effect by influencing the number of available binding sites for monomeric immunoglobulin G (Fc receptors) on monocytes. Another study[14] showed that sex, age (in women only), and the status of the spleen influenced the response of autoimmune thrombocytopenia to danazol. Thrombocytopenia associated with systemic lupus erythematosus[15] and the antiphospholipid antibody syndrome,[16] as well as rheumatoid arthritis[17] has also been reported to respond to treatment with danazol. For mention of the use of danazol in Henoch-Schönlein purpura see Hypersensitivity Vasculitis, p.1022.

Additionally there have been reports of response to danazol therapy in patients with auto-immune haemolytic anaemia,[18,19] myelodysplastic syndromes,[20,21] and paroxysmal cold haemoglobinuria,[22] hereditary haemorrhagic telangiectasia,[23] and Evan's syndrome due to systemic lupus erythematosus.[24]

1. Gralnick HR, Rick ME. Danazol increases factor VIII and factor IX in classic hemophilia and Christmas disease. *N Engl J Med* 1983; **308:** 1393–5.
2. Gralnick HR, *et al.* Benefits of danazol treatment in patients with hemophilia A (classic hemophilia). *JAMA* 1985; **253:** 1151–3.
3. Garewal HS, *et al.* Effect of danazol on coagulation parameters and bleeding in hemophilia. *JAMA* 1985; **253:** 1154–6.
4. Ambriz R, *et al.* Danazol in hemophilia. *JAMA* 1985; **254:** 754.
5. Kasper CK, Boylen AL. Poor response to danazol in hemophilia. *Blood* 1985; **65:** 211–13.
6. Heaton DC, *et al.* Danazol therapy in haemophilia. *N Z Med J* 1986; **99:** 185–7.
7. Henke WJ. Protein C and S response to Danacrine in end-stage renal disease. *Ann Intern Med* 1988; **108:** 910.
8. Ahn YS, *et al.* Danazol for the treatment of idiopathic thrombocytopenic purpura. *N Engl J Med* 1983; **308:** 1396–9.
9. Buelli M, *et al.* Danazol for the treatment of idiopathic thrombocytopenic purpura. *Acta Haematol (Basel)* 1985; **74:** 97–8.
10. McVerry BA, *et al.* The use of danazol in the management of chronic immune thrombocytopenic purpura. *Br J Haematol* 1985; **61:** 145–8.
11. Mylvaganam R, *et al.* Very low dose danazol in idiopathic thrombocytopenic purpura and its role as an immune modulator. *Am J Med Sci* 1989; **298:** 215–20.
12. Edelmann DZ, *et al.* Danazol in non-splenectomised patients with refractory idiopathic thrombocytopenic purpura. *Postgrad Med J* 1990; **66:** 827–30.
13. Schreiber AD, *et al.* Effect of danazol in immune thrombocytopenic purpura. *N Engl J Med* 1987; **316:** 503–8.
14. Ahn YS, *et al.* Long-term danazol therapy in autoimmune thrombocytopenia: unmaintained remission and age-dependent response in women. *Ann Intern Med* 1989; **111:** 723–9.
15. West SG, Johnson SC. Danazol for the treatment of refractory autoimmune thrombocytopenia in systemic lupus erythematosus. *Ann Intern Med* 1988; **108:** 703–6.
16. Kavanaugh A. Danazol therapy in thrombocytopenia associated with the antiphospholipid antibody syndrome. *Ann Intern Med* 1994; **121:** 767–8.
17. Dasgupta B, Grahame R. Treatment with danazol for refractory thrombocytopenia in rheumatoid arthritis. *Br J Rheumatol* 1989; **28:** 550–1.
18. Ahn YS, *et al.* Danazol therapy for autoimmune hemolytic anemia. *Ann Intern Med* 1985; **102:** 298–301.
19. Tan AM, *et al.* Danazol for treatment of refractory autoimmune hemolytic anaemia. *Ann Acad Med Singapore* 1989; **18:** 707–9.
20. Cines DB, *et al.* Danazol therapy in myelodysplasia. *Ann Intern Med* 1985; **103:** 58–60.
21. Kornberg A, *et al.* Danazol and myelodysplastic syndromes. *Ann Intern Med* 1986; **104:** 445–6.
22. Gertz MA. Possible response of paroxysmal cold hemoglobinuria to danazol. *Ann Intern Med* 1987; **106:** 635.
23. Haq AU, *et al.* Hereditary hemorrhagic telangiectasia and danazol. *Ann Intern Med* 1988; **109:** 171.
24. Aranegui P, *et al.* Danazol for Evan's syndrome due to SLE. *DICP Ann Pharmacother* 1990; **24:** 641–2.

Endometriosis. Endometriosis is a condition affecting women in their reproductive years,[1] in which clusters of oestrogen-dependent cells, histologically indistinguishable from endometrium, develop outside their usual location in the uterine cavity. They occur most commonly in the pelvis, less commonly in the peritoneal cavity,[2] and occasionally elsewhere such as the thoracic cavity.[1,3] The aetiology is uncertain, although an immunological defect which permits endometrial cells carried in menstrual blood to implant and grow following reflux of menstrual blood has been suggested. The advent of laparoscopy has indicated that the condition is more common than was previously thought, and not all women with endometriosis are symptomatic.[4,5]

The most common symptom is pain, usually manifesting as secondary dysmenorrhoea, dyspareunia or cyclical back or pelvic pain. Associated adenomyosis may cause menorrhagia; fibrosis and adhesions may develop. Endometriosis is also strongly associated with infertility, although whether it causes infertility is unclear. Management will depend in part on whether the presenting complaint leading to evaluation and diagnosis of endometriosis was pelvic pain or infertility, or if the condition was discovered secondary to laparoscopy for other purposes.[2,6-11] Minimal asymptomatic disease may resolve spontaneously, and there is little evidence that conservative surgery or medical therapy improves fertility. In women wishing to conceive, infertility treatments may be used as appropriate (see p.1239). For more extensive disease, the most commonly used initial treatment is conservative surgery followed by drugs to suppress the endometriosis if pain was the principal complaint or if removal of endometriotic deposits was incomplete. Because available drugs also tend to suppress ovulation they are potentially contraceptive, and their use will defer opportunities for conception in women wishing to conceive. Commonly used drugs include danazol, progestogens such as medroxyprogesterone acetate, combined oral contraceptives, and gonadorelin analogues.

One of the most widely used treatments is *danazol*, which has been shown to produce subjective improvement in symptoms of pain and reduction of some pelvic abnormalities and tissue implants. Its androgenic effects can be a problem and there is concern about its effect on blood lipids, therefore therapy is restricted to 6 months. Gestrinone, has been shown to be equally effective and may be a useful alternative. *Progestogens* such as medroxyprogesterone acetate or norethisterone acetate are also commonly used. They appear to be as effective as danazol in relieving pain symptoms but there is a suggestion that they are less effective in eliminating endometriotic deposits.[6] Despite this, some consider them to be the drugs of first choice for endometriosis.[2,9]

Combined oral contraceptives have been used in a continuous fashion, but such use is associated with a high incidence of breakthrough bleeding. However, it is now apparent that the usual cyclical use of combined oral contraceptives is associated with a decreased incidence of endometriosis,[12] and cyclical use is being investigated as a treatment.

The other major group of drugs that are used in endometriosis are *gonadorelin* and its analogues such as buserelin, goserelin, leuprorelin, and nafarelin. They are as effective as danazol and their adverse effects, which resemble menopausal symptoms, may be better tolerated than the androgenic effects of danazol.[6,13] Long-term use is limited by the risk of osteoporosis, but the use of concomitant low-dose oestrogen and progestogen hormone replacement therapy[8,10] or tibolone[14] ('add-back' therapy) to prevent this is under investigation. Parathyroid hormone[15] may also be effective for 'add-back' therapy. It has been suggested that the gonadorelin analogues should be reserved for patients unable to tolerate conventional treatments,[13] or where rapid initial control is desired, or to facilitate laparoscopic procedures.[8,11]

Investigational drugs include the *antiprogestogens* such as mifepristone.[10]

There is a relatively high recurrence rate of endometriosis after conservative surgery and drug therapy. In women who can accept loss of childbearing potential, definitive therapy is surgical oophorectomy and hysterectomy with complete excision or ablation of endometrial deposits. Oestrogen replacement therapy is given, but carries a risk of recurrence of the disease; some have suggested that combined hormone replacement therapy may be preferable (see p.1437).

1. Rock JA, Markham SM. Pathogenesis of endometriosis. *Lancet* 1992; **340:** 1264–7.
2. Wardle PG. Management of endometriosis. *Prescribers' J* 1994; **34:** 221–6.
3. Joseph J, Sahn SA. Thoracic endometriosis syndrome: new observations from an analysis of 110 cases. *Am J Med* 1996; **100:** 164–70.
4. Anonymous. Endometriosis: time for re-appraisal. *Lancet* 1992; **340:** 1073.
5. Thomas ES. Endometriosis. *Br Med J* 1993; **306:** 158–9.
6. Shaw RW. Treatment of endometriosis. *Lancet* 1992; **340:** 1267–71.
7. Olive DL, Schwartz LB. Endometriosis. *N Engl J Med* 1993; **328:** 1759–69.
8. Shaw RW. A risk/benefit assessment of drugs used in the treatment of endometriosis. *Drug Safety* 1994; **11:** 104–13.
9. Lu PY, Ory SJ. Endometriosis: current management. *Mayo Clin Proc* 1995; **70:** 453–63.
10. Kettel LM, Hummel WP. Modern medical management of endometriosis. *Obstet Gynecol Clin North Am* 1997; **24:** 361–73.
11. Adamson GD, Nelson HP. Surgical treatment of endometriosis. *Obstet Gynecol Clin North Am* 1997; **24:** 375–409.
12. Vessey MP, *et al.* Epidemiology of endometriosis in women attending family planning clinics. *Br Med J* 1993; **306:** 182–4.
13. Anonymous. Gonadotropin releasing hormone analogues for endometriosis. *Drug Ther Bull* 1993; **31:** 21–2.
14. Lindsay PC, *et al.* The effect of add-back treatment with tibolone (Livial) on patients treated with the gonadotropin-releasing hormone agonist triptorelin (Decapeptyl). *Fertil Steril* 1996; **65:** 342–8.
15. Finkelstein JS, *et al.* Parathyroid hormone for the prevention of bone loss induced by estrogen deficiency. *N Engl J Med* 1994; **331:** 1618–23.

Gynaecomastia. Gynaecomastia is a benign glandular enlargement of the male breast, caused either by increased oestrogenic activity or decreased androgenic activity. Examples of gynaecomastia caused by increased oestrogenic activity include oestrogen-secreting malignancies, increased aromatisation of androgens into oestrogens (associated with an increase in adipose tissue), and exposure to drugs with oestrogenic activity such as digitoxin. Neonatal and pubertal gynaecomastia (the former due to exposure to maternal oestrogens, the latter because oestrogen levels increase before androgens do) come into this category. Examples of gynaecomastia caused by decreased androgenic activity include the various forms of hypogonadism, increased metabolism of androgens (for example in alcoholism), and exposure to drugs with anti-androgenic properties such as spironolactone, cimetidine, ketoconazole, cyproterone acetate, or flutamide. Some systemic disorders may also be associated with gynaecomastia, including cirrhosis of the liver, hyperthyroidism, and renal failure; it may also occur on refeeding after starvation.

Gynaecomastia has a high rate of spontaneous regression, and specific therapy (other than the removal of any cause) need only be considered if the enlarged breast tissue causes sufficient pain, embarrassment, or emotional discomfort to interfere with the patient's daily life.[1] Drug therapy is only likely to be of benefit while tissue is still proliferating; once glandular tissue has become inactive and fibrotic (usually after more than 12 months) a complete response is unlikely.

Testosterone itself is unlikely to be of benefit (and may be aromatised to oestradiol, exacerbating the situation), but a non-aromatisable androgen such as *stanolone* (dihydrotestosterone) may produce some benefit.[1] *Danazol* has produced marked responses in some patients.[2] Quite good responses have also been reported with *tamoxifen*,[3-5] and this has been recommended as a drug of choice.[1] Clomiphene[6,7] and testolactone,[8] have also been tried. Where drug therapy is unsuccessful, or the breast enlargement is long-standing, surgical removal of breast tissue is advocated.[1]

1. Braunstein GD. Gynecomastia. *N Engl J Med* 1993; **328:** 490–5.
2. Buckle R. Danazol therapy in gynaecomastia: recent experience and indications for therapy. *Postgrad Med J* 1979; **55** (suppl 5): 71–8.
3. Jefferys DB. Painful gynaecomastia treated with tamoxifen. *Br Med J* 1979; **1:** 1119–20.
4. Hooper PD. Puberty gynaecomastia. *J R Coll Gen Pract* 1985; **35:** 142.
5. McDermott MT, *et al.* Tamoxifen therapy for painful idiopathic gynecomastia. *South Med J* 1990; **83:** 1283–5.
6. LeRoith D, *et al.* The effect of clomiphene citrate on pubertal gynaecomastia. *Acta Endocrinol (Copenh)* 1980; **95;** 177–80.
7. Plourde PV, *et al.* Clomiphene in the treatment of adolescent gynecomastia: clinical and endocrine studies. *Am J Dis Child* 1983; **137:** 1080–2.
8. Zachmann M, *et al.* Treatment of pubertal gynaecomastia with testolactone. *Acta Endocrinol (Copenh)* 1986; **279** (suppl): 218–26.

Hereditary angioedema. Danazol has been used successfully to prevent attacks of hereditary angioedema (p.729); the doses used have ranged from the recommended dose of 200 mg two or three times daily to much lower ones.[1-8] The following studies illustrate the wide dose variation.

In 9 patients with hereditary angioedema there were 44 attacks during 47 courses of treatment with placebo and 1 attack during 46 courses of treatment with danazol 200 mg three times daily given for 28 days or until an attack occurred.[1] In another 10 patients with hereditary angioedema danazol 300 to 600 mg daily with a gap of 5 or 7 days every 7 days was effective.[2] Of 56 patients with hereditary angioedema receiving danazol in a reducing dosage, 95% were free from attacks on danazol 600 mg daily, 88% on 400 mg daily, 68% on 300 mg daily, and 11% on 200 mg daily.[3] Effective short-term prophylaxis before dental procedures was achieved in these patients with 600 mg daily for 10 days. In an 8-year-old boy 200 mg of danazol every other day was effective in preventing attacks[4] and doses gradually reduced to 200 mg three times a week or 300 mg once weekly were effective in 2 other adult patients.[5]

Patients with lupus erythematosus-like syndromes associated with hereditary angioedema have also benefited from danazol therapy.[6-8]

1. Gelfand JA, *et al.* Treatment of hereditary angioedema with danazol: reversal of clinical and biochemical abnormalities. *N Engl J Med* 1976; **295:** 1444–8.
2. Agostoni A, *et al.* Intermittent therapy with danazol in hereditary angioedema. *Lancet* 1978; **i:** 453.
3. Hosea SW, Frank MM. Danazol in the treatment of hereditary angioedema. *Drugs* 1980; **19:** 370–2.
4. Tappeiner G, *et al.* Hereditary angio-oedema: treatment with danazol: report of a case. *Br J Dermatol* 1979; **100:** 207–12.
5. MacFarlane JT, Davies D. Management of hereditary angio-oedema with low-dose danazol. *Br Med J* 1981; **282:** 1275.
6. Masse R, *et al.* Reversal of lupus-erythematosus-like disease with danazol. *Lancet* 1980; **ii:** 651.
7. Donaldson VH, Hess EV. Effect of danazol on lupus-erythematosus-like disease in hereditary angioneurotic oedema. *Lancet* 1980; **ii:** 1145.
8. Duhra P, *et al.* Discoid lupus erythematosus associated with hereditary angioneurotic oedema. *Br J Dermatol* 1990; **123:** 241–4.

Mastalgia. Mastalgia is often associated with nodularity or other fibrocystic changes in the female breast, and is sometimes divided into cyclical mastalgia, which accounts for about two-thirds of all cases, non-cyclical mastalgia, and chest-wall or costochondral pain (Tietze's syndrome). Cyclical mastalgia is most common in the third decade of life, following a chronic relapsing course thereafter, and usually resolving at the menopause. Non-cyclical mastalgia tends to present later in life and the duration of symptoms is usually shorter, with spontaneous resolution occurring in 50% of cases; it tends to be more refractory to drug treatment.

Once clear pathological causes of pain have been excluded most patients can be managed by simple reassurance.[1-5] Drug treatment should rarely be considered unless pain has been present for about 6 months.[2] Patients who are receiving an oral contraceptive or hormone replacement therapy may find that symptoms improve on stopping treatment.[1,2,4] It has been suggested that reducing the intake of saturated fat in the diet may be worthwhile, and there is evidence that a low fat diet reduces symptoms of tenderness and swelling.[6]

Danazol is probably the most effective drug for mastalgia,[3] and produces the most rapid response;[2,5] open studies suggest that it is of benefit in about 70% or more of patients with cyclical mastalgia,[1-4] and somewhat fewer with the non-cyclical form.[1,3,4] However, adverse effects may require dosage reduction. *Gestrinone* has also been reported to be effective in cyclical mastalgia.[5,7]

Other drugs for cyclical mastalgia are *bromocriptine* or *gamolenic acid* (as evening primrose oil in most cases). Both are reported to produce a response in about 50% of cases, and appear to be equally effective.[1-3] However, gamolenic acid produces fewer adverse effects.[1,2,4,5] Again these drugs are less effective in non-cyclical mastalgia.[1,3]

A good response to danazol or bromocriptine would be expected within 2 months; gamolenic acid may take 3 to 4 months to show an effect.[1,4,5] When a response is achieved, therapy is be withdrawn after 6 months to see if continued treatment is needed; even if pain recurs it may be less severe and therapy may be unnecessary.[1,2,5]

In refractory cyclical or non-cyclical mastalgia *tamoxifen*[8,9] has been shown to be effective; however, the concept of using tamoxifen in otherwise healthy premenopausal women has produced some concern.[10-12] *Goserelin* has also been shown to be effective.[13]

Other drugs that have been prescribed for cyclical mastalgia include antibiotics, diuretics, pyridoxine, and the progestogens, but there is no evidence that they are any better than placebo.[1,2,5]

1. Gateley CA, Mansel RE. Management of the painful and nodular breast. *Br Med Bull* 1991; **47:** 284–94.
2. Anonymous. Cyclical breast pain—what works and what doesn't. *Drug Ther Bull* 1992; **30:** 1–3.
3. Gateley CA, *et al.* Drug treatments for mastalgia: 17 years experience in the Cardiff mastalgia clinic. *J R Soc Med* 1992; **85:** 12–15.
4. Mansel RE. Breast pain. *Br Med J* 1994; **309:** 866–8.
5. Holland PA, Gateley CA. Drug therapy of mastalgia: what are the options. *Drugs* 1994; **48:** 709–16.
6. Boyd NF, *et al.* Effect of a low fat high-carbohydrate diet on symptoms of cyclical mastopathy. *Lancet* 1988; **ii:** 128–32.
7. Peters F. Multicentre study of gestrinone in cyclical breast pain. *Lancet* 1992; **339:** 205–8.
8. Fentiman IS, *et al.* Double-blind controlled trial of tamoxifen therapy for mastalgia. *Lancet* 1986; **i:** 287–8.
9. Fentiman IS, *et al.* Studies of tamoxifen in women with mastalgia. *Br J Clin Pract* 1989; **43** (suppl 68): 34–6.
10. Anonymous. Tamoxifen for benign breast disease. *Lancet* 1986; **i:** 305.
11. Smallwood JA, Taylor I. Tamoxifen for mastalgia. *Lancet* 1986; **i:** 680–1.
12. Fentiman IS, *et al.* Tamoxifen for mastalgia. *Lancet* 1986; **i:** 681.
13. Hamed H, *et al.* LHRH analogue for treatment of recurrent and refractory mastalgia. *Ann R Coll Surg Engl* 1990; **72:** 221–4.

Menorrhagia. Danazol is effective in the treatment of menorrhagia (p.1461)[1-3] but it is only used short term because of its adverse effects.

1. Chimbira TH, *et al.* Reduction of menstrual blood loss by danazol in unexplained menorrhagia: lack of effect of placebo. *Br J Obstet Gynaecol* 1980; **87:** 1152–8.
2. Dockeray CJ, *et al.* Comparison between mefenamic acid and danazol in the treatment of established menorrhagia. *Br J Obstet Gynaecol* 1989; **96:** 840–4.
3. Bonduelle M, *et al.* A comparative study of danazol and norethisterone in dysfunctional uterine bleeding presenting as menorrhagia. *Postgrad Med J* 1991; **67:** 833–6.

Premenstrual syndrome. Danazol may be useful in the management of the premenstrual syndrome (p.1456), but adverse effects limit its long-term use. Some references to the use of danazol in this condition are given below.[1,2]

1. Halbreich U, *et al.* Elimination of ovulation and menstrual cyclicity (with danazol) improves dysphoric premenstrual syndromes. *Fertil Steril* 1991; **56:** 1066–9.
2. Deeny M, *et al.* Low dose danazol in the treatment of the premenstrual syndrome. *Postgrad Med J* 1991; **67:** 450–4.

Skin disorders. A patient with a skin condition involving cholinergic pruritus, erythema, and urticaria that was unresponsive to treatment with antihistamines and anti-inflammatory drugs was successfully treated with danazol 600 mg daily.[1] This dose of danazol also resolved a case of chronic actinic dermatitis.[2] In both of these patients, the skin disorder had been associated with low plasma concentrations of antiprotease.

1. Berth-Jones J, Graham-Brown RAC. Cholinergic pruritus, erythema and urticaria: a disease spectrum responding to danazol. *Br J Dermatol* 1989; **121:** 235–7.
2. Humbert P, *et al.* Chronic actinic dermatitis responding to danazol. *Br J Dermatol* 1991; **124:** 195–7.

Preparations

USP 23: Danazol Capsules.

Proprietary Preparations (details are given in Part 3)
Aust.: Danokrin; ***Austral.:*** Azol; Danocrine; ***Belg.:*** Danatrol; ***Canad.:*** Cyclomen; ***Fr.:*** Danatrol; Mastodanatrol†; ***Ger.:*** Winobanin; ***Irl.:*** Danazant; Danol; ***Ital.:*** Danatrol; ***Neth.:*** Danatrol; ***Norw.:*** Danocrine; ***S.Afr.:*** Ladazol; ***Spain:*** Danatrol; ***Swed.:*** Danocrine; ***Switz.:*** Danatrol; ***UK:*** Danol; ***USA:*** Danocrine.

Delmadinone Acetate (12628-y)

Delmadinone Acetate *(BANM, USAN, rINNM).*

RS-1301. 6-Chloro-17α-hydroxypregna-1,4,6-triene-3,20-dione acetate.

$C_{23}H_{27}ClO_4$ = 402.9.

CAS — 15262-77-8 (delmadinone); 13698-49-2 (delmadinone acetate).

Delmadinone acetate is a progestogen with anti-androgenic and anti-oestrogenic activity. It is used as an anti-androgen in veterinary practice.

Demegestone (12629-j)

Demegestone *(rINN).*

R-2453. 17α-Methyl-19-norpregna-4,9-diene-3,20-dione.

$C_{21}H_{28}O_2$ = 312.4.

CAS — 10116-22-0.

Demegestone is a progestogen structurally related to progesterone (p.1459). It has been given cyclically in doses of 1 to 2 mg daily by mouth.

Preparations

Proprietary Preparations (details are given in Part 3)
Fr.: Lutionex.

Desogestrel (12633-w)

Desogestrel *(BAN, USAN, rINN).*

Org-2969. 13β-Ethyl-11-methylene-18,19-dinor-17α-pregn-4-en-20-yn-17β-ol.

$C_{22}H_{30}O$ = 310.5.

CAS — 54024-22-5.

Pharmacopoeias. In Br.

A white, crystalline powder. Practically **insoluble** in water; slightly soluble in alcohol and in ethyl acetate; sparingly soluble in hexane.

Adverse Effects and Precautions

As for progestogens in general (see Progesterone, p.1459). See also under Hormonal Contraceptives, p.1426. Desogestrel is reported to have few androgenic effects, and to have less adverse effect on the serum lipid profile than older 19-nortestosterone derivatives. However, there has been concern that desogestrel-containing combined oral contraceptives are associated with an increased risk of venous thrombo-embolism (see p.1430, and for precautions, see p.1432).

Interactions

As for progestogens in general (see Progesterone, p.1460). See also under Hormonal Contraceptives, p.1432.

Pharmacokinetics

After oral administration, desogestrel undergoes oxidative transformation to its active metabolite 3-keto-desogestrel (see also Etonogestrel, p.1446) in the intestinal mucosa and liver. In the blood, about 32% of 3-keto-desogestrel is bound to sex hormone binding globulin, and 66% to albumin.

References.

1. Madden S, *et al.* Metabolism of the contraceptive steroid desogestrel by the intestinal mucosa. *Br J Clin Pharmacol* 1989; **27:** 295–9.
2. Madden S, *et al.* Metabolism of the contraceptive steroid desogestrel by human liver in vitro. *J Steroid Biochem* 1990; **35:** 281–8.
3. Kuhnz W, *et al.* Protein binding of the contraceptive steroids gestodene, 3-keto-desogestrel and ethinyloestradiol in human serum. *J Steroid Biochem* **35:** 313–18.

Uses and Administration

Desogestrel is a progestogen (see Progesterone, p.1460) structurally related to levonorgestrel that is used as the progestogenic component of combined oral contraceptive preparations (see p.1433); a typical daily dose is 150 μg.

Reviews.

1. Anonymous. Marvelon—an OC with a new progestagen. *Drug Ther Bull* 1984; **22:** 69–70.
2. Anonymous. Mercilon—a new low-dose combined oral contraceptive. *Drug Ther Bull* 1989; **27:** 51–2.
3. Anonymous. Desogestrel—a new progestin for oral contraception. *Med Lett Drugs Ther* 1993; **35:** 73–4.

Preparations

Proprietary Preparations (details are given in Part 3)

Multi-ingredient: ***Aust.:*** Gracial; Marvelon; Mercilon; ***Austral.:*** Marvelon; ***Belg.:*** Gracial; Marvelon; Mercilon; Ovidol; ***Canad.:*** Marvelon; Ortho-Cept; ***Fr.:*** Cycleane; Mercilon; Varnoline; ***Ger.:*** Biviol; Cyclosa; Lovelle; Marvelon; Oviol; ***Irl.:*** Marviol; Mercilon; ***Ital.:*** Mercilon; Planum; Practil; Securgin; ***Neth.:*** Marvelon; Mercilon; Ovidol; ***Norw.:*** Marvelon; ***S.Afr.:*** Marvelon; Mercilon; ***Spain:*** Microdiol; Suavuret; ***Swed.:*** Desolett; Mercilon; ***Switz.:*** Gracial; Lovelle†; Marvelon; Mercilon; Ovidol; Varnoline†; ***UK:*** Marvelon; Mercilon; ***USA:*** Desogen; Ortho-Cept.

Dienoestrol (9037-q)

Dienoestrol *(BAN).*

Dienestrol *(rINN)*; Dehydrostilbestrol; Dienestrolum; Dienoestrolum; Oestrodienolum. *(E,E)*-4,4′-[Di(ethylidene)ethylene]diphenol; 4,4′-(1,2-Diethylidene-1,2-ethanediyl)bisphenol.

$C_{18}H_{18}O_2$ = 266.3.

CAS — 84-17-3 (dienoestrol); 13029-44-2 ((E,E)-dienoestrol).

Pharmacopoeias. In *Eur.* (see p.viii) and *US.*

Aust. also includes dienoestrol diacetate, $C_{22}H_{22}O_4$.

White or almost white, odourless, crystals or crystalline powder. Practically **insoluble** in water; soluble to freely soluble in alcohol and in acetone; soluble in ether, in methyl alcohol, and in propylene glycol; slightly soluble in chloroform and in fatty oils; dissolves in dilute solutions of alkali hydroxides. **Protect** from light.

Dienoestrol is a synthetic nonsteroidal oestrogen structurally related to stilboestrol (p.1462). It is used as a 0.01% cream in the treatment of menopausal atrophic vaginitis. If used on a long-term basis in women with a uterus a progestogen is required.

Dienoestrol diacetate has been used as an ingredient of topical preparations for skin disorders.

Preparations

USP 23: Dienestrol Cream.

Proprietary Preparations (details are given in Part 3)

Belg.: Ortho-Dienoestrol; ***Irl.:*** Ortho; ***USA:*** DV.

Multi-ingredient: ***Canad.:*** AVC/Dienestrol†; ***Ital.:*** Sebohermal†; ***Switz.:*** Crinohermal FEM†.

Dienogest (1999-c)

Dienogest *(rINN).*

STS-557. 17-Hydroxyl-3-oxo-19-nor-17α-pregna-4,9-diene-21-nitrite.

$C_{20}H_{25}NO_2$ = 311.4.

CAS — 65928-58-7.

Dienogest is a nonethinylated progestogen (see Progesterone, p.1459) structurally related to nortestosterone. It is reported to have anti-androgenic properties. Dienogest is used as the progestogen component of some combined oral contraceptives (see p.1426); a typical daily dose is 2 mg.

Preparations

Proprietary Preparations (details are given in Part 3)

Multi-ingredient: ***Ger.:*** Certostat†; Valette.

Drospirenone (14636-g)

Drospirenone *(rINN).*

Dihydrospirenone; ZK-30595.

(6*R*,7*R*,8*R*,9*S*,10*R*,13*S*,14*S*,15*S*,16*S*,17*S*)-1,3′,4′,6,6a,7,8,9,10,11,12,13,14,15,15a,16-Hexadecahydro-10,13-dimethylspiro-[17*H*-dicyclopropa[6,7:15,16]cyclopenta[*a*]phenanthrene-17,2′(5′*H*)-furan]-3,5′(2*H*)-dione.

$C_{24}H_{30}O_3$ = 366.5.

CAS — 67392-87-4.

Drospirenone is a progestogen (see Progesterone, p.1459) with antimineralocorticoid and anti-androgenic activity, under investigation as a component of a combined oral contraceptive.

References.

1. Muhn P, *et al.* Drospirenone: a novel progestogen with antimineralocorticoid and anti-androgenic activity. *Ann N Y Acad Sci* 1995; **761:** 311–35.
2. Oelkers W, *et al.* Effects of a new oral contraceptive containing an antimineralocorticoid progestogen, drospirenone, on the renin-aldosterone system, body weight, blood pressure, glucose tolerance, and lipid metabolism. *J Clin Endocrinol Metab* 1995; **80:** 1816–21.

Drostanolone Propionate (9039-s)

Drostanolone Propionate *(BANM, rINNM).*

Compound 32379; Dromostanolone Propionate *(USAN)*; 2α-Methyldihydrotestosterone Propionate; NSC-12198. 17β-Hydroxy-2α-methyl-5α-androstan-3-one propionate.

$C_{23}H_{36}O_3$ = 360.5.

CAS — 58-19-5 (drostanolone); 521-12-0 (drostanolone propionate).

Pharmacopoeias. In *Jpn.*

Drostanolone has anabolic and androgenic properties (see Testosterone, p.1464) and was formerly used in the treatment of advanced malignant neoplasms of the breast in postmenopausal women.

Preparations

Proprietary Preparations (details are given in Part 3)

Belg.: Masteron†.

Dydrogesterone (9040-h)

Dydrogesterone *(BAN, USAN, rINN).*

Dehydroprogesterone; 6-Dehydro-*retro*-progesterone; 6-Dehydro-9β,10α-progesterone; Didrogesteron; Isopregnenone; NSC-92336. 9β,10α-Pregna-4,6-diene-3,20-dione.

$C_{21}H_{28}O_2$ = 312.4.

CAS — 152-62-5.

Pharmacopoeias. In *Br., Jpn,* and *US.*

A white to pale yellow crystalline powder; odourless or almost odourless. Practically **insoluble** in water; soluble 1 in 40 of alcohol, 1 in 2 of chloroform, and 1 in 200 of ether; soluble in acetone; sparingly soluble in methyl alcohol; slightly soluble in fixed oils. **Protect** from light.

Adverse Effects and Precautions

As for progestogens in general (see Progesterone, p.1459).

Pregnancy. Anomalies (non-virilising) of the genito-urinary tract were found in a 4-month-old baby whose mother had taken dydrogesterone 20 mg daily from the 8th to 20th week of pregnancy and 10 mg daily from then until term.[1] She had also been given hydroxyprogesterone hexanoate 250 mg by intramuscular injection weekly from the 8th to the 20th week.

1. Roberts IF, West RJ. Teratogenesis and maternal progesterone. *Lancet* 1977; **ii:** 982.

Interactions

As for progestogens in general (see Progesterone, p.1460).

Uses and Administration

Dydrogesterone is a progestogen structurally related to progesterone (p.1460). It does not have oestrogenic or androgenic properties.

Dydrogesterone is given by mouth in the treatment of menstrual disorders such as menorrhagia (p.1461), usually in a dose of 10 mg twice daily in a cyclical regimen, and for the treatment of endometriosis (p.1442) at a dose of 10 mg two or three times daily. It is also given cyclically in doses of 10 mg once or twice daily for endometrial protection during menopausal hormone replacement therapy (p.1434).

In threatened abortion suggested doses have been 40 mg initially followed by 10 mg or more every 8 hours, continued for a week after symptoms cease. In habitual abortion suggested doses have been 10 mg twice daily. However, such use is not recommended unless there is proven progesterone deficiency. Cyclical dydrogesterone has also been used in infertility (p.1239) in doses of 10 mg twice daily.

Preparations

BP 1998: Dydrogesterone Tablets;
USP 23: Dydrogesterone Tablets.

Proprietary Preparations (details are given in Part 3)

Aust.: Duphaston; ***Austral.:*** Duphaston; ***Belg.:*** Duphaston; ***Fr.:*** Duphaston; ***Ger.:*** Duphaston; ***Irl.:*** Duphaston; ***Ital.:*** Dufaston; ***Neth.:*** Duphaston; ***S.Afr.:*** Duphaston; ***Spain:*** Duphaston; ***Swed.:*** Duphaston; ***Switz.:*** Duphaston; ***UK:*** Duphaston.

Multi-ingredient: ***Austral.:*** Femoston; ***Belg.:*** Femoston; ***Neth.:*** Femoston; Zumeston†; ***UK:*** Femapak; Femoston.

Epimestrol (12693-f)

Epimestrol *(BAN, USAN, rINN).*

NSC-55975; Org-817. 3-Methoxyestra-1,3,5(10)-triene-16α,17α-diol.

$C_{19}H_{26}O_3$ = 302.4.

CAS — 7004-98-0.

Epimestrol is the 3-methyl ether of the naturally occurring oestrogenic hormone 17-epioestriol. It has been used in the treatment of female infertility due to anovulation and amenorrhoea in doses of 5 to 20 mg given for 10 days.

Preparations

Proprietary Preparations (details are given in Part 3)

Ger.: Stimovul†; ***Ital.:*** Stimovul†; ***Neth.:*** Stimovul†; ***Spain:*** Alene†.

Equilin (18357-p)

3-Hydroxyestra-1,3,5(10),7-tetraen-17-one.

$C_{18}H_{20}O_2$ = 268.4.

CAS — 474-86-2.

Pharmacopoeias. In *US.*

Store in airtight containers. Protect from light.

Equilin is a natural oestrogenic hormone found in horses. Sodium equilin sulphate is one of the components of both conjugated and esterified oestrogens (p.1457) used for menopausal hormone replacement therapy.

Estrapronicate (13426-e)

Estrapronicate *(rINN).*

Oestradiol 17-nicotinate 3-propionate.

$C_{27}H_{31}NO_4$ = 433.5.

CAS — 4140-20-9.

Estrapronicate is a derivative of oestradiol (p.1455) with nicotinic acid. It has been used as an ingredient of a combined preparation with an anabolic steroid and a progestogen for osteoporosis.

Preparations

Proprietary Preparations (details are given in Part 3)

Multi-ingredient: ***Mon.:*** Trophobolene.

Estropipate (9042-b)

Estropipate *(BAN).*

Piperazine Estrone Sulfate; Piperazine Oestrone Sulphate. Piperazine 17-oxoestra-1,3,5-(10)-trien-3-yl hydrogen sulphate.

$C_{18}H_{22}O_5S,C_4H_{10}N_2$ = 436.6.

CAS — 7280-37-7.

Pharmacopoeias. In *Br.* and *US.*

A white to yellowish-white fine crystalline powder, odourless or with a slight odour. Very slightly **soluble** in water, in alcohol, in chloroform, and in ether; soluble 1 in 500 of warm alcohol; soluble in warm water. **Store** in airtight containers.

Adverse Effects and Precautions

As for oestrogens in general (see Oestradiol, p.1455). See also under Hormone Replacement Therapy, p.1435.

Interactions

See under Hormone Replacement Therapy, p.1437.

Uses and Administration

Estropipate is a semisynthetic conjugate of oestrone with piperazine that is used for menopausal hormone replacement therapy (see p.1434). Its action is due to oestrone (p.1458) to which it is hydrolysed in the body.

Estropipate is given by mouth for the short-term treatment of menopausal symptoms; suggested doses have ranged from 0.75 to 6 mg daily, given cyclically or continuously. When used longer term for the prevention of postmenopausal osteoporosis a daily dose of 0.75 or 1.5 mg is given cyclically or continuously. In women with a uterus estropipate should be used in conjunction with a progestogen. Estropipate is also used short term for menopausal atrophic vaginitis as a vaginal cream containing 0.15%; 2 to 4 g of cream is applied daily. It is also given by mouth in the treatment of female hypogonadism, castration, and primary ovarian failure in doses of 1.5 to 9 mg daily, in a cyclical regimen.

Preparations

BP 1998: Estropipate Tablets;
USP 23: Estropipate Tablets; Estropipate Vaginal Cream.

Proprietary Preparations (details are given in Part 3)

Austral.: Genoral; Ogen; ***Canad.:*** Ogen; ***Irl.:*** Harmogen; ***S.Afr.:*** Ortho-Est; ***UK:*** Harmogen; ***USA:*** Ogen; Ortho-Est.

Multi-ingredient: ***UK:*** Improvera.

Ethinyloestradiol (9043-v)

Ethinyloestradiol *(BAN)*.

Ethinylestradiol *(rINN)*; Aethinyloestradiolum; Ethinyl Estradiol; Etinilestradiol; NSC-10973. 17α-Ethynylestra-1,3,5(10)-triene-3,17β-diol; 19-Nor-17α-pregna-1,3,5(10)-trien-20-yne-3,17β-diol.

$C_{20}H_{24}O_2$ = 296.4.

CAS — 57-63-6.

Pharmacopoeias. In *Chin., Eur.* (see p.viii), *Int., Jpn,* and *US.*

A white to slightly yellowish-white, odourless, crystalline powder. Practically **insoluble** in water; soluble to freely soluble in alcohol and in ether; soluble in chloroform and in vegetable oils; dissolves in solutions of alkali hydroxides. **Store** in non-metallic airtight containers. Protect from light.

Adverse Effects and Precautions

As for oestrogens in general (see Oestradiol, p.1455). See also under Hormonal Contraceptives, p.1426.

Effects on calcium homoeostasis. Two patients with metastatic breast cancer given ethinyloestradiol developed rapidly progressive irreversible and fatal hypercalcaemia, considered to be due to stimulation of osteolysis by the oestrogen.[1]

1. Cornbleet M, *et al.* Fatal irreversible hypercalcaemia in breast cancer. *Br Med J* 1977; **1:** 145.

Effects on the liver. Cholestasis and pruritus developed in a liver transplant recipient receiving ethinyloestradiol at a dose of 50 μg daily for the treatment of menorrhagia.[1] Symptoms subsided on withdrawal of ethinyloestradiol but returned on its re-introduction.

1. Fedorkow DM, *et al.* Cholestasis induced by oestrogen after liver transplantation. *Br Med J* 1989; **299:** 1080–1.

Interactions

See under Hormonal Contraceptives, p.1432.

Pharmacokinetics

Ethinyloestradiol is rapidly and well absorbed from the gastro-intestinal tract. The presence of an ethinyl group at the 17-position greatly reduces hepatic first-pass metabolism compared with oestradiol, enabling the compound to be much more active by mouth, but there is some initial conjugation by the gut wall, and the systemic bioavailability is only about 40%. Ethinyloestradiol is highly protein bound, but unlike naturally occurring oestrogens, which are mainly bound to sex-hormone binding globulin, it is principally bound to albumin. It is metabolised in the liver, and excreted in urine and faeces. Metabolites undergo enterohepatic recycling.

References.

1. Back DJ, *et al.* The gut wall metabolism of ethinyloestradiol and its contribution to the pre-systemic metabolism of ethinyloestradiol in humans. *Br J Clin Pharmacol* 1982; **13:** 325–30.

Uses and Administration

Ethinyloestradiol is a synthetic oestrogen with actions similar to those of oestradiol (see p.1456).

It is frequently used as the oestrogenic component of combined oral contraceptive preparations; a typical daily dose is 20 to 50 μg (for guidance on appropriate dose levels, see p.1433). A combined preparation of ethinyloestradiol with the anti-androgen cyproterone (p.1440) is used for the hormonal treatment of acne (p.1072), particularly when contraception is also required.

Ethinyloestradiol has also been used for menopausal hormone replacement therapy (p.1434); doses of 10 to 20 μg daily were given (in conjunction with a progestogen in women with a uterus), but natural oestrogens are usually preferred.

For the treatment of female hypogonadism, 50 μg has been given up to three times daily for 14 consecutive days in every 4 weeks, followed by a progestogen for the next 14 days.

For the palliative treatment of malignant neoplasms of the prostate (p.491) doses of 150 μg to 3 mg have been given daily. For palliation of malignant neoplasms of the breast (p.485) in postmenopausal women doses of 100 μg to 1 mg three times daily have been used.

Preparations

BP 1998: Ethinylestradiol Tablets; Levonorgestrel and Ethinylestradiol Tablets;
USP 23: Ethinyl Estradiol Tablets; Ethynodiol Diacetate and Ethinyl Estradiol Tablets; Levonorgestrel and Ethinyl Estradiol Tablets; Norethindrone Acetate and Ethinyl Estradiol Tablets; Norethindrone and Ethinyl Estradiol Tablets; Norgestrel and Ethinyl Estradiol Tablets.

Proprietary Preparations (details are given in Part 3)

Aust.: Progynon C; ***Austral.:*** Estigyn; Primogyn C†; ***Canad.:*** Estinyl; ***Ger.:*** Progynon C; Turisteron; ***Neth.:*** Lynoral; ***Norw.:*** Etifollin; ***S.Afr.:*** Estinyl; ***Switz.:*** Progynon C†; ***USA:*** Estinyl.

Multi-ingredient: ***Aust.:*** Cileste; Diane; Etalontin; Gracial; Gynovin; Levlen; Liogynon; Lyndiol; Marvelon; Mercilon; Microgynon; Minulet; Monogestin; Myvlar; Neo-Stediril; Neogynon; Neorlest; Orlest; Ostro-Primolut†; Ovanon; Ovranette†; Ovysmen; Perikursal; Primosiston; Restovar; Sequilar; Stediril D; Tri-Minulet; TriCilest; Trigynon; Trinordiol; Trinovum; Triodena; Triogestena; Triogestin; Yermonil; ***Austral.:*** Biphasil; Brenda-35 ED; Brevinor; Diane ED; Femoden ED; Improvil; Levlen ED; Logynon ED; Marvelon; Microgynon; Minulet; Monofeme; Nordette; Nordiol; Norimin; Ovulen; Sequilar ED; Synphasic; Tri-Minulet; Trifeme; Trioden ED; Triphasil; Triquilar; ***Belg.:*** Binordiol; Cilest; Conova; Diane; Femodene; Fysioquens; Gracial; Harmonet; Lyndiol; Marvelon; Meliane; Mercilon; Microgynon; Minestril; Ministat; Minulet; Neo-Stediril; Ovanon; Ovidol; Ovostat; Ovulen; Ovysmen; Stediril; Stediril 30; Stediril D; Tri-Minulet; Trigynon; Trinordiol; Trinovum; Triodene; ***Canad.:*** Brevicon; Cyclen; Demulen; Loestrin 1.5/30; Marvelon; Min-Ovral; Minestrin; Norlestrin†; Ortho 0.5/35; Ortho 1/35; Ortho 10/11; Ortho 7/7/7; Ortho-Cept; Ovral; Synphasic; Tri-Cyclen; Triphasil; Triquilar; ***Fr.:*** Adepal; Cilest; Cycleane; Diane; Effiprev; Gynophase†; Gynovlane†; Harmonet; Lutestral; Meliane; Mercilon; Milli Anovlar; Minidril; Miniphase; Minulet; Moneva; Norquentiel†; Ortho-Novum 1/35; Ovanon; Phaeva; Physiostat; Planor; Stediril; Trentovlane†; Tri-Minulet; Triella; Trinordiol; Varnoline; ***Ger.:*** Anacyclin; Anacyclin 28†; Biviol; Certostat†; Cilest; Conceplan M; Cyclosa; Depositon†; Diane; Duoluton†; Ediwal†; Etalontin†; Eugynon†; Eve; Femigoa; Femovan; Femranette mikro; Gravistat; Leios; Lovelle; Lyn-ratiopharm; Lyn-ratiopharm-Sequenz; Lyndiol; Marvelon; Menova†; Microgynon; Minisiston; Minulet; Miranova; MonoStep; Neo-Eunomin; Neo-Stediril; Neogynon; Neogynon 28†; Neorlest; Non-Ovlon; Nuriphasic; Oestro-Gynaedron†; Orlest†; Ostro-Primolut; Ovanon; Oviol; Ovoresta; Ovoresta M; Ovowop†; Ovysmen; Perikursal; Poly-Gynaedron†; Pramino; Pregnon L; Primosiston; Progylut†; Prosiston; Sequilar; Sequostat; Sinovula; Stediril; Stediril 30; Stediril D; Synphasec; Tetragynon; Triette; Trigoa; Trinordiol; Trinovum; Triquilar; Trisiston; TriStep; Valette; Yermonil; ***Irl.:*** Binovum; Brevinor; Cilest; Conova†; Dianette; Eugynon 30†; Femodene; Logynon; Marviol; Mercilon; Microgynon 30; Minulet; Normin; Ovran; Ovran 30; Ovranette; Ovysmen; Tri-Minulet; Trinordiol; Trinovum; Triodene; ***Ital.:*** Anovlar†; Binordiol†; Bivlar†; Cilest†; Diane; Egogyn 30; Estro-Primolut†; Eugynon; Evanor-D; Fedra; Ginoden; Harmonet; Lyndiol E†; Mercilon; Microgynon; Milvane; Miniluteolas†; Minulet; Novogyn; Ovranet; Planum; Practil; Primosiston†; Securgin; Tri-Minulet; Trigynon; Trinordiol; Trinovum; ***Neth.:*** Binordiol; Cilest; Diane; Femodeen; Fysioquens; Harmonet; Lyndiol†; Marvelon; Meliane; Mercilon; Microgynon; Mini Pregnon; Ministat; Minulet; Modicon; Neo-Stediril; Neocon; Neogynon; Ovanon; Ovidol; Ovostat; Ovulen†; Pregnon†; Primosiston†; Stediril; Tri-Minulet; Trigynon; Trinordiol; Trinovum; Triodeen; ***Norw.:*** Diane; Eugynon; Follimin; Lyndiol†; Marvelon; Microgynon; Synfase; Tetragynon; Trinordiol; Trionetta; ***S.Afr.:*** Biphasil; Brevinor; Demulen†; Diane; Femodene ED; Logynon ED; Lyndiol†; Marvelon; Menoflush; Menoflush + ¼; Mercilon; Minovlar ED†; Minulette; Mixogen†; Nordette; Nordiol; Normovlar ED; Ovanon†; Ovostat; Ovral; Restovar†; Tri-Minulet; Trinovum; Triodene; Triphasil; ***Spain:*** Diane; Eugynon; Gynovin; Microdiol; Microgynon; Minulet; Neo Lyndiol; Neogynona; Ovoplex; Ovoresta Micro†; Primosiston; Suavuret; Tri-Minulet; Triagynon; Triciclor; Trigynovin; ***Swed.:*** Desolett; Follimin; Follinett; Lyndiol†; Lyndiolett; Mercilon; Neovletta; Nordette†; Orthonett Novum; Regunon; Restovar; Sequilarum†; Synfase; Tetragynon†; Trinordiol; Trinovum; Trionetta; ***Switz.:*** Binordiol; Cilest; Diane; Gracial; Gynera; Lovelle†; Marvelon; Mercilon; Microgynon; Milvane; Minulet; Neo-Eunomine; Neo-Stediril; Neogynon; Normophasic; Oestro-Gynaedron†; Ologyn; Ovanon; Ovidol; Ovostat; Ovulen; Ovysmen; Primosiston; Sequilar; Stediril 30; Stediril D; Tetragynon; Tri-Minulet†; Trinordiol; Trinovum; Triquilar; Varnoline†; Yermonil; ***UK:*** Binovum; Brevinor; Cilest; Conova†; Dianette; Eugynon 30; Femodene; Loestrin; Logynon; Marvelon; Mercilon; Microgynon 30; Minulet; Neocon 1/35†; Norimin; Ovran; Ovran 30; Ovranette; Ovysmen; Schering PC4; Synphase; Tri-Minulet; Triadene; Trinordiol; Trinovum; Trinovum ED†; ***USA:*** Alesse; Brevicon; Demulen; Desogen; Estrostep; Estrostep Fe; GenCept 0.5/35; GenCept 10/11; Genora 0.5/35; Jenest; Levlen; Levora; Lo/Ovral; Loestrin; Loestrin Fe; Modicon; Necon; NEE 1/35; Nelova 0.5/35E; Nelova 10/11; Nelulen†; Norcept-E†; Nordette; Norethin 1/35E; Norinyl 1 + 35; Ortho Cyclen; Ortho Tri-Cyclen; Ortho-Cept; Ortho-Novum 1/35; Ortho-Novum 10/11; Ortho-Novum 7/7/7; Ovcon 35; Ovral; Preven; Tri-Levlen; Tri-Norinyl; Triphasil; Zovia.

Ethisterone (9044-g)

Ethisterone *(BAN, rINN)*.

Anhydrohydroxyprogesterone; Ethinyltestosterone; Ethisteronum; Etisterona; NSC-9565; Praegninum; Pregneninolone; Pregnin. 17β-Hydroxy-17α-pregn-4-en-20-yn-3-one.

$C_{21}H_{28}O_2$ = 312.4.

CAS — 434-03-7.

Pharmacopoeias. In *Pol.*

Ethisterone is a progestogen (see Progesterone, p.1459) that also has oestrogenic and androgenic properties.

Pregnancy. Ethisterone, administered to pregnant women, has been associated with masculinisation of female fetuses.[1] Meningomyelocele and hydrocephalus in infants have also been associated with exposure *in utero* to ethisterone.[2]

1. Wilkins L. Masculinization of female fetus due to use of orally given progestins. *JAMA* 1960; **172:** 1028–32.
2. Gal I, *et al.* Hormonal pregnancy tests and congenital malformation. *Nature* 1967; **216:** 83.

Ethyloestrenol (9045-q)

Ethyloestrenol *(BAN)*.

Ethylestrenol *(USAN, rINN)*. 17α-Ethylestr-4-en-17β-ol; 19-Nor-17α-pregn-4-en-17β-ol.

$C_{20}H_{32}O$ = 288.5.

CAS — 965-90-2.

Pharmacopoeias. In *Br.*

A white or almost white, odourless or almost odourless, crystalline powder. Practically **insoluble** in water; freely soluble in alcohol, in chloroform, and in ether. **Store** at a temperature not exceeding 15°. Protect from light.

Ethyloestrenol is a 17α-alkylated anabolic steroid (see Testosterone, p.1464) with little androgenic effect and slight progestational activity. It has been used for the promotion of growth in boys with short stature or delayed bone growth.

Preparations

BP 1998: Ethylestrenol Tablets.

Proprietary Preparations (details are given in Part 3)
Austral.: Orabolin†; ***Belg.:*** Orabolin†; ***S.Afr.:*** Orabolin†.

Ethynodiol Diacetate (9046-p)

Ethynodiol Diacetate *(BANM, USAN)*.

Etynodiol Diacetate *(pINNM)*; Aethynodiolum Diaceticum; SC-11800. 19-Nor-17α-pregn-4-en-20-yne-3β,17β-diol diacetate.

$C_{24}H_{32}O_4$ = 384.5.

CAS — 1231-93-2 (ethynodiol); 297-76-7 (ethynodiol diacetate).

Pharmacopoeias. In *Br., Pol.,* and *US.*

A white or almost white, odourless or almost odourless, crystalline powder. Very slightly **soluble** to practically insoluble in water; soluble in alcohol; freely to very soluble in chloroform; freely soluble in ether; sparingly soluble in fixed oils. **Protect** from light.

Adverse Effects and Precautions

As for progestogens in general (see Progesterone, p.1459). See also under Hormonal Contraceptives, p.1426.

Pregnancy. Fetal adrenal cytomegaly in a 17-week-old fetus was associated with the maternal ingestion of an oral contraceptive containing ethynodiol diacetate 2 mg and mestranol 100 μg from the sixth to the fourteenth week of pregnancy.[1]

1. Gau GS, Bennett MJ. Fetal adrenal cytomegaly. *J Clin Pathol* 1979; **32:** 305–6.

Interactions

As for progestogens in general (see Progesterone, p.1460). See also under Hormonal Contraceptives, p.1432.

Pharmacokinetics

Ethynodiol diacetate is readily absorbed from the gastro-intestinal tract and rapidly metabolised, largely to norethisterone. Following administration of a radiolabelled dose of ethynodiol diacetate about 60% of the radioactivity is stated to be excreted in urine and about 30% in faeces; half-life in plasma was about 25 hours.

Uses and Administration

Ethynodiol diacetate is a progestogen (see Progesterone, p.1460) that is used as the progestogenic component of combined oral contraceptives and also alone as an oral progestogen-only contraceptive (see p.1433); typical daily doses are 2 mg in combination products and 500 μg for progestogen-only contraceptives.

Preparations

USP 23: Ethynodiol Diacetate and Ethinyl Estradiol Tablets; Ethynodiol Diacetate and Mestranol Tablets.

Proprietary Preparations (details are given in Part 3)
Fr.: Lutometrodiol; *Ital.:* Luteonorm†; *S.Afr.:* Femulen†; *UK:* Femulen.

Multi-ingredient: *Austral.:* Ovulen; *Belg.:* Conova; Ovulen; *Canad.:* Demulen; *Irl.:* Conova†; *Ital.:* Luteolas†; Miniluteolas†; Ovaras†; *Neth.:* Ovulen†; *S.Afr.:* Demulen†; *Switz.:* Ovulen; *UK:* Conova†; *USA:* Demulen; Nelulen†; Zovia.

Etonogestrel (15428-g)

Etonogestrel *(BAN, USAN, rINN).*

3-keto-Desogestrel; Org-3236. 13-Ethyl-17-hydroxy-11-methylene-18,19-dinor-17α-pregn-4-en-20-yn-3-one; 17β-Hydroxy-11-methylene-18-homo-19-nor-17α-pregn-4-en-20-yn-3-one.

$C_{22}H_{28}O_2$ = 324.5.

CAS — 54048-10-1.

Etonogestrel, the active metabolite of desogestrel (p.1443), is under investigation as the progestogen component of a combined contraceptive delivered via a vaginal ring device.

References.

1. Roumen FJ, *et al.* The cervico-vaginal epithelium during 20 cycles' use of a combined contraceptive vaginal ring. *Hum Reprod* 1996; **11:** 2443–8.

Finasteride (5502-q)

Finasteride *(BAN, USAN, rINN).*

MK-0906; MK-906. N-*tert*-Butyl-3-oxo-4-aza-5α-androst-1-ene-17β-carboxamide.

$C_{23}H_{36}N_2O_2$ = 372.5.

CAS — 98319-26-7.

Adverse Effects

The most commonly reported adverse effects of finasteride are decreased libido, impotence, and reduced volume of ejaculate.

Breast tenderness and enlargement (gynaecomastia) may occur, and there have been reports of hypersensitivity reactions such as lip swelling and rashes.

In a study using prescription event monitoring data,[1] the most commonly reported adverse effects of finasteride in 14 772 patients were impotence or ejaculatory failure (2.1% of patients), reduced libido (1%), and breast disorders such as gynaecomastia (0.4%). Adverse effects reported in a single patient each, and verified on rechallenge, were exfoliative dermatitis, perioral numbness, and swollen glands. Finasteride appeared to be associated with ataxia in 1 patient and wheeziness in another.

1. Wilton L, *et al.* The safety of finasteride used in benign prostatic hypertrophy: a non-interventional observational cohort study in 14 772 patients. *Br J Urol* 1996; **78:** 379–84.

Effects on the breast. Gynaecomastia was the adverse effect of finasteride most frequently reported to the FDA between June 1992 and February 1995 (a total of 214 reports).[1] The onset after therapy ranged from 14 days to 2.5 years, and the condition could be unilateral or bilateral. Mastectomy was performed in 12 men. Of the 86 men for whom information after discontinuation was available, partial or complete remission of gynaecomastia occurred in 80%, and no change occurred in 20%. In 2 of the cases, primary intraductal breast carcinoma was subsequently found, although 1 probably had breast cancer before finasteride therapy. Continued surveillance of the relationship between finasteride and breast cancer is required.

1. Green L, *et al.* Gynecomastia and breast cancer during finasteride therapy. *N Engl J Med* 1996; **335:** 823.

Precautions

Finasteride should be used with caution in men at risk of obstructive uropathy. Patients should be evaluated for prostatic carcinoma before and during therapy. However, it should be noted that use of finasteride decreases concentrations of serum markers of prostate cancer such as prostate specific antigen even when cancer is present.

Studies in *animals* suggest finasteride could produce feminisation (hypospadia) of a male fetus if used in pregnant women; therefore, its use is contra-indicated in women who are or may become pregnant. In addition, it is recommended that women in this category should not handle crushed or broken finasteride tablets. Finasteride has been detected in semen, therefore use of a condom is recommended if the patient's sexual partner is, or may become, pregnant.

Pharmacokinetics

Finasteride is absorbed following oral administration, and peak plasma concentrations are achieved in 1 to 2 hours. The mean bioavailability has variously been reported as 63% and 80%. It is about 90% bound to plasma protein. Finasteride is metabolised in the liver and excreted in urine and faeces as metabolites. Mean half-life is 6 hours in patients under 60 years of age but may be prolonged to about 8 hours in those 70 years of age or older.

References.

1. Steiner JF. Clinical pharmacokinetics and pharmacodynamics of finasteride. *Clin Pharmacokinet* 1996; **30:** 16–27.

Uses and Administration

Finasteride is an azasteroid that inhibits 5α-reductase, the enzyme responsible for conversion of testosterone to the more active dihydrotestosterone, and therefore has anti-androgenic properties. It is given by mouth in a dose of 5 mg daily in the management of benign prostatic hyperplasia; it is reported to cause regression of the enlarged prostate and to improve symptoms. Response may be delayed and treatment for 6 months or more may be required to assess whether benefit has been achieved.

In the treatment of male-pattern baldness, finasteride is given by mouth in a dose of 1 mg daily. In general use for 3 months or more is required before benefit is seen, and effects are reversed within 12 months of ceasing therapy.

Benign prostatic hyperplasia. Hypertrophy of the prostate gland is common in men with increasing age: as many as 70% of men aged over 75 have histological evidence of hyperplasia.[1] Men with an enlarged prostate may exhibit overt symptoms of obstruction, such as acute or chronic urinary retention, or irritative symptoms such as frequency, urgency, nocturia, or occasionally urge incontinence, resulting from secondary bladder instability.[1-3] Symptoms can fluctuate, and do not necessarily deteriorate with time; furthermore, they do not seem to relate directly to prostatic volume.

In men with mild or moderate symptoms no treatment may be required, although symptoms need to be monitored ('watchful waiting').[4,5] In those with more severe symptoms or complications the mainstay of treatment is *transurethral resection of the prostate* (TURP).[3-7] This is the most effective treatment, but is associated with the greatest risk of complications and morbidity, including potential impotence. In consequence other methods may be tried first in men with more severe symptoms but no definite indications for surgery.[5]

Therapy with an *alpha₁-adrenoceptor blocker* (such as alfuzosin, doxazosin, prazosin, tamsulosin, or terazosin) can produce rapid symptomatic relief, apparently by an action on smooth muscle in the hyperplastic tissue and in the bladder.[2,6,7] However, the results are not as good as with surgery,[8] and adverse effects include orthostatic hypotension.

In recent years the *5α-reductase inhibitor* finasteride has offered an alternative approach.[2,6,7,9-15] Finasteride produces moderate reductions in prostate volume, although this takes a number of months and is not always associated with much symptomatic improvement.[7,9] Like the alpha blockers, therapy must be continued indefinitely for benefit to be maintained. A recent 12-month study[16] found the alpha blocker terazosin to be more effective than finasteride in relieving symptoms and improving peak urine flow rates; the combination of finasteride plus terazosin was no more effective than terazosin alone. Moreover, although finasteride reduced prostatic volume, it was no more effective than placebo, a finding that is at odds with previous placebo-controlled studies. It has been suggested that the smaller median prostate size in this study may explain the negative findings,[17] and that men with larger prostates do benefit from finasteride. However, others consider that the findings indicate that decreasing muscle tone may be more important than reducing prostate size, and that alpha blockers remain the drugs of first choice for the medical management of benign prostatic hyperplasia although finasteride may be useful in gross enlargement.[18] More recently, a 4-year study found that finasteride reduces the probability of surgery and acute urinary retention in men with symptomatic benign prostate hyperplasia with prostatic enlargement.[19] For every 100 men treated, 7 finasteride and 13 placebo recipients required surgery (a 55% reduction).[20]

Other drug therapies exist but are largely unproven or unsuitable for general use. Gonadorelin analogues such as leuprorelin or nafarelin can produce a reduction in prostate size, but it rapidly returns to its former volume on ceasing treatment, and adverse effects make these drugs unsuitable for indefinite therapy. The antifungal mepartricin has been reported to produce symptomatic improvement, possibly by binding to oestrogen in the intestinal lumen and lowering plasma-oestrogen concentrations. A number of plant extracts such as saw palmetto and *Pygeum africanum* are also in use,[21,22] and the phytosterol sitosterol, which is a constituent of these, is reported to be effective.[21] However, the aromatase inhibitor atamestane, which can inhibit the rise in oestrogen biosynthesis, appears not to be of benefit.[23]

Various non-drug therapies other than resection are under investigation: these include transurethral microwave thermotherapy, laser prostatectomy, and the insertion of stents to physically hold the urethra open.[7,24]

1. Abrams P. Benign prostatic hyperplasia. *Br Med J* 1993; **307:** 201.
2. Gingell JC. Review of current and future approaches to the management of benign prostatic hyperplasia. *Postgrad Med J* 1992; **68:** 702–6.
3. Kirk D. How should new treatments for benign prostatic hyperplasia be assessed? *Br Med J* 1993; **306:** 1283–4.
4. McCarthy M. BPH guidelines. *Lancet* 1994; **343:** 473.
5. Cockett AT, *et al.* Recommendations of the International Consensus Committee In: Cockett AT, *et al,* eds. *The 2nd international consultation on benign prostatic hyperplasia (BPH).* Jersey: Scientific Communication International, 1993: 553–64.
6. Monda JM, Oesterling JE. Medical treatment of benign prostatic hyperplasia: 5α-reductase inhibitors and α-adrenergic antagonists. *Mayo Clin Proc* 1993; **68:** 670–9.
7. Oesterling JE. Benign prostatic hyperplasia: medical and minimally invasive treatment options. *N Engl J Med* 1995; **332:** 99–109.
8. Chapple CR, *et al.* Comparative study of selective α₁-adrenoceptor blockade versus surgery in the treatment of prostatic obstruction. *Br J Urol* 1993; **72:** 822–5.
9. Anonymous. Finasteride and benign prostatic hyperplasia. *Drug Ther Bull* 1995; **33:** 19–21.
10. Peters DH, Sorkin EM. Finasteride: a review of its potential in the treatment of benign prostatic hyperplasia. *Drugs* 1993; **46:** 177–208.
11. Rittmaster RS. Finasteride. *N Engl J Med* 1994; **330:** 120–5.
12. Neal DE. Drugs in focus 16: finasteride. *Prescribers' J* 1995; **35:** 89–94.
13. Gormley GJ, *et al.* The effect of finasteride in men with benign prostatic hyperplasia. *N Engl J Med* 1992; **327:** 1185–91.
14. Finasteride Study Group. Finasteride (MK-906) in the treatment of benign prostatic hyperplasia. *Prostate* 1993; **22:** 291–9.
15. Nickel JC, *et al.* Efficacy and safety of finasteride for benign prostatic hyperplasia: results of a 2-year randomized controlled trial (the PROSPECT study). *Can Med Assoc J* 1996; **155:** 1251–9.
16. Lepor H, *et al.* The efficacy of terazosin, finasteride, or both in benign prostatic hyperplasia. *N Engl J Med* 1996; **335:** 533–9.
17. Walsh PC. Treatment of benign prostatic hyperplasia. *N Engl J Med* 1996; **335:** 586–7.
18. Farmer A, Noble J. Drug treatment for benign prostatic hyperplasia. *Br Med J* 1997; **314:** 1215–16.
19. McConnell JD, *et al.* The effect of finasteride on the risk of acute urinary retention and the need for surgical treatment among men with benign prostate hyperplasia. *N Engl J Med* 1998; **338:** 557–63.
20. Wasson JH. Finasteride to prevent morbidity from benign prostatic hyperplasia. *N Engl J Med* 1998; **338:** 612–13.
21. Lowe FC, Ku JC. Phytotherapy in treatment of benign prostatic hyperplasia: a critical review. *Urology* 1996; **48:** 12–20.
22. Buck AC. Phytotherapy for the prostate. *Br J Urol* 1996; **78:** 325–36.
23. Gingell JC, *et al.* Placebo controlled double-blind study to test the efficacy of the aromatase inhibitor atamestane in patients with benign prostatic hyperplasia not requiring operation. *J Urol (Baltimore)* 1995; **154:** 399–401.
24. Lee M, Sharifi R. Benign prostatic hyperplasia: diagnosis and treatment guideline. *Ann Pharmacother* 1997; **31:** 481–6.

Hirsutism and male-pattern alopecia. Finasteride is under investigation for the treatment of hirsutism (p.1441) in women.[1] It is also used in the treatment of alopecia androgenetica (baldness, p.1073) in men.[2,3]

1. Wong IL, *et al.* A prospective randomized trial comparing finasteride to spironolactone in the treatment of hirsute women. *J Clin Endocrinol Metab* 1995; **80:** 233–8.
2. Mazzerella F, *et al.* Topical finasteride in the treatment of androgenic alopecia. *J Dermatol Treat* 1997; **8:** 189–92.
3. Anonymous. Propecia and Rogaine Extra Strength for alopecia. *Med Lett Drugs Ther* 1998; **40:** 25–7.

Malignant neoplasms of the prostate. Finasteride appears to have little effect in men with established prostate cancer,[1,2] but is under investigation for the prevention of prostate cancer (see also p.491).

1. Presti JC, *et al.* Multicenter, randomized, double-blind placebo controlled study to investigate the effect of finasteride (MK-906) on stage D prostate cancer. *J Urol (Baltimore)* 1992; **148:** 1201–4.
2. Rittmaster RS. Finasteride. *N Engl J Med* 1994; **330:** 120–5.

Preparations

Proprietary Preparations (details are given in Part 3)
Aust.: Proscar; *Austral.:* Proscar; *Belg.:* Proscar; *Canad.:* Proscar; *Fr.:* Chibro-Proscar; *Ger.:* Proscar; *Irl.:* Proscar; *Ital.:* Finastid; Proscar; Prostide; *Neth.:* Proscar; *Norw.:* Proscar; *S.Afr.:* Proscar; *Spain:* Proscar; Urprosan; *Swed.:* Proscar; *Switz.:* Proscar; *UK:* Proscar; *USA:* Propecia; Proscar.

Flugestone Acetate (9047-s)

Flugestone Acetate *(BANM)*.

Flurogestone Acetate *(USAN)*; NSC-65411; SC-9880; SC 9880. 9α-Fluoro-11β,17α-dihydroxypregn-4-ene-3,20-dione 17-acetate.

$C_{23}H_{31}FO_5$ = 406.5.

CAS — 337-03-1 (flugestone); 2529-45-5 (flugestone acetate).

Flugestone acetate is a progestogen (see Progesterone, p.1459) used in veterinary medicine.

Fluoxymesterone (9049-e)

Fluoxymesterone *(BAN, rINN)*.

NSC-12165. 9α-Fluoro-11β,17β-dihydroxy-17α-methylandrost-4-en-3-one.

$C_{20}H_{29}FO_3$ = 336.4.

CAS — 76-43-7.

Pharmacopoeias. In *Jpn* and *US*.

A white or almost white, odourless, crystalline powder. Practically **insoluble** in water; sparingly soluble in alcohol; slightly soluble in chloroform. **Protect** from light.

Adverse Effects and Precautions

As for androgens and anabolic steroids in general (see Testosterone, p.1464).

As with other 17α-alkylated compounds fluoxymesterone may cause hepatotoxicity, and is probably best avoided in patients with hepatic impairment, and certainly if this is severe. Hepatic function should be monitored during therapy.

Uses and Administration

Fluoxymesterone has androgenic properties (see Testosterone, p.1465). It is effective when given by mouth and is more potent than methyltestosterone.

In the treatment of male hypogonadism, fluoxymesterone has been given in a dosage of 5 to 20 mg daily. In the treatment of delayed puberty in the male it has been given in usual daily doses of 2.5 to 10 mg, adjusted according to response; care was necessary because of the risk of epiphyseal closure and treatment was generally only given for 4 to 6 months. In the palliation of inoperable neoplasms of the breast in postmenopausal women, it has been given in daily doses of up to 40 mg.

Growth retardation. Fluoxymesterone has been used to increase final adult height in boys with constitutional delay of growth associated with delayed puberty (see p.1237).

Preparations

USP 23: Fluoxymesterone Tablets.

Proprietary Preparations (details are given in Part 3)
Austral.: Halotestin†; ***Canad.:*** Halotestin; ***Fr.:*** Halotestin; ***Ital.:*** Halotestin; ***Neth.:*** Halotestin; ***Norw.:*** Halotestin; ***S.Afr.:*** Halotestin; ***Swed.:*** Halotestin†; ***USA:*** Halotestin.

Formebolone (9051-v)

Formebolone *(BAN, rINN)*.

Formyldienolone. 11α,17β-Dihydroxy-17β-methyl-3-oxoandrosta-1,4-diene-2-carbaldehyde.

$C_{21}H_{28}O_4$ = 344.4.

CAS — 2454-11-7.

Formebolone has anabolic properties (see Testosterone, p.1464) and has been given by mouth or by intramuscular injection.

Preparations

Proprietary Preparations (details are given in Part 3)
Ital.: Esiclene†.

Fosfestrol (9052-g)

Fosfestrol *(BAN, rINN)*.

Diethylstilbestrol Diphosphate; Phosphoestrolum; Stilboestrol Diphosphate. (*E*)-αα′-Diethylstilbene-4,4′-diol bis(dihydrogen phosphate); (*E*)-4,4′-(1,2-Diethylvinylene)bis(phenyl dihydrogen orthophosphate).

$C_{18}H_{22}O_8P_2$ = 428.3.

CAS — 522-40-7.

Pharmacopoeias. In *Jpn* and *US*.

An off-white odourless crystalline powder. Sparingly **soluble** in water; soluble in alcohol and in dilute alkalis. **Store** at a temperature not exceeding 21° in airtight containers.

Fosfestrol Sodium (9053-q)

Fosfestrol Sodium *(BANM, rINNM)*.

$C_{18}H_{18}Na_4O_8P_2$ = 516.2.

CAS — 23519-26-8 (fosfestrol tetrasodium xH₂O); 4719-75-9 (fosfestrol tetrasodium, anhydrous).

Pharmacopoeias. In *Br.*, which specifies xH_2O.

A white or almost white powder. Anhydrous fosfestrol sodium 100 mg is approximately equivalent to 83 mg of fosfestrol. Freely **soluble** in water; practically insoluble in dehydrated alcohol and in ether. A 5% solution has a pH of 7 to 9. **Protect** from light.

Adverse Effects and Precautions

As for Stilboestrol, see p.1463.

Following intravenous injection of fosfestrol sodium there may be temporary local pain in the perineal region and at the site of bony metastases. Slow infusion is not recommended as cytotoxic concentrations of the drug may not be achieved.

Uses and Administration

Fosfestrol is a synthetic nonsteroidal oestrogen that requires dephosphorylation to stilboestrol (p.1462) before it is active. It is used in the treatment of malignant neoplasms of the prostate (p.491).

Expressed in terms of fosfestrol sodium, initial therapy for at least the first 5 days may range from 600 to 1200 mg daily by slow intravenous injection. In terms of fosfestrol, these doses are equivalent to 500 to 1000 mg. Injections should be given preferably with the patient lying down. Maintenance intravenous therapy may be with 300 mg fosfestrol sodium one to four times a week or 300 to 600 mg fosfestrol sodium (250 to 500 mg fosfestrol) once or twice a week. Fosfestrol sodium may also be given by mouth, in a dose of up to 240 mg (200 mg of fosfestrol) three times daily for 7 days then reducing over 14 days to 120 to 360 mg (100 to 300 mg of fosfestrol) daily in divided doses.

Fosfestrol disodium has also been used.

Preparations

USP 23: Diethylstilbestrol Diphosphate Injection.

Proprietary Preparations (details are given in Part 3)
Aust.: Honvan; ***Austral.:*** Honvan; ***Belg.:*** Honvan; ***Canad.:*** Honvol; ***Fr.:*** ST-52; ***Ger.:*** Honvan; ***Ital.:*** Honvan†; ***Neth.:*** Honvan; ***Norw.:*** Honvan; ***S.Afr.:*** Honvan†; ***Spain:*** Honvan; ***Swed.:*** Honvan†; ***Switz.:*** Honvan; ***UK:*** Honvan; ***USA:*** Stilphostrol.

Gestodene (18649-x)

Gestodene *(BAN, USAN, rINN)*.

SH-B-331. 13β-Ethyl-17β-hydroxy-18,19-dinor-17α-pregna-4,15-dien-20-yn-3-one.

$C_{21}H_{26}O_2$ = 310.4.

CAS — 60282-87-3.

Adverse Effects and Precautions

As for progestogens in general (see Progesterone, p.1459). See also under Hormonal Contraceptives, p.1426. Gestodene is reported to have few androgenic effects, and to have less adverse effect on the serum lipid profile than older 19-nortestosterone derivatives. However, there has been concern that gestodene-containing combined oral contraceptives are associated with an increased risk of venous thrombo-embolism (see p.1430, and for precautions, see p.1432).

Interactions

As for progestogens in general (see Progesterone, p.1460). See also under Hormonal Contraceptives, p.1432.

Antiepileptics. *Felbamate* treatment significantly increased gestodene clearance from a low-dose combined oral contraceptive, and might decrease contraceptive efficacy.[1] See also, p.1433.

1. Saano V, *et al.* Effects of felbamate on the pharmacokinetics of a low-dose combination oral contraceptive. *Clin Pharmacol Ther* 1995; **58:** 523–31.

Pharmacokinetics

Gestodene is well absorbed with a high bioavailability when administered by mouth. It is extensively bound to plasma proteins (75 to 87% to sex hormone binding globulin, and 13 to 24% to albumin). Gestodene is metabolised in the liver, less than 1% of a dose being excreted in the urine unchanged.

Uses and Administration

Gestodene is a progestogen (see Progesterone, p.1459) structurally related to levonorgestrel. It is used as the progestogenic component of combined oral contraceptive preparations (see p.1433); a typical daily dose is 75 µg.

Reviews.

1. Anonymous. Femodene/Minulet—how different is gestodene? *Drug Ther Bull* 1990; **28:** 41–2.
2. Wilde MI, Balfour JA. Gestodene: a review of its pharmacology, efficacy and tolerability in combined contraceptive preparations. *Drugs* 1995; **50:** 364–95.

Preparations

Proprietary Preparations (details are given in Part 3)

Multi-ingredient: ***Aust.:*** Gynovin; Minulet; Monogestin; Myvlar; Tri-Minulet; Triodena; Triogestena; Triogestin; ***Austral.:*** Femoden ED; Minulet; Tri-Minulet; Trioden ED; ***Belg.:*** Femodene; Harmonet; Meliane; Minulet; Tri-Minulet; Triodene; ***Fr.:*** Harmonet; Meliane; Minulet; Moneva; Phaeva; Tri-Minulet; ***Ger.:*** Femovan; Minulet; ***Irl.:*** Femodene; Minulet; Tri-Minulet; Triodene; ***Ital.:*** Fedra; Ginoden; Harmonet; Milvane; Minulet; Tri-Minulet; ***Neth.:*** Femodeen; Harmonet; Meliane; Minulet; Tri-Minulet; Triodeen; ***S.Afr.:*** Femodene ED; Minulette; Tri-Minulet; Triodene; ***Spain:*** Gynovin; Minulet; Tri-Minulet; Trigynovin; ***Switz.:*** Gynera; Milvane; Minulet; Tri-Minulet†; ***UK:*** Femodene; Minulet; Tri-Minulet; Triadene.

Gestrinone (12782-d)

Gestrinone *(BAN, USAN, rINN)*.

A-46745; Ethylnorgestrienone; R-2323; RU-2323. 13β-Ethyl-17β-hydroxy-18,19-dinor-17α-pregna-4,9,11-trien-20-yn-3-one.

$C_{21}H_{24}O_2$ = 308.4.

CAS — 16320-04-0; 40542-65-2.

Adverse Effects

As for Danazol, p.1441. Gestrinone may inhibit ovulation, and menstrual irregularities such as breakthrough bleeding may occur during treatment. Androgenic side-effects include acne, oily skin, fluid retention, weight gain, hirsutism, and voice change. Headache, gastro-intestinal disturbances, increased liver enzyme values, altered libido, hot flushes, decreased breast size, nervousness, change in appetite, muscle cramp, and depression may also occur.

Precautions

As for Danazol, p.1441.

Interactions

Antiepileptic drugs and rifampicin may accelerate the metabolism of gestrinone.

Pharmacokinetics

Gestrinone is well absorbed after oral administration with negligible first-pass hepatic metabolism. Peak plasma concentrations occur about 3 hours after administration. The plasma half-life is about 24 hours. Gestrinone is metabolised in the liver with the formation of conjugated metabolites.

Uses and Administration

Gestrinone is a synthetic steroidal hormone reported to have androgenic, anti-oestrogenic, and antiprogestogenic properties. It is used in the treatment of endometriosis (p.1442) in doses of 2.5 mg twice weekly by mouth; the first dose is taken on the first day of the menstrual cycle with the second dose taken three days later; thereafter the doses should be taken on the same two days of each week, usually for a period of 6 months.

References.

1. Thomas EJ, Cooke ID. Impact of gestrinone on the course of asymptomatic endometriosis. *Br Med J* 1987; **294:** 272–4.
2. Hornstein MD, *et al.* A randomized double-blind prospective trial of two doses of gestrinone in the treatment of endometriosis. *Fertil Steril* 1990; **53:** 237–41.
3. Brosens IA, *et al.* The morphologic effect of short-term medical therapy of endometriosis. *Am J Obstet Gynecol* 1987; **157:** 1215–21.
4. Coutinho EM, Azadian-Boulanger G. Treatment of endometriosis by vaginal administration of gestrinone. *Fertil Steril* 1988; **49:** 418–22.
5. Coutinho EM, Gonçalves MT. Long-term treatment of leiomyomas with gestrinone. *Fertil Steril* 1989; **51:** 939–46.

Preparations

Proprietary Preparations (details are given in Part 3)
Austral.: Dimetriose; ***Belg.:*** Dimetrose; ***Irl.:*** Dimetriose†; ***Ital.:*** Dimetrose; ***Neth.:*** Nemestran; ***S.Afr.:*** Tridomose; ***Spain:*** Nemestran; ***Switz.:*** Nemestran; ***UK:*** Dimetriose.

Gestronol Hexanoate (9055-s)

Gestronol Hexanoate *(BANM)*.

Gestonorone Caproate *(USAN, rINN)*; NSC-84054; SH-582.
17α-Hydroxy-19-norpregn-4-ene-3,20-dione hexanoate.

$C_{26}H_{38}O_4$ = 414.6.

CAS — 1253-28-7.

Adverse Effects and Precautions

As for progestogens in general (see Progesterone, p.1459). Local reactions have occurred at the site of injection. Rarely, coughing, dyspnoea, and circulatory disturbances may develop during or immediately after injection but can be avoided by injecting gestronol very slowly. In males, spermatogenesis is temporarily inhibited.

Interactions

As for progestogens in general (see Progesterone, p.1460).

Uses and Administration

Gestronol hexanoate is a long-acting potent progestogen structurally related to progesterone (p.1460). It is given in an oily solution by intramuscular injection in doses of 200 to 400 mg every 5 to 7 days for the adjunctive treatment of endometrial carcinoma (p.487). It has also been used in the management of benign prostatic hyperplasia (p.1446) in doses of 200 mg weekly, increased to 300 to 400 mg weekly if necessary.

Preparations

Proprietary Preparations (details are given in Part 3)
Aust.: Depostat; ***Belg.:*** Depostat†; ***Ger.:*** Depostat; ***Ital.:*** Depostat; ***Neth.:*** Depostat†; ***Spain:*** Depostat; ***Switz.:*** Depostat; ***UK:*** Depostat.

Hydroxyestrone Diacetate (12833-a)

16α-Hydroxyoestrone Diacetate. 3,16α-Dihydroxyestra-1,3,5(10)-trien-17-one diacetate.

$C_{22}H_{26}O_5$ = 370.4.

CAS — 566-76-7 (hydroxyestrone); 1247-71-8 (hydroxyestrone diacetate).

Hydroxyestrone diacetate is an oestrogen (see Oestradiol, p.1455). It has been given by mouth in usual doses of 200 to 300 μg daily in vulvo-vaginal disorders; doses of up to 700 μg daily have been used for female infertility.

Preparations

Proprietary Preparations (details are given in Part 3)
Fr.: Colpormon.

Hydroxyprogesterone Hexanoate (9057-e)

Hydroxyprogesterone Hexanoate *(BANM)*.

Hydroxyprogesterone Caproate *(rINN)*; 17-AHPC; NSC-17592. 3,20-Dioxopregn-4-en-17α-yl hexanoate; 17α-Hydroxypregn-4-ene-3,20-dione hexanoate.

$C_{27}H_{40}O_4$ = 428.6.

CAS — 68-96-2 (hydroxyprogesterone); 630-56-8 (hydroxyprogesterone hexanoate).

Pharmacopoeias. In Br., Chin., and US.

A white or creamy-white, odourless or almost odourless, crystalline powder. Practically **insoluble** in water; freely soluble in alcohol and in ether; very soluble in chloroform; dissolves in fixed oils and esters. **Protect** from light.

Adverse Effects and Precautions

As for progestogens in general (see Progesterone, p.1459). There may be local reactions at the site of injection. Rarely, coughing, dyspnoea, and circulatory disturbances may occur during or immediately after injection of hydroxyprogesterone hexanoate but can be avoided by injecting the drug very slowly.

Pregnancy. Abnormalities reported in infants born to mothers who had received hydroxyprogesterone during pregnancy have included tetralogy of Fallot in one infant,[1] genito-urinary abnormalities in 2 infants,[2] and adrenocortical carcinoma in one infant.[3]

1. Heinonen OP, *et al.* Cardiovascular birth defects and antenatal exposure to female sex hormones. *N Engl J Med* 1977; **296:** 67–70.
2. Evans ANW, *et al.* The ingestion by pregnant women of substances toxic to the foetus. *Practitioner* 1980; **224:** 315–19.
3. Mann JR, *et al.* Transplacental carcinogenesis (adrenocortical carcinoma) associated with hydroxyprogesterone hexanoate. *Lancet* 1983; **ii:** 580.

Interactions

As for progestogens in general (see Progesterone, p.1460).

Uses and Administration

Hydroxyprogesterone hexanoate is a progestogen structurally related to progesterone (p.1460) that has been used for habitual abortion and various menstrual disorders. In habitual abortion associated with proven progesterone deficiency, suggested doses have been 250 to 500 mg weekly by intramuscular injection during the first half of pregnancy.

Hydroxyprogesterone enanthate has also been used.

Preparations

BP 1998: Hydroxyprogesterone Injection;
USP 23: Hydroxyprogesterone Caproate Injection.

Proprietary Preparations (details are given in Part 3)
Aust.: Proluton; ***Austral.:*** Proluton; ***Belg.:*** Proluton†; ***Fr.:*** Progesterone-retard Pharlon; ***Ger.:*** Proluton Depot; ***Irl.:*** Primolut Depot†; ***Ital.:*** Lentogest; Proluton Depot; ***Neth.:*** Proluton Depot; ***Norw.:*** Primolut Depot†; ***S.Afr.:*** Primolut Depot; ***Spain:*** Proluton Depot; ***Switz.:*** Proluton Depot; ***UK:*** Proluton Depot; ***USA:*** Duralutin†; Hylutin; Hyprogest†; Prodrox 250†.

Multi-ingredient: ***Aust.:*** Gravibinon; Ostrolut; ***Fr.:*** Gravibinan†; ***Ger.:*** Gravibinon; Primosiston†; Syngynon; ***Ital.:*** Gravibinan; ***Mon.:*** Tocogestan; Trophobolene; ***Switz.:*** Gravibinon†; Primosiston.

Lynoestrenol (9059-y)

Lynoestrenol *(BAN)*.

Lynestrenol *(USAN, rINN)*; Ethinylestrenol; Linestrenol; Lynenol; Lynestrenolum; NSC-37725. 19-Nor-17α-pregn-4-en-20-yn-17β-ol.

$C_{20}H_{28}O$ = 284.4.

CAS — 52-76-6.

Pharmacopoeias. In Eur. (see p.viii).

A white or almost white crystalline powder. Practically **insoluble** in water; soluble in alcohol, in acetone, and in ether. **Protect** from light.

Lynoestrenol is a progestogen (see Progesterone, p.1459) structurally related to norethisterone that is used alone or as the progestogenic component of some oral contraceptives (see p.1426). Typical oral daily doses for contraception are 0.5 mg when used as a progestogen-only preparation, and 1 to 2.5 mg when combined with an oestrogen. When used alone for menstrual disorders, doses of 5 to 10 mg per day are used, often as cyclical regimens.

Preparations

Proprietary Preparations (details are given in Part 3)
Aust.: Orgametril; ***Belg.:*** Exluton; Orgametril; ***Fr.:*** Exluton; Orgametril; ***Ger.:*** Exlutona; Orgametril; ***Neth.:*** Exluton; Orgametril; ***Norw.:*** Exlutona; ***S.Afr.:*** Exluton†; ***Spain:*** Orgametril; ***Swed.:*** Exlutena; Orgametril; ***Switz.:*** Exlutona; Orgametril.

Multi-ingredient: ***Aust.:*** Lyndiol; Ovanon; Restovar; Yermonil; ***Belg.:*** Fysioquens; Lyndiol; Ministat; Ovanon; Ovostat; ***Fr.:*** Ovanon; Physiostat; ***Ger.:*** Anacyclin; Anacyclin 28†; Lyn-ratiopharm; Lyn-ratiopharm-Sequenz; Lyndiol; Nuriphasic; Ovanon; Ovoresta; Ovoresta M; Pregnon L; Yermonil; ***Ital.:*** Franovul†; Lyndiol E†; ***Neth.:*** Fysioquens; Lyndiol†; Mini Pregnon; Ministat; Ovanon; Ovostat; Pregnon†; ***Norw.:*** Lyndiol†; ***S.Afr.:*** Lyndiol†; Ovanon†; Ovostat; Restovar†; ***Spain:*** Lyndiol 2.5†; Neo Lyndiol; Ovoresta Micro†; ***Swed.:*** Lyndiol†; Lyndiolett; Restovar; ***Switz.:*** Normophasic; Ovanon; Ovostat; Yermonil.

Medrogestone (9061-q)

Medrogestone *(BAN, USAN, rINN)*.

AY-62022; Metrogestone; NSC-123018; R-13-615. 6,17α-Dimethylpregna-4,6-diene-3,20-dione.

$C_{23}H_{32}O_2$ = 340.5.

CAS — 977-79-7.

Medrogestone is a progestogen structurally related to progesterone (p.1459) that is used in the treatment of menstrual disorders, and as the progestogen in menopausal hormone replacement therapy (see p.1434). It is usually administered in daily doses of 5 to 10 mg by mouth, generally in a cyclical regimen. It may also be used in the treatment of endometrial hyperplasia or carcinoma, prostatic hyperplasia, and breast disorders including carcinoma when higher doses are employed. It has been used for threatened or habitual abortion, but such use is not recommended unless there is proven progesterone deficiency.

Preparations

Proprietary Preparations (details are given in Part 3)
Aust.: Colpron; ***Belg.:*** Colpro; ***Canad.:*** Colprone; ***Fr.:*** Colprone; ***Ger.:*** Prothil; ***Ital.:*** Colprone; ***Neth.:*** Colpro; ***S.Afr.:*** Colpro; ***Spain:*** Colpro; ***Switz.:*** Colpro.

Multi-ingredient: ***Aust.:*** Premarin compositum; Premarin Plus†; ***Belg.:*** Premplus; ***Ger.:*** Presomen compositum; ***Neth.:*** Premarin Plus; ***S.Afr.:*** Prempak N; ***Switz.:*** Premarin Plus.

Medroxyprogesterone Acetate

(9062-p)

Medroxyprogesterone Acetate *(BANM, rINNM)*.

Medroxyprogesteroni Acetas; Methylacetoxyprogesterone; Metipregnone; NSC-26386. 6α-Methyl-3,20-dioxopregn-4-en-17α-yl acetate; 17α-Hydroxy-6α-methylpregn-4-ene-3,20-dione acetate.

$C_{24}H_{34}O_4$ = 386.5.

CAS — 520-85-4 (medroxyprogesterone); 71-58-9 (medroxyprogesterone acetate).

Pharmacopoeias. In Eur. (see p.viii), Int., and US.

A white, or off-white odourless, crystalline powder. Practically **insoluble** in water; sparingly soluble in alcohol and in methyl alcohol; slightly soluble in ether; freely soluble in chloroform and in dichloromethane; soluble in acetone and in dioxan. **Store** in airtight containers. Protect from light.

Adverse Effects and Precautions

As for progestogens in general (see Progesterone, p.1459). See also under Hormonal Contraceptives, p.1426. Medroxyprogesterone acetate may have glucocorticoid effects when administered long term at high doses.

Carcinogenicity. The risk of various cancers associated with the use of depot medroxyprogesterone acetate as a contraceptive has been evaluated by WHO.[1] Overall, there was no increase in risk of breast cancer, although there is some evidence that current or recent use may be associated with a slight increase in risk (see also p.1427). There was no increased risk of cervical cancer (see also p.1428), and a protective effect against endometrial cancer (see p.1428). In contrast to combined oral contraceptives, there was no evidence of a protective effect against ovarian cancer (p.1428).

1. Anonymous. Depot-medroxyprogesterone acetate (DMPA) and cancer: memorandum from a WHO meeting. *Bull WHO* 1993; **71:** 669–76.

Effects on bone density. Use of medroxyprogesterone acetate as a parenteral progestogen-only contraceptive has been associated with reductions in bone density (see under Effects on the Musculoskeletal System, p.1431). This effect has also been reported after oral administration for menstrual disorders,[1] and is thought to be due to medroxyprogesterone-induced oestrogen deficiency.

1. Cundy T, *et al.* Short-term effects of high dose oral medroxyprogesterone acetate on bone density in premenopausal women. *J Clin Endocrinol Metab* 1996; **81:** 1014–17.

Glucocorticoid effects. There have been reports of Cushing's syndrome induced by medroxyprogesterone acetate in patients receiving long-term therapy with high doses for the treatment of malignant neoplasms.[1-5] Cushingoid symptoms regressed when treatment was stopped. Medroxyprogesterone possesses glucocorticoid activity and there is a risk of adrenal insufficiency during periods of stress or after sudden withdrawal of treatment. Some[4] consider that patients should be monitored for glucose intolerance and adrenal insufficiency during treatment.

1. Siminoski K, *et al.* The Cushing syndrome induced by medroxyprogesterone acetate. *Ann Intern Med* 1989; **111:** 758–60.
2. Donckier JE, *et al.* Cushing syndrome and medroxyprogesterone acetate. *Lancet* 1990; **335:** 1094.
3. Grenfell A, *et al.* Cushing's syndrome and medroxyprogesterone acetate. *Lancet* 1990; **336:** 256.
4. Merrin PK, Alexander WD. Cushing's syndrome induced by medroxyprogesterone. *Br Med J* 1990; **301:** 345.
5. Shotliff K, Nussey SS. Medroxyprogesterone acetate induced Cushing's syndrome. *Br J Clin Pharmacol* 1997; **44:** 304.

Interactions

As for progestogens in general (see Progesterone, p.1460). It should be noted that aminoglutethimide markedly reduces the plasma concentrations of medroxyprogesterone so that an increase in medroxyprogesterone dosage is likely to be required.

Pharmacokinetics

Medroxyprogesterone is absorbed from the gastro-intestinal tract. In the blood, it is highly protein bound, principally to albumin. It is metabolised in the liver and excreted mainly as glucuronide conjugates in the faeces. It has a half-life of 24 to 30 hours after oral administration; the half-life may be as long as 50 days after intramuscular injection. Medroxyprogesterone is reported to be distributed into breast milk.

Uses and Administration

Medroxyprogesterone acetate is a progestogen structurally related to progesterone, with actions and uses similar to those of the progestogens in general (see Progesterone, p.1460). It is administered by mouth or, for prolonged action, by intramuscular injection as an aqueous suspension.

It is used for the treatment of **menorrhagia**, (p.1461) and **secondary amenorrhoea** in doses of 2.5 to 10 mg daily by mouth for 5 to 10 days starting on the assumed or calculated 16th to 21st day of the cycle, although some sources suggest that treatment may begin on any day in secondary amenorrhoea.

In the treatment of mild to moderate **endometriosis** (p.1442) usual doses are 10 mg three times daily by mouth, or 50 mg weekly or 100 mg every 2 weeks by intramuscular injection. In the UK it is recommended that treatment continue for 90 consecutive days; US sources recommend treatment for at least 6 months.

Medroxyprogesterone acetate is also given by intramuscular injection as a **progestogen-only contraceptive** at a dose of 150 mg every 12 weeks (see under Hormonal Contraceptives, p.1433).

When used as the progestogen component of **menopausal hormone replacement therapy** (see p.1437), medroxyprogesterone acetate is administered orally in a variety of regimens including 2.5 or 5 mg daily continuously, 5 or 10 mg daily for 12 to 14 days of a 28-day cycle, and 20 mg daily for 14 days of a 91-day cycle.

Medroxyprogesterone acetate may also be used in the palliative treatment of some hormone-dependent malignant neoplasms. In **breast carcinoma** (see below) recommended doses have ranged from 0.4 to 1.5 g daily by mouth and from 0.5 g twice weekly to 1 g daily by intramuscular injection. In **endometrial** and **renal carcinoma** (p.487 and p.489, respectively) recommended doses have ranged from 100 to 500 mg daily by mouth and from 0.4 to 1 g weekly by intramuscular injection. Alternative regimens using intramuscular injections have started with twice-weekly or alternate-day dosing before reducing to the weekly dosage interval or have started treatment with weekly doses and reduced to a maintenance schedule of as little as 400 mg monthly. In **prostatic carcinoma** (p.491) recommended doses have been 100 to 500 mg daily by mouth and 0.5 g weekly or twice weekly by intramuscular injection.

Cachexia. Medroxyprogesterone may improve appetite and prevent loss of body-weight in cachexia associated with severe chronic disorders.[1]

1. Simons JPFHA, *et al.* Effects of medroxyprogesterone acetate on appetite, weight, and quality of life in advanced-stage non-hormone-sensitive cancer: a placebo-controlled multicenter study. *J Clin Oncol* 1996; **14:** 1077–84.

Epilepsy. Preliminary findings[1] suggested that medroxyprogesterone acetate might be of value in the management of catamenial epilepsy (p.335). In a more recent review[2] it was suggested that hormonal manipulation with drugs such as medroxyprogesterone be reserved for highly selected groups under close supervision.

1. Mattson RH, *et al.* Treatment of seizures with medroxyprogesterone acetate: preliminary report. *Neurology* 1984; **34:** 1255–8.
2. Herkes GK. Drug treatment of catamenial epilepsy. *CNS Drugs* 1995; **3:** 260–6.

Male hypersexuality. The anti-androgenic action of medroxyprogesterone has been used for suppression of libido in the control of men with deviant or disinhibited sexual behaviour[1-3] (see p.636).

1. Kiersch TA. Treatment of sex offenders with Depo-Provera. *Bull Am Acad Psychiatry Law* 1990; **18:** 179–87.
2. Weiner MF, *et al.* Intramuscular medroxyprogesterone acetate for sexual aggression in elderly men. *Lancet* 1992; **339:** 1121–2.
3. Kravitz HM, *et al.* Medroxyprogesterone treatment for paraphiliacs. *Bull Am Acad Psychiatry Law* 1995; **23:** 19–33.

Malignant neoplasms. BREAST. Progestogens are used as second or third choice drugs in the hormonal therapy of breast cancer (p.485). Some references to the use of medroxyprogesterone acetate in advanced breast cancer are cited below.[1-6] Comparative studies have shown that patients respond equally well to medroxyprogesterone and either mepitiostane,[4] aminoglutethimide,[5] or oophorectomy.[6]

1. Guarnieri A, *et al.* Oral route administration of medroxyprogesterone acetate (MAP) at high doses in the treatment of advanced breast cancer: clinical results. *Chemioterapia* 1984; **3:** 320–3.
2. Pannuti F, *et al.* A possible new approach to the treatment of metastatic breast cancer: massive doses of medroxyprogesterone acetate. *Cancer Treat Rep* 1978; **62:** 499–504.
3. Hedley D, *et al.* Advanced breast cancer: response to high dose oral medroxyprogesterone acetate. *Aust N Z J Med* 1984; **14:** 251–4.
4. Izuo M, *et al.* A phase III trial of oral high-dose medroxyprogesterone acetate (MPA) versus mepitiostane in advanced postmenopausal breast cancer. *Cancer* 1985; **56:** 2576–9.
5. Canney PA, *et al.* Randomized trial comparing aminoglutethimide with high-dose medroxyprogesterone acetate in therapy for advanced breast carcinoma. *J Natl Cancer Inst* 1988; **80:** 1147–51.
6. Martoni A, *et al.* High-dose medroxyprogesterone acetate versus oophorectomy as first-line therapy of advanced breast cancer in premenopausal patients. *Oncology* 1991; **48:** 1–6.

ENDOMETRIUM. Progestogens are well established in the treatment of endometrial carcinoma (p.487). Medroxyprogesterone acetate was also effective in a rare case of low-grade endometrial stromal sarcoma.[1]

1. Rand RJ, Lowe JW. Low-grade endometrial stromal sarcoma treated with a progestogen. *Br J Hosp Med* 1990; **43:** 154–6.

Porphyria. Progestogens are usually considered contra-indicated in porphyria. However, for a reference to the use of medroxyprogesterone acetate with buserelin acetate in the prevention of premenstrual exacerbations of porphyria in 2 women, see p.1243.

Respiratory disorders. In a review of the use of medroxyprogesterone acetate in obstructive sleep apnoea[1] it was concluded that it had no role in the treatment of normocapnic patients and that it was not a first-line treatment in those with hypercapnia.

Medroxyprogesterone was not effective in the treatment of pulmonary lymphangioleiomyomatosis[2] although patients with chylous effusions or chylous ascites might respond.

Medroxyprogesterone acetate was reported to be effective in treating congenital central hypoventilation syndrome in 2 children.[3]

1. Millman RP. Medroxyprogesterone and obstructive sleep apnea. *Chest* 1989; **96:** 225–6.
2. Taylor JR, *et al.* Lymphangioleiomyomatosis: clinical course in 32 patients. *N Engl J Med* 1990; **323:** 1254–60.
3. Milerad J, *et al.* Alveolar hypoventilation treated with medroxyprogesterone. *Arch Dis Child* 1985; **60:** 150–5.

Sickle-cell disease. Intramuscular medroxyprogesterone reduced the frequency of painful crises in patients with homozygous sickle-cell disease (p.703),[1] and is considered a suitable contraceptive in women with the condition[2,3] in whom combined oral contraceptives should probably be avoided (see also p.1432).

1. de Ceulaer K, *et al.* Medroxyprogesterone acetate and homozygous sickle-cell disease. *Lancet* 1982; **ii:** 229–31.
2. Guillebaud J. Sickle cell disease and contraception. *Br Med J* 1993; **307:** 506–7.
3. Kirkman REJ, Elstein M. Management of sickle cell disease: contraception with medroxyprogesterone may be beneficial. *Br Med J* 1998; **316:** 935.

Preparations

USP 23: Medroxyprogesterone Acetate Injectable Suspension; Medroxyprogesterone Acetate Tablets.

Proprietary Preparations (details are given in Part 3)

Aust.: Depo-Provera; Depocon; Farlutal; Prodafem; Provera; ***Austral.:*** Depo-Provera; Depo-Ralovera; Farlutal†; Provera; Ralovera; ***Belg.:*** Depo-Provera; Farlutal; Provera; ***Canad.:*** Depo-Provera; Provera; ***Fr.:*** Depo-Prodasone; Depo-Provera; Farlutal; Gestoral; Prodasone; ***Ger.:*** Clinofem; Clinovir; Depo-Clinovir; Farlutal; G-Farlutal; MPA; ***Irl.:*** Depo-Provera; Provera; ***Ital.:*** Depo-Provera; Farlutal; Lutoral; Provera; ***Neth.:*** Depo-Provera; Farlutal; Provera; ***Norw.:*** Depo-Provera; Farlutal; Perlutex; Provera; ***S.Afr.:*** Depo-Provera; Farlutal; Petogen; Provera; ***Spain:*** Depo-Progevera; Farlutal; Progevera; Progevera 250; ***Swed.:*** Cykrina; Depo-Provera; Farlutal; Gestapuran; Provera; ***Switz.:*** Depo-Provera; Farlutal; Prodafem; Provera; ***UK:*** Depo-Provera; Farlutal; Provera; ***USA:*** Amen; Curretab; Cycrin; Depo-Provera; Provera.

Multi-ingredient: ***Aust.:*** Cyclo-Premarin-MPA; Cyclo-Premella; Dilena†; Filena; Perennia; Premarin-MPA; Premella; Sequennia; Tri-Filena; ***Austral.:*** Divina; Estrapak; Menoprem; Provelle; ***Belg.:*** Diviva; ***Fr.:*** Divina; Precyclan; ***Ger.:*** Osmil; Procyclo; Sisare; ***Irl.:*** Premique Cycle; Tridestra; ***Ital.:*** Filena; Premelle S; ***Neth.:*** Divina; Premelle; Premelle Cycle; ***S.Afr.:*** Divina; Trivina; ***Spain:*** Medricol; Medrivas; Medrivas Antib; ***Swed.:*** Divina; Premelle; Prempac Sekvens; Trivina; ***Switz.:*** Cyclo-Premella; Premella; Triaval; ***UK:*** Improvera; Premique Cycle; Tridestra; ***USA:*** Premphase; Prempro.

Megestrol Acetate (9063-s)

Megestrol Acetate *(BANM, USAN, pINNM).*

BDH-1298; Compound 5071; NSC-71423; SC-10363. 6-Methyl-3,20-dioxopregna-4,6-dien-17α-yl acetate; 17α-Hydroxy-6-methylpregna-4,6-diene-3,20-dione acetate.

$C_{24}H_{32}O_4$ = 384.5.

CAS — 3562-63-8 (megestrol); 595-33-5 (megestrol acetate).

Pharmacopoeias. In *Br.* and *US.*

An odourless or almost odourless, white to creamy-white, crystalline powder. Practically **insoluble** in water; sparingly soluble in alcohol; very soluble in chloroform; soluble in acetone; slightly soluble in ether and in fixed oils. **Protect** from light.

Adverse Effects and Precautions

As for progestogens in general (see Progesterone, p.1459). The weight gain that may be observed with megestrol acetate appears to be associated with an increased appetite and food intake rather than with fluid retention.

Severe pain of the hands reminiscent of carpal tunnel syndrome occurred in 4 women while taking megestrol acetate and melphalan;[1] megestrol appeared to be responsible.

1. DiSaia PJ, Morrow CP. Unusual side effect of megestrol acetate. *Am J Obstet Gynecol* 1977; **129:** 460–1.

Effects on carbohydrate metabolism. Megestrol therapy has been associated with hyperglycaemia[1,2] or diabetes mellitus[3] in AIDS patients being treated for cachexia. It has been suggested that megestrol produces peripheral insulin resistance due to a glucocorticoid action.[4]

1. Panwalker AP. Hyperglycemia induced by megestrol acetate. *Ann Intern Med* 1992; **116:** 878.
2. Bornemann M, Johnson AC. Endocrine effects of HIV infection. *N Engl J Med* 1993; **328:** 890.
3. Henry K, *et al.* Diabetes mellitus induced by megestrol acetate in a patient with AIDS and cachexia. *Ann Intern Med* 1992; **116:** 53–4.
4. Leinung MC, *et al.* Induction of adrenal suppression by megestrol acetate in patients with AIDS. *Ann Intern Med* 1995; **122:** 843–5.

Effects on the respiratory system. Two cases of hyperpnoea in patients receiving megestrol acetate 80 mg three times daily.[1]

1. Fessel WJ. Megestrol acetate and hyperpnea. *Ann Intern Med* 1989; **110:** 1034–5.

Glucocorticoid effects. Megestrol appears to have glucocorticoid-like properties which can result in adrenocortical insufficiency severe enough to require replacement therapy with hydrocortisone.[1-4]

1. Leinung MC, *et al.* Induction of adrenal suppression by megestrol acetate in patients with AIDS. *Ann Intern Med* 1995; **122:** 843–5.
2. Maurer M. Megestrol for AIDS-related anorexia. *Ann Intern Med* 1995; **122:** 880.
3. Stoffer SS, Krakauer JC. Induction of adrenal suppression by megestrol acetate. *Ann Intern Med* 1996; **124:** 613–14.
4. Mann M, *et al.* Glucocorticoidlike activity of megestrol: a summary of Food and Drug Administration experience and a review of the literature. *Arch Intern Med* 1997; **157:** 1651–6.

Interactions

As for progestogens in general (see Progesterone, p.1460).

Pharmacokinetics

Absorption of megestrol acetate from the gastro-intestinal tract is variable following oral administration; peak drug concentrations in plasma occur 1 to 3 hours after a dose by mouth. Megestrol acetate is highly protein bound in plasma. It undergoes hepatic metabolism, with 57 to 78% of a dose being excreted in the urine and 8 to 30% in the faeces.

Uses and Administration

Megestrol acetate is a progestogen structurally related to progesterone (p.1460) that is used for the palliative treatment of various cancers.

It is given by mouth in endometrial carcinoma in doses of 40 to 320 mg daily in divided doses, and in doses of 40 mg four times daily or 160 mg once daily in breast cancer.

Megestrol acetate is used in the treatment of anorexia and cachexia in patients with cancer or AIDS. The usual dose is 800 mg daily, as oral suspension, for one month, followed by a maintenance dose of 400 to 800 mg daily.

Anorexia and cachexia. Double-blind, placebo-controlled trials have confirmed the efficacy of high dose megestrol (800 mg per day) in patients with cancer-related cachexia[1] and HIV-related cachexia (p.601).[2,3] Megestrol was also associated with weight gain in children with HIV infection.[4]

1. Loprinzi CL, *et al.* Controlled trial of megestrol acetate for the treatment of cancer anorexia and cachexia. *J Natl Cancer Inst* 1990; **82:** 1127–32.
2. Von Roenn JH, *et al.* Megestrol acetate in patients with AIDS-related cachexia. *Ann Intern Med* 1994; **121:** 393–9.
3. Oster MH, *et al.* Megestrol acetate in patients with AIDS and cachexia. *Ann Intern Med* 1994; **121:** 400–8.
4. Clarick RH, *et al.* Megestrol acetate treatment of growth failure in children infected with human immunodeficiency virus. *Pediatrics* 1997; **99:** 354–7.

Hot flushes. Megestrol has been used in female patients with breast cancer who were experiencing hot flushes (to avoid the potentially tumour-stimulating effects of an oestrogen—see p.1437), as well as in men with hot flushes after orchidectomy or anti-androgen therapy for prostate cancer.[1] Therapy, which involved low doses of 20 mg twice daily, was associated with a decrease in frequency of flushes of 50% or more in about three-quarters of all patients.

1. Loprinzi CL, *et al.* Megestrol acetate for the prevention of hot flashes. *N Engl J Med* 1994; **331:** 347–52.

Malignant neoplasms. Like some other progestogens megestrol acetate is used in endometrial cancer (p.487), and it has been reported to have similar efficacy to anastrozole[1] and tamoxifen[2] in postmenopausal women with advanced breast cancer (p.485).

1. Buzdar A, *et al.* Anastrozole, a potent and selective aromatase inhibitor, versus megestrol acetate in postmenopausal women with advanced breast cancer: results of overview analysis of two phase III trials. *J Clin Oncol* 1996; **14:** 2000–11.
2. Stuart NSA, *et al.* A randomised phase III cross-over study of tamoxifen versus megestrol acetate in advanced and recurrent breast cancer. *Eur J Cancer* 1996; **32A:** 1888–92.

Preparations

BP 1998: Megestrol Tablets;
USP 23: Megestrol Acetate Tablets.

Proprietary Preparations (details are given in Part 3)
Aust.: Megace; Nia; ***Austral.:*** Megostat; ***Belg.:*** Niagestine†; ***Canad.:*** Megace; ***Fr.:*** Megace; ***Ger.:*** Megestat; Niagestin†; ***Irl.:*** Megace; ***Ital.:*** Megace; Megestil; ***Neth.:*** Megace; ***Norw.:*** Megace; ***Spain:*** Borea; Maygace; Megefren; Megostat; ***Swed.:*** Megace; Niagestin†; ***Switz.:*** Megestat; Niagestine†; ***UK:*** Megace; ***USA:*** Megace.

Mepitiostane (12930-t)

Mepitiostane *(rINN).*

S-10364. 17β-(1-Methoxycyclopentyloxy)-2α,3α-epithio-5α-androstane; Cyclopentanone 2α,3α-epithio-5α-androstan-17β-yl methyl acetal.

$C_{25}H_{40}O_2S$ = 404.6.

CAS — 21362-69-6.

Pharmacopoeias. In *Jpn.*

Mepitiostane has androgenic and anabolic properties (see Testosterone, p.1464) and is used by mouth in treating neoplasms of the breast and anaemia associated with renal failure.

Preparations

Proprietary Preparations (details are given in Part 3)
Jpn: Thioderon.

Mesterolone (9064-w)

Mesterolone *(BAN, USAN, rINN).*

NSC-75054; SH-723. 17β-Hydroxy-1α-methyl-5α-androstan-3-one.

$C_{20}H_{32}O_2$ = 304.5.

CAS — 1424-00-6.

Adverse Effects and Precautions

As for androgens in general (see Testosterone, p.1464).

Mesterolone is reported not to inhibit gonadotrophin secretion or spermatogenesis.

Uses and Administration

Mesterolone has androgenic properties (see Testosterone, p.1465) but is reported to have less inhibitory effect on intrinsic testicular function than testosterone.

Mesterolone is given by mouth in the treatment of male hypogonadism (p.1239) in initial doses of 75 to 100 mg daily followed by doses of 50 to 75 mg daily for maintenance. Doses of 100 mg daily have been used in male infertility (p.1239) due to oligospermia.

Preparations

Proprietary Preparations (details are given in Part 3)
Aust.: Proviron; ***Austral.:*** Proviron; ***Belg.:*** Proviron; ***Fr.:*** Proviron; ***Ger.:*** Proviron; Vistimon; ***Ital.:*** Proviron; ***Neth.:*** Proviron; ***Norw.:*** Mestoranum; ***S.Afr.:*** Proviron; ***Spain:*** Proviron; ***Swed.:*** Mestoranum; ***Switz.:*** Proviron; ***UK:*** Proviron.

Multi-ingredient: ***Ger.:*** Pluriviron†.

Mestranol (9065-e)

Mestranol *(BAN, USAN, rINN).*

Compound 33355; EE3ME; EE_3ME; Ethinyloestradiol-3-methyl Ether; Mestranolum. 3-Methoxy-19-nor-17α-pregna-1,3,5(10)-trien-20-yn-17β-ol.

$C_{21}H_{26}O_2$ = 310.4.

CAS — 72-33-3.

Pharmacopoeias. In *Eur.* (see p.viii), *Jpn, Pol.,* and *US.*

A white to creamy-white, odourless, crystalline powder. Practically **insoluble** in water; sparingly soluble in alcohol; soluble in dioxan and in ether; freely soluble in chloroform; slightly soluble in methyl alcohol. **Protect** from light.

Adverse Effects and Precautions

As for oestrogens in general (see Oestradiol, p.1455). See also under Hormonal Contraceptives, p.1426.

Interactions

See under Hormonal Contraceptives, p.1432.

Pharmacokinetics

Mestranol is readily absorbed from the gastro-intestinal tract. It is metabolised in the liver to ethinyloestradiol and its glucuronide. Excretion is via the kidneys and bile; metabolites undergo enterohepatic recycling. Compared with many other oestrogens, its metabolism is slow. The biological half-life is about 50 hours.

Uses and Administration

Mestranol is a synthetic oestrogen with actions similar to those of oestradiol (see p.1456). It is a component of high-strength combined oral contraceptive preparations (dose 50 μg daily—see under Hormonal Contraceptives p.1433). The progestogen component is often norethisterone. Mestranol is also the oestrogen component of some preparation for menopausal hormone replacement therapy (see p.1434), although natural oestrogens are often preferred. Administration is usually in a sequential regimen with doses ranging from 12.5 to 50 μg daily, in combination with a cyclical progestogen.

Preparations

USP 23: Ethynodiol Diacetate and Mestranol Tablets; Norethindrone and Mestranol Tablets.

Proprietary Preparations (details are given in Part 3)
Multi-ingredient: ***Aust.:*** Ortho-Novum; ***Austral.:*** Norinyl-1; Ortho-Novum 1/50†; ***Belg.:*** Ortho-Novum 1/50; Ortho-Novum SQ†; ***Canad.:*** Norinyl 1/50; Ortho-Novum 0.5 mg†; Ortho-Novum 1/50; Ortho-Novum 1/80†; Ortho-Novum 2 mg†; ***Ger.:*** Eunomin†; Gestamestrol N; Ortho-Novum 1/50; Ovosiston; ***Irl.:*** Menophase; Norinyl-1; Ortho-Novin; ***Ital.:*** Franovul†; Luteolas†; Ovaras†; ***Neth.:*** Ortho-Novum 1/50†; ***S.Afr.:*** Norinyl-1/28; ***Spain:*** Lyndiol 2.5†; ***Switz.:*** Ortho-Novum 1/50; ***UK:*** Menophase; Norinyl-1; Ortho-Novin 1/50†; ***USA:*** Enovid†; Genora 1/50; Nelova 1/50M; Norethin 1/50M; Norinyl 1 + 50; Norinyl 2 mg†; Ortho-Novum 1/50.

Methandienone (9067-y)

Methandienone *(BAN).*

Metandienone *(pINN)*; Methandrostenolone; NSC-42722. 17β-Hydroxy-17α-methylandrosta-1,4-dien-3-one.

$C_{20}H_{28}O_2$ = 300.4.

CAS — 72-63-9.

Pharmacopoeias. In *Pol.*

Adverse Effects and Precautions

As for androgens and anabolic steroids in general (see Testosterone, p.1464).

As with other 17α-alkylated compounds, methandienone is associated with hepatotoxicity and hepatic function should be monitored during therapy. It should probably be avoided in patients with hepatic impairment, and certainly if this is severe.

Effects on the liver. References to carcinoma of the liver in one patient[1] given methandienone and benign liver-cell adenoma in another.[2]

1. Johnson FL, *et al.* Association of androgenic-anabolic steroid therapy with development of hepatocellular carcinoma. *Lancet* 1972; **ii:** 1273–6.
2. Hernandez-Nieto L, *et al.* Benign liver-cell adenoma associated with long-term administration of an androgenic-anabolic steroid (methandienone). *Cancer* 1977; **40:** 1761–4.

Uses and Administration

Methandienone has anabolic and some androgenic properties (see Testosterone, p.1465). It has little progestogenic activity. Methandienone has been given by mouth as an anabolic drug.

Preparations

Proprietary Preparations (details are given in Part 3)
Multi-ingredient: ***Canad.:*** Metaboline†.

Methenolone Acetate (9069-z)

Methenolone Acetate *(BANM, USAN).*

Metenolone Acetate *(rINNM)*; NSC-74226; SH-567; SQ-16496. 17β-Hydroxy-1-methyl-5α-androst-1-en-3-one acetate.

$C_{22}H_{32}O_3$ = 344.5.

CAS — 153-00-4 (methenolone); 434-05-9 (methenolone acetate).

Pharmacopoeias. In *Jpn.*

Methenolone Enanthate (9070-p)

Methenolone Enanthate *(BANM, USAN).*

Metenolone Enantate *(rINNM)*; Metenolone Enanthate; Methenolone Oenanthate; NSC-64967; SH-601; SQ-16374. 17β-Hydroxy-1-methyl-5α-androst-1-en-3-one heptanoate.

$C_{27}H_{42}O_3$ = 414.6.

CAS — 303-42-4.

Pharmacopoeias. In *Jpn.*

Adverse Effects and Precautions

As for androgens and anabolic steroids in general (see Testosterone, p.1464).

Uses and Administration

Methenolone is an anabolic steroid (see Testosterone, p.1465) that has been used in treating aplastic anaemia, breast cancer, and postmenopausal osteoporosis. It has been given by mouth as the acetate in usual doses of 10 to 20 mg daily (although higher doses have been given), and intramuscularly as the enanthate in doses of 100 mg every 2 to 4 weeks.

Preparations

Proprietary Preparations (details are given in Part 3)
Aust.: Primobolan; ***Austral.:*** Primobolan; ***Belg.:*** Primobolan†; ***Ger.:*** Primobolan; ***Ital.:*** Primobolan Depot; ***Neth.:*** Primobolan S; ***Norw.:*** Primobolan; ***S.Afr.:*** Primobolan; ***Spain:*** Primobolan Depot; ***Switz.:*** Primobolan Depot†.

Multi-ingredient: ***Ger.:*** AntiFocal N; NeyChondrin "N" (Revitorgan-Dilutionen "N" Nr. 68); NeyGeront "N" (Revitorgan-Dilutionen "N" Nr. 64); NeyPulpin "N" (Revitorgan-Dilutionen "N" Nr. 10); NeyTumorin "N" (Revitorgan-Dilutionen Nr. 66).

Methyltestosterone (9071-s)

Methyltestosterone *(BAN, rINN).*

Methyltestosteronum; NSC-9701. 17β-Hydroxy-17α-methylandrost-4-en-3-one.

$C_{20}H_{30}O_2$ = 302.5.

CAS — 58-18-4.

Pharmacopoeias. In *Chin., Eur.* (see p.viii), *Int., Jpn, Pol.,* and *US.*

White or slightly yellowish-white, odourless, slightly hygroscopic, crystals or crystalline powder. Practically **insoluble** in water; soluble to freely soluble in alcohol; soluble in methyl alcohol; sparingly soluble in vegetable oils; Ph. Eur. states that it is slightly soluble in ether, while the USP states soluble in ether. **Protect** from light.

Adverse Effects and Precautions

As for androgens and anabolic steroids in general (see Testosterone, p.1464).

As with other 17α-alkylated compounds, methyltestosterone can produce a cholestatic hepatitis with jaundice, and has caused peliosis hepatis and hepatic neoplasms (see below). Methyltestosterone should be used with caution in patients with liver impairment, and is probably best avoided if this is severe. Liver function should be monitored during therapy.

Effects on the liver. Reports of peliosis hepatis[1] and liver damage[2-4] associated with methyltestosterone.

See also under Malignant Neoplasms, below.

1. Bagheri SA, *et al.* Peliosis hepatis associated with androgenic-anabolic steroid therapy: a severe form of hepatic injury. *Ann Intern Med* 1974; **81:** 610–18.
2. Westaby D, *et al.* Liver damage from long-term methyltestosterone. *Lancet* 1977; **ii:** 261–3.
3. Lowdell CP, Murray-Lyon IM. Reversal of liver damage due to long term methyltestosterone and safety of non-17 α-alkylated androgens. *Br Med J* 1985; **291:** 637.
4. Borhan-Manesh F, Farnum JB. Methyltestosterone-induced cholestasis: the importance of disproportionately low serum alkaline phosphatase level. *Arch Intern Med* 1989; **124:** 2127–9.

MALIGNANT NEOPLASMS. Reports of hepatocellular carcinoma[1-6] and hepatic adenoma[5,7] associated with methyltestosterone.

1. Johnson FL, *et al.* Association of androgenic-anabolic steroid therapy with development of hepatocellular carcinoma. *Lancet* 1972; **ii:** 1273–6.
2. Henderson JT, *et al.* Androgenic-anabolic steroid therapy and hepatocellular carcinoma. *Lancet* 1973; **i:** 934.
3. Farrell GC, *et al.* Androgen-induced hepatoma. *Lancet* 1975; **i:** 430–2.
4. Goodman MA, Laden AMJ. Hepatocellular carcinoma in association with androgen therapy. *Med J Aust* 1977; **1:** 220–1.
5. Boyd PR, Mark GJ. Multiple hepatic adenomas and a hepatocellular carcinoma in a man on oral methyl testosterone for eleven years. *Cancer* 1977; **40:** 1765–70.
6. Gleeson D, *et al.* Androgen associated hepatocellular carcinoma with an aggressive course. *Gut* 1991; **32:** 1084–6.
7. Coombes GB, *et al.* An androgen-associated hepatic adenoma in a trans-sexual. *Br J Surg* 1978; **65:** 869–70.

Pregnancy. For reference to virilisation of a female fetus whose mother received methyltestosterone during pregnancy, see p.1465.

Interactions

As for androgens and anabolic steroids in general (see Testosterone, p.1465).

Pharmacokinetics

Methyltestosterone is absorbed from the gastro-intestinal tract and from the oral mucosa. It undergoes less extensive first-pass hepatic metabolism than testosterone following oral administration, and has a longer half-life.

Uses and Administration

As for androgens and anabolic steroids in general (see Testosterone, p.1465).

Methyltestosterone is effective when given by mouth; its effect is increased about twofold when given buccally, as this avoids first-pass hepatic metabolism.

Suggested doses of methyltestosterone for androgen replacement therapy in male hypogonadism (p.1239) have been 10 to 50 mg daily by mouth or 5 to 25 mg daily buccally. Doses of 50 to 200 mg daily by mouth or 25 to 100 mg daily buccally have been given for metastatic breast carcinoma (p.485) in postmenopausal women.

Preparations

USP 23: Methyltestosterone Capsules; Methyltestosterone Tablets.

Proprietary Preparations (details are given in Part 3)
Canad.: Metandren; ***Ital.:*** Testovis; ***USA:*** Android; Oreton Methyl; Testred; Virilon.

Multi-ingredient: ***Aust.:*** Pasuma-Dragees; ***S.Afr.:*** Mixogen†; Pasuma†; ***UK:*** Prowess; ***USA:*** Estratest; Menogen; Premarin with Methyltestosterone; Tylosterone†.

Mifepristone (19516-z)

Mifepristone *(BAN, rINN)*.

RU-486; RU-38486. 11β-(4-Dimethylaminophenyl)-17β-hydroxy-17α-prop-1-ynylestra-4,9-dien-3-one.

$C_{29}H_{35}NO_2$ = 429.6.

CAS — 84371-65-3.

Adverse Effects

In a small proportion of patients given mifepristone uterine bleeding may be severe enough to warrant transfusion and curettage. Few patients have experienced pain after mifepristone administration although uterine pain is often experienced after subsequent prostaglandin administration. Malaise, faintness, nausea, vomiting, and skin rashes have been reported. Uterine and urinary tract infections have occurred in a small number of patients.

Effects on the cardiovascular system. A 31-year-old woman died from cardiovascular shock during an abortion induced by mifepristone followed by sulprostone.[1] She was a heavy cigarette smoker.

1. Anonymous. A death associated with mifepristone/sulprostone. *Lancet* 1991; **337:** 969–70.

Precautions

Mifepristone should not be given to women with a suspected ectopic pregnancy, to those with chronic adrenal failure or haemorrhagic disorders, or to those receiving anticoagulants or long-term corticosteroid therapy. Use in those with renal or hepatic impairment is also not recommended. Women over 35 years of age who are smokers should not receive mifepristone in combination with a prostaglandin for pregnancy termination. Mifepristone should be given with care to patients with asthma or chronic obstructive airways diseases, and to patients with cardiovascular disease or associated risk factors. Patients with prosthetic heart valves or those with a history of infective endocarditis should be given chemoprophylaxis when undergoing pregnancy termination. As with other means of terminating pregnancy, rhesus-negative women who have not been rhesus immunised will require protection with anti-D immunoglobulin.

Pregnancy. Studies in *rabbits*, but not *rats* or *mice*, suggest mifepristone causes fetal malformation. There have been reports of normal fetal development following the use of mifepristone alone in mothers who subsequently decided to continue their pregnancy.[1,2] However, in one woman, use of mifepristone was possibly related to malformations of the fetus including sirenomelia.[2]

1. Lim BH. *et al.* Normal development after exposure to mifepristone in early pregnancy. *Lancet* 1990; **336:** 257–8.
2. Pons J-C, *et al.* Development after exposure to mifepristone in early pregnancy. *Lancet* 1991; **338:** 763.

Interactions

Aspirin and NSAIDs should be avoided until complete termination of pregnancy has been confirmed, because of a theoretical risk that these prostaglandin synthetase inhibitors may alter the efficacy of mifepristone.

Pharmacokinetics

Following administration by mouth peak plasma concentrations of mifepristone are reported to be obtained after 1.3 hours; bioavailability is about 70%. Elimination is biphasic; an initial slow phase is followed by a more rapid terminal phase, with an elimination half-life of about 18 hours. Mifepristone undergoes hepatic metabolism, and metabolites are excreted in the bile and eliminated in the faeces. Only a small fraction is detected in the urine. Mifepristone is about 98% bound to plasma proteins, predominantly α_1-acid glycoprotein.

Uses and Administration

Mifepristone is a steroid derived from norethisterone that has potent antiprogestogenic activity, and is used for the medical termination of pregnancy (see p.1412). When used for the termination of pregnancies of up to 63 days' duration, the recommended procedure is to give a single oral dose of 600 mg of mifepristone followed by the prostaglandin gemeprost 1 mg vaginally 36 to 48 hours later, unless abortion has already been completed. However, lower doses of mifepristone have been employed effectively in some studies as have different prostaglandins (see also below). For the termination of pregnancy between 13 and 20 weeks' gestation, a single oral dose of mifepristone 600 mg may be given 36 to 48 hours prior to scheduled prostaglandin termination of pregnancy, thus shortening the duration of the procedure and reducing the dose of prostaglandin required. Mifepristone may also be used for softening and dilatation of the cervix prior to surgical termination of pregnancy; a single 600-mg dose is given 36 to 48 hours before the procedure.

Mifepristone has been used as a postcoital contraceptive. It has also been investigated for use in endometriosis and leiomyomas, and for progestogen-dependent neoplasms such as meningiomas. Mifepristone also has anti-glucocorticoid activity and has been used in the treatment of Cushing's syndrome.

General references.

1. Baulieu E-E. RU-486 as an antiprogesterone steroid: from receptor to contragestion and beyond. *JAMA* 1989; **262:** 1808–14.
2. Brogden RN, *et al.* Mifepristone: a review of its pharmacodynamic and pharmacokinetic properties, and therapeutic potential. *Drugs* 1993; **45:** 384–409.
3. Glasier A. Mifepristone. *Prescribers' J* 1993; **33:** 156–60.
4. Spitz IM, Bardin CW. Mifepristone (RU 486)—a modulator of progestin and glucocorticoid action. *N Engl J Med* 1993; **329:** 404–12.
5. Heikinheimo O. Clinical pharmacokinetics of mifepristone. *Clin Pharmacokinet* 1997; **33:** 7–17.

Administration. Although a study involving 1151 women found that mifepristone 200 mg was as effective as the currently recommended dose of 600 mg when combined with gemeprost by the vaginal route for termination of early pregnancy,[1] the manufacturers commented that there was no evidence that a lower dose was better tolerated, and that early studies using mifepristone without a prostaglandin had indicated a significantly higher risk of ongoing pregnancy with lower doses.[2] A similar study found mifepristone 200 mg to be as effective as 600 mg when combined with misoprostol for second trimester termination.[3]

1. WHO Task Force on Post-ovulatory Methods of Fertility Regulation. Termination of pregnancy with reduced doses of mifepristone. *Br Med J* 1993; **307:** 532–7.
2. Ulmann A, Barnard J. Termination of pregnancy with mifepristone. *Br Med J* 1993; **307:** 684.
3. Webster D, *et al.* A comparison of 600 and 200 mg mifepristone prior to second trimester abortion with the prostaglandin misoprostol. *Br J Obstet Gynaecol* 1996; **103:** 706–9.

Contraception. Mifepristone is an effective emergency contraceptive (p.1434) when administered within 72 hours postcoitally (pre-implantation),[1,2] and has also been used 2 to 3 weeks postcoitally (post-implantation).[3] The development of a mifepristone-based standard contraceptive (p.1434) has been less successful,[4,5] as yet, because mifepristone alters the length of the menstrual cycle.[3,5]

1. Glasier A, *et al.* Mifepristone (RU 486) compared with high-dose estrogen and progestogen for emergency postcoital contraception. *N Engl J Med* 1992; **327:** 1041–4.
2. Webb AMC, *et al.* Comparison of Yuzpe regimen, danazol, and mifepristone (RU 486) in oral postcoital contraception. *Br Med J* 1992; **305:** 927–31.
3. Lähteenmäki P, *et al.* Late postcoital treatment against pregnancy with antiprogesterone RU 486. *Fertil Steril* 1988; **50:** 36–8.
4. Luukkainen T, *et al.* Inhibition of folliculogenesis and ovulation by the antiprogesterone RU 486. *Fertil Steril* 1988; **49:** 961–3.
5. Swahn ML, *et al.* Contraception with mifepristone. *Lancet* 1991; **338:** 942–3.

Endometriosis. Preliminary results[1,2] have suggested that mifepristone, which is capable of suppressing ovarian function, may be of benefit in patients with endometriosis (p.1442).

1. Kettel LM, *et al.* Endocrine responses to long-term administration of the antiprogesterone RU486 in patients with pelvic endometriosis. *Fertil Steril* 1991; **56:** 402–7.
2. Kettel LM, *et al.* Preliminary report on the treatment of endometriosis with low-dose mifepristone (RU 486). *Am J Obstet Gynecol* 1998; **178:** 1151–6.

Fibroids. Mifepristone has been reported to produce significant decreases in tumour volume when given to patients with uterine leiomyomas,[1] and produced comparable results to a gonadorelin analogue (p.1248) as an adjunct to surgery.

1. Murphy AA, *et al.* Regression of uterine leiomyomata in response to the antiprogesterone RU 486. *J Clin Endocrinol Metab* 1993; **76:** 513–17.

Induction of labour. Some references to the use of mifepristone to induce labour, or facilitate induction of labour, where intra-uterine fetal death has occurred,[1] or when complications necessitate induction at term.[2] See also p.1411.

1. Cabrol D. *et al.* Induction of labor with mifepristone (RU 486) in intrauterine fetal death. *Am J Obstet Gynecol* 1990; **163:** 54–2.
2. Frydman R, *et al.* Labor induction in women at term with mifepristone (RU486): a double-blind, randomized, placebo-controlled study. *Obstet Gynecol* 1992; **80:** 972–5.

Malignant neoplasms. Mifepristone has been used successfully in the treatment of inoperable meningioma,[1-3] a brain tumour that may be progestogen-receptor positive (see p.485). Preliminary data on mifepristone in patients with breast cancer (p.485) were encouraging,[4] but in a more recent study response rates were low.[5]

1. Haak HR, *et al.* Successful mifepristone treatment of recurrent, inoperable meningioma. *Lancet* 1990; **336:** 124–5.
2. Grunberg SM, *et al.* Treatment of unresectable meningiomas with the antiprogesterone agent mifepristone. *J Neurosurg* 1991; **74:** 861–6.
3. Lamberts SWJ, *et al.* Mifepristone (RU 486) treatment of meningiomas. *J Neurol Neurosurg Psychiatry* 1992; **55:** 486–90.
4. Bakker G, *et al.* Treatment of breast cancer with different antiprogestins: preclinical and clinical studies. *J Steroid Biochem Mol Biol* 1990; **37:** 789–94.
5. Perrault D, *et al.* Phase II study of the progesterone antagonist mifepristone in patients with untreated metastatic breast carcinoma: a National Cancer Institute of Canada Clinical Trials Group study. *J Clin Oncol* 1996; **14:** 2709–12.

Termination of pregnancy. Mifepristone is an effective alternative to surgical methods for the termination of early pregnancy, when it is combined with a prostaglandin,[1-12] since it is not always effective when given alone. It is also used to ripen the cervix prior to surgical termination of pregnancy,[13-17] and in combination with a prostaglandin for second trimester termination.[18-22] For a discussion of the termination of pregnancy, see p.1412.

1. Rodger MW, Baird DT. Induction of therapeutic abortion in early pregnancy with mifepristone in combination with prostaglandin pessary. *Lancet* 1987; **ii:** 1415–18.
2. Rodger MW, *et al.* Induction of early abortion with mifepristone (RU486) and two different doses of prostaglandin pessary (gemeprost). *Contraception* 1989; **39:** 497–502.
3. Swahn M-L, Bygdeman M. Termination of early pregnancy with RU486 (mifepristone) in combination with a prostaglandin analogue (sulprostone). *Acta Obstet Gynecol Scand* 1989; **68:** 293–300.
4. Urquhart DR, *et al.* The efficacy and tolerance of mifepristone and prostaglandin in first trimester termination of pregnancy: UK multicentre trial. *Br J Obstet Gynaecol* 1990; **97:** 480–6.
5. Silvestre L, *et al.* Voluntary interruption of pregnancy with mifepristone (RU486) and a prostaglandin analogue: a large-scale French experience. *N Engl J Med* 1990; **322:** 645–8.
6. Hill NCW, *et al.* The efficacy of oral mifepristone (RU38,486) with a prostaglandin E_1 analog vaginal pessary for the termination of early pregnancy: complications and patient acceptability. *Am J Obstet Gynecol* 1990; **162:** 414–17.
7. Norman JE, *et al.* Uterine contractility and induction of abortion in early pregnancy by misoprostol and mifepristone. *Lancet* 1991; **338:** 1233–6.
8. Peyron R, *et al.* Early termination of pregnancy with mifepristone (RU 486) and the orally active prostaglandin misoprostol. *N Engl J Med* 1993; **328:** 1509–13.
9. WHO Task Force on Post-ovulatory Methods of Fertility Regulation. Termination of pregnancy with reduced doses of mifepristone. *Br Med J* 1993; **307:** 532–7.
10. El-Refaey H, *et al.* Induction of abortion with mifepristone (RU 486) and oral or vaginal misoprostol. *N Engl J Med* 1995; **332:** 983–7.
11. Urquhart DR, *et al.* The efficacy and tolerance of mifepristone and prostaglandin in termination of pregnancy of less than 63 days gestation; UK multicentre study final results. *Contraception* 1997; **55:** 1–5.
12. Spitz IM, *et al.* Early pregnancy termination with mifepristone and misoprostol in the United States. *N Engl J Med* 1998; **338:** 1241–7.
13. Rådestad A, *et al.* Induced cervical ripening with mifepristone in first trimester abortion: a double-blind randomized biomechanical study. *Contraception* 1988; **38:** 301–12.
14. Gupta JK, Johnson N. Effect of mifepristone on dilatation of the pregnant and non-pregnant cervix. *Lancet* 1990; **335:** 1238–40.
15. Lefebvre Y, *et al.* The effects of RU-38486 on cervical ripening. *Am J Obstet Gynecol* 1990; **162:** 61–5.
16. WHO. The use of mifepristone (RU 486) for cervical preparation in first trimester pregnancy termination by vacuum aspiration. *Br J Obstet Gynaecol* 1990: **97:** 260–6.
17. Henshaw RC, Templeton AA. Pre-operative cervical preparation before first trimester vacuum aspiration: a randomized controlled comparison between gemeprost and mifepristone (RU 486). *Br J Obstet Gynaecol* 1991; **98:** 1025–30.
18. Gottlieb C, Bygdeman M. The use of antiprogestin (RU 486) for termination of second trimester pregnancy. *Acta Obstet Gynecol Scand* 1991; **70:** 199–203.
19. Urquhart DR, Templeton AA. The use of mifepristone prior to prostaglandin-induced mid-trimester abortion. *Hum Reprod* 1990; **5:** 883–6.
20. Rodger M, Baird D. Pretreatment with mifepristone (RU486) reduces interval between prostaglandin administration and expulsion in second trimester abortion. *Br J Obstet Gynaecol* 1990; **97:** 41–5.
21. Thong KJ, Baird DT. Induction of second trimester abortion with mifepristone and gemeprost. *Br J Obstet Gynaecol* 1993; **100:** 758–61.
22. Webster D, *et al.* A comparison of 600 and 200 mg mifepristone prior to second trimester abortion with the prostaglandin misoprostol. *Br J Obstet Gynaecol* 1996; **103:** 706–9.

Preparations

Proprietary Preparations (details are given in Part 3)
Fr.: Mifegyne; *Swed.:* Mifegyne; *UK:* Mifegyne.

Nandrolone (13507-l)

Nandrolone *(BAN, rINN).*

19-Nortestosterone. 17β-Hydroxyestr-4-en-3-one; 3-Oxoestr-4-en-17β-yl.

$C_{18}H_{26}O_2$ = 274.4.

CAS — 434-22-0.

Nandrolone Cyclohexylpropionate (9072-w)

Nandrolone Cyclohexylpropionate *(BANM, rINNM).*

Nandrolone Cyclotate *(USAN)*; Nortestosterone Cyclohexylpropionate; RS-3268R. 3-Oxoestr-4-en-17β-yl 3-cyclohexylpropionate; 17β-Hydroxyestr-4-en-3-one cyclohexylpropionate.

$C_{27}H_{40}O_3$ = 412.6.

CAS — 912-57-2.

Nandrolone Decanoate (9073-e)

Nandrolone Decanoate *(BANM, USAN, rINNM).*

Nortestosterone Decanoate; Nortestosterone Decylate. 3-Oxoestr-4-en-17β-yl decanoate; 17β-Hydroxyestr-4-en-3-one decanoate.

$C_{28}H_{44}O_3$ = 428.6.

CAS — 360-70-3.

Pharmacopoeias. In Br. and US.

A white to creamy-white fine crystalline powder, odourless or with a faint characteristic odour. Practically **insoluble** in water; soluble to freely soluble in alcohol and in chloroform; freely soluble in ether, in fixed oils, and in esters; soluble in acetone and in vegetable oils. **Store** at 2° to 8° in an atmosphere of nitrogen in airtight containers. Protect from light.

Nandrolone Laurate (12998-c)

Nandrolone Laurate *(BANM, rINNM).*

Nandrolone Dodecanoate; Nortestosterone Laurate. 3-Oxoestr-4-en-17β-yl dodecanoate; 17β-Hydroxyestr-4-en-3-one dodecanoate.

$C_{30}H_{48}O_3$ = 456.7.

CAS — 26490-31-3.

Pharmacopoeias. In BP(Vet).

A white to creamy-white crystalline powder with a faint characteristic odour. Practically **insoluble** in water; freely soluble in alcohol, in chloroform, in ether, in fixed oils, and in esters of fatty acids. **Store** at 2° to 8°. Protect from light.

Nandrolone Phenylpropionate (9074-l)

Nandrolone Phenylpropionate *(BANM, rINNM).*

Nandrolone Hydrocinnamate; Nandrolone Phenpropionate; 19-Norandrostenolone Phenylpropionate; Nortestosterone Phenylpropionate; NSC-23162. 3-Oxoestr-4-en-17β-yl 3-phenylpropionate; 17β-Hydroxyestr-4-en-3-one 3-phenylpropionate.

$C_{27}H_{34}O_3$ = 406.6.

CAS — 62-90-8.

Pharmacopoeias. In Br., Chin., Pol., and US.

A white to creamy-white crystalline powder with a slight characteristic odour. Practically **insoluble** in water; soluble in alcohol. **Store** in airtight containers. Protect from light.

Nandrolone Sodium Sulphate (16489-b)

Nandrolone Sodium Sulphate *(BANM, rINNM).*

Nortestosterone Sodium Sulphate. 3-Oxoestr-4-en-17β-yl sodium sulphate; 17β-Hydroxyestr-4-en-3-one sodium sulphate.

$C_{18}H_{25}O_5SNa$ = 376.4.

CAS — 60672-82-4.

Nandrolone Undecanoate (10062-r)

Nandrolone Undecanoate *(BANM, rINNM).*

Nortestosterone Undecanoate. 3-Oxoestr-4-en-17β-yl undecanoate; 17β-Hydroxyestr-4-en-3-one undecanoate.

$C_{29}H_{46}O_3$ = 442.7.

CAS — 862-89-5.

Adverse Effects and Precautions

As for androgens and anabolic steroids in general (see Testosterone, p.1464).

Effects on the liver. Intrahepatic cholestasis occurred in a patient receiving nandrolone cyclohexylpropionate.[1]

1. Gil VG, *et al.* A non-C17-alkylated steroid and long-term cholestasis. *Ann Intern Med* 1986; **104:** 135–6.

Interactions

As for androgens and anabolic steroids in general (see Testosterone, p.1465).

Uses and Administration

Nandrolone is an anabolic steroid with anabolic and some androgenic properties (see Testosterone, p.1465). It is usually administered as the decanoate or phenylpropionate esters in the form of oily intramuscular injections.

Suggested doses of nandrolone decanoate and phenylpropionate are generally the same but the decanoate ester is usually given once every 3 or 4 weeks while the phenylpropionate is usually given each week. Doses of 25 to 100 mg have been used as an anabolic after debilitating illness. Doses of 50 mg have been suggested for use in postmenopausal osteoporosis and doses of 25 to 100 mg for postmenopausal metastatic breast carcinoma. The undecanoate has been used similarly in doses of about 80 mg.

Doses of between 50 and 200 mg weekly have been suggested for nandrolone decanoate in the treatment of anaemias.

Nandrolone sodium sulphate has been used topically in the treatment of corneal damage.

Nandrolone cyclohexylpropionate, laurate, and phenylpropionate are used in veterinary medicine.

Nandrolone hexyloxyphenylpropionate and nandrolone propionate have also been used.

Male contraception. Preliminary findings showed that nandrolone suppressed spermatogenesis,[1,2] suggesting it may have potential as a male contraceptive (p.1434).

1. Schürmeyer T, *et al.* Reversible azoospermia induced by the anabolic steroid 19-nortestosterone. *Lancet* 1984; **i:** 417–20.
2. Knuth UA, *et al.* Combination of 19-nortestosterone-hexyloxyphenyl-propionate (Anadur) and depot-medroxyprogesterone-acetate (Clinovir) for male contraception. *Fertil Steril* 1989; **51:** 1011–18.

Preparations

BP 1998: Nandrolone Decanoate Injection; Nandrolone Phenylpropionate Injection;
USP 23: Nandrolone Decanoate Injection; Nandrolone Phenpropionate Injection.

Proprietary Preparations (details are given in Part 3)
Aust.: Anadur; Deca-Durabolin; *Austral.:* Deca-Durabolin; Durabolin†; *Belg.:* Anadur†; Deca-Durabolin; Durabolin†; *Canad.:* Deca-Durabolin; Durabolin†; *Fr.:* Anador†; Deca-Durabolin†; Durabolin†; Keratyl; *Ger.:* Anadur†; Deca-Durabolin; Keratyl; *Irl.:* Deca-Durabolin; *Ital.:* Deca-Durabolin; Durabolin†; Dynabolon; Stenabolin†; *Mon.:* Dynabolon; *Neth.:* Anadur†; Deca-Durabolin; Durabolin†; *Norw.:* Deca-Durabolin; *S.Afr.:* Deca-Durabolin; Durabolin†; *Spain:* Deca-Durabolin; Durabolin†; Fherbolico†; *Swed.:* Anadur†; Deca-Durabol; *Switz.:* Anadur†; Deca-Durabolin; Keratyl; *UK:* Deca-Durabolin; Durabolin†; *USA:* Androlone-D; Deca-Durabolin; Durabolin; Hybolin; Kabolin†; Neo-Durabolic.

Multi-ingredient: *Ger.:* Dexatopic†; Docabolin†; *Ital.:* Dexatopic†; *Mon.:* Trophobolene; *Neth.:* Dexatopic; *Spain:* Dexatopic†; Dinatrofon†; Docabolina†.

Nomegestrol Acetate (3147-e)

Nomegestrol Acetate *(rINNM).*

17-Hydroxy-6-methyl-19-norpregna-4,6-diene-3,20-dione acetate.

$C_{23}H_{30}O_4$ = 370.5.

CAS — 58691-88-6 (nomegestrol); 58652-20-3 (nomegestrol acetate).

Nomegestrol acetate is a progestogen structurally related to progesterone (p.1459) that has been used in the treatment of menstrual disorders. Typical doses are 5 mg daily by mouth for 10 days of a 28-day cycle. A subdermal implant is under investigation as a long-acting progestogen-only contraceptive.

Preparations

Proprietary Preparations (details are given in Part 3)
Ital.: Lutenyl; *Mon.:* Lutenyl.

Norethandrolone (9075-y)

Norethandrolone *(BAN, rINN).*

17α-Ethyl-17β-hydroxyestr-4-en-3-one; 17β-Hydroxy-19-nor-17α-pregn-4-en-3-one.

$C_{20}H_{30}O_2$ = 302.5.

CAS — 52-78-8.

Pharmacopoeias. In It.

Adverse Effects and Precautions

As for androgens and anabolic steroids in general (see Testosterone, p.1464). As with other 17α-alkylated compounds, norethandrolone may produce hepatotoxicity and liver function should be monitored. It should probably be avoided in patients with impaired liver function, and certainly if this is severe.

Uses and Administration

Norethandrolone is an anabolic steroid (see Testosterone, p.1465). It is given by mouth in the treatment of anaemia in a dose of 0.25 to 1 mg per kg body-weight daily.

Preparations

Proprietary Preparations (details are given in Part 3)
Fr.: Nilevar.

Norethisterone (9078-c)

Norethisterone *(BAN, pINN)*.

Ethinylnortestosterone; Norethindrone; Norethisteronum; Noretisterona; Noretisterone; Norpregneninolone; NSC-9564. 17β-Hydroxy-19-nor-17α-pregn-4-en-20-yn-3-one.

$C_{20}H_{26}O_2$ = 298.4.

CAS — 68-22-4.

Pharmacopoeias. In *Chin., Eur.* (see p.viii), *Int., Jpn,* and *US.*

A white or yellowish-white odourless crystalline powder. Practically **insoluble** in water; slightly to sparingly soluble in alcohol; soluble in chloroform and in dioxan; slightly soluble in ether. **Protect** from light.

Norethisterone Acetate (9077-z)

Norethisterone Acetate *(BANM, pINNM)*.

Norethindrone Acetate; Norethisteroni Acetas. 17β-Hydroxy-19-nor-17α-pregn-4-en-20-yn-3-one acetate; 3-Oxo-19-nor-17α-pregn-4-en-20-yn-17β-yl acetate.

$C_{22}H_{28}O_3$ = 340.5.

CAS — 51-98-9.

Pharmacopoeias. In *Eur.* (see p.viii), *Int.,* and *US.*

A white or yellowish-white odourless crystalline powder. Practically **insoluble** in water; soluble 1 in 10 of alcohol, 1 in less than 1 of chloroform, 1 in 2 of dioxan, and 1 in 18 of ether. **Protect** from light.

Norethisterone Enanthate (9076-j)

Norethisterone Enanthate *(BANM)*.

Norethisterone Enantate *(pINNM)*; Norethindrone Enanthate; Norethisterone Heptanoate. 17β-Hydroxy-19-nor-17α-pregn-4-en-20-yn-3-one heptanoate.

$C_{27}H_{38}O_3$ = 410.6.

CAS — 3836-23-5.

Pharmacopoeias. In *Int.*

Adverse Effects and Precautions

As for progestogens in general (see Progesterone, p.1459). See also under Hormonal Contraceptives, p.1426.

Effects on the liver. There were 6 cases of jaundice among 107 patients with breast cancer treated with high-dose norethisterone acetate;[1] the jaundice was reversible and of an obstructive type.

1. Langlands AO, Martin WMC. Jaundice associated with norethisterone-acetate treatment of breast cancer. *Lancet* 1975; **i:** 584–5.

Pregnancy. Abnormalities seen in the offspring of women who had received norethisterone during pregnancy (either alone or in combination with ethinyloestradiol) included hypospadias,[1] masculinisation of female infants,[2] meningomyelocele or hydrocephalus,[3] and neonatal choreoathetosis associated with oral contraceptive use.[4] For reference to the fact that oral contraceptives have not generally been associated with teratogenicity, even when used inadvertently in pregnancy, see p.1432.

1. Aarskog D. Clinical and cytogenetic studies in hypospadias. *Acta Paediatr Scand* 1970; (suppl 203): 1–62.
2. Wilkins L. Masculinization of female fetus due to use of orally given progestins. *JAMA* 1960; **172:** 1028–32.
3. Gal I, *et al.* Hormonal pregnancy tests and congenital malformation. *Nature* 1967; **216:** 83.
4. Profumo R, *et al.* Neonatal choreoathetosis following prenatal exposure to oral contraceptives. *Pediatrics* 1990; **86:** 648–9.

Venous thrombo-embolism. For mention that combined oral contraceptives containing older progestogens such as norethisterone appear to be associated with a lower incidence of venous thrombo-embolism than desogestrel- or gestodene-containing preparations, see p.1430.

Interactions

As for progestogens in general (see Progesterone, p.1460). See also under Hormonal Contraceptives, p.1432.

Pharmacokinetics

Norethisterone is absorbed from the gastro-intestinal tract, undergoing first-pass hepatic metabolism, with peak plasma concentrations occurring 1 to 2 hours after a dose by mouth. It exhibits biphasic pharmacokinetics; an initial distribution phase is followed by a prolonged elimination phase with a half-life of about 8 hours or more. Norethisterone is highly protein bound; about 60% to albumin and 35% to sex hormone binding globulin. Administration with an oestrogen increases the proportion bound to sex hormone binding globulin. It is metabolised in the liver with 50 to 80% of a dose being excreted in the urine and up to 40% in the faeces.

Norethisterone acetate is reported to show a more prolonged elimination than norethisterone following oral administration. It is hydrolysed to norethisterone, principally by intestinal tissue.

Following intramuscular injection of norethisterone enanthate peak concentrations of norethisterone in plasma are not attained for several days.

Uses and Administration

Norethisterone and its acetate and enanthate esters are progestogens (see Progesterone, p.1460) derived from nortestosterone that have weak oestrogenic and androgenic properties. They are commonly used as **hormonal contraceptives** (see p.1433). Norethisterone and norethisterone acetate are both administered by mouth. Typical daily doses are 0.35 mg for norethisterone and 0.6 mg for norethisterone acetate when used alone, or 0.5 to 1 mg for norethisterone and 1.0 to 1.5 mg for norethisterone acetate when combined with an oestrogen. Norethisterone enanthate is administered by intramuscular injection; a dose of 200 mg provides contraception for 8 weeks.

Norethisterone and norethisterone acetate are used as the progestogen component of **menopausal hormone replacement therapy** (p.1437) to oppose the effects of oestrogens on the endometrium. Typical regimens have included either continuous daily doses of norethisterone 0.7 mg or norethisterone acetate 1 mg, or cyclical regimens of norethisterone or norethisterone acetate 1 mg daily for 10 to 12 days of a 28-day cycle, or 0.75 to 1.5 mg daily of norethisterone cyclically from multiphasic preparations. Norethisterone acetate is also available as a transdermal patch supplying 250 μg per 24 hours that is applied twice weekly for 2 weeks of a 4-week cycle.

Norethisterone and norethisterone acetate may be given by mouth for the treatment of conditions such as **menorrhagia** (p.1461) and **endometriosis** (p.1442). In menorrhagia (dysfunctional uterine bleeding), norethisterone is given in usual doses of 10 to 15 mg daily and norethisterone acetate in doses of 2.5 to 10 mg daily, in a cyclical regimen. In endometriosis the dosage of norethisterone is 10 to 25 mg daily and of norethisterone acetate 5 to 15 mg daily. Treatment of endometriosis is usually continuous for 4 to 9 months.

Norethisterone has been used in daily doses of up to 15 mg by mouth in a cyclical regimen in the treatment of **premenstrual syndrome** (p.1456).

In **breast cancer** (p.485) doses of up to 60 mg daily by mouth of either norethisterone or norethisterone acetate have been used.

Menorrhagia. Although cyclical norethisterone has been widely used for menorrhagia (p.1461), it is of limited efficacy during ovulatory cycles being most effective for anovulatory bleeding, which occurs in a minority of women with menorrhagia. References to the use of norethisterone are given below.[1,2]

1. Cameron IT, *et al.* The effects of mefenamic acid and norethisterone on measured menstrual blood loss. *Obstet Gynecol* 1990; **76:** 85–8.
2. Preston JT, *et al.* Comparative study of tranexamic acid and norethisterone in the treatment of ovulatory menorrhagia. *Br J Obstet Gynaecol* 1995; **102:** 401–6.

Preparations

BP 1998: Norethisterone Tablets;

USP 23: Norethindrone Acetate and Ethinyl Estradiol Tablets; Norethindrone Acetate Tablets; Norethindrone and Ethinyl Estradiol Tablets; Norethindrone and Mestranol Tablets; Norethindrone Tablets.

Proprietary Preparations (details are given in Part 3)

Aust.: Micronovum; Primolut-Nor; ***Austral.:*** Locilan; Micronor; Noriday; Primolut N; ***Belg.:*** Primolut-Nor; ***Canad.:*** Micronor; Norlutate; ***Fr.:*** Milligynon; Norfor†; Noristerat; Norluten; Primolut-Nor; ***Ger.:*** Gestakadin; Micronovum; Noristerat; Primolut-Nor; Sovel; ***Irl.:*** Micronor; Noriday; Primolut N; ***Ital.:*** Noristerat†; Primolut-Nor; ***Neth.:*** Primolut N; ***Norw.:*** Conludag; Primolut N; ***S.Afr.:*** Micronovum; Nur-Isterate; Primolut N; ***Spain:*** Primolut-Nor; ***Swed.:*** Mini-Pe; Primolut-Nor; ***Switz.:*** Micronovum; Primolut N; Primolut-Nor; ***UK:*** Menzol†; Micronor; Micronor.HRT; Noriday; Noristerat; Primolut N; SH 420†; Utovlan; ***USA:*** Aygestin; Micronor; Nor-QD; Norlutate†.

Multi-ingredient: ***Aust.:*** Estracomb; Estragest; Etalontin; Kliogest; Neorlest; Orlest; Ortho-Novum; Ostro-Primolut†; Ovysmen; Primosiston; Trinovum; Trisequens; ***Austral.:*** Brevinor; Estracombi; Improvil; Kliogest; Norimin; Norinyl-1; Ortho-Novum 1/50†; Synphasic; Trisequens; ***Belg.:*** Estracombi; Kliogest; Minestril; Ortho-Novum 1/50; Ortho-Novum SQ†; Ovysmen; Trinovum; Trisequens; ***Canad.:*** Brevicon; Estracomb; Loestrin 1.5/30; Minestrin; Norinyl 1/50; Norlestrin†; Ortho 0.5/35; Ortho 1/35; Ortho 10/11; Ortho 7/7/7; Ortho-Novum 0.5 mg†; Ortho-Novum 1/50; Ortho-Novum 1/80†; Ortho-Novum 2 mg†; Synphasic; ***Fr.:*** Gynophase†; Gynovlane†; Kliogest; Milli Anovlar; Miniphase; Norquentiel†; Ortho-Novum 1/35; Trentovlane†; Triella; Trisequens; ***Ger.:*** Conceplan M; Deposiston†; Estracomb; Etalontin†; Eve; Kliogest N; Neorlest; Non-Ovlon; Orlest†; Ortho-Novum 1/50; Ostro-Primolut; Ovysmen; Primosiston; Progylut†; Prosiston; Sequostat; Sinovula; Synphasec; Trinovum; Trisequens; ***Irl.:*** Binovum; Brevinor; Estracombi; Estrapak; Kliogest; Menophase; Norinyl-1; Normin; Ortho-Novin; Ovysmen; Trinovum; Trisequens; ***Ital.:*** Ablacton†; Anovlar†; Estracomb; Estro-Primolut†; Kliogest; Primosiston†; Trinovum; Trisequens; ***Neth.:*** Estracomb; Kliogest; Modicon; Neocon; Ortho-Novum 1/50†; Primosiston†; Trinovum; Trisequens; ***Norw.:*** Estracomb; Kliogest; Synfase; Trisekvens; ***S.Afr.:*** Brevinor; Estracombi; Kliogest; Minovlar ED†; Norinyl-1/28; Trinovum; Trisequens; ***Spain:*** Absorlent Plus; Estracomb; Primosiston; ***Swed.:*** Estracomb; Femanor; Femasekvens; Kliogest; Orthonett Novum; Synfase; Trinovum; Trisekvens; ***Switz.:*** Estracomb; Kliogest; Ortho-Novum 1/50; Ovysmen; Primosiston; Trinovum; Trisequens; ***UK:*** Binovum; Brevinor; Climagest; Climesse; Elleste Duet Conti; Elleste-Duet; Estracombi; Estrapak; Evorel Conti; Evorel Sequi; Evorel.Pak; Kliofem; Kliovance; Loestrin; Menophase; Neocon 1/35†; Norimin; Norinyl-1; Ortho-Novin 1/50†; Ovysmen; Synphase; Trinovum; Trinovum ED†; Trisequens; ***USA:*** Brevicon; Estrostep; Estrostep Fe; GenCept 0.5/35; GenCept 10/11; Genora 0.5/35; Genora 1/50; Jenest; Loestrin; Loestrin Fe; Modicon; Necon; NEE 1/35; Nelova 0.5/35E; Nelova 1/50M; Nelova 10/11; Norcept-E†; Norethin 1/35E; Norethin 1/50M; Norinyl 1 + 35; Norinyl 1 + 50; Norinyl 2 mg†; Ortho-Novum 1/35; Ortho-Novum 1/50; Ortho-Novum 10/11; Ortho-Novum 7/7/7; Ovcon 35; Tri-Norinyl.

Norethynodrel (9079-k)

Norethynodrel *(BAN, USAN)*.

Noretynodrel *(rINN)*; NSC-15432; SC-4642. 17β-Hydroxy-19-nor-17α-pregn-5(10)-en-20-yn-3-one.

$C_{20}H_{26}O_2$ = 298.4.

CAS — 68-23-5.

Pharmacopoeias. In *It.* and *US.*

A white or almost white, odourless, crystalline powder. Very slightly **soluble** in water; freely soluble in chloroform; soluble in acetone; sparingly soluble in alcohol.

Norethynodrel is a progestogen (see Progesterone, p.1459) structurally related to norethisterone that has been given by mouth in conjunction with an oestrogen such as mestranol for the treatment of various menstrual disorders and endometriosis. Typical doses are 5 to 10 mg daily, often in a cyclical regimen.

Pregnancy. A woman who had received norethynodrel during pregnancy to prevent threatened abortion gave birth to a female infant showing evidence of masculinisation.[1]

1. Wilkins L. Masculinization of female fetus due to use of orally given progestins. *JAMA* 1960; **172:** 1028–32.

Preparations

Proprietary Preparations (details are given in Part 3)

Multi-ingredient: ***USA:*** Enovid†.

Norgestimate (13031-z)

Norgestimate *(BAN, USAN, rINN)*.

D-138; Dexnorgestrel Acetime; ORF-10131; RWJ-10131. 13β-Ethyl-3-hydroxyimino-18,19-dinor-17α-pregn-4-en-20-yn-17β-yl acetate.

$C_{23}H_{31}NO_3$ = 369.5.

CAS — 35189-28-7.

Norgestimate is a progestogen (see Progesterone, p.1459) structurally related to levonorgestrel (to which it is partly metabolised) that is used as the progestogenic component of combined oral contraceptives (see p.1426). A typical daily dose is 250 μg in monophasic preparations, and 180 to 250 μg in sequential preparations.

Preparations

Proprietary Preparations (details are given in Part 3)

Multi-ingredient: ***Aust.:*** Cileste; TriCilest; ***Belg.:*** Cilest; ***Canad.:*** Cyclen; Tri-Cyclen; ***Fr.:*** Cilest; Effiprev; ***Ger.:*** Cilest; Pramino; ***Irl.:*** Cilest; ***Ital.:*** Cilest†; ***Neth.:*** Cilest; ***Switz.:*** Cilest; ***UK:*** Cilest; ***USA:*** Ortho Cyclen; Ortho Tri-Cyclen.

Norgestomet (6340-y)

Norgestomet *(BAN, USAN, rINN).*

SC-21009. 11β-Methyl-3,20-dioxo-19-norpregn-4-en-17α-yl acetate.

$C_{23}H_{32}O_4$ = 372.5.

CAS — 25092-41-5.

Norgestomet is a progestogen (see Progesterone, p.1459) used in veterinary medicine in combination with oestradiol.

Norgestrel (9080-w)

Norgestrel *(BAN, USAN, rINN).*

dl-Norgestrel; DL-Norgestrel; Norgestrelum; Wy-3707. (±)-13-Ethyl-17β-hydroxy-18,19-dinor-17α-pregn-4-en-20-yn-3-one.

$C_{21}H_{28}O_2$ = 312.4.

CAS — 6533-00-2.

Pharmacopoeias. In *Chin., Eur.* (see p.viii), *Jpn*, and *US.*

A white or almost white, almost odourless crystalline powder. Practically **insoluble** in water; slightly to sparingly soluble in alcohol; sparingly soluble in dichloromethane; freely soluble in chloroform. **Protect** from light.

Levonorgestrel (9081-e)

Levonorgestrel *(BAN, USAN, rINN).*

Levonorgestrelum; D-Norgestrel; WY-5104. (−)-13β-Ethyl-17β-hydroxy-18,19-dinor-17α-pregn-4-en-20-yn-3-one.

CAS — 797-63-7.

NOTE. The name Dexnorgestrel has also been used.

Pharmacopoeias. In *Eur.* (see p.viii), *Int.*, and *US.*

The (−)-isomer of norgestrel. A white or almost white, odourless crystalline powder. Practically **insoluble** in water; slightly soluble in alcohol; soluble in chloroform; sparingly soluble in dichloromethane. **Protect** from light.

Adverse Effects and Precautions

As for progestogens in general (see Progesterone, p.1459). See also under Hormonal Contraceptives, p.1426.

Following the introduction of levonorgestrel in a subdermal implant formulation in February 1991, the US Food and Drug Administration had received about 5800 reports of adverse effects as of December 1993 (out of an estimated 891 000 implants distributed).[1] Serious adverse effects associated with the implant included 24 cases of infection related to insertion of the implant, 15 cases of stroke and 39 of benign intracranial hypertension, 3 cases of thrombocytopenic purpura and 6 of thrombocytopenia (1 fatal). None of the reporting rates for these disorders exceeded the expected rate in this population.

1. Wysowski DK, Green L. Serious adverse events in Norplant users reported to the Food and Drug Administration's MedWatch Spontaneous Reporting System. *Obstet Gynecol* 1995; **85:** 538–42.

Benign intracranial hypertension. Intracranial hypertension, presenting as headaches, vomiting, and visual obscuration associated with florid bilateral papilloedema developed in 2 patients four to five months after subdermal implantation of levonorgestrel.[1] Despite a further 56 cases reported to various drug monitoring centres, and 70 cases known to the manufacturers,[2] it remained unclear whether the drug actually caused intracranial hypertension, but removal of implants in patients in whom intracranial pressure increased was recommended.[1]

1. Alder JB, *et al.* Levonorgestrel implants and intracranial hypertension. *N Engl J Med* 1995; **332:** 1720–1.
2. Weber ME, *et al.* Levonorgestrel implants and intracranial hypertension. *N Engl J Med* 1995; **332:** 1721.

Effects on the blood. A long-term study of the use of levonorgestrel subdermal implants (Norplant) in 100 Singaporean women indicated that during 12 months of use patients possibly had an increased tendency for thrombosis and an increased potential for hypercoagulation.[1] It was felt, however, that further investigation was required since some of the haematological changes observed after 1 year persisted throughout the second year of the study whereas others returned to normal.[2]

1. Viegas OAC, *et al.* The effects of Norplant on clinical chemistry in Singaporean acceptors after 1 year of use I: haemostatic changes. *Contraception* 1988; **38:** 313–23.
2. Singh K, *et al.* Two-year follow-up of changes in clinical chemistry in Singaporean Norplant-2 rod acceptors: haemostatic changes. *Contraception* 1989; **39:** 155–64.

Effects on carbohydrate metabolism. For a mention that levonorgestrel has been reported to be the most potent progestogen in decreasing glucose tolerance when used as a combined oral contraceptive, see p.1428.

Glucocorticoid effects. Reference to the minimal suppressive effect of subdermal levonorgestrel on adrenal function.[1]

1. Toppozada MK, *et al.* Effect of Norplant implants on the pituitary-adrenal axis function and reserve capacity. *Contraception* 1997; **55:** 7–10.

Myasthenia gravis. Myasthenia gravis occurring after insertion of a levonorgestrel implant improved on removal of the implant.[1]

1. Brittain J, Lange LS. Myasthenia gravis and levonorgestrel implant. *Lancet* 1995; **346:** 1556.

Pregnancy. Adverse effects in infants whose mothers had received oral contraceptives containing norgestrel during early pregnancy have included tracheo-oesophageal fistula in one infant[1] and inoperable hepatoblastoma in another.[2] However, for mention of the fact that many epidemiological studies have failed to show any association between fetal malformations and oral contraceptives, even when used inadvertently during pregnancy, see p.1432.

1. Frost O. Tracheo-oesophageal fistula associated with hormonal contraception during pregnancy. *Br Med J* 1976; **2:** 978.
2. Otten J, *et al.* Hepatoblastoma in an infant after contraceptive intake during pregnancy. *N Engl J Med* 1977; **297:** 222.

Venous thrombo-embolism. For mention that levonorgestrel-containing combined oral contraceptives appeared to be associated with a lower incidence of venous thrombo-embolism than desogestrel- or gestodene-containing preparations, see p.1430.

Interactions

As for progestogens in general (see Progesterone, p.1460). See also under Hormonal Contraceptives, p.1432.

Pharmacokinetics

Levonorgestrel is rapidly and almost completely absorbed after administration by mouth, and undergoes little first-pass hepatic metabolism. It is highly bound to plasma proteins; 42 to 68% to sex hormone binding globulin and 30 to 56% to albumin. The proportion bound to sex hormone binding globulin is higher when it is administered with an oestrogen. Levonorgestrel and norgestrel are metabolised in the liver to sulphate and glucuronide conjugates, which are excreted in the urine and to a lesser extent in the faeces.

References.

1. Fotherby K. Levonorgestrel: clinical pharmacokinetics. *Clin Pharmacokinet* 1995; **28:** 203–15.

Uses and Administration

Norgestrel and its active isomer levonorgestrel are progestogens (see Progesterone, p.1460) derived from nortestosterone. They are more potent inhibitors of ovulation than norethisterone and have androgenic activity. Levonorgestrel is more commonly used than norgestrel and is twice as potent. For example, levonorgestrel 37.5 μg is equivalent to norgestrel 75 μg.

They are both used as **hormonal contraceptives** (see p.1433). The typical daily dose when used as an oral progestogen-only contraceptive is the equivalent of 30 or 37.5 μg of levonorgestrel, and when used as a combined oral contraceptive, is the equivalent of 150 to 250 μg of levonorgestrel in monophasic preparations, and 50 to 125 μg of levonorgestrel in sequential preparations. Levonorgestrel is also used as a long-acting progestogen-only contraceptive administered by subcutaneous implantation; 6 implants each containing 38 mg levonorgestrel are inserted under the skin on the first day of the cycle and are replaced at intervals of up to 5 years. A 2-implant preparation providing 3 years of contraception is being investigated. Uterine, cervical, and vaginal devices containing levonorgestrel have also been investigated, and an intra-uterine device is available for contraception, containing a total of 52 mg of levonorgestrel which is released at an initial rate of 20 μg per 24 hours. The device is effective for 5 years.

For **emergency contraception** (p.1434) levonorgestrel may be given by mouth in a dose of 750 μg within 72 hours of coitus (and preferably as soon as possible), repeated after 12 hours.

Both levonorgestrel and norgestrel are used as the progestogenic component of **menopausal hormone replacement therapy** (see p.1437). Typical regimens are the equivalent of 75 to 250 μg of levonorgestrel by mouth for 10 to 12 days of a 28-day cycle. The intra-uterine levonorgestrel device is under investigation for use in combination with oestrogen for this indication. Levonorgestrel may also be given via a combined transdermal patch, releasing 20 μg per 24 hours together with an oestrogen.

Administration. IMPLANTS. Some references to the use of levonorgestrel by subcutaneous implant for hormonal contraception.[1-11]

1. Sivin I, *et al.* Three-year experience with Norplant™ subdermal contraception. *Fertil Steril* 1983; **39:** 799–808.
2. Roy S, *et al.* Long-term reversible contraception with levonorgestrel-releasing Silastic rods. *Am J Obstet Gynecol* 1984; **148:** 1006–13.
3. Shaaban MM, Salah M. A two-year experience with Norplant™ implants in Assiut, Egypt. *Contraception* 1984; **29:** 335–43.
4. The International Committee for Contraception Research (ICCR) of the Population Council. Contraception with long-acting subdermal implants: a five-year clinical trial with Silastic covered rod implants containing levonorgestrel. *Contraception* 1985; **31:** 351–9.
5. Holma P. Long term experience with Norplant contraceptive implants in Finland. *Contraception* 1985; **31:** 231–41.
6. Lopez G, *et al.* Two-year prospective study in Colombia of Norplant implants. *Obstet Gynecol* 1986; **68:** 204–8.
7. Shoupe D, Mishell DR. Norplant: subdermal implant system for long-term contraception. *Am J Obstet Gynecol* 1989; **160:** 1286–92.
8. Brache V, *et al.* Ovarian endocrine function through five years of continuous treatment with Norplant™ subdermal contraceptive implants. *Contraception* 1990; **41:** 169–77.
9. Polaneczky M, *et al.* The use of levonorgestrel implants (Norplant) for contraception in adolescent mothers. *N Engl J Med* 1994; **331:** 1201–6.
10. Anonymous. Long-acting progestogen-only contraception. *Drug Ther Bull* 1996; **34:** 93–6.
11. Coukell AJ, Balfour JA. Levonorgestrel subdermal implants: a review of contraceptive efficacy and acceptability. *Drugs* 1998; **55:** 861–87.

INTRA-UTERINE DEVICES. Some references to the use of levonorgestrel-releasing intra-uterine contraceptive devices.[1-3]

1. Anonymous. Randomized clinical trial with intrauterine devices (levonorgestrel intrauterine device (LNG), CuT 380 Ag, CuT 220C and CuT 200B): 36-month study. *Contraception* 1989; **39:** 37–52.
2. Toivonen J, *et al.* Protective effect of intrauterine release of levonorgestrel on pelvic infection: three years' comparative experience of levonorgestrel- and copper-releasing intrauterine devices. *Obstet Gynecol* 1991; **77:** 261–4.
3. Sturridge F, Guillebaud J. A risk-benefit assessment of the levonorgestrel-releasing intrauterine system. *Drug Safety* 1996; **15:** 430–40.

Menorrhagia. Although oral cyclical progestogens have limited efficacy in the treatment of menorrhagia (p.1461), the levonorgestrel-containing intra-uterine device appears to be particularly useful in reducing menstrual blood loss. References to the use of levonorgestrel are given below.[1-4]

1. Andersson JK, Rybo G. Levonorgestrel-releasing intrauterine device in the treatment of menorrhagia. *Br J Obstet Gynaecol* 1990; **97:** 690–4.
2. Milsom I, *et al.* A comparison of flurbiprofen, tranexamic acid, and a levonorgestrel-releasing intrauterine contraceptive device in the treatment of idiopathic menorrhagia. *Am J Obstet Gynecol* 1991; **164:** 879–83.
3. Crosignani PC, *et al.* Levonorgestrel releasing intrauterine device versus hysteroscopic endometrial resection in the treatment of dysfunctional uterine bleeding. *Obstet Gynecol* 1997; **90:** 257–63.
4. Lähteenmäki P, *et al.* Open randomised study of use of levonorgestrel releasing intrauterine system as alternative to hysterectomy. *Br Med J* 1998; **316:** 1122–6.

Preparations

BP 1998: Levonorgestrel and Ethinylestradiol Tablets;
USP 23: Levonorgestrel and Ethinyl Estradiol Tablets; Norgestrel and Ethinyl Estradiol Tablets; Norgestrel Tablets.

Proprietary Preparations (details are given in Part 3)
Austral.: Microlut; Microval; ***Belg.:*** Microlut; Microval; Mirena; ***Canad.:*** Norplant; ***Fr.:*** Microval; ***Ger.:*** 28 Mini; Microlut; Mikro-30; ***Irl.:*** Microlut†; Microval†; ***Ital.:*** Microlut; ***Neth.:*** Mirena; ***Norw.:*** Levonova; Microluton; ***S.Afr.:*** Microval; ***Swed.:*** Follistrel; Levonova; Norplant; ***Switz.:*** Microlut; Mirena; ***UK:*** Microval; Mirena; Neogest; Norgeston; Norplant; Postinor-2; ***USA:*** Norplant; Ovrette.

Multi-ingredient: ***Aust.:*** Cyclacur; Levlen; Liogynon; Microgynon; Neo-Stediril; Neogynon; Ovranette†; Perikursal; Sequilar; Stediril D; Trigynon; Trinordiol; ***Austral.:*** Biphasil; Levlen ED; Logynon ED; Microgynon; Monofeme; Nordette; Nordiol; Sequilar ED; Trifeme; Triphasil; Triquilar; ***Belg.:*** Binordiol; Cyclocur; Microgynon; Neo-Stediril; Stediril; Stediril 30; Stediril D; Trigynon; Trinordiol; ***Canad.:*** Min-Ovral; Ovral; Triphasil; Triquilar; ***Fr.:*** Adepal; Minidril; Stediril; Trinordiol; ***Ger.:*** Cyclo-Menorette; Cyclo-Progynova; CycloOstrogynal; Duoluton†; Ediwal†; Eugynon†; Femigoa; Femranette mikro; Gravistat; Klimonorm; Leios; Microgynon; Minisiston; Miranova; MonoStep; Neo-Stediril; Neogynon; Neogynon 28†; Ostronara; Perikursal; Sequilar; Stediril;

Stediril 30; Stediril D; Tetragynon; Triette; Trigoa; Trinordiol; Triquilar; Trisiston; TriStep; ***Irl.:*** Cyclo-Progynova†; Eugynon 30†; Logynon; Microgynon 30; Nuvelle; Ovran; Ovran 30; Ovranette; Prempak-C; Trinordiol; ***Ital.:*** Binordiol†; Bivlar†; Cyclacur†; Egogyn 30; Eugynon; Evanor-D; Microgynon; Novogyn; Nuvelle; Ovranet; Trigynon; Trinordiol; ***Neth.:*** Binordiol; Cyclocur; Microgynon; Neo-Stediril; Neogynon; Prempak-C; Stediril; Trigynon; Trinordiol; ***Norw.:*** Cyclabil; Eugynon; Follimin; Microgynon; Tetragynon; Trinordiol; Trionetta; ***S.Afr.:*** Biphasil; Logynon ED; Nordette; Nordiol; Normovlar ED; Ovral; Postoval; Triphasil; ***Spain:*** Eugynon; Microgynon; Neogynona; Ovoplex; Progyluton; Triagynon; Triciclor; ***Swed.:*** Cyclabil; Follimin; Follinett; Neovletta; Nordette†; Regunon; Sequilarum†; Tetragynon†; Trinordiol; Trionetta; ***Switz.:*** Binordiol; Cyclacur; Microgynon; Neo-Stediril; Neogynon; Ologyn; Sequilar; Stediril 30; Stediril D; Tetragynon; Trinordiol; Triquilar; ***UK:*** Cyclo-Progynova 1 mg; Cyclo-Progynova 2 mg; Eugynon 30; Logynon; Microgynon 30; Nuvelle; Nuvelle TS; Ovran; Ovran 30; Ovranette; Prempak-C; Schering PC4; Trinordiol; ***USA:*** Alesse; Levlen; Levora; Lo/Ovral; Nordette; Ovral; Preven; Tri-Levlen; Triphasil.

Norgestrienone (13032-c)

Norgestrienone *(rINN)*.

17β-Hydroxy-19-nor-17α-pregna-4,9,11-trien-20-yn-3-one.

$C_{20}H_{22}O_2$ = 294.4.

CAS — 848-21-5.

Norgestrienone is a progestogen (see Progesterone, p.1459) structurally related to norethisterone that is used as an oral contraceptive (see p.1426). Typical doses are 2 mg daily when combined with an oestrogen, and 350 μg daily when used alone.

Preparations

Proprietary Preparations (details are given in Part 3)
Fr.: Ogyline.

Multi-ingredient: ***Fr.:*** Planor.

Oestradiol (9083-y)

Oestradiol *(BAN)*.

Estradiol *(rINN)*; Beta-oestradiol; Dihydrofolliculin; Dihydrotheelin; Dihydroxyoestrin; Estradiolum; NSC-9895; NSC-20293 (alpha-oestradiol). Estra-1,3,5(10)-triene-3,17β-diol.

$C_{18}H_{24}O_2$ = 272.4.

CAS — 50-28-2 (anhydrous).

Pharmacopoeias. In *Aust., Fr.,* and *US.*
Eur. (see p.viii) includes the hemihydrate.

White or creamy-white, odourless, hygroscopic crystals or crystalline powder. Practically **insoluble** in water; soluble 1 in 28 of alcohol, 1 in 435 of chloroform, and 1 in 150 of ether; soluble in acetone, in dioxan, and in solutions of fixed alkali hydroxides; sparingly soluble in vegetable oils. **Store** in airtight containers. Protect from light.

The hemihydrate is a white or almost white crystalline powder or colourless crystals. Practically insoluble in water; sparingly soluble in alcohol; soluble in acetone; slightly soluble in dichloromethane and in ether. **Protect** from light. Oestradiol hemihydrate 1.03 g is approximately equivalent to 1 g of the anhydrous substance.

Oestradiol Benzoate (9084-j)

Oestradiol Benzoate *(BANM)*.

Estradiol Benzoate *(rINN)*; Beta-oestradiol Benzoate; Dihydroxyoestrin Monobenzoate; Estradioli Benzoas; NSC-9566. Estra-1,3,5(10)-triene-3,17β-diol 3-benzoate.

$C_{25}H_{28}O_3$ = 376.5.

CAS — 50-50-0.

Pharmacopoeias. In *Chin., Eur.* (see p.viii), *Jpn,* and *Pol.*

Colourless crystals or an almost white crystalline powder. Practically **insoluble** in water; slightly soluble in alcohol and in fatty oils; sparingly soluble in acetone. **Protect** from light.

Oestradiol Cypionate (9085-z)

Oestradiol Cypionate *(BANM)*.

Estradiol Cipionate *(rINNM)*; Estradiol Cypionate; Oestradiol Cyclopentylpropionate. Estra-1,3,5(10)-triene-3,17β-diol 17-(3-cyclopentylpropionate).

$C_{26}H_{36}O_3$ = 396.6.

CAS — 313-06-4.

Pharmacopoeias. In *US.*

A white or practically white crystalline powder, odourless or with a slight odour. Practically **insoluble** in water; soluble 1 in 40 of alcohol, 1 in 7 of chloroform, and 1 in 2800 of ether; soluble in acetone and in dioxan; sparingly soluble in vegetable oils. **Store** in airtight containers. Protect from light.

Oestradiol Dipropionate (9086-c)

Oestradiol Dipropionate *(BANM)*.

Estradiol Dipropionate *(rINNM)*; Dihydroxyoestrin Dipropionate. Estra-1,3,5(10)-triene-3,17β-diol dipropionate.

$C_{24}H_{32}O_4$ = 384.5.

CAS — 113-38-2.

Pharmacopoeias. In *Aust.* and *Swiss.*

Oestradiol Enanthate (9087-k)

Oestradiol Enanthate *(BANM)*.

Estradiol Enantate *(rINNM)*; Estradiol Enanthate *(USAN)*; Oestradiol 17-Heptanoate; SQ-16150. Estra-1,3,5(10)-triene-3,17β-diol 17-heptanoate.

$C_{25}H_{36}O_3$ = 384.6.

CAS — 4956-37-0.

Oestradiol Hexahydrobenzoate (13039-d)

Oestradiol Hexahydrobenzoate *(BANM)*.

Estradiol Hexahydrobenzoate *(rINNM)*. Estra-1,3,5(10)-triene-3,17β-diol 17-cyclohexanecarboxylate.

$C_{25}H_{34}O_3$ = 382.5.

CAS — 15140-27-9.

Oestradiol Phenylpropionate (10064-d)

Oestradiol Phenylpropionate *(BANM)*.

Estra-1,3,5(10)-triene-3,17β-diol 17-(3-phenylpropionate).

$C_{27}H_{32}O_3$ = 404.5.

Oestradiol Undecanoate (9088-a)

Oestradiol Undecanoate *(BANM)*.

Estradiol Undecylate *(USAN, rINN)*; SQ-9993. Estra-1,3,5(10)-triene-3,17β-diol 17-undecanoate.

$C_{29}H_{44}O_3$ = 440.7.

CAS — 3571-53-7; 33613-02-4.

Oestradiol Valerate (9089-t)

Oestradiol Valerate *(BANM)*.

Estradiol Valerate *(rINN)*; NSC-17590. Estra-1,3,5(10)-triene-3,17β-diol 17-valerate.

$C_{23}H_{32}O_3$ = 356.5.

CAS — 979-32-8.

Pharmacopoeias. In *Chin.* and *US.*

A white crystalline powder which is odourless or has a faint fatty odour. Practically **insoluble** in water; soluble in benzyl benzoate, in dioxan, in methyl alcohol, and in castor oil; sparingly soluble in arachis oil and sesame oil. **Store** in airtight containers. Protect from light.

Adverse Effects

The adverse effects of oestradiol and other oestrogens are related, in part, to dose and duration of therapy, and to the gender and age of the recipient. In addition, adverse effects may be modified by concomitant administration of a progestogen in menopausal hormone replacement therapy (HRT) or combined oral contraceptives. Whether adverse effects of natural and synthetic oestrogens differ, and the effect of route of administration, is less clear.

The adverse effects of oestrogens used in HRT are considered in detail starting on p.1435. Those of oestrogens used in hormonal contraceptives are considered in detail starting on p.1426.

The use of oestrogens in girls may cause premature closure of the epiphyses resulting in decreased final adult height.

Large doses of oestrogens used in palliation of cancers have additionally been associated with nausea, fluid retention, venous and arterial thrombosis, and hepatic impairment. In men, they cause impotence and feminising effects such as gynaecomastia. In women, they may cause withdrawal bleeding, and, when used for breast cancer, they have caused hypercalcaemia and bone pain.

Effects on the skin. There is some evidence[1] that transdermal patches in which oestradiol is dissolved in the adhesive matrix cause fewer skin reactions than those employing release of oestradiol from an alcoholic reservoir.

1. Ross D. Randomised crossover comparison of skin irritation with two transdermal oestradiol patches. *Br Med J* 1997; **315:** 288.

Precautions

The precautions for the use of oestradiol and other oestrogens used as menopausal hormone replacement therapy (HRT) are considered in detail starting on p.1437. Those for oestrogens used in hormonal contraceptives are considered in detail starting on p.1431.

High doses of oestrogen used in treating malignant disease should be used cautiously in patients with cerebrovascular disorders, coronary artery disease, or venous thrombo-embolism. They may exacerbate hypercalcaemia of malignancy.

Oestrogens should be used with caution in children because premature closure of the epiphyses may occur resulting in inhibited linear growth and small stature.

Oestrogens have been reported to increase the plasma concentrations of cortisol- and thyroxine-binding globulin and hence may interfere with diagnostic tests.

Cosmetic use. Some cosmetic products contain oestrogens and their use has led to adverse effects such as precocious puberty in children and gynaecomastia or postmenopausal bleeding in adults.[1]

1. Anonymous. Estrogens in cosmetics. *Med Lett Drugs Ther* 1985; **27:** 54–5.

Pregnancy. Although gross abnormalities of the genito-urinary tract have been reported in the male offspring of women who took stilboestrol during pregnancy there is conflicting evidence as to whether the oestrogen produced an increased risk of abnormalities, infertility, or testicular cancer in such offspring (see p.1463). The male fetus is normally protected from the feminising effects of the natural oestrogens in the uterine environment by the early development of the testes and the secretion of male hormones.[1] However, there has been considerable concern about a rising incidence of disorders of the male reproductive tract, and a reduction in sperm counts, which has been noted in the last 20 to 30 years. It has been hypothesised that overexposure of male fetuses to environmental oestrogens derived from pollutants such as pesticides and plastics may be responsible for this decline,[2,3] although some dispute this.[4]

For discussion of the lack of effects of hormonal contraceptives on the fetus, including evidence that they are unlikely to increase the risk of hypospadia in the male fetus, see p.1432.

1. Mittwoch U, *et al.* Male sexual development in "a sea of oestrogen". *Lancet* 1993; **342:** 123–4.
2. Sharpe RM, Skakkebaek NE. Are oestrogens involved in falling sperm counts and disorders of the male reproductive tract? *Lancet* 1993; **341:** 1392–5.
3. de Kretser DM. Declining sperm counts. *Br Med J* 1996; **312:** 457–8.
4. Thomas JA. Falling sperm counts. *Lancet* 1995; **346:** 635.

Veterinary use. An FAO/WHO expert committee considered it unnecessary to establish an acceptable daily intake or acceptable residual level in food for endogenous hormones such as oestradiol.[1] Residues resulting from the use of oestradiol as a growth promoter in accordance with good animal husbandry practice were thought unlikely to pose a hazard to human health. However, it should be noted that, in the European Union the use of steroidal hormones such as oestrogens in veterinary practice is restricted, and their use as growth promoters is banned.

There is concern about the effect of environmental oestrogens on male fertility and development, see above.

1. FAO/WHO. Evaluation of certain veterinary drug residues in food: thirty-second report of the joint FAO/WHO expert committee on food additives. *WHO Tech Rep Ser 763* 1988.

Interactions

Interactions involving oestradiol and other oestrogens used in menopausal hormone replacement therapy are covered on p.1437. Interactions for oestrogens used in hormonal contraceptives are covered on p.1432.

Pharmacokinetics

In general, oestradiol and other oestrogens are readily absorbed from the gastro-intestinal tract and through the skin or mucous membranes. However, the natural unconjugated oestrogens such as oestradiol undergo extensive first-pass metabolism in the gastro-intestinal tract and liver following oral administration. They are, therefore, generally not orally active, although a micronised preparation of oestradiol has sufficient bioavailability (3 to 5%) to be orally active. Oestradiol is metabolised in part to less active oestrogens such as oestriol and oestrone. Synthetic oestrogens produced by alkylation of the C17 position, such as ethinyloestradiol, are more slowly metabolised and are therefore orally active. Conjugated oestrogens, which are essentially oestrogen metabolites, are also orally active because they are hydrolysed by enzymes in the lower gastro-intestinal tract allowing absorption of the active oestrogen. Vaginal, transdermal, or parenteral administration of oestrogens also avoids first-pass hepatic metabolism. Plasma-oestradiol concentrations are reported to reach a peak 1.5 to 2 hours after oral administration, and again at about 8 hours due to enterohepatic recycling. Oestradiol esters are rapidly hydrolysed to free oestradiol when administered by mouth. Following intramuscular administration of the esters, absorption is prolonged.

Oestrogens are extensively bound to plasma proteins. Naturally occurring oestrogens such as oestradiol are principally bound to sex-hormone binding globulin. Conversely, ethinyloestradiol is mostly bound to albumin.

Oestrogens are metabolised in the liver. A variety of sulphate and glucuronide conjugates are formed, and these are excreted in the urine and the bile. Those excreted in the bile undergo enterohepatic recycling or are excreted in the faeces.

Some references to the pharmacokinetics of oestradiol[1-4] and other oestrogens[5,6] are cited below.

1. Kuhnz W, *et al.* Pharmacokinetics of estradiol, free and total estrone, in young women following single intravenous and oral administration of 17β-estradiol. *Arzneimittelforschung* 1993; **43:** 966–73.
2. Schubert W, *et al.* Pharmacokinetic evaluation of oral 17β-oestradiol and two different fat soluble analogues in ovariectomized women. *Eur J Clin Pharmacol* 1993; **44:** 563–8.
3. Baker VL. Alternatives to oral estrogen replacement: transdermal patches, percutaneous gels, vaginal creams and rings, implants, other methods of delivery. *Obstet Gynecol Clin North Am* 1994; **21:** 271–9.
4. Price TM, *et al.* Single-dose pharmacokinetics of sublingual versus oral administration of micronized 17β-estradiol. *Obstet Gynecol* 1997; **89:** 340–5.
5. Stumpf PG. Pharmacokinetics of estrogen. *Obstet Gynecol* 1990; **75** (suppl): 9S–14S.
6. O'Connell MB. Pharmacokinetic and pharmacologic variation between different estrogen products. *J Clin Pharmacol* 1995; **35** (suppl): 18S–24S.

Uses and Administration

Oestradiol is the most active of the naturally occurring oestrogens (for further details, see p.1426). Oestradiol and its semisynthetic esters and other natural oestrogens are primarily used as menopausal hormone replacement therapy (HRT) (see p.1437) whereas synthetic derivatives such as ethinyloestradiol and mestranol have a major role as components of combined oral contraceptives (see Hormonal Contraceptives, p.1433). Oestradiol may also be used as replacement therapy for female hypogonadism or primary ovarian failure (see p.1240). Replacement therapy ('add-back' therapy) may also be given to women in whom the pituitary-ovarian axis is suppressed by therapy with gonadorelin or its analogues.

For HRT orally administered preparations of oestradiol are commonly used, as are transdermal patches. Transdermal gels and subcutaneous implants are also available. Intramuscular injections were also formerly used. In women with a uterus, associated administration of a progestogen is required, given cyclically or continuously and usually administered by mouth although some transdermal preparations are available. Local vaginal oestradiol preparations are used specifically for the treatment of menopausal atrophic vaginitis; these are generally recommended for short-term use only, if given without a progestogen in women with a uterus, although specific recommendations vary between products.

For administration by mouth oestradiol or oestradiol valerate are normally employed; doses of 1 to 2 mg daily are given cyclically or more often continuously.

Oestradiol may be used topically as transdermal skin patches to provide a systemic effect; a variety of patches are available which release between 25 and 100 μg of oestradiol every 24 hours. Depending on the preparation, patches are replaced once or twice weekly. Each new patch is applied to a different area of skin in rotation, usually below the waistline; patches should not be applied on or near the breasts. Topical gel preparations are also applied for systemic effect: the usual dose is 0.5 to 1.5 mg of oestradiol daily. The gel should not be applied on or near the breasts or on the vulval region.

In order to prolong the duration of action subcutaneous implants of oestradiol may be employed. The dose of oestradiol is generally 25 to 100 mg with a new implant being administered after about 4 to 8 months according to oestrogen concentrations.

Oestradiol may be applied locally either as 25-μg vaginal tablets, at an initial dose of one tablet daily for 2 weeks followed by a maintenance dose of two tablets weekly, or as a 0.01% vaginal cream, in initial amounts of up to 4 g of cream daily followed by a maintenance dose of 1 to 3 g weekly. Another local delivery system employs a 3-month vaginal ring containing 2 mg of oestradiol hemihydrate, which delivers about 7.5 μg of oestradiol per 24 hours.

Intramuscular injections of oestradiol benzoate or valerate esters have been used as oily solutions to provide a depot, usually administered once every 3 to 4 weeks. The cypionate, dipropionate, enanthate, hexahydrobenzoate, phenylpropionate, and undecanoate esters have been used similarly.

Oestradiol and other oestrogens have sometimes been used in higher doses for palliative treatment in prostate cancer (p.491) and breast cancer in men and postmenopausal women (p.485).

Administration. IMPLANTS. There may be a striking interpatient variation in blood-oestradiol concentrations in women receiving oestradiol implants.[1] In addition, Gangar *et al.*[2] noted that symptoms of oestrogen deficiency re-appeared in some patients even though serum-oestradiol concentrations were within or above the physiological range. This has led to debate on the appropriateness of using serum concentrations of oestradiol as a guide to implant administration, rather than symptoms.[3-7] Some felt that withholding an implant while a patient suffered symptoms of oestrogen deficiency was unacceptable[3,4] and that other oestrogens or routes of administration may be more suitable.[3,5] Although Gangar *et al.*[2] thought that high oestradiol concentrations were probably not harmful, others[6,7] have pointed out that there was evidence to the contrary, lending weight to the suggestion that oestradiol concentration should be monitored during therapy with implants and this is now recommended by the manufacturers.

Cyclical progestogen may be required for a prolonged period after discontinuation of oestradiol implants in women with a uterus.[7]

1. Guirgis RR. Oestradiol implants: what dose, how often? *Lancet* 1987; **ii:** 856.
2. Gangar K, *et al.* Symptoms of oestrogen deficiency associated with supraphysiological plasma oestradiol concentrations in women with oestradiol implants. *Br Med J* 1989; **299:** 601–2.
3. Ginsburg J, Hardiman P. Oestrogen deficiency and oestradiol implants. *Br Med J* 1989; **299:** 1031.
4. Studd J, *et al.* Symptoms of oestrogen deficiency in women with oestradiol implants. *Br Med J* 1989; **299:** 1400–1.
5. Swyer GIM. Symptoms of oestrogen deficiency in women with oestradiol implants. *Br Med J* 1989; **299:** 854.
6. Tobias JH. Chambers TJ. Symptoms of oestrogen deficiency in women with oestradiol implants. *Br Med J* 1989; **299:** 854.
7. Wardle P, Fox R. Symptoms of oestrogen deficiency in women with oestradiol implants. *Br Med J* 1989; **299:** 1102.

TRANSDERMAL ADMINISTRATION. The transdermal administration of oestradiol via patches applied to the skin has been reviewed.[1-7] This method of delivery has certain advantages over oral administration in that gastro-intestinal and hepatic first-pass metabolism is avoided, liver enzymes are not stimulated (although this may also mean that beneficial effects on serum lipids are absent), and the prolonged drug release from the patch means less frequent application is necessary and hence patient compliance may be improved. For oestrogen replacement in menopausal and postmenopausal women oestradiol patches are administered continuously or in a cyclical manner, with added progestogen for part of the cycle in those women with an intact uterus. This does not lead to drug accumulation and produces blood-oestradiol concentrations and oestradiol to oestrone ratios similar to those normally observed in premenopausal women. Administration of oestradiol via a skin patch is well tolerated with skin irritation being the main problem. The patches are as effective as orally administered oestrogens in treating menopausal and postmenopausal symptoms such as flushing and vaginal atrophy and also appear to be as effective in preventing osteoporosis, but further study is needed to determine whether this holds true for reductions in cardiovascular disease risk.

1. Anonymous. Transdermal estrogen. *Med Lett Drugs Ther* 1986; **28:** 119–20.
2. Ridout G, *et al.* Pharmacokinetic considerations in the use of newer transdermal formulations. *Clin Pharmacokinet* 1988; **15:** 114–31.
3. Utian WH. Transdermal oestradiol: a recent advance in oestrogen therapy. *Drugs* 1988; **36:** 383–6.
4. Bauwens SF. Transdermal versus oral estrogen for postmenopausal replacement therapy. *Clin Pharm* 1989; **8:** 364–6.
5. Balfour JA, Heel RC. Transdermal estradiol: a review of its pharmacodynamic and pharmacokinetic properties, and therapeutic efficacy in the treatment of menopausal complaints. *Drugs* 1990; **40:** 561–82.
6. Cheang A, *et al.* A risk-benefit appraisal of transdermal estradiol therapy. *Drug Safety* 1993; **9:** 365–79.
7. Jewelewicz R. New developments in topical estrogen therapy. *Fertil Steril* 1997; **67:** 1–12.

Gender reassignment. Oestrogens such as ethinyloestradiol and conjugated oestrogens are used in male-to-female transsexuals to develop and maintain secondary sexual characteristics. There is some evidence this use improves vascular function.[1]

1. New G, *et al.* Long-term estrogen therapy improves vascular function in male to female transsexuals. *J Am Coll Cardiol* 1997; **29:** 1437–44.

Growth disorders. A discussion on the effects of oestrogens on growth.[1] Early researchers found that supraphysiological doses of oestrogens inhibited somatic growth and from this experience oestrogens, such as ethinyloestradiol in oral doses of over 200 μg daily, came to be used for the treatment of acromegaly and for the arrest of growth in tall girls. One study has reported that treatment with conjugated oestrogens 7.5 to 11.25 mg daily resulted in average decrease of about 5 cm from final predicted height.[2] However, treatment with physiological doses causes growth stimulation, not inhibition, and such physiological doses have been used to promote growth in girls with conditions such as female hypogonadism and Turner's syndrome (see p.1240). Oestrogen therapy has occasionally been used in girls with delayed puberty (see p.1237).

1. Rosenfield RL. Toward optimal estrogen-replacement therapy. *N Engl J Med* 1983; **309:** 1120–1.
2. Weimann E, *et al.* Oestrogen treatment of constitutional tall stature: a risk-benefit ratio. *Arch Dis Child* 1998; **78:** 148–51.

Haemorrhagic disorders. Limited evidence supports the use of oestrogens in various bleeding disorders such as hereditary haemorrhagic telangiectasia, and those associated with chronic renal failure and gastro-intestinal vascular malformations. Some references to these uses are cited below.[1-3]

1. Vase P. Estrogen treatment of hereditary hemorrhagic telangiectasia. *Acta Med Scand* 1981; **209:** 393–6.
2. Livio M, *et al.* Conjugated estrogens for the management of bleeding associated with renal failure. *N Engl J Med* 1986; **315:** 731–5.
3. van Cutsem E, *et al.* Treatment of bleeding gastrointestinal vascular malformations with oestrogen-progesterone. *Lancet* 1990; **335:** 953–5.

Lactation inhibition. Synthetic oestrogens (e.g. quinestrol) and nonsteroidal oestrogens (e.g. stilboestrol) were formerly employed to suppress lactation (p.1240). However, such use is now considered inappropriate because of an increased risk of puerperal thrombo-embolism.

Premenstrual syndrome. Premenstrual syndrome (PMS) presents as a variable combination of psychological and somatic symptoms occurring during the luteal phase of the menstrual cycle, which resolve during, and immediately following, menstruation.[1,2] A further term, premenstrual dysphoric disorder, has been proposed to cover severe cyclical mood disorder that is functionally incapacitating.[2,3] Whereas about 20 to 30% of women have complaints that may be classified as PMS, only 3 to 5% meet criteria for premenstrual dysphoric disorder.[3] The term premenstrual tension (PMT) has sometimes been applied to the psychological symptoms. Many symptoms of PMS are the same as normal premenstrual symptoms, but are more severe. Premenstrual syndrome is not fully understood although it is thought to be due to the effects of the normal luteal phase release of progesterone on CNS neurotransmitter function; the syndrome is abolished by surgical or medical suppression of ovarian function. A recent study has shown that oestrogens, as well as progestogens, can induce symptoms.[4] Findings from another study demonstrated that women with PMS may metabolise progesterone differently to those without PMS.[5]

Initial management includes non-medical interventions such as education and support, counselling, stress management, and relaxation techniques; exercise, and caffeine and salt restriction are of unproven benefit. For patients with moderate to severe symptoms, a number of drugs have been tried with varying degrees of success; objective assessment of efficacy has been hampered by varying diagnostic criteria, a marked placebo response, and difficulties in obtaining reproducible responses. Treatment may be aimed at modifying the menstrual cycle or treating specific symptoms.[2]

In women with predominantly psychological symptoms, increasing evidence suggests that *selective serotonin reuptake inhibitors* (SSRIs) may be helpful.[1,2,6-8] Fluoxetine and sertraline have been shown in controlled trials to alleviate both the psychological and somatic symptoms in women with premenstrual syndrome. Buspirone, a serotonin receptor agonist, and clomipramine, a nonselective serotonin reuptake inhibitor, have also been tried with some success. The anxiolytic *alprazolam* has also been used, but use of this and other benzodiazepines should be restricted to the luteal phase of the cycle in selected patients to minimise the risk of dependence and tolerance.[2,6]

Abdominal bloating and swelling associated with PMS has traditionally been thought to be due to sodium and water retention. However, in most women with these symptoms there is no evidence of an increase in body-weight or in body sodium or total water, and use of *diuretics* is therefore not justified.[1] Nevertheless, in women with appreciable weight gain in the luteal phase diuretics may be useful.[1,6] Another symptom of PMS, cyclical mastalgia, is discussed on p.1443.

Pyridoxine has been tried on the basis that it is a cofactor in neurotransmitter (specifically serotonin) synthesis, and has been found to relieve depression induced by oral contraceptives in selected patients. However, its efficacy in premenstrual syndrome is equivocal, and high daily doses have been associated with neurotoxicity.[2,6]

Treatments that modify the menstrual cycle have often been used in women with PMS. In general, drugs with proven efficacy such as danazol, oestrogen implants, and gonadorelin analogues are reserved for women with severe PMS unresponsive to other treatments, because of their adverse effects. *Progestogen* therapy was once popular, but beneficial responses have not been universally achieved and the theory that progesterone was necessary to correct a hormone imbalance is now losing ground. Combined oral contraceptives have met with limited success[1,2,6,8] and in some women, PMS is caused or exacerbated by them. Young women with severe symptoms and women approaching the menopause may benefit from *oestrogen* delivered either as implants or transdermal patches. In women with a uterus, administration with a cyclical progestogen is required to avoid endometrial hyperplasia which unfortunately, may be associated with the return of symptoms, although they may be milder.[1,2] *Danazol* can be useful, but there is concern over its adverse effects on lipids during long-term use and over the risk of masculinisation of a female fetus should pregnancy occur. For patients with severe symptoms not amenable to other treatments, gonadorelin analogues such as *goserelin* can be used to eliminate ovarian function, 'add-back' treatment with oestrogen plus progestogen being given to protect against the side-effects of oestrogen deficiency including osteoporosis. This treatment is very effective for both physical and psychological symptoms. Short-term use (3 months) of a gonadorelin analogue alone has been used to confirm the diagnosis of PMS, or to predict the response to bilateral oophorectomy.[1,2] Immunological control using an analogue of *luteinising hormone-releasing hormone* (LHRH) to raise antibodies against natural LHRH and thus suppress ovarian function has also been proposed.

1. O'Brien PMS. Helping women with premenstrual syndrome. *Br Med J* 1993; **307:** 1471–5.
2. Severino SK, Moline ML. Premenstrual syndrome: identification and management. *Drugs* 1995; **49:** 71–82.
3. Gold JH. Premenstrual dysphoric disorder. *JAMA* 1997; **278:** 1024–5.
4. Schmidt PJ, *et al.* Differential behavioral effects of gonadal steroids in women with and those without premenstrual syndrome. *N Engl J Med* 1998; **338:** 209–16.
5. Rapkin AJ, *et al.* Progesterone metabolite allopregnanolone in women with premenstrual syndrome. *Obstet Gynecol* 1997; **90:** 709–14.
6. Mortola JF. A risk-benefit appraisal of drugs used in the management of premenstrual syndrome. *Drug Safety* 1994; **10:** 160–9.
7. Barnhart KT, *et al.* A clinician's guide to the premenstrual syndrome. *Med Clin North Am* 1995; **79:** 1457–72.
8. Steiner M. Premenstrual syndromes. *Annu Rev Med* 1997; **48:** 447–55.

Preparations

BP 1998: Estradiol Injection;
USP 23: Estradiol Cypionate Injection; Estradiol Injectable Suspension; Estradiol Pellets; Estradiol Tablets; Estradiol Vaginal Cream; Estradiol Valerate Injection.

Proprietary Preparations (details are given in Part 3)
Aust.: Climara; Estraderm; Estring; Estrofem; Linoladiol; Progynon; Progynova; Substitol; Systen; Vagifem; Zumenon; ***Austral.:*** Climara; Dermestril; Estraderm; Estring; Femtran; Menorest; Primogyn Depot; Progynova; Vagifem; ***Belg.:*** Dermestril; Estraderm; Estrofem; Oestrogel; Progynova; Systen; Vagifem; Zumenon; ***Canad.:*** Delestrogen; Estrace; Estraderm; Estring; Femogex; Vivelle; ***Fr.:*** Benzo-Gynoestryl; Estraderm; Estrofem; Menorest; Oesclim; Oestrodose; Oestrogel; Oromone; Progynova; Provames; Systen; ***Ger.:*** Dermestril; Estraderm; Estrifam; Estring; Evorel; Gynokadin; Linoladiol N; Menorest; Progynon Depot 10; Progynon Depot 100†; Progynon Depot 40†; Progynova; Tradella; Vagifem; ***Irl.:*** Climara; Divigel; Estraderm; Estrofem; Evorel; Fematab; Fematrix; Menorest; Oestrogel; Progynova†; Vagifem; ***Ital.:*** Benztrone; Climara; Dermestril; Epiestrol; Estraderm; Estroclim; Menorest; Progynon Depot; Progynova; Systen; Vagifem; ***Mon.:*** Estreva; ***Neth.:*** Climara; Dermestril; Dimenformon†; Estraderm; Estring; Estrofem; Meno-implant; Menorest; Progynon Depot 10; Progynon Depot 100†; Progynova; Systen; Vagifem; Zumenon; ***Norw.:*** Estraderm; Estring; Evorel; Menorest; Progynova; ***S.Afr.:*** Climara; Estraderm; Estring; Estro-Pause; Estrofem; Evorel; Femigel; Menorest; Primogyn Depot; Progynova; Vagifem; ***Spain:*** Absorlent; Esotran; Estraderm; Evopad; Menorest; Oestraclin; Progynon Depot; Progynova; ***Swed.:*** Climara; Divigel; Estraderm; Evorel; Femanest; FemSeven; Menorest; Oestring; Progynon; Vagifem; ***Switz.:*** Climara; Estraderm; Estring; Estrofem N; Menorest; Oestrogel; Progynon Depot 10; Progynon Depot 100†; Progynova; Systen; Vagifem; ***UK:*** Climaval; Dermestril; Elleste-Solo; Estraderm; Estring; Evorel; Fematrix; FemSeven; Menorest; Oestradiol Implants; Oestrogel; Progynova; Sandrena; Vagifem; Zumenon; ***USA:*** Alora; Climara; Deladiol†; Delestrogen; depGynogen; Depogen; Dioval; Dura-Estrin†; Duragen†; E-Cypionate†; Esclim; Estra-D†; Estra-L; Estrace; Estraderm; Estring; Estro-Cyp; Estroject†; FemPatch; Gynogen†; Menaval†; Valergen†; Vivelle.

Multi-ingredient: ***Aust.:*** Climen; Cyclacur; Dilena†; Estandron; Estracomb; Estragest; Filena; Gravibinon; Gynodian; Ichth-Oestren; Kliogest; Ostrolut; Primodian Depot; Tri-Filena; Trisequens; ***Austral.:*** Climen; Divina; Estracombi; Estrapak; Femoston; Kliogest; Primodian Depot†; Trisequens; ***Belg.:*** Climen; Cyclocur; Dimenformon; Diviva; Estracombi; Femoston; Kliogest; Trisequens; ***Canad.:*** Climacteron; Estracomb; Neo-Pause†; ***Fr.:*** Climene; Divina; Fadiamone; Gravibinan†; Kliogest; TOM†; Trisequens; ***Ger.:*** Acetonal Vaginale†; Aknefug-Emulsion N; Alpicort F; Climen; Crinohermal fem neu; Cyclo-Menorette; Cyclo-Progynova; CycloOstrogynal; Ell-Cranell; Estracomb; Fissan-Brustwarzensalbe†; Gravibinon; Gynodian Depot; Jephagynon; Klimonorm; Kliogest N; Linoladiol-H N; Lynandron†; Malun†; NeoOstrogynal; NeyNormin "N" (Revitorgan-Dilutionen "N" Nr. 65); Osmil; Ostronara; Ovatest†; Primodian Depot†; Primosiston†; Procyclo; Sebohermal†; Sisare; Syngynon; Trisequens; ***Irl.:*** Cyclo-Progynova†; Estracombi; Estrapak; Kliogest; Nuvelle; Tridestra; Trisequens; ***Ital.:*** Ablacton†; Biormon; Climen; Clym-Depositum†; Cyclacur†; Duo-Ormogyn; Estandron†; Estiamen B†; Estiamen†; Estracomb; Filena; Gravibinan; Gynodian Depot; Kliogest; Menovis; Nuvelle; Primodian Depot†; Trisequens; ***Neth.:*** Climene; Cyclocur; Divina; Estracomb; Femoston; Kliogest; Trisequens; Zumeston†; ***Norw.:*** Cyclabil; Estracomb; Kliogest; Trisekvens; ***S.Afr.:*** Climen; Divina; Estracombi; Kliogest; Mixogen; Postoval; Primodian Depot; Trisequens; Trivina; ***Spain:*** Absorlent Plus; Dinatrofon†; Estandron Prolongado†; Estracomb; Gynodian Depot; Progyluton; Topasel; ***Swed.:*** Cyclabil; Divina; Estracomb; Femanor; Femasekvens; Kliogest; Trisekvens; Trivina; ***Switz.:*** Alpicort F; Climen†; Cyclacur; Estandron Prolongatum†; Estracomb; Gravibinon†; Gynodian Depot; Kliogest; Linoladiol; Primodian Depot†; Primosiston; Triaval; Trisequens; Tyliculine†; ***UK:*** Climagest; Climesse; Cyclo-Progynova 1 mg; Cyclo-Progynova 2 mg; Elleste Duet Conti; Elleste-Duet; Estracombi; Estrapak; Evorel Conti; Evorel Sequi; Evorel.Pak; Femapak; Femoston; Hormonin; Kliofem; Kliovance; Nuvelle; Nuvelle TS; Tridestra; Trisequens; ***USA:*** Andro/Fem†; Deladumone†; depAndrogyn; Depo-Testadiol; Depotestogen; Duo-Cyp; Duratestrin; Estra-Testrin†; T-E Cypionate†; Test-Estro; Testaval 90/4†; Valertest.

Oestriol (9090-l)

Oestriol *(BAN)*.

Estriol; Follicular Hormone Hydrate; Theelol. Estra-1,3,5(10)-triene-3,16α,17β-triol.

$C_{18}H_{24}O_3$ = 288.4.

CAS — 50-27-1.

Pharmacopoeias. In *Eur.* (see p.viii), *Jpn,* and *US.*

A white or practically white, odourless, crystalline powder. Practically **insoluble** in water; sparingly soluble in alcohol; soluble in acetone, in chloroform, in dioxan, in ether, and in vegetable oils. **Store** in airtight containers.

Oestriol Sodium Succinate (10345-s)

Oestriol Sodium Succinate *(BAN)*.

Disodium 3-hydroxyestra-1,3,5(10)-triene-16α,17β-diyl disuccinate.

$C_{26}H_{30}Na_2O_9$ = 532.5.

CAS — 113-22-4.

Oestriol Succinate (10068-b)

Oestriol Succinate *(BAN)*.

Estriol Succinate *(rINN)*. 3-Hydroxyestra-1,3,5(10)-triene-16α,17β-diyl di(hydrogen succinate).

$C_{26}H_{32}O_9$ = 488.5.

CAS — 514-68-1.

Oestriol is a naturally occurring oestrogen with actions and uses similar to those described for oestradiol (p.1455). It is claimed to have only a mild proliferative effect on the endometrium.

It is used for menopausal hormone replacement therapy (HRT) (see p.1434). When oestrogens are administered to women with a uterus, a progestogen is required, particularly if used long-term. For short-term treatment, doses by mouth have been 500 μg to 3 mg daily given for one month followed by 500 μg to 1 mg daily. Oestriol has also been given in combination with other natural oestrogens such as oestradiol and oestrone (p.1458); usual doses of oestriol have ranged from about 250 μg to 2 mg daily. It has also been administered intravaginally for the short-term treatment of menopausal atrophic vaginitis as a 0.01% or 0.1% cream or as pessaries containing 500 μg.

Oestriol succinate has also been given by mouth in the treatment of menopausal disorders. The sodium succinate salt has been administered parenterally in the treatment of haemorrhage and thrombocytopenia.

Preparations

Proprietary Preparations (details are given in Part 3)
Aust.: Ortho-Gynest; Ovestin; Styptanon; ***Austral.:*** Ovestin; ***Belg.:*** Aacifemine; Ortho-Gynest; ***Fr.:*** Ovestin†; Physiogine; Synapause†; Trophicreme; ***Ger.:*** Cordes Estriol; Gynasan; Hormomed†; Klimax-E†; OeKolp; Oestrilir N†; Oestro-Gynaedron M; Orgastyptin†; Ortho-Gynest; Ovestin; Ovo-Vinces; Synapause E; Synapause†; Vago-med†; Xapro; ***Irl.:*** Ortho-Gynest; Ovestin; ***Ital.:*** Colpogyn; Ortho Gynest Depot; Ovestin; ***Jpn:*** Estriel†; ***Neth.:*** Ortho-Gynest†; Ovestin†; Synapause-E$_3$; ***Norw.:*** Ovesterin; ***S.Afr.:*** Synapause; ***Spain:*** Ovestinon; Synapause; ***Swed.:*** Ovesterin; Triovex†; ***Switz.:*** Klimadoral†; Oestro-Gynaedron Nouveau; Ortho-Gynest; Ovestin; Styptanon†; ***UK:*** Ortho-Gynest; Ovestin.

Multi-ingredient: ***Aust.:*** Gynoflor; ***Belg.:*** Gynoflor; ***Fr.:*** Trophigil; ***Ger.:*** Cyclo-Menorette; CycloOstrogynal; Gynoflor; NeoOstrogynal; OestroTricho N†; Oestrugol N; ***Ital.:*** Estiamen B†; Estiamen†; ***Switz.:*** Gynoflor E; Trisequens; ***UK:*** Hormonin.

Conjugated Oestrogens (9091-y)

Conjugated Estrogens.

Pharmacopoeias. In *US.*

A mixture of sodium oestrone sulphate and sodium equilin sulphate, derived wholly or in part from equine urine or synthetically from oestrone and equilin. It contains other oestrogenic substances of the type excreted by pregnant mares. The USP substance contains 52.5 to 61.5% of sodium oestrone sulphate and 22.5 to 30.5% of sodium equilin sulphate; the total of the two combined should comprise not less than 79.5% of the labelled content of conjugated oestrogens. The USP also states that it should contain, as sulphate conjugates, 13.5 to 19.5% of 17α-dihydroequilin, 2.5 to 9.5% of 17α-oestradiol, and 0.5 to 4.0% of 17β-dihydroequilin, relative to the labelled content of conjugated oestrogens.

If it is obtained from natural sources it is a buff-coloured amorphous powder which is odourless or has a slight characteristic odour; the synthetic form is a white to light buff-coloured crystalline or amorphous powder, odourless or with a slight odour. **Store** in airtight containers.

Adverse Effects and Precautions

As for oestrogens in general (see Oestradiol, p.1455). See also under Hormone Replacement Therapy, p.1435.

Effects on the cardiovascular system. Treatment of men with a previous myocardial infarction with conjugated oestrogens 5 mg daily in the USA Coronary Drug Project was discontinued because of a higher incidence of subsequent coronary events.[1] Moreover, treatment with the lower 2.5 mg dose was later also discontinued because of suggestions of adverse trends including a greater incidence of venous thrombo-embolism.[2] However, observational studies of menopausal hormone replacement therapy indicate that in postmenopausal women there is a reduction in risk of coronary heart disease (see p.1436).

1. Coronary Drug Project Research Group. The Coronary Drug Project: initial findings leading to modifications of its research protocol. *JAMA* 1970; **214:** 1303–13.
2. Coronary Drug Project Research Group. The Coronary Drug Project: findings leading to discontinuation of the 2.5-mg/day estrogen group. *JAMA* 1973; **226:** 652–7.

Effects on the gallbladder. Analysis of data obtained during the Coronary Drug Project indicated a significant increase in the development of gallbladder disease among men treated with conjugated oestrogens 2.5 and 5 mg daily, compared with those treated with placebo.[1]

1. The Coronary Drug Project Research Group. Gallbladder disease as a side effect of drugs influencing lipid metabolism: experience in the Coronary Drug Project. *N Engl J Med* 1977; **296:** 1185–90.

Effects on the nervous system. Reversible chorea developed in a 57-year-old woman receiving conjugated oestrogens and norgestrel;[1] the woman had a history of migraine and Sydenham's chorea.

1. Steiger MJ, Quinn NP. Hormone replacement therapy induced chorea. *Br Med J* 1991; **302:** 762.

Hypersensitivity. A report of an anaphylactic reaction following the intravenous administration of conjugated oestrogens.[1]

1. Searcy CJ, *et al.* Anaphylactic reaction to intravenous conjugated estrogens. *Clin Pharm* 1987; **6:** 74–6.

Interactions

See under Hormone Replacement Therapy, p.1437.

Pharmacokinetics

Orally administered conjugated oestrogens are hydrolysed by enzymes present in the intestine that remove the sulphate group and allow absorption of the unconjugated oestrogen. Metabolism occurs primarily in the liver; there is some enterohepatic recycling (see also p.1455).

Uses and Administration

Conjugated oestrogens have actions and uses similar to those described for oestradiol (see p.1456).

When used as menopausal hormone replacement therapy (p.1437) doses of 0.3 to 1.25 mg daily are given by mouth either cyclically or continuously, in conjunction with a progestogen either cyclically or continuously in women with a uterus. Topical vaginal therapy may be used specifically for menopausal atrophic vaginitis; 0.5 to 2 g of a 0.0625% cream may be employed daily for 3 weeks of a 4-week cycle. If used long-term in a woman with a uterus, cyclical progestogen is required.

Doses of 1.25 mg daily by mouth are used as replacement therapy for primary ovarian failure and doses of 2.5 to 7.5 mg daily administered on a cyclical basis are used for female hypogonadism.

For the palliative treatment of prostatic carcinoma (p.491), a dose of 1.25 to 2.5 mg three times daily has been employed. A dose of 10 mg three times daily for at least 3 months has been used for palliative treatment of breast carcinoma in postmenopausal women (p.485).

Abnormal uterine bleeding has been treated acutely by giving 25 mg of conjugated oestrogens by slow intravenous injection, repeated if required after 6 to 12 hours; the intramuscular route has also been used.

Haemorrhagic disorders. Some references to the use of high-dose intravenous or oral conjugated oestrogens in the management of haemorrhagic disorders (p.707).[1-5]

1. Liu YK, *et al.* Treatment of uraemic bleeding with conjugated oestrogen. *Lancet* 1984; **ii:** 887–90.
2. Livio M, *et al.* Conjugated estrogens for the management of bleeding associated with renal failure. *N Engl J Med* 1986; **315:** 731–5.
3. Bronner MH, *et al.* Estrogen-progesterone therapy for bleeding gastrointestinal telangiectasias in chronic renal failure: an uncontrolled trial. *Ann Intern Med* 1986; **105:** 371–4.
4. Seth S, Geier TM. Use of conjugated estrogens to control gastrointestinal tract bleeding in two patients with chronic renal failure. *Clin Pharm* 1988; **7:** 906–9.
5. Shemin D, *et al.* Oral estrogens decrease bleeding time and improve clinical bleeding in patients with renal failure. *Am J Med* 1990; **89:** 436–40.

Preparations

USP 23: Conjugated Estrogens Tablets.

Proprietary Preparations (details are given in Part 3)
Aust.: Conjugen; Oestro-Feminal; Premarin; ***Austral.:*** Premarin; ***Belg.:*** Premarin; ***Canad.:*** CES; Congest; Premarin; ***Fr.:*** Premarin; ***Ger.:*** Climarest; Conjugen; Femavit; Oestrofeminal; Presomen spezial†; Presomen†; Transannon; ***Irl.:*** Premarin; ***Ital.:*** Emopremarin; Premarin; Prempak; ***Neth.:*** Dagynil; Premarin; ***S.Afr.:*** Premarin; ***Spain:*** Carentil; Equin; Premarin; ***Swed.:*** Premarina; ***Switz.:*** Conjugen; Premarin; ***UK:*** Premarin; ***USA:*** Mannest†; Premarin.

Multi-ingredient: ***Aust.:*** Cyclo-Premarin-MPA; Cyclo-Premella; Perennia; Premarin compositum; Premarin Plus†; Premarin-MPA; Premella; Sequennia; ***Austral.:*** Menoprem; Provelle; ***Belg.:*** Premplus; ***Irl.:*** Premique Cycle; Prempak-C; ***Ital.:*** Premelle S; ***Neth.:*** Premarin Plus; Premelle; Premelle Cycle; Prempak-C; ***S.Afr.:*** PMB†; Prempak N; ***Swed.:*** Premelle; Prempac Sekvens; ***Switz.:*** Cyclo-Premella; Premarin Plus; Premella; Transannon; ***UK:*** Premique Cycle; Prempak-C; ***USA:*** PMB; Premarin with Methyltestosterone; Premphase; Prempro.

Esterified Oestrogens (10069-v)

Esterified Estrogens.

Pharmacopoeias. In *US.*

A mixture of the sodium salts of the sulphate esters of the oestrogenic substances, principally oestrone. It contains 75 to 85% of sodium oestrone sulphate and 6 to 15% of sodium equilin sulphate, in such a proportion that the total of these two components is not less than 90%.

A white or buff-coloured amorphous powder; odourless or with a slight characteristic odour. **Store** in airtight containers.

Esterified oestrogens have actions and uses similar to those described for oestradiol (see p.1455). They are used for the same purposes (principally menopausal hormone replacement therapy) and in a similar dosage by mouth as conjugated oestrogens (see above).

Preparations

USP 23: Esterified Estrogens Tablets.

Proprietary Preparations (details are given in Part 3)
Canad.: Neo-Estrone†; ***Switz.:*** Oestro-Feminal; ***USA:*** Estratab; Menest.

Multi-ingredient: ***USA:*** Estratest; Menogen; Menrium†.

Oestrone (9092-j)

Oestrone *(BAN).*

Estrone *(rINN)*; Follicular Hormone; Folliculin; Ketohydroxyoestrin. 3-Hydroxyestra-1,3,5(10)-trien-17-one.

$C_{18}H_{22}O_2$ = 270.4.

CAS — 53-16-7.

Pharmacopoeias. In *Aust., It.,* and *US.*

Odourless, small white crystals or white to creamy-white crystalline powder. Practically **insoluble** in water; soluble 1 in 250 of alcohol and 1 in 110 of chloroform at 15°; soluble 1 in 50 of boiling alcohol, 1 in 33 of boiling acetone, and 1 in 80 of boiling chloroform; soluble 1 in 50 of acetone at 50°; soluble in dioxan and in vegetable oils; slightly soluble in solutions of fixed alkali hydroxides. **Store** in airtight containers. Protect from light.

Oestrone is a naturally occurring oestrogen with actions and uses similar to those described for oestradiol (see p.1455).

For menopausal hormone replacement therapy (see p.1434) oestrone has been given by mouth at a dose of 1.4 to 2.8 mg daily in a cyclical or continuous regimen, as a combination product with oestradiol and oestriol. Oestrone has also been administered by intramuscular injection in oily solutions and aqueous suspensions; the usual dose range for menopausal symptoms is 100 to 500 μg given 2 or 3 times a week cyclically or continuously. When used specifically for menopausal atrophic vaginitis, oestrone has been administered vaginally. If used in women with a uterus, oestrone by any route should be given with a progestogen.

Preparations

USP 23: Estrone Injectable Suspension; Estrone Injection.

Proprietary Preparations (details are given in Part 3)
Austral.: Kolpon†; ***Canad.:*** Oestrilin; ***USA:*** Aquest; Kestrone; Theelin†; Wehgen†.

Multi-ingredient: ***Fr.:*** Fadiamone; Synergon; ***Ger.:*** Ovowop†; ***Ital.:*** Estiamen B†; Estiamen†; ***Spain:*** Cicatral; Grietalgen; Grietalgen Hidrocort; Risunal B†; ***UK:*** Hormonin.

Ormeloxifene (18929-v)

Ormeloxifene *(rINN).*

Centchroman. *trans*-1-{2-[4-(3,4-Dihydro-7-methoxy-2,2-dimethyl-3-phenyl-2*H*-1-benzopyran-4-yl)phenoxy]ethyl}pyrrolidine.

$C_{30}H_{35}NO_3$ = 457.6.

CAS — 31477-60-8.

Ormeloxifene is a nonsteroidal benzopyran derivative with anti-oestrogenic and antiprogestogenic actions, which has been administered weekly as an oral contraceptive. Ormeloxifene has also been investigated in the management of osteoporosis. The *l*-isomer, levormeloxifene, has also been investigated.

References.[1,2]

1. Kamboj VP, *et al.* New products: centchroman. *Drugs Today* 1992; **28:** 227–32.
2. Paliwal JK, *et al.* Excretion of centchroman in breast milk. *Br J Clin Pharmacol* 1994; **38:** 485–6.

Ovary Extracts (11486-q)

Ovarian Extracts.

Ovary extracts of animal origin (usually porcine or bovine) have been used for a variety of disorders including gynaecological and menopausal disorders. They are often used in preparations containing other mammalian tissue extracts.

Preparations

Proprietary Preparations (details are given in Part 3)
Aust.: Ovibion; ***Fr.:*** Crinex†; Gynecrise†; ***Ger.:*** Glanoide†; Ovibion†.

Multi-ingredient: ***Ger.:*** Intradermi N.

Oxabolone Cypionate (13050-a)

Oxabolone Cipionate *(rINN)*; FI-5852. 4,17β-Dihydroxyestr-4-en-3-one 17-(β-cyclopentylpropionate).

$C_{26}H_{38}O_4$ = 414.6.

CAS — 1254-35-9.

Oxabolone cypionate has anabolic properties.

Preparations

Proprietary Preparations (details are given in Part 3)
Ger.: Steranabol-Depot†; ***Ital.:*** Steranabol Ritardo.

Oxandrolone (9093-z)

Oxandrolone *(BAN, USAN, rINN).*

NSC-67068; SC-11585. 17β-Hydroxy-17α-methyl-2-oxa-5α-androstan-3-one.

$C_{19}H_{30}O_3$ = 306.4.

CAS — 53-39-4.

Pharmacopoeias. In *US*.

A white odourless crystalline powder. **Soluble** 1 in 5200 of water, 1 in 57 of alcohol, 1 in 69 of acetone, 1 in less than 5 of chloroform, and 1 in 860 of ether. **Protect** from light.

Adverse Effects and Precautions

As for androgens and anabolic steroids in general (see Testosterone, p.1464). As with other 17α-alkylated compounds, oxandrolone may cause hepatotoxicity, and liver function should be monitored. It should be avoided if hepatic impairment is severe.

Pharmacokinetics

Oxandrolone is rapidly absorbed from the gastro-intestinal tract. It is excreted mainly in the urine as metabolites and unchanged oxandrolone. A small amount is excreted in the faeces.

Investigations in 6 healthy male subjects demonstrated that following oral ingestion of oxandrolone 10 mg there was rapid absorption resulting in a maximum plasma concentration of 417 ng per mL between 30 and 90 minutes.[1] Plasma concentrations then declined in 2 phases: from 90 minutes to 4 hours with a half-life of about 33 minutes; from 4 to 48 hours the half-life was about 9 hours. Only 2.8% of the dose was excreted in the faeces whereas 60.4% was excreted in the urine within 96 hours (43.6% in the first 24 hours). Unchanged oxandrolone in the urine accounted for 28.7% of the administered dose.

1. Karim A, *et al.* Oxandrolone disposition and metabolism in man. *Clin Pharmacol Ther* 1973; **14:** 862–9.

Uses and Administration

Oxandrolone has anabolic and androgenic properties (see Testosterone, p.1465) and is given in doses of 2.5 to 20 mg daily by mouth; the usual anabolic dose is 5 to 10 mg daily in divided doses for 2 to 4 weeks. In the promotion of growth in constitutional delayed growth and puberty in boys, daily doses of up to 0.1 mg per kg body-weight have been given (see also below). Courses of treatment are short (generally about 3 to 4 months) to avoid the risk of epiphyseal closure.

Oxandrolone has also been used in treating osteoporosis, breast cancer, anaemias, and hypogonadism and has been tried in patients with alcoholic hepatitis. It is under investigation for the treatment of patients with muscular dystrophy.

Alcoholic hepatitis. Reference to the benefits of oxandrolone as an adjunct to nutritional support in severe alcoholic liver disease and moderate malnutrition.[1]

1. Mendenhall CL, *et al.* A study of oral nutritional support with oxandrolone in malnourished patients with alcoholic, hepatitis: results of a Department of Veterans Affairs Cooperative Study. *Hepatology* 1993; **17:** 564–76.

Growth retardation. A beneficial effect of oxandrolone on growth rate in *boys* with constitutional delay of growth and puberty (p.1237) has been shown in various studies,[1-5] two of which[2,5] were placebo-controlled. Doses used have included 1.25 or 2.5 mg daily[1-3] and 0.05 or 0.1 mg per kg body-weight daily,[4,5] generally for 3 to 12 months. Although a slight advance in bone age has been noted,[1,4,5] final predicted height[5] and actual adult height[3] was not compromised by oxandrolone therapy. Oxandrolone did not affect the rate of pubertal progression and as the aim of such therapy is primarily to relieve psychosocial difficulties associated with short stature and sexual immaturity, it is not clear that it achieves this.[5]

Oxandrolone is also under investigation for the promotion of growth in *girls* with Turner's syndrome (p.1240) in daily doses of 0.05 to 0.125 mg per kg.

1. Stanhope R, Brook CGD. Oxandrolone in low dose for constitutional delay of growth and puberty in boys. *Arch Dis Child* 1985; **60:** 379–81.
2. Stanhope R, *et al.* Double blind placebo controlled trial of low dose oxandrolone in the treatment of boys with constitutional delay of growth and puberty. *Arch Dis Child* 1988; **63:** 501–5.
3. Tse W-Y, *et al.* Long-term outcome of oxandrolone treatment in boys with constitutional delay of growth and puberty. *J Pediatr* 1990; **117:** 588–91.
4. Papadimitriou A, *et al.* Treatment of constitutional growth delay in prepubertal boys with a prolonged course of low dose oxandrolone. *Arch Dis Child* 1991; **66:** 841–3.
5. Wilson DM, *et al.* Oxandrolone therapy in constitutionally delayed growth and puberty. *Pediatrics* 1995; **96:** 1095–1100.

Preparations

USP 23: Oxandrolone Tablets.

Proprietary Preparations (details are given in Part 3)
Austral.: Lonavar; ***USA:*** Oxandrin.

Oxymetholone (9095-k)

Oxymetholone *(BAN, USAN, rINN)*.

CI-406; HMD. 17β-Hydroxy-2-hydroxymethylene-17α-methyl-5α-androstan-3-one.

$C_{21}H_{32}O_3$ = 332.5.

CAS — 434-07-1.

Pharmacopoeias. In Br., Jpn, and US.

A white to creamy-white, odourless or almost odourless, crystalline powder. Practically **insoluble** in water; soluble 1 in 40 of alcohol, 1 in 5 of chloroform, 1 in 82 of ether, and 1 in 14 of dioxan. **Protect** from light. Avoid contact with ferrous metals.

Adverse Effects and Precautions

As for androgens and anabolic steroids in general (see Testosterone, p.1464).

Liver disturbances and jaundice are common with normal doses and hepatic neoplasms have also been reported (see below). Liver function should be monitored during therapy. As with other 17α-alkylated compounds, oxymetholone should probably be avoided in patients with liver impairment, and certainly if this is severe.

Effects on the blood. Leukaemia developed in 4 patients given oxymetholone for aplastic anaemia.[1] Although a causal relationship had not been established,[1] other cases have been cited.[2] It has also been pointed out that of patients who present with aplastic anaemia, 1 to 5% actually have leukaemia.[3]

1. Delamore IW, Geary CG. Aplastic anaemia, acute myeloblastic leukaemia, and oxymetholone. *Br Med J* 1971; **2:** 743–5.
2. Ginsburg AD. Oxymetholone and hematologic disease. *Ann Intern Med* 1973; **79:** 914.
3. Camitta BM, *et al.* Aplastic anemia (first of two parts): pathogenesis, diagnosis, treatment, and prognosis. *N Engl J Med* 1982; **306:** 645–52.

Effects on carbohydrate metabolism. Pronounced hyperglucagonaemia developed in 6 patients receiving oxymetholone.[1]

1. Williams G, *et al.* Severe hyperglucagonaemia during treatment with oxymetholone. *Br Med J* 1986; **292:** 1637–8.

Effects on the liver. Reports of peliosis hepatis[1-4] and various liver tumours[4-11] associated with oxymetholone.

1. Bagheri SA, Boyer JL. Peliosis hepatis associated with androgenic-anabolic steroid therapy: a severe form of hepatic injury. *Ann Intern Med* 1974; **81:** 610–18.
2. Groos G, *et al.* Peliosis hepatis after long-term administration of oxymetholone. *Lancet* 1974; **i:** 874.
3. McDonald EC, Speicher CE. Peliosis hepatis associated with administration of oxymetholone. *JAMA* 1978; **240:** 243–4.
4. Bernstein MS, *et al.* Hepatoma and peliosis hepatis developing in a patient with Fanconi's anemia. *N Engl J Med* 1971; **284:** 1135–6.
5. Johnson FL, *et al.* Association of androgenic-anabolic steroid therapy with development of hepatocellular carcinoma. *Lancet* 1972; **ii:** 1273–6.
6. Henderson JT, *et al.* Androgenic-anabolic steroid therapy and hepatocellular carcinoma. *Lancet* 1973; **i:** 934.
7. Farrell GC, *et al.* Androgen-induced hepatoma. *Lancet* 1975; **i:** 430–2.
8. Anthony PP. Hepatoma associated with androgenic steroids. *Lancet* 1975; **i:** 685–6.
9. Bruguera M. Hepatoma associated with androgenic steroids. *Lancet* 1975; **i:** 1295.
10. Lesna M, *et al.* Liver nodules and androgens. *Lancet* 1976; **i:** 1124.
11. Mokrohisky ST, *et al.* Fulminant hepatic neoplasia after androgen therapy. *N Engl J Med* 1977; **296:** 1411–12.

Effects on the nervous system. Toxic confusional state and choreiform movements developed in an elderly man given oxymetholone 200 to 300 mg daily.[1]

1. Tilzey A, *et al.* Toxic confusional state and choreiform movements after treatment with anabolic steroids. *Br Med J* 1981; **283:** 349–50.

Uses and Administration

Oxymetholone has anabolic and androgenic properties (see Testosterone, p.1465). It has been used mainly in the treatment of anaemias such as aplastic anaemia at a usual dosage by mouth of 1 to 5 mg per kg body-weight daily. Treatment for 3 to 6 months has been suggested, with the drug either withdrawn gradually on remission or reduced to an appropriate maintenance dose.

Anaemia. There have been mixed results[1-5] with oxymetholone in the treatment of aplastic anaemia (p.701); generally, the response and survival rates have been disappointing.

1. Davis S, Rubin AD. Treatment and prognosis in aplastic anaemia. *Lancet* 1972; **i:** 871–3.
2. Mir MA, Delamore IW. Oxymetholone in aplastic anaemia. *Postgrad Med J* 1974; **50:** 166–71.
3. Mir MA, Geary CG. Aplastic anaemia: an analysis of 174 patients. *Postgrad Med J* 1980; **56:** 322–9.
4. Camitta BM, *et al.* A prospective study of androgens and bone marrow transplantation for treatment of severe aplastic anemia. *Blood* 1979; **53:** 504–14.
5. Webb DKH, *et al.* Acquired aplastic anaemia: still a serious disease. *Arch Dis Child* 1991; **66:** 858–61.

Preparations

BP 1998: Oxymetholone Tablets;
USP 23: Oxymetholone Tablets.

Proprietary Preparations (details are given in Part 3)
Austral.: Adroyd†; Anapolon†; ***Belg.:*** Synasteron†; ***Canad.:*** Anapolon†; ***S.Afr.:*** Anapolon†; ***UK:*** Anapolon; ***USA:*** Anadrol.

Polyestradiol Phosphate (9097-t)

Polyestradiol Phosphate *(BAN, rINN)*.

Leo-114; Polyoestradiol Phosphate. A water-soluble polymeric ester of oestradiol and phosphoric acid with a molecular weight of about 26 000.

CAS — 28014-46-2.

Adverse Effects and Precautions

As for oestrogens in general (see Oestradiol, p.1455). Pain may occur at the site of injection, and mepivacaine is included in some preparations to minimise this.

Pharmacokinetics

Following intramuscular injection polyestradiol phosphate is released slowly into the bloodstream where it is slowly metabolised to oestradiol.

Uses and Administration

Polyestradiol phosphate is a polymer of oestradiol (see p.1455) which has a prolonged duration of action, and is used in the treatment of prostatic carcinoma (p.491). It has been given by deep intramuscular injection in initial doses of 80 to 160 mg every 4 weeks for 2 to 3 months, reduced to 40 to 80 mg every 4 weeks for maintenance.

Preparations

Proprietary Preparations (details are given in Part 3)
Aust.: Estradurin; ***Belg.:*** Estradurine; ***Ger.:*** Estradurin; ***Ital.:*** Estradurin†; ***Neth.:*** Estradurin; ***Norw.:*** Estradurin; ***Spain:*** Estradurin; ***Swed.:*** Estradurin; ***Switz.:*** Estradurin; ***UK:*** Estradurin†; ***USA:*** Estradurin†.

Polyoestriol Phosphate (10067-m)

Polyestriol Phosphate.

CAS — 37452-43-0.

Polyoestriol phosphate is a polymer of oestriol (see p.1457) and phosphoric acid and has the properties of oestrogens in general (see Oestradiol, p.1455). It has been given by intramuscular injection in the treatment of menopausal disorders in doses of 80 mg every 4 to 8 weeks.

Preparations

Proprietary Preparations (details are given in Part 3)
Aust.: Triodurin.

Multi-ingredient: ***Swed.:*** Triodurin†.

Prasterone (9036-g)

Prasterone *(rINN)*.

Dehydroandrosterone; Dehydroepiandrosterone; Dehydroisoandrosterone; DHEA. 3β-Hydroxyandrost-5-en-17-one.

$C_{19}H_{28}O_2$ = 288.4.

CAS — 53-43-0.

Prasterone Enanthate (11513-k)

Prasterone Enantate *(rINNM)*. 3β-Hydroxyandrost-5-en-17-one heptanoate.

$C_{26}H_{40}O_3$ = 400.6.

CAS — 23983-43-9.

Prasterone Sodium Sulphate (14252-y)

Prasterone Sodium Sulphate *(rINNM)*.

Dehydroepiandrosterone Sulphate Sodium; DHA-S; DHEAS; Prasterone Sodium Sulfate. 3β-Hydroxyandrost-5-en-17-one hydrogen sulphate sodium.

$C_{19}H_{27}NaO_5S$ = 390.5.

CAS — 651-48-9 (prasterone sulphate); 1099-87-2 (prasterone sodium sulphate).

Pharmacopoeias. In Jpn.

Prasterone is a naturally occurring adrenal androgen that is a precursor of androgens and oestrogens. Prasterone enanthate is given by intramuscular depot injection as menopausal hormone replacement therapy in association with oestradiol valerate. Prasterone is also being investigated in systemic lupus erythematosus, and the sodium sulphate is under investigation for the treatment of burns.

AIDS. Plasma concentrations of prasterone are reported to be abnormally low in patients with AIDS, and it has been suggested that prasterone administration might be of benefit; however controlled studies are lacking.[1]

1. Centurelli MA, *et al.* The role of dehydroepiandrosterone in AIDS. *Ann Pharmacother* 1997; **31:** 639–42.

Replacement therapy. There has been much speculation about the physiological role and importance of prasterone, which is the most abundant steroid hormone in the circulation. Ebeling and Koivisto[1] have proposed that it has both oestrogenic and androgenic properties, depending on the hormonal milieu, and suggested that in men its oestrogenic properties might predominate and protect against cardiovascular disease. Herbert has pointed out in a short review[2] that blood concentrations of the sulphate conjugate, very high at about 20 years, gradually decline with age and that there is some suggestion that certain age-related diseases are linked to this decline; such a hypothesis offers the prospect that replacement therapy with prasterone might alleviate some of the problems of ageing. However, there is insufficient evidence of safety and efficacy to recommend such use.[3] A review[4] of the use of prasterone as a 'food supplement' noted that although it was being taken in the belief that it could reverse some of the effects of ageing there was no good evidence of this. Various androgenic effects, including hirsutism and voice changes, have been reported in women taking prasterone and there is a theoretical possibility that it might promote growth of hormone-sensitive tumours in both sexes. It was concluded that patients would be well advised not to take prasterone in this way.[4]

1. Ebeling P, Koivisto VA. Physiological importance of dehydroepiandrosterone. *Lancet* 1994; **343:** 1479–81.
2. Herbert J. The age of dehydroepiandrosterone. *Lancet* 1995; **345:** 1193–4. Correction. *ibid.*; 1648.
3. Weksler ME. Hormone replacement for men. *Br Med J* 1996; **312:** 859–60.
4. Anonymous. Dehydroepiandrosterone (DHEA). *Med Lett Drugs Ther* 1996; **38:** 91–2.

Systemic lupus erythematosus. Symptomatic improvement was seen in 8 of 10 women with systemic lupus erythematosus (p.1029) who received prasterone 200 mg daily by mouth for several months.[1] Improvement permitted a reduction in the dosage of concomitant corticosteroids. Similar findings were reported in a small 3-month placebo-controlled trial,[2] but have not been confirmed by preliminary results of much larger study.

1. van Vollenhoven RF, *et al.* An open study of dehydroepiandrosterone in systemic lupus erythematosus. *Arthritis Rheum* 1994; **37:** 1305–10.
2. van Vollenhoven RF, *et al.* Dehydroepiandrosterone in systemic lupus erythematosus. *Arthritis Rheum* 1995; **38:** 1826–31.

Preparations

Proprietary Preparations (details are given in Part 3)
Ital.: Astenile†.

Multi-ingredient: ***Aust.:*** Gynodian; ***Ger.:*** Gynodian Depot; ***Ital.:*** Gynodian Depot; Sinsurrene; ***Spain:*** Gynodian Depot; ***Switz.:*** Gynodian Depot.

Progesterone (9098-x)

Progesterone *(BAN, rINN)*.

Corpus Luteum Hormone; Luteal Hormone; Luteine; Luteohormone; NSC-9704; Pregnenedione; Progesteronum. Pregn-4-ene-3,20-dione.

$C_{21}H_{30}O_2$ = 314.5.

CAS — 57-83-0.

Pharmacopoeias. In Chin., Eur. (see p.viii), Int., Jpn, Pol., and US.

Colourless crystals or a white or creamy-white, odourless, crystalline powder. Practically **insoluble** in water; soluble in alcohol; freely soluble in dehydrated alcohol; soluble to sparingly soluble in acetone; sparingly soluble in ether and in fatty oils; soluble in dioxan. **Store** in airtight containers. Protect from light.

Adverse Effects

Progesterone and the progestogens may cause gastro-intestinal disturbances, changes in appetite or weight, fluid retention, oedema, acne, chloasma (melasma), allergic skin rashes, urticaria, mental depression, breast changes including discomfort or occasionally gynaecomastia, changes in libido, hair loss, hirsutism, fatigue, drowsiness or insomnia, fever, headache, premenstrual syndrome-like symptoms, and altered menstrual cycles or irregular menstrual bleeding. Anaphylaxis or anaphylactoid reactions may occur rarely. Alterations in the serum lipid profile may occur, and rarely alterations in liver-function tests and jaundice.

Adverse effects vary depending on the dose and type of progestogen. For example, androgenic effects such as acne and hirsutism are more likely to occur with nortestosterone derivatives such as norethisterone and norgestrel. These derivatives may also be more likely to adversely affect serum lipids. Conversely, adverse effects on serum lipids appear less likely with gestodene and desogestrel, but these 2 drugs have been associated with a higher incidence of thrombo-embolism than norethisterone and norgestrel when used in combined oral contraceptives (see p.1430). High doses of progestogens such as those used in treating cancer have also been associated with thrombo-embolism. For a discussion of the effect of progestogens on the cardiovascular risk profile of menopausal hormone replacement therapy see p.1436. Breakthrough uterine bleeding is more common with oral progestogen-only contraceptives than when progestogens are used for menstrual irregularities or as part of menopausal hormone replacement therapy.

Some progestogens when given during pregnancy have been reported to cause virilisation of a female fetus. This appears to have been associated with those progestogens with more pronounced androgenic activity such as norethisterone; the natural progestogenic hormone progesterone and its derivatives such as dydrogesterone and medroxyprogesterone do not appear to have been associated with such effects.

For the adverse effects of progestogens when administered either alone or with oestrogens as contraceptives, see p.1426. For those of menopausal hormone replacement therapy, see p.1435.

Effects on the skin. A case report and discussion of progesterone-induced urticaria.[1]

1. Wilkinson SM, *et al.* Progesterone-induced urticaria—need it be autoimmune? *Br J Dermatol* 1995; **133:** 792–4.

Precautions

Progesterone and the progestogens should be used with caution in patients with cardiovascular or renal impairment, diabetes mellitus, asthma, epilepsy, and migraine, or other conditions which may be aggravated by fluid retention. They should also be used with care in persons with a history of mental depression.

Progesterone and the progestogens should not be given to patients with undiagnosed vaginal bleeding, nor to those with a history or current high risk of arterial disease and should generally be avoided in hepatic impairment, especially if severe. Unless progestogens are being used as part of the management of breast carcinoma they should not be given to patients with this condition.

Although progestogens have been given as hormonal support during early pregnancy such use is not now generally advised and many authorities now recommend that progestogens should not be used at all in early pregnancy. Some, however, allow the use of a progesterone-type progestogen for women who are progesterone-deficient. Such use may prevent spontaneous evacuation of a dead fetus, therefore careful monitoring of pregnancy is required. Progestogens should not be used diagnostically for pregnancy testing and should not be given in missed or incomplete abortion.

For precautions to be observed when progestogens are used as contraceptives, see p.1431. For those to be observed when progestogens are used in preparations for menopausal hormone replacement therapy, see p.1437.

Abuse. A case report of abuse of and dependency on progesterone.[1]

1. Keefe DL, Sarrel P. Dependency on progesterone in woman with self-diagnosed premenstrual syndrome. *Lancet* 1996; **347:** 1182.

Porphyria. Progesterone and progestogens have been associated with acute attacks of porphyria and are considered unsafe in patients with acute porphyria[1] (but medroxyprogesterone has been used with buserelin to suppress premenstrual exacerbations of porphyria, see p.1243).

1. Moore MR, McColl KEL. *Porphyria: drug lists.* Glasgow: Porphyria Research Unit, University of Glasgow, 1991.

Pregnancy. In Hungary where 30% of all pregnant women were given hormonal support therapy with progestogens during the early 1980s, a case-control study suggested that there was a causal relationship between such treatment and hypospadias in their offspring.[1] Reports of abnormalities in infants following exposure *in utero* to progestogens have included hypospadias[2] with norethisterone and hydroxyprogesterone; other genito-urinary anomalies with dydrogesterone[3] and hydroxyprogesterone;[4] tetralogy of Fallot[5] and adrenocortical carcinoma[6] with hydroxyprogesterone; fetal masculinisation[7] with norethisterone, norethynodrel, and ethisterone; and meningomyelocele or hydrocephalus[8] with norethisterone and ethisterone. For further details see under Pregnancy in the individual monographs. For the effects on the fetus when progestogens are used as contraceptives, see p.1432. For the risk of ectopic pregnancy with progestogen-only contraceptives, see p.1428.

1. Czeizel A. Increasing trends in congenital malformations of male external genitalia. *Lancet* 1985; **i:** 462–3.
2. Aarskog D. Clinical and cytogenetic studies in hypospadias. *Acta Paediatr Scand* 1970; (suppl 203): 1–62.
3. Roberts IF, West RJ. Teratogenesis and maternal progesterone. *Lancet* 1977; **ii:** 982.
4. Evans ANW, *et al.* The ingestion by pregnant women of substances toxic to the foetus. *Practitioner* 1980; **224:** 315–19.
5. Heinonen OP, *et al.* Cardiovascular birth defects and antenatal exposure to female sex hormones. *N Engl J Med* 1977; **296:** 67–70.
6. Mann JR, *et al.* Transplacental carcinogenesis (adrenocortical carcinoma) associated with hydroxyprogesterone hexanoate. *Lancet* 1983; **ii:** 580.
7. Wilkins L. Masculinization of female fetus due to use of orally given progestins. *JAMA* 1960; **172:** 1028–32.
8. Gal I, *et al.* Hormonal pregnancy tests and congenital malformation. *Nature* 1967; **216:** 83.

Veterinary use. An expert committee of the FAO and WHO considered it unnecessary to establish an acceptable daily intake or acceptable residue level in food for endogenous hormones such as progesterone.[1] Residues resulting from the use of progesterone as a growth promoter in accordance with good animal husbandry practice are unlikely to pose a hazard to human health. However, it should be noted that, in the European Union the use of steroidal hormones such as progestogens in veterinary practice is restricted, and their use as growth promoters is banned.

1. FAO/WHO. Evaluation of certain veterinary drug residues in food: thirty-second report of the joint FAO/WHO expert committee on food additives. *WHO Tech Rep Ser 763* 1988.

Interactions

Enzyme-inducing drugs such as carbamazepine, griseofulvin, phenobarbitone, phenytoin, and rifampicin may enhance the clearance of progesterone and the progestogens. These interactions are likely to reduce the efficacy of progestogen-only contraceptives (see p.1432), and additional or alternative contraceptive measures are recommended.

Aminoglutethimide markedly reduces the plasma concentrations of medroxyprogesterone acetate and megestrol, possibly through a hepatic enzyme-inducing effect; an increase in progestogen dose is likely to be required.

Since progesterone and other progestogens can influence diabetic control an adjustment in antidiabetic dosage could be required. Progestogens may inhibit cyclosporin metabolism leading to increased plasma-cyclosporin concentrations and a risk of toxicity (see p.522).

Pharmacokinetics

Progesterone has a short elimination half-life and undergoes extensive first-pass hepatic metabolism when given by mouth; oral bioavailability is very low although it may be increased somewhat by administration in an oily vehicle and by micronisation. It is absorbed when administered buccally, rectally, or vaginally, and rapidly absorbed from the site of an oily intramuscular injection.

Various derivatives have been produced to extend the duration of action and to improve oral activity. Esters of progesterone derivatives such as hydroxyprogesterone hexanoate are used intramuscularly, and megestrol acetate is orally active. The ester medroxyprogesterone acetate is used orally and parenterally. 19-Nortestosterone progestogens have good oral activity because the 17-ethinyl substituent slows hepatic metabolism.

Progesterone and the progestogens are highly protein bound; progesterone is bound to albumin and corticosteroid binding globulin; esters such as medroxyprogesterone acetate are principally bound to albumin; and 19-nortestosterone analogues are bound to sex-steroid binding globulin and albumin. Progesterone is metabolised in the liver to various metabolites including pregnanediol, which are excreted in the urine as sulphate and glucuronide conjugates. Similarly, progestogens undergo hepatic metabolism to various conjugates, which are excreted in the urine.

Reviews.

1. Kuhl H. Comparative pharmacology of newer progestogens. *Drugs* 1996; **51:** 188–215.
2. Stanczyk FZ. Structure-function relationships, metabolism, pharmacokinetics and potency of progestins. *Drugs Today* 1996; **32** (suppl H): 1–14.

Uses and Administration

Progesterone is a natural hormone whereas progestogens are synthetic compounds, derived from progesterone or 19-nortestosterone, with actions similar to those of progesterone (for further details, see p.1426).

Progestogens derived from 19-nortestosterone are used as **hormonal contraceptives** (see p.1433), either alone or combined with an oestrogen. The progesterone derivative medroxyprogesterone acetate is also used, and progesterone itself has been used.

Both progesterone and 19-nortestosterone derivatives are used in combination with oestrogens for **menopausal hormone replacement therapy** (see p.1437) to reduce the increased risk of endometrial hyperplasia and carcinoma which occurs when unopposed long-term oestrogen therapy is employed. Progesterone itself is under investigation for such use.

Progestogens, and sometimes progesterone, may be used in **menstrual disorders** such as dysmenorrhoea (p.9) and menorrhagia associated with dysfunctional uterine bleeding (below). Progestogens may also be used in the management of endometriosis (p.1442). Although progestogens and progesterone have been used for the management of the premenstrual syndrome, such a practice is of debatable value (p.1456).

Progestogens may be valuable in **endometrial cancer** (p.487) and have been tried in some other malignancies. The progestogens typically used for malignant disease include medroxyprogesterone acetate, megestrol, and norethisterone. Some progestogens such as megestrol and medroxyprogesterone are used for the **cachexia** or wasting associated with severe illness including cancer and AIDS.

Progestogens have been widely advocated for either the prevention of **habitual abortion** or the treatment of threatened abortion. However, many authorities now consider that there is little evidence of any benefit from such a practice and recommend against the use of progestogens in early pregnancy, with exception of the use of progesterone or a progesterone derivative in women who are progesterone deficient (see also under Precautions above).

USES AND ADMINISTRATION OF PROGESTERONE. Progesterone is usually administered as an oily intramuscular injection or as pessaries or suppositories. An oral micronised preparation of progesterone is under investigation for a variety of disorders, as is a vaginal gel.

In dysfunctional uterine bleeding 5 to 10 mg daily of progesterone is normally given by intramuscular injection for about 5 to 10 days before the anticipated onset of menstruation. A similar regimen has been used in the treatment of amenorrhoea.

In women with a history of habitual abortion and proven progesterone deficiency, twice weekly intramuscular injection (increased to daily if necessary) of 25 to 100 mg of progesterone from approximately day 15 of the pregnancy until 8 to 16 weeks has been used. A similar schedule has been used in *in vitro* fertilisation or gamete intra-fallopian transfer techniques with treatment beginning on the day of transfer of embryo or gametes. The dose may be increased to 200 mg daily if necessary.

Progesterone may be given vaginally or rectally in doses of 200 mg daily to 400 mg twice daily for the management of the premenstrual syndrome. Treatment usually starts on day 12 to 14 of the menstrual cycle and continues until the onset of menstruation. Similar intravaginal or intrarectal doses have also been used in the treatment of puerperal (post-natal) depression.

A progesterone-releasing intra-uterine device has also been used as a hormonal contraceptive; the device contains 38 mg of progesterone and is effective for up to 12 months.

Menorrhagia. Menorrhagia, or excessive menstrual bleeding, is usually defined as a blood loss exceeding 80 mL per menstrual period,[1-4] compared with a normal loss of about 30 mL. However, many women consider losses below 80 mL to be excessive particularly if 'flooding' occurs. Although not life-threatening, menorrhagia can lead to iron deficiency anaemia as well as considerably impairing quality of life. Menorrhagia may be a symptom of pelvic disorders such as fibroids or endometriosis, or of systemic disorders such as hypothyroidism or clotting defects, or be associated with the use of copper intra-uterine devices.[2,4] However, most commonly it is associated with dysfunctional uterine bleeding; a term used to denote frequent, prolonged or heavy uterine bleeding for which no specific cause is found.[3] In this situation, it may be referred to as essential,[2] idiopathic,[4] or primary menorrhagia.

Dysfunctional uterine bleeding is thought to be associated with abnormalities of prostaglandin production, and treatment with *NSAIDs* such as ibuprofen, mefenamic acid, or naproxen is often employed. These reduce menstrual blood loss by about 30%, and relieve dysmenorrhoea (p.9). There does not appear to be any evidence to suggest that any one NSAID is more effective than any other. An alternative in women who require contraception is a *combined oral contraceptive* which appears to be as effective as an NSAID.[2,4]

In women who are anaemic or who do not respond to NSAIDs or oral contraceptives, or for whom these are not appropriate, the antifibrinolytic *tranexamic acid* may be tried.[2-4] When administered during menstruation, it reduces blood loss by about 50%. However, gastro-intestinal adverse effects are common, and (as with combined oral contraceptives) it is contra-indicated in women with thrombo-embolic disorders. *Ethamsylate* has been reported to have similar efficacy to an NSAID in 1 study,[5] but to be ineffective in another.[6]

More recently, a *levonorgestrel-containing intra-uterine device* has been shown to be very effective in reducing menstrual blood loss,[7,8] and to be an alternative to hysterectomy in menorrhagia.[9] It has been suggested that this may become the preferred long-term medical treatment for menorrhagia.[4]

Danazol is also effective, but has significant adverse effects and treatment is usually limited to 3 to 6 months.[3] Traditional therapy with *progestogens* is of limited efficacy in menorrhagia occurring during ovulatory cycles. However it is suitable for anovulatory bleeding;[3] norethisterone, medroxyprogesterone, or dydrogesterone have been suggested for such use. *Gonadorelin analogues* are effective for menorrhagia associated with fibroids (p.1248), but can only be used short term because of the resultant ovarian suppression.[3,4]

In patients who fail to respond to drug treatment, or in whom such therapy is inappropriate, various *surgical options* exist. Conservative surgical techniques, where the endometrium is ablated or resected, are increasingly being used, and appear to be an effective alternative to hysterectomy.[10,11] Hysterectomy is the ultimate therapy, but is associated with significant morbidity; given that menorrhagia is not life-threatening some consider that hysterectomy has been overused.[2]

1. Macdonald R. Modern treatment of menorrhagia. *Br J Obstet Gynaecol* 1990; **97:** 3–7.
2. van Eijkeren MA, *et al.* Menorrhagia: current drug treatment concepts. *Drugs* 1992; **43:** 201–9.
3. West CP. Dysfunctional uterine bleeding. *Prescribers' J* 1994; **34:** 215–20.
4. Wood CE. Menorrhagia: a clinical update. *Med J Aust* 1996; **165:** 510–14.
5. Chamberlain G, *et al.* A comparative study of ethamsylate and mefenamic acid in dysfunctional uterine bleeding. *Br J Obstet Gynaecol* 1991; **98:** 707–11.
6. Bonnar J, Sheppard BL. Treatment of menorrhagia during menstruation: randomised controlled trial of ethamsylate, mefenamic acid, and tranexamic acid. *Br Med J* 1996; **313:** 579–82.
7. Andersson JK, Rybo G. Levonorgestrel-releasing intrauterine device in the treatment of menorrhagia. *Br J Obstet Gynaecol* 1990; **97:** 690–4.
8. Milsom I, *et al.* A comparison of flurbiprofen, tranexamic acid, and a levonorgestrel-releasing intrauterine contraceptive device in the treatment of idiopathic menorrhagia. *Am J Obstet Gynecol* 1991; **164:** 879–83.
9. Lähteenmäki P, *et al.* Open randomised study of use of levonorgestrel releasing intrauterine system as alternative to hysterectomy. *Br Med J* 1998; **316:** 1122–6.
10. Coulter A. Managing menorrhagia with endometrial resection. *Lancet* 1993; **341:** 1185–6.
11. Carlson KJ, Schiff I. Alternatives to hysterectomy for menorrhagia. *N Engl J Med* 1996; **335:** 198–9.

Premenstrual syndrome. Progestogen therapy was once popular for premenstrual syndrome, but beneficial responses have not been universally achieved and the theory that progesterone was necessary to correct a hormone imbalance is now losing ground (see p.1456). A double-blind, placebo-controlled crossover study[1] involving 168 women showed that progesterone 0.4 or 0.8 g daily by the vaginal route did not significantly improve symptoms of the premenstrual syndrome. However, the view has been expressed[2] that since absorption of progesterone from the vagina or rectum may vary between patients, the dose and frequency of administration needs to be individualised and that if the response to treatment is inadequate the intramuscular route should be tried. A more recent study found oral micronised progesterone, in an initial dose of 1.2 g daily in divided doses, increased as required to 3.6 g daily, to be no better than placebo in the management of severe premenstrual syndrome.[3]

1. Freeman E, *et al.* Ineffectiveness of progesterone suppository treatment for premenstrual syndrome. *JAMA* 1990; **264:** 349–53.
2. Dalton K. Treating the premenstrual syndrome. *Br Med J* 1988; **297:** 490.
3. Freeman EW, *et al.* A double-blind trial of oral progesterone, alprazolam, and placebo in treatment of severe premenstrual syndrome. *JAMA* 1995; **274:** 51–7.

Preparations

BP 1998: Progesterone Injection;
USP 23: Progesterone Injectable Suspension; Progesterone Injection; Progesterone Intrauterine Contraceptive System.

Proprietary Preparations (details are given in Part 3)
Austral.: Proluton; ***Belg.:*** Progestogel; Utrogestan; ***Canad.:*** Gesterol; Prometrium; ***Fr.:*** Progestasert; Progestogel; Progestosol; Utrogestan; ***Ger.:*** Progestogel; ***Irl.:*** Utrogestan; ***Ital.:*** Esolut; Progestogel; Progestol; Proluton†; Prontogest; ***Neth.:*** Progestan; ***S.Afr.:*** Cyclogest; ***Spain:*** Cutifitol; Progeffik; Progestogel; Utrogestan; ***Switz.:*** Progestogel; Progestosol†; Utrogestan; ***UK:*** Crinone; Cyclogest; Gestone; ***USA:*** Crinone; Progestasert; Prometrium.

Multi-ingredient: ***Fr.:*** Synergon; Trophigil; ***Ger.:*** Jephagynon; ***Ital.:*** Biormon; Duo-Ormogyn; Lutex-E†; Menovis; ***Mon.:*** Tocogestan; ***Spain:*** Dinatrofon†; Risunal B†.

Proligestone (8219-v)

Proligestone *(BAN, rINN).*

14a,17α-Propylidene dioxypregn-4-ene-3,20-dione.

$C_{24}H_{34}O_4$ = 386.5.

CAS — 23873-85-0.

Proligestone is a progestogen (see Progesterone, p.1459) used in veterinary medicine.

Promegestone (3871-c)

Promegestone *(rINN).*

R-5020. 17α-Methyl-17-propionylestra-4,9-dien-3-one.

$C_{22}H_{30}O_2$ = 326.5.

CAS — 34184-77-5.

Promegestone is a progestogen structurally related to progesterone (p.1459). It has been given by mouth on a cyclical basis, in doses of 125 to 500 µg daily, in the treatment of menstrual disorders and mastalgia, and as the progestogen component of menopausal hormone replacement therapy.

Preparations

Proprietary Preparations (details are given in Part 3)
Fr.: Surgestone.

Promestriene (13176-s)

Promestriene *(rINN).*

17β-Methoxy-3-propoxyestra-1,3,5(10)-triene.

$C_{22}H_{32}O_2$ = 328.5.

CAS — 39219-28-8.

Promestriene is a derivative of oestradiol (see p.1455) that has been used topically in menopausal atrophic vaginitis, and in seborrhoea.

Preparations

Proprietary Preparations (details are given in Part 3)
Ital.: Colpotrophine; ***Mon.:*** Colpotrophine; Delipoderm; ***Spain:*** Colpotrofin; Delipoderm; ***Switz.:*** Colpotrophine.

Multi-ingredient: ***Mon.:*** Colposeptine; ***Spain:*** Colposeptina†.

Pygeum Africanum (13542-z)

African Prune.

An extract of the bark of the African prune tree, *Pygeum africanum* (Rosaceae), is used in the treatment of benign prostatic hyperplasia (p.1446). Like some other phytotherapies for this disorder, it appears to contain various sitosterols. A usual dosage is 100 mg daily by mouth.

References.

1. Andro M-C, Riffaud J-P. Pygeum africanum extract for the treatment of patients with benign prostatic hyperplasia: a review of 25 years of published experience. *Curr Ther Res* 1995; **56:** 796–817.
2. Buck AC. Phytotherapy for the prostate. *Br J Urol* 1996; **78:** 325–36.

Preparations

Proprietary Preparations (details are given in Part 3)
Aust.: Tadenan; ***Fr.:*** Tadenan; ***Ital.:*** Pigenil; Tadenan; ***Switz.:*** Tadenan.

Multi-ingredient: ***Aust.:*** Prostatonin; ***Switz.:*** Prostatonin.

Quinestradol (9100-r)

Quinestradol *(BAN, rINN).*

Oestriol 3-Cyclopentyl Ether; Quinestradiol. 3-Cyclopentyloxyestra-1,3,5(10)-triene-16α,17β-diol.

$C_{23}H_{32}O_3$ = 356.5.

CAS — 1169-79-5.

Quinestradol is a synthetic oestrogen that has been given by mouth for the treatment of menopausal vaginal symptoms in a dosage of 1 to 2 mg daily.

Preparations

Proprietary Preparations (details are given in Part 3)
Ital.: Colpovis.

Quinestrol (9101-f)

Quinestrol *(BAN, USAN, rINN).*

17α-Ethinyloestradiol 3-cyclopentyl Ether; W-3566. 3-Cyclopentyloxy-19-nor-17α-pregna-1,3,5(10)-trien-20-yn-17β-ol.

$C_{25}H_{32}O_2$ = 364.5.

CAS — 152-43-2.

Quinestrol is a synthetic oestrogen that has a prolonged duration of action and is metabolised to ethinyloestradiol (p.1445). Quinestrol has been given by mouth for the treatment of menopausal symptoms and other conditions arising from oestrogen deficiency.

Preparations

Proprietary Preparations (details are given in Part 3)
Ger.: Estrovis†; ***USA:*** Estrovis†.

Raloxifene Hydrochloride (19377-x)

Raloxifene Hydrochloride *(BANM, USAN, rINNM).*

Keoxifene Hydrochloride; LY-139481 (keoxifene); LY-156758 (raloxifene). 6-Hydroxy-2-(*p*-hydroxyphenyl)benzo[*b*]thien-3-yl-*p*-(2-piperidinoethoxy)phenyl ketone hydrochloride.

$C_{28}H_{27}NO_4S,HCl$ = 510.0.

CAS — 84449-90-1 (raloxifene); 82640-04-8 (raloxifene hydrochloride).

Adverse Effects

The most common adverse effects of raloxifene are hot flushes and leg cramps. Raloxifene is associated with an increased risk of venous thrombo-embolic events, particularly during the first 4 months of treatment. Peripheral oedema has also been reported.

Precautions

Raloxifene should be avoided in women with active venous thrombo-embolism, or a history of thrombo-embolic disorders. It should be discontinued at least 72 hours prior to periods of prolonged immobilisation, such as post-surgical recovery. Raloxifene should be used with caution in women with congestive heart failure or active malignancy, who may be at increased risk of thrombo-embolic disease. It should be used with caution in hepatic impairment; the UK manufacturers recommend it be avoided in hepatic and severe renal impairment.

Raloxifene had adverse effects in *animal* teratogenicity studies and should not be used in women who are or may become pregnant. It should not be given to women with undiagnosed vaginal bleeding.

Interactions

Cholestyramine reduces the absorption and enterohepatic recycling of raloxifene, and should not be given concomitantly. Raloxifene may decrease the efficacy of warfarin.

Pharmacokinetics

Raloxifene is absorbed from the gastro-intestinal tract and undergoes extensive first-pass hepatic metabolism to the glucuronide conjugates. It is highly bound to plasma proteins, principally albumin and α_1-acid glycoprotein. Raloxifene undergoes enterohepatic recycling, and has a half-life of about 27 hours. It is excreted almost entirely in the faeces.

Uses and Administration

Raloxifene is a benzothiophene nonsteroidal antioestrogen related to clomiphene and tamoxifen. It is used, in doses of 60 mg daily by mouth, for the prevention of postmenopausal osteoporosis (p.731).

It is also under investigation for the prophylaxis of breast cancer (p.486).

References.

1. Fuchs-Young R, *et al.* Raloxifene is a tissue-selective agonist/antagonist that functions through the estrogen receptor. *Ann N Y Acad Sci* 1995; **761:** 355–60.
2. Draper MW, *et al.* A controlled trial of raloxifene (LY139481) HCl: impact on bone turnover and serum lipid profile in healthy postmenopausal women. *J Bone Miner Res* 1996; **11:** 835–42.
3. Delmas PD, *et al.* Effects of raloxifene on bone mineral density, serum cholesterol concentrations, and uterine endometrium in postmenopausal women. *N Engl J Med* 1997; **337:** 1641–7.
4. Anonymous. Raloxifene for postmenopausal osteoporosis. *Med Lett Drugs Ther* 1998; **40:** 29–30. Correction. *ibid.*; 54.
5. Walsh BW, *et al.* Effects of raloxifene on serum lipids and coagulation factors in healthy postmenopausal women. *JAMA* 1998; **279:** 1445–51.
6. Balfour JA, Goa KL. Raloxifene. *Drugs Aging* 1998; **12:** 335–41.

Preparations

Proprietary Preparations (details are given in Part 3)
UK: Evista; ***USA:*** Evista.

Saw Palmetto (921-s)

Serenoa repens; *Serenoa serrulatum*; *Sabal serrulata*; *Brahea serrulata*; American Dwarf Palm; PA-109.

Pharmacopoeias. In *USNF.*

The dried fruit of the American dwarf palm, *Serenoa repens* (Arecaceae). **Store** in airtight containers. Protect from light.

Saw palmetto contains various steroidal compounds with anti-androgenic and oestrogenic activities, one of which is sitosterol (p.1279). Saw palmetto is used for the treatment of men with benign prostatic hyperplasia. Preparations of alcoholic or lipophilic extracts have typically been administered in doses of 160 mg twice daily, or 320 mg once daily, by mouth.

Adverse effects. EFFECTS ON THE LIVER. Cholestatic hepatitis occurred in a man who took a herbal preparation containing saw palmetto for 2 weeks to treat nocturia and hesitancy.[1]

1. Hamid S, *et al.* Protracted cholestatic hepatitis after the use of Prostata. *Ann Intern Med* 1997; **127:** 169–70.

Uses. BENIGN PROSTATIC HYPERPLASIA. A lipid hexane extract of saw palmetto has been shown to be generally superior to placebo,[1,2] and of similar efficacy to finasteride[3] in the treatment of benign prostatic hyperplasia (p.1446).

1. Champault G, *et al.* A double-blind trial of an extract of the plant Serenoa repens in benign prostatic hyperplasia. *Br J Clin Pharmacol* 1984; **18:** 461.
2. Plosker GL, Brogden RN. Serenoa repens (Permixon): a review of its pharmacology and therapeutic efficacy in benign prostatic hyperplasia. *Drugs Aging* 1996; **9:** 379–95.
3. Carraro J-C, *et al.* Comparison of phytotherapy (Permixon) with finasteride in the treatment of benign prostate hyperplasia: a randomized international study of 1,098 patients. *Prostate* 1996; **29:** 231–40.

Preparations

Proprietary Preparations (details are given in Part 3)
Aust.: Permixon; Talso; ***Austral.:*** Prosta; ***Belg.:*** Prosta-Urgenin; Prostaserene; ***Fr.:*** Capistan; Permixon; ***Ger.:*** Eviprostat-S; Horphagen uno†; Prosta-Urgenin; Prostamol uno†; Prostess; Remigeron†; Remiprostan Uno; Sita; Steiprostat; Strogen; Talso; ***Ital.:*** Permixon; Proser; Rilaprost; Saba; Sere-Mit; Serpens; ***Spain:*** Permixon; Sereprostat; ***Switz.:*** Permixon Novum; Prosta-Urgenine; Prostasan N; ***UK:*** Sabalin.

Multi-ingredient: ***Aust.:*** Prostagutt; Spasmo-Urgenin; Urgenin; ***Austral.:*** Serenoa Complex; Urgenin; Urinase; ***Belg.:*** Urgenin; ***Fr.:*** Sabal; ***Ger.:*** Cefasabal; Nephroselect M; Prosta Fink N; Prostagutt Tropfen†; Prostatin N Liquidum†; Protitis†; Saburlan†; Salus Kurbis-Tonikum Compositum†; Serrulatum†; Urgenin†; ***S.Afr.:*** Spasmo-Urgenin; ***Spain:*** Fagolitos Renal†; Neo Urgenin; Spasmo-Urgenin; Spasmo-Urgenin Rectal†; Urgenin; ***Switz.:*** Phytomed Prosta; Prosta-Caps Chassot N; Prosta-Caps Fink; Prostagutt-F; Urgenine; ***UK:*** Antiglan; Regina Royal Concorde; Serenoa-C; Strength.

Stanolone (9103-n)

Stanolone *(BAN).*

Androstanolone *(rINN)*; Dihydrotestosterone. 17β-Hydroxy-5α-androstan-3-one.

$C_{19}H_{30}O_2$ = 290.4.

CAS — 521-18-6.

Stanolone (dihydrotestosterone) is formed naturally in the body from testosterone (p.1464) by the action of 5α-reductase, and is more active than the parent compound. It has anabolic and androgenic properties and is applied topically in the form of a gel for male hypogonadism and for vulvar lichen sclerosus. It has been used as an eye ointment for corneal disorders.

Lichen sclerosus. Reference to the use of topical stanolone in vulvar lichen sclerosus.[1] For mention of the use of corticosteroids in this condition see p.1024.

1. Paslin D. Treatment of lichen sclerosus with topical dihydrotestosterone. *Obstet Gynecol* 1991; **78:** 1046–9.

Preparations

Proprietary Preparations (details are given in Part 3)
Belg.: Andractim; ***Fr.:*** Andractim; ***Spain:*** Gelovit.

Multi-ingredient: ***Ger.:*** Ophtovitol†.

Stanozolol (9104-h)

Stanozolol *(BAN, USAN, rINN).*

Androstanazole; Methylstanazole; NSC-43193; Win-14833. 17α-Methyl-2′*H*-5α-androst-2-eno[3,2-c]pyrazol-17β-ol.

$C_{21}H_{32}N_2O$ = 328.5.

CAS — 10418-03-8.

Pharmacopoeias. In *Br., It.,* and *US.*

A white or almost white, odourless crystalline powder. There are 2 forms; needles melt at about 155° and prisms at about 235°. Practically **insoluble** in water; soluble 1 in 41 of alcohol, 1 in 74 of chloroform, and 1 in 370 of ether; soluble in dimethylformamide; slightly soluble in acetone and ethyl acetate. **Store** in airtight containers. Protect from light.

Adverse Effects and Precautions

As for androgens and anabolic steroids in general (see Testosterone, p.1464). As with other 17α-alkylated compounds stanozolol may produce hepatotoxicity, and liver function should be monitored. It is probably best avoided in patients with hepatic impairment, and certainly if this is severe.

Because of its androgenic effects some recommend that it should not be used to treat hereditary angioedema in premenopausal women except in life-threatening situations.

Effects on the liver. Some reports of jaundice associated with stanozolol.[1,2]

1. Slater SD, *et al.* Jaundice induced by stanozolol hypersensitivity. *Postgrad Med J* 1976; **52:** 229–32.
2. Evely RS, *et al.* Severe cholestasis associated with stanozolol. *Br Med J* 1987; **294:** 612–13.

Effects on the nervous system. Benign intracranial hypertension developed in an elderly woman receiving stanozolol; CSF pressure returned to normal after stanozolol was discontinued.[1]

1. Tully MP, *et al.* Intracranial hypertension associated with stanozolol. *DICP Ann Pharmacother* 1990; **24:** 1234.

Interactions

As mentioned under Testosterone, p.1465, anabolic steroids may enhance the activity of a number of drugs. For the effect of stanozolol on some anticoagulants, see p.969.

Uses and Administration

Stanozolol has anabolic and androgenic properties (see Testosterone, p.1465). It is used in the treatment of vascular manifestations of Behçet's syndrome in usual doses of 10 mg daily by mouth. In the management of hereditary angioedema, an initial dose of 2.5 to 10 mg daily by mouth is given to prevent attacks. The dosage may then be reduced, according to the patient's response; maintenance doses of 2 mg daily or on alternate days, or 2.5 mg three times weekly have been used successfully. A suggested initial daily dose by mouth for children is 2.5 mg for those aged 1 to 6 years and 2.5 to 5 mg for those aged 6 to 12 years. However, in the USA doses of 1 mg daily for children under 6 years and up to 2 mg in those aged 6 to 12 years have been suggested. As with other anabolic steroids, stanozolol has been used for breast cancer in postmenopausal women, and for anaemias, osteoporosis, and catabolic disorders.

Stanozolol has also been given by intramuscular injection in doses of 50 mg every 2 or 3 weeks.

Hereditary angioedema. Stanozolol has been used successfully to prevent attacks of hereditary angioedema (p.729).

References.

1. Sheffer AL, *et al.* Hereditary angioedema: a decade of management with stanozolol. *J Allergy Clin Immunol* 1987; **80:** 855–60.

Turner's syndrome. Growth hormone has been suggested to improve the short stature in patients with Turner's syndrome (p.1240) and combination with an anabolic steroid such as stanozolol can improve the response, but there is now some doubt as to whether any marked increase in final height is produced.

Vascular disorders. Stanozolol is used in the treatment of vascular manifestations of Behçet's syndrome (p.1018). It has also been reported to promote fibrinolysis in vascular disorders, including long-standing liposclerosis of the leg,[1-3] necrobiosis lipoidica,[4] Raynaud's syndrome,[5,6] systemic sclerosis,[6] idiopathic recurrent superficial thrombophlebitis,[7] leg ulcers due to cryofibrinogenaemia,[8] and venous ulceration.[9-11] Most of these studies were noncomparative and in small numbers of patients, and results have been variable.

1. Browse NL, *et al.* Treatment of liposclerosis of the leg by fibrinolytic enhancement: a preliminary report. *Br Med J* 1977; **2:** 434–5.
2. Burnand K, *et al.* Venous lipodermatosclerosis: treatment by fibrinolytic enhancement and elastic compression. *Br Med J* 1980; **280:** 7–11.
3. Muston HL. Treatment of liposclerosis. *Br Med J* 1980; **280:** 254–5 [criticism].
4. Rhodes EL. Fibrinolytic agents in the treatment of necrobiosis lipoidica. *Br J Dermatol* 1976; **95:** 673–4.
5. Jarrett PEM, *et al.* Treatment of Raynaud's phenomenon by fibrinolytic enhancement. *Br Med J* 1978; **2:** 523–5.
6. Jayson MIV, *et al.* A controlled study of stanozolol in primary Raynaud's phenomenon and systemic sclerosis. *Ann Rheum Dis* 1991; **50:** 41–7.
7. Jarrett PEM, *et al.* Idiopathic recurrent superficial thrombophlebitis: treatment with fibrinolytic enhancement. *Br Med J* 1977; **1:** 933–4.
8. Falanga V, *et al.* Stanozolol in treatment of leg ulcers due to cryofibrinogenaemia. *Lancet* 1991; **338:** 347–8.
9. Anonymous. Does stanozolol prevent venous ulceration? *Drug Ther Bull* 1985; **23:** 91–2.
10. Browse NL, Burnand KG. Getting the balance right. *Br Med J* 1986; **292:** 825 [criticism].
11. Herxheimer A. Getting the balance right. *Br Med J* 1986; **292:** 1014 [reply].

Preparations

BP 1998: Stanozolol Tablets;
USP 23: Stanozolol Tablets.

Proprietary Preparations (details are given in Part 3)
Belg.: Stromba; Strombaject; ***Irl.:*** Stromba; ***Ital.:*** Winstrol†; ***Neth.:*** Stromba; ***Spain:*** Winstrol; ***UK:*** Stromba; ***USA:*** Winstrol.

Stilboestrol (9106-b)

Stilboestrol *(BAN).*

Diethylstilbestrol *(rINN)*; DES; Diethylstilbestrolum; Diethylstilboestrol; NSC-3070; Stilbestrol. (*E*)-αβ-Diethylstilbene-4-4′-diol.

$C_{18}H_{20}O_2$ = 268.4.

CAS — 56-53-1.

Pharmacopoeias. In *Chin., Eur.* (see p.viii), and *US.*

A white or almost white, odourless, crystalline powder. Practically **insoluble** in water; soluble to freely soluble in alcohol and in ether; soluble in chloroform and in fatty oils; dissolves in solutions of alkali hydroxides. **Store** in airtight containers. Protect from light.

Stilboestrol Dipropionate (9105-m)

Stilboestrol Dipropionate *(BANM).*

Diethylstilbestrol Dipropionate *(rINNM).* (*E*)-αβ-Diethylstilbene-4,4′-diol dipropionate.

$C_{24}H_{28}O_4$ = 380.5.

CAS — 130-80-3.

Pharmacopoeias. In *Aust.*

Adverse Effects and Precautions

Dose-related adverse effects of stilboestrol include nausea, fluid retention, and arterial and venous thrombosis, and these effects are common at the doses used for palliation of cancer. Impotence and gynaecomastia occur in men, and withdrawal bleeding may occur in women, as may hypercalcaemia and bone pain in women treated for breast cancer. Stilboestrol should be used with caution in those with cardiovascular disease or hepatic impairment. Use of stilboestrol is contra-indicated if pregnancy is suspected.

Adverse effects and precautions of oestrogens in general (steroidal compounds) are covered under Oestradiol, on p.1455.

Historically, high doses of stilboestrol and related substances were used for 'hormonal support' in pregnant women to try to prevent miscarriages and preterm births, most commonly in the USA. This practice was later shown to be ineffective. Adverse effects on the genito-urinary tract of offspring of these women have been noted. In particular, an increased incidence of changes in the cervix and vagina including adenosis and rarely clear-cell adenocarcinoma has been seen in postpubertal daughters of women who received stilboestrol or related substances during pregnancy (see below). A possible increased incidence of abnormalities of the genital tract and of abnormal spermatozoa has been reported in male offspring similarly exposed (see below). The recipients themselves appear to be at a small increased risk of breast cancer (see below).

Carcinogenicity. BREAST. In a report by Bibbo *et al.*[1] no statistically significant difference in the incidence of breast cancer was found among a group of 693 women who had received stilboestrol during pregnancy 25 years earlier compared with a control group of 668 who had not. This finding was, however, criticised by Clark and Portier[2] on the basis that the study lacked the statistical power to reject the null hypothesis. In another study Greenberg *et al.*[3] compared the incidence of breast cancer in 3033 women who had taken stilboestrol in pregnancy during the period 1940 to 1960 with the incidence in a comparable group of unexposed women. This study involved over 85 000 women-years of follow-up in each group and it was found that the incidence of breast cancer per 100 000 women-years was 134 in the exposed group and 93 in the unexposed group (a relative risk of 1.4). The authors concluded that in those women given stilboestrol there was a moderately increased incidence of breast cancer but that some unrecognised concomitant of exposure could not be excluded as a possibility for the increase. Although this study suggested that the risk increased over time, subsequent follow-up,[4] while confirming a modest increase in risk overall, did not confirm a higher risk in these women as time went on. Two recent cases of breast cancer[5] in premenopausal women exposed to stilboestrol *in utero* have raised the possibility that the risk of breast cancer may be increased in these women, in addition to the known genito-urinary risk (see below under Pregnancy, Effects on Female Offspring). However, a cohort study[6] involving 4536 women exposed *in utero* found no increased risk of other cancers overall, and did not show an increased risk of breast cancer (relative risk 1.18; 95% confidence intervals 0.56 to 2.49). Nonetheless, since these women were relatively young, continued follow-up was considered necessary.

1. Bibbo M, *et al.* A twenty-five-year follow-up study of women exposed to diethylstilbestrol during pregnancy. *N Engl J Med* 1978; **298:** 763–7.
2. Clark LC, Portier KM. Diethylstilbestrol and the risk of cancer. *N Engl J Med* 1979; **300:** 263–4.
3. Greenberg ER, *et al.* Breast cancer in mothers given diethylstilbestrol in pregnancy. *N Engl J Med* 1984; **311:** 1393–8.
4. Colton T, *et al.* Breast cancer in mothers prescribed diethylstilbestrol in pregnancy. *JAMA* 1993; **269:** 2096–2100.
5. Huckell C, *et al.* Premenopausal breast cancer after in-utero exposure to stilboestrol. *Lancet* 1996; **348:** 331.
6. Hatch EE, *et al.* Cancer risk in women exposed to diethylstilbestrol in utero. *JAMA* 1998; **280:** 630–4.

GENITO-URINARY TRACT. See below under Pregnancy, Effects on Female Offspring.

KIDNEY. Renal carcinoma associated with the long-term use of stilboestrol for prostate cancer in 2 men.[1]

1. Nissenkorn I, *et al.* Oestrogen-induced renal carcinoma. *Br J Urol* 1979; **51:** 6–9.

LIVER. Hepatic angiosarcoma developed in a 76-year-old man who had received stilboestrol 3 mg daily for 12 years.[1] Hepatoma developed in another elderly man who had received a similar dose for 4.5 years.[2]

1. Hoch-Ligeti C. Angiosarcoma of the liver associated with diethylstilbestrol. *JAMA* 1978; **240:** 1510–11.
2. Brooks JJ. Hepatoma associated with diethylstilbestrol therapy for prostate carcinoma. *J Urol (Baltimore)* 1982; **128:** 1044–5.

Effects on the blood. Adverse haematological effects reported with stilboestrol include severe bone-marrow changes in a 71-year-old man given stilboestrol in a massive dose of 150 mg daily for 7 years[1] and fatal immune haemolytic anaemia in a 69-year-old man given weekly infusions of stilboestrol 1 g for 9 weeks.[2] The latter reaction was due to an IgG antibody specific for stilboestrol.

1. Anderson AL, Lynch EC. Myelodyspoietic syndrome associated with diethylstilbestrol therapy. *Arch Intern Med* 1980; **140:** 976–7.
2. Rosenfeld CS, *et al.* Diethylstilbestrol-associated hemolytic anemia with a positive direct antiglobulin test result. *Am J Med* 1989; **86:** 617–18.

Pregnancy. EFFECTS ON FEMALE OFFSPRING. The DESAD (Diethylstilbestrol and Adenosis) Project carried out by the National Cancer Institute in the USA led to several reports linking exposure to stilboestrol *in utero* to adverse genital-tract effects.[1-3] It was reported that of nearly 300 young females with clear-cell adenocarcinoma of the genital tract, more than 80% had been exposed *in utero* to stilboestrol-type hormones.[1] Patients had been aged 7 to 28 years at the time of diagnosis. Doses and duration of treatment varied widely; 1.5 mg of stilboestrol daily throughout pregnancy or varying amounts for a week or more during the first trimester had shown an association. Vaginal adenosis, rare in unexposed young women, was present in about a third of those exposed in the first 4 months of pregnancy, and cervical ectropion in more than two-thirds. Vaginal epithelial changes were most closely associated with early exposure to stilboestrol, with the total dose, and with the duration of exposure; their incidence decreased with age. The risk of cancer in the first 25 years after exposure was small.[2] Fertility did not appear to be impaired in women who had been exposed *in utero* to stilboestrol but the relative risk of an unfavourable outcome of pregnancy in such a group was 1.69. However, of the women who became pregnant, 81% of those exposed to stilboestrol and 95% of control subjects had at least one full-term live birth.[3] In a review of vaginal adenosis and its association with maternal stilboestrol ingestion during pregnancy[4] it was noted that the link between stilboestrol and particularly the benign changes in the vagina and cervix (adenosis) seemed well established. The association between this drug and the development of genital malignancies was less clear, and the very low incidence in the prospective studies in the USA supported this concept. The size of the problem in the UK was small, but clinicians should be aware that it exists. Cases of vaginal adenosis in young women should be investigated and screened appropriately, and preferably referred to centres where colposcopic expertise is available. Treatment of simple vaginal adenosis should be avoided.

More recent reviews[5,6] have highlighted the fact that adverse effects are still emerging in women who had been exposed to stilboestrol *in utero* several decades ago. The need for thorough medical screening of such women was emphasised; genital-tract examination was particularly important. It was pointed out[6] that many women exposed to stilboestrol *in utero* were now in the reproductive stage of their lives and warranted special observation since a stilboestrol-damaged genital tract posed a potential problem during pregnancy.[5,6] It has also been suggested, for example, that such women are at increased risk of developing pre-eclampsia.[7]

Further information on the adverse effects of stilboestrol in females exposed to the drug *in utero* can be obtained from the references listed below.[8-18] For mention of the possible increased risk of breast cancer in these women, see Carcinogenicity, above.

1. Professional and Public Relations Committee of the DESAD (Diethylstilbestrol and Adenosis) Project of the Division of Cancer Control and Rehabilitation. Exposure in utero to diethylstilbestrol and related synthetic hormones: association with vaginal and cervical cancers and other abnormalities. *JAMA* 1976; **236:** 1107–9.
2. O'Brien PC, *et al.* Vaginal epithelial changes in young women enrolled in the National Cooperative Diethylstilbestrol Adenosis (DESAD) Project. *Obstet Gynecol* 1979; **53:** 300–8.
3. Barnes AB, *et al.* Fertility and outcome of pregnancy in women exposed in utero to diethylstilbestrol. *N Engl J Med* 1980; **302:** 609–13.
4. Emens M. Vaginal adenosis and diethylstilboestrol. *Br J Hosp Med* 1984; **31:** 42–8.
5. Anonymous. Diethylstilboestrol—effects of exposure in utero. *Drug Ther Bull* 1991; **29:** 49–50.
6. Wingfield M. The daughters of stilboestrol. *Br Med J* 1991; **302:** 1414–15.
7. Mittendorf R, Williams MA. Stilboestrol exposure in utero and risk of pre-eclampsia. *Lancet* 1995; **345:** 265–6.
8. Herbst AL, *et al.* Prenatal exposure to stilbestrol: a prospective comparison of exposed female offspring with unexposed controls. *N Engl J Med* 1975; **292:** 334–9.
9. Herbst AL, *et al.* Age-incidence and risk of diethylstilbestrol-related clear cell adenocarcinoma of the vagina and cervix. *Am J Obstet Gynecol* 1977; **128:** 43–50.
10. Kaufman RH, *et al.* Upper genital tract changes associated with in-utero exposure to diethylstilbestrol. *Am J Obstet Gynecol* 1977; **128:** 51.
11. Fowler WC, Edelman DA. In utero exposure to DES: evaluation and followup of 199 women. *Obstet Gynecol* 1978; **51:** 459–63.
12. Anderson B, *et al.* Development of DES-associated clear-cell carcinoma: the importance of regular screening. *Obstet Gynecol* 1979; **53:** 293–9.
13. Noller KL, *et al.* Maturation of vaginal and cervical epithelium in women exposed in utero to diethylstilbestrol (DESAD project). *Am J Obstet Gynecol* 1983; **146:** 279–85.
14. Robboy SJ, *et al.* Increased incidence of cervical and vaginal dysplasia in 3980 diethylstilbestrol-exposed young women: experience of the National Collaborative Diethylstilbestrol Adenosis Project. *JAMA* 1984; **252:** 2979–83.
15. Kaufman RH, *et al.* Upper genital tract changes and infertility in diethylstilbestrol-exposed women. *Am J Obstet Gynecol* 1986; **154:** 1312–18.
16. Melnick S, *et al.* Rates and risks of diethylstilbestrol-related clear-cell adenocarcinoma of the vagina and cervix—an update. *N Engl J Med* 1987; **316:** 514–16.
17. Helmerhorst TJM, *et al.* Colposcopic findings and intraepithelial neoplasia in diethylstilbestrol-exposed offspring: the Dutch experience. *Am J Obstet Gynecol* 1989; **161:** 1191–4.
18. Giusti RM, *et al.* Diethylstilbestrol revisited: a review of the long-term health effects. *Ann Intern Med* 1995; **122:** 778–88.

EFFECTS ON MALE OFFSPRING. The effects of exposure to stilboestrol *in utero* have been studied in male offspring.[1-4] Problems in passing urine and abnormalities of the penile urethra were found to be more common in young males exposed to stilboestrol *in utero* than in controls in one study.[1] In another,[2] genital tract abnormalities such as epididymal cysts, capsular induration, and defective testicles occurred in 41 of 163 stilboestrol-exposed men compared with 11 of 168 controls; sperm counts and motility were also reduced in exposed males. In contrast, comparison of 828 men exposed to stilboestrol *in utero* with 676 unexposed men suggested that, overall, stilboestrol exposure did not result in an increased risk of genito-urinary abnormalities, infertility, or testicular cancer.[3] It was suggested that previously reported increased frequencies of such abnormalities may have resulted from a selection bias and/or from a difference in stilboestrol usage. Another study[4] in 253 exposed men found that although there was an increased incidence of congenital malformations of the genitalia (18 cases compared with 5 of 241 controls), this was not associated with any decrease in fertility or impairment of sexual function.

Isolated reports of adverse effects occurring in young men who were exposed to stilboestrol *in utero* have included seminoma and epididymal cysts in one man.[5]

1. Henderson BE, *et al.* Urogenital tract abnormalities in sons of women treated with diethylstilbestrol. *Pediatrics* 1976; **58:** 505–7.
2. Anonymous. Offspring of women given DES remains under study. *JAMA* 1977; **238:** 932.
3. Leary FJ, *et al.* Males exposed in utero to diethylstilbestrol. *JAMA* 1984; **252:** 2984–9.
4. Wilcox AJ, *et al.* Fertility in men exposed prenatally to diethylstilbestrol. *N Engl J Med* 1995; **332:** 1411–16.
5. Conley GR, *et al.* Seminoma and epididymal cysts in a young man with known diethylstilbestrol exposure in utero. *JAMA* 1983; **249:** 1325–6.

Veterinary use. In the European Union, the use of stilboestrol or other stilbenes in veterinary medicine is banned unless prior steps are taken to ensure the treated animal and its products are not available for human or animal consumption.

Pharmacokinetics

Stilboestrol is readily absorbed from the gastro-intestinal tract. It is slowly inactivated in the liver and excreted in the urine and faeces, mainly as the glucuronide.

Uses and Administration

Stilboestrol is a synthetic nonsteroidal oestrogen that has been used in the palliation of breast and prostate cancer.

Daily doses of 10 to 20 mg are occasionally used by mouth in the palliative treatment of malignant neoplasms of the breast in postmenopausal women or in men (p.485). The usual dose in carcinoma of the prostate (p.491) is 1 to 3 mg daily by mouth; higher doses were formerly given. Stilboestrol has also been used in the treatment of prostatic carcinoma in the form of its diphosphate salts (see Fosfestrol, p.1447).

Stilboestrol has been used as pessaries in the short-term management of menopausal atrophic vaginitis at a dose of 0.5 to 1 mg daily.

Preparations

BP 1998: Diethylstilbestrol Pessaries; Diethylstilbestrol Tablets; ***USP 23:*** Diethylstilbestrol Injection; Diethylstilbestrol Tablets.

Proprietary Preparations (details are given in Part 3)
Fr.: Distilbene; ***Irl.:*** Boestrol†; ***UK:*** Apstil.

Multi-ingredient: ***S.Afr.:*** Oestro-Gynedron†; Poly-Gynedron†; ***Spain:*** Cilinavagin Neomicina; ***UK:*** Tampovagan; ***USA:*** Tylosterone†.

Testis Extracts (11567-p)

Testicular Extracts.

Testis extracts are usually of bovine origin and have been used in a variety of disorders. They have been given parenterally to elderly men as androgenic supplements. They have also been used topically, often in preparations containing other mammalian tissue extracts, in the treatment of peripheral circulatory or musculoskeletal disorders.

Preparations

Proprietary Preparations (details are given in Part 3)
Aust.: Testiculi; ***Ger.:*** Glanoide testoidale†; Nervauxan†; Testes-Uvocal†.

Multi-ingredient: ***Canad.:*** Heracline; Revitonus C; ***Ger.:*** cortotact†; Glandulatherm†; Intradermi N; poliomyelan; rheumamed†; tactu-nerval.

Testosterone (9108-g)

Testosterone *(BAN, rINN).*

17β-Hydroxyandrost-4-en-3-one.

$C_{19}H_{28}O_2$ = 288.4.

CAS — 58-22-0.

Pharmacopoeias. In *Eur.* (see p.viii) and *US.*

White or slightly creamy-white, odourless or almost odourless, crystals or crystalline powder. Practically **insoluble** in water; freely soluble in alcohol and in dichloromethane; soluble 1 in 6 of dehydrated alcohol, 1 in 2 of chloroform, and 1 in 100 of ether; slightly soluble in ethyl oleate; soluble in dioxan. The USP states that it is soluble in vegetable oils but Ph. Eur. has practically insoluble in fatty oils. **Protect** from light.

Testosterone Acetate (9109-q)

Testosterone Acetate *(BANM, rINNM).*

3-Oxoandrost-4-en-17β-yl acetate; 17β-Hydroxyandrost-4-en-3-one acetate.

$C_{21}H_{30}O_3$ = 330.5.

CAS — 1045-69-8.

Testosterone Cypionate (9110-d)

Testosterone Cypionate *(BANM).*

Testosterone Cipionate *(rINNM)*; Testosterone Cyclopentylpropionate. 3-Oxoandrost-4-en-17β-yl 3-cyclopentylpropionate; 17β-Hydroxyandrost-4-en-3-one cyclopentanepropionate; 17β-(3-Cyclopentyl-1-oxopropoxy)androst-4-en-3-one.

$C_{27}H_{40}O_3$ = 412.6.

CAS — 58-20-8.

Pharmacopoeias. In *US.*

A white or creamy-white, crystalline powder, odourless or with a slight odour. Practically **insoluble** in water; freely soluble in alcohol, chloroform, dioxan, and ether; soluble in vegetable oils. **Protect** from light.

Testosterone Decanoate (9111-n)

Testosterone Decanoate *(BANM, rINNM).*

3-Oxoandrost-4-en-17β-yl decanoate; 17β-Hydroxyandrost-4-en-3-one decanoate.

$C_{29}H_{46}O_3$ = 442.7.

CAS — 5721-91-5.

Pharmacopoeias. In *Br.*

White or creamy-white crystals or crystalline powder. Practically **insoluble** in water; very soluble in alcohol and in chloroform. **Store** at a temperature not exceeding 15°. Protect from light.

Testosterone Enanthate (9112-h)

Testosterone Enanthate *(BANM).*

Testosterone Enantate *(rINNM)*; NSC-17591; Testosterone Heptanoate; Testosteroni Enantas. 3-Oxoandrost-4-en-17β-yl heptanoate; 17β-Hydroxyandrost-4-en-3-one heptanoate.

$C_{26}H_{40}O_3$ = 400.6.

CAS — 315-37-7.

Pharmacopoeias. In *Eur.* (see p.viii), *Int., Jpn, Pol.,* and *US.*

A white or creamy-white crystalline powder. It is odourless or has a faint odour characteristic of heptanoic acid. Practically **insoluble** in water; very soluble in dehydrated alcohol and in ether; freely soluble in fatty oils. **Store** at a temperature of 2° to 8°. Protect from light.

Testosterone Isocaproate (9113-m)

Testosterone Isocaproate *(BANM, rINNM).*

Testosterone Isohexanoate. 3-Oxoandrost-4-en-17β-yl 4-methylpentanoate; 17β-Hydroxyandrost-4-en-3-one 4-methylpentanoate.

$C_{25}H_{38}O_3$ = 386.6.

CAS — 15262-86-9.

Pharmacopoeias. In *Br.*

White to creamy-white crystals or crystalline powder. Practically **insoluble** in water; very soluble in alcohol and chloroform. **Store** at a temperature not exceeding 15°. Protect from light.

Testosterone Phenylpropionate (9114-b)

Testosterone Phenylpropionate *(BANM, rINNM).*

3-Oxoandrost-4-en-17β-yl 3-phenylpropionate; 17β-Hydroxyandrost-4-en-3-one 3-phenylpropionate.

$C_{28}H_{36}O_3$ = 420.6.

CAS — 1255-49-8.

Pharmacopoeias. In *BP(Vet).*

A white to almost white crystalline powder with a characteristic odour. Practically **insoluble** in water; sparingly soluble in alcohol. **Protect** from light.

Testosterone Propionate (9115-v)

Testosterone Propionate *(BANM, rINNM).*

NSC-9166; Testosteroni Propionas. 3-Oxoandrost-4-en-17β-yl propionate; 17β-Hydroxyandrost-4-en-3-one propionate.

$C_{22}H_{32}O_3$ = 344.5.

CAS — 57-85-2.

Pharmacopoeias. In *Chin., Eur.* (see p.viii), *Int., Jpn, Pol.,* and *US.*

A white or creamy-white odourless crystalline powder or colourless to white or creamy-white crystals. Practically **insoluble** in water; freely soluble in alcohol, in acetone, in dioxan, in ether, and in methyl alcohol; soluble in fatty oils. **Protect** from light.

Testosterone Undecanoate (9116-g)

Testosterone Undecanoate *(BANM, rINNM).*

3-Oxoandrost-4-en-17β-yl undecanoate; 17β-Hydroxyandrost-4-en-3-one undecanoate.

$C_{30}H_{48}O_3$ = 456.7.

CAS — 5949-44-0.

Adverse Effects

Testosterone and other **androgens** may give rise to side-effects which can be related to their androgenic or anabolic activities. They include increase in retention of nitrogen, sodium, and water, oedema, increased vascularity of the skin, hypercalcaemia, impaired glucose tolerance, and increased bone growth and skeletal weight. Other effects include increased low-density-lipoprotein cholesterol, decreased high-density-lipoprotein cholesterol, increased haematocrit, and increased fibrinolytic activity.

Abnormal liver function tests may occur and there have been reports of liver toxicity including jaundice and cholestatic hepatitis. There have also been reports of peliosis hepatis and hepatic tumours in patients who have received high doses over prolonged periods. These adverse hepatic effects have occurred primarily with the 17α-alkylated derivatives (e.g. methyltestosterone, stanozolol).

In men, large doses suppress spermatogenesis and cause degenerative changes in the seminiferous tubules. Priapism is a sign of excessive dosage and may occur especially in elderly males. Gynaecomastia may occur. Androgens may cause prostatic hyperplasia and accelerate the growth of malignant neoplasms of the prostate.

In women, the inhibitory action of androgens on the activity of the anterior pituitary results in the suppression of ovarian activity and menstruation. Continued administration produces symptoms of virilism, such as hirsutism or male-pattern baldness, deepening of the voice, atrophy of the breasts and endometrial tissue, oily skin, acne, and hypertrophy of the clitoris; libido is increased and lactation suppressed. Virilisation may not be reversible, even after discontinuation of therapy.

Large and repeated doses in early puberty may cause closure of the epiphyses and stop linear growth. Children may experience symptoms of virilisation: in boys there may be precocious sexual development with phallic enlargement and increased frequency of erection, and in girls, clitoral enlargement. Gynaecomastia may also occur in boys.

Masculinisation of the external genitalia of the female fetus may occur if androgens are administered during pregnancy.

Following transdermal application of testosterone, skin reactions may include irritation, erythema, allergic contact dermatitis, and sometimes burn-like lesions. Skin reactions are more common with patches that contain permeation enhancers.

The **anabolic steroids**, because they generally retain some androgenic activity, share the adverse effects of the androgens described above, but their virilising effects, especially in women, are usually less. There have been reports of adverse psychiatric effects in athletes taking large doses to try and improve performance.

Carcinogenicity. Reports of malignant neoplasms occurring in association with testosterone therapy have included prostatic cancer (with testosterone cypionate therapy),[1] and renal cell carcinoma (testosterone ester unspecified).[2] Concern has been expressed[3] about the possibility that long-term administration of testosterone esters for male contraception may lead to an increase in the number of cases of prostatic cancer or benign prostatic hyperplasia. For reference to hepatic malignancies associated with androgens and anabolic steroids, see Effects on the Liver, below.

1. Jackson JA, *et al.* Prostatic complications of testosterone replacement therapy. *Arch Intern Med* 1989; **149:** 2365–6.
2. Rosner F, Khan MT. Renal cell carcinoma following prolonged testosterone therapy. *Arch Intern Med* 1992; **152:** 426, 429.
3. Schally AV, Comaru-Schally AM. Male contraception involving testosterone supplementation: possible increased risks of prostate cancer? *Lancet* 1987; **i:** 448–9.

Effects on the cardiovascular system. A cerebrovascular accident has been reported in a young man following the overzealous self-administration of testosterone enanthate intramuscularly for hypogonadism.[1] It was noted that thromboembolic complications are not generally recognised as side-effects of androgen therapy although there is some experimental evidence that testosterone stimulates thrombus formation. Death has been reported due to chronic heart failure secondary to long-term abuse of anabolic steroids.[2]

1. Nagelberg SB, *et al.* Cerebrovascular accident associated with testosterone therapy in a 21-year-old hypogonadal man. *N Engl J Med* 1986; **314:** 649–50.
2. Madea B, Grellner W. Long-term cardiovascular effects of anabolic steroids. *Lancet* 1998; **352:** 33.

Effects on the liver. As mentioned above, hepatotoxicity including elevations in liver enzymes, hepatic cholestasis and jaundice, and rarely peliosis hepatis and hepatic tumours has occurred on administration of androgens and anabolic steroids, particularly the 17α-alkylated derivatives. Prolonged treatment and high doses may be significant contributory factors. Tumours have included hepatocellular carcinomas, benign adenomas, and less commonly angiosarcomas and cholangiocarcinomas. Tumours and peliosis may regress on discontinuation of therapy, but they can also progress to liver failure and death. Some reviews of the hepatic effects of androgens and anabolic steroids are cited below.[1-4] There has been a specific report of benign hepatic adenoma in a patient treated with testosterone enanthate for 11 years,[5] and of hepatocellular carcinoma in a patient receiving testosterone enanthate and methyltestosterone.[6] Further specific references may be found under individual drug monographs.

1. Bagheri SA, Boyer JL. Peliosis hepatis associated with androgenic-anabolic steroid therapy. *Ann Intern Med* 1974; **81:** 610–18.
2. Ishak KG, Zimmerman HJ. Hepatotoxic effects of the anabolic/androgenic steroids. *Semin Liver Dis* 1987; **7:** 230–6.
3. Søe KL, *et al.* Liver pathology associated with the use of anabolic-androgenic steroids. *Liver* 1992; **12:** 73–9.
4. Touraine RL, *et al.* Hepatic tumours during androgen therapy in Fanconi anaemia. *Eur J Pediatr* 1993; **152:** 691–3.
5. Carrasco D, *et al.* Hepatic adenomata and androgen treatment. *Ann Intern Med* 1984; **100:** 316.
6. Johnson FL. *et al.* Association of androgenic-anabolic steroid therapy with development of hepatocellular carcinoma. *Lancet* 1972; **ii:** 1273–6.

Effects on sexual function. Reports of severe priapism following the administration of testosterone for the management of delayed puberty.[1,2]

1. Zelissen PMJ, Stricker BHC. Severe priapism as a complication of testosterone substitution therapy. *Am J Med* 1988; **85:** 273–4.
2. Ruch W, Jenny P. Priapism following testosterone administration for delayed male puberty. *Am J Med* 1989; **86:** 256.

Precautions

Testosterone and other androgens and anabolic steroids should be used cautiously in patients with cardiovascular disorders, renal or hepatic impairment, epilepsy, migraine, diabetes mellitus or other conditions which may be aggravated by the possible fluid retention or oedema caused. They should not be given to patients with hypercalcaemia or hypercalciuria, and should be used cautiously in conditions in which there is a risk of these developing such as skeletal metastases. The use of the 17α-alkylated derivatives, which are associated with an increased risk of hepatotoxicity, is probably best avoided in patients with hepatic impairment, and certainly if this is severe. Hepatic function should be monitored during therapy. Some androgens and anabolic steroids are considered to be unsafe in patients with porphyria.

In men, androgens and anabolic steroids should not be given to those with carcinoma of the breast or prostate (although in women they have been used in the treatment of certain breast carcinomas).

Androgens and anabolic steroids should not be given during pregnancy because of the risk of virilisation of the female fetus. They should be avoided in women who are breast feeding.

Androgens and anabolic steroids should be used with extreme care in children because of the masculinising effects and also because premature closure of the epiphyses may occur resulting in inhibited linear growth and small stature. Skeletal maturation should be monitored during therapy.

Androgens and anabolic steroids may interfere with a number of clinical laboratory tests such as those for glucose tolerance and thyroid function.

Abuse. The adverse effects arising from the illicit use of androgens and anabolic steroids by athletes, often taken together at doses well in excess of those used therapeutically, have been discussed.[1-4] Effects have included abnormal liver function and hepatic neoplasms (see also Effects on the Liver, above), an atherogenic blood lipid profile[5] and increased risk of cardiovascular disease, and reduced glucose tolerance. Hypogonadal states are commonly induced (azoospermia or oligospermia and testicular atrophy in men, and amenorrhoea or oligomenorrhoea in women). Gynaecomastia is relatively common in men, and virilisation in women. Psychiatric disturbances such as mania, hypomania, depression, aggression, and emotional lability, have been described.[6,7] There is also some evidence that dependence associated with an acute withdrawal syndrome can occur.[8,9] Rare reports include alterations in immune response,[10,11] bleeding oesophageal varices,[12] tendon damage,[13] renal cell carcinoma,[14] and peliosis hepatis.[15]

1. American Medical Association Council on Scientific Affairs. Drug abuse in athletes: anabolic steroids and human growth hormone. *JAMA* 1988; **259:** 1703–5.
2. Hallagan JB, *et al.* Anabolic-androgenic steroid use by athletes. *N Engl J Med* 1989; **321:** 1042–5.
3. Graham S, Kennedy M. Recent developments in the toxicology of anabolic steroids. *Drug Safety* 1990; **5:** 458–76.
4. Kennedy M. Drugs and athletes—an update. *Adverse Drug React Bull* 1994; (Dec): 639–42.
5. Glazer G. Atherogenic effects of anabolic steroids on serum lipid levels. *Arch Intern Med* 1991; **151:** 1925–33.
6. Su T-P, *et al.* Neuropsychiatric effects of anabolic steroids in male normal volunteers. *JAMA* 1993; **269:** 2760–4.
7. Pope HG, Katz DL. Psychiatric and medical effects of anabolic-androgenic steroid use: a controlled study of 160 athletes. *Arch Gen Psychiatry* 1994; **51:** 375–82.
8. Kashkin KB, Kleber HD. Hooked on hormones: an anabolic steroid addiction hypothesis. *JAMA* 1989; **262:** 3166–70.
9. Brower KJ, *et al.* Evidence for physical and psychological dependence on anabolic androgenic steroids in eight weight lifters. *Am J Psychiatry* 1990; **147:** 510–12.
10. Widder RA, *et al.* Candida albicans endophthalmitis after anabolic steroid abuse. *Lancet* 1995; **345:** 330–1.
11. Johnson AS, *et al.* Severe chickenpox in an anabolic steroid user. *Lancet* 1995; **345:** 1447–8.
12. Winwood PJ, *et al.* Bleeding oesophageal varices associated with anabolic steroid use in an athlete. *Postgrad Med J* 1990; **66:** 864–5.
13. Laseter JT, Russell JA. Anabolic steroid-induced tendon pathology: a review of the literature. *Med Sci Sports Exerc* 1991; **23:** 1–3.
14. Bryden AAG, *et al.* Anabolic steroid abuse and renal-cell carcinoma. *Lancet* 1995; **346:** 1306–7.
15. Cabasso A. Peliosis hepatis in a young adult bodybuilder. *Med Sci Sports Exerc* 1994; **26:** 2–4.

Pregnancy. Reports of female fetal virilisation following maternal administration of testosterone[1] and methyltestosterone[2] during pregnancy.

1. Reschini E, *et al.* Female pseudohermaphroditism due to maternal androgen administration: 25-year follow-up. *Lancet* 1985; **i:** 1226.
2. Dewhurst J, Gordon RR. Fertility following change of sex. *Lancet* 1984; **ii:** 1461.

Veterinary use. It was considered unnecessary to establish an acceptable daily intake or acceptable residual level in food for endogenous hormones such as testosterone. Residues resulting from the use of testosterone as a growth promoter in accordance with good animal husbandry practice are unlikely to pose a hazard to human health.[1] However, it should be noted that, in the European Union the use of androgens in veterinary practice is restricted and their use as growth promoters is banned. In addition, the use of anabolic steroids is banned in animals intended for human consumption.

1. FAO/WHO. Evaluation of certain veterinary drug residues in food: thirty-second report of the joint FAO/WHO expert committee on food additives. *WHO Tech Rep Ser 763* 1988.

Interactions

Testosterone and other androgens and anabolic steroids have been reported to enhance the activity of a number of drugs, with resulting increases in toxicity. Drugs affected include cyclosporin (see p.522), antidiabetics, thyroxine (see p.1498), and anticoagulants such as warfarin (see p.969). Resistance to the effects of neuromuscular blockers (p.1307) has also been reported.

Pharmacokinetics

Testosterone is absorbed from the gastro-intestinal tract, the skin, and the oral mucosa. However, testosterone undergoes extensive first-pass hepatic metabolism when administered by mouth and is therefore usually administered intramuscularly, subcutaneously, or transdermally. In addition, the basic molecule of testosterone has been modified to produce orally active compounds and to extend the duration of action. Alkylation of the 17α position produces compounds that are more slowly metabolised by the liver, and hence may be administered orally. Esterification of the 17β hydroxyl group increases lipid solubility and results in slower systemic absorption following intramuscular administration. The rate of absorption of the esters is related to the size of the ester group. The undecanoate ester undergoes less complete inactivation after oral administration due to distribution into the lymphatic system. Testosterone esters are hydrolysed to testosterone following absorption.

Testosterone is about 80% bound to sex-hormone binding globulin. Derivatives of 19-nortestosterone and 17-α-methylated compounds have reduced binding to this globulin. The plasma half-life of testosterone is reported to range from about 10 to 100 minutes. It is largely metabolised in the liver via oxidation at the 17-OH group with the formation of androstenedione, which is further metabolised to the weakly androgenic androsterone and inactive etiocholanolone which are excreted in the urine mainly as glucuronides and sulphates. About 6% is excreted unchanged in the faeces after undergoing enterohepatic recirculation. Testosterone is converted to the more active dihydrotestosterone in some target organs by 5α-reductase. 19-Nortestosterone derivatives appear to be less susceptible to this enzyme. Small amounts of testosterone are aromatised to form oestrogenic derivatives in the body. Compounds with a saturated A-ring, such as mesterolone, appear to be less likely to be aromatised to oestrogen.

References to the pharmacokinetics of subcutaneous testosterone pellets,[1] and scrotal[2,3] and non-scrotal[4,5] transdermal patches are given below.

1. Handelsman DJ, *et al.* Pharmacokinetics and pharmacodynamics of testosterone pellets in man. *J Clin Endocrinol Metab* 1990; **71:** 216–22.
2. Findlay JC, *et al.* Transdermal delivery of testosterone. *J Clin Endocrinol Metab* 1987; **64:** 266–8.
3. Cunningham GR, *et al.* Testosterone replacement with transdermal therapeutic systems: physiological serum testosterone and elevated dihydrotestosterone levels. *JAMA* 1989; **261:** 2525–30.
4. Meikle AW, *et al.* Pharmacokinetics and metabolism of a permeation-enhanced testosterone transdermal system in hypogonadal men: influence of application site. *J Clin Endocrinol Metab* 1996; **81:** 1832–40.
5. Yu Z, *et al.* Transdermal testosterone administration in hypogonadal men: comparison of pharmacokinetics at different sites of application and at the first and fifth days of application. *J Clin Pharmacol* 1997; **37:** 1129–38.

Uses and Administration

The natural hormone testosterone and its derivatives have anabolic and androgenic properties (for further details, see p.1426).

The primary indication for androgens, such as testosterone or its esters, is as replacement therapy in **male hypogonadal disorders** (p.1239) caused by either pituitary or testicular disorders or in hypogonadism following orchidectomy. Testosterone may be used as a subcutaneous implant in a dose of 100 to 600 mg; plasma concentrations of testosterone are usually maintained within the physiological range for 4 to 5 months with a dose of 600 mg. It may also be administered by transdermal delivery systems. The scrotal patch contains 10 or 15 mg of testosterone and supplies approximately 4 or 6 mg of testosterone in 24 hours. Non-scrotal patches are also available. These are applied to the back, abdomen, thighs or upper arms nightly to supply 2.5 to 7.5 mg daily (see also below). Testosterone has also been given by intramuscular injection in a dose of up to 50 mg 2 or 3 times weekly, but testosterone esters are generally preferred by this route.

The testosterone esters are usually formulated as oily solutions for intramuscular use to give a prolonged duration of action. Suggested doses for the various esters are: 50 to 400 mg every 2 to 4 weeks for the cypionate; 50 to 400 mg every 2 to 4 weeks for the enanthate (or an initial dose of 250 mg every 2 to 3 weeks followed by maintenance dosing every 3 to 6 weeks may be employed); and up to 50 mg 2 to 3 times weekly for the propionate. The isocaproate, phenylpropionate, and propionate esters may be given as a combined intramuscular preparation, sometimes also containing testosterone decanoate. Testosterone hexahydrobenzoate and testosterone hexahydrobenzylcarbonate have also been used. The undecanoate ester is given by mouth in an initial dose of 120 to 160 mg daily for 2 to 3 weeks, followed by a maintenance dose of 40 to 120 mg daily.

Androgens and anabolic steroids have also been used in adolescent males with constitutionally delayed puberty or growth, and anabolic steroids have been used in the treatment of short stature in girls with Turner's syndrome. However, great care is necessary when using androgens for such conditions as bone growth may be inhibited by the early fusion of the epiphyses. This effect has been utilised by the administration of supraphysiological doses of androgens to reduce final height in boys with constitutionally tall stature.

In postmenopausal women androgens, and sometimes anabolic steroids are occasionally used in the hormonal therapy of disseminated breast carcinoma but care should be taken to choose a compound with a lower masculinising effect; the short-acting synthetic compounds are usually preferred for such purposes. Androgens and anabolic steroids have also sometimes been used in conjunction with oestrogens in the management of certain menopausal disorders, but the use of androgens and anabolic steroids in women with osteoporosis is no longer advocated because their adverse effects essentially outweigh any benefit they may produce.

Anabolic steroids, and sometimes androgens, have been used in the treatment of refractory anaemias characterised by deficient red cell production, such as aplastic anaemia. Anabolic steroids and synthetic androgens with an attenuated action (sometimes known as 'attenuated androgens') such as danazol are also used in the management of hereditary angioedema.

Topical androgens may be used in the treatment of vulvar lichen sclerosus. Anabolic steroids may be useful to relieve the itching associated with obstructive jaundice.

Androgens and anabolic steroids have been used for their anabolic properties in various catabolic states.

Some testosterone esters are being investigated as male contraceptives.

Testosterone hemisuccinate is an ingredient of preparations promoted for the management of cataracts.

General reviews of androgens and anabolic steroids.

1. Hickson RC, *et al.* Adverse effects of anabolic steroids. *Med Toxicol Adverse Drug Exp* 1989; **4:** 254–71.
2. Bagatell CJ, Bremner WJ. Androgens in men—uses and abuses. *N Engl J Med* 1996; **334:** 707–14.

Anabolic effects. The androgens generally possess anabolic activity and were formerly used to increase weight in patients suffering from emaciation or debilitating diseases but effectiveness was doubtful. The anabolic steroids were developed in order to enhance the ability to build proteins and diminish the virilising and masculinising effects of the natural androgens, but all anabolics retain some androgenic activity. The anabolic steroids have again, like the androgens, been used in an attempt to produce weight gain in cachexia and wasting diseases.

The anabolic steroids and androgens have been the subject of much misuse and abuse by athletes, sports persons, and body builders (see under Precautions, above) in an attempt to increase muscle mass and body-weight but such use cannot be justified.

References to the anabolic effects of testosterone.

1. Bhasin S, *et al.* The effects of supraphysiologic doses of testosterone on muscle size and strength in normal men. *N Engl J Med* 1996; **335:** 1–7.
2. Grinspoon S, *et al.* Effects of androgen administration in men with the AIDS wasting syndrome: a randomized, double-blind, placebo-controlled trial. *Ann Intern Med* 1998; **129:** 18–26.

Antineoplastic-induced infertility. For reference to the use of testosterone to preserve gonadal function during cyclophosphamide therapy, see p.516.

Aphthous ulcers. A woman with intractable recurrent premenstrual orogenital aphthous ulcers was successfully treated with 100 mg testosterone implanted subcutaneously at intervals of about 9 months.[1] The only adverse effect was growth of a few hairs on the chin and breasts.

1. Misra R, Anderson DC. Treatment of recurrent premenstrual orogenital aphthae with implants of low doses of testosterone. *Br Med J* 1989; **299:** 834.

Constitutionally delayed puberty. Testosterone enanthate administered by intramuscular injection every one to two months for periods ranging from 3 months to several years, produced beneficial effects in boys with constitutionally delayed puberty and growth;[1,2] growth rate increased, sexual and skeletal maturation were stimulated, and full height potential did not appear to be compromised. However it has been pointed out that repeated intramuscular injections are painful and are disliked by adolescents;[3] oral testosterone undecanoate or oxandrolone have been shown to be effective in the treatment of delayed puberty and growth in boys,[4,5] and may be preferred.[3] It should be noted that administration of androgens to boys with constitutional delay of growth and puberty is controversial (see p.1237). For reference to the use of testosterone in boys with delayed puberty due to hypogonadism see below.

1. Donaldson MDC, Savage DCL. Testosterone therapy in boys with delayed puberty. *Arch Dis Child* 1987; **62:** 647–8.
2. Richman RA, Kirsch LR. Testosterone treatment in adolescent boys with constitutional delay in growth and development. *N Engl J Med* 1988; **319:** 1563–7.
3. Kelnar CJH. Treatment of the short, sexually immature adolescent boy. *Arch Dis Child* 1994; **71:** 285–7.
4. Albanese A, *et al.* Oral treatment for constitutional delay of growth and puberty in boys: a randomised trial of an anabolic steroid or testosterone undecanoate. *Arch Dis Child* 1994; **71:** 315–17.
5. Brown DC, *et al.* A double blind, placebo controlled study of the effects of low dose testosterone undecanoate on the growth of small for age, prepubertal boys. *Arch Dis Child* 1995; **73:** 131–5.

Constitutionally tall stature. Supraphysiological doses of androgens have been used to *reduce* final height in tall adolescent boys. Testosterone esters in monthly doses of up to 1000 mg have been used. Preliminary evidence after a mean of 10 years follow-up suggests that there was no long-term effect on reproductive function.[1] For reference to the use of testosterone to *increase* growth rate, see above.

1. de Waal WJ, *et al.* Long term sequelae of sex steroid treatment in the management of constitutionally tall stature. *Arch Dis Child* 1995; **73:** 311–15.

Gender reassignment. Testosterone is used in female-to-male transsexuals to develop and maintain secondary sexual characteristics. Suggested doses of the cypionate and enanthate esters are 200 mg intramuscularly every 2 weeks.

Hypogonadism. Replacement therapy with testosterone or a testosterone ester is the standard treatment for primary hypogonadism in men (see p.1239). The androgen is often given as an intramuscular depot injection of one of the esters, although subcutaneous implants and oral formulations are also employed, and, more recently, transdermal systems have been developed (for doses see above).[1-5] A sublingual testosterone tablet, and a topical testosterone gel are under investigation. Testosterone is also used to promote masculinisation in hypogonadal adolescent boys.[6,7] Testosterone is also of value in the treatment of osteoporosis in hypogonadal men.[8] Testosterone has a negative feedback effect on gonadotrophin secretion, therefore any remaining spermatogenesis is generally suppressed; androgens are thus rarely useful in reversing male infertility (p.1239).

1. Bals-Pratch M, *et al.* Transdermal testosterone substitution therapy for male hypogonadism. *Lancet* 1986; **ii:** 943–6.
2. Korenman SG, *et al.* Androgen therapy of hypogonadal men with transscrotal testosterone systems. *Am J Med* 1987; **83:** 471–8.
3. Findlay JC, *et al.* Treatment of primary hypogonadism in men by the transdermal administration of testosterone. *J Clin Endocrinol Metab* 1989; **68:** 369–73.
4. Anonymous. Testosterone patches for hypogonadism. *Med Lett Drugs Ther* 1996; **38:** 49–50.
5. Arver S, *et al.* Improvement of sexual function in testosterone deficient men treated for 1 year with a permeation enhanced testosterone transdermal system. *J Urol (Baltimore)* 1996; **155:** 1604–8.
6. Moorthy B, *et al.* Depot testosterone in boys with anorchia or gonadotrophin deficiency: effect on growth rate and adult height. *Arch Dis Child* 1991; **66:** 197–9.
7. Zacharin MR, Warne GL. Treatment of hypogonadal adolescent boys with long acting subcutaneous testosterone pellets. *Arch Dis Child* 1997; **76:** 495–9.
8. Finkelstein JS, *et al.* Increases in bone density during treatment of men with idiopathic hypogonadotropic hypogonadism. *J Clin Endocrinol Metab* 1989; **69:** 776–83.

Lichen sclerosus. Topical testosterone has been used to treat pruritus associated with vulvar lichen sclerosus in postmenopausal women.[1] For reference to the use of corticosteroids in this condition, see p.1024.

1. Friedrich EG, Kalra PS. Serum levels of sex hormones in vulvar lichen sclerosus, and the effect of topical testosterone. *N Engl J Med* 1984; **310:** 488–91.

Male contraception. In male contraceptive trials it was found that high-dose testosterone severely reduced sperm production.[1] In those in whom azoospermia was not induced there was oligozoospermia with remaining sperm having a markedly diminished fertilising capacity. In a multicentre study carried out by the WHO[2] involving 271 healthy fertile men, weekly intramuscular injection of testosterone enanthate 200 mg produced azoospermia in 157 men within 6 months. In a subsequent 12-month study of these azoospermic men, during which time testosterone enanthate was the only contraceptive measure used, there was only 1 pregnancy. Spermatogenesis was re-established on withdrawal of testosterone. These findings have been confirmed in a larger trial of the same regimen, which additionally assessed contraceptive efficacy in men who achieved oligozoospermic (less than 3×10^6 per mL).[3] No pregnancies occurred in couples where the man was azoospermic. However, the pregnancy rate was 8.1 per 100-person-years in the subgroup of couples where the man was oligozoospermic. This rate is sixfold higher than is generally seen with hormonal contraceptives in women.[4] Both studies found that consistent azoospermia was achieved in a higher percentage of Asian men (95%) than Western men (70%).[4]

For a general discussion on choice of contraceptive method, including mention of androgens for male contraception, see p.1434.

1. Matsumoto AM. Is high dosage testosterone an effective male contraceptive agent? *Fertil Steril* 1988; **50:** 324–8.
2. WHO Task Force on Methods for the Regulation of Male Fertility. Contraceptive efficacy of testosterone-induced azoospermia in normal men. *Lancet* 1990; **336:** 955–9.
3. WHO Task Force on Methods for the Regulation of Male Fertility. Contraceptive efficacy of testosterone-induced azoospermia and oligozoospermia in normal men. *Fertil Steril* 1996; **65:** 821–9.
4. Anonymous. An androgen contraceptive for men: preliminary findings. *WHO Drug Inf* 1996; **10:** 50–3.

Menopausal hormone replacement therapy. In the UK menopausal women are sometimes given implants of testosterone (in a dose of 50 to 100 mg every 4 to 8 months) as an adjunct to menopausal hormone replacement therapy (p.1434). In the USA, preparations containing an androgen and an oestrogen are available for the treatment of menopausal vasomotor symptoms, but there is conflicting opinion as to their usefulness, and further data are needed.[1]

1. Abraham D, Carpenter PC. Issues concerning androgen replacement therapy in postmenopausal women. *Mayo Clin Proc* 1997; **72:** 1051–5.

Porphyria. A female patient with acute intermittent porphyria (p.983) who suffered from severe attacks pre-menstrually was successfully managed with subcutaneous implants of testosterone when suppression of the menstrual cycle with buserelin met with limited success.[1]

1. Savage MW, *et al.* Acute intermittent porphyria treated by testosterone implant. *Postgrad Med J* 1992; **68:** 479–81.

Rheumatoid arthritis. A hypogonadic condition characterised by low serum-testosterone concentrations appears to be associated with at least the active stages of rheumatoid arthritis (p.2) in men.[1] Clinical improvement and reductions in IgM rheumatoid factor concentration, tender joint count, and the daily dosage of NSAIDs required, were observed in men with rheumatoid arthritis given oral testosterone undecanoate 40 mg three times daily for 6 months. Improvements in rheumatoid arthritis were also seen in 12 of 36 postmenopausal women treated with intramuscular testosterone 50 mg plus progesterone 2.5 mg once every 2 weeks compared with 2 of 32 women receiving placebo.[2]

1. Cutolo M, *et al.* Androgen replacement therapy in male patients with rheumatoid arthritis. *Arthritis Rheum* 1991; **34:** 1–5.
2. Booij A, *et al.* Androgens as adjuvant treatment in postmenopausal female patients with rheumatoid arthritis. *Ann Rheum Dis* 1996; **55:** 811–15.

Preparations

BP 1998: Testosterone Implants; Testosterone Propionate Injection;

USP 23: Testosterone Cypionate Injection; Testosterone Enanthate Injection; Testosterone Injectable Suspension; Testosterone Propionate Injection.

Proprietary Preparations (details are given in Part 3)

Aust.: Andriol; Testotop; Testoviron 250; ***Austral.:*** Andriol; Primoteston Depot; ***Belg.:*** Testoviron Depot; Undestor; ***Canad.:*** Andriol; Delatestryl; Malogen Aqueous; Malogen in Oil; Malogex; Scheinpharm Testone-Cyp; ***Fr.:*** Androtardyl; Pantestone; ***Ger.:*** Andriol; Testoviron Depot 250; ***Irl.:*** Andropatch; Restandol; Testoviron Depot; ***Ital.:*** Andriol; Testo-Enant; Testoviron†; Testovis; ***Neth.:*** Andriol; Testoviron Depot; ***Norw.:*** Androxon; ***S.Afr.:*** Androxon; Depotrone; Primoteston Depot†; ***Spain:*** Testex; Testoviron Depot 250; ***Swed.:*** Atmos; Testoviron Depot; Undestor; ***Switz.:*** Andriol; Testoviron Depot; ***UK:*** Andropatch; Primoteston Depot; Restandol; Testosterone Implants; Testotop†; Virormone; ***USA:*** Andro; Androderm; Andropository; Delatestryl; depAndro; Depotest; Duratest; Durathate; Everone; Histerone; T-Cypionate†; Tesamone; Testandro; Testoderm; Testopel; Testred†; Virilon†.

Multi-ingredient: ***Aust.:*** Estandron; Primodian Depot; Testoviron 100; ***Austral.:*** Primodian Depot†; Sustanon 100; Sustanon 250; ***Belg.:*** Sustanon; ***Canad.:*** Neo-Pause†; ***Fr.:*** Fadiamone; ***Ger.:*** Lynandron†; Primodian Depot†; Tachynerg N; Testoviron Depot 100; Testoviron Depot 50; ***Irl.:*** Sustanon 100; Sustanon 250; ***Ital.:*** Ablacton†; Clym-Depositum†; Estandron†; Facovit; Homosten†; Primodian Depot†; Rubidiosin Composto; Sustanon; Testoviron Depot; Tevit†; ***Neth.:*** Sustanon 100; Sustanon 250; Testoviron Depot 100†; ***Norw.:*** Primoteston Depot; ***S.Afr.:*** Mixogen; Pasuma†; Primodian Depot; Sustanon 250; ***Spain:*** Estandron Prolongado†; Testoviron Depot 100; ***Swed.:*** Triolandren†; ***Switz.:*** Estandron Prolongatum†; Primodian Depot†; Testoviron Depot 100†; Triolandren†; ***UK:*** Sustanon 100; Sustanon 250; ***USA:*** Andro/Fem†; Deladumone†; depAndrogyn; Depo-Testadiol; Depotestogen; Duo-Cyp; Duratestrin; Estra-Testrin†; T-E Cypionate†; Test-Estro; Testaval 90/4†; Valertest.

Tibolone (13342-q)

Tibolone *(BAN, USAN, rINN).*

7α-Methylnorethynodrel; Org-OD-14. 17β-Hydroxy-7α-methyl-19-nor-17α-pregn-5(10)-en-20-yn-3-one.

$C_{21}H_{28}O_2$ = 312.4.

CAS — 5630-53-5.

Adverse Effects

Irregular vaginal bleeding or spotting may occur with tibolone, mainly during the first few months of treatment, and particularly in women undergoing a natural menopause who use tibolone within 12 months of their last menstrual period. Unlike cyclical, but similar to continuous, combination hormone replacement therapy (p.1435), tibolone does not produce regular withdrawal bleeding. Other adverse effects have included changes in body-weight, ankle oedema, dizziness, skin reactions, headache, migraine, visual disturbances, gastro-intestinal disturbances, increased growth of facial hair, altered liver function, depression, and arthralgia or myalgia.

The UK Committee on Safety of Medicines had received reports of 2796 suspected adverse reactions with tibolone over 3 years, out of about 666 000 prescriptions.[1] The commonest reported effects were headache, dizziness, nausea, rash, itching, and weight gain. Vaginal bleeding appeared to occur in about 8 to 9% of recipients. There had also been 52 reports of migraine, and 4 of exacerbation of migraine, and 49 reports of visual disturbances, some of which had features suggestive of migraine.

1. Committee on Safety of Medicines/Medicines Control Agency. Tibolone (Livial). *Current Problems* 1994; **20:** 14.

Effects on the endometrium. Endometrial hyperplasia and endometrial carcinoma have been rarely reported after investigation of uterine bleeding in women receiving tibolone therapy,[1,2] as has exacerbation of adenomyosis.[3] Some of these women had previously received oestrogens. The authors of 1 report concluded that it was unclear whether tibolone was an aetiological agent or a cofactor in these cases,[1] and they emphasised that, although tibolone has progestogenic properties, it cannot be expected to reverse pre-existing endometrial hyperplasia or to protect against the development of endometrial malignancy.[1]

1. von Dadelszen P, *et al.* Endometrial hyperplasia and adenocarcinoma during tibolone (Livial) therapy. *Br J Obstet Gynaecol* 1994; **101:** 158–61.
2. Ginsburg J, Prelevic GM. Cause of vaginal bleeding in postmenopausal women taking tibolone. *Maturitas* 1996; **24:** 107–110.
3. Prys Davies A, Oram D. Exacerbation of adenomyosis in a postmenopausal woman taking tibolone associated with an elevation in serum CA 125. *Br J Obstet Gynaecol* 1994; **101:** 632–3.

Precautions

Tibolone is contra-indicated in women with hormone-dependent tumours, cardiovascular or cerebrovascular disorders including thrombophlebitis, thrombo-embolic processes, or a history of these conditions, undiagnosed vaginal bleeding, and severe liver disorders. It should not be given to pregnant or lactating women and should not be used prior to the menopause because menstrual regularity may be disturbed. Use of tibolone within 12 months of a natural menopause is also not recommended because irregular vaginal bleeding is likely. In postmenopausal women, vaginal bleeding starting after 3 months or more of treatment, or recurrent or persistent bleeding should be investigated. Care should be taken when administering tibolone to patients with disorders that may be exacerbated by fluid retention such as kidney dysfunction, epilepsy, or migraine, or with a history of these conditions. It should also be given with caution to patients with hypercholesterolaemia and impaired glucose tolerance. Tibolone should be discontinued if there are signs of thrombo-embolism or if abnormal liver function tests or cholestatic jaundice occur.

In women transferring from another form of hormone replacement therapy to tibolone it is suggested that a withdrawal bleed be induced with a progestogen prior to starting tibolone treatment since the endometrium may already be stimulated.

Interactions

On theoretical grounds, it is anticipated that compounds that induce liver enzymes such as phenytoin, carbamazepine, and rifampicin may speed the metabolism of tibolone and thus reduce its activity.

Pharmacokinetics

After oral administration, peak-plasma concentrations are attained in 1 to 4 hours. Tibolone is rapidly metabolised into 3 active metabolites, 2 of which have predominantly oestrogenic activity while the third, like the parent compound, has predominantly progestogenic activity. Metabolites are excreted in the bile and eliminated in the faeces. A small amount is excreted in the urine.

Uses and Administration

Tibolone is a steroid derived from norethynodrel that has oestrogenic, progestogenic, and weak androgenic properties. It is used as menopausal hormone replacement therapy (see p.1437) in the treatment of menopausal vasomotor symptoms and the prevention of postmenopausal osteoporosis. The usual dose is 2.5 mg daily by mouth.

'Add-back' therapy. Tibolone reduces vasomotor symptoms associated with the use of gonadorelin analogues for endometriosis (p.1442) or fibroids.[1]

1. Lindsay PC, *et al.* The effect of add-back treatment with tibolone (Livial) on patients treated with the gonadotropin-releasing hormone agonist triptorelin (Decapetyl). *Fertil Steril* 1996; **65:** 342–8.

Menopausal disorders. References to the use of tibolone for menopausal symptoms[1,2] and prevention of postmenopausal bone loss.[3,4]

1. Anonymous. Tibolone (Livial) – a new steroid for the menopause. *Drug Ther Bull* 1991; **29:** 77–8.
2. Egarter C, *et al.* Tibolone versus conjugated estrogens and sequential progestogen in the treatment of climacteric complaints. *Maturitas* 1996; **23:** 55–62.
3. Berning B, *et al.* Effects of two doses of tibolone on trabecular and cortical bone loss in early postmenopausal women: a two-year randomized, placebo-controlled study. *Bone* 1996; **19:** 395–9.
4. Lippuner K, *et al.* Prevention of postmenopausal bone loss using tibolone or conventional peroral or transdermal hormone replacement therapy with 17β-estradiol and dydrogesterone. *J Bone Miner Res* 1997; **12:** 806–12.

Preparations

Proprietary Preparations (details are given in Part 3)
Aust.: Liviel; ***Belg.:*** Livial; ***Irl.:*** Livial; ***Ital.:*** Livial; ***Neth.:*** Livial; ***S.Afr.:*** Livifem; ***Spain:*** Boltin; ***UK:*** Livial.

Trenbolone Acetate (9117-q)

Trenbolone Acetate *(BANM, USAN, rINNM).*

RU-1697; Trienbolone Acetate. 17β-Hydroxyestra-4,9,11-trien-3-one acetate.

$C_{20}H_{24}O_3$ = 312.4.

CAS — 10161-33-8 (trenbolone); 10161-34-9 (trenbolone acetate).

Pharmacopoeias. In US, for veterinary use only.

Store in airtight containers at a temperature of 2° to 8°.

Trenbolone acetate has been used as an anabolic agent in veterinary practice. The hexahydrobenzylcarbonate has also been used for its anabolic properties.

WHO specifies an acceptable daily intake of trenbolone acetate as a residue in foods, and recommend maximum residue limits in various animal tissues.[1] However, it should be noted that, in the European Union the use of trenbolone acetate and other anabolic steroids is restricted to certain therapeutic indications in non-food producing animals and their use as growth promoters is banned.

1. FAO/WHO. Evaluation of certain veterinary drug residues in food: thirty-fourth report of the joint FAO/WHO expert committee on food additives. *WHO Tech Rep Ser 788* 1989.

Preparations

Proprietary Preparations (details are given in Part 3)
Fr.: Parabolan.

Trimegestone (15930-x)

Trimegestone *(BAN, USAN, rINN).*

RU-27987. 17β-(S)-Lactoyl-17-methylestra-4,9-dien-3-one; 17β-[(S)-2-Hydroxypropionyl]-17α-methylestra-4,9-dien-3-one.

$C_{22}H_{30}O_3$ = 342.5.

CAS — 74513-62-5.

Trimegestone is a progestogen (see Progesterone, p.1459) under investigation in combination with oestradiol for menopausal hormone replacement therapy.

References.

1. Ross D. Endometrial effects of three doses of trimegestone, a new orally active progestogen, on the postmenopausal endometrium. *Maturitas* 1997; **28:** 83–8.

Zeranol (14027-b)

Zeranol *(BAN, USAN, rINN).*

MK-188; P-1496; THFES (HM); Zearalanol. (3S,7R)-3,4,5,6,7,8,9,10,11,12-Decahydro-7,14,16-trihydroxy-3-methyl-1*H*-2-benzoxacyclotetradecin-1-one.

$C_{18}H_{26}O_5$ = 322.4.

CAS — 26538-44-3.

Zeranol is a nonsteroidal oestrogen that has been used for the management of menopausal and menstrual disorders. It has also been used as a growth promoter in veterinary practice.

WHO specifies an acceptable daily intake of zeranol as a residue in foods and recommended maximum residue limits in various animal tissues.[1] However, it should be noted that, in the European Union the use of zeranol in veterinary medicine is prohibited. Certain other steroidal hormones are permitted for restricted use but their use as growth promoters is banned.

1. FAO/WHO. Evaluation of certain veterinary drug residues in food: thirty-second report of the joint FAO/WHO expert committee on food additives. *WHO Tech Rep Ser 763* 1988.

Preparations

Proprietary Preparations (details are given in Part 3)
Spain: Ralone†.

Soaps and Other Anionic Surfactants

Soaps and other anionic surfactants dissociate in aqueous solution to form an anion, which is responsible for the surface activity, and a cation which is devoid of surface-active properties. They are widely used for their emulsifying and cleansing properties. The term detergent is used to describe a surface-active agent that concentrates at oil-water interfaces and possesses emulsifying and cleansing properties. The principal groups of anionic surfactants used in pharmaceutical preparations include:

Alkali-metal and **ammonium soaps** (monovalent alkyl carboxylates) which are the sodium, potassium, and ammonium salts of the higher fatty acids.

Metallic soaps (polyvalent alkyl carboxylates) are the calcium, zinc, magnesium, and aluminium salts of the higher fatty acids and produce water-in-oil emulsions; the soaps are often made by chemical reaction during the preparation of the emulsion.

Amine soaps are salts of amines with fatty acids.

Alkyl sulphates or **sulphated fatty alcohols** are salts of the sulphuric acid esters of the higher fatty alcohols.

Alkyl ether sulphates or **ethoxylated alkyl sulphates** are formed by sulphating ethoxylated alcohols.

Sulphated oils are prepared by treating fixed oils with sulphuric acid and neutralising with sodium hydroxide solution.

Many **sulphonated compounds** have been produced which possess surface-active properties and are used as detergents; they include alkyl sulphonates, alkyl aryl sulphonates, and amide sulphonates. Docusate sodium (p.1189), a sulphonated dibasic acid ester, is used in medicine and pharmacy.

Ampholytic (or amphoteric) surfactants possess at least one anionic group and at least one cationic group in the molecule and can therefore have anionic, nonionic, or cationic properties depending on the pH. When the strength of the cationic portion of the molecule is equivalent to that of the anionic portion the isoelectric point occurs at pH 7 and the molecule is said to be balanced. Ampholytic surfactants have the detergent properties of anionic surfactants and the disinfectant properties of cationic surfactants. Their activity depends on the pH of the media in which they are used. Compounds used include aminocarboxylic acids, aminopropionic acid derivatives, imidazoline derivatives, dodicin, and pendecamaine. Long-chain betaines are sometimes classed as ampholytic surfactants.

Balanced ampholytic surfactants are reputed to be non-irritant to the eyes and skin and have therefore been used in baby shampoos.

Soft Soap (6014-f)

Green Soap; Jabon Blando; Medicinal Soft Soap; Potassium Soap; Sabão Mole; Sapo Mollis.

Pharmacopoeias. In *Br., Chin.,* and *US.*

Soft Soap (BP 1998) is prepared by the interaction of potassium hydroxide or sodium hydroxide with a suitable vegetable oil or oils or their fatty acids. It may be coloured with chlorophyll or not more than 0.015% of a suitable green soap dye.

Green Soap (USP 23) is made by the saponification of suitable vegetable oils, excluding coconut oil and palm kernel oil, without the removal of glycerol. The method given in the USP involves mixing the oil with oleic acid and to the heated mixture adding potassium hydroxide dissolved in glycerol and water. The homogeneous emulsion is then adjusted to weight with hot water.

A yellowish-white to green or brown transparent, soft, unctuous substance with a slight, characteristic odour. **Soluble** in water and in alcohol.

Adverse Effects and Treatment

Soaps and anionic detergents, in general, may be irritant to the skin by removing natural oils and may produce redness, soreness, cracking and scaling, and papular dermatitis. There may be some irritation of the eyes and mucous membranes and this limits the use of soap enemas. Ingestion of anionic detergents may cause gastro-intestinal irritation with nausea, diarrhoea, intestinal distension, and occasionally vomiting. Treatment is symptomatic.

Uses

Soft soap is used to remove incrustations in chronic scaly skin diseases such as psoriasis (see p.1075) and to cleanse the scalp before the application of lotions. A solution in industrial methylated spirit, with the addition of solvent ether, has been used to cleanse the skin. A solution of soft soap in warm water has been used as an enema to soften impacted faeces but should be avoided as it may inflame the colonic mucosa and other measures are employed (see Constipation, p.1168). Soft soap is an ingredient of Soap Spirit (BP 1998) and Green Soap Tincture (USP 23).

Potash soap (linseed oil soap) has been used in the preparation of liquid soaps. Hard soap (castile soap) and curd soap were formerly used as pill excipients and hard soap was also formerly used in the preparation of plasters.

Preparations

BP 1998: Soap Spirit *(Sp. Sap.; Spiritus Saponatus; Spiritus Saponis);*
USP 23: Green Soap; Green Soap Tincture.

Proprietary Preparations (details are given in Part 3)
USA: Fleet Bagenema.

Multi-ingredient: ***Aust.:*** Abfuhrdragees; Abfuhrdragees mild; ***Ger.:*** Ilioton†; ***Spain:*** Linimento Naion; ***USA:*** Therevac Plus; Therevac SB.

Aluminium Monostearate (6015-d)

Aluminii Monostearas; Aluminum Monostearate. Dihydroxy(octadecanoato-*O*-)aluminium; Dihydroxy(stearato)aluminium.

CAS — 7047-84-9.

Pharmacopoeias. In *Jpn* and *Pol.* Also in *USNF.*

A compound of aluminium with a mixture of solid organic acids obtained from fats and consisting mainly of variable proportions of aluminium monostearate and aluminium monopalmitate.

A fine, white to yellowish-white, bulky powder with a faint characteristic odour. Practically **insoluble** in water, alcohol, and ether.

Aluminium monostearate forms gels with fixed or mineral oils when heated to about 60°; such gels are used to suspend medicaments in oily injections.

Calcium Stearate (6016-n)

Calcii Stearas. Octadecanoic Acid, Calcium Salt.

CAS — 542-42-7 (calcium palmitate); 1592-23-0 (calcium stearate).

Pharmacopoeias. In *Eur.* (see p.viii), *Int.*, and *Jpn.* Also in *USNF.*

A compound of calcium with a mixture of solid organic acids obtained from fats, consisting mainly of variable proportions of calcium stearate ($C_{36}H_{70}CaO_4$ = 607.0) and calcium palmitate ($C_{32}H_{62}CaO_4$ = 550.9).

A fine, white to yellowish-white, crystalline, bulky, unctuous powder, free from grittiness with a slight characteristic odour. Practically **insoluble** in water, alcohol, and ether.

Calcium stearate is added to granules as a lubricant in the manufacture of tablets and capsules.

Sulphated Castor Oil (6017-h)

Ol. Ricin. Sulphat.; Oleum Ricini Sulphatum; Sulphonated Castor Oil.

CAS — 8002-33-3.

Sulphated castor oil is a detergent and wetting agent that has been used as a skin cleanser and emulsifying agent.

Sulphated hydrogenated castor oil (hydroxystearin sulphate) has been used in the manufacture of hydrophilic ointment bases and other emulsions.

Sodium ricinoleate has been used for its surfactant properties.

Magnesium Stearate (6022-f)

572; Estearato de Magnésio; Magnesii Stearas.

CAS — 1555-53-9 (magnesium oleate); 2601-98-1 (magnesium palmitate); 557-04-0 (magnesium stearate).

Pharmacopoeias. In *Chin., Eur.* (see p.viii), *Int., Jpn,* and *Pol.* Also in *USNF.*

A compound of magnesium with a mixture of solid organic acids obtained from fats, and consisting mainly of magnesium stearate ($C_{36}H_{70}MgO_4$ = 591.2) with variable proportions of magnesium palmitate ($C_{32}H_{62}MgO_4$ = 535.1); Ph. Eur. also allows magnesium oleate ($C_{36}H_{66}MgO_4$ = 587.2).

It is a fine, white, light powder, slippery to touch, and odourless or with a faint odour of stearic acid. Practically **insoluble** in water, dehydrated alcohol, alcohol, and ether.

Magnesium stearate is added as a lubricant to the granules in tablet-making and has been used as a dusting-powder and in barrier creams.

Sodium Cetostearyl Sulphate (6023-d)

Cetylstearylschwefelsaures Natrium; Natrii Cetylo- et Stearylosulfas; Natrium Cetylosulphuricum; Natrium Cetylstearylosulphuricum.

CAS — 1120-01-0 (sodium cetyl sulphate); 1120-04-3 (sodium stearyl sulphate).

Pharmacopoeias. In *Eur.* (see p.viii) and *Pol.*

A mixture of sodium cetyl sulphate ($C_{16}H_{33}NaO_4S$=344.5) and sodium stearyl sulphate ($C_{18}H_{37}NaO_4S$=372.5).

A white or pale yellow, amorphous or crystalline powder. **Soluble** in hot water giving an opalescent solution; practically insoluble in cold water; partly soluble in alcohol.

Sodium cetostearyl sulphate is used for similar purposes to sodium lauryl sulphate (see below).

Sodium Lauryl Sulphate (6024-n)

Sodium Laurilsulfate *(pINNM)*; Laurilsulfato de Sódio; Natrii Laurilsulfas; Natrium Lauryl Sulphuricum; Sodium Dodecyl Sulphate; Sodium Lauryl Sulfate.

CAS — 151-21-3.

Pharmacopoeias. In *Eur.* (see p.viii), *Jpn,* and *Pol.* Also in *USNF.*

A mixture of sodium alkyl sulphates, consisting mainly of sodium lauryl sulphate ($C_{12}H_{25}O.SO_2.ONa$ = 288.4). The Ph. Eur. specifies that the mixture contains not less than 85% of sodium alkyl sulphates and both the Ph. Eur. and the USNF specify not more than a total of 8% of sodium chloride and sodium sulphate.

A white or pale yellow powder or crystals with a slight, characteristic odour. **Soluble** 1 in 10 of water giving an opalescent solution; partly soluble in alcohol.

Incompatibilities. Sodium lauryl sulphate interacts with cationic surfactants such as cetrimide, resulting in a loss of activity. It is also incompatible with salts of polyvalent metal ions (e.g. aluminium, lead, tin, or zinc) and with acids of pH below 2.5. It is not affected by hard water on account of the solubility of the corresponding calcium and magnesium salts.

Sodium lauryl sulphate is an anionic emulsifying agent. It is a detergent and wetting agent, effective in both acid and alkaline solution and in hard water. It is used in medicated shampoos and as a skin cleanser and in toothpastes. It is used in the preparation of Emulsifying Wax (see p.1383).

Other salts of lauryl sulphate have been used for their surfactant properties. These include mono-, di-, and triethanolamine lauryl sulphates, and magnesium and ammonium lauryl sulphates. Similar surfactants include sodium lauryl ether sulphate and sodium alkyl sulphoacetates such as sodium lauryl sulphoacetate.

Sodium lauryl sulphate and related surfactants are also included in some combination preparations used rectally for the management of constipation.

Preparations

BP 1998: Emulsifying Wax.

Proprietary Preparations (details are given in Part 3)
Spain: Anticerumen; ***UK:*** Empicols.

Multi-ingredient: ***Aust.:*** Microklist; ***Austral.:*** Microlax; ***Belg.:*** Dermacide†; Microlax; Neo-Sabenyl; ***Canad.:*** Microlax; Plax; ***Fr.:*** Bactident; Microlax; Vitaclair†; Ysol 206; ***Ger.:*** Dermofug; Microklist; Nephulon E†; ***Irl.:*** Micolette; Microlax; ***Ital.:*** Florigien; Novilax; Si-Cliss; ***Neth.:*** Microlax; ***Norw.:*** Microlax; ***S.Afr.:*** Medigel; Microlax; ***Spain:*** Micralax; ***Swed.:*** Fleet Micro; Microlax; ***Switz.:*** Microklist; Stellisept; ***UK:*** Dentinox Cradle Cap; Fleet Micro-Enema; Micolette; Micralax; Relaxit; ***USA:*** Maxilube; Summer's Eve Post-Menstrual; Trichotine; Trimo-San.

Sodium Oleate (6025-h)

CAS — 143-19-1.

Sodium oleate is an anionic surfactant used as an ingredient in preparations for the symptomatic relief of haemorrhoids and pruritus ani.

Zinc oleate and potassium oleate have also been used in skin preparations, while the sodium, potassium, and calcium salts have applications as food additives.

Preparations

Proprietary Preparations (details are given in Part 3)

Multi-ingredient: ***Austral.:*** Alcos-Anal†; ***Belg.:*** Neo-Alcos-Anal; ***Fr.:*** Bilifluine; ***Ger.:*** Alcos-Anal; ***Neth.:*** Epianal; ***Norw.:*** Alcos-Anal; ***Swed.:*** Alcos-Anal; ***Switz.:*** Alcos-Anal†.

Sodium Stearate (6027-b)

Estearato de Sodio.

CAS — 408-35-5 (sodium palmitate); 822-16-2 (sodium stearate).

Pharmacopoeias. In *It.*, *Pol.*, *Port.*, and *Swiss.* Also in *USNF.*

A mixture containing not less than 90% of sodium stearate ($C_{18}H_{35}NaO_2$ = 306.5) and sodium palmitate ($C_{16}H_{31}NaO_2$ = 278.4); the content of sodium stearate is not less than 40% of the total. It contains small amounts of the sodium salts of other fatty acids.

A fine white powder, soapy to the touch, with a slight tallow-like odour. Slowly **soluble** in water and alcohol; readily soluble in hot water and hot alcohol. **Protect** from light.

Sodium stearate is an emulsifying and stiffening agent used in a variety of topical preparations. It is an ingredient of Glycerin Suppositories (USP 23).

Sodium Stearyl Fumarate (18350-n)

$C_{22}H_{39}NaO_4$ = 390.5.

Pharmacopoeias. In *USNF.*

A fine white powder. Slightly **soluble** in methyl alcohol; practically insoluble in water.

Sodium stearyl fumarate is used as a lubricant in the manufacture of tablets and capsules.

Sodium Tetradecyl Sulphate (6028-v)

Sodium Tetradecyl Sulfate *(rINN)*. Sodium 4-ethyl-1-isobutyloctyl sulphate.

$C_{14}H_{29}NaO_4S$ = 316.4.

CAS — 139-88-8.

Pharmacopoeias. Br. has a monograph for Sodium Tetradecyl Sulphate Concentrate.

Store the concentrate, which is a clear colourless aqueous gel, at a temperature not exceeding 25°. Protect from light.

Adverse Effects and Precautions

The complications of injection sclerotherapy with sclerosants such as sodium tetradecyl sulphate are discussed under Ethanolamine Oleate, p.1576.

Uses and Administration

Sodium tetradecyl sulphate is an anionic surfactant. It has sclerosing properties (see under Ethanolamine Oleate, p.1576) and is used in the treatment of varicose veins. It has also been given in the management of bleeding oesophageal varices.

Sclerotherapy for varicose veins is a specialised technique. A solution of sodium tetradecyl sulphate is injected slowly into the lumen of an isolated segment of an emptied superficial vein, followed by compression. Solutions are available in a variety of strengths (0.2 to 3%); doses depend on the site and condition being treated. A test dose is advisable in patients with a history of allergy. Facilities for treating anaphylaxis should be available.

Preparations

BP 1998: Sodium Tetradecyl Sulphate Injection.

Proprietary Preparations (details are given in Part 3)
Austral.: STD; ***Canad.:*** Thrombojecti†; Trombovar; ***Fr.:*** Trombovar; ***Irl.:*** Fibro-Vein; ***Ital.:*** Trombovar; ***Neth.:*** Trombovar†; ***S.Afr.:*** STD; ***UK:*** Fibro-Vein; ***USA:*** Sotradecol.

Zinc Stearate (6030-f)

Zinci Stearas.

CAS — 4991-47-3 (zinc palmitate); 557-05-1 (zinc stearate).

Pharmacopoeias. In *Eur.* (see p.viii), *Pol.*, and *US.*

A compound of zinc with a mixture of solid organic acids obtained from fats and consisting mainly of zinc stearate [$(C_{17}H_{35}CO_2)_2Zn$ = 632.3] with variable proportions of zinc palmitate [$(C_{15}H_{31}CO_2)_2Zn$ = 576.2]; Ph. Eur. also allows zinc oleate [$(C_{17}H_{33}CO_2)_2Zn$ = 628.3].

It is a light, white, amorphous powder, free from gritty particles, with a faint characteristic odour. Practically **insoluble** in water, alcohol, and ether.

Adverse Effects

Zinc stearate inhalation has caused fatal pneumonitis, particularly in infants.

Uses

Zinc stearate is used as a soothing and protective application in the treatment of skin inflammation. It is used either alone or with other powders or in the form of a cream.

Zinc stearate is also added as a lubricant to the granules in tablet-making.

Preparations

USP 23: Compound Clioquinol Topical Powder.

Proprietary Preparations (details are given in Part 3)

Multi-ingredient: ***Aust.:*** Mykozem; ***Belg.:*** Baseler Haussalbe; Pelsano; ***Ital.:*** Neo Zeta-Foot; Silicogamma†; Steril Zeta; Zeta-Foot†; ***Switz.:*** Adrectal; Hydrocortisone comp; Rocanal Permanent Gangrene; Rocanal Permanent Vital; ***UK:*** Simpsons.

Stabilising and Suspending Agents

The stabilising and suspending agents described in this chapter have the property of increasing the viscosity of water when dissolved or dispersed. The rheological properties of the dispersions can vary widely from thin liquids to thick gels.

These agents have wide applications both in pharmaceutical manufacturing and in the food industry. As well as being used as thickening and suspending agents many are used in emulsions as stabilisers and in some cases as emulsifying agents; some are also used in the manufacture of tablets as disintegrants, binding and granulating agents, and for film or enteric coating.

Some of the agents in this chapter are used in artificial tear and artificial saliva preparations which are employed in the management of dry eye and dry mouth respectively. The agents most commonly used are carbomers; cellulose ethers such as carmellose and hypromellose; polyvinyl alcohol; and povidone. Some agents, such as the alginates and methylcellulose, are also used in gastro-intestinal disorders.

Dry eye

Dry eye is a chronic condition caused by instability of the tear film covering the eye; the tear film breaks up into dry spots rather than being maintained between blinks. Tears consist of a slightly alkaline fluid that is spread across the eye by blinking and is lost via the lachrymal ducts or by evaporation. Mucus secreted by the conjunctiva is also required to maintain tear film stability and dry eye can result from reduced production of either tears or conjunctival mucus. Reduced tear secretion is common in the elderly, but also occurs in some systemic disorders or as an adverse effect of drugs such as those, like tricyclic antidepressants, that have antimuscarinic effects. Tear film instability may also result from increased tear evaporation, for example due to corneal exposure in thyroid disease, or from lid, corneal, or other eye disorders.

The main symptoms of dry eye are discomfort, typically with a chronic gritty sensation, visual disturbances, and sometimes photophobia. If left untreated corneal ulceration and eventual loss of sight may occur. Keratoconjunctivitis sicca (corneal inflammation) may result from severe dry eye in Sjögren's syndrome (see below).

Treatment of dry eye is primarily symptomatic using 'artificial tears' preparations; eye drops containing hypromellose or other cellulose ethers (carmellose, hydroxyethylcellulose, methylcellulose); polyvinyl alcohol; or povidone are used. Carbomer, in liquid gel formulations, and ointments containing soft or liquid paraffins are also employed. Ointments have a longer duration of action than drops, but tend to blur the vision and are most suitable for use at night. Drops should be used as frequently as required, up to hourly or more often if necessary. Frequent use of eye drops may cause sensitivity to the preservative, in which case preservative-free preparations should be considered. An alternative in patients requiring very frequent instillation of drops is a slow-release ophthalmic insert of hydroxypropylcellulose. Punctal occlusion with gelatin rods or collagen implants is used diagnostically to block tear outflow and treatment by permanent occlusion may be considered. Mucus build-up due to reduced tear production may respond to mucolytics applied topically such as acetylcysteine or bromhexine.

Sjögren's syndrome is an auto-immune inflammatory disease primarily affecting the lachrymal and salivary glands, and manifests as dry eye and dry mouth. The condition may be primary, but is often secondary to an auto-immune disorder such as rheumatoid arthritis. Treatment is mainly symptomatic using artificial tears and topical mucolytics for dry eye; dry mouth is treated with artificial saliva as outlined below. Systemic treatment with the mucolytic bromhexine has produced conflicting results.[1-3]

1. Frost-Larsen K, *et al.* Sjögren's syndrome treated with bromhexine: a randomised clinical study. *Br Med J* 1978; **i:** 1579–81.
2. Tapper-Jones LM, *et al.* Sjögren's syndrome treated with bromhexine: a reassessment. *Br Med J* 1980; **280:** 1356.
3. Prause JU, *et al.* Lacrimal and salivary secretion in Sjögren's syndrome: the effect of systemic treatment with bromhexine. *Acta Ophthalmol (Copenh)* 1984; **62:** 489–97.

Dry mouth

Dryness of the mouth (xerostomia) resulting from decreased salivary secretion is often an adverse effect of therapy with drugs such as antimuscarinics, antihistamines, tricyclic antidepressants, and diuretics. Other causes include dehydration, anxiety, Sjögren's syndrome (see Dry Eye, above), and radiotherapy of the head and neck. Dry mouth can cause eating difficulties and lead to oral disease such as candidiasis, dental caries, and bacterial infections.[1,2] Where possible any underlying disorder should be treated first. It may be possible to stimulate saliva production with sialogogues such as sugarless chewing gum or citrus products but the low pH of the latter can damage the teeth. Malic acid has also been used as a sialogogue.

Artificial saliva products are important in the symptomatic treatment of dry mouth. They aim to mimic normal saliva and generally contain the viscosity-increasing agents mucins or cellulose derivatives such as carmellose[3,4] as well as electrolytes, including fluoride; they seldom relieve symptoms for more than one or two hours.

A number of systemic therapies have also been tried. Pilocarpine is an effective sialogogue, increasing salivary production where some function remains,[5] and is used in dry mouth following radiotherapy; it may also be effective in Sjögren's syndrome and in dry mouth due to other causes. Adverse effects, particularly increased sweating, may, however, limit its use. Carbachol has been suggested as an alternative to pilocarpine with one study[6] reporting comparable efficacy but less sweating. Anethole trithione has also been used similarly. Amifostine is being investigated for dry mouth associated with radiotherapy.

1. Navazesh M, Ship II. Xerostomia: diagnosis and treatment. *Am J Otol* 1983; **4:** 283–92.
2. Anonymous. Xerostomia. *Lancet* 1989; **i:** 884.
3. Vissink A, *et al.* A clinical comparison between commercially available mucin- and CMC-containing saliva substitutes. *Int J Oral Surg* 1983; **12:** 232–8.
4. Duxbury AJ, *et al.* A double-blind cross-over trial of a mucin-containing artificial saliva. *Br Dent J* 1989; **166:** 115–20.
5. Wiseman LR, Faulds D. Oral pilocarpine: a review of its pharmacological properties and clinical potential in xerostomia. *Drugs* 1995; **49:** 143–55.
6. Joensuu H. Treatment for post-irradiation xerostomia. *N Engl J Med* 1994; **330:** 141–2.

Acacia (5402-m)

Acac.; Acaciae Gummi; E414; Gomme Arabique; Gomme de Sénégal; Gum Acacia; Gum Arabic; Gummi Africanum; Gummi Arabicum; Gummi Mimosae.

CAS — 9000-01-5.

Pharmacopoeias. In *Eur.* (see p.viii), *Int., Jpn,* and *Pol.* Also in *USNF.*

The air-hardened gummy exudate from the stem and branches of *Acacia senegal* (Leguminosae) and other species of *Acacia* of African origin.

Practically odourless, white or yellowish-white to pale amber, brittle tears. It may also appear as a powder, granules, or flakes and a spray-dried form is available.

Very slowly but almost completely **soluble** 1 in 2 of water leaving only a very small residue of vegetable particles; practically insoluble in alcohol and in ether. **Store** in airtight containers.

Incompatibilities have been reported with a number of substances including: alcohol, amidopyrine, apomorphine, cresol, ferric salts, morphine, phenol, physostigmine, tannins, thymol, and vanillin. Acacia contains an oxidising enzyme which may affect preparations containing easily oxidised substances; the enzyme may be inactivated by heating at 100° for a short time.

Adverse Effects

Hypersensitivity reactions have occurred rarely after inhalation or ingestion of acacia.

Uses

Acacia is used in pharmaceutical manufacturing as a suspending and emulsifying agent, as a tablet binder, and in pastilles. It is often used with tragacanth.

It is used as an emulsifier and stabiliser in the food industry.

Preparations

Proprietary Preparations (details are given in Part 3)

Multi-ingredient: ***Fr.:*** Edulcor sans sucre†; ***Ger.:*** Kalantol-A†; Kalantol-B†; ***UK:*** Salivix.

Agar (5403-b)

Agar-agar; Colle du Japon; E406; Gelosa; Gélose; Japanese Isinglass; Layor Carang.

CAS — 9002-18-0.

Pharmacopoeias. In *Chin., Eur.* (see p.viii), and *Jpn.* Also in *USNF.*

Polysaccharides obtained by extracting various species of Rhodophyceae algae. The Ph. Eur. specifies mainly those belonging to the genus *Gelidium*; the USNF specifies *Gelidium cartilagineum, Gracilaria confervoides,* and related red algae of this class.

Odourless or almost odourless, thin, colourless to pale yellow, yellowish orange, or yellowish grey, translucent strips, flakes, or granules; tough when damp but becoming more brittle on drying. It is also available in a powdered form. **Soluble** in boiling water to produce a clear solution that gels on cooling; practically insoluble in cold water.

Uses and Administration

Agar is used as a suspending or thickening agent in pharmaceutical manufacturing and as an emulsifying and stabilising agent in the food industry.

It was formerly used similarly to methylcellulose (p.1473) as a bulk laxative. Preparations containing agar together with liquid paraffin and phenolphthalein are available to treat constipation, but the relatively small amount of agar in these probably acts solely as an emulsion stabiliser.

Preparations

Proprietary Preparations (details are given in Part 3)

Multi-ingredient: ***Austral.:*** Diet Fibre Complex 1500†; Lexat; ***Belg.:*** Agarol; ***Canad.:*** Agarol; Agarol Plain; ***Fr.:*** Molagar†; Pseudophage; ***Irl.:*** Agarol; ***Ital.:*** Agarbil†; Agarol†; Emulsione Lassativa†; ***Neth.:*** Agarol†; ***S.Afr.:*** Agarol; ***Spain:*** Lactolaxine†; ***Switz.:*** Agarol; Demosvelte N; Falqui; Paragar; ***UK:*** Agarol; ***USA:*** Agoral.

Alginic Acid (12341-r)

Acidum Alginicum; E400; Polymannuronic Acid.

CAS — 9005-32-7.

Pharmacopoeias. In *Eur.* (see p.viii) and *Int.* Also in *USNF.*

A mixture of polyuronic acids composed of residues of D-mannuronic and L-guluronic acids extracted from algae belonging to the Phaeophyceae. A white to pale yellowish-brown, odourless or almost odourless, crystalline, fibrous, or amorphous powder.

It swells in water but does not dissolve. Very slightly **soluble** or practically insoluble in alcohol; practically insoluble in organic solvents; dissolves in solutions of alkali hydroxides. A 3% dispersion in water has a pH of 1.5 to 3.5.

Propylene Glycol Alginate (10233-n)

E405. Propane-1,2-diol Alginate.

Pharmacopoeias. In *USNF.*

A white to yellowish, practically odourless, fibrous or granular powder. **Soluble** in water and in solutions of dilute organic acids.

Sodium Alginate (5459-x)

Algin; E401; Natrii Alginas; Sodium Polymannuronate.

CAS — 9005-38-3.

Pharmacopoeias. In *Eur.* (see p.viii). Also in *USNF.*

It consists chiefly of the sodium salt of alginic acid. A white to pale yellowish-brown, practically odourless powder.

Slowly **soluble** in water, forming a viscous colloidal solution; alginic acid is precipitated below pH 3. Practically insoluble in alcohol, chloroform, and ether, and in aqueous solutions containing more than 30% of alcohol. **Store** in airtight containers.

Incompatibilities have been observed with acridine derivatives, crystal violet, phenylmercuric acetate and nitrate, calcium salts, alcohol in concentrations greater than 5%, and heavy metals. High concentrations of electrolytes cause an increase in viscosity until salting-out of sodium alginate occurs; salting-out occurs if more than 4% of sodium chloride is present.

Uses and Administration

Alginic acid and alginates such as propylene glycol alginate and sodium alginate are used in pharmaceutical manufacturing as suspending and thickening agents. They may be used as stabilisers for oil-in-water emulsions and as binding and disintegrating agents in tablets. Various grades are usually available commercially for different applications and yield solutions of varying viscosity. A reduction in viscosity has been said to occur following sterilisation by autoclaving of sodium alginate solutions.

Alginic acid and alginates (ammonium alginate, calcium alginate, potassium alginate, propylene glycol alginate, and sodium alginate) are also employed as emulsifiers and stabilisers in the food industry.

Alginic acid or the alginates, magnesium alginate and sodium alginate, are used with an antacid or a histamine H_2-receptor antagonist such as cimetidine in the management of gastro-oesophageal reflux disease (p.1170). Alginic acid or the alginate reacts with gastric acid to form a viscous gel (often termed a raft) which floats on top of the gastric contents. This raft then acts as a mechanical barrier to reduce reflux.

Sodium alginate is used in the form of a mixed calcium-sodium salt of alginic acid as a haemostatic and wound dressing; it is employed in the form of a fibre made into a dressing or packing material.

Preparations

Proprietary Preparations (details are given in Part 3)
Irl.: Kaltostat; ***Ital.:*** Kaltostat; Sazio†; ***S.Afr.:*** Kaltostat; ***UK:*** Comfeel Seasorb.

Multi-ingredient: ***Aust.:*** Cimetalgin; Sodinon; ***Austral.:*** Algicon; Digest-eze†; Gavigrans†; Gaviscon; Meracote; Mylanta Plus; ***Belg.:*** Gaviscon; ***Canad.:*** Algicon†; Gastrifom; Gastrocote; Gaviscon Heartburn Relief; Gaviscon Heartburn Relief Aluminium-Free; Heartburn Relief; Maalox HRF; Rafton; ***Fr.:*** Algicon†; Gaviscon; Pseudophage; Topaal; ***Ger.:*** Gaviscon; Nu-Gel; ***Irl.:*** Algicon; Algitec; Gaviscon; Pyrogastrone; ***Ital.:*** Digerall; Gaviscon; Ulcotris†; ***Neth.:*** Aciflux; Algicon; Gaviscon; ***Norw.:*** Algicon; Gaviscon; ***S.Afr.:*** Gastrocote†; Gaviscon; Infant Gaviscon; ***Spain:*** Gaviscon; ***Swed.:*** Algicon†; Gaviscon; ***Switz.:*** Demosvelte N; Gaviscon; Refluxine; ***UK:*** Algicon; Algitec; Asilone Heartburn; Bisodol Heartburn; Gastrocote; Gastron†; Gaviscon; Gaviscon Advance; Gaviscon Infant; Peptac; Pyrogastrone; Tagamet Dual Action†; Topal; ***USA:*** Foamicon; Gaviscon; Genaton; Pretts Diet Aid.

Aluminium Magnesium Silicate (5405-g)

Magnesium Aluminium Silicate; Magnesium Aluminum Silicate; Saponite.

CAS — 1327-43-1; 12511-31-8.

Pharmacopoeias. In *Br.* and *Int.* Also in *USNF.*

A hydrated native colloidal saponite freed from gritty particles. It is an odourless or almost odourless, creamy-white powder or small flakes. Practically **insoluble** in water and alcohol; swells to form a colloidal dispersion in water and glycerol; practically insoluble in organic solvents. A dispersion in water (4 or 5%) has a pH of about 9.0.

The USNF describes several types with varying ranges of aluminium:magnesium content and varying viscosity ranges for dispersions of approximately 5%.

Store in airtight containers.

Uses

Aluminium magnesium silicate has a variety of pharmaceutical uses, including use as a suspending and thickening agent, as an emulsion stabiliser, and as a binder and disintegrating agent in tablets.

Other forms of aluminium magnesium silicate include an artificial hydrate known as almasilate (p.1177), which is used as an antacid, and attapulgite (p.1178), a purified native hydrated magnesium aluminium silicate that is highly adsorbent and is used in a wide range of products including fertilisers and pesticides. Activated attapulgite, which is attapulgite that has been carefully heated to increase its adsorptive capacity, is used in combination preparations for diarrhoea.

Preparations

Proprietary Preparations (details are given in Part 3)
Ger.: Akne-Pyodron Kur†; Mucal; Sicco-Gynaedron†.

Multi-ingredient: ***Fr.:*** Mucal; ***Ger.:*** Akne-Pyodron lokal†; ***Switz.:*** TRI-OM.

Bentonite (5407-p)

558; Bentonitum; Mineral Soap; Soap Clay; Wilkinite.

CAS — 1302-78-9.

Pharmacopoeias. In *Eur.* (see p.viii), *Int., Jpn,* and *Pol.* Also in *USNF* which includes additionally Purified Bentonite.

A native colloidal hydrated aluminium silicate consisting mainly of montmorillonite, $Al_2O_3,4SiO_2,H_2O$; it may also contain calcium, magnesium, and iron.

An odourless, hygroscopic, very fine, homogeneous, greyish-white powder with a yellowish or pinkish tint.

Practically **insoluble** in water and in aqueous solutions, but swells with a little water forming a malleable mass. Practically insoluble, and does not swell, in organic solvents. A 2% suspension in water has a pH of 9.5 to 10.5; a 5% suspension of purified bentonite in water has a pH of 9.0 to 10.0. **Store** in airtight containers.

Uses

Bentonite absorbs water readily to form sols or gels, depending on its concentration. It is used in pharmaceutical manufacturing as a suspending and stabilising agent and as an adsorbent or clarifying agent. It is also used as an anticaking agent in the food industry.

Bentonite may be used as an oral adsorbent in paraquat poisoning (p.1409).

Preparations

BP 1998: Calamine Lotion;
USNF 18: Bentonite Magma.

Carbomers (5409-w)

Acrylic Acid Polymers; Carbopols; Carboxypolymethylene; Carboxyvinyl Polymers; Polyacrylic Acid.

CAS — 9003-01-4; 54182-57-9.

NOTE. Carbomer is *BAN, USAN,* and *rINN.*

Pharmacopoeias. In *Eur.* (see p.viii), and *Int. USNF* has separate monographs for Carbomer 910, Carbomer 934, Carbomer 934P, Carbomer 940, Carbomer 941, and Carbomer 1342.

Generally synthetic high molecular weight polymers of acrylic acid cross-linked with polyalkenyl ethers of sugars or polyalcohols. They are produced in several grades characterised by the viscosity of a defined solution.

White, fluffy, acidic, hygroscopic powders with a slight characteristic odour. After dispersion and neutralisation with sodium hydroxide they swell in water and in other polar solvents.

Store in airtight containers.

Uses and Administration

Carbomers are used in pharmaceutical manufacturing as suspending agents, gel bases, emulsifiers, and binding agents in tablets.

Carbomers, in liquid gel formulations containing typically 0.2 or 0.3%, are used topically as tear substitutes in the management of dry eye (p.1470).

Preparations

Proprietary Preparations (details are given in Part 3)
Aust.: Lacrisic; Vidisic; ***Austral.:*** Viscotears; ***Belg.:*** Thilo Tears; Vidisic; ***Canad.:*** Tear-Gel; ***Fr.:*** Gel-Larmes; Lacrinorm; Lacryvisc; ***Ger.:*** Thilo-Tears; Vidisic; ***Irl.:*** Geltears; Vidisic; ***Ital.:*** Dacriogel; Lacrigel; Lacrinorm; Viscotirs; ***Mon.:*** Lacrigel; ***Neth.:*** Dry Eye Gel†; Thilo-Tears†; Vidisic; ***Norw.:*** Viscotears; ***S.Afr.:*** Teargel; ***Spain:*** Revic; Viscotears; ***Swed.:*** Viscotears; ***Switz.:*** Lacrinorm; Thilo-Tears; Viscotears; ***UK:*** Geltears; Viscotears.

Multi-ingredient: ***Belg.:*** Alcon Eye Gel; ***Ital.:*** Dropyal; ***USA:*** Maxilube.

Carmellose (14163-l)

Carmellose *(rINN).*

Carboxymethylcellulose; CMC.

Pharmacopoeias. In *Jpn.*

Carmellose Calcium (5410-m)

Carmellose Calcium *(rINNM).*

Calcium Carboxymethylcellulose; Carboxymethylcellulose Calcium; Carmellosum Calcicum.

CAS — 9050-04-8.

Pharmacopoeias. In *Eur.* (see p.viii) and *Jpn.* Also in *USNF.*

A white to yellowish-white hygroscopic powder. It swells in water to form a suspension; practically **insoluble** in acetone, alcohol, chloroform, ether, and toluene. A 1% suspension in water has a pH of 4.5 to 6.0. **Store** in airtight containers.

Carmellose Sodium (5411-b)

Carmellose Sodium *(BAN, rINNM).*

Carboxymethylcellulose Sodium; Carboxymethylcellulosum Natricum; Cellulose Gum; E466; SCMC; Sodium Carboxymethylcellulose; Sodium Cellulose Glycollate.

CAS — 9004-32-4.

Pharmacopoeias. In *Eur.* (see p.viii), *Int., Jpn, Pol.,* and *US. USNF* also includes Carboxymethylcellulose Sodium 12.

A white to almost white, hygroscopic granular powder. The Ph. Eur. specifies a sodium content of 6.5 to 10.8%, and the USP 6.5 to 9.5%, both calculated on the dry substance. Ph. Eur. also has standards for Low-substituted Carmellose Sodium which has a sodium content of 2.0 to 4.5%. Carboxymethylcellulose Sodium 12 (USNF) has a sodium content of 10.5 to 12.0%, calculated on the dry substance.

Easily **dispersed** in water forming colloidal solutions; practically insoluble in acetone, dehydrated alcohol, ether, toluene, and most other organic solvents. A 1% dispersion in water has a pH of 6.0 to 8.5. **Store** in airtight containers.

Incompatibilities have been reported with strongly acidic solutions, with soluble salts of iron and some other metals, and with xanthan gum.

Croscarmellose Sodium (10208-d)

Croscarmellose Sodium *(USAN).*

Carmellosum Natricum Conexum; Crosslinked Carboxymethylcellulose Sodium; Modified Cellulose Gum.

Pharmacopoeias. In *Eur.* (see p.viii). Also in *USNF.*

A cross-linked polymer of carmellose sodium. It has a sodium content of 5 to 9% calculated with reference to the dried substance. A white or greyish white, free flowing, powder. Partially **soluble** in water; practically insoluble in acetone, in dehydrated alcohol, in ether, in toluene, and in most other organic solvents. A 1% suspension in water has a pH of 5 to 7. **Store** in airtight containers.

Uses and Administration

Carmellose calcium and carmellose sodium have a variety of pharmaceutical uses, including use as suspending, thickening, and emulsifying agents, and as disintegrants, binders, and coating agents in tablets. Carmellose sodium is also used as an emulsifier or stabiliser in the food industry. Croscarmellose sodium is employed as a tablet disintegrant.

Carmellose sodium is used topically as an ingredient of protective preparations for stoma care, in the management of wounds, and for the mechanical protection of oral and perioral lesions, such as mouth ulceration (p.1172). It is also used, in concentrations of up to 1%, in artificial saliva preparations for the treatment of dry mouth (p.1470), and in eye drops for the management of dry eye (p.1470).

Carmellose sodium given orally absorbs water and acts as a bulk-forming agent; the volume of faeces is increased and peristalsis promoted. It is used in the treatment of constipation (p.1168). Carmellose sodium has been included in preparations to control appetite in the management of obesity (p.1476) but there is little evidence of efficacy. For precautions to be observed with bulk-forming agents, see under Methylcellulose, p.1473.

Preparations

USP 23: Carboxymethylcellulose Sodium Paste; Carboxymethylcellulose Sodium Tablets.

Proprietary Preparations (details are given in Part 3)
Austral.: Cellufresh; Celluvisc; ***Canad.:*** Cellufresh; Celluvisc; ***Fr.:*** Aquacel; Askina; Celluvisc; Comfeel; Urgomed; ***Ger.:*** Celluvisc; ***Ital.:*** Celluvisc; ***S.Afr.:*** Celluvisc; ***Spain:*** Celluvisc; ***Swed.:*** Celluvisc; ***Switz.:*** Celluvisc; Comfeel; ***UK:*** Comfeel; Intrasite; Revive; ***USA:*** Cellufresh; Celluvisc; Refresh Plus.

Multi-ingredient: ***Aust.:*** Glandosane; Sialin; ***Austral.:*** Aquae; Diet-Trim†; Orabase; Orahesive; SoloSite; Stomahesive; United Soft Guard†; ***Canad.:*** Appedrine; Dexatrim; Moi-Stir; Orabase; Orahesive; Salivart; ***Fr.:*** Artisial; Sureskin; Syaline-spray†; Tegasorb; ***Ger.:*** Artisial; Glandosane; Nu-Gel; ***Irl.:*** Luborant; Orabase; ***Ital.:*** Agena; Flamlax†; Idrum; Placacid†; ***Spain:*** Laxvital; ***Switz.:*** Glandosane; Varihesive Hydroactive; ***UK:*** Comfeel Plus; Glandosane; Luborant; Orabase; Orahesive; Salivace; Seprafilm; Stomahesive; Varihesive; ***USA:*** Dieutrim; Disolan Forte; Disoplex; Glandosane; Moi-Stir; Pretts Diet Aid; Salivart; Surgel.

Carrageenan (5412-v)

Carrageenin; Carraghénates; Chondrus Extract; E407; Irish Moss Extract.

CAS — 9000-07-1 (carrageenan); 11114-20-8 (κ-carrageenan); 9064-57-7 (λ-carrageenan).

Pharmacopoeias. In *Fr.* Also in *USNF.*

The USNF defines carrageenan as the hydrocolloid obtained by extraction with water or aqueous alkali from some members of the class Rhodophyceae (red seaweeds). It consists chiefly of a mixture of the ammonium, calcium, magnesium, potassium, and sodium sulphate esters of galactose and 3,6-anhydrogalactose copolymers. The prevalent copolymers in the hydrocolloids are κ-carrageenan, ι-carrageenan, and λ-carrageenan.

A white to yellowish or tan, coarse or fine, practically odourless powder. **Soluble** in water at 80° forming a viscous clear or slightly opalescent solution. It disperses more readily if first mixed with alcohol, glycerol, or syrup.

Store in airtight containers in a cool place.

Uses and Administration

Carrageenan is used in pharmaceutical manufacturing and the food industry as a suspending and gelling agent.

It is included for its effect as a bulk-forming laxative in several preparations used to treat constipation (p.1168). For precautions to be observed with bulk-forming laxatives, see under Methylcellulose, p.1473. Carrageenan is also included in topical preparations for the symptomatic relief of anorectal disorders.

A degraded form of carrageenan also used to be given in gastro-intestinal disorders but it was associated with lesions in *animals* and is no longer used.

An acceptable daily intake (ADI) of 'not specified' was allocated to refined non-degraded carrageenan as a food additive since the total daily intake of this form of carrageenan (arising from its use at the levels necessary to achieve the desired effect and from its acceptable background in food) was not considered to represent a hazard to health. The toxic effects associated with degraded carrageenan and of the use of 'semi-refined' carrageenan as a food in some countries were considered and the ADI of 'not specified' was not applied to these forms of carrageenan. The ADI did, however, apply to furcellaran [a similar extract from Rhodophyceae] which is included in the specifications for food-grade carrageenan.[1]

In the UK the Food Advisory Committee has recommended that carrageenan should not be permitted as an additive for infant formulas because of the possibility of immunological consequences following absorption from the immature gut.[2] Carrageenans were known to affect the immune system of experimental *animals* after parenteral administration and immune effects have been noted in *rats* after oral administration of undegraded carrageenan. Small amounts of food-grade carrageenan cross the intestinal epithelium in *rats* and are taken up by gut-associated lymphoid tissue.[3]

1. FAO/WHO. Evaluation of certain food additives and contaminants: twenty-eighth report of the joint FAO/WHO expert committee on food additives. *WHO Tech Rep Ser 710* 1984.
2. MAFF. Food Advisory Committee: report on the review of the use of additives in foods specially prepared for infants and young children. FdAC/REP/12. London: HMSO, 1992.
3. MAFF. Food Advisory Committee: report on the review of the emulsifiers and stabilisers in food regulations. FdAC/REP/11. London: HMSO, 1992.

Preparations

Proprietary Preparations (details are given in Part 3)
Aust.: Coreine; ***Fr.:*** Coreine†.

Multi-ingredient: ***Aust.:*** Anoreine; Anoreine mit Lidocain; ***Austral.:*** Bonnington's Irish Moss; Irish Moss Cough Syrup†; ***Belg.:*** Tisane Pectorale; ***Fr.:*** Anoreine; Rectolax†; Titanoreine; ***Spain:*** Emuliquen Antiespasmodic†; Laxante Bescansa; ***Switz.:*** Flogecyl; Titanoreine; ***UK:*** Biobalm; Liminate.

Cellacephate (5413-g)

Cellacephate *(BAN)*.

Cellacefate *(rINN)*; CAP; Cellulose Acetate Phthalate; Cellulosi Acetas Phthalas; Cellulosum Acetylphthalicum; Celophthalum.

CAS — 9004-38-0.

Pharmacopoeias. In *Eur.* (see p.viii), *Int.*, *Jpn*, and *Pol.* Also in *USNF.*

Cellulose in which some of the hydroxyl groups are acetylated (21.5 to 26.0%) and some are esterified by hydrogen phthaloyl groups (30.0 to 36.0%).

A hygroscopic, white, free-flowing powder or colourless flakes, odourless or with a slight odour of acetic acid. Practically **insoluble** in water, in dehydrated alcohol, and in dichloromethane; freely soluble in acetone; soluble in diethylene glycol and dioxan; it dissolves in dilute solutions of alkalis. **Store** in airtight containers.

Uses

Cellacephate is unaffected by immersion in acid media in the stomach but softens and swells in intestinal fluid. It is used in pharmaceutical manufacturing as an enteric-coating material for tablets and capsules, usually with a plasticiser. Films of cellacephate are reported to be permeable to some ionic substances such as ammonium chloride and potassium iodide, and such substances require a sealing coat.

Cellulose (15824-a)

An unbranched polysaccharide polymer consisting of 1,4-β-linked glucopyranose units. It is the chief constituent of fibrous plant material.

Dispersible Cellulose (5415-p)

Dispersible Cellulose *(BAN)*.

Microcrystalline Cellulose and Carboxymethylcellulose Sodium.

Pharmacopoeias. In *Br.* Also in *USNF.*

An odourless or almost odourless, white to off-white coarse to fine powder consisting of a colloid-forming attrited mixture of microcrystalline cellulose and carmellose sodium.

Dispersible in water, with swelling, to produce a white, opaque dispersion or gel; practically insoluble in organic solvents and dilute acids. **Store** in airtight containers and at a temperature between 8° and 15°.

Microcrystalline Cellulose (5414-q)

Cellulosa Microgranulare; Cellulose Gel; Cellulosum Microcrystallinum; Crystalline Cellulose; E460.

CAS — 9004-34-6.

Pharmacopoeias. In *Eur.* (see p.viii), *Int.*, *Jpn*, and *Pol.* Also in *USNF.*

A purified, partly depolymerised cellulose, prepared by treating alpha-cellulose, obtained as a pulp from fibrous plant materials, with mineral acids. It is a white or almost white, odourless, fine or granular powder.

Practically **insoluble** in water, dilute acids, sodium hydroxide solution (1 in 20), acetone, dehydrated alcohol, toluene, and most organic solvents. **Store** in airtight containers.

Powdered Cellulose (5416-s)

Cellulose Powder; Cellulosi Pulvis; E460.

Pharmacopoeias. In *Eur.* (see p.viii) and *Jpn.* Also in *USNF.*

A purified mechanically disintegrated cellulose prepared from alpha-cellulose obtained as a pulp from fibrous plant materials. It is a white or almost white, odourless, fine, granular, or fluffy powder.

Practically **insoluble** in water, dilute acids, acetone, dehydrated alcohol, toluene, and most organic solvents; slightly soluble in sodium hydroxide solution (1 in 20). **Store** in airtight containers.

Uses and Administration

Powdered cellulose and microcrystalline cellulose are used in pharmaceutical manufacturing as tablet binders and disintegrants and as capsule and tablet diluents. These two forms of cellulose are also used in the food industry. Dispersible cellulose (which also contains some carmellose sodium) forms a thixotropic gel with water and is used pharmaceutically as a suspending and thickening agent.

Various forms of cellulose have been included in preparations employed in the management of constipation and obesity. Cellulose is also used in adsorbent powder preparations used for skin disorders including hyperhidrosis.

Preparations

Proprietary Preparations (details are given in Part 3)
Ger.: Deshisan†; ***UK:*** Nasaleze; Sterigel; ***USA:*** Unifiber.

Multi-ingredient: ***Austral.:*** ZeaSorb; ***Canad.:*** ZeaSorb; ***Fr.:*** Gelopectose; ZeaSorb; ***Ger.:*** ZeaSorb; ***Irl.:*** ZeaSorb; ***Switz.:*** Fiblet†; ***UK:*** Nilstim†.

Ceratonia (5417-w)

Carob Bean Gum; Carob Gum; Cerat.; Ceratonia Gum; E410; Gomme de Caroube; Locust Bean Gum.

CAS — 9000-40-2.

The endosperms separated from the seeds of the locust bean tree, *Ceratonia siliqua* (Leguminosae).

Uses and Administration

Ceratonia is used as a thickening agent and stabiliser in the food industry.

Preparations

Proprietary Preparations (details are given in Part 3)
Aust.: Arobon; ***Austral.:*** Carobel†; ***Irl.:*** Carobel; ***Ital.:*** Arobon; Piantanol†; ***Norw.:*** Arobon; ***S.Afr.:*** Nestargel†; ***Switz.:*** Arobon†; Nestargel; ***UK:*** Arobon; Carobel; Nestargel.

Multi-ingredient: ***Aust.:*** China-Eisenwein; ***Austral.:*** Diet Fibre Complex 1500†; ***Belg.:*** Kestomatine Baby; ***Fr.:*** Gumilk; Polysilane Joullie; ***Switz.:*** Gastricure; Kestomatine Bebe.

Dextrates (5420-v)

Dextrates *(USAN)*.

CAS — 39404-33-6.

Pharmacopoeias. In *USNF.*

A purified anhydrous or hydrated mixture of saccharides obtained by the controlled enzymatic hydrolysis of starch. Free-flowing, porous, white odourless spherical granules. Freely **soluble** in water (solubility increases in hot water); soluble in dilute acids and alkalis and in basic organic solvents; practically insoluble in the common organic solvents. A 20% solution in water has a pH of 3.8 to 5.8. **Store** in a cool dry place.

Uses

Dextrates is used as a capsule and tablet diluent and as a tablet binding agent.

Ethylcellulose (5421-g)

E462; Ethylcellulosum.

CAS — 9004-57-3.

Pharmacopoeias. In *Eur.* (see p.viii) and *Int.* Also in *USNF.*

A partly *O*-ethylated cellulose. It contains 44 to 51% of ethoxy ($-OC_2H_5$) groups, calculated on the dried basis.

A free-flowing white to yellowish-white, odourless or almost odourless, powder or granular powder. Solutions of ethylcellulose may show a slight opalescence.

Practically **insoluble** in water, glycerol, and propylene glycol; soluble in dichloromethane and in a mixture of 20 parts alcohol and 80 parts toluene (w/w); slightly soluble in ethyl acetate and methyl alcohol. Ethylcellulose containing less than 46.5% of ethoxy groups is freely soluble in chloroform, methyl acetate, tetrahydrofuran, and in mixtures of aromatic hydrocarbons with alcohol; ethylcellulose containing not less than 46.5% of ethoxy groups is freely soluble in alcohol, chloroform, ethyl acetate, methyl alcohol, and toluene.

Uses

Ethylcellulose is used as a binder in tablets and as a coating material for tablets, granules, and microcapsules. It is also used as a thickening agent.

Preparations

USNF 18: Ethylcellulose Aqueous Dispersion.

Gastric Mucin (2492-x)

Gastric Mucin *(BAN)*.

Gastric mucin is a high molecular weight glycoprotein precipitated by alcohol (60%) after digestion of hogs' stomach linings by pepsin and hydrochloric acid.

Uses and Administration

Gastric mucin is used in artificial saliva formulations for dry mouth, the overall management of which is discussed on p.1470. An aerosol spray containing 3.5% is employed; lozenges are also available.

Preparations

Proprietary Preparations (details are given in Part 3)

Multi-ingredient: ***Austral.:*** Saliva Orthana†; ***Ital.:*** Enzygaster†; ***UK:*** Saliva Orthana.

Hydroxyethylcellulose (5429-j)

Hydroxyethyl Cellulose; Hydroxyethylcellulosum.

CAS — 9004-62-0.

NOTE. HECL is a code approved by the BP for use on single unit doses of eye drops containing hydroxyethylcellulose and sodium chloride where the individual container may be too small to bear all the appropriate labelling information.

Pharmacopoeias. In *Eur.* (see p.viii), *Int.*, and *Pol.* Also in *USNF.*

A partially substituted 2-hydroxyethyl ether of cellulose. Various grades are available and are distinguished by appending a number indicative of the apparent viscosity in millipascal seconds of a 2% solution measured at 20°.

A white, yellowish-white, or greyish-white, practically odourless powder or granules; hygroscopic after drying. **Soluble** in cold or hot water, forming colloidal solutions; practically insoluble in alcohol, in acetone, in ether, in toluene, and in most other organic solvents. A 1% dispersion in water has a pH of 5.5 to 8.5.

Uses and Administration

Hydroxyethylcellulose is used in pharmaceutical manufacturing as a thickener and stabiliser and as a tablet coating and binding agent. It is present in lubricant preparations for dry eye (p.1470), contact lens care (p.1097), and dry mouth (p.1470).

Preparations

Proprietary Preparations (details are given in Part 3)
Austral.: Comfortcare GP Comfort Drops†; ***Ger.:*** Lacrigel; ***USA:*** Comfort Tears; Gonioscopic; TearGard.

Multi-ingredient: ***Austral.:*** Barnes-Hind Wetting and Soaking Solution†; Minims Artificial Tears; ***Ger.:*** Nu-Gel; ***Irl.:*** Minims Artificial Tears; ***UK:*** Minims Artificial Tears; ***USA:*** Adsorbotear; Optimoist.

Hydroxyethylmethylcellulose (5430-q)

HEMC; Hydroxyethyl Methylcellulose; Methylhydroxyethylcellulose; Methylhydroxyethylcellulosum.

CAS — 9032-42-2.

Pharmacopoeias. In *Eur.* (see p.viii).

A partially substituted ether of cellulose containing methoxyl and 2-hydroxyethyl groups. Various grades are available and are distinguished by appending a number indicative of the apparent viscosity in millipascal seconds of a 2% w/w solution measured at 20°.

A white, yellowish-white, or greyish-white, powder or granules; hygroscopic after drying.

Practically **insoluble** in hot water, dehydrated alcohol, acetone, ether, and toluene; dissolves in cold water forming a colloidal solution. A 1% w/w solution in water has a pH of 5.5 to 8.0.

Uses

Hydroxyethylmethylcellulose is used similarly to the other cellulose ethers as a pharmaceutical excipient.

Preparations

Proprietary Preparations (details are given in Part 3)

Multi-ingredient: ***Fr.:*** Pharmatex.

Hydroxypropylcellulose (5431-p)

E463; Hydroxypropyl Cellulose; Hydroxypropylcellulosum; Hyprolose.

CAS — 9004-64-2.

Pharmacopoeias. In *Chin., Eur.* (see p.viii), *Int.,* and *Jpn.* Also in *USNF* which has two separate monographs, for Hydroxypropyl Cellulose (not more than 80.5% of hydroxypropoxy groups), and for Low-Substituted Hydroxypropyl Cellulose (5 to 16%).

A partially substituted 2-hydroxypropyl ether of cellulose. Various grades are available and may be distinguished by appending a number indicative of the apparent viscosity in millipascal seconds of a 2% w/w solution measured at 20°.

White or yellowish-white, practically odourless granules or powder; hygroscopic after drying.

Soluble in cold water, glacial acetic acid, dehydrated alcohol, chloroform, methyl alcohol, propylene glycol, and in a mixture of 1 part methyl alcohol and 9 parts dichloromethane, forming colloidal solutions; practically insoluble in hot water, ethylene glycol, and toluene; sparingly soluble or slightly soluble in acetone. A 1% w/w solution in water has a pH of 5.0 to 8.5.

Low-Substituted Hydroxypropyl Cellulose (USNF 18) is a hygroscopic fibrous or granular powder. Practically insoluble in alcohol and in ether; dissolves in a solution of sodium hydroxide (1 in 10) and produces a viscous solution; swells in water. A 1% suspension in water has a pH of 5.0 to 7.5. Store in airtight containers.

Adverse Effects

Hydroxypropylcellulose used as a solid ocular insert may result in blurred vision and ocular discomfort or irritation including hypersensitivity and oedema of the eyelids.

Allergic contact dermatitis was reported in one patient, associated with the hydroxypropylcellulose present in the reservoir layer of a transdermal oestradiol patch.[1]

1. Schwartz BK, Clendenning WE. Allergic contact dermatitis from hydroxypropyl cellulose is a transdermal estradiol patch. *Contact Dermatitis* 1988; **18:** 106–7.

Uses and Administration

Hydroxypropylcellulose is used in pharmaceutical manufacturing in the film coating of tablets, as a tablet excipient, as a thickener, and in microencapsulation. It is used as an emulsifier and stabiliser in the food industry.

Hydroxypropylcellulose is also used as a slow-release solid ophthalmic insert in the management of dry eye (p.1470).

Preparations

USP 23: Hydroxypropyl Cellulose Ocular System.

Proprietary Preparations (details are given in Part 3)
Austral.: Lacrisert; ***Canad.:*** Lacrisert; ***Fr.:*** Lacrisert; ***Ital.:*** Lacrisert; ***Neth.:*** Lacrisert; ***Norw.:*** Lacrisert; ***S.Afr.:*** Lacrisert; ***Swed.:*** Lacrisert; ***USA:*** Lacrisert.

Hypromellose (5432-s)

Hypromellose *(BAN, rINN).*

E464; Hydroxypropyl Methylcellulose; Hydroxypropylmethylcellulose; Hypromellosum; Methyl Hydroxypropyl Cellulose; Methylcellulose Propylene Glycol Ether; Methylhydroxypropylcellulose; Methylhydroxypropylcellulosum.

CAS — 8063-82-9; 9004-65-3.

NOTE. HPRM is a code approved by the BP for use on single unit doses of eye drops containing hypromellose where the individual container may be too small to bear all the appropriate labelling information.

Pharmacopoeias. In *Chin., Eur.* (see p.viii), *Int., Jpn, Pol.,* and *US.*

A mixed ether of cellulose containing a variable proportion of methoxy and 2-hydroxypropoxy groups. Several grades are available. In the UK these are distinguished by appending a number indicative of the apparent viscosity in millipascal seconds of a 2% w/w solution measured at 20° (e.g. hypromellose 4500). In the USA they are distinguished by appending a number in which the first 2 digits represent the approximate percentage content of methoxy groups, and the third and fourth digits the approximate percentage content of hydroxypropoxy groups. Standards for hypromellose 1828, hypromellose 2208, hypromellose 2906, and hypromellose 2910 are given in the USP.

A white, yellowish-white, or greyish-white, practically odourless fibrous powder or granules; hygroscopic after drying. **Dissolves** in cold water, forming a colloidal solution; practically insoluble in hot water, dehydrated alcohol, acetone, chloroform, ether, and toluene. A 1% w/w solution in water has a pH of 5.5 to 8.0.

Hypromellose Phthalate (5436-y)

Hypromellose Phthalate *(BANM, rINNM).*

Hydroxypropyl Methylcellulose Phthalate; Hypromellosi Phthalas; Methylhydroxypropylcellulose Phthalate; Methylhydroxypropylcellulosi Phthalas.

Pharmacopoeias. In *Eur.* (see p.viii) and *Jpn.* Also in *USNF.*

A cellulose with some of the hydroxy groups in the form of the methyl ether, some in the form of the 2-hydroxypropyl ether, and some in the form of the phthalyl ester (21 to 35% phthalyl). Different grades in the USA are distinguished by appending a number in which the first 2 digits represent the approximate percentage content of the methoxy groups, the next 2 digits the approximate percentage content of hydroxypropoxy groups, and the last 2 digits the approximate percentage content of the phthalyl groups. Standards for hypromellose phthalate 200731 and hypromellose phthalate 220824 are given in the USNF. Another system of nomenclature involves appending a number which indicates the pH value (x10) at which the polymer dissolves in aqueous buffer solutions; letters such as S or F may also be used to indicate grades of high molecular-weight or small particle size respectively.

White to slightly off-white free-flowing flakes or a granular powder, odourless or with a slight acidic odour.

Practically **insoluble** in water, dehydrated alcohol, and petroleum spirit; very slightly soluble in acetone and toluene; soluble in a mixture of equal volumes of acetone and methyl alcohol, of dehydrated alcohol and acetone, and of dichloromethane and methyl alcohol. Dissolves in 1*N* sodium hydroxide. **Store** in airtight containers.

Uses and Administration

Hypromellose has properties similar to those of methylcellulose (below). It is used in pharmaceutical manufacturing for film-coating tablets, as a tablet binder, as an extended-release matrix, and as an emulsifier, suspending agent, and stabiliser in topical gels and ointments. Hypromellose may also be used as an emulsifier and stabiliser in the food industry.

Hypromellose phthalate is used to provide enteric coating for tablets and granules, for the preparation of sustained-release granules, and as a coating to mask the unpleasant taste of some tablets.

Hypromellose is widely used clinically in ophthalmic solutions; it is preferred to methylcellulose since mucilages of hypromellose have greater clarity and usually contain fewer undispersed fibres. Hypromellose is used to prolong the action of medicated eye drops and, either alone or in combination with other viscosity-increasing agents, in artificial tears preparations for the management of dry eye (p.1470); solutions containing 0.3 to 1% of hypromellose are commonly used. Solutions for contact lens care (p.1097) and for lubricating artificial eyes contain similar concentrations. Hypromellose is also administered intra-ocularly, usually as a 2% solution, as an adjunct in ophthalmic surgery (below) and concentrations of up to 2.5% may be used topically to protect the cornea during gonioscopy procedures.

Hypromellose has been included in artificial saliva preparations used in the management of dry mouth (p.1470), but other drugs are usually preferred.

Ophthalmic surgery. Intra-ocular hypromellose may be used as a visco-elastic agent to protect the eye during surgery. In cataract extraction it is employed to maintain the anterior chamber and to coat the intra-ocular lens to facilitate its implantation. Although intra-ocular hypromellose is generally considered to be well tolerated, some workers[1] reported an increased incidence of pupil abnormalities (non-reactive semi-dilated pupils) following such use; others[2] did not confirm this.

1. Tan AKK, Humphry RC. The fixed dilated pupil after cataract surgery—is it related to intraocular use of hypromellose? *Br J Ophthalmol* 1993; **77:** 639–41.
2. Eason J, Seward HC. Pupil size and reactivity following hydroxypropyl methylcellulose and sodium hyaluronate. *Br J Ophthalmol* 1995; **79:** 541–3.

Preparations

BP 1998: Hypromellose Eye Drops *(Alkaline Eye Drops; Artificial Tears);*
USP 23: Hydroxypropyl Methylcellulose Ophthalmic Solution.

Proprietary Preparations (details are given in Part 3)
Aust.: Artelac; Okuzell; Puroptal; ***Austral.:*** Isopto Tears; Lacril†; Methopt; ***Belg.:*** Artelac; Isopto Tears; Ocucoat; ***Canad.:*** Eyelube; Isopto Tears; Lacril; M C†; ***Fr.:*** Contactol; Ocucoat†; ***Ger.:*** Artelac; Hymecel; Isopto Fluid; Methocel; Methocel Dispersa; Sic-Ophtal; Sicca-Stulln; Visc-Ophtal sine†; ***Irl.:*** Artelac; Isopto Alkaline; Isopto Plain; ***Ital.:*** Lacrimill; Lacrisifi; Lacrisol; Methocel; ***Norw.:*** Ocucoat†; ***S.Afr.:*** Isopto Plain†; Methocel; Spersatear; Viscotraan; ***Swed.:*** Isopto Plain; Ocucoat†; ***Switz.:*** Hymecel†; Isopto Tears; Ultra-Tears; ***UK:*** BJ6†; Isopto Alkaline; Isopto Plain; Moisture Eyes; Ocucoat; ***USA:*** Gonak; Goniosoft; Goniosol; Isopto Alkaline; Isopto Plain; Isopto Tears; Lacril; Ocucoat; Tearisol; Tears Again MC; Ultra Tears.

Multi-ingredient: ***Austral.:*** Bausch & Lomb Sensitive Eyes Lens Lubricant; Murine Sore Eyes; Poly-Tears; Tears Naturale; ***Belg.:*** Lacrystat; Tears Naturale; ***Canad.:*** Bion Tears; Moisture Drops; Ocutears; Tears Naturale; ***Ger.:*** Isopto Naturale; Lacrisic; ***Irl.:*** Ilube; Tears Naturale; ***Ital.:*** Dacriosol; Hamamilla; Tirs; ***Neth.:*** Cromovist†; Duratears†; ***S.Afr.:*** Tears Naturale; ***Spain:*** Dacrolux; Tears Humectante; ***Switz.:*** Tears Naturale; ***UK:*** Ilube; Tears Naturale; ***USA:*** Bion Tears; Estivin; LubriTears; Maximum Strength Allergy Drops; Moisture Drops; Muro's Opcon; Nature's Tears; Ocucoat; Tears Naturale; Tears Renewed.

Magnesium Silicate (5443-l)

553(a) (synthetic magnesium silicate).

CAS — 1343-88-0.

Pharmacopoeias. In *Jpn.* Also in *USNF.*

A compound of magnesium oxide and silicon dioxide. It is a fine white odourless powder free from grittiness. Practically **insoluble** in water, and in alcohol. It is readily decomposed by mineral acids. A 10% suspension in water has a pH of 7.0 to 10.8.

Uses

Magnesium silicate is used in the food industry and in pharmaceutical manufacturing as an anticaking agent.

Preparations

Proprietary Preparations (details are given in Part 3)
Multi-ingredient: ***Belg.:*** Mucal; ***Fr.:*** Phytemag; ZeaSorb; ***Ital.:*** Babigoz Crema Protettiva; Crema Protettiva†; ***Switz.:*** Aloplastine Acide†; Aloplastine simple†; Bigasan.

Methylcellulose (5401-h)

Methylcellulose *(rINN).*

E461; Methylcellulosum; Metilcelulosa.

CAS — 9004-67-5.

Pharmacopoeias. In *Eur.* (see p.viii), *Int., Jpn, Pol.,* and *US.*

A cellulose having some of the hydroxyl groups in the form of the methyl ether.

Various grades of methylcellulose are available and are distinguished by appending a number indicating the apparent viscosity in millipascal seconds of a 2% w/w solution at 20°. It is a white, yellowish-white, or greyish-white, fibrous powder or granules; hygroscopic after drying.

Practically **insoluble** in hot water, dehydrated alcohol, acetone, chloroform, ether, and toluene; dissolves in cold water, forming a colloidal solution; soluble in glacial acetic acid and in a mixture of equal volumes of alcohol and chloroform. A 1% w/w solution in water has a pH of 5.5 to 8.0.

Incompatibilities have been reported with a number of compounds including chlorocresol, hydroxybenzoates, and phenol. Large amounts of electrolytes increase the viscosity of methylcellulose mucilages owing to salting-out of the methylcellulose; in very high concentrations of electrolytes, the methylcellulose may be completely precipitated.

Adverse Effects

Large quantities of methylcellulose may temporarily increase flatulence and distension and there is a risk of intestinal obstruction. Oesophageal obstruction may occur if compounds like methylcellulose are swallowed dry.

Precautions

Methylcellulose and other bulk-forming agents should not be given to patients with intestinal obstruction or conditions likely to lead to intestinal obstruction. They should be taken with sufficient fluid to prevent faecal impaction or oesophageal obstruction, and should not be taken immediately before going to bed.

Interactions

Bulk laxatives such as methylcellulose lower the transit time through the gut and could affect the absorption of other drugs. Incompatibilities that have been reported *in vitro* with methylcellulose are listed above.

Uses and Administration

The various grades of methylcellulose are widely used in pharmaceutical manufacturing as emulsifying, suspending, and thickening agents and as binding, disintegrating, and coating agents in tablet manufacturing. Low-viscosity grades are preferred for use as emulsifying agents as the surface tension produced is lower than with the higher-viscosity grades. Low-viscosity grades may also be used as suspending or thickening agents for liquid oral dosage forms and solutions of methylcellulose may be used as replacements for sugar-based syrups or other suspension bases. For thickening topically applied products such as gels and creams a high-viscosity grade is usually employed. In tablet technology low- or medium-viscosity grades are used as binding agents while high-viscosity grades act as tablet disintegrants by swelling on contact with the disintegration medium. For tablet coating, highly substituted low-viscosity grades are usually used. Methylcellulose may also be included in sustained-release tablet formulations.

Methylcellulose is also employed as an emulsifier and stabiliser in the food industry.

Methylcellulose is also used clinically as a bulk-forming agent. Medium- or high-viscosity grades are used as bulk laxatives in the treatment of constipation (p.1168); by taking up moisture they increase the volume of the faeces and promote peristalsis. Methylcellulose is usually given in a dosage of up to 6 g daily in divided doses, taken with plenty of fluid. It is also given in similar doses but with a minimum amount of water for the control of diarrhoea (p.1168) and for the control of faecal consistency in ostomies. It is also used in the management of diverticular disease (p.1169). Methylcellulose has also been used as an aid to appetite control in the management of obesity (p.1476) but there is little evidence of efficacy.

A 0.5 to 1% solution of a high-viscosity grade of methylcellulose has been used as a vehicle for eye drops, as artificial tears, and in contact lens care, but hypromellose (p.1473) is now generally preferred for this purpose.

Preparations

BP 1998: Methylcellulose Granules; Methylcellulose Tablets; ***USP 23:*** Methylcellulose Ophthalmic Solution; Methylcellulose Oral Solution; Methylcellulose Tablets.

Proprietary Preparations (details are given in Part 3)
Aust.: Bulk; ***Austral.:*** Cellulone; ***Canad.:*** Citrucel†; Murocel; ***Fr.:*** Dacryolarmes; ***Irl.:*** Celevac; ***Ital.:*** Lacrimart; ***Spain:*** Muciplasma; ***UK:*** Celevac; ***USA:*** Citrucel; Murocel.

Multi-ingredient: ***Aust.:*** Cellobexon; ***Austral.:*** Le Trim-BM; Parachoc; ***Canad.:*** Slim Mint; ***Ital.:*** Conta-Lens Wetting; ***S.Afr.:*** Kolantyl; Medigel; Merasyn; ***Spain:*** Humectante; ***UK:*** Nilstim†.

Pectin (5447-c)

E440(i); E440(ii) (amidated pectin or pectin extract).

CAS — 9000-69-5.

Pharmacopoeias. In *Aust.* and *US.*

A purified carbohydrate product obtained from the dilute acid extract of the inner portion of the rind of citrus fruits or from apple pomace; it consists mainly of partially methoxylated polygalacturonic acids.

A coarse or fine, yellowish-white, almost odourless powder. Almost completely **soluble** 1 in 20 of water, forming a viscous, opalescent, colloidal solution which flows readily and is acid to litmus; practically insoluble in alcohol and other organic solvents. It dissolves more readily in water if first moistened with alcohol, glycerol, or syrup, or if mixed with 3 or more parts of sucrose. **Store** in airtight containers.

Interactions

Bulk-forming agents such as dietary fibre lower the transit time through the gut and may affect the absorption of other drugs.

Pectin, employed as a source of fibre, together with a lipid-lowering diet and lovastatin has resulted in a paradoxical increase in low-density lipoprotein (LDL)-cholesterol in patients with hypercholesterolaemia. It was believed the pectin reduced the absorption of lovastatin from the gut.[1]

1. Richter WO, *et al.* Interaction between fibre and lovastatin. *Lancet* 1991; **338:** 706.

Uses and Administration

Pectins are used as emulsifiers and stabilisers in the food industry. They are non-starch polysaccharide constituents of dietary fibre (see Bran, p.1181).

Pectin is an adsorbent and bulk-forming agent and is present in multi-ingredient preparations for the management of diarrhoea, constipation, and obesity. Pectin has also been tried for reducing or slowing carbohydrate absorption in the dumping syndrome (p.1169).

Preparations

Proprietary Preparations (details are given in Part 3)
Fr.: Arhemapectine Antihemorragique.

Multi-ingredient: ***Aust.:*** Diarrhoesan; ***Austral.:*** Betaine Digestive Aid; Diaguard Forte†; Diaguard†; Diarcalm; Diareze; Diet Fibre Complex 1500†; Diet-Trim†; Donnagel; Glucomagma†; Kaomagma with Pectin; Kaopectate; Orabase; Orahesive; PC Regulax; Stomahesive; United Soft Guard†; ***Belg.:*** Kaopectate; Tanalone; ***Canad.:*** Diarex; Diban; Donnagel-MB†; Donnagel-PG; Donnagel†; Kaomycin†; Orabase; Orahesive; ***Fr.:*** Carbonaphtine Pectinee†; Gelopectose; Sureskin; ***Ger.:*** Diarrhoesan; Kaopectate N†; Kaoprompt-H; Noventerol†; ***Irl.:*** Kaopectate; Orabase; Pekolin†; ***Ital.:*** Cruscasohn; Streptomagma; ***S.Afr.:*** Bipectinol; Biskapect; Chloropect; Collodyne; Diastat†; Enterolyte; Gastropect; Kantrexil; Kao; Kaomagma†; Kaomycin†; Kaoneo†; Kaopectin; Kaostatex; Medipect†; Neopect†; Pectikon; Pectin-K; Pectolin†; Pectrolyte; Peterpect†; ***Spain:*** Bio Hubber; Bio Hubber Fuerte; Dextricea; Estreptoenterol; Estreptosirup†; Salvacolina NN†; Sorbitoxin†; ***Switz.:*** Demosvelte N; Fiblet†; Geli-Stop†; HEC; Kaopectate; Varihesive Hydroactive; ***UK:*** Kaopectate†; KLN; Orabase; Orahesive; Stomahesive; Varihesive; ***USA:*** Donnagel-PG†; K-C; Kao-Spen; Kaodene Non-Narcotic; Parepectolin.

Polyethylene Oxide (3271-z)

Pharmacopoeias. In *USNF.*

A nonionic homopolymer of ethylene oxide, represented by the formula $(OCH_2CH_2)_n$, in which n represents the average number of oxyethylene groups (about 2000 to over 100 000). It is obtainable in several grades, varying in viscosity profile. It may contain not more than 3% of silicon dioxide. A white to off-white powder. **Miscible** with water; freely soluble in acetonitrile, in dichloromethane, in ethylene dichloride, and in trichloroethylene; practically insoluble in aliphatic hydrocarbons, in ethylene glycol, in diethylene glycol, and in glycerol. **Store** in airtight containers. Protect from light.

Uses

Polyethylene oxide is used as a tablet binder and as a suspending and thickening agent in pharmaceutical preparations. Polyethylene oxide is also used in a hydrogel wound dressing.

Preparations

Proprietary Preparations (details are given in Part 3)
UK: Vigilon.

Polyvinyl Acetate Phthalate (18369-l)

Pharmacopoeias. In *USNF.*

Polyvinyl acetate phthalate is a reaction product of phthalic anhydride and a partially hydrolysed polyvinyl acetate, containing 55 to 62% of phthalyl ($C_8H_5O_3$) groups, calculated on an anhydrous acid-free basis.

It is a free-flowing white powder and may have a slight odour of acetic acid. Practically **insoluble** in water, in chloroform and in dichloromethane; soluble in alcohol and in methyl alcohol. **Store** in airtight containers.

Uses

Polyvinyl acetate phthalate is a viscosity-modifying agent which is used in the manufacture of enteric coating for tablets.

Polyvinyl Alcohol (468-b)

CAS — 9002-89-5.

Pharmacopoeias. In *Pol.* and *US.*

A synthetic resin represented by the formula $(-CH_2CHOH-)_n$, where the average value of n is 500 to 5000. It is prepared by 85 to 89% hydrolysis of polyvinyl acetate.

White to cream-coloured odourless granules or powder. Freely **soluble** in water; more rapidly soluble at higher temperatures. A 4% solution in water has a pH of 5.0 to 8.0.

A range of polyvinyl alcohols of varying viscosity and saponification value is available commercially.

Uses and Administration

Polyvinyl alcohol is a nonionic surfactant that is used in pharmaceutical manufacturing as a stabilising agent and as a viscosity-increasing agent and lubricant.

Polyvinyl alcohols have also been used in the preparation of jellies which dry rapidly when applied to the skin to form a soluble plastic film.

Polyvinyl alcohols of various grades are used for a wide variety of industrial applications.

Polyvinyl alcohol has been used to increase the viscosity of ophthalmic preparations thus prolonging contact of the active ingredient with the eye. It is included in artificial tears preparations used for dry eye (p.1470) and in contact lens solutions (p.1097). For dry eye it is often used in a concentration of 1.4% with or without povidone.

Preparations

Proprietary Preparations (details are given in Part 3)
Aust.: Liquifilm; ***Austral.:*** Barnes-Hind Wetting Solution; Liquifilm; ***Belg.:*** Liquifilm; ***Canad.:*** Cooper Tears; Hypotears; Liquifilm; Optilube PVA; PMS-Artificial Tears; Revitaleyes; RO-Dry Eyes; Scheinpharm Artificial Tears; ***Fr.:*** Liquifilm; ***Ger.:*** Alltotal; Contafilm; Lacrimal; Liquifilm; Vistofilm; ***Irl.:*** Liquifilm; Sno Tears; ***Ital.:*** Lacrilux; ***Neth.:*** Liquifilm†; ***Norw.:*** Ocufri; ***S.Afr.:*** Liquifilm; ***Spain:*** Hypo Tears; Liquifilm Lagrimas; ***Swed.:*** Sincon; ***Switz.:*** Liquifilm; ***UK:*** Liquifilm Tears; Sno Tears; ***USA:*** Akwa Tears; Dry Eyes; Liquifilm; Nu-Tears; Puralube; Tear Drop; Tears Again.

Multi-ingredient: ***Aust.:*** Siccaprotect; ***Austral.:*** Barnes-Hind Wetting and Soaking Solution†; Refresh; Teardrops; Tears Plus; ***Canad.:*** Murine; PMS-Artificial Tears Plus; Refresh; Scheinpharm Artificial Tears Plus; Teardrops; Tears Plus; ***Ger.:*** Dispatenol; Duracare; Lacrimal OK; Siccaprotect; ***Irl.:*** Hypotears†; ***Ital.:*** Collyria; Hypotears; ***Neth.:*** Tears Plus†; ***S.Afr.:*** Refresh; Tears Plus; ***Spain:*** Liquifresh; ***Switz.:*** Collylarm; Tears Plus; ***UK:*** Hypotears; Refresh; ***USA:*** Hypotears; Murine; Murine Plus; Nu-Tears II; Nutra Tear†; Refresh; Tears Plus; VasoClear.

Povidone (5450-e)

Povidone *(BAN, USAN, rINN).*

Polyvidone; Polyvidonum; Polyvinylpyrrolidone; Povidonum; PVP; Vinylpyrrolidinone Polymer. Poly (2-oxopyrrolidin-1-ylethylene).

$(C_6H_9NO)_n$.

CAS — 9003-39-8.

Pharmacopoeias. In *Eur.* (see p.viii), *Int., Jpn, Pol.,* and *US.*

A mixture of essentially linear synthetic polymers of 1-vinylpyrrolidin-2-one of different chain lengths and molecular weights.

A white or yellowish-white, hygroscopic powder or flakes. Freely **soluble** in water, in alcohol, and in methyl alcohol; slightly soluble in acetone; practically insoluble in ether. A 5% solution in water has a pH of 3 to 7. **Store** in airtight containers.

Copovidone (17698-r)

Copolyvidone; Copolyvidonum; Copovidonum.

Pharmacopoeias. In *Eur.* (see p.viii).

A copolymer of 1-vinylpyrrolidin-2-one and vinyl acetate in the mass proportion 3:2.

A white or yellowish-white, hygroscopic powder or flakes. Freely **soluble** in water, in alcohol, and in dichloromethane; practically insoluble in ether. **Store** in airtight containers.

Crospovidone (10229-v)

Crospovidone *(rINN).*

Crospovidonum; Polyplasdone XL.

CAS — 9003-39-8.

Pharmacopoeias. In *Eur.* (see p.viii). Also in *USNF.*

A cross-linked homopolymer of 1-vinylpyrrolidin-2-one.

A white or yellowish-white, hygroscopic powder or flakes with a faint odour. Practically **insoluble** in water, in alcohol, and in dichloromethane. A 1% suspension in water has a pH of 5 to 8. **Store** in airtight containers.

Adverse Effects

Some products intended for parenteral administration contain povidone as an excipient and injection has led to deposition of povidone in various tissues with consequent lesions and pain. There have been occasional reports of liver involvement.

Reviews of adverse effects associated with pharmaceutical excipients including povidone.

1. Golightly LK, *et al.* Pharmaceutical excipients: adverse effects associated with 'inactive ingredients' in drug products (part II). *Med Toxicol* 1988; **3:** 209–40.

Uses and Administration

Povidone is used in pharmaceutical manufacturing as a suspending and dispersing agent and as a tablet binding, granulating, and coating agent. It is used as a carrier for iodine (see Povidone-Iodine, p.1123). An insoluble cross-linked form of povidone known as crospovidone is used as a tablet disintegrant. Copovidone, a copolymer with vinyl acetate, is used as a tablet binding and coating agent.

Povidone is included in artificial tears preparations used in the management of dry eye (p.1470) and in solutions for contact lens care (p.1097). For dry eye it is often used in a concentration of 0.6% together with other viscosity-increasing agents (such as polyvinyl alcohol); it may also be used alone in solutions containing 1.5 to 5%.

Povidone has also been used as an adsorbent in gastro-intestinal disorders.

Povidone was formerly used as a plasma expander but other compounds are now preferred.

Preparations

Proprietary Preparations (details are given in Part 3)
Aust.: Oculotect; Protagent; ***Austral.:*** Clerz Moisturising Drops; In A Wink Moisturing; ***Belg.:*** Protagent; Siccagent; ***Fr.:*** Bolinan†; Dulcilarmes; Nu-Gel; ***Ger.:*** Arufil; Lac-Ophtal; Lacri-Stulln; Oculotect Fluid; Protagent; Vidirakt S; Vidisept N; ***Neth.:*** Duratears Free†; Oculotect; Protagens†; ***Switz.:*** Bolinan†; Dulcilarmes†; Protagent.

Multi-ingredient: ***Austral.:*** Barnes-Hind Wetting and Soaking Solution†; Bausch & Lomb Sensitive Eyes Lens Lubricant; Refresh; Teardrops; Tears Plus; ***Canad.:*** Moisture Drops; Murine; PMS-Artificial Tears Plus; Refresh; Scheinpharm Artificial Tears Plus; Teardrops; Tears Plus; ***Fr.:*** Poly-Karaya; ***Ger.:*** Lacrimal OK; Lacrisic; ***Neth.:*** Tears Plus†; ***S.Afr.:*** Refresh; Tears Plus; ***Spain:*** Liquifresh; Plasmoid†; ***Switz.:*** Collylarm; Poly-Karaya; Tears Plus; ***UK:*** Refresh; ***USA:*** Adsorbotear; Murine; Murine Plus; Refresh; Tears Plus.

Silica (4000-d)

Silica or silicon dioxide is available in various forms.

Purified Siliceous Earth (5456-k)

Diatomaceous Earth; Diatomite; Purified Infusorial Earth; Purified Kieselguhr; Terra Silicea Purificada.

CAS — 7631-86-9.

Pharmacopoeias. In *USNF.*

An amorphous form of silicon dioxide consisting chiefly of frustules and fragments of diatoms purified by calcining.

A very fine, white, light grey, or pale buff, gritty powder. Practically **insoluble** in water, acids, and in dilute solutions of alkali hydroxides. It absorbs about 4 times its weight of water without becoming fluid.

Silicon Dioxide (5455-c)

551; Colloidal Hydrated Silica; Precipitated Silica; Silica Colloidalis Hydrica; Silica Gel.

SiO_2,xH_2O = 60.08 (anhydrous).

CAS — 63231-67-4; 7631-86-9.

Pharmacopoeias. In *Eur.* (see p.viii). Also in *USNF.*

Silicon Dioxide (USNF 18) is obtained by insolubilising the dissolved silica in sodium silicate solution. Where obtained by the addition of sodium silicate to a mineral acid, the product is termed silica gel; where obtained by the destabilisation of a solution of sodium silicate in such a manner as to yield very fine particles, the product is termed precipitated silica. Dental-Type Silica (USNF 18) is obtained from sodium silicate solution by destabilising with acid in such a way as to yield very fine particles.

The Ph. Eur. monograph is entitled Colloidal Hydrated Silica.

A light, fine, white or almost white, odourless, hygroscopic, amorphous powder in which the diameter of the average particles ranges from 2 to 10 μm.

Practically **insoluble** in water, in alcohol and other organic solvents, and in mineral acids except hydrofluoric acid; dissolves in hot solutions of alkali hydroxides. A 5% suspension in water has a pH of 4 to 8. **Store** in airtight containers.

Colloidal Silicon Dioxide (5457-a)

Acidum Silicicum Colloidale; Colloidal Anhydrous Silica; Colloidal Silica; Hochdisperses Silicumdioxid; Silica Colloidalis Anhydrica.

SiO_2 = 60.08.

CAS — 7631-86-9.

Pharmacopoeias. In *Eur.* (see p.viii). Also in *USNF.*

The USNF describes a submicroscopic fumed silica, prepared by the vapour-phase hydrolysis of a silicon compound. The Ph. Eur. monograph is entitled Colloidal Anhydrous Silica.

A light, fine, white, odourless, amorphous, non-gritty powder. It has a particle size of about 15 nm. Practically **insoluble** in water and in mineral acids except hydrofluoric acid; dissolves in hot solutions of alkali hydroxides. A dispersion in water (3.3 to 4%) has a pH of 3.5 to 5.5.

Adverse Effects

Prolonged inhalation of some forms of silica dust may be associated with the development of fibrosis of the lung (silicosis). The forms of silica described here and used as pharmaceutical excipients may cause irritation of the respiratory tract if inhaled but do not appear to be associated with silicosis.

Uses

The different forms of silica have various pharmaceutical uses. Purified siliceous earth is used as a filtering medium and adsorbent. Silicon dioxide is used as a suspending and thickening agent and, as silica gel, as a desiccant. Colloidal silicon dioxide is used as a suspending agent and thickener, as a stabiliser in emulsions, and as an anticaking agent and desiccant. Silicon dioxide is also used as an anticaking agent in the food industry.

Silicon dioxide (Silicea) is used in homoeopathic medicine.

Preparations

Proprietary Preparations (details are given in Part 3)
Austral.: Celloids S 79; ***Ger.:*** Aktiv-Puder; Entero-Teknosal; Sklerosol; ***Mon.:*** Dissolvurol.

Multi-ingredient: ***Aust.:*** CO_2 Granulat; Kephalodoron; ***Austral.:*** Bio-Disc; Duo Celloids SCF; Duo Celloids SPS; Duo Celloids SSS; Hair and Nail Formula†; Silicic Complex; ***Belg.:*** Trisibam†; ***Canad.:*** Topol Gel with Fluoride†; Topol with Fluoride†; ***Fr.:*** Gastralugel†; Gelopectose; Topaal; ***Ger.:*** Adsorgan†; Aplona; Atmulen E†; Azulon compositum Homburg†; Biosilit-Heilsalbe†; CO_2 Granulat; Equisil; Gastrovison†; Rowarolan; Tectivit†; Vobaderm Basiscreme†; ***Ital.:*** Belsar†; Gastrovison; Lacalut; ***Spain:*** Sales Gras†; ***Switz.:*** Acne Creme; Balsafissan†; Cicafissan; Fissan; Globase†; ***UK:*** Bidor; New Era Hymosa; New Era Zief; WCS Dusting Powder.

Sodium Starch Glycollate (5460-y)

Carboxymethylamylum Natricum; Sodium Carboxymethyl Starch; Sodium Starch Glycolate; Starch Sodium Glycollate.

CAS — 9063-38-1.

Pharmacopoeias. In *Chin.* Also in *USNF.*

Eur. (see p.viii) includes Sodium Starch Glycollate (Type A) and Sodium Starch Glycollate (Type B).

The sodium salt of a carboxymethyl ether of starch.

Sodium Starch Glycollate (Type A) (Ph. Eur.) and Sodium Starch Glycolate (USNF 18) contain 2.8 to 4.2% of sodium. Sodium Starch Glycollate (Type B) (Ph. Eur.) contains 2.0 to 3.4% of sodium.

A fine, odourless, white or almost white, very hygroscopic, free-flowing powder. Practically **insoluble** in dichloromethane. Forms a translucent suspension in water. A 2% dispersion in cold water settles, on standing, to give a highly hydrated layer. **Store** in airtight containers. Protect from light, and from variations in temperature and humidity which may cause caking.

Uses

Sodium starch glycollate is used as a disintegrating agent in tablet manufacture.

Tragacanth (5463-c)

E413; Goma Alcatira; Gomme Adragante; Gum Dragon; Gum Tragacanth; Trag.; Tragacantha; Tragacanto; Tragant.

CAS — 9000-65-1.

Pharmacopoeias. In *Eur.* (see p.viii), *Jpn,* and *Pol.* Also in *USNF.*

The dried gummy exudation flowing naturally or obtained by incision from the trunk and branches of *Astragalus gummifer* and some other species of *Astragalus* (Leguminosae) from western Asia.

It occurs as thin, flattened, more or less curved, ribbon-like, white or pale yellow, translucent, horny odourless strips; it may also appear as a powder. When reduced to a powder it forms a mucilaginous gel with about ten times its weight of water.

Store in airtight containers. Protect from light.

Adverse Effects

Hypersensitivity reactions, sometimes severe, have occurred rarely after the ingestion of products containing tragacanth. Contact dermatitis has been reported following the external use of tragacanth.

Uses

Tragacanth forms viscous solutions or gels with water, depending on the concentration. It is used in pharmaceutical manufacturing as a suspending agent and as an emulsifying agent. In dispensing aqueous preparations of tragacanth, the powdered tragacanth is first dispersed in a wetting agent, such as alcohol, to prevent agglomeration on the addition of water.

Tragacanth is also used for similar purposes in the food industry.

Xanthan Gum (5465-a)

Corn Sugar Gum; E415; Polysaccharide B 1459; Xantham Gum; Xanthani Gummi.

CAS — 11138-66-2.

Pharmacopoeias. In *Eur.* (see p.viii). Also in *USNF.*

A gum produced by a pure-culture fermentation of a carbohydrate with *Xanthomonas campestris* and purified. It is the sodium, potassium, or calcium salt of a high molecular weight polysaccharide containing D-glucose, D-mannose, and D-glucuronic acid. It also contains not less than 1.5% of pyruvic acid.

A white or yellowish-white, free-flowing powder. **Soluble** in hot and cold water; practically insoluble in organic solvents. A 1% solution in water has a pH of 6 to 8.

Uses

Xanthan gum is used in pharmaceutical manufacturing as a suspending, stabilising, thickening, and emulsifying agent. It is also used similarly in the food industry.

Suspensions of crushed tablets or insoluble powders made with xanthan gum were reported to be preferable to those made with tragacanth.[1]

The stability was generally good and only a small number of drugs had been found to be incompatible (amitriptyline, tamoxifen, and verapamil).[1] For extemporaneous dispensing, a 1% solution of xanthan gum with hydroxybenzoate, prepared in advance, was diluted to 0.5% with water when preparing the suspension.

Xanthan gum was found to be a suitable suspending vehicle for delivering antispasmodics topically along the length of the oesophagus in patients with oesophageal spasm.[2] Coagulation of the gum had been observed when it was used for suspensions of certain film-coated tablets.

1. Anonymous. "Extremely useful" new suspending agent. *Pharm J* 1986; **237:** 665.
2. Evans BK, Fenton-May V. Keltrol. *Pharm J* 1986; **237:** 736–7.

Preparations

Proprietary Preparations (details are given in Part 3)
UK: Keltrol.

Stimulants and Anorectics

This chapter includes compounds used for their central stimulant or their anorectic effects. Many are sympathomimetics and are subject to extensive abuse, which has led to strict limitations on their availability. The use of central stimulants and anorectics is now generally restricted to a few indications that require specialist supervision such as hyperactivity, the narcoleptic syndrome, and obesity.

Hyperactivity

Attention deficit hyperactivity disorder (ADHD) is a heterogeneous behaviour disorder which first becomes evident during childhood and consists of developmentally inappropriate and socially disruptive behaviour characterised by varying degrees of hyperactivity, inattention, and impulsiveness. Children with this disorder are easily distracted and have difficulty in completing tasks. Associated features may include low frustration tolerance, mood lability, and defiance. Some children continue to have symptoms throughout adolescence and into adulthood. The terms hyperkinesis, hyperkinetic syndrome, minimal brain dysfunction, attention deficit disorder, and attention deficit disorder with hyperactivity have sometimes been used synonymously for ADHD but patients described as having these disorders do not necessarily satisfy the diagnostic criteria.

Treatment depends on the severity of the disorder. In the USA drug treatment for ADHD is quite common even in mild forms but in the UK it is generally only used under specialist supervision for the more severely affected child who fails to respond to counselling and behaviour therapy. When drug therapy is indicated treatment should initially be with a central stimulant.[1-7] They are useful for the management of symptoms but are not curative. Dexamphetamine and methylphenidate are usually the drugs of first choice but there is no consensus on which is the most effective. Pemoline has been used but is associated with hepatotoxicity. Prolonged administration of central stimulants can retard growth and it is advised that drug holidays should be given occasionally to determine the continued need for therapy. It is generally recommended that children under 5 or 6 years of age should not receive stimulants. Stimulants also appear to be of use when the disorder persists into adulthood.[8] Tricyclic antidepressants such as imipramine and desipramine are also used for ADHD and their effect in this condition appears to be independent of their antidepressant action. However, because of their lower efficacy and adverse effects, they are reserved as second-line drugs for patients who fail to respond to or are intolerant of central stimulants; they may be a useful alternative in patients with Tourette's syndrome[9] or in those with a family history of the disorder as stimulants are believed to precipitate or exacerbate associated tics (see p.636). Tricyclic antidepressants might also be preferred in patients with additional disorders such as depression, anxiety, or enuresis. Combined therapy with tricyclic antidepressants and central stimulants has been studied[10,11] but careful monitoring is advised. MAOIs have been used successfully but problems with dietary restriction and potential drug interactions have limited their use. For further information concerning potential interactions between stimulants and tricyclic antidepressants or MAOIs, see under Dexamphetamine, p.1479. Fluoxetine has produced beneficial results as an adjunct to central stimulants in a small number of patients with associated depression or obsessive-compulsive disorder.[12,13] Venlafaxine has been effective in open trials in a small number of adult patients.[14,15] Clonidine has produced some promising results but again numbers have been small.[16] A meta-analysis of a small number of trials has provided preliminary evidence that carbamazepine may be an effective alternative to central stimulants.[17] Antipsychotics can produce severe adverse effects and are probably rarely indicated in ADHD. Their use might be warranted as adjunctive therapy to central stimulants in severe cases or when there is also extremely violent or destructive behaviour. Lithium is not considered to be effective in ADHD but might be useful as an adjunct in selected patients with coexisting bipolar disorder.

Much controversy has surrounded the hypothesis that certain synthetic food additives including preservatives and artificial flavours and colours are aetiological agents in ADHD. Diets such as the 'Feingold diet' which eliminate these additives appear to help only a few hyperactive children and require considerable parental effort to prepare. It has been considered that few children who react to diet would react to additives alone; there seemed to be no justification in using diets that excluded additives, although it was worthwhile paying attention to parental comments that implicated certain foods.[3]

1. Elia J. Drug treatment for hyperactive children: therapeutic guidelines. *Drugs* 1993; **46:** 863–71.
2. Fox AM, Rieder MJ. Risks and benefits of drugs used in the management of the hyperactive child. *Drug Safety* 1993; **9:** 38–50.
3. Anonymous. Adderall and other drugs for attention-deficit/hyperactivity disorder. *Med Lett Drugs Ther* 1994; **36:** 109–10.
4. Anonymous. The management of hyperactive children. *Drug Ther Bull* 1995; **33:** 57–60.
5. Carrey NJ, *et al.* Pharmacological treatment of psychiatric disorders in children and adolescents: focus on guidelines for the primary care practitioner. *Drugs* 1996; **51:** 750–9.
6. Barbaresi WJ. Primary-care approach to the diagnosis and management of attention-deficit hyperactivity disorder. *Mayo Clin Proc* 1996; **71:** 463–71.
7. Committee on Children With Disabilities and Committee on Drugs. Medication for children with attention disorders. *Pediatrics* 1996; **98:** 301–4.
8. Wender PH, *et al.* A controlled study of methylphenidate in the treatment of attention deficit disorder, residual type, in adults. *Am J Psychiatry* 1985; **142:** 547–52.
9. Singer HS, *et al.* The treatment of attention-deficit hyperactivity disorder in Tourette's syndrome: a double-blind placebo-controlled study with clonidine and desipramine. *Pediatrics* 1995; **95:** 74–81.
10. Rapport MD, *et al.* Methylphenidate and desipramine in hospitalized children I: separate and combined effects on cognitive function. *J Am Acad Child Adolesc Psychiatry* 1993; **32:** 333–42.
11. Pataki CS, *et al.* Side effects of methylphenidate and desipramine alone and in combination in children. *J Am Acad Child Adolesc Psychiatry* 1993; **32:** 1065–72.
12. Gammon GD, Brown TE. Fluoxetine and methylphenidate in combination for treatment of attention deficit disorder and comorbid depressive disorder. *J Child Adolesc Psychopharmacol* 1993; **3:** 1–10.
13. Bussing R, Levin GM. Methamphetamine and fluoxetine treatment of a child with attention-deficit hyperactivity disorder and obsessive-compulsive disorder. *J Child Adolesc Psychopharmacol* 1993; **3:** 53–8.
14. Hedges D, *et al.* An open trial of venlafaxine in adult patients with attention deficit hyperactivity disorder. *Psychopharmacol Bull* 1995; **31:** 779–83.
15. Adler LA, *et al.* Open-label trial of venlafaxine in adults with attention deficit disorder. *Psychopharmacol Bull* 1995; **31:** 785–8.
16. Anonymous. Clonidine for treatment of attention-deficit/hyperactivity disorder. *Med Lett Drugs Ther* 1996; **38:** 109–10.
17. Silva RR, *et al.* Carbamazepine use in children and adolescents with features of attention-deficit hyperactivity disorder: a meta-analysis. *J Am Acad Child Adolesc Psychiatry* 1996; **35:** 352–8.

Narcoleptic syndrome

Narcolepsy is characterised by excessive daytime sleepiness and irresistible sleep attacks that last from a few minutes to hours. The term narcoleptic syndrome is sometimes used, as narcolepsy is often accompanied by other symptoms such as cataplexy, sleep paralysis, hypnagogic hallucinations, or disturbed sleep. Most patients with narcolepsy experience **cataplexy**, a sudden short-lived loss of muscle tone and paralysis of voluntary muscles induced by strong emotions. The severity of the attack can vary and some patients may experience complete collapse but there is no loss of consciousness. **Sleep paralysis** consists of transient episodes of complete paralysis that occur while falling asleep or during waking; respiration is unaffected. Some patients may complain of vivid auditory or visual hallucinations while falling asleep (**hypnagogic hallucinations**).

In the treatment of narcoleptic syndrome the patient is initially encouraged to take planned regular short periods of sleep during the day[1,2] and to avoid stressful events that may provoke attacks. If drug treatment is required then central stimulants are the main drugs used for the sleep attacks of narcolepsy.[1-4] However, they are ineffective against cataplexy. The selection, dose, and timing of administration of these drugs needs to be titrated for each patient[5] and drug holidays have been suggested to reduce the risk of developing tolerance.[1,4] Amphetamines were the first drugs used. However, methylphenidate is often preferred to dexamphetamine as it has a rapid action and is considered to have fewer adverse effects.[2,3] Alternative stimulants include mazindol and modafinil. Selegiline has been reported to improve excessive daytime sleepiness and cataplexy.[6,7] There is a wide range of other drugs for which there is anecdotal or other limited evidence of efficacy in narcolepsy but there appears to be no evidence that they are superior to the central stimulants.[1,4]

Tricyclic antidepressants are the primary treatment for cataplexy and sleep paralysis.[1] Imipramine appears to be one of the most widely used and has been reported to act more rapidly and to require a lower dose for cataplexy than when used as an antidepressant.[2,4] The daily dose may be given once daily or in divided doses but should be titrated to provide maximal protection for the time of day when symptoms usually occur; evening doses may need to be avoided to minimise nocturnal arousal.[2] Clomipramine is also commonly used. Protriptyline has been reported to be effective;[8] it may also be beneficial for sleepiness in patients who remain symptomatic when given central stimulants or who cannot tolerate them.[1] Other antidepressants that have been tried for cataplexy include femoxetine[9] and fluoxetine.[10] The use of sodium oxybate at night with stimulants during the day has been reported to improve the symptoms of patients with narcoleptic syndrome.[11]

Patients requiring treatment for both narcolepsy and cataplexy may be given central stimulants and tricyclic antidepressants but require careful monitoring as the combination may produce serious adverse effects such as cardiac arrhythmias or hypertension;[2] see also Interactions, under Dexamphetamine, p.1479.

1. Aldrich MS. Narcolepsy. *N Engl J Med* 1990; **323:** 389–94.
2. Kales A, *et al.* Sleep disorders: sleep apnea and narcolepsy. *Ann Intern Med* 1987; **106:** 434–43.
3. Eisen J, *et al.* Psychotropic drugs and sleep. *Br Med J* 1993; **306:** 1331–4.
4. Richardson JW, *et al.* Narcolepsy update. *Mayo Clin Proc* 1990; **65:** 991–8.
5. Parkes JD. Daytime sleepiness. *Br Med J* 1993; **306:** 772–5.
6. Hublin C, *et al.* Selegiline in the treatment of narcolepsy, *Neurology* 1994; **44:** 2095–2101.
7. Mayer G, *et al.* Selegiline hydrochloride treatment in narcolepsy: a double-blind, placebo-controlled study. *Clin Neuropharmacol* 1995; **18:** 306–19.
8. Schmidt HS, *et al.* Protriptyline: an effective agent in the treatment of the narcolepsy-cataplexy syndrome and hypersomnia. *Am J Psychiatry* 1977; **134:** 183–5.
9. Schrader H, *et al.* The treatment of accessory symptoms in narcolepsy: a double-blind cross-over study of a selective serotonin re-uptake inhibitor (femoxetine) versus placebo. *Acta Neurol Scand* 1986; **74:** 297–303.
10. Langdon N, *et al.* Fluoxetine in the treatment of cataplexy. *Sleep* 1986; **9:** 371–3.
11. Mamelak M, *et al.* Treatment of narcolepsy with γ-hydroxybutyrate: a review of clinical and sleep laboratory findings. *Sleep* 1986; **9:** 285–9.

Obesity

Obesity is an important medical problem as those who are obese are at risk of many medical complications including cardiovascular disease, diabetes mellitus, gallstones, respiratory disease, osteoarthritis, and some forms of cancer. It occurs when there is an imbalance between energy intake and energy expenditure. A commonly used measure for body fatness is the body mass index. It is the weight (kg) divided by the square of the height (m^2). Values of 18.5 to 24.9 are considered to be the normal range; 25.0 to 29.9 to be overweight; and 30.0 or more to be obesity with 30.0 to 34.9 considered a moderate, 35.0 to 39.9 a severe, and 40.0 or more a very severe, risk of co-morbidity.

The management of obesity includes dietary modification, behaviour modification, and exercise, with adjunctive drug therapy, where indicated. Weight loss appears to improve control of diabetes mellitus and hypertension, and to reduce cardiovascular risk factors but the long-term health effects are less clear as weight is often regained.

The initial stage in management is dietary modification and includes calorie restriction and changes in the dietary proportions of fat, protein, and carbohydrates. Physical activity should also be increased and excess alcohol avoided and smoking stopped. These measures should be followed for at least 3 months and if at this stage there has been less than 10% reduction in weight and body mass index is still above 30, drug treatment may be considered. For patients with associated risk factors such as diabetes mellitus, ischaemic heart disease, hyperlipidaemias, hypertension, or sleep apnoea drugs may be considered when the body mass index is

27 or 28. Combination drug therapy is not recommended. Drugs should be given initially for 12 weeks. If weight loss is less than 5% then they should be considered a failure and discontinued. If weight loss is more than 5% they may be continued and the patient monitored at monthly intervals. Treatment should be stopped once the body mass index falls below 30 (or 27/28 as appropriate), if weight is regained, or if there is any suspicion of toxicity.

Many drugs are capable of reducing appetite and have been used as such in the treatment of obesity. However, toxicity has been a major problem and very few are still in current use.

Appetite suppressants or anorectics can be divided into two main groups: central (CNS) stimulants that act on central catecholamine pathways and drugs acting on central serotonin pathways. Stimulants such as the amphetamines and phenmetrazine are no longer recommended because of their addictive potential. Other stimulants that have been used include diethylpropion, phentermine, mazindol, and phenylpropanolamine but they are also no longer recommended. The serotonergic drugs dexfenfluramine and fenfluramine were formerly used in long-term therapy (up to 1 year) but have both been associated with valvular heart defects and have now been withdrawn worldwide.

Two drugs recently introduced for use in obesity are orlistat (a gastric lipase inhibitor) and sibutramine (a serotonin and noradrenaline reuptake inhibitor).

Investigative drugs have included fluoxetine, which has been tried with some success, and opioid antagonists such as naloxone and naltrexone but their value is limited and their routine use cannot be justified. Bulk-forming drugs such as methylcellulose and sterculia have been used in an attempt to control appetite by the local effect they might exert when they swell in the gastro-intestinal tract, but there is little evidence of efficacy.

Thyroid drugs were formerly tried in the treatment of obesity in euthyroid patients, but they produce only temporary weight loss, mainly of lean body mass, and can produce serious complications, especially cardiac complications. Hypothyroidism has also been reported on withdrawal.

The control of appetite and the mechanisms of obesity are under investigation. A gene, called the ob-gene, and its protein product, leptin, have been identified and appear to regulate food intake. Further studies will clarify their role in obesity and may influence future treatment options.

References.

1. Rosenbaum M, *et al.* Obesity. *N Engl J Med* 1997; **337:** 396–407.
2. Björntorp P. Obesity. *Lancet* 1997; **350:** 423–6.
3. Wilding J. Obesity treatment. *Br Med J* 1997; **315:** 997–1000.
4. Auwerx J, Staels B. Leptin. *Lancet* 1998; **351:** 737–42.
5. Epstein LH, *et al.* Treatment of pediatric obesity. *Pediatrics* 1998; **101:** 554–70.
6. National Institutes of Health. *Clinical guidelines on the identification, evaluation, and treatment of overweight and obesity in adults: the evidence report.* Betheseda: National Heart, Lung, and Blood Institute, 1998.
7. Royal College of Physicians of London. *Clinical management of overweight and obese patients with particular reference to the use of drugs.* London: Royal College of Physicians of London, 1998.

Prader-Willi syndrome

Compulsive eating and a voracious appetite are two of the many clinical features of Prader-Willi syndrome, a congenital disorder characterised by infantile hypotonia, hypogonadism, and facial dysmorphism, with subsequent development of abnormalities of behaviour and intellect.[1] Supervision and restricted access to food are the mainstay in preventing obesity, but are commonly not sufficient. Anorectics such as fenfluramine have been tried but this drug, along with dexfenfluramine, was withdrawn worldwide following reports of valvular heart defects.

1. Donaldson MDC, *et al.* The Prader-Willi syndrome. *Arch Dis Child* 1994; **70:** 58–63.

Adrafinil (3018-h)

Adrafinil *(rINN).*

CRL-40048. 2-[(Diphenylmethyl)sulfinyl]acetohydroxamic acid.

$C_{15}H_{15}NO_3S$ = 289.4.
CAS — 63547-13-7.

Adrafinil is a central stimulant and $alpha_1$-adrenergic agonist chemically related to modafinil (p.1483). It is given by mouth for mental function impairment in the elderly in doses of 600 mg to 1.2 g daily.

Preparations

Proprietary Preparations (details are given in Part 3)
Fr.: Olmifon.

Almitrine Dimesylate (12342-f)

Almitrine Dimesylate *(BANM).*

Almitrine Dimesilate *(rINNM)*; Almitrine Bismesylate; S-2620 (almitrine). *NN'*-Diallyl-6-[4-(4,4'-difluorobenzhydryl)piperazin-1-yl]-1,3,5-triazine-2,4-diyldiamine bis(methanesulphonate).

$C_{26}H_{29}F_2N_7,2CH_4SO_3$ = 669.8.
CAS — 27469-53-0 (almitrine).

Almitrine dimesylate has been used as a respiratory stimulant in acute respiratory failure associated with conditions such as chronic obstructive pulmonary disease. Usual oral doses range from 50 to 100 mg daily and treatment may be intermittent. Up to 3 mg per kg body-weight has been given daily by intravenous infusion in 2 or 3 divided doses, each dose being infused over 2 hours. It is also available in a compound preparation with raubasine for mental function impairment in the elderly.

Mental impairment. References.

1. Poitrenaud J, *et al.* Almitrine-raubasine and cognitive impairment in the elderly: results of a 6-month controlled multicenter study. *Clin Neuropharmacol* 1990; **13** (suppl 3): S100–S108.
2. Poitrenaud J, *et al.* Time course of age-associated memory impairment in 8037 patients treated with Duxil for 6 months. *Rev Geriatr* 1994; **19:** 531–8.
3. Poitrenaud J, *et al.* Memory disorders in 8037 elderly patients with age-associated memory impairment: multicenter trial with a 6-month follow-up under almitrine-raubasine. *Eur Neurol* 1995; **35** (suppl 1): 43–6.

Respiratory system disorders. Respiratory stimulants (such as almitrine) have a limited and short-term role in acute respiratory failure in chronic obstructive pulmonary disease (p.747). Almitrine has been reported[1-6] to improve ventilation and blood oxygenation, and to decrease the number of episodes of dyspnoea and hospital admissions. There is also a report of beneficial effects when used with inhaled nitric oxide in patients with severe hypoxaemic acute respiratory distress syndrome[7] (p.1017). However, these modest benefits may be outweighed by the adverse effects, which have included peripheral paraesthesia and weight loss,[4] and headache, urticaria, breathlessness, diarrhoea, chest pain, nausea, and vomiting.[6] The peripheral neuropathy which sometimes occurs during long-term use of almitrine[8,9] may be due to an underlying feature of the pulmonary disease being treated,[10-12] although some disagree with this.[13]

1. Huchon G. Advances in treatment of chronic obstructive lung disease with almitrine bis-mesylate. *Postgrad Med J* 1983; **59** (suppl 3): 66–7.
2. Bell RC, *et al.* The effect of almitrine bismesylate on hypoxemia in chronic obstructive pulmonary disease. *Ann Intern Med* 1986; **105:** 342–6.
3. Chung KF, Barnes PJ. Respiratory and allergic disease II: chronic obstructive airways disease and respiratory infections. *Br Med J* 1988; **296:** 111–5.
4. Watanabe S, *et al.* Long-term effect of almitrine bismesylate in patients with hypoxemic chronic obstructive pulmonary disease. *Am Rev Respir Dis* 1989; **140:** 1269–73.
5. Daskalopoulou E, *et al.* Comparison of almitrine bismesylate and medroxyprogesterone acetate on oxygenation during wakefulness and sleep in patients with chronic obstructive lung disease. *Thorax* 1990; **45:** 666–9.
6. Bakran I, *et al.* Double-blind placebo controlled clinical trial of almitrine bismesylate in patients with chronic respiratory insufficiency. *Eur J Clin Pharmacol* 1990; **38:** 249–53.
7. Payen D, *et al.* Almitrine magnifies the beneficial effect of inhaled NO in severe hypoxemic ARDS. *Br J Anaesth* 1994; **72** (suppl 1): 111.
8. Chedru F, *et al.* Peripheral neuropathy during treatment with almitrine. *Br Med J* 1985; **290:** 896.
9. Gherardi R, *et al.* Peripheral neuropathy in patients treated with almitrine dimesylate. *Lancet* 1985; **i:** 1247–50.
10. Suggett AJ, *et al.* Almitrine and peripheral neuropathy. *Lancet* 1985; **ii:** 830–1.
11. Alani SM, *et al.* Almitrine and peripheral neuropathy. *Lancet* 1985; **ii:** 1251.
12. Moore N, *et al.* Peripheral neuropathy in chronic obstructive lung disease. *Lancet* 1985; **ii:** 1311.
13. Louarn F, Gherardi R. Almitrine and peripheral neuropathy. *Lancet* 1985; **ii:** 1068.

Preparations

Proprietary Preparations (details are given in Part 3)
Belg.: Vectarion; ***Fr.:*** Vectarion; ***Ger.:*** Vectarion; ***Irl.:*** Vectarion; ***Spain:*** Sovarel; Vectarion.

Multi-ingredient: ***Fr.:*** Duxil; ***Spain:*** Duxor; Salvalion.

Amiphenazole Hydrochloride (1411-a)

Amiphenazole Hydrochloride *(BANM, rINNM).*

Amiphenazole Chloride. 5-Phenylthiazole-2,4-diamine hydrochloride.

$C_9H_9N_3S,HCl$ = 227.7.
CAS — 490-55-1 (amiphenazole); 942-31-4 (amiphenazole hydrochloride).

Amiphenazole has properties similar to those of doxapram hydrochloride (p.1480) and has been used as a respiratory stimulant in usual doses of 100 to 150 mg intramuscularly or intravenously.

Lichenoid reactions have been reported in addition to those reactions expected from its central activity.

Preparations

Proprietary Preparations (details are given in Part 3)
Aust.: Daptazole†; ***Ger.:*** Daptazile†.

Ammonium Camphocarbonate (14455-n)

$C_{11}H_{19}NO_3$ = 213.3.
CAS — 5972-75-8.

Ammonium camphocarbonate has been used in preparations for the treatment of respiratory-tract disorders.

Preparations

Proprietary Preparations (details are given in Part 3)

Multi-ingredient: ***Spain:*** Pulmofasa; Pulmofasa Antihist.

Amphetamine (1412-t)

Amphetamine *(BAN).*

Amfetamine *(rINN)*; Anfetamina; Racemic Desoxynorephedrine. *(R,S)*-α-Methylphenethylamine.

$C_9H_{13}N$ = 135.2.
CAS — 300-62-9 (amphetamine); 139-10-6 (amphetamine phosphate).

Amphetamine Sulphate (1414-r)

Amphetamine Sulphate *(BANM).*

Amfetamine Sulphate *(rINNM)*; Amphetamine Sulfate; Amphetamini Sulfas; Phenaminum; Phenylaminopropanum Racemicum Sulfuricum. *(R,S)*-α-Methylphenethylamine sulphate.

$(C_9H_{13}N)_2,H_2SO_4$ = 368.5.
CAS — 60-13-9.

Pharmacopoeias. In *Eur.* (see p.viii) and *US.*

A white odourless crystalline powder. Freely **soluble** in water; slightly soluble in alcohol; practically insoluble in ether. Aqueous solutions have a pH of 5 to 6. **Protect** from light. **Incompatible** with alkalis and calcium salts.

Amphetamine is an indirect-acting sympathomimetic with actions and uses similar to those of its isomer dexamphetamine (below). Amphetamine, amphetamine sulphate, and amphetamine aspartate are given by mouth in doses similar to those of dexamphetamine sulphate. The laevo-isomer, levamphetamine was formerly used in a similar manner. Amphetamine, being volatile, was formerly employed by inhalation.

Preparations

USP 23: Amphetamine Sulfate Tablets.

Proprietary Preparations (details are given in Part 3)
Norw.: Dexamin†; ***Spain:*** Centramina.

Multi-ingredient: ***Belg.:*** Epipropane; ***Fr.:*** Ortenal; ***Ital.:*** Dintospina†; ***USA:*** Adderall; Obetrol.

Amphetaminil (1415-f)

Amfetaminil *(rINN).* α-(α-Methylphenethylamino)-α-phenylacetonitrile.

$C_{17}H_{18}N_2$ = 250.3.
CAS — 17590-01-1.

Amphetaminil is a central stimulant given by mouth in doses of 10 to 30 mg daily in the treatment of narcolepsy.

Preparations

Proprietary Preparations (details are given in Part 3)
Ger.: AN 1.

Multi-ingredient: ***Ger.:*** Ton-O_2 (Tonozwei)†; Vit-O_2 (Vitozwei)†.

Bemegride (1416-d)

Bemegride *(BAN, rINN)*.

Bemegridum. 3-Ethyl-3-methylglutarimide; 4-Ethyl-4-methylpiperidine-2,6-dione.

$C_8H_{13}NO_2$ = 155.2.

CAS — 64-65-3.

Bemegride has properties similar to those of doxapram (p.1480). It has been given intravenously as a respiratory stimulant.

Porphyria. Bemegride has been associated with acute attacks of porphyria and is considered unsafe in patients with acute porphyria.[1]

1. Moore MR, McColl KEL. *Porphyria: drug lists.* Glasgow: Porphyria Research Unit, University of Glasgow, 1991.

Preparations

Proprietary Preparations (details are given in Part 3)
Spain: Megimide†.

Benzphetamine Hydrochloride (1471-q)

Benzphetamine Hydrochloride *(BANM)*.

Benzfetamine Hydrochloride *(rINNM)*. (+)-*N*-Benzyl-*N*,α-dimethylphenethylamine hydrochloride.

$C_{17}H_{21}N,HCl$ = 275.8.

CAS — 156-08-1 (benzphetamine); 5411-22-3 (benzphetamine hydrochloride).

Benzphetamine hydrochloride is a central stimulant and sympathomimetic with properties similar to those of dexamphetamine (below). It has been used as an anorectic administered by mouth in the treatment of obesity (p.1476), although amphetamines are no longer recommended for this indication. The usual initial dose is 25 to 50 mg once daily, subsequently adjusted, according to requirements, to a dose of 25 to 50 mg once to three times daily.

Preparations

Proprietary Preparations (details are given in Part 3)
USA: Didrex.

Catha (12537-w)

Abyssinian, African, or Arabian Tea; Kat; Kath; Khat; Miraa.

The leaves of *Catha edulis* (Celastraceae), containing cathine, cathinone, celastrin, choline, tannins, and inorganic salts.

Cathine (12538-e)

Cathine *(pINN)*.

(+)-Norpseudoephedrine. *threo*-2-Amino-1-phenylpropan-1-ol.

$C_9H_{13}NO$ = 151.2.

CAS — 492-39-7; 36393-56-3.

Cathinone (10136-d)

Cathinone *(pINN)*.

(*S*)-2-Aminopropiophenone.

$C_9H_{11}NO$ = 149.2.

CAS — 71031-15-7.

Catha is used for its stimulant properties among some cultures of Africa and the Middle East, usually by chewing the leaves. Its effects are reported to resemble those of the amphetamines (see Dexamphetamine Sulphate, below), and are thought to be largely due to the content of cathinone. Dependence and psychotic reactions have been reported. Cathine, another constituent, is used as the hydrochloride as an anorectic.

References to the pharmacology and pharmacokinetics of catha and its constituents[1-6] and reports of adverse effects.[7-11]

1. Kalix P. Pharmacological properties of the stimulant khat. *Pharmacol Ther* 1990; **48:** 397–416.
2. Kalix P. Cathinone, a natural amphetamine. *Pharmacol Toxicol* 1992; **70:** 77–86.
3. Kalix P. Chewing khat, an old drug habit that is new in Europe. *Int J Risk Safety Med* 1992; **3:** 143–56.
4. Widler P, *et al.* Pharmacodynamics and pharmacokinetics of khat: a controlled study. *Clin Pharmacol Ther* 1994; **55:** 556–62.
5. Brenneisen R, *et al.* Metabolism of cathinone to (−)-norephedrine and (−)-norpseudoephedrine. *J Pharm Pharmacol* 1986; **38:** 298–300.
6. Brenneisen R, *et al.* Amphetamine-like effects in humans of the khat alkaloid cathinone. *Br J Clin Pharmacol* 1990; **30:** 825–8.
7. Rumpf KW, *et al.* Rhabdomyolysis after ingestion of an appetite suppressant. *JAMA* 1983; **250:** 2112.
8. Gough SP, Cookson IB. Khat-induced schizophreniform psychosis in UK. *Lancet* 1984; **i:** 455.
9. Roper JP. The presumed neurotoxic effects of Catha edulis—an exotic plant now available in the United Kingdom. *Br J Ophthalmol* 1986; **70:** 779–81.
10. Zureikat N, *et al.* Chewing khat slows the orocaecal transit time. *Gut* 1992; **33** (suppl): S23.
11. Yousef G, *et al.* Khat chewing as a cause of psychosis. *Br J Hosp Med* 1995; **54:** 322–6.

Preparations

Proprietary Preparations (details are given in Part 3)
Ger.: Amorphan†; Antiadipositum X-112 S; Exponcit N†; Miraprront N; Vita-Schlanktropfen; ***S.Afr.:*** Appetrol; Dietene; Eetless; Laser Slim 'n Trim†; Nobese No. 1; Slenz†; Slim 'n Trim; Thinz; ***Switz.:*** Adistop; Antiadipositum X-112; Belloform nouvelle formule; Limit-X; Miniscap.

Multi-ingredient: ***Ger.:*** Recatol†; ***S.Afr.:*** Slendoll†.

Chlorphentermine Hydrochloride (1472-p)

Chlorphentermine Hydrochloride *(BANM, USAN, rINNM)*.

NSC-76098; S-62; W-2426. 4-Chloro-α,α-dimethylphenethylamine hydrochloride.

$C_{10}H_{14}ClN,HCl$ = 220.1.

CAS — 461-78-9 (chlorphentermine); 151-06-4 (chlorphentermine hydrochloride).

Pharmacopoeias. In *Fr.*

Chlorphentermine hydrochloride is a sympathomimetic with properties similar to those of dexamphetamine (below). It was formerly used as an anorectic and has been implicated in lipid storage disorders and pulmonary hypertension.

Clobenzorex Hydrochloride (1473-s)

Clobenzorex Hydrochloride *(rINNM)*.

SD-271-12. (+)-*N*-(2-Chlorobenzyl)-α-methylphenethylamine hydrochloride.

$C_{16}H_{18}ClN,HCl$ = 296.2.

CAS — 13364-32-4 (clobenzorex); 5843-53-8 (clobenzorex hydrochloride).

Clobenzorex hydrochloride is a central stimulant and sympathomimetic with properties similar to those of dexamphetamine (below). It has been used as an anorectic in the treatment of obesity (p.1476) in usual doses of 30 mg twice daily by mouth, before meals.

Preparations

Proprietary Preparations (details are given in Part 3)
Fr.: Dinintel; ***Spain:*** Finedal.

Deanol (12624-s)

Deanol *(BAN)*.

Démanol. 2-Dimethylaminoethanol.

$C_4H_{11}NO$ = 89.14.

CAS — 108-01-0 (deanol); 3342-61-8 (deanol aceglumate); 968-46-7 (deanol benzilate); 71-79-4 (deanol benzilate hydrochloride).

NOTE. Deanol Aceglumate is *pINN*.

Deanol, a precursor of choline, may enhance central acetylcholine formation. It has been employed as a central stimulant in the treatment of hyperactivity in children but its efficacy has not been substantiated. It is included in preparations used as tonics and for the management of impaired mental function.

It has been used as a variety of salts and esters including deanol aceglumate, deanol acetamidobenzoate, deanol bisorcate, deanol cyclohexylpropionate (cyprodenate; cyprodemanol), deanol hemisuccinate, deanol pidolate, and deanol tartrate. Deanol benzilate (deanol diphenylglycolate; benzacine) has been used as the hydrochloride in antispasmodic preparations.

Preparations

Proprietary Preparations (details are given in Part 3)
Belg.: Actebral; ***Fr.:*** Actebral; Astyl; Cleregil; Tonibral Adulte; ***Ger.:*** Medacaps N; Risatarun; ***Ital.:*** Pabenol†; Rischiaril.

Multi-ingredient: ***Aust.:*** Prospervital; ***Fr.:*** Debrumyl; Tonuvital†; ***Ger.:*** Dimaestad†; Rowachol comp.; Seniosan†; ***Spain:*** Acticinco; Anti Anorex Triple; Denubil; ***Switz.:*** Vigoran.

Dexamphetamine Sulphate (1419-m)

Dexamphetamine Sulphate *(BANM)*.

Dexamfetamine Sulphate *(pINNM)*; Dexamphetamini Sulfas; Dextro Amphetamine Sulphate; Dextroamphetamine Sulfate; NSC-73713 (dexamphetamine). (*S*)-α-Methylphenethylammonium sulphate; (+)-α-Methylphenethylamine sulphate.

$(C_9H_{13}N)_2,H_2SO_4$ = 368.5.

CAS — 51-64-9 (dexamphetamine); 7528-00-9 (dexamphetamine phosphate); 51-63-8 (dexamphetamine sulphate).

Pharmacopoeias. In *Br., Swiss,* and *US.*

A white or almost white, odourless or almost odourless, crystalline powder. **Soluble** 1 in 10 of water and 1 in 800 of alcohol; practically insoluble in ether. A 5% solution in water has a pH of 5.0 to 6.0.

Adverse Effects

The side-effects of dexamphetamine are commonly symptoms of overstimulation of the CNS and include insomnia, night terrors, nervousness, restlessness, irritability, and euphoria that may be followed by fatigue and depression. There may be dryness of the mouth, anorexia, abdominal cramps and other gastro-intestinal disturbances, headache, dizziness, tremor, sweating, tachycardia, palpitations, increased or sometimes decreased blood pressure, altered libido, and impotence. Psychotic reactions have occurred as has muscle damage with associated rhabdomyolysis and renal complications. Rarely, cardiomyopathy has occurred with chronic use. In children, growth retardation may occur during prolonged treatment.

In *acute overdosage*, the adverse effects are accentuated and may be accompanied by hyperpyrexia, mydriasis, hyperreflexia, chest pain, cardiac arrhythmias, confusion, panic states, aggressive behaviour, hallucinations, delirium, convulsions, respiratory depression, coma, circulatory collapse, and death. Individual patient response may vary widely and toxic manifestations may occur at relatively low overdoses.

Tolerance can develop to some of dexamphetamine's central effects leading to increased doses and habituation. Abrupt cessation after prolonged treatment or abuse of amphetamines has been associated with extreme fatigue, hyperphagia, and depression. However, it is generally accepted that the amphetamines, although widely abused, are not associated with substantial physical dependence.

Amphetamines are abused for their euphoriant effects. *Abuse* has resulted in personality changes, compulsive and stereotyped behaviour, and may induce a toxic psychosis with auditory and visual hallucinations and paranoid delusions.

Abuse. Abuse of amphetamines can lead to toxicity affecting many organs or body systems. There have been reports of *intracerebral haemorrhage*[1-3] and of *cardiomyopathy*.[4-6]

Kendrick *et al.*[7] described a syndrome characterised by *circulatory collapse, fever, leukaemoid reaction, disseminated intravascular coagulation*, and *rhabdomyolysis* with *diffuse myalgias* and *muscle tenderness* in 5 drug abusers who had administered amphetamines or phenmetrazine intravenously. Scandling and Spital[8] reported a 30-year-old man who had ingested 50 amphetamine sulphate tablets and developed *rhabdomyolysis* and *myoglobinuric renal failure*, possibly secondary to a crush syndrome, but in the absence of prolonged coma or other major myotoxic factors. In contrast, Foley *et al.*[9] reported a patient who developed *acute interstitial nephritis* and *acute renal failure* after oral amphetamine abuse without the associated factors of rhabdomyolysis, hyperpyrexia, or necrotising angiitis. In an earlier study, Citron *et al.*[10] had found *necrotising angiitis* to be associated with intravenous methylamphetamine abuse.

Chronic use may result in adverse effects such as *hallucinations*, a *delusional disorder* resembling *paranoid schizophrenia, stereotyped behaviour*, and *movement disorders*.[11] Although chronic intoxication is the most common precondition for psychosis, individual sensitivities are an important aspect of the drug reaction.

Increased serum concentrations of *thyroxine* have been associated with heavy amphetamine abuse in 4 psychiatric patients.[12]

Abrupt cessation after prolonged treatment or abuse of amphetamines may cause *extreme fatigue, hyperphagia,* and *depression. Depressive stupor* has been reported in 3 long-term abusers of amphetamine after sudden withdrawal.[13]

1. Delaney P, Estes M. Intracranial hemorrhage with amphetamine abuse. *Neurology* 1980; **30:** 1125–8.
2. Harrington H, *et al.* Intracerebral hemorrhage and oral amphetamine. *Arch Neurol* 1983; **40:** 503–7.
3. Salanova V, Taubner R. Intracerebral haemorrhage and vasculitis secondary to amphetamine use. *Postgrad Med J* 1984; **60:** 429–30.
4. Smith HJ, *et al.* Cardiomyopathy associated with amphetamine administration. *Am Heart J* 1976; **91:** 792–7.
5. Call TD, *et al.* Acute cardiomyopathy secondary to intravenous amphetamine abuse. *Ann Intern Med* 1982; **97:** 559–60.
6. Hong R, *et al.* Cardiomyopathy associated with the smoking of crystal methamphetamine. *JAMA* 1991; **265:** 1152–4.
7. Kendrick WC, *et al.* Rhabdomyolysis and shock after intravenous amphetamine administration. *Ann Intern Med* 1977; **86:** 381–7.
8. Scandling J, Spital A. Amphetamine-associated myoglobinuric renal failure. *South Med J* 1982; **75:** 237–40.
9. Foley RJ, *et al.* Amphetamine-induced acute renal failure. *South Med J* 1984; **77:** 258–60.
10. Citron BP, *et al.* Necrotizing angiitis associated with drug abuse. *N Engl J Med* 1970; **283:** 1003–11.
11. Ellinwood EH, Kilbey MM. Fundamental mechanisms underlying altered behavior following chronic administration of psychomotor stimulants. *Biol Psychiatry* 1980; **15:** 749–57.
12. Morley JE, *et al.* Amphetamine-induced hyperthyroxinemia. *Ann Intern Med* 1980; **93:** 707–9.
13. Tuma TA. Depressive stupor following amphetamine withdrawal. *Br J Hosp Med* 1993; **49:** 361–3.

Effects on growth. The Pediatric Subcommittee of the FDA Psychopharmacologic Drugs Advisory Committee reviewed the growth-suppressing effects of stimulant medication in hyperkinetic children.[1] There was reasonable evidence that stimulant drugs, particularly in higher doses, moderately suppressed growth in weight and might have a minor suppressing effect on growth in stature. There were indications that some growth caught up during drug holidays, and that early growth suppression was not evident in adulthood. Careful monitoring during treatment was recommended.

See also under Methylphenidate Hydrochloride, p.1483.

1. Roche AF, *et al.* The effects of stimulant medication on the growth of hyperkinetic children. *Pediatrics* 1979; **63:** 847–50.

Treatment of Adverse Effects

In general the management of overdosage with amphetamines involves supportive and symptomatic therapy. Sedation is usually sufficient. Forced acid diuresis has been advocated to increase amphetamine excretion but is seldom necessary and should only be considered in severely poisoned patients; it requires close supervision and monitoring.

Precautions

Dexamphetamine is contra-indicated in patients with cardiovascular disease including moderate to severe hypertension, and in patients with hyperthyroidism, glaucoma, hyperexcitability, or agitated states. It should not be given to patients with a history of drug abuse and it should be avoided in pregnant women or breast-feeding mothers. It should be given with caution to patients with mild hypertension, impaired kidney function, or unstable personality. Height and weight in children should be monitored as growth retardation may occur. Prolonged high doses may need gradual withdrawal as abrupt cessation may produce fatigue and mental depression.

Care may be needed in certain patients predisposed to tics or Tourette's syndrome as symptoms may be provoked. Dexamphetamine is likely to reduce the convulsive threshold; caution is therefore advised in patients with epilepsy. However, it appears that in some countries amphetamines are included in antiepileptic preparations containing phenytoin or phenobarbitone in an attempt to increase their antiepileptic action. Amphetamines may impair patients' ability to drive or to operate machinery.

Diabetic control should be monitored when central stimulants are used for the control of obesity.

Abuse. Dexamphetamine is subject to extensive abuse and for this reason its availability needs to be severely curtailed. For adverse effects associated with abuse, see above.

Porphyria. Amphetamines were considered to be unsafe in patients with acute porphyria although there is conflicting experimental evidence on porphyrinogenicity.[1] Methylamphetamine has been associated with clinical exacerbations of porphyria.

1. Moore MR, McColl KEL. *Porphyria: drug lists.* Glasgow: Porphyria Research Unit, University of Glasgow, 1991.

Pregnancy. No difference was found in the incidence of severe congenital anomalies between 1824 children of mothers prescribed amphetamines or phenmetrazine during pregnancy and 8989 children of mothers who had not received these drugs.[1] Though an excess of oral clefts was noted in the offspring of mothers prescribed amphetamines, there was no excess of congenital heart disease.[1] This was contrary to a previous suggestion[2] in which congenital heart disease in 184 infants had been studied and a link to maternal dexamphetamine exposure postulated. There has been a report of a bradycardia followed by death in a fetus due to maternal intravenous self-administration of 500 mg of amphetamine.[3]

1. Milkovich L, van den Berg BJ. Effects of antenatal exposure to anorectic drugs. *Am J Obstet Gynecol* 1977; **129:** 637–42.
2. Nora JJ, *et al.* Dexamphetamine: a possible environmental trigger in cardiovascular malformations. *Lancet* 1970; **i:** 1290–1.
3. Dearlove JC, Betteridge TJ. Stillbirth due to intravenous amphetamine. *Br Med J* 1992; **304:** 548.

Tourette's syndrome. In a review of clinical reports, Shapiro and Shapiro[1] concluded that there was virtually no evidence that central stimulants caused or provoked Tourette's syndrome and weak or inadequate evidence that clinically appropriate doses of central stimulants caused tics in previously asymptomatic patients or exacerbated pre-existing symptoms. However, they suggested that there was evidence that high or toxic doses might exacerbate or provoke tics in predisposed patients. Lowe *et al.*[2] reported on 15 children who developed Tourette's syndrome while receiving stimulant medication for attention deficit disorders; 13 of these children had either pre-existing tics or a family history of tics or of Tourette's syndrome. They considered that stimulant therapy for hyperactivity was contra-indicated in children with motor tics or diagnosed Tourette's syndrome and should be used with caution in children with a family history of these symptoms. In addition, they suggested that the development of motor tic symptoms in any child receiving stimulants should be a clear indication for immediate discontinuation to minimise the possibility of eliciting a full-blown Tourette's syndrome.

1. Shapiro AK, Shapiro E. Do stimulants provoke, cause, or exacerbate tics and Tourette syndrome? *Compr Psychiatry* 1981; **22:** 265–73.
2. Lowe TL, *et al.* Stimulant medications precipitate Tourette's syndrome. *JAMA* 1982; **247:** 1729–31.

Interactions

Dexamphetamine is an indirect-acting sympathomimetic and may interact with a number of other drugs. To avoid precipitating a hypertensive crisis, it should not be given to patients being treated with an MAOI or within 14 days of stopping such treatment. Concurrent use of beta blockers and amphetamines may produce severe hypertension. Dexamphetamine may also diminish the effects of other antihypertensives, including guanethidine and similar drugs, and concurrent use should be avoided. Patients receiving amphetamines and tricyclic antidepressants require careful monitoring as the risk of cardiovascular effects including arrhythmias may be increased. The urinary excretion of amphetamines is reduced by urinary alkalinisers which may enhance or prolong their effects; excretion is increased by urinary acidifiers.

Amphetamines may delay the absorption of ethosuximide, phenobarbitone, and phenytoin. The stimulant effects of amphetamines are inhibited by chlorpromazine, haloperidol, and lithium. Disulfiram may inhibit the metabolism and excretion of amphetamines.

Concurrent use of sympathomimetics with volatile liquid anaesthetics such as halothane is associated with an increased risk of cardiac arrhythmias.

Pharmacokinetics

Amphetamines are readily absorbed from the gastro-intestinal tract and are distributed into most body tissues with high concentrations in the brain and CSF. They are partially metabolised in the liver but a considerable fraction may be excreted in the urine unchanged. Urinary elimination is pH-dependent and enhanced in acid urine. Amphetamines are distributed into breast milk.

References.

1. Steiner E, *et al.* Amphetamine secretion in breast milk. *Eur J Clin Pharmacol* 1984; **27:** 123–4.

Uses and Administration

Dexamphetamine, the dextrorotatory isomer of amphetamine, is an indirect-acting sympathomimetic with alpha- and beta-adrenergic agonist activity. It has a marked stimulant effect on the CNS, particularly the cerebral cortex.

Dexamphetamine is used in the treatment of narcolepsy (p.1476) and as an adjunct in the management of refractory hyperactivity disorders in children above the age of 6 years (p.1476).

Dexamphetamine has been given in the treatment of obesity (p.1476), although amphetamines are no longer recommended for this indication. Amphetamines have also been used to overcome fatigue but, again, such use is considered undesirable.

In some countries amphetamines have been included in antiepileptic preparations but the practice is not recommended.

Dexamphetamine is used as the sulphate and is given by mouth.

In the treatment of narcolepsy, the usual starting dose is 5 to 10 mg daily in divided doses, increased if necessary by 5 to 10 mg at weekly intervals to a maximum of 60 mg daily. The lower initial starting dose of 5 mg daily is suggested for the elderly and any weekly increments should also be restricted to 5 mg in such patients.

In hyperactive children individualisation of treatment is especially important; children aged 6 years and over usually start with a dose of 5 mg once or twice daily, increased if necessary by 5 mg at weekly intervals to an upper limit of 20 mg daily, though older children might require up to 40 mg daily.

Dexamphetamine has also been given as the saccharate.

Preparations

BP 1998: Dexamfetamine Tablets;
USP 23: Dextroamphetamine Sulfate Capsules; Dextroamphetamine Sulfate Elixir; Dextroamphetamine Sulfate Tablets.

Proprietary Preparations (details are given in Part 3)
Canad.: Dexedrine; ***Switz.:*** Dexamin; ***UK:*** Dexedrine; ***USA:*** Dexedrine; Dextrostat; Oxydess II; Spancap No. 1.

Multi-ingredient: ***USA:*** Adderall; Obetrol.

Dexfenfluramine Hydrochloride (18628-z)

Dexfenfluramine Hydrochloride *(BANM, USAN, rINNM).*

S-5614 (dexfenfluramine). (*S*)-*N*-Ethyl-α-methyl-3-trifluoromethylphenethylamine hydrochloride.

$C_{12}H_{16}F_3N,HCl = 267.7.$

CAS — 3239-44-9 (dexfenfluramine); 3239-45-0 (dexfenfluramine hydrochloride).

Pharmacopoeias. In Fr.

Adverse Effects, Treatment, and Precautions

As for Fenfluramine Hydrochloride, p.1480.

Interactions

As for Fenfluramine Hydrochloride, p.1481.

Pharmacokinetics

Dexfenfluramine is absorbed from the gastro-intestinal tract and peak plasma concentrations are achieved within 4 hours. It is widely distributed in the body. It is metabolised mainly in the liver to an active metabolite, nordexfenfluramine. It is excreted in the urine, mostly as 3-trifluoromethylhippuric acid.

References.

1. Cheymol G, *et al.* The pharmacokinetics of dexfenfluramine in obese and non-obese subjects. *Br J Clin Pharmacol* 1995; **39:** 684–7.

Uses and Administration

Dexfenfluramine is the *S*-isomer of fenfluramine (p.1480). It stimulates the release of serotonin and selectively inhibits its reuptake, but differs from fenfluramine in not possessing any catecholamine agonist activity.

Dexfenfluramine was formerly given by mouth as the hydrochloride in the long-term (up to one year) treatment of obesity (p.1476) but, like fenfluramine, was withdrawn worldwide following reports of valvular heart defects.

Preparations

Proprietary Preparations (details are given in Part 3)
Aust.: Isomeride†; ***Austral.:*** Adifax†; ***Belg.:*** Isomeride†; ***Fr.:*** Isomeride†; ***Ger.:*** Isomeride†; ***Irl.:*** Adifax†; ***Ital.:*** Glypolix†; Isomeride†; ***Neth.:*** Isomeride†; ***S.Afr.:*** Adifax†; ***Spain:*** Dipondal†; ***Switz.:*** Isomeride†; ***UK:*** Adifax†.

Diethylaminoethanol (12648-k)

2-Diethylaminoethanol.

$C_6H_{15}NO = 117.2.$

CAS — 100-37-8.

Diethylaminoethanol is an analogue of deanol (p.1478) and has been used similarly as the malate. The hydrochloride has also been used.

Preparations

Proprietary Preparations (details are given in Part 3)
Fr.: Cerebrol.

Multi-ingredient: ***Aust.:*** Barokaton†; Thrombion.

Diethylpropion Hydrochloride (1475-e)

Diethylpropion Hydrochloride *(BANM).*

Amfepramone Hydrochloride *(pINNM).* *N*-(1-Benzoylethyl)-*NN*-diethylammonium chloride; 2-Diethylaminopropiophenone hydrochloride; (*RS*)-α-Diethylaminopropiophenone hydrochloride.

$C_{13}H_{19}NO,HCl = 241.8.$

CAS — 90-84-6 (diethylpropion); 134-80-5 (diethylpropion hydrochloride).

Pharmacopoeias. In US.

A white to off-white fine crystalline powder, odourless or with a slight characteristic odour. It may contain tartaric acid as a stabilising agent. **Soluble** 1 in 0.5 of water, 1 in 3 of alcohol, and 1 in 3 of chloroform; practically insoluble in ether. **Protect** from light.

Adverse Effects, Treatment, and Precautions

As for Dexamphetamine Sulphate, p.1478. In addition gynaecomastia has been reported rarely. The incidence of central adverse effects may be lower with diethylpropion than with dexamphetamine. Diethylpropion should not be given to patients with emotional instability or a history of psychiatric illness. It should be avoided in children and the elderly and it should be given with caution to patients with peptic ulceration or prostatic hyperplasia. Diethylpropion hydrochloride is subject to abuse.

Interactions

Diethylpropion is an indirect-acting sympathomimetic and, similarly to dexamphetamine (p.1479), may interact with a number of other drugs.

Pharmacokinetics

Diethylpropion is readily absorbed from the gastro-intestinal tract. It is extensively metabolised in the liver and possibly the gastro-intestinal tract and is excreted in the urine. Diethylpropion crosses the blood-brain barrier and the placenta. Diethylpropion and its metabolites are distributed into breast milk.

References.

1. Beckett AH. A comparative study of the pharmacokinetics of fenfluramine, ethylamphetamine, diethylpropion and their metabolites. *Curr Med Res Opin* 1979; **6** (suppl 1): 107–17.

Uses and Administration

Diethylpropion hydrochloride is a central stimulant and indirect-acting sympathomimetic with the actions of dexamphetamine (p.1479). It has been used as an anorectic administered by mouth in the treatment of obesity (p.1476), although stimulants are not generally recommended for this indication.

The usual dose is 25 mg three times daily 1 hour before meals or 75 mg, as a modified-release preparation, once daily in mid-morning. To reduce the risk of dependence it is preferably given intermittently, a period of 4 to 8 weeks' treatment being followed by a similar period without treatment.

Preparations

USP 23: Diethylpropion Hydrochloride Tablets.

Proprietary Preparations (details are given in Part 3)
Aust.: Regenon; ***Austral.:*** Tenuate; ***Belg.:*** Atractil; Dietil; Menutil; Prefamone; Regenon; Tenuate Dospan; ***Canad.:*** Tenuate; ***Fr.:*** Anorex†; Moderatan; Prefamone Chronules; Tenuate Dospan; ***Ger.:*** Regenon; Tenuate Retard; ***Ital.:*** Linea; Tenuate Dospan; ***S.Afr.:*** Tenuate Dospan; ***Spain:*** Delgamer; ***Switz.:*** Prefamone Chronules; Regenon; Tenuate Retard; ***UK:*** Tenuate Dospan†; ***USA:*** Tenuate; Tepanil†.

Multi-ingredient: ***Ger.:*** Regenon A†; ***Irl.:*** Apisate†; ***UK:*** Apisate†.

Dimefline Hydrochloride (1420-t)

Dimefline Hydrochloride *(BANM, USAN, rINNM).*

DW-62; NSC-114650; Rec-7/0267. 8-Dimethylaminomethyl-7-methoxy-3-methyl-2-phenylchromen-4-one hydrochloride.

$C_{20}H_{21}NO_3,HCl = 359.8.$

CAS — 1165-48-6 (dimefline); 2740-04-7 (dimefline hydrochloride).

Dimefline has actions similar to those of doxapram (below) and has been used by mouth and parenterally as the hydrochloride as a respiratory stimulant.

Preparations

Proprietary Preparations (details are given in Part 3)
Ital.: Remeflin; ***Spain:*** Remeflin†.

Doxapram Hydrochloride (1421-x)

Doxapram Hydrochloride *(BANM, USAN, rINNM).*

AHR-619; Doxaprami Hydrochloridum. 1-Ethyl-4-(2-morpholinoethyl)-3,3-diphenyl-2-pyrrolidinone hydrochloride monohydrate.

$C_{24}H_{30}N_2O_2,HCl,H_2O = 433.0.$

CAS — 309-29-5 (doxapram); 113-07-5 (anhydrous doxapram hydrochloride); 7081-53-0 (doxapram hydrochloride monohydrate).

Pharmacopoeias. In *Eur.* (see p.viii), *Jpn,* and *US.*

A white to off-white, odourless, crystalline powder. **Soluble** 1 in 50 of water; soluble in chloroform; sparingly soluble in alcohol and in dichloromethane; practically insoluble in ether. A 1% solution in water has a pH of 3.5 to 5.0. The commercial injection is reported to be **incompatible** with alkaline solutions such as aminophylline, frusemide, or thiopentone sodium. **Store** in airtight containers.

Adverse Effects

As with other respiratory stimulants, there is a risk that doxapram will produce adverse effects due to general stimulation of the CNS.

Doxapram may produce dyspnoea and other respiratory problems such as coughing, bronchospasm, laryngospasm, hiccup, hyperventilation, and rebound hypoventilation. Muscle involvement may range from fasciculations to spasticity. Convulsions may occur. Headache, dizziness, hyperactivity, and confusion can occur as can sweating, flushing, hyperpyrexia or a sensation of warmth, particularly in the genital or perineal regions. Hallucinations may occur rarely. There may be nausea, vomiting, diarrhoea, and problems with urination. Cardiovascular effects include alterations in blood pressure and various arrhythmias.

Thrombophlebitis may follow extravasation of doxapram during injection.

Effects on the liver. Acute hepatic necrosis in one patient was attributed to a 24-hour infusion of doxapram.[1] Liver function tests returned to normal over 3 weeks.

1. Fancourt GJ, *et al.* Hepatic necrosis with doxapram hydrochloride. *Postgrad Med J* 1985; **61:** 833–5.

Precautions

Doxapram should be given cautiously to patients with heart diseases or obstructive airway disease; where these conditions are severe its use is contra-indicated. It should be given with care to patients with liver dysfunction. Doxapram should not be administered to patients with epilepsy or other convulsive disorders, cerebral oedema, cerebrovascular accident, head injury, acute severe asthma, physical obstruction of the airway, severe hypertension, ischaemic heart disease, hyperthyroidism, or phaeochromocytoma.

Patients should be carefully supervised during administration of doxapram; special attention should be paid to changes in blood gas measurements.

Interactions

Additive pressor effects may occur when doxapram is administered concurrently with sympathomimetics or MAOIs. Cardiac arrhythmias may occur when doxapram is given with anaesthetics known to sensitise the myocardium, such as halothane, enflurane, and isoflurane; it has been recommended that doxapram should not be given for at least 10 minutes after discontinuation of these anaesthetics. Doxapram may temporarily mask the residual effects of muscle relaxants. The manufacturers have reported that there may be an interaction between doxapram and aminophylline manifested by agitation and increased skeletal muscle activity.

Pharmacokinetics

Doxapram is extensively metabolised in the liver after intravenous injection. Metabolites and a small amount of unchanged drug are excreted in the urine. Some absorption has been demonstrated when doxapram is given by mouth.

References.

1. Robson RH, Prescott LF. A pharmacokinetic study of doxapram in patients and volunteers. *Br J Clin Pharmacol* 1978; **7:** 81–7.
2. Baker JR, *et al.* Normal pharmacokinetics of doxapram in a patient with renal failure and hypothyroidism. *Br J Clin Pharmacol* 1981; **11:** 305–6.

Uses and Administration

Doxapram hydrochloride is a central and respiratory stimulant with a brief duration of action. It acts by stimulation of peripheral chemoreceptors and central respiratory centres; at higher doses, it stimulates other parts of the brain and spinal cord. Doxapram has a pressor action and may also increase catecholamine release. It improves opioid-induced respiratory depression without affecting analgesia.

Doxapram is used in the treatment of acute respiratory failure and of postoperative respiratory depression (see Respiratory Failure, p.1166).

For postoperative respiratory depression it is usually given in a dose of 0.5 to 1.5 mg per kg body-weight by intravenous injection over a period of at least 30 seconds. This dose may be repeated at hourly intervals. It may also be given by intravenous infusion, initially administered at a rate of 2 to 5 mg per minute and then reduced, according to the patient's response, to 1 to 3 mg per minute; a recommended maximum total dosage is 4 mg per kg.

Doxapram hydrochloride may be infused at a rate of 1.5 to 4.0 mg per minute in the treatment of acute respiratory failure.

Doxapram hydrochloride has also been used to treat respiratory and CNS depression following drug overdose but its use for this indication is no longer recommended.

Chronic obstructive pulmonary disease. Respiratory stimulants such as doxapram have a limited and short-term role in hypercapnic respiratory failure in patients with chronic obstructive pulmonary disease (p.747). Benefit has been reported in 3 such patients in whom doxapram was used as an alternative to intubation.[1]

1. Hirshberg AJ, *et al.* Use of doxapram hydrochloride injection as an alternative to intubation to treat chronic obstructive pulmonary disease patients with hypercapnia. *Ann Emerg Med* 1994; **24:** 701–3.

Neonatal apnoea. Doxapram is effective in neonatal apnoea (p.773) and may be considered as an alternative, or in addition, to xanthines in infants with apnoea that does not respond to xanthine therapy alone. However, it is less convenient to use as it must be administered by continuous intravenous infusion and blood pressure must be monitored. Additionally, some preparations may contain benzyl alcohol as a preservative making them unsuitable for use in neonates. It has been used in doses of 2.5 mg per kg body-weight per hour.[1-3] Adverse CNS effects have been reported.[3] Lower doses of 0.25 or 1.5 mg per kg per hour have been shown to be effective.[4,5]

1. Sagi E, *et al.* Idiopathic apnoea of prematurity treated with doxapram and aminophylline. *Arch Dis Child* 1984; **59:** 281–3.
2. Eyal F, *et al.* Aminophylline versus doxapram in idiopathic apnea of prematurity: a double-blind controlled study. *Pediatrics* 1985; **75:** 709–13.
3. Dear PRF, Wheeler D. Doxapram and neonatal apnoea. *Arch Dis Child* 1984; **59:** 903–4.
4. Bairam A, Vert P. Low-dose doxapram for apnoea of prematurity. *Lancet* 1986; **i:** 793–4.
5. Peliowski A, Finer NN. A blinded, randomized, placebo-controlled trial to compare theophylline and doxapram for the treatment of apnea of prematurity. *J Pediatr* 1990; **116:** 648–53.

Respiratory depression. References to the use of doxapram in postoperative or opioid-induced respiratory depression.

1. Gupta PK, Dundee JW. Morphine combined with doxapram or naloxone: a study of post-operative pain relief. *Anaesthesia* 1974; **29:** 33–9.
2. Gupta PK, Dundee JW. The effect of an infusion of doxapram on morphine analgesia. *Anaesthesia* 1974; **29:** 40–3.
3. Gawley TH, *et al.* Role of doxapram in reducing pulmonary complications after major surgery. *Br Med J* 1976; **1:** 122–4.
4. Allen CJ, Gough KR. Effect of doxapram on heavy sedation produced by intravenous diazepam. *Br Med J* 1983; **286:** 1181–2.
5. Jansen JE, *et al.* Effect of doxapram on postoperative pulmonary complications after upper abdominal surgery in high-risk patients. *Lancet* 1990; **335:** 936–8.
6. Thangathurai D, *et al.* Doxapram for respiratory depression after epidural morphine. *Anaesthesia* 1990; **45:** 64–5.
7. Sajjad T. Comparison of the effects of doxapram or carbon dioxide on ventilatory frequency and tidal volume during induction of anaesthesia with propofol, *Br J Anaesth* 1994; **73:** 266P.
8. Alexander-Williams M, *et al.* Doxapram and the prevention of postoperative hypoxaemia. *Br J Anaesth* 1995; **75:** 233P.

Shivering. For references to the use of doxapram in postoperative shivering, see p.1219.

Preparations

BP 1998: Doxapram Injection;
USP 23: Doxapram Hydrochloride Injection.

Proprietary Preparations (details are given in Part 3)
Aust.: Dopram; ***Austral.:*** Dopram; ***Belg.:*** Dopram; ***Canad.:*** Dopram; ***Ger.:*** Dopram†; ***Irl.:*** Dopram; ***Ital.:*** Doxapril†; ***Neth.:*** Dopram; ***Norw.:*** Dopram; ***S.Afr.:*** Dopram; ***Spain:*** Docatone; ***Switz.:*** Dopram; ***UK:*** Dopram; ***USA:*** Dopram.

Ethamivan (1422-r)

Ethamivan *(BAN, USAN).*

Etamivan *(rINN)*; NSC-406087; Vanillic Acid Diethylamide; Vanillic Diethylamide. *N,N*-Diethylvanillamide.

$C_{12}H_{17}NO_3 = 223.3.$

CAS — 304-84-7.

Pharmacopoeias. In *Br.*

A white crystalline powder; odourless or almost odourless. Slightly **soluble** in water; freely soluble in alcohol, in acetone, and in chloroform; sparingly soluble in ether. A 1% solution in water has a pH of 5.5 to 7.0.

Ethamivan has actions similar to those of doxapram (above). It was formerly used as a respiratory stimulant, but its use for this indication has largely been abandoned as the risk of toxicity associated with effective doses is now considered to be unacceptable.

Ethamivan is available in compound preparations for administration by mouth in cerebrovascular and circulatory disorders and hypotension, but such use is not recommended.

Preparations

BP 1998: Etamivan Oral Solution.

Proprietary Preparations (details are given in Part 3)
UK: Clairvan†.

Multi-ingredient: ***Aust.:*** Cinnarplus; Instenon; ***Ger.:*** Card-Instenon†; Instenon†; Normotin-P†; Normotin-R; ***Spain:*** Vasperdil.

Fencamfamin Hydrochloride (1423-f)

Fencamfamin Hydrochloride *(BANM, rINNM).*

H-610. *N*-Ethyl-3-phenylbicyclo[2.2.1]hept-2-ylamine hydrochloride.

$C_{15}H_{21}N,HCl = 251.8.$

CAS — 1209-98-9 (fencamfamin); 2240-14-4 (fencamfamin hydrochloride).

Fencamfamin hydrochloride has been given by mouth as a central stimulant.

Preparations

Proprietary Preparations (details are given in Part 3)
Multi-ingredient: ***Ger.:*** Reactivan†; ***S.Afr.:*** Reactivan.

Fenethylline Hydrochloride (12738-t)

Fenethylline Hydrochloride *(BANM, USAN).*

Fenetylline Hydrochloride *(rINNM)*; Amfetyline Hydrochloride; 7-Ethyltheophylline Amphetamine Hydrochloride; H-814; R-720-11. 7-[2-(α-Methylphenethylamino)ethyl]theophylline hydrochloride.

$C_{18}H_{23}N_5O_2,HCl = 377.9.$

CAS — 3736-08-1 (fenethylline); 1892-80-4 (fenethylline hydrochloride).

Fenethylline is a theophylline derivative of amphetamine with properties similar to those of dexamphetamine (p.1478). It has been given by mouth in the management of hyperactivity disorders in children. Fenethylline is subject to abuse.

Preparations

Proprietary Preparations (details are given in Part 3)
Belg.: Captagon; ***Ger.:*** Captagon.

Fenfluramine Hydrochloride (1478-j)

Fenfluramine Hydrochloride *(BANM, USAN, rINNM).*

AHR-3002; S-768. *N*-Ethyl-α-methyl-3-trifluoromethylphenethylamine hydrochloride.

$C_{12}H_{16}F_3N,HCl = 267.7.$

CAS — 458-24-2 (fenfluramine); 404-82-0 (fenfluramine hydrochloride).

Pharmacopoeias. In *Fr.*

Adverse Effects and Treatment

Fenfluramine has been associated with serious cardiovascular toxicity. Pulmonary hypertension led to certain precautions being imposed upon its use and subsequent reports of valvular heart defects led to its withdrawal worldwide.

At therapeutic doses fenfluramine usually depresses rather than stimulates the CNS, although some CNS excitation may occur with higher doses. The most common adverse effects of fenfluramine are drowsiness, diarrhoea, dizziness, and lethargy. Headache, gastro-intestinal disturbances, dry mouth, changes in blood pressure (most often hypotension), altered libido, impotence, sweating, palpitations, restlessness, incoordination, chills, anxiety, irritability, elevated mood, fatigue, insomnia, bad dreams, depression (particularly after withdrawal), urinary frequency, dysuria, and visual disturbances may also occur. Skin rashes and blood disorders may occur rarely, as may dependence and psychotic reactions including schizophrenia.

Since the non-CNS effects and some of the CNS effects of fenfluramine are similar to those of dexamphetamine sulphate, the adverse effects may be treated similarly (see p.1479).

Effects on the cardiovascular system. The association of primary *pulmonary hypertension* with the use of anorectics including fenfluramine, dexfenfluramine, and phentermine is well recognised.[1-3] Both reversible and irreversible cases have been reported and in some cases it has proved fatal.[1,4-9] The condition appears to be linked to prolonged or repeated therapy.[1,10] In 1992 the Committee on Safety of Medicines in the UK advised that treatment should not exceed 3 months[1] but later in 1997 it revised its recommendations for fenfluramine and dexfenfluramine allowing treatment for up to 12 months under certain conditions.[2] The CSM stated that treatment could be continued beyond 3 months only if there had been a satisfactory response (more than 10% weight loss) and that this loss was maintained. Patients should also be monitored for symptoms of pulmonary hypertension. The Committee did not apply these revisions to other anorectics such as phentermine the duration of treatment still standing at 3 months.

However, shortly after this, a report was published[11] that outlined an association between the use of a fenfluramine-phentermine combination and the development of *valvular heart disease* in 24 patients. Initially, the response by the CSM in the UK was to advise against the use of combinations of anorectics[12] although subsequently fenfluramine, along with dexfenfluramine, was withdrawn from the world market after more cases became known.[13,14] By September 1997 the FDA in the USA[14] had received 144 reports of valvulopathy, including the original 24, associated with fenfluramine or dexfenfluramine, with or without phentermine; none were associated with phentermine treatment alone. As a consequence the US authorities made recommendations[14] for the screening of all patients who had previously received fenfluramine or dexfenfluramine in order to detect heart valve lesions and to provide optimal care. Three further studies[15-17] supported the association with valvular abnormalities. Although it was noted[18] that precise comparison between all studies was impossible, prolonged exposure or exposure to high doses of dexfenfluramine or fenfluramine did appear to increase the risk; clinically important disease would probably not develop in most patients with only short-term exposure.

1. Committee on Safety of Medicines. Fenfluramine (Ponderax Pacaps), dexfenfluramine (Adifax) and pulmonary hypertension. *Current Problems 34* 1992.
2. Committee on Safety of Medicines/Medicines Control Agency. Anorectic agents: risks and benefits. *Current Problems* 1997; **23:** 1–2.
3. Abenhaim L, *et al.* Appetite-suppressant drugs and the risk of primary pulmonary hypertension. *N Engl J Med* 1996; **335:** 609–16.
4. Douglas JG, *et al.* Pulmonary hypertension and fenfluramine. *Br Med J* 1981; **283:** 881–3.
5. McMurray J, *et al.* Irreversible pulmonary hypertension after treatment with fenfluramine. *Br Med J* 1986; **292:** 239–40.
6. Fotiadis I, *et al.* Fenfluramine-induced irreversible pulmonary hypertension. *Postgrad Med J* 1991; **67:** 776–7.
7. Atanassoff PG, *et al.* Pulmonary hypertension and dexfenfluramine. *Lancet* 1992; **339:** 436.
8. Cacoub P, *et al.* Pulmonary hypertension and dexfenfluramine. *Eur J Clin Pharmacol* 1995; **48:** 81–3.
9. Roche N, *et al.* Pulmonary hypertension and dexfenfluramine. *Lancet* 1992; **339:** 436–7.
10. Thomas SHL, *et al.* Appetite suppressants and primary pulmonary hypertension in the United Kingdom. *Br Heart J* 1995; **74:** 600–63.
11. Connolly HM, *et al.* Valvular heart disease associated with fenfluramine-phentermine. *N Engl J Med* 1997; **337:** 581–8. Correction. *ibid.*; 1783.
12. Committee on Safety of Medicines/Medicines Control Agency. Anorectic agents and valvular heart disease. *Current Problems* 1997; **23:** 12.
13. Committee on Safety of Medicines/Medicines Control Agency. Fenfluramine and dexfenfluramine withdrawn. *Current Problems* 1997; **23:** 13–14.
14. Anonymous. Cardiac valvulopathy associated with exposure to fenfluramine or dexfenfluramine: US Department of Health and Human Services interim public health recommendations, November 1997. *MMWR* 1997; **46:** 1061–6.
15. Khan MA, *et al.* The prevalence of cardiac valvular insufficiency assessed by transthoracic echocardiography in obese patients treated with appetite-suppressant drugs. *N Engl J Med* 1998; **339:** 713–18.
16. Jick H, *et al.* A population-based study of appetite-suppressant drugs and the risk of cardiac-valve regurgitation. *N Engl J Med* 1998; **339:** 719–24.
17. Weissman NJ, *et al.* An assessment of heart-valve abnormalities in obese patients taking dexfenfluramine, sustained-release dexfenfluramine, or placebo. *N Engl J Med* 1998; **339:** 725–32.
18. Devereux RB. Appetite suppressants and valvular heart disease. *N Engl J Med* 1998; **339:** 765–6.

Overdosage. In a review[1] of 53 cases of fenfluramine poisoning, the most commonly observed symptoms were mydriasis, sluggish or absent pupillary response to light, and tachycardia; additional signs included nystagmus, elevated blood pressure, hypertonia, trismus, hyperreflexia, clonus, tremor, excitation, hyperthermia, facial flushing, tachypnoea, and sweating; in severe intoxication coma and convulsions were frequently present. Onset was rapid and symptoms could persist for several days. Nine patients died following cardiac and respiratory arrest that occurred 1 to 4 hours after ingestion.

1. Von Mühlendahl KE, Krienke EG. Fenfluramine poisoning. *Clin Toxicol* 1979; **14:** 97–106.

Precautions

Fenfluramine should not be given to patients with pulmonary hypertension or current or past history of cardiovascular or cerebrovascular disease. Patients should also be advised to report immediately chest pain, palpitations, oedema, dyspnoea, or deterioration in exercise tolerance as this may indicate the development of pulmonary hypertension. For further details concerning the adverse effects of pulmonary hypertension and valvular heart defects, and precautions to be observed, see Effects on the Cardiovascular System, above. It should not be given to those with a psychiatric illness (including anorexia nervosa and depression), glaucoma, epilepsy, a history of drug abuse, alcoholism, or emotional instability. It should be given with caution, if at all, to the elderly or to pregnant or breast-feeding women. Fenfluramine can produce mood changes and abrupt withdrawal can provoke severe depression. Therefore withdrawal should be gradual.

Patients should also be advised that fenfluramine can cause drowsiness and that if affected they should not drive or operate machinery and should avoid alcoholic drink.

Abuse. The risk of drug abuse with fenfluramine has been considered to be virtually non-existent.[1] However, there have been reports of fenfluramine abuse involving large doses.[2-4] In the sample of young men surveyed in one study,[2] single oral doses of fenfluramine 80 to 500 mg were used to elicit a psychotomimetic state consisting of euphoria, relaxation, and inane laughter, often accompanied by perceptual alterations, including visual hallucinations, alterations in sense of temperature, derealisation, and depersonalisation.

1. Anonymous. Appetite suppressants reassessed. *Drug Ther Bull* 1982; **20:** 35–6.
2. Levin A. The non-medical misuse of fenfluramine by drug-dependent young South Africans. *Postgrad Med J* 1975; **51** (suppl 1): 186–8.
3. Rosenvinge HP. Abuse of fenfluramine. *Br Med J* 1975; **1:** 735.
4. Dare GL, Goldney RD. Fenfluramine abuse. *Med J Aust* 1976; **2:** 537–40.

Interactions

Fenfluramine should not be given to patients being treated with an MAOI or within at least 14 days of stopping such treatment. Antipsychotics and other anorectics should also not be used concomitantly. Fenfluramine may potentiate the effects of antidiabetics and may also slightly enhance the effect of antihypertensives and sedatives.

General anaesthetics. A possible interaction between fenfluramine and halothane anaesthesia resulting in cardiac arrest has been reported.[1] Despite severe criticism of this report it was still considered that potent anaesthetics should be administered with caution to patients taking fenfluramine.[2]

1. Bennett JA, Eltringham RJ. Possible dangers of anaesthesia in patients receiving fenfluramine: results of animal studies following a case of human cardiac arrest. *Anaesthesia* 1977; **32:** 8–13.
2. Winnie AP. Fenfluramine and halothane. *Anaesthesia* 1979; **34:** 79–80.

Pharmacokinetics

Fenfluramine is readily absorbed from the gastro-intestinal tract. It is extensively metabolised; initial metabolism involves de-ethylation to active norfenfluramine. Fenfluramine is widely distributed into body tissues; it crosses the blood-brain barrier. Excretion is via the urine in the form of unchanged drug and metabolites. The rate of excretion is influenced by urinary pH being somewhat increased in acid urine.

Studies by Hossain and Campbell[1] and by Innes *et al.*[2] indicated a significant correlation between weight loss and plasma concentrations of fenfluramine and its active metabolite norfenfluramine. In contrast, Pietrusko *et al.*[3] found no such correlation in a group of 36 obese women treated with fenfluramine and behaviour therapy.

1. Hossain M, Campbell DB. Fenfluramine and methylcellulose in the treatment of obesity: the relationship between plasma drug concentrations and therapeutic efficacy. *Postgrad Med J* 1975; **51** (suppl 1): 178–82.
2. Innes JA, *et al.* Plasma fenfluramine levels, weight loss, and side effects. *Br Med J* 1977; **2:** 1322–5.
3. Pietrusko R, *et al.* Plasma fenfluramine levels, weight loss and side effects: a failure to find a relationship. *Int J Obes* 1982; **6:** 567–71.

Uses and Administration

Fenfluramine is an indirect-acting sympathomimetic related to amphetamine, but at standard doses it usually depresses rather than stimulates the CNS. It appears to stimulate the release of serotonin and selectively inhibits its reuptake resulting in increased CNS serotonin concentrations. It may also increase glucose utilisation and lower blood-glucose concentrations.

Fenfluramine was formerly given by mouth as the hydrochloride in the treatment of obesity (p.1476) but was withdrawn worldwide following reports of valvular heart defects.

Preparations

Proprietary Preparations (details are given in Part 3)
Aust.: Ponderax†; ***Austral.:*** Ponderax†; ***Belg.:*** Fentrate†; Ponderal†; ***Canad.:*** Ponderal†; Pondimin†; ***Fr.:*** Ponderal†; ***Ger.:*** Ponderax†; ***Irl.:*** Ponderax†; ***Ital.:*** Dima-Fen†; Pesos†; Ponderal†; ***Neth.:*** Ponderal†; ***S.Afr.:*** Fenured†; Ponderax†; ***Spain:*** Ponderal†; ***Switz.:*** Adipomin†; Ponflural†; ***UK:*** Ponderax†; ***USA:*** Pondimin†.

Fenozolone (12741-j)

Fenozolone *(rINN)*.

LD-3394; Phenozolone. 2-Ethylamino-5-phenyl-2-oxazolin-4-one.

$C_{11}H_{12}N_2O_2$ = 204.2.
CAS — 15302-16-6.

Fenozolone is a central stimulant and indirect-acting sympathomimetic with actions similar to those of dexamphetamine (p.1478). It has been given by mouth in the treatment of symptoms of intellectual impairment in a daily dose of 20 to 30 mg in divided doses.

Preparations

Proprietary Preparations (details are given in Part 3)
Fr.: Ordinator.

Fenproporex Hydrochloride (1479-z)

Fenproporex Hydrochloride *(rINNM)*.

N-2-Cyanoethylamphetamine Hydrochloride. (±)-3-(α-Methylphenethylamino)propionitrile hydrochloride.

$C_{12}H_{16}N_2$,HCl = 224.7.
CAS — 15686-61-0 (fenproporex); 18305-29-8 (fenproporex hydrochloride).

Fenproporex is a central stimulant and indirect-acting sympathomimetic with actions similar to those of dexamphetamine (p.1478). Following administration by mouth it is reported to be metabolised to amphetamine. Fenproporex has been given as the hydrochloride, the diphenylacetate, and as a resinate.

Fenproporex hydrochloride has been used as an anorectic in the treatment of obesity (p.1476) in doses of 20 mg daily by mouth, usually in divided doses before meals; it has also been given in the form of a modified-release preparation in a dose of 20 mg daily before breakfast.

Preparations

Proprietary Preparations (details are given in Part 3)
Spain: Antiobes; Dicel; Falagan†; Grasmin; Tegisec.

Lobelia (1426-h)

Indian Tobacco.

Pharmacopoeias. In *Aust.*

The dried aerial parts of *Lobelia inflata* (Lobeliaceae). Lobeline is the main alkaloidal constituent.

Lobeline Hydrochloride (1427-m)

Lobeline Hydrochloride *(rINNM)*.

Alpha-lobeline Hydrochloride; Lobelini Hydrochloridum. 2-[6-(β-Hydroxyphenethyl)-1-methyl-2-piperidyl]acetophenone hydrochloride.

$C_{22}H_{27}NO_2$,HCl = 373.9.
CAS — 90-69-7 (lobeline); 134-63-4 (lobeline hydrochloride).

Pharmacopoeias. In *Aust., Belg.,* and *It.*

Lobeline Sulphate (1428-b)

Lobeline Sulphate *(rINNM)*.

$(C_{22}H_{27}NO_2)_2,H_2SO_4$ = 773.0.
CAS — 134-64-5.

Adverse Effects

Side-effects of lobelia and lobeline include nausea and vomiting, coughing, tremor, and dizziness. Symptoms of overdosage include profuse diaphoresis, paresis, tachycardia, hypothermia, hypotension, and coma; fatalities have occurred.

Uses and Administration

Lobeline, which chiefly accounts for the activity of lobelia, has peripheral and central effects similar to those of nicotine (p.1607).

Lobelia has been used mainly in preparations aimed at relieving respiratory-tract disorders. Lobeline has been given by mouth as the hydrochloride or sulphate as a smoking deterrent. Lobelia has been used similarly given either by mouth or incorporated into herbal cigarettes.

Reviews of anti-smoking therapy generally consider lobeline to have little benefit compared with placebo.[1,2]

1. Nunn-Thompson CL, Simon PA. Pharmacotherapy for smoking cessation. *Clin Pharm* 1989; **8:** 710–20.
2. Gourlay SG, McNeil JJ. Antismoking products. *Med J Aust* 1990; **153:** 699–707.

Preparations

Proprietary Preparations (details are given in Part 3)
Austral.: Cig-Ridettes; ***Spain:*** Nofum; Smokeless; ***UK:*** Anti-Smoking Tablets; ***USA:*** Bantron.

Multi-ingredient: ***Austral.:*** Potassium Iodide and Stramonium Compound; ***Belg.:*** Kamfeine; Sirop Toux du Larynx; ***Fr.:*** Asthmasedine†; Broncorinol toux seches; Cigarettes Berthiot†; Pulmothiol†; ***Ger.:*** Citotal†; ***Spain:*** Bronquiasmol†; Iodocafedrina†; Pazbronquial; ***UK:*** Antibron; Balm of Gilead; Chest Mixture; Herbelix; Hill's Balsam Expectorant Pastilles; Horehound and Aniseed Cough Mixture; Iceland Moss Compound†; Lobelia Compound; Vegetable Cough Remover.

Mazindol (1482-w)

Mazindol *(BAN, USAN, rINN)*.

42-548; AN-448; SaH-42548. 5-(4-Chlorophenyl)-2,5-dihydro-3*H*-imidazo[2,1-*a*]isoindol-5-ol.

$C_{16}H_{13}ClN_2O$ = 284.7.

CAS — 22232-71-9.

Pharmacopoeias. In US.

A white to off-white crystalline powder, having not more than a faint odour. Practically **insoluble** in water; slightly soluble in methyl alcohol and in chloroform. **Store** in airtight containers.

Adverse Effects, Treatment, and Precautions

As for Dexamphetamine Sulphate, p.1478.

Effects on the testes. A report of 8 men who developed testicular pain after taking mazindol.[1]

1. McEwen J, Meyboom RHB. Testicular pain caused by mazindol. *Br Med J* 1983; **287:** 1763–4.

Interactions

As for Dexamphetamine Sulphate, p.1479.

Lithium. For a report of mazindol interacting with lithium to cause lithium toxicity, see p.294.

Pharmacokinetics

Mazindol is readily absorbed from the gastro-intestinal tract and is excreted in the urine, partly unchanged and partly as metabolites.

Uses and Administration

Mazindol is a central stimulant with actions similar to those of dexamphetamine (p.1479), although structurally the two compounds are unrelated. It appears to inhibit reuptake of dopamine and noradrenaline. It has been used as an anorectic, given by mouth in the treatment of obesity (p.1476). The usual initial dose is 1 mg once daily before food adjusted as required up to a maximum of 1 mg three times a day.

Mazindol has been investigated in the treatment of Duchenne muscular dystrophy.

Narcolepsy. Mazindol has been reported[1-4] to be beneficial in patients with narcolepsy (p.1476). A wide range of doses has been employed: 3 to 8 mg daily in one study,[1] 1 mg weekly to 16 mg daily in another;[3] children have been given 1 to 2 mg daily.[4]

1. Parkes JD, Schachter M. Mazindol in the treatment of narcolepsy. *Acta Neurol Scand* 1979; **60:** 250–4.
2. Shindler J, *et al.* Amphetamine, mazindol, and fencamfamin in narcolepsy. *Br Med J* 1985; **290:** 1167–70.
3. Alvarez B, *et al.* Mazindol in long-term treatment of narcolepsy. *Lancet* 1991; **337:** 1293–4.
4. Allsopp MR, Zaiwalla Z. Narcolepsy. *Arch Dis Child* 1992; **67:** 302–6.

Preparations

USP 23: Mazindol Tablets.

Proprietary Preparations (details are given in Part 3)
Austral.: Sanorex†; ***Canad.:*** Sanorex; ***Irl.:*** Teronac†; ***Jpn:*** Sanorex; ***Neth.:*** Teronac; ***S.Afr.:*** Teronac†; ***Switz.:*** Teronac; ***UK:*** Teronac†; ***USA:*** Mazanor; Sanorex.

Mefenorex Hydrochloride (1483-e)

Mefenorex Hydrochloride *(USAN, pINNM)*.

Ro-4-5282. *N*-(3-Chloropropyl)-α-methylphenethylamine hydrochloride.

$C_{12}H_{18}ClN,HCl$ = 248.2.

CAS — 17243-57-1 (mefenorex); 5586-87-8 (mefenorex hydrochloride).

Mefenorex hydrochloride is a central stimulant and indirect-acting sympathomimetic with actions similar to those of dexamphetamine (p.1478). It has been used as an anorectic in the treatment of obesity in a dose equivalent to 40 mg of mefenorex once or twice daily by mouth before food.

Preparations

Proprietary Preparations (details are given in Part 3)
Fr.: Incital†; ***Ger.:*** Rondimen; ***Switz.:*** Pondinil†.

Mepixanox (12931-x)

Mepixanox *(rINN)*.

Mepixantone. 3-Methoxy-4-piperidinomethyl-9*H*-xanthen-9-one.

$C_{20}H_{21}NO_3$ = 323.4.

CAS — 17854-59-0.

Mepixanox has been used as a respiratory stimulant in doses of 50 mg three times daily or more by mouth, 50 to 100 mg once or twice daily by slow intravenous injection, or 50 mg two or three times daily by intramuscular injection.

Preparations

Proprietary Preparations (details are given in Part 3)
Ital.: Pimexone.

Methylamphetamine Hydrochloride (1431-f)

Metamfetamine Hydrochloride *(rINNM)*; *d*-Deoxyephedrine Hydrochloride; *d*-Desoxyephedrine Hydrochloride; Methamphetamine Hydrochloride; Methamphetamini Hydrochloridum; Phenylmethylaminopropane Hydrochloride. (+)-*N*,α-Dimethylphenethylamine hydrochloride.

$C_{10}H_{15}N,HCl$ = 185.7.

CAS — 537-46-2 (methylamphetamine); 51-57-0 (methylamphetamine hydrochloride).

NOTE. Methylamphetamine in a smokeable form has been known as Crank, Crystal, Crystal Meth, Ice, Meth, and Speed.

Pharmacopoeias. In *Aust., Jpn, Swiss,* and *US.*

White, odourless or almost odourless, crystals or crystalline powder. Freely **soluble** in water, in alcohol, and in chloroform; very slightly soluble in ether. Solutions have a pH of about 6. **Store** in airtight containers. Protect from light.

Adverse Effects, Treatment, and Precautions

As for Dexamphetamine Sulphate, p.1478.

Methylamphetamine has been subject to extensive abuse, in particular by injection.

Abuse. Pulmonary oedema,[1,2] cardiomyopathy,[2] and choreoathetosis and rhabdomyolysis[3] have occurred following smoking of methylamphetamine crystals.

1. Nestor TA, *et al.* Acute pulmonary oedema caused by crystalline methamphetamine. *Lancet* 1989; **ii:** 1277–8.
2. Hong R, *et al.* Cardiomyopathy associated with the smoking of crystal methamphetamine. *JAMA* 1991; **265:** 1152–4.
3. Sperling LS, Horowitz JL. Methamphetamine-induced choreoathetosis and rhabdomyolysis. *Ann Intern Med* 1994; **121:** 986.

Porphyria. Methylamphetamine has been associated with clinical exacerbations of porphyria and is considered unsafe in porphyric patients.[1]

1. Moore MR, McColl KEL. *Porphyria: drug lists.* Glasgow: Porphyria Research Unit, University of Glasgow, 1991.

Interactions

As for Dexamphetamine Sulphate, p.1479.

Pharmacokinetics

Like most amphetamines (see Dexamphetamine Sulphate, p.1479) methylamphetamine is readily absorbed from the gastro-intestinal tract and is distributed into most body tissues. It is partially metabolised in the liver and excreted in the urine.

References.

1. Shappell SA, *et al.* Chronopharmacokinetics and chronopharmacodynamics of dextromethamphetamine in man. *J Clin Pharmacol* 1996; **36:** 1051–63.

Uses and Administration

Methylamphetamine hydrochloride is a central stimulant and indirect-acting sympathomimetic with actions and uses similar to those of dexamphetamine (p.1479).

It has been given by mouth in the treatment of hyperactivity disorders in children aged 6 years and over although dexamphetamine and methylphenidate are the main stimulants used (p.1476). Initial doses are 5 mg once or twice daily, increased if necessary by 5 mg at weekly intervals to the optimum effective dose, usually 20 to 25 mg daily. The maintenance dose may be given once daily if a modified-release preparation is used.

Methylamphetamine hydrochloride has also been used as an anorectic in the management of obesity (p.1476), although amphetamines are no longer recommended for this indication. A dose of 10 or 15 mg has been given by mouth as a modified-release preparation once daily in the morning.

Methylamphetamine hydrochloride has also been used parenterally as a pressor agent.

The laevo-rotatory form, levmetamfetamine (*l*-desoxyephedrine), is used as a nasal decongestant.

Preparations

USP 23: Methamphetamine Hydrochloride Tablets.

Proprietary Preparations (details are given in Part 3)
USA: Desoxyn; Vicks Vapor Inhaler.

Methylenedioxymethamphetamine (19493-n)

MDMA; 3,4-Methylenedioxymethamphetamine. *N*,α-Dimethyl-1,3-benzodioxole-5-ethanamine.

$C_{11}H_{15}NO_2$ = 193.2.

CAS — 42542-10-9.

NOTE. Methylenedioxymethamphetamine has also been known as Adam, E, Ecstasy, M&M, MDM, and XTC.

Methylenedioxymethamphetamine is a phenylethylamine compound structurally related to amphetamine and mescaline and is an analogue of tenamfetamine (p.1485). It is subject to abuse. Its adverse effects are similar to those of dexamphetamine (p.1478) and may be treated similarly.

Abuse. The toxicity associated with abuse of methylenedioxymethamphetamine has been the subject of a number of discussions.[1-6] Acute effects can be severe and symptoms associated with fatalities have included cardiac arrhythmias, fulminant hyperthermia, convulsions, disseminated intravascular coagulation, rhabdomyolysis, and acute renal failure. Repeated use may cause hepatic damage. Psychiatric effects reported include psychosis[7-9] and depression.[8-10] Damage to central serotonergic nerves has been implicated[7-10] and hence there is some concern regarding the long-term effects of methylenedioxymethamphetamine abuse.[11] Hyponatraemia, inappropriate antidiuretic hormone secretion, and cerebral oedema have also been reported;[12-17] the severity may be increased by excessive fluid intake that is frequently advocated to prevent dehydration and hyperthermia.[15-18] Urinary retention has also been reported.[19]

Concern has been expressed regarding abuse during pregnancy. Eight congenital malformations, including two cases of congenital heart disease, have been noted among 51 liveborn infants whose mothers had taken methylenedioxymethamphetamine, often with other drugs of abuse, during their pregnancies.[20]

For mention of the treatment of hyperthermia, see p.1.

For reviews of the properties of other phenylethylamine compounds, see under Tenamfetamine, p.1485.

1. Henry JA. Ecstasy and the dance of death. *Br Med J* 1992; **305:** 5–6.
2. Henry JA, *et al.* Toxicity and deaths from 3,4-methylenedioxymethamphetamine ("ecstasy"). *Lancet* 1992; **340:** 384–7.
3. O'Connor B. Hazards associated with the recreational drug 'ecstasy'. *Br J Hosp Med* 1994; **52:** 507–14.
4. McCann UD, *et al.* Adverse reactions with 3,4-methylenedioxymethamphetamine (MDMA; 'Ecstasy'). *Drug Safety* 1996; **15:** 107–115.
5. Hall AP. Ecstasy and the anaesthetist. *Br J Anaesth* 1997; **79:** 697–8.
6. Schwartz RH, Miller NS. MDMA (ecstasy) and the rave: a review. *Pediatrics* 1997; **100:** 705–8.
7. McGuire P, Fahy T. Chronic paranoid psychosis after misuse of MDMA ("ecstasy"). *Br Med J* 1991; **302:** 697.
8. Winstock AR. Chronic paranoid psychosis after misuse of MDMA. *Br Med J* 1991; **302:** 1150–1.
9. Schifano F. Chronic atypical psychosis associated with MDMA ("ecstasy") abuse. *Lancet* 1991; **338:** 1335.
10. Benazzi F, Mazzoli M. Psychiatric illness associated with "ecstasy". *Lancet* 1991; **338:** 1520.
11. Green AR, Goodwin GM. Ecstasy and neurodegeneration. *Br Med J* 1996; **312:** 1493–4.
12. Maxwell DL, *et al.* Hyponatraemia and catatonic stupor after taking "ecstasy". *Br Med J* 1993; **307:** 1399.
13. Kessel B. Hyponatraemia after ingestion of "ecstasy". *Br Med J* 1994; **308:** 414.
14. Satchell SC, Connaughton M. Inappropriate antidiuretic hormone secretion and extreme rises in serum creatinine kinase following MDMA ingestion. *Br J Hosp Med* 1994; **51:** 495.
15. Holden R, Jackson MA. Near-fatal hyponatraemic coma due to vasopressin over-secretion after ecstasy (3,4-MDMA). *Lancet* 1996; **347:** 1052.
16. Matthai SM, *et al.* Cerebral oedema after ingestion of MDMA (ecstasy) and unrestricted intake of water. *Br Med J* 1996; **312:** 1359.
17. Parr MJA, *et al.* Hyponatraemia and death after ecstasy ingestion. *Med J Aust* 1997; **166:** 136–7.
18. Cook TM. Cerebral oedema after MDMA ('ecstasy') and unrestricted water intake. *Br Med J* 1996; **313:** 689.
19. Bryden AA, *et al.* Urinary retention with misuse of 'ecstasy'. *Br Med J* 1995; **310:** 504.
20. McElhatton PR, *et al.* Does prenatal exposure to ecstasy cause congenital malformations? A prospective follow-up of 92 pregnancies. *Br J Clin Pharmacol* 1998; **45:** 184P.

Interactions. A patient receiving *phenelzine* and lithium therapy experienced a serotonin syndrome after ingesting methylenedioxymethamphetamine.[1] Symptoms included markedly increased muscle tension, tremulousness, abnormal posturing, limited pain response, tachycardia, hypertension, hyperthermia, increased white blood cell count, increased creatine phosphokinase concentration, respiratory acidosis, metabolic acidosis, delirium, and agitation. Within 15 minutes of methylenedioxymethamphetamine ingestion the patient was comatose; within 5 hours the patient was alert with a normal muscle tone. An interaction between phenelzine and methylenedioxymethamphetamine was suggested as the cause of the serotonin syndrome.

A fatal serotoninergic reaction to methylenedioxymethamphetamine possibly due to an interaction with *ritonavir* has been described.[2]

1. Kaskey GB. Possible interaction between an MAOI and "ecstasy". *Am J Psychiatry* 1992; **149:** 411–12.
2. Henry JA, Hill IR. Fatal interaction between ritonavir and MDMA. *Lancet* 1998; **352:** 1751–2.

Methylphenidate Hydrochloride (1433-n)

Methylphenidate Hydrochloride *(BANM, rINNM).*

Methyl Phenidate Hydrochloride. Methyl α-phenyl-2-piperidylacetate hydrochloride.

$C_{14}H_{19}NO_2,HCl = 269.8.$

CAS — 113-45-1 (methylphenidate); 298-59-9 (methylphenidate hydrochloride).

Pharmacopoeias. In *Chin., Swiss,* and *US.*

Odourless fine white crystalline powder. Freely **soluble** in water and in methyl alcohol; soluble in alcohol; slightly soluble in acetone and in chloroform. Solutions are acid to litmus.

Adverse Effects, Treatment, and Precautions

As for Dexamphetamine Sulphate, p.1478. Hypersensitivity reactions have been reported.

References.

1. Ahmann PA, *et al.* Placebo-controlled evaluation of Ritalin side effects. *Pediatrics* 1993; **91:** 1101–6.
2. Efron D, *et al.* Side effects of methylphenidate and dexamphetamine in children with attention deficit hyperactivity disorder: a double-blind, crossover trial. *Pediatrics* 1997; **100:** 662–6.
3. Rappley MD. Safety issues in the use of methylphenidate: an American perspective. *Drug Safety* 1997; **17:** 143–8.

Abuse. Reports of adverse effects following the abuse of methylphenidate by injecting solutions of crushed tablets.[1-3]

See also under Effects on the Liver, below.

1. Wolf J, *et al.* Eosinophilic syndrome with methylphenidate abuse. *Ann Intern Med* 1978; **89:** 224–5.
2. Gunby P. Methylphenidate abuse produces retinopathy. *JAMA* 1979; **241:** 546.
3. Parran TV, Jasinski DR. Intravenous methylphenidate abuse: prototype for prescription drug abuse. *Arch Intern Med* 1991; **151:** 781–3.

Effects on growth. Concern has been expressed about the effects of central stimulants such as methylphenidate on growth rate when used to treat hyperactivity in children. One study showed that methylphenidate treatment resulted in decreases in weight percentiles after one year of treatment and progressive decrement in height percentiles that became significant after 2 years of treatment.[1] However, another suggested that moderate doses might have a lower risk for long-term height suppression than dexamphetamine.[2] There has also been a study which showed that, even when methylphenidate had an adverse effect on growth rate during active treatment, final height was not compromised and that a compensatory rebound of growth appeared to occur following discontinuation of the stimulant treatment.[3]

See also under Dexamphetamine Sulphate, p.1478.

1. Mattes JA, Gittelman R. Growth of hyperactive children on maintenance regimen of methylphenidate. *Arch Gen Psychiatry* 1983; **40:** 317–21.
2. Greenhill LL, *et al.* Prolactin, growth hormone and growth responses in boys with attention deficit disorder and hyperactivity treated with methylphenidate. *J Am Acad Child Psychiatry* 1984; **23:** 58–67.
3. Klein RG, Mannuzza S. Hyperactive boys almost grown up III: methylphenidate effects on ultimate height. *Arch Gen Psychiatry* 1988; **45:** 1131–4.

Effects on the liver. Hepatotoxicity with raised liver enzyme values in a 67-year-old woman was associated with the administration of methylphenidate hydrochloride 30 mg daily by mouth.[1] Methylphenidate-induced hepatocellular injury was reported in a 19-year old woman who developed jaundice, fever, and malaise after intravenous abuse of methylphenidate hydrochloride tablets.[2]

1. Goodman CR. Hepatotoxicity due to methylphenidate hydrochloride. *N Y State J Med* 1972; **72:** 2339–40.
2. Mehta H, *et al.* Hepatic dysfunction due to intravenous abuse of methylphenidate hydrochloride. *J Clin Gastroenterol* 1984; **6:** 149–51.

Effects on the skin. A fixed drug eruption of the scrotum has been reported in 2 children treated with methylphenidate for attention deficit disorder.[1]

1. Cohen HA, *et al.* Fixed drug eruption of the scrotum due to methylphenidate. *Ann Pharmacother* 1992; **26:** 1378–9.

Tourette's syndrome. For a discussion on central stimulants provoking Tourette's syndrome, see Dexamphetamine Sulphate, p.1479.

Interactions

As for Dexamphetamine Sulphate, p.1479.

For specific mention of interactions involving methylphenidate, see under Amitriptyline Hydrochloride, p.276, Phenylbutazone, p.79, Phenytoin, p.356, and Warfarin, p.968.

Pharmacokinetics

Methylphenidate is readily absorbed from the gastro-intestinal tract. The presence of food in the stomach accelerates the rate of absorption but not the total amount absorbed. Peak plasma concentrations are reached about 2 hours after oral administration; methylphenidate undergoes extensive first-pass metabolism. Protein binding is low. It is excreted as metabolites mainly in the urine with small amounts appearing in the faeces; less than 1% appears in the urine as unchanged methylphenidate. The major metabolite is ritalinic acid (2-phenyl-2-piperidyl acetic acid). The plasma elimination half-life is about 2 hours.

References.

1. Aoyama T, *et al.* Nonlinear kinetics of threo-methylphenidate enantiomers in a patient with narcolepsy and in healthy volunteers. *Eur J Clin Pharmacol* 1993; **44:** 79–84.
2. Aoyama T, *et al.* Pharmacokinetics and pharmacodynamics of (+)-threo-methylphenidate enantiomer in patients with hypersomnia. *Clin Pharmacol Ther* 1994; **55:** 270–6.

Uses and Administration

Methylphenidate hydrochloride is a central stimulant and indirect-acting sympathomimetic with actions and uses similar to those of dexamphetamine (p.1479). It is used in the treatment of narcolepsy (p.1476) and as an adjunct to psychological, educational, and social measures in the treatment of hyperactivity disorders in children (below and p.1476).

In the treatment of narcolepsy, the usual dose is 20 to 30 mg daily by mouth in divided doses, normally 30 to 45 minutes before meals, but the effective dose may range from 10 to 60 mg daily.

In hyperactivity disorders, children aged 6 years and over usually start with a dose of 5 mg once or twice daily by mouth, increased if necessary by 5 to 10 mg at weekly intervals to a maximum of 60 mg daily in divided doses. Methylphenidate may be given before breakfast and lunch. A bedtime dose may be considered if the effect wears off in the evening causing rebound hyperactivity. The dosage of methylphenidate in the treatment of hyperactivity in children has sometimes been expressed in terms of body-weight; usual doses are 0.25 mg per kg daily, doubled each week, if necessary, to 2 mg per kg. Methylphenidate should be discontinued if there is no improvement in symptoms after appropriate adjustments in dosage over one month. It needs to be discontinued from time to time in those who do respond to assess the patient's condition; treatment is not usually continued beyond puberty.

Methylphenidate hydrochloride is also administered as a modified-release preparation.

A single isomer form of methylphenidate, *d-threo*-methylphenidate (D2785), is being investigated for hyperactivity disorders.

Depression. Stimulants are no longer recommended as sole treatment for depression (p.271), although they have been tried in augmenting the effect of standard antidepressants such as the selective serotonin reuptake inhibitors (SSRIs)[1] in patients with refractory depressive disorders.

1. Stoll AL, *et al.* Methylphenidate augmentation of serotonin selective reuptake inhibitors: a case series. *J Clin Psychiatry* 1996; **57:** 72–6.

Disturbed behaviour. Disturbed behaviour can have a number of causes and is usually treated with an antipsychotic or benzodiazepine (see p.636). However, a study of methylphenidate in patients who had sustained serious brain injury found that methylphenidate 30 mg daily reduced anger and temper outbursts and improved memory and general measure of psychopathological outcome.[1]

1. Mooney GF, Haas LJ. Effect of methylphenidate on brain injury-related anger. *Arch Phys Med Rehabil* 1993; **74:** 153–60.

Hyperactivity. Methylphenidate is one of the main drugs used in hyperactivity, including attention deficit hyperactivity disorder (p.1476).

Small studies have indicated that different aspects of attention deficit disorders in children might respond to different doses of methylphenidate.[1-4] In addition to the morning and noon doses commonly used in hyperactivity disorders, studies[5,6] have shown improved clinical outcome with little adverse effect on sleep patterns if a third late afternoon dose is given.

1. Sprague RL, Sleator EK. Methylphenidate in hyperkinetic children: differences in dose effects on learning and social behavior. *Science* 1977; **198:** 1274–6.
2. Tannock R, *et al.* Dose-response effects of methylphenidate on academic performance and overt behavior in hyperactive children. *Pediatrics* 1989; **84:** 648–57.
3. Sebrechts MM, *et al.* Components of attention, methylphenidate dosage, and blood levels in children with attention deficit disorder. *Pediatrics* 1986; **77:** 222–8.
4. Barkley RA, *et al.* Attention deficit disorder with and without hyperactivity: clinical response to three dose levels of methylphenidate. *Pediatrics* 1991; **87:** 519–31.
5. Kent JD, *et al.* Effects of late-afternoon methylphenidate administration on behavior and sleep in attention-deficit hyperactivity disorders. *Pediatrics* 1995; **96:** 320–5.
6. Stein MA, *et al.* Methylphenidate dosing: twice daily versus three times daily. *Pediatrics* 1996; **98:** 748–56.

Preparations

USP 23: Methylphenidate Hydrochloride Extended-release Tablets; Methylphenidate Hydrochloride Tablets.

Proprietary Preparations (details are given in Part 3)
Austral.: Ritalin; ***Belg.:*** Rilatine; ***Canad.:*** Ritalin; ***Fr.:*** Ritaline; ***Ger.:*** Ritalin; ***Irl.:*** Ritalin†; ***Neth.:*** Ritalin; ***Norw.:*** Ritalin; ***S.Afr.:*** Ritalin; ***Spain:*** Rubifen; ***Switz.:*** Ritaline; ***UK:*** Ritalin; ***USA:*** Ritalin.

Modafinil (2963-l)

Modafinil *(USAN, rINN).*

CEP-1538; CRL-40476. 2-[(Diphenylmethyl)sulfinyl]acetamide.

$C_{15}H_{15}NO_2S = 273.4.$

CAS — 68693-11-8.

Adverse Effects, Treatment, and Precautions

Adverse effects of modafinil may be a result of CNS stimulation and effects such as nervousness, insomnia, excitation, aggressive tendencies, personality disorder, tremor, and euphoria have been noted. There may also be gastro-intestinal disturbances, including nausea and abdominal pain, dry mouth, headache, anorexia, and cardiovascular effects such as hypertension, palpitations, and tachycardia. Pruritic skin rashes, dose-related increases in alkaline phosphatase and, very rarely, bucco-facial dyskinesia have been observed.

Modafinil is contra-indicated in patients with moderate to severe hypertension or cardiac arrhythmias. It is not recommended in patients with a history of left ventricular hypertrophy or ischaemic ECG changes, chest pain, or other signs of mitral valve prolapse.

As with other stimulants, there is the possibility of dependence with long-term use.

Interactions

Modafinil has enzyme-inducing activity and may impair the effectiveness of drugs such as oral contraceptives and antiepileptics when given concomitantly.

Pharmacokinetics

Modafinil is well absorbed from the gastro-intestinal tract following oral administration with peak plasma concentrations occurring after 2 to 3 hours. Plasma protein binding is 62%. Modafinil is metabolised in the liver, the major metabolite being acid modafinil. Excretion is mainly through the kidneys with less than 10% of the dose being eliminated unchanged. The elimination half-life is 10 to 12 hours.

Uses and Administration

Modafinil is a central stimulant and alpha$_1$-adrenergic agonist chemically related to adrafinil (p.1477). It is used in the treatment of the narcoleptic syndrome (p.1476). Modafinil is given by mouth in a dose of 200 to 400 mg daily, administered in two divided doses, in the morning and at midday, or as a single dose in the morning. An initial dose of 100 mg daily should be used in the elderly and adjusted as necessary. The total dose should be reduced to 100 to 200 mg daily in any patient with severe hepatic or renal impairment.

References.

1. Saletu B, *et al.* Differential effects of a new central adrenergic agonist–modafinil–and d-amphetamine on sleep and early morning behaviour in young healthy volunteers. *Int J Clin Pharmacol Res* 1989; **9:** 183–95.
2. Saletu B, *et al.* Differential effects of the new central adrenergic agonist modafinil and d-amphetamine on sleep and early morning behaviour in elderlies. *Arzneimittelforschung* 1989; **39:** 1268–73.
3. Saletu B, *et al.* Treatment of the alcoholic organic brain syndrome: double-blind, placebo-controlled clinical, psychometric and electroencephalographic mapping studies with modafinil. *Neuropsychobiology* 1993; **27:** 26–39.
4. Lamberg L. Narcolepsy researchers barking up the right tree. *JAMA* 1996; **276:** 765–6.

Preparations

Proprietary Preparations (details are given in Part 3)
Fr.: Modiodal; ***UK:*** Provigil.

Nikethamide (1434-h)

Nikethamide *(BAN, rINN).*

Nicethamidum; Nicotinic Acid Diethylamide; Nicotinoyldiaethylamidum; Nikethylamide. *N,N*-Diethylnicotinamide; *N,N*-Diethylpyridine-3-carboxamide.

$C_{10}H_{14}N_2O = 178.2.$

CAS — 59-26-7.

Pharmacopoeias. In *Chin., Eur.* (see p.viii), and *Pol.*

A colourless or slightly yellow oily liquid or crystalline mass. **Miscible** with water, with alcohol, and with ether. A 25% solution in water has a pH of 6.0 to 7.8.

Nikethamide has actions similar to those of doxapram (p.1480). It was formerly given parenterally or by mouth as a respiratory stimulant but its use for this indication has largely been abandoned as the risk of toxicity associated with effective doses is now considered to be unacceptable.

Nikethamide and its calcium thiocyanate salt have been given by mouth in some countries as central stimulants and in preparations for hypotensive disorders.

Porphyria. Nikethamide has been associated with acute attacks of porphyria and is considered unsafe in patients with acute porphyria.[1]

1. Moore MR, McColl KEL. *Porphyria: drug lists*. Glasgow: Porphyria Research Unit, University of Glasgow, 1991.

Preparations

BP 1998: Nikethamide Injection.

Proprietary Preparations (details are given in Part 3)
Spain: Coramina†.

Multi-ingredient: ***Fr.:*** Coramine Glucose; ***Ger.:*** Felsol Neo; Hypotonin forte†; Poikiloton†; Zellaforte N Plus; ***Switz.:*** Gly-Coramin.

Pemoline (1436-b)

Pemoline *(BAN, USAN, rINN)*.

LA-956; NSC-25159; Phenoxazole; Phenylisohydantoin; Phenylpseudohydantoin. 2-Imino-5-phenyl-4-oxazolidinone.

$C_9H_8N_2O_2$ = 176.2.

CAS — 2152-34-3 (pemoline); 68942-31-4 (pemoline hydrochloride); 18968-99-5 (magnesium pemoline).

Adverse Effects, Treatment, and Precautions

As for Dexamphetamine Sulphate, p.1478; however, the effects of over-stimulation and sympathomimetic activity are considered to be less with pemoline. There are reports of liver toxicity in patients taking pemoline (see Effects on the Liver, below); its use is contra-indicated in patients with liver disorders. There have also been rare or isolated reports of chorea, tics, mania, and neutropenia.

Abuse. Paranoid psychosis was observed in a 38-year-old man taking pemoline 75 to 225 mg daily.[1] The patient's compulsive use of the drug, development of tolerance, depressive withdrawal syndrome, and inability to abstain indicated dependence and it was evident that the patient was addicted to pemoline.

Choreoathetosis and rhabdomyolysis developed in a patient following a marked increase in intake of pemoline.[2] Abnormal movements responded to diazepam.

1. Polchert SE, Morse RM. Pemoline abuse. *JAMA* 1985; **254:** 946–7.
2. Briscoe JG, *et al.* Pemoline-induced choreoathetosis and rhabdomyolysis. *Med Toxicol* 1988; **3:** 72–6.

Effects on growth. Results of a study in 24 hyperkinetic children suggested that growth suppression was a potential side-effect of prolonged treatment with clinically effective doses of pemoline and that this effect might be dose-related.[1]

See also under Dexamphetamine Sulphate, p.1478.

1. Dickinson LC, *et al.* Impaired growth in hyperkinetic children receiving pemoline. *J Pediatr* 1979; **94:** 538–41.

Effects on the liver. Pemoline has been associated with hepatotoxicity.

Elevated concentrations of serum aspartate aminotransferase (SGOT) and serum alanine aminotransferase (SGPT) have been noted in 2% of children taking pemoline for hyperactivity; the effect was stated to be transient and reversible.[1]

However, more serious reactions have also occurred. Acute hepatitis was associated with pemoline in a 10-year-old boy[2] and the drug was believed to be the cause of fatal fulminant liver failure in a 14-year-old boy and in 2 previously published cases.[3] The Committee on Safety of Medicines in the UK[4] subsequently became aware of 33 reports of serious hepatic reactions in the USA, including a total of 6 fatalities and the need for liver transplantation in 2 cases. This prompted the withdrawal of pemoline for the treatment of hyperactivity in the UK.

1. Anonymous. 'Hyperkinesis' can have many causes, symptoms. *JAMA* 1975; **232:** 1204–16.
2. Patterson JF. Hepatitis associated with pemoline. *South Med J* 1984; **77:** 938.
3. Berkovitch M, *et al.* Pemoline-associated fulminant liver failure: testing the evidence for causation. *Clin Pharmacol Ther* 1995; **57:** 696–8.
4. Committee on Safety of Medicines/Medicines Control Agency. Volital (pemoline) has been withdrawn. *Current Problems* 1997; **23:** 10.

Effects on the prostate. Experience in one patient suggested that pemoline might adversely affect the prostate gland or interfere with tests for prostatic acid phosphatase used in the diagnosis of prostatic carcinoma.[1]

1. Lindau W, de Girolami E. Pemoline and the prostate. *Lancet* 1986; **i:** 738.

Interactions

A possibility of hypertensive crisis when pemoline is administered with MAOIs has been suggested. Reduced seizure threshold has been reported in epileptic patients receiving pemoline and antiepileptics.

Pharmacokinetics

Pemoline is readily absorbed from the gastro-intestinal tract. About 50% is bound to plasma protein. It is partially metabolised in the liver and excreted in the urine as unchanged pemoline and metabolites.

References.

1. Vermeulen NPE, *et al.* Pharmacokinetics of pemoline in plasma, saliva and urine following oral administration. *Br J Clin Pharmacol* 1979; **8:** 459–63.
2. Sallee F, *et al.* Oral pemoline kinetics in hyperactive children. *Clin Pharmacol Ther* 1985; **37:** 606–9.
3. Collier CP, *et al.* Pemoline pharmacokinetics and long term therapy in children with attention deficit disorder and hyperactivity. *Clin Pharmacokinet* 1985; **10:** 269–78.

Uses and Administration

Pemoline is a central stimulant with actions similar to those of dexamphetamine (p.1479).

It has been used in the management of hyperactivity disorders in children (p.1476). In the USA 37.5 mg is given by mouth each morning initially, increased gradually at weekly intervals by 18.75 mg; the usual range is 56.25 to 75 mg daily and the maximum recommended daily dose is 112.5 mg. In the UK, pemoline was withdrawn from use for hyperactivity in children after reports of serious hepatotoxicity in the USA.

Pemoline has also been used in the narcoleptic syndrome (p.1476).

Pemoline has been included in preparations also containing yohimbine hydrochloride and methyltestosterone that are claimed to combat failure of sexual desire and functioning in males and females; such preparations are not recommended.

Pemoline has been given with magnesium hydroxide (magnesium pemoline) in an attempt to increase its absorption.

Preparations

Proprietary Preparations (details are given in Part 3)
Canad.: Cylert; ***Ger.:*** Senior; Tradon†; ***S.Afr.:*** Dynalert; ***Switz.:*** Stimul; ***UK:*** Volital†; ***USA:*** Cylert.

Multi-ingredient: ***Ital.:*** Deadyn†; ***S.Afr.:*** Lentogesic; ***Spain:*** Neurocordin†; ***UK:*** Prowess.

Pentetrazol (1437-v)

Pentetrazol *(BAN, rINN)*.

Corazol; Leptazol; Pentamethazol; 1,5-Pentamethylenetetrazole; Pentazol; Pentetrazolum; Pentylenetetrazol. 6,7,8,9-Tetrahydro-5*H*-tetrazoloazepine.

$C_6H_{10}N_4$ = 138.2.

CAS — 54-95-5.

Pharmacopoeias. In *Aust.* and *It.*

Pentetrazol is a central and respiratory stimulant similar to doxapram (p.1480). It has been used in respiratory depression and in multi-ingredient preparations intended for the treatment of respiratory-tract disorders including cough, cardiovascular disorders including hypotension, and for the treatment of pruritus. Administration has been by mouth and by injection.

Porphyria. Pentetrazol has been associated with acute attacks of porphyria and is considered unsafe in patients with acute porphyria.[1]

1. Moore MR, McColl KEL. *Porphyria: drug lists*. Glasgow: Porphyria Research Unit, University of Glasgow, 1991.

Preparations

Proprietary Preparations (details are given in Part 3)
Spain: Cardiorapide†.

Multi-ingredient: ***Aust.:*** Prospervital; ***Ger.:*** Cardaminol†; Jasivita†; Poikiloton†; Sympatocard†; ***Ital.:*** Cardiazol-Paracodina; ***Spain:*** Cardiorapide Efed†; Espectona Compositum†.

Phendimetrazine Tartrate (1486-j)

Phendimetrazine Tartrate *(BANM, rINNM)*.

Phendimetrazine Acid Tartrate; Phendimetrazine Bitartrate. (+)-3,4-Dimethyl-2-phenylmorpholine hydrogen tartrate.

$C_{12}H_{17}NO,C_4H_6O_6$ = 341.4.

CAS — 634-03-7 (phendimetrazine); 7635-51-0 (phendimetrazine hydrochloride); 50-58-8 (phendimetrazine tartrate).

Pharmacopoeias. In *US.*

A white odourless crystalline powder. Freely **soluble** in water; sparingly soluble in warm alcohol; practically insoluble in acetone, in chloroform, and in ether. A 2.5% solution in water has a pH of 3 to 4. **Store** in airtight containers.

Adverse Effects, Treatment, and Precautions

As for Dexamphetamine Sulphate, p.1478.

Interactions

Phendimetrazine is an indirect-acting sympathomimetic and, similarly to dexamphetamine (p.1479), may interact with a number of other drugs.

Pharmacokinetics

Phendimetrazine tartrate is readily absorbed from the gastro-intestinal tract and is excreted in the urine, partly unchanged and partly as metabolites, including phenmetrazine.

Uses and Administration

Phendimetrazine tartrate is a central stimulant and indirect-acting sympathomimetic with actions similar to those of dexamphetamine (p.1479). It has been used as an anorectic in the treatment of obesity (p.1476). The usual dose is 35 mg two or three times daily by mouth before food. An alternative dose is 105 mg once daily in the morning as a modified-release preparation.

Phendimetrazine hydrochloride has been used similarly in doses of 15 to 40 mg daily.

Preparations

USP 23: Phendimetrazine Tartrate Capsules; Phendimetrazine Tartrate Tablets.

Proprietary Preparations (details are given in Part 3)
Belg.: Anoran; Antapentan†; ***Ital.:*** Plegine; ***S.Afr.:*** Obesan-X; Obex-LA; ***Switz.:*** Antapentan†; ***USA:*** Adphen†; Anorex; Bacarate†; Bontril; Dital†; Dyrexan-OD; Melfiat†; Metra†; Obalan; Obeval†; Phenazine†; Phenzine†; Plegine†; Prelu-2; PT 105†; Rexigen Forte; Statobex†; Trimstat; Weh-less; Weightrol; X-trozine.

Phenmetrazine Hydrochloride (1487-z)

Phenmetrazine Hydrochloride *(BANM, rINNM)*.

Oxazimédrine. (±)-*trans*-3-Methyl-2-phenylmorpholine hydrochloride.

$C_{11}H_{15}NO,HCl$ = 213.7.

CAS — 134-49-6 (phenmetrazine); 1707-14-8 (phenmetrazine hydrochloride); 13931-75-4 (phenmetrazine theoclate).

Pharmacopoeias. In *US.*

A white to off-white crystalline powder. **Soluble** 1 in 0.4 of water, 1 in 2 of alcohol, and 1 in 2 of chloroform. A 2.5% solution in water has a pH of 4.5 to 5.5. **Store** in airtight containers.

Phenmetrazine hydrochloride is a central stimulant and indirect-acting sympathomimetic with actions similar to those of dexamphetamine (p.1479). It has been used as an anorectic in the treatment of obesity. It has been subject to extensive abuse.

Abuse. For reference to a serious syndrome involving rhabdomyolysis following intravenous abuse of phenmetrazine, see Dexamphetamine Sulphate, p.1478.

Preparations

USP 23: Phenmetrazine Hydrochloride Tablets.

Proprietary Preparations (details are given in Part 3)
USA: Preludin Endurets†.

Phentermine (1490-w)

Phentermine *(BAN, USAN, rINN)*.

α,α-Dimethylphenethylamine.

$C_{10}H_{15}N$ = 149.2.

CAS — 122-09-8.

Phentermine Hydrochloride (1489-k)

Phentermine Hydrochloride *(BANM, rINNM)*.

$C_{10}H_{15}N,HCl$ = 185.7.

CAS — 1197-21-3.

Pharmacopoeias. In *US.*

A white, odourless, hygroscopic, crystalline powder. Phentermine hydrochloride 1.24 mg is approximately equivalent to 1 mg of phentermine. **Soluble** in water, and in the lower alcohols; slightly soluble in chloroform; practically insoluble in ether. A 2% solution in water has a pH of 5 to 6. **Store** in airtight containers.

Adverse Effects, Treatment, and Precautions

As for Dexamphetamine Sulphate, p.1478. Urticaria may occur with use of phentermine.

Pulmonary hypertension has been reported in patients receiving phentermine and valvular heart defects in patients receiving the drug in combination with either fenfluramine or dexfenfluramine; these adverse effects, together with the relevant precautions to be observed, are discussed under Fenfluramine Hydrochloride, p.1481.

Interactions

Phentermine is an indirect-acting sympathomimetic and, similarly to dexamphetamine (p.1479), may interact with a number of other drugs.

Pharmacokinetics

Phentermine is readily absorbed from the gastro-intestinal tract and is excreted in the urine, partly unchanged and partly as metabolites.

Uses and Administration

Phentermine is a central stimulant and indirect-acting sympathomimetic with actions similar to those of dexamphetamine (p.1479). It is used as an anorectic and is administered by mouth as the base or hydrochloride in the treatment of moderate to severe obesity (p.1476).

The usual dose of phentermine is 15 to 30 mg once daily before breakfast given as an ion-exchange resin complex that provides modified-release. A suggested dose for phentermine hydrochloride is 8 mg three times daily before meals or 15 to 37.5 mg once daily in the morning. To reduce the risk of dependence phentermine is preferably given intermittently, a period of several weeks' treatment being followed by a similar period without treatment. In the UK the Committee on Safety of Medicines has recommended that treatment should not exceed 3 months.

Preparations

USP 23: Phentermine Hydrochloride Capsules; Phentermine Hydrochloride Tablets.

Proprietary Preparations (details are given in Part 3)
Aust.: Adipex; Mirapront; ***Austral.:*** Duromine; ***Belg.:*** Panbesy; ***Canad.:*** Fastin; Ionamin; ***Irl.:*** Ionamin; ***Ital.:*** Lipopill†; ***S.Afr.:*** Duromine; Minobese; ***Switz.:*** Adipex; Ionamine; Normaform; ***UK:*** Duromine; Ionamin; ***USA:*** Adipex-P; Fastin; Ionamin; Obe-Nix; Obephen†; Oby-Cap; Oby-Trim 30; Phentrol†; T-Diet†; Teramine†; Zantryl.

Pipradrol Hydrochloride (1440-d)

Pipradrol Hydrochloride *(BANM, rINNM).*

α-2-Piperidylbenzhydrol hydrochloride; α,α-Diphenyl-2-piperidinemethanol hydrochloride.

$C_{18}H_{21}NO,HCl = 303.8.$

CAS — 467-60-7 (pipradrol); 71-78-3 (pipradrol hydrochloride).

Pipradrol hydrochloride has been given by mouth in tonic preparations as a stimulant of the central nervous system.

Preparations

Proprietary Preparations (details are given in Part 3)

Multi-ingredient: ***Austral.:*** Alertonic; ***Canad.:*** Alertonic; ***S.Afr.:*** Alertonic.

Prethcamide (1443-m)

G-5668. *N,N*-Dimethyl-2-(*N*-propylcrotonamido)butyramide (cropropamide, $C_{13}H_{24}N_2O_2$ = 240.3);
2-(*N*-Ethylcrotonamido)-*N,N*-dimethylbutyramide (crotethamide, $C_{12}H_{22}N_2O_2$ = 226.3).

CAS — 8015-51-8 (prethcamide); 633-47-6 (cropropamide); 6168-76-9 (crotethamide).

NOTE. Cropropamide is *pINN*, Crotetamide is *rINN*.

A mixture of equal parts by weight of cropropamide and crotethamide.

Prethcamide has actions similar to those of doxapram (p.1480) and has been used as a respiratory stimulant. Doses of 100 mg have been given three times daily by mouth.

Preparations

Proprietary Preparations (details are given in Part 3)
Ital.: Micoren.

Prolintane Hydrochloride (1444-b)

Prolintane Hydrochloride *(BANM, USAN, rINNM).*

SP-732. 1-(α-Propylphenethyl)pyrrolidine hydrochloride.

$C_{15}H_{23}N,HCl = 253.8.$

CAS — 493-92-5 (prolintane); 1211-28-5 (prolintane hydrochloride).

Prolintane hydrochloride is a mild central stimulant and has properties similar to those of dexamphetamine (p.1478). It has been available mainly in tonic preparations that also contained vitamin supplements. Doses have ranged up to 30 mg daily by mouth. It has also been used in narcolepsy (p.1476) in doses of up to 40 mg daily.

Preparations

Proprietary Preparations (details are given in Part 3)
Belg.: Catorid; ***Ger.:*** Katovit N†.

Multi-ingredient: ***Austral.:*** Catovit†; ***Ger.:*** Katovit†; ***S.Afr.:*** Catovit; ***Spain:*** Katovit; ***Switz.:*** Katovit†; ***UK:*** Villescon†.

Propylhexedrine (1445-v)

Propylhexedrine *(BAN, rINN).*

Hexahydrodesoxyephedrine; Propylhexed. 2-Cyclohexyl-1-methylethyl-(methyl)amine; (±)-*N*-α-Dimethylcyclo-hexane-ethylamine.

$C_{10}H_{21}N = 155.3.$

CAS — 101-40-6; 3595-11-7 ((±)-propylhexedrine).

Pharmacopoeias. In *US.*

A clear colourless liquid with a characteristic amine-like odour. It slowly volatilises at room temperature and absorbs carbon dioxide from the air. Slightly **soluble** in water; soluble 1 in 0.4 of alcohol, 1 in 0.2 of chloroform, and 1 in 0.1 of ether. Solutions in water are alkaline to litmus. **Store** in airtight containers.

Propylhexedrine Hydrochloride (1446-g)

Propylhexedrine Hydrochloride *(BANM, rINNM).*

$C_{10}H_{21}N,HCl = 191.7.$

CAS — 1007-33-6; 6192-95-6 ((±)-propylhexedrine hydrochloride).

Adverse Effects, Treatment and Precautions

As for Dexamphetamine Sulphate, p.1478.

Nasal inhalation may cause transient burning, stinging, mucosal dryness, and sneezing. Prolonged use can cause rebound congestion, redness, swelling, and rhinitis. Systemic effects such as headache, hypertension, nervousness, and increased heart rate may occur.

Propylhexedrine is subject to abuse; fatalities following oral and intravenous use have been reported due to myocardial infarction, heart failure, or pulmonary hypertension. Psychosis may occur.

Abuse. References.

1. White L, DiMaio VJM. Intravenous propylhexedrine and sudden death. *N Engl J Med* 1977; **297:** 1071.
2. Anderson RJ, *et al.* Intravenous propylhexedrine (Benzedrex®) abuse and sudden death. *Am J Med* 1979; **67:** 15–20.
3. Cameron J, *et al.* Possible association of pulmonary hypertension with an anorectic drug. *Med J Aust* 1984; **140:** 595–7.

Uses and Administration

Propylhexedrine is a central stimulant and indirect-acting sympathomimetic with actions similar to those of dexamphetamine (p.1479). It has been used as an inhalant for nasal decongestion (p.1052).

Propylhexedrine hydrochloride has been given by mouth as an anorectic in the treatment of obesity (p.1476). The (−)-isomer, levopropylhexedrine hydrochloride, has been used similarly.

Preparations

USP 23: Propylhexedrine Inhalant.

Proprietary Preparations (details are given in Part 3)
Austral.: Eventin†; ***Ger.:*** Eventin†; ***USA:*** Benzedrex.

Multi-ingredient: ***Ger.:*** Soventol C†; ***S.Afr.:*** Reducealin.

Sibutramine (1677-r)

Sibutramine *(BAN, rINN).*

BTS-54524 (sibutramine hydrochloride). (±)-1-(*p*-Chlorophenyl)-α-isobutyl-*N,N*-dimethylcyclobutanemethylamine.

$C_{17}H_{26}ClN = 279.8.$

CAS — 106650-56-0 (sibutramine); 84485-00-7 (anhydrous sibutramine hydrochloride); 125494-59-9 (sibutramine hydrochloride monohydrate).

NOTE. Sibutramine Hydrochloride is *USAN*.

Adverse Effects

Commonly reported side-effects of sibutramine are dry mouth, headache, insomnia, and constipation; diarrhoea, dizziness, drowsiness, and rhinitis have also occurred. Less frequently reported side-effects include dysmenorrhoea, oedema, influenza-like symptoms, and depression. Abnormal bleeding, acute interstitial nephritis, emotional lability, migraine, seizures, and skin rashes have been reported rarely. Clinically significant increases in heart rate and blood pressure may occur. Sibutramine may decrease salivary flow and therefore increase the risk of dental caries, periodontal disease, or other oral disorders. It may also produce mydriasis. Increases in liver enzymes have been reported.

Precautions

Sibutramine should be avoided in anorexia nervosa or in uncontrolled or poorly controlled hypertension; it should be used with caution in patients with a history of or with well-controlled hypertension. Blood pressure and heart rate should be monitored before starting therapy and at regular intervals during therapy. In the event of sustained elevations, the dose should be reduced or treatment discontinued.

Sibutramine should be used with caution in patients with a history of seizures, stroke, or cardiovascular disorders such as cardiac arrhythmias, heart failure, and coronary artery disease. It should also be used cautiously in patients with angle-closure glaucoma, severe hepatic or renal impairment, or with a history of gallstones (which may be precipitated or exacerbated by weight loss).

Ability to perform tasks requiring judgement or motor or cognitive skills may be impaired by sibutramine, and patients, if affected, should not drive or operate machinery.

Interactions

Sibutramine should not be given concurrently with, or within at least two weeks of stopping an MAOI; at least two weeks should elapse between discontinuation of sibutramine and starting therapy with an MAOI. There is a risk of the serotonin syndrome (p.303) developing if sibutramine is administered together with other serotonergic drugs such as selective serotonin reuptake inhibitors (SSRIs), sumatriptan, lithium, pethidine, fentanyl, dextromethorphan, and pentazocine. Sibutramine should not be used with other drugs that may increase heart rate or blood pressure such as ephedrine, phenylpropanolamine, and pseudoephedrine (which may be ingredients of some cough and cold remedies). Alcohol should be avoided.

Inhibitors of the cytochrome P450 isoenzyme CYP3A4, such as ketoconazole and erythromycin, may increase plasma concentrations of sibutramine.

Pharmacokinetics

Sibutramine is well-absorbed from the gastro-intestinal tract; peak plasma concentrations appear after 1.2 hours (parent drug) and 3 to 4 hours (metabolites). It undergoes extensive first-pass hepatic metabolism, principally by the cytochrome P450 isoenzyme CYP3A4. Biotransformation pathways are demethylation to produce mono- and di-desmethylsibutramine (both of which are pharmacologically active) followed by hydroxylation and conjugation to inactive metabolites. Protein binding is 97%. Plasma-elimination half-life is 14 to 16 hours. Elimination is mainly in the urine as inactive metabolites, and partly in the faeces.

Uses and Administration

Sibutramine, which is structurally related to amphetamine (p.1477), is a serotonin and noradrenaline reuptake inhibitor; it also inhibits dopamine reuptake but to a lesser extent. Sibutramine is used in the management of obesity (p.1476). It may also be used in overweight patients (body mass index of 27 kg per m^2 or more) if other risk factors such as hypertension (but see Precautions, above), diabetes mellitus, or hyperlipidaemias are present.

Sibutramine is given as the hydrochloride in an initial daily dose of 10 mg, usually taken in the morning. Patients who cannot tolerate 10 mg daily may benefit from a dose of 5 mg daily. Treatment with sibutramine should be re-evaluated if the patient does not lose at least 1.8 kg in the first 4 weeks of therapy. The dose may be increased if necessary to a maximum of 15 mg daily, taking into consideration effects on heart rate and blood pressure.

Preparations

Proprietary Preparations (details are given in Part 3)
USA: Meridia.

Tenamfetamine (1432-d)

Tenamfetamine *(rINN).*

MDA; Methylenedioxyamphetamine; 3,4-Methylenedioxyamphetamine; SKF-5. α-Methyl-3,4-methylenedioxyphenethylamine.

$C_{10}H_{13}NO_2 = 179.2.$

CAS — 4764-17-4; 51497-09-7.

NOTE. Tenamfetamine has also been known as Love Drug, Love Pill, and Mellow Drug of America.

Tenamfetamine is a phenylethylamine compound, structurally related to amphetamine and mescaline, with hallucinogenic effects. It has been subject to abuse and dependence. A number of similar compounds are known because of their abuse and include:

- brolamfetamine (4-bromo-2,5-dimethoxyamphetamine; bromo-DMA; bromo-DOM; 2,5-dimethoxy-4-bromoamphetamine; DOB);
- 4-bromo-2,5-methoxyphenylethylamine (afterburner; 2-CB; MFT);
- 2,5-dimethoxy-4-methylamphetamine (DOM; methyl-2,5-dimethoxyamphetamine; Serenity, Tranquillity and Peace; STP);
- *N*-ethyltenamfetamine (Eve; MDE; MDEA; 3,4-methylenedioxyethamphetamine);
- *N*-hydroxytenamfetamine (*N*-hydroxy MDA; 3,4-methylenedioxy-*N*-hydroxyamphetamine);
- methoxyamphetamine (4-methoxyamphetamine; *p*-methoxyamphetamine; PMA);
- methylenedioxymethamphetamine (see p.1482);
- 2,4,5-trimethoxyamphetamine (TMA; TMA-2).

In large doses the side-effects of tenamfetamine and related compounds are similar to those of dexamphetamine and may be treated similarly (see p.1478). Fatalities have been associated with the abuse of some of these compounds.

Reviews of the properties of some designer drugs, including phenylethylamine compounds.

1. Buchanan JF, Brown CR. 'Designer drugs': a problem in clinical toxicology. *Med Toxicol* 1988; **3:** 1–17.
2. Chesher G. Designer drugs—the "whats" and the "whys". *Med J Aust* 1990; **153:** 157–61.

Sunscreens

In normal healthy individuals **exposure to sunlight** causes an increase in pigmentation (tanning). However, excessive exposure to strong sunlight causes erythema and sunburn. Immediate tanning may occur resulting from the oxidation of melanin precursors in the uppermost layers of the skin. There may also be a delayed and indirect pigmentation due to the formation of new melanin. The ability of an individual to form a tan is genetically predetermined. Melanin provides some protection against further exposure, but the main protection is provided by thickening of the corneous layer.

Excessive and prolonged exposure to intense sunlight may lead to degenerative changes in the skin (premature ageing of the skin or photoageing), actinic (solar) keratoses (which are risk factors or precursors of skin cancers), and some skin cancers such as basal-cell or squamous-cell carcinomas and malignant melanomas (see Malignant Neoplasms of the Skin, p.492).

Ultraviolet (UV) light has different properties according to its wavelength.

- UVA (wavelengths 320 to 400 nm) produces immediate direct tanning of the skin with little erythema although it does contribute to the long-term harmful effects of photoageing and cancers.
- UVB (wavelengths 290 to 320 nm) is about 1000 times stronger than UVA in producing erythema and is that part of the sun's spectrum that is responsible for producing sunburn and it too contributes to long-term effects. UVB also produces tanning by indirect pigmentation.
- UVC (wavelengths 200 to 290 nm) produces erythema without tanning. The earth's surface is usually screened by the ozone layer from UVC radiation although UVC may be emitted by artificial sources such as bactericidal lamps and industrial welding arcs.

Reflected ultraviolet light from snow, white sand, or water adds to direct irradiation.

In some persons brief exposure to sunlight can induce a variety of skin complaints. *Polymorphic light eruption* is characterised by pruritic erythematous lesions which develop some hours after exposure to sunlight. *Chronic actinic dermatitis* is manifested by a persistent eczematous eruption which usually only affects the exposed areas although in a small number of patients the whole skin can be affected. Photosensitivity can also be produced by drugs administered either systemically or applied topically (p.1073). Such photosensitivity can be either phototoxic or photoallergic in nature. In *phototoxicity*, tissues are damaged when the drug is energised by absorbing radiation. In *photoallergy*, a hypersensitivity reaction is produced when the drug is chemically altered after exposure to light. Other conditions that can be exacerbated by sunlight include the *cutaneous porphyrias, lupus erythematosus, solar urticaria, xeroderma pigmentosum*, and sometimes *herpes labialis*. In many of these cases the photosensitivity is particularly associated with the longer UVA wavelengths.

Protection against sunlight is therefore beneficial, both in healthy people to prevent skin damage, and in patients with the disorders mentioned above. Protection may also be necessary in patients with *hypopigmentation disorders* such as vitiligo or albinism and medical personnel exposed to ultraviolet bactericidal lamps may need protection against the whole of the UV spectrum.

Sunscreens are of 2 types: *chemical* agents that because of their chromophore groups absorb a particular range of wavelengths within the UV spectrum and *physical* agents that are opaque and reflect most UV radiation. A classification of the chemical sunscreens included in this chapter is given in Table 1, below. Triethanolamine salicylate (p.91) is a chemical sunscreen that is also used as a topical analgesic. Physical sunscreens include titanium dioxide (p.1093) and zinc oxide (p.1096). Many of the available products combine sunscreens from the different groups in order to widen the protection afforded. Other agents used as physical sunscreens include calcium carbonate, kaolin, magnesium oxide, red veterinary petroleum, and talc. Powders may be dusted onto the skin or applied in an aqueous or oily basis but these types of sunscreens are usually cosmetically unappealing.

The efficacy of a particular sunscreen preparation is often expressed as its **sun protection factor (SPF)**. This is a ratio of the time required for irradiation to produce minimal perceptible erythema (minimal erythemal dose; MED) with the skin protected with the sunscreen compared with the MED without protection. Thus the SPF is predominantly an indication of efficacy against UVB light. Various systems have been suggested for classifying the relative efficacies of sunscreens against UVA light but none appears, as yet, to be universally accepted.

Sunscreens are used topically. Adverse effects such as photosensitisation may occur with chemical agents, and skin irritation has also been reported. Sunscreens in highly alcoholic vehicles should not be used on patients with inflamed skin.

Several other agents including betacarotene (p.1335) and psoralens (see Methoxsalen, p.1086), which are neither chemical nor physical sunscreens, have been used to increase tolerance to sunlight in various diseases characterised by photosensitivity. Dihydroxyacetone (p.1081) and lawsone (p.1594) when employed together appear to provide some protection against UV light although neither is effective when used alone.

General references to sunscreens.

1. Council on Scientific Affairs, American Medical Association. Harmful effects of ultraviolet radiation. *JAMA* 1989; **262:** 380–4.
2. Anonymous. Measuring sunscreen protection against UVA. *Lancet* 1990; **336:** 472.
3. Taylor CR, *et al.* Photoaging/photodamage and photoprotection. *J Am Acad Dermatol* 1990; **22:** 1–15.
4. Ratnavel RC, Norris PG. Sunscreens and their medical uses. *Prescribers' J* 1993; **33:** 63–71.
5. McGregor JM, Young AR. Sunscreens, suntans, and skin cancer. *Br Med J* 1996; **312:** 1621–2.

Table 1. Chemical sunscreens.

UVA absorbers	UVB absorbers
Anthranilates	*Aminobenzoates*
Menthyl anthranilate	Aminobenzoic acid
Dibenzoylmethanes	Lisadimate
Avobenzone	Padimate
Dibenzoylmethane	Padimate O
Isopropyldibenzoylmethane	Roxadimate
	Camphor derivatives
UVA and UVB absorbers	3-(4-Methylbenzylidene)bornan-2-one
	Cinnamates
Benzophenones	Cinoxate
Benzophenone-6	Ethylhexyl *p*-methoxycinnamate
Dioxybenzone	Octocrylene
Mexenone	*Salicylates*
Oxybenzone	Homosalate
Sulisobenzone	Octyl salicylate

Aminobenzoic Acid (7871-h)

Amben; PAB; PABA; Pabacidum; Para-aminobenzoic Acid; Vitamin H'. 4-Aminobenzoic acid.

$C_7H_7NO_2$ = 137.1.

CAS — 150-13-0.

Pharmacopoeias. In *Aust., Br., Swiss,* and *US.*

White or slightly yellow odourless or almost odourless crystals or crystalline powder. It gradually darkens on exposure to air and light. Slightly **soluble** in water and in chloroform; sparingly soluble in ether; freely soluble in alcohol; dissolves in solutions of alkali hydroxides and carbonates. **Store** in airtight containers. Protect from light.

Adverse Effects

Contact and photocontact allergic dermatitis has been reported following the topical administration of aminobenzoate sunscreens.

Adverse skin reactions have been reported following the topical use[1-6] of aminobenzoic acid or its esters. Skin reactions (vitiligo) have also been reported following the oral administration of aminobenzoic acid[7] and the adverse effects associated with the former use of high oral doses for various conditions have been highlighted.[8]

1. Parrish JA, *et al.* Facial irritation due to sunscreen products. *Arch Dermatol* 1975; **111:** 525.
2. Mathias CGT, *et al.* Allergic contact photodermatitis to para-aminobenzoic acid. *Arch Dermatol* 1978; **114:** 1665–6.
3. Horio T, Higuchi T. Photocontact dermatitis from p-aminobenzoic acid. *Dermatologica* 1978; **156:** 124–8.
4. Marmelzat J, Rapaport MJ. Photodermatitis with PABA. *Contact Dermatitis* 1980; **6:** 230–1.
5. Thune P. Contact and photocontact allergy to sunscreens. *Photodermatology* 1984; **1:** 5–9.
6. English JSC, *et al.* Sensitivity to sunscreens. *Contact Dermatitis* 1987; **17:** 159–62.
7. Hughes CG. Oral PABA and vitiligo. *J Am Acad Dermatol* 1983; **9:** 770.
8. Worobec S, LaChine A. Dangers of orally administered para-aminobenzoic acid. *JAMA* 1984; **251:** 2348.

Precautions

Aminobenzoate sunscreens should not be used by patients with previous experience of photosensitivity or hypersensitivity reactions to chemically related drugs such as sulphonamides, thiazide diuretics, and certain local anaesthetics, particularly benzocaine.

Aminobenzoic acid may stain clothing.

Pharmacokinetics

If administered by mouth, aminobenzoic acid is absorbed from the gastro-intestinal tract. It is metabolised in the liver and excreted in the urine as unchanged drug and metabolites.

Uses and Administration

Aminobenzoic acid is used by topical application as a sunscreen; a concentration of 5% is commonly used. Aminobenzoic acid and its derivatives effectively absorb light throughout the UVB range but absorb little or no UVA light (for definitions, see above). Aminobenzoate sunscreens may therefore be used to prevent sunburn, but are unlikely to prevent drug-related or other photosensitivity reactions associated with UVA light; combination with a benzophenone may give some added protection against such photosensitivity.

Aminobenzoic acid has sometimes been included as a member of the vitamin-B group, but deficiency of aminobenzoic acid in man or animals has not been demonstrated.

Aminobenzoic acid has been used in conjunction with bentiromide (p.1552) in the PABA or BTPABA test of pancreatic function.

Preparations

USP 23: Aminobenzoic Acid Gel; Aminobenzoic Acid Topical Solution.

Proprietary Preparations

Some preparations are listed in Part 3.

Avobenzone (10926-q)

Avobenzone *(USAN, rINN).*

Butylmethoxydibenzoylmethane; 4-*tert*-Butyl-4'-methoxydibenzoylmethane; Parsol 1789. 1-(*p*-*tert*-Butylphenyl)-3-(*p*-methoxyphenyl)-1,3-propanedione; 1-[4-(1,1-dimethylethyl)phenyl]-3-(4-methoxyphenyl)-1,3-propanedione.

$C_{20}H_{22}O_3$ = 310.4.

CAS — 70356-09-1.

Avobenzone is a substituted dibenzoylmethane used by topical application as a sunscreen. Dibenzoylmethanes absorb light in the UVA range (for definitions, see above) and may therefore be used in conjunction with other sunscreens that absorb UVB light to prevent sunburn; they will also provide some protection against drug-related or other photosensitivity reactions associated with UVA light.

Contact and photocontact allergic dermatitis has occasionally been reported following the topical use of dibenzoylmethane sunscreens.

Preparations

Proprietary Preparations
Numerous preparations are listed in Part 3.

Benzophenone-6 (9318-c)

2,2′-Dihydroxy-4,4′-dimethoxybenzophenone.

$C_{15}H_{14}O_5$ = 274.3.

CAS — 131-54-4.

Benzophenone-6 is a sunscreen with actions similar to those of oxybenzone (below). It is effective against UVB and some UVA light (for definitions, see above).

Cinoxate (9302-p)

Cinoxate *(USAN, rINN).*

2-Ethoxyethyl *p*-methoxycinnamate.

$C_{14}H_{18}O_4$ = 250.3.

CAS — 104-28-9.

Pharmacopoeias. In *US.*

A slightly yellow, practically odourless, viscous liquid. Very slightly **soluble** in water; slightly soluble in glycerol; soluble in propylene glycol; miscible with alcohol and vegetable oils. **Store** in airtight containers. Protect from light.

Cinoxate, a substituted cinnamate, is a sunscreen with actions similar to those of ethylhexyl *p*-methoxycinnamate (below). It is effective against UVB light (for definitions, see above).

Preparations

USP 23: Cinoxate Lotion.

Proprietary Preparations
Some preparations are listed in Part 3.

Dibenzoylmethane (13410-m)

1,3-Diphenyl-1,3-propanedione.

$C_{15}H_{12}O_2$ = 224.3.

CAS — 120-46-7.

Dibenzoylmethane is a sunscreen with actions similar to those of avobenzone (p.1486). It absorbs UVA light (for definitions, see above).

Dioxybenzone (9303-s)

Dioxybenzone *(USAN, rINN).*

Benzophenone-8; NSC-56769. 2,2′-Dihydroxy-4-methoxybenzophenone.

$C_{14}H_{12}O_4$ = 244.2.

CAS — 131-53-3.

Pharmacopoeias. In *US.*

A yellow powder. Practically **insoluble** in water; freely soluble in alcohol and toluene. **Store** in airtight containers. Protect from light.

Dioxybenzone, a substituted benzophenone, is a sunscreen with actions similar to those of oxybenzone (below). It is effective against UVB and some UVA light (for definitions, see above).

Preparations

USP 23: Dioxybenzone and Oxybenzone Cream.

Proprietary Preparations
Some preparations are listed in Part 3.

Ethylhexyl *p*-Methoxycinnamate (9324-j)

Octyl methoxycinnamate; Parsol MCX. 2-Ethylhexyl-*p*-methoxycinnamate.

$C_{18}H_{26}O_3$ = 290.4.

CAS — 5466-77-3.

Ethylhexyl *p*-methoxycinnamate, a substituted cinnamate, is used by topical application as a sunscreen. Cinnamate sunscreens effectively absorb light throughout the UVB range but absorb little or no UVA light (for definitions, see above). Cinnamate sunscreens may therefore be used to prevent sunburn but are unlikely to prevent drug-related or other photosensitivity reactions associated with UVA light; combination with a benzophenone may give some added protection against such photosensitivity. Cinnamates may occasionally produce photosensitivity reactions.

Preparations

Proprietary Preparations
Numerous preparations are listed in Part 3.

Homosalate (9306-l)

Homosalate *(USAN, rINN).*

Homomenthyl Salicylate. 3,3,5-Trimethylcyclohexyl salicylate.

$C_{16}H_{22}O_3$ = 262.3.

CAS — 118-56-9.

Homosalate, a substituted salicylate, is a sunscreen with actions similar to those of octyl salicylate (below). It is effective against UVB light (for definitions, see above).

Preparations

Proprietary Preparations
Some preparations are listed in Part 3.

Isopropyldibenzoylmethane (15708-j)

1-[4-(1-Methylethyl)phenyl]-3-phenyl-1,3-propanedione.

$C_{18}H_{18}O_2$ = 266.3.

CAS — 63250-25-9.

Isopropyldibenzoylmethane, a substituted dibenzoylmethane, is a sunscreen with actions similar to those of avobenzone (above). It absorbs UVA light (for definitions, see above).

Lisadimate (9305-e)

Lisadimate *(USAN, rINN).*

Glyceryl Aminobenzoate; Glyceryl PABA. Glyceryl 1-(4-aminobenzoate).

$C_{10}H_{13}NO_4$ = 211.2.

CAS — 136-44-7.

Lisadimate is a sunscreen with actions similar to those of aminobenzoic acid (above). It is effective against UVB light (for definitions, see above).

Menthyl Anthranilate (19515-j)

Menthyl *O*-Aminobenzoate. 5-Methyl-2-(1-methylethyl)-cyclohexyl 2-aminobenzoate.

$C_{17}H_{25}NO_2$ = 275.4.

CAS — 134-09-8.

Menthyl anthranilate is used as a sunscreen. It is effective against UVA light (for definitions, see above).

Preparations

Proprietary Preparations
Some preparations are listed in Part 3.

3-(4-Methylbenzylidene)bornan-2-one (9327-k)

3-(4-Methylbenzylidene)camphor. 1,7,7-Trimethyl-3-[(4-methylphenyl)methylene]bicyclo[2.2.1]heptan-2-one.

$C_{18}H_{22}O$ = 254.4.

*CAS — 36861-47-9 (*D,L*-form); 38102-62-4 (form unspecified).*

3-(4-Methylbenzylidene)bornan-2-one is a camphor derivative used as a sunscreen. It is effective against UVB light (for definitions, see above).

A case report of allergic contact dermatitis from 3-(4-methylbenzylidene)bornan-2-one.[1]

1. Hunloh W, Goerz G. Contact dermatitis form Eusolex® 6300. *Contact Dermatitis* 1983; **9:** 333–4.

Preparations

Proprietary Preparations
Some preparations are listed in Part 3.

Mexenone (9310-p)

Mexenone *(BAN, pINN).*

Benzophenone-10. 2-Hydroxy-4-methoxy-4′-methylbenzophenone.

$C_{15}H_{14}O_3$ = 242.3.

CAS — 1641-17-4.

Pharmacopoeias. In *Br.*

A pale yellow odourless or almost odourless crystalline powder. Practically **insoluble** in water; sparingly soluble in alcohol; freely soluble in acetone.

Mexenone, a substituted benzophenone, is a sunscreen with actions similar to those of oxybenzone (below). It is effective against UVB and some UVA light (for definitions, see above)

Preparations

BP 1998: Mexenone Cream.

Proprietary Preparations
Some preparations are listed in Part 3.

Octocrylene (9328-a)

Octocrylene *(USAN).*

Octocrilene *(rINN)*; 2-Ethylhexyl α-cyano-β-phenylcinnamate. 2-Ethylhexyl 2-cyano-3,3-diphenylacrylate.

$C_{24}H_{27}NO_2$ = 361.5.

CAS — 6197-30-4.

Octocrylene, a substituted cinnamate, is a sunscreen with actions similar to those of ethylhexyl *p*-methoxycinnamate (above). It is effective against UVB light (for definitions, see above).

Preparations

Proprietary Preparations
Some preparations are listed in Part 3.

Octyl Salicylate (18470-s)

Octyl salicylate is a substituted salicylate used by topical application as a sunscreen. Salicylates effectively absorb light throughout the UVB range but absorb little or no UVA light (for definitions, see above). Salicylate sunscreens may therefore be used to prevent sunburn, but are unlikely to prevent drug-related or other photosensitivity reactions associated with UVA light; combination with a benzophenone may give some added protection.

Salicylates may occasionally produce photosensitivity reactions.

Preparations

Proprietary Preparations
Numerous preparations are listed in Part 3.

Oxybenzone (9312-w)

Oxybenzone *(USAN, rINN).*

Benzophenone-3. 2-Hydroxy-4-methoxybenzophenone.

$C_{14}H_{12}O_3$ = 228.2.

CAS — 131-57-7.

Pharmacopoeias. In *US.*

A pale yellow powder. Practically **insoluble** in water; freely soluble in alcohol and in toluene. **Store** in airtight containers. Protect from light.

Oxybenzone is a substituted benzophenone used by topical application as a sunscreen. Benzophenones effectively absorb light throughout the UVB range (wavelengths 290 to 320 nm) and also absorb some UVA light with wavelengths of 320 to about 360 nm and some UVC light with wavelengths of about 250 to 290 nm (for definitions, see above). Benzophenones may therefore be used to prevent sunburn and may also provide some protection against drug-related or other photosensitivity reactions associated with UVA light; in practice they are usually combined with a sunscreen from another group.

Contact and photocontact allergic dermatitis has occasionally been reported following the topical administration of benzophenone sunscreens.

References to allergic and photoallergic reactions in a few patients using oxybenzone sunscreens.[1-4]

1. Thompson G, *et al.* Allergic contact dermatitis from sunscreen preparations complicating photodermatitis. *Arch Dermatol* 1977; **113:** 1252–3.
2. Thune P. Contact and photocontact allergy to sunscreens. *Photodermatology* 1984; **1:** 5–9.
3. Knoler E, *et al.* Photoallergy to benzophenone. *Arch Dermatol* 1989; **125:** 801–4.
4. Collins P, Ferguson J. Photoallergic contact dermatitis to oxybenzone. *Br J Dermatol* 1994; **131:** 124–9.

Preparations

USP 23: Dioxybenzone and Oxybenzone Cream.

Proprietary Preparations
Numerous preparations are listed in Part 3.

Padimate (9313-e)

Padimate *(BAN, rINN).*

Amyl Dimethylaminobenzoate; Isoamyl Dimethylaminobenzoate; Padimate A *(USAN)*. A mixture of pentyl, isopentyl, and 2-methylbutyl 4-dimethylaminobenzoates.

$C_{14}H_{21}NO_2$ = 235.3.

CAS — 14779-78-3 (pentyl 4-dimethylaminobenzoate); 21245-01-2(isopentyl 4-dimethylaminobenzoate).

Padimate, a substituted aminobenzoate, is a sunscreen with actions similar to those of aminobenzoic acid (above). It is effective against UVB light (for definitions, see above).

Padimate O (9314-l)

Padimate O *(BANM, USAN)*.

Octyl dimethyl PABA. 2-Ethylhexyl 4-(dimethylamino)benzoate.

$C_{17}H_{27}NO_2$ = 277.4.

CAS — 21245-02-3.

Pharmacopoeias. In US.

A light yellow, mobile liquid with a faint aromatic odour. Practically **insoluble** in water, in glycerol, and in propylene glycol; soluble in alcohol, in isopropyl alcohol, and in liquid paraffin. **Store** in airtight containers. Protect from light.

Padimate O, a substituted aminobenzoate, is a sunscreen with actions similar to those of aminobenzoic acid (above). It is effective against UVB light (for definitions, see above).

References to contact or photocontact allergy to padimate O.

1. Weller P, Freeman S. Photocontact allergy to octyldimethyl PABA. *Australas J Dermatol* 1984; **25:** 73–6.
2. Thune P. Contact and photocontact allergy to sunscreens. *Photodermatology* 1984; **1:** 5–9.
3. English JSC, *et al.* Sensitivity to sunscreens. *Contact Dermatitis* 1987; **17:** 159–62.

Preparations

USP 23: Padimate O Lotion.

Proprietary Preparations

Numerous preparations are listed in Part 3.

2-Phenyl-1*H*-benzimidazole-5-sulphonic Acid (9329-t)

$C_{13}H_{10}N_2O_3S$ = 274.3.

CAS — 27503-81-7.

2-Phenyl-1*H*-benzimidazole-5-sulphonic acid is used topically as a sunscreen.

Preparations

Proprietary Preparations

Some preparations are listed in Part 3.

Roxadimate (9322-l)

Roxadimate *(USAN, rINN)*.

Ethyl Dihydroxypropyl PABA. Ethyl (±)-4-[bis(2-hydroxypropyl)amino]benzoate.

$C_{15}H_{23}NO_4$ = 281.3.

CAS — 58882-17-0.

Roxadimate, a substituted aminobenzoate, is a sunscreen with actions similar to those of aminobenzoic acid (above). It is effective against UVB light (for definitions, see above).

Sodium 3,4-Dimethoxyphenylglyoxylate (9330-l)

$C_{10}H_9NaO_5$ = 232.2.

CAS — 37891-88-6.

Sodium 3,4-dimethoxyphenylglyoxylate has been used topically as a sunscreen.

Sulisobenzone (9316-j)

Sulisobenzone *(USAN, rINN)*.

Benzophenone-4; NSC-60584. 5-Benzoyl-4-hydroxy-2-methoxybenzenesulphonic acid.

$C_{14}H_{12}O_6S$ = 308.3.

CAS — 4065-45-6.

Sulisobenzone, a substituted benzophenone, is a sunscreen with actions similar to those of oxybenzone (above). It is effective against UVB and some UVA light (for definitions, see above).

Thyroid and Antithyroid Drugs

This chapter describes the drugs used to treat the endocrine disorders associated with the thyroid gland including hyperthyroidism, Graves' disease and thyroid storm (thyroid crisis), and hypothyroidism and myxoedema.

The principal role of the thyroid gland is to regulate tissue metabolism through production of the **thyroid hormones** 3,5,3′,5′-tetra-iodo-L-thyronine (L-thyroxine; T_4) and, in smaller amounts, 3,5,3′-tri-iodo-L-thyronine (liothyronine; T_3). In infants and children thyroid hormones are also necessary for the development of the CNS and for normal growth and bone maturation.

The production of hormones by the thyroid gland is dependent on an adequate supply of dietary iodine. Iodide is actively transported into the gland and undergoes oxidation. Oxidised iodide is incorporated into the tyrosyl residues of the glycoprotein thyroglobulin to form L-mono-iodotyrosine (MIT) and L-di-iodotyrosine (DIT). Coupling of these inactive iodotyrosines yields the hormonally active iodothyronines, L-thyroxine and L-tri-iodothyronine in peptide linkage with thyroglobulin for storage in the follicular colloid. The secretion of thyroid hormones is mediated by the release of proteolytic enzymes from lysosomes to degrade the thyroglobulin into its constituent amino acids releasing L-thyroxine and L-tri-iodothyronine into the circulation; iodide resulting from this reaction is recycled.

Thyroid hormones are extensively protein bound, principally to thyroxine-binding globulin (TBG) but also to a lesser extent to thyroxine-binding pre-albumin (TBPA) or to albumin.

Whereas L-thyroxine enters the circulation only by direct glandular secretion, very little L-tri-iodothyronine is secreted by a normal thyroid gland and most of the extra-thyroid L-tri-iodothyronine is produced by the mono-deiodination of L-thyroxine in the peripheral tissues. About 35% of secreted L-thyroxine is converted to L-tri-iodothyronine and about 40% is converted to inactive reverse tri-iodothyronine (rT_3). The metabolic activity of L-tri-iodothyronine is about 3 to 5 times that of L-thyroxine and it has been suggested that L-tri-iodothyronine is the active thyroid hormone with L-thyroxine acting primarily as a prohormone.

Thyroid hormone homoeostasis is maintained by a large intraglandular store of hormone, autoregulatory mechanisms within the gland, and complex feedback mechanisms. Feedback is mediated by thyroid-stimulating hormone (thyrotrophin, TSH—see p.1262), which is produced by the anterior pituitary gland and acts on the thyroid gland to stimulate hormone production. The release and synthesis of TSH are stimulated by thyrotrophin-releasing hormone (protirelin, TRH—see p.1259) secreted from the hypothalamus and inhibited by the unbound thyroid hormones circulating in the blood. Thus when thyroid hormone concentrations in blood are increased the secretion of TSH and possibly TRH will be suppressed and conversely when decreased the secretion of TSH will be stimulated. The term euthyroidism is used when the thyroid gland is functioning normally and there are normal amounts of thyroid hormone in the blood.

The main drugs used for **thyroid replacement** and described in this chapter are thyroxine and liothyronine. The main **antithyroid drugs** included in this chapter are the thiourea derivatives (thiocarbamides, thionamides, or thioureylenes); this group comprises the imidazole derivatives (carbimazole and methimazole) and the thiouracils (benzylthiouracil, methylthiouracil, and propylthiouracil). The thiourea compounds block the production of thyroid hormones through inhibition of thyroid peroxidase. This leads to inhibition of oxidation of iodide and of iodination of tyrosyl groups of thyroglobulin. There is also inhibition of the coupling of the iodotyrosines to form iodothyronines. The place of immunosuppression in the antithyroid activity of these drugs is subject to debate. Antithyroid drugs do not block the release of stored thyroid hormones and it is only when the preformed hormones are depleted and concentrations of circulating hormones decline that clinical effects become apparent. An additional action of propylthiouracil is inhibition of the peripheral deiodination of thyroxine to tri-iodothyronine. Other antithyroid drugs in this chapter include perchlorates (potassium and sodium perchlorate), tyrosine derivatives (dibromotyrosine, diiodotyrosine, and fluorotyrosine), and iodine and iodides.

Goitre and thyroid nodules

Goitre is the enlargement of the thyroid gland. This may be focal (as in a solitary thyroid nodule, adenoma, or cyst) or generalised, in which case it is usually diffuse at first, later becoming multinodular. The general aims in the management of thyroid masses are:

- the detection and treatment of malignancy
- the reduction of goitre or prevention of further enlargement, and the relief of obstructive symptoms
- the maintenance of a euthyroid state.

Toxic goitres are associated with the hypersecretion of thyroid hormone and their management is discussed under Hyperthyroidism, below.

Non-toxic goitres may be associated with hypothyroidism (below) or euthyroidism, and are generally attributed to impaired synthesis of thyroid hormones due to intrinsic defects in hormone production or to extrinsic factors such as dietary-iodine deficiency in endemic goitre (see Iodine Deficiency Disorders, p.1494). This decreased secretion of thyroid hormone results in an excessive output of thyroid-stimulating hormone (TSH) from the pituitary which stimulates thyroid-hormone production but also leads to hypertrophy and hyperplasia of the thyroid gland; if the response to TSH overcomes the deficiency in thyroid-hormone synthesis then the patient is goitrous and euthyroid but if the compensatory response to TSH is inadequate then goitre with hypothyroidism is observed. However, other factors such as autoantibodies might stimulate thyroid growth; thyroid autonomy where the gland functions independently of TSH control can also occur.

Ultrasound or radionuclide imaging may be employed to determine the number and size of any nodules present but cannot distinguish a benign from a malignant nodule. Cytological analysis is the most reliable means of diagnosing malignancy.[1-3] Thyroxine has been given short-term in an attempt to distinguish benign from malignant nodules, with failure of the nodule to shrink being regarded as an indication of malignancy, but it is much less reliable.[2]

In established **malignancy**, surgery, followed by thyroxine replacement therapy, is the usual course (for further discussion of the treatment of thyroid cancer, see p.494).

The treatment of **benign solitary** non-toxic nodules is a matter of dispute. Suppressive therapy with doses of thyroxine (or, less often, liothyronine) sufficient to suppress TSH production and reduce the size of the nodule has been widely practised, but results conflict as to whether such therapy is effective,[2,3,8] and there has been some concern about the possible risk of osteoporosis[1,2,4] (see Effects on the Bones, p.1497). An alternative to thyroxine is treatment with potassium iodide, although it is somewhat less effective,[5] and has adverse effects of its own.[4] In a preliminary study alcohol sclerotherapy reduced the size of benign solitary solid nodules apparently without serious side-effects or changes in thyroid function.[6] However, many workers now prefer simply to observe patients with benign solitary nodules.[1,2] Thyroxine suppression therapy is effective in patients with **diffuse** non-toxic goitre, and may be of benefit in some patients with **multinodular** disease.[3] However, many patients with large multinodular goitres have autonomous thyroid hormone production, and in such patients thyroxine is of no benefit and may cause overt hyperthyroidism. Radio-iodine (^{131}I) treatment of multinodular non-toxic goitre has been a useful alternative to surgery in selected cases.[3,7]

1. Mazzaferri EL. Management of a solitary thyroid nodule. *N Engl J Med* 1993; **328:** 553–9.
2. Giuffrida D, Gharib H. Controversies in the management of cold, hot, and occult thyroid nodules. *Am J Med* 1995; **99:** 642–50.
3. Hermus AR, Huysmans DA. Treatment of benign nodular thyroid disease. *N Engl J Med* 1998; **338:** 1438–47.
4. Blum M. Why do clinicians continue to debate the use of levothyroxine in the diagnosis and management of thyroid nodules? *Ann Intern Med* 1995; **122:** 63–4.
5. La Rosa GL, *et al.* Levothyroxine and potassium iodide are both effective in treating benign solitary cold nodules of the thyroid. *Ann Intern Med* 1995; **122:** 1–8.
6. Bennedbaek FN, Hegedüs L. Alcohol sclerotherapy for benign solitary solid cold thyroid nodules. *Lancet* 1995; **346:** 1227.
7. Nygaard B, *et al.* Radio iodine treatment of multinodular non-toxic goitre. *Br Med J* 1993; **307:** 828–32.
8. Gharib H, Mazzaferri EL. Thyroxine suppressive therapy in patients with nodular thyroid disease. *Ann Intern Med* 1998; **128:** 386–94.

Hyperthyroidism

Hyperthyroidism is overactivity of the thyroid gland with consequent excess secretion of hormones. The terms thyrotoxicosis and hyperthyroidism are used interchangeably, although some apply 'thyrotoxicosis' to the *effects* of excessive thyroid hormone whether exogenous or endogenous. The most common causes of hyperthyroidism are Graves' disease and hyperactivity arising from thyroidal nodules (toxic nodular goitre) which may be either single or multiple. Graves' disease (or Basedow's disease) is an auto-immune condition characterised by the presence of thyroid-stimulating antibodies in the plasma which are directed against the thyroid-stimulating hormone (TSH) receptor or a closely associated protein on the thyroid cell. Graves' disease, which is more prevalent in females, frequently occurs in association with other auto-immune diseases such as rheumatoid arthritis and there may be a genetic predisposition. Iodine or its salts, as well as iodine-containing drugs such as amiodarone, can also be a cause of hyperthyroidism as well as hypothyroidism. Subclinical hyperthyroidism is characterised by normal thyroid hormone concentrations, decreased TSH concentrations, but no clinical symptoms. It has been reported to occur less frequently than subclinical hypothyroidism. Thyroid storm, an extreme form of hyperthyroidism, is discussed later.

The major symptoms associated with hyperthyroidism include goitre, nervousness, agitation, tremor, tachycardia or atrial fibrillation, weight loss (often despite increased appetite), emotional lability, muscle weakness, fatigue, heat intolerance and excessive perspiration, and increased bowel frequency. Exaggerated growth may occur in children. Females may occasionally experience amenorrhoea or oligomenorrhoea and males may develop gynaecomastia. Occasionally there is subcutaneous deposition of mucopolysaccharides around the ankles and/or feet.

In Graves' ophthalmopathy, oedematous swelling of the muscles around the eyes produces exophthalmos or proptosis and diplopia. On rare occasions patients may develop papilloedema and loss of vision.

A **diagnosis** of hyperthyroidism may be confirmed by demonstration of a high concentration of free T_4 or T_3 in the circulation. Determination of thyroid-stimulating hormone (TSH) concentration, which is low in hyperthyroidism due to negative feedback, allows differential diagnosis of hyperthyroidism from pituitary tumour and is the test of choice in the elderly as physiological changes and non-thyroidal illness present problems with interpretation of T_4 and T_3 concentrations.

There are three forms of **treatment**: drug therapy, use of radio-iodine, or surgery.

Drug therapy. Initially, many patients are given an antithyroid drug. The thiourea derivatives carbimazole (in the UK) or methimazole (in the USA), or propylthiouracil, are the mainstays of such treatment. Patients usually receive fairly high doses initially until they become euthyroid, generally within 1 to 2 months. Once a response to the antithyroid drug has been obtained, patients with more severe or recurrent disease may require ablative treatment with either radio-iodine or surgery (see below), while those with mild to moderate disease may be best managed with lower maintenance doses of antithyroid drug therapy, either indefinitely, or usually for at least a year, and often for 18 months, followed by observation to see if remission is maintained in the absence of therapy.[1-5] Relapse at some stage following cessation of therapy is fairly common but unpredictable. Addition of thyroxine to the maintenance dose of methimazole has been reported to reduce the rate of relapse in patients with Graves' disease when therapy was subsequently withdrawn.[6,7] However, results conflict as to the real benefit of adding thyroxine to the treatment regimen.[8-10] An alternative maintenance regimen is to add the thyroid hormone while maintaining the high initial doses of antithyroid drug. This 'blocking-replacement therapy' has been suggested to help to prevent hypothyroidism which may be induced when antithyroid drugs are used alone. Because of the high doses of thioureas required the blocking-replacement regimen should not be used in pregnancy.

More rapid relief of the symptoms of hyperthyroidism can be achieved with beta blockers or iodide.[1-3] Beta blockers usually achieve a response within 48 hours, and are given as short-term adjuncts to antithyroid drugs to control severe sympathetic overactivity in patients such as those with thyroid storm (see below), but their use in heart failure associated with thyrotoxicosis is controversial because of the risk of cardiac deterioration.[11] The use of beta blockers in patients with mild to moderate hyperthyroidism is usually unnecessary.

Iodine and iodides are given in conjunction with antithyroid drugs for 7 to 14 days as pre-operative preparation for patients who are to undergo thyroidectomy (but see also under Surgical Therapy, below); a combination of iodide and a beta blocker has also been used. Iodide has been used in conjunction with antithyroid drugs, for control of thyroid storm. It is suggested that the antithyroid drugs should always be given first to prevent incorporation of iodide into new hormone stores.[3]

Other drugs tried in hyperthyroidism have included lithium, though its practical value is a matter of debate.[1,3] Potassium and sodium perchlorate have been used and by increasing responsiveness to conventional antithyroid drugs they may be useful in patients with iodine-induced hyperthyroidism.[1]

In those patients in whom drug therapy fails to achieve long-term remission, ablative therapy may be considered in the form of radio-iodine therapy or surgery.

Radio-iodine therapy. Radio-iodine therapy with ^{131}I as oral ^{131}I-sodium iodide cures hyperthyroidism by destroying the functioning cells of the thyroid gland. It is especially useful for patients who have not responded to antithyroid drug therapy or who have relapsed following it.[2,4,5,12,13] It is also increasingly used as initial therapy.[2,3,12]

Pretreatment of patients with an antithyroid drug for 2 to 8 weeks before radio-iodine therapy has been advocated,[13] to avoid the risk of precipitating thyroid storm. However, many no longer consider this to be necessary for all patients,[2,3,14] although it is generally agreed that the elderly or those with severe disease or increased risk of cardiac symptoms should receive some form of pretreatment. In younger patients, a study has suggested that antithyroid pretreatment may exacerbate the risks when the drugs are withdrawn.[15] Such withdrawal, 2 to 4 days before radio-iodine is given, is standard practice to maximise the latter's effect, although some consider it unnecessary.[3] There is also some evidence that pretreated patients respond less well, and an increased dose of radio-iodine has been advocated in such patients.[14] Pretreatment or ancillary treatment with a beta blocker is a possible alternative to antithyroid drugs in patients receiving radio-iodine.[2,3]

The dose of radio-iodine required to achieve euthyroidism is difficult to predict and there is little agreement on the most appropriate dosage schedule.[2,4,13] Radio-iodine therapy may take up to 10 weeks to achieve a clinical response, and cover with an antithyroid drug may be required during this period. Radio-iodine is not generally considered to increase the risk of malignancy,[2,3,12,13,26] but it is contra-indicated in pregnancy. The commonest unwanted effect of radio-iodine therapy is hypothyroidism and all patients require long-term follow-up and possible thyroxine replacement therapy. Iodide may be given after radio-iodine therapy to help the return of normal thyroid function.[3] Controversy exists as to whether radio-iodine therapy exacerbates Graves' ophthalmopathy.[2,3,16-18]

Surgical therapy. Surgical treatment is usually reserved for patients with severe hyperthyroidism or for those with extreme thyroid enlargement or a single nodule. Euthyroidism is first established using antithyroid drugs and then iodide is given for 7 to 14 days before surgery to reduce the vasculature of the gland. Alternatively, a beta blocker and iodide may be used together for pre-operative preparation. However, a consensus view[19] suggested that pre-operative iodine probably has no beneficial effect. Thyroxine replacement therapy may be required following surgical treatment.

Failure to control symptoms of hyperthyroidism with antithyroid drugs during **pregnancy** may indicate the need for surgery which is most safely performed in the second trimester.[20] Iodide and radio-iodine should not be used during pregnancy.[2,20] **Neonatal hyperthyroidism** may occur rarely due to transfer of thyroid-stimulating immunoglobulins across the placenta, and should be treated with antithyroid drugs, iodide, and appropriate therapy for cardiovascular complications.

There is currently no consensus on whether patients with **subclinical hyperthyroidism** should receive antithyroid treatment.[4,19]

Thyroid storm (also known as thyroid crisis or thyrotoxic crisis) is an extreme accentuation of the hyperthyroid state and should be treated as a medical emergency. It is usually abrupt in onset and is often related to some precipitating factor such as inadequate preparation for thyroidectomy or radio-iodine therapy, or infection in previously unrecognised hyperthyroid subjects. The most common symptoms are hyperpyrexia and extreme tachycardia; others may include arrhythmia, heart failure, shock, agitation, tremor, mania, delirium, stupor, coma, abdominal pain, diarrhoea, vomiting, jaundice, and hepatomegaly. Treatment consists of high-dose antithyroid drugs, gradually reduced as the condition improves, along with a beta blocker and iodide to control cardiovascular symptoms and prevent thyroid hormone release from the thyroid gland. Additional symptomatic treatment may also be required.

The symptoms of **Graves' ophthalmopathy** may not occur in conjunction with signs of systemic hyperthyroidism, and it has been characterised as an independent manifestation of the immunological abnormality in Graves' disease.[21] The treatment of Graves' ophthalmopathy is generally unsatisfactory and signs of disease may persist indefinitely.[22] Opinions differ as to whether controlling associated hyperthyroidism improves ocular symptoms.[21-23] Reports that radio-iodine therapy may exacerbate Graves' ophthalmopathy are disputed,[2,3,16-18] but some workers prefer to avoid its use in active ocular disease.[2,4] Most patients with mild ocular involvement in hyperthyroidism require no specific therapy; artificial tears and a lubricant eye ointment such as yellow soft paraffin at night may relieve irritation. Patients with moderate to severe ophthalmopathy may be treated with high-dose systemic corticosteroids such as oral prednisone or prednisolone or intravenous methylprednisolone, or with orbital radiotherapy, which appears to be equally effective.[24] Other immunosuppressants, particularly cyclosporin, have also been used and have produced equivocal results, although there have been encouraging results from the use of cyclosporin and prednisone in combination.[25] Surgical decompression may be required if patients do not respond to such therapy or cannot tolerate its adverse effects, or if vision is threatened by severe optic nerve compression.

1. Stockigt JR, Topliss DJ. Hyperthyroidism: current drug therapy. *Drugs* 1989; **37:** 375–81.
2. Franklyn JA. The management of hyperthyroidism. *N Engl J Med* 1994; **330:** 1731–8. Correction. *ibid.*; **331:** 559.
3. Klein I, *et al.* Treatment of hyperthyroid disease. *Ann Intern Med* 1994; **121:** 281–8.
4. Gittoes NJL, Franklyn JA. Hyperthyroidism: current treatment guidelines. *Drugs* 1998; **55:** 543–53.
5. Cheetham TD, *et al.* Treatment of hyperthyroidism in young people. *Arch Dis Child* 1998; **78:** 207–9.
6. Hashizume K, *et al.* Administration of thyroxine in treated Graves' disease: effects on the level of antibodies to thyroid-stimulating hormone receptors and on the risk of recurrence of hyperthyroidism. *N Engl J Med* 1991; **324:** 947–53.
7. Ladenson PW. Treatments for Graves' disease: letting the thyroid rest. *N Engl J Med* 1991; **324:** 989–90.
8. Tamai H, *et al.* Lack of effect of thyroxine administration on elevated thyroid stimulating hormone receptor antibody levels in treated Graves' disease patients. *J Clin Endocrinol Metab* 1995; **80:** 1481–4.
9. Hershman JM. Does thyroxine therapy prevent recurrence of Graves' hyperthyroidism? *J Clin Endocrinol Metab* 1995; **80:** 1479–80.
10. McIver B, *et al.* Lack of effect of thyroxine in patients with Graves' hyperthyroidism who are treated with an antithyroid drug. *N Engl J Med* 1996; **334:** 220–4.
11. Ko GTC, *et al.* Should β-blocking agents be used in thyrotoxic heart disease? *Med J Aust* 1995; **162:** 426–7.
12. Franklyn J, Sheppard M. Radioiodine for hyperthyroidism. *Br Med J* 1992; **305:** 727–8.
13. Anonymous. Radioiodine for the treatment of thyroid disease. *Drug Ther Bull* 1993; **31:** 39–40.
14. Cooper DS. Antithyroid drugs and radioiodine therapy: a grain of (iodized) salt. *Ann Intern Med* 1994; **121:** 612–14.
15. Burch HB, *et al.* Discontinuing antithyroid drug therapy before ablation with radioiodine in Graves disease. *Ann Intern Med* 1994; **121:** 553–9.
16. Tallstedt L, *et al.* Occurrence of ophthalmopathy after treatment for Graves' hyperthyroidism. *N Engl J Med* 1992; **326:** 1733–8.
17. Sridama V, DeGroot L. Treatment of Graves' disease and the course of ophthalmopathy. *Am J Med* 1989; **87:** 70–3.
18. Bartalena L, *et al.* Relation between therapy for hyperthyroidism and the course of Graves' ophthalmopathy. *N Engl J Med* 1998; **338:** 73–8.
19. Vanderpump MPJ, *et al.* Consensus statement for good practice and audit measures in the management of hypothyroidism and hyperthyroidism *Br Med J* 1996; **313:** 539–44.
20. Rodin A, Rodin A. Thyroid disease in pregnancy. *Br J Hosp Med* 1989; **41:** 234–42.
21. Larkins R. Treatment of Graves' ophthalmopathy. *Lancet* 1993; **342:** 941.
22. Fleck BW, Toft AD. Graves' ophthalmopathy. *Br Med J* 1990; **300:** 1352–3.
23. Munro D. Thyroid eye disease. *Br Med J* 1993; **306:** 805–6.
24. Prummel MF, *et al.* Randomised double-blind trial of prednisone versus radiotherapy in Graves' ophthalmopathy. *Lancet* 1993; **342:** 949–54.
25. Prummel MF, *et al.* Prednisone and cyclosporine in the treatment of severe Graves' ophthalmopathy. *N Engl J Med* 1989; **321:** 1353–9.
26. Ron E, *et al.* Cancer mortality following treatment for adult hyperthyroidism. *JAMA* 1998; **280:** 347–55.

Hypothyroidism

Hypothyroidism is the clinical syndrome resulting from deficiency of thyroid hormones. The term myxoedema is usually reserved for severe or advanced hypothyroidism associated with deposition of a mucopolysaccharide in subcutaneous tissues with consequent thickening of the skin and nonpitting oedema. Subclinical hypothyroidism is a condition in which there are normal concentrations of thyroid hormones, raised concentrations of thyroid-stimulating hormone (TSH), but no clinical symptoms.

Hypothyroidism is usually primary, resulting from malfunction of the thyroid gland. In areas where iodine intake is sufficient the commonest cause of hypothyroidism is auto-immune lymphocytic thyroiditis of which there are two major variants. In Hashimoto's thyroiditis there is also goitre whereas in idiopathic or primary myxoedema (atrophic thyroiditis) there is no thyroid enlargement. Hypothyroidism can also be caused by either an excess or a deficiency of iodine. An excess may result from intake of iodine or its salts or iodine-containing drugs such as amiodarone. Drugs that decrease thyroid hormone synthesis such as lithium can also be a cause of hypothyroidism. In some patients hypothyroidism may be secondary to disorders of the hypothalamus or pituitary gland.

Hypothyroidism, like hyperthyroidism, predominantly affects women; it is also more prevalent in the middle-aged and elderly. The symptoms of hypothyroidism may be due to general deceleration of metabolism or to accumulation of mucopolysaccharide in the subcutaneous tissues and vocal cords. Common symptoms include weakness, fatigue, lethargy, physical and mental slowness, and weight gain. Menstrual disorders and constipation can occur. Hyperlipidaemia may be seen which may be more atherogenic in secondary than primary hypothyroidism due to lower high-density lipoprotein cholesterol levels. Goitre may occur despite associated cell destruction. Hypothyroid patients commonly exhibit puffy, nonpitted swelling of the subcutaneous tissue, particularly around the eyes. In severely affected patients, progressive somnolence and torpor combine with cold intolerance and bradycardia to induce a state of coma often known as 'myxoedema coma' (see below). In children, untreated hypothyroidism results in retardation of growth and mental development. Endemic cretinism is a result of maternal, and hence fetal, iodine deficiency and consequent lack of thyroid hormone production (see Iodine Deficiency Disorders, p.1494).

The **diagnosis** of hypothyroidism is essentially clinical but, given the non-specific nature of many of the symptoms, biochemical tests are performed for confirmation.[1,2] Protirelin and thyrotrophin have also been used for the differential diagnosis of hypothyroidism. Patients with subclinical hypothyroidism are at a greater risk of developing clinical hypothyroidism if they also have thyroid antibodies against thyroid peroxidase/microsomal antigen although the best strategy for identifying those at risk is not yet known.[2-4]

Hypothyroidism is readily **treated** by lifelong replacement therapy with thyroxine.[1-3,5,6] Although the thyroid gland produces both T_3 (liothyronine) and T_4 (thyroxine), T_3 is mainly produced by peripheral monodeiodination of circulating T_4 and it is therefore sufficient to administer thyroxine alone. There is no rationale for the administration of combined preparations containing liothyronine and thyroxine, or of dried thyroid hormone extracts, which may lead to elevated serum concentrations of T_3 and thyrotoxic symptoms. Liothyronine may, however, be used initially for its rapid onset of action in severe hypothyroid states such as myxoedema coma (see below). There is a need to check that thyroid replacement treatment is restoring deficiencies in thyroid hormone, but is not providing an excess. While most workers accept that this is best done by monitoring hormone concentrations, there has been considerable debate as to whether T_3, T_4, TSH, or a combination of these should be measured, and whether the free or the total hormone concentrations should be used. Extremely sensitive assays for TSH have been developed and the goal of replacement therapy has been advocated as a normal TSH value together with a normal free T_4 value.[7]

In **subclinical hypothyroidism**, treatment with thyroxine is recommended[2-4] if thyroid peroxidase antibodies are present or if TSH levels are above 10 milliunits per litre.

It has generally been believed that during **pregnancy** hypothyroid women do not require any modification to their thyroxine maintenance therapy, although they experience an oestrogen-stimulated increase in serum concentrations of thyroxine-binding globulin.[8,9] However, some studies have indicated that thyroxine requirements may be increased[10,11] and it is now recommended that serum TSH be checked in each trimester and the thyroxine dose adjusted if necessary.[1-3,5]

The diagnosis of **congenital hypothyroidism** (neonatal hypothyroidism) is now most commonly made on the basis of screening programmes.[12] Early treatment with adequate doses of thyroxine is required to minimise the effects of hypothyroidism on mental and physical development. Although some studies have reported complete normalisation of IQ, other studies,[13] and clinical experience,[5,14] suggest that in those with more severe hypothyroidism at diagnosis some small degree of deficit and incoordination remains, although they should be mild enough to permit a normal life. One study reported that commencing treatment at 14 days of age with a relatively high initial dose of thyroxine eliminated the developmental gap in severe congenital hypothyroidism.[15] Others warned that doses above 10 µg per kg body-weight daily may be linked to behaviour problems, such as anxiety, later in childhood.[16]

Myxoedema coma (hypothyroid coma) is a medical emergency requiring prompt treatment usually with liothyronine given by intravenous injection because of its rapid action, although some centres use intravenous thyroxine. Alternatively, the nasogastric route may be employed. In some patients, liothyronine given intravenously is followed by oral thyroxine. Other treatment includes intravenous hydrocortisone (because of the likelihood of adrenocortical insufficiency) and intravenous fluids (to maintain plasma-glucose and electrolyte concentrations). Respiratory function should be supported by assisted ventilation and oxygen administration.

1. Singer PA, *et al.* Treatment guidelines for patients with hyperthyroidism and hypothyroidism. *JAMA* 1995; **273:** 808–12.
2. Lindsay RS, Toft AD. Hypothyroidism. *Lancet* 1997; **349:** 413–17. Correction. *ibid.*; 1023.
3. Vanderpump MPJ, *et al.* Consensus statement for good practice and audit measures in the management of hypothyroidism and hyperthyroidism. *Br Med J* 1996; **313:** 539–44.
4. Weetman AP. Hypothyroidism: screening and subclinical disease. *Br Med J* 1997; **314:** 1175–78.
5. Toft AD. Thyroxine therapy. *N Engl J Med* 1994; **331:** 174–80.
6. Mandel SJ, *et al.* Levothyroxine therapy in patients with thyroid disease. *Ann Intern Med* 1993; **119:** 492–502.
7. Surks MI, *et al.* American Thyroid Association guidelines for use of laboratory tests in thyroid disorders. *JAMA* 1990; **263:** 1529–32.
8. Burr W. Thyroid disease. *Clin Obstet Gynecol* 1986; **13:** 277–90.
9. Hague WM. Treatment of endocrine diseases. *Br Med J* 1987; **294:** 297–300.
10. Mandel SJ, *et al.* Increased need for thyroxine during pregnancy in women with primary hypothyroidism. *N Engl J Med* 1990; **323:** 91–6.
11. Tamaki H, *et al.* Thyroxine requirement during pregnancy for replacement therapy of hypothyroidism. *Obstet Gynecol* 1990; **76:** 230–3.
12. American Academy of Pediatrics/American Thyroid Association. Newborn screening for congenital hypothyroidism: recommended guidelines. *Pediatrics* 1993; **91:** 1203–9.
13. Tillotson SL, *et al.* Relation between biochemical severity and intelligence in early treated congenital hypothyroidism: a threshold effect. *Br Med J* 1994; **309:** 440–5.
14. Grant DB. Congenital hypothyroidism: optimal management in the light of 15 years' experience of screening. *Arch Dis Child* 1995; **72:** 85–9.
15. Dubuis J-M, *et al.* Outcome of severe congenital hypothyroidism: closing the developmental gap with early high dose levothyroxine treatment. *J Clin Endocrinol Metab* 1996; **81:** 222–7.
16. Rovet JF, Ehrlich RM. Long-term effects of L-thyroxine therapy for congenital hypothyroidism. *J Pediatr* 1995; **126:** 380–6.

Benzylthiouracil (832-p)

6-Benzyl-2,3-dihydro-2-thioxopyrimidin-4(1*H*)-one; 6-Benzyl-2-mercaptopyrimidin-4-ol; 6-Benzyl-2-thiouracil.

$C_{11}H_{10}N_2OS$ = 218.3.

CAS — 33086-27-0; 6336-50-1.

Benzylthiouracil is a thiourea antithyroid drug. It is given by mouth in the treatment of hyperthyroidism (p.1489) in an initial dose of 150 to 200 mg daily, reducing to a maintenance dose of 100 mg daily after several weeks.

Preparations

Proprietary Preparations (details are given in Part 3)
Fr.: Basdene.

Carbimazole (831-q)

Carbimazole (*BAN, rINN*).

Carbimazolum. Ethyl 3-methyl-2-thioxo-4-imidazoline-1-carboxylate.

$C_7H_{10}N_2O_2S$ = 186.2.

CAS — 22232-54-8.

Pharmacopoeias. In *Chin.* and *Eur.* (see p.viii).

A white or yellowish-white crystalline powder. Slightly **soluble** in water; soluble in acetone and in alcohol.

Adverse Effects and Precautions

Adverse effects from carbimazole and other thiourea antithyroid drugs occur most frequently during the first 8 weeks of treatment. The most common minor adverse effects are nausea and vomiting, gastric discomfort, headache, arthralgia, skin rashes, and pruritus. Abnormal hair loss has also been reported.

Bone-marrow depression may occur and mild leucopenia is common. In severe cases agranulocytosis can develop and this is the most serious adverse reaction associated with this class of drugs. Patients or their carers should be told how to recognise such toxicity and should be advised to seek immediate medical attention if mouth ulcers or sore throat, fever, bruising, malaise, or non-specific illness develop; treatment should be discontinued immediately if there is any clinical or laboratory evidence of neutropenia. Aplastic anaemia has been reported rarely, as has hypoprothrombinaemia.

There have been several reports of liver damage in patients taking thiourea antithyroid drugs.

Other adverse effects sometimes observed with the thiourea antithyroid compounds include fever, a lupus-like syndrome, vasculitis and nephritis, and taste disturbances.

Excessive doses of antithyroid drugs may cause hypothyroidism and goitre. High doses in pregnancy may result in fetal hypothyroidism and goitre (see Pregnancy and Breast Feeding, below).

An immune mechanism has been implicated in many of these reactions and cross-sensitivity between the thiourea antithyroid drugs may occur.

Effects on the blood. While leucopenia is considered to be a common adverse effect of the thiourea antithyroid drugs, occurring in up to a quarter of patients, it is usually mild and improves as treatment continues.[1,2]

The incidence of agranulocytosis, a more serious hazard, is usually reported to be between 0.1 and 1.0%,[1,3-5] but may be much lower.[6] Fatalities have been reported;[3,7,8] the Committee on Safety of Medicines in the UK was aware of 62 cases of agranulocytosis and 44 reports of neutropenia with antithyroid drugs at January 1993, of which 16 and 2 respectively were fatal.[8] The onset of agranulocytosis is usually rapid and monitoring of the white cell count is not always of predictive value.[1,9] Agranulocytosis has occurred in patients receiving propylthiouracil for a second time who had no such complications in their first course of therapy.[10] A dose-dependent effect has been suggested for methimazole though not propylthiouracil.[4] While agranulocytosis has occurred with doses of methimazole less than 30 mg daily,[11,12] the likelihood of this adverse effect occurring may be reduced with doses below 30 mg daily. An age-dependent effect has also been suggested for the thiourea drugs;[4] the risk of developing agranulocytosis is possibly reduced in patients under 40 years.[4,5] Although a direct toxic effect had been suggested, the agranulocytosis associated with the thiourea drugs is now generally considered to be immunologically mediated.[1,4-6]

There have been some case reports of aplastic anaemia being produced by antithyroid drugs, but the excess risk associated with their use is considered to be very low[6,13,14] and complete recovery has been reported following withdrawal of the antithyroid drug. An immune mechanism has been implicated.

Carbimazole has produced haemolytic anaemia.[15] In this case the immune reaction was specific to carbimazole and could not be demonstrated with methimazole.

On very rare occasions patients taking propylthiouracil have experienced a reduction in prothrombin values and bleeding.[16-18] In one patient bleeding was linked to propylthiouracil-induced thrombocytopenia.[19]

1. Cooper DS. Antithyroid drugs. *N Engl J Med* 1984; **311:** 1353–62.
2. Amrhein JA, *et al.* Granulocytopenia, lupus-like syndrome, and other complications of propylthiouracil therapy. *J Pediatr* 1970; **76:** 54–63.
3. Reidy TJ, *et al.* Propylthiouracil-induced vasculitis: a fatal case. *South Med J* 1982; **75:** 1297–8.
4. Cooper DS, *et al.* Agranulocytosis associated with antithyroid drugs. *Ann Intern Med* 1983; **98:** 26–9.
5. Guffy MM, *et al.* Granulocytotoxic antibodies in a patient with propylthiouracil-induced agranulocytosis. *Arch Intern Med* 1984; **144:** 1687–8.
6. International Agranulocytosis and Aplastic Anaemia Study. Risk of agranulocytosis and aplastic anaemia in relation to use of antithyroid drugs. *Br Med J* 1988; **297:** 262–5.
7. Böttiger LE, *et al.* Drug-induced blood dyscrasias. *Acta Med Scand* 1979; **205:** 457–61.
8. Committee on Safety of Medicines/Medicines Control Agency. Drug-induced neutropenia and agranulocytosis. *Current Problems* 1993; **19:** 10–11.
9. Tajiri J, *et al.* Antithyroid drug-induced agranulocytosis: the usefulness of routine white blood cell count monitoring. *Arch Intern Med* 1990; **150:** 621–4.
10. Shiran A, *et al.* Propylthiouracil-induced agranulocytosis in four patients previously treated with the drug. *JAMA* 1991; **266:** 3129–30.
11. Cooper DS, *et al.* Agranulocytosis and dose of methimazole. *Ann Intern Med* 1984; **101:** 283.
12. Fincher ME, *et al.* Agranulocytosis and a small dose of methimazole. *Ann Intern Med* 1984; **101:** 404–5.
13. Aksoy M, Erdem S. Aplastic anaemia after propylthiouracil. *Lancet* 1968; **i:** 1379.
14. Bishara J. Methimazole-induced aplastic anemia. *Ann Pharmacother* 1996; **30:** 684.
15. Salama A, *et al.* Carbimazole-induced immune haemolytic anaemia: role of drug-red blood cell complexes for immunization. *Br J Haematol* 1988; **68:** 479–82.
16. D'Angelo G, Le Gresley LP. Severe hypoprothrombinaemia after propylthiouracil therapy. *Can Med Assoc J* 1959; **81:** 479–81.
17. Naeye RL, Terrien CM. Hemorrhagic state after therapy with propylthiouracil. *Am J Clin Pathol* 1960; **34:** 254–7.
18. Gotta AW, *et al.* Prolonged intraoperative bleeding caused by propylthiouracil-induced hypoprothrombinemia. *Anesthesiology* 1972; **37:** 562–3.
19. Ikeda S, Schweiss JF. Excessive blood loss during operation in the patient treated with propylthiouracil. *Can Anaesth Soc J* 1982; **29:** 477–80.

Effects on the ears. Earache, high-frequency hearing loss, and tinnitus in a patient with Graves' disease were considered to be associated with hypersensitivity to carbimazole therapy;[1] hearing loss, but not the tinnitus, resolved when carbimazole was replaced with propylthiouracil.

1. Hill D, *et al.* Hearing loss and tinnitus with carbimazole *Br Med J* 1994; **309:** 929.

Effects on the kidneys. Nephritis associated with vasculitis has occurred in some patients taking thiourea antithyroid drugs.[1,2] An immune mechanism has been proposed. There has also been the rare report of acute glomerulonephritis[3,4] or the nephrotic syndrome.[5]

1. Griswold WR, *et al.* Vasculitis associated with propylthiouracil. *West J Med* 1978; **128:** 543–6.
2. Cassorla FG, *et al.* Vasculitis, pulmonary cavitation, and anemia during antithyroid drug therapy. *Am J Dis Child* 1983; **137:** 118–22.

3. Amrhein JA, *et al.* Granulocytopenia, lupus-like syndrome, and other complications of propylthiouracil therapy. *J Pediatr* 1970; **76:** 54–63.
4. Vogt BA, *et al.* Antineutrophil cytoplasmic autoantibody-positive crescentic glomerulonephritis as a complication of treatment with propylthiouracil in children. *J Pediatr* 1994; **124:** 986–8.
5. Reynolds LR, Bhathena D. Nephrotic syndrome associated with methimazole therapy. *Arch Intern Med* 1979; **139:** 236–7.

Effects on the liver. Jaundice, usually cholestatic has been reported with methimazole and carbimazole.[1-6] An immune-mediated mechanism rather than a toxic reaction has been proposed. Hepatitis (sometimes progressing to cirrhosis[7]) and hepatic necrosis have been associated with propylthiouracil,[7-13] sometimes with fatal consequences.[10,11,13] However, in one study[14] almost 30% of patients being treated with propylthiouracil developed asymptomatic liver changes (increased alanine aminotransferase values) that were mostly reversible as treatment continued at a reduced dose.

Despite reports of liver damage, propylthiouracil has been investigated in the treatment of patients with alcoholic liver disease (see p.1496).

The elimination half-life of methimazole and of propylthiouracil may be prolonged in patients with liver damage.[15,16]

1. Becker CE, *et al.* Hepatitis from methimazole during adrenal steroid therapy for malignant exophthalmos. *JAMA* 1968; **206:** 1787–9.
2. Fischer MG, *et al.* Methimazole-induced jaundice. *JAMA* 1973; **223:** 1028–9.
3. Dinsmore WW, *et al.* Postanesthetic carbimazole jaundice. *N Engl J Med* 1983; **309:** 438.
4. Wheeler DC, *et al.* Carbimazole-induced jaundice. *J R Soc Med* 1985; **78:** 75–6.
5. Blom H, *et al.* A case of carbimazole-induced intrahepatic cholestasis. *Arch Intern Med* 1985; **145:** 1513–15.
6. Schmidt G, *et al.* Methimazole-associated cholestatic liver injury: case report and brief literature review. *Hepatogastroenterology* 1986; **33:** 244–6.
7. Özemirler S, *et al.* Propylthiouracil-induced hepatic damage. *Ann Pharmacother* 1996; **30:** 960–3.
8. Amrhein JA, *et al.* Granulocytopenia, lupus-like syndrome, and other complications of propylthiouracil therapy. *J Pediatr* 1970; **76:** 54–63.
9. Parker LN. Hepatitis and propylthiouracil. *Ann Intern Med* 1975; **82:** 228–9.
10. Safani MM, *et al.* Fatal propylthiouracil-induced hepatitis. *Arch Intern Med* 1982; **142:** 838–9.
11. Hanson JS. Propylthiouracil and hepatitis. Two cases and a review of the literature. *Arch Intern Med* 1984; **144:** 994–6.
12. Mihas AA, *et al.* Fulminant hepatitis and lymphocyte sensitization due to propylthiouracil. *Gastroenterology* 1976; **70:** 770–4.
13. Limaye A, Ruffolo PR. Propylthiouracil-induced fatal hepatic necrosis. *Am J Gastroenterol* 1987; **82:** 152–4.
14. Liaw Y-F, *et al.* Hepatic injury during propylthiouracil therapy in patients with hyperthyroidism. *Ann Intern Med* 1993; **118:** 424–8.
15. Kampmann JP, Hansen JM. Clinical pharmacokinetics of antithyroid drugs. *Clin Pharmacokinet* 1981; **6:** 401–28.
16. Cooper DS, *et al.* Methimazole pharmacology in man: studies using a newly developed radioimmunoassay for methimazole. *J Clin Endocrinol Metab* 1984; **58:** 473–9.

Effects on the lungs. A report of a diffuse interstitial pneumonitis in 2 patients who had received propylthiouracil.[1] A hypersensitivity reaction to propylthiouracil was suggested.

1. Miyazono K, *et al.* Propylthiouracil-induced diffuse interstitial pneumonitis. *Arch Intern Med* 1984; **144:** 1764–5.

Effects on the muscles. Myositis with pain, weakness, and increased creatine kinase concentrations has been reported with carbimazole.[1,2] This effect might be explained by 'tissue hypothyroidism', and might respond to dosage reduction.[3]

1. Page SR, Nussey SS. Myositis in association with carbimazole therapy. *Lancet* 1989; **i:** 964.
2. Pasquier E, *et al.* Biopsy-proven myositis with microvasculitis in association with carbimazole. *Lancet* 1991; **338:** 1082–3.
3. O'Malley B. Carbimazole-induced cramps. *Lancet* 1989; **i:** 1456.

Hypersensitivity. Many of the adverse effects associated with the thiourea antithyroid drugs, such as those involving the blood, kidneys, or liver, appear to have an immune basis.

There have been rare reports of allergic cutaneous vasculitis. It may be a severe multisystem condition and a fatal case of cutaneous vasculitis with agranulocytosis has been reported.[1] Anaemia, arthralgia, arthritis, nephritis, and thrombocytopenia are some of the other adverse effects associated with thiourea antithyroid drugs considered to have an immune basis; they may sometimes be associated with cutaneous vasculitis.[2-9] A lupus-like syndrome may also be associated very rarely with thiourea antithyroid drugs. Anaemia, arthralgia, arthritis, cutaneous vasculitis, fever, leucopenia, liver impairment, renal impairment, and positive tests for antinuclear factor and lupus erythematosus cells have been associated with the syndrome.[2,10,11] Serum sickness with arthralgias and raised immunoglobulin M (IgM) concentrations has been reported with methimazole[12] and the production of antibodies to insulin resulting in episodes of hypoglycaemia has been associated with methimazole[13] and carbimazole.[14]

The thiourea antithyroid drugs all contain a thioamide group and cross-sensitivity between them might be expected. In cases of drug reactions to methimazole, complete cross-reactivity may be expected with carbimazole since its antithyroid activity is attributable to its *in-vivo* conversion to methimazole. Cross-sensitivity between propylthiouracil and carbimazole[15] or methimazole[1,2,16] has been reported but the incidence and clinical importance is not clear. Although it has been suggested that carbimazole or methimazole may be substituted for propylthiouracil in hypersensitive patients, it is safer to discontinue antithyroid drugs in such patients.[3,15]

1. Reidy TJ, *et al.* Propylthiouracil-induced vasculitis: a fatal case. *South Med J* 1982; **75:** 1297–8.
2. Amrhein JA, *et al.* Granulocytopenia, lupus-like syndrome, and other complications of propylthiouracil therapy. *J Pediatr* 1970; **76:** 54–63.
3. Griswold WR, *et al.* Vasculitis associated with propylthiouracil. *West J Med* 1978; **128:** 543–6.
4. Vasily DB, Tyler WB. Propylthiouracil-induced cutaneous vasculitis: case presentation and review of the literature. *JAMA* 1980; **243:** 458–61.
5. Gammeltoft M, Kristensen JK. Propylthio-uracil-induced cutaneous vasculitis. *Acta Derm Venereol (Stockh)* 1982; **62:** 171–3.
6. Cassorla FG, *et al.* Vasculitis, pulmonary cavitation, and anemia during antithyroid drug therapy. *Am J Dis Child* 1983; **137:** 118–22.
7. Shabtai R, *et al.* The antithyroid arthritis syndrome reviewed. *Arthritis Rheum* 1984; **27:** 227–9.
8. Wing SS, Fantus IG. Adverse immunologic effects of antithyroid drugs. *Can Med Assoc J* 1987; **136:** 121–7.
9. Dolman KM, *et al.* Vasculitis and antineutrophil cytoplasmic autoantibodies associated with propylthiouracil therapy. *Lancet* 1993; **342:** 651–2.
10. Oh BK, *et al.* Polyarthritis induced by propylthiouracil. *Br J Rheumatol* 1983; **22:** 106–8.
11. Horton RC, *et al.* Propylthiouracil-induced systemic lupus erythematosus. *Lancet* 1989; **ii:** 568.
12. Van Kuyk M, *et al.* Methimazole-induced serum sickness. *Acta Clin Belg* 1983; **38:** 68–9.
13. Hirata Y. Methimazole and insulin autoimmune syndrome with hypoglycaemia. *Lancet* 1983; **ii:** 1037–8.
14. Burden AC, Rosenthal FD. Methimazole and insulin autoimmune syndrome. *Lancet* 1983; **ii:** 1311.
15. Smith A, *et al.* Cross sensitivity to antithyroid drugs. *Br Med J* 1989; **298:** 1253.
16. De Weweire A, *et al.* Failure to control hyperthyroidism with a thionamide after potassium perchlorate withdrawal in a patient with amiodarone associated thyrotoxicosis. *J Endocrinol Invest* 1987; **10:** 529.

Pregnancy and breast feeding. Thiourea antithyroid drugs have been used successfully in pregnancy (see Hyperthyroidism, p.1489).

Methimazole (the metabolite of carbimazole) has been the antithyroid drug most frequently involved in the few reports of **congenital defects** following maternal use of such compounds. Several infants exposed to methimazole *in utero* have been born with scalp defects (aplasia cutis congenita—a localised absence of skin at birth)[1,2] although hyperthyroidism itself may give rise to such defects.[3] Individual case reports of other congenital defects associated with methimazole have included choanal atresia (an upper respiratory-tract defect), oesophageal atresia, and tracheo-oesophageal fistula[3] but the incidence of congenital abnormalities is not increased compared with the general population.[4] There have been some reports of neonates exposed to thiourea antithyroid drugs *in utero* displaying signs of **hypothyroidism** including goitre.[5-7]

The safety of **breast feeding** during maternal treatment depends partly on how much drug is distributed into the breast milk. Thiourea antithyroid drugs may be used with care in breast-feeding mothers; neonatal development and thyroid function of the infant should be closely monitored and the lowest effective dose used. Propylthiouracil has been preferred to carbimazole or methimazole since it enters breast milk less readily.[8,9] The infant's intake of methimazole following administration of carbimazole [or methimazole] might be greatly reduced by discarding the breast milk produced 2 to 4 hours after a dose,[10] since the highest concentration was found at this time. One study found no adverse effects on thyroid function or thyroid hormone levels in breast-fed infants during up to 6 months of maternal treatment with methimazole.[11]

1. Milham S. Scalp defects in infants of mothers treated for hyperthyroidism with methimazole or carbimazole during pregnancy. *Teratology* 1985; **32:** 321.
2. Vogt T, *et al.* Aplasia cutis congenita after exposure to methimazole: a causal relationship? *Br J Dermatol* 1995; **133:** 994–6.
3. Johnsson E, *et al.* Severe malformations in infant born to hyperthyroid woman on methimazole. *Lancet* 1997; **350:** 1520.
4. Wing DA, *et al.* A comparison of propylthiouracil versus methimazole in the treatment of hyperthyroidism in pregnancy. *Am J Obstet Gynecol* 1994; **170:** 90–5.
5. Refetoff S, *et al.* Neonatal hypothyroidism and goiter in one infant of each of two sets of twins due to maternal therapy with antithyroid drugs. *J Pediatr* 1974; **85:** 240–4.
6. Mujtaba Q, Burrow GN. Treatment of hyperthyroidism in pregnancy with propylthiouracil and methimazole. *Obstet Gynecol* 1975; **46:** 282–6.
7. Sugrue D. Drury MI. Hyperthyroidism complicating pregnancy: results of treatment by antithyroid drugs in 77 pregnancies. *Br J Obstet Gynaecol* 1980; **87:** 970–5.
8. Kampmann JP, *et al.* Propylthiouracil in human milk: revision of a dogma. *Lancet* 1980; **i:** 736–8.
9. Johansen K, *et al.* Excretion of methimazole in human milk. *Eur J Clin Pharmacol* 1982; **23:** 339–41.
10. Rylance GW, *et al.* Carbimazole and breastfeeding. *Lancet* 1987; **i:** 928.
11. Azizi F. Effect of methimazole treatment of maternal thyrotoxicosis on thyroid function in breast-feeding infants. *J Pediatr* 1996; **128:** 855–8.

Pharmacokinetics

The pharmacokinetics of carbimazole and methimazole can be considered together since carbimazole is rapidly and completely metabolised to methimazole in the body. The antithyroid activity of carbimazole is dependent upon this conversion to methimazole.

Carbimazole and other thiourea antithyroid drugs are rapidly absorbed from the gastro-intestinal tract with peak plasma concentrations occurring about 1 to 2 hours following administration by mouth.

They are concentrated in the thyroid gland and, since their duration of action is more closely related to the intrathyroidal drug concentration than their plasma half-life, this results in a prolongation of antithyroid activity such that single daily doses are possible. Methimazole is not bound to plasma proteins.

Methimazole has an elimination half-life from plasma of about 3 to 6 hours and is metabolised, probably by the liver, and excreted in the urine. Less than 12% of a dose of methimazole may be excreted as unchanged drug. 3-Methyl-2-thiohydantoin has been identified as a metabolite of methimazole. The elimination half-life may be increased in hepatic and renal impairment.

Methimazole crosses the placenta and is distributed into breast milk.

References to the pharmacokinetics of carbimazole and methimazole.

1. Skellern GG, *et al.* The pharmacokinetics of methimazole after oral administration of carbimazole and methimazole, in hyperthyroid patients. *Br J Clin Pharmacol* 1980; **9:** 137–43.
2. Kampmann JP, Hansen JM. Clinical pharmacokinetics of antithyroid drugs. *Clin Pharmacokinet* 1981; **6:** 401–28.
3. Jansson R, *et al.* Intrathyroidal concentrations of methimazole in patients with Graves' disease. *J Clin Endocrinol Metab* 1983; **57:** 129–32.
4. Cooper DS, *et al.* Methimazole pharmacology in man: studies using a newly developed radioimmunoassay for methimazole. *J Clin Endocrinol Metab* 1984; **58:** 473–9.
5. Jansson R, *et al.* Pharmacokinetic properties and bioavailability of methimazole. *Clin Pharmacokinet* 1985; **10:** 443–50.

Uses and Administration

Carbimazole is a thiourea antithyroid drug that acts by blocking the production of thyroid hormones (see p.1489). It is used in the management of hyperthyroidism (p.1489), including the treatment of Graves' disease, the preparation of hyperthyroid patients for thyroidectomy, use as an adjunct to radio-iodine therapy, and the treatment of thyroid storm.

Carbimazole is completely metabolised to methimazole and it is this metabolite that is responsible for the clinical antithyroid activity of carbimazole.

Carbimazole is given by mouth usually in an initial dosage of 20 to 60 mg daily. It has often been given in divided daily doses but once daily administration is also possible. Improvement is usually seen in 1 to 3 weeks and control of symptoms is achieved in 1 to 2 months. When the patient is euthyroid the dose is gradually reduced to the smallest amount that will maintain the euthyroid state. Typical maintenance doses are 5 to 15 mg daily. Alternatively, the dose may be continued at the initial level in combination with supplemental thyroxine as a blocking-replacement regimen. Either form of maintenance treatment is usually continued for at least a year, and often for 18 months. A suggested initial dose for children is 15 mg daily.

Action. There is evidence to suggest that thiourea antithyroid drugs suppress the immune response. However, it is not clear whether this immunosuppressive effect contributes to their antithyroid action or has any clinical significance in the treatment of auto-immune thyroid disorders.[1-5] Increasing the daily dose of methimazole with the aim of immunosuppression was of no benefit in a large study of patients with Graves' disease.[6]

A number of the adverse effects of the thiourea drugs are considered to have an immune basis (see under Adverse Effects, above).

1. Kendall-Taylor P. Are antithyroid drugs immunosuppressive? *Br Med J* 1984; **288:** 509–11.
2. Ludgate ME, *et al.* Analysis of T cell subsets in Graves' disease: alterations associated with carbimazole. *Br Med J* 1984; **288:** 526–30.

3. Jansson R, *et al.* Thyroxine, methimazole, and thyroid microsomal autoantibody titres in hypothyroid Hashimoto's thyroiditis. *Br Med J* 1985; **290:** 11–12.
4. Tötterman TH, *et al.* Induction of circulating activated suppressor-like T cells by methimazole therapy for Graves' disease. *N Engl J Med* 1987; **316:** 15–22.
5. Volpé R. Immunoregulation in autoimmune thyroid disease. *N Engl J Med* 1987; **316:** 44–6.
6. Reinwein D, *et al.* A prospective randomised trial of antithyroid drug dose in Graves' disease therapy. *J Clin Endocrinol Metab* 1993; **76:** 1516–21.

Preparations

BP 1998: Carbimazole Tablets.

Proprietary Preparations (details are given in Part 3)
Austral.: Neo-Mercazole; ***Fr.:*** Neo-Mercazole; ***Ger.:*** neo-morphazole†; Neo-Thyreostat; ***Irl.:*** Neo-Mercazole; ***Norw.:*** Neo-Mercazole; ***S.Afr.:*** Neo-Mercazole; ***Spain:*** Neo Tomizol; ***Swed.:*** Neo-Mercazole†; ***Switz.:*** Neo-Mercazole; ***UK:*** Neo-Mercazole.

Dibromotyrosine (12643-l)

3,5-Dibromo-L-tyrosine.
$C_9H_9Br_2NO_3$ = 339.0.
CAS — 300-38-9.

Dibromotyrosine is an antithyroid drug used in the treatment of hyperthyroidism.

Preparations

Proprietary Preparations (details are given in Part 3)
Ital.: Bromotiren.

Multi-ingredient: ***Ital.:*** Bromazolo; Sirenitas†.

Diiodotyrosine (9005-f)

Diotyrosine; Iodogorgoic Acid. 3,5-Di-iodo-L-tyrosine dihydrate.
$C_9H_9I_2NO_3,2H_2O$ = 469.0.
CAS — 66-02-4 (anhydrous); 300-39-0 (L, anhydrous).
Pharmacopoeias. In *Aust.*

Diiodotyrosine is an antithyroid drug. It is given by mouth for the treatment of hyperthyroidism and iodine deficiency disorders.

Preparations

Proprietary Preparations (details are given in Part 3)
Ger.: Strumedical 400.

Multi-ingredient: ***Spain:*** Endofren†; Neo Endofren†; Normosedin†.

Fluorotyrosine (19714-r)

Fluorotyrosinum; Fluortyrosine. 3-Fluorotyrosine.
$C_9H_{10}FNO_3$ = 199.2.
CAS — 139-26-4.

Fluorotyrosine is an antithyroid drug used in the treatment of hyperthyroidism.

Preparations

Proprietary Preparations (details are given in Part 3)
Aust.: Fluorthyrin.

Iodine (4571-l)

Iode; Iodum; Jodum; Yodo.
I_2 = 253.80894.
CAS — 7553-56-2.
Pharmacopoeias. In *Chin.*, *Eur.* (see p.viii), *Int.*, *Jpn*, *Pol.*, and *US.*

Greyish-violet or greyish-black brittle plates or small crystals, with a metallic sheen and a distinctive penetrating irritant odour. It is slowly volatile at room temperature.

Soluble 1 in 3000 of water, 1 in 13 of alcohol, 1 in 80 of glycerol, and 1 in 4 of carbon disulphide; freely soluble in chloroform and in ether; soluble in solutions of iodides. With acetone iodine forms a pungent irritating compound. **Store** in airtight ground-glass-stoppered containers.

Potassium Iodide (4579-x)

Iodeto de Potássio; Kalii Iodetum; Kalii Iodidum; Kalii Jodidum; Kalium Iodatum; Kalium Jodatum; Pot. Iod.; Potassii Iodidum; Potassium (Iodure de).
KI = 166.0.
CAS — 7681-11-0.
Pharmacopoeias. In *Chin.*, *Eur.* (see p.viii), *Int.*, *Jpn*, *Pol.*, and *US.*

Odourless, colourless, transparent or somewhat opaque crystals or white granular powder. It is slightly hygroscopic. Each g represents 6 mmol of potassium and of iodide.

Soluble 1 in 0.7 of water and 1 in 0.5 of boiling water, 1 in 22 of alcohol, and 1 in 2 of glycerol. Solutions in water are neutral or alkaline to litmus. **Protect** from light.

Sodium Iodide (4581-j)

Iodeto de Sódio; Natrii Iodetum; Natrii Iodidum; Natrii Jodidum; Natrium Iodatum; Sod. Iod.; Sodii Iodidum; Sodium (Iodure de).
NaI = 149.9.
CAS — 7681-82-5.
Pharmacopoeias. In *Chin.*, *Eur.* (see p.viii), *Jpn*, *Pol.*, and *US.*

Colourless crystals or white odourless crystalline powder. It is deliquescent in moist air and develops a brown tint upon decomposition. **Soluble** 1 in 0.6 of water, 1 in 2 of alcohol, and 1 in 1 of glycerol.

Store in airtight containers. Protect from light.

Adverse Effects and Treatment

Iodine and iodides, whether applied topically or administered systemically, can give rise to hypersensitivity reactions which may include urticaria, angioedema, cutaneous haemorrhage or purpuras, fever, arthralgia, lymphadenopathy, and eosinophilia.

Iodine and iodides have variable effects on the thyroid (see below) and can produce goitre and hypothyroidism as well as hyperthyroidism (the Iod-Basedow or Jod-Basedow phenomenon). Goitre and hypothyroidism have also occurred in infants born to mothers who had taken iodides during pregnancy.

Prolonged administration may lead to a range of adverse effects, often called 'iodism' although some of the effects could be considered to be due to hypersensitivity. These include adverse effects on the mouth such as metallic taste, increased salivation, burning or pain; there may be acute rhinitis and swelling and inflammation of the throat. Eyes may be irritated and swollen and there may be increased lachrymation. Pulmonary oedema and bronchitis may develop. Skin reactions include acneform or, more rarely, severe eruptions (ioderma). Other reported effects include depression, insomnia, impotence, headache, and gastro-intestinal disturbances, notably diarrhoea (which may be bloody).

Inhalation of iodine vapour is very irritating to mucous membranes.

The symptoms of acute poisoning from ingestion of iodine are mainly due to its corrosive effects on the gastro-intestinal tract; a disagreeable metallic taste, vomiting, abdominal pain, and diarrhoea occur. Renal failure and anuria may occur 1 to 3 days later; death may be due to circulatory failure, oedema of the epiglottis resulting in asphyxia, aspiration pneumonia, or pulmonary oedema. Oesophageal stricture may occur if the patient survives the acute stage.

Victims of acute poisoning have been given copious draughts of milk or starch mucilage; lavage may be attempted if there is no oesophageal damage. Other treatments include activated charcoal and sodium thiosulphate solution 1% or 5% to reduce iodine to the less toxic iodides.

Effects on the thyroid. While the thyroid is dependent on iodine for the production of thyroid hormones, an excess of iodine can lead to goitre and hypothyroidism (more usually seen in iodine deficiency) as well as to hyperthyroidism.

The normal daily requirement ranges from 100 to 300 µg. Quantities of 500 µg to 1 mg daily probably have no untoward effects on thyroid function in most cases. When progressively larger doses are given there is an initial rise in thyroid hormone production, but at still higher doses, production decreases (the Wolff-Chaikoff effect). This effect is usually seen with doses of more than about 2 mg daily, but is normally transient, adaptation occurring on repeated administration. In certain individuals a lack of adaptation produces a chronic inhibition of thyroid hormone synthesis leading to goitre and **hypothyroidism**. This has been seen in patients exposed to iodine from a variety of sources, including an iodine-rich diet[1] or drugs containing iodine[2-4] (see also under Amiodarone, p.821).

Excess iodine may also induce **hyperthyroidism** (the Iod-Basedow or Jod-Basedow phenomenon). This has followed exposure to iodine from a variety of drugs, iodinated preparations for water purification, and an iodine-rich diet.[5-13] Iodine-induced hyperthyroidism has been associated with iodine prophylaxis programmes in developing countries and it may be an increasing problem.[14,15] The highest incidence of hyperthyroidism has been reported to occur 1 to 3 years after supplementation commences, with the incidence returning to normal within 3 to 10 years despite continued iodine exposure.[10] Elderly subjects and those with nodular goitres have been found to be at greatest risk.

In **pregnancy**, congenital goitre and hypothyroidism have followed maternal ingestion of iodides,[16,17] and neonates have been affected following maternal application of povidone-iodine[18-20] as well as following direct application to the neonate.[21-24] To overcome any adverse effects on thyroid function as a result of iodine prophylaxis during pregnancy, WHO has issued guidelines on the safe use of iodised oil during gestation.[25,26]

1. Li M, *et al.* Endemic goitre in central China caused by excessive iodine intake. *Lancet* 1987; **ii:** 257–9.
2. Murray IPC, Stewart RDH. Iodide goitre. *Lancet* 1967; **i:** 922–6.
3. Dolan TF, Gibson LE. Complications of iodide therapy in patients with cystic fibrosis. *J Pediatr* 1971; **79:** 684–7.
4. Gomolin IH. Iodinated glycerol-induced hypothyroidism. *Drug Intell Clin Pharm* 1987; **21:** 726–7.
5. Stewart JC, Vidor GI. Thyrotoxicosis induced by iodine contamination of food—a common unrecognised condition? *Br Med J* 1976; **1:** 372–5.
6. Fisher JR. Effect of iodide treatment on thyroid function. *N Engl J Med* 1977; **297:** 171.
7. Sobrinho LG, *et al.* Thyroxine toxicosis in patients with iodine induced thyrotoxicosis. *J Clin Endocrinol Metab* 1977; **45:** 25–9.
8. Miller HA, *et al.* Topical iodine and hyperthyroidism. *Ann Intern Med* 1981; **95:** 121.
9. Jacobson JM, *et al.* Self-limited hyperthyroidism following intravaginal iodine administration. *Am J Obstet Gynecol* 1981; **140:** 472–3.
10. Fradkin JE, Wolff J. Iodide-induced thyrotoxicosis. *Medicine (Baltimore)* 1983; **62:** 1–20.
11. Shilo S, Hirsch HJ. Iodine-induced hyperthyroidism in a patient with a normal thyroid gland. *Postgrad Med J* 1986; **62:** 661–2.
12. Hall R, Lazarus JH. Changing iodine intake and the effect on thyroid disease. *Br Med J* 1987; **294:** 721–2.
13. Liel Y, Alkan M. Travelers' thyrotoxicosis: transitory thyrotoxicosis induced by iodinated preparations for water purification. *Arch Intern Med* 1996; **156:** 807–10.
14. Todd CH, *et al.* Increase in thyrotoxicosis associated with iodine supplements in Zimbabwe. *Lancet* 1995; **346:** 1563–4.
15. Bourdoux, *et al.* Iodine-induced thyrotoxicosis in Kivu, Zaire. *Lancet* 1996; **347:** 552–3.
16. Galina MP, *et al.* Iodides during pregnancy: an apparent cause of neonatal death. *N Engl J Med* 1962; **267:** 1124–7.
17. Carswell F, *et al.* Congenital goitre and hypothyroidism produced by maternal ingestion of iodides. *Lancet* 1970; **i:** 1241–3.
18. Danziger Y, *et al.* Transient congenital hypothyroidism after topical iodine in pregnancy and lactation. *Arch Dis Child* 1987; **62:** 295–6.
19. Delange F, *et al.* Topical iodine, breast feeding, and neonatal hypothyroidism. *Arch Dis Child* 1988; **63:** 106–7.
20. Chanoine JP, *et al.* Increased recall rate at screening for congenital hypothyroidism in breast fed infants born to iodine overloaded mothers. *Arch Dis Child* 1988; **63:** 1207–10.
21. Wuilloud A, *et al.* Erworbene hypothyreose bei einem neugeborenen durch anwendung einer jodhaltigen salbe. *Z Kinderchir* 1977; **20:** 181–5.
22. Jackson HJ, Sutherland RM. Effect of povidone-iodine on neonatal thyroid function. *Lancet* 1981; **ii:** 992.
23. Lyen KR, *et al.* Transient thyroid suppression associated with topically applied povidone-iodine. *Am J Dis Child* 1982; **136:** 369–70.
24. Smerdely P, *et al.* Topical iodine-containing antiseptics and neonatal hypothyroidism in very-low-birthweight infants. *Lancet* 1989; **ii:** 661–4.
25. WHO. Safe use of iodized oil to prevent iodine deficiency in pregnant women. *Bull WHO* 1996; **74:** 1–3.
26. Delange F. Administration of iodized oil during pregnancy: a summary of the published evidence. *Bull WHO* 1996; **74:** 101–8.

Precautions

Caution is necessary if preparations containing iodine or iodides are taken for prolonged periods, and such preparations should not be taken regularly during pregnancy except when iodine supplementation is required. Iodine or iodides are contra-indicated during breast feeding. Caution is also required when giving iodine or iodides to children. Patients over the age of 45 years or with nodular goitres are especially susceptible to hyperthyroidism when given iodine supplementation. Reduced doses should therefore be employed and supplementation with iodised oil may not be appropriate.

Solutions of iodine applied to the skin should not be covered with occlusive dressings. The disinfectant activity of iodine is reduced by alkalis as well as by protein.

As iodine and iodides can affect the thyroid gland the administration of such preparations may interfere with tests of thyroid function.

Interactions

The effects of iodine and iodides on the thyroid may be altered by other compounds including amiodarone and lithium.

Pharmacokinetics

Iodine is slightly absorbed when applied to the skin. When taken by mouth iodine preparations (which are converted to iodide) and iodides are trapped by the thyroid gland (see p.1489). Iodides not taken up by the thyroid are excreted mainly in the urine, with smaller amounts appearing in the faeces, saliva, and sweat. They cross the placenta and are distributed into breast milk.

Uses and Administration

Iodine is an essential trace element in the human diet, necessary for the formation of thyroid hormones (see p.1489), and consequently it is used in iodine deficiency and thyroid disorders. It also has antimicrobial activity.

For the prophylaxis and treatment of **iodine deficiency disorders** (below) it may be administered as potassium or sodium iodide, as iodised oil, or as potassium iodate.

In the pre-operative management of **hyperthyroidism** (p.1489) iodine and iodides are used in conjunction with antithyroid drugs such as carbimazole, methimazole, or propylthiouracil. Iodine may be given as a solution with potassium iodide (Aqueous Iodine Oral Solution BP 1998: Lugol's Solution or Strong Iodine Solution USP 23) which contains in each mL 130 mg of free and combined iodine; a dose of 0.1 to 0.3 mL in milk or water three times daily for 7 to 14 days renders the thyroid firm and avoids the increased vascularity and friability with increased risk of haemorrhage that may result from the use of an antithyroid agent alone. Alternatively, suggested doses of potassium iodide have been up to 250 mg three times daily with food. Solutions of potassium iodide intended for oral administration should be given well diluted to avoid gastric irritation. Potassium iodide may also be given as part of the management of thyroid storm one hour after administration of an antithyroid drug; doses of 50 to 100 mg have been given twice daily; higher doses have sometimes been employed. Sodium iodide has been given by intravenous injection as part of the management of thyroid storm.

Potassium iodide has been tried in the treatment of benign **thyroid nodules** (p.1489).

Potassium iodide or potassium iodate are taken by mouth for **radiation protection** (below) to saturate the thyroid when uptake of radio-iodine by the gland is not desired.

Iodine has a powerful bactericidal action. It is also active against fungi, viruses, protozoa, cysts, and spores. Iodine is used as an **antiseptic** and **disinfectant** generally as a 2.0% or 2.5% solution. Its activity is reduced in the presence of organic matter, though not to the same extent as with the other halogen disinfectants. Also if industrial methylated spirit is used for the solution, it should be free from acetone with which iodine forms an irritant and lachrymatory compound. Iodine solutions may be applied to small wounds or abrasions as well as to unbroken skin, but an iodophore such as povidone-iodine (p.1123) may be preferred.

Iodine may also be used to sterilise drinking water; 5 drops of a 2% alcoholic solution added to about one litre (one US quart) of water is reported to kill amoebae and bacteria within 15 minutes. Water contaminated with *Giardia* requires 12 drops of a 2% alcoholic solution for each litre which may take one hour to achieve its effect.

Iodine stains the skin a deep reddish-brown; the stain can readily be removed by dilute solutions of alkalis or sodium thiosulphate. A dilute solution of iodine (Schiller's Iodine) has been used as a **diagnostic** stain in colposcopy.

When iodine combines chemically it is decolorised and so-called colourless iodine preparations do not have the disinfectant properties of iodine.

There have been numerous other uses of iodine and iodides. Potassium iodide has been used in the treatment of fungal infections such as sporotrichosis (below). Iodides have long been used as ingredients of expectorant mixtures but there is little evidence of their effectiveness. A diatomic iodine formulation is under investigation for the treatment of fibrocystic breast disease. Iodinated organic compounds including iodised oil are used as X-ray contrast media (p.1002). Iodine radionuclides are often administered as preparations of sodium iodide.

Fungal infections. Potassium iodide is used in the treatment of cutaneous sporotrichosis (p.371), although how it acts is unclear since antifungal activity was not demonstrated *in vitro* against *Sporothrix schenkii*.[1] It is usually given in a gradually increasing dosage up to the limit of tolerance. Recommendations for the initial dose vary from 250 mg to 1 g or more three times daily; treatment should be continued for at least 1 month after the disappearance or stabilisation of the lesions.

Potassium iodide has also been found to be effective in the treatment of phycomycosis caused by *Basidiobolus haptosporus*;[2,3] once again the mode of action is unclear.[4]

Potassium iodide and sodium iodide have been tried by local intracavitary instillation for the treatment of life-threatening haemoptysis from pulmonary aspergillomas.[5] Mechanical factors may have accounted for a beneficial effect rather than any antifungal action. Aspergillomas are usually managed conservatively or, in more severe disease, with antifungals or surgery (see p.367).

1. Hay RJ. Managing fungal infections. *Br J Hosp Med* 1984; **31:** 278–82.
2. Kelly S, *et al.* Subcutaneous phycomycosis in Sierra Leone. *Trans R Soc Trop Med Hyg* 1980; **74:** 396–7.
3. Kamalam A, Thambiah AS. Muscle invasion by Basidiobolus haptosporus. *Sabouraudia* 1984; **22:** 273–7.
4. Yangco BG, *et al.* In vitro susceptibilities of human and wild-type isolates of Basidiobolus and Conidiobolus species. *Antimicrob Agents Chemother* 1984; **25:** 413–16.
5. Rumbak M, *et al.* Topical treatment of life threatening haemoptysis from aspergillomas. *Thorax* 1996; **51:** 253–5.

Iodine deficiency disorders. Iodine is an essential trace element required for thyroid hormone production. Daily adult requirements are about 100 to 300 μg. In the UK the reference nutrient intake (RNI) for adults is 140 μg (1.1 μmol) of iodine daily[1] and in the USA the recommended dietary allowance (RDA) is 150 μg daily.[2] A full explanation of the terms RNI and RDA can be found under Human Requirements of Vitamins, p.1332.

When iodine requirements are not met, a range of disorders can develop. These iodine deficiency disorders (IDD) include endemic goitre (enlargement of the thyroid), endemic cretinism (a syndrome characterised by deaf-mutism, intellectual deficit, spasticity, and sometimes hypothyroidism), impaired mental function in children and adults, and an increased incidence of still-births as well as perinatal and infant mortality.[3]

Iodine deficiency disorders can be prevented by iodine supplementation. The incidence of endemic goitre[4-7] and endemic cretinism[8-11] can be reduced and some of the effects of established iodine deficiency ameliorated.[12-15]

Although various methods of iodine supplementation, including iodination of water and bread as well as the administration of potassium iodide tablets, have been investigated, the two methods generally used are iodination of culinary salt and the administration of iodised oil.[3] Salt may be iodinated by the addition of potassium iodide. However, in countries where impurities or environmental factors such as moisture and temperature are likely to cause a reduction in the iodine content of the salt, potassium iodate is the preferred compound since it is more stable than iodide under varying climatic conditions.[16] The concentration used in different countries varies over a wide range from 10 to 80 ppm of elemental iodine.[16]

The chief alternative to supplementation with iodinated salt is iodised oil, usually by intramuscular injection; it is useful where salt consumption is unreliable or inadequate or where immediate action is necessary to correct severe iodine deficiency.[3] A commonly used type of iodised oil has been a poppyseed oil containing about 38% w/w of iodine (see Iodised Oil, p.1006). The Pan American Health Organization has proposed[17] that children in the first year of life receive a dose of 0.5 mL with 1.0 mL being given to all other subjects. Single intramuscular doses of 1 mL can provide adequate protection from iodine deficiency for at least 3 years while a dose of 2 mL provides adequate coverage for 3½ to 5 years.

Subjects over the age of 45 years and those with nodular goitre are susceptible to hyperthyroidism when given iodine, and iodised oil may not be a suitable means of supplementation. If it is used then doses of 0.2 mL should be employed.[17]

Iodised oil has been tried by mouth. A single dose of 1 mL is reported to provide protection for 1 year and 2 mL for 2 years[17] although there is some evidence that much smaller doses of 0.1 or 0.25 mL can provide protection for about 1 year.[18]

Indirect iodine supplementation, by addition of potassium iodate to the water used to irrigate crops, has been tried in areas of iodine deficiency where other methods had proved difficult to implement.[19]

Iodine or iodides may suppress neonatal thyroid function and it is generally recommended that iodine compounds should be avoided during **pregnancy**. However, where it is essential to prevent neonatal goitre and cretinism, iodine supplementation should not be withheld from pregnant women.[20,21] Iodine supplementation has been found to be effective in preventing brain-damage in the fetus provided it is given to the mother in the first or second trimester;[20] treatment later in pregnancy was not effective in improving neurological status, although some developmental improvement was seen and hypothyroidism will be corrected. WHO has stated that in areas where iodine deficiency disorders are moderate to severe, iodised oil given either before or at any stage of gestation is beneficial.[21] A dose of 480 mg iodine intramuscularly each year or 300 to 480 mg iodine by mouth each year or 100 to 300 mg iodine by mouth every 6 months is recommended for pregnant women and for at least one year postpartum. Similar intramuscular doses are recommended for non-pregnant fertile women with oral doses being 400 to 960 mg iodine every year or 200 to 480 mg every 6 months.

1. DoH. Dietary reference values for food energy and nutrients for the United Kingdom: report of the panel on dietary reference values of the Committee on Medical Aspects of Food Policy. *Report on health and social subjects 41*. London: HMSO, 1991.
2. Subcommittee on the Tenth Edition of the RDAs, Food and Nutrition Board, Commission on Life Sciences, National Research Council. *Recommended dietary allowances*. 10th ed. Washington, DC: National Academy Press, 1989.
3. Hetzel BS. An overview of the prevention and control of iodine deficiency disorders. In: Hetzel BS, *et al.*, eds. *The prevention and control of iodine deficiency disorders*. Amsterdam: Elsevier, 1987: 7–31.
4. Clements FW, *et al.* Goitre studies in Tasmania. *Bull WHO* 1968; **38:** 297–318.
5. Clements FW, *et al.* Goitre prophylaxis by addition of potassium iodate to bread: experience in Tasmania. *Lancet* 1970; **i:** 489–92.
6. Sooch SS, *et al.* Prevention of endemic goitre with iodized salt. *Bull WHO* 1973; **49:** 307–12.
7. Maberly GF, *et al.* Effect of iodination of a village water-supply on goitre size and thyroid function. *Lancet* 1981; **ii:** 1270–2.
8. Pharoah POD, *et al.* Neurological damage to the fetus resulting from severe iodine deficiency during pregnancy. *Lancet* 1971; **i:** 308–10.
9. Fierro-Benitez R, *et al.* The role of iodine in intellectual development in an area of endemic goiter. In: Dunn JT, Medeiros-Neto GA, eds. *Endemic goiter and cretinism: continuing threats to world health*. Washington: Pan American Health Organization, 1974: 135–42.
10. Connolly KJ, *et al.* Fetal iodine deficiency and motor performance during childhood. *Lancet* 1979; **ii:** 1149–51.
11. Ma T, *et al.* The present status of endemic goitre and endemic cretinism in China. *Food Nutr Bull* 1982; **4:** 13–19.
12. Buttfield IH, Hetzel BJ. Endemic goitre in eastern New Guinea. *Bull WHO* 1967; **36:** 243–62.
13. Bantista A, *et al.* The effects of oral iodized oil on intelligence, thyroid status, and somatic growth in school-age children from an area of endemic goiter. *Am J Clin Nutr* 1982; **35:** 127–34.
14. Wang Y-Y, Yang S-H. Improvement in hearing among otherwise normal schoolchildren in iodine-deficient areas of Guizhou, China, following use of iodised salt. *Lancet* 1985; **ii:** 518–20.
15. Vanderpas JB, *et al.* Reversibility of severe hypothyroidism with supplementary iodine in patients with endemic cretinism. *N Engl J Med* 1986; **315:** 791–5.
16. Mannar MGV. Control of iodine deficiency disorders by iodination of salt: strategy for developing countries. In: Hetzel BS, *et al.*, eds. *The prevention and control of iodine deficiency disorders*. Amsterdam: Elsevier, 1987: 111–25.
17. Dunn JT. Iodized oil in the treatment and prophylaxis of IDD. In: Hetzel BS, *et al.*, eds. *The prevention and control of iodine deficiency disorders*. Amsterdam: Elsevier, 1987: 127–34.
18. Tonglet R, *et al.* Efficacy of low oral doses of iodized oil in the control of iodine deficiency in Zaire. *N Engl J Med* 1992; **326:** 236–41.
19. Cao X-Y, *et al.* Iodination of irrigation water as a method of supplying iodine to a severely iodine-deficient population in Xinjiang, China. *Lancet* 1994; **344:** 107–10.
20. Delange F. Administration of iodized oil during pregnancy: a summary of the published evidence. *Bull WHO* 1996; **74:** 101–8.
21. WHO. Safe use of iodized oil to prevent iodine deficiency in pregnant women. *Bull WHO* 1996; **74:** 1–3.

Radiation protection. The administration of a radiologically stable form of iodine to saturate the thyroid gland confers thyroid protection from iodine radionuclides, be they nuclides being used medically or nuclides released as a result of a nuclear accident.[1,2]

When thyroid protection from a medical procedure involving radio-iodine is needed, a dose of 100 to 150 mg of potassium iodide may be given 24 hours before the procedure and daily for up to 10 days following it.

In the USA a dose of 130 mg of potassium iodide given daily for 10 days has been recommended following a nuclear accident.[1,3] In the UK the Department of Health[4] recommend, in the event of a nuclear accident, a single dose of 100 mg of stable iodine (as 170 mg of potassium iodate) for adults (including pregnant women and women who are breast feeding) as soon as possible after exposure and before evacuation. Dosages for children are: 3 to 12 years, 50 mg of stable iodine (85 mg of potassium iodate); 1 month to 3 years, 25 mg of stable iodine (42.5 mg of potassium iodate); and for neonates, 12.5 mg of stable iodine (21.25 mg of potassium iodate) given as a single dose. When evacuation is delayed, repeated daily administration is recommended.

1. Halperin JA. Potassium iodide as a thyroid blocker— Three Mile Island today. *Drug Intell Clin Pharm* 1989; **23:** 422–7.
2. Nauman J, Wolff J. Iodide prophylaxis in Poland after the Chernobyl reactor accident: benefits and risks. *Am J Med* 1993; **94:** 524–32.
3. Schleien B, *et al.* Recommendations on the use of potassium iodide as a thyroid-blocking agent in radiation accidents: an FDA update. *Bull N Y Acad Med* 1983; **59:** 1009–19.
4. DoH. Nuclear accident countermeasures: iodine prophylaxis: report of the United Kingdom working group on iodine prophylaxis following nuclear accidents. *Report on health and social subjects 39.* London: HMSO, 1991.

Preparations

BP 1998: Alcoholic Iodine Solution *(Weak Iodine Solution)*; Aqueous Iodine Oral Solution *(Lugol's Solution)*; Sodium Iodide Injection;
BPC 1968: Compound Iodine Paint *(Mandl's Paint)*;
USP 23: Iodine Tincture; Iodine Topical Solution; Potassium Iodide Delayed-release Tablets; Potassium Iodide Oral Solution; Potassium Iodide Tablets; Strong Iodine Solution; Strong Iodine Tincture.

Proprietary Preparations (details are given in Part 3)
Aust.: Jodonorm; Leukona-Jod-Bad; ***Belg.:*** Iodex; ***Canad.:*** Iodaminol†; Micro I; Thyro-Block; ***Fr.:*** Axyol; ***Ger.:*** Jodetten; Jodid; jodminerase; Kaliklora Jod med; Kataraktont†; Leukona-Jod-Bad; Mikroplex Jod†; Strumex; Thyrojod depot†; ***Ital.:*** Goccemed; Iodosan Collutorio; Sol-Jod; ***Norw.:*** Idu-Phor; ***USA:*** Iodopen; Pima; Roma-nol†; SSKI; Thyro-Block.

Multi-ingredient: ***Aust.:*** Jodthyrox; Jopinol; ***Austral.:*** ASA Tones; Ayrton's Iodised†; Elixophyllin-KI†; Potassium Iodide and Stramonium Compound; ***Belg.:*** Aperop; Iodex MS†; ITC; Pneumogenol†; Richelet†; ***Canad.:*** Diodine; IDM Solution; Iode; Mathieu Cough Syrup; Sclerodine†; Theo-Bronc; Vito Bronches; ***Fr.:*** Asthmasedine†; Cataridol; Cristopal; Ioducyl†; Marinol; Nitrol; Pneumogeine; Sommieres Au Pentavit B†; Vita-Iodurol; Vita-Iodurol ATP; ***Ger.:*** Adelheid-Jodquelle, Tolzer; Akseka-pseln†; Diaporin†; Ger N in der Ophtiole†; Jodthyrox; Krophan N; Mandrorhinon†; Pherajod†; Prolugol-liquid N†; Thyreocomb N; Thyronajod; Tolzer, Jodquell-Dragees†; Varigloban; Vidirakt N†; Vitreolent N†; ***Ital.:*** Calcio Jodico†; Esoform Jod 20; Facovit; Fertomcidina-U†; Jodo-Calcio-Vitaminico; Polijodurato; Rubidiosin Composto; Rubistenol; Rubjovit; Ultimex†; ***S.Afr.:*** Efcospect†; ***Spain:*** Adiod; Angiofiline†; Audione; Balsamo Germano†; Bronquiasmol†; Callicida Rojo; Depurativo Richelet; Diptol Antihist†; Elixifilin; Encialina; Iodocafedrina†; Lasa Antiasmatico; Nitroina; Otogen†; Yodo Tio Calci; ***Switz.:*** Dental-Phenjoca; Perpector; Varigloblin; Vitreolent; ***UK:*** TCP; ***USA:*** Elixophyllin-KI; Iodex with Methyl Salicylate; Iodo-Niacin†; KIE; Mudrane; Mudrane-2†; ORA5; Pediacof; Pedituss Cough; Phylorinol; Quadrinal.

Liothyronine Sodium (9006-d)

Liothyronine Sodium *(BANM, rINNM)*.

Liothyroninum Natricum; Sodium Liothyronine; L-Tri-iodothyronine Sodium; 3,5,3′-Tri-iodo-L-thyronine Sodium. Sodium 4-*O*-(4-hydroxy-3-iodophenyl)-3,5-di-iodo-L-tyrosine.

$C_{15}H_{11}I_3NNaO_4$ = 673.0.

CAS — 6893-02-3 (liothyronine); 55-06-1 (liothyronine sodium); 8065-29-0 (liotrix).

NOTE. The abbreviation T_3 is often used for endogenous tri-iodothyronine in medical and biochemical reports. Liotrix is the *USAN* name for a mixture of liothyronine sodium with thyroxine sodium.

Pharmacopoeias. In *Eur.* (see p.viii), *Jpn*, and *US*.

A white to light tan, odourless, crystalline, powder. Liothyronine sodium 10.3 μg is approximately equivalent to 10 μg of liothyronine.

Very slightly **soluble** to practically insoluble in water; slightly soluble in alcohol; practically insoluble in ether, and most other organic solvents. It dissolves in dilute solutions of alkali hydroxides. **Store** at 2° to 8° in airtight containers. Protect from light.

Adverse Effects, Treatment, and Precautions

As for Thyroxine Sodium, p.1497.

Interactions

As for Thyroxine Sodium, p.1498.

Pharmacokinetics

Liothyronine is readily and almost completely absorbed from the gastro-intestinal tract following oral administration. Once in the circulation, liothyronine is extensively protein bound, principally to thyroxine-binding globulin (TBG) but also to a lesser extent to thyroxine-binding pre-albumin (TBPA) or to albumin. Liothyronine has a plasma half-life in euthyroidism of about 1 to 2 days; the half-life is prolonged in hypothyroidism and reduced in hyperthyroidism.

Liothyronine is metabolised by deiodination to inactive di-iodothyronine and mono-iodothyronine. Iodine released by deiodination is largely reused within the thyroid cells. Further metabolites result from deamination and decarboxylation to tiratricol (triac).

Uses and Administration

Liothyronine is a thyroid hormone (see p.1489 for a description of the endogenous hormones). It has actions similar to those of thyroxine (p.1498) and is used in the treatment of hypothyroidism (p.1490). The onset of action of liothyronine is rapid, developing within a few hours of administration, and therefore liothyronine tends to be used in circumstances where this, and its short duration of action, are useful, particularly in myxoedema (hypothyroid) coma.

With regular dosing the peak therapeutic effect is usually achieved by 3 days; on withdrawal its effects may persist for 1 to 3 days.

The dose of liothyronine should be individualised on the basis of clinical response and biochemical tests and should be monitored regularly. Although liothyronine is administered as the sodium salt, doses can be expressed in terms of liothyronine sodium or liothyronine; the doses below are in terms of liothyronine sodium. Liothyronine sodium 20 to 25 μg is generally considered to be approximately equivalent in activity to thyroxine sodium 100 μg.

In hypothyroidism a usual initial adult dose is 20 μg daily by mouth increased gradually to a maintenance dose of 60 μg daily in 2 to 3 divided doses, although up to 100 μg daily may be required in some patients. In elderly patients, in those with cardiovascular disorders, or in those with severe long-standing hypothyroidism, treatment should be introduced more gradually using lower initial doses, smaller increments, and longer intervals between increases, as necessary.

In myxoedema coma liothyronine sodium may be given intravenously in a dose of 5 to 20 μg by slow intravenous injection, repeated as necessary, usually at intervals of 12 hours; the minimum interval between doses is 4 hours. Some authorities have advocated an initial dose of 50 μg intravenously followed by further injections of 25 μg every 8 hours until improvement occurs; the dosage may then be reduced to 25 μg intravenously twice daily.

Liothyronine has also been given in the diagnosis of hyperthyroidism in adults. Failure to suppress the take up of radio-iodine after several days of receiving liothyronine sodium suggests a diagnosis of hyperthyroidism.

Liothyronine hydrochloride has also been used.

Preparations

BP 1998: Liothyronine Tablets;
USP 23: Liothyronine Sodium Tablets; Liotrix Tablets.

Proprietary Preparations (details are given in Part 3)
Austral.: Tertroxin; ***Belg.:*** Cytomel; ***Canad.:*** Cytomel; ***Fr.:*** Cynomel; ***Ger.:*** Thybon; Thyrotardin; ***Irl.:*** Tertroxin†; ***Ital.:*** Dispon; Ti-Tre; ***Neth.:*** Cytomel; ***S.Afr.:*** Tertroxin; ***UK:*** Tertroxin; Triiodothyronine Injection; ***USA:*** Cytomel; Triostat.

Multi-ingredient: ***Aust.:*** Combithyrex; Novothyral; Prothyrid†; ***Belg.:*** Novothyral; ***Fr.:*** Euthyral; ***Ger.:*** AntiFocal N; NeyNormin "N" (Revitorgan-Dilutionen "N" Nr. 65); NeyTumorin "N" (Revitorgan-Dilutionen Nr. 66); Novothyral; Prothyrid; Thyreotom; ***S.Afr.:*** Diotroxin; ***Switz.:*** Novothyral; ***USA:*** Thyrolar.

Methimazole (835-e)

Methimazole *(BAN)*.

Thiamazole *(rINN)*; Mercazolylum; Methylmercaptoimidazole; Tiamazol. 1-Methylimidazole-2-thiol.

$C_4H_6N_2S$ = 114.2.

CAS — 60-56-0.

Pharmacopoeias. In *Chin., It., Jpn, Pol.,* and *US.*

A white to pale buff crystalline powder with a faint characteristic odour. **Soluble** 1 in 5 of water, 1 in 5 of alcohol, 1 in 4.5 of chloroform, and 1 in 125 of ether. Solutions in water are practically neutral to litmus. **Protect** from light.

Adverse Effects and Precautions

As for Carbimazole, p.1491.

Pharmacokinetics

The pharmacokinetics of methimazole can be considered together with those of carbimazole (p.1492) since the latter is rapidly and completely metabolised to methimazole in the body.

Uses and Administration

Methimazole is a thiourea antithyroid drug that acts by blocking the production of thyroid hormones (see p.1489). It is used in the management of hyperthyroidism (p.1489), including the treatment of Graves' disease, the preparation of hyperthyroid patients for thyroidectomy, use as an adjunct to radio-iodine therapy, and the treatment of thyroid storm.

Methimazole is given by mouth usually in an initial dosage of 15 to 60 mg daily. It has often been given in divided doses but once daily administration is also possible. Improvement is usually seen in 1 to 3 weeks and control of symptoms in 1 to 2 months. When the patient is euthyroid the dose is gradually reduced to a maintenance dose, usually 5 to 15 mg daily. Alternatively, the dose may be continued at the initial level in combination with supplemental thyroxine as a blocking-replacement regimen. Either form of maintenance treatment is usually continued for at least a year, and often for 18 months. A suggested initial dose for children is 400 μg per kg body-weight daily; for maintenance this dose may be halved.

Action. For reference to the possible immunosuppressant effects of thiourea antithyroid drugs, see Carbimazole, p.1492.

Preparations

USP 23: Methimazole Tablets.

Proprietary Preparations (details are given in Part 3)
Aust.: Favistan; ***Belg.:*** Strumazol; ***Canad.:*** Tapazole; ***Ger.:*** Favistan; Thyrozol; ***Ital.:*** Antitiroide†; Tapazole; ***Neth.:*** Strumazol; ***S.Afr.:*** Tapazole†; ***Spain:*** Tirodril; ***Swed.:*** Thacapzol; ***Switz.:*** Tapazole; ***USA:*** Tapazole.

Multi-ingredient: ***Ital.:*** Bromazolo; Sirenitas†; ***Spain:*** Neo Endofren†.

Methylthiouracil (836-l)

Methylthiouracil *(rINN)*.

2,3-Dihydro-2-thioxo-6-methylpyrimidin-4(1*H*)-one; 2-Mercapto-6-methylpyrimidin-4-ol; 6-Methyl-2-thiouracil.

$C_5H_6N_2OS$ = 142.2.

CAS — 56-04-2.

Pharmacopoeias. In *Aust., It.,* and *Pol.*

Methylthiouracil is a thiourea antithyroid drug that has been used in the treatment of hyperthyroidism.

Preparations

Proprietary Preparations (details are given in Part 3)
Ger.: Thyreostat†.

Potassium Iodate (13154-m)

KIO_3 = 214.0.

CAS — 7758-05-6.

Pharmacopoeias. In *Br.* and *It.*

A white crystalline powder with a slight odour. Slowly **soluble** in water; practically insoluble in alcohol. A 5% solution in water has a pH of 5.0 to 8.0.

Potassium iodate has the actions of iodine (p.1493) and the iodides. It is used for the prophylaxis and treatment of iodine deficiency disorders (p.1494).

It may be used similarly to potassium iodide as an adjunct to antithyroid drugs in the pre-operative management of hyperthyroidism (p.1489) and for radiation protection to prevent the uptake of radio-iodine by the thyroid (see p.1494 for suggested doses).

Preparations

BP 1998: Potassium Iodate Tablets.

Proprietary Preparations (details are given in Part 3)
UK: Bioiodine.

Potassium Perchlorate (837-y)

$KClO_4$ = 138.5.
CAS — 7778-74-7.

WARNING. *Potassium perchlorate has been used for the illicit preparation of explosives or fireworks; care is required with its supply.*

Adverse Effects

Potassium perchlorate seldom produces adverse effects when given as a single dose for diagnostic purposes. Prolonged administration of potassium perchlorate as an antithyroid drug has been associated with serious dose-related adverse effects. Aplastic anaemia (with some fatalities), agranulocytosis, leucopenia, pancytopenia, and the nephrotic syndrome have been reported. Fever and rashes have also been observed. Some patients may experience nausea and vomiting. Excessive doses may cause hypothyroidism and goitre.

Effects on the blood. Reports of fatal aplastic anaemia[1,2] and of leucopenia and agranulocytosis[2] associated with the use of potassium perchlorate for the treatment of hyperthyroidism.

1. Krevans JR, *et al.* Fatal aplastic anemia following use of potassium perchlorate in thyrotoxicosis. *JAMA* 1962; **181:** 182–4.
2. Anonymous. Potassium perchlorate and aplastic anaemia. *Br Med J* 1961; **i:** 1520–1.

Uses and Administration

Potassium perchlorate reduces the uptake and concentration of iodide, pertechnetate, and other anions by the thyroid, choroid plexus, gastric mucosa, and salivary glands probably by competitive inhibition of active transport mechanisms.

It is used diagnostically as an adjunct to pertechnetate (^{99m}Tc) to enhance visualisation of the brain, Meckel's diverticulum, or the placenta by reducing unwanted images of other organs. The usual adult dose is 200 to 400 mg by mouth given 30 to 60 minutes before the administration of pertechnetate (^{99m}Tc). For children aged 2 to 12 years, a dose of 200 mg by mouth has been recommended; for children younger than 2 years of age, 100 mg may be given by mouth.

Potassium perchlorate is also used in conjunction with sodium iodide (^{131}I) in the perchlorate discharge test of thyroid function. The release of radioiodine from the gland following an oral dose of potassium perchlorate indicates a defect in the binding of iodide by the thyroid and thus a defect in thyroid hormone synthesis. The test has also been used to investigate the action of antithyroid drugs.

Potassium perchlorate has been used in the treatment of hyperthyroidism (p.1489), but because of its toxicity it has been largely replaced by alternative treatments. However, it may be useful in patients with iodine-induced hyperthyroidism such as that associated with amiodarone therapy, by increasing responsiveness to conventional antithyroid drugs. An adult dose of 800 mg to 1 g daily by mouth in 3 or 4 divided doses is used as initial therapy with maintenance doses of 200 to 500 mg daily in divided doses. The total daily dose should not exceed 1 g.

References.

1. Wolff J. Perchlorate and the thyroid gland. *Pharmacol Rev* 1998; **50:** 89–105.

Preparations

Proprietary Preparations (details are given in Part 3)
Ital.: Pertiroid; ***USA:*** Perchloracap.

Prolonium Iodide (13175-p)

Prolonium Iodide *(rINN).*
NN-(2-Hydroxytrimethylene)bis(trimethylammonium) di-iodide.
$C_9H_{24}I_2N_2O$ = 430.1.
CAS — 123-47-7.
Pharmacopoeias. In *Chin.*

Prolonium iodide has been given by injection as a source of iodine (p.1493) as part of the treatment of thyroid storm and for the pre-operative management of hyperthyroidism.

Propylthiouracil (838-j)

Propylthiouracil *(BAN, rINN).*
Propylthiouracilum. 2,3-Dihydro-6-propyl-2-thioxopyrimidin-4(1*H*)-one; 2-Mercapto-6-propylpyrimidin-4-ol; 6-Propyl-2-thiouracil.
$C_7H_{10}N_2OS$ = 170.2.
CAS — 51-52-5.
Pharmacopoeias. In *Chin., Eur.* (see p.viii), *Int., Jpn,* and *US.*

White or practically white crystals or crystalline powder. Slightly or very slightly **soluble** in water and in ether; sparingly soluble in alcohol; slightly soluble in chloroform; dissolves in ammonium hydroxide and aqueous solutions of alkali hydroxides. **Protect** from light.

Adverse Effects and Precautions

As for Carbimazole, p.1491.

Propylthiouracil has been associated with greater hepatotoxicity than other thiourea antithyroid drugs (such as carbimazole or methimazole). Rarely hepatitis, hepatic necrosis, encephalopathy, and death have occurred; asymptomatic liver damage is more common (see Effects on the Liver, p.1492).

Propylthiouracil should be given with care, and in reduced doses, to patients with renal impairment.

Pharmacokinetics

Propylthiouracil is rapidly absorbed from the gastro-intestinal tract with peak plasma concentrations occurring about 1 to 2 hours following administration by mouth. It is concentrated in the thyroid gland and, since its duration of action is more closely related to the intrathyroidal drug concentration than its plasma half-life, this results in a prolongation of antithyroid activity such that single daily doses are possible. Propylthiouracil is 75 to 80% bound to plasma proteins.

Propylthiouracil has an elimination half-life of about 1 to 2 hours and is metabolised, probably by the liver, and excreted in the urine as unchanged drug (less than 2% of a dose) and metabolites; more than 50% of a dose is excreted as the glucuronic acid conjugate. The elimination half-life may be increased in renal and hepatic impairment.

Propylthiouracil crosses the placenta and is distributed into breast milk.

References.

1. Kampmann JP, Hansen JM. Clinical pharmacokinetics of antithyroid drugs. *Clin Pharmacokinet* 1981; **6:** 401–28.
2. Giles HG, *et al.* Disposition of intravenous propylthiouracil. *J Clin Pharmacol* 1981; **21:** 466–71.
3. Kampmann JP, Hansen JEM. Serum protein binding of propylthiouracil. *Br J Clin Pharmacol* 1983; **16:** 549–52.

Uses and Administration

Propylthiouracil is a thiourea antithyroid drug that acts by blocking the production of thyroid hormones (see p.1489); it also inhibits the peripheral deiodination of thyroxine to tri-iodothyronine. It is used in the management of hyperthyroidism (p.1489), including the treatment of Graves' disease, preparation of hyperthyroid patients for thyroidectomy, use as an adjunct to radio-iodine therapy, and the treatment of thyroid storm.

Propylthiouracil is given by mouth usually in an initial dosage of 300 to 600 mg daily. It has often been given in divided daily doses but once daily administration is also possible. Improvement is usually seen in 1 to 3 weeks and control of symptoms is achieved in 1 to 2 months. When the patient is euthyroid the dose is gradually reduced to a maintenance dose, usually 50 to 150 mg daily. Treatment is usually continued for at least a year, and often for 18 months. A suggested initial dose for children aged 6 to 10 years is 50 to 150 mg daily, and for children over 10 years 150 to 300 mg daily.

Doses should be reduced by 25% in mild to moderate renal impairment and by 50% in severe renal impairment. Doses may also need to be reduced in hepatic impairment.

Alcoholic liver disease. Propylthiouracil has been said to reduce hyperoxic liver injury in hypermetabolic *animals* and despite reports of hepatotoxicity, including some fatalities, associated with propylthiouracil (p.1492), it has been investigated in the treatment of patients with alcoholic liver disease. In a 2-year double-blind study Orrego *et al.*[1] found the 13% mortality rate in patients receiving propylthiouracil 300 mg daily to be significantly lower than the 25% mortality rate in patients receiving placebo. The main effect of propylthiouracil appeared to be on acute alcoholic hepatitis as the difference in mortality rate was greatest during the first 12 weeks. However, Sherlock commented[2] that propylthiouracil had never gained general acceptance for the treatment of alcoholic liver disease.

1. Orrego H, *et al.* Long-term treatment of alcoholic liver disease with propylthiouracil. *N Engl J Med* 1987; **317:** 1421–7.
2. Sherlock S. Alcoholic liver disease. *Lancet* 1995; **345:** 227–9.

Psoriasis. Propylthiouracil has been tried orally[1] and topically[2] in a few patients with psoriasis (p.1075). The beneficial effects may be due to its immunomodulatory properties.

1. Elias AN, *et al.* Propylthiouracil in psoriasis: results of an open trial. *J Am Acad Dermatol* 1993; **29:** 78–81.
2. Elias AN, *et al.* A controlled trial of topical propylthiouracil in the treatment of patients with psoriasis. *J Am Acad Dermatol* 1994; **31:** 455–8.

Preparations

BP 1998: Propylthiouracil Tablets;
USP 23: Propylthiouracil Tablets.

Proprietary Preparations (details are given in Part 3)
Aust.: Prothiucil; ***Canad.:*** Propyl-Thyracil; ***Ger.:*** Propycil; Thyreostat II; ***Swed.:*** Tiotil.

Sodium Perchlorate (13255-p)

$NaClO_4$ = 122.4.
CAS — 7601-89-0 (anhydrous); 7791-07-3 (monohydrate).

WARNING. *Sodium perchlorate has been used for the illicit preparation of explosives or fireworks; care is required with its supply.*

Sodium perchlorate has actions and uses similar to those of potassium perchlorate (p.1496). A dose of 200 to 400 mg by mouth has been given 30 to 60 minutes before radionuclide brain scanning.

It has been used to treat hyperthyroidism (p.1489) in an initial dose of 800 mg to 1 g daily by mouth in divided doses, reduced as required to a maintenance dose of 400 mg daily. Because of their toxicity the perchlorates have largely been replaced by other antithyroid drugs.

Preparations

Proprietary Preparations (details are given in Part 3)
Aust.: Irenat; ***Ger.:*** Irenat.

Thyroglobulin (9007-n)

Thyroglobulin *(USAN, rINN).*
CAS — 9010-34-8.

Thyroglobulin is an extract obtained by the fractionation of porcine thyroid glands, which yields thyroxine and liothyronine on hydrolysis. It has been used in the treatment of hypothyroidism, but such treatment with mixtures of thyroid hormones and preparations of animal extracts is not recommended.

Preparations

Proprietary Preparations (details are given in Part 3)
S.Afr.: Proloid†; ***Spain:*** Proloide†.

Thyroid (9001-a)

Dry Thyroid; Getrocknete Schilddrüse; NSC-26492; Thyreoidin; Thyroid Extract; Thyroid Gland; Thyroidea; Thyroideum Siccum; Tiroide Secca.
Pharmacopoeias. In *Aust., Chin., Fr., Jpn,* and *US.*

Thyroid is the cleaned, dried, and powdered thyroid gland, previously deprived of connective tissue and fat, obtained from domesticated animals used for food by man. On hydrolysis it yields not less than 90% and not more than 110% each of the labelled amounts of thyroxine and liothyronine calculated on the dried basis. It is free from iodine in inorganic form or any combination other than that peculiar to the thyroid gland. It loses not more than 6% of its weight on drying. It may contain a suitable diluent such as glucose, lactose, sodium chloride, starch, or sucrose.

A yellowish to buff-coloured amorphous powder with a slight characteristic meat-like odour. **Store** in airtight containers.

Thyroid has been used in the treatment of hypothyroidism, but such treatment with mixtures of thyroid hormones and preparations of animal extracts is not recommended.

Preparations

USP 23: Thyroid Tablets.

Proprietary Preparations (details are given in Part 3)
Fr.: Tetrapongyl†; ***Ger.:*** Thyreoid-Dispert†; ***Ital.:*** Cinetic; ***Spain:*** Thyranon†; ***USA:*** S-P-T; Thyrar.

Multi-ingredient: ***Fr.:*** Iodorganine T†; ***Ger.:*** AntiFocal; ***Ital.:*** Moloco T†; Obesaic†.

Thyroxine Sodium (9008-h)

Thyroxine Sodium *(BANM)*.

Levothyroxine Sodium *(rINN)*; Levothyroxinnatrium; Levothyroxinum Natricum; 3,5,3′,5′-Tetra-iodo-L-thyronine Sodium; L-Thyroxine Sodium; Thyroxinum Natricum; Tirossina; Tiroxina Sodica. Sodium 4-*O*-(4-hydroxy-3,5-di-iodophenyl)-3,5-di-iodo-L-tyrosine hydrate.

$C_{15}H_{10}I_4NNaO_4,xH_2O$ = 798.9 (anhydrous).

CAS — 51-48-9 (L-thyroxine); 55-03-8 (thyroxine sodium, anhydrous); 25416-65-3 (thyroxine sodium, hydrate); 8065-29-0 (liotrix).

NOTE. The abbreviation T_4 is often used for endogenous thyroxine in medical and biochemical reports. Liotrix is the *USAN* name for a mixture of liothyronine sodium with thyroxine sodium.

Pharmacopoeias. In *Eur.* (see p.viii), *Int.*, *Jpn*, and *US.*
Int. includes the anhydrous. *Aust.* also includes a monograph on DL-thyroxine.

An odourless almost white to pale brownish-yellow, hygroscopic, amorphous or crystalline powder. It may assume a slight pink colour on exposure to light. It may be obtained from the thyroid gland of domesticated animals used for food by man or be prepared synthetically.

Very slightly **soluble** in water; slightly soluble in alcohol (1 in 300); practically insoluble in acetone, in chloroform, and in ether. It dissolves in aqueous solutions of alkali hydroxides and in hot solutions of alkali carbonates. A saturated solution in water has a pH of about 8.9. **Store** at 2° to 8° in airtight containers. Protect from light.

Adverse Effects and Treatment

The adverse effects of thyroxine are generally associated with excessive dosage and correspond to symptoms of hyperthyroidism. They may include tachycardia, palpitations, anginal pain, headache, nervousness, excitability, insomnia, tremors, muscle weakness and cramps, heat intolerance, sweating, flushing, fever, weight loss, menstrual irregularities, diarrhoea, and vomiting. These adverse reactions usually disappear after dosage reduction or temporary withdrawal of treatment. Thyroid storm has occasionally been reported following massive or chronic intoxication and convulsions, cardiac arrhythmias, heart failure, coma, and death have occurred.

In acute overdosage, gastric lavage or emesis induction should be considered to reduce gastro-intestinal absorption. Treatment is usually symptomatic and supportive; propranolol may be useful in controlling the symptoms of sympathetic overactivity. Thyroxine overdosage requires an extended follow-up period as symptoms may be delayed for several days due to the gradual peripheral conversion of thyroxine to tri-iodothyronine.

Carcinogenicity. An association between the use of thyroid hormones and an increased risk of breast cancer in women was proposed by Kapdi and Wolfe.[1] A further analysis by Mustacchi and Greenspan[2] of the data from the same group of patients did not confirm such an association nor did later studies by Wallace *et al.*,[3] Shapiro *et al.*,[4] and Hoffman *et al.*[5]

1. Kapdi CC, Wolfe JN. Breast cancer. Relationship to thyroid supplements for hypothyroidism. *JAMA* 1976; **236:** 1124–7.
2. Mustacchi P, Greenspan F. Thyroid supplementation for hypothyroidism. An iatrogenic cause of breast cancer? *JAMA* 1977; **237:** 1446–7.
3. Wallace RB, *et al.* Thyroid hormone use in patients with breast cancer. Absence of an association. *JAMA* 1978; **239:** 958.
4. Shapiro S, *et al.* Use of thyroid supplements in relation to the risk of breast cancer. *JAMA* 1980; **244:** 1685–7.
5. Hoffman DA, *et al.* Breast cancer in hypothyroid women using thyroid supplements. *JAMA* 1984; **251:** 616–19.

Effects on the bones. Hyperthyroidism is a known risk factor for osteoporosis and some studies have indicated that women receiving long-term thyroxine therapy may have decreased bone density or accelerated bone mineralisation and thus be at greater risk of developing osteoporosis.[1-5] The bone changes were greatest in those who had some degree of overtreatment resulting in subclinical hyperthyroidism (usually indicated by low TSH concentrations) and therefore strict attention to monitoring of therapy by using sensitive TSH assays, and possibly the use of bone studies, has been advised.[1-7] Conversely, Franklyn *et al.*[8] found no effect of long-term thyroxine treatment on bone density and neither did Ross[9] when he gave thyroxine short term to postmenopausal women with subclinical hypothyroidism. However, in another study[10] loss of bone density did occur in postmenopausal women taking relatively high doses of thyroxine (1.6 μg or more per kg body-weight daily) long term and appeared to be prevented by oestrogen replacement therapy.

1. Paul TL, *et al.* Long-term L-thyroxine therapy is associated with decreased hip bone density in premenopausal women. *JAMA* 1988; **259:** 3137–41.
2. Stall GM, *et al.* Accelerated bone loss in hypothyroid patients overtreated with L-thyroxine. *Ann Intern Med* 1990; **113:** 265–9.
3. Adlin EV, *et al.* Bone mineral density in postmenopausal women treated with L-thyroxine. *Am J Med* 1991; **90:** 360–6.
4. Kung AWC, Pun KK. Bone mineral density in premenopausal women receiving long-term physiological doses of levothyroxine. *JAMA* 1991; **265:** 2688–91.
5. Greenspan SL, *et al.* Skeletal integrity in premenopausal and postmenopausal women receiving long-term L-thyroxine therapy. *Am J Med* 1991; **91:** 5–14.
6. Anonymous. Thyroxine replacement therapy—too much of a good thing? *Lancet* 1990; **336:** 1352–3.
7. Ross DS. Monitoring L-thyroxine therapy: lessons from the effects of L-thyroxine on bone density. *Am J Med* 1991; **91:** 1–4.
8. Franklyn JA, *et al.* Long-term thyroxine treatment and bone mineral density. *Lancet* 1992; **340:** 9–13.
9. Ross DS. Bone density is not reduced during the short-term administration of levothyroxine to postmenopausal women with subclinical hypothyroidism: a randomized prospective study. *Am J Med* 1993; **95:** 385–8.
10. Schneider DL, *et al.* Thyroid hormone use and bone mineral density in elderly women: effects of estrogen. *JAMA* 1994; **271:** 1245–9.

Effects on the nervous system. Two children aged 8 and 11 years developed pseudotumour cerebri (benign intracranial hypertension) shortly after the initiation of thyroxine therapy for hypothyroidism.[1] There have been further reports on individual children[2,3] and infants.[4]

Partial complex status epilepticus, with confusion, agitation, and continuous myoclonic jerks in the left side of the face and left hand, was seen in a hypothyroid patient with Turner's syndrome who was receiving treatment with thyroxine for myxoedema coma.[5] The condition responded to anticonvulsant therapy; the patient subsequently remained seizure-free on a reduced dose of thyroxine and concomitant phenytoin.

1. Van Dop C, *et al.* Pseudotumor cerebri associated with initiation of levothyroxine therapy for juvenile hypothyroidism. *N Engl J Med* 1983; **308:** 1076–80.
2. McVie R. Pseudotumor cerebri and thyroid-replacement therapy. *N Engl J Med* 1983; **309:** 731.
3. Hymes LC, *et al.* Pseudotumor cerebri and thyroid-replacement therapy. *N Engl J Med* 1983; **309:** 732.
4. Raghavan S, *et al.* Pseudotumor cerebri in an infant after L-thyroxine therapy for transient neonatal hypothyroidism. *J Pediatr* 1997; **130:** 478–80.
5. Duarte J, *et al.* Thyroxine-induced partial complex status epilepticus. *Ann Pharmacother* 1993; **27:** 1139.

Hypersensitivity. A hypersensitivity reaction to synthetic thyroid hormones was reported in a 63-year-old hypothyroid woman with Hashimoto's thyroiditis.[1] Fever, eosinophilia, and liver dysfunction developed after replacement treatment with liothyronine or thyroxine, but disappeared when therapy was discontinued. After an interval of 4 months liothyronine was gradually reintroduced without adverse effect.

Urticaria and angioedema has been described in one patient who received thyroid and thyroxine.[2] In a further case similar reactions were attributed to the presence of sunset yellow as colouring agent in the proprietary thyroxine preparation.[3]

1. Shibata H, *et al.* Hypersensitivity caused by synthetic thyroid hormones in a hypothyroid patient with Hashimoto's thyroiditis. *Arch Intern Med* 1986; **146:** 1624–5.
2. Pandya AG, *et al.* Chronic urticaria associated with exogenous thyroid use. *Arch Dermatol* 1990; **126:** 1238–9.
3. Lévesque H, *et al.* Reporting adverse drug reactions by proprietary name. *Lancet* 1991; **338:** 393.

Overdosage. The clinical features and management of overdosage with thyroid drugs have been reviewed.[1] Although aggressive therapy is not normally justified in asymptomatic patients, various regimens have been tried.

Binimelis and colleagues have described six adults who ingested massive doses of thyroxine ranging from 70 to 1200 mg over 2 to 12 days due to an error in the pharmaceutical preparation.[2] All the patients developed symptoms of thyrotoxicosis within 3 days of taking the first dose. Treatment to reduce the conversion of L-thyroxine to L-tri-iodothyronine was tried using propranolol 120 to 140 mg daily, with hydrocortisone 400 mg daily, and in 3 patients, propylthiouracil 400 to 1200 mg daily, but the benefits of such therapy were considered doubtful. Seven to 10 days after the first dose of thyroxine, all 6 patients developed neurological complications and 5 went into coma. Cardiac disturbances were also noted; 2 had left ventricular failure and 3 developed severe arrhythmias. As clinical status deteriorated, plasmapheresis and charcoal haemoperfusion were both found to increase the elimination of L-thyroxine from serum. Plasmapheresis appeared to be the more effective procedure, though the magnitude of the extraction of L-thyroxine depended on the serum concentration of L-thyroxine. One patient died of septic shock and acute renal failure; the other 5 recovered after troubled courses.

In a further study[3] of 41 children aged 1 to 5 years who had accidentally ingested estimated amounts of thyroxine sodium ranging from 0.05 to 13 mg, symptoms of hyperthyroidism occurred in only 11 between 12 hours and 11 days after ingestion. Treatment was limited to initial measures to decrease absorption; no adverse effect was considered severe enough to warrant specific symptomatic treatment and all symptoms fully resolved within 14 days. These findings appeared to be consistent with previous reports, although Kulig *et al.*[4] had described a 2-year-old boy who developed clinical signs of hyperthyroidism and suffered 2 episodes of tonic-clonic seizures 7 days after the ingestion of up to 18 mg of thyroxine sodium. However, since serious complications appeared to be uncommon and most symptoms remitted without treatment, a conservative approach to the management of acute thyroxine overdosage in children was recommended.[3]

1. Lin T-H, *et al.* Clinical features and management of overdosage with thyroid drugs. *Med Toxicol* 1988; **3:** 264–72.
2. Binimelis J, *et al.* Massive thyroxine intoxication: evaluation of plasma extraction. *Intensive Care Med* 1987; **13:** 33–8.
3. Golightly LK, *et al.* Clinical effects of accidental levothyroxine ingestion in children. *Am J Dis Child* 1987; **141:** 1025–7.
4. Kulig K, *et al.* Levothyroxine overdosage associated with seizures in a young child. *JAMA* 1985; **254:** 2109–10.

Precautions

Thyroxine is contra-indicated in untreated hyperthyroidism. It should be used with extreme caution in patients with cardiovascular disorders including angina, heart failure, myocardial infarction, and hypertension; lower initial doses, smaller increments, and longer intervals between increases should be used as necessary. An ECG performed before starting treatment with thyroxine may help to distinguish underlying myocardial ischaemia from changes induced by hypothyroidism. Thyroxine should also be introduced very gradually in elderly patients and those with long-standing hypothyroidism to avoid any sudden increase in metabolic demands. It should not be given to patients with adrenal insufficiency without adequate corticosteroid cover otherwise the thyroid replacement therapy might precipitate an acute adrenal crisis. Care is also required when thyroxine is given to patients with diabetes mellitus or diabetes insipidus.

Tests of thyroid function are subject to alteration by a number of nonthyroidal clinical conditions and by a wide variety of drugs, some of which are mentioned under Interactions, below.

Adrenocortical insufficiency. Thyroid-hormone replacement without concomitant treatment with corticosteroids may precipitate acute adrenocortical insufficiency in patients with impaired adrenocortical function, including those with subclinical or unrecognised adrenocortical disease.[1] Adrenocortical insufficiency should be suspected in patients who develop symptoms of lassitude, malaise, weight loss, and hypotension; prompt diagnosis and replacement of corticosteroids could prevent the development of a potentially fatal crisis. In commenting on this report, Davis and Sheppard[2] point out that a raised concentration of thyroid-stimulating-hormone alone may not necessarily imply hypothyroidism in patients with chronic adrenocortical insufficiency. Even confirmed hypothyroidism in these patients may not be permanent.

1. Fonseca V, *et al.* Acute adrenal crisis precipitated by thyroxine. *Br Med J* 1986; **292:** 1185–6.
2. Davis J, Sheppard M. Acute adrenal crisis precipitated by thyroxine. *Br Med J* 1986; **292:** 1595.

Cardiovascular disorders. There is a complex relationship between the heart and thyroid.[1] Cardiovascular abnormalities may be associated with hypothyroidism as well as with thyroxine replacement therapy, hence the need for caution.

1. Gammage M, Franklyn J. Hypothyroidism, thyroxine treatment, and the heart. *Heart* 1997; **77:** 189–90.

Myasthenia. Thyroid hormones may occasionally precipitate or exacerbate a pre-existing myasthenic syndrome.[1,2]

1. Mastaglia FL. Adverse effects of drugs on muscle. *Drugs* 1982; **24:** 304–21.
2. Lane RJM, Routledge PA. Drug-induced neurological disorders. *Drugs* 1983; **26:** 124–47.

Pregnancy and breast feeding. Most authorities consider that thyroid hormones do not readily cross the placenta. Placental transfer has been reported,[1] but in amounts so limited that a mother with physiological concentrations of thyroxine and tri-iodothyronine would not provide normal thyroid hormone concentrations to a fetus with congenital hypothyroidism.[2-4]

Minimal amounts of thyroid hormones are distributed into breast milk.[5] There is insufficient thyroid hormone to meet the biological needs of a suckling infant with a nonfunctioning thyroid gland but it has been suggested that thyroxine in breast milk might mask any hypothyroidism in the suckling newborn.[6]

1. Vulsma T, *et al.* Maternal-fetal transfer of thyroxine in congenital hypothyroidism due to a total organification defect or thyroid agenesis. *N Engl J Med* 1989; **321:** 13–16.
2. Sack J, *et al.* Maternal-fetal transfer of thyroxine. *N Engl J Med* 1989; **321:** 1549–50.
3. Bachrach LK, Burrow GN. Maternal-fetal transfer of thyroxine. *N Engl J Med* 1989; **321:** 1549.
4. Vulsma T, *et al.* Maternal-fetal transfer of thyroxine. *N Engl J Med* 1989; **321:** 1550.
5. Bennett PN, ed. *Drugs and human lactation.* Amsterdam: Elsevier, 1988.
6. Anonymous. Can a woman on thyroxine safely breast-feed her baby? *Br Med J* 1977; **2:** 1589.

Interactions

As thyroid status influences metabolic activity and most body systems, correction of hypothyroidism with thyroid agents may affect other disease states and their treatment. In hypothyroid diabetics for instance, the initiation of thyroid replacement therapy may increase their *insulin* or *oral hypoglycaemic* requirements.[1] Thyroid status can also affect drug metabolism and clearance. Studies have indicated that plasma concentrations of *propranolol* are reduced in hyperthyroidism compared with the euthyroid state, probably due to increased clearance[2-5] and hypothyroid patients receiving chronic propranolol therapy have had a reduction in plasma-propranolol concentrations when given thyroxine treatment[3] (propranolol can also reduce the activity of thyroxine, see below). Similarly, serum-digoxin concentrations appear to be lower in hyperthyroidism and higher in hypothyroidism[6] which may contribute in part to the observed insensitivity of hyperthyroid patients to *digoxin* therapy[7] although other mechanisms have been proposed.[8]

Thyroid status can itself be altered by a number of disease states such as chronic active liver disorders[9] and by a range of drugs. Some drugs such as *lithium* and *iodide* act directly on the thyroid gland and inhibit the release of thyroid hormones leading to clinical hypothyroidism.[10]

Enzyme-induction by drugs such as *chloroquine*,[11] *rifampicin*,[12] *carbamazepine*,[13,14] *phenytoin*,[14,15] or *barbiturates*[12] enhances thyroid hormone metabolism resulting in reduced serum concentrations of thyroid hormones. Therefore, patients on thyroid replacement therapy may require an increase in their dose of thyroid hormone if these drugs are given concurrently[16] and a decrease if the enzyme-inducing drug is withdrawn.[17]

Other drugs such as *amiodarone*[18] and *propranolol*[19,20] may inhibit the de-iodination of thyroxine to tri-iodothyronine resulting in a decreased concentration of tri-iodothyronine with a concomitant rise in the concentration of inactive reverse tri-iodothyronine.

The protein binding of thyroid hormones may be altered by drug treatment. For example, *oral contraceptives*[10] may induce an oestrogen-dependent rise in thyroxine-binding globulin and the total thyroid hormone bound to it, whereas androgen administration reduces the concentration of the binding globulin, and has resulted in clinical hyperthyroidism when given to postmenopausal women maintained on thyroxine replacement therapy.[21] Drugs such as *phenytoin*,[15] *carbamazepine*, and *fenclofenac*[22] may reduce protein binding by displacing the thyroid hormones from their plasma-binding sites. As thyroid hormones are highly protein bound, changes in binding might be expected to influence requirements in thyroid replacement therapy, but in practice there is little clinical evidence of any problems except with thyroid-function testing (see below).

Cholestyramine, an anionic exchange resin, significantly reduces the absorption of ingested thyroxine by binding with thyroid hormones in the gastro-intestinal tract. The malabsorption of thyroxine is minimised by allowing an interval of 4 to 5 hours to elapse between the ingestion of the two drugs.[23] A similar effect has been observed with *sodium polystyrene sulphonate*.[24] *Sucralfate* also reduces absorption of thyroxine from the gastro-intestinal tract[25,26] as does *aluminium hydroxide*,[27] *calcium carbonate*,[28] and *ferrous sulphate*.[29]

Thyroid hormones enhance the effects of *oral anticoagulants*. Patients on anticoagulant therapy therefore require careful monitoring when treatment with thyroid agents is initiated or altered as the oral anticoagulant dose may need to be adjusted (see under the interactions of Warfarin, p.969).

Thyroid agents increase metabolic demands and should therefore be used with caution with drugs known to influence cardiac function, such as the *sympathomimetics*, as they may enhance this effect. In addition, thyroid hormones may increase receptor sensitivity to catecholamines. Such a mechanism has been proposed to explain the increase in response to *tricyclic antidepressants* observed when thyroid agents are given concurrently.[30,31]

Isolated reports of drugs interacting with thyroid agents include *ketamine* (severe hypertension and tachycardia)[32] and *lovastatin*.[33,34]

1. Refetoff S. Thyroid hormone therapy. *Med Clin North Am* 1975; **59:** 1147–62.
2. Feely J, *et al.* Increased clearance of propranolol in thyrotoxicosis. *Ann Intern Med* 1981; **94:** 472–4.
3. Feely J, *et al.* Plasma propranolol steady state concentrations in thyroid disorders. *Eur J Clin Pharmacol* 1981; **19:** 329–33.
4. Aro A, *et al.* Pharmacokinetics of propranolol and sotalol in hyperthyroidism. *Eur J Clin Pharmacol* 1982; **21:** 373–7.
5. Hallengren B, *et al.* Influence of hyperthyroidism on the kinetics of methimazole, propranolol, metoprolol, and atenolol. *Eur J Clin Pharmacol* 1982; **21:** 379–84.
6. Croxson MS, Ibbertson HK. Serum digoxin in patients with thyroid disease. *Br Med J* 1975; **3:** 566–8.
7. Huffman DH, *et al.* Digoxin in hyperthyroidism. *Clin Pharmacol Ther* 1977; **22:** 533–7.
8. Lawrence JR, *et al.* Digoxin kinetics in patients with thyroid dysfunction. *Clin Pharmacol Ther* 1977; **22:** 7–13.
9. Schussler GC, *et al.* Increased serum thyroid hormone binding and decreased free hormone in chronic active liver disease. *N Engl J Med* 1978; **299:** 510–15.
10. Ramsay I. Drugs and non-thyroid induced changes in thyroid function tests. *Postgrad Med J* 1985; **61:** 375–7.
11. Munera Y, *et al.* Interaction of thyroxine sodium with antimalarial drugs. *Br Med J* 1997; **314:** 1593.
12. Ohnhaus EE, Studer H. A link between liver microsomal enzyme activity and thyroid hormone metabolism in man. *Br J Clin Pharmacol* 1983; **15:** 71–6.
13. Connell JMC, *et al.* Changes in circulating thyroid hormones during short-term hepatic enzyme induction with carbamazepine. *Eur J Clin Pharmacol* 1984; **26:** 453–6.
14. Larkin JG, *et al.* Thyroid hormone concentrations in epileptic patients. *Eur J Clin Pharmacol* 1989; **36:** 213–6.
15. Franklyn JA, *et al.* Measurement of free thyroid hormones in patients on long-term phenytoin therapy. *Eur J Clin Pharmacol* 1984; **26:** 633–4.
16. Blackshear JL, *et al.* Thyroxine replacement requirements in hypothyroid patients receiving phenytoin. *Ann Intern Med* 1983; **99:** 341–2.
17. Hoffbrand BI. Barbiturate/thyroid-hormone interaction. *Lancet* 1979; **ii:** 903–4.
18. Hershman JM, *et al.* Thyroxine and triiodothyronine kinetics in cardiac patients taking amiodarone. *Acta Endocrinol (Copenh)* 1986; **111:** 193–9.
19. Chambers JB, *et al.* The effects of propranolol on thyroxine metabolism and triiodothyronines production in man. *J Clin Pharmacol* 1982; **22:** 110–16.
20. Wilkins MR, *et al.* Effect of propranolol on thyroid homeostasis of healthy volunteers. *Postgrad Med J* 1985; **61:** 391–4.
21. Arafah BM. Decreased levothyroxine requirement in women with hypothyroidism during androgen therapy for breast cancer. *Ann Intern Med* 1994; **121:** 247–51.
22. Humphrey MJ, *et al.* Fenclofenac and thyroid hormone concentrations. *Lancet* 1980; **i:** 487–8.
23. Northcutt RC, *et al.* The influence of cholestyramine on thyroxine absorption. *JAMA* 1969; **208:** 1857–61.
24. McLean M, *et al.* Cation-exchange resin and inhibition of intestinal absorption of thyroxine. *Lancet* 1993; **341:** 1286.
25. Sherman SI, *et al.* Sucralfate causes malabsorption of L-thyroxine. *Am J Med* 1994; **96:** 531–5.
26. Campbell JA, *et al.* Sucralfate and the absorption of L-thyroxine. *Ann Intern Med* 1994; **121:** 152.
27. Liel Y, *et al.* Nonspecific intestinal adsorption of levothyroxine by aluminium hydroxide. *Am J Med* 1994; **97:** 363–5.
28. Schneyer CR. Calcium carbonate and reduction of levothyroxine efficacy. *JAMA* 1998; **279:** 750.
29. Campbell NRC, *et al.* Ferrous sulfate reduces thyroxine efficacy in patients with hypothyroidism. *Ann Intern Med* 1992; **117:** 1010–13.
30. Banki CM. Cerebrospinal fluid amine metabolites after combined amitriptyline-triiodothyronine treatment of depressed women. *Eur J Clin Pharmacol* 1977; **11:** 311–15.
31. Goodwin FK, *et al.* Potentiation of antidepressant effects by L-triiodothyronine in tricyclic nonresponders. *Am J Psychiatry* 1982; **139:** 34–8.
32. Kaplan JA, Cooperman LH. Alarming reactions to ketamine in patients taking thyroid medication-treatment with propranolol. *Anesthesiology* 1971; **35:** 229–30.
33. Demke DM. Drug interaction between thyroxine and lovastatin. *N Engl J Med* 1989; **321:** 1341–2.
34. Gormley GJ, Tobert JA. Drug interaction between thyroxine and lovastatin. *N Engl J Med* 1989; **321:** 1342.

Pharmacokinetics

Thyroxine is variably but adequately absorbed from the gastro-intestinal tract following oral administration. Fasting increases absorption. Once in the circulation, thyroxine is extensively protein bound, principally to thyroxine-binding globulin (TBG) but also to a lesser extent to thyroxine-binding pre-albumin (TBPA) or to albumin. Thyroxine has a plasma half-life in euthyroidism of about 6 to 7 days; the half-life is prolonged in hypothyroidism and reduced in hyperthyroidism.

Thyroxine is primarily metabolised in the liver and kidney to tri-iodothyronine (liothyronine) and, about 40%, to inactive reverse tri-iodothyronine, both of which undergo further deiodination to inactive metabolites. Further metabolites result from the deamination and decarboxylation of thyroxine to tetrac.

Thyroxine is reported to undergo enterohepatic recycling and excretion in the faeces.

The distribution of thyroid hormones across the placenta and into breast milk is discussed under Pregnancy and Breast Feeding (above).

Uses and Administration

Thyroxine is a thyroid hormone (see p.1489 for a description of the endogenous hormones) used as replacement therapy in the treatment of hypothyroidism (p.1490). It is given in conditions such as diffuse non-toxic goitre (see Goitre and Thyroid Nodules, p.1489) and Hashimoto's thyroiditis (see Hypothyroidism, p.1490) to suppress the secretion of thyroid-stimulating hormone (TSH) and hence prevent or reverse enlargement of the thyroid gland. Thyroxine is also used to suppress TSH production in the treatment of thyroid carcinoma (p.494) and as a diagnostic agent for the differential diagnosis of hyperthyroidism. It is given with antithyroid drugs in the management of hyperthyroidism (p.1489).

The peak therapeutic effect of regular oral administration of thyroxine may not be achieved until after several weeks and there is a slow response to changes in dosage. Similarly, effects may persist for several weeks after withdrawal. Thyroxine is given as the sodium salt in a single daily dose. Its absorption can be irregular and it is probably best taken on an empty stomach, usually before breakfast.

The dose of thyroxine sodium for the treatment of any thyroid disorder should be individualised on the basis of clinical response and biochemical tests and should be monitored regularly.

In **hypothyroidism** the initial adult dose of thyroxine sodium is 50 to 100 μg daily by mouth increased by increments of 25 to 50 μg every 4 weeks or more until the thyroid deficiency is corrected and a maintenance dose is established. The adult maintenance dose is usually between 100 and 200 μg daily. In elderly patients, in those with cardiovascular disorders, or in those with severe hypothyroidism of long standing, treatment should be introduced more gradually: an initial dose of 25 to 50 μg daily increased by increments of 25 μg at intervals of 4 weeks may be appropriate.

In children, individualisation of dosage and monitoring of treatment is especially important. One suggested regimen for the treatment of congenital hypothyroidism is 25 μg initially and increased by increments of 25 μg every 2 to 4 weeks until mild toxic symptoms appear, at which time the dosage is slightly reduced. Similar doses may be used for juvenile myxoedema except that children over 1 year of age may be given 2.5 to 5 μg per kg body-weight daily initially.

Thyroxine sodium may also be given by the nasogastric route or by intravenous injection. It has also been given intramuscularly. In myxoedema (hypothyroid) coma a suggested dose by intravenous injection is 200 to 500 μg initially, followed by daily supplements of 100 to 200 μg until the patient is euthyroid and can tolerate administration by mouth.

General references.

1. Mandel SJ, *et al.* Levothyroxine therapy in patients with thyroid disease. *Ann Intern Med* 1993; **119:** 492–502.
2. Toft AD. Thyroxine therapy. *N Engl J Med* 1994; **331:** 174–80. Correction. *ibid.*; 1035.

Administration. There has been controversy over the bioequivalence or otherwise of different brands of thyroxine. Most studies and reports have come from the USA and results may have depended to some extent on the particular brands compared. Formulations may also have changed which makes comparison of results difficult. A recently published study[1] concluded that 2 generic thyroxine products were bioequivalent and interchangeable with 2 branded products.

1. Dong BJ, *et al.* Bioequivalence of generic and brand-name levothyroxine products in the treatment of hypothyroidism. *JAMA* 1997; **277:** 1205–13.

Depression. While thyroid hormones may increase the activity of tricyclic antidepressants, as mentioned under Interactions (see above), the benefits in the treatment of refractory depression (p.271) are debatable. A meta-analysis[1] of 8 studies involving 292 patients treated with liothyronine in addition to tricyclic antidepressants indicated that such therapy was effective in a subgroup of cases but that the small number of patients studied made additional placebo-controlled data desirable. It was also noted that current trends in the treatment of depression favoured drugs other than tricyclics, so that future trials with liothyronine may need to investigate combination treatment with selective serotonin reuptake inhibitors.

1. Aronson R, *et al.* Triiodothyronine augmentation in the treatment of refractory depression: a meta-analysis. *Arch Gen Psychiatry* 1996; **53:** 842–8.

Obesity. Thyroid drugs have been tried in the treatment of obesity (p.1476) in euthyroid patients, but they produce only temporary weight loss, mainly of lean body-mass, and can produce serious adverse effects, especially cardiac complications.[1] Hypothyroidism has also been reported[2] when these drugs were withdrawn from previously euthyroid patients being treated for simple obesity. It has also been noted that thyroxine is probably being abused by some athletes to promote weight loss.[3]

1. Rivlin RS. Therapy of obesity with hormones. *N Engl J Med* 1975; **292:** 26–9.
2. Dornhorst A, *et al.* Possible iatrogenic hypothyroidism. *Lancet* 1981; **i:** 52.
3. MacAuley D. Drugs in sport. *Br Med J* 1996; **313:** 211–15.

Urticaria. There is some suggestion that chronic urticaria (p.1076) may be associated with thyroid autoimmunity and that treatment with thyroid hormones may result in clinical remission.[1] In one study, a nine-year-old boy was successfully treated for chronic urticaria with thyroxine therapy at doses of 50 to 100 μg daily.[2] The workers advised screening for thyroid function and anti-thyroid microsomal antibodies in cases of chronic urticaria as these patients may benefit from thyroid hormone therapy.

1. Rumbyrt JS, *et al.* Resolution of chronic urticaria in patients with thyroid autoimmunity. *J Allergy Clin Immunol* 1995; **96:** 901–5.
2. Dreyfus DH, *et al.* Steroid-resistant chronic urticaria associated with anti-thyroid microsomal antibodies in a nine-year-old boy. *J Pediatr* 1996; **128:** 576–8.

Preparations

BP 1998: Levothyroxine Tablets;
USP 23: Levothyroxine Sodium Tablets; Liotrix Tablets.

Proprietary Preparations (details are given in Part 3)
Aust.: Euthyrox; Thyrex; ***Austral.:*** Oroxine; ***Belg.:*** Elthyrone; Euthyrox; Thyrax; ***Canad.:*** Eltroxin; Levo-T; Synthroid; ***Fr.:*** Levothyrox; Percutacrine Thyroxinique†; ***Ger.:*** Berlthyrox; Eferox; Euthyrox; Thevier; ***Irl.:*** Eltroxin; ***Ital.:*** Eutirox; Levotirox†; ***Neth.:*** Eltroxin; Euthyrox; Thyrax; ***S.Afr.:*** Eltroxin; ***Spain:*** Dexnon; Levothroid; Thyrax; ***Swed.:*** Levaxin; ***Switz.:*** Eltroxine; ***UK:*** Eltroxin; ***USA:*** Eltroxin; Levo-T; Levothroid; Levoxyl; Synthroid.

Multi-ingredient: ***Aust.:*** Combithyrex; Jodthyrox; Novothyral; Prothyrid†; ***Belg.:*** Novothyral; ***Fr.:*** Euthyral; ***Ger.:*** Jodthyrox; Novothyral; Prothyrid; Thyreocomb N; Thyreotom; Thyronajod; ***Ital.:*** Dermocinetic; Somatoline; ***S.Afr.:*** Diotroxin; ***Switz.:*** Novothyral; ***USA:*** Thyrolar.

Tiratricol (9009-m)

Tiratricol (*rINN*).

Triac; Triiodothyroacetic Acid. [4-(4-Hydroxy-3-iodophenoxy)-3,5-di-iodophenyl]acetic acid.

$C_{14}H_9I_3O_4$ = 621.9.

CAS — 51-24-1.

NOTE. Tri-ac has also been used as a name for proprietary preparations containing other drugs.

Tiratricol, a metabolite of tri-iodothyronine, is reported to be less active than the thyroid hormones but is given by mouth to suppress the secretion of thyroid-stimulating hormone.

Preparations

Proprietary Preparations (details are given in Part 3)
Fr.: Teatrois; Triacana.

Vaccines Immunoglobulins and Antisera

Described in this section are immunological agents used for both active immunisation and passive immunisation.

Active immunisation is a process of increasing resistance to infection whereby micro-organisms or products of their activity act as antigens and stimulate certain body cells to produce antibodies with a specific protective capacity. It may be a natural process following recovery from an infection, or an artificial process following the administration of *vaccines*. It is inevitably a slow process dependent upon the rate at which the antibody formation can be developed. Although the terms vaccination and immunisation are often used synonymously and interchangeably, *vaccination* simply refers to the administration of a vaccine whereas *immunisation* implies the development of protective levels of antibodies confirmed usually by serological testing.

Passive immunisation, which results in immediate protection of short duration, may be achieved by the administration of the antibodies themselves usually in the form of *antisera* (of animal origin) or *immunoglobulins*.

Antisera (7931-r)

Antisera (immunosera) are sterile preparations containing immunoglobulins obtained from the serum of immunised animals by purification. The term antisera includes antitoxins, which are antibodies that combine with and neutralise specific toxins, and antivenins, which are antitoxins directed against the toxic principle of the venoms of poisonous animals such as certain snakes and arthropods.

Antisera are obtained from healthy animals immunised by injections of the appropriate toxins or toxoids, venins, or suspensions of micro-organisms or other antigens. The specific immunoglobulins may be obtained from the serum by fractional precipitation and enzyme treatment or by other chemical or physical means. A suitable antimicrobial preservative may be added, and is invariably added if the product is issued in multidose containers. The Ph. Eur. directs that when antisera contain phenol, the concentration is not more than 0.25%. The antiserum is distributed aseptically into sterile containers which are sealed so as to exclude micro-organisms. Alternatively they may be supplied as freeze-dried preparations for reconstitution immediately before use.

Adverse Effects and Precautions

Reactions are liable to occur after the injection of any serum of animal origin. Anaphylaxis (type I hypersensitivity reaction, p.397) may occur, with hypotension, dyspnoea, urticaria, and shock which requires management as a medical emergency (see p.816).

Serum sickness (type III hypersensitivity reaction, see p.397) may occur, frequently 7 to 10 days after the injection of serum of animal origin.

Before injecting serum, information should be obtained whenever possible as to whether previous injections of serum have been received and whether the patient is subject to hypersensitivity disorders. Sensitivity testing should be performed before the administration of antisera. The patient must be kept under observation after the administration of full doses of antisera. Adrenaline injection and resuscitation facilities should be available.

Uses and Administration

Antisera have the specific power of neutralising venins or bacterial toxins, or combining with the bacterium, virus, or other antigen used for their preparation. Most antisera in current use are antitoxins or antivenins. The use of antisera to induce passive immunity has declined; immunoglobulins are preferred. Although antisera are defined as being of animal origin (see above), the term antisera has been used in some countries to describe antitoxins of human origin (immunoglobulins).

Immunoglobulins (3893-f)

Immunoglobulins are produced by B lymphocytes as part of the humoral response to foreign antigens. Immunoglobulins used in clinical practice are preparations containing antibodies, usually prepared from human plasma or serum, and mainly comprise IgG. Normal immunoglobulin, prepared from material from blood donors, contains several antibodies against infectious diseases prevalent in the general population, whereas specific immunoglobulins contain minimum specified levels of one antibody. Antibodies may also be prepared by genetic engineering techniques.

Adverse Effects

Local reactions with pain and tenderness at the site of intramuscular injection may follow the administration of immunoglobulins. Hypersensitivity reactions, including, rarely, anaphylactic reactions, have also been reported; such reactions, though, are far less frequent than following the use of antisera of animal origin.

Some immunoglobulins are available as intravenous preparations. Systemic reactions with fever, chills, facial flushing, headache, and nausea may occur following their administration, particularly at high rates of infusion.

Precautions

Strenuous efforts are made to screen human donor material used in the preparation of immunoglobulins; the transmission of infections (including hepatitis B and HIV) which has been associated with the use of certain blood products (see p.713) does not appear to be a problem with the immunoglobulins currently in use.

IgA, present in some immunoglobulin preparations, may give rise to the production of anti-IgA antibodies in patients with IgA deficiencies with the consequent risk of anaphylactic reactions. For precautions in such patients see Hypersensitivity under Adverse Effects and Precautions in Normal Immunoglobulins, p.1522.

Interactions

Immunoglobulins may interfere with the ability of live vaccines to induce an immune response and a suitable interval should separate administration of the two (see p.1501).

Reviews of possible interactions between immunoglobulins and other drugs.

1. Grabenstein JD. Drug interactions involving immunologic agents. Part I. Vaccine-vaccine, vaccine-immunoglobulin, and vaccine-drug interactions. *DICP Ann Pharmacother* 1990; **24:** 67–81.
2. Grabenstein JD. Drug interactions involving immunologic agents. Part II. Immunodiagnostic and other immunologic drug interactions. *DICP Ann Pharmacother* 1990; **24:** 186–93.

Uses and Administration

Immunoglobulins are used for passive immunisation, thus conferring immediate protection against some infectious diseases. They are preferred to antisera of animal origin as the incidence of adverse reactions is less.

It is generally important to follow the conferment of passive immunity, which is largely an emergency procedure, by the injection of suitable antigens to produce active immunity.

Monoclonal antibodies. While the use of specific immunoglobulins provides a safer method of delivering antibodies than the use of animal-derived antisera, there are still problems with availability, safety, and efficacy. The development of monoclonal antibodies (MAbs) provides an alternative and possibly superior source of antibodies for clinical use. Potential advantages over immunoglobulins include lower doses, greater specificity, and freedom from the risk of transmission of blood-borne infections. Not least is the ability to produce antibodies not only against infective agents but also against a wide range of antigens with potential applications including cardiovascular disease, transplantation, malignancies, and auto-immune disorders. Murine MAbs have been used clinically, but their use is limited by the production of human anti-murine antibodies. The preparation of human MAbs has presented some technical difficulties although these are now being overcome, and the use of genetic manipulation to produce humanised murine MAbs has met with some success.

Vaccines (7930-x)

Vaccines are traditionally preparations of antigenic materials which are administered with the object of inducing in the recipient active immunity to specific infecting agents or toxins or antigens produced by them. They may contain living or killed micro-organisms, bacterial toxoids, or antigenic material from particular parts of the infecting organism which may be derived from the organism or produced by recombinant DNA technology. Vaccines may be single-component vaccines or mixed combined vaccines. Vaccines against non-infective diseases are being developed.

Storage. Advice concerning the effects of temperature on vaccines.

1. Miller LG, Loomis JH. Advice of manufacturers about effects of temperature on biologicals. *Am J Hosp Pharm* 1985; **42:** 843–8.
2. Longland PW, Rowbotham PC. Stability at room temperature of medicines normally recommended for cold storage. *Pharm J* 1987; **238:** 147–51 and 220 (correction).
3. Anonymous. Stability of vaccines. *Bull WHO* 1990; **68:** 118–20.
4. Casto DT, Brunell PA. Safe handling of vaccines. *Pediatrics* 1991; **87:** 108–12.
5. André FE. Stability of vaccines. *Br Med J* 1993; **307:** 939.

Adverse Effects

Administration of a vaccine by injection may be followed by a local reaction, possibly with inflammation and lymphangitis. An induration or sterile abscess may develop at the site of injected vaccine. Administration may be followed by fever, headache, and malaise starting a few hours after injection and lasting for 1 or 2 days. Hypersensitivity reactions may occur and anaphylaxis has been reported rarely.

Further details, if appropriate, of adverse effects of vaccines may be found in the respective individual monographs.

The introduction of routine childhood vaccination has been accompanied by concerns over the safety and possible long term sequelae of some commonly used vaccines. Difficulties have arisen in distinguishing temporal and causal associations and in some cases the perceived dangers of vaccination have impeded uptake. Among the disorders temporally associated with childhood vaccination are neurological disorders, sudden infant death syndrome, and demyelinating disorders. Information on adverse effects associated with specific vaccines can be found under individual monographs.

References.

1. Stratton KR, *et al.* Adverse events associated with childhood vaccines other than pertussis and rubella: summary of a report from the Institute of Medicine. *JAMA* 1994; **271:** 1602–5.
2. Mitchell EA, *et al.* Immunisation and the sudden infant death syndrome. *Arch Dis Child* 1995; **73:** 498–501.
3. Freed GL, *et al.* Safety of vaccinations: Miss America, the media, and public health. *JAMA* 1996; **276:** 1869–72.

4. Centers for Disease Control. Update: vaccine side effects, adverse reactions, contraindications, and precautions: recommendations of the Advisory Committee on Immunization Practices (ACIP). *MMWR* 1996; **45** (RR-12): 1–45.
5. Braun MM, Ellenberg SS. Descriptive epidemiology of adverse events after immunization: reports to the vaccine adverse event reporting system (VAERS), 1991-1994. *J Pediatr* 1997; **131:** 529–35.
6. Jefferson T. Vaccination and its adverse effects: real or perceived. *Br Med J* 1998; **317:** 159–60.
7. Ball LK, *et al.* Risky business: challenges in vaccine risk communication. *Pediatrics* 1998; **101:** 453–8.

Effects of contaminating cytokines. Cytokines, including interleukin-6, interleukin-1, granulocyte colony-stimulating factor, and granulocyte-macrophage colony-stimulating factor were detected in some viral vaccines produced from mammalian cell lines.[1] Significant levels of interleukin-6 were found in several vaccines, particularly rabies vaccines. Although interleukin-6 may act beneficially as an adjuvant potentiating the immune response to vaccines, the possibility of adverse effects of cytokines such as inflammatory reactions and the induction of anti-cytokine antibodies, albeit slight, should be considered.

1. Gearing AJH, *et al.* Demonstration of cytokines in biological medicines produced in mammalian cell lines. *Lancet* 1989; **ii:** 1011–12.

Effects on the nervous system. GUILLAIN-BARRÉ SYNDROME. Guillain-Barré syndrome (see p.1524) has occasionally been associated with vaccination, although causal relationships have been difficult to evaluate. Vaccines implicated include a swine influenza vaccine, diphtheria and tetanus vaccines, some rabies vaccines, and oral poliomyelitis vaccines.[1] A report by the Institute of Medicine in the USA, summarised by Stratton and colleagues,[2] concluded that there was evidence favouring a causal relation with tetanus or diphtheria and tetanus vaccines (mainly in immunocompromised patients), and with oral poliomyelitis vaccines, but that the evidence was inadequate for measles vaccines, inactivated poliomyelitis vaccines, hepatitis B vaccines, or haemophilus influenzae vaccines. See individual monographs for further details.

1. Awong IE, *et al.* Drug-associated Guillain-Barré syndrome: a literature review. *Ann Pharmacother* 1996; **30:** 173–80.
2. Stratton KR, *et al.* Adverse events associated with childhood vaccines other than pertussis and rubella: summary of a report from the Institute of Medicine. *JAMA* 1994; **271:** 1602–5.

Effects on the skin. Granuloma, in 3 patients, at the injection site of adsorbed vaccines.[1] Biopsy and microscopy suggested the granuloma to be due to aluminium used as the adsorbant in the vaccines.

1. Fawcett HA, Smith NP. Injection-site granuloma due to aluminum. *Arch Dermatol* 1984; **120:** 1318–22.

Febrile reactions. A discussion of the administration of paracetamol with childhood immunisations for prophylaxis against febrile reactions.[1] It was considered that such a practice could not be justified routinely unless it could be shown to decrease the incidence of post-immunisation seizures or collapse (hypotonic hyporesponsive episodes); studies to date were deemed inconclusive. Prophylactic oral paracetamol may, however, be considered for infants at higher than normal risk with each of the 3 primary diphtheria-tetanus-pertussis and polio immunisations. Parents should be advised to treat common minor reactions, such as fever or painful swelling at the site of injection, with paracetamol when they occur (see also Fever and Hyperthermia, p.1).

1. Anonymous. Prophylactic paracetamol with childhood immunisation? *Drug Ther Bull* 1990; **28:** 73–4.

Precautions

Vaccination should be postponed in patients suffering from any acute illness although minor infections without fever or systemic upset are not regarded as contra-indications.

Enquiry regarding previous hypersensitivity, either local or generalised, should precede the administration of a vaccine and measures to treat hypersensitivity reactions up to and including anaphylactic shock (p.816) should be immediately available. Immunisation should not be carried out in individuals who have previously had a severe local or generalised reaction to the vaccine. Reactions which should be regarded as severe include extensive redness and swelling with induration involving large areas of the vaccinated limb, fever of 39.5° or more within 48 hours of vaccination, anaphylaxis, bronchospasm, laryngeal oedema, generalised collapse, prolonged unresponsiveness, prolonged inconsolable or high-pitched screaming (more than 4 hours), convulsions, or encephalopathy within 72 hours. Some vaccines contain small amounts of antibiotics and should not be given to patients with a history of anaphylaxis to the agent used. Caution should be observed in patients with less severe manifestations of antibiotic hypersensitivity. Additionally some vaccines are prepared using hens' eggs and a history of anaphylaxis to the ingestion of eggs is a contra-indication to the use of such vaccines. Similarly, caution should be observed in patients with less severe manifestations of egg hypersensitivity. Asthma, eczema, hay fever, or a history of other allergies, should not be regarded as contra-indications to vaccination.

Before injection of a vaccine any alcohol or disinfectant used for cleansing the skin should be allowed to evaporate otherwise inactivation of live vaccines may occur.

It is recommended that immunisation of infants should not be postponed because of prematurity and that the normal schedules and timings based on the actual birth date should be adhered to.

Certain precautions and contra-indications apply specifically to vaccines containing live attenuated micro-organisms.

Live vaccines should not be given to patients receiving immunosuppressive therapy (see under Interactions, below); to patients suffering from certain malignant conditions such as lymphoma, leukaemia, Hodgkin's disease, or other tumours of the reticuloendothelial system; to patients who have received bone-marrow transplants within the previous 6 months (after which time they should have their immune status checked and be immunised appropriately); or to patients with other types of impaired immunological responses, such as hypogammaglobulinaemia.

It should be remembered that the immune response to all vaccines (live or inactivated) may be diminished in immunocompromised patients.

Live vaccines should not be administered during pregnancy because of a theoretical risk to the fetus, unless it is considered there is a significant risk of exposure to infection.

HIV. A review[1] of experience of the safety and efficacy of vaccines in patients infected with HIV found that the theoretical risk of accelerating HIV infection by immunisation is not supported by the limited clinical information available and the risks may be trivial compared with other natural sources of antigenic stimulation especially in areas of the world with high levels of endemic infectious diseases.

Recommendations for immunisation of HIV-positive individuals vary, particularly with regard to the use of live vaccines[2] (see Immunisation of Immunocompromised Patients, below for UK recommendations). Where an alternative is available an inactivated vaccine may be preferred to a live one (for example, poliomyelitis vaccines), but in general vaccines recommended for routine immunisation in childhood may be given to HIV-positive individuals. For HIV-positive children, WHO and UNICEF[3] recommend that routine immunisation should be carried out according to the usual schedule in asymptomatic infants. In addition, an extra dose of measles vaccine should be given at 6 months of age. BCG vaccine should not be given to children with symptomatic disease. See individual monographs for further information.

1. von Reyn CF, *et al.* Human immunodeficiency virus infection and routine childhood immunisation. *Lancet* 1987; **ii:** 669–72.
2. Centers for Disease Control. Recommendations of the Advisory Committee on Immunization Practices (ACIP): use of vaccines and immune globulins for persons with altered immunocompetence. *Clin Pharm* 1993; **12:** 675–84.
3. WHO. *Global programme on AIDS: guidelines for the clinical management of HIV infection in children.* Geneva: WHO 1993.

Premature infants. References.

1. Anonymous. Routine immunisation of preterm infants. *Lancet* 1990; **335:** 23–4.
2. Khalak R, *et al.* Three-year follow-up of vaccine response in extremely preterm infants. *Pediatrics* 1998; **101:** 597–603.

Interactions

The ability of vaccines to induce an immune response can be influenced by the recent administration of other vaccines or immunoglobulins. Live vaccines should either be administered simultaneously (but at different sites) or an interval of at least 3 weeks allowed between administration. Live vaccines should normally be given at least 2 to 3 weeks before or at least 3 months after the administration of immunoglobulin. However, travellers should receive appropriate vaccines regardless of these limitations if time is short.

Patients receiving immunosuppressant therapy, including antineoplastics or therapeutic doses of corticosteroids, may also display a reduced response to vaccines, and there is a possibility of generalised infections with live viral vaccines. In the UK, the Department of Health suggest that immunosuppression may be expected in children receiving the equivalent of 2 mg prednisolone per kg body-weight daily for at least 1 week or 1 mg per kg daily for 1 month, and in adults receiving the equivalent of 40 mg prednisolone daily for more than 1 week. Vaccination should also be postponed for at least 6 months after the cessation of antineoplastic chemotherapy and for at least 3 months after high-dose systemic corticosteroid therapy.

Any agent which is active against the bacterial or viral strain present in the vaccine may interfere with development of a protective immune response but treatment with antibiotics should not be considered to be a contra-indication to immunisation.

References.

1. Grabenstein JD. Drug interactions involving immunologic agents. Part I. Vaccine-vaccine, vaccine-immunoglobulin, and vaccine-drug interactions. *DICP Ann Pharmacother* 1990; **24:** 67–81.
2. Grabenstein JD. Drug interactions involving immunologic agents. Part II. Immunodiagnostic and other immunologic drug interactions. *DICP Ann Pharmacother* 1990; **24:** 186–93.

Uses and Administration

Vaccines are used for active immunisation as a prophylactic measure against some infectious diseases. They provide partial or complete protection for months or years. For inactivated vaccines a slight and rather slow antibody response of primarily immunoglobulin M (IgM) (the primary response) is produced after the first or second dose but, when a further dose is given after a suitable interval, a prompt antibody response follows and high concentrations of IgG occur in the blood (the secondary response). Though the antibody concentration may later fall, a further dose of vaccine promptly restores it. For most live vaccines only one dose is required although 3 doses of live (oral) poliomyelitis vaccines are needed to achieve complete immunisation. Some inactivated vaccines contain an adjuvant such as aluminium hydroxide or aluminium phosphate to enhance the immune response.

Protection against several infectious diseases may be provided in early life by active immunisation and national schedules for childhood immunisation are regularly reviewed and updated. Schedules for routine immunisation of infants and children are generally designed to fit in with routine health checks and landmark events such as school starting and leaving ages. National immunisation schedules should be consulted for full details of local recommendations.

In the UK the following schedule of vaccination and immunisation is recommended:

- at 2, 3, and 4 months of age, doses of an adsorbed diphtheria, tetanus, and pertussis vaccine (p.1509) together with a *Haemophilus influenzae* vaccine (p.1511) and a live (oral) poliomyelitis vaccine (p.1528). If pertussis vaccine is contra-indicated an adsorbed diphtheria and tetanus vaccine (p.1508) should be given
- at 12 to 15 months of age, measles, mumps, and rubella vaccine (p.1519)
- at 3 to 5 years, reinforcing doses of an adsorbed diphtheria and tetanus vaccine and a live (oral) poliomyelitis vaccine and a second dose of measles, mumps, and rubella vaccine
- between 10 and 14 years of age, BCG vaccine (p.1504) may be given to tuberculin-negative children if it has not been given in infancy

- before leaving school (age 13 to 18 years), reinforcing doses of an adsorbed tetanus with low-dose diphtheria vaccine (p.1535) and a live (oral) poliomyelitis vaccine
- a further reinforcing dose of tetanus vaccine may be given after 10 years. Adults who have received 5 doses of tetanus should not require further routine boosters.

Similar immunisation schedules are recommended in other countries. For example, the following schedule is recommended in the USA:

- at birth or up to 2 months of age, the first dose of hepatitis B vaccine (p.1513)
- at age 1 to 4 months, a second dose of hepatitis B vaccine, not less than 1 month after the first
- at 2 months and 4 months of age, diphtheria, tetanus, and pertussis vaccine, together with a *Haemophilus influenzae* vaccine and a poliomyelitis vaccine
- at 6 months, the third dose of *Haemophilus influenzae* vaccine if necessary (depending on the type of vaccine used) and a third dose of diphtheria, tetanus, and pertussis vaccine
- at 6 to 18 months, the third doses of hepatitis B and poliomyelitis vaccines
- at 12 to 15 months, a reinforcing dose of *Haemophilus influenzae* vaccine and the first dose of measles, mumps, and rubella vaccine
- at 12 to 18 months (or at age 11 to 12 years), a varicella-zoster vaccine (p.1538)
- at 15 to 18 months the fourth dose of diphtheria, tetanus, and pertussis vaccine
- at 4 to 6 years of age, the fifth dose of diphtheria, tetanus, and pertussis vaccine and the fourth dose of poliomyelitis vaccine; the second dose of measles, mumps, and rubella vaccine may be given at this age (or at age 11 to 12 years)
- at 11 to 12 years, varicella-zoster vaccine (if not previously given), the second dose of measles, mumps, and rubella vaccine, and a 3-dose course of hepatitis B vaccine if not given earlier
- at age 11 to 16 years, tetanus and low-dose diphtheria toxoids. Susceptible children 13 years of age and older should receive 2 doses of varicella vaccine, at least 1 month apart
- subsequently routine booster doses of tetanus vaccine are recommended every 10 years.

Immunisation schedules for older children and adults are also produced, along with recommendations for vaccination of high risk groups, including the immunocompromised and the elderly, and of travellers.

In addition to vaccines directed against bacteria and viruses, advances are being made in producing vaccines against fungi, protozoa, and helminths, and for non-infective diseases including cancer and autoimmune disorders.

Development of novel vaccine formulations and delivery methods is continuing, including transdermal and transmucosal systems. Genetic manipulations of foodstuffs is being investigated with the aim of producing edible vaccines.

Some general references to vaccines and immunisation including vaccine development and research.

1. Moxon ER. The scope of immunisation. *Lancet* 1990; **335:** 448–51.
2. Ada GL. The immunological principles of vaccination. *Lancet* 1990; **335:** 523–6.
3. Anderson RM, May RM. Immunisation and herd immunity. *Lancet* 1990; **335:** 641–5.
4. Swedish Agency for Research Cooperation with Developing Countries. Prospects for public health benefits in developing countries from new vaccines against enteric infections. *J Infect Dis* 1991; **163:** 503–6.
5. Gilligan CA, Li Wan Po A. Oral vaccines: design and delivery. *Int J Pharmaceutics* 1991; **75:** 1–24.
6. O'Hagan DT. Oral delivery of vaccines: formulation and clinical pharmacokinetic considerations. *Clin Pharmacokinet* 1992; **22:** 1–10.
7. Gilsdorf JR. Vaccines: moving into the molecular era. *J Pediatr* 1994; **125:** 339–44.
8. André F, *et al.*, eds. 2nd European conference on vaccinology: combined vaccines for Europe, pharmaceutical, regulatory and policy-making aspects. *Biologicals* 1994; **22:** 297–436.
9. Leclerc C, ed. Live DNA recombinant vaccines. *Biologicals* 1995; **23:** 111–78.
10. Corbel MJ. New mechanisms for developing vaccines. *Br J Hosp Med* 1996; **56:** 4–6.
11. McDonnell WM, Askari FK. Molecular medicine: DNA vaccines. *N Engl J Med* 1996; **334:** 42–5.
12. McCarthy M. DNA vaccination: a direct line to the immune system. *Lancet* 1996; **348:** 1232.
13. Various. Vaccine series. *Lancet* 1997; **350.**
14. McDonnell WM, Askari FK. Immunization. *JAMA* 1997; **278:** 2000–2007.
15. Lambert P-H, Siegrist C-A. Vaccines and vaccination. *Br Med J* 1997; **315:** 1595–8
16. Eskola J. Childhood immunisation today. *Drugs* 1998; **55:** 759–66.

Eradication of infections. Eradication of infectious diseases has proved more difficult than was hoped, and smallpox is the only disease to have been officially eradicated so far. Eradication is defined as the extinction of the pathogen that causes the infectious disease in question whereas in elimination the disease disappears but the causative agent remains. Of the 6 target diseases of WHO's Expanded Programme on Immunization, many of the factors necessary for elimination are present for each of the diseases, but some are not.[1] *Measles* is so highly communicable a disease that a vaccine efficacy rate of about 95% is probably not high enough even to eliminate, much less eradicate the disease.[1] However, immunisation campaigns have produced substantial reductions of infection rate in some countries although repeated vaccination may be necessary.[2] *Pertussis* is also highly infectious and the vaccine is almost certainly not effective enough. *Tetanus* is not eradicable as the causative organism is ubiquitous. However, elimination of neonatal tetanus may be possible although it depends on protection of more than 80% of infants at birth. This depends not only on maternal vaccination but also on delivery practices.[2] For *poliomyelitis*, countries that are efficient at giving vaccines have proved remarkably successful not only in practically eliminating the disease but also in virtually eradicating the organism. *Tuberculosis* is clearly not eradicable at present and *diphtheria* has many features that suggest it cannot be easily eradicated. Prospects for eradicating *congenital rubella syndrome* are more encouraging and the prospects for elimination or eradication of *mumps* are probably similar to those of rubella.

Other factors which may contribute to the failure of vaccination policies in eradicating disease include: concern over the safety of vaccines, often unfounded and the perpetuation of invalid contra-indications; the use of inappropriate indicators for the effectiveness of vaccines; the suitability of different types of vaccine and of vaccination schedules; difficulties in vaccine supply; and social and behavioural pressures which reduce compliance with vaccination schedules.[2,3]

1. Noah ND, Begg NT. Smallpox ten years gone: what next? *Br Med J* 1987; **295:** 1013–14.
2. Stanwell-Smith R. Immunization: celebrating the past and injecting the future. *J R Soc Med* 1996; **89:** 509–13.
3. Preston NW. Smallpox could be but one of many diseases that vaccination confines to the history of medicine. *Trop Dis Bull* 1994; **91:** R151–R165.

Immunisation schedules. Recommendations and discussions of routine immunisation schedules in the UK,[1,2] the USA[3-8] and the developed world in general.[9] See below for discussion of the Expanded Programme on Immunization.

1. Salisbury DM, Begg NT (eds), Joint Committee on Vaccination and Immunisation. *Immunisation against infectious disease.* London: HMSO, 1996.
2. Mayon-White RT. Vaccination for the elderly. *Br J Hosp Med* 1994; **51:** 265–7.
3. Fedson DS, National Vaccine Advisory Committee. Adult immunization: summary of the National Vaccine Advisory Committee report. *JAMA* 1994; **272:** 1133–7.
4. Halsey NA, Hall CB. Workshop on conflicting guidelines for the use of vaccines. *Pediatrics* 1995; **95:** 938–41.
5. Somani J, *et al.* Reimmunization after allogeneic bone marrow transplantation. *Am J Med* 1995; **98:** 389–98.
6. Gardner P, *et al.* Adult immunizations. *Ann Intern Med* 1996; **124:** 35–40.
7. American Academy of Pediatrics Committee on Infectious Diseases. Immunization of adolescents: recommendations of the Advisory Committee on Immunization Practices, the American Academy of Pediatrics, the American Academy of Family Physicians, and the American Medical Association. *Pediatrics* 1997; **99:** 479–88.
8. American Academy of Pediatrics Committee on Infectious Diseases. Recommended childhood immunization schedule—United States, January-December 1998. *Pediatrics* 1998; **101:** 154–7.
9. Hinman AR, Onenstein WA. Immunisation practice in developed countries. *Lancet* 1990; **335:** 707–10.

EXPANDED PROGRAMME ON IMMUNIZATION. In 1974 the World Health Assembly adopted a resolution creating the Expanded Programme on Immunization, the aim of which was to provide immunisation against six target diseases (diphtheria, measles, pertussis, poliomyelitis, tetanus, and tuberculosis) for all children throughout the world by 1990. Although the attention of WHO had been focussed primarily on the developing countries, it was emphasised that the programme was not created exclusively for these countries. Besides WHO, many other organisations, including UNICEF, were involved. Vaccine uptake was around 70% in 1990 compared with less than 5% in 1974. Although many cases of the target diseases and many deaths have been prevented, vaccine coverage, especially for measles and neonatal tetanus is still low. It is particularly important to immunise children as early in life as possible and not to withhold vaccines from those suffering from minor illness or malnutrition.

A schedule designed to provide protection at the earliest possible age consists of: trivalent oral poliomyelitis vaccine together with BCG vaccine at birth; trivalent oral poliomyelitis vaccine together with diphtheria, tetanus, and pertussis vaccine at 6, 10, and 14 weeks of age; and measles vaccine at 9 months of age. Tetanus vaccine is also administered to all women of child-bearing age. Other vaccines included in the programme are: yellow fever vaccine in parts of Africa and Japanese encephalitis vaccine in parts of the Far East. Further expansion to include vaccination against other diseases, particularly hepatitis B, (see p.1514) is under continued consideration.

Some references to the Expanded Programme on Immunization.

1. Hayden GF, *et al.* Progress in worldwide control and elimination of disease through immunization. *J Pediatr* 1989; **114:** 520–7.
2. Hall AJ, *et al.* Practice in developing countries. *Lancet* 1990; **335:** 774–7.

Immunisation of immunocompromised patients. Immunocompromised and asplenic patients and recipients of bone marrow transplants may require immunisation against opportunistic infections. As discussed under Precautions, above, immune response to vaccination may be impaired, and there is a risk of disseminated infection with live vaccines.

In the UK, the Department of Health recommends that HIV-positive individuals (whether symptomatic or asymptomatic) may receive, where appropriate, live vaccines against measles, mumps, poliomyelitis, and rubella and inactivated vaccines against cholera, diphtheria, *Haemophilus influenzae* type b infections, hepatitis B, pertussis, poliomyelitis, tetanus, and typhoid. Hepatitis A, meningococcal, pneumococcal, and rabies vaccines may also be given. In the UK it is recommended that BCG vaccine not be given to HIV-positive individuals; WHO have, however, advised immunisation of asymptomatic infants when the risk of tuberculosis is high. There is as yet insufficient data on the safety of yellow fever vaccine in HIV-positive individuals. In the UK administration of yellow fever vaccine to such individuals is not recommended. WHO advise that the vaccine should be administered if the risk of infection is high.

As with other causes of immunosuppression, the efficacy of vaccines may be reduced in HIV-positive individuals. Administration of normal immunoglobulins is suggested for HIV-positive individuals exposed to measles.

Further references.

1. Kaplan JE, *et al.* USPHS/IDSA guidelines for the prevention of opportunistic infections in persons infected with human immunodeficiency virus: an overview. *Clin Infect Dis* 1995; **21** (suppl 1): S12–S31.
2. Ljungman P, Hammarström V. Immunisation of transplant recipients. *Clin Immunother* 1995; **3:** 330–7.
3. Henning KJ, *et al.* A national survey of immunization practices following allogeneic bone marrow transplantation. *JAMA* 1997; **277:** 1148–51.
4. Loutan L. Vaccination of the immunocompromised patient. *Biologicals* 1997; **25:** 231–6.
5. Pirofski L-A, Casadevall A. Use of licensed vaccines for active immunization of the immunocompromised host. *Clin Microbiol Rev* 1998; **11:** 1–26.

Immunisation for travellers. A booklet entitled *International Travel and Health: Vaccination Requirements and Health Advice* is published annually by WHO. In the 1997 edition the following information regarding certification of vaccination was given.

A *yellow fever* vaccination certificate is now the only one that should be required in international travel, and then only for a limited number of travellers. The vaccine used must be approved by WHO and administered at a designated vaccinating centre. Vaccination is strongly recommended for travel outside the urban areas of countries in the yellow fever endemic zone even if these countries have not officially reported the disease and do not require evidence of vaccination on entry. Many countries require a certificate from travellers arriving from infected areas or from countries with infected areas, or who have been in transit through those areas. Some countries require a certificate from all entering travellers including those in transit; although there is no epidemiological justification for this requirement, and it is clearly in excess of the International Health Regulations (WHO recommendations for prevention of the international spread of diseases), travellers may find that it is strictly enforced, particularly for persons going to Asia from Africa or South America. The validity period of international certificates of vaccination against yellow fever is 10 years, beginning 10 days after vaccination.

No country or territory any longer requires a certificate of *cholera* immunisation as the introduction of cholera into any country cannot be prevented by cholera vaccination.

Now that *smallpox* has been eradicated, smallpox vaccination is no longer required by any country.

Apart from vaccinations required by countries for entry to their territory, other vaccinations are either recommended by WHO for general protection against certain diseases or advised in certain circumstances. A vaccination plan should be established, taking into account the traveller's destination, overall state of health and current immune status, the duration and type of travel, and the time available.

Further information for international travellers is also often provided by national authorities. In the UK the Department of Health issues *Health Advice for Travellers* for the public and *Health Information for Overseas Travel* for the medical profession. In the USA guidelines are produced by the Centers for Disease Control.

AIDS Immunoglobulins (11739-l)

HIV Immunoglobulins.

AIDS immunoglobulin preparations containing HIV-neutralising antibodies have been prepared from the plasma of asymptomatic HIV-positive subjects. They are being tried for passive immunisation in patients with AIDS or AIDS-related complex.

References.

1. Jackson GG, *et al.* Passive immunoneutralisation of human immunodeficiency virus in patients with advanced AIDS. *Lancet* 1988; **ii:** 647–52.
2. Lambert JS, *et al.* Pediatric AIDS Clinical Trials Group Protocol 185 Pharmacokinetic Study Group. Safety and pharmacokinetics of hyperimmune anti-human immunodeficiency virus (HIV) immunoglobulin administered to HIV-infected pregnant women and their newborns. *J Infect Dis* 1997; **175:** 283–91.
3. Fletcher CV, *et al.* Pharmacokinetics of hyperimmune anti-human immunodeficiency virus immunoglobulins in persons with AIDS. *Antimicrob Agents Chemother* 1997; **41:** 1571–4.

AIDS Vaccines (18734-k)

HIV Vaccines.

Many prototype vaccines against the acquired immunodeficiency syndrome have been or are being developed but the results of clinical studies have generally been disappointing.

Research into AIDS vaccines has continued into both therapeutic vaccines, aimed at reducing the rate of disease progression in HIV-infected individuals, and prophylactic vaccines, aimed at preventing primary infection. It is now appreciated that both humoral and cell-mediated immune mechanisms play a vital role in controlling HIV infection. Among a number of possible approaches, subunit recombinant viral envelope proteins (gp120 or gp160) have been candidates for both therapeutic and prophylactic vaccines, either as monovalent or polyvalent formulations. They mainly produce a humoral (antibody) response although cell-mediated responses, possibly to other components of the vaccine, have been detected. Clinical studies have not demonstrated a delay in disease progression. Attenuated live viral vaccines are potentially useful for prophylaxis but were initially dismissed because the risk of reversion to virulent strains was felt to be too great. However, they are now being re-examined since they are capable of producing both cell-mediated and humoral immune responses, although the problem of safety remains to be resolved. Another recent development is investigation of nucleic acid vaccines. Free DNA encoding for viral antigens injected into the muscle results in expression of the encoded antigens promoting a humoral and cell-mediated response. Although these vaccines are still at an early stage of development, they may represent a safer alternative to live viral vaccines.

Reviews.

1. Graham BS, Wright PF. Candidate AIDS vaccines. *N Engl J Med* 1995; **333:** 1331–9.
2. Anonymous. Update on AIDS: vaccines and genetic manipulation. *WHO Drug Inf* 1995; **9:** 201–9.
3. Esparaza J, *et al.* HIV prospective vaccines: progress to date. *Drugs* 1995; **50:** 792–804.
4. Stott EJ, Schild GC. Strategies for AIDS vaccines. *J Antimicrob Chemother* 1996: **37** (suppl B): 185–98.
5. Haynes BF. HIV vaccines: where we are and where we are going. *Lancet* 1996; **348:** 933–7.
6. Bangham CRM, Phillips RE. What is required of an HIV vaccine? *Lancet* 1997; **350:** 1617–21.

Anthrax Vaccines (7933-d)

Adverse Effects and Precautions

As for vaccines in general, p.1500.

Interactions

As for vaccines in general, p.1501.

Uses and Administration

In the UK an anthrax vaccine which is an alum precipitate of the antigen found in the sterile filtrate of suitable cultures of the Sterne strain of *Bacillus anthracis* is available for human use. It is used for active immunisation against anthrax and is recommended for persons working with potentially infected animals or animal products. It is given in 4 doses, each of 0.5 mL, administered by intramuscular injection. The first 3 doses are separated by intervals of 3 weeks and the fourth dose follows after an interval of 6 months. In the USA, where an anthrax vaccine is also available, 6 doses, each of 0.5 mL, are given subcutaneously, the first 3 at intervals of 2 weeks and the last 3 at intervals of 6 months. Reinforcing doses are required each year. Anthrax vaccine has no role in the management of a case or outbreak.

References.

1. Hambleton P, *et al.* Anthrax: the disease in relation to vaccines. *Vaccine* 1984; **2:** 125–32.
2. Turnbull PCB. Thoroughly modern anthrax. *Abstr Hyg* 1986; **61:** R1–R13.
3. Turnbull PCB. Anthrax vaccines: past, present and future. *Vaccine* 1991; **9:** 533–9.
4. Farrar WE. Anthrax: virulence and vaccines. *Ann Intern Med* 1994; **121:** 379–80.

Anti-D Immunoglobulins (1234-k)

Human Anti-D Immunoglobulin (Ph. Eur.) (Anti-D (Rh_o) Immunoglobulin (BP 1998); Immunoglobulinum Humanum Anti-D) is a liquid or freeze-dried preparation containing immunoglobulins, mainly immunoglobulin G (IgG). It is obtained from plasma from D-negative donors who have been immunised against the D-antigen. It contains specific antibodies against the erythrocyte D-antigen and may also contain small quantities of other blood group antibodies, such as anti-C, anti-E, anti-A, and anti-B. Normal immunoglobulin may be added. The liquid and freeze-dried preparations should be stored, protected from light, in a colourless, glass container. The freeze-dried preparation should be stored under vacuum or under an inert gas.

Rh_o (D) Immune Globulin (USP 23) is a sterile solution of globulins derived from human plasma containing antibody to the erythrocyte factor Rh_o (D). It contains 10 to 18% of protein, of which not less than 90% is gamma globulin. It contains glycine as a stabilising agent, and a suitable preservative. It should be stored at 2° to 8°.

Adverse Effects and Precautions

As for immunoglobulins in general, p.1500.

Anti-D immunoglobulin should be administered with caution to rhesus-positive persons for the treatment of blood disorders; the resultant haemolysis may exacerbate pre-existing anaemia.

Interactions

As for immunoglobulins in general, p.1500.

Uses and Administration

Anti-D immunoglobulin is used to prevent a rhesus-negative mother actively forming antibodies to fetal rhesus-positive red blood cells that may pass into the maternal circulation during childbirth, abortion, or certain other sensitising events. In subsequent rhesus-positive pregnancies these antibodies could produce haemolytic disease of the newborn (erythroblastosis foetalis). The injection of anti-D immunoglobulin is not effective once the mother has formed anti-D antibodies. Anti-D immunoglobulin is also used in the management of some blood disorders, primarily idiopathic thrombocytopenic purpura.

Anti-D immunoglobulin should always be given to rhesus-negative mothers with no anti-D antibodies in their serum and who have just delivered rhesus-positive infants. It should be given as soon as possible after delivery but may give some protection even if administration is delayed beyond 72 hours. In the UK, the Blood Transfusion Services recommend a dose of 500 units (100 μg) by intramuscular injection although an additional dose may be required depending on the amount of transplacental bleeding as assessed by the Kleihauer test; for bleeds exceeding 4 to 5 mL an additional 100 to 125 units is given for each mL.

For routine antenatal prophylaxis 500 units of anti-D immunoglobulin may be given at 28 and 34 weeks gestation. Alternatively a single dose, usually of 1500 units, may be given at 28 to 30 weeks. Postnatal prophylaxis is still necessary.

There is also a risk of sensitisation during pregnancy from spontaneous, induced, or threatened abortion, amniocentesis, or external version. Any rhesus-negative woman at risk of transplacental haemorrhage during pregnancy and not known to be sensitised should be given 250 units at up to 20 weeks gestation and 500 units of anti-D immunoglobulin after 20 weeks gestation.

Anti-D immunoglobulin is also given to rhesus-negative women of child-bearing potential after the inadvertent transfusion of Rh-incompatible blood, or after receiving blood components containing rhesus-positive red cells or organ donations from rhesus-positive donors. The dose is based on the amount of red blood cells transfused.

In Europe and the USA doses of anti-D immunoglobulins have traditionally been higher than in the UK; WHO and the European Commissions Committee for Proprietary Medicinal Products have recommended a standard dose of 200 to 300 μg (1000 to 1500 units) but do not include a requirement for Kleihauer screening. A dose of approximately 250 μg (1250 units) will suppress the immune response to up to 10 mL of red blood cells. In the USA the dosage recommendations are based on a standard dose which is capable of suppressing the immune response to 15 mL of incompatible red blood cells. One sixth of this dose may be used up to 12 weeks of gestation for sensitising episodes.

For idiopathic thrombocytopenic purpura, an initial dose of 250 units (50 μg) per kg body-weight of anti-D immunoglobulin by intravenous injection has been suggested. Maintenance doses will depend on the clinical response.

Haemolytic disease of the newborn. Rhesus (Rh) incompatibility, in particular Rh(D) incompatibility, is a major cause of potentially severe haemolytic disease of the newborn, although other blood group antibodies may also cause the disease.[1] The use of anti-D immunoglobulin to suppress the production of anti-D antibodies in a Rh(D)-negative mother in response to leakage of red blood cells across the placenta from a Rh(D)-positive fetus has produced a major reduction in the incidence of this disorder.[1]

Postnatal prophylaxis of Rh(D)-negative mothers following the birth of a Rh(D)-positive infant is well established. In 1971 WHO[2] suggested a standard dose of 200 to 300 μg but stated that a 100-μg dose is likely to have a success rate only slightly inferior to that of a 200-μg dose, thus allowing optimum use to be made of a limited resource. Clinical experience in the UK has confirmed the efficacy of the 100-μg dose and this is the amount officially recommended in the UK in such situations.[3]

Despite the success of anti-D prophylaxis, sensitisations have continued to occur.[4] There are several possible reasons for this. Failures may occur when an inadequate dose has been administered or when anti-D prophylaxis is omitted following a sensitising event.[5,6] Postpartum doses may be omitted due to oversight or loss to follow-up. Sensitisation may occur spontaneously during the first pregnancy without any identifiable event causing feto-maternal haemorrhage. Inadequate dosing can be avoided by application of the Kleihauer test to estimate the size of any transplacental haemorrhage.[1]

Significant feto-maternal transfusion may also occur following still-birth, abortion (both therapeutic and spontaneous), threatened abortion, external fetal version, abdominal injury, or amniocentesis.

The efficacy of postpartum prophylaxis is not in question but opinions differ on the need for prophylaxis during pregnancy. It is generally agreed that prophylaxis is necessary following therapeutic terminations at any stage of pregnancy,[7,8] including medical termination utilising mifepristone,[9] but there is no generally accepted policy for other possibly sensitising events. A study of 655 Rh(D)-negative women in Denmark,[10] where antepartum prophylaxis is not common practice, suggested that the sensitisation rate following amniocentesis was no higher than the spontaneous sensitisation rate. Surveys of general medical practitioners and consultant obstetricians and haematologists in the UK[11,12] have suggested that many do not recommend routine prophylaxis following early complete or threatened miscarriages; 74% of general practitioners in one survey[12] never gave anti-D after threatened miscarriages. Spontaneous miscarriages during early pregnancy might not cause sensitisation so long as there is no surgical intervention.[7,8,13] Nonetheless some authorities[4] in the UK urge routine antenatal prophylaxis for all Rh(D)-negative women. Everett[14] and Hussey[15] represent the alternative opinion that, with the shortage of anti-D, indiscriminate use of anti-D should be avoided[14] and attention should be focussed upon administration of adequate doses following term deliveries and terminations of pregnancy in Rh(D)-negative women.[5,15] Further debate arises over the significance of spontaneous sensitisation during the first pregnancy. Tovey and colleagues[16] found that administration of anti-D to 2069 Rh(D)-negative primigravidas at 28 and 34 weeks as well as standard postpartum administration was more effective at preventing immunisation than standard postpartum prophylaxis in 2000 primigravidas. In a subsequent analysis of women from this study[17] following further pregnancies, comparison with a group of Rh(D)-positive mothers showed no detrimental effects to mothers or infants. In addition antenatal prophylaxis may not need to be given beyond the first pregnancy. Nevertheless, concerns have been expressed[18] over the consequent unnecessary administration of anti-D to women who are carrying Rh(D)-negative fetuses and the possible long-term effects, although anti-D has had a good safety record.[19] Both factions agree[18,20] on the desirability of identifying high-risk women to reduce the indiscriminate use of anti-D. A remaining major stumbling block, in the UK at least, is the continuing expense and scarcity of anti-D immunoglobulin. Supplies are derived from plasma collected from Rh-negative donors who have to undergo potentially hazardous sensitisation with Rh-positive red blood cells. The development of genetically-engineered anti-D should help to improve availability. The UK[3] and WHO[2] guidelines may represent a counsel of perfection, but until difficulties with supply are overcome, prophylaxis during the first pregnancy for Rh(D)-negative women, thus ensuring the possibility of two unaffected infants, would seem a reasonable priority.

Treatment. In mild cases, the resultant hyperbilirubinaemia can be managed with phototherapy. In severe cases, exchange transfusions may be necessary and intra-uterine transfusions may be considered in pregnancies of less than about 34 weeks gestation; beyond this, premature delivery is often preferable.[21] Some clinicians[22] have reported treatment failures with intra-uterine transfusions but have found the intravenous administration of normal immunoglobulin 400 mg per kg body-weight daily for 5 days every 2 to 3 weeks to the mother to be effective. There are several case reports[23,24] of beneficial responses using similar doses, but no benefit was seen in 4 patients receiving 1000 mg per kg once a week.[25] This dose, however, appeared to reduce the severity of the disease in a patient with Kell sensitisation.[25] Reductions in bilirubin concentrations have been reported following intravenous administration of normal immunoglobulin 500 mg per kg as a single dose to newborn infants.[26] Preliminary studies in small numbers of infants[27,28] suggest that epoetins may be of value in controlling anaemia which develops 2 to 8 weeks after birth.

1. Tovey LAD. Haemolytic disease of the newborn and its prevention. *Br Med J* 1990; **300:** 313–16.
2. WHO. Prevention of Rh sensitization: report of a WHO scientific group. *WHO Tech Rep Ser 468* 1971.
3. National Blood Transfusion Service Immunoglobulin Working Party. Recommendations for the use of anti-D immunoglobulin. *Prescribers' J* 1991; **31:** 137–45.
4. Robson SC, *et al.* Anti-D immunoglobulin in RhD prophylaxis. *Br J Obstet Gynaecol* 1998; **105:** 129–34.
5. James D. Anti-D prophylaxis in 1997: the Edinburgh consensus statement. *Arch Dis Child* 1998; **78:** F161–F165.
6. Howard HL, *et al.* Preventing rhesus D haemolytic disease of the newborn by giving anti-D immunoglobulin: are the guidelines being adequately followed? *Br J Obstet Gynaecol* 1997; **104:** 37–41.
7. Contreras M. Is anti-D immunoglobulin unnecessary in the domiciliary treatment of miscarriages? *Br Med J* 1988; **297:** 733.
8. Tovey LAD. Anti-D and miscarriages. *Br Med J* 1988; **297:** 977–8.
9. Lee D. Recommendations for the use of anti-D immunoglobulin. *Prescribers' J* 1991; **31:** 262–3.
10. Tabor A, *et al.* Incidence of rhesus immunisation after genetic amniocentesis. *Br Med J* 1986; **293:** 533–6.
11. Contreras M, *et al.* Why women are not receiving anti-Rh prophylaxis. *Br Med J* 1986; **293:** 1373.
12. Everett C, *et al.* Reported management of threatened miscarriage by general practitioners in Wessex. *Br Med J* 1987; **295:** 583–6.
13. Everett CB. Is anti-D immunoglobulin unnecessary in the domiciliary treatment of miscarriages? *Br Med J* 1988; **297:** 732.
14. Everett CB. Anti-D immunoglobulin for bleeding in early pregnancy. *Br Med J* 1990; **301:** 1329.
15. Hussey RM. Why women are not receiving anti-Rh prophylaxis. *Br Med J* 1987; **294:** 119.
16. Tovey LAD, *et al.* The Yorkshire antenatal anti-D immunoglobulin trial in primigravidae. *Lancet* 1983; **ii:** 244–6.
17. Thornton JG, *et al.* Efficacy and long term effects of antenatal prophylaxis with anti-D immunoglobulin. *Br Med J* 1989; **298:** 1671–3.
18. Hussey R. Antenatal prophylaxis with anti-D immunoglobulin. *Br Med J* 1989; **299:** 568.
19. Lee D. Antenatal prophylaxis with anti-D immunoglobulin. *Br Med J* 1989; **299:** 920.
20. Thornton JG, Tovey LAD. Antenatal prophylaxis with anti-D immunoglobulin. *Br Med J* 1989; **299:** 919–20.
21. Whittle MJ. Rhesus haemolytic disease. *Arch Dis Child* 1992; **67:** 65–8.
22. Margulies M, Voto LS. High-dose intravenous gamma globulin: does it have a role in the treatment of severe erythroblastosis fetalis? *Obstet Gynecol* 1991; **77:** 804–5.
23. Berlin G, *et al.* Rhesus haemolytic disease treated with high-dose intravenous immunoglobulin. *Lancet* 1985; **i:** 1153.
24. de la Cámara C, *et al.* High-dose intravenous immunoglobulin as the sole prenatal treatment for severe Rh immunization. *N Engl J Med* 1988; **318:** 519–20.
25. Chitkara U, *et al.* High-dose intravenous gamma globulin: does it have a role in the treatment of severe erythroblastosis fetalis? *Obstet Gynecol* 1990; **76:** 703–8.
26. Rübo J, *et al.* High-dose intravenous immune globulin therapy for hyperbilirubinemia caused by Rh hemolytic disease. *J Pediatr* 1992; **121:** 93–7.
27. Ohls RK, *et al.* Recombinant erythropoietin as treatment for the late hyporegenerative anemia of Rh hemolytic disease. *Pediatrics* 1992; **90:** 678–80.
28. Scaradavou A, *et al.* Suppression of erythropoiesis by intrauterine transfusions in hemolytic disease of the newborn: use of erythropoietin to treat the late anemia. *J Pediatr* 1993; **123:** 279–84.

Idiopathic thrombocytopenic purpura. Although corticosteroids or splenectomy are established as the usual therapy for chronic idiopathic thrombocytopenic purpura (p.1023), normal immunoglobulin is also used in some circumstances, and anti-D immunoglobulin has been found to have similar properties.[1] Treatment of an Rh(D)-positive patient with a long history of severe immune thrombocytopenic purpura with a single dose of 500 units (100 μg) of anti-D immunoglobulin intravenously was reported to result in a steady rise in platelet count and rapid resolution of a cephalic haematoma.[2] Responses to anti-D immunoglobulin were reported in 23 of 25 children with chronic idiopathic thrombocytopenia[3] following treatment with 25 μg per kg body-weight on each of two consecutive days. However, in children with acute disease,[4] a similar dose of anti-D immunoglobulin was less effective in restoring platelet count and produced a greater fall in haemoglobin than either normal immunoglobulin or corticosteroids. (Most children with the acute form do not in any case require therapy.)

Beneficial results in both rhesus-positive and rhesus-negative patients with HIV-related thrombocytopenia were reported[5-8] with doses in the order of 1 to 3 mg daily, given intravenously.

1. Anonymous. Rho(D) immunoglobulin iv for prevention of Rh isoimmunization and for treatment of ITP. *Med Lett Drugs Ther* 1996; **38:** 6–8.
2. Baglin TP, *et al.* Rapid and complete response of immune thrombocytopenic purpura to a single injection of rhesus anti-D immunoglobulin. *Lancet* 1986; **i:** 1329–30.
3. Andrew M, *et al.* A multicenter study of the treatment of childhood chronic idiopathic thrombocytopenic purpura with anti-D. *J Pediatr* 1992; **120:** 522–7.
4. Blanchette V, *et al.* Randomised trial of intravenous immunoglobulin G, intravenous anti-D, and oral prednisone in childhood acute immune thrombocytopenic purpura. *Lancet* 1994; **344:** 703–7.
5. Durand JM, *et al.* Anti-Rh(D) immunoglobulin for immune thrombocytopenic purpura. *Lancet* 1986; **ii:** 49–50.
6. Biniek R, *et al.* Anti-Rh(D) immunoglobulin for AIDS-related thrombocytopenia. *Lancet* 1986; **ii:** 627.
7. Bierling P, *et al.* Anti-rhesus antibodies, immune thrombocytopenia, and human immunodeficiency virus infection. *Ann Intern Med* 1987; **106:** 773–4.
8. Landonio G, *et al.* HIV-related severe thrombocytopenia in intravenous drug users: prevalence, response to therapy in a medium-term follow-up, and pathogenic evaluation. *AIDS* 1990; **4:** 29–34.

Preparations

Ph. Eur.: Human Anti-D Immunoglobulin;
USP 23: Rh_o (D) Immune Globulin.

Proprietary Preparations (details are given in Part 3)
Aust.: Partobulin; Partogloman†; ***Belg.:*** Rhesuman; ***Canad.:*** HypRho-D; WinRho; ***Ger.:*** HypRho-D†; Partobulin; Rhesogam; Rhesonativ†; ***Ital.:*** Gamma-Men; Haima-D; Immunorho; Parto-Gamma; Partobulin; Rhesogamma†; Rhesonativ†; Rhesuman; Venogamma Anti-Rho (D); ***Norw.:*** Rhesogamma; Rhesonativ; ***S.Afr.:*** Rhesugam; ***Spain:*** Beriglobina Anti D-P; Gamma Glob Anti D; Gamma Glob Anti Rh; Globulina Lloren Anti RH; Inmunogamma Anti D†; Inmunoglob Anti D†; Rhesuman; ***Swed.:*** Rhesogamma; Rhesonativ; ***Switz.:*** Partobuline†; Rhesuman; Rhophylac; ***UK:*** Partobulin; ***USA:*** Gamulin Rh; HypRho-D; MICRhoGAM; Mini-Gamulin Rh; Rhesonativ†; RhoGAM.

Argentine Haemorrhagic Fever Vaccines

(14682-l)

Junin Haemorrhagic Fever Vaccines.

A live attenuated vaccine is under investigation for active immunisation against Argentine haemorrhagic fever.

References.

1. Maiztegui JI, *et al.* Protective efficacy of a live attenuated vaccine against Argentine hemorrhagic fever. *J Infect Dis* 1998; **177:** 277–83.

BCG Vaccines (7936-m)

Bacillus Calmette-Guérin Vaccines.

Freeze-dried BCG Vaccine (Ph. Eur.) (Bacillus Calmette-Guérin Vaccine (BP 1998); BCG Vaccine; Dried Tub/Vac/BCG; Vaccinum Tuberculosis (BCG) Cryodesiccatum) is a freeze-dried preparation containing live bacteria obtained from a strain derived from the bacillus of Calmette and Guérin (*Mycobacterium bovis* BCG) and known to protect man against tuberculosis. It may contain a stabiliser. The dried vaccine should be stored at 2° to 8° and be protected from sunlight.

BCG Vaccine (USP 23) is a dried living culture of the bacillus Calmette-Guérin strain of *Mycobacterium tuberculosis* var. *bovis*; it is grown from a strain that has been maintained to preserve its capacity for conferring immunity. It contains an amount of viable bacteria such that inoculation, in the recommended dose, of tuberculin-negative persons results in an acceptable tuberculin conversion rate. It contains a suitable stabiliser and no antimicrobial agent. The dried vaccine should be stored at 2° to 8°. The reconstituted vaccine should be used immediately after preparation and any portion not used within 2 hours should be discarded.

Percutaneous Bacillus Calmette-Guérin Vaccine (BP 1998) (Percut. BCG Vaccine) is a suspension of living cells of an authentic strain of the bacillus of Calmette and Guérin with a higher viable bacterial count than Bacillus Calmette-Guérin Vaccine. It is supplied as a dried vaccine (Tub/Vac/BCG(Perc)) and is reconstituted immediately before use by the addition of a suitable sterile liquid. The dried vaccine should be stored at 2° to 8°, not be allowed to freeze, and be protected from light.

Adverse Effects

As for vaccines in general, p.1500.

Side-effects occur rarely with BCG vaccines. They include ulceration of the inoculation site, lymphadenitis, and keloid formation. Serious local reactions are usually due to faulty injection techniques. Very rarely, a lupoid type of reaction has occurred. Generalised, possibly hypersensitivity, reactions with a few fatalities have been reported. Disseminated BCG infection may occur. Osteitis has been reported with some BCG vaccines.

Reviews and studies of the adverse effects of BCG vaccines.[1-3] An increased incidence of local effects has followed intradermal injection of high doses of BCG vaccines.[4,5]

1. Lotte A, *et al.* Second IUATLD study on complications induced by intradermal BCG-vaccination. *Bull Int Union Tuberc Lung Dis* 1988; **63:** 47–59.
2. Milstien JB, Gibson JJ. Quality control of BCG vaccine by WHO: a review of factors that may influence vaccine effectiveness and safety. *Bull WHO* 1990; **68:** 93–108.
3. Grange JM. Complications of bacille Calmette-Guérin (BCG) vaccination and immunotherapy and their management. *Commun Dis Public Health* 1998; **1:** 84–8.
4. Miles MM, Shaw RJ. Effect of inadvertent intradermal administration of high dose percutaneous BCG vaccine. *Br Med J* 1996; **312:** 1014.
5. Puliyel JM, *et al.* Adverse local reactions from accidental BCG overdose in infants. *Br Med J* 1996; **313:** 528–9.

Effects on the bones and joints. The risk of osteitis following BCG vaccination varies from country to country and appears to be linked to the strain of bacillus used.[1]

Osteitis or arthritis has also been reported following intravesicular administration of BCG (see below).

1. Milstien JB, Gibson JJ. Quality control of BCG vaccine by WHO: a review of factors that may influence vaccine effectiveness and safety. *Bull WHO* 1990; **68:** 93–108.

Effects on the eyes. Follicular conjunctivitis occurred following accidental contamination of the eye with BCG vaccine.[1] The conjunctivitis responded to topical corticosteroid therapy, but a course of isoniazid was given as a precautionary measure.

1. Pollard AJ, George RH. Ocular contamination with BCG vaccine. *Arch Dis Child* 1994; **70:** 71.

Effects on the lymphatic system. Increases in the incidence and severity of lymphadenitis have been reported following changes in BCG vaccine to one containing more virulent strains or with different dosage recommendations.[1,2]

1. Hengster P, *et al.* Occurrence of suppurative lymphadenitis after a change of BCG vaccine. *Arch Dis Child* 1992; **67:** 952–5.
2. Kabra SK, *et al.* BCG-associated adenitis. *Lancet* 1993; **341:** 970.

Intravesicular administration. Intravesicular instillation of BCG can give rise to both localised and systemic adverse effects.[1] Local effects include bladder irritation and urinary-tract infections. A case of local infection with vaccine-derived *Mycobacterium bovis* has been reported.[2] Symptoms of hypersensitivity reactions include malaise, fever, and chills. The most serious reactions are severe sepsis with cardiorespiratory manifestations and a disseminated mycobacterial infection with lung granulomas and impaired liver function; both require prompt treatment with antimycobacterial agents.[1] There have been case reports of arthritis and osteitis as a rare complication of intravesicular BCG.[3-5]

1. Lamm DL, *et al.* Incidence and treatment of complications of bacillus Calmette-Guerin intravesical therapy in superficial bladder cancer. *J Urol (Baltimore)* 1992; **147:** 596–600.
2. Ribera M, *et al.* Mycobacterium bovis-BCG infection of the glans penis: a complication of intravesical administration of bacillus Calmette-Guerin. *Br J Dermatol* 1995; **132:** 309–10.
3. Puett DW, Fuchs HA. Arthritis after bacillus Calmette-Guerin therapy. *Ann Intern Med* 1992; **117:** 537.
4. Devlin M, *et al.* Arthritis as a complication of intravesical BCG vaccine. *Br Med J* 1994; **308:** 1638.
5. Morgan MB, Iseman MD. Mycobacterium bovis vertebral osteomyelitis as a complication of intravesical administration of Bacille Calmette-Guérin. *Am J Med* 1996; **100:** 372–3.

Precautions

As for vaccines in general, p.1501. BCG vaccines may be given concomitantly with other live vaccines, but if they are not given at the same time it is preferable to allow an interval of 3 weeks between administration although the period may be reduced to 10 days if absolutely necessary. However, routine immunisation with live poliomyelitis vaccine need not be delayed. No further vaccination should be given in the arm used for BCG vaccination for at least 3 months because of the risk of lymphadenitis. Because of the possible risk of disseminated infections, it is recommended in the UK that BCG vaccines should not be given to HIV-positive persons or those with impaired immune systems from other causes. WHO has, however, advised immunisation of asymptomatic HIV-positive children when the risk of tuberculosis is high. In patients with eczema, BCG vaccines should be given at a site free from lesions. They should not be given to patients receiving antimycobacterial therapy.

Immunocompromised patients. Like other live vaccines, BCG vaccine should not be given to immunocompromised patients including those with symptomatic HIV infections and AIDS. However, the risk of possible adverse effects in patients with asymptomatic HIV infections may be outweighed by the possible advantages of vaccination (see under Uses, below). Disseminated BCG infections have been reported in children with HIV infections,[1] but large studies have shown that infants born to HIV-positive mothers had only a slightly increased risk of adverse reactions, and many of these were generally mild.[2,3]

1. Ryder RW, *et al.* Safety and immunogenicity of bacille Calmette-Guérin, diphtheria-tetanus-pertussis, and oral polio vaccines in newborn children in Zaire infected with human immunodeficiency virus type 1. *J Pediatr* 1993; **122:** 697–702.
2. Besnard M, *et al.* Bacillus Calmette-Guérin infection after vaccination of human immunodeficiency virus-infected children. *Pediatr Infect Dis J* 1993; **12:** 993–7.
3. O'Brien KL, *et al.* Bacillus Calmette-Guérin complications in children born to HIV-1-infected women with a review of the literature. *Pediatrics* 1995; **95:** 414–18.

Interactions

As for vaccines in general, p.1501.

Theophylline. For a report of increased theophylline half-life and serum concentrations after BCG vaccination, see under Theophylline Hydrate, p.770.

Uses and Administration

BCG vaccines are used for active immunisation against tuberculosis, principally for the vaccination of selected groups of the population and of persons likely to be exposed to infection. In some countries it is administered only to persons who give a negative tuberculin reaction, but in countries with a high prevalence of tuberculosis, routine vaccination in infancy is recommended (see below under Tuberculosis for further details). It is also used locally in the treatment of bladder cancers.

In the UK vaccination is recommended in the following groups of persons, if there is *no evidence of previous immunisation* and they are found to be *tuberculin-negative* (see under Tuberculins, p.1640):

- school children aged 10 to 14 years (as part of the standard schedule for immunisation—see p.1501)
- contacts of persons suffering from active respiratory tuberculosis
- immigrants in whose communities there is known to be a high incidence of tuberculosis and all their children wherever born
- health service staff at high risk of infection
- veterinary and other staff who handle animals known to be susceptible to tuberculosis
- staff in any institution where the incidence of tuberculosis is high
- persons intending to stay in Asia, Africa, or Central or South America for more than a month
- any other individual upon request.

Sensitivity testing to tuberculin need not be performed for infants less than 3 months old.

The BCG vaccine is given intradermally (intracutaneously) at the insertion of the deltoid muscle in a dose of 0.1 mL; infants under 3 months of age are given 0.05 mL. For cosmetic reasons, the injection may be given into the upper and lateral surface of the thigh.

A BCG vaccine approximately 10 times the strength of the intradermal vaccine may be given percutaneously using a multiple-puncture device, but such administration is only recommended in infants and young children (up to 5 years of age).

Contacts of patients with active pulmonary tuberculosis may require chemoprophylaxis in addition to vaccination (see under Tuberculosis, p.146). Neonates and children under 2 years of age should be given chemoprophylaxis and immunised, if appropriate, once the course is completed. An isoniazid-resistant form of the vaccine has been produced for use in patients who have received isoniazid, but is not considered necessary.

General references and reviews.

1. Lugosi L. Theoretical and methodological aspects of BCG vaccine from the discovery of Calmette and Guérin to molecular biology: a review. *Tubercle Lung Dis* 1992; **73:** 252–61.

Diabetes mellitus. Although some have reported that BCG vaccination can retard the development[1] of diabetes mellitus (p.313), others have failed to note any benefit.[2]

1. Shehadeh N, *et al.* Effect of adjuvant therapy on development of diabetes in mouse and man. *Lancet* 1994; **343:** 706–7.
2. Pozzilli P, *et al.* BCG vaccines in insulin-dependent diabetes mellitus. *Lancet* 1997; **349:** 1520–1.

Leishmaniasis. For reference to the use of BCG vaccines in leishmaniasis, see Leishmaniasis Vaccines, p.1516.

Leprosy. BCG vaccination has been shown to protect recipients against leprosy[1] and is considered to be one of the factors responsible for the decrease in the incidence of leprosy. As in tuberculosis considerable variation has been noted in the efficacy of BCG in leprosy, and it appears to be more effective in Africa[2-4] and South America than in Asia.[5,6] Protection appears to be afforded against both multibacillary and paucibacillary leprosy[7,8] and a second dose may provide additional protection.[9] Adding killed *Mycobacterium leprae* did not improve the response further.[9] BCG is considered to be an important addition to multidrug treatment in long-term eradication programmes.[1] Specific vaccines against leprosy are under development (see p.1516).

1. Lienhardt C, Fine PEM. Controlling leprosy. *Br Med J* 1992; **305:** 206–7.
2. Stanley SJ, *et al.* BCG vaccination of children against leprosy in Uganda: final results. *J Hyg (Camb)* 1981; **87:** 233–48.
3. Fine PEM, *et al.* Protective efficacy of BCG against leprosy in northern Malawi. *Lancet* 1986; **ii:** 499–502.
4. Baker DM, Nguyen-Van-Tam JS. BCG vaccine and leprosy. *Lancet* 1992; **339:** 1236.
5. Lwin KW, *et al.* BCG vaccination of children against leprosy: fourteen-year findings of the trial in Burma. *Bull WHO* 1985; **63:** 1069–78.
6. Tripathy SP. The case for BCG. *Ann Natl Med Sci (India)* 1983; **19:** 11–21.
7. Pönnighaus JM, *et al.* Efficacy of BCG vaccine against leprosy and tuberculosis in northern Malawi. *Lancet* 1992; **339:** 636–9.
8. Muliyil J, *et al.* Effect of BCG on the risk of leprosy in an endemic area: case control study. *Int J Lepr* 1991; **59:** 229–36.
9. Karonga Prevention Trial Group. Randomised controlled trial of single BCG, repeated BCG, or combined BCG and killed mycobacterium leprae vaccine for prevention of leprosy and tuberculosis in Malawi. *Lancet* 1996; **348:** 17–24.

Malignant neoplasms. Immunotherapy with BCG vaccines has been tried in various malignant disorders and is most successful when administered locally. The possibility that BCG vaccination might protect children against malignancies has been discussed.[1]

1. Grange JM, Stanford JL. BCG vaccination and cancer. *Tubercle* 1990; **71:** 61–4.

BLADDER. Immunotherapy with intravesicular BCG is used in the management of bladder cancers and is the treatment of choice for carcinoma *in situ* (p.484). Local and systemic adverse effects, although rarely severe, are relatively common[1,2] and in the UK, intravesicular BCG has been reserved for advanced tumours which have failed to respond to other drugs.[2] However, in North America, where BCG instillation has been shown to be superior to doxorubicin,[3] it appears to be used more commonly as an alternative to intravascular chemotherapy.[4]

A number of regimens have been tried. BCG is commonly instilled into the bladder once weekly for 6 weeks. Patients at high risk may receive a second course of 6 instillations[1] or maintenance therapy of instillations at monthly or 3-monthly intervals for up to 24 months. Treatment is not started until 7 to 14 days after bladder biopsy or transurethral resection. Urine voided for 6 hours after instillation of BCG vaccines should be disinfected with sodium hypochlorite solution.

1. Witjes JA. Current recommendations for the management of bladder cancer: drug therapies. *Drugs* 1997; **53:** 404–14.
2. Hall RR. Superficial bladder cancer. *Br Med J* 1994; **308:** 910–13.
3. Lamm DL, *et al.* A randomized trial of intravesical doxorubicin and immunotherapy with bacille Calmette-Guérin for transitional-cell carcinoma of the bladder. *N Engl J Med* 1991; **325:** 1205–9.
4. Moss JT, Kadmon D. BCG and the treatment of superficial bladder cancer. *DICP Ann Pharmacother* 1991; **25:** 1355–67.

SKIN. Several studies have reported that BCG vaccine injected into intradermal metastases of melanoma can result in regression of the injected, and sometimes also the uninjected nodules. BCG therapy has been disappointing for visceral metastases. Many anecdotal reports and nonrandomised studies have shown benefit from BCG vaccine as adjuvant therapy, but these results have not been confirmed in large randomised, controlled studies.[1] More specific immunological interventions such as therapeutic vaccines are now being investigated in the treatment of melanomas (p.492).

1. Ho VC, Sober AJ. Therapy for cutaneous melanoma: an update. *J Am Acad Dermatol* 1990; **22:** 159–76.

Tuberculosis. Studies from many parts of the world have evaluated the efficacy of BCG vaccine to protect against tuberculosis. Levels of protection have varied from 0 to over 80%.[1] Many explanations for such variability have been proposed: interaction with the immune response to other mycobacterial infections; antigenic, microbiological, or formulation differences between BCG vaccines; differences in the natural history of infection and disease; variations in host genetics or nutrition; methodological differences between studies.[1,2] It has been noted that in general the efficacy of BCG vaccine in any region is proportional to its distance from the equator and this possibly reflects differences in exposure to environmental mycobacteria.[3] This could be the strongest influence on efficacy,[3] with the implication that BCG may be least effective in areas of the world where the risk of tuberculosis is greatest. BCG also appears to be more effective against systemic (miliary and meningitic tuberculosis) than against pulmonary tuberculosis. It is likely that BCG cannot produce complete protection against infection, and the development of new vaccines is underway.[4]

National policies of BCG vaccination vary widely. In the USA vaccination is recommended only for tuberculin-negative infants and children at high risk of tuberculosis.[5] Most other countries recommend routine vaccination (the UK recommendations are described above).[1] Schedules vary from single vaccination at birth (as recommended by WHO),[6] to single vaccination at age 10 to 14 (as in the UK), to repeated vaccination every few years (particularly in eastern Europe). These policy differences appear to be related as much to differences of opinion about the mechanism of action and effectiveness of vaccines as to local differences in the epidemiology of tuberculosis.[1] WHO considers BCG vaccination to be an adjunct to case detection and treatment in the control of tuberculosis,[6] and recommends that neither tuberculin skin testing nor repeat vaccination should be used.

1. Fine PEM, Rodrigues LC. Modern vaccines: mycobacterial diseases. *Lancet* 1990; **335:** 1016–20.
2. Fine PEM. BCG vaccination against tuberculosis and leprosy. *Br Med Bull* 1988; **44:** 691–703.
3. Fine PEM. Variation in protection by BCG: implications of and for heterologous immunity. *Lancet* 1995; **346:** 1339–45. Correction. *ibid.*; **347:** 340.
4. Malin AS, Young DB. Designing a vaccine for tuberculosis. *Br Med J* 1996; **312:** 1495.
5. Centers for Disease Control. The role of BCG vaccine in the prevention and control of tuberculosis in the United States: a joint statement by the Advisory Council for the Elimination of Tuberculosis and the Advisory Committee on Immunization Practices. *MMWR* 1996; **45** (RR-4): 1–18.
6. Anonymous. WHO statement on BCG revaccination for the prevention of tuberculosis. *Bull WHO* 1995; **73:** 805–6.

HIV-INFECTED PATIENTS. Like other live vaccines, BCG vaccine should not be given to immunocompromised patients including patients with symptomatic HIV infection or AIDS. Doubts about the safety (see under Precautions, above) and efficacy of BCG vaccines in patients with asymptomatic HIV infection have resulted in differing national policies. WHO recommends that the national policy should depend on the local prevalence of tuberculosis.[1] In countries where prevalence is high, the possible benefits of immunisation outweigh the possible disadvantages, and routine BCG vaccination should be given to all children except those with symptomatic HIV infection or AIDS. In countries with low tuberculosis prevalence, BCG vaccination should not be given to children with HIV infections. In the UK[2] and USA,[3] BCG vaccination is not recommended for HIV-positive patients. Similar policies apply to infants born to HIV-positive mothers, although it is not necessary to screen mothers for HIV infection before giving routine BCG vaccination.[2]

1. WHO. *TB/HIV: a clinical manual.* Geneva: WHO, 1996.
2. Salisbury DM, Begg NT, eds. *Immunisation against infectious diseases.* London: HMSO, 1996.
3. Centers for Disease Control. The role of BCG vaccine in the prevention and control of tuberculosis in the United States: a joint statement by the Advisory Council for the Elimination of Tuberculosis and the Advisory Committee on Immunization Practices. *MMWR* 1996; **45** (RR-4) 1–18.

Preparations

BP 1998: Percutaneous Bacillus Calmette-Guérin Vaccine;
Ph. Eur.: Freeze-dried BCG Vaccine;
USP 23: BCG Vaccine.

Proprietary Preparations (details are given in Part 3)
Aust.: ImmuCyst; OncoTICE; ***Austral.:*** ImmuCyst; OncoTICE; ***Belg.:*** Pastimmun; ***Canad.:*** ImmuCyst; OncoTICE; Pacis; ***Fr.:*** Monovax; ***Ger.:*** ImmuCyst; OncoTICE; ***Ital.:*** ImmuCyst; Imovax BCG; OncoTICE; ***Neth.:*** OncoTICE; ***Norw.:*** OncoTICE; ***Spain:*** ImmuCyst; ***Swed.:*** OncoTICE; ***Switz.:*** ImmuCyst; OncoTICE; ***USA:*** TheraCys; Tice.

Botulism Antitoxins (7939-g)

Botulinum Antitoxin (Ph. Eur.) (Bot/Ser; Immunoserum Botulinicum) is a sterile preparation containing the specific antitoxic globulins that have the power of neutralising the toxins formed by type A, type B, type E, or any mixture of types A, B, and E, of *Clostridium botulinum.* It contains not less than 500 international units of each of type A and type B and not less than 50 units of type E per mL. It should be stored at 2° to 8°, and not be allowed to freeze. The BP states that when Mixed Botulinum Antitoxin or Botulinum Antitoxin is prescribed or demanded and the types to be present are not stated, Botulinum Antitoxin prepared from types A, B, and E shall be dispensed or supplied. It should be noted, however, that some antitoxins available in the UK have not conformed to the requirements of the BP and Ph. Eur. (having a higher phenol content than the pharmacopoeias allow), and thus have been referred to as botulism rather than botulinum antitoxin.

Botulism Antitoxin (USP 23) is a sterile solution of the refined and concentrated antitoxic antibodies, chiefly globulins, obtained from the blood of healthy horses that have been immunised against the toxins produced by type A and type B and/or E strains of *Clostridium botulinum.* It contains a suitable antimicrobial agent. It should be stored at 2° to 8° in single-use containers.

Adverse Effects and Precautions

As for antisera in general, p.1500.

Uses and Administration

Botulism antitoxins are used in the postexposure prophylaxis and treatment of botulism. Treatment should be given as early as possible in the course of the disease. Botulism antitoxins are generally not effective for infant botulism.

Since the type of botulism toxin is seldom known the polyvalent antitoxin is usually given. Sensitivity testing should always be performed before administration of the antitoxin.

In the UK a trivalent antitoxin containing not less than 500 units per mL of each of antitoxins types A, B, and E is employed. For the treatment of botulism, 20 mL of this antitoxin should be diluted to 100 mL with sodium chloride 0.9% and given by slow intravenous infusion over at least 30 minutes; another 10 mL may be given 2 to 4 hours later if necessary, and further doses at 12- to 24-hour intervals if indicated. Persons who have been exposed to the toxin and in whom symptoms have not developed should be given 20 mL intramuscularly as a prophylactic measure.

In some countries the mixed antitoxin contains differing amounts of type A, B, and E antitoxin.

Botulism. Botulism is caused by the exotoxin of *Clostridium botulinum*, a spore-forming, Gram-positive anaerobe which occurs in soil and mud. The disease usually follows ingestion of contaminated preserved foodstuffs, but may develop from infected wounds or following gastro-intestinal colonisation in infants. The toxin is heat labile, but the spores can survive temperatures of up to 100°. Eight types of *C. botulinum* can be distinguished, each producing a different exotoxin; human disease is usually caused by types A, B and E.

Symptoms are due to the prevention of acetylcholine-mediated neurotransmission and include descending weakness or paralysis, gastro-intestinal symptoms, postural hypotension, dry mouth, and dilated pupils. Death is usually from respiratory arrest.

Treatment of botulism is with antitoxins and intensive respiratory and supportive therapy. Antitoxins should be given as early as possible but may still be beneficial if treatment is delayed.

Drug therapy aimed at reversing the neuromuscular blockade has included fampridine, guanidine, and guanoxan, and some patients may benefit from this treatment.

Oral penicillins have been tried to eliminate any organisms remaining in the gastro-intestinal tract.

Infant botulism is of increasing importance, especially in the USA where it is reported to be the most commonly occurring form of botulism, with honey (see p.1345) reputed to be the most frequent source of infection. Treatment is with intensive supportive care; antitoxins are not considered to be effective.

Preparations

Ph. Eur.: Botulinum Antitoxin;
USP 23: Botulism Antitoxin.

Proprietary Preparations (details are given in Part 3)
Ital.: Liosiero.

Bovine Colostrum (3802-m)

Bovine colostrum has been used similarly to antisera and human immunoglobulin preparations to provide passive immunity against infectious diseases. Hyperimmune bovine colostra have been prepared from cows previously immunised with specific antigens. In particular, these specific hyperimmune bovine colostra have been tried in cryptosporidiosis.

Preparations

Proprietary Preparations (details are given in Part 3)
Ger.: Lactobin†.

Brucellosis Vaccines (5171-b)

A brucellosis vaccine prepared from an antigenic extract of *Brucella abortus* has been used for active immunisation against brucellosis in persons at high risk of contracting the disease.

Cancer Vaccines (3041-n)

Vaccines are being developed for therapeutic use in a variety of neoplastic diseases including breast, colorectal, and prostate cancers and melanoma. BCG vaccine (p.1505) is used locally in the treatment of bladder cancer and has been tried in other neoplastic diseases.

Melanoma vaccines. References.

1. Morton DL, *et al.* Prolongation of survival in metastatic melanoma after active specific immunotherapy with a new polyvalent melanoma vaccine. *Ann Surg* 1992; **216:** 463–82.
2. Livingston PO, *et al.* Improved survival in stage III melanoma patients with GM2 antibodies: a randomized trial of adjuvant vaccination with GM2 ganglioside. *J Clin Oncol* 1994; **12:** 1036–44.
3. Mitchell MS. Active specific immunotherapy of melanoma. *Br Med Bull* 1995; **51:** 631–46.
4. Bonn D. Getting under the skin with melanoma vaccines. *Lancet* 1996; **348:** 396.
5. Berd D, *et al.* Autologous hapten-modified melanoma vaccine as postsurgical adjuvant treatment after resection of nodal metastases. *J Clin Oncol* 1997; **15:** 2359–70.

Cholera Vaccines (7941-d)

Cholera Vaccine (Ph. Eur.) (Cho/Vac; Vaccinum Cholerae) is a sterile homogeneous suspension of a suitable killed strain or strains of *Vibrio cholerae.* It consists of a mixture of equal parts of vaccines prepared from smooth strains of 2 main serological types, Inaba and Ogawa of the classical biotype with or without the El Tor biotype. A single strain or several strains of each type may be included. All strains must contain, in addition to their type O antigens, the heat-stable O antigen common to the Inaba and Ogawa types. If more than one strain each of Inaba and Ogawa are used they may be selected to contain other O antigens. It contains not less than 8000 million *V. cholerae* per dose, which does not exceed 1 mL. It contains not more than 0.5% of phenol. It should be stored at 2° to 8° and protected from light. It may also be supplied as a dried vaccine (Dried Cho/Vac; Freeze-dried Cholera Vaccine (Ph. Eur.); Vaccinum Cholerae Cryodesiccatum) which is reconstituted immediately before use by the addition of a suitable sterile liquid. Phenol may not be used in the preparation of the dried vaccine. It should be stored at 2° to 8° and be protected from light.

Cholera Vaccine (USP 23) is a sterile suspension, in sodium chloride injection or other suitable diluent, of killed *Vibrio cholerae* selected for high antigenic efficiency. It is prepared from equal parts of suspensions of cholera vibrios of the Inaba and Ogawa strains. It has a labelled potency of 8 units per serotype per mL. It contains a suitable antimicrobial agent. It should be stored at 2° to 8° and not be allowed to freeze.

Adverse Effects and Precautions

As for vaccines in general, p.1500.

Slight swelling, erythema, and tenderness occasionally occur at the injection site. Fever and malaise have been reported and general reactions, including anaphylaxis and hypersensitivity reactions, have occurred. Neurological and psychiatric reactions have occasionally occurred.

Interactions

As for vaccines in general, p.1501.

For reference to the effect of cholera vaccination on the response to yellow fever vaccines, see under Yellow Fever Vaccines, p.1539.

Uses and Administration

Injectable inactivated whole-cell cholera vaccines have been used for active immunisation against cholera but are not considered to be very effective and the immunity conferred is short-lived. They have no role in the management of contacts of cases or in controlling the spread of infection. The WHO International Health Regulations do not require cholera vaccination for travellers as the introduction of cholera into any country cannot be prevented by cholera vaccination. However, travellers may still be asked for evidence of immunisation at some borders.

In the UK a vaccine containing not less than 8000 million *V. cholerae* per mL has been used and a primary prophylactic course of 2 injections at an interval of at least a week and preferably 4 weeks has been given. Further doses should be given at intervals of 6 months.

Oral vaccines containing either live attenuated or inactivated strains are available in some countries and appear to be more effective than parenteral vaccines (see below).

Oral cholera vaccines. Since parenteral cholera vaccines are not considered to be very effective, providing at best 50% protection and confer immunity lasting only 3 to 6 months, attention has been turned towards oral vaccines which stimulate intestinal immunity. Both killed and living oral vaccines have been developed, and both types have been shown to be non-toxic and immunogenic.

Killed vaccines contain inactivated whole *V. cholerae* O1 either alone or with B subunit component of cholera toxin.[1-6] These vaccines produce a protective efficacy of about 60 to 70%[1,2,6] and both modify established infections and prevent new ones. Although the vaccines are effective in areas where El Tor predominates,[5,6] they are more effective against classical strains.[1] Immunity particularly against El Tor may be less sustained in children under 5 years of age than in older children and adults.[1,2,7] The main drawback is the need to administer two or more doses at 1- to 2-week intervals to achieve a protective effect.[4,5,8] The protective effect is rapidly established[5] but wanes over time[1,7] and booster doses after 1 year may be necessary to maintain a high level of immunity.[9]

The most widely investigated live attenuated vaccine is CVD 103-HgR in which the genes encoding the toxic A subunit are deleted by recombinant techniques.[10-14] This vaccine is effective 8 days after a single dose but less so against El Tor than against classical strains. Live oral vaccines effective against El Tor are now being developed,[15,16] and promising responses have also been reported with a live attenuated O139 vaccine.[17]

The efficacy and cost-effectiveness of oral vaccines to control cholera outbreaks in refugee populations remains uncertain.[18,19]

1. Clemens JD, *et al.* Field trial of oral cholera vaccines in Bangladesh: results from three-year follow-up. *Lancet* 1990; **335:** 270–3.
2. Clemens JD, *et al.* Evidence that inactivated oral cholera vaccines both prevent and mitigate Vibrio cholerae O1 infections in a cholera-endemic area. *J Infect Dis* 1992; **166:** 1029–34.
3. Jertborn M, *et al.* Evaluation of different immunization schedules for oral cholera B subunit-whole cell vaccine in Swedish volunteers. *Vaccine* 1993; **11:** 1007–12.
4. Sanchez JL, *et al.* Safety and immunogenicity of the oral, whole cell/recombinant B subunit cholera vaccine in North American volunteers. *J Infect Dis* 1993; **167:** 1446–9.
5. Sanchez JL, *et al.* Protective efficacy of oral whole-cell/recombinant-B-subunit cholera vaccine in Peruvian military recruits. *Lancet* 1994; **344:** 1273–6.
6. Trach DD, *et al.* Field trial of a locally produced, killed, oral cholera vaccine in Vietnam. *Lancet* 1997; **349:** 231–5.
7. van Loon FPL, *et al.* Field trial of inactivated oral cholera vaccines in Bangladesh: results from 5 years of follow-up. *Vaccine* 1996; **14:** 162–6.
8. Sanchez JL, *et al.* Immunological response to Vibrio cholerae O1 infection and an oral cholera vaccine among Peruvians. *Trans R Soc Trop Med Hyg* 1995; **89:** 542–5.
9. Begue RE, *et al.* Immunogenicity in Peruvian volunteers of a booster dose of oral cholera vaccine consisting of whole cells plus recombinant B subunit. *Infect Immun* 1995; **63:** 3726–8.

10. Levine MM, *et al.* Safety, immunogenicity, and efficacy of recombinant live oral cholera vaccines, CVD 103 and CVD 103-HgR. *Lancet* 1988; **ii:** 467–70.
11. Suharyono, *et al.* Safety and immunogenicity of single-dose live oral cholera vaccine CVD 103-HgR in 5-9-year-old Indonesian children. *Lancet* 1992; **340:** 689–94.
12. Su-Arehawaratana P, *et al.* Safety and immunogenicity of different immunization regimens of CVD 103-HgR live oral cholera vaccine in soldiers and civilians in Thailand. *J Infect Dis* 1992; **165:** 1042–8.
13. Barrett P, *et al.* Oral cholera vaccine well tolerated. *Br Med J* 1993; **307:** 1425.
14. Tacket CO, *et al.* Onset and duration of protective immunity in challenged volunteers after vaccination with live oral cholera vaccine CVD 103-HgR. *J Infect Dis* 1992; **166:** 837–41.
15. Tacket CO, *et al.* Volunteer studies investigating the safety and efficacy of live El Tor Vibrio cholerae O1 vaccine strain CVD 111. *Am J Trop Med Hyg* 1997; **56:** 533–7.
16. Sack DA, *et al.* Evaluation of Peru-15, a new live oral vaccine for cholera, in volunteers. *J Infect Dis* 1997; **176:** 201–5.
17. Coster TS, *et al.* Safety, immunogenicity, and efficacy of live attenuated Vibrio cholerae O139 vaccine prototype. *Lancet* 1995; **345:** 949–52.
18. Naficy A, *et al.* Treatment and vaccination strategies to control cholera in sub-Saharan refugee settings: a cost-effectiveness analysis. *JAMA* 1998; **279:** 521–5.
19. Waldman RJ. Cholera vaccination in refugee settings. *JAMA* 1998; **279:** 552–3.

Preparations

Ph. Eur.: Cholera Vaccine; Freeze-dried Cholera Vaccine;
USP 23: Cholera Vaccine.

Proprietary Preparations (details are given in Part 3)
Ital.: Imovax Colera†; ***Spain:*** Vac Anticolerica†; ***Swed.:*** Dukoral; ***Switz.:*** Orochol.

Contraceptive Vaccines (3865-a)

Various approaches to development of a contraceptive vaccine are under investigation. A synthetic contraceptive vaccine which stimulates the production of an antibody against human chorionic gonadotrophin has been studied in human trials.

A safety and immunogenicity study in 30 sterilised women of a potential contraceptive vaccine.[1] The vaccine was based on a synthetic peptide antigen representing the amino-acid sequence 109 to 145 of the carboxy-terminal region of the beta subunit of human chorionic gonadotrophin (HCG). It was postulated that the vaccine would stimulate the production of antibodies against the hormone thus preventing implantation of the fertilised ovum.

In a study in India,[2] contraceptive efficacy was maintained in women who had HCG-antibody titres of over 50 μg per litre. However, adequate antibody titres were attained in only 80% of 148 recipients, and frequent booster injections were required to maintain antibody concentrations.

1. Jones WR, *et al.* Phase I clinical trial of a World Health Organisation birth control vaccine. *Lancet* 1988; **i:** 1295–8.
2. Talwar GP, *et al.* A vaccine that prevents pregnancy in women. *Proc Natl Acad Sci U S A* 1994; **91:** 8532–6.

Crimean-Congo Haemorrhagic Fever Immunoglobulins (14731-v)

Preparations containing antibodies against Crimean-Congo haemorrhagic fever are available in some countries for passive immunisation against the disease.

References.

1. Vassilenko SM, *et al.* Specific intravenous immunoglobulin for Crimean-Congo haemorrhagic fever. *Lancet* 1990; **335:** 791–2.

Cytomegalovirus Immunoglobulins (3896-h)

Cytomegalovirus immunoglobulins containing high levels of specific antibody against cytomegalovirus have been prepared from human plasma.

Adverse Effects and Precautions

As for immunoglobulins in general, p.1500.

Interactions

As for immunoglobulins in general, p.1500.

Uses and Administration

Cytomegalovirus immunoglobulins are used for passive immunisation against cytomegalovirus infection. They may be used prophylactically, especially in patients undergoing certain transplant procedures, or therapeutically for the treatment of established cytomegalovirus infections. For therapeutic use, they are commonly given with ganciclovir.

In the USA a cytomegalovirus immunoglobulin G is available for use in recipients of kidney transplants from cytomegalovirus seropositive donors. The recommended dosage schedule is 150 mg per kg body-weight by intravenous infusion within 72 hours of transplantation, then 100 mg per kg once every 2 weeks for 4 doses, then 50 mg per kg every 4 weeks for 2 doses. The rate of infusion should start at 15 mg per kg per hour increasing to a maximum rate of 60 mg per kg per hour.

The name sevirumab is applied to a χ-chain human monoclonal cytomegalovirus immunoglobulin G1.

Preparations

Proprietary Preparations (details are given in Part 3)
Aust.: Cytotect; ***Austral.:*** CMV Immunoglobulin; ***Canad.:*** CMV Iveegam; ***Ger.:*** Cytoglobin; Cytotect; ***Irl.:*** Megalotect; ***Ital.:*** Cytotect; Uman-Cig; ***S.Afr.:*** Megalotect; ***Swed.:*** Megalotect; ***Switz.:*** Cytotect; Globuman iv Anti-CMV; ***USA:*** CytoGam.

Cytomegalovirus Vaccines (16597-p)

A live attenuated cytomegalovirus vaccine containing human cytomegalovirus Towne strain has been investigated in humans since the late 1970s, particularly for the prevention of cytomegalovirus infection in renal transplant recipients. However, there are doubts over its safety. Vaccines produced by recombinant technology are also being studied.

In a placebo-controlled study involving 237 renal transplant patients Plotkin *et al.*[1] could demonstrate no effect of the cytomegalovirus vaccine (Towne strain) (administered subcutaneously) on overall incidence of cytomegalovirus infection or disease, but there was less severe disease in seronegative recipients who received kidneys from seropositive donors. The vaccine also appeared to prolong graft survival in this subset of patients. However, the Towne vaccine failed to prevent infection in immunocompetent women exposed to young infectious children.[2]

Early studies of subunit vaccines have produced some promising results.[3]

1. Plotkin SA, *et al.* Effect of Towne live virus vaccine on cytomegalovirus disease after renal transplant. *Ann Intern Med* 1991; **114:** 525–31.
2. Adler SP, *et al.* Immunity induced by primary human cytomegalovirus infection protects against secondary infection among women of childbearing age. *J Infect Dis* 1995; **171:** 26–32.
3. Britt WJ. Vaccines against human cytomegalovirus: time to test. *Trends Microbiol* 1996; **4:** 34–8.

Dengue Fever Vaccines (16601-e)

Live attenuated vaccines under study for active immunisation against dengue fever contain dengue virus types 1, 2, and 4 alone or in various combinations. The ultimate aim is to produce a vaccine active against dengue virus types 1, 2, 3, and 4.

References.

1. Bhamarapravati N, *et al.* Immunization with a live attenuated dengue 2 virus candidate vaccine (16681-PDK 53): clinical, immunological and biological responses in adult volunteers. *Bull WHO* 1987; **65:** 189–95.
2. Bhamarapravati N, Yoksan S. Study of bivalent dengue vaccine in volunteers. *Lancet* 1989; **i:** 1077.
3. Brandt WE (WHO). Development of dengue and Japanese encephalitis vaccines. *J Infect Dis* 1990; **162:** 577–83.
4. Barrett ADT. Japanese encephalitis and dengue vaccines. *Biologicals* 1997; **25:** 27–34.

Dental Caries Vaccines (1883-b)

A dental caries vaccine consisting of purified protein from the surface of *Streptococcus mutans* has been investigated.

References.

1. Russell RRB, Johnson NW. The prospects for vaccination against dental caries. *Br Dent J* 1987; **162:** 29–34.
2. Russell MW. Immunization against dental caries. *Curr Opin Dent* 1992; **2:** 72–80.

Diphtheria Antitoxins (7951-h)

Diphtheria Antitoxin (Ph. Eur.) (Dip/Ser; Immunoserum Diphthericum) is a sterile preparation containing the specific antitoxic globulins that have the power of neutralising the toxin formed by *Corynebacterium diphtheriae*. It has a potency of not less than 1000 international units per mL when obtained from horse serum and not less than 500 international units per mL when obtained from other mammals. It should be stored at 2° to 8°, and not be allowed to freeze.

Diphtheria Antitoxin (USP 23) is a sterile solution of the refined and concentrated proteins, chiefly globulins, containing antitoxic antibodies obtained from the serum or plasma of healthy horses that have been immunised against diphtheria toxin or toxoid. It contains not less than 500 units per mL. It should be stored at 2° to 8°.

Adverse Effects and Precautions

As for antisera in general, p.1500.

Uses and Administration

Diphtheria antitoxins neutralise the toxin produced by *Corynebacterium diphtheriae* locally at the site of infection and in the circulation.

Diphtheria antitoxin is used for passive immunisation in suspected cases of diphtheria and should be given without waiting for bacteriological confirmation of the infection. An antibacterial is usually given concomitantly (see p.120). Diphtheria antitoxin is generally not used for the prophylaxis of diphtheria because of the risk of provoking a hypersensitivity reaction. Contacts of a diphtheria case should be promptly investigated, given antibacterial prophylaxis and active immunisation with a suitable diphtheria-containing vaccine as appropriate (see p.1507), and kept under observation.

A test dose of diphtheria antitoxin should always be given to exclude hypersensitivity. For the treatment of diphtheria of mild or moderate severity doses of 10 000 to 30 000 units of diphtheria antitoxin may be given intramuscularly; doses of 40 000 to 100 000 units may be given in severe cases. Higher doses have been used in some countries. For doses of more than 40 000 units a portion of the dose is given intramuscularly followed by the bulk of the dose intravenously after about 0.5 to 2 hours.

Preparations

Ph. Eur.: Diphtheria Antitoxin;
USP 23: Diphtheria Antitoxin.

Diphtheria Immunoglobulins (3894-d)

A diphtheria immunoglobulin containing high levels of specific antibody to the toxin of *Corynebacterium diphtheriae* has been prepared from human plasma. It is used similarly to diphtheria antitoxins (above) in suspected cases of diphtheria. It has also been suggested for prophylaxis in subjects exposed to diphtheria. It should be given in conjunction with a suitable antibacterial.

Preparations

Proprietary Preparations (details are given in Part 3)
Switz.: Diphuman.

Diphtheria Vaccines (7961-b)

Diphtheria Vaccine (Adsorbed) (Ph. Eur.) (Adsorbed Diphtheria Vaccine (BP 1998); Adsorbed Diphtheria Prophylactic; Dip/Vac/Ads(Child); Vaccinum Diphtheriae Adsorbatum) is a preparation of diphtheria formol toxoid adsorbed on a mineral carrier. The formol toxoid is prepared from the toxin produced by the growth of *Corynebacterium diphtheriae*. The mineral carrier may be hydrated aluminium hydroxide, aluminium phosphate, or calcium phosphate and the resulting mixture is approximately isotonic with blood. The antigenic properties are adversely affected by certain antimicrobial preservatives, particularly those of the phenolic type. It contains not less than 30 international units per dose. It should be stored at 2° to 8°, not be allowed to freeze, and be protected from light.

Diphtheria Vaccine (Adsorbed) for Adults and Adolescents (Ph. Eur.) (Dip/Vac/Ads(Adults); Adsorbed Diphtheria Vaccine for Adults and Adolescents (BP 1998); Vaccinum Diphtheriae Adulti et Adulescentis Adsorbatum; Adsorbed Diphtheria Prophylactic for Adults and Adolescents) is adsorbed diphtheria vaccine containing not less than 2 international units per dose. For use in the UK, it contains not more than 2 Lf per dose.

Diphtheria Toxoid (USP 23) is a sterile solution of the formaldehyde-treated products of growth of *Corynebacterium diphtheriae*. It contains a non-phenolic preservative. It should be stored at 2° to 8° and not be allowed to freeze.

Diphtheria Toxoid Adsorbed (USP 23) is a sterile preparation of plain diphtheria toxoid that has been precipitated or adsorbed by alum, aluminium hydroxide, or aluminium phosphate adjuvants. It should be stored at 2° to 8° and not be allowed to freeze.

Units

0.5 mL of the injection of absorbed diphtheria vaccine available in the UK for use in children is equivalent to 30 international units; 0.5 mL of the diluted vaccine for use in adults and older children is equivalent to 2 international units. The toxoid content is represented by flocculation equivalents or Limes flocculationis (Lf). There is no simple correlation between international units and Lf equivalents.

Adverse Effects and Precautions

As for vaccines in general, p.1500.

Local reactions may occur but are generally not severe in young children; the frequency and severity of reactions is reported to be less in children under 2 years of age than in older children and adults.

If diphtheria vaccines or vaccines containing a diphtheria component need to be given to children over the age of 10 years or to adults, vaccines with a reduced content of diphtheria toxoid and intended for adults and adolescents should be used. For further details see under Uses and Administration, below.

Uses and Administration

Diphtheria vaccines are used for active immunisation against diphtheria. The non-adsorbed vaccine has poor immunogenic properties and its effects are enhanced by administration as an adsorbed preparation. For primary immunisation combined diphtheria, tetanus, and pertussis vaccines (p.1509) or combined diphtheria and tetanus vaccines (p.1508) are usually used. For discussion of immunisation schedules see under Vaccines, p.1501.

A single-component diphtheria vaccine may sometimes be used for example in the event of contact with an infected patient or a carrier. In the UK a single-component adsorbed vaccine suitable for infants and children and one containing a low dose of toxoid suitable for children over 10 years of age and adults are available and are given by deep subcutaneous or by intramuscular injection in usual doses of 0.5 mL. For primary immunisation three doses are given at intervals of one month. For children who receive primary immunisation during infancy reinforcing doses should be given at school entry (preferably at least 3 years after primary immunisation) and again on leaving school, using the low-dose preparation.

Individuals coming into contact with a case of diphtheria or carriers of a toxigenic strain, or those travelling to an endemic or epidemic area should receive a complete primary course or a reinforcing dose according to age and immunisation history; those not previously immunised should receive a 3-dose primary course using the appropriate vaccine as outlined above, those previously immunised should receive a single 0.5 mL dose. Unimmunised contacts of a case of diphtheria should in addition receive a prophylactic course of a suitable antibacterial (see p.120). Individuals at repeated risk of exposure to infection may be offered booster doses every 10 years.

If the low-dose vaccine for adults is not available, it has been suggested that 0.1 mL of the standard paediatric vaccine may be given as an alternative for both primary and reinforcing doses.

Schick testing (p.1627) to ascertain immune status is no longer considered necessary before administering diphtheria vaccine to adults provided that a low dose is given; antibody testing is used to check immunity in those regularly exposed to diphtheria.

In some countries, booster doses of diphtheria in combination with tetanus vaccine are recommended every 10 years (see under Diphtheria and Tetanus Vaccines, p.1508).

Conjugation to diphtheria toxoid has been used to increase the immunogenicity of other vaccines (see Haemophilus Influenzae Vaccines, p.1511).

Preparations

Ph. Eur.: Diphtheria Vaccine (Adsorbed); Diphtheria Vaccine (Adsorbed) for Adults and Adolescents;
USP 23: Diphtheria Toxoid; Diphtheria Toxoid Adsorbed.

Proprietary Preparations (details are given in Part 3)
Ital.: H-Adiftal; ***Spain:*** Alun Difter†; Anatoxal Di†; ***Switz.:*** Anatoxal Di.

Diphtheria and Tetanus Vaccines

(7949-p)

Diphtheria and Tetanus Vaccine (Adsorbed) (Ph. Eur.) (Adsorbed Diphtheria-Tetanus Prophylactic; DT/Vac/Ads(Child); Adsorbed Diphtheria and Tetanus Vaccine (BP 1998); Vaccinum Diphtheriae et Tetani Adsorbatum) is a preparation of diphtheria formol toxoid and tetanus formol toxoid adsorbed on a mineral carrier. The mineral carrier may be hydrated aluminium hydroxide, aluminium phosphate, or calcium phosphate and the resulting mixture is approximately isotonic with blood. The antigenic properties are adversely affected by certain antimicrobial preservatives particularly those of the phenolic type. It contains not less than 30 international units of diphtheria toxoid and not less than 40 international units of tetanus toxoid per dose. It should be stored at 2° to 8°, not be allowed to freeze, and be protected from light.

Diphtheria and Tetanus Vaccine (Adsorbed) for Adults and Adolescents (Ph. Eur.) (Adsorbed Diphtheria-Tetanus Prophylactic for Adults and Adolescents; DT/Vac/Ads(Adult); Adsorbed Diphtheria and Tetanus Vaccine for Adults and Adolescents (BP 1998); Vaccinum Diphtheriae et Tetani Adulti et Adulescentis Adsorbatum) is adsorbed diphtheria and tetanus vaccine containing not less than 2 units of diphtheria toxoid and not less than 20 units of tetanus toxoid per dose. For use in the UK, it contains not more than 2 Lf per dose.

Diphtheria and Tetanus Toxoids (USP 23) is a sterile solution prepared by mixing suitable quantities of fluid diphtheria toxoid and fluid tetanus toxoid. The antigenicity or potency and the proportions of the toxoids are such as to provide an immunising dose of each toxoid in the labelled dose. It should be stored at 2° to 8° and not be allowed to freeze.

Diphtheria and Tetanus Toxoids Adsorbed (USP 23) is a sterile suspension prepared by mixing suitable quantities of plain or adsorbed diphtheria toxoid and plain or adsorbed tetanus toxoid and, if plain toxoids are used, an aluminium adsorbing agent. The antigenicity or potency and the proportions of the toxoids are such as to provide an immunising dose of each toxoid in the labelled dose. It should be stored at 2° to 8° and not be allowed to freeze.

Tetanus and Diphtheria Toxoids Adsorbed for Adult Use (USP 23) is a sterile suspension prepared by mixing suitable quantities of adsorbed diphtheria toxoid and adsorbed tetanus toxoid using the same precipitating or adsorbing agent for both toxoids. The antigenicity or potency and the proportions of the toxoids are such as to provide, in the labelled dose, an immunising dose of adsorbed tetanus toxoid and one-tenth of the immunising dose of adsorbed diphtheria toxoid specified for children and not more than 2 Lf of diphtheria toxoid. It should be stored at 2° to 8° and not be allowed to freeze.

Units

0.5 mL of the injection of adsorbed diphtheria and tetanus vaccine available in the UK for use in children is equivalent to not less than 30 international units of diphtheria toxoid and not less than 40 international units of tetanus toxoid. The BP and Ph. Eur. injections for adults and adolescents contain the equivalent of not less than 2 international units of diphtheria toxoid and not less than 20 international units of tetanus toxoid per dose. However, the available UK preparation for adults and children over 10 years of age contains in each 0.5-mL dose not less than 4 international units of diphtheria toxoid and not less than 40 international units of tetanus toxoid.

Adverse Effects and Precautions

As for vaccines in general, p.1500. See also under Diphtheria Vaccines, p.1507, and Tetanus Vaccines, p.1535. Diphtheria and tetanus vaccines are reported to produce fewer adverse effects than diphtheria, tetanus, and pertussis vaccines (p.1509).

Dose-related effects. A high incidence of adverse effects was reported in teenagers inadvertently given a high-dose diphtheria and tetanus vaccine intended for use in infants.[1] Most reactions were classified as mild or moderately severe, but severe local or systemic reactions occurred in a third of those reporting reactions.

1. Sidebotham PD, Lenton SW. Incidence of adverse reactions after administration of high dose diphtheria with tetanus vaccine to school leavers: retrospective questionnaire study. *Br Med J* 1996; **313:** 533–4.

Effects on the nervous system. Encephalopathy more commonly follows vaccination with diphtheria, tetanus, and pertussis vaccine than with diphtheria and tetanus vaccine (p.1509). However, several cases of encephalopathy have occurred in a small region in Italy in children following immunisation against diphtheria and tetanus,[1] although it was not possible to infer a causal relationship. A case of polyradiculoneuritis has been reported in a patient following the use of a diphtheria-tetanus vaccine and was considered most likely to have been due to the tetanus component.[2]

1. Greco D. Case-control study on encephalopathy associated with diphtheria-tetanus immunization in Campania, Italy. *Bull WHO* 1985; **63:** 919–25.
2. Holliday PL, Bauer RB. Polyradiculoneuritis secondary to immunization with tetanus and diphtheria toxoids. *Arch Neurol* 1983; **40:** 56–7.

GUILLAIN-BARRÉ SYNDROME. Evidence mainly from case reports and uncontrolled studies favoured a causal relationship between vaccination with diphtheria and tetanus vaccines or single-antigen tetanus vaccines and Guillain-Barré syndrome. The data came primarily from immunocompromised patients.[1]

1. Stratton KR, *et al.* Adverse events associated with childhood vaccines other than pertussis and rubella: summary of a report from the Institute of Medicine. *JAMA* 1994; **271:** 1602–5.

Uses and Administration

Combined adsorbed diphtheria and tetanus vaccines are used for active immunisation against diphtheria and tetanus; they are used in the UK for reinforcing doses following primary immunisation with diphtheria, tetanus, and pertussis vaccine, and also for primary immunisation. For discussion of immunisation schedules see under Vaccines, p.1501.

In the UK a combined adsorbed diphtheria and tetanus vaccine suitable for use in infants and young children and one with a lower dose of diphtheria toxoid suitable for use in children over 10 years of age and adults are each given in usual doses of 0.5 mL by deep subcutaneous or intramuscular injection. For primary immunisation 3 injections of 0.5 mL of the appropriate vaccine are given at intervals of not less than 4 weeks. For children who receive primary immunisation during infancy reinforcing doses are given at school entry (preferably at least 3 years after primary immunisation) and again on leaving school, using the low-dose preparation. For adults a reinforcing dose may be given after 10 years.

The non-adsorbed combined diphtheria and tetanus vaccines have weaker immunogenic properties than adsorbed vaccines and are no longer recommended.

As, in some countries, booster doses of combined diphtheria and tetanus vaccines are recommended every 10 years, studies have been conducted to assess whether this is necessary. Until relatively recently it had been considered that since the incidence of clinical diphtheria in many countries in western Europe and North America approaches zero, there was no need for booster doses in adults despite low antibody titres, so long as the policy of immunisation during infancy was maintained.[1,2]

However, following a report[3] of an outbreak of clinical diphtheria in Sweden after a period of many years when no indigenous cases of diphtheria had occurred and the disease was regarded as being eliminated from the country the question of immunity in adults and the need for revaccination again arose. Addressing the question with regard to the situation in the USA Karzon and Edwards,[4] considered that re-immunisation every 10 years with a diphtheria and tetanus combined vaccine was mandatory and that this combined vaccine should be used whenever, as in treating emergency wounds, a tetanus vaccine was indicated. Recent outbreaks of diphtheria in Russia and neighbouring countries[5] have prompted recommendations for booster doses in travellers to these countries, and, in the UK, for an additional dose to be added to the routine immunisation schedule at school-leaving age.[6]

A study has shown that an intranasal formulation could produce an adequate booster response and may be advantageous in some patients.[7]

1. Mathias RG, Schechter MT. Booster immunisation for diphtheria and tetanus: no evidence of need in adults. *Lancet* 1985; **i:** 1089–91.
2. Anonymous. Diphtheria and tetanus boosters. *Lancet* 1985; **i:** 1081–2.
3. Rappuoli R, *et al.* Molecular epidemiology of the 1984–1986 outbreak of diphtheria in Sweden. *N Engl J Med* 1988; **318:** 12–14.
4. Karzon DT, Edwards KM. Diphtheria outbreaks in immunized populations. *N Engl J Med* 1988; **318:** 41–3.
5. Anonymous. Diphtheria immunisation—advice from the Chief Medical Officer. *Commun Dis Rep* 1993; **3:** 27.
6. Chief Medical Officer, Department of Health. Immunisation update. *CMO's Update 2* 1994.
7. Aggerbeck H, *et al.* Intranasal booster vaccination against diphtheria and tetanus in man. *Vaccine* 1997; **15:** 307–16.

Preparations

Ph. Eur.: Diphtheria and Tetanus Vaccine (Adsorbed); Diphtheria and Tetanus Vaccine (Adsorbed) for Adults and Adolescents;
USP 23: Diphtheria and Tetanus Toxoids; Diphtheria and Tetanus Toxoids Adsorbed; Tetanus and Diphtheria Toxoids Adsorbed for Adult Use.

Proprietary Preparations (details are given in Part 3)
Aust.: Anatoxal Di Te; Ditanrix; DT-reduct; ***Austral.:*** ADT Vaccine; CDT Vaccine; ***Belg.:*** Anatoxal Di Te; Ditemer; Tedivax; ***Fr.:*** DT Bis; DT Vax; ***Ger.:*** DT-Impfstoff; DT-Rix; DT-Vaccinol; DT-Wellcovax†; Td-Impfstoff; Td-Rix; Td-Vaccinol; ***Irl.:*** Diftavax; ***Ital.:*** Anatoxal Di Te; Dif-Tet-All; Ditanrix; H-Adiftetal; Imovax DT; Vaccino Difto Tetano; ***Spain:*** Alutoxoide D T†; Anatoxal Di Te; Diftavax; Ditanrix; Divacuna TD; Tetano Difter†; Vac Antidift Tet Llte Ev†; ***Swed.:*** Duplex; ***Switz.:*** Anatoxal Di Te; ***UK:*** Diftavax.

Diphtheria, Tetanus, and Haemophilus Influenzae Vaccines (17901-p)

Combined adsorbed diphtheria, tetanus, and *Haemophilus influenzae* type b vaccines are available in some countries for active immunisation of infants. For discussion of immunisation schedules see under Vaccines, p.1501. For concern over the antigenicity of *Haemophilus influenzae* type b vaccine in combined vaccines, see p.1511.

Preparations

Proprietary Preparations (details are given in Part 3)
Swed.: DT-HIB†.

Diphtheria, Tetanus, and Pertussis Vaccines (7955-g)

Diphtheria, Tetanus and Pertussis Vaccine (Adsorbed) (Ph. Eur.) (Adsorbed-Diphtheria-Tetanus-Whooping-cough Prophylactic; DTPer/Vac/Ads; Adsorbed Diphtheria, Tetanus and Pertussis Vaccine (BP 1998); Vaccinum Diphtheriae, Tetani et Pertussis Adsorbatum) is a preparation of diphtheria formol toxoid and tetanus formol toxoid on a mineral carrier to which a suspension of killed *Bordetella pertussis* has been added. The mineral carrier may be hydrated aluminium hydroxide, aluminium phosphate, or calcium phosphate and the resulting mixture is approximately isotonic with blood. The antigenic properties are adversely affected by certain antimicrobial preservatives particularly those of the phenolic type. It contains not less than 30 international units of diphtheria toxoid, not less than 40 international units if the test is performed in *guinea-pigs*, or 60 international units if the test is performed in *mice*, of tetanus toxoid, and not less than 4 international units of the pertussis component per dose. It should be stored at 2° to 8°, not be allowed to freeze, and be protected from light.

Diphtheria and Tetanus Toxoids and Pertussis Vaccine (USP 23) is a sterile suspension prepared by mixing suitable quantities of pertussis vaccine component of killed *Bordetella pertussis*, or a fraction of this organism, fluid diphtheria toxoid, and fluid tetanus toxoid. The antigenicity or potency and the proportions of the components are such that the labelled dose provides an immunising dose of each component. It should be stored at 2° to 8° and not be allowed to freeze.

Diphtheria and Tetanus Toxoids and Pertussis Vaccine Adsorbed (USP 23) is a sterile suspension prepared by mixing suitable quantities of plain or adsorbed diphtheria toxoid, plain or adsorbed tetanus toxoid, plain or adsorbed pertussis vaccine, and, if plain antigen components are used, an aluminium adsorbing agent. The antigenicity or potency and the proportions of the components are such that the labelled dose provides an immunising dose of each component. It should be stored at 2° to 8° and not be allowed to freeze.

Units

0.5 mL of the injection of adsorbed diphtheria, tetanus, and pertussis vaccine available in the UK is equivalent to not less than 30 international units of diphtheria toxoid, not less than 40 international units (or 60 international units if the *mouse* assay is employed) of tetanus toxoid, and not less than 4 international units of the *Bordetella pertussis* component.

Adverse Effects and Precautions

As for vaccines in general, p.1500. See also under Diphtheria Vaccines, p.1507, Pertussis Vaccines, p.1526, and Tetanus Vaccines, p.1535.

The incidence of local reactions and fever is reported to be lower with the accelerated immunisation schedule currently used in the UK than schedules spreading primary immunisation over 6 months. Local reactions and pyrexia occur less commonly after acellular pertussis vaccines, especially in children older than 6 months.

In infants with a personal or close family history of seizures, precautions should be taken to avoid pyrexia. See under Pertussis Vaccines for further details of precautions and contraindications in individuals with a history of neurological problems.

As with other vaccines immunisation should not be carried out in individuals with a definite history of severe reactions. However, in individuals with a history of a less severe general reaction to a preceding dose, immunisation should be completed using diphtheria and tetanus vaccine.

Local and systemic reactions are more common following diphtheria, tetanus, and pertussis (DTP) vaccines than diphtheria and tetanus (DT) vaccines. However, they are generally mild and self-limiting.[1] Infrequently, high fever, persistent or inconsolable crying (possibly as a reaction to pain), hypotonic-hyporesponsive collapse, or short-lived convulsions (frequently febrile convulsions) may occur, and have been reported after both DT and DTP vaccines.[2] These reactions do not appear to have any long-term consequences.[1] Rare but serious acute neurological complications including encephalopathy and prolonged seizures have been reported after DTP and have been attributed to the whole-cell pertussis component (see p.1526) but the association could be coincidental. Epidemiological studies have shown that such events are exceedingly rare and only occasionally followed by long-term neurological damage. Analysis of these studies has been difficult but the National Vaccine Advisory Committee and the Advisory Committee on Immunization Practices[1] concluded that the evidence was insufficient for a link, and this was also the view of the Joint Committee on Vaccination and Immunisation in the UK.[2]

The risk of febrile convulsions following DTP vaccination is reported not to be increased in children immunised before 6 months of age,[2] but there appears to be an increased risk beyond this. Children with a personal or close family history of epilepsy may also be at increased risk of seizures after DTP vaccination. Current recommendations are that immunisation should be given to children with stable neurological conditions, using precautions (such as paracetamol administration and tepid sponging) to prevent pyrexia.

Children experiencing a seizure during the course of immunisation should be carefully assessed before deciding whether to continue immunisation with DTP or DT vaccine. A causal relationship between DTP vaccination and sudden infant death syndrome (SIDS) has not been established and any temporal relationship is likely to be due to chance.[3,4] There is evidence that the risk of SIDS is lower in infants who have been vaccinated.[5]

Immediate anaphylactic reactions have been reported and are regarded as a contra-indication to further use of DTP vaccine. However, the appearance of a rash is not generally regarded as a contra-indication to further doses.

1. Centers for Disease Control. Update: vaccine side effects, adverse reactions, contraindications, and precautions: recommendations of the Advisory Committee on Immunization Practices (ACIP). *MMWR* 1996; **45** (RR-12): 1–45.
2. Salisbury DM, Begg NT (eds), Joint Committee on Vaccination and Immunisation. *Immunisation against infectious disease.* London: HMSO, 1996.
3. Hoffman HJ, *et al.* Diphtheria-tetanus-pertussis immunization and sudden infant death: results of the National Institute of Child Health and Human Development Cooperative Epidemiological Study of Sudden Infant Death Syndrome Risk Factors. *Pediatrics* 1987; **79:** 598–611.
4. Griffin MR, *et al.* Risk of sudden infant death syndrome after immunization with the diphtheria-tetanus-pertussis vaccine. *N Engl J Med* 1988; **319:** 618–23.
5. Mitchell EA, *et al.* Immunisation and the sudden infant death syndrome. *Arch Dis Child* 1995; **73:** 498–501.

Interactions

As for vaccines in general, p.1501.

For a report of a diminished immune response to the pertussis component of diphtheria, tetanus, and pertussis vaccine when mixed with inactivated poliomyelitis vaccine, see Pertussis Vaccines, p.1526.

For a report of a diminished immune response to *Haemophilus influenzae* conjugated vaccine when mixed with diphtheria, tetanus, and acellular pertussis vaccine, see Haemophilus Influenzae Vaccines, p.1511.

Uses and Administration

Combined diphtheria, tetanus, and pertussis vaccines are used for active immunisation of children against diphtheria, tetanus, and pertussis (whooping cough). For discussion of immunisation schedules see below.

In the UK a combined adsorbed vaccine is given by deep subcutaneous or intramuscular injection in usual doses of 0.5 mL. For primary immunisation of infants and children under 10 years of age three doses are given at intervals of one month. The combined vaccine is not suitable for older children or adults. In the USA, three doses are given at intervals of 2 months, a fourth dose at least 6 months after the third, and a fifth dose at school entry. A vaccine containing an acellular pertussis component rather than the standard whole-cell component is now preferred in some countries (see under Uses and Administration of Pertussis Vaccines, p.1527). The non-adsorbed type of combined diphtheria, tetanus, and pertussis vaccines have weaker immunogenic properties than adsorbed vaccines and are no longer recommended.

Immunisation schedules. In 1990 the schedule for primary immunisation of infants for diphtheria, tetanus, pertussis, and polio in the UK changed[1] from three injections at 3, 4½ to 5, and 8½ to 11 months to 2, 3, and 4 months, with no further doses recommended until the child was 4 years of age (see also under Vaccines, p.1501). The aim was to improve compliance and to provide protection against pertussis at a younger age. An improvement of vaccine coverage has been achieved[2] and fewer adverse effects are associated with this accelerated schedule.[3] However, the accelerated schedule has been shown to be less immunogenic for diphtheria and tetanus than the old schedule at a month after completion of the vaccination course.[4] This could be due partly to the immaturity of the immune system at 2 months of age and an inhibitory effect of maternal tetanus toxoid antibodies. Nevertheless, differences in antibody concentrations produced by the two schedules were less marked at 12 months[5] and it was considered that adequate immunity would be maintained until the booster dose when the child is 4 years of age.

1. Department of Health. *Immunisation against infectious disease.* London: HMSO, 1990.
2. White JM, *et al.* Vaccine coverage: recent trends and future prospects. *Br Med J* 1992; **304:** 682–4.
3. Ramsay MEB, *et al.* Symptoms after accelerated immunisation. *Br Med J* 1992; **304:** 1534–6.
4. Booy R, *et al.* Immunogenicity of combined diphtheria, tetanus, and pertussis vaccine given at 2, 3, and 4 months versus 3, 5, and 9 months of age. *Lancet* 1992; **339:** 507–10.
5. Ramsay MEB, *et al.* Antibody response to accelerated immunisation with diphtheria, tetanus, and pertussis vaccine. *Lancet* 1993; **342:** 203–5.

Preparations

Ph. Eur.: Diphtheria, Tetanus and Pertussis Vaccine (Adsorbed); ***USP 23:*** Diphtheria and Tetanus Toxoids and Pertussis Vaccine; Diphtheria and Tetanus Toxoids and Pertussis Vaccine Adsorbed.

Proprietary Preparations (details are given in Part 3)
Aust.: Anatoxal Di Te Per; Infanrix; Tritanrix-DTPw; ***Austral.:*** Infanrix; Triple Antigen; ***Belg.:*** Anatoxal Di Te Per; Combivax; Infanrix; Triamer; ***Canad.:*** Tri-Immunol; Tripacel; ***Fr.:*** DT Coq; ***Ger.:*** DPT Merieux; DPT-Impfstoff; DPT-Vaccinol; DTP-Rix; Infanrix DTPa; ***Irl.:*** Infanrix; Trivax; Trivax-AD; ***Ital.:*** Adifteper; Anatoxal Di Te Per; Dif-Per-Tet-All†; Imovax DTP; Infanrix; Triacelluvax; Tritanrix; Vaccino DPT; ***S.Afr.:*** DTP-Merieux; ***Spain:*** Alutoxoide D T P†; Anatoxal Di Te Per; Imovax DPT†; Neo Diftepertus†; Trivacuna; Welltrivax†; ***Swed.:*** Di-Te Kik; Infanrix; ***Switz.:*** Acel-Imune; Anatoxal Di Te Per; Infanrix DTPa; ***UK:*** Trivax-AD; Trivax†; ***USA:*** Acel-Imune; Certiva; Infanrix; Tri-Immunol; Tripedia.

Diphtheria, Tetanus, Pertussis, and Haemophilus Influenzae Vaccines (17266-x)

Combined adsorbed diphtheria, tetanus, whole-cell or acellular pertussis, and *Haemophilus influenzae* type b vaccines are used for active immunisation of infants. For discussion of immunisation schedules, see under Vaccines, p.1501. For concern over the antigenicity of *Haemophilus influenzae* type b vaccine in combined vaccines, see p.1511.

Preparations

Proprietary Preparations (details are given in Part 3)
Belg.: Tetract-HIB; ***Canad.:*** Tetramune; ***Ger.:*** Infanrix DTPa + Hib; ***Ital.:*** Tetract-HIB; ***S.Afr.:*** TetraTITER; ***Swed.:*** DT-HIB†; ***Switz.:*** ProHIBiT-DPT; Tetramune; ***UK:*** Act-HIB DTP; Trivax-Hib; ***USA:*** Tetramune; TriHIBit.

Diphtheria, Tetanus, Pertussis, and Poliomyelitis Vaccines (7957-p)

Diphtheria, tetanus, pertussis, and poliomyelitis vaccines are available in some countries for active immunisation of infants against diphtheria, tetanus, pertussis, and poliomyelitis. Preparations containing acellular pertussis vaccine are also available.

For discussion of immunisation schedules see under Vaccines, p.1501.

Preparations

Proprietary Preparations (details are given in Part 3)
Fr.: Tetracoq; Vaccin DTCP; ***Switz.:*** DiTePerPol Vaccin†.

Diphtheria, Tetanus, and Poliomyelitis Vaccines (7956-q)

An adsorbed diphtheria, tetanus, and poliomyelitis vaccine may be used for both primary immunisation against diphtheria, tetanus, and poliomyelitis and to reinforce the immunity of those who have previously been immunised. For discussion of immunisation schedules see under Vaccines, p.1501.

In some countries a preparation with a low dose of diphtheria vaccine is available for use in older children and adults.

Preparations

Proprietary Preparations (details are given in Part 3)
Fr.: DT Polio; Vaccin DTP.

Diphtheria, Tetanus, and Rubella Vaccines (13415-p)

Diphtheria, tetanus, and rubella vaccines have been used in some countries for active immunisation against diphtheria, tetanus, and rubella.

Japanese Encephalitis Vaccines (16619-r)

Adverse Effects and Precautions

As for vaccines in general, p.1500.

Hypersensitivity reactions including urticaria, angioedema, hypotension, and dyspnoea have been reported mainly in travellers from non-endemic areas.

References.

1. Andersen MM, Rønne T. Side-effects with Japanese encephalitis vaccine. *Lancet* 1991; **337:** 1044.
2. Ruff TA, *et al.* Adverse reactions to Japanese encephalitis vaccine. *Lancet* 1991; **338:** 881–2.
3. Plesner A-M, *et al.* Neurological complications and Japanese encephalitis vaccination. *Lancet* 1996; **348:** 202–3.
4. Nothdurft HD, *et al.* Adverse reactions to Japanese encephalitis vaccine in travellers. *J Infect* 1996; **32:** 119–22.
5. Jelinek T, Nothdurft HD. Japanese encephalitis vaccine in travellers: is wider use prudent? *Drug Safety* 1997; **16:** 153–6.

Interactions

As for vaccines in general, p.1501.

Uses and Administration

Two types of inactivated Japanese encephalitis vaccine are being used for active immunisation against encephalitis due to Japanese encephalitis virus, an infection against which there is currently no specific treatment. One type of vaccine is derived from mouse brain and the other from primary hamster kidney cells. The vaccines are widely used in Japan and other parts of Asia and may form part of the World Health Organization's Expanded Programme on Immunization.

Vaccination is recommended for visitors to rural areas of South East Asia and the Far East where infection is endemic and where the visit is to be for more than one month; it is also recommended for shorter visits in individuals likely to be at exceptional risk. Adults are usually given 3 doses each of 1 mL of the inactivated vaccine subcutaneously at 0, 7 to 14, and 28 to 30 days; full immunity will take up to one month to develop. A two-dose schedule with doses given 7 to 14 days apart is suggested to provide short-term immunity but is effective in only 80% of recipients; in the USA an abbreviated dosage schedule with administration at 0, 7, and 14 days is suggested if time is not available for the standard schedule. Children under 3 years of age may be given a dose of 0.5 mL; in the USA the vaccine is not recommended for children under 1 year. A reinforcing dose is given after 2 years.

Live attenuated Japanese encephalitis vaccines are used in some countries.

Inactivated Japanese encephalitis vaccines have been widely used in Asia for some years. In Japan the incidence of the disease has decreased since the introduction of nationwide vaccination in the mid-1960s.[1] A study in Thailand in 1984–5 compared a monovalent Nakayama strain vaccine (21 628 subjects), a bivalent Nakayama-Beijing 1 strain vaccine (22 080 subjects), and a tetanus toxoid placebo (21 516 subjects) in children aged 1 to 14 years.[2] Two subcutaneous 1-mL doses (0.5 mL for children under 3 years of age) were given seven days apart. The attack rate for encephalitis caused by Japanese encephalitis virus was 51 per 100 000 in the placebo group and 5 per 100 000 in both vaccine groups. Vaccine efficacy in both groups combined was calculated to be 91%. Results suggested that Japanese encephalitis vaccine does not prevent virus infection but protects against symptomatic Japanese encephalitis. Immunisation had no significant effect on the incidence of dengue haemorrhagic fever although the severity of episodes may be decreased. The vaccines were associated with minimal short-term side-effects. Findings suggested that post-vaccine encephalomyelitis does not occur or is very rare with these vaccines.

A case-control study of a live attenuated vaccine (SA14-14-2) indicated that 2 doses given a year apart were 97% effective in an endemic region of rural China.[3] Similar results were obtained when the interval between doses was reduced to 1 to 3 months.[4]

Other vaccines are at early stages of development.[5]

1. Denning DW, Kaneko Y. Should travellers to Asia be vaccinated against Japanese encephalitis? *Lancet* 1987; **i:** 853–4.
2. Hoke CH, *et al.* Protection against Japanese encephalitis by inactivated vaccines. *N Engl J Med* 1988; **319:** 608–14.
3. Hennessy S, *et al.* Effectiveness of live-attenuated Japanese encephalitis vaccine (SA14-14-2): a case-control study. *Lancet* 1996; **347:** 1583–6.
4. Tsai TF, *et al.* Immunogenicity of live attenuated SA14-14-2 Japanese encephalitis vaccine—a comparison of 1- and 3-month immunization schedules. *J Infect Dis* 1998; **177:** 221–3.
5. Barrett ADT. Japanese encephalitis and dengue vaccines. *Biologicals* 1997; **25:** 27–34.

Preparations

Proprietary Preparations (details are given in Part 3)
Canad.: JE-Vax; *USA:* JE-Vax.

Tick-borne Encephalitis Immunoglobulins (11616-n)

Preparations containing antibodies against tick-borne encephalitis are available in some countries for passive immunisation against the disease.

Preparations

Proprietary Preparations (details are given in Part 3)
Aust.: FSME-Bulin; *Canad.:* FSME-Immun†; *Ger.:* Encegam; FSME-Bulin s; FSME-Immunoglobulin†; *Switz.:* FSME-Bulin.

Tick-borne Encephalitis Vaccines (3869-f)

Tick-borne Encephalitis Vaccine (Inactivated) (Ph. Eur.) (Vaccinum Encephalitidis Ixodibus Advectae Inactivatum) is a liquid preparation of a suitable strain of tick-borne encephalitis virus grown in cultures of chick-embryo cells or other suitable cell cultures and inactivated by a suitable method. It should be stored at 2° to 8°, not be allowed to freeze, and be protect from light.

Adverse Effects and Precautions

As for vaccines in general, p.1500.

Effects on the nervous system. Severe progressive sensorimotor spastic paralysis occurred in a 54-year-old man after a second booster dose of tick-borne encephalitis vaccine.[1] Partial recovery was noted after about 6 months.

1. Bohus M, *et al.* Myelitis after immunisation against tick-borne encephalitis. *Lancet* 1993; **342:** 239–40.

Interactions

As for vaccines in general, p.1501.

Uses and Administration

A vaccine is available for active immunisation against tick-borne viral encephalitis.

In the UK, vaccination against tick-borne encephalitis is recommended for those who anticipate prolonged exposure to the infective agent, for example persons visiting or working in the warm forested parts of Europe and Scandinavia. The vaccine is given by intramuscular injection in a dose of 0.5 mL. A two-dose regimen with an interval of 4 to 12 weeks will provide protection for 1 year. A third dose 9 to 12 months after the second will give protection for up to 3 years. A further reinforcing dose may be given up to six years later if required. Reinforcing doses every 3 years are recommended for those at continued risk of exposure.

Preparations

Ph. Eur.: Tick-borne Encephalitis Vaccine (Inactivated).

Proprietary Preparations (details are given in Part 3)
Aust.: FSME-Immun; *Belg.:* FSME-Immun; *Ger.:* Encepur; FSME-Immun; *Switz.:* FSME-Immun.

Endotoxin Antibodies (19133-d)

Antibodies against the endotoxin of Gram-negative bacteria have been tried as adjunctive therapy for the treatment and prevention of Gram-negative bacteraemia and shock.

Early preparations consisted of antisera prepared from the sera of donors immunised with *Escherichia coli* J5; these were superseded by human and murine IgM monoclonal antibodies. Nebacumab (HA-1A) is a human monoclonal IgM antibody that binds specifically to the lipid A domain of endotoxin. Lipid A in the circulation releases tumour necrosis factor and other cytokines from macrophages and endothelial cells which may ultimately culminate in physiological effects such as multiple organ failure. Despite early promising results of clinical studies the safety of nebacumab in patients without Gram-negative septicaemia has been questioned and the product has been withdrawn from the European market pending the results of further studies. A single dose of nebacumab 100 mg administered by intravenous infusion over 15 to 30 minutes was used.

A murine monoclonal IgM antibody (edobacomab; E5) has also undergone clinical trials.

Initial promising results in patients with Gram-negative infections given antibodies against the endotoxin core glycolipid of Gram-negative bacteria[1,2] prompted further investigations using monoclonal antibodies to these endotoxins in the management of septicaemia (p.141).

Studies concentrated on preparations of either human or murine IgM monoclonal antibodies to the endotoxin of Gram-negative organisms. A study[3] of nebacumab in 543 patients with sepsis showed a reduction in mortality from 49 to 30% in patients with Gram-negative bacteraemia. However, the study was severely criticised on the grounds that this group of patients could only be identified retrospectively, and overall nebacumab had no effect on mortality. A subsequent study involving 2199 patients with septic shock[4] was stopped when the mortality rate in patients without Gram-negative bacteraemia was found to be higher in those receiving nebacumab than in those receiving the placebo. The mortality rate was unchanged in patients with Gram-negative bacteraemia. Doubts about the safety and clinical efficacy of nebacumab were sufficient to lead to its withdrawal from the European market[5] although some clinical studies have continued, including a study in children.[6] In the meantime, doubts over the role of endotoxins in the development of the sepsis syndrome have been raised[7] although there has been a report[8] of the development of full clinical manifestations of septic shock in a man following self-administration of a single large dose of endotoxin in an attempt to treat a tumour.

An initial study of the murine monoclonal antibody edobacomab showed some benefit in patients with Gram-negative infections but not in shock, although there was no overall improvement in survival at 30 days.[9] A subsequent study of patients with similar characteristics to those who had responded in the first study also failed to show an improvement in survival at 30 days[10] although some beneficial responses were seen in patients with organ failure.

1. Ziegler EJ, *et al.* Treatment of Gram-negative bacteremia and shock with human antiserum to a mutant Escherichia coli. *N Engl J Med* 1982; **307:** 1225–30.
2. Baumgartner J-D, *et al.* Prevention of Gram-negative shock and death in surgical patients by antibody to endotoxin core glycolipid. *Lancet* 1985; **ii:** 59–63.
3. Ziegler EJ, *et al.* Treatment of Gram-negative bacteremia and septic shock with HA-1A human monoclonal antibody against endotoxin. *N Engl J Med* 1991; **324:** 429–36.
4. McCloskey RV, *et al.* Treatment of septic shock with human monoclonal antibody HA-1A: a randomized, double-blind, placebo-controlled trial. *Ann Intern Med* 1994; **121:** 1–5.
5. Horton R. Voluntary suspension of Centoxin. *Lancet* 1993; **341:** 298.
6. Romano MJ, *et al.* Single-dose pharmacokinetics and safety of HA-1A, a human IgM anti-lipid-A monoclonal antibody, in pediatric patients with sepsis syndrome. *J Pediatr* 1993; **122:** 974–81.
7. Hurley JC. Reappraisal of the role of endotoxin in the sepsis syndrome. *Lancet* 1993; **341:** 1133–5.
8. da Silva AMT, *et al.* Brief report: shock and multiple-organ dysfunction after self-administration of salmonella endotoxin. *N Engl J Med* 1993; **328:** 1457–60.
9. Greenman RL, *et al.* A controlled clinical trial of E5 murine monoclonal IgM antibody to endotoxin in the treatment of Gram-negative sepsis. *JAMA* 1991; **266:** 1097–1102.
10. Bone RC, *et al.* A second large controlled clinical study of E5, a monoclonal antibody to endotoxin: results of a prospective, multicenter, randomized controlled trial. *Crit Care Med* 1995; **23:** 994–1005.

Preparations

Proprietary Preparations (details are given in Part 3)
Fr.: Centoxin†; *Neth.:* Centoxin†; *UK:* Centoxin†.

Epstein-Barr Virus Vaccines (1742-j)

Several Epstein-Barr virus vaccines are under investigation for active immunisation against infectious mononucleosis and post-transplant lymphoproliferative disorders.

References.

1. Moss DJ, *et al.* Candidate vaccines for Epstein-Barr virus. *Br Med J* 1998; **317:** 423–4.

Escherichia Coli Vaccines (3067-e)

Vaccines against enterotoxigenic strains of *Escherichia coli* are under study. Vaccine candidates include toxoids, inactivated whole bacteria, purified surface antigens, and live oral vaccines.

References.

1. Levine MM. Modern vaccines: enteric infections. *Lancet* 1990; **335:** 958–61.
2. Cross A, *et al.* Safety and immunogenicity of a polyvalent Escherichia coli vaccine in human volunteers. *J Infect Dis* 1994; **170:** 834–40.
3. Tacket CO, *et al.* Enteral immunization and challenge of volunteers given enterotoxigenic E. coli CFA/II encapsulated in biodegradable microspheres. *Vaccine* 1994; **12:** 1270–4.
4. Konadu EY, *et al.* Investigational vaccine for Escherichia coli O157: phase 1 study of O157 O-specific polysaccharide-Pseudomonas aeruginosa recombinant exoprotein A conjugates in adults. *J Infect Dis* 1998; **177:** 383–7.
5. Savarino SJ, *et al.* Safety and immunogenicity of an oral, killed enterotoxigenic Escherichia coli-cholera toxin B subunit vaccine in Egyptian adults. *J Infect Dis* 1998; **177:** 796–9.

Gas-gangrene Antitoxins (8039-n)

Gas-gangrene Antitoxin (Novyi) (Ph. Eur.) (Gas-gangrene Antitoxin (Oedematiens); Immunoserum Gangraenicum (Clostridium Novyi); Nov/Ser) is a sterile preparation containing the specific antitoxic globulins that have the power of neutralising the alpha toxin formed by *Clostridium novyi*. It has a potency of not less than 3750 international units (iu) per mL.

Gas-gangrene Antitoxin (Perfringens) (Ph. Eur.) (Immunoserum Gangraenicum (Clostridium Perfringens); Perf/Ser) is a sterile preparation containing the specific antitoxic globulins that have the power of neutralising the alpha toxin formed by *Clostridium perfringens*. It has a potency of not less than 1500 iu per mL.

Gas-gangrene Antitoxin (Septicum) (Ph. Eur.) (Immunoserum Gangraenicum (Clostridium Septicum); Sep/Ser) is a sterile preparation containing the specific antitoxic globulins that have the power of neutralising the alpha toxin formed by *Clostridium septicum*. It has a potency of not less than 1500 iu per mL.

Mixed Gas-gangrene Antitoxin (Ph. Eur.) (Immunoserum Gangraenicum Mixtum; Gas/Ser) is prepared by mixing Gas-gangrene Antitoxin (Novyi), Gas-gangrene Antitoxin (Perfringens), and Gas-gangrene Antitoxin (Septicum) in appropriate quantities. It has a potency of not less than 1000 iu of Gas-gangrene Antitoxin (Novyi), not less than 1000 iu of Gas-gangrene Antitoxin (Perfringens), and not less than 500 iu of Gas-gangrene Antitoxin (Septicum) per mL.

The above antitoxins should be stored at 2° to 8°, and not be allowed to freeze.

Gas-gangrene antitoxins have been used for the treatment of gas gangrene and for prophylaxis in patients at risk following injury. They are now seldom used and have been superseded by antibacterials.

Suggested doses for a mixed gas-gangrene antitoxin were 25 000 units intravenously or intramuscularly for prophylaxis and 75 000 units intravenously for treatment; these doses might have been repeated or larger doses given initially. Monovalent gas-gangrene antitoxins have been little used in practice owing to the difficulty of rapidly identifying the infecting organism.

Preparations

Ph. Eur.: Gas-gangrene Antitoxin (Novyi); Gas-gangrene Antitoxin (Perfringens); Gas-gangrene Antitoxin (Septicum); Mixed Gas-gangrene Antitoxin.

Proprietary Preparations (details are given in Part 3)
Ger.: Gasbrand-Antitoxin.

Gonococcal Vaccines (19267-j)

Gonorrhoea Vaccines.

Several experimental gonococcal vaccines produced usually from the surface antigens of *Neisseria gonorrhoeae* have been investigated. A polyvalent bacterial vaccine with activity against Gonococcus is available in some countries.

Haemophilus Influenzae Immunoglobulins

(14704-h)

A bacterial polysaccharide immunoglobulin has been prepared from the plasma of individuals immunised with *Haemophilus influenzae* type b, pneumococcal, and meningococcal capsular polysaccharide vaccines. This has been tried for passive immunisation against *H. influenzae* type b infections.

References.

1. Santosham M, *et al.* Prevention of Haemophilus influenzae type b infections in high-risk infants treated with bacterial polysaccharide immune globulin. *N Engl J Med* 1987; **317:** 923–9.
2. Santosham M, *et al.* Passive immunization for infection with Haemophilus influenzae type b. *Pediatrics* 1990; **85** (suppl): 662–6.

Haemophilus Influenzae Vaccines

(16828-q)

Haemophilus Type b Conjugate Vaccine (Ph. Eur.) (Vaccinum Haemophili Stirpe b Conjugatum) is a liquid or freeze-dried preparation of a polysaccharide, polyribosylribitol phosphate (PRP), derived from a suitable strain of *Haemophilus influenzae* type b, covalently bound to a carrier protein. It should be stored at 2° to 8° and protected from light.

Haemophilus Influenzae Conjugate Vaccine (Diphtheria Toxoid Conjugate) (PRP-D) consists of the purified capsular polysaccharide of *Haemophilus influenzae* type b covalently linked to diphtheria toxoid.

Haemophilus Influenzae Conjugate Vaccine (Diphtheria CRM_{197} Protein Conjugate) (HbOC) consists of oligosaccharides derived from the purified capsular polysaccharide of *Haemophilus influenzae* type b covalently linked to a non-toxic variant of diphtheria toxin isolated from *Corynebacterium diphtheriae.*

Haemophilus Influenzae Conjugate Vaccine (Meningococcal Protein Conjugate) (PRP-OMP or PRP-OMPC) consists of the purified capsular polysaccharide of *Haemophilus influenzae* type b covalently linked to an outer membrane protein complex of *Neisseria meningitidis* group B.

Haemophilus Influenzae Conjugate Vaccine (Tetanus Toxoid Conjugate) (PRP-T) consists of the purified capsular polysaccharide of *Haemophilus influenzae* type b covalently linked to tetanus toxoid.

Haemophilus Influenzae Polysaccharide Vaccine. Non-conjugate vaccines (formerly used).

Adverse Effects and Precautions

As for vaccines in general, p.1500.

Erythema multiforme, convulsions, and transient cyanosis of the lower limbs have been reported rarely in children receiving haemophilus influenzae vaccines.

Effects on the nervous system. A report of Guillain-Barré syndrome in 3 infants,[1] with onset of symptoms within one week of vaccination with haemophilus influenzae conjugate vaccine (diphtheria toxoid conjugate).

1. D'Cruz OF, *et al.* Acute inflammatory demyelinating polyradiculoneuropathy (Guillain-Barré syndrome) after immunization with Haemophilus influenzae type b conjugate vaccine. *J Pediatr* 1989; **115:** 743–6.

Interactions

As for vaccines in general, p.1501.

Antineoplastics. Haemophilus influenzae infection occurred in a child who had received antineoplastic therapy despite having completed a primary course of immunisation before the neoplasia was diagnosed.[1] A subsequent booster dose produced an adequate antibody response. Antineoplastic therapy may have impaired the T-cell response to infection.

1. Jenkins DR, *et al.* Childhood neoplasia and Haemophilus influenzae type b vaccine failure. *Lancet* 1996; **348:** 131.

Diphtheria, tetanus, and pertussis vaccines. Some haemophilus influenzae conjugated vaccines may be mixed with diphtheria, tetanus, and pertussis vaccines before administration without adversely affecting the immunogenicity of the components.[1,2] However the immunogenicity of a haemophilus influenzae conjugated vaccine was reduced when mixed with a diphtheria, tetanus, and acellular pertussis vaccine.[3]

1. Miller MA, *et al.* Safety and immunogenicity of PRP-T combined with DTP: excretion of capsular polysaccharide and antibody response in the immediate post-vaccination period. *Pediatrics* 1995; **95:** 522–7.
2. Mulholland EK, *et al.* The use of Haemophilus influenzae type b-tetanus toxoid conjugate vaccine mixed with diphtheria-tetanus-pertussis vaccine in Gambian infants. *Vaccine* 1996; **14:** 905–9.
3. Eskola J, *et al.* Randomised trial of the effect of co-administration with acellular pertussis DTP vaccine on immunogenicity of Haemophilus influenzae type b conjugated vaccine. *Lancet* 1996; **348:** 1688–92.

Uses and Administration

Haemophilus influenzae (Hib) vaccines are used for active immunisation against *Haemophilus influenzae* type b infections, one of the major causes of meningitis and other severe systemic illnesses in young children. Vaccines have been prepared from the capsular polysaccharide of *H. influenzae* type b and immunogenicity, especially in young children, has been shown to be improved by linking the polysaccharide to a protein carrier to form a conjugate vaccine (see above for description of different conjugate vaccines). For discussion of immunisation schedules see below.

Different proprietary vaccines may be conjugated to differing proteins (see above) but are generally regarded as interchangeable.

In the UK a conjugate vaccine is given by deep subcutaneous or intramuscular injection in doses of 0.5 mL. For primary immunisation of infants from 2 months of age, three doses are given at intervals of one month. The vaccine may be administered at the same time as combined diphtheria, tetanus, and pertussis vaccines of the primary immunisation schedule. Children aged under 13 months who have already commenced or completed their primary immunisation schedule should receive three doses of Hib vaccine at intervals of one month. Children aged 13 to 48 months should be given a single dose as they are at lower risk and the vaccine is effective after a single dose in this age group. Routine use in older children or adults is not recommended in the UK. Unimmunised household contacts of a case of invasive disease who are under 4 years of age, and asplenic children and adults, should receive a single dose of Hib vaccine, or three doses for children under 1 year of age.

In the USA, primary immunisation is also carried out in conjunction with diphtheria, tetanus, and pertussis vaccination. If a meningococcal protein conjugate vaccine is used, only 2 doses are given for the primary course. A reinforcing dose using any of the available vaccines is given at 12 to 15 months of age.

Where compatibility has been demonstrated, Hib vaccines may be administered as mixtures with diphtheria, tetanus, and pertussis vaccines (but see Interactions, above).

Immunisation schedules. Various regimens for vaccination against *Haemophilus influenzae* type b infection (Hib) have been tried. In the USA a reinforcing dose is given at 12 to 15 months of age to children who have received a primary course and studies in other countries have shown that a booster dose substantially reduces the risk of infection.[1] In the UK this is considered unnecessary[2] and a reinforcing dose is not included in the routine schedule (see under Vaccines, p.1501). Follow-up of children vaccinated using this schedule have shown that satisfactory serum-antibody concentrations persist at 4.5 years of age.[3] This difference in recommendations may reflect the high vaccine uptake, the use of a three-dose primary schedule, and the use of a highly immunogenic vaccine in the UK.[1] Studies have shown that two-dose schedules[4,5] or giving one-half or one-third of the full dose at 2, 4, and 6 months of age[6] can produce an adequate immune response although the usual three-dose schedule produces higher antibody concentrations.[5]

Differing immunogenicity of conjugate vaccines led to concern over the interchangeability of vaccines during primary immunisation.[7] In general, studies have shown that, despite some differences in antibody concentrations when different vaccines are used for doses during the primary course, the immune response was usually adequate.[8-11]

Response to some Hib vaccines may be diminished in premature infants,[12,13] although adequate responses even in very premature infants have been reported.[14] Raised antibody titres have been reported in infants following maternal immunisation during the third trimester of pregnancy.[15]

1. Böhm O, von Kries R. Are Hib booster vaccinations redundant? *Lancet* 1997; **350:** 68.
2. Booy R, *et al.* Vaccine failures after primary immunisation with Haemophilus influenzae type-b conjugate vaccine without booster. *Lancet* 1997; **349:** 1197–1202.
3. Heath PT, *et al.* Antibody persistence and Haemophilus influenzae type b carriage after infant immunisation with PRP-T. *Arch Dis Child* 1997; **77:** 488–92.
4. Kurikka S, *et al.* Immunologic priming by one dose of Haemophilus influenzae type b conjugate vaccine in infancy. *J Infect Dis* 1995; **172:** 1268–72.
5. Kurikka S, *et al.* Comparison of five different vaccination schedules with Haemophilus influenzae type b-tetanus toxoid conjugate vaccine. *J Pediatr* 1996; **128:** 524–30.
6. Lagos R, *et al.* Economisation of vaccination against Haemophilus influenzae type b: a randomised trial of immunogenicity of fractional-dose and two-dose regimens. *Lancet* 1998; **351:** 1472–6.
7. Granoff DM, *et al.* Differences in the immunogenicity of three Haemophilus influenzae type b vaccines in infants. *J Pediatr* 1992; **121:** 187–94.
8. Anderson EL, *et al.* Interchangeability of conjugated Haemophilus influenzae type b vaccines in infants. *JAMA* 1995; **273:** 849–53.
9. Greenberg DP, *et al.* Enhanced antibody responses in infants given different sequences of Haemophilus influenzae type b conjugate vaccines. *J Pediatr* 1995; **126:** 206–11.
10. Goldblatt D, *et al.* Interchangeability of conjugated Haemophilus influenzae type b vaccines during primary immunisation of infants. *Br Med J* 1996; **312:** 817–18.
11. Bewley KM, *et al.* Interchangeability of Haemophilus influenzae type b vaccines in the primary series: evaluation of a two-dose mixed regimen. *Pediatrics* 1996; **98:** 898–904.
12. Munoz A, *et al.* Antibody response of low birth weight infants to Haemophilus influenzae type b polyribosylribitol phosphate-outer membrane protein conjugate vaccine. *Pediatrics* 1995; **96:** 216–19.
13. Kristensen K, *et al.* Antibody response to Haemophilus influenzae type b capsular polysaccharide conjugated to tetanus toxoid in preterm infants. *Pediatr Infect Dis J* 1996; **15:** 525–9.
14. D'Angio CT, *et al.* Immunologic response of extremely premature infants to tetanus, Haemophilus influenzae, and polio immunizations. *Pediatrics* 1995; **96:** 18–22.
15. Englund JA, *et al.* Haemophilus influenzae type b-specific antibody in infants after maternal immunization. *Pediatr Infect Dis J* 1997; **16:** 1122–30.

Preparations

Ph. Eur.: Haemophilus Type b Conjugate Vaccine.

Proprietary Preparations (details are given in Part 3)
Aust.: Act-HIB; HibTITER; ProHIBiT; ***Austral.:*** Act-HIB†; Hiberix; HibTITER; PedvaxHIB; ProHIBiT†; ***Belg.:*** Act-HIB; HibTITER; Pediavax†; ***Canad.:*** Act-HIB; HibTITER; PedvaxHIB; ***Fr.:*** Act-HIB; HIBest; ***Ger.:*** Act-HIB; HIB-Vaccinol; HibTITER; PedvaxHIB; ***Irl.:*** HibTITER; ***Ital.:*** Act-HIB; Hiberix; HibTITER†; Vaxem Hib†; ***Neth.:*** Act-HIB; PedvaxHIB†; ***Norw.:*** Act-HIB; ***S.Afr.:*** Act-HIB; HibTITER; ***Spain:*** Act-HIB; HibTITER; ***Swed.:*** Act-HIB; HibTITER; PedvaxHIB; ProHIBiT†; ***Switz.:*** Act-HIB; HibTITER; PedvaxHIB†; ProHIBiT; ***UK:*** Act-HIB; HibTITER; ***USA:*** Act-HIB; HibTITER; OmniHIB; PedvaxHIB; ProHIBiT.

Haemophilus Influenzae and Hepatitis B Vaccines (9796-d)

Haemophilus influenzae type b (Hib) conjugate and hepatitis B vaccines are available in some countries for active immunisation as part of the primary immunisation of infants.

Preparations

Proprietary Preparations (details are given in Part 3)
USA: Comvax.

Haemorrhagic Fever with Renal Syndrome Vaccines (9466-v)

HFRS Vaccine; Vaccinum Haemorrhagia Febris cum Renis Sindronum.

A fluid or freeze-dried preparation of a suitable hantavirus grown in the neural tissue of suckling rodents or in cell cultures and inactivated. The fluid vaccine should be stored at 2° to 8° and not allowed to freeze. The freeze-dried form should be stored below 10°.

Inactivated viral vaccines against haemorrhagic fever with renal syndrome are being developed in several countries.

References.

1. Lee HW, *et al.* Field trial of an inactivated vaccine against hemorrhagic fever with renal syndrome in humans. *Arch Virol* 1990; (suppl 1): 35–47.
2. Song G, *et al.* Preliminary trials of inactivated vaccine against haemorrhagic fever with renal syndrome. *Lancet* 1991; **337:** 801.
3. Zhu Z-Y, *et al.* Investigation on inactivated epidemic hemorrhagic fever tissue culture vaccine in humans. *Chin Med J* 1994; **107:** 167–70.

Helicobacter Pylori Vaccines (10802-a)

Vaccines against *Helicobacter pylori* are being developed for prophylaxis of peptic ulcer disease and gastric cancer.

References.

1. Kreiss C, *et al.* Safety of oral immunisation with recombinant urease in patients with Helicobacter pylori infection. *Lancet* 1996; **347:** 1630–1.
2. Telford JL, Ghiara P. Prospects for the development of a vaccine against Helicobacter pylori. *Drugs* 1996; **52:** 799–804.
3. Haas R, Meyer TF. Vaccine development against Helicobacter pylori infections. *Biologicals* 1997; **25:** 175–7.

Hepatitis A Immunoglobulins (15378-l)

Human Hepatitis A Immunoglobulin (Ph. Eur.) (Hepatitis A Immunoglobulin (BP 1998); Immunoglobulinum Humanum Hepatitidis A) is a liquid or freeze-dried preparation containing human immunoglobulins, mainly immunoglobulin G (IgG). It is obtained from plasma from selected donors having specific antibodies against the hepatitis A virus. Normal immunoglobulin may be added. It contains not less than 600 international units per mL. The liquid preparation should be stored, protected from light, in a sealed, colourless, glass container. The freeze-dried preparation should be stored, protected from light, in a colourless, glass container under vacuum or under an inert gas.

Immunoglobulins containing high levels of specific antibodies against hepatitis A are available in some countries for passive immunisation against hepatitis A infection; in the UK, normal immunoglobulin is usually given.

Preparations

Ph. Eur.: Human Hepatitis A Immunoglobulin.

Proprietary Preparations (details are given in Part 3)
Aust.: Globuman; ***Belg.:*** Globuman Hepatite A; ***Ger.:*** Gammabulin A; ***S.Afr.:*** Globuman Hepatitis A; ***Switz.:*** Globuman Hepatite A.

Hepatitis A Vaccines (19290-y)

Hepatitis A Vaccine (Inactivated, Adsorbed) (Ph. Eur.) (Inactivated Hepatitis A Vaccine (BP 1998); Hep A/Vac; Vaccinum Hepatitidis A Inactivatum) is a liquid preparation of a suitable strain of hepatitis A virus grown in cell cultures, inactivated by a validated method, and adsorbed on a mineral carrier. It should be stored at 2° to 8°, not be allowed to freeze, and be protected from light.

Adverse Effects and Precautions

As for vaccines in general, p.1500.

General references.

1. Niu MT, *et al.* Two-year review of hepatitis A vaccine safety: data from the Vaccine Adverse Event Reporting System (VAERS). *Clin Infect Dis* 1998; **26:** 1475–6.

Effects on the blood. WHO has received reports of 5 cases of thrombocytopenia, 3 with purpura, associated with hepatitis A vaccine.[1]

1. Meyboom RHB, *et al.* Thrombocytopenia reported in association with hepatitis B and A vaccines. *Lancet* 1995; **345:** 1638.

Effects on the nervous system. Neurological symptoms resembling encephalitis have followed a third dose of hepatitis A vaccine.[1] Other serious neurological reactions reported in patients receiving inactivated hepatitis A vaccine include transverse myelitis, Guillain-Barré syndrome, and neuralgic amyotrophy.[2] Such reactions appear to be very rare, and, since other vaccines have often been given simultaneously, may not be directly attributable to hepatitis A vaccine.

1. Hughes PJ, *et al.* Probable post-hepatitis A vaccination encephalopathy. *Lancet* 1993; **342:** 302.
2. Committee on Safety of Medicines/Medicines Control Agency. Hepatitis A vaccination (Havrix). *Current Problems* 1994; **20:** 16.

Interactions

As for vaccines in general, p.1501.

Uses and Administration

Hepatitis A vaccines are used for active immunisation against hepatitis A infections.

In the UK the use of an inactivated vaccine is recommended as an alternative to normal immunoglobulin for frequent travellers to areas of high or moderate hepatitis A endemicity or for those staying for more than 3 months in such areas; in some countries a hepatitis A immunoglobulin (p.1512) is available for those making shorter or less frequent journeys. Immunisation is also recommended in haemophiliacs and in those at risk of exposure to hepatitis A by virtue of their occupation, and should be considered in persons whose lifestyle is likely to place them at risk. The vaccine is given intramuscularly in the deltoid region, except in haemophiliacs in whom it should be given subcutaneously. In the UK vaccines containing 1440 ELISA units per mL (derived from the HM175 strain of virus), or 320 antigen units per mL (GBM strain) may be used: adult doses are 1 mL of the former, or 0.5 mL of the latter. The dose is repeated 6 to 12 months later. Alternatively a formulation containing 50 antigen units per 1-mL dose may be given, and repeated after an interval of 6 months. Children under the age of 15 years may be given a dose of 0.5 mL containing 720 ELISA units with a booster dose of 0.5 mL 6 to 12 months later. Alternatively 0.5 mL of a preparation containing 50 antigen units per mL may be given to adolescents or children over 2 years of age, and repeated after 6 to 18 months.

Immunity is provided for up to 10 years following these doses.

Commercially available hepatitis A vaccines are usually produced from inactivated hepatitis A virus strains propagated in cell culture, commonly of human diploid fibroblast cells. Live attenuated hepatitis A vaccines have also been developed, although an oral live vaccine does not appear to have yet been produced. 'Virosome' hepatitis A vaccines consisting of inactivated hepatitis A virus epitopes formulated into liposomes are under investigation.

References.

1. Mao JS, *et al.* Primary study of attenuated live hepatitis A vaccine (H2 strain) in humans. *J Infect Dis* 1989; **159:** 621–4.
2. Loutan L, *et al.* Inactivated virosome hepatitis A vaccine. *Lancet* 1994; **343:** 322–4.
3. Strader DB, Seeff LB. New hepatitis A vaccines and their role in prevention. *Drugs* 1996; **51:** 359–66.
4. Committee on Infectious Diseases of the American Academy of Pediatrics. Prevention of hepatitis A infections: guidelines for use of hepatitis A vaccines and immune globulin. *Pediatrics* 1996; **98:** 1207–15.
5. Holzer BR, *et al.* Immunogenicity and adverse effects of inactivated virosome versus alum-adsorbed hepatitis A vaccine: a randomized controlled trial. *Vaccine* 1996; **14:** 982–6.
6. Lemon SM, Thomas DL. Vaccines to prevent viral hepatitis. *N Engl J Med* 1997; **336:** 196–204.

Preparations

Ph. Eur.: Hepatitis A Vaccine (Inactivated, Adsorbed).

Proprietary Preparations (details are given in Part 3)
Aust.: Havrix; ***Austral.:*** Havrix; VAQTA; ***Belg.:*** Havrix; ***Canad.:*** Havrix; ***Fr.:*** Havrix; ***Ger.:*** Havrix; VAQTA; ***Irl.:*** Havrix; ***Ital.:*** Havrix; ***Neth.:*** Avaxim; Havrix; ***Norw.:*** Havrix; ***S.Afr.:*** Havrix; ***Spain:*** Havrix; ***Swed.:*** Avaxim; Epaxal; Havrix; ***Switz.:*** Epaxal; Havrix; ***UK:*** Avaxim; Havrix; VAQTA; ***USA:*** Havrix; VAQTA.

Hepatitis B Immunoglobulins

(1235-a)

Human Hepatitis B Immunoglobulin (Ph. Eur.) (Hepatitis B Immunoglobulin (BP 1998); Immunoglobulinum Humanum Hepatitidis B) is a liquid or freeze-dried preparation containing immunoglobulins, mainly immunoglobulin G (IgG). It is obtained from plasma from selected and/or immunised donors having specific antibodies against hepatitis B surface antigen. Normal immunoglobulin may be added. It contains not less than 100 international units per mL. The liquid preparation should be stored, protected from light, in a sealed, colourless, glass container. The freeze-dried preparation should be stored, protected from light, in a colourless, glass container, under vacuum or under an inert gas.

Human Hepatitis B Immunoglobulin for Intravenous Use (Ph. Eur.) (Hepatitis B Immunoglobulin for Intravenous Use (BP 1998); Immunoglobulinum Humanum Hepatitidis B ad Usum Intravenosum) is a liquid or freeze-dried preparation containing immunoglobulins, mainly immunoglobulin G (IgG). It is obtained from plasma from selected and/or immunised donors having antibodies against hepatitis B surface antigen. Normal immunoglobulin for intravenous use may be added. It contains not less than 50 international units per mL. Storage requirements are similar to those for Hepatitis B Immunoglobulin, except that the freeze-dried preparation is stored at a temperature not exceeding 25°.

Hepatitis B Immune Globulin (USP 23) is a sterile solution consisting of globulins derived from the plasma of human donors who have high titres of antibodies against hepatitis B surface antigen. It contains 10 to 18% of protein, of which not less than 80% is monomeric immunoglobulin G. It contains glycine as a stabilising agent, and a suitable preservative. It should be stored at 2° to 8°.

Adverse Effects and Precautions

As for immunoglobulins in general, p.1500.

For a warning concerning possible lack of equivalence between different preparations of hepatitis B immunoglobulins see under Uses and Administration, below.

Uses and Administration

Hepatitis B immunoglobulins are used for passive immunisation of persons exposed or possibly exposed to hepatitis B virus, including by sexual contact. They are not appropriate for treatment. Active immunisation with hepatitis B vaccine should always be commenced in conjunction with administration of hepatitis B immunoglobulins in patients exposed to hepatitis B virus.

In the UK a hepatitis B immunoglobulin containing 100 international units per mL is available for intramuscular use. The recommended dose in adults and children over 10 years of age is a single dose of 500 international units by intramuscular injection given preferably within 48 hours of exposure and not more than 1 week after exposure. Children aged 5 to 9 years may be given 300 international units, and children under 5 years 200 international units. Hepatitis B immunoglobulin should also be given to newborn infants at risk whose mothers are persistent carriers of hepatitis B surface antigen or whose mothers are HBsAg-positive as a result of recent infection. The recommended dose is 200 international units by intramuscular injection preferably at birth, and certainly within 48 hours of birth.

There is now a UK and European standard for a preparation for intravenous use containing not less than 50 international units per mL.

In the USA a hepatitis B immunoglobulin containing 15 to 18% of protein is available for intramuscular use. The recommended dose for adults is 0.06 mL per kg body-weight. A dose of 0.5 mL is given to infants perinatally exposed to hepatitis B; this appears to be equivalent to approximately half the dose employed in the UK.

The US Immunization Practices Advisory Committee has issued recommendations on the use of hepatitis B vaccines and hepatitis B immunoglobulins.[1]

The content of hepatitis B immunoglobulin may vary between countries and between manufacturers. Care should be taken in interpreting dosage recommendations which are not given in terms of international units.[2] Products available in the USA have their strength expressed with reference to an FDA standard but are considered to contain the equivalent of at least 200 international units per mL.[3]

1. Immunization Practices Advisory Committee. Hepatitis B virus: a comprehensive strategy for eliminating transmission in the United States through universal childhood vaccination. *MMWR* 1991; **40** (RR-13).
2. Vegnente A, *et al.* Universal hepatitis B immunization: the dose of HBIg that should be administered at birth. *Pediatrics* 1994; **94:** 242.
3. Halsey NA, Hall CB. Universal hepatitis B immunization: the dose of HBIg that should be administered at birth. *Pediatrics* 1994; **94:** 242–3.

Monoclonal antibodies. The name tuvirumab is applied to a human hepatitis B monoclonal antibody. A murine monoclonal antibody has been tried in a few patients with primary antibody deficiency.[1]

1. Lever AML, *et al.* Monoclonal antibody to HBsAg for chronic hepatitis B virus infection with hypogammaglobulinaemia. *Lancet* 1990; **335:** 1529

Organ transplantation. A study[1] in 110 patients positive for hepatitis B surface antigen undergoing liver transplantation suggested that long-term passive immunisation with hepatitis B immunoglobulin could reduce hepatitis B re-infection and improve survival in these patients.

1. Samuel D, *et al.* Passive immunoprophylaxis after liver transplantation in HBsAg-positive patients. *Lancet* 1991; **337:** 813–15.

Postexposure prophylaxis. For discussion of the use of hepatitis B immunoglobulins in patients exposed to hepatitis B virus, see under Hepatitis B Vaccines, below.

Preparations

Ph. Eur.: Human Hepatitis B Immunoglobulin; Human Hepatitis B Immunoglobulin for Intravenous Use;
USP 23: Hepatitis B Immune Globulin.

Proprietary Preparations (details are given in Part 3)
Aust.: Aunativ; Hepatect; ***Belg.:*** Hepuman; ***Canad.:*** HyperHep; ***Ger.:*** Aunativ; Gammaprotect†; Hepaglobin†; Hepatect; ***Irl.:*** Hepatect; ***Ital.:*** Haimabig; Hepatect; Hepuman B; ImmunoHBs; Uman-Big; Venbig; ***Norw.:*** Aunativ; ***S.Afr.:*** Hebagam IM; ***Spain:*** Aunative†; Gamma Glob Antihepa B; Gammaglob Antihep B; Glogama Antihepatitis B; Hepuman; ***Swed.:*** Aunativ; ***Switz.:*** Hepatect; Hepuman; ***USA:*** H-BIG; Hep-B-Gammagee†; Hyper-Hep.

Hepatitis B Vaccines (12818-t)

Hepatitis B Vaccine (rDNA) (Ph. Eur.) (Hep B/Vac); (Vaccinum Hepatitidis B (ADNr)) is a preparation of hepatitis B surface antigen, that is obtained by recombinant DNA technology. It should be stored at a temperature of 2° to 8°, not be allowed to freeze, and be protected from light. Under these storage conditions it may be expected to retain its potency for 24 months.

Hepatitis B Virus Vaccine Inactivated (USP 23) is a sterile preparation consisting of a suspension of particles of hepatitis B surface antigen (HBsAg) isolated from the plasma of HBsAg carriers; it is treated so as to inactivate any hepatitis B virus and other viruses. It is adsorbed onto aluminium hydroxide and contains thiomersal as a preservative. It should be stored at 2° to 8° and not be allowed to freeze.

Adverse Effects

As for vaccines in general, p.1500.

In addition, hepatitis B vaccines have been reported to cause abdominal pain and gastro-intestinal disturbance, and musculoskeletal and joint pain and inflammation. There may also be dizziness and sleep disturbance. Cardiovascular effects include occasional hypotension and, rarely, tachycardia. Other rare adverse effects include dysuria, visual disturbances, and earache.

Hepatitis B vaccines were generally well tolerated in 2 surveys[1,2] of adverse reactions following vaccination. The most frequent adverse reactions were local reactions at the injection site, other skin reactions, fever and myalgias or arthralgias. Serious reactions were very rare.

1. McMahon BJ, *et al.* Frequency of adverse reactions to hepatitis B vaccine in 43,618 persons. *Am J Med* 1992; **92:** 254–6.
2. Anonymous. Adverse events after hepatitis B vaccination. *Can Med Assoc J* 1992; **147:** 1023–6.

Effects on the blood. Rare cases of thrombocytopenia associated with hepatitis B vaccination have been reported.[1-3]

1. Poullin P, Gabriel B. Thrombocytopenic purpura after recombinant hepatitis B vaccine. *Lancet* 1994; **344:** 1293.
2. Meyboom RHB, *et al.* Thrombocytopenia reported in association with hepatitis B and A vaccines. *Lancet* 1995; **345:** 1638.
3. Ronchi F, *et al.* Thrombocytopenic purpura as adverse reaction to recombinant hepatitis B vaccine. *Arch Dis Child* 1998; **78:** 273–4.

Effects on bones and joints. Reactive arthritis[1,2] and Reiter's syndrome[2] have been reported after hepatitis B vaccination. A number of reports of arthralgia have been received by the Committee on Safety of Medicines in the UK and by the manufacturers of Engerix B, SmithKline Beecham Pharmaceuticals.[2]

1. Rogerson SJ, Nye FJ. Hepatitis B vaccine associated with erythema nodosum and polyarthritis. *Br Med J* 1990; **301:** 345.
2. Hassan W, Oldham R. Reiter's syndrome and reactive arthritis in health care workers after vaccination. *Br Med J* 1994; **309:** 94–5

Effects on the eyes. Acute posterior uveitis occurred in a patient[1] after the booster doses of hepatitis B vaccines. Visual loss associated with eosinophilia was reported in a patient[2] following hepatitis B vaccination. There have also been reports of acute posterior multifocal placoid pigment epitheliopathy[3] and central retinal vein occlusion[4] following vaccination against hepatitis B.

For mention of optic neuritis in patients receiving hepatitis B vaccine, see under Effects on the Nervous System, below.

1. Fried M, *et al.* Uveitis after hepatitis B vaccination. *Lancet* 1987; **ii:** 631–2.
2. Brézin AP, *et al.* Visual loss and eosinophilia after recombinant hepatitis B vaccine. *Lancet* 1993; **342:** 563–4.
3. Brézin AP, *et al.* Acute posterior multifocal placoid pigment epitheliopathy after hepatitis B vaccine. *Arch Ophthalmol* 1995; **113:** 297–300.
4. Devin F, *et al.* Occlusion of central retinal vein after hepatitis B vaccination. *Lancet* 1996; **347:** 1626.

Effects on the kidneys. Acute glomerulonephritis was reported in 1 patient following the third injection of hepatitis B vaccine.[1]

1. Carmeli Y, Oren R. Hepatitis B vaccine side-effect. *Lancet* 1993; **341:** 250–1.

Effects on the liver. There have been occasional reports of transient abnormalities in liver function associated with hepatitis B vaccine.[1-3] Lilic and Ghosh[2] reported the appearance of autoantibodies in 1 patient, and severe cytolysis consistent with an allergic mechanism was present in the patient reported by Germanaud and colleagues.[3]

1. Rajendran V, Brooks AP. Symptomatic reaction to hepatitis B vaccine with abnormal liver function values. *Br Med J* 1985; **290:** 1476.
2. Lilic D, Ghosh SK. Liver Dysfunction and DNA antibodies after hepatitis B vaccination. *Lancet* 1994; **344:** 1292–3.
3. Germanaud J, *et al.* A case of severe cytolysis after hepatitis B vaccination. *Am J Med* 1995; **98:** 595.

Effects on the nervous system. In the 3 years 1982 to 1985 the Centers for Disease Control, the FDA, and the manufacturer of plasma-derived hepatitis B vaccine received 41 reports of adverse neurological effects.[1] It was estimated that about 850 000 persons had received the vaccine in this time. Neurological events were convulsions (5 cases), Bell's palsy (10), Guillain-Barré syndrome (9), lumbar radiculopathy (5), brachial plexus neuropathy (3), optic neuritis (5), and transverse myelitis (4). In some analyses Guillain-Barré syndrome was reported significantly more often than expected. However, no conclusive epidemiological association could be made between any neurological adverse effect and the vaccine.

Additional case reports of neurological symptoms following hepatitis B vaccination include CNS demyelination in 2 patients,[2] one of whom had pre-existing multiple sclerosis, and acute cerebellar ataxia in 1 patient.[3]

1. Shaw FE, *et al.* Postmarketing surveillance for neurologic adverse events reported after hepatitis B vaccination: experience of the first three years. *Am J Epidemiol* 1988; **127:** 337–52.
2. Herroelen L, *et al.* Central-nervous-system demyelination after immunisation with recombinant hepatitis B vaccine. *Lancet* 1991; **338:** 1174–5.
3. Deisenhammer F, *et al.* Childhood immunizations. *N Engl J Med* 1993; **328:** 1421.

Effects on the skin. Skin reactions which have been reported in a few individuals after hepatitis B vaccination include erythema multiforme,[1,2] erythema nodosum,[3-5] lichen planus,[6] and vasculitis.[7]

1. Feldshon SD, Sampliner RE. Reaction to hepatitis B virus vaccine. *Ann Intern Med* 1984; **100:** 156–7.
2. Wakeel RA, White MI. Erythema multiforme associated with hepatitis B vaccine. *Br J Dermatol* 1992; **126:** 94–5.
3. Di Giusto CA, Bernhard JD. Erythema nodosum provoked by hepatitis B vaccine. *Lancet* 1986; **ii:** 1042.
4. Goolsby PL. Erythema nodosum after Recombivax HB hepatitis B vaccine. *N Engl J Med* 1989; **321:** 1198–9.
5. Rogerson SJ, Nye FJ. Hepatitis B vaccine associated with erythema nodosum and polyarthritis. *Br Med J* 1990; **301:** 345.
6. Ciaccio M, Rebora A. Lichen planus following HBV vaccination: a coincidence? *Br J Dermatol* 1990; **122:** 424.
7. Cockwell P, *et al.* Vasculitis related to hepatitis B vaccine. *Br Med J* 1990; **301:** 1281.

Hypersensitivity. Acute exacerbation of eczema[1] in a patient on the day after vaccination against hepatitis B; the pruritus experienced and the exacerbation of the eczema was probably due to the formaldehyde contained in the vaccine. Hypersensitivity to thiomersal included in recombinant hepatitis B vaccine has also been reported.[2]

There has also been a report of a hypersensitivity reaction after administration of a yeast-derived recombinant DNA hepatitis B vaccine to a patient with a history of reactions to mouldy foods.[3] The clinical history and skin-prick testing suggested a type I hypersensitivity reaction to small quantities of *Saccharomyces cerevisiae* remaining in the vaccine.

1. Ring J. Exacerbation of eczema by formalin-containing hepatitis B vaccine in formaldehyde-allergic patient. *Lancet* 1986; **ii:** 522–3.
2. Noel I, *et al.* Hypersensitivity to thiomersal in hepatitis B vaccine. *Lancet* 1991; **338:** 705.
3. Brightman CAJ, *et al.* Yeast-derived hepatitis B vaccine and yeast sensitivity. *Lancet* 1989; **i:** 903.

Precautions

As for vaccines in general, p.1501.

Reduced immune response. The immune response to hepatitis B vaccine is dependent on both host- and immunisation-related factors.[1] Host-related factors that appear to diminish the response include increasing age, increasing body-weight, smoking,[1,2] and male sex;[3] particular HLA haplotypes may also be associated with poor response.[4] Failure of hepatitis B immunisation in infants could be related to high perinatal maternal viraemia[5] rather than to inherent resistance to the vaccine.

Some studies have observed a defective response in chronic alcoholics[6,7] whereas others have not;[8] the degree of liver impairment may be a significant factor. It has been suggested that an increased dose of hepatitis B vaccine may be appropriate in those with a history of alcoholism.[9] Active infection with *Schistosoma mansoni* also appears to decrease the response to hepatitis B vaccination.[10] A diminished response occurs in HIV-positive patients[11-13] and in patients on haemodialysis;[1] an increased dose of hepatitis B vaccine is recommended in these patients. In patients with haemophilia who are not HIV-positive[14] immunity is reported to wane rapidly after vaccination and frequent booster doses may be required. Biological response modifiers such as thymopentin[15] and interferon,[16] have been used successfully in some patients on haemodialysis to overcome the immune deficit. Administration of interleukin-2 has met with variable success[17,18] (see p.543).

The immune response to hepatitis B vaccine is affected by the site of intramuscular injection. The deltoid region is recommended for adults and the anterolateral thigh for infants. A diminished response has been associated with administration in the gluteal region (buttock).[1]

A related problem is posed by subjects who become infected with hepatitis B despite mounting an adequate response to immunisation. Evidence of viral replication was detected in 44 of 1590 hepatitis B vaccinees despite development of protective titres of antibody.[19] Acute hepatitis occurred in one patient. Although the infection may have been incubating at the time of vaccination, the virus isolated from the child with acute disease was an escape mutant with a different DNA sequence from that isolated from the mother.

1. Hollinger FB. Factors influencing the immune response to hepatitis b vaccine, booster dose guidelines, and vaccine protocol recommendations. *Am J Med* 1989; **87** (suppl 3A): 36S–40S.
2. Horowitz MM, *et al.* Duration of immunity after hepatitis B vaccination: efficacy of low-dose booster vaccine. *Ann Intern Med* 1988; **108:** 185–9.
3. Morris CA, *et al.* Intradermal hepatitis B immunization with yeast-derived vaccine: serological response by sex and age. *Epidemiol Infect* 1989; **103:** 387–94.
4. Alper CA, *et al.* Genetic prediction of nonresponse to hepatitis B vaccine. *N Engl J Med* 1989; **321:** 708–12.
5. del Canho R, *et al.* Failure of neonatal hepatitis B vaccination: the role of HBV-DNA levels in hepatitis B carrier mothers and HLA antigens in neonates. *J Hepatol* 1994; **20:** 483–6.
6. Degos F, *et al.* Hepatitis B vaccination and alcoholic cirrhosis. *Lancet* 1983; **ii:** 1498.
7. Mendenhall C, *et al.* Hepatitis B vaccination: response of alcoholic with and without liver injury. *Dig Dis Sci* 1988; **33:** 263–9.
8. McMahon BJ, *et al.* Response to hepatitis B vaccine in Alaska Natives with chronic alcoholism compared with non-alcoholic control subjects. *Am J Med* 1990; **88:** 460–4.
9. Rosman AS, *et al.* Efficacy of a high and accelerated dose of hepatitis B vaccine in alcoholic patients: a randomized clinical trial. *Am J Med* 1997; **103:** 217–22.
10. Ghaffar YA, *et al.* Response to hepatitis B vaccine in infants born to mothers with schistosomiasis. *Lancet* 1989; **ii:** 272.
11. Carne CA, *et al.* Impaired responsiveness of homosexual men with HIV antibodies to plasma derived hepatitis B vaccine. *Br Med J* 1987; **294:** 866–8.
12. Collier AC, *et al.* Antibody to human immunodeficiency virus (HIV) and suboptimal response to hepatitis B vaccination. *Ann Intern Med* 1988; **109:** 101–5.

13. Chan W, *et al.* Response to hepatitis B immunization in children with hemophilia: relationship to infection with human immunodeficiency virus type 1. *J Pediatr* 1990; **117:** 427–30.
14. Maris JM, *et al.* Loss of detectable antibody to hepatitis B surface antigen in immunized patients with hemophilia but without human immunodeficiency virus infection. *J Pediatr* 1995; **126:** 269–71.
15. Donati D, Gastaldi L. Controlled trial of thymopentin in hemodialysis patients who fail to respond to hepatitis B vaccination. *Nephron* 1988; **50:** 133–6.
16. Quiroga JA, Carreño V. Interferon and hepatitis B vaccine in haemodialysis patients. *Lancet* 1989; **i:** 1264.
17. Meuer SC, *et al.* Low-dose interleukin-2 induces systemic immune responses against HBsAg in immunodeficient non-responders to hepatitis B vaccination. *Lancet* 1989, **i:** 15–18.
18. Jungers P, *et al.* Randomized placebo-controlled trial of recombinant interleukin-2 in chronic uraemic patients who are non-responders to hepatitis B vaccine. *Lancet* 1994; **344:** 856–7.
19. Carman WF, *et al.* Vaccine-induced escape mutant of hepatitis B virus. *Lancet* 1990; **336:** 325–9.

Uses and Administration

Hepatitis B vaccines are used for active immunisation against hepatitis B infections. Two types of vaccine are available each containing hepatitis B surface antigen (HBsAg) adsorbed onto aluminium hydroxide. In one type of vaccine the surface antigen is obtained from plasma after purification and inactivation processes and in the second type the surface antigen is produced in yeast cells using recombinant DNA techniques. This second type of vaccine is now widely used and there has been considerable interest in further developments to improve immunogenicity.

WHO had recommended that national immunisation policies should include routine hepatitis B immunisation for the whole population by 1997 and this has been implemented in some countries including the USA (see below). The current recommendations in the UK are for immunisation of persons at high risk of contracting hepatitis B. High-risk groups include: health care personnel, laboratory workers, or any other personnel who have direct contact with patients or their body fluids; staff and residents of accommodation for the mentally handicapped; patients with chronic renal failure including those requiring haemodialysis; haemophiliacs and those receiving regular blood transfusions or blood products; close family contacts or sexual partners of cases or carriers of hepatitis B; families adopting children from countries with a high prevalence of hepatitis B; individuals who frequently change sexual partners; parenteral drug abusers; inmates of custodial institutions; and some travellers to areas where hepatitis B is endemic. Immunisation should also be performed in infants born to women who are persistent carriers of hepatitis B surface antigen or infants born to women who are HBsAg-positive as a result of recent infection.

The basic immunisation schedule consists of 3 doses of a hepatitis B vaccine, with the second and third doses 1 and 6 months, respectively, after the first. Doses should be given intramuscularly, with the deltoid region being the preferred site in adults and the anterolateral thigh the preferred site in infants; the gluteal region (buttock) should not be used as efficacy may be reduced. The dose of the recombinant vaccine depends on the product used. Typical doses for adults are 10 or 20 μg and for children 2.5 to 10 μg. However, *the dose of one recombinant preparation should not be seen as equivalent to the dose of another.* Plasma-derived vaccines are less widely available now but the recommended dose of the plasma-derived vaccine, expressed in terms of content of the hepatitis B surface antigen, has been 10 μg for all those under 10 years of age and 20 μg for older children and adults.

The recombinant vaccine has also been used where more rapid immunisation, for instance with travellers, is required. This schedule has involved the administration of the third dose 2 months after the initial dose with a further booster at 1 year.

For newborn infants at risk combined active and passive immunisation against hepatitis B is recommended. The first dose of vaccine should preferably be given at birth, and certainly within 48 hours of birth. A single dose of hepatitis B immunoglobulin (200 international units) should be administered at the same time into a different site. Additionally, in any patient in whom immediate protection is required, combined active and passive immunisation may be considered with a single dose of 500 international units of hepatitis B immunoglobulin being the suggested dose for adults. See under Hepatitis B Immunoglobulins, p.1512, for children's doses.

The subcutaneous route should be used in patients with haemophilia. Some authorities suggest that intradermal administration, in a dose of about 2 μg, may be considered for haemophiliacs, but the likelihood of effective antibody response is reduced and the risk of local adverse effects may be increased.

General references.

1. Buynak EB, *et al.* Vaccine against human hepatitis B. *JAMA* 1976; **235:** 2832–4.
2. Douglas RG. The heritage of hepatitis B vaccine. *JAMA* 1996; **276:** 1796–8.
3. Lemon SM, Thomas DL. Vaccines to prevent viral hepatitis. *N Engl J Med* 1997; **336:** 196–204.

Administration. The major public health burden of hepatitis B infection in the developing world is due to the consequences of chronic carriage of hepatitis B virus (hepatocellular carcinoma and chronic cirrhosis) rather than acute infection. WHO[1] considered that the most important means of controlling hepatitis B on a global scale and of reducing mortality from its sequelae was mass immunisation of infants. It stated that hepatitis B vaccine should be incorporated into the Expanded Programme on Immunization (EPI) and many countries have since done so. WHO later reiterated this aim[2] stating that hepatitis B vaccine should be integrated into national immunisation programmes in all countries with a hepatitis B carrier prevalence (HBsAg) of 8% or greater by 1995 and in all countries by 1997. WHO's current aim is to reduce the incidence of new child carriers of hepatitis B by 80% by 2001. Results from Taiwan, where mass immunisation of infants has been in place for over a decade have shown a marked decline in the number of child carriers under 10 years of age.[3] The incidence of hepatocellular carcinoma in children has also been reduced.[4,5]

Opinion remains divided in the UK regarding implementation of universal hepatitis B immunisation,[6-8] with some advising increased emphasis on alternative strategies already in place such as antenatal screening.[6,7]

The optimum vaccination strategy depends on the pattern of hepatitis B viral transmission in a particular country. In hyperendemic regions where most infections are acquired early in life, the vaccine should be administered shortly after birth and hepatitis B immunisation integrated into the EPI. Immunisation of all infants should be considered for population groups with chronic hepatitis B virus carrier rates greater than 2% and should be a public health priority where carrier rates are greater than 10%. Countries with a lower carrier rate might opt to immunise all adolescents as an alternative to infant immunisation. Immunisation of individuals at high risk of infection should be continued in addition to routine vaccination schedules[2] and, if hepatitis B is not integrated into infant vaccination schedules, screening pregnant women for HBsAg and immunising the infants of HBsAg-positive mothers should continue.[1]

If use of hepatitis vaccine is integrated into the EPI, three doses should be given intramuscularly, the first dose being given as soon as possible after birth concomitantly with the first EPI immunisation. The exact timing of these doses will depend on the EPI schedule in operation. In the USA, these recommendations have been implemented by immunisation of all infants and of adolescents aged 11 to 12 years who have not previously received three doses of vaccine. The recommended schedule[9] is: infants of HBsAg-negative mothers, the initial dose is given at birth or at up to 2 months of age, a second dose at 1 to 4 months of age but at least 1 month after the first dose and the third dose at 6 to 18 months of age; infants of HBsAg-positive mothers or of mothers whose HBsAg status is unknown, hepatitis B vaccine plus immunoglobulin at birth, then additional doses of vaccine at age 1 month and 6 months. Adolescents aged 11 to 12 years who have not received immunisation as an infant should be given three doses with the second dose given at least one month after the first and third given at least 4 months after the first and 2 months after the second. For further details, see p.1501. For premature infants of HBsAg-negative mothers, it has been suggested that the initial dose of vaccine could be delayed until the infant weighs at least 2000 g or until about 2 months of age.[10]

1. WHO. Progress in the control of viral hepatitis: memorandum from a WHO meeting. *Bull WHO* 1988; **66:** 443–55.
2. Anonymous. Hepatitis B vaccine. *WHO Drug Inf* 1993; **7:** 130–1.
3. Chen H-L, *et al.* Seroepidemiology of hepatitis B virus infection in children: ten years of mass vaccination in Taiwan. *JAMA* 1996; **276:** 906–8.
4. Lee C-L, Ko Y-C. Hepatitis B vaccination and hepatocellular carcinoma in Taiwan. *Pediatrics* 1997; **99:** 351–3.
5. Chang M-H, *et al.* Universal hepatitis B vaccination in Taiwan and the incidence of hepatocellular carcinoma in children. *N Engl J Med* 1997; **336:** 1855–9.
6. Mortimer PP, Miller E. Commentary: antenatal screening and targeting should be sufficient in some countries. *Br Med J* 1997; **314:** 1036–7.
7. Dunn J, *et al.* Integration of hepatitis B vaccination into national immunisation programmes: alternative strategies must be considered before universal vaccination is adopted. *Br Med J* 1997; **315:** 121–2.
8. Goldberg D, McMenamin J. The United Kingdom's hepatitis B immunisation strategy—where now? *Commun Dis Public Health* 1998; **1:** 79–83.
9. Committee on Infectious Diseases of the American Academy of Pediatrics. Immunization of adolescents: recommendations of the Advisory Committee on Immunization Practices, the American Academy of Pediatrics, the American Academy of Family Physicians, and the American Medical Association. *Pediatrics* 1997; **99:** 479–88.
10. Committee on Infectious Diseases. Update on timing of hepatitis B vaccination for premature infants and for children with lapsed immunization. *Pediatrics* 1994; **94:** 403–4.

ALTERNATIVE ROUTES. Hepatitis B vaccine is usually given by intramuscular injection. Smaller doses may be given by intradermal injection and this has commercial attractions. However, the antibody response may be less with the intradermal route and it is not as convenient as the intramuscular route. The use of smaller intramuscular doses has also been investigated.

References.

1. Horowitz MM, *et al.* Duration of immunity after hepatitis B vaccination: efficacy of low-dose booster vaccine. *Ann Intern Med* 1988; **108:** 185–9.
2. Milne A, *et al.* Low dose hepatitis B vaccination in children: benefit of low dose boosters. *N Z Med J* 1988; **101:** 370–1.
3. Clarke JA, *et al.* Intradermal inoculation with Heptavax-B: immune response and histologic evaluation of injection sites. *JAMA* 1989; **262:** 2567–71.
4. Mok Q, *et al.* Intradermal hepatitis B vaccine in thalassaemia and sickle cell disease. *Arch Dis Child* 1989; **64:** 535–40.
5. Morris CA, *et al.* Intradermal hepatitis B immunization with yeast-derived vaccine: serological response by sex and age. *Epidemiol Infect* 1989; **103:** 387–94.
6. Lee C-Y, *et al.* Low-dose hepatitis B vaccine. *Lancet* 1989; **ii:** 860–1.
7. Wilkins TD, Cossart YE. Low-dose intradermal vaccination of medical and dental students. *Med J Aust* 1990; **152:** 140–3.
8. Zuckerman AJ. Immunization against hepatitis B. *Br Med Bull* 1990; **46:** 383–98.
9. Wiström J, *et al.* Intradermal vs intramuscular hepatitis B vaccinations. *JAMA* 1990; **264:** 181–2.
10. Leonardi S, *et al.* Intradermal hepatitis B vaccination in thalassaemia. *Arch Dis Child* 1990; **65:** 527–9.
11. Guan R, *et al.* The immune response of low dose recombinant DNA hepatitis B vaccine in teenagers in Singapore. *Trans R Soc Trop Med Hyg* 1990; **84:** 731–2.
12. Catterall AP, Murray-Lyon IM. Strategies for hepatitis B immunisation. *Gut* 1992; **33:** 576–9.
13. Payton CD, *et al.* Vaccination against hepatitis B: comparison of intradermal and intramuscular administration of plasma derived and recombinant vaccines. *Epidemiol Infect* 1993; **110:** 177–80.

BOOSTER DOSES. There has been considerable interest in the duration of immunity conferred by hepatitis B vaccination and the possible need for booster doses. However there are no official guidelines yet on administering booster doses after the recommended schedules, apart from recommendations that health care workers who have already been successfully vaccinated should be given a booster dose of vaccine after contamination of skin or eyes with blood from a HBsAg-positive person, unless they are known to have protective concentrations of antibody.

References.

1. Hollinger FB. Factors influencing the immune response to hepatitis B vaccine, booster dose guidelines, and vaccine protocol recommendations. *Am J Med* 1989; **87** (suppl 3A): 36S–40S.
2. Hadler SC. Are booster doses of hepatitis B vaccine necessary? *Ann Intern Med* 1988; **108:** 457–8.
3. Nommensen FE, *et al.* Half-life of HBs antibody after hepatitis B vaccination: an aid to timing of booster vaccination. *Lancet* 1989; **ii:** 847–9.
4. Gilks WR, *et al.* Timing of booster doses of hepatitis B vaccine. *Lancet* 1989; **ii:** 1273–4.
5. Coursaget P, *et al.* Scheduling of revaccination against hepatitis B virus. *Lancet* 1991; **337:** 1180–3.
6. Prince AM. Revaccination against hepatitis B. *Lancet* 1991; **338:** 61.
7. Hall AJ. Hepatitis B vaccination: protection for how long and against what? *Br Med J* 1993; **307:** 276–7.
8. Tilzey AJ. Hepatitis B vaccine boosting: the debate continues. *Lancet* 1995; **345:** 1000–1.
9. Simó Miñana J, *et al.* Hepatitis B vaccine immunoresponsiveness in adolescents: a revaccination proposal after primary vaccination. *Vaccine* 1996; **14:** 103–6.
10. Edmunds WJ, *et al.* Vaccination against hepatitis B virus in highly endemic areas: waning vaccine-induced immunity and the need for booster doses. *Trans R Soc Trop Med Hyg* 1996; **90:** 436–40.

Postexposure prophylaxis. A combination of passive immunisation with a hepatitis B immunoglobulin and active immunisation with a hepatitis B vaccine is generally recommended for postexposure prophylaxis against hepatitis B.

One group of patients who should be considered for postexposure prophylaxis are infants born to mothers who are persistent carriers of hepatitis B surface antigen (HBsAg). The risk is particularly high if the mother has detectable hepatitis B e antigen (HBeAg) or hepatitis B virus DNA or absence of detectable antibody to hepatitis e antigen (anti-HBe). Postexposure prophylaxis is also recommended in the UK for persons accidentally inoculated, or who contaminate the eye or mouth or breaks to the skin with blood from a known HBsAg-positive person, as well as in sexual contacts (and sometimes close family contacts) of sufferers from acute hepatitis B and who are seen within a week of the onset of jaundice in the contact.

In the UK, the recommended schedule for postexposure prophylaxis is the first dose of vaccine given preferably within 48 hours of exposure and no later than one week after exposure, or, for babies exposed to hepatitis B at birth, no later than 48 hours after birth, in conjunction with a single dose of hepatitis B immunoglobulin given at a separate site. The second and third doses of vaccine are given one and two months after the first dose, with a booster dose at 12 months. Health care workers who have been successfully immunised should be given a booster dose following subsequent contamination with blood from an infected person, unless they are known to have adequate antibody concentration.

Some references to postexposure prophylaxis against hepatitis B, including variations in the combined regimens used, the use of vaccine alone, and the use of accelerated regimens, are given below.

1. Polakoff S. Public Health Laboratory Service surveillance of prophylaxis by specific hepatitis B immunoglobulin in England and Wales during the period 1975-1987. *J Infect* 1990; **21:** 213–20.
2. O'Grady JG, Williams R. Liver transplantation for viral hepatitis. *Br Med Bull* 1990; **46:** 481–91.
3. Polakoff S, Vandervelde EM. Immunisation of neonates at high risk of hepatitis B in England and Wales: national surveillance. *Br Med J* 1988; **297:** 249–53.
4. WHO. Progress in the control of viral hepatitis: memorandum from a WHO meeting. *Bull WHO* 1988; **66:** 443–55.
5. Iwarson S. Post-exposure prophylaxis for hepatitis B: active or passive? *Lancet* 1989; **ii:** 146–8.
6. Vodopija I, *et al.* Post-exposure prophylaxis for hepatitis B. *Lancet* 1989; **ii:** 1161–2.
7. Ip HMH, *et al.* Prevention of hepatitis B virus carrier state in infants according to maternal serum levels of HBV DNA. *Lancet* 1989; **i:** 406–10.
8. Poovorawan Y, *et al.* Protective efficacy of a recombinant DNA hepatitis B vaccine in neonates of HBe antigen-positive mothers. *JAMA* 1989; **261:** 3278–81.

Preparations

Ph. Eur.: Hepatitis B Vaccine (rDNA);
USP 23: Hepatitis B Virus Vaccine Inactivated.

Proprietary Preparations (details are given in Part 3)
Aust.: Engerix-B; Gen H-B-Vax; Hevac B; ***Austral.:*** Engerix-B; H-B-Vax II; ***Belg.:*** Engerix-B; H-B-Vax II; Hevac†; ***Canad.:*** Engerix-B; Recombivax HB; ***Fr.:*** Engerix-B; GenHevac B; HB-Vax-DNA; ***Ger.:*** Engerix-B; Gen H-B-Vax; Hevac B†; ***Irl.:*** Engerix-B; H-B-Vax II; ***Ital.:*** Engerix-B; H-B-Vax†; Recombivax HB; ***Neth.:*** Engerix-B; ***Norw.:*** Engerix-B; ***S.Afr.:*** Engerix-B; H-B-Vax II; Hepaccine-B; ***Spain:*** Engerix-B; Recombivax HB; ***Swed.:*** Engerix-B; H-B-Vax; ***Switz.:*** Engerix-B; Gen H-B-Vax; Heprecomb; Hevac B†; ***UK:*** Engerix-B; H-B-Vax II; ***USA:*** Engerix-B; Recombivax HB.

Hepatitis A and B Vaccines (6339-x)

Adverse Effects and Precautions

As for vaccines in general, p.1500.

See also under Hepatitis A Vaccines, p.1512, and Hepatitis B Vaccines, p.1513.

Uses and Administration

Combined hepatitis A and B vaccines are used for active immunisation against hepatitis A and hepatitis B.

In the UK, a hepatitis A and B vaccine is available containing not less than 720 ELISA units of inactivated hepatitis A virus and not less than 20 µg of recombinant hepatitis B surface antigen (HBsAg) protein in 1 mL. For primary immunisation, three doses of 1 mL are given by intramuscular injection, with the second and third doses 1 and 6 months after the first. For children up to the age of 16 years a 0.5-mL dose is given.

Booster doses may be given as appropriate with the monovalent component vaccines since protection against hepatitis A and B declines at different rates, or a booster dose of the combined vaccine may be given after 5 years.

References.

1. Leroux-Roels G, *et al.* Safety and immunogenicity of a combined hepatitis A and hepatitis B vaccine in young healthy adults. *Scand J Gastroenterol* 1996; **31:** 1027–31.
2. Bruguera M, *et al.* Immunogenicity and reactogenicity of a combined hepatitis A and B vaccine in young adults. *Vaccine* 1996; **14:** 1407–11.

Preparations

Proprietary Preparations (details are given in Part 3)
Austral.: Twinrix; ***Fr.:*** Twinrix; ***Ger.:*** Twinrix; ***Irl.:*** Twinrix; ***Ital.:*** Twinrix; ***Neth.:*** Twinrix; ***Swed.:*** Twinrix; ***UK:*** Twinrix.

Herpes Simplex Vaccines (16841-b)

Several types of vaccines against herpes simplex virus types 1 and 2 have been developed. They have been tried in patients with both oral and genital herpes infections. They are also being studied for the prevention of infection in sexual partners of patients with genital herpes.

Reviews and references.

1. Rooney JF, *et al.* Vaccinia virus recombinants as potential herpes simplex virus vaccines. *Adv Exp Med Biol* 1992; **327:** 183–9.
2. Whitly RJ, Meignier B. Herpes simplex vaccines. *Biotechnology* 1992; **20:** 223–54.
3. Straus SE, *et al.* Induction and enhancement of immune responses to herpes simplex virus type 2 in humans by use of a recombinant glycoprotein D vaccine. *J Infect Dis* 1993; **167:** 1045–52.
4. Langenberg AGM, *et al.* A recombinant glycoprotein vaccine for herpes simplex type 2: safety and efficacy. *Ann Intern Med* 1995; **122:** 889–98. Correction. *ibid.*; **123:** 395.
5. Straus SE, *et al.* Placebo-controlled trial of vaccination with recombinant glycoprotein D of herpes simplex virus type 2 for immunotherapy of genital herpes. *Lancet* 1994; **343:** 1460–3.
6. Ashley RL, *et al.* Cervical antibody responses to a herpes simplex virus type 2 glycoprotein subunit vaccine. *J Infect Dis* 1998; **178:** 1–7.

Preparations

Proprietary Preparations (details are given in Part 3)
Ital.: Lupidon G; Lupidon H.

Influenza Vaccines (7967-w)

Influenza Vaccine (Whole Virion, Inactivated) (Ph. Eur.); (Vaccinum Influenzae Inactivatum ex Viris Integris Praeparatum; Inactivated Influenza Vaccine (Whole Virion) (BP 1998); Flu/Vac) is a sterile aqueous suspension of a suitable strain or strains of influenza virus types A and B, either individually or mixed, grown individually in embryonated hen eggs and inactivated so that they retain their antigenic properties. The stated amount of haemagglutinin antigen for each strain present is usually 15 µg per dose. Suitable strains of influenza virus are those recommended by WHO. An antimicrobial preservative may be added. The vaccine should be stored at 2° to 8°, not be allowed to freeze, and be protected from light. Under these conditions it may be expected to be suitable for use for 1 year, provided that the strains of virus continue to be appropriate.

Influenza Vaccine (Split Virion, Inactivated) (Ph. Eur.) (Flu/Vac/Split; Inactivated Influenza Vaccine (Split Virion) (BP 1998); Vaccinum Influenzae Inactivatum ex Virorum Fragmentis Praeparatum) is a sterile aqueous suspension of a suitable strain or strains of influenza virus types A and B, either individually or mixed, grown individually in embryonated hen eggs and inactivated so that the integrity of the virus particles has been disrupted without diminishing their antigenic properties. The stated amount of haemagglutinin antigen for each strain present is usually 15 µg per dose. Suitable strains of influenza virus are those recommended by WHO. An antimicrobial preservative may be added. The vaccine should be stored at 2° to 8°, not be allowed to freeze, and be protected from light. Under these conditions it may be expected to be suitable for use for 1 year, provided that the strains of virus continue to be appropriate.

Influenza Vaccine (Surface Antigen, Inactivated) (Ph. Eur.) (Flu/Vac/SA; Inactivated Influenza Vaccine (Surface Antigen) (BP 1998); Vaccinum Influenzae Inactivatum ex Corticis Antigeniis Praeparatum) is a sterile aqueous suspension consisting predominantly of haemagglutinin and neuraminidase antigens of a suitable strain or strains of influenza virus types A and B either individually or mixed, grown individually in embryonated hen eggs and inactivated so that they retain their antigenic properties. The stated amount of haemagglutinin antigen for each strain is usually 15 µg per dose. Suitable strains of influenza virus are those recommended by WHO. An antimicrobial preservative may be added. The vaccine should be stored at 2° to 8°, not be allowed to freeze, and be protected from light. Under these conditions it may be expected to be suitable for use for 1 year, provided that the strains of virus continue to be appropriate.

The BP directs that when Inactivated Influenza Vaccine or Influenza Vaccine is prescribed or demanded and the form is not stated, Inactivated Influenza Vaccine (Whole Virion), (Split Virion), or (Surface Antigen) may be dispensed or supplied.

Influenza Virus Vaccine (USP 23) is a sterile aqueous suspension of suitably inactivated influenza virus types A and B, either individually or combined, or virus subunits prepared from the extra-embryonic fluid of virus-infected chick embryos. Suitable strains of influenza virus are those designated by the US Government's Expert Committee on Influenza and recommended by the Surgeon General of the US Public Health Service. It may contain a suitable antimicrobial agent. It should be stored at 2° to 8° and not be allowed to freeze.

Nomenclature of strains. The strain designation for influenza virus types A, B, and C contains: a description of the antigenic specificity of the nucleoprotein antigen (types A, B, or C) (an internal antigen, the matrix antigen, has also been described); the host of origin (if not man, including, if appropriate, the inanimate source); the geographical origin; the strain number; and the year of isolation; e.g. A/lake water/Wisconsin/1/79. For type A viruses the antigenic description follows (in parenthesis) including the antigenic character of the haemagglutinin (e.g. H1) and the antigenic character of the neuraminidase (e.g. N1). There is no provision for describing subtypes of B and C viruses. Recombination between viruses within a type is readily accomplished; the letter R should be added after the strain description to indicate the recombinant nature of the virus, e.g. A/Hong Kong/1/68(H3N2)R. In addition the strain of origin of the H and N antigens of antigenic hybrid recombinant A and B viruses should be given, e.g. A/BEL/42(H1)—Singapore/1/57(N2)R.[1]

1. Assaad FA, *et al.* Revision of the system of nomenclature for influenza viruses: a WHO Memorandum. *Bull WHO* 1980; **58:** 585–91.

Adverse Effects

As for vaccines in general, p.1500.

Local and systemic reactions may occur but are usually mild. Fever and malaise sometimes occur and severe febrile reactions have been reported particularly after administration of whole-virion vaccine to children.

Various neurological syndromes have been temporally associated with administration of influenza vaccine, the most notable report being of the Guillain-Barré syndrome occurring after vaccination with inactivated swine influenza vaccine in 1976 (see below).

Effects on the nervous system. GUILLAIN-BARRÉ SYNDROME. Comment on the Guillain-Barré syndrome associated with influenza vaccination.[1] In 1976 a limited outbreak of influenza in the USA caused by a virus closely resembling the swine influenza virus led to the use of a killed swine influenza virus vaccine. After about 45 million doses of the vaccine had been administered the vaccination programme ceased because there was some evidence of a temporal association between vaccination and the onset of a paralytic polyneuropathy of the Guillain-Barré type. An epidemiologic and clinical evaluation of these cases suggested a definite link between vaccination and the onset of the syndrome with extensive paralysis but no association with the onset of limited motor lesions. Influenza virus vaccines which lack a swine influenza virus component seem not to raise the risk of paralysis above background levels.

1. Anonymous. Influenza and the Guillain-Barré syndrome. *Lancet* 1984; **ii:** 850–1.

MULTIPLE SCLEROSIS. Analysis[1] indicating there was no association between the use in the USA during 1976 of influenza vaccines containing a swine virus component and the development of multiple sclerosis.

1. Kurland LT, *et al.* Swine flu vaccine and multiple sclerosis. *JAMA* 1984; **251:** 2672–5.

Henoch-Schönlein purpura. Influenza vaccination has been associated with both development[1] and exacerbation[2] of Henoch-Schönlein purpura.

1. Patel U, *et al.* Henoch-Schönlein purpura after influenza vaccination. *Br Med J* 1988; **296:** 1800.
2. Damjanov I, Amato JA. Progression of renal disease in Henoch-Schönlein purpura after influenza vaccination. *JAMA* 1979; **242:** 2555–6.

Precautions

As for vaccines in general, p.1501.

Whole-virion influenza vaccine is not recommended for use in children because of the increased risk of febrile reactions.

Influenza vaccines should not be given to individuals with a known anaphylactic hypersensitivity to egg products.

Vaccination should be postponed in patients with active infection or acute febrile illness.

Asthma. There have been reports of exacerbations of asthma following influenza vaccination[1,2] but reviews[3,4] have concluded that evidence of a causal relationship is lacking and that any risk of exacerbation which might exist is outweighed by the risk of influenza itself. Chronic respiratory disease, including asthma, is an indication for influenza vaccination in both the UK and USA.

1. Hassan WU, *et al.* Influenza vaccination in asthma. *Lancet* 1992; **339:** 194.
2. Nicholson KG, *et al.* Randomised placebo-controlled crossover trial on effect of inactivated influenza vaccine on pulmonary function in asthma. *Lancet* 1998; **351:** 326–31.
3. Watson JM, *et al.* Does influenza immunisation cause exacerbations of chronic airflow obstruction or asthma? *Thorax* 1997; **52:** 190–4.
4. Park CL, Frank A. Does influenza vaccination exacerbate asthma? *Drug Safety* 1998; **19:** 83–8.

Diagnostic tests. False-positive screening enzyme-linked immunosorbent assays (ELISAs) for antibodies to HIV-1, HTLV-1 and hepatitis C virus were reported in blood donors who had recently received influenza vaccine.[1] The reaction was attributed to cross-reactivity of the test kit in use at the time with nonspecific IgM.

1. Anonymous. False-positive serologic tests for human T-cell lymphotropic virus type 1 among blood donors following influenza vaccination, 1992. *JAMA* 1993; **269:** 2076 and 2078.

Interactions

For the effect of influenza vaccination on some other drugs see under Phenobarbitone Sodium, p.351, Phenytoin Sodium, p.357, Theophylline Hydrate, p.770, and Warfarin Sodium, p.969.

Uses and Administration

Influenza vaccines are used for active immunisation against influenza.

Three types of the influenza virus occur, namely types A, B, and C, and the formulation and composition of influenza vaccines is constantly reviewed with changes made to accommodate the antigenic shifts and drifts of the influenza virus. Recommendations concerning the antigenic nature of influenza vaccines are made annually by WHO. Currently, influenza vaccines are of the inactivated type and may be available in three forms, as a whole-virion vaccine, as a split-virion vaccine, or as a surface-antigen vaccine.

Influenza vaccination is recommended for persons considered to be at special risk, particularly the elderly, those with chronic cardiac disease, chronic pulmonary disease including asthma (see above), chronic renal disease, diabetes or other endocrine disorders, and patients who are immunosuppressed. Vaccination should also be considered for residents, particularly elderly persons and children, in closed institutions. Medical personnel and other persons at risk from infection through contact with infected patients should also receive vaccination. Influenza vaccines are administered in the UK by deep subcutaneous injection or intramuscular injection. The preferred site for injection is the deltoid muscle in adults and older children and, in infants and young children, the anterolateral aspect of the thigh. Vaccination usually produces immunity after about 14 days, lasting for about 6 months to 1 year. Injections are therefore scheduled annually so that the period of maximum immunity coincides with the usual period of influenza infection. In the UK and USA they are generally given in October or November. The recommended dose is 0.5 mL for adults and children aged over 4 years. In children aged 6 months to 4 years doses of 0.25 or 0.5 mL have been used. Children under 13 years of age should be given a second dose 4 to 6 weeks after the first if receiving the vaccine for the first time.

Reviews.

1. Palache AM. Influenza vaccines: a reappraisal of their use. *Drugs* 1997; **54:** 841–56.

Haemagglutinin on the surface of the influenza virus allows the virus to attach to the host cells, and antibody against it is the main form of immunity to influenza. Antibody to neuraminidase on the virus surface and cell-mediated immunity may be important as well. Adults with previous exposure to the relevant subtype usually get a fourfold or greater increase in haemagglutinin antibody after vaccination with 20 to 30 μg of haemagglutinin [approximately equivalent to one 0.5-mL dose], but in some cases most of the new antibody is against the original strain rather than the variant in the vaccine. Children and unprimed adults need two injections of a much larger dose of haemagglutinin (60 μg or more) for an adequate antibody response. The level of antibody falls by about 75% over 8 months after split-virus vaccine and by 50% over 6 months after whole-virus vaccine. Because of this decrease in antibody level, and antigenic drift, **immunisation** against influenza is required each year. After one or two doses of killed vaccine, clinical infection rates are reduced by 60 to 80% in children and young adults. Vaccination reduces clinical infection by only about 30% in elderly patients in institutions, but serious illness and death are probably cut by about 70%. The effectiveness of vaccination has varied widely in different studies, probably because of differences in previous exposure to the influenza subtype, vaccine dose, interval between vaccination and challenge, and matching of vaccine and challenge antigens.[1]

Various live influenza vaccines, all administered by the **intranasal** route, have been investigated.[1-8] They are produced by reassortment of the viral genes. The 2 genes that code for haemagglutinin and neuraminidase from a current infectious strain are combined with the 6 genes that code for the internal proteins from an attenuated strain.[1] Cold-adapted and avian attenuated virus strains are considered to be potentially useful.[2,3,7-9] The intranasal route has also produced promising results with an inactivated split virion vaccine.[5] Preliminary *animal* studies are also under way[10] using microencapsulated inactivated influenza virus for **oral** administration.

A vaccine produced by inserting influenza haemagglutinin into **liposomes** produced higher concentrations of antibodies than conventional vaccines in a study in 126 elderly nursing-home residents,[11] an age group traditionally considered to respond poorly to the vaccine.

1. Shann F. Modern vaccines: pneumococcus and influenza. *Lancet* 1990; **335:** 898–901.
2. Clements ML, *et al.* Evaluation of the infectivity, immunogenicity, and efficacy of live cold-adapted influenza B/Ann Arbor/1/86 reassortant virus vaccine in adult volunteers. *J Infect Dis* 1990; **161:** 869–77.
3. Steinhoff MC, *et al.* Comparison of live attenuated cold-adapted and avian-human influenza A/Bethesda/85 (H3N2) reassortant virus vaccines in infants and children. *J Infect Dis* 1990; **162:** 394–401.
4. Clover RD, *et al.* Comparison of heterotypic protection against influenza A/Taiwan/86 (H1N1) by attenuated and inactivated vaccines to A/Chile/83-like viruses. *J Infect Dis* 1991; **163:** 300–4.
5. Oh Y, *et al.* Local and systemic influenza haemagglutinin-specific antibody responses following aerosol and subcutaneous administration of inactivated split influenza vaccine. *Vaccine* 1992; **10:** 506–11.
6. Gruber WC, *et al.* Evaluation of bivalent live attenuated influenza A vaccines in children 2 months to 3 years of age: safety, immunogenicity and dose-response. *Vaccine* 1997; **15:** 1379–84.
7. Belshe RB, *et al.* The efficacy of live attenuated, cold-adapted, trivalent, intranasal influenzavirus vaccine in children. *N Engl J Med* 1998; **338:** 1405–12.
8. King JC, *et al.* Safety and immunogenicity of low and high doses of trivalent live cold-adapted influenza vaccine administered intranasally as drops or spray to healthy children. *J Infect Dis* 1998; **177:** 1394–7.
9. Rudenko LG, *et al.* Clinical and epidemiological evaluation of a live, cold-adapted influenza vaccine for 3–14-year-olds. *Bull WHO* 1996; **74:** 77–84.
10. Moldoveanu Z, *et al.* Oral immunization with influenza virus in biodegradable microspheres. *J Infect Dis* 1993; **167:** 84–90.
11. Glück R, *et al.* Immunogenicity of new virosome influenza vaccine in elderly people. *Lancet* 1994; **344:** 160–3.

Preparations

Ph. Eur.: Influenza Vaccine (Split Virion, Inactivated); Influenza Vaccine (Surface Antigen, Inactivated); Influenza Vaccine (Whole Virion, Inactivated);
USP 23: Influenza Virus Vaccine.

Proprietary Preparations (details are given in Part 3)
Aust.: Begrivac; Inflexal; Influvac; Sandovac; Vaxigrip; ***Austral.:*** Fluvax; Vaxigrip†; Xflu; ***Belg.:*** α-Rix; Influvac; Mutagrip; Vaxigrip; ***Canad.:*** Fluviral; Fluzone; ***Fr.:*** Fluarix; Fluvirine; Immugrip; Influvac; Mutagrip; Previgrip; Vaxigrip; ***Ger.:*** Alorbat†; Begrivac; Influsplit SSW; Influvac; Mutagrip; ***Irl.:*** Begrivac-F†; Fluarix; Fluvirin; Fluzone; Influvac; ***Ital.:*** Agrippal; Biaflu; Biaflu-Zonale SU; Fluad; Fluarix; Fluvirin; Inflexal; Influmix†; Influpozzi; Influvac S; Influvirus; Isiflu Zonale; Miniflu†; Mutagrip; Vaxigrip; ***Neth.:*** Fluarix; Influvac; Mutagrip†; Vaxigrip; ***Norw.:*** Fluarix; Fluvirin; Fluzone; Vaxigrip; ***S.Afr.:*** Agrippal; Fluvirin; Inflexal; Influvac; Vaxigrip; Xflu; ***Spain:*** Evagrip; Fluarix; Gripavac; Imuvac†; Inflexal; Mutagrip; Vac Antigripal; ***Swed.:*** Begrivac; Fluarix; Fluvaccin†; Fluvirin; Fluzone†; Influvac; Vaxigrip; ***Switz.:*** Alorbat†; Fluarix; Inflexal; Influvac; ***UK:*** Begrivac; Fluarix; Fluvirin; Fluzone; Influvac; MFV-Ject; ***USA:*** Flu-Imune; Flu-Shield; Fluogen; Fluvirin; Fluzone.

Jellyfish Venom Antisera (10837-g)

Jellyfish Antivenins; Jellyfish Antivenoms.

Adverse Effects and Precautions

As for antisera in general, p.1500.

Uses and Administration

An antiserum for use in the management of severe stings by the box jellyfish or sea wasp (*Chironex fleckeri*) is available in Australia. The preparation contains the specific antitoxic globulins that have the power of neutralising the venom of *Chironex fleckeri*. The globulins are obtained from the serum of sheep that have been immunised with the venom of the box jellyfish.

Box jellyfish antivenom is usually given by the intravenous route in a dose of 20 000 units. Alternatively, 60 000 units may be injected intramuscularly.

Box jellyfish sting. The sting of the box jellyfish (*Chironex fleckeri*) can be rapidly fatal so immediate first aid is vital. Fragments of tentacle adhering to the skin should be inactivated by the application of vinegar or 3 to 10% acetic acid solution. Artificial respiration and external cardiac massage may be necessary. The antiserum can be effective if administered quickly and in adequate dosage.[1-3] (Some have suggested its use for severe envenomation by related species.[4]) Studies in *rodents*[5] suggest that verapamil may be useful for treatment of the cardiotoxic effects of the venom and allow more time for the antiserum to exert its action.

1. Lumley J, *et al.* Fatal envenomation by Chironex fleckeri, the north Australian box jellyfish: the continuing search for lethal mechanisms. *Med J Aust* 1988; **148:** 527–34.
2. Horne TW. Box-jellyfish envenomation. *Med J Aust* 1988; **148:** 540.
3. Fenner PJ, *et al.* Successful use of chironex antivenom by members of the Queensland Ambulance Transport Brigade. *Med J Aust* 1989; **151:** 708–10.
4. Fenner PJ, Williamson JA. Worldwide deaths and severe envenomation from jellyfish stings. *Med J Aust* 1996; **165:** 658–61.
5. Burnett JW. The use of verapamil to treat box-jellyfish stings. *Med J Aust* 1990; **153:** 363.

Leishmaniasis Vaccines (16872-e)

Vaccines containing *Leishmania* spp. are under investigation in an attempt to prevent cutaneous leishmaniasis.

The inoculation of an infective strain of a *Leishmania* sp. into the skin, a technique known as leishmanisation, has been used to protect against cutaneous leishmaniasis.[1] Although the technique has been standardised it is not generally recommended since large, slow-healing lesions have occurred in some patients.

Vaccines containing strains of killed leishmanial promastigotes have been developed and have conferred some protection against cutaneous leishmaniasis[1,2] although this has waned relatively quickly in some cases.[1] The safety and efficacy of killed *Leishmania* vaccines is under clinical investigation.[3] Killed vaccines combined with BCG as an adjuvant have also been tried.[4,5] Also under development are live vaccines containing stable mutants of *Leishmania* or recombinant subunit and synthetic vaccines.[3]

Immunotherapy with a mixture of heat-killed promastigotes of *Leishmania mexicana amazonensis* and live BCG has compared favourably with meglumine antimonate treatment in patients with cutaneous leishmaniasis.[6] Immunotherapy resulted in fewer side-effects than chemotherapy. For a discussion of the difficulties in treating cutaneous leishmaniasis, see p.575.

1. Playfair JHL, *et al.* Modern vaccines: parasitic diseases. *Lancet* 1990; **335:** 1263–6.
2. Nascimento E, *et al.* Vaccination of humans against cutaneous leishmaniasis: cellular and humoral immune responses. *Infect Immun* 1990; **58:** 2198–2203.
3. Modabber F. Vaccines against leishmaniasis. *Ann Trop Med Parasitol* 1995; **89:** 83–8.
4. Armijos RX, *et al.* Field trial of a vaccine against New World cutaneous leishmaniasis in an at-risk child population: safety, immunogenicity, and efficacy during the first 12 months of follow-up. *J Infect Dis* 1998; **177:** 1352–7.
5. Sharifi I, *et al.* Randomised vaccine trial of single dose of killed Leishmania major plus BCG against anthroponotic cutaneous leishmaniasis in Bam, Iran. *Lancet* 1998; **351:** 1540–3.
6. Convit J, *et al.* Immunotherapy of localized, intermediate, and diffuse forms of American cutaneous leishmaniasis. *J Infect Dis* 1989; **160:** 104–15.

Leprosy Vaccines (16874-y)

Vaccines against leprosy including those using *Mycobacterium leprae* as well as other mycobacteria are under investigation. A killed vaccine has been developed in India for use as an adjunct to standard multidrug therapy in the treatment of leprosy. Although studies of new vaccines are continuing, BCG vaccine (p.1505) also appears to be effective.

Attempts to develop a vaccine against leprosy are based on the assumption that induction of a cell-mediated immune response to *Mycobacterium leprae* will lead to protection against the bacillus.[1-4] Considerable protection against leprosy is afforded by BCG vaccination (see p.1505), and a study in Malawi showed that repeated vaccination provided additional protection.[5] However, the addition of killed *M. leprae* did not produce any further improvement, confirming preliminary results of a study in Venezuela.[6] The fortuitous finding that BCG vaccine, which is inexpensive and widely available, is effective against leprosy has important implications for leprosy control programmes.[7] Vaccines from non-pathogenic species of mycobacteria, *Mycobacterium w,* have been developed in India.

Leprosy vaccines are being studied both to prevent infection with *M. leprae* (immunoprophylaxis) and to prevent disease in infected individuals (immunotherapeutic). Beneficial responses have been reported[8,9,14,15] from the immunotherapeutic use of *Mycobacterium w* vaccine in combination with standard multidrug therapy (p.128) although a small increase in Type 1 lepra reactions has been observed.[10] A similar, and possibly identical, vaccine based on the ICRC bacillus is also being evaluated.[11,12] WHO has suggested that the immunotherapeutic use of vaccines may ultimately prove to be more clinically relevant than the immunoprophylactic use,[11] and high compliance with immunotherapy appears to be attainable.[13]

1. Anonymous. Vaccines against leprosy. *Lancet* 1987; **i:** 1183–4.
2. WHO. WHO expert committee on leprosy: sixth report. *WHO Tech Rep Ser 768* 1988.
3. Fine PEM, Ponnighaus JM. Leprosy in Malawi 2: background, design and prospects of the Karonga Prevention Trial, a leprosy vaccine trial in northern Malawi. *Trans R Soc Trop Med Hyg* 1988; **82:** 810–17.
4. Anonymous. Bettering BCG. *Lancet* 1992; **339:** 462–3.
5. Karonga Prevention Trial Group. Randomised controlled trial of single BCG, repeated BCG, or combined BCG and killed Mycobacterium leprae vaccine for prevention of leprosy and tuberculosis in Malawi. *Lancet* 1996; **348:** 17–24.
6. Convit J, *et al.* Immunoprophylactic trial with combined Mycobacterium leprae/BCG vaccine against leprosy: preliminary results. *Lancet* 1992; **339:** 446–50.
7. Fine PEM, Smith PG. Vaccination against leprosy—the view from 1996. *Lepr Rev* 1996; **67:** 249–52.
8. Zaheer SA, *et al.* Combined multidrug and Mycobacterium w vaccine therapy in patients with multibacillary leprosy. *J Infect Dis* 1993; **167:** 401–10.
9. Zaheer SA, *et al.* Immunotherapy with Mycobacterium w vaccine decreases the incidence and severity of type 2 (ENL) reactions. *Lepr Rev* 1993; **64:** 7–14.
10. Kar HK, *et al.* Reversal reaction in multibacillary leprosy patients following MDT with and without immunotherapy with a candidate for an antileprosy vaccine, Mycobacterium w. *Lepr Rev* 1993; **64:** 219–26.
11. Mangla B. Leprosy vaccine debate in India re-ignited. *Lancet* 1993; **342:** 233.
12. Jayaraman KS. Charges fly over rival leprosy vaccines. *Nature* 1994: **367:** 403.
13. Walia R, *et al.* Field trials on the use of Mycobacterium w vaccine in conjunction with multidrug therapy in leprosy patients for immunotherapeutic and immunoprophylactic purposes. *Lepr Rev* 1993; **64:** 302–11.
14. Zaheer SA, *et al.* Addition of immunotherapy with Mycobacterium w vaccine to multi-drug therapy benefits multibacillary leprosy patients. *Vaccine* 1995; **13:** 1102–10.
15. Katoch K, *et al.* Treatment of bacilliferous BL/LL cases with combined chemotherapy and immunotherapy. *Int J Lepr* 1995; **63:** 202–12.

Leptospirosis Vaccines (7688-m)

Leptospira Vaccines.

Leptospirosis vaccines prepared from killed *Leptospira interrogans* are available in some countries. They are used for active immunisation against leptospirosis icterohaemorrhagica (spirochaetal jaundice; Weil's disease) in persons at high risk of contracting the disease.

Lyme Disease Vaccines (14348-r)

Vaccines based on recombinant outer surface proteins of *Borrelia burgdorferi* are being investigated for active immunisation against Lyme disease.

References.

1. Keller D, *et al.* Safety and immunogenicity of a recombinant outer surface protein A Lyme vaccine. *JAMA* 1994; **271:** 1764–8.
2. Wormser GP. Prospects for a vaccine to prevent Lyme disease in humans. *Clin Infect Dis* 1995; **21:** 1267–74.
3. van Hoecke C, *et al.* Evaluation of the safety, reactogenicity and immunogenicity of three recombinant outer surface protein (OspA) Lyme vaccines in healthy adults. *Vaccine* 1996; **14:** 1620–6.
4. Steere AC, *et al.* Vaccination against Lyme disease with recombinant Borrelia burgdorferi outer-surface lipoprotein A with adjuvant. *N Engl J Med* 1998; **339:** 209–15.
5. Sigal LH, *et al.* A vaccine consisting of recombinant Borrelia burgdorferi outer-surface protein A to prevent Lyme disease. *N Engl J Med* 1998; **339:** 216–22.

Malaria Vaccines (16882-y)

Malaria vaccines acting against the sporozoite, asexual, and sexual stages of the *Plasmodium falciparum* life cycle are under investigation, as well as multicomponent vaccines consisting of combined antigens from various stages.

Chemoprophylaxis of malaria is becoming increasingly problematical (see p.422), resulting in the increased desirability of effective malaria vaccines, several of which have been or are being studied clinically. The various approaches to malaria vaccine development have been reviewed.[1,2] Malaria vaccines can be categorised into 3 main groups:

- vaccines against pre-erythrocytic forms of the parasite or specifically sporozoites would prevent development of clinical disease and interrupt transmission by insect vectors. However, infection acquired by blood transfusion would not be prevented. RTS/S, a recombinant circumsporozoite protein fused with the more immunogenic adjuvant hepatis B surface antigen, produced encouraging results in a recent preliminary study[3]
- vaccines against asexual stages of the parasite would inhibit development of clinical disease but would not interrupt transmission. Infection of the liver would not be impeded
- vaccines against the sexual stages of the life cycle (so called 'altruistic' vaccines) would interrupt malaria transmission but would not prevent infection with sporozoites or development of asexual forms in the blood or liver.

A further approach that has been studied involves the development of vaccines to induce production of cytotoxic T-lymphocytes which confer immunity from malaria via destruction of parasite-infected hepatocytes.[4]

WHO envisages that different types of vaccine could be used in combination. Various malarial antigens have been identified and studied in the hope of developing a multicomponent vaccine. One such vaccine, SPf66, was developed in Colombia where it was shown to be effective in semi-immune populations in endemic areas.[5,6] The vaccine consists of a synthetic preparation of three antigens from the asexual phase of the parasite in the blood linked by a sporozoite antigen. Subsequent studies in Ecuador[7] and Venezuela[8] demonstrated efficacy of 67 and 55% respectively. However, the reproducibility of the results and the efficacy of this vaccine in highly endemic regions was the cause of considerable controversy[9-11] which, it was hoped, had been resolved by the results of a clinical study from Tanzania[12,13] which reported vaccine efficacy to be 31%. Although low, it was thought that this degree of efficacy could substantially reduce mortality.[14] Unfortunately, however, SPf66 did not protect against clinical falciparum malaria in studies from The Gambia[15] and Thailand.[16]

Another multicomponent vaccine, NYVAC-Pf7, utilising a recombinant vaccinia viral vector that expresses 7 proteins from different stages of malarial infection, has also been studied.[17]

1. Riley E. Malaria vaccines: current status and future prospects. *J Pharm Pharmacol* 1997; **49:** (suppl 2): 21–7.
2. Kwiatkowski D, Marsh K. Development of a malaria vaccine. *Lancet* 1997; **350:** 1696–1701.
3. Stoute JA, *et al.* A preliminary evaluation of a recombinant circumsporozoite protein vaccine against Plasmodium falciparum malaria. *N Engl J Med* 1997; **336:** 86–91.
4. Aidoo M, *et al.* Identification of conserved antigenic components for a cytotoxic T lymphocyte-inducing vaccine against malaria. *Lancet* 1995; **345:** 1003–7.
5. Valero MV, *et al.* Vaccination with SPf66, a chemically synthesised vaccine, against Plasmodium falciparum malaria in Colombia. *Lancet* 1993; **341:** 705–10.
6. Amador R, *et al.* The first field trials of the chemically synthesized malaria vaccine SPf66: safety, immunogenicity and protectivity. *Vaccine* 1992; **10:** 179–84.
7. Sempertergui F, *et al.* Safety, immunogenicity and protective effect of the SPf66 malaria synthetic vaccine against Plasmodium falciparum infection in a randomised double-blind placebo-controlled field trial in an endemic area of Ecuador. *Vaccine* 1994; **12:** 337–42.
8. Noya O, *et al.* A population based clinical trial with the SPf66 synthetic Plasmodium falciparum malaria vaccine in Venezuela. *J Infect Dis* 1994; **170:** 396–402.
9. Anonymous. Towards a malarial vaccine. *Lancet* 1992; **339:** 586–7.
10. Marsh K. Patarroyo's vaccine. *Lancet* 1993; **341:** 729–30.
11. Anonymous. Malaria: a first stride towards effective vaccination? *WHO Drug Inf* 1993; **7:** 45–7.
12. Teuscher T, *et al.* SPf66, a chemically synthesized subunit malaria vaccine, is safe and immunogenic in Tanzanians exposed to intense malaria transmission. *Vaccine* 1994; **12:** 328–36.
13. Alonso PL, *et al.* Randomised trial of efficacy of SPf66 vaccine against Plasmodium falciparum malaria in children in southern Tanzania. *Lancet* 1994; **344:** 1175–81.
14. White NJ. Tough test for malaria vaccine. *Lancet* 1994; **344:** 1172–3.
15. D'Alessandro U, *et al.* Efficacy trial of malaria vaccine SPf66 in Gambian infants. *Lancet* 1995; **346:** 462–7.
16. Nosten F, *et al.* Randomised double-blind placebo-controlled trial of SPf66 malaria vaccine in children in northwestern Thailand. *Lancet* 1996; **348:** 701–7.
17. Ockenhouse CF, *et al.* Phase I/IIa safety, immunogenicity, and efficacy trial of NYVAC-Pf7, a pox-vectored, multiantigen, multistage vaccine candidate for Plasmodium falciparum malaria. *J Infect Dis* 1998; **177:** 1664–73.

Measles Immunoglobulins (1236-t)

Human Measles Immunoglobulin (Ph. Eur.) (Immunoglobulinum Humanum Morbillicum; Measles Immunoglobulin (BP 1998)) is a liquid or freeze-dried preparation containing immunoglobulins, mainly immunoglobulin G (IgG). It is obtained from plasma containing specific antibodies against the measles virus. Normal immunoglobulin may be added. It contains not less than 50 international units per mL. Both the liquid and freeze-dried preparations should be stored, protected from light, in a colourless, glass container. The freeze-dried preparation should be stored under vacuum or under an inert gas.

Adverse Effects and Precautions

As for immunoglobulins in general, p.1500.

Interactions

As for immunoglobulins in general, p.1500.

Uses and Administration

Measles immunoglobulins may be used for passive immunisation against measles. They have been used to prevent or modify measles in susceptible persons who have been exposed to infection; in the UK, normal immunoglobulin is usually given.

Preparations

Ph. Eur.: Human Measles Immunoglobulin.

Proprietary Preparations (details are given in Part 3)
Ital.: Haima-Morbil†; Immunomorb; Morbil; Morbulin†; Moruman; ***S.Afr.:*** Measlegam; ***Spain:*** Glogama Antisarampion†; ***Switz.:*** Moruman.

Measles Vaccines (7976-e)

Measles Vaccine (Live) (Ph. Eur.) (Meas/Vac (Live); Measles Vaccine, Live (BP 1998); Vaccinum Morbillorum Vivum) is a freeze-dried preparation of a suitable live attenuated strain of measles virus grown in cultures of chick-embryo cells or human diploid cells. It is prepared immediately before use by reconstitution from the dried vaccine. The virus titre is not less than 1×10^3 $CCID_{50}$ per dose. The dried vaccine should be stored at 2° to 8° and be protected from light.

Measles Virus Vaccine Live (USP 23) is a bacterially sterile freeze-dried preparation of a suitable live strain of measles virus grown in cultures of chick-embryo cells. It contains not less than the equivalent of 1×10^3 $TCID_{50}$ in each immunising dose, and may contain suitable antimicrobial agents. It should be stored at 2° to 8° and be protected from light.

Adverse Effects

As for vaccines in general, p.1500.

Fever and skin rashes may occur following the administration of measles vaccines. The fever generally starts 5 to 10 days after the injection, lasts for about 1 or 2 days, and has sometimes been accompanied by convulsions. More serious effects reported rarely include encephalitis and thrombocytopenia.

Some brief comments on side-effects and adverse reactions to standard measles vaccines made by the Advisory Committee on Immunization in the USA.[1] An excellent safety record of measles vaccines has been indicated by the experience gained through the use of more than 160 million doses up to 1986. Fever with a temperature of 39.4° or more may develop in 5 to 15% of vaccinees beginning about the fifth day after vaccination and usually lasts several days. Transient rashes have been reported in about 5% of vaccinees. CNS disorders, including encephalitis and encephalopathy, have been reported with a frequency of less than one case per million doses administered. The incidence of encephalitis or encephalopathy following vaccination is lower than the incidence rate of encephalitis of unknown origin suggesting that such events following vaccination may be only temporally related to, rather than due to, vaccination.

1. Immunization Practices Advisory Committee. Measles prevention. *JAMA* 1987; **258:** 890–5.

Atypical measles. The atypical-measles syndrome has occurred in persons vaccinated against measles and later exposed to the natural infection. The syndrome has been characterised by high fever and atypical rash; abdominal pain has been common and pneumonia almost universal.[1] Although atypical measles has occurred particularly in patients given the no-longer used killed vaccine[1] it has been reported in recipients of live measles vaccines.[2-4]

Measles occurring in patients previously vaccinated with live measles vaccines may be mild and go unrecognised. However, secondary vaccine failure does not appear to be a major problem (see Immunisation Schedules under Uses, below).

1. Anonymous. The atypical-measles syndrome. *Lancet* 1979; **i:** 962–3.
2. Chatterji M, Mankad V. Failure of attenuated viral vaccine in prevention of atypical measles. *JAMA* 1977; **238:** 2635.

3. Henderson JAM, Hammond DI. Delayed diagnosis in atypical measles syndrome. *Can Med Assoc J* 1985; **133:** 211–13.
4. Hirose M, *et al.* Five cases of measles secondary vaccine failure with confirmed seroconversion after live measles vaccination. *Scand J Infect Dis* 1997; **29:** 187–90.

Effects on hearing. There have been individual case reports of sensorineural hearing loss after measles vaccination.[1,2] Similar reports have been made after vaccination with measles and rubella vaccines (p.1519) and measles, mumps, and rubella vaccines (p.1520).

1. Watson JG. Bilateral hearing loss in a 3-year-old girl following measles immunisation at the age of 15 months. *Int J Pediatr Otorhinolaryngol* 1990; **19:** 189–90.
2. Jayarajan V, Sedler PA. Hearing loss following measles vaccination. *J Infect* 1995; **30:** 184–5.

Effects on the nervous system. Subacute sclerosing panencephalitis (SSPE) is a rare complication of measles infection (p.602) and has been reported in children who have received measles vaccine but have no history of clinical disease. Nevertheless mass measles vaccination has been effective in reducing the incidence of SSPE in both developing and industrialised countries,[1] and the risks of remaining unimmunised are considered to be greater than those arising from immunisation.

1. Anonymous. SSPE in the developing world. *Lancet* 1990; **336:** 600.

GUILLAIN-BARRÉ SYNDROME. No association was found between measles vaccination and Guillain-Barré syndrome in an analysis of 2296 cases.[1]

1. da Silveira CM, *et al.* Measles vaccination and Guillain-Barré syndrome. *Lancet* 1997; **349:** 14–16.

OPTIC NEURITIS. For a report of optic neuritis in 2 children following administration of measles and rubella vaccine, see p.1519.

Effects on the skin. Stevens-Johnson syndrome was associated with measles vaccination in a 10-month-old infant.[1]

1. Hazir T, *et al.* Stevens-Johnson syndrome following measles vaccination. *J Pakistan Med Assoc* 1997; **47:** 264–5.

High-titre vaccines and mortality. Following reports of excess mortality, especially among girls, in children who received high-titre Edmonston-Zagreb (EZ) measles vaccine,[1] the WHO reversed its recommendation for the use of this vaccine in its Expanded Programme on Immunization in developing countries.[2,3] Subsequent study[4] of children who had received high-titre EZ vaccine showed adverse effects on the nutritional status in either sex, confirming a generally deleterious effect of the vaccine.

1. Knudsen KM, *et al.* Child mortality following standard, medium or high titre measles immunization in West Africa. *Int J Epidemiol* 1996; **25:** 665–73.
2. Anonymous. High-titre measles vaccines dropped. *Lancet* 1992; **340:** 232.
3. WHO. Expanded Programme on Immunization; safety of high-titre measles vaccines. *Wkly Epidem Rec* 1992; **67:** 357–61.
4. Garenne M. Effect of Edmonston-Zagreb high-titre vaccine on nutritional status. *Lancet* 1994; **344:** 261–2.

Precautions

As for vaccines in general, p.1501.

In the UK it was formerly recommended that children with a personal history of convulsions or those whose parents or siblings have a history of idiopathic epilepsy should receive measles vaccine but simultaneously with a specially diluted human normal immunoglobulin; it is now, however, recommended that such children be vaccinated with combined measles, mumps, and rubella vaccine in the same manner as normal healthy children. The parents should understand that a febrile reaction is possible and that suitable prophylactic treatment against febrile convulsions be undertaken (see Fever and Hyperthermia, p.1 for comments on the prevention of fever following immunisation). Immunoglobulin should not be given with the combined vaccine.

Measles vaccines are not generally recommended for children below the age of 1 year in whom maternal antibodies might prevent a response, but they have been administered to younger infants when the risk of measles is particularly high (see under Uses, below, for further discussion).

Hypersensitivity. For discussion of precautions to be taken on administration of measles vaccines to egg-allergic children, see Measles, Mumps, and Rubella Vaccines, p.1520.

Immunocompromised patients. For a discussion of the use of live vaccines in immunocompromised patients including those with HIV infections see under Uses on p.1502.

As with other live vaccines, measles vaccine is generally not recommended for use in patients with impaired immunity, although combined measles, mumps, and rubella vaccine may be given to HIV-positive individuals in the absence of other contra-indications. The WHO and UNICEF[1] recommend that children with suspected or confirmed HIV infection should receive a dose of measles vaccine at 6 months of age in addition to the scheduled dose at 9 to 15 months. The immunogenicity of measles vaccine in children with HIV infections has been shown to be low[2,3] although immunisation at 6 months of age was more effective than at 12 months of age.[3] Immunodeficient patients who come into contact with measles should be given normal immunoglobulin. Specific measles immunoglobulins are available in some countries. Although measles vaccines have been given to immunocompromised patients without causing adverse effects[2] there have been some reports of severe reactions; disseminated measles infection was reported in a child with severe congenital immunodeficiency,[4] and fatal giant-cell pneumonitis was reported in an adult with AIDS.[5] As a consequence of reports of adverse effects in severely immunocompromised individuals, the Advisory Committee on Immunization Practices in the USA is re-evaluating its recommendations for immunising patients with advanced HIV infection.[6]

1. WHO. *Global programme on AIDS: guidelines for the clinical management of HIV infection in children.* Geneva: WHO, 1993.
2. Krasinski K, Borkowsky W. Measles and measles immunity in children infected with human immunodeficiency virus. *JAMA* 1989; **261:** 2512–16.
3. Rudy BJ, *et al.* Responses to measles immunization in children infected with human immunodeficiency virus. *J Pediatr* 1994; **125:** 72–4.
4. Monafo WJ, *et al.* Disseminated measles infection after vaccination in a child with a congenital immunodeficiency. *J Pediatr* 1994; **124:** 273–6.
5. Angel JB, *et al.* Vaccine-associated measles pneumonitis in an adult with AIDS. *Ann Intern Med* 1998; **129:** 104–6.
6. Centers for Disease Control. Update: vaccine side effects, adverse reactions, contraindications, and precautions: recommendations of the Advisory Committee on Immunization Practices (ACIP). *MMWR* 1996; **45:** (RR-12): 1–35.

Inflammatory bowel disease. Measles vaccination has been suggested as a possible factor in the development of inflammatory bowel disease.[1] However a case-control study involving 140 patients with inflammatory bowel disease provided no support for this hypothesis,[2] and measles virus has not been detected in biopsy specimens from patients with inflammatory bowel disease.[3] A suggested link between measles vaccine-associated inflammatory bowel disease and autism has proved controversial (see p.1520).

1. Thompson NP, *et al.* Is measles vaccination a risk factor for inflammatory bowel disease? *Lancet* 1995; **345:** 1071–4.
2. Feeney M, *et al.* A case-control study of measles vaccination and inflammatory bowel disease. *Lancet* 1997; **350:** 764–6.
3. Afzal MA, *et al.* Absence of measles-virus genome in inflammatory bowel disease. *Lancet* 1998; **351:** 646–7.

Interactions

As for vaccines in general, p.1501

Vitamin A. Supplementation with vitamin A (p.1359) is now included as part of WHO's Expanded Programme on Immunization. There is conflicting evidence of the effects of such supplementation on the response to measles vaccination. Semba *et al.*[1] reported a reduced response if vaccination occurs at 6 months while Benn *et al.*[2] found the response to be unaffected in children vaccinated at 9 months. This difference, if confirmed, could be due to the influence of maternal antibodies, which would still be present at 6 months but not at 9 months of age.[3]

1. Semba RD, *et al.* Reduced seroconversion to measles in infants given vitamin A with measles vaccination. *Lancet* 1995; **345:** 1330–2.
2. Benn CS, *et al.* Randomised trial of effect of vitamin A supplementation on antibody response to measles vaccine in Guinea-Bissau, West Africa. *Lancet* 1997; **350:** 101–5.
3. Semba RD. Vitamin A supplementation. *Lancet* 1997; **350:** 1031–2.

Uses and Administration

Measles vaccines are used for active immunisation against measles.

For primary immunisation a combined measles, mumps, and rubella vaccine (p.1519) is usually used. For discussion of immunisation schedules see below.

In the UK single-antigen measles vaccine prepared from the Schwarz strain of the measles virus is no longer used. It was formerly given in a dose of 0.5 mL by deep subcutaneous or intramuscular injection.

Measles vaccines are not generally recommended for children below the age of 1 year in whom maternal antibodies might prevent a response. However, they have been administered to infants at 6 to 9 months in developing countries and in the USA in certain circumstances (see also below). A high-potency measles vaccine prepared from the Edmonston-Zagreb strain of measles virus was formerly used but was discontinued following evidence of increased mortality (see under Adverse Effects above).

Single-antigen measles vaccines have also been used for prophylaxis after exposure to measles provided they are given within 72 hours of contact.

Administration. Several alternative routes of administration of measles vaccines have been investigated in an attempt to overcome some of the disadvantages of subcutaneous or intramuscular injection.[1] Intradermal injection is effective if a needle is used but carries the same risk of secondary infection; the use of a jet injector has produced less reliable results. The conjunctival and oral routes are not sufficiently effective, and the intranasal route produced variable responses and could be influenced by concurrent upper respiratory tract infections. Aerosol administration has produced good responses in children over 9 months of age, with the Edmonston-Zagreb strain generally producing higher rates of seroconversion than the Schwarz strain, although this route was not so effective in younger children. Aerosol could be potentially useful for mass immunisation campaigns.

1. Cutts FT, *et al.* Alternative routes of measles immunization: a review. *Biologicals* 1997; **25:** 323–38.

Immunisation schedules. In the developed world measles vaccine (usually as measles, mumps, and rubella vaccine) is usually given in the second year of life.[1] As a result of concern that measles vaccine would not elicit an appropriate immune response in young infants due to the persistence of maternal antibodies in circulation, vaccination has generally not been attempted in children under 12 months old. Studies have shown that seroconversion rates are similar following vaccination at 12, 13, 14, and 15 to 18 months.[2] However, infants born to vaccinated mothers tend to have lower levels of maternal antibodies and are susceptible to measles infection at under 12 months of age; vaccination has been shown to be effective at 6 to 9 months of age in such children,[3-5] although antibody titres were lower in infants vaccinated at 6 months of age than in those vaccinated later.[3,6]

In the UK and USA[7] routine vaccination is given at 12 to 15 months, with a second dose given at 3 to 6 years or 11 to 12 years of age (see the immunisation schedules summarised under Vaccines, p.1501). Similar schedules are used in other countries. There is evidence that these 2-dose strategies will produce high levels of immunity in the community.[8] During an outbreak of measles, vaccination may be given as early as 6 months of age;[9] revaccination is recommended in any child who is vaccinated before their first birthday. Vaccine may be given to non-immune persons of any age considered to be at risk of infection even if their immune status is uncertain.

Immunisation strategies involving a single dose of measles vaccine have not been successful in eradicating or eliminating the disease in developed countries.[10,11] Immunisation has changed the epidemiology of measles and several isolated outbreaks have occurred among both unvaccinated and vaccinated persons.[10] Primary vaccine failure (approximately 2 to 10% of vaccinees fail to seroconvert after measles vaccination) has played a substantial role in transmission of measles.[10] Furthermore, waning of immunity in the vaccinated cohort coupled with a reduction in the prevalence of the natural infection has resulted in increasing numbers of young adults with low concentrations of antibodies.[12,13] As these young adults reach child-bearing age, their children in turn have lower, faster-waning immunity and are susceptible to infection before the usual age of immunisation.[14] Immunisation schedules which include a second dose of measles vaccine in adolescence would boost immunity in young adults and hence in their offspring, but there is evidence that revaccination is ineffective in a proportion of recipients.[15,16] The alternative is to give the first dose of vaccine earlier, for example at 6 months of age, and a second dose in early childhood. However this too would not overcome the problem of secondary vaccine failures in young adults. This dilemma over the most appropriate schedule is most pressing in developing countries where transmission rates are usually high. For discussion of immunisation schedules in the developing world, see under Expanded Programme on Immunization, below.

1. Isaacs D, Menser M. Modern vaccines: measles, mumps, rubella, and varicella. *Lancet* 1990; **335:** 1384–7.
2. Kakakios AM, *et al.* Optimal age for measles and mumps vaccination in Australia. *Med J Aust* 1990; **152:** 472–4.
3. Johnson CE, *et al.* Measles vaccine immunogenicity in 6- versus 15-month-old infants born to mothers in the measles vaccine era. *Pediatrics* 1994; **93:** 939–44.
4. Carson MM, *et al.* Measles vaccination of infants in a well-vaccinated population. *Pediatr Infect Dis J* 1995; **14:** 17–22.
5. Markowitz LE, *et al.* Changing levels of measles antibody titers in women and children in the United States: impact on response to vaccination. *Pediatrics* 1996; **97:** 53–8.
6. Gans HA, *et al.* Deficiency of the humoral immune response to measles vaccine in infants immunized at age 6 months. *JAMA* 1998; **280:** 527–32.
7. American Academy of Pediatrics Committee on Infectious Diseases. Recommended childhood immunization schedule—United States, January-December 1997. *Pediatrics* 1997; **99:** 136–8.
8. Poland GA, *et al.* Measles reimmunization in children seronegative after initial immunization. *JAMA* 1997; **277:** 1156–8.

9. De Serres G, *et al.* Effectiveness of vaccination at 6 to 11 months of age during an outbreak of measles. *Pediatrics* 1996; **97:** 232–5.
10. Immunization Practices Advisory Committee. Measles prevention: supplementary statement. *JAMA* 1989; **261:** 827 and 831.
11. Levy MH, Bridges-Webb C. "Just one shot" is not enough — measles control and eradication. *Med J Aust* 1990; **152:** 489–91.
12. Mulholland K. Measles and pertussis in developing countries with good vaccine coverage. *Lancet* 1995; **345:** 305–7.
13. McLean AR. After the honeymoon in measles control. *Lancet* 1995; **345:** 272.
14. Maldonado YA, *et al.* Early loss of passive measles antibody in infants of mothers with vaccine-induced immunity. *Pediatrics* 1995; **96:** 447–50.
15. Markowitz LE, *et al.* Persistence of measles antibody after revaccination. *J Infect Dis* 1992; **166:** 205–8.
16. Cohn ML, *et al.* Measles vaccine failures: lack of sustained measles-specific immunoglobulin G responses in revaccinated adolescents and young adults. *Pediatr Infect Dis J* 1994; **13:** 34–8.

EXPANDED PROGRAMME ON IMMUNIZATION. In the developed world measles vaccine (usually as measles, mumps, and rubella vaccine) is usually given in the second year of life. If given earlier, passively-acquired maternal antibodies against measles may interfere with development of protective immunity although this situation is changing as vaccinated women reach child-bearing age (see above). In the developing world, protection given by maternal antibodies is often rapidly lost.[1] Thus in hyperendemic areas, such as urban and peri-urban areas, clinical measles may occur in children as young as 5 to 6 months of age. Immunisation against measles is part of WHO's Expanded Programme on Immunization.[2] It is given as a single-antigen vaccine generally at 9 months of age. However control of measles in children less than 9 months of age is a major concern in some countries, in particular in areas of high population density.[3] WHO no longer recommends the use of high-titre Edmonston-Zagreb measles vaccine which, unlike conventional vaccines, was shown to be effective at 6 months of age following the observation of increased mortality despite the resulting increase in immunity (see under Adverse Effects, above). For comments on the possibility of a resurgence of measles infection in young adults and infants in countries with good vaccine coverage, see under Immunisation Schedules, above. WHO recognises that vaccination strategies will need to be formulated to cope with local disease patterns and available resources.[3]

In some situations high coverage with a single dose of vaccine can produce a high degree of immunity[3] and standard titre vaccines have been shown to be as effective as high-titre vaccines.[4,5] Mass immunisation campaigns can also be very effective[6] but can be expensive when a large proportion of the community is already immune.[7,8]

Early 2-dose schedules[3] may be more applicable in areas with high transmission rates among young infants. The first dose is typically given at 9 months of age and the second dose 3 to 6 months later. In very high risk situations, such as refugee camps and following disasters, the first dose may be given at 6 months of age and the second dose as soon as possible after the child reaches 9 months of age.

Late 2-dose schedules[3] may be more appropriate in industrialised countries in which measles transmission among young infants is limited. The schedule is aimed at preventing infection in older children following primary or secondary vaccine failure. The first dose is typically given at 9 to 12 months of age, and the second dose at school entry.

Several studies have examined the effect of measles immunisation on mortality and morbidity in developing countries.[9] Data suggest that the reduction in mortality following immunisation is greater than that expected simply from a reduction in death from acute measles. Measles immunisation may protect children dying not only from an acute measles attack but also from late causes which may be attributable to measles. It is also possible that measles vaccine has an immunostimulant effect.

For discussion of the link between vitamin A status and measles see Vitamin A Substances, p.1359.

1. Toole MJ, *et al.* Measles prevention and control in emergency settings. *Bull WHO* 1989; **67:** 381–8.
2. Hall AJ, *et al.* Modern vaccines: practice in developing countries. *Lancet* 1990; **335:** 774–7.
3. Rosenthal SR, Clements CJ. Two-dose measles vaccination schedules. *Bull WHO* 1993; **71:** 421–8.
4. Garenne M, *et al.* Efficacy of measles vaccines after controlling for exposure. *Am J Epidemiol* 1993; **138:** 182–95.
5. Diaz-Ortega J-L, *et al.* The relationship between dose and response of standard measles vaccines. *Biologicals* 1994; **22:** 35–44.
6. de Quadros CA, *et al.* Measles elimination in the Americas: evolving strategies. *JAMA* 1996; **275:** 224–9.
7. Cutts FT. Measles control in young infants: where do we go from here? *Lancet* 1993; **341:** 290–1.
8. Global Programme for Vaccines of the World Health Organization. Role of mass campaigns in global measles control. *Lancet* 1994; **344:** 174–5.
9. Aaby P, Clements CJ. Measles immunization research: a review. *Bull WHO* 1989; **67:** 443–8.

Immunisation for travellers. The Immunization Practices Advisory Committee in the USA has recommended that administration of measles vaccine be considered for all persons travelling abroad who were born after 1956, regardless of their vaccination status.[1] Travellers who have had measles or were born before 1957 are considered immune secondary to natural infection.[2] Single-antigen measles vaccine or measles, mumps, and rubella vaccine may be used.[1] Children aged 6 to 11 months should receive a dose of single-antigen vaccine if travelling to areas where measles is endemic or epidemic.[1] A dose of measles, mumps, and rubella vaccine is given at 15 months, or 12 months if the child remains in a high-risk area.

1. Immunization Practices Advisory Committee. Measles prevention. *JAMA* 1987; **258:** 890–5.
2. Hill DR, Pearson RD. Measles prophylaxis for international travel. *Ann Intern Med* 1989; **111:** 699–701.

Preparations

Ph. Eur.: Measles Vaccine (Live);
USP 23: Measles Virus Vaccine Live.

Proprietary Preparations (details are given in Part 3)
Aust.: Attenuvax; Rimevax; ***Austral.:*** Attenuvax†; Rimevax†; ***Belg.:*** Attenuvax†; Rimevax; ***Fr.:*** Rouvax; ***Ger.:*** Masern-Impfstoff Merieux; Masern-Lebend-Impfstoff; Masern-Vaccinol; Masern-Virus-Impfstoff; ***Ital.:*** Attenuvax; Lio-Morbillo; Moraten; Morbilvax; Rimevax; Rouvax; ***Neth.:*** Attenuvax†; ***S.Afr.:*** Diplovax; Moraten; Morbilvax; Rimevax; Rouvax; ***Spain:*** Amunovax; Moraten†; Rimevax; Rouvax†; Vac Antisaramp†; ***Switz.:*** Attenuvax; Moraten; Rimevax; ***UK:*** Measavax†; Mevilin-L; ***USA:*** Attenuvax.

Measles and Mumps Vaccines (7971-g)

Measles and Mumps Virus Vaccine Live (USP 23) is a bacterially sterile freeze-dried preparation of a suitable live strain of measles virus and a suitable live strain of mumps virus. It may contain suitable antimicrobial agents. Each labelled dose provides an immunising dose of each component. It should be stored at 2° to 8° and be protected from light.

Adverse Effects and Precautions

As for vaccines in general, p.1500.

See also under Measles Vaccines, p.1517, and Mumps Vaccines, p.1521.

Effects on the bones and joints. For a reference to arthritis occurring after administration of measles and mumps vaccine, see under Adverse Effects and Precautions of Measles, Mumps, and Rubella Vaccines, p.1520.

Interactions

As for vaccines in general, p.1501.

See also under Measles Vaccines, p.1518.

Uses and Administration

Measles and mumps vaccines may be used for active immunisation against measles and mumps. Vaccination against measles and mumps is normally performed using a combined measles, mumps, and rubella vaccine (p.1519) but the bivalent measles and mumps vaccine may be employed when vaccination against rubella is not indicated. For discussion of immunisation schedules see under Vaccines, p.1501.

Two types of vaccine have been used. That usually available now is prepared from a more attenuated line of measles virus derived from Enders' attenuated Edmonston strain and the Jeryl Lynn (B level) strain of mumps virus. The second type of vaccine is prepared from the attenuated Schwarz strain of measles virus and the attenuated Urabe Am 9 strain of mumps virus. For both types, a 0.5 mL dose is given by intramuscular or subcutaneous injection.

Measles and mumps vaccines may also be used for prophylaxis after exposure to measles provided it is given within 72 hours of contact.

Preparations

USP 23: Measles and Mumps Virus Vaccine Live.

Proprietary Preparations (details are given in Part 3)
Aust.: M-M Vax; ***Austral.:*** M-M Vax†; ***Belg.:*** Duovax; ***Ger.:*** M-M Vax; Rimparix†; ***S.Afr.:*** Bivaraten; ***Spain:*** Inmunivirus Doble†; ***Switz.:*** Biviraten; M-M Vax; Rimparix†.

Measles and Rubella Vaccines (7972-q)

Measles and Rubella Virus Vaccine Live (USP 23) is a bacterially sterile freeze-dried preparation of suitable live strains of measles virus and live rubella virus. It may contain suitable antimicrobial agents. Each labelled dose provides an immunising dose of each component. It should be stored at 2° to 8° and be protected from light.

Adverse Effects and Precautions

As for vaccines in general, p.1500.

See also under Measles Vaccines, p.1517, and Rubella Vaccines, p.1532.

Eight million children aged between 5 and 16 years were immunised with a measles and rubella vaccine in 1994 in the UK. By October 1995 the Committee on Safety of Medicines had received reports on 2735 suspected adverse reactions most of which were minor and self-limiting.[1] Serious suspected reactions were rare and generally the number of reported cases was consistent with the background frequency of the particular disorder.

1. Committee on Safety of Medicines/Medicines Control Agency. Adverse reactions to measles rubella vaccine. *Current Problems* 1995; **21:** 9–10.

Effects on hearing. Profound, irreversible sensorineural deafness was reported in a 27-year-old woman following administration of a measles and rubella vaccine.[1] Sensorineural deafness has also been reported following administration of measles, mumps, and rubella vaccine (p.1520), and monovalent measles vaccine (p.1518).

1. Hulbert TV, *et al.* Bilateral hearing loss after measles and rubella vaccination in an adult. *N Engl J Med* 1991; **325:** 134.

Effects on the nervous system. Optic neuritis was reported in two children who had received measles and rubella vaccine two to three weeks previously.[1]

1. Stevenson VL, *et al.* Optic neuritis following measles/rubella vaccination in two 13-year-old children. *Br J Ophthalmol* 1996; **80:** 1110–11.

Interactions

As for vaccines in general, p.1501.

See also under Measles Vaccines, p.1518.

Uses and Administration

Measles and rubella vaccines may be used for active immunisation against measles and rubella. For primary immunisation a combined measles, mumps, and rubella vaccine (p.1519) is usually used but the bivalent measles and rubella vaccine may be employed when vaccination against mumps is not indicated. For discussion of immunisation schedules see under Vaccines, p.1501.

Vaccines have been prepared from either a more attenuated line of measles virus derived from Enders' attenuated Edmonston strain or attenuated Schwarz strain, and the Wistar RA 27/3 strain of rubella virus. The vaccine is generally given in a dose of 0.5 mL by subcutaneous or intramuscular injection to infants or to other susceptible children or adults considered to be at risk.

Measles and rubella vaccine was successfully used in a mass immunisation campaign in children aged 5 to 16 years in the UK in order to avert an anticipated measles epidemic.[1,2]

1. Cutts FT. Revaccination against measles and rubella. *Br Med J* 1996; **312:** 589–90.
2. Anonymous. Measles/rubella vaccine: a favourable balance of risk and benefit. *WHO Drug Inf* 1996; **10:** 43.

Preparations

USP 23: Measles and Rubella Virus Vaccine Live.

Proprietary Preparations (details are given in Part 3)
Canad.: MoRu-Viraten; ***Fr.:*** Rudi-Rouvax; ***Ital.:*** Morubel†; ***UK:*** Eolarix†; ***USA:*** M-R-Vax II.

Measles, Mumps, and Rubella Vaccines (7973-p)

Measles, Mumps and Rubella Vaccine (Live) (Ph. Eur.) (MMR/Vac (Live); Measles, Mumps and Rubella Vaccine, Live (BP 1998); Vaccinum Morbillorum, Parotitidis et Rubellae Vivum) is a freeze-dried preparation containing suitable live attenuated strains of measles virus, mumps virus (*Paramyxovirus parotitidis*), and rubella virus. The vaccine is prepared immediately before use by reconstitution from the dried vaccine. It contains in each dose not less than 1×10^3 $CCID_{50}$ of infective measles virus, not less than 5×10^3 $CCID_{50}$ of infective mumps virus, and not less than 1×10^3 $CCID_{50}$ of infective rubella virus. The dried vaccine should be stored at 2° to 8° and be protected from light.

Measles, Mumps, and Rubella Virus Vaccine Live (USP 23) is a bacterially sterile freeze-dried preparation of suitable live strains of measles virus, mumps virus, and rubella virus. It may contain suitable antimicrobial agents. Each labelled dose provides an immunising dose of each component. It should be stored at 2° to 8° and be protected from light.

Adverse Effects and Precautions

As for vaccines in general, p.1500.

See also under Measles Vaccines, p.1517, Mumps Vaccines, p.1521, and Rubella Vaccines, p.1532.

Adverse effects tend to be less frequent after the second dose of vaccine than after the first dose.

Measles, mumps, and rubella vaccines should not be given to individuals hypersensitive to neomycin; in the UK hypersensitivity to kanamycin is also regarded as a contra-indication.

Recommendations on vaccination in persons with egg allergy are being modified (see below). A history of mild reactions to egg is not regarded as a contra-indication.

Children with a history of convulsions should receive measles, mumps, and rubella vaccination, but advice should be given on controlling fever.

A double-blind placebo-controlled crossover study[1] in 581 pairs of twins showed that the true frequency of side-effects was between 0.5 and 4.0%, indicating that adverse reactions are much less common than was previously thought.

A study in the USA[2] showed that children receiving the vaccine at age 4 to 6 years had fewer adverse effects than those receiving it at 10 to 12 years.

1. Peltola H, Heinonen OP. Frequency of true adverse reactions to measles-mumps-rubella vaccine: a double-blind placebo-controlled trial in twins. *Lancet* 1986; **i:** 939–42.
2. Davis RL, *et al.* MMR2 immunization at 4 to 5 years and 10 to 12 years of age: a comparison of adverse clinical events after immunization in the vaccine safety datalink project. *Pediatrics* 1997; **100:** 767–71.

Effects on the blood. Thrombocytopenia occurs rarely in children receiving measles, mumps, and rubella vaccine and usually resolves spontaneously. An increased incidence of thrombocytopenia following the second dose of the vaccine has been reported in children who developed thrombocytopenia after the first dose.[1]

1. Vlacha V, *et al.* Recurrent thrombocytopenic purpura after repeated measles-mumps-rubella vaccination. *Pediatrics* 1996; **97:** 738–9.

Effects on the bones and joints. Arthralgia and arthritis occurring in patients receiving mumps, measles, and rubella vaccines have generally been attributed to the rubella component.[1] However, arthritis has been reported in 1 infant following vaccination with measles and mumps vaccine.[2]

1. Benjamin CM, *et al.* Joint and limb symptoms in children after immunisation with measles, mumps, and rubella vaccine. *Br Med J* 1992; **304:** 1075–8.
2. Nussinovitch M, *et al.* Arthritis after mumps and measles vaccination. *Arch Dis Child* 1995; **72:** 348–9.

Effects on hearing. Nine cases of sensorineural hearing loss following measles, mumps, and rubella (MMR) vaccine administration were reported to the Committee on Safety of Medicines (CSM) in the UK between 1988 and 1993.[1] Of these, three cases were judged not to have been associated with MMR vaccine. In the remaining 6, the mumps virus component was considered to be the most likely cause of deafness if the vaccine was to blame, but the risk was considered to be small compared with the risks of natural infection. However, sensorineural deafness has also been reported following administration of measles and rubella vaccine (see p.1519), and monovalent measles vaccine (see p.1518).

1. Stewart BJA, Prabhu PU. Reports of sensorineural deafness after measles, mumps, and rubella immunisation. *Arch Dis Child* 1993; **69:** 153–4.

Effects on the nervous system. Guillain-Barré syndrome was reported[1] in a 16-month-old girl following vaccination with measles, mumps, and rubella vaccine.

Prolonged tonic-clonic seizures were associated with prolonged hemiparesis in a 16-month-old girl six days after measles, mumps, and rubella vaccination.[2] There was evidence of transient encephalopathy. However, a causal relationship between measles-containing vaccines and encephalitis is generally considered to be unlikely. Other reported neurological effects following vaccination include gait disturbances[3] and transverse myelitis.[4]

For discussion of meningitis and encephalitis occurring after measles, mumps, and rubella vaccination, see under Mumps Vaccines, p.1521.

1. Morris K, Rylance G. Guillain-Barré syndrome after measles, mumps, and rubella vaccine. *Lancet* 1994; **343:** 60.
2. Sackey AH, Broadhead RL. Hemiplegia after measles, mumps, and rubella vaccination. *Br Med J* 1993; **306:** 1169.
3. Plesner A-M. Gait disturbances after measles, mumps, and rubella vaccine. *Lancet* 1995; **345:** 316.
4. Joyce KA, Rees JE. Transverse myelitis after measles, mumps, and rubella vaccine. *Br Med J* 1995; **311:** 422.

Hypersensitivity. Since the measles and mumps components of measles, mumps, and rubella vaccines are grown in cell cultures of chick embryos the vaccine has in the past been contra-indicated in individuals with a history of anaphylactic reactions to egg. It is generally agreed that the vaccine can be given safely to children with less severe reactions to eggs. In the USA the American Academy of Pediatrics (AAP) has recommended[1] that children with a history of severe reactions to eggs should have a series of skin tests to assess sensitivity to the vaccine followed by desensitisation in those showing a positive result. Although skin tests have predicted hypersensitivity reactions to the vaccine in some patients[2,3] there are doubts over their predictive value.[4] The vaccine has been given to patients with allergy to eggs without provoking hypersensitivity reactions[5] and it is possible that hypersensitivity may be provoked by other allergenic components of the vaccine, for example gelatin[6] or antibiotics. The US Advisory Committee on Immunization Practices (ACIP) is re-evaluating the need for skin testing and desensitisation protocols in patients with a history of hypersensitivity to egg[7] and in the UK severe allergy to eggs is no longer regarded as an absolute contra-indication.[8]

1. American Academy of Pediatrics. *Report of the committee of infectious diseases* (red book). 22nd ed. Elk Grove Village, Illinois: American Academy of Pediatrics Publications, 1991.
2. Lavi S, *et al.* Administration of measles, mumps, and rubella virus vaccine (live) to egg-allergic children. *JAMA* 1990; **263:** 269–71.
3. Trotter AC, *et al.* Measles, mumps, rubella (MMR) vaccine administration in egg-sensitive children: systemic reactions during vaccine desensitization. *Ann Allergy* 1994; **72:** 25–8.
4. Aickin R, *et al.* Measles immunisation in children with allergy to egg. *Br Med J* 1994; **309:** 223–5.
5. James JM, *et al.* Safe administration of the measles vaccine to children allergic to eggs. *N Engl J Med* 1995; **332:** 1262–6.
6. Kelso JM, *et al.* Anaphylaxis to measles, mumps, and rubella vaccine mediated by IgE to gelatin. *J Allergy Clin Immunol* 1993; **91:** 867–72.
7. Centers for Disease Control. Update: vaccine side effects, adverse reactions, contraindications, and precautions: recommendations of the Advisory Committee on Immunization Practices (ACIP). *MMWR* 1996; **45:** (RR-12): 1–45.
8. Salisbury DM, Begg NT (eds), Joint Committee on Vaccination and Immunisation. *Immunisation against infectious disease.* London: HMSO, 1996.

Inflammatory bowel disease and autism. A controversial report[1] linking measles, mumps, and rubella vaccination with the development of inflammatory bowel disease and behavioural abnormalities including autism was not supported by epidemiological evidence[2,3] and provoked concern over a reduction in vaccine uptake as a result of media coverage.[4-6] Other suggestions of links between measles vaccines and inflammatory bowel disease have not been substantiated (see p.1518).

1. Wakefield AJ, *et al.* Ileal-lymphoid-nodular hyperplasia, non-specific colitis, and pervasive developmental disorder in children. *Lancet* 1998; **351:** 637–41.
2. Peltola H, *et al.* No evidence for measles, mumps, and rubella vaccine-associated inflammatory bowel disease or autism in a 14-year prospective study. *Lancet* 1998; **351:** 1327–8.
3. Roberts R. There is no causal link between MMR vaccine and autism. *Br Med J* 1998; **316:** 1824.
4. Chen RT, DeStefano F. Vaccine adverse events: causal or coincidental? *Lancet* 1998; **351:** 611–12.
5. Nicoll A, *et al.* MMR vaccination and autism 1998. *Br Med J* 1998; **316:** 715–16. Correction. *ibid.*; 796.
6. Lee JW, *et al.* Autism, inflammatory bowel disease, and MMR vaccine. *Lancet* 1998; **351:** 905.

Interactions

As for vaccines in general, p.1501.

See also under Measles Vaccines, p.1518.

Uses and Administration

Measles, mumps, and rubella vaccines are used for active immunisation against measles, mumps, and rubella. They are used for primary immunisation in children 12 months of age or older and to protect susceptible contacts during an outbreak of measles. For discussion of immunisation schedules see under Vaccines, p.1501.

In the UK and USA the vaccine is prepared from an attenuated line of measles virus derived from Enders' attenuated Edmonston strain, the Jeryl Lynn (B level) strain of mumps virus, and the Wistar RA 27/3 strain of rubella virus. Another type, no longer used in several countries because of an increased risk of meningoencephalitis (see under Adverse Effects of Mumps Vaccines, p.1521), has been prepared from the Schwarz strain of measles virus, the Urabe Am 9 strain of mumps virus, and the Wistar RA 27/3 strain of rubella virus.

In the UK it is recommended that all children receive two doses of 0.5 mL of a measles, mumps, and rubella vaccine by deep subcutaneous or intramuscular injection. These are usually given shortly after the first birthday and before school entry, but may be given at any age if routine administration has been omitted, allowing 3 months between doses. The combined vaccine may also be used for prophylaxis after exposure to measles provided it is given within 72 hours of contact. However, it is not considered to be effective for postexposure prophylaxis against either mumps or rubella. If the vaccine is given before 12 months of age, re-immunisation will be necessary.

In the USA, the second dose is recommended at age 4 to 6 years. Children who have not previously received the second dose should complete the vaccination schedule by age 11 to 12 years.

Preparations

Ph. Eur.: Measles, Mumps, and Rubella Vaccine (Live);
USP 23: Measles, Mumps, and Rubella Virus Vaccine Live.

Proprietary Preparations (details are given in Part 3)
Aust.: MMR Vax; ***Austral.:*** MMR II; Pluserix†; ***Belg.:*** MMR Vax; ***Canad.:*** MMR II; ***Fr.:*** R.O.R.; Trimovax†; ***Ger.:*** MMR Triplovax; MMR Vax; Pluserix†; ***Irl.:*** MMR II; Pluserix†; ***Ital.:*** MMR II; Morupar; Pluserix†; Trimovax; Triviraten; ***S.Afr.:*** MMR II; Trimovax; Triviraten; ***Spain:*** Inmunovirus Triple†; Triviraten; Vac Triple MSD; ***Swed.:*** MMR II; Virivac; ***Switz.:*** MMR II; Pluserix†; Trimovax†; Triviraten; ***UK:*** MMR II; Priorix; ***USA:*** MMR II.

Meningococcal Vaccines (7979-j)

Meningococcal Polysaccharide Vaccine (Ph. Eur.) (Neimen/Vac; Vaccinum Meningitidis Cerebrospinalis) consists of one or more purified capsular polysaccharides obtained from one or more suitable strains of *Neisseria meningitidis* group A, group C, group Y, and group W135; it may contain a single type of polysaccharide or any mixture of the types. It is prepared immediately before use by reconstitution from the stabilised freeze-dried vaccine with a suitable sterile liquid. The freeze-dried vaccine should be stored at 2° to 8° and be protected from light.

Meningococcal Polysaccharide Vaccine Group A (USP 23) is a sterile preparation of the group-specific polysaccharide antigen from *Neisseria meningitidis* group A.

Meningococcal Polysaccharide Vaccine Group C (USP 23) is a sterile preparation of the group-specific polysaccharide antigen from *Neisseria meningitidis* group C.

Meningococcal Polysaccharide Vaccine Groups A and C Combined (USP 23) is a sterile preparation of meningococcal polysaccharide group A and C specific antigens (see above). All three USP vaccines are supplied as dried vaccines which are reconstituted before use with bacteriostatic sodium chloride injection containing thiomersal. The dried vaccines should be stored at 2° to 8° and the reconstituted vaccines should be used immediately after preparation, or within 8 hours if stored at 2° to 8°.

Adverse Effects and Precautions

As for vaccines in general, p.1500.

Immunity to some meningococcal vaccines may be insufficient to confer adequate protection against infection in infants under about 2 years of age (for further discussion see under Uses, below).

Pregnancy and the neonate. A mixed meningococcal vaccine (A and C) was evaluated in pregnant women and infants during an epidemic of meningitis in Brazil.[1] Antibodies were detected in the women and there was some placental transfer of antibody although this was irregular. Vaccination of children in the first 6 months of life was unsuccessful.

These results were supported by a subsequent study in the Gambia.[2] Maternal antibodies were high in all women at the time of delivery, but only a proportion of the antibody crossed the placenta. There was considerable individual variation in the cord blood: maternal blood antibody ratios. Antibody concentrations declined rapidly in the infants and had effectively disappeared by 3 to 4 months of age.

1. Carvalho A de A, *et al.* Maternal and infant antibody response to meningococcal vaccination in pregnancy. *Lancet* 1977; **ii:** 809–11.
2. O'Dempsey TJD, *et al.* Meningococcal antibody titres in infants of women immunised with meningococcal polysaccharide vaccine during pregnancy. *Arch Dis Child* 1996; **74:** F43–6.

Interactions

As for vaccines in general, p.1501.

Uses and Administration

Meningococcal vaccines are used for active immunisation against *Neisseria meningitidis* infections which include meningitis and septicaemia. They are preparations of purified polysaccharide antigens from *N. meningitidis* and may be monovalent, containing the antigen of only one serotype of *N. meningitidis* or polyvalent, containing antigens of two or more serotypes. Commonly available vaccines appear to be a bivalent vaccine from groups A and C (in the UK) and a tetravalent vaccine from groups A, C, Y, and W135 (in the USA), both given in a dose of 0.5 mL by subcutaneous or intramuscular injection.

Meningococcal vaccines are indicated in persons at risk, in epidemic or endemic areas, of meningococcal disease caused by the specific serotypes contained in the vaccine. It is given as an adjunct to chemoprophylaxis in close contacts of persons with the disease and should be considered for persons travelling to countries where the risk of infection is high, particularly for visits of 1 month or more and for those backpacking or living or working with local residents. Asplenic persons or those who have terminal complement component deficiencies are at higher than normal risk of acquiring meningococcal infection. The minimum recommended age for administration of meningococcal vaccines has varied from 2 months to 2 years because of reports of poor immune response in younger infants (see below for further discussion). Immunity following vaccination lasts for about 3 to 5 years except in young children in whom it declines more rapidly.

Reviews.

1. Peltola H. Meningococcal vaccines: current status and future possibilities. *Drugs* 1998; **55:** 347–66.

Immunisation. *Neisseria meningitidis* is an important cause of meningitis. About 60% of meningococcal infections (p.131) in the UK and the USA are caused by *Neisseria meningitidis* of group B serotype. However, there is no available vaccine against these organisms because the purified group B polysaccharide is only poorly immunogenic, even after conjugation with proteins.[1] A number of avenues of research are being followed in the development of an effective vaccine against the group B serotype.[2-4] A number of candidate vaccines based on class 1 outer membrane proteins have been field-tested but efficacy has been variable. Favourable results with a fairly crude vaccine in Cuba were not confirmed by a study in Brazil using the same vaccine,[5] and the response in young children was especially disappointing. Similarly, a vaccine produced in Norway gave a protection rate of about 60%, judged to be too low for use in a general immunisation programme.[6] A direct comparison of the two vaccines[7] found that the Norwegian vaccine produced greater immunity in adolescents than the Cuban vaccine. Other strategies have included vaccines based on other outer membrane proteins and lipopolysaccharide derivatives.[2-4]

Outbreaks of meningococcal infections are more commonly caused by group A or C meningococci. Epidemics of group A infection occur particularly in the meningitis belt of Africa in the dry season. Polysaccharide vaccines of meningococci of groups A, C, W135, and Y have been successful in producing short-term immunity (up to about 5 years) and controlling epidemics and outbreaks, although vaccination does not influence nasopharyngeal carriage of the organism.[1,8] Antibody response to group A polysaccharide vaccine is reduced in infants under 2 years of age, but it is still sufficient to confer protection from infection in infants over 3 months.[9] Response can be improved in infants and young children by giving a second dose after 3 months. Infants and children do, however, show a poor immune response in areas where malaria is holoendemic.[10] Immunity to group C meningococcal vaccine is low in infants below the age of 2 years and has been stated to be unlikely to persist for more than 1 to 2 years. However, a partial response has been demonstrated in children as young at 6 months of age following a mass vaccination campaign during an epidemic.[11] Therefore, the minimum age for administration recommended by manufacturers of polyvalent polysaccharide meningococcal vaccines varies from 2 months to 2 years. Attempts to enhance passive protection of infants by immunising their mothers during pregnancy has not been successful (see above).

Conjugate vaccines against group A and C meningococci are being developed in an attempt to improve the immunogenicity,[3,4] and the results of clinical studies are encouraging.[12]

No country is at present regularly vaccinating children with meningococcal vaccines.[13] The relative infrequency of epidemics and the necessity to give vaccine at an age not included in the immunisation schedule of the Expanded Programme on Immunization have hampered the development of a uniform vaccination policy.

1. Anonymous. Preventing meningococcal infection. *Drug Ther Bull* 1990; **28:** 34–6.
2. Zollinger WD, Moran E. Meningococcal vaccines—present and future. *Trans R Soc Trop Med Hyg* 1991; **85** (suppl 1): 37–43.
3. Herbert MA, *et al.* Meningococcal vaccines for the United Kingdom. *Commun Dis Rep* 1995; **5** (review 9): R130–5.
4. Ala'Aldeen DAA, Cartwright KAV. Neisseria meningitidis: vaccines and vaccine candidates. *J Infect* 1996; **33:** 153–7.
5. de Morales JC, *et al.* Protective efficacy of a serogroup B meningococcal vaccine in Sao Paulo, Brazil. *Lancet* 1992; **340:** 1074–8.
6. Bjune G, *et al.* Effect of outer membrane vesicle vaccine against group B meningococcal disease in Norway. *Lancet* 1991; **338:** 1093–6.
7. Perkins BA, *et al.* Immunogenicity of two efficacious outer membrane protein-based serogroup B meningococcal vaccines among young adults in Iceland. *J Infect Dis* 1998; **177:** 683–91.
8. Anonymous. Meningococcal meningitis. *Lancet* 1989; **i:** 647–8. Correction. *ibid.*; 742.
9. Peltola H, *et al.* Clinical efficacy of meningococcus group A capsular polysaccharide vaccine in children three months to five years of age. *N Engl J Med* 1977; **297:** 686–91.
10. Moxon ER, Rappuoli R. Modern vaccines: Haemophilus influenzae infections and whooping cough. *Lancet* 1990; **335:** 1324–9.
11. King WJ, *et al.* Total and functional antibody response to a quadrivalent meningococcal polysaccharide vaccine among children. *J Pediatr* 1996; **128:** 196–202.
12. Lieberman JM, *et al.* Safety and immunogenicity of a serogroups A/C Neisseria meningitidis oligosaccharide-protein conjugate vaccine in young children: a randomized controlled trial. *JAMA* 1996; **275:** 1499–1503.
13. Wright PF. Approaches to prevent acute bacterial meningitis in developing countries. *Bull WHO* 1989; **67:** 479–86.

Preparations

Ph. Eur.: Meningococcal Polysaccharide Vaccine;
USP 23: Meningococcal Polysaccharide Vaccine Group A; Meningococcal Polysaccharide Vaccine Group C; Meningococcal Polysaccharide Vaccine Groups A and C Combined.

Proprietary Preparations (details are given in Part 3)
Aust.: Mencevax ACWY; ***Austral.:*** Mencevax ACWY; Menomune; ***Belg.:*** Mencevax ACWY; ***Ger.:*** Mencevax ACWY; Meningokokken-Impfstoff A + C; ***Irl.:*** Mengivac (A+C); ***Ital.:*** Mencevax ACWY; Menomune; Menpovax 4†; Menpovax A+C†; ***Neth.:*** Meningovax A+C; ***Norw.:*** Meningovax A+C; ***S.Afr.:*** Imovax Meningo A & C; ***Spain:*** Vac Antimenin AC†; ***Swed.:*** Meningovax A+C; ***UK:*** AC Vax; Mengivac (A+C); ***USA:*** Menomune.

Multiple Sclerosis Vaccines (18390-s)

Vaccines based on T cells are under investigation for the management of multiple sclerosis.

References.

1. Medaer R, *et al.* Depletion of myelin-basic-protein autoreactive T cells by T-cell vaccination: pilot trial in multiple sclerosis. *Lancet* 1995; **346:** 807–8.

Mumps Immunoglobulins (14232-s)

Preparations containing antibodies against mumps virus are available in some countries for passive immunisation against mumps.

Preparations

Proprietary Preparations (details are given in Part 3)
Ital.: Haima-Parot; Immunoparot; Par-Gamma; Paruman; ***Spain:*** Gamma Glob Antiparot†; Glogama Antiparotiditis†; ***Switz.:*** Paruman.

Mumps Vaccines (7982-s)

Mumps Vaccine (Live) (Ph. Eur.) (Mump/Vac (Live); Mumps Vaccine, Live (BP 1998); Vaccinum Parotitidis Vivum) is a freeze-dried preparation containing a suitable live attenuated strain of mumps virus (*Paramyxovirus parotitidis*) grown in cultures of human diploid cells or chick-embryo cells or the amniotic cavity of chick embryos. It is prepared immediately before use by reconstitution from the dried vaccine. The cell-culture medium may contain the lowest effective concentration of a suitable antibiotic. The virus titre is not less than 5×10^3 $CCID_{50}$ per dose. The dried vaccine should be stored at 2° to 8° and be protected from light.

Mumps Virus Vaccine Live (USP 23) is a bacterially sterile freeze-dried preparation of a suitable strain of mumps virus grown in cultures of chick-embryo cells. It contains not less than the equivalent of 5×10^3 $TCID_{50}$ in each immunising dose. It may contain suitable antimicrobial agents. It should be stored at 2° to 8° and be protected from light.

Adverse Effects and Precautions

As for vaccines in general, p.1500.

Parotid swelling may occur. Unilateral nerve deafness, meningitis, and encephalitis have occurred rarely (see below for further discussion).

Mumps vaccines are not generally recommended for children below the age of 1 year in whom maternal antibodies might prevent a response.

Effects on hearing. For a report of sensorineural hearing loss following measles, mumps, and rubella vaccination, see p.1520.

Effects on the nervous system. There have been a few reports of neurological reactions including meningitis and encephalitis after vaccination with measles, mumps, and rubella vaccines. These reactions have been attributed to the mumps component. However, it has not been possible to isolate the virus from the CSF in every case and identify it as either the vaccine strain or a wild-type strain. Meningitis develops up to 35 days after immunisation, is mild, and sequelae are rare.[1,2] A study by Miller and colleagues[3] found the incidence of virus-positive post-immunisation meningitis from the Urabe strain of mumps vaccine to be approximately 1 in 11 000 immunised children with the incidence following Jeryl Lynn mumps vaccine being much lower. This result is supported by the incidence of 1 in about 4000 reported by Colville and Pugh,[4] making it less likely that this was a chance result, and much higher than the estimates of up to 1 in 1 million reported previously.[5] Subsequent research by Forsey and colleagues[6] identified the Urabe vaccine strain in CSF samples from all of 20 children with post-vaccination meningitis in the UK, and no isolates of the Jeryl Lynn strain in patients with meningitis among 80 samples tested. Thus, vaccines containing the Urabe strain, including combined measles, mumps, and rubella vaccines are no longer used in the UK and some other countries.[7] A relatively high incidence of about 1 in 1000 has also been observed after use of a measles and mumps vaccine prepared from the Leningrad-3 strain of mumps virus.[8,9]

Encephalitis has been associated with mumps vaccination less frequently than meningitis, but may be more serious.[1] The Immunization Practices Advisory Committee in the USA have reported that the incidence of encephalitis within 30 days of receiving a mumps-containing vaccine is 0.4 per one million doses.[10] This is no higher than the observed background incidence for CNS dysfunction in the general population.

In considering the above data it should be remembered that mumps is the most common cause of meningoencephalitis in children under 15 years of age in the UK and an important cause of permanent sensorineural deafness in childhood.[1] Meningitis after natural mumps infection is estimated to occur in 1 in 400 cases, an incidence that is very considerably above any reported with vaccination.

1. Anonymous. Mumps meningitis and MMR vaccination. *Lancet* 1989; **ii:** 1015–16.
2. Maguire HC, *et al.* Meningoencephalitis associated with MMR vaccine. *Commun Dis Rep* 1991; **1** (review 6): R60–R61.
3. Miller E, *et al.* Risk of aseptic meningitis after measles, mumps, and rubella vaccine in UK children. *Lancet* 1993; **341:** 979–82.
4. Colville A, Pugh S. Mumps meningitis and measles, mumps, and rubella vaccine. *Lancet* 1992; **340:** 786. Correction. *ibid.*: 986.
5. McDonald JC, *et al.* Clinical and epidemiologic features of mumps meningoencephalitis and possible vaccine-related disease. *Pediatr Infect Dis J* 1989; **8:** 751–5.
6. Forsey T, *et al.* Mumps vaccine and meningitis. *Lancet* 1992; **340:** 980.
7. Anonymous. Two MMR vaccines withdrawn. *Lancet* 1992; **340:** 722.
8. Čižman M, *et al.* Aseptic meningitis after vaccination against measles and mumps. *Pediatr Infect Dis J* 1989; **8:** 302–8.
9. Tešović G, *et al.* Aseptic meningitis after measles, mumps, and rubella vaccine. *Lancet* 1993; **341:** 1541.
10. Immunization Practices Advisory Committee. Mumps prevention. *MMWR* 1989; **38:** 388–400.

Interactions

As for vaccines in general, p.1501.

Uses and Administration

Mumps vaccines are used for active immunisation against mumps.

For primary immunisation a combined measles, mumps, and rubella vaccine (p.1519) is usually used. For discussion of immunisation schedules see under Vaccines, p.1501.

In the UK and USA a vaccine prepared from the Jeryl Lynn (B level) strain of mumps virus is available. It may be given in a dose of 0.5 mL by subcutaneous injection.

Preparations

Ph. Eur.: Mumps Vaccine (Live);
USP 23: Mumps Virus Vaccine Live.

Proprietary Preparations (details are given in Part 3)
Aust.: Mumpsvax; Pariorix†; ***Austral.:*** Mumpsvax†; Pariorix†; ***Belg.:*** Mumpsvax†; ***Canad.:*** Mumpsvax; ***Fr.:*** Imovax; ***Ger.:*** Mumpsvax; ***Irl.:*** Mumpsvax; ***Ital.:*** Mumaten; Mumpsvax; Vaxipar; ***S.Afr.:*** Mumaten; ***Spain:*** Imovax Antiparotiditis†; Vac Antiparotiditis; ***Switz.:*** Mumaten; Mumpsvax; Pariorix†; ***UK:*** Mumpsvax; ***USA:*** Mumpsvax.

Normal Immunoglobulins (1232-z)

Human Normal Immunoglobulin (Ph. Eur.) (Normal Immunoglobulin Injection; Normal Immunoglobulin (BP 1998); Immunoglobulinum Humanum Normale) is a liquid or freeze-dried preparation containing immunoglobulins, mainly immunoglobulin G (IgG) antibodies, of normal subjects. Other proteins may be present; it contains not less than 10 and not more than 18% of total protein. It is intended for intramuscular injection. It is obtained from the pooled plasma collected from at least 1000 donors who must be healthy, must not have been treated with substances of human pituitary origin, and as far as can be ascertained be free from detectable agents of infection transmissible by transfusion of blood or blood components. No antibiotic is added to the plasma used. It is prepared as a stabilised solution and passed through a bacteria-retentive filter. Multidose, but not single dose, preparations contain an antimicrobial preservative. The pH of a solution in sodium chloride 0.9% containing 1% of protein is 6.4 to 7.2. The liquid preparation should be stored, protected from light, in a sealed, colourless, glass container. The freeze-dried preparation should be stored, protected from light, under vacuum or under an inert gas.

Human Normal Immunoglobulin for Intravenous Administration (Ph. Eur.) (Normal Immunoglobulin for Intravenous Use (BP 1998); Immunoglobulinum Humanum Normale ad Usum Intravenosum) is a liquid or freeze-dried preparation containing immunoglobulins, mainly immunoglobulin G (IgG); other proteins may be present and the total protein content is not less than 3%. It contains IgG antibodies of normal subjects; the standard does not apply to products intentionally prepared to contain fragments or chemically modified IgG. It is prepared as a stabilised solution and passed through a bacteria-retentive filter. It does not contain an antimicrobial preservative. The pH of a solution in sodium chloride 0.9% containing 1% of protein is 4.0 to 7.4. Storage requirements are similar to those for Human Normal Immunoglobulin, except that the freeze-dried preparation is stored at a temperature not exceeding 25°.

Immune Globulin (USP 23) is a sterile solution of globulins that contains many antibodies normally present in human adult blood. It is prepared from pooled material (approximately equal quantities of blood, plasma, serum, or placentas) from not fewer than 1000 donors. It contains 15 to 18% of protein, of which not less than 90% is gamma globulin. It contains glycine as a stabiliser, and a suitable preservative. It contains antibodies against diphtheria, measles, and poliomyelitis. It should be stored at 2° to 8°.

Adverse Effects and Precautions

As for immunoglobulins in general, p.1500.

Antibody titres for some common pathogens can vary widely not only between products from different manufacturers, but also from lot to lot. Formulations of intravenous immunoglobulins should therefore not be regarded as equivalent.

Reviews.

1. Misbah SA, Chapel HM. Adverse effects of intravenous immunoglobulin. *Drug Safety* 1993; **9:** 254–62.

Effects on the blood. Adverse effects on the blood have occasionally been reported following intravenous administration of normal immunoglobulin to increase the platelet count in patients with idiopathic thrombocytopenic purpura. Reduced platelet adhesiveness with multiple subcutaneous haematomas occurred in one patient.[1] Thrombotic events in 4 elderly subjects (fatal in 3) suggested that a rising platelet count during normal immunoglobulin treatment may represent a risk in patients with severe atherosclerotic disease.[2] A review in Scotland of 34 patients over 60 years of age treated with normal immunoglobulin could not, however, confirm the association.[3]

Passive transfer of anti-A, anti-B, or anti-D antibodies or active immunisation by blood group substances from normal immunoglobulin preparations has been implicated in the production of haemolytic reactions including a case of haemolytic disease of the newborn.[4,5] Nicholls *et al.*[5] suggested that blood phenotyping be carried out before treatment with normal immunoglobulin is commenced.

Transient neutropenia has been observed after administration of normal immunoglobulin to patients with thrombocytopenic purpura, but the clinical significance of this effect has been disputed.[6-8]

1. Ljung R, Nilsson IM. High-dose intravenous gammaglobulin: a cautionary note. *Lancet* 1985; **i:** 467.
2. Woodruff RK, *et al.* Fatal thrombotic events during treatment of autoimmune thrombocytopenia with intravenous immunoglobulin in elderly patients. *Lancet* 1986; **ii:** 217–18.
3. Frame WD, Crawford RJ. Thrombotic events after intravenous immunoglobulin. *Lancet* 1986; **ii:** 468.
4. Potter M, *et al.* ABO alloimmunisation after intravenous immunoglobulin infusion. *Lancet* 1988; **i:** 932–3.
5. Nicholls MD, *et al.* Haemolysis induced by intravenously-administered immunoglobulin. *Med J Aust* 1989; **150:** 404–6.
6. Majer RV, Green PJ. Neutropenia caused by intravenous immunoglobulin. *Br Med J* 1988; **296:** 1262.
7. Veys PA, *et al.* Neutropenia following intravenous immunoglobulin. *Br Med J* 1988; **296:** 1800.
8. Ben-Chetrit E, Putterman C. Transient neutropenia induced by intravenous immune globulin. *N Engl J Med* 1992; **326:** 270–1.

Effects on the kidneys. Barton *et al.*[1] reported the development of acute renal failure after intravenous administration of normal immunoglobulin to a patient who had demonstrable serum rheumatoid factor associated with lymphoma. They recommended that normal immunoglobulin should not be given to such patients. Schifferli *et al.*[2] noted a symptomless, transient rise in plasma-creatinine concentrations in 6 patients with nephrotic syndrome after administration of intravenous normal immunoglobulin. A similar rise in plasma creatinine was observed in two other patients with pre-existing renal impairment but no nephrotic syndrome. More recently,[3] an elderly patient with lymphoproliferative disorder and idiopathic thrombocytopenic purpura received normal immunoglobulin and developed acute renal failure within 48 hours, with subsequently fatal heart failure and pulmonary oedema.

1. Barton JC, *et al.* Acute cryoglobulinemic renal failure after intravenous infusion of gamma globulin. *Am J Med* 1987; **82:** 624–9.
2. Schifferli J, *et al.* High-dose intravenous IgG treatment and renal function. *Lancet* 1991; **337:** 457–8.
3. Winward DB, Brophy MT. Acute renal failure after administration of intravenous immunoglobulin: review of the literature and case report. *Pharmacotherapy* 1995; **15:** 765–72.

Effects on the nervous system. Reports of aseptic meningitis after intravenous administration of normal immunoglobulin.[1-4]

Migraine was associated with intravenous immunoglobulin therapy in a patient on two occasions.[5] Migraine did not recur after prophylaxis with propranolol was instituted.

1. Kato E, *et al.* Administration of immune globulin associated with aseptic meningitis. *JAMA* 1988; **259:** 3269–71.
2. Casteels-Van Daele M, *et al.* Intravenous immune globulin and acute aseptic meningitis. *N Engl J Med* 1990; **323:** 614–15.
3. Sekul EA, *et al.* Aseptic meningitis associated with high-dose intravenous immunoglobulin therapy: frequency and risk factors. *Ann Intern Med* 1994; **121:** 259–62.
4. Picton P, Chisholm M. Aseptic meningitis associated with high dose immunoglobulin: case report. *Br Med J* 1997; **315:** 1203–4.
5. Constantinescu CS, *et al.* Recurrent migraine and intravenous immune globulin therapy. *N Engl J Med* 1993; **329:** 583–4.

Effects on the skin. A report[1] of 3 women experiencing diffuse alopecia within 1 to 4 weeks of treatment with intravenous normal immunoglobulin. There have been reports[2,3] of severe and extensive eczema in elderly patients up to 3 weeks after receiving normal immunoglobulin intravenously. There has also been a report of cutaneous vasculitic rash on the face of a woman receiving intravenous normal immunoglobulin.[4]

For mention of a patient with AIDS who developed erythema characteristic of fifth disease following intravenous normal immunoglobulin, see Infection, below.

1. Chan-Lam D, *et al.* Alopecia after immunoglobulin infusion. *Lancet* 1987; **i:** 1436.
2. Barucha C, McMillan JC. Eczema after intravenous infusion of immunoglobulin. *Br Med J* 1987; **295:** 1141.
3. Whittam LR, *et al.* Eczematous reactions to human immune globulin. *Br J Dermatol* 1997; **137:** 481–2.
4. Howse M, *et al.* Facial vasculitic rash associated with intravenous immunoglobulin. *Br Med J* 1998; **317:** 1291.

Hypersensitivity. Hypersensitivity reactions may occasionally occur after intramuscular or intravenous administration of normal immunoglobulins particularly in hypogammaglobulinaemic or agammaglobulinaemic patients. Both immediate and late[1] reactions have occurred.

The IgA content of normal immunoglobulins can result in the development of IgE and IgG anti-IgA antibodies in immunodeficient patients with IgA deficiency. Burks *et al.*[2] have suggested that the IgE anti-IgA antibodies are responsible for anaphylaxis although others have disagreed.[3] The two patients reported by Burks *et al.* who had reactions to conventional normal immunoglobulin preparations tolerated preparations with a low content of IgA.[2] Some manufacturers of normal immunoglobulin preparations recommend that they not be used in patients with selective IgA deficiencies who have known antibody against IgA.

The IgE content of some preparations has also been suggested as causing hypersensitivity reactions[4] although this has been disputed.[5] Complement-activating IgG aggregates may also be involved although the anticomplementary activity of the products does not appear to be related to the incidence of side-effects.[5]

1. Hachimi-Idrissi S, *et al.* Type III allergic reaction after infusion of immunoglobulins. *Lancet* 1990; **336:** 55.
2. Burks AW, *et al.* Anaphylactic reactions after gamma globulin administration in patients with hypogammaglobulinemia. *N Engl J Med* 1986; **314:** 560–4.
3. Hammarström L, Smith CIE. Anaphylaxis after administration of gamma globulin for hypogammaglobulinemia. *N Engl J Med* 1986; **315:** 519.
4. Tovo P-A, *et al.* IgE content of commercial intravenous IgG preparations. *Lancet* 1984; **i:** 458.
5. Newland AC, *et al.* IgE in intravenous IgG. *Lancet* 1984; **i:** 1406–7.

Infection. An association between administration of certain intravenous immunoglobulin preparations and hepatitis C infections has led to changes in manufacturing procedures and withdrawal of the affected products from the market.[1-3]

In addition, there has been a report[4] of a patient with AIDS who developed fifth disease (erythema infectiosum) following intravenous normal immunoglobulin treatment for infection with parvovirus.

1. Quinti I, *et al.* Intravenous gammaglobulin may still infect patients. *Br Med J* 1994; **308:** 856.
2. Bader J-M. HCV and Gammagard in France. *Lancet* 1994; **343:** 1628. Corrections. *ibid.*; **344:** 201 and 206.
3. Anonymous. Outbreak of hepatitis C associated with intravenous immunoglobulin administration—United States, October 1993–June 1994. *JAMA* 1994; **272:** 424–5.
4. French AL, *et al.* Fifth disease after immunoglobulin administration in an AIDS patient with parvovirus-induced red cell aplasia. *Am J Med* 1996; **101:** 108–9.

Interactions

Administration of normal immunoglobulin may interfere with the immune response to live viral vaccines. Such vaccines should therefore be given at least 3 weeks before or 3 months after normal immunoglobulins. This does not apply to yellow fever vaccine for immunoglobulins prepared in the UK, nor for booster doses of oral poliomyelitis vaccines. Where such an interval is impractical for immunisation preceding foreign travel it may have to be ignored.

For a study indicating that normal immunoglobulin has no effect on the antibody response to oral poliomyelitis vaccine, see p.1529.

Uses and Administration

Normal immunoglobulin is available as two distinct preparations and formulations. One type of injection generally containing 16% of protein is used for passive immunisation, and sometimes also for primary antibody deficiencies, and should only be given intramuscularly; Human Normal Immunoglobulin (Ph. Eur.) and Immune Globulin (USP 23) are intended for intramuscular use only. The second type of preparation is formulated for intravenous administration (Human Normal Immunoglobulin for Intravenous Administration (Ph. Eur.)) and is used in disorders such as primary antibody deficiencies and idiopathic thrombocytopenic purpura; solutions generally contain about 3 to 6% of protein, although some may contain up to 12%. Doses of normal immunoglobulin often appear confusing, being expressed variously in terms of weight (protein or immunoglobulin G content) or in terms of volume to be administered; the two do not always appear to correspond. It should be remembered that there may be differences between intravenous preparations of normal immunoglobulin including differing IgA content and IgG subclass distribution.

Normal immunoglobulin, being derived from the pooled plasma of blood donors, contains antibodies to bacteria and viruses currently prevalent in the general population; in the UK, and also in some other countries, typical antibodies present include those against hepatitis A, measles, mumps, rubella, and varicella. Normal immunoglobulin, therefore, may be used to provide passive immunisation against such diseases.

For the pre-exposure prophylaxis against **hepatitis A** in travellers going to endemic areas doses recommended in the UK for intramuscular injection are: for short-term exposure of up to 2 months, 125 mg for children under 10 years of age and 250 mg for older children and adults; for longer-term exposure, 250 mg for children under 10 years of age and 500 mg for older children and adults. Alternative doses, expressed in terms of volume administered, have been 0.02 to 0.04 mL per kg body-weight for short-term exposure in both adults and children and 0.06 to 0.12 mL per kg for longer-term exposure. Hepatitis A vaccine (p.1512) may be preferred in adults visiting endemic countries frequently or staying for over 3 months or hepatitis A immunoglobulin (p.1512) for shorter or less frequent journeys.

Normal immunoglobulin may also be used to control outbreaks of hepatitis A, the recommended dose for close contacts being 250 mg in those under 10 years of age and 500 mg in older children and adults.

Normal immunoglobulin may be used to prevent or possibly modify an attack of **measles** in children and adults at special risk (such as those who are immunocompromised) but should be given as soon as possible after contact with measles. In the UK recommended doses, administered intramuscularly, for the prevention of an attack are 250 mg for those under 1 year of age, 500 mg for those aged 1 to 2 years, and 750 mg for those aged 3 years and over; to modify an attack, recommended doses are 100 mg for those under 1 year of age and 250 mg for older children. Alternatively, doses (expressed in terms of volume) of 0.2 mL per kg have been suggested to prevent an attack and 0.04 mL per kg to modify an attack. The dose should be repeated after 3 weeks in the case of continued exposure to measles.

Normal immunoglobulin may reduce the likelihood of a clinical attack in pregnant women exposed to **rubella** but should be given as soon as possible after exposure. The recommended dose is 750 mg by intramuscular injection. A dose of 20 mL has also been suggested.

Normal immunoglobulin may be used in the management of patients with **primary antibody deficiencies** such as congenital agammaglobulinaemia, hypogammaglobulinaemia, or **immunocompromised patients** including those with immunodeficiency syndromes; the immunoglobulin is given to provide protection against infectious diseases that such patients may suffer. The intramuscular preparation may be used but the intravenous route is usually preferred since administration is less painful for the doses required. For intravenous infusion, the dose, expressed in terms of weight (protein or immunoglobulin G content), is usually 400 to 800 mg per kg body-weight initially, then 200 mg per kg every 3 weeks adjusted as necessary according to trough-immunoglobulin concentrations; the maintenance dose is usually 200 to 800 mg per kg per month. In patients with secondary immunodeficiency syndromes doses of 200 to 400 mg per kg every 3 to 4 weeks have been recommended. Other dosage regimens have been used. When infused intravenously, normal immunoglobulin should always be given very carefully and slowly with gradual increases in the rate of administration. For the intramuscular type of preparation the usual initial dose, expressed in terms of volume, is 1.3 to 1.8 mL per kg in divided doses over 48 hours; the maximum recommended total initial dose is 60 mL. For maintenance, doses of 0.6 to 0.65 mL per kg (maximum 30 mL) may be given every 3 to 4 weeks.

For prophylaxis of infection after **bone marrow transplantation**, normal immunoglobulin is given intravenously in a dose of 500 mg per kg weekly, adjusted according to response.

Intravenous infusion of normal immunoglobulin is also employed to raise the platelet count in patients with **idiopathic thrombocytopenic purpura**. Doses of 400 mg per kg are given daily for 2 to 5 consecutive days. Alternatively doses of 800 to 1000 mg per kg may be given on day 1 and repeated on day 3 if necessary. Further doses may be given as necessary.

For **Kawasaki disease**, normal immunoglobulin is given intravenously in a dose of 1.6 to 2 g per kg in divided doses over 2 to 5 days, or 2 g per kg given as a single dose. Similar doses of intravenous normal immunoglobulin have been tried in a range of disorders believed to have an auto-immune origin. The precise mode of action of normal immunoglobulin in such disorders is unknown.

Normal immunoglobulin is also given intramuscularly as an adjunct to plasma and blood in the treatment of burns.

Reviews and discussions of the actions and uses of intravenous normal immunoglobulins.

1. National Institutes of Health Consensus Conference. Intravenous immunoglobulin: prevention and treatment of disease. *JAMA* 1990; **264:** 3189–93.
2. Anonymous. Consensus on IVIG. *Lancet* 1990; **336:** 470–2.
3. ASHP Commission on Therapeutics. ASHP therapeutic guidelines for intravenous immune globulin. *Clin Pharm* 1992; **11:** 117–36.
4. Dwyer JM. Manipulating the immune system with immune globulin. *N Engl J Med* 1992; **326:** 107–16.
5. Pirofsky B, Kinzey DM. Intravenous immune globulins: a review of their uses in selected immunodeficiency and autoimmune diseases. *Drugs* 1992; **43:** 6–14.
6. Keller T, *et al.* Indications for the use of intravenous immunoglobulin: recommendations of the Australasian Society of Blood Transfusion consensus symposium. *Med J Aust* 1993; **159:** 204–6.
7. Blasczyk R, *et al.* Soluble CD4, CD8, and HLA molecules in commercial immunoglobulin preparations. *Lancet* 1993; **341:** 789–90.
8. Ratko TA, *et al.* Recommendations for off-label use of intravenously administered immunoglobulin preparations. *JAMA* 1995; **273:** 1865–70.
9. Stiehm ER. Appropriate therapeutic use of immunoglobulin. *Transfus Med Rev* 1996; **10:** 203–21.

Administration. In order to overcome some of the problems associated with ensuring regular venous access necessary for long term intravenous immunoglobulin therapy, administration by rapid subcutaneous infusion has been evaluated. Subcutaneous infusion of approximately 16% preservative-free solutions or solutions not containing a mercurial preservative were administered to adults[1] through 2 pumps at a rate of 17 to 20 mL per hour at each pump and to children[2,3] at a rate of 10 to 20 mL per hour. Adequate immunoglobulin concentrations were achieved and this route of administration was generally well tolerated. A subsequent review[4] of subcutaneous infusion therapy in 165 patients receiving doses of between 80 and 800 mg per kg body-weight per month in divided doses supported these results.

Oral administration of normal immunoglobulins has been proposed to reduce the incidence and severity of gastro-intestinal infections,[5,6] particularly in patients with defective immune systems including neonates. Although the predominant immunoglobulin secreted into the gastro-intestinal tract in subjects with a normal immune system is IgA, a species not present in large quantities in commercial normal immunoglobulins, beneficial responses, especially in viral infections,[7] have been reported following oral administration. Preparations of immunoglobulin A are available in some countries and have been tried, mainly in bacterial gastro-intestinal infections.[8,9]

1. Gardulf A, *et al.* Home treatment of hypogammaglobulinaemia with subcutaneous gammaglobulin by rapid infusion. *Lancet* 1991; **338:** 162–6.
2. Thomas MJ, *et al.* Rapid subcutaneous immunoglobulin infusions in children. *Lancet* 1993; **342:** 1432–3.
3. Gaspar J, *et al.* Immunoglobulin replacement treatment by rapid subcutaneous infusion. *Arch Dis Child* 1998; **79:** 48–51.
4. Gardulf A, *et al.* Subcutaneous immunoglobulin replacement in patients with primary antibody deficiencies: safety and costs. *Lancet* 1995; **345:** 365–9.
5. Dattani SJ, Connelly JF. Oral immunoglobulins for gastroenteritis. *Ann Pharmacother* 1996; **30:** 1323–4.
6. Reilly RM, *et al.* Oral delivery of antibodies: future pharmacokinetic trends. *Clin Pharmacokinet* 1997; **32:** 313–23.
7. Guarino A, *et al.* Oral immunoglobulins for treatment of acute rotaviral gastroenteritis. *Pediatrics* 1994; **93:** 12–16.
8. Tjellström B, *et al.* Oral immunoglobulin A supplement in treatment of Clostridium difficile enteritis. *Lancet* 1993; **341:** 701–2.
9. Hammarström V, *et al.* Oral immunoglobulin treatment in Campylobacter jejuni enteritis. *Lancet* 1993; **341:** 1036.

Blood disorders. Intravenous normal immunoglobulins are used in the treatment of symptomatic severe acute and chronic idiopathic thrombocytopenic purpura (p.1023). Other blood disorders in which normal immunoglobulins have been tried include agranulocytosis[1] and haemolytic disease of the newborn (p.1503), aplastic and haemolytic anaemias (p.701), red-cell aplasia caused by parvovirus B19 infections (below), thrombotic thrombocytopenic purpura and haemolytic-uraemic syndrome (see Thrombotic Microangiopathies p.726), and thrombocytopenia with a variety of causes.[2-8]

1. Fasth A. Immunoglobulin for neonatal agranulocytosis. *Arch Dis Child* 1986; **61:** 86–7.
2. Hoffman DM, *et al.* Human immunodeficiency virus-associated thrombocytopenia. *DICP Ann Pharmacother* 1989; **23:** 157–160.
3. Landonio G, *et al.* HIV-related severe thrombocytopenia in intravenous drug users: prevalence, response to therapy in a medium-term follow-up, and pathogenic evaluation. *AIDS* 1990; **4:** 29–34.
4. Goulder P, *et al.* Intravenous immunoglobulin in virus associated haemophagocytic syndrome. *Arch Dis Child* 1990; **65:** 1275–7.
5. Larner AJ, *et al.* Life threatening thrombocytopenia in sarcoidosis: response to vincristine, human immunoglobulin, and corticosteroids. *Br Med J* 1990; **300:** 317–19.
6. Frame JN, *et al.* Correction of severe heparin-associated thrombocytopenia with intravenous immunoglobulin. *Ann Intern Med* 1989; **111:** 946–7.
7. Howrie DL, *et al.* Use of iv immune globulin for treatment of phenytoin-induced thrombocytopenia. *Clin Pharm* 1989; **8:** 734–7.
8. Ray JB, *et al.* Intravenous immune globulin for the treatment of presumed quinidine-induced thrombocytopenia. *DICP Ann Pharmacother* 1990; **24:** 693–5.

Epilepsy. Normal immunoglobulins have sometimes been of benefit[1,2] in the treatment of children with epilepsy unresponsive to conventional therapy (p.335). More recently, 13 of 15 children with intractable Lennox-Gastaut syndrome or West's syndrome[3] responded to high doses of intravenous immunoglobulins.

1. Ariizumi M, *et al.* High dose gammaglobulin for intractable childhood epilepsy. *Lancet* 1983; **ii:** 162–3.
2. Sandstedt P, *et al.* Intravenous gammaglobulin for post-encephalitic epilepsy. *Lancet* 1984; **ii:** 1154–5.
3. van Engelen BGH, *et al.* High-dose intravenous immunoglobulin treatment in cryptogenic West and Lennox-Gastaut syndrome: an add-on study. *Eur J Pediatr* 1994; **153:** 762–9.

Hypogammaglobulinaemia. See under Primary Antibody Deficiency, below.

Immunocompromised patients. Immunodeficiency states may arise from primary disorders of the immune system, or, more commonly, they are secondary to immunosuppressive therapy, HIV infection, or haematological malignancies. Premature neonates may have deficits in their immune systems due to their immaturity; placental transfer of maternal antibodies usually occurs after about 32 weeks of gestation. Such immunodeficient patients and neonates may be deficient in gammaglobulins which increases their susceptibility to infections, and they could potentially benefit from the administration of normal immunoglobulins. For information on the use of immunoglobulins in specific conditions, see the following sections and under Neonatal Sepsis, below.

BONE-MARROW TRANSPLANTATION. In patients undergoing allogeneic bone-marrow transplantation (p.498), intravenous normal immunoglobulin has decreased the incidence of both bacterial infections[1] and of symptomatic cytomegalovirus infection, particularly interstitial pneumonia.[1,2] Overall survival[1] or overall incidence of cytomegalovirus infection[1,2] was not decreased. A combination of normal immunoglobulin and ganciclovir appears to improve the outcome of cytomegalovirus pneumonia subsequent to bone-marrow transplantation.[3] No patients treated with normal immunoglobulin alone survived. Cytomegalovirus immunoglobulins (p.1507) may be more appropriate for the specific prophylaxis and treatment of cytomegalovirus infections.

Intravenous immunoglobulin therapy has been found to be ineffective in preventing infections in patients receiving autologous bone-marrow transplants[4] and may have contributed to an increased incidence of fatal hepatic veno-occlusive disease.

Normal immunoglobulin administration has been associated with a reduced frequency of acute graft-versus-host disease, possibly as a result of a direct immunomodulatory effect.

1. Sullivan KM, *et al.* Immunomodulatory and antimicrobial efficacy of intravenous immunoglobulin in bone marrow transplantation. *N Engl J Med* 1990; **323:** 705–12.
2. Winston DJ, *et al.* Intravenous immune globulin for prevention of cytomegalovirus infection and interstitial pneumonia after bone marrow transplantation. *Ann Intern Med* 1987; **106:** 12–18.
3. Emanuel D, *et al.* Cytomegalovirus pneumonia after bone marrow transplantation successfully treated with the combination of ganciclovir and high-dose intravenous immune globulin. *Ann Intern Med* 1988; **109:** 777–82.
4. Wolff SN, *et al.* High-dose weekly intravenous immunoglobulin to prevent infections in patients undergoing autologous bone marrow transplantation or severe myelosuppressive therapy: a study of the American Bone Marrow Transplant Group. *Ann Intern Med* 1993; **118:** 937–42.

HIV INFECTION AND AIDS. Immunoglobulin levels are typically raised in patients with AIDS, but hypogammaglobulinaemia has been observed and, even in the presence of hypergammaglobulinaemia, patients behave as though they were hypogammaglobulinaemic. Normal immunoglobulin has therefore been administered to some symptomatic HIV-positive children. A significant improvement was noted[1] in 8 children given intravenous normal immunoglobulin, in terms of weight gain, number of infectious episodes, and diarrhoea. HIV core antigen was detected in 4 children before treatment. All became core-antigen negative after treatment was commenced although the effect was only maintained in 3. The validity of these results was questioned.[2] Larger studies have reported improvements in the rate of decline of the CD4+ T lymphocyte count[3] and the incidence of serious bacterial infections[4,5] but could not demonstrate improved survival. However, a further controlled study[6] in adult patients with AIDS given intravenous normal immunoglobulin demonstrated both an increase in the time free from bacterial or viral infection and also an improvement in survival rate after 31 weeks, and a small study in 24 patients[7] has reported improved survival at up to 12 months in patients who received normal immunoglobulin.

1. Hague RA, *et al.* Intravenous immunoglobulin in HIV infection: evidence for the efficacy of treatment. *Arch Dis Child* 1989; **64:** 1146–50.
2. Gibb D, Levin M. Intravenous immunoglobulin in HIV infection. *Arch Dis Child* 1990; **65:** 247–8.
3. Mofenson LM, *et al.* Effect of intravenous immunoglobulin (IVIG) on CD4+ lymphocyte decline in HIV-infected children in a clinical trial of IVIG infection prophylaxis. *J Acquir Immune Defic Syndr* 1993; **6:** 1103–13.
4. The National Institute of Child Health and Human Development Intravenous Immunoglobulin Study Group. Intravenous immune globulin for the prevention of bacterial infections in children with symptomatic human immunodeficiency virus infection. *N Engl J Med* 1991; **325:** 73–80.
5. Spector SA, *et al.* A controlled trial of intravenous immune globulin for the prevention of serious bacterial infections in children receiving zidovudine for advanced human immunodeficiency virus infection. *N Engl J Med* 1994; **331:** 1181–7.
6. Kiehl MG, *et al.* A controlled trial of intravenous immune globulin for the prevention of serious infections in adults with advanced human immunodeficiency virus infection. *Arch Intern Med* 1996; **156:** 2545–50.
7. Saint-Marc T, *et al.* Beneficial effects of intravenous immunoglobulins in AIDS. *Lancet* 1992; **340:** 1347.

MALIGNANCIES. Hypogammaglobulinaemia and the effects of treatment may increase the susceptibility to infection of patients with *chronic lymphocytic leukaemia*.[1] In a study of 81 patients with chronic lymphocytic leukaemia considered to be at an increased risk of infection, intravenous normal immunoglobulin 400 mg per kg body-weight given every 3 weeks for one year reduced the incidence of bacterial infection compared with saline placebo. The incidence of viral and fungal infections was not affected. A study in 34 patients[2] suggested that a dose of normal immunoglobulin 250 mg per kg per month was adequate for routine prophylaxis in most patients. Beneficial effects on infection rates have been reported in patients with *multiple myeloma* receiving normal immunoglobulins.[3]

1. Cooperative Group for the Study of Immunoglobulin in Chronic Lymphocytic Leukemia. Intravenous immunoglobulin for *N Engl J Med* 1988; **319:** 902–7.
2. Chapel H, *et al.* Immunoglobulin replacement in patients with chronic lymphocytic leukaemia: a comparison of two dose regimes. *Br J Haematol* 1994; **88:** 209–12.
3. Chapel HM, *et al.* Randomised trial of intravenous immunoglobulin as prophylaxis against infection in plateau-phase multiple myeloma. *Lancet* 1994; **343:** 1059–63.

PRIMARY ANTIBODY DEFICIENCY. There are three major forms of primary antibody deficiency: X-linked agammaglobulinaemia (XLA, Bruton's agammaglobulinaemia), common variable immunodeficiency (CVID) which includes IgG subclass and specific antibody deficiencies, and selective IgA deficiency. The disease is characterised by a wide range of infective complications as well as auto-immune disorders. Management is by replacement therapy with normal immunoglobulin accompanied by appropriate antimicrobial therapy for breakthrough infections. Immunisation against infection is of no value and is contra-indicated for live viral vaccines.

Normal immunoglobulin was traditionally administered by the intramuscular route. However, the maximum dose that can be reasonably given by this route is 25 mg per kg bodyweight weekly, and it is therefore only satisfactory for patients with mild disease.[1] The introduction of intravenous preparations of normal immunoglobulin allows high doses to be given to those with severe disease. This route should therefore be used for all patients with XLA and for patients with CVID who have more than mild disease. The use of intravenous normal immunoglobulin in IgG subclass deficiency, with or without IgA deficiency, or in specific antibody deficiency is successful, though less well established. The dose and frequency of administration of intravenous normal immunoglobulin is variable and should be adjusted to prevent breakthrough infection. Most patients require 200 to 600 mg per kg every 2 or 3 weeks to maintain optimum protection.[1] Surgical procedures should be covered with additional normal immunoglobulin and appropriate prophylactic antibacterials. Home treatment with intravenous normal immunoglobulin has been used successfully in several countries in both adults and children.[1-5] Adverse reactions have been few and generally mild.[1,3,4] They are most likely to occur during the first infusion and during intercurrent illness, and may be precipitated by a high infusion rate.[5] Long-term treatment of children with antibody deficiencies with intravenous normal immunoglobulin has been shown to lead to normal growth and similar rates of infection to those found in non-immunodeficient children.[6]

Some patients have been successfully treated with subcutaneous infusion of normal immunoglobulin (see Administration, above) and the intraventricular route may be of benefit to some patients with echovirus encephalitis.[1,7]

In a pilot study, normal immunoglobulin given subcutaneously to 10 patients with selective IgA deficiency was safe and reduced the rate of respiratory-tract infections.[8]

1. Spickett GP, *et al.* Primary antibody deficiency in adults. *Lancet* 1991; **337:** 281–4.
2. Ochs HD, *et al.* Intravenous immunoglobulin home treatment for patients with primary immunodeficiency diseases. *Lancet* 1986; **i:** 610–11.
3. Ryan A, *et al.* Home intravenous immunoglobulin therapy for patients with primary hypogammaglobulinaemia. *Lancet* 1988; **ii:** 793.
4. Kobayashi RH, *et al.* Home self-administration of intravenous immunoglobulin therapy in children. *Pediatrics* 1990; **85:** 705–9.
5. Chapel HM. Consensus on diagnosis and management of primary antibody deficiencies. *Br Med J* 1994; **308:** 581–5.
6. Skull S, Kemp A. Treatment of hypogammaglobulinaemia with intravenous immunoglobulin, 1973-93. *Arch Dis Child* 1996; **74:** 527–30.
7. Erlendsson K, *et al.* Successful reversal of echovirus encephalitis in x-linked hypogammaglobulinemia by intraventricular administration of immunoglobulin. *N Engl J Med* 1985; **312:** 351–30.
8. Gustafson R, *et al.* Prophylactic therapy for selective IgA deficiency. *Lancet* 1997; **350:** 865.

Inflammatory bowel diseases. High-dose intravenous normal immunoglobulin may be beneficial[1,2] in inducing remission of Crohn's disease and ulcerative colitis and has been tried[3] in antibiotic-associated colitis.

1. Rohr G, *et al.* Treatment of Crohn's disease and ulcerative colitis with 7S-immunoglobulin. *Lancet* 1987; **i:** 170.
2. Knoflach P, *et al.* Crohn disease and intravenous immunoglobulin G. *Ann Intern Med* 1990; **112:** 385–6.
3. Leung DYM, *et al.* Treatment with intravenously administered gamma globulin of chronic relapsing colitis induced by Clostridium difficile toxin. *J Pediatr* 1991; **118:** 633–7.

Kawasaki disease. Kawasaki disease, also known as mucocutaneous lymph node syndrome of childhood, occurs mainly in children under 5 years of age. It is epidemic and endemic worldwide but is a particular problem in Japan. Kawasaki disease presents with high fever which persists for at least 5 days and may be followed by bilateral conjunctival injection, changes in the oropharyngeal mucosa, signs of vasculitis in the extremities, rash, and cervical lymphadenopathy. The major complications of Kawasaki disease are cardiac effects including coronary artery aneurysm, aortic or mitral incompetence, myocarditis, and pericarditis with effusion. The cause of the disease is unknown, although an infective aetiology has been suggested. Early diagnosis, expert cardiac assessment, and immediate treatment are essential for improved outcome.

Initial treatment aims to reduce inflammation, particularly in the coronary arterial wall and myocardium, and therefore prevent the development of cardiac complications.[1] Long-term treatment is given as necessary to prevent coronary thrombosis.[2]

Initial treatment is with aspirin and normal immunoglobulin. Newburger *et al.* demonstrated a decreased incidence of coronary-artery abnormalities after such a combination as compared with aspirin alone.[3] Normal immunoglobulin has generally been given by intravenous infusion in divided doses over 2 to 5 days, although administration as a single dose is recommended as an alternative,[1,4] and has been associated with a lower incidence of coronary abnormalities after 30 days than multiple-dose treatment.[5] The optimum dosage and duration of treatment with aspirin is not yet established, but the usual practice is to use an anti-inflammatory regimen until the fever has settled and then to convert to an antithrombotic regimen. Some recommend an anti-inflammatory regimen until the fourteenth day of illness.[1] A few patients fail to respond to treatment with aspirin and normal immunoglobulin. A small study[6] suggested that re-treatment with normal immunoglobulin may be considered for those with persistent or recurring fever. Oxpentifylline, which may moderate the inflammatory response, is being investigated as adjunctive therapy to aspirin and normal immunoglobulin.[7] Corticosteroids are not routinely used in Kawasaki disease as there is a risk that they may exacerbate coronary artery aneurysms.

Long-term management. Aspirin should be continued for 6 to 8 weeks after the onset of illness and then discontinued if there are no coronary abnormalities. Some practitioners use aspirin and dipyridamole as antithrombotic therapy although it is not known whether this combination provides benefit over aspirin alone.[2] Dipyridamole may be used as an alternative antithrombotic agent for patients who cannot tolerate aspirin. Aspirin is usually continued for at least one year if coronary abnormalities are present and should be continued indefinitely if coronary aneurysms persist. Anticoagulation with warfarin or heparin in addition to aspirin may be necessary in some patients such as those with giant or multiple aneurysms.

1. Dajani AS, *et al.* Diagnosis and therapy of Kawasaki disease in children. *Circulation* 1993; **87:** 1776–80.
2. Dajani AS, *et al.* Guidelines for long-term management of patients with Kawasaki disease: report from the Committee on Rheumatic Fever, Endocarditis, and Kawasaki Disease, Council on Cardiovascular Disease in the Young, American Heart Association. *Circulation* 1994; **89:** 916–22.
3. Newburger JW, *et al.* The treatment of Kawasaki syndrome with intravenous gamma globulin. *N Engl J Med* 1986; **315:** 341–7.
4. Newburger JW, *et al.* A single intravenous infusion of gamma globulin as compared with four infusions in the treatment of acute Kawasaki syndrome. *N Engl J Med* 1991; **324:** 1633–9.
5. Durongpisitkul K, *et al.* The prevention of coronary artery aneurysm in Kawasaki disease: a meta-analysis on the efficacy of aspirin and immunoglobulin treatment. *Pediatrics* 1995; **96:** 1057–61.
6. Sundel RP, *et al.* Gamma globulin re-treatment in Kawasaki disease. *J Pediatr* 1993; **123:** 657–9.
7. Matsubara T, *et al.* Treatment of Kawasaki disease with pentoxifylline, an inhibitor of TNF-α transcription. *Clin Res* 1994; **42:** 1A.

Kidney disorders. Treatment with normal immunoglobulin has been of benefit in some patients with haemolytic-uraemic syndrome (see under Blood Disorders, above) and with lupus nephritis (see under Musculoskeletal and Nerve Disorders, below). For mention of the use of normal immunoglobulin in IgA nephropathy see Glomerular Kidney Disease, p.1021.

Musculoskeletal and nerve disorders. High-dose intravenous normal immunoglobulin has been tried with some benefit in various disorders of the nerves, muscles, joints, and connective tissues which may have an auto-immune basis. These include multiple sclerosis,[1] chronic inflammatory demyelinating polyneuropathy,[2] polymyositis and dermatomyositis,[3-7] myasthenia gravis,[8] stiff-man syndrome,[9-11] chronic systemic juvenile arthritis,[12-14] systemic lupus erythematosus[15] including lupus nephritis,[16] Guillain-Barré syndrome (see below), and motor neurone disease (see also below).

1. Fazekas F, *et al.* Randomised placebo-controlled trial of monthly intravenous immunoglobulin therapy in relapsing-remitting multiple sclerosis. *Lancet* 1997; **349:** 589–93.
2. van Doorn PA, *et al.* High-dose intravenous immunoglobulin treatment in chronic inflammatory demyelinating polyneuropathy: a double-blind, placebo-controlled, crossover study. *Neurology* 1990; **40:** 209–12.
3. Cherin P, *et al.* Efficacy of intravenous gammaglobulin therapy in chronic refractory polymyositis and dermatomyositis: an open study with 20 adult patients. *Am J Med* 1991; **91:** 162–8.
4. Lang BA, *et al.* Treatment of dermatomyositis with intravenous gammaglobulin. *Am J Med* 1991; **91:** 169–72.
5. Dalakas MC, *et al.* A controlled trial of high-dose intravenous immune globulin infusions as treatment for dermatomyositis. *N Engl J Med* 1993; **329:** 1993–2000.
6. Brownell AKW. Intravenous immune globulin for dermatomyositis. *N Engl J Med* 1994; **330:** 1392.
7. Collet E, *et al.* Juvenile dermatomyositis: treatment with intravenous gammaglobulin. *Br J Dermatol* 1994; **130:** 231–4.
8. Gajdos P. Intravenous immune globulin in myasthenia gravis. *Clin Exp Immunol* 1994; **97** (suppl 1): 49–51.
9. Karlson EW, *et al.* Treatment of stiff-man syndrome with intravenous immune globulin. *Arthritis Rheum* 1994; **37:** 915–18.
10. Amato AA, *et al.* Treatment of stiff-man syndrome with intravenous immunoglobulin. *Neurology* 1994; **44:** 1652–4.
11. Barker RA, Marsden CD. Successful treatment of stiff man syndrome with intravenous immunoglobulin. *J Neurol Neurosurg Psychiatry* 1997; **62:** 426–7.
12. Groothoff JW, van Leeuwen EF. High dose intravenous gammaglobulin in chronic systemic juvenile arthritis. *Br Med J* 1988; **296:** 1362–3.
13. Giannini EH, *et al.* Intravenous immunoglobulin in the treatment of polyarticular juvenile rheumatoid arthritis: a phase I/II study. *J Rheumatol* 1996; **23:** 919–24.
14. Uziel Y, *et al.* Intravenous immunoglobulin therapy in systemic onset juvenile rheumatoid arthritis: a followup study. *J Rheumatol* 1996; **23:** 910–18.
15. Francioni C, *et al.* Long term IV Ig treatment in systemic lupus erythematosus. *Clin Exp Rheumatol* 1994; **12:** 163–8.
16. Lin C-Y, *et al.* Improvement of histological and immunological change in steroid and immunosuppressive drug-resistant lupus nephritis by high-dose intravenous gamma globulin. *Nephron* 1989; **53:** 303–10.

GUILLAIN-BARRÉ SYNDROME. Guillain-Barré syndrome (acute idiopathic inflammatory polyneuropathy; acute idiopathic demyelinating neuropathy; acute infectious polyneuropathy) may follow an infection or, more rarely, immunisation, but very often no predisposing factor can be identified.[1-4] There may be an association with infection with *Campylobacter jejuni*.[5] Reversible demyelination results in pain and progressive flaccid paralysis. An autoimmune aetiology seems likely.[6] Severely affected patients require cardiovascular monitoring and respiratory support if respiratory muscles are affected or autonomic instability is present. Corticosteroids have been given but are generally considered to be of little value (see Polyneuropathies, p.1028).[6-9] Plasma exchange (see p.726) is effective if given early,[1,7,10,11] but is not universally available and is not suitable for all patients.[7] Administration of immunoglobulins has been shown to be at least as effective as plasma exchange in a study of 150 patients[12] although the response to plasma exchange in this study was lower than would be expected.[1,7] A more recent study[13] has confirmed the equivalent efficacy of plasma exchange and immunoglobulins and has also demonstrated no advantage from combining the two forms of treatment. Deterioration has also been noted in some patients following immunoglobulin therapy[14,15] and further evaluation of the use of immunoglobulins is awaited.

1. Howard RS. Neurology. *Br Med J* 1994; **309:** 392–5.
2. Morris K, Rylance G. Guillain-Barré syndrome after measles, mumps, and rubella vaccine. *Lancet* 1994; **343:** 60.
3. Hadden RDM, Hughes RAC. Guillain-Barré syndrome: recent advances. *Hosp Med* 1998; **59:** 55–60.
4. Hahn AF. Guillain-Barré syndrome. *Lancet* 1998; **352:** 635–41.
5. Rees JH, *et al.* Campylobacter jejuni infection and Guillain-Barré syndrome. *N Engl J Med* 1995; **333:** 1374–9.
6. Anonymous. Guillain-Barré syndrome: immunoglobulins or steroids? *WHO Drug Inf* 1993; **7:** 110–11.
7. Rees J. Guillain-Barré syndrome: the latest on treatment. *Br J Hosp Med* 1993; **50:** 226–9.

8. Guillain-Barré Syndrome Steroid Trial Group. Double-blind trial of intravenous methylprednisolone in Guillain-Barré syndrome. *Lancet* 1993; **341:** 586–90.
9. Korinthenberg R, Mönting JS. Natural history and treatment effects in Guillain-Barré syndrome: a multicentre study. *Arch Dis Child* 1996; **74:** 281–7.
10. The Guillain-Barré Syndrome Study Group. Plasmapheresis and acute Guillain-Barré syndrome. *Neurology* 1985; **35:** 1096–1104.
11. French Cooperative Group on Plasma Exchange in Guillain-Barré syndrome. Efficacy of plasma exchange in Guillain-Barré syndrome: role of replacement fluids. *Ann Neurol* 1987; **22:** 753–61.
12. van der Meché FGA, *et al.* A randomized trial comparing intravenous immune globulin and plasma exchange in Guillain-Barré syndrome. *N Engl J Med* 1992; **326:** 1123–9.
13. Plasma Exchange/Sandoglobulin Guillain-Barré Syndrome Trial Group. Randomised trial of plasma exchange, intravenous immunoglobulin, and combined treatments in Guillain-Barré syndrome. *Lancet* 1997; **349:** 225–30.
14. Irani DN, *et al.* Relapse in Guillain-Barré syndrome after treatment with human immune globulin. *Neurology* 1993; **43:** 872–5.
15. Castro LHM, Ropper AH. Human immune globulin infusion in Guillain-Barré syndrome: worsening during and after treatment. *Neurology* 1993; **43:** 1034–6.

MOTOR NEURONE DISEASE. Normal immunoglobulins have been tried in the treatment of motor neurone disease, in particular multifocal motor neuropathy.[1-3]

1. Chaudhry V, *et al.* Multifocal motor neuropathy: response to human immune globulin. *Ann Neurol* 1993; **33:** 237–42.
2. Nobile-Orazio E, *et al.* High-dose intravenous immunoglobulin therapy in multifocal motor neuropathy. *Neurology* 1993; **43:** 537–44.
3. Azulay J-P, *et al.* Intravenous immunoglobulin treatment in patients with motor neuron syndromes associated with anti-GM_1 antibodies: a double-blind, placebo-controlled study. *Neurology* 1994; **44:** 429–32.

Neonatal disorders. HAEMOLYTIC DISEASE OF THE NEWBORN. For a discussion of haemolytic disease of the newborn and its management, including the use of intravenous immunoglobulin as an alternative to exchange transfusions in affected pregnancies, see p.1503.

NEONATAL SEPSIS. Sepsis is a serious problem in premature infants despite appropriate antimicrobial therapy.[1] Preterm infants are born with low serum-immunoglobulin concentrations which decrease over the next several weeks of life.[1,2] There is also a deficiency of antibodies to specific organisms such as group B streptococci, *Staphylococcus epidermidis*, and *Escherichia coli*.[1,2]

Some, but not all studies, suggest that prophylactic administration of intravenous normal immunoglobulin to premature infants shortly after birth can decrease the incidence of septicaemia.[1] Aspects of the methodology of these studies have, however, been criticised.[2] Some benefit has been observed after administration of intravenous immunoglobulin to treat infants ill with suspected sepsis,[1] and may improve the response to antibacterials.[3]

The optimum effective dosage of intravenous immunoglobulin is not established. A prophylactic dose of 500 mg per kg body-weight on admission repeated every one to two weeks has been suggested for units where infection is common in very low birth-weight infants.[1] Others have suggested adjusting the dose to maintain a specified serum-immunoglobulin concentration.[4,5] Alternatively, normal immunoglobulin could be administered only to infants with immunoglobulin concentrations below a certain level, or be reserved for immediate use in those who become ill with suspected sepsis.[1]

Normal immunoglobulin cannot protect against all types of infection. Givner[6] has shown that normal immunoglobulin preparations from different manufacturers demonstrate, for a specific pathogen (group B streptococcus), differing levels of specific antibody and differing levels of functional activity both *in vitro* and in *animals*. Lot-to-lot variability in functional activity was also observed for normal immunoglobulin from a specific manufacturer. Such variability, resulting in low concentrations of functional antibodies in the 4 batches of immunoglobulins used in the National Institute of Child Health Study,[7] was held responsible for the lack of demonstrable effectiveness of immunoglobulins in that study, one of the largest to date. Kohl *et al.*[8] considered that normal immunoglobulin would probably not be effective for the prevention of serious *Herpes simplex* virus infection in neonates at risk.

The use of fresh frozen plasma as an alternative to normal immunoglobulin could not be recommended following a study[9] which showed that it did not produce the beneficial effects on humoral immune markers seen with normal immunoglobulin.

Human immunoglobulin preparations hyperimmune for a specific pathogen[6] or human monoclonal antibody preparations against common perinatal pathogens[1,10] are possible future strategies.

1. Whitelaw A. Treatment of sepsis with IgG in very low birth-weight infants. *Arch Dis Child* 1990; **65:** 347–8.
2. Noya FJD, Baker CJ. Intravenously administered immune globulin for premature infants: a time to wait. *J Pediatr* 1989; **115:** 969–71.
3. Christensen RD, *et al.* Effect on neutrophil kinetics and serum opsonic capacity of intravenous administration of immune globulin to neonates with clinical signs of early-onset sepsis. *J Pediatr* 1991; **118:** 606–14.
4. Clapp DW, *et al.* Use of intravenously administered immune globulin to prevent nosocomial sepsis in low birth weight infants: report of a pilot study. *J Pediatr* 1989; **115:** 973–8.
5. Kyllonen KS, *et al.* Dosage of intravenously administered immune globulin and dosing interval required to maintain target levels of immunoglobulin G in low birth weight infants. *J Pediatr* 1989; **115:** 1013–16.
6. Givner LB. Human immunoglobulins for intravenous use: comparison of available preparations for group B streptococcal antibody levels, opsonic activity, and efficacy in animal models. *Pediatrics* 1990; **86:** 955–62.
7. Fanaroff AA, *et al.* A controlled trial of intravenous immune globulin to reduce nosocomial infections in very-low-birth-weight infants. *N Engl J Med* 1994; **330:** 1107–13.
8. Kohl S, *et al.* Effect of intravenously administered immune globulin on functional antibody to herpes simplex virus in low birth weight neonates. *J Pediatr* 1989; **115:** 135–9.
9. Acunas BA, *et al.* Effect of fresh frozen plasma and gammaglobulin on humoral immunity in neonatal sepsis. *Arch Dis Child* 1994; **70:** F182–7.
10. Weisman LE, *et al.* Comparison of group B streptococcal hyperimmune globulin and standard intravenously administered immune globulin in neonates. *J Pediatr* 1993; **122:** 929–37.

Passive immunisation. CYTOMEGALOVIRUS INFECTION. See under Bone Marrow Transplantation, above.

HEPATITIS. *Hepatitis A.* With the decreasing incidence of hepatitis A in the UK, a reduction in the concentration of hepatitis A antibodies in normal immunoglobulin has been observed. In the future, normal immunoglobulin could become unsuitable for hepatitis A prophylaxis.[1,2] However, hepatitis A vaccines (p.1512) have been developed and specific hepatitis A immunoglobulins (p.1512) are available in some countries.

1. Higgins G, *et al.* Hepatitis A virus antibody in East Anglian blood donors. *Lancet* 1990; **336:** 1330.
2. Behrens RH, Doherty JF. Severe hepatitis A despite passive immunisation. *Lancet* 1993; **341:** 972.

Hepatitis C. In a randomised, placebo-controlled study[1] in seronegative sexual partners of patients positive for antibody to hepatitis C, normal immunoglobulin administered intramuscularly every 2 months was found to significantly reduce the incidence of subsequent seroconversion. One of 450 subjects who received normal immunoglobulin became seropositive during follow-up compared with 6 of 449 who had received placebo.

1. Piazza M, *et al.* Sexual transmission of the hepatitis C virus and efficacy of prophylaxis with intramuscular immune serum globulin: a randomized controlled trial. *Arch Intern Med* 1997; **157:** 1537–44.

PARVOVIRUS B19 INFECTION. Persistent infection with human parvovirus B19 can cause red-cell aplasia with resultant anaemia particularly in immunocompromised patients. Kurtzman *et al.* reported resolution of anaemia and clearance of parvovirus B19 from the circulation after administration of normal immunoglobulin to a patient who had had red-cell aplasia for 10 years.[1] Normal immunoglobulin was given by intravenous infusion in a dose of 400 mg per kg body-weight daily for 10 days and then periodically for several months. Ramage *et al.* have described successful treatment of anaemia due to parvovirus B19-induced red-cell aplasia with plasmapheresis and intravenous immunoglobulin in a liver transplant recipient.[2] Clearance of parvovirus B19 from the circulation has been reported in patients who also have AIDS, but the presence of concomitant opportunistic infections may prevent resolution of the anaemia.[3,4]

Beneficial responses to intravenous immunoglobulin have also been reported in a few patients with parvovirus B19 infections associated with vasculitic syndromes.[5]

1. Kurtzman G, *et al.* Pure red-cell aplasia of 10 years' duration due to persistent parvovirus B19 infection and its cure with immunoglobulin therapy. *N Engl J Med* 1989; **321:** 519–23.
2. Ramage JK, *et al.* Parvovirus B19-induced red cell aplasia treated with plasmapheresis and immunoglobulin. *Lancet* 1994; **343:** 667–8.
3. Frickhofen N, *et al.* Persistent B19 parvovirus infection in patients infected with human immunodeficiency virus type 1 (HIV-1): a treatable cause of anemia in AIDS. *Ann Intern Med* 1990; **113:** 926–33.
4. Bowman CA, *et al.* Red cell aplasia associated with human parvovirus B19 and HIV infection: failure to respond clinically to intravenous immunoglobulin. *AIDS* 1990; **4:** 1038–9.
5. Finkel TH, *et al.* Chronic parvovirus B19 infection and systemic necrotising vasculitis: opportunistic infection or aetiological agent? *Lancet* 1994; **343:** 1255–8.

RUBELLA. One of the uses of normal immunoglobulin involves the administration to pregnant women recently exposed to rubella. It does not prevent infection in non-immune contacts, but may reduce the risk to the fetus and may be used when termination of pregnancy is unacceptable.

TOXIC SHOCK SYNDROME. For a discussion of toxic shock syndrome and its treatment, including reference to clinical improvement in one patient after administration of intravenous normal immunoglobulins, see p.146.

Skin disorders. Normal immunoglobulins have been tried in a few patients with blistering skin diseases. The usual treatment for pemphigoid is with systemic corticosteroids; normal immunoglobulins in high doses have produced generally transient improvement when used alone,[1] although steroid-sparing effects have been reported.[2] A patient with severe epidermolysis bullosa responded to therapy with high-dose intravenous immunoglobulins.[3] Clinical benefit was noted in 9 of 10 patients with auto-immune chronic urticaria who were given a 5-day course of intravenous immunoglobulins, 2 of whom experienced prolonged remission over 3 years of follow-up.[4]

1. Godard W, *et al.* Bullous pemphigoid and intravenous gammaglobulin. *Ann Intern Med* 1985; **103:** 965.
2. Beckers RCY, *et al.* Adjuvant high-dose intravenous gammaglobulin in the treatment of pemphigus and bullous pemphigoid: experience in six patients. *Br J Dermatol* 1995; **133:** 289–93.
3. Mohr C, *et al.* Successful treatment of epidermolysis bullosa acquisita using intravenous immunoglobulins. *Br J Dermatol* 1995; **132:** 824–6.
4. O'Donnell BF, *et al.* Intravenous immunoglobulin in autoimmune chronic urticaria. *Br J Dermatol* 1998; **138:** 101–6.

Spontaneous abortion. Fetal loss has been attributed in some cases to the presence of antiphospholipid antibodies (lupus anticoagulant and anticardiolipin) in the mother. Successful pregnancy outcome has been reported after administration of intravenous normal immunoglobulin during pregnancy to a few such women.[1-5]

1. Carreras LO, *et al.* Lupus anticoagulant and recurrent fetal loss: successful treatment with gammaglobulin. *Lancet* 1988; **ii:** 393–4.
2. Francois A, *et al.* Repeated fetal losses and the lupus anticoagulant. *Ann Intern Med* 1988; **109:** 993–4.
3. Parke A, *et al.* Intravenous gamma-globulin, antiphospholipid antibodies, and pregnancy. *Ann Intern Med* 1989; **110:** 495–6.
4. Katz VL, *et al.* Human immunoglobulin therapy for preeclampsia associated with lupus anticoagulant and anticardiolipin antibody. *Obstet Gynecol* 1990; **76:** 986–8.
5. Mueller-Eckhardt G, *et al.* IVIG to prevent recurrent spontaneous abortion. *Lancet* 1991; **337:** 424–5.

Preparations

Ph. Eur.: Human Normal Immunoglobulin; Human Normal Immunoglobulin for Intravenous Administration;
USP 23: Immune Globulin.

Proprietary Preparations (details are given in Part 3)
Aust.: Beriglobin; Endobulin; Gamma-Venin; Gammabulin; Gammonativ; Igabulin; Intragam; Intraglobin; Octagam; Pentaglobin; Venimmun; ***Austral.:*** Intragam; Sandoglobulin; ***Belg.:*** Gamma 16†; Gammagard; Globuman; Sandoglobuline; Veinoglobuline†; ***Canad.:*** Gamimune N; Gammabulin†; Iveegam†; ***Fr.:*** Allergamma†; Polygamma†; Sandoglobuline; Tegeline; Veinoglobuline†; ***Ger.:*** Alphaglobin; Beriglobin; Cutterglobin†; Endobulin; Gamma-Venin; Gammabulin; Gammagard; Gammonativ; Intraglobin F; Intraglobin†; Kabiglobin†; Octagam; Pentaglobin; Polyglobin N; Purimmun†; Sandoglobulin; Venimmun; ***Irl.:*** Gammabulin; Sandoglobulin; ***Ital.:*** Alphaglobin; Biaven; Endobulin; Gamma-Venin P; Gammabulin; Globuman; Haimagamma†; Haimaven; Ig Vena N; Intraglobin; Isiven; Kabigamma†; Normogamma; Pentaglobin; Sandoglobulina; Uman-Gamma; Venimmun; Venogamma Polivalente; Venoglobulina†; ***Neth.:*** Gamma 16†; Veinoglobuline†; ***Norw.:*** Gammaglobulin; Gammanorm; Gammonativ; Octagam; Sandoglobulin; ***S.Afr.:*** Beriglobin; Endobulin; Gamma-Veinine†; Globuman; Intragam; Intraglobin F; Polygam; Sandoglobulin†; ***Spain:*** Alerglobulina†; Alergogamma†; Artroglobina†; Beriglobina; Endobulin; Flebogamma; Gamma Glob; Gamma Glob Antial†; Gamma-Venin†; Gammabion†; Gammagard; Globuman; Glogama Antialergica†; Glogama†; Gloinar†; Inglobin†; Inmunogamma†; Poliglobin N; ***Swed.:*** Beriglobin; Endobulin; Gammabulin†; Gammagard; Gammanorm; Gammonativ; Nordimmun†; Octagam; Polyglobin†; Rhodiglobin†; Sandoglobulin; ***Switz.:*** Endobulin; Gamma-Globuline†; Gammabuline†; Gammagard; Globuman; Intraglobin F; Octagam; Pentaglobin; Sandoglobuline; ***UK:*** Alphaglobin; Endobulin†; Gamimune N†; Gammabulin; Kabiglobulin; Octagam; Sandoglobulin; Venoglobulin†; Vigam S; ***USA:*** Gamastan†; Gamimune N; Gammagard; Gammar-P; Iveegam†; Polygam†; Sandoglobulin; Venoglobulin.

Pertussis Immunoglobulins (1237-x)

Pertussis Immune Globulin (USP 23) is a sterile solution of globulins derived from the plasma of adult human donors who have been immunised with pertussis vaccine. It may contain glycine as a stabilising agent, and a suitable preservative. It should be stored at 2° to 8°.

Adverse Effects and Precautions

As for immunoglobulins in general, p.1500.

Interactions

As for immunoglobulins in general, p.1500.

Uses and Administration

Pertussis immunoglobulins may be used for passive immunisation against pertussis (whooping cough). They have been used to prevent or modify pertussis in susceptible persons who have been exposed to infection.

References.

1. Granström M, *et al.* Specific immunoglobulin for treatment of whooping cough. *Lancet* 1991; **338:** 1230–3.

Preparations

USP 23: Pertussis Immune Globulin.

Proprietary Preparations (details are given in Part 3)
Fr.: Gamma Coq†; ***Ger.:*** Tussoglobin†; ***Ital.:*** Haimapertus; Immunopertox; Pertoglobulin; Pertus-Gamma; Tosuman; Tussoglobin†; ***Spain:*** Gamma Glob Antiper†; Glogama Antipertusis†; ***Switz.:*** Tosuman.

Pertussis Vaccines (7985-l)

Pertussis Vaccine (Ph. Eur.) (Per/Vac; Vaccinum Pertussis; Whooping-cough Vaccine) is a sterile suspension of inactivated whole cells of one or more strains of *Bordetella pertussis* in saline. The estimated potency is not less than 4 international units per dose. It may contain a suitable antimicrobial preservative. It should be stored at 2° to 8°, not be allowed to freeze, and be protected from light.

Pertussis Vaccine (Adsorbed) (Ph. Eur.) (Per/Vac/Ads; Vaccinum Pertussis Adsorbatum) is a sterile suspension of inactivated whole cells of one or more strains of *Bordetella pertussis* in saline to which hydrated aluminium hydroxide, aluminium phosphate, or calcium phosphate has been added. It may contain a suitable antimicrobial preservative. The estimated potency is not less than 4 units per dose. It should be stored at 2° to 8°, not be allowed to freeze, and be protected from light. The BP directs that when Pertussis Vaccine is prescribed or demanded and the form is not stated, either the plain or the adsorbed vaccine may be dispensed or supplied.

Pertussis Vaccine (Acellular, Component, Adsorbed) (Ph. Eur.) (Vaccinum Pertussis sine Cellulis ex Elementis Praeparatum Adsorbatum) is a preparation of individually prepared and purified antigenic components of *Bordetella pertussis* adsorbed on a mineral carrier such as aluminium hydroxide or hydrated aluminium phosphate. It contains either a suitably prepared pertussis toxoid or a pertussis toxin-like protein free from toxic properties produced by expression of a genetically modified form of the corresponding gene. It may also contain filamentous haemagglutinin, pertactin, and other defined antigens such as fimbrial-2 and fimbrial-3 antigens. The final vaccine contains not more than 100 units of bacterial endotoxin per dose. It may contain a suitable antimicrobial preservative. It should be stored at 2° to 8°, not be allowed to freeze, and be protected from light.

Pertussis Vaccine (USP 23) is a sterile bacterial fraction or suspension of killed *Bordetella pertussis* of a strain or strains selected for high antigenicity. It contains a preservative. It contains 12 protective units per immunising dose. It should be stored at 2° to 8° and not be allowed to freeze.

Pertussis Vaccine Adsorbed (USP 23) is a sterile bacterial fraction or suspension of killed *Bordetella pertussis* of a strain or strains selected for high antigenicity, precipitated or adsorbed by the addition of aluminium hydroxide or aluminium phosphate. It contains a preservative. It contains 12 protective units per immunising dose. It should be stored at 2° to 8° and not be allowed to freeze.

Adverse Effects

As for vaccines in general, p.1500.

Local reactions may occur at the site of injection of pertussis vaccines or pertussis-containing vaccines and administration may be followed by fever and irritability. Local reactions and fever occur less frequently following use of the acellular vaccine than after whole cell vaccine, especially in children over 6 months of age and adults.

Severe reactions which have been reported include persistent screaming and generalised collapse but these effects were generally associated with an earlier type of vaccine and the reactions are stated to be rarely observed with the currently available vaccines.

Rare neurological adverse reactions have included convulsions and encephalopathy. There has been much debate, however, on the causal role of pertussis vaccine in such reactions (see below for detailed discussion). It should be remembered that neurological complications occur more frequently as a consequence of pertussis infection than in association with vaccination.

Asthma. A higher incidence of asthma was reported in 243 children who had received pertussis vaccine than in 203 children who had not.[1] However, follow-up of a large Swedish study[2] showed no difference in the incidence of wheezing or allergic reactions between children who had received diphtheria, tetanus, and pertussis vaccines and those who had not.

1. Odent MR, *et al.* Pertussis vaccination and asthma: is there a link? *JAMA* 1994; **272:** 592–3.
2. Nilsson L, *et al.* Lack of association between pertussis vaccination and symptoms of asthma and allergy. *JAMA* 1996; **275:** 760.

Effects on the nervous system. There has been continuing debate over several decades concerning the perceived link between pertussis vaccination and brain damage. Anxiety among both the public and health care professionals in the UK in the mid-1970s over the safety of pertussis vaccines led to a fall in the acceptance rates for infant vaccination and major epidemics of pertussis in 1977/79 and 1981/83. Since that time confidence has been restored, and by 1995 94% of infants were receiving the vaccine before their second birthday.

The consensus of opinion now seems to be that there is a temporal but not necessarily causal relationship between pertussis vaccine and acute neurological illness which may occasionally lead to long-term dysfunction, and that risks of not immunising are greater than the potential risks associated with the vaccine.

The difficulty in ascertaining whether a causal relationship exists between pertussis vaccine (usually given as diphtheria, tetanus, and pertussis (DTP) vaccine) and acute neurological reactions arises partly because primary vaccination is given at an age when neurological dysfunction with other causes is often first manifested. The observed temporal relationship may be entirely coincidental, or may result from indirect factors such as pyrexia following vaccination, or may represent a direct effect of DTP vaccine. Much of the evidence is based on large epidemiological studies,[1-6] in particular the National Childhood Encephalopathy Study (NCES)[7] from the UK and its 10-year follow-up.[8] Serious acute neurological illnesses reported to the NCES[7] were found to be more common in infants immunised within 7 days (relative risk 2.4), and especially within 72 hours of onset, than in unimmunised children. For previously normal children irrespective of outcome the risk was estimated as 1 in 110 000 injections. In a subset of cases diagnosed as infantile spasms,[9] no link with vaccination was found overall, but there was a small excess of cases of infantile spasm in previously normal children who had received either DTP or diphtheria and tetanus (DT) vaccines during the previous 7 days (relative risk 2.0-2.5) followed by a corresponding deficit during the next 3 weeks. This suggested that vaccination may trigger the onset of spasms in a child with an underlying predisposition.

In 1991, the Institute of Medicine (IOM) in the USA reviewed the available data, including the NCES results, and concluded that a causal relationship between DTP vaccine and acute encephalopathy probably existed, with an estimated risk of zero to 10.5 per million vaccinations.[10] They concurred with the conclusion that a causal relationship between vaccination and infantile spasm was unlikely.

The NCES 10-year follow-up found that children who had had a serious acute neurological illness (excluding infantile spasms) had an increased risk of death or long-term dysfunction, but the risk was no greater in children who had received DTP vaccine in the 7 days before the original acute illness.[8] The National Vaccines Advisory Committee concluded that the results were insufficient to determine whether DTP vaccine influenced the development of chronic neurological dysfunction, and this conclusion has been accepted by both the Advisory Committee on Immunization Practices (ACIP)[11] and the American Academy of Pediatrics.[12]

1. Pollock TM, Morris J. A 7-year survey of disorders attributed to vaccination in North West Thames Region. *Lancet* 1983; **i:** 753–7.
2. Pollock TM, *et al.* Symptoms after primary immunisation with DTP and with DT vaccine. *Lancet* 1984; **ii:** 146–9.
3. Walker AM, *et al.* Neurologic events following diphtheria-tetanus-pertussis immunization. *Pediatrics* 1988; **81:** 345–9.
4. Shields WD, *et al.* Relationship of pertussis immunization to the onset of neurologic disorders: a retrospective epidemiologic study. *J Pediatr* 1988; **113:** 801–5.
5. Griffin MR, *et al.* Risk of seizures and encephalopathy after immunization with the diphtheria-tetanus-pertussis vaccine. *JAMA* 1990; **263:** 1641–5.
6. Gale JL, *et al.* Risk of serious acute neurological illness after immunization with diphtheria-tetanus-pertussis vaccine: a population-based case-control study. *JAMA* 1994; **271:** 37–41.
7. Miller DL, *et al.* Pertussis immunisation and serious acute neurological illness in children. *Br Med J* 1981; **282:** 1595–9.
8. Miller D, *et al.* Pertussis immunisation and serious acute neurological illnesses in children. *Br Med J* 1993; **307:** 1171–6.
9. Bellman MH, *et al.* Infantile spasms and pertussis immunisation. *Lancet* 1983; **i:** 1031–4.
10. Howson CP, Fineberg HV. Adverse events following pertussis and rubella vaccines: summary of a report of the Institute of Medicine. *JAMA* 1992; **267:** 392–6.
11. Centers for Disease Control. Update: vaccine side effects, adverse reactions, contraindications, and precautions: recommendations of the Advisory Committee on Immunization Practices (ACIP). *MMWR* 1996; **45** (RR-12): 1–45.
12. Committee on Infectious Disease, American Academy of Pediatrics. The relationship between pertussis vaccine and central nervous system sequelae: continuing assessment. *Pediatrics* 1996; **97:** 279–81.

Precautions

As for vaccines in general, p.1501. Because of the controversy concerning the potential adverse effects, especially neurotoxicity, of pertussis vaccines (see under Adverse Effects, above) the precautions and contra-indications to the use of these vaccines have sometimes been more stringent than is now considered necessary. As with other vaccines, immunisation should not be carried out in individuals with a definite history of a severe local or general reaction to a preceding dose. In children who have a history of less severe general reactions, immunisation may be completed omitting the pertussis component, or, in the case of local reactions or pyrexia, substituting an acellular pertussis vaccine.

Whether children with a personal or family history of convulsions or epilepsy or who have suffered cerebral damage in the neonatal period should receive pertussis vaccines appears to have been the most difficult question to resolve in the past. In the UK the Department of Health now recommends that children with a personal or family history of febrile convulsions and children with a close family history of idiopathic epilepsy should be immunised and children whose epilepsy is well controlled may receive pertussis vaccine; advice on the prevention of fever should be given at the time of immunisation (see Fever and Hyperthermia, p.1 for comments on the prevention of fever following immunisation). Immunisation should also be carried out in children with a history of cerebral damage in the neonatal period unless there is evidence of an evolving neurological abnormality. In children with a neurological problem that is still evolving it is recommended that immunisation should be deferred until the condition is stable.

A personal or family history of hypersensitivity reactions is not generally considered to be a contra-indication to the use of pertussis vaccines, nor are stable neurological conditions such as cerebral palsy or spina bifida.

Although collapse (hypotonic-hyporesponsive episode) after pertussis vaccination remains a contra-indication to further doses of the whole cell vaccine in the UK, a follow-up study of infants who had experienced such an episode in the Netherlands showed a very low incidence of recurrence on second and subsequent doses.[1]

1. Vermeer-de Bondt PE, *et al.* Rate of recurrent collapse after vaccination with whole cell pertussis vaccine: follow up study. *Br Med J* 1998; **316:** 902–3.

Interactions

As for vaccines in general, p.1501.

Poliomyelitis vaccines. A diminished immune response to pertussis vaccine was reported in infants given inactivated poliomyelitis vaccine mixed with diphtheria, tetanus, and pertussis vaccine compared with infants given the two vaccines as separate injections on the same visit.[1]

1. Halperin SA, *et al.* Effect of inactivated poliovirus vaccine on the antibody response to Bordetella pertussis antigens when combined with diphtheria-pertussis-tetanus vaccine. *Clin Infect Dis* 1996; **22:** 59–62.

Uses and Administration

Pertussis vaccines are used for active immunisation against pertussis (whooping cough) (p.137).

For primary immunisation combined diphtheria, tetanus, and whole cell pertussis vaccines (p.1509) are usually used. For discussion of immunisation schedules, see below. Acellular pertussis vaccines are taking the place of whole cell vaccines in several countries including the USA and are being incorporated into primary immunisation schedules for infants and children and for reinforcing doses in older children and adults. In the UK a single-component acellular vaccine is available only for use when the pertussis component has been omitted from all or part of the primary immunisation schedule; if doses of diphtheria and tetanus remain to be given, diphtheria, tetanus, and whole cell pertussis vaccine should be used followed by acellular pertussis at monthly intervals to complete three doses. A primary course may also be given with the pre-school tetanus and diphtheria booster in a similar way. Acellular vaccines may also be substituted in individuals who have a moderate local reaction or pyrexia following diphtheria, tetanus, and whole cell pertussis vaccine. Acellular vaccines are given in a dose of 0.5 mL by deep subcutaneous or intramuscular injection.

Acellular vaccines. Vaccination using whole-cell pertussis vaccines has been effective but adverse reactions are common (see above). The immunogenicity of the UK whole-cell vaccine is estimated at about 90% using the current accelerated three-dose schedule.[1] Dissatisfaction with whole-cell vaccines in the 1970s led to reduced uptake and a resurgence of pertussis in several countries. In Japan, research into less reactogenic pertussis vaccines resulted in the introduction of acellular vaccines for routine vaccination in the early 1980s.

The antigenic components of acellular pertussis vaccines are pertussis toxin (PT; also formerly known as lymphocytosis-promoting factor, LPF) either alone or more usually in combination with filamentous haemagglutinin (FHA), the 69 kilodalton outer membrane protein pertactin, and/or fimbrial agglutinogens (with 3 major serotypes; also referred to as fimbrial antigens). Adverse reactions to acellular vaccines are less frequent and less severe than those associated with whole-cell vaccines.[2] The acellular vaccines have successfully controlled pertussis infections but formal comparisons of efficacy with whole-cell vaccines have only been reported more recently. For studies of primary immunisation pertussis vaccine is used in combination with diphtheria and tetanus toxoids (DTP), and diphtheria and tetanus vaccines (DT) are used in the placebo groups.

As with whole-cell vaccines,[3,4] acellular vaccines varied in their efficacy. Multivalent vaccines were generally more effective than monovalent vaccines.[5] It has been argued that a monovalent pertussis toxoid, while providing incomplete protection for the individual, may nevertheless produce adequate herd immunity to inhibit disease transmission.[6] However, the use of multivalent vaccines seems preferable.[7,8]

In general, acellular vaccines approached the efficacy of and were better tolerated than whole-cell vaccines.[5,9,10] A surprising result of large studies in Sweden[5] and Italy,[10] in which the acellular vaccines were considerably more effective than the whole-cell vaccines, was the low efficacy of the US whole-cell vaccine (less than 50%). This was attributed to a rapidly waning effect after 3 doses given at 2, 4, and 6 months of age, suggesting that the booster doses at age 12 to 18 months and at school entry are essential to the US schedule. The UK whole-cell vaccine was found to be as effective as a pentavalent acellular vaccine and both were more effective than a trivalent vaccine in a large study in Sweden.[11]

In the UK, confidence in the whole-cell vaccine has been largely restored, and uptake of primary immunisation in infants is approximately 90%.[1] Under these circumstances it is unlikely that there would be any benefit from switching to the use of the more expensive acellular vaccines.[12] However, there is some concern over the incidence of pertussis infection in adults[13] and it is possible that acellular vaccines, which are better tolerated in older recipients than whole-cell vaccines, would be more acceptable if booster doses are added at school entry and in school leavers. In the USA, however, acellular pertussis vaccines are now recommended for both primary immunisation in infants and for the booster doses at 12 to 18 months and at school entry.

1. White JM, *et al.* The effect of an accelerated immunisation schedule on pertussis in England and Wales. *Commun Dis Rep* 1996; **6** (review 6): R86–R91.
2. Decker MD, *et al.* Comparison of 13 acellular pertussis vaccines: adverse reactions. *Pediatrics* 1995; **96** (suppl): 557–66.
3. Edwards KM, *et al.* Differences in antibody response to whole-cell pertussis vaccines. *Pediatrics* 1991; **88:** 1019–23.
4. Baker JD, *et al.* Antibody response to Bordetella pertussis antigens after immunization with American and Canadian whole-cell vaccines. *J Pediatr* 1992; **121:** 523–7.
5. Gustafsson L, *et al.* A controlled trial of a two-component acellular, five-component acellular, and a whole-cell pertussis vaccine. *N Engl J Med* 1996; **334:** 349–55. Correction. *ibid.;* 1207.
6. Schneerson R, *et al.* A toxoid vaccine for pertussis as well as diphtheria? Lessons to be relearned. *Lancet* 1996; **348:** 1289–92.
7. Wirsing von König CH, Schmitt HJ. Toxoid vaccine for pertussis. *Lancet* 1997; **349:** 136.
8. He Q, *et al.* Toxoid vaccine for pertussis. *Lancet* 1997; **349:** 136–7.
9. Schmitt H-J, *et al.* Efficacy of acellular pertussis vaccine in early childhood after household exposure. *JAMA* 1996; **275:** 37–41.
10. Greco D, *et al.* A controlled trial of two acellular vaccines and one whole-cell vaccine against pertussis. *N Engl J Med* 1996; **334:** 341–8.
11. Olin P, *et al.* Randomised controlled trial of two-component, three-component, and five-component acellular pertussis vaccines compared with whole-cell pertussis vaccine. *Lancet* 1997; **350:** 1569–77. Correction. *ibid.;* **351:** 454.
12. Miller E. Acellular pertussis vaccines. *Arch Dis Child* 1995; **73:** 390–1.
13. Nenning ME. Prevalence and incidence of adult pertussis in an urban population. *JAMA* 1996; **275:** 1672–4.

Immunisation schedules. A review of the epidemiology and control of pertussis.[1] Pertussis is a common, highly infectious, respiratory disease, predominantly affecting children, and for which there is no effective treatment. WHO has estimated that 60 million cases of pertussis occur annually and that the disease is responsible for half a million to one million deaths each year. The highest incidence of pertussis is observed in developing countries where immunisation is low.

A combined adsorbed diphtheria, tetanus, and pertussis vaccine is now used in most countries but both the strength of the pertussis component and production methods vary, leading to vaccines of different potencies.

Depending upon the country, the age at which a child is given the first dose of the combined vaccine varies from 5 weeks to 6 months. (For summaries of immunisation schedules in the UK and USA, see under Vaccines, p.1501.) In countries with a high incidence of pertussis WHO recommends that immunisation should start at 6 weeks of age and that the schedule involve three doses at monthly intervals. A booster dose should be given one year after the end of the primary series of 3 injections and in some countries a second booster at entry to school is given. Several reports have described the use of a two-dose widely-spaced primary immunisation schedule and this would indeed simplify procedures in developing countries; however, the limitation of such a schedule is the long period of risk between doses without adequate protection and unless the interval can be shortened to 4 weeks, the wide use of such a schedule is not advisable in endemic areas.

1. Muller AS, *et al.* Pertussis: epidemiology and control. *Bull WHO* 1986; **64:** 321–31.

Preparations

Ph. Eur.: Pertussis Vaccine; Pertussis Vaccine (Acellular, Component, Adsorbed); Pertussis Vaccine (Adsorbed);
USP 23: Pertussis Vaccine; Pertussis Vaccine Adsorbed.

Proprietary Preparations (details are given in Part 3)

Fr.: Vaxicoq; ***Ger.:*** Acel-P; Pa-Vaccinol; Pac Merieux; Pertuvac; ***Ital.:*** Acelluvax; ***Switz.:*** Acel-P.

Pigbel Vaccines (16951-w)

A vaccine against pigbel (necrotising enteritis), a disease occurring predominantly in children in the highlands of Papua New Guinea, is used for active immunisation against the disease. The vaccine consists of an adsorbed *Clostridium perfringens* type C toxoid.

Subsequent to a study indicating that pigbel vaccine could confer protection against the disease, an immunisation programme was introduced in Papua New Guinea in 1980.[1] Pigbel vaccine was given to children at 2, 4, and 6 months of age and, initially, to older children. A survey has shown a sustained overall fall in the incidence of severe pigbel in children coincident with the increased induced immunity. However, protection may be relatively short-lived and boosters may be necessary for full protection of young children.

1. Lawrence GW, *et al.* Impact of active immunisation against enteritis necroticans in Papua New Guinea. *Lancet* 1990; **336:** 1165–7.

Plague Vaccines (7987-j)

Plague Vaccine (USP 23) is a sterile suspension of formaldehyde-killed *Yersinia pestis* (strain 195/P). It should be stored at 2° to 8° and not be allowed to freeze.

Adverse Effects and Precautions

As for vaccines in general, p.1500.

Interactions

As for vaccines in general, p.1501.

Uses and Administration

Plague vaccines are used for active immunisation against plague in those occupationally exposed to the organism and in some field workers in infected areas. They may reduce morbidity and mortality in bubonic plague but their activity against pneumonic plague is unknown.

A plague vaccine containing 2000 million inactivated *Yersinia pestis* (strain 195/P) per mL is administered by intramuscular injection. The initial dose for adults and children over 10 years of age is usually 1 mL, and is followed by two further doses, each of 0.2 mL, given 1 to 3 months after the first dose and 5 to 6 months after the second respectively. Booster doses of 0.1 to 0.2 mL may be given at 6-monthly intervals; the interval between booster doses may be extended to every 1 to 2 years in persons who have received 3 or more boosters at intervals of 6 months. Suggested first, second, third, and booster doses for children are: under one year of age, 0.2, 0.04, 0.04, and 0.02 to 0.04 mL respectively; aged 1 to 4 years, 0.4, 0.08, 0.08, and 0.04 to 0.08 mL respectively; 5 to 10 years, 0.6, 0.12, 0.12, and 0.06 to 0.12 mL respectively.

Preparations

USP 23: Plague Vaccine.

Pneumococcal Vaccines (7988-z)

Pneumococcal Polysaccharide Vaccine (Ph. Eur.) (Pneumo/Vac; Vaccinum Pneumococcale Polysaccharidum) is a mixture of purified polysaccharide capsular antigens from 23 differing serotypes of *Streptococcus pneumoniae*. Each 0.5-mL dose contains 25 μg of each of the 23 polysaccharide types. An antimicrobial preservative may be added. The vaccine has a pH of 4.5 to 7.4. It should be stored at 2° to 8°, not be allowed to freeze, and be protected from light.

Adverse Effects and Precautions

As for vaccines in general, p.1500.

Revaccination of adults is not generally recommended because of the increased incidence and severity of adverse reactions. For details of patient groups in whom revaccination may be considered and timings, see under Uses and Administration, below.

Pneumococcal vaccination is relatively ineffective in patients with multiple myeloma, Hodgkin's and non-Hodgkin's lymphoma, especially during treatment, and in chronic alcoholism. In patients with Hodgkin's disease the use of pneumococcal vaccines is not recommended in those who have received extensive chemotherapy or nodal irradiation. Pneumococcal vaccines should be given at least 10 days before starting immunosuppressive therapy or be delayed until at least 6 months after completion of therapy.

A satisfactory response to pneumococcal vaccines is not obtained in children less than 2 years of age and therefore immunisation of this age group is not recommended.

Effects on the blood. The manufacturer reports that on rare occasions, relapses have occurred in patients with stabilised idiopathic thrombocytopenic purpura at 2 to 14 days after vaccination against pneumococcal infections, lasting for up to 2 weeks. One such case was reported[1] following revaccination less than 2.5 years after an uneventful primary vaccination with pneumococcal vaccine.

1. Neil VS. Long term management after splenectomy: revaccination may cause relapse. *Br Med J* 1994; **308:** 339.

Effects on the kidneys. Glomerulonephritis was described[1] in a splenectomised patient following administration of pneumococcal vaccine. It was postulated that high antibody titres from a recent pneumococcal infection could have contributed.

1. Tan SY, Cumming AD. Vaccine related glomerulonephritis. *Br Med J* 1993; **306:** 248.

Effect of nutritional status. An impaired antibody response to pneumococcal vaccine was reported[1] in elderly patients with low serum concentrations of vitamin B_{12}.

1. Fata FT, *et al.* Impaired antibody responses to pneumococcal polysaccharide in elderly patients with low serum vitamin B12 levels. *Ann Intern Med* 1996; **124:** 299–304.

Interactions

As for vaccines in general, p.1501.

Uses and Administration

Of the many serotypes of *Streptococcus pneumoniae* the 23 from which antigens are obtained for the most commonly available pneumococcal vaccine are considered to cause about 90% of pneumococcal disease.

Pneumococcal vaccines are used for active immunisation in those at increased risk from infection with the types of *Streptococcus pneumoniae* contained in the vaccine. In the UK it is recommended that immunisation should be considered in persons over 2 years of age who have undergone splenectomy and those with splenic dysfunction due to sickle-cell anaemia or other causes; patients with immunodeficiency or immunosuppression due to disease or treatment including HIV infection at all stages; and persons with chronic cardiac, pulmonary, hepatic, or renal impairment including nephrotic syndrome, or diabetes mellitus.

An antibody response develops by the third week, and usually lasts about 5 years. The antibody response is less reliable and declines more rapidly in young children and persons with impaired immune function.

A single dose of 0.5 mL of the 23-type vaccine, containing 25 μg of each of the 23 polysaccharide types, is given by subcutaneous or intramuscular injection. The vaccine should be given at least 2 weeks before elective splenectomy or chemotherapy. Revaccination is not generally recommended except, after 5 to 10 years, in patients likely to have rapidly declining antibody concentrations; see below for further discussion.

Although pneumococcal vaccines are effective in protecting against *Streptococcus pneumoniae* infection in healthy subjects there has been much debate over their **efficacy** in patients at increased risk of infection.[1-4] There are several frequently-cited studies demonstrating adequate[5-7] and inadequate[8,9] protection in high-risk groups of patients. Most of these studies used the now discontinued 14-valent pneumococcal vaccine. They have also been criticised for various aspects of their methodology including the suitability of the chosen end-point.[1,4] It has been suggested that the divergent results are a consequence of the varying type and degree of risk of infection in the populations studied.[1] Most[10-13] but not all[14] studies using the current 23-valent pneumococcal vaccines have demonstrated that they provide a useful degree of protection against pneumococcal infections in high-risk groups including the elderly.

One major consequence of the doubts over the efficacy and safety of pneumococcal vaccines has been a low **uptake** of vaccination in persons at risk of infection. It has been estimated that as few as 10% of subjects for whom vaccination is recommended have received it,[15] and surveys in splenectomised patients in the UK in 1993[16,17] showed that, although the situation was improving, vaccine coverage remained inadequate. Doubts are still occasionally expressed[18] over the necessity to vaccinate any but those at highest risk, despite evidence of efficacy of the 23-valent vaccine in all patient groups covered by current recommendations.[19]

The **recommendations** of the Department of Health in the UK are outlined under Uses and Administration, above. Similar recommendations have been made elsewhere. The Immunization Practices Advisory Committee in the USA (ACIP)[20] and WHO[21] recommend in addition vaccination of all persons aged 65 years or more. Vaccination of the healthy elderly has also been advocated in the UK[22-24] although the topic remains controversial.[25] Pneumococcal vaccine is also recommended for persons living in environments or social settings with an identified increased risk of pneumococcal disease. Pneumococcal vaccine is not indicated for children with recurrent upper respiratory tract disease including otitis media and sinusitis.

Routine **revaccination** of adults with pneumococcal vaccines is not recommended. The ACIP[20] and the Department of Health in the UK suggest that revaccination be considered after 5 to 10 years for individuals likely to have a rapid decline in antibody titre such as asplenic patients or those with dysfunction of the spleen, severely immunosuppressed patients, or those with nephrotic syndrome. However there is some evidence that earlier revaccination may be needed in these groups.[24] Revaccination may be considered after 3 to 5 years for children at highest risk of pneumococcal infection who would be aged 10 years or under at revaccination.[20]

The increase in pneumococci resistant to antibacterials makes the development of vaccines with improved immunogenicity, especially in young children, more important.[26] Of the possible **new vaccines**, conjugate vaccines are at the most advanced stage of development. Technical difficulties in conjugation mean that most conjugate vaccines currently being studied use a subset of the 23 serotypes present in the polysaccharide vaccine.[26] Nevertheless clinical studies have shown that conjugate vaccines can produce an immune response in children under 2 years of age,[27,28] but immunogenicity in a group of healthy adults was no better than that obtained with conventional vaccines.[29]

1. LaForce FM, Eickhoff TC. Pneumococcal vaccine: an emerging consensus. *Ann Intern Med* 1988; **108:** 757–9.
2. Noah ND. Vaccination against pneumococcal infection. *Br Med J* 1988; **297:** 1351–2.
3. Anonymous. When to use the new pneumococcal vaccine. *Drug Ther Bull* 1990; **28:** 31–2.
4. Shann F. Modern vaccines: pneumococcus and influenza. *Lancet* 1990; **335:** 898–901.
5. Gaillat J, *et al.* Essai clinique du vaccin antipneumococcique chez des personnes âgées vivant en institution. *Rev Epidemiol Sante Publique* 1985; **33:** 437–44.
6. Bolan G, *et al.* Pneumococcal vaccine efficacy in selected populations in the United States. *Ann Intern Med* 1986; **104:** 1–6.
7. Sims RV, *et al.* The clinical effectiveness of pneumococcal vaccine in the elderly. *Ann Intern Med* 1988; **108:** 653–7.
8. Forrester HL, *et al.* Inefficacy of pneumococcal vaccine in a high-risk population. *Am J Med* 1987; **83:** 425–30.
9. Simberkoff MS, *et al.* Efficacy of pneumococcal vaccine in high-risk patients: results of a Veterans Administration Cooperative Study. *N Engl J Med* 1986; **315:** 1318–27.
10. Lee H, *et al.* Immunogenicity and safety of a 23-valent pneumococcal polysaccharide vaccine in healthy children and in children at increased risk of pneumococcal infection. *Vaccine* 1995; **13:** 1533–8.
11. Farr BM, *et al.* Preventing pneumococcal bacteremia in patients at risk. *Arch Intern Med* 1995; **155:** 2336–8.
12. Sankilampi U, *et al.* Antibody response to pneumococcal capsular polysaccharide vaccine in the elderly. *J Infect Dis* 1996; **173:** 387–93.
13. Furth SL, *et al.* Pneumococcal polysaccharide vaccine in children with chronic renal disease: a prospective study of antibody response and duration. *J Pediatr* 1996; **128:** 99–101.
14. Örtqvist Å, *et al.* Randomised trial of 23-valent pneumococcal capsular polysaccharide vaccine in prevention of pneumonia in middle-aged and elderly people. *Lancet* 1998; **351:** 399–403.
15. Williams WW, *et al.* Immunization policies and vaccine coverage among adults: the risk for missed opportunities. *Ann Intern Med* 1988; **108:** 616–25.
16. Kinnersley P, *et al.* Pneumococcal vaccination after splenectomy: survey of hospital and primary care records. *Br Med J* 1993; **307:** 1398–9.
17. Deodhar HA, *et al.* Increased risk of sepsis after splenectomy. *Br Med J* 1993; **307:** 1408–9.
18. Hirschman JV, Lipsky BA. The pneumococcal vaccine after 15 years of use. *Arch Intern Med* 1994; **154:** 373–7.
19. Butler JC, *et al.* Pneumococcal polysaccharide vaccine efficacy: an evaluation of current recommendations. *JAMA* 1993; **270:** 1826–31.
20. Centers for Disease Control. Prevention of pneumococcal disease: recommendations of the Advisory Committee on Immunization Practices (ACIP). *MMWR* 1997; **46** (RR-8): 1–24.
21. Fedson D, *et al.* WHO recommendations on pneumococcal vaccination: immunization of elderly people with polyvalent pneumococcal vaccine. *Infection* 1989; **17:** 437–41.
22. Steven N, Wright P. Pneumococcal immunisation and the healthy elderly. *Lancet* 1992; **340:** 1036–7. Correction. *ibid.*: 1236.
23. Neal K. Pneumococcal immunisation and the healthy elderly. *Lancet* 1993; **341:** 319.
24. Anonymous. The place of pneumococcal vaccination. *Drug Ther Bull* 1998; **36:** 73–6.
25. Bruyn GAW. Pneumococcal immunisation and the healthy elderly. *Lancet* 1992; **340:** 1418.
26. Stephenson J. Conjugate vaccines hold hope for countering resistant pneumococcus. *JAMA* 1995; **274:** 1327–8.
27. Anderson EL, *et al.* Immunogenicity of heptavalent pneumococcal vaccine in infants. *J Pediatr* 1996; **128:** 649–53.
28. King JC, *et al.* Safety and immunogenicity of three doses of a five-valent pneumococcal vaccine in children younger than two years with and without human immunodeficiency virus infection. *Pediatrics* 1997; **99:** 575–80.
29. Powers DC, *et al.* Reactogenicity and immunogenicity of a protein-conjugated pneumococcal oligosaccharide vaccine in older adults. *J Infect Dis* 1996; **173:** 1014–18.

Preparations

Ph. Eur.: Pneumococcal Polysaccharide Vaccine.

Proprietary Preparations (details are given in Part 3)
Aust.: Pneumovax; ***Austral.:*** Pneumovax 23; ***Belg.:*** Pneumovax 23; Pneumune; ***Canad.:*** Pneumovax 23; ***Fr.:*** Pneumo 23; ***Ger.:*** Pneumovax 23; ***Irl.:*** Pneumovax II; ***Ital.:*** Pneumo 23; ***Neth.:*** Pneumune; ***Norw.:*** Pneumovax; ***S.Afr.:*** Pneumovax 23; ***Swed.:*** Pneumovax; Pnu-Imune; ***Switz.:*** Pneumovax 23; ***UK:*** Pneumovax II; Pnu-Imune; ***USA:*** Pneumovax 23; Pnu-Imune 23.

Poliomyelitis Vaccines (7992-e)

Polio Vaccines; Poliovirus Vaccines.

NOTE. Inactivated poliomyelitis vaccines are sometimes termed Salk Vaccine and live (oral) poliomyelitis vaccines are sometimes termed Sabin Vaccine.

Poliomyelitis Vaccine (Inactivated) (Ph. Eur.) (Pol/Vac(Inact); Inactivated Poliomyelitis Vaccine (BP 1998); Vaccinum Poliomyelitidis Inactivatum) is a sterile aqueous suspension of suitable strains of poliomyelitis virus, types 1, 2, and 3, grown in suitable cell cultures and inactivated by a suitable method. Permitted antibiotics may be used in its production and it may contain preservatives. It should be stored at 2° to 8°, not be allowed to freeze, and be protected from light.

Poliovirus Vaccine Inactivated (USP 23) is a sterile aqueous suspension of poliomyelitis virus, types 1, 2, and 3, grown in cultures of monkey kidney tissue and inactivated. Suitable antimicrobial agents may be used during production. It should be stored at 2° to 8°.

Poliomyelitis Vaccine (Oral) (Ph. Eur.) (OPV; Pol/Vac (Oral); Poliomyelitis Vaccine, Live (Oral) (BP 1998); Vaccinum Poliomyelitidis Perorale) is an aqueous suspension of suitable live attenuated strains of poliomyelitis virus, types 1, 2, or 3, grown in suitable, approved cell cultures; it may contain any one of the 3 virus types or combinations of them. The trivalent vaccine is standardised for virus titre which is not less than 1×10^6 $CCID_{50}$ for type 1, not less than 1×10^5 $CCID_{50}$ for type 2, and not less than $1 \times 10^{5.5}$ $CCID_{50}$ for type 3 per dose. Permitted antibiotics may be used in its production. It should be stored at 2° to 8°, not be allowed to freeze, and be protected from light.

Poliovirus Vaccine Live Oral (USP 23) is a preparation of a combination of the 3 types of suitable live attenuated polioviruses, grown in cultures of monkey kidney tissue. It contains not less than $10^{5.4}$ to $10^{6.4}$ virus titre for type 1, not less than $10^{4.5}$ to $10^{5.5}$ for type 2, and not less than $10^{5.2}$ to $10^{6.2}$ for type 3 per dose. It should be stored at 2° to 8° or in the frozen state. The vaccine should not be thawed and refrozen more than 10 times.

Adverse Effects

As for vaccines in general, p.1500.

Vaccine-associated poliomyelitis has been reported in a small number of recipients of oral poliomyelitis vaccines and in contacts of recipients.

Effects on the nervous system. Case reports of the isolation of poliovaccine virus from the CSF after administration of oral poliomyelitis vaccine.

1. Rantala H, *et al.* Poliovaccine virus in the cerebrospinal fluid after oral polio vaccination. *J Infect* 1989; **19:** 173–6.
2. Gutierrez K, Abzug MJ. Vaccine-associated poliovirus meningitis in children with ventriculoperitoneal shunts. *J Pediatr* 1990; **117:** 424–7.

GUILLAIN-BARRÉ SYNDROME. A small cluster of cases of Guillain-Barré syndrome has been observed in children after a mass poliomyelitis vaccination campaign in Finland in 1985.[1] An increased frequency of Guillain-Barré syndrome was also seen in adults. However, a direct link with poliovaccine virus infection could not be established and no link between Guillain-Barré syndrome and oral polio vaccine was revealed by a subsequent, epidemiological study in California.[2]

1. Uhari M, *et al.* Cluster of childhood Guillain-Barré cases after an oral poliovaccine campaign. *Lancet* 1989; **ii:** 440–1.
2. Rantala H, *et al.* Epidemiology of Guillain-Barré syndrome in children: relationship of oral polio vaccine administration to occurrence. *J Pediatr* 1994; **124:** 220–3.

PARALYTIC POLIOMYELITIS. A survey of the incidence of paralytic poliomyelitis following vaccination conducted by WHO[1] reported that, in all but one of the 13 participating countries, the risk was 0.03 per million vaccine recipients. The incidence was least with the use of type 1 strains and greatest with type 3 strains. Paralytic poliomyelitis in contacts of vaccine recipients could be further reduced by ensuring that parents without evidence of previous immunisation receive the vaccine at the same time as their children. The risk of vaccine-associated paralytic poliomyelitis may be increased in immunocompromised patients.

Until recently there has been no satisfactory explanation of the high risk of paralytic poliomyelitis found in Romania by the WHO survey.[1] A case-control study[2] identified intramuscular injections given within 30 days of polio vaccination as a risk factor in the development of paralytic poliomyelitis. This phenomenon, known as provocation paralysis or provocation poliomyelitis has been described with the wild virus[3] and more recently has been recognised as a factor in vaccine-associated paralysis in the UK and USA.[4] Romanian children may be further predisposed to vaccine-associated paralysis because the first dose of polio vaccine is delayed until two to seven months of age, by which time they possess little or no residual maternal antibody.[5]

In the USA, where the majority of cases of clinical poliomyelitis are associated with vaccination, there is evidence that the incidence is still falling.[6-8]

1. Esteves K. Safety of oral poliomyelitis vaccine: results of a WHO enquiry. *Bull WHO* 1988; **66:** 739–46.
2. Strebel PM, *et al.* Intramuscular injections within 30 days of immunization with oral poliovirus vaccine—a risk factor for vaccine-associated paralytic poliomyelitis. *N Engl J Med* 1995; **332:** 500–6.
3. Anonymous. Provocation paralysis. *Lancet* 1992; **340:** 1005–6.
4. Wyatt HV. Vaccine-associated poliomyelitis. *Lancet* 1994; **343:** 610.
5. Wright PF, Karzon DT. Minimizing the risks associated with the prevention of poliomyelitis. *N Engl J Med* 1995; **332:** 529–30.
6. Nkowane BM, *et al.* Vaccine-associated paralytic poliomyelitis. United States: 1973 through 1984. *JAMA* 1987; **257:** 1335–40.
7. Centers for Disease Control. Paralytic poliomyelitis—United States, 1980-1994. *MMWR* 1997; **46:** 79–83.
8. Sepkowitz S. Vaccine-associated paralytic poliomyelitis. *Pediatrics* 1997; **99:** 145.

Precautions

As for vaccines in general, p.1501.

Oral poliomyelitis vaccine may contain trace amounts of penicillin, neomycin, polymyxin, and streptomycin and the inactivated vaccine may contain trace amounts of neomycin and polymyxin: both should be used with caution in patients with severe hypersensitivity to these antibiotics.

Oral poliomyelitis vaccines should not be given to patients with diarrhoea or vomiting.

Because the vaccine virus of oral poliomyelitis vaccines is excreted in the faeces for up to 6 weeks, the contacts of recently vaccinated babies and infants should be advised of the need for strict personal hygiene, particularly hand washing after napkin changing, in order to reduce the possibility of infection in unimmunised contacts. Unimmunised adults can be immunised at the same time as their children.

Immunocompromised patients are at increased risk of developing vaccine-associated paralytic poliomyelitis. Oral poliomyelitis vaccines should not be given to immunosuppressed patients or their household contacts and in these persons an inactivated vaccine should be used (see under Uses and Administration, below). Asymptomatic HIV-positive persons may receive oral poliomyelitis vaccines but faecal excretion of the vaccine virus may continue for longer than in uninfected individuals. For symptomatic HIV-positive persons the use of inactivated poliomyelitis vaccine may be considered.

Intramuscular injections given after the oral vaccine may also increase the risk of vaccine-associated paralytic poliomyelitis (see above).

Pregnancy. Live vaccines such as *oral poliomyelitis vaccines* are generally contra-indicated in pregnancy because of a theoretical risk to the fetus. Population-wide mass vaccination programmes become impossible, however, if pregnant mothers and women of childbearing age are to be excluded.[1] In February 1985 mass vaccination with live oral poliomyelitis vaccine was started during a poliomyelitis outbreak in Finland.[1] Pregnant women were advised to take the vaccine. An analysis of all reported congenital malformations in the years 1982 to 1986 suggested that oral poliomyelitis vaccine had no harmful effects on fetal development as measured by overall prevalence of malformations or as the incidence of either CNS or orofacial defects. The results do not, however, exclude an effect measurable by other criteria of fetal development; further analysis will examine the possible increase in rare types of congenital defect.

The incidence of spontaneous abortions was measured during a mass poliomyelitis vaccination campaign in Israel.[2] The number of spontaneous abortions did not differ between controls and women vaccinated during the first trimester of pregnancy; the percentage of spontaneous abortions in relation to live births was also similar. Microscopic examination of placentas from spontaneous abortions indicated no effect of oral poliomyelitis vaccine on the frequency or type of pathological changes. In addition, subsequent epidemiological study[3] found no increases in congenital malformations or in premature births during the period of and immediately following the vaccination campaign compared with those born before the campaign.

The Collaborative Perinatal Project in the USA followed up 50 897 pregnancies to examine risk factors for the development of malignancies in offspring born between 1959 and 1966.[4] In 18 342 children whose mothers were vaccinated during pregnancy with *inactivated poliomyelitis vaccines* there were 14 malignancies (7.6 per 10 000) and in 32 555 non-exposed children there were 10 malignancies (3.1 per 10 000). There were 7 tumours derived from neural tissue in the exposed children (3.8 per 10 000) and one in non-exposed children (0.3 per 10 000). Thus there was an excess of neural tumours but not of leukaemias or other malignancies in children exposed *in utero* to inactivated poliomyelitis vaccine. No malignancies occurred among the children born to 3056 women who received oral poliomyelitis vaccine. Serum samples collected from mothers on entry into the Collaborative Perinatal Project and at delivery have subsequently been analysed for the presence of antibodies to Simian virus 40 (SV40).[5] None of the serum samples from 8 mothers of infants with neural tumours had antibodies to SV40. Two of the 7 mothers of infants with leukaemia had SV40 antibodies, but only one had conversion during pregnancy. None of the samples from the 7 mothers of children with other types of cancer had antibodies. Three of 36 controls had antibodies, but in both the first and second samples. The association between administration of inactivated poliomyelitis vaccine to mothers and neural tumours in their offspring could not be attributed to contamination of vaccine with SV40.

1. Harjulehto T, *et al.* Congenital malformations and oral poliovirus vaccination during pregnancy. *Lancet* 1989; **i:** 771–2.
2. Ornoy A, *et al.* Spontaneous abortions following oral poliovirus vaccination in first trimester. *Lancet* 1990; **i:** 800.
3. Ornoy A, Ben Ishai P. Congenital anomalies after oral poliovirus vaccination during pregnancy. *Lancet* 1993; **341:** 1162.
4. Heinonen OP, *et al.* Immunization during pregnancy against poliomyelitis and influenza in relation to childhood malignancy. *Int J Epidemiol* 1973; **2:** 229–35.
5. Rosa FW, *et al.* Absence of antibody response to simian virus 40 after inoculation with killed-poliovirus vaccine of mothers of offspring with neurologic tumors. *N Engl J Med* 1988; **318:** 1469.

Interactions

As for vaccines in general, p.1501.

Normal immunoglobulins. Although the concurrent administration of live vaccines and immunoglobulins is generally not recommended, normal immunoglobulin had no effect on the antibody response to oral poliomyelitis vaccine when the 2 preparations were given simultaneously to 50 subjects.[1]

1. Green MS, *et al.* Response to trivalent oral poliovirus vaccine with and without immune serum globulin in young adults in Israel in 1988. *J Infect Dis* 1990; **162:** 971–4.

Pertussis vaccines. For a report of a diminished immune response to the pertussis component of diphtheria, tetanus, and pertussis vaccine when mixed with inactivated poliomyelitis vaccine, see Pertussis Vaccines, p.1526.

Uses and Administration

Poliomyelitis vaccines are used for active immunisation against poliomyelitis. For discussion of immunisation schedules see under Vaccines, p.1501. Both live (oral) poliomyelitis vaccines and inactivated poliomyelitis vaccines are available. The oral vaccine stimulates the formation of antibodies both in the blood and in the mucosal tissues of the gastro-intestinal tract.

In the UK an oral poliomyelitis vaccine, containing the three types of poliovirus (trivalent), is recommended for the primary immunisation of all age groups, given as a course of 3 doses at intervals of 4 weeks. The dose of the oral poliomyelitis vaccine is dropped directly into the mouth of an infant or given on a sugar lump to older children and adults. For children who received primary immunisation during infancy reinforcing doses of the oral vaccine are recommended at school entry and before leaving school. Further reinforcing doses are necessary only in adults exposed to infection including travellers to countries where poliomyelitis is epidemic or endemic and health care workers in contact with poliomyelitis cases. A single dose is given, repeated every 10 years if necessary.

In the USA, either the oral or the inactivated vaccine may be used for primary immunisation. In 1997, the controversial decision was made to recommend the use of inactivated vaccine for the first two doses given at 2 and 4 months of age, completing immunisation with two doses of oral vaccine given at between 12 and 18 months, and at 4 to 6 years of age. See below for further discussion.

On the occurrence of a single case of paralytic poliomyelitis from wild virus, a single dose of the oral vaccine is recommended for all persons in the neighbourhood, regardless of whether they have previously been immunised. A primary course should be completed in previously unimmunised individuals. Immunisation of contacts is unnecessary in the case of vaccine-associated infections.

Inactivated poliomyelitis vaccine is recommended in the UK for the immunisation of persons in whom the use of the live oral vaccine is contra-indicated; inactivated vaccine, rather than the live oral vaccine, is also recommended for contacts of immunosuppressed persons and may be considered for symptomatic HIV-positive individuals. The inactivated vaccine is given by subcutaneous injection in a dose of 0.5 mL using a similar dosage schedule to the oral vaccine.

Choice of vaccine. In the USA, both oral and inactivated poliomyelitis vaccines (OPV and IPV respectively) are available for primary immunisation. Three schedule options, each involving a total of four doses of vaccine at or before school entry, are available to physicians:[1]

- sequential IPV and OPV (2 doses of IPV at 2 and 4 months of age, followed by 2 doses of OPV at 12 to 18 months and 4 to 6 years) is intended to minimise the risk of vaccine associated paralytic poliomyelitis (VAPP) while producing adequate intestinal immunity
- IPV only (dose intervals as above) is recommended when OPV is contra-indicated and to reduce the risk of VAPP in unimmunised household contacts of the vaccine recipient
- OPV only (when the third dose may be given 2 months after the second dose) is recommended when rapid immunisation is necessary, for example in older children, or in areas where vaccine uptake is low. It also has the advantage of requiring no injections.

In 1996, the Advisory Committee on Immunization Practices of the Centers for Disease Control and Prevention recommended that the sequential IPV and OPV schedule should be preferred on the basis that, while there had been no cases of poliomyelitis from wild poliovirus in the USA since 1979, 8 to 10 cases of VAPP continued to occur each year.[2,3] This decision has been criticised by commentators both in the USA and elsewhere. Objections raised include the lack of experience with the recommended combined schedule, the lack of evidence that it will reduce the incidence of VAPP, and a possible reduction in compliance because of the increased number of injections needed.[4] Added to this is the greater cost of IPV than OPV which may further reduce compliance and has raised doubts over the cost-effectiveness of the strategy.[5,6]

Commenting on the change for WHO, Hull and Lee[7] stressed the necessity of the continued use of OPV for global eradication of poliomyelitis (see below). WHO was concerned that the change in US policy could be interpreted as implying that OPV alone is ineffective or unsafe, and might lead to the adoption of inappropriate vaccine policies in countries where wild polio still exists. The continued use of OPV for the global eradication strategy was endorsed by the American Academy of Pediatrics.[2]

1. Committee on Infectious Diseases, American Academy of Pediatrics. Poliomyelitis prevention: recommendations for use of inactivated poliovirus vaccine and live oral poliovirus vaccine. *Pediatrics* 1997; **99:** 300–305.
2. Marwick C. Switch to inactivated polio vaccine recommended. *JAMA* 1996; **276:** 89.
3. Katz SL. Poliovaccine policy—time for a change. *Pediatrics* 1996; **98:** 116–17.
4. Judelsohn R. Changing the US polio immunization schedule would be bad public health policy. *Pediatrics* 1996; **98:** 115–16.
5. Miller MA, *et al.* Cost-effectiveness of incorporating inactivated poliovirus vaccine into the routine childhood immunization schedule. *JAMA* 1996; **276:** 967–71.
6. Schneider S. The new immunization debate. *Pediatrics* 1996; **98:** 795.
7. Hull HF, Lee JW. Sabine, Salk, or sequential? *Lancet* 1996; **347:** 630.

Eradication of infection. Considerable progress has been made towards the WHO goal of eradicating poliomyelitis by the year 2000.[1] Nevertheless, sporadic outbreaks of disease in unimmunised or inadequately immunised populations[2,3] are reminders of the importance of maintaining the momentum of the WHO campaign.

The WHO campaign depends on four strategies:[1]

- routine immunisation—although routine immunisation alone cannot eliminate polio, it remains the foundation of eradication policy
- national immunisation days—regular (usually annual) nationwide immunisation of all children under 5 years of age regardless of immunisation history
- immunisation after an outbreak—all children under 5 years of age living in the vicinity of a suspected case receive one dose of oral vaccine
- mopping-up immunisation—house-to-house immunisation of children in high-risk areas to reach children missed during routine immunisation or national immunisation days.

WHO has consistently argued for the continued use of oral poliomyelitis vaccine (OPV) rather than inactivated vaccine (IPV) in immunisation schedules. The main argument must be the proven efficacy of repeated doses of OPV to abort outbreaks[4] and eliminate wild virus entirely, notably in South America.[1] Other advantages include the rapid induction of both humoral and intestinal immunity which is necessary to interrupt wild virus transmission; passive transfer of vaccine virus to non-immunised individuals improving population immunity; ease of administration by non-medical personnel; and the low cost of OPV.[5]

OPV produces a lower rate of seroconversion in developing countries than in developed countries, typically needing at least 5 doses to produce an adequate response.[1] There have been reports of poliomyelitis occurring in children who have completed a three-dose course of OPV.[6-8] Possible reasons for this suboptimal response include high levels of maternal antibodies, inhibition of types 1 and 3 viruses by type 2, interference from competing enteroviruses, and diarrhoea.[1,9] Mass immunisation campaigns are reported to produce a higher immune response than equivalent doses given in the routine schedule, and are seen as an essential adjunct to routine immunisation.[10] Seroconversion rates are highest when the vaccine is administered during mass campaigns in the cool and dry season.[1]

There have been several advocates of IPV either as an alternative or in addition to OPV. Most cite the higher immunogenicity of IPV and its successful use in some (mainly industrialised) countries.[11,12] Combined IPV and OPV schedules have been shown to produce high levels of humoral immunity, with intestinal immunity equivalent to that produced by OPV alone.[13] The use of combined IPV and OPV schedules in countries which have not eliminated the wild virus could improve the effectiveness of routine vaccination schedules.[11,14] In the USA, a combined schedule is advocated to reduce vaccine associated paralytic poliomyelitis while still providing protection against transmission of imported wild virus (see above).

However, most cases of poliomyelitis in endemic countries occur among unimmunised children and the main priority remains to improve vaccine uptake rather than to alter immunisation schedules.[1,15] There is concern that uncertainty fostered by a change in vaccination policy could be interpreted as implying that OPV alone is ineffective or unsafe, and the central message that high uptake of vaccine is essential could be lost.[5]

1. Hull HF, *et al.* Paralytic poliomyelitis: seasoned strategies, disappearing disease. *Lancet* 1994; **343:** 1331–7.
2. van Niekerk ABW, *et al.* Outbreak of paralytic poliomyelitis in Namibia. *Lancet* 1994; **344:** 661–4.
3. Oostvogel PM, *et al.* Poliomyelitis outbreak in an unvaccinated community in the Netherlands, 1992-93. *Lancet* 1994; **344:** 665–70.
4. Greco D, *et al.* Poliomyelitis vaccination strategies for Europe. *Lancet* 1997; **349:** 437.
5. Hull HF, Lee JW. Sabine, Salk, or sequential? *Lancet* 1996; **347:** 630.
6. Sutter RW, *et al.* Outbreak of paralytic poliomyelitis in Oman: evidence for widespread transmission among fully vaccinated children. *Lancet* 1991; **338:** 715–20.
7. Samuel R, *et al.* Persisting poliomyelitis after high coverage with oral poliovaccine. *Lancet* 1993; **341:** 903.
8. Mudur G. Flawed immunisation policies in India led to polio paralysis. *Br Med J* 1998; **316:** 1264.
9. WHO Collaborative Study Group on Oral Poliovirus Vaccine. Factors affecting the immunogenicity of oral poliovirus vaccine: a prospective evaluation in Brazil and the Gambia. *J Infect Dis* 1995; **171:** 1097–1106.
10. Richardson G, *et al.* Immunogenicity of oral poliovirus vaccine administered in mass campaigns versus routine immunization programmes. *Bull WHO* 1995; **73:** 769–77.
11. Patriarca PA, *et al.* Progress in polio eradication. *Lancet* 1993; **342:** 1461–4.
12. Preston NW. Polio eradication. *Lancet* 1994; **344:** 1163
13. WHO Collaborative Study Group on Oral and Inactivated Poliovirus Vaccines. Combined immunization of infants with oral and inactivated poliovirus vaccines: results of a randomized trial in the Gambia, Oman, and Thailand. *Bull WHO* 1996; **75:** 253–68.
14. Moriniere BJ, *et al.* Immunogenicity of a supplemental dose of oral versus inactivated poliomyelitis vaccine. *Lancet* 1993; **341:** 1545–50.
15. Chander J, Subrahmanyan S. Mass polio vaccination. *Br Med J* 1996; **312:** 1178–9.

Preparations

Ph. Eur.: Poliomyelitis Vaccine (Inactivated); Poliomyelitis Vaccine (Oral);
USP 23: Poliovirus Vaccine Inactivated; Poliovirus Vaccine Live Oral.

Proprietary Preparations (details are given in Part 3)
Aust.: Buccapol†; ***Austral.:*** Enpovax HDC; Ipol; ***Belg.:*** Imovax Polio; Sabin; ***Ger.:*** Oral-Virelon; Polio-Vaccinol; Virelon C; ***Ital.:*** Imovax Polio; Polio Sabin (Orale); Polioral; ***Norw.:*** Imovax Polio; ***S.Afr.:*** OPV-Merieux; Polioral; ***Spain:*** Vac Antipolio Or; Vac Antipolio Oral; Vac Polio Sabin; Vac Poliomielitica; ***Swed.:*** Imovax Polio; ***Switz.:*** Poloral; ***USA:*** Ipol; Orimune.

Pseudomonas Immunoglobulins (11611-t)

Preparations containing antibodies against *Pseudomonas aeruginosa* are available in some countries for passive immunisation against severe pseudomonal infections.

Preparations

Proprietary Preparations (details are given in Part 3)
Ger.: Psomaglobin N†.

Pseudomonas Vaccines (7993-l)

A number of polyvalent *Pseudomonas aeruginosa* conjugate vaccines are under investigation for the prevention of pseudomonal infections in a variety of disease states.

References.

1. Schaad UB, *et al.* Safety and immunogenicity of Pseudomonas aeruginosa conjugate A vaccine in cystic fibrosis. *Lancet* 1991; **338:** 1236–7.
2. Cryz SJ, *et al.* Immunization of noncolonized cystic fibrosis patients against Pseudomonas aeruginosa. *J Infect Dis* 1994; **169:** 1159–62.
3. Lang AB, *et al.* Effect of high-affinity anti-Pseudomonas aeruginosa lipopolysaccharide antibodies induced by immunization on the rate of Pseudomonas aeruginosa infection in patients with cystic fibrosis. *J Pediatr* 1995; **127:** 711–17.
4. Campbell WN, *et al.* Immunogenicity of a 24-valent Klebsiella capsular polysaccharide vaccine and an eight-valent Pseudomonas O-polysaccharide conjugate vaccine administered to victims of acute trauma. *Clin Infect Dis* 1996; **23:** 179–81.

Q Fever Vaccines (16972-z)

A Q fever vaccine consisting of a purified killed suspension of *Coxiella burnetii* is available in Australia. It is prepared from Phase I Henzerling strain of *C. burnetii* grown in the yolk sacs of embryonated eggs. A single 0.5-mL subcutaneous dose is given for active immunisation in individuals at high risk of Q fever. These include abattoir workers, veterinarians, and laboratory workers handling potentially infected tissue.

References.

1. Kazár J, *et al.* Immunogenicity and reactogenicity of a Q fever chemovaccine in persons professionally exposed to Q fever in Czechoslovakia. *Bull WHO* 1982; **60:** 389–94.
2. Marmion BP, *et al.* Vaccine prophylaxis of abattoir-associated Q fever. *Lancet* 1984; **ii:** 1411–14.

Preparations

Proprietary Preparations (details are given in Part 3)
Austral.: Q-Vax.

Rabies Antisera (7995-j)

Antirabies Serum (USP 23) is a sterile solution containing antiviral substances obtained from the serum or plasma of a healthy animal, usually the horse, that has been immunised by vaccine against rabies. It contains a suitable antimicrobial agent. It should be stored at 2° to 8°.

Adverse Effects and Precautions

As for antisera in general, p.1500.

A skin test should be carried out before rabies antisera are administered.

Hypersensitivity. In a retrospective study[1] of 3156 patients who received rabies antisera, 51 (1.6%) developed one or more symptoms or signs characteristic of serum sickness. All patients recovered within 7 days of the onset of the reaction. There was a higher incidence of serum-sickness-like reactions in females and individuals aged over 21 years. An immediate hypersensitivity reaction occurred in only one patient. The low incidence of adverse reactions compared with earlier studies may be attributed to the reduced protein content of the preparation used.

1. Wilde H, *et al.* Purified equine rabies immune globulin: a safe and affordable alternative to human rabies immune globulin. *Bull WHO* 1989; **67:** 731–6.

Uses and Administration

Rabies antisera have been used to provide passive immunisation against rabies but the use of rabies immunoglobulins (see below) is preferred.

Preparations

USP 23: Antirabies Serum.

Rabies Immunoglobulins (1239-f)

Human Rabies Immunoglobulin (Ph. Eur.) (Antirabies Immunoglobulin Injection; Rabies Immunoglobulin (BP 1998); Immunoglobulinum Humanum Rabicum) is a liquid or freeze-dried preparation containing human immunoglobulins, mainly immunoglobulin G (IgG). It is obtained from plasma from donors immunised against rabies and contains specific antibodies that neutralise the rabies virus. Normal immunoglobulin may be added. It contains not less than 150 international units per mL. The liquid preparation should be stored, protected from light, in a colourless, glass container. The freeze-dried preparation should be stored, protected from light, in a colourless, glass container, under vacuum or under an inert gas.

Rabies Immune Globulin (USP 23) is a sterile solution of globulins derived from plasma or serum from selected adult human donors who have been immunised with rabies vaccine and have developed high titres of rabies antibody. It contains 10 to 18% of protein of which not less than 80% is monomeric immunoglobulin G. It contains glycine as a stabilising agent, and a suitable preservative. A solution diluted to contain 1% of protein has a pH of 6.4 to 7.2. It should be stored at 2° to 8°.

Adverse Effects and Precautions

As for immunoglobulins in general, p.1500.

Uses and Administration

Rabies immunoglobulins are used for passive immunisation against rabies. They are used in conjunction with active immunisation with rabies vaccines (see below) as part of the postexposure treatment for the prevention of rabies in previously unimmunised persons who have been bitten by rabid animals or animals suspected of being rabid. The recommended dose of rabies immunoglobulin is 20 international units per kg body-weight, up to half of which should be infiltrated around the wound with the remainder being given intramuscularly at a different site to that at which the vaccine was administered.

Preparations

Ph. Eur.: Human Rabies Immunoglobulin;
USP 23: Rabies Immune Globulin.

Proprietary Preparations (details are given in Part 3)
Aust.: Berirab; Lyssagam†; Rabuman; ***Austral.:*** Hyperab†; Imogam; ***Canad.:*** Hyperab; Imogam; ***Ger.:*** Berirab; Hyperab†; Tollwutglobulin; ***Ital.:*** Haimarab; Rabuman; ***S.Afr.:*** Rabigam; ***Spain:*** Imogam Rabia; Inmunogamma Antirrabica†; Lyssuman; ***Switz.:*** Rabuman; ***USA:*** Hyperab; Imogam Rabies.

Rabies Vaccines (7997-c)

Rabies Vaccine for Human Use Prepared in Cell Cultures (Ph. Eur.) (Rab/Vac; Rabies Vaccine (BP 1998); Vaccinum Rabiei ex Cellulis ad Usum Humanum) is a sterile freeze-dried suspension of inactivated rabies virus; a suitable strain is grown in an approved cell culture. The cell-culture medium may contain suitable antibiotics at the smallest effective concentration. The vaccine is prepared immediately before use by the addition of a suitable sterile liquid. The estimated potency is not less than 2.5 international units per dose. The dried vaccine should be stored at 2° to 8°, not be allowed to freeze, and be protected from light.

Rabies Vaccine (USP 23) is a sterile preparation, in dried or liquid form, of inactivated rabies virus obtained from inoculated diploid cell cultures. It has a potency of not less than 2.5 units per dose. It should be stored at 2° to 8°.

Adverse Effects and Precautions

As for vaccines in general, p.1500.

Patients may experience pain, erythema, and induration at the injection site after the use of any type of rabies vaccine; nausea, headache, fever, malaise, or myalgia may also occur. Hypersensitivity reactions including anaphylaxis occur more commonly with vaccines prepared from non-human sources than with human diploid-cell vaccine.

Neuroparalytic reactions (transverse myelitis, neuropathy, or encephalopathy) have been associated with the use of animal brain-tissue vaccines and, to a lesser extent with duck-embryo vaccines.

There are only isolated reports of neurological reactions after administration of human diploid-cell vaccines.

Effects on the nervous system. The incidence of neuroparalytic accidents following a course of nerve-tissue vaccines is known to vary from country to country.[1] The risk of CNS damage associated with the use of rabies vaccines prepared in the brains of adult animals has been stated to be about 1 in 2000 doses administered.[2] Paralytic accidents have occurred much less frequently with vaccines produced from brain tissue of mice younger than 9 days of age compared with older animals[1] and a particularly high risk of neurological complications has been observed with a sheep-brain vaccine.[3]

Neuroparalytic reactions occur less frequently with duck-embryo than nerve-tissue vaccines.[1] In an estimated 424 000 patients receiving duck-embryo rabies vaccine in the USA from 1958 to 1971 there were 137 reports of minor transient neurological reactions, 4 of transverse myelitis, 5 of neuropathy, and 4 of encephalopathy (2 fatal).[4]

There are only isolated reports of neuroparalytic reactions associated with human diploid-cell vaccines.[5,6]

1. WHO. WHO expert committee on rabies: seventh report. *WHO Tech Rep Ser 709* 1984.
2. WHO. WHO expert committee on biological standardization: thirty-seventh report. *WHO Tech Rep Ser 760* 1987.
3. Swaddiwuthipong W, *et al.* A high rate of neurological complications following Semple anti-rabies vaccine. *Trans R Soc Trop Med Hyg* 1988; **82:** 472–5.
4. Rubin RH, *et al.* Adverse reactions to duck embryo rabies vaccine: range and incidence. *Ann Intern Med* 1973; **78:** 643–9.
5. Knittel T, *et al.* Guillain-Barré syndrome and human diploid cell rabies vaccine. *Lancet* 1989; **i:** 1334–5.
6. Tornatore CS, Richert JR. CNS demyelination associated with diploid cell rabies vaccine. *Lancet* 1990; **335:** 1346–7.

Hypersensitivity. An analysis of cases of systemic hypersensitivity reactions following immunisation with human diploid-cell rabies vaccine reported to the Centers for Disease Control in the USA over the period June 1980 to March 1984.[1] Of the 108 reports received, classification, on the basis of clinical observation, revealed 9 cases of presumed type I immediate hypersensitivity (incidence of 1 in 10 000 vaccinees), 87 cases of presumed type III hypersensitivity (9 in 10 000 vaccinees), and 12 cases of indeterminate type. All the reactions presumed to be type I occurred during either primary pre- or postexposure immunisation whereas 93% of the presumed type III reactions were observed following booster immunisations. Presenting features of the type III reaction included generalised or pruritic rash or urticaria, angioedema, arthralgias, fever, nausea, vomiting, and malaise.

1. Centers for Disease Control. Systemic allergic reactions following immunization with HDCV. *JAMA* 1984; **251:** 2194–5.

Spongiform encephalopathies. Possible transmission of Creutzfeldt-Jakob disease associated with sheep-brain rabies vaccine has been reported from India.[1] It was suggested that transmission of the abnormal prion protein from sheep with scrapie could be implicated.

1. Arya SC. Acquisition of spongiform encephalopathies in India through sheep-brain rabies vaccination. *Natl Med J India* 1992; **4:** 311–12.

Interactions

As for vaccines in general, p.1501.

Antimalarials. Studies suggesting that continuous antimalarial chemoprophylaxis with chloroquine during primary immunisation with human diploid-cell rabies vaccine administered intradermally for pre-exposure prophylaxis may be associated with a poor antibody response.[1,2]

1. Taylor DN, *et al.* Chloroquine prophylaxis associated with a poor antibody response to human diploid cell rabies vaccine. *Lancet* 1984; **i:** 1405.
2. Pappaioanou M, *et al.* Antibody response to preexposure human diploid-cell rabies vaccine given concurrently with chloroquine. *N Engl J Med* 1986; **314:** 280–4.

Uses and Administration

Rabies vaccines are used for active immunisation against rabies. They are used as part of postexposure treatment to prevent rabies in patients who have been bitten by rabid animals or animals suspected of being rabid. Infection does not take place through unbroken skin but it is possible through uninjured mucous membranes and has been reported after the inhalation of virus in the laboratory. Rabies vaccines are also used for pre-exposure prophylaxis against rabies in persons exposed to a high risk of being bitten by rabid or potentially rabid animals.

Schedules for prophylaxis and treatment of rabies are recommended by WHO (see below) and many countries have immunisation schedules based on these.

In the UK a rabies vaccine prepared from inactivated Wistar rabies virus strain PM/WI38 1503-3M cultured on human diploid cells is used. It contains not less than 2.5 international units per mL. The vaccine should be given by deep subcutaneous or intramuscular injection into the deltoid region, or in a child, the anterolateral aspect of the thigh.

For **pre-exposure prophylaxis** against rabies the recommended schedule in the UK for the human diploid-cell vaccine is 3 doses, each of 1 mL, by deep subcutaneous or intramuscular injection on days 0, 7, and 28; alternatively a dose of 0.1 mL has been given intradermally on the same days. Booster doses may be given every 2 to 3 years depending upon the risk of exposure, but where postexposure treatment is readily available booster doses are not normally required in individuals who have received three doses of vaccine.

A 2-dose schedule has also been employed for travellers to enzootic areas who are not animal handlers: doses of 1 mL by deep subcutaneous or intramuscular injection, or 0.1 mL intradermally, are given 4 weeks apart. This schedule is somewhat less effective than the 3-dose schedule and should only be used where postexposure treatment will be readily available.

It has been suggested that rapid immunisation of personnel engaged in the care of a patient with rabies may be achieved by the intradermal administration of 0.1 mL into each limb (total of 0.4 mL) on the first day of exposure to the patient.

For **postexposure treatment**, thorough cleansing of the wound with soap and water is imperative. The recommended schedule in the UK for the human diploid-cell vaccine is 5 doses, each of 1 mL, by deep subcutaneous or intramuscular injection on days 0, 3, 7, 14, and 30. The UK manufacturers also recommend a further dose on day 90. Vaccination should be started as soon as possible after exposure, and may be discontinued if it is proved that the patient was not at risk. In previously unimmunised patients at high risk, rabies immunoglobulin (see above) should also be given at the same time as the first dose of vaccine; the recommended dose is 20 international units per kg body-weight, up to half of which should be infiltrated around the wound with the remainder being given intramuscularly but at a different site to that at which the vaccine was administered. A modified course of vaccine administration may be employed in previously immunised persons consisting of 2 doses on day 0 and between days 3 to 7; rabies immunoglobulins are not required in these patients.

Rabies. Rabies is caused by infection with a rhabdovirus of the genus Lyssavirus which also contains a number of related viruses some of which have caused disease in man. The rabies virus is usually transmitted by the bite of an infected animal or contamination of broken skin by saliva. Infection is possible via intact mucous membranes and by aerosol transmission, but infection is unlikely following contamination of intact skin. Other body fluids such as urine and tears should be regarded as potentially infectious.

Human rabies is almost always fatal once symptoms have appeared. After an incubation period of about 30 to 90 days there is a prodrome lasting up to about 10 days of generally nonspecific symptoms. This prodrome is followed by the onset of acute neurological symptoms. Periods of hyperexcitability accompanied by severe agitation and bizarre behaviour alternate with periods of lucidity. Severe spasms of the larynx and pharynx may be provoked by attempts at swallowing leading to hydrophobia or by air blown at the face (aerophobia). Other symptoms include hypersalivation, fever, and convulsions. An alternative presentation of nervous system involvement is a progressive flaccid paralysis. Patients not dying through respiratory or cardiac arrest during the acute phase may develop any of a number of complications culminating in coma and death or (very rarely) recovery; only 3 patients are documented as having survived after the onset of coma, and all had received either pre- or postexposure immunisation.

Rabies has a worldwide distribution, primarily in domesticated and wild dogs but also in bats and other warm-blooded animals, although some countries, including the UK, most of Australasia, and Antarctica are designated as rabies-free areas. National control programmes involve epidemiological surveillance, mass canine immunisation campaigns, and dog population management. The recent development of oral animal vaccines delivered on baited food has met with considerable success in a number of areas and has become an essential tool for eliminating rabies in wild animals. Rigorously applied controls of international transfer of animals including certification of vaccination and quarantine for animals entering rabies-free areas are necessary to prevent re-introduction of rabies.

Although a number of treatments have been tried including various antiviral drugs, interferon, high doses of rabies immunoglobulin, and corticosteroids, none has shown evidence of effectiveness. Avoidance of rabies after contact with a suspected or confirmed rabid animal depends upon prompt and thorough cleansing of the contaminated site and administration of rabies vaccine with or without rabies immunoglobulins immediately. For a brief outline of postexposure treatment, see below; however, readers are strongly advised to consult the complete guidelines published by WHO if they are likely to be involved with the management of patients exposed to rabies.

Prophylaxis is recommended in persons at high risk of exposure, either due to their occupation or those travelling in enzootic areas. The main obstacle to mass pre-exposure vaccination appears to be the high cost of cell culture vaccines. See under Pre-exposure Immunisation (below) for outlines of recommended vaccination schedules.

CHOICE OF VACCINES. Many different rabies vaccines are available for human use. There are: those derived from nerve tissue of animals; those derived from avian tissues (duck embryos); and those prepared in cell cultures. Originally the only source of rabies virus available for vaccine production was infected brain tissue from adult animals; such vaccines contain neuroparalytic and encephalitogenic substances and WHO supports the trend to limit, or abandon completely, their production.[1] Vaccines prepared from virus grown in duck embryos have been developed and a purified duck-embryo vaccine (PDEV) may provide similar efficacy and safety to vaccines produced from cell cultures.[1] Improvements in biotechnology may reduce the costs of cell-culture production. Among the vaccines prepared in this way is one developed from an adapted Pasteur strain of virus grown in a human diploid cell strain (HDCV), a purified chick embryo-cell vaccine (PCECV), and a purified Vero-cell vaccine (PVRV).[2] There appears to be little difference in terms of safety and antigenicity between HDCV, PCECV, PVRV, and PDEV in recommended regimens.[2] The incidence of severe hypersensitivity reactions should, however, be lower with PVRV and PCECV than with HDCV since the purification process removes most human serum albumin in the cell-growth medium before virus inactivation.[2]

There is little data concerning the efficacy of rabies vaccines.[2] It appears that nerve-tissue vaccines afford limited protection after minor exposures to rabies virus, are less effective after head bites, and are of little use after very severe exposures. Failure rates for HDCV, PCECV, and PVRV (including cases with less than the recommended therapy) has been estimated as less than 1 in 80 000 treatments in the USA, Canada, and Europe, 1 in 12 000 to 20 000 in Thailand, and 1 in 30 000 in the remaining tropical countries. Reported failures of these vaccines are often accounted for by deviation from recommendations, incorrect site of vaccine administration, or delay in treatment.

The cost of cell-culture rabies vaccines is prohibitively high in the developing world. Although the adverse effects of nerve-tissue vaccines preclude their use for pre-exposure prophylaxis, they are still used for postexposure prophylaxis.[2] WHO is anxious that nerve-tissue vaccines should be replaced with affordable cell-culture vaccines as soon as possible. Rabies vaccines for veterinary use have been produced in cell culture at low cost and there are moves to apply the advances made in this field to human vaccines.[3] In the meantime, cost-cutting regimens have been devised for use of cell-culture rabies vaccines by the intradermal route. Rapid immunisation is achieved by the use of several sites of injection; fewer injections are required than with traditional intramuscular regimens.[2,4,5]

1. WHO. WHO expert committee on rabies: eighth report. *WHO Tech Rep Ser 824* 1992.
2. Nicholson KG. Modern vaccines: rabies. *Lancet* 1990; **335:** 1201–5. Correction. *ibid.*; 1540.
3. Petricciani JC. Ongoing tragedy of rabies. *Lancet* 1993; **342:** 1067–8.
4. Warrell MJ, *et al.* Economical multiple-site intradermal immunisation with human diploid-cell-strain vaccine is effective for post-exposure rabies prophylaxis. *Lancet* 1985; **i:** 1059–62.
5. Chutivongse S, *et al.* Postexposure prophylaxis for rabies with antiserum and intradermal vaccination. *Lancet* 1990; **335:** 896–8.

PRE-EXPOSURE IMMUNISATION. Pre-exposure prophylaxis with rabies vaccine is generally recommended for use in persons at high risk of infection with rabies virus. Where available, the vaccines produced in cell culture are preferred over the vaccines produced in animal tissues (see under Choice of Vaccines, above). WHO recommends[1] pre-exposure prophylaxis for persons regularly at high risk of exposure, such as certain laboratory workers, veterinarians, animal handlers, and wildlife officers, and those living in or travelling to areas where rabies is endemic. The immunisation schedule should preferably consist of 3 injections of a tissue-culture rabies vaccine of potency at least 2.5 international units given on days 0, 7, and 28, but a few days' variation is unimportant. Administration should be into the deltoid area of the arm or for young children into the anterolateral area of the thigh. Titres of virus-neutralising antibodies can be checked in serum samples collected 1 to 3 weeks after the last dose. Those who work with the live virus should have their antibody titres checked every 6 months and if the figure falls below 0.5 IU per mL they should receive a booster. Other individuals at continuing risk should have their titres checked every 12 months and a booster given if the titre is below 0.5 IU per mL.

The intradermal administration of rabies vaccine in doses of 0.1 mL on days 0, 7, and 28 has also been shown to induce seroconversion.

National policies vary somewhat from that of WHO, depending on the local risk of contracting rabies and the vaccines available.

In the UK the schedule for primary immunisation (see above) is similar to that recommended by WHO.

In the USA, immunisation with either a human diploid cell vaccine or a vaccine adsorbed onto an aluminium salt is carried out similarly to the WHO schedule, with serum-antibody titres determined at 6 months to 2 years, depending upon the level of exposure, and booster doses given as necessary.[2]

1. WHO. WHO expert committee on rabies: eighth report. *WHO Tech Rep Ser 824* 1992.
2. Immunization Practices Advisory Committee. Rabies prevention—United States, 1984. *JAMA* 1984; **252:** 883–93.

POSTEXPOSURE TREATMENT. WHO[1] emphasises the importance of prompt local treatment for all bite wounds and scratches that may be contaminated with rabies virus and that, depending on the category of animal contact, rabies vaccine on its own or with rabies immunoglobulin should be given. The combination of these measures immediately after exposure is considered virtually to guarantee complete protection. Pregnancy and infancy are not contra-indications to postexposure vaccination. Also these measures should be instituted in patients who present even months after having been bitten.

First aid or local treatment consists of immediate thorough flushing and washing of the wound with water, or soap and water, or detergent followed by the application of alcohol 70% or tincture or aqueous solution of iodine. Medical care may then consist of the instillation of rabies immunoglobulin into the depth of the wound and infiltration around the wound. Ideally the wound should not be sutured, but if suturing is necessary then it is essential that it be preceded by the administration of rabies immunoglobulin as above.

The administration of rabies vaccine and of rabies immunoglobulin depends on the category of animal contact. WHO classifies the type of contact with a suspect or rabid animal into 3 categories. Category I covers touching or feeding of animals and licks on intact skin. Category II covers nibbling of uncovered skin, minor scratches or abrasions without bleeding, and licks on broken skin. Category III covers single or multiple transdermal bites or scratches and contamination of mucous membranes with the animal's saliva. Generally no treatment is required for category I contact. Patients who have experienced category II contact should be given rabies vaccine but the course may be stopped if the contact has been with a cat or dog that remains healthy throughout an observation period of 10 days or if postmortem study of the contact animal shows it to be negative for rabies. Patients who have experienced category III contact should also be given rabies vaccine. It should be preceded by rabies immunoglobulin infiltrated around the wound and instilled into it as described above.

The dose for rabies immunoglobulin is 20 international units per kg body-weight; as much as possible of the dose should be infiltrated into and around the wound with the remainder being injected intramuscularly into the gluteal region.

The potency of rabies vaccines should be at least 2.5 international units per single human dose. For intramuscular vaccination schedules one dose should be administered on days 0, 3, 7, 14, and 30 into the deltoid region or, for small children, into the anterolateral area of the thigh. An abbreviated multisite schedule (the 2-1-1 regimen) induces an early antibody response and may be particularly effective when postexposure treatment has not included a rabies immunoglobulin. This schedule consists of one dose given in the right arm and one in the left arm on day 0, and one dose intramuscularly into the deltoid region on days 7 and 21. For intradermal vaccination one dose (0.1 mL) should be given at each of two sites, either the forearm or the upper arm, on days 0, 3, and 7, and one dose at one site on days 30 and 90.

In the UK, rabies immunoglobulin is given if the patient is previously unimmunised and at high risk. Human diploid cell vaccine is given on days 0, 3, 7, 14, and 30 (five doses) in unimmunised persons (although the UK manufacturers also recommend a sixth dose on day 90), and on days 0 and 3 to 7 (two doses) in previously fully immunised persons.

In the USA, human diploid cell vaccine or adsorbed rabies vaccine may be used for postexposure treatment. In previously unimmunised individuals, a 1 mL dose of either vaccine is given intramuscularly on days 0, 3, 7, 14, and 28 together with rabies immunoglobulin as in the WHO schedule. In previously immunised individuals, two doses of vaccine are given on days 0 and 3, and rabies immunoglobulin is not required.

1. WHO. WHO expert committee on rabies: eighth report. *WHO Tech Rep Ser 824* 1992.

Preparations

Ph. Eur.: Rabies Vaccine for Human Use Prepared in Cell Cultures;
USP 23: Rabies Vaccine.

Proprietary Preparations (details are given in Part 3)
Aust.: Rabipur; ***Ger.:*** Rabipur; Rabivac; Tollwut-Impfstoff (HDC); ***Ital.:*** Imovax Rabbia; Lyssavac N; Rasilvax; ***S.Afr.:*** Verorab; ***Spain:*** Vac Antirrabica; ***Swed.:*** Rabies-Imovax; ***Switz.:*** Lyssavac N; ***UK:*** Merieux Inactivated Rabies Vaccine; ***USA:*** Imovax Rabies; RabAvert.

Respiratory Syncytial Virus Immunoglobulins (14725-q)

Adverse Effects and Precautions

As for immunoglobulins in general, p.1500.

Uses and Administration

Respiratory syncytial virus immunoglobulin is available in some countries for the passive immunisation of infants against lower respiratory-tract infections caused by respiratory syncytial virus. It is prepared from the pooled plasma of adults selected for high titres of antibodies that neutralise the virus. Each mL of respiratory syncytial virus immunoglobulin contains approximately 50 mg of protein.

In the USA at-risk children under 2 years of age with bronchopulmonary dysplasia or a history of premature birth may receive a prophylactic intravenous infusion once a month during the respiratory syncytial virus season (typically November to April). The drug is given in a dose of up to 750 mg per kg body-weight at an initial rate of 75 mg per kg per hour for 15 minutes, followed by 150 mg per kg per hour for a further 15 minutes, and then 300 mg per kg per hour until the end of the infusion.

A human monoclonal antibody to respiratory syncytial virus (palivizumab) is available in some countries and is used intramuscularly for similar purposes, in a dose of 15 mg per kg monthly.

References.

1. Wandstrat TL. Respiratory syncytial virus immune globulin intravenous. *Ann Pharmacother* 1997; **31:** 83–8.
2. The Prophylaxis of Respiratory Syncytial Virus in Elevated-Risk Neonates (PREVENT) Study Group. Reduction of respiratory syncytial virus hospitalization among premature infants and infants with bronchopulmonary dysplasia using respiratory syncytial virus immune globulin prophylaxis. *Pediatrics* 1997; **99:** 93–9.
3. Rodriguez WJ, *et al.* Respiratory syncytial virus (RSV) immune globulin intravenous therapy for RSV lower respiratory tract infection in infants and young children at high risk for severe RSV infections. *Pediatrics* 1997; **99:** 454–61.
4. Committee on Infectious Diseases/Committee on Fetus and Newborn of the American Academy of Pediatrics. Respiratory syncytial virus immune globulin intravenous: indications for use. *Pediatrics* 1997; **99:** 645–50.
5. Meissner HC, Groothuis JR. Immunoprophylaxis and the control of RSV disease. *Pediatrics* 1997; **100:** 260–3.

Preparations

Proprietary Preparations (details are given in Part 3)
USA: RespiGam; Synagis.

Respiratory Syncytial Virus Vaccines (499-e)

Vaccines containing respiratory syncytial virus protein subunit are being studied for active immunisation.

References.

1. Tristram DA, *et al.* Immunogenicity and safety of respiratory syncytial virus subunit vaccine in seropositive children 18–36 months old. *J Infect Dis* 1993; **167:** 191–5.
2. Tristram DA, *et al.* Second-year surveillance of recipients of a respiratory syncytial virus (RSV) F protein subunit vaccine, PFP-1: evaluation of antibody persistence and possible disease enhancement. *Vaccine* 1994; **12:** 551–6.
3. Toms GL. Respiratory syncytial virus—how soon will we have a vaccine? *Arch Dis Child* 1995; **72:** 1–5.
4. Falsey AR, Walsh EE. Safety and immunogenicity of a respiratory syncytial virus subunit vaccine (PFP-2) in ambulatory adults over age 60. *Vaccine* 1996; **14:** 1214–18.
5. Piedra PA, *et al.* Purified fusion protein vaccine protects against lower respiratory tract illness during respiratory syncytial virus season in children with cystic fibrosis. *Pediatr Infect Dis J* 1996; **15:** 23–31.
6. Falsey AR, Walsh EE. Safety and immunogenicity of a respiratory syncytial virus subunit vaccine (PFP-2) in the institutionalized elderly. *Vaccine* 1997; **15:** 1130–2.
7. Groothuis JR, *et al.* Safety and immunogenicity of a purified F protein respiratory syncytial virus (PFP-2) vaccine in seropositive children with bronchopulmonary dysplasia. *J Infect Dis* 1998; **177:** 467–9.

Rift Valley Fever Vaccines (8290-l)

An inactivated rift valley fever vaccine has been developed for the active immunisation of persons at high risk of contracting the disease.

Rotavirus Vaccines (16981-c)

Several live oral rotavirus vaccines for use in the prevention of childhood diarrhoea have been developed.

Rotaviruses are an important cause of severe diarrhoea in both developed and developing countries (see Viral Gastroenteritis, p.595), being most prevalent among children 6 to 24 months of age.[1] Human rotavirus diarrhoea is caused by group A, B, or C rotaviruses.[2] Development of a suitable vaccine has been made difficult by the diversity of rotaviruses.[2] Initial attempts at vaccine development used single bovine or rhesus monkey strains but these were associated with variable efficacy and adverse effects.[1,3-5]

To overcome these problems reassortant rotavirus (RRV) strains have been constructed. These combine animal rotavirus strains with human rotavirus genes coding for serotype-specific antigens, enabling polyvalent vaccines to be produced against the major rotavirus serotypes causing disease. A tetravalent vaccine (RRV-TV) produced a 57% protection rate against all rotavirus-induced diarrhoea and 82% protection against severe forms in a multicentre study in the USA.[6] Results in developing countries have, however, been comparatively disappointing with protection rates of only 20%[7] and 35%[8] against all rotavirus diarrhoea and 50 to 60% against severe diarrhoea.

A higher titre version of RRV-TV has also produced encouraging results[9-11] and may prove suitable for use in developing countries. Monovalent reassortant vaccines have also been studied.[12]

Another approach to production of a rotavirus vaccine is to use a naturally attenuated human rotavirus strain that causes asymptomatic rotavirus infection in infants, but with induction of immunity.[13]

1. Anonymous. Rotavirus vaccines. *Bull WHO* 1989; **67:** 583–4.
2. Anonymous. Puzzling diversity of rotaviruses. *Lancet* 1990; **335:** 573–5.
3. Levine MM. Modern vaccines: enteric infections. *Lancet* 1990; **335:** 958–61.
4. Bernstein DI, *et al.* Evaluation of WC3 rotavirus vaccine and correlates of protection in healthy infants. *J Infect Dis* 1990; **162:** 1055–62.
5. Flores J, *et al.* Protection against severe rotavirus diarrhoea by rhesus rotavirus vaccine in Venezuelan infants. *Lancet* 1987; **i:** 882–4.
6. Bernstein DI, *et al.* Evaluation of rhesus rotavirus monovalent and tetravalent reassortant vaccines in US children. *JAMA* 1996; **273:** 1191–6.
7. Lanata CF, *et al.* Safety, immunogenicity, and protective efficacy of one and three doses of the tetravalent rhesus rotavirus vaccine in infants in Lima, Peru. *J Infect Dis* 1996; **174:** 268–75.
8. Linhares AC, *et al.* Immunogenicity, safety and efficacy of tetravalent rhesus-human, reassortant rotavirus vaccine in Belém, Brazil. *Bull WHO* 1996; **74:** 491–500.
9. Rennels MB, *et al.* Safety and efficacy of high-dose rhesus-human reassortant rotavirus vaccines—report of the national multicenter trial. *Pediatrics* 1996; **97:** 7–13.
10. Joensuu J, *et al.* Randomised placebo-controlled trial of rhesus-human reassortant rotavirus vaccine for prevention of severe rotavirus gastroenteritis. *Lancet* 1997; **350:** 1205–9.
11. Perez-Schael I, *et al.* Efficacy of the rhesus rotavirus-based quadrivalent vaccine in infants and young children in Venezuela. *N Engl J Med* 1997; **337:** 1181–7.
12. Treanor JJ, *et al.* Evaluation of the protective efficacy of a serotype 1 bovine-human rotavirus reassortant vaccine in infants. *Pediatr Infect Dis J* 1995; **14:** 301–7.
13. Midthun K, *et al.* Safety and immunogenicity of human rotavirus vaccine strain M37 in adults, children, and infants. *J Infect Dis* 1991; **164:** 792–6.

Preparations

Proprietary Preparations (details are given in Part 3)
USA: RotaShield.

Rubella Immunoglobulins (11051-m)

Human Rubella Immunoglobulin (Ph. Eur.) (Antirubella Immunoglobulin Injection; Rubella Immunoglobulin (BP 1998); Immunoglobulinum Humanum Rubellae) is a liquid or freeze-dried preparation containing immunoglobulins, mainly immunoglobulin G (IgG). It is obtained from plasma containing specific antibodies against the rubella virus. Normal immunoglobulin may be added. It contains not less than 4500 international units per mL. Both the liquid and freeze-dried preparations should be stored, protected from light, in a colourless, glass container. The freeze-dried preparation should be stored under vacuum or under an inert gas.

Adverse Effects and Precautions

As for immunoglobulins in general, p.1500.

Interactions

As for immunoglobulins in general, p.1500.

Uses and Administration

Rubella immunoglobulins may be used for passive immunisation against rubella (German measles). They have been used to prevent or modify rubella in susceptible persons, although if such a measure is used then normal immunoglobulin is often employed instead.

Preparations

Ph. Eur.: Human Rubella Immunoglobulin.

Proprietary Preparations (details are given in Part 3)
Ital.: Haimaros†; Immunoros; Rosol-Gamma; Rubellabulin†; Rubeuman; ***S.Afr.:*** Rubegam†; ***Spain:*** Gamma Glob Antirub†; Glogama Antirubeola†; Rubeuman†; ***Switz.:*** Rubeuman.

Rubella Vaccines (8001-w)

Rubella Vaccine (Live) (Ph. Eur.) (Rub/Vac (Live); Rubella Vaccine, Live (BP 1998); Vaccinum Rubellae Vivum) is a freeze-dried preparation of a suitable live attenuated strain of rubella virus grown in human diploid cell cultures. It is reconstituted immediately before use. The cell-culture medium may contain a permitted antibiotic at the smallest effective concentration, and a suitable stabiliser may be added to the bulk vaccine. The final vaccine contains not less than 1×10^3 $CCID_{50}$ per dose. The dried vaccine should be stored at 2° to 8° and be protected from light.

Rubella Virus Vaccine Live (USP 23) is a bacterially sterile freeze-dried preparation of a suitable live strain of rubella virus grown in cultures of duck-embryo tissue or human tissue. It contains the equivalent of not less than 1×10^3 $TCID_{50}$ in each immunising dose. It should be stored at 2° to 8° and be protected from light.

Adverse Effects

As for vaccines in general, p.1500.

Generally, side-effects have not been severe. Those occurring most commonly are skin rashes, pharyngitis, fever, and lymphadenopathy; arthralgia and arthritis may also occur and are reported to be more common in women than young girls. Thrombocytopenia and neurological symptoms including neuropathy and paraesthesia have been reported rarely.

Effects on bones and joints. Although acute arthralgia or arthritis occurs in up to 30% of women following rubella vaccination,[1] a retrospective analysis found no evidence of an increased risk of chronic arthropathies.[2]

1. Tingle AJ, *et al.* Randomised double-blind placebo-controlled study on adverse effects of rubella immunisation in seronegative women. *Lancet* 1997; **349:** 1277–81.
2. Ray P, *et al.* Risk of chronic arthropathy among women after rubella vaccination. *JAMA* 1997; **278:** 551–6.

Effects on the nervous system. For a report of optic neuritis in 2 children following administration of measles and rubella vaccine, see p.1519.

Precautions

As for vaccines in general, p.1501.

Rubella vaccines should not be given during pregnancy and in the UK it is recommended that patients should be advised not to become pregnant within one month of vaccination. However, no case of congenital rubella syndrome has been reported following the inadvertent administration of rubella vaccines shortly before or during pregnancy and it is thus considered that there is no evidence that the vaccines are teratogenic. Inadvertent administration of rubella vaccines during pregnancy should not therefore result in a routine recommendation to terminate the pregnancy. There is no risk to a pregnant woman from contact with recently vaccinated persons as the vaccine virus is not transmitted.

Rubella vaccines are not generally recommended for children below the age of 1 year in whom maternal antibodies might prevent a response.

The vaccine available in the UK contains traces of neomycin and/or polymyxin. Rubella vaccine should therefore not be given to individuals with a history of anaphylaxis to these antibiotics.

Pregnancy. Since 1971 the Centers for Disease Control in the USA has followed up women who received rubella vaccines within 3 months before or after conception.[1] Up to 1979 vaccines containing either the Cendehill or HPV-77 strains of rubella virus were available. None of the 290 infants born to the 538 women who had received these vaccines had defects indicative of congenital rubella syndrome; this included 94 live-born infants of women who were known to be susceptible to rubella before receiving the vaccine. In 1979 a rubella vaccine containing the Wistar RA 27/3 strain was introduced. None of 212 infants born live to 254 women known to be susceptible to rubella and who had received the RA 27/3 rubella vaccine from 1979 to 1988 had defects indicative of congenital rubella syndrome. These results are consistent with experiences in Germany[2] and the UK.[3,4] However, because of evidence that rubella vaccine viruses can cross the placenta and infect the fetus a theoretical risk to the fetus cannot be completely ruled out.[1] Thus in both the UK and USA pregnancy is considered a contra-indication to rubella vaccination. In the UK patients are also advised not to become pregnant within one month of vaccination; in the USA a period of 3 months is advised.[1] However, in neither country is termination of pregnancy routinely recommended if the vaccine is inadvertently administered during pregnancy.

1. Anonymous. Rubella vaccination during pregnancy—United States, 1971–1988. *JAMA* 1989; **261:** 3374–83.
2. Enders G. Rubella antibody titers in vaccinated and nonvaccinated women and results of vaccination during pregnancy. *Rev Infect Dis* 1985; **7** (suppl 1): S103–S107.
3. Sheppard S, *et al.* Rubella vaccination and pregnancy: preliminary report of a national survey. *Br Med J* 1986; **292:** 727.
4. Tookey PA, *et al.* Rubella vaccination in pregnancy. *Commun Dis Rep* 1991; **1** (review 7): R86–R88.

Interactions

As for vaccines in general, p.1501.

Uses and Administration

Rubella vaccines are used for active immunisation against rubella (German measles). The symptoms of rubella infection are generally mild except in the early stages of pregnancy when it leads to fetal damage in most infants.

For primary immunisation combined measles, mumps, and rubella vaccine (p.1519) is usually given. For discussion of immunisation schedules see under Vaccines, p.1501.

In the UK administration of a single-antigen rubella vaccine to girls aged 10 to 14 years has been discontinued following the mass immunisation campaign in 1994 and the introduction of a two-dose immunisation schedule in all children. Vaccine should still be given to women of child-bearing age if they are seronegative; women who are found to be seronegative during pregnancy should be vaccinated in the early postpartum period. Effective precautions against pregnancy must be observed for at least one month following vaccination. To avoid the risk of transmitting rubella to pregnant patients, all health service staff, both male and female, should be screened and those found to be seronegative should be vaccinated.

The rubella vaccine available in the UK contains the Wistar RA 27/3 strain and is given by deep subcutaneous or intramuscular injection in a dose of 0.5 mL.

The rubella vaccine available in the USA is similar to that used in the UK. Vaccines containing other strains of rubella virus, such as the Cendehill strain, are available in other countries.

Preparations

Ph. Eur.: Rubella Vaccine (Live);
USP 23: Rubella Virus Vaccine Live.

Proprietary Preparations (details are given in Part 3)
Aust.: Ervevax; Rubeaten; ***Austral.:*** Ervevax; Meruvax II; ***Belg.:*** Ervevax; Meruvax II†; ***Fr.:*** Rudivax; ***Ger.:*** Ervevax; Rot-Wellcovax†; Rubellovac; ***Irl.:*** Almevax; Ervevax; ***Ital.:*** Ervevax; Gunevax; Meruvax II†; Rosovax; Rubeaten; Rudivax; ***Neth.:*** Ervevax†; ***S.Afr.:*** Rubeaten; Rudivax; ***Spain:*** Rubeaten; Vac Antirub†; Vac Antirrubeola; Vac Antirubeola†; ***Swed.:*** Almevax†; Meruvax; ***Switz.:*** Ervevax; Meruvax II; Rubeaten; ***UK:*** Almevax; Ervevax; Meruvax II†; Rubavax†; ***USA:*** Meruvax II.

Rubella and Mumps Vaccines (7999-a)

Rubella and Mumps Virus Vaccine Live (USP 23) is a bacterially sterile preparation of a suitable live strain of rubella virus and a suitable live strain of mumps virus. It may contain suitable antimicrobial agents. The dried vaccine should be stored at 2° to 8° and be protected from light.

Adverse Effects and Precautions

As for vaccines in general, p.1500.

See also under mumps vaccines, p.1521, and rubella vaccines, p.1532.

Interactions

As for vaccines in general, p.1501.

Uses and Administration

Rubella and mumps vaccines may be used for active immunisation against mumps and rubella. Vaccination against mumps and rubella is normally performed using a combined measles, mumps, and rubella vaccine (p.1519) but the bivalent rubella and mumps vaccine may be employed when vaccination against measles is not indicated. For discussion of immunisation schedules see under Vaccines, p.1501.

A vaccine used in the USA is prepared from the Wistar RA 27/3 strain of rubella virus and the Jeryl Lynn (B level) strain of mumps virus. It is generally given in a dose of 0.5 mL by subcutaneous injection to infants during the second year of life or to other children or adults considered to be at risk.

Preparations

USP 23: Rubella and Mumps Virus Vaccine Live.

Proprietary Preparations (details are given in Part 3)
USA: Biavax II.

Schistosomiasis Vaccines (1795-b)

Bilharzia Vaccines.

Vaccines against schistosomiasis are in early stages of development.

References.

1. Playfair JHL, *et al.* Modern vaccines: parasitic diseases. *Lancet* 1990; **335:** 1263–6.
2. Anonymous. From Bilharz to B cells. *Lancet* 1991; **337:** 421–2.
3. Cherfas J. New hope for vaccine against schistosomiasis. *Science* 1991; **251:** 630–1.
4. Butterworth AE. Vaccines against schistosomiasis: where do we stand? *Trans R Soc Trop Med Hyg* 1992; **86:** 1–2.
5. Dunne DW, *et al.* Prospects for immunological control of schistosomiasis. *Lancet* 1995; **345:** 1488–92.
6. Waine GJ, McManus DP. Schistosomiasis vaccine development—the current picture. *Bioessays* 1997; **19:** 435–43.

Scorpion Venom Antisera (8006-z)

Scorpion Antivenins; Scorpion Antivenoms.

Scorpion Venom Antiserum (BP 1998) is a sterile preparation containing the specific antitoxic globulins that have the power of neutralising the venom of one or more species of scorpion. The species of scorpion against whose venom or venoms the antiserum is intended to be used varies according to the geographical region and for any particular region should include those species prevalent in the region. The potency should be such that the dose stated on the label will completely neutralise the maximum amount of venom likely to be delivered by a single sting. It should be stored at 2° to 8°, and not be allowed to freeze.

Adverse Effects and Precautions

As for antisera in general, p.1500.

Uses and Administration

Some scorpion stings are dangerous and even fatal. The use of a scorpion antiserum suitable for the species of scorpion can prevent symptoms provided it is given with the least possible delay; other general supportive measures and symptomatic treatment are also needed. The effectiveness of antisera is disputed by some clinicians.

Scorpion stings. Scorpion stings are common throughout the tropics, but the most dangerous and potentially fatal species are found in India, North Africa and the Middle East, the southern states of North America and Mexico, Latin America and the Caribbean, and southern Africa. Local symptoms following scorpion stings include intense pain and swelling. Systemic symptoms result from excitation of nerve and muscle cells by the venom: the pattern of symptoms depends upon the species of scorpion. Symptoms of parasympathetic stimulation such as dilatation of pupils, hypersalivation, vomiting and diarrhoea are generally followed by adrenergic features, with release of catecholamines producing hypertension, toxic myocarditis, arrhythmias, heart failure, and pulmonary oedema. The cardiotoxic effects are prominent features of stings in India, North Africa and the Middle East. Neurotoxic effects such as fasciculations, spasms, and respiratory paralysis are seen with stings from North American species. Stings by the black scorpion of Trinidad may also produce pancreatitis.

Pain is treated with local infiltration or peripheral nerve block with local anaesthetics; opioid analgesics may be necessary, but are regarded as dangerous following stings by some North American species. An appropriate antiserum should be administered as soon as possible after envenomation, although the effectiveness of some antisera has been questioned. Supportive treatment for cardiotoxic effects includes alpha blockers, calcium-channel blockers, and ACE inhibitors. The use of cardiac glycosides, beta blockers, and atropine is controversial. Phenobarbitone has been suggested for neurotoxic effects.

References.

1. Warrell DA, Fenner PJ. Venomous bites and stings. *Br Med Bull* 1993; **49:** 423–39.
2. Karalliedde L. Animal toxins. *Br J Anaesth* 1995; **74:** 319–27.
3. el Amin EO, *et al.* Scorpion sting: a management problem. *Ann Trop Paediatr* 1991; **11:** 143–8.
4. Bond GR. Antivenin administration for Centruroides scorpion sting: risks and benefits. *Ann Emerg Med* 1992; **21:** 788–91.
5. Müller GJ. Scorpionism in South Africa: a report of 42 serious scorpion envenomations. *S Afr Med J* 1993; **83:** 405–11.
6. Gateau T, *et al.* Response to specific centruroides sculpturatus antivenom in 151 cases of scorpion stings. *Clin Toxicol* 1994; **32:** 165–71.
7. Sofer S, *et al.* Scorpion envenomation and antivenom therapy. *J Pediatr* 1994; **124:** 973–8.

Preparations

BP 1998: Scorpion Venom Antiserum.

Shigella Vaccines (19113-t)

Dysentery Vaccines; Shigellosis Vaccines.

Live attenuated shigella vaccines have been under investigation since the 1960s but early prototypes were unsatisfactory. A live oral vaccine and a conjugated vaccine are now under development.

References.

1. Levine MM. Modern vaccines: enteric infections. *Lancet* 1990; **335:** 958–61.
2. Taylor DN, *et al.* Outpatient studies of the safety and immunogenicity of an auxotrophic Escherichia coli K-12-Shigella flexneri 2a hybrid vaccine candidate, EcSf2a-2. *Vaccine* 1994; **12:** 565–8.
3. Cohen D, *et al.* Safety and immunogenicity of the oral E coli K12-S flexneri 2a vaccine (EcSf2a-2) among Israeli soldiers. *Vaccine* 1994; **12:** 1436–42.
4. Kärnell A, *et al.* Safety and immunogenicity study of the auxotrophic Shigella flexneri 2a vaccine SFL1070 with a deleted aroD gene in adult Swedish volunteers. *Vaccine* 1995; **13:** 88–99.
5. Cohen D, *et al.* Double-blind vaccine-controlled randomised efficacy trial of an investigational Shigella sonnei conjugate vaccine in young adults. *Lancet* 1997; **349:** 155–9.

Smallpox Vaccines (8008-k)

Smallpox Vaccine (USP 23) is a suspension or solid containing a suitable strain of the living virus of vaccinia grown in the skin of bovine calves; it may contain a suitable preservative. The liquid vaccine should be stored below 0° and the dried vaccine at 2° to 8°.

Uses and Administration

Following the global eradication of smallpox, vaccination against smallpox (using vaccinia virus) has been indicated only for investigators at special risk such as laboratory workers handling certain orthopoxviruses.

WHO has recommended that all stocks of smallpox (variola) virus be destroyed. This is to be followed by destruction of all remaining doses of smallpox vaccine.

Recombinant vaccinia viruses are being investigated as vectors of foreign antigens, for example in a candidate AIDS vaccine (p.1503).

References.

1. Jezek Z, *et al.* Smallpox and its post-eradication surveillance. *Bull WHO* 1987; **65:** 425–34.
2. Barquet N, Domingo P. Smallpox: the triumph over the most terrible of the ministers of death. *Ann Intern Med* 1997; **127:** 635–42.

Preparations

USP 23: Smallpox Vaccine.

Snake Venom Antisera (8011-l)

Snake Antivenins; Snake Antivenoms.

European Viper Venom Antiserum (Ph. Eur.), (Immunoserum Contra Venena Viperarum Europaearum) is a preparation containing the specific antitoxic globulins that have the power of neutralising the venom of one or more species of viper (*Vipera ammodytes, V. aspis, V. berus*, or *V. ursinii*). The globulins are obtained by fractionation of the serum of animals that have been immunised against the venom or venoms. Each mL neutralises the venoms in not less than 100 mouse LD_{50} of *V. ammodytes*, 100 of *V. aspis*, 50 of *V. berus*, or 50 of *V. ursinii*. It should be stored at 2° to 8°, and not be allowed to freeze.

Antivenin (Crotalidae) Polyvalent (USP 23) is a sterile freeze-dried preparation of specific venom-neutralising globulins obtained from the serum of healthy horses immunised against 4 species of pit vipers, *Crotalus atrox* (Western diamondback), *Crotalus adamanteus, Crotalus durissus terrificus* (South American rattlesnake), and *Bothrops atrox* (South American fer de lance). One dose neutralises the venoms in not less than 180 mouse LD_{50} of *C. atrox*, 1320 of *C. durissus terrificus*, and 780 of *B. atrox*. It may contain a suitable preservative. It should be preserved in single-dose containers and stored at a temperature not exceeding 40°.

Antivenin (Micrurus Fulvius) (USP 23) is a sterile freeze-dried preparation of specific venom-neutralising globulins obtained from the serum of healthy horses immunised against venom of *Micrurus fulvius* (Eastern Coral snake). One dose neutralises the venom in not less than 250 mouse LD_{50} of *M. fulvius*. It may contain a suitable preservative. It should be preserved in single-dose containers and stored at a temperature not exceeding 40°.

Adverse Effects and Precautions

As for antisera in general, p.1500.

Serum sickness is not uncommon and anaphylactic reactions may occur.

A study[1] on the prediction, prevention, and mechanism of early (anaphylactic) snake venom antiserum reactions in victims of snake bites in Nigeria with systemic envenoming by the saw-scaled or carpet viper (*Echis carinatus*) and in Thailand with local or systemic envenoming by green pit vipers (*Trimeresurus albolabris* and *T. macrops*), the monocellate Thai cobra (*Naja kaouthia*), or the Malayan pit viper (*Calloselasma rhodostoma*). Conjunctival or cutaneous (intradermal or subcutaneous) hypersensitivity testing was performed before the administration of the antisera but failed to predict reactions to the antivenom. It was considered that conventional hypersensitivity testing has no predictive value for the occurrence of allergic reactions to antivenom and that it is not justifiable to delay treatment for 20 or 30 minutes to read the results of these tests. It was also considered that although the rate of administration of the antiserum can be more easily controlled by intravenous infusion this method has serious practical disadvantages in the rural tropics where most cases of snake bite occur and that an advantage of the intravenous push injection is that the person administering the antiserum must remain with the patient during the period when most severe anaphylactic reactions develop.

1. Malasit P, *et al.* Prediction, prevention, and mechanism of early (anaphylactic) antivenom reactions in victims of snake bites. *Br Med J* 1986; **292:** 17–20.

Uses and Administration

Venomous snakes comprise the Viperidae (vipers), Elapidae (cobras, kraits, and mambas), and the Hydrophiidae (sea snakes).

The venom of snakes is a complex mixture chiefly of proteins, many of which have enzymatic activity, and may also provoke local inflammatory reactions. The venom may have profound effects on tissue, blood vessels and other organs, blood cells, coagulation, and myotoxic or neurotoxic effects with sensory, motor, cardiac, renal, and respiratory involvement.

Snake venom antisera are the only specific treatment available for venomous snake bites, but can produce severe adverse reactions. They are generally only used if there are clear indications of systemic involvement, severe local involvement, or, in regions where supplies are not limited, in patients at high risk of systemic or severe local involvement.

In Great Britain the only indigenous poisonous snake is the adder, *Viperus berus*, and European Viper Venom Antiserum (or Zagreb antivenom) may sometimes be indicated as part of the overall treatment. The usual dose for adults and children is 10 mL by intravenous injection over 10 to 15 minutes or by intravenous infusion over 30 minutes after diluting in 5 mL per kg body-weight of sodium chloride 0.9%; the dose may be repeated after about 1 to 2 hours if symptoms of systemic envenoming persist. Resuscitation facilities should be available.

In the USA a polyvalent crotaline antiserum against *Bothrops atrox, Crotalus adamanteus, C. atrox*, and *C. durissus terrificus*, and an antiserum against the North American coral snake, *Micrurus fulvius*, are available. In Australia a polyvalent antiserum against the black snake, brown snake, death adder, taipan, and tiger snake is available. In many countries a wide variety of other antisera are also available.

Snake bites. Most snake species are non-venomous and belong to the colubrid family although a few colubrids are technically venomous. The three families of venomous front-fanged snakes are the elapids, vipers, and sea snakes. Elapids include cobras, mambas, kraits, coral snakes, and the Australasian venomous land snakes. Vipers are subdivided into crotalids (pit vipers) and viperids. Viper bites are much more common than elapid bites, except in Australasia, where vipers do not occur naturally. Sea snake bites occur among fishermen of the Asian and western Pacific coastal areas. Although there are some notable exceptions, viper bites tend to cause vasculotoxicity, elapids cause neurotoxicity, and sea snakes cause myotoxicity.

Only a few snakes are known to be of medical importance. Of the vipers these include *Bothrops atrox* (Central and South America), *Bitis arietans* (Africa), *Echis carinatus* (Africa and Asia), *Vipera russelli* (Asia), and *Agkistrodon rhodostoma* (south-east Asia). In a few restricted areas of Africa and Asia, cobra bites are common; bites by mambas (Africa) and kraits (Asia) are rare. The carpet or saw-scaled viper, *Echis carinatus*, can justifiably be labelled the most dangerous snake in the world and it causes more deaths and serious poisoning than any other snake.

Management of snake bite involves general supportive care and monitoring of vital functions but in a systemic snake-bite poisoning, specific snake venom antiserum is the most effective therapeutic agent available. If used correctly, it can reverse systemic poisoning when given hours or even days after the bite. It is highly desirable to wait for clear clinical evidence of systemic poisoning before giving an antiserum and therefore it should not be given routinely in all cases of snake bite. Monospecific antisera are more effective, and less likely to cause reactions, than polyvalent antisera. The dosage of antiserum to be used is dependent on the species of snake and the consequent potency of the requisite antiserum. The antiserum should be given intravenously diluted in isotonic saline, either by infusion or bolus injection (see under Adverse Effects and Precautions, above). First aid measures including incisions and suction to remove the venom and application of tourniquets are generally to be discouraged. In most cases, the bitten limb should be immobilised and the victim transferred to a medical facility, together with the snake if possible. For bites by elapids, when respiratory failure may occur before the patient reaches hospital, a tourniquet may be justified to delay the onset of neurotoxicity. Supportive treatment is necessary even in patients who have received an adequate dose of antiserum. Local pain may be treated with a suitable analgesic. Artificial respiration may be required in patients with symptoms of neurotoxicity. Anticholinesterases may be of benefit against the neurotoxic effects of some snake venoms and it has been recommended that an intravenous test dose of edrophonium preceded by atropine should be tried in patients with severe symptoms of neurotoxicity. For those patients who respond, treatment with neostigmine should be started but anticholinesterases are unlikely to affect outcome in patients who already require assisted respiration. Hypovolaemia should be corrected cautiously with parenteral fluids. Hypotension may be treated with subcutaneous adrenaline or, in patients bitten by Russell's viper, has responded to dopamine. Patients with impaired renal function may require dialysis if they do not respond to rehydration, diuretics, and dopamine. Broad spectrum antibiotics and tetanus toxoid should be given as prophylactic measures. Surgical decompression and debridement of necrotic tissue may be necessary once normal haemostasis has been restored.

References.

1. Reid HA, Theakston RDG. The management of snake bite. *Bull WHO* 1983; **61:** 885–95.
2. Nelson BK. Snake envenomation: incidence, clinical presentation and management. *Med Toxicol* 1989; **4:** 17–31.
3. Warrell DA. Snake venoms in science and clinical medicine: 1. Russell's viper: biology, venom and treatment of bites. *Trans R Soc Trop Med Hyg* 1989; **83:** 732–40.
4. Theakston RDG. Snakes venoms in science and clinical medicine: 2. applied immunology in snake venom research. *Trans R Soc Trop Med Hyg* 1989; **83:** 741–4.
5. Hulton RA, *et al.* Arboreal green pit vipers (genus Trimeresurus) of South-east Asia: bites by T. albolabris and T. macrops in Thailand and a review of the literature. *Trans R Soc Trop Med Hyg* 1990; **84:** 866–74.
6. Smith TA, Figge HL. Treatment of snakebite poisoning. *Am J Hosp Pharm* 1991; **48:** 2190–6.
7. Warrell DA, Fenner PJ. Venomous bites and stings. *Br Med Bull* 1993; **49:** 423–39.
8. Tibballs J. Premedication for snake antivenom. *Med J Aust* 1994; **160:** 4–7.
9. Caiaffa WT, *et al.* Snake bite and antivenom complications in Belo Horizonate, Brazil. *Trans R Soc Trop Med Hyg* 1994; **88:** 81–5.
10. Trevett AJ, *et al.* The efficacy of antivenom in the treatment of bites by the Papuan taipan (Oxyuranus scutellatus canni). *Trans R Soc Trop Med Hyg* 1995; **89:** 322–5.
11. Jorge MT, *et al.* A randomized 'blinded' comparison of two doses of antivenom in the treatment of Bothrops envenoming in Sao Paulo, Brazil. *Trans R Soc Trop Med Hyg* 1995; **89:** 111–14.
12. Otero R, *et al.* A randomized double-blind clinical trial of two antivenoms in patients bitten by Bothrops atrox in Colombia. *Trans R Soc Trop Med Hyg* 1996; **90:** 696–700.
13. Mead HJ, Jelinek GA. Suspected snakebite in children: a study of 156 patients over 10 years. *Med J Aust* 1996; **164:** 467–70.
14. Paret G, *et al.* Vipera palaestinae snake envenomations: experience in children. *Hum Exp Toxicol* 1997; **16:** 683–7.

Preparations

Ph. Eur.: European Viper Venom Antiserum;
USP 23: Antivenin (Crotalidae) Polyvalent; Antivenin (Micrurus Fulvius).

Proprietary Preparations (details are given in Part 3)
Austral.: Polyvalent Snake Antivenom; Snake Bite; ***Canad.:*** Antivenin; ***Fr.:*** Ipser Europe; ***Ital.:*** Siero Antiofidico.

Spider Venom Antisera (8035-x)

Spider Antivenins; Spider Antivenoms.

Antivenin (Latrodectus Mactans) (USP 23) a sterile freeze-dried preparation of specific venom-neutralising globulins obtained from the serum of healthy horses immunised against venom of black widow spiders (*Latrodectus mactans*). One dose neutralises the venom in not less than 6000 mouse LD_{50} of *L. mactans*. It contains thiomersal as preservative. It should be preserved in single-dose containers and stored at a temperature not exceeding 40°.

Adverse Effects and Precautions

As for antisera in general, p.1500.

Uses and Administration

The use of a spider venom antiserum suitable for the species of spider can prevent symptoms provided it is done with the least possible delay; other general supportive measures and symptomatic treatment may also be needed.

An antiserum against the black widow spider (*Latrodectus mactans*) is available in the USA and the contents of a vial containing at least 6000 antivenin units is the usual dose for adults and children. In severe cases and children under 12 years of age it is given by intravenous infusion in sodium chloride 0.9% over 15 minutes; in less severe cases, it may be given by intramuscular injection.

An antiserum against the funnel-web spider (*Atrax robustus*) is available in Australia.

Spider bites. Although many species of spider are venomous, relatively few pose a danger to man. Two main clinical syndromes are recognised; necrotic araneism, produced mainly by members of the genus *Loxosceles* which includes the brown recluse spider *L. reclusa*, and neurotoxic araneism produced by members of the genera *Latrodectus* (including the black widow and red-back spiders), *Phoneutria* (South American banana spiders), and *Atrax* (funnel-web spiders).

Necrotic araneism presents as local pain and erythema at the site of the bite, commonly developing into a necrotic lesion with a black eschar which sloughs after a few weeks, sometimes leaving an ulcer which heals gradually. The area affected can be extensive. Rarely, systemic symptoms including intravascular coagulation, haemolytic anaemia, respiratory distress, and renal failure, occur and may be life-threatening. A number of therapies have been suggested, but conservative management is usually adequate with surgical repair of any persistent defects if necessary. Dapsone is reported to produce beneficial effects on healing. Treatment for systemic manifestations is supportive. Antisera are available in some countries.

Neurotoxic araneism may involve severe pain, headache, vomiting, tachycardia, hypertension, muscle spasms, and occasionally pulmonary oedema, and coma, depending upon the species. Antisera are available and reported to be more effective than those for necrotic araneism, but should be reserved for serious envenomation. Intravenous injection of calcium gluconate 10% has been suggested to relieve muscle spasm as an alternative to conventional muscle relaxants.

References.

1. King LE, Rees RS. Dapsone treatment of a brown recluse bite. *JAMA* 1983; **250:** 648.
2. Hartman LJ, Sutherland SK. Funnel-web spider (Atrax robustus) antivenom in the treatment of human envenomation. *Med J Aust* 1984; **141:** 796–9.
3. Rees RS, *et al.* Brown recluse spider bites: a comparison of early surgical excision versus dapsone and delayed surgical excision. *Ann Surg* 1985; **202:** 659–63.
4. Dieckmann J, *et al.* Efficacy of funnel-web spider antivenom in human envenomation by Hadronyche species. *Med J Aust* 1989; **151:** 706–7.
5. Binder LS. Acute arthropod envenomation: incidence, clinical features and management. *Med Toxicol Adverse Drug Exp* 1989; **4:** 163–73.
6. Clark RF, *et al.* Clinical presentation and treatment of black widow spider envenomation: a review of 163 cases. *Ann Emerg Med* 1992; **21:** 782–7.
7. Warrell DA, Fenner PJ. Venomous bites and stings. *Br Med Bull* 1993; **49:** 423–39.

Preparations

USP 23: Antivenin (Latrodectus Mactans).

Proprietary Preparations (details are given in Part 3)
Canad.: Antivenin (Latrodectus Mactans).

Staphylococcal Vaccines (8013-j)

Staphylococcal vaccines, prepared from inactivated *Staphylococcus* spp. are used for the prophylaxis and treatment of staphylococcal infections. They have been administered orally, topically, and by injection.

Preparations

Proprietary Preparations (details are given in Part 3)
Ital.: Duplovac†; *Spain:* Duplovac†; *USA:* SPL.

Stone Fish Venom Antisera (12230-j)

Stone Fish Antivenins; Stone Fish antivenoms.

Adverse Effects and Precautions

As for antisera in general, p.1500.

Uses and Administration

An antiserum for use in the management of stings by the stone fish (*Synanceja trachynis*) is available in Australia. The antiserum is prepared from the serum of horses that have been immunised with the venom of the stone fish. Other symptomatic and supportive treatments are given in addition.

Stone fish venom antiserum may be given by intramuscular injection or, in more severe cases, by intravenous infusion.

References.

1. Sutherland SK. Stone fish bite. *Br Med J* 1990; **300:** 679–80.
2. Lehmann DF, Hardy JC. Stonefish envenomation. *N Engl J Med* 1993; **329:** 510–11.

Streptococcus Group B Vaccines (11716-v)

Vaccines for active immunisation against group B streptococcal infections are being developed. Administration of a vaccine to pregnant women to prevent neonatal infection has been proposed.

References.

1. Baker CJ, *et al.* Immunization of pregnant women with a polysaccharide vaccine of group B streptococcus. *N Engl J Med* 1988; **319:** 1180–5.
2. Coleman RT, *et al.* Prevention of neonatal group B streptococcal infections: advances in maternal vaccine development. *Obstet Gynecol* 1992; **80:** 301–9.
3. Kasper DL, *et al.* Immune response to type III group B streptococcal polysaccharide-tetanus toxoid conjugate vaccine. *J Clin Invest* 1996; **98:** 2308–14.
4. Kotloff KL, *et al.* Safety and immunogenicity of a tetravalent group B streptococcal polysaccharide vaccine in healthy adults. *Vaccine* 1996; **14:** 446–50.

Tetanus Antitoxins (8016-k)

Tetanus Antitoxin for Human Use (Ph. Eur.) (Tetanus Antitoxin (BP 1998); Immunoserum Tetanicum ad Usum Humanum; Tet/Ser) is a sterile preparation containing the specific antitoxic globulins that have the power of neutralising the toxin formed by *Clostridium tetani*. It is obtained by fractionation from the serum of horses, or other mammals, that have been immunised against tetanus toxin. For prophylactic use, it has a potency of not less than 1000 international units per mL, and for therapeutic use not less than 3000 international units per mL. It should be stored at 2° to 8°, and not be allowed to freeze.

Tetanus Antitoxin (USP 23) is a sterile solution of the refined and concentrated proteins, chiefly globulins, containing antitoxic antibodies obtained from the serum or plasma of healthy horses that have been immunised against tetanus toxin or toxoid. It contains not less than 400 units per mL. It should be stored at 2° to 8°.

Tetanus antitoxins neutralise the toxin produced by *Clostridium tetani* and have been used to provide temporary passive immunity against tetanus, but tetanus immunoglobulins (below) are preferred. A test dose of tetanus antitoxin should always be given to identify those who might suffer hypersensitivity reactions.

Whenever a non-immune patient is seen because of injury opportunity should be taken to institute a course of active immunisation (see Tetanus Vaccines, p.1535).

Preparations

Ph. Eur.: Tetanus Antitoxin for Human Use;
USP 23: Tetanus Antitoxin.

Tetanus Immunoglobulins (1241-c)

Human Tetanus Immunoglobulin (Ph. Eur.) (Antitetanus Immunoglobulin Injection; Tetanus Immunoglobulin (BP 1998); Immunoglobulinum Humanum Tetanicum) is a liquid or freeze-dried preparation containing immunoglobulins, mainly immunoglobulin G (IgG). It is obtained from plasma containing specific antibodies against the toxin of *Clostridium tetani*. Normal immunoglobulin may be added. It contains not less than 100 international units per mL. Both the liquid and freeze-dried preparations should be stored, protected from light, in a colourless, glass container. The freeze-dried preparation should be stored under vacuum or under an inert gas.

Tetanus Immune Globulin (USP 23) is a sterile solution of globulins derived from the plasma of adult human donors who have been immunised with tetanus vaccine. It contains not less than 50 units of tetanus antitoxin per mL. It contains 10 to 18% of protein of which not less than 90% is gamma globulin. It contains glycine as a stabilising agent, and a suitable preservative. It should be stored at 2° to 8°.

Adverse Effects and Precautions

As for immunoglobulins in general, p.1500.

Interactions

As for immunoglobulins in general, p.1500.

Tetanus immunoglobulins will neutralise tetanus toxoid and should not be injected into the same site or in the same syringe as a tetanus vaccine.

Uses and Administration

Tetanus immunoglobulins are used for passive immunisation against tetanus.

The use of tetanus immunoglobulins is recommended in the UK and the USA as part of the management of tetanus-prone wounds in persons unimmunised or incompletely immunised against tetanus, in persons whose immunisation history is unknown, in persons who received the last dose of tetanus vaccine more than 10 years previously, and in patients with impaired immunity. Active immunisation with a tetanus vaccine (p.1535) should also be started simultaneously, and antibacterials and symptomatic therapy given as appropriate (see p.145 and p.1304). The usual dose of tetanus immunoglobulin is 250 units by intramuscular injection but if more than 24 hours have elapsed since the wound was sustained, if there is a risk of heavy contamination, or following burns 500 units should be given irrespective of the immunisation history.

Tetanus immunoglobulin is also used in the treatment of tetanus, a recommended dose being 150 units per kg body-weight given intramuscularly into multiple sites. Doses in the range 30 to 300 units per kg are suggested by the manufacturer in the UK.

A preparation suitable for intravenous use is available in some countries. It is given for the treatment of tetanus in a dose of 5000 to 10 000 units by intravenous infusion.

Preparations

Ph. Eur.: Human Tetanus Immunoglobulin;
USP 23: Tetanus Immune Globulin.

Proprietary Preparations (details are given in Part 3)
Aust.: T-GAM†; Tetabulin; Tetagam; Tetagloman†; Tetanosimultan; Tetavenin; Tetuman; *Belg.:* Tetabuline; Tetaglobuline†; Tetuman; *Canad.:* Hyper-Tet; *Fr.:* Gamma Tetanos†; *Ger.:* Hyper-Tet†; Tetagam N; Tetaglobulin S†; Tetanobulin S; TIG Horm†; WellcoTIG†; *Irl.:* Humotet†; Tetabulin; *Ital.:* Gamma-Tet P; Haima-Tetanus; Immunotetan; Imogam 16†; Imogam Tetano; Tetabulin; Tetagamma; Tetanus-Gamma; Tetaven; Tetuman; *S.Afr.:* Tetagam; Tetuman; *Spain:* Gamma Glob Antite; Glogama Antitetanica†; Imogam Tetanos†; Inmunogamma Antitet†; Noviserum Antitet†; Tetuman; Torlanbulina Antitenani; *Switz.:* Tetabuline; Tetavenine†; Tetuman; *UK:* Tetabulin; *USA:* Hyper-Tet.

Tetanus Vaccines (8020-y)

Tetanus Vaccine (BP 1998) (Tet/Vac/FT) is prepared from tetanus toxin produced by the growth of *Clostridium tetani*. The toxin is converted to tetanus formol toxoid by treatment with formaldehyde solution. It should be stored at 2° to 8°, not be allowed to freeze, and be protected from light. The BP directs that when Tetanus Vaccine is prescribed or demanded and the form is not stated, Adsorbed Tetanus Vaccine may be dispensed or supplied.

Tetanus Vaccine (Adsorbed) (Ph. Eur.) (Tet/Vac/Ads; Adsorbed Tetanus Vaccine (BP 1998); Vaccinum Tetani Adsorbatum) is prepared from tetanus formol toxoid adsorbed on a mineral carrier which may be hydrated aluminium hydroxide, aluminium phosphate, or calcium phosphate. The resulting mixture is isotonic with blood. Suitable antimicrobial preservatives may be added. The antigenic properties are adversely affected by certain antimicrobial preservatives particularly those of the phenolic type and these should not be added to the vaccine. It contains not less than 40 units per dose. It should be stored at 2° to 8°, not be allowed to freeze, and be protected from light.

Tetanus Toxoid (USP 23) is a sterile solution of the formaldehyde-treated products of growth of *Clostridium tetani*. It contains a non-phenolic preservative. It should be stored at 2° to 8° and not be allowed to freeze.

Tetanus Toxoid Adsorbed (USP 23) is a sterile preparation of plain tetanus toxoid precipitated or adsorbed by alum, aluminium hydroxide, or aluminium phosphate adjuvants. It should be stored at 2° to 8° and not be allowed to freeze.

Adverse Effects and Precautions

As for vaccines in general, p.1500.

Local reactions, usually following the use of adsorbed vaccines, and mild systemic reactions may occur. The incidence and severity of reactions increases with the number of doses given.

Anaphylaxis and neurological reactions have occasionally been reported.

Although vaccination is usually postponed in patients suffering from an acute febrile illness, tetanus vaccine should be given to such patients in the presence of a tetanus-prone wound.

Booster doses of tetanus vaccine should not generally be given at intervals of less than 10 years because of an increased risk of severe local reactions.

Effects of purification. In a double-blind comparative study[1] involving 205 healthy subjects there was no difference in side-effects in those given a standard (commercial) tetanus vaccine and those given an antibody-affinity-purified vaccine. The results confirmed that side-effects to tetanus vaccines are not eliminated by purification.

1. Leen CLS, *et al.* Double-blind comparative trial of standard (commercial) and antibody-affinity-purified tetanus toxoid vaccines. *J Infect* 1987; **14:** 119–24.

Effects on the nervous system. Neuropathies have been reported rarely following tetanus vaccination. Optic neuritis and myelitis occurred[1] in an 11-year-old girl following a routine booster dose. Corticosteroids and immunoglobulin were given, and both vision and muscle power were restored after 11 months. Acute transverse myelitis was reported[2] in a 50-year-old man who received tetanus toxoid and immunoglobulin following an injury. Neurological deficits were unchanged after 1 month despite treatment with corticosteroids. Other causes could not be ruled out in either case. Brachial neuritis which developed in 2 infants following immunisation with diphtheria, tetanus, and pertussis vaccine was attributed to the tetanus component.[3]

1. Topaloglu H, *et al.* Optic neuritis and myelitis after booster tetanus toxoid vaccination. *Lancet* 1992; **339:** 178–9.
2. Read SJ, *et al.* Acute transverse myelitis after tetanus toxoid vaccination. *Lancet* 1992; **339:** 1111–12.
3. Hamati-Haddad A, Fenichel GM. Brachial neuritis following routine childhood immunization for diphtheria, tetanus, and pertussis (DTP): report of two cases and review of the literature. *Pediatrics* 1997; **99:** 602–3.

GUILLAIN-BARRÉ SYNDROME. A possible causal relationship between tetanus-containing vaccines and Guillain-Barré syndrome has been proposed (see Diphtheria and Tetanus Vaccines, p.1508).

Pregnancy. No connection has been found between administration of tetanus toxoid during pregnancy and either congenital malformations[1] or spontaneous abortion.[2]

1. Silveira CM, *et al.* Safety of tetanus toxoid in pregnant women: a hospital-based case-control study of congenital anomalies. *Bull WHO* 1995; **73:** 605–8.
2. Catindig N, *et al.* Tetanus toxoid and spontaneous abortions: is there epidemiological evidence of an association? *Lancet* 1996; **348:** 1098–9.

Interactions

As for vaccines in general, p.1501.

Tetanus immunoglobulins will neutralise tetanus toxoid and should not be injected into the same site or in the same syringe as a tetanus vaccine.

Uses and Administration

Tetanus vaccines are used for active immunisation against tetanus.

For primary immunisation a combined diphtheria, tetanus, and pertussis vaccine (p.1509) or a combined diphtheria and tetanus vaccine (p.1508) is usually used. For discussion of immunisation schedules see under Vaccines, p.1501. In adults requiring primary immunisation, single component adsorbed tetanus vaccine or, if appropriate, combined tetanus and low-dose diphtheria vaccine may be used. The non-adsorbed type of tetanus vaccine is less potent as an antigen than the adsorbed type and the adsorbed vaccine is generally preferred. The primary immunisation course in the UK consists of 3 doses, each of 0.5 mL, administered at intervals of one month by deep subcutaneous or intramuscular injection. In children who complete the primary course in infancy, reinforcing doses are given at school entry and on leaving school in combination with the appropriate diphtheria vaccine. In adults, a reinforcing dose is desirable 10 years later with a further dose after a further 10 years. Further booster doses are not recommended for adults who have received 5 doses, other than at the time of injury, since they are unnecessary and can cause considerable local reactions. However, in some countries, including the USA, reinforcing doses are given every 10 years.

The need for tetanus vaccines in wound management depends on both the condition of the wound and the patient's immunisation history. If primary immunisation or a reinforcing dose has been given within the last 10 years, tetanus vaccine should not be given but the patient should receive tetanus immunoglobulin if the risk of infection is considered especially high. If more than 10 years has elapsed, a reinforcing dose of adsorbed vaccine should be given. For tetanus-prone wounds tetanus immunoglobulin (see above) may also be required. Tetanus vaccine and tetanus immunoglobulin may be given concomitantly, but not at the same site. In the event of injury in non-immunised persons or if immunisation status is uncertain opportunity is usually taken to initiate a course of primary immunisation. Since this provides no immediate protection, prophylactic treatment with tetanus immunoglobulin is recommended for tetanus-prone wounds. Suitable antibacterial therapy may also be given (see p.145).

Anergy testing. For reference to the use of tetanus vaccines for anergy testing in HIV-positive patients, see Tuberculins, p.1640.

Bone-marrow transplant recipients. In a study[1] of 48 recipients of bone-marrow transplants immunity to tetanus was not transferred from seropositive donors to seronegative patients. An unexpected finding was that pre-transplant antibody level of the patient, and not the donor, strongly influenced the antibody level one year after transplantation. Immunity quickly waned, however, after transplantation. Reimmunisation with tetanus vaccine is therefore required in long-term survivors of bone-marrow transplants. The study suggested that 3 doses are needed to obtain adequate protection. The necessity for further doses requires study.

1. Ljungman P, *et al.* Response to tetanus toxoid immunization after allogeneic bone marrow transplantation. *J Infect Dis* 1990; **162:** 496–500.

Neonatal tetanus. Responding to an estimated 800 000 deaths of newborn infants from neonatal tetanus each year world-wide (but excluding China), accounting for approximately 50% of all deaths in the neonatal period in developing countries, WHO adopted a resolution in 1989 to eliminate neonatal tetanus. Control of neonatal tetanus may be achieved by ensuring adequate hygiene during delivery and by ensuring protective immunity of the mother in late pregnancy.

Tetanus vaccine is administered to all women of childbearing age as part of WHO's Expanded Programme on Immunization. For pregnant women, two doses of toxoid, the second dose at least 4 weeks after the first and at least 2 weeks before delivery, provide the newborn infant with approximately 80% protection against tetanus. For all women of childbearing age, three doses of toxoid, with at least 4 weeks between the first two doses and 6 months between the second and third doses, provide 95% protection for up to 5 years. Fourth and fifth doses, each at least one year after the previous dose, ensure lifelong protection.

Immunisation of pregnant women with tetanus toxoid lags well behind levels achieved for childhood vaccines in the Expanded Programme on Immunization. In June 1987, it was estimated that fewer than 20% of all pregnant women had received two doses of toxoid.[1] By 1993 this had increased to 45%, and the estimated number of deaths had decreased to 515 000 (including 98 000 in China, where immunisation began in 1992).[2]

1. Hayden GF, *et al.* Progress in worldwide control and elimination of disease through immunization. *J Pediatr* 1989; **114:** 520–7.
2. Centers for Disease Control. Progress toward the global elimination of neonatal tetanus, 1989-1993. *MMWR* 1994; **43:** 885–94.

Reinforcing doses in adults. Although the current recommendation in the UK is that 5 doses of tetanus toxoid (as a 3-dose primary course and 2 reinforcing doses at 10-year intervals) is sufficient to produce life-long immunity to tetanus, there is still concern about immunity in the elderly, and in particular women. Routine primary immunisation against tetanus was introduced in the UK in 1961, so individuals born before that year would not have been immunised in infancy, and unless they had been in the armed forces, may never have received a full primary course.[1] Unless there is a clear immunisation history immunity to tetanus may be difficult to assess.

Studies in the USA,[2] Australia,[3] and Austria[4] have shown that at least half of healthy people over 50 years of age did not have adequate circulating tetanus antibodies. However, the level of circulating antibodies in the absence of an antigen challenge may not be an appropriate measure of the immune status. The low incidence of clinical tetanus in adults provides circumstantial evidence of an adequate inducible antibody response on exposure to tetanus despite a decline in antibody concentrations with increasing age.[5,6] Conversely, there have been reports of tetanus occurring despite high antibody concentrations.[7,8] There have been calls for the introduction of regular booster injections in adults,[4,8-10] as is standard practice in the USA or alternatively a single booster in late middle age[11,12] or administering a primary course to elderly persons who have never received one.[2]

1. Salisbury DM, Begg NT (eds), Joint Committee on Vaccination and Immunisation. *Immunisation against infectious disease.* London: HMSO, 1996.
2. Gergen PJ, *et al.* A population-based serologic survey of immunity to tetanus in the United States. *N Engl J Med* 1995; **332:** 761–6.
3. Heath TC, *et al.* Tetanus immunity in an older Australian population. *Med J Aust* 1996; **164:** 593–6.
4. Steger MM, *et al.* Vaccination against tetanus in the elderly: do recommended vaccination strategies give sufficient protection? *Lancet* 1996; **348:** 762.
5. Bowie C. Tetanus toxoid for adults—too much of a good thing. *Lancet* 1996; **348:** 1185–6.
6. Baily G. Are the elderly inadequately protected against tetanus? *Lancet* 1996; **348:** 1389–90.
7. Passen EL, Andersen BR. Clinical tetanus despite a 'protective' level of toxin-neutralising antibody. *JAMA* 1986; **255:** 1171–3.
8. Bowman C, *et al.* Tetanus toxoid for adults. *Lancet* 1996; **348:** 1664.
9. Rethy LA, Rethy L. Can tetanus boosting be rejected? *Lancet* 1997; **349:** 359–60.
10. Sehgal R. Tetanus toxoid for adults. *Lancet* 1997; **349:** 573.
11. Balestra DJ, Littenberg B. Tetanus immunization in adults. *JAMA* 1994; **272:** 1900.
12. Gardner P, LaForce FM. Protection against tetanus. *N Engl J Med* 1995; **333:** 599.

Preparations

BP 1998: Tetanus Vaccine;
Ph. Eur.: Tetanus Vaccine (Adsorbed);
USP 23: Tetanus Toxoid; Tetanus Toxoid Adsorbed.

Proprietary Preparations (details are given in Part 3)
Aust.: T-Immun; Tanrix; Te Anatoxal; Tetanol; ***Austral.:*** Tet-Tox; ***Belg.:*** Anatoxal Te; Tetamer; Tevax; ***Fr.:*** Tetavax; ***Ger.:*** T-Immun; T-Medevax; T-Rix†; T-Vaccinol†; T-Wellcovax†; Tet-Aktiv†; Tetamun SSW; Tetanol; Tetasorbat SSW; Tetavax; ***Ital.:*** Anatetall; H-Atetal; Imovax Tetano; Tanrix; Tetanol†; Tetatox; ***Neth.:*** Tetavax; ***S.Afr.:*** Tetavax; ***Spain:*** Alutoxoide T†; Anatoxal Te; Tetanibys†; Vac Antitet†; Vac Antitetanica; ***Switz.:*** Anatoxal Te; ***UK:*** Clostet; Tetavax.

Tetanus and Influenza Vaccines (13574-d)

Tetanus and influenza vaccines are available in some countries for active immunisation against tetanus and influenza.

Preparations

Proprietary Preparations (details are given in Part 3)
Fr.: Tetagrip.

Tetanus and Poliomyelitis Vaccines (13575-n)

Tetanus and poliomyelitis (inactivated) vaccines are available in some countries for active immunisation against tetanus and poliomyelitis.

Preparations

Proprietary Preparations (details are given in Part 3)
Fr.: T. Polio; Vaccin TP.

Tick Venom Antisera (19671-m)

Tick antivenins; Tick Antivenoms.

Adverse Effects and Precautions

As for antisera in general, p.1500.

Uses and Administration

An antiserum is available in Australia for treatment of the neurotoxic effects of envenomation by the tick *Ixodes holocyclus*. The antiserum is prepared from the serum of dogs that have been immunised with tick venom.

Tick venom antiserum is given by slow intravenous infusion.

Trichomoniasis Vaccines (3870-z)

A trichomoniasis vaccine containing inactivated *Lactobacillus acidophilus* is available in some countries for the prophylaxis of recurrent vaginal trichomoniasis in women. The vaccine is reported to stimulate production of antibodies against the aberrant coccoid forms of the lactobacilli associated with trichomoniasis and also, by cross-reaction, against the trichomonads themselves.

Preparations

Proprietary Preparations (details are given in Part 3)
Aust.: Solco-Trichovac†; ***Ger.:*** Gynatren; ***Ital.:*** Ginatren.

Tularaemia Vaccines (1330-k)

A tularaemia vaccine prepared from a live attenuated strain of *Francisella tularensis* is available in some countries. It is used for active immunisation against tularaemia in persons at high risk of contracting the disease.

Typhoid Vaccines (8027-x)

Typhoid Vaccine (Ph. Eur.) (Typhoid/Vac; Vaccinum Febris Typhoidi) is a sterile suspension of inactivated *Salmonella typhi* containing not less than 500 million and not more than 1000 million bacteria per dose which does not exceed 1 mL. It is prepared from a suitable strain of *S. typhi* such as Ty 2. The bacteria are inactivated by heat, or by treatment with acetone, formaldehyde, or phenol, or by phenol and heat. It may also be supplied as a freeze-dried vaccine (Dried Typhoid/Vac) which is reconstituted immediately before use by the addition of suitable sterile liquid. Phenol may not be used in the preparation of the dried vaccine. Ph. Eur. includes the dried vaccine as Typhoid Vaccine, Freeze-dried (Vaccinum Febris Typhoidi Cryodesiccatum). Both the liquid vaccine and the dried vaccine should be stored at 2° to 8°, and be protected from light; the liquid vaccine should not be allowed to freeze. Under these conditions the liquid vaccine may be expected to retain its potency for at least 2 years and the dried vaccine for at least 5 years.

Typhoid Vaccine (Live, Oral, Strain Ty 21a) (Ph. Eur.) (Vaccinum Febris Typhoidis Vivum Perorale (Stirpe Ty 21a); Typhoid (Strain Ty 21a) Vaccine, Live (Oral) (BP 1998); Typhoid/Vac(Oral)) is a freeze-dried preparation of live *S. typhi* strain Ty 21a grown in a suitable medium. It contains not less than 2×10^9 bacteria per dose. It should be stored at 2° to 8°, and be protected from light. Under these conditions it may be expected to retain its potency for at least 18 months.

Typhoid Polysaccharide Vaccine (BP 1998, Ph. Eur.) (Typhoid/Vi/Vac; Vaccinum Febris Typhoidis Polysaccharidicum) is a preparation of purified Vi capsular polysaccharide obtained from *S. typhi* Ty2 strain or some other suitable strain that has the capacity to produce Vi polysaccharide. It contains 25 μg of polysaccharide per dose. It should be stored at 2° to 8°, not be allowed to freeze, and be protected from light.

Typhoid Vaccine (USP 23) is a sterile suspension or solid containing killed typhoid bacilli (*S. typhi*) of the Ty 2 strain. It has a labelled potency of 8 units per mL. Dried vaccine contains no preservative; aqueous vaccine and reconstituting fluid contain a preservative. It should be stored at 2° to 8° and not be allowed to freeze.

Adverse Effects and Precautions

As for vaccines in general, p.1500.

Oral live typhoid and parenteral polysaccharide vaccines have been associated with fewer adverse effects than parenteral killed typhoid vaccines.

Interactions

As for vaccines in general, p.1501. Oral typhoid vaccine should not be given to individuals receiving antibacterials since the development of immunity may be impaired. Individuals receiving mefloquine for malaria prophylaxis should not take oral typhoid vaccine on the same day or, if this is unavoidable, within 12 hours of the mefloquine dose.

Uses and Administration

Typhoid vaccines are used for active immunisation against typhoid fever. As with many vaccines, the efficacy of typhoid vaccine is not complete and the importance of maintaining attention to hygiene should be emphasised to those travelling to endemic areas.

Typhoid vaccination is advised for laboratory workers handling specimens which may contain typhoid organisms and for persons travelling to areas where typhoid fever is endemic. In the UK, vaccination of contacts of a known typhoid carrier is not recommended; in the USA such persons are advised to receive the vaccine. Typhoid vaccine is not useful in controlling outbreaks of the disease.

In the UK two vaccines are available: a capsular polysaccharide vaccine for parenteral use, and a live oral vaccine.

The capsular polysaccharide typhoid vaccine contains 25 μg of the Vi polysaccharide antigen per dose. A single dose of 0.5 mL is given by deep subcutaneous or intramuscular injection. Booster doses may be given every 3 years to those who remain at risk. The response in children under 18 months of age may be suboptimal, and the decision to vaccinate will be governed by the risk of exposure to infection.

The live oral typhoid vaccine contains an attenuated strain of *Salmonella typhi*, Ty 21a, and is administered as enteric-coated capsules containing not less than 2×10^9 bacteria per dose. A primary immunisation schedule of one capsule every other day for 3 doses is recommended. The capsule should be taken on an empty stomach with a cold or luke-warm drink. This oral vaccine is not considered suitable for children under 6 years of age. Immunity persists for about 3 years under conditions of continuous or repeated exposure. For less frequent visitors to endemic regions, a 3-dose booster may be given annually.

A monovalent whole-cell killed vaccine was also formerly available, and was given parenterally in 2 doses at an interval of 4 to 6 weeks. The first dose was given by intramuscular or deep subcutaneous injection, although subsequent doses could be given intradermally to reduce adverse reactions.

In the USA, whole cell parenteral, capsular polysaccharide, and live oral vaccines are available. The former is given in a primary course of 2 injections of 0.5 mL, given subcutaneously at an interval of 4 or more weeks to adults and children over 10 years of age; children from 6 months to 10 years may be given 2 doses of 0.25 mL. An additional alternative accelerated schedule of three doses at weekly intervals is suggested, although this may be less effective than the standard 2-dose schedule. Booster doses should be given every 3 years. The capsular polysaccharide vaccine is given similarly to the UK, with a booster dose suggested every 2 years. For the oral vaccine, 4 doses on alternate days is recommended for both primary immunisation and boosters, which are given every 5 years if exposure continues.

Attenuated *Salmonella typhi* strains are being investigated as live delivery systems for other foreign antigens. They are attractive candidates as live carriers because they are administered orally and they elicit a broad immune response in human beings. Techniques have been developed for incorporation of foreign genes in the chromosome or plasmids of the *S. typhi* organism.[1]

1. Levine MM. Modern vaccines: enteric infections. *Lancet* 1990; **335:** 958–61.

Immunisation for travellers. In most developed countries where typhoid is not endemic, the major use for typhoid vaccine is for non-immune travellers visiting endemic areas. Doubts have been raised over the necessity for typhoid vaccination for the majority of travellers because of the rarity of the disease in travellers and the unproven efficacy of the available vaccines in this population.[1] The highest incidence of the disease is associated with travel to the Indian subcontinent and parts of tropical South America although immunisation is also recommended for travellers to lower risk areas of Africa, Asia, and south-east Europe.[1,2] By far the most important form of protection against gastro-intestinal infection is strict attention to personal, food, and water hygiene, although in practice this advice is often difficult to follow.

None of the vaccines currently available is 100% effective in preventing disease. The effectiveness of the vaccines has generally been assessed in field trials in the populations of endemic areas. Such populations acquire a degree of natural immunity due to continued exposure and it may not be possible to equate protection rates in these populations to non-immune travellers.[1] The whole-cell vaccine has been evaluated in non-immune subjects[3] and was shown to confer partial protection against a relatively low inoculum compared with that likely to be encountered from foodborne transmission.[1] The live oral vaccine has been shown to confer a useful degree of immunity in field trials[4,5] but the dose used may have been insufficient to protect non-immune individuals. The degree of immunity induced may be increased by the use of higher inocula[6] or liquid preparations.[5,7] In addition, compliance with dosing and storage requirements may further limit the effectiveness of this dosage form.[8]

Two large field studies[9,10] have verified the effectiveness of the capsular polysaccharide vaccine but its efficacy has not been assessed in non-immune populations. However, it does have the advantage of being administered as a single dose.

A recent meta-analysis[11] of randomised studies has concluded that whole-cell vaccines are more efficacious than the capsular polysaccharide and oral vaccines, but are more frequently associated with adverse effects. Thus the decision over which vaccine to use will essentially be based on cost, availability, severity of adverse effects, route, and dosage schedules.[2] For individuals who have previously received the whole-cell vaccine without difficulty, there is no need to change to the newer vaccines, especially since booster doses can be given intradermally to reduce adverse reactions. The single dose required for the capsular polysaccharide vaccine may recommend it for primary immunisation. The oral vaccine may have obvious advantages in patient acceptability but it is expensive and the importance of correct storage and dosing should be stressed.[2]

1. Anonymous. Typhoid vaccination: weighing the options. *Lancet* 1992; **340:** 341–2.
2. Anonymous. Typhoid vaccines—which one to choose? *Drug Ther Bull* 1993; **31:** 9–10.
3. Hornick RB, *et al.* Typhoid fever: pathogenesis and immunologic control, part 2. *N Engl J Med* 1970; **283:** 739–46.
4. Levine MM, *et al.* Large-scale field trial of Ty21a live oral typhoid vaccine in enteric-coated capsule formulation. *Lancet* 1987; **i:** 1049–52.
5. Simanjuntak CH, *et al.* Oral immunisation against typhoid fever in Indonesia with Ty21a vaccine. *Lancet* 1991; **338:** 1055–9.
6. Ferreccio C, *et al.* Comparative efficacy of two, three, or four doses of Ty21a live oral typhoid vaccine in enteric-coated capsules: a field trial in an endemic area. *J Infect Dis* 1989; **159:** 766–9.
7. Levine MM, *et al.* Comparison of enteric-coated capsules and liquid formulation of Ty21a typhoid vaccine in randomised controlled field trial. *Lancet* 1990; **336:** 891–4.
8. Kaplan DT, *et al.* Compliance with live, oral Ty21a typhoid vaccine. *JAMA* 1992; **267:** 1074.
9. Acharya IL, *et al.* Prevention of typhoid fever in Nepal with the Vi capsular polysaccharide of Salmonella typhi: a preliminary report. *N Engl J Med* 1987; **317:** 1101–4.
10. Klugman KP, *et al.* Protective activity of Vi capsular polysaccharide vaccine against typhoid fever. *Lancet* 1987; **ii:** 1165–9.
11. Engels EA, *et al.* Typhoid fever vaccines: a meta-analysis of studies on efficacy and toxicity. *Br Med J* 1998; **316:** 110–16.

Preparations

Ph. Eur.: Freeze-dried Typhoid Vaccine; Typhoid Polysaccharide Vaccine; Typhoid Vaccine; Typhoid Vaccine (Live, Oral, Strain Ty 21a);
USP 23: Typhoid Vaccine.

Proprietary Preparations (details are given in Part 3)
Aust.: Typhim Vi; Vivotif; ***Austral.:*** Typh-Vax; Typhim Vi; ***Belg.:*** Typhim Vi; Vivotif; ***Canad.:*** Typhim Vi; Vivotif; ***Fr.:*** Typhim Vi; ***Ger.:*** Typhim Vi; Typhoral L; Vivotif; ***Irl.:*** Typhim Vi; Vivotif; ***Ital.:*** Enterovaccino ISI (Antitifico); Enterovaccino Nuovo ISM; Neotyf; Typhim Vi; Vivotif; ***Neth.:*** Typhim Vi; ***Norw.:*** Typhim Vi; Vivotif; ***S.Afr.:*** Typhim Vi; Vivotif; ***Spain:*** Vac Antitifica†; Vac Tab Berna†; Vivotif; ***Swed.:*** Typhim Vi; Vivotif; ***Switz.:*** Vaccin Tab; Vivotif; ***UK:*** Typherix; Typhim Vi; Vivotif; ***USA:*** Typhim Vi; Vivotif.

Typhoid and Tetanus Vaccines (8025-a)

Typhoid and Tetanus Vaccine (BP 1998) (Typhoid/Tet/Vac) is a sterile mixture of a suspension of killed *Salmonella typhi* and tetanus formol toxoid, containing 1000 million or 2000 million typhoid bacteria per mL. The suspension is prepared from a strain or strains of *S. typhi* that are smooth and have a full complement of H, O, and Vi antigens. The bacteria are killed by heat or by treatment with formaldehyde or phenol. It should be stored at 2° to 8°, not be allowed to freeze, and be protected from light.

A combined typhoid and tetanus vaccine has been used by subcutaneous injection for primary immunisation against typhoid fever and tetanus and by intramuscular injection to reinforce immunity.

Preparations

BP 1998: Typhoid and Tetanus Vaccine.

Proprietary Preparations (details are given in Part 3)
Ital.: Vaccino Tab Te.

Typhus Vaccines (8034-t)

Typhus Vaccine (BP 1998) (Typhus/Vac) is a sterile suspension of killed epidemic typhus rickettsiae [*Rickettsia prowazekii*] prepared in the yolk sacs of embryonated eggs, rodent lungs, or the peritoneal cavity of gerbils. It should be stored at 2° to 8°, not be allowed to freeze, and be protected from light. Under these conditions it may be expected to retain its potency for at least 1 year.

Adverse Effects and Precautions

As for vaccines in general, p.1500.

Interactions

As for vaccines in general, p.1501.

Uses and Administration

Typhus vaccines may be used for active immunisation against louse-borne typhus. Their use may be considered for those living in or visiting the few endemic areas who are likely to have close contact with the indigenous population, including health care workers, and for laboratory workers. They do not provide protection against scrub typhus.

Preparations

BP 1998: Typhus Vaccine.

Vaccinia Immunoglobulins (1243-a)

Vaccinia Immune Globulin (USP 23) is a sterile solution of globulins derived from the plasma of adult human donors who have been immunised with vaccinia virus (smallpox vaccine). It contains 15 to 18% of protein, of which not less than 90% is gamma globulin. It contains glycine as a stabilising agent, and a suitable antimicrobial agent. It should be stored at 2° to 8°.

Adverse Effects and Precautions

As for immunoglobulins in general, p.1500.

Uses and Administration

Vaccinia immunoglobulins have been used for the treatment of clinical complications of smallpox vaccination. They are not effective for postviral encephalitis.

Preparations

USP 23: Vaccinia Immune Globulin.

Varicella-Zoster Immunoglobulins (17024-h)

Human Varicella Immunoglobulin (Ph. Eur.) (Varicella Immunoglobulin (BP 1998); Immunoglobulinum Humanum Varicellae) is a liquid or freeze-dried preparation containing immunoglobulins, mainly immunoglobulin G (IgG). It is obtained from plasma from selected donors having specific antibodies against *Herpesvirus varicellae*. Normal immunoglobulin may be added. It contains not less than 100 international units per mL. The liquid and freeze-dried preparations should be stored, protected from light, in a colourless, glass container. The freeze-dried preparation should be stored under vacuum or under inert gas.

Varicella-Zoster Immune Globulin (USP 23) is a sterile solution of globulins derived from the plasma of adult donors selected for high titres of varicella-zoster antibodies. It contains 15 to 18% of globulins, of which not less than 99% is immunoglobulin G with traces of immunoglobulin A and immunoglobulin M. It contains glycine as a stabilising agent and thiomersal as a preservative. It contains not less than 125 units of specific antibody in not more than 2.5 mL of solution. It should be stored at 2° to 8°.

Adverse Effects and Precautions

As for immunoglobulins in general, p.1500.

Interactions

As for immunoglobulins in general, p.1500.

Uses and Administration

Varicella-zoster immunoglobulins are used for passive immunisation against varicella (chickenpox) in susceptible persons considered to be at high risk of developing varicella-associated complications after exposure to varicella or herpes zoster (shingles).

In the UK varicella-zoster immunoglobulins are recommended for individuals who are at high risk of severe varicella and who have no antibodies to varicella-zoster virus and who have significant exposure to chickenpox or herpes zoster. Those at increased risk include immunosuppressed patients; neonates including those whose mothers develop chickenpox (but not herpes zoster) in the period 7 days before to 28 days after delivery; and pregnant women. Varicella-zoster immunoglobulin does not prevent infection when given after exposure but may modify the course of disease. Treatment with antivirals may be necessary in severe disease (see p.598).

The recommended doses, given by deep intramuscular injection, of the varicella-zoster immunoglobulin available in the UK are: 250 mg for children up to 5 years of age; 500 mg for those aged 6 to 10 years; 750 mg for those aged 11 to 14 years; and 1 g for all those 15 years of age or older. A further dose is required if a second exposure occurs more than 3 weeks later. Varicella-zoster immunoglobulin should be given as soon as possible and not later than 10 days after exposure. Preparations of normal immunoglobulin for intravenous use may be used to provide an immediate source of antibody.

Recommendations in the USA are similar to those in the UK. Suggested doses are 125 units per 10 kg body-weight by intramuscular injection up to a maximum of 625 units. Adults may be given 625 units but higher doses may be required in immunocompromised patients. Administration should start within 96 hours of exposure.

Preparations

Ph. Eur.: Human Varicella Immunoglobulin;
USP 23: Varicella-Zoster Immune Globulin.

Proprietary Preparations (details are given in Part 3)

Aust.: Varitect; ***Ger.:*** Gammaprotect Varizellen†; Varicellon; Varitect; ***Irl.:*** Varitect; ***Ital.:*** Immunozig; Intrazig; Uman-Vzig; Var-Zeta; Varitect; ***S.Afr.:*** Vazigam; ***Spain:*** Gammalonga Varicela-Zona†; ***Switz.:*** Varitect.

Varicella-Zoster Vaccines (14011-t)

Varicella Vaccine (Live) (Ph. Eur.) (Var/Vac (Live); Varicella Vaccine, Live (BP 1998); Vaccinum Varicellae Vivum) is a freeze-dried preparation of the OKA attenuated strain of *Herpesvirus varicellae* grown in cultures of human diploid cells. The culture medium may contain suitable antibiotics at the smallest effective concentration. It is prepared immediately before use by reconstitution from the dried vaccine; it may contain a stabiliser. The vaccine contains not less than 2000 plaque-forming units per dose. The dried vaccine should be stored at 2° to 8°. Protect from light.

Adverse Effects and Precautions

As for vaccines in general, p.1500.

Rashes at the injection site and varicella-like rashes elsewhere have been reported. It is not known whether the virus becomes latent which could result in late development of zoster infections although there are early indications that the incidence of herpes zoster is lower following vaccination than in an unvaccinated population.

Transmission of the vaccine strain of varicella virus has been reported from a young child to his pregnant mother.[1] After elective termination of the pregnancy, no virus was detected in the fetus.

1. Salzman MB, *et al.* Transmission of varicella-vaccine virus from a healthy 12-month-old child to his pregnant mother. *J Pediatr* 1997; **131:** 151–4.

Interactions

As for vaccines in general, p.1501.

Uses and Administration

Varicella-zoster vaccines may be used for active immunisation against varicella (chickenpox) in persons considered to be at high risk of either contracting the infection or to be highly susceptible to any complications it may cause; such patients include those with leukaemia or those receiving immunosuppressant therapy.

In the USA, vaccination against varicella is recommended as part of the primary immunisation schedule (see under Vaccines, p.1501). A single dose of 0.5 mL is given subcutaneously at 12 to 18 months of age to healthy children unless there is a reliable history of varicella although children may receive the vaccine at any time during childhood after the first birthday. Persons over the age of 13 years at increased risk of exposure or complications should receive two doses at an interval of 4 to 8 weeks.

Although the results of studies of varicella-zoster vaccines in healthy and leukaemic children have been largely favourable,[1,2] until recently, these vaccines have not been recommended for routine use in the UK or USA. Protective **efficacy** in healthy children appears to be over 90%.[1-4] In healthy adolescents and adults, adding a second dose 4 or 8 weeks after the first increased seroconversion rates from about 70 to 80% to 97% or better.[5] A protective efficacy of about 85% has been reported in leukaemic children given one dose of varicella-zoster vaccine.[6,7] A two-dose regimen (doses separated by 3 months) has been tried. Although a second dose is probably of benefit to those who do not seroconvert after one dose, its additional benefit to those who do seroconvert is doubtful.[7] Interruption of chemotherapy for vaccination does not appear necessary in terms of immunogenicity of the vaccine.[6,8] A higher rate of vaccine-associated rashes has, however, been observed in leukaemic children when chemotherapy was suspended for 2 weeks compared with those whose chemotherapy had previously been terminated; this only occurred with certain lots of vaccine.[6]

The **duration of immunity** after varicella-zoster vaccination is also under debate. Studies indicate that the immunity induced by natural infection with wild type virus is superior to that induced by the vaccine. In one study,[7] about one-quarter of all vaccinees (both leukaemic children and healthy adults) were seronegative one year after a second dose of vaccine, but none were seronegative after up to 6 years after breakthrough varicella infection. However, immunity to varicella-zoster is complex, depending not only on circulating antibody but also on cellular immunity and secretory antibody.[1] Thus, although a person may become seronegative after vaccination, protection from varicella may remain, albeit partial.[6] Both humoral and cell mediated immunity have been shown to persist for up to 20 years after vaccination.[9] Leukaemic children observed up to 6 years after immunisation have continued to be well protected[6] and varicella in previously-vaccinated persons is usually mild.[6,7]

There is some controversy over vaccinating healthy children, mainly due to uncertainties over long-term consequences and the impact vaccination may have on unimmunised members of the population. Two studies[10,11] in the USA have suggested that inclusion of varicella vaccines into routine **immunisation schedules** in infants could be cost effective, particularly if work time lost by parents caring for sick children is included in the calculation. This view has been rigorously opposed by clinicians who think such a step would be premature.[12-14] Nevertheless, the American Academy of Pediatrics Committee on Infectious Diseases recommends universal vaccination of healthy children at age 12 to 18 months, and in susceptible older children and adolescents.[15]

Varicella-zoster vaccine may prevent or modify varicella if given within 3 days of exposure to the infection. It may be useful as an **adjunct** to varicella-zoster immunoglobulin.[2] The treatment of varicella-zoster infections with antivirals is discussed on p.598.

One concern of varicella-zoster vaccination has been the possibility of an **increased risk of herpes zoster** (shingles) in immunised children. Although herpes zoster has been reported in vaccinated persons, a study involving 346 leukaemic children and 84 matched controls concluded that the incidence of herpes zoster following varicella-zoster vaccine was no greater than that following natural varicella infection.[16] The study did suggest that the risk of herpes zoster may be lowered by vaccination but this must be confirmed by long-term follow-up. The vaccine strain of varicella-zoster virus is transmissible, particularly from vaccinees who develop a rash (see also under Adverse Effects, above).[1] There is no evidence of reversion to virulence of the vaccine strain with secondary transmission.[1]

Another concern is that vaccination of children could result in more severe infections in later life after immunity has waned. However, studies have shown that in general varicella is less severe in previously immunised than in non-immunised patients.[17,18]

1. Isaacs D, Menser M. Modern vaccines: measles, mumps, rubella, and varicella. *Lancet* 1990; **335:** 1384–7.
2. National Institutes of Health Conference. Varicella-zoster virus infections: biology, natural history, treatment, and prevention. *Ann Intern Med* 1988; **108:** 221–37.
3. White CJ, *et al.* Varicella vaccine (Varivax) in healthy children and adolescents: results from clinical trials, 1987 to 1989. *Pediatrics* 1991; **87:** 604–10.
4. Dennehy PH, *et al.* Immunogenicity of subcutaneous versus intramuscular Oka/Merck varicella vaccination in healthy children. *Pediatrics* 1991; **88:** 604–7.
5. Kuter BJ, *et al.* Safety, tolerability, and immunogenicity of two regimens of Oka/Merck varicella vaccine (Varivax) in healthy adolescents and adults. *Vaccine* 1995; **13:** 967 72.
6. Gershon AA, *et al.* Persistence of immunity to varicella in children with leukemia immunized with live attenuated varicella vaccine. *N Engl J Med* 1989; **320:** 892–7.
7. Gershon AA, *et al.* Live attenuated varicella vaccine: protection in healthy adults compared with leukemic children. *J Infect Dis* 1990; **161:** 661–6.
8. Arbeter AM, *et al.* Immunization of children with acute lymphoblastic leukemia with live attenuated varicella vaccine without complete suspension of chemotherapy. *Pediatrics* 1990; **85:** 338–44.
9. Asano Y, *et al.* Experience and reason: twenty-year follow-up of protective immunity of the Oka strain live varicella vaccine. *Pediatrics* 1994; **94:** 524–6.
10. Huse DM, *et al.* Childhood vaccination against chickenpox: an analysis of benefits and costs. *J Pediatr* 1994; **124:** 869–74.
11. Lieu TA, *et al.* Cost-effectiveness of a routine varicella vaccination program for US children. *JAMA* 1994; **271:** 375–81.
12. Bader M, Oswego L. Varicella vaccine. *JAMA* 1994; **271:** 1744–5.
13. Smukler M. Routine childhood varicella vaccination. *JAMA* 1994; **271:** 1906.
14. Ross LF, Lantos JD. Immunisation against chickenpox. *Br Med J* 1995; **310:** 2–3.
15. Committee on Infectious Diseases. Recommendations for the use of live attenuated varicella vaccine. *Pediatrics* 1995; **95:** 791–6. Correction. *ibid.*; **96** (1).
16. Lawrence R, *et al.* The risk of zoster after varicella vaccination in children with leukemia. *N Engl J Med* 1988; **318:** 543–8.
17. Watson BM, *et al.* Modified chickenpox in children immunized with the Oka/Merck varicella vaccine. *Pediatrics* 1993; **91:** 17–22.
18. Bernstein HH, *et al.* Clinical survey of natural varicella compared with breakthrough varicella after immunization with live attenuated Oka/Merck varicella vaccine. *Pediatrics* 1993; **92:** 833–7.

Preparations

Ph. Eur.: Varicella Vaccine (Live).

Proprietary Preparations (details are given in Part 3)

Aust.: Varicella; ***Belg.:*** Varilrix; ***Ger.:*** Varilrix; ***Swed.:*** Varilrix; ***Switz.:*** Varicella†; Varilrix; ***USA:*** Varivax.

Yellow Fever Vaccines (8038-d)

Yellow Fever Vaccine (Live) (Ph. Eur.) (Yel/Vac; Yellow Fever Vaccine, Live (BP 1998); Vaccinum Febris Flavae Vivum) is a freeze-dried preparation of the 17D strain of yellow fever virus (*Flavivirus hominis*) grown in fertilised hen eggs. It is reconstituted before use. It should be stored at 2° to 8° and be protected from light.

Yellow Fever Vaccine (USP 23) is a freeze-dried preparation of a selected attenuated strain of live yellow fever virus cultured in chick embryos. It is reconstituted, just prior to use, by the addition of sodium chloride injection containing no antimicrobial agent. It should be stored under nitrogen preferably below 0° but not above 5°.

Adverse Effects and Precautions

As for vaccines in general, p.1500.

Local and general reactions are not common after vaccination for yellow fever. Very rarely encephalitis has followed vaccination, generally in infants under 9 months of age. Therefore, yellow fever vaccine is not usually given to infants under 9 months (but see below).

There is as yet insufficient data on the safety of yellow fever vaccine in HIV-positive individuals. In the UK administration of yellow fever vaccine to such individuals is not recommended. WHO advises that the vaccine should be administered to HIV-positive individuals who are asymptomatic if the risk of infection is high.

Effects on the nervous system. Encephalitis may occur very rarely following vaccination against yellow fever, but WHO in 1986 stated[1] that not more than 17 cases of encephalitis had been recorded over a period of 40 years and all occurred in children; although it was possible that some cases may have gone unrecorded, the number would be very small in proportion to the tens of millions of immunisations performed without known encephalitic complications. As a precaution against possible encephalitic complications, infants under 9 months of age are not generally immunised but it may be advisable to immunise children at 6 months of age if they live in rural areas with a history of yellow fever epidemics, and even at 4 months in an active epidemic focus; no child less than 4 months old should receive yellow fever vaccine.

1. WHO. *Prevention and control of yellow fever in Africa*. Geneva: WHO, 1986.

Pregnancy. Although yellow fever vaccine has been given to women during pregnancy without adverse effects in the infants,[1] fetal infection has been reported.[2]

1. Nasidi A, *et al.* Yellow fever vaccination and pregnancy: a four-year prospective study. *Trans R Soc Trop Med Hyg* 1993; **87:** 337–9.
2. Tsai TF, *et al.* Congenital yellow fever virus infection after immunization in pregnancy. *J Infect Dis* 1993; **168:** 1520–3.

Interactions

As for vaccines in general, p.1501.

There have been several studies on the combined use of yellow fever vaccine and other vaccines.[1] The administration of smallpox vaccine (now no longer in use), measles vaccine, and yellow fever vaccine at the same site has resulted in a decrease in the rate of seroconversions to yellow fever but the injection was made intradermally. When given at different sites, and when diphtheria, tetanus, and pertussis vaccine was also added, no interference was shown. Cholera vaccines should not be given together with yellow fever vaccine, or in the preceding 3 weeks, since the yellow fever neutralising antibody response is reduced at least temporarily. Pooled human immunoglobulin given before, at the same time as, or after yellow fever vaccine does not impair the rate of serological conversion. The UK manufacturers do, however, state that it is advisable to avoid administration of yellow fever vaccine within 6 weeks following administration of normal immunoglobulin and, conversely, to avoid administration of normal immunoglobulin for at least 2 weeks after vaccination.

1. WHO. *Prevention and control of yellow fever in Africa*. Geneva: WHO, 1986.

Uses and Administration

Yellow fever vaccines are used for active immunisation against yellow fever. Immunity is usually established within about 10 days of administration and persists for many years. Only one dose is required for immunisation and is given by subcutaneous injection; the dose (0.5 mL) is the volume containing at least 1000 mouse LD_{50} units.

In the UK, immunisation against yellow fever is recommended for laboratory workers handling infected material, for persons travelling through or living in areas of infection, and for travellers entering countries which require an International Certificate of Vaccination. The immunity produced may last for life although officially an International Certificate of Vaccination against yellow fever is valid only for 10 years starting 10 days after the primary immunisation and only if the vaccine used has been approved by WHO and administered at a designated vaccinating centre.

Vaccination under 9 months of age is not generally recommended (but see under Adverse Effects and Precautions, above).

In the USA vaccination of children aged 6 to 9 months is recommended only for travel to an area of ongoing yellow fever epidemic, or when travel cannot be postponed and a high level of protection against mosquito bites is not feasible. Infants under 4 months of age should not be vaccinated.

General references.

1. Barrett ADT. Yellow fever vaccines. *Biologicals* 1997; **25:** 17–25.

Immunisation schedules. The 17D (Rockefeller) yellow fever vaccine is now the only yellow fever vaccine produced.[1] The quantity at present available in the world is limited and its relatively short half-life does not permit the accumulation of large stocks. The demand for the vaccine is also somewhat irregular, being suddenly high during epidemics and low during inter-epidemic periods.

During the past 40 years in Africa two different strategies for yellow fever immunisation have been followed.[1] Firstly, an emergency immunisation programme takes place once an outbreak has begun, in an attempt to limit the spread of infection by immunising all persons in the focus, regardless of their former immune status. One disadvantage is that immunity does not appear until 7 days after immunisation and deaths may be expected to occur in the interim period. Secondly, a routine mass immunisation programme for yellow fever is aimed at immunising in advance all populations considered to be at risk. Yellow fever vaccine may be considered for inclusion in a national Expanded Programme on Immunization; there are obvious logistic advantages in administering it at the age of 9 months at the same time as measles vaccine. In rural areas of the endemic zone that are considered at high risk, the minimum age for routine immunisation may be lowered to 6 months (see under Adverse Effects and Precautions, above). Studies have suggested that immunisation with a combined yellow fever and measles vaccine may be possible.[2]

1. WHO. *Prevention and control of yellow fever in Africa*. Geneva: WHO, 1986.
2. Lhuillier M, *et al.* Study of combined vaccination against yellow fever and measles in infants from six to nine months. *J Biol Stand* 1989; **17:** 9–15.

Recommendations of the Advisory Committee on Immunization Practices for the prevention of yellow fever in the USA.[1]

1. Immunization Practices Advisory Committee. Yellow fever vaccine. *MMWR* 1990; **39** (RR-6): 1–6.

Immunisation for travellers. A booklet entitled *International Travel and Health: Vaccination Requirements and Health Advice* is published annually by WHO. Information is provided concerning the countries in Africa and South America where yellow fever is endemic and also countries requiring a traveller to hold a valid vaccination certificate. For some further details, see p.1502.

Preparations

Ph. Eur.: Yellow Fever Vaccine (Live);
USP 23: Yellow Fever Vaccine.

Proprietary Preparations (details are given in Part 3)
Belg.: Arilvax†; Stamaril; ***Fr.:*** Stamaril; ***Irl.:*** Arilvax; ***Ital.:*** Stamaril; ***Neth.:*** Arilvax; ***S.Afr.:*** Arilvax; Stamaril; ***Swed.:*** Arilvax; Stamaril; ***Switz.:*** Arilvax†; Stamaril; ***UK:*** Arilvax; ***USA:*** YF-Vax.

Part 2

Supplementary Drugs and Other Substances

Abrus (12303-z)

Abrus Seed; Indian Liquorice; Jequirity Bean; Jumble Beads; Prayer Beads; Rosary Beans.

The seeds of *Abrus precatorius* (Leguminosae), one of whose constituents is abrin.

Abrin is considered responsible for the toxic effects of abrus seeds. It is closely related to ricin. Deaths of children have occurred from eating one or more seeds. Toxic effects may occur within a few hours or may be delayed for several days following ingestion and include gastro-enteritis, circulatory collapse, haemorrhages, oliguria, agglutination and haemolysis of the red blood cells, and convulsions. Treatment is symptomatic following removal of ingested beans by gastric lavage; activated charcoal may be given.

Absinthium (521-c)

Absinthii Herba; Assenzio; Losna; Pelin; Wermutkraut; Wormwood.

CAS — 546-80-5 (α-thujone); 471-15-8 (β-thujone).

Pharmacopoeias. In *Eur.* (see p.viii) and *Pol.*

The fresh or dried leaves and flowering tops of wormwood, *Artemisia absinthium* (Compositae). It contains not less than 2 mL per kg of essential oil, calculated with reference to the dried drug. Thujone, related to camphor, is the major constituent of the essential oil derived from absinthium.

Absinthium has been used as a bitter. It is also used in small quantities as a flavouring agent in alcoholic beverages although it is considered in some countries not to be safe for use in foods, beverages, or drugs. Habitual use or large doses cause absinthism, which is characterised by restlessness, vomiting, vertigo, tremors, and convulsions. Absinthium has been used in homoeopathic medicine.

References.

1. Weisbord SD, *et al.* Poison on line—acute renal failure caused by oil of wormwood purchased through the Internet. *N Engl J Med* 1997; **337:** 825–7.

Preparations

Proprietary Preparations (details are given in Part 3)

Multi-ingredient: ***Aust.:*** Abdomilon†; Amara; Amylatin; Bio-Garten Tee fur Leber und Galle; Bio-Garten Tropfen fur Galle und Leber; Eryval; Felidon neu; Gallogran; Krauterdoktor Gallentreibende Tropfen; Krauterdoktor Verdauungsfordernde Tropfen; Krauterhaus Mag Kottas Tee fur die Verdauung; Krautertee Nr 17; Krautertee Nr 28; Krautertee Nr 30; Leber- und Galletee; Magentee EF-EM-ES; Mariazeller; Pepsiton; Sigman-Haustropfen; St Radegunder Verdauungstee; Vinopepsin; Virgilocard; ***Ger.:*** Abdomilon N; Agrimonas N; Amara-Tropfen-Pascoe; Anore X N; Aristochol N; Aruto-Magenpulver-forte†; Asgocholan†; Cefagastrin; Cheihepar†; Chol-Truw S; Doppelherz Magenstarkung; Dr. Klinger's Bergischer Krautertee, Leber- und Gallentee†; entero sanol†; Floradix Multipretten; Gallemolan forte; Gallemolan G; Gallemolan N†; Gallexier; Gastralon N; Gastritol; Gastrol S; Heparchofid S†; Hepaticum novo; Hepatofalk Neu; Hevert-Magen-Galle-Leber-Tee; Kneipp Gastropressan†; Kneipp Magentrost†; Lomatol; Majocarmin mite†; Majocarmin†; Marianon; Montana; Nervosana; Neurochol C; Novo Mandrogallan N; Pascopankreat†; Pascopnakreat novo; Phonix Gastriphon; Presselin 214†; Presselin 52 N; rohasal; Stomachysat Burger; Stovalid N; Stullmaton; Unex Amarum; ventri-loges; Ventrimarin Novo; ***Switz.:*** Baume†; Kernosan Heidelberger Poudre; Phytomed Hepato; Tisane gastrique "H"†; Tisane hepatique et biliaire "H"†.

Acedoben (11903-p)

Acedoben *(pINN).*

p-Acetamidobenzoic acid.

$C_9H_9NO_3$ = 179.2.

CAS — 556-08-1.

Acedoben is a component of inosine pranobex (p.615) which has been given by mouth as the potassium salt in the treatment of skin disorders. Acedoben and its sodium salt have been applied topically.

Preparations

Proprietary Preparations (details are given in Part 3)

Multi-ingredient: ***Spain:*** Amplidermis; Fibroderm; Hongosan; Perlinsol Cutaneo; S 13†.

Aceglutamide (12306-a)

Aceglutamide *(rINN).*

N^2-Acetyl-L-glutamine; 2-Acetylamino-L-glutaramic acid.

$C_7H_{12}N_2O_4$ = 188.2.

CAS — 2490-97-3.

Aceglutamide has been given in an attempt to improve memory and concentration.

Preparations

Proprietary Preparations (details are given in Part 3)

Multi-ingredient: ***Ital.:*** Fosfoglutil†; Memovisus; Tonoplus; ***Spain:*** Levaliver; Neurocordin†; Teovit.

Acemannan (9340-j)

Acemannan *(USAN, rINN).*

Polymanoacetate.

CAS — 110042-95-0.

Acemannan is a highly acetylated, polydispersed, linear mannan obtained from the mucilage of *Aloe barbadensis* (=*A. vera*). It has immunomodulating properties.

Glacial Acetic Acid (1306-k)

Acide Acetique Cristallisable; Acidum Aceticum Glaciale; Concentrated Acetic Acid; E260 (acetic acid); Eisessig; Etanoico; Ethanoic Acid; Glac. Acet. Acid; Konzentrierte Essigsäure.

$C_2H_4O_2$ = 60.05.

CAS — 64-19-7.

Pharmacopoeias. In *Chin., Eur.* (see p.viii), *Jpn, Pol.,* and *US.*

A translucent crystalline mass or a clear colourless volatile liquid with a pungent odour. B.p. about 118°. F.p. not lower than 14.8°. **Miscible** with water, alcohol, dichloromethane, ether, and glycerol. **Store** in airtight containers.

Acetic Acid (1305-c)

NOTE. The nomenclature of acetic acid often leads to confusion as to whether concentrations are expressed as percentages of glacial acetic acid ($C_2H_4O_2$) or of this diluted form. In *Martindale*, the percentage figures given against acetic acid represent the amount of $C_2H_4O_2$.

Pharmacopoeias. In *Br.* (33%), *Aust.* (33.7 to 35.5%), *Jpn* (30 to 32%), *Pol.* (30%), and *Swiss* (30%). Also in *USNF* (36 to 37%). The following pharmacopoeias include weaker solutions under the titles or synonyms Dilute Acetic Acid or Diluted Acetic Acid: *Aust.* (11.5 to 12.2%), *Br.* (6%), and *It.* (10%).

A clear colourless liquid with a pungent odour. **Miscible** with water, alcohol, and glycerol. **Store** in airtight containers.

Adverse Effects and Treatment

Local or topical application of acetic acid preparations may produce stinging or burning. Ingestion of glacial acetic acid can produce similar adverse effects to those of hydrochloric acid (p.1588), and these may be treated similarly.

Uses and Administration

Glacial acetic acid has been used as an escharotic. Diluted forms have been used as an antibacterial (it is reported to be effective against *Haemophilus* and *Pseudomonas* spp.), antifungal, and antiprotozoal in vaginal gels and douches, irrigations, topical preparations for the skin and nails, and in ear drops. Diluted forms have also been used as an expectorant, an astringent lotion, and as treatments for warts (p.1076), callosities, and for certain jelly-fish stings.

A solution containing 4% w/v $C_2H_4O_2$ is known as artificial vinegar or non-brewed condiment. Vinegar is a product of fermentation.

Jellyfish sting. Vinegar or 3 to 10% acetic acid solution is applied to box jellyfish stings to inactivate any fragments of adherent tentacle[1,2] (see p.1516). Acetic acid solutions have been reported to be useful in stings by related species[3] although they may produce further discharge of venom in some jellyfish.[4]

1. Hartwick RJ, *et al.* Disarming the box jellyfish. *Med J Aust* 1980; **1:** 15–20.
2. Fenner PJ, Williamson JA. Worldwide deaths and severe envenomation from jellyfish stings. *Med J Aust* 1996; **165:** 658–61.
3. Fenner PJ, *et al.* "Morbakka", another cubomedusan. *Med J Aust* 1985; **143:** 550–5.
4. Fenner PJ, Fitzpatrick PF. Experiments with the nematocysts of Cyanea capillata. *Med J Aust* 1986; **145:** 174.

Stoma care. Crystalline phosphatic deposits that build up on the stoma of a urostomy can be dissolved by dabbing vinegar onto the stoma.[1] A few drops of vinegar into the appliance will reduce the odour of stale urine.

1. Smith JC, *et al.* Management of stoma. *Prescribers' J* 1983; **23:** 21–8.

Wounds and burns. Infection of wounds (p.1076) and burns (p.1073) with *Pseudomonas aeruginosa* may delay healing. Acetic acid has been used, in concentrations of up to 5%,[1] to eradicate these infections.

1. Milner SM. Acetic acid to treat Pseudomonas aeruginosa in superficial wounds and burns. *Lancet* 1992; **340:** 61.

Preparations

BP 1998: Strong Ammonium Acetate Solution;
USP 23: Acetic Acid Irrigation; Acetic Acid Otic Solution; Hydrocortisone and Acetic Acid Otic Solution.

Proprietary Preparations (details are given in Part 3)
Austral.: Summer's Eve Disposable; ***Canad.:*** Midol Douche; ***Fr.:*** Para Lentes; ***Irl.:*** Aci-Jel; ***UK:*** Aci-Jel; Baby Cough Syrup†; Meltus Baby; Wart Solvent†; ***USA:*** Feminique; Massengill Disposable; Summer's Eve Disposable.

Multi-ingredient: ***Aust.:*** Onycho Phytex; Phytex; ***Austral.:*** Aci-Jel; Aquaear; Ear Clear for Swimmer's Ear; Emidote APF†; Phytex†; ***Belg.:*** Aporil; Ysol†; ***Canad.:*** Aci-Jel†; SH-206; Viron Wart Lotion; VoSoL; VoSoL HC; ***Fr.:*** Marie Rose†; Nitrol; Ysol 206; ***Ger.:*** Chol-Truw S; Gehwol Huhneraugen Tinktur; Solco-Derman; ***Irl.:*** Phytex; ***Ital.:*** Silvana; ***Neth.:*** Hexoll; ***Spain:*** Callicida Cor Pik; Callicida Cor Pik Stick†; Callicida Durcall; Callicida Rojo; Calloverk†; Nitroina; Quocin; ***Swed.:*** Aci-Jel†; ***Switz.:*** Onycho Phytex†; Solcoderm; Solcogyn; ***UK:*** Ellimans; Galloway's Cough Syrup; Goddards White Oil Embrocation; Hill's Balsam Adult Expectorant; Hill's Balsam Adult Suppressant; Phytex; Sanderson's Throat Specific; ***USA:*** AA-HC Otic; Acetasol; Acetasol HC; Aci-Jel; Borofair Otic; Burow's; New Freshness†; Otic Domeboro; Renalin Dialyzer Reprocessing Concentrate; Star-Otic; Tridesilon†; VoSoL; VoSoL HC.

Acetohydroxamic Acid (12310-j)

Acetohydroxamic Acid *(USAN, rINN).*

N-Acetyl Hydroxyacetamide; AHA.

$C_2H_5NO_2$ = 75.07.

CAS — 546-88-3.

Pharmacopoeias. In *US.*

White, slightly hygroscopic, crystalline powder. Freely **soluble** in water and in alcohol; very slightly soluble in chloroform. **Store** in airtight containers at a temperature between 8° and 15°.

Adverse Effects and Precautions

Phlebitis, thrombo-embolism, haemolytic anaemia, and iron-deficiency anaemia have occurred. Other adverse effects include headache, gastro-intestinal disturbances, alopecia, rash (particularly following ingestion of alcohol), trembling, and mental symptoms including anxiety and depression. Blood counts and renal function should be monitored regularly during treatment. Patients with acute renal failure should not be given acetohydroxamic acid.

Studies in *animals* indicate that acetohydroxamic acid is teratogenic and may cause bone-marrow depression.

Interactions

Acetohydroxamic acid chelates iron administered orally, resulting in reduced absorption of both. Concomitant consumption of alcohol may precipitate skin rash.

Pharmacokinetics

Acetohydroxamic acid is rapidly absorbed from the gastro-intestinal tract with peak serum concentrations being reached within 1 hour. The plasma half-life is reported to be up to 10 hours, but may be longer in patients with impaired renal function. Acetohydroxamic acid is partially metabolised in the liver to acetamide, which is inactive; up to about two-thirds of a dose may be excreted unchanged in the urine.

Uses and Administration

Acetohydroxamic acid acts by inhibiting bacterial urease, thus decreasing urinary ammonia concentration and alkalinity. It is used in the prophylaxis of renal calculi formed as a result of bacterial urease and as an adjunct in the treatment of chronic urinary-tract infection due to urease-splitting bacteria.

Acetohydroxamic acid is given by mouth in a usual dose of 250 mg three or four times a day. The dose should not exceed 1.5 g daily. Children aged over 8 years have been given 10 mg per kg body-weight daily in 2 or 3 divided doses.

In patients with impaired renal function the dosage interval should be increased to 12 hours and the dose may need to be reduced.

References.

1. Martelli A, *et al.* Acetohydroxamic acid therapy in infected renal stones. *Urology* 1981; **17**: 320–2.
2. Griffith DP. Infection-induced renal calculi. *Kidney Int* 1982; **21**: 422–30.
3. Rodman JS, *et al.* Partial dissolution of struvite calculus with oral acetohydroxamic acid. *Urology* 1983; **22**: 410–12.
4. Williams JJ, *et al.* A randomized double-blind study of acetohydroxamic acid in struvite nephrolithiasis. *N Engl J Med* 1984; **311**: 760–4.
5. Smith LH. New treatment for struvite urinary stones. *N Engl J Med* 1984; **311**: 792–4.
6. Burr RG, Nuseibeh I. The effect of oral acetohydroxamic acid on urinary saturation in stone-forming spinal cord patients. *Br J Urol* 1983; **55**: 162–5.
7. El Nujumi AM, *et al.* Effect of inhibition of Helicobacter pylori urease activity by acetohydroxamic acid on serum gastrin in duodenal ulcer subjects. *Gut* 1991; **32**: 866–70.

Preparations

USP 23: Acetohydroxamic Acid Tablets.

Proprietary Preparations (details are given in Part 3)
Belg.: Uronefrex; ***Fr.:*** Uronefrex; ***Spain:*** Uronefrex; ***USA:*** Lithostat.

Acetylcarnitine Hydrochloride (3015-f)

Acetyl-L-carnitine Hydrochloride; ST-200. (3-Carboxy-2-hydroxypropyl)trimethylammonium acetate (ester) chloride.

$C_9H_{17}NO_4,HCl$ = 239.7.

CAS — 5080-50-2.

Acetylcarnitine hydrochloride has been given by mouth and by injection in the treatment of cerebrovascular insufficiency and peripheral neuropathies. It is under investigation in Alzheimer's disease (p.1386).

References.

1. Thal LJ, *et al.* A 1-year multicenter placebo-controlled study of acetyl-L-carnitine in patients with Alzheimer's disease. *Neurology* 1996; **47**: 705–11.
2. Bella R, *et al.* Effect of acetyl-L-carnitine on geriatric patients suffering from dysthymic disorders. *Int J Clin Pharmacol Res* 1990; **10**: 355–60.

Preparations

Proprietary Preparations (details are given in Part 3)
Ital.: Acilen; Branigen; Ceredor†; Nicetile; Normobren; Zibren.

Acetylleucine (12313-k)

Acetylleucine *(rINN).*

RP-7542. *N*-Acetyl-DL-leucine.

$C_8H_{15}NO_3$ = 173.2.

CAS — 99-15-0.

Acetylleucine has been used in the treatment of vertigo (p.401) in usual doses of up to 2 g daily by mouth, in divided doses, or 1 g daily by slow intravenous injection. Higher doses are occasionally employed.

Preparations

Proprietary Preparations (details are given in Part 3)
Fr.: Tanganil; ***Neth.:*** Tanganil†.

Acexamic Acid (12315-t)

Acexamic Acid *(BAN, rINN).*

CY-153; Epsilon Acetamidocaproic Acid. 6-Acetamidohexanoic acid.

$C_8H_{15}NO_3$ = 173.2.

CAS — 57-08-9 (acexamic acid); 70020-71-2 (zinc acexamate).

Acexamic acid is related structurally to the antifibrinolytic agent aminocaproic acid (p.711). Acexamic acid, usually as the calcium or sodium salt, has been administered topically or systemically to promote the healing of ulcers and various other lesions. Zinc acexamate has been given for peptic ulcer disease.

Preparations

Proprietary Preparations (details are given in Part 3)
Belg.: Plastenan; ***Fr.:*** Plastenan; ***Spain:*** Copinal; Plastenan†.

Multi-ingredient: ***Belg.:*** Plastenan Neomycine†; ***Fr.:*** Plastenan Neomycine; ***Spain:*** Linitul Antibiotico; Plaskine Neomicina; Plasmutan†; Plastenan Neomicina†; Unitul Complex.

Achillea (4601-h)

Achillée Millefeuille; Milfoil; Millefolii Herba; Schafgarbe; Yarrow.

Pharmacopoeias. In *Eur.* (see p.viii) and *Pol.*

The dried flowering tops of yarrow, *Achillea millefolium* (Compositae). It contains not less than 2 mL per kg of essential oil and not less than 0.02% of proazulenes, expressed as chamazulene ($C_{14}H_{16}$ = 184.3), both calculated with reference to the dried drug. **Protect** from light.

Achillea has been used mainly in herbal and homoeopathic medicine for a great variety of purposes. It has been stated to have diaphoretic, anti-inflammatory, and other miscellaneous properties. It has been reported to cause contact dermatitis.

References.

1. Phillipson JD, Anderson LA. Herbal remedies used in sedative and antirheumatic preparations: part 2. *Pharm J* 1984; **233**: 111–15.
2. Chandler RF. Yarrow. *Can Pharm J* 1989; **122**: 41–3.

Preparations

Proprietary Preparations (details are given in Part 3)
Ger.: Kneipp Schafgarbe-Pflanzensaft Frauentost N.

Multi-ingredient: ***Aust.:*** Abfuhrtee EF-EM-ES; Aktiv Leber- und Gallentee; Aktiv milder Magen- und Darmtee; Amersan; Bio-Garten Tee gegen Blahungen; Bio-Garten Tee zur Starkung und Kraftigung; Bio-Garten Tropfen fur Galle und Leber; Chol-Grandelat; Citochol; Felidon neu; Gallen- und Lebertee; Gallogran; Krauterdoktor Gallentreibende Tropfen; Krauterhaus Mag Kottas Blutreinigungstee; Krauterhaus Mag Kottas Fruhjahrs- und Herbstkurtee; Krauterhaus Mag Kottas Magen- und Darmtee; Krauterhaus Mag Kottas Tee gegen Blahungen; Krauterhaus Mag Kottas Wechseltee; Krautertee Nr 124; Krautertee Nr 16; Krautertee Nr 44; Mag Kottas Wechseltee; Magentee; Mariazeller; Menodoron; Sidroga Leber-Galle-Tee; Sidroga Magen-Darm-Tee; Windtreibender Tee; ***Austral.:*** Cholagogum†; Crataegus Complex; Flavons; ***Canad.:*** Cystoforce†; ***Fr.:*** Cicaderma; Tisane Digestive Weleda; Tisanes de l'Abbe Hamon no 14; ***Ger.:*** Abfuhr-Tee Depuraflux†; Alasenn; Aristochol N; Aruto-Magenpulver-forte†; Asgocholan†; Befelka-Tinktur; Cha-mill†; Cheihepar†; Cheiranthol; Cholaflux N†; Cholaflux†; Dr. Hotz Vollbad; Dr. Kleinschrod's Cor-Insuffin†; Dr. Kleinschrod's Spasmi Tropfen†; Dr. Klinger's Bergischer Krautertee, Herz- und Kreislauftee†; Floradix Multipretten; Gallen-Tee Cholaflux S†; Gallexier; Hevert-Gicht-Rheuma-Tee comp; Hevert-Magen-Galle-Leber-Tee; Hovnizym†; Kamillan plus; Kneipp Magentrost†; Knufinke Gastrobin Magen- und Darm-Tee†; Magen-Tee Stada N; Marianon; Nervosana; Phytpulmon†; Presselin 214†; Salus Leber-Galle-Tee Nr.18; Salus Rheuma-Tee Krautertee Nr. 12; Sedovent; Stomachysat Burger; Tonsilgon-N; Worishofener Leber- und Gallenstein-mittel Dr. Kleinschrod†; Worishofener Nervenpflege Dr. Kleinschrod†; ***Ital.:*** Fluiven; Forticrin; ***Switz.:*** Baume†; Enveloppements ECR; Gastrosan; Kernosan Heidelberger Poudre; Tisane gastrique "H"†; Tisane hepatique et biliaire; Tisane pour l'estomac; Tisane relaxante; Tisane sedative et somnifere "H"†; Viola Pommade a l'huile d'amandes†; ***UK:*** Carminative Tea; Catarrh; Catarrh-eeze; Laxadoron; Liverguard; Menodoron; Rheumatic Pain Remedy; Tabritis; Wellwoman.

Acid Fuchsine (2247-q)

Acid Magenta; Acid Roseine; Acid Rubine; CI Acid Violet 19; Colour Index No. 42685.

The disodium or diammonium salt of the trisulphonic acid of magenta.

Acid fuchsine is used as a microscopic stain and a pH indicator.

Aconite (12320-c)

Acetylbenzoylaconine (aconitine); Aconit.; Aconit Napel; Aconite Root; Aconiti Tuber; Monkshood Root; Radix Aconiti; Wolfsbane Root. 8-Acetoxy-3,11,18-trihydroxy-16-ethyl-1,6,19-trimethoxy-4-methoxymethylaconitan-10-yl benzoate (aconitine).

$C_{34}H_{47}NO_{11}$ (aconitine) = 645.7 (aconitine).

CAS — 8063-12-5 (aconite); 302-27-2 (aconitine).

NOTE. Wolfsbane is also used as a common name for arnica flower.

Pharmacopoeias. In *Belg. Chin.* includes *Aconitum carmichaeli* and *A. kusnezoffii. Aust.* also includes aconitine.

The dried tuberous root of *Aconitum napellus* agg. (Ranunculaceae). It contains a number of alkaloids, the main pharmacologically active one being aconitine.

Adverse Effects

Aconite has variable effects on the heart leading to heart failure. It also affects the central nervous system.

Symptoms of aconite poisoning may appear almost immediately and are rarely delayed beyond an hour; in fatal poisoning death usually occurs within 6 hours, although with larger doses it may be instantaneous.

Moderately toxic doses produce a tingling of the tongue, mouth, stomach, and skin (this is the most important diagnostic feature) followed by numbness and anaesthesia. Other symptoms include gastro-intestinal disturbances; irregular pulse; difficult respiration; cold, clammy, and livid skin; muscular weakness, incoordination, and vertigo.

Treatment of aconite poisoning is symptomatic; atropine sulphate may be given in severe cases.

Reports of poisoning with aconite.

1. Kelly SP. Aconite poisoning. *Med J Aust* 1990; **153**: 499.
2. Tai Y-T, *et al.* Cardiotoxicity after accidental herb-induced aconite poisoning. *Lancet* 1992; **340**: 1254–6.
3. Kolev ST, *et al.* Toxicity following accidental ingestion of Aconitum containing Chinese remedy. *Hum Exp Toxicol* 1996; **15**: 839–42.

Uses and Administration

Aconite liniments have been used in the treatment of neuralgia, sciatica, and rheumatism. Sufficient aconitine may be absorbed through the skin to cause serious poisoning; liniments should never be applied to wounds or abraded surfaces. Aconite should not be used internally because of its low therapeutic index and variable potency; however it is reported to be a common ingredient in traditional Chinese remedies and is also an ingredient of some cough mixtures.

A preparation of aconite is used in homoeopathic medicine.

Preparations

Proprietary Preparations (details are given in Part 3)
Belg.: Bromofotyl†; ***Ger.:*** Aconitysat†; Herbadon.

Multi-ingredient: ***Aust.:*** Rheuma; ***Belg.:*** Bronchosedal; Captol†; Colimax; Eucalyptine Le Brun; Eucalyptine Pholcodine Le Brun; Euphon; Folcodex; Gloceda; Glottyl†; Inalpin; Pectocalmine Junior†; Sirop Toux du Larynx; Solucamphre; ***Fr.:*** Broncorinol toux seches; Bronpax; Campho-Pneumine Aminophylline†; Camphodionyl; Clarix; Codotussyl; Creme Rap; Curibronches†; Euphon; Gaiarsol; Grippony l†; Nican†; Pastilles Monleon; Pecto 6†; Pectospir†; Pectovox†; Peter's Sirop; Polery; Premidan Adult†; Premidan Infant†; Pulmonase; Pulmospir†; Pulmothiol†; Quintopan Adult; Sedophon; Sirop Adrian a la pholcodine adulte†; Sirop Boin; Sirop Famel†; Sirop Pectoral adulte; Tuberol†; ***Ger.:*** Bryonia-Strath†; Diaporin†; Expectorans Solucampher†; ***Ital.:*** Creosolactol Adulti†; Lactocol; ***Spain:*** Encialina; Etermol; Pectoral Brum; Pulmosepta†; Sanovox†; ***Switz.:*** Neo-Codion Adultes†.

Acridine Orange (18717-c)

3,6-Bis(dimethylamino)acridine.

$C_{17}H_{19}N_3$ = 265.4.

CAS — 494-38-2.

Acridine orange is a dye with antiseptic properties. It has been used as a diagnostic stain in microbiology.

For details of the antiseptic properties of acridine derivatives, see p.1098.

A report of the use of acridine orange for the rapid diagnostic staining of malarial parasites,[1] and discussions of the potential of this procedure.[2-5]

1. Rickman LS, *et al.* Rapid diagnosis of malaria by acridine orange staining of centrifuged parasites. *Lancet* 1989; **i**: 68–71.
2. White NJ, Silamut K. Rapid diagnosis of malaria. *Lancet* 1989; **i**: 435.
3. Spielman A, Perrone JB. Rapid diagnosis of malaria. *Lancet* 1989; **i**: 727.
4. Wongsrichanalai C, *et al.* Rapid diagnosis of malaria by acridine orange staining of centrifuged parasites. *Lancet* 1989; **i**: 967.
5. Zimmerman R, Gathecha E. Rapid test for malaria. *Lancet* 1989; **i** 1013–14.

Acrolein (12322-a)

Acraldehyde; Acrylaldehyde; Acrylic Aldehyde. Prop-2-enal.

C_3H_4O = 56.06.

CAS — 107-02-8.

Acrolein is irritant to the skin and may cause vesiculation. Ingestion of acrolein produces severe gastro-intestinal distress. The vapour causes lachrymation and nasal irritation. Inhalation may cause pulmonary oedema, nephritis, or pneumonia. It has various industrial uses.

References.

1. Acrolein. *Environmental Health Criteria 127.* Geneva: WHO, 1992.
2. Acrolein. *IPCS Health and Safety Guide 67.* Geneva: WHO, 1991.

Acrylamide (12324-x)

Propenamide.
$C_3H_5NO = 71.08$.
CAS — 79-06-1.

Acrylamide is highly toxic and moderately irritant; it can be absorbed through unbroken skin. Symptoms of poisoning include cold sweating hands and peripheral neuropathies with numbness, paraesthesias and weakness, especially associated with the lower limbs.

Acrylamide has various industrial applications, including use as a plasticiser and a waterproof 'chemical grout'.

References to acrylamide toxicity.

1. Kesson CM, *et al.* Acrylamide poisoning. *Postgrad Med J* 1977; **53:** 16–17.
2. Acrylamide health and safety guide. *IPCS Health and Safety Guide 45.* Geneva: WHO, 1991.

Actinoquinol (12281-h)

Actinoquinol *(rINN).*
8-Ethoxy-5-quinolinesulphonic acid.
$C_{11}H_{11}NO_4S = 253.3$.
CAS — 15301-40-3 (actinoquinol); 7246-07-3 (actinoquinol sodium).

NOTE. Actinoquinol Sodium is *USAN.*

Actinoquinol is administered as an ingredient of eye drop preparations intended to protect eyes from the effects of light. Actinoquinol sodium is also used.

Preparations

Proprietary Preparations (details are given in Part 3)
Aust.: Ultra Augenschutz.

Multi-ingredient: ***Fr.:*** Uvicol; ***Ger.:*** duraultra; duraultra forte†; Idril; Tele-Stulln; ***Ital.:*** Fotofil.

Ademetionine (12326-f)

Ademetionine *(rINN).*
Ademethionine; *S*-Adenosyl-L-methionine; Methioninyl adenylate; SAMe. (S)-5′-[(3-Amino-3-carboxypropyl)methylsulphonio]-5′-deoxyadenosine hydroxide, inner salt.
$C_{15}H_{22}N_6O_5S = 398.4$.
CAS — 29908-03-0; 485-80-3; 17176-17-9.

S-Adenosyl-L-methionine is a naturally occurring molecule found in virtually all body tissues and fluids. It acts as a methyl group donor in many transmethylation reactions and therefore is involved in the synthesis or metabolism of a wide range of compounds that maintain normal cell function. Ademetionine is a stable form of *S*-adenosyl-L-methionine that has been used for the treatment of liver disorders and in depression. It has also been investigated for the treatment of osteoarthritis.

Reviews.

1. Friedel HA, *et al.* S-Adenosyl-L-methionine: a review of its pharmacological properties and therapeutic potential in liver dysfunction and affective disorders in relation to its physiological role in cell metabolism. *Drugs* 1989; **38:** 389–416.
2. Bottiglieri T, *et al.* The clinical potential of ademetionine (S-adenosylmethionine) in neurological disorders. *Drugs* 1994; **48:** 137–52.

Depression. Ademetionine has been given by mouth or parenterally in the management of depression (p.271); it appears to be of similar efficacy to the tricyclic antidepressants.

References.

1. Baldessarini RJ. Neuropharmacology of S-adenosyl-L-methionine. *Am J Med* 1987; **83** (suppl 5A): 95–103.
2. Bressa GM. S-adenosyl-l-methionine (SAMe) as antidepressant: meta-analysis of clinical studies. *Acta Neurol Scand* 1994; **154** (suppl): 7–14.

Liver disorders. Administration of ademetionine in doses of 800 mg daily intravenously or 800 mg twice daily by mouth has produced clinical improvement in patients with intrahepatic cholestasis,[1,2] including that associated with pregnancy.[3] Pruritus associated with the condition has also been relieved. Ademetionine given by intramuscular injection in a dose of 100 mg daily for one month, followed by 100 mg every other day for a further month, produced a good or excellent clinical response in 21 of 28 patients with hepatic steatosis.[4]

1. Frezza M, *et al.* Oral S-adenosylmethionine in the symptomatic treatment of intrahepatic cholestasis: a double-blind, placebo-controlled study. *Gastroenterology* 1990; **99:** 211–15.
2. Almasio P, *et al.* Role of S-adenosyl-L-methionine in the treatment of intrahepatic cholestasis. *Drugs* 1990; **40** (suppl 3): 111–23.
3. Bonfirraro G, *et al.* S-Adenosyl-L-methionine (SAMe)-induced amelioration of intrahepatic cholestasis of pregnancy: results of an open study. *Drug Invest* 1990; **2:** 125–8.
4. Caballeria E, Moreno J. Therapeutic effects of S-adenosylmethionine (SAMe) in hepatic steatosis. *Acta Ther* 1990; **16:** 253–64.

Osteoarthritis. Ademetionine has been reported to possess therapeutic efficacy in the treatment of osteoarthritis (p.2) and similar conditions[1-3] possibly due to an effect on cartilage metabolism and formation of anti-inflammatory mediators within the cell; it may also inhibit leukotrienes but does not appear markedly to interfere with prostaglandin synthesis.

1. DiPadova C. S-Adenosylmethionine in the treatment of osteoarthritis. *Am J Med* 1987; **83** (suppl 5A): 60–4.
2. Anonymous. Ademetionine—a new approach to the treatment of degenerative joint diseases. *Drugs Today* 1988; **24:** 165–8.
3. Domljan Z, *et al.* A double-blind trial of ademethionine vs naproxen in activated gonarthrosis. *Int J Clin Pharmacol Ther Toxicol* 1989; **27:** 329–33.

Preparations

Proprietary Preparations (details are given in Part 3)
Ger.: Gumbaral; ***Ital.:*** Donamet; Samyr; Transmetil; ***Spain:*** S Amet.

Adenine (12325-r)

Adeninum; Vitamin B_4. 6-Aminopurine; 1,6-Dihydro-6-iminopurine.
$C_5H_5N_5 = 135.1$.
CAS — 73-24-5.
Pharmacopoeias. In *Eur.* (see p.viii) and *US.*

Odourless white crystals or crystalline powder. Very slightly **soluble** in water; sparingly soluble in boiling water; very slightly to slightly soluble in alcohol; practically insoluble in ether and in chloroform; dissolves in dilute mineral acids and in dilute solutions of alkali hydroxides.

Adenine is a constituent of coenzymes and nucleic acids and has been used to extend the storage life of whole blood (p.713). It has also been given for the management of white blood-cell disorders. Adenine hydrochloride has also been used.

Preparations

USP 23: Anticoagulant Citrate Phosphate Dextrose Adenine Solution.

Proprietary Preparations (details are given in Part 3)
Fr.: Leuco-4†; ***Spain:*** B4 Hemosan†.

Multi-ingredient: ***Fr.:*** Leuco-4†; TTD-B_3-B_4; ***Spain:*** Hepacomplet B12 1000; Hepadif.

Adenosine Phosphate (9201-m)

Adenosine Phosphate *(BAN, USAN, rINN).*
Adenosine 5′-Monophosphate; Adenosine-5′-(dihydrogen phosphate); Adenosine-5′-phosphoric Acid; 5′-Adenylic Acid; AMP; A-5MP; Monophosadénine; Muscle Adenylic Acid; NSC-20264. 6-Amino-9-β-D-ribofuranosylpurine 5′-(dihydrogen phosphate).
$C_{10}H_{14}N_5O_7P = 347.2$.
CAS — 61-19-8.
Pharmacopoeias. Ger. includes the disodium salt under the title Adenosinmonophosphat-dinatrium-hydrat ($C_{10}H_{12}N_5Na_2O_7P,xH_2O$).

Adenosine is an endogenous nucleoside involved in many biological processes. As well as the base it is present as various phosphates. The monophosphate, adenosine phosphate has been tried in a variety of disorders including the complications of varicose veins, peripheral neuropathies, and inflammation.

Unlike adenosine (p.812) and adenosine triphosphate (below), adenosine phosphate is not used in supraventricular tachycardias.

Preparations

Proprietary Preparations (details are given in Part 3)
Fr.: Adenyl; ***USA:*** Kaysine†.

Multi-ingredient: ***Ger.:*** Laevadosin†; ***Ital.:*** Adeneurina†; Nucleodoxina†; ***S.Afr.:*** Lipostabil; ***Spain:*** Artri; Taurobetina.

Adenosine Triphosphate (9203-v)

Adenosine 5′-Triphosphate; 5′-Adenyldiphosphoric Acid; Adenylpyrophosphoric Acid; ATP; Triphosadénine. Adenosine 5′-(tetrahydrogen triphosphate).
$C_{10}H_{16}N_5O_{13}P_3 = 507.2$.
CAS — 56-65-5.
Pharmacopoeias. Ger. includes the disodium salt ($C_{10}H_{14}N_5Na_2O_{13}P_3 = 551.1$).

Adenosine triphosphate is a nucleotide constituent of animal cells with a fundamental role in biological energy transformations, being concerned with the storage and release of energy; it is converted to adenosine diphosphate, release of energy occurring during the process.

Adenosine triphosphate and its sodium salt are used as a source of nucleotides. The disodium salt has been given in the treatment of supraventricular tachycardia, but adenosine base (p.812) is the form generally used as an antiarrhythmic agent. The triphosphate is being investigated for use in cystic fibrosis (p.119).

Preparations

Proprietary Preparations (details are given in Part 3)
Fr.: Atepadene; Striadyne†; ***Ger.:*** ATP-Uvocal N†; Bio-Regenerat; ***Spain:*** Atepodin.

Multi-ingredient: ***Aust.:*** Laevadosin; ***Belg.:*** Vitathion; ***Canad.:*** Vitathion-ATP; ***Fr.:*** Betriphos-C; Myoviton; RhinATP; Triphosmag; Vita-Iodurol ATP; ***Ger.:*** Dimaestad†; Laevadosin†; Movicard†; Seda-Movicard†; ***Ital.:*** Citicortex†; ***Spain:*** Biomax†; Bronquiasmol†; Refulgin; Sedionbel†.

Adipic Acid (12328-n)

355; Adipinsäure; Hexanedioic Acid.
$C_6H_{10}O_4 = 146.1$.
CAS — 124-04-9.
Pharmacopoeias. In *Ger.*

Adipic acid is an acidifier that is used in foods and may also be included in preparations for the treatment of urinary-tract infections.

Preparations

Proprietary Preparations (details are given in Part 3)
Multi-ingredient: ***Ger.:*** Extin; ***Ital.:*** Aflogine.

Adonis Vernalis (5805-f)

Adonide; Adonis; Adoniskraut; False Hellebore; Herba Adonidis; Vernal Pheasant's Eye.
Pharmacopoeias. In *Ger.*

The dried aerial roots of *Adonis vernalis* (Ranunculaceae).

Adonis vernalis contains cardiac glycosides which have actions similar to those of digoxin (p.849). Adonis vernalis is used in herbal and homoeopathic medicine.

Preparations

Proprietary Preparations (details are given in Part 3)
Multi-ingredient: ***Canad.:*** Hepax†; ***Ger.:*** Asthmacolat†; Baldronit cum Nitro†; Baldronit forte N†; Baldronit N†; Card-Ompin S†; Cardalept†; Cardaminol†; Castrophan†; Cor-myocrat†; Corguttin + Magnesium†; Corguttin N plus; Corguttin†; Digaloid†; Gelsadon†; Hocura-Diureticum†; Miroton; Miroton N; Oxacant N; Oxacant-forte N; Oxacant-Khella N; Raufuncton N; Szillosan†; Venopyronum N triplex; Verus†.

Adrenalone Hydrochloride (1711-q)

Adrenalone Hydrochloride *(pINNM).*
3′,4′-Dihydroxy-2-(methylamino)acetophenone hydrochloride.
$C_9H_{11}NO_3,HCl = 217.6$.
CAS — 99-45-6 (adrenalone); 62-13-5 (adrenalone hydrochloride).

NOTE. Adrenalone is *USAN.*

Adrenalone hydrochloride is used as a local haemostatic and vasoconstrictor. It has also been used in combination with adrenaline as eye drops for glaucoma.

Preparations

Proprietary Preparations (details are given in Part 3)
Ger.: Stryphnasal.

Multi-ingredient: ***Ger.:*** Links-Glaukosan†.

Aesculus (12329-h)

Aesculus hippocastanum; Horse-chestnut; Marron d'Inde; Rosskastaniensamen.
CAS — 6805-41-0 (aescin); 11072-93-8 (β-aescin); 531-75-9 (esculoside, anhydrous).
Pharmacopoeias. In *Fr.* and *Ger.*
Ger. also includes esculoside in the sesquihydrate form.

The horse-chestnut, *Aesculus hippocastanum* (Hippocastanaceae) contains several active principles including esculoside (aesculin or esculin; 6-β-D-glucopyranosyloxy-7-hydroxycoumarin, $C_{15}H_{16}O_9 = 340.3$) and aescin (escin), which is a mixture of saponins.

Aesculus hippocastanum and other species of horse-chestnut may be poisonous.

Aescin and esculoside (aesculin or esculin), the major active principles of aesculus, have been used in the prevention and treatment of various peripheral vascular disorders including haemorrhoids (p.1170). They have been given by mouth, by intravenous injection (in the form of sodium aescinate), by rectal suppository, and applied topically. Aescin has also been administered intravenously in the prevention and treatment of post-operative oedema. The maximum dose for intravenous administration in adults for such conditions has been stated to be 20 mg daily; acute renal failure has been reported in patients given higher doses, sometimes in conjunction with other nephrotoxic drugs. Other derivatives such as sodium aescin polysulphate have also been used.

Aesculus hippocastanum has been used in homoeopathic medicine.

Effects on the kidneys. A report of the incidence of acute renal failure in patients following cardiac surgery and implicating high-dose intravenous aescin therapy.[1] In 70 patients receiving a mean maximum daily dose of 340 μg per kg body-weight no alteration of renal function was observed; in 16 receiving 360 μg per kg mild renal impairment was observed; and in 40 receiving 510 μg per kg acute renal failure developed.

1. Hellberg K, *et al.* Drug induced acute renal failure after heart surgery. *Thoraxchirurgie* 1975; **23:** 396–400.

Poisoning. There have been reports of poisoning in children from eating the seeds, or drinking infusions made from the leaves and twigs of horse-chestnut trees.[1] The toxic substance is considered to be esculoside. Symptoms of poisoning were muscle twitching, weakness, lack of coordination, dilated pupils, vomiting, diarrhoea, paralysis, and stupor.

1. Nagy M. Human poisoning from horse chestnuts. *JAMA* 1973; **226:** 213.

Preparations

Proprietary Preparations (details are given in Part 3)
Aust.: Reparil; Traumaparil; Venoplant; Venosin; Venostasin†; ***Austral.:*** Tecura†; ***Belg.:*** Reparil; ***Fr.:*** Flogencyl; Hemorrogel; Reparil†; ***Ger.:*** Aescorin N; Aescusan; Aescuven; Concentrin; Essaven Mono; Hamos-Tropfen-S; Hoevenol; Noricaven novo; opino N; Perivar; Plissamur forte; Proveno N; Reparil; Rexiluven S; Rhenus; Sanaven Venentabletten; Vasoforte N; Vasotonin; Venen-Dragees; Venen-Fluid; Venen-Tabletten; Venen-Tropfen; Venentabs; Veno-biomo; Venogal S; Venoplant; Venoplant plus†; Venoplant†; Venopyronum; Venopyronum N; Venostasin; Venotrulan N; ***Ital.:*** Curaven; Flebostasin; Ginoven; Reparil; Venoplant†; ***S.Afr.:*** Reparil†; ***Spain:*** Feparil; Flebostasin; ***Switz.:*** Aesculaforce; Phlebostasin; Reparil; Venostasin special†.

Multi-ingredient: ***Aust.:*** Aesrutan; Alpha-Apoplectal; Amphodyn; Apoplectal; Augentropfen Stulln; Dilaescol; Opino; Reparil; Sandoven; Urelium Neu; Venosin; Venostasin†; ***Austral.:*** Bioglan Fingers & Toes; Cirflo†; Herbal Capillary Care; Proflo; ***Belg.:*** Hemocoavit†; Mictasol; Paracodine†; Rectovasol; Reparil; ***Canad.:*** Pommade Midy; Proctosedyl; Proctosone; ***Fr.:*** Actisane Hemorroides, Jambes Lourdes; Anti-Hemorroidaires; Aphloine P; Arterase; Bioveinal†; Cepevit; Circularine; Climaxol; Creme Rap; Curoveinyl; Escinogel; Fluon; Fluxival†; Fragonal; Hemoluol; Hemorrogel; Histo-Fluine P; Hyalurectal†; Intrait de Marron D'Inde P; Mediflor Tisane Circulation du Sang No 12; Opo-Veinogene†; P. Veinos; Phlebogel; Phytomelis; Pommade Midy†; Preparation H; Reparil; Sedorrhoide; Suppositoires Midy†; Tisane Phlebosedol; Veinostase; Veinotonyl; Vivene; ***Ger.:*** Aescorin N; Aescusan; Alpha-Apoplectal†; Amphodyn; Anisan; Apoplectal N; Arnika plus; Augentropfen Stulln Mono; Bryonia-Strath†; Carito†; Cefadysbasin; Cefasabal; Clemenzil†; Comforte†; Conjunctisan-A; Conjunctisan-B; Cycloven Forte N; Diu Venostasin; Duoform†; Essaven; Essaven 50 000†; Essaven N; Essaven ultra; Ger N in der Ophtiole†; Hametum-N; Hamoagil†; Hamos N; Haven†; Heparin Comp; Heweven P 3; Heweven P 7; Hoevenol; Hoevenol A; Intradermi Fluid N; Intradermi N; Jatamansin†; Jossathromb†; JuPhlebon S; Lindigoa S; Mastu NH†; Maudor†; Medivarsin†; Nephrubin; Neuro-Demoplas†; Nicoplectal†; opino heparinoid†; opino N spezial; Pascovenol novo; Pascovenol S†; PC 30 V; Pe-Ce Ven N; Pentavenon†; Phlebex†; Posti N; Praecivenin†; Protitis†; Rectosellan; Reparil-Gel N; Rephastasan†; Revicain Comp; Revicain Comp Plus; Rheumex†; RR-plus†; Salhumin Teilbad N; Salus Venen Krauter Dragees N; Sklerovenol N; Sportupac N; Tamposit†; Trauma-cyl; Urol†; varico sanol Beincreme†; varico sanol forte†; Varicylum S; Vasesana-Vasoregulans; Vasotonin forte; Vasotonin S†; Vasotonin Serol†; Venacton; Venen-Salbe; Venen-Salbe N; Veno-Kattwiga N; Venoplant; Venopyronum N triplex; Venostasin; Venothromb†; Venotrulan Compositum†; ventri-loges; ***Irl.:*** Proctosedyl; ***Ital.:*** Bres; Castindia; Dermocinetic; Dermoprolyn; Elisir Depurativo Ambrosiano; Essaven; Ginkgo Plus; Hirudex; Nitesco S; Opino†; Pomata Midy HC; Pomata Midy†; Premium†; Proctosedyl; Recto-Reparil; Reparil; Sandoven†; Somatoline; Supposte Midy†; Tioscina; Varicogel; Venoplant†; Venoplus; Venotrauma; Venovit; Zeta-Bat†; ***Neth.:*** Venoplant†; ***Norw.:*** Proctosedyl; ***S.Afr.:*** Essaven; Proctosedyl; Reparil; Sandovene†; ***Spain:*** Caprofides Hemostatico; Circovenil; Circovenil Fuerte; Essavenon; Feparil; Flebo Stop; Hemodren Compuesto; Hemorrane; Killpan; Liviane Compuesto; Roidhemo; Uralyt Urato; Urgenin; Venacol; Venoplant; ***Swed.:*** Proctosedyl; ***Switz.:*** Amphodyn special†; Augentonicum; Demoven N; Dolo-Veniten; Flavovenyl; Flogecyl; Optazine; Proctosedyl†; Reparil; Reparil N; Ruvenas†; Sandovene f†; Venoplant N; Venostasin comp†; ***UK:*** Catarrh Cream.

Aflatoxins (12330-a)

CAS — 1162-65-8 (aflatoxin B_1); 7220-81-7 (aflatoxin B_2); 1165-39-5 (aflatoxin G_1); 7241-98-7 (aflatoxin G_2).

Aflatoxins are toxic metabolites produced by many strains of *Aspergillus flavus*, growing on many vegetable foods, notably peanuts. A number of forms, including aflatoxins B_1, B_2, G_1, G_2, and M_1 have been identified.

Aflatoxins have been implicated in liver cancer. Aflatoxin B_1 is reported to be one of the most potent carcinogens known in *animals*.

References.

1. Denning DW, *et al.* Measurement of aflatoxin in Nigerian sera by enzyme-linked immunosorbent assay. *Trans R Soc Trop Med Hyg* 1988; **82:** 169–71.
2. Lamplugh SM, *et al.* Aflatoxins in breast milk, neonatal cord blood, and serum of pregnant women. *Br Med J* 1988; **296:** 968.
3. Nyathi CB, *et al.* Human exposure to aflatoxins in Zimbabwe. *Cent Afr J Med* 1989; **35:** 542–5.
4. Wild CP, *et al.* In-utero exposure to aflatoxin in West Africa. *Lancet* 1991; **337:** 1602.
5. Ross RK, *et al.* Urinary aflatoxin biomarkers and risk of hepatocellular carcinoma. *Lancet* 1992; **339:** 943–6.

Agnus Castus (14089-a)

Keuschlamm; Mönchspfeffer.

The dried fruits of *Vitex agnus castus* (Verbenaceae).

Agnus castus is reported to stimulate the secretion of luteinising hormone and prolactin by the pituitary and to inhibit the release of follicle stimulating hormone. It is included in herbal preparations for menstrual and menopausal disorders but should be avoided in patients receiving exogenous sex hormones including oral contraceptives.

It is also used in homoeopathic medicine.

References.

1. Houghton P. Agnus castus. *Pharm J* 1994; **253:** 720–1.

Preparations

Proprietary Preparations (details are given in Part 3)
Aust.: Agnumens; ***Ger.:*** Agnolyt; Agnucaston; Agnufemil; Castufemin N; Cefanorm; Gynocastus; Kytta-Femin; Strotan; ***Switz.:*** Emoton; ***UK:*** Agnolyt.

Multi-ingredient: ***Austral.:*** Dong Quai Complex; Lifesystem Herbal Formula 4 Women's Formula; PMT Complex; Women's Formula Herbal Formula 3; ***Ger.:*** Femisana N.

Alfalfa (12026-w)

Lucerne; Purple medick.

The plant *Medicago sativa* (Leguminosae) which is cultivated as an animal feedstuff.

The seeds and sprouts of alfalfa contain canavanine (2-amino-4-(guanidinooxy)butyric acid), a toxic amino acid structurally related to arginine; content is reported to represent about 1.5% of the dry weight. A syndrome resembling systemic lupus erythematosus has been recorded in *monkeys* fed alfalfa.

Alfalfa is used in herbal preparations for a variety of disorders and in homoeopathic medicine.

Preparations

Proprietary Preparations (details are given in Part 3)
Ger.: Schneckensirup.

Multi-ingredient: ***Austral.:*** Neo-Cleanse; Panax Complex; Plantiodine Plus; Zinc Zenith; ***UK:*** Fat-Solv.

Alglucerase (5252-v)

Alglucerase *(BAN, USAN, rINN).*

Glucosylceramidase; Macrophage-targeted β-Glucocerebrosidase.

CAS — 143003-46-7.

A modified form of human placental β-glucocerebrosidase (ceramide glucosidase; β-D-glucosyl-*N*-acylsphingosine glucohydrolase). It is a monomeric glycoprotein of 497 amino acids with glycosylation making up about 6% of the molecule.

Imiglucerase (17703-h)

Imiglucerase *(BAN, USAN, rINN).*

Recombinant Macrophage-targeted β-Glucocerebrosidase; r-GCR.

CAS — 154248-97-2.

A recombinant human-derived β-glucocerebrosidase. It is a monomeric glycoprotein of 497 amino acids glycosylated at 4 asparagine residues.

Units

One unit is defined as the amount of alglucerase or imiglucerase required to hydrolyse one micromole of *p*-nitrophenyl-β-D-glucopyranoside in one minute at 37°.

Adverse Effects, Treatment, and Precautions

Fever, chills, pruritus, flushing, and gastro-intestinal symptoms, including cramps, diarrhoea, nausea, and vomiting have been reported following administration of alglucerase or imiglucerase. Some of these may be hypersensitivity reactions; other hypersensitivity reactions, including urticaria and angioedema, respiratory symptoms, and hypotension have also occurred. Caution is required in patients who have exhibited signs of hypersensitivity; reduction of the rate of infusion, and pretreatment with antihistamines and/or corticosteroids may permit further treatment. Antibodies have developed in about 15% of patients receiving a glucocerebrosidase enzyme during the first year of therapy. Patients who develop antibodies are at increased risk of hypersensitivity reactions and periodic assessment for antibody formation is recommended.

Pain and irritation at the injection site may occur. Other adverse effects reported include fatigue, dizziness, headache, backache, peripheral oedema, mouth ulcers, and disturbances in sense of smell.

Alglucerase is prepared from human placentas and its infusion therefore carries a risk of transmission of infections although this is minimised by the manufacturing process. Chorionic gonadotrophin, a naturally occurring hormone in human placentas, has been detected in alglucerase. The presence of this hormone may produce early virilisation in young boys when high doses of alglucerase are used and false positive results of pregnancy tests that are performed within 48 hours after administration. Alglucerase should be used with caution, if at all, in patients with androgen-sensitive malignancies.

Effects on the lungs. Pulmonary hypertension developed in two patients with Gaucher disease after initiation of treatment with alglucerase.[1] Neither patient had evidence of parenchymal lung infiltration with Gaucher cells.

1. Dawson A, *et al.* Pulmonary hypertension developing after alglucerase therapy in two patients with type 1 Gaucher disease complicated by the hepatopulmonary syndrome. *Ann Intern Med* 1996; **125:** 901–4.

Uses and Administration

Alglucerase and imiglucerase are forms of β-glucocerebrosidase given as enzyme replacement therapy to patients with symptomatic type 1 Gaucher disease (see below). The enzyme is given in a mannose-containing form to ensure uptake into macrophages.

Alglucerase and imiglucerase are administered by intravenous infusion over 1 to 2 hours. Up to 60 units of alglucerase or imiglucerase per kg body-weight may be given as a single infusion. The frequency of administration depends on the severity of symptoms and can vary from once every four weeks to alternate days. Once the patient's condition is stabilised the dose should be reduced at intervals of 3 to 12 months to a maintenance dose.

References.

1. Anonymous. Alglucerase for Gaucher's disease. *Med Lett Drugs Ther* 1991; **33:** 82.
2. Whittington R, Goa KL. Alglucerase; a review of its therapeutic use in Gaucher's disease. *Drugs* 1992; **44:** 72–93.

Gaucher disease. Gaucher disease[1-3] (glucocerebrosidosis) is a rare disease although it is the commonest lysosomal storage disease. It is caused by a deficiency of the lysosomal enzyme β-glucocerebrosidase (acid β-glucosidase, ceramide glucosidase, β-D-glucosyl-*N*-acylsphingosine glucohydrolase, or glucosylceramidase) which catalyses the hydrolysis of glucocerebroside, a lipid component of cell membranes, to glucose and ceramide. Deficiency of β-glucocerebrosidase results in accumulation of glucocerebroside in the lysosomes of reticuloendothelial cells, particularly macrophages. These large lipid-laden macrophages (termed Gaucher cells) eventually infiltrate the liver, spleen, bone, and bone marrow leading to hepatomegaly, splenomegaly, splenic infarction, anaemia, thrombocytopenia, leucopenia, and bone disorders including osteoporosis and osteonecrosis. In some cases infiltration of brain tissue also occurs producing neurological impairment and seizures. Rarely, infiltration of lung parenchymal tissue occurs leading to pulmonary infections.

Gaucher disease is an autosomal recessive disorder that has been classified into three main forms on the basis of clinical signs and symptoms. Hepatosplenomegaly occurs in all forms. Type 1 Gaucher disease, also known as chronic adult non-neuronopathic disease, accounts for 99% of cases and occurs especially in Ashkenazi Jews. The disease follows a chronic course of variable severity and onset, with hepatosplenomegaly and blood and bone disorders being the main features; there is no neurological involvement. In type 2 Gaucher disease (acute infantile neuronopathic disease) neurological involvement predominates. Patients show developmental delay by the age of 6 months, suffer seizures, pulmonary infections, and usually die during the first year of life. Type 3 Gaucher disease (subacute juvenile neuronopathic disease or Norrbotten disease) is a more slowly progressive form that presents later in childhood than type 2 disease and varies in severity. As in type 2 disease, there is neurological involvement. Patients may survive into early adulthood, although death by age 10 to 15 is frequent.

Treatment of Gaucher disease was previously limited to symptomatic management. In some cases bone-marrow transplantation was required for life-threatening bone-marrow involvement. Preparations of β-glucocerebrosidase, the deficient enzyme, are now available. Due to the rarity of Gaucher disease, clinical studies have been limited mainly to small case series of patients with type 1 disease. Administration of alglucerase or imiglucerase has been shown to reverse hepatosplenomegaly and the haematological abnormalities;[4] effects may be seen within a few months although in many the response is poor during the first 6 to 9 months and then improves rapidly.[2] Bone symptoms respond more slowly. Decreases in bone pain during the first year of treatment have been reported although there was no radiological improvement.[5] Normalised growth velocity has been reported in children[6] and radiographical assessments have shown improvements in bone density and mineralisation.[7] The efficacy of enzyme replacement therapy in managing neurological symptoms in patients with type 2 or type 3 disease[8] has yet to be established. It is not yet known whether enzyme replacement is able to prevent the development of symptoms in asymptomatic patients.

There is some controversy over the optimal dosage regimen. Doses of alglucerase as low as 2.3 units per kg body-weight three times a week[9] or 1.15 units per kg three times a week[10] may be sufficient to produce improvement, even in patients with severe symptoms. Doses of imiglucerase of 15 units per kg every two weeks or 2.5 units per kg three times a week have produced satisfactory clinical responses.[11] Patients vary considerably in their response to enzyme replacement therapy, and dosages must be individualised. Antibodies to the enzyme do not generally affect enzyme activity; neutralising antibodies have been reported in a very few patients.[2]

Possible future therapies that are under investigation include gene therapy and L-cycloserine. L-Cycloserine may inhibit or reduce the synthesis of glucocerebroside by inhibiting one of the early enzymes in the sphingolipid pathway. Other modified forms of β-glucocerebrosidase are also under investigation to improve uptake into the affected macrophages.

1. NIH Technology Assessment Panel on Gaucher Disease. Gaucher disease: current issues in diagnosis and treatment. *JAMA* 1996; **275:** 548–53.
2. Grabowski GA. Current issues in enzyme therapy for Gaucher disease. *Drugs* 1996; **52:** 159–67.
3. Morales LE. Gaucher's disease: a review. *Ann Pharmacother* 1996; **30:** 381–8.
4. Grabowski GA, *et al.* Enzyme therapy in type 1 Gaucher disease: comparative efficacy of mannose-terminated glucocerebrosidase from natural and recombinant sources. *Ann Intern Med* 1995; **122:** 33–9.
5. Pastores GM, *et al.* Enzyme therapy in Gaucher disease type 1: dosage efficacy and adverse effects in 33 patients treated for 6 to 24 months. *Blood* 1993; **82:** 408–16.
6. Kaplan P, *et al.* Acceleration of retarded growth in children with Gaucher disease after treatment with alglucerase. *J Pediatr* 1996; **129:** 149–53.
7. Rosenthal DI, *et al.* Enzyme replacement therapy for Gaucher disease: skeletal responses to macrophage-targeted glucocerebrosidase. *Pediatrics* 1995; **96:** 629–37.
8. Bembi B, *et al.* Enzyme replacement treatment in type 1 and type 3 Gaucher's disease. *Lancet* 1994; **344:** 1679–82.
9. Zimran A, *et al.* Low-dose enzyme replacement therapy for Gaucher's disease: effects of age, sex, genotype, and clinical features on response to treatment. *Am J Med* 1994; **97:** 3–13.
10. Hollak CEM, *et al.* Individualised low-dose alglucerase therapy for type 1 Gaucher's disease. *Lancet* 1995; **345:** 1474–8.
11. Zimran A, *et al.* Replacement therapy with imiglucerase for type 1 Gaucher's disease. *Lancet* 1995; **345:** 1479–80.

Preparations

Proprietary Preparations (details are given in Part 3)
Ger.: Ceredase; ***Ital.:*** Ceredase; ***Spain:*** Ceredase; ***UK:*** Ceredase; Cerezyme; ***USA:*** Ceredase; Cerezyme.

Alibendol (18738-r)

Alibendol *(rINN)*.

5-Allyl-*N*-(2-hydroxyethyl)-3-methoxysalicylamide.

$C_{13}H_{17}NO_4$ = 251.3.

CAS — 26750-81-2.

A choleretic used in the treatment of gastro-intestinal disorders.

Preparations

Proprietary Preparations (details are given in Part 3)
Fr.: Cebera.

Allergen Products (6175-c)

Pharmacopoeias. In *Eur.* (see p.viii).

Adverse Effects and Treatment

Adverse effects to prepared allergens can range from mild local reactions to severe generalised reactions which may be fatal. Severe reactions may be seen after skin tests in sensitive individuals as well as at any time during hyposensitisation. Aqueous solutions are more likely to provoke systemic reactions than preparations designed to give slower release rates. Severe reactions have been associated with tyrosine-adsorbed vaccines which have a relatively short half-life.

Hypersensitivity reactions may be immediate or delayed. Local reactions are normally limited to swelling and irritation. Systemic reactions include rhinitis, conjunctivitis, urticaria, bronchospasm, laryngeal oedema, generalised anaphylaxis, and shock. Severe reactions normally occur within 30 minutes and should be treated promptly with intramuscular adrenaline injection 1 in 1000, which should be immediately available when hyposensitising injections are being administered. Full supportive measures should be implemented and treatment with antihistamines and corticosteroids may be required (for a discussion of the treatment of anaphylactic shock, see p.816). Further hyposensitisation should be stopped or continued at reduced dosage depending on the severity of the reaction and in accordance with the manufacturer's recommendations.

In 1986 the UK Committee on Safety of Medicines (CSM) reported that hyposensitising vaccines have the potential to induce severe bronchospasm and anaphylaxis, and that these reactions had caused 26 deaths in the UK since 1957.[1] The majority of patients had no reaction to previous hyposensitising injections. In view of the risks, the CSM recommended that hyposensitising agents should be used only where facilities for full cardiopulmonary resuscitation are immediately available, that desensitising vaccines should only be used for seasonal allergic hay fever not responding to anti-allergic drugs and for hypersensitivity to Hymenoptera stings, that treatment should usually be avoided in patients with asthma, and that patients should be kept under medical observation for 1 hour after injection, or, if symptoms of hypersensitivity develop, until they are completely resolved.[1,2] A working group of the WHO and the International Union of Immunological Societies stated that a waiting period of 30 minutes after allergen injection was widely used throughout the world, since there was no convincing evidence that a longer wait can alter the fatality rate.[3,4] The working group considered that the observation period should be extended if the patient developed symptoms, even mild, of a general reaction. Since 1980, the American Academy of Allergy and Immunology had received 14 reports of death following hyposensitisation, and 4 deaths following skin testing for allergies.[5] The most common clinical factor in these patients was a prior history of asthma.

Active and passive immunotherapy have been used in combination to decrease the incidence of adverse effects to insect venoms (see under Hyposensitisation, below).

There have been anecdotal reports of persistent worsening of the original condition after hyposensitisation and rarely of the development of connective tissue disorders.[3,4]

Of twelve samples of *Aspergillus* extract used for hyposensitisation, 4 were found to contain aflatoxin (p.1544), one being highly mutagenic as determined by the Ames' test. The results suggested that careful screening of commercially available mould extracts was warranted.[6]

1. Committee on Safety of Medicines. Desensitising vaccines. *Br Med J* 1986; **293:** 948.
2. Committee on Safety of Medicines/Medicines Control Agency. Desensitising vaccines: new advice. *Current Problems* 1994; **20:** 5.
3. WHO/International Union of Immunological Societies. Current status of allergen immunotherapy: shortened version of a World Health Organisation/International Union of Immunological Societies Working Group Report. *Lancet* 1989; **i:** 259–61.
4. WHO/International Union of Immunological Societies. Current status of allergen immunotherapy (hyposensitization): memorandum from a WHO/IUIS meeting. *Bull WHO* 1989; **67:** 263–72.
5. Food and Drug Administration. Fatality risk with allergenic extract use. *JAMA* 1989; **261:** 3368.
6. Legator MS, *et al.* Aflatoxin B_1 in mould extracts used for desensitisation. *Lancet* 1983; **ii:** 915.

Precautions

Hyposensitising injections should not be given to patients with febrile conditions, serious immunological illness, or acute asthma. Allergen preparations should be avoided during pregnancy because of the risk to the fetus of any systemic reactions. Hyposensitising injections should only be administered where facilities for full cardiopulmonary resuscitation are immediately available. It has been recommended that patients should be observed for at least 1 hour after each injection (see under Adverse Effects, above). Patients with asthma may be more susceptible to hypersensitivity reactions with allergen extracts and in the UK it is considered that hyposensitising injections should be avoided in patients with asthma with the possible exception of those at risk of severe hypersensitivity reactions to Hymenoptera stings. Hyposensitising injections should also be avoided in children under 5 years of age.

Whenever possible, the same batch of allergen should be used throughout the treatment course. Injections should be given subcutaneously and not by intravenous or intramuscular injection.

Hyposensitising injections should be avoided in patients taking beta blockers since adrenaline will be ineffective if hypersensitivity reactions occur in these patients. Severe anaphylactoid reactions have been reported in patients undergoing hyposensitisation who are also receiving ACE inhibitors (p.806). Some manufacturers suggest that the reaction could be avoided by temporarily withholding ACE inhibitor therapy during each desensitisation.

Antihistamines should be avoided for at least 24 hours before sensitivity testing is carried out since they may mask skin reactivity; they have been given, during hyposensitisation, to very sensitive patients. Long-term topical use of potent corticosteroids may also mask skin reactivity.

Uses

Allergen extracts are used diagnostically in skin tests and provocation tests to confirm the cause of a suspected hypersensitivity reaction. They are also administered for hyposensitisation of certain patients with hypersensitivity reactions, particularly to insect venoms, pollens, or house-dust mite.

Diagnostic use. Sensitivity testing can be used to confirm that suspected allergens are predominantly responsible for the symptoms of a suspected hypersensitivity reaction. However, sensitivity testing should not form the sole basis of the treatment of hypersensitivity reactions.

Type IV (delayed) hypersensitivity reactions such as contact dermatitis are normally diagnosed using patch tests. A number of standard techniques are available, but in general they all involve maintaining a standard amount of the test substance in contact with the skin for 48 to 72 hours. A positive response is shown by erythema, swelling, or vesiculation. The sensitivity of different parts of the body varies, and this should be accounted for in applying test substances and controls. The test results are normally read half to one hour after removal of the patches to allow any pressure effects of the patches to subside. Patch testing with mixtures of allergens may be necessary to diagnose contact dermatitis in patients hypersensitive to multiple allergens.

Type I (immediate) hypersensitivity reactions such as allergic rhinitis, allergic asthma, and insect-sting hypersensitivity are tested using prick or intradermal tests. Since the allergen is introduced through the skin in these tests the risk of systemic reactions is greater, and adrenaline injection should be kept available. The test involves pricking the skin through a drop of allergen in solution, and comparing the result after 15 to 20 minutes with positive and negative controls. The intradermal test is used if the prick test result does not agree with a strong clinical suspicion. Skin testing is unreliable for evaluating hypersensitivity to drugs, except for penicillins and for certain macromolecules. Skin test titration, that is testing with a series of dilutions, has been used to determine a safe starting dose for hyposensitisation.

Provocation tests are designed to reproduce symptoms of hypersensitivity by controlled exposure to a suspected allergen. Provocation may be by the bronchial, oral, nasal, or ocular routes. Facilities for full cardiopulmonary resuscitation should be immediately available.

In-vitro methods for measuring antigen-specific IgE include the radioallergosorbent test (RAST).

1. VanArsdel PP, Larson EB. Diagnostic tests for patients with suspected allergic disease: utility and limitations. *Ann Intern Med* 1989; **110:** 304–12.
2. VanArsdel PP, Larson EB. Allergy testing. *Ann Intern Med* 1989; **110:** 317–20.
3. McLelland J, Shuster S. Contact dermatitis with negative patch tests: the additive effects of allergens in combination. *Br J Dermatol* 1990; **122:** 623–30.
4. Anonymous. Allergen testing in patients with type I hypersensitivity. *Drug Ther Bull* 1995; **33:** 45–7. Correction. *ibid.*: 55.

Hyposensitisation. Hyposensitisation (desensitisation or allergen immunotherapy) is the administration of gradually increasing quantities of allergen extract to ameliorate the effects of subsequent exposure to the allergen. Such therapy has become less popular following reports of severe and fatal anaphylactic reactions during therapy and should only be carried out in specialist centres. Hyposensitisation with a specific allergen has been found to be useful in hypersensitivities to pollens and insect venom, particularly that of Hymenoptera. For further discussion of the mechanisms of and indications for hyposensitisation, see below.

Allergen extracts are administered as aqueous extracts or as depot preparations bound to aluminium or calcium salts or to tyrosine; allergens modified to reduce side-effects while retaining immunogenicity have also been used. Whenever possible, the same batch of allergen should be used during a course of treatment because of possible differences in potency between batches. Allergen extracts are administered by subcutaneous injection in dosage regimens as recommended by the manufacturers and depending on the sensitivity of the patient. Skin test titration has been used to determine a safe starting dose. In conventional regimens, increasing doses are given once or twice weekly for aqueous extracts, or every one to two weeks for depot preparations until a maintenance dose is reached. Maintenance doses are given every 4 to 6 weeks. Modified dosage schedules have been used where maintenance needs to be achieved more quickly; such regimens may, however, be associated with an increased risk of adverse reactions. Aqueous extracts should be used for modified schedules until the maintenance dose is reached. In rush schedules, several injections are given daily on consecutive days. Semi-rush, modified rush, or cluster regimens involve the administration of several injections on a single day separated by an interval of several days.

The optimal duration of hyposensitisation therapy is unknown, but a period of 3 to 5 years is usually recommended.

Oral, nasal, sublingual, and bronchial routes of administration have sometimes been used for hyposensitisation.

Hyposensitisation is indicated exclusively for Type I (immediate) hypersensitivity reactions mediated by IgE antibodies.[1-4] Various authorities have published recommendations on the use of hyposensitisation;[1-3,5] there have also been several reviews.[4,6-10] Hyposensitisation may be used for the treatment of bee and wasp sting hypersensitivity, allergic rhinitis and conjunctivitis, and allergic asthma. Reports of severe and sometimes fatal hypersensitivity reactions to allergen extracts (see under Adverse Effects, above) produced recommendations that hyposensitisation should be carried out only in specialist centres with immediate access to adrenaline, oxygen, and intravenous fluids.[1-3] The UK Committee on Safety of Medicines considers that facilities for full cardiopulmonary resuscitation should be available.[8] However, a recent WHO report states that oral and nasal formulations may be administered at home. The restrictions on use of hyposensitisation in the UK have meant that this treatment is much less widely used there than in other parts of Europe and the US.

Hyposensitisation is generally more effective in children than adults.[1-4] It is less well tolerated, however, in young children and seldom recommended below the age of 5 years.[1-3]

Hyposensitisation for severe anaphylaxis following insect stings, particularly those of Hymenoptera, is achieved using purified extracts of insect venom.[1-5,7,8,11] Whole-body extracts of insects were formerly used but are ineffective.[3,7] A combined approach of passive and active immunotherapy has been used in patients demonstrating intolerable side-effects to hyposensitisation;[3,4] patients have been pretreated with specific venom IgG before commencing hyposensitisation.[4]

Hyposensitisation for seasonal allergic hay fever has generally been reserved for severely affected patients when anti-allergic drugs have failed.[5] However, there is some evidence that hyposensitisation for allergies such as hay fever may prevent the development of asthma and thus earlier use of hyposensitisation may be warranted. Hyposensitisation for rhinoconjunctivitis due to house-dust mite, animal danders, or fungi is generally less effective.[1-4,6-8] The use of hyposensitising injections is not generally recommended in patients with asthma[5] (see under Adverse Effects, above). However, some[12,13] consider that it may be tried as an adjunct to conventional treatment in highly selected patients with demonstrated sensitisation to an unavoidable allergen.

Hyposensitisation to a drug may be warranted on the rare occasions when hypersensitivity has developed and continued use is considered essential, possibly with penicillins or insulin.[1,3,4,14] Such regimens produce clinical tolerance, lost on cessation of therapy, without immunological change.[2,3]

Studies in a few patients have demonstrated some benefit from hyposensitisation in hypersensitivity disorders of the skin,[15,16] but further studies are required. Hyposensitisation appears to have no role in the routine management of hypersensitivity reactions to foods.[1-4]

Rush hyposensitisation has been successful in a woman hypersensitive to seminal plasma.[17]

Hyposensitisation with a single intradermal injection of an enzyme-potentiated allergen extract has been tried.[18]

1. Immunotherapy Subcommittee of the European Academy of Allergology and Clinical Immunology. Immunotherapy: position paper. *Allergy* 1988; **43** (suppl 6): 1–33.
2. WHO/International Union of Immunological Societies. Current status of allergen immunotherapy: shortened version of a World Health Organisation/International Union of Immunological Societies Working Group Report. *Lancet* 1989; **i:** 259–61.
3. WHO/International Union of Immunological Societies. Current status of allergen immunotherapy (hyposensitization): memorandum from a WHO/IUIS meeting. *Bull WHO* 1989; **67:** 263–72.
4. Eiser N. Desensitisation today. *Br Med J* 1990; **300:** 1412–13.
5. Frew AJ, British Society for Allergy and Clinical Immunology Working Party. Injection Immunotherapy. *Br Med J* 1993; **307:** 919–23.
6. Creticos PS, Norman PS. Immunotherapy with allergens. *JAMA* 1987; **258:** 2874–80.
7. Bush RK. Immunotherapy for the treatment of allergic diseases: clinical applications reviewed. *Hosp Formul* 1988; **23:** 245–67.
8. Naish PF. The place of hyposensitisation. *Prescribers' J* 1988; **28:** 37–43.
9. Loblay RH. Allergen immunotherapy: when is it useful? *Drugs* 1990; **40** 493–7.
10. Weber RW. Immunotherapy with allergens. *JAMA* 1997; **278:** 1881–7.
11. Valentine MD, Lichtenstein LM. Anaphylaxis and stinging insect hypersensitivity. *JAMA* 1987; **258:** 2881–5.
12. Abramson MJ, *et al.* Is allergen immunotherapy effective in asthma? A meta-analysis of randomized controlled trials. *Am J Respir Crit Care Med* 1995; **151:** 969–74.
13. Thoracic Society of Australia and New Zealand and Australasian Society of Clinical Immunology and Allergy. Specific allergen immunotherapy for asthma. *Med J Aust* 1997; **167:** 540–44.
14. Anderson JA, Adkinson NF. Allergic reactions to drugs and biologic agents. *JAMA* 1987; **258:** 2891–9.
15. August PJ, O'Driscoll J. Urticaria successfully treated by desensitization with grass pollen extract. *Br J Dermatol* 1989; **120:** 409–10.
16. Jacquemin MG, *et al.* Successful treatment of atopic dermatitis with complexes of allergen and specific antibodies. *Lancet* 1990; **i:** 1468–9.
17. Frisch C, *et al.* Rush hyposensitisation for allergy to seminal plasma. *Lancet* 1984; **i:** 1073.
18. Fell P, Brostoff J. A single dose desensitization for summer hay fever. *Eur J Clin Pharmacol* 1990; **38:** 77–9.

Preparations

Proprietary Preparations (details are given in Part 3)
Aust.: Alavac†; ALK†; Alutard†; Depot-Hal†; HAL†; Novo-Helisen†; Pangramin†; Pharmalgen†; ***Austral.:*** Albay; Allpyral; ***Belg.:*** Pollinex; ***Canad.:*** Pollinex-R; ***Fr.:*** Albay; Allpyral; Alpha-R†; Alphatest†; Alyostal; ASAD; Candidine; ***Ger.:*** ADL; Alk; Allergovit; Allerset†; Conjuvac†; Depot-Hal; Hal-oral; Heligoid†; Novo-Helisen; Oralvac; Purethal; SDL; TA Baumpollen; TA Graserpollen; TA MIX; True Test; Tyrosin S; Venomil; ***Ital.:*** Alavac†; Allergodex†; Alludex†; Bencard DP6†; Oraldex†; Pollinex†; Tirodex†; ***Neth.:*** Alavac-S; Allerset; Artoid; Baclysar†; Depot-Hal; Haloral; Immunovac; Oralgen; Oralgen β†; Pollalin; Pollinex Boompollen; Pollinex Graspollen; Purethal; Sublivac B.E.S.T.; ***Norw.:*** Alutard; ***S.Afr.:*** Albay; Allpyral Pure Mite; Allpyral Special Grass; Diagnostic Skin Testing Kit; ***Swed.:*** Alutard SQ; Aquagen SQ; Pharmalgen; Soluprick SQ; ***Switz.:*** Alavac-P†; Alavac-S; Allergovit; Alutard SQ; Alyostal; ASAD; Novo-Helisen; Pharmalgen; Polvac; SDV; Stallergenes†; Stallerpatch†; Staloral; ***UK:*** Bencard Skin Testing Solutions; Merck Skin Testing Solutions†; Pharmalgen; Spectralgen 3 Tree Mix†; Spectralgen 4 Grass Mix†; Spectralgen Single Species†; ***USA:*** Albay; Allpyral; Center-Al; Pharmalgen; True Test; Venomil.

Almond Oil (7352-h)

Aceite de Almendra; Amygdalae Oleum; Bitter Almond Oil; Expressed Almond Oil; Huile d'Amande; Mandelöl; Ol. Amygdal.; Oleo de Amêndoas; Olio di Mandorla; Sweet Almond Oil.

Pharmacopoeias. In *Eur.* (see p.viii), which specifies *Prunus dulcis* var. *dulcis* or var. *amara*. or a mixture of the two varieties. *Eur.* also includes Refined Almond Oil (Amygdalae Oleum Raffinatum).
Also in *USNF* which specifies oil from varieties of *Prunus amygdalus.*
Fr. also specifies Huile de Noyaux, an oil obtained from various species of *Prunus.*

A clear colourless or pale yellow oil with a bland nutty taste, consisting of glycerides chiefly of oleic acid, with smaller amounts of linoleic and palmitic acids. It is expressed, without the application of heat, from the seeds of the bitter or the sweet almond, *Prunus dulcis (Prunus amygdalus; Amygdalus communis)* var. *amara* or var. *dulcis* (Rosaceae). Slightly **soluble** in alcohol; miscible with chloroform, ether, and petroleum spirit. **Store** in well-filled airtight containers. Protect from light.

Almond oil has nutritive and demulcent properties. It is used as an emollient and to soften ear wax. It is also employed as a vehicle in some injections.

Preparations

BP 1998: Almond Oil Ear Drops;
USP 23: Rose Water Ointment.

Proprietary Preparations (details are given in Part 3)
Fr.: Karelyne.

Multi-ingredient: ***Irl.:*** Balmandol†; ***Ital.:*** Babysteril; Otosan Gocce Auricolari; ***Spain:*** Crema Antisolar Evanesce†; Pasta Lassar Imba; ***Switz.:*** Antidry; Balmandol; Ceralba†; Premandol; Viola Pommade a l'huile d'amandes†; Woloderma†; ***UK:*** Balmandol†; Earex; Imuderm; Infaderm.

Alpha Glucosidase (19670-h)

Alpha glucosidase is a therapeutic enzyme under investigation for the treatment of glycogen storage disease type II (Pompe's disease).

Preparations

Proprietary Preparations (details are given in Part 3)

Multi-ingredient: ***Austral.:*** Bioglan Active Enzyme Complex†; Digestaid; Zinc Zenith.

Alpha$_1$-proteinase Inhibitor (16516-j)

Alpha$_1$ Antitrypsin.

Adverse Effects and Precautions

Intravenous administration of alpha$_1$-proteinase inhibitor may produce flu-like symptoms, chills, dyspnoea, hypotension, tachycardia, or rashes. Allergic-type reactions have been reported. Preparations derived from pooled human plasma carry a risk of transmission of infection (see Blood, p.713). Vaccination against hepatitis B is recommended before starting treatment with alpha$_1$-proteinase inhibitor.

Uses and Administration

Endogenous alpha$_1$-proteinase inhibitor is a serum glycoprotein synthesised in the liver that acts as an elastase inhibitor, primarily inhibiting neutrophil elastase. Alpha$_1$-proteinase inhibitor, prepared from pooled human plasma, is used as replacement therapy in patients with emphysema who have congenital alpha$_1$ antitrypsin deficiency (see below). It is given in a dose of 60 mg per kg body-weight once a week by intravenous infusion over about 30 minutes.

Alpha$_1$ antitrypsin deficiency. Alpha$_1$ antitrypsin deficiency is a rare genetic disorder characterised by the development of emphysema usually in the third or fourth decade of life. Patients with this disorder lack alpha$_1$-proteinase inhibitor that acts in the lungs as an inhibitor of neutrophil elastase, an enzyme that is released in response to inflammation. A deficiency of this inhibitor thus leaves the lungs vulnerable to destruction by elastase and leads to the development of emphysema (p.747).

Management of alpha$_1$ antitrypsin deficiency involves avoidance of factors (mainly cigarette smoking) that cause pulmonary inflammation and supportive treatment with bronchodilators and oxygen as appropriate. Replacement therapy with alpha$_1$-proteinase inhibitor by intravenous infusion has been shown to correct the biochemical abnormality[1] and has been recommended in those patients with some deterioration of lung function.[2,3] However, studies have not yet shown that alpha$_1$-proteinase inhibitor can prevent the development of emphysema[4] and it has limited value in patients with very severe emphysema as replacement therapy cannot reverse established lung damage.[2]

A dosage regimen of 250 mg per kg body-weight intravenously once a month produces adequate alpha$_1$-proteinase inhibitor-serum concentrations and may be an alternative to the recommended weekly injections.[5] Recombinant forms of alpha$_1$-proteinase inhibitor[2] and administration by aerosol[6] have also been investigated.

Patients with alpha$_1$ antitrypsin deficiency may also have some liver involvement. This may present as neonatal jaundice or in adults as cirrhosis. The liver disease is managed symptomatically; it does not respond to treatment with alpha$_1$-proteinase inhibitor.

1. Wewers MD, *et al.* Replacement therapy for alpha$_1$-antitrypsin deficiency associated with emphysema. *N Engl J Med* 1987; **316:** 1055–62.
2. MacDonald JL, Johnson CE. Pathophysiology and treatment of α_1-antitrypsin deficiency. *Am J Health-Syst Pharm* 1995; **52:** 481–9.
3. American Thoracic Society. Guidelines for the approach to the patient with severe hereditary alpha-1-antitrypsin deficiency. *Am Rev Respir Dis* 1989; **140:** 1494–7.
4. Burdon JGW, *et al.* Antiproteinase deficiency, emphysema and replacement therapy. *Aust N Z J Med* 1996; **26:** 769–71.
5. Hubbard RC, *et al.* Biochemical efficacy and safety of monthly augmentation therapy for α_1-antitrypsin deficiency. *JAMA* 1988; **260:** 1259–64.
6. Hubbard RC, *et al.* Anti-neutrophil-elastase defenses of the lower respiratory tract in α1-antitrypsin deficiency directly augmented with an aerosol of α1-antitrypsin. *Ann Intern Med* 1989; **111:** 206–12.

Cystic fibrosis. Some of the inflammatory damage that occurs in the lungs of patients with cystic fibrosis is thought to result from locally released elastase. Alpha$_1$-proteinase inhibitor given by nebuliser is therefore under investigation[1] in patients with cystic fibrosis (p.119).

1. McElvaney NG, *et al.* Aerosol α1-antitrypsin treatment for cystic fibrosis. *Lancet* 1991; **337:** 392–4.

Preparations

Proprietary Preparations (details are given in Part 3)
Canad.: Prolastin; ***Ger.:*** Prolastin HS; ***Spain:*** Prolastina; ***USA:*** Prolastin.

Althaea (5404-v)

Alteia; Alth.; Althaeae Radix; Eibischwurzel; Marshmallow; Marshmallow Root; Racine de Guimauve; Raiz de Altea.

Pharmacopoeias. In *Eur.* (see p.viii) and *Pol.*
Althaea Leaf is also included in *Aust., Fr.,* and *Pol.* and Althaea Flower in *Fr.*

The peeled or unpeeled, whole or cut, dried root of *Althaea officinalis* (Malvaceae). **Protect** from light.

Althaea is demulcent and emollient and has been used for irritation and inflammation of the mucous membranes of the mouth and pharynx. It has also been used in traditional remedies for a variety of disorders including gastro-intestinal disturbances.

Preparations

Proprietary Preparations (details are given in Part 3)
Ger.: Phytobronchin†.

Multi-ingredient: ***Aust.:*** Aktiv Husten- und Bronchialtee; Anifer Hustentee; Bio-Garten Tee gegen Erkaltung; Bronchostop; Erkaltungstee; Heumann's Bronchialtee; Krauterhaus Mag Kottas Husten- und Bronchialtee; Krautertee Nr 11; Krautertee Nr 7; Mag Kottas Husten-Bronchialtee; Mediplant Krauter; Paracodin; Sidroga Brust-Husten-Tee; St Radegunder Hustentee; The Chambard-Tee; ***Austral.:*** Althaea Complex; Cough Relief; Garlic and Horseradish + C Complex; Garlic and Horseradish Complex 1000†; Hydrastis Complex; Respatona; Respatona Plus with Echinacea; ***Belg.:*** Eugiron; Paracodine; Sedemol†; Sulfa-Sedemol†; Tisane Antibiliaire et Stomachique; Tisane Pectorale; Tisane Purgative; ***Fr.:*** Elixir Contre La Toux Weleda; Mediflor Tisane Diuretique†; Mediflor Tisane Pectorale d'Alsace†; Tisane des Familles†; Tisane Grande Chartreuse; ***Ger.:*** Atmulen K†; Biotuss N; Bronchangin†; Bronchialtee†; Bronchitussin SC†; Bronchostad†; Dr. Klinger's Bergischer Krautertee, Husten- u. Bronchialtee†; Heumann Bronchialtee Solubifix; Infantussin N; Junisana;

Knufinke Broncholind K†; Priatan†; Thymitussin†; Tonsilgon-N; *Ital.:* Cura; *Switz.:* DemoAngina†; Dipect†; Malveol; Melior†; Sirop antitussif Wyss a base de codeine; Sirop pectoral DP1; Sirop pectoral DP2; Sirop Wyss contre la toux; Tisane antitussive et pectorale "H"†; Tisane pectorale et antitussive; Tuscalman; *UK:* Bio-balm; Cough Elixir; Digest; Garlodex; Golden Seal Compound; Herb and Honey Cough Elixir; Herbheal Ointment; Potter's Pastilles; Sinotar.

Alum (294-r)

Alaun; Allume; Aluin; Alumbre; Alumen; Aluminium Kalium Sulfuricum; Aluminium Potassium Sulphate; Alun; Potash Alum; Potassium Alum. Potassium aluminium sulphate dodecahydrate.

$KAl(SO_4)_2,12H_2O$ = 474.4.

CAS — 7784-24-9 (dodecahydrate); 10043-67-1 (anhydrous).

Pharmacopoeias. In *Chin., Eur.* (see p.viii), *Jpn, Pol.,* and *US.*
US also includes the anhydrous form and both anhydrous and dodecahydrated ammonia alum (Ammonium Alum). *Belg.* and *Jpn* also include dried alum.

Colourless, transparent, odourless, crystalline masses or a granular powder. **Soluble** 1 in 7 of water and 1 in 0.3 of boiling water; soluble in glycerol; practically insoluble in alcohol. A 10% solution in water has a pH of 3.0 to 3.5.

Adverse Effects

Large doses of alum are irritant and may be corrosive; gum necrosis and gastro-intestinal haemorrhage have occurred. Adverse effects on muscle and kidneys have been reported.

Uses and Administration

Alum precipitates proteins and is a powerful astringent. It is often included in preparations used as mouthwashes or gargles and in dermatological preparations.

Alum, either as a solid or as a solution, may be used as a haemostatic.

Alum is also used as a mordant in the dyeing industry.

Haemorrhage associated with malignant disease can be difficult to control and some success in bladder haemorrhage[1,2] or rectal haemorrhage[3] has been described with the use of an alum 1% solution.

1. Kennedy C, *et al.* Use of alum to control intractable vesical haemorrhage. *Br J Urol* 1984; **56:** 673–5.
2. Goel AK, *et al.* Intravesical irrigation with alum for the control of massive bladder hemorrhage. *J Urol (Baltimore)* 1985; **133:** 956–7.
3. Paes TRF, *et al.* Alum solution in the control of intractable haemorrhage from advanced rectal carcinoma. *Br J Surg* 1986; **73:** 192.

Preparations

Proprietary Preparations (details are given in Part 3)

Multi-ingredient: *Aust.:* EST; *Austral.:* BFI; *Canad.:* Fletchers Sore Mouth Medicine; *Fr.:* Denisoline; Stom-Antiba†; *Ger.:* Dr. Hotz Vollbad; Retterspitz Ausserlich; Retterspitz Gelee; Retterspitz Innerlich; Trachitol; *Irl.:* Pedamed†; *Ital.:* Emoplast; Gineosepta†; Lavanda Sofar; *Spain:* Cloroboral; Co Bucal; Faderma†; Lindemil; *USA:* BFI; Mycinette.

Aluminium (5261-g)

Aluminum; E173.

Al = 26.981538.

CAS — 7429-90-5.

Pharmacopoeias. Br. includes Aluminium Powder.

Aluminium is a malleable and ductile soft silvery-white metal, becoming coated with a thin layer of oxide.

Aluminium powder is an odourless or almost odourless, silvery-grey powder. It consists mainly of metallic aluminium in very small flakes, usually with an appreciable quantity of aluminium oxide. It is lubricated with stearic acid to protect the metal from oxidation. The powder is practically **insoluble** in water and in alcohol; it dissolves in dilute acids and solutions of alkali hydroxides, with the evolution of hydrogen.

WARNING. *Aluminium powder has been used for the illicit preparation of explosives or fireworks; care is required with its supply.*

Incompatibility. Incompatibilities have been reported between aluminium in injection equipment and metronidazole[1,2] and between aluminium and various antineoplastic agents including cisplatin, daunorubicin, and doxorubicin.[3-6] The suitability of aluminium caps for sugar-containing liquids has also been questioned. Abrasion of the aluminium cap by sugar from Ceporex Syrup has resulted in the formation of a black slime.[7]

1. Schell KH, Copeland JR. Metronidazole hydrochloride-aluminum interaction. *Am J Hosp Pharm* 1985; **42:** 1040, 1042.
2. Struthers BJ, Parr RJ. Clarifying the metronidazole hydrochloride-aluminum interaction. *Am J Hosp Pharm* 1985; **42:** 2660.
3. Bohart RD, Ogawa G. An observation on the stability of cis-dichlorodiammineplatinum (II): a caution regarding its administration. *Cancer Treat Rep* 1979; **63:** 2117–18.
4. Gardiner WA. Possible incompatibility of doxorubicin hydrochloride with aluminum. *Am J Hosp Pharm* 1981; **38:** 1276.
5. Williamson MJ, *et al.* Doxorubicin hydrochloride-aluminum interaction. *Am J Hosp Pharm* 1983; **40:** 214.
6. Ogawa GS, *et al.* Dispensing-pin problems. *Am J Hosp Pharm* 1985; **42:** 1042.
7. Tressler LJ. Medicine bottle caps. *Pharm J* 1985; **235:** 99.

Adverse Effects, Treatment, and Precautions

Aluminium toxicity is well recognised in patients with renal impairment. Patients undergoing dialysis have experienced encephalopathy, osteodystrophy, and anaemia associated with an aluminium salt taken as a phosphate binder or with aluminium present in the water supply. For this reason, aluminium-free phosphate binders are often used in dialysis patients (see Renal Osteodystrophy, p.732); also the concentration of aluminium in dialysis fluid has been limited to not more than 10 μg per litre. Serum-aluminium concentrations should be monitored regularly in patients undergoing dialysis.

Aluminium toxicity has followed the administration of parenteral fluids and infant feeds with a high concentration of aluminium.

Aluminium toxicity may be treated by removal of the aluminium with desferrioxamine (p.976).

The adverse effects of aluminium salts and precautions to be observed are described under Aluminium Hydroxide, p.1177.

A review of aluminium toxicity[1] lists possible sources of aluminium including water, antacids, phosphate-binding gels, total parenteral nutrition solutions, processed human serum albumin, fluids used in infants, and environmental pollution; cooking utensils and beverages such as tea have also been suggested as possible sources of aluminium. Toxicity tends to occur when the gastro-intestinal barrier to aluminium absorption is circumvented, as in intravenous fluid administration or dialysis, or if the excretion of aluminium is reduced, as in renal impairment. Infants, especially preterm infants, form a special risk group.[2-5]

Accidental deposition of a large amount of aluminium sulphate in a reservoir in Cornwall in 1988 led to contamination of a nearby town's water supply.[6] Symptoms reported included diarrhoea, mouth ulcers or blisters, malaise, joint symptoms (mainly deterioration of existing symptoms), and memory defects (usually beginning 2 to 3 months after the incident). Although some medical experts considered that no long-term toxic effects were to be expected,[6] aluminium deposits were found in the bones of 2 individuals 6 to 7 months later.[7]

1. Monteagudo FSE, *et al.* Recent developments in aluminium toxicology. *Med Toxicol* 1989; **4:** 1–16.
2. Bishop N, *et al.* Aluminium in infant formulas. *Lancet* 1989; **i:** 490.
3. Lawson M, *et al.* Aluminium and infant formulae. *Lancet* 1989; **i:** 614–15.
4. Anonymous. Aluminium content of parenteral drug products. *WHO Drug Inf* 1990; **4:** 70.
5. American Academy of Pediatrics Committee on Nutrition. Aluminum toxicity in infants and children. *Pediatrics* 1996; **97:** 413–16.
6. Anonymous. Camelford two years on. *Lancet* 1990; **336:** 366.
7. Eastwood JB, *et al.* Aluminium deposition in bone after contamination of drinking water supply. *Lancet* 1990; **336:** 462–4.

Effects on mental function. Encephalopathy with seizures has been associated with the use of aluminium-containing materials used for bone reconstruction.[1,2] In each case, reconstruction of areas of the skull resulted in high concentrations of aluminium in the cerebrospinal fluid.

1. Renard JL, *et al.* Post-otoneurosurgery aluminium encephalopathy. *Lancet* 1994; **344:** 63–4.
2. Hantson P, *et al.* Encephalopathy with seizures after use of aluminium-containing bone cement. *Lancet* 1994; **344:** 1647.

ALZHEIMER'S DISEASE. Aluminium has been implicated in the aetiology of Alzheimer's disease (p.1386), although a causative link has yet to be proved.[1-6] Circumstantial evidence of a positive association arises from *animal* and *in-vitro* data together with clinical observations that aluminium is present in senile plaques and neurofibrillary tangles occurring in Alzheimer's disease, the administration of aluminium chelators to Alzheimer patients may slow the progression of the disease, and the risk of brain changes is increased in people living in areas that have a high aluminium content in the drinking water supply. Some of these findings have been criticised or unconfirmed by other workers. Listed below are some of the studies which point to an association between aluminium intake and Alzheimer's disease,[7-12] some criticisms,[13-17] and some negative findings.[18,19]

There does not appear to be a risk of aluminium accumulation from normal use of aluminium-containing antacids by patients with normal renal function, consequently use of these antacids by such patients should not be considered to put them at risk of Alzheimer's disease if aluminium is implicated in it.[20,21]

1. Deary IJ, Whalley LJ. Recent research on the causes of Alzheimer's disease. *Br Med J* 1988; **297:** 807–10.
2. Birchall JD, Chappell JS. Aluminium, chemical physiology, and Alzheimer's disease. *Lancet* 1988; **ii:** 1008–10.
3. Anonymous. Aluminium and Alzheimer's disease. *Lancet* 1989; **i:** 82–3.
4. Moody GH, Drummond JR. Alzheimer's disease. *Br Dent J* 1990; **169:** 45–7.
5. Crapper McLachlan DR, *et al.* Would decreased aluminum ingestion reduce the incidence of Alzheimer's disease? *Can Med Assoc J* 1991; **145:** 793–804.
6. Anonymous. Is aluminium a dementing ion? *Lancet* 1992; **339:** 713–14.
7. Martyn CN, *et al.* Geographical relation between Alzheimer's disease and aluminium in drinking water. *Lancet* 1989; **i:** 59–62.
8. Cowburn JD, Blair JA. Aluminium chelator (transferrin) reverses biochemical deficiency in Alzheimer brain preparations. *Lancet* 1989; **i:** 99.
9. Neri LC, Hewitt D. Aluminium, Alzheimer's disease, and drinking water. *Lancet* 1991; **338:** 390.
10. Crapper McLachlan DR, *et al.* Intramuscular desferrioxamine in patients with Alzheimer's disease. *Lancet* 1991; **337:** 1304–8.
11. Good PF, *et al.* Selective accumulation of aluminum and iron in the neurofibrillary tangles of Alzheimer's disease: a laser microprobe (LAMMA) study. *Ann Neurol* 1992; **31:** 286–92.
12. Harrington CR, *et al.* Alzheimer's-disease-like changes in tau protein processing: association with aluminium accumulation in brains of renal dialysis patients. *Lancet* 1994; **343:** 993–7.
13. Ebrahim S. Aluminium and Alzheimer's disease. *Lancet* 1989; **i:** 267.
14. Schupf N, *et al.* Aluminium and Alzheimer's disease. *Lancet* 1989; **i:** 267.
15. Lindesay J. Aluminium and Alzheimer's disease. *Lancet* 1989; **i:** 268.
16. Birchall JD, Chappell JS. Aluminium, water chemistry, and Alzheimer's disease. *Lancet* 1989; **i:** 953.
17. Whalley LJ, *et al.* Aluminium and dementia. *Lancet* 1992; **339:** 1235–6.
18. Markesbery WR, *et al.* Instrumental neutron activation analysis of brain aluminum in Alzheimer's disease and aging. *Ann Neurol* 1981; **10:** 511–16.
19. Wettstein A, *et al.* Failure to find a relationship between mnestic skills of octogenarians and aluminum in drinking water. *Int Arch Occup Environ Health* 1991; **63:** 97–103.
20. Anonymous. Aluminium salts and Alzheimer's disease. *Pharm J* 1991; **246:** 809.
21. Flaten TP, *et al.* Mortality from dementia among gastroduodenal ulcer patients. *J Epidemiol Community Health* 1991; **45:** 203–6.

Uses and Administration

Aluminium is used in packaging and in injection equipment. The foil is also used as a dressing and for insulation. Aluminium may also be employed as a colouring agent for some foodstuffs.

Aluminium powder alone and in paste form with zinc oxide has been used as a dressing.

Astringent aluminium salts are used as antiperspirants. Aluminium hydroxide is used as an antacid. Aluminium is used in homoeopathic medicine.

Preparations

BP 1998: Compound Aluminium Paste *(Baltimore Paste).*

Aluminium Acetate (296-d)

Aluminum Acetate.

$C_6H_9AlO_6$ = 204.1.

CAS — 139-12-8.

Aluminium acetate is prepared from aluminium sulphate and acetic acid. The BP includes Aluminium Acetate Ear Drops which correspond to a solution of aluminium acetotartrate in that they are prepared from aluminium sulphate with the aid of acetic acid and tartaric acid. The USP includes Aluminum Acetate Topical Solution which is prepared from glacial acetic acid and Aluminum Subacetate Topical Solution (which is itself prepared from aluminium sulphate and acetic acid); it does not involve tartaric acid.

Solutions containing aluminium acetate are astringent. Ear drops containing aluminium acetates reduce oedema and inflammation of the ear by producing an acidic environment hostile to pathogenic bacteria; they are also hygroscopic. Solutions are also used in dermatology as astringent lotions for irritating skin conditions.

Various preparations containing aluminium acetates have been known as Burow's creams, emulsions, lotions, or solutions.

Aluminium acetotartrate and aluminium subacetate (basic aluminium acetate) are also used as topical astringents.

Preparations

BP 1998: Aluminium Acetate Ear Drops;
USP 23: Aluminum Subacetate Topical Solution.

Proprietary Preparations (details are given in Part 3)

Canad.: Acid Mantle†; *Ger.:* Alsol; Alsol N; Essigsaure Tonerde-Salbe; Essitol; *Ital.:* Euceta; *Neth.:* Euceta†; *Switz.:* Euceta; *USA:* Buro-Sol.

Multi-ingredient: *Aust.:* Acetonal; Euceta mit Kamille; Methyment; Nasanal; Neo-Phlogicid; *Austral.:* Xyloproct; *Belg.:* Xyloproct; *Canad.:* Buro Derm; Buro-Sol; *Fr.:* Gel a l'Acetotartrate d'Alumine Defresne†; *Ger.:* Acetonal Vaginale†; Alsol†; Anisan; *Irl.:* Xyloproct; *Ital.:* Betaderm; Neo Zeta-Foot; Vegetallumina; Xyloproct; Zeta-Foot†; *Neth.:* Xyloproct; *Norw.:* Xyloproct; *Spain:* Agua Germana†; Avril; *Swed.:* Xyloproct; *Switz.:* Anginesin; Cetona; Euceta avec camomille et arnica; Euceta Pic†; Frigoplasma; Fungex; Mikutan N; Realderm; *UK:* Xyloproct; *USA:* Borofair Otic; Burow's; Otic Domeboro; Star-Otic.

Aluminium Lactate (12347-b)

Tris(lactato)aluminium.
$C_9H_{15}AlO_9$ = 294.2.
CAS — 537-02-0; 18917-91-4.

Aluminium lactate is used in the local treatment of various disorders of the mouth.

Preparations

Proprietary Preparations (details are given in Part 3)
Fr.: Aluctyl; Etiaxil†; ***Ital.:*** Aluctyl.

Multi-ingredient: ***Ger.:*** Hexomedin transkutan†; ***Ital.:*** Lacalut; ***Switz.:*** Deaftol avec lidocaine; Gynasol; Lurgyl†.

Aluminium Sulphate (301-b)

Aluminii Sulfas; Aluminium Sulfuricum; Aluminium Trisulphate; Aluminum Sulfate.
$Al_2(SO_4)_3,xH_2O$ = 342.2 (anhydrous).
CAS — 10043-01-3 (anhydrous aluminium sulphate); 17927-65-0 (aluminium sulphate hydrate).
Pharmacopoeias. In *Eur.* (see p.viii), *Int.*, *Pol.*, and *US.*

Colourless or white odourless lustrous crystals or crystalline masses. The Ph. Eur. specifies 51 to 59% of $Al_2(SO_4)_3$; the USP specifies 54 to 59% of $Al_2(SO_4)_3$.

Ph. Eur. **solubilities** are: soluble in water; freely soluble in hot water; practically insoluble in alcohol. USP solubilities are: soluble 1 in 1 of water; insoluble in alcohol. A 2% solution in water has a pH of 2.5 to 4.0. **Store** in airtight containers.

Aluminium sulphate has an action similar to that of alum (p.1547) but is more astringent. A 20% solution is employed for the treatment of envenomation by certain insects and marine organisms. The aluminium may cause precipitation of the proteins contained within the venoms thus reducing local toxicity. Aluminium sulphate is also included in astringent preparations intended for irritating skin conditions.

Aluminium sulphate is also used in the preparation of aluminium acetate solutions.

Possible adverse effects or toxicity associated with aluminium, or aluminium salts such as aluminium sulphate, in the public water supply are discussed under Aluminium, p.1547.

Preparations

USP 23: Aluminum Subacetate Topical Solution; Aluminum Sulfate and Calcium Acetate Tablets for Topical Solution.

Proprietary Preparations (details are given in Part 3)
Austral.: Stingose; ***S.Afr.:*** Stingose; ***UK:*** Stingose.

Multi-ingredient: ***Aust.:*** Citoburol; ***Canad.:*** Boropak†; ***Ger.:*** Schupps Kohlensaurebad; Silvapin Kohlensaurebad F mit Fichtennadelol†; Silvapin Kohlensaurebad†; Tannolil; ***Ital.:*** Cepral; ***Spain:*** Sales Gras†; ***Switz.:*** Gynasol; ***USA:*** Bluboro; Boropak; Domeboro; Ostiderm; Pedi-Boro Soak Paks.

Alverine Citrate (5226-m)

Alverine Citrate *(BANM, USAN, rINNM).*
Dipropyline Citrate; Phenpropamine Citrate. *N*-Ethyl-3,3′-diphenyldipropylamine citrate.
$C_{20}H_{27}N,C_6H_8O_7$ = 473.6.
CAS — 150-59-4 (alverine); 5560-59-8 (alverine citrate).

Alverine citrate 67.3 mg is approximately equivalent to 40 mg of alverine.

Adverse Effects and Precautions

Nausea, headache, pruritus, rash, and dizziness have been reported. Allergic reactions, including anaphylaxis, have also occurred. Alverine is contra-indicated in patients with intestinal obstruction or paralytic ileus.

Pharmacokinetics

Alverine is absorbed from the gastro-intestinal tract following oral administration and is rapidly metabolised to an active metabolite, peak plasma concentrations of which occur 1 to 1.5 hours after an oral dose. Further metabolism to inactive metabolites occurs; metabolites are excreted in the urine by active renal secretion.

Uses and Administration

Alverine is an antispasmodic that acts on intestinal and uterine smooth muscle. It is used for the relief of smooth muscle spasm in the treatment of gastro-intestinal disorders such as irritable bowel syndrome (p.1172). It is also used in the treatment of dysmenorrhoea (p.9).

Alverine is given by mouth as the citrate in doses of 60 to 120 mg one to three times daily or by suppository as alverine in doses of 80 mg two or three times daily. It has also been given by intramuscular or slow intravenous injection.

Preparations

Proprietary Preparations (details are given in Part 3)
Fr.: Spasmaverine; ***Irl.:*** Spasmonal; ***UK:*** Relaxyl; Spasmonal.

Multi-ingredient: ***Austral.:*** Alvercol; ***Belg.:*** Normacol Antispasmodique; ***Fr.:*** Meteospasmyl; Normacol a la Dipropyline†; Schoum; Spasmaverine; ***Irl.:*** Alvercol; ***S.Afr.:*** Alvercol; ***UK:*** Alvercol.

Ambucetamide (5227-b)

Ambucetamide *(BAN, rINN).*
A-16; Dibutamide. 2-Dibutylamino-2-(4-methoxyphenyl)acetamide.
$C_{17}H_{28}N_2O_2$ = 292.4.
CAS — 519-88-0.

Ambucetamide is used as an antispasmodic and has been given for the relief of dysmenorrhoea. The hydrochloride is also used.

Preparations

Proprietary Preparations (details are given in Part 3)

Multi-ingredient: ***Belg.:*** Neomeritine; ***Ger.:*** Bersicaran N†; ***Neth.:*** Femerital.

Amikhelline Hydrochloride (12356-v)

Amikhelline Hydrochloride *(rINNM).*
9-(2-Diethylaminoethoxy)-4-hydroxy-7-methyl-5*H*-furo[3,2-g][1]benzopyran-5-one hydrochloride.
$C_{18}H_{21}NO_5,HCl$ = 367.8.
CAS — 4439-67-2 (amikhelline); 40709-23-7 (amikhelline hydrochloride).

Amikhelline hydrochloride has been used as an antispasmodic.

Preparations

Proprietary Preparations (details are given in Part 3)
Spain: Nokhel†.

Aminohippuric Acid (2122-k)

p-Aminobenzoylglycine; *p*-Aminohippuric Acid; PAHA; Para-aminohippuric Acid. *N*-4-Aminobenzoylaminoacetic acid.
$C_9H_{10}N_2O_3$ = 194.2.
CAS — 61-78-9 (aminohippuric acid); 94-16-6 (sodium aminohippurate).
Pharmacopoeias. In *US.*

A white crystalline powder which discolours on exposure to light. **Soluble** 1 in 45 of water, 1 in 50 of alcohol, and 1 in 5 of 3N hydrochloric acid; very slightly soluble in carbon tetrachloride, chloroform, and ether; freely soluble, with decomposition, in alkaline solutions. **Store** in airtight containers. Protect from light.

Adverse Effects

Sodium aminohippurate may cause nausea and vomiting, vasomotor disturbances, flushing, tingling, cramps, and a feeling of warmth. Patients may develop an urge to urinate or defaecate after infusion.

Interactions

The estimation of sodium aminohippurate may be affected in patients taking procaine, sulphonamides, or thiazosulphone. Probenecid diminishes the excretion of aminohippuric acid. Clearance is also affected by penicillins, salicylates, sulphinpyrazone, and other drugs that compete for the same excretory pathways.

Uses and Administration

Aminohippuric acid is excreted mainly by proximal tubular secretion, with some glomerular filtration. It is given by intravenous infusion, as the sodium salt, sodium aminohippurate (aminohippurate sodium; $C_9H_9N_2NaO_3$ = 216.2) for the estimation of effective renal plasma flow. Doses are aimed at producing a plasma concentration of 20 µg per mL; at these concentrations approximately 90% of aminohippurate is cleared from the renal blood stream in a single circuit in patients with normal renal function. Sodium aminohippurate has also been used for the assessment of the renal tubular secretory mechanism. Doses for this purpose are infused slowly to achieve a plasma concentration of 400 to 600 µg per mL to saturate the tubular secretion. These tests are used mainly in research procedures.

Preparations

USP 23: Aminohippurate Sodium Injection.

Amiprilose Hydrochloride (1207-j)

Amiprilose Hydrochloride *(USAN, pINNM).*
SM-1213 (amiprilose). 3-*O*-[3-(Dimethylamino)propyl]-1,2-*O*-isopropylidene-α-D-glucofuranose hydrochloride.
$C_{14}H_{27}NO_6,HCl$ = 341.8.
CAS — 56824-20-5 (amiprilose); 60414-06-4 (amiprilose hydrochloride).

Amiprilose hydrochloride is an immunomodulator that has been investigated in the treatment of rheumatoid arthritis.

Strong Ammonia Solution (201-d)

Ammoniaca; Ammoniacum; Ammoniae Solutio Concentrata; Ammoniaque Officinale; Liquor Ammoniae Fortis; Solutio Ammoniaci Concentrata; Stronger Ammonia Water; Stronger Ammonium Hydroxide Solution.
CAS — 7664-41-7 (NH_3).

NOTE. The food additive number 527 is used for ammonium hydroxide.

Pharmacopoeias. In *Chin.* (25 to 28%) and *Eur.* (see p.viii) (25 to 30%). Also in *USNF* which has 27 to 31%.

A clear colourless liquid with a strongly pungent characteristic odour. Very caustic. **Miscible** with water and with alcohol. '0.880 ammonia' contains about 35% w/w. **Store** at a temperature not exceeding 20° in airtight containers.

CAUTION. *Strong Ammonia Solution should be handled with great care because of the caustic nature of the solution and the irritating properties of the vapour. Cool the container well before opening and avoid inhalation of the vapour.*

Dilute Ammonia Solution (202-n)

Ammonia Water; Ammoniaque Officinale Diluée; Ammonium Hydricum Solutum; Diluted Ammonium Hydroxide Solution; Liquor Ammoniae; Liquor Ammoniae Dilutus.

Pharmacopoeias. In *Br.*, *Ger.*, *Jpn*, *Pol.*, and *Swiss* (all about 10%); in *Aust.* (10.2 to 11%).

Prepared by diluting Strong Ammonia Solution with freshly boiled and cooled Purified Water. It contains 9.5 to 10.5% w/w of NH_3.

NOTE. The BP directs that when Ammonia Solution is prescribed or demanded, Dilute Ammonia Solution shall be dispensed or supplied.

Adverse Effects

Ingestion of strong solutions of ammonia causes severe pain in the mouth, throat, and gastro-intestinal tract, severe local oedema and salivation, with cough, vomiting, and shock. Burns to the oesophagus and stomach may result in perforation. Stricture formation usually in the oesophagus can occur weeks or months later. Ingestion may also cause oedema of the respiratory tract and pneumonitis, though this may not develop for a few hours.

Inhalation of ammonia vapour causes sneezing and coughing and in high concentration causes pulmonary oedema. Asphyxia has been reported following oedema or spasm of the glottis. Ammonia vapour is irritant to the eyes and causes weeping; there may be conjunctival swelling and temporary blindness. Strong solutions on the conjunctiva cause a severe reaction with conjunctival oedema, corneal damage, and acute glaucoma. Late complications include angle-closure glaucoma, opaque corneal scars, atrophy of the iris, and formation of cataracts. Ammonia burns have resulted from treating insect bites and stings with the strong solution, and even with the dilute solution, especially if a dressing is subsequently applied.

References.

1. Beare JDL, *et al.* Ammonia burns of the eye: an old weapon in new hands. *Br Med J* 1988; **296:** 590.
2. Payne MP, Delic JI. Ammonia. In: *Toxicity Review 24.* London: HMSO, 1991: 1–12.
3. Payne MP, *et al. Toxicology of substances in relation to major hazards: ammonia.* London: HMSO, 1991.

Treatment of Adverse Effects

Ingestion should not be treated by lavage or emesis. Give copious drinks of water and follow this with demulcents. Appropriate measures should be taken to alleviate pain, shock and pulmonary oedema, and maintain an airway.

Contaminated skin and eyes should be flooded immediately with water and the washing continued for at least 15 minutes. Any affected clothing should be removed while flooding is being carried out.

Uses and Administration

Dilute solutions of ammonia have been used as reflex stimulants either as smelling salts or solutions for oral administration. They have also been used as rubefacients and counter-irritants (see p.7) and to neutralise insect stings. Users should always be aware of the irritant properties of ammonia.

Hartshorn and Oil was sometimes used as a name for an ammonia liniment. Household ammonia and cloudy ammonia have been used as names for cleaning preparations of ammonia with oleic acid or soap respectively.

Stings. Bathers who were stung after intercepting an armada of Portuguese men-of-war (*Physalia physalis*) were rapidly and effectively relieved of discomfort, paresis, irritation, and other symptoms by the application of aromatic ammonia spirit compresses.[1]

1. Frohman IG. Treatment of physalia stings. *JAMA* 1966; **197:** 733.

Preparations

BP 1998: Aromatic Ammonia Solution; Aromatic Ammonia Spirit *(Sal Volatile Spirit)*; Strong Ammonium Acetate Solution; White Liniment *(White Embrocation)*.

Proprietary Preparations (details are given in Part 3)
Spain: After Bite; Calmapica; Traspica†; ***UK:*** After Bite.

Multi-ingredient: ***Aust.:*** Apotheker Bauer's Franzbranntwein-Gel; Rowalind; ***Austral.:*** Respatona; Senega and Ammonia; ***Canad.:*** Bronchex; Bronchisaft; SJ Liniment; ***Ger.:*** Laryngsan N; Optipect mit Kodein†; Optipect†; Rowalind; Soledum Hustensaft N†; ***Irl.:*** Rowalind; ***S.Afr.:*** Enterodyne; Famstim; Peter Pote's†; ***Spain:*** Analgesico Ut Asens Fn; Licor Amoniacal; Linimento Sloan; Masagil; ***Swed.:*** Sloan's liniment†; ***UK:*** Blisteze; BN; Goddards White Oil Embrocation; Mackenzies; ***USA:*** Emergent-Ez.

Ammonium Iodide (4572-y)

Ammonii Iodetum; Ammonii Iodidum; Ammonium Iodatum.
NH_4I = 144.9.
CAS — 12027-06-4.

Ammonium iodide has the actions of iodine and iodides (p.1493). Former uses included its topical application for disinfection or easing inflammation.

Ammonium Phosphate (12369-w)

545 (ammonium polyphosphates); Diammonium Hydrogen Phosphate; Dibasic Ammonium Phosphate. Diammonium hydrogen orthophosphate.
$(NH_4)_2HPO_4$ = 132.1.
CAS — 7783-28-0.
Pharmacopoeias. In *USNF.*

Colourless or white granules or powder. Freely **soluble** in water; practically insoluble in acetone and alcohol. A 1% solution in water has a pH of 7.6 to 8.2. **Store** in airtight containers.

Ammonium phosphate was formerly used as a diuretic. It may be used as a buffering agent in pharmaceutical preparations.

Ammonium biphosphate (monobasic ammonium phosphate; $(NH_4)H_2PO_4$ = 115.0) has been used to acidify urine and as a phosphate supplement.

Preparations

Proprietary Preparations (details are given in Part 3)
Multi-ingredient: ***Fr.:*** Phosphore-Sandoz; ***USA:*** pHos-pHaid†.

Amnion (16505-e)

Human extra-embryonic fetal membranes comprising an inner amniotic membrane and an outer membrane, the chorion. Amnion has been used as a dressing for raw wounds including chronic ulcers and burns.

Preparations

Proprietary Preparations (details are given in Part 3)
Ital.: Amniex.

Amylase (3702-f)

Diastase; Glucogenase; Ptyalin.
CAS — 9000-92-4 (amylase); 9000-85-5 (bacterial α-amylase); 9000-90-2 (porcine α-amylase, pancreatic).
Pharmacopoeias. In *Fr.* and *Jpn.*

An enzyme catalysing the hydrolysis of α-1,4-glucosidic linkages of polysaccharides such as starch, glycogen, or their degradation products. Amylases may be classified according to the manner in which the glucosidic bond is attacked. Endoamylases attack the α-1,4-glucosidic linkage at random. Alpha-amylases are the only types of endoamylases known and yield dextrins, oligosaccharides, and monosaccharides. The more common alpha-amylases include those isolated from human saliva, mammalian pancreas, *Bacillus subtilis*, *Aspergillus oryzae*, and barley malt. Exoamylases attack the α-1,4-glucosidic linkage only from the non-reducing outer polysaccharide chain ends. They include beta-amylases and glucoamylases (amyloglucosidases or gamma-amylases) and are of vegetable or microbial origin. Beta-amylases yield beta-limit dextrins and maltose and glucoamylases yield glucose.

Adverse Effects

Hypersensitivity reactions have been reported.

A report of allergic responses in workers exposed to fungal α-amylase derived from *Aspergillus oryzae*.[1] These responses were not obtained with α-amylase derived from *Bacillus subtilis*. These findings have implications for workers in the flour milling and bakery industries.

1. Flindt MLH. Allergy to α-amylase and papain. *Lancet* 1979; **i:** 1407–8.

Uses and Administration

Amylase is used in the production of predigested starchy foods and for the conversion of starch to fermentable sugars in the baking, brewing, and fermentation industries.

Amylase from various sources has been used as an ingredient of preparations of digestive enzymes, and has been given by mouth for its supposed activity in reducing respiratory tract inflammation and local swelling and oedema.

Preparations

Proprietary Preparations (details are given in Part 3)
Fr.: Amylodiastase; Maxilase; ***Spain:*** Maxilase.

Multi-ingredient: ***Aust.:*** Festal; Ozym; Wobenzym; ***Austral.:*** Bioglan Vegetable Enzymes†; Enzyme; ***Belg.:*** Digestomen; ***Canad.:*** Festal†; Ku-Zyme†; ***Fr.:*** Febrectol; Hepatoum; Maxilase-Bacitracine; Tridigestine Hepatoum†; ***Ger.:*** dichronase†; Enzym-Wied; Tri Viaben†; ***Ital.:*** Digestopan; Digestozim†; Enzygaster†; Essen Enzimatico; Essen†; Kilozim†; Luizym; Pepto Pancreasi Composta†; Quanto†; Trimalcina†; ***Spain:*** Demusin; Digestibys†; Digestomen Complex; Espasmo Digestomen; Gastrosindrom†; Maxilase Antibiotica†; Paidozim; Polidasa; Takadispep Complex; Trizima†; ***Switz.:*** Zymoplex; ***UK:*** Enzyme Digest; ***USA:*** Arco-Lase; Arco-Lase Plus; Bilezyme†; Enzyme; Festalan†; Gustase; Gustase Plus; Ku-Zyme; Kutrase; Medazyme†; Papaya Enzyme; Prevenzyme†.

Anagrelide Hydrochloride (12375-p)

Anagrelide Hydrochloride *(BANM, USAN, rINNM).*
BL-4162A; BL-4162a. 6,7-Dichloro-1,5-dihydroimidazo[2,1-*b*]quinazolin-2(3*H*)-one hydrochloride.
$C_{10}H_7Cl_2N_3O,HCl$ = 292.5.
CAS — 68475-42-3 (anagrelide); 58579-51-4 (anagrelide hydrochloride).

Adverse Effects

Anagrelide may cause headache, diarrhoea, abdominal pain, nausea, oedema, and palpitations. Cardiovascular effects include vasodilatation and positive inotropic effects; myocardial infarction and heart failure have also been reported. Anagrelide has been shown to be embryotoxic and fetotoxic in *animal* studies.

Precautions

Anagrelide should not be used during pregnancy. It should be used with caution in patients with cardiovascular disease. Platelet counts should be monitored closely, especially during the initial stages of treatment (see below). Liver and kidney function should also be monitored while the platelet count is being lowered.

Pharmacokinetics

Anagrelide is rapidly absorbed from the gastro-intestinal tract. It is extensively metabolised before elimination in the urine; less than 1% of a dose is excreted unchanged. The terminal elimination half-life has been reported to be about 3 days.

Uses and Administration

Anagrelide reduces platelet production and at higher doses inhibits platelet aggregation. It was formerly investigated for its platelet anti-aggregation effects, but is now used to reduce platelet production in patients with essential thrombocythaemia (p.496).

Anagrelide is given by mouth as the hydrochloride but doses are expressed in terms of the base. The initial dose is 2 mg daily divided into 2 or 4 doses. After at least a week, the dose is adjusted, by increasing the daily dose by not more than 0.5 mg in any one week, until the platelet count is maintained within the normal range. The usual maintenance dose is 1.5 to 3.0 mg daily. The dose should not exceed 10 mg per day or 2.5 mg as a single dose.

Platelet counts should be measured every 2 days during the first week of treatment and then at least weekly until the maintenance dose is reached.

References.

1. Silverstein MN, *et al.* Anagrelide: a new drug for treating thrombocytosis. *N Engl J Med* 1988; **318:** 1292–4.
2. Anagrelide Study Group. Anagrelide, a therapy for thrombocythemic states: experience in 577 patients. *Am J Med* 1992; **92:** 69–76.
3. Spencer CM, Brogden RN. Anagrelide: a review of its pharmacodynamic and pharmacokinetic properties, and therapeutic potential in the treatment of thrombocythaemia. *Drugs* 1994; **47:** 809–22.
4. Chintagumpala MM, *et al.* Treatment of essential thrombocythemia with anagrelide. *J Pediatr* 1995; **127:** 495–8. [Study in children].
5. Anonymous. Anagrelide for essential thrombocythemia. *Med Lett Drugs Ther* 1997; **39:** 120.

Preparations

Proprietary Preparations (details are given in Part 3)
USA: Agrylin.

Anethole (4606-q)

Anethol; Anetol; *p*-Propenylanisole. (*E*)-1-Methoxy-4-(prop-1-enyl)benzene.
$C_{10}H_{12}O$ = 148.2.
CAS — 104-46-1; 4180-23-8 (E isomer).

NOTE. Distinguish from Anethole Trithione (below).
Pharmacopoeias. In *Ger.* Also in *USNF.*

At or above 23° anethole is a colourless or faintly yellow liquid with a sweet taste and the characteristic aromatic odour of aniseed. It is obtained from anise oil or other sources or prepared synthetically. Very slightly **soluble** in water; soluble 1 in 2 by volume of alcohol; readily miscible with chloroform and with ether. **Store** in airtight containers. Protect from light.

Anethole has similar properties to anise oil (below).

Preparations

Proprietary Preparations (details are given in Part 3)
Multi-ingredient: ***Aust.:*** Rowatinex; ***Belg.:*** Calmant Martou; ***Canad.:*** Beech Nut Cough Drops; Bentasil; Bronco Asmol; ***Ger.:*** Medichol†; Pinimenthol-Oral N; Rowatinex; Tussipect; ***Irl.:*** Rowatinex; ***Ital.:*** Rowatin†; ***Spain:*** Mabogastrol; Pulmofasa; Pulmofasa Antihist; Rowanefrin; Vicks Formula 44; ***Switz.:*** Dental-Phenjoca; Neo-Angin exempt de sucre; Pectocalmine Junior; Spirogel; ***UK:*** Rowatinex.

Anethole Trithione (3703-d)

SKF-1717; Trithioparamethoxyphenylpropene. 5-(4-Methoxyphenyl)-3*H*-1,2-dithiole-3-thione.
$C_{10}H_8OS_3$ = 240.4.
CAS — 532-11-6 (anethole trithione).

NOTE. Distinguish from Anethole (above).

Anethole trithione has been given orally in the management of dry mouth (p.1470) and as a choleretic. The usual daily dose is 37.5 to 75 mg, generally in divided doses before meals. Anethole trithione may cause discoloration of the urine.

Preparations

Proprietary Preparations (details are given in Part 3)
Belg.: Sulfarlem; Sulfarlem S 25; ***Canad.:*** Sialor; Sulfarlem; ***Fr.:*** Sulfarlem; ***Ger.:*** Mucinol; ***Ital.:*** Sulfarlem†; ***S.Afr.:*** Sulfarlem; ***Spain:*** Sonicur; ***Switz.:*** Sulfarlem.

Multi-ingredient: ***Belg.:*** Sulfarlem Choline.

Aniracetam (16511-s)

Aniracetam *(USAN, rINN).*
Ro-13-5057. 1-(4-Methoxybenzoyl)-2-pyrrolidinone.
$C_{12}H_{13}NO_3$ = 219.2.
CAS — 72432-10-1.

Aniracetam is a nootropic drug which has been tried in senile dementia (p.1386). It is given by mouth in usual doses of 1500 mg daily.

References.

1. Sourander LB, *et al.* Senile dementia of the Alzheimer type treated with aniracetam: a new nootropic agent. *Psychopharmacology (Berl)* 1987; **91:** 90–5.
2. Parnetti L, *et al.* Aniracetam (Ro 13-5057) for the treatment of senile dementia of Alzheimer type: results of a multicentre clinical study. *Dementia* 1991; **2:** 262–7.

Preparations

Proprietary Preparations (details are given in Part 3)
Ital.: Ampamet; Draganon; Reset.

Aniseed (4607-p)

Anice; Anis Verde; Anis Vert; Anise; Anise Fruit; Anisi Fructus; Fructus Anisi Vulgaris.

NOTE. The names Anís Estrellado, Anis Étoilé, Anisum Badium, Anisum Stellatum, Badiana, Badiane de Chine, Star Anise Fruit, and Sternanis are synonyms for Star Anise.
Pharmacopoeias. In *Eur.* (see p.viii) and *Pol.*
Eur. also includes a monograph for Star Anise (Anisi Stellati Fructus).

Aniseed is the dried ripe fruit of *Pimpinella anisum* (Umbelliferae), containing not less than 2% v/w of volatile oil. Star anise is the dried composite fruit of *Illicium verum* (Magnoliaceae). **Protect** from light.

Aniseed is carminative and mildly expectorant; it is used mainly as anise oil or as preparations of the oil. It may cause contact dermatitis, probably due to its anethole content.

Aniseed and star anise are the source of anise oil (below).

A brief review of aniseed and anise oil.[1]

1. Chandler RF, Hawkes D. Aniseed—a spice, a flavor, a drug. *Can Pharm J* 1984; **117:** 28–9.

Preparations

Proprietary Preparations (details are given in Part 3)

Multi-ingredient: ***Aust.:*** Aktiv Husten- und Bronchialtee; Aktiv milder Magen- und Darmtee; Anifer Hustentee; Asthmatee; Brady's-Magentropfen; Euka; Krauterdoktor Krampf- und Reizhustensirup; Krauterhaus Mag Kottas Tee gegen Durchfall; Krautertee Nr 10; Krautertee Nr 107; Krautertee Nr 11; Krautertee Nr 126; Krautertee Nr 211; Krautertee Nr 7; Mag Kottas Husten-Bronchialtee; Nesthakchen; Sidroga Brust-Husten-Tee; Spasmo-Granobil-Krampf- und Reizhusten; Species Carvi comp; Teekanne Husten- und Brusttee; ***Austral.:*** Neo-Cleanse; ***Belg.:*** Eugiron; Tisane Antibiliaire et Stomachique; Tisane pour le Foie; Tisane Purgative; ***Canad.:*** Pectothymin; ***Fr.:*** Elixir Bonjean; Elixir Contre La Toux Weleda; Herbesan; Mediflor Tisane Digestive No 3; Mucinum; Mucinum a l'Extrait de Cascara; Peter's Sirop; Santane D_5; Soker; Tisane Clairo; Tisane des Familles†; Tisane Digestive Weleda; ***Ger.:*** Abfuhr-Tee Depuraflux†; Abfuhr-Tee Stada†; Broncholind†; Cholaflux N†; Dr. Klinger's Bergischer Krautertee, Nerven- und Beruhigungstee†; Dr. Maurers Magen-Apotheke†; Echtroferment-N; Friosmin†; Grunlicht Hingfong Essenz; Knufinke Broncholind K†; Majocarmin-Tee; Orbis Husten-und Bronchial-tee†; Pascopankreat†; Phytpulmon†; Ramend Krauter; Rheumex†; rohasal; Stern Biene Fencheltee†; Stovalid N; Thymitussin†; Ventrodigest†; Vier-Winde-Tee†; ***Ital.:*** Dicalmir; Florerbe Lassativa; Lassatina; Tisana Kelemata; Tonactiv; ***Neth.:*** Hoestsiroop†; ***S.Afr.:*** Misfans†; ***Spain:*** Broncomicin Bals; Bronquinflamatoria; Crislaxo; Digestol Sanatorium; Digestovital; Laxante Sanatorium; ***Switz.:*** Bronchocodin; Kernosan Elixir; Kernosan Heidelberger Poudre; Radix†; The Franklin; Tisane d'allaitement "H"†; Tisane diuretique "H"†; Tisane gastrique "H"†; Tisane laxative H; Tisane laxative Natterman no 13; ***UK:*** Carminative Tea; Clairo Tea; Cough Elixir; Laxadoron; Revitonil.

Anise Oil (4609-w)

Aniseed Oil; Anisi Aetheroleum; Esencia de Anís; Essence d'Anis; Oleum Anisi.

Pharmacopoeias. In *Chin.*, *Eur.* (see p.viii), and *Pol.*

A clear, colourless or pale yellow volatile oil obtained by distillation from aniseed or star anise; anethole is the major constituent. It has a characteristic odour and a sweet aromatic taste. Solidifies on cooling; f.p. 15° to 19°. Practically **insoluble** in water; miscible with alcohol, with dichloromethane, with ether, and with petroleum spirit. If the oil has crystallised it should be melted completely and mixed before use. **Store** at a temperature not exceeding 25° in airtight containers. Protect from light.

Incompatibility. PVC bottles softened and distorted fairly rapidly in the presence of anise oil, which should not be stored or dispensed in such bottles.[1]

1. Department of Pharmaceutical Sciences of the Pharmaceutical Society of Great Britain. Plastics medicine bottles of rigid PVC. *Pharm J* 1973; **210:** 100.

Anise oil is carminative and mildly expectorant and is a common ingredient of cough preparations. It is also a flavouring agent.

It may cause contact dermatitis, probably due to its anethole content.

For a brief review of aniseed and anise oil, see Aniseed, above.

Preparations

BP 1998: Camphorated Opium Tincture *(Paregoric)*; Compound Orange Spirit; Concentrated Anise Water; Concentrated Camphorated Opium Tincture.

Proprietary Preparations (details are given in Part 3)

Multi-ingredient: ***Aust.:*** Bradosol; Bronchostop; Embrocation; Expectal-Tropfen; Expigen; Heumann's Bronchialtee; Medizinalbad†; Neo-Angin; Nesthakchen; Red Point†; SynPharma Bronchial; ***Austral.:*** Cough Relief; Digestive Aid; Gartech; Respatona; Respatona Plus with Echinacea; ***Canad.:*** Babys Own Gripe Water; Beech Nut Cough Drops; Herbal Cough Expectorant; ***Fr.:*** Biphedrine Huileuse†; Paregorique; ***Ger.:*** Abfuhr-Tee Depuraflux†; Abfuhr-Tee Stada†; Anastil†; Aspasmon N; Benium; Bisolvomed mit Codein†; Bisolvomed†; Bronchicum Hustentee; Broncho Sanol†; Bronchocedin N; Bronchoforton; Dorex Hustensaft N mit Oxeladin†; Ephepect; Floradix Multipretten; Frubibalsam†; Grunlicht Hingfong Essenz; Guakalin†; Heumann Bronchialtee Solubifix; Hevertopect; Infantussin N; Kamillosan Mundspray; Kneipp Brustkaramellen†; Neo-Ballistol; Optipect†; Orbis Husten- und Bronchial-tee†; Pulmocordio mite SL; Pulmotin-N; Repha-Os; Salviathymol N; Sinuforton; Solamin†; Stern Biene Fencheltee†; ***Neth.:*** Bronchicum; ***Spain:*** Carminativo Ibys; Carminativo Juventus; H Tussan; Magnesia Validada†; Odontocromil c Sulfamida; ***Switz.:*** Bronchol N; Bronchosan; Capsules laxatives Nattermann Nr. 13; Carmol "blanche"†; Carmol "thermogene"†; Carmol†; Delica-Sol†; Demo pates pectorales; Endomethasone; GEM†; Graminflor†; Kamillosan; Makatussin; Makatussin forte; ***UK:*** Fisherman's Friend Honey Cough Syrup†; Hill's Balsam Adult Expectorant; Hill's Balsam Adult Suppressant; Honey & Molasses; Lightning Cough Remedy; Venos Dry Cough; Venos Expectorant.

Apis mellifera (12386-e)

The honey bee.

A preparation containing the venom of *Apis mellifera* is used in homoeopathic medicine where it is known as Apis mellifica or Apis mel. Apis mellifera is a source of purified honey (p.1345) and royal jelly (p.1626).

For reference to the use of whole body extracts or venom from *Hymenoptera* spp. in hyposensitisation procedures in allergic subjects see under Allergen Products, p.1545.

There have been a number of anecdotal reports of successful treatment of chronic inflammatory disease such as arthritis with bee venom.[1] Studies *in vitro* have shown that bee venom has anti-inflammatory activity similar to that of cyclophosphamide. Melittin appears to be the active constituent, and seems to act by interfering with superoxide radical production from human leucocytes.

1. Somerfield SD. Bee venom and arthritis: magic, myth or medicine? *N Z Med J* 1986; **99:** 281–3.

Preparations

Proprietary Preparations (details are given in Part 3)

Multi-ingredient: ***Aust.:*** Forapin; ***UK:*** Bolus Eucalypti Comp.

Aptiganel (14951-k)

Aptiganel (*pINN*).

CNS-1102 (aptiganel hydrochloride). 1-(*m*-Ethylphenyl)-1-methyl-3-(1-naphthyl)guanidine.

$C_{20}H_{21}N_3$ = 303.4.

CAS — 137159-92-3 (aptiganel); 137160-11-3 (aptiganel hydrochloride).

NOTE. Aptiganel Hydrochloride is *USAN*.

Aptiganel is a guanidine derivative which antagonises the effects of the excitatory amino-acid neurotransmitter glutamate at the *N*-methyl D-aspartate (NMDA) receptor. It is under investigation for the prevention of ischaemic brain damage in patients with traumatic head injury or stoke.

References.

1. Muir KW, *et al.* Pharmacological effects of the non-competitive NMDA antagonist CNS 1102 in normal volunteers. *Br J Clin Pharmacol* 1994; **38:** 33–8.
2. Block GA, *et al.* Final results from a dose-escalating safety and tolerance study of the non-competitive NMDA antagonist CNS1102 in patients with acute cerebral ischaemia. *Stroke* 1995; **26:** 185.

Arachis Oil (7353-m)

Arachidis Oleum; Earth-nut Oil; Erdnussöl; Ground-nut Oil; Huile d'Arachide; Nut Oil; Ol. Arach.; Óleo de Amendoim; Oleum Arachis; Peanut Oil.

Pharmacopoeias. In *Eur.* (see p.viii), *Int.*, and *Pol.* Also in *USNF* (Peanut Oil) which specifies oil from the seed kernels of one or more of the cultivated varieties of *A. hypogaea*.

Eur. also includes Hydrogenated Arachis Oil.

Arachis oil is the refined fixed oil obtained from the shelled seeds of *Arachis hypogaea* (Leguminosae). It is a clear, colourless or pale yellow viscous oil; odourless or with a faint nutty odour and a bland nutty taste consisting of glycerides, chiefly of oleic and linoleic acids, with smaller amounts of other acids. Very slightly **soluble** in alcohol; miscible with carbon disulphide, chloroform, ether, and petroleum spirit. **Store** at a temperature not exceeding 40° in well-filled airtight containers. Protect from light.

Hydrogenated arachis oil is arachis oil (as above) that has been bleached, hydrogenated, and deodorised. It is a white or faintly yellowish soft mass that melts to a clear pale yellow liquid when heated. Practically **insoluble** in water; very slightly soluble in alcohol; freely soluble in dichloromethane and in petroleum spirit. **Protect** from light.

Uses

Emulsions containing arachis oil are used in nutrition. Arachis oil is given as an enema for softening impacted faeces. It is used in drops for softening ear wax and in emollient creams. Arachis oil is given by mouth, usually with sorbitol, as a gallbladder evacuant prior to cholecystography.

Precautions. It has been suggested that the use during infancy of preparations containing arachis oil, including infant formulae and topical preparations, may be responsible for sensitisation to peanut, with a subsequent risk of hypersensitivity reactions.[1,2] However, the arachis oil used in such preparations is refined oil and it has been pointed out that such oil should not contain the proteins that produce allergic reactions in susceptible people.[3]

1. de Montis G, *et al.* Sensitisation to peanut and vitamin D oily preparations. *Lancet* 1993; **341:** 1411.
2. Lever LR. Peanut and nut allergy: creams and ointments containing peanut oil may lead to sensitisation. *Br Med J* 1996; **313:** 299.
3. Hourihane J O'B, *et al.* Randomised, double blind, crossover challenge study of allergenicity of peanut oil in subjects allergic to peanuts. *Br Med J* 1997; **314:** 1084–8.

Preparations

BP 1998: Arachis Oil Enema.

Proprietary Preparations (details are given in Part 3)

Austral.: Calogen; ***Fr.:*** Matiga; ***Ger.:*** Olbad Cordes F; ***Irl.:*** Calogen; Oilatum Cream; ***S.Afr.:*** Oilatum Soap†; ***UK:*** Calogen; Fletchers Arachis Oil Retention Enema; Oilatum Cream.

Multi-ingredient: ***Aust.:*** Balneum Hermal F; ***Austral.:*** Cerumol; Emtobil†; Medevac; ***Fr.:*** Balneum surgras; ***Ger.:*** Balneum F; Dr. Hotz Vollbad; Hoecutin Olbad F; Paradiol†; Parfenac Basisbad; ***Irl.:*** Hydromol; ***S.Afr.:*** Cerumol; ***Switz.:*** Balneum F; ***UK:*** Cerumol; Earex; Eczederm†; Hewletts; Hydromol Cream; Red Oil.

Arnica (303-g)

Wolfsbane.

NOTE. Wolfsbane is also used as a common name for aconite.

Pharmacopoeias. In *Aust.*, *Fr.*, *Ger.*, *Pol.*, and *Swiss.*

Aust. also includes arnica root.

Arnica is generally employed in the form of the flowerheads of *Arnica montana* (Compositae).

Arnica flower is irritant to mucous membranes and when ingested has produced severe symptoms including gastro-intestinal and nervous system disturbances, both tachycardia and bradycardia, and collapse. Tincture of arnica may cause dermatitis when applied to the skin of sensitive persons.

Preparations of arnica flower and arnica root are used as astringents for topical application to unbroken skin in conditions such as sprains and bruises; such preparations are not considered suitable for internal use.

Herbal and homoeopathic preparations containing arnica are available for oral use.

Preparations

Proprietary Preparations (details are given in Part 3)

Fr.: Arnican; Pharmadose teinture d'arnica; ***Ger.:*** Arniflor-N; Arthrosenex AR; Hoevenol A; Hyzum N; Vasotonin; ***Ital.:*** Venustas Lozione Caduta; ***Neth.:*** Arniflor†.

Multi-ingredient: ***Aust.:*** Arnicet; Asthmatee; Berggeist; Cional; Dynexan; Embrocation; Red Point†; Rheuma; Varicylum; ***Fr.:*** Arnicadol; Creme Rap; Elastocapsil†; Lelong Contusions; Stom-Antiba†; ***Ger.:*** ABC Warme-Pflaster N; Arnica Kneipp Salbe; Arnika plus; Arnika-Balsam†; Arnikamill; Asthmacolat†; Befelka-Tinktur; Blend-a-med Fluid†; Bryonia-Strath†; Castrophan†; Cefacutan†; Cefagastrin; Ceprovit; Combudoron; derma-loges N; Dolocyl; Dr. Kleinschrod's Cor-Insuffin†; Dr. Klinger's Bergischer Krautertee, Magentee†; Dynexan†; Echtrosept-GT†; Essaven 50 000†; Essaven Sportgel; Grunlicht Hingfong Essenz; Heparchofid S†; Heparin Comp; Hoevenol A; Hovnizym†; Jatamansin†; Kalantol-A†; Kalantol-B†; Lindofluid N; Myonasan†; Palatol†; Phonix Kalophon†; Rephastasan†; Rheumex†; Rhoival; Secerna†; Sportino Akut; Sportofit†; Stullmaton; Trauma-cyl; Turgostad†; Varicylum S; Vasesana-Vasoregulans; Vasotonin Serol†; Venen-Salbe; Ventrodigest†; Verus†; Vitosal; Warondo-Wundsalbe†; ***Ital.:*** Elisir Depurativo Ambrosiano; Herbavit; ***S.Afr.:*** Dynexan; ***Spain:*** Arnicon; Encialina; Killpan; Pentoderm†; Uralyt; ***Switz.:*** Alpina Gel a l'arnica avec spilanthes; Cetona; Cional†; Dynexan; Eubucal†; Euceta avec camomille et arnica; Mucosan†; ***UK:*** Frost Cream; Rheumadoron; WCS Dusting Powder.

Arsenic Trioxide (12396-y)

Acidum Arsenicosum Anhydricum; Arseni Trioxydum; Arsenic; Arsenicum Album; Arsenious Acid; Arsenous Oxide; White Arsenic.

As_2O_3 = 197.8.

CAS — 1327-53-3 (arsenic trioxide); 7784-45-4 (arsenic triiodide).

Pharmacopoeias. In *Jpn.*

Adverse Effects

The toxicity of inorganic arsenic increases with increasing solubility, and trivalent compounds are considered to be more toxic than pentavalent compounds. The symptoms of acute poisoning due to arsenic usually occur within one hour of ingestion but may be delayed for up to 12 hours, especially in the presence of food. In severe poisoning the principle toxic effect is haemorrhagic gastro-enteritis which can result in profound dehydration, collapse, shock, and death. Cardiac arrhythmias, convulsions, or muscle cramps may also occur. From 70 to 300 mg of arsenic trioxide may be fatal depending on the physical form and the rate of absorption. In the absence of adequate treatment death can occur within one hour but a period of 12 to 48 hours is more usual. Patients who survive the initial effects of arsenic trioxide may develop severe peripheral neuropathies and encephalopathy. Other effects following acute poisoning resemble those seen in chronic poisoning. Acute systemic effects may also be seen following inhalation or contact with the skin. Ingested arsenic salts cause oral irritation and a sensation of burning in the mouth and throat; pulmonary irritation may follow inhalation.

Chronic poisoning or occupational exposure typically produces varied skin afflictions, particularly hyperkeratosis, especially affecting the palms and soles, skin pigmentation, eczematous or follicular dermatitis, oedema especially affecting the eyelids, and alopecia. Muscle aching and weakness, and stomatitis may also occur. Gastro-intestinal disturbances are generally mild. The breath and perspiration may have an odour of garlic. Patients may also experience excessive salivation, lachrymation, and inflammation of the conjunctiva and nasal mucosa resembling coryza. Chronic inhalation of arsenic salts may result in perforation of the nasal septum. Characteristic deposits of arsenic may appear in the nails 6 weeks after absorption. Obstructive jaundice may occur as a result of hepatomegaly and portal hypertension may eventually develop. Cirrhosis has been reported rarely. Proteinuria, haematuria, and anuria may occur secondary to renal damage. In advanced poisoning neurological effects are prominent. Encephalopathy has been reported but peripheral neuropathies are more common. There is both sensory and motor involvement and patients may at first experience paraesthesia, and numbness and burning in the extremities, but eventually muscular atrophy and paralysis occur. The legs are usually more affected than the arms. Arsenic is toxic to the bone marrow and produces a wide range of blood disorders including leucopenia, thrombocytopenia, and various anaemias.

Chronic exposure to arsenic has been associated with neoplasms of the skin, lungs, and liver and possibly other organs.

Reviews.

1. Arsenic. *Environmental Health Criteria 18.* Geneva: WHO, 1981.
2. Health and Safety Executive. Inorganic arsenic compounds. *Toxicity Review 16.* London: HMSO, 1986.
3. Shannon RL, Strayer DS. Arsenic-induced skin toxicity. *Hum Toxicol* 1989; **8:** 99–104.

Arsenical compounds have reportedly been used to "cut" cocaine and symptoms of arsenic poisoning may occur in cocaine abusers.[1] Toxicity due to the presence of arsenic in various ethnic remedies has also been reported.[2]

1. Lombard J, *et al.* Arsenic intoxication in a cocaine abuser. *N Engl J Med* 1989; **320:** 869.
2. Kew J, *et al.* Arsenic and mercury intoxication due to Indian ethnic remedies. *Br Med J* 1993; **306:** 506–7.

Treatment of Adverse Effects

Acute poisoning due to the ingestion of arsenic compounds should be treated by immediate gastric lavage if the patient has not already vomited. Activated charcoal may be of use to reduce absorption. Chelation therapy with intramuscular dimercaprol (p.979) should be started immediately the cause of poisoning is suspected. Prompt treatment is necessary to prevent or reduce the severity of neuropathy. It has been suggested that administration of dimercaprol should continue until abdominal symptoms subside and the gut is clear of ingested arsenic. Unithiol (p.998) given intravenously may be used as an alternative. Oral treatment with succimer (p.997) or penicillamine (p.991) may then be substituted. A second course of treatment with penicillamine may be required if symptoms recur. Intravenous replacement of fluids and electrolytes should be undertaken as necessary to correct dehydration and electrolyte imbalance and to prevent shock; pressor agents and oxygen may be required. Morphine has been suggested for the control of severe abdominal pain but care should be taken that this does not lead to colonic retention of arsenic compounds.

If renal failure occurs haemodialysis may be required to remove any absorbed or chelated arsenic. Exchange blood transfusion may be required for severe liver damage.

Dimercaprol may also be used in the treatment of chronic poisoning, but penicillamine, succimer, or unithiol (all given orally) may be preferred.

Pharmacokinetics

Water-soluble arsenic acids and their salts are more rapidly absorbed from the gastro-intestinal tract than poorly soluble arsenicals such as arsenic trioxide. The absorption of arsenic trioxide is dependent upon the physical form of the compound and coarsely powdered material may be eliminated in the faeces before significant dissolution and absorption can occur. Soluble arsenic salts may also be absorbed following inhalation and through skin.

Once absorbed arsenic is stored mainly in the liver, kidney, heart, and lung, with smaller amounts in the muscles and nervous tissue. About two weeks after ingestion, arsenic is deposited in the hair and nails and remains fixed to the keratin for years. It is also deposited in the bones and teeth.

Although pentavalent arsenic is reduced to some degree *in vivo* to the more toxic trivalent form, trivalent arsenic is slowly and extensively oxidised to pentavalent arsenic. Both forms are methylated to relatively non-toxic derivatives and excreted in the urine mainly as dimethylarsinic acid with smaller amounts appearing as monomethylarsonic acid and inorganic arsenic compounds. Although 50% of a dose may be eliminated in the urine within 3 to 5 days small amounts may continue to be excreted for several weeks after a single dose. Less significant amounts of arsenic are excreted in the faeces and sweat and via the lungs and skin. It is also excreted in breast milk and readily crosses the placenta.

Uses and Administration

The therapeutic use of inorganic arsenical preparations is generally no longer recommended. Arsenic trioxide and arsenic triiodide were formerly used internally as solutions or externally as ointments in the treatment of various skin diseases.

Externally, arsenic trioxide has a caustic action.

Arsenic trioxide is used in homoeopathic medicine and in certain Asian herbal remedies. Arsenic anhydride has also been used.

Arsenic trioxide has been widely employed as a constituent of weedkillers and sheepdips and as a rodenticide.

Acute non-lymphoblastic leukaemia. Low doses of arsenic trioxide have been used successfully to induce remission in a few patients with acute promyelocytic leukaemia[1] who had relapsed despite conventional therapy (see p.479) with retinoids and antineoplastics.

1. Soignet SL, *et al.* Complete remission after treatment of acute promyelocytic leukemia with arsenic trioxide. *N Engl J Med* 1998; **339:** 1341–8.

Arsine (12397-j)

Arsenic Trihydride; Hydrogen Arsenide.

AsH_3 = 77.95.

CAS — 7784-42-1.

Arsine gas has no clinical uses but is an environmental or occupational hazard. It is highly toxic and causes severe haemolysis which may result in acute renal failure. Exposure to as little as 3 ppm may cause symptoms, after a latent period of 2 to 24 hours, including headache, abdominal pain, nausea, vomiting, anorexia, jaundice, haemolytic anaemia, haematuria, oliguria, and anuria. Pulmonary oedema, ECG abnormalities, and neurological disorders have also been reported. Treatment involves exchange transfusions and haemodialysis; dimercaprol has been used but does not prevent haemolysis.

References.

1. Fowler BA, Weissberg JB. Arsine poisoning. *N Engl J Med* 1974; **291:** 1171–4.
2. Hesdorffer CS, *et al.* Arsine gas poisoning: the importance of exchange transfusions in severe cases. *Br J Ind Med* 1986; **43:** 353–5.

Asafetida (272-z)

Asafoetida; Asant; Devil's Dung; Gum Asafetida.

Pharmacopoeias. In *Chin.*

An oleo-gum-resin obtained from various species of *Ferula* (Umbelliferae).

Asafetida has been used as a carminative and antispasmodic. It was also formerly used as an expectorant. It is used in cooking and is an ingredient of certain foods.

References.

1. Kelly KJ, *et al.* Methemoglobinemia in an infant treated with the folk remedy glycerited asafoetida. *Pediatrics* 1984; **73:** 717–19.

Asarabacca (12401-k)

Hazelwort; Rhizoma Asari; Wild Nard.

The dried rhizome, roots, and leaves of *Asarum europaeum* (Aristolochiaceae).

Asarabacca is an ingredient of snuffs. It is also an irritant emetic and has been used in rodent poisons. Asarabacca has been used in homoeopathic medicine and is an ingredient of preparations given for respiratory disorders.

Preparations

Proprietary Preparations (details are given in Part 3)
Ger.: Escarol.

Asbestos (12402-a)

The name asbestos is applied to several naturally occurring and widely distributed fibrous mineral silicates of the serpentine and amphibole groups. They include amosite (brown asbestos), anthophyllite, chrysotile (white asbestos), and crocidolite (blue asbestos).

Asbestos has properties of heat resistance, insulation, and reinforcement and has been used extensively for heat or electrical insulation, fire protection, in friction materials, and in the construction industry in a wide variety of materials including cement, pipes, and tiles.

When inhaled, asbestos fibres can cause asbestosis (pulmonary fibrosis), lung cancer, and mesothelioma of the pleura and peritoneum. Mesothelioma has been reported in persons exposed to relatively small amounts of asbestos after an average latent period of 30 to 40 years. Occupational exposure has sometimes been associated with an increased incidence of gastro-intestinal, laryngeal, and other cancers. Some types of asbestos are more hazardous than others; crocidolite (a member of the amphibole group) is considered to be the most dangerous.

References.

1. Wagner GR. Asbestosis and silicosis. *Lancet* 1997; **349:** 1311–15.

Avena (12408-n)

Aven; Cultivated White Oats; Oatmeal; Oats.

Pharmacopoeias. US includes Colloidal Oatmeal.

The grain of *Avena sativa* (Gramineae).

Avena has been used in homoeopathic medicine and is reputed to have sedative activity; an extract or tincture has been claimed to be of value in the treatment of drug dependence.

A colloidal fraction extracted from avena has been used in the preparation of emollient dermatological preparations.

Avenin, a protein present in oats, might be harmful to patients with coeliac disease.

Preparations

Proprietary Preparations (details are given in Part 3)
Austral.: Aveeno Preparations†; DermaVeen Bath; DermaVeen Dry Skin; ***Canad.:*** Aveeno Preparations; ***Fr.:*** Aveeno Preparations; Emulave; Sensifluid; ***Irl.:*** Aveeno; ***Ital.:*** Aveeno Preparations; Emulave; Micaveen; ***Switz.:*** Avenaforce; ***UK:*** Aveeno Preparations; ***USA:*** ActiBath.

Multi-ingredient: ***Austral.:*** Aveenobar (for acne)†; Avena Complex; Calmo; DermaVeen Acne; DermaVeen Moisturising; DermaVeen Shower and Bath; Dong Quai Complex; Glycyrrhiza Complex; Pacifenity; Panax Complex; Vitaglow Herbal Stress†; ***Canad.:*** Aveeno Acne Bar; Cystoforce†; ***Fr.:*** Acnaveen; Aveenoderm; Biocarde; Dermalibour; Epitheliale; Exomega; Septalibour; ***Ger.:*** Aureal†; Esberi-Nervin†; Eupronerv†; Mistelan†; Nervoregin; Requiesan; Somnium†; Vollmers praparierter gruner; ***Ital.:*** Acnaveen; Sebaveen; ***Switz.:*** Dormeasan†; Mucilar Avena; Sebodermt†; ***UK:*** Avena sativa comp.; ***USA:*** Aveeno Cleansing Bar.

Azadirachta (523-a)

Margosa; Neem.

The dried stem bark, root bark, and leaves of *Azadirachta indica* (=*Melia azadirachta*) (Meliaceae).

Azadirachta has been used as a bitter. It is widely used in Asia and has been reported to have insecticidal, antimalarial, and spermicidal properties.

Severe poisoning in Indian children given margosa oil as a remedy for minor ailments.[1]

1. Sinniah D, Baskaran G. Margosa oil poisoning as a cause of Reye's syndrome. *Lancet* 1981; **i:** 487–9.

Azintamide (4119-z)

Azintamide *(rINN).*

Azinthiamide; ST-9067. 2-[(6-Chloro-3-pyridazinyl)thio]-*N,N*-diethylacetamide.

$C_{10}H_{14}ClN_3OS$ = 259.8.

CAS — 1830-32-6.

Azintamide has been used as a choleretic.

Preparations

Proprietary Preparations (details are given in Part 3)
Aust.: Ora-Gallin purum.

Multi-ingredient: ***Aust.:*** Ora-Gallin; Ora-Gallin compositum; ***Ger.:*** Oragallin S; Oragallin†; ***Spain:*** Oragalin Espasmolitico; Oragalin†.

Azovan Blue (2123-a)

Azovan Blue *(BAN).*

Azovanum Caeruleum; CI Direct Blue 53; Colour Index No. 23860; Evans Blue; T-1824. Tetrasodium 1,1′-diamino-8,8′-dihydroxy-7,7′-(2,2′-dimethylbiphenyl-4,4′-diylbisdiazo)di-(naphthalene-2,4-disulphonate); Tetrasodium 6,6′-[3,3′-dimethylbiphenyl-4,4′-diylbis(azo)]bis[4-amino-5-hydroxy-naphthalene-1,3-disulphonate].

$C_{34}H_{24}N_6Na_4O_{14}S_4$ = 960.8.

CAS — 314-13-6.

Azovan blue is a dye that has been given intravenously for the determination of blood volume; it is firmly bound to plasma proteins and is slow to leave the circulation. Some patients may experience staining of the skin.

Azulene (1594-a)

Cyclopentacycloheptene.

$C_{10}H_8$ = 128.2.

CAS — 275-51-4.

NOTE. The name 'Azulene' has also been used for a number of derivatives of azulene including azulene sodium sulphonate, chamazulene, guaiazulene, and sodium gualenate.

Azulene has been used in preparations for anorectal disorders. The sodium sulphonate salt has been used in preparations for oral hygiene and for dyspepsia; sodium gualenate has also been used in gastro-intestinal disorders.

Allergic cheilitis in one patient following long-term use of a toothpaste containing azulene.[1]

1. Balato N, *et al.* Allergic cheilitis to azulene. *Contact Dermatitis* 1985; **13:** 39–40.

Preparations

Proprietary Preparations (details are given in Part 3)

Multi-ingredient: ***Aust.:*** Emser Nasensalbe; ***Ger.:*** Emser Balsam echt†; Emser Nasensalbe N; ***Ital.:*** AZ 15 Gengidentifricio; Otazul; ***Switz.:*** Azulene†.

Bactericidal Permeability Increasing Protein (11623-d)

Bactericidal permeability increasing protein is produced by human leucocytes and possesses both bactericidal and endotoxin-neutralising properties. It has been investigated for the treatment of meningococcal septicaemia. The use of recombinant fragments has also been investigated in a range of endotoxin-related disorders including complications of haemorrhagic trauma.

Bactericidal permeability increasing protein also possesses antifungal activity.

References.

1. Giroir BP, *et al.* Preliminary evaluation of recombinant amino-terminal fragment of human bactericidal/permeability-increasing protein in children with severe meningococcal sepsis. *Lancet* 1997; **350:** 1439–43.

Barium (5263-p)

Ba = 137.327.

CAS — 7440-39-3.

A soft highly reactive silvery-white metal.

Adverse Effects and Treatment

The symptoms of barium poisoning from soluble barium salts arise from stimulation of all forms of muscle and include vomiting, excess salivation, colic, diarrhoea, slow or irregular pulse, hypertension, dysarthria, confusion, somnolence, headache, paraesthesias, tinnitus, giddiness, vertigo, muscle twitching, convulsive tremors, and muscular paralysis. Hypokalaemia is common. A case of renal failure due to barium poisoning has been reported. Death from cardiac or respiratory failure may occur.

Treatment of poisoning with soluble barium salts may involve emptying the stomach by lavage, unless vomiting is severe. Magnesium or sodium sulphate may be given to convert barium to insoluble barium sulphate. Hypokalaemia should be corrected. Assisted ventilation may be necessary. Excretion may be increased by diuresis.

Reports of barium intoxication.

1. Lewi Z, Bar-Khayim Y. Food poisoning from barium carbonate. *Lancet* 1964; **ii:** 342–3.
2. Diengott D, *et al.* Hypokalaemia in barium poisoning. *Lancet* 1964; **ii:** 343–4.
3. Berning J. Hypokalaemia of barium poisoning. *Lancet* 1975; **i:** 110.
4. Gould DB, *et al.* Barium sulfide poisoning: some factors contributing to survival. *Arch Intern Med* 1973; **132:** 891–4.
5. Wetherill SF, *et al.* Acute renal failure associated with barium chloride poisoning. *Ann Intern Med* 1981; **95:** 187–8.
6. Phelan DM, *et al.* Is hypokalaemia the cause of paralysis in barium poisoning? *Br Med J* 1984; **289:** 882.
7. Barium. *Environmental Health Criteria 107.* Geneva: WHO, 1990.

Uses and Administration

The soluble barium salts are not used in therapeutics but are widely used in industry. Barium sulphide has been used as a depilatory and barium carbonate was used as a rodenticide. The insoluble barium sulphate (p.1003) is used as a contrast medium.

Barium Hydroxide Lime (203-h)

CAS — 17194-00-2 (barium hydroxide, anhydrous); 12230-71-6 (barium hydroxide, octahydrate).

Pharmacopoeias. In *US.*

A mixture of barium hydroxide octahydrate [$Ba(OH)_2,8H_2O$=315.5] and calcium hydroxide; it may also contain potassium hydroxide. White or greyish-white granules, or coloured with an indicator to show when absorptive power is exhausted. It absorbs not less than 19% of its weight of carbon dioxide. **Store** in airtight containers.

Barium hydroxide lime is used similarly to soda lime to absorb carbon dioxide in closed-circuit anaesthetic apparatus. Barium hydroxide lime contains a soluble form of barium and is toxic if swallowed.

Excessive drying out of barium hydroxide lime in anaesthetic apparatus, which may occur if oxygen flow through the equipment is left on for prolonged periods, can lead to the production of carbon monoxide and the risk of inducing carboxyhaemoglobinaemia in patients undergoing anaesthesia using the apparatus.[1]

1. Committee on Safety of Medicines/Medicines Control Agency. Safety issues in anaesthesia: volatile anesthetic agents and carboxyhaemoglobinaemia. *Current Problems* 1997; **23:** 7.

Bay Oil (4611-b)

Myrcia Oil; Oleum Myrciae.

NOTE. Distinguish from Laurel Leaf Oil (Bay Leaf Oil) which is obtained from the leaves of *Laurus nobilis* (Lauraceae).

A yellow volatile oil, darkening rapidly on exposure to air, with a pleasant odour and spicy taste, obtained by distillation from the leaves of Pimenta racemosa (Myrtaceae) and probably other allied species.

The principal use of bay oil is in the preparation of bay rum, which is used as a hair lotion and as an astringent application.

Preparations

Proprietary Preparations (details are given in Part 3)

Multi-ingredient: ***UK:*** Adiantine.

Bearberry (12420-x)

Bärentraubenblätter; Bearberry Leaves; Busserole; Ptarmiganberry Leaves; Uva Ursi; Uvae Ursi Folium.

Pharmacopoeias. In *Eur.* (see p.viii) and *Jpn.*

The whole or cut dried leaves of the bearberry, *Arctostaphylos uva-ursi* (Ericaceae). It contains not less than 8% of hydroquinone derivatives, expressed as anhydrous arbutin and calculated with reference to the dried drug. **Protect** from light.

Bearberry has been reported to be a diuretic, bacteriostatic, and astringent and has been used in the treatment of urinary-tract disorders. It has also been used in homoeopathic medicine.

Preparations

Proprietary Preparations (details are given in Part 3)

Ger.: Cystinol Akut; Uvalysat; ***Ital.:*** Ginocap.

Multi-ingredient: ***Aust.:*** Aktiv Blasen- und Nierentee; Apotheker Bauer's Nieren- und Blasentee; Bio-Garten Tee fur Niere und Blase; Blasen- und Nierentee; Blasen-Tee; Krautertee Nr 204; Krautertee Nr 3; Krautertee Nr 31; Mag Kottas Nieren-Blasentee; Sidroga Nieren- und Blasentee; Solisan; St Radegunder Nierentee; Uropurat; ***Austral.:*** Althaea Complex; De Witt's Pills; Fluid Loss; Herbal Diuretic Formula; Medinat PMT-Eze; New De Witt's Pills; PMT-EZE†; Profluid; Protemp; Urinase; Uva-Ursi Complex; Uva-Ursi Plus; ***Belg.:*** Tisane Contre la Tension; Tisane Diuretique; ***Canad.:*** Cystoforce†; Hepax†; ***Fr.:*** Mediflor Tisane Antirhumatismale No 2; Mediflor Tisane Diuretique†; Santane O_1; Santane R_8; Saprol†; Tisane Orientale Soker; ***Ger.:*** Arctuvan N; Blasen-Nieren-Tee Uroflux S†; Blasen-Nieren-Tee Uroflux†; Cefanephrin N; Cystinol; Cysto Fink; Harntee 400; Hernia-Tee; Herniol; Hevert-Blasen- und Nieren- Tee; Kneipp Nieren- und Blasen-Tee N†; Liruptin†; NB-tee Siegfried†; Nephrisol†; Nieren-Tee†; Prostatin F; Prostatin N Liquidum†; Prostatin N†; Salus Nieren-Blasen-Tee Nr.23; Salusan; Solvefort N†; Uro Fink; Urodil N†; Urodil S†; Worishofener Nieren- und Blasenmittel Dr. Kleinschrod†; ***Spain:*** Fagolitos Renal†; Vegetalin; ***Switz.:*** Cystinol N†; Cysto Fink; Cysto-Caps Chassot; Demonatur Dragees pour les reins et la vessie; Dragees pour reins et vessie S; Tisane antirhumatismale "H"†; Tisane antiseptique diuretique†; Tisane diuretique "H"†; Tisane pour les reins et la vessie; Tisane pour les reins et la vessie "H"†; Urinex (nouvelle formule); ***UK:*** Antitis; Backache Tablets; Boldo; Buchu Compound; Cascade; Diuretabs; HealthAid Boldo-Plus; Herbal Powder No.8†; Kas-Bah; Premental; Sciargo; Tabritis; Uvacin; Waterlex; Wellwoman; ***USA:*** Tri-Aqua.

Bentiromide (1957-g)

Bentiromide *(BAN, USAN, rINN).*

BTPABA; BT-PABA; E-2663; PFT; Ro-11-7891. 4-(N-Benzoyl-L-tyrosylamino)benzoic acid.

$C_{23}H_{20}N_2O_5$ = 404.4.

CAS — 37106-97-1.

Adverse Effects and Precautions

Reported adverse effects of bentiromide include headache, diarrhoea, and other gastro-intestinal effects. There may be hypersensitivity and transient increases in the values obtained in liver function studies.

Misleading results may be obtained in patients with gastro-intestinal, liver, or kidney disorders, or in patients receiving certain foods or drugs that are excreted as arylamines. Some of these drugs include benzocaine, chloramphenicol, lignocaine, paracetamol, procaine, procainamide, sulphonamides, and some diuretics.

Pharmacokinetics

Following administration by mouth, bentiromide is hydrolysed by chymotrypsin in the gut to release *p*-aminobenzoic acid and benzoyl-tyrosine. The aminobenzoic acid is absorbed, metabolised in the liver, and excreted in the urine as *p*-aminobenzoic acid and metabolites.

Uses and Administration

Bentiromide is used as a noninvasive test of exocrine pancreatic function, the amount of *p*-aminobenzoic acid and its metabolites being excreted in the urine being taken as a measure of the chymotrypsin-secreting activity of the pancreas.

The usual dose is 500 mg by mouth. Children aged 6 to 12 years may be given 14 mg per kg body-weight up to a maximum dose of 500 mg.

References.

1. Hoek FJ, *et al.* Improved specificity of the PABA test with p-aminosalicylic acid (PAS). *Gut* 1987; **28:** 468–73.
2. Puntis JWL, *et al.* Simplified oral pancreatic function test. *Arch Dis Child* 1988; **63:** 780–4.
3. Lang C, *et al.* Value of serum PABA as a pancreatic function test. *Gut* 1984; **25:** 508–12.

Preparations

Proprietary Preparations (details are given in Part 3)

USA: Chymex.

Benzaldehyde (4612-v)

$C_6H_5.CHO$ = 106.1.

CAS — 100-52-7.

Pharmacopoeias. In *Belg.* and *Br.* Also in *USNF.*

A clear colourless strongly refractive liquid with a characteristic odour of bitter almonds and a burning aromatic taste. Slightly **soluble** in water; miscible with alcohol, with ether, and with fixed and volatile oils. It becomes yellowish on keeping and oxidises in air to benzoic acid. **Store** at a temperature not exceeding 15° in airtight containers. Protect from light.

Benzaldehyde is used as a flavouring agent in the place of volatile bitter almond oil. It may cause contact dermatitis.

Preparations

BP 1998: Benzaldehyde Spirit;
USNF 18: Compound Benzaldehyde Elixir.

Benzarone (12432-n)

Benzarone *(rINN).*

L-2197. 2-Ethylbenzofuran-3-yl 4-hydroxyphenyl ketone.

$C_{17}H_{14}O_3$ = 266.3.

CAS — 1477-19-6.

Benzarone has been given by mouth and applied topically in the treatment of various peripheral vascular disorders. Hepatitis has been reported in patients given benzarone.

Preparations

Proprietary Preparations (details are given in Part 3)

Belg.: Fragivix†; ***Ger.:*** Fragivix†; Vasoc†; ***Ital.:*** Venagil†.

Benzyl Isothiocyanate (12434-m)

Benzyl Mustard Oil; Benzylsenföl; Oleum Tropaeoli.

C_8H_7NS = 149.2.

CAS — 622-78-6.

Pharmacopoeias. In *Fr.* which also includes Capucine (*Tropaeolum majus*).

An oil obtained from Capuchin cress, *Tropaeolum majus* (Tropaeolaceae).

Benzyl isothiocyanate has been given as an antibacterial agent.

Tropaeolum majus has been used in homoeopathic medicine.

Preparations

Proprietary Preparations (details are given in Part 3)

Ger.: Tromacaps†.

Multi-ingredient: ***Ger.:*** Soledexin†.

Berberine (524-t)

5,6-Dihydro-9,10-dimethoxybenzo[g]-1,3-benzodioxolo[5,6-*a*]quinolizinium.

$C_{20}H_{18}NO_4$ = 336.4.

CAS — 2086-83-1 (berberine); 633-66-9 (berberine sulphate).

Pharmacopoeias. Jpn includes berberine chloride and berberine tannate.

A quaternary alkaloid present in hydrastis, in various species of *Berberis*, and in many other plants.

Berberine has been used as a bitter. It possesses antimicrobial activity and has been tried as various salts in a number of infections. Berberine may also be used as a flavouring agent in food and alcoholic drinks.

References.

1. Khin-Maung-U, *et al.* Clinical trial of berberine in acute watery diarrhoea. *Br Med J* 1985; **291**: 1601–5.
2. Rabbani GH, *et al.* Randomized controlled trial of berberine sulfate therapy for diarrhea due to enterotoxigenic Escherichia coli and Vibrio cholerae. *J Infect Dis* 1987; **155**: 979–84.
3. Vennerstrom JL, *et al.* Berberine derivatives as antileishmanial drugs. *Antimicrob Agents Chemother* 1990; **34**: 918–21.
4. Phillipson JD, Wright CW. Medicinal plants in tropical medicine: 1 Medicinal plants against protozoal diseases. *Trans R Soc Trop Med Hyg* 1991; **85**: 18–21.

Preparations

Proprietary Preparations (details are given in Part 3)
Austral.: Murine.

Multi-ingredient: ***Fr.:*** Pastilles Jessel†; Sedacollyre.

Bergamot Oil (4613-g)

Bergamot Essence; Oleum Bergamottae.

Pharmacopoeias. In *Fr.*

A greenish or brownish-yellow volatile oil with a characteristic fragrant odour and a bitter aromatic taste, obtained by expression from the fresh peel of fruit of *Citrus bergamia* (Rutaceae). Constituents include linalyl acetate and 5-methoxypsoralen.

Bergamot oil is employed in perfumery. It is included in some preparations for upper respiratory-tract disorders. It is also used as a flavouring in Earl Grey tea. It contains 5-methoxypsoralen (p.1088). Photosensitivity reactions have occurred following the topical use of preparations containing bergamot oil.

Preparations

Proprietary Preparations (details are given in Part 3)

Multi-ingredient: ***Belg.:*** Ebexol†; ***Fr.:*** Balsamorhinol; Ephydrol; Humex; ***Ger.:*** Nephulon E†; ***Ital.:*** Cura; Sanaderm.

Betahistine Hydrochloride (9213-q)

Betahistine Hydrochloride *(USAN, rINNM).*

Betahistine Dihydrochloride *(BANM)*; PT-9. *N*-Methyl-2-(2-pyridyl)ethylamine dihydrochloride.

$C_8H_{12}N_2,2HCl = 209.1.$

CAS — 5638-76-6 (betahistine); 5579-84-0 (betahistine hydrochloride).

Betahistine Mesylate (10085-v)

Betahistine Mesilate; Betahistini Mesilas. *N*-Methyl-2-(2-pyridyl)ethylamine bismethanesulphonate.

$C_8H_{12}N_2,(CH_4O_3S)_2 = 328.4.$

CAS — 54856-23-4.

Pharmacopoeias. In *Eur.* (see p.viii) and *Jpn.*

A white, crystalline, very hygroscopic powder. Very **soluble** in water; freely soluble in alcohol; very slightly soluble in isopropyl alcohol. A 10% solution in water has a pH of 2 to 3. **Store** in airtight containers.

Adverse Effects

Gastro-intestinal disturbances, headache, and skin rashes have been reported.

Precautions

Betahistine should not be given to patients with phaeochromocytoma. It should be given with care to patients with asthma, peptic ulcer disease or a history of peptic ulcer disease.

Uses and Administration

Betahistine is an analogue of histamine and is claimed to improve the microcirculation of the labyrinth resulting in reduced endolymphatic pressure. It is used to reduce the symptoms of Ménière's disease (p.400).

Betahistine is given by mouth as the hydrochloride or mesylate. The usual initial dose (of the hydrochloride) is 16 mg three times daily taken preferably with meals; maintenance doses are generally in the range of 24 to 48 mg daily. Betahistine mesylate is used in similar doses.

Preparations

Proprietary Preparations (details are given in Part 3)
Aust.: Betaserc; ***Austral.:*** Serc; ***Belg.:*** Betaserc; Lobione; ***Canad.:*** Serc; ***Fr.:*** Extovyl; Lectil; Serc; ***Ger.:*** Aequamen; Melopat; Ribrain; Vasomotal; ***Irl.:*** Serc; ***Ital.:*** Microser; Vertiserc; ***Jpn:*** Merislon; ***Neth.:*** Betaserc; ***S.Afr.:*** Serc; ***Spain:*** Fidium; Serc; ***Switz.:*** Betaserc; ***UK:*** Serc.

Betaine (16532-j)

Glycine Betaine; Glycocoll Betaine; Lycine; Trimethylglycine. (Carboxymethyl)trimethylammonium hydroxide inner salt.

$C_5H_{11}NO_2 = 117.1.$

CAS — 107-43-7.

Betaine Hydrochloride (1303-j)

Trimethylglycine Hydrochloride. (Carboxymethyl)trimethylammonium hydroxide inner salt hydrochloride.

$C_5H_{11}NO_2,HCl = 153.6.$

CAS — 590-46-5.

Pharmacopoeias. In *Aust., Belg.,* and *US.*

A 25% solution has a pH of 0.8 to 1.2.

Uses and Administration

Betaine is used as a methyl donor to remethylate homocysteine to methionine in the treatment of patients with homocystinuria (p.1330). It is given by mouth in a usual dose of 3 g of anhydrous betaine twice daily. Doses are adjusted according to homocysteine-plasma concentrations; up to 20 g daily has been required in some patients. In children under 3 years old, an initial dose of 100 mg per kg body-weight daily may be used.

Betaine has also been used as a variety of salts in preparations for liver and gastro-intestinal disorders. The hydrochloride has been given as a source of hydrochloric acid in the treatment of hypochlorhydria.

References to betaine use in homocystinuria.

1. Smolin LA, *et al.* The use of betaine for the treatment of homocystinuria. *J Pediatr* 1981; **99**: 467–72.
2. Wilcken DEL, *et al.* Homocystinuria—the effects of betaine in the treatment of patients not responsive to pyridoxine. *N Engl J Med* 1983; **309**: 448–53.
3. Holme E, *et al.* Betaine for treatment of homocystinuria caused by methylenetetrahydrofolate reductase deficiency. *Arch Dis Child* 1989; **64**: 1061–4.
4. Anonymous. Betaine for homocystinuria. *Med Lett Drugs Ther* 1997; **39**: 12.

Preparations

Proprietary Preparations (details are given in Part 3)
Austral.: Cystadane; ***Fr.:*** Hepagrume; ***Ital.:*** Ascorbeta†; Somatyl.

Multi-ingredient: ***Aust.:*** CO_2 Granulat; Oroacid; ***Austral.:*** Betaine Digestive Aid; Bioglan Digestive Zyme†; Digestaid; Vitaplex Digestive Enzyme Formula†; ***Belg.:*** Digestomen; Gastrobul†; ***Fr.:*** Citrarginine; Citro-B_6†; Gastrobul; Liporex†; Nivabetol; Ornitaine; Scorbo-Betaine†; ***Ger.:*** CO_2 Granulat; Flacar; Unexym MD; Unexym N†; ***Ital.:*** Beta-Cortex B12†; Betascor B12; Citicortex†; Citroepatina; Epabetina; Equipar†; Fruttidasi†; Glutestere B-Complesso†; Ietepar; ***S.Afr.:*** Kloref; ***Spain:*** Digestomen Complex; Espasmo Digestomen; Levaliver; ***UK:*** Digezyme; Enzyme Digest; Fat-Solv; Kloref; Kloref-S; ***USA:*** Prevenzyme†.

Bibrocathol (5267-l)

Bibrocathol *(rINN).*

Bibrocathin; Bibrokatol; Bismuth Tetrabrompyrocatechinate; Tetrabromopyrocatechol Bismuth. 4,5,6,7-Tetrabromo-2-hydroxy-1,3,2-benzodioxabismole.

$C_6HBiBr_4O_3 = 649.7.$

CAS — 6915-57-7.

Practically **insoluble** in water.

Bibrocathol is a bismuth-containing compound that has been applied topically in the treatment of eye disorders, wounds, and burns.

Preparations

Proprietary Preparations (details are given in Part 3)
Belg.: Keraform†; ***Ger.:*** Noviform; Posiformin; ***Swed.:*** Noviform; ***Switz.:*** Noviform; Noviforme.

Multi-ingredient: ***Ger.:*** Lucrusanum†; Noviform-Aethylmorphin†; Novifort.

Bifemelane (1962-m)

Bifemelane *(rINN).*

N-Methyl-4-[(α-phenyl-*o*-tolyl)oxy]butylamine.

$C_{18}H_{23}NO = 269.4.$

CAS — 90293-01-9.

Bifemelane is a nootropic that has been used in the treatment of senile dementia.

Bile Acids and Salts (998-q)

CAS — 81-25-4 (cholic acid); 11006-55-6 (sodium tauroglycocholate).

Pharmacopoeias. Aust. includes cholic acid. *Jpn* includes bear bile.

The principal primary bile acids, cholic acid and chenodeoxycholic acid (p.1562), are produced in the liver from cholesterol and are conjugated with glycine or taurine to give glycocholic acid, taurocholic acid, glycochenodeoxycholic acid, and taurochenodeoxycholic acid before being secreted into the bile where they are present as the sodium or potassium salts (bile salts). Secondary bile acids are formed in the colon by bacterial deconjugation and 7α-dehydroxylation of cholic acid and chenodeoxycholic acid producing deoxycholic acid and lithocholic acid respectively. Ursodeoxycholic acid (p.1642) is a minor bile acid in man although it is the principal bile acid in *bears*. Dehydrocholic acid (p.1570) is a semisynthetic bile acid.

The total body pool of bile salts is about 3 g, and most of the secreted bile salts are reabsorbed in a process of enterohepatic recycling, so that only a small fraction of this amount must be synthesised *de novo* each day.

Bile salts are strongly amphiphilic; with the aid of phospholipids they form micelles and emulsify cholesterol and other lipids in bile. Oral administration of chenodeoxycholic acid also reduces the synthesis of cholesterol in the liver, while ursodeoxycholic acid reduces biliary cholesterol secretion apparently by increasing conversion of cholesterol to other bile acids. The bile acids (but not the bile salts) also have a choleretic action, increasing the secretion of bile, when given by mouth.

Chenodeoxycholic acid and ursodeoxycholic acid are given by mouth in the management of cholesterol-rich gallstones (p.1642) in patients unsuited to, or unwilling to undergo, surgery. Ursodeoxycholic acid is also under investigation in some liver disorders.

Preparations containing bile salts have been used to assist the emulsification of fats and absorption of fat-soluble vitamins in conditions in which there is a deficiency of bile in the gastro-intestinal tract. Ox bile has also been used in the treatment of chronic constipation.

Preparations

Proprietary Preparations (details are given in Part 3)
Austral.: Proslim-Lipid; ***Fr.:*** Antimucose; ***Ger.:*** Cholecysmon; ***S.Afr.:*** Bilron; ***USA:*** Bilron†.

Multi-ingredient: ***Aust.:*** Arca-Enzym; Buccalin; Combizym Compositum; Dragees Neunzehn; Euflat; Festal; Helopanzym; Hylakombun; Nutrizym†; Ozym; Pankreon compositum; Peribilan†; Silberne; Spasmo Gallosanol; ***Austral.:*** Combizym Co†; Digestaid; Enzyme; Lexat; ***Belg.:*** Buccaline; Grains de Vals; Pankreon compositum†; Trizymal†; ***Canad.:*** Aid-Lax; Alsiline; Bicholate; Caroid; Festal†; Herbalax; Herbalax Forte; Laxa; Phytolax; Regubil; Triolax; Vesilax; ***Fr.:*** Bilifluine; Bilkaby; Festale†; Grains de Vals; Mucinum; Rectopanbiline; ***Ger.:*** Bilgast†; Bilicombin sp†; Bilipeptal forte†; Cholosom†; Combizym Compositum; Divinal-Bohnen†; Enterotropin†; enzym gallo sanol N†; Enzym-Hepaduran†; Eupond; Gallemolan N†; Gallitophen†; Gallo sanol N†; Gastrocaps†; Glissitol†; Helopanzym†; Hepabionta comp†; Heparaxal†; Hepasteril†; Hepaticum-Divinal†; Hepatofalk Neu; Hylakombun N†; Ludoxin†; Mandrogallan†; Meteophyt-V†; Meteophyt†; Neo-Gallonorm†; Omnadin†; Opobyl†; Pankreatin comp. N†; Pankreon compositum†; Panzynorm forte†; Panzynorm†; Pascopankreat†; Spasmo Gallo Sanol N; Spasmo-Bilicura†; Stomachiagil†; ***Ital.:*** Bilagar†; Boldosten†; Cheliboldo†; Combizym Compositum†; Enteroton Lassativo†; Enzygaster†; Menabil Complex†; Onoton†; Pancreon Compositum; Reolina†; ***Neth.:*** Combizym Compositum; Cotazym Forte†; Opobyl†; ***S.Afr.:*** Nutrizym†; ***Spain:*** Digestomen Complex; Espasmo Digestomen; Kneipp Pildoras†; Laxante Richelet†; Menabil Complex; Pankreon Fuerte†; Secrebil B†; Tornacin†; ***Swed.:*** Combizym Compositum; Festal†; Pankreon comp. forte†; ***Switz.:*** Buccaline; Combizym Compositum†; Digestofluid†; Digestozym†; Festal†; Globase†; Nutrizym†; Opobyl; ***UK:*** Digezyme; ***USA:*** Digepepsin; Entozyme†.

Birch Leaf (9616-m)

Betulae Folium; Birkenblätter; Bouleau.

Pharmacopoeias. In *Eur.* (see p.viii) and *Pol.*

The whole or fragmented dried leaves of *Betula pendula (B. verrucosa)* and/or *B. pubescens* as well as hybrids of both species. It contains not less than 1.5% of flavonoids, calculated as hyperoside, with reference to the dried drug. **Protect** from light.

Birch leaf is used in herbal medicine.

Preparations

Proprietary Preparations (details are given in Part 3)
Aust.: Bakanasan Entwasserungs; Galama; Sanhelios-Entwasserungsdragees; ***Ger.:*** Kneipp Birkenblatter-Pflanzensaft.

Multi-ingredient: ***Aust.:*** Aktiv Blasen- und Nierentee; Apotheker Bauer's Nieren- und Blasentee; Bio-Garten Entschlackungstee; Bio-Garten Tee fur Niere und Blase; Bio-Garten Tee zur Erhohung der Harnmenge; Bio-Garten Tropfen fur Niere und Blase; Blasen- und Nierentee; Blasentee; Brennesseltonikum; Drogimed; Ehrmann's Entschlackungstee; Entschlackungstee; Fruhjahrs-Elixier ohne Alkohol; Harntreibender Tee; Kneipp Entwasserungstee; Kneipp Nieren- und Blasen-Tee; Krauterdoktor Entwasserungs-Elixier; Krauterhaus Mag Kottas Blasentee; Krauterhaus Mag Kottas Entschlackungstee; Krautertee Nr 19; Krautertee Nr 2; Krautertee Nr 204; Krautertee Nr 25; Krautertee Nr 29; Krautertee Nr 30; Mag Doskar's Nieren- und Blasentonikum; Mag Kottas Entschlackungstee; Rheuma; Sanvita-Entschlackungstonikum; Sidroga Nieren- und Blasentee; Solubitrat; St Radegunder Entwasserungs-Elixier; St Radegunder Entwasserungstee; Synpharma Instant-Blasen-und-Nierentee; Teekanne Blasen- und

Nierentee; **Austral.:** Natural Vegetable Alkaliniser†; **Fr.:** B.O.P.; Drainactil; **Ger.:** Agamadon; Antihypertonicum S; Blasen-Nieren-Tee Stada; Blasen-Nieren-Tee Uroflux S†; Blasen-Nieren-Tee Uroflux†; Buccotean TF†; Buccotean†; Discmigon; Entwasserungs-Tee†; Etmoren; Eupond; Gallitophen†; Harntee; Harntee 400; Hevert-Blasen- und Nieren- Tee; Hevert-Entwasserungs-Tee; Hevert-Gicht-Rheuma-Tee comp; Kneipp Blasen- und Nieren-Tee; Kneipp Blutreinigungs-Tee†; Kneipp Entschlackungs-Tee; Kneipp Nieren- und Blasen-Tee N†; Liruptin†; NB-Tee N; NB-tee Siegfried†; Nephro-Pasc; Nephronorm Med; Nephropur tri; Nephroselect M; Nephrubin; Nierentee 2000; Original-Hico-Gallenheil†; Reducelle; Renob Blasen- und Nierentee; Rheumex†; Ullus Blasen-Nieren-Tee N; Uro Fink; Urodil Blasen-Nieren Arzneitee; Urodil N†; Urodil phyto; Urodil S†; Urostei; Worishofener Nieren- und Blasenmittel Dr. Kleinschrod†; **Ital.:** Artoxan; Betullosin†; Depurfat; Fluend; Ginoday; Prexene; Slim-Linea; **Switz.:** Cystinol N†; Nephrosolid N; Phytomed Nephro; Solubitrat†; Tisane antirhumatismale "H"†; Tisane antiseptique diuretique†; Tisane diuretique; Tisane diuretique "H"†; Tisane pour le coeur et la circulation; Tisane pour les reins et la vessie; Tisane pour les reins et la vessie "H"†; Urinex (nouvelle formule); **UK:** Erysidoron 2; Massage Balm Calendula; Rheumadoron.

Black Nightshade (12449-w)

Morelle Noire.

The leaves and flowering tops of the black or garden nightshade, *Solanum nigrum* (Solanaceae). It contains solanine and its allied alkaloids.

Black nightshade is distributed throughout most of the world as a weed of cultivation. It appears to have little medicinal value but was used in liniments, poultices, and decoctions for external application. Ingestion can cause typical antimuscarinic effects that may require treatment as described under Atropine, p.455.

Bladderwrack (5408-s)

Fucus; Kelpware; Seawrack; Tang.

Pharmacopoeias. In *Fr.* and *Pol.*

Bladderwrack is the dried seaweed *Fucus vesiculosus* (Fucaceae). It is an ingredient of a number of herbal preparations given for various disorders including obesity, constipation, and iodine deficiency. Kelp (p.1593) is another preparation of dried seaweeds.

Bladderwrack is used in homoeopathic medicine.

Preparations

Proprietary Preparations (details are given in Part 3)

Multi-ingredient: Belg.: Feves De Fuca†; **Fr.:** Actisane Minceur; Aminsane; AMK; Dellova; Dragees Fuca; Mediflor Tisane Dietetique†; Phytotherpie Boribel no 9; Promincil; Reduligne†; Tisane Obeflorine; Tisanes de l'Abbe Hamon no 11; **Ger.:** Krophan N; Lipozet†; Viscophyll; **Ital.:** Fave di Fuca; Fitolinea; SlimLinea; **Spain:** Lipograsil; **UK:** Boldo; HealthAid Boldo-Plus; Water Naturtabs; Water Relief Tablets.

Boldo (2309-v)

Boldo Leaves; Peumus.

CAS — 476-70-0 (boldine); 1398-22-7 (boldoglucin).

Pharmacopoeias. In *Fr.*, *It.*, and *Swiss.*

Fr. also includes Boldine.

The dried leaves of *Peumus boldus* (Monimiaceae). It contains the alkaloid boldine, the glycoside boldoglucin, and about 2% of volatile oil.

Boldo is employed in herbal medicine as a diuretic and in the treatment of gallstones and gastro-intestinal disorders such as constipation. The alkaloid boldine is also used.

Preparations

Proprietary Preparations (details are given in Part 3)

Multi-ingredient: Aust.: St Bonifatius-Tee; **Austral.:** Berberis Complex; Lexat; **Belg.:** Boldolaxine Aloes†; Stago†; Tisane pour le Foie; **Canad.:** Alsilax; Hepax†; **Fr.:** Actisane Digestion; Aromabyl; Bolcitol; Boldoflorine†; Boldolaxine†; Drainactil; Elixir Spark; Gastralsan; Gripponyl†; Hepaclem; Hepatorex†; Hepax; Jecopeptol; Mediflor Tisane Hepatique No 5; Mucinum; Mucinum a l'Extrait de Cascara; Neo-Boldolaxine†; Opobyl; Oxyboldine; Palmi; Petites Pilules Carters pour le Foie; Romarinex-Choline; Santane C_6; Santane F_{10}; Saprol†; Solution Stago Diluee; Spark; Tisane des Familles†; Tisane Mexicaine; Vegelax; **Ger.:** Boldo "Dr. Eberth"†; Cholapret; Cynarzym N; Divinal-Bohnen†; Dr. Klinger's Bergischer Krautertee, Leber- und Gallentee†; Gallemolan G; Gallemolan N†; Heparaxal†; Hepaticum-Divinal†; Hepatofalk Neu; Heumann Leber- und Gallentee Solu-Hepar NT; Hevert-Gall S; Losapan†; Ludoxin†; Nephrisol†; Opobyl†; Pankreaticum; Solu-Hepar N†; Stomachiagil†; **Ital.:** Amaro Lassativo†; Amaro Medicinale; Bilarvis†; Boldina He; Boldosten†; Caramelle alle Erbe Digestive; Certobil; Cheliboldo†; Coladren; Colax; Confetti Lassativi†; Confetto Complex†; Critichol; Dis-Cinil Complex; Enteroton Digestivo†; Enteroton Lassativo†; Epaglutone†; Epar Euchessina†; Eparema; Eparema-Levul; Eupatol; Fitodorf Rabarbaro; Florerbe Digestiva†; Florerbe Lassativa; Frangulina; Heparbil†; Hepasil Composto; Hepatos; Hepatos B12; Magisbile; Menabil Complex†; Mepalax; Ormobyl†; Pillole Schias†; Politintura Schias†; Prid con Boldo†; Raboldo; Regular†; Schias-Amaro Medicinale; Sedonerva†; Sintobil; Solvobil; Tisana Arnaldi; Vegebyl; Vitabil Composto†; **Neth.:** Opobyl†; **Spain:** Boldolaxin; Boldosal; Ibsesal†; Laxante Richelet†; Menabil Complex; Nico Hepatocyn; Opobyl; Resolutivo Regium; Sambil; Secrebil B†; Sol Schoum; **Switz.:** Amaro†; Boldocynara N; Boldoflorine; Dragees pour reins et vessie S; Grains de Vals; Laxativum Nouvelle Formule; Laxativum†; Livartil†; Opobyl; Stago†; The Franklin; Tisane antiseptique diuretique†; Tisane hepatique et biliaire; Tisane hepatique et biliaire "H"†; Tisane pour les reins et la vessie; **UK:** Boldo; HealthAid Boldo-Plus.

Bone Morphogenetic Proteins (11757-j)

BMP.

Bone morphogenetic proteins (BMPs) are growth factors which promote ectopic bone formation and can be extracted from demineralised bone matrix. At least 7 have been identified, including osteogenin (BMP-3) and osteogenic protein 1 (OP-1, BMP-7), and some have been produced by recombinant technology. They are under investigation for use in orthopaedic and reconstructive surgery.

References.

1. Anonymous. New bone? *Lancet* 1992; **339:** 463–4.
2. Reddi AH. Bone morphogenetic proteins, bone marrow stromal cells, and mesenchymal cells: Maureen Owen revisited. *Clin Orthop* 1995; (313): 115–19.

Borax (261-l)

Disodium Tetraborate; E241; Natrii Tetraboras; Natrium Boricum; Purified Borax; Sodium Biborate or Pyroborate; Sodium Borate; Sodium Tetraborate.

$Na_2B_4O_7,10H_2O = 381.4.$

CAS — 1330-43-4; 61028-24-8 (both anhydrous borax); 1303-96-4 (borax decahydrate).

Pharmacopoeias. In *Chin., Eur.* (see p.viii), *Jpn,* and *Pol.* Also in *USNF.*

Odourless transparent colourless crystals, crystalline masses, or white crystalline powder. It effloresces in dry air. **Soluble** 1 in 16 of water, 1 in less than 1 of boiling water, and 1 in 1 of glycerol; practically insoluble in alcohol. A 4% solution in water has a pH of 9.0 to 9.6. **Store** in airtight containers.

For a warning on the supply of preparations of borax see under boric acid, below.

Boric Acid (260-e)

Acidum Boricum; Boracic Acid; Borsäure; E240; Orthoboric Acid; Sal Sedativa de Homberg.

$H_3BO_3 = 61.83.$

CAS — 10043-35-3.

Pharmacopoeias. In *Chin., Eur.* (see p.viii), *Jpn,* and *Pol.* Also in *USNF.*

Odourless colourless brilliant plates, or white crystals, somewhat pearly lustrous scales, or white crystalline powder, unctuous to the touch. It volatilises in steam. **Soluble** 1 in 18 of water, 1 in 4 of boiling water, 1 in 18 of alcohol, 1 in 6 of boiling alcohol, and 1 in 4 of glycerol. Boric acid forms a complex with glycerol which is a stronger acid than boric acid. A 3.3% solution in water has a pH of 3.8 to 4.8.

CAUTION. *Pharmacists are advised not to sell boric acid as such for use as a dusting-powder. Dusting-powders containing more than 5% of boric acid should be labelled: 'not to be applied to raw or weeping surfaces'. Pharmacists are also advised not to supply Borax Glycerin or Honey of Borax, even with an appropriate warning, because of the hazards associated with the use of these preparations in infants.*

Adverse Effects and Treatment

The main symptoms of acute boric acid poisoning are vomiting and diarrhoea, abdominal pain, an erythematous rash involving both skin and mucous membranes, followed by desquamation, and stimulation or depression of the central nervous system. There may be convulsions and hyperpyrexia. There may also be renal tubular damage. Abnormal liver function and jaundice have been reported rarely. Death, resulting from circulatory collapse and shock, may occur within 3 to 5 days.

The slow excretion of boric acid can lead to cumulative toxicity during repeated use. Symptoms of chronic intoxication include anorexia, gastro-intestinal disturbances, debility, confusion, dermatitis, menstrual disorders, anaemia, convulsions, and alopecia.

Fatalities have occurred most frequently in young children after the accidental ingestion of solutions of boric acid or after the application of boric acid powder to abraded skin. The concentration of boric acid in talcs and products for oral hygiene is limited in the UK to 5 and 0.5% respectively and talcs must be labelled 'not to be used for children less than 3 years old'. In the UK the concentration of boric acid in other cosmetic products is limited to 3%. Topical preparations of boric acid should not be applied to extensive areas of abraded or damaged skin.

Deaths have resulted from absorption following lavage of body cavities with solutions of boric acid, and this practice is no longer recommended.

Inhaled boric acid and borax are pulmonary irritants.

Treatment of poisoning is symptomatic. The stomach should be emptied if a large amount of boric acid has been ingested; activated charcoal is not effective. Peritoneal dialysis or haemodialysis may be of value.

Pharmacokinetics

Boric acid is absorbed from the gastro-intestinal tract, from damaged skin, from wounds, and from mucous membranes. It does not readily penetrate intact skin. About 50% of the amount absorbed is excreted in the urine within 12 hours; the remainder is probably excreted over 5 to 7 days.

Uses and Administration

Boric acid possesses weak bacteriostatic and fungistatic properties; it has generally been superseded by more effective and less toxic disinfectants. It is used as a pesticide against ants and cockroaches.

Boric acid is used, usually with borax, as a buffer and antimicrobial in eye drops and was formerly used as a soluble lubricant in solution-tablets. Boric acid and borax are not used internally.

In the UK the use of boric acid in cosmetics and toiletries is restricted.

Borax is used similarly to boric acid and has also been used externally as a mild astringent and as an emulsifier in creams. Borax Glycerin and Honey of Borax were formerly used as paints for the throat, tongue, and mouth, but should not be used due to the risk of toxicity.

Other salts of boric acid, including potassium and zinc salts, have been used.

A preparation of borax is used in homoeopathic medicine.

Antimicrobial activity. Evaluation of the antimicrobial activity of 1.22% borate buffer.[1]

1. Houlsby RD, *et al.* Antimicrobial activity of borate-buffered solutions. *Antimicrob Agents Chemother* 1986; **29:** 803–6.

Urine preservation. Boric acid in concentrations of about 2% may be a suitable preservative for urine samples in transit requiring bacteriological examination.[1,2]

1. Porter IA, Brodie J. Boric acid preservation of urine samples. *Br Med J* 1969; **2:** 353–5.
2. Lum KT, Meers PD. Boric acid converts urine into an effective bacteriostatic transport medium. *J Infect* 1989; **18:** 51–8.

Vaginitis. Satisfactory clinical and mycological responses to boric acid were reported in 2 patients with *Candida glabrata* vaginitis (p.367) who had not responded to repeated courses of azole antifungals.[1]

1. Redondo-Lopez V, *et al.* Torulopsis glabrata vaginitis: clinical aspects and susceptibility of antifungal agents. *Obstet Gynecol* 1990; **76:** 651–5.

Preparations

BP 1998: Kaolin Poultice;
BPC 1973: Magenta Paint; Surgical Chlorinated Soda Solution;
USP 23: Rose Water Ointment.

Proprietary Preparations (details are given in Part 3)

Canad.: RO-Eyewash; **Fr.:** Hydralin; **Spain:** Jabon Borico†.

Multi-ingredient: Aust.: Coldophthal; Ophtaguttal; Polyrinse-Augenelement; **Austral.:** Anusol-HC†; Blinx†; Boz†; Floraquin; Phytex†; **Belg.:** Alcasol; Amazyl; Baseler Haussalbe; Boradrine; Borostyrol; Inotyol; Ocal†; Osmoleine; Peneytol†; Sedemol†; Sulfa-Sedemol†; Tablettes pour la Gorge Medica†; Tercinol†; **Canad.:** British Army Foot Powder; Eye Eze; Ingrown Toe Nail Salve; **Fr.:** Antiseptique-Calmante; Baume Disalgyl†; Boroclarine; Borostyrol; Buccawalter; Chibro-Boraline†; Dacryoboraline; Dacryoserum; Eau Precieuse Depensier; Genola; Glyco-Thymoline; Gynescal; Gynoplix†; Hydralin; Mucosodine†; Ophtalmine; Optrex; Oxy-thymoline†; Paps; Pastilles M.B.C†; Pate a l'Eau Roche-Posay; Phylarm; Posine; Pulveol†; Sophtal; Uvicol; **Ger.:** Boro-Hexamin†; Ophtopur-N; **Irl.:** Phytex; **Ital.:** Adrenosin Composto†; Bagno Oculare; Borossigeno Plus Stomatologico; Collirium Geymonat; Fotofil; Gineosepta†; Lucisan; Optrex; Otocaina†; **S.Afr.:** Anugesic; Anusol-HC; Gynedron†; Moni-Gynedron†; Oestro-Gynedron†; Poly-Gynedron†; Tricho-Gynedron†; Universal Eye Drops; Vagarsol; **Spain:** Acnosan; Amidoyina†; Banoftal; Boradren; Clor Hemi; Cloroboral; Coliriocilina Adren Astr; Dermomycose; Detergente Cusi Acido†; Elixir Dental Formahina†; Euboral; Floraquin†; Fungusol; Grinal Hidrocortisona†; Lamnotyl; Lema C; Mentol Sedans Sulfamidad†; Milrosina; Milrosina Hidrocort†; Natusan; Oftalmol Dexa; Oftalmol Ocular; Pentoderm†; Pomada Infantil Vera; Pomada Oftalm Antisep†; Sanovox†; Talquissar; Talquistina; Topico Denticion Vera; Vaselina Boricada; Zolina; **Swed.:** Antasten-Privin; **Switz.:** Chibro-Boraline; **UK:** Natusan†; Oxy Clean Facial Scrub; Phytex; **USA:** Auro-Dri; BFI; Castaderm; Collyrium for Fresh Eyes; Dri/Ear; Ear-Dry; Fostex Medicated Cleansing Bar†; Neo-Castaderm†; Oxy Clean Soap†; Phenaseptic†; Phylorinol; RA Lotion; Saratoga; Seale's Lotion; Star-Otic; Succus Cineraria Maritima; Trichotine; Trimo-San; Wyanoids.

Bornyl Acetate (9377-b)

Bornyl Acetate *(USAN)*.

Borneol Acetate. 1,7,7-Trimethylbicyclo[2.2.1]heptan-2-ol acetate.

$C_{12}H_{20}O_2$ = 196.3.
CAS — 76-49-3.

Bornyl acetate is a constituent of some essential oils. It has been used in aromatic preparations in the treatment of coughs, other respiratory-tract disorders, and musculoskeletal and joint disorders.

Preparations

Proprietary Preparations (details are given in Part 3)

Multi-ingredient: ***Ger.:*** Lindofluid N; ***Ital.:*** Balsamico F. di M.†; ***Spain:*** Vicks Inhalador.

Bromelains (3705-h)

Bromelains *(BAN, USAN, rINN)*.

Bromelins; Plant Protease Concentrate.
CAS — 9001-00-7.

A concentrate of proteolytic enzymes derived from the pineapple plant, *Ananas comosus* (=*A. sativus*) (Bromeliaceae).

Units

One Rorer unit of protease activity has been defined as that amount of enzyme which hydrolyses a standardised casein substrate at pH 7 and 25° so as to cause an increase in absorbance of 0.00001 per minute at 280 nm.

One FIP unit of bromelain activity is reported to be contained in that amount of a standard preparation, which hydrolyses a suitable preparation of casein (FIP controlled) under the standard conditions at an initial rate such that there is liberated per minute an amount of peptides, not precipitated by a specified protein precipitation reagent which gives the same absorbance as 1 μmol of tyrosine at 275 nm.

Activity has also been described in terms of milk-clotting units.

Adverse Effects

Bromelains may cause nausea, vomiting, and diarrhoea. Metrorrhagia and menorrhagia have occasionally occurred. Hypersensitivity reactions have been reported and have included skin reactions and asthma.

Effects on the respiratory system. Bronchial asthma was experienced by 2 patients after exposure to bromelains.[1] Of 6 workers sensitised to papain 5 showed positive skin tests to bromelains and 2 of them also showed immediate asthmatic reactions after bronchial challenge with bromelains.[2]

1. Galleguillos F, Rodriguez JC. Asthma caused by bromelin inhalation. *Clin Allergy* 1978; **8:** 21–4.
2. Baur X, Fruhmann G. Allergic reactions, including asthma, to the pineapple protease bromelain following occupational exposure. *Clin Allergy* 1979; **9:** 443–50.

Precautions

Bromelains should be given with care to patients with coagulation disorders or with severely impaired hepatic or renal function.

Uses and Administration

Bromelains are used as an adjunct in the treatment of soft tissue inflammation and oedema associated with trauma and surgery. Bromelains have also been given as an aid to digestion.

Preparations

Proprietary Preparations (details are given in Part 3)
Belg.: Extranase†; ***Fr.:*** Extranase; ***Ger.:*** Proteozym; Traumanase; ***Irl.:*** Ananase; ***Ital.:*** Ananase; Proteolis†; Rogorin†; ***S.Afr.:*** Ananase; ***Switz.:*** Traumanase; ***USA:*** Dayto-Anase.

Multi-ingredient: ***Aust.:*** Arca-Enzym; Nutrizym†; Wobenzym; ***Austral.:*** Bio-Disc; Bioglan Discone†; Digestaid; Digestive Aid; Prost-1; Prost-2; Prozyme; Vita Disc†; Vitaplex Digestive Enzyme Formula†; ***Fr.:*** Tetranase; ***Ger.:*** Enzym-Hepaduran†; Enzym-Wied; Esberizym N; Floradix Multipretten; Meteophyt-V†; Mulsal N; Phlogenzym; Traumanase-cyclin†; Wobenzym N; ***Ital.:*** Bres; Convivial†; Debridat Enzimatico†; Derinase Plus; Kilozim†; Plasil Enzimatico†; Prandium†; ***Jpn:*** Kimotab†; ***S.Afr.:*** Haemonase P†; Nutrizym†; ***Spain:*** Bequipecto; Flebo Stop; Tornacin†; Trizima†; ***Switz.:*** Globase†; Nutrizym†; ***UK:*** Cardeymin; Cellbloc†; Digezyme; Enzyme Digest.

Bromine (1022-v)

Bromum.

Br_2 = 159.808.
CAS — 7726-95-6.

A dark reddish-brown, heavy, mobile liquid which gives off intensely irritating brown fumes.

Adverse Effects

Bromine is intensely irritating and corrosive to mucous membranes and, even in dilute solution, may cause fatal gastroenteritis if swallowed. Contact with the skin can produce severe burns and inhalation of the vapour causes violent irritation of the respiratory tract and pulmonary oedema.

Treatment of Adverse Effects

Milk, white of egg, or starch mucilage, taken as soon as possible, have been recommended following ingestion of bromine. If bromine vapour has been inhaled, give assisted respiration, if necessary, and oxygen. Splashes on the skin and eyes should be immediately washed off; washing under running water should continue for at least 15 minutes.

Uses and Administration

Bromine is widely used in industry. It was formerly used, in the form of an adduct with a quaternary ammonium compound in the treatment of plantar warts.

Preparations

Proprietary Preparations (details are given in Part 3)

Multi-ingredient: ***UK:*** Callusolve†.

Bryonia (12460-v)

The root of *Bryonia alba* or *B. dioica* (Cucurbitaceae).

Bryonia is an ingredient of preparations used in respiratory-tract infections and inflammatory disorders. It is also used in homoeopathic medicine.

Preparations

Proprietary Preparations (details are given in Part 3)

Multi-ingredient: ***Austral.:*** Cough Relief; Harpagophytum Complex; Respatona; Respatona Plus with Echinacea; ***Fr.:*** Quintopan Adult; ***Ger.:*** B 10-Strath†; Bryonia-Strath†; Dolo-Arthrosetten†.

Buchu (12461-g)

Bucco; Buchu Leaves; Diosma; Folia Bucco.

Pharmacopoeias. In *Fr.*

The dried leaves of 'short' or 'round' buchu, *Agathosma betulina* (=*Barosma betulina*) (Rutaceae).

Buchu is a weak diuretic and urinary antiseptic and has been used in multi-ingredient preparations for the treatment of urinary-tract disorders.

Buchu has been used in homoeopathic medicine.

Preparations

Proprietary Preparations (details are given in Part 3)

Multi-ingredient: ***Austral.:*** Althaea Complex; De Witt's Pills; Fluid Loss; Herbal Diuretic Complex†; Medinat PMT-Eze; New De Witt's Pills; PMS Support; Serenoa Complex; Urinase; Uva-Ursi Complex; Vitaplex PMT†; ***Belg.:*** Stago†; ***Canad.:*** Herbal Laxative; ***Fr.:*** Saprol†; ***Ger.:*** Buccotean TF†; Buccotean†; Entwasserungs-Tee†; Hevert-Entwasserungs-Tee; Salus Kurbis-Tonikum Compositum†; Urodil N†; Urodil S†; ***S.Afr.:*** Docrub; ***Spain:*** Fagolitos Renal†; ***Switz.:*** Stago†; Urinex (nouvelle formule); ***UK:*** Antitis; Backache Tablets; Buchu Compound; Diuretabs; Herbal Powder No.8†; Kas-Bah; Skin Eruptions Mixture; ***USA:*** Aqua-Rid; Fluidex; Tri-Aqua.

Bucillamine (2897-a)

Bucillamine *(rINN)*.

DE-019; SA-96; Tiobutarit. *N*-(2-Mercapto-2-methylpropionyl)-L-cysteine.

$C_7H_{13}NO_3S_2$ = 223.3.
CAS — 65002-17-7.

Bucillamine is reported to be an immunomodulator used in rheumatoid arthritis.

Preparations

Proprietary Preparations (details are given in Part 3)
Jpn: Rimatil†.

Bucladesine Sodium (18881-v)

Bucladesine Sodium *(rINNM)*.

N-(9-β-D-Ribofuranosyl-9*H*-purin-6-yl)butyramide cyclic 3′,5′-(hydrogen phosphate) 2′-butyrate sodium.

$C_{18}H_{24}N_5O_8PNa$ = 492.4.
CAS — 362-74-3 (bucladesine).

Bucladesine sodium has been reported to have cardiotonic properties. It has been given intravenously. It has also been applied topically for the treatment of bedsores.

Bufotenine (5012-l)

NN-Dimethylserotonin; 5-Hydroxy-*NN*-dimethyltryptamine; Mappine. 3-(2-Dimethylaminoethyl)indol-5-ol.

$C_{12}H_{16}N_2O$ = 204.3.
CAS — 487-93-4.

An indole alkaloid obtained from the seeds and leaves of *Piptadenia peregrina* from which the hallucinogenic snuff, cohoba is prepared, and *P. macrocarpa* (Mimosaceae). It was first isolated from the skin glands of toads (*Bufo* spp.) and has also been isolated from species of *Amanita* (Agaricaceae).

Bufotenine has serotonergic activity and is reported to have hallucinogenic properties. It has no therapeutic use.

Buphenine Hydrochloride (9214-p)

Buphenine Hydrochloride *(BANM)*.

Nylidrin Hydrochloride; Nylidrinium Chloride. 1-(4-Hydroxyphenyl)-2-(1-methyl-3-phenylpropylamino)propan-1-ol hydrochloride.

$C_{19}H_{25}NO_2,HCl$ = 335.9.
CAS — 447-41-6 (buphenine); 849-55-8 (buphenine hydrochloride).

Pharmacopoeias. In *US.*

An odourless, white, crystalline powder. **Soluble** 1 in 65 of water and 1 in 40 of alcohol; slightly soluble in chloroform and ether. A 1% solution in water has a pH of 4.5 to 6.5. **Store** in airtight containers.

Adverse Effects and Precautions

For the adverse effects of sympathomimetics and precautions to be observed, see p.951.

Uses and Administration

Buphenine produces peripheral vasodilatation through beta-adrenoceptor stimulation and a direct action on the arteries and arterioles of the skeletal muscles.

Buphenine has been used in the treatment of disorders of peripheral and cerebral circulatory insufficiency. It has also been used in preparations for rhinitis and nasal congestion. The usual dose of buphenine hydrochloride was 3 to 12 mg by mouth three or four times daily.

An intravenous infusion of buphenine hydrochloride has been used to arrest premature labour. It has also been given orally as a prophylactic tocolytic agent.

Preparations

Proprietary Preparations (details are given in Part 3)
Aust.: Dilatol; Dilydrin; ***Canad.:*** Arlidin; ***Ger.:*** Dilatol†; Penitardon†; ***S.Afr.:*** Dilatol†; ***Spain:*** Diatolil; ***Switz.:*** Dilydrine Retard; Tocodrine; ***USA:*** Arlidin†.

Multi-ingredient: ***Aust.:*** Apoplectal; Arbid; Dilaescol; Dilatol-Chinin; Opino; Tropoderm; ***Belg.:*** Agyrax; ***Fr.:*** Ophtadil; Phlebogel; ***Ger.:*** Apoplectal N; Arbid†; opino heparinoid†; opino N spezial; Rhinoinfant†; ***Ital.:*** Opino†; ***Spain:*** Circovenil; Circovenil Fuerte; Spasmo-Urgenin Rectal†; ***Switz.:*** Arbid; Symfona†; Visaline.

Butinoline Phosphate (11282-a)

Butinoline Phosphate *(rINNM)*.

1,1-Diphenyl-4-pyrrolidino-1′-yl but-2-yn-l-ol phosphate.

$C_{20}H_{21}NO,H_3PO_4$ = 389.4.
CAS — 54118-66-0 (butinoline phosphate); 968-63-8 (butinoline).

Butinoline phosphate is used as an antispasmodic in preparations for gastro-intestinal disorders.

Preparations

Proprietary Preparations (details are given in Part 3)

Multi-ingredient: ***Aust.:*** Spasmo-Solugastril; ***Ger.:*** Azulon compositum Homburg†; Jasicholin N; Spasmo-Nervogastrol; Spasmo-Solugastril.

Butyl Nitrite (12483-l)

$C_4H_9NO_2$ = 103.1.

Butyl nitrite is not used medicinally but, as with other volatile nitrites, is abused for its vasodilating and related effects following inhalation (see p.974).

Cadmium (1596-x)

Cd = 112.411.
CAS — 7440-43-9.

Cadmium is employed in a wide range of manufacturing processes and cadmium poisoning presents a recognised industrial hazard. Inhalation of cadmium fume during welding procedures may not produce symptoms until 4 to 10 hours have passed and these symptoms include respiratory distress leading to pulmonary oedema; kidney toxicity is also a feature of cadmium poisoning. Ingestion of cadmium or its salts has the additional hazard of severe gastro-intestinal effects. Cadmium has a long biological half-life and accumulates in body tissues, particularly the liver and kidneys. Chelation therapy is not generally recommended for cadmium poisoning; although *animal* studies have suggested that chelators may be effective in acute poisoning they do not increase cadmium elimination in chronic poisoning and administration of dimercaprol may increase cadmium toxicity. Chronic exposure to cadmium results in progressive renal insufficiency.

Cadmium sulphide has been used topically in some countries for the treatment of skin conditions. Cadmium sulphate has been included in some preparations for the treatment of eye irritation.

The toxicity of cadmium has been reviewed.[1] Environmental or occupational exposure to cadmium has been associated with renal dysfunction,[2-4] and fatalities due to industrial exposure or self-poisoning have also been reported.[5,6] No effect on testicular endocrine function was observed in 77 industrial workers exposed to cadmium.[3]

1. Fielder RJ, Dale EA. Cadmium and its compounds. *Toxicity Review 7*. London: HMSO, 1983.
2. Buchet JP, *et al.* Renal effects of cadmium body burden of the general population. *Lancet* 1990; **336:** 699–702. Correction. *ibid.* 1991; **337:** 1554.
3. Mason HJ. Occupational cadmium exposure and testicular endocrine function. *Hum Exp Toxicol* 1990; **9:** 91–4.
4. Cai S, *et al.* Renal dysfunction from cadmium contamination of irrigation water: dose-response analysis in a Chinese population. *Bull WHO* 1998; **76:** 153–9.
5. Taylor A, *et al.* Poisoning with cadmium fumes after smelting lead. *Br Med J* 1984; **288:** 1270–1.
6. Buckler HM, *et al.* Self poisoning with oral cadmium chloride. *Br Med J* 1986; **292:** 1559–60. Correction. *ibid.*; **293:** 236.

Malignant neoplasms. An increased incidence of cancer of the prostate has been reported in subjects exposed to high levels of cadmium but the evidence is not conclusive.[1] There may be an association between cadmium exposure and lung cancer, although observations on this type of cancer are difficult to interpret because of exposure to other hazards such as smoking.

1. Bell GM. Carcinogenicity of cadmium and its compounds. *Toxicity Review 24*. London: HMSO, 1991.

Preparations

Proprietary Preparations (details are given in Part 3)
Spain: Biocadmio.

Multi-ingredient: ***Aust.:*** Ichtho-Cadmin; ***Fr.:*** Visiolyre; ***Ger.:*** Ichtho-Cadmin†; ***Switz.:*** Cadmiofrine†; Ichtho-Cadmin†.

Cajuput Oil (4616-s)

Cajeput Oil; Cajuput Essence; Oleum Cajuputi.

A colourless, yellow, or green volatile oil with an agreeable camphoraceous odour and a bitter, aromatic, camphoraceous taste, obtained by distillation from the fresh leaves and twigs of *Melaleuca cajuputi* (*M. leucadendron*) (Myrtaceae). It contains cineole. **Store** in a cool place in airtight containers. Protect from light.

Cajuput oil obtained from the leaves of *Melaleuca cajuputi* contained about 10% of a crystalline phenolic compound 3,5-dimethyl-4,6-di-*O*-methylphloroacetophenone ($C_{12}H_{16}O_4$).[1] This would explain its reputed antiseptic properties and the green colour due to chelation of copper distillation vessels.

1. Lowry JB. A new constituent of biogenetic, pharmacological and historical interest from Melaleuca cajeputi oil. *Nature* 1973; **241:** 61–2.

Cajuput oil has been applied externally as a stimulant and mild rubefacient in rheumatism. It is also used with other volatile agents in preparations for the relief of respiratory congestion. It has been given internally as a carminative.

Niaouli oil (p.1607) is also prepared from *Melaleuca* spp.

Preparations

Proprietary Preparations (details are given in Part 3)

Multi-ingredient: ***Aust.:*** Babix; Luuf-Heilpflanzenol; Tiger Balsam Rot; ***Austral.:*** Capsolin†; Methyl Salicylate Ointment Compound; Tiger Balm Red; Tiger Balm White; ***Belg.:*** Vegebom†; ***Canad.:*** Broncho Rub; Capsolin†; Penetrating Rub; Tiger Balm Red; Tiger Balm White; ***Fr.:*** Balseptol†; Phytocoltar†; Tuberol†; Vegebom; ***Ger.:*** Kalantol-A†; Kalantol-B†; Liniplant; Palatol; Palatol N; Palatol†; Segmentocut†; ***Ital.:*** Kindian†; Otosan Gocce Auricolari; ***Neth.:*** Tijgerbalsem†; ***Switz.:*** Frigoplasma; Olbas; ***UK:*** Olbas; Penetrol; Tiger Balm Liquid; Tiger Balm Red; Tiger Balm White; ***USA:*** Dermal-Rub; Ponaris†.

Calamus (525-x)

Acore Vrai; Calamus Rhizome; Kalmus; Sweet Flag Root.
CAS — 8015-79-0 (calamus oil).
Pharmacopoeias. In Aust. and Swiss.

The dried rhizome of the sweet flag, *Acorus calamus* (Araceae).

Calamus has been used as a bitter and carminative; it is also used as a source of calamus oil which is employed in perfumery. In the USA the FDA has prohibited marketing calamus as a food or food additive; the oil (Jammu variety) is reported to be a carcinogen.

Preparations

Proprietary Preparations (details are given in Part 3)

Multi-ingredient: ***Aust.:*** Abdomilon†; Bio-Garten Tee fur Leber und Galle; Leber- und Galletee; Mag Kottas Magen-Darmtee; Sidroga Magen-Darm-Tee; ***Belg.:*** Roter†; ***Fr.:*** Caved-S†; Depuratum; Jouvence de l'Abbe Soury; ***Ger.:*** "Mletzko" Tropfen†; Abdomilon N; Aureal†; Azupanthenol†; Friosmin†; Gallexier; Gastrol S; Grunlicht Hingfong Essenz; Hevert-Gall S; Hevert-Magen-Galle-Leber-Tee; Majocarmin mite†; Majocarmin†; Montana; Presselin 214†; Sedovent; Stacho N†; Stoffwechseldragees†; Stomasal Med; Stomasal†; Stovalid N; ventri-loges; ***Ital.:*** Amaro Maffioli†; Frerichs Maldifassi; Pillole Frerichs Maldifassi†; ***Spain:*** Caved-S; Kneipp Pildoras†; Melisana†; Roter Complex; Roter†; ***Switz.:*** Caved-S; Kernosan Elixir; Tisane gastrique "H"†; Tisane pour l'estomac; Urinex (nouvelle formule).

Calcium Carbimide (2732-x)

Calcium Carbimide *(rINN).*
Calcium Cyanamide; Cyanamide.
$CCaN_2$ = 80.1.
CAS — 156-62-7 (calcium carbimide); 8013-88-5 (citrated calcium carbimide).

NOTE. The name cyanamide is also used to designate carbimide, which is used in veterinary medicine.

Adverse Effects and Precautions

Calcium carbimide may cause drowsiness, dizziness, fatigue, skin rash, tinnitus, mental depression, impotence, and urinary frequency. There may be a reversible increase in the white cell count. It should be used with caution in patients with asthma, coronary artery disease, or myocardial disease. Calcium carbimide causes a reaction in patients who have consumed alcohol similar to that seen with disulfiram (see p.1573).

Effects on the heart. Hypotension and tachycardia were reported during the carbimide-alcohol reaction.[1]

1. Peachey JE, *et al.* Cardiovascular changes during the calcium carbimide-ethanol interaction. *Clin Pharmacol Ther* 1981; **29:** 40–6.

Effects on the liver. Reports[1,2] of hepatic lesions in patients receiving calcium carbimide.

1. Vázquez JJ, Cervera S. Cyanamide-induced liver injury in alcoholics. *Lancet* 1980; **i:** 361–2.
2. Moreno A, *et al.* Structural hepatic changes associated with cyanamide treatment: cholangiolar proliferation, fibrosis and cirrhosis. *Liver* 1984; **4:** 15–21.

Uses and Administration

Calcium carbimide has actions and uses similar to those of disulfiram (p.1573). It is an aversive agent used as an adjunct in the treatment of chronic alcoholism (p.1099). An alcohol challenge reaction will occur between 9 and 15 hours after administration of calcium carbimide. It is given in doses of 50 to 100 mg twice daily by mouth. Citrated calcium carbimide has been used similarly.

A comparative review of the alcohol deterrents calcium carbimide and disulfiram.[1] Both drugs inhibit aldehyde dehydrogenase to produce raised acetaldehyde concentrations in the blood, and the ensuing adverse reaction, when alcohol is consumed during treatment. However, in *animals* inhibition with calcium carbimide is reported to be maximal 1 to 2 hours after administration and aldehyde dehydrogenase activity restored to 80% of control activity within 24 hours, whereas disulfiram inhibition develops slowly over 12 hours and is irreversible with restoration of activity dependent on synthesis of new enzyme over several days. It has been assumed that calcium carbimide produces a less intense interaction with alcohol than disulfiram, but appreciable cardiovascular changes have been observed. Behavioural and some other effects associated with disulfiram have been attributed to its inhibition of dopamine-β-hydroxylase; calcium carbimide does not inhibit this enzyme.

1. Peachey JE, *et al.* A comparative review of the pharmacological and toxicological properties of disulfiram and calcium carbimide. *J Clin Psychopharmacol* 1981; **1:** 21–6.

Preparations

Proprietary Preparations (details are given in Part 3)
Aust.: Colme; ***Austral.:*** Dipsan†; ***Canad.:*** Temposil; ***Irl.:*** Abstem; ***Neth.:*** Dipsan†; ***S.Afr.:*** Dipsan†; ***Spain:*** Colme; ***Swed.:*** Dipsan†.

Calcium Dihydrogen Phosphate (1167-f)

Acid Calcium Phosphate; Calcium Dihydrogenphosphoricum; E341; Monobasic Calcium Phosphate; Monocalcium Phosphate. Calcium tetrahydrogen diorthophosphate monohydrate.
$Ca(H_2PO_4)_2,H_2O$ = 252.1.
CAS — 7758-23-8 (anhydrous calcium dihydrogen phosphate).
Pharmacopoeias. In *Jpn* and Swiss.

Calcium dihydrogen phosphate is used in fertilisers. It is also used as an antoxidant in baking powders and flours and as a source of calcium in some mineral supplement preparations.

Preparations

Proprietary Preparations (details are given in Part 3)

Multi-ingredient: ***Austral.:*** Hypol; ***Fr.:*** Marinol; Phosphoneuros.

Calcium Dobesilate (12506-m)

Calcium Dobesilate *(rINN).*
Calcii Dobesilas; Calcium Doxybenzylate; 205E. Calcium 2,5-dihydroxybenzenesulphonate.
$C_{12}H_{10}CaO_{10}S_2$ = 418.4.
CAS — 88-46-0 (dobesilic acid); 20123-80-2 (calcium dobesilate).
Pharmacopoeias. In *Eur.* (see p.viii) which specifies the monohydrate.

A white or almost white hygroscopic powder. Very **soluble** in water; freely soluble in dehydrated alcohol; very slightly soluble in isopropyl alcohol; practically insoluble in dichloromethane. A 10% solution in water has a pH of 4.5 to 6.0. **Store** in airtight containers. Protect from light.

Calcium dobesilate is claimed to reduce capillary permeability and has been used in various peripheral circulatory disorders including diabetic retinopathy and haemorrhoids. Gastro-intestinal disturbances have occurred with its use, and there are also reports of hypersensitivity reactions.

Calcium dobesilate is given by mouth in usual doses of 500 to 1000 mg daily in divided doses. It is also given rectally for haemorrhoids and is applied topically.

Effects on the blood. Agranulocytosis developed on 2 occasions in a woman following treatment with calcium dobesilate.[1]

1. Kulessa W, *et al.* Wiederholte agranulozytose nach einnahme von calciumdobesilat. *Dtsch Med Wochenschr* 1992; **117:** 372–4.

Preparations

Proprietary Preparations (details are given in Part 3)
Aust.: Doxium; ***Belg.:*** Doxium; ***Fr.:*** Doxium; ***Ger.:*** Dexium; Dobica; ***Ital.:*** Dobesifar†; Doxium; ***Spain:*** Doxium; ***Switz.:*** Doxium.

Multi-ingredient: ***Aust.:*** Doxiproct mit Dexamethason†; Doxiproct†; ***Ital.:*** Doxiproct Plus; Doxiproct†; Doxivenil†; ***Spain:*** Acnisdin; Acnisdin Retinoico; Ederal; Proctium; ***Switz.:*** Doxiproct; Doxiproct Plus; Doxivenil.

Calcium Fluoride (12507-b)

CaF_2 = 78.07.
CAS — 7789-75-5.
Pharmacopoeias. In *Ger.*

Calcium fluoride is used similarly to sodium fluoride (p.742) for the prevention of dental caries. Calcium fluoride is also used as a source of calcium.

Native calcium fluoride (Calcarea Fluorica; Calc. Fluor.) is used in homoeopathic medicine.

Preparations

Proprietary Preparations (details are given in Part 3)

Multi-ingredient: ***Austral.:*** Cirflo†; ***Fr.:*** Fluopate; ***Ger.:*** Calcipot F†; ***Spain:*** Calcio Faes DYC; ***UK:*** New Era Elasto.

Calcium Hopantenate (12509-g)

Calcium Hopantenate *(rINNM).*
Calcium Homopantothenate. The hemihydrate of the calcium salt of D(+)-4-(2,4-dihydroxy-3,3-dimethylbutyramido)butyric acid.
$Ca(C_{10}H_{18}NO_5)_2,\frac{1}{2}H_2O$ = 513.6.
CAS — 18679-90-8 (hopantenic acid); 17097-76-6 (anhydrous calcium hopantenate).

Calcium hopantenate is a homologue of pantothenic acid (p.1352) and has been tried in the treatment of various behavioural and extrapyramidal disorders. Its use is limited by severe metabolic side-effects and fatalities have been reported.

Calcium Hydroxide (204-m)

526; Calcii Hydroxidum; Calcium Hydrate; Slaked Lime.
$Ca(OH)_2$ = 74.09.
CAS — 1305-62-0.
Pharmacopoeias. In *Eur.* (see p.viii), *Jpn*, and *US*.

A fine white powder with a slightly bitter alkaline taste.

Ph. Eur. **solubility** is: practically insoluble in water. USP solubilities are: soluble 1 in 630 of water, and 1 in 1300 of boiling water; soluble in glycerol and in syrup; insoluble in alcohol. A solution in water is alkaline to phenolphthalein and readily absorbs carbon dioxide.

Store in airtight containers.

Calcium hydroxide is a weak alkali. It is used in the form of Calcium Hydroxide Solution (lime water) in some skin lotions and oily preparations to form calcium soaps of fatty acids which produce water-in-oil emulsions.

Calcium hydroxide pastes are used in dentistry. A paste made from a mixture of calcium hydroxide and potassium hydroxide and known as Vienna paste was used as an escharotic. Soda lime (p.1630) is a mixture of calcium hydroxide and potassium hydroxide and/or sodium hydroxide.

For the use of disodium edetate in treatment of lime burns of the eye, see p.980.

Preparations

BP 1998: Calcium Hydroxide Solution *(Lime Water)*; ***USP 23:*** Calcium Hydroxide Topical Solution.

Proprietary Preparations (details are given in Part 3)
Ger.: Dermi-cyl; ***Ital.:*** Stomidros.

Multi-ingredient: ***Belg.:*** Oxyplastine; ***Spain:*** Balsamo BOI†; Cremsol; ***Swed.:*** Calasept†; ***Switz.:*** Calcipulpe.

Calcium Oxide (12510-f)

529; Calcium Oxydatum; Calx; Calx Usta; Chaux Vive; Gebrannter Kalk; Lime; Quicklime.

CaO = 56.08.

CAS — 1305-78-8.

Pharmacopoeias. In *Belg., Jpn, Pol., Swiss,* and *US.*

Hard, odourless, white or greyish-white masses, granules, or powder. When it is moistened with water a reaction occurs, heat being evolved and calcium hydroxide formed. Slightly **soluble** in water, very slightly soluble in boiling water. **Store** in airtight containers.

Adverse Effects and Treatment

Calcium oxide may cause burns on contact with moist skin and mucous membranes; it is particularly irritant to the eyes. Washing or flooding of affected areas may need to be prolonged. Pneumonitis may follow inhalation.

For the use of disodium edetate in treatment of lime burns of the eye, see p.980.

Uses and Administration

Calcium oxide has been used in various dermatological preparations. With sulphur it forms sulphurated lime (p.1091). A paste made from a mixture of calcium oxide and sodium hydroxide and known as London paste was used as an escharotic.

Preparations

Proprietary Preparations (details are given in Part 3)
Ital.: Stomylex†.

Multi-ingredient: ***UK:*** Mijex.

Calcium Saccharate (1163-a)

Calcium Saccharate *(rINN).*

Calcii Saccharas; Calcium D-Saccharate. Calcium D-glucarate tetrahydrate.

$C_6H_8CaO_8,4H_2O$ = 320.3.

CAS — 5793-88-4 (anhydrous calcium saccharate); 5793-89-5 (calcium saccharate tetrahydrate).

Pharmacopoeias. In *US* which specifies the tetrahydrate.

A white, odourless, crystalline powder. Each g represents approximately 3.1 mmol of calcium. Calcium saccharate 8 g is approximately equivalent to 1 g of calcium. Very slightly **soluble** in cold water; slightly soluble in boiling water; very slightly soluble in alcohol; practically insoluble in chloroform and ether; soluble in dilute mineral acids and in solutions of calcium gluconate.

Calcium saccharate is employed as a stabilising agent in solutions of calcium gluconate for injection.

Preparations

Proprietary Preparations (details are given in Part 3)

Multi-ingredient: ***Ger.:*** Calciject†; Calcitrans; Calcium Braun; Calcium Truw; Calcium Verla; Calcium-Gluconicum-Losung Phytopharma†; ***S.Afr.:*** Sabax Calcium†; ***Switz.:*** C-Calcium.

Calcium Sulphate (1165-x)

516; Calcii Sulfas; Calcium Sulfate; Gypsum (dihydrate).

$CaSO_4$ = 136.1.

CAS — 7778-18-9 (anhydrous calcium sulphate); 10101-41-4 (calcium sulphate dihydrate).

Pharmacopoeias. In *Chin., Eur.* (see p.viii), *Int.,* and *Jpn* which specify the dihydrate. Also in *USNF* which specifies the dihydrate or the anhydrous material.

A white to yellowish-white odourless fine powder. Ph. Eur. **solubilities** are: very slightly soluble in water; practically insoluble in alcohol. USP solubilities are: soluble 1 in 375 of water and 1 in 485 of boiling water; practically insoluble in alcohol.

Calcium sulphate is used as an excipient for the preparation of tablets or capsules.

Preparations

Proprietary Preparations (details are given in Part 3)
Austral.: Celloids CS 36.

Multi-ingredient: ***Austral.:*** Duo Celloid CSIP†; ***Ger.:*** Durasol-Badesalz†; ***Switz.:*** Sulfoxyl†; ***UK:*** New Era Hymosa.

Dried Calcium Sulphate (1166-r)

Calcii Sulfas Hemihydricus; Calcined Gypsum; Calcium Sulfuricum ad Usum Chirurgicum; Calcium Sulphuricum Ustum; Exsiccated Calcium Sulphate; Gebrannter Gips; Gêsso; Gypsum Siccatum; Plaster of Paris; Plâtre Cuit; Sulphate of Lime; Yeso Blanco.

$CaSO_4,\frac{1}{2}H_2O$ = 145.1.

CAS — 7778-18-9 (anhydrous calcium sulphate); 10034-76-1 (calcium sulphate hemihydrate); 26499-65-0 (calcium sulphate hemihydrate).

Pharmacopoeias. In *Aust., Br., Ger.,* and *Jpn.*

A white or almost white, odourless or almost odourless hygroscopic powder. The BP permits the presence of suitable setting accelerators or decelerators. Slightly **soluble** in water; more soluble in dilute mineral acids; practically insoluble in alcohol.

Dried calcium sulphate is used for the preparation of Plaster of Paris Bandage which is used for the immobilisation of limbs and fractures. It is also employed for making dental casts.

Preparations

Proprietary Preparations (details are given in Part 3)
Fr.: Biplatrix; Gypsona†; Platrix†.

Calumba (526-r)

Calumba Root; Colombo.

Pharmacopoeias. In *Jpn.*

The dried root of *Jateorhiza palmata (=J. columba)* (Menispermaceae).

Calumba has been used as a bitter and as a flavouring agent.

Preparations

Proprietary Preparations (details are given in Part 3)

Multi-ingredient: ***Belg.:*** Richelet†; ***Fr.:*** Ducase; ***Ital.:*** Amaro Maffioli†; Bitteridina; ***Switz.:*** Padma-Lax; ***UK:*** Appetiser Mixture; Travel-Caps.

Camostat Mesylate (3922-e)

Camostat Mesilate *(pINNM)*; FOY-305. *N,N*-Dimethylcarbamoylmethyl 4-(4-guanidinobenzoyloxy)phenylacetate mesylate.

$C_{20}H_{22}N_4O_5,CH_4O_3S$ = 494.5.

CAS — 59721-28-7 (camostat); 59721-29-8 (camostat mesylate).

Pharmacopoeias. In *Jpn.*

Camostat is a protease inhibitor that has been given by mouth in the treatment of pancreatitis and postoperative reflux oesophagitis.

Preparations

Proprietary Preparations (details are given in Part 3)
Jpn: Foipan.

Camphor (263-j)

Alcanfor; 2-Camphanone; Camphora; Camphre Droit (natural); Camphre du Japon (natural); Cânfora; Kamfer. Bornan-2-one; 1,7,7-Trimethylbicyclo[2.2.1]heptan-2-one.

$C_{10}H_{16}O$ = 152.2.

CAS — 76-22-2; 464-49-3 (+); 464-48-2 (−); 21368-68-3 (±).

Pharmacopoeias. In *Chin., Eur.* (see p.viii), *Jpn, Pol.,* and *US*; some only describe natural camphor and some only synthetic camphor; *Jpn* has separate monographs for natural and racemic or synthetic camphor.

Camphor is a ketone obtained from *Cinnamomum camphora* (Lauraceae) and purified by sublimation, or it may be prepared synthetically. The natural product is dextrorotatory and the synthetic product is the optically inactive racemic form.

Colourless transparent or white crystals, crystalline masses, blocks, or powdery masses known as 'flowers of camphor', with a penetrating characteristic aromatic odour.

Soluble 1 in 800 of water, 1 in 1 of alcohol, 1 in 1 of ether, and 1 in 0.5 of chloroform; very slightly soluble in glycerol; freely soluble in fixed and volatile oils; very soluble in petroleum spirit. **Store** at a temperature not exceeding 25° in airtight containers.

A liquid or soft mass is formed when camphor is triturated with chloral hydrate, menthol, phenol, and many other substances. Camphor is readily powdered by triturating with a few drops of alcohol, ether, or chloroform. It volatilises at ordinary temperatures.

Adverse Effects

In addition to accidental ingestion of preparations containing camphor, poisoning has also occurred from administration of camphorated oil (camphor liniment) to children in mistake for castor oil. The symptoms include nausea, vomiting, colic, headache, dizziness, a feeling of warmth, delirium, muscle twitching, epileptiform convulsions, depression of the central nervous system, and coma. Breathing is difficult and the breath has a characteristic odour; anuria may occur. Death from respiratory failure or status epilepticus may occur; fatalities in children have been recorded from 1 g. There have been reports of instant collapse in infants following the local application of camphor to their nostrils.

Treatment of Adverse Effects

Empty the stomach by gastric lavage. Administer a saline laxative and activated charcoal by mouth. Convulsions may be controlled by the slow intravenous administration of diazepam or, if necessary, a short-acting barbiturate such as thiopentone sodium. Haemodialysis with a lipid dialysate has been employed; the use of haemoperfusion, however, has been criticised.

Precautions

It is dangerous to place camphor, for instance as an ointment, into the nostrils of an infant. A small quantity applied in this way may cause immediate collapse.

Pharmacokinetics

Camphor is readily absorbed from all administration sites. It is hydroxylated in the liver to yield hydroxycamphor metabolites which are then conjugated with glucuronic acid and excreted in the urine. Camphor crosses the placenta.

Uses and Administration

Applied externally, camphor acts as a rubefacient and mild analgesic (see p.7) and is employed in liniments as a counter-irritant in fibrositis, neuralgia, and similar conditions. It is also an ingredient of many inhaled nasal decongestant preparations but it is of doubtful efficacy. The use of camphor liniment (camphorated oil) is discouraged because of its potential toxicity. It has been withdrawn from the market in both the UK and the USA. In the USA the concentration of camphor in preparations for external use may not exceed 11%.

Taken internally camphor has irritant and carminative properties and has been used as a mild expectorant. It has also been used in mixed preparations for cardiovascular disorders.

Camphor-related monoterpene compounds have been used in the treatment of urolithiasis, renal disorders, and urinary-tract infections, and also with menthol in combination with chenodeoxycholic acid as adjunct therapy for the dispersal of bile duct stones.

It has been recommended by the Committee on the Review of Medicines[1] that camphor should not be included in products intended for the treatment of hepatic and biliary disorders, gallstones, colic, renal disorders, urinary tract infections, or ureteral stones. The administration of camphor parenterally or as irrigants was undesirable due to the associated safety hazard.

1. Anonymous. Camphorated oil: licensing authority takes action on camphor products. *Pharm J* 1984; **232:** 792.

Preparations

BP 1998: Camphorated Opium Tincture *(Paregoric)*; Concentrated Camphor Water; Concentrated Camphorated Opium Tincture; ***USP 23:*** Camphor Spirit; Camphorated Parachlorophenol; Flexible Collodion.

Proprietary Preparations (details are given in Part 3)
Austral.: Campholinct†; ***Fr.:*** Camphrice Du Canada; ***Ger.:*** Camphoderm N; Divinal Rheuma; Mulmicor; Pectocor N; Rheunervol N; Trauma-Salbe Rodler 303 N; ***Ital.:*** Resina Carbolica Dentilin.

Multi-ingredient: ***Aust.:*** Asthma-Frenon; Baby Luuf; Bronchiplant; Bronchostop; Caladryl; Carl Baders Divinal; Cehasol; China; Claim; Colda; Corodyn; DDD; Derivon; Dolex; Dolothricin; Dracodermalin; Emser Nasensalbe; Endrine mild†; Endrine†; Erkaltungsbalsam; Euka; Expectal-Balsam; Forapin; Igitur-antirheumatische; Igitur-Rheumafluid†; Inno Rheuma; Isosal; Kinder Luuf; Leukona-Rheuma-Bad; Luuf Balsam; Makatussin; Mayfit akut; Mediplant; Mediplant Inhalations; Medizinalbad†; Mentopin; Neo-Phlogicid; Pe-Ce; Perozon Erkaltungsbad; Piniment; Pinimenthol†; Piniol†; Pulmex†; Red Point†; Resol; Rheumasan†; Rhinospray Plus; Rowalind; Rubizon-Rheumagel; Rubriment; Salhumin; Scottopect; Spasmo Claim; Sulgan 99; Tetesept; Tiger Balsam Rot; Trafuril†; Tussamag; Tussimont; Wick Sinex; Wick Vaporub; ***Austral.:*** Alcusal Sport; Analgesic Rub†; Ayrton's Chilblain; Biosal; Blistex Medicated Lip Ointment; Bonnington's Irish Moss; Caladryl; Camphor Linctus Compound; Capsolin†; Cold Sore Cream†; Cold Sore Lotion†; Coso; Cremor Menthol†; Dencorub; Dentese†; Euky Bearub; Irish Moss Cough Syrup†; Logicin Chest Rub; Nyal Cold Sore; Painguard†; Quelfas A†; Radian-B; Rubesal; Sacsol; Sacsol NF; Sarna; Senamon†; Senega and Ammonia; Sigma Relief Chest Rub†; Solarub†; Tiger Balm Red; Tiger Balm White; Turpentine White Liniment; Vicks Inhaler; Vicks Sinex; Vicks Vaporub; Zam-Buk; ***Belg.:*** Beogaze; Campho-Pneumine†; Ebexol†; Endrine; Endrine

Doux; Eucalyptine Le Brun; Eucalyptine Pholcodine Le Brun; Inopectol†; Pelarol†; Pinthym†; Pulmex; Rado-Salil; Reflexspray; Revocyl†; Vegebom†; Vicks Vaporub; Ysol†; ***Canad.:*** Absorbine Analgesic; Anbesol; Antiphlogistine Rub A-535; Aurisan; Balminil Nasal Ointment; Baume Analgesique; Baume Analgesique Medicamente; Ben-Gay Ultra; Blistex DCT Lip Balm; Blistex Lip Ointment; Blistex Medicated Lip Conditioner Jar; Blistex Medicated Lip Conditioner Tube; Boil Ease; Broncho Rub; Bronchodex Vapo; Bronco Asmol; Buckley's Mixture; Buckley's White Rub; Bunion Salve; Cal Mo Dol; Camphre Compose; Capsolin†; Carmatis; Chapstick Medicated Lip Balm; Cherry Chest Rub; Cold Sore Lotion; Creo Grippe; Creo-Rectal; Demo-Cineol; Dentalgar; Eptico; Gouttes Dentaires; Gouttes pour Mal d'Orreilles; Heet; Ingrown Toe Nail Salve; Jack & Jill Rub; Kinot; Kiro Rub; Lip Medex; Lotion pour Feux Sauvages; Marco Rub Camphorated; Marco Rub Camphorated Ointment; Mecca; Medi-Quik; Medicated Analgesic Cream; Medicated Chest Rub; Mentholatum Extra Strength Ointment; Mentholatum Ointment; Minard's Liniment; MRX; Noivy; Oralgar; Pain Buster; Pommade au The des Bois; Rheumalan; Rheumatisme; Sarna-P; Savex; Savex 15; Savex with PABA; Savex with Sunscreen; Sea Breeze; SH-206; Therapeutic Soothing Ice; Thermo-Gel; Thunas Salve for Rheumatic Pains; Tiger Balm Red; Tiger Balm White; Triaminic Night Time Rub; Vap Air; Vaporisateur Medicamente; Vaporizing Colds Rub; Vaporizing Ointment; Vicks Inhaler; Vicks Vaporub; Webber Antibiotic Cold Sore Ointment; ***Fr.:*** Balsofletol†; Baume Disalgyl†; Baume du Tigre†; Baume Saint-Bernard; Bi-Qui-Nol; Biocarde; Biphedrine Huileuse†; Bismurectol; Campho-Pneumine; Capsic; Circulatonic; Coquelusedal; Disalgyl; Ephydrol; Eucalyptine Le Brun; Eucalyptine Pholcodine; Eutalgic; Euvanol; Inongan; Kamol; Laccoderme Dalibour†; Lao-Dal; Lumbalgine; Mysca†; Paps; Paregorique; Pectoderme; Pholcones; Pholcones Bismuth-Quinine†; Pholcones Guaiphenesine-Quinine†; Pinorhinol; Pulmax; Rectophedrol; Sedartryl; Sinex; Tigidol; Valda Septol; Vegebom; Vicks Pastilles†; Vicks Vaporub; Vicks vitamine C pastilles†; Ysol 206; ***Ger.:*** A + B Balsam N; Akne-Medice Kombipackung†; Anastil N; Anastil†; Anginasin N; Angocin percutan; Arnika-Balsam†; Arthrodestal N; Arthrodynat P; Aspecton-Balsam; Asthma-Frenon-S†; Bartelin N; Bormelin†; Bronchicum Balsam mit Eukalyptusol; Broncholind Balsam†; Camphopin; Capsamol; Cardaminol†; Cardiagen; Cardisetten†; Cefarheumin N; Cobed†; Concardisett†; Cor-Select; Cor-Vel; Denosol; Dermalid†; Divinal-Broncho-Balsam; Dolo-Menthoneurin CreSa; Dolorsan-Balsam; Dorex Hustensaft N mit Oxeladin†; Dracodermalin†; Emser Balsam echt†; Emser Erkaltungsgel; Emser Nasensalbe N; Endrine mild†; Endrine†; Erkaltungsbalsam-ratiopharm E; Euflux-N; Expectal Balsam†; Extropin†; Franzbranntwein; Glutisal-buton-Salbe†; Goldtropfen-Hetterich; Grune Nervensalbe†; Grunlicht Hingfong Essenz; Guakalin†; Guttacor-Balsam N; Heilit; Heilit Rheuma-Bad N-Kombi†; Heilit Rheuma-Olbad; Hocura-Spondylose novo; Hyperiagil†; Hypotonin†; Influsanbalm†; Infrotto†; Iosimitan†; Jossathromb†; Kalantol-B†; Keldrin†; Kelofibrase; Kneipp Erkaltungsbad Spezial; Kneipp Herzsalbe Unguentum Cardiacum Kneipp; Kneipp Kreislauf-Bad Rosmarin-Aquasan; Kneipp Latschernkiefer Franzbranntwein; Korodin; Koryn mild†; Koryn†; Kyaugutt N†; Laryngsan N; Latschenkiefer Franzbranntwein; Leukona-Kreislauf-Bad; Leukona-Rheumasalbe; Leukona-Sauna-Konzentrat†; Leukona-Tonikum-Bad†; Logomed Erkaltungs-Balsam; Lyobalsam; Lyobalsam N ohne Menthol†; Lyobalsam N†; Marament Balsam W; Mediment†; Mentholon Original N; Monapax N†; Mucidan†; Myonasan†; Nasenol-ratiopharm†; Nasivin Intensiv-Bad N; Nasivin Intensiv-Balsam†; Nervfluid S; Optipect mit Kodein†; Optipect N; Optipect Neo; Optipect†; Pectolitan mit Codein†; Phardol N Balsam†; Phlebex†; Pinimenthol Bad N; Piniol N; Pinoidal-Bad†; Plantmobil; Pro-Pecton Balsam†; Pulmotin-N; Rectosellan N†; Retterspitz Quick; Rheubalmin Bad; Rheubalmin Thermo; Rheuma Bad; Rheuma-Salbe Lichtenstein; Rheumaliment N; Rheumaliment†; Rheumasan†; Rhinotussal E Balsam†; Rhinotussal S Balsam†; Risocon†; Riwa Franzbranntwein; Rowalind; Rubriment-N; Salhumin Gel N; Sanato-Rhev; Schupps Heilkrauter Rheumabad; Schwedentrunk; Schwedentrunk mit Ginseng; Schwefel-Diasporal; Segmentocut†; Silvapin Franzbranntwein†; Spondylon; Stas Erkaltungs-Salbe; Steinhoff's Fluid Esco Pin†; Tachynerg N; Terbintil†; Thermosenex; Thymipin N; Thymitussin†; Transpulmin E; Transpulmin†; Trauma-Salbe Rodler 301 N; Trauma-Salbe Rodler 302 N; Tumarol-N; Tussipect; Vaxicum N; Vipracutan†; Vipratox; Wick Inhalierstift N; Wick Vaporub; Zynedo-B†; Zynedo-K†; ***Irl.:*** Caladryl; Purporent†; Radian-B; Rowalind; Vicks Inhaler; Vicks Vaporub; ***Ital.:*** Abiostil; Balsamico F. di M.†; Balsamo Italstadium; Bronchenolo Balsamo†; Bronco Valda†; Broncopulmin; Capsolin; Cloristamina†; Disalgil; Donatiol; Efedrocanfine†; Eucalipto Composto; Kindian†; Linimento Bertelli†; Neo Eubalsamina†; Remy; Rinogutt Eucalipto-Fher; Rinostil; Salonpas; Termobalsamo†; Transpulmina Gel†; Transpulmina Tosse; Vegetallumina; Vicks Gola†; Vicks Inalante; Vicks Sinex; Vicks Vaporub; ***Neth.:*** Bronchoforton†; Dampo; Rhinocaps; Sloan's balsem; Sloan's liniment†; Tijgerbalsem†; Tijgerolie†; Vicks Sinex; Vicks Vaporub; ***Norw.:*** Allcocks Plaster†; ***S.Afr.:*** Caladryl; Docrub; Histamed; Radian; Zam-Buk; ***Spain:*** Acnosan; Aerospray Analgesico†; Amidoyina†; Analgesico Ut Asens Fn; Balsamo Analgesic Karmel; Balsamo Germano†; Bartal†; Bellacanfor†; Bronquimar; Bronquimar Vit A; Brota Rectal Bals; Caladryl; Dentol Topico; Dimayon; Dolokey; Edusan Fte Rectal; Halogedol; Homocodeina Timol†; Inhalador; Killpan; Kneipp Balsamo; Lapiz Termo Compositum†; Liderflex; Linimento Klari; Linimento Naion; Linimento Sloan; Maboterpen; Masagil; Mentobox; Mentol Sedans Sulfamidad†; Mostazola†; Pastillas Vicks Mentol†; Pinimenthol†; Pomada Balsamica; Pomada Revulsiva; Porosan†; Pulmo Grey Balsam; Radio Salil; Reflex; Respir Balsamico; Sartol; Sinus Inhalaciones; Termosan; Vicks Inhalador; Vicks Spray; Vicks Vaporub; Vitavox Pastillas; Xibornol Prodes; ***Swed.:*** Trafuril†; Vicks Vaporub; ***Switz.:*** Alginex†; Alphastria; Anginol; Artragel; Asba; Asphaline; Baume de Chine Temple of Heaven blanc; Bisolvex; Brachialin†; Bronchol N; Caladryl; Caprisana; Capsolin; Carmol "blanche"†; Carmol "thermogene"†; Carmol†; Collyre Alpha; Cresophene; Demo baume; Demo pommade contre les refroidissements; Dental-Phenjoca; Dolo-Arthrosenex; Dolorex; Embropax; Forapin†; Fortalis; Frigoplasma; Furodermal; Histacyl Cutane†; Huile analgesique "Polar-Bar"; Incutin; Kernosan Huile de Massage; Kreuzlinger Klosterliniment; Liberol; Makatussin; Makatussin forte; Marament-N; Massorax; Methylan†; Mirocor†; Nasello; Neo-Liniment†; Pate Iodoforme du Prof Dr Walkhoff; Phlogantine†; Pinimenthol; Pirom; Pommade nasale Ruedi; Pulmex; Rapura; Resorbane; Roliwol; Roliwol B; Sloan Baume; Sloan Liniment; Solin S†; Solution ChKM du Prof Dr Walkhoff; Spirogel; Sportusal Spray sine heparino; Sulgan; Tumarol; Vicks Inhaler N; Vicks Sinex; Vicks Vaporub; ***UK:*** Aleevex; Antiseptic Throat Pastilles; Aspellin; Balmosa; Balto Foot Balm; Boots Vapour Rub; Caladryl; Catarrh Cream; Cold Sore Ointment†; Corn & Callous Removal Liquid; Dragon Balm; Flurex Inhalant†; Gonne Balm; Kleer Cream; Menthol and Wintergreen Heat Product†; Mentholatum Balm†; Mentholatum Nasal Inhaler; Nicobrevin; Nosor Nose Balm; PR Heat Spray; Radian-B; Salonair; Seal & Heal; Skintex; Sunspot; TCP; Tiger Balm Liquid; Tiger Balm Red; Tiger Balm White; Tixylix Inhalant; Vapour Rub; Venos Dry Cough; Venos Expectorant; Vicks Inhaler; Vicks Sinex; Vicks Vaporub; Zam-Buk†; ***USA:*** Anbesol; Arthricare Double Ice; Aveeno Anti-Itch; Babee; Banalg; Ben-Gay Ultra; Betuline; Blistex; Blistex Lip Balm; Boil Ease; Cala-gen; Calamatum; Campho-Phenique; Chapstick Medicated Lip Balm; Chiggerex; Dasin†; Deep-Down Rub; Dermal-Rub; Dermolin; Florida Sunburn Relief; Gordobalm; Heet; Lip Medex; Medacote; Medadyne†; Mentholatum Cherry Chest Rub; Mentholatum Natural Ice Lip Protectant; Mentholatum Ointment; MenthoRub; Methalgen; Mexsana; Minit-Rub; Musterole Extra; Nasal Jelly; Orabase Lip; Ostiderm; Pain X; Panalgesic Gold; Paralgesic; Pazo; Pfeiffer's Cold Sore; Rhuli Gel; Rhuli Spray; Sarna Anti-Itch; Soltice; Sports Spray†; Sting-Eze; Topic; Vicks Menthol Cough Drops; Vicks Vaporub; Ziradryl.

Camylofin Hydrochloride (5230-f)

Camylofin Hydrochloride *(rINNM)*.

Acamylophenine Hydrochloride; Camylofin Dihydrochloride. Isopentyl 2-(2-diethylaminoethylamino)-2-phenylacetate dihydrochloride.

$C_{19}H_{32}N_2O_2,2HCl = 393.4$.

CAS — 54-30-8 (camylofin); 5892-41-1 (camylofin hydrochloride).

Camylofin is used as an antispasmodic, usually in combination with other agents. It is usually used as the hydrochloride; the bis(noramidopyrine mesylate) and the sodium salts have also been used.

Overdosage. Ingestion of large doses of camylofin by two infants resulted in symptoms similar to those produced by opioid intoxication.[1] Both infants responded to treatment with naloxone.

1. Schvartsman S, *et al.* Camylofin intoxication reversed by naloxone. *Lancet* 1988; **ii:** 1246.

Preparations

Proprietary Preparations (details are given in Part 3)
S.Afr.: Avacan†.

Multi-ingredient: ***Aust.:*** Avamigran; Spasmo-Urolong; ***Fr.:*** Avafortan; ***Ger.:*** Spasmo-Urolong†; ***Switz.:*** Spasmo-Urolong†.

Cannabis (842-w)

Cáñamo Indiano; Cannab.; Cannabis Indica; Chanvre; Hanfkraut; Indian Hemp.

CAS — 8063-14-7.

NOTE. Cannabis has also been known as: Ait makhlif, Aliamba, Anassa, Anhascha, Assyuni, Bambalacha, Bambia, Bangi-Aku, Bango, Bangue, Bhang, Bhangaku, Canapa, Cangonha, Canhama, Cannacoro, Can-Yac, Caroçuda, Chur ganja, Chutras, Chutsao, Da-boa, Dacha, Dagga, Darakte-Bang, Diamba, Dirijo, Djamba, Djoma, Dokka, Donajuanita, Dormilona, Durijo, Elva, Erva maligna, Erva do norte, Esrar, Fêmea, Fininha, Finote, Fokkra, Fumo brabo, Fumo de caboclo, Gandia, Ganga, Ganja, Ganjila, Gnaoui, Gongo, Gozah, Grahni Sherdool, Greefe, Grifa, Guabza, Guaza, Gunjah, Gunza, Hamp, Haouzi, Hen-Nab, Hursini, Hashish, Igbo, Indische-hennepkruid, Indisk hampa, Intianhamppu, Intsangu, Isangu, Janjah, Jatiphaladya churna, Jea, Juana, Kanab, Karpura rasa, Khanh-Chha, Khanje, Kif, Kif Ktami, Kinnab, Liamba, Lianda, Maconha, Maconia, Madi, Magiyam, Makhlif, Malva, Maraguango, Marajuana, Marigongo, Marihuana, Marijuana, Mariquita, Maruamba, Matekwane, Mbanje, Meconha, Misari, Mnoana, Momea, Mota, Mulatinha, Mundyadi vatika, Namba, Ntsangu, Nwonkaka, Peinka, Penek, Penka, Pito, Pot, Pretinha, Rafe, Rafi, Rafo, Riamba, Rongony, Rora, Rosa Maria, Sabsi, Sadda, Siddhi, Soñadora, Soussi, Subji, Summitates cannabis, Suruma, Tahgalim, Takrouri, Tedrika, Teloeut, Teriaki, Tronadora, Umya, Urumogi, Wee, Wewe, Yamba, Yoruba, Zacate chino, Zerouali, and Ziele konopi indyjskich.

Synonyms and approximate synonyms for cannabis resin included: Bheng, Charas, Charris, Chira, Churrus, Chus, Garaouich, Garawiche, Garoarsch, Gauja, Hachiche, Hascisc, Hashish, Hasis, Hasji's, Hasjisj, Haszysz, Haxixe, Heloua, Kamonga, Malak, Manzul, Momeka, N'rama, and Sighirma.

Pharmacopoeias. In *Chin.*

The dried flowering or fruiting tops of the pistillate plant of *Cannabis sativa* (Cannabinaceae). In the UK cannabis is defined by law as any part of any plant of the genus *Cannabis*. *Marihuana* usually refers to a mixture of the leaves and flowering tops. *Bhang, dagga, ganja, kif,* and *maconha* are commonly used in various countries to describe similar preparations. *Hashish* and *charas* are names often applied to the resin, although in some countries *hashish* is applied to any cannabis preparation.

A series of cannabinoids has been extracted from the drug, the most important being Δ^9-tetrahydrocannabinol (dronabinol), Δ^8-tetrahydrocannabinol, Δ^9-tetrahydrocannabinolic acid, cannabinol, and cannabidiol. Cannabinol and cannabidiol may be present in large amounts but have little activity. The amount of Δ^9-tetrahydrocannabinol may average 1, 3, and 5% in marihuana, ganja, and hashish respectively.

Dependence

It has been reported that the prolonged heavy use of cannabis could lead to tolerance and psychic dependence but that physical dependence had not been demonstrated. There have been occasional reports of non-specific symptoms such as anorexia, anxiety, insomnia, irritability, restlessness, sweating, headache, and mild gastro-intestinal upsets occurring when cannabis is withdrawn.

Adverse Effects, Treatment, and Precautions

Nausea and vomiting may be the first effects of cannabis taken by mouth. The most frequent physical effects of cannabis intoxication are an increase in heart rate with alterations in blood-pressure, injected conjunctival vessels, dry mouth, and increased appetite. Deterioration in motor coordination is common and cannabis has been reported to affect driving. The psychological effects include elation, distortion of time and space, irritability, and disturbances of memory and judgement. Anxiety or panic reactions may occur, particularly in inexperienced users. These reactions do not usually require specific therapy; diazepam may be necessary for severe reactions. Psychotic episodes of a paranoid or schizophrenic nature, and usually acute, have occurred in subjects taking cannabis, especially in large doses or after the use of varieties bred for a high yield of cannabinoids (so-called skunk).

Some reviews of the adverse effects of cannabis.

1. Nahas GG. Cannabis: toxicological properties and epidemiological aspects. *Med J Aust* 1986; **145**: 82–7.
2. Johnson BA. Psychopharmacological effects of cannabis. *Br J Hosp Med* 1990; **43**: 114–22.
3. American Academy of Pediatrics. Marijuana: a continuing concern for pediatricians. *Pediatrics* 1991; **88**: 1070–2.
4. Wills S. Cannabis and cocaine. *Pharm J* 1993; **251:** 483–5.
5. Hall W, Solowij N. Adverse effects of cannabis. *Lancet* 1998; **352:** 1611–16.

Coma. Coma that was reversed by flumazenil has been reported in 2 children who had ingested cannabis.[1]

1. Rubio F, *et al.* Flumazenil for coma reversal in children after cannabis. *Lancet* 1993; **341:** 1028–9.

Effects on the eyes. A report of persistent visual abnormalities in a patient, following discontinuation of heavy abuse of hashish.[1] No organic cause for the effects, which were accompanied by less persistent mental changes, could be found.

1. Laffi GL, Safran AB. Persistent visual changes following hashish consumption. *Br J Ophthalmol* 1993; **77:** 601–2.

Hyperthermia. Life-threatening hyperthermia was reported[1] in a 24-year-old man who went jogging after smoking cannabis.

1. Walter FG, *et al.* Marijuana and hyperthermia. *J Toxicol Clin Toxicol* 1996; **34:** 217–21.

Pregnancy. Cannabis has effects on sperm and can alter reproductive hormonal systems. Infants born to mothers exposed to cannabis during pregnancy tend to have a lower birth-weight[1,2] and may suffer from increased excitation in the postnatal period.[3]

1. Zuckerman B, *et al.* Effects of maternal marijuana and cocaine use on fetal growth. *N Engl J Med* 1989; **320**: 762–8.
2. Frank DA, *et al.* Neonatal body proportionality and body composition after in utero exposure to cocaine and marijuana. *J Pediatr* 1990; **117:** 622–6.
3. Silverman S. Interaction of drug-abusing mother, fetus, types of drugs examined in numerous studies. *JAMA* 1989; **261**: 1689, 1693.

Psychosis. References to psychosis associated with cannabis.

1. Rottanburg D, *et al.* Cannabis-associated psychoses with hypomanic features. *Lancet* 1982; **ii:** 1364–6.
2. Andréasson S, *et al.* Cannabis and schizophrenia: a longitudinal study of Swedish conscripts. *Lancet* 1987; **ii**: 1483–6.
3. Wylie AS, *et al.* Psychosis due to "skunk". *Br Med J* 1995; **311:** 125.

Interactions

Cannabis and alcohol have additive effects. Additive antimuscarinic effects, for example tachycardia, may occur with concomitant use of drugs such as tricyclic antidepressants. Cannabis induces microsomal enzymes and therefore interactions with a wide range of drugs that are metabolised by these enzymes might be expected. See, for example, Theophylline, p.769.

Disulfiram. Limited evidence indicates that a combination of disulfiram and cannabis may produce a hypomanic state.[1]

1. Lacoursiere RB, Swatek R. Adverse interaction between disulfiram and marijuana: a case report. *Am J Psychiatry* 1983; **140:** 243–4.

Pharmacokinetics

The active principles of cannabis are absorbed from the gastro-intestinal tract and the lungs.

About 50% of the Δ^9-tetrahydrocannabinol available in cannabis is present in the smoke inhaled from a whole cannabis cigarette. This produces an effect almost immediately, reaches a peak in 20 to 30 minutes, and is dissipated in about 3 to 4 hours. When cannabis is taken by mouth absorption may be slow and irregular. Effects are not seen for 30 minutes to 1 hour and persist for about 8 hours.

Tetrahydrocannabinol is lipophilic and becomes widely distributed in the body. It crosses the placenta and is distributed into breast milk. It is extensively metabolised, primarily in the liver, to the active 11-hydroxy derivative; both are extensively bound to plasma proteins. It is excreted in the urine and faeces, sometimes over prolonged periods. Excretion may be more rapid in chronic users.

Uses and Administration

Cannabis was formerly employed as a sedative or narcotic. Its main active constituent Δ^9-tetrahydrocannabinol (dronabinol, p.1191) and a synthetic cannabinol (nabilone, p.1203) are used as antiemetics in patients receiving cancer chemotherapy; they are also being investigated for a number of other potential therapeutic uses. Cannabis has analgesic, muscle relaxant, and appetite stimulant effects and reduces intra-ocular pressure. Anecdotal reports exist of benefit from cannabis in a variety of disorders including glaucoma, multiple sclerosis, and wasting in patients with AIDS and malignant neoplasms.

References to the potential medical uses of cannabis.

1. Doyle E, Spence AA. Cannabis as a medicine? *Br J Anaesth* 1995; **74:** 359–61.
2. Gray C. Cannabis—the therapeutic potential. *Pharm J* 1995; **254:** 771–3.
3. Grinspoon L, Bakalar JB. Marihuana as a medicine: a plea for reconsideration. *JAMA* 1995; **273:** 1875–6.
4. Wills S. The use of cannabis in multiple sclerosis. *Pharm J* 1995; **225:** 237–8.
5. Voth EA, Schwartz RH. Medicinal applications of delta-9-tetrahydrocannabinol and marijuana. *Ann Intern Med* 1997; **126:** 791–8.
6. British Medical Association. *Therapeutic uses of cannabis.* Amsterdam: Harwood Academic, 1997.
7. Robson P. Cannabis as medicine: time for the phoenix to rise? *Br Med J* 1998; **316:** 1034–5.

Canola Oil (17665-l)

Canola oil is a form of rape oil (p.1624) from strains selected for low erucic acid content. It is used as an edible oil and in pharmaceutical manufacturing and cosmetics.

Cantharides (12517-g)

Blistering Beetle; Cantharis; Insectes Coléoptères Hétéromères; Lytta; Méloides; Russian Flies; Spanish Fly.

The dried beetle *Cantharis vesicatoria* (=*Lytta vesicatoria*) (Meloidae) or other spp., containing not less than 0.6% of cantharidin.

Adverse Effects

Following ingestion of cantharides there is burning pain in the throat and stomach, with difficulty in swallowing; nausea, vomiting, haematemesis, abdominal pain, bloody diarrhoea, and tenesmus; renal pain, frequent micturition, haematuria, uraemia; severe hypotension and circulatory failure. Oral doses of cantharidin (the active ingredient of cantharides) of less than 65 mg have been lethal. A dose of 1 mg or contact with one insect can produce distressing symptoms. Skin contact results in blisters.

References.

1. Hundt HKL, *et al.* Post-mortem serum concentration of cantharidin in a fatal case of cantharides poisoning. *Hum Exp Toxicol* 1990; **9**: 35–40.

Uses and Administration

Preparations of cantharides have been employed externally as rubefacients, counter-irritants, and vesicants. They should not be taken internally or applied over large surfaces owing to the risk of absorption. The use of cantharides in cosmetic products is prohibited in the UK by law.

Cantharides is used in homoeopathic medicine.

Mylabris (Chinese blistering beetle; Chinese cantharides; Indian blistering beetle), the dried beetles of the species *Mylabrus sidae* (= *M, phalerata*), *M. cichorii*, and *M. pustulator*, has been used as a substitute for cantharides and as a source of cantharidin (see below) in the East.

Preparations

Proprietary Preparations (details are given in Part 3)
Multi-ingredient: ***Spain:*** Frikton†.

Cantharidin (12518-q)

Hexahydro-3aα,7aα-dimethyl-4β,7β-epoxyisobenzofuran-1,3-dione.

$C_{10}H_{12}O_4$ = 196.2.
CAS — 56-25-7.

Cantharidin is obtained from cantharides or mylabris (see under Cantharides, above).

Cantharidin in flexible collodion has been applied for the removal of warts. It has also been used in veterinary medicine. Owing to the high toxicity of cantharidin it is recommended that preparations containing it should not be used medicinally. Adverse effects are those described for cantharides (see above).

Preparations

Proprietary Preparations (details are given in Part 3)
Canad.: Canthacur; Cantharone; ***USA:*** Cantharone†; Verr-Canth†.

Multi-ingredient: ***Canad.:*** Canthacur-PS; Cantharone Plus; ***USA:*** Cantharone Plus†; Verrusol†.

Capsicum (4617-w)

Capsic.; Capsici Fructus; Chillies; Piment Rouge; Pimentão; Spanischer Pfeffer.

CAS — 404-86-4 (capsaicin).

NOTE. Ground cayenne pepper of commerce is normally a blend of varieties. Paprika is from *Capsicum annuum* var. *longum*; it is milder than capsicum.

Pharmacopoeias. In Aust., Ger., It., Jpn, and Swiss.
US includes capsicum oleoresin.

The dried ripe fruits of *Capsicum annuum* var. *minimum* and small-fruited varieties of *C. frutescens* (Solanaceae). Some pharmacopoeias allow different varieties. It contains not less than 0.5% of the pungent principle capsaicin. **Store** in a cool dry place. Protect from light.

Capsicum Oleoresin (USP 23) is an alcoholic extract of capsicum. It is a dark red oily liquid. **Soluble** in alcohol, in acetone, in ether, in chloroform, and in volatile oils; soluble with opalescence in fixed oils. **Store** in airtight containers.

Capsicum has a carminative action but it is mainly used externally, often in the form of capsicum oleoresin, as a counter-irritant (see p.7). It is also included in preparations for the management of cough and cold symptoms. However, preparations of capsicum and capsicum oleoresin can be very irritant. Capsaicin (p.24), the active ingredient of capsicum, is also used in topical preparations in the treatment of painful skin conditions.

Capsicum is also used in homoeopathic medicine and in cookery.

Effects on the gastro-intestinal tract. The initial response to the ingestion of a hot pepper is a hot or burning sensation in the mouth which is attributed to the binding of capsaicin to receptors in the oral cavity.[1] Casein containing substances such as milk can reverse this burning sensation, apparently by displacing capsaicin due to their lipophilicity.

Spicy meals have long been associated with gastro-intestinal discomfort and ingestion of meals containing 1.5 g of red or black pepper have been shown to cause signs of gastric mucosal damage comparable to those caused by a 625-mg dose of aspirin.[2] However, other studies in *animals*[3] and humans[4,5] suggest that capsaicin may have a protective effect on gastric mucosa. Ingestion of approximately 30 g of jalapeño peppers (a capsicum fruit) caused no visible damage to the duodenal or gastric mucosa of 12 healthy subjects[6] and daily ingestion of meals containing a total of 3 g of chilli powder did not affect the clinical progress of patients with duodenal ulcers receiving antacids.[7]

1. Henkin R. Cooling the burn from hot peppers. *JAMA* 1991; **266**: 2766.
2. Myers BM, *et al.* Effect of red pepper and black pepper on the stomach. *Am J Gastroenterol* 1987; **82:** 211–14.
3. Holzer P. Peppers, capsaicin, and the gastric mucosa. *JAMA* 1989; **261:** 3244.
4. Kang JY, *et al.* Chili—protective factor against peptic ulcer? *Dig Dis Sci* 1995; **40:** 576–9.
5. Yeoh KG, *et al.* Chili protects against aspirin-induced gastroduodenal mucosal injury in humans. *Dig Dis Sci* 1995; **40:** 580–3.
6. Graham DY, *et al.* Spicy food and the stomach: evaluation by videoendoscopy. *JAMA* 1988; **260:** 3473–5.
7. Kumar N, *et al.* Do chillies influence healing of duodenal ulcer? *Br Med J* 1984; **288:** 1803–4.

Preparations

Proprietary Preparations (details are given in Part 3)
Aust.: ABC; ***Ger.:*** Capsamol; Thermo Burger.

Multi-ingredient: ***Aust.:*** Mayfit chronisch; Mentopin; Munari†; Salhumin; Traumasalbe; ***Austral.:*** For Peripheral Circulation Herbal Plus Formula 5; Lifesystem Herbal Formula 6 For Peripheral Circulation; Valerian; ***Belg.:*** Revocyl†; ***Fr.:*** Baume Saint-Bernard; Capsic; Dolpyc; Elastocapsil†; ***Ger.:*** Caye Balsam; Hewedolor; Mydalgan†; Rheumasalbe Capsicum†; Segmentocut†; ***Neth.:*** Sloan's balsem; Sloan's liniment†; ***Norw.:*** Allcocks Plaster†; ***Spain:*** Balsamo Midalgan; Bellacanfor†; Dolokey; Killpan; Linimento Klari; Linimento Naion; Linimento Sloan; ***Switz.:*** Embropax; Incutin; Massorax; Midalgan; ***UK:*** Backache Tablets; Buttercup Syrup; Catarrh Mixture; Hill's Balsam Adult Expectorant; Hill's Balsam Adult Suppressant; Hill's Balsam Junior Expectorant; Honey & Molasses; Indian Brandee; Jamaica Sarsaparilla; Life Drops; Sanderson's Throat Specific; Venos Dry Cough; Venos Expectorant; ***USA:*** Throat Discs.

Caraway (4619-l)

Alcaravia; Caraway Fruit; Caraway Seed; Carum; Cumin des Prés; Fructus Carvi; Kümmel.

Pharmacopoeias. In Eur. (see p.viii) and Pol.

The dried ripe fruits of *Carum carvi* (Umbelliferae); when crushed they have a characteristic aromatic odour and taste. Ph. Eur. specifies not less than 3.0% v/w of volatile oil. **Protect** from light.

Powdered caraway contains not less than 2.5% v/w of volatile oil.

Caraway is an aromatic carminative, and is used as a flavouring agent. The seeds are used in cookery. It is the source of caraway oil.

Preparations

Proprietary Preparations (details are given in Part 3)
Multi-ingredient: ***Aust.:*** Abbiofort; Absimed; Aktiv milder Magen- und Darmtee; Apotheker Bauer's Magentee; Bio-Garten Tee fur den Magen; Bio-Garten Tee gegen Blahungen; Bio-Garten Tropfen gegen Blahungen; Carminative; Karvisin; Krauterdoktor Magen-Darmtropfen; Krauterhaus Mag Kottas Babytee; Krauterhaus Mag Kottas Tee fur die Verdauung; Krauterhaus Mag Kottas Tee gegen Blahungen; Krautertee Nr 107; Krautertee Nr 126; Krautertee Nr 14; Krautertee Nr 17; Krautertee Nr 217; Mag Kottas Baby-Tee; Mag Kottas Blahungs-Verdauungstee; Mag Kottas Tee fur stillende Mutter; Magentee; Midro-Tee; Montana; Myrtilen; Nesthakchen; Sanvita Verdauungstropfen; Sidroga Leber-Galle-Tee; Species Carvi comp; St Radegunder Blahungstreibender Tee; St Radegunder Verdauungstee; Windtreibender Tee; ***Austral.:*** Cholagogum†; ***Fr.:*** Santane C_6; Santane D_5; Santane F_{10}; Santane O_1; Tisane des Familles†; Tisane Digestive Weleda; ***Ger.:*** Abfuhr-Tee Depuraflux†; Agamadon N; Aruto-Magenpulver-forte†; Basofer forte†; Basofer†; Carminat†; Carminativum-Hetterich N; Carminativum-Pascoe; Cholaflux N†; Cholaflux†; Cholosom-Tee; Divinal Gastro; Dr. Kleinschrod's Spasmi Tropfen†; Echtroferment-N; Floradix Multipretten; Friosmin†; Gallen-Leber-Tee Stada†; Gastrol S; Gastrosecur; Hepa-L†; Iberogast; Ilioton†; Kneipp Flatuol; Knufinke Gastrobin Magen- und Darm-Tee†; Lomatol; Majocarmin-Tee; Meteophyt S; Meteophyt†; Montana; Presselin 214†; Presselin 52 N; Rheumex†; Stern Biene Fencheltee†; Stoffwechseldragees†; Stomachicon N; Stovalid N; Ventrodigest†; Vier-Winde-Tee†; Worishofener Dronalax†; Worishofener Leber- und Gallensteinmittel Dr. Kleinschrod†; ***Ital.:*** Florelax; Midro; ***Switz.:*** Adistop Lax; Ajaka; Digestofluid†; Kernosan Heidelberger Poudre; Phytomed Gastro; Tisane d'allaitement "H"†; Tisane gastrique "H"†; Tisane laxative Natterman no 13; ***UK:*** Carminative Tea; Laxadoron.

Caraway Oil (4620-v)

Kümmelöl; Oleum Cari; Oleum Carui; Oleum Carvi.

Pharmacopoeias. In Aust., Br., and Ger.

A clear colourless or pale yellow volatile oil with a characteristic odour and taste, obtained by distillation from caraway. The BP specifies that it contains 53 to 63% w/w of ketones calculated as carvone ($C_{10}H_{14}O$).

At 20° it is **soluble** 1 in 7 of alcohol (80%). **Store** at a temperature not exceeding 25°. Protect from light.

Caraway oil is an aromatic carminative and is used as a flavouring agent. It is also employed as caraway water for the flatulent colic of infants (p.1170).

Preparations

BP 1998: Aromatic Cardamom Tincture; Compound Cardamom Tincture.

Proprietary Preparations (details are given in Part 3)
Multi-ingredient: ***Aust.:*** Nesthakchen; Parodontax; Pascopankreat; Sabatif†; Sanvita Magen; Sigman-Haustropfen; Spasmo Claim; ***Ger.:*** Abfuhr-Tee Depuraflux†; Aspasmon N; Benium; Cholaktol-L†; Choldestal†; Cholosom†; Cholosum N†; dichronase†; Divinal-Bohnen†; Enteroplant; Euflat I; Flatus-Pillen N Andreae†; Floradix Multipretten; Gallen-Leber-Tee Stada†; Galloselect M; Gastricard N; Hepaticum-Divinal†; Hevert-Gall S; Ilioton†; Kneipp Rheuma Stoffwechsel-Bad Heublumen-Aquasan; Lomatol; Majocarmin†; Meteophyt-V†; Meteophyt†; Neo-Ballistol; Obstinoletten†; Pascopankreat S; Pascopnkreat novo; Roflatol Phyto (Rowo-146); Sirmia Abfuhrkapseln; ***Switz.:*** Ajaka; Capsules laxatives Nattermann Nr. 13; Digestozym†; Flatulex;

Globase†; Huile Po-Ho A. Vogel; Tirgon†; *UK:* Nurse Harvey's Gripe Mixture.

Cardamom Fruit (4621-g)

Cardam. Fruit; Cardamom Seed; Cardamomi Fructus.

Pharmacopoeias. In *Br.* and *Jpn.*

The dried, nearly ripe fruit of *Elettaria cardamomum* var. *minuscula* (Zingiberaceae). Only the seeds are used in making preparations of cardamom and they are used immediately after removal from the fruit. The seeds should not be stored after removal from the fruit. They have a strongly aromatic odour and an aromatic slightly bitter taste and contain not less than 4% v/w of volatile oil.

Preparations of cardamom fruit are used as carminatives and as flavours. The seeds are used in cookery.

Cardamom fruit is the source of cardamom oil.

Preparations

Proprietary Preparations (details are given in Part 3)

Multi-ingredient: *Aust.:* Mariazeller; *Austral.:* Travelaide; Vitaglow Herbal Laxative†; *Ger.:* Carminat†; Cholongal plus†; Cholongal†; Dr. Maurers Magen-Apotheke†; Montana; Presselin 214†; Presselin 52 N; *Ital.:* Sedobex; *S.Afr.:* Alma; Carminex; Enterodyne; *Spain:* Digestovital; *Switz.:* Radix†; Stomacine; *UK:* Aluminium Free Indigestion; Indian Brandee.

Cardamom Oil (4622-q)

Ol. Cardamom.

Pharmacopoeias. In *Br.*

A clear colourless or pale yellow oil with an aromatic pungent odour and taste, distilled from crushed cardamom fruit. It contains cineole. At 20° it is **soluble** 1 in 6 of alcohol (70%). **Store** at a temperature not exceeding 25°. Protect from light.

Preparations of cardamom oil are used as carminatives and as flavours.

Preparations

BP 1998: Aromatic Cardamom Tincture; Compound Cardamom Tincture; Compound Rhubarb Tincture.

Proprietary Preparations (details are given in Part 3)

Multi-ingredient: *Belg.:* Melisana†.

Carnauba Wax (12527-p)

903; Caranda Wax; Cera Carnauba; Cera Coperniciae.

Pharmacopoeias. In *Eur.* (see p.viii), *Int.*, and *Jpn.* Also in *USNF.*

It is obtained from the leaves of *Copernicia cerifera* (Palmae).

Light brown to pale yellow or yellow moderately coarse powder, or flakes or irregular lumps, with a characteristic bland odour free from rancidity. Sp. gr. about 0.99. M.p. 80° to 88°. Practically **insoluble** in water and in alcohol; slightly soluble in boiling alcohol; soluble in warm chloroform, warm ethyl acetate, warm toluene, and in warm xylene. **Protect** from light.

Carnauba wax is used in pharmacy as a coating agent. Various types and grades are used industrially in the manufacture of polishes. Its use is also permitted in certain foods.

Caroverine (19682-g)

Caroverine (*pINN*).

1-[2-(Diethylamino)ethyl]-3-(*p*-methoxybenzyl)-2(1*H*)-quinoxalinone.

$C_{22}H_{27}N_3O_2$ = 365.5.

CAS — 23465-76-1.

Caroverine is a smooth muscle relaxant with calcium-channel blocking and glutamate-antagonist properties. It is used as the base or the hydrochloride in conditions associated with painful smooth muscle spasm; typical doses (expressed as the base) are 20 or 40 mg by mouth three or four times daily, 40 to 80 mg by slow intravenous or intramuscular injection, up to a maximum of 200 mg daily, or 40 mg by rectal administration up to four times daily. It is also used in cerebral circulatory disorders.

Preparations

Proprietary Preparations (details are given in Part 3)

Aust.: Spasmium; *Switz.:* Calmaverine.

Multi-ingredient: *Aust.:* Spagall; Spasmium comp.

Carzenide (11597-j)

Carzenide (*rINN*).

p-Sulphamoylbenzoic acid.

$C_7H_7NO_4S$ = 201.2.

CAS — 138-41-0.

Carzenide is an antispasmodic which has been used in the treatment of dysmenorrhoea. It is also reported to be an inhibitor of carbonic anhydrase.

Preparations

Proprietary Preparations (details are given in Part 3)

Multi-ingredient: *Spain:* Nefrolit†; *Switz.:* Dismenol†.

Cassia Oil (4624-s)

Chinese Cinnamon Oil; Oleum Cassiae; Oleum Cinnamomi; Oleum Cinnamomi Cassiae.

Pharmacopoeias. In *Chin.* and *Jpn*, which also include cassia bark which may be known as cinnamon bark. In some countries Cassia Oil is known as Cinnamon Oil.

A yellowish or brownish volatile oil with a fragrant pungent odour and a sweetish, spicy, burning taste, obtained by steam distillation from the leaves and twigs of *Cinnamomum cassia* (Lauraceae), and rectified by distillation. It darkens with age or exposure to light, and becomes more viscous. It contains not less than 80% v/v of aldehydes; cinnamaldehyde is the major constituent. **Soluble** 1 in 2 of alcohol (70%) and 1 in 1 of glacial acetic acid. **Store** at a temperature not exceeding 40° in airtight containers. Protect from light.

Cassia oil has properties resembling those of cinnamon oil (p.1564) and is used similarly as a carminative and flavour. There have been a number of reports of hypersensitivity to cinnamaldehyde, the main constituent of cassia oil.

Preparations

Proprietary Preparations (details are given in Part 3)

Multi-ingredient: *Austral.:* Tiger Balm Red; *Ger.:* Grunlicht Hingfong Essenz; *UK:* Dragon Balm.

Castor Oil (7355-v)

Aceite de Ricino; Huile de Ricin; Ol. Ricin.; Oleum Ricini; Ricini Oleum; Rizinusöl.

NOTE. CASOIL is a code approved by the BP for use on single unit doses of eye drops containing castor oil where the individual container may be too small to bear all the appropriate labelling information.

Pharmacopoeias. In *Chin., Eur.* (see p.viii), *Jpn*, and *US.*
Ger., It., and *USNF* also include hydrogenated castor oil.

The fixed oil expressed, without the application of heat, from the seeds of *Ricinus communis* (Euphorbiaceae). It is a nearly colourless or slightly yellow transparent viscid oil with a slight odour and taste which is bland at first, but afterwards slightly acrid.

Soluble in alcohol; miscible with dehydrated alcohol, chloroform, ether, and glacial acetic acid; slightly soluble in petroleum spirit. **Store** at a temperature not exceeding 15° in well-filled airtight containers. Protect from light.

Adverse Effects and Precautions

The administration of castor oil by mouth, particularly in large doses, may produce nausea, vomiting, colic, and severe purgation. Castor oil should not be given when intestinal obstruction is present.

The seeds of *Ricinus communis* contain a toxic protein, ricin (p.1625). Allergic reactions have been reported in subjects handling the seeds.

Uses and Administration

Castor oil has been used for its laxative action, but other agents are now generally preferred (see p.1168).

Castor oil is a soothing application to the conjunctiva and allays irritation due to foreign bodies in the eye.

It is used externally for its emollient effect. Castor oil may be employed as the solvent in some injections.

Hydrogenated castor oil is used as a stiffening agent. Polyoxyl castor oils (p.1326) are used as emulsifying and solubilising agents.

Preparations

BP 1998: Chloroxylenol Solution *(Roxenol)*; Flexible Collodion; Zinc and Castor Oil Ointment;

USP 23: Aromatic Castor Oil; Castor Oil Capsules; Castor Oil Emulsion; Flexible Collodion.

Proprietary Preparations (details are given in Part 3)

Canad.: Neoloid; Unisoil; *Ger.:* Laxopol; *Spain:* Palmil; Ricino Koki; *USA:* Emulsoil; Fleet Castor Oil Emulsion†; Neoloid; Purge.

Multi-ingredient: *Aust.:* Endrine mild†; Endrine†; *Austral.:* Egozite Cradle Cap; Seda-Rash; *Ger.:* Consablitz†; *Ital.:* Bal Tar; Herbatar; *S.Afr.:* Episeal†; *Spain:* Otocerum; *Switz.:* Warz-ab Extor; *UK:* Exzem Oil; Panda Baby Cream; *USA:* Dermuspray; Dr Dermi-Heal; Granulderm; Granulex; GranuMed; Mammol; Medicone Rectal; Proderm.

Catalase (3044-b)

Caperase; Equilase; Optidase.

A protein composed of 4 polypeptide subunits, the precise composition of which varies according to the source, and having a molecular weight of about 240 000.

Catalase is an enzyme obtained from a wide variety of biological sources including animal liver (hepatocatalase) and certain bacteria and fungi. It has the ability to promote the decomposition of hydrogen peroxide to water and oxygen.

It has been applied to wounds and skin ulcers and has also been used in the treatment of eczema. It has sometimes been used with glucose oxidase (p.1585) in food preservation to break down hydrogen peroxide produced during oxidation of glucose, and is also included in preparations for contact lens care to neutralise hydrogen peroxide.

Catalase is a free-radical scavenger and has been investigated for its ability to limit reperfusion injury thought to be related to free-radical production. Combinations of catalase with superoxide dismutase have also been investigated.

Preparations

Proprietary Preparations (details are given in Part 3)

Aust.: Lensan B; Les Yeux 2; Oxysept Quick; Titmus Losung 2; *Ger.:* Oxysept Quick†; *Ital.:* Citrizan; *Spain:* Biocatalase.

Multi-ingredient: *Aust.:* Omnicare; Oxysept; Oxysept Comfort; *Belg.:* Pulvo 47; Pulvo Neomycine; *Canad.:* UltraCare; *Fr.:* Pulvo 47; Pulvo 47 Neomycine; *Ger.:* Oxysept Comfort; Oxysept Light†; Pulvo; Pulvo Neomycin; *Ital.:* Citrizan Antibiotico; *Neth.:* Rheumajecta†; *USA:* UltraCare.

Catechu (306-s)

Gambier; Gambir; Pale Catechu.

CAS — 8001-48-7; 8001-76-1 (black catechu).

Pharmacopoeias. In *Jpn*, which also allows Powdered Catechu. *Chin.* includes Ramulus Uncariae cum Uncis and Black Catechu from *Acacia catechu* (Leguminosae). Also in *BP(Vet).*

Usually a dried aqueous extract of the leaves and young shoots of *Uncaria gambier* (Rubiaceae) occurring as dull pale greyish-brown to dark reddish-brown cubes or pale brown powder.

Catechu is an astringent and has been included in preparations for the treatment of diarrhoea and other gastro-intestinal disorders.

Preparations

Proprietary Preparations (details are given in Part 3)

Multi-ingredient: *Austral.:* Acacia Complex†; Diarcalm; *Fr.:* Elixir Bonjean; *S.Afr.:* Enterodyne; *UK:* Spanish Tummy Mixture.

CD4 Antibodies (14392-h)

Anti-CD4 Monoclonal Antibodies; CD4mAb; Monoclonal CD4 Antibodies.

Monoclonal antibodies raised against CD4 receptors are under investigation in the treatment of immunologically mediated disorders, such as rheumatoid arthritis, multiple sclerosis, inflammatory bowel disease, and various skin disorders, with the aim of decreasing and eliminating circulating helper T lymphocytes. One such antibody, keliximab, has also been investigated in asthma.

References.

1. Horneff G, *et al.* Treatment of rheumatoid arthritis with an anti-CD4 monoclonal antibody. *Arthritis Rheum* 1991; **34:** 129–40.
2. Wendling D, *et al.* Therapeutic use of monoclonal anti-CD4 antibody in rheumatoid arthritis. *J Rheumatol* 1991; **18:** 325–7.
3. Robinet E, *et al.* CD4 monoclonal antibody administration in atopic dermatitis. *J Am Acad Dermatol* 1997; **36:** 582–8.
4. van Oosten BW, *et al.* Treatment of multiple sclerosis with the monoclonal anti-CD4 antibody CM-T412: results of a randomized, double-blind, placebo-controlled, MR-monitored phase II trial. *Neurology* 1997; **49:** 351–7.
5. van der Lubbe PA, *et al.* Anti-CD4 monoclonal antibody for relapsing polychondritis. *Lancet* 1991; **337:** 1349.
6. Choy EHS, *et al.* Chimaeric anti-CD4 monoclonal antibody for relapsing polychondritis. *Lancet* 1991; **338:** 450.
7. Heipe F, *et al.* Treatment of severe systemic lupus erythematosus with anti-CD4 monoclonal antibody. *Lancet* 1991; **338:** 1529–30.
8. Mathieson PW, *et al.* Monoclonal-antibody therapy in systemic vasculitis. *N Engl J Med* 1990; **323:** 250–4.
9. Poizot-Martin I, *et al.* Are CD4 antibodies and peptide T new treatments for psoriasis? *Lancet* 1991; **337:** 1477.
10. Prinz J, *et al.* Chimaeric CD4 monoclonal antibody in treatment of generalised pustular psoriasis. *Lancet* 1991; **338:** 320–1.
11. Nicolas JF, *et al.* CD4 antibody treatment of severe psoriasis. *Lancet* 1991; **338:** 321.

12. Stronkhorst A, *et al.* CD4 antibody treatment in patients with active Crohn's disease: a phase I dose finding study. *Gut* 1997; **40:** 320–7.
13. Kon OM, *et al.* Randomised, dose-ranging, placebo-controlled study of chimeric antibody to CD4 (keliximab) in chronic severe asthma. *Lancet* 1998; **352:** 1109–13.

Celery (4626-e)

Apium; Celery Fruit; Celery Seed.
CAS — 8015-90-5 (celery oil).

The dried ripe fruits of celery, *Apium graveolens* (Umbelliferae). Other parts of the plant are also used.

Celery is reported to have diuretic properties and has been included in herbal preparations for rheumatic disorders. Celery oil has also been used as a spasmolytic. Allergic and phototallergic reactions have been reported.

Celery is also used in homoeopathic medicine.

References.

1. Houghton P. Bearberry, dandelion and celery. *Pharm J* 1995; **255:** 272–3.

Interactions. For a report of severe phototoxicity occurring in a patient who had consumed celery soup before undergoing PUVA therapy, see Interactions under Methoxsalen, p.1087.

Preparations

Proprietary Preparations (details are given in Part 3)

Multi-ingredient: ***Austral.:*** Arthritic Pain Herbal Formula 1; Devils Claw Plus; Fluid Loss; Herbal Diuretic Complex†; Lifesystem Herbal Formula 1 Arthritic Aid; Natural Vegetable Alkaliniser†; ***Ger.:*** Nephrubin; ***UK:*** Rheumatic Pain; Rheumatic Pain Tablets; Vegetex.

Cellobiose (18926-h)

4-*O*-β-D-Glucopyranosyl-D-glucose.
$C_{12}H_{22}O_{11}$ = 342.3.
CAS — 528-50-7.

Cellobiose is a disaccharide that has been used to assess intestinal permeability. It has been used as an alternative to lactulose in the differential sugar absorption test (p.1196).

References.

1. Hodges S, *et al.* Cellobiose: mannitol differential permeability in small bowel disease. *Arch Dis Child* 1989; **64:** 853–74.
2. Juby LD, *et al.* Cellobiose/mannitol sugar test—a sensitive tubeless test for coeliac disease: results on 1010 unselected patients. *Gut* 1989; **30:** 476–80.

Cellulase (18473-l)

Cellulase *(USAN).*
CAS — 9012-54-8.

Cellulase is a concentrate of cellulose-splitting (cellulolytic) enzymes derived from *Aspergillus niger* or other sources. It is used in food processing and has been given by mouth in combination with other digestive enzymes for its supposed benefit in minor digestive disorders such as dyspepsia and flatulence. Hemicellulase has been given for similar purposes.

Preparations

Proprietary Preparations (details are given in Part 3)

Multi-ingredient: ***Aust.:*** Arca-Enzym; Festal; Gallo Merz; Ora-Gallin; ***Austral.:*** Bioglan Active Enzyme Complex†; Bioglan Vegetable Enzymes†; ***Belg.:*** Digestomen; ***Canad.:*** Festal†; Ku-Zyme†; ***Fr.:*** Festale†; Pancrelase; ***Ger.:*** Cholspasminase†; Oragallin†; ***Ital.:*** Canulase†; Convivial†; Digestopan; Digestozim†; Enzygaster†; Essen Enzimatico; Essen†; Kilozim†; Luizym; Onoton†; Trimalcina†; ***Spain:*** Digestomen Complex; Espasmo Canulasa; Espasmo Digestomen; Lidobama Complex; Lidobama Plus†; Oragalin†; Paidozim; Polidasa; Trizima†; ***Swed.:*** Festal†; ***Switz.:*** Pantozyme†; Spasmo-Canulase; Zymoplex; ***USA:*** Arco-Lase; Arco-Lase Plus; Enzyme; Gustase; Gustase Plus; Ku-Zyme; Kutrase; Medazyme†.

Centaury (527-f)

Centaurii Minoris Herba; Petite Centaurée; Tausendgüldenkraut.

Pharmacopoeias. In *Eur.* (see p.viii).

The dried flowering tops of the common centaury, *Centaurium erythraea* (=*C.minus; C. umbellatum; Erythraea centaurium*), and other species of *Centaurium* (Gentianaceae). **Protect** from light.

Centaury is used as a bitter.

Preparations

Proprietary Preparations (details are given in Part 3)

Multi-ingredient: ***Aust.:*** Amylatin; Apotheker Bauer's Magentee; China-Eisenwein; Eryval; Grippogran; Kneipp Verdauungs-Tee; Krauterdoktor Erkaltungstropfen; Krauterdoktor Harnstein- und Nieren-griesstropfen; Krauterdoktor Verdauungsfordernde Tropfen; Krautertee Nr 14; Krautertee Nr 17; Krautertee Nr 20; Krautertee Nr 9; Mag Kottas Blahungs-Verdauungstee; Mag Kottas Magen-Darmtee; Magentee EF-EM-ES; Mariazeller; Sidroga Magen-Darm-Tee; Solisan; St Radegunder Verdauungstee; ***Fr.:*** Copaltra; Diacure; Tisanes de l'Abbe Hamon no 16; ***Ger.:*** Abfuhr-Tee Depuraflux†; Alsicur; Aranidorm-S; Canephron N; Cefagastrin; Cholaflux†; Gastro-Vial†; Hepaticum-Divinal†; Hevert-Magen-Galle-Leber-Tee; JuGrippan; Kneipp Magentrost†; Kneipp Verdauungs-Tee N; Losapan†; Montana; Nephrubin; Phonix Gastriphon; Stullmaton; Ventrodigest†; Zettagall V†; ***Ital.:*** Fluxoten; ***Spain:*** Digestol Sanatorium; ***Switz.:*** Gastrosan; Phytomed Gastro; Tisane pour l'estomac; ***UK:*** Digest; Laxadoron.

Ceruletide (2124-t)

Ceruletide *(BAN, USAN, rINN).*
Caerulein.
$C_{58}H_{73}N_{13}O_{21}S_2$ = 1352.4.
CAS — 17650-98-5 (ceruletide); 71247-25-1 (ceruletide diethylamine).

NOTE. The name Ceruleinum has been applied to Indigo Carmine (p.1590).

Ceruletide is a decapeptide amide originally isolated from the skin of the Australian frog, *Hyla caerulea*, and other amphibians. Ceruletide compound with diethylamine (ceruletide diethylamine) may exist as a salt with 1 to 3 moles of diethylamine.

Adverse Effects

Ceruletide stimulates gallbladder contraction and gastro-intestinal muscle and may give rise to abdominal discomfort. Hypotensive reactions may also occur.

Uses and Administration

Ceruletide is structurally related to pancreozymin (p.1613) and has similar actions. When administered parenterally it stimulates gallbladder contraction and relaxes the sphincter of Oddi; it also causes an increase in the secretion of pancreatic enzymes and stimulates intestinal muscle.

As ceruletide diethylamine it is used as an aid to diagnostic radiology and in the management of paralytic ileus. It is also used in tests of pancreatic exocrine function, sometimes in combination with secretin (p.1628); these studies generally require duodenal intubation of the patient and examination of duodenal aspirate and are rarely performed.

For most radiographic procedures of the biliary and digestive tracts and for treatment of postoperative ileus, ceruletide diethylamine is given by intramuscular injection in a dose equivalent to 300 ng per kg body-weight of ceruletide. Doses of 1 to 2 ng per kg per minute are given by intravenous infusion in pancreatic function tests and in the treatment of other causes of paralytic ileus.

References.

1. Vincent ME, *et al.* Pharmacology, clinical uses, and adverse effects of ceruletide, a cholecystokinetic agent. *Pharmacotherapy* 1982; **2:** 223–34.
2. Gullo L, *et al.* Caerulein induced plasma amino acid decrease: a simple, sensitive, and specific test of pancreatic function. *Gut* 1990; **31:** 926–9.

Preparations

Proprietary Preparations (details are given in Part 3)
Fr.: Cerulex†; ***Ger.:*** Takus.

Chamomile (4628-y)

NOTE. The name Chamomile is used for the dried flowerheads from 2 species of *Compositae* having similar medicinal properties:

Chamomile from *Anthemis nobilis* (*Chamaemelum nobile*) is known as **Roman Chamomile Flower** (Ph. Eur.) (Chamomile Flowers, Chamomillae Romanae Flos, or Manzanilla Romana).

Chamomile from *Matricaria recutita* (*Chamomilla recutita*) is known as **Matricaria Flower** (Ph. Eur.) (Camomile Allemande, Camomilla, Chamomilla, Chamomillae Anthodium, Flos Chamomillae, Flos Chamomillae Vulgaris, German Chamomile, Hungarian Chamomile, Kamillenblüten, Manzanilla Ordinaria, or Matricariae Flos).

Pharmacopoeias. Eur. (see p.viii) includes chamomile from *Anthemis nobilis* and *Matricaria recutita*. *Pol.* and *USNF* include chamomile from *Matricaria recutita*.
Aust. and *Ger.* also include Matricaria Oil.

Roman Chamomile Flower (Ph. Eur.) consists of the dried flowerheads obtained from the cultivated double variety of *Anthemis nobilis* (= *Chamaemelum nobile*), containing not less than 0.7% v/w of volatile oil. Matricaria Flower (Ph. Eur.) consists of the dried flowerheads obtained from *Matricaria recutita* (=*Chamomilla recutita*), containing not less than 0.4% v/w of volatile oil. Chamomile (USNF 18) consist of the dried flowerheads of *M. recutita* containing not less than 0.4% of blue volatile oil and not less than 0.3% of apigenin-7-glucoside.

Protect from light.

Chamomile has been applied externally as a poultice in the early stages of inflammation, and ointments containing chamomile or extracts of chamomile have been used for the prevention and treatment of cracked nipples and nappy rash. It is also used in homoeopathic medicine. 'Chamomile tea' is a domestic remedy for indigestion and has also been reported to have hypnotic properties.

There have been reports of contact sensitivity and anaphylaxis.

Reviews.

1. Berry M. The chamomiles. *Pharm J* 1995; **254:** 191–3.

Hypersensitivity. A report of contact dermatitis, in a 62-year-old florist, due to matricaria flowers.[1]

1. Van Ketel WG. Allergy to Matricaria chamomilla. *Contact Dermatitis* 1987; **16:** 50–1.

Preparations

Proprietary Preparations (details are given in Part 3)

Aust.: Kamillomed; Markalakt; ***Belg.:*** Kamillosan; ***Ger.:*** Azulon; Chamo; Eukamillat; Kamillan supra; Kamille N; Kamillen Spuman†; Kamilloderm; Kamillosan; Markalakt; Matmille; PC 30 N; Perkamillon; Rekomill†; Silvapin Kamillenbluten-Extrakt†; ***Irl.:*** Kamillosan; ***Ital.:*** Ceru Spray; Milla; ***Neth.:*** Kamillosan†; ***Switz.:*** Edmilla; Kamillen-Bad; Kamillex†; Kamillofluid; Kamillosan; Perkamillon; ***UK:*** Ashton & Parsons Infants Powders; Kamillosan.

Multi-ingredient: ***Aust.:*** Abfuhrtee; Aktiv milder Magen- und Darmtee; Apotheker Bauer's Blahungstee; Bio-Garten Tee fur den Magen; Bio-Garten Tee gegen Blahungen; Bio-Garten Tee gegen Durchfall; Bio-Garten Tee gegen Verstopfung; Bio-Garten Tropfen fur Magen und Darm; Bogumil-tassenfertiger milder Abfurtee; Bronchostop; Carminativum Babynos; Chol-Grandelat; Cional; Dentinox; Diarrhoesan; Dynexan; Ehrmann's Entschlackungstee; Eogran; Gastregan; Illings Bozner Maycur-Tee; Karvisin; Kneipp Grippe-Tee; Kneipp Verdauungs-Tee; Krauterhaus Mag Kottas Babytee; Krauterhaus Mag Kottas Entschlackungstee; Krauterhaus Mag Kottas Magen- und Darmtee; Krauterhaus Mag Kottas Tee gegen Durchfall; Krauterhaus Mag Kottas Wechseltee; Krautertee Nr 1; Krautertee Nr 124; Krautertee Nr 17; Krautertee Nr 209; Krautertee Nr 217; Krautertee Nr 311; Krautertee Nr 8; Krautertee Nr 9; Laxalpin; Laxolind; Mag Doskar's Magentonikum; Mag Doskar's Nerventonikum; Mag Kottas Baby-Tee; Mag Kottas Leber-Gallentee; Mag Kottas Magen-Darmtee; Mag Kottas Wechseltee; Magentee; Mariazeller; May-Cur-Tee; Nesthakchen; Paididont; Paradenton; Parodontax; Planta Lax; Robugen-Kamillensalbe†; Sidroga Erkaltungstee; Sidroga Kindertee; Sidroga Magen-Darm-Tee; Sigman-Haustropfen; St Radegunder Blahungstreibender Tee; St Radegunder Fiebertee; St Radegunder Reizmildernder Magentee; St Radegunder Tee gegen Durchfall; Sulgan 99; Tee gegen Durchfall nach Dr Bohmig†; Teekanne Leber- und Galletee; Teekanne Magen- und Darmtee; Windtreibender Tee; ***Austral.:*** Cough Relief; Digest-eze†; Goodnight Formula; Herbal Anxiety Formula; Hydrastis Complex; Nappy Rash Relief Cream; Perpain†; Respatona; Respatona Plus with Echinacea; ***Belg.:*** Stago†; Tisane pour Dormir; ***Fr.:*** Activox; Calmophytum; Dologyne; Santane A_4; Santane D_5; Santane F_{10}; Solution Stago Diluee; Tisane Digestive Weleda; ***Ger.:*** Ad-Muc; Agamadon; Agamadon N; Anisan; Aranidorm-S; Arnikamill; Aruto-Magenpulver-forte†; Batkaletta†; Befelka-Tinktur; Bilisan forte†; bioplant-Kamillenfluid; Broncholind†; Carminativum Babynos; Carminativum-Hetterich N; Carminativum-Pascoe; Cefadiarrhon†; Cefagastrin; Cha-mill†; Dentinox N; derma-loges N; Diarrhoesan; Dr. Kleinschrod's Spasmi Tropfen†; Dr. Klinger's Bergischer Krautertee, Leber- und Gallentee†; Dr. Klinger's Bergischer Krautertee, Magentee†; Dr. Maurers Magen-Apotheke†; Dynexan†; Echtrosept-GT†; Esberigal N; Gallemolan G; Gallemolan N†; Gallen-Leber-Tee Stada†; Gallexier; Gallitophen†; Galloselect M; Gastralon N; Gastrarctin N; Gastricholan-L; Gastritol; Gastro-Vial†; Gastrol S; Grippe-Tee Stada†; Grunlicht Hingfong Essenz; Guakalin†; Gutnacht; Hamo-ratiopharm; Helago-oel N; Hepa-L†; Hevert-Gall S; Hovnizym†; Iberogast; JuGrippan; Kamillan plus; Kamillen-Bad-Robugen; Kamillobad; Kamillosan Mundspray; Kamistad†; Kneipp Gastropressan†; Kneipp Verdauungs-Tee N; Knufinke Blasen- und Nieren-Tee Uro-K†; Knufinke Gastrobin Magen- und Darm-Tee†; Magen-Tee Stada N; Majocarmin-Tee; Matmille; Medosalgon†; Meteophyt S; Meteophyt†; Myrrhinil-Intest; Nephulon E†; Nervosana; Odala wern; Parodontal; Pascoletten N; Pascomag; PC 30 V; Presselin 214†; Presselin 52 N; Presselin Stoffwechseltee†; Roflatol Phyto (Rowo-146); Salus Abfuhr-Tee Nr. 2; Salus Leber-Galle-Tee Nr.18; Salus Nerven-Schlaf-Tee Nr.22; Secerna†; Seda-Pasc N†; Stacho N†; Stomachicon N; Stovalid N; Stullmaton; Thymitussin†; Tonsilgon-N; Transpulmin†; Ulcotruw N; Ulcu-Pasc; Ullus Kapseln N; Valeriana comp; Ventrodigest†; Vier-Winde-Tee†; ***Ital.:*** Babygella; Bio Notte Baby†; Bramserene†; Dicalmir; Donalg; Florelax; Florerbe Digestiva†; Gocce D'Erbe†; Hamamilla; Heparbil†; Herbatar; Lycia Luminique; Nebris; Normalax; Otosan Gocce Auricolari; Parvisedil; Relaten; Sedatol; Sedonerva†; Sideck Shampoo Antiforfora†; Valeromill†; Vegebyl; Videorelax; ***S.Afr.:*** Dynexan; Kamillosan; ***Spain:*** Agua del Carmen; Digestol Sanatorium; Encialina; Ginejuvent; Jarabe Manceau; Laxante Sanatorium; ***Switz.:*** Bain extra-doux dermatologique; Beclonarin; Cetona; Cional†; Dentinox; Digestofluid†; Dynexan; Enveloppements ECR; Eubucal†; Euceta avec camomille et arnica; Frigoplasma; Iberogast; Kamillosan; Korodin; Mucosan†; Narifresh; Optilax; Perkamillon; Phytomed Gastro; Rhinocure; Riccomycine; Riccovitan; Saltrates Rodell; Solin S†; Spuman a la camomille†; Stago†; Sulgan; Tavolax; Tisane contre les refroidissements; Tisane gastrique "H"†; Tisane hepatique et biliaire "H"†; Tisane pour l'estomac; Tisane pour les enfants; Tisane sedative et somnifere "H"†; Tonex; Transpulmine†; ***UK:*** Appetiser Mixture; Carminative Tea; Travel-Caps.

Chaparral (3046-g)

Chaparral is derived from the leaves of the creosote bush, *Larrea tridentata* (Zygophyllaceae). It has been taken as an ingredient of various herbal preparations but such use has been associated with severe hepatotoxicity. Recommendations that products containing chaparral should not be consumed have been made in several countries.

References.

1. Gordon DW, *et al.* Chaparral ingestion: the broadening spectrum of liver injury caused by herbal medications. *JAMA* 1995; **273:** 489–90.

Preparations

Proprietary Preparations (details are given in Part 3)

Multi-ingredient: ***Austral.:*** Proyeast.

Chenodeoxycholic Acid (3706-m)

Chenodeoxycholic Acid *(BAN, rINN).*

Acidum Chenodeoxycholicum; CDCA; Chenic Acid; Chenodiol *(USAN).* 3α,7α-Dihydroxy-5β-cholan-24-oic acid.

$C_{24}H_{40}O_4$ = 392.6.

CAS — 474-25-9.

Pharmacopoeias. In *Eur.* (see p.viii).

A white or almost white powder. Very slightly **soluble** in water; freely soluble in alcohol; soluble in acetone; slightly soluble in dichloromethane.

Adverse Effects

Chenodeoxycholic acid may cause diarrhoea, especially at the start of treatment, and pruritus. A transient rise in liver-function test values and hypercholesterolaemia (low-density lipoprotein) have been reported.

Chenodeoxycholic acid is embryotoxic in some *animals.*

Precautions

Chenodeoxycholic acid should not be administered to patients with chronic liver disease, peptic ulcers, or inflammatory bowel disease. It is ineffective for the dissolution of calcified and pigment gallstones and is of no value in patients without a patent and functioning gallbladder. Its use should be avoided in pregnancy.

Interactions

Chenodeoxycholic acid should not be used with drugs, such as oestrogenic hormones, that increase bile cholesterol. Concomitant administration with bile-acid binding drugs including antacids, charcoal, and cholestyramine should be avoided since this may reduce the effectiveness of therapy with chenodeoxycholic acid.

Pharmacokinetics

Chenodeoxycholic acid is absorbed from the gastro-intestinal tract and undergoes first-pass metabolism and enterohepatic recycling. It is partly conjugated in the liver before being excreted into the bile and under the influence of intestinal bacteria the free and conjugated forms undergo 7α-dehydroxylation to lithocholic acid some of which is excreted directly in the faeces and the rest absorbed mainly to be conjugated and sulphated by the liver before excretion in the faeces. Chenodeoxycholic acid also undergoes epimerisation to ursodeoxycholic acid.

References.

1. Crosignani A, *et al.* Clinical pharmacokinetics of therapeutic bile acids. *Clin Pharmacokinet* 1996; **30:** 333–58.

Uses and Administration

Chenodeoxycholic acid is a naturally occurring bile acid (see p.1553). When given by mouth it reduces hepatic synthesis of cholesterol and provides additional bile salts to the pool available for solubilisation of cholesterol and lipids. It is used for the dissolution of cholesterol-rich gallstones (p.1642) in patients with a functioning gallbladder.

Chenodeoxycholic acid is given by mouth in usual doses of 10 to 15 mg per kg body-weight daily in a single dose given at bedtime or in divided doses; obese patients may require doses of up to 20 mg per kg daily. The daily dose may be divided unequally and the larger dose given before bedtime to counteract the increase in biliary cholesterol concentrations seen overnight.

Chenodeoxycholic acid is also used in combination with ursodeoxycholic acid in the management of gallstones and lower doses of 5 to 7.5 mg per kg daily may then be given. Treatment may need to be given for up to 2 years, depending on the size of the stone. It should be continued for about 3 months after radiological disappearance of the stones.

Preparations

Proprietary Preparations (details are given in Part 3)
Aust.: Chenofalk; ***Austral.:*** Chendol†; ***Belg.:*** Chenofalk; ***Fr.:*** Chenodex; ***Ger.:*** Chenofalk; Cholit-Chenosan†; ***Irl.:*** Chendol; Chenofalk; ***Ital.:*** Chenocol†; Chenofalk†; Chenossil†; Fluibil†; ***Jpn:*** Regalen; ***Neth.:*** Chenofalk; ***Spain:*** Chelobil†; Quenobilan; Quenocol; ***Switz.:*** Chenofalk; ***UK:*** Chendol†; Chenofalk; ***USA:*** Chenix†.

Multi-ingredient: ***Aust.:*** Lithofalk†; ***Ger.:*** Lithofalk; Urso Mix; Ursofalk + Chenofalk; ***Ital.:*** Bilenor; Litobile; ***Switz.:*** Cumulit†; Lithofalk; ***UK:*** Combidol†; Lithofalk†.

Chlorindanol (3423-z)

Chlorindanol *(USAN).*

Clorindanol *(rINN)*; NSC-158565. 7-Chloro-4-indanol; 7-Chloro-2,3-dihydro-1*H*-inden-4-ol.

C_9H_9ClO = 168.6.

CAS — 145-94-8.

Chlorindanol is reported to have antiseptic and spermicidal properties.

Preparations

Proprietary Preparations (details are given in Part 3)

Multi-ingredient: ***Ger.:*** Poly-Gynaedron†.

Chloroacetophenone (12553-w)

CN; Phenacyl Chloride. 2-Chloroacetophenone.

C_8H_7ClO = 154.6.

CAS — 532-27-4.

NOTE. The name mace is applied to solutions of chloroacetophenone.

Chloroacetophenone is a lachrymatory which is irritant to the skin and eyes. It has been used in a riot-control gas.

References.

1. Hu H, *et al.* Tear gas—harassing agent or toxic chemical weapon? *JAMA* 1989; **262:** 660–3.

Chloroplatinic Acid (12555-l)

Kloroplatinasyra. Hexachloroplatinic acid hexahydrate.

$H_2PtCl_6,6H_2O$ = 517.9.

CAS — 16941-12-1 (anhydrous chloroplatinic acid); 18497-13-7 (chloroplatinic acid hexahydrate).

Aqueous solutions of platinic chloride ($PtCl_4$=336.9) are used in corneal tattooing solutions.

Chondroitin Sulphate A (12558-z)

Chondroitin 4-Sulphate; CSA.

CAS — 24967-93-9 (chondroitin sulphate A); 39455-18-0 (chondroitin sulphate A sodium).

Chondroitin sulphate A is an acid mucopolysaccharide which is a constituent of most mammalian cartilaginous tissues. It is a component of the heparinoid danaparoid (p.846). It has been used in osteoporosis, osteoarthritis, ischaemic heart disease, and hyperlipidaemias. It is also used as an adjunct to ocular surgery. A medium containing chondroitin sulphate A has been used to preserve corneas for transplantation. It may also be used as the sodium salt.

Preparations

Proprietary Preparations (details are given in Part 3)
Aust.: Condrosulf; ***Belg.:*** Lacrypos†; ***Fr.:*** Chondrosulf; Lacrypos; Structum; ***Spain:*** Turkadon; ***Switz.:*** Condrosulf; Lacrypos†; Structum.

Multi-ingredient: ***Aust.:*** Viscoat; ***Austral.:*** Duovisc; Viscoat; ***Belg.:*** Viscoat; ***Fr.:*** Viscoat; ***Ger.:*** Duovisc; Viscoat; ***Ital.:*** Viscoat; ***S.Afr.:*** Viscoat; ***Swed.:*** Viscoat†; ***Switz.:*** Viscoat; ***UK:*** Viscoat; ***USA:*** Viscoat.

Chrome Alum (12559-c)

Chromium Potassium Sulphate.

$KCr(SO_4)_2,12H_2O$ = 499.4.

CAS — 10141-00-1 (anhydrous chrome alum).

Chrome alum is used in tanning, as a mordant in dyeing, and for hardening gelatin in photographic materials. It has been used as a sclerosant in medicine.

Preparations

Proprietary Preparations (details are given in Part 3)

Multi-ingredient: ***Fr.:*** Scleremo.

Chromium Trioxide (307-w)

Anhídrido Crómico; Chromic Acid; Chromic Anhydride.

CrO_3 = 99.99.

CAS — 1333-82-0.

CAUTION. *Chromium trioxide is a powerful oxidising agent and is liable to explode in contact with small quantities of alcohol, ether, glycerol, and other organic substances.*

Chromium trioxide and other chromium compounds are used in industry. Solutions of chromium trioxide are corrosive, acting by oxidation. Repeated contact with chromium and its salts may cause eczematous dermatitis, particularly in hypersensitive persons and can also cause deep perforating ulcers known as 'chrome holes'. If inhaled, chromic dusts cause rhinitis and painless ulcers which may perforate the nasal septum; inhalation may cause severe lung damage and inflammation of the eyes. There may also be involvement of the central nervous system and there is an increased risk of lung cancer. Hexavalent chromium compounds are more dangerous than di- or trivalent compounds.

Acute symptoms of poisoning from the ingestion of chromium salts include intense thirst, dizziness, abdominal pain with vomiting and diarrhoea, hepatic injury, anuria or oliguria, and peripheral vascular collapse. Kidney damage may lead to fatal uraemia.

Treatment is symptomatic and supportive. Protective measures should be taken when handling or working with chromium and its salts.

Chromium trioxide was formerly used as a caustic and astringent.

Chromium is an essential trace element as described on p.1337.

General references[1,2] to chromium toxicity including reports of poisoning with sodium dichromate[3] and potassium dichromate.[4]

1. Chromium. *Environmental Health Criteria 61.* Geneva: WHO, 1988.
2. Health and Safety Executive. The toxicity of chromium and inorganic chromium compounds. *Toxicity Review 21.* London: HMSO, 1989.
3. Ellis EN, *et al.* Effects of hemodialysis and dimercaprol in acute dichromate poisoning. *J Toxicol Clin Toxicol* 1982; **19:** 249–58.
4. Michie CA, *et al.* Poisoning with a traditional remedy containing potassium dichromate. *Hum Exp Toxicol* 1991; **10:** 129–31.

Chromocarb Diethylamine (12561-w)

The diethylamine salt of 4-oxo-4*H*-1-benzopyran-2-carboxylic acid.

$C_{14}H_{17}O_4N$ = 263.3.

CAS — 4940-39-0 (chromocarb).

NOTE. Chromocarb is *rINN.*

Chromocarb diethylamine is used to reduce capillary haemorrhage (including conjunctival haemorrhage) associated with various disorders, and for venous insufficiency. It is given by mouth in doses of 600 to 1200 mg daily in divided doses. It is also used as eye drops; 1 or 2 drops of a 10% solution have been instilled up to 6 times daily.

Preparations

Proprietary Preparations (details are given in Part 3)
Belg.: Angiophtal; ***Fr.:*** Angiophtal; Campel; ***Ital.:*** Fludarene; ***Spain:*** Activadone.

Chrysoidine Hydrochloride Citrate

(12562-e)

4-Phenylazobenzene-1,3-diamine hydrochloride citrate; Azobenzene-2,4-diamine hydrochloride citrate.

$C_{12}H_{12}N_4,HCl,C_6H_8O_7$ = 440.8.

CAS — 532-82-1 (chrysoidine hydrochloride); 5909-04-6 (chrysoidine hydrochloride citrate).

Chrysoidine hydrochloride citrate has been used as a dye but has been associated with tumours of the bladder.

Mention that the development of tumours of the urinary bladder in anglers was possibly associated with the use of chrysoidine hydrochloride (chrysoidine Y; CI Basic Orange 2; Colour Index No. 11270) for colouring the maggots used as bait.[1-3]

1. Searle CE, Teale J. Chrysoidine-dyed bait: a possible carcinogenic hazard to anglers? *Lancet* 1982; **i:** 564.
2. Sole GM. Maggots dyed with chrysoidine: a possible risk to anglers. *Br Med J* 1984; **289:** 1043–4.
3. Massey JA, *et al.* Maggots dyed with chrysoidine. *Br Med J* 1984; **289:** 1451–2.

Chymopapain (3708-v)

Chymopapain *(BAN, USAN, rINN).*

Bax-1526; NSC-107079; Quimopapaina.

CAS — 9001-09-6.

A proteolytic enzyme isolated from the latex of papaya (*Carica papaya*), differing from papain in electrophoretic mobility, solubility, and substrate specificity. Molecular weight approximately 27 000.

Units

One nanokatal (nKat) is defined as the amount of chymopapain which produces 1 nanomole of *p*-nitroaniline per second from DL-benzoylarginine-*p*-nitroanilide substrate at pH 6.4 and 37°.

In some countries CTE units have been used, defined as the amount of chymopapain which produces a hydrolysate from acid-denatured haemoglobin at pH 4.0 in one minute with an optical density at 275 nm equivalent to that of a tyrosine solution 0.0001%.

Adverse Effects

The most important adverse effect of chymopapain is anaphylaxis which can occur in up to about 1% of patients. It has resulted in fatalities and restricts use to a single treatment session per patient. Typical symptoms include angioedema, hypotension, laryngeal oedema and bronchospasm, shock and cardiac arrest. Allergic skin reactions may also occur. Other reported reactions include headache, nausea and vomiting, paralytic ileus, urinary retention, thrombophlebitis, paraesthesias, foot-drop, and discitis. Severe muscle spasm and an increase in back pain are common. Paraplegia, acute transverse myelitis, and intracerebral and subarachnoid haemorrhage have occurred.

In a postmarketing surveillance study on a chymopapain preparation for intradiscal injection (Chymodiactin) data was received on 29 075 patients by January 1984 (representing about 50% of the total number of vials sold by that USA manufacturer to that date).[1] Anaphylactic reactions were confirmed in 194 patients (0.67%), 2 of whom died. The incidence was higher in women than in men. In 52 cases the reaction occurred after the test dose.

Neurological reactions of a serious nature were reported in 22 patients. Six patients had cerebral haemorrhage and 3 died; autopsy revealed that they had underlying cerebrovascular abnormalities. Eleven patients were reported to have developed paraplegia; in 5 of these cases this may have been due to incorrect needle placement. Two patients suddenly developed transverse myelitis with paraplegia after 2 and 3 weeks, with subsequent recovery. Two patients had seizures after the injection of chymopapain, and in another patient this reaction occurred several days after the procedure. Hypersensitivity to the contrast medium and underlying epilepsy may have played a role in 2 of these cases. Twenty-two patients had discitis with severe back pain and spasm. In 9 cases bacteria could be cultured. There were 11 deaths. In addition to the 5 deaths mentioned above 1 patient developed a fatal *Staphylococcus aureus* meningitis following discitis at the site of injection. Three patients apparently died of an underlying disease and in 2 other cases the relationship to the administration of chymopapain was not clear.

Another review[2] of serious reactions associated with chymopapain administration reported between 1982 and 1991 (including the earlier postmarketing study) found 121 reactions among approximately 135 000 patients. They included fatal anaphylaxis (7), infections (24), haemorrhage (32), and neurological reactions (32).

Both reviews concluded that careful attention to proper patient selection and correct techniques of intradiscal needle placement are the most important factors in avoiding adverse effects with chymopapain.

1. Agre K, *et al*. Chymodiactin postmarketing surveillance: demographic and adverse experience data in 29075 patients. *Spine* 1984; **9:** 479–85.
2. Nordby EJ, *et al*. Safety of chemonucleolysis: adverse effects reported in the United States, 1982–1991. *Clin Orthop* 1993; **293:** 122–34.

Precautions

Chymopapain should not be used in those patients with a known sensitivity to papaya proteins or in patients with progressive paralysis, or tumours of the spinal cord, or lesions of the cauda equina. Severe spondylolisthesis is also a contra-indication. It should not be given to patients with heart failure, coronary artery disease, or respiratory failure who may be at increased risk if anaphylaxis occurs, nor to patients receiving beta blockers.

Care is required in administering chymopapain to ensure that the injection is into the disc and not intrathecal. However, discography is not recommended since the use of contrast media may exacerbate neurotoxicity and may inactivate the enzyme.

The risk of allergic reactions associated with chymopapain is so high that no patient should ever receive it more than once. Tests to identify those most at risk and pretreatment with antihistamines (H_1 and H_2) and corticosteroids may be employed, but drugs and equipment for the emergency management of anaphylactic reactions should always be to hand when giving patients chymopapain. The risk of anaphylaxis is higher in women.

Injection of more than one disc is associated with an increased frequency of neurological reactions therefore such injection should only be carried out following confirmation of definite further disc involvement.

Uses and Administration

Chymopapain is used as an injection into the intervertebral disc in the treatment of sciatic pain secondary to herniation of intervertebral discs of the lumbar spine (chemonucleolysis). Chymopapain injection should preferably be administered under local anaesthesia rather than under general anaesthesia. A recommended dose for a single intervertebral disc is 2 to 4 nanokatals, with a maximum dose per patient of 8 nanokatals.

The use of chymopapain for the treatment of discogenic sciatica remains controversial. While some clinicians consider it when conservative management of low back pain (p.10) has failed and before proceeding to surgery[1] others are reported to have largely abandoned the technique in view of its serious adverse effects.[2]

1. Williams F. Chemonucleolysis for treating sciatica. *Br J Hosp Med* 1994; **52:** 52.
2. Bush K. Chemonucleolysis for treating sciatica. *Br J Hosp Med* 1994; **52:** 52–3.

Preparations

Proprietary Preparations (details are given in Part 3)
Austral.: Chymodiactin; ***Belg.:*** Discase; ***Canad.:*** Chymodiactin; ***Fr.:*** Chymodiactine; ***Irl.:*** Chymodiactin; ***Spain:*** Chymodiactin; ***UK:*** Chymodiactin; ***USA:*** Chymodiactin.

Chymotrypsin (3709-g)

Chymotrypsin *(BAN, rINN)*.

α-Chymotrypsin; Chymotrypsinum; Quimotripsina.

CAS — 9004-07-3.

Pharmacopoeias. In *Chin., Eur.* (see p.viii), and *US.*

A proteolytic enzyme obtained by the activation of chymotrypsinogen extracted from the pancreas of beef (ox).

Chymotrypsin (Ph. Eur.) contains not less than 5 microkatals in each mg. Chymotrypsin (USP 23) contains not less than 1000 USP units in each mg, calculated on the dry basis.

A white to yellowish-white odourless crystalline or amorphous powder; the amorphous form is hygroscopic. Sparingly **soluble** in water. A 1% solution has a pH of 3.0 to 5.0. Solutions have a maximum stability at pH 3 and a maximum activity at about pH 8. **Store** at 2° to 8° in airtight containers. Protect from light.

Units

Chymotrypsin (Ph. Eur.) is assayed for potency, by comparison with a reference standard, in terms of its ability to digest ethyl *N*-acetyl-L-tyrosinate at 25° and the hydrolysis is followed potentiometrically. The activity is expressed in terms of microkatals and Chymotrypsin (Ph. Eur.) contains not less than 5.0 microkatals per mg.

Chymotrypsin (USP 23) is assayed for potency, by comparison with a reference standard, in terms of its ability to digest ethyl *N*-acetyl-L-tyrosinate at 25°. The hydrolysis is followed spectrophotometrically by measurement of the light absorption at 237 nm and the potency is determined by the average change in absorption per minute. The activity is expressed in terms of USP units and Chymotrypsin (USP 23) contains not less than 1000 units per mg.

Other units that may be encountered are FIP units, 60 of which have been taken to be equivalent to about one microkatal, Armour units and Denver (or Wallace or Wampole) units.

Adverse Effects

Chymotrypsin is antigenic and severe allergic reactions have occasionally followed its intramuscular injection; where hypersensitivity is suspected, a sensitivity test should be made before injection.

Increased intra-ocular pressure, corneal oedema, striation, and moderate uveitis have occurred following its use in ophthalmology.

Precautions

It is inadvisable to use chymotrypsin in ocular surgery for patients under 20 years of age or for patients with congenital cataracts or high vitreous pressure and a gaping incisional wound.

Uses and Administration

Chymotrypsin is used in ophthalmology for the dissection of the zonule of the lens, thus facilitating intracapsular cataract extraction and reducing trauma to the eye. For this purpose a solution of chymotrypsin in a sterile diluent such as sodium chloride injection (0.9%) is injected to irrigate the posterior chamber.

Chymotrypsin is also given, usually by mouth or topically, for its supposed action in reducing soft tissue inflammation and oedema associated with surgery or traumatic injuries, and in patients suffering from upper respiratory-tract disorders.

Preparations

USP 23: Chymotrypsin for Ophthalmic Solution.

Proprietary Preparations (details are given in Part 3)
Canad.: Catarase†; ***Fr.:*** Alphacutanee; ***Ger.:*** Alpha-Chymocutan; Alpha-Chymotrase; ***Irl.:*** Chymar†; ***Ital.:*** Zonulasi†; ***S.Afr.:*** Zonulysin†; ***Spain:*** Quimotrase; ***Switz.:*** Zolyse†; ***UK:*** Zonulysin†.

Multi-ingredient: ***Aust.:*** Wobenzym; ***Fr.:*** Alpha-Kadol†; Alphintern; Aphlomycine†; ***Ger.:*** Alphintern†; Enzym-Wied; Wobe-Mugos E; Wobenzym N; ***Irl.:*** Chymoral†; ***Ital.:*** Chimotetra†; Chymoral†; Chymoser Balsamico†; Chymoser†; Essen Enzimatico; Essen†; Flogozym†; Kilozim†; Quanto†; Ribociclina; Trimalcina†; ***Spain:*** Bristaciclina Dental; Chymar†; Chymocyclar†; Dertrase; Dosil Enzimatico; Doxiten Enzimatico; Duo Gobens; Epixian; Hemotripsin†; Quimodril; Sinus†; Solupen Enzimatico; Terranilo; Tetralfa†.

Cianidanol (12563-l)

Cianidanol *(rINN)*.

(+)-Catechin; (+)-Catechol; (+)-Cyanidanol-3; Dexcyanidanol. *trans*-2-(3,4-Dihydroxyphenyl)-3,4-dihydro-2*H*-1-benzopyran-3,5,7-triol.

$C_{15}H_{14}O_6$ = 290.3.

CAS — 154-23-4.

NOTE. The name cianidol has been used for this compound.

Cianidanol was formerly used in the treatment of hepatic disorders. Its use has been associated with severe haemolytic anaemia; fatalities have been reported.

Cicloxilic Acid (12569-a)

Cicloxilic Acid *(rINN)*.

cis-2-Hydroxy-2-phenylcyclohexanecarboxylic acid.

$C_{13}H_{16}O_3$ = 220.3.

CAS — 57808-63-6.

Cicloxilic acid has been used in the treatment of hepatic disorders.

Preparations

Proprietary Preparations (details are given in Part 3)
Ital.: Plecton†.

Multi-ingredient: ***Ital.:*** Pleiabil†.

Ciliary Neurotrophic Factor (11770-e)

CNTF.

Ciliary neurotrophic factor is a nerve growth factor produced in neural tissues and released in response to injury. Recombinant ciliary neurotrophic factor is under investigation in motor neurone disease (p.1625) and peripheral neuropathy.

References.

1. Miller RG, *et al*. A placebo-controlled trial of recombinant human ciliary neurotrophic (rhCNTF) factor in amyotrophic lateral sclerosis. *Ann Neurol* 1996; **39:** 256–60.

Cimicifuga (12570-e)

Black Cohosh; Black Snakeroot.

Pharmacopoeias. Chin. includes the rhizome of *C. heracleifolia, C. dahurica,* and *C. foetida. Jpn* includes the rhizome of *C. simplex* (=*C. foetida*) or other species of the same genus.

The roots of *Cimicifuga racemosa* (Ranunculaceae).

Cimicifuga is included in a number of preparations for coughs and for gynaecological disorders. It is reported that it may cause vertigo, headache, prostration, and gastro-intestinal irritation when taken in large doses.

It is used in homoeopathic medicine where it is known as Actaea racemosa or Actaea rac.

Preparations

Proprietary Preparations (details are given in Part 3)
Aust.: Agnukliman; ***Ger.:*** Cefakliman mono; Cimisan; Cirkufemal; Femilla N; Klimadynon; ***Switz.:*** Remifemin.

Multi-ingredient: ***Austral.:*** Dong Quai Complex; Esten†; Harpagophytum Complex; Herbal PMS Formula; Lifesystem Herbal Formula 4 Women's Formula; Medinat Esten; Perpain†; PMT Complex; Proesten; Salagesic; Viburnum Complex; Women's Formula Herbal Formula 3; ***Ger.:*** Femisana N; Remifemin plus; ***S.Afr.:*** Bronchicough; Bronchicum; Bronchicum SB†; ***Spain:*** Iodocafedrina†; ***UK:*** Biophylin; Helonias Compound; Ligvites; Super Mega B+C; Vegetable Cough Remover; Vegetex.

Cinametic Acid (3711-d)

Cinametic Acid *(rINN)*.

Acidum Cinameticum. 4-(2-Hydroxyethoxy)-3-methoxycinnamic acid.

$C_{12}H_{14}O_5$ = 238.2.

CAS — 35703-32-3.

Cinametic acid has been used as a choleretic in doses of 500 to 750 mg daily in divided doses.

Preparations

Proprietary Preparations (details are given in Part 3)
Fr.: Transoddi.

Cinchona Bark (529-n)

Chinae Cortex; Chinarinde; Cinchona; Cinchonae Cortex; Cinchonae Succirubrae Cortex; Jesuit's Bark; Peruvian Bark; Quina; Quina Vermelha; Quinquina; Quinquina Rouge; Red Cinchona Bark.

Pharmacopoeias. In *Eur.* (see p.viii), which permits other species of Cinchona.

The dried bark of *Cinchona pubescens* (=*Cinchona succirubra*) or of its varieties or hybrids. It contains not less than 6.5% of total alkaloids, of which 30% to 60% are quinine-type alkaloids. **Protect** from light and moisture.

Cinchona contains a number of alkaloids including two pairs of optical isomers quinine (p.439) and quinidine (p.938) and cinchonine and cinchonidine. Cinchona alkaloids have long been used for their antimalarial activity either singly, as quinine or quinidine, or in mixtures, such as totaquine. Quinidine is also used for its antiarrhythmic properties.

Cinchona bark is used as a bitter and is also employed in herbal remedies and in homoeopathic medicine.

Preparations

Proprietary Preparations (details are given in Part 3)
Ital.: Venustas Lozione Antiforfora.

Multi-ingredient: ***Aust.:*** Amara; Brady's-Magentropfen; China Eisenwein; China-Eisenwein; Ferrovin-Chinaeisenwein; Mariazeller; ***Belg.:*** Aperop; Stago†; ***Fr.:*** Gripponyl†; Phospharome; Quintonine; ***Ger.:*** "Mletzko" Tropfen†; Amara-Tropfen-Pascoe; Cardibisana; Castrophan†; Chinavit†; Dr. Maurers Magen-Apotheke†; Friosmin†; Gastrol S; Hepaticum "Mletzko"†; Hepaticum-Medice H; Hepaton†; Hicoton; Majocarmin mite†; Majocarmin†; Pascopankreat†; Sedovent; ***Ital.:*** Amaro Maffioli†; Bitteridina; Chinoidina; Crisolax†; Prid con Boldo†; Prid†; Rabarbaroni; ***Spain:*** Pildoras Ferrug Sanatori; ***Switz.:*** Phytomed Rhino; Stago†; Valverde contre les douleurs†; Vin Tonique de Vial.

Cineole (4629-j)

Cajuputol; Cineol; Eucalyptol *(USAN)*. 1,8-Epoxy-*p*-menthane; 1,3,3-Trimethyl-2-oxabicyclo[2.2.2]octane.
$C_{10}H_{18}O$ = 154.2.
CAS — 470-82-6.

Pharmacopoeias. In *Belg., Fr., Swiss,* and *US.*

A colourless liquid with an aromatic camphoraceous odour obtained from eucalyptus oil, cajuput oil, and other oils. **Soluble** 1 in 2 of alcohol (70%). **Store** in a cool place in airtight containers. Protect from light.

Cineole has the actions and uses of eucalyptus oil (p.1578). It has been used in counter-irritant ointments and in dentifrices. It has also been used in nasal preparations, but oily solutions inhibit ciliary movement and may cause lipoid pneumonia. Preparations containing cineole with other volatile substances have been used in the treatment of renal and biliary calculi.

Preparations

Proprietary Preparations (details are given in Part 3)
Ger.: Soledum; Soledum Balsam.

Multi-ingredient: ***Aust.:*** Asthma-Frenon; Endrine mild†; Endrine†; Rhinospray Plus; Rowachol; Rowatinex; ***Austral.:*** BFI; Euky Bear Nasex; Euky Bearub; Methyl Salicylate Ointment Compound; Tixylix Chest Rub; Vasylox; Vicks Sinex; ***Belg.:*** Balsoclase; Calyptol†; Campho-Pneumine†; Captol†; Endrine; Endrine Doux; Eucalyptine Le Brun; Eucalyptine Pholcodine Le Brun; Inhalene; Inopectol†; Pinthym†; Vegebom†; ***Canad.:*** Alsirub; Antiseptic Mouthwash; Balminil Nasal Ointment; Balminil Suppositoires; Bentasil; Cal Mo Dol; Calmomusc; Camphre Compose; Carboseptol; Creo Grippe; Demo-Cineol; Inarub; Infraline; Jack & Jill Rub; Listerine; Marco Rub Camphorated; Marco Rub Camphorated Ointment; Mielocol; Pastilles Valda; Physio-Rub; Pommade au The des Bois; Thermo Rub; Valda; Vaporisateur Medicamente; ***Fr.:*** Atussil-Eucalyptol†; Balseptol†; Bi-Qui-Nol; Biocalyptol; Biolau; Biphedrine Huileuse†; Bismurectol; Broncho-Tulisan Eucalyptol; Bronchodermine; Bronchospray; Campho-Pneumine; Dinacode; Essence Algerienne; Eucalyptine Le Brun; Eucalyptine Pholcodine; Glyco-Thymoline; Hexapneumine; Lyptocodine; Neo-Codion; Pectoderme; Pholcones; Pholcones Bismuth; Pholcones Bismuth-Quinine†; Pholcones Guaiphenesine-Quinine†; Pinorhinol; Pulmofluide Ephedrine†; Pulmofluide Simple; Pulveol†; Rectophedrol; Rhino-Sulforgan†; Thiopheol†; Tuberol†; Valda; Valda Septol; Vapo-Myrtol; Vegebom; ***Ger.:*** Asthma-Frenon-S†; Bisolvomed mit Codein†; Bisolvomed†; Bronchicum Inhalat†; Choldestal†; Denosol; Eufimenth-Balsam N; Franzbragil "F"†; Influsanbalm†; Parodontal F5 med; Pinimenthol-Oral N; Rowachol; Rowachol comp.; Rowachol-Digestiv; Rowatinex; Sedotussin Expectorans; Soledexin†; Transpulmin E; Transpulmin†; Wick Vaporub; Zynedo-B†; Zynedo-K†; ***Irl.:*** Listerine; Rowachol; Rowatinex; Valda†; ***Ital.:*** Abiostil; Antalgola†; Balsamico F. di M.†; Balta Intimo Soluzione; Bronchenolo Balsamo†; Broncopulmin; Calyptol; Codetilina-Eucaliptolo He; Efedrocanfine†; Eucaliptina; Lacrime; Linimento Bertelli†; Lipobalsamo; Neo Soluzione Sulfo Balsamica; Otormon F (Femminile)†; Paidorinovit; Pastiglie Valda; Pulmarin; Respiro; Rinogutt Eucalipto-Fher; Rinos; Rinovit; Rowachol†; Rowatin†; Sedopulmina†; Transpulmina Gel†; Transpulmina Gola; Transpulmina Gola Nebulizzatore†; Transpulmina Tosse; Vapor Sol†; Vicks Sinex; ***Mon.:*** Calyptol; ***Neth.:*** Balsoclase Compositum; Balsoclase-E; Rhinocaps; ***S.Afr.:*** Respisniffers; ***Spain:*** Amidoyina†; Angi†; Broncosolvente EP†; Broncovital; Bronquimar; Bronquimar Vit A; Brota Rectal Bals; Caltoson Balsamico; Caramelos Agua del Carmen; Caramelos Balsam; Combitorax Ampicilina†; Complexobiotico Bals†; Dimayon; Diminex Antitusigeno; Diminex Balsamico; Doctomitil; Dolmitin; Edusan Fte Rectal; Etro Balsamico; Eucalyptospirine; Eucalyptospirine Lact; Eufipulmo†; Eupnol; Exapenil Mucolitico†; Homocodeina Timol†; Kneipp Balsamo; Maboterpen; Mentobox; Orto Nasal; Pastillas Juanola; Pastillas Pectoral Kely; Pinimenthol†; Piorlis; Pomada Balsamica; Pulmo Grey Balsam; Pulmofasa; Pulmofasa Antihist; Pulmonilo Synergium; Queratil; Respir Balsamico; Retarpen Balsamico; Rinobanedif; Rinotiazol Fenilefri†; Rowachol; Rowanefrin; Sinus Inhalaciones; Tifell; Trophires; Trophires Rectal Lact†; Vicks Spray; Vitavox Pastillas; Yoguito†; ***Swed.:*** Otrivin Menthol; ***Switz.:*** Bisolvex; Bronchodermine†; Bronchol N; Demotussil; Mucosan†; Neo-Codion†; Olbas; Rectoquintyl; Rectoquintyl-Promethazine; Rectoseptal-Neo bismuthe; Rectoseptal-Neo Pholcodine; Rectoseptal-Neo simple; Resorbane; Sedasept; Sedotussin; Transpulmine†; Vicks Sinex; ***UK:*** Copholco†; Copholcoids†; Covonia Bronchial Balsam; Dubam; Fisherman's Friend Honey Cough Syrup†; Listerine Antiseptic Mouthwash; Rowachol; Rowatinex; Valda; Vicks Sinex; ***USA:*** Babee; BFI; Cool-Mint Listerine; FreshBurst Listerine; Listerine; Pfeiffer's Cold Sore; Rid-a-Pain†; Saratoga; Sting-Eze; Vitanumonyl.

Cinnamaverine (13340-v)

Cinnamaverine *(rINN)*.
2-(Diethylamino)ethyl 2,3-diphenylacrylate.
$C_{21}H_{25}NO_2$ = 323.4.
CAS — 1679-75-0.

Cinnamaverine has been used for its relaxant effect on smooth muscle. The hydrochloride is an ingredient in some cough preparations.

Cinnamon (4630-q)

Canela; Canela do Ceilão; Cannelle Dite de Ceylan; Ceylon Cinnamon; Ceylonzimt; Cinnam.; Cinnamomi Cortex; Cinnamon Bark; Zimt.

Pharmacopoeias. In *Eur.* (see p.viii).

The dried bark of the shoots of coppiced trees of *Cinnamomum zeylanicum* (Lauraceae) containing not less than 1.2% v/w of volatile oil. It has a characteristic, aromatic odour and a characteristic, slightly sweet, warm and fragrant taste.

Powdered cinnamon contains not less than 1% v/w of volatile oil. **Protect** from light.

Cinnamon is carminative and slightly astringent and is included in preparations for gastro-intestinal disorders. It is also used as a flavour. There have been a number of reports of hypersensitivity to cinnamaldehyde and other constituents of cinnamon oil.

Preparations

Proprietary Preparations (details are given in Part 3)

Multi-ingredient: ***Aust.:*** Brady's-Magentropfen; China-Eisenwein; Mariazeller; Montana; Teekanne Magen- und Darmtee; ***Belg.:*** Richelet†; ***Fr.:*** Elixir Grez; Polypirine; Quintonine; Santane D_5; Santane F_{10}; Santane R_8; ***Ger.:*** Amara-Tropfen-Pascoe; Doppelherz Melissengeist; Dr. Maurers Magen-Apotheke†; Gastrosecur; Majocarmin†; Montana; Presselin 214†; Sedovent; ***Ital.:*** Dam; ***Spain:*** Agua del Carmen; Melisana†; ***Switz.:*** Baume†; ***UK:*** Aluminium Free Indigestion; Cough Drops; Melissa comp..

Cinnamon Oil (4631-p)

Aetheroleum Cinnamomi Zeylanici; Ceylon Cinnamon Bark Oil; Cinnam. Oil; Esencia de Canela; Essence de Cannelle de Ceylan; Oleum Cinnamomi; Zimtöl.

Pharmacopoeias. In *Aust., Br., Fr.,* and *Swiss.* Cinnamon oil has been used as the name for Cassia Oil in some countries. Cinnamon Oil (*Jpn P.*) is obtained from either *Cinnamomum cassia* or *Cinnamomum zeylanicum*.

A clear yellow volatile oil with a characteristic odour obtained by distillation from cinnamon. It becomes reddish-brown with age. It contains 60 to 80% w/w of aldehydes, calculated as cinnamaldehyde (C_9H_8O). It also contains eugenol. **Store** at a temperature not exceeding 25°. Protect from light.

Cinnamon oil has properties and uses similar to those of cinnamon (above). It is also included in preparations for musculoskeletal and joint disorders and for respiratory-tract disorders. There have been a number of reports of sensitivity to cinnamaldehyde, a constituent of cinnamon oil.

Preparations

BP 1998: Aromatic Cardamom Tincture; Compound Cardamom Tincture; Concentrated Cinnamon Water; Tolu-flavour Solution.

Proprietary Preparations (details are given in Part 3)

Multi-ingredient: ***Aust.:*** Dr Fischers Melissengeist; Tiger Balsam Rot; ***Belg.:*** Calmant Martou; Melisana†; ***Canad.:*** Tiger Balm Red; ***Fr.:*** Aromasol; Baume du Tigre†; Gouttes aux Essences; Tigidol; ***Ger.:*** Amol Heilkrautergeist N; Salviathymol N; ***Neth.:*** Tijgerbalsem†; ***S.Afr.:*** Enterodyne; Karvol; ***Spain:*** Depurativo Richelet; ***Switz.:*** Baume de Chine Temple of Heaven blanc; Carmol†; Hederka†; Pirom; ***UK:*** Slippery Elm Stomach Tablets; Tiger Balm Liquid; Tiger Balm Red.

Citicoline (12576-k)

Citicoline *(pINN)*.
CDP-Choline; Citidoline; Cytidine Diphosphate Choline; IP-302. Choline cytidine-5′-pyrophosphate.
$C_{14}H_{26}N_4O_{11}P_2$ = 488.3.
CAS — 987-78-0.

NOTE. Citicoline Sodium is *USAN*.

Citicoline is a derivative of choline and cytidine involved in the biosynthesis of lecithin. It is claimed to increase blood flow and oxygen consumption in the brain and has been given in the treatment of cerebrovascular disorders, including ischaemic stroke (p.799), and head injury. It is given by intravenous or intramuscular injection in doses of up to 1000 mg daily or by mouth in divided doses of 200 to 600 mg daily. Citicoline sodium has also been used.

References.

1. Cubells JM, Hernando C. Clinical trial on the use of cytidine diphosphate choline in Parkinson's disease. *Clin Ther* 1988; **10:** 664–71.
2. Tazaki Y, *et al.* Treatment of acute cerebral infarction with a choline precursor in a multicenter double-blind placebo-controlled study. *Stroke* 1988; **19:** 211–16.
3. Clark WM, *et al.* A randomized dose-response trial of citicoline in acute ischemic stroke patients. *Neurology* 1997; **49:** 671–8.

Preparations

Proprietary Preparations (details are given in Part 3)
Aust.: Startonyl; ***Fr.:*** Rexort; ***Ital.:*** Acticolin; Actomin; Brassel; Cebroton; Cidifos†; Cidilin; Citidel; Citifar; Citsav; Difosfocin; Encelin; Flussorex; Gerolin; Kemodyn; Logan; Neurex; Neuroton; Nicholin; Nicolsint; Polineural; Sinkron; Sintoclar; ***Jpn:*** Nicholin; ***Spain:*** Neurodynamicum; Numatol; Sauran; Somazina; ***Switz.:*** Somazina†.

Citiolone (12577-a)

Citiolone *(rINN)*.
BO-714. *N*-(Perhydro-2-oxo-3-thienyl)acetamide.
$C_6H_9NO_2S$ = 159.2.
CAS — 1195-16-0.

Citiolone has been used in the treatment of hepatic disorders and as a mucolytic. Hypersensitivity reactions have been reported.

Preparations

Proprietary Preparations (details are given in Part 3)
Ital.: Citiolase; ***Spain:*** Mucorex.

Multi-ingredient: ***Ger.:*** Mederma†; Reducdyn†; Sterofundin CH compositum†; Tutofusin LC†; ***Spain:*** Exapenil Mucolitico†; Hubergrip; Juven Tos†; Muco Teolixir†; Mucorex Ampicilina; Mucorex Ciclin; Tosdetan.

Anhydrous Citric Acid (1307-a)

Acidum Citricum Anhydricum; Citronensäure; E330. 2-Hydroxypropane-1,2,3-tricarboxylic acid.
$C_6H_8O_7$ = 192.1.
CAS — 77-92-9.

NOTE. Anhydrous citric acid was formerly known as citric acid.

Pharmacopoeias. In *Eur.* (see p.viii) and *Jpn. US* allows either the anhydrous or monohydrate form.

Odourless or almost odourless, colourless crystals or granules or white crystalline powder. **Soluble** 1 in 0.5 of water and 1 in 2 of alcohol; sparingly soluble in ether. **Store** in airtight containers.

Citric Acid Monohydrate (1308-t)

Acido del Limón; Acidum Citricum Monohydricum; Hydrous Citric Acid.
$C_6H_8O_7,H_2O$ = 210.1.
CAS — 5949-29-1.

Pharmacopoeias. In *Chin., Eur.* (see p.viii), *Jpn,* and *Pol. US* allows either the anhydrous or monohydrate form.

Odourless or almost odourless, efflorescent, colourless crystals or granules or white crystalline powder. **Soluble** 1 in 0.5 of water and 1 in 2 of alcohol; sparingly soluble in ether. **Store** in airtight containers.

Adverse Effects and Precautions

Citric acid ingested frequently or in large quantities may cause erosion of the teeth and have a local irritant action.

Interactions

Aluminium hydroxide. Intestinal absorption of aluminium ions may be enhanced by concurrent administration of citrates. Caution is needed in patients with chronic renal disease receiving aluminium hydroxide as a phosphate binder who are given a calcium supplement in the form of effervescent tablets which contain citric acid.[1]

1. Mees EJD, Basçi A. Citric acid in calcium effervescent tablets may favour aluminium intoxication. *Nephron* 1991; **59:** 322.

Uses and Administration

Citric acid is used in effervescing mixtures; citric acid monohydrate is used in the preparation of effervescent granules.

Citric acid monohydrate is used as a synergist to enhance the effectiveness of antioxidants.

Preparations containing citric acid are used in the management of dry mouth (p.1470) and to dissolve renal calculi, alkalinise the urine, and prevent encrustation of urinary catheters. Citric acid is an ingredient of citrated anticoagulant solutions. Citric acid has also been used in preparations for the treatment of gastro-intestinal disturbances and metabolic acidosis.

In Great Britain, citric acid 1 in 500 of water is an approved disinfectant for foot and mouth disease.

Preparations

BP 1998: Lemon Syrup; Paediatric Compound Tolu Linctus; Paediatric Simple Linctus; Potassium Citrate Mixture; Simple Linctus;
Ph. Eur.: Anticoagulant Acid-Citrate-Glucose Solutions (ACD); Anticoagulant Citrate-Phosphate-Glucose Solution (CPD);
USP 23: Anticoagulant Citrate Dextrose Solution; Anticoagulant Citrate Phosphate Dextrose Adenine Solution; Anticoagulant Citrate Phosphate Dextrose Solution; Citric Acid, Magnesium Oxide, and Sodium Carbonate Irrigation; Magnesium Carbonate and Citric Acid for Oral Solution; Magnesium Citrate Oral Solution; Potassium and Sodium Bicarbonates and Citric Acid Effervescent Tablets for Oral Solution; Potassium Citrate And Citric Acid Oral Solution; Sodium Citrate and Citric Acid Oral Solution; Tricitrates Oral Solution.

Proprietary Preparations (details are given in Part 3)
Ger.: Citrosteril; ***UK:*** Uriflex†.

Multi-ingredient: ***Aust.:*** Alka-Seltzer; Duplotrast Z; Helo-acid; Kalioral; ***Austral.:*** Alka-Seltzer; Citralite; Citravescent; Durolax X-Pack; Eno; Ural; ***Belg.:*** Andrews; Uro-Tainer Solutio R†; Uro-Tainer Suby G†; ***Canad.:*** Alka-Seltzer; Bromo Madelon; Citrocarbonate; PMS-Dicitrate; Renacidin†; ***Fr.:*** Aerophagyl†; Alka-Seltzer; Citro-B_6†; Citrocholine; Elixir Grez; Foncitril; Gastrilax; Hepargitol; Ornitaine; ***Ger.:*** Alka-Seltzer; Blemaren N; Citropepsin; Gastrovison†; Hanooxygen†; Helo-acid compositum†; Helo-acid†; Lithurex; Pepzitrat; Presselin Osmo†; Retterspitz Ausserlich; Retterspitz Gelee; Retterspitz Innerlich; Syracerin†; Unibaryt; Uralyt-Kalium†; Uricedin†; ***Irl.:*** Andrews†; Cymalon; Mictral; ***Ital.:*** Alka-Seltzer; Citroepatina; Duogas; Eno; Gastrovison; Geffer; Lavanda Sofar; Limonal; Nuovo Andrews†; Roge; ***Neth.:*** Alka-Seltzer; Hexoll; ***Norw.:*** Pico-Salax; ***S.Afr.:*** Adco-Sodasol; Alkafizz; Betasoda; Citro-Soda; Citrocit; Citrovescent†; Effersol; Pneucid; ***Spain:*** Alka-Seltzer; Alquil Dermol†; Eno†; Justegas; Sal de Frutas Eno; Salcedogen; Sales de Frutas P G; Sales Orto; Uralyt Urato; ***Swed.:*** Alka-Seltzer; Pico-Salax; Renapur; ***Switz.:*** Alka-Seltzer; Aloplastine Acide†; Andrews†; E-Z-Gas II; Pico-Salax; Siesta-1; Uro-Tainer Solutio R; Uro-Tainer Suby G; ***UK:*** Alka-Seltzer; Andrews; Carbex; Collins Elixir Pastilles; Dinneford's†; Effercitrate; Eno; Fisherman's Friend Honey Cough Syrup†; Hill's Balsam Junior Expectorant; Jackson's Children's Cough Pastilles; Lemsip Linctus†; Melissin; Mictral; Tancolin†; Throaties Family Cough Linctus; Uriflex G; Uriflex R; Uro-Tainer Solution R; Uro-Tainer Suby G; ***USA:*** Alka-Seltzer Antacid; Alka-Seltzer Effervescent Tablets; Alka-Seltzer with Aspirin; Bicitra; Bromo Seltzer Effervescent Granules; Cytra-2; Cytra-3; Cytra-K; Cytra-LC; Extra Strength Alka-Seltzer Effervescent Tablets; Gold Alka-Seltzer; Oracit; Original Alka-Seltzer Effervescent Tablets; Polycitra; Polycitra-K; Polycitra-LC; Renacidin; Sparkles; Summer's Eve Disposable.

Citronella Oil (4633-w)

Oleum Citronellae.

Pharmacopoeias. In *Aust., Belg.,* and *Swiss.*
Aust. gives Oleum Melissae Indicum as a synonym for citronella oil.

A pale to deep yellow volatile oil with a pleasant characteristic odour, obtained by distillation from *Cymbopogon nardus* or *C. winterianus* (Gramineae) or varietal or hybrid forms of these species. The chief constituents are geraniol ($C_{10}H_{18}O$) and citronellal ($C_{10}H_{18}O$).

Citronella oil is used as a perfume and insect repellent. Hypersensitivity has been reported.

Preparations

Proprietary Preparations (details are given in Part 3)
Ger.: Valmarin Bad N.

Multi-ingredient: ***Aust.:*** Dr Fischers Melissengeist; Embrocation; Medizinalbad†; Red Point†; Valin Baldrian; ***Fr.:*** Ysol 206; ***Ger.:*** Kneipp Beruhigungs-Bad A; Kneipp Krauter Taschenkur Nerven und Schlaf N; Kneipp Sedativ-Bad†; Schupps Baldrian Sedativbad; Silvapin Aktiv-Tonic MMP†; ***Ital.:*** Citrosystem; Natural Zanzy; Pungino; ***UK:*** Snowfire; ***USA:*** Treo.

Clivers (12130-w)

Cleavers; Galii Aparinis Herba; Galium; Goosegrass.

Clivers is the dried aerial parts of *Galium aparine* (Rubiaceae). It has been used in herbal medicine, principally as a diuretic.

Preparations

Proprietary Preparations (details are given in Part 3)

Multi-ingredient: ***Austral.:*** Galium Complex; Herbal Cleanse; Uva-Ursi Complex; ***UK:*** Antitis; Athera; Boldo; Buchu Compound; Cascade; HealthAid Boldo-Plus; Kas-Bah; Psorasolv; Sciargo; Skin Cleansing; Tabritis; Water Naturtabs; Water Relief Tablets.

Clove (4634-e)

Caryoph.; Caryophylli Flos; Caryophyllum; Clou de Girofle; Cloves; Cravinho; Cravo-da-Índia; Gewürznelke; Giroflier; Tropical Myrtle.

Pharmacopoeias. In *Chin., Eur.* (see p.viii), and *Jpn.*

The dried flower-buds of *Syzygium aromaticum* (=*Eugenia caryophyllus*) (Myrtaceae), containing not less than 15% v/w of volatile oil.

Powdered clove contains not less than 12% v/w of volatile oil. Clove is reddish-brown and has a characteristic odour and an aromatic pungent taste. **Protect** from light.

Clove is a carminative and is used as a flavour. It is the source of clove oil (below).

Clove and clove oil have been abused in the form of cigarettes.

Abuse. Smoking of cigarettes composed of a mixture of tobacco and cloves is a habit which originated in Indonesia and has spread to the USA. There have been a number of reports of severe and sometimes fatal respiratory illness related to smoking clove cigarettes and there is also evidence from *animal* studies that clove cigarette smoke and eugenol (the principal constituent of clove oil) have harmful pulmonary effects. The Council on Scientific Affairs of the American Medical Association considers that in addition to the hazards associated with smoking tobacco, clove cigarettes may also produce severe lung injury in certain susceptible individuals and could also induce pulmonary aspiration in healthy individuals due to diminution of the gag reflex produced by the local anaesthetic action of eugenol.[1] The American Academy of Pediatrics has also alerted paediatricians in the USA to clove-cigarette smoking by young people and warned of the risks.[2]

1. American Medical Association Council on Scientific Affairs. Evaluation of the health hazard of clove cigarettes. *JAMA* 1988; **260:** 3641–4.
2. Committee on Substance Abuse. Hazards of clove cigarettes. *Pediatrics* 1991; **88:** 395–6.

Preparations

Proprietary Preparations (details are given in Part 3)

Multi-ingredient: ***Aust.:*** Apotheker Bauer's Kindertee; Drovitol; Mariazeller; ***Belg.:*** Eugiron; ***Fr.:*** Tisane Clairo; ***Ger.:*** Discmigon; Doppelherz Melissengeist; Dr. Maurers Magen-Apotheke†; Echtrosept-GT†; Inconturina; Presselin 214†; Ventrovis†; ***Ital.:*** Saugella Uomo; ***Switz.:*** Tisane sedative et somnifere "H"†; ***UK:*** Aluminium Free Indigestion; Clairo Tea; Cough Drops; Laxadoron; Revitonil.

Clove Oil (4635-l)

Caryophylli Floris Aetheroleum; Esencia de Clavo; Essence de Girofle; Nelkenöl; Ol. Caryoph.; Oleum Caryophylli.

Pharmacopoeias. In *Eur.* (see p.viii) and *Jpn.*

A clear colourless or pale yellow volatile oil with the characteristic odour and taste of clove, obtained by distillation from clove. It darkens and thickens with age and on exposure to air. It contains phenolic substances, chiefly eugenol. **Soluble** 1 in 2 of alcohol (70%). **Miscible** with dichloromethane, with ether, with fatty oils, and with toluene. **Store** at a temperature not exceeding 25° in airtight containers. Protect from light.

Incompatibility. PVC bottles softened and distorted fairly rapidly in the presence of clove oil, which should not be stored or dispensed in such bottles.[1]

1. Department of Pharmaceutical Sciences of the Pharmaceutical Society of Great Britain. Plastics medicine bottles of rigid PVC. *Pharm J* 1973; **210:** 100.

Clove oil is a carminative that is sometimes used in the treatment of flatulent colic. It is also used as a flavour. Eugenol, a constituent of clove oil, may cause hypersensitivity.

Applied externally clove oil is irritant but can produce local anaesthesia. It is used as a domestic remedy for toothache, a plug of cotton wool soaked in the oil being inserted in the cavity of the carious tooth; repeated application may damage the gingival tissues. Mixed with zinc oxide, it is used as a temporary anodyne dental filling, though eugenol (p.1578) is often preferred.

Adverse effects. A report of severe toxicity following ingestion of clove oil in a child.[1] Adverse effects included coma, acidosis, a generalised seizure, disordered blood clotting, and acute liver damage.

For reference to the harmful effects of smoking clove cigarettes, see under Clove, above.

1. Hartnoll G, *et al.* Near fatal ingestion of oil of cloves. *Arch Dis Child* 1993; **69:** 392–3.

Preparations

BP 1998: Aromatic Cardamom Tincture.

Proprietary Preparations (details are given in Part 3)
UK: Dentogen.

Multi-ingredient: ***Aust.:*** China; Dr Fischers Melissengeist; Fittydent; Parodontax; Tiger Balsam Rot; ***Austral.:*** Dentese†; Logicin Chest Rub; Sigma Relief Chest Rub†; Tiger Balm Red; Tiger Balm White; ***Canad.:*** Dentalgar; Gouttes Dentaires; Tiger Balm Red; Tiger Balm White; ***Fr.:*** Aromasol; Baume Aroma; Baume du Tigre†; Gouttes aux Essences; Tigidol; ***Ger.:*** Amol Heilkrautergeist N; GA-301-Redskin 301; Hustagil Erkaltungsbalsam; Menthol-Balsam†; Parodontal F5 med; Repha-Os; Salviathymol N; ***Ital.:*** Dentosan "Pagni" Collutorio†; Dentosan Mese†; Fialetta Odontalgica Dr Knapp; Ondroly-A; ***Neth.:*** Tijgerbalsem†; ***S.Afr.:*** Enterodyne; ***Spain:*** Dentol Topico; Elixir Dental Formahina†; Otogen Calmante; ***Switz.:*** Baume de Chine Temple of Heaven blanc; Carmol "blanche"†; Carmol "thermogene"†; Carmol†; Olbas; Osa Gel de dentition aux plantes; ***UK:*** 9 Rubbing Oils; Eftab; Medicinal Gargle; Olbas; Pickles Toothache Tincture; Red Oil; Slippery Elm Stomach Tablets; Snowfire; Soothake Toothache Gel; Tiger Balm Liquid; Tiger Balm Red; Tiger Balm White; ***USA:*** Numzit; Toothache Gel.

Cnicus Benedictus (530-k)

Blessed Thistle; Cardo Santo; Carduus Benedictus; Chardon Bénit; Holy Thistle; Kardobenediktenkraut.
CAS — 24394-09-0 (cnicin).
Pharmacopoeias. In *Aust.*

The flowering tops of *Cnicus benedictus* (=*Carbenia benedicta; Carduus benedictus*) (Compositae).

Cnicus benedictus has been used as a bitter.

Preparations

Proprietary Preparations (details are given in Part 3)

Multi-ingredient: ***Aust.:*** Mag Kottas Leber-Gallentee; Mariazeller; ***Belg.:*** Tisane Antibiliaire et Stomachique; ***Ger.:*** Asgocholan†; Bilisan forte†; Bomagall forte S; Carvomin; Cheiranthol; Esberigal N; Friosmin†; Gallexier; Gallitophen†; Gastritol; Hepaticum-Divinal†; Hevert-Gall S; Losapan†; Ventrodigest†; ***Switz.:*** Gastrosan; Rasayana†; Tisane pour le coeur et la circulation "H"†; ***UK:*** Gladlax.

Cobalt Chloride (12597-f)

Cobaltous Chloride.
$CoCl_2,6H_2O$ = 237.9.
CAS — 7646-79-9 (anhydrous).
Pharmacopoeias. In *Aust.*

Adverse Effects

Reactions to cobalt have included anorexia, nausea and vomiting, diarrhoea, precordial pain, cardiomyopathy, flushing of the face and extremities, skin rashes, tinnitus, temporary nerve deafness, renal injury, diffuse thyroid enlargement, and hypothyroidism. In large doses it may reduce the production of erythrocytes.

References.

1. Kennedy A, *et al.* Fatal myocardial disease associated with industrial exposure to cobalt. *Lancet* 1981; **i:** 412–4.
2. Cugell DW, *et al.* The respiratory effects of cobalt. *Arch Intern Med* 1990; **150:** 177–83.
3. Evans P, *et al.* Cobalt and cobalt compounds. *Toxicity Review 29.* London: HMSO, 1993.

Uses and Administration

Cobalt chloride, when administered to both normal and anaemic subjects, produces reticulocytosis and a rise in the erythrocyte count. This property suggested its use in the treatment of certain types of anaemia, but its general therapeutic use is, however, unjustified and not without danger.

In veterinary medicine, cobalt chloride has been given as a dietary supplement to ruminants.

Preparations

Proprietary Preparations (details are given in Part 3)
Multi-ingredient: ***Ital.:*** Ferrlecit†.

Cobalt Oxide (12598-d)

Tricobalt Tetroxide.
Co_3O_4 = 240.8.
CAS — 1308-06-1.
Pharmacopoeias. In *BP(Vet).*

It consists of cobalt (II, III) oxide (tricobalt tetroxide) with a small proportion of cobalt (III) oxide (dicobalt trioxide). A black odourless powder. Practically **insoluble** in water; dissolves in mineral acids and in solutions of the alkali hydroxides.

Cobalt oxide is used in veterinary practice for the prevention of cobalt deficiency in ruminants. The sulphate has been used similarly. For the adverse effects of cobalt, see Cobalt Chloride, above.

Coccidioidin (7942-n)

Pharmacopoeias. In US.

A sterile solution containing the antigens obtained from the byproducts of mycelial growth or from the spherules of the fungus *Coccidioides immitis*; it contains a suitable antimicrobial. It should be stored at 2° to 8° and any dilutions should be used within 24 hours. The expiry date is not later than 3 years (mycelial product) or 18 months (spherule-derived product) after release from the manufacturer's cold storage.

Coccidioidin is used as an aid to the diagnosis of coccidioidomycosis and, in conjunction with other antigens, to assess the status of cell-mediated immunity. The usual dose is 0.1 mL of a 1 in 100 dilution by intradermal (intracutaneous) injection.

For reference to the use of coccidioidin for anergy testing in HIV-positive patients, see Tuberculins, p.1640.

Preparations

USP 23: Coccidioidin.

Proprietary Preparations (details are given in Part 3)
USA: BioCox; Spherulin.

Co-dergocrine Mesylate (1503-f)

Co-dergocrine Mesylate *(BAN)*.

Co-dergocrine Mesilate; Co-dergocrine Methanesulphonate; Dihydroergotoxine Mesylate; Dihydroergotoxine Methanesulphonate; Dihydrogenated Ergot Alkaloids; Ergoloid Mesylates *(USAN)*; Hydrogenated Ergot Alkaloids.

CAS — 11032-41-0 (co-dergocrine); 8067-24-1 (co-dergocrine mesylate).

Pharmacopoeias. In Br., Fr., Swiss, and US.

A mixture in equal proportions of dihydroergocornine mesylate ($C_{31}H_{41}N_5O_5,CH_4O_3S$ = 659.8), dihydroergocristine mesylate, and dihydroergocryptine mesylate, the dihydroergocryptine being present as both the α and β forms in the ratio 1.5 to 2.5:1.

A white to yellowish-white odourless or almost odourless powder. Slightly to sparingly **soluble** in water; soluble in alcohol and in methyl alcohol; soluble to sparingly soluble in acetone; slightly soluble in chloroform; practically insoluble in ether. A 0.5% solution in water has a pH of 4.2 to 5.2. **Store** in airtight containers at a temperature not exceeding 25°. Protect from light.

Adverse Effects

Side-effects occasionally reported with co-dergocrine mesylate include abdominal cramps, nausea, vomiting, headache, blurred vision, skin rashes, nasal stuffiness, flushing of the skin, dizziness, bradycardia, and orthostatic hypotension.

Local irritation has been reported following sublingual administration.

Effects on the cardiovascular system. Of 8 patients given co-dergocrine mesylate 1.5 mg three times daily for the treatment of dementia, 3 developed severe sinus bradycardia associated with general deterioration in their condition, necessitating withdrawal of the treatment.[1] However, Cohen[2] reported that no sinus bradycardia had been observed in 40 elderly patients in whom the dose was built up to 1.5 mg three times daily over 3 weeks.

1. Cayley ACD, *et al.* Sinus bradycardia following treatment with Hydergine for cerebrovascular insufficiency. *Br Med J* 1975; **4:** 384–5.
2. Cohen C. Sinus bradycardia following treatment with Hydergine. *Br Med J* 1975; **4:** 581.

Precautions

Co-dergocrine mesylate should be used with caution in patients with severe bradycardia.

Pharmacokinetics

Bioavailability of co-dergocrine after administration by mouth is low; this has been attributed to incomplete absorption from the gastro-intestinal tract and extensive first-pass metabolism of the portion that is absorbed. The half-life has been reported to be 2 to 5 hours.

Uses and Administration

Unlike the natural ergot alkaloids, co-dergocrine mesylate has only limited vasoconstrictor effects.

It is used with the intention of treating symptoms of mild to moderate dementia in the elderly in doses of 3 or 4.5 mg daily by mouth, preferably before meals. Higher doses have also been used. It is also given sublingually in similar doses. Doses of 300 to 600 μg have been given intramuscularly; it has also been given subcutaneously or by intravenous infusion.

In some countries, co-dergocrine mesylate has been used in the treatment of hypertension (p.788), migraine (p.443), and in peripheral vascular disease (p.794).

Co-dergocrine esylate has been used similarly to the mesylate.

Dementia. Co-dergocrine has been used for many years in dementia (p.1386) but its value is not established.[1-3] Originally its effects were thought to be mediated through peripheral and cerebral vasodilatation but it is now classified as a metabolic enhancer.

1. Hollister LE, Yesavage J. Ergoloid mesylates for senile dementias: unanswered questions. *Ann Intern Med* 1984; **100:** 894–8.
2. Wadworth AN, Chrisp P. Co-dergocrine mesylate: a review of its pharmacodynamic and pharmacokinetic properties and therapeutic use in age-related cognitive decline. *Drugs Aging* 1992; **2:** 153–73.
3. Schneider LS, Olin JT. Overview of clinical trials of Hydergine in dementia. *Arch Neurol* 1994; **51:** 787–98.

Erectile dysfunction. A cream containing aminophylline, co-dergocrine mesylate, and isosorbide dinitrate produced satisfactory erections following topical application in 21 of 36 men with erectile dysfunction (p.1614) due to various causes.[1] Eight out of 9 men with erectile dysfunction of psychogenic origin reported a satisfactory response. However, another study was abandoned after the cream produced no effect in 10 consecutive patients.[2]

1. Gomaa A, *et al.* Topical treatment of erectile dysfunction: randomised double blind placebo controlled trial of cream containing aminophylline, isosorbide dinitrate, and co-dergocrine mesylate. *Br Med J* 1996; **312:** 1512–15.
2. Naude JH, Le Roux PJ. Topical treatment of erectile dysfunction did not show results. *Br Med J* 1998; **316:** 1318.

Preparations

BP 1998: Co-dergocrine Tablets;
USP 23: Ergoloid Mesylates Capsules; Ergoloid Mesylates Oral Solution; Ergoloid Mesylates Tablets.

Proprietary Preparations (details are given in Part 3)
Aust.: Aramexe; Dorehydrin; Ergomed; Ergoplex; Hydergin; ***Belg.:*** Hydergine; Ibexone; Stofilan; ***Canad.:*** Hydergine; ***Fr.:*** Capergyl; Dulcion†; Ergodose; Ergokod†; Hydergine; Optamine; Perenan; Simactil†; ***Ger.:*** Circanol; Dacoren; DCCK; Defluina N; DH-Tox†; Enirant; Ergodesit; Ergoplus; Ergotox; Hydergin; Hydro-Cebral; Nehydrin N; Novofluen†; Orphol; Sponsin; ***Irl.:*** Hydergine; ***Ital.:*** Coristin†; Hydergina; Ischelium; Progeril†; Tredilat†; ***Neth.:*** Hydergine; Hydroxium†; ***S.Afr.:*** Hydergine†; ***Spain:*** Artedil†; Ergodilat; Hydergina; ***Swed.:*** Hydergin; ***Switz.:*** Ergohydrine; Hydergine; Progeril; ***UK:*** Hydergine; ***USA:*** Gerimal; Hydergine.

Multi-ingredient: ***Aust.:*** Pontuc; ***Ger.:*** Pontuc; Sinedyston; ***Ital.:*** Ischelium Papaverina; Progeril Papaverina†; Visergil; ***Spain:*** Clinadil Compositum; Neorgine; Piracetam Complex; Visergil.

Coenzyme A (12604-v)

CoA; CoASH. 5′-*O*-{3-Hydroxy-3-[2-(2-mercaptoethylcarbamoyl)ethylcarbamoyl]-2,2-dimethylpropyl}adenosine-3′-dihydrogenphosphate-5′-trihydrogendiphosphate.

$C_{21}H_{36}N_7O_{16}P_3S$ = 767.5.

CAS — 85-61-0.

Formed from adenosine triphosphate, cysteine, and pantothenic acid, coenzyme A is involved in the body in many physiological roles, including the formation of citrate, the oxidation of pyruvate, the oxidation and synthesis of fatty acids, the synthesis of triglycerides, cholesterol, and phospholipids, and the acetylation of amines, choline, and glucosamine. It has been given by injection in a variety of metabolic disorders. Coenzyme A is contra-indicated in acute myocardial infarction.

Preparations

Proprietary Preparations (details are given in Part 3)
Ital.: Coalip; ***Spain:*** Aluzime.

Multi-ingredient: ***Fr.:*** Co-A†; ***Ital.:*** Bio-Biol; Piruvasi†.

Cogalactoisomerase Sodium (12605-g)

UDPG; Uridine-5′-diphosphoglucose Sodium.

$C_{15}H_{22}N_2Na_2O_{17}P_2,3H_2O$ = 664.3.

CAS — 133-89-1 (cogalactoisomerase).

Cogalactoisomerase sodium is used in various hepatic disorders.

Preparations

Proprietary Preparations (details are given in Part 3)
Ital.: Anatox†; Atoxepan†; Bivitox; Detoxasi†; Epatoxil; Evident†; Liotoxid†; Liverasi; Netox†; Toxepasi; Udepasi-50†; Udetox†; Udicit†; Urepasina†; Uridasi†; Zimeton†.

Multi-ingredient: ***Ital.:*** Toxepasi Complex†; ***Spain:*** Toxepasi Complex Forte†.

Colforsin (16542-c)

Colforsin *(USAN, rINN)*.

Boforsin; Forscolin; Forskolin; HL-362; L-75-1362B. (3*R*,4a*R*,5*S*,6*S*,6a*S*,10*S*,10a*R*,10b*S*)-Dodecahydro-5,6,10,10b-tetrahydroxy-3,4a,7,7,10a-pentamethyl-3-vinyl-1*H*-naphtho[2,1-*b*]pyran-1-one, 5-acetate.

$C_{22}H_{34}O_7$ = 410.5.

CAS — 66575-29-9.

Colforsin is an adenylate cyclase stimulator derived from *Coleus forskholii* that has been investigated for a number of conditions, including glaucoma and impotence. It is reported to have positive inotropic and bronchodilator effects.

Collagen (15335-n)

A fibrous protein component of mammalian connective tissue making up almost one third of the total body protein.

Collagen, processed in a variety of ways, has been used in surgery as a haemostatic and as a repair and suture material. For cosmetic purposes it has been injected into the dermis to correct scars and other contour deformities of the skin. Collagen implants have been used to block tear outflow in the management of dry eye (p.1470).

Intraurethral administration of collagen has been used in the treatment of stress incontinence (p.454). There has also been interest in the use of collagen by mouth to suppress the inflammatory process in rheumatoid arthritis (p.2).

References.

1. Herschorn S, *et al.* Early experience with intraurethral collagen injections for urinary incontinence. *J Urol (Baltimore)* 1992; **148:** 1797–1800.
2. Sieper J, *et al.* Oral type II collagen treatment in early rheumatoid arthritis: a double-blind, placebo-controlled, randomized trial. *Arthritis Rheum* 1996; **39:** 41–51.
3. Stanton SL, Monga AK. Incontinence in elderly women: is periurethral collagen an advance? *Br J Obstet Gynaecol* 1997; **104:** 154–7.
4. Anonymous. GAX collagen for genuine stress incontinence. *Drug Ther Bull* 1997; **35:** 86–7.

Preparations

Proprietary Preparations (details are given in Part 3)
Aust.: Avitene; Instat; Urgo Pangen; Zyderm; Zyplast; ***Austral.:*** Ionil Rinse; Zyderm; Zyplast; ***Belg.:*** Colgen; ***Fr.:*** Collafilm; Lenidermyl; Zyderm; Zyplast; ***Ger.:*** Opragen; Pangen; Surgicoll; Tachotop N; TissuVlies; Zyderm; Zyplast; ***Ital.:*** Alfagen; Condress; Idroskin; Instat; Neopelle; Skinat; Stimtes; ***Neth.:*** Willospon Forte; ***Switz.:*** Instat; Lyostypt; ***UK:*** Contigen; Fibracol; Instat; Lyodura†; Lyostypt; Tutoplast Dura†; ***USA:*** Avitene; Helistat; Hemopad†; Hemotene; Instat.

Multi-ingredient: ***Aust.:*** TachoComb; ***Austral.:*** John Plunkett's Protective Day Cream; John Plunkett's Super Wrinkle Cream; ***Belg.:*** Duracoll; ***Ger.:*** TachoComb; ***Ital.:*** Katoderm; Sulfadeck†; Unidermo; ***Switz.:*** Gorgonium; ***USA:*** PDP Liquid Protein.

Collagenase (12606-q)

Clostridiopeptidase A.

CAS — 9001-12-1.

An enzyme derived from the fermentation of *Clostridium histolyticum*.

Collagenase is a proteolytic enzyme with the ability to break down collagen. Preparations containing collagenase are used topically for the debridement of dermal ulcers and burns, and possibly other necrotic lesions, to facilitate granulation and epithelialisation. It has also been given by injection into the intervertebral disc for chemonucleolysis in the treatment of low back pain (p.10).

Hypersensitivity reactions may occur. Local burning, erythema, and pain have been reported at the site of application. It has been suggested that debridement of infected wounds may increase the risk of bacteraemia and that patients should be watched for signs of systemic bacterial infection. The activity of collagenase may be reduced by concomitant use of antiseptics containing detergents, hexachlorophane, and heavy metal ions.

Collagenase potency is expressed in units based on the amount of enzyme required to degrade a standard preparation of undenatured collagen.

Peyronie's disease. Beneficial effects of intralesional collagenase in men with Peyronie's disease.[1]

1. Gelbard MK, *et al.* The use of collagenase in the treatment of Peyronie's disease. *J Urol (Baltimore)* 1985; **134:** 280–3.

Preparations

Proprietary Preparations (details are given in Part 3)
Belg.: Varilisin; ***Canad.:*** Santyl; ***Ital.:*** Noruxol; ***Neth.:*** Novuxol; ***USA:*** Santyl.

Multi-ingredient: ***Ger.:*** Iruxol; ***Irl.:*** Iruxol Mono; Iruxol†; ***Ital.:*** Iruxol; ***S.Afr.:*** Iruxol Mono; ***Spain:*** Iruxol Mono; Iruxol Neo; ***Switz.:*** Iruxol Mono.

Colophony (276-t)

Coloph.; Colophane; Colophonium; Resin; Resina Pini; Resina Terebinthinae; Rosin.

Pharmacopoeias. In *Aust., Br., Jpn, Pol.,* and *Swiss.*

The residue left after distilling the volatile oil from the oleoresin obtained from various species of *Pinus* (Pinaceae). Translucent, pale yellow or brownish-yellow, angular, brittle, readily fusible, glassy masses, with a faint terebinthinate odour.

Practically **insoluble** in water; soluble in alcohol, in carbon disulphide, and in ether; partially soluble in petroleum spirit. It should be **stored** preferably in the unground condition.

Colophony is an ingredient of some collodions and plaster-masses. It has been used as an ingredient of ointments and dressings for wounds and minor skin disorders. Skin sensitisation and allergic respiratory symptoms have been reported.

Preparations

BP 1998: Flexible Collodion.

Proprietary Preparations (details are given in Part 3)

Multi-ingredient: ***Aust.:*** Ehrenhofer-Salbe; Vulpuran; ***Austral.:*** Zam-Buk; ***Ital.:*** Fialetta Odontalgica Dr Knapp; ***Spain:*** Empapol; ***UK:*** Herbheal Ointment; Pickles Corn Caps; Secaderm†; Zam-Buk†.

Comfrey (12607-p)

Comfrey Root; Consolidae Radix; Symphytum.

The dried root and rhizome of *Symphytum officinale* (Boraginaceae). It contains about 0.7% of allantoin, large quantities of mucilage, and some tannin. It may also contain pyrrolizidine alkaloids.

Comfrey was formerly used as an application to wounds and ulcers to stimulate healing and was also given internally for gastric ulceration. It has been applied topically in the treatment of inflammatory disorders. The healing action of comfrey has been attributed to the presence of allantoin (p.1078). Comfrey is used in homoeopathic medicine.

There are reports of hepatotoxicity attributed to pyrrolizidine alkaloids present in comfrey preparations and such preparations have been withdrawn or banned in a number of countries.

Pyrrolizidine alkaloids occur in at least 8 plant families including *Symphytum*. Toxic alkaloids have been isolated from several species of comfrey plants including common comfrey (*S. officinale*), prickly comfrey (*S. asperum*), and Russian comfrey (*S. uplandicum*). Ingestion of plants containing pyrrolizidine alkaloids is a common cause of hepatic veno-occlusive disease in developing countries[1] and pyrrolizidine alkaloid hepatotoxicity presumably due to comfrey has been reported in North America and Europe.[1,2] Pulmonary endothelial hyperplasia and carcinogenic activity have also been reported in *animals*.[1,2]

1. Ridker PM, McDermott WV. Comfrey herb tea and hepatic veno-occlusive disease. *Lancet* 1989; **i:** 657–8.
2. Bach N, *et al.* Comfrey herb tea-induced hepatic veno-occlusive disease. *Am J Med* 1989; **87:** 97–9.

Preparations

Proprietary Preparations (details are given in Part 3)

Canad.: Procomfrin; ***Ger.:*** Kytta-Plasma f; Kytta-Salbe f; Traumaplant.

Multi-ingredient: ***Fr.:*** Tisanes de l'Abbe Hamon no 15; ***Ger.:*** Bronchangin†; Kytta-Balsam f; Kytta-Nagelsalbe†; Rhus-Rheuma-Gel N; Symphytum Ro-Plex (Rowo-777)†; Syviman N; ***Switz.:*** Alpina Gel a la consoude; Baume Kytta†; Cetona; Keppur; Kytta Baume; Kytta Pommade; Pommade Kytta†.

Complement Blockers (12038-j)

A number of compounds are under investigation for their ability to inhibit activation of the complement system. Such compounds include soluble forms of the complement receptors such as sCR1, or its derivatives; naturally-occurring complement blockers such as CD59; and synthetic complement blockers. The potential clinical applications of such compounds are being investigated in various conditions, including the prevention of acute respiratory distress syndrome, and for the prevention of reperfusion injury following myocardial infarction or lung transplantation.

References.

1. Makrides SC. Therapeutic inhibition of the complement system. *Pharmacol Rev* 1998; **50:** 59–87.
2. McGeer EG, McGeer PL. The future use of complement inhibitors for the treatment of neurological diseases. *Drugs* 1998; **55:** 739–46.

Complement C1 Esterase Inhibitor

(16557-d)

C_1 Esterase Inhibitor.

Complement C1 esterase inhibitor is prepared from human plasma and has been used as replacement therapy in the management of life-threatening attacks of hereditary angioedema (p.729).

Complement C1 esterase inhibitor may be effective in both the prevention and treatment of acute hereditary angioedema.[1] It has also been tried in the management of sepsis[2,3] (p.141).

1. Waytes AT, *et al.* Treatment of hereditary angioedema with a vapor-heated C1 inhibitor concentrate. *N Engl J Med* 1996; **334:** 1630–4.
2. Hack CE, *et al.* C1-esterase inhibitor substitution in sepsis. *Lancet* 1992; **339:** 378.
3. Nürnberger W, *et al.* C1-inhibitor concentrate for sepsis-related capillary leak syndrome. *Lancet* 1992; **339:** 990.

Preparations

Proprietary Preparations (details are given in Part 3)

Aust.: Berinert; ***Ger.:*** Berinert; ***Ital.:*** C1 Inattivatore Umano; ***Switz.:*** Berinert HS; ***UK:*** Berinert P.

Condurango (531-a)

Condurango Bark; Eagle-vine Bark.

CAS — 1401-98-5 (condurangin).

Pharmacopoeias. In *Aust., Belg., Jpn,* and *Swiss.*

The dried stem bark of *Marsdenia condurango* (=*Gonolobus condurango*) (Asclepiadaceae).

Condurango has been used as a bitter. It has also been used in homoeopathic medicine.

Preparations

Proprietary Preparations (details are given in Part 3)

Multi-ingredient: ***Aust.:*** Pascopankreat; Sigman-Haustropfen; ***Belg.:*** Valeria-Fordine†; ***Fr.:*** Soker; ***Ger.:*** Dr. Klinger's Bergischer Krautertee, Magentee†; Gastrocaps†; Majocarmin†; Nervogastrol; Pankreaplex N†; Pankreaplex Neu; Pascopankreat†; Pascopnakreat novo; Stomaform†; ***Switz.:*** Padma-Lax; Stomacine.

Congo Red (2125-x)

CI Direct Red 28; Colour Index No. 22120; Rubrum Congoensis. Disodium 3,3′-[biphenyl-4,4′-diylbis(azo)]bis[4-aminonaphthalene-1-sulphonate].

$C_{32}H_{22}N_6Na_2O_6S_2 = 696.7$.

CAS — 573-58-0.

Congo red is used as a stain in the diagnosis of amyloidosis deposits in tissue samples causing amyloid to fluoresce under polarised light.

Convallaria (5806-d)

Lily of the Valley; Maiblume; Maiglöckchenkraut; May Lily; Muguet.

CAS — 3253-62-1 (convallatoxol); 13473-51-3 (convalloside); 13289-19-5 (convallatoxoloside); 508-75-8 (convallatoxin).

Pharmacopoeias. In *Aust.* and *Ger.* (from *C. majalis* or closely related species).

The dried flowers, herb, or the rhizomes and roots of lily of the valley, *Convallaria majalis* (Liliaceae). Several crystalline glycosides have been obtained from the plant including convallarin, convalloside, convallatoxoloside, and convallatoxin.

Convallaria contains cardiac glycosides and has actions on the heart similar to those of digoxin (p.849). Convallaria is used in herbal and homoeopathic medicine.

Convallaria majalis has been designated unsafe for inclusion in foods, beverages, or drugs by the Food and Drug Administration in the USA.[1]

1. Larkin T. *FDA Consumer* 1983; **17** (Oct.): 5.

Preparations

Proprietary Preparations (details are given in Part 3)

Ger.: Convacard; Valdig-N Burger.

Multi-ingredient: ***Aust.:*** Cardiofrik; Omega; ***Fr.:*** Biocarde; Tisanes de l'Abbe Hamon no 16; Tisanes de l'Abbe Hamon no 3; ***Ger.:*** Aesrutal S; Card-Ompin S†; Cardalept†; Cardiacum I S†; Cardiacum II S†; Cardibisana; Castrophan†; Cefascillan N; Concardisett†; Convallocor-SL; Convastabil; Cor-loges; Cor-myocrat†; Cor-Vel N; Corguttin + Magnesium†; Corguttin N plus; Corguttin†; Digaloid†; Dr. Kleinschrod's Cor-Insuffin†; Goldtropfen-Hetterich; Guttacor; Hypercard; Hypotonin†; Laco-erdin-N; Miroton; Miroton N; Oxacant N; Oxacant-forte N; Oxacant-Khella N; Raufuncton N; RR-plus†; Strophanon†; Strophanthus-Strath†; Szillosan†; Venopyronum N triplex; Verus†; Viscorapas Duo; ***Spain:*** Nefrolit†; Uralyt.

Coriander (4637-j)

Coentro; Coriand.; Coriander Fruit; Coriander Seed; Coriandri Fructus; Fruto de Cilantro.

Pharmacopoeias. In *Eur.* (see p.viii) and *Pol.*

The dried cremocarp of *Coriandrum sativum* (Umbelliferae), containing not less than 3 mL per kg of volatile oil. **Protect** from light.

Coriander is the source of coriander oil. It is a carminative and is used as a flavour.

Preparations

Proprietary Preparations (details are given in Part 3)

Multi-ingredient: ***Aust.:*** Apotheker Bauer's Blahungstee; Bio-Garten Tropfen gegen Blahungen; Brady's-Magentropfen; Carminative; Carminativum Babynos; Mariazeller; Planta Lax; ***Belg.:*** Tamarine; ***Fr.:*** Mediflor Tisane Digestive No 3; Tisane Grande Chartreuse; ***Ger.:*** Abfuhr-Tee Depuraflux†; Carminat†; Carminativum Babynos; Drix Richter's Krautertee†; Floradix Multipretten; Friosmin†; Gastrol S; Hacko-Kloster-Krautertee†; Knufinke Gastrobin Magen- und Darm-Tee†; Presselin 214†; Presselin 52 N; Ramend Krauter; Rheumex†; Stern Biene Fencheltee†; ***Ital.:*** Dicalmir; Tamarine; Tisana Cisbey; ***Spain:*** Agua del Carmen; Jarabe Manceau; Jarabe Manzanas Siken; Pruina; Vegetalin; ***Switz.:*** Boldoflorine; Tamarine; Tisane laxative Natterman no 13; ***UK:*** Cough Drops.

Coriander Oil (4638-z)

Ol. Coriand; Oleum Coriandri.

Pharmacopoeias. In *Br.*

A clear colourless or pale yellow volatile oil with the characteristic odour and taste of coriander, obtained by distillation from coriander. It contains linalol.

Soluble 1 in 3 of alcohol (70%). **Store** at a temperature not exceeding 25°. Protect from light.

Coriander oil is aromatic and carminative and is used as a flavour.

Preparations

BP 1998: Compound Orange Spirit; Compound Rhubarb Tincture.

Proprietary Preparations (details are given in Part 3)

Multi-ingredient: ***Belg.:*** Melisana†; ***Ger.:*** Abfuhr-Tee Depuraflux†; Floradix Multipretten; Gastricard N; Stern Biene Fencheltee†.

Cottonseed Oil (7358-p)

Aceite de Algodon; Cotton Oil; Ol. Gossyp. Sem.; Oléo de Algodoeiro; Oleum Gossypii Seminis.

Pharmacopoeias. In *USNF*. *Eur.* (see p.viii) includes Hydrogenated Cottonseed Oil.

The refined fixed oil obtained by expression or solvent extraction from the seeds of the cotton plant, *Gossypium hirsutum*, and other cultivated species of *Gossypium* (Malvaceae).

It is a pale yellow odourless or nearly odourless oil with a bland taste. Slightly **soluble** in alcohol; miscible with carbon disulphide, chloroform, ether, and petroleum spirit. **Store** at a temperature not exceeding 40° in well-filled airtight containers. Protect from light. At temperatures below 10° particles of solid fat may separate from the oil and at temperatures between 0° and −5° it congeals.

Hydrogenated Cottonseed Oil (Ph. Eur.) consists mainly of triglycerides of palmitic and stearic acids. It is a white mass or powder which melts to a clear pale yellow liquid when heated. Practically **insoluble** in water; very slightly soluble in alcohol; freely soluble in dichloromethane and in toluene. **Protect** from light.

Cottonseed oil is used as an oily vehicle.

An extract of cottonseed oil, gossypol (p.1586), has been tried as a contraceptive in males.

Preparations

Proprietary Preparations (details are given in Part 3)

Canad.: Neo-Cholex†.

Couch-grass (2322-h)

Agropyron; Chiendent; Dogs Grass; Graminis Rhizoma; Quackgrass; Twitch.

Pharmacopoeias. In *Eur.* (see p.viii) and *Pol.*

The rhizome of *Agropyron repens* (=*Elymus repens*; *Triticum repens*) (Gramineae). It contains glucose, mannitol, inositol, and triticin (a carbohydrate resembling inulin).

Couch-grass is a mild diuretic which has been used in herbal medicine in the treatment of cystitis.

Preparations

Proprietary Preparations (details are given in Part 3)
Ger.: Acorus.

Multi-ingredient: ***Aust.:*** Abfuhrtee; Brostalin; Krauterhaus Mag Kottas Blasentee; Krauterhaus Mag Kottas Entwasserungstee; Krautertee Nr 2; Sidroga Nieren- und Blasentee; ***Fr.:*** Alpha Renol†; Herbesan; Mediflor Tisane Antirhumatismale No 2; Mediflor Tisane Diuretique†; Mediflor Tisane Pectorale d'Alsace†; Tisane Orientale Soker; Tisanes de l'Abbe Hamon no 11; ***Ger.:*** Blasen-Nieren-Tee Stada; Blasen-Nieren-Tee Uroflux S†; Blasen-Nieren-Tee Uroflux†; Buccotean TF†; Buccotean†; Harntee 400; Hevert-Blasen- und Nieren- Tee; NB-tee Siegfried†; Presselin Stoffwechseltee†; Renob Blasen- und Nierentee; ***Ital.:*** Depurativo; Tisana Arnaldi; Tisana Cisbey; Tisana Kelemata; ***Switz.:*** The Franklin; Tisane antirhumatismale "H"†; Viola Pommade a l'huile d'amandes†; ***UK:*** Antitis; Herbal Powder No.8†; Kas-Bah; ***USA:*** Aqua-Rid; Fluidex.

Coumarin (2388-x)

1,2-Benzopyrone; 5,6-Benzo-α-pyrone; Cumarin; Tonka Bean Camphor. 2*H*-1-Benzopyran-2-one.

$C_9H_6O_2$ = 146.1.

CAS — 91-64-5.

Pharmacopoeias. In *Ger.*

Coumarin is the odorous principle of Tonka seed (Tonka or Tonquin bean); it may be prepared synthetically.

Coumarin is used in the treatment of lymphoedema. It is also used as a fixative in perfumery and as a flavour. It is reported to be an immunostimulant and has been tried in the treatment of malignant neoplasms.

Coumarin derivatives are used as anticoagulants.

Effects on the liver. Coumarin has been classified as hepatotoxic based on studies in *animals*. Liver toxicity ranging from elevated liver enzymes to serious organ damage has been reported in humans. Seventeen of 2173 patients enrolled in a clinical/toxicological study of coumarin developed elevated liver enzyme values;[1] the majority of patients were given 100 mg coumarin daily for 1 month followed by 50 mg daily for 2 years. However, none of the patients developed permanent liver damage and liver enzyme values returned to normal in 5 patients who continued taking coumarin. Results from 5 studies supported by the Lymphoedema Association of Australia in which patients received 400 mg daily, for a mean duration of 14.6 months showed 2 cases of hepatotoxicity among 1106 patients.[2] In the period of 14 months up to May 1995 the Australian Drug Evaluation Committee received 10 reports of suspected adverse reactions to coumarin,[3] including 6 cases of jaundice in women who had taken 400 mg daily for one to four months. Periportal and lobular necrosis were found on biopsy in one case and another had a fatal outcome due to massive hepatic necrosis.

Reports of hepatotoxicity have led to the withdrawal of coumarin in a number of countries.

1. Cox D, *et al.* The rarity of liver toxicity in patients treated with coumarin (1,2-benzopyrone). *Hum Toxicol* 1989; **8:** 501–6.
2. Casley-Smith JR, Casley-Smith JR. Frequency of coumarin hepatotoxicity. *Med J Aust* 1995; **162:** 391.
3. Anonymous. Lodema and the liver. *Aust Adverse Drug React Bull* 1995; **14:** 11.

Lymphoedema. Benzopyrones such as coumarin are reported to reduce excess protein in tissues with high-protein oedema, hence coumarin's use in lymphoedema. However, the action is slow and treatment may need to be continued for 6 months to 2 years before benefit is seen. Some references to its use in lymphoedema of various causes, including postmastectomy, and filarial lymphoedema and elephantiasis (p.95) are given below.

1. Turner CS. Congenital lymphedema. *JAMA* 1990; **264:** 518.
2. Jamal S, *et al.* The effects of 5,6 benzo-[a]-pyrone (coumarin) and DEC on filaritic lymphoedema and elephantiasis in India: preliminary results. *Ann Trop Med Parasitol* 1989; **83:** 287–90.
3. Casley-Smith JR, *et al.* Treatment of lymphedema of the arms and legs with 5,6-benzo-[α]-pyrone. *N Engl J Med* 1993; **329:** 1158–63.
4. Casley-Smith JR, *et al.* Treatment of filarial lymphoedema and elephantiasis with 5,6-benzo-α-pyrone (coumarin). *Br Med J* 1993; **307:** 1037–41.

Preparations

Proprietary Preparations (details are given in Part 3)
Austral.: Lodema; ***Fr.:*** Lysedem; ***Ger.:*** Venalot mono; ***Switz.:*** Lymphex; Venalot; Venium.

Multi-ingredient: ***Belg.:*** Venalot†; ***Ger.:*** Caye Balsam; Cycloarthrin†; Kneipp Rheuma Stoffwechsel-Bad Heublumen-Aquasan; Theokal†; Venalot.

Cowberry (308-e)

Red Whortleberry.

Pharmacopoeias. In *Aust.*

The leaves of the cowberry, *Vaccinium vitis-idaea* (Ericaceae), have astringent properties and have been used as a domestic remedy for diarrhoea.

CR Gas (12615-p)

EA-3547. Dibenz[*b,f*][1,4]oxazepine.

$C_{13}H_9NO$ = 195.2.

CAS — 257-07-8.

A riot-control gas with properties similar to those of CS gas (p.1569); it is described as a tear gas. CR gas is reported not to be hydrolysed by water and therefore to be capable of use in water cannons.

Cranberry (9415-k)

The fruit of *Vaccinium macrocarpon*, the American cranberry.

Cranberry juice has been reported to reduce the incidence of urinary tract infections.

References.

1. Ofek I, *et al.* Anti-Escherichia coli adhesin activity of cranberry and blueberry juices. *N Engl J Med* 1991; **324:** 1599.
2. Avorn J, *et al.* Reduction of bacteriuria and pyuria after ingestion of cranberry juice. *JAMA* 1994; **271:** 751–4 [with comments from several authors—*ibid.*; **272:** 588–90.]

Preparations

Proprietary Preparations (details are given in Part 3)
Multi-ingredient: ***USA:*** Uro-pH Control.

Crataegus (5807-n)

Aubépine; Biancospino; Crataegus Oxyacantha; English Hawthorn; Haw; Pirliteiro; Weissdorn; Whitethorn.

Pharmacopoeias. In *Chin., Eur.* (see p.viii), and *Pol.*

The dried flowers, fruit, or leaves, or mixtures of these parts of *Crataegus oxyacantha* (*C. laevigata*), *C. monogyna*, or other spp.

Crataegus contains flavonoid glycosides with cardiotonic properties similar to those of digoxin (p.849). Crataegus is used in herbal and homoeopathic medicine.

General references.

1. Hamon NW. Hawthorns: the genus Crataegus. *Can Pharm J* 1988; **121:** 708–9 and 724.

Preparations

Proprietary Preparations (details are given in Part 3)
Aust.: Born†; Cardiphyt; Crataegan; Crataegutt; Esbericard; Neo-Cratylen; Sanadorn; Senecard; ***Fr.:*** Aubeline; Crataegol; Divane†; ***Ger.:*** Adenylocrat; Arte Rutin C; Basticrat; Born; Chronocard; Cordapur; Corocrat; Coronator; Craegium; Crataegutt; Crataegysat; Crataepas; Crataesan†; Crataezyma; Cratamed novo; Cratecor; Craviscum mono; Esbericard; Faros; Kneipp Pflanzendragees Weissdorn; Kneipp Weissdorn-Pflanzensaft Sebastianeum; Knufinke Herz- und Kreislauf-Tee Arterio-K†; Kyaugutt; Kytta-Cor; Liquicard; Logomed Herz; Melicedin†; Naranocor; Neo-Cratylen; Normotin V1; Optocor; Orthangin N; Orthangin Novo; Orthocardon-N; Oxacant mono; Poikilocard N; Regulacor; Rephacratin; Senicor; Steicorton; Tensitruw; Tonoplantin Mono; ***Ital.:*** Cardiplant†; ***Neth.:*** Crataegutt†; ***Spain:*** Crataegutt; ***Switz.:*** Cardiplant; Crataegisan N; Crataegitan; Esbericard; Eurhyton.

Multi-ingredient: ***Aust.:*** Apotheker Bauer's Grippetee; Cardalept; Cardiofrik; Corodyn; Coroverlan; Doppelherz Tonikum; Herz- und Kreislauftonikum Bioflora; Kneipp Herz- und Kreislauf-Unterstutzungs-Tee; Krautertee Nr 20; Krautertee Nr 32; Krautertee Nr 44; Mag Kottas Herz- und Kreislauftee; Omega; Sanvita Herz; Sidroga Herz-Kreislauf-Tee; St Radegunder Herz-Kreislauf-Tonikum; St Radegunder Herz-Kreislauf-unterstutzender Tee; Teekanne Herz- und Kreislauftee; Virgilocard; Wechseltee; ***Austral.:*** ASA Tones; Crataegus Complex; For Peripheral Circulation Herbal Plus Formula 5; Gingo A; Ginkgo Complex; Lifesystem Herbal Formula 6 For Peripheral Circulation; ***Belg.:*** Sedinal; Spasmosedine; Tisane Contre la Tension; Tisane pour Dormir; Valeria-Fordine†; ***Canad.:*** Hepax†; ***Fr.:*** Achisane Troubles du Sommeil; Actisane Nervosite; Aeine†; Anxoral; Astresane; Biocarde; Canteine Bouteille†; Cardiocalm; Epanal†; Euphytose; Felisedine†; Germose; Insomnyl†; Kaneuron; Lenicalm; Mediflor Tisane Calmante Troubles du Sommeil No 14; Mediflor Tisane Circulation du Sang No 12; Mediflor Tisane Hypotensive†; Mensuosedyl†; Natudor; Neuroflorine; Neuropax†; Neurotensyl; Nicoprive; Noctisan; Nocvalene; Nuidor†; Passiflorine; Passinevryl†; Phytocalm; Pulmothiol†; Quinisedine; Santane H_7; Santane N_9; Santane V_3; Sedalozia; Sedatif Tiber; Sedatonyl; Sedibaine; Sedopal; Serenival; Spasmidenal; Spasmine; Spasmosedine; Sympaneurol; Sympathyl; Sympavagol; Tranquital; Vagostabyl; Vericardine; ***Ger.:*** Aesrutal S; Antihypertonicum S; Antisklerosin S; Ardeycordal N; Asgoviscum N; Aureal†; Befelka Herz-Dragees†; Belladonna-Valobonin†; Biovital Forte N; Biovital N; Bomacorin; Bunetten†; Card-Ompin S†; Cardalept†; Cardaminol†; Cardiacum I S†; Cardiacum II S†; Cardiagen; Cardibisana; Cardio-Longoral; Cardisetten†; Cefasedativ; Concardisett†; Convallocor-SL; Convastabil; Cor-myocrat†; Cor-Select; Cor-Vel N; Corguttin N plus; Corguttin†; Coroverlan; Coroverlan-Digoxin†; Crataegutt-Strophanthin†; Crataelanat; Crataezyma N†; Cratylen†; Craviscum†; Diawern; Digaloid†; Diureticum-Medice†; Dr. Hotz Vollbad; Dr. Kleinschrod's Cor-Insuffin†; Dr. Klinger's Bergischer Krautertee, Herz- und Kreislauftee†; Drix Richter's Krautertee†; Eupronerv†; Euvalon; Fovysat†; Fovysatum†; Gastricard N; Ginseng-Complex "Schuh"; Goldtropfen-Hetterich; Guttacor; Herz-Plus Nerven†; Herz-plus†; Herz-Starkung N; Hypotonin†; JuViton; Kneipp Drei-Pflanzen-Dragees; Korodin; Kyaugutt N†; Lacoerdin-N; Lipozet†; Manns Knoblauch Pillen Plus†; Mistelan†; Movicard†; Myonasan†; Nervoregin; Nitro-Crataegutt; Noricaven†; Orbis Nerven- und Beruhigungstee†; Oxacant N; Oxacant-forte N; Oxacant-Khella N; Oxacant-sedativ; Passiorin N; Passiorin†; Protecor; Rauwoplant; Rhythmochin I†; Rhythmochin II (cum sedativo)†; RR-plus†; Salus Herz-Schutz-Kapseln; Salusan; Seda-Movicard†; Seda-Pasc N†; Seda-Stenocrat-N†; Septacord; Stenocrat; Strophanon†; Strophanthus-Strath†; Szillosan forte; Szillosan†; Tornix; Valeriana-Strath†; Valobonin†; Vasesana-Vasoregulans; Verus†; Viscorapas Duo; Worishofener Nervenpflege Dr. Kleinschrod†; ***Ital.:*** Anevrasi; Bianco Val; Blandonal; Fiorlin†; Florerbe Calmante†; Lenicalm; Neurobiol; Nicoprive; Noctis; Parvisedil; Passiflorine; Prexene; Quietan; Relaten; Sedatol; Sedonerva†; Sedopuer F; Tauma; ***Spain:*** Desinto†; Iodocafedrina†; Passiflorine; ***Switz.:*** Arterosan Plus; Cardiaforce; Demonatur Capsules ailaubepine†; Dragees pour le coeur et les nerfs; Ginkovit†; Gouttes pour le coeur et les nerfs Concentrees; Korodin; Mirocor†; Passiorin†; Phytomed Cardio; Radacor†; Sedosan; Sedovalin†; Sirop Passi-Par; Tai Ginseng N; Tisane pour le coeur et la circulation; Tisane pour le coeur et la circulation "H"†; Valverde Dragees pour le coeur; Valverde Gouttes pour le coeur; ***UK:*** Tranquil.

Creatine Phosphate (6828-j)

Creatine Phosphoric Acid; Phosphocreatine. *N*-[Imino(phosphonoamino)-methyl]-*N*-methylglycine.

$C_4H_{10}N_3O_5P$ = 211.1.

CAS — 67-07-2 (creatine phosphate); 922-32-7 (creatine phosphate disodium).

Creatine phosphate is an endogenous substance found mainly in skeletal muscle of vertebrates. It has been tried in the treatment of cardiac disorders and has been added to cardioplegic solutions. Creatine monohydrate has been tried in metabolic disorders and as a dietary supplement.

References.

1. Pedone V, *et al.* An assessment of the activity of creatine phosphate (Neoton) on premature ventricular beats by continuous ECG monitoring in patients with coronary cardiac disease. *Clin Trials J* 1984; **21:** 91.
2. Ferraro S, *et al.* Acute and short-term efficacy of high doses of creatine phosphate in the treatment of cardiac failure. *Curr Ther Res* 1990; **47:** 917–23.
3. Mastoroberto P, *et al.* Creatine phosphate protection of the ischemic myocardium during cardiac surgery. *Curr Ther Res* 1992; **51:** 37–45.
4. Stöckler S, *et al.* Creatine replacement therapy in guanidinoacetate methyltransferase deficiency, a novel inborn error of metabolism. *Lancet* 1996; **348:** 789–90.
5. Mujika I, Padilla S. Creatine supplementation as an ergogenic aid for sports performance in highly trained athletes: a critical review. *Int J Sports Med* 1997; **18:** 491–6.

Preparations

Proprietary Preparations (details are given in Part 3)
Ital.: Creatile.

Creatinine (14445-f)

2-Amino-1-methyl-4-imidazolidinone.

$C_4H_7N_3O$ = 113.1.

CAS — 60-27-5.

Pharmacopoeias. In *Ger.* and *USNF.*

Creatinine is used as a bulking agent for freeze-drying.

Plasma concentrations or clearance of endogenous creatinine are used as an index of renal function.

Creatinolfosfate Sodium (12616-s)

Creatinolfosfate Sodium *(rINNM).*

The sodium salt of 1-(2-hydroxyethyl)-1-methylguanidine *O*-phosphate.

$C_4H_{11}N_3NaO_4P$ = 219.1.

CAS — 6903-79-3 (creatinolfosfate).

Creatinolfosfate is used as an adjuvant in the treatment of cardiac disorders.

Preparations

Proprietary Preparations (details are given in Part 3)
Ital.: Aplodan; Gipron†; ***Spain:*** Dragosil.

Crotalaria (12021-v)

Crotalaria spp. have been used in the preparation of herbal teas but liver damage has been reported following their ingestion possibly due to their content of pyrrolizidine alkaloids.

CS Gas (12618-e)

α-(o-Chlorobenzylidene)malononitrile.

$C_{10}H_5ClN_2$ = 188.6.

CAS — 2698-41-1.

CS gas has been used as a riot-control gas.

It is known as a tear gas and its toxic effects include irritation of the eyes and nose, with copious lachrymation and rhinorrhoea; a burning sensation of the mouth and throat; pain in the chest, with difficulty in breathing; coughing; an increase in salivation; and retching and vomiting. These effects usually disappear a few minutes after exposure ends. The effects of pre-existing disease of the chest may be exacerbated. Erythema and blistering of the skin may occur.

Exposed persons should be removed to a well ventilated area. Treatment is symptomatic. Contaminated skin may be washed with soap and water, although exposure to water may initially exacerbate symptoms. If contamination of the eyes has been severe they should be irrigated with physiological saline or water and a local anaesthetic instilled to relieve pain.

References.

1. Hu H, *et al.* Tear gas—harassing agent or toxic chemical weapon? *JAMA* 1989; **262:** 660–3.
2. Yih J-P. CS gas injury to the eye. *Br Med J* 1995; **311:** 276.
3. Gray PJ. Treating CS gas injuries to the eye: exposure at close range is particularly dangerous. *Br Med J* 1995; **311:** 871.
4. Jones GRN. CS sprays: antidote and decontaminant. *Lancet* 1996; **347:** 968–9.
5. Anderson PJ, *et al.* Acute effects of the potent lacrimator o-chlorobenzylidene malonitrile (CS) tear gas. *Hum Exp Toxicol* 1996; **15:** 461–5.
6. Anonymous. "Safety" of chemical batons. *Lancet* 1998; **352:** 159.

Cucurbita (769-k)

Abóbora; Kürbissamen; Melon Pumpkin Seeds; Pepo; Semence de Courge.

Pharmacopoeias. In *Ger.* which specifies seeds of *Cucurbita pepo.*

The seeds of *Cucurbita pepo* (Cucurbitaceae) or related species.

Cucurbita was formerly used for the expulsion of tapeworms (*Taenia*).

It is an ingredient of several herbal preparations used in urinary-tract disorders.

Preparations

Proprietary Preparations (details are given in Part 3)
Ger.: Granufink Kurbiskern; Nomon Mono; Prosta Fink forte; Prostaherb Cucurbitae; Prostalog; Turiplex.

Multi-ingredient: ***Ger.:*** Alsicur; Carito†; Granufink N; Prosta Fink N; Prostamed; Prostata-Kurbis S; Saburlan†; Salus Kurbis-Tonikum Compositum†; Uvirgan Mono; Uvirgan N; ***Switz.:*** Cysto-Caps Chassot; Prosta-Caps Chassot N; Prosta-Caps Fink.

Cusparia (532-t)

Angostura Bark; Carony Bark; Cusparia Bark.

The bark of *Galipea officinalis* (Rutaceae).

Cusparia has been used as a bitter.

It should be noted that 'Angostura Bitters' (*Dr. J.G.B. Siegert & Sons Ltd*) contain gentian and various aromatic ingredients but no cusparia; they are named after the town in which they were first made.

Cyanoacrylate Adhesives (12619-l)

CAS — 1069-55-2 (bucrylate); 6606-65-1 (enbucrilate); 137-05-3 (mecrylate).

A number of cyanoacrylate compounds have been used as surgical tissue adhesives. They include bucrylate (isobutyl 2-cyanoacrylate, $C_8H_{11}NO_2$=153.2), enbucrilate (butyl 2-cyanoacrylate, $C_8H_{11}NO_2$=153.2), mecrylate (methyl 2-cyanoacrylate, $C_5H_5NO_2$=111.1), and octylcyanoacrylate. Some cyanoacrylates are used for household purposes and as nail fixatives and others have been investigated as tubal occlusive agents for female sterilisation, for sclerotherapy in bleeding gastric varices (p.1576), and for embolisation of intracranial vascular lesions.

In the event of accidental adhesion of the skin or lips the bonded surfaces should be immersed in warm soapy water, the surfaces peeled or rolled apart with the aid of a spatula, and the adhesive removed from the skin with soap and water; attempts should not be made to pull the surfaces apart. Eyelids stuck together or bonded to the eyeball should be washed thoroughly with warm water and a gauze patch applied; the eye will open without further action in 1 to 4 days. Manipulative attempts to open the eyes should not be made. Although cyanoacrylate introduced into the eyes may cause double vision and lachrymation there is usually no residual damage. If lips are accidentally stuck together plenty of warm water should be applied and maximum wetting and pressure from saliva inside the mouth encouraged. Lips should be peeled or rolled apart and not pulled. Adhesive introduced into the mouth solidifies and adheres, but saliva will lift the adhesive in ½ to 2 days. Care should be taken to avoid choking.

Heat is evolved on solidification of cyanoacrylate and in rare cases may cause burns.

Reports of inadvertent application of cyanoacrylate adhesives to the eyes[1,2] and mouth.[3]

1. Lyons C, *et al.* Superglue inadvertently used as eyedrops. *Br Med J* 1990; **300:** 328.
2. DeRespinis PA. Cyanoacrylate nail glue mistaken for eye drops. *JAMA* 1990; **263:** 2301.
3. Cousin GCS. Accidental application of cyanoacrylate to the mouth. *Br Dent J* 1990; **169:** 293–4.

Preparations

Proprietary Preparations (details are given in Part 3)
UK: Histoacryl.

Cyclobutyrol Sodium (3712-n)

Cyclobutyrol Sodium *(rINNM).*

Sodium 2-(1-hydroxycyclohexyl)butyrate.

$C_{10}H_{17}NaO_3$ = 208.2.

CAS — 512-16-3 (cyclobutyrol); 1130-23-0 (cyclobutyrol sodium).

Cyclobutyrol sodium is a choleretic. It has been given in doses of 0.5 to 1 g daily in divided doses with meals. Cyclobutyrol betaine and cyclobutyrol calcium have been used similarly.

Preparations

Proprietary Preparations (details are given in Part 3)
Fr.: Hebucol; ***Ital.:*** Epa-Bon.

Multi-ingredient: ***Aust.:*** Tromgallol; ***Ital.:*** Menabil Complex†; Tribilina†; ***Spain:*** Hepadigest; Levaliver; Liberbil; Lidobama Complex; Lidobama Plus†; Menabil Complex; Prodessal; Salcemetic; Sugarbil.

Cyclodextrins (16595-g)

NOTE. Alfadex is *rINN* for α-cyclodextrin (alpha cyclodextrin). Betadex is *pINN* for β-cyclodextrin (beta cyclodextrin).

Pharmacopoeias. Eur. (see p.viii) and *USNF* include betadex.

Betadex is a white or almost white amorphous or crystalline powder. Sparingly **soluble** in water; freely soluble in propylene glycol; practically insoluble in alcohol and in dichloromethane. **Store** in airtight containers.

Uses

Cyclodextrins, such as alfadex and betadex, are produced by the enzymatic degradation of starch and are used as carrier molecules for drug delivery systems.

References.

1. Ridgway K. Drug release rates: cyclodextrin complexes. *Pharm J* 1990; **245:** 344–5.
2. Szejtli J. Cyclodextrins: properties and applications. *Drug Invest* 1990; **2** (suppl 4): 11–21.
3. El Shaboury MH. Physical properties and dissolution profiles of tablets directly compressed with β-cyclodextrin. *Int J Pharmaceutics* 1990; **63:** 95–100.
4. Abosehmah-Albidy AZM, *et al.* Improved bioavailability and clinical response in patients with chronic liver disease following the administration of a spironolactone:β-cyclodextrin complex. *Br J Clin Pharmacol* 1997; **44:** 35–9.

Cyclovalone (3713-h)

Cyclovalone *(rINN).*

Divanillidenecyclohexanone. 2,6-Divanillylidenecyclohexanone.

$C_{22}H_{22}O_5$ = 366.4.

CAS — 579-23-7.

Cyclovalone is a choleretic. It has been given in doses of 300 to 900 mg daily in divided doses.

Preparations

Proprietary Preparations (details are given in Part 3)
Belg.: Vanidene; ***Fr.:*** Vanilone.

Cynara (3714-m)

Alcachôfra; Artichaut; Artichoke Leaf.

Pharmacopoeias. In *Fr.*

The leaves of the globe artichoke, *Cynara scolymus* (Compositae).

Cynara is reputed to have diuretic and choleretic properties.

Preparations

Proprietary Preparations (details are given in Part 3)
Belg.: Cynarol; ***Fr.:*** Chophytol; Hepanephrol; ***Ger.:*** Cyna Bilisan; Cynacur; Cynafol; Divinal Galle; Hekbilin Kapseln; Hepa-POS; Hepagallin N; Hepar SL; Hepar-POS; Hewechol Artischockendragees; Maquil; ***Switz.:*** Chophytol.

Multi-ingredient: ***Aust.:*** Agnuchol; Cynarix; Cynarix comp; Mag Doskar's Leber-Galletonikum; Sanvita Leber-Galle; ***Austral.:*** Lifesystem Herbal Formula 7 Liver Tonic; Liver Tonic Herbal Formula 6; ***Belg.:*** Tisane pour le Foie; ***Canad.:*** Hepax†; ***Fr.:*** Actibil; Actisane Digestion; Aromabyl; Canol; Elixir Spark; Gastralsan; Hepaclem; Hepatorex†; Hepax; Romarinex-Choline; Tisane des Familles†; Vegelax; ***Ger.:*** Bilicura Forte; Boldo "Dr. Eberth"†; Carminagal N; Cynarix†; Cynarzym N; Dr. Maurers Magen-Apotheke†; Gallexier; Galloselect M; Heparaxal†; Heparchofid S†; Hepaticum "Mletzko"†; Hepatofalk Neu; Ludoxin†; Orotofalk†; Pascobilin novo; Salus Leber-Galle-Tee Nr.18; Sirmia Artischockenelixier N; Spasmo-Bilicura†; Stomachiagil†; Ullus Galle-Tee N; ***Ital.:*** Boldosten†; Cinarbile†; Colax; Epaglutone†; Florerbe Lassativa; Fluend; Hepacolina†; Heparbil†; Laxygocce†; Lievistar; Lievital†; Menabil Complex†; Vadolax; Vegebyl; Vitabil Composto†; ***Spain:*** Cinaro Bilina; Lipograsil; Menabil Complex; Nico Hepatocyn; ***Switz.:*** Bilifuge; Boldocynara N; Demonatur Gouttes pour le foie et la bile; Gouttes bile†; Livartil†; Phytomed Hepato; Stago†; Tisane hepatique et biliaire.

Cynarine (3715-b)

Cynarin; 1,5-Dicaffeoylquinic Acid. 1-Carboxy-4,5-dihydroxy-1,3-cyclohexylene bis(3,4-dihydroxycinnamate).

$C_{25}H_{24}O_{12}$ = 516.5.

CAS — 1182-34-9; 1884-24-8.

Cynarine is an active ingredient of cynara (above). It is used as a choleretic.

Preparations

Proprietary Preparations (details are given in Part 3)

Multi-ingredient: ***Aust.:*** Tromgallol; ***Ital.:*** Bilarvis†; Liverchin†; Neo-Epa†.

Cysteamine Hydrochloride (1041-p)

Cysteamine Hydrochloride *(BANM, USAN).*

Mercaptamine Hydrochloride *(rINNM)*; CI-9148; L-1573 (cysteamine); MEA (cysteamine); Mercamine Hydrochloride. 2-Aminoethanethiol hydrochloride.

C_2H_7NS,HCl = 113.6.

CAS — 60-23-1 (cysteamine); 156-57-0 (cysteamine hydrochloride).

Adverse Effects and Precautions

When taken by mouth cysteamine can be unpalatable. It may cause gastro-intestinal side-effects including anorexia, nausea, vomiting, and abdominal pain; other side-effects reported include drowsiness, malaise, rashes, fever, flushing, and ventricular tachycardia. Cysteamine may precipitate hepatic coma in patients with overt hepatic damage.

Three patients with nephropathic cystinosis developed fever, maculopapular eruption, leucopenia, or headache within 2 weeks of starting cysteamine at doses of 53, 67, and 75 mg per kg body-weight daily by mouth.[1] These side-effects resolved within 48 hours of drug withdrawal and all 3 patients were able to tolerate cysteamine when restarted at a dose of 10 mg per kg daily, slowly increased to therapeutic levels over 2 to 3 months. Higher doses of cysteamine had been associated with lethargy and seizures.

1. Schneider JA, *et al.* Cysteamine therapy in nephropathic cystinosis. *N Engl J Med* 1981; **304:** 1172.

Uses and Administration

Cysteamine reduces intracellular cystine levels and is used in the treatment of cystinosis (see below); it has been given orally as the hydrochloride or as the bitartrate. Phosphocysteamine, a phosphorothioester of cysteamine, is more palatable being odourless and tasteless, and is used similarly.

Cysteamine facilitates glutathione synthesis and was formerly used in the treatment of severe paracetamol poisoning to prevent hepatic damage, but other forms of treatment are now preferred (see p.72). A suggested regimen was to give the equivalent of 2 g of cysteamine (as the hydrochloride) by intravenous infusion over 10 minutes, followed by 3 doses of 400 mg infused over 4, 8, and 8 hours.

Cystinosis. Cysteamine and phosphocysteamine (which appears to be rapidly hydrolysed to cysteamine after administration) have been reported to be of benefit in children with cystinosis, a rare autosomal recessive metabolic disorder characterised by the intracellular accumulation of cystine. Cystinosis is marked by growth retardation, rickets, Fanconi syndrome, and renal failure; acute episodes of acidosis and dehydration may develop, and there may be photophobia associated with deposition of cystine in the eye. Treatment, which results in a reduction in the concentrations of cystine in leucocytes, has been shown to be effective in controlling many of the symptoms,[1-3] especially if begun early, although it is not clear from the present contradictory results[3,4] how much benefit is seen on renal function. Compliance may be a problem, due to the unpalatable taste and odour of cysteamine, and the more palatable prodrug phosphocysteamine has been developed as an alternative;[5,6] more palatable formulations of cysteamine are also being investigated. Typical oral doses have been equivalent to 50 to 60 mg of cysteamine free base per kg body-weight daily or in later studies cysteamine or phosphocysteamine at a randomly assigned dose of either 1.3 or 1.95 g per m^2 body-surface daily.[4] Cysteamine eye drops are reportedly of benefit in reversing or preventing deposition of corneal cystine crystals.[7]

1. Yudkoff M, *et al.* Effects of cysteamine therapy in nephropathic cystinosis. *N Engl J Med* 1981; **304:** 141–5.
2. Gahl WA, *et al.* Cysteamine therapy for children with nephropathic cystinosis. *N Engl J Med* 1987; **316:** 971–7.
3. Reznik VM, *et al.* Treatment of cystinosis with cysteamine from early infancy. *J Pediatr* 1991; **119:** 491–3.
4. Markello TC, *et al.* Improved renal function in children with cystinosis treated with cysteamine. *N Engl J Med* 1993; **328:** 1157–62.
5. Gahl WA, *et al.* Cystinosis: progress in a prototypic disease. *Ann Intern Med* 1988; **109:** 557–69.
6. van't Hoff WG, *et al.* Effects of oral phosphocysteamine and rectal cysteamine in cystinosis. *Arch Dis Child* 1991; **66:** 1434–7.
7. Kaiser-Kupfer MI, *et al.* A randomized placebo-controlled trial of cysteamine eye drops in nephropathic cystinosis. *Arch Ophthalmol* 1990; **108;** 689–93.

Preparations

Proprietary Preparations (details are given in Part 3)
Austral.: Cystagon; ***Swed.:*** Cystagon; ***UK:*** Cystagon.

Cytochrome C (12622-q)

Pharmacopoeias. Chin. includes Cytochrome C Solution and preparations for injection.

A haemoprotein occurring in the body and involved in electron and hydrogen transport in biological oxidation processes.

Cytochrome C has been given intravenously in various hypoxic conditions.

It is an ingredient of some eye drops used for the treatment of cataract but its actions, if any, are unclear. Surgery is usually the preferred treatment for cataract once established.

Preparations

Proprietary Preparations (details are given in Part 3)
Ger.: Cytochrom C-Uvocal†; ***Jpn:*** Cytorest†.

Multi-ingredient: ***Fr.:*** Vitaphakol; ***Ger.:*** Vitaphakol N†; Vitreolent Plus; ***Spain:*** Vitaphakol; ***Switz.:*** Vitaphakol.

Cytokines (230-v)

Cytokines are a group of endogenous peptide regulatory molecules with the ability to affect cellular differentiation and/or proliferation. In contrast to peptide hormones, cytokines tend to act locally. Most cytokines are multifunctional molecules with a range of biological effects; they act primarily as mediators of inflammation or as growth factors. Cytokines that are being used clinically include erythropoietin (p.717), thrombopoietin (p.728), granulocyte and granulocyte-macrophage colony-stimulating factors (p.714), interferons (p.615), interleukin-1 (p.1591), interleukin-2 (p.541), interleukin-3 (p.724), oprelvekin (p.725), tumour necrosis factor (p.568), somatomedins (p.1260), and urogastrone (p.1218); those under investigation include fibroblast growth factor, nerve growth factor, platelet-derived growth factor, and transforming growth factor. Some cytokines are involved in the pathophysiology of diseases and a number of cytokine antagonists are also being studied.

References.

1. Green AR. Peptide regulatory factors: multifunctional mediators of cellular growth and differentiation. *Lancet* 1989; **i:** 705–7.
2. Sporn MB, Roberts AB. Transforming growth factor-β: multiple actions and potential clinical applications. *JAMA* 1989; **262:** 938–41.
3. Ross R. Platelet-derived growth factor. *Lancet* 1989; **i:** 1179–82.
4. Anonymous. Fibroblast growth factors: time to take note. *Lancet* 1990; **336:** 777–8.
5. Robson MC, *et al.* Platelet-derived growth factor BB for the treatment of chronic pressure ulcers. *Lancet* 1992; **339:** 23–5.
6. Rowe PM. Clinical potential for TGF-β. *Lancet* 1994; **344:** 72–3.
7. Sheeran P, Hall GM. Cytokines in anaesthesia. *Br J Anaesth* 1997; **78:** 201–19.
8. Lambiase A, *et al.* Topical treatment with nerve growth factor for corneal neurotrophic ulcers. *N Engl J Med* 1998; **338:** 1174–80.
9. Fu X, *et al.* Randomised placebo-controlled trial of use of topical recombinant bovine basic fibroblast growth factor for second-degree burns. *Lancet* 1998; **352:** 1661–4.

Damiana (14088-k)

Turnera.

Damiana is the dried leaves and stem of *Turnera diffusa* var. *aphrodisiaca* (Turneraceae) and possibly other species of *Turnera*. Damiana is drunk as a tea, and is used in herbal medicine for a variety of indications. It has a reputation as an aphrodisiac, but there is no evidence for this. It is also used in homoeopathic medicine.

Preparations

Proprietary Preparations (details are given in Part 3)
UK: Curzon.

Multi-ingredient: ***Austral.:*** Medinat Esten; ***Ger.:*** Carito†; ***Ital.:*** Dam; Four-Ton; ***UK:*** Regina Royal Concorde; Strength.

Dapiprazole Hydrochloride (19035-r)

Dapiprazole Hydrochloride *(USAN, rINNM).*

AF-2139. 5,6,7,8-Tetrahydro-3-[2-(4-*o*-tolyl-1-piperazinyl)ethyl]-s-triazolo[4,3-*a*]pyridine monohydrochloride.

$C_{19}H_{27}N_5,HCl = 361.9.$

CAS — 72822-12-9 (dapiprazole); 72822-13-0 (dapiprazole hydrochloride).

Dapiprazole hydrochloride is an alpha-adrenoceptor blocker administered as eye drops to reverse mydriasis; it is also used in some countries in the management of glaucoma. Dapiprazole may also have antipsychotic activity.

References.

1. Pini LA, *et al.* Dapiprazole compared with clonidine and a placebo in detoxification of opiate addicts. *Int J Clin Pharmacol Res* 1991; **11:** 99–105.
2. Bonomi L, *et al.* Effects of the association of alpha and beta-blocking agents in glaucoma. *J Ocul Pharmacol* 1992; **8:** 279–83.
3. Mastropasqua L, *et al.* Effect of dapiprazole, an alpha-adrenergic blocking agent, on aqueous humor dynamics in pigmentary glaucoma. *Ophthalmic Res* 1996; **28:** 312–18.

Reversal of mydriasis. Dapiprazole is used to reverse the effects of mydriatics (sympathomimetics, and to some extent tropicamide) following surgery or ophthalmoscopic examination (p.1388). It also appears to enhance recovery of accommodation after the use of cycloplegics and may be effective for reversing mydriasis after cataract extraction.

References.

1. Allinson RW, *et al.* Reversal of mydriasis by dapiprazole. *Ann Ophthalmol* 1990; **22:** 131–8.
2. Ponte F, *et al.* Intraocular dapiprazole for the reversal of mydriasis after extracapsular cataract extraction with intraocular lens implantation: Part II: comparison with acetylcholine. *J Cataract Refract Surg* 1991; **17:** 785–9.
3. Johnson ME, *et al.* Efficacy of dapiprazole with hydroxyamphetamine hydrobromide and tropicamide. *J Am Optom Assoc* 1993; **64:** 629–33.
4. Molinari JF, *et al.* Dapiprazole clinical efficacy for counteracting tropicamide 1%. *Optom Vis Sci* 1994; **71:** 319–22.
5. Wilcox CS, *et al.* Comparison of the effects on pupil size and accommodation of three regimens of topical dapiprazole. *Br J Ophthalmol* 1995; **79:** 544–8.

Preparations

Proprietary Preparations (details are given in Part 3)
Aust.: Benglau; ***Canad.:*** Rev-Eyes†; ***Ger.:*** Remydrial; ***Ital.:*** Glamidolo; ***USA:*** Rev-Eyes.

Dectaflur (3487-p)

Dectaflur *(USAN, rINN).*

SKF-38094. 9-Octadecenylamine hydrofluoride.

$C_{18}H_{38}NF = 287.5.$

CAS — 36505-83-6 (nonstereospecific); 1838-19-3 (9-octadecenylamine).

Dectaflur has been used in the prevention of dental caries.

Preparations

Proprietary Preparations (details are given in Part 3)

Multi-ingredient: ***Aust.:*** Elmex; ***Ger.:*** Elmex; Multifluorid; ***Ital.:*** Elmex; ***Switz.:*** Elmex.

Dehydrocholic Acid (3716-v)

Dehydrocholic Acid *(BAN, rINN).*

Chologon; Triketocholanic Acid. 3,7,12-Trioxo-5β-cholan-24-oic acid.

$C_{24}H_{34}O_5 = 402.5.$

CAS — 81-23-2 (dehydrocholic acid); 145-41-5 (sodium dehydrocholate).

Pharmacopoeias. In *Aust., It., Jpn,* and *US.*

A white fluffy odourless powder with a bitter taste. Practically **insoluble** in water; soluble 1 in 100 of alcohol and 1 in 35 of chloroform; soluble 1 in 130 of acetone, 1 in 135 of acetic acid and ethyl acetate, and 1 in 2200 of ether at 15°; solutions in alcohol and chloroform are usually slightly turbid; soluble in glacial acetic acid and in solutions of alkali hydroxides and carbonates.

Dehydrocholic acid is a semisynthetic bile acid (p.1553) which is used for its hydrocholeretic properties, increasing the volume and water content of the bile without appreciably altering the content of bile acids. It has been used to improve biliary drainage and has also been given for the temporary relief of constipation. Usual doses of 250 to 500 mg three times daily by mouth have been employed.

Dehydrocholic acid is contra-indicated in complete mechanical biliary obstruction and in severe hepatitis.

Preparations

USP 23: Dehydrocholic Acid Tablets.

Proprietary Preparations (details are given in Part 3)
Canad.: Dycholium; ***Ital.:*** Deidroepar†; Didrocolo†; ***USA:*** Cholan-HMB; Decholin.

Multi-ingredient: ***Aust.:*** Gallo Merz; ***Canad.:*** Regubil; ***Ger.:*** Enzymed†; Eupond; Hepavis†; Migranex†; ***Ital.:*** Agarbil†; Canulase†; Certobil; Cheliboldo†; Cinarbile†; Debridat Enzimatico†; Heparbil†; Kilozim†; Plasil Enzimatico†; Prandium†; Vasofilo†; ***S.Afr.:*** Spasmo-Canulase; ***Spain:*** Espasmo Canulasa; Gastrosindrom†; Nulacin Fermentos; Trizima†; ***Swed.:*** Fellesan; ***Switz.:*** Dessertase†; Feloflux compose†; Feloflux†; Gillazyme; Gillazyme plus; Spasmo-Canulase; ***USA:*** Bilezyme†.

Denatonium Benzoate (533-x)

Denatonium Benzoate *(BAN, USAN, rINN).*

NSC-157658. Benzyldiethyl(2,6-xylylcarbamoylmethyl)ammonium benzoate monohydrate.

$C_{28}H_{34}N_2O_3,H_2O = 464.6.$

CAS — 3734-33-6 (anhydrous denatonium benzoate); 86398-53-0 (denatonium benzoate monohydrate).

Pharmacopoeias. In *USNF.*

A white odourless crystalline powder with an intensely bitter taste. **Soluble** 1 in 20 of water, 1 in about 2 of alcohol, and 1 in about 3 of chloroform; very slightly soluble in ether. A 3% solution in water has a pH of 6.5 to 7.5. **Store** in airtight containers.

Denatonium benzoate is used where an intensely bitter taste is required for medicinal or industrial purposes and as a partial denaturant for alcohol in toiletries. It is known commercially as Bitrex.

Deoxyribonucleic Acid (12632-s)

ADN; Animal Nucleic Acid; Desoxypentose Nucleic Acid; Desoxyribonucleic Acid; Desoxyribose Nucleic Acid; DNA; Thymus Nucleic Acid.

A nucleotide polymer, and 1 of the 2 distinct varieties of nucleic acid (p.1609). It is found in the cell nuclei of living tissues.

Proprietary preparations of deoxyribonucleic acid are marketed in some countries and are advocated for a variety of debilitated and convalescent conditions. The sodium and magnesium salts are also used.

Preparations

Proprietary Preparations (details are given in Part 3)
Ital.: Placentex; Polides; Poliplacen†.

Multi-ingredient: ***Fr.:*** Adena C; Nutrigene; Osteogen.

Dexpanthenol (7869-p)

Dexpanthenol *(BAN, USAN, rINN).*

Dexpanthenolum; Dextro-Pantothenyl Alcohol; Pantothenol. (*R*)-2,4-Dihydroxy-*N*-(3-hydroxypropyl)-3,3-dimethylbutyramide.

$C_9H_{19}NO_4 = 205.3.$

CAS — 81-13-0.

Pharmacopoeias. In *Eur.* (see p.viii) and *US. US* also includes a racemic mixture under the title Panthenol.

A clear, colourless or slightly yellowish, hygroscopic, viscous liquid, or a white, crystalline powder, with a slight characteristic odour.

Very **soluble** to freely soluble in water; freely soluble in alcohol, in methyl alcohol, and in propylene glycol; soluble in chloroform; soluble to slightly soluble in ether; slightly soluble in glycerol. Some crystallisation may occur on standing. **Store** in airtight containers.

Adverse Effects and Precautions

There have been a few reports of allergic reactions associated with the administration of dexpanthenol although these have not been confirmed. Dexpanthenol is contra-indicated in haemophiliacs and in patients with ileus due to mechanical obstruction.

Uses and Administration

Dexpanthenol is the alcoholic analogue of D-pantothenic acid (p.1352). It has been given intramuscularly in doses of 250 to 500 mg to prevent or control gastro-intestinal atony but its value has not been established. It has also been given by slow intravenous infusion.

Dexpanthenol has been used topically as an ointment, cream, or solution, usually in a strength of 2%, for the treatment of various minor skin disorders.

Dexpanthenol and the racemate panthenol are included in some vitamin preparations.

Preparations

USP 23: Dexpanthenol Preparation; Oil- and Water-soluble Vitamins Capsules; Oil- and Water-soluble Vitamins Oral Solution; Water-soluble Vitamins Capsules.

Proprietary Preparations (details are given in Part 3)
Aust.: Bepanthen; Pantothen; ***Austral.:*** Bepanthen; ***Belg.:*** Bepanthene; ***Fr.:*** Bepanthene; ***Ger.:*** Bepanthen; Corneregel; Cutemul; Frio Augentropfen "B"†; Logomed Wund-Heilbalsam†; Marolderm; Pan-Ophtal; Panthenol; Panthogenat; Pelina; Ucee D; Urupan; Wund- und Heilsalbe; ***Ital.:*** Bepanten; ***S.Afr.:*** Bepantol; ***Spain:*** Bepanthene; ***Swed.:*** Bepanthen†; ***Switz.:*** Bepanthene; ***USA:*** Dexol 250†; Ilopan; Panthoderm.

Multi-ingredient: ***Aust.:*** Beneuran Vit B-Komplex; Bepanthen; Bepanthen plus; Colda; Coldistan; Felix; Hansamed†; Hermalind†; Hermasept; Keratosis; Keratosis forte; Oleovit; Pelsano; Pilowal†; Siccaprotect; Sigman-Haustropfen; Sunsan-Heillotion; Venobene; ***Austral.:*** Le Tan Burn Relief†; Macro Natural Vitamin E Cream; Sebirinse; Superfade; Z-Acne†; ***Belg.:*** Romilar†; ***Canad.:*** Aquasol A; ***Ger.:*** Aknelan Lotio†; Aknelan Milch†; Bepanthen V†; Corneregen N†; Dexabiotan in der Ophtiole†; Dispatenol; Dolobene; Dreisalind†; Essaven Tri-Complex; Hansamed Balsam†; Heparin 30 000-ratiopharm/ Heparin 50 000-ratiopharm†; Hermalind; Hewekzem novo; Hydro Cordes; K_5 "spezial"†; Lipo Cordes; Lygal; Pan†; Pantederm; PC 30 V; Proculens N†; Rectoparin N†; Rectoparin†; Remederm; Ricolind†; Siccaprotect; Thrombocutan†; Vetren†; Vulneral†; Vulnoagil†; Vulnostad†; Wund- und Brand-Gel Eu Rho; ***Ital.:*** Alfa Acid; Dry-Tar†; Emazian B12; Emoantitossina; Gliviton†; Globuleno†; Herbavit; Lenirose; Rinopanteina; ***S.Afr.:*** Broncol; ***Spain:*** Anasilpiel; Neo Visage; Pentoderm†; Romilar Expectorante†; Tododermil Compuesto; Tododermil Simple†; Vigencial; ***Switz.:*** Alphastria; Bepanthene Plus; Cetona; Cortimycine; Creme Carbamide; Creme Carbamide + VAS; Demo gouttes pour les yeux No 1†; Demo-Rhinil†; Dermacalm-d; DermaSept-d†; Dexa Loscon†; Dolobene; Galamila; Gingivitol†; Gorgonium; Hepathrombine; Leniderm†; Lyman; Pelsano; Pigmanorm; Roll-bene; Siccalix; Sportusal; Sportusal Spray sine heparino; Stilex; Turexan Capilla; Turexan Lotion; Unatol; Undex†; Wulnasin†; ***UK:*** Vipsogal; ***USA:*** Ilopan-Choline.

Dextran Sulphate (4810-e)

Dextran Sulfate Sodium; Dextran Sulphate Sodium.
CAS — 9011-18-1.
Pharmacopoeias. In Jpn.

The sodium salt of sulphuric acid esters of dextran.

Dextran sulphate has been used as an anticoagulant and as a lipid regulating drug, and has been investigated for its antiviral activity.

Interactions. As mentioned on p.806, anaphylactoid reactions have occurred in patients receiving ACE inhibitors during low-density lipoprotein apheresis using a dextran sulphate-cellulose column.[1,2] Withdrawal of the ACE inhibitor for 1 to 3 days before apheresis may prevent the reaction.[2]

1. Olbricht CJ, *et al.* Anaphylactoid reactions, LDL apheresis with dextran sulphate, and ACE inhibitors. *Lancet* 1992; **340:** 908–9.
2. Agishi T. Anion-blood contact reaction (ABC reaction) in patients treated by LDL apheresis with dextran sulfate-cellulose column while receiving ACE inhibitors. *JAMA* 1994; **271:** 195–6.

Preparations

Proprietary Preparations (details are given in Part 3)

Multi-ingredient: ***Fr.:*** Avene†; Dextrarine Phenylbutazone; ***Ger.:*** Phlebodril N; ***Ital.:*** Doxivenil†; Stranoval; ***Spain:*** Fabroven; ***Switz.:*** Doxivenil.

Dextrorphan (5614-z)

Dextrorphan *(BAN, pINN).*
Ro-01-6794/706 (dextrorphan hydrochloride). (+)-9a-Methylmorphinan-3-ol.
$C_{17}H_{23}NO = 257.4.$
CAS — 125-73-5 (dextrorphan); 69376-27-8 (dextrorphan hydrochloride).

NOTE. Dextrorphan Hydrochloride is *USAN.*

Dextrorphan, a metabolite of dextromethorphan (p.1057), is an antagonist of the excitatory neurotransmitter *N*-methyl-D-aspartate (NMDA). It possesses some cough suppressant activity and is under investigation as a neuroprotective agent in the management of stroke.

References.

1. Albers GW, *et al.* Safety, tolerability, and pharmacokinetics of the N-methyl-D-aspartate antagonist dextrorphan in patients with acute stroke. *Stroke* 1995; **26:** 254–8.

Dibutyl Sebacate (11142-g)

$C_{18}H_{34}O_4 = 314.5.$
CAS — 109-43-3.
Pharmacopoeias. In USNF.

A colourless oily liquid with a mild odour. Practically **insoluble** in water; soluble in alcohol, in isopropyl alcohol, and in liquid paraffin; very slightly soluble in propylene glycol; practically insoluble in glycerol.

Dibutyl sebacate is a plasticiser.

Dichlorodiethylsulphide (1830-j)

Mustard Gas; Sulphur Mustard; Yellow Cross Liquid. Bis(2-chloroethyl)sulphide.
$C_4H_8Cl_2S = 159.1.$
CAS — 505-60-2.

Dichlorodiethylsulphide was developed for use in chemical warfare and has even more severe vesicant and irritant properties than its nitrogen analogue, mustine (p.555). It was formerly used topically in the treatment of psoriasis.

A report of 11 cases of exposure to dichlorodiethylsulphide in fishermen who accidentally retrieved corroded and leaking gas shells from underwater dumps.[1] The patients presented with very inflamed skin, especially in the axillary and genitofemoral regions, yellow blisters on the hands and legs, painful irritation of the eyes, and transient blindness. Two developed pulmonary oedema. There was evidence of a mutagenic effect and in view of the increased risk of lung cancer in soldiers and workers exposed to the gas it is reasonable to assume that fishermen heavily exposed to dichlorodiethylsulphide also have an increased cancer risk.

1. Wulf HC, *et al.* Sister chromatid exchanges in fishermen exposed to leaking mustard gas shells. *Lancet* 1985; **i:** 690–1.

A review of the toxicology of dichlorodiethylsulphide,[1] and debate on the management of casualties injured by dichlorodiethylsulphide and other chemical warfare agents.[2-8] Most patients exposed to dichlorodiethylsulphide recover completely and only a small proportion will have long-term eye or lung damage,[9] although death from respiratory, renal, and bone-marrow failure may occur.[8]

1. Dacre JC, Goldman M. Toxicology and pharmacology of the chemical warfare agent sulfur mustard. *Pharmacol Rev* 1996; **48:** 289–326.
2. Heyndrickx A, Heyndrickx B. Management of war gas injuries. *Lancet* 1990; **ii:** 1248–9.
3. Fouyn T, *et al.* Management of chemical warfare injuries. *Lancet* 1991; **337:** 121.
4. Willems JL, *et al.* Management of chemical warfare injuries. *Lancet* 1991; **337:** 121–2.
5. Maynard RL, *et al.* Management of chemical warfare injuries. *Lancet* 1991; **337:** 122.
6. Newman-Taylor AJ, Morris AJR. Experience with mustard gas casualties. *Lancet* 1991; **337:** 242.
7. Heyndrickx A. Chemical warfare injuries. *Lancet* 1991; **337:** 430.
8. Rees J, *et al.* Mustard gas casualties. *Lancet* 1991; **337:** 430.
9. Murray VSG, Volans GN. Management of injuries due to chemical weapons. *Br Med J* 1991; **302:** 129–30.

Diethanolamine (205-b)

Diolamine *(pINN)*; Diaethanolamin. Bis(2-hydroxyethyl)amine; 2,2′-Iminobisethanol.
$C_4H_{11}NO_2 = 105.1.$
CAS — 111-42-2.
Pharmacopoeias. In USNF, which specifies a mixture of ethanolamines consisting largely of diethanolamine.

Diethanolamine (USNF 18) consists of white or clear, colourless crystals, deliquescing in moist air, or a colourless liquid. **Miscible** with water, with alcohol, with acetone, with chloroform, and with glycerol; slightly soluble to practically insoluble in ether and in petroleum spirit. **Store** in airtight containers. Protect from light.

Diethanolamine is an organic base which is used as an emulsifier and dispersant.

It is used to solubilise fusidic acid by the formation of the diethanolamine salt. It has been used for the preparation of salts of iodinated organic acids used as contrast media. It may be irritating to the skin and mucous membranes.

Digitalin (5811-x)

Amorphous Digitalin; Digitalinum Purum Germanicum.

A standardised mixture of glycosides from *Digitalis purpurea.*

Digitalin has actions similar to those of digoxin (p.849). Because of its ready solubility in water it was formerly used for the preparation of solutions for injection. It is also present in several ophthalmic preparations.

Digitalin must be distinguished from digitoxin (Digitaline Cristallisée) which is very much more potent.

Preparations

Proprietary Preparations (details are given in Part 3)
Multi-ingredient: ***Ger.:*** Augentonikum; durajod†; ***Ital.:*** Digifar.

Dihydroergocristine Mesylate (12007-q)

Dihydroergocristine Methanesulphonate.
$C_{35}H_{41}N_5O_5,CH_4O_3S = 707.8.$
CAS — 17479-19-5 (dihydroergocristine); 24730-10-7 (dihydroergocristine mesylate).

Dihydroergocristine mesylate is a component of co-dergocrine mesylate (p.1566) and has similar actions. In some countries it has been given by mouth in the symptomatic treatment of mental deterioration associated with cerebrovascular insufficiency and in peripheral vascular disease. It has also been given by intramuscular injection.

References.

1. de Aloysio D, *et al.* Dihydroergocristine in stopping lactation: double-blind study vs bromocriptine. *Gynecol Endocrinol* 1988; **2:** 67–71.
2. Franciosi A, Zavattini G. Dihydroergocristine in the treatment of elderly patients with cognitive deterioration: a double-blind, placebo-controlled, dose-response study. *Curr Ther Res* 1994; **55:** 1391–1401.

Preparations

Proprietary Preparations (details are given in Part 3)
Aust.: Diertina; Nehydrin; ***Ger.:*** Decme†; Nehydrin†; ***Ital.:*** Defluina; Diertina; Difluid; Ergo†; Ergocris; Ergotina†; Gral; Unergol; Vasoton; ***Spain:*** Diertine; Ergodavur; ***Switz.:*** Diertina.

Multi-ingredient: ***Aust.:*** Brinerdin; Defluina; Pressimedin; Sandoven; Supergan; ***Fr.:*** Cervilane; Cristanyl†; Iskedyl; ***Ital.:*** Brinerdina; Diertina Ipotensiva†; Sandoven†; ***Neth.:*** Brinerdin†; ***S.Afr.:*** Brinerdin; Sandovene†; ***Spain:*** Brinerdina; Clinadil; Diemil; Dipervina; Iskedyl; Isquebral; ***Switz.:*** Brinerdine; Pressimed; Sandovene f†.

Dihydroergocryptine Mesylate (12008-p)

Dihydroergocryptine Methanesulphonate; Dihydroergokryptine Mesylate.
$C_{32}H_{43}N_5O_5,CH_4O_3S = 673.8.$
CAS — 25447-66-9 (dihydroergocryptine, α-isomer); 19467-62-0 (dihydroergocryptine, β-isomer); 14271-05-7 (dihydroergocryptine mesylate, α-isomer); 65914-79-6 (dihydroergocryptine mesylate, β-isomer).

Dihydroergocryptine mesylate is a component of co-dergocrine mesylate (p.1566) and has similar actions. In some countries it has been given by mouth, often in combination with caffeine, in the symptomatic treatment of mental deterioration associated with cerebrovascular insufficiency and in peripheral vascular disease. It has also been used in the management of hyperprolactinaemia.

References.

1. Faglia G, *et al.* Dihydroergocriptine in management of microprolactinomas. *J Clin Endocrinol Metab* 1987; **65:** 779–84.

Preparations

Proprietary Preparations (details are given in Part 3)
Ger.: Almirid; ***Ital.:*** Daverium; Myrol.
Multi-ingredient: ***Fr.:*** Vasobral; ***Ital.:*** Vasobral.

Dihydroxydibutylether (12654-z)

Hydroxybutyloxide. 4,4′-Oxybis(butan-2-ol).
$C_8H_{18}O_3 = 162.2.$
CAS — 821-33-0.

Dihydroxydibutylether is a choleretic.

Preparations

Proprietary Preparations (details are given in Part 3)
Fr.: Dyskinebyl; ***Ital.:*** Dis-Cinil Ilfi; Diskin.
Multi-ingredient: ***Ital.:*** Dis-Cinil Complex; Fluidobil†.

Diiodhydrin (12655-c)

Iodazone; Iothion. 1,3-Di-iodopropan-2-ol.
$C_3H_6I_2O$ = 311.9.
CAS — 534-08-7.

Diiodhydrin is an organic iodine-containing compound that has been used with aromatic oils in nose drops for the treatment of rhinitis and pharyngitis.

Preparations

Proprietary Preparations (details are given in Part 3)
Multi-ingredient: ***Ital.:*** Bronco Valda†.

Diisopropanolamine (206-v)

1,1′-Iminobis(propan-2-ol).
$C_6H_{15}NO_2$ = 133.2.
CAS — 110-97-4.

Diisopropanolamine is an organic base which is used as a neutralising agent in cosmetics and toiletries.

Dill Oil (4642-e)

European Dill Seed Oil; Oleum Anethi.
CAS — 8016-06-6.
Pharmacopoeias. In Br.

A clear colourless or pale yellow volatile oil obtained by distillation from the dried ripe fruits of dill, *Anethum graveolens* (Umbelliferae). It darkens with age and has a characteristic odour. It contains 43 to 63% of carvone ($C_{10}H_{14}O$).
Soluble 1 in 1 of alcohol (90%) and 1 in 10 of alcohol (80%). **Store** at a temperature not exceeding 25°. Protect from light.

Dill oil, usually in the form of dill water, is used as an aromatic carminative, although the efficacy of such traditional remedies in infantile colic is considered dubious (see Gastro-intestinal Spasm, p.1170).

Preparations

Proprietary Preparations (details are given in Part 3)
Multi-ingredient: ***Canad.:*** Babys Own Gripe Water; Chase Kolik Gripe Water; Woodwards Gripe Water; ***UK:*** Atkinson & Barker's Gripe Mixture; Neo; Nurse Harvey's Gripe Mixture; Woodwards Gripe Water.

Dimepropion Hydrochloride (1476-l)

Dimepropion Hydrochloride *(BANM).*
Metamfepramone Hydrochloride *(pINNM)*; Metamfepyramone Hydrochloride. 2-Dimethylaminopropiophenone hydrochloride.
$C_{11}H_{15}NO,HCl$ = 213.7.
CAS — 15351-09-4 (dimepropion); 10105-90-5 (dimepropion hydrochloride).

Dimepropion, the dimethyl analogue of diethylpropion (p.1479), is a sympathomimetic that has been used as the hydrochloride in the treatment of hypotension and in preparations for the relief of the symptoms of the common cold. It was formerly used as an anorectic agent.

Preparations

Proprietary Preparations (details are given in Part 3)
Multi-ingredient: ***Ger.:*** Tempil N.

Dimethoxymethane (19847-e)

Formal; Formaldehyde Dimethyl Acetal; Methylal.
$CH_2(OCH_3)_2$ = 76.09.
CAS — 109-87-5.

Dimethoxymethane has been used in perfumery. It has been included in preparations for topical anaesthesia.

Preparations

Proprietary Preparations (details are given in Part 3)
Multi-ingredient: ***UK:*** PR Freeze Spray.

Dimethyltryptamine (5013-y)

Businessman's Trip; DMT; N,N-Dimethyltryptamine. 3-(2-Dimethylaminoethyl)indole.
$C_{12}H_{16}N_2$ = 188.3.
CAS — 61-50-7.

An active principle obtained from the seeds and leaves of *Piptadenia peregrina* (Mimosaceae) from which the hallucinogenic snuff cohoba is prepared, and other South American plants. It has been reported to be present in the tropical legume *Mucuna pruriens.*

Dimethyltryptamine produces hallucinogenic and sympathomimetic effects which are similar to those of lysergide (p.1597), but of shorter duration. It has no therapeutic use. Diethyltryptamine (DET) and dipropyltryptamine (DPT) are related synthetic hallucinogens with longer actions but are less potent than dimethyltryptamine.

2,4-Dinitrochlorobenzene (12666-t)

DNCB. 1-Chloro-2,4-dinitrobenzene.
$C_6H_3ClN_2O_4$ = 202.6.
CAS — 97-00-7.

2,4-Dinitrochlorobenzene is used in photography. It is a potent sensitiser and has been applied topically in the evaluation of delayed hypersensitivity. It has also been used as an immunostimulant in leprosy, AIDS, and some forms of cancer and in the treatment of alopecia and warts.

2,4-Dinitrochlorobenzene has been reported to be mutagenic *in vitro.*

References.

1. Happle R. The potential hazards of dinitrochlorobenzene. *Arch Dermatol* 1985; **121:** 330–2.
2. Stricker RB, Goldberg B. Host-directed therapy for AIDS. *Ann Intern Med* 1995; **123:** 471–2.
3. Todd DJ. Topical treatment with dinitrochlorobenzene. *Lancet* 1995; **346:** 975.
4. Stricker RB, Goldberg B. Safety of topical dinitrochlorobenzene. *Lancet* 1995; **346:** 1293.

Dioxethedrin Hydrochloride (11600-c)

Dioxethedrin Hydrochloride *(rINNM).*
Dioxethedrine Hydrochloride. α-(1-Ethylaminoethyl)protocatechuyl alcohol hydrochloride.
$C_{11}H_{17}NO_3,HCl$ = 247.7.
CAS — 497-75-6 (dioxethedrin).

Dioxethedrin hydrochloride is a sympathomimetic used in combination with antitussive agents in preparations intended for the relief of coughs and associated respiratory-tract disorders.

Preparations

Proprietary Preparations (details are given in Part 3)
Multi-ingredient: ***Belg.:*** Quintex; Quintex Pediatrique; ***Fr.:*** Quintopan Enfant.

Dioxins (13301-r)

NOTE. The name Dioxin has also been applied to dimethoxane.

The term 'dioxins' encompasses a large group of closely related chemicals known as polychlorinated dibenzo-*p*-dioxins (PCDDs) and polychlorinated dibenzofurans (PCDFs). The most toxic is 2,3,7,8-tetrachlorodibenzo-*p*-dioxin (TCDD).

Dioxins are byproducts in the manufacture of commercial chemical products such as chlorinated phenols and polychlorinated biphenyls (PCBs), and can also be produced in smaller quantities by combustion processes and industrial waste. They first came to public attention during the Vietnam War, when they were found to be present in the herbicide Agent Orange used as a defoliant. They are incriminated as causing chloracne (a severe and persistent acne caused by chlorinated compounds). They are potent teratogens and carcinogens in *animals.* An increased incidence of cancer at different organs due to dioxins has been claimed but this has not been substantiated by clinical and follow-up studies. An effect on cell-mediated immunity has been observed.

Exposure should be limited to the lowest feasible concentration.

The impact of dioxins in food and the environment has been reviewed.[1-3]

An excess of soft tissue sarcomas was found in workers exposed to chlorophenoxy herbicides including those contaminated with TCDD,[4] but cautious interpretation of these results was advised.[5] In Vietnam veterans the risk for non-Hodgkin's lymphoma was approximately 50% higher than control subjects, but was not related to exposure to Agent Orange, nor was there evidence for an increase in other cancers.[6] Exposure to TCDD was implicated in an increase in cancer mortality in chemical workers[7,8] but confounding factors such as smoking may have been present.[8,9] Other studies[10,11] have not shown an association between dioxin exposure and an increase in the incidence of human cancer and epidemiological studies following occupational or accidental exposures have found no clear persistent systemic effects except for chloracne and no clear association with carcinogenesis or reproductive disorders.[1,2]

In the USA, the National Academy of Sciences' Institute of Medicine is reported to have carried out an evaluation of publications on herbicide exposure, largely in industrial and agricultural workers.[12] They concluded that exposure to herbicides or dioxin was associated with soft-tissue sarcomas, Hodgkin's disease, non-Hodgkin lymphoma, chloracne, and porphyria cutanea tarda, and that there was limited evidence of an association with respiratory and prostate cancers and multiple myeloma. An update to the report has also suggested a link between Agent Orange exposure and spina bifida in veterans' offspring.[13]

1. Polychlorinated dibenzo-para-dioxins and dibenzofurans. *Environmental Health Criteria 88.* Geneva: WHO, 1989.
2. Department of the Environment. Dioxins in the environment. *Pollution Paper 27.* London: HMSO, 1989.
3. MAFF. Dioxins in food. *Food Surveillance Paper 31.* London: HMSO, 1992.
4. Saracci R, *et al.* Cancer mortality in workers exposed to chlorophenoxy herbicides and chlorophenols. *Lancet* 1991; **338:** 1027–32.
5. Peto R. Occupational exposure to chlorophenoxy herbicides and chlorophenols. *Lancet* 1991; **338:** 1392.
6. Suskind R. The association of selected cancers with service in the US military in Vietnam. *Arch Intern Med* 1990; **150:** 2449–50.
7. Manz A, *et al.* Cancer mortality among workers in chemical plant contaminated with dioxin. *Lancet* 1991; **338:** 959–64.
8. Fingerhut MA, *et al.* Cancer mortality in workers exposed to 2,3,7,8-tetrachlorodibenzo-p-dioxin. *N Engl J Med* 1991; **324:** 212–18.
9. Triebig G. Is dioxin carcinogenic? *Lancet* 1991; **338:** 1592.
10. Coggon O, *et al.* Mortality and incidence of cancer at four factories making phenoxy herbicides. *Br J Ind Med* 1991; **48:** 173–80.
11. Green LM. A cohort mortality study of forestry workers exposed to phenoxy acid herbicides. *Br J Ind Med* 1991; **48:** 234–8.
12. McCarthy M. Agent Orange. *Lancet* 1993; **342:** 362.
13. Stephenson J. New IOM report links Agent Orange Exposure to risk of birth defect in Vietnam vets' children. *JAMA* 1996; **275:** 1066–7.

Diphenyl (6644-g)

E230; Phenylbenzene. Biphenyl.
$C_{12}H_{10}$ = 154.2.
CAS — 92-52-4.

Diphenyl is fungistatic against a limited number of moulds and has been employed for impregnating the material used for wrapping citrus fruits.

Workers exposed to high concentrations of diphenyl (up to 128 mg per m^3) developed toxic symptoms which included irritation of the throat and eyes, headache, nausea, diffuse abdominal pain, numbness, aching of limbs, and general fatigue.[1] One of the workers who also had somnolence, icterus, ascites, and oedema of the legs, died; at autopsy, the liver showed necrosis.

1. Häkkinen I, *et al.* Diphenyl poisoning in fruit paper production. *Arch Environ Health* 1973; **26:** 70–4.

Dipivefrine Hydrochloride (12670-z)

Dipivefrine Hydrochloride *(BANM, rINNM).*
Dipivalyl Adrenaline Hydrochloride; Dipivalyl Epinephrine Hydrochloride; Dipivefrin Hydrochloride; DPE (dipivefrine). (*RS*)-4-[1-Hydroxy-2-(methylamino)ethyl]-*o*-phenylene dipivalate hydrochloride.
$C_{19}H_{29}NO_5,HCl$ = 387.9.
CAS — 52365-63-6 (dipivefrine); 64019-93-8 (dipivefrine hydrochloride).

NOTE. Dipivefrin is *USAN.*
Pharmacopoeias. In US.

White crystals or crystalline powder, with a faint odour. Very **soluble** in water. **Store** in airtight containers.

Dipivefrine is an ester and prodrug of adrenaline (p.813). A 0.1% solution of the hydrochloride is used topically as eye drops to reduce intra-ocular pressure in patients with open-angle glaucoma or ocular hypertension (p.1387).

References.

1. Parrow KA, *et al.* Is it worthwhile to add dipivefrin HCl 0.1% to topical β_1-, β_2-blocker therapy? *Ophthalmology* 1989; **96:** 1338–41.
2. Drake MV, *et al.* Levobunolol compared to dipivefrin in African American patients with open angle glaucoma. *J Ocul Pharmacol* 1993; **9:** 91–5. Correction. *ibid.*; 385.
3. Albracht DC, *et al.* A double-masked comparison of betaxolol and dipivefrin for the treatment of increased intraocular pressure. *Am J Ophthalmol* 1993; **116:** 307–13.

Preparations

USP 23: Dipivefrin Hydrochloride Ophthalmic Solution.

Proprietary Preparations (details are given in Part 3)
Aust.: Glaucothil; ***Austral.:*** Propine; ***Belg.:*** Propine; ***Canad.:*** Propine; ***Fr.:*** Propine; ***Ger.:*** d Epifrin; Glaucothil; ***Irl.:*** Propine; ***Ital.:*** Propine; ***Neth.:*** Diopine†; ***Norw.:*** Propine; ***S.Afr.:*** Propine; ***Spain:*** Diopine; Glaudrops; ***Swed.:*** Diprin; Oftapinex; Propine; ***Switz.:*** Diopine; Diphemin; ***UK:*** Propine; ***USA:*** AkPro; Propine.

Multi-ingredient: ***Aust.:*** Thiloadren; Thilodigon; ***Canad.:*** Probeta; ***Ger.:*** Thiloadren N; Thilodigon.

Disodium Guanylate (12675-x)

627; Disodium Guanosine-5′-monophosphate; Sodium 5′-Guanylate. Guanosine 5′-(disodium phosphate).

$C_{10}H_{12}N_5Na_2O_8P,xH_2O$.

CAS — 5550-12-9 (anhydrous disodium guanylate).

Disodium guanylate has been used as a flavour enhancer in foods. It has also been used in eye drops containing other nucleosides in the treatment of corneal damage. The term sodium 5′-ribonucleotide has been used to refer to a mixture of disodium guanylate with disodium inosinate (below).

Preparations

Proprietary Preparations (details are given in Part 3)

Multi-ingredient: ***Aust.:*** Vitasic; ***Fr.:*** Vitacic; ***Ger.:*** Vitasic†; ***Ital.:*** Emazian Cortex†.

Disodium Inosinate (12676-r)

631; Disodium Inosine-5′-monophosphate; Sodium 5′-Inosinate. Inosine 5′-(disodium phosphate).

$C_{10}H_{11}N_4Na_2O_8P,xH_2O$.

CAS — 4691-65-0 (anhydrous disodium inosinate).

Disodium inosinate has been used as a flavour enhancer in foods. It has also been given by mouth and been applied topically in the treatment of visual disturbance.

Preparations

Proprietary Preparations (details are given in Part 3)

Fr.: Catacol; Correctol; ***Ger.:*** Antikataraktikum N; ***Switz.:*** Catacol.

Multi-ingredient: ***Ital.:*** Emazian Cortex†.

Disulfiram (2731-t)

Disulfiram *(BAN, rINN).*

Dissulfiramo; Disulfiramum; Éthyldithiourame; TTD. Tetraethylthiuram disulphide; Bis(diethylthiocarbamoyl) disulfide.

$C_{10}H_{20}N_2S_4 = 296.5$.

CAS — 97-77-8.

Pharmacopoeias. In *Eur.* (see p.viii), *Jpn, Pol.,* and *US.*

A white or almost white, odourless crystalline powder. Practically **insoluble** to very slightly soluble in water; soluble 1 in 30 of alcohol and 1 in 15 of ether; soluble in acetone, in carbon disulphide, and in chloroform; freely soluble in dichloromethane. **Store** in airtight containers. Protect from light.

Stability. Studies on the stability of disulfiram preparations.

1. Gupta VD. Stability of aqueous suspensions of disulfiram. *Am J Hosp Pharm* 1981; **38:** 363–4.
2. Philips M, *et al.* Stability of an injectable disulfiram formulation sterilized by gamma irradiation. *Am J Hosp Pharm* 1985; **42:** 343–5.

Adverse Effects

Drowsiness and fatigue are common during initial treatment with disulfiram. Other side-effects reported include a garlic-like or metallic after-taste, gastro-intestinal upsets, body odour, bad breath, headache, impotence, and allergic dermatitis. Peripheral and optic neuropathies, psychotic reactions, and hepatotoxicity may occur.

Disulfiram-alcohol reaction. The use of disulfiram in the management of alcoholism is based on the extremely unpleasant, but generally self-limiting, systemic effects which occur when a patient receiving the drug ingests alcohol. These effects begin with flushing of the face and, as vasodilatation spreads, throbbing in the head and neck and a pulsating headache may develop. Respiratory difficulties, nausea, copious vomiting, sweating, thirst, chest pain, tachycardia, palpitations, marked hypotension, giddiness, weakness, blurred vision, and confusion may follow. The intensity and duration of symptoms is very variable and even small quantities of alcohol may result in alarming reactions. In addition to the above effects, severe reactions have included respiratory depression, cardiovascular collapse, cardiac arrhythmias, myocardial infarction, acute congestive heart failure, unconsciousness, convulsions, and sudden death. Severe reactions require intensive supportive therapy; oxygen and intravenous fluids may be necessary. Potassium concentrations should be monitored. The intravenous administration of ascorbic acid or antihistamines has been suggested but no benefit has been established.

Effects on the blood. There were isolated reports of blood dyscrasias associated with disulfiram in the 1960s. The US manufacturer recommends that blood counts should be performed every 6 months during treatment.

Effects on the liver. A review of 18 cases of hepatitis in patients receiving disulfiram.[1] Symptoms have appeared between 10 days and six months after initiating disulfiram, and clinical improvement has been seen within 2 weeks of discontinuing disulfiram although liver enzyme values may not return to normal for several months. Fatal hepatic coma had been reported in 7 patients. The clinical picture of disulfiram-induced hepatitis is consistent with a hypersensitivity reaction.

1. Mason NA. Disulfiram-induced hepatitis: case report and review of the literature. *DICP Ann Pharmacother* 1989; **23:** 872–4.

Effects on the nervous system. ENCEPHALOPATHY. A 2% incidence of reversible toxic encephalopathy has been reported in patients receiving disulfiram.[1] Onset varies from days to months following the start of therapy and early signs include impaired concentration, memory deficits, anxiety, depression, and somnolence. Confusion and disorientation follow, often accompanied by paranoid delusions and sometimes hallucinations. Other symptoms may include ataxia, loss of fine motor coordination, slurred speech, and intention tremor. The encephalopathy usually resolves within 3 days to 2 weeks of stopping disulfiram, although symptoms may persist for 6 weeks. There are conflicting opinions on whether this psychosis is a toxic reaction to disulfiram or a response to abstinence from alcohol, but the authors suspect that most cases represent a toxic encephalopathy. However, psychosis without any suggestion of encephalopathy has been reported.[2]

1. Hotson JR, Langston JW. Disulfiram-induced encephalopathy. *Arch Neurol* 1976; **33:** 141–2.
2. Rossiter SK. Psychosis with disulfiram prescribed under probation order. *Br Med J* 1992; **305:** 763.

PERIPHERAL NEUROPATHY. A report of peripheral neuropathy associated with disulfiram in 4 patients and reference to 25 reported cases.[1] Onset of neuropathy varied from days to months after starting disulfiram treatment and could develop with doses of 250 or 500 mg daily. The most common symptom reported was pins and needles, but numbness, pain/burning, and weakness were frequently described; usually both muscle weakness and sensory loss were noted. Optic atrophy has also been described. Although there might be some improvement immediately after disulfiram withdrawal, the neurological deficit only improved slowly and symptoms might persist for as long as 2 years.

1. Watson CP, *et al.* Disulfiram neuropathy. *Can Med Assoc J* 1980; **123:** 123–6.

Effects on the respiratory tract. Bronchospasm and hypertension were observed in an asthmatic patient taking disulfiram following an alcohol challenge test.[1]

1. Zapata E, Orwin A. Severe hypertension and bronchospasm during disulfiram-ethanol test reaction. *Br Med J* 1992; **305:** 870.

Effects on the skin. Orange-coloured palms and soles, provoking an initial diagnosis of jaundice, developed in a 55-year-old man who had been taking disulfiram for about 2 months.[1] It was postulated that the discoloration was due to accumulation of carotenes in the skin as a result of inhibition of vitamin A metabolism by disulfiram. The discoloration disappeared soon after disulfiram was stopped.

1. Santonastaso M, *et al.* Yellow palms with disulfiram. *Lancet* 1997; **350:** 266.

Overdosage. Disulfiram intoxication has been reported in a 6-year-old boy who recovered after receiving disulfiram 250 mg four times daily to a total of 13 doses.[1] Of 6 previous reports one child died and 3 had moderate or severe brain damage. The syndrome of disulfiram intoxication in children is distinct from the disulfiram-alcohol interaction or acute disulfiram intoxication in adults. It is characterised by lethargy or somnolence, weakness, hypotonia, and vomiting, beginning approximately 12 hours after ingestion and progressing to stupor or coma. Dehydration, moderate tachycardia, and marked tachypnoea occur frequently, muscle tone is greatly decreased, and deep-tendon reflexes may be weak or absent.

Severe neurological damage has also been reported[2] in a 5-year-old girl following acute disulfiram intoxication which was initially diagnosed as diabetic ketoacidosis.

1. Benitz WE, Tatro DS. Disulfiram intoxication in a child. *J Pediatr* 1984; **105:** 487–9.
2. Mahajan P, *et al.* Basal ganglion infarction in a child with disulfiram poisoning. *Pediatrics* 1997; **99:** 605–8.

Precautions

Disulfiram is contra-indicated in the presence of cardiovascular disease or psychosis or severe personality disorders, and should not be given to patients known to be hypersensitive to it or to other thiuram compounds, such as those used in rubber vulcanisation or pesticides. It should be used with caution in the presence of diabetes mellitus, epilepsy, impaired hepatic or renal function, respiratory disorders, cerebral damage, or hypothyroidism. Caution is also advised when administering disulfiram to drug addicts. It is probably best avoided in pregnancy.

Disulfiram should not be given until at least 24 hours after the last ingestion of alcohol. Patients beginning therapy should be fully aware of the disulfiram-alcohol reaction and should be warned to avoid alcohol in any form, including alcohol-containing medicines and alcohol-based topical preparations. Reactions to alcohol may occur as long as 2 weeks after the cessation of disulfiram.

The US manufacturers have recommended that regular blood counts and liver function tests should be performed during long-term therapy.

Pregnancy. A report of 2 infants with severe limb-reduction anomalies whose mothers had taken disulfiram during pregnancy.[1] Only 2 similar cases had previously been reported.

1. Nora AH, *et al.* Limb-reduction anomalies in infants born to disulfiram-treated alcoholic mothers. *Lancet* 1977; **ii:** 664.

Interactions

Disulfiram inhibits hepatic enzymes and may interfere with the metabolism of other drugs taken at the same time. It enhances the effects of phenytoin and coumarin anticoagulants and their dosage may need to be reduced. It inhibits the metabolism and excretion of rifampicin, and may similarly affect pethidine, morphine, and amphetamines. Toxic reactions have occurred following the concomitant administration of disulfiram and isoniazid or metronidazole. Disulfiram may inhibit the metabolism of paraldehyde leading to an accumulation of acetaldehyde and these drugs should not be given concomitantly.

The potential of disulfiram to impair drug metabolism was demonstrated by Vesell *et al.*[1] who found that it prolonged the plasma half-life of phenazone, probably by inhibiting the hepatic microsomal mixed function oxidases. They also suggested that disulfiram alters catecholamine metabolism since urinary excretion of vanilmandelic acid (VMA) was significantly reduced and that of homovanillic acid (HVA) was increased.

Although *chlorpromazine* was once given to reduce the nausea and vomiting associated with the disulfiram-alcohol reaction,[2] Kwentus and Major[3] considered that phenothiazine antiemetics such as chlorpromazine might increase hypotension because of their α-adrenoceptor blocking activity and should therefore be contra-indicated. Sellers *et al.*[4] also noted that clinically serious pharmacodynamic interactions could be anticipated during the disulfiram-alcohol reaction in patients taking other drugs that impair blood pressure regulation, such as α- and β-adrenoceptor blocking agents and vasodilators. MacCallum[5] reported that *amitriptyline* appeared to enhance the disulfiram-alcohol reaction. Sellers *et al.*[4] pointed out the potential for serious interactions during the disulfiram-alcohol reaction with drugs having CNS actions mediated by noradrenaline or dopamine, such as *tricyclic antidepressants* and *phenothiazines*, or those inhibiting the same enzymes as disulfiram, such as *MAOIs*. Conversely, *diazepam* was reported by MacCallum[5] to reduce the intensity of the disulfiram-alcohol reaction.

Reports of the effects of disulfiram on the following drugs may be found in their respective monographs: Amitriptyline Hydrochloride, Cannabis, Diazepam, Enflurane, Ethylene Dibromide, Isoniazid, Metronidazole, Paraldehyde, Perphenazine, Phenytoin Sodium, and Warfarin Sodium.

1. Vesell ES, *et al.* Impairment of drug metabolism by disulfiram in man. *Clin Pharmacol Ther* 1971; **12:** 785–92.
2. Cummins JF, Friend DG. Use of chlorpromazine in chronic alcoholics. *Am J Med Sci* 1954; **227:** 561–4.
3. Kwentus J, Major LF. Disulfiram in the treatment of alcoholism: a review. *J Stud Alcohol* 1979; **40:** 428–46.
4. Sellers EM, *et al.* Drugs to decrease alcohol consumption. *N Engl J Med* 1981; **305:** 1255–62.
5. MacCallum WAG. Drug interactions in alcoholism treatment. *Lancet* 1969; **i:** 313.

Pharmacokinetics

Disulfiram is absorbed from the gastro-intestinal tract and is rapidly reduced to diethyldithiocarbamate, principally by the glutathione reductase system in the erythrocytes; reduction may also occur in the liver. Diethyldithiocarbamate is metabolised in the liver to its glucuronide and methyl ester and to diethylamine, carbon disulphide, and sulphate ions. Metabolites are excreted primarily in the urine; carbon disulphide is exhaled in the breath.

There was marked intersubject variability in plasma concentrations of disulfiram and its metabolites in a study of 15 male alcoholics given single 250-mg doses of disulfiram by mouth and repeated dosing with 250 mg daily for 12 days.[1] Variability might result from the marked lipid solubility of disulfiram, differences in plasma protein binding, or enterohepatic cycling. Average times to reach peak plasma concentrations after single or repeated doses were 8 to 10 hours for disulfiram, diethyldithiocarbamate, diethyldithiocarbamate-methyl ester, and diethylamine, and for carbon disulphide in breath; peak plasma concentrations of carbon disulphide occurred after 5 to 6 hours. Plasma concentrations of disulfiram were negligible within 48 hours of a dose although concentrations of some metabolites were still raised. In urine, 1.7 and 8.3% of a disulfiram dose was eliminated as diethyldithiocarbamate-glucuronide in the 24 hours after a single and repeated dose, while diethylamine accounted for 1.6 and 5.7%, respectively. In the 24 hours after a single and repeated dose 22.4 and 31.3%, respectively, was eliminated as carbon disulphide in the breath.

1. Faiman MD, *et al.* Elimination kinetics of disulfiram in alcoholics after single and repeated doses. *Clin Pharmacol Ther* 1984; **36:** 520–6.

Uses and Administration

Disulfiram is used as an adjunct in the treatment of chronic alcoholism (p.1099). Disulfiram is not a cure and the treatment is likely to be of little value unless it is undertaken with the willing cooperation of the patient and is employed in conjunction with supportive psychotherapy.

Disulfiram inhibits aldehyde dehydrogenase, the enzyme responsible for the oxidation of acetaldehyde, a metabolite of alcohol. The resulting accumulation of acetaldehyde in the blood is widely believed to be responsible for many of the unpleasant symptoms of the disulfiram-alcohol reaction which occur when alcohol is taken, even in small quantities, after the administration of disulfiram (see Adverse Effects, above). Symptoms can arise within 10 minutes of the ingestion of alcohol and last from half an hour in mild cases to several hours in severe cases. It is advisable to carry out the initial treatment in hospital where the patient can be kept under close supervision.

Disulfiram is given by mouth. A suggested dose is 800 mg, taken as a single dose, on the first day of treatment, reduced by 200 mg daily to a maintenance dose which is usually 100 to 200 mg daily. In the USA, where doses above 500 mg daily are not recommended, an initial dose of 500 mg daily for 1 to 2 weeks is suggested, followed by a maintenance dose of 250 mg daily or within the range of 125 to 500 mg daily.

A test dose of alcohol has been given under close supervision when the patient is receiving maintenance doses of disulfiram, in order to demonstrate the nature of the disulfiram-alcohol reaction. However, these challenge tests have generally been abandoned, and should not in any case be used in patients over 50 years of age. Many authorities consider that an explicit description of the reaction is sufficient.

Disulfiram implants have been used in an attempt to overcome problems of patient compliance but have been largely abandoned due to lack of clinical efficacy.

Alcoholism. Some references.

1. Wright C, Moore RD. Disulfiram treatment of alcoholism. *Am J Med* 1990; **88:** 647–55.
2. Hughes JC, Cook CCH. The efficacy of disulfiram: a review of outcome studies. *Addiction* 1997; **92:** 381–95.

Preparations

BP 1998: Disulfiram Tablets;
USP 23: Disulfiram Tablets.

Proprietary Preparations (details are given in Part 3)
Aust.: Antabus; ***Austral.:*** Antabuse; ***Belg.:*** Antabuse; Esperal†; ***Canad.:*** Antabuse; ***Fr.:*** Esperal; ***Ger.:*** Antabus; ***Irl.:*** Antabuse; ***Ital.:*** Antabuse; Etiltox; ***Neth.:*** Antabus†; Refusal; ***Norw.:*** Antabus; ***S.Afr.:*** Antabuse; ***Spain:*** Antabus; ***Swed.:*** Antabus; ***Switz.:*** Antabus; ***UK:*** Antabuse; ***USA:*** Antabuse.

Multi-ingredient: ***Fr.:*** TTD-B_3-B_4; ***Swed.:*** Tenutex.

Dizocilpine Maleate (9426-x)

Dizocilpine Maleate *(USAN, rINNM).*

MK-801. (+)-10,11-Dihydro-5-methyl-5*H*-dibenzo[*a*,*d*]cyclohepten-5,10-imine maleate.

$C_{16}H_{15}N,C_4H_4O_4$ = 337.4.

CAS — 77086-21-6 (dizocilpine); 77086-22-7 (dizocilpine maleate).

Dizocilpine is an antagonist of the excitatory neurotransmitter *N*-methyl-D-aspartate (NMDA), and has been investigated in *animals* for its antiepileptic properties as well as for a potential role in various other neurological disorders including preventing damage due to cerebral ischaemia.

Dizocilpine has good anticonvulsant activity but as it causes alarming psychotropic effects it had been abandoned as a possible therapy for epilepsy.[1] Interest in its use as a possible therapy for stroke continued.

1. Richens A. New antiepileptic drugs. *Br J Hosp Med* 1990; **44:** 241.

Drosera (12681-a)

Droserae Herba; Herba Rorellae; Rorela; Ros Solis; Sundew.

Pharmacopoeias. In *Belg.*

The air-dried entire plant *Drosera rotundifolia* (Droseraceae) and other *Drosera* spp.

Preparations of drosera have been used for its reputed value in respiratory disorders but it is of doubtful value.

It has been used in homoeopathic medicine.

Preparations

Proprietary Preparations (details are given in Part 3)
Ger.: Makatussin Saft Drosera; Makatussin Tropfen Drosera.

Multi-ingredient: ***Aust.:*** Erkaltungstee; Grippetee Dr Zeidler; Heumann Hustenstiller; Krauterdoktor Krampf- und Reizhustensirup; Krautertee Nr 211; Pilka; Pilka Forte; ***Austral.:*** ASA Tones; Pertussin†; ***Belg.:*** Gloceda; Glottyl†; Sirop Toux du Larynx; ***Fr.:*** Desbly†; Humex; Passedyl; Pastilles Monleon; Pecto 6†; Premidan Infant†; Pulmonase; Sirop Pectoral adulte; Sirop Pectoral enfant; ***Ger.:*** Atmulen E†; Biotuss N; Bronchicum Pflanzlicher; Drosithym-N; Makatussin Saft forte†; Makatussin Tropfen forte; Mintetten Truw; Pertussin†; Primotussin N mit Codein†; Thymitussin†; ***Neth.:*** Abdijsiroop (Akker-Siroop)†; ***Spain:*** Broncovital; Mentobox; Pazbronquial; Pilka; ***Switz.:*** Bromocod N; Bronchalin; Bronchofluid; Demo elixir pectoral; Demo gouttes contre la toux; Demo pates pectorales; Demo sirop contre la toux; Dipect†; Drosinula N; Escotussin; Famel; Gouttes contre la toux "S"; Makatussin; Makatussin forte; Neo-Codion Enfants†; Neo-Codion Nourrisons†; Nican; Pilka; Rectopyrine†; Sirop S contre la toux et la bronchite; Thymodrosin; Tussanil Compositum.

Drotaverine (12682-t)

Drotaverine *(rINN).*

1-(3,4-Diethoxybenzylidene)-6,7-diethoxy-1,2,3,4-tetrahydroisoquinoline.

$C_{24}H_{31}NO_4$ = 397.5.

CAS — 14009-24-6.

Pharmacopoeias. Pol. includes Drotaverine Hydrochloride.

Drotaverine has been used as an antispasmodic.

Preparations

Proprietary Preparations (details are given in Part 3)
Hung.: No-spa.

Multi-ingredient: ***Aust.:*** Lenticor†; ***Hung.:*** Bispan; Neotroparin; Quarelin; Triospan.

Dulcamara (12684-r)

Bittersweet; Douce-Amère; Dulcamarae Caulis; Woody Nightshade.

The dried stems and branches of *Solanum dulcamara* (Solanaceae).

Dulcamara was formerly a popular remedy for chronic rheumatism and skin eruptions and was administered as an infusion. It has been used in homoeopathic medicine.

All parts of the plant are poisonous due to the presence of solanaceous alkaloids. The berries have caused poisoning in children. Adverse effects are treated as described under Atropine, p.455.

Preparations

Proprietary Preparations (details are given in Part 3)
Ger.: Cefabene; Dolexaderm H.

Multi-ingredient: ***Aust.:*** Dermatodoron; ***Fr.:*** Elixir Contre La Toux Weleda; ***Ger.:*** Kneipp Rheuma Tee N; Rheumex†; ***Ital.:*** Depurativo; Tisana Arnaldi; ***UK:*** Dermatodoron.

Ebselen (2036-t)

Ebselen *(rINN).*

2-Phenyl-1,2-benzisoselenazolin-3-one.

$C_{13}H_9NOSe$ = 274.2.

CAS — 60940-34-3.

Ebselen is under investigation as a neuroprotectant in stroke.

Echinacea (7140-y)

Black Sampson; Brauneria; Coneflower; Sonnenhutkraut.

The dried roots of *Echinacea angustifolia* (Compositae). *E. pallida* or *E. purpura* are sometimes substituted.

Echinacea is reported to have non-specific stimulant effects on the immune system and is used in preparations given for the prophylaxis of bacterial and viral infections. It is also used in homoeopathic medicine.

References.

1. Houghton P. Echinacea. *Pharm J* 1994; **253:** 342–3.

Preparations

Proprietary Preparations (details are given in Part 3)
Aust.: Echinaforce; Myo-Echinacin; ***Austral.:*** Echinacin; Proechina; ***Canad.:*** Echina Pro; ***Ger.:*** Bilgast echinac; Cefasept; Cefasept mono; Contra Infekt†; Echan; Echiherb; Echinacea Hevert purp. forte; Echinacin; Echinaforce; Echinapur; Echinatruw†; Episcorit; Esberitox mono; Fudimun; Immunopret; Logopharm Immun; Mentopin Echinacea; Pascotox forte-Injektopas; Pascotox mono; Resplant; Wiedimmun; ***Switz.:*** Echinaforce; ***UK:*** Skin Clear.

Multi-ingredient: ***Aust.:*** Parodontax; Spasmo-Urgenin; Urgenin; ***Austral.:*** Cold and Flu Symptoms Relief; Cough Relief; Echinacea & Antioxidants; Echinacea ACE Plus Zinc; Echinacea Herbal Plus Formula; Echinacea Plus; Flavons; Galium Complex; Gartech; Herbal Cleanse; Herbal Cold & Flu Relief; Lifesystem Herbal Plus Formula 8 Echinacea; Odourless Garlic; Proyeast; Respatona Plus with Echinacea; Sambucus Complex; Urgenin; Urinase; ***Belg.:*** Urgenin; ***Canad.:*** Cystoforce†; ***Ger.:*** Alsicur; Bagnisan med Heilbad; Bagnisan S med Rheumabad†; Bomagall forte S; Bryonia-Strath†; Carito†; Cefaktivon "novum"; Choanol†; Echtromint†; Echtrosept-GT†; Ermsech; Esberitox N; Ferrum-Strath†; Galleb†; Hewenephron duo; Hovnizym†; JuGrippan; Liruptin†; Lymphozil; Mederma†; Nasalgon†; Noricaven†; Palatol†; Pascotox; Pascotox-Injektopas†; Protitis†; RH 50 Antirheumatikum†; RH 50 percutan†; Salus Kurbis-Tonikum Compositum†; Serrulatum†; Toxorephan†; Urgenin†; ***Ital.:*** Aclon Lievit; Allergenid; Enertonic; Probigol; Ribovir; Sanaderm; ***S.Afr.:*** Spasmo-Urgenin; ***Spain:*** Neo Urgenin; Spasmo-Urgenin; Spasmo-Urgenin Rectal†; Uralyt; Urgenin; ***Switz.:*** Alpina Gel a la consoude; Demonatur Capsules contre les refroidissements; Demonatur Dragees pour les reins et la vessie; Esberitox N; Phytomed Prosta; Phytomed Rhino; Prosta-Caps Chassot N; Rectopyrine†; Urgenine; ***UK:*** Antifect; Buttercup Pol'N'Count; Catarrh Cream; Cold-eeze; Herbal Booster; Kleer; Revitonil; Sinotar; WCS Dusting Powder.

Eledoisin (3898-b)

Eledoisin *(pINN).*

ELD-950. 5-Oxo-Pro-Pro-Ser-Lys-Asp-Ala-Phe-Ile-Gly-Leu-Met-NH_2.

$C_{54}H_{85}N_{13}O_{15}S$ = 1188.4.

CAS — 69-25-0.

Eledoisin is a peptide extracted from the posterior salivary glands of certain small octopi (*Eledone* spp., Mollusca), or obtained by synthesis. Its actions resemble those of substance P; it is a potent vasodilator and increases capillary permeability. It has been given as eye drops to stimulate lachrymal secretion in Sjögren's syndrome and other dry eye conditions (p.1470).

Preparations

Proprietary Preparations (details are given in Part 3)
Spain: Eloisin.

Entsufon Sodium (3541-r)

Entsufon Sodium *(USAN, rINNM).*

Sodium 2-{2-[2-[*p*-1,3,3-tetramethylbutylphenoxy]ethoxy]ethoxy}ethanesulfonate.

$C_{20}H_{33}NaO_6S$ = 424.5.

CAS — 55837-16-6 (entsufon); 2917-94-4 (entsufon sodium).

Entsufon sodium is a detergent used as a soap substitute for cleansing the skin and mucous membranes.

Preparations

Proprietary Preparations (details are given in Part 3)
Canad.: pHisoDerm†; ***USA:*** pHisoHex.

Multi-ingredient: ***Canad.:*** pHisoHex; ***Ital.:*** pHisoHex†.

Epomediol (12695-n)

1,8-Epoxy-4-isopropyl-1-methylcylohexane-2,6-diol.

$C_{10}H_{18}O_3$ = 186.2.

Epomediol has been given by mouth in the treatment of hepatic disorders.

References.

1. Capurso L, *et al.* Activity of epomediol in the treatment of hepatopathies: a double-blind multi-centre study. *J Int Med Res* 1987; **15:** 134–47.

Preparations

Proprietary Preparations (details are given in Part 3)
Ital.: Clesidren.

Epostane (19144-m)

Epostane *(BAN, USAN, rINN).*

Win-32729. 4α,5α-Epoxy-3,17β-dihydroxy-4β,17α-dimethyl-5α-androst-2-ene-2-carbonitrile.

$C_{22}H_{31}NO_3$ = 357.5.

CAS — 80471-63-2.

Epostane has antiprogestogenic activity and has been investigated for use as an abortifacient in conjunction with prostaglandins and as a uterine stimulant for the induction of labour.

References.

1. Webster MA, *et al.* Interruption of first trimester human pregnancy following epostane therapy: effect of prostaglandin E_2 pessaries. *Br J Obstet Gynaecol* 1985; **92:** 963–8.
2. Birgerson L, Odlind V. Early pregnancy termination with antiprogestins: a comparative clinical study of RU 486 given in two dose regimens and epostane. *Fertil Steril* 1987; **48:** 565–70.
3. Crooij MJ, *et al.* Termination of early pregnancy by the 3β-hydroxysteroid dehydrogenase inhibitor epostane. *N Engl J Med* 1988; **319:** 813–17.

Eprozinol Hydrochloride (12697-m)

Eprozinol Hydrochloride *(rINNM).*

3-[4-(β-Methoxyphenethyl)piperazin-1-yl]-1-phenylpropan-1-ol dihydrochloride.

$C_{22}H_{30}N_2O_2$,2HCl = 427.4.

CAS — 32665-36-4 (eprozinol).

Eprozinol hydrochloride is given by mouth in doses of 50 mg three times daily for its mucolytic or expectorant properties.

Convulsions and coma were reported in a 19-year-old patient following administration of eprozinol.[1]

1. Merigot P, *et al.* Les convulsions avec trois antitussifs dérivés substitués de la pipérazine: (zipéprol, éprazinone, éprozinol). *Ann Pediatr (Paris)* 1985; **32:** 504–11.

Preparations

Proprietary Preparations (details are given in Part 3)
Fr.: Eupneron; ***Ital.:*** Brovel†; ***Spain:*** Asmisul†.

Equisetum (12699-v)

Herba Equiseti; Horsetail; Prêle; Schachtelhalmkraut.

Pharmacopoeias. In *Aust., Fr., Ger., Pol.,* and *Swiss.*

The dried sterile green stems of the common horsetail, *Equisetum arvense* (Equisetaceae).

Equisetum is an ingredient of herbal preparations that have been used in the treatment of genito-urinary and respiratory disorders. Similar preparations have been used in the treatment of cardiovascular disorders, rheumatic disorders, liver disorders, constipation, and as a tonic.

Equisetum is used in homoeopathic medicine.

The related species *Equisetum hiemale* is used in China for the treatment of eye disorders.

Preparations

Proprietary Preparations (details are given in Part 3)
Fr.: Siliprele; ***Ger.:*** Biolavan; Kneipp Zinnkraut-Pflanzensaft; Pulvhydrops D; Redaxa Fit; Salus Zinnkraut; ***Ital.:*** Bioequiseto; Osteosil.

Multi-ingredient: ***Aust.:*** Bio-Garten Tee fur Niere und Blase; Bio-Garten Tropfen fur Niere und Blase; Blasen- und Nierentee; Blasentee; Blutreinigungstee†; Bogumil-tassenfertiger milder Abfurtee; Drogimed; Droxitop; Ehrmann's Entschlackungstee; Entschlackungstee; Kneipp Nieren- und Blasen-Tee; Krauterdoktor Entwasserungs-Elixier; Krauterhaus Mag Kottas Entwasserungstee; Krauterhaus Mag Kottas Fruhjahrs- und Herbstkurtee; Krauterhaus Mag Kottas Nierentee; Krautertee Nr 3; Krautertee Nr 32; Krautertee Nr 4; Mag Doskar's Nieren- und Blasentonikum; Mag Kottas Entwasserungstee; Mag Kottas Nieren-Blasentee; Nierentee; Pneumopan; St Bonifatius-Tee; St Radegunder Entwasserungs-Elixier; St Radegunder Entwasserungstee; St Radegunder Nierentee; Synpharma Instant-Blasen-und-Nierentee; Teekanne Blasen- und Nierentee; Uropurat; ***Austral.:*** Adenas; Adrenas†; Cal-Alkyline; Hair and Nail Formula†; Herbal Diuretic Complex†; Medinat Esten; Serenoa Complex; Silicic Complex; ***Fr.:*** Alpha Renol†; Arterase; Circulatonic; Promincil; Reduligne†; Tisane des Familles†; Tisanes de l'Abbe Hamon no 3; ***Ger.:*** Abfuhr-Tee Depuraflux†; Agamadon; Blasen-Nieren-Tee Uroflux†; Buccotean TF†; Buccotean†; Cystinol; Dr. Boether Bronchitten S†; Dr. Klinger's Bergischer Krautertee, Blasen- u. Nierentee†; Equisil; Eviprostat N; Gallitophen†; Harntee 400; Hernia-Tee; Hevert-Blasen- und Nieren- Tee; Kneipp Blasen- und Nieren-Tee; Kneipp Nieren- und Blasen-Tee N†; Knufinke Blasen- und Nieren-Tee Uro-K†; Liruptin†; Mistelan†; NB-tee Siegfried†; nephro-loges; Nephroselect M; Nieren-Tee†; Nieron-Tee N; Original-Hico-Gallenheil†; Presselin Stoffwechseltee†; Protitis†; Rheumex†; Salus Nieren-Blasen-Tee Nr.23; Salus Rheuma-Tee Krautertee Nr. 12; Salusan; Silphoscalin†; Soledum Hustensaft N†; Soledum Hustentropfen N†; Solidagoren N; Solvefort N†; Thymitussin†; Tonsilgon-N; Tussiflorin N; Worishofener Nieren- und Blasenmittel Dr. Kleinschrod†; ***Ital.:*** Boldosten†; Heparbil†; Nosenil; ***Spain:*** Resolutivo Regium; Uralyt; ***Switz.:*** Cystinol N†; Enveloppements ECR; Eviprostat; Nephrosolid N; Solubitrat†; Tisane antiseptique diuretique†; Tisane diuretique; Tisane diuretique "H"†; Tisane pour les reins et la vessie; Tisane pour les reins et la vessie "H"†; Urinex (nouvelle formule); ***UK:*** Antiglan; Antitis; Aqualette; Kas-Bah; Waterlex.

Ergometrine Maleate (1506-h)

Ergometrine Maleate *(BANM, rINNM).*

Ergobasine Maleate; Ergometrinhydrogenmaleat; Ergometrini Maleas; Ergonovine Bimaleate; Ergonovine Maleate; Ergostetrine Maleate; Ergotocine Maleate; Maleato de Ergonovina. *N*-[(*S*)-2-Hydroxy-1-methylethyl]-D-lysergamide hydrogen maleate; 9,10-Didehydro-*N*-[(*S*)-2-hydroxy-1-methylethyl]-6-methylergoline-8β-carboxamide hydrogen maleate.

$C_{19}H_{23}N_3O_2,C_4H_4O_4 = 441.5.$

CAS — 60-79-7 (ergometrine); 129-51-1 (ergometrine maleate).

Pharmacopoeias. In *Chin., Eur.* (see p.viii), *Int., Jpn,* and *US.*

A white or yellowish, odourless, crystalline powder. It darkens with age and on exposure to light. Sparingly **soluble** in water; slightly soluble in alcohol; practically insoluble in chloroform and ether. A 1% solution in water has a pH of 3.6 to 4.4. **Store** in airtight glass containers at a temperature of 2° to 8°. Protect from light.

Stability. Reports of deterioration and degradation of ergometrine-containing injections when exposed to high temperatures in the tropics.[1-3] The mean loss in one study[3] of ergometrine injection under shipment to the tropics was 5.8%, but in some individual samples the loss was more marked: 18 of 80 test samples contained less than 80% of the stated content, and in 3 cases the content was less than 60% of the stated amount. A similar but much less significant pattern was seen with methylergometrine: the content varied from 98.6 to 99.5% of the labelled amount.

1. Walker GJA, *et al.* Potency of ergometrine in tropical countries. *Lancet* 1988; **ii:** 393.
2. Abu-Reid IO, *et al.* Stability of drugs in the tropics. *Int Pharm J* 1990; **4:** 6–10.
3. Hogerzeil HV, *et al.* Stability of essential drugs during shipment to the tropics. *Br Med J* 1992; **304:** 210–12.

Adverse Effects and Treatment

Nausea and vomiting, abdominal pain, diarrhoea, headache, dizziness, tinnitus, chest pain, palpitations, bradycardia, and dyspnoea have been reported after administration of ergometrine. Hypertension has occurred, particularly after rapid intravenous administration. Hypersensitivity reactions have occurred. Ergometrine shows less tendency to produce gangrene than ergotamine, but ergotism has been reported and symptoms of acute poisoning are similar (see p.445).

Adverse effects should be treated as for ergotamine, p.446.

Effects on the cardiovascular system. For reference to cardiovascular effects, including arrhythmias and myocardial infarction, associated with the administration of ergometrine maleate, see Diagnosis and Testing under Uses, below.

Effects on the respiratory system. Bronchospasm has been reported after administration of ergometrine.[1] Although studies *in vitro* on *canine* bronchi have suggested a direct action on smooth muscle, this could not be confirmed in studies using human bronchi.

1. Hill H, *et al.* Ergometrine and bronchospasm. *Anaesthesia* 1987; **42:** 1115–16.

Overdosage. There have been reports of accidental administration of adult doses of ergometrine maleate to neonates, sometimes instead of vitamin K.[1-4] Symptoms have included peripheral vasoconstriction, convulsions, respiratory failure, acute renal failure, and temporary lactose intolerance. After administration of ergometrine with oxytocin, water intoxication has also been reported.[3] In all of these cases recovery occurred after intensive symptomatic treatment including assisted ventilation and anticonvulsants.

1. Pandey SK, Haines CI. Accidental administration of ergometrine to newborn infant. *Br Med J* 1982; **285:** 693.
2. Mitchell AA, *et al.* Accidental administration of ergonovine to a newborn. *JAMA* 1983; **250:** 730–1.
3. Whitfield MF, Salfield SAW. Accidental administration of Syntometrine in adult dosage to the newborn. *Arch Dis Child* 1980; **55:** 68–70.
4. Donatini B, *et al.* Inadvertent administration of uterotonics to neonates. *Lancet* 1993; **341:** 839–40.

Precautions

As for Ergotamine Tartrate, p.446. Ergometrine maleate should not be used for the induction of labour or during the first stage of labour. If used at the end of the second stage of labour, prior to delivery of the placenta, there must be expert obstetric supervision. Its use should be avoided in patients with eclampsia.

Porphyria. Ergometrine maleate has been associated with clinical exacerbations of porphyria and is considered unsafe in porphyric patients.[1]

1. Moore MR, McColl KEL. *Porphyria: drug lists.* Glasgow: Porphyria Research Unit, University of Glasgow, 1991.

Interactions

Halothane has been considered to diminish the effects of ergometrine on the uterus.

Sympathomimetics. Use of dopamine in a patient treatment with ergometrine was associated with subsequent development of gangrene in both hands and feet.[1]

1. Buchanan N, *et al.* Symmetrical gangrene of the extremities associated with the use of dopamine subsequent to ergometrine administration. *Intensive Care Med* 1977; **3:** 55–6.

Pharmacokinetics

Ergometrine is reported to be rapidly absorbed after administration by mouth and by intramuscular injection, with onset of uterine contractions in about 5 to 15 minutes after an oral dose and 2 or 3 minutes after an intramuscular dose. Elimination appears to be principally by metabolism in the liver.

Uses and Administration

Ergometrine has a much more powerful action on the uterus than most of the other alkaloids of ergot, especially on the puerperal uterus. Its main action is the production of intense contractions, which at higher doses are sustained, in contrast to the more physiological rhythmic uterine contractions induced by oxytocin; its action is more prolonged than that of oxytocin.

Ergometrine maleate may be used in the prevention and treatment of postpartum haemorrhage caused by uterine atony; by maintaining uterine contraction and tone, blood vessels in the uterine wall are compressed, and blood flow reduced. In the UK it is generally given with oxytocin. Following intramuscular injection of ergometrine with oxytocin contractions are reported to occur within 2 or 3 minutes. Ergometrine and oxytocin are administered under full obstetric supervision in the active management of the third stage of labour of normal confinements. A dose of ergometrine maleate 500 μg and oxytocin 5 units is injected intramuscularly after delivery of the anterior shoulder of the infant. Delivery of the placenta is actively assisted while the uterus is firmly contracted. Alternatively, a similar dose may be given following delivery of the placenta to prevent or treat postpartum haemorrhage. In patients considered at high risk of postpartum haemorrhage ergometrine maleate may be given intravenously in a dose of 125 to 250 μg. Oxytocin may be used as an alternative but intravenous administration of the combined preparation is no longer recommended. In the treatment of mild secondary postpartum haemorrhage ergometrine maleate has been given by mouth in a dose of 500 μg three times daily for 3 days.

In the USA ergometrine maleate is usually given alone and is not generally recommended before delivery of the placenta. Doses have generally been lower than those used in the UK. A typical regimen is 200 μg intramuscularly or by slow intravenous injection every 2 to 4 hours as needed, for up to 5 doses. This may be followed by 200 to 400 μg by mouth two to four times a day for up to 7 days, until the danger of atony and haemorrhage has passed.

Ergometrine maleate has been administered by the sublingual and rectal routes.

Ergometrine tartrate was formerly used.

Diagnosis and testing. Ergometrine maleate[1-3] or methylergometrine maleate[2,4] have been used in a provocation test for the diagnosis of variant angina (Prinzmetal's angina) (p.780). Ergometrine maleate has also been used in the diagnosis of oesophageal spasm.[5]

1. Waters DD, *et al.* Ergonovine testing in a coronary care unit. *Am J Cardiol* 1980; **46:** 922–30.
2. Anonymous. Provocation of coronary spasm: research or diagnostic test? *Lancet* 1982; **ii:** 805.
3. Health and Public Policy Committee, American College of Physicians. Performance of ergonovine provocative testing for coronary artery spasm. *Ann Intern Med* 1984; **100:** 151–2.
4. Bertrand ME, *et al.* Frequency of provoked coronary arterial spasm in 1089 consecutive patients undergoing coronary arteriography. *Circulation* 1982; **65:** 1299–1306.
5. Richter JE, *et al.* Esophageal chest pain: current controversies in pathogenesis, diagnosis, and therapy. *Ann Intern Med* 1989; **110:** 66–78.

Postpartum haemorrhage. In normal labour, once the child is born myometrial retraction and strong uterine contractions cause shortening and kinking of the uterine blood vessels and a retraction of the placental bed: these changes operate to minimise blood loss. However, if the uterus fails to contract adequately (uterine atony) or if retained placental remnants prevent retraction of the placental bed, postpartum haemorrhage may occur. These two causes account for about 80% of cases of postpartum haemorrhage; in the remainder it is usually due to trauma of the genital tract.

Postpartum haemorrhage may well be fatal to the mother unless promptly dealt with: management generally involves removal of the placenta if this has not been expelled, the use of oxytocics to contract the uterus, and, if blood loss is severe, transfusion. Prophylactic management is favoured in some countries but in others may be reserved for women at greater risk, including those who have undergone prolonged labour, those who have an overdistended uterus (for example in multiple pregnancy), or after antepartum haemorrhage, or deep general anaesthesia.

A policy of active management of the third stage of labour (prophylactic administration of an oxytocic, cord clamping before placental delivery, and cord traction) is common in the UK. The rationale for such management has been examined.[1-4] A meta-analysis of all known, randomised, controlled studies of routine prophylactic oxytocics has shown that, when labour is actively managed, routine oxytocics (usually with crowning of the head, delivery of the anterior shoulder, or after delivery of the placenta) reduced the risk of postpartum haemorrhage by about 40%.[2] These studies were further analysed[3] to compare the efficacy and safety of the different oxytocic agents: ergot alkaloids, oxytocin, prostaglandins, and a mixture of ergometrine and oxytocin (Syntometrine). Comparison of oxytocin and ergot alkaloids suggested that, although they may be of similar efficacy in decreasing postpartum haemorrhage, oxytocin is less likely to predispose to delayed placental delivery and also less likely to cause hypertension. Syntometrine and ergot alkaloids also appeared to be of similar efficacy, but Syntometrine may be less likely to be associated with a prolonged third stage of labour. The available evidence from two studies comparing Syntometrine (used preferentially in the UK) and oxytocin (used preferentially in North America) suggests that Syntometrine is the more effective prophylactic, but possibly at the expense of a higher risk of hypertension. A subsequent Australian study involving 3497 women found no significant difference in efficacy between intramuscular oxytocin and Syntometrine for active management of third stage labour,[5] but a higher incidence of adverse effects (nausea, vomiting, hypertension) with the latter. This group concluded that there were no advantages to the use of Syntometrine, but their analysis has been criticised on the grounds that there was a lower incidence of postpartum haemorrhage in the group given Syntometrine, which would be clinically significant even if it failed to achieve statistical significance.[6,7]

There are numerous reports suggesting the efficacy of prostaglandins such as carboprost, dinoprostone, or sulprostone in the treatment of established postpartum haemorrhage but there is little evidence of their role in active management of third stage labour.[3] However, prophylactic use of misoprostol, given orally immediately after delivery was effective in one study,[8] although comparative trials are needed.

1. Prendiville WJ, *et al.* The Bristol third stage trial: active versus physiological management of third stage of labour. *Br Med J* 1988; **297:** 1295–1300.
2. Prendiville W, *et al.* The effects of routine oxytocic administration in the management of the third stage of labour: an overview of the evidence from controlled trials. *Br J Obstet Gynaecol* 1988; **95:** 3–16.
3. Elbourne D, *et al.* Choice of oxytocic preparation for routine use in the management of the third stage of labour: an overview of the evidence from controlled trials. *Br J Obstet Gynaecol* 1988; **95:** 17–30.
4. Rogers J, *et al.* Active versus expectant management of third stage of labour: the Hinchingbrooke randomised controlled trial. *Lancet* 1998; **351:** 693–9.
5. McDonald SJ, *et al.* Randomised controlled trial of oxytocin alone versus oxytocin and ergometrine in active management of third stage of labour. *Br Med J* 1993; **307:** 1167–71.
6. Dwyer N. Managing the third stage of labour. *Br Med J* 1994; **308:** 59.
7. Macintosh MCM, Erskine KJ. Managing the third stage of labour. *Br Med J* 1994; **308:** 59.
8. El-Refaey H, *et al.* Use of oral misoprostol in the prevention of postpartum haemorrhage. *Br J Obstet Gynaecol* 1997; **104:** 336–9.

Preparations

BP 1998: Ergometrine and Oxytocin Injection; Ergometrine Injection; Ergometrine Tablets;
USP 23: Ergonovine Maleate Injection; Ergonovine Maleate Tablets.

Proprietary Preparations (details are given in Part 3)
Canad.: Ergotrate; ***Ger.:*** Secalysat EM; ***S.Afr.:*** Ergometron†; Ergotrate†; ***USA:*** Ergotrate.

Multi-ingredient: ***Austral.:*** Syntometrine; ***Irl.:*** Syntometrine; ***S.Afr.:*** Syntometrine; ***UK:*** Syntometrine.

Ergot (1501-x)

Secale Cornutum.

Pharmacopoeias. In *Aust.*, which also includes Prepared Ergot.

The sclerotium of the fungus *Claviceps purpurea* (Hypocreaceae) developed in the ovary of the rye, *Secale cereale* (Gramineae), containing not less than 0.15% of total alkaloids, calculated as ergotoxine, and not less than 0.01% of water-soluble alkaloids, calculated as ergometrine. Some authorities have expressed alkaloidal content in terms of ergotamine and ergometrine.

Adverse Effects and Treatment

As for Ergotamine Tartrate, p.445.

Epidemic ergot poisoning, arising from the ingestion of ergotised rye bread, is now seldom seen. Two forms of epidemic toxicity, which rarely occur together, have been described: a gangrenous form characterised by agonising pain of the extremities of the body followed by dry gangrene of the peripheral parts, and a rarer nervous type giving rise to paroxysmal epileptiform convulsions.

A report of an outbreak of ergotism, attributed to the ingestion of infected wild oats (*Avena abyssinica*), in Wollo, Ethiopia.[1]

1. King B. Outbreak of ergotism in Wollo, Ethiopia. *Lancet* 1979; **ii:** 1411.

Uses and Administration

Ergot has the vasoconstricting and oxytocic actions of its constituent alkaloids, especially ergotamine (p.445) and ergometrine (above). A liquid extract or tablets of prepared ergot were formerly used as an oxytocic. Preparations containing ergot extracts have been promoted for use in dyspepsia and nervous disorders.

Preparations

Proprietary Preparations (details are given in Part 3)

Multi-ingredient: ***Ger.:*** Bellaravil†; Secafobell†.

Ergotoxine (1509-v)

CAS — 8006-25-5 (ergotoxine); 8047-28-7 (ergotoxine esylate); 8047-29-8 (ergotoxine phosphate); 564-36-3 (ergocornine); 511-08-0 (ergocristine); 511-09-1 (ergocryptine).

A mixture in equal proportions of ergocornine ($C_{31}H_{39}N_5O_5$ = 561.7), ergocristine ($C_{35}H_{39}N_5O_5$ = 609.7), and ergocryptine, as the α- and β-isomers ($C_{32}H_{41}N_5O_5$ = 575.7).

Ergotoxine is a mixture of naturally occurring ergot alkaloids. The esylate was formerly used as an oxytocic and in the treatment of migraine. Ergotoxine phosphate has also been used.

Preparations

Proprietary Preparations (details are given in Part 3)

Multi-ingredient: ***Ger.:*** Circovegetalin compositum†; Circovegetalin†.

Ethanolamine Oleate (207-g)

Ethanolamine Oleate *(USAN).*

Monoethanolamine Oleate *(rINN)*; Aethanolaminum. 2-Hydroxyethylamine compound with oleic acid; 2-Aminoethanol compound with oleic acid.

$C_2H_7NO,C_{18}H_{34}O_2$ = 343.5.

CAS — 141-43-5 (ethanolamine); 2272-11-9 (ethanolamine oleate).

Pharmacopoeias. Aust., Br., and *USNF* include Ethanolamine.

Ethanolamine is a clear colourless or pale yellow moderately viscous liquid with a slight ammoniacal odour. It is alkaline to litmus.

Miscible with water, alcohol, acetone, chloroform, and glycerol; it is immiscible with petroleum spirit and fixed oils but it will dissolve many essential oils. Ph. Eur. has slightly soluble in ether while USNF has immiscible with ether. **Store** in airtight containers. Protect from light.

Adverse Effects and Precautions

Ethanolamine oleate is irritant to skin and mucous membranes. Local injection may cause sloughing, ulceration, and, in severe cases, necrosis. Pain may occur at the site of injection. Patients receiving treatment for oesophageal varices may develop pleural effusion or infiltration. Hypersensitivity reactions have been reported.

When used to treat varicose veins of the legs, ethanolamine oleate and other sclerotherapeutic agents should not be used in patients with thrombosis or a tendency to thrombosis; acute phlebitis; marked arterial, cardiac, or renal disease; local or systemic infections; or uncontrolled metabolic disorders such as diabetes mellitus. In the USA ethanolamine oleate is not recommended for the treatment of varicose leg veins.

Effects on the kidneys. Acute renal failure, which cleared spontaneously within 3 weeks, occurred in 2 obese women given sclerosing injections of 15 to 20 mL of a solution containing ethanolamine oleate 5% and benzyl alcohol 2%.[1]

1. Maling TJB, Cretney MJ. Ethanolamine oleate and acute renal failure. *N Z Med J* 1975; **82:** 269–70.

Uses and Administration

Ethanolamine oleate is used as a sclerosing agent in the injection treatment of varicose veins and oesophageal varices. For sclerotherapy of varicose veins, 2 to 5 mL of a 5% solution of ethanolamine oleate is injected into empty isolated sections of vein, divided between 3 or 4 sites. Injection into full veins is also possible. For sclerotherapy of oesophageal varices, a suggested dose is 1.5 to 5 mL of a 5% solution per varix to a maximum total dose of 20 mL per treatment session. Treatment may be repeated at intervals until the varices are occluded.

Sclerotherapy. Sclerosants are used in the management of varicosities including varicose veins and oesophageal varices (see below). The mechanisms by which injection sclerotherapy works are not completely understood but are thought to involve damage to the intima, intraluminal thrombosis, and intravascular fibrous organisation, resulting in occlusion of the vein. Sclerosants used include ethanolamine oleate, laureth 9 (p.1325), sodium tetradecyl sulphate (p.1469), and sodium morrhuate (p.1631). Direct intravariceal injection of sclerosant is less likely to cause local necrosis, ulcer or stricture formation than paravariceal injection.

Variceal haemorrhage. Portal hypertension, one definition of which is an increase in resting portal venous pressure above 12 mmHg, may occur in many pathological conditions affecting the liver. and leads to the development of collateral channels linking the portal and systemic circulations. Enlargement of such blood vessels beneath the oesophageal and gastric mucosa produces varices which have about a 30% risk of rupture and bleeding. Oesophageal varices are more often a cause of haemorrhage than gastric varices. Capillaries and veins in the gastric mucosa may also become swollen, a condition known as portal hypertensive gastropathy, and clinically important bleeding may occur in severe cases.

Variceal haemorrhage is usually severe with mortality as high as 50% for the initial episode and the recurrence rate may be as high as 100% within two years. Bleeding stops spontaneously in many patients, but in those who continue to bleed control of haemorrhage is difficult and patients should be referred to a centre with appropriate specialist facilities. Treatment to stabilise the patient may be necessary before they can be safely transferred.

Acute management. Initially treatment is supportive and requires measures to prevent aspiration and maintain a clear airway, and volume replacement with colloid and blood. Emergency endoscopy should be performed to establish the site of haemorrhage and exclude non-variceal sources of bleeding. The choice of treatment depends on the site of haemorrhage.[1-6] **Endoscopic methods** are favoured for initial management with injection sclerotherapy or banding ligation being used in bleeding oesophageal varices. The optimum management of bleeding gastric varices remains to be defined. Injection sclerotherapy is a suitable method for controlling bleeding from varices on the lesser curve of the stomach or within a hiatus hernia, but is not so effective in haemorrhaging fundal gastric varices. Intravariceal injection of bovine thrombin and cyanoacrylate tissue adhesives has been used in such cases. Where the source of haemorrhage is non-variceal and due to gastropathy, portal decompressive surgery is effective although it is associated with a high incidence of encephalopathy in cirrhotic patients. Small studies have shown propranolol to be effective in arresting haemorrhage.[7]

Injection sclerotherapy for variceal haemorrhage may be performed during the emergency endoscopy procedure.[1,2,8] Intravariceal injection, paravariceal injection or a combination of the two have been used. The most widely-used sclerosants are ethanolamine oleate and sodium tetradecyl sulphate for intravariceal injection and laureth 9 for paravariceal injection. Sclerotherapy controls bleeding in up to 95% of cases. Ulceration and stricture formation occur frequently following injection sclerotherapy.

An alternative technique is **endoscopic banding ligation**[1,2,8,9] where elastic bands are placed around the varices. The tissue subsequently necroses to leave a superficial ulcer. This technique has a similar efficacy to injection sclerotherapy but may be more difficult to perform if active bleeding is occurring. Procedures may be repeated if bleeding continues or restarts.

Where endoscopy is unavailable drug therapy or balloon tamponade may be used until the patient can be transferred to a specialist centre. These techniques may also have a role when sclerotherapy fails. **Drug therapy** using vasoconstrictors is ineffective in massive haemorrhage and its effects cease once the drug is stopped. Drugs that are used include vasopressin and its analogue terlipressin and, more recently, somatostatin and its analogue octreotide. Vasopressin controls haemorrhage in 60 to 70% of patients. It is given by continuous intravenous infusion together with glyceryl trinitrate which counteracts the adverse cardiac effects of vasopressin, while potentiating its reduction of portal pressure. Terlipressin, has the advantage of a longer therapeutic action enabling bolus doses to be given. However, somatostatin and particularly octreotide, which may be given by bolus injection, are now generally preferred as they have similar efficacy to vasopressin but fewer side effects.[4] Octreotide is as effective as injection sclerotherapy in the control of acute variceal bleeding.[10] Octreotide[11] or somatostatin[12] may also have a role as adjuncts to sclerotherapy or ligation but no mortality benefit has yet been shown.

Balloon tamponade controls bleeding by direct pressure on the varices. Although it is a very effective means of controlling haemorrhage there is a high incidence of rebleeding once pressure is removed and the incidence of complications is high. It is useful in cases of massive haemorrhage when drug therapy is ineffective and sclerotherapy is difficult.

Surgery, such as the formation of a shunt or oesophageal transection, may be necessary if the above measures fail to control the bleeding. However, such techniques have been associated with high mortality in some series. Formation of a transjugular intrahepatic portal-systemic shunt is now generally preferred.[6] It may be particularly useful in candidates for liver transplantation.

Long-term management. Once the acute bleeding has been controlled measures are needed to prevent rebleeding. Endoscopic therapy is widely used, with injection sclerotherapy or banding ligation being repeated until the varices are obliterated. Banding ligation is now the treatment of choice; it eradicates varices in fewer treatment sessions than injection sclerotherapy and reduces the risk of ulceration and stricture formation.[9] Sucralfate has been given following sclerotherapy as it may reduce the frequency of stricture formation and reduce bleeding from treatment-related ulcers. It seems to have no influence on ulcer healing following banding ligation.[13] Some practitioners carry out regular endoscopic checks and repeat sclerotherapy or banding ligation when varices reappear, although this approach is no more effective in terms of improving survival than giving treatment once bleeding occurs. Drug therapy may be an alternative to endoscopic methods. Beta blockers (mainly propranolol) reduce the incidence of recurrent variceal bleeding in some patients[14] although patients with poor liver function, who form a large proportion of the population with variceal haemorrhage, do not seem to benefit. A combination of nadolol with isosorbide mononitrate has been reported to reduce the risk of rebleeding more than repeated sclerotherapy, although there was no significant effect on mortality.[15] Drug therapy has also been used as an adjunct to endoscopic methods to control rebleeding in the period before variceal obliteration has occurred, or for long-term management following endoscopic therapy. Several studies[16-18] have compared transjugular intrahepatic portosystemic shunting with endoscopic treatment but no clear benefit has been demonstrated and there may be an increased risk of encephalopathy with the use of shunts. Surgery, including liver transplantation, should be considered in patients with recurrent life-threatening haemorrhage. Propranolol may also have a role in patients with portal hypertensive gastropathy. In a controlled study propranolol reduced the incidence of recurrent bleeding from portal hypertensive gastropathy in patients with cirrhosis.[19]

Prophylaxis of a first bleed in patients with portal hypertension is controversial since about 70% of patients who have varices will never bleed, but should probably be given to patients with cirrhosis and varices thought to be at high risk of bleeding. A reliable system that will identify those at high risk of haemorrhage has yet to be devised. The NIEC (North Italian Endoscopic Club) system is probably the best so far.[20] Sclerotherapy had been considered as a method of prophylaxis, but its value has not been clearly established. Studies show that beta blockers decrease the incidence of a first bleed[21] and are probably the treatment of choice if prophylaxis is to be given.

It is postulated that a reduction in portal pressure to below 12 mmHg is necessary to reduce the incidence of variceal bleeding and that treatment with beta blockers alone does not achieve this. More effective drugs are being sought and isosorbide mononitrate[22,23] (as adjunctive therapy with a beta blocker) and clonidine[24] are under investigation for the prophylaxis of a first bleed and prevention of recurrent haemorrhage in patients with portal hypertension.

1. Bornman PC, *et al.* Management of oesophageal varices. *Lancet* 1994; **343:** 1079–84.
2. Williams SGJ, Westaby D. Management of variceal haemorrhage. *Br Med J* 1994; **308:** 1213–17.
3. Parks RW, Diamond T. Emergency and long-term management of bleeding oesophageal varices. *Br J Hosp Med* 1995; **54:** 161–8.
4. Roberts LR, Kamath PS. Pathophysiology and treatment of variceal hemorrhage. *Mayo Clin Proc* 1996; **71:** 973–83.
5. Sung JJY. Non-surgical treatment of variceal haemorrhage. *Br J Hosp Med* 1997; **57:** 162–6.
6. Stanely AJ, Haynes PC. Portal hypertension and variceal haemorrhage. *Lancet* 1997; **350:** 1235–9.
7. Anonymous. Portal hypertensive gastropathy. *Lancet* 1991; **338:** 1045–6.
8. Anonymous. Bleeding oesophageal varices: IST, EVL, or TIPS. *Lancet* 1992; **340:** 515–16.
9. Laine L, Cook D. Endoscopic ligation compared with sclerotherapy for treatment of esophageal variceal bleeding: a meta-analysis. *Ann Intern Med* 1995; **123:** 280–7.
10. Jenkins SA, *et al.* A multicentre randomised trial comparing octreotide and injection sclerotherapy in the management and outcome of acute variceal haemorrhage. *Gut* 1997; **41:** 526–33.
11. Sung JJY, *et al.* Prospective randomised study of effect of octreotide on rebleeding from oesophageal varices after endoscopic ligation. *Lancet* 1995; **346:** 1666–9.
12. Avgerinos A, *et al.* Early administration of somatostatin and efficacy of sclerotherapy in acute oesophageal variceal bleeds: the European Acute Bleeding Oesophageal Variceal Episodes (ABOVE) randomised trial. *Lancet* 1997; **350:** 1495–9.
13. Nijhawan S, Rai RR. Does post-ligation oesophageal ulcer healing require treatment? *Lancet* 1994; **343:** 116–17.
14. Hayes PC, *et al.* Meta-analysis of value of propranolol in prevention of variceal haemorrhage. *Lancet* 1990; **336:** 153–6. Correction. *ibid.*; 324.
15. Villanueva C, *et al.* Nadolol plus isosorbide mononitrate compared with sclerotherapy for the prevention of variceal rebleeding. *N Engl J Med* 1996; **334:** 1624–9.
16. Sanyal AJ, *et al.* Transjugular intrahepatic portosystemic shunts compared with endoscopic sclerotherapy for the prevention of recurrent variceal hemorrhage: a randomized, controlled trial. *Ann Intern Med* 1997; **126:** 849–57.
17. Cello JP, *et al.* Endoscopic sclerotherapy compared with percutaneous transjugular intrahepatic portosystemic shunt after initial sclerotherapy in patients with acute variceal hemorrhage: a randomized, controlled trial. *Ann Intern Med* 1997; **126:** 858–65.
18. Rössle M, *et al.* Randomised trial of transjugular-intrahepatic-portosystemic shunt versus endoscopy plus propranolol for prevention of variceal rebleeding. *Lancet* 1997; **349:** 1043–9.
19. Pérez-Ayuso RM, *et al.* Propranolol in prevention of recurrent bleeding from severe portal hypertensive gastropathy in cirrhosis. *Lancet* 1991; **337:** 1431–4.
20. The North Italian Endoscopic Club for the Study and Treatment of Esophageal Varices. Prediction of the first variceal hemorrhage in patients with cirrhosis of the liver and esophageal varices: a prospective multicenter study. *N Engl J Med* 1988; **319:** 983–9.
21. Pagliaro L, *et al.* Prevention of first bleeding in cirrhosis: a meta-analysis of randomised trials of nonsurgical treatment. *Ann Intern Med* 1992; **117:** 59–70.
22. Angelico M, *et al.* Isosorbide-5-mononitrate versus propranolol in the prevention of first bleeding in cirrhosis. *Gastroenterology* 1993; **104:** 1460–5.
23. Merkel C, *et al.* Randomised trial of nadolol alone or with isosorbide mononitrate for primary prophylaxis of variceal bleeding in cirrhosis. *Lancet* 1996; **348:** 1677–81.
24. Blendis LM. Clonidine for portal hypertension: a sympathetic solution? *Ann Intern Med* 1992; **116:** 515–17.

Preparations

BP 1998: Ethanolamine Oleate Injection.

Proprietary Preparations (details are given in Part 3)
Austral.: Ethamolin†; ***Canad.:*** Ethamolin; ***Jpn:*** Oldamin; ***USA:*** Ethamolin.

Ethaverine Hydrochloride (5232-n)

Ethaverine Hydrochloride (*rINNM*).

6,7-Diethoxy-1-(3,4-diethoxybenzyl)isoquinoline hydrochloride.

$C_{24}H_{29}NO_4,HCl = 432.0.$

CAS — 486-47-5 (ethaverine); 985-13-7 (ethaverine hydrochloride).

Ethaverine is the tetraethoxy analogue of papaverine (p.1614). Ethaverine hydrochloride has been used as an antispasmodic in biliary, gastro-intestinal, and genito-urinary disorders. It has also been used in vascular disorders and as an antiarrhythmic.

Ethaverine sulphamate has also been used.

Preparations

Proprietary Preparations (details are given in Part 3)
USA: Ethaquin†; Ethatab†; Ethavex†; Isovex†; Pasmol†.

Multi-ingredient: ***Aust.:*** Asthma Efeum†; Gastripan; Hylakombun; ***Belg.:*** Migraine-Kranit†; ***Ger.:*** Adenopurin†; Adenovasin†; Coropar†; Gallolingual†; Gentil†; Hylakombun N†; Ilioton†; Keldrin†; Lioftal s. T.†; Migrane-Kranit N; Olren†; Solamin†; Spasmo-Bilicura†; Spasmo-Gentarol N†; Thymitussin†; Ventrodynat†; ***Switz.:*** Elzym.

Ethoxyphenyldiethylphenylbutylamine Hydrochloride (11368-n)

1-(4-Ethoxyphenyl)-*N*,*N*-diethyl-3-phenylbutylamine hydrochloride.

$C_{22}H_{31}NO,HCl = 361.9.$

CAS — 10535-87-2 (ethoxyphenyldiethylphenylbutylamine hydrochloride); 13988-32-4 (ethoxyphenyldiethylphenylbutylamine).

Ethoxyphenyldiethylphenylbutylamine hydrochloride is used as an antispasmodic.

Preparations

Proprietary Preparations (details are given in Part 3)

Multi-ingredient: ***Ger.:*** Agevis†; ***Spain:*** Spasmalfher†.

Ethoxyquin (6646-p)

6-Ethoxy-1,2-dihydro-2,2,4-trimethylquinoline.

$C_{14}H_{19}NO = 217.3.$

CAS — 91-53-2.

Ethoxyquin has been used as an antoxidant for the prevention of common scald of apples and pears during storage and as an additive to animal feeds. Concern has been expressed over the toxicity of ethoxyquin and its residues on foodstuffs and its use is limited or restricted in some countries.

Ethyl Cinnamate (18370-v)

Ethyl (*E*)-3-phenylprop-2-enoate.

$C_{11}H_{12}O_2 = 176.2.$

CAS — 103-36-6.

Pharmacopoeias. In *Br.*

A clear, colourless or almost colourless liquid with a fruity, balsamic odour. Practically **insoluble** in water; miscible with most organic solvents.

Ethyl cinnamate is used as a flavour and perfume; it is an ingredient of Tolu-flavour Solution (BP 1998).

Preparations

BP 1998: Tolu-flavour Solution.

Ethyl Oleate (7359-s)

Aethylis Oleas; Ethylis Oleas.

$C_{20}H_{38}O_2 = 310.5.$

CAS — 111-62-6.

Pharmacopoeias. In *Eur.* (see p.viii). Also in *USNF.*

An almost colourless or pale yellow oily mobile liquid with a slight but not rancid odour. It consists of the ethyl esters of oleic acid and related high molecular weight fatty acids.

Practically **insoluble** in water; miscible with alcohol, chloroform, dichloromethane, ether, fixed oils, liquid paraffin, and most other organic solvents. Ethyl oleate dissolves some types of rubber and causes others to swell. It oxidises on exposure to air; the air in partially filled containers should be replaced by nitrogen or other suitable inert gas. **Store** in small well-filled airtight containers or in an atmosphere of nitrogen. Protect from light.

Ethyl oleate is used as an oily vehicle.

Ethyl Vanillin (2393-k)

3-Ethoxy-4-hydroxybenzaldehyde.

$C_9H_{10}O_3 = 166.2.$

CAS — 121-32-4.

Pharmacopoeias. In *USNF.*

Fine white or slightly yellowish crystals with a vanilla-like odour and taste.

Soluble 1 in 100 of water at 50°; soluble 1 in 2 of alcohol; freely soluble in chloroform, ether, and solutions of alkali hydroxides. **Store** in airtight containers. Protect from light.

Ethyl vanillin is used as a flavour and in perfumery to impart the odour and taste of vanilla.

Ethylene Glycol (1907-t)

Ethylene Alcohol; Glycol. Ethane-1,2-diol.

$C_2H_6O_2 = 62.07.$

CAS — 107-21-1.

Adverse Effects

Toxic effects arising from ingestion of ethylene glycol result from its major metabolites: aldehydes, glycolate, lactate, and oxalate. The patient may show signs of drunkenness and experience nausea and vomiting. Convulsions and neurological defects may occur. There may be tachycardia and pulmonary oedema. Severe ethylene glycol poisoning may involve decreased plasma concentrations of calcium and bicarbonate, metabolic acidosis, deposition of oxalate in tissues and kidney tubules, proteinuria, oxaluria, haematuria, renal failure, respiratory failure, cardiovascular collapse, and sometimes coma and death. The fatal dose is reported to be about 100 mL.

Skin irritation and penetration have been reported following topical application.

Diethylene glycol produces similar toxicity except that there is no conversion to oxalate and there is greater nephrotoxicity. Poisoning has followed adulteration of medicinal products with diethylene glycol.

References.

1. Anonymous. Some wine to break the ice. *Lancet* 1985; **ii:** 254.
2. Vale JA, Buckley BM. Metabolic acidosis in diethylene glycol poisoning. *Lancet* 1985; **ii:** 394.
3. Buckley BM, Vale JA. Poisoning by alcohols and ethylene glycol. *Prescribers' J* 1986; **26:** 110–15.
4. Hanif M, *et al.* Fatal renal failure caused by diethylene glycol in paracetamol elixir: the Bangladesh epidemic. *Br Med J* 1995; **311:** 88–91.
5. Lewis LD, *et al.* Delayed sequelae after acute overdoses or poisonings: cranial neuropathy related to ethylene glycol ingestion. *Clin Pharmacol Ther* 1997; **61:** 692–9.
6. O'Brien KL, *et al.* Epidemic of pediatric deaths from acute renal failure caused by diethylene glycol poisoning. *JAMA* 1998; **279:** 1175–80.

Treatment of Adverse Effects

Following ethylene glycol ingestion the stomach should be emptied by aspiration and lavage or emesis. Severe metabolic acidosis should be corrected with sodium bicarbonate intravenously and hypocalcaemia corrected with calcium gluconate. Haemodialysis or peritoneal dialysis may be of value. Alcohol may be given by mouth or intravenously as it is a competitor of ethylene glycol's metabolism.

Fomepizole (p.982), an alcohol-dehydrogenase inhibitor has also been proposed for the treatment of ethylene glycol poisoning.

References.

1. Vale JA, *et al.* Treatment of ethylene glycol poisoning with peritoneal dialysis. *Br Med J* 1982; **284:** 557.
2. Baud FJ, *et al.* Treatment of ethylene glycol poisoning with intravenous 4-methylpyrazole. *N Engl J Med* 1988; **319:** 97–100.
3. Porter GA. The treatment of ethylene glycol poisoning simplified. *N Engl J Med* 1988; **319:** 109–10.
4. Harry P, *et al.* Efficacy of 4-methylpyrazole in ethylene glycol poisoning: clinical and toxokinetic aspects. *Hum Exp Toxicol* 1994; **13:** 61–4.

Pharmacokinetics

Ethylene glycol is absorbed from the gastro-intestinal tract and is metabolised, chiefly in the liver, by alcohol dehydrogenase. Its breakdown products account for its toxicity and include aldehydes, glycolate, oxalate, and lactate.

Uses

Ethylene glycol is commonly encountered in antifreeze solutions and has been used illicitly to sweeten some wines. Diethylene glycol has been used similarly.

Ethylenediamine (208-q)

Edamine (*USAN, pINN*); Ethylendiaminum.

$C_2H_8N_2 = 60.10.$

CAS — 107-15-3 (anhydrous ethylenediamine); 6780-13-8 (ethylenediamine monohydrate).

Pharmacopoeias. In *Eur.* (see p.viii), *Jpn,* and *US.*

A clear, colourless or slightly yellow, strongly alkaline, hygroscopic liquid with an ammoniacal odour. On exposure to air it absorbs carbon dioxide with the evolution of white fumes. **Miscible** with water and alcohol; slightly soluble in ether. **Store** in airtight glass containers. Protect from light.

Adverse Effects

Ethylenediamine is irritant to the skin and to mucous membranes. Severe exfoliative dermatitis has been reported following systemic use of preparations containing ethylenediamine. Hypersensitivity reactions are common. Concentrated solutions cause skin burns. Headache, dizziness, shortness of breath, nausea, and vomiting have also been reported following exposure to fumes. Ethylenediamine splashed onto the skin or eyes should be removed by flooding with water for a prolonged period.

A review of allergy to ethylenediamine and aminophylline.[1]

1. Anonymous. Allergy to aminophylline. *Lancet* 1984; **ii :** 1192–3.

Precautions

Skin reactions may occur in patients given aminophylline after they have become sensitised to ethylenediamine. Cross-sensitivity with edetic acid and with some antihistamines has been reported.

It was reported that some topical corticosteroid creams including Tri-Adcortyl in the UK[1] and Kenacomb, Halcicomb, and Viaderm in Canada[2] contained ethylenediamine and could cause unexpected cross-sensitivity reactions with piperazine[1] or aminophylline.[2]

1. Wright S, Harman RRM. Ethylenediamine and piperazine sensitivity. *Br Med J* 1983; **287**: 463–4.
2. Hogan DJ. Excipients in topical corticosteroid preparations in Canada. *Can Med Assoc J* 1989; **141**: 1032.

Uses and Administration

Ethylenediamine or ethylenediamine hydrate forms a stable mixture with theophylline to produce aminophylline or aminophylline hydrate. It is widely used in the chemical and pharmaceutical industries and as an ingredient of some topical creams.

Eucalyptus Oil (4644-y)

Esencia de Eucalipto; Essence d'Eucalyptus Rectifiée; Eucalypti Aetheroleum; Oleum Eucalypti.

Pharmacopoeias. In *Chin., Eur.* (see p.viii), which also includes Eucalyptus Leaf from *E. globulus*, *Jpn*, and *Pol.*

A colourless or pale yellow volatile oil with a characteristic aromatic camphoraceous odour and a pungent camphoraceous cooling taste, obtained by rectifying the oil distilled from the fresh leaves and terminal branches of various species of *Eucalyptus* (Myrtaceae) (*E. globulus, E. fructicetorum*, and *E. smithii* are used). It contains not less than 70% w/w of cineole (eucalyptol). **Soluble** 1 in 5 of alcohol (70%). **Store** at a temperature not exceeding 25° in airtight containers.

Adverse Effects and Precautions

The symptoms of poisoning with eucalyptus oil include gastro-intestinal symptoms such as epigastric burning, nausea and vomiting, and CNS depression, including coma. Cyanosis, ataxia, miosis, pulmonary damage, delirium, and convulsions may occur. Deaths have been reported.

Oily solutions of eucalyptus oil are unsuitable for use in nasal sprays as the vehicle inhibits ciliary movements and may cause lipoid pneumonia.

References.

1. Patel S, Wiggins J. Eucalyptus oil poisoning. *Arch Dis Child* 1980; **55:** 405.
2. Spoerke DG, *et al.* Eucalyptus oil: 14 cases of exposure. *Vet Hum Toxicol* 1989; **31:** 166–8.
3. Webb NJA, Pitt WR. Eucalyptus oil poisoning in childhood: 41 cases in south-east Queensland. *J Paediatr Child Health* 1993; **29:** 368–71.
4. Tibballs J. Clinical effects and management of eucalyptus oil ingestion in infants and young children. *Med J Aust* 1995; **163:** 177–80.

Uses and Administration

Eucalyptus oil has been taken by mouth for catarrh and coughs and is an ingredient of many preparations. It has been used as an inhalation often in combination with other volatile substances. Eucalyptus oil has also been applied as a rubefacient and is used as a flavour.

Preparations

Proprietary Preparations (details are given in Part 3)
Austral.: Bosisto's Eucalyptus Spray; ***Fr.:*** Edulcor eucalyptus†; ***Ger.:*** Bronchodurat Eucalyptusol; Bronchomed; Eucalyptrol L; Gelodurat†; Nasivin Kinderbad; Tussidermil N.

Multi-ingredient: ***Aust.:*** Allgauer; Anifer Hustenbalsam; Anifer Krauterol; Apotheker Bauer's Inhalationsmischung; Babix; Baby Luuf; Berggeist; Bradosol; Bronchiplant; Bronchoforton; Bronchostop; Cehasol; Claim; Colda; Diphlogen; Embrocation; Emser Nasensalbe; Emser Pastillen mit Menthol; Erkaltungsbad; Erkaltungsbalsam; Euka; Expectal-Balsam; Fittydent; Kinder Luuf; Luuf Balsam; Luuf-Erkaltungsol; Luuf-Heilpflanzenol; Makatussin; Mediplant; Mediplant Inhalations; Medizinalbad†; Neo-Phlogicid; Pe-Ce; Perozon Erkaltungsbad; Pertussin†; Piniment; Pinimenthol†; Piniol†; Pulmex†; Red Point†; Resol; Rheumasan†; Salhumin; Sanvita Bronchial; Scottopect; St Radegunder Bronchialtee; SynPharma Bronchial; Tetesept; Tineafax; Tussamag; Tussimont; Wick Vaporub; ***Austral.:*** Alcusal Sport; Analgesic Rub†; Biosal; Bosisto's Eucalyptus Inhalant; Bosisto's Eucalyptus Rub; Cremor Menthol†; Dencorub; Dentese†; Euclean Eucalyptus Hand Cleaner†; Euky Bear Eu-Clear Inhalant; Euky Bear Limberub†; Euky Bearub; Genuine Australian Eucalyptus Drops; Logicin Chest Rub; Mentholyptus Vaporiser Fluid†; Methyl Salicylate Compound Liniment; Metsal; Metsal AR Heat Rub; Metsal Heat Rub; Painguard†; Quelfas A†; Sigma Relief Chest Rub†; Solarub†; Vicks Vapodrops; Vicks Vaporub; Zam-Buk; ***Belg.:*** Eugiron; Pulmex; Pulmex Baby; Vicks Vaporub; ***Canad.:*** Absorbine Analgesic; Analgesic Balm; Antiphlogistine Rub A-535; Baume Analgesique Medicamente; Beech Nut Cough Drops; Bronchodex Vapo; Cepastat; Cherry Chest Rub; EM Eukal; Eucalyptamint†; Eucamenth; Fisherman's Friend Original; Franzbranns; Halls; Herbal Cold Relief; Herbal Cough Expectorant; Kiro Rub; Medicated Analgesic Cream; Medicated Chest Rub; Mentholatum Cough Drops; Mentholatum Extra Strength Ointment; Mouthwash Antiseptic & Gargle; Pain Buster; Penetrating Rub; Rheumalan; Therapeutic Soothing Ice; Triaminic Night Time Rub; Vap Air; Vaporisateur Medicamente; Vaporizing Colds Rub; Vaporizing Ointment; Vicks Vaporub; ***Fr.:*** Balsofletol†; Balsofumine; Balsofumine Mentholee; Balsolene; Baume du Tigre†; Broncorinol toux seches; Campho-Pneumine Aminophylline†; Curibronches†; Edulcor eucalyptus et menthol†; Inongan; Kamol; Merol; Nazophyl; Pecto 6†; Pulmax; Pulmoll au menthol et a l'eucalyptus; Pulmothiol†; Santane O_1; Sirop Pectoral adulte; Sirop Pectoral enfant; Terpone; Thiopon Balsamique; Tigidol; Tisanes de l'Abbe Hamon no 15; Trophires; Trophires Compose; Tussipax a l'Euquinine; Vicks Pastilles†; Vicks Vaporub; Vicks vitamine C pastilles†; ***Ger.:*** A + B Balsam N; Aerosol Spitzner N; Alformin†; Angocin percutan; Aspecton-Balsam; Babiforton; Babix-Inhalat N; Baby-Transpulmin; Baokang†; Bergauf†; Bronchicum Balsam mit Eukalyptusol; Bronchicum Sekret-Loser; Bronchocedin N; Bronchocedin†; Bronchodurat; Bronchoforton; Bronchoforton Infant†; Bronchoforton Kinderbalsam; Bronchoforton N†; Broncholind Balsam†; Broncholind†; Cefabronchin N; Divinal-Broncho-Balsam; Dolexamed N; Dolo-cyl; Dorex Hustensaft N mit Oxeladin†; Dorex†; Emser Balsam echt†; Emser Erkaltungsgel; Emser Nasensalbe N; Emsilat; Endrine mild†; Endrine†; Ephepect; Erkaltungs-Balsam†; Erkaltungsbalsam-ratiopharm E; Eucabal-Balsam S; Eucafluid N; Eufimenth N mild; Expectal Balsam†; Extropin†; Frubibalsam†; Hevertopect; Hoemarin Rheuma; Hustagil Erkaltungsbalsam; Inspirol Mundwasser konzentrat; Iosimitan†; Ipalat; Kneipp Erkaltungs-Balsam N; Kneipp Erkaltungsbad Spezial; Kneipp Tonikum-Bad Fichtennadel-Aquasan; Leukona-Eukalpin-Bad; Leukona-Kreislauf-Bad; Leukona-Sauna-Konzentrat†; Leukona-Tonikum-Bad†; Liniplant; Logomed Erkaltungs-Balsam; Lyobalsam N ohne Menthol†; Lyobalsam N†; Makatussin Balsam Mild†; Makatussin Balsam mit Menthol; Makatussin Inhalat Menthol†; Makatussin Inhalat Mild†; Melrosum Inhalationstropfen†; Mentholon Original N; Mentopin Erkaltungsbalsam; Mintetten S†; Monapax N†; Nasenol-ratiopharm†; Nasivin Intensiv-Bad N; Nasivin Intensiv-Balsam†; Nervencreme S; Nervfluid S; Night-Care; Optipect mit Kodein†; Optipect†; Palatol; Palatol N; Palatol†; Phardol N Balsam†; Pinimenthol Bad N; Pinimenthol N; Pinimenthol-S; Piniol N; Plantmobil; Pro-Pecton Balsam†; Pulmotin-N; Pumilen-Balsam†; Pumilen-N; Repha-Os; Retterspitz Aerosol; Rheumaliment N; Rheumasalbe; rhino-loges N†; Rhinotussal E Balsam†; Rhinotussal S Balsam†; Salviathymol N; Sanopinwern; Schupps Fichte-Menthol Olbad; Schupps Heilkrauter Erkaltungsbad; Sinuforton; Soledum Nasentropfen N†; Stas Erkaltungs-Salbe; Stas Erkaltungs-Salbe Mild; Thymipin N; Transpulmin Kinderbalsam S; Trauma-Salbe Rodler 302 N; Tumarol Kinderbalsam; Tumarol-N; Tussamag Erkaltungsbalsam N; Tussamag Halstabletten; Tussipect; Wick Vaporub; ***Irl.:*** Purporent†; Vicks Vaporub; ***Ital.:*** Anacufen†; Antipulmina†; Capsolin; Eucalipto Composto; Florerbe Balsamica†; Fomentil; Fosfoguaiacol; Ingro; Kindian†; Neo Eubalsamina†; Rinopaidolo; Rinostil; Sloan; Vicks Gola†; Vicks Vaporub; ***Neth.:*** Bronchicum; Bronchoforton†; Dampo; Strepsils Menthol en Eucalyptus; Tijgerolie†; Vicks Sinex; Vicks Vaporub; ***S.Afr.:*** Bronchicough; Bronchicum; Bronchicum SB†; Docrub; Warm-Up; Zam-Buk; ***Spain:*** Bellacanfor†; Calyptol Inhalante; Dolokey; Gartricin; Lapiz Termo Compositum†; Pastillas Vicks Mentol†; Porosan†; Sinus Inhalaciones; Termosan; Vapores Pyt; Vicks Vaporub; ***Swed.:*** Vicks Vaporub; ***Switz.:*** Antiphlogistine; Baby Liberol; Baume de Chine Temple of Heaven blanc; Baume Kytta†; Bismorectal; Bradoral†; Bronchoforton; Capsolin; Carmol "blanche"†; Carmol "thermogene"†; Carmol†; Demo pates pectorales; Demo pommade contre les refroidissements; Demo pommade contre les refroidissements pour bebes; Dipect†; Embropax; GEM†; Huile analgesique "Polar-Bar"; Huile Po-Ho A. Vogel; Kemeol; Kemerhine; Kernosan Huile de Massage; Liberol; Makatussin; Makatussin forte; Massorax; Nasobol; Neo-Liniment†; Olbas; Pasta boli; Phlogantine†; Pinimenthol; Pirom; Pulmex; Pulmex Baby; Pulmex†; Rhinothricinol; Roliwol; Sloan Baume; Tumarol; Tussanil Compositum; Vicks Vaporub; ***UK:*** 9 Rubbing Oils; Aleevex; Antiseptic Lozenges; Baby Chest Rub†; Bolus Eucalypti Comp; Boots Vapour Rub; Cabdrivers Adult Linctus; Catarrh Cream; Catarrh Pastilles; Chymol Emollient Balm; Deep Heat Rub; Dragon Balm; Flurex Inhalant†; Gonne Balm; Kleer Cream; Mackenzies; Medicinal Gargle; Mentho-lyptus; Menthol and Wintergreen Heat Product†; Mentholatum Balm†; Mentholease; Merothol; Nasal Inhaler; Nicobrevin; Nosor Nose Balm; Olbas; Oleum Rhinale; Penetrol; Potter's Pastilles; Proctor's Pinelyptus; Revitonil; Sanderson's Throat Specific; Snufflebabe; Throaties Catarrh Pastilles; Tixylix Inhalant; Vapour Rub; Vicks Vaporub; Woodwards Baby Chest Rub; Zam-Buk†; ***USA:*** Boil Ease; Cepastat; Eucalyptamint; Hall's Sugar Free Mentho-Lyptus; Massengill; Maximum Strength Flexall 454; Mentholatum Cherry Chest Rub; Mentholatum Ointment; Mexsana; Nasal Jelly; Ponaris†; Robitussin Cough Drops; Unguentine; Vicks Menthol Cough Drops; Vicks Vaporub; Vicks Victors Dual Action Cough Drops.

Eugenol (4645-j)

4-Allylguaiacol; Eugen.; Eugenic Acid; Eugenolum. 4-Allyl-2-methoxyphenol.

$C_{10}H_{12}O_2$ = 164.2.
CAS — 97-53-0.

Pharmacopoeias. In *Eur.* (see p.viii), *Pol.*, and *US.*

A colourless or pale yellow liquid with a strongly aromatic odour of clove and a spicy pungent taste; it may be obtained from clove oil.

Practically **insoluble** to slightly soluble in water; freely soluble in alcohol (70%); practically insoluble in glycerol; miscible with acetic acid, with alcohol, with chloroform, with dichloromethane, with ether, and with fixed oils. Eugenol darkens in colour and becomes more viscous on exposure to air. **Store** in well-filled airtight containers. Protect from light.

Eugenol is a constituent of clove oil (p.1565) and some other essential oils. It is employed in dentistry, often mixed with zinc oxide, as a temporary anodyne dental filling, and is an ingredient in oral hygiene preparations. Eugenol has been used as a flavour.

Eugenol is an irritant and sensitiser and can produce local anaesthesia. It is reported to inhibit prostaglandin synthesis.

For the pulmonary effects of eugenol inhalation from clove cigarettes, see Abuse, under Clove, p.1565.

Preparations

Proprietary Preparations (details are given in Part 3)
Ital.: Bastoncino; ***USA:*** Red Cross Toothache.

Multi-ingredient: ***Aust.:*** Ledermix; ***Belg.:*** Calmant Martou; Dentophar; ***Canad.:*** Jiffy Toothache Drops; ***Fr.:*** Alodont; Pectoderme; ***Irl.:*** Ledermix; Rovaktivit†; ***S.Afr.:*** Counterpain; Ledermix; ***Spain:*** Alvogil; Neodesfila; Piorlis; Pomada Revulsiva; Tangenol; Tifell; ***Switz.:*** Alodont nouvelle formule; Alvogyl; Benzocaine PD; Dental-Phenjoca; Endomethasone; Ledermix; Rocanal Permanent Gangrene; Rocanal Permanent Vital; Spirogel; ***UK:*** Aezodent; Ledermix.

Exifone (3929-a)

Exifone *(rINN).*

2,3,3',4,4',5'-Hexahydroxybenzophenone.

$C_{13}H_{10}O_7$ = 278.2.
CAS — 52479-85-3.

Exifone was formerly used in the treatment of cognitive memory problems in the elderly but was withdrawn from the market following reports of fatal cytolytic hepatitis.

Exiproben Sodium (12726-z)

Exiproben Sodium *(rINNM).*

DCH-21. Sodium 2-(3-hexyloxy-2-hydroxypropoxy)benzoate.

$C_{16}H_{23}NaO_5$ = 318.3.
CAS — 26281-69-6 (exiproben); 3478-44-2 (exiproben sodium).

Exiproben sodium is a choleretic which has been used in the treatment of hepatic disorders.

Preparations

Proprietary Preparations (details are given in Part 3)
Ital.: Droctil†.

Febuprol (16800-a)

Febuprol *(rINN).*

1-Butoxy-3-phenoxy-2-propanol.

$C_{13}H_{20}O_3$ = 224.3.
CAS — 3102-00-9.

Febuprol is a choleretic used in the treatment of biliary-tract disorders.

Preparations

Proprietary Preparations (details are given in Part 3)
Aust.: Valbil†; ***Ger.:*** Valbil.

Fenalamide (12731-l)

Fenalamide *(USAN, pINN).*

Ethyl *N*-(2-diethylaminoethyl)-2-ethyl-2-phenylmalonamate.

$C_{19}H_{30}N_2O_3$ = 334.5.
CAS — 4551-59-1.

Fenalamide and its citrate are used as antispasmodics.

Preparations

Proprietary Preparations (details are given in Part 3)
Ital.: Spasmamide Semplice†.

Multi-ingredient: ***Ital.:*** Diarstop†; Rectocoricidin†; Spasmamide Composta†.

Fencibutirol (12735-c)

Fencibutirol *(USAN, rINN).*

Mg-4833. 2-(1-Hydroxy-4-phenylcyclohexyl)butyric acid.

$C_{16}H_{22}O_3$ = 262.3.
CAS — 5977-10-6.

Fencibutirol is a choleretic which has been used in the treatment of hepatic and gastro-intestinal disorders.

Preparations

Proprietary Preparations (details are given in Part 3)
Ital.: Hepasil†.

Multi-ingredient: ***Ital.:*** Epar Euchessina†; Hepasil Composto; Magisbile; Neo-Heparbil; Sintobil; Verecolene Complesso†; Verecolene†.

Fenclonine (12736-k)

Fenclonine *(USAN, rINN)*.

CP-10188; NSC-77370; Parachlorophenylalanine. 2-Amino-3-(4-chlorophenyl)propionic acid; DL-3-(*p*-Chlorophenyl)alanine.

$C_9H_{10}ClNO_2$ = 199.6.

CAS — 7424-00-2.

Fenclonine is an inhibitor of the biosynthesis of serotonin. It has been given to patients with carcinoid syndrome and some relief of symptoms, especially of flushing and diarrhoea, has been reported. Hypothermia, bone marrow depression, and psychiatric side-effects such as confusion and depression have occurred during treatment.

Fenipentol (3722-m)

Fenipentol *(rINN)*.

1-Phenylpentan-1-ol; α-Butylbenzyl alcohol.

$C_{11}H_{16}O$ = 164.2.

CAS — 583-03-9.

Fenipentol is a choleretic used in the treatment of hepatic and biliary-tract disorders. The hemisuccinate and sodium hemisuccinate are also used.

Preparations

Proprietary Preparations (details are given in Part 3)
Ger.: Febichol; ***Ital.:*** Pentabil.

Multi-ingredient: ***Belg.:*** Cholipin†; ***Ital.:*** Critichol; Menabil Complex†; Quanto†; ***Spain:*** Cholipin†; Menabil Complex.

Fennel (4646-z)

Fenchel; Fennel Fruit; Fennel Seed; Fenouil; Fenouil Amer; Foeniculum; Fruto de Hinojo; Funcho.

Pharmacopoeias. In *Chin., Eur.* (see p.viii), *Jpn,* and *Pol.*

Bitter Fennel (Ph. Eur.) (Foeniculi Amari Fructus) consists of the dry, whole cremocarps and mericarps of *Foeniculum vulgare*, subsp. *vulgare*, var. *vulgare*. It contains not less than 4.0% v/w of volatile oil, calculated with reference to the anhydrous drug. The oil contains not less than 60.0% of anethole and not less than 15.0% of fenchone.

Sweet Fennel (Ph. Eur.) (Foeniculi Dulcis Fructus) consists of the dry, whole cremocarps and mericarps of *Foeniculum vulgare*, subsp. *vulgare*, var. *dulce*. It contains not less than 2.0% v/w of essential oil, calculated with reference to the anhydrous drug. The oil contains not less than 80.0% of anethole.

Store protected from light and moisture.

Fennel is the source of fennel oil. It is used as a carminative and flavouring agent although the efficacy of such traditional remedies in infantile colic is considered dubious (see Gastrointestinal Spasm, p.1170). It is also used in herbal remedies for respiratory-tract disorders.

Preparations

Proprietary Preparations (details are given in Part 3)

Multi-ingredient: ***Aust.:*** Aktiv Leber- und Gallentee; Aktiv milder Magen- und Darmtee; Apotheker Bauer's Blahungstee; Apotheker Bauer's Brust- und Hustentee; Apotheker Bauer's Kindertee; Bio-Garten Tee gegen Blahungen; Bio-Garten Tee gegen Verstopfung; Brady's-Magentropfen; Carminativum Babynos; Caved-S; Euka; Granobil; Illings Bozner Maycur-Tee; Karvisin; Kneipp Husten- und Bronchial-Tee; Kneipp Verdauungs-Tee; Krauterdoktor Hustentropfen; Krauterhaus Mag Kottas Babytee; Krauterhaus Mag Kottas milder Abfuhrtee; Krauterhaus Mag Kottas Tee gegen Blahungen; Krautertee Nr 10; Krautertee Nr 11; Krautertee Nr 126; Krautertee Nr 14; Krautertee Nr 217; Krautertee Nr 8; Krautertee Nr 9; Laxalpin; Mag Kottas Baby-Tee; Mag Kottas Blahungs-Verdauungstee; Mag Kottas Magen-Darmtee; Mag Kottas Tee fur stillende Mutter; May-Cur-Tee; Nesthakchen; Pascopankreat; Planta Lax; Sidroga Kindertee; Sinolax-Milder; Species Carvi comp; St Radegunder Abfuhrtee mild; St Radegunder Blahungstreibender Tee; St Radegunder Bronchialtee; St Radegunder Magenberuhigungstee; St Radegunder Reizmildernder Magentee; St Radegunder Tee gegen Durchfall; Teekanne Herz- und Kreislauftee; Teekanne Husten- und Brusttee; Teekanne Leber- und Galletee; Windtreibender Tee; ***Austral.:*** Digestaid; Digestive Aid; ***Belg.:*** Eugiron; Tisane Antibiliaire et Stomachique; Tisane Depurative "les 12 Plantes"; Tisane Diuretique; Tisane Purgative; ***Canad.:*** Thunas Laxative; ***Fr.:*** Bolcitol; Colominthe; Mediflor Tisane Contre la Constipation Passagere No 7; Mediflor Tisane Digestive No 3; Mediflor Tisane Diuretique†; Santane D_5; Santane H_7; Tisane des Familles†; Tisane Digestive Weleda; ***Ger.:*** Abfuhr-Tee Depuraflux†; Abfuhr-Tee Stada†; Aruto-Magenpulver-forte†; Atmulen K†; Bronchialtee†; Broncholind†; Brust- und Husten-Tee Stada N; Carminativum Babynos; Carminativum-Hetterich N; Cefabronchin N; Cefagastrin; Cholaflux N†; Divinal Gastro; Dr. Kleinschrod's Spasmi Tropfen†; Dr. Klinger's Bergischer Krautertee, Abfuhr- und Verdauungstee†; Dr. Klinger's Bergischer Krautertee, Magentee†; Dr. Klinger's Bergischer Krautertee, Nerven- und Beruhigungstee†; Echtroferment-N; Floradix Maskam; Floradix Multipretten; Friosmin†; Gallen-Leber-Tee Stada†; Gallexier; Gastricholan-L; Gastrol S; Grunlicht Hingfong Essenz; Guakalin†; Hacko-Kloster-Krautertee†; Harntee 400; Hevert-Magen-Galle-Leber-Tee; Ilioton†; Kneipp Flatuol; Kneipp Husten- und Bronchial-Tee; Kneipp Verdauungs-Tee N; Kneipp Worisetten†; Knufinke Broncholind K†; Knufinke Gastrobin Magen- und Darm-Tee†; Lomatol; Majocarmin-Tee; Meteophyt†; Orbis Husten- und Bronchialtee†; Pascopankreat†; Pascopnakreat novo; Presselin 214†; Presselin 52 N; Presselin Stoffwechseltee†; Ramend Krauter; Rheumex†; Salus Abfuhr-Tee Nr. 2; Salus Bronchial-Tee Nr.8; Salus Leber-Galle-Tee Nr.18; Salus Nerven-Schlaf-Tee Nr.22; Salus Rheuma-Tee Krautertee Nr. 12; Stacho N†; Stern Biene Fencheltee†; Stovalid N; Ullus Magen-Tee N; Urodil Blasen-Nieren Arzneitee; Ventrodigest†; Worisetten†; Worishofener Dronalax†; ***Ital.:*** Dicalmir; Normalax; Tisana Cisbey; Tonactiv; ***Spain:*** Crislaxo; Jarabe Manzanas Siken; ***Swed.:*** Cavedess†; ***Switz.:*** Adistop Lax; Ajaka; Comprimes laxatifs de Worishofen†; Digestofluid†; Kernosan Elixir; Kernosan Heidelberger Poudre; Radix†; The Brioni; The Franklin; Tisane d'allaitement "H"†; Tisane gastrique "H"†; Tisane laxative; Tisane laxative H; Tisane laxative Natterman no 13; Tisane pectorale et antitussive; Tisane pour les enfants; ***UK:*** Carminative Tea; Cleansing Herb Tablets; Gladlax; Herbal Indigestion Naturtabs; Herbalene; Indigestion and Flatulence; Out-of-Sorts; Priory Cleansing Herbs†; Revitonil.

Fennel Oil (4647-c)

Aetheroleum Foeniculi; Esencia de Hinojo; Essência de Funcho; Oleum Foeniculi.

Pharmacopoeias. In *Aust., Ger., Jpn, Neth.,* and *Swiss.*

A colourless or pale yellow volatile oil with the characteristic aromatic odour and taste of fennel, obtained by distillation from dried ripe fennel fruit. It contains anethole. **Soluble** 1 in 1 of alcohol (90%). If solid matter separates it should be melted and mixed before use. **Store** in airtight containers. Protect from light.

Fennel oil is used as an aromatic carminative and flavour (but see the comment under Fennel, above). It is also used in herbal remedies for respiratory-tract disorders.

Preparations

Proprietary Preparations (details are given in Part 3)
Aust.: Sternbiene-Fenchelhonig; ***Ger.:*** Stern Biene Fenchelhonig N; Stern Biene Fenchelhonig N Sirup.

Multi-ingredient: ***Aust.:*** Eucarbon; Nesthakchen; Sabatif†; Solubitrat; Spasmo Claim; Thierry; Zeller-Augenwasser†; ***Belg.:*** Eucarbon; ***Canad.:*** Babys Own Gripe Water; Chase Kolik Gripe Water Alcohol-Free; ***Ger.:*** Abfuhr-Tee Depuraflux†; Azupanthenol†; Benium; Bisolvomed mit Codein†; Bisolvomed†; Bronchicum Hustentee; Broncho Sanol†; Cystium; Divinal-Bohnen†; Dr. Klinger's Bergischer Krautertee, Blasen- u. Nierentee†; Ephepect; Euflat I; Flatus-Pillen N Andreae†; Floradix Multipretten; Gastricard N; Gastrocaps†; Grunlicht Hingfong Essenz; Hepaticum-Divinal†; Heumann Blasen- und Nierentee Solubitrat N; Hevertopect; Ilioton†; Infantussin N; Kretussot†; Majocarmin†; Meteophyt-V†; Meteophyt†; Neo-Lapitrypsin; Nierentee 2000; Obstinoletten†; Orbis Husten- und Bronchial-tee†; Pulmocordio mite SL; Roflatol Phyto (Rowo-146); Salviathymol N; Stacho N†; Stern Biene Fencheltee†; Stoffwechseldragees†; ***Switz.:*** Ajaka; Caved-S; Delica-Sol†; Digestozym†; Eucarbon; Flatulex; Globase†; Hederka†; Huile Po-Ho A. Vogel; Lapidar 10 plus; Laxasan; Solubitrat†; ***UK:*** Atkinson & Barker's Gripe Mixture; Indigestion and Flatulence Tablets.

Fenoverine (12019-e)

Fenoverine *(rINN)*.

10-[(4-Piperonyl-1-piperazinyl)acetyl]phenothiazine.

$C_{26}H_{25}N_3O_3S$ = 459.6.

CAS — 37561-27-6.

Fenoverine has been used as an antispasmodic but has been withdrawn in some countries following reports of rhabdomyolysis.

Reports of rhabdomyolysis associated with fenoverine administration,[1,2] including one fatality.[1] A genetic predisposition has been suggested.[2]

1. Chariot P, *et al.* Fenoverine-induced rhabdomyolysis. *Hum Exp Toxicol* 1995; **14:** 654–6.
2. Jouglard J, *et al.* Research into individual predisposition to develop acute rhabdomyolysis attributed to fenoverine. *Hum Exp Toxicol* 1996; **15:** 815–20.

Preparations

Proprietary Preparations (details are given in Part 3)
Fr.: Spasmopriv†; ***Ital.:*** Spasmopriv†.

Fenpipramide Hydrochloride (16444-j)

Fenpipramide Hydrochloride *(BANM, rINNM)*.

2,2-Diphenyl-4-piperidinobutyramide hydrochloride.

$C_{21}H_{26}N_2O,HCl$ = 358.9.

CAS — 77-01-0 (fenpipramide); 14007-53-5 (fenpipramide hydrochloride).

Fenpipramide hydrochloride has been used as an antispasmodic.

Fenpiverinium Bromide (13439-c)

Fenpiverinium Bromide *(rINN)*.

Fenpipramide Methobromide; Fenpipramide Methylbromide. 1-(3-Carbamoyl-3,3-diphenylpropyl)-1-methylpiperidinium bromide; 2,2-Diphenyl-4-piperidinobutyramide methyl bromide.

$C_{22}H_{29}BrN_2O$ = 417.4.

CAS — 125-60-0.

Fenpiverinium bromide has been used as an antispasmodic.

Preparations

Proprietary Preparations (details are given in Part 3)

Multi-ingredient: ***Aust.:*** Baralgin†; ***Belg.:*** Baralgin†; ***Fr.:*** Baralgine†; ***Ital.:*** Baralgina†; ***S.Afr.:*** Baralgan†; ***Spain:*** Baralgin†; ***Switz.:*** Baralgine†.

Fenspiride Hydrochloride (12746-t)

Fenspiride Hydrochloride *(USAN, rINNM)*.

Decaspiride; JP-428; NAT-333; NDR-5998A. 8-Phenethyl-1-oxa-3,8-diazaspiro[4.5]decan-2-one hydrochloride.

$C_{15}H_{20}N_2O_2,HCl$ = 296.8.

CAS — 5053-06-5 (fenspiride); 5053-08-7 (fenspiride hydrochloride).

Fenspiride is reported to have bronchodilator and anti-inflammatory properties. It has been given in asthma (p.745) and other respiratory disorders in usual doses of 160 to 240 mg daily by mouth in divided doses before meals. It has also been administered rectally and by intramuscular or intravenous injection.

References.

1. Montes B, *et al.* Single dose pharmacokinetics of fenspiride hydrochloride: phase I clinical trial. *Eur J Clin Pharmacol* 1993; **45:** 169–72.

Preparations

Proprietary Preparations (details are given in Part 3)
Belg.: Pneumorel; ***Fr.:*** Pneumorel; ***Ital.:*** Decaspir†; Espiran; Fenspir; Fluiden; Pneumorel; Respiride†.

Fenugreek (12748-r)

Bockshornsame; Faenum-Graecum; Semen Foenugraeci; Semen Trigonellae.

Pharmacopoeias. In *Chin.* and *Eur.* (see p.viii).

The dried ripe seeds of *Trigonella foenum-graecum* (Leguminosae). **Protect** from light.

Fenugreek has been used as an appetite stimulant and as an ingredient in preparations for respiratory disorders. It has also been used in veterinary medicine as an aromatic.

Preparations

Proprietary Preparations (details are given in Part 3)
Fr.: Fenugrene.

Multi-ingredient: ***Austral.:*** Bilberry Plus; Garlic and Horseradish + C Complex; Garlic and Horseradish Complex 1000†; Panax Complex; Sinus and Hayfever; ***UK:*** Fenulin.

Ferric Chloride (5036-x)

Ferr. Perchlor.; Ferrum Sesquichloratum; Iron Perchloride; Iron Sesquichloride; Iron Trichloride.

$FeCl_3,6H_2O$ = 270.3.

CAS — 7705-08-0 (anhydrous ferric chloride); 10025-77-1 (ferric chloride hexahydrate).

Pharmacopoeias. In *Aust.* and *Swiss.*

Ferric chloride has the general properties of iron salts (see p.1346) but is exceptionally astringent. It has been used mainly by local application for its styptic and astringent properties. Local application of ferric chloride or other iron salts may cause permanent discoloration of the skin.

Preparations

Proprietary Preparations (details are given in Part 3)

Multi-ingredient: ***Belg.:*** Ouate Hemostatique; ***Ger.:*** Sepso†.

Ferritin (3934-z)

Ferritin is the major iron storage protein of vertebrates found mainly in the liver, spleen, intestinal mucosa, and bone marrow and consisting of a soluble protein shell (apoferritin) with a core of crystalline ferric hydroxyphosphate complex.

Ferritin has been given by mouth as a source of iron in various anaemias.

Preparations

Proprietary Preparations (details are given in Part 3)
Ital.: Anemial†; Bios Ferro†; Emodisintox†; Epadora†; Ferrofolin Venti Simplex†; Ferrostar†; Sideros†; ***Spain:*** Ferro Morgens†; Ferroprotina; Hierco; Profer; Protoferron†.

Multi-ingredient: ***Ital.:*** Epaplex†; Ferro-Tre; Ferrofolin Venti†; Fevital†; Rekord B12 Ferro†; Tonoliver Ferro†.

Fibronectin (16809-b)

Cold-insoluble Globulin.

Fibronectin is an endogenous polypeptide with a molecular weight of 440 000 to 550 000 whose roles include attachment of cells to the extracellular matrix and stimulation of phagocytosis. It is used in combination with other blood products in wound-sealant preparations. Infusion of fibronectin or fibronectin-rich plasma has been tried in patients with sepsis, infection, burns or other trauma, or severe malnutrition. Eye drops of fibronectin have been used in the treatment of corneal erosions.

References.

1. Anonymous. Fibronectins and vitronectin. *Lancet* 1989; **i:** 474–6.

Preparations

Ph. Eur.: Fibrin Sealant Kit.

Proprietary Preparations (details are given in Part 3)

Multi-ingredient: ***Aust.:*** Tissucol; Tissucol Duo Quick; ***Canad.:*** Tisseel†; ***Fr.:*** Biocol; ***Ger.:*** Tissucol Duo S; Tissucol Fibrinkleber tiefgefroren; Tissucol-Kit; ***Spain:*** Tissucol; ***Swed.:*** Tisseel Duo Quick; ***Switz.:*** Tissucol; ***UK:*** Tisseel.

Flavodate Sodium (12752-k)

Flavodate Disodium. Disodium (4-oxo-2-phenyl-4*H*-chromene-5,7-diyldioxy)diacetate.

$C_{19}H_{12}Na_2O_8$ = 414.3.
CAS — 37470-13-6 (flavodic acid); 13358-62-8 (flavodate disodium).

NOTE. Flavodic Acid is rINN.

Flavodate sodium is stated to increase the resistance of capillaries and to reduce their permeability. It has been given in the treatment of vascular disorders in usual doses of 200 to 600 mg daily by mouth; doses of up to 2 g daily have been given. It has also been administered by intravenous or intramuscular injection.

References.

1. Schmidt C, *et al.* Etude pléthysmographique et pharmacocinétique d'un phlébotrope: le flavodate disodique. *Therapie* 1985; **40:** 221–4.

Preparations

Proprietary Preparations (details are given in Part 3)
Fr.: Intercyton; Squad; ***Ital.:*** Pericel; ***Spain:*** Intercyton.

Flavonoid Compounds (7910-c)

Bioflavonoids; Vitamin P Substances.

Benzquercin (12493-j)

Benzquercin *(rINN).*

3,3′,4′,5,7-Pentakis(benzyloxy)flavone.

$C_{50}H_{40}O_7$ = 752.8.
CAS — 13157-90-9.

Diosmin (12667-x)

Diosmin *(pINN).*

Barosmin; Buchu Resin; Diosmetin 7-Rutinoside. 3′,5,7-Trihydroxy-4′-methoxyflavone 7-[6-*O*-(6-deoxy-α-L-mannopyranosyl)-β-D-glucopyranoside].

$C_{28}H_{32}O_{15}$ = 608.5.
CAS — 520-27-4.

Ethoxazorutoside (11367-d)

Ethoxazorutoside *(rINN).*

Aethoxazorutin; Aethoxazorutoside; Ethoxazorutin.

$C_{33}H_{41}NO_{17}$ = 723.7.
CAS — 30851-76-4.

Hesperidin (12821-j)

5-Hydroxy-2-(3-hydroxy-4-methoxyphenyl)-4-oxo-4*H*-chromen-7-yl rutinoside.

$C_{28}H_{34}O_{15}$ = 610.6.
CAS — 520-26-3 (hesperidin); 24292-52-2 (hesperidin methyl chalcone).

A flavonoid isolated from the rind of certain citrus fruits.

Leucocianidol (12894-p)

Leucocianidol *(rINN).*

Leucocyanidin; Leucocyanidol. 2-(3,4-Dihydroxyphenyl)chroman-3,4,5,7-tetrol.

$C_{15}H_{14}O_7$ = 306.3.
CAS — 480-17-1.

Monoxerutin (11467-b)

Monoxerutin *(rINN).*

Monohydroxyethylrutosides. 7-(β-Hydroxyethyl)rutoside.

$C_{29}H_{34}O_{17}$ = 654.6.
CAS — 23869-24-1.

Oxerutins (12020-b)

Oxerutins *(BAN).*

Hydroxyethylrutosides.

A mixture of 5 different *O*-(β-hydroxyethyl)rutosides, not less than 45% of which is troxerutin (trihydroxyethylrutoside, below), but which also includes monohydroxyethylrutoside, dihydroxyethylrutoside, and tetrahydroxyethylrutoside.

Quercetin (488-p)

3,3′,4′,5,7-Pentahydroxyflavone. 2-(3,4-Dihydroxyphenyl)-3,5,7-trihydroxy-4*H*-1-benzopyran-4-one.

$C_{15}H_{10}O_7$ = 302.2.
CAS — 117-39-5.

Rutin (15304-k)

Rutoside *(BAN, rINN).* 2-(3,4-Dihydroxyphenyl)-3,5,7-trihydroxy-4-oxo-4*H*-chromen-3-yl rutinoside trihydrate; 2-(3,4-Dihydroxyphenyl)-5,7-dihydroxy-4-oxo-4*H*-chromen-3-yl 6-*O*-(α-L-rhamnosyl)-β-D-glucoside.

$C_{27}H_{30}O_{16},3H_2O$ = 664.6.
CAS — 153-18-4 (anhydrous).

Pharmacopoeias. In *Aust., Fr., Ger., Pol.,* and *Swiss.*

A flavonoid obtained from buckwheat, *Fagopyrum esculentum* (Polygonaceae), or from other sources which include the flower buds of the Japanese pagoda-tree, *Sophora japonica*, and the leaves of several species of *Eucalyptus*.

Troxerutin (13386-t)

Troxerutin *(BAN, rINN).*

THR; Trihydroxyethylrutoside; Trioxyethylrutin. 3′,4′,7-Tris[*O*-(2-hydroxyethyl)]rutin; 5-Hydroxy-7-(2-hydroxyethoxy)-2-[3,4-bis(2-hydroxyethoxy)phenyl]-4-oxo-4*H*-chromen-3-yl rutinoside.

$C_{33}H_{42}O_{19}$ = 742.7.
CAS — 7085-55-4.

Pharmacopoeias. In *Ger.*

The principal component of oxerutins, above.

Uses and Administration

Flavonoids are naturally occurring antoxidants that are widely distributed in plants. Preparations containing natural or semisynthetic flavonoids are thought to improve capillary function by reducing abnormal leakage. They have been given to relieve capillary impairment and venous insufficiency of the lower limbs, and for haemorrhoids.

It has been suggested that flavonoids present in some foods, such as fruit, vegetables, tea, and red wine may protect against the development of atherosclerosis (p.782).

References.

1. Anonymous. Paroven: not much effect in trials. *Drug Ther Bull* 1992; **30:** 7–8.
2. Wadworth AN, Faulds D. Hydroxyethylrutosides: a review of its pharmacology, and therapeutic efficacy in venous insufficiency and related disorders. *Drugs* 1992; **44:** 1013–32.
3. Knekt P, *et al.* Flavonoid intake and coronary mortality in Finland: a cohort study. *Br Med J* 1996; **312:** 478–81.
4. Hertog MGL, *et al.* Antioxidant flavonols and coronary heart disease risk. *Lancet* 1997; **349:** 699.

Preparations

Proprietary Preparations (details are given in Part 3)
Aust.: Venoruton; ***Austral.:*** Paroven; Varemoid; ***Belg.:*** Veinamitol; Ven-Detrex; Venoruton; ***Fr.:*** Daflon; Diamoril; Dio; Diosmil; Diovenor; Flavan; Flebosmil; Litosmil; Mediveine; Preparation H Veinotonic; Relvene; Resivit†; Rheoflux; Veinamitol; ***Ger.:*** Drisi-Ven; Pherarutin; Posorutin; Rutinion; Tovene; Trirutin N; Troxeven; Vastribil; Veno SL; Venoruton; ***Irl.:*** Paroven; ***Ital.:*** Alven; Arvenum; Daflon†; Diosven; Doven; Flebil; Venolen; Venoruton; Venosmine; ***Mon.:*** Endium; ***Neth.:*** Venoruton; ***S.Afr.:*** Paroven; Varemoid; ***Spain:*** Daflon; Diosminil; Insuven; Okavena†; Pentovena; Venoruton; ***Switz.:*** Daflon; Hemerven; Neorutin; Pur-Rutin; Varemoid; Ven-Detrex†; Veniten; Venoruton; ***UK:*** Paroven; ***USA:*** Citro-Flav.

Multi-ingredient: ***Aust.:*** Aesrutan; Calcipot C; Daflon; Helopyrin; Influvidon; Ruticalzon; Rutiscorbin; Sandoven; Sklerovitol; Sterofundin R; Tetesept; Trimedil; Veno; Venotop; Wobenzym; ***Austral.:*** Acerola Complex†; B-Complex Threshold; Beta A-C; Bio-C Complex; Biocitrin†; Bioglan Fingers & Toes; Bioglan Super Cal C; Bioglan Zn-A-C; Biosor-C; C Supa + Bioflavonoids; Cirflo†; Cold & Flu Tablets; Crataegus Complex; Devils Claw Plus; Extra C 1000 Non Acid with Bioflavonoids†; Eye Health Herbal Plus Formula 4; Flavonoid C†; Flavonoid Complex; Flavons; For Peripheral Circulation Herbal Plus Formula 5; Ginkgo ACE†; Hamamelis Complex; Harpagophytum Complex; Lifesystem Herbal Formula 6 For Peripheral Circulation; Lifesystem Herbal Plus Formula 5 Eye Relief; Macro C; Min-Detox-C†; Proflo; Rubus Complex; Sinuguard N/F Without Antihistamine†; Sinuguard With Antihistamine†; Super Cal-C Bio; ***Belg.:*** Agruton-C†; Daflon; Ex'ail; Hemocoavit†; Mictasol; Trimedil†; Venalot†; ***Canad.:*** Duo-CVP; Duo-CVP with Vitamin K†; Rose Hips C†; ***Fr.:*** Acti 5; Cemaflavone; Cepevit; Circularine; Cirkan; Cyclo 3 Fort; Dilpavan†; Ercevit; Esberiven Forte; Ex'ail; Fragiprel†; Ginkor; Ginkor Fort; Hamamelide P†; Ophtadil; Rheobral; Rutovincine†; Solurutine Papaverine F. Retard; Trisolvit; Vascocitrol; Vascumine†; Veliten; Venyl; Video; Vincarutine; Vita 3; Vitarutine; Vivene; ***Ger.:*** Aescorin N; Antihypertonicum S; Antimyopikum; Antisklerosin S; Calcium-Rutinion; Coropar†; Cratylen†; Cycloven Forte N; Daflon†; dehydro sanol†; Echtrovit-K; Emocrat forte; Enzym-Wied; Essaven N; Essaven ultra; Eukalisan forte; Eukalisan N; Euvitan; Fagorutin Buchweizen; Hepabionta†; Hepasteril A†; Herz-plus†; Heweven P 7†; Intradermi N; Jatamansin†; Jossathromb†; Lindigoa S; Movicard; Pascovenol S†; Paveron†; Pentavenon†; Perivar N; Phlebodril; Phlogenzym; Posti N; Praecivenin†; Ruticalzon N†; Seda-Movicard†; Seniosan†; Sklerovenol N; Styptobion†; Theokal†; Tornix; varico sanol forte†; Vaso-E-Bion; Venalot; Venelbin; Veno-Hexanicit; Veno-Tebonin N; Venosan†; Venothromb†; Venotrulan Compositum†; Vitosal; Wobenzym N; ***Ital.:*** Angiopan†; Askarutina†; Biodyn†; Blunorm; Bo-Gum; C-Plus†; CVP; Daflon 500; Dermoangiopan; Digifar; Emorril; Essaven; Flavone 500; Fleboside; Nevanil†; Premium†; Proctocort†; Rutisan CE; Sandoven†; Traumal; ***Neth.:*** Venalot†; ***S.Afr.:*** Essaven; Sandovene†; Vitaforce 21-Plus†; ***Spain:*** Caprofides Hemostatico; Ciclotres†; Circovenil Fuerte; Citroflavona; Citroflavona Mag; Citroflavona Solu†; Daflon 500; Duvaline Flebo†; Epistaxol; Esberiven; Essavenon†; Fabroven; Flebeside; Gingilone; Gingilone Comp†; Nasopomada; Prosanon†; Quercetol Hemostatico; Quercetol K; Rutice Fuerte; Venosan; Vitaendil C K P; ***Switz.:*** Daflon 500; Demoven N; Flavovenyl; Geriavit; No Grip; Optazine; Phlebodril; Ruvenas†; Sandovene f†; Trimedil†; Varecort†; Venalot†; Venosan; Video-Net; Vita 3; ***UK:*** Flavorola C; ***USA:*** Ak-Bicholine; Akoline†; Amino-Opti-C; Bio-Acerola C Complex; C Factors "1000" Plus; C Speridin; Cholinoid; Citrus-flav C; Ester-C Plus; Ester-C Plus Multi-Mineral; Flavons; HY-C†; Lipoflavonoid; Pan C; Peridin-C; Span C; Super Citro Cee; Super Complex C.

Flopropione (5234-m)

Flopropione *(rINN).*

Fluropropiofenone; Phloropropiophenone; RP-13907. 2′,4′,6′-Trihydroxypropiophenone.

$C_9H_{10}O_4$ = 182.2.
CAS — 2295-58-1.

Pharmacopoeias. In *Jpn.*

Flopropione is used by mouth as an antispasmodic.

Preparations

Proprietary Preparations (details are given in Part 3)
Jpn: Cospanon.

Multi-ingredient: ***Spain:*** Espasmo Digestomen.

Flumecinol (19184-e)

Flumecinol *(rINN).*

RGH-3332. α-Ethyl-3-(trifluoromethyl)benzhydrol.

$C_{16}H_{15}F_3O$ = 280.3.
CAS — 56430-99-0.

Flumecinol has been investigated for treatment of neonatal hyperbilirubinaemia and has been tried for cholestatic pruritus.

References.

1. Turner IB, *et al.* Flumecinol for the treatment of pruritus associated with primary biliary cirrhosis. *Aliment Pharmacol Ther* 1994; **8:** 337–42.

Flumedroxone Acetate (9048-w)

Flumedroxone Acetate *(BANM, rINNM).*

6α-Trifluoromethyl-17α-acetoxyprogesterone; WG-537. 17α-Hydroxy-6α-trifluoromethylpregn-4-ene-3,20-dione acetate.

$C_{24}H_{31}F_3O_4$ = 440.5.
CAS — 15687-21-5 (flumedroxone); 987-18-8 (flumedroxone acetate).

Flumedroxone acetate is a derivative of progesterone that is reported to possess no anabolic, androgenic, oestrogenic, or progestogenic activity. It was once given by mouth in the treatment of migraine and was an ingredient of a preparation for the premenstrual syndrome.

Fluorescein (2129-n)

Fluorescein *(BAN)*.

3′,6′-Dihydroxyspiro[isobenzofuran-1(3*H*),9′(9*H*)xanthen]-3-one.

$C_{20}H_{12}O_5$ = 332.3.

CAS — 2321-07-5.

Pharmacopoeias. In *US.*

An odourless yellowish-red to red powder. Practically **insoluble** in water; soluble in dilute alkali hydroxides. **Store** in airtight containers.

Fluorescein Dilaurate (1956-v)

Fluorescein Dilaurate *(BANM)*.

$C_{44}H_{56}O_7$ = 696.9.

CAS — 7308-90-9.

Fluorescein Sodium (2130-k)

Fluorescein Sodium *(BANM)*.

CI Acid Yellow 73; Colour Index No. 45350; D & C Yellow No. 8; Fluorescein Natrium; Fluoresceinum Natricum; Obiturin; Resorcinolphthalein Sodium; Sodium Fluorescein; Soluble Fluorescein; Uranin. Disodium fluorescein.

$C_{20}H_{10}Na_2O_5$ = 376.3.

CAS — 518-47-8.

NOTE. FLN is a code approved by the BP for use on single unit doses of eye drops containing fluorescein sodium where the individual container may be too small to bear all the appropriate labelling information. LIDFLN is a similar code approved for eye drops containing lignocaine hydrochloride and fluorescein sodium and PROXFLN a code for eye drops containing proxymetacaine hydrochloride and fluorescein sodium.

Pharmacopoeias. In *Chin., Eur.* (see p.viii), *Int., Jpn,* and *US.*

An orange-red, odourless, fine hygroscopic powder. Freely **soluble** in water; soluble in alcohol; practically insoluble in hexane and in dichloromethane. A 2% solution in water has a pH of 7.0 to 9.0. **Store** in airtight containers. Protect from light.

Adverse Effects and Precautions

The intravenous injection of fluorescein sodium may produce nausea and vomiting. Extravasation is painful. Hypersensitivity reactions range from urticaria to occasional instances of severe anaphylaxis. Cardiac arrests and fatalities have occurred rarely. Concern that impurities or a defect in manufacturing processes might be responsible for the serious reactions led to a review of the BP specification in the early 1980s and a reduction in the permitted level of impurities.

The skin and urine may be coloured yellow but this is transient. Fluorescein sodium can stain skin, clothing, and soft contact lenses on contact.

Facilities for resuscitation should be available whenever fluorescein sodium is administered intravenously.

Oral fluorescein dilaurate should not be given to patients with acute necrotising pancreatitis. Sulphasalazine may interfere with estimations of fluorescein in the fluorescein dilaurate test.

Two large studies have examined the incidence of adverse reactions following intravenous fluorescein angiography. An international survey[1] collected information concerning 594 687 angiographic procedures; the incidence of serious reactions was 1 in 18 020, and that of fatal reactions, 1 in 49 557. Reactions included anaphylactic shock, cardiac arrest, myocardial infarction, and shock with hypotension or respiratory distress. A USA survey of 221 781 fluorescein angiograms[2] reported frequency rates of 1 in 63 for a moderate reaction (urticaria, syncope, thrombophlebitis, pyrexia, tissue necrosis, or nerve palsy) and 1 in 1900 for severe reactions (respiratory or cardiac events or tonic-clonic seizures); there was one death.

Individual reports of adverse reactions to intravenous fluorescein sodium include pancreatitis,[3] painful crises in patients with sickle-cell disease,[4] and photoallergy[5] and phototoxicity.[6]

1. Zografos L. Enquête internationale sur l'incidence des accidents graves ou fatals pouvant survenir lors d'une angiographie fluorescéinique. *J Fr Ophtalmol* 1983; **6:** 495–506.
2. Yannuzzi LA, *et al.* Fluorescein angiography complication survey. *Ophthalmology* 1986; **93:** 611–17.
3. Morgan LH, Martin JM. Acute pancreatitis after fluorescein. *Br Med J* 1983; **287:** 1596.
4. Acheson R, Serjeant G. Painful crises in sickle cell disease after fluorescein angiography. *Lancet* 1985; **i:** 1222.
5. Hochsattel R, *et al.* Photoallergic reaction to fluorescein. *Contact Dermatitis* 1990; **22:** 42–4.
6. Kearns GL, *et al.* Fluorescein phototoxicity in a premature infant. *J Pediatr* 1985; **107:** 796–8.

Uses and Administration

Fluorescein sodium stains damaged cornea and ocular fluids and is applied to the eye for the detection of corneal lesions and foreign bodies, as an aid to the fitting of hard contact lenses, and in various other diagnostic ophthalmic procedures. It is applied as a 1 or 2% solution as eye drops or as sterile papers impregnated with fluorescein sodium.

Fluorescein sodium may be given by rapid intravenous injection, usually as a 10 to 25% solution in a dose of 500 mg, for the examination of the ophthalmic vasculature by retinal angiography. A dose of 7.5 mg per kg body-weight has been suggested for children. The oral route has been tried for this purpose. Other uses of intravenous fluorescein sodium have included the differentiation of healthy from diseased or damaged tissue and visualisation of the biliary tract.

Fluorescein dilaurate is given by mouth for the assessment of exocrine pancreatic function (see below). Pancreatic enzymes hydrolyse the ester and the amount of free fluorescein excreted in the urine can therefore be taken as a measure of pancreatic activity. A dose of 348.5 mg of fluorescein dilaurate, equivalent to 0.5 mmol of fluorescein, is given with a standard meal, and urine collected for the following 10 hours. The manufacturers give instructions concerning the type and amount of liquid and food which may be taken during this period. A control dose of 188.14 mg of fluorescein sodium, also equivalent to 0.5 mmol of fluorescein, is given on the following day under the same conditions.

Pancreatic function test. Studies of the fluorescein dilaurate test have considered it to be a useful noninvasive screening test for the exclusion of pancreatic exocrine failure in outpatients, particularly those presenting with steatorrhoea.[1-3] The need for tests such as the pancreozymin-secretin test which requires duodenal intubation may thus be avoided. However, low specificity (a relatively high rate of false-positive responses) has been reported with the fluorescein dilaurate test in some patient populations[2,4] and the need for careful patient instruction in performance of the test has been emphasised.[3]

The test has been used successfully in children,[5] particularly when the doses of fluorescein dilaurate and fluorescein sodium are reduced and fluid intake modified,[6] although the manufacturers recommend that the commercially available test is not used for this age group. In children, a simplified, single day test using dual markers, fluorescein dilaurate and mannitol, has been investigated with encouraging results.[7]

1. Barry RE, *et al.* Fluorescein dilaurate—tubeless test for pancreatic exocrine failure. *Lancet* 1982; **ii:** 742–4.
2. Boyd EJS, *et al.* Prospective comparison of the fluorescein-dilaurate test with the secretin-cholecystokinin test for pancreatic exocrine function. *J Clin Pathol* 1982; **35:** 1240–3.
3. Gould SR, *et al.* Evaluation of a tubeless pancreatic function test in patients with steatorrhoea in a district general hospital. *J R Soc Med* 1988; **81:** 270–3.
4. Braganza JM. Fluorescein dilaurate test. *Lancet* 1982; **ii:** 927–8.
5. Cumming JGR, *et al.* Diagnosis of exocrine pancreatic insufficiency in cystic fibrosis by use of fluorescein dilaurate test. *Arch Dis Child* 1986; **61:** 573–5.
6. Dalzell AM, Heaf DP. Fluorescein dilaurate test of exocrine pancreatic function in cystic fibrosis. *Arch Dis Child* 1990; **65:** 788–9.
7. Green MR, *et al.* Dual marker one day pancreolauryl test. *Arch Dis Child* 1993; **68:** 649–52.

Pediculosis. Infestation of the eye lashes or brows with pubic lice (p.1401) has been successfully treated with a single application of a 20% solution of fluorescein.[1]

1. Mathew M, *et al.* A new treatment of pthiriasis palpebrarum. *Ann Ophthalmol* 1982; **14:** 439–41.

Retinal angiography. Fluorescein is usually given intravenously for retinal angiography but a study in 20 healthy subjects concluded that an oral dose of fluorescein sodium 25 mg per kg body-weight could produce good quality retinal angiograms in the majority of subjects.[1] This study used specially prepared 500-mg capsules of fluorescein sodium; the authors commented that previous oral studies had used the liquid preparation intended for intravenous use. Only mild reactions, possibly due to hypersensitivity, appear to have been reported with oral fluorescein.

1. Watson AP, Rosen ES. Oral fluorescein angiography: reassessment of its relative safety and evaluation of optimum conditions with use of capsules. *Br J Ophthalmol* 1990; **74:** 458–61.

Preparations

BP 1998: Fluorescein Eye Drops; Fluorescein Injection;
USP 23: Fluorescein Injection; Fluorescein Sodium and Benoxinate Hydrochloride Ophthalmic Solution; Fluorescein Sodium and Proparacaine Hydrochloride Ophthalmic Solution; Fluorescein Sodium Ophthalmic Strips.

Proprietary Preparations (details are given in Part 3)
Aust.: Fluoftal; ***Austral.:*** Disclo-Plaque; Fluorescite; Fluorets; Ful-Glo; ***Canad.:*** Diofluor; Fluor-I-Strip AT; Fluorescite; Fluorets; Funduscein; ***Irl.:*** Fluorets; ***Ital.:*** Fluoralfa; Pancreolauryl-Test; ***S.Afr.:*** Fluores†; Fluorescite; Fluorets; ***UK:*** Fluorets; ***USA:*** Ak-Fluor; Fluor-I-Strip; Fluorescite; Fluorets; Ful-Glo; Funduscein; Ophthifluor.

Multi-ingredient: ***Aust.:*** Healonid Yellow; Pancreolauryl-Test; ***Austral.:*** Fluress; ***Canad.:*** Dioflur-P†; Fluoracaine; Fluress; Healon Yellow†; ***Ger.:*** Pancreolauryl-Test N; Thilorbin; ***Ital.:*** Healon Yellow; ***Spain:*** Fluotest; Pancreolauryl†; ***Swed.:*** Fluress; Healon Yellow†; ***UK:*** Pancreolauryl-Test; ***USA:*** Flu-Oxinate; Fluoracaine; Flurate; Fluress; Flurox; Healon Yellow.

Formic Acid (1309-x)

Ameisensäure; Aminic Acid; E236; E238 (calcium formate); E237 (sodium formate).

CH_2O_2 = 46.03.

CAS — 64-18-6.

Pharmacopoeias. In *Aust.* and *Pol.*

Formic acid resembles acetic acid in its properties (see p.1541) but is more irritating and pungent. The acid and its sodium and calcium salts are used as preservatives in food. Solutions containing about 60% formic acid have been marketed for the removal of lime scales from kettles. Formic acid has also been used for the removal of tattoos. It is an ingredient of some external preparations promoted for the relief of musculoskeletal and joint disorders, and has been applied in conjunction with benzyl alcohol to aid the removal of nits.

There has been a report of 3 patients who swallowed descaling agents containing 40 or 55% formic acid in which the major complications included local corrosive effects, metabolic acidosis, derangement of blood-clotting mechanisms, and acute onset of respiratory and renal failure.[1] All 3 patients died between 5 to 14 days after admission to hospital. A report of 53 cases of formic acid ingestion included 15 fatalities.[2]

1. Naik RB, *et al.* Ingestion of formic acid-containing agents — report of three fatal cases. *Postgrad Med J* 1980; **56:** 451–6.
2. Rajan N, *et al.* Formic acid poisoning with suicidal intent: a report of 53 cases. *Postgrad Med J* 1985; **61:** 35–6.

Preparations

Proprietary Preparations (details are given in Part 3)
Multi-ingredient: ***Aust.:*** Aciforin; Berggeist; ***Belg.:*** Euphon; ***Fr.:*** Euphon; ***Ger.:*** Discmigon; Schwefel-Diasporal†; ***Ital.:*** Rubistenol; Rubjovit; ***Switz.:*** Fortalis; ***USA:*** Step 2.

Fosfocreatinine (3794-t)

Fosfocreatinine *(rINN)*.

(1-Methyl-4-oxo-2-imidazolidinylidene)phosphoramidic acid.

$C_4H_8N_3O_4P$ = 193.1.

CAS — 5786-71-0 (fosfocreatinine); 19604-05-8 (fosfocreatinine sodium).

Fosfocreatinine or fosfocreatinine sodium has been used in muscle disorders.

Preparations

Proprietary Preparations (details are given in Part 3)
Ital.: Creatergyl†; Sustenium.
Multi-ingredient: ***Fr.:*** Ergadyl†.

Fosforylcholine (12771-x)

Phosphorylcholine. (2-Hydroxyethyl)trimethylammonium chloride dihydrogen phosphate.

$C_5H_{15}ClNO_4P$ = 219.6.

CAS — 107-73-3.

Fosforylcholine is a choleretic that has been used in the treatment of hepatic disorders. The calcium and magnesium salts have also been used.

Preparations

Proprietary Preparations (details are given in Part 3)
Fr.: Heparexine; ***Ital.:*** Epaspes†.
Multi-ingredient: ***Ital.:*** Analip†; Fosfolip†.

Fumitory (8880-e)

Erdrauchkraut; Herba Fumariae.

Pharmacopoeias. In *Ger.*

Fumitory comprises the dried or fresh flowering plant *Fumaria officinalis* (Papaveraceae) and is used in herbal medicine. It is an ingredient of preparations used mainly for gastro-intestinal and biliary-tract disorders. Fumitory is also used in homoeopathic medicine.

Preparations

Proprietary Preparations (details are given in Part 3)
Aust.: Bilobene; Oddibil; Oddispasmol; ***Fr.:*** Oddibil; ***Ger.:*** Bilobene; Bomagall mono; Oddibil; ***Spain:*** Colambil.
Multi-ingredient: ***Aust.:*** Hepabene; ***Belg.:*** Tisane Depurative "les 12 Plantes"; ***Fr.:*** Actibil; Actisane Digestion; Bolcitol; Campho-Pneumine Aminophylline†; Depuratif Parnel; Depuratum; Gastralsan; Mediflor Tisane Hypotensive†; Schoum; ***Ger.:*** Choldestal†; Cholongal plus†; Cholongal†; ***Ital.:*** Depurativo; Soluzione Schoum; ***Spain:*** Sol Schoum; ***Switz.:*** Rasayana†; ***UK:*** Skin Cleansing.

Gabexate Mesylate (12777-m)

Gabexate Mesilate *(rINNM)*. Ethyl 4-(6-guanidinohexanoyloxy)benzoate methanesulphonate.

$C_{16}H_{23}N_3O_4,CH_4SO_3$ = 417.5.

CAS — 39492-01-8 (gabexate); 56974-61-9 (gabexate mesylate).

Pharmacopoeias. In *Jpn.*

Gabexate mesylate is a proteolytic enzyme inhibitor which has been tried in the treatment of pancreatitis (p.1613), although results do not appear to be promising, and in the prevention of pancreatitis following endoscopic retrograde cholangiopancreatography. It has also been tried as an anticoagulant for haemodialysis. Hypersensitivity reactions including anaphylaxis have occurred.

References.

1. Scuro LA, *et al.* Gabexate mesilate (Foy) treatment of acute pancreatitis: an Italian multicentre pilot study. *Clin Trials J* 1990; **27:** 39–49.
2. Messori A, *et al.* Effectiveness of gabexate mesilate in acute pancreatitis: a metaanalysis. *Dig Dis Sci* 1995; **40:** 734–8.
3. Cavallini G, *et al.* Gabexate for the prevention of pancreatic damage related to endoscopic retrograde cholangiopancreatography. *N Engl J Med* 1996; **335:** 919–23.
4. Matsukawa Y, *et al.* Anaphylaxis induced by gabexate mesylate. *Br Med J* 1998; **317:** 1563.

Preparations

Proprietary Preparations (details are given in Part 3)
Ital.: Foy; ***Jpn:*** Foy.

Gall (310-v)

Aleppo Galls; Blue Galls; Galla; Galläpfel; Galls; Noix de Galle; Nutgall.

Pharmacopoeias. In *Aust.*

Excrescences on the twigs of *Quercus infectoria* (Fagaceae), resulting from the stimulus given to the tissues of the young twigs by the development of the larvae of the gall-wasp, *Adleria gallae-tinctoriae*(=*Cynips gallae-tinctoriae*) (Cynipidae). It contains about 50 to 70% of gallotannic acid.

Gall is an astringent and has been used in ointments and suppositories for the treatment of haemorrhoids. It is a source of tannic acid (p.1634).

Preparations

Proprietary Preparations (details are given in Part 3)
Spain: Litiax.

Gamma-aminobutyric Acid (12359-p)

Aminobutyric Acid; GABA; Piperidic Acid. 4-Aminobutyric acid.

$C_4H_9NO_2$ = 103.1.

CAS — 56-12-2.

Gamma-aminobutyric acid is a principal inhibitory neurotransmitter in the CNS. It has been claimed to be of value in cerebral disorders and to have an antihypertensive effect.

Preparations

Proprietary Preparations (details are given in Part 3)
Multi-ingredient: ***Spain:*** Cefabol; Gamalate B6; Neurocordin†.

Gamolenic Acid (11660-v)

Gamolenic Acid *(BAN, rINN)*.

GLA; γ-Linolenic Acid. (*Z,Z,Z*)-Octadeca-6,9,12-trienoic acid.

$C_{18}H_{30}O_2$ = 278.4.

CAS — 506-26-3.

Borage Oil (12114-w)

Starflower Oil.

An oil derived from the seeds of borage (*Borago officinalis*, Boraginaceae).

Evening Primrose Oil (9808-e)

King's Cureall.

A fixed oil obtained from the seeds of *Oenothera biennis* or other spp. (Onagraceae) and containing linoleic acid with some gamolenic acid.

Linoleic Acid (9748-z)

Linolic Acid. (*Z,Z*)-Octadeca-9,12-dienoic acid.

$C_{18}H_{32}O_2$ = 280.4.

Adverse Effects and Precautions

Evening primrose oil, and presumably other sources of gamolenic and linoleic acids, can produce minor gastro-intestinal disturbances and headache. It can precipitate symptoms of undiagnosed temporal lobe epilepsy and should be used with caution in patients with a history of epilepsy or those taking epileptogenic drugs, in particular phenothiazines. Hypersensitivity reactions may also occur.

Effects on the nervous system. Temporal lobe epilepsy was diagnosed following treatment with evening primrose oil in 3 patients who had previously been diagnosed as schizophrenic.[1] Grand mal seizures occurred in 2 additional schizophrenic patients during treatment with evening primrose oil.[2] All of these patients had received or were taking phenothiazine neuroleptics.

1. Vaddadi KS. The use of gamma-linolenic acid and linoleic acid to differentiate between temporal lobe epilepsy and schizophrenia. *Prostaglandins Med* 1981; **6:** 375–9.
2. Holman CP, Bell AFJ. A trial of evening primrose oil in the treatment of chronic schizophrenia. *J Orthomol Psychiatry* 1983; **12:** 302–4.

Uses and Administration

Linoleic and gamolenic acid are essential fatty acids of the omega-6 series which act as prostaglandin precursors; endogenous gamolenic acid is derived from linoleic acid which is an essential constituent of the diet. Evening primrose oil, which contains these acids, is used for symptomatic relief of atopic eczema and mastalgia. Typical doses expressed as gamolenic acid are 320 to 480 mg daily in divided doses in eczema, and 240 to 320 mg daily in divided doses for mastalgia. Evening primrose oil has been investigated in a variety of other disorders including multiple sclerosis, diabetic neuropathy, rheumatoid arthritis, chronic fatigue syndrome, and the premenstrual syndrome, as indicated by the cross references given below. Mixtures of essential fatty acids (including EF-4, EF-12, and EF-27) derived from evening primrose oil and other oils have also been investigated in various conditions, including diabetic neuropathy, restenosis following angioplasty, and skin damage following radiotherapy.

Other plant oils which have been used similarly to evening primrose oil as sources of gamolenic acid include blackcurrant seed oil, and borage oil (starflower oil). Products containing gamolenic acid-rich plant oils are promoted in many countries as dietary supplements, often in combination with fish oils or other sources of omega-3 triglycerides (see p.1276).

A derivative of gamolenic acid, lithium gamolenate (p.544), is under investigation in pancreatic cancer.

General references.

1. Kleijnen J. Evening primrose oil. *Br Med J* 1994; **309:** 824–5.

Eczema. Atopic eczema (p.1073) may be due to a defect in essential fatty acid metabolism[1] and some beneficial symptomatic effects have been reported with evening primrose oil.[1,2] Meta-analysis of 9 studies involving 311 patients[3] has reported improvement in disease symptoms, especially itching, but a more recent study in 123 patients found no therapeutic effect of evening primrose oil, alone or with fish oil.[4] Although the design and interpretation of this study has been criticised by the manufacturers of evening primrose oil,[5] the authors consider such criticism invalid,[6] and point out that an earlier large study yielded similar results.[7] No difference was found between placebo and evening primrose oil in a further study[8] in children with eczema, and there was also no effect on asthma symptoms in those patients suffering from both disorders. Benefit has been reported in infants with seborrhoeic dermatitis from local application of borage oil.[9]

1. Wright S. Essential fatty acids and the skin. *Br J Dermatol* 1991; **125:** 503–15.
2. Rustin MHA. Dermatology. *Postgrad Med J* 1990; **66:** 894–905.
3. Morse PF, *et al.* Meta-analysis of placebo-controlled studies of the efficacy of Epogam in the treatment of atopic eczema: relationship between plasma essential fatty acid changes and clinical response. *Br J Dermatol* 1989; **121:** 75–90.
4. Berth-Jones J, Graham-Brown RAC. Placebo-controlled trial of essential fatty acid supplementation in atopic dermatitis. *Lancet* 1993; **341:** 1557–60. Correction. *ibid.*; **342:** 564.
5. Shield MJ, *et al.* Essential fatty acid supplementation in atopic dermatitis. *Lancet* 1993; **342:** 377.
6. Berth-Jones J, *et al.* Essential fatty acid supplementation in atopic dermatitis. *Lancet* 1993; **342:** 377–8. Correction. *ibid.*; 752.
7. Bamford JTM, *et al.* Atopic eczema unresponsive to evening primrose oil (linoleic and gamma-linolenic acids). *J Am Acad Dermatol* 1985; **13:** 959–65.
8. Hederos C-A, Berg A. Epogam evening primrose oil treatment in atopic dermatitis and asthma. *Arch Dis Child* 1996; **75:** 494–7.
9. Tollesson A, Frithz A. Borage oil, an effective new treatment for infantile seborrhoeic dermatitis. *Br J Dermatol* 1993; **129:** 95.

Mastalgia. Gamolenic acid (usually given in the form of evening primrose oil) has fewer adverse effects than drugs such as danazol or bromocriptine and some authorities prefer it for mastalgia (p.1443), especially in patients with less severe symptoms or those who require prolonged or repeated treatment.

Menopausal disorders. For reference to a study suggesting that evening primrose oil is of no benefit in preventing menopausal vasomotor symptoms, see under Benefits and Risks of HRT, p.1437.

Multiple sclerosis. There is some evidence that modifying the intake of dietary fats and supplementing the diet with omega-6 polyunsaturated fatty acids, such as linoleic acid, could influence the clinical course of multiple sclerosis (p.620) and many patients practice dietary modification, including taking evening primrose oil. Some studies have shown a reduction in severity and duration of relapse in patients taking linoleic acid supplements (as sunflower oil)[1] and another[2] has reported benefit in patients who limited their intake of dietary saturated fatty acids and supplemented their diet with polyunsaturated fatty acids. However, the relationship between dietary fat and multiple sclerosis cannot be considered proven.

1. Millar JHD, *et al.* Double-blind trial of lineoleate supplementation of the diet in multiple sclerosis. *Br Med J* 1973; **1:** 765–8.
2. Swank RL, Dugan BB. Effect of low saturated fat diet in early and late cases of multiple sclerosis. *Lancet* 1990; **336:** 37–9.

Premenstrual syndrome. Progressive improvement in premenstrual syndrome was reported over 5 cycles in an open pilot study in 19 patients receiving evening primrose only.[1] However, subsequent results have not demonstrated any benefit.[2-4] Evening primrose oil may be considered for cyclical mastalgia associated with premenstrual syndrome, but other drugs are preferred if other symptoms predominate (see p.1456).

1. Larsson B, *et al.* Evening primrose oil in the treatment of premenstrual syndrome: a pilot study. *Curr Ther Res* 1989; **46:** 58–63.
2. Khoo SK, *et al.* Evening primrose oil and treatment of premenstrual syndrome. *Med J Aust* 1990; **153:** 189–92.
3. Collins A, *et al.* Essential fatty acids in the treatment of premenstrual syndrome. *Obstet Gynecol* 1993; **81:** 93–8.
4. Budeiri DJ, *et al.* Is evening primrose oil of value in the treatment of premenstrual syndrome? *Control Clin Trials* 1996; **17:** 60–8.

Rheumatoid arthritis. In a study by Belch *et al.*[1] patients with rheumatoid arthritis (p.2) taking NSAIDs showed subjective improvement following 12 months' treatment with evening primrose oil with or without fish oil, compared with placebo. A clinically important reduction in signs and symptoms of disease activity has also been seen in patients treated with gamolenic acid in the form of borage oil.[2] Jäntti *et al.*[3] have demonstrated that during treatment with evening primrose oil patients with rheumatoid arthritis have an increased plasma concentration of gamolenic, dihomo-gamma-linolenic, and arachidonic acids and a decreased plasma concentration of oleic and eicosapentaenoic acids and apolipoprotein B. The increase in plasma-arachidonic acid and decrease in eicosapentaenoic acid may be unfavourable in patients with rheumatoid arthritis since arachidonic acid is the precursor of inflammatory prostaglandins and eicosapentaenoic acid may have an anti-inflammatory role.

1. Belch JJF, *et al.* Effects of altering dietary essential fatty acids on requirements for non-steroidal anti-inflammatory drugs in patients with rheumatoid arthritis: a double blind placebo controlled study. *Ann Rheum Dis* 1988; **47:** 96–104.
2. Leventhal LJ, *et al.* Treatment of rheumatoid arthritis with gammalinolenic acid. *Ann Intern Med* 1993; **119:** 867–73.
3. Jäntti J, *et al.* Evening primrose oil in rheumatoid arthritis: changes in serum lipids and fatty acids. *Ann Rheum Dis* 1989; **48:** 124–7.

Preparations

Proprietary Preparations (details are given in Part 3)
Austral.: Bioglan Primrose Micelle; Efamol†; Epogam; Eviprim†; Naudicelle; ***Canad.:*** Boracelle; Efamol; Gamma Oil; Naudicelle; Onagre; Primanol; ***Fr.:*** Bioleine; Bionagrol; Gamatol; Omegaline; ***Ger.:*** Epogam; Gammacur; Linola-Fett 2000; Neobonsen; Unigamol; ***Irl.:*** Epogam; Naudicelle; ***Ital.:*** Efamol†; Epogam; Normogam; ***S.Afr.:*** Epogam; ***Spain:*** Epogam; ***Switz.:*** Cremol-P; Efamol; ***UK:*** Boracelle; E.P.O. & E; Efamast; Efamol; EPOC; Epogam; Evening Gold; Evoprim; Floresse; Galanol GLX; Gamma Oil; GammaOil Premium; Naudicelle; PowerLean; Super Galanol; Super GLA; Unigam.

Multi-ingredient: ***Austral.:*** Bioglan E-Plus; Bioglan Primrose-E; Efamol Marine Capsules†; Epo + Maxepa + Vitamin E Herbal Plus Formula 8; Lifesystem Herbal Plus Formula 9 Fatty Acids And Vitamin E; Maxepa & EPO; Medinat PMT-Eze; Naudicelle Marine; Naudicelle plus Epanoil†; Naudicelle Plus†; Naudicelle Super†; PMS Support; ***Canad.:*** Bionagre plus E; Gamma Oil Marine; Primanol-Borage; ***Fr.:*** Bionagrol Plus; Elteans; Exomega; Ichtyosoft; Phytophanere; ***Ger.:*** Linola; Linola-Fett N; ***Ital.:*** Dermana; Efagel; Granoleina; ***S.Afr.:*** Efamol G; ***Switz.:*** Linola; Linola gras; Linola mi-gras; Linoladiol; Vitafissan; ***UK:*** Efacal; Efalex; Efamarine; Efamol Plus Coenzyme Q10; Efamol PMP; Efamol Safflower & Linseed; Efanatal; EPOC Marine; Epopa; Exzem Oil; Galanol Gold; Galmarin; Gamma Marine; Naudicelle Forte; Naudicelle Plus; PMT Formula; Royal Galanol; Super GammaOil Marine; ***USA:*** Efamol PMS†.

Gangliosides (16820-f)

Gangliosides are endogenous substances present in mammalian cell membranes, especially in the cortex of the brain. They are glycosphingolipids composed of a hydrophilic oligosaccharide chain, characterised by sialic acid residues, attached to a lipophilic moiety. The four major gangliosides found in the mammalian brain are referred to as G_{M1}, G_{D1a}, G_{D1b}, and G_{T1b}.

Preparations of gangliosides from bovine brain were given for peripheral neuropathies and cerebrovascular disorders and their role in spinal cord injury has also been investigated. The modified ganglioside siagoside is being studied in patients with Parkinson's disease.

Concern has been expressed by several authorities about the development of Guillain-Barré syndrome and other motor neurone disorders in some patients and it was suggested that gangliosides were contra-indicated in Guillain-Barré syndrome and all autoimmune disorders. Subsequently these concerns over safety as well as of efficacy led to the withdrawal of ganglioside preparations in many countries.

References.

1. Geisler FH, *et al.* Recovery of motor function after spinal-cord injury—a randomized, placebo-controlled trial with GM-1 ganglioside. *N Engl J Med* 1991; **324:** 1829–38.
2. Raschetti R, *et al.* Guillain-Barré syndrome and ganglioside therapy in Italy. *Lancet* 1992; **340:** 60.
3. Figueras A, *et al.* Bovine gangliosides and acute motor polyneuropathy. *Br Med J* 1992; **305:** 1330–1.
4. Roberts JW, *et al.* Iatrogenic hyperlipidaemia with GM-1 ganglioside. *Lancet* 1993; **342:** 115.
5. Landi G, *et al.* Guillain-Barré syndrome after exogenous gangliosides in Italy. *Br Med J* 1993; **307:** 1463–4.
6. Nobile-Orazio E, *et al.* Gangliosides: their role in clinical neurology. *Drugs* 1994; **47:** 576–85.

Preparations

Proprietary Preparations (details are given in Part 3)
Ital.: Biosinax†; Cronassial†; Sygen†; ***Spain:*** Nevrotal†.

Garlic (2014-y)

Ajo; Allium.

CAS — 8008-99-9 (extract).

Pharmacopoeias. In *USNF*, which also includes Powdered Garlic. *Eur.* (see p.viii) includes Garlic Powder.

The fresh or dried bulb of *Allium sativum* (Liliaceae). Constituents of garlic include Alliin, Allicin, diallyl disulphide, and Ajoene.

Garlic Powder (Ph. Eur.) is a light yellowish powder containing not less than 0.45% of allicin, calculated with reference to the dried drug.

Powdered Garlic (USNF) contains not less than 0.3% of allicin, calculated with references to the dried drug.

Protect from light.

Garlic has traditionally been reported to have expectorant, diaphoretic, disinfectant, and diuretic properties. More recently, it has been investigated for antimicrobial, lipid-lowering, fibrinolytic, antiplatelet, and cancer protective effects. It is used in homoeopathic medicine.

There have been some reports of contact dermatitis or burns associated with garlic.

Adverse effects. Reports of burns or skin lesions following topical application of garlic to children,[1,2] and to adults.[3]

1. Garty B-Z. Garlic burns. *Pediatrics* 1993; **91:** 658–9.
2. Canduela V, *et al.* Garlic: always good for the health? *Br J Dermatol* 1995; **132:** 161–2.
3. Farrell AM, Staughton RCD. Garlic burns mimicking herpes zoster. *Lancet* 1996; **347:** 1195.

Uses. References.

1. Kleijnen J, *et al.* Garlic, onions and cardiovascular risk factors: a review of the evidence from human experiments with emphasis on commercially available preparations. *Br J Clin Pharmacol* 1989; **28:** 535–44.
2. Mansell P, Reckless JPD. Garlic. *Br Med J* 1991; **303:** 379–80.
3. McElnay JC, Po ALW. Garlic. *Pharm J* 1991; **246:** 324–6.
4. Jain AK, *et al.* Can garlic reduce levels of serum lipids? A controlled clinical study. *Am J Med* 1993; **94:** 632–5.
5. Kenzelmann R, Kade F. Limitation of the deterioration of lipid parameters by a standardized garlic-ginkgo combination product: a multicenter placebo-controlled double-blind study. *Arzneimittelforschung* 1993; **43:** 978–81.
6. Warshafsky S, *et al.* Effect of garlic on total serum cholesterol: a meta-analysis. *Ann Intern Med* 1993; **119:** 599–605.
7. Kiesewetter H, *et al.* Effect of garlic on platelet aggregation in patients with increased risk of juvenile ischaemic attack. *Eur J Clin Pharmacol* 1993; **45:** 333–6.
8. Deshpande RG, *et al.* Inhibition of Mycobacterium avium complex isolates from AIDS patients by garlic (Allium sativum). *J Antimicrob Chemother* 1993; **32:** 623–6.
9. Dorant E, *et al.* Garlic and its significance for the prevention of cancer in humans: a critical review. *Br J Cancer* 1993; **67:** 424–9.
10. Neil HAW, *et al.* Garlic powder in the treatment of moderate hyperlipidaemia: a controlled trial and a meta-analysis. *J R Coll Physicians Lond* 1996; **30:** 329–34.
11. Berthold HK, *et al.* Effect of a garlic oil preparation on serum lipoproteins and cholesterol metabolism: a randomized controlled trial. *JAMA* 1998; **279:** 1900–2.

Preparations

Proprietary Preparations (details are given in Part 3)
Aust.: Kwai; ***Austral.:*** Cirkulin†; Kwai†; Macro Garlic; ***Fr.:*** Kwai†; Past Ail; Thirial; ***Ger.:*** Beni-cur; Carisano; Ilja Rogoff†; Kneipp Knoblauch Dragees N; Kneipp Knoblauch-Pflanzensaft; Kwai N; Sapec; Sirmia Knoblauchsaft N; Strongus; Venotrulan compt†; ***Ital.:*** Kwai; ***Switz.:*** A Vogel Capsules a l'ail; Kwai; ***UK:*** Cirkulin†; Garlimega; Kwai; Kyolic.

Multi-ingredient: ***Austral.:*** Crataegus Complex; Echinacea & Antioxidants; Echinacea ACE Plus Zinc; Esten†; Garlic Allium Complex; Garlic and Horseradish + C Complex; Garlic and Horseradish Complex 1000†; Gartech; Herbal Cold & Flu Relief; Horse Radish and Garlic Tablets; Lifesystem Herbal Formula 7 Liver Tonic; Liver Tonic Herbal Formula 6; Macro C + Garlic with Zinc; Odourless Garlic; Procold; Proesten; Protol; Proyeast; Silybum Complex; Vitalyt†; ***Belg.:*** Ex'ail; ***Fr.:*** Arterase; Ex'ail; ***Ger.:*** Asgoviscum N; Discmigon; Dynamol†; Gelovitall†; Hanoartin†; Kneipp Drei-Pflanzen-Dragees; Manns Knoblauch Pillen Plus†; ***Ital.:*** Prexene; ***Switz.:*** Allium Plus; Ginkovit†; Keli-med; Tisane pour le coeur et la circulation "H"†; ***UK:*** Antifect; Brewers Yeast with Garlic; Buttercup Pol'N'Count; Cold-eeze; Kincare.

Gavestinel (3223-q)

Gavestinel *(BAN, rINN).*

GV-150526X. 4,6-Dichloro-3-[2-(phenylcarbamoyl)vinyl]indole-2-carboxylic acid.

$C_{18}H_{12}Cl_2N_2O_3$ = 375.2.

CAS — 153436-22-7.

Gavestinel is a glycine antagonist under investigation as a neuroprotectant in stroke.

Gelsemium (12781-f)

Gelsemium Root; Jessamine; Yellow Jasmine Root.

CAS — 509-15-9 (gelsemine).

The dried rhizome and roots of *Gelsemium sempervirens* (Loganiaceae) containing not less than 0.32% of total alkaloids, calculated as gelsemine ($C_{20}H_{22}N_2O_2$ = 322.4).

Gelsemium depresses the central nervous system and has been used mainly in neuralgic conditions, particularly trigeminal neuralgia and migraine.

Gelsemium is used in homoeopathic medicine.

Preparations

Proprietary Preparations (details are given in Part 3)

Multi-ingredient: ***Austral.:*** Migran-eze†; ***Fr.:*** Campho-Pneumine Aminophylline†; Coquelusedal; Coquelusedal Paracetamol; ***Ger.:*** Dystomin forte†; Gelsadon†; Migranex spezial N†; Migranex†; Pan-Nerventonikum†.

Gene Therapy (10553-k)

Gene therapy is a product of the increasing knowledge of genetic function and the availability of methods to examine and manipulate the genome. It comprises the administration of exogenous genetic material into body cells (transfection) in such a way that the cells are able to express the products of the new genes. It should be distinguished from the administration of products themselves derived from organisms (usually micro-organisms) whose genome has been manipulated by similar recombinant DNA technology, for example the use of recombinant cytokines, monoclonal antibodies, or antisense products.

Gene therapy is under investigation in three main areas: the replacement of abnormal or defective genes in patients with inherited disease; the alteration of the characteristics of cells to change their relative susceptibility to other therapies (for example by making haematopoietic stem cells more resistant to the adverse effects of antineoplastics, or by making tumour cells selectively express an enzyme which converts an otherwise non-toxic prodrug into a cytotoxic agent); or to permit the localised production of a biologically-active substance that cannot be administered directly or without the effects that would result from its systemic administration. To date, all gene therapy in humans has been of differentiated somatic cells; alteration of the human genome in a manner transmissible to offspring, either by treating the germ cells or the early embryo, is considered at present to pose insuperable ethical problems.

An efficient means of delivery for genetic material is necessary for effective gene therapy. Various methods have been investigated, none of which is yet completely satisfactory. Although removal of donor cells from the patient followed by *ex vivo* transfer of the new gene (by physical or viral methods) and return of the modified cells may be feasible for modifying haematopoietic stem cells, for most tissues, methods of *in vivo* transfer are required. Modified viruses rendered incapable of replicating have been widely studied as vectors for gene therapy. Retroviruses have the advantage that the DNA they carry is integrated into the host genome, resulting in permanent expression of the gene, but there is some concern that they may disrupt existing genetic material with possibly oncogenic effect; in addition, their small size limits the size of gene that they can carry, and they are largely ineffective in infecting non-dividing cells. Adenoviruses are more stable and can infect non-dividing as well as dividing cells, but their genetic freight is not integrated into the chromosome and transmitted to the cell's progeny, and the gene products are therefore only expressed transiently; they are also highly immunogenic which limits repeated administration. Some other viral types, including herpes simplex viruses, adeno-associated viruses, and lentiviruses, are also under investigation. Viruses with tropisms for a particular tissue may be useful in producing localised effects.

Chemical or physical methods for DNA delivery have been extensively investigated *in vitro* and in *animals*, and have been studied in small numbers of patients. Such methods include direct injection of DNA, the use of DNA complexes bound to a ligand which can be taken up by cells, formulation of DNA in liposomes which can fuse with cell membranes and allow the DNA to enter the cell, and more exotic methods such as 'gene guns' in which DNA-coated gold particles are fired into the cells. Although gene expression can be achieved following such methods it is again transient because the new genetic material is not integrated with that of the host, and physical methods are currently less efficient and more limited in scope than viral ones.

Numerous clinical studies are being carried out although, at present, relatively few patients have actually received gene therapy. The first successful therapy was for severe combined immunodeficiency, a single-gene disorder due to deficiency of the enzyme adenosine deaminase. Transfection of the gene for this enzyme into the patient's T-cells *ex vivo* and re-infusion of the modified T-cells has been shown to produce substantial clinical improvement, although therapy must be repeated periodically because of the limited lifespan of the lymphocytes.

Studies in patients with cystic fibrosis have also shown some success, and a number of other single-gene disorders, including alpha$_1$ antitrypsin deficiency, familial hypercholesterolaemia, Gaucher disease, the haemoglobinopathies and haemophilias, and Duchenne muscular dystrophy are being studied or have been proposed as possible candidates.

Gene therapy is also under investigation in various acquired diseases, particularly in the management of various types of cancer. Strategies being studied include modification of tumour cells either to increase their immunogenicity or to render them selectively sensitive to antineoplastics, and transfection of tumour cells with tumour suppressor genes. Other disorders being studied clinically include HIV infection, rheumatoid arthritis, and atherosclerosis.

Some reviews and references concerning gene therapy are listed below. See also under the discussions of individual diseases for comments on gene therapy in the context of their conventional treatment.

1. Morsy MA, *et al.* Progress toward human gene therapy. JAMA 1993; **270:** 2338–45.
2. Brooks G. Gene therapy. *Pharm J* 1994; **252:** 256–60.
3. Sikora K. Genes, dreams, and cancer. *Br Med J* 1994; **308:** 1217–21.
4. Coutelle C. Gene therapy approaches for cystic fibrosis. *Biologicals* 1995; **23:** 21–5.
5. Hoeben RC. Gene therapy for the haemophilias: current status. *Biologicals* 1995; **23:** 27–9.
6. Lever AML, Goodfellow P, eds. Gene therapy. *Br Med Bull* 1995; **51:** 1–242.
7. Hanania EG, *et al.* Recent advances in the application of gene therapy to human disease. *Am J Med* 1995; **99:** 537–52.
8. Blau HM, Spinger ML. Gene therapy—a novel of drug delivery. *N Engl J Med* 1995; **333:** 1204–7.
9. Whartenby KA, *et al.* Gene therapy: clinical potential and relationships to drug treatment. *Drugs* 1995; **50:** 951–8.
10. Dorin J. Somatic gene therapy. *Br Med J* 1996; **312:** 323–4.
11. Southern KW. Gene therapy for cystic fibrosis: current issues. *Br J Hosp Med* 1996; **55:** 495–9.
12. Weichselbaum RR, Kufe D. Gene therapy of cancer. *Lancet* 1997; **349** (suppl II): 10–12.
13. Alton EWFW, Geddes DM. Prospects for respiratory gene therapy. *Br J Hosp Med* 1997; **58:** 47–9.
14. Knoell DL, Yiu IM. Human gene therapy for hereditary diseases: a review of trials. *Am J Health-Syst Pharm* 1998; **55:** 899–904.

Gentian (534-r)

Bitter Root; Enzianwurzel; Gentian Root; Gentiana; Gentianae Radix; Genziana; Raiz de Genciana.

Pharmacopoeias. In *Eur.* (see p.viii), *Jpn*, and *Pol.*

Jpn includes also Japanese Gentian, from *G. scabra. Chin.* specifies *G. scabra* and other species.

The dried underground organs of *Gentiana lutea* (Gentianaceae), yielding not less than 33% of water-soluble extractive. Protect from light.

Gentian is used as a bitter. An alcoholic infusion of gentian, bitter-orange peel, and lemon peel has been used as an ingredient in a number of bitter mixtures.

Gentian has been used in homoeopathic medicine.

Preparations

BP 1998: Acid Gentian Mixture; Alkaline Gentian Mixture; Compound Gentian Infusion; Concentrated Compound Gentian Infusion.

Proprietary Preparations (details are given in Part 3)
Ger.: Digestivum-Hetterich S; Enziagil Magenplus.

Multi-ingredient: ***Aust.:*** Abdomilon†; Amara; Bio-Garten Tee zur Starkung und Kraftigung; Brady's-Magentropfen; China-Eisenwein; Digestol; Krautertee Nr 20; Magentee; Mariazeller; Montana; Sanvita Magen; Sanvita Verdauungstropfen; Schwedenjorg mild; Sigman-Haustropfen; Sinupret; Sinusol; St Radegunder Verdauungstee; ***Austral.:*** Calmo; Digest-eze†; Digestaid; Digestive Aid; Pacifenity; Plantago Complex†; Relaxaplex; Waterbury's Compound†; ***Canad.:*** Herbal Laxative; Herbal Nerve; ***Fr.:*** Ducase; Elixir Grez; Elixir Grez Chlorhydropepsique†; Palmi; Phospharome; Quintonine; Triogene; ***Ger.:*** "Mletzko" Tropfen†; Abdomilon N; Amara-Tropfen-Pascoe; Anore X N; Aruto-Magenpulver-forte†; Choldestal†; Discmigon; Divinal-Bohnen†; Dr. Hotz Vollbad; Dr. Klinger's Bergischer Krautertee, Magentee†; Gallen-Leber-Tee Stada†; Gallexier; Gastralon N; Gastricard N; Gastrol S; Gastrosecur; Hepaticum "Mletzko"†; Hepaticum-Divinal†; Hepaticum-Medice H; Hepaton†; Infi-tract N; Kneipp Abfuhr Dragees N†; Kneipp Flatuol; Kneipp Magentrost†; Majocarmin mite†; Majocarmin†; Montana; Phonix Gastriphon; Presselin 214†; Schwedentrunk; Schwedentrunk mit Ginseng; Sedovent; Sinupret; Stomaform†; Stovalid N; Unex Amarum; ventriloges; Ventrimarin Novo; Ventrodigest†; Worishofener Nieren-und Blasenmittel Dr. Kleinschrod†; ***Ital.:*** Amaro Maffioli†; Amaro Medicinale; Amaro Padil; Bilarvis†; Caramelle alle Erbe Digestive; Chinoidina; Depurativo; Elisir Depurativo Ambrosiano; Epaglutone†; Florerbe Digestiva†; Frerichs Maldifassi; Pillole Frerichs Maldifassi†; Pillole Schias†; ***Spain:*** Depurativo Richelet; Digestol Sanatorium; ***Switz.:*** Amaro†; Demonatur Gouttes pour le foie et la bile; Gastrosan; Padma-Lax; Tisane gastrique "H"†; ***UK:*** Appetiser Mixture; Indigestion Mixture; Kalms; Quiet Tyme; Serenity; Stomach Mixture.

Gentisic Acid Ethanolamide (3272-c)

2,5-Dihydroxybenzoic acid ethanolamide.

$C_9H_{11}NO_4$ = 197.2.

Pharmacopoeias. In *USNF.*

A white to tan powder. Sparingly **soluble** in water; freely soluble in acetone, in alcohol, and in methyl alcohol; very slightly soluble in ether; practically insoluble in chloroform.

Gentisic acid ethanolamide is used as a complexing agent in the manufacture of pharmaceutical preparations.

Geranium Oil (4652-y)

Aetheroleum Pelargonii; Oleum Geranii; Pelargonium Oil; Rose Geranium Oil.

A volatile oil obtained by distillation from the aerial parts of various species and hybrid forms of *Pelargonium* (Geraniaceae). It contains geraniol. **Store** in airtight containers. Protect from light.

Geranium oil is used to perfume various preparations. Hypersensitivity reactions have been associated with geraniol.

Preparations

Proprietary Preparations (details are given in Part 3)
Ital.: Entom Nature.

Multi-ingredient: ***Fr.:*** Acarcid; Euvanol; ***Ital.:*** Dentosan "Pagni" Collutorio†; Dentosan Mese†; Natural Zanzy; Otosan Gocce Auricolari; Sanaderm; Vapor Flay; ***Spain:*** Synthol†; ***UK:*** Medicinal Gargle.

Germanium (5251-b)

Ge = 72.61.

CAS — 7440-56-4.

Germanium compounds have been used in dietary supplements promoted as beneficial in a wide range of conditions including cancer, chronic fatigue syndrome, and immunodeficiency disorders. However, germanium compounds can produce severe renal damage and their use should be discouraged.

Germanium has also been used in dental alloys and has various industrial uses.

In the UK the Department of Health has recommended that germanium should not be taken as a dietary supplement due to a significant incidence of renal toxicity. There have been a number of reports of severe renal damage resulting from germanium ingestion, of which a few are given below.

1. Okada K, *et al.* Renal failure caused by long-term use of a germanium preparation as an elixir. *Clin Nephrol* 1989; **31:** 219–24.
2. van der Spoel JI, *et al.* Dangers of dietary germanium supplements. *Lancet* 1990; **336:** 117. Correction. *ibid.* 1991; **337:** 864.
3. Schauss AG. Nephrotoxicity in humans by the ultratrace element germanium. *Ren Fail* 1991; **13:** 1–4.
4. Hess B, *et al.* Tubulointerstitial nephropathy persisting 20 months after discontinuation of chronic intake of germanium lactate citrate. *Am J Kidney Dis* 1993; **21:** 548–52.

Ginkgo Biloba (19248-e)

EGB-761; Fossil Tree; GBE-761; Kew Tree; Maidenhair Tree; *Salisburia Adiantifolia.*

Pharmacopoeias. In *USNF. Chin.* includes the seeds.

An extract from the leaves of *Ginkgo biloba* has been used in cerebrovascular and peripheral vascular disorders. It is also being investigated in Alzheimer's disease and multi-infarct dementia (p.1386).

Adverse effects include headaches, dizziness, palpitations, gastro-intestinal disturbances, bleeding disorders, and skin hypersensitivity reactions.

Ginkgo biloba is used in homoeopathic medicine.

Ginkgolides (p.754) have been investigated for the management of asthma and various inflammatory and immune disorders.

References.

1. Kleijnen J, Knipschild P. Ginkgo biloba. *Lancet* 1992; **340:** 1136–9.
2. Houghton P. Ginkgo. *Pharm J* 1994; **253:** 122–3.
3. Kanowski S, *et al.* Proof of efficacy of the ginkgo biloba special extract EGb 761 in outpatients suffering from mild to moderate primary degenerative dementia of the Alzheimer type or multi-infarct dementia. *Pharmacopsychiatry* 1996; **29:** 47–56.
4. Le Bars PL, *et al.* A placebo-controlled, double-blind, randomized trial of an extract of Ginkgo biloba for dementia. *JAMA* 1997; **278:** 1327–32.
5. Anonymous. Ginkgo biloba for dementia. *Med Lett Drugs Ther* 1998; **40:** 63–4.

Preparations

Proprietary Preparations (details are given in Part 3)
Aust.: Ceremin; Tebofortan; Tebonin; ***Austral.:*** Proginkgo; ***Fr.:*** Ginkogink; Tanakan; Tramisal; ***Ger.:*** Duogink; Gingiloba; Gingium; Gingobeta; Gingopret; Ginkobil N; Ginkodilat; Ginkopur; Isoginkgo; Kaveri; Rokan; Tebonin; ***Ital.:*** Vasan†; ***Neth.:*** Tavonin; ***Spain:*** Tanakene; ***Switz.:*** Geriaforce; Oxivel; Symfona N; Tanakene; Tebofortin; Valverde Ginkgo Vital; ***UK:*** Ginkovital; Mentor.

Multi-ingredient: ***Austral.:*** Bioglan Fingers & Toes; Eye Health Herbal Plus Formula 4; For Peripheral Circulation Herbal Plus Formula 5; Gingo A; Ginkgo ACE†; Ginkgo Complex; Ginkgo Plus Herbal Plus Formula 10; Ginzing G; Herbal Arthritis Formula; Herbal Capillary Care; Lifesystem Herbal Formula 6 For Peripheral Circulation; Lifesystem Herbal Plus Formula 11 Ginkgo; Lifesystem Herbal Plus Formula 5 Eye Relief; Prophthal; Vig; ***Fr.:*** Ginkor; Ginkor Fort; Ginkor Procto; ***Ger.:*** Perivar N; Veno-Tebonin N; ***Ital.:*** Alvear Sport; Enertonic; Forticrin; Ginkgo Plus; Nosenil; Nutrex; ***Switz.:*** Allium Plus; Arterosan Plus; Gincosan; Ginkovit†.

Ginseng (12784-h)

Ginseng Radix; Jintsam; Ninjin; Panax; Pannag; Schinsent.

Pharmacopoeias. In *Aust., Chin., Fr., Ger., Jpn,* and *Swiss.* Also in *USNF* as Oriental Ginseng. *Chin.* and *Jpn* also include Rhizoma Panacis Japonica from *Panax japonicus. Chin.* also includes Radix Notoginseng from *P. notoginseng,* and Rhizoma Panacis Majoris from *P. japonicus* var. *major* and *P. japonicus* var. *bipinnatifidus.* Red Ginseng (*Jpn P.*) is the dried root of *P. ginseng* which has been steamed.

The dried root of *Panax ginseng* (= *P. schinseng*) (Araliaceae). Other varieties of ginseng include *Panax quinquefolium* (North America) and *P. pseudoginseng.* The root commonly known as Siberian or Russian ginseng belongs to the same family, Araliaceae, but is an entirely different plant, *Eleutherococcus senticosis.* Ginseng contains complex mixtures of saponins termed ginsenosides or panaxosides. At least 13 saponins have been isolated from extracts of *P. ginseng* roots.

Some material supplied as Siberian ginseng may be *Periploca sepium* (Asclepiadaceae), a plant unrelated to either *Panax ginseng* or *Eleutherococcus senticosis,* due to the similarity of the chinese names for these plants.[1] Brazilian ginseng is reported to be derived from another unrelated plant, *Pfaffia paniculata.*[2]

1. Awang DVC. Maternal use of ginseng and neonatal androgenization. *JAMA* 1991; **266:** 363.
2. Walker AF. What is in ginseng? *Lancet* 1994; **344:** 619.

Ginseng is reported to enhance the natural resistance and recuperative power of the body and to reduce fatigue. Its toxicity at usual dosages appears to be low. It is available commercially as roots, powdered roots, tablets, capsules, teas, oils, or extracts. Siberian or Russian ginseng is used similarly.

Adverse Effects. A 2-year study of ginseng in 133 subjects who had used a wide variety of commercial preparations including roots, capsules, tablets, teas, extracts, cigarettes, chewing gum, and candies. The majority of preparations were taken by mouth but a few subjects had experimented with intranasal or parenteral routes and topical preparations had also been used. The stimulant effects of ginseng were confirmed but there was also a high incidence of side-effects including morning diarrhoea (47 subjects), skin eruptions (33), sleeplessness (26), nervousness (25), hypertension (22), euphoria (18), and oedema (14). The 'ginseng abuse syndrome' defined as hypertension together with nervousness, sleeplessness, skin eruptions, and morning diarrhoea was experienced by 14 subjects who took ginseng by mouth in an average daily dose of 3 g. Abrupt withdrawal precipitated hypotension, weakness, and tremor in one user. About 50% of the subjects had discontinued the use of ginseng within 2 years.[1] Oestrogenic effects have also been reported,[2-4] and a case of Stevens-Johnson syndrome has also occurred in association with ginseng.[5]

1. Siegel RK. Ginseng abuse syndrome: problems with the panacea. *JAMA* 1979; **241:** 1614–15.
2. Palmer BV, *et al.* Gin Seng and mastalgia. *Br Med J* 1978; **1:** 1284.
3. Punnonen R, Lukola A. Oestrogen-like effect of ginseng. *Br Med J* 1980; **281:** 1110.
4. Greenspan EM. Ginseng and vaginal bleeding. *JAMA* 1983; **249:** 2018.
5. Dega H, *et al.* Ginseng as a cause for Stevens-Johnson syndrome? *Lancet* 1996; **347:** 1344.

Interactions. For a report of raised serum-digoxin concentrations in a patient taking digoxin and Siberian ginseng, see under Digoxin, Interactions, p.852.

Preparations

Proprietary Preparations (details are given in Part 3)
Aust.: Ginsana; ***Austral.:*** Ginzing; Herbal Stress Relief; ***Fr.:*** Ginsana; Ginsatonic; Lyoginseng†; ***Ger.:*** Ardey aktiv; Eleu-Kokk; Eleutheroforce; Eleutherokokk-Aktiv-Kapseln SenticoMega; Gerivit; Ginroy; Ginsana; Hevert-Aktivon Mono; Kaukafin†; Kneipp Ginsenetten; Konstitutin; Orgaplasma; Vital-Kapseln; ***Ital.:*** Neo Ginsana†; ***S.Afr.:*** Ginsana†; ***Spain:*** Bio Star; Ginsana; ***Switz.:*** Ginsana; ***UK:*** Elagen; Red Kooga.

Multi-ingredient: ***Austral.:*** Bolo; Gingo A; Ginkgo Complex; Ginzing E; Ginzing G; Glycyrrhiza Complex; Infant Tonic; Irontona; Medinat Esten; Panax Complex; Trillium Complex; Tyroseng; Vig; Vitatona; Zestabs†; ***Fr.:*** Actisane Fatigue Passagere; Ginzinc†; Tonactil; Tonisan; ***Ger.:*** Alsiroyal; Cardibisana; Ginseng-Complex "Schuh"; Hypercard; Neuraston†; Schwedentrunk mit Ginseng; ***Ital.:*** Apergan; Bio-Real Complex; Bio-Real Plus; Bioton; Cocktail Reale; Enertonic; Fitostress; Fon Wan Eleuthero; Fon Wan Ginsenergy; Fon Wan Pocket Energy; Fon Wan Pollen; Forticrin; Fosfarsile Forte; Four-Ton; Gincola; Neo Trefogel†; Neoplus; Nosenil; Nutrex; Ottovis; Royal Mille†; Vitalmix; ***S.Afr.:*** Activex 40 Plus; ***Spain:*** Farmacola; Micebrina Ginseng; Minadex Mix Ginseng; Ton Was; ***Switz.:*** Biorganic Geri; Biovital Ginseng; Cimexon G†; Gincosan; Ginkovit†; Imuvit; Tai Ginseng N; Vigoran; ***UK:*** Regina Royal Concorde.

Glatiramer Acetate (6806-p)

Glatiramer Acetate *(BAN, USAN).*

COP-1; Cop 1; Copolymer 1. L-Glutamic acid polymer with L-alanine, L-lysine and L-tyrosine, acetate.

CAS — 28704-27-0; 147245-92-9.

Adverse Effects

Transient systemic effects including chest pain, palpitations, dyspnoea, urticaria, flushing, and anxiety may follow injection of glatiramer acetate. Pain, erythema, pruritus, and induration may occur at the injection site.

Uses and Administration

Glatiramer acetate, a random polymer of L-alanine, L-glutamic acid, L-lysine, and L-tyrosine, is a peptide which has some structural resemblance to myelin basic protein. It is administered by subcutaneous injection in a dose of 20 mg daily, to prevent relapses in the management of relapsing-remitting multiple sclerosis (p.620).

References.

1. Bornstein MB, *et al.* A pilot trial of Cop 1 in exacerbating-remitting multiple sclerosis. *N Engl J Med* 1987; **317:** 408–14.
2. Bornstein MB, *et al.* A placebo-controlled, double-blind, randomized, two-centre, pilot trial of Cop 1 in chronic progressive multiple sclerosis. *Neurology* 1991; **41:** 533–9.
3. Johnson KP, *et al.* Copolymer 1 reduces relapse rate and improves disability in relapsing-remitting multiple sclerosis: results of a phase III multicenter, double-blind, placebo-controlled study. *Neurology* 1995; **45:** 1268–76.
4. Anonymous. Glatiramer acetate for relapsing multiple sclerosis. *Med Lett Drugs Ther* 1997; **39:** 61–2.
5. Johnson KP, *et al.* Extended use of glatiramer acetate (Copaxone) is well tolerated and maintains its clinical effect on multiple sclerosis relapse rate and degree of disability. *Neurology* 1998; **50:** 701–8.

Preparations

Proprietary Preparations (details are given in Part 3)
USA: Copaxone.

Glicofosfopeptical (3905-w)

Fosfoglicopeptical.

Glicofosfopeptical is reported to possess immunostimulant properties and has been given in doses of 1000 mg by mouth every eight hours.

Preparations

Proprietary Preparations (details are given in Part 3)
Spain: Inmunoferon.

Glucomannan (16823-h)

Konjac Flour; Konjac Mannan.

Glucomannan, a powdered extract from the tubers of *Amorphophallus konjac,* has been promoted as an anorectic. It has been claimed to reduce the appetite by absorbing liquid in the gastro-intestinal tract. Glucomannan has also been investigated as a dietary adjunct in the management of diabetes mellitus.

There is a risk of intestinal or oesophageal obstruction and faecal impaction, especially if it is swallowed dry. Therefore, it should always be taken with sufficient fluid and should not be taken immediately before going to bed. It should be avoided in patients who have difficulty swallowing.

References.

1. Henry DA, *et al.* Glucomannan and risk of oesophageal obstruction. *Br Med J* 1986; **292:** 591–2.
2. Renard E, *et al.* Noninsulin-dependent diabetes and glucose intolerance: effect of glucomannan fibre on blood glucose and serum insulin. *Sem Hop Paris* 1991; **67:** 153–7.

Preparations

Proprietary Preparations (details are given in Part 3)
Fr.: Konjax; ***Ital.:*** Dicoplus; Dietoman; NormaLine.

Multi-ingredient: ***Fr.:*** AMK; ***Ital.:*** Ecamannan; Glucoman.

Glucosamine (12790-d)

Glucosamine *(USAN, rINN).*

Chitosamine; NSC-758. 2-Amino-2-deoxy-β-D-glucopyranose.

$C_6H_{13}NO_5$ = 179.2.

CAS — 3416-24-8.

Glucosamine is found in chitin, mucoproteins, and mucopolysaccharides; it is isolated from chitin or prepared synthetically.

Glucosamine sulphate and hydriodide have been given in the treatment of rheumatic disorders including osteoarthritis (p.2).

References.

1. Anonymous. Glucosamine for osteoarthritis. *Med Lett Drugs Ther* 1997; **39:** 91–2.
2. Barclay TS, *et al.* Glucosamine. *Ann Pharmacother* 1998; **32:** 574–9.
3. da Camara CC, Donless GV. Glucosamine sulfate for osteoarthritis. *Ann Pharmacother* 1998; **32:** 580–7.

Preparations

Proprietary Preparations (details are given in Part 3)
Ger.: Dona 200-S; ***Ital.:*** Dona; ***Spain:*** Hespercorbin; Xicil.

Multi-ingredient: ***Ital.:*** Viartril†; ***Spain:*** Anartril.

Glucose Oxidase (10555-t)

Corylophyline; β-D-Glucopyranose aerodehydrogenase; Microcide; Notatin; P-FAD.

CAS — 9001-37-0.

Glucose oxidase is an enzyme obtained from certain fungi which catalyses the oxidation of glucose to gluconic acid, with the concomitant production of hydrogen peroxide. It is used for its preservative properties as an additive in certain foods, sometimes in combination with catalase (p.1560). It is also used in fertility tests and tests of diabetic control. It has been used as an ingredient of toothpastes for its supposed benefits in the prophylaxis of dental caries.

Preparations

Proprietary Preparations (details are given in Part 3)

Multi-ingredient: ***Austral.:*** Biotene†.

Glucose Tests (1958-q)

Several tests are available so that patients with diabetes mellitus (p.313) can monitor their disease. Tests can be employed to detect the presence of glucose in the urine and some of the preparations are used to detect several substances in the urine. These tests are easy to carry out but are not considered reliable enough for insulin-dependent patients who should ideally check their blood-glucose concentrations using one of the available blood tests. Diabetic clinics often measure the degree of haemoglobin glycosylation as an indicator of mean blood-glucose control over a period of weeks.

Urine tests generally employ either the copper-reduction method or the glucose-oxidase method and both methods produce a colour change in the presence of glucose. Blood tests generally employ the glucose-oxidase method; they may be read visually or by means of a meter. A meter gives the more precise reading. Patients should be properly trained in the use of these tests and in the interpretation of the results; they should be aware that concomitant drug therapy might affect the result.

Preparations

USP 23: Glucose Enzymatic Test Strip.

Proprietary Preparations (details are given in Part 3)
Austral.: Advantage; Ames-BG†; BM-Test BG; BM-Test Glycemie 20-800; Clinistix; Clinitest; Diabur-Test 5000; Diastix; Esprit; Glucofilm; Glucometer; Glucostix; Medi-Test Glucose; Tes-Tape; ***Canad.:*** Accu-Check III/Chemstrip bG; Accutrend GC; Chemstrip bG; Chemstrip uG; Clinistix; Clinitest; Companion 2; Diastix; Easy Strip; Glucofilm; Glucostix; Pen 2†; Tes-Tape; ***Fr.:*** Accu-Chek; BM-Test Glycemie; Clinistix; Clinitest; Dextrostix; Glucofilm; Glucostix; Glucotide; One Touch; Tracer Glucose; ***Irl.:*** BM-Accutest; BM-Test 1-44; Clinistix; Clinitest; Dextrostix; Diabur-Test 5000; Diastix; Glucostix; Glucotide; Hypoguard; Tes-Tape; ***Ital.:*** Accutrend Glucose; BM-Test BG; Clinistix; Clinitest; Dextrostix; Diabe Strip†; Diabur-Test 5000; Diastix; Glico Test; Glico Urine B; Glucofilm; Glucometer; Glucosan; Glucostix; Glukurtest; Haemoglukotest 20-800; Reflocheck; Tes-Tape; ***S.Afr.:*** Clinistix; Clinitest; Dextrostix; Glucose Medi-Test; Glucostix; Glycaemie Medi-Test; Haemo-Glukotest 20-800R; Lenstrip B.G.2; Lenstrip Glucose; Lenstrip Glyco; Tes-Tape; ***Switz.:*** Tes-Tape; ***UK:*** BM-Accutest; BM-Test 1-44; BM-Test BG†; Clinistix; Clinitest; Dextrostix†; Diabur-Test 5000; Diastix; Easistix BG; Easistix UG; Exactech; Glucostix; Glucotide; Hypoguard GA; Medi-Test Glucose; Medi-Test Glycaemie C; Medisense G2; Reflocheck†; Visidex II†; ***USA:*** Accu-Check Advantage; Biotel diabetes; Chemstrip bG; Chemstrip uG; Clinistix; Clinitest; Dextrostix; Diascan; Diastix; First Choice; Glucofilm; Glucostix; One Touch; Tes-Tape†; Tracer bG.

Gluten (12792-h)

A mixture of 2 proteins, gliadin and glutenin, present in wheat flour and to a lesser extent in barley, oats, and rye. Gliadin is a prolamine, one of the 2 chief groups of plant proteins, and glutenin belongs to the other main group termed glutelins

Gluten is of medicinal and pharmaceutical interest in that patients with coeliac disease (p.1330) are sensitive to the gliadin fraction of gluten contained in the normal diet. Treatment consists of the use of gluten-free diets; gluten-free foods are available.

A gluten-free diet may also be beneficial in patients with dermatitis herpetiformis (p.1073).

References to the gluten content of pharmaceutical products and 'gluten-free' foods.

1. Olson GB, Gallo GR. Gluten in pharmaceutical and nutritional products. *Am J Hosp Pharm* 1983; **40:** 121–2.
2. Patel DG, *et al.* Gluten in pills: a hazard for patients with celiac disease. *Can Med Assoc J* 1985; **133**: 114–15.
3. Golightly LK, *et al.* Pharmaceutical excipients: adverse effects associated with 'inactive' ingredients in drug products (part II). *Med Toxicol* 1988; **3**: 209–40.

Glycerol (1901-y)

Glycerol *(rINN).*

E422; Glicerol; Glycerin; Glycerolum. Propane-1,2,3-triol.

$C_3H_8O_3$ = 92.09.

CAS — 56-81-5.

Pharmacopoeias. In *Chin., Eur.* (see p.viii), *Int., Jpn,* and *US.*
Eur. and *Int.* also include Glycerol (85 per cent).
Pol. includes Glycerol (86 per cent).

A clear, colourless or almost colourless, hygroscopic, syrupy liquid, odourless or with a slight odour and with a sweet taste. **Miscible** with water and with alcohol; slightly soluble in acetone; practically insoluble in chloroform, in ether, and in fixed and essential oils. Solutions in water are neutral to litmus. **Store** in airtight containers.

Strong oxidising agents form explosive mixtures with glycerol. Black discoloration has been reported with glycerol and bismuth subnitrate or zinc oxide when exposed to light.

Adverse Effects and Precautions

Glycerol's adverse effects are primarily due to its dehydrating action.

When taken by mouth glycerol may cause headache, nausea, and vomiting; less frequently diarrhoea, thirst, dizziness, and mental confusion can occur. Cardiac arrhythmias have been reported.

Glycerol increases plasma osmolality resulting in the withdrawal of water from the extravascular spaces. The consequent expansion of extracellular fluid, especially if sudden, can lead to circulatory overload, pulmonary oedema, and congestive heart failure; glycerol must therefore be used with caution in patients at risk, such as those with hypervolaemia, cardiac failure, or renal disease. Severe dehydration can occur and glycerol should be used cautiously in dehydrated patients. Patients with diabetes mellitus as well as being at risk through any dehydration may develop hyperglycaemia and glycosuria following glycerol's metabolism. Nonketotic hyperosmolar hyperglycaemic coma is rare, but fatalities have been reported.

Haemolysis, haemoglobinuria, and acute renal failure have also been associated with glycerol when administered intravenously.

Glycerol when given topically or rectally can cause irritation. A local anaesthetic may be administered before application of glycerol to the cornea to reduce the likelihood of a painful response.

See above for incompatibilities with glycerol including the risk of explosive mixtures.

Effects on the cardiovascular system. A 73-year-old man, free of cardiac complaints but who had previously experienced an acute myocardial infarction, developed severe pulmonary oedema following the administration of glycerol by mouth for elevated intra-ocular pressure.[1] The necessity for detailed cardiac evaluation before the use of oral glycerol was emphasised.

1. Almog Y, *et al.* Pulmonary edema as a complication of oral glycerol administration. *Ann Ophthalmol* 1986; **18:** 38–9.

Effects on the ears. A report of temporary hearing loss in the noninvolved ear of a 56-year-old man following the ingestion of 100 mL of glycerol and 100 mL of normal saline solution as part of a glycerol test for Ménière's disease, and a review of two previous reports associating the glycerol test with a deterioration in hearing.[1]

1. Mattox DE, Goode RL. Temporary loss of hearing after a glycerin test. *Arch Otolaryngol* 1978; **104:** 359–61.

Effects on the eyes. Studies in *animals*[1] and in *man*[2] have indicated that the topical application of glycerol to the eye can damage the endothelial cells of the cornea. Caution in applying glycerol to the cornea has been recommended.

1. Sherrard ES. The corneal endothelium in vivo: its response to mild trauma. *Exp Eye Res* 1976; **22:** 347–57.
2. Goldberg MH, *et al.* The effects of topically applied glycerin on the human corneal endothelium. *Cornea* 1982; **1:** 39–44.

Hyperosmolar nonketotic coma. Hyperosmolar nonketotic coma have been associated with the administration of glycerol by mouth[1] and deaths have occurred.[2] The most susceptible patients are maturity-onset elderly diabetics with acute or chronic disease predisposing to fluid deprivation, and in these patients oral glycerol may be best avoided.[1] If glycerol is used in patients with predisposing conditions, adequate measures should be taken to recognise the development of hyperosmolar nonketotic hyperglycaemia and prevent dehydration.[1,2]

1. Oakley DE, Ellis PP. Glycerol and hyperosmolar nonketotic coma. *Am J Ophthalmol* 1976; **81:** 469–72.
2. Sears ES. Nonketotic hyperosmolar hyperglycemia during glycerol therapy for cerebral edema. *Neurology* 1976; **26:** 89–94.

Pharmacokinetics

Glycerol is readily absorbed from the gastro-intestinal tract and undergoes extensive metabolism, principally in the liver; it may be used in the synthesis of lipids, metabolised to glucose or glycogen, or oxidised to carbon dioxide and water. It may also be excreted in the urine unchanged.

References.

1. Nahata MC, *et al.* Variations in glycerol kinetics in Reye's syndrome. *Clin Pharmacol Ther* 1981; **29:** 782–7.
2. Heinemeyer G. Clinical pharmacokinetic considerations in the treatment of increased intracranial pressure. *Clin Pharmacokinet* 1987; **13:** 1–25.

Uses and Administration

Glycerol is an osmotic dehydrating agent with hygroscopic and lubricating properties. When administered by mouth or parenterally, glycerol increases the plasma osmolality resulting in the movement of water by osmosis from the extravascular spaces into the plasma. There can be problems of palatability when glycerol solutions are given by mouth; chilling or flavouring the solutions may help.

Glycerol is given by mouth for the short-term reduction of vitreous volume and intra-ocular pressure before and after ophthalmic surgery and as an adjunct in the management of acute glaucoma (p.1387). Its onset of action is rapid with a maximal reduction in intra-ocular pressure occurring approximately 1 to 1½ hours after administration; the duration of action is about 5 hours. The usual initial dose of glycerol is 1 to 1.5 g per kg body-weight administered as a 50% or 75% solution; further doses of 0.5 g per kg may be given if necessary.

Glycerol may be applied topically to reduce corneal oedema but as the effect is only transient its use is primarily limited to facilitating ocular examination and diagnosis. Glycerol eye drops can be painful on instillation and the prior application of a local anaesthetic has been recommended.

Glycerol has also been given by mouth or intravenously to reduce intracranial pressure (see below).

Glycerol may be administered rectally as suppositories or a solution in single doses to promote faecal evacuation in the management of constipation (p.1168). It usually acts within 15 to 30 minutes. Glycerol is commonly classified as an osmotic laxative but may act additionally or alternatively through its local irritant effects; it may also have lubricating and faecal softening actions.

Glycerol is used as a demulcent in cough preparations (p.1052).

It has a wide range of applications in pharmaceutical formulation; these include the use of glycerol as a vehicle and solvent, a sweetening agent, a preservative in some liquid medications, a plasticiser in tablet film-coating, and as a tonicity adjuster. It is often included in topical preparations such as eye drops, creams, and lotions as a lubricant and also for its moisturising properties since when absorbed, its hygroscopic action may enhance moisture retention. Ear drops for the removal of ear wax often contain glycerol as a lubricating and softening agent.

Glycerol is also used as a cryoprotectant in cryopreservation.

Diagnosis of Ménière's disease. Glycerol has been used in the diagnosis of Ménière's disease, although the test can have problems.[1-3] The aim is to distinguish potentially reversible cochlear dysfunction from the relatively irreversible pathology found in the advanced stages of the disease or to predict the hearing results following endolymphatic sac surgery. The test involves the administration of glycerol by mouth to reduce the endolymphatic fluid volume and pressure and the measurement of any transient improvement in hearing. However, the side-effects of glycerol such as headache, nausea, and vomiting can be a problem and the test has been reported to have low sensitivity and to give false-positive results. See also under Effects on the Ears under Adverse Effects, above.

1. Brookes GB. Ménière's disease: a practical approach to management. *Drugs* 1983; **25:** 77–89.
2. Skalabrin TA, Mangham CA. Analysis of the glycerin test for Meniere's disease. *Otolaryngol Head Neck Surg* 1987; **96:** 282–8.
3. Norris CH. Drugs affecting the inner ear: a review of their clinical efficacy, mechanisms of action, toxicity, and place in therapy. *Drugs* 1988; **36:** 754–72.

Raised intracranial pressure. Glycerol has been given intravenously or by mouth for its osmotic diuretic effect to reduce cerebral oedema and hence decrease the intracranial pressure (p.796). It is also reported to be able to increase blood flow to areas of brain ischaemia. It has been used in a variety of clinical conditions[1] including cerebral infarction or stroke,[2-6] Reye's syndrome,[7] and meningitis;[8] it has been reported to be ineffective in hepatic coma.[9] Some patients have experienced serious adverse effects including haemolysis, haemoglobinuria, and renal failure.[10,11]

1. Frank MSB, *et al.* Glycerol: a review of its pharmacology, pharmacokinetics, adverse reactions, and clinical use. *Pharmacotherapy* 1981; **1:** 147–60.
2. Meyer JS, *et al.* Treatment with glycerol of cerebral oedema due to acute cerebral infarction. *Lancet* 1971; **ii:** 993–7.
3. Mathew NT, *et al.* Double-blind evaluation of glycerol therapy in acute cerebral infarction. *Lancet* 1972; **ii:** 1327–9.
4. Gilsanz V, *et al.* Controlled trial of glycerol versus dexamethasone in the treatment of cerebral oedema in acute cerebral infarction. *Lancet* 1975; **i:** 1049–51.
5. Larsson O, *et al.* Double-blind trial of glycerol therapy in early stroke. *Lancet* 1976; **i:** 832–4.
6. Bayer AJ, *et al.* Double-blind randomised trial of intravenous glycerol in acute stroke. *Lancet* 1987; **i:** 405–8.
7. Nahata MC, *et al.* Variations in glycerol kinetics in Reye's syndrome. *Clin Pharmacol Ther* 1981; **29:** 782–7.
8. Kilpi T, *et al.* Oral glycerol and intravenous dexamethasone in preventing neurologic and audiologic sequelae of childhood bacterial meningitis. *Pediatr Infect Dis J* 1995; **14:** 270–8.
9. Record CO, *et al.* Glycerol therapy for cerebral oedema complicating fulminant hepatic failure. *Br Med J* 1975; **ii:** 540.
10. Hägnevik K, *et al.* Glycerol-induced haemolysis with haemoglobinuria and acute renal failure: report of three cases. *Lancet* 1974; **i:** 75–7.
11. Welch KMA, *et al.* Glycerol-induced haemolysis. *Lancet* 1974; **i:** 416–17.

Trigeminal neuralgia. Selective destruction of pain bearing nerves is reserved for patients who do not respond to conventional drug therapy for trigeminal neuralgia (p.12). This may be achieved by the instillation of glycerol among the trigeminal rootlets (percutaneous retrogasserian glycerol rhizolysis).[1-4] However, the efficacy and safety of this procedure are debatable.[1,4] It has been suggested that variations in viscosity and osmolality may influence results.[2]

1. Sweet WH. The treatment of trigeminal neuralgia (tic douloureux). *N Engl J Med* 1986; **315:** 174–7.
2. Waltz TA, Copeland BR. Treatment of trigeminal neuralgia. *N Engl J Med* 1987; **316:** 693.
3. Young RF. Glycerol rhizolysis for treatment of trigeminal neuralgia. *J Neurosurg* 1988; **69:** 39–45.
4. Burchiel KJ. Percutaneous retrogasserian glycerol rhizolysis in the management of trigeminal neuralgia. *J Neurosurg* 1988; **69:** 361–6.

Preparations

BP 1998: Glycerol Suppositories; Phenol and Glycerol Injection; ***USP 23:*** Calamine Lotion; Glycerin Ophthalmic Solution; Glycerin Oral Solution; Glycerin Suppositories.

Proprietary Preparations (details are given in Part 3)
Aust.: Babylax; ***Canad.:*** Alpha Keri; Gly-Rectal; ***Fr.:*** Bebegel; Glycerotone; ***Ger.:*** Babylax; Glycerosteril; Glycilax; Milax; ***Irl.:*** Babylax; ***Ital.:*** Microclisma Evacuante AD-BB; Microclismi Marco Viti; Microclismi Sella; Verolax; ***Jpn:*** Glyceol; ***S.Afr.:*** Babylax†; Regard; ***Spain:*** Glicerotens; Obifax†; Supo Gliz; Supo Kristal; Vitrosups; ***Switz.:*** Bulboid; Cristal; Practomil; ***USA:*** Dry Eye Therapy; Eye-Lube-A; Fleet Babylax; Glyrol; Listermint Arctic Mint Mouthwash; Ophthalgan; Osmoglyn; Sani-Supp.

Multi-ingredient: ***Austral.:*** Aci-Jel; Acnederm Wash; Anusol; Auralgan; Cleansing Lotion; Egozite Cream†; Emidote APF†; Hamilton Skin Lotion; Magnoplasm; Nutrasorb; Soothe'n Heal; ***Belg.:*** Laxavit; ***Canad.:*** Aci-Jel†; Agarol; Agarol Plain; Auralgan; Bronchex; Bronchisaft; Collyrium; Epi-Lyt; Moisture Drops; Swim-Ear; Tucks; ***Fr.:*** Aloplastine; Aloplastine Acide†; Aloplastine Ichthyolee†; Denisoline; Edulcor sans sucre†; Glyco-Thymoline; Humex†; Pharmatex; Rectopanbiline; Scleremo; ***Ger.:*** Adebilan†; Akne-Pyodron lokal†; Duoform-Balsam†; Lacrisic; Lotio Hermal†; Pero; Tussinfantum†; Warondo-Flechtensalbe†; ***Irl.:*** Micolette; ***Ital.:*** Dropyal; Evasen Dischetti; Glicerolax; Novilax; Salviette H; Solecin; ***S.Afr.:*** Plastolin Poultice†; ***Spain:*** Boydenex†; Fagolitos Renal†; ***Swed.:*** Aci-Jel†; ***Switz.:*** Aloplastine Acide†; Aloplastine simple†; Astroglide†; Decongestine†; Neo-Decongestine†; Realderm; ***UK:*** Adiantine; Audinorme†; Bronal†; Codella; Collins Elixir Pastilles; Earex Plus; Honey & Molasses; Imuderm; Lemsip Chesty Cough; Lemsip Dry Tickly Cough; Lemsip Linctus†; Melissin; Meltus Honey & Lemon; Micolette; Neutrogena Dermatological Cream; Relaxit; Throaties Family Cough Linctus; ***USA:*** Aci-Jel; Allergen; Americaine Otic; Astroglide; Auralgan; Clearasil Antibacterial; Collyrium Fresh; Dermasil; Epilyt; Hemorid For Women; Lubrin; Maxilube; Moisture Drops; N'ice; Numzit; Phenaseptic†; Surgel; Swim-Ear; Therevac Plus; Therevac SB; Trimo-San; Triple Care Cleanser; Tucks.

Glycerophosphoric Acid (1935-d)

Glycerylphosphoric Acid; Monoglycerylphosphoric Acid.

$C_3H_9O_6P$ = 172.1.

CAS — 27082-31-1; 57-03-4 (α-form); 17181-54-3 (β-form); 5746-57-6 (L-α-form); 1509-81-5 (DL-α-form).

Glycerophosphoric acid and various glycerophosphates have been used in tonics. They were once considered as a suitable means of providing phosphorus. Calcium and magnesium glycerophosphates are described in the Electrolytes chapter as they may be considered as a source of calcium and magnesium respectively.

References to the use of sodium glycerophosphate as a source of phosphorus in infant parenteral nutrition.[1]

1. Costello I, *et al.* Sodium glycerophosphate in the treatment of neonatal hypophosphataemia. *Arch Dis Child* 1995; **73:** F44–5.

Preparations

Proprietary Preparations (details are given in Part 3)
Aust.: Glycophos; ***Neth.:*** Glycophos†; ***Swed.:*** Glycophos†; ***Switz.:*** Glycophos.

Multi-ingredient: ***Belg.:*** Neo Genyl†; Verrulyse-Methionine; ***Fr.:*** Biotone; Ionyl; Phosphore-Sandoz; Verrulyse-Methionine; ***Ger.:*** B 12 Nervinfant†; Eupronerv†; Nervinfant†; ***Ital.:*** Calciofix; Cobalton†; Glicero-Valerovit; Gliviton†; Neuroftal; Neurol; Nevrostenina B12†; Piruvasi†; ***S.Afr.:*** Nervade; ***Switz.:*** Glutadouze†.

Glyceryl Palmitostearate (17666-y)

A mixture of mono- di- and triglycerides of C_{16} and C_{18} fatty acids.

CAS — 8067-32-1.

Glyceryl palmitostearate is used in pharmaceutical manufacturing as a diluent and lubricant for tablets and capsules.

Gold (5292-y)

E175.

Au = 196.96655.

CAS — 7440-57-5.

A bright-yellow, malleable, and ductile metal; the finely divided powder may be black, ruby, or purple.

The main use of metallic gold in health care is now in dentistry. Gold may also be employed as a colouring agent for some foodstuffs. In the treatment of rheumatoid arthritis, gold is used in the form of compounds such as auranofin (p.19), aurothioglucose (p.20), and sodium aurothiomalate (p.83). The radionuclide gold-198 is described in the chapter on radiopharmaceuticals (p.1423). There have been rare reports of hypersensitivity reactions to metallic gold.

Gold is used (as Aurum or Aurum Met.) in homoeopathic medicine. Gold salts are also used in homoeopathy.

References.

1. Merchant B. Gold, the noble metal and the paradoxes of its toxicology. *Biologicals* 1998; **26:** 49–59.

Preparations

Proprietary Preparations (details are given in Part 3)
USA: Aurasol.

Multi-ingredient: ***Fr.:*** Biocarde; ***Ger.:*** Cefossin H.

Gossypol (12798-p)

2,2′-Bis(1,6,7-trihydroxy-3-methyl-5-isopropylnaphthalene-8-carboxaldehyde).

$C_{30}H_{30}O_8$ = 518.6.

CAS — 303-45-7.

Gossypol is a pigment extracted from cottonseed oil (p.1567).

Because of its antispermatogenic activity, gossypol has been studied, especially in China, as a male contraceptive. It has also been investigated for its antineoplastic, antiprotozoal, antiviral, and spermicidal activity and has been studied in women in the treatment of certain gynaecological disorders.

Side-effects have included fatigue, changes in appetite, gastro-intestinal effects, burning sensation of the face and hands, some loss of libido, and persistent oligospermia. Hypokalaemia has occurred.

The pharmacology and therapeutic potential of gossypol have been reviewed.[1] Controlled studies have shown gossypol to be an effective male contraceptive.[2,3] These studies involved administration of gossypol in an initial dose of 20 mg daily by mouth for 2.5 or 4 months followed by weekly maintenance doses of 50 or 60 mg respectively. Unfortunately hypokalaemia may be a problem that neither the use of potassium supplements nor potassium-conserving diuretics can remedy.[4] Development of an acceptable and effective male oral contraceptive has yet to achieve comparable success to that in women (p.1434).

1. Wu D. An overview of the clinical pharmacology and therapeutic potential of gossypol as a male contraceptive agent and in gynaecological disease. *Drugs* 1989; **38:** 333–41.
2. Coutinho EM, *et al.* Antispermatogenic action of gossypol in men. *Fertil Steril* 1984; **42:** 424–30.
3. Liu G, *et al.* Clinical trial of gossypol as a male contraceptive drug part I: efficacy study. *Fertil Steril* 1987; **48:** 459–61.
4. Liu G, Lyle KC. Clinical trial of gossypol as a male contraceptive drug part II: hypokalemia study. *Fertil Steril* 1987; **48:** 462–5.

Green-lipped Mussel (12983-s)

An extract from the green-lipped mussel *Perna canaliculata* (Mytilidae), stated to contain amino acids, fats, carbohydrates, and minerals, has been promoted for the treatment of rheumatic disorders including rheumatoid arthritis (p.2).

A review of the investigation of green-lipped mussel in the treatment of arthritis has not revealed conclusive evidence of its usefulness.[1]

1. Li Wan Po A, Maguire T. Green-lipped mussel. *Pharm J* 1990; **244:** 640–1

Preparations

Proprietary Preparations (details are given in Part 3)
UK: Lyprinol; Oceantone; Seatone.

Multi-ingredient: ***Austral.:*** Green Lipped Mussel†; Prost-1; Prost-2.

Guaiacum Resin (278-r)

Guaiac; Guaiacum; Guajakharz.

Guaiacum resin is obtained from guaiacum wood (lignum vitae; *Guaiacum officinale* or *G. sanctum*) and has been used in the treatment of rheumatism. It is used in herbal and homoeopathic medicine.

Guaiacum resin is used in the detection of occult blood in the faeces. The accuracy of the guaiacum test has been questioned and some drugs may interfere with the result.

Preparations

Proprietary Preparations (details are given in Part 3)

Multi-ingredient: ***UK:*** Ligvites; Rheumasol; Rheumatic Pain; Rheumatic Pain Remedy; Rheumatic Pain Tablets.

Guaiazulene (1611-m)

1,4-Dimethyl-7-isopropylazulene.

$C_{15}H_{18}$ = 198.3.

CAS — 489-84-9.

Guaiazulene has been reported to have anti-allergic, anti-inflammatory, antipyretic, and antiseptic properties.

Preparations

Proprietary Preparations (details are given in Part 3)
Aust.: Azulen; Azulenal; Garmastan; ***Fr.:*** Azulene†; ***Ger.:*** Garmastan.

Multi-ingredient: ***Aust.:*** Piniment; Piniol†; Spasmo Claim; Tampositorien mit Belladonna; Thrombocid; ***Belg.:*** Agiolax; ***Fr.:*** Cicatryl; Pepsane; ***Ger.:*** Azupanthenol; bioplant-Kinderol†; Blend-a-med Fluid†; Divinal-Bohnen†; Fissan-Azulenpaste†; Hepaticum-Divinal†; Kneipp Gastropressan†; Protitis†; Pulvicrus†; Quartan†; Rectosellan N†; rhino-loges N†; Rhinotussal S Balsam†; Spasmo-Bilicura†; Suczulen compositum†; Suczulen†; Tampositorien B†; Thrombocid; ***Ital.:*** Citroen Action 2 Collutorio†; Citroen Action 2 Dentrificio†; Collyria; ***Spain:*** Anticatarral Alcala Farm; Balneogel; Nani Pre Dental; Predni Azuleno; ***Switz.:*** Pepsane†; Phlogidermil; Phytoberidin; Tampositoires B†; Thrombocid.

Gutta Percha (12809-a)

Gummi Plasticum; Gutt. Perch.

Pharmacopoeias. In US.

The coagulated, dried, purified latex of trees of the genera *Palaquium* and *Payena* and most commonly *Palaquium gutta* (Sapotaceae).

It occurs in lumps or blocks with a slight characteristic odour and is of a brown or greyish-brown to greyish-white colour externally and reddish-yellow or reddish-grey internally with a laminated or fibrous appearance; it is flexible, but only slightly elastic. Practically **insoluble** in water; partly soluble in carbon disulphide and turpentine oil; about 90% soluble in chloroform. **Store** under water. Protect from light.

Gutta percha has been used in various dressings. In dentistry, gutta percha has been used as a filling material and as the basis of compounds for taking dental impressions.

Haematoporphyrin (12811-l)

$C_{34}H_{38}N_4O_6$ = 598.7.
CAS — 14459-29-1.

A red pigment free from iron obtained from haematin.

Haematoporphyrin is an ingredient of preparations promoted as tonics, particularly for the elderly, and has been used in the treatment of mental depression; it has been given by mouth and by intramuscular injection. Derivatives of haematoporphyrin have been used as photosensitisers in the phototherapy of malignant neoplasms (see Porfimer Sodium, p.559).

Preparations

Proprietary Preparations (details are given in Part 3)
Fr.: Hemedonine; ***Ital.:*** Porphyrin†.

Multi-ingredient: ***Aust.:*** KH3; ***Fr.:*** Novitan; ***Ger.:*** KH3; Revicain Comp Plus; ***Ital.:*** Porfirin 12; Tonogen; Vit-Porphyrin; ***S.Afr.:*** Revaton; ***Spain:*** Actilevol C†; Actilevol Orex; KH3 Powel; ***UK:*** KH3.

Hamamelis (311-g)

Amamelide; Hamamelidis; Witch Hazel.

Pharmacopoeias. In *Eur.* (see p.viii).

The dried leaves of *Hamamelis virginiana* (Hamamelidaceae) containing not less than 7% tannins, calculated with reference to the dried drug. It also contains gallic acid, a bitter principle, and a trace of volatile oil. **Protect** from light.

Hamamelis has astringent properties. It is used in ointments and suppositories in the treatment of haemorrhoids (p.1170). Hamamelis water is used as a cooling application and has been applied as a haemostatic.

Hamamelis, from various parts of the plant, is used in herbal or homoeopathic preparations for a variety of disorders.

Preparations

USP 23: Witch Hazel.

Proprietary Preparations (details are given in Part 3)
Aust.: Hametum; ***Austral.:*** Optrex; Witch Doctor; Witch Stik; ***Canad.:*** Preparation H Cleansing Pads; ***Ger.:*** Aescorin N; F 99 Sulgan N; Haemo Duoform; Hamasana; Hametum; Hamevis†; Pellit Sonnenbrand; Posterine; Tampositorien H; Venoplant; Virgamelis; ***Irl.:*** Optrex; ***Ital.:*** Acqua Virginiana; ***Spain:*** Optrex; ***Switz.:*** Hametum; Hametum-N; ***UK:*** I-Doc; Optrex; Witch Doctor; Witch Sunsore; ***USA:*** A-E-R; Fleet Medicated Pads; Mediconet; Neutrogena Drying; Tucks†.

Multi-ingredient: ***Aust.:*** Arnicet; Felix; Inotyol; Mirfulan; Robugen-Kamillensalbe†; St Radegunder Tee gegen Durchfall; Sulgan 99; Tampositorien mit Belladonna; Varicylum; ***Austral.:*** Acacia Complex†; Anusol; Bioglan Fingers & Toes; Cirflo†; Gentlees; Hamamelis Complex; Hemocane; John Plunkett's Vita-Pore; Optrex Medicated; Proflo; Septacene†; ***Belg.:*** Inotyol; Rectovasol; ***Canad.:*** Onrectal; Penaten; Pommade Midy; Tucks; ***Fr.:*** Aphloine P; Bioveinal†; Canteine Bouteille†; Climaxol; Curoveinyl; Fluon; Hamamelide P†; HEC; Histo-Fluine P; Hyalurectal†; Inotyol; Jouvence de l'Abbe Soury; Mediflor Tisane Circulation du Sang No 12; Mediflor Tisane Hypotensive†; Ophtalmine; Optrex; P. Veinos; Pastilles Monleon; Phytomelis; Pommade Midy†; Posine; Sacnel†; Suppositoires Midy†; Tisane Phlebosedol; Veinostase; Vitalgine; ***Ger.:*** Aescusan; Anisan; Bagnisan med Heilbad; Bagnisan S med Rheumabad†; Bryonia-Strath†; Chlorophyllin Salbe "Schuh"; Chlortesin-N†; derma-loges N; Duoform-Balsam†; Eulatin NN; Hametum-N; Heparchofid S†; Heweven P 3; Heweven P 7; Jatamansin†; Jossathromb†; Kneipp Gastropressan†; Leukona-Wundsalbe; Mirfulan; Palatol N; Palatol†; Pascovenol novo; Pascovenol S†; Perkamillon†; Rephastasan†; Rheuma-Pasc N; Sagittaproct; Secerna†; Siozwo N; Tamposit†; Tampositorien B†; Thermazet†; Trauma-cyl; Ulcotest†; varico sanol Beincreme†; varico sanol forte†; Varicylum S; Vasesana-Vasoregulans; Venacton; Vulnoagil†; ***Ital.:*** Betullosin†; Castindia; Dermitina; Dermoprolyn; Elisir Depurativo Ambrosiano; Emocicatrol†; Facocinerin†; Fluiven; Ginkgo Plus; Gocce D'Erbe†; Hamamilla; Herbe; Inotyol; Lucisan; Lycia Luminique; Milupa Neo†; Neo Topico Giusto; Optrex; Otazul; Pomata Midy HC; Pomata Midy†; Sacnel; Salviette H; Steril Zeta; Supposte Midy†; Varicogel; Venoplant†; Venoplus; Venotrauma; Venovit; ***Neth.:*** Venoplant†; ***S.Afr.:*** Lacto Calamine; ***Spain:*** Antihemorroidal†; Banoftal; Hemodren Compuesto; Hemostatico Antisep Asen; Inotyol†; Lamnotyl; Ojosbel; Ojosbel Azul; Roidhemo; Sol Schoum; Venoplant; ***Switz.:*** Anal-Gen; Collypan; Demo gouttes pour les yeux No 1†; Escothyol†; Frigoplasma; Haemocortin; Haemolan; HEC; Oculosan; Oculosan forte; Optazine; Optrex; Perkamillon; Phlogidermil; Pommade Po-Ho N A Vogel; Proctalgen; Riccomycine; Riccovitan; Sulgan; Tampositoires B†; ***UK:*** Adiantine; Heemex; Kleer Cream; Lacto Calamine; Optrex Clear Eyes; Optrex Eye Dew; Pennine†; Swarm; Varicose Ointment; Vital Eyes; ***USA:*** Clearasil Double Clear; Gentz†; Succus Cineraria Maritima; Tucks.

Harmaline (5015-z)

3,4-Dihydroharmine.
$C_{13}H_{14}N_2O$ = 214.3.
CAS — 304-21-2.

An alkaloid obtained from peganum, the dried seeds of *Peganum harmala* (Zygophyllaceae).

Harmine (5016-c)

7-Methoxy-1-methyl-9*H*-pyrido[3,4-*b*]indole.
$C_{13}H_{12}N_2O$ = 212.2.
CAS — 442-51-3.

An alkaloid obtained from peganum, the dried seeds of *Peganum harmala* (Zygophyllaceae).

Harmine is identical with an alkaloid known as banisterine or telepathine obtained from *Banisteria caapi* (Malpighiaceae).

A hallucinogenic drink which is known in the Western Amazonian regions as 'caapi' (Brazil and Colombia), 'Yagé' (Colombia), and 'ayahuasca' (Ecuador, Peru, and Bolivia), is made from closely related plants of the family Malpighiaceae. The main active principles are harmine and harmaline. It has no therapeutic use.

Helonias (12135-z)

Blazing Star; Chamaelirium; False Unicorn; Starwort.

Helonias is the root of *Chamaelirium luteum* (*Helonias dioica*)(Liliaceae). It is used in herbal medicine.

Preparations

Proprietary Preparations (details are given in Part 3)

Multi-ingredient: ***UK:*** Helonias Compound.

Henna (12817-a)

Henna Leaf; Lawsonia.

The dried leaves of *Lawsonia inermis* (= *L. alba*) (Lythraceae), containing lawsone (see p.1594).

Powdered henna is used for dyeing the hair and skin.

Heptaminol Hydrochloride (12819-x)

Heptaminol Hydrochloride *(BANM, rINNM).*

RP-2831. 6-Amino-2-methylheptan-2-ol hydrochloride.

$C_8H_{19}NO,HCl$ = 181.7.

CAS — 372-66-7 (heptaminol); 543-15-7 (heptaminol hydrochloride).

Pharmacopoeias. In *Fr.*

Heptaminol hydrochloride is a cardiac stimulant and vasodilator and has been given in the treatment of cardiovascular disorders. Heptaminol and heptaminol adenosine phosphate have also been used.

Preparations

Proprietary Preparations (details are given in Part 3)
Belg.: Hept-A-Myl; ***Fr.:*** Ampecyclal; Hept-A-Myl; ***Ger.:*** eoden†; ***Ital.:*** Coreptil.

Multi-ingredient: ***Aust.:*** Thilocombin; ***Fr.:*** Debrumyl; Ginkor Fort; ***Ger.:*** Normotin-P†; Normotin-R; Orthoheptamin†; Perivar N; Ton-O_2 (Tonozwei)†; Veno-Hexanicit; Veno-Tebonin N; ***Spain:*** Denubil; Largatrex.

Herniaria (12820-y)

Bruchkraut; Herba Herniariae; Herniary; Rupture-wort.

Pharmacopoeias. In *Aust.*

The dried leaves and flowering tops of various species of rupture-wort, chiefly *Herniaria glabra* and *H. hirsuta* (Caryophyllaceae).

Herniaria has astringent and diuretic properties and has been given by mouth, usually as an infusion, in urinary-tract disorders.

Preparations

Proprietary Preparations (details are given in Part 3)

Multi-ingredient: ***Aust.:*** Blasen-Tee; Blasentee; Krauterhaus Mag Kottas Blasentee; Krauterhaus Mag Kottas Nierentee; Mag Kottas Entwasserungstee; Mag Kottas Nieren-Blasentee; St Radegunder Nierentee; Uropurat; ***Ger.:*** Buccotean TF†; Buccotean†; Diureticum-Medice†; Hernia-Tee; Herniol; Nephrisol†; Nephrubin; Nieren-Tee†; Urodil N†; Urodil S†.

Hexylene Glycol (18345-b)

2-Methyl-2,4-pentanediol.
$C_6H_{14}O_2$ = 118.2.
CAS — 107-41-5.
Pharmacopoeias. In *USNF.*

A clear, colourless, viscous liquid which absorbs moisture when exposed to moist air. **Miscible** with water, alcohol, ether, chloroform, acetone, and many other organic solvents. **Store** in airtight containers.

Hexylene glycol has properties similar to those of propylene glycol (p.1622). It is used as a pharmaceutical aid.

Histamine (2132-t)

2-(Imidazol-4-yl)ethylamine.
$C_5H_9N_3$ = 111.1.
CAS — 51-45-6.

Histamine Dihydrochloride (2133-x)

Histamine Dihydrochloride *(USAN).*

Histamine Hydrochloride; Histamini Dihydrochloridum.

$C_5H_9N_3,2HCl$ = 184.1.
CAS — 56-92-8.

Pharmacopoeias. In *Eur.* (see p.viii).

Hygroscopic, colourless crystals or white crystalline powder. Histamine hydrochloride 1.66 mg is approximately equivalent to 1 mg of histamine. Very **soluble** in water; soluble in alcohol; practically insoluble in ether. A 5% solution in water has a pH of 2.85 to 3.60. **Protect** from light.

Histamine Phosphate (2134-r)

Histamine Acid Phosphate; Histamine Diphosphate; Histamini Phosphas.

$C_5H_9N_3,2H_3PO_4,H_2O$ = 325.2.

CAS — 51-74-1 (anhydrous histamine phosphate).

Pharmacopoeias. In *Eur.* (see p.viii). *US* specifies the anhydrous substance.

Colourless, odourless, long prismatic crystals; stable in air but affected by light. Histamine phosphate (anhydrous) 2.76 mg or histamine phosphate monohydrate 2.93 mg is approximately equivalent to 1 mg of histamine.

Soluble 1 in 4 of water; slightly soluble in alcohol. A 5% solution in water has a pH of 3.75 to 3.95.

Store in airtight containers. Protect from light.

Stability. A study concluded that solutions of histamine phosphate could be sterilised by heating in an autoclave with little degradation.[1] Autoclaved solutions could be stored for a minimum of 4 months.

1. McDonald C, *et al.* Stability of solutions of histamine acid phosphate after sterilization by heating in an autoclave. *J Clin Pharm Ther* 1990; **15:** 41–4.

Adverse Effects and Treatment

Injection of histamine salts can produce a range of adverse effects that includes headache, flushing of the skin, general vasodilatation with a fall in blood pressure, tachycardia, bronchial constriction and dyspnoea, visual disturbances, vomiting, diarrhoea, and other gastro-intestinal effects. These reactions may be serious and excessive dosage can produce collapse and shock, and may be fatal. Reactions may occur at the injection site.

Some of these effects may be relieved by an antihistamine, but adrenaline may be required and should always be available.

Precautions

Histamine salts should be used with care in patients with asthma or other hypersensitivity disorders, in elderly patients, and in patients with cardiovascular disorders.

Pharmacokinetics

Histamine salts exert a rapid, though transient, effect when given parenterally. Histamine is rapidly metabolised by methylation and oxidation; the metabolites are excreted in the urine.

Uses and Administration

Histamine causes stimulation of smooth muscle, especially of the bronchioles, and lowers blood pressure by dilating the arterioles and capillaries. It also stimulates exocrine gland secretion, especially the gastric glands.

Intradermal injection of histamine produces the characteristic 'triple response' of erythema, flare, and wheal. This is utilised as a control response in skin testing for hypersensitivity. Also, since it is mediated in part by axon reflexes, it has been used to test the integrity of sensory nerves, for example in leprosy.

Inhalation of histamine causes bronchoconstriction and is used as a test of bronchial reactivity.

Histamine has also been given subcutaneously to identify the causes of achlorhydria and intravenously in the diagnosis of phaeochromocytoma, but safer tests are generally preferred.

Histamine is included in some combination topical preparations for musculoskeletal disorders.

Preparations

USP 23: Histamine Phosphate Injection.

Proprietary Preparations (details are given in Part 3)

Multi-ingredient: ***Aust.:*** Histaglobin; ***Belg.:*** Algext†; ***Canad.:*** Midalgan; ***Fr.:*** Algipant†; Histaglobinet†; Pneumoplasme a l'Histamine; ***Ger.:*** Algonergt†; GA-301-Redskin 301; Histadestal; Midysalb; Mydalgant†; ***Ital.:*** Istaglobinat†; ***Neth.:*** Cremes Tegen Spierpijnt†; ***S.Afr.:*** Histaglobin; ***Spain:*** Histaglobinet†; ***Switz.:*** Histaglobint†; Methylant†; Midalgan; Radalgin.

Histoplasmin (8040-k)

Pharmacopoeias. In *US.*

A sterile solution containing standardised culture filtrates of the fungus *Histoplasma capsulatum* grown on a synthetic liquid medium; it may contain a suitable antimicrobial. It should be stored at 2° to 8°. The expiry date is not later than 2 years after release from the manufacturer's cold storage.

Histoplasmin, in an intradermal (intracutaneous) dose of 0.1 mL of a 1 in 100 dilution, may be used as an aid to the diagnosis of histoplasmosis. However, the diagnostic value of the test has been questioned and it may interfere with serological tests for histoplasmosis.

Histoplasmin has also been used, in conjunction with other antigens, to assess cell-mediated immunity.

For reference to the use of histoplasmin for anergy testing in HIV-positive patients, see Tuberculins, p.1640.

Preparations

USP 23: Histoplasmin.

Proprietary Preparations (details are given in Part 3)
USA: Histolyn-CYL.

Hyaluronidase (3724-v)

Hyaluronidase *(BAN, rINN).*

Hyaluronidasum.

CAS — 9001-54-1.

Pharmacopoeias. In *Chin., Eur.* (see p.viii), and *US.*

An enzyme which depolymerises the mucopolysaccharide hyaluronic acid. It is prepared from the testes of mammals by a method that has been shown to reduce contamination by known infections agents to acceptable limits; a suitable stabilising agent may be added to the purified preparation.

A white or yellowish-white, powder; Ph. Eur. states that it contains not less than 300 International units per mg. The USP specifies not more than 0.25 μg of tyrosine for each unit of hyaluronidase, i.e. not less than 4000 units of hyaluronidase for each mg of tyrosine.

Soluble in water; practically insoluble in alcohol, in acetone, and in ether. A 0.3% solution in water has a **Store** at 2° to 8° in airtight containers.

Units

The International and USP units are equivalent. One International or USP unit is equivalent to one turbidity-reducing unit or about 3.3 viscosity-reducing units.

Adverse Effects and Precautions

Sensitivity to hyaluronidase occasionally occurs. Hyaluronidase should be administered with caution to patients with infections; because of the danger of spreading infection, the enzyme generally should not be injected into or around an infected area. It has been suggested that the presence of malignancy may similarly be a contra-indication to the use of hyaluronidase. It should not be administered by intravenous injection nor should it be used for anaesthetic procedures in cases of unexplained premature labour. Hyaluronidase should not be applied directly to the cornea. It should not be used to reduce the swelling of bites or stings.

Uses and Administration

Hyaluronidase is an enzyme which reversibly depolymerises hyaluronic acid, a component of the ground substance or tissue cement surrounding cells, thereby temporarily reducing its viscosity and rendering the tissues more readily permeable to injected fluids.

Therapeutically, hyaluronidase is employed to increase the speed of absorption and to diminish discomfort due to subcutaneous or intramuscular injection of fluids, to promote resorption of excess fluids and extravasated blood in the tissues, and to increase the effectiveness of local anaesthesia.

In the UK the usual dose of hyaluronidase to facilitate subcutaneous or intramuscular injection is 1500 units, added directly to the injection. To aid the dispersal of extravasated fluids or blood the same dose is given in 1 mL of Water for Injections into the affected area. Lower doses of hyaluronidase are used in some countries; in the USA the usual dose is one-tenth the UK dose, i.e. 150 units.

In hypodermoclysis, hyaluronidase is used to aid the subcutaneous administration of relatively large volumes of fluids, especially in infants and young children, where intravenous injection is difficult. Care should be taken in the treatment of children to control the speed and total volume administered and to avoid over-hydration. Hyaluronidase may be added to the injection fluid or may be injected into the site before the fluid is administered. In the UK 1500 units of hyaluronidase is generally used for each 500 to 1000 mL of fluid for subcutaneous administration, but again, in the USA 150 units of hyaluronidase is considered adequate for each litre of hypodermoclysis solution.

The diffusion of local anaesthetics is accelerated by the addition of 1500 units (in the USA, 150 units) of hyaluronidase to the anaesthetic solution. This is of value in the reduction of fractures and in pudendal block in midwifery. It has also been used in ophthalmology as an aid to local anaesthesia at recommended doses of 15 units per mL of local anaesthetic solution.

Hyalosidase (GL enzyme) is a highly purified form of hyaluronidase that has been studied in the treatment of myocardial infarction but without much apparent success.

General references.

1. Watson D. Hyaluronidase. *Br J Anaesth* 1993; **71:** 422–5.

Ophthalmic surgery. In a study[1] involving 150 consecutive patients undergoing surgery for senile cataract, retrobulbar anaesthesia with lignocaine 2% solution plus adrenaline 1:100 000 and hyaluronidase 15 units per mL produced successful anaesthesia in 69 of 75 cases (92%), which was significantly better than 42 of 75 treated with lignocaine plus adrenaline alone. Although poor results have been reported from hyaluronidase and a local anaesthetic without adrenaline to restrict local anaesthetic absorption, the use of the enzyme and adrenaline was recommended as an aid to achieving complete ocular akinesia and anaesthesia in cataract surgery. Hyaluronidase has also been used in conjunction with a mixture of bupivacaine and lignocaine for peribulbar anaesthesia, but conflicting results have been reported. In a study[2] in 50 patients, addition of hyaluronidase 25 units per mL of local anaesthetic mixture had no significant effect on time to satisfactory anaesthesia. However, in a second study[3] involving 200 patients, addition of hyaluronidase 50 or 300 units per mL improved the quality of the peribulbar block and, in the case of the higher concentration, also increased the speed of onset.

1. Thomson I. Addition of hyaluronidase to lignocaine with adrenaline for retrobulbar anaesthesia in the surgery of senile cataract. *Br J Ophthalmol* 1988; **72:** 700–2.
2. Prosser DP, *et al.* Re-evaluation of hyaluronidase in peribulbar anaesthesia. *Br J Ophthalmol* 1996; **80:** 827–30.
3. Dempsey GA, *et al.* Hyaluronidase and peribulbar block. *Br J Anaesth* 1997; **78:** 671–4.

Preparations

BP 1998: Hyaluronidase Injection;
USP 23: Hyaluronidase for Injection; Hyaluronidase Injection.

Proprietary Preparations (details are given in Part 3)
Aust.: Neopermease; Permease; ***Austral.:*** Hyalase; ***Canad.:*** Wydase; ***Ger.:*** Hylase; Kinetint†; ***Ital.:*** Jalovist†; Jaluran; ***Neth.:*** Hyason; ***S.Afr.:*** Hyalase; ***UK:*** Hyalase; ***USA:*** Wydase.

Multi-ingredient: ***Aust.:*** Lasonil; Lemuval; ***Austral.:*** Lasonil; ***Belg.:*** Lasonil; ***Fr.:*** Hyalurectalt†; Lasonil; ***Ger.:*** Lasonil; Neurotropan-Hyt†; ***Ital.:*** Algolisina; Jalovis; Lasonil; Lasonil H; Laso-proct; Lido-Hyal; ***Neth.:*** Lasonil; ***Spain:*** Lasonil; Oto Difusor; Otocusi Enzimaticot†; ***Switz.:*** Lasonilt†; Lido-Hyal; ***UK:*** Lasonil.

Hydrastine Hydrochloride (12828-r)

6,7-Dimethoxy-3-(5,6,7,8-tetrahydro-6-methyl-1,3-dioxolo[4,5-*g*]isoquinolin-5-yl)isobenzofuran-1(3*H*)-one hydrochloride.

$C_{21}H_{21}NO_6,HCl = 419.9.$

CAS — 118-08-1 (hydrastine); 5936-28-7 (hydrastine hydrochloride).

Hydrastine hydrochloride, the hydrochloride of an alkaloid obtained from *Hydrastis canadensis* (Ranunculaceae), has been reputed to cause uterine contractions and arrest uterine haemorrhage but it is of doubtful value. It was also formerly used in gastro-intestinal disorders. Toxic doses are reported to cause strychnine-like convulsions and relaxation of the gut. Hydrastine has also been used.

Hydrastis (12830-z)

Golden Seal; Hidraste; Hydrast.; Idraste; Yellow Root.

Pharmacopoeias. In *Fr.*

The dried rhizome and roots of golden seal, *Hydrastis canadensis* (Ranunculaceae), containing not less than 1.5% of hydrastine; it also contains the alkaloids berberine and canadine.

Hydrastis was formerly used to check excessive uterine haemorrhage. It is included in some herbal preparations for gastro-intestinal disorders and peripheral vascular disorders. It is used in homoeopathic medicine.

Preparations

Proprietary Preparations (details are given in Part 3)
Ger.: Gingivitol N.

Multi-ingredient: ***Austral.:*** Bilberry Plus; Herbal Cleanse; Hydrastis Complex; Sambucus Complex; Trillium Complex; Urinase; ***Fr.:*** Aphloine P; Climaxol; Curoveinyl; ***Ger.:*** Hepatimed N; ***Spain:*** Sol Schoum; ***Switz.:*** Gingivitolt†; ***UK:*** Fenulin; Golden Seal Compound; Papaya Plus.

Hydrazine Sulphate (12831-c)

$H_6N_2O_4S = 130.1.$

CAS — 302-01-2 (hydrazine); 10034-93-2 (hydrazine sulphate).

Hydrazine sulphate is employed in various industrial processes. It is used in the preparation of hydrazine hydrate which is applied after a solution of platinic chloride for corneal tattooing. It has been tried in the management of cancer-related anorexia and cachexia.

Adverse effects and treatment. References to adverse effects resulting from exposure to hydrazine.[1-4] Pyridoxine has been used in the management of hydrazine intoxication.[5,6]

1. Albert DM, Puliafito CA. Choroidal melanoma: possible exposure to industrial toxins. *N Engl J Med* 1977; **296:** 634–5.
2. Durant PJ, Harris RA. Hydrazine and lupus. *N Engl J Med* 1980; **303:** 584–5.
3. Hydrazine. *Environmental Health Criteria 68.* Geneva: WHO, 1987.
4. Hydrazine health and safety guide. *IPCS Health and Safety Guide 56.* Geneva: WHO, 1991.
5. Kirklin JK, *et al.* Treatment of hydrazine-induced coma with pyridoxine. *N Engl J Med* 1976; **294:** 938–9.
6. Harati Y, Niakan E. Hydrazine toxicity, pyridoxine therapy, and peripheral neuropathy. *Ann Intern Med* 1986; **104:** 728–9.

Anorexia and cachexia. References[1,2] to the use of hydrazine sulphate in patients with anorexia or cachexia associated with cancer.

1. Tayek JA, *et al.* Effect of hydrazine sulphate on whole-body protein breakdown measured by ^{14}C-lysine metabolism in lung cancer patients. *Lancet* 1987; **ii:** 241–4.
2. Loprinzi CL, *et al.* Cancer-associated anorexia and cachexia: implications for drug therapy. *Drugs* 1992; **43:** 499–506.

Hydrochloric Acid (1301-l)

507; Acidum Hydrochloricum; Acidum Hydrochloricum Concentratum; Concentrated Hydrochloric Acid; Salzsäure.

$HCl = 36.46.$

CAS — 7647-01-0.

Pharmacopoeias. In *Chin., Eur.* (see p.viii), *Int.,* and *Jpn* (all specify approximately 35 to 39% w/w). *USNF* specifies 36.5 to 38.0% w/w. *Swiss* also has Acidum Hydrochloricum 25%. *Aust.* also has Acidum Hydrochloricum (19 to 21%). The impure acid of commerce is known as Spirits of Salt and as Muriatic Acid.

A clear, colourless, fuming aqueous solution of hydrogen chloride with a pungent odour. **Store** below 30° in airtight containers of glass or other inert material.

Dilute Hydrochloric Acid (1302-y)

Acidum Hydrochloricum Dilutum; Diluted Hydrochloric Acid; Verdünnte Salzsäure.

Pharmacopoeias. In *Eur.* (see p.viii), *Int., Jpn,* and *Pol.* (all approximately 9.5 to 10.5% w/w). Also in *USNF* (9.5 to 10.5% w/v).

Ph. Eur. specifies 9.5 to 10.5% w/w of HCl prepared by mixing hydrochloric acid 274 g with water 726 g. The USNF specifies 9.5 to 10.5% w/v prepared by mixing hydrochloric acid 226 mL with sufficient water to make 1000 mL. **Store** in airtight containers.

Adverse Effects

Hydrochloric acid is highly irritant and corrosive and ingestion has proved fatal. The corrosive effect causes severe pain. There may be violent vomiting, haematemesis, and circulatory collapse; acids can also produce intravascular coagulation and haemolysis. Ulceration may lead to perforation and patients can suffer strictures and pyloric stenosis. Asphyxiation may result from laryngeal oedema. Inhalation of acid fumes or aspiration of ingested acids may cause pneumonitis.

References.

1. Chlorine and hydrogen chloride. *Environmental Health Criteria 21.* Geneva: WHO, 1982.

Treatment of Adverse Effects

Treatment following ingestion is mainly symptomatic. Careful gastric lavage or aspiration may be performed but emetics must *not* be used. The use of large amounts of water or milk for dilution or neutralising agents such as aluminium hydroxide is controversial; carbonates and bicarbonates should not be used as release of carbon dioxide distends the stomach. Opioid analgesia may be required for pain. Endoscopy should be performed and surgical intervention may be necessary. There is little evidence to support the value of corticosteroids in preventing stricture formation.

Acid burns of the skin should be flooded immediately with water and the washing should be copious and prolonged. Any affected clothing should be removed while flooding is being carried out. For burns in the eye, the lids should be kept open and the eye flushed with a steady stream of water. A few drops of a local anaesthetic solution will relieve lid spasm and facilitate irrigation.

Uses and Administration

Hydrochloric acid has been used as an escharotic. It has been used in the diluted form for the treatment of achlorhydria and other gastro-intestinal disorders. It has also been given intravenously in the management of metabolic alkalosis (p.1147). An acid perfusion test using hydrochloric acid has been used in the diagnosis of oesophageal disorders. When taken orally, it should be sipped through a straw to protect the teeth.

Hydrochloride acid (muriaticum acidum) is used in homoeopathic medicine.

Diagnosis and testing. References and comments on the use of an acid perfusion test in the diagnosis of oesophageal disorders,[1-5] such as gastro-oesophageal reflux disease (p.1170) and oesophageal motility disorders (p.1174). The test involves intra-oesophageal perfusion of 0.1M hydrochloric acid; subsequent development of pain indicates an acid-sensitive oesophagus. This test has also been used in the diagnosis of angina.[2]

1. Sladen GE, *et al.* Oesophagoscopy, biopsy, and acid perfusion test in diagnosis of "reflux oesophagitis". *Br Med J* 1975; **1:** 71–6.
2. Anonymous. Angina and oesophageal disease. *Lancet* 1986; **i:** 191–2.
3. Hewson EG, *et al.* Acid perfusion test: does it have a role in the assessment of non cardiac chest pain? *Gut* 1989; **30:** 305–10.
4. de Caestecker JS, Heading RC. Acid perfusion in the assessment of non-cardiac chest pain. *Gut* 1989; **30:** 1795–7.
5. Howard PJ, *et al.* Acid perfusion is a good screening test for symptomatic oesophageal reflux. *Gut* 1989; **30:** A1445.

Pregnancy. Heartburn during pregnancy may be due to reflux of alkaline duodenal contents. A dilute solution of hydrochloric acid (pH 2) taken after meals and at bedtime produced improvements in heartburn in pregnant women.[1]

1. Anonymous. Heartburn in pregnancy. *Drug Ther Bull* 1990; **28:** 11–12.

Preparations

Proprietary Preparations (details are given in Part 3)
Multi-ingredient: ***Fr.:*** Chloridia†; Elixir Grez Chlorhydropepsique†; ***Ital.:*** Gastro-Pepsin; ***Spain:*** Acidona†.

Hydrofluoric Acid (1311-j)

Fluohydric Acid; Fluoric Acid.

HF = 20.01.

CAS — 7664-39-3.

A solution of hydrogen fluoride in water. Various strengths are used. It attacks glass strongly.

Adverse Effects

As for Hydrochloric Acid, p.1588. Although the corrosive effects of hydrofluoric acid tend to predominate, absorption may produce systemic fluoride poisoning as described under Sodium Fluoride, p.742.

The pain from contact with weak solutions may be delayed, so that the patient is not aware of being burned until some hours later, when the area begins to smart; intense pain then sets in and this may persist for several days. Destruction of tissue proceeds under the toughened coagulated skin, so that the ulcers extend deeply, heal slowly, and leave a scar.

The fumes of hydrofluoric acid are highly irritant.

Treatment of Adverse Effects

For the treatment of hydrofluoric acid burns in the eye, immediate and prolonged flooding of the eye with water is recommended while the eye lids are held open. Anaesthetic eye drops may facilitate lid retraction. In the event of skin burns contaminated clothing or articles should be removed and the skin washed with copious cold water or sodium chloride 0.9%. Irrigation with a solution of a calcium salt, e.g. 1% calcium gluconate, is carried out to convert the fluoride to an insoluble form and so prevent absorption. Milk may be tried if such solutions are not available. A calcium gluconate gel is sometimes used and it may be necessary to infiltrate the affected areas with calcium gluconate intradermally or subcutaneously. Other first-aid measures reported to be effective include prolonged soaks in iced solutions of benzalkonium chloride or benzethonium chloride; iced water has sometimes been used as has iced magnesium sulphate solution. Calcium gluconate should also be given intravenously. Local, or even general, anaesthesia may be needed. Burn eschars should be excised and necrotic tissue debrided.

Hydrofluoric acid passes through finger- and toe-nails without causing any apparent damage; nails will therefore have to be removed or perforated to be able to treat the underlying tissues.

References to the treatment of hydrofluoric acid burns.

1. Browne TD. The treatment of hydrofluoric acid burns. *J Soc Occup Med* 1974; **24:** 80–9.
2. MacKinnon MA. Hydrofluoric acid burns. *Dermatol Clin* 1988; **6:** 67–74.
3. McIvor ME. Acute fluoride toxicity: pathophysiology and management. *Drug Safety* 1990; **5**; 79–85.

Uses

Hydrofluoric acid is used in industry. Its main use has been for the production of fluorocarbons for use as refrigerants and propellants. It has also been used as an ingredient of preparations for glass etching and rust removal.

Hydroquinine Hydrobromide (7850-x)

Dihydrochinin Hydrobromide; Dihydroquinine Hydrobromide; Hydrochinin Hydrobromide; Methylhydrocupreine Hydrobromide. 8α,9R-10,11-Dihydro-6′-methoxycinchonan-9-ol hydrobromide.

$C_{20}H_{26}N_2O_2$,HBr = 407.3.

CAS — 522-66-7 (hydroquinine).

NOTE. Do not confuse with Hydroquinone (p.1083).

Hydroquinine is a derivative of quinine (p.439) used similarly in the treatment of nocturnal muscle cramps. It is given as the hydrobromide in a dose of 200 mg with the evening meal and a further 100 mg at bedtime for 14 days.

Muscle spasm. Quinine and its derivatives such as hydroquinine have traditionally been used for the prevention of nocturnal cramps (p.1303) but there has been concern over their efficacy and potential for adverse effects, especially in the elderly.

References.

1. Jansen PHP, *et al.* Randomised controlled trial of hydroquinine in muscle cramps. *Lancet* 1997; **349:** 528–32.

Preparations

Proprietary Preparations (details are given in Part 3)
Neth.: Inhibin.

Hydroxyamphetamine Hydrobromide

(2067-m)

Hydroxyamphetamine Hydrobromide *(BANM)*.

Hydroxyamfetamine Hydrobromide *(rINNM)*; Bromhidrato de Hidroxianfetamina; Oxamphetamine Hydrobromide. (±)-4-(2-Aminopropyl)phenol hydrobromide.

$C_9H_{13}NO$,HBr = 232.1.

CAS — 103-86-6 (hydroxyamphetamine); 1518-86-1 ((±)-hydroxyamphetamine); 306-21-8 (hydroxyamphetamine hydrobromide); 140-36-3 ((±)-hydroxyamphetamine hydrobromide).

Pharmacopoeias. In US.

A white crystalline powder. Freely **soluble** in water and in alcohol; slightly soluble in chloroform; practically insoluble in ether. Solutions in water have a pH of about 5. **Protect** from light.

Hydroxyamphetamine hydrobromide is a sympathomimetic with an action similar to that of ephedrine (p.1060), but it has little or no stimulant effect on the central nervous system. It was formerly used as a vasopressor and in the management of some cardiac disorders.

In ophthalmology, hydroxyamphetamine hydrobromide has been used in a 1% solution as a mydriatic and in the diagnosis of Horner's syndrome.

Preparations

USP 23: Hydroxyamphetamine Hydrobromide Ophthalmic Solution.

Proprietary Preparations (details are given in Part 3)
USA: Paredrine.

Multi-ingredient: ***USA:*** Paremyd.

Hydroxyapatite (1168-d)

Hydroxyapatite *(BAN)*.

542 (edible bone phosphate). Decacalcium dihydroxide hexakis(orthophosphate).

$3Ca_3(PO_4)_2,Ca(OH)_2$ = 1004.6.

CAS — 1306-06-5.

A natural mineral with composition similar to that of the mineral in bone.

Hydroxyapatite for therapeutic purposes is prepared from bovine bone and contains, in addition to calcium and phosphate, trace elements, fluoride and other ions, proteins, and glycosaminoglycans. It is administered by mouth to patients requiring both calcium and phosphorus supplementation.

Hydroxyapatite with tricalcium phosphate has been used in bone grafts.

Hydroxyapatite derived from marine coral has been used in the construction of orbital implants for use following surgical removal of the eye.

Reference to problems associated with the use of coral-derived orbital implants.[1]

1. Shields CL, *et al.* Problems with the hydroxyapatite orbital implant: experience with 250 consecutive cases. *Br J Ophthalmol* 1994; **78:** 702–6.

A mixture of calcium phosphates with calcium carbonate could be combined to form a paste which could be injected into acute fractures;[1] under physiological conditions the paste hardened within minutes, due to the formation of dahllite, a carbonated apatite, and held the bones in place as it was progressively replaced by living bone.

1. Constantz BR, *et al.* Skeletal repair by in situ formation of the mineral phase of bone. *Science* 1995; **267:** 1796–9.

Preparations

Proprietary Preparations (details are given in Part 3)
Aust.: Ossopan; Ossyl†; Osteogenon; ***Belg.:*** Ossopan†; ***Fr.:*** Ossopan; ***Ger.:*** Allotropat†; Ossopan; ***Irl.:*** Ossopan; ***Ital.:*** Apagen; ***Spain:*** Ossopan; Osteopor; ***Switz.:*** Ossopan; ***UK:*** Ossopan.

Multi-ingredient: ***Spain:*** Osspulvit Vitaminado†.

Hydroxymethylnicotinamide (12835-x)

N-Hydroxymethylnicotinamide; Nicotinylmethylamide. *N*-Hydroxymethylpyridine-3-carboxamide.

$C_7H_8N_2O_2$ = 152.2.

CAS — 3569-99-1.

Pharmacopoeias. In *Pol.*

Hydroxymethylnicotinamide is a cholagogue and has been used in the treatment of various disorders of the gallbladder.

Preparations

Proprietary Preparations (details are given in Part 3)
Multi-ingredient: ***Spain:*** Sambil.

Hydroxyquinoline Sulphate (1614-g)

Chinosolum; Oxichinolini Sulfas; Oxine Sulphate; Oxyquinol; Oxyquinoline Sulfate *(USAN)*; Sulfate d'Orthoxyquinoléine. Quinolin-8-ol sulphate; 8-Quinolinol sulphate.

$(C_9H_7NO)_2,H_2SO_4$ = 388.4.

CAS — 148-24-3 (hydroxyquinoline); 134-31-6 (hydroxyquinoline sulphate).

Pharmacopoeias. In *Fr.* and *Swiss.* Also in *USNF.*

A yellow powder. Very **soluble** in water; slightly soluble in alcohol; freely soluble in methyl alcohol; practically insoluble in acetone and in ether.

Hydroxyquinoline sulphate has properties similar to those of potassium hydroxyquinoline sulphate (p.1621) and has been used similarly in the topical treatment of skin, oropharyngeal, and vaginal disorders.

Hydroxyquinoline salicylate, hydroxyquinoline benzoate, hydroxyquinoline hydrofluoride, and hydroxyquinoline silicofluoride have been used similarly.

Preparations

Proprietary Preparations (details are given in Part 3)
Fr.: Rivacide†; ***Ger.:*** Leioderm; ***Ital.:*** Aftir Shampoo; Bio-Frin†; Oxynol†; ***Neth.:*** Superol.

Multi-ingredient: ***Aust.:*** Racestyptin; ***Austral.:*** Aci-Jel; ***Canad.:*** Aci-Jel†; Dermoplast; ***Fr.:*** Chromargon; Dermacide; Dermster†; Nestosyl; ***Ger.:*** Antimycoticum†; Chinomint Plus†; Chinosol; Chinosol S Vaseline; Leioderm P; Nasalgon†; ***Ital.:*** Foille; Leucorsan; Neo Foille Pomata Disinfettante†; Polvere Disinfettante†; Viderm; ***Neth.:*** Creme bij Wondjes†; ***S.Afr.:*** Dermoplast†; ***Spain:*** Neodesfila; ***Swed.:*** Aci-Jel†; ***Switz.:*** Benzocaine PD; Nasello; Racestyptine; ***USA:*** Aci-Jel; Analgesic Otic Solution; Cuticura†; Medicone Derma; Medicone Dressing; Medicone Rectal; Oxyzal; Sanitube†; Stypto-Caine; Trimo-San; Triv.

Hymecromone (3725-g)

Hymecromone *(USAN, rINN)*.

Imecromone; LM-94. 7-Hydroxy-4-methylcoumarin.

$C_{10}H_8O_3$ = 176.2.

CAS — 90-33-5.

Pharmacopoeias. In *Jpn.*

Hymecromone is a choleretic and biliary antispasmodic. Diarrhoea may occasionally occur. It has been given in doses of 400 mg three times daily before meals. It has also been given by slow intravenous injection as an adjunct to diagnostic procedures.

Preparations

Proprietary Preparations (details are given in Part 3)
Aust.: Cholonerton†; Unichol; ***Belg.:*** Cantabiline; ***Fr.:*** Cantabiline; ***Ger.:*** Biliton H†; Chol-Spasmoletten; Cholonerton†; Chol-

spasmin; Gallo Merz Spasmo; Logomed Galle-Dragees; ***Ital.:*** Cantabilin; ***Spain:*** Bilicanta; ***Switz.:*** Bilicante†.

Multi-ingredient: ***Ger.:*** Cholspasminase†.

Hypericum (314-s)

Millepertuis; St. John's Wort.

CAS — 548-04-9 (hypericin).

Pharmacopoeias. In *Fr., Pol.,* and *Swiss.* Also in *USNF.*

The dried flowering tops or aerial parts of St John's Wort, *Hypericum perforatum* (Hypericaceae), gathered shortly before or during flowering. It contains not less than 0.04% of total hypericins, calculated as hypericin ($C_{30}H_{16}O_8$ = 504.4). **Store** in airtight containers. Protect from light.

Hypericum, in the form of an infusion has been used as an astringent and diuretic. Hypericum is also used in depression (see below).

Hypericum, as well as an oil from the plant, is used in herbal and homoeopathic preparations for a variety of disorders.

The herb contains a red pigment, hypericin, which causes photosensitisation. *Animals* are also sensitive and hypericum poses problems in agriculture. Hypericin has been investigated as an antiviral in the management of AIDS.

Depression. Hypericum extracts are widely used in Germany for the treatment of depression (p.271).

A meta-analysis[1] of randomised trials found hypericum extracts to be more effective than placebo in mild to moderately severe depressive disorders. However, there was insufficient evidence available to establish relative efficacy and tolerability compared with standard antidepressants,[1] although experience from those populations in whom hypericum extracts are widely used suggests that the herb may offer an advantage in terms of relative safety and tolerability.[2] Longer term studies are required before the herb can be recommended in major depression.[2] The mechanism of action of hypericum extracts in the treatment of depression is unclear. Extracts contain at least 10 active principles. Hypericin is one of the major constituents[3] and has been used to standardise hypericum extracts.[2] Hypericin has been shown experimentally to have monoamine oxidase inhibitory activity, although the clinical relevance of this is not clear.[2] Hypericum extracts have also been demonstrated to inhibit the synaptic reuptake of serotonin *in vitro*.[3]

1. Linde K, *et al.* St John's wort for depression—an overview and meta-analysis of randomised clinical trials. *Br Med J* 1996; **313:** 253–8.
2. de Smet PAGM, Nolen WA. St John's wort as an antidepressant. *Br Med J* 1996; **313:** 241–2.
3. Perovic S, Müller WEG. Pharmacological profile of hypericum extract—effect on serotonin uptake by postsynaptic receptors. *Arzneimittelforschung* 1995; **45:** 1145–8.

Preparations

Proprietary Preparations (details are given in Part 3)
Aust.: Psychotonin; ***Ger.:*** Aristoforat; Cesradyston; Divinal Seda; Esbericum; Felis; Herbaneurin; Hewepsychon uno; Hyperforat; Hypericaps; Jarsin; Kira; Kneipp Johanniskrasut-Pflanzensaft N; Kneipp Johanniskraut-Ol N; Kneipp Pflanzendragees Johanniskraut; Lomahypericum; mct Psycho Dragees N; Neuroplant; Neurotisan; Neurovegetalin; Psychatrin†; Psychotonin forte; Psychotonin M; Remotiv; Rephahyval; Rotol; Sedovegan; Spilan; Tonizin; Turineurin; Viviplus; ***Switz.:*** Remotiv; Valverde Hyperval; ***UK:*** Kira.

Multi-ingredient: ***Aust.:*** Eryval; Magentee EF-EM-ES; Nerventee; Species nervinae; Vulpuran; Wechseltee; ***Austral.:*** Infant Tonic; Irontona; Nappy Rash Relief Cream; Vitatona; ***Canad.:*** Cystoforce†; ***Fr.:*** Cicaderma; ***Ger.:*** anabol-loges; Anisan; Arthrodynat P; Befelka-Oel; Castrophan†; Cefaktivon "novum"; Cheihepar†; Cheiranthol; Chelidonium-Strath†; Discmigon; Dolo-cyl; Echtromint†; Gastritol; Gastrol S; Gutnacht; Hepaticum-Divinal†; Hewepsychon duo; Hocura-Spondylose novo; Hyperesa; Hyperforat-forte; Johanniskrautol mit Lecithin; JuCholan S; JuDorm; JuNeuron S; JuViton; Kalantol-A†; Kalantol-B†; Kneipp Krauter Taschenkur Nerven und Schlaf N; Kneipp Magentrost†; Losapan†; Marianon; Menstrualin†; Migranex†; Neurapas; Neuro-Presselin†; Oxacant N; Pan-Nerventonikum†; Phonix Kalophon†; Phytogran; Presselin K 1 N; Psychotonin-sed.; Remifemin plus; Rhoival; Salus Nerven-Schlaf-Tee Nr.22; Salusan; Sedariston; Sedariston Konzentrat; Sinedyston; Ucee†; Valena N; Venacton; Vollmers praparierter gruner; Warondo-Wundsalbe†; Worishofener Nervenpflege Dr. Kleinschrod†; ***Ital.:*** Elisir Depurativo Ambrosiano; ***Switz.:*** Alpina Gel a la consoude; Cetona; Huile de millepertuis A. Vogel (huile de St. Jean); Hyperiforce; Keppur; Malvedrin; Phytoberidin; Phytogran†; Pommade Po-Ho N A Vogel; Saltrates; Saltrates Rodell; Solin S†; Tai Ginseng N; Yakona N.

Hypoglycin A (12837-f)

L-2-Amino-3-(2-methylenecyclopropyl)propionic acid.

$C_7H_{11}NO_2$ = 141.2.

CAS — 156-56-9.

A toxic substance present in the arillus of unripe akee, the fruit of *Blighia sapida* (Sapindaceae).

Hypoglycin A is responsible for Jamaican vomiting sickness, with symptoms of acute and severe vomiting, hypoglycaemia, muscular weakness, CNS depression, convulsions, and coma, frequently fatal. Glycine has been suggested for the management of hypoglycin A toxicity.

Hypophosphorous Acid (1936-n)

Acidum Hypophosphorosum; Phosphinic Acid.

H_3PO_2 = 66.0.

CAS — 6303-21-5; 14332-09-3.

Pharmacopoeias. In *USNF.*

A colourless or slightly yellow odourless liquid, containing 30 to 32% of H_3PO_2. **Store** in airtight containers.

Hypophosphorous acid is used as an antoxidant. Hypophosphates were used in tonics; like the glycerophosphates they are not a suitable source of phosphorus.

Ibogaine (17207-s)

NIH-10567.

Ibogaine is a hallucinogenic indole alkaloid extracted from the West African shrub *Tabernanthe iboga* (Apocynaceae). It has been investigated as an aid to withdrawal from drug addiction.

References.

1. Popik P, *et al.* 100 years of ibogaine: neurochemical and pharmacological actions of a putative anti-addictive drug. *Pharmacol Rev* 1995; **47:** 235–53.

Idazoxan Hydrochloride (16846-s)

Idazoxan Hydrochloride *(BANM, pINNM).*

RX-781094. 2-(2,3-Dihydro-1,4-benzodioxin-2-yl)-2-imidazoline hydrochloride.

$C_{11}H_{12}N_2O_2HCl$ = 240.7.

CAS — 79944-58-4 (idazoxan); 79944-56-2 (idazoxan hydrochloride).

Idazoxan hydrochloride is an α_2-adrenoceptor antagonist under investigation in neurological disorders including depression, dementia, and parkinsonism.

References.

1. Ghika J, *et al.* Idazoxan treatment in progressive supranuclear palsy. *Neurology* 1991; **41:** 986–91.
2. Litman RE, *et al.* Idazoxan, an alpha2 antagonist, augments fluphenazine in schizophrenic patients: a pilot study. *J Clin Psychopharmacol* 1993; **13:** 264–7.
3. Schmidt ME, *et al.* Regional brain glucose metabolism after acute α_2-blockade by idazoxan. *Clin Pharmacol Ther* 1995; **57:** 684–95.

Idebenone (19336-e)

Idebenone *(rINN).*

CV-2619. 2-(10-Hydroxydecyl)-5,6-dimethoxy-3-methyl-*p*-benzoquinone.

$C_{19}H_{30}O_5$ = 338.4.

CAS — 58186-27-9.

Idebenone has been given by mouth in doses of 90 mg daily in divided doses after food in the treatment of mental impairment associated with cerebrovascular disorders. It has also been tried in Alzheimer's disease (p.1386).

References.

1. Weyer G, *et al.* Efficacy and safety of idebenone in the long-term treatment of Alzheimer's disease: a double-blind, placebo controlled multicentre study. *Hum Psychopharmacol Clin Exp* 1996; **11:** 53–65.

Preparations

Proprietary Preparations (details are given in Part 3)
Ital.: Daruma; Mnesis; ***Jpn:*** Avan.

Indeloxazine Hydrochloride (15324-r)

Indeloxazine Hydrochloride *(USAN, rINNM).*

CI-874. (±)-2-[(Inden-7-yloxy)methyl]morpholine hydrochloride.

$C_{14}H_{17}NO_2$,HCl = 267.8.

CAS — 60929-23-9 (indeloxazine); 65043-22-3 (indeloxazine hydrochloride).

Indeloxazine hydrochloride has been reported to improve cerebral function. It has been promoted for the treatment of hypobulia (a lack of volition or drive) and for emotional disturbances associated with cerebrovascular disorders.

Preparations

Proprietary Preparations (details are given in Part 3)
Jpn: Elen.

Indigo Carmine (2135-f)

Blue X; Ceruleinum; CI Food Blue 1; Colour Index No. 73015; Disodium Indigotin-5,5′-disulphonate; E132; FD & C Blue No. 2; Indicarminum; Indigotindisulfonate Sodium; Indigotine; Sodium Indigotindisulphonate. Disodium 3,3′-dioxo-2,2′-bi-indolinylidene-5,5′-disulphonate.

$C_{16}H_8N_2Na_2O_8S_2$ = 466.4.

CAS — 483-20-5 (indigotin-5,5′-disulphonic acid); 860-22-0 (indigo carmine).

NOTE. The name Caerulein has been applied to Ceruletide (p.1561).

Pharmacopoeias. In *Fr., It., Jpn,* and *US.*

A purplish-blue powder or blue granules with a coppery lustre. **Soluble** 1 in 100 of water; slightly soluble in alcohol; practically insoluble in most other organic solvents. **Store** in airtight containers. Protect from light.

Adverse Effects and Precautions

Indigo carmine may cause nausea, vomiting, hypertension, and bradycardia, and occasionally, hypersensitivity reactions such as skin rash, pruritus, and bronchoconstriction. Skin discoloration may occur following administration of large parenteral doses.

A report of fatal cardiac arrest in 2 elderly patients following the administration of indigo carmine 80 mg intravenously.[1] Both had a history of asthmatic bronchitis.

1. Voiry AM, *et al.* Deux accidents mortels lors d'une injection per-opératoire de carmin d'indigo. *Ann Med Nancy* 1976; **15:** 413–19.

Uses and Administration

Following injection indigo carmine is rapidly excreted, principally by the kidneys. It has been used in a test of renal function, but has largely been replaced by agents which give more precise results. It is used as a marker dye, particularly in urological procedures, when it is administered in a usual dose of 40 mg, preferably by intravenous injection but sometimes intramuscularly. It has also been used as a marker dye in amniocentesis.

Indigo carmine has been used as a blue dye in medicinal preparations but it is relatively unstable. It is used as a food colour.

Preparations

USP 23: Indigotindisulfonate Sodium Injection.

Indocyanine Green (2136-d)

Sodium 2-{7-[1,1-dimethyl-3-(4-sulphobutyl)benz[*e*]indolin-2-ylidene]hepta-1,3,5-trienyl}-1,1-dimethyl-1*H*-benz[*e*]indolio-3-(butyl-4-sulphonate).

$C_{43}H_{47}N_2NaO_6S_2$ = 775.0.

CAS — 3599-32-4.

Pharmacopoeias. In *US.*

An olive-brown, dark green, blue-green, dark blue, or black powder, odourless or with a slight odour. It contains not more than 5% of sodium iodide. **Soluble** in water and methyl alcohol; practically insoluble in most other organic solvents. A 0.5% solution in water has a pH of about 6. Aqueous solutions are deep emerald green in colour and are stable for about 8 hours.

Adverse Effects and Precautions

Indocyanine green is reported to be well tolerated. Solutions contain a small amount of sodium iodide and should be used with caution in patients hypersensitive to iodine. Clearance of indocyanine green may be altered by drugs that interfere with liver function.

Hypersensitivity. A report of anaphylactoid reactions to indocyanine green in 3 patients.[1] The authors commented that of 20 reactions that had been reported 9 involved anaphylactoid shock (with 2 subsequent deaths) and 11 involved hypotension or bronchospasm; they suggested that such reactions were dose-dependent and had a non-immune mechanism.

1. Speich R, *et al.* Anaphylactoid reactions after indocyanine-green administration. *Ann Intern Med* 1988; **109:** 345–6.

Pharmacokinetics

After intravenous injection indocyanine green is almost completely bound to plasma protein. It is taken up by the liver and is rapidly excreted unchanged into the bile.

Uses and Administration

Indocyanine green is an indicator dye used for assessing cardiac output and liver function, and for examining the choroidal vasculature in ophthalmic angiography. It is also used to assess blood flow and haemodynamics in various organs including the liver.

The usual dose for cardiac assessment is 5 mg injected rapidly via a cardiac catheter. A suggested dose for children is 2.5 mg, and for infants 1.25 mg. Several doses need to be given to obtain a number of dilution curves. However, the total dose should not exceed 2 mg per kg body-weight.

The usual dose of indocyanine green for testing liver function is 500 μg per kg body-weight intravenously.

Indocyanine green has been employed to assess blood flow to various organs and in other haemodynamic studies. However, some methods of determination of indocyanine green clearance as a measure of liver blood flow have been questioned on the grounds that extraction of the dye by the liver is not complete as is often assumed.[1] Interindividual variability in indocyanine clearance may introduce further error.[2]

There have been reports of the use of indocyanine green to assess cerebral blood flow in children during cardiopulmonary bypass[3] and to measure plasma volume in neonates.[4] In ophthalmology, indocyanine green angiography may have a role in visualising the choroidal circulation.[5]

1. Skak C, Keiding S. Methodological problems in the use of indocyanine green to estimate hepatic blood flow and ICG clearance in man. *Liver* 1987; **7:** 155–62.
2. Bauer LA, *et al.* Variability of indocyanine green pharmacokinetics in healthy adults. *Clin Pharm* 1989; **8:** 54–5.
3. Roberts I, *et al.* Estimation of cerebral blood flow with near infrared spectroscopy and indocyanine green. *Lancet* 1993; **342:** 1425.
4. Anthony MY, *et al.* Measurement of plasma volume in neonates. *Arch Dis Child* 1992; **67:** 36–40.
5. Owens SL. Indocyanine green angiography. *Br J Ophthalmol* 1996; **80:** 263–6.

Preparations

USP 23: Indocyanine Green for Injection.

Proprietary Preparations (details are given in Part 3)
Canad.: Cardio-Green†; ***Ger.:*** Cardio-Green; ICG-Pulsion; ***USA:*** Cardio-Green.

Inhibin (19345-l)

Inhibin is a glycoprotein secreted by the testes and ovaries which has been investigated as a potential contraceptive in both men and women, because of its ability to suppress secretion of follicle-stimulating hormone by the pituitary.

Inosine (12852-r)

Inosine *(rINN)*.

Hypoxanthine Riboside. 6,9-Dihydro-9-β-D-ribofuranosyl-1*H*-purin-6-one.

$C_{10}H_{12}N_4O_5$ = 268.2.

CAS — 58-63-9.

Inosine has been used in the treatment of anaemias and cardiovascular, liver, and skin disorders and has been used as a tonic.

Preparations

Proprietary Preparations (details are given in Part 3)
Spain: Tebertin.

Multi-ingredient: ***Aust.:*** Laevadosin; ***Ger.:*** Dreisalind†; Inosin comp.†; Laevadosin†; ***Ital.:*** Adinepar†; Biocortex†; Emonucleosina Cortex†; Fitepar Cortex†; For Liver; Fruttocal; Liver-Atox Dus†; Liverest†; NE 300†; Neo-Eparbiol; Nucleodoxina†; Redinon Cortex†; Ribocort B12†; Ricoliver†; Ricortex†; Rossocorten†; Rubrocortex†; Vitalion†; ***Spain:*** Boldosal; Duvaline Compositum†; Ibsesal†; Nutracel; Rubrocortin.

Inositol (7877-p)

i-Inositol; *meso*-Inositol. *myo*-Inositol.

$C_6H_{12}O_6$ = 180.2.

CAS — 87-89-8.

Pharmacopoeias. In *Aust., Belg.,* and *Fr.*

Inositol, an isomer of glucose, has traditionally been considered to be a vitamin B substance although it has an uncertain status as a vitamin and a deficiency syndrome has not been identified in man. Sources of inositol include whole-grain cereals, fruits, and plants, in which it occurs as the hexaphosphate, phytic acid. It also occurs in both vegetables and meats in other forms. The usual daily intake of inositol from the diet is about 1 g.

Inositol appears to be involved physiologically in lipid metabolism and has been tried, with little evidence of efficacy, in disorders associated with fat transport and metabolism. It has been investigated in the treatment of depression and anxiety, in diabetic neuropathy, and in respiratory distress syndrome and retinopathy of prematurity. Inositol is an ingredient of numerous vitamin preparations and dietary supplements, and of preparations promoted for a wide variety of disorders.

Neonatal respiratory distress syndrome. Inositol, in quantities equivalent to those supplied in breast milk, has been tried in premature infants with respiratory distress syndrome (p.1025);[1] infants given inositol had improved survival and lower rates of bronchopulmonary dysplasia and retinopathy of prematurity than those given placebo.

1. Hallman M, *et al.* Inositol supplementation in premature infants with respiratory distress syndrome. *N Engl J Med* 1992; **326:** 1233–9.

Preparations

Proprietary Preparations (details are given in Part 3)
Fr.: Hepagrume.

Multi-ingredient: ***Aust.:*** Aslavital†; Lemazol; ***Austral.:*** Ginkgo ACE†; Hair and Skin Formula; Liv-Detox; ***Canad.:*** Amino-Cerv; ***Fr.:*** Liporex†; ***Ger.:*** Hepabionta†; Hepalipon N; Lemazol†; Prohepar†; ***Ital.:*** Boldosten†; Cebran†; Detoxicon†; Enteroton Lassativo†; Equipar†; Glutestere B-Complesso†; Hepatos B12; Neo-Epa†; Pillole Schias†; Politintura Schias†; Porfirin 12; Protidepar 100†; Protidepar†; Vitabil Composto†; ***S.Afr.:*** Hepavite; ***Spain:*** Complidermol; Dertrase; Policolinosil; Tri Hachemina; ***UK:*** Fat-Solv; Lipotropic Factors; ***USA:*** Amino-Cerv.

Interleukin-1 (16853-p)

Catabolin; Endogenous Pyrogen; Haematopoietin-1; IL-1; Leucocyte Endogenous Mediator; Lymphocyte Activating Factor.

A protein produced by monocytes and a variety of other cell types *in vivo* and which may also be produced by recombinant DNA technology.

Two distinct forms interleukin-1α and interleukin-1β are known to exist which interact with the same receptor and appear to have similar biological activities.

Interleukin-1 is one of a number of polypeptides produced by lymphocytes, monocytes, and other cells which are involved in the complex hormonal regulation of immune response, and which are known collectively as cytokines. The term lymphokines has also been used to describe these compounds but is more properly restricted to products of the various lymphocyte subsets, such as interleukin-2 (p.541).

It has been suggested that interleukin-1 may be of value in a wide variety of conditions including burn and wound healing, as an adjuvant to enhance the response to vaccines, and as an adjunct to cancer chemotherapy or radiotherapy for its haematopoietic and possible antitum or activity. Adverse effects include fever, chills, headache, gastro-intestinal disturbances, local erythema at the injection site, hypotension, and CNS effects.

Interleukin-2 is described in the chapter on Antineoplastics and Immunosuppressants (p.541). Other interleukins under investigation include interleukin-3 (p.724) as a haematopoietic; interleukin-4 (IL-4) and interleukin-6 (IL-6) for malignant neoplasms and thrombocytopenia; interleukin-10 for inflammatory disorders; and interleukin-12 for malignant neoplasms and infections. Oprelvekin (p.725) is a recombinant interleukin-11 under investigation in thrombocytopenia.

Pharmacokinetics of some interleukins.

1. Bocci V. Interleukins: clinical pharmacokinetics and practical implications. *Clin Pharmacokinet* 1991; **21:** 274–84.

Interleukin-1 Receptor Antagonists

(19857-y)

IL-1ra; IL-1i; Interleukin-1 Inhibitors.

Anakinra (10702-j)

Anakinra *(USAN, rINN)*.

rhIL-1ra.

CAS — 143090-92-0.

Interleukin-1 (p.1591) is a polypeptide that is involved in the hormonal regulation of immune response. Antagonism of interleukin-1 is under investigation in a range of disorders where interleukin-1 is thought to play a role. A recombinant interleukin-1 antagonist, anakinra, is under investigation in rheumatoid arthritis and has been suggested for the management of graft-versus-host disease in transplant recipients. It was tried in septic shock, but results were disappointing.

References.

1. Fisher CJ, Recombination human interleukin 1 receptor antagonist in the treatment of patients with sepsis syndrome: results from a randomized, double-blind, placebo-controlled trial. *JAMA* 1994; **271:** 1836–43.
2. Campion GV, *et al.* Dose-range and dose-frequency study of recombinant human interleukin-1 receptor antagonist in patients with rheumatoid arthritis. *Arthritis Rheum* 1996; **39:** 1092–1101.

Interleukin-2 Fusion Toxins (19769-y)

Recombinant technology has permitted the production of a number of products in which protein sequences from natural growth factors or cytokines are combined with a toxin. Such products include fusion toxins in which the receptor binding domain of diphtheria toxin is replaced with sequences from interleukin-2, thus producing specific cytotoxicity in cells expressing the interleukin-2 receptor. The interleukin-2 fusion toxins denileukin diftitox (DAB_{389} interleukin-2) and DAB_{486} interleukin-2 are under investigation in a variety of disorders including diabetes mellitus, psoriasis, rheumatoid arthritis, cutaneous T-cell lymphoma and other malignancies, and HIV infection.

References to the use of interleukin-2 fusion toxins.

1. LeMaistre CF, *et al.* Therapeutic effects of genetically engineered toxin (DAB_{486}IL-2) in patient with chronic lymphocytic leukaemia. *Lancet* 1991; **337:** 1124–5.
2. Sewell KL, *et al.* DAB-486-IL-2 fusion toxin in refractory rheumatoid arthritis. *Arthritis Rheum* 1993; **36:** 1223–33.
3. Platanias LC, *et al.* Phase I trial of a genetically engineered interleukin-2 fusion toxin (DAB[486]IL-2) as a 6 hour intravenous infusion in patients with hematologic malignancies. *Leukemia Lymphoma* 1994; **14:** 257–62.
4. Foss FM, *et al.* Chimeric fusion protein toxin DAB(486)IL-2 in advanced mycosis fungoides and the Sezary syndrome: correlation of activity and interleukin-2 receptor expression in a phase II study. *Blood* 1994; **84:** 1765–74.
5. Gottlieb SL, *et al.* Response of psoriasis to a lymphocyte-selective toxin (DAB389IL-2) suggests a primary immune, but not keratinocyte, pathogenic basis. *Nature Med* 1995; **1:** 442–7.

Inulin (2137-n)

Inulin *(BAN)*.

Alant Starch.

CAS — 9005-80-5.

Pharmacopoeias. In *Br.* and *US.*

A polysaccharide obtained from the tubers of *Dahlia variabilis*, *Helianthus tuberosus*, and other genera of the family Compositae. On hydrolysis it yields mainly fructose. It is a white, odourless or almost odourless, hygroscopic, amorphous, granular powder. Slightly **soluble** in cold water, but freely soluble in hot water; slightly soluble in organic solvents. A 10% solution in water has a pH of 4.5 to 7.0. Crystals of inulin may be deposited on storage of the injection; they should be dissolved by heating for not more than 15 minutes before use and the injection cooled to a suitable temperature before administration.

Pharmacokinetics

Inulin is rapidly removed from the circulation following intravenous administration but is not metabolised. A trace may be found in the bile and may cross the placenta, but it is predominantly eliminated in the urine by glomerular filtration without secretion or reabsorption in the renal tubule.

Uses and Administration

Inulin is used intravenously as a diagnostic agent to measure the glomerular filtration rate. Although an accurate test, it is complex to perform and is generally reserved for research purposes.

Polyfructosan, an inulin analogue of lower average molecular weight has been used similarly.

Preparations

BP 1998: Inulin Injection;
USP 23: Inulin in Sodium Chloride Injection.

Proprietary Preparations (details are given in Part 3)
Aust.: Inutest; ***Swed.:*** Inutest; ***Switz.:*** Inutest†.

Iris Versicolor (14052-v)

Blue Flag; Iris Virginica.

The rhizomes of *Iris versicolor* (Iridaceae) are used in herbal and homoeopathic medicine.

Preparations

Proprietary Preparations (details are given in Part 3)

Multi-ingredient: ***UK:*** Blue Flag Root Compound; Catarrh Mixture; Skin Eruptions Mixture.

Isospaglumic Acid (2547-t)

Isospaglumic Acid *(rINN)*.

N-(*N*-Acetyl-L-α-aspartyl)-L-glutamic acid.

$C_{11}H_{16}N_2O_8$ = 304.3.

CAS — 3106-85-2.

Isospaglumic acid is used as the sodium or the magnesium salt in eye drops for allergic eye conditions and in nasal solutions for allergic rhinitis.

Preparations

Proprietary Preparations (details are given in Part 3)
Aust.: Rhinaaxia; ***Belg.:*** Naaxia†; Rhinaaxia†; ***Fr.:*** Naabak; Naaxia; Rhinaaxia; ***Ger.:*** Naaxia; ***Spain:*** Naaxia; ***Switz.:*** Rhinaaxia.

Multi-ingredient: ***Switz.:*** Naaxia Nouvelle formule.

Isoxsuprine Hydrochloride (9246-c)

Isoxsuprine Hydrochloride *(BANM, rINNM)*.

Caa-40; Isoxsuprini Hydrochloridum; Phenoxyisopropylnorsuprifen. 1-(4-Hydroxyphenyl)-2-(1-methyl-2-phenoxyethylamino)propan-1-ol hydrochloride.

$C_{18}H_{23}NO_3,HCl = 337.8$.

CAS — 395-28-8 (isoxsuprine); 579-56-6 (isoxsuprine hydrochloride).

Pharmacopoeias. In *Eur.* (see p.viii) and *US.*

A white or almost white odourless or almost odourless crystalline powder. **Soluble** 1 in 500 of water, 1 in 100 of alcohol and dilute sodium hydroxide solution, and 1 in 2500 of dilute hydrochloric acid; practically insoluble in dichloromethane and ether. A 1% solution in water has a pH of 4.5 to 6.0. **Store** in airtight containers. Protect from light.

Adverse Effects

Isoxsuprine may cause transient flushing, hypotension, tachycardia, rashes, and gastro-intestinal disturbances. Maternal pulmonary oedema and fetal tachycardia have been reported following intravenous administration in premature labour.

Pulmonary oedema. Pulmonary oedema has been reported in mothers given isoxsuprine for premature labour.[1,2]

1. Nagey DA, Crenshaw MC. Pulmonary complications of isoxsuprine therapy in the gravida. *Obstet Gynecol* 1982; **59** (suppl): 38S–42S.
2. Nimrod C, *et al.* Pulmonary edema associated with isoxsuprine therapy. *Am J Obstet Gynecol* 1984; **148:** 625–9.

Precautions

Isoxsuprine is contra-indicated following recent arterial haemorrhage. It should not be administered immediately post partum, nor should it be used for premature labour if there is infection.

In *women being treated for premature labour* the risk of pulmonary oedema means that extreme caution is required and the precautions and risk factors discussed under Salbutamol Sulphate, p.759, apply.

Pregnancy. Ileus was found to be more common in the offspring of mothers who received isoxsuprine than in matched controls.[1] The incidence of respiratory distress syndrome also rose as the isoxsuprine concentration in cord blood exceeded 10 ng per mL; likewise the incidence of hypocalcaemia and hypotension rose progressively with increasing concentrations. The cord concentrations correlated inversely with the drug-free interval before delivery and it was suggested that with frequent assessment of uterine response it should be possible to avoid delivering infants at a time when they have high plasma-isoxsuprine concentrations.[1]

In another study[2] of the association between ruptured membranes, beta-adrenergic therapy and respiratory distress syndrome, it was found that both therapy with isoxsuprine and premature rupture of membranes were individually associated with a lowered incidence of respiratory distress syndrome, but when present together they resulted in an increased risk of respiratory distress syndrome. It was suggested that therapy with beta-adrenergic drugs including isoxsuprine should be restricted to patients with intact membranes.[1]

1. Brazy JE, *et al.* Isoxsuprine in the perinatal period II: relationships between neonatal symptoms, drug exposure, and drug concentration at the time of birth. *J Pediatr* 1981; **98:** 146–51.
2. Curet LB, *et al.* Association between ruptured membranes, tocolytic therapy, and respiratory distress syndrome. *Am J Obstet Gynecol* 1984; **148:** 263–8.

Pharmacokinetics

Isoxsuprine hydrochloride is well absorbed from the gastro-intestinal tract. The peak plasma concentration occurs about 1 hour after administration by mouth. A plasma half-life of 1.5 hours has been reported. Isoxsuprine is excreted in the urine mainly as conjugates.

Uses and Administration

Isoxsuprine is a vasodilator which also stimulates beta-adrenergic receptors. It causes direct relaxation of vascular and uterine smooth muscle and its vasodilating action is greater on the arteries supplying skeletal muscles than on those supplying skin. Isoxsuprine also produces positive inotropic and chronotropic effects.

For use as a vasodilator isoxsuprine hydrochloride is given by mouth in doses of 10 to 20 mg 3 or 4 times daily.

Isoxsuprine hydrochloride has been used to arrest premature labour (p.760) but drugs with a more selective action on $beta_2$ receptors such as ritodrine are now generally preferred. It has also been given in the treatment of cerebral and peripheral vascular disease.

To arrest premature labour, isoxsuprine hydrochloride is given initially by intravenous infusion (200 μg per mL) in doses of 200 to 500 μg per minute, adjusted according to the patient's response, until control is achieved. It is now common practice to administer beta agonists by syringe pump when using them to delay premature labour. Maternal blood pressure and hydration, and maternal and fetal heart rates should be monitored during the infusion. Subsequent treatment when labour has been arrested consists of intramuscular injections of 10 mg every 3 to 8 hours for several days. Prophylaxis may be continued by mouth with 30 to 90 mg daily in divided doses.

The resinate has also been used.

Preparations

USP 23: Isoxsuprine Hydrochloride Injection; Isoxsuprine Hydrochloride Tablets.

Proprietary Preparations (details are given in Part 3)
Aust.: Xuprin; ***Austral.:*** Duvadilan; ***Belg.:*** Duvadilan; ***Fr.:*** Duvadilan; ***Ger.:*** Duvadilan†; ***Irl.:*** Duvadilan; ***Ital.:*** Duvadilan; Fenam; Vasosuprina Ilfi; ***Neth.:*** Duvadilan; ***Spain:*** Duvadilan; ***UK:*** Duvadilan†; ***USA:*** Vasodilan; Voxsuprine.

Java Tea (11483-b)

Orthosiphonblätter; Orthosiphonis Folium.

Pharmacopoeias. In *Eur.* (see p.viii).

The fragmented, dried leaves and tops of stems of *Orthosiphon stamineus* (*O. aristatus*; *O. spicatus*). **Protect** from light.

Java tea is used in herbal medicine.

Preparations

Proprietary Preparations (details are given in Part 3)
Aust.: Carito mono; ***Fr.:*** Urosiphon; ***Ger.:*** Aquacaps; Carito mono; Folindor†; Late Orphon†; Nephronorm Med; Repha Orphon.

Multi-ingredient: ***Aust.:*** Apotheker Bauer's Harntreibender Tee; Apotheker Bauer's Nieren- und Blasentee; Blasen- und Nierentee; Droxitop; Krauterhaus Mag Kottas Blasentee; Krauterhaus Mag Kottas Nierentee; Krautertee Nr 31; Mag Kottas Entwasserungstee; Mag Kottas Nieren-Blasentee; Sidroga Nieren- und Blasentee; Solubitrat; ***Belg.:*** Tisane Contre la Tension; ***Fr.:*** Actisane Minceur; Aminsane; Aromalgyl; Dellova; Tealine; ***Ger.:*** Aqualibra; Buccotean TF†; Buccotean†; Canephron novo; Diureticum-Medice†; Dr. Klinger's Bergischer Krautertee, Blasen- u. Nierentee†; Etmoren; Harntee; Harntee 400; Hepaduran†; Heumann Blasen- und Nierentee Solubitrat N; Hevert-Blasen- und Nieren- Tee; Heweberberol-Tee; Knufinke Blasen- und Nieren-Tee Uro-K†; Knufinke Sanguis-L†; Lipozet†; NB-Tee N; NB-tee Siegfried†; Nephro-Pasc; Nephronorm Med; Nephropur tri; Nephrubin; Nieren-Tee†; Nierentee 2000; Nieron Blasen- und Nieren-Tee VI; Orbis Blasen- und Nierentee†; Salus Nieren-Blasen-Tee Nr.23; Solvefort N†; Uro Fink; Urodil Blasen-Nieren Arzneitee; Urodil phyto; Urostei; Worishofener Nieren- und Blasenmittel Dr. Kleinschrod†; ***Ital.:*** Enteroton Lassativo†; ***Switz.:*** Bilifuge; Demonatur Dragees pour les reins et la vessie; Dragees pour reins et vessie S; Livartil†; Phytomed Nephro; Prosta-Caps Chassot N; Solubitrat†; Tisane antiseptique diuretique†; Tisane diuretique "H"†; Tisane pour les reins et la vessie.

Jin Bu Huan (17753-l)

Jin bu huan is a traditional Chinese remedy used as a sedative and analgesic and variously stated to contain *Lycopodium serratum* or *Polygala chinensis*. Adverse effects including CNS depression and acute hepatotoxicity have been attributed to its alkaloidal content of L-tetrahydropalmatine.

A report of acute hepatitis in 7 previously healthy patients following ingestion of jin bu huan; symptoms recrudesced in 2 following re-use.[1] It was noted that the content of plant material did not seem to correspond to the labelled species. Hepatitis and extreme fatigue have also been reported in 3 adults after taking jin bu huan for periods ranging from 6 days to 6 months.[2]

Accidental ingestion of jin bu huan by 3 children[2] produced profound lethargy and muscle weakness. Two of the children also developed respiratory depression and bradycardia.

1. Woolf GM, *et al.* Acute hepatitis associated with the Chinese herbal product Jin Bu Huan. *Ann Intern Med* 1994; **121:** 729–35.
2. Horowitz RS, *et al.* The clinical spectrum of Jin Bu Huan toxicity. *Arch Intern Med* 1996; **156:** 899–903.

Juniper (4654-z)

Baccae Juniperi; Genièvre; Juniper Berry; Juniper Fruit; Juniperi Fructus; Juniperi Galbulus; Wacholderbeeren; Zimbro.

Pharmacopoeias. In *Aust., Ger.,* and *Swiss.*

The dried ripe fruits of *Juniperus communis* (Cupressaceae).

Juniper is the source of juniper oil. It has carminative, diuretic, antiseptic, and anti-inflammatory properties. It is used in herbal and homoeopathic medicine and as a flavour in gin.

Preparations

Proprietary Preparations (details are given in Part 3)
Ger.: Kneipp Wacholderbeer-Pflanzensaft.

Multi-ingredient: ***Aust.:*** Aktiv Blasen- und Nierentee; Apotheker Bauer's Harntreibender Tee; Blasen-Tee; Kneipp Entwasserungstee; Krautertee Nr 18; Krautertee Nr 19; Krautertee Nr 29; Krautertee Nr 30; Krautertee Nr 4; Mariazeller; St Bonifatius-Tee; ***Austral.:*** Arthritic Pain Herbal Formula 1; Fluid Loss; Herbal Diuretic Complex†; Lifesystem Herbal Formula 1 Arthritic Aid; PMT-EZE†; Profluid; Protemp; ***Belg.:*** Tisane Diuretique; ***Canad.:*** Arthrisan; Herbal Laxative; ***Fr.:*** Alpha Renol†; Depuratum; Mediflor Tisane Antirhumatismale No 2; Santane A_4; Santane R_8; ***Ger.:*** Atmulen E†; Befelka-Tinktur; Blasen-Nieren-Tee Uroflux†; Buccotean†; Discmigon; Entwasserungs-Tee†; Gastrol S; Harntee 400; Hevert-Entwasserungs-Tee; Hevert-Gicht-Rheuma-Tee comp; Hocura-Diureticum†; Imbak; Junisana; Kneipp Blutreinigungs-Tee†; Kneipp Entschlackungs-Tee; Kneipp Magentrost†; Kneipp Rheuma Tee N; Knufinke Blasen- und Nieren-Tee Uro-K†; Montana; NB-tee Siegfried†; Nieren-Tee†; Presselin 214†; Presselin Stoffwechseltee†; Rheumex†; Salus Nieren-Blasen-Tee Nr.23; Salus Rheuma-Tee Krautertee Nr. 12; Verus†; Worishofener Nieren- und Blasenmittel Dr. Kleinschrod†; ***Ital.:*** Broncosedina; Depurfat; ***Spain:*** Kneipp Pildoras†; ***Switz.:*** Ajaka; Cystinol N†; Kernosan Heidelberger Poudre; Phytomed Nephro; Radix†; Tisane antirhumatismale "H"†; Tisane antiseptique diuretique†; Tisane diuretique "H"†; Tisane laxative Natterman no 13; Tisane pour les reins et la vessie.

Juniper Oil (4655-c)

Essence de Genièvre; Juniper Berry Oil; Oleum Juniperi; Wacholderöl.

Pharmacopoeias. In *Aust., Fr., Pol.,* and *Swiss.*

The volatile oil distilled from juniper (above). **Store** in a cool place in airtight containers. Protect from light.

Juniper oil has been used as a carminative and as an ingredient of herbal remedies for urinary-tract disorders and muscle and joint pain. Prolonged use may cause gastro-intestinal irritation and there may be a risk of renal damage from high doses.

Preparations

Proprietary Preparations (details are given in Part 3)
Ger.: Leukona-Stoffwechsel-Bad; Roleca Wacholder.

Multi-ingredient: ***Aust.:*** Apotheker Bauer's Inhalationsmischung; Berggeist; ***Austral.:*** Medinat PMT-Eze; ***Fr.:*** Baume Aroma; ***Ger.:*** Buccotean TF†; Dolo-cyl; GA-301-Redskin 301; Kneipp Rheuma Bad; Neo-Lapitrypsin; Nierentee 2000; Nieroxin N; Optipect†; Schupps Heilkrauter Rheumabad; Schupps Latschenkiefer Olbad; ***Ital.:*** Otosan Gocce Auricolari; ***S.Afr.:*** Slendoll†; ***Spain:*** Emolytar; ***Switz.:*** Ajaka; Baby Liberol; Caprisana; Demo pommade contre les refroidissements pour bebes; Huile Po-Ho A. Vogel; Methylan†; Olbas; Solubitrat†; ***UK:*** Diuretabs; HealthAid Boldo-Plus; Juno Junipah; Olbas; Sciargo.

Kallidinogenase (9248-a)

Kallidinogenase *(BAN, rINN)*.

Callicrein; Kalléone; Kallikrein.

CAS — 9001-01-8.

An enzyme isolated from the pancreas and urine of mammals.

Kallidinogenase converts kininogen into the kinin, kallidin. It has vasodilating properties and has been used in the treatment of peripheral vascular disorders (p.794). It has also been used in the treatment of male infertility (p.1239) since the kallikrein-kinin system has a physiological role in the male genital tract.

A discussion of the treatment of male fertility disturbances, including the use of kallidinogenase.[1]

1. Haidl G, Schill W-B. Guidelines for drug treatment of male infertility. *Drugs* 1991; **41:** 60–8.

Preparations

Proprietary Preparations (details are given in Part 3)
Aust.: Padutin; ***Ger.:*** Depot-Padutin†; Padutin.

Multi-ingredient: ***Ger.:*** Nico-Padutin†.

Kava (12878-p)

Kava-Kava.

CAS — 500-64-1 (kawain); 495-85-2 (methysticin); 500-62-9 (yangonin).

The rhizome of *Piper methysticum* (Piperaceae), a shrub indigenous to islands of the South Pacific. It contains pyrones including kawain, methysticin, and yangonin.

Kava has been used in the South Pacific to produce an intoxicating beverage used for recreational purposes and during convalescence. It is reported to have skeletal muscle relaxing and anaesthetic properties. It is given in some anxiety- and stress-related disorders. It was formerly used as an antiseptic and diuretic in inflammatory conditions of the genito-urinary tract in the form of a liquid extract. Kawain has also been used.

A characteristic rash resembling that of pellagra occurs in some heavy consumers of kava. Extrapyramidal effects have been reported.

References.

1. Anonymous. Kava. *Lancet* 1988; **ii:** 258–9.
2. Anonymous. Tonga trouble. *Pharm J* 1990; **245:** 288.
3. Ruze P. Kava-induced dermopathy: a niacin deficiency? *Lancet* 1990; **335:** 1442–5.

4. Schelosky L, *et al.* Kava and dopamine antagonism. *J Neurol Neurosurg Psychiatry* 1995; **58:** 639–40.
5. Spillane PK, *et al.* Neurological manifestations of kava intoxication. *Med J Aust* 1997; **167:** 172–3.

Preparations

Proprietary Preparations (details are given in Part 3)
Aust.: Largon; Mosaro†; ***Ger.:*** Aigin; Antares; Ardeydystin; Cefakava; Eukavan; Kavacur; Kavaform N; Kavasedon; Kavatino; Kavosporal forte; Laitan; Limbao; Nervonocton N†; Neuronika; Sedalint Kava; ***Switz.:*** Laitan.

Multi-ingredient: ***Aust.:*** Kavaform; Kavavit; ***Ger.:*** Bilicura Forte; Cysto Fink; Dolo-Arthrosetten†; Hewepsychon duo; Hyposedon N; Kavain Harras Plus; Kavosporal comp; Somnuvis S; Spasmo-Bilicura†; Valeriana comp; ***Spain:*** Bleukawine; ***Switz.:*** Cysto Fink; Cysto-Caps Chassot; Kawaform; Yakona N; ***UK:*** Antiglan; GB Tablets; Protat.

Kelp (12137-k)

Kelp is a preparation of dried seaweed of various species that is present as an ingredient of several dietary supplements and herbal preparations. It has been used as a source of iodine.

Kelp can concentrate various heavy metals; auto-immune thrombocytopenic purpura with dyserythropoiesis in a patient who had been taking kelp tablets for 6 weeks was attributed to the arsenic content of the preparation.[1]

There has also been a report of clinical hyperthyroidism in a patient taking a kelp-containing preparation as part of a slimming regimen.[2]

The FDA has advised that preparations containing compounds such as kelp that may be taken by mouth in bulk laxatives or weight-control preparations should be taken with a full glass of water or, if the patient has difficulty in swallowing, they should be avoided. Such compounds swell into masses that may obstruct the oesophagus if not taken with sufficient water.

1. Pye KG, *et al.* Severe dyserythropoiesis and autoimmune thrombocytopenia associated with ingestion of kelp supplements. *Lancet* 1992; **339:** 1540.
2. de Smet PA, *et al.* Hyperthyreoidie tijdens het gebruik van kelp tabletten. *Ned Tijdschr Geneeskd* 1990; **134:** 1058–9.

Preparations

Proprietary Preparations (details are given in Part 3)

Multi-ingredient: ***Austral.:*** Herbal Diuretic Complex†; Plantiodine Plus; PMT Complex; ***S.Afr.:*** Activex 40 Plus; Vitaforce 21-Plus†; Vitaforce Forti-Plus†; ***UK:*** Cellbloc†; Fat-Solv; Kelp Plus 3; ***USA:*** KLB6.

Keracyanin (12879-s)

Keracyanin (*rINN*).

3-[6-*O*-(6-Deoxy-α-L-mannopyranosyl)-β-D-glucopyranosyloxy]-3′,4′,5,7-tetrahydroxyflavylium chloride.

$C_{27}H_{31}ClO_{15}$ = 631.0.

CAS — 18719-76-1.

Keracyanin is claimed to improve visual function in poor light conditions. It has been given by mouth in usual doses of 400 to 600 mg daily.

Preparations

Proprietary Preparations (details are given in Part 3)
Fr.: Meralops; ***Ital.:*** Meralop; ***Spain:*** Meralop.

Keratinase (7377-e)

CAS — 9025-41-6.

Keratinase is a proteolytic enzyme which has been obtained from cultures of *Streptomyces fradiae*. It can digest keratin, which is resistant to most proteolytic enzymes, in the presence of trace amounts of metal ions. It is used in the commercial separation of hair from animal hides, and has been tried as a depilatory; it is also an ingredient of some topical antibiotic ointments, presumably to aid penetration of the active substances.

Preparations

Proprietary Preparations (details are given in Part 3)

Multi-ingredient: ***Spain:*** Deltasiton.

Khellin (9249-t)

Khellin (*rINN*).

Khelline; Khellinum; Visammin. 4,9-Dimethoxy-7-methyl-5*H*-furo[3,2-g]chromen-5-one.

$C_{14}H_{12}O_5$ = 260.2.

CAS — 82-02-0.

Pharmacopoeias. In *Aust.*

Khellin is obtained by extraction from the dried ripe fruit of *Ammi visnaga* (Umbelliferae) or by synthesis.

Khellin is a vasodilator which also has a bronchodilatory action. It has been employed in the treatment of angina pectoris, in the treatment of asthma, and, in conjunction with ultraviolet A light, has been tried in the treatment of vitiligo. Extracts of *Ammi visnaga* fruit are used similarly.

References.

1. Morliere P, *et al.* Phototherapeutic, photobiologic, and photosensitizing properties of khellin. *J Invest Dermatol* 1988; **90:** 720–4.
2. Antoniou C, Katsambas A. Guidelines for the treatment of vitiligo. *Drugs* 1992; **43:** 490–8.

Preparations

Proprietary Preparations (details are given in Part 3)
Ger.: Carduben; Khellangan N; steno-loges N.

Multi-ingredient: ***Aust.:*** Urelium Neu; ***Ger.:*** Aesrutal S; Cardaminol†; Cardisetten†; Cefedrin N; Coropar†; Hepatofalk Neu; Hevertopect; Iosimitan†; Keldrin†; Oxacant-Khella N; Salusan; Seda-Stenocrat-N†; Silphoscalin†; Stenocrat; Urol†; ***Spain:*** Nefrolit†.

Kinkeliba (12883-v)

Combreti Folium.

Pharmacopoeias. In *Fr.*

The dried leaves of *Combretum micranthum* (=*C. altum; C. raimbaultii*) (Combretaceae), a shrub indigenous to West Africa.

Kinkeliba has been used as an ingredient of herbal remedies given for the treatment of biliary, liver, and gastro-intestinal disorders. Other species of *Combretum* are also used.

Kinkeliba is used in homoeopathic medicine.

Preparations

Proprietary Preparations (details are given in Part 3)

Multi-ingredient: ***Belg.:*** Stago†; Tisane pour le Foie; ***Canad.:*** Hepax†; ***Fr.:*** Hepaclem; Hepatorex†; Hepax; Jecopeptol; Mediflor Tisane Hepatique No 5; Palmi; Romarene; Romarinex-Choline; Solution Stago Diluee; Uremiase; ***Ital.:*** Boldosten†; Cheliboldo†; Heparbil†; ***Switz.:*** Bilifuge; Livartil†; Stago†.

Klebsiella pneumoniae Glycoprotein

(3028-b)

RU-41740.

Klebsiella pneumoniae glycoprotein has been used for its immunomodulating activity in the management of respiratory-tract infections, wounds, burns, and soft-tissue disorders, and has been used in immunotherapy.

Preparations

Proprietary Preparations (details are given in Part 3)
Fr.: Biostim; ***Ital.:*** Acintor; Biostim; ***S.Afr.:*** Biostim†.

Multi-ingredient: ***Ger.:*** Biomunyl†.

Krebiozen (12884-g)

CAS — 9008-19-9.

Krebiozen is the name of a preparation that was formerly promoted as a 'cancer cure' in the USA, but totally discredited by the FDA. It was stated to be obtained from the blood of horses previously injected with an extract of *Actinomyces bovis*.

Kveim Antigen (12885-q)

Kveim antigen is a fine suspension in physiological saline of sarcoid tissue prepared from spleens taken from patients with active sarcoidosis. It is used as an intradermal injection in the Kveim-Siltzbach test for the diagnosis of sarcoidosis (p.1028).

References.

1. James DG, Williams WJ. Kveim-Siltzbach test revisited. *Sarcoidosis* 1991; **8:** 6–9.

The safety of the Kveim test has been questioned, particularly with reference to the risk of transmission of sarcoidosis, and of hepatitis B, human immunodeficiency virus, and Creutzfeldt-Jakob disease.[1] However, the procedure to identify acceptable sarcoid spleens and the method of preparation were considered sufficient to reduce the risk of transmission of infections[2] and of Creutzfeldt-Jakob disease.[3]

1. Wigly RD. Moratorium on Kveim tests. *Lancet* 1993; **341:** 1284.
2. du Bois RM, *et al.* Moratorium on Kveim tests. *Lancet* 1993; **342:** 173.
3. de Silva RN, Will RG. Moratorium on Kveim tests. *Lancet* 1993; **342:** 173.

Laburnum (12886-p)

Golden Chain; Golden Rain.

Laburnum anagyroides (= *L. vulgare; Cytisus laburnum*) (Leguminosae).

All parts of laburnum are toxic. The toxic principle is cytisine which has actions similar to nicotine.

Lactic Acid (1312-z)

Acidum Lacticum; E270; E326 (potassium lactate); Milchsäure. 2-Hydroxypropionic acid.

$C_3H_6O_3$ = 90.08.

CAS — 50-21-5; 79-33-4 (+); 10326-41-7 (−); 598-82-3 (±).

Pharmacopoeias. In *Chin., Eur.* (see p.viii), *Int., Jpn, Pol.,* and *US.*

A colourless or slightly yellow, syrupy, hygroscopic, practically odourless liquid.

The Ph. Eur. specifies a mixture of lactic acid, its condensation products such as lactoyl-lactic acid and other polylactic acids, and water. In most cases lactic acid is in the form of the racemate (*RS*-lactic acid), but in some cases the (+)-(*S*)-isomer is predominant. It contains the equivalent of 88 to 92% w/w of $C_3H_6O_3$.

The USP specifies a mixture of lactic acid and lactic acid lactate equivalent to 85 to 90% w/w of $C_3H_6O_3$. Lactic acid prepared by fermentation of sugars is laevorotatory; that prepared synthetically is racemic.

Miscible with water, with alcohol, and with ether; practically insoluble in chloroform. **Store** in airtight containers.

Adverse Effects and Treatment

As for Hydrochloric Acid, p.1588, although in the concentrations used it is less corrosive.

There was evidence that neonates had difficulty in metabolising *R*-(−)-lactic acid and this isomer and the racemate should not be used in foods for infants less than 3 months old.[1]

1. FAO/WHO. Toxicological evaluation of certain food additives with a review of general principles and of specifications: seventeenth report of the joint FAO/WHO expert committee on food additives. *WHO Tech Rep Ser 539* 1974.

Uses and Administration

Lactic acid has actions similar to those of acetic acid (see p.1541) and has been used similarly in the treatment of infective skin and vaginal disorders. It has been used in the preparation of lactate injections and infusions to provide a source of bicarbonate for the treatment of metabolic acidosis (for the problems of using lactate in metabolic acidosis see p.1147). It is also employed in the treatment of warts, often in combination with salicylic acid, a topic discussed further on p.1076, and in emollient creams.

Lactic acid is also used as a food preservative and as an ingredient of cosmetics.

References to the use of lactic acid in the treatment of bacterial vaginosis,[1,2] warts,[3] and dry[4,5] and photodamaged[6] skin.

1. Andersch B, *et al.* Treatment of bacterial vaginosis with an acid cream: a comparison between the effect of lactate-gel and metronidazole. *Gynecol Obstet Invest* 1986; **21:** 19–25.
2. Holst E, Brandberg Å. Treatment of bacterial vaginosis in pregnancy with a lactate gel. *Scand J Infect Dis* 1990; **22:** 625–6.
3. Bunney MH, *et al.* An assessment of methods of treating viral warts by comparative treatment trials based on a standard design. *Br J Dermatol* 1976; **94:** 667–79.
4. Dahl MV, Dahl AC. 12% Lactate lotion for the treatment of xerosis: a double-blind clinical evaluation. *Arch Dermatol* 1983; **119:** 27–30.
5. Rogers RS, *et al.* Comparative efficacy of 12% ammonium lactate lotion and 5% lactic acid lotion in the treatment of moderate to severe xerosis. *J Am Acad Dermatol* 1989; **21:** 714–16.
6. Stiller MJ, *et al.* Topical 8% glycolic acid and 8% L-lactic acid creams for the treatment of photodamaged skin: a double-blind vehicle-controlled clinical trial. *Arch Dermatol* 1996; **132:** 631–6.

Preparations

BP 1998: Lactic Acid Pessaries;
USP 23: Compound Clioquinol Topical Powder.

Proprietary Preparations (details are given in Part 3)
Aust.: Espritin; Warzin; ***Austral.:*** Avecyde; ***Belg.:*** Lacta-Gynecogel; ***Canad.:*** Calmurid; Lubriderm AHA; Penederm; pHygiene†; ***Ger.:*** Lactisan; RMS; Tampovagan c. Acid. lact.; Tonsillosan†; Unguentum Lactisol; ***Ital.:*** Unigyn; ***Neth.:*** Calmurid; ***Spain:*** Keratisdin; ***Swed.:*** Calmuril; ***Switz.:*** Lactovagan†; Vagoclyss; ***USA:*** Lactinol.

Multi-ingredient: ***Aust.:*** Anthozym; Apotheker Bauer's Huhneraugentinktur; Calmurid; Calmurid HC; Duofilm; Helo-acid; Hylak; Hylak forte; Lavagin; ***Austral.:*** Aussie Tan Skin Moisturiser; Calmurid; Collomack†; Cornkil; Dermadrate; Dermatech Wart Treatment; Duofilm; Lacticare†; Wart-Off†; Wartkil†; ***Belg.:*** Aporil; Calmurid; ***Canad.:*** Calmurid HC; Cuplex; Duofilm; Duoplant; Epi-Lyt; Lacticare; Penederm; Soluver Plus; Tiacid; Viron Wart Lotion; ***Fr.:*** Duofilm; Kerafilm; Lactacyd; Lacticare†; Verrufilm; ***Ger.:*** Aknederm N; Anthozym N; Bepanthen V†; Calmurid; Calmurid HC; Clabin†; Collomack; Consablitz†; Dr. Hotz Vollbad; Duofilm; Echtrosept-GT†; Efasit N; Gehwol Huhneraugenpflaster N; Gelum-Tropfen; Kneipp Milch-Molke-Bad; Lactacyd†; Sagrosept; Solco-Derman; Warzen-Alldahin; ***Irl.:*** Calmurid; Calmurid HC; Cuplex; Duofilm; Lacticare; Salactol; Salatac; ***Ital.:***

Aflogine; Bruciaporri; Creosolactol Adulti†; Creosolactol Bambini†; Dose†; Euzymina I Bambini†; Gastro-Pepsin; Geroderm Zolfo; Lactacyd Derma; Lactacyd Intimo; Lactocol; Pluriderm; Saugella Salviettine; Unidermo; Unigal Solido†; Verel; Verucid; Verunec 3; Violgen; ***Neth.:*** Tintorine; ***Norw.:*** Verucid; ***S.Afr.:*** Duofilm; Lacticare†; ***Spain:*** Aknedertim†; Antiverrugas; Callicida Brujo; Callicida Cor Pik; Callicida Durcall; Callix D; Calloverk†; Cusiter; Dermijabon Acido†; Ginejuvent; Roidhemo; Unguento Callicida Naion; Verufil; ***Swed.:*** Lactal; Vartmedel†; ***Switz.:*** Acne Lotion; Acnidazil†; Aloplastine Acide†; Calmurid; Calmurid HC; Clabin; Delica-Sol†; Duofilm; Elle-care; Gynogella†; Lactacyd†; Solcoderm; Vin Tonique de Vial; Warz-ab Extor; ***UK:*** Bazuka; Calmurid; Calmurid HC; Cuplex; Duofilm; Lacticare; Salactol; Salatac Gel; Tampovagan; Variclene†; ***USA:*** Epilyt; Feminique; Lacticare-HC; Lactinol-E; Lactisol†; Massengill; Massengill Disposable; Paplex†; SLT; Viranol†.

Lactic-acid-producing Organisms (1313-c)

Lactic-acid-producing organisms were introduced as a therapeutic agent by Metchnikoff with the idea of acidifying the intestinal contents and thus preventing the growth of putrefactive organisms. The organism chosen by him for this purpose was *Lactobacillus bulgaricus*, which occurs in naturally soured milk, but many workers found it difficult to produce a growth of this organism in the intestines and preferred *L. acidophilus* which is an inhabitant of the human intestine. Natural yoghurt is a common source of lactic-acid-producing organisms.

Preparations containing various *Lactobacillus* spp. and other lactic-acid-producing organisms have been used in the treatment of vaginal and gastro-intestinal disorders but evidence to support this use is limited. Other organisms which have been tried include *Bifidobacterium bifidum, Enterococcus* and *Streptococcus* spp., and the yeast *Saccharomyces boulardii*.

A vaccine from strains of lactobacillus found in women with trichomoniasis has been used in the prophylaxis of recurrent trichomoniasis (see p.1536).

Some reviews[1-4] and references[5-15] to the use of lactic-acid-producing organisms including *Lactobacillus* spp., *Bifidobacterium bifidum*, and *Streptococcus thermophilus*. However, some preparations have been found to contain smaller quantities or different species of organisms to those specified on the label.[16]

Metabolic acidosis has occurred following use of tablets containing *Lactobacillus acidophilus*.[17]

1. Scott E, Li Wan Po A. Lactobacillus. *Pharm J* 1990; **245:** 698–9.
2. Fuller R. Probiotics in human medicine. *Gut* 1991; **32:** 439–42.
3. Drutz DJ. Lactobacillus prophylaxis for Candida vaginitis. *Ann Intern Med* 1992; **116:** 419–20.
4. Roffe C. Biotherapy for antibiotic-associated and other diarrhoeas. *J Infect* 1996; **32:** 1–10.
5. Gotz V, *et al.* Prophylaxis against ampicillin-associated diarrhea with a lactobacillus preparation. *Am J Hosp Pharm* 1979; **36:** 754–7.
6. Clements ML, *et al.* Exogenous lactobacilli fed to man—their fate and ability to prevent diarrheal disease. *Prog Food Nutr Sci* 1983; **7:** 29–37.
7. Gorbach SL, *et al.* Successful treatment of relapsing Clostridium difficile colitis with Lactobacillus GG. *Lancet* 1987; **ii:** 1519.
8. Wunderlich PF, *et al.* Double-blind report on the efficacy of lactic acid-producing Enterococcus SF68 in the prevention of antibiotic-associated diarrhoea and in the treatment of acute diarrhoea. *J Int Med Res* 1989; **17:** 333–8.
9. Tankanow RM, *et al.* Double-blind, placebo-controlled study of the efficacy of Lactinex in the prophylaxis of amoxicillin-induced diarrhea. *DICP Ann Pharmacother* 1990; **24:** 382–4.
10. Isolauri E, *et al.* A human Lactobacillus strain (Lactobacillus casei sp strain GG) promotes recovery from acute diarrhea in children. *Pediatrics* 1991; **88:** 90–7.
11. Hilton E, *et al.* Ingestion of yogurt containing Lactobacillus acidophilus as prophylaxis for candidal vaginitis. *Ann Intern Med* 1992; **116:** 353–7.
12. Hallén A, *et al.* Treatment of bacterial vaginosis with lactobacilli. *Sex Transm Dis* 1992; **19:** 146–8.
13. Saavedra JM, *et al.* Feeding of Bifidobacterium bifidum and Streptococcus thermophilus to infants in hospital for prevention of diarrhoea and shedding of rotavirus. *Lancet* 1994; **344:** 1046–9.
14. Reid G, *et al.* Implantation of Lactobacillus casei var rhamnosus into vagina. *Lancet* 1994; **344:** 1229.
15. Kaila M, *et al.* Viable versus inactivated lactobacillus strain GG in acute rotavirus diarrhoea. *Arch Dis Child* 1995; **72:** 51–3.
16. Hamilton-Miller JMT, *et al.* "Probiotic" remedies are not what they seem. *Br Med J* 1996; **312:** 55–6.
17. Oh MS, *et al.* D-lactic acidosis in a man with short-bowel syndrome. *N Engl J Med* 1979; **301:** 249–52.

Preparations

Proprietary Preparations (details are given in Part 3)

Aust.: Antibiophilus; Bioflorin; Doederlein; Symbioflor I; ***Austral.:*** Acidophilus Tablets; Bioglan Acidophilus; Bioglan Superdophilus; Candi-Biffidus†; ***Belg.:*** Bioflorin†; Lacteol; ***Canad.:*** Bacid; ***Fr.:*** Antibiophilus; Diarlac; Lacteol; Lyo-Bifidus; Rhino-Lacteol; Ultra-Levure; Ultraderme; ***Ger.:*** Acidophilus; Hamadin; Hylak N; Omnisept; Paidoflor; Perenterol; Perocur; Santax S; Symbioflor 1; Vagiflor; Yomogi†; ***Ital.:*** Bioflorin; Codex; Dicoflor; Ecoflorina; Fermenturto-Lio; Fermenturto†; Hygine In; Lab/A; Lacteol; Lactomicina-R†; Ramno-Flor; ***S.Afr.:*** Actiflora†; Enpac†; Inteflora; ***Spain:*** Electrolactil Sol†; Lacteol; Lactofilus; Lactoliofil; Ultra Levura; ***Swed.:*** Precosa; Trevis†; ***Switz.:*** Bioflorin; Fiormil; Lacteol; Lactoferment nouvelle formule; Perenterol; Solco-Trichovac; Ultra-Levure; Ventrux; ***UK:*** Bio Acidophilus; Biodophilus; ***USA:*** Bacid; Kala; Lactinex; MoreDophilus; Pro-Bionate; Superdophilus.

Multi-ingredient: ***Aust.:*** Gynoflor; Hylak; Hylak forte; Hylakombun; Infloran; Omniflora; Prosymbioflor; ***Austral.:*** Acidophilus Complex; Cyto-Biffidus; ***Belg.:*** Gynoflor; ***Canad.:*** Fermalac; Fermalac Vaginal; Sisu-Dophilus Plus†; ***Fr.:*** Ampho-Vaccin intestinal; Imudon; Trophigil; ***Ger.:*** Antiprurit; Ferro-Kombun N†; Gynoflor; Hylak forte N; Imbak; IRS 19; Kolpicortin†; Omniflora†; Pro-Symbioflor; Ribolac†; SolcoUrovac†; ***Ital.:*** Alvear Complex; Bifilact; Biolactine; Coli-Fagina S; Ecoendocilli Testimonia; Ecofermenti; Ergozim Lactis†; Flar; Florelax; Infloran; Lactipan; Lactisporin; Lactivis; Lactogermine; Lactolife; Lactonorm; Lactovit; Liozim; Neo Lactoflorene; Yovis; ***S.Afr.:*** Eksalb†; ***Spain:*** Acidona†; Antibiofilus; Infloran; Lactolaxine†; ***Switz.:*** Gynoflor E; Infloran; Ribolac; SolcoUrovac†; ***UK:*** Acidophilus Plus; Biosym†; Natudophilus; ***USA:*** Entrin Acidophilus; Entrin Bifidus.

Lactomicin (3907-l)

Gamma-lactomicin.

Lactomicin is described as a protein supplement and co-adjuvant for use in the treatment of bacterial and viral infections; it has also been advocated in the treatment of hepatitis and other liver disorders.

Laetrile (12887-s)

CAS — 1332-94-1 (laetrile); 29883-15-6 (amygdalin).

The term laetrile is used for a product consisting chiefly of amygdalin, which is the major cyanogenic glycoside of apricot kernels. Amygdalin is *R*-α-cyanobenzyl-6-*O*-β-D-glucopyranosyl-β-D-glucopyranoside ($C_{20}H_{27}NO_{11}$=457.4). Laetrile is also used as a term for *R*-α-cyanobenzyl-6-*O*-β-D-glucopyranosiduronic acid ($C_{14}H_{15}NO_7$=309.3).

Laetrile was claimed to be preferentially hydrolysed in cancer cells by β-glucosidases to benzaldehyde and hydrogen cyanide, which killed the cell, but amygdalin does not appear to be absorbed from the gastro-intestinal tract, and both normal and malignant cells contain only traces of β-glucosidases. Laetrile has also been claimed to be 'vitamin B_{17}', the deficiency of which is said to result in cancer; there is no evidence for accepting this view and laetrile is of no known value in human nutrition.

There have been several reports of cyanide poisoning and other adverse reactions associated with the use of laetrile, especially when taken by mouth.

A review of the sources, chemistry, metabolism, claims for efficacy, and toxicity of laetrile.[1]

1. Chandler RF, *et al.* Controversial laetrile. *Pharm J* 1984; **232:** 330–2.

Laminaria (12888-w)

Stipites Laminariae; Styli Laminariae; Thallus Eckloniae; Thallus Laminariae.

Pharmacopoeias. In *Chin.*

The dried stalks of the seaweeds *Laminaria japonica, L. digitata*, and possibly other species of *Laminaria*.

Laminaria stalks swell in water to about 6 times their volume and have been used surgically to dilate cavities and to dilate the cervix in labour or abortion induction.

An extract of laminaria has been used as a dietary supplement.

Preparations

Proprietary Preparations (details are given in Part 3)

Fr.: Bio Soufre†.

Lappa (12889-e)

Bardanae Radix; Bardane (Grande); Burdock; Burdock Root; Lappa Root.

Pharmacopoeias. In *Fr.*
Chin. includes the fruits.

The dried root of the great burdock, *Arctium lappa* (= *A. majus*), and other species of *Arctium* (Compositae).

Lappa was formerly used in the form of a decoction as a diuretic and diaphoretic but there is little evidence of its efficacy. Herbal preparations containing lappa have been used in the treatment of skin, musculoskeletal, and gastro-intestinal disorders. The leaves and fruits of *Arctium* spp. have also been used.

Lappa is used in homoeopathic medicine.

Preparations

Proprietary Preparations (details are given in Part 3)

Fr.: Anthraxivore.

Multi-ingredient: ***Austral.:*** Herbal Cleanse; Trifolium Complex; ***Belg.:*** Stanno-Bardane; Tisane Depurative "les 12 Plantes"; ***Fr.:*** Arbum; Aromabyl; Depuratif Parnel; Fitacnol; Tisanes de l'Abbe Hamon no 16; ***Ital.:*** Cheliboldo†; Depurativo; ***UK:*** Blue Flag Root Compound; Cascade; Catarrh Mixture; GB Tablets; Kleer; Rheumatic Pain Remedy; Skin Cleansing; Skin Eruptions Mixture; Skin Tablets; Tabritis; Water Naturtabs; Water Relief Tablets.

Lavender Oil (4659-x)

English Lavender Oil (from *L. intermedia*); Esencia de Alhucema; Esencia de Espliego; Essência de Alfazema; Foreign Lavender Oil (from *L. officinalis*); Huile Essentielle de Lavande; Lavandulae Aetheroleum; Lavendelöl; Lavender Flower Oil; Oleum Lavandulae.

Pharmacopoeias. In *Eur.* (see p.viii) and *Pol.* Some pharmacopoeias include Lavender Flower.

A colourless or pale yellow or yellowish-green volatile oil with a characteristic fragrant odour reminiscent of the flowers, obtained by distillation from the fresh flowering tops of *Lavandula angustifolia* (=*L. spica* = *L. vera* = *L. officinalis*) (Labiatae) or *L. intermedia.*

Lavender oil has been used as a carminative and as a flavour. It is sometimes applied externally as an insect repellent. Its chief use is in perfumery and it is occasionally used in ointments and other pharmaceutical preparations to cover disagreeable odours. It has been suggested that lavender oil may have sedative properties following inhalation.

Lavender oil has been reported to produce nausea, vomiting, headache, and chills when inhaled or absorbed through the skin. It may cause contact allergy and phototoxicity.

Adverse effects. A report of contact dermatitis associated with lavender oil in a shampoo.[1]

1. Brandão FM. Occupational allergy to lavender oil. *Contact Dermatitis* 1986; **15:** 249–50.

Insomnia. Ambient exposure to lavender oil produced similar sleep patterns to conventional sedatives in 4 elderly patients.[1]

1. Hardy M, *et al.* Replacement of drug treatment for insomnia by ambient odour. *Lancet* 1995; **346:** 701.

Preparations

Proprietary Preparations (details are given in Part 3)

Multi-ingredient: ***Aust.:*** Baldrian-Krautertonikum; Berggeist; Beruhigungstee; Bio-Garten Tee zur Beruhigung; Euka; Herz- und Kreislauftonikum Bioflora; Inno Rheuma; Krautertee Nr 1; Krautertee Nr 141; Krautertee Nr 201; Mentopin; Rowalind; St Radegunder Herz-Kreislauf-unterstutzender Tee; Teekanne Schlaf- und Nerventee; ***Belg.:*** Cigarettes Anti-asthmatiques†; ***Fr.:*** Aromasol; Balsofletol†; Balsofumine; Balsofumine Mentholee; Bronchospray; Citrosil; Ephydrol; Gouttes aux Essences; Mediflor Tisane Digestive No 3; Pectoderme; Perubore; Santane N_9; Santane R_8; Tisane Sedative Weleda; ***Ger.:*** "Topfer" Kinderbad mit Teer†; "Topfer" Teerkleiebad†; Amol Heilkrautergeist N; Aranidorm-S; Beruhigungs-Tee Nervoflux†; Dolo-cyl; Dr. Klinger's Bergischer Krautertee, Nerven- und Beruhigungstee†; Euviterin; Iosimitan†; Pan-Nerventonikum†; Presselin 214†; Presselin 52 N; Rowalind; Salus Nerven-Schlaf-Tee Nr.22; Valeriana-Strath†; Ventrovis†; ***Irl.:*** Rowalind; ***Ital.:*** Citrosystem; Natural Zanzy; Sanaderm; ***Neth.:*** Tijgerolie†; ***Spain:*** Bellacanfor†; Dolokey; Lapiz Termo Compositum†; Linimento Naion; Mostazola†; Porosan†; Termosan; ***Switz.:*** Baume du Chalet; Baume Kytta†; Carmol†; Demo baume; Dolorex; Embropax; Escothyol†; Hygiodermil; Kernosan Huile de Massage; Kytta Pommade; Lyman; Massorax; Muco-Sana; Nasobol; Oculosan; Perubare; Phlogidermil; Pommade Kytta†; Saltrates; Seracalm; Tisane antirhumatismale "H"†; Tisane Natterman instantanee no 6 pour calmer les nerfs et lutter contre l'insomnie†; Tisane relaxante; Tisane sedative et somnifere "H"†; ***UK:*** Larch Resin comp.; Massage Balm Arnica; Massage Balm Calendula; Medicinal Gargle; Penetrol; Vital Eyes; ***USA:*** Nasal Jelly.

Lawsone (9307-y)

2-Hydroxy-1,4-naphthoquinone.

$C_{10}H_6O_3$ = 174.2.

CAS — 83-72-7.

Lawsone is a dye present in henna, the leaves of *Lawsonia* spp., and may also be prepared synthetically.

Lawsone has been used with dihydroxyacetone in sunscreen preparations. There appears to be no evidence that it has any sunscreening properties when used alone.

Observation that lawsone causes oxidative damage to red blood cells *in vitro* supported a suggestion that percutaneous absorption of henna could contribute to unexplained neonatal hyperbilirubinaemia in countries where the ceremonial use of henna is widespread.[1]

1. Zinkham WH, Oski FA. Henna: a potential cause of oxidative hemolysis and neonatal hyperbilirubinemia. *Pediatrics* 1996; **97:** 707–9.

Lead (5298-t)

Pb = 207.2.
CAS — 7439-92-1.

A grey, malleable and ductile metal.

Adverse Effects

Lead poisoning (plumbism) may be due to inorganic or organic lead and may be acute or more often chronic. It has followed exposure to a wide range of compounds and objects from which lead may be absorbed following ingestion or inhalation. Some of those incriminated include paint, pottery glazes, crystal glassware, domestic water supplies, petrol and poteen, cosmetics, herbal or folk remedies, newsprint, and even bullets. Children are often the victims of accidental poisoning and may be vulnerable to chronic exposure to lead from environmental pollution. Symptoms of poisoning with inorganic lead include anorexia, colic, vomiting, anaemia, peripheral neuropathy, and encephalopathy with convulsions and coma. There may be kidney damage and impairment of mental function. Children with elevated lead concentrations may be asymptomatic apart from intellectual deficits and behavioural disorders.

Organic lead poisoning produces mainly CNS symptoms; there can be gastro-intestinal and cardiovascular effects, and renal and hepatic damage.

General references.

1. WHO. Recommended health-based limits in occupational exposure to heavy metals: report of a WHO study group. *WHO Tech Rep Ser 647* 1980.
2. Ibels LS, Pollock CA. Lead intoxication. *Med Toxicol* 1986; **1:** 387–410.
3. Lead—environmental aspects. *Environmental Health Criteria 85.* Geneva: WHO, 1989.
4. Inorganic lead. *Environmental Health Criteria 165.* Geneva: WHO, 1995.

Acute poisoning. Acute lead intoxication following the intravenous injection of lead acetate.[1]

1. Sixel-Dietrich F, *et al.* Acute lead intoxication due to intravenous injection. *Hum Toxicol* 1985; **4:** 301–9.

Chronic poisoning. References to the adverse effects of chronic exposure to lead.

1. Needleman HL, Gatsonis CA. Low-level lead exposure and the IQ of children: a meta-analysis of modern studies. *JAMA* 1990; **263:** 673–8.
2. Needleman HL, *et al.* The long-term effects of exposure to low doses of lead in childhood: an 11-year follow-up report. *N Engl J Med* 1990; **322:** 83–8.
3. Bellinger D, *et al.* Low-level lead exposure and children's cognitive function in the preschool years. *Pediatrics* 1991; **87:** 219–27.
4. Shukla R, *et al.* Lead exposure and growth in the early preschool child: a follow-up report from the Cincinnati lead study. *Pediatrics* 1991; **88:** 886–92.
5. Shannon MW, Graef JW. Lead intoxication in infancy. *Pediatrics* 1992; **89:** 87–90.
6. Huseman CA, *et al.* Neuroendocrine effects of toxic and low blood lead levels in children. *Pediatrics* 1992; **90:** 186–9.
7. Piomelli S. Childhood lead poisoning in the '90s. *Pediatrics* 1994; **93:** 508–10.
8. Mason HJ, *et al.* Effects of occupational lead exposure on serum 1,25-hydroxyvitamin D levels. *Hum Exp Toxicol* 1990; **9:** 29–34.
9. Koo WWK, *et al.* Serum vitamin D metabolites and bone mineralization in young children with chronic low to moderate lead exposure. *Pediatrics* 1991; **87:** 680–7.
10. Hu H, *et al.* The relationship of bone and blood lead to hypertension: the Normative Aging Study. *JAMA* 1996; **275:** 1171–6. Correction. *ibid.*; **276:** 1038.
11. Kim R, *et al.* A longitudinal study of low-level lead exposure and impairment of renal function: the Normative Aging Study. *JAMA* 1996; **275:** 1177–81.
12. Staessen JA, *et al.* Lead exposure and conventional and ambulatory blood pressure: a prospective population study. *JAMA* 1996; **275:** 1563–70.
13. González-Cossío T, *et al.* Decrease in birth weight in relation to maternal bone-lead burden. *Pediatrics* 1997; **100:** 856–62.

Treatment of Adverse Effects

Treatment of lead poisoning is aimed at controlling symptoms and reducing the concentration of lead in the body with chelating agents. Sodium calciumedetate (p.994) in conjunction with dimercaprol (p.979) is given for the initial management of symptomatic lead poisoning. Sodium calciumedetate, succimer (p.997), or penicillamine (p.988) are used for chelation therapy in asymptomatic patients.

Treatment of lead poisoning is aimed primarily at alleviating acute symptoms, and then at reducing the body-lead stores.[1] Initial therapy of acute symptomatic poisoning entails supportive therapy including intravenous fluids and antiepileptics if necessary. Encephalopathy is rare in adults but more common in children and requires urgent treatment; combined therapy with sodium calciumedetate in combination with dimercaprol has substantially reduced mortality rates.[2] In this case, only the minimum fluid should be administered to avoid overload. Chelation therapy with both sodium calciumedetate and dimercaprol should be continued for 5 days and may be repeated if necessary.[1-4] For symptomatic patients without encephalopathy it may be possible to discontinue the dimercaprol after 3 days. Patients who are asymptomatic may be treated with sodium calciumedetate alone[1,3,4] or succimer.[4] Penicillamine may be used as an alternative.[4] Long-term management involves eliminating environmental exposure.[5] Contained chelation with oral penicillamine may be necessary until the desired tissue levels are achieved.[2,3]

A provocation test that measures urinary excretion of lead following administration of a standard dose of sodium calciumedetate has been widely used as a means of assessing the need for therapy. However, sodium calciumedetate is associated with nephrotoxicity and the test is cumbersome to perform, thus guidelines recommend blood-lead concentrations as a guide to treatment.[4]

Finally, it should be noted that chelation therapy is not a substitute for environmental controls in those suffering occupational exposure.[6] Chelation therapy is generally not appropriate for long-term lead exposure in asymptomatic individuals in whom a significant proportion of the total body lead is tightly bound to compact bone and brain. A provocation test may be useful in identifying patients with mild symptoms who may respond to chelation therapy.[6]

1. Ibels LS, Pollock CA. Lead intoxication. *Med Toxicol* 1986; **1:** 387–410.
2. Chisholm JJ. The use of chelating agents in the treatment of acute and chronic lead intoxication in childhood. *J Pediatr* 1968; **73:** 1–38.
3. Chisholm JJ, Barltrop D. Recognition and management of children with increased lead absorption. *Arch Dis Child* 1979; **54:** 249–62.
4. Committee on Drugs of the American Academy of Pediatrics. Treatment guidelines for lead exposure in children. *Pediatrics* 1995; **96:** 155–60.
5. Committee on Environmental Health of the American Academy of Pediatrics. Lead poisoning: from screening to primary prevention. *Pediatrics* 1993; **92:** 176–83.
6. Rempel D. The lead-exposed worker. *JAMA* 1989; **262:** 532–4.

Lead in the Environment

Many countries have taken action to reduce lead exposure from environmental sources, including food, paint, and petrol, by limiting or banning altogether the use of lead compounds in such sources. Such measures have been of value in reducing childhood exposure to lead. Screening of all children to detect those at risk of chronic lead poisoning and developmental deficit has been advocated, but selective screening in areas perceived as high risk may be appropriate in countries where the overall level of lead contamination is low.

References.

1. MAFF. Survey of lead in food: second supplementary report. *Food Surveillance Paper 10.* London: HMSO, 1982.
2. MAFF. Lead in food: progress report. *Food Surveillance Paper 27.* London: HMSO, 1989.
3. Brody DJ, *et al.* Blood lead levels in the US population: phase 1 of the Third National Health and Nutrition Examination Survey (NHANES III, 1988 to 1991). *JAMA* 1994; **272:** 277–83.
4. Pirkle JL, *et al.* The decline in blood lead levels in the United States: the National Health and Nutrition Examination Surveys (NHANES). *JAMA* 1994; **272:** 284–91.
5. Diermayer M, *et al.* Backing off universal childhood lead screening in the USA: opportunity or pitfall? *Lancet* 1994; **344:** 1587–8.

Pharmacokinetics

Lead is absorbed from the gastro-intestinal tract. Lead is also absorbed by the lungs from dust particles.

Inorganic lead is not absorbed through intact skin, but organic lead compounds may be absorbed rapidly.

Lead is distributed in the soft tissues, with higher concentrations in the liver and kidneys. In the blood it is associated with the erythrocytes. Over a period of time lead accumulates in the body and is deposited in calcified bone, hair, and teeth. Lead crosses the placental barrier. It is excreted in the faeces, urine, in sweat, and in milk.

Uses and Administration

Lead compounds were formerly employed as astringents, but the medicinal use of preparations containing lead is no longer recommended. The lead salts or compounds that have been used have included lead acetate and lead subacetate (for lead lotion, still known sometimes as lotio plumbi), lead carbonate, lead monoxide, and lead oleate (for lead plaster-mass).

Preparations

Proprietary Preparations (details are given in Part 3)
Aust.: Pasta Plumbi.

Multi-ingredient: ***Aust.:*** Vulpuran.

Lecithin (596-l)

E322.

Pharmacopoeias. In *Aust.* and *Ger.* Also in *USNF.*

A phospholipid composed of a complex mixture of acetone-insoluble phosphatidyl esters (phosphatides) which consist chiefly of phosphatidyl choline, phosphatidyl ethanolamine, phosphatidyl serine, and phosphatidyl inositol, combined with various amounts of other substances such as triglycerides, fatty acids, and carbohydrates, as separated from the crude vegetable oil source.

The consistency of both natural grades and refined grades of lecithin may vary from plastic to fluid, depending upon the content of free fatty acid and oil, and upon the presence or absence of other diluents. Its colour varies from light yellow to brown, depending on the source, on crop variations, and on whether it is bleached or unbleached.

It is odourless or has a characteristic, slight nutlike odour. It is partially **soluble** in water, but readily hydrates to form emulsions. The oil-free phosphatides are soluble in fatty acids, but are practically insoluble in fixed oils. When all phosphatide fractions are present, lecithin is partially soluble in alcohol and practically insoluble in acetone.

Lecithin is an emulsifying and stabilising agent used in both the pharmaceutical and the food industries.

Lecithin has also been used as a source of choline and tried in the treatment of dementia (p.1386) with little evidence of clinical benefit. It has also been tired in various extrapyramidal disorders. Phosphatidyl serine (p.1618) has been used similarly.

Preparations

Proprietary Preparations (details are given in Part 3)
Aust.: Buerlecithin Compact; Dermo WAS; ***Austral.:*** Buerlecithin; ***Ger.:*** Buerlecithin; ***Ital.:*** Cholsoy L†; ***Switz.:*** Buerlecithine Compact†.

Multi-ingredient: ***Aust.:*** Bilatin; Buerlecithin; Colagain; Lecithin comp†; Lecivital; Sanvita Enerlecit; Sanvita Enerlecit-Tonikum mit Rosmarin; ***Austral.:*** Berberis Complex; Bioglan E-Plus; Esten†; ML 20; Plantiodine Plus; ***Canad.:*** Complex 15; ***Fr.:*** Arkotonic; Cholegerol; Ginzinc†; ***Ger.:*** Balneoconzen; Haut-Vital; Hepsan†; Hicoton; Johanniskrautol mit Lecithin; Kola-Dallmann mit Lecithin; Lotio Hermal†; tissula-N†; Vita Buerlecithin; ***Irl.:*** Rovaktivit†; ***Ital.:*** Lemivit; Mnemo Organico Plus†; Nutrigel; Ottovis; Solecin; Tricortin; ***S.Afr.:*** Vitaforce 21-Plus†; ***Switz.:*** Biovital Ginseng; Geriavit; Vita Buerlecithine†; ***UK:*** All In One Plus Grapefruit; Kelp Plus 3; Naudicelle SL; S.P.H.P.; ***USA:*** KLB6.

Leishmanin (4333-r)

Leishmanin is a suspension of *Leishmania* promastigotes used in an intradermal test to indicate previous exposure to leishmanial antigens. Its chief use is in epidemiological studies of leishmaniasis (p.575). The Leishmanin skin test has also been known as the Montenegro test.

Lemon Grass Oil (4661-j)

Essência de Capim-Limão; Indian Melissa Oil; Indian Verbena Oil; Lemongrass Oil; Oleum Graminis Citrati.

The volatile oil is obtained by distillation from *Cymbopogon flexuosus* or *C. citratus* (Gramineae). It contains citral and citronellal. **Store** in airtight containers. Protect from light.

Lemon grass oil was formerly given as a carminative. It has been used in perfumery and as a flavour.

Preparations

Proprietary Preparations (details are given in Part 3)

Multi-ingredient: ***Ger.:*** Kneipp Krauter Taschenkur Nerven und Schlaf N; ***Switz.:*** Carmol†.

Lemon Oil (4662-z)

Aetheroleum Citri; Citronenöl; Esencia de Cidra; Essence de Citron; Essência de Limão; Limonis Aetheroleum; Ol. Limon.; Oleum Citri; Oleum Limonis.

Pharmacopoeias. In *Eur.* (see p.viii).
Br. also includes a monograph on dried lemon peel; *Fr.* also includes fresh lemon peel.

A clear mobile pale yellow to greenish-yellow liquid. It is obtained without the aid of heat from the fresh peel of *Citrus limon* (Rutaceae) and contains not less than 2.2% w/w and not more than 4.5% w/w of carbonyl compounds calculated as citral ($C_{10}H_{16}O$=152.2); limonene is the major constituent. It may become cloudy at low temperatures. **Miscible** with dehydrated alcohol, with ether, and with glacial acetic acid. **Store** in well-filled airtight containers and protect from light. The Ph. Eur. directs that where appropriate the label should state that the contents are Italian-type Lemon Oil.

Lemon oil is chiefly used in perfumery and as a flavour. It is used in the preparation of terpeneless lemon oil. It has also been used with other volatile agents in rubefacient preparations and preparations for respiratory-tract disorders. Photosensitivity reactions have been reported.

An oil extracted from the leaves of *Citrus medica* was a simple and effective repellent against sandfly bites.[1]

1. Rojas E, Scorza JV. The use of lemon essential oil as a sandfly repellent. *Trans R Soc Trop Med Hyg* 1991; **85:** 803.

Preparations

BP 1998: Aromatic Ammonia Spirit *(Sal Volatile Spirit).*

Proprietary Preparations (details are given in Part 3)

Multi-ingredient: ***Aust.:*** Spasmo Claim; ***Austral.:*** Genuine Australian Eucalyptus Drops; ***Belg.:*** Melisana†; ***Fr.:*** Balsofletol†; Biphedrine Huileuse†; Citrosil; Ephydrol; ***Ger.:*** Amol Heilkrautergeist N; Babix-Wundsalbe N; Ceprovit; Tachynerg N; ***Spain:*** Alquil Dermol†; Synthol†; ***Switz.:*** Carmol†; Neo-Angin au miel et citron; Pommade Po-Ho N A Vogel; ***UK:*** Collins Elixir Pastilles; Cough Drops; Famel Catarrh & Throat Pastilles; Throaties Catarrh Pastilles; ***USA:*** Mexsana.

Terpeneless Lemon Oil (4663-c)

Oleum Limonis Deterpenatum.

Pharmacopoeias. In Br.

A clear colourless or pale yellow liquid with the characteristic odour and taste of lemon, prepared by concentrating lemon oil under reduced pressure until most of the terpenes have been removed, or by solvent partition. It contains not less than 40% w/w of aldehydes calculated as citral. **Soluble** 1 in 1 of alcohol (80%). **Store** at a temperature not exceeding 25° in well-filled containers. Protect from light.

Terpeneless lemon oil is used as a flavour. It has the advantages of being stronger in taste and odour and more readily soluble than the natural oil and is the oil used in the preparation of lemon spirit and lemon syrup. Photosensitivity is associated with citrus oils.

Preparations

BP 1998: Compound Orange Spirit; Lemon Spirit; Lemon Syrup.

Proprietary Preparations (details are given in Part 3)

Multi-ingredient: ***UK:*** Lemsip Chesty Cough; Lemsip Dry Tickly Cough; Lemsip Linctus†; Meltus Honey & Lemon; Throaties Family Cough Linctus.

Lentinan (19404-q)

LC-33.

A glucan extracted from the mushroom *Lentinus edodes.*

Lentinan appears to act as an immunostimulant. It has been tried in the treatment of malignant neoplasms and in AIDS.

Lepromin (12892-g)

Lepromin is a suspension of killed *Mycobacterium leprae* prepared from the skin of heavily infected patients suffering from lepromatous leprosy (lepromin H) or from armadillo tissue infected with *M. leprae* (lepromin A). It is used in an intradermal skin test for the classification of leprosy (p.128) and the assessment of immune responsiveness to *M. leprae.* The test is not diagnostic for leprosy.

The original lepromin (of Mitsuda and Hayashi), a suspension of the whole autoclaved homogenised leproma including some tissue elements, is sometimes called integral lepromin, whereas purified bacillary suspensions are sometimes called bacillary lepromins.[1] Leprolins are the soluble proteins of the bacilli with or without proteins of the lepra, not coagulated by heating, and do not elicit the early reaction. The Dharmendra antigen is neither a lepromin nor a leprolin and is used especially for testing the early reactions; it gives only a weak late reaction. Purified protein derivatives of *Mycobacterium leprae,* such as leprosin A,[2] have also been developed.

1. Abe M, *et al.* Immunological problems in leprosy research. *Lepr Rev* 1974; **45:** 244–72.
2. Stanford JL. Skin testing with mycobacterial reagents in leprosy. *Tubercle* 1984; **65:** 63–74.

Leptin (1669-r)

Leptin is an endogenous protein that is involved in the control of body weight. A recombinant form is under investigation in the management of obesity.

Reviews.

1. Auwerx J, Staels B. Leptin. *Lancet* 1998; **351:** 737–42.

Levomenol (9734-s)

Levomenol *(rINN).*

(−)-α-Bisabolol. (−)-6-Methyl-2-(4-methyl-3-cyclohexen-1-yl)-5-hepten-2-ol.

$C_{15}H_{26}O$ = 222.4.

CAS — 23089-26-1.

Levomenol has been tried as a transepidermal penetration enhancer.

References.

1. Kadir R, Barry BW. α-Bisabolol, a possible safe penetration enhancer for dermal and transdermal therapeutics. *Int J Pharmaceutics* 1991; **70:** 87–94.

Preparations

Proprietary Preparations (details are given in Part 3)

Multi-ingredient: ***Fr.:*** Apaisance; ***Ger.:*** Elbozon†; Mirfulan Spray N; Sensicutan; ***Ital.:*** Broxo al Fluoro; ***Switz.:*** Antidry; Dermophil Indien.

Levonordefrin (2076-b)

Corbadrine *(rINN)*; *l*-3,4-Dihydroxynorephedrine; *l*-Nordefrin. (−)-2-Amino-1-(3,4-dihydroxyphenyl)propan-1-ol.

$C_9H_{13}NO_3$ = 183.2.

CAS — 829-74-3 (levonordefrin); 6539-57-7 (nordefrin); 61-96-1 (nordefrin hydrochloride).

Pharmacopoeias. In US.

Aust. includes Nordefrin Hydrochloride, which is the salt of the racemic substance.

A white to buff-coloured, odourless, crystalline solid. Practically **insoluble** in water; slightly soluble in alcohol, acetone, chloroform, and ether; freely soluble in aqueous solutions of mineral acids.

Levonordefrin is a sympathomimetic (p.951) which has been used as a vasoconstrictor in dentistry in a concentration of 1 in 20 000 in solutions of local anaesthetics.

Preparations

USP 23: Mepivacaine Hydrochloride and Levonordefrin Injection; Procaine and Tetracaine Hydrochlorides and Levonordefrin Injection; Propoxycaine and Procaine Hydrochlorides and Levonordefrin Injection.

Proprietary Preparations (details are given in Part 3)

Used as an adjunct in: ***S.Afr.:*** Carbocaine; ***USA:*** Carbocaine with Neo-Cobefrin; Isocaine.

Lexipafant (15459-y)

Lexipafant *(BAN, USAN, rINN).*

BB-882; DO-6. Ethyl *N*-methyl-*N*-[α-(2-methylimidazo[4,5-c]pyridin-1-yl)tosyl]-L-leucinate.

$C_{23}H_{30}N_4O_4S$ = 458.6.

CAS — 139133-26-9.

Lexipafant is a platelet-activating factor antagonist that is being investigated in pancreatitis (p.1613). It has also been studied for possible applications in asthma, sepsis, and reperfusion injury.

References.

1. Ventresca GP, *et al.* The effects of oral lexipafant on ex vivo platelet aggregation and intradermal PAF challenge in healthy subjects. *Br J Clin Pharmacol* 1995; **39:** 546P.
2. Olsson P, *et al.* Pharmacokinetics of lexipafant after single and repeat oral doses and in fasted/fed conditions. *Br J Clin Pharmacol* 1995; **39:** 561P–562P.
3. McKay C, Imrie CW. Intravenous lexipafant reduces mortality and morbidity in acute pancreatitis. *Gut* 1997; **41** (suppl 3): A75.
4. Kingsnorth AN, *et al.* Early treatment with lexipafant, a platelet-activating factor antagonist, reduces mortality in acute pancreatitis: a double-blind, randomised, placebo controlled study. *Gastroenterology* 1997; **112:** A453.

Linseed (5441-w)

Flaxseed; Leinsamen; Lin; Linho; Lini Semen; Lini Semina; Linum; Semilla de Lino.

Pharmacopoeias. In *Chin., Eur.* (see p.viii), and *Pol.*

The dried ripe seeds of *Linum usitatissimum* (Linaceae). **Protect** from light.

Uses and Administration

Preparations of linseed have been administered for their demulcent action. Crushed linseed has been used as a poultice. See also Linseed Oil, below.

Preparations

Proprietary Preparations (details are given in Part 3)

Aust.: Linusit Gold; ***Ger.:*** Linusit Creola; Linusit Darmaktiv Leinsamen; ***Ital.:*** Linusit†.

Multi-ingredient: ***Canad.:*** Linoforce†; ***Ger.:*** Dralinsa; Duoventrin; Pascomag; ***Switz.:*** Enveloppements ECR; Linoforce; Optilax.

Linseed Oil (7360-h)

Aceite de Linaza; Flaxseed Oil; Huile de Lin; Leinöl; Oleum Lini.

Pharmacopoeias. In *Aust., Br., Pol.,* and *Swiss.*

The fixed oil expressed from the ripe seeds of linseed (above), *Linum usitatissimum* (Linaceae). A clear, yellowish brown oil. Gradually thickens on exposure to air forming, when spread in a thin film, a hard transparent varnish. Slightly **soluble** in alcohol; miscible with chloroform, ether, and petroleum spirit. **Store** in well-filled well-closed containers.

Linseed oil is used in veterinary medicine as a purgative for horses and cattle. In man, linseed oil is included in topical preparations for a variety of skin disorders. It has been tried as a vegetable source of omega-3 fatty acids (p.1276).

Boiled linseed oil ('boiled oil') is linseed oil heated with litharge, manganese resinate, or other driers, to a temperature of about 150° so that metallic salts of the fatty acids are formed and cause the oil to dry more rapidly. It must not be used for medicinal purposes.

Preparations

Proprietary Preparations (details are given in Part 3)

Multi-ingredient: ***Aust.:*** Dermowund; ***Fr.:*** Huile de Haarlem; ***Switz.:*** Epithelial†; Malvedrin; Vulna†; ***UK:*** 9 Rubbing Oils; Efamol Safflower & Linseed; Vericap†.

Lithium Benzoate (2337-s)

$C_7H_5LiO_2$ = 128.1.

CAS — 553-54-8.

Each g represents 7.8 mmol (7.8 mEq) of lithium.

Lithium benzoate has been used as a diuretic and urinary disinfectant. Its use cannot be recommended because of the pharmacological effect of the lithium ion (p.290).

Preparations

Proprietary Preparations (details are given in Part 3)

Multi-ingredient: ***Fr.:*** Antigoutteux Rezall; Uraseptine Rogier†.

Lobenzarit Sodium (16879-a)

Lobenzarit Sodium *(USAN, rINNM).*

CCA. 4-Chloro-2,2′-iminodibenzoate disodium.

$C_{14}H_8ClNNa_2O_4$ = 335.6.

CAS — 63329-53-3 (lobenzarit); 64808-48-6 (lobenzarit sodium).

Lobenzarit sodium is used as an immunomodulator in rheumatoid arthritis.

References.

1. Shiokawa Y, *et al.* A multicenter double-blind controlled study of lobenzarit, a novel immunomodulator, in rheumatoid arthritis. *J Rheumatol* 1984; **11:** 615–23.
2. Ueo T, *et al.* Changes of IL-2 receptor expression of lymphocytes in the peripheral blood and synovial fluid of patients with rheumatoid arthritis treated by a new immunomodulator, disodium 4-chloro-2-2′-iminodibenzoate. *Int J Immunother* 1988; **4:** 145–50.
3. Hirohata S, *et al.* Regulation of B cell function by lobenzarit, a novel disease-modifying antirheumatic drug. *Arthritis Rheum* 1992; **35:** 168–75.

Preparations

Proprietary Preparations (details are given in Part 3)

Jpn: Carfenil.

Lofexidine Hydrochloride (12901-j)

Lofexidine Hydrochloride *(BANM, USAN, rINNM).*

Ba-168; MDL-14042; MDL-14042A; RMI-14042A. 2-[1-(2,6-Dichlorophenoxy)ethyl]-2-imidazoline hydrochloride.

$C_{11}H_{12}Cl_2N_2O,HCl$ = 295.6.

CAS — 31036-80-3 (lofexidine); 21498-08-8 (lofexidine hydrochloride).

Adverse Effects

Lofexidine has central alpha-adrenergic effects and may cause drowsiness, and dryness of the mouth, throat, and nose. Symptoms of overdosage with lofexidine include hypotension, bradycardia, sedation, and coma.

Sudden withdrawal of lofexidine may produce rebound hypertension.

Precautions

Lofexidine should be used with caution in patients with cerebrovascular disease, ischaemic heart disease including recent myocardial infarction, bradycardia, renal impairment, or a history of depression.

It can cause drowsiness and if affected, patients should not drive or operate machinery. The effects of other CNS depressants, including alcohol, may be enhanced.

Withdrawal of lofexidine therapy should be gradual over 2 to 4 days or more to reduce the risk of rebound hypertension.

Interactions

Lofexidine may enhance the central depressant effects of sedative agents. Tricyclic antidepressants administered concomitantly may reduce the efficacy of lofexidine.

Uses and Administration

Lofexidine is an alpha$_2$-adrenoceptor agonist structurally related to clonidine (p.841). It has antihypertensive activity, but is used mainly in the control of opioid withdrawal symptoms.

In opioid withdrawal lofexidine is given as the hydrochloride in an initial dose of 0.2 mg twice daily by mouth. The dose may be increased gradually by 0.2 to 0.4 mg daily to a maximum of 2.4 mg daily. After 7 to 10 days, or longer in some cases, treatment is withdrawn gradually over at least 2 to 4 days.

Opioid dependence. Washton and colleagues found that 10 of 15 methadone addicts managed with a regimen including lofexidine in doses of 100 μg twice daily to 400 μg four times daily were successfully withdrawn without unacceptable withdrawal symptoms.[1] The findings were similar to those with clonidine but lofexidine appeared to be less sedating and hypotensive. Similar results have been reported by Gold and colleagues,[2] and in a further report by Washton *et al.*[3] A commentary on lofexidine at the time of its launch on the UK market[4] pointed to the lack of clinical data from studies other than from those cited above and hinted at the need for controlled studies on a larger scale.

For a discussion of the treatment of opioid dependence, see p.67.

1. Washton AM, *et al.* Lofexidine, a clonidine analogue effective in opiate withdrawal. *Lancet* 1981; **i:** 991–2.
2. Gold MS, *et al.* Lofexidine, a clonidine analogue effective in opiate withdrawal. *Lancet* 1981; **i:** 992–3.
3. Washton AM, *et al.* Opiate withdrawal using lofexidine, a clonidine analogue with fewer side-effects. *J Clin Psychiatry* 1983; **44:** 335–7.
4. Cox S, Alcorn R. Lofexidine and opioid withdrawal. *Lancet* 1995; **345:** 1385–6.

Preparations

Proprietary Preparations (details are given in Part 3)
UK: Britlofex.

Lorenzo's Oil (14102-f)

Lorenzo's oil is a liquid containing glyceryl trierucate (a source of erucic acid) and glyceryl trioleate (a source of oleic acid), in the ratio one part to four parts respectively. It has been used in conjunction with dietary modification for the treatment of adrenoleucodystrophy, a genetic disorder characterised by demyelination, adrenal cortical insufficiency, and accumulation of saturated 'very-long-chain fatty acids'.

Adrenoleucodystrophy. Adrenoleucodystrophy is a rare X-linked metabolic disorder in which accumulation of saturated very-long-chain fatty acids results in diffuse and multifocal demyelination of the nervous system and adrenocortical insufficiency. The most common form usually affects children and is characterised primarily by cerebral demyelination; it is usually fatal within a few years. In the adult variant, called adrenomyeloneuropathy, demyelination of the spinal cord and peripheral neuropathy progress slowly over many years.

There appears to be no effective treatment for adrenoleucodystrophy or its variants. A high dietary intake of long-chain monounsaturated fatty acids, as provided by the mixture Lorenzo's oil (glyceryl trierucate with glyceryl trioleate), has been tried, the idea being to monopolise the specific enzyme involved in the conversion of long-chain fatty acids to very-long-chain fatty acids. Although dietary therapy with Lorenzo's oil has reduced plasma concentrations of saturated very-long-chain fatty acids there is no evidence that this improves or delays progression of adrenoleucodystrophy or adrenomyeloneuropathy.[1-3] However, it has been suggested that these disorders may not respond to correction of the biochemical abnormality once neurological damage has occurred.[3] The effectiveness of treatment before the appearance of neurological symptoms is currently being studied. There is some evidence to suggest that the childhood form may have an immunological component but results using immunosuppressive agents or immunoglobulins have been reported to be disappointing.[3] Lovastatin can also reduce plasma concentrations of very-long-chain fatty acids.[4]

1. Aubourg P, *et al.* A two-year trial of oleic and erucic acids ("Lorenzo's oil") as treatment for adrenomyeloneuropathy. *N Engl J Med* 1993; **329:** 745–52.
2. Kaplan PW, *et al.* Visual evoked potentials in adrenoleukodystrophy: a trial with glycerol trioleate and Lorenzo oil. *Ann Neurol* 1993; **34:** 169–74.
3. Rizzo WB. Lorenzo's oil—hope and disappointment. *N Engl J Med* 1993; **329:** 801–2.
4. Singh I, *et al.* Lovastatin for X-linked adrenoleukodystrophy. *N Engl J Med* 1998; **339:** 702–3.

Adverse effects. Thrombocytopenia has been reported in patients receiving Lorenzo's oil, although patients are often asymptomatic.[1] It is possible that giant platelets which retain most of their function are produced and that these are not counted by automatic counting procedures giving a false impression of thrombocytopenia.[2]

Lymphocytopenia with an increased incidence of infection has also been reported in few patients.[3]

1. Zinkham WH, *et al.* Lorenzo's oil and thrombocytopenia in patients with adrenoleukodystrophy. *N Engl J Med* 1993; **328:** 1126–7.
2. Stöckler S, *et al.* Giant platelets in erucic acid therapy for adrenoleukodystrophy. *Lancet* 1993; **341:** 1414–15.
3. Unkrig CJ, *et al.* Lorenzo's oil and lymphocytopenia. *N Engl J Med* 1994; **330:** 577.

Preparations

Proprietary Preparations (details are given in Part 3)
Multi-ingredient: ***UK:*** Lorenzo's Oil.

Lovage Root (11834-e)

Levistici Radix.

Pharmacopoeias. In *Eur.* (see p.viii) and *Pol.*

The whole or cut, dried rhizome and root of *Levisticum officinale*. The whole drug contains not less than 4.0 mL per kg of essential oil and the cut drug not less than 3.0 mL per kg of essential oil, calculated with reference to the anhydrous drug. **Protect** from light.

Lovage root is used in herbal medicine.

Preparations

Proprietary Preparations (details are given in Part 3)
Multi-ingredient: ***Aust.:*** Ehrenhofer-Salbe; Kneipp Stoffwechsel-Unterstutzungs-Tee; Krautertee Nr 19; Krautertee Nr 2; Krautertee Nr 31; ***Ger.:*** Canephron N; Castrophan†; Dr. Kleinschrod's Cor-Insuffin†; Entwasserungs-Tee†; Hevert-Entwasserungs-Tee; Kneipp Schlankheits-Unterstutzungstee†; Nephroselect M; Rheumex†; ***Switz.:*** Tisane antiseptique diuretique†; Tisane diuretique "H"†; ***UK:*** Fragador.

Lupulus (535-f)

Hop Strobile; Hopfenzapfen; Hops; Houblon; Humulus; Lupuli Flos; Lupuli Strobulus; Strobili Lupuli.

Pharmacopoeias. In *Eur.* (see p.viii).

The dried, generally whole, female inflorescences (strobiles) of the hop plant *Humulus lupulus* (Cannabinaceae). **Protect** from light.

Lupulus has been used as a bitter, and supplies the characteristic flavour of beers. It is used in herbal and folk medicine as a sedative. It is also used in homoeopathic medicine.

Preparations

Proprietary Preparations (details are given in Part 3)
Aust.: Zirkulin Beruhigungs-Tee; ***Ger.:*** Bonased-L; Lactidorm.

Multi-ingredient: ***Aust.:*** Aktiv Nerven- und Schlaftee; Bakanasan Einschlaf; Baldracin; Baldrian AMA; Baldrian Dispert Compositum; Baldrian-Elixier; Baldrian-Krautertonikum; Baldriparan Beruhigungs; Beruhigungskapseln; Beruhigungstee; Bio-Garten Tee zur Beruhigung; Bio-Garten Tropfen zur Beruhigung; Biogelat Schlaf; Doppelherz Tonikum; Einschlafkapseln; Hova; Hovaletten†; Krauterdoktor Beruhigungstropfen; Krauterdoktor Entspannungs- und Einschlaftropfen; Krauterdoktor Nerven-Tonikum; Krauterhaus Mag Kottas Nerven- und Schlaftee; Krautertee Nr 1; Krautertee Nr 141; Krautertee Nr 16; Krautertee Nr 201; Luvased; Mag Doskar's Nerventonikum; Mag Kottas Krauterexpress-Nerven-Schlaf-Tee; Mag Kottas Schlaftee; Montana; Nervendragees; Nervenruh; Nerventee; Nervifloran; Phytogran; Sanhelios Einschlaf; Seda-Grandelat; Sidroga Nerven- und Schlaftee; St Radegunder Beruhigungs- und Einschlaftee; St Radegunder Nerven-Tonikum; St Radegunder Nerventee; Vivinox; Wechseltee; ***Austral.:*** Kavosporal†; Migran-eze†; Pacifenity; Passiflora Complex; Passionflower Plus; Prosed-X; Relaxaplex; Vitaglow Executive Anti Stress†; Vitaglow Herbal Stress†; ***Canad.:*** Herbal Sleep Well†; ***Fr.:*** Santane D_5; Santane N_9; ***Ger.:*** Aranidorm-S; Ardeysedon N; Avedorm; Avedorm N; B 12 Nervinfant†; Baldrian-Dispert Nacht; Baldrianox S; Baldriparan N; Baldriparan stark N; Belladonna-Valobonin†; Beruhigungs-Tee Nervoflux†; Biosedon S; Boxocalm; Bunetten†; Cefasedativ; Cysto Fink; Discmigon; Dormeasan; Dormoverlan; Dr. Klinger's Bergischer Krautertee, Nerven- und Beruhigungstee†; Einschlaf-Kapseln biologisch; Euvegal N†; Gutnacht; Herz-plus Forte N†; Herz-Plus Nerven†; Herz-plus†; Hicoton; Hova†; Hovaletten N; Ivel Schlaf; JuDorm; JuNeuron S; Knufinke Nervenruh Beruhigungs-Tee†; Kytta-Sedativum f; Leukona-Sedativ-Bad; Leukona-Sedativ-Bad sine Chloralhydrat; Luvased; Luvased-Tropfen N; Manns Knoblauch Pillen Plus†; Moradorm S; Nervendragees; Nervenruh†; Nerviguttum†; Nervinetten; Nervinfant N; Nervinfant†; Nervisal†; Nervo.opt†; Nervoregin forte; Neuraston†; Orbis Nerven- und Beruhigungstee†; Pan-Nerventonikum†; Pascosedon S; Phytogran; Presselin K 1 N; Salus Nerven-Schlaf-Tee Nr.22; Salusan; Schupps Baldrian Sedativbad; Seda Kneipp N; Seda-Pasc N†; Seda-Plantina; Sedacur; Sedahopf; Sedaselect N; Sedasyx; Sedatruw S; Sedinfant N; Sediomed S†; Selon; Sensinerv forte; Somnium†; Somnuvis S; Steno-Valocordin†; Stomasal Med; Stomasal†; Valdispert comp; Valeriana comp; Valeriana forte; Valeriana mild; Valeriana-Strath†; Valobonin†; Visinal; Vivinox; Vivinox-Schlafdragees; Worishofener Nervenpflege Dr. Kleinschrod†; ***Switz.:*** Baldriparan; Cysto Fink; Cysto-Caps Chassot; Demonatur Dragees calmantes†; Dicalm†; Dormeasan N; Dormeasan†; Dragees pour le coeur et les nerfs; Dragees pour le sommeil nouvelle formule; Dragees relaxantes et tranquillisantes†; Hyperiforce; Phytoberidin; Phytomed Somni; Soporin; Tisane Natterman instantanee no 6 pour calmer les nerfs et lutter contre l'insomnie†; Tisane pour le coeur et la circulation "H"†; Tisane pour le sommeil et les nerfs; Valobonin†; Valverde Dragees pour le coeur; Valverde Dragees pour le sommeil N; ***UK:*** Ana-Sed; Avena sativa comp.; Becalm; Gerard 99; Kalms; Natrasleep; Newrelax; Night Time; Nytol Herbal; Quiet Days; Quiet Life; Quiet Night; Quiet Nite; Quiet Tyme; Relax B+; Serenity; Somnus; Super Mega B+C; Valerian Compound; Valerina Night-Time.

Lysergide (5011-e)

Lysergide *(BAN, rINN)*.

LSD; LSD-25; Lysergic Acid Diethylamide. (+)-*NN*-Diethyl-D-lysergamide; (6a*R*,9*R*)-*NN*-Diethyl-4,6,6a,7,8,9-hexahydro-7-methylindolo[4,3-*fg*]quinoline-9-carboxamide.

$C_{20}H_{25}N_3O$ = 323.4.

CAS — 50-37-3.

Lysergide was formerly used therapeutically but is now encountered as a drug of abuse for its hallucinogenic and psychedelic properties.

There is considerable variation in individual reaction to lysergide. Disorders of visual perception are among the first and most constant reactions to lysergide. Subjects may be hypersensitive to sound. Extreme alterations of mood, depression, distortion of body image, depersonalisation, disorders of thought and time sense, and synaesthesias may be experienced. Anxiety, often amounting to panic, may occur (a 'bad trip'). The effects of lysergide may recur months after ingestion of lysergide; the recurrence or 'flashback' may be spontaneous or induced by alcohol, other drugs, stress, or fatigue.

The subjective effects of lysergide may be preceded or accompanied by somatic effects which are mainly sympathomimetic in nature and include mydriasis, tremor, hyperreflexia, hyperthermia, piloerection, muscle weakness, and ataxia. There may be nausea and vomiting and increased heart rate and blood pressure. Derangement of blood clotting mechanisms has been described. In addition, respiratory arrest, convulsions, and coma may result from overdoses. There is no evidence of fatal reactions to lysergide in man, although accidental deaths, suicides, and homicides have occurred during lysergide intoxication.

Tolerance develops to the behavioural effects of lysergide after several days and may be lost over a similar period. There is cross-tolerance between lysergide, mescaline, and psilocybin and psilocin, but not to amphetamine or to cannabis.

Physical dependence on lysergide does not seem to occur.

Mace Oil (4667-x)

NOTE. Mace has also been used as a name for a tear gas.

A volatile oil obtained by distillation from mace, the arillus of the seed of *Myristica fragrans* (Myristicaceae). **Store** in airtight containers. Protect from light.

Nutmeg (p.1609) is the dried kernel of the seed of *M. fragrans*.

Mace is used as a flavour and carminative similarly to nutmeg (p.1609). It has also been used with herbal substances and other volatile agents in preparations for musculoskeletal and respiratory-tract disorders. As with nutmeg, large doses of mace may cause epileptiform convulsions and hallucinations.

Preparations

Proprietary Preparations (details are given in Part 3)
Multi-ingredient: ***Ger.:*** Bormelin†; Reflex-Zonen-Salbe (RZS) (Rowo-333)†; ***Switz.:*** Carmol "blanche"†; Carmol†.

Macrogols (1922-a)

Macrogols *(BAN, rINN)*.

PEGs; Polyethylene Glycols; Polyoxyethylene Glycols.

$CH_2(OH)(CH_2OCH_2)_mCH_2OH$. Alternatively some authorities use the general formula $H(OCH_2CH_2)_nOH$ when the number assigned to *n* for a specified macrogol is 1 more than that of *m* in the first formula.

CAS — 25322-68-3 (macrogols); 37361-15-2 (macrogol 300).

Pharmacopoeias. Macrogols of various molecular weights are included in many pharmacopoeias.

Eur. (see p.viii) specifies macrogol 300, 400, 1000, 1500, 3000, 4000, 6000, 20 000, and 35 000. *USNF* has a general monograph describing Polyethylene Glycol which requires that it be labelled with the average nominal molecular weight as part of the official title.

Macrogols are condensation polymers of ethylene oxide and water. Each macrogol name is followed by a number indicating its approximate average molecular weight; thus macrogol 300 has an average molecular weight of about 300 (*m*=5 or 6 giving a molecular weight of 282.3 or 326.4).

Macrogols with an average molecular weight of 200 to 600 are clear to slightly hazy, colourless or almost colourless, viscous liquids with a slight characteristic odour; those with an average molecular weight of more than 1000 are white to off-white solids, also with a slight characteristic odour, which vary in consistency between soft unctuous pastes and hard waxy flakes, beads, or powder. Viscosity increases with increasing molecular weight but hygroscopicity decreases and at average molecular weights above 4000, hygroscopicity is low. Solid macrogols are very or freely **soluble** in water; liquid macrogols are miscible with water. Macrogols dissolve in alcohol, acetone, chloroform, ethoxyethanol, ethyl acetate, dichloromethane, and toluene, their solubility decreasing with increasing molecular weight. They are insoluble in ether and in fixed or mineral oils.

Macrogols can demonstrate oxidising activity leading to **incompatibilities**. The activity of bacitracin or benzylpenicillin may be reduced in a macrogol basis. Some plastics are softened by macrogols.

The pH of a 5% solution of a macrogol in water is about 4.5 to 7.5. Aqueous solutions can be **sterilised** by autoclaving or filtration.

Store in airtight containers.

Adverse Effects and Precautions

Macrogols appear to have relatively low toxicity, although any toxicity appears to be greatest with the macrogols of low molecular weight. They may cause stinging when administered topically, especially to mucous membranes, and have been associated with hypersensitivity reactions such as urticaria. Hyperosmolality, metabolic acidosis, and renal failure have been reported following the topical application of macrogols to burn patients. Topical preparations with a macrogol base should therefore be used with caution in patients with renal impairment and/or large areas of raw surfaces, burns, or open wounds.

Patients undergoing bowel cleansing with mixtures of macrogols (3350 or 4000) and electrolytes commonly experience local gastro-intestinal discomfort, bloating, and nausea. Abdominal cramps, vomiting, and anal irritation may also occur and there have been rare reports of possible hypersensitivity reactions. These colonic lavage solutions are contra-indicated in gastro-intestinal obstruction or perforation, ileus, gastric retention, peptic ulceration, and toxic megacolon; caution is advisable in patients with ulcerative colitis. Since aspiration may be a problem, they should be used with caution in patients with an impaired gag reflex, reflux oesophagitis, or diminished levels of consciousness. They should be given with caution to diabetic patients. Drugs taken within one hour of starting colonic lavage with an orally administered macrogol and electrolyte mixture may be flushed from the gastro-intestinal tract unabsorbed.

Effects on the kidneys. Macrogol 400 in lorazepam injection could have contributed to renal damage suggestive of acute tubular necrosis in a patient who received large doses of lorazepam injection (averaging lorazepam 95 mg per day) for 43 days.[1] The cumulative dose of macrogol 400 during this period was about 220 mL.

1. Laine GA, *et al.* Polyethylene glycol nephrotoxicity secondary to prolonged high-dose intravenous lorazepam. *Ann Pharmacother* 1995; **29:** 1110–14.

Fluid and electrolyte homoeostasis. A syndrome of elevated total serum calcium (with a concomitant decrease in ionised calcium), hyperosmolality, metabolic acidosis, and renal failure has been observed in *animals*[1] and in burn patients[2] following the topical application of preparations with a macrogol base. The FDA has recommended that topical preparations containing macrogols should be used with caution in burn patients with known or suspected renal impairment, as macrogols absorbed through denuded skin and not excreted normally by a compromised kidney could lead to symptoms of progressive renal impairment.[3]

The use of macrogol and electrolyte solutions for bowel preparation has also been associated with sodium and water retention resulting in exacerbation of heart failure in a patient with diabetic gastroparesis[4] and with the development of pulmonary oedema possibly due to aspiration in a child without cardiac or renal disease.[5]

1. Herold DA, *et al.* Toxicity of topical polyethylene glycol. *Toxicol Appl Pharmacol* 1982; **65:** 329–35.
2. Bruns DE, *et al.* Polyethylene glycol intoxication in burn patients. *Burns* 1982; **9:** 49–52.
3. Anonymous. Topical PEG in burn ointments. *FDA Drug Bull* 1982; **12:** 25–6.
4. Granberry MC, *et al.* Exacerbation of congestive heart failure after administration of polyethylene glycol-electrolyte lavage solution. *Ann Pharmacother* 1995; **29:** 1232–5.
5. Paap CM, Ehrlich R. Acute pulmonary edema after polyethylene glycol intestinal lavage in a child. *Ann Pharmacother* 1993; **27:** 1044–7.

Hypersensitivity. Hypersensitivity to macrogols is uncommon but both immediate urticarial reactions and delayed allergic contact dermatitis have been reported following the topical application of preparations with a macrogol vehicle or base.[1] An anaphylactic reaction has been associated with the ingestion of macrogols in a multivitamin tablet.[2] The manufacturers of preparations containing macrogols and electrolytes for bowel cleansing have reported isolated instances of skin reactions and rhinorrhoea.

1. Fisher AA. Immediate and delayed allergic contact reactions to polyethylene glycol. *Contact Dermatitis* 1978; **4:** 135–8.
2. Kwee YN, Dolovich J. Anaphylaxis to polyethylene glycol (PEG) in a multivitamin tablet. *J Allergy Clin Immunol* 1982; **69:** 138.

Overdosage. Ingestion of 2 litres of a colonic lavage solution containing macrogol 400 instead of macrogol 4000 resulted in the patient developing severe metabolic acidosis due to systemic absorption of the macrogol and rapidly becoming comatose.[1] The patient was successfully treated with intravenous bicarbonate and dialysis.

1. Bélaïche J, *et al.* Coma acidosique après préparation colique par du polyèthylène glycol. *Gastroenterol Clin Biol* 1983; **7:** 426–7.

Pharmacokinetics

Liquid macrogols may be absorbed when taken by mouth but macrogols of high molecular weight, such as macrogol 3350, are not significantly absorbed from the gastro-intestinal tract. There is evidence of absorption of macrogols when applied to damaged skin. Macrogols entering the systemic circulation are predominantly excreted unchanged in the urine; low-molecular-weight macrogols may be partly metabolised.

References.

1. DiPiro JT, *et al.* Absorption of polyethylene glycol after administration of a PEG-electrolyte lavage solution. *Clin Pharm* 1986; **5:** 153–5.

Uses and Administration

Macrogols are relatively stable, non-toxic compounds which have a range of properties depending on their molecular weight. They are widely used in pharmaceutical manufacturing as water-soluble bases for topical preparations and suppositories, as solvents and vehicles, and as solubilising agents, tablet binders, plasticisers in film coating, and tablet lubricants. They have also been reported to have antibacterial properties.

A mixture of macrogol 3350 or 4000 with electrolytes is used to empty the bowel before colonoscopy, radiological procedures, or surgery. These preparations have been formulated so that the osmotic activity of the macrogol and concentrations of the electrolytes result in a minimum net effect on the fluid and electrolyte balance. Adults are given 200 to 300 mL of the reconstituted aqueous solution (containing about 59 or 60 g or 105 g of the macrogol per litre) which they have to swallow rapidly and this is repeated every 10 to 15 minutes until the rectal effluent is clear or until a total of 4 litres of the solution has been consumed. A suggested dose for children is 25 to 40 mL per kg body-weight per hour. Bowel evacuation usually begins about one hour after starting administration and is complete in about 4 hours. Patients should fast for at least 2 or 3 hours before drinking the solution. Flavourings such as clear fruit cordials may be added as advised by the manufacturer or palatability may be improved by chilling the solution but sugar or other sweeteners should not be added. If distension or pain occur, administration should be temporarily stopped or the interval between drinks extended. For administration by nasogastric tube a rate of 20 to 30 mL per minute has been suggested. Similar preparations are used as routine laxatives in a usual dose of 125 mL of a solution containing 105 g of the macrogol per litre two or three times daily.

Macrogols of high molecular weight such as macrogol 4000 have been used as inert markers in studies on intestinal absorption and excretion.

The protection of therapeutic proteins from the human immune system by conjugation with macrogols is under investigation.

Drug delivery systems. References to the use of macrogols in delivery systems for drugs and proteins.

1. Duncan R, Spreafico F. Polymer conjugates: pharmacokinetic considerations for design and development. *Clin Pharmacokinet* 1994; **27:** 290–306.

Phenol poisoning. Washing with liquid macrogols has been recommended in the emergency treatment of skin contamination with phenol, see under Treatment of Adverse Effects in Phenol, p.1121.

Preparations

BP 1998: Macrogol Ointment;
USP 23: PEG 3350 and Electrolytes for Oral Solution.

Proprietary Preparations (details are given in Part 3)
Canad.: Visatear; Visine True Tears; ***Fr.:*** Forlax.

Multi-ingredient: ***Aust.:*** Klean-Prep; ***Austral.:*** Blink-N-Clean†; Colonlytely; GoLytely; Visine Revive; ***Belg.:*** Colopeg; Klean-Prep; Precosol; Transipeg; ***Canad.:*** Aquasite; CoLyte; Cytospray†; GoLytely; Klean-Prep; Peglyte; Pro-Lax; Rhinaris; Salinol; Secaris; Visine Moisturizing; ***Fr.:*** Colopeg; Fortrans; Klean-Prep; Movicol; Transipeg; ***Ger.:*** Delcoprep; Klean-Prep; Lens Fresh; Movicol; Oralav; ***Irl.:*** Colocler†; Hypotears†; Klean-Prep; ***Ital.:*** Agena; Gofreely; Hypotears; Isocolan; Movicol; Selg; Selg-Esse; ***Norw.:*** Laxabon; ***S.Afr.:*** GoLytely; Klean-Prep; Movicol; ***Spain:*** Evacuante; ***Swed.:*** Klean-Prep; Laxabon; ***Switz.:*** Cololyt; Colopeg†; Fordtran; Gelee lubrifiante simple; Isocolan; Klean-Prep; Tracheo Fresh; ***UK:*** Hypotears; Klean-Prep; Movicol; ***USA:*** Aquasite; Co-Lav; Colovage; CoLyte; Go-Evac; GoLytely; Hypotears; Nu-Tears II; NuLytely; OCL; Tetrasine Extra; Visine Moisturizing.

Magnesium Ferulate (12908-r)

Magnesium 4-hydroxy-3-methoxycinnamate.
$(C_{10}H_9O_4)_2Mg$ = 410.7.
CAS — 32179-46-7.

Magnesium ferulate has been used as a choleretic agent.

Preparations

Proprietary Preparations (details are given in Part 3)
Fr.: Frucol†.

Magnesium Glutamate Hydrobromide

(12910-z)

Magnesium α-Aminoglutarate Hydrobromide; Magnesium Bromoglutamate.
$(C_5H_8NO_4)_2Mg,HBr$ = 397.5.

Magnesium glutamate hydrobromide has been used as a sedative and hypnotic in the treatment of insomnia, neuroses, and behavioural disorders.

Preparations

Proprietary Preparations (details are given in Part 3)
Ger.: Psicosoma†; Psychoverlan†; ***Spain:*** Psicosoma†.

Multi-ingredient: ***Spain:*** Cefabol; Gamalate B6.

Maize Oil (7361-m)

Corn Oil; Huile de Maïs; Ol. Mayd.; Oleum Maydis.

Pharmacopoeias. In *Eur* (see p.viii) and *Jpn*. Also in *USNF*.

The refined fixed oil obtained from the embryos of maize, *Zea mays* (Gramineae). It is a clear light yellow oil with a faint characteristic odour and taste. Slightly **soluble** or practically insoluble in alcohol; miscible with chloroform, dichloromethane, ether, and petroleum spirit. **Store** at a temperature not exceeding 25° in airtight containers. Protect from light.

Maize oil has a high content of unsaturated acids and has been used in patients with familial hypercholesterolaemia and as a high-calorie nutritional supplement. It is also used as an oily vehicle.

Preparations

Proprietary Preparations (details are given in Part 3)

Multi-ingredient: ***USA:*** Lipomul.

Maleic Acid (1314-k)

Acidum Maleicum; Toxilic Acid. *cis*-Butenedioic acid.
$C_2H_2(CO_2H)_2$ = 116.1.
CAS — 110-16-7.

Pharmacopoeias. In *Eur.* (see p.viii).

A white crystalline powder. **Soluble** 1 in 1.5 of water and 1 in 2 of alcohol; sparingly soluble in ether. **Store** in glass containers. Protect from light.

Maleic acid is used in the preparation of Ergometrine Injection (BP 1998) and Ergometrine and Oxytocin Injection (BP 1998).

Malic Acid (1315-a)

296 (DL-malic acid or L-malic acid); Apple Acid; Hydroxysuccinic Acid. Hydroxybutanedioic acid.
$C_4H_6O_5$ = 134.1.
CAS — 6915-15-7; 636-61-3 ((+)-form); 97-67-6 ((−)-form); 617-48-1 ((±)-form).

Pharmacopoeias. In *Ger.* Also in *USNF*.

An acid present in apples, pears, and many other fruits. It occurs as a white or practically white crystalline powder or granules. Very **soluble** in water; freely soluble in alcohol.

Malic acid is used in pharmaceutical formulations as an acidifier, flavour, and as an alternative to citric acid in effervescent powders. It is used in combination with butylated hydroxytoluene as an antioxidant in vegetable oils. It has been used topically in combination with benzoic acid and salicylic acid for desloughing of ulcers, burns, and wounds, and systemically in combination with arginine (p.1334) in preparations for the treatment of liver disorders. Pastilles containing malic acid are also used in the management of dry mouth (p.1470).

Preparations

Proprietary Preparations (details are given in Part 3)

Multi-ingredient: ***Aust.:*** Acerbine; Leberinfusion; Rocmaline; ***Fr.:*** Rocmaline; ***Ger.:*** Hepasteril†; Rocmalat†; ***Irl.:*** Aserbine†; ***S.Afr.:*** Aserbine; ***Spain:*** Acerbiol; ***Swed.:*** Salivin†; ***Switz.:*** Acerbine; ***UK:*** Aserbine; Malatex†; Salivix; ***USA:*** Super Malic.

Malotilate (17039-s)

Malotilate (USAN, rINN).

NKK-105. Diisopropyl 1,3-dithiole-$\Delta^{2,\alpha}$-malonate.

$C_{12}H_{16}O_4S_2$ = 288.4.

CAS — 59937-28-9.

Malotilate has been investigated for its reported hepato-protective effects on liver function in patients with chronic hepatic disease.

References.

1. A European Multicentre Study Group. The results of a randomized double blind controlled trial evaluating malotilate in primary biliary cirrhosis. *J Hepatol* 1993; **17:** 227–35.

Mammalian Tissue Extracts (12913-a)

Many medicinal preparations with definite pharmacological activity and valid clinical uses are of mammalian origin and are described under their appropriate monographs—for example, calcitonin, corticotrophin, hydrocortisone (cortisol), some enzymes, heparin, insulin, parathyroid, pituitary hormones, some sex hormones, thyroid.

Many other preparations of animal origin have been promoted for a wide variety of disorders. Evidence of pharmacological activity is often lacking, and such preparations are of doubtful benefit.

Preparations

Proprietary Preparations (details are given in Part 3)
Aust.: Cerebrolysin; Epiphysan; ***Ger.:*** Alvinorm†; Ardeyceryl†; Cerebral-Uvocal†; Cerebrolysin; Glanoide cerebrale†; Glanoide diencephale†; Placentormon†; ***Ital.:*** Liposom; ***Spain:*** Artrodif†.

Multi-ingredient: ***Canad.:*** Revitonus C; ***Fr.:*** Pro-Nat; ***Ger.:*** AntiFocal; Conjunctisan-A; Conjunctisan-B; NeyChondrin "N" (Revitorgan-Dilutionen "N" Nr. 68); NeyTumorin "N" (Revitorgan-Dilutionen Nr. 66); NeyTumorin-Tropfen (Revitorgan-Lingual Nr. 66); rheumamed†; Ribo-Wied; ***Ital.:*** Diamantil†; ***Switz.:*** Glutadouze†; ***UK:*** S.P.H.P..

Mastic (280-z)

Almáciga; Mastiche; Mastix.

Pharmacopoeias. In *Aust.* and *Swiss.*

A resinous exudation from certain forms or varieties of *Pistacia lentiscus* (Anacardiaceae).

Solutions of mastic in alcohol, chloroform, or ether have been used, applied on cotton wool, as temporary fillings for carious teeth. Compound Mastic Paint (BP 1980) was formerly used as a protective covering for wounds and to hold gauze in position.

Meadowsweet (13569-m)

Filipendula; Reine des Prés; Spiraeae Herba; Ulmaria.

Meadowsweet comprises the dried, aerial flowering parts of *Filipendula ulmaria* (*Spiraea ulmaria*) (Rosaceae). It is used in herbal medicine as a diuretic and in gastro-intestinal and rheumatic disorders. It is also used in homoeopathic medicine.

Preparations

Proprietary Preparations (details are given in Part 3)
Fr.: Spireadosa†.

Multi-ingredient: ***Belg.:*** Tisane Diuretique; ***Fr.:*** Actisane Douleurs Articulaires; Actisane Minceur; Aminsane; Artival†; Artrosan; Mediflor Tisane Antirhumatismale No 2; Mediflor Tisane Diuretique†; Mediflor Tisane Pectorale d'Alsace†; Promincil; Santane A_4; Santane O_1; Santane R_8; Tisane des Familles†; Tisane Touraine; Tisanes de l'Abbe Hamon no 3; ***Ger.:*** Grippe-Tee Stada†; Rheumex†; ***Ital.:*** Artoxan; Sambuco (Specie Composta); ***Switz.:*** Tisane antirhumatismale "H"†; Urinex (nouvelle formule); ***UK:*** Acidosis; Indigestion Mixture; Natraleze.

Meclofenoxate Hydrochloride (1429-v)

Meclofenoxate Hydrochloride (BANM, rINNM).

Centrophenoxine Hydrochloride; Clofenoxine Hydrochloride; Clophenoxate Hydrochloride; Deanol 4-Chlorophenoxyacetate Hydrochloride; Meclofenoxane Hydrochloride. 2-Dimethylaminoethyl 4-chlorophenoxyacetate hydrochloride.

$C_{12}H_{16}ClNO_3,HCl$ = 294.2.

CAS — 51-68-3 (meclofenoxate); 3685-84-5 (meclofenoxate hydrochloride).

Pharmacopoeias. In *Jpn.*

Meclofenoxate hydrochloride has been claimed to aid cellular metabolism in the presence of diminished oxygen concentrations. It has been given mainly for mental changes in the elderly, or following strokes or head injury.

References.

1. Pék G, *et al.* Gerontopsychological studies using NAI ('Nürnberger Alters-Inventar') on patients with organic psychosyndrome (DSM III, Category 1) treated with centrophenoxine in a double-blind, comparative, randomized clinical trial. *Arch Gerontol Geriatr* 1989; **9:** 17–30.

Preparations

Proprietary Preparations (details are given in Part 3)
Aust.: Lucidril; ***Fr.:*** Lucidril; ***Ger.:*** Cerutil; Helfergin; ***Jpn:*** Lucidril†.

Medium-chain Triglycerides (7357-q)

Triglycerida Saturata Media.

Pharmacopoeias. In *Eur.* (see p.viii).

They are prepared from the fixed oil obtained from the dried solid part of the endosperm of the coconut, the fruit of *Cocos nucifera* (Palmae) when they may be termed Fractionated Coconut Oil, or from the dried endosperm of *Elaeis guineensis*. They consist of a mixture of triglycerides of saturated fatty acids, mainly of octanoic acid (p.1609) and of capric acid ($C_{10}H_{20}O_2$), of which not less than 95% are saturated fatty acids with 8 and 10 carbon atoms.

They are colourless or pale yellow oily liquids. Practically **insoluble** in water; miscible with alcohol, with dichloromethane, with petroleum spirit, and with fatty oils. **Store** in well-filled containers. Protect from light.

Medium-chain triglycerides are given parenterally and enterally for nutritional purposes in conditions associated with malabsorption of fat, such as cystic fibrosis, enteritis, and steatorrhoea, and following intestinal resection. Medium-chain triglycerides are more readily hydrolysed than long-chain triglycerides and are not dependent upon biliary or pancreatic secretions for absorption from the gastro-intestinal tract. They provide 35 kJ (8.3 kcal) per g. They do not provide essential fatty acids.

Medium-chain triglycerides have also been used as bases for pharmaceutical preparations.

Preparations

Proprietary Preparations (details are given in Part 3)
UK: Alembicol D.

Multi-ingredient: ***UK:*** Imuderm.

Meglumine (209-p)

Meglumine (BAN, rINN).

N-Methylglucamine; 1-Methylamino-1-deoxy-D-glucitol.

$C_7H_{17}NO_5$ = 195.2.

CAS — 6284-40-8.

Pharmacopoeias. In *Br., Chin., Fr., Int., Jpn,* and *US.*

A white to faintly yellowish microcrystalline powder or crystals, odourless or with a slight odour. Freely **soluble** in water; slightly or sparingly soluble in alcohol; practically insoluble in chloroform and ether.

Meglumine is an organic base used for the preparation of salts of organic acids including many used as contrast media.

Preparations

Proprietary Preparations (details are given in Part 3)

Multi-ingredient: ***Ital.:*** Rubrocortex†; ***Spain:*** Toxepasi Complex Forte†.

Melaleuca Oil (4669-f)

Australian Tea Tree Oil; Oleum Melaleucae; Tea Tree Oil.

CAS — 8022-72-8.

NOTE. Though the synonym Ti-tree Oil has been used for melaleuca oil (e.g. in BPC 1949), the name Ti-tree is also applied to species of *Cordyline* (Liliaceae) indigenous to New Zealand.

A colourless or pale yellow volatile oil with a pleasant characteristic odour and a terebinthinate taste, obtained by distillation from the leaves of the Australian tea tree, *Melaleuca alternifolia* (Myrtaceae). It contains about 50 to 60% of terpenes, cineole (up to 10%), and terpineol. **Soluble** 1 in 3 of alcohol. **Store** in airtight containers. Protect from light.

Melaleuca oil has been reported to have bactericidal and fungicidal properties and is used topically for various skin disorders.

References.

1. Altman PM. Australian tea tree oil. *Aust J Pharm* 1988; **69:** 276–8.
2. Altman PM. Australian tea tree oil—a natural antiseptic. *Aust J Biotechnol* 1989; **3:** 247–8.
3. Bassett IB, *et al.* A comparative study of tea-tree oil versus benzoylperoxide in the treatment of acne. *Med J Aust* 1990; **153:** 455–8.
4. Blackwell AL. Tea tree oil and anaerobic (bacterial) vaginosis. *Lancet* 1991; **337:** 300.
5. Carson CF, *et al.* Susceptibility of methicillin-resistant Staphylococcus aureus to the essential oil of melaleuca alternifolia. *J Antimicrob Chemother* 1995; **35:** 421–4.

Preparations

Proprietary Preparations (details are given in Part 3)
Austral.: Clean Skin Anti Acne; ***Canad.:*** Ti-Bi†; ***UK:*** Amber Gold.

Multi-ingredient: ***Austral.:*** Clean Skin Face Wash; ***Fr.:*** Mycogel†; Tuberol†; ***UK:*** Kleer Cream; Secaderm†.

Melatonin (12924-r)

N-Acetyl-5-methoxytryptamine. N-[2-(5-Methoxyindol-3-yl)ethyl]acetamide.

$C_{13}H_{16}N_2O_2$ = 232.3.

CAS — 73-31-4.

Melatonin is a hormone produced in the pineal gland. Results mainly from *animal* studies indicate that melatonin increases the concentration of aminobutyric acid and serotonin in the midbrain and hypothalamus and enhances the activity of pyridoxal-kinase, an enzyme involved in the synthesis of aminobutyric acid, dopamine, and serotonin. Melatonin is involved in the inhibition of gonadal development and in the control of oestrus. It is also involved in protective changes in skin coloration. There appears to be a diurnal rhythm of melatonin secretion; it is secreted during hours of darkness and may affect sleep pattern. Because of its possible role in influencing circadian rhythm, melatonin has been tried in the alleviation of jet lag and other disorders resulting from delay of sleep. It is also being studied in insomnia and various depressive disorders including seasonal affective disorder, and in large doses for its contraceptive activity.

A number of melatonin analogues are being developed.

Adverse effects. An increase in seizure activity was noted in 4 of 6 children with severe neurological deficits during treatment with melatonin for sleeping disorders.[1] Seizure activity returned to base-line values when melatonin was stopped and recurred on rechallenge.

1. Sheldon SH. Pro-convulsant effects of oral melatonin in neurologically disabled children. *Lancet* 1998; **351:** 1254.

Uses. Melatonin has been tried in a number of disorders including, in large doses, as an adjunct to interleukin-2 therapy for malignant neoplasms,[1-3] and, in combination with norethisterone, as a contraceptive.[4] It is possible that contraceptive use of melatonin may be associated with a reduced risk of breast cancer.[5] (For mention of response to melatonin in 2 patients with sarcoidosis see p.1028.) However, the effects of long-term administration have yet to be assessed. Preliminary studies have also suggested that melatonin may be beneficial in hyperlipidaemias[6] and cluster headaches.[7] Claims for its value as an anti-aging treatment and for use in conditions such as Alzheimer's disease and AIDS are unfounded.[8]

1. Lissoni P, *et al.* Subcutaneous therapy with low-dose interleukin-2 plus the neurohormone melatonin in metastatic gastric cancer patients with low performance status. *Tumori* 1993; **79:** 401–4.
2. Lissoni P, *et al.* A randomised study with subcutaneous low-dose interleukin 2 alone vs interleukin 2 plus the pineal neurohormone melatonin in advanced solid neoplasms other than renal cancer and melanoma. *Br J Cancer* 1994; **69:** 196–9.
3. Bregani ER, *et al.* Prevention of interleukin-2-induced thrombocytopenia during the immunotherapy of cancer by a concomitant administration of the pineal hormone melatonin. *Recenti Prog Med* 1995; **86:** 231–3.
4. Short RV. Melatonin. *Br Med J* 1993; **307:** 952–3.
5. Cohen M, *et al.* Hypotheses: melatonin/steroid combination contraceptives will prevent breast cancer. *Breast Cancer Res Treat* 1995; **33:** 257–64.
6. Pittalis S, *et al.* Effect of a chronic therapy with the pineal hormone melatonin on cholesterol levels in idiopathic hypercholesterolemic patients. *Recenti Prog Med* 1997; **88:** 401–2.
7. Leone M, *et al.* Melatonin versus placebo in the prophylaxis of cluster headache; a double-blind pilot study with parallel groups. *Cephalalgia* 1996; **16:** 494–6.
8. Brzezinski A. Melatonin in humans. *N Engl J Med* 1997; **336:** 186–95.

INSOMNIA. Although melatonin is considered[1-5] to be potentially useful in the management of various forms of insomnia (p.638), especially those associated with circadian rhythm disturbances, there is little evidence of efficacy from large studies and its long term safety remains to be established. In healthy subjects melatonin has been reported[6,7] to reduce the time to onset of sleep and to increase the time spent asleep. Whether this is due to adjustment of the body clock or any hypnotic action of melatonin is unclear. Improved quality of sleep has been reported in elderly patients treated with melatonin for insomnia,[8] and it might be of use in delayed sleep phase syndrome[9] and insomnia in shift workers and totally blind people. There has also been a report[10] of a patient with somnolence associated with melatonin deficiency after pinealectomy who responded to treatment with melatonin. However, melatonin might have a deleterious effect on sleep patterns in some circumstances.[11]

1. Haimov I, Lavie P. Potential of melatonin replacement therapy in older patients with sleep disorders. *Drugs Aging* 1995; **7:** 75–8.

2. Brown GM. Melatonin in psychiatric and sleep disorders: therapeutic implications. *CNS Drugs* 1995; **3:** 209–26.
3. Anonymous. Melatonin. *Med Lett Drugs Ther* 1995; **37:** 111–12.
4. Arendt J. Melatonin. *Br Med J* 1996; **312:** 1242–3.
5. Lamberg L. Melatonin potentially useful but safety, efficacy remain uncertain. *JAMA* 1996; **276:** 1011–14.
6. Zhdanova IV, *et al.* Sleep-inducing effects of low doses of melatonin ingested in the evening. *Clin Pharmacol Ther* 1995; **57:** 552–8.
7. Attenburrow MEJ, *et al.* Low dose melatonin improves sleep in middle-aged subjects. *Psychopharmacology (Berl)* 1996; **126:** 179–81.
8. Garfinkel D, *et al.* Improvement of sleep quality in elderly people by controlled-release melatonin. *Lancet* 1995; **346:** 541–4.
9. Dahlitz M, *et al.* Delayed sleep phase syndrome response to melatonin. *Lancet* 1991; **337:** 1121–4.
10. Lehmann ED, *et al.* Somnolence associated with melatonin deficiency after pinealectomy. *Lancet* 1996; **347:** 323.
11. Middleton BA, *et al.* Melatonin and fragmented sleep patterns. *Lancet* 1996; **348:** 551–2.

JET LAG. Melatonin has been reported to alleviate jet lag following long flights.[1-3] The most appropriate dosing schedule has yet to be determined but will depend on both the direction of travel and the distance travelled.[1,4]

1. Waterhouse J, *et al.* Jet-lag. *Lancet* 1997; **350:** 1611–16.
2. Arendt J. Melatonin. *Br Med J* 1996; **312:** 1242–3.
3. Petrie K, *et al.* A double-blind trial of melatonin as a treatment for jet lag in international cabin crew. *Biol Psychiatry* 1993; **33:** 526–30.
4. Arendt J. Jet-lag. *Lancet* 1998; **351:** 293–4.

Preparations

Proprietary Preparations (details are given in Part 3)
Multi-ingredient: ***UK:*** Rapi-snooze.

Melissa (4670-z)

Balm; Lemon Balm; Melissae Folium; Melissenblatt.

Pharmacopoeias. In *Aust., Fr., Ger., Pol.,* and *Swiss.*

The leaves or leaves and tops of *Melissa officinalis* (Labiatae). The chief constituent is citral.

Melissa has been used as a carminative and sedative. It is an ingredient of herbal remedies used for a variety of disorders. It is also reported to have virustatic activity. Hypersensitivity reactions have been reported.

References.

1. Wölbling RH, Milbradt R. Klinik und therapie des Herpes simplex: vorstellung eines neuen phytotherapeutischen wirkstoffes. *Therapiewoche* 1984; **34:** 1193–1200.

Preparations

Proprietary Preparations (details are given in Part 3)
Aust.: Lomaherpan; ***Ger.:*** Gastrovegetalin; Kneipp Melissen-Pflanzensaft; Lomaherpan.

Multi-ingredient: ***Aust.:*** Abdomilon†; Absimed; Aktiv Nerven- und Schlaftee; Baldracin; Baldrian-Elixier; Baldrian-Krautertonikum; Baldriparan Beruhigungs; Beruhigungstee; Bio-Garten Tee zur Beruhigung; Bio-Garten Tropfen zur Beruhigung; Cardalept; Doppelherz Tonikum; Gastregan; Herz- und Kreislauftonikum Biofora; Kneipp Nerven- und Schlaf-Tee; Krauterdoktor Beruhigungstropfen; Krauterdoktor Entspannungs- und Einschlaftropfen; Krauterdoktor Magen-Darmtropfen; Krauterdoktor Nerven-Tonikum; Krauterdoktor Rosmarin-Wein; Krauterhaus Mag Kottas Babytee; Krauterhaus Mag Kottas Magen- und Darmtee; Krauterhaus Mag Kottas Nerven- und Schlaftee; Krauterhaus Mag Kottas Wechseltee; Krautertee Nr 1; Krautertee Nr 141; Krautertee Nr 16; Krautertee Nr 201; Krautertee Nr 209; Krautertee Nr 9; Mag Doskar's Magentonikum; Mag Doskar's Nerventonikum; Mag Kottas Beruhigungstee; Mag Kottas Krauterexpress-Nerven-Schlaf-Tee; Mag Kottas Magen-Darmtee; Mag Kottas Nerven-Beruhigungstee; Mag Kottas Schlaftee; Mag Kottas Tee fur stillende Mutter; Mag Kottas Wechseltee; Mariazeller; Nervendragees; Nerviforan; Passedan; Passelyt; Phytogran; Seda-Grandelat; Sedogelat; Sidroga Herz-Kreislauf-Tee; Sidroga Kindertee; Sidroga Magen-Darm-Tee; Sidroga Nerven- und Schlaftee; Species nervinae; St Radegunder Beruhigungs- und Einschlaftee; St Radegunder Fiebertee; St Radegunder Herz-Kreislauf-Tonikum; St Radegunder Herz-Kreislauf-unterstutzender Tee; St Radegunder Magenberuhigungstee; St Radegunder Nerven-Tonikum; St Radegunder Nerventee; St Radegunder Reizmildernder Magentee; St Radegunder Rosmarin-Wein; Synpharma Instant-Nerventee; Teekanne Magen- und Darmtee; Teekanne Schlaf- und Nerventee; The Chambard-Tee; Wechseltee; ***Belg.:*** Seneuval; Tisane pour le Foie; Tisane Purgative; ***Canad.:*** Herbal Sleep Well†; Nyrene; ***Fr.:*** Colominthe; Elixir Bonjean; Mediflor Tisane Calmante Troubles du Sommeil No 14; Mediflor Tisane Circulation du Sang No 12; Mediflor Tisane Pectorale d'Alsace†; Quietival†; Santane D_5; Santane N_9; Tisane des Familles†; Tisane Grande Chartreuse; Tisane Touraine; Vagostabyl; ***Ger.:*** Abdomilon N; Aranidorm-S; Avedorm; Baldriparan stark N; Befelka-Tinktur; Beruhigungs-Tee Nervoflux†; bioplant-Kinderol†; Cardalept†; Castrophan†; Doppelherz Melissengeist; Dormarist; Dr. Kleinschrod's Cor-Insuffin†; Dr. Kleinschrod's Spasmi Tropfen†; Dr. Klinger's Bergischer Krautertee, Herz- und Kreislauftee†; Dr. Klinger's Bergischer Krautertee, Nerven- und Beruhigungstee†; Esberi-Nervin†; Eupronerv†; Euvegal forte; Euvegal N; Euviterin; Gastrol S; Gutnacht; Hacko-Kloster-Krautertee†; Herz-Plus Nerven†; Herz-plus†; Heumann Beruhigungsdragees Tenerval N†; Heumann Beruhigungstee Tenerval N; Iberogast; JuDorm; JuNeuron S; Kneipp Krauter Taschenkur Nerven und Schlaf N; Kneipp Nerven- und Schlaf-Tee N; Knufinke Nervenruh Beruhigungs-Tee†; Lindofluid N; Luvased-Tropfen N; Majocarmin†; Myonasan†; Nerven-Tee Stada N; Nerviguttum†; Nervosana; Orbis Blasen- und Nierentee†; Orbis Nerven- und Beruhigungstee†; Oxacant N; Oxacant-sedativ; Pan-Nerventonikum†; Pascosedon S; Phytonoctu; Plantival Novo; Pronervon N†; Pronervon Phyto; Salus Nerven-Schlaf-Tee Nr.22; Salusan; Seda-Pasc N†; Seda-Plantina; Sedacur; Sedariston; Sedaselect N; Sedasyx; Sedatruw S; Sirmiosta Nervenelixier N; Stullmaton; Valeriana-Strath†; Worishofener Nervenpflege Dr. Kleinschrod†; ***Irl.:*** Rovaktivit†; ***Ital.:*** Cura; Fluxoten; Sedatol; Tisana Arnaldi; Tisana Cisbey; Tisana Kelemata; ***Spain:*** Agua del Carmen; Caramelos Agua del Carmen; Digestol Sanatorium; Melisana†; Resolutivo Regium; Sol Schoum; ***Switz.:*** Arterosan Plus; Baldriparan; Cardiaforce; Carmol†; Demonatur Dragees calmantes†; Dormeasan†; Dormiplant; Dragees pour la detente nerveuse; Gastrosan; Hyperiforce; Iberogast; Melissa Tonic; Phytoberidin; Radacor†; Seracalm; Soporin; The Brioni; The Franklin; Tisane gastrique "H"†; Tisane Natterman instantanee no 6 pour calmer les nerfs et lutter contre l'insomnie†; Tisane pour l'estomac; Tisane pour le coeur et la circulation; Tisane pour le coeur et la circulation "H"†; Tisane pour le sommeil et les nerfs; Tisane pour les enfants; Tisane relaxante; Tisane sedative et somnifere "H"†; Valobonin†; Valverde Dragees pour la detente nerveuse; ***UK:*** Cough Drops; Melissa comp.; Melissin; Valerina Day Time; Valerina Night-Time.

Menthol (266-k)

Hexahydrothymol; Mentholum; Mentol. p-Menthan-3-ol; 2-Isopropyl-5-methylcyclohexanol.

$C_{10}H_{20}O = 156.3.$

CAS — 89-78-1; 1490-04-6; 15356-60-2 (+); 2216-51-5 (−); 15356-70-4 (±).

NOTE. Levomenthol and racementhol are *rINN* and *BAN*.

Pharmacopoeias. In *Chin., Eur.* (see p.viii), *Jpn, Pol.,* and *US.*

Eur. and *Jpn* have separate monographs for laevo-menthol (levomenthol) and racemic menthol (racementhol).

Natural laevo-menthol obtained from the volatile oils of various species of *Mentha* (Labiatae) or synthetic laevo-menthol or racemic menthol.

It occurs as colourless, acicular or prismatic crystals or crystalline powder with a penetrating odour resembling that of peppermint. M.p. of natural or synthetic (−)-menthol 41° to 44° and racemic menthol, about 34°. Ph. Eur. states that it is practically **insoluble** and USP that it is slightly soluble in water; very soluble in alcohol, in chloroform, in ether, and in petroleum spirit; freely soluble in glacial acetic acid, in fixed and volatile oils, and in liquid paraffin; very slightly soluble in glycerol. **Store** in airtight containers in a cool place.

A liquid or soft mass is formed when menthol is triturated with camphor, chloral hydrate, phenol, and many other substances.

Stability. A formulation of menthol 1% in aqueous cream was reported to be stable for up to 18 months when stored at room temperature.[1]

1. Gallagher P, Jones S. A stability and validation study of 1% w/w menthol in aqueous cream. *Int J Pharm Pract* 1997; **5:** 101–4.

Adverse Effects

Menthol may give rise to hypersensitivity reactions including contact dermatitis. There have been reports of apnoea and instant collapse in infants following the local application of menthol to their nostrils. Ingestion of menthol is reported to cause severe abdominal pain, nausea, vomiting, vertigo, ataxia, drowsiness, and coma.

Effects on the nervous system. Ataxia, confusion, euphoria, nystagmus, and diplopia developed in a 13-year-old boy following the inhalation of 5 mL of Olbas oil instead of the recommended few drops.[1] It was considered probable that the menthol in the preparation was responsible for the symptoms; the amount of menthol inhaled was approximately 200 mg.

1. O'Mullane NM, *et al.* Adverse CNS effects of menthol-containing Olbas oil. *Lancet* 1982; **i:** 1121.

Treatment of Adverse Effects and Precautions

As for Camphor, p.1557.

Instillation of decongestant preparations containing menthol directly into the nostrils of infants and young children has resulted in acute respiratory distress with cyanosis[1] and respiratory arrest.[2] In one case,[1] nasal application was associated with concurrent chemical conjunctivitis.

1. Wyllie JP, Alexander FW. Nasal instillation of 'Olbas Oil' in an infant. *Arch Dis Child* 1994; **70:** 357–8.
2. Blake KD. Dangers of common cold treatments in children. *Lancet* 1993; **341:** 640.

Pharmacokinetics

After absorption, menthol is excreted in the urine and bile as a glucuronide.

Uses and Administration

Menthol is chiefly used to relieve symptoms of bronchitis, sinusitis, and similar conditions. For this purpose it may be used as an inhalation, usually with benzoin, as pastilles, or as an ointment with camphor and eucalyptus oil for application to the chest or nostrils (but see Adverse Effects above). However, as mentioned under the section on the management of cough (p.1052) the use of menthol in inhalations is unlikely to provide any additional benefit to that from the steam inhalation.

When applied to the skin menthol dilates the blood vessels, causing a sensation of coldness followed by an analgesic effect. It relieves itching and is used in creams, lotions, or ointments in pruritus and urticaria.

In small doses by mouth menthol has a carminative action.

Action. It has been suggested that the apparent benefits of menthol in nasal congestion may be due to an effect on calcium channels of sensory nerves.[1] This mechanism has also been implicated in its muscle relaxant action (as peppermint oil) on the gastro-intestinal tract (p.1208).

1. Anonymous. How does menthol work? *Pharm J* 1993; **251:** 480.

Preparations

BP 1998: Menthol and Benzoin Inhalation;
USP 23: Benzocaine and Menthol Topical Aerosol; Menthol Lozenges; Tetracaine and Menthol Ointment.

Proprietary Preparations (details are given in Part 3)
Aust.: Nifint; Wick Vapo Sirup; ***Austral.:*** Dencorub Ice; Ice Gel; Kaz; Vicks Throat Drops; Vicks Vapodrops with Butter and Menthol; ***Canad.:*** Absorbine Jr; Absorbine Power Gel; Antiphlogistine Rub A-535 Ice; Ben-Gay Ice; Big V Cough Lozenge; Cough Drops; Deep Cold; Direct Formulary Cough Lozenges; Fisherman's Friend; Flex-All; Honey Lemon Cough Lozenges; Ice Gel; Ice Gel Therapy; Ice Therapy; Life Brand Cough Lozenges; Meggezones; Myoflex Ice; No Name Cough Lozenge; Physiomenthol; Polar Ice; Safeway Cough Lozenges; Vicks Throat Drops; Vicks Vaposyrup; ***Fr.:*** Matiga; ***Ger.:*** Bormelin N†; Franzbragil "M"†; Nifint; Novopin MIG; Wick Vaposyrup; ***Spain:*** Icespray; Nopika; ***Switz.:*** Perskindol; ***UK:*** Deep Freeze Cold Gel†; Meggezones; Nostroline†; ***USA:*** Absorbine Jr; Absorbine Power Gel; Ben-Gay Vanishing; Blue Gel Muscular Pain Reliever; Extra Strength Vicks Cough Drops; Halls-Plus Maximum Strength; Kof-Eze; N'ice; N'ice 'n Clear; Pain Gel Plus; Pain Patch; Soothers†; Sportscreme Ice; Therapeutic Mineral Ice; Vicks Cough Drops; Wonder Ice.

Multi-ingredient: ***Aust.:*** Asthma-Frenon; Benadryl; Benadryl mit Codein; Berggeist; Bronchostop; Carl Baders Divinal; Cehasol; China; Claim; Corodyn; Delta-Hadensa; Diphlogen; Dolo-Menthoneurin; Embrocation; Emser Pastillen mit Menthol; Endrine†; Erkaltungsbad; Erkaltungsbalsam; Eryval; Etrat; Everon; Gallesyn; Hadensa; Haemanal; Inno Rheuma; Kinder Luuf; Lemuval; Luuf Balsam; Makatussin; Mayfit akut; Mediplant; Mediplant Inhalations; Menthoneurin; Mentopin; Neo-Angin; Neo-Phlogicid; Parodontax; Perozon Erkaltungsbad; Piniment; Pinimenthol†; Prurimix; Rectosan; Resol; Rheumasan†; Rhinospray Plus; Rowachol; Rowalind; Scottopect; Sulgan 99; Tetesept; Tiger Balsam Rot; Trafuril†; Tussimont; Wick Sinex; Wick Vaporub; ***Austral.:*** Alcusal Sport; Analgesic Balm†; Analgesic Rub†; Avil Decongestant; Ayrton's Iodised†; BFI; Bidramine†; Biosal; Bonnington's Irish Moss; Bosisto's Eucalyptus Inhalant; Bosisto's Eucalyptus Rub; Cepacol Cough and Sore Throat; Cold Sore Cream†; Cold Sore Lotion†; Coso; Cremor Menthol†; Deep Heat; Dencorub; Dencorub Extra Strength; Dermocaine; Euky Bear Eu-Clear Inhalant; Euky Bear Limberub†; Euky Bear Nasex; Euky Bearub; Formicare Skin Relief†; Genuine Australian Eucalyptus Drops; Irish Moss Cough Syrup†; Karvol; Logicin Chest Rub; Menalation; Mentholyptus Vaporiser Fluid†; Methyl Salicylate Compound Liniment; Methyl Salicylate Ointment Compound; Metsal; Metsal Analgesic; Metsal AR Heat Rub; Metsal Heat Rub; Nutrasorb; Nyal Cold Sore; Painguard†; Phenephrin†; Quelfas A†; Radian-B; Rubesal; Sarna; Seda-Gel; Sigma Relief Chest Rub†; SM-33; Solarub†; Soov Bite; Tiger Balm Red; Tiger Balm White; Vasylox; Vicks Blue Drops; Vicks Cough Syrup; Vicks Decongestive Cough Syrup†; Vicks Inhaler; Vicks Sinex; Vicks Vapodrops; Vicks Vaporub; ***Belg.:*** Baume Dalet; Borostyrol; Dentophar; Endrine; Inhalene; Inopectol†; Pelarol†; Pinthym†; Procto-Synalar; Rado-Salil; Reflexspray; Revocyl†; Strepsils Menthol; Synthol; Tablettes pour la Gorge Medica†; Vegebom†; Vicks Vaporub; ***Canad.:*** Absorbine Analgesic; Absorbine Jr Antifungal; Alsirub; Analgesic Balm; Analgesic Rub (NCP)†; Anbesol; Antiphlogistine Rub A-535; Antiseptic Mouthwash; Arthricare Odor Free; Arthricare Triple Medicated; Artritol; Balminil Nasal Ointment; Balminil Suppositoires; Banana Boat Sooth-A-Caine; Baume Analgesique Medicamente; Beech Nut Cough Drops; Ben-Gay Original; Ben-Gay Ultra; Bentasil; Blistex DCT Lip Balm; Blistex Medicated Lip Conditioner Jar; Bronchex; Bronchisaft; Broncho Rub; Bronchodex DM; Bronchodex Vapo; Bronchozone; Buckley's Mixture; Buckley's White Rub; Buckleys Pain Relief; Bunion Salve; Bye Bye Bite; Cal Mo Dol; Calmomusc; Camphre Compose; Carboseptol; Carmatis; Cepastat; Chapstick Medicated Lip Balm; Cherry Chest Rub; Chloraseptic Lozenges; Cold Sore Lotion; Deep Heating; Denorex; Dentalgar; Dermolan†; Dermoplast; Ease Pain Away; EM Eukal; Eucalyptamint†; Eucamenth; Fisherman's Friend Original; Franzbranns; Gold Bond; Gouttes Dentaires; Halls; Inarub; Infraline; Instant Rub; Jack & Jill Rub; Kiro Rub; Listerine; Lotion pour Feux Sauvages; Marco Rub Camphorated; Marco Rub Camphorated Ointment; Medicated Analgesic Cream; Medicated Chest Rub; Mentholatum Cough Drops; Mentholatum Extra Strength Ointment; Mentholatum Ointment; Methacin; Mouthwash Antiseptic & Gargle; Myoflex Ice Plus; Noivy; Pain Buster; Pastilles Valda; Penetrating Rub; Physio-Rub; Polytar AF; Pommade au The des Bois; PrameGel; Rheila Medicated Cough Drops; Rheumalan; Sarna-P; Savex; Savex with PABA; Savex with Sunscreen; Scalpicin Anti-Dandruff Anti-Itch; SJ Liniment; Sore Throat Lozenges; Therapeutic Soothing Ice; Thermo Rub; Thermo-Gel; Thunas Salve for Rheumatic Pains; Tiger Balm Red; Tiger Balm White; Triaminic Night Time Rub; Valda; Vap Air; Vaporisateur Medicamente; Vaporizing Colds Rub; Vaporizing Ointment; Vicks Inhaler; Vicks Vaporub; Webber Antibiotic Cold Sore Ointment; X-Seb T Plus; X-Tar; Z-Plus; ***Fr.:*** Arnicadol; Bain de Bouche Lipha†; Balsamorhinol; Balsofumine Mentholee; Balsolene; Baume Bengue; Baume Dalet; Baume du Tigre†; Baume

Saint-Bernard; Borostyrol; Bronpax; Circulatonic; Eau Precieuse Depensier; Edulcor eucalyptus et menthol†; Ephydrol; Essence Algerienne; Eutalgic; Glyco-Thymoline; Hemagene Tailleur; Inongan; Kamol; Lao-Dal; Lini-Bombe; Lumbalgine; Lysocalm; Mysca†; Paps; Pastilles M.B.C†; Pinorhinol; Pulmoll; Pulmoll au menthol et a l'eucalyptus; Pulveol†; Sacnel†; Sedartryl; Sinex; Sirop Boin; Strepsils Menthol Eucalyptus†; Synthol; Tigidol; Valda; Vapo-Myrtol; Vegebom; Vicks Pastilles†; Vicks Soulagil†; Vicks Vaporub; Vicks vitamine C pastilles†; ***Ger.:*** A + B Balsam N; Alferm; Amol Heilkrautergeist N; Anastil†; Anginasin N; Anginetten†; Animbo-N†; Anisan; Asthma-Frenon-S†; Bisolvomed mit Codein†; Bisolvomed†; Bormelin N-Adrenalin†; Bormelin†; Bronchicum Tropfen mit Codein†; Bronchodurat; Bronchoforton N†; Broncholind Balsam†; Cobed†; Colomba N†; Cor-Vel; Dalet-Balsam; Denosol; Dolo-Menthoneurin; Dolorsan-Balsam; Dorex†; Efisalin N†; Emser Pastillen echt "Stark"†; Emser Pastillen mit Menthol N; Endrine†; Erkaltungs-Balsam†; Etrat Sportgel; Eufimenth-Balsam N; Fibraflex N†; Fibraflex†; Franzbranntwein; Glutisal-buton-Salbe†; Grunlicht Hingfong Essenz; Guakalin†; Hamos N; Heilit Rheuma-Bad N-Kombi†; Heilit Rheuma-Olbad; Hustenstiller N; Influsanbalm†; Inspirol Mundwasser konzentrat; Iosimitan†; Keldrin†; Kneipp Brustkaramellen†; Kneipp Fichtennadel Franzbranntwein; Kneipp Herzsalbe Unguentum Cardiacum Kneipp; Koryn†; Leukona-Sauna-Konzentrat†; Lyobalsam N†; Makatussin Balsam mit Menthol; Makinil†; Medichol†; Mentholon Original N; Menthoneurin-Salbe; Mintetten S†; Mucidan†; Nasenol-ratiopharm†; Nasivin Intensiv-Balsam†; Neo-Angin N; Nephulon E†; Nervpin N; Night-Care; Optipect mit Kodein†; Optipect N; Optipect Neo; Optipect†; Perflamint†; Pfefferminz-Lysoform; Pin-Alcol; Pinimenthol Bad N; Pinimenthol N; Pinofit†; Pinoidal-Bad†; Praecordin S; Pro-Pecton Balsam†; Probaphen†; Pumilen-Balsam†; Rectosellan N†; Repha-Os; Retterspitz Aerosol; Retterspitz Quick; Rowachol; Rowachol comp.; Rowachol-Digestiv; Rowalind; Salviathymol N; Schupps Fichte-Menthol Olbad; Sedotussin Expectorans; Segmentocut†; Silvapin Aktiv-Tonic MMP†; Sorot-comp†; Stas Halstabletten†; sulfopecticept†; Tachynerg N; Thymitussin†; Transpulmin E; Trauma-Puren; Trauma-Salbe Rodler 301 N; Tumarol-N; Tussamag Halstabletten; Tussipect; Valometten†; Vipracutan†; Wick Inhalierstift N; Wick Vaporub; Zynedo-K†; ***Irl.:*** Bengue's Balsam; Benylin; Benylin Chesty Cough†; Benylin Childrens Cough; Benylin Decongestant†; Benylin Dry Cough; Benylin Non-Drowsy Chesty Coughs; Benylin with Codeine; Bexalin†; Clonalin; Denorex; Expulin; Karvol; Leotuss†; Listerine; Radian-B; Rowachol; Rowalind; Rowatanal; Valda†; Vicks Inhaler; Vicks Vaporub; ***Ital.:*** Abiostil; Antalgola†; Balsamico F. di M.†; Balsamo Italstadium; Balta Intimo Soluzione; Benadryl; Benadryl Complex; Benagol Mentolo-Eucaliptolo; Blefarolin; Bronchenolo Balsamo†; Bronco Valda†; Broncopulmin; Donalg; Efedrocanfine†; Essaproct†; Eucalipto Composto; Fomentil; Golosan†; Herbavit; Lacrime; Lasonil H; Lasoproct; Neo Foille Pomata Disinfettante†; Ondroly-A; Pastiglie Valda; Pinselina Dr. Knapp; Pulmarin; Remy; Respiro; Rinobalsamiche; Rinofil†; Rinogutt Eucalipto-Fher; Rinostil; Rowachol†; Salonpas; Selsun Trattamento†; Sloan; Transpulmina Gel†; Transpulmina Gola; Transpulmina Tosse; Via Mal Trauma Gel; Vicks Cetamium Vit/C†; Vicks Gola†; Vicks Inalante; Vicks Sinex; Vicks Vaporub; ***Mon.:*** Blackoids du Docteur Meur; ***Neth.:*** Agre-Gola; Bronchicum; Bronchoforton†; Dampo; Denorex; Menthoneurin; Resdan Rx†; Rhinocaps; Strepsils Menthol en Eucalyptus; Tijgerbalsem†; Tijgerolie†; Vicks Sinex; Vicks Vaporub; ***Norw.:*** Cosylan; ***S.Afr.:*** Allergin; Benylin; Benylin with Codeine; Betalin; Bronchicough; Bronchicum; Bronchicum SB†; Bronchiflu; Bronchilate†; Bronchistop; Cocilix†; Cocillana Co; Coff-Up; Counterpain; Dermoplast†; Diatussin; Difco†; Docrub; Elixirol†; Karvol; Lennamine†; Linctosan; Medituss; Nasomixin; Numzit; Oramond†; Pernicream†; Radian; Respisniffers; Strepsils Eucalyptus Menthol; Strepsils Orange-C; Tussimed; Tussimed Expectorant†; Warm-Up; ***Spain:*** Aerospray Analgesico†; Aerospray Antialergico†; Amidoyina†; Analgesico Ut Asens Fn; Angi†; Angiofiline†; Antiseptico Dent Donner†; Arnicon; Balsamo Analgesic Karmel; Bartal†; Bellacanfor†; Benadryl Expectorante; Bronquimar; Bronquimar Vit A; Buco Regis; Caltoson Balsamico; Caramelos Agua del Carmen; Caramelos Balsam; Cloroboral; Dentikrisos; Dentol Topico; Dermomycose Talco; Descongestivo Cuve Nasal†; Dol.S Regaliz†; Dolokey; Elixir Dental Formahina†; Eupnol; Gargaril Sulfamida†; Gargaril†; Gartricin; Gingilone Comp†; Hadensa; Ictiomen; Inhalador; Killpan; Kneipp Balsamo; Lapiz Termo Compositum†; Liderflex; Linimento Naion; Magnesia Validada†; Masagil; Mentobox; Mentobox Antitusivo; Mentol Sedans Sulfamidad†; Nani Pre Dental; Orto Nasal; Otogen Calmante; Pastillas Juanola; Pastillas Koki Ment Tivo; Pastillas Vicks Limon†; Pastillas Vicks Mentol†; Pazbronquial; Pinimenthol†; Radio Salil; Reflex; Regal; Respir Balsamico; Rowachol; Ruscus; Sabanotropico; Sartol; Scheriproct; Sinus Inhalaciones; Super Koki†; Synalar Rectal; Synthol†; Talco Antihistam Calber; Termosan; Tyropenicilin R†; Vaselina Mentolada; Vicks Formula 44; Vicks Inhalador; Vicks Spray; Vicks Vaporub; Vitavox Pastillas; Yoguito†; ***Swed.:*** Cosylan; Munvatten†; Otrivin Menthol; Trafuril†; Vicks Vaporub; ***Switz.:*** Alginex†; Alphastria; Angina MCC; Anginol; Artragel; Baume de Chine Temple of Heaven blanc; Baume Esco; Baume Esco Forte; Borostyrol N; Bradoral†; Broncho-Rivo; Bronchocodin; Carmol "blanche"†; Carmol "thermogene"†; Carmol†; Contugel†; Deca; Demo baume; Demo pates pectorales; Demostan; Diabetosan†; Dolo-Menthoneurin†; Eau-de-vie de France avec huile de pin nain du Tirol; Eubucal†; Euproctol; Expectorant Cough Syrup†; Expectoryn Paediatric†; Expectoryn†; Flavangin; Flavovenyl; GEM†; Haemocortin; Haemolan; Histacyl Cutane†; Huile analgesique "Polar-Bar"; Hygiodermil; Makatussin; Makatussin forte; Mirocor†; Nasello; Neo-Angin avec vitamin C exempt de sucre; Neo-Angin exempt de sucre; Noscalin†; Novomint N; Olbas; Pate Iodoforme du Prof Dr Walkhoff; Pectramin; Pharmalyn†; Pinimenthol; Pirom; Pulmex†; Rivolyn†; Roliwol; Saltrates; Sedasept; Sedodermil; Sedotussin; Sloan Baume; Solin S†; Solution ChKM du Prof Dr Walkhoff; Sportusal Spray sine heparino; Stilex; Stix†; Sulgan; Synthol†; Tonex; Tumarol; Tyrothricin; Vicks Formel 44; Vicks Inhaler N; Vicks Sinex; Vicks Vaporub; ***UK:*** Aezodent; Aleevex; Antiseptic Foot Balm; Antiseptic Lozenges; Antiseptic Throat Pastilles; Aspellin; Baby Chest Rub†; Balmosa; Balto Foot Balm; Bengue's Balsam; Benylin Chesty Cough; Benylin Childrens Night Coughs; Benylin Cough & Congestion; Benylin Dry Cough; Benylin Mentholated Linctus; Benylin Non-Drowsy; Benylin Non-Drowsy Chesty Coughs; Benylin with Codeine; Bonjela; Boots Vapour Rub; Buttercup Syrup (Blackcurrant flavour); Buttercup Syrup (Honey and Lemon flavour); Cabdrivers Adult Linctus; Catarrh Pastilles; Chloraseptic†; Colsor; Copholco†; Copholcoids†; Covonia Bronchial Balsam; DDD; Deep Heat Massage; Deep Heat Maximum Strength; Deep Heat Rub; Deep Relief; Denorex; Dermacreme; Dragon Balm; Dubam; Eftab; Expulin; Expulin Paediatric; Expurhin†; Famel Catarrh & Throat Pastilles; Fisherman's Friend Honey Cough Syrup†; Flurex Inhalant†; Frador; Germoloids; Gonne Balm; Guanor; Hill's Balsam Expectorant Pastilles; Hills Balsam Extra Strong; Histalix; Karvol; Lanacane Medicated Powder; Liqufruta Cough Medicine; Listerine Antiseptic Mouthwash; Mac; Melissin; Meltus Expectorant with Decongestant; Mentho-lyptus; Menthol and Wintergreen Heat Product†; Mentholatum Balm†; Mentholatum Nasal Inhaler; Mentholease; Merothol; Nasal Inhaler; Nigroids; Nirolex for Chesty Coughs; Nosor Nose Balm; Olbas; Owbridges for Children†; Penetrol; Phytocil†; Potter's Pastilles; Proctor's Pinelyptus; Radian-B; Ralgex; Rinstead; Rowachol; Salonair; Sanderson's Throat Specific; Snufflebabe; Throaties Catarrh Pastilles; Tiger Balm Liquid; Tiger Balm Red; Tiger Balm White; Tixylix Catarrh; Tixylix Inhalant; Valda; Vapex†; Vapour Rub; Vicks Inhaler; Vicks Sinex; Vicks Vaporub; Vocalzone; Woodwards Baby Chest Rub; ***USA:*** Absorbine Athletes Foot Care; Analgesic Balm; Anbesol; Arthricare Double Ice; Arthricare Odor Free; Arthricare Triple Medicated; Arthritis Hot Creme; Babee; Banadyne-3; Banalg; Ben-Gay; Ben-Gay Ultra; Betuline; BFI; Boil Ease; Calamatum; Campho-Phenique Sting Relief Formula†; Cepacol Maximum Strength; Cepacol Regular Strength; Cepastat; Cepastat Cherry; Chapstick Medicated Lip Balm; Chiggerex; Cool-Mint Listerine; Deep Heating Lotion; Deep Heating Rub; Deep-Down Rub; Denorex; Dermacoat; Dermal-Rub; Dermarest Plus; Dermolin; Eucalyptamint; Flex-all 454; Florida Sunburn Relief; FreshBurst Listerine; Gordobalm; Hall's Sugar Free Mentho-Lyptus; Hawaiian Tropic Cool Aloe with I.C.E.; Icy Hot; Improved Analgesic; infraRUB; Legatrin Rub; Listerine; Massengill; Maximum Strength Flexall 454; Medacote; Medadyne†; Medatussin Plus†; Medicone Derma; Medicone Dressing; Medicone Rectal; Menthacin; Mentholatum Cherry Chest Rub; Mentholatum Natural Ice Lip Protectant; Mentholatum Ointment; MenthoRub; Methalgen; MG Cold Sore Formula; Minit-Rub; MouthKote O/R; Muscle Rub; Musterole; Musterole Extra; N'ice; Nasal Jelly; Orabase Lip; Orasept; Pain Bust-R II; Pain Doctor; Pain X; Panalgesic; Panalgesic Gold; Paralgesic; Pedi-Dri; Pedi-Pro; Pfeiffer's Cold Sore; Phenaseptic†; PrameGel; Rhuli Gel; Rid-a-Pain†; Robitussin Cough Drops; Sarna Anti-Itch; Scalpicin; Schamberg†; Soltice; Sports Spray†; Sting-Kill; Thera-gesic; TiSol; Topic; Tussirex; Vicks Chloraseptic Sore Throat; Vicks Menthol Cough Drops; Vicks Vaporub; Vicks Victors Dual Action Cough Drops; X-Seb T Plus; Ziks; Zonite.

Menyanthes (537-n)

Bitterklee; Bogbean; Buckbean; Folia Trifoli Fibrini; Marsh Trefoil; Trèfle d'Eau.

Pharmacopoeias. In *Aust.*, *Fr.*, and *Pol.*

The dried leaves of the buckbean, *Menyanthes trifoliata* (Menyanthaceae).

Menyanthes has been used as a bitter. It is used in herbal medicine for rheumatic disorders. It is also used in homoeopathic and folk medicine.

Preparations

Proprietary Preparations (details are given in Part 3)

Multi-ingredient: ***Aust.:*** Krauterhaus Mag Kottas Gallen- und Lebertee; Krautertee Nr 9; Mag Kottas Leber-Gallentee; Magentee; Mariazeller; ***Belg.:*** Richelet†; ***Ger.:*** Cefaktivon "novum"; Gallexier; Montana; Nervigutum†; Ventrodigest†; ***UK:*** Rheumatic Pain; Rheumatic Pain Remedy; Rheumatic Pain Tablets; Vegetex.

Mercuric Chloride (5307-b)

Bicloruro de Mercurio; Cloreto Mercúrico; Corrosive Sublimate; Hydrarg. Perchlor.; Hydrargyri Dichloridum; Hydrargyri Perchloridum; Hydrargyrum Bichloratum; Mercuric Chlor.; Mercurique (Chlorure); Mercury Bichloride; Mercury Perchloride; Quecksilberchlorid.

$HgCl_2$ = 271.5.

CAS — 7487-94-7.

Pharmacopoeias. In *Eur.* (see p.viii).

A heavy, colourless or white, crystalline powder or crystalline masses. **Soluble** 1 in 15 of water, 1 in 3 of alcohol, 1 in 25 of ether, and 1 in 15 of glycerol. A solution in water is acid to litmus. **Protect** from light.

The use of mercuric chloride as an antibacterial substance is limited by its toxicity, its precipitating action on proteins, its irritant action on raw surfaces, its corrosive action on metals, and by the fact that its activity is greatly reduced in the presence of excreta or body fluids.

Details of the adverse effects of mercury compounds are provided under Mercury, below.

Preparations

Proprietary Preparations (details are given in Part 3)

Multi-ingredient: ***Spain:*** Lucil†; Oxido Amari; Pantenil; Pomada Pptado Blanc Brum†; Pomada Pptado Blanc Orra†; Resorpil†.

Yellow Mercuric Oxide (5311-d)

Gelbes Quecksilberoxyd; Hydrargyri Oxidum Flavum; Hydrargyri Oxydum Flavum; Mercurique (Oxyde) Jaune; Oxido Amarillo de Mercurio; Yellow Precipitate.

HgO = 216.6.

CAS — 21908-53-2.

Pharmacopoeias. In *Belg.*, *Fr.*, and *It.*

An odourless orange-yellow, amorphous powder. Practically **insoluble** in water and in alcohol; soluble in acids.

Yellow mercuric oxide has been used in eye ointments for the local treatment of minor infections including the eradication of pubic lice from the eyelashes. Absorption can occur and produce the adverse effects of inorganic mercury (see below).

Mercuric oxide has been associated with clinical exacerbations of porphyria and is considered unsafe in porphyric patients.[1]

1. Moore MR, McColl KEL. *Porphyria: drug lists.* Glasgow: Porphyria Research Unit, University of Glasgow, 1991.

Pediculosis. Yellow mercuric oxide 1% eye ointment was considered to be a safe and effective treatment in pediculosis (p.1401) of the eyelashes caused by pubic lice (pthiriasis palpebrarum).[1]

1. Ashkenazi I, *et al.* Yellow mercuric oxide: a treatment of choice for phthiriasis palpebrarum. *Br J Ophthalmol* 1991; **75:** 356–8.

Preparations

Proprietary Preparations (details are given in Part 3)

Austral.: Golden Eye Ointment; ***Fr.:*** Ophtergine†; ***Spain:*** Pomada Mercurial†; ***USA:*** Stye†.

Multi-ingredient: ***Spain:*** Oxido Amari; Pomada Orravan Prec Amar†.

Mercurous Chloride (5314-m)

Calomel; Calomelanos; Cloreto Mercuroso; Hydrarg. Subchlor.; Hydrargyri Subchloridum; Hydrargyrosi Chloridum; Hydrargyrum Chloratum (Mite); Mercureux (Chlorure); Mercurius Dulcis; Mercury Monochloride; Mercury Subchloride; Mild Mercurous Chloride; Protocloruro de Mercurio; Quecksilberchlorür.

HgCl = 236.0.

CAS — 7546-30-7 (HgCl); 10112-91-1 (Hg_2Cl_2).

Pharmacopoeias. In *Chin.*

Some pharmacopoeias also include Precipitated Mercurous Chloride (Hydrargyri Subchloridum Praecipitatum), a white amorphous powder, to which the synonym 'White Precipitate' (Praecipitatum Album) may be applied. White Precipitate has also been used as a name for Ammoniated Mercury.

Mercurous chloride was formerly given as a laxative and was applied topically as an antibacterial. It was one of the mercury compounds employed in the management of syphilis in the pre-antibiotic era.

The mercurous form of mercury does not possess the corrosive properties of the mercuric form and is not absorbed to any great extent. However, the mercurous form can be converted to the mercuric with consequent toxicity as described under mercury (see below).

Preparations

Proprietary Preparations (details are given in Part 3)

Multi-ingredient: ***USA:*** Sanitube†.

Mercury (5306-m)

Hydrarg.; Hydrargyrum; Hydrargyrum Depuratum; Mercure; Mercurio; Quecksilber; Quicksilver.

Hg = 200.59.

CAS — 7439-97-6.

Pharmacopoeias. In *Aust.* and *Fr.*

A shining, silvery white, very mobile liquid, easily divisible into globules, which readily volatilises on heating.

Adverse Effects

Liquid mercury if ingested is poorly absorbed and, unless there is aspiration or pre-existing gastro-intestinal disorders, is not considered to be a severe toxicological hazard.

The greatest dangers from liquid mercury arise from the inhalation of mercury vapour. On acute exposure, it can cause various gastro-intestinal effects including nausea, vomiting, and diarrhoea; more importantly it is toxic to the respiratory system and this effect can be fatal. Some CNS involvement has also been reported. Liquid mercury is not without its dangers when injected and there have been a number of reports of accidental or intentional parenteral administration. Inorganic salts such as mercuric chloride are corrosive when ingested causing severe nausea, vomiting, pain, bloody diarrhoea, and necrosis. The kidney is also involved and tubular necrosis may develop. Mercurous salts are considered to be less hazardous, but the mercurous form can be converted to the mercuric.

Chronic mercury poisoning may result from inhalation of mercury vapour, skin contact with mercury or mercury compounds, or ingestion of mercury salts over prolonged periods. It is characterised by many symptoms including tremor, motor and sensory disturbances, mental deterioration, gastro-intestinal symptoms, dermatitis, kidney damage, salivation, and loosening of teeth. A blue line may be present on the gums.

Poisoning with mercury or inorganic mercury salts has arisen from a variety of sources such as batteries, cosmetics, dental materials, medical equipment, and jewellery manufacture. Barometers, sphygmomanometers, and thermometers are still sources of liquid mercury. Trace amounts of organic and inorganic mercury may also be ingested in the diet.

The syndrome of acrodynia (pink disease), with symptoms of sweat, rash, oedema of the extremities, photophobia, wasting, weakness, tachycardia, and diminished reflexes, occurred in children given mercury in teething powders or in ointments or dusting powders. Such preparations have long since been withdrawn from use. However, the syndrome is still a feature of mercury poisoning from other sources.

Organic mercurial compounds produce similar toxic effects to inorganic compounds, but they have a more selective action on the CNS that has proved difficult to treat. The degree of toxicity varies with the different groups of organic mercurials; those used as preservatives or disinfectants being less toxic than the ethyl or methyl compounds that are not used pharmaceutically or clinically. Methylmercury is notorious for its toxicity; there have been cases of fetal neurotoxicity during outbreaks of methylmercury poisoning. There is little difference between acute and chronic poisoning with organic mercurials.

Hypersensitivity to mercury and mercurial compounds has been reported.

Mercurialentis has been reported in patients treated with eye drops containing an organomercurial preservative.

Acute occupational exposure to mercury vapour in 53 men resulted in an initial phase described as metal fume fever, an intermediate phase of severe symptoms with CNS, gastro-intestinal, respiratory, and urological involvement, and a late phase with persistent CNS symptoms, dysuria, and pain on ejaculation.[1,2] Although persistent hyperchloraemia was noted in the 11 patients with the highest mercury levels, renal impairment tended to be temporary.[2] Long-term follow-up of a patient who had an intravenous injection of mercury 12 years previously also revealed no persistent renal impairment,[3] despite the presence of mercury microemboli in lungs, kidneys, liver, and subcutaneous tissues and high concentrations in the urine. At this time, the patient had residual reductions in respiratory function, polyneuropathy, and marked asthenozoospermia. Spermatozoal abnormalities may also have contributed to his wife's miscarriage. Fetal neurotoxicity following maternal exposure to methylmercury is well recognised, and has been shown to cause delays in neurological development in affected children up to the age of 7 years.[4]

There has been considerable concern over the systemic absorption of mercury from *dental amalgam*, which typically contains between 40 and 70% of mercury. However, the quantities absorbed from amalgam fillings is reported to be relatively small[5,6] and current evidence suggests that the use of dental amalgam for tooth restoration is both safe and effective.[7,8] The main risks appear to be occupational exposure of dental staff and environmental concerns. Some patients with hypersensitivity to mercury may benefit from removal of amalgam fillings.[9]

The symptoms of acrodynia have been mistaken for those of phaeochromocytoma.[10,11]

1. Bluhm RE, *et al.* Elemental mercury vapour toxicity, treatment, and prognosis after acute, intensive exposure in chloralkali plant workers part I: history, neuropsychological findings and chelator effects. *Hum Exp Toxicol* 1992; **11:** 201–10.
2. Bluhm RE, *et al.* Elemental mercury vapour toxicity, treatment, and prognosis after acute, intensive exposure in chloralkali plant workers part II: hyperchloraemia and genitourinary symptoms. *Hum Exp Toxicol* 1992; **11:** 211–15.
3. dell'Omo M, *et al.* Long-term toxicity of intravenous mercury injection. *Lancet* 1996; **348:** 64.
4. Grandjean P, *et al.* Cognitive deficit in 7-year-old children with prenatal exposure to methylmercury. *Neurotoxicol Teratol* 1997; **19:** 417–28.
5. Eley BM. The future of dental amalgam: a review of the literature. Part 3: mercury exposure from amalgam restorations in dental patients. *Br Dent J* 1997; **182:** 333–8.
6. Eley BM. The future of dental amalgam: a review of the literature. Part 4: mercury exposure hazards and risk assessment. *Br Dent J* 1997; **182:** 373–81.
7. FDI/WHO. Consensus statement on dental amalgam. *FDI World* 1995; **4** (July/Aug): 9–10.
8. Eley BM. The future of dental amalgam: a review of the literature. Part 6: possible harmful effects of mercury from dental amalgam. *Br Dent J* 1997; **182:** 455–9.
9. Ibbotson SH, *et al.* The relevance and effect of amalgam replacement in subjects with oral lichenoid reactions. *Br J Dermatol* 1996; **134:** 420–3.
10. Henningsson C, *et al.* Acute mercury poisoning (acrodynia) mimicking pheochromocytoma in an adolescent. *J Pediatr* 1993; **122:** 252–3.
11. Velzeboer SCJM, *et al.* A hypertensive toddler. *Lancet* 1997; **349:** 1810.

Treatment of Adverse Effects

Ingestion of liquid mercury seldom requires active treatment. Acute poisoning due to other inorganic mercury sources should be treated if appropriate by immediate emesis or gastric lavage; a 5% solution of sodium formaldehyde sulphoxylate may be used with the aim of converting the mercuric form to the mercurous. Large quantities of milk or charcoal may also be given. Dimercaprol (see p.979) therapy should be started immediately. Other chelating agents that may be used include penicillamine (see p.991), succimer (see p.997), or unithiol (p.998).

Some centres institute haemodialysis at the beginning of treatment; others wait until renal failure develops when either haemodialysis or peritoneal dialysis is used.

Symptomatic measures should be used to alleviate the potentially wide range of toxic effects.

Mercurials on the skin should be removed by copious washing with soap and water.

Poisoning due to organic mercury is difficult to treat. The same measures as above should be adopted, except that it is recommended by some that dimercaprol should not be used since *animal* evidence indicates that it may increase the brain concentrations of mercury. An additional measure that has been tried is the administration of a resin complex to prevent the reabsorption of mercury from the bile.

References to the treatment of mercury poisoning,[1-6] including the use of chelating agents during haemodialysis procedures.[2,3]

1. Florentine MJ, Sanfilippo DJ. Elemental mercury poisoning. *Clin Pharm* 1991; **10:** 213–21.
2. Kostyniak PJ, *et al.* Extracorporeal regional complexing haemodialysis treatment of acute inorganic mercury intoxication. *Hum Toxicol* 1990; **9:** 137–41.
3. Ferguson L, Cantilena LR. Enhanced mercury clearance during hemodialysis with chelating agents. *Clin Pharmacol Ther* 1991; **49:** 131.
4. Houeto P, *et al.* Elemental mercury vapour toxicity: treatment and levels in plasma and urine. *Hum Exp Toxicol* 1994; **13:** 848–52.
5. Toet AE, *et al.* Mercury kinetics in a case of severe mercuric chloride poisoning treated with dimercapto-1-propane sulphonate (DMPS). *Hum Exp Toxicol* 1994; **13:** 11–16.
6. Bluhm RE, *et al.* Elemental mercury vapour toxicity, treatment, and prognosis after acute, intensive exposure in chloralkali plant workers part I: history, neuropsychological findings and chelator effects. *Hum Exp Toxicol* 1992; **11:** 201–10.

Pharmacokinetics

There is little absorption of mercury from globules in the gastro-intestinal tract. The main hazard of liquid mercury is from absorption following inhalation of mercury vapour; this mercury is widely distributed before being oxidised to the mercuric form. Concentrations can be detected in the brain.

Soluble inorganic mercuric salts are absorbed from the gastro-intestinal tract and can also be absorbed through the skin. The mercury is distributed throughout the soft tissues with high concentrations in the kidneys; it is mainly excreted in the urine and through the colon with an elimination half-life of about 60 days, although it may take years to eliminate mercury from the brain; elimination from other tissues may take several months.

Alkyl mercury compounds are more readily absorbed from both the gastro-intestinal and the respiratory tracts. They are widely distributed and can produce high concentrations in the brain. Alkyl mercury compounds are excreted in urine and in the faeces with extensive enterohepatic recycling. The biological half-life varies but is longer than that of inorganic mercury.

Organic mercury, and to some extent inorganic mercury, diffuse across the placenta and are distributed into breast milk.

Uses and Administration

The hazards associated with mercury generally outweigh any therapeutic benefit and its clinical use has largely been abandoned. The use of mercurial diuretics such as mersalyl (p.902) has generally been superseded by other diuretics. Ointments containing mercurials, such as ammoniated mercury (p.1086) have also generally been replaced by less toxic preparations. Mercurials were formerly used as spermicides.

The ionisable mercury salts and certain organic compounds of mercury have been used as disinfectants, and some mercury salts are effective parasiticides and fungicides. Organic mercurials such as phenylmercuric acetate, borate, and nitrate are also used as preservatives (p.1122). Mercury is a component of dental amalgams.

Other mercury salts which have been used for their antibacterial activity include mercuric chloride, yellow mercuric oxide and mercurous chloride (above).

Some mercury compounds have been used in homoeopathic medicine.

Preparations

Proprietary Preparations (details are given in Part 3)
Ger.: Farco-Oxicyanid-Tupfer; ***Spain:*** Jabon Oxician Merc†.

Multi-ingredient: ***Aust.:*** Coldophthal; ***Belg.:*** Ocal†; ***Spain:*** Oftalmol Dexa; Oftalmol Ocular; Riosol F†.

Mescaline (5017-k)

3,4,5-Trimethoxyphenethylamine.

$C_{11}H_{17}NO_3$ = 211.3.

CAS — 54-04-6.

An alkaloid obtained from the cactus *Lophophora williamsii* (=*Anhalonium williamsii*=*A. lewinii*) (Cactaceae), which grows in the northern regions of Mexico. The cactus is known in those areas by the Aztec name 'peyote' or 'peyotl' and dried slices of the cactus are called 'mescal buttons'. Both Mexican and North American Indians have used peyote in religious ceremonies on account of its hallucinogenic activity.

Mescaline produces hallucinogenic and sympathomimetic effects similar to those produced by lysergide (see p.1597), but it is less potent. Its effects last for up to 12 hours. It has no therapeutic use.

Mesoglycan Sodium (14224-s)

A mucopolysaccharide complex extracted from calf aorta.

Mesoglycan sodium has been claimed to have antithrombotic, antiplatelet, and antihyperlipidaemic properties.

References.

1. Forconi S, *et al.* A randomized, ASA-controlled trial of mesoglycan in secondary prevention after cerebral ischemic events. *Cerebrovasc Dis* 1995; **5:** 334–41.

Preparations

Proprietary Preparations (details are given in Part 3)
Ital.: Perclar; Prisma.

Metescufylline (12934-d)

Metescufylline (*rINN*).

7-(2-Diethylaminoethyl)theophylline (7-hydroxy-4-methyl-2-oxo-2*H*-1-benzopyran-6-yloxy)acetate.

$C_{25}H_{31}N_5O_8$ = 529.5.

CAS — 15518-82-8.

Metescufylline is a compound of metesculetol (below) and etamiphylline (p.753) that has been given by mouth for its reputed vasoprotectant effect.

Metesculetol Sodium (13490-t)

Metesculetol Sodium (*rINNM*).

[(7-Hydroxy-4-methyl-2-oxo-2*H*-1-benzopyran-6-yl)oxy]acetate sodium.

$C_{12}H_9NaO_6$ = 272.2.

CAS — 52814-39-8 (metesculetol); 53285-61-3 (metesculetol sodium).

Metesculetol is contained in preparations for peripheral vascular disorders and haemorrhoids.

Preparations

Proprietary Preparations (details are given in Part 3)

Multi-ingredient: ***Fr.:*** Cirkan; Fluon; Intrait de Marron D'Inde P; Veinotonyl.

Methallibure (12935-n)

Methallibure (*BAN, USAN*).

Metallibure (*rINN*); AY-61122; ICI-33828; NSC-69536. 1-Methyl-6-(1-methylallyl)-2,5-dithiobiurea.

$C_7H_{14}N_4S_2$ = 218.3.

CAS — 926-93-2.

Methallibure has the property of modifying certain hypothalamic and anterior pituitary functions. It has been used in veterinary medicine.

Methiosulfonium Chloride (12939-v)

Methylmethionine Sulfonium Chloride; Vitamin U. (3-Amino-3-carboxypropyl)dimethylsulphonium chloride.

$C_6H_{14}ClNO_2S$ = 199.7.

CAS — 1115-84-0.

Methiosulfonium chloride has been used for its reputed protective effect on the liver and gastro-intestinal mucosa.

Preparations

Proprietary Preparations (details are given in Part 3)

Multi-ingredient: ***Ger.:*** Medosalgon†.

Methyl Fluorosulphate (12951-n)

Methyl Fluorosulphonate.

$CH_3O.SO_2F$ = 114.1.

Methyl fluorosulphate has been used as a laboratory methylating agent. Pulmonary oedema has occurred after inhalation, and concern has been expressed concerning possible carcinogenicity.

Methylergometrine Maleate (1512-d)

Methylergometrine Maleate *(BANM, rINNM).*

Methylergobasine Maleate; Methylergonovine Maleate. *N*-[(*S*)-1-(Hydroxymethyl)propyl]-D-lysergamide hydrogen maleate; 9,10-Didehydro-*N*-[(*S*)-1-(hydroxymethyl)propyl]-6-methylergoline-8β-carboxamide hydrogen maleate.

$C_{20}H_{25}N_3O_2,C_4H_4O_4$ = 455.5.

CAS — 113-42-8 (methylergometrine); 57432-61-8 (methylergometrine maleate).

Pharmacopoeias. In *Jpn* and *US.*

A white to pinkish-tan, odourless, microcrystalline powder. **Soluble** 1 in 100 of water, 1 in 175 of alcohol, 1 in 1900 of chloroform, and 1 in 8400 of ether. A 0.02% solution in water has a pH of 4.4 to 5.2.

Store in airtight containers at a temperature not exceeding 8°. Protect from light. Solutions for injection should not be used if discoloured.

Stability. For mention of slight variations in the methylergometrine content of the injection following transport to a tropical climate, see under Ergometrine Maleate, p.1575.

Adverse Effects, Treatment, and Precautions

As for Ergometrine Maleate, p.1575.

Pharmacokinetics

Methylergometrine maleate is reported to be rapidly absorbed after administration by mouth and by intramuscular injection. It undergoes extensive first-pass hepatic metabolism. It is mainly excreted in the urine as metabolites.

The pharmacokinetics of methylergometrine maleate has been studied following oral administration in healthy subjects[1] and in postpartum women.[2] Small amounts of methylergometrine have been detected in breast milk.[3]

1. Mäntylä R, *et al.* Methylergometrine (methylergonovine) concentrations in the human plasma and urine. *Int J Clin Pharmacol Biopharm* 1978; **16:** 254–7.
2. Allonen H, *et al.* Methylergometrine: comparison of plasma concentrations and clinical response of two brands. *Int J Clin Pharmacol Biopharm* 1978; **16:** 340–2.
3. Erkkola R, *et al.* Excretion of methylergometrine (methylergonovine) into the human breast milk. *Int J Clin Pharmacol Biopharm* 1978; **16:** 579–80.

Uses and Administration

Methylergometrine maleate has an action on the uterus similar to that of ergometrine maleate (p.1575) and is used similarly in the prevention and treatment of postpartum haemorrhage. It is given after delivery of the anterior shoulder or on completion of the third stage of labour in a dose of 200 µg intramuscularly, repeated for up to 5 doses if necessary at intervals of 2 to 4 hours. In emergencies 200 µg may be given by slow intravenous injection over at least 60 seconds. In the USA its use before delivery of the placenta is not generally recommended. During the puerperium 200 µg may be given by mouth 3 or 4 times daily for up to 7 days.

Methylergometrine is a metabolite of methysergide (p.448).

Diagnosis and testing. For reference to the use of methylergometrine maleate in the diagnosis of variant angina, see Ergometrine Maleate, p.1575.

Preparations

USP 23: Methylergonovine Maleate Injection; Methylergonovine Maleate Tablets.

Proprietary Preparations (details are given in Part 3)

Aust.: Methergin; ***Belg.:*** Methergin; ***Fr.:*** Methergin; ***Ger.:*** Methergin; Methylergobrevin; ***Ital.:*** Methergin; ***Neth.:*** Methergin; ***Norw.:*** Methergin; ***Spain:*** Methergin; ***Swed.:*** Methergin; ***Switz.:*** Methergin; ***USA:*** Methergine.

Multi-ingredient: ***Ger.:*** Syntometrin.

Methylhydroxyquinoline Methylsulphate

(12949-q)

1-Methyl-8-hydroxyquinolinium methyl sulphate.

$C_{10}H_{10}NO,CH_3O_4S$ = 271.3.

Methylhydroxyquinoline methylsulphate has been used topically for eye irritation.

Preparations

Proprietary Preparations (details are given in Part 3)

Belg.: Uvestat; ***Fr.:*** Uveline; ***Ger.:*** Chibro-Uvelin†; ***Spain:*** Chibro-Uvelina.

Methylmethacrylate (12950-d)

Methyl 2-methylacrylate; Methyl 2-methylpropenoate.

$C_5H_8O_2$ = 100.1.

CAS — 80-62-6.

Adverse Effects

Methylmethacrylate monomer vapour may irritate the respiratory tract, eyes, and skin. Cases of occupational asthma have been reported. Contact dermatitis, dizziness, nausea and vomiting may also occur. Methylmethacrylate monomer may be harmful to the liver. It acts as a peripheral vasodilator and has caused hypotension and, rarely, cardiac arrest and death when absorbed during the use of polymethylmethacrylate (PMMA) as a bone cement during orthopaedic surgery.

Other adverse effects associated with the use of polymethylmethacrylate as a bone cement include thrombophlebitis, pulmonary embolism, haemorrhage, haematoma, short-term irregularities in cardiac conduction, and cerebrovascular accident.

Uses and Administration

Methylmethacrylate forms the basis of acrylic bone cements used in orthopaedic surgery. A liquid consisting chiefly of methylmethacrylate monomer with a polymerisation initiator is mixed with a powder consisting of polymethylmethacrylate (PMMA) or a methylmethacrylate ester copolymer. Barium sulphate or zirconium dioxide may be added as a contrast medium. The reaction is exothermic. Beads of polymethylmethacrylate containing gentamicin have been implanted in the prophylaxis and treatment of bone infections and some soft-tissue infections. A bone cement containing gentamicin is also available.

Polymethylmethacrylate has also been used as a material for intra-ocular lenses, for denture bases, as a cement for dental prostheses, and in composite resins for dental restoration.

A number of polymers based on methacrylic acid are used in pharmaceutical technology mainly as film coating agents and binders. The Ph. Eur. includes Methacrylic Acid-Methyl Methacrylate Copolymer (1:1), Methacrylic Acid-Ethyl Acrylate Copolymer (1:1), Methacrylic Acid-Methyl Methacrylate Copolymer (1:2), and Polyacrylate Dispersion 30 per cent (a dispersion of an ethylacrylate-methyl methacrylate copolymer in water). The USNF includes Methacrylic Acid Copolymer (a copolymer of methacrylic acid and an acrylic or methacrylic ester) and Ammonio Methacrylate Copolymer (a copolymer of acrylic and methacrylic acid esters).

Percutaneous vertebral injection of methylmethacrylate bone cement relieved pain in 17 of 20 patients with metastatic vertebral bone lesions within 48 hours.[1] No adverse effects from the cement were encountered. This technique may be a useful alternative to surgery for the early treatment of the pain associated with metastatic bone disease (p.484).

1. Kaemmerlen P, *et al.* Percutaneous injection of orthopedic cement in metastatic vertebral lesions. *N Engl J Med* 1989; **321:** 121.

Preparations

Proprietary Preparations (details are given in Part 3)

Aust.: Knochenzement; Sulfix; ***Ger.:*** Flint; Hansaplast; Palacos R; ***Ital.:*** Septopal†; ***Switz.:*** Palacos; ***UK:*** Palacos R.

Multi-ingredient: ***Aust.:*** AKZ; Refobacin-Palacos R; Septopal; ***Austral.:*** Palacos E with Garamycin; Palacos R with Garamycin; Septopal; ***Belg.:*** Septopal; ***Fr.:*** Palacos avec Gentamicine; Palacos R Gentamicine; ***Ger.:*** Refobacin-Palacos R; Septopal; ***Irl.:*** Palacos R with Gentamicin; Septopal; ***Neth.:*** Palacos R met gentamicine; Septopal; ***Norw.:*** Palacos cum gentamicin; Septopal; ***S.Afr.:*** Palacos R with Garamycin; Septopal; ***Swed.:*** Palacos cum gentamicin; Septopal; ***Switz.:*** AKZ; Palacos avec Garamycin; Septopal; ***UK:*** Palacos LV with Gentamicin; Palacos R with Gentamicin; Septopal.

Metochalcone (3727-p)

Metochalcone *(rINN).*

CB1314; Methochalcone; Trimethoxychalcone. 2′,4,4′-Trimethoxychalcone.

$C_{18}H_{18}O_4$ = 298.3.

CAS — 18493-30-6.

Metochalcone is a choleretic.

Preparations

Proprietary Preparations (details are given in Part 3)

Ital.: Auxibilina†; Megalip†.

Multi-ingredient: ***Ital.:*** Lebersana†; ***Spain:*** Neocolan.

Metyrapone (2139-m)

Metyrapone *(BAN, USAN, rINN).*

SU-4885. 2-Methyl-1,2-di(3-pyridyl)propan-1-one.

$C_{14}H_{14}N_2O$ = 226.3.

CAS — 54-36-4.

Pharmacopoeias. In *Br., Jpn,* and *US.*

A white to light amber, fine, crystalline powder with a characteristic odour. M.p. 50° to 53°. It darkens on exposure to light. Sparingly **soluble** in water; freely soluble in alcohol; freely soluble to soluble in chloroform; soluble in methyl alcohol; dissolves in dilute mineral acids. **Store** in airtight containers. Protect from heat and light.

Adverse Effects

Metyrapone may give rise to nausea and vomiting, abdominal pain, headache, sedation, dizziness, hypotension, and hypersensitivity rashes. Hypoadrenalism, hirsutism, and bone marrow depression may occur rarely. Long-term use of metyrapone can cause hypertension.

Reports of alopecia[1,2] associated with administration of metyrapone for Cushing's syndrome.

1. Harris PL. Alopecia associated with long-term metyrapone use. *Clin Pharm* 1986; **5:** 66–8.
2. Harries-Jones R, Overstall P. Metyrapone-induced alopecia. *Postgrad Med J* 1990; **66:** 584.

Precautions

Metyrapone should be used with extreme caution, if at all, in patients with gross hypopituitarism or with reduced adrenal secretory activity because of the risk of precipitating acute adrenal failure. Thyroid dysfunction or liver cirrhosis may alter the response to metyrapone.

Interaction

Phenytoin is reported to increase the metabolism of metyrapone; doubling the dose of metyrapone may counteract the interaction. However, as many other drugs may interfere with the steroid assessment, medication is best avoided where possible during the metyrapone test. Drugs reported to interfere with the metyrapone test include antidepressants such as amitriptyline, antithyroid drugs, antipsychotics such as chlorpromazine, barbiturates, corticosteroids, and hormones that affect the hypothalamic-pituitary axis such as oestrogens and progestogens.

Pharmacokinetics

Metyrapone is rapidly absorbed from the gastro-intestinal tract. It is metabolised by rapid reduction to metyrapol and excreted in the urine as glucuronide conjugates of metyrapone and metyrapol.

Uses and Administration

Metyrapone inhibits the enzyme 11β-hydroxylase responsible for the synthesis of the glucocorticoids cortisone and hydrocortisone (cortisol) as well as aldosterone from their precursors. The consequent fall in the plasma concentrations of circulating glucocorticoids stimulates the anterior pituitary gland to produce more corticotrophin. This, in turn, stimulates the production of more 11-deoxycortisol and other precursors which are metabolised in the liver and excreted in the urine where they can be measured. Metyrapone is therefore used as a test of the feedback hypothalamic-pituitary mechanism in the diagnosis of Cushing's syndrome, although the dexamethasone suppression test (p.1038) may be preferred.

After demonstration of the responsiveness of the adrenal cortex, metyrapone is given by mouth, usually in a dose of 750 mg every 4 hours for 6 doses. Administration with milk or after a meal may minimise the gastro-intestinal side-effects of metyrapone. A suggested dose by mouth for children is 15 mg per kg body-weight, with a minimum dose of 250 mg, every 4 hours for 6 doses. In patients with a normally functioning pituitary gland excretion of 17-hydroxycorticosteroids is increased two- to fourfold and that of 17-ketosteroids about twofold.

Metyrapone is also used in the management of Cushing's syndrome (p.1236) when doses may range from 250 mg to 6 g daily.

Since metyrapone inhibits the synthesis of aldosterone it has been used to treat some cases of resistant oedema in conjunction with a glucocorticoid to suppress the normal corticotrophin response to low plasma concentrations of glucocorticoids. The suggested usual dosage of metyrapone in resistant oedema is 3 g daily in divided doses.

Metyrapone tartrate has also been used.

References.

1. Atkinson AB. The treatment of Cushing's syndrome. *Clin Endocrinol (Oxf)* 1991; **34:** 507–13.
2. Avgerinos PC, *et al.* The metyrapone and dexamethasone suppression tests for the differential diagnosis of the adrenocorticotropin-dependent Cushing syndrome: a comparison. *Ann Intern Med* 1994; **121:** 318–27.

Preparations

BP 1998: Metyrapone Capsules;
USP 23: Metyrapone Tablets.

Proprietary Preparations (details are given in Part 3)
Austral.: Metopirone; ***Canad.:*** Metopirone†; ***Fr.:*** Metopirone; ***Ger.:*** Metopiron†; ***Irl.:*** Metopirone; ***Neth.:*** Metopiron; ***Norw.:*** Metopiron; ***Swed.:*** Metopiron; ***Switz.:*** Metopirone; ***UK:*** Metopirone; ***USA:*** Metopirone.

Dementholised Mint Oil (3268-x)

Pharmacopoeias. In *Br.* and *Fr.*
Mint oil or Mentha oil is in *Ger.* and *Jpn.*

A clear colourless to pale yellow volatile oil with a characteristic odour obtained by steam distillation followed by partial dementholisation and processing from the flowering tops of *Mentha arvensis* var. *piperascens* (Labiatae). The BP describes Brazilian-type oil and Chinese-type oil which differ in their optical rotation, refractive index, and pulegone content.

Soluble 1 in 4 of alcohol (70%); there may be some opalescence on further dilution. **Store** in well-filled containers at a temperature not exceeding 25°. Protect from light.

Dementholised mint oil is used as a flavour. *Mentha arvensis* is used in herbal medicine as a febrifuge and for rheumatic disorders. Peppermint oil (p.1208) and spearmint oil (p.1632) are used as carminatives and flavouring agents.

Preparations

Proprietary Preparations (details are given in Part 3)
Aust.: Physiomint; ***Ger.:*** Japanol; JHP Rodler Japanisches Heilpflanzenol; Kneipp Minzol; Minx-med†.

Multi-ingredient: ***Aust.:*** Parodontax; ***Austral.:*** Tiger Balm White; ***Belg.:*** Calmant Martou; Pinthym†; ***Fr.:*** Pastilles M.B.C†; ***Ger.:*** Pinofit†; Silvapin Aktiv-Tonic MMP†; ***Ital.:*** Broncosedina; Transpulmina Gola Nebulizzatore†; ***Switz.:*** Acidodermil; Carmol†; Huile analgesique "Polar-Bar"; Kernosan Huile de Massage; Lapidar 10 plus; Malveol; Neo-Angin au miel et citron; Neo-Angin exempt de sucre; Onguent nasal Ruedi; Osa Gel de dentition aux plantes; Pommade nasale Ruedi; Roliwol; Stago†; Tonex; Tyrothricin; ***UK:*** Olbas.

Miracle Fruit (12965-q)

The fruit of *Synsepalum dulcificum* (=*Richardella dulcifica*) (Sapotaceae)

Miracle fruit contains a glycoprotein 'miraculin' with no apparent taste of its own but able to make sour substances taste sweet and to improve the flavour of foods. Its activity is reduced by heating.

Mistletoe (885-r)

European Mistletoe; Gui; Mistelkraut; Tallo de Muérdago; Visci Caulis; Viscum; Viscum Album.

Pharmacopoeias. In *Ger.*

The dried, evergreen, dioecious semi-parasite, *Viscum album* (Loranthaceae), which grows on the branches of deciduous trees, chiefly apple, poplar, and plum. It occurs as a mixture of broken stems and leaves and occasional fruits.

Mistletoe has a vasodilator action and has been used in herbal preparations for hypertension and cardiovascular disorders although its activity when taken orally is questionable. It has also been used in nervous disorders, and in homoeopathic medicines. Mistletoe contains lectins with cytotoxic and immunomodulatory actions *in vitro* and preparations have been given by injection in a number of neoplastic diseases. Ingestion of the berries and other parts has been reported to cause nausea, vomiting, diarrhoea, and bradycardia.

A review of mistletoe.[1] There are about 1300 species of mistletoe representing 36 genera of the Loranthaceae, and what is called the "common mistletoe" varies from country to country: in Europe the term describes *Viscum album* while in the USA it describes *Phoradendron flavescens*. The toxicity of aqueous extracts of mistletoe has been found to depend upon the nature of the host plant. Three classes of cytotoxic compounds are present in the leaves and stems of *V. album* although the berries are generally considered to be the most toxic part of the plant. These are alkaloids, viscotoxins, and lectins. The viscotoxins have been shown to cause hypotension, bradycardia, arterial vasoconstriction, and a negative inotropic effect, and may act as acetylcholine agonists. The lectins show toxic effects in *animals* similar to those seen with ricin.

1. Anderson LA, Phillipson JD. Mistletoe—the magic herb. *Pharm J* 1982; **229:** 437–9.

Reports of hepatitis following the ingestion of herbal remedies containing mistletoe.[1,2]

1. Harvey J, Colin-Jones DG. Mistletoe hepatitis. *Br Med J* 1981; **282:** 186–7.
2. Weeks GR, Proper JS. Herbal medicines—gaps in our knowledge. *Aust J Hosp Pharm* 1989; **19:** 155–7.

Preparations

Proprietary Preparations (details are given in Part 3)
Aust.: Apotheker Bauer's Misteltinktur; Eurixor; Helixor; Iscador; Isorel; Isugran; ***Ger.:*** Abnobaviscum; Eurixor; Helixor; Iscador; Kneipp Mistel-Pflanzensaft; Kneipp Pflanzendragees Mistel; Lektinol; Mistel Curarina; Mistel-Krautertabletten; Mistelol-Kapseln; Plenosol N; Viscysat; Vysorel.

Multi-ingredient: ***Aust.:*** Herz- und Kreislauftonikum Bioflora; Krautertee Nr 20; Krautertee Nr 32; Mag Kottas Nerven-Beruhigungstee; Vivinox; Wechseltee; ***Austral.:*** Calmo; Pacifenity; Vitaglow Herbal Stress†; ***Belg.:*** Tisane Contre la Tension; ***Fr.:*** Mediflor Tisane Circulation du Sang No 12; Mediflor Tisane Hypotensive†; Santane H_7; Tisanes de l'Abbe Hamon no 6; ***Ger.:*** Antihypertonicum S; Antisklerosin S; Asgoviscum N; B 12 Nerv-infant†; Baldronit forte N†; Castrophan†; Craviscum†; Dr. Kleinschrod's Cor-Insuffin†; Fovysatum†; Herz-Plus Nerven†; Herz-plus†; Hypercard; Kneipp Drei-Pflanzen-Dragees; Manns Knoblauch Pillen Plus†; Mistelan†; Movicard†; Nervinfant†; Salusan; Seda-Movicard†; Syviman N; Vasesana-Vasoregulans; Verus†; Viscophyll; Worishofener Nervenpflege Dr. Kleinschrod†.

Monoctanoin (12794-b)

Monoctanoin *(BAN, USAN).*
Monooctanoin; Mono-octanoin.
CAS — 26402-26-6 (glyceryl mono-octanoate).

A semisynthetic mixture of glycerol esters, containing 80 to 85% of glyceryl mono-octanoate ($C_{11}H_{22}O_4$ = 218.3), 10 to 15% of glyceryl mono-decanoate ($C_{13}H_{26}O_4$=246.3) and glyceryl di-octanoate ($C_{19}H_{36}O_5$=344.5), and a maximum of 2.5% of free glycerol ($C_3H_8O_3$=92.09)

Adverse Effects and Precautions

Abdominal pain, nausea, vomiting, and diarrhoea may occur particularly if monoctanoin is infused rapidly or in large doses; it has been recommended that perfusion pressure should not exceed 20 cm of water. Minor irritation of the gastric and duodenal mucosa has been reported. Acidosis may occur, particularly in patients with impaired hepatic function and leucopenia has been reported. Monoctanoin should not be administered to patients with impaired hepatic function, biliary tract infection, cholestatic jaundice, jejunitis, duodenal ulcer, or pancreatitis. It should not be administered by the intravenous or intramuscular routes.

Side-effects[1] occurred in 67% of 343 patients treated with monoctanoin perfusion, with multiple side-effects in 41%. Abdominal pain was the most common adverse effect occurring in 40% of patients. Nausea, vomiting, and diarrhoea were usually dose related, occurring in 25%, 15%, and 16% of patients respectively. Fever, attributed to cholangitis, was noted in 5%. Severe side-effects occurred in 12 patients; a patient with cirrhosis developed acidosis and encephalopathic signs.

1. Palmer KR, Hofmann AF. Intraductal mono-octanoin for the direct dissolution of bile duct stones: experience in 343 patients. *Gut* 1986; **27:** 196–202.

Uses and Administration

Monoctanoin is used to dissolve cholesterol gallstones (p.1642) retained following cholecystectomy. It is administered by continuous perfusion through a catheter inserted directly into the common bile duct at a rate of 3 to 5 mL per hour at a pressure of 10 cm of water. Perfusion may be suspended during meals. The solution should be warmed prior to perfusion, and the temperature should be maintained at 37° during administration. Treatment is continued for 2 to 10 days. If no reduction in the size of the stones is detectable after 7 to 10 days of treatment, further treatment is unlikely to be effective.

Reviews[1,2] and studies[3] of the use of monoctanoin.

1. Abate MA, Moore TL. Monooctanoin use for gallstone dissolution. *Drug Intell Clin Pharm* 1985; **19:** 708–13.
2. Anonymous. Monooctanoin for gallstones. *Med Lett Drugs Ther* 1987; **29:** 52.
3. Palmer KR, Hofmann AF. Intraductal mono-octanoin for the direct dissolution of bile duct stones: experience in 343 patients. *Gut* 1986; **27:** 196–202.

Preparations

Proprietary Preparations (details are given in Part 3)
USA: Moctanin.

Motherwort (11430-j)

Herba Leonuri Cardiacae; Leonurus; Motherwort Herb.

Pharmacopoeias. In *Ger.*

Motherwort is the dried aerial parts of *Leonurus cardiaca* (Labiatae). It is given in herbal medicine for nervous and cardiac disorders; it is also used in products promoted for mild hyperthyroidism.

Preparations

Proprietary Preparations (details are given in Part 3)
Ger.: Thyreogutt mono.

Multi-ingredient: ***Aust.:*** Thyreogutt; ***Austral.:*** Pacifenity; Valerian; Vitaplex PMT†; ***Canad.:*** Thunas Tab for Menstrual Pain; ***Ger.:*** Aureal†; Befelka Herz-Dragees†; Biovital N; Cardisetten†; Concardisett†; Crataezyma N†; Dr. Klinger's Bergischer Krautertee, Herz- und Kreislauftee†; Knufinke Nervenruh Beruhigungs-Tee†; Mutellon; Oxacant N; Oxacant-sedativ; Thyreogutt-N†; ***Switz.:*** Demonatur Capsules ail-aubepine†; Tisane pour le coeur et la circulation; Tisane pour le coeur et la circulation "H"†; ***UK:*** Motherwort Compound; Prementaid; Quiet Life; SuNerven; Wellwoman.

Moxaverine Hydrochloride (5237-g)

Moxaverine Hydrochloride *(BANM, rINNM).*
Meteverine Hydrochloride. 1-Benzyl-3-ethyl-6,7-dimethoxyisoquinoline hydrochloride.
$C_{20}H_{21}NO_2$,HCl = 343.8.
CAS — 10539-19-2 (moxaverine); 1163-37-7 (moxaverine hydrochloride).

Moxaverine hydrochloride has a similar structure to papaverine (p.1614) and has been given by mouth and injection as an antispasmodic and in vascular disorders. The base is also used as an antispasmodic.

Doses of moxaverine hydrochloride of up to 300 mg three times daily have been suggested for the treatment of vasospastic disorders, although much lower doses are recommended for the treatment of gastro-intestinal and biliary-tract spasm.

Preparations

Proprietary Preparations (details are given in Part 3)
Ger.: Certonal; Kollateral; ***Ital.:*** Eupaverina†; ***Swed.:*** Eupaverin†.

Multi-ingredient: ***Aust.:*** Hedonin; ***Ger.:*** Ichthospasmin N†; Kollateral A + E; Sorbosan†.

Mumps Skin Test Antigen (7980-q)

Pharmacopoeias. In *US.*

A sterile aqueous suspension of formaldehyde-inactivated mumps virus prepared from the extra-embryonic fluid of virus-infected chick embryos, concentrated and purified by differential centrifugation, and diluted with isotonic sodium chloride solution. It contains a preservative and glycine as a stabilising agent. Each mL contains not less than 20 complement-fixing units. It should be stored at 2° to 8°. The expiry date is not later than 18 months after date of manufacture or of release from manufacturer's cold storage.

Recovery from mumps produces skin hypersensitivity to mumps virus. Mumps skin test antigen, 0.1 mL intradermally (intracutaneously), is used in conjunction with other antigens to assess the status of cell-mediated immunity. A positive reaction may indicate previous infection with mumps virus but it is not considered to be very reliable. It should not be given to patients hypersensitive to egg protein.

For reference to the use of mumps skin test antigen for anergy testing in HIV-positive patients, see Tuberculins, p.1640.

Preparations

USP 23: Mumps Skin Test Antigen.

Proprietary Preparations (details are given in Part 3)
USA: MSTA.

Muramidase Hydrochloride (11469-g)

N-Acetylmuramide Glycanohydrolase Hydrochloride; Globulin G_1 Hydrochloride; Lysozyme Hydrochloride.

Muramidase is a mucopolysaccharidase which is active against Gram-positive bacteria, possibly by transforming the insoluble polysaccharides of the cell wall to soluble mucopeptides. It is also thought to be active against some viruses and some Gram-negative bacteria.

Muramidase has been given, usually as the hydrochloride, to patients with herpes zoster and other painful viral infections and for mouth and respiratory-tract disorders. It has been used in combination with antibacterial agents in an attempt to enhance their activity. Sensitivity reactions have been reported.

Preparations

Proprietary Preparations (details are given in Part 3)
Belg.: Murazyme; ***Ital.:*** Debizima†; Fisiozima†; Immunozima; ***Jpn:*** Neuzym; ***Switz.:*** Eyebel†.

Multi-ingredient: ***Aust.:*** Sanoral; Tongill; ***Fr.:*** Cantalene; Eufosyl†; Glossithiase; Hexalyse; Lyso-6; Lysocalm; Lysopaine; Oroseptol Lysozyme; ***Ger.:*** Enzym-Tyrosolvetten†; Frubienzym; Tonsilase†; ***Ital.:*** Narlisim; ***Spain:*** Anticatarral Alcala Farm; Egarone; Espectral; Espectral Balsamico; Finegosan†; Indosolona†;

Inexfal; Lizipaina; Lysokana; Normo Nar; Polirino†; Pulmotropic; Rino Dexa; Trofalgon; *Switz.:* Arbid-top; GEM†; Larocal†; Lyso-6; Lysocline†; Lysopaine; Sangerol.

Poisonous Mushrooms or Toadstools

(12350-f)

CAS — 23109-05-9 (α-amanitin); 21150-22-1 (β-amanitin); 21150-23-2 (γ-amanitin); 58919-61-2 (coprine); 16568-02-8 (gyromitrin); 2552-55-8 (ibotenic acid); 60-34-4 (methylhydrazine); 300-54-9 (muscarine); 2763-96-4 (muscimol); 37338-80-0 (orellanine); 17466-45-4 (phalloidin); 28227-92-1 (phalloin); 39412-56-1 (phallolysin).

This monograph describes poisonous mushrooms often known as toadstools, their toxins, toxic effects, and the treatment of those effects. Their only use is in homoeopathic medicine which employs *Amanita muscaria* as Agaricus muscarius. *A. muscaria* and *Psilocybe* spp. are abused for their psychoactive properties (see also Psilocin, p.1622).

Mushrooms can be classified into 8 groups according to their principal toxins and toxic effects:

Group I. Most deaths due to mushroom poisoning follow the ingestion of mushrooms containing cyclopeptides and among these mushrooms *Amanita phalloides* or 'death cap' has been reported to be responsible for 90% of all mushroom fatalities. The cyclopeptides are a group of heat-stable cyclic polypeptides with molecular weights ranging from 800 to 1100 and include the amatoxins (α-, β-, γ-amanitin) and phallotoxins (phalloidin, phaloin, phallolysin). Other mushrooms containing cyclopeptides include *A. verna* ('deadly agaric', fool's mushroom), *A. virosa*, and *A. bisporigera* (known as the 'destroying angel'), and *Galerina autumnalis*, *G. marginata*, and *G. venenata*.

Group II. Although *A. muscaria* ('fly agaric') and *A. pantherina* ('panther cap') may contain small amounts of muscarine, the antimuscarinic effects of the hallucinogenic agent muscimol and the insecticidal agent ibotenic acid usually predominate.

Group III. Many species of *Gyromitra* contain toxins known as gyromitrins that decompose to release methylhydrazine (monomethylhydrazine; MMH) an inhibitor of the coenzyme pyridoxal phosphate.

Group IV. Mushrooms whose principal toxin is muscarine include many of the *Clitocybe* and *Inocybe* spp. *A. muscaria* and *A. pantherina* (see above) may also contain small amounts.

Group V. Coprinus atramentarius ('ink cap') contains the compound coprine, one of whose metabolites is an inhibitor of acetaldehyde dehydrogenase and it may therefore produce 'disulfiram-like' symptoms after drinking alcohol.

Group VI. Mushrooms which may contain the hallucinogenic indoles psilocin and psilocybin include species of *Psilocybe*, *Panaeolus*, *Gymnopilus*, *Stropharia*, and *Conocybe*.

Group VII. Many mushrooms which only act as gastro-intestinal irritants and do not produce systemic effects are included in this group.

Group VIII. A further group has sometimes been used to classify some species of *Cortinarius* that contain a renal toxin whose exact nature remains to be determined. It is thought by some to be orellanine.

Adverse Effects

The clinical course of poisoning due to mushrooms containing cyclopeptides may be divided into three phases. Initial symptoms may occur 4 to 24 hours after ingestion and usually consist of gastro-intestinal effects such as abdominal pain, nausea, severe vomiting, and profuse diarrhoea similar to that in cholera. The patient may then appear to recover and be symptom-free for 2 to 3 days, but liver-enzyme values may be increasing. Following this phase, the more serious toxic effects of the amatoxins become apparent and there are signs of liver, renal, cardiac, and CNS toxicity. Symptoms include jaundice, oliguria, anuria, hypoglycaemia, coagulopathies, circulatory collapse, convulsions, and coma. The mortality rate is high in this phase with death usually being due to liver failure following hepatic necrosis. Up to 90% of untreated patients may die, though the rate may be as low as 15 to 30% following treatment.

The adverse effects of mushrooms containing ibotenic acid and muscimol usually occur within 2 hours of ingestion. Symptoms may include ataxia, euphoria, delirium, and hallucinations associated with other antimuscarinic effects. Fatalities are rare.

Patients who have ingested mushrooms containing gyromitrins usually develop symptoms of poisoning within 6 to 24 hours. These consist initially of nausea, vomiting, abdominal pain, and muscle cramps, headache, dizziness and fatigue. Delirium, convulsions, coma, methaemoglobinaemia and haemolysis may also occur. Occasionally jaundice and hepatic necrosis may lead to hepatic failure and death. Up to 40% of patients may die.

Symptoms typical of 'cholinergic crisis' (see Neostigmine Methylsulphate, p.1394) may appear about 30 minutes to 2 hours after ingestion of mushrooms containing muscarine. These may include bradycardia, bronchospasm, salivation, perspiration, lachrymation, rhinorrhoea, involuntary urination and defaecation, and diarrhoea. Miosis, hypotension, and cardiac arrhythmias may also occur. Rarely death may follow due to cardiac arrest or respiratory-tract obstruction.

Since one of the metabolites of coprine is an acetaldehyde dehydrogenase inhibitor, drinking alcohol, even up to several days after ingestion of mushrooms containing this compound, will produce symptoms similar to those of the 'disulfiram-alcohol' interaction (see Disulfiram, p.1573). Fatalities are rare.

The adverse effects of ingestion of mushrooms containing psilocin and psilocybin are similar to those described under Lysergide (p.1597). Symptoms usually occur within about 30 minutes to 2 hours. Fatalities are rare.

There may be a delay of as long as 14 to 20 days before symptoms of poisoning due to *Cortinarius* appear. Patients will develop an intense thirst. Other symptoms usually include nausea, vomiting, diarrhoea, and anorexia. Muscle aching and spasms and a feeling of coldness may also occur. In severe cases renal failure may lead to death. It has been reported that up to 15% of patients may die.

Pregnancy. α-Amanitine does not appear to cross the placental barrier, even during the acute phase of intoxication.[1]

1. Belliardo F, *et al.* Amatoxins do not cross the placental barrier. *Lancet* 1983; **i:** 1381.

Treatment of Adverse Effects

As there are no specific antidotes for the majority of cases of mushroom poisoning, treatment consists primarily of symptomatic and supportive measures. The stomach should be emptied by inducing emesis or by gastric lavage if the patient has not already vomited spontaneously. However, if the onset of symptoms is delayed this is unlikely to be productive. Activated charcoal may be of use in binding toxins in the gastro-intestinal tract. Determining the interval between ingestion and the onset of symptoms may help to identify the type of mushrooms ingested. If possible specimens of the mushrooms or a sample of the stomach contents should be sent to an expert mycologist for identification. Particular attention should be paid to intravenous replacement of fluids and electrolytes especially if vomiting and diarrhoea are severe. If the ingestion of hepatotoxic or nephrotoxic mushrooms is suspected liver and renal function should be monitored. Although there is little evidence of efficacy, exchange transfusions, haemodialysis, or charcoal haemoperfusion may be of value to remove amatoxins. The removal of bile via a duodenal tube left *in situ* has been suggested to reduce enterohepatic circulation of amatoxins. Forced diuresis has also been advocated by some for amatoxin poisoning.

Since some mushrooms contain a wide range of toxins and patients may have ingested more than one species, specific therapy should only be instituted following positive identification.

Group I. There is little clinical evidence to support the efficacy of specific agents used in the treatment of cyclopeptide poisoning. A variety of agents including benzylpenicillin and silymarin or silybin (silibinin) have been administered to try to protect the liver against the hepatotoxic effects of the amatoxins. Liver transplantation may be required in patients with progressive liver failure. A radioimmunoassay for the detection of amatoxins is available in some countries to confirm a diagnosis of cyclopeptide poisoning.

Group II. Specific treatment is usually only required if symptoms are severe. Physostigmine should only be used if definite antimuscarinic symptoms are present. As mushrooms containing ibotenic acid and muscimol may also contain small amounts of muscarine, atropine may be required to control muscarinic symptoms.

Group III. Pyridoxine hydrochloride 25 mg per kg body-weight given as an intravenous infusion and repeated as required has been recommended as specific therapy to overcome the inhibition of pyridoxal phosphate by methylhydrazine. However, concern has been expressed that the use of such large doses of pyridoxine can itself produce adverse neurological effects. Methylene blue may be required if methaemoglobinaemia is severe.

Group IV. Atropine sulphate may be required to control the symptoms of muscarine poisoning but it should only be used if definite muscarinic symptoms are present.

Group V. There is no specific treatment for the 'disulfiram-alcohol' reaction except for the maintenance of blood pressure.

Group VI. If symptoms are severe some patients may require sedation with diazepam.

General reviews.

1. Köppel C. Clinical symptomatology and management of mushroom poisoning. *Toxicon* 1993; **31:** 1513–40.

Amanita phalloides. The use of specific antidotes in the treatment of poisoning due to *Amanita phalloides* remains controversial. Agents such as benzylpenicillin, sulphamethoxazole, thioctic acid, cytochrome C, ascorbic acid, insulin, growth hormone, silymarin or silybin, and corticosteroids have all been used or suggested. However, at present there is limited clinical evidence to support the use of only benzylpenicillin and silymarin or silybin.[1,2] Liver transplantation should be considered in patients with progressive liver failure.[2]

1. Floersheim GL. Treatment of human amatoxin mushroom poisoning: myths and advances in therapy. *Med Toxicol* 1987; **2:** 1–9.
2. Klein AS, *et al.* Amanita poisoning: treatment and the role of liver transplantation. *Am J Med* 1989; **86:** 187–93.

Musk (12982-p)

Almíscar; Deer Musk; Mosc.; Moschus.

CAS — 541-91-3 (muskone).

Pharmacopoeias. In *Chin.*

The dried secretions from the preputial follicles of the musk deer, *Moschus moschiferus* or some other spp. of *Moschus* (Cervidae).

Musk is used as a fragrance and fixative in perfumery.

A series of nitrated tertiary butyl toluenes or xylenes, or related compounds, are used as artificial musks. Musk ambrette, a synthetic nitromusk compound used in perfumery and as a food flavouring, has been reported to cause contact dermatitis and photosensitivity.

Musk is used in homoeopathic medicine.

References.

1. Golightly LK, *et al.* Pharmaceutical excipients: adverse effects associated with inactive ingredients in drug products (part I). *Med Toxicol* 1988; **3:** 128–65.

Preparations

Proprietary Preparations (details are given in Part 3)

Multi-ingredient: *Ital.:* Balsamico F. di M.†.

Black Mustard (4672-k)

Graine de Moutarde Noire; Mostarda Preta; Moutarde Jonciforme; Schwarzer Senfsame; Semen Sinapis; Semilla de Mostaza; Sinapis Nigra.

Pharmacopoeias. In *Aust.* and *Swiss.*

Swiss allows *B. nigra*, *B. juncea*, and other species.

The dried ripe seeds of *Brassica nigra* (= *B. sinapioides*) (Cruciferae).

White Mustard (4673-a)

Sinapis Alba.

Pharmacopoeias. Chin. allows *B. alba* or *B. juncea* under the title Semen Sinapis.

The dried ripe seeds of *Brassica alba* (Cruciferae).

Volatile Mustard Oil (4675-x)

Allylsenföl; Essence of Mustard; Oleum Sinapis Volatile.

CAS — 57-06-7 (allyl isothiocyanate).

NOTE. Allyl Isothiocyanate is *USAN.*

Pharmacopoeias. In *Aust.* and *Pol.*

Fr. and *US* include allyl isothiocyanate.

It may be prepared synthetically or distilled from black mustard seeds after expression of the fixed oil and is largely composed of allyl isothiocyanate (C_3H_5CNS = 99.16). Allyl isothiocyanate is slightly **soluble** in water; miscible with alcohol, with carbon disulphide, and with ether.

Black and white mustard seeds have been used as emetics, in counter-irritant and rubefacient preparations, and as a condiment. Volatile mustard oil is an extremely powerful irritant that has been used as a counter-irritant and rubefacient. Expressed mustard oil contains a smaller proportion of volatile oil and was used as a less powerful counter-irritant.

A report of 2 cases of IgE-mediated anaphylaxis to mustard condiment.[1]

1. Vidal C, *et al.* Anaphylaxis to mustard. *Postgrad Med J* 1991; **67:** 404.

Preparations

Proprietary Preparations (details are given in Part 3)

Fr.: Autoplasme Vaillant; Pneumoplasme; Sinapisme Rigollot.

Multi-ingredient: *Aust.:* Munari†; Red Point†; *Canad.:* Kinot; Penetrating Rub; Rheumalan; *Fr.:* Pneumoplasme a l'Histamine; Sedartryl; *Ger.:* Cor-Select; Infrotto†; Rheumaliment†; *Spain:* Bellacanfor†; Dolokey; Mostazola†; *Switz.:* Liberol; *UK:* 9 Rubbing Oils; Menthol and Wintergreen Heat Product†; Red Oil; *USA:* Dermolin; Methalgen; Musterole Extra.

Myristyl Alcohol (7190-d)

1-Tetradecanol.

$C_{14}H_{30}O$ = 214.4.

Pharmacopoeias. In *USNF.*

A white wax-like mass. M.p. 36° to 42°. Practically **insoluble** in water; slightly soluble in alcohol; soluble in ether.

Myristyl alcohol is used as an oleaginous vehicle.

Myrrh (281-c)

Gum Myrrh; Myrrha.

Pharmacopoeias. In *Eur.* (see p.viii).

A gum-resin obtained from the stem of *Commiphora molmol* and possibly other species of *Commiphora* (Burseraceae). **Protect** from light.

Myrrh is astringent to mucous membranes; the tincture is used in mouthwashes and gargles for inflammatory disorders of the mouth and pharynx. It has been used internally as a carminative.

Preparations

Proprietary Preparations (details are given in Part 3)
Ger.: Inspirol P; Lomasatin M.

Multi-ingredient: ***Aust.:*** Brady's-Magentropfen; Dentinox; Drovitol; Paradenton; Parodontax; ***Austral.:*** Formula 1†; ***Canad.:*** Cold Sore Lotion; Lotion pour Feux Sauvages; ***Ger.:*** Ad-Muc; Blend-a-med Fluid†; Echtrosept-GT†; Fluomint; Infi-tract N; Kalantol-A†; Kalantol-B†; Majocarmin†; Myrrhinil-Intest; Para Muc†; Repha-Os; Schwedentrunk; Schwedentrunk mit Ginseng; ***Ital.:*** Gengivario; ***Norw.:*** Allcocks Plaster†; ***Spain:*** Antiseptico Dent Donner†; Buco Regis; Nani Pre Dental; Regal; ***Switz.:*** Baume†; Eubucal†; ***UK:*** Herbal Indigestion Naturtabs; Indigestion and Flatulence; Medicinal Gargle; Vocalzone; ***USA:*** Astring-O-Sol.

Myrtillus (12987-y)

Baccae Myrtilli; Bilberry; Blaeberry; Heidelbeere; Huckleberry; Hurtleberry; Myrtilli Fructus; Whortleberry.

Pharmacopoeias. In *Aust., Fr.,* and *Swiss.*

The dried fruits of *Vaccinium myrtillus* (Ericaceae).

Myrtillus has diuretic and astringent properties. It has been used for ophthalmic and circulatory disorders and for non-specific diarrhoea.

Myrtillus is used in homoeopathic medicine.

Preparations

Proprietary Preparations (details are given in Part 3)
Austral.: Herbal Eye Care Formula; ***Ger.:*** Difrarel; ***Ital.:*** Alcodin; Angiorex; Antocin; Mirtilene Forte; Retinol; Tegens; ***Spain:*** Difrarel; Largitor; ***Switz.:*** Myrtaven.

Multi-ingredient: ***Aust.:*** Amersan; Krauterhaus Mag Kottas Tee gegen Durchfall; Myrtilen; ***Austral.:*** Bilberry Plus; Herbal PMS Formula; Prophthal; Pykno; St Mary's Thistle Plus; ***Fr.:*** Diacure; Difrarel; Difrarel E; Santane H_7; ***Ger.:*** Salus Augenschutz-Kapseln; ***Ital.:*** Alfa Mirtillo†; Alvear Sport; Api Baby; Bebimix; Biolactine; Biophil; Difravit†; Fluiven; Fotoretin†; Lactovit; Memovisus; Mirtilene; Neomyrt Plus; Nerex; Premium†; Ultravisin; Vitalmix; ***Spain:*** Antomiopic; Difrarel E; Mirtilus; ***Switz.:*** Difrarel†; ***UK:*** Se-Power.

Nadide (12991-s)

Nadide (*BAN, USAN, rINN*).

Codehydrogenase I; Coenzyme I; Co-I; Diphosphopyridine Nucleotide; DPN; NAD; Nicotinamide Adenine Dinucleotide; NSC-20272. 1-(3-Carbamoylpyridinio)-β-D-ribofuranoside 5-(adenosine-5'-pyrophosphate).

$C_{21}H_{27}N_7O_{14}P_2$ = 663.4.

CAS — 53-84-9.

Nadide is a naturally occurring coenzyme claimed to be of value in the treatment of alcohol and opioid addiction.

The reduced form of nadide, NADH (β-NADH; reduced DPN) and its phosphate derivative (NADPH) are being investigated in the management of Parkinson's disease (p.1128). It has been given in an attempt to enhance endogenous dopamine synthesis by stimulating the enzyme tyrosine hydroxylase; some beneficial effects have been reported.[1,2]

1. Birkmayer GJD, Birkmayer W. Stimulation of endogenous L-dopa biosynthesis—a new principle for the therapy of Parkinson's disease: the clinical effect of nicotinamide adenine dinucleotide (NADH) and nicotinamide adenine dinucleotidephosphate (NADPH). *Acta Neurol Scand* 1989; **80** (suppl 126): 183–7.
2. Birkmayer JGD, *et al.* Nicotinamide adenine dinucleotide (NADH)—a new therapeutic approach to Parkinson's disease: comparison of oral and parenteral application. *Acta Neurol Scand* 1993; **87** (suppl 146): 32–5.

Preparations

Proprietary Preparations (details are given in Part 3)
Ital.: Nicodrasi†; ***S.Afr.:*** DPN; ***Spain:*** Nad.

Multi-ingredient: ***Ital.:*** Piruvasi†.

Nafamostat (1775-d)

Nafamostat (*rINN*).

FUT-175 (nafamostat mesylate). 6-Amidino-2-naphthyl *p*-guanidinobenzoate.

$C_{19}H_{17}N_5O_2$ = 347.4.

CAS — 81525-10-2 (nafamostat); 82956-11-4 (nafamostat mesylate).

NOTE. Nafamostat Mesylate is *USAN.*

Like aprotinin (p.711) nafamostat is a proteolytic enzyme inhibitor. It is used as the mesylate in the treatment of acute pancreatitis and is under investigation for use in other conditions including shock and the prevention of surgical blood loss, and for cerebral vasospasm.

Hyperkalaemia has been reported.

References.

1. Yanamoto H, *et al.* Therapeutic trial of cerebral vasospasm with the serine protease inhibitor, FUT-175, administered in the acute stage after subarachnoid hemorrhage. *Neurosurgery* 1992; **30:** 358–63.
2. Akizawa T, *et al.* Nafamostat mesilate: a regional anticoagulant for haemodialysis in patients at high risk for bleeding. *Nephron* 1993; **64:** 376–81.
3. Miyata T, *et al.* Effectiveness of nafamostat mesilate on glomerulonephritis in immune-complex diseases. *Lancet* 1993; **341:** 1353.
4. Murase M, *et al.* Nafamostat mesilate reduces blood loss during open heart surgery. *Circulation* 1993; **88:** 432–6.
5. Kitagawa H, *et al.* Hyperkalaemia due to nafamostat mesylate. *N Engl J Med* 1995; **332:** 687.

Nafiverine Hydrochloride (12994-l)

Nafiverine Hydrochloride (*rINNM*).

DA-914 (base). *NN'*-Bis{2-[2-(1-naphthyl)propionyloxy]ethyl}piperazine dihydrochloride.

$C_{34}H_{38}N_2O_4.2HCl$ = 611.6.

CAS — 5061-22-3 (nafiverine); 5051-16-1 (nafiverine hydrochloride).

Nafiverine hydrochloride is used as an antispasmodic.

Preparations

Proprietary Preparations (details are given in Part 3)

Multi-ingredient: ***Ital.:*** Gefarnil Compositum†.

Naphthylacetic Acid (14833-e)

1-Naphthaleneacetic Acid; 1-Naphthylacetic Acid.

$C_{12}H_{10}O_2$ = 186.2.

CAS — 86-87-3.

Naphthylacetic acid has been used as a choleretic.

Preparations

Proprietary Preparations (details are given in Part 3)

Multi-ingredient: ***Aust.:*** Galle-Donau; Spagall; ***Spain:*** Genebilina†; ***Switz.:*** Bilipax.

Nebracetam (6489-e)

Nebracetam (*rINN*).

WEB-1881-FU. (±)-4-(Aminomethyl)-1-benzyl-2-pyrrolidinone.

$C_{12}H_{16}N_2O$ = 204.3.

CAS — 116041-13-5.

Nebracetam acts on the CNS and is under investigation as a cognition adjuvant in the treatment of Alzheimer's disease.

Nefiracetam (15298-l)

Nefiracetam (*rINN*).

DM-9384; DZL-221. 2-Oxo-1-pyrrolidineaceto-2',6'-xylidide.

$C_{14}H_{18}N_2O_2$ = 246.3.

CAS — 77191-36-7.

Nefiracetam acts on the CNS and has been described as a 'nootropic'. It has been investigated in some cerebrovascular disorders and for the treatment of Alzheimer's disease.

Neroli Oil (4676-r)

Aurantii Amari Floris Aetheroleum; Bitter-orange Flower Oil; Esencia de Azahar; Essência de Flor de Laranjeira; Oleum Neroli; Orange Flower Oil; Orange-flower Oil.

Pharmacopoeias. In *Eur.* (see p.viii).
Aust. also includes a monograph on the dried flowers.

A clear, pale yellow or dark yellow, volatile oil. It has a characteristic fragrant odour and a sweet aromatic taste with a bitter after-taste and is obtained by steam distillation from the fresh flowers of the bitter-orange tree, *Citrus aurantium* subsp. *amara* (=*C. aurantium* subsp. *aurantium*) (Rutaceae). **Soluble** 1 in 2 of alcohol (80%), the solution becoming turbid on the addition of more of the alcohol; miscible with alcohol (96%), ether, fatty oils, liquid paraffin, and petroleum spirit. **Store** in well-filled airtight containers. Protect from light and heat.

Neroli oil is used as a flavour and in perfumery. Photosensitivity reactions have been reported.

Preparations

Proprietary Preparations (details are given in Part 3)

Multi-ingredient: ***Fr.:*** Balsamorhinol; ***Switz.:*** Hygiodermil; Oculosan; Seracalm.

Nerve Agents (15575-k)

Sarin (8370-l)

GB. Isopropyl methylphosphonofluoridate.

$C_4H_{10}FO_2P$ = 140.1.

CAS — 107-44-8.

Soman (11059-e)

GD. Pinacolyl methylphosphonofluoridate.

$C_7H_{16}FO_2P$ = 182.2.

CAS — 96-64-0.

Tabun (11062-g)

GA. Ethyl *N*-dimethylphosphoramidocyanidate.

$C_5H_{11}N_2O_2P$ = 162.1.

CAS — 77-81-6.

VX (11080-p)

Methylphosphonothioic acid *S*-{2-[bis(1-methylethyl)amino]ethyl} *O*-ethyl ester.

$C_{11}H_{26}NO_2PS$ = 267.4.

CAS — 50782-69-9.

The nerve agents, sarin, soman, tabun, and vx (also referred to as 'nerve gases') used in chemical warfare are extremely potent inhibitors of cholinesterase activity. The effects of poisoning due to these agents, and their treatment, are similar to those for organophosphorus insecticides (p.1408) but as the nerve agents have a much greater intrinsic toxicity the symptoms of poisoning are more severe. Pyridostigmine has been administered prophylactically to personnel at risk from exposure to nerve agents (see p.1398).

References.

1. Dunn MA, Sidell FR. Progress in medical defense against nerve agents. *JAMA* 1989; **262:** 649–52.
2. Ministry of Defence. *Medical manual of defence against chemical agents.* London: HMSO, 1987. (JSP312)
3. Suzuki T, *et al.* Sarin poisoning in Tokyo subway. *Lancet* 1995; **345:** 980.
4. Masuda N, *et al.* Sarin poisoning in Tokyo subway. *Lancet* 1995; **345:** 1446.
5. World MJ. Toxic gas trauma. *Lancet* 1995; **346:** 260–1.
6. Morita H, *et al.* Sarin poisoning in Matsumoto, Japan. *Lancet* 1995; **346:** 290–3.
7. Yokoyama K, *et al.* Blood purification for severe sarin poisoning after the Tokyo subway attack. *JAMA* 1995; **274:** 379.
8. Nozaki H, *et al.* A case of VX poisoning and the difference from sarin. *Lancet* 1995; **346:** 698–9.
9. Yokoyama K, *et al.* Clinical profiles of patients with sarin poisoning after the Tokyo subway attack. *Am J Med* 1996; **100:** 586.
10. Nohara M, Segawa K. Ocular symptoms due to organophosphorus gas (sarin) poisoning in Matsumoto. *Br J Ophthalmol* 1996; **80:** 1023.
11. Sekijima Y, *et al.* Follow-up of sarin poisoning in Matsumoto. *Ann Intern Med* 1997; **127:** 1042.

Neutral Red (13005-y)

CI Basic Red 5; Colour Index No. 50040; Neutral Red Chloride; Nuclear Fast Red; Toluylene Red. 3-Amino-7-dimethylamino-2-methylphenazine hydrochloride.

$C_{15}H_{16}N_4.HCl$ = 288.8.

CAS — 553-24-2.

Neutral red is used as an indicator for alkalinity and for preparing neutral-red paper. It is also used as a stain in microscopy.

It is a photoactive dye that has been tried in the treatment of recurrent herpes simplex infections with limited success.

Niaouli Oil (4677-f)

Essence de Niaouli.

Pharmacopoeias. In *Fr.* and *Neth.*

A volatile oil, obtained by distillation from the fresh leaves of *Melaleuca viridiflora* or *Melaleuca quinquenervia* (Myrtaceae). **Store** in airtight containers. Protect from light.

Niaouli oil contains cineole and has similar actions to eucalyptus oil (p.1578). Cajuput oil (p.1556) is also prepared from *Melaleuca* spp.

Preparations

Proprietary Preparations (details are given in Part 3)
Fr.: Gomenol; Gomenoleo; Huile Gomenolee.

Multi-ingredient: ***Aust.:*** Expigen; Medizinalbad†; Red Point†; ***Belg.:*** Beogaze; Ebexol†; ***Canad.:*** Balminil Suppositoires; ***Fr.:*** Anthelox†; Balseptol†; Balsolene; Biogaze; Coquelusedal; Coquelusedal Paracetamol; Dinacode; Euvanol; Gomenol-Syner-Penicilline; Hexaquine; Terpone; Thiopon Balsamique; Tuberol†; Vapo-Myrtol; Vaseline Gomenolee; ***Ger.:*** Palatol; Palatol N; Palatol†; ***Ital.:*** Anacufen†; Auricovit†; Balsamico F. di M.†; Biopulmin†; Broncopulmin; Otormon F (Femminile)†; Paidorinovit; Rinantipiol; Rinobalsamiche; Rinofil†; Rinopaidolo; Rinovit; Rinovit Nube; ***Spain:*** Amidoyina†; Brisfirina Balsamica; Broncosolvente EP†; Broncovital; Bronquimar; Bronquimar Vit A; Brota Rectal Bals; Combitorax Ampicilina†; Complexobiotico Bals†; Dimayon; Diminex Balsamico; Edusan Fte Rectal; Electopen Balsam Retard; Etro Balsamico; Eufipulmo†; Exapenil Mucolitico†; Gartricin; Homocodeina Timol†; Juven Tos†; Maboterpen; Neumobiot; Pastillas Pectoral Kely; Pulmo Grey Balsam; Pulmonilo Synergium; Rinobanedif; Rinotiazol Fenilefri†; Sanaden Reforzado; Ultrabion Balsamico; Vapores Pyt; Vitavox Pastillas; Xibornol Prodes; ***Switz.:*** Bisolvex; Demo baume; Resorbane.

Nicaraven (10338-w)

Nicaraven *(rINN).*

(±)-*N*,*N'*-Propylenebis[nicotinamide].

$C_{15}H_{16}N_4O_2$ = 284.3.

CAS — 79455-30-4.

Nicaraven is under investigation as a cerebral vasodilator.

Nicergoline (1514-h)

Nicergoline *(BAN, USAN, rINN).*

FI-6714. 10α-Methoxy-1,6-dimethylergolin-8β-ylmethyl 5-bromonicotinate.

$C_{24}H_{26}BrN_3O_3$ = 484.4.

CAS — 27848-84-6.

Pharmacopoeias. In *Fr.*

Adverse Effects and Precautions

Adverse effects which may occur after nicergoline include gastro-intestinal disturbances and, particularly after parenteral administration, hypotension.

Of 359 patients with cerebrovascular insufficiency treated with nicergoline for 1 month[1] side-effects occurred in 25, necessitating withdrawal of therapy in 11. The reactions included hot flushes (6), general malaise (8), agitation (2), hyperacidity (3), nausea (1), diarrhoea (3), and dizziness and somnolence (2).

1. Dauverchain J. Bedeutung von nicergolin bei der symptomatischen behandlung des arteriellen hochdrucks und der chronischen, zerebro-vaskulären insuffizienz. *Arzneimittelforschung* 1979; **29:** 1308–10.

Interactions

For a study indicating that nicergoline enhances the cardiac depressant action of propranolol, see Beta Blockers, p.830.

Uses and Administration

Nicergoline is an ergot derivative. It has been used similarly to co-dergocrine mesylate (p.1566) to treat symptoms of mental deterioration associated with cerebrovascular insufficiency (see Dementia, p.1386) and has also been used in peripheral vascular disease (p.794). Nicergoline has been given in doses of up to 60 mg daily by mouth in divided doses, and by intramuscular injection in doses of 2 to 4 mg twice daily; 4 to 8 mg has been given by slow intravenous infusion. Nicergoline tartrate has been used in preparations for parenteral administration.

References.

1. Borgioli M, *et al.* Therapeutische wirksamkeit von nicergolin in der ophthalmologie. Fluoreszenzretinographischer beitrag. *Arzneimittelforschung* 1979; **29:** 1311–16.
2. Aliprandi G, Tantalo V. Physiopathologie des innenohres und therapie der perzeptionstaubheit. *Arzneimittelforschung* 1979; **29:** 1287–95.
3. Ronchi F, *et al.* Symptomatic treatment of benign prostatic obstruction with nicergoline: a placebo controlled clinical study and urodynamic evaluation. *Urol Res* 1982; **10:** 131–4.
4. Bousquet J, *et al.* Double-blind, placebo-controlled study of nicergoline in the treatment of pruritus in patients receiving maintenance hemodialysis. *J Allergy Clin Immunol* 1989; **83:** 825–8.
5. Saletu B, *et al.* Nicergoline in senile dementia of Alzheimer type and multi-infarct dementia: a double-blind, placebo-controlled, clinical and EEG/ERP mapping study. *Psychopharmacology (Berl)* 1995; **117:** 385–95.
6. Herrmann WM, *et al.* A multicenter randomized double-blind study on the efficacy and safety of nicergoline in patients with multi-infarct dementia. *Dementia Geriatr Cogn Disord* 1997; **8:** 9–17.

Preparations

Proprietary Preparations (details are given in Part 3)
Aust.: Ergotop; Sermion; ***Fr.:*** Sermion; ***Ger.:*** Circo-Maren; duracebrol; ergobel; Memoq; Nicerium; Sermion; ***Ital.:*** Cebran; Neugen; Nicer; Nicergolyn†; Sermion; ***Spain:*** Fisifax; Sermion; Varson; ***Switz.:*** Sermion.

Multi-ingredient: ***Ital.:*** Sermidrina†.

Nicofetamide (3938-t)

C-1065. *N*-(1,2-Diphenylethyl)-3-pyridinecarboxamide.

$C_{20}H_{18}N_2O$ = 302.4.

CAS — 553-06-0.

Nicofetamide has been used as an antispasmodic.

Preparations

Proprietary Preparations (details are given in Part 3)
Ital.: Lyspamin†.

Nicotine (15303-c)

(*S*)-3-(1-Methylpyrrolidin-2-yl)pyridine.

$C_{10}H_{14}N_2$ = 162.2.

CAS — 54-11-5.

Pharmacopoeias. In *Swiss* and *US.*

US also includes Nicotine Polacrilex (a complex of nicotine with a methacrylic acid polymer).

A liquid alkaloid obtained from the dried leaves of the tobacco plant, *Nicotiana tabacum* and related species (Solanaceae). Tobacco leaves contain 0.5 to 8% of nicotine combined as malate or citrate. **Store** under nitrogen at a temperature below 25°. Protect from light and moisture.

The USP includes Nicotine Polacrilex, a weak carboxylic cation exchange resin prepared from methacrylic acid and divinylbenzene, in complex with nicotine. It should be **stored** in airtight containers.

Dependence

Nicotine dependence is most commonly associated with cigarette smoking. Such dependence is characterised by a strong desire to continue taking the agent, a physical and psychological dependence on it, and a characteristic abstinence syndrome on withdrawal. The management of smoking cessation is discussed under Uses and Administration, below.

Mild withdrawal symptoms have been reported following the use of nicotine gum to aid smoking cessation.

References.

1. Benowitz NL, Henningfield JE. Establishing a nicotine threshold for addiction: the implications for tobacco regulation. *N Engl J Med* 1994; **331:** 123–5.
2. Keenan RM, *et al.* Pharmacodynamic effects of cotinine in abstinent cigarette smokers. *Clin Pharmacol Ther* 1994; **55:** 581–90.
3. Slade J, *et al.* Nicotine and addiction: the Brown and Williamson documents. *JAMA* 1995; **274:** 225–33.
4. Kessler DA. Nicotine addiction in young people. *N Engl J Med* 1995; **333:** 186–9.
5. Hatsukami D, *et al.* Physical dependence on nicotine gum: effect of duration of use. *Psychopharmacology (Berl)* 1993; **111:** 449–56.
6. Doll R, Crofton J, eds. Tobacco and health. *Br Med Bull* 1996; **52:** 1–223.

Adverse Effects and Treatment

Nicotine is a highly toxic substance and in acute poisoning death may occur within a few minutes due to respiratory failure arising from paralysis of the muscles of respiration. The fatal dose of nicotine for an adult is from 30 to 60 mg.

Less severe poisoning causes initial stimulation followed by depression of the autonomic nervous system. Typical symptoms include burning of the mouth and throat, nausea and salivation, abdominal pain, vomiting, diarrhoea, dizziness, hypertension followed by hypotension, mental confusion, headache, disturbed hearing and vision, dyspnoea, faintness, convulsions, sweating, and prostration. Transient cardiac standstill or paroxysmal atrial fibrillation may occur.

Nicotine is rapidly absorbed through the skin or by inhalation as well as by ingestion and nicotine poisoning may occur due to careless handling when it is employed as a horticultural insecticide.

Prompt treatment of nicotine poisoning is essential. If contact was with the skin, contaminated clothing should be removed and the skin washed thoroughly with cold water without rubbing. If the patient has swallowed nicotine, gastric lavage and administration of activated charcoal may be beneficial. Treatment is supportive and includes support of respiration and control of convulsions. Atropine may be used to suppress features of parasympathomimetic stimulation.

Apart from effects such as dizziness, headache, and gastro-intestinal disturbances mentioned above, adverse effects associated with nicotine replacement preparations have also included cold and flu-like symptoms, palpitations, insomnia, vivid dreams, myalgia, chest pain, blood pressure changes, anxiety, irritability, somnolence, and dysmenorrhoea. Allergic reactions have been reported. Adverse effects associated with specific preparations include skin reactions with transdermal patches; nasal irritation, epistaxis, lachrymation, and sensations in the ear with the nasal spray; throat irritation with the spray or chewing gum and increased salivation, aphthous ulceration and sometimes swelling of the tongue with chewing gum.

References.

1. Greenland S, *et al.* A meta-analysis to assess the incidence of adverse effects associated with the transdermal nicotine patch. *Drug Safety* 1998; **18:** 297–308.

In addition to the adverse effects listed above, a case of hiccups has been reported following use of nicotine gum[1] and vasculitis in 2 patients was associated with transdermal patches.[2] Hyperinsulinaemia and insulin resistance have been associated with long-term use of nicotine gum.[3]

1. Einarson TR, Einarson A. Hiccups following nicotine gum use. *Ann Pharmacother* 1997; **31:** 1263–4.
2. van der Klauw MM, *et al.* Vasculitis attributed to the nicotine patch (Nicotinell). *Br J Dermatol* 1996; **134:** 361–4.
3. Eliasson B, *et al.* Long-term use of nicotine gum is associated with hyperinsulinemia and insulin resistance. *Circulation* 1996; **94:** 878–81.

Adverse effects of tobacco products. Chronic use of tobacco is linked to a variety of diseases. By the mid-1960s, epidemiological data established tobacco smoking as a cause of lung cancer. Smoking is also associated with other cancers including cervical, oesophageal, and oral cancer, and cancers of the larynx, bladder, pancreas, stomach, and kidneys, and leukaemia.[1] Smoking is a risk factor in cardiovascular, respiratory, and peripheral and cerebral vascular diseases.[1,2] Maternal smoking in pregnancy is associated with low birth-weight infants and increased risk of abortion, still-birth, and neonatal death. Smoking also increases the risk of developing peptic ulcer and may affect other gastro-intestinal disorders.

Passive smoking refers to inhalation of secondhand tobacco smoke or environmental tobacco smoke. Risks to health from passive exposure are lower than those from active smoking. However, studies have established passive smoking as a cause of lung cancer;[3] passive smoking is also associated with increased risk of heart disease[4] and chronic respiratory disease.[5,6] Smokeless tobacco products also carry risks to health.

1. Wald NJ, Hackshaw AK. Cigarette smoking: an epidemiological overview. *Br Med Bull* 1996; **52:** 3–11.
2. Ashton H. Adverse effects of nicotine. *Adverse Drug React Bull* 1991; **149:** 560–3.
3. Lam TH. Passive smoking in perspective. *Med Toxicol Adverse Drug Exp* 1989; **4:** 153–62.
4. Steenland K. Passive smoking and the risk of heart disease. *JAMA* 1992; **267:** 94–9.
5. Law MR, Hackshaw AK. Environmental tobacco smoke. *Br Med Bull* 1996; **52:** 22–34.
6. DiFranza JR, Lew RA. Mortality and morbidity in children associated with the use of tobacco products by other people. *Pediatrics* 1996; **97:** 560–8.

Effects on the cardiovascular system. As mentioned above, nicotine from tobacco products is associated with increased risk of cardiovascular disease. It would not be surprising, therefore, if nicotine replacement preparations were also associated with cardiovascular adverse effects, and there are anecdotal reports of cardiovascular events, including myocardial infarction,[1,2] stroke,[3] and cerebral haematoma,[4] associated with use of such products. However, in studies in patients with cardiovascular disease, 5- or 10-week courses of transdermal nicotine were not associated with an increase in cardiovascular events compared to placebo.[5,6]

1. Warner JG, Little WC. Myocardial infarction in a patient who smoked while wearing a nicotine patch. *Ann Intern Med* 1994; **120:** 695.
2. Arnaot MR. Nicotine patches may not be safe. *Br Med J* 1995; **310:** 663–4.
3. Pierce JR. Stroke following application of a nicotine patch. *Ann Pharmacother* 1994; **28:** 402.
4. Riche G, *et al.* Intracerebral haematoma after application of nicotine patch. *Lancet* 1995; **346:** 777–8.
5. Working Group for the Study of Transdermal Nicotine in Patients with Coronary Artery Disease. Nicotine replacement therapy for patients with coronary artery disease. *Arch Intern Med* 1994; **154:** 989–95.
6. Joseph AM, *et al.* The safety of transdermal nicotine as an aid to smoking cessation in patients with cardiac disease. *N Engl J Med* 1996; **335:** 1792–8.

Precautions

Nicotine should not be used in patients who have experienced recent cerebrovascular accident. It should be used with caution in patients with cardiovascular disease and should be avoided in severe cardiovascular disease including during the immediate postmyocardial infarction period, and in patients with severe arrhythmias or unstable angina pectoris. It should be used with caution in those with endocrine disorders including hyperthyroidism and diabetes mellitus, in peptic ulcer disease, or renal or hepatic impairment. Its use is contra-indicated during pregnancy or breast feeding.

Nicotine should not be used in patients who continue to smoke.

Skin patches should not be used on broken skin.

Exercise. Physical exercise increased mean peak plasma concentrations of nicotine in 8 healthy subjects treated with a transdermal nicotine patch.[1] The effect was thought to be most likely due to increased skin perfusion resulting in increased uptake.

1. Klemsdal TO, *et al.* Physical exercise increases plasma concentrations of nicotine during treatment with a nicotine patch. *Br J Clin Pharmacol* 1995; **39:** 677–9.

Myasthenia gravis. A patient with myasthenia gravis noted worsening of his symptoms following application of transdermal nicotine patches, the effects being most severe about 1 hour after application, and resolving within 3 hours once the patch was removed.[1] Previous heavy smoking had not produced similar adverse effects, despite the fact that blood-nicotine concentrations are typically higher just after finishing a cigarette than when using the patch.[2]

1. Moreau T, *et al.* Nicotine-sensitive myasthenia gravis. *Lancet* 1994; **344:** 548–9.
2. Pethica D. Nicotine-sensitive myasthenia gravis. *Lancet* 1994; **344:** 961.

Interactions

Tobacco smoking induces hepatic metabolic enzymes and the pharmacokinetics of many drugs are altered in smokers, as discussed under their individual monographs.

References.

1. Miller LG. Cigarettes and drug therapy: pharmacokinetic and pharmacodynamic considerations. *Clin Pharm* 1990; **9:** 125–35.

Nicotinic acid. As described on p.1352, a possible interaction between nicotinic acid and nicotine from a transdermal patch has been reported.

Pharmacokinetics

Nicotine is readily absorbed through mucous membranes and the skin; bioavailability of oral nicotine is low due to extensive first-pass metabolism. Nicotine is widely distributed; it crosses the placenta and is found in breast milk. The elimination half-life is about 1 to 2 hours. Nicotine is metabolised mainly in the liver to cotinine and nicotine-*N*-oxide. Nicotine and its metabolites are excreted in the urine.

References.

1. Gorsline J, *et al.* Steady-state pharmacokinetics and dose relationship of nicotine delivered from Nicoderm (nicotine transdermal system). *J Clin Pharmacol* 1993; **33:** 161–8.
2. Gupta SK, *et al.* Bioavailability and absorption kinetics of nicotine following application of a transdermal system. *Br J Clin Pharmacol* 1993; **36:** 221–7.
3. Schneider NG, *et al.* Clinical pharmacokinetics of nasal nicotine delivery: a review and comparison to other nicotine systems. *Clin Pharmacokinet* 1996; **31:** 65–80.
4. Benowitz NL, *et al.* Sources of variability in nicotine and cotinine levels with the use of nicotine nasal spray, transdermal nicotine and cigarette smoking. *Br J Clin Pharmacol* 1997; **43:** 259–67.
5. Zins BJ, *et al.* Pharmacokinetics of nicotine tartrate after single-dose liquid enema, oral, and intravenous administration. *J Clin Pharmacol* 1997; **37:** 426–36.

Uses and Administration

The main physiological action of nicotine is paralysis of all autonomic ganglia, preceded by stimulation. Centrally, small doses cause respiratory stimulation, while larger doses produce convulsions of the medullary type and cause arrest of respiration. The effects on skeletal muscle are similar to those on ganglia.

Nicotine chewing gum, adhesive patches, lozenges, sublingual tablets, a nasal spray, or inhaler are used as aids to giving up smoking. *Chewing gum* is available in strengths of 2 mg and 4 mg; the nicotine may be present in the gum in the form of a complex with methacrylic acid polymer (nicotine polacrilex). It is recommended that treatment should be started with 2 mg chewed slowly over about 30 minutes when the urge to smoke occurs. If more than fifteen 2-mg pieces of chewing gum are required each day patients should transfer to the 4-mg strength. Not more than fifteen 4-mg pieces should be used per day.

Sublingual tablets containing the equivalent of 2 mg of nicotine as a β-cyclodextrin complex may also be used: the recommended dose is 1 or 2 tablets sublingually every hour, increased to a maximum of 40 tablets daily if necessary, for at least 3 months. The dose should then be gradually reduced until it can be withdrawn.

Adhesive *transdermal patches* are designed to be worn for 16 or 24 hours and are available in different strengths which deliver from 5 to 22 mg during the recommended wearing time. One patch should be applied daily to the trunk or upper arm, usually beginning with the highest strength or with a dose determined by the previous daily consumption of cigarettes. A different site of application should be used each day with several days elapsing before the patch is applied to the same area of skin. Treatment is usually withdrawn gradually by reducing the dose every 2 to 8 weeks.

A suggested initial dosage for a *nasal spray* containing 500 μg per spray is one spray administered into each nostril as required up to twice hourly for 16 hours (a maximum of 64 sprays daily) for the first 8 weeks and reduced gradually thereafter.

Nicotine *inhaler cartridges* contain nicotine 10 mg for use in an appropriate inhaler mouthpiece. The initial dose is 6 to 12 cartridges daily for up to 8 weeks and is reduced gradually over a further 4 weeks.

It has been recommended that the use of nicotine therapy for smoking cessation should be reviewed if abstinence has not been achieved in 3 months.

Nicotine has been used as a horticultural insecticide either as a vapour or as a spray.

Alzheimer's disease. The use of nicotine as a cholinergic agonist is one of a number of methods being studied[1] to overcome brain cholinergic deficits in patients with Alzheimer's disease (p.1386). Preliminary studies[2,3] using nicotine patches have been of limited duration and are inconclusive.

1. Baldinger SL, Schroeder DJ. Nicotine therapy in patients with Alzheimer's disease. *Ann Pharmacother* 1995; **29:** 314–15.
2. Wilson AL, *et al.* Nicotine patches in Alzheimer's disease: pilot study on learning, memory, and safety. *Pharmacol Biochem Behav* 1995; **51:** 509–14.
3. Snaedal J, *et al.* The effects of nicotine in dermal plaster on cognitive functions in patients with Alzheimer's disease. *Dementia* 1996; **7:** 47–52.

Blepharospasm. Nicotine nasal spray was reported to be of benefit in a patient with blepharospasm (p.1311) refractory to botulinum A toxin.[1]

1. Dursun SM, *et al.* Treatment of blepharospasm with nicotine nasal spray. *Lancet* 1996; **348:** 60.

Extrapyramidal disorders. Nicotine transdermal patches have been reported to produce beneficial effects[1] in schizophrenic patients with antipsychotic-induced akathisia (p.650).

1. Anfang MK, Pope HG. Treatment of neuroleptic-induced akathisia with nicotine patches. *Psychopharmacology (Berl)* 1997; **134:** 153–6.

Skin disorders. There have been anecdotal reports of nicotine producing beneficial effects in various skin disorders, including pyoderma gangrenosum[1] and dermatitis due to fluorouracil therapy.[2]

1. Kanekura T, *et al.* Nicotine for pyoderma gangrenosum. *Lancet* 1995; **345:** 1058.
2. Kingsley EC. 5-Fluorouracil dermatitis prophylaxis with a nicotine patch. *Ann Intern Med* 1994; **120:** 813.

Smoking cessation. The cessation of cigarette smoking often results in the development of a nicotine withdrawal syndrome.[1] Nicotine dependence may be treated with behavioural or psychological counselling, but pharmacotherapy has also been used alone or as an adjunct to alleviate symptoms of nicotine withdrawal and achieve smoking cessation.[2-4] Meta-analyses[5-10] indicate that nicotine replacement can alleviate withdrawal symptoms and can help patients to quit smoking. It is most effective when used in a setting providing intensive support and counselling[11] but is still of value in general practice providing more limited support.[12,13] Although many patients relapse, resulting in only a modest increase in long-term abstinence,[14,15] even small increases in the rate of cessation have been considered to be clinically useful.[14] A need for higher doses and/or longer therapy with nicotine has been suggested,[16-19] but others have found no particular advantage from high-dose transdermal treatment.[20] Repeated treatments for relapsed smokers might provide incremental benefits for those wishing to cease smoking.[21]

Most studies have involved the use of transdermal patches or chewing gum but intranasal administration[22,23] or inhalation[24,25] also appears to be of benefit. The use of transdermal patches has been the subject of a number of reviews.[26-29] Transdermal patches which supply nicotine over 16 or 24 hours are considered to be equally effective[30,31] but as mentioned above the benefits of high versus low doses are as yet uncertain.[18,20] Combined use of patches and chewing gum may be of help to some patients.[31] Although long-term nicotine maintenance therapy has been proposed,[32] adverse metabolic effects may limit this application.[33]

Following reports of cardiovascular reactions associated with nicotine replacement there has been concern over its safety in patients with cardiovascular disease (see above), although nicotine patches appear to produce less platelet activation and catecholamine release than smoking and would be less likely to cause coronary ischaemia or thrombosis.[34] Some studies[35,36] also found that nicotine replacement therapy could safely be used by smokers with less severe cardiovascular disease. Nicotine nasal spray did not aggravate the effects of smoking on myocardial oxygen demand or coronary artery dimensions,[37] but it has been stressed that patients should not smoke while wearing nicotine patches.

Clonidine has been tried orally and transdermally to alleviate withdrawal symptoms but results have been conflicting and its use may be limited by a high incidence of adverse effects;[31,38] it might be of use in selected patients who experience severe agitation and anxiety on cessation of smoking.[38] Other agents that have been tried with varying degrees of success including bupropion, buspirone, tricyclic antidepressants, and mecamylamine. There is little evidence to support the use of silver compounds such as silver acetate, and lobeline appears to be no more effective than placebo.[2,4]

1. Benowitz NL. Pharmacologic aspects of cigarette smoking and nicotine addiction. *N Engl J Med* 1988; **319:** 1318–30.
2. Nunn-Thompson CL, Simon PA. Pharmacotherapy for smoking cessation. *Clin Pharm* 1989; **8:** 710–20.
3. Glassman AH, Corey LS. Future trends in the pharmacological treatment of smoking cessation. *Drugs* 1990; **40:** 1–5.
4. Gourlay SG, McNeil JJ. Antismoking products. *Med J Aust* 1990; **153:** 699–707.
5. Lam W, *et al.* Meta-analysis of randomised controlled trials of nicotine chewing-gum. *Lancet* 1987; **ii:** 27–30.
6. Li Wan Po, A. Transdermal nicotine in smoking cessation: a meta-analysis. *Eur J Clin Pharmacol* 1993; **45:** 519–28.
7. Tang JL, *et al.* How effective is nicotine replacement therapy in helping people to stop smoking? *Br Med J* 1994; **308:** 21–6. Correction. *ibid.*: 626.
8. Silagy C, *et al.* Meta-analysis on efficacy of nicotine replacement therapies in smoking cessation. *Lancet* 1994; **343:** 139–42.
9. Fiore MC, *et al.* The effectiveness of the nicotine patch for smoking cessation: a meta-analysis. *JAMA* 1994; **271:** 1940–7.
10. Silagy C, *et al.* Nicotine replacement therapy for smoking cessation. Tobacco Addiction Module of The Cochrane Database of Systematic Reviews (updated 1 December 1997). Available in The Cochrane Library; Issue 1. Oxford: Update Software; 1998.
11. Fiore MC, *et al.* Two studies of the clinical effectiveness of the nicotine patch with different counseling treatments. *Chest* 1994; **105:** 524–323.
12. Imperial Cancer Research Fund General Practice Research Group. Effectiveness of a nicotine patch in helping people stop smoking: results of a randomised trial in general practice. *Br Med J* 1993; **306:** 1304–8.
13. Russell MAH, *et al.* Targeting heavy smokers in general practice: randomised controlled trial of transdermal nicotine patches. *Br Med J* 1993; **306:** 1308–12.
14. Fowler G, *et al.* Randomised trial of nicotine patches in general practice: results at one year. *Br Med J* 1994; **308:** 1476–7.
15. Stapleton JA, *et al.* How much does relapse after one year erode effectiveness of smoking cessation treatment? Long term follow up of randomised trial of nicotine nasal spray. *Br Med J* 1998; **316:** 830–1.
16. Benowitz NL. Nicotine replacement therapy: what has been accomplished—can we do better? *Drugs* 1993; **45:** 157–70.
17. Hurt RD, *et al.* Nicotine patch therapy for smoking cessation combined with physician advice and nurse follow-up: one-year outcome and percentage of nicotine replacement. *JAMA* 1994; **271:** 595–600.
18. Dale LC, *et al.* High-dose nicotine patch therapy: percentage of replacement and smoking cessation. *JAMA* 1995; **274:** 1353–8.
19. Sachs DPL. Effectiveness of the 4-mg dose of nicotine polacrilex for the initial treatment of high-dependent smokers. *Arch Intern Med* 1995; **155:** 1973–80.
20. Jorenby DE, *et al.* Varying nicotine patch dose and type of smoking cessation counseling. *JAMA* 1995; **274:** 1347–52.
21. Gourlay SG, *et al.* Double blind trial of repeated treatment with transdermal nicotine for relapsed smokers. *Br Med J* 1995; **311:** 363–6.
22. Sutherland G, *et al.* Randomised controlled trial of nasal nicotine spray in smoking cessation. *Lancet* 1992; **340:** 324–9.
23. Perkins KA, *et al.* Nasal spray nicotine replacement suppresses cigarette smoking desire and behavior. *Clin Pharmacol Ther* 1992; **52:** 627–34.
24. Tønnesen P, *et al.* A double-blind trial of a nicotine inhaler for smoking cessation. *JAMA* 1993; **269:** 1268–71.
25. Lunell E, *et al.* Effect of nicotine vapour inhalation on the relief of tobacco withdrawal symptoms. *Eur J Clin Pharmacol* 1995; **48:** 235–40.
26. Palmer KJ, *et al.* Transdermal nicotine: a review of its pharmacodynamic and pharmacokinetic properties, and therapeutic efficacy as an aid to smoking cessation. *Drugs* 1992; **44:** 498–529.
27. Fiore MC, *et al.* Tobacco dependence and the nicotine patch: clinical guidelines for effective use. *JAMA* 1992; **268:** 2687–94.
28. Gora ML. Nicotine transdermal systems. *Ann Pharmacother* 1993; **27:** 742–50.
29. Gourlay S. The pros and cons of transdermal nicotine therapy. *Med J Aust* 1994; **160:** 152–9.
30. Anonymous. Nicotine patches. *Drug Ther Bull* 1993; **31:** 95–6.
31. Anonymous. Use of nicotine to stop smoking. *Med Lett Drugs Ther* 1995; **37:** 6–8.
32. Warner KE, *et al.* The emerging market for long-term nicotine maintenance. *JAMA* 1997; **278:** 1087–92.
33. Eliasson B, *et al.* Long-term use of nicotine gum is associated with hyperinsulinemia and insulin resistance. *Circulation* 1996; **94:** 878–81.
34. Benowitz NL, *et al.* Nicotine effects on eicosanoid formation and hemostatic function: comparison of transdermal nicotine and cigarette smoking. *J Am Coll Cardiol* 1993; **22:** 1159–67.
35. Working Group for the Study of Transdermal Nicotine in Patients with Coronary Artery Disease. Nicotine replacement therapy for patients with coronary artery disease. *Arch Intern Med* 1994; **154:** 989–95.
36. Joseph AM, *et al.* The safety of transdermal nicotine as an aid to smoking cessation in patients with cardiac disease. *N Engl J Med* 1996; **335:** 1792–8.
37. Keeley EC, *et al.* Intranasal nicotine spray does not augment the adverse effects of cigarette smoking on myocardial oxygen demand or coronary artery dimensions. *Am J Med* 1996; **171:** 357–63.
38. Gourlay SG, Benowitz NL. Is clonidine an effective smoking cessation therapy? *Drugs* 1995; **50:** 197–207.

Spasticity. There have been anecdotal reports[1] of beneficial responses to nicotine in spastic dystonia (see Spasticity, p.1303).

1. Vaughan CJ, *et al.* Treatment of spastic dystonia with transdermal nicotine. *Lancet* 1997; **350:** 565.

Tics. Tourette's syndrome (p.636) is characterised by motor and vocal tics and behavioural disturbances. Nicotine[1-3] has been reported to be of benefit when used alone or with haloperidol in patients with Tourette's syndrome whose symptoms were not satisfactorily controlled with usual treatment with haloperidol. It is hoped that the use of transdermal nicotine patches will avoid the reported problems of compliance associated with the taste and gastro-intestinal effects of nicotine gum.

1. McConville BJ, *et al.* The effects of nicotine plus haloperidol compared to nicotine only and placebo nicotine only in reducing tic severity and frequency to Tourette's disorder. *Biol Psychiatry* 1992; **31:** 832–40.
2. Silver AA, Sanberg PR. Transdermal nicotine patch and potentiation of haloperidol in Tourette's syndrome. *Lancet* 1993; **342:** 182.
3. Dursun SM, *et al.* Longlasting improvement of Tourette's syndrome with transdermal nicotine. *Lancet* 1994; **344:** 1577.

Ulcerative colitis. The mainstays of treatment for inflammatory bowel disease (p.1171) remain aminosalicylates and corticosteroids. Investigation of the use of nicotine in ulcerative colitis has been prompted by the observation that this condition is rare in smokers. Preliminary results from one study[1] suggested that transdermal nicotine added to conventional maintenance therapy could improve symptoms but a later study[2] found that when used alone nicotine was no more effective than placebo in maintaining remission. Some consider[3] that if further trials do confirm any therapeutic value for nicotine in ulcerative colitis its adverse effects are likely to limit its use in some patients, particularly those who have never smoked. Rectal administration of nicotine is under investigation.[4]

1. Pullan RD, *et al.* Transdermal nicotine for active ulcerative colitis. *N Engl J Med* 1994; **330:** 811–15.
2. Thomas GAO, *et al.* Transdermal nicotine as maintenance therapy for ulcerative colitis. *N Engl J Med* 1995; **332:** 988–92.
3. Rhodes J, Thomas G. Nicotine treatment in ulcerative colitis. *Drugs* 1995; **49:** 157–60.
4. Sandborn WJ, *et al.* Nicotine tartrate liquid enemas for mildly to moderately active left-sided ulcerative colitis unresponsive to first-line therapy: a pilot study. *Aliment Pharmacol Ther* 1997; **11:** 663–71.

Preparations

USP 23: Nicotine Polacrilex Gum; Nicotine Transdermal System.

Proprietary Preparations (details are given in Part 3)
Aust.: Nicolan; Nicorette; Nicotinell; Nicotrol; ***Austral.:*** Nicabate; Nicorette; Nicotinell; Prostep; ***Belg.:*** Nicorette; Nicotinell; ***Canad.:*** Habitrol; Nicoderm; Nicorette; Nicotrol; Prostep; ***Fr.:*** Nicopatch; Nicorette; Nicotinell; Tabazur†; ***Ger.:*** Nicorette; Nicotinell; nikofrenon; ***Irl.:*** Niconil; Nicorette; Nicotinell; ***Ital.:*** Nicorette; Nicotinell TTS; Nicotrans; ***Neth.:*** Nicorette; Nicotinell; ***Norw.:*** Nicorette; Nicotinell; ***S.Afr.:*** Nicorette; Nicotinell TTS; ***Spain:*** Nicodisc; Nicomax; Nicorette; Nicotinell TTS; Nicotrans; Nicotrol; ***Swed.:*** Nicolan; Nicorette; Nicotinell; Nikotugg; Quitt†; ***Switz.:*** Nicorette; Nicostop TTS; Nicotinell; ***UK:*** Nicabate†; Niconil; Nicorette; Nicotinell; NiQuitin CQ; Stubit; ***USA:*** Habitrol; Nicoderm; Nicorette; Nicotrol; Prostep.

Multi-ingredient: ***UK:*** Resolution.

Nitric Acid (1318-r)

Aqua Fortis; Azotic Acid; Nit. Acid; Salpetersäure.

$HNO_3 = 63.01$.

CAS — 7697-37-2.

Pharmacopoeias. In *Br.* (approximately 70%) and *Pol.* (10%). *Aust.* has Acidum Nitricum Concentratum (64.3 to 66.4%) and Acidum Nitricum (31.1 to 32.2%). Also in *USNF* (69 to 71%).

A clear, colourless or almost colourless, highly corrosive fuming liquid, with a characteristic irritating odour. **Store** in airtight containers.

Adverse Effects and Treatment

As for Hydrochloric Acid, p.1588.

There may be methaemoglobinaemia. Nitric acid stains the skin yellow.

Uses and Administration

Nitric acid has a powerful corrosive action and has been used to remove warts (p.1076), but it should be applied with caution, and less corrosive substances are available. It has also been used for the removal of tattoos.

Preparations

Proprietary Preparations (details are given in Part 3)

Multi-ingredient: ***Ger.:*** Solco-Derman; ***Switz.:*** Solcoderm; Solcogyn.

Nitrobenzene (13025-k)

Nitrobenzol; Oil of Mirbane.

$C_6H_5NO_2 = 123.1$.

CAS — 98-95-3.

A pale yellow liquid with an almond-like odour.

Adverse Effects

Nitrobenzene is highly toxic and the ingestion of 1 g may be fatal. Toxic effects from ingestion are usually delayed for several hours and may include nausea, prostration, burning headache, methaemoglobinaemia with cyanosis, haemolytic anaemia, vomiting (with characteristic odour), convulsions, and coma, ending in death after a few hours. Poisoning may also occur from absorption through the skin, or by inhalation.

Treatment of Adverse Effects

After ingestion of nitrobenzene the stomach should be emptied. Methaemoglobinaemia may be treated with methylene blue. Blood transfusions or haemodialysis may be necessary. Oxygen should be given if cyanosis is severe.

If the skin or eyes are splashed with nitrobenzene, contaminated clothing should be removed immediately and the affected areas washed with running water for at least 15 minutes.

Uses

Nitrobenzene is used in the manufacture of aniline, as a preservative in polishes, and in perfumery and soaps.

Nizofenone (19584-b)

Nizofenone *(rINN).*

Y-9179. 2′-Chloro-2-[2-[(diethylamino)methyl]imidazol-1-yl]-5-nitrobenzophenone.

$C_{21}H_{21}ClN_4O_3 = 412.9$.

CAS — 54533-85-6.

Nizofenone has been used as a nootropic.

Nucleic Acid (15306-t)

Acide Zymonucléique; Acidum Nucleicum; Nucleinic Acid.

A complex mixture of phosphorus-containing organic acids present in living cells.

Nucleic acids are of 2 types, ribonucleic acids (RNA) (see p.1624) and deoxyribonucleic acids (DNA) (see p.1570). They are composed of chains of nucleotides (phosphate esters of purine or pyrimidine bases and pentose sugars).

Since the administration of nucleic acid gives rise to a marked temporary leucocytosis (usually preceded by a short period of leucopenia) it was formerly given in the treatment of a variety of bacterial infections in the hope of enhancing the natural defence mechanisms. Its therapeutic value, however, was never established.

Preparations

Proprietary Preparations (details are given in Part 3)
Ger.: Embran†.

Nutmeg (4679-n)

Muscade; Myristica; Noz Moscada; Nuez Moscada; Nux Moschata.

Pharmacopoeias. In *Chin.*

The dried kernels of the seeds of *Myristica fragrans* (Myristicaceae), containing not less than 5% v/w of volatile oil; the powdered drug contains not less than 4% v/w. Mace (p.1597) is the dried arillus of the seed of *M. fragrans.*

Adverse Effects

Nutmeg, taken in large doses may cause nausea and vomiting, flushing, dry mouth, tachycardia, stimulation of the central nervous system possibly with epileptiform convulsions, miosis, mydriasis, euphoria, and hallucinations. Myristicin and elimicin are thought to be the constituents responsible for the psychotic effects of nutmeg, possibly following metabolism to amphetamine-like compounds.

Some references to the adverse effects of nutmeg.

1. Panayotopoulos DJ, Chisholm DD. Hallucinogenic effect of nutmeg. *Br Med J* 1970; **1:** 754.
2. Faguet RA, Rowland KF. "Spice cabinet" intoxication. *Am J Psychiatry* 1978; **135:** 860–1.
3. Venables GS, *et al.* Nutmeg poisoning. *Br Med J* 1976; **1:** 96.
4. Dietz WH, Stuart MJ. Nutmeg and prostaglandins. *N Engl J Med* 1976; **294:** 503.

Uses and Administration

Nutmeg is the source of nutmeg oil. It is aromatic and carminative and is used as a flavour. Nutmeg has been reported to inhibit prostaglandin synthesis.

It is used in homoeopathic medicine.

Preparations

Proprietary Preparations (details are given in Part 3)

Multi-ingredient: ***Aust.:*** Mariazeller; Schwedenjorg mild; ***Ger.:*** Doppelherz Melissengeist; ***Spain:*** Agua del Carmen; Melisana†; Vicks Vaporub; ***UK:*** Aluminium Free Indigestion; Cough Drops; Melissa comp..

Nutmeg Oil (4678-d)

Ätherisches Muskatöl; Esencia de Nuez Moscada; Essence de Muscade; Essência de Moscada; Myristica Oil; Oleum Myristicae.

Pharmacopoeias. In *Aust., Br., Fr.,* and *Swiss.*

A volatile oil obtained by distillation from nutmeg. It is a clear, colourless, pale yellow or pale green liquid with an odour of nutmeg. It is available as East Indian Nutmeg Oil and West Indian Nutmeg Oil.

East Indian oil is **soluble** 1 in 3 of alcohol (90%), West Indian 1 in 4. **Store** in well-filled containers at a temperature not exceeding 25°. Protect from light.

Nutmeg oil is aromatic and carminative and is used as a flavour. Nutmeg oil and expressed nutmeg oil, a solid fat, are rubefacient.

Preparations

BP 1998: Aromatic Ammonia Spirit *(Sal Volatile Spirit).*

Proprietary Preparations (details are given in Part 3)

Multi-ingredient: ***Aust.:*** Dr Fischers Melissengeist; Emser Nasensalbe; Expectal-Balsam; Pe-Ce; Wick Vaporub; ***Austral.:*** Vicks Vaporub; ***Belg.:*** Melisana†; Vegebom†; Vicks Vaporub; ***Canad.:*** Vaporizing Ointment; ***Fr.:*** Vegebom; Vicks Vaporub; ***Ger.:*** Emser Balsam echt†; Emser Nasensalbe N; Expectal Balsam†; ***S.Afr.:*** Enterodyne; ***Swed.:*** Vicks Vaporub; ***Switz.:*** Carmol "thermogene"†; Carmol†; Roliwol; Vicks Vaporub; ***UK:*** Dragon Balm.

Nux Vomica (538-h)

Brechnuss; Neuz Vómica; Noce Vomica; Noix Vomique; Strychni Semen.

CAS — 357-57-3 (anhydrous brucine).

Pharmacopoeias. In *Aust., Chin., Fr.,* and *Jpn.*
Chin. and *Fr.* also include Powdered Nux Vomica.
Chin. also allows *Strychnos pierriana.*

The dried ripe seeds of *Strychnos nux-vomica* (Loganiaceae).

Nux vomica has the actions of strychnine (see p.1633). Extracts of nux vomica have been used for a wide variety of disorders including those of digestion or debility.

As well as containing strychnine, nux vomica contains brucine which has similar properties.

Nux vomica (Nux vom.) is used in herbal and homoeopathic medicine. Ignatia, the dried seed of *Strychnos ignatii,* is also used in homoeopathic medicine where it is known as Ignatia amara or Iamara.

Preparations

Proprietary Preparations (details are given in Part 3)

Multi-ingredient: ***Belg.:*** Aperop; Digestobiase†; Sanicolax; ***Fr.:*** Creme Rap; Curoveinyl; Digestobiase†; Elixir Grez Chlorhydropepsique†; Quintonine; YSE; YSE Glutamique; ***Ital.:*** Amaro Maffioli†; Enteroton Digestivo†; Lassatina; Pillole Schias†; ***S.Afr.:*** Peter Pote's†; ***Spain:*** Alofedina; ***Switz.:*** Padma-Lax.

Oak Bark (317-l)

Écorce de Chêne; Eichenrinde; Quercus; Quercus Cortex.

Pharmacopoeias. In *Aust., Pol.,* and *Swiss.*

The dried bark from the smaller branches and young stems of the common oak, *Quercus robur* (=*Q. pedunculata*), or the durmast oak, *Q. petraea* (=*Q. sessiliflora*) (Fagaceae).

Oak bark contains quercitannic acid. It has astringent properties and is used in some herbal and homoeopathic preparations. It was formerly used for haemorrhoids and as a gargle.

Preparations

Proprietary Preparations (details are given in Part 3)
Ger.: Silvapin Eichenrinden-Extrakt†; Traxaton.

Multi-ingredient: ***Aust.:*** Menodoron; ***Fr.:*** Tisanes de l'Abbe Hamon no 14; ***Ger.:*** entero sanol†; Pektan N†; Tonsilgon-N; ***Switz.:*** Kernosan Elixir; ***UK:*** Conchae comp.; Menodoron; Peerless Composition Essence.

Octanoic Acid (2597-g)

Octanoic Acid *(USAN, rINN).*

Caprylic Acid.

$CH_3.(CH_2)_6.CO_2H = 144.2$.

CAS — 124-07-2.

Pharmacopoeias. In *Br.* and *Ger.*

A colourless oily liquid with a characteristic odour. Very slightly **soluble** in water; freely soluble in alcohol; very soluble in acetone and in ether; it dissolves in dilute alcohols.

Sodium Octanoate (3004-t)

Sodium Caprylate.

$C_8H_{15}NaO_2 = 166.2$.

CAS — 1984-06-1.

Pharmacopoeias. In *Ger.*

Octanoic acid and its salts have antifungal activity.

Sodium octanoate is used to stabilise albumin solution against the effects of heat.

Preparations

Proprietary Preparations (details are given in Part 3)
Canad.: Capricin.

Multi-ingredient: ***Austral.:*** Caprilate; ***Ital.:*** Undetin†.

Octaverine Hydrochloride (13037-r)

Octaverine Hydrochloride *(BANM, rINNM).*

6,7-Dimethoxy-1-(3,4,5-triethoxyphenyl)isoquinoline hydrochloride.

$C_{23}H_{27}NO_5,HCl = 433.9.$

CAS — 549-68-8 (octaverine); 6775-26-4 (octaverine hydrochloride).

Octaverine hydrochloride is an analogue of papaverine (p.1614) which has been used as an antispasmodic.

Olaflur (2496-n)

Olaflur *(BAN, USAN, rINN).*

GA-297; SKF-38095. 2,2′-(3-[N-(2-Hydroxyethyl)octadecylamino]propylimino)diethanol dihydrofluoride.

$C_{27}H_{60}F_2N_2O_3 = 498.8.$

CAS — 6818-37-7.

Olaflur has been used in the prevention of dental caries.

Preparations

Proprietary Preparations (details are given in Part 3)

Multi-ingredient: ***Aust.:*** Elmex; ***Ger.:*** Elmex; Multifluorid; ***Ital.:*** Elmex; ***Switz.:*** Elmex.

Olaquindox (16936-e)

Olaquindox *(BAN, rINN).*

Bay-Va-9391. 2-(2-Hydroxyethylcarbamoyl)-3-methylquinoxaline 1,4-dioxide.

$C_{12}H_{13}N_3O_4 = 263.2.$

CAS — 23696-28-8.

Olaquindox is an antibacterial added to animal feedstuffs as a growth promoter.

Oleander (16134-d)

Oleanderblätter; Oleandri Folium; Rose Bay.

The dried leaves of the shrub *Nerium oleander* (Apocynaceae), which contain cardioactive glycosides, including oleandrin, have been used in the treatment of heart disorders. The flowers and bark have been used similarly. Toxicity may occur following ingestion of any part of the plant; fatalities have been reported.

Oleander has also been used in homoeopathic medicine.

Preparations

Proprietary Preparations (details are given in Part 3)

Multi-ingredient: ***Ger.:*** Miroton; Venopyronum N triplex.

Olive Oil (7363-v)

Azeite; Olivae Oleum.

Pharmacopoeias. In *Eur.* (see p.viii) and *Jpn.* Also in *USNF. Fr.* also includes olive leaves.

The fatty oil expressed from the ripe fruits of *Olea europaea* (Oleaceae). It is a clear, yellow or greenish-yellow transparent liquid with a slight characteristic odour and taste and a faintly acrid after-taste. At low temperatures it may be solid or partly solid.

Practically **insoluble** in alcohol; miscible with carbon disulphide, chloroform, ether, and petroleum spirit. **Store** at a temperature not exceeding 25° in well-filled containers. Protect from light. Olive oil intended for use in the preparation of a parenteral dosage form should be kept in a glass container.

Internally, olive oil is nutrient, demulcent, and mildly laxative. It may also be given rectally (100 to 500 mL warmed to about 32°) to soften impacted faeces, which require manual disimpaction when laxative enemas fail (p.1168).

Externally, olive oil is emollient and soothing to inflamed surfaces, and is employed to soften the skin and crusts in eczema (p.1073) and psoriasis (p.1075), and as a lubricant for massage. It is used to soften ear wax.

Olive oil is used in the preparation of liniments, ointments, plasters, and soaps; it is also used as a vehicle for oily suspensions for injection.

Epidemiological evidence points to the cardiovascular benefits of olive oil in the diet.

Preparations

BP 1998: Olive Oil Ear Drops.

Proprietary Preparations (details are given in Part 3)

Multi-ingredient: ***Austral.:*** Boz†; Egozite Cradle Cap; Egozite Cream†; ***Fr.:*** Clinoleic; Parlax Compose†; ***Ger.:*** Baran-mild N; Befelka-Oel; Dr. Hotz Vollbad; Paradiol†; ***Ital.:*** Prexene; ***Spain:*** Aceite Acalorico; ***UK:*** Exzem Oil.

Ololiuqui (5018-a)

CAS — 2889-26-1 (isoergine); 478-94-4 (ergine); 2390-99-0 (chanoclavine); 548-43-6 (elymoclavine); 602-85-7 (lysergol).

The seeds of *Rivea corymbosa* or *Ipomoea tricolor* (=*I. violacea*) both convolvulaceous plants similar to the garden plant 'morning glory', *Ipomoea purpurea*. The brown seeds of *R. corymbosa* are known as 'badoh' and the black seeds of *I. tricolor* as 'badoh negro'.

Ololiuqui has hallucinogenic properties and is considered to be sacred by some Mexican Indians. Alkaloidal fractions contain at least 5 closely related individual components, viz. D-isolysergic acid amide (isoergine), D-lysergic acid amide (ergine), chanoclavine, elymoclavine, and lysergol.

The name 'ololiuqui' has been erroneously applied to seeds of *Datura meteloides* (Solanaceae).

Onion (13040-c)

The bulb of *Allium cepa* (Liliaceae).

Onion has been reported to reduce platelet aggregation, lower serum cholesterol, and to enhance fibrinolysis. It has been used in preparations for the treatment of urinary-tract disorders and topical preparations for scars and contractures.

Onion is used in homoeopathic medicine.

A review of controlled studies purporting to show beneficial effects of garlic and/or onion on cardiovascular risk factors found those studies to have severe methodological failings.[1]

1. Kleijnen J, *et al.* Garlic, onions and cardiovascular risk factors: a review of the evidence from human experiments with emphasis on commercially available preparations. *Br J Clin Pharmacol* 1989; **28:** 535–44.

Preparations

Proprietary Preparations (details are given in Part 3)

Multi-ingredient: ***Aust.:*** Contractubex; ***Austral.:*** Garlic Allium Complex; ***Belg.:*** Pelvo Magnesium; ***Fr.:*** Pelvo Magnesium†; ***Ger.:*** Carito†; Contractubex; ***Switz.:*** Contractubex.

Ononis (13041-k)

Arrête-Boeuf; Hauhechelwurzel; Racine de Bugrane; Radix Ononidis; Restharrow Root.

Pharmacopoeias. In *Aust.*

The dried roots of *Ononis spinosa* (Leguminosae), containing saponins.

Ononis has diuretic activity and has been used in herbal preparations for the treatment of oedema, urinary-tract disorders, rheumatic disorders, and constipation.

Preparations

Proprietary Preparations (details are given in Part 3)

Multi-ingredient: ***Aust.:*** Aktiv Blasen- und Nierentee; Bio-Garten Tee zur Erhohung der Harnmenge; Blasen-Tee; Harntreibender Tee; Kneipp Nieren- und Blasen-Tee; Krauter Hustensaft†; Krauterdoktor Harnstein- und Nieren-griesstropfen; Krauterhaus Mag Kottas Blasentee; Krauterhaus Mag Kottas Entschlackungstee; Krauterhaus Mag Kottas Nierentee; Krautertee Nr 18; Krautertee Nr 204; Krautertee Nr 25; Krautertee Nr 30; Mag Kottas Nieren-Blasentee; Nierentee; Sanvita-Entschlackungstonikum; Solisan; St Radegunder Entwasserungstee; St Radegunder Nierentee; Teekanne Blasen- und Nierentee; Uropurat; ***Fr.:*** Depuratum; Schoum; ***Ger.:*** Abfuhr-Tee Stada†; Alasenn; Aqualibra; Befelka-Tinktur; Blasen-Nieren-Tee Stada; Blasen-Nieren-Tee Urolux†; Buccotean†; Diureticum-Medice†; Dr. Klinger's Bergischer Krautertee, Abfuhr- und Verdauungstee†; Dr. Klinger's Bergischer Krautertee, Blasen- u. Nierentee†; Entwasserungs-Tee†; Eupond; Gallen-Leber-Tee Stada†; Harntee 400; Hevert-Blasen- und Nieren- Tee; Hevert-Entwasserungs-Tee; Hevert-Gicht-Rheuma-Tee comp; Heweberberol-Tee; Kneipp Blasen- und Nieren-Tee; Knufinke Blasen- und Nieren-Tee Uro-K†; Liruptin†; NB-tee Siegfried†; nephro-loges; Nephronorm Med; Nephroselect M; Nieren-Tee†; Nieron Blasen- und Nieren-Tee VI; Nieron-Tee N; Protitis†; Reducelle; Renob Blasen- und Nierentee; Rheumex†; Ullus Blasen-Nieren-Tee N; Urodil Blasen-Nieren Arzneitee; Urodil N†; Urodil S†; Uvirgan N; ***Ital.:*** Soluzione Schoum; ***Switz.:*** Demonatur Dragees pour les reins et la vessie; Dragees pour reins et vessie S; Nephrosolid N; Phytomed Nephro; Prosta-Caps Chassot N; Tisane pour les reins et la vessie "H"†.

Orange Oil (4680-k)

Arancia Dolce Essenza; Essence of Orange; Essence of Portugal; Essência de Laranja; Sweet Orange Oil.

NOTE. The oil from the flowers of *Citrus aurantium* var. *amara* is known as neroli oil or orange flower oil (p.1606).

Pharmacopoeias. In *Br., Fr., It.,* and *Jpn.*

A yellow to yellowish-brown volatile oil obtained by mechanical means from the fresh peel of the sweet orange *Citrus aurantium* var. *sinensis* (=*C. sinensis*) (Rutaceae), containing not less than 1% w/w of aldehydes calculated as decanal ($C_{10}H_{20}O$). It has the characteristic odour and taste of orange.

Soluble 1 in 7 of alcohol (90%) but rarely with the formation of bright solutions on account of the presence of waxy nonvolatile substances. **Store** at a temperature not exceeding 25° in well-filled containers. Protect from light.

Orange oil is used as a flavour and in perfumery. It is used in the preparation of terpeneless orange oil. Photosensitivity reactions have been reported.

Preparations

Proprietary Preparations (details are given in Part 3)

Multi-ingredient: ***Fr.:*** Balsamorhinol; ***Ger.:*** Contrheuma flussig†; Meteophyt-V†; Meteophyt†; ***Switz.:*** Globase†; Kemeol; Kemerhine; Pinimenthol; ***UK:*** Hill's Balsam Junior Expectorant.

Terpeneless Orange Oil (4681-a)

Oleum Aurantii Deterpenatum.

Pharmacopoeias. In *Br.*

A clear yellow or orange-yellow volatile oil with the characteristic odour and taste of orange, prepared by concentrating orange oil under reduced pressure until most of the terpenes have been removed, or by solvent partition. It consists chiefly of the free alcohols (+)-linalol and (+)-terpineol and contains not less than 18% w/w of aldehydes calculated as decanal, $C_{10}H_{20}O$.

Soluble 1 in 1 of alcohol (90%). **Store** at a temperature not exceeding 25° in well-filled containers. Protect from light.

Terpeneless orange oil is used as a flavour. It is stronger in flavour and more readily soluble than the natural oil. Photosensitivity is associated with citrus oils.

Preparations

BP 1998: Compound Orange Spirit.

Dried Bitter-Orange Peel (4682-t)

Aurantii Amari Cortex; Aurantii Cortex Siccatus; Corteza de Naranja Amarga; Écorce de Bigaradier; Flavedo Aurantii Amara; Pericarpium Aurantii; Pomeranzenschale.

Pharmacopoeias. In *Br., Fr., Ger., Jpn,* and *Swiss.*

The dried outer part of the pericarp of the ripe or nearly ripe fruit of the bitter orange, *Citrus aurantium* (Rutaceae), containing not less than 2.5% v/w volatile oil. It has an aromatic odour and an aromatic and bitter taste.

Dried bitter-orange peel is used as a flavour and for its bitter and carminative properties. Photosensitivity is associated with citrus oils.

Citrus aurantium was one of the most frequently used herbal remedies in Puerto Rico.[1] Indications included sleep disorders, gastro-intestinal disorders, respiratory ailments, and raised blood pressure.

1. Hernández L, *et al.* Use of medicinal plants by ambulatory patients in Puerto Rico. *Am J Hosp Pharm* 1984; **41:** 2060–4.

Preparations

BP 1998: Concentrated Compound Gentian Infusion; Concentrated Orange Peel Infusion; Orange Peel Infusion; Orange Syrup; Orange Tincture.

Proprietary Preparations (details are given in Part 3)
Ger.: Carvomin Magentropfen mit Pomeranze.

Multi-ingredient: ***Aust.:*** Bio-Garten Tee zur Starkung und Kraftigung; Bronchiplant; Bronchiplant light; China-Eisenwein; Digestol; Ferrovin-Eisenelixier; Krauterdoktor Entschlackungs-Elixier; Krauterhaus Mag Kottas Tee fur die Verdauung; Krauterhaus Mag Kottas Tee gegen Durchfall; Krautertee Nr 210; Krautertee Nr 217; Mariazeller; Montana; Sigman-Haustropfen; St Radegunder Entschlackungs-Elixier; St Radegunder Verdauungstee; ***Belg.:*** Aperop; ***Fr.:*** Antigoutteux Rezall; Elixir Bonjean; Elixir Grez; Elixir Grez Chlorhydropepsique†; Mediflor Tisane Calmante Troubles du Sommeil No 14; Merol; Quintonine; Santane V_3; ***Ger.:*** Carminativum-Hetterich N; Doppelherz Melissengeist; Dr. Maurers Magen-Apotheke†; Eupronerv†; Gastrosecur; Meteophyt S; Meteophyt†; Salus Kurbis-Tonikum Compositum†; Salusan; Sedovent; Stomachicon N; Valeriana comp; Worishofener Nervenpflege Dr. Kleinschrod†; ***Ital.:*** Depurativo; Rabarbaroni; Regular†; ***Spain:*** Agua del Carmen.

Orazamide (13042-a)

Orazamide *(rINN)*.

AICA Orotate; Oroxamide. 5-Aminoimidazole-4-carboxamide orotate dihydrate.

$C_9H_{10}N_6O_5,2H_2O = 318.2.$

CAS — 2574-78-9 (anhydrous orazamide); 60104-30-5 (orazamide dihydrate).

Orazamide has been given by mouth in the treatment of liver disorders. AICA riboside, a ribonucleoside analogue, has been investigated for its cardioprotective activity.

References.

1. Dixon R, *et al.* AICA-riboside: safety, tolerance, and pharmacokinetics of a novel adenosine-regulating agent. *J Clin Pharmacol* 1991; **31:** 342–7.

Preparations

Proprietary Preparations (details are given in Part 3)
Belg.: Aicamin; ***Ger.:*** Aicorat†.

Orlistat (10352-p)

Orlistat *(BAN, USAN, rINN)*.

Orlipastat; Ro-18-0647; Ro-18-0647/002; Tetrahydrolipstatin. *N*-Formyl-L-leucine, ester with (3*S*,4*S*)-3-hexyl-4-[(2*S*)-2-hydroxytridecyl]-2-oxetanone; (*S*)-1-[(2*S*,3*S*)-3-Hexyl-4-oxo-oxetan-2-ylmethyl]dodecyl *N*-formyl-L-leucinate.

$C_{29}H_{53}NO_5 = 495.7.$

CAS — 96829-58-2.

Adverse Effects

Gastro-intestinal disturbances, including faecal urgency and incontinence, flatulence, and fatty stools or discharge, are the most frequently reported adverse effects during treatment with orlistat. They may be minimised by limiting the amount of fat in the diet. There have been concerns about an increased risk of breast cancer in patients taking orlistat but the manufacturers consider that there is no evidence of a causal link.

Precautions

Orlistat should not be given to patients with chronic malabsorption syndrome or cholestasis. It should be given with caution to diabetic patients, and the manufacturer recommends that it should be avoided during pregnancy and breast feeding. Supplements of fat-soluble vitamins may be necessary during long-term therapy.

Interactions

Concomitant administration of orlistat and pravastatin may result in elevated pravastatin plasma concentrations with a consequent increase in adverse effects. Orlistat may reduce the absorption of fat-soluble vitamins. The manufacturer recommends that concomitant administration with acarbose, biguanide antidiabetics, fibric acid derivatives, or anorectic drugs should be avoided. In patients receiving warfarin, international normalised ratio should be monitored during treatment with orlistat.

Pharmacokinetics

Orlistat is not absorbed following oral administration.

Uses and Administration

Orlistat is a gastric and pancreatic lipase inhibitor that limits the absorption of dietary fat. It is used in conjunction with dietary modification, in the management of obesity, in a usual dose of 120 mg by mouth three times daily, immediately before, during, or up to 1 hour after meals.

References.

1. McNeely W, Benfield P. Orlistat. *Drugs* 1998; **56:** 241–9.
2. Sjöström L, *et al.* Randomised placebo-controlled trial of orlistat for weight loss and prevention of weight regain in obese patients. *Lancet* 1998; **352:** 167–72.

Preparations

Proprietary Preparations (details are given in Part 3)
UK: Xenical.

Ornicarbase (13044-x)

Ornithine Carbamoyltransferase.

CAS — 9001-69-8.

Ornicarbase has been used in hepatic disorders. Hypersensitivity reactions have occurred occasionally.

Preparations

Proprietary Preparations (details are given in Part 3)
Ital.: Enzimepar†; Ociter†.

Orotic Acid (13045-r)

Orotic Acid *(BAN, pINN)*.

Animal Galactose Factor; Uracil-6-carboxylic Acid; Whey Factor. 1,2,3,6-Tetrahydro-2,6-dioxopyrimidine-4-carboxylic acid.

$C_5H_4N_2O_4 = 156.1.$

CAS — 65-86-1 (anhydrous orotic acid); 50887-69-9 (orotic acid monohydrate).

Orotic acid occurs naturally in the body; it is found in milk. It is an intermediate in the biosynthesis of pyrimidine nucleotides. Orotic acid and its calcium, carnitine, choline, lithium, lysine, magnesium, and potassium salts have been used in liver disorders. Some of these salts, chromium orotate, cyproheptadine orotate, and deanol orotate, have been given as tonics or dietary supplements. Magnesium and ferrous orotates have been used as mineral sources.

Preparations

Proprietary Preparations (details are given in Part 3)
Belg.: Dioron†; ***Ger.:*** Lactinium†; Magnerot Classic.

Multi-ingredient: ***Aust.:*** Kavaform; Lemazol; Prospervital; ***Austral.:*** Magnesium Plus; ***Ger.:*** Antisklerosin S; Divinal-Bohnen†; emagnesit†; Enterotropin†; Hepabionta comp†; Hepabionta†; Heparaxal†; Hepaticum "Mletzko"†; Hepaticum-Divinal†; Hepatofalk; Hepatofalk Neu; Hepavis†; Lemazol†; Orotofalk†; Oxygenabund†; Pantona†; Sklerocedin N†; Xanpervit†; ***Ital.:*** Epa-Treis; Itahepar†; Oro B12; Oromag B12†; Oroticon Lisina†; ***S.Afr.:*** Hepabionta; ***Spain:*** Antibiofilus; Hepadif; Hepato Fardi; Histiotone†; Tres Orix Forte; ***Switz.:*** Ginkovit†; Kawaform; Magnesium Complexe; Vigoran; ***UK:*** Cardeymin; Sugar Bloc.

Orthodichlorobenzene (3598-z)

1,2-Dichlorobenzene.

$C_6H_4Cl_2 = 147.0.$

CAS — 95-50-1.

Orthodichlorobenzene has been used as a wood and furniture preservative. It has also been used as an ingredient of solutions for dissolving ear wax. It is an irritant volatile liquid; lens opacities have occurred.

Preparations

Proprietary Preparations (details are given in Part 3)
Multi-ingredient: ***Switz.:*** Cerumenol.

Oryzanol (13046-f)

Gamma Oryzanol; γ-Oryzanol; γ-OZ. Triacontanyl 3-(4-hydroxy-3-methoxyphenyl)prop-2-enoate.

$C_{40}H_{58}O_4 = 602.9.$

CAS — 11042-64-1.

A substance extracted from rice bran oil and rice embryo bud oil.

Oryzanol has been given by mouth in the treatment of hyperlipidaemias (p.1265). It has also been used for its supposed effects on autonomic and endocrine function.

References.

1. Yoshino G, *et al.* Effects of gamma-oryzanol on hyperlipidemic subjects. *Curr Ther Res* 1989; **45:** 543–52.
2. Yoshino G, *et al.* Effects of gamma-oryzanol and probucol on hyperlipidemia. *Curr Ther Res* 1989; **45:** 975–82.

Preparations

Proprietary Preparations (details are given in Part 3)
Jpn: Hi-Z.

Multi-ingredient: ***Ital.:*** Lenirose; Mavipiu.

Osalmid (3729-w)

Osalmid *(rINN)*.

L-1718; Oxaphenamide. 4′-Hydroxysalicylanilide.

$C_{13}H_{11}NO_3 = 229.2.$

CAS — 526-18-1.

Osalmid is a choleretic.

Preparations

Proprietary Preparations (details are given in Part 3)
Belg.: Driol.

Otilonium Bromide (13048-n)

Otilonium Bromide *(BAN, rINN)*.

SP-63. Diethylmethyl{2-[4-(2-octyloxybenzamido)benzoyloxy]ethyl}ammonium bromide.

$C_{29}H_{43}BrN_2O_4 = 563.6.$

CAS — 26095-59-0.

Otilonium bromide is used in the symptomatic treatment of gastro-intestinal disorders associated with smooth muscle spasms.

Preparations

Proprietary Preparations (details are given in Part 3)
Belg.: Spasmomen; ***Ital.:*** Spasen; Spasmomen; ***Spain:*** Spasmoctyl.

Multi-ingredient: ***Ital.:*** Spasen; Spasen Somatico; Spasmomen Somatico.

Oxaceprol (13051-t)

Oxaceprol *(rINN)*.

Acetylhydroxyproline; C061. (−)-1-Acetyl-4-hydroxy-L-proline.

$C_7H_{11}NO_4 = 173.2.$

CAS — 33996-33-7.

Oxaceprol is reported to affect connective-tissue metabolism and has been used in dermatology, to promote wound healing, and in rheumatic disorders. Adverse effects have included gastric pain, nausea, diarrhoea, dizziness, headache, and skin rashes.

Preparations

Proprietary Preparations (details are given in Part 3)
Fr.: Jonctum; ***Ger.:*** AHP 200; ***Spain:*** Tejuntivo.

Multi-ingredient: ***Spain:*** Robervital.

Oxalic Acid (1320-z)

$HO_2C.CO_2H,2H_2O = 126.1.$

CAS — 144-62-7 (anhydrous oxalic acid); 6153-56-6 (oxalic acid dihydrate).

Adverse Effects

In dilute solution oxalic acid and its salts are toxic owing to withdrawal of ionisable calcium from the blood and tissues. Strong solutions of the acid are corrosive and produce adverse effects similar to those of hydrochloric acid (p.1588). There may be muscular tremors and convulsions. Death may occur within a few minutes. After apparent recovery acute renal failure may occur from blocking of the renal tubules by calcium oxalate crystals.

References to fatalities resulting from ingestion of oxalic acid[1] or intravenous administration of sodium oxalate.[2]

1. Farré M, *et al.* Fatal oxalic acid poisoning from sorrel soup. *Lancet* 1989 **ii:** 1524.
2. Dvořáčková I. Tödliche Vergiftung nach intravenöser Verabreichung von Natriumoxalat. *Arch Toxikol* 1966; **22:** 63–7.

Treatment of Adverse Effects

Following ingestion of oxalic acid, a dilute solution of any soluble calcium salt should be given to precipitate the oxalate. If mucosal corrosion has not occurred the stomach should be carefully emptied by lavage using large quantities of diluted lime water or dilute solutions of other calcium salts. Calcium gluconate 10% should be given intravenously in doses of 10 to 20 mL to prevent tetany. If renal function is not impaired, 4 to 5 litres of fluid should be given daily to prevent crystalluria.

Uses

Oxalic acid has varied industrial uses and has been used in escharotic preparations. Oxalic acid salts have been administered by mouth and the urinary excretion of oxalate used as a screening test for lipid malabsorption.

References.

1. Rampton DS, *et al.* Screening for steatorrhoea with an oxalate loading test. *Br Med J* 1984; **288:** 1419. Correction. *ibid.*; 1728.
2. Sangaletti O, *et al.* Urinary oxalate recovery after oral oxalic acid load: an alternative method to the quantitative determination of stool fat for the diagnosis of lipid malabsorption. *J Int Med Res* 1989; **17:** 526–31.

Preparations

Proprietary Preparations (details are given in Part 3)
Multi-ingredient: ***Ger.:*** Solco-Derman; ***Switz.:*** Solcoderm; Solcogyn.

Oxiracetam (16922-v)

Oxiracetam *(BAN, rINN)*.

CGP-21690E; ISF-2522. 4-Hydroxy-2-oxo-1-pyrrolidineacetamide.

$C_6H_{10}N_2O_3 = 158.2.$

CAS — 62613-82-5.

Oxiracetam has been used as a nootropic in organic brain syndromes and senile dementia.

Clinical benefit has been reported in patients with dementia (p.1386) given oxiracetam,[1] but in the USA it has been withdrawn from phase II clinical studies in patients with Alzheimer's disease due to lack of efficacy.[2]

1. Maina G, *et al.* Oxiracetam in the treatment of primary degenerative and multi-infarct dementia: a double-blind, placebo-controlled study. *Neuropsychobiology* 1990; **21:** 141–5.
2. Parnetti L. Clinical pharmacokinetics of drugs for Alzheimer's disease. *Clin Pharmacokinet* 1995; **29:** 110–29.

Preparations

Proprietary Preparations (details are given in Part 3)
Ital.: Neupant†; Neuractiv; Neuromet.

Oxybromonaftoic Acid (13069-g)

4-Bromo-3-hydroxy-2-naphthoic acid.
$C_{11}H_7BrO_3$ = 267.1.
CAS — 2208-15-3.

Oxybromonaftoic acid has been used by mouth in hepatic disorders.

Preparations

Proprietary Preparations (details are given in Part 3)
Ital.: Naftocol†.

Ozagrel (19602-y)

Ozagrel *(rINN).*
OKY-046 (hydrochloride). *(E)-p-*(imidazol-1-ylmethyl)cinnamic acid.
$C_{13}H_{12}N_2O_2$ = 228.2.
CAS — 82571-53-7.

Ozagrel is a thromboxane synthetase inhibitor which has been used as the hydrochloride in the treatment of asthma and as the sodium salt in cerebrovascular disorders.

References.

1. Nagatsuka K, *et al. Stroke* 1985; **16:** 806–9.
2. Fujimura M, *et al.* Effects of aerosol administration of a thromboxane synthetase inhibitor (OKY-046) on bronchial responsiveness to acetylcholine in asthmatic subjects. *Chest* 1990; **98:** 276–9.
3. Fujimura M, *et al.* Attenuating effect of a thromboxane synthetase inhibitor (OKY-046) on bronchial responsiveness to methacholine is specific to bronchial asthma. *Chest* 1990; **98:** 656–60.

Preparations

Proprietary Preparations (details are given in Part 3)
Jpn: Cataclot; Domenan; Vega; Xanbon.

Palmidrol (14843-y)

Palmidrol *(rINN).*
N-(2-Hydroxyethyl)palmitamide.
$C_{18}H_{37}NO_2$ = 299.5.
CAS — 544-31-0.

Palmidrol is a naturally occurring lipid compound which has been used as an immunostimulant. It is given by mouth for the treatment of respiratory tract infections.

Pancreatin (3731-b)

Pancreatin *(BAN).*
Pancreatinum.
CAS — 8049-47-6.
Pharmacopoeias. In *Chin., Eur.* (see p.viii), *Jpn,* and *US* as pancreatin or another pancreatic extract or both.

A preparation of mammalian pancreas containing enzymes having protease, lipase, and amylase activity. Its greatest activity is in neutral or slightly alkaline media; more than a trace of mineral acid, or large amounts of alkali hydroxide, render it inert.

The BP describes pancreatin as a white or buff-coloured amorphous powder free from unpleasant odour. Each g of pancreatin contains not less than 1400 units of free protease activity, not less than 20 000 units of lipase activity, and not less than 24 000 units of amylase activity. It may contain sodium chloride. **Soluble** or partly soluble in water forming a slightly turbid solution; practically insoluble in alcohol and ether. **Store** at a temperature not exceeding 15°.

The Ph. Eur. describes Pancreas Powder (Pancreatic Extract (BP), Pancreatis Pulvis), a slightly brown, amorphous powder, prepared from fresh or frozen mammalian pancreases. Each g of Pancreatic Extract contains not less than 1000 Ph. Eur. units of total proteolytic activity, not less than 15 000 Ph. Eur. units of lipolytic activity, and not less than 12 000 Ph. Eur. units of amylolytic activity. Partly **soluble** in water; practically insoluble in alcohol and in ether. It should be stored in airtight containers at a temperature not exceeding 15°.

The USP includes Pancreatin, a cream-coloured amorphous powder with a faint characteristic not offensive odour, prepared from the pancreas of the hog or the ox. Each g contains not less than 25 000 USP units of protease activity, not less than 2000 USP units of lipase activity, and not less than 25 000 USP units of amylase activity. It may be labelled as a whole-number multiple of the 3 minimum activities, or may be diluted with lactose, sucrose containing up to 3.25% of starch, or pancreatin of lower digestive power. Store at a temperature not exceeding 30° in airtight containers.

Units

The Ph. Eur. and USP units of protease activity depend upon the rate of hydrolysis of casein, those of lipase activity depend upon the rate of hydrolysis of olive oil, and those of amylase activity depend upon the rate of hydrolysis of starch. Because of differences in the assay conditions, the Ph. Eur. and USP units are not readily comparable.

FIP units of protease, lipase, and amylase activity are equivalent to Ph. Eur. units.

Adverse Effects and Precautions

Pancreatin may cause buccal and perianal soreness, particularly in infants. Colonic strictures (fibrosing colonopathy) have occurred, mainly in children with cystic fibrosis receiving high doses of pancreatin preparations; the use of high doses in patients with cystic fibrosis should preferably be avoided (see below). Hypersensitivity reactions have been reported; these may be sneezing, lachrymation, or skin rashes. Hyperuricaemia or hyperuricosuria have occurred with high doses. There have been occasional reports of the contamination of pancreatin preparations with *Salmonella* spp.

Effects on folic acid. Pancreatic extract significantly inhibited folate absorption in healthy subjects and in pancreatic insufficient patients.[1] Testing *in vitro* showed that pancreatic extract formed insoluble complexes with folate. Patients being treated for pancreatic insufficiency should be monitored for folate status or given folic acid supplementation, particularly if pancreatic enzymes and bicarbonate (or cimetidine) were being used together in the treatment regimen.

1. Russell RM, *et al.* Impairment of folic acid absorption by oral pancreatic extracts. *Dig Dis Sci* 1980; **25:** 369–73.

Effects on the gastro-intestinal tract. Following the introduction of high-strength pancreatic enzyme preparations, there have been a number of reports[1-6] of colonic strictures in children with cystic fibrosis who received these formulations, and the problem has been reviewed by Taylor.[7,8] The pathogenesis and aetiology of this condition remain unclear. Dose-related thickening of the colon wall has been described,[9] and an inflammatory or immune-mediated mechanism has been suggested.[10,11] It has been suggested that the presence of intact enteric-coated granules in the colon[12] and possibly a direct effect of components of the methylacrylic acid copolymer used in the enteric coating could be responsible[12,13] but at least one case of fibrosing colonopathy has been reported in a child receiving a standard strength preparation which did not contain this coating material.[14] An analysis[15] of cases of fibrosing colonopathy occurring in the UK between 1984 and 1994 demonstrated that there was a dose-related association between the high-strength preparations and this adverse effect, and the results were confirmed by a case-control study of patients in the US presenting between 1990 and 1994.[16] As a result of these problems, high-strength preparations have been withdrawn in the USA, while in the UK, the Committee on Safety of Medicines has recommended[17] that unless special reasons exist, patients with cystic fibrosis should not use high-strength pancreatin preparations, and that all patients treated with these products should be monitored carefully for gastro-intestinal obstruction. The Committee subsequently elaborated on these recommendations:[18] they advised that Nutrizym 22, Pancrease HL, and Panzytrat 25 000 should not be used in children with cystic fibrosis who were aged 15 years or less; that the total daily dose of pancreatic enzyme supplements for patients with cystic fibrosis should not exceed 10 000 units of lipase activity per kg body-weight; and that patients on any pancreatin preparation should be reviewed to exclude colonic damage if new abdominal symptoms or a change in symptoms occurred. The US Cystic Fibrosis Foundation has made recommendations for the management of patients who do not respond adequately to moderate doses of pancreatic enzymes,[19] and similar recommendations have been made in the UK.[20]

1. Smyth RL, *et al.* Strictures of ascending colon in cystic fibrosis and high-strength pancreatic enzymes. *Lancet* 1994; **343:** 85–6.
2. Oades PJ, *et al.* High-strength pancreatic enzyme supplements and large-bowel stricture in cystic fibrosis. *Lancet* 1994; **343:** 109.
3. Campbell CA, *et al.* High-strength pancreatic enzyme supplements and large-bowel stricture in cystic fibrosis. *Lancet* 1994; **343:** 109–110.
4. Mahony MJ, Corcoran M. High-strength pancreatic enzymes. *Lancet* 1994; **343:** 599–600.
5. Knabe N, *et al.* Extensive pathological changes of the colon in cystic fibrosis and high-strength pancreatic enzymes. *Lancet* 1994; **343:** 1230.
6. Pettei MJ, *et al.* Pancolonic disease in cystic fibrosis and high-dose pancreatic enzyme therapy. *J Pediatr* 1994; **125:** 587–9.
7. Taylor CJ. Colonic strictures in cystic fibrosis. *Lancet* 1994; **343:** 615–16. Correction. *ibid.*; 1108.
8. Taylor CJ. The problems with high dose pancreatic enzyme preparations. *Drug Safety* 1994; **11:** 75–9.
9. MacSweeney EJ, *et al.* Relationship of thickening of colon wall to pancreatic-enzyme treatment in cystic fibrosis. *Lancet* 1995; **345:** 752–6.
10. Croft NM, *et al.* Gut inflammation in children with cystic fibrosis on high-dose enzyme supplements. *Lancet* 1995; **346:** 1265–7.
11. Lee J, *et al.* Is fibrosing colonopathy an immune mediated disease? *Arch Dis Child* 1997; **77:** 66–70.
12. Jones R, *et al.* Colonic strictures in children with cystic fibrosis on low-strength pancreatic enzymes. *Lancet* 1995; **346:** 499.
13. van Velzen D. Colonic strictures in children with cystic fibrosis on low-strength pancreatic enzymes. *Lancet* 1995; **346:** 499–500.
14. Taylor CJ, Steiner GM. Fibrosing colonopathy in a child on low-dose pancreatin. *Lancet* 1995; **345:** 1106–7
15. Smyth RL, *et al.* Fibrosing colonopathy in cystic fibrosis: results of a case-control study. *Lancet* 1995; **346:** 1247–51.
16. FitzSimmons SC, *et al.* High-dose pancreatic-enzyme supplements and fibrosing colonopathy in children with cystic fibrosis. *N Engl J Med* 1997; **336:** 1283–9.
17. Committee on Safety of Medicines/Medicines Control Agency. Update: bowel strictures and high-potency pancreatins. *Current Problems* 1994; **20:** 13.
18. Committee on Safety of Medicines/Medicines Control Agency. Fibrosing colonopathy associated with pancreatic enzymes. *Current Problems* 1995; **21:** 11.
19. Borowitz DS, *et al.* Use of pancreatic enzyme supplements for patients with cystic fibrosis in the context of fibrosing colonopathy. *J Pediatr* 1995; **127:** 681–4.
20. Littlewood JM. Fibrosing colonopathy in cystic fibrosis: commentary, implications of the Committee on Safety of Medicines 10 000 IU lipase/kg/day recommendation for use of pancreatic enzymes in cystic fibrosis. *Arch Dis Child* 1996; **74:** 466–8.

MOUTH ULCERATION. In 3 children taking preparations of pancreatic extracts (Pancrex V powder, Pancrex V Forte), severe mouth ulceration and angular stomatitis, causing dysphagia, loss of weight, and pyrexia, were attributed to digestion of the mucous membrane due to retention of the preparations in the mouth before swallowing.[1]

1. Darby CW. Pancreatic extracts. *Br Med J* 1970; **2:** 299–300.

Uses and Administration

Pancreatin hydrolyses fats to glycerol and fatty acids, breaks down protein into peptides, proteoses and derived substances, and converts starch into dextrins and sugars. It is given by mouth in conditions of pancreatic exocrine deficiency such as pancreatitis and cystic fibrosis. It is available in the form of powder, capsules containing powder or enteric-coated granules (which may be opened before use and the contents sprinkled on the food), enteric-coated tablets, or granules. If pancreatin is mixed with liquids or food the resulting mixture should not be allowed to stand for more than 1 hour prior to use. Antacids and histamine H_2-receptor antagonists, such as cimetidine, have been given in conjunction with pancreatin in an attempt to lessen destruction of pancreatin by the gastric acids.

The dose of pancreatin is adjusted according to the needs of the individual patient and will also depend on the dosage form. In the UK doses of up to about 3300 units of protease activity, 60 000 units of amylase activity, and 56 000 units of lipase activity have been given with each meal. So-called high-strength or high-potency preparations are available for those receiving high doses, but their use has been associated with the development of fibrosing colonopathy in children with cystic fibrosis (see above). Such preparations are consequently not recommended for children in the UK and the total daily dose of pancreatic supplements for patients with cystic fibrosis should not exceed 10 000 units of lipase activity per kg body-weight. In the USA doses providing up to 45 000 USP units of lipase activity have been given with each meal.

Pancreatin is also used to remove protein deposits from the surface of soft contact lenses (p.1097).

Administration. Available preparations of pancreatin have varied widely in their activity. This may be due both to variation in their enzyme content and an apparent reduction in clinical activity due to enteric coating.[1,2] It has been suggested that the theoretical basis for enteric-coating pancreatin may be in error,[3] although Gow and colleagues found an enteric-coated preparation to have advantages over conventional therapy.[4] Such preparations were introduced in order to try to overcome the substantial loss of activity that may occur when uncoated pancreatic enzymes are given, because of the denaturing effect of stomach acid.[5,6] It has been suggested following an *in vitro* study that pancreatin powder may be particularly affected by stomach pH,[7] although the relevance of this to *in vivo* conditions has been criticised.[8,9] Administration of antacids or histamine H_2 antagonists before pancreatin has also been tried, in an attempt to reduce gastric pH;[2,4,6,10-12]omeprazole has also been used as an adjunct to pancreatin therapy.[13]

Recently it was suggested that, in the UK at least, recommended doses of some enteric-coated pancreatic enzyme preparations might be too low for some patients with cystic fibrosis.[14,15] Since then higher strength preparations have become available; however, although initially welcomed,[16] concern has since arisen about an association between their use and colonic stricture formation (see Effects on the Gastro-intestinal Tract, above).

1. Graham DY. Enzyme replacement therapy of exocrine pancreatic insufficiency in man: relation between in vitro enzyme activities and in vivo potency in commercial pancreatic extracts. *N Engl J Med* 1977; **296:** 1314–17.
2. Marotta F, *et al.* Pancreatic enzyme replacement therapy: importance of gastric acid secretion, H_2-antagonists, and enteric coating. *Dig Dis Sci* 1989; **34:** 456–61.
3. Meyer JH. The ins and outs of oral pancreatic enzymes. *N Engl J Med* 1977; **296:** 1347–8.

4. Gow R, *et al.* Comparative study of varying regimens to improve steatorrhoea and creatorrhoea in cystic fibrosis: effectiveness of an enteric-coated preparation with and without antacids and cimetidine. *Lancet* 1981; **ii:** 1071–4.
5. DiMagno EP, *et al.* Fate of orally ingested enzymes in pancreatic insufficiency: comparison of two dosage schedules. *N Engl J Med* 1977; **296:** 1318–22.
6. Maguire S, Goodchild MC. Enzyme contents of pancreatic extract preparations: are they optimal? *Drugs* 1992; **44:** 685–9.
7. Graham DT, *et al.* Stability of oral pancreatin powders. *Med J Aust* 1979; **1:** 45–6.
8. Barnes GL, Phelan PD. Stability of oral pancreatic powders. *Med J Aust* 1979; **1:** 282.
9. Allen B, Giles G. Stability of oral pancreatic powders. *Med J Aust* 1979; **1:** 282–3.
10. Saunders JHB, *et al.* Inhibition of gastric secretion in treatment of pancreatic insufficiency. *Br Med J* 1977; **1:** 418–19.
11. Regan PT, *et al.* Comparative effects of antacids, cimetidine and enteric coating on the therapeutic response to oral enzymes in severe pancreatic insufficiency. *N Engl J Med* 1977; **297:** 854–8.
12. Chalmers DM, *et al.* Influence of long term cimetidine as an adjuvant to pancreatic enzyme therapy in cystic fibrosis. *Gut* 1983; **24:** A978.
13. Heijerman HG, *et al.* Omeprazole enhances the efficacy of pancreatin (Pancrease) in cystic fibrosis. *Ann Intern Med* 1991; **114:** 200–201.
14. Owen G, *et al.* Pancreatic enzyme supplement dosage in cystic fibrosis. *Lancet* 1991; **338:** 1153.
15. Morrison G, *et al.* Pancreatic enzyme supplements in cystic fibrosis. *Lancet* 1991; **338:** 1596.
16. Anonymous. High-potency preparations of pancreatin. *Drug Ther Bull* 1993; **31:** 63–4.

Cystic fibrosis. Patients with cystic fibrosis (p.119) suffer from pancreatic insufficiency and consequent malabsorption. Pancreatin or pancrelipase may therefore play a role in the management of the disorder, being taken before or with each meal or snack.

Pancreatitis. Pancreatitis is an inflammatory process affecting the pancreas. Acute pancreatitis comprises necrosis of pancreatic tissue occurring in an otherwise healthy gland, whereas chronic pancreatitis is the manifestation of pathological processes resulting in inflammation and progressive fibrosis of pancreatic tissue. Acute disease may be superimposed on a background of chronic pancreatitis.

Acute pancreatitis is frequently associated with either biliary tract disorders (such as gallstones or cholecystitis) or the intake of large amounts of alcohol, or less frequently with abdominal surgery, pancreatic trauma, hyperparathyroidism, hyperlipidaemia, infection, or the adverse effects of drugs. Symptoms include pain, which ranges from mild to extremely severe and which typically persists for several days, nausea and vomiting, ileus, and hypovolaemic shock. In severe disease there may ensue pulmonary, renal, and hepatic failure, encephalopathy, and death. A mortality rate of about 10% has been reported.

The management of acute disease is essentially supportive. Adequate analgesia for pain is important (see Pancreatic Pain, p.10), and in mild cases analgesia, adequate hydration, and temporary interruption of oral intake of food to 'rest' the pancreas may be adequate. Since most patients suffer from hypoxaemia it has been recommended that they should receive additional humidified oxygen by mask, with mechanical ventilation if blood gases indicate the development of severe pulmonary failure. Shock should be managed with blood or plasma, and electrolyte solutions, while insulin may be required for disturbances of glucose homoeostasis.

The value of other interventions is mostly doubtful. As an extension of the concept of 'pancreatic rest' inhibitors of pancreatic secretion such as somatostatin or octreotide have been tried but without significant effect, while protease inhibitors such as aprotinin or gabexate mesylate have also proven disappointing,[1] perhaps because activation of pancreatic proteases (thought to play a significant role in pathogenesis) has already taken place by the time therapy is begun.[1] Preliminary studies of the platelet-activating factor antagonist lexipafant have been more promising. Although prophylactic antibiotics are often given, there has been some uncertainty about their value.[2] However, a study in patients with acute necrotising pancreatitis indicated markedly reduced mortality in those given prophylactic antibiotics (initially cefuroxime),[3] and a retrospective study[4] reported a reduction in the incidence of infection in those receiving prophylactic antibiotics but not in the time of onset. Peritoneal dialysis reduces early complications of acute pancreatitis but increases the risk of subsequent infection and has no overall effect on survival.[2] The role of surgery has been and continues to be somewhat controversial; it is accepted for complications or where a potential surgical emergency exists, and surgery to remove gallstones may be carried out once pancreatitis has resolved, but surgical intervention during acute episodes may increase morbidity and mortality. Early endoscopic decompression of the obstructed bile duct may be beneficial in patients with cholangitis or progressive jaundice but not in those without biliary obstruction.[5]

Chronic pancreatitis is frequently associated with high alcohol-intake although a tropical form, associated with malnutrition, also exists, and some cases are idiopathic. Symptoms include, most prominently, recurrent episodes of pain (often less excruciating and of shorter duration than in acute pancreatitis) which normally become less severe and frequent over the years with the inexorable progression of fibrosis. Loss of exocrine tissue eventually leads in many patients to pancreatic exocrine insufficiency, with maldigestion and steatorrhoea, and in some to diabetes mellitus due to islet cell loss. Other symptoms may include cholestatic jaundice, fatty degeneration of the liver, stenosis of the bile duct, and hepatic cirrhosis (although this may also be due to alcohol intake). The prognosis is poor. It has been estimated that more than 50% of patients die within 20 years of diagnosis, with those who continue to drink alcohol being at greatest risk.

Adequate analgesia with opioids is essential (see Pancreatic Pain, p.10). Nerve blocks of the coeliac plexus with phenol or alcohol may be helpful, and there is one report of a response to danazol.[6] Patients should be advised to abstain from alcohol which can exacerbate the frequency and severity of painful episodes. Steatorrhoea requires replacement of pancreatic enzymes with preparations of pancreatin or pancrelipase. Because the enzymes are inactivated by gastric acid they may be taken after histamine H_2 antagonists or with a sodium-containing antacid such as sodium bicarbonate (magnesium-, calcium-, and, according to some authorities, aluminium-containing antacids may further interfere with fat absorption). Alternatively, enteric-coated enzyme preparations may be used. In some patients with mild disease pancreatic enzyme replacement may also improve pain. Supplements of fat-soluble vitamins are not normally necessary, but may be given intravenously if required. Diabetes should be managed appropriately once steatorrhoea is under control.

Surgery, up to and including total pancreatectomy, has an important role in the relief of intractable pain, and may also be necessary for the management of complications. Endoscopic decompression using contrast media containing prednisolone and ulinastatin has been reported to produce beneficial responses.[7] Anecdotal results suggest that some patients with pancreatic pseudocysts, which usually require surgical drainage, may respond to octreotide.[8]

1. Steinberg W, Tenner S. Acute pancreatitis. *N Engl J Med* 1994; **330:** 1198–1210.
2. Fernández-del Castillo C, *et al.* Acute pancreatitis. *Lancet* 1993; **342:** 475–9.
3. Sainio V, *et al.* Early antibiotic treatment in acute necrotising pancreatitis. *Lancet* 1995; **346:** 663–7.
4. Ho HS, Frey CF. The role of antibiotic prophylaxis in severe acute pancreatitis. *Arch Surg* 1997; **132:** 487–93.
5. Baillie J. Treatment of acute biliary pancreatitis. *N Engl J Med* 1997; **336:** 286–7.
6. Hardo PG, Axon ATR. Danazol improves chronic pancreatic pain. *J R Soc Med* 1993; **86:** 359.
7. Ohwada M, *et al.* New endoscopic treatment for chronic pancreatitis, using contrast media containing ulinastatin and prednisolone. *J Gastroenterol* 1997; **32:** 216–21.
8. Gullo L, Barbara L. Treatment of pancreatic pseudocysts with octreotide. *Lancet* 1991; **338:** 540–1.

Preparations

BP 1998: Pancreatin Granules; Pancreatin Tablets;
USP 23: Pancreatin Capsules; Pancreatin Tablets.

Proprietary Preparations (details are given in Part 3)
Aust.: Kreon; Opti-Free; Pancrin; Pankreon forte; Panzynorm; Polyzym; ***Austral.:*** Bioglan Panazyme†; Opti-Free Enzymatic; Opti-Plus; Pancrex V†; Polyzym; Viokase; ***Belg.:*** Creon; ***Canad.:*** Creon; Opti-Zyme; ***Fr.:*** Creon; Opti-Plus; Pancreal Kirchner; Polyzym; ***Ger.:*** Bilipeptal Mono; Carzodelan; Cholspasminase N; Cotazym; Digest Merz forte†; Enzymed N†; Euflat-E; Festal N†; Hevertozym; Kreon; Meteophyt forte; Mezym F; Nutrizym N; Ozym; Pancholtruw N; Pangrol; Pankreatan; Pankreon; Pankreon forte; Panpeptal N; Panpur; Panzynorm forte-N; Panzytrat; Tryptoferm; ***Irl.:*** Creon; Nutrizym; Pancrease; Pancrex; Panzytrat; ***Ital.:*** Atezym†; Creon; Enzipan; Festal N; Pancreon; Pancrex; Pancrotanon; ***Neth.:*** Creon; Pancrease HL; Panzytrat; ***Norw.:*** Pankreon; ***S.Afr.:*** Creon; Viokase; ***Spain:*** Kreon; Pankreon; ***Swed.:*** Pankreon; ***Switz.:*** Creon; Pankrotanon†; Panzytrat; ***UK:*** Clen-Zym; Creon; Nutrizym; Pancrease HL; Pancrex; Panzytrat†; ***USA:*** Creon; Donnazyme; Enzymatic Cleaner; Opti-Zyme; Viokase; Vision Care Enzymatic Cleaner.

Multi-ingredient: ***Aust.:*** Arca-Enzym; Aristochol; Combizym; Combizym Compositum; Digestif Rennie; Enzyflat; Euflat; Gallo Merz; Helopanflat; Helopanzym; Intestinol; Nutrizym†; Ora-Gallin; Ozym; Pankreoflat; Pankreon compositum; Paspertase; Recessan; Wobenzym; ***Austral.:*** Combizym Co†; Combizym†; Digesteze†; Digestaid; Enzyme; Lexat; Prozyme; Vitaplex Digestive Enzyme Formula†; ***Belg.:*** Combizym; Digestobiase†; Digestomen; Pankreon compositum†; Trizymal†; ***Canad.:*** Alsilax; Entozyme†; Vesilax; ***Fr.:*** Digestobiase†; Hepatoum; Pancrelase; Tridigestine Hepatoum†; ***Ger.:*** Bilipeptal forte†; Cholongal†; Cholspasminase†; Combizym; Combizym Compositum; dichronase†; Digest Merz†; Divinal-Bohnen†; Enterotropin†; enzym gallo sanol N†; Enzym-Hepaduran†; Enzym-Lefax; Enzym-Lefax forte; Enzym-Wied; Enzymed†; Esberizym N; Euflat-N†; Fermento duodenal; Helo-acid compositum†; Helopanflat N; Helopanzym†; Hepa-Merz†; Hepabionta comp†; Hepasteril†; Hevert Enzym Novo; Hylakombun N†; Mederma†; Meteophyt-V†; Meteophyt†; Meteozym; Neo-Gallonorm†; Oragallin†; Pankreaplex N†; Pankreas S†; Pankreatin comp. N†; Pankreoflat; Pankreon compositum†; Pankreon fur Kinder†; Panzynorm forte†; Panzynorm†; Pascopankreat†; Pascopnakreat novo; Paspertase; Pepsaldra compositum N†; Spasmo-Canulase N†; Stacho-Zym N; Unexym MD; Unexym N†; Ventracid N; Wobenzym N; ***Ital.:*** Canulase†; Combizym; Combizym Compositum†; Convivial†; Debridat Enzimatico†; Digestopan; Digestozim†; Digestum†; Ede 6; Enteroton Digestivo†; Enzygaster†; Eudigestio; Onoton†; Pancreoflat; Pancreon Compositum; Pancresil; Pepto Pancreasi Compostat†; Pepto-Pancreasi; Plasil Enzimatico†; Prandium†; Taka-Diastase; ***Neth.:*** Combizym; Combizym Compositum; ***Norw.:*** Combizym; ***S.Afr.:*** Nutrizym†; Pankreoflat; Spasmo-Canulase; ***Spain:*** Digestibys†; Digestomen Complex; Edym Sedante; Espasmo Canulasa; Espasmo Digestomen; Lidobama Complex; Lidobama Plus†; Nulacin Fermentos; Oragalin†; Paigastrol; Pankreoflat; Pankreoflat Sedante†; Pankreon Fuerte†; Takadispep Complex; Tornacin†; Trizima†; Wobenzimal; ***Swed.:*** Combizym; Combizym Compositum; Pankreon comp. forte†; ***Switz.:*** Chymocycline†; Combizym; Combizym Compositum†; Dessertase†; Digestozym†; Fermento duodenal; Festal†; Gillazyme; Gillazyme plus; Globase†; Helopanflat; Nutrizym†; Pankreoflat†; Pantozyme†; Spasmo-Canulase; ***USA:*** Digepepsin; Entozyme†; Hi-Vegi-Lip; Pancrezyme 4X; Prevenzyme†.

Pancrelipase (3732-v)

Pancrelipase *(USAN)*.
CAS — 53608-75-6.
Pharmacopoeias. In US.

A preparation obtained from the pancreas of the hog. It is a cream amorphous powder with a faint characteristic, not offensive odour, containing lipase, with protease and amylase. Its lipase activity is greater weight for weight than pancreatin; it contains in each g not less than 100 000 USP units of protease activity, not less than 24 000 USP units of lipase activity, and not less than 100 000 USP units of amylase activity. Its greatest activity is exhibited in neutral or faintly alkaline media. It is inactivated by more than traces of acids, by large amounts of alkali hydroxides, or by excess of alkali carbonate. **Store** in airtight containers.

Units

See Pancreatin, p.1612.

Uses and Administration

Pancrelipase has the actions and uses of pancreatin (see p.1612). Various doses are employed. In the USA the equivalent of 4000 to 48 000 USP units of lipase activity may be given before each meal or snack, adjusted according to the patient's needs. In the UK a preparation may be used that provides 5000 Ph. Eur. units of lipase activity in each capsule; one to three capsules may be given with each meal.

Three patients with cystic fibrosis whose gastro-intestinal symptoms had been well controlled with pancrelipase developed symptoms following substitution of generic pancrelipase for their previous brand.[1] The generic product had a different lipase content and was almost inactive at stomach pH *in vitro*, apparently because of a defective enteric coating. Different brands of pancrelipase may not be therapeutically equivalent and should not be routinely substituted.

1. Hendeles L, *et al.* Treatment failure after substitution of generic pancrelipase capsules: correlation with in vitro lipase activity. *JAMA* 1990; **263:** 2459–61.

Preparations

USP 23: Pancrelipase Capsules; Pancrelipase Delayed-release Capsules; Pancrelipase Tablets.

Proprietary Preparations (details are given in Part 3)
Aust.: Prolipase; ***Austral.:*** Cotazym S Forte; Pancrease; ***Belg.:*** Pancrease; Viokase; ***Canad.:*** Cotazym; Digess; Pancrease; Ultrase; Viokase; ***Fr.:*** Alipase; ***Ital.:*** Krebsilasi; Luitase; Pancrease; Pankreaden; ***Neth.:*** Pancrease; ***Norw.:*** Pancrease; ***S.Afr.:*** Pankrease; ***Spain:*** Pancrease; ***Swed.:*** Pancrease; ***Switz.:*** Prolipase; ***UK:*** Pancrease; ***USA:*** Cotazym; Entolase†; Ilozyme; Ku-Zyme HP; Pancrease; Protilase; Ultrase; Zymase.

Multi-ingredient: ***Belg.:*** Digestomen; ***UK:*** Digezyme; ***USA:*** Hi-Vegi-Lip; Pancrezyme 4X.

Pancreozymin (2141-x)

Pancreozymin *(BAN)*.
CCK-PZ.

NOTE. The endogenous hormone is known as cholecystokinin (CCK).

Units

The potency of pancreozymin may be expressed as Crick-Harper-Raper units based on the pancreatic secretion in *cats* or as Ivy *dog* units based on the increase in gallbladder pressure. One Ivy dog unit is considered to be approximately equivalent to 1 Crick-Harper-Raper unit.

Adverse Effects

Flushing of the skin and other vasomotor effects may occur, particularly after rapid intravenous injection of pancreozymin. Hypersensitivity reactions may occasionally occur. Gallbladder contraction may give rise to abdominal discomfort.

Uses and Administration

Pancreozymin is a polypeptide hormone prepared from the duodenal mucosa of *pigs*. When administered by intravenous injection it causes an increase in the secretion of pancreatic enzymes and stimulates gallbladder contraction.

Pancreozymin has been used, usually in conjunction with secretin, as a test for exocrine pancreatic function and in the diagnosis of biliary-tract disorders; these tests generally involved duodenal intubation of the patient and examination of duodenal aspirate. Pancreozymin has also been used as an adjunct to cholecystography.

The dose of pancreozymin used has varied, but a common dose is 1 to 2 Crick-Harper-Raper units per kg body-weight given by slow intravenous injection.

Pangamic Acid (13074-m)

The name pangamic acid has been applied variously to gluconic acid 6-[bis(diisopropylamino)acetate] ($C_{20}H_{40}N_2O_8$=436.5), gluconic acid, 6-ester with N,N-dimethylglycine ($C_{10}H_{19}NO_8$=281.3), gluconic acid, 6-ester with N,N-diisopropylglycine ($C_{14}H_{27}NO_8$=337.4), and a substance or mixture of substances isolated from apricot kernels and rice bran. It has also been known as vitamin B_{15} although it seems unlikely that pangamic acid is a vitamin. Preparations containing the vasoactive substance di-isopropylammonium dichloroacetate (p.854) have sometimes been described as pangamic acid or vitamin B_{15}. There is much uncertainty about the identity of products sold in health food stores as 'vitamin B_{15}', pangamic acid, or sodium or calcium pangamate and different brands have been reported to have completely different compositions.

Claims for the activity of pangamic acid as a promoter of tissue oxygenation and its alleged value in numerous disorders have not been substantiated. There is no evidence that pangamic acid is a vitamin.

Preparations

Proprietary Preparations (details are given in Part 3)
Ger.: Oyo.

Multi-ingredient: ***Ger.:*** Vitamin B 15†; Zettaviran†; ***Spain:*** Bronquiasmol†; Policolinosil; Sedionbel†.

Papain (3733-g)

Papayotin.

CAS — 9001-73-4.

Pharmacopoeias. In *US.*

A proteolytic enzyme or mixture of enzymes prepared from the juice of the unripe fruit of *Carica papaya* (Caricaceae). The USP specifies not less than 6000 USP units per mg.

An amorphous, white to light tan powder. **Soluble** in water, the solution being colourless to light yellow and more or less opalescent; practically insoluble in alcohol, chloroform, and ether. A 2% solution in water has a pH of 4.8 to 6.2. **Store** below 15° in airtight containers. Protect from light.

Units

One USP unit of papain activity is the activity that releases the equivalent of 1 µg of tyrosine from a specified casein substrate under the conditions of the assay, using the enzyme concentration that liberates 40 µg of tyrosine per mL of test solution.

One FIP unit of papain is defined as the enzyme activity which under specified conditions hydrolyses 1 µmol of *N*-benzoyl-L-arginine ethyl ester per minute.

The Warner-Chilcott unit, based on the quantity of enzyme required to clot 2.64 µL of milk substrate in 2 minutes at 40°, under specified conditions, has also been used for papain.

Adverse Effects

Hypersensitivity reactions have occurred.

Extensive destruction of the oesophageal wall, with perforation, resulted from the use of a papain suspension given to treat an obstruction caused by impacted meat.[1] The patient had been given 1.2 g of papain over a 12-hour period. Ten days after a thoracotomy, the descending thoracic aorta ruptured, and she died from haemorrhage.

1. Holsinger JW, *et al.* Esophageal perforation following meat impaction and papain ingestion. *JAMA* 1968; **204:** 734–5.

A case report of ocular and periorbital angioedema within 4 hours of use of a contact lens cleansing solution containing papain.[1]

1. Bernstein DI, *et al.* Local ocular anaphylaxis to papain enzyme contained in a contact lens cleansing solution. *J Allergy Clin Immunol* 1984; **74:** 258–60.

Uses and Administration

Papain consists chiefly of a mixture of papain and chymopapain, proteolytic enzymes which hydrolyse polypeptides, amides, and esters, especially at bonds involving basic amino acids, or leucine or glycine, yielding peptides of lower molecular weight. It is used as a topical debriding agent in conjunction with urea. It is also used for the removal of protein deposits from the surface of soft contact lenses (p.1097).

Preparations of papain, alone or combined with antibacterial agents and/or other substances, have been taken by mouth for their supposed anti-inflammatory properties, and it has also been used as an ingredient of various mixtures claimed to aid digestion.

Papain is widely used as a meat tenderiser and in the clarification of beverages.

Preparations

USP 23: Papain Tablets for Topical Solution.

Proprietary Preparations (details are given in Part 3)
Austral.: Hydrocare Enzymatic Protein Remover; ***Canad.:*** Solarcaine Stop Itch; ***S.Afr.:*** Tromasin SA†; ***Spain:*** Cacital; ***USA:*** Allergan Enzymatic; ProFree.

Multi-ingredient: ***Aust.:*** Digestif Rennie; Ozym; Wobe-Mugos; Wobenzym; ***Austral.:*** Betaine Digestive Aid; Bio-Disc; Bioglan Active Enzyme Complex†; Bioglan Discone†; Digestaid; Digestive Aid; Enzyme; Prost-1; Prost-2; Prozyme; Vita Disc†; Vitaplex Digestive Enzyme Formula†; ***Belg.:*** Digestomen; ***Canad.:*** Herbalax Forte; Phytolax; Vesilax; ***Fr.:*** Digestobiase†; Penetradol†; ***Ger.:*** Basofer†; Choldestal†; Divinal-Bohnen†; Enzym-Tyrosolvetten†; Enzym-Wied; Katulcin†; Meteophyt-V†; Meteophyt†; Mulsal N; Pascopankreat†; Stoffwechseldragees†; Tonsilase†; Unexym MD; Unexym N†; Wobe-Mugos E; Wobe-Mugos Th; Wobenzym N; ***Ital.:*** Digestopan; Digestozim†; Enteroton Digestivo†; Enzygaster†; ***Spain:*** Digestomen Complex; Espasmo Digestomen; Gastrosindrom†; Lizipaina; Lysokana; Nasotic Oto; Prosanon†; Takadispep Complex; Trizima†; ***Switz.:*** Digestozym†; Globase†; Lysopaine; ***UK:*** Enzyme Digest; Herbal Indigestion Naturtabs; Indigestion and Flatulence; Papaya Plus; ***USA:*** Panafil; Panafil-White; Papaya Enzyme; Prevenzyme†.

Papaverine (5221-r)

Papaverine *(BAN).*

6,7-Dimethoxy-1-(3,4-dimethoxybenzyl)isoquinoline.

$C_{20}H_{21}NO_4$ = 339.4.

CAS — 58-74-2.

NOTE. Do not confuse papaverine with papaveretum (p.71).

Papaverine Hydrochloride (5224-n)

Papaverine Hydrochloride *(BAN).*

Papaverini Hydrochloridum; Papaverinii Chloridum; Papaverinium Chloride. 6,7-Dimethoxy-1-(3,4-dimethoxybenzyl)isoquinoline hydrochloride.

$C_{20}H_{21}NO_4$,HCl = 375.8.

CAS — 63817-84-5 (papaverine cromesilate); 61-25-6 (papaverine hydrochloride); 39024-96-9 (papaverine monophosadenine); 2053-26-1 (papaverine sulphate, anhydrous).

Pharmacopoeias. In *Chin., Eur.* (see p.viii), *Int., Jpn, Pol.,* and *US.*

Odourless white or almost white crystals or crystalline powder.

Soluble 1 in 30 of water and 1 in 120 of alcohol; soluble in chloroform; practically insoluble in ether. A 2% solution in water has a pH of 3.0 to 4.5; precipitation may occur if mixed with alkaline solutions. **Store** in airtight containers. Protect from light.

Adverse Effects

Side-effects of papaverine given by mouth include gastro-intestinal disturbance, flushing of the face, headache, malaise, drowsiness, skin rash, sweating, orthostatic hypotension, and dizziness. Jaundice, eosinophilia, and signs of altered liver function may occur, sometimes due to hypersensitivity. In addition parenteral administration of high doses can result in cardiac arrhythmias; a slow rate of intravenous or intramuscular administration is recommended. Thrombosis has been reported at the injection site.

Intracavernosal injection can cause dose-related priapism and local fibrosis has been reported following long-term therapy.

Systemic adverse effects occurring after intracavernosal injection of papaverine are infrequent but include dizziness and syncope,[1,2] probably related to the hypotensive effects of papaverine, and abnormal liver function test results.[1-3]

The most serious acute adverse effect is priapism[1,2,4] and patients should be instructed to seek medical help if an erection lasts for more than 4 hours. Detumescence can be effected by aspiration of blood from the corpus or by local injection of an alpha-adrenergic agonist such as adrenaline, metaraminol, or phenylephrine (see Priapism under Alprostadil, p.1413). Other local effects include haematoma, infection, and, on long-term therapy, fibrosis and penile distortion.[1,2]

Dispensing errors have resulted in inadvertent injection of *papaveretum* with potentially fatal consequences.[2,5,6]

1. Krane RJ, *et al.* Impotence. *N Engl J Med* 1989; **321:** 1648–59.
2. Bénard F, Lue TF. Self-administration in the pharmacological treatment of impotence. *Drugs* 1990; **39:** 394–8.
3. Levine SB, *et al.* Side effects of self-administration of intracavernous papaverine and phentolamine for the treatment of impotence. *J Urol (Baltimore)* 1989; **141:** 54–7.
4. Virag R. About pharmacologically induced prolonged erection. *Lancet* 1985; **i:** 519–20.
5. Robinson LQ, Stephenson TP. Self injection treatment for impotence. *Br Med J* 1989; **299:** 1568.
6. Gregoire A. Self injection treatment for impotence. *Br Med J* 1990; **300:** 537.

Precautions

Papaverine should be given with caution to patients with reduced gastro-intestinal motility. Caution is also advised in the presence of cardiac conduction disorders or unstable cardiovascular disease, especially when papaverine is administered parenterally. Intravenous administration is contra-indicated in patients with complete atrioventricular block.

There appeared to be no basis for the manufacturers' recommendation that papaverine be used with caution in patients with glaucoma.[1] There was no obvious mechanism for such a warning and only one report of an adverse reaction had been received by the FDA. The author had given papaverine intracavernosally to patients with glaucoma and had observed no deterioration.

1. Swartz DA, Todd MW. Intracavernous papaverine and glaucoma. *JAMA* 1990; **264:** 570.

Papaveretum (p.71) has been confused with papaverine and in one such case[1] a patient became unconscious after self-injection of papaveretum in mistake for papaverine.

1. Robinson LQ, Stephenson TP. Self injection treatment for impotence. *Br Med J* 1989; **299:** 1568.

Interactions

For a report of papaverine decreasing the effectiveness of levodopa, see Levodopa, p.1140.

Pharmacokinetics

The biological half-life of papaverine given by mouth is reported to be between one and two hours, but there is wide interindividual variation. It is extensively bound (about 90%) to plasma proteins.

Papaverine is mainly metabolised in the liver and excreted in the urine, almost entirely as glucuronide-conjugated phenolic metabolites.

The reports of infrequent systemic effects following intracavernosal injection of papaverine indicate that there is some distribution to the systemic circulation from the corpus cavernosus.

Uses and Administration

Papaverine is an alkaloid present in opium, although it is not related chemically or pharmacologically to the other opium alkaloids. Papaverine has a direct relaxant effect on smooth muscle which is attributed in part to its ability to inhibit phosphodiesterase. It has been given in the management of cerebral, peripheral, and coronary vascular disorders; it is also given as an antispasmodic for gastro-intestinal disorders and coughs. However, there is little evidence to justify its clinical use in these conditions.

Papaverine has been given by mouth as the hydrochloride in doses of up to 600 mg daily although doses of up to 1500 mg daily have been suggested. Sustained-release preparations have been used. The codecarboxylate, cromesilate, hydrobromide, monophosadenine, nicotinate, sulphate, and teprosilate have also been used. Papaverine hydrochloride has also been given in doses of 30 to 120 mg by slow intramuscular or intravenous injection (but see Adverse Effects, above).

Papaverine hydrochloride is given by injection into the corpus cavernosus of the penis for the diagnosis and treatment of erectile dysfunction (below). The initial dose is 7.5 mg and is increased according to response to a range of 30 to 60 mg. Phentolamine may be added if the response is inadequate. It has been recommended that the injection should not be given more than three times a week or on two successive days.

Mention[1] of the injection of papaverine into the superior mesenteric artery as one of the protective measures in intensive care units for patients with acute intestinal ischaemia.

1. Marston A. Acute intestinal ischaemia. *Br Med J* 1990; **301:** 1174–6.

Erectile dysfunction. Erectile dysfunction or impotence signifies inability of a male to achieve satisfactory erection of the penis during sexual intercourse. Estimates of prevalence depend to some extent upon the definitions that are used, and are in any case difficult to come by, but the problem is thought to be not uncommon, particularly in older men.

In a normal erection parasympathetic stimulation, usually initiated by the central nervous system and enhanced by sensory stimuli from the penis, dilates penile arteries and relaxes trabecular smooth muscle via a second messenger, probably nitric oxide. This favours flow of blood into the spaces of the corpora cavernosa, increasing pressure in the penis and leading to tumescence. The increased pressure compresses the venules against the fibrous tissue layer called the tunica albuginea, thus preventing outflow of the blood and leading to rigidity.

The causes of impotence may be psychological, including factors such as stress, mental depression, and anxieties about sexual performance; or organic, or a mixture of the two. Organic causes include androgen deficiency due to hypogonadism, neurological dysfunction (including central or peripheral lesions due to malignancy or trauma), peripheral vascular disorders, and penile abnormalities such as Peyronie's disease or microphallus. Sometimes organic dysfunction may be secondary to another disease, such as in diabetes mellitus where neurological and vascular damage lead to impotence in over a third of all patients. In addition, a number of drugs include impotence among their adverse effects.

Approaches to the management of erectile dysfunction depend to some extent upon the causative factors, and it is important to determine whether dysfunction is primarily psychogenic, organic, or of mixed origin, and to check the medical history for possible contributory factors such as hypertension, diabetes, smoking, pelvic trauma or surgery, or endocrine or neurological dysfunction.

Psychotherapy or behavioural therapy alone may be adequate in patients in whom no organic cause is detected,[1,2] but even where organic factors play a role psychosocial factors are also important and should be addressed by appropriate counselling.

Where causes of erectile dysfunction are partly or primarily organic, two main options are in common use: the use of a vacuum pump to induce erection by negative pressure, followed by constriction of the base of the penis with a band to maintain tumescence; and the injection of vasoactive substances into the corpora cavernosa.[1,2] The third option, implantation of a penile prosthesis is often reserved for patients in whom other therapy fails or is refused, but it may be a suitable first-line choice for some patients.[3] In those few patients where impotence is secondary to androgen deficiency in hypogonadism, androgen replacement, preferably by the intramuscular injection of a suitable testosterone ester, may be of value.[1] Androgen replacement therapy is inappropriate in patients with normal testosterone concentrations and may carry significant health risks. In patients with hypogonadism secondary to hyperprolactinaemia addition of bromocriptine is often effective in improving sexual function.[1]

Intracavernosal injection therapy has become more common in recent years, and because of the difficulties in establishing the causes of erectile dysfunction has been tried in dysfunction due to a variety of causes; neurogenic and psychogenic dysfunction usually respond well, but dysfunction of vascular origin is less likely to give a satisfactory response.

The three drugs most commonly used for injection therapy are alprostadil, papaverine, and phentolamine. High response rates have been reported with papaverine, with or without phentolamine,[4-9] in a number of studies, and alprostadil appears to be equally effective.[10-16] Early studies used relatively high doses of papaverine, which resulted in frequent priapism requiring assisted detumescence,[17] but this is somewhat less frequent with current doses, and with lower doses used when combined with phentolamine. Long-term use of intracavernosal papaverine may result in fibrosis, and it has been suggested that its use should be restricted to once or twice weekly;[6,7] fibrosis has not been reported to be a problem with alprostadil injection but such injection is frequently painful. As with papaverine, priapism can occur, although there is a report that it will respond to oral terbutaline.[18] Triple therapy, involving the combination of papaverine, phentolamine, and alprostadil has been reported to be effective and to have a relatively low incidence of adverse effects.[19] Other agents which have been used for intracavernosal therapy of impotence include thymoxamine, and peptides such as vasoactive intestinal peptide or calcitonin gene-related peptide (combined with other agents).[20,21] Unfortunately studies of injection therapy to date suggest that the long-term drop-out rate is high, implying that problems of patient acceptability have yet to be overcome.

One of the major hurdles to patient acceptance of intracavernosal drugs is the requirement for repeated self-injection of the penis, and a number of studies have investigated topical therapies. Transurethral alprostadil is now available in several countries and is reported to be effective.[22] Urethral instillation of dinoprostone cream produced erections in a few men in a small pilot study[23] and glyceryl trinitrate, applied either as ointment or as a transdermal delivery system, has also been investigated.[24-27]

Oral therapy for impotence has had a checkered history, and most of the drugs tried have proved little better than placebo. Yohimbine may work in some patients[30] but is not recommended by the American Urological Association.[3] Recently, good results have been reported with sildenafil,[28] which has aroused great attention, and other oral therapies are under investigation.[29]

Vascular surgery may have a limited application, in vasogenic dysfunction, but its role is not clearly defined and there are some doubts about its long-term effectiveness.

1. NIH Consensus Development Panel on Impotence. Impotence. *JAMA* 1993; **270:** 83–90.
2. Krane RJ, *et al.* Impotence. *N Engl J Med* 1989; **321:** 1648–59.
3. Skolnick AA. Guidelines for treating erectile dysfunction issued. *JAMA* 1997; **277:** 7–8.
4. Sidi AA, *et al.* Intracavernous drug-induced erections in the management of male erectile dysfunction: experience with 100 patients. *J Urol (Baltimore)* 1986; **135:** 704–6.
5. Williams G, *et al.* Impotence: treatment by autoinjection of vasoactive drugs. *Br Med J* 1987; **295:** 595–6.
6. Anonymous. Help for erectile impotence. *Drug Ther Bull* 1989; **27:** 61–3.
7. Bénard F, Lue TF. Self-administration in the pharmacological treatment of impotence. *Drugs* 1990; **39:** 394–8.
8. Watters GR, *et al.* Prolonged erections following intracorporeal injection of medications to overcome impotence. *Br J Urol* 1988; **62:** 173–5.
9. Brindley GS. Maintenance treatment of erectile impotence by cavernosal unstriated muscle relaxant injection. *Br J Psychiatry* 1986; **149:** 210–15.
10. Stackl W, *et al.* Intracavernous injection of prostaglandin E1 in impotent men. *J Urol (Baltimore)* 1988; **140:** 66–8.
11. Waldhauser M, Schramek P. Efficiency and side effects of prostaglandin E1 in the treatment of erectile dysfunction. *J Urol (Baltimore)* 1988; **140:** 525–7.
12. Schramek P, Waldhauser M. Dose-dependent effect and side-effect of prostaglandin E_1 in erectile dysfunction. *Br J Clin Pharmacol* 1989; **28:** 567–71.
13. Ishii N, *et al.* Intracavernous injection of prostaglandin E1 for the treatment of erectile impotence. *J Urol (Baltimore)* 1989; **141:** 323–5.
14. Lee LM, *et al.* Prostaglandin E1 versus phentolamine/papaverine for the treatment of erectile impotence: a double-blind comparison. *J Urol (Baltimore)* 1989; **141:** 549–50.
15. Sarosdy MF, *et al.* A prospective double-blind trial of intracorporeal papaverine versus prostaglandin E1 in the treatment of impotence. *J Urol (Baltimore)* 1989; **141:** 551–3.
16. Linet OI, *et al.* Efficacy and safety of intracavernosal alprostadil in men with erectile dysfunction. *N Engl J Med* 1996; **334:** 873–7.
17. Virag R. About pharmacologically induced prolonged erection. *Lancet* 1985; **i:** 519–20.
18. Lowe FC, Jarow JP. Placebo-controlled study of oral terbutaline and pseudoephedrine in management of prostaglandin E1-induced prolonged erections. *Urology* 1993; **42:** 51–4.
19. Govier FE, *et al.* Experience with triple-drug therapy in a pharmacological erection program. *J Urol (Baltimore)* 1993; **150:** 1822–4.
20. Montorsi F, *et al.* Pharmacological management of erectile dysfunction. *Drugs* 1995; **50:** 465–79.
21. Chaudhuri A, Wiles P. Optimal treatment of erectile failure in patients with diabetes. *Drugs* 1995; **49:** 548–54.
22. Padma-Nathan H, *et al.* Treatment of men with erectile dysfunction with transurethral alprostadil. *N Engl J Med* 1997; **336:** 1–7.
23. Wolfson B, *et al.* Intraurethral prostaglandin E-2 cream: a possible alternative treatment for erectile dysfunction. *Urology* 1993; **42:** 73–5.
24. Heaton JPW, *et al.* Topical glyceryltrinitrate causes measurable penile arterial dilation in impotent men. *J Urol (Baltimore)* 1990; **143:** 729–31.
25. Meyhoff HH, *et al.* Non-invasive management of impotence with transcutaneous nitroglycerin. *Br J Urol* 1992; **69:** 88–90.
26. Nunez BD, Anderson DC. Nitroglycerin ointment in the treatment of impotence. *J Urol (Baltimore)* 1993; **150:** 1241–3.
27. Anderson DC, Seifert CF. Topical nitrate treatment of impotence. *Ann Pharmacother* 1993; **27:** 1203–5.
28. Goldstein I, *et al.* Oral sildenafil in the treatment of erectile dysfunction. *N Engl J Med* 1998; **338:** 1397–1404. Correction. *ibid.*; **339:** 59.
29. Eardley I. New oral therapies for the treatment of erectile dysfunction. *Br J Urol* 1998; **81:** 122–7.
30. Ernst E, Pittler MH. Yohimbine for erectile dysfunction: a systematic review and meta-analysis of randomised clinical trials. *J Urol (Baltimore)* 1998; **159:** 433–6.

Preparations

USP 23: Papaverine Hydrochloride Injection; Papaverine Hydrochloride Tablets.

Proprietary Preparations (details are given in Part 3)
Fr.: Albatran; ***Ger.:*** Opdensit†; Optenyl†; Panergon†; Paveron†; ***Ital.:*** Pameion†; ***Spain:*** Sustein†; ***UK:*** Papaverine Hydrochloride; ***USA:*** Cerespan†; Genabid†; Pavabid; Pavarine; Pavased†; Pavatine†; Paverolan.

Multi-ingredient: ***Aust.:*** Androskat; Asthma; Asthma 23 D; Euflat; Myocardon; Normensan; Ora-Gallin compositum; Perphyllon; ***Belg.:*** Asperal-B†; Perphyllone†; ***Fr.:*** Acticarbine; Dilpavan†; Garaspirine†; Oxadilene; Solurutine Papaverine F. Retard; Vasocalm†; ***Ger.:*** Broncho-Binotal†; Bronchovydrin†; Brox-Aerosol N†; BTH-N Broncho-Tetra-Holz†; Euflat-N†; Makatussin Tetra†; Mandrogallan†; Mandros-forte†; Migranex spezial N†; Myocardetten†; Neutromil†; Paveron†; Ribbeck†; Spasdilat N†; ***Ital.:*** Anacufen†; Antispasmina Colica; Bilancen†; Entero-V†; Farmospasmina Colica†; Ischelium Papaverina; Monotrean; Progeril Papaverina†; Teofilcolina Sedativa†; ***Neth.:*** Androskat; ***Spain:*** Aletor Compositum; Analgilasa; Angiosedante; Biocortison†; Bonciclol†; Gastrosindrom†; Rubia Paver; Sulmetin Papaver; Sulmetin Papaverina; ***Swed.:*** Spasmofen; ***Switz.:*** Dolopyrine; Feloflux compose†; Monotrean†; Spasmanodine†; Spasmosol; Supadol†; ***USA:*** Copavin†.

Paradichlorobenzene (3599-c)

Dichlorbenzol. 1,4-Dichlorobenzene.
$C_6H_4Cl_2$ = 147.0.
CAS — 106-46-7.

Paradichlorobenzene has general properties similar to those of orthodichlorobenzene (see p.1611) but is considered to be less toxic. It is present in several preparations intended for the removal of ear wax (see p.1190). It has been used as a furniture preservative and in mothballs and lavatory deodorant blocks.

Preparations

Proprietary Preparations (details are given in Part 3)
Multi-ingredient: ***Austral.:*** Cerumol; ***Canad.:*** Cerumol; ***Irl.:*** Cerumol; ***S.Afr.:*** Cerumol; ***Switz.:*** Cerumenol; ***UK:*** Cerumol; Wax Aid†.

Paraphenylenediamine (13078-q)

$C_6H_4(NH_2)_2$ = 108.1.
CAS — 106-50-3.

NOTE. Commonly known in the hairdressing trade as *'para'*.

Paraphenylenediamine is used as a hair dye.

It is estimated that about 4% of apparently normal subjects are sensitive to paraphenylenediamine, and 1% acutely sensitive; oedema and severe dermatitis may follow application in such persons. Effects on the eye may include chemosis, lachrymation, exophthalmos, and sometimes permanent blindness.

Following ingestion severe angioedema-like symptoms with respiratory difficulty and dyspnoea may occur and may require emergency tracheostomy; vomiting, massive oedema, gastritis, rise in blood pressure, vertigo, tremors, convulsions, and coma have been reported.

Some studies have linked hair dyes with mutagenicity and carcinogenicity, although such findings have often been refuted.

Paratoluenediamine (13080-n)

2-Methyl-1,4-phenylenediamine.
$C_7H_{10}N_2$ = 122.2.
CAS — 95-70-5.

Paratoluenediamine is used as a hair dye.

Like paraphenylenediamine, above, paratoluenediamine may be associated with sensitivity reactions.

Paroxypropione (13083-b)

Paroxypropione *(rINN).*
B-360; H-365; NSC-2834. 4′-Hydroxypropiophenone.
$C_9H_{10}O_2$ = 150.2.
CAS — 70-70-2.

Paroxypropione is a pituitary gonadotrophic hormone inhibitor which has been used for the control of pituitary hyperactivity.

Parsley (4686-d)

Persil; Petroselinum.

Parsley (*Petroselinum crispum*, Umbelliferae) is used in herbal medicine, where it is mainly given as a diuretic. It is also used as a culinary herb and flavouring.

Preparations

Proprietary Preparations (details are given in Part 3)
Ger.: Kneipp Petersilie N.

Multi-ingredient: ***Aust.:*** Apotheker Bauer's Harntreibender Tee; Blasen-Tee; Krauterhaus Mag Kottas Entwasserungstee; Krautertee Nr 126; Krautertee Nr 18; Krautertee Nr 25; Krautertee Nr 3; Krautertee Nr 4; Magentee; Sanvita-Entschlackungstonikum; ***Austral.:*** Fluid Loss; Garlic and Horseradish Complex 1000†; Herbal Diuretic Complex†; Medinat PMT-Eze; Natural Vegetable Alkaliniser†; PMT-EZE†; Protemp; Uva-Ursi Plus; ***Ger.:*** Asparagus-P; Diureticum-Medice†; Eupond; nephro-loges; Nephrubin; ***Switz.:*** Tisane pour les reins et la vessie "H"†; ***UK:*** Athera; Digest; Garlodex; Helonias Compound; Kincare.

Passion Flower (13086-q)

Grenadille; May-pop; Pasionari; Passiflora; Passiflorae Herba.
CAS — 486-84-0 (harman).
Pharmacopoeias. In *Fr., Ger.,* and *Swiss.*

The dried aerial parts of *Passiflora incarnata* (Passifloraceae) containing flavonoids and varying quantities of harman alkaloids.

Passion flower is reputed to have antispasmodic and sedative properties and has been used widely as an ingredient of herbal remedies, chiefly in the form of a liquid extract tincture.

Passion flower is used in homoeopathic medicine.

Preparations

Proprietary Preparations (details are given in Part 3)
UK: Natracalm; Naturest.

Multi-ingredient: ***Aust.:*** Nervenruh; Passedan; Passelyt; Sedogelat; Wechseltee; ***Austral.:*** Calmo; Esten†; Euphorbia Complex; Executive B; Goodnight Formula; Herbal Anxiety Formula; Infant Calm; Lifesystem Herbal Plus Formula 2 Valerian; Naturest; Pacifenity; Passiflora Complex; Passionflower Plus; Proesten; Prosed-X; Relaxaplex; Tranquiplex†; Valerian Plus Herbal Plus Formula 12; Vitaglow Executive Anti Stress†; Vitaglow Herbal Stress†; ***Belg.:*** Sedinal; Tisane Contre la Tension; Valeria-Fordine†; ***Canad.:*** Herbal Sleep Well†; ***Fr.:*** Actisane Nervosite; Anxoral; Astressane; Biocarde; Canteine Bouteille†; Euphytose; Kaneuron; Mediflor Tisane Calmante Troubles du Sommeil No 14; Natisedine; Natudor; Neuroflorine; Neuropax†; Neurotensyl; Nocvalene; Nuidor†; Panxeol; Parlax Compose†; Passiflorine; Passinevryl†; Phytocalm; Phytotherapie Boribel no 8; Quietival†; Sedatif Tiber; Serenival; Sympaneurol; Sympavagol; Tisanes de l'Abbe Hamon no 6; ***Ger.:*** Aranidorm-S; Aureal†; Avedorm; B 12 Nervinfant†; Belladonna-Valobonin†; Biosedon S; Biral; Bunetten†; Cardaminol†; Dormo-Sern; Dormoverlan; Eupronerv†; Euvegal N; Gutnacht; Habstal-Nerv N; Hyposedon N; JuNeuron S; Kytta-Sedativum f; Luvased-Tropfen N; Moradorm; Moradorm S; Nerven-Tee Stada N; Nervendragees; Nervinfant N; Nervinfant†; Nervoregin; Nervoregin forte; Neurapas; Neuraston†; Neuro-Presselin†; Passiorin N; Passiorin†; Phytonoctu; Plantival N†; Plantival plus†; Presselin K 1 N; Pronervon N†; Pronervon Phyto;

Salusan; Seda-Pasc N†; Seda-Plantina; Sedaselect N; Sedinfant N; Sediomed S†; Sirmiosta Nervenelixier N; Somnium†; Somnuvis S; Tornix; Valena N; Valeriana mild; Valobonin†; Visinal; Vivinox; *Ital.:* Anevrasi; Bio Notte Baby†; Bio-Strath; Blandonal; Calmactiv†; Fiorlin†; Fitosonno; Florerbe Calmante†; Neurobiol; Noctis; Parvisedil; Passiflorine; Quietan; Reve; Sedatol; Sedonerva†; Sedopuer F; Tauma; Val-Plus; *S.Afr.:* Biral; *Spain:* Brevilon; Decima Nil†; Passiflorine; *Switz.:* Dicalm†; Dipect†; Dormeasan†; Dragees antirhumatismales fortes; Dragees pour la detente nerveuse; Dragees pour le coeur et les nerfs; Dragees relaxantes et tranquillisantes†; Epizon†; Gouttes pour le coeur et les nerfs Concentrees; Melissa Tonic; Passiorin†; Phytoberidin; Phytomed Cardio; Phytomed Somni; Plantival; Sedosan; Sirop Passi-Par; Soporin; Tisane antirhumatismale; Tisane relaxante; Valobonin†; Valverde Dragees pour la detente nerveuse; Valverde Dragees pour le coeur; Valverde Gouttes pour le coeur; *UK:* Ana-Sed; Avena sativa comp.; Becalm; Gerard 99; Herbal Pain Relief; Motherwort Compound; Night Time; Nytol Herbal; PMT Formula; Quiet Life; Quiet Night; Quiet Nite; Quiet Tyme; Relax B+; Serenity; SuNerven; Super Mega B+C; Valerian Compound.

Patent Blue V (2142-r)

Acid Blue 3; CI Food Blue 5; Colour Index No. 42051; E131. Calcium α-(4-diethylaminophenyl)-α-(4-diethyliminiocyclohexa-2,5-dienylidene)-5-hydroxytoluene-2,4-disulphonate.

$(C_{27}H_{31}N_2O_7S_2)_2Ca$ = 1159.4.
CAS — 3536-49-0.

NOTE. The name Patent Blue V is also used as a synonym for Sulphan Blue (CI No. 42045) (p.1633).

Pharmacopoeias. In *Fr.*

Adverse Effects and Precautions

Hypersensitivity reactions may occur immediately or a few minutes after injection of patent blue V; on rare occasions they may be severe and include shock, dyspnoea, laryngeal spasm, and oedema. Nausea, hypotension, and tremor have been reported.

Administration of a small dose to test for hypersensitivity has been suggested.

An urticarial rash occurred in a 5-year-old girl after use of disclosing tablets containing patent blue V to demonstrate the presence of dental plaque.[1]

1. Chadwick BL, *et al.* Allergic reaction to the food dye patent blue. *Br Dent J* 1990; **168:** 386–7.

Uses and Administration

Patent blue V is injected subcutaneously to colour the lymph vessels so that they can be injected with a contrast medium. The usual dose of 0.25 mL of the 2.5% solution diluted with an equal volume of sodium chloride 0.9% or 1% lignocaine hydrochloride is injected subcutaneously in each interdigital web space. Additional injections at different sites may be required when the lower limbs are to be examined. The bluish skin colour which may develop after injection usually disappears after 24 to 48 hours.

Patent blue V is used as a food colour.

Intradermal injection of patent blue V at the site of a primary breast tumour has been used to identify the associated lymph nodes,[1] but concern has been expressed regarding possible long-term staining of the skin.[2]

1. Borgstein PJ, *et al.* Intradermal blue dye to identify sentinel lymphnode in breast cancer. *Lancet* 1997; **349:** 1668–9.
2. Giuliano AE. Intradermal blue dye to identify sentinel lymph node in breast cancer. *Lancet* 1997; **350:** 958.

Pegademase (14397-q)

Pegademase *(rINN).*
PEG-ADA; PEG-Adenosine Deaminase.

NOTE. Pegademase Bovine is *USAN.*

Pegademase is adenosine deaminase, an endogenous enzyme which converts adenosine to inosine, conjugated with polyethylene glycol. Pegademase bovine is used in the treatment of severe combined immunodeficiency disease (SCID) associated with a deficiency of adenosine deaminase. It is administered by intramuscular injection once every 7 days in an initial dose of 10 units per kg body-weight increasing by increments of 5 units per kg to a weekly maintenance dose of 20 units per kg. A single dose of 30 units per kg should not be exceeded.

Gene therapy (p.1583) has also been tried successfully in this deficiency syndrome.

References.

1. Hershfield MS, *et al.* Treatment of adenosine deaminase deficiency with polyethylene glycol-modified adenosine deaminase. *N Engl J Med* 1987; **316:** 589–96.
2. Anonymous. Pegademase. *Med Lett Drugs Ther* 1990; **32:** 87–8.
3. Lee CR, *et al.* Pegademase bovine: replacement therapy for severe combined immunodeficiency disease. *DICP Ann Pharmacother* 1991; **25:** 1092–5.
4. Shovlin CL, *et al.* Adult presentation of adenosine deaminase deficiency. *Lancet* 1993; **341:** 1471.

Preparations

Proprietary Preparations (details are given in Part 3)
USA: Adagen.

Penicilloyl-polylysine (2143-f)

Benzylpenicilloyl-polylysine; PO-PLL; PPL.
CAS — 53608-77-8.

Pharmacopoeias. In *US.*

A polypeptide compound formed by the interaction of a penicillanic acid and polylysine of an average degree of polymerisation of 20 lysine residues per molecule.

Adverse Effects and Precautions

Severe hypersensitivity reactions have occasionally been reported following administration of penicilloyl-polylysine; a scratch test is recommended before intradermal administration.

Uses and Administration

Penicilloyl-polylysine is used to detect penicillin hypersensitivity. It is generally indicated only for adults with a history of penicillin hypersensitivity. After a preliminary scratch test it is given by intradermal injection. The development, usually within 15 minutes, of a wheal, erythema, and pruritus is generally judged a positive reaction. The incidence of penicillin hypersensitivity is stated to be less than 5% in patients showing a negative reaction. Penicilloyl-polylysine does not detect those liable to suffer late reactions or reactions due to minor antigen determinants; these reactions require other tests. False-positive reactions to penicilloyl-polylysine also occur.

Preparations

USP 23: Benzylpenicilloyl Polylysine Injection.

Proprietary Preparations (details are given in Part 3)
Canad.: Pre-Pen; *Swed.:* Pre-Pen; *USA:* Pre-Pen.

Pentachlorophenol (6655-s)

PCP; Penta.
C_6HCl_5O = 266.3.
CAS — 87-86-5.

NOTE. The name PCP has also been used as a synonym for phencyclidine hydrochloride.

Adverse Effects, Treatment, and Precautions

Pentachlorophenol may be absorbed in toxic amounts through the skin or by inhalation, as well as by ingestion. Pentachlorophenol and its aqueous solutions are irritant to the eyes, mucous membranes, and to the skin and may produce caustic burns. The systemic effects are due to uncoupling of oxidative phosphorylation with consequent stimulation of cellular metabolism. Acute poisoning with pentachlorophenol increases metabolic rate, leading to raised temperature with copious sweating and thirst, restlessness, fatigue, increased rate and depth of respiration, and tachycardia. There may be abdominal pain and nausea, and death has occurred from respiratory failure. Symptoms of subacute or chronic poisoning include hyperpyrexia, and central nervous system, haematological, renal, reproductive, respiratory, and skin disorders.

Treatment is symptomatic; it has been suggested that forced alkaline diuresis may be useful. The use of antipyretics is not recommended since they can increase toxicity.

Reviews of the toxicity of pentachlorophenol.

1. Health and Safety Executive. Pentachlorophenol. *Toxicity Review 5.* London: HMSO, 1982.
2. Pentachlorophenol. *Environmental Health Criteria 71.* Geneva: WHO, 1987.
3. Pentachlorophenol health and safety guide. *Health and Safety Guide 19.* Geneva: WHO, 1989.
4. Jorens PG, Schepens PJC. Human pentachlorophenol poisoning. *Hum Exp Toxicol* 1993; **12:** 479–95.

There have been reports of malignant neoplasms,[1,2] aplastic anaemia,[3] pancreatitis,[4] intravascular haemolysis,[5] and urticaria[6] associated with exposure to pentachlorophenol.

1. Greene MH, *et al.* Familial and sporadic Hodgkin's disease associated with occupational wood exposure. *Lancet* 1978; **ii:** 626–7.
2. Hardell L. Malignant lymphoma of histiocytic type and exposure to phenoxyacetic acids or chlorophenols. *Lancet* 1979; **i:** 55–6.
3. Roberts HJ. Aplastic anemia due to pentachlorophenol. *N Engl J Med* 1981; **305:** 1650–1.
4. Cooper RG, Macaulay MB. Pentachlorophenol pancreatitis. *Lancet* 1982; **i:** 517.
5. Hassan AB, *et al.* Intravascular haemolysis induced by pentachlorophenol. *Br Med J* 1985; **291:** 21–2.
6. Kentor PM. Urticaria from contact with pentachlorophenate. *JAMA* 1986; **256:** 3350.

Pharmacokinetics

Pentachlorophenol may be absorbed after ingestion or inhalation or through the skin. Following ingestion the majority of a dose is eliminated in the urine as unchanged pentachlorophenol and its glucuronide with small amounts appearing in the faeces.

Uses

Pentachlorophenol has been used mainly as the sodium salt (C_6Cl_5NaO = 288.3), as a preservative for a wide range of industrial and agricultural products, including wood and other building materials, textiles, glues and starch. It has also been used for the control of slime and algae, and as a molluscicide, fungicide, and herbicide.

Pentagastrin (2144-d)

Pentagastrin *(BAN, USAN, rINN).*
AY-6608; ICI-50123. *tert*-Butyloxycarbonyl-[β-Ala[1]3]gastrin-(13-17)-pentapeptide amide; Boc-βAla-Trp-Met-Asp-Phe—NH_2.
$C_{37}H_{49}N_7O_9S$ = 767.9.
CAS — 5534-95-2.

Pharmacopoeias. In *Br.*

A white or almost white powder. Practically **insoluble** in water; slightly soluble in alcohol; soluble in dimethylformamide and in dilute ammonia solution. **Protect** from light.

Adverse Effects

Pentagastrin may cause a number of gastro-intestinal effects including nausea and abdominal cramps. Cardiovascular effects including flushing of the skin, tachycardia, bradycardia, and hypotension have occasionally been reported. There may be headache, drowsiness, dizziness, and altered sensations in the extremities. Hypersensitivity reactions are rare.

Some individual reports of adverse effects of pentagastrin.

1. Drucker D. Atrial fibrillation after administration of calcium and pentagastrin. *N Engl J Med* 1981; **304:** 1427–8.
2. Goldman M. Acute interstitial nephritis after administration of pentagastrin. *Br Med J* 1984; **289:** 470.
3. Arnved J, *et al.* Pentagastrin-induced thrombocytopenia. *Lancet* 1985; **ii:** 1068–9.

Precautions

Pentagastrin should be given with care to patients with acute peptic ulceration or with active pancreatic, hepatic, or biliary-tract disease.

Uses and Administration

Pentagastrin is a synthetic pentapeptide which is not active when given by mouth but when given parenterally has effects similar to those of natural gastrin. Since it stimulates the secretion of gastric acid, pepsin, and intrinsic factor, it is used as a diagnostic agent to test the secretory action of the stomach. It has been used to diagnose disorders associated with increased or decreased gastric acid secretion and in the evaluation of gastric acid secretion following vagotomy or gastric resection. The usual dose is 6 μg per kg body-weight by subcutaneous injection; by intravenous infusion the dose is 0.6 μg per kg per hour, in sodium chloride 0.9%. It has also been given intramuscularly and by nasal inhalation.

Pentagastrin stimulates the secretion of pancreatic enzymes and thus has been used as a test for pancreatic function. It has also been tried in the diagnosis of medullary carcinoma of the thyroid.

Preparations

BP 1998: Pentagastrin Injection.

Proprietary Preparations (details are given in Part 3)
Aust.: Peptavlon; *Canad.:* Peptavlon; *Fr.:* Peptavlon; *Ger.:* Gastrodiagnost†; *Irl.:* Peptavlon†; *Norw.:* Peptavlon†; *Swed.:* Peptavlon†; *Switz.:* Peptavlon; *UK:* Peptavlon; *USA:* Peptavlon.

Pentanobornamide (13746-b)

N-[(3-Methylbicyclo[2.2.1]-hept-2-yl)methyl]-*N*-(3-methylbutyl)-4-oxopentanamide.
$C_{19}H_{33}NO_2$ = 307.5.
CAS — 18966-39-7.

Pentanobornamide has been used as an antispasmodic.

Preparations

Proprietary Preparations (details are given in Part 3)
Ital.: Bornamid†.

Pepsin (3736-s)

Pepsina; Pepsini Pulvis.
CAS — 9001-75-6.

Pharmacopoeias. In *Eur.* (see p.viii). In *Chin.* and *Jpn* as Saccharated Pepsin.

A substance containing proteolytic enzymes present in the gastric juice of animals and active at acid pH, obtained from the gastric mucosa of pigs, cattle, or sheep. The Ph. Eur. specifies an activity of not less than 0.5 Ph. Eur. units per mg of dried substance. A hygroscopic, white or slightly yellow, crystalline or amorphous powder. **Soluble** in water; practically insoluble in alcohol and in ether. A solution in water may be slightly opalescent with a weak acidic reaction. **Store** at 2° to 8° in airtight containers. Protect from light.

Units

The activity of pepsin is determined by comparing the quantity of peptides not precipitable by a 4.0% w/v solution of trichloroacetic acid released per minute from a substrate of haemoglobin solution, with that released by the FIP Standard Preparation of pepsin from the same substrate under the same conditions. The peptides are assayed using phosphomolybdotungstic reagent.

Uses and Administration

Pepsin contains proteolytic enzymes secreted by the stomach which control the degradation of proteins into proteoses and peptones. It hydrolyses polypeptides including those with bonds adjacent to aromatic or dicarboxylic L-amino-acid residues.

Pepsin has been given with dilute hydrochloric acid, or with substances such as glutamic acid hydrochloride, or betaine hydrochloride, as an adjunct in the treatment of gastric hypochlorhydria, or to treat deficiencies of digestive enzyme secretion. It has also been given for its supposed benefit as an ingredient of mixtures for dyspepsia and other gastro-intestinal disorders.

Preparations

Proprietary Preparations (details are given in Part 3)
Canad.: Fermentol.

Multi-ingredient: ***Aust.:*** Everon; Helo-acid; Helopanzym; Oro-acid; Pansan; Pepsiton; Vinopepsin; ***Austral.:*** Betaine Digestive Aid; Bioglan Digestive Zyme†; Digestaid; Enzyme; Prozyme; ***Belg.:*** Digestobiase†; Digestomen; ***Fr.:*** Chloridia†; Digestobiase†; Elixir Grez Chlorhydropepsique†; Hepatoum; Tridigestine Hepatoum†; ***Ger.:*** Bilipeptal forte†; Citropepsin; dichronase†; Dr. Maurers Magen-Apotheke†; Enzymed†; Helopanzym†; Hepasteril†; Pansan†; Pepsaldra compositum N†; Pepsaldra†; Pepzitrat; Tri Viaben†; Unexym N†; ***Ital.:*** Canulase†; Convivial†; Digestopan; Digestozim†; Digestum†; Enteroton Digestivo†; Enzygaster†; Essen Enzimatico; Essen†; Eudigestio; Euzymina I Bambini†; Euzymina II Adulti†; Gastro-Pepsin; Kilozim†; Pepto Pancreasi Composta†; Pepto-Pancreasi; Quanto†; Taka-Diastase; Trimalcina†; ***S.Afr.:*** Peter Pote's†; Spasmo-Canulase; ***Spain:*** Acidona†; Digestibys†; Digestomen Complex; Digestonico†; Espasmo Canulasa; Espasmo Digestomen; Euzymina Lisina; Gastrosindrom†; Paigastrol; Troforex Pepsico; ***Switz.:*** Pantozyme†; Spasmo-Canulase; Stomacine; ***UK:*** Digezyme; ***USA:*** Digepepsin; Entozyme†; Prevenzyme†.

Perflubron (15914-x)

Perflubron *(USAN, rINN).*

Perfluorooctylbromide; PFOB. 1-Bromoheptadecafluorooctane.

C_8BrF_{17} = 499.0.

CAS — 423-55-2.

Pharmacopoeias. In *US.*

Clear, colourless, practically odourless liquid. **Store** in airtight containers. Protect from light.

Perflubron is a perfluorocarbon that has been given by mouth to enhance delineation of the bowel during magnetic resonance imaging.

Emulsions of perfluorocarbons can absorb, transport, and release oxygen and carbon dioxide and perflubron is under investigation for use in partial liquid ventilation in patients with respiratory failure and also as an alternative to red blood cell preparations to improve gaseous transport and in particular oxygen supply to the tissues.

Other perfluorocarbons have also been used. A mixture of perfluamine (perfluorotripropylamine) and perflunafene (perfluorodecahydronaphthalene, perfluorodecalin) has been used to prevent myocardial ischaemia during percutaneous transluminal coronary angioplasty.

Perfluorocarbons have been used in eye surgery.

Blood substitutes. References to the use of perflubron and other perfluorocarbons as blood substitutes.

1. Ravis WR, *et al.* Perfluorochemical erythrocyte substitutes: disposition and effects on drug distribution and elimination. *Drug Metab Rev* 1991; **23:** 375–411.
2. Urbaniak SJ. Artificial blood. *Br Med J* 1991; **303:** 1348–50.
3. Garrelts JC. Fluosol: an oxygen-delivery fluid for use in percutaneous transluminal coronary angioplasty. *DICP Ann Pharmacother* 1990; **24:** 1105–12.
4. Jones JA. Red blood cell substitutes: current status. *Br J Anaesth* 1995; **74:** 697–703.

Respiratory distress syndrome. Partial liquid ventilation using perflubron has been tried in a few neonates[1,2] (p.1025), children,[1] and adults[1,3] (p.1017) with respiratory distress syndrome. These preliminary studies suggest that perflubron may improve lung function in these patients.

1. Hirschl RB, *et al.* Liquid ventilation in adults, children, and full-term neonates. *Lancet* 1995; **346:** 1201–2.
2. Leach CL, *et al.* Partial liquid ventilation with perflubron in premature infants with severe respiratory distress syndrome. *N Engl J Med* 1996; **335:** 761–7.
3. Hirschl RB, *et al.* Initial experience with partial liquid ventilation in adult patients with acute respiratory distress syndrome. *JAMA* 1996; **275:** 383–9.

Preparations

Proprietary Preparations (details are given in Part 3)
USA: Imagent GI†.

Multi-ingredient: ***UK:*** Fluosol†; ***USA:*** Fluosol†.

Persic Oil (7364-g)

Oleum Persicorum; Peach or Apricot Kernel Oil.

Pharmacopoeias. Jpn and *Chin.* include Peach Kernel (Persicae Semen) and also Apricot Kernel (Armeniacae Semen).

The fixed oil expressed from the kernels of varieties of *Prunus persica* (peach) or *P. armeniaca* (apricot) (Rosaceae). It is a clear, colourless or pale straw-coloured, almost odourless oil with a bland taste. Slightly **soluble** in alcohol; miscible with chloroform, ether, and petroleum spirit. **Store** in airtight containers.

Persic oil closely resembles almond oil in its general characteristics and is used as an oily vehicle.

Peru Balsam (282-k)

Bals. Peruv.; Balsamum Pieruvianum; Baume du Pérou; Baume du San Salvador; Peruvian Balsam.

Pharmacopoeias. In *Eur.* (see p.viii).

A balsam exuded from the trunk of *Myroxylon balsamum* var. *pereirae* (Leguminosae). It contains not less than 45.0% w/w and not more than 70.0% w/w of esters, mainly benzyl benzoate and benzyl cinnamate.

A dark brown, viscous liquid which is not sticky, is non-drying, and does not form threads. It is transparent and yellowish brown when viewed in a thin layer. Practically **insoluble** in water, freely soluble in dehydrated alcohol; not miscible with fatty oils except for castor oil. **Protect** from light.

Peru balsam has a very mild antiseptic action by virtue of its content of cinnamic and benzoic acids. Diluted with an equal part of castor oil, it has been used as an application to bedsores and chronic ulcers; it has also been used in topical preparations for the treatment of superficial skin lesions and pruritus. It is an ingredient of some rectal preparations used for the symptomatic relief of haemorrhoids (see p.1170).

Peru balsam is an ingredient of some preparations used in the treatment of respiratory congestion.

Skin sensitisation has been reported.

Preparations

Proprietary Preparations (details are given in Part 3)
Aust.: Perudent; ***Belg.:*** Tulle Gras Lumiere; ***Fr.:*** Tulle Gras Lumiere; ***Ger.:*** Branolind N; Tulle Gras Lumiere; ***Switz.:*** Branolind†; ***USA:*** Flanders Buttocks.

Multi-ingredient: ***Aust.:*** Mamellin; Pudan-Lebertran-Zinksalbe; Pulmex†; Rombay; Vulpuran; ***Austral.:*** Anusol; Anusol-HC†; Ayrton's Chilblain; ***Belg.:*** Dermophil Indien†; Oxyplastine; Perubore; Pulmex; Pulmex Baby; Rectovasol; ***Canad.:*** Dera; ***Fr.:*** Agathol; Anaxeryl; Balsofumine; Balsofumine Mentholee; Brulex; Hyalurectal†; Oxyperol; Perubore; Pommade Lelong; Pulmax; ***Ger.:*** Anusol; Anusol + H†; Branolind L†; Claudemor†; derma-loges N; Duoform-Balsam†; Ekzevowen; Kalantol-A†; Kalantol-B†; Kremulsion†; Peru-Lenicet; ***Irl.:*** Anugesic-HC; Anusol; Anusol-HC; ***Ital.:*** Anusol; Fomentil; Paneraj†; ***Norw.:*** Anusol†; ***S.Afr.:*** Anugesic; Anusol-HC; Episeal†; Rectosan 'A'†; Ung Vernleigh; ***Spain:*** Antigrietun; Antihemorroidal†; Anusol†; Cicatral; Grietalgen; Kneipp Balsamo; Linitul; Sarnical†; Vapores Pyt; Vitamina F99 Topica; Xilorroidal†; ***Swed.:*** Anusol; ***Switz.:*** Anginol; Anusol; Demo pommade contre les refroidissements; Demo pommade contre les refroidissements pour bebes; Dermophil Indien; Escothyol†; Furodermil; Haemocortin; Haemolan; HEC; Nasobol; Perubare; Pulmex; Pulmex Baby; Pulmex†; Rapura; Solin S†; ***UK:*** Anugesic-HC; Anusol; Anusol-HC; Balsamicum; Dragon Balm; Frost Cream; ***USA:*** Anocaine†; Anumed; Anumed HC; Anuprep Hemorrhoidal†; Anusol; Balmex Baby; Dermuspray; Dr Dermi-Heal; Granulderm; Granulex; GranuMed; Hemril; Mammol; Medicone Rectal; Proderm; Rectagene II†; Saratoga; Wyanoids.

Phencyclidine Hydrochloride (13100-l)

Phencyclidine Hydrochloride *(BANM, USAN, rINNM).*

CI-395; CN-25253-2; GP-121; NSC-40902; PCP. 1-(1-Phenylcyclohexyl)piperidine hydrochloride.

$C_{17}H_{25}N,HCl$ = 279.8.

CAS — 77-10-1 (phencyclidine); 956-90-1 (phencyclidine hydrochloride).

NOTE. The name PCP has also been used as a synonym for pentachlorophenol.

Phencyclidine used illicitly has been known as: angel dust, angel hair, angel mist, crystal, cyclone, dust, elephant tranquilliser, embalming fluid, goon, hog, horse tranquilliser, killer weed, KW, mint weed, mist, monkey dust, monkey gland, peace pills, peace weed, rocket fuel, scuffle, sheets, super weed, surfer, and T.

Adverse Effects and Treatment

Phencyclidine can induce a psychosis clinically indistinguishable from schizophrenia. Adverse effects reported include bizarre and violent behaviour, hallucinations, euphoria, agitation, catatonic rigidity, disorientation, incoordination, nystagmus, hypersalivation, vomiting, convulsions, numbness, hypertension, and tachycardia, rhabdomyolysis leading to renal failure, acidosis, and occasionally, malignant hyperthermia. Severe intoxication may result in respiratory depression, coma, and death.

Treatment of the adverse effects of phencyclidine is symptomatic; if agitated the patient should be kept quiet in a darkened room, and diazepam given if necessary. Hyperthermia should be treated. Repeated doses of charcoal should be given. Acidification of the urine is no longer recommended since acidosis may be exacerbated and renal failure precipitated. Haloperidol or a similar butyrophenone may be preferable to chlorpromazine in the management of psychotic symptoms.

Uses and Administration

Phencyclidine is related chemically to ketamine (see p.1226) and is a potent analgesic and anaesthetic. It was formerly given intravenously to produce an amnesic trance-like state, with analgesia, but severe adverse effects, especially postoperative psychoses, precluded its use. It was formerly used in veterinary medicine as an immobilising agent and is widely used in some countries as a hallucinogenic drug of abuse. When used illicitly phencyclidine has been taken by mouth, sniffed, injected or smoked.

Numerous analogues of phencyclidine have been similarly abused and include PHP (rolicyclidine; 1-(1-phenylcyclohexyl)pyrrolidine), PCC (1-piperidinocyclohexanecarbonitrile), PCE (*N*-ethyl-1-phenylcyclohexylamine), and TCP (1-[1-(2-thienyl)cyclohexyl]piperidine).

Phenolsulphonphthalein (2145-n)

Phenolsulphonphthalein *(BAN).*

Fenolsolfonftaleina; Phenol Red; Phenolsulfonphthalein; Phenolsulfonphthaleinum; PSP. 4,4′-(3*H*-2,1-Benzoxathiol-3-ylidene)diphenol *S,S*-dioxide.

$C_{19}H_{14}O_5S$ = 354.4.

CAS — 143-74-8.

Pharmacopoeias. In *Chin., Eur.* (see p.viii), and *Jpn.*

A bright to dark red, crystalline powder. Very slightly **soluble** in water; slightly soluble in alcohol.

Adverse Effects and Precautions

Hypersensitivity reactions to phenolsulphonphthalein may occasionally occur. Excretion may be altered in patients with gout.

Interactions

Excretion of phenolsulphonphthalein may be affected in patients taking aminohippuric acid, atropine, penicillin, probenecid, salicylates, sulphinpyrazone, some sulphonamides, diuretics, or contrast media.

Pharmacokinetics

After intravenous injection, phenolsulphonphthalein is in part bound to plasma proteins, and in a patient with normal kidney function is rapidly excreted, mainly in the urine; some is excreted by the liver. Renal clearance is predominantly by tubular secretion, only a small amount being eliminated by glomerular filtration.

Uses and Administration

Phenolsulphonphthalein has been used as a test of renal function by estimating the rate of urinary excretion after intravenous administration. It has also been given intramuscularly.

Alkaline urine is coloured red to violet.

Phenolsulphonphthalein has also been used as a drug ingestion indicator, a marker in drug absorption studies, and in a test of residual urine.

Phenylpropanol (3737-w)

Ethyl Phenyl Carbinol; α-Hydroxypropylbenzene; SH-261. 1-Phenylpropan-1-ol; α-Ethylbenzyl alcohol.

$C_9H_{12}O$ = 136.2.

CAS — 93-54-9.

Pharmacopoeias. In *Chin.*

Phenylpropanol is a choleretic.

Preparations

Proprietary Preparations (details are given in Part 3)
Aust.: Gallenperlen.

Multi-ingredient: ***Aust.:*** Hedonin; ***Ger.:*** Medichol†.

Phloroglucinol (13104-c)

Phloroglucin. Benzene-1,3,5-triol.

$C_6H_6O_3$ = 126.1.

CAS — 108-73-6.

Pharmacopoeias. In *Fr.*

Phloroglucinol is used as an antispasmodic sometimes in combination with trimethylphloroglucinol.

Preparations

Proprietary Preparations (details are given in Part 3)
Fr.: Spasfon-Lyoc; ***Ital.:*** Spasmex.

Multi-ingredient: ***Belg.:*** Spasfon; ***Fr.:*** Foncitril; Meteoxane; Spasfon; ***Ital.:*** Spasmex.

Phosgene (13105-k)

Carbonyl Chloride; Chloroformyl Chloride.

$COCl_2$ = 98.92.

CAS — 75-44-5.

Adverse Effects

Poisoning may occur from industrial use or from the generation of phosgene from chlorinated compounds such as chloroform or carbon tetrachloride in the presence of heat. Symptoms of poisoning, which may be delayed for up to 24 hours, include burning of the eyes and throat, cough, dyspnoea, cyanosis, and pulmonary congestion and oedema. Death may result from anoxia. Exposure to 50 ppm may be rapidly fatal. Massive exposure may cause intravascular haemolysis, thrombus formation, and immediate death.

Treatment of Adverse Effects

After inhalation of phosgene or absorption from the skin, treatment consists of complete rest and the administration of oxygen. The mouth, eyes, nose, and skin should be irrigated with water; a 1% solution of sodium bicarbonate has also been advocated. Corticosteroids may reduce tissue damage. Antibacterials may reduce respiratory infections. Further treatment is symptomatic.

Uses and Administration

Phosgene is used in the chemical industry. It has been used as a war gas.

Phosphatidyl Choline (11497-w)

Phosphatidylcholine.

Phosphatidyl choline is a phospholipid and a constituent of lecithin (p.1595). Phosphatidyl choline is an ingredient of preparations that have been promoted for liver disorders, peripheral vascular disorders, and hyperlipidaemias.

Preparations

Proprietary Preparations (details are given in Part 3)
Ital.: Essentiale; Lipostabil; ***USA:*** PhosChol; Ultracholine†.

Multi-ingredient: ***Austral.:*** Tyroseng; ***Ital.:*** Essaven.

Phosphatidyl Serine (3918-z)

Phosphatidylserine.

Phosphatidyl serine is a phospholipid which has been tried in the treatment of organic psychiatric syndromes. It is under investigation as a cognition adjuvant. Phosphatidyl serine is a constituent of lecithin (p.1595).

References.

1. Amaducci L, *et al.* Phosphatidylserine in the treatment of Alzheimer's disease: results of a multicenter study. *Psychopharmacol Bull* 1988; **24:** 130–4.
2. Crook TH, *et al.* Effects of phosphatidylserine in age-associated memory impairment. *Neurology* 1991; **41:** 644–9.

Preparations

Proprietary Preparations (details are given in Part 3)
Ital.: Bros†; Keras†; Senefor; ***UK:*** Cognito.

Phosphoric Acid (1321-c)

Acido Fosfórico; Acidum Phosphoricum Concentratum; Concentrated Phosphoric Acid; E338; Orthophosphoric Acid; Phosph. Acid; Phosphorsäure.

H_3PO_4 = 98.00.

CAS — 7664-38-2.

Pharmacopoeias. In *Eur.* (see p.viii) (84 to 90%). Also in *USNF* (85 to 88%).

Odourless, clear, colourless, corrosive, syrupy liquid.

Miscible with water or alcohol. When stored at a low temperature it may solidify, forming a mass of colourless crystals which do not melt until the temperature reaches 28°. **Store** in airtight glass containers.

Dilute Phosphoric Acid (1322-k)

Acidum Phosphoricum Dilutum; Diluted Phosphoric Acid.

Pharmacopoeias. In *Eur.* (see p.viii) and *Pol.* Also in *USNF.*

Dilute Phosphoric Acid (Ph. Eur.) contains 9.5 to 10.5% w/w H_3PO_4 and may be prepared by mixing phosphoric acid 115 g with water 885 g. Diluted Phosphoric Acid (USNF) contains 9.5 to 10.5% w/w H_3PO_4 and may be prepared by mixing phosphoric acid 115 g with 885 g of water. **Store** in airtight containers.

Adverse Effects and Treatment

As for Hydrochloric Acid, p.1588.

Uses and Administration

Phosphoric acid has industrial uses. Dilute phosphoric acid has been used well diluted in preparations intended for the management of nausea and vomiting (p.1172). Phosphoric acid 35% gel has been used in dentistry to etch tooth enamel. In Great Britain, a technical grade of orthophosphoric acid 1 in 330 of water is an approved disinfectant for foot-and-mouth disease.

Phosphoric acid is used in homoeopathic medicine.

Preparations

USP 23: Sodium Fluoride and Phosphoric Acid Gel; Sodium Fluoride and Phosphoric Acid Topical Solution.

Proprietary Preparations (details are given in Part 3)

Multi-ingredient: ***Austral.:*** Anvatrol†; Emetrol; Floraquin; ***Belg.:*** Frubiase†; ***Fr.:*** Acti 5; Actiphos; Arphos; Biotone; Ionyl; Marinol; Phosoforme; Phosoveol Vitamine C†; Phosphoneuros; Pulmoserum; Triphosmag; ***Ger.:*** Alinda†; ***S.Afr.:*** Emetrol; Emex; ***Switz.:*** Frubiose Calcium; Phosoforme†; ***USA:*** Emecheck†; Emetrol; Naus-A-Way†.

Phosphorus (13106-a)

Fósforo; White Phosphorus; Yellow Phosphorus.

P = 30.973761.

CAS — 7723-14-0.

It is unstable in air and should be **stored** under water.

WARNING. *Phosphorus has been used for the illicit preparation of explosives or fireworks; care is required with its supply.*

Adverse Effects

Acute poisoning by phosphorus, a general protoplasmic poison, occurs in three distinct stages. The first stage represents local gastro-intestinal irritation with intense thirst, pain, nausea, vomiting, and diarrhoea. The breath may smell of garlic and vomitus and excreta are luminescent. Shock, delirium, convulsions, coma, and death may occur. In patients who survive, a second, asymptomatic stage may be present lasting for up to several days. The third stage represents systemic toxicity and is characterised by hepatic and renal damage, haemorrhage due to hypoprothrombinaemia and low fibrinogen concentrations, cardiovascular collapse, and CNS involvement including confusion, convulsions, and coma. Death may occur during either the first or third stages.

The fatal dose is about 1 mg per kg body-weight.

Symptoms of chronic poisoning are very slow in onset and are associated with lowered resistance to infection and defective tissue repair. They include periostitis and necrosis of the mandible ('phossy jaw').

Externally, phosphorus causes severe burns to the skin. Phosphorus is absorbed following skin contamination and systemic symptoms may occur.

Treatment of Adverse Effects

After ingestion of phosphorus the stomach should be washed out with copious amounts of water; a 1 in 5000 solution of potassium permanganate (very pale pink) or a 0.2% solution of copper sulphate have also been advocated.

Liquid paraffin may be introduced into the stomach following lavage and left there. The use of digestible fats and oils should be avoided.

Further treatment is symptomatic and supportive and may include: fluid and electrolyte replacement; blood transfusion or vitamin K to correct coagulation disorders; and management of convulsions and renal and hepatic dysfunctions. Treat burns by copious irrigation with water or a 1% copper sulphate solution.

Uses and Administration

Elemental phosphorus is no longer used in medicine. Inorganic phosphates are given in deficiency states and bone diseases (see Sodium Phosphate, p.1160). Phosphorus has been used in the manufacture of rat and cockroach poisons.

It is used in homoeopathic medicine.

Physalis (13109-r)

Alkekengi; Bladder Cherry; Chinese Lantern; Ground Cherry; Strawberry Tomato; Winter Cherry.

Pharmacopoeias. In *Chin.*

The berries of *Physalis alkekengi* (Solanaceae), reputed to have diuretic properties.

Cape gooseberry is the edible fruit of *P. peruviana.*

Picibanil (19659-q)

OK-432.

Picibanil, which is derived from *Streptococcus pyogenes,* is an immunomodulator which has been tried in the treatment of malignant neoplasms and viral infections.

References.

1. Shirai M, *et al.* Intratumoural injection of OK-432 and lymphokine-activated killer activity in peripheral blood of patients with hepatocellular carcinoma. *Eur J Cancer* 1990; **26:** 965–9.
2. Imarura T, *et al.* Intrapericardial OK-432 instillation for the management of malignant pericardial effusion. *Cancer* 1991; **68:** 259–63.
3. Tanaka N, *et al.* Intratumoral injection of a streptococcal preparation, OK-432, before surgery for gastric cancer: a randomized trial. *Cancer* 1994; **74:** 3097–3103.

Pidotimod (14649-e)

Pidotimod *(rINN).*

(*R*)-3-[(*S*)-5-Oxoprolyl]-4-thiazolidinecarboxylic acid.

$C_9H_{12}N_2O_4S$ = 244.3.

CAS — 121808-62-6.

Pidotimod is an immunostimulant used in patients with cell-mediated immunodepression during respiratory- and urinary-tract infections.

References.

1. Various. Pidotimod: a new biological response modifier. *Arzneimittelforschung* 1994; **44** (12a): 1399–1530.

Preparations

Proprietary Preparations (details are given in Part 3)
Ital.: Axil†; Onaka; Pigitil; Polimod.

Pinaverium Bromide (13119-d)

Pinaverium Bromide *(rINN).*

4-(6-Bromoveratryl)-4-{2-[2-(6,6-dimethyl-2-norpinyl)ethoxy]ethyl}morpholinium bromide.

$C_{26}H_{41}Br_2NO_4$ = 591.4.

CAS — 59995-65-2 (pinaverium); 53251-94-8 (pinaverium bromide).

Pinaverium bromide is a quaternary ammonium smooth muscle relaxant with some antimuscarinic-like effects. It is used as an antispasmodic.

Two patients experienced heartburn and dysphagia after taking pinaverium bromide by mouth between meals; endoscopy revealed acute oesophageal ulceration which healed on discontinuation of treatment.[1] The manufacturers recommendation to take pinaverium bromide during meals was emphasised.

1. André J-M, *et al.* Ulcères oesophagiens après prise de bromure de pinaverium. *Acta Endosc* 1980; **10:** 289–91.

Preparations

Proprietary Preparations (details are given in Part 3)
Aust.: Dicetel; ***Belg.:*** Dicetel; ***Canad.:*** Dicetel; ***Fr.:*** Dicetel; ***Ital.:*** Dicetel; ***Neth.:*** Dicetel; ***Spain:*** Eldicet; ***Switz.:*** Dicetel.

Pipoxolan (5240-n)

Pipoxolan *(BAN, pINN).*

5,5-Diphenyl-2-(2-piperidinoethyl)-1,3-dioxolan-4-one.

$C_{22}H_{25}NO_3$ = 351.4.

CAS — 23744-24-3 (pipoxolan); 18174-58-8 (pipoxolan hydrochloride).

NOTE. Pipoxolan Hydrochloride is *USAN.*

Pipoxolan is used as a smooth muscle relaxant. Pipoxolan hydrochloride has also been used.

Preparations

Proprietary Preparations (details are given in Part 3)
Ger.: Rowapraxin; ***Irl.:*** Rowapraxin.

Multi-ingredient: ***Irl.:*** Migranat; Rowacylat†.

Piprozolin (3738-e)

Piprozolin *(USAN, rINN).*

Gö-919; W-3699. Ethyl (3-ethyl-4-oxo-5-piperidinothiazolidin-2-ylidene)acetate.

$C_{14}H_{22}N_2O_3S$ = 298.4.

CAS — 17243-64-0.

Piprozolin is a choleretic.

Preparations

Proprietary Preparations (details are given in Part 3)
Ger.: Probilin†; ***Ital.:*** Probilin†; Secrebil†.

Piracetam (13124-x)

Piracetam *(BAN, USAN, rINN).*

CI-871; Pyrrolidone Acetamide; UCB-6215. 2-(2-Oxopyrrolidin-1-yl)acetamide.

$C_6H_{10}N_2O_2$ = 142.2.

CAS — 7491-74-9.

Pharmacopoeias. In *Fr.*

Adverse Effects and Precautions

Piracetam is reported to produce insomnia or somnolence, weight gain, nervousness, and depression. Diarrhoea and rashes may occur at a lower frequency. Piracetam should not be given to patients with hepatic dysfunction or severe renal impairment; dosage reductions are recommended for patients with lesser degrees of renal impairment. Therapy with piracetam should not be withdrawn abruptly.

Interactions

Anticoagulants. Prothrombin time was increased in a patient stabilised on warfarin when treatment with piracetam was started.[1]

1. Pan HYM, Ng RP. The effect of Nootropil in a patient on warfarin. *Eur J Clin Pharmacol* 1983; **24:** 711.

Uses and Administration

Piracetam acts on the CNS and has been described as a 'nootropic' and is said to protect the cerebral cortex against hypoxia. It is used as an adjunct in the treatment of myoclonus of cortical origin. It has also been used in dementia. Other so-called cerebro-cortical insufficiency disorders or states in which it has been tried include after trauma or surgery, alcoholism, vertigo, cerebrovascular accidents, and behavioural disorders in children.

Piracetam has been given for cerebro-cortical insufficiency disorders in doses of 800 to 1000 mg three times daily by mouth. In severe disorders it has been given by intramuscular or intravenous injection. In myoclonus, piracetam is given in doses of 7.2 g daily increasing by 4.8 g per day every 3 to 4 days up to a maximum of 20 g daily. It is given by mouth in 2 or 3 divided doses. Once the optimal dose of piracetam has been established, attempts should be made to reduce the dose of concurrent therapy.

Piracetam is reported to inhibit platelet aggregation and reduce blood viscosity at high doses.

References to the effects of piracetam on the blood.

1. Moriam M, *et al.* Platelet anti-aggregant and rheological properties of piracetam: a pharmacodynamic study in normal subjects. *Arzneimittelforschung* 1993; **43:** 110–18.

Neurological disorders. DEMENTIA. Although piracetam has been used in the treatment of senile dementia[1] and Alzheimer's disease[2] (p.1386) there is little convincing evidence of efficacy.

1. Kendall MJ, *et al.* Therapeutic progress—review XVIII: Alzheimer's disease. *J Clin Hosp Pharm* 1985; **10:** 327–36.
2. Croisile B, *et al.* Long-term and high-dose piracetam treatment of Alzheimer's disease. *Neurology* 1993; **43:** 301–5.

MYOCLONUS. In a review[1] of case reports (62), open studies (3), and double-blind studies (2), the authors concluded that piracetam is beneficial in the treatment of disabling myoclonus (p.338) either as adjunctive treatment or as monotherapy.

1. Van Vleymen B, Van Zandijcke M. Piracetam in the treatment of myoclonus: an overview. *Acta Neurol Belg* 1996; **96:** 270–80.

Preparations

Proprietary Preparations (details are given in Part 3)
Aust.: Cerebryl; Nootropil; Pirabene; ***Belg.:*** Braintop; Geratam; Noodis; Nootropil; ***Fr.:*** Axonyl; Gabacet; Geram; Nootropyl; ***Ger.:*** Avigilen; Cerebroforte; Cerebrosteril†; Cerepar N; Cuxabrain; durapitrop; Encetrop; Memo-Puren; Nootrop; Normabrain; Novocetam; Piracebral; Piracetrop; Sinapsan; ***Ital.:*** Cerebropan; Cetam†; Cleveral; Flavis; Nootropil; Norzetam; Psycoton; ***Neth.:*** Nootropil; ***S.Afr.:*** Nootropil; ***Spain:*** Ciclofalina; Genogris; Nootropil; ***Switz.:*** Nootropil; ***UK:*** Nootropil.

Multi-ingredient: ***Spain:*** Anacervix; Devincal; Diemil; Memorino; Peobe†; Piracetam Complex.

Pirenoxine Sodium (13131-t)

Pirenoxine Sodium *(rINNM).*

Catalin Sodium; Pirfenoxone Sodium. Sodium 1-hydroxy-5-oxo-5*H*-pyrido[3,2-*a*]phenoxazine-3-carboxylate.

$C_{16}H_7N_2NaO_5$ = 330.2.

CAS — 1043-21-6 (pirenoxine); 51410-30-1 (pirenoxine sodium).

Pharmacopoeias. Jpn includes Pirenoxine.

Pirenoxine sodium has been used in the treatment of cataracts, usually as eye drops.

Preparations

Proprietary Preparations (details are given in Part 3)
Ger.: Clarvisor; ***Ital.:*** Clarvisan; Pirfalin; ***Spain:*** Clarvisan.

Pirfenidone (6383-n)

Pirfenidone *(USAN, rINN).*

AMR-69. 5-Methyl-1-phenyl-2(1*H*)-pyridone.

$C_{12}H_{11}NO$ = 185.2.

CAS — 53179-13-8.

Pirfenidone is an antifibrotic drug under investigation in fibrosing disorders such as idiopathic pulmonary fibrosis and in multiple sclerosis.

Pirglutargine (13132-x)

Arginine Pidolate; Arginine Pyroglutamate. L-Arginine DL-pyroglutamate.

$C_{11}H_{21}N_5O_5$ = 303.3.

CAS — 64855-91-0.

Pirglutargine has been used for its reputed cerebral stimulant effect.

Preparations

Proprietary Preparations (details are given in Part 3)
Ital.: Adiuvant.

Multi-ingredient: ***Ital.:*** Detoxergon.

Piridoxilate (13133-r)

Piridoxilate *(BAN, rINN).*

Pyridoxine α_5-Hemiacetal Glyoxylate; Pyridoxylate. The reciprocal salt of 2-(5-hydroxy-4-hydroxymethyl-6-methyl-3-pyridylmethoxy)glycolic acid with 2-[4,5-bis(hydroxymethyl)-2-methyl-3-pyridyloxy]glycolic acid (1:1).

$C_{10}H_{13}NO_6,C_{10}H_{13}NO_6$ = 486.4.

CAS — 24340-35-0.

Piridoxilate was formerly used in the treatment of various circulatory disorders.

Pirisudanol Maleate (13192-s)

Pirisudanol Maleate *(rINNM).*

Pyrisuccideanol Maleate. 2-Dimethylaminoethyl 5-hydroxy-4-hydroxymethyl-6-methyl-3-pyridylmethyl succinate maleate.

$C_{16}H_{24}N_2O_6,(C_4H_4O_4)_2$ = 572.5.

CAS — 33605-94-6 (pirisudanol); 53659-00-0 (pirisudanol maleate).

Pirisudanol is the succinic acid ester of pyridoxine and of deanol.

Pirisudanol has been given as the maleate in the treatment of cerebrovascular and similar disorders in doses of up to 1200 mg daily.

Preparations

Proprietary Preparations (details are given in Part 3)
Belg.: Nadex; ***Fr.:*** Stivane; ***Ital.:*** Mentium; ***Spain:*** Mentis; ***Switz.:*** Nadex.

Pitofenone Hydrochloride (5241-h)

Pitofenone Hydrochloride *(rINNM).*

Methyl 2-[4-(2-piperidinoethoxy)benzoyl]benzoate hydrochloride.

$C_{22}H_{25}NO_4,HCl$ = 403.9.

CAS — 54063-52-4 (pitofenone); 1248-42-6 (pitofenone hydrochloride).

Pitofenone hydrochloride has been used as an antispasmodic.

Preparations

Proprietary Preparations (details are given in Part 3)

Multi-ingredient: ***Aust.:*** Baralgin†; ***Belg.:*** Baralgin†; ***Fr.:*** Baralgine†; ***Ital.:*** Baralgina†; ***S.Afr.:*** Baralgan†; ***Spain:*** Baralgin†; ***Switz.:*** Baralgine†.

Plastics (13141-r)

Pharmacopoeias. Many pharmacopoeias include standards for plastic containers and closures.

Adverse Effects

Plastic materials used in medicine and pharmacy may give rise to various adverse effects, either by direct contact of the plastic with tissues or by indirect contact as when a solution stored in a plastic container, such as a disposable syringe, is injected. Adverse effects may also arise among workers through handling the materials or by inhaling fumes during manufacture.

Pure polymeric plastics appear to be of low toxicity, though carcinogenic effects have been produced by prolonged implantation of some pure plastics. However, some monomers are toxic, as may be substances added during manufacture to impart specific physical properties. These additives include plasticisers added to reduce brittleness, ultraviolet-ray absorbers to prevent degradation by light, and antioxidants and lubricants which are sometimes needed for satisfactory processing. Monomer residues or additives can leach out from the finished plastic materials, have been the main causes of adverse effects. These may include haemolysis of blood cells, thrombosis, hypersensitivity reactions, precancerous changes, and local tissue necrosis. Silicone particles have been shed from dialysis tubing resulting in hypersplenism, pancytopenia, and occasionally in the production of a granulomatous hepatitis.

See also under Vinyl Chloride, p.1644, Methylmethacrylate, p.1603, and Polytef, below.

Polacrilin Potassium (5006-j)

Polacrilin Potassium *(USAN, rINNM).*

Polacrilinum Kalii.

CAS — 54182-62-6 (polacrilin); 50602-21-6 (polacrilin).

Pharmacopoeias. In *USNF.*

The potassium salt of a carboxylic cation-exchange resin prepared from methacrylic acid and divinylbenzene. An odourless or almost odourless, white to off-white, free-flowing powder. Practically **insoluble** in water and in most liquids.

Polacrilin potassium is used as a tablet disintegrant.

Poly A.poly U (13143-d)

Polyadenylic-polyuridylic Acid.

CAS — 24936-38-7.

Poly A.poly U is a double-stranded polyribonucleotide comprising polyadenylic and polyuridylic acids, and is believed to be a stimulant of the immune system. It has been studied as an adjuvant in the management of operable solid tumours.

Poly I.poly C (13144-n)

Polyinosinic-polycytidylic Acid.

CAS — 24939-03-5.

Poly I.poly C is a synthetic double-stranded polyribonucleotide complex of equimolar concentrations of polyinosinic and polycytidylic acids, described as a mismatched double-strand RNA.

Poly I.poly C and the complex of poly I.poly C stabilised with poly-L-lysine in carboxymethylcellulose [poly(ICLC)] have been found to induce the production of interferon and have been investigated in the treatment of malignant neoplasms and viral infections. Poly(ICLC) has orphan drug status in the USA for the treatment of primary brain tumours.

Preparations

Proprietary Preparations (details are given in Part 3)
USA: Ampligen.

Polysaccharide-K (3850-e)

PSK; PS-K.

A protein-bound polysaccharide isolated from a fungus and claimed to have immunostimulant and antineoplastic properties.

References:

1. Tsukagoshi S, *et al.* Krestin (PSK). *Cancer Treat Rev* 1984; **11:** 131–55.
2. Go P, Chung C-H. Adjuvant PSK immunotherapy in patients with carcinoma of the nasopharynx. *J Int Med Res* 1989; **17:** 141–9.
3. Torisu M, *et al.* Significant prolongation of disease-free period gained by oral polysaccharide K (PSK) administration after curative surgical operation of colorectal cancer. *Cancer Immunol Immunother* 1990; **31:** 261–8.
4. Nakazato H, *et al.* Efficacy of immunochemotherapy as adjuvant treatment after curative resection of gastric cancer. *Lancet* 1994; **343:** 1122–6.

Preparations

Proprietary Preparations (details are given in Part 3)
Jpn: Krestin†.

Polytef (13150-f)

Polytef *(USAN)*.
Politef *(pINN)*; PTFE. Poly(tetrafluoroethylene).
$(C_2F_4)_n$.
CAS — 9002-84-0.

Polytef has numerous industrial applications. As 'Teflon' it is used on 'non-stick' cooking utensils.

A paste of polytef has been used for a variety of purposes including the treatment of aphonia, for replacement grafts in vascular surgery, and in the correction of some forms of urinary incontinence (p.454). The main concern with these procedures is migration of polytef particles.

Adverse effects. Brain injury in a child was possibly associated with migration of polytef particles from a periureteral injection performed 1 year earlier.[1]

1. Borgatti R, *et al.* Brain injury in a healthy child one year after periureteral injection of Teflon. *Pediatrics* 1996; **98:** 290–1.

Uses. References.

1. O'Donnell B, Puri P. Endoscopic correction of primary vesicoureteric reflux: results in 94 ureters. *Br Med J* 1986; **293:** 1404–6.
2. Puri P. Endoscopic correction of primary vesicoureteric reflux by subureteric injection of polytetrafluoroethylene. *Lancet* 1990; **335:** 1320–2.
3. Maskell R, *et al.* Correction of vesicoureteric reflux by endoscopic injection. *Lancet* 1991; **338:** 1460–1.
4. Kidson IG. Prosthetic implants: arterial prostheses. *Br J Hosp Med* 1983; **30:** 248–54.
5. Schulman CC, *et al.* Endoscopic injections of Teflon to treat urinary incontinence in women. *Br Med J* 1984; **288:** 192.
6. Polley JW, *et al.* The use of Teflon in orbital floor reconstruction following blunt facial trauma: a 20-year experience. *Plast Reconstr Surg* 1987; **79:** 39–43.
7. Anonymous. Use of Teflon preparations for urinary incontinence and vesicoureteral reflux. *JAMA* 1993; **269:** 2975–80.

Poplar Buds (8199-k)

Balm of Gilead Buds.

The buds of various species of *Populus*, including *P. nigra*, *P. candicans*, *P. gileadensis*, and *P. tacamahacca* (*P. balsamifera*) have been used for the analgesic properties conveyed by their salicin content, as well as in preparations for a variety of other disorders. They also contain volatile oil, resin, and other substances. The resin from poplar buds is one of the major sources of propolis (p.1621).

Preparations

Proprietary Preparations (details are given in Part 3)

Multi-ingredient: ***Aust.:*** Phytodolor; Prostagutt; ***Austral.:*** Valerian; ***Canad.:*** Mielocol; Wampole Bronchial Cough Syrup; ***Ger.:*** Carito†; Eviprostat N; Phytodolor; Prostagutt Tropfen†; Prostamed; Salus Kurbis-Tonikum Compositum†; ***Switz.:*** Eviprostat; Phytomed Prosta; ***UK:*** Balm of Gilead; Ligvites; Peerless Composition Essence; Tabritis.

Poppy-seed Oil (7365-q)

Huile d'Oeillette; Maw Oil; Oleum Papaveris; Oleum Papaveris Seminis.

The fixed oil expressed from the ripe seeds of the opium poppy, *Papaver somniferum* (Papaveraceae).

Poppy-seed oil is used as a substitute for olive oil for culinary and pharmaceutical purposes. It is also used in the preparation of Iodised Oil Fluid Injection (BP 1998). Commercial grades are used in making soaps, paints, and varnishes.

Preparations

Proprietary Preparations (details are given in Part 3)

Multi-ingredient: ***Ger.:*** Reflex-Zonen-Salbe (RZS) (Rowo-333)†.

Potassium Aminobenzoate (7872-m)

Aminobenzoate Potassium. Potassium 4-aminobenzoate.
$C_7H_6KNO_2$ = 175.2.
CAS — 138-84-1.
Pharmacopoeias. In *US.*

A white crystalline powder. Very **soluble** in water; soluble in alcohol; practically insoluble in ether. A 1% solution in water has pH of about 7, while a 5% solution has a pH of 8 to 9. **Store** in airtight containers.

Adverse Effects and Precautions

Anorexia, nausea, fever, and skin rash have been reported.

Potassium aminobenzoate should be given with caution to patients with renal impairment.

Interactions

Potassium aminobenzoate will inactivate sulphonamides given concurrently.

Uses and Administration

Potassium aminobenzoate has been used in the treatment of various disorders associated with excessive fibrosis, such as scleroderma (p.501) and Peyronie's disease. The usual dose is 12 g daily in 4 to 6 divided doses.

Peyronie's disease. Variable results have been achieved with potassium aminobenzoate in the treatment of Peyronie's disease.[1,2] It has been suggested that a successful response is more likely if treatment is commenced in the acute stage.[2]

1. Gingell JC, Desai KM. Peyronie's disease. *Br Med J* 1988; **298:** 1489–90.
2. Mohanty KC, Strachan RG. Peyronie's disease. *Br Med J* 1989; **298:** 254.

Preparations

USP 23: Aminobenzoate Potassium Capsules; Aminobenzoate Potassium for Oral Solution; Aminobenzoate Potassium Tablets.

Proprietary Preparations (details are given in Part 3)
Aust.: Potaba; ***Canad.:*** Potaba; ***Ger.:*** Potaba; ***Switz.:*** Potaba; ***UK:*** Potaba; ***USA:*** Potaba.

Multi-ingredient: *USA:* Pabalate-SF†.

Potassium Borotartrate (13152-n)

Potassium Sodium Borotartrate; Soluble Cream of Tartar.

Potassium borotartrate is reported to have similar properties to those of bromides. It has been used in nervous disorders and is used in photography as a retarder for alkaline developers. Chronic boron poisoning (see under Boric Acid, p.1554) has been reported following the use of potassium borotartrate internally.

Preparations

Proprietary Preparations (details are given in Part 3)
Fr.: Neurobore Pur†.

Multi-ingredient: ***Fr.:*** Dinacode.

Potassium Bromate (13153-h)

924.
$KBrO_3$ = 167.0.
CAS — 7758-01-2.

Adverse Effects

Ingestion of potassium bromate is followed by nausea, vomiting, severe abdominal pain, and diarrhoea. Deafness may also occur. The patient becomes apathetic or lethargic but very irritable; loss of consciousness, central nervous depression, and loss of tendon reflexes ensue, but convulsions may occur. Methaemoglobinaemia may possibly occur rarely. Kidney damage, with albuminuria and oliguria or anuria may arise. Respiration becomes shallow and rapid, the heart rate increases, and the blood pressure falls. Death from renal failure may occur within 1 to 2 weeks.

Potassium bromate is carcinogenic in *animals*.

Reports of bromate poisoning.

1. Lue JN, *et al.* Bromate poisoning from ingestion of professional hair-care neutralizer. *Clin Pharm* 1988; **7:** 66–70.
2. Lichtenberg R, *et al.* Bromate poisoning. *J Pediatr* 1989; **114:** 891–4.

Treatment of Adverse Effects

After the ingestion of potassium bromate the stomach should be emptied by lavage. Thiosulphate solutions have been used for lavage, although there is a view that they should not be left in the stomach as hydrogen sulphide may be evolved. Pain is relieved by the injection of pethidine. An intravenous infusion of 100 to 500 mL of a 1% sodium thiosulphate solution or intravenous injection of 1 mL per kg body-weight of a 10% solution has sometimes been given. Attention to the patient's fluid, acid-base, and electrolyte status is important and acute renal failure may require treatment with fluids and diuretics. Oxygen may be indicated.

The prompt use of haemodialysis or peritoneal dialysis has been suggested.

The use of intravenous sodium thiosulphate for the treatment of bromate poisoning has been questioned.[1]

1. McElwee NE, Kearney TE. Sodium thiosulfate unproven as bromate antidote. *Clin Pharm* 1988; **7:** 570–2.

Uses

Potassium bromate is an oxidising agent. It has no therapeutic uses but it has been widely used as the 'neutraliser' of thioglycollate hair-waving lotions. It has been used in the preparation of barley malt for beer. It has also been used as a flour-maturing agent but such use is no longer considered appropriate and is prohibited in some countries.

Potassium bromate is a genotoxic carcinogen and should not be present in foods as consumed. Its use for the treatment of flour for bread-making is not appropriate.

1. FAO/WHO. Evaluation of certain food additives and contaminants: forty-fourth report of the joint FAO/WHO expert committee on food additives. *WHO Tech Rep Ser 859* 1995.

Potassium Bromide (1026-s)

Brometo de Potássio; Bromure de Potassium; Kalii Bromidum; Kalium Bromatum; Pot. Brom.; Potassii Bromidum.
KBr = 119.0.
CAS — 7758-02-3.
Pharmacopoeias. In *Chin., Eur.* (see p.viii), *Jpn,* and *Pol.*

Colourless crystals or a white crystalline powder. Each g represents 8.4 mmol of potassium and of bromide.

Freely **soluble** in water and in glycerol; slightly soluble in alcohol.

Adverse Effects

During prolonged exposure bromide accumulation may occur giving rise to bromide intoxication or bromism. Symptoms include nausea and vomiting, slurred speech, memory impairment, drowsiness, irritability, ataxia, tremors, hallucinations, mania, delirium, psychoses, stupor, coma, and other manifestations of central nervous system depression. Skin rashes of various types may occur and toxic epidermal necrolysis has been reported. Death after acute poisoning appears to be rare as vomiting follows the ingestion of large doses.

There have been reports of neonatal bromide intoxication and growth defects associated with maternal bromide ingestion during pregnancy. Symptoms of bromide intoxication have also been reported in breast-fed infants whose mothers were taking bromides.

Treatment of Adverse Effects

In acute poisoning the stomach should be emptied by emesis (if this has not already occurred) or lavage, and sodium chloride should be given by intravenous infusion. Glucose may also be administered and frusemide may be given to aid diuresis.

In chronic poisoning, bromide administration is stopped and sodium chloride, up to 2 to 3 g three or four times daily, is given by mouth with adequate amounts of fluid. Ammonium chloride has been given but is no longer recommended as it may precipitate metabolic acidosis. Diuretics are of value. In severe cases of bromide intoxication or when the usual treatments cannot be used, haemodialysis may be of value.

Pharmacokinetics

Bromides are readily absorbed from the gastro-intestinal tract. They displace chloride in extracellular body fluids and have a half-life in the body of about 12 days. They may be detected in the milk of nursing mothers and in the fetus.

Uses and Administration

Bromides depress the central nervous system. Potassium bromide has been used as a sedative and anticonvulsant but has generally been replaced by more effective less toxic agents. Ammonium, calcium, sodium, and strontium bromide have been used similarly, as have bromoform and dilute hydrobromic acid. They have also been used in multi-ingredient preparations for the treatment of coughs.

Potassium bromide has been used in homoeopathic medicine.

Preparations

Proprietary Preparations (details are given in Part 3)
Belg.: Bromofotyl†; ***Ger.:*** Dibro-Be Mono.

Multi-ingredient: ***Belg.:*** Babygencal; Captol†; Eucalyptine Le Brun; Eucalyptine Pholcodine Le Brun; Inalpin; Normogastryl; Pectocalmine Baby†; ***Fr.:*** Aerophagyl†; Campho-Pneumine Aminophylline†; Campho-Pneumine†; Curibronches†; Desbly†; Dinacode; Eucalyptine Le Brun; Galirene; Lyptocodine; Neurocalcium; Nican†; Passedyl; Pectosan; Pectospir†; Pectovox†; Pneumopan; Polery; Pulmosodyl; Pulmothiol†; Quintopan Adult; Sedatif Tiber; Sirop Adrian a la pholcodine adulte†; Sirop Adrian a la pholcodine enfant†; Sirop Pectoral adulte; Sirop Pectoral enfant; Sirop Teyssedre†; Tuberol†; Vermifuge; ***Ger.:*** Antisacer comp.†; Priatan†; Silvapin Brombaldrianbad†; ***Ital.:*** Bromocodeina†; Bronchised†; Fertomcidina-U†; Neo Soluzione Sulfo Balsamica; Neurobiol; ***S.Afr.:*** Bronchicum; ***Spain:*** Medecitral; Otogen†; Stomosan; Topico Denticion Vera; ***Switz.:*** Neo-Codion Adultes†; Neo-Codion Enfants†; Neo-Codion Nourrissons†.

Potassium Chlorate (318-y)

Kalium Chloricum; Potassii Chloras.
$KClO_3$ = 122.5.
CAS — 3811-04-9.
Pharmacopoeias. In *Belg.* and *Swiss.*

CAUTION. *Potassium chlorate is unstable and, in contact with organic or readily oxidisable substances such as charcoal, phosphorus, or sulphur it is liable to explode especially if heated or subjected to friction or percussion. It should not be allowed to come into contact with matches or surfaces containing phosphorus compounds. Reasonable steps should be taken before supplying potassium chlorate to ensure that it will not be used for the illicit preparation of explosives or fireworks.*

Potassium chlorate has been used as an astringent, usually as a mouthwash or gargle. Concentrated solutions are irritant.

Acute poisoning from ingestion requires prompt symptomatic treatment. Symptoms include nausea, vomiting, diarrhoea, abdominal pain, haemolytic anaemia, haemorrhage, methaemoglobinaemia, and renal failure. There may be liver damage and central effects with convulsions and coma.

If methaemoglobinaemia is severe, poisoned patients may require exchange transfusion with whole blood; the use of methylene blue should be avoided as it may enhance toxicity.

Preparations

Proprietary Preparations (details are given in Part 3)

Multi-ingredient: ***Belg.:*** Tablettes pour la Gorge Medica†; ***Canad.:*** Fletchers Sore Mouth Medicine; ***Fr.:*** Pastaba†; Pastilles M.B.C†; ***Ger.:*** Gargarisma; ***Spain:*** Cloroboral; Solurrinol; Tyroneomicin; Tyropenicilin R†.

Potassium Hydroxide (211-h)

525; Ätzkali; Caustic Potash; Kalii Hydroxidum; Kalii Hydroxydum; Kalium Hydroxydatum; Potash Lye.

KOH = 56.11.

CAS — 1310-58-3.

Pharmacopoeias. In *Eur.* (see p.viii) and *Jpn.* Also in *USNF.*

White, crystalline, deliquescent sticks, pellets, or irregular masses. It rapidly absorbs moisture and carbon dioxide.

Soluble or almost completely soluble 1 in 1 of water, 1 in 3 of alcohol, and 1 in 2.5 of glycerol; very soluble in boiling alcohol. **Store** in airtight, non-metallic containers.

Adverse Effects

The ingestion of caustic alkalis causes immediate burning pain in the mouth, throat, substernal region, and epigastrium, and the lining membranes become swollen and detached. There is dysphagia, hypersalivation, vomiting with the vomitus becoming blood-stained, diarrhoea, and shock. In severe cases, asphyxia due to oedema of the glottis, circulatory failure, oesophageal or gastric perforation, peritonitis, or pneumonia may occur. Stricture of the oesophagus can develop weeks or months later.

Caustic alkalis on contact with the eyes cause conjunctival oedema and corneal destruction.

Treatment of Adverse Effects

Ingestion should not be treated by lavage or emesis. Give copious drinks of water and follow this with demulcents. Maintain an airway and alleviate shock and pain.

Contaminated skin and eyes should be flooded immediately with water and the washing continued for about 30 minutes. Any affected clothing should be removed while flooding is being carried out.

Uses and Administration

Potassium hydroxide is a powerful caustic which has been used to remove warts (see p.1076). A 2.5% solution in glycerol has been used as a cuticle solvent. An escharotic preparation of potassium hydroxide and calcium hydroxide was known as Vienna paste.

Preparations

BP 1998: Chloroxylenol Solution *(Roxenol)*; Potassium Hydroxide Solution *(Potash Solution)*.

Proprietary Preparations (details are given in Part 3)
Spain: Cerumenol; Kuson.

Multi-ingredient: ***Aust.:*** Leberinfusion; ***Ger.:*** Acarex; Glutarsin E; Kalium-Magnesium-Asparaginat; KMA; Sekudrill; ***Ital.:*** Sekudrill; ***S.Afr.:*** Peter Pote's†; ***UK:*** Acarex†.

Potassium Hydroxyquinoline Sulphate (1630-g)

Oxyquinol Potassium; Potassii Hydroxyquinolini Sulphas; Potassium Oxyquinoline Sulphate.

Pharmacopoeias. In *Aust.*, *Br.*, and *Fr.*

An equimolecular mixture of potassium sulphate and quinolin-8-ol sulphate monohydrate. A pale yellow odourless or almost odourless microcrystalline powder. Freely **soluble** in water; practically insoluble in ether.

Potassium hydroxyquinoline sulphate has antibacterial, antifungal, and deodorant properties and is used, often in conjunction with benzoyl peroxide, in the topical treatment of fungal infections, minor bacterial infections, and acne.

Preparations

BP 1998: Potassium Hydroxyquinoline Sulphate and Benzoyl Peroxide Cream.

Proprietary Preparations (details are given in Part 3)

Multi-ingredient: ***Belg.:*** Aseptosyl; ***Irl.:*** Quinocort; Quinoderm; Valderma; ***S.Afr.:*** Auralgicin; Oto-Phen Forte; Quinoderm-H; Quinoderm†; Universal Earache Drops; ***Spain:*** Stoma Anestesia Dental; ***Switz.:*** Quinoderm; Quinoderm Hydrocortisone†; Rectoseptal-Neo bismuthe; Rectoseptal-Neo simple; ***UK:*** Quinocort; Quinoderm; Quinoderm with Hydrocortisone†; Quinoped; Valderma Cream.

Potassium Metaphosphate (1182-r)

E450(c); Potassium Kurrol's Salt; Potassium Polymetaphosphate.

$(KPO_3)_x$.

CAS — 7790-53-6.

Pharmacopoeias. In *USNF.*

A straight-chain polyphosphate, having a high degree of polymerisation, containing the equivalent of 59 to 61% of P_2O_5. It is a white odourless powder. Practically **insoluble** in water; soluble in dilute solutions of sodium salts.

Potassium metaphosphate is used as a buffer.

Pramiracetam Sulphate (16967-a)

Pramiracetam Sulphate *(rINNM)*.

Amacetam Sulphate; CI-879; Pramiracetam Sulfate *(USAN)*. *N*-[2-(Diisopropylamino)ethyl]-2-oxo-1-pyrrolidineacetamide sulphate.

$C_{14}H_{27}N_3O_2,H_2SO_4$ = 367.5.

CAS — 68497-62-1 (pramiracetam); 72869-16-0 (pramiracetam sulphate).

Pramiracetam sulphate is used in age-related memory impairment and senile dementia (p.1386), in doses equivalent to 600 mg of pramiracetam twice daily by mouth. It has also been tried, without much success, as an adjunct to electroconvulsive therapy in severe depression.

References.

1. Chang T, *et al.* Pharmacokinetics of oral pramiracetam in normal volunteers. *J Clin Pharmacol* 1985; **25:** 291–5.
2. Dejong R. Safety of pramiracetam. *Curr Ther Res* 1987; **41:** 254–7.
3. Scarpazza P, *et al.* Multicenter evaluation of pramiracetam for the treatment of memory impairment of probable vascular origin. *Adv Therapy* 1993; **10:** 217–25.

Preparations

Proprietary Preparations (details are given in Part 3)
Ital.: Neupramir; Pramistar; Remen.

Pramiverine Hydrochloride (5242-m)

Pramiverine Hydrochloride *(BANM, rINNM)*.

EMD-9806 (pramiverine); HSP-2986 (pramiverine). *N*-Isopropyl-4,4-diphenylcyclohexylamine hydrochloride.

$C_{21}H_{27}N,HCl$ = 329.9.

CAS — 14334-40-8 (pramiverine); 14334-41-9 (pramiverine hydrochloride).

Pramiverine hydrochloride has been used as an antispasmodic.

Preparations

Proprietary Preparations (details are given in Part 3)

Multi-ingredient: ***Ital.:*** Sistalgin Compositum†; ***Spain:*** Syntaverin†.

Pregnancy and Fertility Tests (1959-p)

There are a number of kits available for simple pregnancy and fertility testing. A common method of detecting pregnancy is to use specific antibodies to measure the increase in chorionic gonadotrophin in the urine. The period of ovulation can be detected by measuring luteinising hormone excretion in similar ways.

These tests can give false results. Those carrying out the tests should be aware of this and of problems such as contaminated specimens, concomitant drug therapy, or other factors that could affect the result.

Preparations

Proprietary Preparations (details are given in Part 3)
Austral.: Clearblue One Step; Clearblue†; Clearplan One Step; Clearview HCG; Discover Onestep; Discover-2†; Easy hCG†; Evaplan; Evatest One Step; First Response; Gonavislide†; Neo-Planotest Duoclon; Neo-Pregnosticon; Planosec†; Predictor; Pregcolor†; Pregnosis; Preview Urine†; Simplicity Plus†; UCG-Beta†; UCG-Slide†; ***Canad.:*** Answer Now; Clearblue; Clearplan; Conceive; Confidelle; Confirm; Denco†; Fact Plus; First Response; Pregnosis†; UCG-Beta†; ***Fr.:*** Bluetest; Clearblue; Clearplan; Discretest†; Elle-Test Beta†; G.Test; Indicatest; Predictor; Revelatest; ***Irl.:*** Fertility Score; Prepurex†; Testpack hCG-Urine; ***Ital.:*** Clearblue Monofase; Clearplan; Confidelle Progress; Diagnosis; Discretest†; Neo-Gravidtest†; PG 53; Predictor; Prevision†; Rivela; ***Jpn:*** Gonacard†; Gonavis†; New-Gonavislide†; ***S.Afr.:*** Event Test Strip HCG; Gonavislide; Planosec†; Pregcolor; Pregstik; Prepurex†; ***Switz.:*** LH-Color†; ***UK:*** Auratek hCG; Clearblue; Clearplan; Clearview HCG; Concept Blue; Concise; Confirm†; Directaclone CG†; Discover; Discretest†; Early Bird; Easy Check†; Fact Plus†; First Response; Gravindex†; HCG-Nostick†; Neo-Planotest; Organon LH Color†; Ovukit; Ovuquick; Predictor; Pregna-Cert; Pregna-Sure HCG; Pregnospia Duoclon; Pregnosticon Planotest†; Pregnosticon 'All In'†; Pregstik†; Prepurex; Ramp; Reveal; Tandem Icon; Test Pack Plus; ***USA:*** Advance; Answer; Clearblue Easy; Clearplan Easy; Clearview HCG†; Conceive Ovulation Predictor; Conceive Pregnancy; Daisy; ept Stick Test; Fact Plus; First Response; Fortel; HCG-Nostick†; Nimbus; One-Step hCG†; OvuGen; Ovukit; Ovuquick; Pregnosis; QTest; QTest Ovulation; QuickVue; RapidVue; TestPack Plus hCG-Urine; UCG-Slide; Unistep hCG.

Prenylamine Lactate (9275-r)

Prenylamine Lactate *(BANM, rINNM)*.

B-436 (prenylamine); Hoechst-12512 (prenylamine); Prenylaminii Lactas. 2-Benzhydrylethyl(α-methylphenethyl)amine lactate.

$C_{24}H_{27}N,C_3H_6O_3$ = 419.6.

CAS — 69-43-2 (prenylamine lactate); 390-64-7 (prenylamine).

NOTE. Prenylamine is *USAN*

Pharmacopoeias. In *Pol.*

Prenylamine depletes myocardial catecholamine stores and has some calcium-channel blocking activity. It was formerly used in the treatment of angina pectoris (p.780) but has been superseded by less toxic drugs. Administration of prenylamine has been associated with the development of ventricular arrhythmias and ECG abnormalities. Tremor and extrapyramidal symptoms have also occurred.

Proadifen Hydrochloride (13169-w)

Proadifen Hydrochloride *(USAN, rINNM)*.

NSC-39690; Propyladiphenine Hydrochloride; RP-5171; SKF-525A; SKF-525-A. 2-Diethylaminoethyl 2,2-diphenylvalerate hydrochloride.

$C_{23}H_{31}NO_2,HCl$ = 390.0.

CAS — 302-33-0 (proadifen); 62-68-0 (proadifen hydrochloride).

Proadifen has been found to enhance the effects of a large number of drugs, possibly by inhibiting metabolism.

Procodazole (13172-v)

Procodazole *(rINN)*.

3-(Benzimidazol-2-yl)propionic acid.

$C_{10}H_{10}N_2O_2$ = 190.2.

CAS — 23249-97-0.

Procodazole is reported to have immunostimulant properties. It is given as the ethyl ester. The sodium salt has also been used.

Preparations

Proprietary Preparations (details are given in Part 3)
Spain: Estimulocel.

Promelase (8399-h)

Promelase *(pINN)*.

Seaprose S.

CAS — 9074-07-1.

An alkaline protease derived from *Aspergillus melleus*. It has been taken by mouth in doses of 30 to 90 mg daily for its supposed benefit in oedema and inflammation associated with trauma, infection, and surgical procedures.

Preparations

Proprietary Preparations (details are given in Part 3)
Ital.: Altan; Flaminase; Mezen; ***Jpn:*** Onoprose.

Propolis (8226-b)

Bee Glue.

Propolis is a resinous substance collected by bees, primarily, at least in Europe, from poplar buds (see also p.1620), and used by them to seal their hives. It has been traditionally used for a wide variety of disorders, in cosmetics, and for the varnishing of Stradivarius violins. Propolis appears to have anti-inflammatory and antimicrobial properties. Hypersensitivity reactions have been reported.

References to the antibacterial and anti-inflammatory properties of propolis.

1. Grange JM, Davey RW. Antibacterial properties of propolis (bee glue). *J R Soc Med* 1990; **83:** 159–60.
2. Krol W, *et al.* Synergistic effect of ethanolic extract of propolis and antibiotics on the growth of Staphylococcus aureus. *Arzneimittelforschung* 1993; **43:** 607–9.
3. Volpert R, Elstner EF. Interactions of different extracts of propolis with leukocytes and leukocytic enzymes. *Arzneimittelforschung* 1996; **46:** 47–51.

Preparations

Proprietary Preparations (details are given in Part 3)
Austral.: Helastop; ***Ital.:*** Dermintact†; Pro-Gola; Propolcream; Propolgel†; Proporal†; ***UK:*** Buttercup Lozenges; ***USA:*** Probax.

Multi-ingredient: ***Austral.:*** Formula 1†; ***Fr.:*** Pollen Royal; Propargile; ***Ital.:*** Apistress; Aprolis†; Cocktail Reale; Fosfarsile Forte; Neo-Stomygen; Probigol; ***Switz.:*** Osa Gel de dentition aux plantes; ***UK:*** Beeline.

Propylene Glycol (1908-x)

Glicol Propilênico; Propilenoglicol; Propylenglycolum. (±)-Propane-1,2-diol.

$CH_3CHOHCH_2OH$ = 76.09.

CAS — 57-55-6; 4254-15-3 (+); 4254-14-2 (−); 4254-16-4 (±).

Pharmacopoeias. In *Eur.* (see p.viii), *Jpn, Pol.*, and *US*.

A clear, colourless, odourless or almost odourless, viscous, hygroscopic liquid with a slight characteristic taste. **Miscible** with water, with acetone, with alcohol, and with chloroform; soluble in ether; immiscible with fixed oils but will dissolve some essential oils. **Store** in airtight containers.

Adverse Effects and Precautions

Propylene glycol may cause some local irritation of the skin and mucous membranes. Hypersensitivity reactions have been reported. Hyperosmolality, lactic acidosis, and central nervous system depression have occurred, particularly in patients with renal impairment. Hyperosmolality has also been reported in burn patients following the topical application of preparations in which the basis is propylene glycol.

Effects on the blood. Studies have indicated that propylene glycol may have a haemolytic effect[1] and haemolysis in one patient has been attributed to the administration of red blood cells and 50% propylene glycol through the same intravenous line.[2]

1. Ruddick JA. Toxicology, metabolism, and biochemistry of 1,2-propanediol. *Toxicol Appl Pharmacol* 1972; **21:** 102–11.
2. Demey H, *et al.* Propylene glycol intoxication due to intravenous nitroglycerin. *Lancet* 1984; **i:** 1360.

Effects on the ears. Chloramphenicol sodium succinate 5% in Ringer's solution and propylene glycol 10% both caused irreversible deafness when instilled into the middle-ear cavity in *guinea-pigs*.[1] It was recommended that propylene glycol should not be used as a solvent for chloramphenicol ear drops.

1. Morizono T, Johnstone BM. Ototoxicity of chloramphenicol ear drops with propylene glycol as solvent. *Med J Aust* 1975; **2:** 634–8.

Effects on the nervous system. Central nervous system toxicity in children has been associated with propylene glycol used as a solvent in some oral vitamin preparations. Stupor has been reported and a 15-month-old boy had episodes of unresponsiveness, tachypnoea, tachycardia, and diaphoresis until the vitamin preparation was discontinued.[1] There have also been isolated reports of seizures associated with ingestion or use in preparations for parenteral nutrition.[2,3]

1. Martin G, Finberg L. Propylene glycol: a potentially toxic vehicle in liquid dosage form. *J Pediatr* 1970; **77:** 877–8.
2. Arulanantham K, Genel M. Central nervous system toxicity associated with ingestion of propylene glycol. *J Pediatr* 1978; **93:** 515–16.
3. MacDonald MG, *et al.* Propylene glycol: increased incidence of seizures in low birth weight infants. *Pediatrics* 1987; **79:** 622–5.

Fluid and electrolyte homoeostasis. Intravenous infusions of preparations containing a high proportion of propylene glycol as a solvent have been associated with increased serum osmolality,[1-6] especially in small infants (for example those under 2kg body-weight) and in patients with diminished renal function.[4] Hyperosmolality following the transdermal absorption of propylene glycol from a topically applied silver sulphadiazine preparation has been reported in patients with extensive burns and toxic epidermal necrolysis.[7,8] The monitoring of osmolality in susceptible patients receiving high doses of propylene glycol has therefore been recommended.[4,8] Patients with renal impairment exposed to propylene glycol have also developed lactic acidosis possibly due to the metabolism of propylene glycol to lactic acid in the liver and its subsequent accumulation.[2,9]

1. Glasgow AM, *et al.* Hyperosmolality in small infants due to propylene glycol. *Pediatrics* 1983; **72:** 353–5.
2. Demey H, *et al.* Propyleneglycol intoxication due to intravenous nitroglycerin. *Lancet* 1984; **i:** 1360.
3. Molter K, *et al.* Serumhyperosmolalität bei Langzeitanwendung von Etomidate (Radenarcon). *Anaesthesiol Reanim* 1987; **12:** 25–34.
4. Demey HE, *et al.* Propylene glycol-induced side effects during intravenous nitroglycerin therapy. *Intensive Care Med* 1988; **14:** 221–6.
5. Huggon I, *et al.* Hyperosmolality related to propylene glycol in an infant treated with enoximone infusion. *Br Med J* 1990; **301:** 19–20.
6. Seay RE, *et al.* Comment: possible toxicity from propylene glycol in lorazepam infusion. *Ann Pharmacother* 1997; **31:** 647–8. Correction. Woycik CL, Walker PC. *ibid.* 1413.
7. Bekeris L, *et al.* Propylene glycol as a cause of an elevated serum osmolality. *Am J Clin Pathol* 1979; **72:** 633–6.
8. Fligner CL, *et al.* Hyperosmolality induced by propylene glycol: a complication of silver sulfadiazine therapy. *JAMA* 1985; **253:** 1606–9.
9. Cate JC, Hedrick R. Propylene glycol intoxication and lactic acidosis. *N Engl J Med* 1980; **303:** 1237.

Hypersensitivity. Skin reactions due to propylene glycol are generally rare.[1] Irritation of the skin may occur,[2] especially under occlusive conditions,[3] and hypersensitivity-type reactions have been reported.[4]

1. Andersen KE, Storrs FJ. Hautreizungen durch Propylenglykol. *Hautarzt* 1982; **33:** 12–14.
2. Trancik RJ, Maibach HI. Propylene glycol: irritation or sensitization? *Contact Dermatitis* 1982; **8:** 185–9.
3. Motoyoshi K, *et al.* The safety of propylene glycol and other humectants. *Cosmet Toilet* 1984; **99** (Oct): 83–91.
4. Hannuksela M, Förström L. Reactions to peroral propylene glycol. *Contact Dermatitis* 1978; **4:** 41–5.

Interactions

Propylene glycol has been reported to decrease the effect of heparin.[1]

1. Col J, *et al.* Propylene glycol-induced heparin resistance during nitroglycerin infusion. *Am Heart J* 1985; **110:** 171–3.

Pharmacokinetics

Propylene glycol is rapidly absorbed from the gastro-intestinal tract. There is evidence of topical absorption when applied to damaged skin.

It is extensively metabolised in the liver primarily by oxidation to lactic and pyruvic acid and is also excreted in the urine unchanged.

References.

1. Yu DK, *et al.* Pharmacokinetics of propylene glycol in humans during multiple dosing regimens. *J Pharm Sci* 1985; **74:** 876–9.
2. Speth PAJ, *et al.* Propylene glycol pharmacokinetics and effects after intravenous infusion in humans. *Ther Drug Monit* 1987; **9:** 255–8.

Uses and Administration

Propylene glycol is widely used in pharmaceutical manufacturing as a solvent and vehicle especially for drugs unstable or insoluble in water. It may also be employed as a stabilising agent in vitamin preparations, a plasticiser, and as a preservative. Propylene glycol is also used extensively in foods and cosmetics.

Propylene glycol has humectant properties and is used similarly to glycerol in topical moisturising preparations.

Propylene glycol is used in veterinary medicine as a glucose precursor.

Preparations

Proprietary Preparations (details are given in Part 3)
Canad.: Seboval†.

Multi-ingredient: ***Aust.:*** Acerbine; ***Austral.:*** Dermatech Liquid; ***Canad.:*** Episec; Gyne-Moistrin; Rhinaris; Salinol; Secaris; ***Ger.:*** Sekudrill; ***Irl.:*** Aserbine†; ***Ital.:*** Dopo Pik; Sekudrill; ***S.Afr.:*** Aserbine; ***Spain:*** Acerbiol; ***Switz.:*** Acerbine; Astroglide†; ***UK:*** Aserbine; Malatex†; ***USA:*** Astroglide; Gyne-Moistrin†; Massengill Disposable; Surgel; Zonite.

Proquamezine Fumarate (13179-l)

Proquamezine Fumarate *(BANM)*.

Aminopromazine Fumarate *(rINNM)*; Bayer-A-124; RP-3828; Tetrameprozine Fumarate. *NNN'N'*-Tetramethyl-3-(phenothiazin-10-yl)propane-1,2-diamine fumarate; Tetramethyl(1-phenothiazin-10-ylmethylethylene)diamine fumarate.

$(C_{19}H_{25}N_3S)_2,C_4H_4O_4$ = 771.0.

CAS — 58-37-7 (proquamezine); 3688-62-8 (proquamezine fumarate).

Pharmacopoeias. In *Fr.*

Proquamezine fumarate is a phenothiazine derivative with antispasmodic properties and has been used in veterinary medicine.

Protoporphyrin IX Disodium (5575-n)

Protoporphyrin Disodium. Disodium 7,12-diethenyl-3,8,13,17-tetramethyl-21*H*,23*H*-porphine-2,18-dipropanoate.

$C_{34}H_{32}N_4Na_2O_4$ = 606.6.

CAS — 50865-01-5 (protoporphyrin IX disodium); 553-12-8 (protoporphyrin IX).

Protoporphyrin IX disodium has been given by mouth for the treatment of impaired hepatic function associated with gallstones and cholecystitis.

Proxazole Citrate (5243-b)

Proxazole Citrate *(USAN, rINNM)*.

AF-634; Propaxoline Citrate; PZ-17105. *NN*-Diethyl-3-(1-phenylpropyl)-1,2,4-oxadiazole-5-ethanamine citrate.

$C_{17}H_{25}N_3O,C_6H_8O_7$ = 479.5.

CAS — 5696-09-3 (proxazole); 132-35-4 (proxazole citrate).

Proxazole citrate is used as an antispasmodic and in vascular disorders. It has been given by mouth, rectally, and by injection.

Preparations

Proprietary Preparations (details are given in Part 3)
Ital.: Toness.

Prozapine Hydrochloride (3740-v)

Prozapine Hydrochloride *(rINNM)*.

Hexadiphane Hydrochloride. 1-(3,3-Diphenylpropyl)cyclohexamethyleneimine hydrochloride.

$C_{21}H_{27}N,HCl$ = 329.9.

CAS — 3426-08-2 (prozapine); 13657-24-4 (prozapine hydrochloride).

Prozapine hydrochloride is an antispasmodic used with sorbitol in biliary and gastro-intestinal disorders. It has been given in doses of 2 to 6 mg daily taken in water before meals.

Preparations

Proprietary Preparations (details are given in Part 3)

Multi-ingredient: ***Fr.:*** Norbiline; ***Ital.:*** Norbiline; Prandium†; ***Spain:*** Norbiline†.

Psilocin (5019-t)

4-Hydroxy-*NN*-dimethyltryptamine; Psilocyn. 3-(2-Dimethylaminoethyl)indol-4-ol.

$C_{12}H_{16}N_2O$ = 204.3.

CAS — 520-53-6.

An indole alkaloid obtained from the sacred Mexican mushroom (Teonanácatl), *Psilocybe mexicana* (Agaricaceae). It has hallucinogenic properties.

Psilocybin (5020-l)

Psilocybin *(BAN)*.

Psilocybine *(rINN)*; CY-39; 4-Phosphoryloxy-*NN*-dimethyltryptamine. 3-(2-Dimethylaminoethyl)indol-4-yl dihydrogen phosphate.

$C_{12}H_{17}N_2O_4P$ = 284.2.

CAS — 520-52-5.

The main indole alkaloid present in the sacred Mexican mushroom (Teonanácatl), *Psilocybe mexicana* (Agaricaceae). In the UK, psilocybin is present in the indigenous mushroom *Psilocybe semilanceata* (magic mushroom; liberty cap). Psilocybin is also present in other species of mushrooms including *Stropharia cubensis* and *Conocybe* spp.

Psilocybin has hallucinogenic and sympathomimetic properties similar to those of lysergide (p.1597). It is less potent than lysergide and its hallucinogenic effects last for up to 6 hours. There is evidence to suggest that psilocybin is converted to the active form psilocin in the body. It has no therapeutic use.

Pulegium Oil (4696-h)

Pennyroyal Oil.

A volatile oil distilled from pennyroyal herb, *Mentha pulegium* (Labiatae), containing pulegone ($C_{10}H_{16}O$).

Pulegium oil was formerly used as an emmenagogue. Severe toxic effects have followed its use as an abortifacient with convulsions, hepatotoxicity, and death. It is reported to have insect repellent activity.

Severe hepatotoxicity accompanied by seizures occurred in 2 infants each of whom had received herbal teas containing pulegium oil.[1] In one of the infants multiple organ failure developed, and fulminant hepatic failure with hepatocellular necrosis and cerebral oedema proved fatal.

1. Bakerink JA, *et al.* Multiple organ failure after ingestion of pennyroyal oil from herbal tea in two infants. *Pediatrics* 1996; **98:** 944–7.

Pulmonary Surfactants (15937-b)

Pulmonary surfactants are used to replace deficient endogenous lung surfactants. A number of preparations have been studied including: natural human surfactant obtained from amniotic fluid or biosynthetic material; natural animal-derived surfactants, which are bovine or porcine lung extracts that may be modified by the addition of synthetic surfactants, as in the case of beractant, or unmodified, as in the case of bovactant and calfactant; and synthetic or semisynthetic preparations, which often contain colfosceril palmitate, a major constituent of endogenous lung surfactant, in combination with other surfactants which aid spreading and absorption.

Beractant (11625-h)

Beractant *(BAN, USAN)*.

A-60386X.

CAS — 108778-82-1.

NOTE. The term Surfactant TA has been applied to a modified bovine lung surfactant.

Beractant is a modified bovine lung extract containing mostly phospholipids, modified by the addition of colfosceril palmitate, palmitic acid, and tripalmitin.

Bovactant (15942-n)

Bovactant *(BAN)*.

SF-R11.

Bovactant is an extract of bovine lung containing about 92% of phospholipids, 3.2% of cholesterol, 0.6% of surfactant-associated hydrophobic proteins, and 0.4% of free fatty acid.

Calfactant (19960-l)

Calfactant *(BAN)*.

Calfactant is an unmodified calf lung extract that includes mostly phospholipids and hydrophobic surfactant-specific proteins (SP-B and SP-C).

Colfosceril Palmitate (13779-y)

Colfosceril Palmitate *(BAN, USAN, rINN)*.

Dipalmitoylphosphatidylcholine; DPPC; 129Y83. 1,2-Dipalmitoyl-*sn*-glycero(3)phosphocholine.

$C_{40}H_{80}NO_8P = 734.0$.

CAS — 63-89-8.

Colfosceril palmitate is a phospholipid which forms an important constituent of endogenous pulmonary surfactant compounds.

Poractant Alfa (17490-v)

Poractant Alfa *(BAN)*.

CAS — 129069-19-8.

Poractant alfa is an extract of porcine lung containing not less than 90% of phospholipids, about 1% of hydrophobic proteins (SP-B and SP-C), and about 9% of other lipids.

Pumactant (11043-m)

Pumactant *(BAN)*.

Artificial Lung Expanding Compound.

Pumactant is a mixture of colfosceril palmitate and phosphatidyl glycerol (2-oleoyl-1-palmitoyl-*sn*-glycero(3)phospho(1)-*sn*-glycerol) in the proportion 7:3.

Adverse Effects and Precautions

Surfactant therapy may be associated with an increased risk of pulmonary haemorrhage, especially in more premature infants. Therapy should only be given where there are adequate facilities for ventilation and monitoring. Rapid chest expansion and improvement of oxygenation may follow successful treatment, and peak ventilatory pressure and inspired oxygen concentration may need to be reduced promptly to avoid the risk of pneumothorax and hyperoxaemia. A transient decrease in brain electrical activity has been reported in neonates given surfactant but its significance is unknown.

While surfactant therapy is clearly associated with an increased risk of pulmonary haemorrhage,[1-4] meta-analysis suggests that the risk is small compared with the benefits of therapy.[1] There is some evidence that haemodynamic changes associated with surfactant therapy may also predispose premature infants to intracranial (periventricular) haemorrhage,[5] though this is less well established. Early use of prophylactic surfactant in very low birth-weight infants may be associated with a poorer long-term neurodevelopmental outcome,[6] although the significance of this finding is as yet uncertain. Decreased brain electrical activity has been reported following surfactant treatment.[7] The rate of instillation of surfactant may be significant: one study[8] found that rapid instillation provoked a transient increase in cerebral blood flow velocity, associated with an increase in carbon dioxide tension. The authors concluded that instillation should take place slowly, over 15 to 20 minutes (most manufacturers suggest a more rapid bolus, since the infant is normally disconnected from the ventilator during administration, but in this study the apparatus was adapted so that mechanical ventilation could continue during administration).

1. Raju TNK, Langenberg P. Pulmonary hemorrhage and exogenous surfactant therapy: a metaanalysis. *J Pediatr* 1993; **123:** 603–10.
2. Majeed-Saidan MA, *et al.* Pulmonary haemorrhage in low-birthweight babies. *Lancet* 1993; **341:** 120.
3. Rogers D. Pulmonary haemorrhage, surfactant, and low-birthweight babies. *Lancet* 1993; **341:** 698.
4. Pappin A, *et al.* Extensive intraalveolar pulmonary hemorrhage in infants dying after surfactant therapy. *J Pediatr* 1994; **124:** 621–6.
5. Gunkel JH, Banks PLC. Surfactant therapy and intracranial hemorrhage: review of the literature and results of new analyses. *Pediatrics* 1993; **92:** 775–86.
6. Vaucher YE, *et al.* Outcome at twelve months of adjusted age in very low birthweight infants with lung immaturity: a randomized placebo-controlled trial of human surfactant. *J Pediatr* 1993; **122:** 126–32.
7. Hellström-Westas L, *et al.* Cerebroelectrical depression following surfactant treatment in preterm neonates. *Pediatrics* 1992; **89:** 643–7.
8. Saliba E, *et al.* Instillation rate effects of Exosurf on cerebral and cardiovascular haemodynamics in preterm neonates. *Arch Dis Child* 1994; **71:** F174–8.

Uses and Administration

Pulmonary surfactants are compounds with surface active properties similar to those natural substances in the lung which help to maintain the patency of the airways by reducing the surface tension of pulmonary fluids. Exogenous pulmonary surfactants are used in the treatment of neonatal respiratory distress syndrome in premature infants (p.1025), and may also be given for prophylaxis in infants considered at risk of developing the syndrome. Doses vary; most agents are given in recommended doses of 100 to 200 mg per kg birthweight, although a suggested dose for colfosceril palmitate is 67.5 mg per kg. For the treatment of overt neonatal respiratory distress syndrome, the initial dose is given as soon as possible after diagnosis, while for prophylaxis it is given as soon as possible after birth. Administration is as a suspension via an endotracheal tube. Repeat doses may be given if necessary, although the number of doses and the interval between them varies.

Pulmonary surfactants have also been investigated in the acute respiratory distress syndrome (p.1017).

Reviews.

1. Dechant KL, Faulds D. Colfosceril palmitate: a review of the therapeutic efficacy and clinical tolerability of a synthetic surfactant preparation (Exosurf Neonatal) in neonatal respiratory distress syndrome. *Drugs* 1991; **42:** 877–94.
2. Jobe AH. Pulmonary surfactant therapy. *N Engl J Med* 1993; **328:** 861–8.
3. Wiseman LR, Bryson HM. Porcine-derived lung surfactant: a review of the therapeutic efficacy and clinical tolerability of a natural surfactant preparation (Curosurf) in neonatal respiratory distress syndrome. *Drugs* 1994; **48:** 386–403.
4. Halliday HL. Natural vs synthetic surfactants in neonatal respiratory distress syndrome. *Drugs* 1996; **51:** 226–37.
5. Ishisaka DY. Exogenous surfactant use in neonates. *Pediatrics* 1996; **30:** 389–98.
6. Morley CJ. Systematic review of prophylactic vs rescue surfactant. *Arch Dis Child* 1997; **77:** F70–F74.
7. Gibson AT. Surfactant and the neonatal lung. *Br J Hosp Med* 1997; **58:** 381–4, 397.

Acute respiratory distress syndrome. Pulmonary surfactants have been investigated in the management of acute respiratory distress syndrome (p.1017) but with largely disappointing results. Some references are given below.

1. Haslam PL, *et al.* Surfactant replacement therapy in late-stage adult respiratory distress syndrome. *Lancet* 1994; **343:** 1009–11.
2. do Campo JL, *et al.* Natural surfactant aerosolisation in adult respiratory distress syndrome. *Lancet* 1994; **344:** 413–14.
3. Weg JG, *et al.* Safety and potential efficacy of an aerosolized surfactant in human sepsis-induced adult respiratory distress syndrome. *JAMA* 1994; **272:** 1433–8.
4. Anzueto A, *et al.* Aerosolized surfactant in adults with sepsis-induced respiratory distress syndrome. *N Engl J Med* 1996; **334:** 1417–21.

Drowning. Reference to the use of artificial surfactant (colfosceril palmitate) in the management of a 9-year-old rescued after near drowning.[1]

1. McBrien M, *et al.* Artificial surfactant in the treatment of near drowning. *Lancet* 1993; **342:** 1485–6.

Neonatal respiratory distress syndrome. Surfactants are effective in reducing the risk of death from respiratory distress syndrome in premature neonates (p.1025), and the development of pneumothorax as indicated by the references below.[1-8] However, whether to give surfactant prophylactically to all infants thought to be at risk, or to wait and treat the syndrome if it develops, remains an unresolved question, and the optimum regimen for administration also remains to be determined. It is also unclear whether any one preparation is better than another, although there is some evidence that surfactants of natural origin are superior to current synthetic surfactants,[9,10] and there are some results that suggest that improvement is more rapid and complications fewer with poractant[7] or surfactant from calf lung[11] rather than beractant.

1. The Osiris Collaborative Group. Early versus delayed neonatal administration of a synthetic surfactant—the judgement of OSIRIS. *Lancet* 1992; **340:** 1363–9.
2. Horbar JD, *et al.* Decreasing mortality associated with the introduction of surfactant therapy: an observational study of neonates weighing 601 to 1300 grams at birth. *Pediatrics* 1993; **92:** 191–6.
3. Ferrara TB, *et al.* Survival and follow-up of infants born at 23 to 26 weeks of gestational age: effects of surfactant therapy. *J Pediatr* 1994; **124:** 119–24.
4. Berry DD, *et al.* Comparison of the effect of three doses of a synthetic surfactant on the alveolar-arterial oxygen gradient in infants weighing not more than 1250 grams with respiratory distress syndrome. *J Pediatr* 1994; **124:** 294–301.
5. Schwartz RM, *et al.* Effect of surfactant on morbidity, mortality, and resource use in newborn infants weighing 500 to 1500 g. *N Engl J Med* 1994; **330:** 1476–80.
6. Corbet A, *et al.* Double-blind, randomized trial of one versus three prophylactic doses of synthetic surfactant in 826 neonates weighing 700 to 1100 grams: effects on mortality rate. *J Pediatr* 1995; **126:** 969–78.
7. Speer CP, *et al.* Randomized clinical trial of two treatment regimens of natural surfactant preparations in neonatal respiratory distress syndrome. *Arch Dis Child* 1995; **72:** F8–13.
8. Walti H, Monset-Couchard M. A risk-benefit assessment of natural and synthetic exogenous surfactants in the management of neonatal respiratory distress syndrome. *Drug Safety* 1998; **18:** 321–37.
9. Halliday HL. Natural vs synthetic surfactants in neonatal respiratory distress syndrome. *Drugs* 1996; **51:** 226–37.
10. Hudak ML, *et al.* A multicenter randomized, masked comparison trial of natural versus synthetic surfactant for the treatment of respiratory distress syndrome. *J Pediatr* 1996; **128:** 396–406.
11. Bloom BT, *et al.* Randomized double-blind multicenter trial of Survanta (SURV) and Infasurf (IS). *Pediatr Res* 1994; **35:** 326.

Preparations

Proprietary Preparations (details are given in Part 3)
Aust.: Alveofact; Curosurf; Exosurf; Survanta; ***Austral.:*** Exosurf; Survanta; ***Belg.:*** Alvofact; Exosurf; Survanta; ***Canad.:*** Exosurf; Survanta; ***Fr.:*** Curosurf; Surfexo Neonatal; Survanta; ***Ger.:*** Alveofact; Curosurf; Exosurf; Survanta; ***Irl.:*** Curosurf; Exosurf; ***Ital.:*** Alveofact; Curosurf; Exosurf; ***Jpn:*** Surfacten; ***Neth.:*** Alvofact; Curosurf; Exosurf; Survanta; ***Norw.:*** Curosurf; Exosurf†; Survanta-Vent; ***S.Afr.:*** Exosurf; Survanta; ***Spain:*** Curosurf; Exosurf; Survanta; ***Swed.:*** Curosurf; Exosurf; Survanta-Vent; ***Switz.:*** Curosurf; Exosurf; Survanta; ***UK:*** Alec; Curosurf; Exosurf; Survanta; ***USA:*** Exosurf†; Infasurf; Survanta.

Pulsatilla (13187-l)

Meadow Anemone; Pasque Flower.

CAS — 62887-80-3.

The whole flowering plant of *Pulsatilla vulgaris* (*Anemone pulsatilla*) or *Pulsatilla pratensis* (Ranunculaceae).

Pulsatilla has been used in herbal preparations for the treatment of a wide variety of conditions including nervous disorders, circulatory disorders, and gynaecological disorders and is used in homoeopathic medicine.

Preparations

Proprietary Preparations (details are given in Part 3)
USA: Yeast-X.

Multi-ingredient: ***Austral.:*** Calmo; Cirflo†; Lifesystem Herbal Formula 4 Women's Formula; Proflo; Viburnum Complex; Women's Formula Herbal Formula 3; ***Fr.:*** Biocarde; Cicaderma; Hepatoum; Histo-Fluine P; Mensuosedyl†; ***Ger.:*** Eviprostat N; ***Switz.:*** Eviprostat; ***UK:*** Ana-Sed; Nytol Herbal; Prementaid.

Pumilio Pine Oil (4697-m)

Dwarf Pine Needle Oil; Essence de Pin de Montagne; Latschenöl; Oleum Pini Pumilionis; Olio di Mugo.

CAS — 8016-46-4.

Pharmacopoeias. In *Aust.* and *Swiss.*

A colourless or yellowish volatile oil with a pleasant aromatic odour, obtained by distillation from the fresh leaves of *Pinus mugo* var. *pumilio* (Pinaceae).

Soluble 1 in 4.5 to 10 of alcohol (90%), often with turbidity. **Store** in airtight containers. Protect from light.

Pumilio pine oil has been inhaled with steam, sometimes with other essential oils, to relieve cough and nasal congestion and has been applied externally as a rubefacient. It has also been used as a perfume.

Preparations

Proprietary Preparations (details are given in Part 3)
Ital.: Recto Mugolio.

Multi-ingredient: ***Aust.:*** Allgauer; Anifer Hustenbalsam; Anifer Krauterol; Apotheker Bauer's Inhalationsmischung; Babix; Berggeist; Bronchostop; Colda; Emser Nasensalbe; Erkaltungsbad; Erkaltungsbalsam; Expectal-Balsam; Jopinol; Leukona-Rheuma-Bad; Luuf Balsam; Luuf-Erkaltungsol; Makatussin; Mentopin; Nasanal; Opino; Piniment; Pinimenthol†; Piniol†; Resol; Tetesept; ***Austral.:*** Analgesic Rub†; Biosal; Karvol; Menalation; Vicks Inhaler; ***Belg.:*** Calyptol†; ***Canad.:*** Vap Air; ***Fr.:*** Febrectol; ***Ger.:*** Aerosol Spitzner N; Atmulen E†; Bormelin†; Cefarheumin N; Dolo-cyl; Emser Balsam echt†; Emser Erkaltungsgel; Emser Nasensalbe N; Euflux-N; Expectal Balsam†; Frubibalsam†; Grune Nervensalbe†; Hevertopect; Inspirol Mundwasser konzentrat; Ipalat; Kneipp Erkaltungs-Balsam N; Kneipp Krauter Hustensaft N; Latschenkiefer Franzbranntwein; Lyobalsam; Lyobalsam N ohne Menthol†; Lyobalsam N†; Monapax N†; Nasivin Intensiv-Balsam†; Neo-Lapitrypsin; Nervfluid S; Night-Care; opino heparinoid†; Optipect†; Ortholan†; Phardol N Balsam†; Pin-Alcol; Pinimenthol-Oral N; Pro-Pecton Balsam†; Pumilen-Balsam†; Pumilen-N; Retterspitz Aerosol; Retterspitz Heilsalbe; Rheumasan†; rhino-loges N†; Rhinotussal E Balsam†; Rosarthron; Schupps Latschenkiefer Olbad; Silvapin Franzbranntwein†; Spolera therm†; Terpestrol-Inhalant†; Thrombocid; ***Irl.:*** Karvol; ***Ital.:*** Abiostil; Antalgola Plus†; Antalgola†; Antipulmina†; Auricovit†; Bronco Valda†; Broncosedina; Opino†; Otormon F (Femminile)†; Pantosse†; Pinedrin; Pinefedrina†; Pumilene†; Sedopulmina†; ***Neth.:*** Bronchoforton†; ***Switz.:*** Baby Liberol; Baume Kytta†; Demo pommade contre les refroidissements; Demo pommade contre les refroidissements pour bebes; Eau-de-vie de France avec huile de pin nain du Tirol; Liberol; Makatussin;

Pinimenthol; Pommade Kytta†; Thrombocid; *UK:* Boots Vapour Rub; Cabdrivers Adult Linctus; Catarrh Pastilles; Karvol; Mentholatum Balm†; Nasal Inhaler; Potter's Pastilles.

Punarnava (13188-y)

Punarnaba.

The fresh or dried plant *Boerhaavia diffusa* (= *B. repens*) (Nyctaginaceae), containing an alkaloid, punarnavine.

Punarnava has been used in India as a diuretic, usually in the form of a liquid extract.

Pyricarbate (13191-p)

Pyricarbate *(rINN)*.

Pyridinolcarbamate. 2,6-Pyridinediyldimethylene bis(methylcarbamate).

$C_{11}H_{15}N_3O_4$ = 253.3.

CAS — 1882-26-4.

Pharmacopoeias. In *Fr.* and *Pol.*

Pyricarbate has been given by mouth in the treatment of atherosclerosis and other vascular disorders, hyperlipidaemias, and thrombo-embolic disorders. Adverse effects have included gastro-intestinal disturbances and liver damage.

Preparations

Proprietary Preparations (details are given in Part 3)
Ital.: Angioxil†; Atover†; Cicloven; Movecil†; Vasagin†; Vasocil†; ***Jpn:*** Anginin; ***Spain:*** Colesterinex; Duvaline†; Esterbiol; Vasmol†.

Multi-ingredient: ***Ital.:*** Clopir†; Ellemger†; S.trat.os†; ***Spain:*** Duvaline Compositum†; Duvaline Flebo†; Esclerobion†.

Pyritinol Hydrochloride (13194-e)

Pyritinol Hydrochloride *(BANM, rINNM)*.

Pyrithioxine Hydrochloride. 5,5-Dihydroxy-6,6-dimethyl-3,3-dithiodimethylenebis(4-pyridylmethanol) dihydochloride monohydrate.

$C_{16}H_{20}N_2O_4S_2,2HCl,H_2O$ = 459.4.

CAS — 1098-97-1 (pyritinol); 10049-83-9 (anhydrous pyritinol hydrochloride).

Pharmacopoeias. In *Pol.*

Pyritinol hydrochloride has been described as a nootropic which promotes the uptake of glucose by the brain and has been used in the treatment of various cerebrovascular and mental function disorders. Pyritinol hydrochloride has also been given as an alternative to penicillamine in rheumatoid arthritis. It is given by mouth in a usual dose of 600 mg daily.

References.

1. Martin KJ. On the mechanism of action of Encephabol. *J Int Med Res* 1983; **11:** 55–65.
2. Knezevic S, *et al.* Pyritinol treatment of SDAT patients: evaluation by psychiatric and neurological examination, psychometric testing and rCBF measurements. *Int Clin Psychopharmacol* 1989; **4:** 25–38.

Preparations

Proprietary Preparations (details are given in Part 3)
Aust.: Encephabol; ***Belg.:*** Encephabol†; ***Fr.:*** Encephabol†; ***Ger.:*** Ardeyceryl P; Encephabol; Logomed Neuro-Aktiv-Tabletten; ***Ital.:*** Cerebrotrofina†; Cervitalin†; Encebrovit†; Encefabol; Encerebron†; Maind†; ***S.Afr.:*** Encephabol; ***Spain:*** Bonifen†; ***Switz.:*** Encephabol†.

Multi-ingredient: ***Spain:*** Bonifen B6†; Bonifen H†; Esclerobion†; Memorino; Plenumil†; Refulgin.

Quassia (539-m)

Bitter Wood; Leño de Cuasia; Quassia Wood; Quassiae Lignum; Quassiaholz.

CAS — 76-78-8 (quassin); 76-77-7 (neoquassin).

Pharmacopoeias. In *Jpn* which allows Jamaican or Surinam quassia.

The dried stem wood of Jamaica quassia, *Picrasma excelsa* (=*Aeschrion excelsa; Picraena excelsa*) (Simaroubaceae) or of Surinam quassia, *Quassia amara* (Simaroubaceae).

Quassia has been used as a bitter. It was formerly given as an enema for the expulsion of threadworms and was applied for pediculosis. It may also be used as a flavour in food, drinks, and confectionery. Extracts of quassia or preparations containing its triterpenoid bitter principle quassin are used to denature alcohol.

Preparations

Proprietary Preparations (details are given in Part 3)

Multi-ingredient: ***Austral.:*** Fisher's Phospherine; ***Belg.:*** Valeria-Fordine†; ***Fr.:*** Ducase; Quintonine; Spevin; ***Ital.:*** Amaro Maffioli†; Cura; ***Switz.:*** Stomacine; ***UK:*** Sanderson's Throat Specific.

Quinine and Urea Hydrochloride (13201-k)

Carbamidated Quinine Dihydrochloride; Chininum Dihydrochloricum Carbamidatum; Urea-Quinine.

$C_{20}H_{24}N_2O_2,CH_4N_2O,2HCl,5H_2O$ = 547.5.

CAS — 549-52-0 (anhydrous).

Quinine and urea hydrochloride is used for the treatment of haemorrhoidal bleeding and anal fissure. It was formerly used as a local anaesthetic and for the therapeutic actions of quinine.

Preparations

Proprietary Preparations (details are given in Part 3)
Fr.: Kinurea H.

Quinine Ascorbate (13202-a)

Quinine Ascorbate *(USAN)*.

Quinine Biascorbate.

$C_{20}H_{24}N_2O_2,2C_6H_8O_6$ = 676.7.

CAS — 146-40-7.

A compound (2 : 1) of ascorbic acid with quinine.

Quinine ascorbate has been used as a smoking deterrent.

Preparations

Proprietary Preparations (details are given in Part 3)

Multi-ingredient: ***Fr.:*** Nicoprive; Paranico; ***Ital.:*** Nicoprive; ***Spain:*** Desinto†.

Rape Oil (7366-p)

Colza Oil; Oleum Rapae; Rapeseed Oil.

Pharmacopoeias. In *Eur.* (see p.viii), *Jpn*, and *Pol.*

The refined fixed oil expressed from the seeds of *Brassica napus* (*Brassica campestris*) var. *oleifera* and certain other species of *Brassica* (Cruciferae). A clear light yellow liquid. Practically **insoluble** in water and in alcohol; miscible with petroleum spirit. It contains not more than 2% of erucic acid. **Store** in well filled airtight containers. Protect from light.

Rape oil has been used in liniments in place of olive oil. It is used in some countries as an edible oil but the erucic acid ($C_{22}H_{42}O_2$=338.6) content of the oil has been implicated in muscle damage. The erucic acid content of oils and fats intended for human consumption and of foodstuffs containing oil or fat is subject to legal control. Contaminated rape oil was the cause of the toxic oil syndrome that affected thousands of Spanish citizens following its distribution in early 1981. There has been some debate as to whether increased frequencies of allergic respiratory symptoms occur in sensitive individuals in areas in which oilseed rape is cultivated.

Raspberry Leaf (13207-d)

Rubi Idaei Folium.

The dried leaflets of *Rubus idaeus* (Rosaceae).

Raspberry leaf contains a principle, readily extracted with hot water, which relaxes the smooth muscle of the uterus and intestine of some *animals.*

Raspberry 'tea' has been a traditional remedy for painful and profuse menstruation and for use before and during confinement. The infusion has also been used as an astringent gargle.

Preparations

Proprietary Preparations (details are given in Part 3)

Multi-ingredient: ***Aust.:*** Bio-Garten Tee gegen Durchfall; Tee gegen Durchfall nach Dr Bohmig†; ***Austral.:*** Rubus Complex; ***Belg.:*** Eugiron; ***Fr.:*** Carbonaphtine Pectinee†; ***Ger.:*** Buccotean†; Salus Bronchial-Tee Nr.8; ***UK:*** Helonias Compound.

Red Clover (12167-d)

Cow Clover; Meadow Clover; Purple Clover; Trefoil.

The flowerheads of red clover, *Trifolium pratense* (Leguminosae) have been used in herbal medicine.

Preparations

Proprietary Preparations (details are given in Part 3)

Multi-ingredient: ***Austral.:*** Trifolium Complex.

Relaxin (13208-n)

CAS — 9002-69-1.

A polypeptide hormone extracted from the corpus luteum of the ovaries of pregnant sows. It is reported to be related structurally to insulin and has a molecular weight of about 6000.

Relaxin acts on connective tissue, including collagen, and causes relaxation of the pubic symphysis and softening of the uterine cervix. In many *animal* species it appears to play a major part in cervical ripening before parturition; significant species difference is shown. Relaxin is secreted by the human corpus luteum during pregnancy and is thought to interact with other reproductive hormones. It has been studied for cervical ripening and is under investigation in scleroderma (p.501).

Rhamnose (3921-w)

L-Rhamnose. 6-Deoxy-L-mannose.

$C_6H_{12}O_5$ = 164.2.

CAS — 3615-41-6.

Rhamnose is a monosaccharide used to assess intestinal permeability.

For reference to the use of rhamnose in the differential sugar absorption test, see Lactulose, p.1196.

Rhatany Root (319-j)

Krameria; Krameria Root; Ratanhiae Radix.

Pharmacopoeias. In *Eur.* (see p.viii).

The dried, usually fragmented, underground organs of *Krameria triandra* (Krameriaceae), containing not less than 10% tannins. It is known in commerce as Peruvian rhatany.

The powder is reddish brown. **Protect** from light and humidity.

Rhatany root has astringent properties and is used in herbal and homoeopathic preparations for a variety of disorders, including oropharyngeal inflammation.

Preparations

Proprietary Preparations (details are given in Part 3)

Multi-ingredient: ***Aust.:*** Parodontax; ***Fr.:*** Oxy-thymoline†; ***Ger.:*** Echtrosept-GT†; Repha-Os; ***Ital.:*** Gengivario; ***Spain:*** Encialina; Regal; ***Switz.:*** Eubucal†; ***UK:*** Medicinal Gargle.

Rhus (13210-a)

Sumach Berries.

The dried fruits of the smooth or Pennsylvanian sumach, *Rhus glabra* (Anacardiaceae).

Rhus has astringent and reputed diuretic properties. Poison ivy (*Rhus radicans*) and poison oak (*R. toxicodendron*), species growing in the USA, contain irritant poisons such as urushiol, producing severe contact dermatitis. Extracts of poison ivy and poison oak have been used for the prophylaxis of poison ivy dermatitis but their effectiveness has not been proved.

Poison oak is used in homoeopathic medicine.

Preparations

Proprietary Preparations (details are given in Part 3)

Multi-ingredient: ***Ger.:*** C 34-Strath†; Colchicum-Strath†; Hewedolor; Hicoton; Rhus-Rheuma-Gel N.

Ribonuclease (13211-t)

RNase.

CAS — 9001-99-4.

An enzyme present in most mammalian tissue.

Ribonuclease is involved in the catalytic cleavage of ribonucleic acid. It has been applied, alone or in combination with other agents, for its supposed anti-inflammatory properties.

Preparations

Proprietary Preparations (details are given in Part 3)
Ital.: Ribalgilasi†.

Multi-ingredient: ***Fr.:*** Ribatran; ***Ital.:*** Ribociclina.

Ribonucleic Acid (15326-d)

ARN; Plant Nucleic Acid; Ribose Nucleic Acid; RNA; Yeast Nucleic Acid.

Ribonucleic acid is a nucleotide polymer, and 1 of the 2 distinct varieties of nucleic acid (see p.1609). It is found in the cytoplasm and in small amounts in the cell nuclei of living tissues and is directly involved in protein synthesis. It can be extracted from beer or bread yeast. Therapeutically, it has been tried in the treatment of mental retardation and to improve memory in senile dementia and proprietary preparations containing various salts of ribonucleic acid have been advocated for a variety of asthenic and convalescent conditions.

Immune RNA (extracted from the spleens and lymph nodes of immunised animals) has been tried in the immunotherapy of hepatitis and cancer.

Preparations

Proprietary Preparations (details are given in Part 3)
Ger.: AU 4 Regeneresen; Osteochondrin S; RN13 Regeneresen.
Multi-ingredient: *Fr.:* Megasthenyl; Nutrigene; Tonuvital†; *Spain:* Dertrase; Nucleserina; Policolinosil.

Ricin (13213-r)

NOTE. The title ricin is used for the castor seed in *Chin.* and *Fr.*

A highly toxic lectin present in castor seeds, the seeds of *Ricinus communis* (Euphorbiaceae).

Ricin is extremely toxic when administered parenterally and the fatal dose by intravenous injection in experimental *animals* has been reported to be as low as 300 ng per kg bodyweight. The toxicity of orally ingested beans depends on how thoroughly they are chewed since the hard seed coat prevents absorption. Ricin conjugated with monoclonal or polyclonal antibodies is being studied in the treatment of cancers; zolimomab aritox (p.572) is an example of such a conjugate.

Ingestion of 5 castor seeds in a child and 20 in an adult has proved fatal; signs and symptoms of poisoning are similar to those described for abrus seeds (p.1541). After expression of the oil from castor seed (see p.1560), the ricin remains in the seed cake or 'pomace', which is subjected to steam treatment to destroy the ricin. The detoxified pomace is used as a fertiliser.

A report of ricin toxicity following partial chewing and ingestion of 10 to 15 castor oil seeds.[1]

1. Aplin PJ, Eliseo T. Ingestion of castor oil plant seeds. *Med J Aust* 1997; **167:** 260–1.

References to the use of ricin and abrin conjugates with monoclonal antibodies in the treatment of cancer.

1. Byers VS, *et al.* Phase I study of monoclonal antibody-ricin A chain immunotoxin XomaZyme-791 in patients with metastatic colon cancer. *Cancer Res* 1989; **49:** 6153–60.
2. Oratz R, *et al.* Antimelanoma monoclonal antibody-ricin A chain immunoconjugate (XMMME-001-RTA) plus cyclophosphamide in the treatment of metastatic malignant melanoma: results of a phase II trial. *J Biol Response Mod* 1990; **9:** 345–54.
3. Anonymous. Application considered for immunotoxin in treatment of graft-vs-host disease. *JAMA* 1991; **265:** 2041–2.
4. Amlot PL, *et al.* A phase I study of an anti-CD22-deglycosylated ricin A chain immunotoxin in the treatment of B-cell lymphomas resistant to conventional therapy. *Blood* 1993; **82:** 2624–33.
5. Senderowicz AM, *et al.* Complete sustained response of a refractory, post-transplantation, large B-cell lymphoma to an anti-CD22 immunotoxin. *Ann Intern Med* 1997; **126:** 882–5.

Ricinoleic Acid (1323-a)

A mixture of fatty acids obtained by the hydrolysis of castor oil.

Ricinoleic acid is an ingredient of some proprietary vaginal jellies used to maintain or restore normal vaginal acidity.

Preparations

Proprietary Preparations (details are given in Part 3)
Multi-ingredient: *Austral.:* Aci-Jel; *Canad.:* Aci-Jel†; *Swed.:* Aci-Jel†; *USA:* Aci-Jel.

Riluzole (10406-g)

Riluzole *(BAN, USAN, rINN).*

PK-26124; RP-54274. 2-Amino-6-(trifluoromethoxy) benzothiazole; 6-Trifluoromethoxy-1,3-benzothiazol-2-ylamine.

$C_8H_5F_3N_2OS$ = 234.2.

CAS — 1744-22-5.

Adverse Effects

Adverse effects associated most commonly with riluzole are asthenia, nausea, elevations in liver enzyme values, headache, and abdominal pain. Other gastro-intestinal effects may include diarrhoea or constipation, anorexia, and vomiting. There may be tachycardia, dizziness, vertigo, or somnolence. Circumoral paraesthesia has been reported and decreased lung function and rhinitis may occur. Anaphylactoid reactions, angioedema, and neutropenia have all been reported rarely.

A report[1] of icteric toxic hepatitis manifested by jaundice and elevated liver enzyme values in an elderly woman receiving riluzole for amyotrophic lateral sclerosis. Symptoms of hepatotoxicity were reversed following discontinuation of riluzole.

1. Castells LI, *et al.* Icteric toxic hepatitis associated with riluzole. *Lancet* 1998; **351:** 648.

Precautions

Riluzole is contra-indicated in patients with hepatic disease or markedly raised liver enzyme values. Liver function tests should be performed before and throughout treatment with riluzole. Extreme caution should be exercised in patients with renal impairment or those with a previous history of liver disorders. Patients or their carers should be told how to recognise signs of neutropenia and should be advised to seek immediate medical attention if symptoms such as fever develop; white blood cell counts should be determined in febrile illness and riluzole discontinued if neutropenia occurs. Riluzole may cause dizziness or vertigo and patients should be warned not to drive or operate machinery if these symptoms occur.

Riluzole has been reported to impair fertility in *animals.*

Pharmacokinetics

Riluzole is rapidly absorbed from the gastro-intestinal tract following oral administration with peak plasma concentrations occurring after 1 to 1½ hours. The rate and extent of absorption are decreased when riluzole is administered with a high-fat meal. Riluzole is widely distributed throughout the body and is approximately 97% bound to plasma proteins. It crosses the blood-brain barrier. Riluzole is extensively metabolised to several inactive metabolites in the liver by cytochrome P450 and subsequent glucuronidation. Riluzole is excreted mainly in the urine predominantly as glucuronides with an elimination half-life of about 12 hours. Approximately 2% is excreted unchanged in the urine. Small amounts are excreted in faeces. There is some evidence that clearance of riluzole might be reduced in Japanese patients.

References.

1. Le Liboux A, *et al.* Single- and multiple-dose pharmacokinetics of riluzole in white subjects. *J Clin Pharmacol* 1997; **37:** 820–7.

Uses and Administration

Riluzole is a glutamate antagonist used for the treatment of amyotrophic lateral sclerosis, a form of motor neurone disease. The precise mechanism of action of riluzole is unknown but it may both inhibit presynaptic glutamate release and interfere with its postsynaptic effects. Riluzole is indicated to slow progression of early disease but efficacy has not been demonstrated in its late stages. The usual adult dose of riluzole is 50 mg twice daily by mouth on an empty stomach. Use in children is not recommended.

Reviews.

1. Wokke J. Riluzole. *Lancet* 1996; **348:** 795–9.
2. Bryson HM, *et al.* Riluzole: a review of its pharmacodynamic and pharmacokinetic properties and therapeutic potential in amyotrophic lateral sclerosis. *Drugs* 1996; **52:** 549–63.
3. Wagner ML, Landis BE. Riluzole: a new agent for amyotrophic lateral sclerosis. *Ann Pharmacother* 1997; **31:** 738–44.
4. Anonymous. Riluzole for amyotrophic lateral sclerosis. *Drug Ther Bull* 1997; **35:** 11–12.

Motor neurone disease. Motor neurone diseases (motoneuron diseases) are fatal progressive degenerative disorders of unknown cause which affect upper and lower motor neurones in the brain and spinal cord. The most common form of motor neurone disease is amyotrophic lateral sclerosis (know in the USA as Lou Gehrig's disease) which produces muscular atrophy and weakness and symptoms of progressive bulbar palsy such as slowness of movement and speech disturbances. Most patients die within 2 to 5 years of disease onset, usually from respiratory failure. There is no completely effective treatment. It is thought that accumulation of the neurotransmitter glutamate in the CNS may be involved in the pathogenesis of the disease. Use of the glutamate antagonist riluzole was reported to slow the progression of early-stage disease and to produce a modest improvement in survival rate after 12 months,[1] but the effect was limited to the subgroup with bulbar symptoms at onset, and the trial and its conclusions have been criticised.[2-5] A much larger multicentre dose-ranging study,[6] however, conducted by the same workers appeared to confirm the efficacy of riluzole and established the optimal daily dose as 100 mg. This study found that riluzole decreased the risk of tracheotomy or death after both 12 and 18 months in all subgroups. The American Academy of Neurology has produced guidelines as to which categories of patients should receive riluzole therapy.[7]

Also under study for the treatment of motor neurone disease are somatomedins, in particular mecasermin (insulin-like growth factor I). Neurotrophic factors have been investigated including brain-derived neurotrophic factor (BDNF) and recombinant ciliary neurotrophic factor (CNTF), but results have been generally inconclusive. Glial-cell-derived neurotrophic factor (GDNF) is also under investigation.

There has also been some interest in the antiepileptic drug gabapentin[8] which may inhibit glutamate formation in the CNS from branched-chain amino acids. Lamotrigine has also been tried but with disappointing results.[9]

Other drugs which have been studied for amyotrophic lateral sclerosis include dextromethorphan and protirelin. Immunoglobulins have been tried in some forms of motor neurone disease such as multifocal motor neuropathy. A small percentage of patients with familial amyotrophic lateral sclerosis have been shown to have a mutation in the gene encoding for the enzyme copper-zinc superoxide dismutase but there is no consensus as to whether patients with this mutation should be given superoxide dismutase supplements.[10]

1. Bensimon G, *et al.* A controlled trial of riluzole in amyotrophic lateral sclerosis. *N Engl J Med* 1994; **330:** 585–91.
2. McKee P, *et al.* Riluzole in amyotrophic lateral sclerosis. *N Engl J Med* 1994; **331:** 272.
3. MacRae KD. Riluzole in amyotrophic lateral sclerosis. *N Engl J Med* 1994; **331:** 272–3.
4. Burgerman RS. Riluzole in amyotrophic lateral sclerosis. *N Engl J Med* 1994; **331:** 273.
5. Rowland LP. Riluzole in amyotrophic lateral sclerosis. *N Engl J Med* 1994; **331:** 274.
6. Lacomblez L, *et al.* Dose-ranging study of riluzole in amyotrophic lateral sclerosis. *Lancet* 1996; **347:** 1425–31.
7. Quality Standards Subcommittee of the American Academy of Neurolory. Practice advisory on the treatment of amyotrophic lateral sclerosis with riluzole: report of the Quality Standard Subcommittee of the American Academy of Neurology. *Neurology* 1997; **49:** 657–9.
8. Miller RG, *et al.* Placebo-controlled trial of gabapentin in patients with amyotrophic lateral sclerosis. *Neurology* 1996; **47:** 1383–8.
9. Eisen A, *et al.* Anti-glutamate therapy in amyotrophic lateral sclerosis: a trial using lamotrigine. *Can J Neurol Sci* 1993; **20:** 297–301.
10. Orrell RW, deBelleroche JS. Superoxide dismutase and ALS. *Lancet* 1994; **344:** 1651–2.

Preparations

Proprietary Preparations (details are given in Part 3)
Aust.: Rilutek; *Fr.:* Rilutek; *Ger.:* Rilutek; *Irl.:* Rilutek; *Ital.:* Rilutek; *Neth.:* Rilutek; *Swed.:* Rilutek; *UK:* Rilutek.

Ritodrine Hydrochloride (2103-j)

Ritodrine Hydrochloride *(BANM, USAN, rINNM).*

DU-21220 (ritodrine). *erythro*-2-(4-Hydroxyphenethylamino)-1-(4-hydroxyphenyl)propan-1-ol hydrochloride.

$C_{17}H_{21}NO_3,HCl$ = 323.8.

CAS — 26652-09-5 (ritodrine); 23239-51-2 (ritodrine hydrochloride).

Pharmacopoeias. In Br. and US.

White, or nearly white, odourless or practically odourless crystalline powder. Freely **soluble** in water and in alcohol; soluble in dehydrated alcohol and in propyl alcohol; practically insoluble in acetone and in ether. A 2% solution has a pH between 4.5 and 6.0.

Store in airtight containers.

Adverse Effects and Precautions

As for Salbutamol Sulphate, p.758. Leucopenia or agranulocytosis has been reported occasionally in association with prolonged administration of ritodrine.

In *women being treated for premature labour* the risk of pulmonary oedema means that extreme caution is required and the precautions and risk factors discussed under Salbutamol Sulphate, p.759, apply.

Effects on the eyes. Ritodrine and to a lesser extent salbutamol have been implicated in retinopathy in the premature infant when used for premature labour.[1]

1. Michie CA, *et al.* Do maternal β-sympathomimetics influence the development of retinopathy in the premature infant? *Arch Dis Child* 1994; **71:** F149.

Effects on the heart. Myocardial ischaemia or signs of myocardial ischaemia have been reported in patients given ritodrine.[1,2]

1. Brosset P, *et al.* Cardiac complications of ritodrine in mother and baby. *Lancet* 1982; **i:** 1468.
2. Ben-Shlomo I, *et al.* Myocardial ischaemia during intravenous ritodrine treatment: is it so rare? *Lancet* 1986; **ii:** 917–18.

Pulmonary oedema. Several cases of pulmonary oedema have been reported in patients given a beta$_2$ agonist, including ritodrine, for premature labour.[1-4] In 1995 the UK Committee on Safety of Medicines[4] (CSM) commented that it had received 10 reports of pulmonary oedema, fatal in 2 patients. The CSM considered that fluid overload was the most important predisposing factor. Other risk factors included multiple pregnancies, a history of cardiac disease, and maternal infection. For further discussion of the precautions necessary in the use of beta$_2$ agonists to treat premature labour, and the risk factors involved, see p.759.

1. Hawker F. Pulmonary oedema associated with β_2-sympathomimetic treatment of premature labour. *Anaesth Intensive Care* 1984; **12:** 143–51.
2. Pisani RJ, Rosenow EC. Pulmonary edema associated with tocolytic therapy. *Ann Intern Med* 1989; **110:** 714–18.
3. Clesham GJ, *et al.* β Adrenergic agonists and pulmonary oedema in preterm labour. *Br Med J* 1994; **308:** 260–2.
4. Committee on Safety of Medicines/Medicines Control Agency. Reminder: ritodrine and pulmonary oedema. *Current Problems* 1995; **21:** 7.

Pharmacokinetics

Ritodrine is rapidly absorbed from the gastro-intestinal tract but is subject to fairly extensive first-pass metabolism; about 30% of an oral dose is bioavailable. It is metabolised in the liver primarily by conjugation with glucuronic acid or sulphate and excreted in urine as unchanged drug and metabolites. About 70 to 90% of a dose is reported to be excreted in the urine within 10 to 12 hours. It crosses the placenta.

References.

1. Gandar R, *et al.* Serum level of ritodrine in man. *Eur J Clin Pharmacol* 1980; **17:** 117–22.
2. Gross AS, Brown KF. Plasma protein binding of ritodrine at parturition and in nonpregnant women. *Eur J Clin Pharmacol* 1985; **28:** 479–81.
3. Pacifici GM, *et al.* Sulphation and glucuronidation of ritodrine in human foetal and adult tissues. *Eur J Clin Pharmacol* 1993; **44:** 259–64.

Uses and Administration

Ritodrine hydrochloride is a direct-acting sympathomimetic with predominantly beta-adrenergic activity and a selective action on $beta_2$ receptors ($beta_2$ agonist). It has general properties similar to those of salbutamol (see p.759). It decreases uterine contractility and is used to arrest premature labour (p.760). Ritodrine hydrochloride is given by intravenous infusion preferably with the aid of a syringe pump when the concentration should be 3 mg per mL, glucose 5% having been used for dilution. A recommended initial rate of infusion is 50 µg per minute increased at intervals of 10 minutes by 50-µg increments until there is evidence of patient response, which is usually at a rate of 150 to 350 µg per minute, the latter figure being the maximum recommended rate. The maternal pulse should be monitored throughout the infusion and the rate adjusted to avoid a maternal heart rate of more than 135 to 140 beats per minute. A close watch should also be kept on the patient's state of hydration since fluid overload is considered to be a key risk factor for pulmonary oedema. The infusion should be continued for 12 to 48 hours after the contractions have stopped. Ritodrine hydrochloride may subsequently be given by mouth in an initial dose of 10 mg every 2 hours for 24 hours starting 30 minutes before the end of the intravenous infusion. Thereafter, 10 to 20 mg may be given every 4 to 6 hours according to the patient's response. The total daily dose by mouth should not exceed 120 mg.

If no syringe pump is available then the infusion may be made using a controlled infusion device to deliver a more dilute solution of 300 µg per mL with glucose 5% being used once again as the diluent. The same dose is employed as with the syringe pump. Where intravenous infusion is inappropriate 10 mg may be given intramuscularly every 3 to 8 hours and continued for 12 to 48 hours after the contractions have stopped.

Ritodrine hydrochloride was also formerly given intravenously to the mother as an emergency means of alleviating fetal asphyxia during labour while other procedures were being arranged for assisted delivery.

Preparations

BP 1998: Ritodrine Injection; Ritodrine Tablets;
USP 23: Ritodrine Hydrochloride Injection; Ritodrine Hydrochloride Tablets.

Proprietary Preparations (details are given in Part 3)
Aust.: Pre-Par†; ***Austral.:*** Yutopar; ***Belg.:*** Pre-Par; ***Canad.:*** Yutopar; ***Fr.:*** Pre-Par; ***Ger.:*** Pre-Par; ***Irl.:*** Yutopar; ***Ital.:*** Miolene; Pre-Par; ***Neth.:*** Pre-Par; ***Norw.:*** Utopar†; ***S.Afr.:*** Yutopar†; ***Spain:*** Pre-Par; ***UK:*** Yutopar; ***USA:*** Yutopar.

Rociverine (13217-h)

Rociverine (*rINN*).

LG-30158. 2-Diethylamino-1-methylethyl *cis*-1-hydroxy(bicyclohexyl)-2-carboxylate.

$C_{20}H_{37}NO_3$ = 339.5.

CAS — 53716-44-2.

Rociverine is used as an antispasmodic. It is given by mouth in doses of 30 to 40 mg or rectally in doses of 50 to 75 mg daily. It has also been given by injection.

Preparations

Proprietary Preparations (details are given in Part 3)
Ital.: Rilaten.

Rose Bengal Sodium (2146-h)

CI Acid Red 94; Colour Index No. 45440; Rose Bengal; Sodium Rose Bengal. The disodium salt of 4,5,6,7-tetrachloro-2′,4′,5′,7′-tetraiodofluorescein.

$C_{20}H_2Cl_4I_4Na_2O_5$ = 1017.6.

CAS — 11121-48-5 (rose bengal); 632-69-9 (rose bengal disodium).

NOTE. The name Rose Bengale has been applied to the substance described in this monograph as well as to dichlorotetraiodofluorescein (CI Acid Red 93; Ext. D & C Reds Nos. 5 and 6; Colour Index No. 45435), a compound used as its disodium or dipotassium salt as a colouring agent.

ROS is a code approved by the BP for use on single unit doses of eye drops containing rose bengal sodium where the individual container may be too small to bear all the appropriate labelling information.

Rose bengal sodium stains devitalised conjunctival and corneal epithelial cells as well as mucus and is used as an aid in the diagnosis of dry eye. It is used to detect or assess ocular damage resulting from Sjögren's syndrome or from ill-fitting contact lenses, and for keratitis, squamous cell carcinomas, and detection of foreign bodies. Rose bengal sodium is applied as 1% eye drops or as sterile papers impregnated with the dye.

Instillation of this dye may be painful. Rose bengal sodium can stain exposed skin, clothing, and soft contact lenses.

Rose bengal sodium is taken up by the liver and excreted in the bile; the iodine-131-labelled compound (p.1424) has been used as a diagnostic aid in the determination of hepato-biliary function.

Preparations

Proprietary Preparations (details are given in Part 3)
Canad.: Ak-Rose; ***USA:*** Rosets.

Rose Oil (4699-v)

Attar of Rose; Esencia de Rosa; Oleum Rosae; Otto of Rose.

Pharmacopoeias. In *USNF* which allows the oil of *R. gallica, R. damascena, R. alba, R. centifolia,* and varieties of these species.

A volatile oil obtained by distillation from the fresh flowers of *Rosa damascena* (Rosaceae) and other species. It is a colourless or yellow liquid with the characteristic odour and taste of rose. At 25° it is a viscous liquid but on cooling becomes a translucent crystalline solid, easily liquefied by warming. It contains citronellol. **Miscible** with an equal volume of chloroform. **Store** in airtight containers. Protect from light.

Rose oil is largely employed in perfumery and toilet preparations and has been used as a flavour. Hypersensitivity reactions have been reported.

Preparations

USNF 18: Stronger Rose Water;
USP 23: Rose Water Ointment.

Rosemary Oil (4700-v)

Esencia de Romero; Essence de Romarin; Essência de Alecrim; Oleum Roris Marini; Oleum Rosmarini; Rosmarinöl.

Pharmacopoeias. In *Aust., Ger., Pol.,* and *Swiss.*

A volatile oil obtained by distillation from the flowering tops or leafy twigs of rosemary, *Rosmarinus officinalis* (Labiatae) containing esters, notably bornyl acetate ($C_{12}H_{20}O_2$) and free alcohols including borneol ($C_{10}H_{18}O$) and linalol ($C_{10}H_{18}O$). It is a colourless or pale yellow oil with a characteristic odour and a warm bitter camphoraceous taste.

Rosemary oil is carminative and mildly irritant. It is used in perfumery and as a flavour and has been employed in hair lotions, inhalations, and liniments.

Preparations

Proprietary Preparations (details are given in Part 3)
Ger.: Perozon Rosmarin-Olbad mono.

Multi-ingredient: ***Aust.:*** Berggeist; Bronchiplant; Carl Baders Divinal; Criniton; Dracodermalin; Embrocation; Inno Rheuma; Medizinalbad†; Opino; Pulmex†; Red Point†; Rheuma; Rowalind; Salhumin; Tetesept; ***Austral.:*** Bioglan E-Plus; Bioglan Fingers & Toes; Euky Bearub; Tixylix Chest Rub; ***Belg.:*** Calyptol†; Perubore; Pinthym†; Pulmex; Pulmex Baby; ***Fr.:*** Aromasol; Balsofletol†; Dinacode; Perubore; Phytocoltar†; Pulmax; ***Ger.:*** "Topfer" Kinderbad mit Teer†; "Topfer" Teerkleiebad†; Algonerg†; Arnika-Balsam†; Arthrodeformat P; Arthrodynat P; Balnostim Bad N; Bergauf†; Bronchicum Inhalat†; Bronchoforton Infant†; Cefarheumin N; Cobed†; Cor-Vel; Criniton; Crinocedin†; Dolexamed N; Dolo-cyl; Dr. Hotz Vollbad; Dracodermalin†; Eucafluid N; Grune Nervensalbe†; Grunlicht Hingfong Essenz; Guttacor-Balsam N; Histajodol N; Hyperiagil†; Infrotto†; Kneipp Erkaltungs-Balsam N; Kneipp Herzsalbe Unguentum Cardiacum Kneipp; Kneipp Kreislauf-Bad Rosmarin-Aquasan; Koryn mild†; Koryn†; Leukona-Kreislauf-Bad; Leukona-Rheumasalbe; Leukona-Tonikum-Bad†; Makinil†; opino heparinoid†; Phardol N Balsam†; Retterspitz Ausserlich; Retterspitz Gelee; Retterspitz Quick; Rheuma-Pasc N; Rheumaliment†; Rheumex†; Rhinotussal E Balsam†; Rosarthron; Rosarthron forte; Rosmarinsalbe†; Rowalind; Schupps Heilkrauter Rheumabad; Silvapin Franzbranntwein†; stadasan Thermo†; thermo-loges; Thrombocid; Vaxicum N; ***Irl.:*** Purporent†; Rowalind; ***Ital.:*** Balsamico F. di M.†; Calyptol; Opino†; ***Mon.:*** Calyptol; ***Spain:*** Bellacanfor†; Calyptol Inhalante; Dolokey; Linimento Klari; Masagil; Porosan†; ***Switz.:*** Acidodermil; Brachialin†; Caprisana; Carmol "thermogene"†; Carmol†; Frigoplasma; Graminflor†; Incutin; Kernosan Huile de Massage; Methylan†; Perubare; Pulmex; Pulmex Baby; Pulmex†; Thrombocid; ***UK:*** Adiantine; Frost Cream; Massage Balm Arnica; Rheumadoron.

Roxarsone (13220-x)

Roxarsone *(BAN, USAN, rINN).*

NSC-2101. 4-Hydroxy-3-nitrophenylarsonic acid.

$C_6H_6AsNO_6$ = 263.0.

CAS — 121-19-7.

Pharmacopoeias. In *US.*

A pale yellow crystalline powder. Slightly **soluble** in cold water; soluble in boiling water; freely soluble in dehydrated alcohol, in acetic acid, in acetone, in alkalis, and in methyl alcohol; sparingly soluble in dilute mineral acids; practically insoluble in ether and in ethyl acetate. It puffs up and deflagrates on heating.

Roxarsone has been used as a growth promoter in animal feeds.

Royal Jelly (13221-r)

Queen Bee Jelly.

A milky-white viscid secretion from the salivary glands of the worker hive bee, *Apis mellifera* (Apidae); it is essential for the development of queen bees.

Royal jelly has been used as a general 'tonic', to ward off the effects of old age, and to ease sufferers from chronic degenerative diseases, but of the many and diverse claims made for the therapeutic value of the jelly, none has been substantiated.

Royal jelly is also incorporated in some cosmetic preparations for its supposed beneficial effect on skin tissue.

Hypersensitivity. There have been a number of cases of anaphylactoid reactions and acute severe exacerbations of asthma[1-3] (one fatal[2]) in atopic individuals who took royal jelly.

1. Thien FCK, *et al.* Royal jelly-induced asthma. *Med J Aust* 1993; **159:** 639.
2. Bullock RJ, *et al.* Fatal royal jelly-induced asthma. *Med J Aust* 1994; **160:** 44.
3. Peacock S, *et al.* Respiratory distress and royal jelly. *Br Med J* 1995; **311:** 1472.

Preparations

Proprietary Preparations (details are given in Part 3)
Fr.: Apiserum; ***Ital.:*** Alvear; Biogel; Biovital; Clinvit; Ecogel†; Ergon 1000†; Gelamel; Magisgel†; Megel†; Opalia; Pa-Real; Ritmogel; Roburvit; Telergon II; Theogel; Trefovital; Trofomed; ***UK:*** Regina Royal One Hundred.

Multi-ingredient: ***Aust.:*** DH 112†; ***Austral.:*** Zestabs†; ***Fr.:*** Arkotonic; Pollen Royal; ***Ger.:*** Alsiroyal; ***Ital.:*** Alvear Complex; Alvear Sport; Apergan; Api Baby; Apiserum con Telergon 1; Apistress; Bebimix; Bio Ritz†; Bio-200; Bio-Real; Bio-Real Complex; Bio-Real Plus; Bioton; Biotrefon Plus; Biovigor; Cocktail Reale; Eurogel; Fon Wan Ginsenergy; Fon Wan Pollen; Fosfarsile Forte; Fosfarsile Yunior; Four-Ton; Granvit; Longevital; Miegel; Mnemo Organico; Mnemo Organico Plus†; Neo Trefogel†; Neoplus; Nerex; Novogel; Nutrex; Nutrigel; Ottovis; Pollingel; Provitamin A-E; Ribovir; Royal E; Royal Mille†; Vigogel; Vitalmix; ***UK:*** Arthrotone; Beeline; Regina Royal Concorde; Regina Royal Five; Royal Galanol.

Rubber (12519-p)

Caoutchouc; India-Rubber.

Rubber consists of the prepared latex of *Hevea brasiliensis* and other species of *Hevea*. It is used as a component of many medical devices such as catheters, syringes, enema tips, ostomy bags, balloons, and surgical gloves. Hypersensitivity reactions have occurred after direct contact of skin and mucous membranes with rubber components of such products and also after indirect contact with preparations stored in or administered by them; deaths have been reported. Reactions have been attributed either to protein components of the rubber or to additives such as preservatives or vulcanisation accelerators. Cross-sensitivity between rubber proteins and those of certain fruits, including bananas and chestnuts, has been reported.

References.

1. Llátser R, *et al.* Anaphylaxis to natural rubber latex in a girl with food allergy. *Pediatrics* 1994; **94:** 736–7.
2. Sussman GL, Beezhold DH. Allergy to latex rubber. *Ann Intern Med* 1995; **122:** 43–6.
3. Kwittken PL, *et al.* Latex hypersensitivity in children: clinical presentation and detection of latex-specific immunoglobulin E. *Pediatrics* 1995; **95:** 693–9.
4. Landwehr LP, Boguniewicz M. Current perspectives on latex allergy. *J Pediatr* 1996; **128:** 305–12.
5. Shah M, *et al.* Delayed and immediate orofacial reactions following contact with rubber gloves during dental treatment. *Br Dent J* 1996; **181:** 137–9.
6. Wilkinson SM, Beck MH. Allergic contact dermatitis from latex rubber. *Br J Dermatol* 1996; **134:** 910–14.
7. Senst BL, Johnson RA. Latex allergy. *Am J Health-Syst Pharm* 1997; **54:** 1071–5.
8. Poole CJM. Hazards of powdered surgical gloves. *Lancet* 1997; **350:** 973–4.
9. Handfield-Jones SE. Latex allergy in health-care workers in an English district general hospital. *Br J Dermatol* 1998; **138:** 273–6.
10. Zaidi Z, *et al.* Latex allergy: a life-threatening complication. *Hosp Med* 1998; **59:** 505–7.

Rubidium Iodide (11529-h)

RbI = 212.4.

CAS — 7790-29-6.

Rubidium iodide has the actions of iodine and the iodides (see p.1493). It is an ingredient of several proprietary ophthalmic preparations promoted for the treatment of eye disorders.

Preparations

Proprietary Preparations (details are given in Part 3)

Multi-ingredient: ***Ger.:*** durajod†; ***Ital.:*** Calcio Jodico†; Facovit; Jodo-Calcio-Vitaminico; Polijodurato; Rubidiosin Composto; Rubistenol; Rubjovit.

Rue Oil (4702-q)

Oleum Rutae.

A volatile oil obtained from rue, *Ruta graveolens* (Rutaceae).

Rue oil and infusions of rue were formerly used as antispasmodics and emmenagogues and are reported to have abortifacient properties. Rue is a photosensitiser and the oil is a powerful local irritant.

Rue (Ruta grav.) is used in homoeopathic medicine.

Ruscogenin (3913-w)

(25*R*)-Spirost-5-ene-1β,3β-diol.

$C_{27}H_{42}O_4$ = 430.6.

CAS — 472-11-7.

A sapogenin obtained from butcher's broom, *Ruscus aculeatus* (Liliaceae).

Ruscogenin has been applied in the local treatment of haemorrhoids as rectal ointment or suppositories.

Preparations

Proprietary Preparations (details are given in Part 3)

Ger.: Ruscorectal; ***Spain:*** Hemodren Simple; Ruscorectal.

Multi-ingredient: ***Fr.:*** Calmoroide; Proctolog; ***Ital.:*** Ruscoroid; ***Spain:*** Abrasone Rectal; Hemodren Compuesto; Neo Analsona; Proctolog; Ruscus; Venacol.

Sabeluzole (2980-y)

Sabeluzole *(BAN, USAN, rINN).*

R-58735. (±)-4-(2-Benzothiazolylmethylamino)-α-[(4-fluorophenoxy)methyl]-1-piperidineethanol.

$C_{22}H_{26}FN_3O_2S$ = 415.5.

CAS — 104153-38-0.

Sabeluzole is a benzothiazole derivative with anticonvulsant and antihypoxic properties. It is under investigation in the treatment of Alzheimer's disease.

Sacrosidase (19809-v)

Sacrosidase is a therapeutic enzyme used for replacement therapy in congenital sucrase-isomaltase deficiency.

Preparations

Proprietary Preparations (details are given in Part 3)

USA: Sucraid.

Sage (4704-s)

Feuilles de Sauge; Salbeiblätter; Salvia.

Pharmacopoeias. In *Eur.* (see p.viii) and *Pol.*

The whole of cut dried leaves of *Salvia officinalis* (Labiatae). The whole drug contains not less that 15 mL per kg and the cut drug not less than 10 mL per kg of an essential oil rich in thujone, both calculated with reference to the anhydrous drug. **Protect** from light.

Sage has carminative, antispasmodic, antiseptic, and astringent properties and is used as a flavour. It is used in preparations for a wide variety of purposes, including respiratory-tract disorders, gastro-intestinal disorders, and in mouthwashes and gargles for disorders of the mouth and throat. It is also used in homoeopathic medicine.

Preparations

Proprietary Preparations (details are given in Part 3)

Aust.: Salvysat; ***Ger.:*** Aperisan; Fichtensirup N; Salvysat; Sweatosan N; Viru-Salvysat.

Multi-ingredient: ***Aust.:*** Apotheker Bauer's Blahungstee; Bronchostop; Cional; Dynexan; Krauterhaus Mag Kottas Wechseltee; Krautertee Nr 10; Krautertee Nr 107; Krautertee Nr 16; Krautertee Nr 311; Krautertee Nr 8; Mentopin; Paradenton; Teekanne Husten- und Brusttee; ***Belg.:*** Cigarettes Anti-asthmatiques†; Tisane pour Dormir; ***Fr.:*** Bolcitol; Phytocoltar†; Santane V_3; Tisanes de l'Abbe Hamon no 6; ***Ger.:*** Agamadon; Bronchialtee†; Broncholind†; Chelidonium-Strath†; Dynexan†; Echtrosept-GT†; entero sanol†; Helago-oel N; Mycatox; Odala wern; Optipect mit Kodein†; Optipect†; Parodontal; Phytpulmon†; Polypharm-Zahnungsgel N; Presselin 214†; Presselin 52 N; Thymitussin†; Ventrovis†; Verus†; Vitosal; Worishofener Leber- und Gallensteinmittel Dr. Kleinschrod†; Worishofener Nieren- und Blasenmittel Dr. Kleinschrod†; ***Ital.:*** Babygella†; Donalg; Saugella Antisettica†; Saugella Salviettine; ***S.Afr.:*** Dynexan; ***Spain:*** Vegetalin; ***Switz.:*** Anginesin; Cional†; Dynexan; Gynogella†; Mucosan†; Tisane pectorale et antitussive; Tonex; ***UK:*** Catarrh; Fragador.

Salverine Hydrochloride (19696-l)

Salverine Hydrochloride *(rINNM).*

M-811 (salverine). 2-[2-(Diethylamino)ethoxy]-benzanilide hydrochloride.

$C_{19}H_{24}N_2O_2,HCl$ = 348.9.

CAS — 6376-26-7 (salverine).

Salverine hydrochloride is used as an antispasmodic, usually in combination with other drugs.

Preparations

Proprietary Preparations (details are given in Part 3)

Multi-ingredient: ***Aust.:*** Cynarix comp; Montamed; Novipec.

Sambucus (320-q)

Elder Flowers; Fleurs de Sureau; Holunderblüten; Sabugueiro; Sambuc.

Pharmacopoeias. In *Eur.* (see p.viii) and *Pol.*

The dried flowers of *Sambucus nigra* (Caprifoliaceae). **Protect** from light.

Sambucus has astringent, diaphoretic, and anticatarrhal properties and is used in herbal and homoeopathic preparations for a variety of disorders, particularly respiratory-tract disorders. Elder-flower water has been used as a vehicle for eye and skin lotions. Elder-flower ointment has been used as a basis for pomades and cosmetic ointments.

Preparations

Proprietary Preparations (details are given in Part 3)

Multi-ingredient: ***Aust.:*** Apotheker Bauer's Grippetee; Bio-Garten Entschlackungstee; Blutreinigungstee†; Bogumil-tassenfertiger milder Abfurtee; Entschlackungstee; Grippetee Dr Zeidler; Grippetee EF-EM-ES; Grippogran; Krauter Hustensaft†; Krauterdoktor Erkaltungstropfen; Krauterhaus Mag Kottas Grippetee; Krautertee Nr 10; Krautertee Nr 2; Krautertee Nr 210; Laxalpin; Mag Kottas Grippe-Tee; Sidroga Erkaltungstee; Sinupret; Sinusol-Schleimlosender Tee; St Radegunder Fiebertee; Teekanne Erkaltungstee; ***Austral.:*** Sambucus Complex; ***Fr.:*** Tisane des Familles†; ***Ger.:*** Abfuhr-Tee Stada†; Grippe-Tee Stada†; Hevert-Erkaltungs-Tee; Hevert-Gicht-Rheuma-Tee comp; Kneipp Rheuma Tee N; Nephrubin; Sinupret; ***Ital.:*** Sambuco (Specie Composta); ***Switz.:*** The Brioni; Tisane contre les refroidissements; Tisane laxative H; ***UK:*** Elder Flowers with Peppermint and Composition Essence; Herb and Honey Cough Elixir; Life Drops; Lifedrops; Sinotar; Tabritis.

Sanguinaria (739-e)

Bloodroot; Red Puccoon; Sanguinaria canadensis; Sanguinarine canadensis; Sanguinaris canadensis.

The dried rhizome of *Sanguinaria canadensis* (Papaveraceae).

Sanguinarine, an alkaloid extracted from *Sanguinaria canadensis*, has been used as an antiplaque agent in toothpaste and mouthwash preparations. Sanguinaria was formerly used as an expectorant but fell into disuse because of its toxicity. Sanguinaria has also been classified by the FDA as a herb that is unsafe for use in foods, beverages, or drugs.

Sanguinaria is used in homoeopathic medicine.

Reviews.

1. Karlowsky JA. Bloodroot: Sanguinaria canadensis L. *Can Pharm J* 1991; **124:** 260, 262–3, 267.

Preparations

Proprietary Preparations (details are given in Part 3)

Canad.: Viadent; ***Ital.:*** Periogard.

Multi-ingredient: ***Austral.:*** Lexat; ***Canad.:*** Mielocol; Viadent; Wampole Bronchial Cough Syrup; ***Ital.:*** Eudent con Glysan; Periogard.

Sarsaparilla (2408-p)

Salsaparilha; Salsepareille; Sarsa; Sarsaparilla Root; Smilacis Rhizoma.

Pharmacopoeias. In *Chin.* and *Jpn.* which specify *Smilax glabra.*

The dried root of various species of *Smilax* (Liliaceae).

Sarsaparilla, usually in the form of a decoction or extract, has been used as a vehicle and flavour for medicaments. It is also an ingredient of herbal and homoeopathic preparations.

Preparations

Proprietary Preparations (details are given in Part 3)

Ger.: Sarsapsor.

Multi-ingredient: ***Austral.:*** Esten†; Herbal Cleanse; Proesten; Zestabs†; ***Belg.:*** Stago†; Tisane Depurative "les 12 Plantes"; ***Fr.:*** Depuratif Parnel; ***Ger.:*** Dr. Klinger's Bergischer Krautertee, Abfuhr- und Verdauungstee†; Montana; Pankreaplex N†; Pankreaplex Neu; Pascopankreat†; ***Ital.:*** Depurativo; Tisana Kelemata; ***UK:*** Blue Flag Root Compound; Jamaica Sarsaparilla; Ligvites; Skin Eruptions Mixture.

Sassafras Oil (4708-y)

Oleum Sassafras.

A volatile oil distilled from the root or root bark of *Sassafras albidum* (Lauraceae), or from the wood of certain species of *Ocotea* (Lauraceae). It contains safrole.

Sassafras oil has rubefacient properties and was formerly used as a pediculicide. Neither sassafras nor the oil should be taken internally; the use of herb teas of sassafras may lead to a large dose of safrole. The use of safrole in foods has been banned because of carcinogenic and hepatotoxic risks. The use of safrole in toilet preparations is also controlled.

A 47-year-old woman experienced 'shakiness', vomiting, anxiety, tachycardia, and raised blood pressure following ingestion of a potentially fatal dose of sassafras oil (5 mL).[1] Treatment was symptomatic following the use of activated charcoal.

1. Grande GA, Dannewitz SR. Symptomatic sassafras oil ingestion. *Vet Hum Toxicol* 1987; **29:** 447.

Preparations

Proprietary Preparations (details are given in Part 3)

Multi-ingredient: ***Austral.:*** Zam-Buk; ***Belg.:*** Vegebom†; ***Fr.:*** Vegebom; ***S.Afr.:*** Zam-Buk; ***Spain:*** Inhalador; Linimento Klari; Vicks Inhalador.

Saxitoxin (746-w)

Saxitoxin is a neurotoxin associated with paralytic shellfish poisoning. It is an endotoxin produced by species of dinoflagellate plankton present in infected molluscs.

References.

1. Halstead BW, Schantz EJ. *Paralytic shellfish poisoning.* Geneva: WHO, 1984.
2. Aquatic (marine and freshwater) biotoxins. *Environmental Health Criteria 37.* Geneva: WHO, 1984.
3. Hartigan-Go K, Bateman DN. Redtide in the Philippines. *Hum Exp Toxicol* 1994; **13:** 824–30.

Schick Test (8005-j)

Pharmacopoeias. Br. and *US* include standards for Schick test toxin and control.

Schick toxin is prepared from the toxic products of *Corynebacterium diphtheriae*. It should be stored at 2° to 8°. Schick control is Schick toxin that has been inactivated by heat. It should be stored at 2° to 8°.

The Schick test has been used for the diagnosis of susceptibility to diphtheria and, more importantly, to detect patients who might experience an adverse reaction to diphtheria vaccines. Children up to the age of about 8 to 10 years rarely suffer from such reactions following diphtheria vaccination and therefore the Schick test is not usually performed in this age group. In older children and adults a Schick test was formerly used before the use of standard diphtheria vaccines. However, diphtheria vaccines for use in adults and adolescents (p.1507) are now formulated with lesser amounts of toxoid so that the need for prior Schick testing is unnecessary.

A dose of 0.2 mL of the Schick toxin was administered intradermally (intracutaneously) into the flexor surface of the forearm. A similar dose of Schick control was injected into the other forearm. The reaction to the injections was read after 24 to 48 hours, and again after 5 to 7 days to detect late reactors and to confirm a reading taken earlier.

A *negative reaction*, indicating that the patient is immune to diphtheria, occurs when there is no redness at either injection site. A *positive reaction*, indicating susceptibility to diphtheria, occurs as a red flush about 10 mm or more in diameter at the site of injection of the test dose with no reaction to the control injection. A *negative-and-pseudo reaction*, also indicating immunity, is shown by a flush which develops rapidly at each injection site but the reaction fades more rapidly than a positive reaction; the reaction is due to non-specific constituents of the injection. A *combined* or *positive-and-pseudo reaction*, also indicating susceptibility, is shown by a flush which develops rapidly at each injection site, but as it fades a positive reaction develops at the site of the test dose.

Preparations

BP 1998: Schick Control; Schick Test Toxin;

USP 23: Diphtheria Toxin for Schick Test; Schick Test Control.

Scoparium (13224-n)

Broom Tops; Genêt; Genêt à Balai; Planta Genista; Scoparii Cacumina.

Pharmacopoeias. In *Fr.*

The dried tops of broom, *Sarothamnus scoparius* (=*Cytisus scoparius*) (Leguminosae).

Scoparium is a mild diuretic, haemostatic, and vasoconstrictor and has been administered as a decoction or infusion. It has oxytocic properties and should be avoided in pregnancy. It contains sparteine (p.1632).

Preparations

Proprietary Preparations (details are given in Part 3)
Ger.: Repowine; Spartiol.

Multi-ingredient: *Fr.:* Creme Rap; Curoveinyl; Santane H_7; Santane R_8; Santane V_3; Tisanes de l'Abbe Hamon no 16; *Ger.:* Aureal†; Cardaminol†; Dr. Kleinschrod's Cor-Insuffin†; Goldtropfen-Hetterich; Intradermi N; JuPhlebon S; Liruptin†; Oxacant N; Venacton; Worishofener Nervenpflege Dr. Kleinschrod†.

Secretin (2147-m)

Secretin *(BAN, rINN).*
CAS — 17034-35-4.

Units

The potency of secretin may be expressed as Crick-Harper-Raper (CHR) units based on the pancreatic secretion in *cats* or as Clinical units, the value of which was amended in the 1960s. One Clinical unit is considered to be approximately equivalent to 4 CHR units.

Adverse Effects

Hypersensitivity reactions may occasionally occur. Diarrhoea has occurred in patients given high doses by intravenous infusion.

Precautions

The secretin test should be avoided in patients with acute pancreatitis. Administration of a test dose has been suggested for patients at particular risk of hypersensitivity reactions.

Uses and Administration

Secretin is a polypeptide hormone involved in the regulation of gastric function; it is prepared from the duodenal mucosa of *pigs*. Following administration by intravenous injection it causes an increase in the secretion by the pancreas of water and bicarbonate into the duodenum. It is used alone, or in conjunction with pancreozymin or other cholecystokinetic agents such as ceruletide (p.1561) or sincalide (p.1630), as a test for exocrine pancreatic function, and in the diagnosis of biliary-tract disorders. These tests usually involve duodenal intubation of the patient and examination of duodenal aspirate. The dose of secretin used has varied but common doses have been 1 Clinical unit per kg body-weight given by slow intravenous injection.

Patients with the Zollinger-Ellison syndrome (p.1176) show an increase in gastrin following the administration of secretin; this is in contrast to a small change or no effect in subjects without the disorder. The usual dose of secretin for the diagnosis of Zollinger-Ellison syndrome is 2 Clinical units per kg by slow intravenous injection. Serum-gastrin concentrations are measured for up to 30 minutes following the test dose.

Preparations

Proprietary Preparations (details are given in Part 3)
Ger.: Sekretolin.

Selfotel (17312-w)

Selfotel *(USAN, rINN).*
CGS-19755. *cis*-4-(Phosphonomethyl)pipecolic acid.
$C_7H_{14}NO_5P$ = 223.2.
CAS — 110347-85-8.

Selfotel is an *N*-methyl-D-aspartate (NMDA) antagonist which has been investigated for use in ischaemic stroke and head trauma.

References.

1. Horton R. Optimism over therapy for stroke. *Lancet* 1994; **343:** 1220.
2. Grotta J, *et al.* Safety and tolerability of the glutamate antagonist CGS 19755 (Selfotel) in patients with acute ischemic stroke: results of a phase IIa randomized trial. *Stroke* 1995; **26:** 602–5.
3. Davis SM, *et al.* Termination of acute stroke studies involving selfotel treatment. *Lancet* 1997; **349:** 32.

Senecio (13229-g)

Liferoot; Squaw Weed.

The ragwort, *Senecio jacobaea*, and, in the USA, the golden ragwort, *Senecio aureus*, in the form of extracts have been used as emmenagogues but are of doubtful value. Ragwort, in the form of a decoction or ointment, has also been applied externally to aid wound healing and in the treatment of peripheral vascular disorders.

Many species of the genus *Senecio* (Compositae), which includes the ragworts and groundsels, are poisonous and have been found to contain pyrrolizidine alkaloids which produce hepatic necrosis. The ragwort, *S. jacobaea*, which is abundant throughout the British Isles, is poisonous to livestock when eaten in quantity. Poisoning has also been reported in humans following ingestion of herbal teas containing pyrrolizidine alkaloids.

Preparations

Proprietary Preparations (details are given in Part 3)

Multi-ingredient: *Canad.:* Thunas Tab for Menstrual Pain; *Fr.:* Fluon; Tisane Phlebosedol; *Ger.:* Senecion; *USA:* Succus Cineraria Maritima.

Sepia (13230-f)

Sepia is the dried inky secretion of the cuttle fish. It is used in homoeopathic medicine.

Preparations

Proprietary Preparations (details are given in Part 3)

Multi-ingredient: *Ger.:* Gastro-Vial†.

Serotonin (15305-a)

Enteramine; 5-HT; 5-Hydroxytryptamine. 3-(2-Aminoethyl)-1*H*-indol-5-ol.
$C_{10}H_{12}N_2O$ = 176.2.
CAS — 50-67-9.

Serotonin is widely distributed in the body; it also occurs in stinging nettles (*Urtica dioica*), bananas, and other fruit, and in the stings of wasps and scorpions.

Serotonin is found in the brain, blood platelets, and throughout the gastro-intestinal tract. It has several actions which include involvement in CNS neurotransmission, haemostasis, vascular spasm, and gastro-intestinal motility. Several types and subtypes of serotonin receptors have been identified and drugs with serotonin-agonist activity and those displaying serotonin-antagonist activity can be used to treat the same condition such as migraine or depression. Many drugs have some action on serotonin receptors. Serotonin *precursors* have been given for the treatment of depression (see Oxitriptan, p.301 and Tryptophan, p.310). *Selective serotonin reuptake inhibitors* are used in depression (see Fluoxetine Hydrochloride, p.284); also *MAOIs* and *tricyclic antidepressants* have some serotonin-agonist activity. *Sumatriptan* (see p.450) is an agonist used in migraine. The *dopaminergic ergot derivatives* such as Bromocriptine Mesylate, p.1132 Lysuride Maleate, p.1142, and Pergolide Mesylate, p.1142 are partial serotonin agonists.

Among the drugs exhibiting serotonin-antagonist activity are the antimigraine *ergot alkaloids*; *antihistamines* such as Cyproheptadine Hydrochloride, p.407, and Pizotifen Malate, p.449; *antihypertensives* such as Ketanserin Tartrate, p.894; and *antiemetics* such as Ondansetron Hydrochloride, p.1206. *Other drugs* with recognised serotonin-antagonist activity include Fenclonine, p.1579, Dexfenfluramine Hydrochloride p.1479, Fenfluramine Hydrochloride, p.1480, Chlorpromazine, p.649, and the tetracyclic antidepressant Mianserin Hydrochloride, p.297.

Serotonin itself is used in the treatment of myoclonus (p.338).

References.

1. Hindle AT. Recent developments in the physiology and pharmacology of 5-hydroxytryptamine. *Br J Anaesth* 1994; **73:** 395–407.
2. Hoyer D, *et al.* International Union of Pharmacology classification of receptors for 5-hydroxytryptamine (serotonin). *Pharmacol Rev* 1994; **46:** 157–203.

Serpentary (541-x)

Serpentaria; Serpentary Rhizome; Texan or Virginian Snakeroot.

NOTE. Snakeroot is also used as a common name to describe poisonous *Eupatorium* spp.

Pharmacopoeias. In *Chin.* which allows various species of *Aristolochia.*

Preparations of serpentary have been employed as bitters. Its active ingredient is aristolochic acid and this and its sodium salt have been tried in a number of inflammatory disorders, mainly in folk medicine. However there is concern over its use since aristolochic acid has been reported to be carcinogenic in animals.

Serrapeptase (13233-h)

Serrapeptase *(rINN).*
CAS — 37312-62-2.

A proteolytic enzyme derived from *Serratia* spp.

Serrapeptase has been taken by mouth for its supposed action in relieving inflammation and oedema associated with trauma, infection, or chronic venous insufficiency, in usual doses of 5 to 10 mg (10 000 to 20 000 units) up to three times daily.

References.

1. Tachibana M, *et al.* A multi-centre, double-blind study of serrapeptase versus placebo in post-antrotomy buccal swelling. *Pharmatherapeutica* 1984; **3:** 526–30.
2. Paparella P, *et al.* Serratia peptidase and acute phase protein behavior following vaginal hysterectomy: results of a randomized double-blind, placebo-controlled trial. *Curr Ther Res* 1989; **45:** 664–76.

Preparations

Proprietary Preparations (details are given in Part 3)
Fr.: Dazen; *Ger.:* Aniflazym; *Ital.:* Danzen; *Jpn:* Dasen.

Sesame Oil (7368-w)

Aceite de Ajonjoli; Benne Oil; Gingelly Oil; Oleum Sesami; Teel Oil.

Pharmacopoeias. In *Chin., Eur.* (see p.viii), and *Jpn.* Also in *USNF.*

The fatty oil obtained from the ripe seeds of *Sesamum indicum* (Pedaliaceae) by expression or extraction and subsequent refining. It is a clear pale yellow oil, almost odourless and with a bland taste with a fatty-acid content consisting mainly of linoleic and oleic acids. It solidifies to a buttery mass at about −4°.

Slightly **soluble** to practically insoluble in alcohol; miscible with carbon disulphide, with chloroform, with ether, and with petroleum spirit. **Store** at a temperature not exceeding 40° in well-filled airtight containers. Protect from light. Sesame oil for use in the manufacture of parenteral dosage forms should be stored under an inert gas in airtight containers.

Sesame oil has been used in the preparation of liniments, plasters, ointments, and soaps. Because it is relatively stable, it is a useful solvent and vehicle for parenteral products. Hypersensitivity reactions have been observed.

Shellac (285-x)

904; Gomme Laque; Lacca; Lacca in Tabulis; Schellack.

Pharmacopoeias. In *Eur.* (see p.viii). Also in *USNF.*
Jpn includes Purified Shellac and White Shellac (Bleached).

Shellac is obtained by purification of the resinous secretion of the female insect *Kerria lacca* Kerr Lindinger (*Laccifer lacca* Kerr) (Coccidae). Ph. Eur. defines 4 types of shellac depending on the nature of the treatment of crude secretion (seedlac): Wax-containing Shellac; Bleached Shellac; Dewaxed Shellac; and Bleached, Dewaxed Shellac. The USNF also describes 4 grades: Orange Shellac; Dewaxed Orange Shellac; Regular Bleached (White) Shellac; and Refined Bleached Shellac.

Brownish-orange or yellow, shining, translucent, hard or brittle flakes, odourless or almost odourless (Wax-containing Shellac; Dewaxed Shellac; Orange Shellac). Creamy-white or brownish-yellow, opaque, amorphous granules or coarse powder, odourless or almost odourless (Bleached Shellac; Bleached, Dewaxed Shellac).

Practically **insoluble** in water; very slowly soluble in alcohol 85% to 95% (w/w); soluble in ether, 13% to 15%; in petroleum spirit, 2% to 6%, and in aqueous solutions of ethanolamines, alkalis, and borax; sparingly soluble in turpentine oil. **Store** preferably at a temperature not exceeding 8°. Protect from light.

Shellac is used as an enteric coating for pills and tablets, but disintegration time has been reported to increase markedly on storage.

Preparations

USNF 18: Pharmaceutical Glaze.

Siam Benzoin (273-c)

Benjoin du Laos; Benzoe Tonkinensis.

Pharmacopoeias. In *Aust., Chin., Fr., It.,* and *Swiss.* Also in many pharmacopoeias under the title benzoin and should not be confused with Sumatra benzoin. *Jpn* and *US* allow both Siam benzoin and Sumatra benzoin under the title Benzoin.

A balsamic resin from *Styrax tonkinensis* (Styracaceae) and containing not more than 10% of alcohol (90%)-insoluble matter.

Yellowish-brown to rusty brown compressed pebble-like tears with an agreeable, balsamic, vanilla-like odour. The tears are separate or very slightly agglutinated, milky white on fracture, and hard and brittle at ordinary temperatures, but softened by heat.

Siam benzoin has been used similarly to Sumatra benzoin (p.1634). It has also been used as a preservative and was formerly used in the preparation of benzoinated lard.

Preparations

USP 23: Compound Benzoin Tincture; Podophyllum Resin Topical Solution.

Proprietary Preparations (details are given in Part 3)

Multi-ingredient: ***Canad.:*** Cold Sore Lotion; ***Fr.:*** Balsolene; Borostyrol; Inotyol; ***Ital.:*** Ondroly-A; ***Switz.:*** Borostyrol N.

Sildenafil Citrate (17680-e)

Sildenafil Citrate *(BANM, USAN, rINNM)*.

UK-92480-10. 5-[2-Ethoxy-5-(4-methylpiperazin-1-ylsulfonyl)phenyl]-1,6-dihydro-1-methyl-3-propylpyrazolo[4,3-*d*]pyrimidin-7-one citrate; 1-{[3-(6,7-Dihydro-1-methyl-7-oxo-3-propyl-1*H*-pyrazolo[4,3-*d*]pyrimidin-5-yl)-4-ethoxyphenyl]sulfonyl}-4-methylpiperazone citrate.

$C_{22}H_{30}N_6O_4S,C_6H_8O_7$ = 666.7.

CAS — 139755-83-2 (sildenafil); 171599-83-0 (sildenafil citrate).

Adverse Effects

Adverse effects most commonly reported from sildenafil are headache, flushing, and dyspepsia. There may be visual disturbances, dizziness, and nasal congestion. Other adverse effects reported include diarrhoea, muscle pain, skin rashes, and urinary- or respiratory-tract infection. Priapism has also occurred.

Effects on the cardiovascular system. Acute myocardial infarction developed about 30 minutes after taking sildenafil in a 65-year-old man with no apparent risk factors for cardiovascular disease and before any attempt at sexual intercourse.[1] In the USA, of 69 patients who had died after taking sildenafil 2 deaths were due to stroke and 46 from some other cardiovascular event, although whether there was an association remains unclear.[2]

1. Feenstra J, *et al.* Acute myocardial infarction associated with sildenafil. *Lancet* 1998; **352:** 957–8.
2. Anonymous. Sildenafil for erectile dysfunction. *Drug Ther Bull* 1998; **36:** 81–4.

Precautions

The cardiovascular risks of sexual activity should be considered before beginning therapy with sildenafil; in some patients, sexual activity may be inadvisable. Caution is required in patients with renal or hepatic impairment, and dosage reduction may be necessary. Care is also needed in patients with anatomical or haematological disorders which may predispose them to priapism, and may be advisable in those with bleeding disorders or active peptic ulceration. The safety of sildenafil is uncertain in patients with hypotension, a recent history of stroke or myocardial infarction, or retinal disorders such as retinitis pigmentosa (a minority of whom have genetic disorders of retinal phosphodiesterases). Patients who experience dizziness or visual disturbances should not drive or operate hazardous machinery.

Interactions

Sildenafil is contra-indicated in anyone taking organic nitrates as it may potentiate their hypotensive effects. Concomitant administration of sildenafil with drugs that inhibit cytochrome CYP3A4, such as cimetidine, may reduce sildenafil clearance.

Pharmacokinetics

Sildenafil is rapidly absorbed following administration by mouth, with a bioavailability of approximately 40%. Peak plasma concentrations are attained within 30 to 120 minutes; the rate of absorption is reduced when sildenafil is administered with food.

Sildenafil is widely distributed into tissues and is approximately 96% bound to plasma proteins. It is metabolised in the liver primarily by cytochrome CYP3A4 and CYP2C9 isoforms. The major metabolite *N*-desmethylsildenafil, also has some activity. The terminal half-lives of sildenafil and the N-desmethyl metabolite are about 4 hours.

Sildenafil is excreted, predominantly as metabolites, in the faeces, and to a lesser extent the urine. Clearance may be reduced in the elderly and in patients with severe renal or hepatic impairment.

Uses and Administration

Sildenafil is a phosphodiesterase type-5 inhibitor used in the management of erectile dysfunction (p.1614). It is given by mouth as the citrate although doses are expressed in terms of the base. The usual dose is 50 mg about one hour before sexual intercourse. The dose may be increased to 100 mg once a day or decreased to 25 mg once a day depending on response. An initial dose of 25 mg is recommended in elderly patients and in those with severe renal or hepatic impairment, increased according to response if appropriate.

References.

1. Boolell M, *et al.* Sildenafil, a novel effective oral therapy for male erectile dysfunction. *Br J Urol* 1996; **78:** 257–61.
2. Muirhead GJ, *et al.* Pharmacokinetics of sildenafil (VIAGRA™), a selective cGMP PDE5 inhibitor, after single oral doses in fasted and fed healthy volunteers. *Br J Clin Pharmacol* 1996; **42:** 268P.
3. Goldstein I, *et al.* Oral sildenafil in the treatment of erectile dysfunction. *N Engl J Med* 1998; **338:** 1397–1404. Correction. *ibid.*; **339:** 59.
4. Anonymous. Sildenafil: an oral drug for impotence. *Med Lett Drugs Ther* 1998; **40:** 51–2.
5. Anonymous. Sildenafil for erectile dysfunction. *Drug Ther Bull* 1998; **36:** 81–4.

Preparations

Proprietary Preparations (details are given in Part 3)
UK: Viagra; ***USA:*** Viagra.

Silver (5316-v)

E174.

Ag = 107.8682.

CAS — 7440-22-4.

Pharmacopoeias. In Swiss.

A pure white, malleable and ductile metal.

Silver possesses antibacterial properties and is used topically either as the metal or as silver salts. It is not absorbed to any great extent and the main problem associated with the metal is argyria, a general grey discoloration. Silver is used as a colouring agent for some types of confectionery. It is also used as Argentum Metallicum in homoeopathy.

Numerous salts or compounds of silver have been employed for various therapeutic purposes, including silver acetate (p.1629), silver allantoinate and silver zinc allantoinate, silver borate, silver carbonate, silver chloride, silver chromate, silver glycerolate, colloidal silver iodide, silver lactate, silver manganite, silver nitrate (p.1629), silver-nylon polymers, silver protein (p.1629), and silver sulphadiazine (p.247).

Coating catheters with silver has been reported to reduce the incidence of catheter-associated bacteriuria,[1,2] but other studies have reported increased infection.[3]

1. Lundeberg T. Prevention of catheter-associated urinary-tract infections by use of silver-impregnated catheters. *Lancet* 1986; **ii:** 1031.
2. Johnson JR, *et al.* Prevention of catheter-associated urinary tract infections with a silver oxide-coated urinary catheter: clinical and microbiologic correlates. *J Infect Dis* 1990; **162:** 1145–50.
3. Riley DK, *et al.* A large randomized clinical trial of a silver-impregnated urinary catheter: lack of efficacy and staphylococcal superinfection. *Am J Med* 1995; **98:** 349–56.

Preparations

Proprietary Preparations (details are given in Part 3)
Austral.: Micropur; ***Canad.:*** Tabanil†; ***Fr.:*** Micropur; ***Ger.:*** Dulcargan†; Silargetten†.

Multi-ingredient: ***Canad.:*** Nova-T; ***Fr.:*** Actisorb Plus; Nova-T; ***Ger.:*** Adsorgan†; Grune Salbe "Schmidt" N; Nova-T; ***Irl.:*** Actisorb Plus; ***Ital.:*** Actisorb Plus; Agipiu; Katoderm; Katoxyn; Nova-T; Silver-Nova T†; ***Neth.:*** Nova-T; ***S.Afr.:*** Nova-T; ***Spain:*** Argentocromo; ***Switz.:*** Nova-T; ***UK:*** Actisorb Plus; Nova-T.

Silver Acetate (5319-p)

Argenti Acetas.

CH_3COOAg = 166.9.

CAS — 563-63-3.

Pharmacopoeias. In Aust.

Silver acetate has been used similarly to silver nitrate as a disinfectant. It has also been used in antismoking preparations.

References.

1. Malcolm R, *et al.* Silver acetate gum as a deterrent to smoking. *Chest* 1986; **90:** 107–11.
2. Jensen EJ, *et al.* Effect of nicotine, silver acetate, and ordinary chewing gum in combination with group counselling on smoking cessation. *Thorax* 1990; **45:** 831–4.
3. Hymowitz N, Eckholdt H. Effects of a 2.5-mg silver acetate lozenge on initial and long-term smoking cessation. *Prev Med* 1996; **25:** 537–46.

Preparations

Proprietary Preparations (details are given in Part 3)
Canad.: Smokerette; ***UK:*** Tabmint†.

Silver Nitrate (5321-h)

Argenti Nitras; Nitrato de Plata; Nitrato de Prata.

$AgNO_3$ = 169.9.

CAS — 7761-88-8.

Pharmacopoeias. In Eur. (see p.viii), Int., Jpn, Pol., and US.

Colourless or white transparent crystals or crystalline odourless powder. On exposure to light in the presence of organic matter, silver nitrate becomes grey or greyish-black. **Soluble** 1 in 0.4 of water and 1 in 30 of alcohol; its solubility is increased in boiling water or alcohol; slightly soluble in ether. A solution in water has a pH of about 5.5.

Silver nitrate is **incompatible** with a range of substances. Although it is unlikely that there will be a need to add any of the interacting substances to silver nitrate solutions considering its current uses, pharmacists should be aware of the potential for incompatibility. **Store** in airtight non-metallic containers. Protect from light.

The reported yellow-brown discoloration of samples of silver nitrate bladder irrigation (1 in 10 000) probably arose from the reaction of the silver nitrate with alkali released from the glass bottle which appeared to be soda-glass.[1]

1. *PSGB Lab Report P/80/6* 1980.

Adverse Effects

Symptoms of poisoning stem from the corrosive action of silver nitrate and include pain in the mouth, sialorrhoea, diarrhoea, vomiting, coma, and convulsions.

A short lived minor conjunctivitis is common in infants given silver nitrate eye drops; repeated use or the use of high concentrations produces severe damage and even blindness. Chronic application to the conjunctiva, mucous surfaces, or open wounds leads to argyria (see Silver, above), which though difficult to treat is mainly a cosmetic hazard.

Although silver nitrate is not readily absorbed, absorption of nitrite following reduction of nitrate may cause methaemoglobinaemia. There is also a risk of electrolyte disturbances.

Effects on the eyes. Silver nitrate from a stick containing 75% was applied to the eyes of a newborn infant instead of a 1% solution.[1] After 1 hour there was a thick purulent secretion, the eyelids were red and oedematous, and the conjunctiva markedly injected. The corneas had a blue-grey bedewed appearance with areas of corneal opacification. After treatment by lavage and topical application of antibiotics and homatropine 2% there was a marked improvement and after 1 week topical application of corticosteroids was started. Residual damage was limited to slight corneal opacity.

1. Hornblass A. Silver nitrate ocular damage in newborns. *JAMA* 1975; **231:** 245.

Uses and Administration

Silver nitrate possesses disinfectant properties and is used in many countries as a 1% solution for the prophylaxis of gonococcal ophthalmia neonatorum (see Neonatal Conjunctivitis, p.132) when 2 drops are instilled into each conjunctival sac of the neonate. However, as it can cause irritation, other agents are often used.

In stick form it has been used as a caustic to destroy warts (p.1076) and other small skin growths. Compresses soaked in a 0.5% solution of silver nitrate have been applied to severe burns to reduce infection. Solutions have also been used as topical disinfectants and astringents in other conditions.

Silver nitrate (Argentum Nitricum; Argent. Nit.) is used in homoeopathic medicine. It is also used in cosmetics to dye eyebrows and eye lashes in a concentration of not more than 4%.

Preparations

USP 23: Silver Nitrate Ophthalmic Solution; Toughened Silver Nitrate.

Proprietary Preparations (details are given in Part 3)
Austral.: Quit†; ***Ger.:*** Mova Nitrat; Pluralane†; ***Spain:*** Argenpal.

Multi-ingredient: ***Austral.:*** Super Banish; ***Spain:*** Argentofenol; ***Switz.:*** Grafco†; ***UK:*** AVOCA.

Silver Protein (5322-m)

Albumosesilber; Argentoproteinum; Argentum Proteinicum; Protargolum; Proteinato de Plata; Proteinato de Prata; Strong Protargin; Strong Protein Silver; Strong Silver Protein.

CAS — 9007-35-6 (colloidal silver).

NOTE. Synonyms for mild silver protein include: Argentoproteinum Mite; Argentum Vitellinicum; Mild Protargin; Mild Silver Proteinate; Silver Nucleinate; Silver Vitellin; Vitelinato de Plata and Vitelinato de Prata.

Pharmacopoeias. In Aust., Belg., Fr., It., Jpn, and Pol. Many of these pharmacopoeias include monographs on mild silver protein as well as on colloidal silver.

Silver protein solutions have antibacterial properties, due to the presence of low concentrations of ionised silver, and have been used as eye drops and for application to mucous membranes. The mild form of silver protein is considered to be less irritating, but less active.

Colloidal silver, which is also a preparation of silver in combination with protein, has also been used topically for its antibacterial activity.

Preparations

Proprietary Preparations (details are given in Part 3)
Fr.: Stillargol; Vitargenol.

Multi-ingredient: ***Aust.:*** Coldargan; ***Fr.:*** Pastabat†; ***Ger.:*** Coldargan†; ***Ital.:*** Arscolloid; Bio-Arscolloid; Corti-Arscolloid; Rikosilver†; Rinantipiol; Rinovit Nube.

Sincalide (2148-b)

Sincalide (*BAN, USAN, rINN*).

CCK-OP; SQ-19844. De-1-(5-oxo-L-proline)-de-2-L-glutamine-5-methionine-caerulein.

$C_{49}H_{62}N_{10}O_{16}S_3$ = 1143.3.

CAS — 25126-32-3.

Adverse Effects

Sincalide stimulates gallbladder contraction and gastro-intestinal muscle and may give rise to abdominal discomfort. Dizziness and flushing may also occur.

Uses and Administration

Sincalide is the synthetic C-terminal octapeptide of cholecystokinin (pancreozymin, p.1613) and when administered by intravenous injection it stimulates gallbladder contraction; it also stimulates intestinal muscle.

Sincalide is used for testing gallbladder function and as an adjunct to cholecystography. It is usually given in doses of 20 ng per kg body-weight by intravenous injection over ½ to 1 minute. It is also used as a diagnostic agent, often in conjunction with secretin (p.1628), for testing the functional capacity of the pancreas; this test generally requires duodenal intubation of the patient and examination of duodenal aspirate. A suggested procedure is to give secretin by intravenous infusion over 1 hour and 30 minutes after starting this infusion, sincalide 20 ng per kg is infused over a 30-minute period.

Sincalide may be given in a usual dose of 40 ng per kg by intravenous injection for the treatment of postoperative ileus or to decrease small-bowel transit time during radiological procedures.

Preparations

Proprietary Preparations (details are given in Part 3)
Canad.: Kinevac; ***USA:*** Kinevac.

Skin Substitutes (13151-d)

A variety of biological and semisynthetic materials have been developed for use as temporary dressings in burns, ulcers, and other injuries associated with skin loss. The rationale is to prevent fluid and heat loss, to reduce infection, to protect exposed structures, to reduce pain, and to prepare the site for grafting (see Burns, p.1073).

Denatured porcine and bovine skin, consisting of the dermal and/or epidermal layers, have been used. More recently bioengineered human skin equivalents have been produced which more closely mimic human skin.

References.

1. Mitchell R. A new biological dressing for areas denuded of mucous membrane. *Br Dent J* 1983; **155:** 346–8.
2. Poskitt KR, *et al.* Pinch skin grafting or porcine dermis in venous ulcers: a randomised clinical trial. *Br Med J* 1987; **294:** 674–6.
3. Muhart M, *et al.* Bioengineered skin. *Lancet* 1997; **350:** 1142.
4. Freedlander E. New forms of skin grafting: from the laboratory to the clinic. *Hosp Med* 1998; **59:** 484–7.

Preparations

Proprietary Preparations (details are given in Part 3)
UK: Corethium.

Slippery Elm (5458-t)

Elm Bark; Slippery Elm Bark; Ulmus; Ulmus Fulva.

Pharmacopoeias. In US.

The dried inner bark of *Ulmus rubra* (=*U. fulva*) (Ulmaceae).

Slippery elm contains much mucilage and has been used as a demulcent.

Preparations

Proprietary Preparations (details are given in Part 3)

Multi-ingredient: ***Austral.:*** Cal-Alkyline; Digestive Aid; Formula 1†; Herbal Cleanse; PC Regulax; Travelaide; ***Canad.:*** Herbal Cough Expectorant; ***UK:*** Biobalm; Fenulin; Natraleze; Papaya Plus; Pileabs; Slippery Elm Stomach Tablets.

Soda Lime (212-m)

Cal Sodada; Calcaria absorbens; Calcaria Compositio; Calx Sodica; Chaux Sodée.

CAS — 8006-28-8.

Pharmacopoeias. In Br. Also in USNF.

The BP specifies a mixture of sodium hydroxide, or sodium hydroxide and potassium hydroxide, with calcium hydroxide. The USNF specifies a mixture of calcium hydroxide with sodium or potassium hydroxide or both.

White or greyish-white granules, or coloured with an indicator to show when absorptive capacity is exhausted. Soda lime absorbs about 20% of its weight of carbon dioxide. Partially **soluble** in water; almost completely soluble in 1M acetic acid. **Incompatible** with trichloroethylene.

Soda lime is used to absorb carbon dioxide for instance in closed-circuit anaesthetic apparatus and in determining the basal metabolic rate. Limits are specified for particle size, and particles should be free from dust.

Soda lime must not be used with trichloroethylene, since this is decomposed by warm alkali to produce a toxic end product that gives rise to lesions of the nervous system.

Sodium Arsenate (13242-m)

Natrium Arsenicicum; Sodium Arseniate.

$Na_2HAsO_4,7H_2O$ = 312.0.

CAS — 7778-43-0 (anhydrous sodium arsenate); 10048-95-0 (sodium arsenate heptahydrate).

Sodium arsenate was formerly used in the treatment of chronic skin diseases, in parasitic diseases of the blood, and in some forms of anaemia. It has the adverse effects of Arsenic Trioxide, p.1550.

Preparations

Proprietary Preparations (details are given in Part 3)

Multi-ingredient: ***Fr.:*** Aromabyl.

Sodium Carbonate Anhydrous (213-b)

500; Cenizas de Soda; Exsiccated Sodium Carbonate; Natrii Carbonas Anhydricus; Natrium Carbonicum Calcinatum; Natrium Carbonicum Siccatum.

Na_2CO_3 = 106.0.

CAS — 497-19-8.

Pharmacopoeias. In *Eur.* (see p.viii), *Jpn*, and *Pol.* NOTE. Sodium Carbonate (*USNF*) is anhydrous or the monohydrate.

A white or almost white hygroscopic granular powder. **Soluble** 1 in 3 of water and 1 in 1.8 of boiling water; practically insoluble in alcohol. A solution in water is strongly alkaline to phenolphthalein. **Store** in airtight containers.

Sodium Carbonate Decahydrate (214-v)

500; Cristales de Sosa; Natrii Carbonas; Natrii Carbonas Decahydricus; Natrium Carbonicum Crystallisatum.

$Na_2CO_3,10H_2O$ = 286.1.

CAS — 6132-02-1.

NOTE. Washing soda is a synonym for the technical grade of sodium carbonate decahydrate.

Pharmacopoeias. In *Eur.* (see p.viii), *Jpn*, and *Pol.*

Odourless, colourless, efflorescent, transparent crystals or white crystalline powder. Freely **soluble** in water; practically insoluble in alcohol. A 10% solution in water is strongly alkaline. **Store** in airtight containers.

Sodium Carbonate Monohydrate (215-g)

500; Natrii Carbonas Monohydricus.

Na_2CO_3,H_2O = 124.0.

CAS — 5968-11-6.

Pharmacopoeias. In *Eur.* (see p.viii).

NOTE. Sodium Carbonate (*USNF*) is anhydrous or the monohydrate.

Odourless, colourless crystals or white crystalline powder or granules. It is stable in air under ordinary conditions but effloresces when exposed to dry air above 50°; at 100° it becomes anhydrous. **Soluble** 1 in 3 of water and 1 in 1.8 of boiling water; practically insoluble in alcohol. A 10% solution in water is strongly alkaline. **Store** in airtight containers.

Anhydrous sodium carbonate and the monohydrate are used as reagents. The decahydrate has been used in alkaline baths and in Great Britain is an approved disinfectant for foot-and-mouth disease. Sodium carbonate in its anhydrous or hydrated form is also used as a water softener.

Preparations

BPC 1973: Surgical Chlorinated Soda Solution;
USP 23: Citric Acid, Magnesium Oxide, and Sodium Carbonate Irrigation.

Proprietary Preparations (details are given in Part 3)

Multi-ingredient: ***Austral.:*** Eno; ***Canad.:*** Carbicarb†; ***Fr.:*** Bactident; Eno†; Hydralin; ***Irl.:*** Cymalon; ***Ital.:*** Eno; ***Spain:*** Cloritines; Eno†; Frutosel†; Sal de Frutas Eno; Samarin Sal de Frutas†; Tanasid; ***Switz.:*** Saltrates Rodell.

Sodium Chlorate (321-p)

Natrium Chloricum; Sodii Chloras.

$NaClO_3$ = 106.4.

CAS — 7775-09-9.

Sodium chlorate closely resembles potassium chlorate (see p.1620) in its properties and has been used as an astringent. Its main use is as a weedkiller and it is therefore a common household chemical. Poor storage conditions can lead to explosions.

Preparations

Proprietary Preparations (details are given in Part 3)

Multi-ingredient: ***Spain:*** Co Bucal; Sanovox†.

Sodium Dichloroacetate (13247-p)

DCA.

$C_2HCl_2NaO_2$ = 150.9.

CAS — 2156-56-1 (sodium dichloroacetate); 79-43-6 (dichloroacetic acid).

Dichloroacetic acid activates pyruvate dehydrogenase, a mitochondrial enzyme which catalyses metabolism of pyruvate and lactate, and it inhibits glycolysis. It also stimulates myocardial contractility. It has been tried by mouth or parenterally as the sodium salt in the treatment of lactic acidosis.

Adverse effects. The chronic oral administration of dichloroacetate was suspended[1] because of adverse effects in *animals* and a polyneuropathy which developed in a patient given dichloroacetate for 16 weeks. Dichloroacetate may also be mutagenic.[2]

1. Stacpoole PW, *et al.* Toxicity of chronic dichloroacetate. *N Engl J Med* 1979; **300:** 372.
2. Herbert V, *et al.* Dichloroacetate a mutagen? *N Engl J Med* 1979; **300:** 625.

Pharmacokinetics. References.

1. Henderson GN, *et al.* Pharmacokinetics of dichloroacetate in adult patients with lactic acidosis. *J Clin Pharmacol* 1997; **37:** 416–25.

Use in lactic acidosis. In a study[1] in 29 patients with lactic acidosis (see p.1147) sodium dichloroacetate 50 mg per kg body-weight given by intravenous infusion over 30 minutes, followed by a second dose 2 hours after beginning the first infusion, produced a metabolic response in 23 patients with a short-term increase in survival. However, subsequent study[2] found that while dichloroacetate infusion did reduce blood-lactate concentrations it did not alter haemodynamics or survival in patients with severe lactic acidosis.

1. Stacpoole PW, *et al.* Dichloroacetate in the treatment of lactic acidosis. *Ann Intern Med* 1988; **108:** 58–63.
2. Stacpoole PW, *et al.* A controlled clinical trial of dichloroacetate for treatment of lactic acidosis in adults. *N Engl J Med* 1992; **327:** 1564–9.

Sodium Dithionite (13248-s)

Sodium Hydrosulphite; Sodium Sulphoxylate.

$Na_2S_2O_4$ = 174.1, or $Na_2S_2O_4,2H_2O$ = 210.1.

CAS — 7775-14-6 (anhydrous).

NOTE. The name sodium hydrosulfite is also applied to $NaHSO_2$ = 88.06.

Pharmacopoeias. In *Pol.*

Sodium dithionite is used as a reducing agent. It may be used in the form of a simple urine test in the detection of paraquat poisoning. A 0.25% solution has been used to remove phenazopyridine stains. It is irritant to the skin.

Sodium Gluconate (3942-z)

E576. Monosodium D-gluconate.

$C_6H_{11}NaO_7$ = 218.1.

CAS — 527-07-1.

Pharmacopoeias. In *US.*

Sodium gluconate is a food additive.

Gluconates act as acceptors of hydrogen ions produced by metabolic processes and are an indirect source of bicarbonate ions.

Sodium Hyaluronate (13251-b)

Sodium Hyaluronate (*BANM*).

Hyaluronate Sodium (*USAN*).

CAS — 9004-61-9 (hyaluronic acid); 9067-32-7 (sodium hyaluronate).

The sodium salt of a high-viscosity mucopolysaccharide of high molecular weight.

Adverse Effects

There have been reports of a transient rise in intra-ocular pressure following the administration of sodium hyaluronate into the eye. When administered to the knee, pain and inflammation may occur at the injection site. There have also been occasional reports of hypersensitivity, including, rarely, anaphylaxis.

Crystalline deposits on intra-ocular lenses have been reported in patients following the use of a high viscosity sodium hyaluronate preparation during cataract surgery.[1]

1. Jensen MK, *et al.* Crystallization on intraocular lens surfaces associated with the use of Healon GV. *Arch Ophthalmol* 1994; **112:** 1037–42.

Uses and Administration

Hyaluronic acid is widely distributed in body tissues and intracellular fluids including the aqueous and vitreous humour; it is a component of the ground substance or tissue cement surrounding cells.

A viscous solution of sodium hyaluronate is used during surgical procedures on the eye, for example for cataract. Introduction of the solution into the anterior or posterior chamber via a fine cannula or needle allows tissues to be separated during surgery and protects them from trauma. Sodium hyaluronate is given in the treatment of osteoarthritis of the knee (p.2) by intra-articular injection in a dose of 20 mg once weekly for 5 weeks, repeated if necessary at intervals of not less than 6 months. Hylans, which are polymers derived from hyaluronan, are used similarly.

Hyaluronic acid is applied topically to promote wound healing. Zinc hyaluronate has also been used. A film containing sodium hyaluronate and carmellose is used to prevent surgical adhesion.

Hyaluronic acid has also been used in topical formulations of diclofenac (CT-1101, AT-2101). The combination is under investigation in the treatment of actinic keratoses.

Reviews.

1. Goa KL, Benfield P. Hyaluronic acid: a review of its pharmacology and use as a surgical aid in ophthalmology, and its therapeutic potential in joint disease and wound healing. *Drugs* 1994; **47:** 536–66.

Dry eye. The usual management of dry eye (p.1470) is with artificial tears. Sodium hyaluronate has also been reported to be of some benefit. Topical application of sodium hyaluronate solution (0.1%) in 10 patients with dry eye increased tear film stability for at least 40 minutes, and alleviated symptoms of burning and grittiness.[1] Application of sodium hyaluronate solution (0.2%) was also reported to be of benefit in 20 patients in the treatment of keratoconjunctivitis sicca.[2] A more recent study[3] found that sodium hyaluronate eye drops (0.1%) offered no advantage over the use of artificial tears for dry eye, although it was suggested that sodium hyaluronate might play a role in maintaining a healthy corneal epithelium.

1. Mengher LS, *et al.* Effect of sodium hyaluronate (0.1%) on break-up time (NIBUT) in patients with dry eyes. *Br J Ophthalmol* 1986; **70:** 442–7.
2. Sand BB, *et al.* Sodium hyaluronate in the treatment of keratoconjunctivitis sicca: a double masked clinical trial. *Acta Ophthalmol (Copenh)* 1989; **67:** 181–3.
3. Shimmura S, *et al.* Sodium hyaluronate eyedrops in the treatment of dry eyes. *Br J Ophthalmol* 1995; **79:** 1007–11.

Preparations

Proprietary Preparations (details are given in Part 3)
Aust.: Amvisc; Artzal; Connettivina; Etamucin†; Healonid; Hyalgan; Provisc; ***Austral.:*** AMO Vitrax; Healon; Ophthalin; Provisc; ***Belg.:*** Healon; Provisc; ***Canad.:*** Amvisc†; Biolon; Cystistat; Eyestil; Healon; Hylashield; Suplasyn; Synvisc; ***Fr.:*** Healon; Healonid†; Hyalgan; Provisc; Vitrax; ***Ger.:*** Dispasan; Healon; Hyalart; Jossalind; Provisc; ***Irl.:*** Healonid; ***Ital.:*** Artz; Biolon; Bionect†; Connettivina; Dropstar; Healon; Hy-Drop; Hyalart; Hyalgan; Hyalistil; Ial; Ialurex; Ocustil; Otoial; Provisc; ***Neth.:*** Healon†; ***Norw.:*** Amvisc†; Healon; Provisc†; ***S.Afr.:*** Amvisc; Healon; Provisc; ***Spain:*** Pandermin Cicatrizante†; ***Swed.:*** AMO Vitrax; Amvisc; Artzal; Healon; Synvisc; ***Switz.:*** AMO Vitrax; Biolon; Ialugen; ***UK:*** Healonid; Hyalgan; Ophthalin; Provisc; ***USA:*** AMO Vitrax; Amvisc; Healon; Healon GV; Hyalgan; Synvisc.

Multi-ingredient: ***Aust.:*** Healonid Yellow; Viscoat; ***Austral.:*** Duovisc; Viscoat; ***Belg.:*** Viscoat; ***Canad.:*** Healon Yellow†; ***Fr.:*** Viscoat; ***Ger.:*** Duovisc; Viscoat; ***Ital.:*** Connettivina Plus; Dropyal; Healon Yellow; Viscoat; ***S.Afr.:*** Viscoat; ***Swed.:*** Healon Yellow†; Provisc; Viscoat†; ***Switz.:*** Alphastria; Ialugen Plus; Viscoat; ***UK:*** Seprafilm; Viscoat; ***USA:*** Healon Yellow; Viscoat.

Sodium Hydroxide (216-q)

524; Ätznatron; Caustic Soda; Hidróxido de Sódio; Natrii Hydroxidum; Natrium Hydricum; Natrium Hydroxydatum; Soda Lye.

NaOH = 40.00.

CAS — 1310-73-2.

Pharmacopoeias. In *Chin., Eur.* (see p.viii), *Int., Jpn,* and *Pol.* Also in *USNF.*

Dry, very deliquescent, white or almost white sticks, pellets, or fused masses. It is hard and brittle and shows a crystalline fracture. Strongly alkaline and corrosive, and rapidly destroys organic tissues. When exposed to air it rapidly absorbs moisture and carbon dioxide. Completely or almost completely **soluble** 1 in 1 of water; freely soluble in alcohol. A 0.01% solution in water has a pH not less than 11.0. **Store** in airtight, non-metallic containers.

Adverse Effects

The ingestion of caustic alkalis causes immediate burning pain in the mouth, throat, substernal region, and epigastrium, and the lining membranes become swollen and detached. There is dysphagia, hypersalivation, vomiting with the vomitus becoming blood-stained, diarrhoea, and shock. In severe cases, asphyxia due to oedema of the glottis, circulatory failure, oesophageal or gastric perforation, peritonitis, or pneumonia may occur. Stricture of the oesophagus can develop weeks or months later.

Caustic alkalis on contact with the eyes cause conjunctival oedema and corneal destruction.

Treatment of Adverse Effects

Ingestion should not be treated by lavage or emesis. Give copious drinks of water and follow this with demulcents. Maintain an airway and alleviate shock and pain.

Contaminated skin and eyes should be flooded immediately with water and the washing continued for about 30 minutes. Any affected clothing should be removed while flooding is being carried out.

Uses and Administration

Sodium hydroxide is a powerful caustic. A 2.5% solution in glycerol has been used as a cuticle solvent. An escharotic preparation of sodium hydroxide and calcium oxide was known as London paste. It is also used for adjusting the pH of solutions. A 1% aqueous solution has been used as an approved disinfectant for swine vesicular disease.

Disinfection. When autoclaving is impractical, exposure to 1N sodium hydroxide for one hour has been found to be effective in the decontamination of the agent causing Creutzfeldt-Jakob disease. Contaminated skin could be disinfected with little hazard by 5 to 10 minutes of exposure to 1N sodium hydroxide, followed by extensive washing with water.[1] Full protection is afforded by autoclaving instruments for one hour at 132° and then immersion in 1N sodium hydroxide for one hour at room temperature.[2]

1. Brown P, *et al.* Sodium hydroxide decontamination of Creutzfeldt-Jakob disease virus. *N Engl J Med* 1984; **310:** 727.
2. Harries-Jones R. Creutzfeldt-Jakob disease. *Br Med J* 1990; **301:** 46.

Preparations

Proprietary Preparations (details are given in Part 3)

Multi-ingredient: ***Aust.:*** Leberinfusion; Sulfo-Schwefelbad; ***Belg.:*** Trisibam†; ***Fr.:*** Coricide Rodell†; ***Ger.:*** Glutarsin E; ***Ital.:*** Gevisol†; ***Switz.:*** Saltrates.

Sodium Iodoheparinate (4820-y)

Iodoheparinate Sodium.

Sodium iodoheparinate is a derivative of heparin (p.879) used topically for the treatment of corneal burns and ulceration.

Preparations

Proprietary Preparations (details are given in Part 3)
Fr.: Dioparine; ***Switz.:*** Dioparine.

Sodium Methylarsinate (13253-g)

Natrium Methylarsonicum; Sodium Metharsinite. Disodium monomethylarsonate hexahydrate.

$CH_3AsNa_2O_3,6H_2O$ = 292.0.

CAS — 5967-62-4.

Sodium methylarsinate is an organic arsenic compound with adverse effects similar to those of arsenic trioxide (p.1550). It was formerly included in some vitamin and mineral preparations. It has also been used as a herbicide.

Preparations

Proprietary Preparations (details are given in Part 3)

Multi-ingredient: ***Belg.:*** Calcigenol Simple†; Neo Genyl†; Neocalcigenol Forte†.

Sodium Morrhuate (9845-c)

Sodium Morrhuate *(rINN).*

Morrhuate Sodium.

CAS — 8031-09-2.

Sodium morrhuate consists of the sodium salts of the fatty acids of cod-liver oil. It is a sclerosant with properties similar to those of ethanolamine (p.1576) and has been used in the treatment of varicose veins by intravenous injection of usual doses of 50 to 100 mg for small veins or 150 to 250 mg for large veins, as a 5% solution.

Preparations

USP 23: Morrhuate Sodium Injection.

Proprietary Preparations (details are given in Part 3)
USA: Scleromate.

Multi-ingredient: ***Ger.:*** Varicocid†.

Sodium Phenylacetate (16986-r)

Sodium Phenylacetate *(USAN).*

$C_8H_7NaO_2$ = 158.1.

CAS — 114-70-5.

Sodium phenylacetate or sodium phenylbutyrate are used for hyperammonaemia in patients with enzymatic deficiencies in the urea cycle (see p.1334). Sodium phenylbutyrate is a prodrug for sodium phenylacetate and has been studied for its effect in increasing fetal haemoglobin.

References.

1. Dover GJ, *et al.* Increased fetal hemoglobin in patients receiving sodium 4-phenylbutyrate. *N Engl J Med* 1992; **327:** 569–70.
2. Maestri NE, *et al.* Long-term survival of patients with argininosuccinate synthetase deficiency. *J Pediatr* 1995; **127:** 929–35.
3. Maestri NE, *et al.* Long-term treatment of girls with ornithine transcarbamylase deficiency. *N Engl J Med* 1996; **335:** 855–9.
4. Anonymous. Sodium phenylbutyrate for urea cycle enzyme deficiencies. *Med Lett Drugs Ther* 1996; **38:** 105–6.

Preparations

Proprietary Preparations (details are given in Part 3)
USA: Buphenyl.

Multi-ingredient: ***USA:*** Ucephan.

Sodium Polymetaphosphate (1640-p)

E450(c) (sodium polyphosphates).

CAS — 50813-16-6.

NOTE. Sodium Hexametaphosphate has been used as a synonym for this substance, but it exists in much higher degrees of polymerisation.

Sodium polymetaphosphate has been used as a 5% dusting-powder in hyperhidrosis and bromhidrosis, and as a prophylactic against athlete's foot.

Sodium polymetaphosphate combines with calcium and magnesium ions to form complex soluble compounds and is used as a water softener.

Sodium Pyruvate (8584-m)

Sodium α-ketopropionate; sodium 2-oxopropanoate.

$C_3H_4O_3,Na$ = 111.1.

CAS — 127-17-3 (pyruvic acid); 113-24-6 (sodium pyruvate).

Sodium pyruvate has been administered intravenously in the diagnosis of disorders of pyruvate metabolism.

Relative serum concentrations of lactate and pyruvate following a 10-minute intravenous infusion of sodium pyruvate 500 mg per kg body-weight have been used as an aid to the diagnosis of disorders of pyruvate metabolism.[1] Death shortly after pyruvate loading in a 9-year-old child with restrictive cardiomyopathy suggests that the test should not be performed when cardiac function is decreased.[2]

1. Dijkstra U, *et al.* Friedreich's ataxia: intravenous pyruvate load to demonstrate a defect in pyruvate metabolism. *Neurology* 1984; **34:** 1493–7.
2. Matthys D, *et al.* Fatal outcome of pyruvate loading test in child with restrictive cardiomyopathy. *Lancet* 1991; **338:** 1020–1.

Preparations

Proprietary Preparations (details are given in Part 3)

Multi-ingredient: ***Ger.:*** Inosin comp.†.

Sodium Silicate (13260-v)

Soluble Glass; Water Glass.

CAS — 1344-09-8.

Concentrated aqueous solutions of sodium silicate are commercially available and have many industrial uses. The solutions vary in composition, viscosity, and density; the greater the ratio of Na_2O to SiO_2 the more tacky and alkaline the solution.

Sodium Silicofluoride (7736-a)

Sodium Fluorosilicate; Sodium Fluosilicate; Sodium Hexafluorosilicate.

Na_2SiF_6 = 188.1.

CAS — 16893-85-9.

Sodium silicofluoride has the actions of sodium fluoride (p.742) and is used in controlled amounts for the fluoridation of drinking water. It has also been considered for inclusion in oral hygiene products.

Other silicofluoride (fluorosilicate) salts permitted for use in oral hygiene products include ammonium silicofluoride, magnesium silicofluoride, and potassium silicofluoride.

Sodium silicofluoride has also been used in insecticides.

Sodium Succinate (13261-g)

E363 (succinic acid); E363 (succinic acid).

$C_4H_4Na_2O_4,6H_2O = 270.1$.

CAS — 150-90-3 (anhydrous sodium succinate); 6106-21-4 (sodium succinate hexahydrate).

Sodium succinate is an ingredient of topical preparations tried in cataract. It is used as a food additive.

Succinic dinitrile ($C_4H_4N_2 = 80.09$) has been used in the treatment of exhaustion and depression.

Preparations

Proprietary Preparations (details are given in Part 3)

Multi-ingredient: ***Fr.:*** Vitaphakol; ***Spain:*** Vitaphakol; ***Switz.:*** Vitaphakol.

Sparteine Sulphate (13264-s)

Sparteine Sulphate *(rINNM)*.

Spart. Sulph.; Sparteine Sulfate *(USAN)*; (−)-Sparteine Sulphate; *l*-Sparteine Sulphate; Sparteinum Sulfuricum; Sulfato de Esparteina. Dodecahydro-7,14-methano-2*H*,6*H*-dipyrido[1,2-*a*:1′,2′-*e*][1,5]diazocine sulphate pentahydrate.

$C_{15}H_{26}N_2,H_2SO_4,5H_2O = 422.5$.

CAS — 90-39-1 (sparteine); 299-39-8 (anhydrous sparteine sulphate); 6160-12-9 (sparteine sulphate pentahydrate).

Pharmacopoeias. In Fr.

Sparteine sulphate is a salt of the dibasic alkaloid, sparteine, obtained from scoparium, *Sarothamnus scoparius* (=*Cytisus scoparius*) (Leguminosae).

Sparteine sulphate has been reported to lessen the irritability and conductivity of cardiac muscle and has been used in the treatment of cardiac arrhythmias. Small doses stimulate and large doses paralyse the autonomic ganglia. Peripherally, it has a fairly strong curare-like action, arresting respiration by paralysing the phrenic endings.

The metabolic oxidation of sparteine exhibits genetic polymorphism and this property has been exploited in *in-vitro* screening tests to identify other drugs that may be subject to similar genetic variations in their metabolism.

Concern has been expressed that sparteine present in a herbal slimming preparation may cause adverse effects in slow metabolisers if excessive doses are ingested; pregnant women may be particularly at risk.[1]

1. Galloway JH, *et al.* Potentially hazardous compound in a herbal slimming remedy. *Lancet* 1992; **340:** 179.

Preparations

Proprietary Preparations (details are given in Part 3)

Ger.: Depasan†.

Multi-ingredient: ***Ger.:*** Digi-Pulsnorma†; Gelsadon†; Hypotonin forte†; Hypotonin†; Jatamansin†; Normotin†; Pulsnorma†; RR-plus†.

Spearmint (4712-s)

Mentha Viridis; Menthae Crispae Folium; Mint.

The dried leaves and flowering tops of common spearmint, *Mentha spicata* (= *M. viridis*) or of scotch spearmint (*M. cardiaca*) (Labiatae).

Spearmint is the source of spearmint oil. It has carminative properties and is used as a flavouring agent.

Preparations

Proprietary Preparations (details are given in Part 3)

Multi-ingredient: ***Aust.:*** Carminative; Mag Kottas Baby-Tee; Mag Kottas Beruhigungstee; Sidroga Herz-Kreislauf-Tee; Sidroga Magen-Darm-Tee; Sidroga Nerven- und Schlaftee; Sidroga Stoffwechseltee; Teekanne Herz- und Kreislauftee; ***Fr.:*** Tisanes de l'Abbe Hamon no 17; Tisanes de l'Abbe Hamon no 18†; ***Switz.:*** Alpina Gel a la consoude; Tisane antirhumatismale; Tisane pour l'estomac; Tisane pour le coeur et la circulation; Tisane pour le sommeil et les nerfs.

Spearmint Oil (4713-w)

Huile Essentielle de Menthe Crépue; Oleum Menthae Crispae; Oleum Menthae Viridis.

Pharmacopoeias. In Br. and Fr.

A clear colourless, pale yellow or greenish-yellow volatile oil with the characteristic odour of spearmint, obtained by distillation from the overground parts of fresh flowering common spearmint (*Mentha spicata*) or scotch spearmint (*Mentha cardiaca* or *Mentha × cardiaca*) (Labiatae). It becomes darker and viscous on keeping. It contains not less than 55% w/w of carvone ($C_{10}H_{14}O$).

Soluble 1 in 1 of alcohol (80%); the solution may become cloudy when diluted. **Store** at a temperature not exceeding 25° in airtight containers. Protect from light.

Spearmint oil has similar properties to peppermint oil and is used as a carminative and as a flavouring agent.

Preparations

Proprietary Preparations (details are given in Part 3)

Multi-ingredient: ***Aust.:*** Euka; ***Ital.:*** Dentosan "Pagni" Collutorio†; Dentosan Mese†; ***Switz.:*** Alvogyl; ***UK:*** Eftab.

Spike Lavender Oil (4660-y)

Huile Essentielle d'Aspic; Ol. Lavand. Spic.; Oleum Lavandulae Spicatae; Spicae Aetheroleum; Spike Oil.

Pharmacopoeias. In Fr.

The volatile oil from *Lavandula latifolia* (= *L. spica*) (Labiatae).

Spike lavender oil resembles lavender oil (p.1594) in its properties and is mainly used in perfumery. Hypersensitivity reactions may occur.

Preparations

Proprietary Preparations (details are given in Part 3)

Aust.: Tavipec; ***Ger.:*** Bronchobest.

Multi-ingredient: ***Aust.:*** Novipec; Tussamag; ***Ger.:*** Neo-Lapitrypsin; Rheumasan†; ***Switz.:*** Baume du Chalet; Carmol†; Gramminflor†.

Spirulina (8599-w)

Spirulina is a species of blue-green algae that has been promoted as an anorectic but there is no convincing evidence that it is safe or effective for this indication.

References.

1. Popovich NG. Spirulina. *Am Pharm* 1982; **NS22** (June): 8–10.

Preparations

Proprietary Preparations (details are given in Part 3)

UK: Biolina.

Multi-ingredient: ***Austral.:*** Cal-Alkyline; Diet-Trim†; Rubus Complex; ***UK:*** Herbal Booster.

Stannous Fluoride (7737-t)

Stannosi Fluoridum. Tin fluoride.

$SnF_2 = 156.7$.

CAS — 7783-47-3.

Pharmacopoeias. In US.

A white crystalline powder with a bitter saline taste. Freely **soluble** in water; practically insoluble in alcohol, in chloroform, and in ether. A 0.4% freshly prepared solution in water has a pH of 2.8 to 3.5. Aqueous solutions decompose within a few hours with the formation of a white precipitate; they slowly attack glass.

Stannous fluoride has similar actions to sodium fluoride (see p.742) and is used for the prophylaxis of dental caries. Dental gels containing concentrations of stannous fluoride 0.4% are available for daily use. Higher concentrations have been applied under professional supervision. Stannous fluoride has also been used in dentifrices and mouth rinses.

Stannous fluoride has been reported to have an unpleasant taste.

Preparations

USP 23: Stannous Fluoride Gel.

Proprietary Preparations (details are given in Part 3)

UK: Fluorigard Gel-Kam; Omnigel†; ***USA:*** Cav-X†; Gel Kam; Gel-Tin; Stop.

Starch Blockers (3920-s)

Inhibitors of alpha-amylase such as phaseolamin and tendamistat (HOE-467) are termed starch blockers and they were proposed as dietary aids, the principle behind this being that they would inhibit the absorption of starch. Various studies have shown that these compounds have no effect on calorie absorption. Alpha-amylase inhibitors have been investigated as an adjunct in the management of diabetes mellitus.

Stearic Acid (1324-t)

570; Acido Esteárico; Acidum Stearicum; Octadecanoic Acid; Stearinsäure.

CAS — 57-11-4 (stearic acid); 57-10-3 (palmitic acid).

Pharmacopoeias. In Aust., Belg., Br., Chin., It., Jpn, Pol., and Swiss. Also in USNF.

USNF also includes Purified Stearic Acid.

White, greasy, flaky crystals or a white or yellowish, glossy crystalline solid or powder, with a slight odour suggesting tallow, consisting of a mixture of fatty acids, chiefly stearic and palmitic acids. BP and USNF specify not less than 40% of stearic acid ($C_{18}H_{36}O_2$), and not less than 90% of stearic and palmitic acids; congealing point not below 54°. It is sometimes wrongly called 'stearine' in commerce.

Practically **insoluble** in water; soluble 1 in 20 of alcohol, 1 in 2 of chloroform, and 1 in 3 of ether; soluble in dehydrated alcohol.

Purified Stearic Acid (USNF) contains not less than 90% stearic acid and not less than 96% of stearic and palmitic acids; congealing point 66° to 69°.

Stearic acid is used as a lubricant in making tablets and capsules. It is also used as an emulsifying and solubilising agent. Various stearates are also used as pharmaceutical aids (see Nonionic Surfactants, p.1324, and Soaps and other Anionic Surfactants, p.1468).

Preparations

Proprietary Preparations (details are given in Part 3)

Multi-ingredient: ***Fr.:*** Abi†.

Storax (286-r)

Balsamum Styrax Liquidus; Estoraque Líquido; Liquid Storax; Styrax.

Pharmacopoeias. In Chin.

US specifies crude storax from *L. orientalis* (Levant storax) or *L. styraciflua* (American storax).

The balsam obtained from the trunk of *Liquidambar orientalis* (Hamamelidaceae). It is a semiliquid grey to greyish-brown opaque mass with a characteristic odour.

Practically **insoluble** in water; soluble in warm alcohol (90%) (usually incompletely), carbon disulphide, and acetone; partly soluble in ether.

Storax has actions similar to those of Peru balsam (p.1617). Purified storax or prepared storax was formerly applied as an ointment in the treatment of parasitic skin diseases. It is an ingredient of Compound Benzoin Tincture and of Benzoin Inhalation. Skin sensitisation has been reported.

Preparations

BP 1998: Benzoin Inhalation; Compound Benzoin Tincture *(Friars' Balsam)*;

BPC 1954: Compound Iodoform Paint;

USP 23: Compound Benzoin Tincture.

Proprietary Preparations (details are given in Part 3)

Multi-ingredient: ***Ital.:*** Lacrime; ***UK:*** Frador.

Streptodornase (3745-w)

Streptodornase *(BAN, rINN)*.

Streptococcal Deoxyribonuclease.

CAS — 37340-82-2.

An enzyme obtained from cultures of various strains of *Streptococcus haemolyticus*.

Uses and Administration

Streptodornase catalyses the depolymerisation of polymerised deoxyribonucleoproteins. It liquefies the viscous nucleoprotein of dead cells; it has no effect on living cells. It is used in conjunction with streptokinase in the topical treatment of lesions, wounds, and other conditions that require the removal of clots or purulent matter.

It has also been given by mouth with streptokinase and sometimes with antibacterial agents, for its supposed benefit in reducing oedema and inflammation associated with trauma and infection.

Preparations

Proprietary Preparations (details are given in Part 3)

Multi-ingredient: ***Aust.:*** Varidase; ***Austral.:*** Varidase; ***Belg.:*** Varidase; ***Ger.:*** Varidase; ***Irl.:*** Varidase; ***Ital.:*** Varibiotic†; Varidase; ***Neth.:*** Varidase; ***Norw.:*** Varidase; ***S.Afr.:*** Varidase; ***Spain:*** Ernodasa; Varibiotic; Varidasa; ***Swed.:*** Varidase; ***UK:*** Varidase.

Strontium Chloride (13270-q)

$SrCl_2,6H_2O$ = 266.6.
CAS — 10476-85-4 (anhydrous strontium chloride).

Strontium chloride is used as a 10% toothpaste for the relief of dental hypersensitivity.

Preparations

Proprietary Preparations (details are given in Part 3)
Aust.: Sensodyne med; ***Canad.:*** Sensodyne; ***Switz.:*** Sensodent; ***USA:*** Original Sensodyne; Sensodyne-SC.

Strychnine (542-r)

Estricnina; Strychnina. Strychnidin-10-one.
$C_{21}H_{22}N_2O_2$ = 334.4.
CAS — 57-24-9.

An alkaloid obtained from the seeds of nux vomica (see p.1609) and other species of *Strychnos.*

Strychnine Hydrochloride (543-f)

Strych. Hydrochlor.; Strychninae Hydrochloridum.
$C_{21}H_{22}N_2O_2,HCl,2H_2O$ = 406.9.
CAS — 1421-86-9 (anhydrous strychnine hydrochloride); 6101-04-8 (strychnine hydrochloride dihydrate).

Strychnine Nitrate (544-d)

Azotato de Estricnina; Nitrato de Estricnina; Strychninae Nitras; Strychninum Nitricum.
$C_{21}H_{22}N_2O_2,HNO_3$ = 397.4.
CAS — 66-32-0.
Pharmacopoeias. In *Aust.* and *Belg.*

Strychnine Sulphate (546-h)

Strychninae Sulphas; Strychninum Sulfuricum; Sulfato de Estricnina.
$(C_{21}H_{22}N_2O_2)_2,H_2SO_4,5H_2O$ = 857.0.
CAS — 60-41-3 (anhydrous strychnine sulphate); 60491-10-3 (strychnine sulphate pentahydrate).
Pharmacopoeias. In *Fr.*

Adverse Effects

The symptoms of strychnine poisoning are mainly those arising from stimulation of the CNS. Early signs occurring within 15 to 30 minutes of ingestion include tremors, slight twitching, and stiffness of the face and legs. Painful convulsions develop and may be triggered by minor sensory stimuli; since consciousness is not impaired patients may be extremely distressed. All forms of sensation are heightened. The body becomes arched backwards in hyperextension with the head retracted, arms and legs extended, fists clenched, and the feet turned inward. The jaw is rigidly clamped and contraction of the facial muscles produces a characteristic grinning expression known as 'risus sardonicus'. The convulsions may recur repeatedly and are interspersed with periods of relaxation. If not treated adequately, few patients survive more than 5 episodes of convulsions, death usually occurring due to respiratory arrest. Fatalities have occurred with doses as little as 16 mg.

Secondary effects arising from the severe spasms include lactic acidosis, rhabdomyolysis, renal failure, hyperthermia, hyperkalaemia, and dehydration.

Some references to strychnine poisoning.

1. O'Callaghan WG, *et al.* Unusual strychnine poisoning and its treatment: report of eight cases. *Br Med J* 1982; **285:** 478.
2. Blain PG, *et al.* Strychnine poisoning: abnormal eye movements. *J Toxicol Clin Toxicol* 1982; **19:** 215–17.
3. Boyd RE, *et al.* Strychnine poisoning: recovery from profound lactic acidosis, hyperthermia, and rhabdomyolysis. *Am J Med* 1983; **74:** 507–12.
4. Burn DJ, *et al.* Strychnine poisoning as an unusual cause of convulsions. *Postgrad Med J* 1989; **65:** 563–4.

Treatment of Adverse Effects

The main object of therapy in strychnine poisoning is the prompt prevention or control of convulsions and asphyxia. Patients should be given activated charcoal. Convulsions should be controlled or prevented by diazepam. Should diazepam fail then muscle relaxants should be tried together with intubation and assisted respiration. Gastric lavage should only be carried out when the patient is no longer at risk from convulsions. All unnecessary external stimuli should be avoided and if possible the patient should be kept in a quiet darkened room. Patients should be monitored for any secondary effects from the convulsions so that appropriate symptomatic treatment can be given.

Uses and Administration

Strychnine competes with glycine which is an inhibitory neurotransmitter; it thus exerts a central stimulant effect through blocking an inhibitory activity.

Strychnine was formerly used as a bitter and analeptic but is now mainly used under strict control as a rodenticide, or as a mole poison. It has been used in multi-ingredient preparations for the treatment of ophthalmic and urinary-tract disorders. It has also been tried in the treatment of nonketotic hyperglycinaemia.

Nonketotic hyperglycinaemia. Nonketotic hyperglycinaemia is an inborn defect in the enzyme system responsible for the metabolism of glycine. It is characterised by raised concentrations of glycine in plasma, CSF, and urine. Symptoms of glycine accumulation include respiratory distress, muscular hypotonia, seizures, vomiting, and extreme lethargy. Mental retardation and early infant death are common.

Sodium benzoate has been reported to be effective in reducing plasma-glycine concentrations to near normal but is relatively ineffective in reducing CSF levels or in preventing mental retardation.[1] Strychnine, a glycine antagonist, has been of some benefit in counteracting the effects of high concentrations of glycine in the CNS.[2-4] However, some reports suggest that even concomitant treatment with sodium benzoate and strychnine may be ineffective in severe forms[5] and may ultimately have little effect on the course of the disease.[6] The combination of strychnine and ketamine (a N-methyl-D-aspartate receptor antagonist) was of some benefit in a newborn infant with severe nonketotic hyperglycinaemia.[7] Addition of low-dose dextromethorphan to treatment with sodium benzoate, arginine, carnitine, diazepam, and phenobarbitone in an infant with nonketotic hyperglycinaemia[8] was associated with resolution of nystagmus and improvement in eye contact and interactive behaviour, without altering serum- or CSF-glycine concentrations. Dextromethorphan with sodium benzoate alone may also be helpful, although the combination is not uniformly effective.[9]

1. Krieger I, *et al.* Cerebrospinal fluid glycine in nonketotic hyperglycinemia: effect of treatment with sodium benzoate and a ventricular shunt. *Metabolism* 1977; **26:** 517–24.
2. Ch'ien LT, *et al.* Glycine encephalopathy. *N Engl J Med* 1978; **298:** 687.
3. Gitzelmann R, *et al.* Strychnine for the treatment of nonketotic hyperglycinaemia. *N Engl J Med* 1978; **298:** 1424.
4. Arneson D, *et al.* Strychnine therapy in nonketotic hyperglycinemia. *Pediatrics* 1979; **63:** 369–73.
5. Sankaran K, *et al.* Glycine encephalopathy in a neonate. *Clin Pediatr (Phila)* 1982; **21:** 636–7.
6. MacDermot KD, *et al.* Attempts at use of strychnine sulfate in the treatment of nonketotic hyperglycinemia. *Pediatrics* 1980; **65:** 61–4.
7. Tegtmeyer-Metzdorf H, *et al.* Ketamine and strychnine treatment of an infant with nonketotic hyperglycinaemia. *Eur J Pediatr* 1995; **154:** 649–53.
8. Alemzadeh R, *et al.* Efficacy of low-dose dextromethorphan in the treatment of nonketotic hyperglycinemia. *Pediatrics* 1996; **97:** 924–6.
9. Hamosh A, *et al.* Long-term use of high-dose benzoate and dextromethorphan for the treatment of nonketotic hyperglycinemia. *J Pediatr* 1998; **132:** 709–13.

Preparations

Proprietary Preparations (details are given in Part 3)
Multi-ingredient: ***Aust.:*** Dysurgal; ***Fr.:*** Pastilles Jessel†; ***Ital.:*** Neuroftal; Retinovix†.

Suanzaorentang (985-h)

Ziziphus Soup.

Suanzaorentang is an ancient Chinese remedy for anxiety and insomnia. It contains five herbs: suanzaoren (*Zizyphus spinosus* of the Rhamnaceae), fuling (*Poria cocos* of the Polyporaceae), gancao (*Glycyrrhiza uralensis* of the Leguminosae), zhimu (*Anemarrhena asphodeloides* of the Liliaceae), and chuanxiong (*Ligusticum chuanxiong* of the Umbelliferae).

Succinimide (13271-p)

Butanimide. Pyrrolidine-2,5-dione.
$C_4H_5NO_2$ = 99.09.
CAS — 123-56-8.

Succinimide has been claimed to inhibit the formation of oxalic acid calculi in the kidney and to reduce hyperoxaluria.

It has been given by mouth in doses of 3 g two or three times daily.

Preparations

Proprietary Preparations (details are given in Part 3)
Spain: Orotric.

Sucrose Octa-acetate (13273-w)

Sucrose Octaacetate.
$C_{28}H_{38}O_{19}$ = 678.6.
CAS — 126-14-7.
Pharmacopoeias. In *USNF.*

A white, practically odourless, hygroscopic powder with an intensely bitter taste. **Soluble** 1 in 1100 of water, 1 in 11 of alcohol, 1 in 0.3 of acetone, and 1 in 0.5 of toluene; soluble in ether; very soluble in chloroform and in methyl alcohol. **Store** in airtight containers.

Sucrose octa-acetate has been used as an alcohol denaturant. It is also incorporated into preparations intended to deter nail biting.

Preparations

Proprietary Preparations (details are given in Part 3)
Multi-ingredient: ***Austral.:*** Bansuk†; ***Spain:*** Morde X; ***USA:*** Don't.

Sulphan Blue (2150-r)

Sulphan Blue *(BAN).*

Acid Blue 1; Alphazurine 2G; Blue VRS; Colour Index No. 42045; Isosulfan Blue *(USAN)*; P-1888; P-4125; Patent Blue V; Sulphanum Caeruleum. Sodium α-(4-diethylaminophenyl)-α-(4-diethyliminiocyclo-hexa-2,5-dienylidene)toluene-2,5-disulphonate.
$C_{27}H_{31}N_2NaO_6S_2$ = 566.7.
CAS — 68238-36-8; 129-17-9 (2,4-disulphonate isomer).

NOTE. The name Patent Blue V is mainly used for CI No. 42051 (p.1616). Sulphan blue was formerly described as the 2,4-disulphonate isomer.

Sulphan blue is reported to be **incompatible** with lignocaine.

Adverse Effects and Precautions

Sulphan blue occasionally causes nausea. Hypersensitivity reactions and attacks of asthma have been reported.

Sulphan blue should not be used during surgical shock. Sulphan blue has been reported to interfere with blood tests for protein and iron.

Hypersensitivity. References.

1. Hepps S, Dollinger M. Anaphylactic death after administration of a triphenylmethane dye to determine burn depth. *N Engl J Med* 1965; **272:** 1281.
2. Longnecker SM, *et al.* Life-threatening anaphylaxis following subcutaneous administration of isosulfan blue 1%. *Clin Pharm* 1985; **4:** 219–21.

Uses and Administration

Changes in skin colour occur 60 to 90 seconds after an intravenous injection of sulphan blue and complete body staining is established in 3 to 5 minutes. This effect has been used as a direct visual test of the state of the circulation in healthy and damaged tissues, particularly in assessing tissue viability in burns and soft-tissue trauma.

Sulphan blue given subcutaneously has been used in lymphangiography to outline the lymph vessels.

Preparations

Proprietary Preparations (details are given in Part 3)
USA: Lymphazurin.

Sulphobromophthalein Sodium (2151-f)

Sulphobromophthalein Sodium *(BANM).*

Bromsulfophthalein Sodium; Bromsulphthalein Sodium; BSP; SBP; Sodium Sulfobromophthalein; Sulfobromophthalein Sodium. Disodium 4,5,6,7-tetrabromophenolphthalein-3′,3″-disulphonate; Disodium 5,5′-(4,5,6,7-tetrabromophthalidylidene)bis(2-hydroxybenzenesulphonate).
$C_{20}H_8Br_4Na_2O_{10}S_2$ = 838.0.
CAS — 297-83-6 (sulphobromophthalein); 71-67-0 (sulphobromophthalein sodium).
Pharmacopoeias. In *It.* and *Jpn.*

In patients with normal hepatic function sulphobromophthalein sodium is rapidly extracted, conjugated, and excreted in bile. It was formerly used intravenously as a diagnostic agent for testing the functional capacity of the liver but may cause severe hypersensitivity reactions.

Sulphuric Acid (1325-x)

513; Acid. Sulph. Conc.; Oil of Vitriol; Schwefelsäure; Sulfuric Acid.
H_2SO_4 = 98.08.
CAS — 7664-93-9.
Pharmacopoeias. In *Aust., Br.,* and *Fr.* Also in *USNF.*

A clear colourless corrosive liquid of oily consistence. **Miscible** with water and with alcohol. Much heat is evolved when sulphuric acid is added to other liquids. Concentrated oil of vitriol of commerce, 'COV', contains about 95 to 98% w/w, and brown oil of vitriol, 'BOV', contains 75 to 85% w/w of H_2SO_4. Nordhausen or fuming sulphuric acid, 'Oleum', is sulphuric acid containing SO_3; battery or accumulator acid is sulphuric acid diluted with distilled water to a specific gravity of 1.2 to 1.26.

Store in airtight containers.

CAUTION. *When sulphuric acid is mixed with other liquids, it should always be added slowly, with constant stirring, to the diluent.*

Dilute Sulphuric Acid (1326-r)

Acid. Sulph. Dil.; Verdünnte Schwefelsäure.

Pharmacopoeias. In *Aust.* (9.1 to 9.4%), *Br.* (9.5 to 10.5%), and *Pol.* (15.5 to 16.3%).

Dilute Sulphuric Acid (BP 1998) is prepared by adding 104 g of sulphuric acid to 896 g of water, with constant stirring and cooling.

Adverse Effects and Treatment

As for Hydrochloric Acid, p.1588.

Uses and Administration

Sulphuric acid has various industrial uses. Dilute sulphuric acid has been used as an astringent in diarrhoea and it has occasionally been prescribed in mixtures with vegetable bitters to stimulate appetite.

Sumatra Benzoin (274-k)

Benjoim; Benzoë; Benzoin; Gum Benjamin; Gum Benzoin.

CAS — 9000-73-1; 9000-05-9 (the first of these numbers is stated to apply to Sumatra benzoin and the second to benzoin).

Pharmacopoeias. In *Br.* and *Jpn.*

US allows both Siam benzoin and Sumatra benzoin.

A balsamic resin from the incised stem of *Styrax benzoin* and of *S. paralleloneurus*. It contains not less than 25% of total balsamic acids, calculated as cinnamic acid and with reference to the dried material, and not more than 20% of alcohol (90%)-insoluble matter.

Hard brittle masses of whitish tears embedded in a greyish-brown to reddish-brown translucent matrix; also as cream-coloured tears. It has an agreeable balsamic odour. **Store** at a temperature not exceeding 25°. Protect from light.

Sumatra benzoin is an ingredient of inhalations which are used in the treatment of catarrh of the upper respiratory tract. Sumatra benzoin is also used in topical preparations for its antiseptic and protective properties. Skin sensitisation has been reported.

Preparations

BP 1998: Benzoin Inhalation; Compound Benzoin Tincture (*Friars' Balsam*);
BPC 1954: Compound Iodoform Paint;
USP 23: Compound Benzoin Tincture; Podophyllum Resin Topical Solution.

Proprietary Preparations (details are given in Part 3)

Multi-ingredient: ***Austral.:*** Cold Sore Lotion†; Nappy-Mate; Nyal Cold Sore; ***Belg.:*** Borostyrol; ***Canad.:*** Cold Sore Lotion; Lotion pour Feux Sauvages; ***Fr.:*** Balsofumine; Balsofumine Mentholee; ***Ital.:*** Citrosil Nubesan; Fomentil; ***Switz.:*** Baume†; ***UK:*** Frador; Hill's Balsam Adult Expectorant; Hills Balsam Extra Strong; Snowfire; Sunspot; ***USA:*** Pfeiffer's Cold Sore.

Sunflower Oil (7370-b)

Helianthi Annui Oleum; Huile de Tournesol; Oleum Helianthi; Sunflowerseed Oil.

Pharmacopoeias. In *Eur.* (see p.viii).

The fixed oil obtained from the fruits (achenes) of the sunflower, *Helianthus annuus* (Compositae) by mechanical expression or extraction and then refined. A clear light yellow liquid. Practically **insoluble** in water and in alcohol; miscible with petroleum spirit. It may contain a suitable antioxidant. **Store** in well filled airtight containers. Protect from light.

Sunflower oil is used as a salad oil and in pharmaceutical preparations. It is rich in linoleic acid.

Multiple sclerosis. As discussed on p.620, the role of dietary lipids in multiple sclerosis remains to be proven,[1] although many patients modify their diets and take supplements of sunflower and other oils. Some studies have shown a reduction in severity and duration of relapse in patients taking linoleic acid supplements (as sunflower oil)[2] and another[3] has reported benefit in patients who limit their intake of dietary saturated fatty acids and supplement their diet with polyunsaturated fatty acids.

1. Anonymous. Lipids and multiple sclerosis. *Lancet* 1990; **336:** 25–6.
2. Millar JHD, *et al.* Double-blind trial of linoleate supplementation of the diet in multiple sclerosis. *Br Med J* 1973; **1:** 765–8.
3. Swank RL, Dugan BB. Effect of low saturated fat diet in early and late cases of multiple sclerosis. *Lancet* 1990; **336:** 37–9.

Preparations

Proprietary Preparations (details are given in Part 3)

Multi-ingredient: ***Aust.:*** Pelsano; Piniment; Piniol†; ***Ger.:*** Aksekapseln†; derma-loges N; ***Switz.:*** Huile de millepertuis A. Vogel (huile de St. Jean); Pelsano.

Surgibone (13290-e)

Surgibone (*USAN*).

Surgibone is sterile, specially processed mature bovine bone, that has been used for grafting procedures in orthopaedic and reconstructive surgery.

Preparations

Proprietary Preparations (details are given in Part 3)
UK: Kiel Bone Graft†.

Sutilains (3748-y)

Sutilains (*BAN, USAN, rINN*).

BAX-1515.

CAS — 12211-28-8.

Pharmacopoeias. In *US.*

A cream-coloured powder containing proteolytic enzymes derived from *Bacillus subtilis*. It contains not less than 2 500 000 USP Casein units of proteolytic activity per g. A 1% solution has a pH of 6.1 to 7.1. **Store** at 2° to 8° in airtight containers.

Sutilains has proteolytic actions in most conditions, and has been used for the debridement of wounds, burns, and decubitus ulcers.

Preparations

USP 23: Sutilains Ointment.

Proprietary Preparations (details are given in Part 3)
Canad.: Travase†; ***USA:*** Travase†.

Tannic Acid (322-s)

Acidum Tannicum; Gallotannic Acid; Gerbstoff; Tanin; Tann. Acid; Tannin.

CAS — 1401-55-4.

Pharmacopoeias. In *Aust., Belg., It., Jpn, Neth., Pol., Swiss,* and *US.*

A tannin usually obtained from nutgalls, the excrescences produced on the young twigs of *Quercus infectoria* and allied species of *Quercus,* from the seed pods of tara (*Caesalpinia spinosa*), or from the nutgalls or leaves of sumac (any of genus *Rhus*).

Commercial grades of tannic acid may contain gallic acid and being less soluble are not suitable for medicinal use.

Yellowish-white or light brown glistening scales, spongy masses, or an amorphous powder, odourless or with a characteristic odour.

Very **soluble** in water, alcohol, and in acetone; soluble 1 in 1 of warm glycerol; practically insoluble in chloroform, ether, and petroleum spirit. **Store** in airtight containers. Protect from light.

Tannic acid has been used as an astringent for the mucous membranes of the mouth and throat. Suppositories containing tannic acid have been used in the treatment of haemorrhoids. It is an ingredient in a number of dermatological preparations. Former uses of tannic acid include its application to burns and its addition to barium sulphate enemas to improve the quality of the pictures in the radiological examination of the colon. Both of these uses were associated with liver toxicity, sometimes fatal.

Although tannic acid may be used by plastic surgeons and dermatologists to produce a controlled partial-thickness burn in tattoo removal[1] it has been pointed out that in unskilled or amateur hands this procedure has resulted in full thickness burns requiring skin grafting to obtain satisfactory healing.[2]

1. Mercer NSG, Davies DM. Tattoos. *Br Med J* 1991; **303:** 380.
2. Scott M, Ridings P. Tattoos. *Br Med J* 1991; **303:** 720.

Preparations

Proprietary Preparations (details are given in Part 3)
Ger.: Tannosynt; ***USA:*** Zilactin.

Multi-ingredient: ***Aust.:*** Haemanal; Onycho Phytex; Paradenton; Phytex; Tebege-Tannin; ***Austral.:*** Phytex†; SM-33; ***Belg.:*** Aperop; ***Canad.:*** Bunion Salve; Outgro; Tanac; ***Fr.:*** Allerbiocid S; Eau Precieuse Depensier; HEC; Marinol; Pancrelase; ***Ger.:*** Akne-Medice Kombipackung†; Bioget; Biosilit-Heilsalbe†; Schwefel-Diasporal†; Tannolil; ***Irl.:*** Phytex; ***Ital.:*** Blefarolin; Emocicatrol†; Neo-Emocicatrol; Tannovit†; ***Spain:*** Antihemorr; Antihemorroidal†; Depurativo Richelet; Faderma†; Queratil; Sabanotropico; Talkosona; Talquissar; Talquistina; Tangenol; ***Switz.:*** Gingivitol†; HEC; Stomaqualine†; ***UK:*** Colsor; Phytex; TCP; ***USA:*** Dermasept Antifungal; Medadyne†; Orasept; Outgro; Res-Q†; Tanac; Tanac Dual Core.

Taraxacum (547-m)

Dandelion Root; Löwenzahnwurzel; Pissenlit; Taraxacum Root.

Pharmacopoeias. In *Aust.* and *Pol.*

Chin. specifies Taraxacum Herb from other species of *Taraxacum.*

The fresh or dried root of the common dandelion, *Taraxacum officinale* (Compositae).

Taraxacum has been used as a bitter, as a diuretic, and as a mild laxative. It has also been used in homoeopathic medicine.

References.

1. Houghton P. Bearberry, dandelion and celery. *Pharm J* 1995; **255:** 272–3.

Preparations

Proprietary Preparations (details are given in Part 3)
Ger.: Cholaktol TR†; Galleb S; Justogen mono; Kneipp Lowenzahn-Pflanzensaft; Taraleon.

Multi-ingredient: ***Aust.:*** Agnuchol; Bio-Garten Entschlackungstee; Bio-Garten Tee zur Erhohung der Harnmenge; Bio-Garten Tropfen fur Galle und Leber; Brennesseltonikum; Citochol; Digestol; Ehrmann's Entschlackungstee; Entschlackungstee; Felidon neu; Fruhjahrs-Elixier ohne Alkohol; Gallen- und Lebertee; Gallogran; Harntreibender Tee; Kneipp Galle- und Leber-Tee; Kneipp Stoffwechsel-Unterstutzungs-Tee; Krauterdoktor Entschlackungs-Elixier; Krauterdoktor Gallentreibende Tropfen; Krauterdoktor Harnstein- und Nieren-griesstropfen; Krauterhaus Mag Kottas Blutreinigungstee; Krauterhaus Mag Kottas Entschlackungstee; Krauterhaus Mag Kottas Gallen- und Lebertee; Krautertee Nr 17; Krautertee Nr 20; Krautertee Nr 25; Krautertee Nr 29; Mag Doskar's Leber-Galletonikum; Mag Kottas Entschlackungstee; Mag Kottas Entwasserungstee; Mag Kottas Leber-Gallentee; Magentee EF-EM-ES; Montana; Sidroga Leber-Galle-Tee; Sidroga Stoffwechseltee; St Radegunder Entschlackungs-Elixier; St Radegunder Leber-Galle-Tee; Teekanne Leber- und Galletee; Urelium Neu; ***Austral.:*** Berberis Complex; Cholagogum†; Digest-eze†; Fluid Loss; Glycoplex; Herbal Cleanse; Herbal Diuretic Complex†; Herbal Diuretic Formula; Lifesystem Herbal Formula 7 Liver Tonic; Liver Tonic Herbal Formula 6; Profluid; Silybum Complex; St Mary's Thistle Plus; Trifolium Complex; Uva-Ursi Complex; Uva-Ursi Plus; ***Fr.:*** Diacure; Lithiabyl; Reduligne†; Romarene; Romarinex-Choline; ***Ger.:*** Agrimonas N; Alasenn; Aristochol N; Asgocholan†; C 34-Strath†; Cefachol N; Cholaflux N†; Cholaflux†; Cholongal plus†; Cholongal†; Cholosolm Phyto; Cholosom SL; Cholosom-Tee; Cholosom†; Cholosum N†; Colchicum-Strath†; Dolo-Arthrosetten†; Dr. Klinger's Bergischer Krautertee, Leber- und Gallentee†; Drix Richter's Krautertee†; Entwasserungs-Tee†; Galleb†; Gallemolan forte; Gallemolan G; Gallemolan N†; Gallen-Leber-Tee Stada†; Gallen-Tee Cholaflux S†; Gallexier; Gallitophen†; Galloselect M; Hepa-L†; Hepafungin†; Hepalixier†; Heparaxal†; Heparchofid S†; Hepaticum-Divinal†; Hepatofalk Neu; Hevert-Entwasserungs-Tee; Hevert-Gall S; JuCholan S; Kneipp Galle- und Leber-Tee N; Legapas comp; Neo-Gallonorm†; Neurochol C; Nieron S; Nieron-Tee N; Novo Mandrogallan N; Original-Hico-Gallenheil†; Pascobilin novo; Pascohepan novo; Presselin Hepaticum P; Rheumex†; Salus Leber-Galle-Tee Nr.18; Salus Rheuma-Tee Krautertee Nr. 12; Sirmia Artischockenelixier N; Tonsilgon-N; Ullus Galle-Tee N; Uro-Pasc; Urol†; ventri-loges; Worishofener Leber- und Gallensteinmittel Dr. Kleinschrod†; Zettagall V†; ***Ital.:*** Boldosten†; Cheliboldo†; Depurfat; ***Switz.:*** Boldocynara N; Demodon†; Demonatur Gouttes pour le foie et la bile; Gastrosan; Maffee N†; Phytomed Hepato; Phytomed Nephro; Tisane hepatique et biliaire; Tisane hepatique et biliaire "H"†; ***UK:*** Aqualette; Boldo; Buchu Compound; Cleansing Herb Tablets; Golden Seal Compound; HealthAid Boldo-Plus; Herbal Powder No.8†; Herbulax; Out-of-Sorts; Rheumatic Pain; Stomach Mixture; Uvacin; Waterlex.

Targinine (3222-g)

Targinine (*BAN*).

BW-546C88; 546C88. N^{ω}-Methyl-L-arginine.

$C_7H_{16}N_4O_2$ = 188.2.

CAS — 17035-90-4.

Targinine is a nitric oxide synthase inhibitor under investigation in the treatment of septic shock and migraine.

References.

1. Lassen LH, *et al.* Nitric oxide synthase inhibition in migraine. *Lancet* 1997; **349:** 401–2.

Tartaric Acid (1327-f)

353 (metatartaric acid); Acidum Tartaricum; E334; Tart. Acid; Tartrique (Acide); Weinsäure. (+)-L-Tartaric acid; (+)-L-2,3-Dihydroxybutanedioic acid; (2*R*,3*R*)-2,3-Dihydroxybutane-1,4-dioic acid.

$C_4H_6O_6$ = 150.1.

CAS — 87-69-4; 526-83-0.

Pharmacopoeias. In *Eur.* (see p.viii), *Jpn,* and *Pol.* Also in *USNF.*

Odourless, colourless or translucent crystals or a white or almost white crystalline powder.

Soluble 1 in 0.8 of water, 1 in 0.5 of boiling water, 1 in 3 of alcohol, 1 in 250 of ether, and 1 in 1.7 of methyl alcohol.

Adverse Effects

Strong solutions of tartaric acid are mildly irritant and if ingested undiluted may cause violent vomiting and diarrhoea, abdominal pain, and thirst. Cardiovascular collapse or acute renal failure may follow.

Pharmacokinetics

Tartaric acid is absorbed from the gastro-intestinal tract but up to 80% of an ingested dose is probably destroyed by micro-organisms in the lumen of the intestine before absorption occurs. Absorbed tartaric acid is excreted unchanged in the urine.

Uses and Administration

Tartaric acid is used in the preparation of effervescent powders, granules, and tablets, as an ingredient of cooling drinks, and as a saline purgative. If not neutralised, it must be taken well diluted. Tartaric acid or metatartaric acid are used in wine-making as de-acidifying agents to assist in the removal of excess malic acid by forming an insoluble double salt with calcium carbonate.

Preparations

Proprietary Preparations (details are given in Part 3)

Multi-ingredient: ***Aust.:*** Helo-acid; Lactolavol; ***Austral.:*** Dexsal; Salvital; Ural; ***Belg.:*** Zoru†; ***Canad.:*** E-Z-Gas II; Unik-Zoru; ***Fr.:*** Dermacide; Eno†; Lithines Magnesies†; ***Ger.:*** Abfuhr-Tee Depuraflux†; Bourget N; Helo-acid compositum†; Helo-acid†; Presselin Osmo†; Retterspitz Ausserlich; Retterspitz Gelee; Retterspitz Innerlich; Sepdelen 7†; ***Ital.:*** Geffer; Magnesia Effervescente Sanitas†; Magnesia Effervescente Sella; Non Acid; Nuovo Andrews†; ***Neth.:*** Zoru†; ***S.Afr.:*** Adco-Sodasol; Alkafizz; Citro-Soda; Citrovescent†; Effersol; ***Spain:*** Agua Germana†; Frutosel†; Hectonona; Lithines†; Litinoides†; Magnesia Validada†; Mucorex Ciclin; Salcedol; Sales de Frutas P G; Sales de Frutas Verkos†; Sales Fruta Mag Viviar; Sales Orto; Salmagne; Starlep; ***Swed.:*** Gastroluft; ***Switz.:*** Gastroluft; Gynasol; Marciderm†; Siesta-1; ***UK:*** Bioglan Effervescent Granules; Bioglan Effervescent Tablets; Eno; Jaaps Health Salt; ***USA:*** Baros.

Taurine (13299-x)

Taurine *(rINN)*.

2-Aminoethanesulphonic acid.

$C_2H_7NO_3S$ = 125.1.

CAS — 107-35-7.

Taurine is an amino acid known to be involved in bile acid conjugation and having other physiological functions. It has been included in preparations for parenteral nutrition of low-birth-weight infants and in infant formulas but its role as an essential nutrient has not been established.

Taurine is included in preparations for cardiovascular and metabolic disorders.

Preparations

Proprietary Preparations (details are given in Part 3)

Ital.: O-Due.

Multi-ingredient: ***Ital.:*** Detoxergon; Nucleodoxina†; ***Spain:*** Taurobetina.

Terpineol (4715-l)

$C_{10}H_{18}O$ = 154.2.

CAS — 8000-41-7; 98-55-5 (α); 2438-12-2 [(±)-α].

Pharmacopoeias. In Br.

A mixture of isomers in which α-terpineol (*p*-menth-1-en-8-ol) predominates.

It is a colourless, slightly viscous liquid which may deposit crystals; it has a pleasant lilac-like odour.

Very slightly **soluble** in water; freely soluble in alcohol (70%); soluble in ether.

Terpineol has disinfectant and solvent properties. It is used with other volatile agents in preparations for respiratory-tract disorders.

Preparations

BP 1998: Chloroxylenol Solution *(Roxenol)*.

Proprietary Preparations (details are given in Part 3)

Multi-ingredient: ***Aust.:*** Resol; Tineafax; ***Austral.:*** Karvol; Tixylix Chest Rub; ***Belg.:*** Balsoclase; Calyptol†; ***Canad.:*** Iba-Cide; ***Fr.:*** Bronchodermine; Bronchospray; Pectoderme; Valda; ***Ger.:*** Bronchicum Inhalat†; Extropin†; ***Irl.:*** Karvol; Valda†; ***Ital.:*** Calyptol; Rikospray; ***Mon.:*** Calyptol; ***Neth.:*** Rhinocaps; ***S.Afr.:*** AF; Karvol; Rikerspray†; ***Spain:*** Caltoson Balsamico; Calyptol Inhalante; Empapol; Eupnol; ***Swed.:*** Munvatten†; ***Switz.:*** Sedotussin; ***UK:*** Biocream; Chymol Emollient Balm; Karvol; Valda; Waxwane.

Tetrachlorodecaoxide (1145-c)

TCDO; Tetrachlorodecaoxygen Anion Complex.

Cl_4O_{10} = 301.8.

Tetrachlorodecaoxide is a water-soluble anion complex containing oxygen in a chlorite matrix. Active oxygen is only released in the presence of biological material. It has been applied as a solution for the stimulation of wound healing.

Wounds. Tetrachlorodecaoxide was reported to promote wound healing (p.1076) compared with saline in a double-blind study of 271 patients,[1] but a smaller study failed to show any benefit over glycerol.[2]

1. Hinz J, *et al.* Rationale for and results from a randomised, double-blind trial of tetrachlorodecaoxygen anion complex in wound healing. *Lancet* 1986; **i:** 825–8.
2. Hughes LE, *et al.* Failure of tetrachlorodecaoxygen anion complex to assist wound healing. *Lancet* 1989; **ii:** 1271.

Preparations

Proprietary Preparations (details are given in Part 3)

Aust.: Oxilium; ***Switz.:*** Oxilium.

Tetrahydrobiopterin (13312-n)

2-Amino-5,6,7,8-tetrahydro-6-(1,2-dihydroxypropyl)pterid-in-4(3*H*)-one.

$C_9H_{15}N_5O_3$ = 241.2.

CAS — 17528-72-2.

Tetrahydrobiopterin has been tried to correct the hyperphenylalaninaemia which may be responsible for neurological symptoms seen in patients receiving treatment for leukaemia.

References.

1. Blau N, *et al.* Hyperphenylalaninemia caused by dihydropteridine reductase deficiency in children receiving chemotherapy for acute lymphoblastic leukemia. *J Pediatr* 1989; **115:** 661–20.
2. Hyland K, *et al.* Reply. *J Pediatr* 1989; **115:** 662.

Tetramethylammonium Iodide (13313-h)

$C_4H_{12}IN$ = 201.0.

CAS — 75-58-1.

Tetramethylammonium iodide is a quaternary ammonium compound that has been used for the emergency disinfection of drinking water. It has also been employed for its ganglion-blocking properties.

Preparations

Proprietary Preparations (details are given in Part 3)

Multi-ingredient: ***Fr.:*** Banikol Vitamine B_1†.

Thalidomide (13316-v)

Thalidomide *(BAN, USAN, rINN)*.

K-17; NSC-66847. 2-Phthalimidoglutarimide.

$C_{13}H_{10}N_2O_4$ = 258.2.

CAS — 50-35-1.

Adverse Effects and Precautions

Thalidomide was withdrawn from use as a hypnotic in the early 1960s after it was discovered that it produced teratogenic effects when administered to women in early pregnancy. These effects involved mainly malformations of the limbs and defects of the ears, eyes, and internal organs. Further abnormalities and problems, including effects on the CNS, continue to appear in affected individuals.

In consequence, thalidomide should not be used in women of child-bearing potential, or if such use is absolutely essential then stringent contraceptive measures are mandatory. If pregnancy occurs during thalidomide therapy the drug must be discontinued immediately and the patient given appropriate evaluation and counselling. Although it is unclear if thalidomide is present in semen, male patients receiving thalidomide should use barrier methods of contraception if their partner is of child-bearing potential.

The other major adverse effect of thalidomide is peripheral neuropathy, which can be severe and irreversible. Other effects have included somnolence, constipation, peripheral oedema, dryness of the mouth and nasal mucosa, and erythema of the face or other rashes. Hypersensitivity reactions have been reported.

Reviews.

1. Günzler V. Thalidomide in human immunodeficiency virus (HIV) patients: a review of safety considerations. *Drug Safety* 1992; **7:** 116–34.

Migraine. Migraine attacks were associated with thalidomide administration in a 36-year-old man.[1]

1. García-Albea E, *et al.* Jaqueca típica y talidomida. *Med Clin (Barc)* 1993; **100:** 557.

Mutagenicity. Reports of the birth of 3 malformed infants to parents who had themselves been exposed to thalidomide *in utero*[1,2] have provoked fears that thalidomide may be a mutagen. However, the limb malformations seen in the infants are not typical of mutagenesis[3] and the teratogenic effect of thalidomide is likely to be associated with interference with angiogenesis in the fetus rather than mutation.[4]

1. McBride WG. Thalidomide may be a mutagen. *Br Med J* 1994; **308:** 1635–6.
2. Tenconi R, *et al.* Amniotic band sequence in child of thalidomide victim. *Br Med J* 1994; **309:** 1442.
3. Read AP. Thalidomide may be a mutagen. *Br Med J* 1994; **308:** 1636.
4. D'Amato RJ, *et al.* Thalidomide is an inhibitor of angiogenesis. *Proc Natl Acad Sci U S A* 1994; **91:** 4082–5.

Pharmacokinetics

References.

1. Chen T-L, *et al.* Plasma pharmacokinetics and urinary excretion of thalidomide after oral dosing in healthy male volunteers. *Drug Metab Dispos* 1989; **17:** 402–5.
2. Piscitelli SC, *et al.* Single-dose pharmacokinetics of thalidomide in human immunodeficiency virus-infected patients. *Antimicrob Agents Chemother* 1997; **41:** 2797–9.

Uses and Administration

Thalidomide has been shown to have immunomodulating activity. It is effective in the control of type 2 (erythema nodosum leprosum) lepra reactions and is usually given in doses of 100 to 300 mg once daily by mouth, preferably at bedtime. In severe cases up to 400 mg daily may be given. The dose should be reduced gradually by 50 mg every 2 to 4 weeks once a satisfactory response has been achieved. Thalidomide is of no value in type 1 lepra reactions.

The immunomodulating activity of thalidomide has led to its investigation in a wide range of conditions (see below) whose aetiology may involve the immune system, including AIDS-related cachexia, diarrhoea, and aphthous ulceration, oral and genital ulceration associated with Behçet's syndrome, and lupus erythematosus. Thalidomide is also being investigated in some malignancies.

Guidelines on the clinical use of thalidomide.

1. Powell RJ, Gardner-Medwin JMM. Guideline for the clinical use and dispensing of thalidomide. *Postgrad Med J* 1994; **70:** 901–4.

Immunological and inflammatory disorders. Thalidomide has become one of the established treatments for type 2 lepra reactions (erythema nodosum leprosum) as described on p.128 under Leprosy. It has also been used in graft-versus-host disease (see p.498) and it has been tried in a number of other immunological disorders. Investigations into its mode of action have shown that thalidomide may produce a decrease in concentrations of tumour necrosis factor, effects on CD4+ cells, and variable effects on other mediators of intercellular reactions.[1]

Beneficial responses to thalidomide have been reported in bone marrow transplant recipients,[2-6] refractory mucus membrane ulcers in immunocompromised patients[7-10] and in Behçet's syndrome,[11] Crohn's disease,[12] lupus erythematosus,[13-17] erythema multiforme,[18,19] rheumatoid arthritis,[20] adult-onset Still's disease,[21] sarcoidosis,[22] pruritus associated with uraemia,[23] Langerhans cell histiocytosis,[24] epidermolysis bullosa,[25] prurigo nodularis,[26] and other inflammatory skin disorders.[27] Clinical studies of thalidomide are also being conducted in cachexia in patients with malignancies or AIDS and in some infections including HIV.[28]

1. Schuler U, Ehninger G. Thalidomide: rationale for renewed use in immunological disorders. *Drug Safety* 1995; **12:** 364–9.
2. Lim SH, *et al.* Successful treatment with thalidomide of acute graft-versus-host disease after bone-marrow transplantation. *Lancet* 1988; **i:** 117.
3. McCarthy DM, *et al.* Thalidomide for graft-versus-host disease. *Lancet* 1988; **ii:** 1135.
4. Heney D, *et al.* Thalidomide for chronic graft-versus-host disease in children. *Lancet* 1988; **ii:** 1317.
5. Vogelsang GB, *et al.* Thalidomide for the treatment of chronic graft-versus-host disease. *N Engl J Med* 1992; **326:** 1055–8.
6. Cole CH, *et al.* Thalidomide in the management of chronic graft-versus-host disease in children following bone marrow transplantation. *Bone Marrow Transplant* 1994; **14:** 937–42.
7. Georghiou PR, Kemp RJ. HIV-associated oesophageal ulcers treated with thalidomide. *Med J Aust* 1990; **152:** 382–3.
8. Solèr RA, *et al.* Thalidomide treatment of mucosal ulcerations in HIV infection. *Arch Dis Child* 1996; **74:** 64–5.
9. Verberkmoes A, *et al.* Thalidomide for genital ulcer in HIV-positive woman. *Lancet* 1996; **347:** 974.
10. Jacobson JM, *et al.* Thalidomide for the treatment of oral aphthous ulcers in patients with human immunodeficiency virus infection. *N Engl J Med* 1997; **336:** 1487–93.
11. Hamuryudan V, *et al.* Thalidomide in the treatment of the mucocutaneous lesions of the Behçet syndrome: a randomized, double-blind, placebo-controlled trial. *Ann Intern Med* 1998; **128:** 443–50.
12. Wettstein AR, Meagher AP. Thalidomide in Crohn's disease. *Lancet* 1997; **350:** 1445–6.
13. Knop J, *et al.* Thalidomide in the treatment of sixty cases of chronic discoid lupus erythematosus. *Br J Dermatol* 1983; **108:** 461–6.
14. Burrows NP, *et al.* Lupus erythematosus profundus with partial C4 deficiency responding to thalidomide. *Br J Dermatol* 1991; **125:** 62–7.
15. Bessis D, *et al.* Thalidomide for systemic lupus erythematosus. *Lancet* 1992; **339:** 549–50.
16. Atra E, Sato EI. Treatment of the cutaneous lesions of systemic lupus erythematosus with thalidomide. *Clin Exp Rheumatol* 1993; **11:** 487–93.
17. Stevens RJ, *et al.* Thalidomide in the treatment of the cutaneous manifestations of lupus erythematosus: experience in sixteen consecutive patients. *Br J Rheumatol* 1997; **36:** 353–9.
18. Bahmer FA, *et al.* Thalidomide treatment of recurrent erythema multiforme. *Acta Derm Venereol (Stockh)* 1982; **62:** 449–50.
19. Moisson YF, *et al.* Thalidomide for recurrent erythema multiforme. *Br J Dermatol* 1992; **126:** 92–3.
20. Gutiérrez-Rodríguez O, *et al.* Treatment of refractory rheumatoid arthritis—the thalidomide experience. *J Rheumatol* 1989; **16:** 158–63.
21. Stambe C, Wicks IP. TNFα and response of treatment-resistant adult-onset Still's disease to thalidomide. *Lancet* 1998; **352:** 544–5.

22. Carlesimo M, *et al.* Treatment of cutaneous and pulmonary sarcoidosis with thalidomide. *J Am Acad Dermatol* 1995; **32:** 866–9.
23. Silva SRB, *et al.* Thalidomide for the treatment of uremic pruritus: a crossover randomized double-blind trial. *Nephron* 1994; **67:** 270–3.
24. Meunier L, *et al.* Adult cutaneous Langerhans cell histiocytosis: remission with thalidomide treatment. *Br J Dermatol* 1995; **132:** 168.
25. Goulden V, *et al.* Linear prurigo simulating dermatitis artefacta in dominant dystrophic epidermolysis bullosa. *Br J Dermatol* 1993; **129:** 443–6.
26. Ferrándiz C, *et al.* Sequential combined therapy with thalidomide and narrow-band (TL01) UVB in the treatment of prurigo nodularis. *Dermatology* 1997; **195:** 359–61.
27. Grosshans E, Illy G. Thalidomide therapy for inflammatory dermatoses. *Int J Dermatol* 1984; **23:** 598–602.
28. Reyes-Terán G, *et al.* Effects of thalidomide on HIV-associated wasting syndrome: a randomized, double-blind, placebo-controlled trial. *AIDS* 1996; **10:** 1501–7.

Preparations

Proprietary Preparations (details are given in Part 3)
USA: Thalomid.

Thallium Acetate (15328-h)

Thallous Acetate.

$C_2H_3O_2Tl$ = 263.4.

CAS — 563-68-8.

Adverse Effects

Thallium salts are toxic when inhaled, ingested, or absorbed through the skin. Symptoms of poisoning may appear within 12 to 24 hours of a single toxic dose and include severe abdominal pain, vomiting, diarrhoea, gastro-intestinal haemorrhage, paralytic ileus, pancreatic damage, and in severe cases cardiovascular collapse, tremors, delirium, convulsions, paralysis, and coma, leading to death in 1 to 2 days. However, the acute reaction may subside to be followed within about 10 days by the development of neurological effects including paraesthesia, myalgia, myopathy, motor neuropathy, and visual disturbances due to optic neuropathy, psychosis, delirium, convulsions, and other signs of encephalopathy, tachycardia, hypertension, skin eruptions, and hepatorenal injury. Alopecia occurs within 15 to 20 days. Death may result from respiratory failure; patients are also predisposed to cardiac arrhythmias and sudden death for several weeks. The usual lethal dose of thallium sulphate is 10 to 15 mg per kg bodyweight.

Smaller repeated doses are also toxic, with symptoms appearing over several weeks. Constipation is a common feature of less severe poisoning.

References.

1. Moeschlin S. Thallium poisoning. *Clin Toxicol* 1980; **17:** 133–46.
2. Heyl T, Barlow RJ. Thallium poisoning: a dermatological perspective. *Br J Dermatol* 1989; **121:** 787–92.
3. Luckit J, *et al.* Thrombocytopenia associated with thallium poisoning. *Hum Exp Toxicol* 1990; **9:** 47–8.
4. Moore D, *et al.* Thallium poisoning. *Br Med J* 1993; **306:** 1527–8.
5. Tabandeh H, Thompson GM. Visual function in thallium toxicity. *Br Med J* 1993; **307:** 324.
6. Questel F, *et al.* Thallium-contaminated heroin. *Ann Intern Med* 1996; **124:** 616.
7. Tromme I, *et al.* Skin signs in the diagnosis of thallium poisoning. *Br J Dermatol* 1998; **138:** 321–5.

Treatment of Adverse Effects

After the acute ingestion of thallium the stomach should be emptied by emesis or lavage and a saline purgative such as magnesium sulphate may be given. Intensive supportive therapy is necessary.

Various methods have been employed in an attempt to increase the faecal and urinary excretion of thallium. A suspension of activated charcoal has been given to reduce intestinal absorption and enteric recycling but is less successful than Prussian blue (see p.993) administered by duodenal tube. Systemic chelating agents have been tried but are of doubtful value and potentially dangerous. The administration of potassium chloride by mouth may mobilise thallium from the tissues but is also hazardous especially if given during the early stage; signs of poisoning may be transiently aggravated.

Haemoperfusion or haemodialysis combined with forced diuresis are reported to be effective in eliminating absorbed thallium if given within 48 hours of ingestion.

Uses and Administration

Thallium acetate was formerly used by mouth for depilation in ringworm and as an ingredient of depilatory creams but owing to numerous fatalities following both systemic and local treatments it is no longer used for such purposes. It has also been used as a rodenticide and insecticide, although its use is strictly regulated in many countries. However, it is used in industry and is therefore still a hazard. Cases of malicious poisoning are still encountered occasionally.

Theobroma (2412-b)

Cacao or Cocoa Powder; Cocoa; Non-alkalised Cocoa Powder; Theobrom.

The roasted seed of theobroma, *Theobroma cacao* (Sterculiaceae), deprived of most of the shell, pressed to remove a portion of its fat, and finely ground.

Prepared theobroma is used as a flavoured basis for tablets and lozenges.

Preparations

Proprietary Preparations (details are given in Part 3)

Multi-ingredient: ***Aust.:*** Asthmatee; Blutreinigungsteet†; ***Ger.:*** Buccotean TF†; Buccotean†; Cholebrine-Reizmahlzeit†; Pektan N†.

Theodrenaline Hydrochloride (13321-h)

Theodrenaline Hydrochloride *(BANM, rINNM).*

H-8352. 7-[2-(3,4,β-Trihydroxyphenethylamino)ethyl]theophylline hydrochloride.

$C_{17}H_{21}N_5O_5,HCl$ = 411.8.

CAS — 13460-98-5 (theodrenaline); 2572-61-4 (theodrenaline hydrochloride).

Theodrenaline is mainly used as the hydrochloride in preparations with cafedrine promoted for the treatment of hypotension.

Preparations

Proprietary Preparations (details are given in Part 3)

Multi-ingredient: ***Aust.:*** Akrinor; ***Fr.:*** Praxinor; ***Ger.:*** Akrinor; ***S.Afr.:*** Akrinor; ***Spain:*** Bifort; ***Switz.:*** Akrinor.

Thioctic Acid (13325-g)

Lipoic Acid. 5-(1,2-Dithiolan-3-yl)valeric acid.

$C_8H_{14}O_2S_2$ = 206.3.

CAS — 62-46-4.

Thioctic acid has been tried in the treatment of liver dysfunction; it has also been tried in subacute necrotising encephalopathy. Beneficial results have been claimed in amanitin poisoning following ingestion of the mushroom *Amanita phalloides,* but its use is controversial (see under Poisonous Mushrooms or Toadstools, p.1605). Ethylenediamine thioctate, sodium thioctate, and thioctic acid amide have been used similarly.

Thioctic acid is also used for the treatment of diabetic neuropathy.

References suggesting thioctic acid may be of benefit in diabetic cardiac autonomic neuropathy.

1. Ziegler D, *et al.* Effects of treatment with the antioxidant α-lipoic acid on cardiac autonomic neuropathy in non-insulin-dependent diabetic patients: a 4-month randomized controlled trial (DEKAN study). *Clin Auton Res* 1995; **5:** 323.

Preparations

Proprietary Preparations (details are given in Part 3)
Aust.: Tioctan; ***Ger.:*** Alpha-Lipon; alpha-Vibolex; Azulipont; Berlithion; Biomo-lipon; duralipon; espa-lipon; Fenint; Neurium; Neurothioct; Pleomix-Alpha; Thioctacid; Thiogamma; Tromlipon; Verla-Lipon; ***Ital.:*** Tioctidasi†; ***Jpn:*** Tioctan.

Multi-ingredient: ***Ger.:*** Hepabionta comp†; Hepabionta†; Sterofundin CH compositum†; Tutofusin CH†; Tutofusin LC†; ***Ital.:*** Atoxan†; Epaplex†; Piruvasi†; Tiobec; ***Spain:*** Policolinosil.

Thiomucase (3903-p)

C-84-04; Chondroitinsulphatase.

Thiomucase is a mucopolysaccharidase with general properties similar to those of hyaluronidase, p.1588, but which also depolymerises chondroitin sulphate. It has been given to assist the diffusion of local anaesthetic injections.

Thiram (13330-m)

Thiram *(USAN, pINN).*

NSC-1771; SQ-1489; TMT; TMTD. Tetramethylthiuram disulphide.

$C_6H_{12}N_2S_4$ = 240.4.

CAS — 137-26-8.

Thiram, the methyl analogue of disulfiram (p.1573), has antibacterial and antifungal activity. It is applied topically as an aerosol in the treatment of wounds and other skin disorders. It has been used as a fungicide in agriculture, and in industry as a rubber accelerator. Occupational exposure to thiram may cause irritation of mucous membranes and skin.

Preparations

Proprietary Preparations (details are given in Part 3)
Belg.: Nobecutane; ***Ger.:*** Nobecutan; ***Ital.:*** Nobecutane†; ***Neth.:*** Nobecutan†; ***Norw.:*** Nobecutan†; ***Switz.:*** Nobecutan†.

Multi-ingredient: ***Spain:*** Sulfiselen.

Thonzonium Bromide (13331-b)

Thonzonium Bromide *(USAN).*

Tonzonium Bromide *(rINN)*; NC-1264; NSC-5648. Hexadecyl[2-(*N*-*p*-methoxybenzyl-*N*-pyrimidin-2-ylamino)ethyl]dimethylammonium bromide.

$C_{32}H_{55}BrN_4O$ = 591.7.

CAS — 553-08-2.

Thonzonium bromide is a cationic surfactant. As an additive in ear drops and aerosol sprays it has been claimed to promote tissue contact by dispersion and penetration of cellular debris and exudate.

Preparations

Proprietary Preparations (details are given in Part 3)

Multi-ingredient: ***Canad.:*** Coly-Mycin Otic†; ***Ital.:*** Rinedrone; ***USA:*** Coly-Mycin S Otic; Cortisporin-TC.

Thorium Dioxide (13332-v)

Thorium Oxide.

ThO_2 = 264.0.

CAS — 1314-20-1.

Colloidal solutions of thorium dioxide were formerly used as X-ray contrast media for examination of the liver and spleen, for arteriography, and occasionally for outlining the cerebral ventricles. Its elimination is very slow and incomplete. It accumulates in the reticulo-endothelial system, especially in the liver and spleen. As it is radioactive (half-life: 1.41×10^{10} years), this accumulation is dangerous and there is strong evidence that the ensuing prolonged exposure to its radiation is a contributing factor in the development of malignant diseases and blood disorders often 20 to 30 years after its administration.

Thuja (13333-g)

The fresh leaves and twigs of *Thuja occidentalis* (Coniferae).

Thuja is included in some topical preparations for warts and herbal antiseptic preparations. It is also used in homoeopathic medicine.

Preparations

Proprietary Preparations (details are given in Part 3)

Multi-ingredient: ***Belg.:*** Aporil; ***Fr.:*** Nitrol; ***Ger.:*** Esberitox N; ***Spain:*** Nitroina; ***Switz.:*** Esberitox N.

Thyme (4716-y)

Common Thyme; Garden Thyme; Rubbed Thyme; Thymi Herba; Timo.

Pharmacopoeias. In *Eur.* (see p.viii) and *Pol.*

The whole leaves and flowers separated from the previously dried stems of the 'garden thyme', *Thymus vulgaris*, or *Thymus zygis* (Labiatae), or a mixture of both species. It contains not less than 12 mL per kg of essential oil and not less than 0.5% m/m of volatile phenols, expressed as thymol, both calculated with reference to the anhydrous drug. **Protect** from light and moisture.

Thyme is the source of thyme oil. It has carminative, antitussive, antiseptic, and expectorant properties and is used chiefly in preparations for respiratory-tract disorders and as a flavour.

Preparations

Proprietary Preparations (details are given in Part 3)
Aust.: Heumann's Bronchial; Pertussin†; Scottopect; ***Ger.:*** Anastil; Antussan; Antussan "T"†; Aspecton; Bronchicum Husten-Pastillen†; Bronchitten; Dr. Boether Bronchial Tropfen†; Expectal N; Fichtensirup N; Hustagil Thymian-Hustensaft; Hustles; Isephca S; Kolton bronchiale Erkaltungssaft; Makatussin Saft; Melrosum Hustensirup Forte; Menthymin Mono; Mirfusot; Nimopect; Pertussin N†; Schneckensirup; Soledum Hustensaft; Soledum Hustentropfen; Thymi-Fips; Thymipin N; Thymiverlan; Tussamag Hustensaft N; Tussamag Hustentropfen N; ***Neth.:*** Daro Thijm; ***Spain:*** Drocorcina†.

Multi-ingredient: ***Aust.:*** Aktiv Husten- und Bronchialtee; Anifer Hustentee; Anifer Hustentropfen; Apotheker Bauer's Brust- und Hustentee; Bio-Garten Tee gegen Erkaltung; Bio-Garten Tropfen gegen Husten; Bronchiplant; Bronchiplant light; Bronchostop; Brust- und Hustentee; Codelum; Codipront cum Expectorans; Erkaltungstee; Expectal-Tropfen; Granobil; Grippetee Dr Zeidler; Heumann Hustenstiller; Hustensaft-Dr Schmidgall†; Jutussin neo; Kneipp Grippe-Tee; Kneipp Husten- und Bronchial-Tee; Krauter Hustensaft†; Krauterdoktor Hustentropfen; Krauterdoktor Krampf- und Reizhustensirup; Krauterhaus Mag Kottas Husten- und Bronchialtee; Krautertee Nr 10; Krautertee Nr 126;

Krautertee Nr 211; Krautertee Nr 311; Krautertee Nr 7; Mag Kottas Husten-Bronchialtee; Mediplant Krauter; Paracodin; Pertussetten†; Pertussin†; Pilka; Pilka Forte; Pneumopan; Pneumopect†; Purianta; Scottopect; Sidroga Brust-Husten-Tee; Spasmo-Granobil-Krampf- und Reizhusten; St Radegunder Bronchialtee; St Radegunder Thorasan-Krauterhustensaft; Teekanne Erkaltungstee; Teekanne Husten- und Brusttee; Thymoval; Tussamag; Tussimont; ***Austral.:*** Cough Relief; Euphorbia Complex; Pertussin†; Respatona; Respatona Plus with Echinacea; ***Belg.:*** Balsoclase; Colimax; Paracodine†; ***Canad.:*** Pectothymin; ***Fr.:*** Depuratum; Elixir Contre La Toux Weleda; Gastropax; Germose; Santane D_5; Santane R_8; ***Ger.:*** Anastil N; Anastil†; Antibex†; Aspecton N; Atmulen E†; Biotuss N; Bronchialtee†; Bronchicum Elixir N; Bronchicum Elixir Plus; Bronchicum Hustentee; Bronchicum Pflanzlicher; Bronchicum Sekret-Loser; Bronchicum Thymian; Bronchicum Tropfen mit Codein†; Bronchicum Tropfen N; Bronchipret; Bronchitten forte K; Bronchitussin SC†; Bronchocedin†; Broncholind†; Bronchosyx N; Brust- und Husten-Tee Stada N; Cefabronchin N; Cefedrin N; Cito-Guakalin†; Codipront cum Expectorans†; Dorex Hustensaft N mit Oxeladin†; Dr. Boether Bronchitten forte N†; Dr. Boether Bronchitten S†; Dr. Klinger's Bergischer Krautertee, Husten- u. Bronchial-tee†; Drosithym-N; Ephepect; Equisil; Eucabal; Eupatal; Expectal S†; Expectysat-N; Expectysat†; Friosmin†; Guakalin†; Guttae 20 Hustentropfen N; Harzer Hustenloser; Hevert-Erkaltungs-Tee; Hevert-Magen-Galle-Leber-Tee; Hevertopect; Infantussin N; Ipalat; Junisana; Kneipp Husten- und Bronchial-Tee; Kneipp Krauter Hustensaft N; Knufinke Broncholind K†; Kolton grippale N†; Kretussot†; Makatussin Tropfen; Melrosum Hustensirup N; Mintetten S†; Mintetten Truw; Mirfusot N mit Kodein†; Optipect mit Kodein†; Optipect†; Perdiphen phyto; Perdiphen-N†; Pertussin†; Phytobronchin; Pinus-Strath†; Praecipect; Priatan†; Primotussan; Primotussin N mit Codein†; Pulmocordio forte; Pulmocordio mite SL; Pulmotin; Salus Bronchial-Tee Nr.8; Schneckensaft N; Sedotussin Expectorans; Sinuforton; Soledum Hustensaft N†; Soledum Hustentropfen N†; Thymipin N; Thymitussin†; Tussiflorin forte; Tussinfant N; Tussinfantum†; Tussipect; Tussipect mit Codein†; Tussipect N†; ***Ital.:*** Broncosedina; Florerbe Balsamica†; Fluend; Pinedrin; Pinefedrina†; Pluriderm; Saugella Antisettica†; Sciroppo Merck all'Efetonina; ***Neth.:*** Balsoclase Compositum; Bronchicum; Hoestsiroop†; ***S.Afr.:*** Bronchicough; Bronchicum; Bronchicum SB†; ***Spain:*** Mentobox; Pazbronquial; Pilka; Wobenzimal; ***Switz.:*** Bronchalin; Bronchofluid; Bronchosan; Codipront cum Expectorans; Demo gouttes bronchiques; Demo sirop bronchique N; Demo sirop contre la toux; Dinacode N; Dipect†; Dragees contre la toux no 536; Expectoran avec codeine†; Expectoran Codein; Expectoran†; Makatussin; Makatussin forte; Nican; Pectoral N; Pilka; Radix†; Sedotussin; Sirop pectoral DP1; Sirop pectoral DP2; Thymodrosin; Tisane pectorale et antitussive; Tisane sedative et somnifere "H"†; ***UK:*** Cough Elixir; Herb and Honey Cough Elixir; Snowfire.

Thyme Oil (4717-j)

Esencia de Tomillo; Essência de Tomilho; Ol. Thym.; Oleum Thymi.

Pharmacopoeias. In *Eur.* (see p.viii) and *Pol.*

A volatile oil obtained by steam distillation from fresh flowering aerial parts of *Thymus vulgaris*, *T. zygis* or a mixture of both species. A clear, yellow or very dark reddish brown, mobile liquid with a characteristic odour. **Miscible** with dehydrated alcohol, with ether, and with petroleum spirit. It contains between 36 and 55% of thymol. **Store** in well filled airtight containers. Protect from light.

Thyme oil is used similarly to thyme (above).

Preparations

Proprietary Preparations (details are given in Part 3)
Ger.: Bronchicum; Fichtensirup N; Kneipp Erkaltungs-Bad.

Multi-ingredient: ***Aust.:*** Bronchostop; Expectal-Balsam; Expigen; Heumann's Bronchialtee; Leukona-Rheuma-Bad; Makatussin; Medizinalbad†; Perozon Heublumen; Pertussin†; Red Point†; Sanvita Bronchial; Scottopect; SynPharma Bronchial; ***Austral.:*** Tixylix Chest Rub; Zam-Buk; ***Belg.:*** Calyptol†; Perubore; Pinthym†; ***Fr.:*** Acarcid; Balsofletol†; Balsofumine; Balsofumine Mentholee; Biogaze; Bronchorectine au Citral; Citrosil; Gouttes aux Essences; Mysca†; Otylol; Perubore; Vapo-Myrtol; ***Ger.:*** Antitussivum Burger; Aspecton-Balsam; Bisolvomed mit Codein†; Bisolvomed†; Bronchicum Inhalat†; Broncho Sanol†; Dorex Hustensaft N mit Oxeladin†; Erkaltungs-Balsam†; Expectal Balsam†; Grunlicht Hingfong Essenz; Heumann Bronchialtee Solubifix; Hoepixin N; Hustagil Erkaltungsbalsam; Kneipp Erkaltungs-Balsam N; Kneipp Rheuma Stoffwechsel-Bad Heublumen-Aquasan; Leukona-Sauna-Konzentrat†; Makatussin Balsam Mild†; Makatussin Balsam mit Menthol; Makatussin Inhalat Menthol†; Makatussin Inhalat Mild†; Melrosum Medizinalbad; Nasivin Intensiv-Bad N; Nasulind; Night-Care; Pulmotin-N; Retterspitz Aerosol; Retterspitz Innerlich; Schupps Heilkrauter Erkaltungsbad; Silvapin Heublumen/Krauter-Extrakt†; ***Ital.:*** Calyptol; Fomentil; Neo Zeta-Foot; Sanaderm; Transpulmina Gola Nebulizzatore†; Vegetallumina; ***Mon.:*** Calyptol; ***S.Afr.:*** Zam-Buk; ***Spain:*** Calyptol Inhalante; H Tussan; Lapiz Termo Compositum†; Termosan; ***Switz.:*** Brosol; Caprisana; Carmol "blanche"†; Carmol "thermogene"†; Carmol†; Demo gouttes contre la toux; Demo pommade contre les refroidissements; Demo pommade contre les refroidissements pour bebes; Demonatur Capsules contre les refroidissements; Dolorex; Frigoplasma; Graminflor†; Hederka†; Kernosan Huile de Massage; Liberol; Makatussin; Neo-Liniment†; Perubare; Sedasept; Tisane pectorale et bechique Natterman instantee no 9†; ***UK:*** 9 Rubbing Oils; Catarrh Cream; Efalex; Snowfire; Snufflebabe; Zam-Buk†; ***USA:*** Unguentine.

Thymidine (13334-q)

NSC-21548; Thymine 2-Desoxyriboside. 1-(2-Deoxy-β-D-ribofuranosyl)-5-methyluracil; 1-(2-Deoxy-β-D-ribofuranosyl)-1,2,3,4-tetrahydro-5-methylpyrimidine-2,4-dione.

$C_{10}H_{14}N_2O_5$ = 242.2.

CAS — 50-89-5.

Thymidine is a nucleoside constituent of cells. It was formerly given by intravenous infusion to modulate the toxicity of methotrexate; it may also have an antineoplastic action of its own. Thymidine is not considered to be a substitute for calcium folinate.

Thymidine is given topically with other nucleosides in preparations for the treatment of corneal damage.

Preparations

Proprietary Preparations (details are given in Part 3)

Multi-ingredient: ***Aust.:*** Vitasic; ***Fr.:*** Vitacic; ***Ger.:*** Vitasic†.

Thymus Hormones (13335-p)

CAS — 69558-55-0 (thymopentin); 69521-94-4 (thymosin α_1); 60529-76-2 (thymopoietin); 63340-72-7 (thymic humoral factor).

The thymus gland controls the development of T-lymphocytes and thereby plays a central role in cell-mediated immunity and the regulation of immune responses. It secretes hormones although the multiplicity of factors isolated has led to some confusion. Several polypeptides characterised in the thymus or serum are able to induce lymphocyte differentiation *in vitro* and *in vivo*. They include: thymosin fraction 5, a crude thymus gland extract; thymosin α_1, a component of fraction 5 which has been synthesised; thymic humoral factor (THF), isolated from crude thymic extract dialysate; nonathymulin (thymulin, serum thymic factor, Facteur Thymique Serique, FTS), a synthetic nonapeptide; thymomodulin, a partially purified extract from calf thymus; thymogene A, extracted from calf thymus; thymopoietin, a polypeptide of known amino acid sequence; thymopentin (thymopoietin pentapeptide, TP-5), a fragment of thymopoietin with 5 amino acids; and thymostimulin (TP-1), extracted from calf thymus.

Various preparations, including crude extracts from calf thymus gland, thymopentin, and thymostimulin have been tried as immunomodulators in autoimmune and immunodeficiency disorders and as adjuncts in the treatment of malignant disease. Thymosin α_1 has been tried as an adjunct to interferons in chronic hepatitis B (p.595).

Thymus hormones have been tried in the treatment of numerous conditions including rheumatoid arthritis,[1-4]diabetes mellitus,[5,6] immunodeficiency disorders,[7-12] skin disorders[13-16] (for mention of their use in scleroderma, see p.501), malignant neoplasms[17-19] and some infections.[20,21] Thymosin α_1, in combination with interferon alfa is under investigation in the treatment of chronic hepatitis C;[22] thymosin may also have potential in hepatitis D.[23]

1. Amor B, *et al.* Nonathymulin in rheumatoid arthritis: two double blind, placebo controlled trials. *Ann Rheum Dis* 1987; **46:** 549–54.
2. Lemmel EM, *et al.* Immunomodulating therapy in chronic polyarthritis with thymopentin: a multicenter placebo-controlled study of 119 patients. *Dtsch Med Wochenschr* 1988; **113:** 172–6.
3. Kantharia BK, *et al.* Thymopentin (TP-5) in the treatment of rheumatoid arthritis. *Br J Rheumatol* 1989; **23:** 118–23.
4. Sundal E, Bertelletti D. Thymopentin treatment of rheumatoid arthritis. *Arzneimittelforschung* 1994; **44:** 1145–9.
5. Giordano C, *et al.* Early administration of an immunomodulator and induction of remission in insulin-dependent diabetes mellitus. *J Autoimmun* 1990; **3:** 611–17.
6. Moncada E, *et al.* Insulin requirements and residual beta-cell function 12 months after concluding immunotherapy in type I diabetic patients treated with combined azathioprine and thymostimulin administration for one year. *J Autoimmun* 1990; **3:** 625–38.
7. Terrizzi A, *et al.* Thymomodulin prevents post-operative immunodepression measured by means of skin tests. *Int J Immunother* 1988; **4:** 193–8.
8. Skotnicki AB. Thymic hormones and lymphokines. *Drugs Today* 1989; **25:** 337–62.
9. Beyer WEP, *et al.* Effect of immunomodulator thymopentin on impaired seroresponse to influenza vaccine in patients on haemodialysis. *Nephron* 1990; **54:** 296–301.
10. Beall G, *et al.* A double-blind, placebo-controlled trial of thymostimulin in symptomatic HIV-infected patients. *AIDS* 1990; **4:** 679–81.
11. Brivio F, *et al.* Effect of thymopentin administered perioperatively on the surgery-induced increase in soluble interleukin-2 receptor blood levels in colon cancer patients. *Curr Ther Res* 1991; **50:** 293–7.
12. Hassner A, Adelman DC. Biologic response modifiers in primary immunodeficiency disorders. *Ann Intern Med* 1991; **115:** 294–307.
13. David TJ. Recent developments in the treatment of childhood atopic eczema. *J R Coll Physicians Lond* 1991; **25:** 95–101.
14. Harper JI, *et al.* A double-blind placebo-controlled study of thymostimulin (TP-1) for the treatment of atopic eczema. *Br J Dermatol* 1991; **125:** 368–72.
15. Giordano N, *et al.* Efficacy and safety of thymopentin in patients suffering from progressive systemic sclerosis. *Curr Ther Res* 1991; **49:** 731–9.
16. Hsieh K-H, *et al.* Thymopentin treatment in severe atopic dermatitis—clinical and immunological evaluations. *Arch Dis Child* 1992; **67:** 1095–1102.
17. Cascinelli N, *et al.* Perinodular injection of thymopentine (TP5) in cutaneous and subcutaneous metastases of melanoma. *Melanoma Res* 1993; **3:** 471–6.
18. Pavesi L, Italian Cooperative Trials Group. Fluorouracil (F), with and without high dose folinic acid (HDFA) plus epirubicin (E) and cyclophosphamide (C): FEC versus HDFA-FEC plus or minus thymostimulin (TS) in metastatic breast cancer: results of a multicenter study. *Eur J Cancer* 1993; **29A:** S77.
19. Mustacchi G, Italian Cooperative Trials Group. High dose folinic acid (HDFA) and fluorouracil (Fu) plus or minus thymostimulin (TS) for treatment of metastatic colorectal cancer (MCRC): a randomized multicentric study. *Eur J Cancer* 1993; **29A:** S89.
20. Periti P, *et al.* Antimicrobial chemoimmunoprophylaxis in colorectal surgery with cefotetan and thymostimulin: prospective, controlled multicenter study. *J Chemother* 1993; **5:** 37–42.
21. Sundal E, Bertelletti D. Management of viral infections with thymopentin. *Arzneimittelforschung* 1994; **44:** 866–71.
22. Rasi G, *et al.* Combination thymosin α_1 and lymphoblastoid interferon treatment in chronic hepatitis C. *Gut* 1996; **39:** 679–83.
23. Zavaglia C, *et al.* A pilot study of thymosin-α1 therapy for chronic hepatitis D. *J Clin Gastroenterol* 1996; **23:** 162–3.

Preparations

Proprietary Preparations (details are given in Part 3)
Ital.: Mepentil†; Sintomodulina; Timosin; Timunox.

Tibezonium Iodide (13341-g)

Tibezonium Iodide *(rINN)*.

Rec-15/0691. Diethylmethyl{2-[4-(4-phenylthiophenyl)-3*H*-1,5-benzodiazepin-2-ylthio]ethyl}ammonium iodide.

$C_{28}H_{32}IN_3S_2$ = 601.6.

CAS — 54663-47-7.

Tibezonium iodide has been used in the treatment of infections of the mouth and throat.

Preparations

Proprietary Preparations (details are given in Part 3)
Ital.: Antoral.

Tilactase (12779-v)

Tilactase *(rINN)*.

β-D-Galactosidase; Lactase.

CAS — 9031-11-2.

Pharmacopoeias. In *US.*

A hydrolytic enzyme derived from *Aspergillus oryzae*. **Store** in airtight containers at room temperature.

Tilactase hydrolyses lactose into glucose and galactose. It has been added to milk and milk products, or taken by mouth before a meal containing dairy products, in order to prevent the symptoms of lactose intolerance (p.1349) in persons deficient in the endogenous enzyme.

α-Galactosidase has also been added to legumes and other vegetables to reduce flatulence associated with their consumption.

Preparations

Proprietary Preparations (details are given in Part 3)
Austral.: Lact-Easy; Lactaid; ***Canad.:*** Dairyaid; Lactaid; Lactrase; PMS-Prolactase†; Prolactase†; ***Irl.:*** Lactaid; ***Ital.:*** Lactaid; Lysolac†; ***Jpn:*** Galantase; ***S.Afr.:*** Galantase; ***UK:*** Lactaid; ***USA:*** Dairy Ease; Lactaid; Lactogest†; Lactrase; SureLac.

Multi-ingredient: ***Spain:*** Lactored; Polidasa.

Tilia (323-w)

Lime Flower; Linden; Tiliae Flos; Tilleul; Tilo.

Pharmacopoeias. In *Eur.* (see p.viii) and *Pol.*

The whole dried inflorescences of *Tilia cordata*, *Tilia platyphyllos*, *Tilia × vulgaris* (Tiliaceae), or a mixture of these species.

Tilia is mildly astringent and is reputed to have antispasmodic and diaphoretic properties. Lime-flower 'tea' is a traditional domestic remedy.

Various species of tilia are used in herbal and homoeopathic preparations for a variety of disorders.

Preparations

Proprietary Preparations (details are given in Part 3)
Belg.: Vibtil; ***Fr.:*** Vibtil; ***Spain:*** Tilaren Midy†.

Multi-ingredient: ***Aust.:*** Apotheker Bauer's Grippetee; Bogumil-tassenfertiger milder Abfurtee; Grippefloran; Grippetee Dr Zeidler; Grippetee EF-EM-ES; Grippogran; Kneipp Grippe-Tee; Krauterdoktor Erkaltungstropfen; Krauterhaus Mag Kottas Grippetee; Krautertee Nr 10; Krautertee Nr 210; Mag Kottas Grippe-Tee; Sidroga Erkaltungstee; Sidroga Kindertee; St Bonifatius-Tee; St Radegunder Fiebertee; Teekanne Erkaltungstee; ***Austral.:*** Crataegus Complex; ***Belg.:*** Eugiron; Tisane Antibiliaire et Stomachique; Tisane Pectorale; Tisane pour le Foie; ***Canad.:*** Herbal Sleep Well†; ***Fr.:*** Achisane Troubles du Sommeil; Apaisance; Assagix; Calmophytum; Lenicalm; Mediflor Tisane Antirhumatismale No 2; Mediflor Tisane Calmante Troubles du Sommeil No 14; Noctisan; Phytotherapie Boribel no 8; Santane N_9; Santane O_1; Tisane des Familles†; Tisanes de l'Abbe Hamon no 6; Vigilia; ***Ger.:*** Bronchialtee†; Dr. Klinger's Bergischer Krautertee, Husten- u. Bronchial-tee†; Grippe-Tee Stada†; Grunlicht Hingfong Essenz; Hevert-Blasen- und Nieren- Tee; Liruptin†; Nephrubin; Nervosana; Salus Bronchial-Tee Nr.8; Silphoscalin†; ***Ital.:*** Alkagin; Bramserene†; Fluend; Lenicalm; Sambuco (Specie Composta); Videorelax; ***Spain:*** Agua del Carmen; ***Switz.:*** Stago†; Tisane antiseptique diuretique†; Tisane contre les refroidissements; Tisane pour les enfants; Tisane pour les reins et la vessie; Tisane pour les reins et la vessie "H"†; Tisane sedative et somnifere "H"†; ***UK:*** Motherwort Compound; Tranquil; Wellwoman.

Timonacic (3749-j)

Timonacic *(rINN)*.

ATC; NSC-25855; Thioproline. Thiazolidine-4-carboxylic acid.

$C_4H_7NO_2S$ = 133.2.

CAS — 444-27-9.

NOTE. The name ATC has also been used for a combination of paracetamol and trichloroethanol (4-acetamidophenyl 2,2,2-trichloroethyl carbonate).

Timonacic is used as an adjuvant in the treatment of acute and chronic hepatic disorders.

Timonacic methyl hydrochloride (carbolidine hydrochloride) has been used as a mucolytic.

Preparations

Proprietary Preparations (details are given in Part 3)
Ital.: Ciliar; Detoxepa†; Muvial; Tiazolidin; ***Switz.:*** Heparegen.

Tin (5326-q)

Sn = 118.71.

CAS — 7440-31-5.

A silver-white, lustrous, malleable, ductile metal.

Owing to their low solubility tin and tin oxide are very poorly absorbed from the gastro-intestinal tract and are not toxic. Chronic inhalation causes a benign form of pneumoconiosis.

Organic compounds of tin are highly toxic and may cause liver and kidney damage as well as severe neurological damage associated with oedema of the white matter of the brain. Treatment has been symptomatic. Contamination of the skin with organic tin compounds can cause severe burning; suitable precautions should be taken to prevent absorption of organic tin compounds through the skin.

Tin and tin oxide have been given in the treatment of boils but there is little evidence of effectiveness; they were also formerly used in some countries for the treatment of tapeworm. Organic tin compounds, especially tributyltin oxide (TBTO) are used as molluscicides.

Excess amounts of tin in food tend to arise from tin-coated cans, especially un-lacquered ones, and may produce gastric irritation. It appears likely that infants and small children consume proportionally greater amounts of tin than adults. Consumers should be advised not to store foods in opened cans.

Concentrations as low as 150 μg per g in canned beverages and 250 μg per g in other canned foods have produced adverse effects in certain individuals but some foods containing up to 700 μg per g have not produced any detectable effects. Further studies were required to identify the chemical forms of tin that cause acute gastric irritation and any possible potentiating or moderating factors.

The previously recommended acceptable daily intake for chronic exposure to tin was re-affirmed as a provisional tolerable weekly intake of 14 mg per kg body-weight.[1]

1. FAO/WHO. Evaluation of certain food additives and contaminants: thirty-third report of the joint FAO/WHO expert committee on food additives. *WHO Tech Rep Ser 776* 1989.

Preparations

Proprietary Preparations (details are given in Part 3)

Multi-ingredient: ***Belg.:*** Stanno-Bardane; ***S.Afr.:*** Metinox†.

Tin-protoporphyrin (1896-s)

(Sn)-protoporphyrin.

Tin-protoporphyrin and the related compound tin-mesoporphyrin are metalloporphyrins which inhibit haem oxygenase, an enzyme involved in the breakdown of haem to bile pigments. They have been investigated as inhibitors of bilirubin production in hyperbilirubinaemia of various causes, and have been tried in porphyria (p.983).

References.

1. Emtestam L, *et al.* Tin-protoporphyrin and long wave length ultraviolet light in treatment of psoriasis. *Lancet* 1989; **i:** 1231–3.
2. Rubaltelli FF, *et al.* Tin-protoporphyrin in the management of children with Crigler-Najjar disease. *Pediatrics* 1989; **84:** 728–31.
3. McDonagh AF. Tin-protoporphyrin in the management of children with Crigler-Najjar disease. *Pediatrics* 1990; **86:** 151–2.
4. Berglund L, *et al.* Studies with the haeme oxygenase inhibitor Sn-protoporphyrin in patients with primary biliary cirrhosis and idiopathic haemochromatosis. *Gut* 1990; **31:** 899–904.
5. Dover SB, *et al.* Tin-protoporphyrin combined with haem arginate—an improved treatment for acute hepatic porphyria. *Gut* 1991; **32:** A597.
6. Dover SB, *et al.* Haem-arginate plus tin-protoporphyrin for acute hepatic porphyria. *Lancet* 1991; **338:** 263.
7. Kappas A, *et al.* Direct comparison of Sn-mesoporphyrin, an inhibitor of bilirubin production, and phototherapy in controlling hyperbilirubinemia in term and near-term newborns. *Pediatrics* 1995; **95:** 468–74.
8. Rubaltelli FF, *et al.* Congenital nonobstructive, nonhemolytic jaundice: effect of tin-mesoporphyrin. *Pediatrics* 1995; **95:** 942–4.
9. Valaes T, *et al.* Control of hyperbilirubinemia in glucose-6-phosphate dehyrogenase-deficient newborns using an inhibitor of bilirubin production, Sn-mesoporphyrin. *Pediatrics* 1998; **101:** 915.

Tiquizium Bromide (1276-b)

Tiquizium Bromide *(pINN)*.

HSR-902. *trans*-3-(Di-2-thienylmethylene)octahydro-5-methyl-2*H*-quinolizinium bromide.

$C_{19}H_{24}BrNS_2$ = 410.4.

CAS — 71731-58-3.

Tiquizium bromide is used as an antispasmodic in daily divided doses of 15 to 30 mg.

Preparations

Proprietary Preparations (details are given in Part 3)
Jpn: Thiaton.

Tiropramide Hydrochloride (17012-r)

Tiropramide Hydrochloride *(rINNM)*.

DL-α-Benzamido-*p*-[2-(diethylamino)ethoxy]-*N*,*N*-dipropylhydrocinnamamide hydrochloride.

$C_{28}H_{41}N_3O_3$,HCl = 504.1.

CAS — 55837-29-1 (tiropramide); 57227-16-4 (tiropramide hydrochloride).

Tiropramide hydrochloride is used as an antispasmodic. Doses of 100 mg have been given two or three times daily by mouth. It has also been given rectally and parenterally.

Preparations

Proprietary Preparations (details are given in Part 3)
Ger.: Alfospas; ***Ital.:*** Alfospas; Maiorad.

Titanium (13355-l)

Ti = 47.867.

CAS — 7440-32-6.

Titanium has been used in the repair of skull damage and for implantation in dental surgery.

References.

1. Brown D. All you wanted to know about titanium, but were afraid to ask. *Br Dent J* 1997; **182:** 393–4.

Tolonium Chloride (2152-d)

Tolonium Chloride *(rINN)*.

CI Basic Blue 17; Colour Index No. 52040; Toluidine Blue O. 3-Amino-7-dimethylamino-2-methylphenazathionium chloride; 3-Amino-7-dimethylamino-2-methylphenothiazin-5-ium chloride.

$C_{15}H_{16}ClN_3S$ = 305.8.

CAS — 92-31-9.

NOTE. Distinguish from Toluidine Blue, Colour Index No. 63340.

Tolonium chloride is a thiazine dye chemically related to methylene blue (p.984). It has been used to stain oral and gastric neoplasms and was given intravenously to stain the parathyroid glands. Other uses have included the treatment of menstrual disorders and methaemoglobinaemia.

Tolonium chloride should be avoided in patients with glucose-6-phosphate dehydrogenase deficiency as haemolysis may occur.

Preparations

Proprietary Preparations (details are given in Part 3)
Canad.: Orascan; ***Ger.:*** Toluidinblau.

Tolynol (13362-e)

1-(*p*-Tolyl)ethanol; *p*,α-Dimethylbenzyl alcohol.

$C_9H_{12}O$ = 136.2.

CAS — 536-50-5.

Tolynol has been used as a choleretic in the treatment of hepatic disorders and is an ingredient of preparations for gastro-intestinal disorders. Tolynol nicotinate has also been used.

Preparations

Proprietary Preparations (details are given in Part 3)

Multi-ingredient: ***Aust.:*** Claim; Galle-Donau; Spagall; Spasmo Claim; ***Ger.:*** Solu-Hepar N†; ***Spain:*** Genebilina†.

Tormentil (324-e)

Consolda Vermelha; Erect Cinquefoil.

Pharmacopoeias. In *Aust., Ger.,* and *Pol.*

Tormentil is the dried rhizome of the common tormentil, *Potentilla erecta* (Rosaceae). It has astringent properties and is used in herbal preparations for diarrhoea and other indications.

Preparations

Proprietary Preparations (details are given in Part 3)
Ger.: Herbatorment.

Multi-ingredient: ***Aust.:*** Bio-Garten Tee gegen Durchfall; Drovitol; Eogran; Krauterhaus Mag Kottas Tee gegen Durchfall; Tee gegen Durchfall nach Dr Bohmig†; ***Ger.:*** Cefadiarrhon†; Duoform-Balsam†; Repha-Os; ***Switz.:*** Baume†.

Transfer Factor (13365-j)

Transfer factor can passively transfer cell-mediated immunity from a sensitised donor to a non-sensitised recipient. It is a peptide constituent of dialysable leucocyte extracts prepared from the leucocytes of the donor, whose sensitivity may have been demonstrated by skin tests.

Transfer factor has been suggested for use in infections due to bacteria, fungi, and viruses, inflammatory disorders, nervous system disorders, immunodeficiency diseases, and malignancies although the response when it has been tried in some of these conditions has not always been satisfactory.

Some reviews[1-6] and references.[7-10]

1. Attallah AM, *et al.* Biological response modifiers and their promise in clinical medicine. *Pharmacol Ther* 1983; **19:** 435–54.
2. Gibson J, *et al.* Clinical use of transfer factor: 25 years on. *Clin Immunol Allergy* 1983; **3:** 331–57.
3. Fudenberg HH. "Transfer factor": an update. *Proc Soc Exp Biol Med* 1985; **178:** 327–32.
4. Tsang KY, Fudenberg HH. Transfer factor and other T cell products. *Springer Semin Immunopathol* 1986; **9:** 19–32.
5. Fudenberg HH, Fudenberg HH. Transfer factor: past, present and future. *Annu Rev Pharmacol Toxicol* 1989; **29:** 475–516.
6. Hassner A, Adelman DC. Biologic response modifiers in primary immunodeficiency disorders. *Ann Intern Med* 1991; **115:** 294–307.
7. Carey JT, *et al.* Augmentation of skin test reactivity and lymphocyte blastogenesis in patients with AIDS treated with transfer factor. *JAMA* 1987; **257:** 651–5.
8. Anonymous. Zidovudine and other drugs against HIV. *Drug Ther Bull* 1988; **26:** 101–4.
9. McBride SJ, McCluskey DR. Treatment of chronic fatigue syndrome. *Br Med Bull* 1991; **47:** 895–907.
10. AUSTIMS Research Group. Interferon-α and transfer factor in the treatment of multiple sclerosis: a double-blind, placebo-controlled trial. *J Neurol Neurosurg Psychiatry* 1989; **52:** 566–74.

Trepibutone (13369-a)

Trepibutone *(rINN)*.

AA-149; Trepionate. 3-(2,4,5-Triethoxybenzoyl)propionic acid.

$C_{16}H_{22}O_6$ = 310.3.

CAS — 41826-92-0.

Pharmacopoeias. In *Jpn.*

Trepibutone has been reported to have spasmolytic and choleretic activity.

Tribenoside (13374-z)

Tribenoside *(USAN, rINN)*.

21401-Ba; Ba-21401. Ethyl 3,5,6-tri-*O*-benzyl-D-glucofuranoside.

$C_{29}H_{34}O_6$ = 478.6.

CAS — 10310-32-4.

Tribenoside has been used in inflammatory and varicose disorders of the veins including for the treatment of haemorrhoids (p.1170). It has been given by mouth in usual doses of 800 mg daily. It has also been administered rectally and topically.

Preparations

Proprietary Preparations (details are given in Part 3)
Aust.: Glyvenol; ***Belg.:*** Glyvenol; ***Fr.:*** Glyvenol†; ***Ger.:*** Glyvenol†; ***Ital.:*** Flebosan†; Glyvenol†; Venalisin; Venex†; Venodin; ***Spain:*** Glyvenol†; ***Switz.:*** Glyvenol.

Multi-ingredient: ***Aust.:*** Procto-Glyvenol; ***Fr.:*** Glyvenol†; ***Switz.:*** Procto-Glyvenol.

Tricaprylin (13375-c)

Caprylic Acid Triglyceride; Glycerin Tricaprylate. Glyceryl trioctanoate; Propane-1,2,3-triyl trioctanoate.

$C_{27}H_{50}O_6$ = 470.7.

CAS — 538-23-8.

Tricaprylin has the general properties of the medium-chain triglycerides (p.1599) and has been similarly used.

Preparations

Proprietary Preparations (details are given in Part 3)

Multi-ingredient: ***USA:*** Lubrin.

Tricarbaurinium (13376-k)

Aluminon; Triammonium Aurintricarboxylate. The triammonium salt of 3-(3,3′-dicarboxy-4,4′-dihydroxybenzhydrylidene)-6-oxocyclohexa-1,4-diene-1-carboxylic acid.

$C_{22}H_{23}N_3O_9$ = 473.4.

CAS — 569-58-4.

Tricarbaurinium has been used topically in the treatment of oropharyngeal disorders.

Preparations

Proprietary Preparations (details are given in Part 3)
Fr.: Lysofon.

Multi-ingredient: ***Fr.:*** Lysofon.

Trichloroacetic Acid (1328-d)

Acidum Trichloraceticum; Trichloracetic Acid; Trichloressigsäure.

$CCl_3.CO_2H$ = 163.4.

CAS — 76-03-9.

Pharmacopoeias. In *Aust., Belg., Fr., Pol.,* and *Port.*

Adverse Effects and Treatment

As for Hydrochloric Acid, p.1588.

Uses and Administration

Trichloroacetic acid is caustic and astringent. It is used as a quick escharotic for warts. It is applied as a strong solution, prepared by adding 10% by weight of water [e.g. trichloroacetic acid 10 g plus water 1 g]; the surrounding parts are usually protected. It has also been used for the removal of tattoos.

Tattoo removal. References to the use of trichloroacetic acid in the removal of tattoos.

1. Hall-Smith P, Bennett J. Tattoos: a lasting regret. *Br Med J* 1991; **303:** 397.

Warts. References to the use of trichloroacetic acid in the treatment of genital warts (p.1076).

1. Godley MJ, *et al.* Cryotherapy compared with trichloroacetic acid in treating genital warts. *Genitourin Med* 1987; **63:** 390–2.
2. Davis AJ, Emans SJ. Human papilloma virus infection in the pediatric and adolescent patient. *J Pediatr* 1989; **115:** 1–9.
3. Boothby RA, *et al.* Single application treatment of human papillomavirus infection of the cervix and vagina with trichloroacetic acid: a randomized trial. *Obstet Gynecol* 1990; **76:** 278–80.

Preparations

Proprietary Preparations (details are given in Part 3)
Ital.: Averuk Bruciaporri; CL 3 Bruciaporri; Porriver; Verrupor; ***USA:*** Tri-Chlor.

Multi-ingredient: ***Fr.:*** ATS†; ***Spain:*** Callicida Brum.

Triethanolamine (218-s)

Trolamine *(pINN).*

CAS — 102-71-6.

Pharmacopoeias. In *Aust., Br., Fr., It., Neth.,* and *Swiss.* Also in *USNF.*

A variable mixture of bases containing mainly 2,2′,2″-nitrilotriethanol, (triethanolamine), $(CH_2OH.CH_2)_3N$, together with 2,2′-iminobisethanol (diethanolamine) and smaller amounts of 2-aminoethanol (monoethanolamine).

It is a clear, colourless or pale yellow, viscous, hygroscopic liquid; odourless or with a slight ammoniacal odour.

Miscible with water and alcohol; soluble in chloroform; slightly soluble in ether. A 10% solution in water is strongly alkaline to litmus. **Store** in airtight containers. Protect from light.

Adverse Effects

It may be irritating to the skin and mucous membranes. Contact dermatitis has been reported following the use of ear drops containing triethanolamine polypeptide oleate-condensate.

Following concern of the possible production of carcinogenic nitrosamines in the stomach, the Swiss authorities restricted the use of triethanolamine to preparations for external use.[1]

1. Anonymous. Trolamine: concerns regarding potential carcinogenicity. *WHO Drug Inf* 1991; **5:** 9.

Uses and Administration

Triethanolamine is used combined with fatty acids such as stearic and oleic acids as an emulsifier and as an alkalinising agent. It has also been used to reduce dithranol-induced staining of the skin.

Ear drops containing triethanolamine polypeptide oleate-condensate 10% are used for the removal of impacted ear wax.

Topical analgesic preparations of triethanolamine combined with salicylic acid have also been used.

Preparations

Proprietary Preparations (details are given in Part 3)
Austral.: Dencorub Arthritis; Metsal AR Analgesic; ***Belg.:*** Xerumenex; ***Canad.:*** Antiphlogistine Rub A-535 No Odour; Aspercreme; Ben-Gay No Odor; Cerumenex; Miosal; Myoflex; Royflex; Sportscreme†; ***Ger.:*** Cerumenex N; ***Ital.:*** Cerumenex; ***Neth.:*** Xerumenex; ***S.Afr.:*** Cerumenex; ***Spain:*** Bexidermil; Topicrem; ***Switz.:*** Cerumenex; ***USA:*** Analgesia Creme; Aspercreme; Cerumenex; Coppertone Tan Magnifier; Curastain; Exocaine Odor Free†; Mobisyl; Myoflex; Pro-gesic; Sportscreme; Tropical Blend Tan Magnifier.

Multi-ingredient: ***Austral.:*** Metsal Analgesic; ***Canad.:*** Ease Pain Away; Myoflex Ice Plus; Soropon; ***Fr.:*** Abi†; Coricide Rodell†; ***Ital.:*** Dopo Pik; ***USA:*** Maxilube.

Triethyl Citrate (18351-h)

2-Hydroxy-1,2,3-propanetricarboxylic acid triethyl ester.

$C_{12}H_{20}O_7$ = 276.3.

CAS — 77-93-0.

Pharmacopoeias. In *USNF.*

An odourless practically colourless oily liquid. Slightly **soluble** in water; miscible with alcohol and with ether. **Store** in airtight containers.

Triethyl citrate is a plasticiser used in pharmaceutical manufacturing, and in the food and cosmetics industries.

Trilostane (13380-y)

Trilostane *(BAN, USAN, pINN).*

Win-24540. 4α,5α-Epoxy-17β-hydroxy-3-oxoandrostane-2α-carbonitrile.

$C_{20}H_{27}NO_3$ = 329.4.

CAS — 13647-35-3.

Adverse Effects

Side-effects associated with trilostane have included flushing, nausea, vomiting, diarrhoea, rhinorrhoea, and oedema of the palate. Skin rashes may occur and, rarely, granulocytopenia in immunocompromised patients.

Precautions

Trilostane is contra-indicated in pregnancy and should be used with caution in patients with renal or hepatic dysfunction. Circulating corticosteroids and blood electrolytes should be monitored. During severe stress, the drug may have to be discontinued and corticosteroid supplements may be required.

Interactions

Trilostane may interfere with the activity of oral contraceptives. Hyperkalaemia may occur if trilostane is given concurrently with potassium-sparing diuretics.

Uses and Administration

Trilostane is an adrenocortical suppressant which inhibits the enzyme system essential for the production of glucocorticoids and mineralocorticoids. It has been used in the treatment of Cushing's syndrome (p.1236) and primary aldosteronism.

The usual dose is 240 mg by mouth in divided doses for at least 3 days and then adjusted, according to the patient's response, within the range of 120 to 480 mg daily. Doses of 960 mg daily have been given.

Trilostane has also been used for hormonal adjuvant treatment in postmenopausal women with breast cancer.

Preparations

Proprietary Preparations (details are given in Part 3)
Jpn: Desopan†; ***UK:*** Modrenal; ***USA:*** Modrastane†.

Trimebutine Maleate (13381-j)

Trimebutine Maleate *(BANM, rINNM).*

2-Dimethylamino-2-phenylbutyl 3,4,5-trimethoxybenzoate hydrogen maleate.

$C_{22}H_{29}NO_5,C_4H_4O_4$ = 503.5.

CAS — 39133-31-8 (trimebutine); 34140-59-5 (trimebutine maleate).

Trimebutine maleate has been used as an antispasmodic in doses of up to 600 mg daily by mouth. It has also been given by injection and rectally. Trimebutine base has also been used.

Irritable bowel syndrome. Trimebutine has been reported to be effective in the treatment of irritable bowel syndrome (p.1172)[1,2] although Ghidini *et al.*[1] observed a considerable placebo response. Schaffstein *et al.*[2] considered that the effectiveness of trimebutine might be related to its action on opioid receptors in the gastro-intestinal tract.

1. Ghidini O, *et al.* Single drug treatment for irritable colon: rociverine versus trimebutine maleate. *Curr Ther Res* 1986; **39:** 541–8.
2. Schaffstein W, *et al.* Comparative safety and efficacy of trimebutine versus mebeverine in the treatment of irritable bowel syndrome. *Curr Ther Res* 1990; **47:** 136–45.

Preparations

Proprietary Preparations (details are given in Part 3)
Aust.: Debridat; ***Canad.:*** Modulon; ***Fr.:*** Debridat; Modulon; Transacalm; ***Ital.:*** Debridat; Digerent; Kalius; Modulase†; Spabucol†; Trimedat; ***Jpn:*** Cerekinon; ***Spain:*** Polibutin; ***Switz.:*** Debridat.

Multi-ingredient: ***Fr.:*** Modulite; Proctolog; ***Ital.:*** Debridat Enzimatico†; Debrum; ***Spain:*** Proctolog.

Trinitrophenol (2288-c)

Carbazotic Acid; Picric Acid; Picrinic Acid. 2,4,6-Trinitrophenol.

$C_6H_3N_3O_7$ = 229.1.

CAS — 88-89-1.

Pharmacopoeias. In *Fr.*

Trinitrophenol should be **stored** in a cool place, mixed with an equal weight of water. It must not be stored in glass-stoppered bottles.

CAUTION. Trinitrophenol burns readily and explodes when heated rapidly or when subjected to percussion. For safety in handling it is usually supplied mixed with not less than half its weight of water. It combines with metals to form salts, some of which are very explosive.

Trinitrophenol has disinfectant properties and was formerly used in the treatment of burns. It is now chiefly used in manufacturing and as a laboratory reagent.

Dermatitis, skin eruptions, and severe itching may occur following contact with trinitrophenol. Systemic toxicity may follow ingestion or absorption through the skin or lungs; symptoms may include vomiting, pain, and diarrhoea, progressing to haemolysis, hepatitis, anuria, convulsions, unconsciousness, and death. The metabolic rate is increased, causing pyrexia.

It has been used in homoeopathy.

Preparations

Proprietary Preparations (details are given in Part 3)

Multi-ingredient: ***Spain:*** Oftalmol Dexa; Oftalmol Ocular; Queratil.

Trometamol (2360-p)

Trometamol *(BAN, rINN).*

NSC-6365; THAM; Trihydroxymethylaminomethane; TRIS; Tris(hydroxymethyl)aminomethane; Trometamolum; Tromethamine *(USAN).* 2-Amino-2-(hydroxymethyl)propane-1,3-diol.

$C_4H_{11}NO_3$ = 121.1.

CAS — 77-86-1.

Pharmacopoeias. In *Eur.* (see p.viii) and *US.*

A white crystalline powder or colourless crystals with a slight characteristic odour.

Soluble 1 in 1.8 of water and 1 in about 45 of alcohol; freely soluble in low-molecular-weight aliphatic alcohols; very slightly soluble in ethyl acetate; practically insoluble in carbon tetrachloride and in chloroform. A 5% solution in water has a pH of 10.0 to 11.5. **Store** in airtight containers.

Adverse Effects and Precautions

Great care must be taken to avoid extravasation at the injection site as solutions may cause tissue damage. Local irritation may follow administration and venospasm and phlebitis have occurred.

Respiratory depression and hypoglycaemia may occur and the respiration may require assistance. Trometamol is contra-indicated in anuria and uraemia and should be administered cautiously in patients with impaired renal function. Hyperkalaemia has been reported in patients with renal impairment. Trometamol is contra-indicated in chronic respiratory acidosis.

Blood concentrations of bicarbonate, glucose, and electrolytes, partial pressure of carbon dioxide, and blood pH should be monitored during infusion of trometamol.

Uses and Administration

Trometamol is an organic amine proton acceptor which is used as an alkalinising agent in the treatment of metabolic acidosis (p.1147). It should not be used in patients with chronic respiratory acidosis. It also acts as a weak osmotic diuretic. Trometamol is mainly used during cardiac bypass surgery and during cardiac arrest. It may also be used to reduce the acidity of citrated blood for use in bypass surgery.

The dose used should be the minimum required to increase the pH of the blood to within normal limits and is based on the body weight and the base deficit. Trometamol is administered by slow intravenous infusion as a 0.3M solution over a period of not less than 1 hour.

Trometamol citrate is given by mouth for the management of urinary calculi and acidosis.

Trometamol acephyllinate and trometamol thioctate have also been used.

References.

1. Nahas GG, *et al.* Guidelines for the treatment of acidaemia with THAM. *Drugs* 1998; **55:** 191–224.

Preparations

USP 23: Tromethamine for Injection.

Proprietary Preparations (details are given in Part 3)
Aust.: Tris; ***Austral.:*** Tham; ***Fr.:*** Thamacetat; ***Ger.:*** Pleomix-Alpha; Thioctacid; Tris; Tromlipon; ***Ital.:*** Thamesol.

Multi-ingredient: ***Fr.:*** Alcaphor; ***Ger.:*** Complete; ***Ital.:*** Ulcotris†; ***Norw.:*** Tribonat; ***Spain:*** Sugarceton; ***Swed.:*** Tribonat; ***Switz.:*** Saltrates.

Trospium Chloride (5246-q)

Trospium Chloride *(rINN)*.

3α-Benziloyloxynortropane-8-spiro-1′-pyrrolidinium chloride.

$C_{25}H_{30}ClNO_3$ = 428.0.

CAS — 10405-02-4.

Trospium chloride has been used as an antispasmodic in doses of up to 15 mg three times daily by mouth. It has also been given by intramuscular or slow intravenous injection, and rectally.

References.

1. Pfeiffer A, *et al.* Effect of trospium chloride on gastrointestinal motility in humans. *Eur J Clin Pharmacol* 1993; **44:** 219–23.
2. Pietzko A, *et al.* Influences of trospium chloride and oxybutynin on quantitative EEG in healthy volunteers. *Eur J Clin Pharmacol* 1994; **47:** 337–43.

Preparations

Proprietary Preparations (details are given in Part 3)
Aust.: Rekont; Spasmolyt; ***Ger.:*** Spasmex; Spasmo-lyt; Spasmo-Rhoival; Spasmo-Urgenin TC; Trospi; ***Spain:*** Spasmosarto; Uraplex; ***Switz.:*** Spasmo-Urgenine Neo.

Multi-ingredient: ***Aust.:*** Spasmo-Urgenin; ***Ger.:*** Optipyrin S†; ***S.Afr.:*** Spasmo-Urgenin; ***Spain:*** Spasmo-Urgenin; Spasmo-Urgenin Rectal†.

Trypsin (3751-p)

Trypsin *(BAN)*.

CAS — 9002-07-7.

Pharmacopoeias. In *Chin., Eur.* (see p.viii), and *US.*

A proteolytic enzyme (protease) obtained by the activation of trypsinogen extracted from mammalian pancreas. Trypsin is assayed for potency on the basis of its proteolytic activity and the potency of commercial products has been expressed in various units based on different methods of assay. Trypsin (Ph. Eur.) contains not less than 0.5 microkatals in each mg, calculated on the dried basis. The USP 23 specifies bovine pancreas and not less than 2500 USP units in each mg.

A white to yellowish-white, odourless, crystalline or amorphous powder; the amorphous form is hygroscopic. Sparingly **soluble** in water. A 1% solution has a pH of 3.0 to 6.0. Solutions have a maximum stability at pH 3 and a maximum activity at pH 8. **Store** at 2° to 8° in airtight containers. Protect from light.

Trypsin is a proteolytic enzyme that has been applied for the debridement of wounds. It has also been taken by mouth, usually in combination with chymotrypsin (p.1563), and sometimes with antibacterial or other agents, for its supposed benefit in relieving oedema and inflammation associated with infection or trauma. Trypsin solutions have been inhaled for the liquefaction of viscous sputum, and trypsin is also an ingredient of mixtures intended to relieve various gastro-intestinal disorders.

Hypersensitivity reactions may occasionally occur.

Preparations

USP 23: Crystallized Trypsin for Inhalation Aerosol.

Proprietary Preparations (details are given in Part 3)

Multi-ingredient: ***Aust.:*** Leukase; Leukase-Kegel; Wobenzym; ***Canad.:*** Festal†; ***Fr.:*** Alphintern; Ribatran; ***Ger.:*** Alphintern†; dichronase†; Enzym-Hepaduran†; Enzym-Wied; Enzymed†; Hevert Enzym Novo; Leukase†; Mulsal N; Phlogenzym; Wobe-Mugos E; Wobe-Mugos Th; Wobenzym N; ***Irl.:*** Chymoral†; ***Ital.:*** Chimotetra†; Chymoral†; Chymoser Balsamico†; Chymoser†; Essen Enzimatico; Essen†; Flogozym†; Kilozim†; Quanto†; Ribociclina; Trimalcina†; ***Jpn:*** Kimotab†; ***S.Afr.:*** Episeal†; ***Spain:*** Bristaciclina Dental; Cavum Pediatrico†; Chymar†; Chymocyclar†; Dertrase; Dosil Enzimatico; Doxiten Enzimatico; Duo Gobens; Epixian; Forunculone†; Hemotripsin†; Kanapomada; Naso Pekamin; Otocusi Enzimatico†; Oxidermiol Enzima; Quimodril; Solupen Enzimatico; ***USA:*** Dermuspray; Granulderm; Granulex; GranuMed.

Tuberculins (8024-k)

Pharmacopoeias. In *Eur.* (see p.viii) and *US.*

Old Tuberculin is a sterile heat-concentrated filtrate from the soluble products of growth and lysis of one or more strains of *Mycobacterium tuberculosis* and/or *M. bovis*. It contains a suitable preservative that does not give rise to false-positive reactions. It may be issued in concentrated or diluted form.

Tuberculin Purified Protein Derivative is a sterile preparation obtained by precipitation from the heat-treated products of growth and lysis of *Mycobacterium tuberculosis* and/or *M. bovis*. It may contain a suitable preservative that does not give rise to a false-positive reaction and a suitable stabiliser. It may be issued in concentrated or diluted form as a liquid and the diluted form may be freeze-dried.

Adverse Effects

Pain and pruritus may occur at the injection site, occasionally with vesiculation, ulceration, or necrosis in highly sensitive persons. If given to patients with tuberculosis a severe reaction may occur. Granuloma has been reported.

Hypersensitivity reactions, including anaphylaxis, to tuberculins have been reported rarely.

Hypersensitivity. There are rare reports,[1-3] occasionally fatal,[1] of severe anaphylactic or anaphylactoid reactions to tuberculin.

1. DiMaio VJM, Froede RC. Allergic reactions to the tine test. *JAMA* 1975; **233:** 769.
2. Spiteri MA, *et al.* Life threatening reaction to tuberculin testing. *Br Med J* 1986; **293:** 243–4.
3. Wright DN, *et al.* Systemic and local allergic reactions to the tine test purified protein derivative. *JAMA* 1989; **262:** 2999–3000.

Lymphangitis. Morrison reported lymphangitis on 5 occasions after the Mantoux test and on 7 occasions after the Heaf test.[1] However, Festenstein commented that performance of a tuberculin test may have been inappropriate in some of these patients, particularly older subjects and those with evidence of healed tuberculous lesions.[2]

1. Morrison JB. Lymphangitis after tuberculin tests. *Br Med J* 1984; **289:** 413.
2. Festenstein F. Lymphangitis after tuberculin tests. *Br Med J* 1984; **289:** 625–6.

Precautions

Sensitivity to tuberculin may be diminished in the following conditions: viral or severe bacterial infection including HIV infection and severe tuberculosis; neoplastic disease particularly lymphoma; sarcoidosis; corticosteroid or immunosuppressive therapy; recent administration of live virus vaccines; ultraviolet light treatment; chronic renal failure; and malnutrition.

Tuberculins may be adsorbed onto the surface of syringes and should therefore be administered immediately.

Uses and Administration

Tuberculins are used to test for hypersensitivity to tuberculoprotein. A person showing a specific sensitivity to tuberculin is considered to have been infected with the tubercle bacillus, though the infection may be inactive. Administration of tuberculin for sensitivity testing is by intradermal injection (as in the Mantoux test) or by multiple-puncture devices (such as the Heaf test or tine tests). The term tine test is generally used for disposable multiple-puncture devices coated with dried old tuberculin or purified protein derivative. However, some authorities consider tine tests to be unreliable and they are not recommended for use in the UK.

In the UK it is recommended that tuberculin testing should always be performed, except in neonates, when BCG vaccination is being considered; either the Mantoux test or the Heaf test is recommended.

For a routine **Mantoux** test, 0.1 mL (10 units) of a diluted solution of tuberculin purified protein derivative (PPD), containing 100 units per mL, is injected intradermally. A positive and a strongly positive result are considered to consist of induration of at least 5 mm and 15 mm respectively in diameter; the results should be read after 48 to 72 hours but may, if necessary, be read for up to 96 hours after the test. If a patient is suspected of having tuberculosis or is known to be hypersensitive to tuberculin, 0.1 mL (1 unit) of a solution of tuberculin PPD containing 10 units per mL should be used. A solution containing 1000 units per mL is also available; it may be used if there is doubt about interpretation when the 100 units per mL solution is used.

For the **Heaf** test a solution of tuberculin purified protein derivative containing 100 000 units per mL is used. The solution is applied to the forearm and a multiple-puncture gun (Heaf gun) is used; a puncture of 1 mm depth is recommended for children under 2 years of age and a puncture of 2 mm for older children and adults. Results may be read 3 to 10 days after the test and a positive result is considered to consist of a palpable induration around at least four puncture points. Positive results are also graded as follows: grade 1, at least 4 small indurated papules; grade 2, an indurated ring formed by confluent papules; grade 3, solid induration 5 to 10 mm wide; and grade 4, induration over 10 mm wide. Grade 3 and 4 reactions are regarded as strongly positive equivalent to an induration of 15 mm or more in the Mantoux test. In individuals with grade 1 reactions who have not previously received BCG vaccines, the reaction is not usually related to infection with *Mycobacterium tuberculosis* and these patients may be offered BCG vaccination. Patients with a grade 2 reaction or more (or an induration of 5 to 14 mm in the Mantoux test) are considered to be hypersensitive to tuberculoprotein and should not be vaccinated. Investigation for the presence of active tuberculosis is generally only indicated for patients showing a strongly positive reaction to a Mantoux or Heaf test. However, there are many factors that should be considered when interpreting the results of a tuberculin skin test. In addition to those listed under Precautions (see above), are the effects of previous BCG vaccination, repeated tuberculin testing, and age. In some areas, a positive reaction may be a result of cross-sensitivity of the test to non-tuberculous mycobacteria.

In some other countries the population tested, the procedures used, and grading of reactions may differ slightly from that outlined above.

Tuberculins are also used, in conjunction with other antigens, to assess the status of cell-mediated immunity.

Anergy testing. Patients with HIV infection are at an increased risk of developing tuberculosis but often show a diminished reactivity to antigens (anergy), making the interpretation of negative tuberculin skin tests difficult.[1-3] Anergy testing has therefore been recommended in patients with HIV infection when tuberculin testing is used in the diagnosis of tuberculosis.[1,2] In general, two additional skin test antigens are used in conjunction with tuberculin purified protein derivative; these may be chosen from *Candida*, mumps, or tetanus antigens, although various other antigens, including coccidioidin, histoplasmin, and trichophyton, have also been used. The test antigens are given, usually by intradermal injection, concurrently with the tuberculin test and the response measured 48 to 72 hours later. Any amount of induration, but not erythema alone, is considered evidence of delayed-type hypersensitivity; failure to elicit a response is considered evidence of anergy.

1. Centers for Disease Control: Division of Tuberculosis Elimination. Purified protein derivative (PPD)-tuberculin anergy and HIV infection: guidelines for anergy testing and management of anergic persons at risk of tuberculosis. *MMWR* 1991; **40:** 27–33.
2. Graham NMH, *et al.* Prevalence of tuberculin positivity and skin test anergy in HIV-1-seropositive and -seronegative intravenous drug users. *JAMA* 1992; **267:** 369–73.
3. Markowitz N, *et al.* Tuberculin and anergy testing in HIV-seropositive and HIV-seronegative persons. *Ann Intern Med* 1993; **119:** 185–93.

Preparations

Ph. Eur.: Old Tuberculin for Human Use; Tuberculin Purified Protein Derivative for Human Use;
USP 23: Tuberculin.

Proprietary Preparations (details are given in Part 3)
Aust.: Monotest; ***Belg.:*** Monovacc-Test; ***Fr.:*** Monotest; Neotest; ***Ger.:*** Tubergen-Test; ***Ital.:*** Monotest; Sclavo-Test P.P.D.†; ***S.Afr.:*** Japan Freeze-Dried Tuberculin; Monotest; PPD Tine Test; ***Spain:*** Tubersol PPD; ***Swed.:*** Monotest; Rhoditest-Tuberkulin†; ***Switz.:*** Monotest†; Neotest normal†; Tubergen-Test†; ***USA:*** Aplisol; Aplitest; Mono-Vacc Test (O.T.); Tine Test PPD; Tubersol.

Multi-ingredient: ***Aust.:*** Immignost; Multitest; ***Austral.:*** Multitest CMI; ***Belg.:*** Multitest; ***Canad.:*** Multitest CMI; ***Fr.:*** Multitest IMC; ***Ger.:*** Immignost; Multitest; ***Ital.:*** Multitest IMC; ***Neth.:*** Multitest CMI; ***S.Afr.:*** Multitest CMI; ***Spain:*** Multitest IMC; ***Switz.:*** Multitest IMC†; ***USA:*** Multitest CMI.

Tucaresol (11118-g)

Tucaresol *(BAN, rINN)*.

BW-589C; 589C; 589C80. α-(2-Formyl-3-hydroxyphenoxy)-*p*-toluic acid.

$C_{15}H_{12}O_5$ = 272.3.

CAS — 84290-27-7.

Tucaresol is reported to interact with haemoglobin to increase oxygen affinity. It has been investigated as an oral drug for the treatment of sickle-cell disease (p.703). Tucaresol is also reported to have immunostimulant properties and is under investigation in HIV infection and hepatitis B. Hypersensitivity reactions have occurred.

References.

1. Rolan PE, *et al.* The pharmacokinetics, tolerability and pharmacodynamics of tucaresol (589C80; 4[2-formyl-3-hydroxyphenoxymethyl]benzoic acid), a potential anti-sickling agent, following oral administration to healthy subjects. *Br J Clin Pharmacol* 1993; **35:** 419–25.
2. Rolan PE, *et al.* Pharmacokinetics and pharmacodynamics of tucaresol, an antisickling agent, in healthy volunteers. *Br J Clin Pharmacol* 1995; **39:** 375–80.
3. Peck RW, *et al.* Effect of food and gender on the pharmacokinetics of tucaresol in healthy volunteers. *Br J Clin Pharmacol* 1998; **46:** 83–6.

Tuftsin (1329-n)

N^2-[1-(N^2-L-threonyl-L-lysyl)-L-prolyl]-L-arginine.

$C_{21}H_{40}N_8O_6$ = 500.6.

CAS — 9063-57-4.

Tuftsin is a naturally occurring tetrapeptide and has been investigated as the acetate for its immunostimulating activity.

Tumour Necrosis Factor Antibodies

(14434-t)

Tumour necrosis factor (p.568) plays an important role in inflammation and consequently antibodies against tumour necrosis factor are under investigation in a variety of autoimmune and inflammatory disorders, including septic shock, rheumatoid arthritis, and Crohn's disease. Tumour necrosis factor antibodies under investigation include afelimomab (MAK-195F), CDP-571 (Bay-10-3356), infliximab (p.1194), and nerelimomab (Bay-X-1351). Soluble tumour necrosis factor receptor (etanercept), and tumour necrosis factor-binding proteins are also under investigation. The name lenercept is *BAN* and *pINN* for a recombinant tumour necrosis factor receptor.

References.

1. Derkx B, *et al.* Tumour-necrosis-factor antibody treatment in Crohn's disease. *Lancet* 1993; **342:** 173–4.
2. Elliott MJ, *et al.* Randomised double-blind comparison of chimeric monoclonal antibody to tumour necrosis factor α (cA2) versus placebo in rheumatoid arthritis. *Lancet* 1994; **344:** 1105–10.
3. Elliott MJ, *et al.* Repeated therapy with monoclonal antibody to tumour necrosis factor α (cA2) in patients with rheumatoid arthritis. *Lancet* 1994; **344:** 1125–7.
4. Abraham E, *et al.* Efficacy and safety of monoclonal antibody to human tumor necrosis factor alpha in patients with sepsis syndrome: a randomized, controlled, double-blind, multicenter clinical trial. *JAMA* 1995; **273:** 934–41.
5. Fisher CJ, *et al.* Treatment of septic shock with the tumor necrosis factor receptor:Fc fusion protein. *N Engl J Med* 1996; **334:** 1697–1702.
6. Fekade D, *et al.* Prevention of Jarisch-Herxheimer reactions by treatment with antibodies against tumor necrosis factor α. *N Engl J Med* 1996; **335:** 311–15.
7. Moreland LW, *et al.* Treatment of rheumatoid arthritis with a recombinant human tumor necrosis factor receptor (p75)-Fc fusion protein. *N Engl J Med* 1997; **337:** 141–7.
8. Targan SR, *et al.* A short-term study of chimeric monoclonal antibody cA2 to tumor necrosis factor α for Crohn's disease. *N Engl J Med* 1997; **337:** 1029–35.
9. Stack WA, *et al.* Randomised controlled trial of CDP571 antibody to tumour necrosis factor-α in Crohn's disease. *Lancet* 1997; **349:** 521–4.
10. Abraham E, *et al.* Double-blind randomised controlled trial of monoclonal antibody to human tumour necrosis factor in treatment of septic shock. *Lancet* 1998; **351:** 929–33.
11. Camussi G, Lupia E. The future role of anti-tumour necrosis factor (TNF) products in the treatment of rheumatoid arthritis. *Drugs* 1998; **55:** 613–20.
12. van Hogezand RA, Verspaget HW. The future role of anti-tumour necrosis factor-α products in the treatment of Crohn's disease. *Drugs* 1998; **56:** 299–305.

Turpentine Oil (4720-s)

Aetheroleum Terebinthinae; Esencia de Trementina; Essence de Térébenthine; Oleum Terebinthinae; Oleum Terebinthinae Depuratum; Rectified Turpentine Oil; Spirits of Turpentine.

Pharmacopoeias. In *Aust., Br., Chin., Fr., Jpn,* and *Swiss.*

The volatile oil obtained by distillation and rectification from turpentine, an oleoresin obtained from various species of *Pinus* (Pinaceae).

It is a clear bright colourless liquid with a characteristic odour. **Soluble** 1 in 7 of alcohol (90%) and 1 in 3 of alcohol (96%). **Store** at a temperature not exceeding 25° in airtight containers. Protect from light.

Adverse Effects

In poisoning with turpentine oil there may be local burning and gastro-intestinal upset, coughing and choking, pulmonary oedema, excitement, coma, fever, tachycardia, liver damage, haematuria, and albuminuria. Fatalities have occurred.

The application to the skin of liniments containing turpentine oil may cause irritation and absorption of large amounts may cause some of the effects listed above. Hypersensitivity reactions and local irritation have been reported.

Uses and Administration

Turpentine oil is widely used as a solvent. It is applied topically as a rubefacient. It is an ingredient of many preparations used in respiratory-tract disorders, but is now judged to be neither safe nor effective.

Myiasis in 14 patients caused by maggots in the ear was treated by turpentine oil, given as ear drops, and douching.[1] The parasite was removed in 6 patients; pain and severe inflammation occurred in 3 patients. Ether ear drops were effective in the remaining 8 patients and caused no pain.

1. Sharan R, Isser DK. Aural myiasis. *J Laryngol Otol* 1978; **92:** 705–8.

Preparations

BP 1998: White Liniment *(White Embrocation).*

Proprietary Preparations (details are given in Part 3)
Fr.: Ozothine; ***Ger.:*** Terpestrol H.

Multi-ingredient: ***Aust.:*** Aciforin; Baby Luuf; Bronchostop; Carl Baders Divinal; Dolex; Dracodermalin; Emser Nasensalbe; Ilon Abszess; Kinder Luuf; Leukona-Rheuma-Bad; Luuf Balsam; Makatussin; Mayfit chronisch; Pe-Ce; Piniment; Pinimenthol†; Piniol†; Rubriment; Salhumin; Scottopect; Tetesept; Traumasalbe; Tussamag; Vulpuran; Wick Vaporub; ***Austral.:*** Capsolin†; Cerumol; Logicin Chest Rub; Sigma Relief Chest Rub†; Turpentine White Liniment; Vicks Vaporub; ***Belg.:*** Reflexspray; Vicks Vaporub; ***Canad.:*** Cal Mo Dol; Capsolin†; Cerumol; ***Fr.:*** Dinacode; Huile de Haarlem; Lao-Dal; Lumbalgine; Ozothine; Ozothine a la Diprophylline; Sedartryl; Tuberol†; Vicks Vaporub; ***Ger.:*** Angocin percutan; Bartelin N; Cobed†; Cuxaflex N; Divinal-Broncho-Balsam; Dracodermalin†; Emser Balsam echt†; Emser Nasensalbe N; Erkaltungsbalsam-ratiopharm E; Extropin†; Fibraflex†; Hevertopect; Hoemarin Rheuma; Ilon Abszess; Influsanbalm†; Infrotto†; Iosimitan†; Kneipp Erkaltungs-Balsam N; Kneipp Tonikum-Bad Fichtennadel-Aquasan; Leukona-Rheuma-Bad N; Leukona-Rheumasalbe; Logomed Erkaltungs-Balsam; Optipect†; Ozothin; Phardol N Balsam†; Plantmobil; Pro-Pecton Balsam†; Pumilen-Balsam†; Rheumaliment N; Rhinotussal S Balsam†; Schupps Latschenkiefer Olbad; Terbintil†; Terpestrol-Inhalant†; Tetra-Ozothin†; Trauma-Salbe Rodler 302 N; Wick Vaporub; ***Irl.:*** Cerumol; Vicks Vaporub; ***Ital.:*** Capsolin; Neo Eubalsamina†; Vicks Vaporub; ***S.Afr.:*** Chisi; Respisniffers; Warm-Up; ***Spain:*** Bartal†; Embrocacion Gras; Killpan; Lapiz Termo Compositum†; Linimento Klari; Linimento Sloan; Masagil; Mostazola†; Otocerum; Ozopulmin Antiasmatico†; Pinimenthol†; Pomada Revulsiva; Porosan†; Reflex; Termosan; ***Swed.:*** Sloan's liniment†; Vicks Vaporub; ***Switz.:*** Alginex†; Artragel; Baume du Chalet; Caprisana; Capsolin; Carmol "blanche"†; Carmol†; Cerumenol; Embropax; Kernosan Huile de Massage; Liberol; Makatussin; Massorax; Olbas; Pinimenthol; Roliwol; Schwefelbad Dr Klopfer; Sloan Baume; Sloan Liniment; Tumarol; Vicks Vaporub; ***UK:*** 9 Rubbing Oils; Baby Chest Rub†; BN; Boots Vapour Rub; Deep Heat Rub; Dragon Balm; Ellimans; Flurex Inhalant†; Goddards White Oil Embrocation; Gonne Balm; Secaderm†; Tixylix Inhalant; Vicks Vaporub; Wax Aid†; Waxwane.

Tyramine Hydrochloride (2153-n)

p-Tyramine Hydrochloride; Tyrosamine Hydrochloride. 4-Hydroxyphenethylamine hydrochloride; 4-(2-Aminoethyl)phenol hydrochloride.

$C_8H_{11}NO,HCl$ = 173.6.

CAS — 51-67-2 (tyramine); 60-19-5 (tyramine hydrochloride).

Tyramine hydrochloride is a sympathomimetic with indirect effects on adrenergic receptors. It has been given by mouth or injection in the tyramine pressor test in the investigation of monoamine oxidase inhibitory activity or of amine uptake blocking activity as well as of various physiological and diseased states.

It has also been tried in the diagnosis of migraine and phaeochromocytoma.

The hazards of taking foods rich in tyramine while under treatment with MAOIs are described in the chapter on Antidepressants (see Phenelzine Sulphate, p.304).

Preparations

Proprietary Preparations (details are given in Part 3)
Multi-ingredient: ***Ger.:*** Mydrial-Atropin†.

Ubidecarenone (14000-c)

Ubidecarenone *(rINN).*

Coenzyme Q10; Ubiquinone-10. 2-Deca(3-methylbut-2-enylene)-5,6-dimethoxy-3-methyl-*p*-benzoquinone.

$C_{59}H_{90}O_4$ = 863.3.

CAS — 303-98-0.

Pharmacopoeias. In *Jpn.*

Ubidecarenone is a naturally occurring coenzyme involved in electron transport in the mitochondria. It is claimed to be a free radical scavenger and to have antoxidant and membrane stabilising properties. It has been given by mouth, in conjunction with standard treatment, in cardiovascular disorders including mild or moderate heart failure. Ubidecarenone is under investigation for the management of Huntington's chorea. It has also been tried in conditions associated with coenzyme deficiency.

For a report of the use of ubidecarenone in muscle weakness, see Lovastatin, p.1275.

For mention of the use of ubidecarenone in the treatment of cardiotoxicity associated with doxorubicin, see p.529.

References.

1. Greenberg S, Frishman WH. Co-enzyme Q_{10}: a new drug for cardiovascular disease. *J Clin Pharmacol* 1990; **30:** 596–608.
2. Spigset O. Reduced effect of warfarin caused by ubidecarenone. *Lancet* 1994; **344:** 1372–3.
3. Garcia Silva MT, *et al.* Improvement of refractory sideroblastic anaemia with ubidecarenone. *Lancet* 1994; **343:** 1039.
4. Gattermann N, *et al.* No improvement of refractory sideroblastic anaemia with ubidecarenone. *Lancet* 1995; **345:** 1121–2.
5. Nagao T, *et al.* Treatment of warfarin-induced hair loss with ubidecarenone. *Lancet* 1995; **346:** 1104–5.

Preparations

Proprietary Preparations (details are given in Part 3)
Ital.: Caomet; Cardioton; Coedieci; Decafar; Decarene†; Decorenone; Dymion; Iuvacor; Miodene; Miotyn; Mitocor; Roburis; Ubicarden; Ubicardio; Ubicor; Ubidenone; Ubidex; Ubifactor; Ubilab; Ubimaior; Ubisan†; Ubisint; Ubiten; Ubivis; Ubixal†; ***Jpn:*** Neuquinon; ***UK:*** Co-Q-10; ***USA:*** Co-Q-10†.

Multi-ingredient: ***Ital.:*** Agedin Plus; Ener-E; ***UK:*** Efamol Plus Coenzyme Q10.

Ulinastatin (2998-d)

Ulinastatin *(rINN).*

Ulinastatin is a glycoprotein proteolytic enzyme inhibitor isolated from human urine. It has been given by injection in acute pancreatitis (p.1613) and in acute circulatory insufficiency.

References.

1. Ohwada M, *et al.* New endoscopic treatment for chronic pancreatitis, using contrast media containing ulinastatin and prednisolone. *J Gastroenterol* 1997; **32:** 216–21.

Preparations

Proprietary Preparations (details are given in Part 3)
Jpn: Miraclid†.

Urazamide (14003-t)

5-Aminoimidazole-4-carboxamide ureidosuccinate.

$C_9H_{14}N_6O_6$ = 302.2.

Urazamide has been used in the treatment of hepatic disorders in doses of 400 to 800 mg daily by mouth. It has also been administered by intramuscular and intravenous injection.

Preparations

Proprietary Preparations (details are given in Part 3)
Ital.: Aicase†; Carbaica.

Uridine (14004-x)

Uracil Riboside. 1-β-D-Ribofuranosyluracil; 1-β-D-Ribofuranosylpyrimidine-2,4(1*H*,3*H*)-dione.

$C_9H_{12}N_2O_6$ = 244.2.

CAS — 58-96-8.

Uridine is one of the four nucleosides present in ribonucleic acid. Uridine has been used in patients with hereditary orotic aciduria. It has also been reported to be of benefit in reducing fluorouracil toxicity (p.535).

References.

1. Girot R, *et al.* Cellular immune deficiency in two siblings with hereditary orotic aciduria. *N Engl J Med* 1983; **308:** 700–4.
2. Becroft DMO, *et al.* Absence of immune deficiency in hereditary orotic aciduria. *N Engl J Med* 1984; **310:** 1333–4.

Preparations

Proprietary Preparations (details are given in Part 3)
Multi-ingredient: ***Aust.:*** Laevadosin; Vitasic; ***Fr.:*** Vitacic; ***Ger.:*** Laevadosin†; Vitasic†; ***Ital.:*** Centrum; Citicortex†; Citoglutar†; Citokrebiol†; Cituridina; Emonucleosina Cortex†; For Liver; Liverasten†; NE 300†; Neo-Epa†; Nucleodoxina†; ***Spain:*** Inexfal; Prodessal.

Uridine Triphosphate (14005-r)

Uridine Triphosphoric Acid; UTP. Uridine 5′-(tetrahydrogen triphosphate).

$C_9H_{15}N_2O_{15}P_3$ = 484.1.

CAS — 63-39-8.

Uridine triphosphate is under investigation for the treatment of cystic fibrosis (p.119). It has also been claimed to be of value in muscular atrophy and muscular weakness.

Uridine triphosphate has been reported to be effective in stimulating chloride secretion in the nasal epithelium of patients with cystic fibrosis.[1] It has been suggested that correction of the ion-transport abnormalities in cystic fibrosis patients may reduce the viscosity of the secretions in the early stages of the disease,[2] and selected nucleotides such as uridine triphosphate should be investigated as therapeutic agents.[1]

The suggestion that uridine might produce improvement in patients with galactosaemia has not been confirmed.[3]

1. Knowles MR, *et al.* Activation by extracellular nucleotides of chloride secretion in the airway epithelia of patients with cystic fibrosis. *N Engl J Med* 1991; **325:** 533–8.
2. Davis PB. Cystic fibrosis from bench to bedside. *N Engl J Med* 1991; **325:** 575–77.
3. Holton JB, Leonard JV. Clouds still gathering over galactosaemia. *Lancet* 1994; **344:** 1242–3.

Preparations

Proprietary Preparations (details are given in Part 3)

Multi-ingredient: ***Ital.:*** Dinamozim†; Fosfoutipi Vitaminico; ***Spain:*** Sedionbel†; Taurobetina.

Ursodeoxycholic Acid (3753-w)

Ursodeoxycholic Acid *(BAN, rINN).*

Acidum Ursodeoxycholicum; UDCA; Ursodesoxycholic Acid; Ursodiol *(USAN).* 3α,7β-Dihydroxy-5β-cholan-24-oic acid.

$C_{24}H_{40}O_4$ = 392.6.

CAS — *128-13-2.*

Pharmacopoeias. In *Chin., Eur.* (see p.viii), *Jpn,* and *US.*

A white or almost white crystalline powder. Practically **insoluble** or very slightly soluble in water; freely soluble in alcohol and in glacial acetic acid; sparingly soluble in chloroform; slightly soluble in acetone, in dichloromethane, and in ether. **Store** in airtight containers.

Stability. References.

1. Mallett MS, *et al.* Stability of ursodiol 25 mg/mL in an extemporaneously prepared oral liquid. *Am J Health-Syst Pharm* 1997; **54:** 1401–4.

Adverse Effects and Precautions

As for Chenodeoxycholic Acid, p.1562. Ursodeoxycholic acid may cause nausea, vomiting, and other gastro-intestinal disturbances but diarrhoea is reported to occur less frequently than with chenodeoxycholic acid. Increased liver enzyme values are also less likely. However, treatment with ursodeoxycholic acid may cause more calcification of cholesterol stones than chenodeoxycholic acid.

Interactions

As for Chenodeoxycholic Acid, p.1562.

Pharmacokinetics

Ursodeoxycholic acid is absorbed from the gastro-intestinal tract and undergoes enterohepatic recycling. It is partly conjugated in the liver before being excreted into the bile. Under the influence of intestinal bacteria the free and conjugated forms undergo 7α-dehydroxylation to lithocholic acid, some of which is excreted directly in the faeces and the rest absorbed and mainly conjugated and sulphated by the liver before excretion in the faeces. However, in comparison with chenodeoxycholic acid, less ursodeoxycholic acid undergoes such bacterial degradation.

References.

1. Crosignani A, *et al.* Clinical pharmacokinetics of therapeutic bile acids. *Clin Pharmacokinet* 1996; **30:** 333–58.

Uses and Administration

Ursodeoxycholic acid is a naturally occurring bile acid (see p.1553) present in small quantities in human bile. Ursodeoxycholic acid suppresses the synthesis and secretion of cholesterol by the liver and inhibits intestinal absorption of cholesterol. It is used for the dissolution of cholesterol-rich gallstones in patients with functioning gallbladders (see below). The usual dose is 6 to 12 mg per kg body-weight daily as a single bedtime dose or in 2 or 3 divided doses; obese patients may require up to 15 mg per kg daily. The daily dose may be divided unequally and the larger dose given before bedtime to counteract the increase in biliary cholesterol concentration seen overnight. The time required for dissolution of gallstones is likely to be between 6 and 24 months depending on stone size and composition. Treatment should be continued for 3 to 4 months after radiological disappearance of the stones. Ursodeoxycholic acid has also been given in combination with chenodeoxycholic acid (p.1562) and lower doses of 5 to 7.5 mg per kg daily may then be given.

Ursodeoxycholic acid is also used in primary biliary cirrhosis. The usual dose is 10 to 15 mg per kg daily in 2 to 4 divided doses.

Ursodeoxycholic acid has been tried in the treatment of primary sclerosing cholangitis.

The more hydrophilic derivative, tauroursodeoxycholic acid, has also been used.

Chronic liver disease. The use of ursodeoxycholic acid in chronic liver diseases has been summarised.[1,2] Although used to slow disease progression[3] in primary biliary cirrhosis (p.497) there have been differing opinions as to its value.[4,5] Response has also been reported in liver disease in cystic fibrosis,[6-8] cholestasis associated with pregnancy,[9] sclerosing cholangitis,[10] chronic active hepatitis,[11] and viral hepatitis.[12,13] Ursodeoxycholic acid has also shown some promise in the treatment of nonalcoholic steatohepatitis,[14] but randomised, controlled studies are required to confirm this. There has also been some interest in the use of ursodeoxycholic acid to treat refractory graft-versus-host disease of the liver in transplant patients,[15] and possibly as an adjuvant to immunosuppressant therapy[16-18] after orthotopic liver transplantation (p.500).

1. de Caestecker JS, *et al.* Ursodeoxycholic acid in chronic liver disease. *Gut* 1991; **32:** 1061–5.
2. Rubin RA, *et al.* Ursodiol for hepatobiliary disorders. *Ann Intern Med* 1994; **121:** 207–18.
3. Poupon RE, *et al.* Ursodiol for the long-term treatment of primary biliary cirrhosis. *N Engl J Med* 1994; **330:** 1342–7.
4. Goddard CJR, Warnes TW. Primary biliary cirrhosis: how should we evaluate new treatments? *Lancet* 1994; **343:** 1305–6.
5. Lim AG, Northfield TC. Ursodeoxycholic acid and primary biliary cirrhosis. *Br Med J* 1994; **309:** 491–2.
6. Colombo C, *et al.* Effects of ursodeoxycholic acid therapy for liver disease associated with cystic fibrosis. *J Pediatr* 1990; **117:** 482–9.
7. Cotting J, *et al.* Effects of ursodeoxycholic acid treatment on nutrition and liver function in patients with cystic fibrosis and longstanding cholestasis. *Gut* 1990; **31:** 918–21.
8. Scher H, *et al.* Ursodeoxycholic acid improves cholestasis in infants with cystic fibrosis. *Ann Pharmacother* 1997; **31:** 1003–5.
9. Palma J, *et al.* Ursodeoxycholic acid in the treatment of cholestasis of pregnancy: a randomized, double-blind study controlled with placebo. *J Hepatol* 1997; **27:** 1022–8.
10. Lindor KD, *et al.* Ursodiol for primary sclerosing cholangitis. *N Engl J Med* 1997; **336:** 691–5.
11. Rolandi E, *et al.* Effects of ursodeoxycholic acid (UDCA) on serum liver damage indices in patients with chronic active hepatitis: a double-blind controlled study. *Eur J Clin Pharmacol* 1991; **40:** 473–6.
12. Puoti C, *et al.* Ursodeoxycholic acid and chronic hepatitis C infection. *Lancet* 1993; **341:** 1413–14.
13. Angelico M, *et al.* Recombinant interferon-α and ursodeoxycholic acid versus interferon-α alone in the treatment of chronic hepatitis C: a randomized clinical trial with long-term follow-up. *Am J Gastroenterol* 1995: **90:** 263–9.
14. Laurin J, *et al.* Ursodeoxycholic acid or clofibrate in the treatment of non-alcohol-induced steatohepatitis: a pilot study. *Hepatology* 1996; **23:** 1464–7.
15. Fried RH, *et al.* Ursodeoxycholic acid treatment of refractory chronic graft-versus-host disease of the liver. *Ann Intern Med* 1992; **116:** 624–9.
16. Persson H, *et al.* Ursodeoxycholic acid for prevention of acute rejection in liver transplant recipients. *Lancet* 1990; **ii:** 52–3.
17. Friman S, *et al.* Adjuvant treatment with ursodeoxycholic acid reduces acute rejection after liver transplantation. *Transplant Proc* 1992; **24:** 389–90.
18. Clavien P-A, *et al.* Evidence that ursodeoxycholic acid prevents steroid-resistant rejection in adult liver transplantation. *Clin Transplant* 1996; **10:** 658–62.

Gallstones. Gallstones (cholelithiasis) occur when mechanisms for the solubilisation of cholesterol or bilirubin fail or are overcome. They may be divided into those formed of pure cholesterol, which are usually solitary; pigment stones, largely made up of bilirubin or its derivatives; and mixed stones of cholesterol, bile pigment, and calcium salts, which form the great majority of cases seen in the West.

Gallstones occur more often in women than men and the prevalence increases with age and obesity. As many as two-thirds of those with gallstones are asymptomatic. When stones impact in the neck of the gallbladder or in the biliary tract patients develop attacks of acute, sometimes very severe, pain in the abdomen, sometimes radiating to the right shoulder or back. If the stone blocks the exit from the gallbladder inflammation and bacterial infection may follow (acute cholecystitis), sometimes leading to perforation and subsequent peritonitis. Less commonly, obstruction of the common bile duct by gallstones (choledocholithiasis) may lead to cholestasis and jaundice, often painless; infection of the bile ducts and septicaemia may follow. Pancreatitis may also be associated with gallstone disease, and there may be an increased risk of developing malignant neoplasms of the gallbladder.

Treatment. Asymptomatic gallstones discovered during other investigations should not be treated,[1-6] and even mildly symptomatic patients may be managed with analgesics and subsequent observation.[4] Glyceryl trinitrate is also reported to be effective in relieving biliary pain[7] (p.8). In symptomatic patients the preferred treatment for gallstones is surgical removal of the gallbladder;[1-6] 'keyhole surgery' (laparoscopic cholecystectomy) is associated with less postoperative morbidity than open surgery, and has largely replaced other methods of treatment.

In patients unsuited to, or unwilling to undergo, surgery for gallbladder stones, drug therapy, alone or in combination with lithotripsy, may be considered.

Administration of exogenous bile acids has been tried in an attempt to dissolve the cholesterol component of gallstones. Chenodeoxycholic acid has largely been replaced by ursodeoxycholic acid, which is more effective and is associated with fewer adverse effects;[1,4,5,8] combination therapy has also been tried,[5,8] given at bedtime since this increases the efficacy of chenodeoxycholic acid.[5] Dissolution of gallstones can be achieved in about one-third of cases,[1,5] but is slow, and about half of all successfully treated patients will develop further gallstones within 10 years,[1,5,6] though not all will be symptomatic. Studies of prophylactic bile acid therapy have mostly yielded disappointing results,[5] although there is a report of benefit from the prophylactic use of ursodeoxycholic acid in patients on very-low-calorie diets.[9]

Somewhat larger stones may respond to extracorporeal shock-wave lithotripsy,[1-6] or fluoroscopically guided laser lithotripsy, which may be more effective.[10] Subsequent treatment with oral bile acids should be given to dissolve the stone fragments.[1-6]

An alternative to bile acid therapy is the direct instillation of a solvent (usually methyl *tert*-butyl ether) into the gallbladder.[1,4,5] This dissolves stones within a matter of hours, and is effective against almost all cholesterol-based stones regardless of size and number;[5] a preliminary CT scan to eliminate patients with hyperdense stones, which do not readily dissolve, has been recommended.[5] Care is required to avoid overflow of the solvent into the common bile duct or the duodenum, where it may cause inflammation.[1,5] Other solvents, such as ethyl propionate[11] have been investigated as potentially less toxic alternatives, and edetic acid has been suggested as a possible solvent for non-cholesterol gallstones.[5] As with bile acid therapy, recurrence is likely.

Patients with stones in the common bile duct or acute cholecystitis require prompt therapy because of the risk of serious complications; endoscopic sphincterotomy and physical retrieval of the stones with a basket or balloon appears to be the preferred treatment, with open surgery as an alternative. Lithotripsy or infusion of a solvent such as monoctanoin[4,12] or methyl *tert*-butyl ether are possible alternatives in patients unfit for surgery,[4] as is insertion of a biliary stent to allow bile flow around the stone.[1]

In patients who develop cholecystitis or cholangitis antibacterial therapy may be required (see p.117).

1. Johnston DE, Kaplan MM. Pathogenesis and treatment of gallstones. *N Engl J Med* 1993; **328:** 412–21.
2. Ransohoff DF, Gracie WA. Treatment of gallstones. *Ann Intern Med* 1993; **119:** 606–19.
3. American College of Physicians. Guidelines for the treatment of gallstones. *Ann Intern Med* 1993; **119:** 620–2.
4. Anonymous. Managing patients with gallstones. *Drug Ther Bull* 1994; **32:** 33–5.
5. Lanzini A, Northfield TC. Pharmacological treatment of gallstones: practical guidelines. *Drugs* 1994; **47:** 458–70.
6. Tait N, Little JM. The treatment of gall stones. *Br Med J* 1995; **311:** 99–105.
7. Hassel B. Treatment of biliary colic with nitroglycerin. *Lancet* 1993; **342:** 1305.
8. May GR, *et al.* Efficacy of bile acid therapy for gallstone dissolution: a meta-analysis of randomized trials. *Aliment Pharmacol Ther* 1993; **7:** 139–48.
9. Shiffman ML, *et al.* Prophylaxis against gallstone formation with ursodeoxycholic acid in patients participating in a very-low-calorie diet program. *Ann Intern Med* 1995; **122:** 899–905.
10. Jakobs R, *et al.* Fluoroscopically guided laser lithotripsy versus extracorporeal shock wave lithotripsy for retained bile duct stones: a prospective randomised study. *Gut* 1997; **40:** 678–82.
11. Hofmann AF, *et al.* Pathogenesis and treatment of gallstones. *N Engl J Med* 1993; **328:** 1854–5.
12. Palmer KR, Hofmann AF. Intraductal mono-octanoin for the direct dissolution of bile duct stones: experience in 343 patients. *Gut* 1986; **27:** 196–202.

Preparations

USP 23: Ursodiol Capsules.

Proprietary Preparations (details are given in Part 3)

Aust.: Ursofalk; ***Belg.:*** Ursochol; Ursofalk; ***Canad.:*** Ursofalk; ***Fr.:*** Arsacol; Delursan; Destolit; Ursolvan; ***Ger.:*** Cholacid; Cholit-Ursan; Cholofalk; Peptarom†; Urso; Ursochol; Ursofalk; ***Irl.:*** Ursofalk; ***Ital.:*** Biliepar; Desocol; Desoxil; Deursil; Fraurs; Galmax; Lentorsil; Litoff; Litursol; Lyeton†; Tauro; Taursol†; Tudcabil; Urdes; Ursacol; Ursilon; Ursobil; Ursodamor; Ursodiol; Ursofalk; Ursoflor; Ursolac; Ursolisin; Urson; Ursoproge; ***Jpn:*** Urso; ***Neth.:*** Ursochol; Ursofalk; ***S.Afr.:*** Ursotan; ***Spain:*** Ursobilane; Ursochol; Ursolite; ***Swed.:*** Ursofalk; ***Switz.:*** Deursil; Ursochol; Ursofalk; ***UK:*** Destolit; Urdox; Ursofalk; Ursogal; ***USA:*** Actigall.

Multi-ingredient: ***Aust.:*** Lithofalk†; ***Ger.:*** Lithofalk; Urso Mix; Ursofalk + Chenofalk; ***Ital.:*** Bilenor; Litobile; ***Switz.:*** Cumulit†; Lithofalk; ***UK:*** Combidol†; Lithofalk†.

Urtica (18427-g)

Stinging Nettle.

Pharmacopoeias. Ger. includes monographs for the leaves and root of *U. dioica. Swiss* includes a monograph for Urtica Herba.

The dried aerial parts or leaves of *Urtica dioica* (Urticaceae), the stinging nettle, have been used in herbal medicine, mainly for urinary-tract and rheumatic disorders. *Urtica urens* has been used similarly.

Preparations

Proprietary Preparations (details are given in Part 3)

Aust.: Urtica Plus; ***Ger.:*** Arthrodynat N; Bazoton; Cirkuprostan; Cletan; Dr. Grandel Brennessel Vital Tonikum†; Kneipp Brennessel-Pflanzensaft; Kneipp Pflanzendragees Brennessel; Logomed Prostata-Kapseln; Prostaforton; Prostagalen; Prostaherb N; Prostaneurin; Prostawern; Reumaless; Rheuma-Hek; Uriginex Urtica; Uro-Pos; Urtica Plus N; Urticaprostat Uno; Urticur; Urtipret; Utk

Uno; ***Ital.:*** Venustas Shampoo per Capelli con Forfora e/o Grassi; ***Switz.:*** Simic.

Multi-ingredient: ***Aust.:*** Anaemodoron; Apotheker Bauer's Harntreibender Tee; Apotheker Bauer's Nieren- und Blasentee; Berggeist; Bio-Garten Tee zur Erhohung der Harnmenge; Bogumil-tassenfertiger milder Abfurtee; Brennesseltonikum; Brostalin; Ehrmann's Entschlackungstee; Fruhjahrs-Elixier ohne Alkohol; Harntreibender Tee; Krauterdoktor Entwasserungs-Elixier; Krauterhaus Mag Kottas Blutreinigungstee; Krauterhaus Mag Kottas Entschlackungstee; Krauterhaus Mag Kottas Entwasserungstee; Krauterhaus Mag Kottas Fruhjahrs- und Herbstkurtee; Krautertee Nr 19; Krautertee Nr 8; Mag Doskar's Nieren- und Blasentonikum; Mag Kottas Entschlackungstee; Menodoron; Mentopin; Prostagutt; Prostatonin; Sidroga Stoffwechseltee; Species Carvi comp; St Radegunder Entwasserungs-Elixier; St Radegunder Entwasserungstee; Synpharma Instant-Blasen-und-Nierentee; ***Austral.:*** Cough Relief; Infant Tonic; Irontona; Respatona; Respatona Plus with Echinacea; Vitatona; ***Fr.:*** Lithiabyl; ***Ger.:*** Befelka-Tinktur; C 34-Strath†; Cholaflux†; Colchicum-Strath†; Combudoron; Crinocedin†; Dr. Klinger's Bergischer Krautertee, Abfuhr- und Verdauungstee†; Heparchofid S†; Liruptin†; Prostagutt forte; Prostagutt Tropfen†; Prostatin F; Prostatin N Liquidum†; Prostatin N†; Rheumex†; Salus Kurbis-Tonikum Compositum†; Salus Rheuma-Tee Krautertee Nr. 12; Secerna†; Stoffwechseldragees†; Uvirgan N; Vollmers praparierter gruner; ***Ital.:*** Herbavit; Nosenil; Omadine; Shamday Antiforfora; ***Switz.:*** Prostagutt-F; Prostatonin; Tisane d'allaitement "H"†; Tisane diuretique; ***UK:*** Fragador; Kleer; Menodoron.

Usnea Barbata (14006-f)

CAS — 125-46-2 (usnic acid).

Usnea barbata is a lichen.

Usnea barbata contains usnic acid which is reported to have antimicrobial activity. *Usnea barbata* extract, usnic acid, and copper usnate have been used in topical preparations.

Preparations

Proprietary Preparations (details are given in Part 3)
Ger.: Dr. Grandel Granobil; ***Ital.:*** Vidermina; Zeta N.

Multi-ingredient: ***Ital.:*** Aseptil; Neo Zeta-Foot; Sideck Shampoo Antiforfora†; Zeta-Foot†.

Valepotriates (14008-n)

CAS — 18296-45-2 (didrovaltrate); 18296-44-1 (valtrate); 25161-41-5 (acevaltrate).

NOTE. Acevaltrate and didrovaltrate are *rINN*; Valtrate is *pINN*.

Epoxy-iridoid esters, isolated from valerian (see below). They include *didrovaltrate* (6-acetoxy-1,4a,5,6,7,7a-hexahydro-1-isovaleryloxy-4-isovaleryloxymethylcyclopenta[*c*]pyran-7-spiro-2′-oxiran, $C_{22}H_{32}O_8$=424.5), *valtrate* (4-acetoxymethyl-1,6-di-isovaleryloxy-1,6,7,7a-tetrahydrocyclopenta[*c*]pyran-7-spiro-2′-oxiran, $C_{22}H_{30}O_8$=422.5), and *acevaltrate* (4-acetoxymethyl-(1 or 6)-3-(acetoxy-3-methylbutyryloxy)-1,6,7,7a-tetrahydro-(6 or 1)-isovaleryloxycyclopenta[*c*]pyran-7-spiro-2′-oxiran, $C_{24}H_{32}O_{10}$=480.5). On prolonged storage and drying they are hydrolysed to yield isovaleric acid.

A mixture stated to contain didrovaltrate, valtrate, and acevaltrate has been used as a sedative and as an anxiolytic. Concern has been expressed over the potential toxicity of valepotriates which have been reported to have cytotoxic properties *in vitro*.

Preparations

Proprietary Preparations (details are given in Part 3)
Aust.: Nervipane; Valmane; ***Ital.:*** Nervipan†; ***S.Afr.:*** Valmane†.

Valerian (14009-h)

Baldrianwurzel; Valer; Valerian Rhizome; Valerian Root; Valerianae Radix.

CAS — 8057-49-6 (valerian extract).

Pharmacopoeias. In *Eur.* (see p.viii) and *Pol.* Also in *USNF*. *Jpn* has Japanese Valerian from *V. fauriei* or allied plants.

The yellowish-grey to pale brownish-grey subterranean organs, including the rhizome, root, and stolon of *Valeriana officinalis* (Valerianaceae), dried below 40°. It has a characteristic, penetrating, odour and a sweet taste with a spicy bitter after-taste. **Store** in airtight containers. Protect from light.

Valerian has sedative properties and is used as an extract, infusion, or tincture, or occasionally as the dried root, in preparations for anxiety states. It has also been used as a carminative. The odour of valerian may be removed from the skin and from hard surfaces with sodium bicarbonate.

Reviews.

1. Houghton P. Valerian. *Pharm J* 1994; **253:** 95–6.

Adverse effects. Report of four cases of liver damage[1] that may have been caused by valerian present in herbal remedies for stress.

1. MacGregor FB, *et al.* Hepatotoxicity of herbal remedies. *Br Med J* 1989; **299:** 1156–7.

Preparations

Proprietary Preparations (details are given in Part 3)
Aust.: Baldrinetten; Gewusst wie Beruhigungs; Psychobald; Valdispert†; ***Austral.:*** Herbal Sleep Formula; ***Belg.:*** Relaxine; Valdispert; Valerial; ***Canad.:*** Nytol Natural Source; ***Fr.:*** Relaxine; ***Ger.:*** Baldrianetten N; Baldrisedon Mono; Benedorm; Hewedormir; Kneipp Baldrian; Kneipp Baldrian-Pflanzensaft Nerventrost; Nervipan; Orasedon†; Recvalysat; Sedalint Baldrian; Sedonium; Silvapin Baldrianwurzel-Extrakt†; Valdispert; Valmane; ***Ital.:*** Ticalma; Val-Uno; ***Neth.:*** Sanox-N†; Valdispert; Valmane†; ***Spain:*** Tauval; Valdispert; Valeriana Orto; ***Swed.:*** Baldrian-Dispert; Neurol; Valerecen; ***Switz.:*** Baldrisedon; Regivital†; Sirop pour le sommeil; Valdispert; Valverde Sirop pour le sommeil.

Multi-ingredient: ***Aust.:*** Absimed; Aktiv Nerven- und Schlaftee; Bakanasan Einschlaf; Baldracin; Baldrian AMA; Baldrian Dispert Compositum; Baldrian-Elixier; Baldrian-Krautertonikum; Baldriparan Beruhigungs; Beruhigungskapseln; Beruhigungstee; Bio-Garten Tee fur den Magen; Bio-Garten Tee zur Beruhigung; Bio-Garten Tropfen fur Magen und Darm; Biogelat Schlaf; Cardiofrik; Einschlafkapseln; Eryval; Hova; Hovaletten†; Kneipp Nerven- und Schlaf-Tee; Krauterdoktor Entspannungs- und Einschlaftropfen; Krauterdoktor Magen-Darmtropfen; Krauterdoktor Nerven-Tonikum; Krauterhaus Mag Kottas Nerven- und Schlaftee; Krauterhaus Mag Kottas Wechseltee; Krautertee Nr 1; Krautertee Nr 124; Krautertee Nr 141; Krautertee Nr 9; Luvased; Mag Doskar's Nerventonikum; Mag Kottas Beruhigungstee; Mag Kottas Krauterexpress-Nerven-Schlaf-Tee; Mag Kottas Nerven-Beruhigungstee; Mag Kottas Schlaftee; Mag Kottas Wechseltee; Magentee; Nervendragees; Nervenruh; Nerventee; Nervifloran; Phytogran; Sanhelios Einschlaf; Sedogelat; Sidroga Nerven- und Schlaftee; Species nervinae; St Bonifatius-Tee; St Radegunder Beruhigungs- und Einschlaftee; St Radegunder Nerven-Tonikum; St Radegunder Nerventee; Synpharma Instant-Nerventee; Teekanne Schlaf- und Nerventee; Thymoval; Valin Baldrian; Vivinox; Wechseltee; ***Austral.:*** Calmo; Executive B; Goodnight Formula; Kavosporal†; Lifesystem Herbal Plus Formula 2 Valerian; Macro Anti-Stress; Naturest; Pacifenity; Passiflora Complex; Passionflower Plus; Prosed-X; Relaxaplex; Tranquiplex†; Valerian; Valerian Plus Herbal Plus Formula 12; Vitaglow Herbal Stress†; ***Belg.:*** Seneuval; Valeria-Fordine†; ***Canad.:*** Herbal Nerve; Herbal Sleep Well†; Nyrene; ***Fr.:*** Achisane Troubles du Sommeil; Anxoral; Biocarde; Euphytose; Felisedine†; Fluon; Mediflor Tisane Calmante Troubles du Sommeil No 14; Mediflor Tisane Circulation du Sang No 12; Neuroflorine; Neurotensyl; Noctisan; Palpipax; Passinevryl†; Phytocalm; Phytotherapie Boribel no 8; Quietival†; Sedalozia; Sedibaine; Serenival; Spasmidenal; Spasmine; Sympaneurol; Tabapax†; Tisane Sedative Weleda; Tranquital; Valerbe; ***Ger.:*** Aranidorm-S; Ardeysedon N; Aureal†; Avedorm; B 10-Strath†; Baldrian-Dispert Nacht; Baldrianox S; Baldriparan N; Baldriparan stark N; Baldronit cum Nitro†; Baldronit forte N†; Baldronit N†; Belladonna-Strath†; Belladonna-Valobonin†; Beruhigungs-Tee Nervoflux†; Biosedon S; Biral; Boxocalm; Bunetten†; Card-Ompin S†; Cardisetten†; Carminat†; Castrophan†; Cefasedativ; Cholongal plus†; Cholongal†; Concardisett†; Cor-Select; Corguttin†; Diawern; Digaloid†; Dormarist; Dormeasan; Dormo-Sern; Dormoverlan; Dr. Kleinschrod's Cor-Insuffin†; Dr. Kleinschrod's Spasmi Tropfen†; Einschlaf-Kapseln biologisch; Esberi-Nervin†; Euchon†; Eupronerv†; Euvalon; Euvegal forte; Euvegal N; Euvitan; Gastrocaps†; Goldtropfen-Hetterich; Grunlicht Hingfong Essenz; Gutnacht; Guttacor; Habstal-Nerv N; Herz-plus Forte N†; Herz-Plus Nerven†; Herz-plus†; Heumann Beruhigungsdragees Tenerval N†; Heumann Beruhigungstee Tenerval N; Hova†; Hovaletten N; Hyperesa; Ivel Schlaf; JuDorm; JuNeuron S; Kavosporal comp; Kneipp Krauter Taschenkur Nerven und Schlaf N; Kneipp Nerven- und Schlaf-Tee N; Knufinke Nervenruh Beruhigungs-Tee†; Kyaugutt N†; Kytta-Sedativum f; Leukona-Sedativ-Bad; Leukona-Sedativ-Bad sine Chloralhydrat; Luvased; Luvased-Tropfen N; Majocarmin mite†; Montana; Moradorm; Moradorm S; Mutellon; Nerven-Tee Stada N; Nervendragees; Nervenruh†; Nerviguttum†; Nervinetten; Nervinfant comp†; Nervinfant†; Nervinum Stada†; Nervisal†; Nervo.opt†; Nervoregin forte; Nervosana; Neurapas; Nitrangin compositum; Oxacant N; Oxacant-sedativ; Pan-Nerventonikum†; Pascosedon S; Phytonoctu; Plantival N†; Plantival Novo; Plantival plus†; Presselin K 1 N; Pronervon N†; Pronervon Phyto; Psychotonin-sed.; Rhoival; Salusan; Schupps Baldrian Sedativbad; Seda Kneipp N; Seda-Pasc N†; Seda-Plantina; Sedacur; Sedahopf; Sedariston; Sedariston Konzentrat; Sedaselect N; Sedasyx; Sedatruw S; Sedinfant N; Sediomed S†; Selon; Sensinerv forte; Sirmiosta Nervenelixier N; Somnium forte†; Somnium†; Somnuvis S; Stacho N†; Tornix; Ulcotest†; Valdispert comp; Valena N; Valeriana comp; Valeriana forte; Valeriana mild; Valeriana-Digitalysat (Valdig)†; Valeriana-Strath†; Valobonin†; Valomenth†; Valomettent†; Ventrodigest†; Visinal; Vivinox; Vivinox-Schlafdragees; Worishofener Nervenpflege Dr. Kleinschrod†; ***Ital.:*** Anevrasi; Antispasmina Colica B†; Bianco Val; Bio-Strath; Bitteridina; Bramserene†; Calmactiv†; Entero-V†; Fitosonno; Florelax; Florerbe Calmante†; Glicero-Valerovit; Noctis; Parvisedil; Quietan; Reve; Sedatol; Sedonerva†; Sedopuer F; Val-Plus; Valeromill†; ***S.Afr.:*** Biral; Restin; ***Spain:*** Brevilon; ***Switz.:*** Baldriparan; Demonatur Dragees calmantes†; Dicalm†; Dormeasan N; Dormeasan†; Dormiplant; Dragees pour la detente nerveuse; Dragees pour le coeur et les nerfs; Dragees pour le sommeil nouvelle formule; Dragees relaxantes et tranquillisantes†; Epizon†; Melissa Tonic; Mirocor†; Perpector; Phytoberidin; Phytomed Somni; Plantival; Sedovalin†; Seracalm; Soporin; Tisane Natterman instantanee no 6 pour calmer les nerfs et lutter contre l'insomnie†; Tisane pour le coeur et la circulation "H"†; Tisane pour le sommeil et les nerfs; Tisane relaxante; Tisane sedative et somnifere "H"†; Valobonin†; Valverde Dragees pour la detente nerveuse; Valverde Dragees pour le coeur; Valverde Dragees pour le sommeil N; ***UK:*** Avena sativa comp.; Becalm; Biophylin; Gerard 99; Gladlax; Herbal Indigestion Naturtabs; Herbal Pain Relief; Indigestion and Flatulence; Kalms; Natrasleep; Newrelax; Night Time; PMT Formula; Prementaid; Quiet Days; Quiet Life; Quiet Night; Quiet Nite; Quiet Tyme; Rapi-snooze; Relax B+; Serenity; Somnus; SuNerven; Super Mega B+C; Valerian Compound; Valerina Day Time; Valerina Night-Time; Wellwoman.

Vanilla (2416-p)

Baunilha; Vainilla; Vanilla Beans; Vanilla Pods.

The cured, fully grown, unripe fruit of Madagascar, Mexican, or Bourbon vanilla, *Vanilla planifolia*, or of Tahiti vanilla, *V. tahitensis* (Orchidaceae). Its odour and flavour are not entirely due to vanillin but depend on the presence of other aromatic substances. **Store** at a temperature not exceeding 8° in airtight containers; vanilla which has become brittle should not be used.

Vanilla is used as a flavour and in perfumery.

Vanillin (2417-s)

Vainillina; Vanillic Aldehyde; Vanillinum. 4-Hydroxy-3-methoxybenzaldehyde.

$C_8H_8O_3$ = 152.1.

CAS — 121-33-5.

Pharmacopoeias. In *Eur.* (see p.viii) and *Pol.* Also in *USNF*.

White or slightly yellow crystalline needles or powder with an odour and taste of vanilla. It can be extracted from vanilla or prepared synthetically. M.p. 81° to 84°.

Soluble 1 in 100 of water at 25°, 1 in 20 of water at 80°, 1 in 20 of glycerol; freely soluble in alcohol, in chloroform, in methyl alcohol, and in solutions of fixed alkali hydroxides; soluble in ether and in fixed and volatile oils. A saturated solution in water is acid to litmus. **Store** in airtight containers. Protect from light.

Vanillin is used as a flavour and in perfumery.

Preparations

BP 1998: Tolu-flavour Solution.

Vasoactive Intestinal Peptide (17025-m)

Aviptadil *(BAN, rINN)*; VIP.

$C_{147}H_{238}N_{44}O_{42}S$ = 3325.8.

CAS — 40077-57-4.

Vasoactive intestinal peptide acts as a hormone and neurotransmitter in various parts of the body; it is a potent relaxant of smooth muscle and has vasodilator and bronchodilator properties as well as stimulating the gastro-intestinal tract to increased secretion. Vasoactive intestinal peptide is under investigation for use in combination with phentolamine for induction of erection in men with erectile dysfunction (p.1614). It also has orphan drug status in the USA in the management of acute oesophageal food impaction.

Hydrogenated Vegetable Oil (7371-v)

Pharmacopoeias. In *Br.* and *Jpn.* Also in *USNF*.

Refined, bleached, hydrogenated, and deodorised vegetable oil stearins consisting mainly of the triglycerides of stearic and palmitic acids. It is a fine white powder at room temperature and a pale yellow, oily liquid above its m.p. of 20° to 70°.

Practically **insoluble** in water; soluble in chloroform, in petroleum spirit, and in hot isopropyl alcohol. **Store** between 8° and 25° in airtight containers.

Hydrogenated vegetable oil is used as a tablet lubricant and as an ointment basis.

Preparations

Proprietary Preparations (details are given in Part 3)
Spain: Blodex.

Velaresol (19217-b)

Velaresol *(BAN, rINN)*.

BW-12C; 12C. 5-(2-Formyl-3-hydroxyphenoxy)pentaenoic acid; 5-(2-Formyl-3-hydroxyphenoxy)valeric acid.

$C_{12}H_{14}O_5$ = 238.2.

CAS — 77858-21-0.

Velaresol is an anti-sickling drug that has been investigated for the treatment of sickle-cell disease.

References.

1. Nicholls A, *et al.* Effect of BW12C on lactate levels during exercise in healthy volunteers. *Br J Clin Pharmacol* 1989; **28:** 747P.
2. Philip PA, *et al.* A phase 1 study of the left-shifting agent BW 12C79 plus mitomycin C and the effect on the skeletal muscle metabolism using 31P magnetic resonance spectroscopy. *Cancer Res* 1993; **53:** 5649–53.

Veratrine (14013-r)

Veratrine.

CAS — 8051-02-3 (mixture).

NOTE. Veratrine should be distinguished from protoveratrines obtained from veratrum.

A mixture of alkaloids from the dried ripe seeds of *Schoenocaulon officinale* (Liliaceae) (sabadilla).

Adverse Effects, Treatment, and Precautions

Veratrine resembles aconite (p.1542) in its action on the peripheral nerve endings and poisoning should be treated similarly. It is an intense local irritant and has a powerful direct stimulating action on all muscle tissues. It has a violent irritant action on mucous membranes, even in minute doses, and must be handled with great care. When ingested it causes violent vomiting, purging, an intense burning sensation in the mouth and throat, and general muscular weakness.

Uses and Administration

Veratrine should not be used internally. It was formerly applied externally for its analgesic properties and as a parasiticide, especially for head lice, but even when used in this way there is danger of systemic poisoning from absorption.

Vetrabutine Hydrochloride (12663-c)

Vetrabutine Hydrochloride *(BANM, rINNM).*

Dimophebumine Hydrochloride; Sp-281. *N,N*-Dimethyl-α-(3-phenylpropyl)veratrylamine hydrochloride.

$C_{20}H_{27}NO_2,HCl$ = 349.9.

CAS — 3735-45-3 (vetrabutine); 5974-09-4 (vetrabutine hydrochloride).

Vetrabutine hydrochloride is a uterine relaxant.

Preparations

Proprietary Preparations (details are given in Part 3)
Ger.: Monzal†.

Vinburnine (14014-f)

Vinburnine *(rINN).*

CH-846; (−)-Eburnamonine; 3α,16α-Eburnamonine; Vincamone. (3α,16α)-Eburnamenin-14(15*H*)-one.

$C_{19}H_{22}N_2O$ = 294.4.

CAS — 4880-88-0.

Vinburnine has been used in conditions associated with cerebral circulatory insufficiency.

Vinburnine phosphate has been used similarly.

Preparations

Proprietary Preparations (details are given in Part 3)
Fr.: Cervoxan; ***Ital.:*** Eburnal; Eubran†; Luvenil†; Scleramin; Tensiplex; ***Spain:*** Cervoxan; Eburnoxin.

Vincamine (14015-d)

Vincamine *(BAN, rINN).*

Methyl (3α,16α)-14,15-dihydro-14β-hydroxyeburnamenine-14-carboxylate.

$C_{21}H_{26}N_2O_3$ = 354.4.

CAS — 1617-90-9.

Pharmacopoeias. In *Belg.* and *Fr.*

An alkaloid obtained from *Vinca minor* (Apocynaceae).

Vincamine is claimed to increase cerebral circulation and utilisation of oxygen and has been used in a variety of cerebral disorders. Vincamine may have adverse effects on the cardiovascular system and care should be taken in patients with hypertension or cardiac dysfunction.

Vincamine salts including vincamine hydrochloride, oxoglurate, teprosilate, and hydrogen tartrate have also been used.

Preparations

Proprietary Preparations (details are given in Part 3)
Aust.: Aethroma; Cetal; Oxygeron; ***Belg.:*** Cerebroxine; Nooxine†; Pervincamine†; ***Fr.:*** Oxovinca†; Pervincamine; Tripervan†; Vinca; Vincafor; Vincimax; ***Ger.:*** Angiopac†; Cetal; Equipur; Esberidin†; Ocu-Vinc†; Ophdilvas N; Vinca-Tablinen; Vincapront; ***Ital.:*** Anasclerol; Ausomina; Cerebraminat; Dilar†; Encevin†; Pervin†; Roiten†; Teproside†; Vasonett; Vinca-Dil†; Vinca-Ri; Vinca-Treis; Vincadar; Vincafarm†; Vincafolina; Vincalen†; Vincamidol†; Vinsal; Vraap; ***Spain:*** Artensen†; Arteriovinca; Ceredilan†; Cetovinca; Dilarterial; Domeni†; Oxicebral†; Tefavinca; Vadicate; Vincacen; Vincamas†; Vincaminol; Vincavix†; ***Switz.:*** Aethroma; Cetal; Oxygeron; Pervincamine†; Vinca minor†.
Multi-ingredient: ***Fr.:*** Rheobral; Vincarutine; ***Ital.:*** Bilancen†; ***Spain:*** Anacervix; Arteriobrate; Devincal; Dipervina.

Vinpocetine (14016-n)

Vinpocetine *(USAN, rINN).*

AY-27255; Ethyl Apovincaminate; Ethyl Apovincaminoate; RGH-4405. Ethyl (3α,16α)-eburnamenine-14-carboxylate.

$C_{22}H_{26}N_2O_2$ = 350.5.

CAS — 42971-09-5.

Vinpocetine 15 to 30 mg daily by mouth in divided doses has been used in cerebrovascular and cognitive disorders.

References.

1. Grandt R, *et al.* Vinpocetine pharmacokinetics in elderly subjects. *Arzneimittelforschung* 1989; **39:** 1599–1602.
2. Blaha L, *et al.* Clinical evidence of the effectiveness of vinpocetine in the treatment of organic psychosyndrome. *Hum Psychopharmacol Clin Exp* 1989; **4:** 103–11.

Preparations

Proprietary Preparations (details are given in Part 3)
Aust.: Cavinton†; Remedial†; ***Ger.:*** Cavinton; ***Jpn:*** Calan.

Vinyl Chloride (14017-h)

VCM; Vinyl Chloride Monomer. Chloroethylene.

C_2H_3Cl = 62.50.

CAS — 75-01-4.

Vinyl chloride is used in the manufacture of polyvinyl chloride (PVC) and other vinyl polymers. Occupational exposure to vinyl chloride in polymerisation plants has been associated with acro-osteolysis, especially in the terminal phalanges of the fingers, a condition resembling Raynaud's phenomenon, and sclerodermatous skin changes. Liver damage and hepatic angiosarcoma, splenomegaly, thrombocytopenia, impaired respiratory function, and chromosomal abnormalities have also occurred.

References.

1. Piratsu R, *et al.* La mortalità dei produttori di cloruro di vinile in Italia. *Med Lav* 1991; **82:** 388–423.
2. Infante PF, *et al.* Genetic risks of vinyl chloride. *Lancet* 1976; **i:** 734–5.
3. Mur JM, *et al.* Spontaneous abortion and exposure to vinyl chloride. *Lancet* 1992; **339:** 127–8.
4. Black CM, *et al.* Genetic susceptibility to scleroderma-like syndrome induced by vinyl chloride. *Lancet* 1983; **i:** 53–5.
5. Riordan SM, *et al.* Vinyl chloride related hepatic angiosarcoma in a polyvinyl chloride autoclave cleaner in Australia. *Med J Aust* 1991; **155:** 125–8.

Viquidil Hydrochloride (14019-b)

Viquidil Hydrochloride *(rINNM).*

LM-192; Mequiverine Hydrochloride; Quinicine Hydrochloride. 1-(6-Methoxy-4-quinolyl)-3-(3-vinyl-4-piperidyl)propan-1-one hydrochloride.

$C_{20}H_{24}N_2O_2,HCl$ = 360.9.

CAS — 84-55-9 (viquidil); 52211-63-9 (viquidil hydrochloride).

Viquidil has been used in various cerebrovascular disorders as the hydrochloride in a daily divided dose of 200 to 300 mg by mouth.

Preparations

Proprietary Preparations (details are given in Part 3)
Fr.: Xitadil†; ***Ger.:*** Desclidium.

Water (7700-g)

Aqua; Aqua Communis; Aqua Fontana; Aqua Potabilis; Eau Potable; Wasser.

H_2O = 18.02.

CAS — 7732-18-5.

Purified Water (7701-q)

Aqua Purificata.

Pharmacopoeias. In *Chin., Eur.* (see p.viii), *Int., Jpn, Pol.,* and *US.*
US also includes Sterile Purified Water.

Some pharmacopoeias only include distilled water or have additional monographs for demineralised water or distilled water.

Purified water is prepared from suitable potable water either by distillation, by treatment with ion-exchange materials, or by any other suitable method. pH 5 to 7. **Store** in airtight containers which do not alter the properties of the water.

PREPARATION BY DEIONISATION. By passing potable water through columns of anionic and cationic ion-exchange resins, ionisable substances can be removed, producing a water of high specific resistance. Colloidal and non-ionisable impurities such as pyrogens may not be removed by this process.

PREPARATION BY DISTILLATION. In this process water is separated as vapour from non-volatile impurities and is subsequently condensed. In practice, non-volatile impurities may be carried into the distillate by entrainment unless a suitable baffle is fitted to the still.

Water for Injections (7702-p)

Aq. pro Inj.; Aqua ad Iniectabilia; Aqua ad Injectionem; Aqua Injectabilis; Aqua pro Injectione; Aqua pro Injectionibus; Eau pour Préparations Injectables; Wasser für Injektionszwecke; Water for Injection.

Pharmacopoeias. In *Chin., Eur.* (see p.viii), *Int., Jpn, Pol.,* and *US.*
Br. also includes Water for Irrigation and *US* also includes Sterile Water for Injection, Sterile Water for Inhalation, Sterile Water for Irrigation, and Bacteriostatic Water for Injection.

Water for Injections (Ph. Eur.) is distilled water free from pyrogens used to produce solutions for injection; it is prepared by distillation of potable water or purified water from a neutral glass, quartz, or suitable metal still fitted with an efficient device for preventing the entrainment of droplets; the first portion of the distillate is discarded and the remainder collected. Sub-monographs cover Water for Injections in Bulk and Sterilised Water for Injections.

Water for Injection (USP 23) is water purified by distillation or by reverse osmosis and contains no added substance. It is intended for use in parenteral solutions which are to be sterilised after preparation. Sterile Water for Injection (USP 23) is the subject of a separate monograph.

There are international standards for the quality of water intended for human consumption. Toxic substances such as arsenic, barium, cadmium, chromium, copper, cyanide, lead, and selenium may constitute a danger to health if present in drinking water in excess of the recommended concentrations. Water-borne infections are also a hazard.

Fluoride is regarded as an essential constituent of drinking water but may endanger health if present in excess—see Sodium Fluoride, p.742. Ingestion of water containing large quantities of nitrates may cause methaemoglobinaemia in infants; many countries have standards for nitrates in water.

The use of tap water containing metal ions (such as aluminium, copper, and lead), fluoride, or chloramine, for dialysis may be hazardous.

A hard water contains soluble calcium and magnesium salts, which cause the precipitation of soap and prevent its lathering and form scale and sludge in boilers, water pipes, and autoclaves. Temporary hardness in water is due to the presence of bicarbonates which are converted to insoluble carbonates on heating. Permanent hardness is due to dissolved chlorides, nitrates, and sulphates, which do not form a precipitate on heating. The presence or absence of such salts can play a part in cardiovascular health.

Without further purification, potable water may be unsuitable for certain pharmaceutical purposes. In such instances, purified water should always be used. Most pharmacopoeias include monographs on various preparations of water, such as water for injection or injections. Potable water should not be used when such preparations of water are specified.

Excessive ingestion of water can lead to water intoxication with disturbances of the electrolyte balance.

Wild Carrot (13990-c)

Dauci Herba; Daucus.

Pharmacopoeias. In *Chin.*

The fruits of the wild carrot, *Daucus carota* (Umbelliferae) have been used as a diuretic and anthelmintic, and are included in herbal preparations for various indications. Other parts of the plant have been used in folk medicine. The root of the cultivated form is a culinary item and a source of carotenoids in the diet.

Preparations

Proprietary Preparations (details are given in Part 3)
Ger.: Infectodyspept.
Multi-ingredient: ***Ital.:*** Pluriderm; ***UK:*** Sciargo.

Wild Cherry Bark (2418-w)

Prunus Serotina; Virginian Prune; Virginian Prune Bark; Wild Black Cherry Bark; Wild Cherry.

The dried bark of the wild or black cherry, *Prunus serotina* (Rosaceae), known in commerce as Thin Natural Wild Cherry Bark, containing not less than 10% of water-soluble extractive. It has a slight odour and an astringent, aromatic, bitter taste, recalling that of bitter almonds. It contains (+)-mandelonitrile glucoside (prunasin) and an enzyme system, which interact in the presence of water yielding benzaldehyde, hydrocyanic acid, and glucose.

Wild cherry bark, in the form of the syrup, has been used in the treatment of cough but it has little therapeutic value. It has also been used as a flavour.

Preparations

Proprietary Preparations (details are given in Part 3)

Multi-ingredient: ***Austral.:*** Waterbury's Compound†; ***Canad.:*** Mielocol; Rophelin; Wampole Bronchial Cough Syrup; ***UK:*** Night Cough Pastilles.

Wild Lettuce (19394-r)

Herba Lactucae Virosae.

The wild lettuce, *Lactuca virosa* (Compositae), has been given in herbal medicine as a sedative and antitussive. The dried sap (lactucarium; lettuce opium) is also used.

Preparations

Proprietary Preparations (details are given in Part 3)

Multi-ingredient: ***Ital.:*** Bio Notte Baby†; ***UK:*** Ana-Sed; Antibron; Nytol Herbal; Quiet Life; Quiet Nite; Somnus; Valerian Compound.

Xanthine-containing Beverages (3874-t)

Adverse Effects

The adverse effects of xanthine-containing beverages are largely due to their caffeine (p.749), theophylline (p.765), and theobromine (p.765) content. Common side-effects are sleeplessness, anxiety, tremor, palpitations, and withdrawal headache.

Effects on the heart. A meta-analysis of published studies found no evidence of an association between coffee consumption and the development of coronary heart disease (CHD),[1] and a large cohort study in women also found no evidence of a link.[2] Expert opinion in the UK[3] is that the evidence that caffeine or coffee consumption contributes to the development of CHD is inconsistent. Coffee prepared by boiling, as is the practice in Scandinavia, does raise serum cholesterol concentrations due to the presence of the diterpenes cafestol and kahweol, and coffee made in a cafetière has a similar effect, but filtered coffee does not, as the hypercholesterolaemic fraction does not pass a paper filter.[4] Others have raised concern that the potential pressor effects of caffeine itself may be a cardiovascular risk factor,[5] but as mentioned above there is little evidence for this.

Tea drinking has not been associated with increased cardiovascular risk[3]—indeed, its polyphenol content has been suggested to have beneficial antoxidant effects.[6]

1. Myers MG, Basinski A. Coffee and coronary heart disease. *Arch Intern Med* 1992; **152:** 1767–72.
2. Willett WC, *et al.* Coffee consumption and coronary heart disease in women: a ten-year follow-up. *JAMA* 1996; **275:** 458–62.
3. Department of Health. Nutritional aspects of cardiovascular disease. Report of the cardiovascular review group committee on medical aspects of food policy. Report on health and social subjects no. 46. London: HMSO, 1994.
4. Urgert R, *et al.* Comparison of effect of cafetière and filtered coffee on serum concentrations of liver aminotransferases and lipids: six month randomised controlled trial. *Br Med J* 1996; **313:** 1362–6.
5. James JE. Is habitual caffeine use a preventable cardiovascular risk factor? *Lancet* 1997; **349:** 279–81.
6. Luo M, *et al.* Inhibition of LDL oxidation by green tea extract. *Lancet* 1997; **349:** 360–1.

Effects on the muscles. Severe myositis in an elderly man who drank around 14 litres of tea daily was attributed to hypokalaemia produced by the xanthine content of the beverage.[1] The patient improved following intravenous potassium replacement and subsequently remained well following a reduction in tea intake.

1. Trewby PN, *et al.* Teapot myositis. *Lancet* 1998; **351:** 1248.

Malignant neoplasms. A review of available data did not suggest a clinically significant association between the regular use of coffee and the development of cancer of the lower urinary tract in men or women.[1]

1. Viscoli CM, *et al.* Bladder cancer and coffee drinking: a summary of case-control research. *Lancet* 1993; **341:** 1432–7.

Interactions

The possibility of synergistic effects in patients receiving xanthines who consume large amounts of xanthine-containing beverages should be borne in mind.

Antipsychotics. Xanthine-containing beverages have been reported to precipitate some antipsychotic drugs from solution *in vitro*, but do not appear to alter antipsychotic concentrations *in vivo*. For references, see p.654.

Uses and Administration

Xanthine-containing beverages including chocolate, coffee, cocoa, cola, maté, and tea are widely consumed and have a mild stimulant effect on the CNS. The primary xanthine constituent is caffeine but other xanthine derivatives may also be present; cocoa and chocolate contain significant amounts of theobromine.

Coffee is the kernel of the dried ripe seeds of *Coffea arabica*, *C. liberica*, *C. canephora* (robusta coffee), and other species of *Coffea* (Rubiaceae), roasted until it acquires a deep brown colour and a pleasant characteristic aroma. It contains about 1 to 2% of caffeine. Coffee has been used in the form of an infusion or decoction as a stimulant and as a flavouring agent in some pharmaceutical preparations. A decoction is used as a beverage containing up to about 100 mg of caffeine per 100 mL. Preparations of instant coffee may contain up to 40% less caffeine while decaffeinated preparations may contain only up to about 3 mg per 100 mL.

Kola (cola, cola seeds, kola nuts) is the dried cotyledons of *Cola nitida* and *C. acuminata* (Sterculiaceae), containing up to about 2.5% of caffeine and traces of theobromine. Kola is used in the preparation of cola drinks which may contain up to 20 mg of caffeine per 100 mL. Kola has been used to treat migraine in homoeopathic medicine.

Maté (Paraguay Tea) is the dried leaves of *Ilex paraguensis* (Aquifoliaceae), containing 0.2 to 2% of caffeine. Maté is less astringent than tea and is extensively used as a beverage in South America.

Tea (thea, chá, thé, tee) is the prepared young leaves and leaf-buds of *Camellia sinensis* (=*C. thea*) (Theaceae). It contains 1 to 5% of caffeine and up to 24% of tannin. Tea is used in an infusion as a beverage containing up to about 60 mg of caffeine per 100 mL.

Guarana consists of the crushed seeds of *Paullinia cupana* var *sorbilis*. Caffeine appears to be its major active ingredient which was once termed guaranine. Herbal preparations include a beverage or liquid extract and may contain 5% caffeine.

Preparations

Proprietary Preparations (details are given in Part 3)

Fr.: Camiline; ***Ger.:*** Carbo Konigsfeld.

Multi-ingredient: ***Aust.:*** Blasen- und Nierentee; Colagain; Euflat; Kneipp Herz- und Kreislauf-Unterstutzungs-Tee; Mag Kottas Herz- und Kreislauftee; ***Austral.:*** Avena Complex; Infant Tonic; Irontona; T & T Antioxidant; Vig; Vitatona; ***Belg.:*** Aperop; ***Canad.:*** Hemarexin†; ***Fr.:*** Actisane Fatigue Passagere; Biotone; Euphytose; Gripponyl†; Mincifit; Phospharome; Quintonine; Santane V_3; Tealine; Tonactil; Tonisan; Triogene; YSE; YSE Glutamique; ***Ger.:*** Cardibisana; Euflat-N†; Kneipp Schlankheits-Unterstutzungstee†; Kola-Dallmann; Kola-Dallmann mit Lecithin; Kola-Traubenzucker Dallmann's†; Myrrhinil-Intest; Nierox-in N; Orbis Blasen- und Nierentee†; Poikiloton†; Ramend Krauter; Repursan ST; Tonamyl†; ***Ital.:*** Amaro Maffioli†; Chinoidina; Dam; Enertonic; Enteroton Digestivo†; Fitostress; Four-Ton; Gincola; Nosenil; Prid con Boldo†; Prid†; ***Spain:*** Elingrip; Fitsovelt; ***Switz.:*** Dragees contre les maux de tete; Valverde contre les douleurs†; ***UK:*** Chlorophyll; Herbal Booster; Koladex; Labiton; S.P.H.P.; Strength.

Xantofyl Palmitate (14020-x)

Xantofyl Palmitate (*rINN*).

Heleniene; Xanthophyl Dipalmitate. β,ε-Carotene-3,3′-diyl dipalmitate.

$C_{72}H_{116}O_4$ = 1045.7.

CAS — 547-17-1.

Xantofyl palmitate has been used by mouth in the treatment of some visual disturbances.

Xylazine (14023-d)

Xylazine (*BAN, rINN*).

BAY-Va-1470 (xylazine hydrochloride). *N*-(5,6-Dihydro-4*H*-1,3-thiazin-2-yl)-2,6-xylidine.

$C_{12}H_{16}N_2S$ = 220.3.

CAS — 7361-61-7 (xylazine); 23076-35-9 (xylazine hydrochloride).

NOTE. Xylazine Hydrochloride is *USAN*.

Xylazine is a sedative, analgesic, and muscle relaxant used in veterinary medicine.

Bradycardia, hypotension, and coma was associated with self-administration of 200 mg xylazine. Treatment was supportive.[1]

1. Samanta A, *et al.* Accidental self administration of xylazine in a veterinary nurse. *Postgrad Med J* 1990; **66:** 244–5.

Xylose (2154-h)

Wood Sugar; D-Xylose; Xylosum. α-D-Xylopyranose.

$C_5H_{10}O_5$ = 150.1.

CAS — 58-86-6; 6763-34-4.

Pharmacopoeias. In *Eur.* (see p.viii) and *US.*

Odourless colourless needles or white crystalline powder. Very **soluble** to freely soluble in water; slightly soluble in alcohol; soluble in hot alcohol. **Store** in airtight containers at a temperature of 15° to 30°.

Adverse Effects and Precautions

Xylose may cause some gastro-intestinal discomfort with large doses. Other drugs may affect the absorption of xylose and interfere with the xylose test.

Pharmacokinetics

Xylose is incompletely absorbed from the gastro-intestinal tract. Part of the absorbed xylose is metabolised in the body mainly to carbon dioxide and water. In the absence of malabsorption, about 35% of a 5-g oral dose and about 25% of a 25-g oral dose are reported to be excreted in the urine within 5 hours.

Uses and Administration

Xylose is used for the investigation of absorption from the gastro-intestinal tract. It is given by mouth, usually in a dose of either 5 or 25 g, with up to 500 mL of water. The amount recovered in the urine is estimated over a certain period and that figure can be used to assess any malabsorption. Adjustment may have to be made for renal impairment.

The test has been adapted to use blood-xylose concentrations.

Preparations

Proprietary Preparations (details are given in Part 3)

Canad.: Xylo-Pfan; ***UK:*** Xylose-BMS; ***USA:*** Xylo-Pfan.

Yohimbine Hydrochloride (14024-n)

Yohimbine Hydrochloride (*rINNM*).

Aphrodine Hydrochloride; Chlorhydrate de Québrachine; Corynine Hydrochloride. Methyl 17α-hydroxy-yohimban-16α-carboxylate hydrochloride.

$C_{21}H_{26}N_2O_3$,HCl = 390.9.

CAS — 146-48-5 (yohimbine); 65-19-0 (yohimbine hydrochloride).

Pharmacopoeias. In *Aust.*

The hydrochloride of the principal alkaloid of the bark of the yohimbe tree, *Pausinystalia yohimbe* (= *Corynanthe yohimbi*) (Rubiaceae).

Yohimbine produces an α_2-adrenoceptor block of short duration. It produces an antidiuretic action, increases in heart rate and blood pressure, and orthostatic hypotension. It has been reported to cause anxiety and manic reactions. It has been given by mouth in the treatment of erectile dysfunction (p.1614) and for its alleged aphrodisiac properties but convincing evidence of such an effect is lacking. It is contra-indicated in renal or hepatic disease.

Adverse effects. A warning as to the potential adverse effects, including anxiety, manic reactions, bronchospasm and a lupus-like syndrome, associated with yohimbine taken in health food products.[1] Interactions with tricyclic antidepressants and with phenothiazines might also occur.

1. De Smet PAGM, Smeets OSNM. Potential risks of health food products containing yohimbe extracts. *Br Med J* 1994; **309:** 958.

Uses. References to the use of yohimbine in erectile dysfunction.

1. Ernst E, Pittler MH. Yohimbine for erectile dysfunction: a systematic review and meta-analysis of randomised clinical trials. *J Urol (Baltimore)* 1998; **159:** 433–6.

Preparations

Proprietary Preparations (details are given in Part 3)

Canad.: Yocon; ***Ger.:*** Yocon; ***UK:*** Prowess Plain; ***USA:*** Aphrodyne; Dayto Himbin; Yocon; Yohimex.

Multi-ingredient: ***Aust.:*** Pasuma-Dragees; ***Ger.:*** Diuraupur sine†; Diuraupur†; Ichtho-Himbin†; Pluriviron†; Sedapon D†; ***S.Afr.:*** Pasuma†; ***UK:*** Prowess.

Zanthoxylum Fruit (14025-h)

Prickly Ash Berries.

Pharmacopoeias. In *Jpn.*

The pericarp of the ripe fruit of *Zanthoxylum piperitum* (= *Xanthoxylum piperitum*) (Rutaceae) or other species of *Zanthoxylum*. It contains about 3.3% v/w of essential oil. It is an ingredient of Bitter Tincture (*Jpn P.*).

Zanthoxylum (BPC 1934) (Toothache Bark; Xanthoxylum) is the dried bark of the northern prickly ash, *Z. americanum*, or the southern prickly ash, *Z. clavaherculis*. Both varieties contain a complex mixture of components, including benzophenanthridine alkaloids; northern prickly ash also contains coumarins.

Zanthoxylum fruit has carminative properties and has been used for rheumatic disorders. Zanthoxylum bark has been used similarly, but there is some concern about the potential toxicity of the benzophenanthridine alkaloids which it contains, and some authorities consider that it should not be recommended.

Preparations

Proprietary Preparations (details are given in Part 3)

Multi-ingredient: ***Austral.:*** For Peripheral Circulation Herbal Plus Formula 5; Lifesystem Herbal Formula 6 For Peripheral Circulation; Uva-Ursi Plus; ***UK:*** Peerless Composition Essence; Rheumasol; Tabritis.

Zein (3925-j)

Pharmacopoeias. In *USNF.*

A prolamine derived from corn, *Zea mays* (Gramineae). A white to yellow powder. Practically **insoluble** in water and in acetone; readily soluble in acetone-water mixtures (acetone 60 to 80% w/v); soluble in aqueous alcohols, in glycols, and in aqueous alkaline solutions of pH 11.5 and above; practically insoluble in all anhydrous alcohols except methyl alcohol. **Store** in airtight containers.

Zein is used as a tablet binder and coating agent for pharmaceutical preparations and foodstuffs. It has been used as a substitute for shellac.

Zinc Acetate (5328-s)

$(CH_3CO_2)_2Zn,2H_2O = 219.5.$

CAS — 557-34-6 (anhydrous zinc acetate); 5970-45-6 (zinc acetate dihydrate).

NOTE. Zinc Acetate, Basic is *rINN.*

Pharmacopoeias. In *US.*

White crystals or granules with a faint acetous odour. It effloresces slightly. **Soluble** 1 in 2.5 of water and 1 in 30 of alcohol. A 5% solution in water has a pH of 6.0 to 8.0.

Store in airtight containers.

A 1.2% solution of zinc acetate is used topically in combination with erythromycin in the treatment of acne vulgaris (p.1072). Zinc acetate, but more commonly zinc sulphate (p.1373), has been used in oral zinc supplements. Zinc acetate is also used for the treatment of Wilson's disease (p.992).

References.

1. Anderson LA, *et al.* Zinc acetate treatment in Wilson's disease. *Ann Pharmacother* 1998; **32:** 78–87.

Preparations

Proprietary Preparations (details are given in Part 3)
UK: Cold-Gard; ***USA:*** Halls Zinc Defense.

Multi-ingredient: ***Belg.:*** Zineryt; ***Ger.:*** Zineryt; ***Irl.:*** Zineryt; ***Ital.:*** Zineryt; ***Neth.:*** Zineryt; ***Switz.:*** Rocanal Permanent Gangrene; Rocanal Permanent Vital; ***UK:*** Zineryt; ***USA:*** Benadryl Itch; Caladryl Clear; Clearly Cala-gel.

Zirconium (15965-p)

Zr = 91.224.
CAS — 7440-67-7.

Zirconium and its compounds e.g. zirconium dioxide, zirconium lactate, and zirconium oxychloride, have been used in deodorant preparations. There have been reports of hypersensitivity reactions with granulomas. Zirconium dioxide has also been used as a contrast medium.

A report[1] of pulmonary fibrosis associated with inhalation of a polishing agent containing mainly zirconium dioxide with quartz.

1. Bartter T, *et al.* Zirconium compound-induced pulmonary fibrosis. *Arch Intern Med* 1991; **151:** 1197–1201.

Part 3

Preparations

This part of Martindale contains brief details of proprietary preparations available in a number of countries and includes those supplied on prescription as well as those sold directly to the public. They are provided to help the reader identify preparations and to suggest their uses. Inclusion is not an endorsement of the activity of any ingredient nor of the preparation's indications.

For this edition we have covered Australia, Austria, Belgium, Canada, France, Germany, Ireland, Italy, the Netherlands, Norway, South Africa, Spain, Sweden, Switzerland, UK, and USA. We have also included some proprietary preparations from Japan. Generally each entry consists of: the proprietary name; manufacturer or source of supply and country; ingredients usually listed by the manufacturer as being active; and a guide to the manufacturer's indications. Where possible, entries from different countries but with the same name and active ingredients have been amalgamated for clarity.

An entry may cover a range of dosage forms and strengths. Dosage forms are only specified when different forms have the same proprietary name but different active ingredients. Specifying all dosage forms and the quantity of each active ingredient would have vastly increased the number of entries. Furthermore, Part 3 is not intended as a guide to prescribing; where a preparation is to be supplied the dose should be appropriate for that preparation and that particular patient, and authoritative local sources should be consulted.

With the exception of homoeopathic preparations the names of the ingredients have been translated into English. Almost all the ingredients listed are described in the monographs in Parts 1 and 2, and readers are directed to an appropriate monograph by the page number provided after the ingredient.

We have tried to include preparations that were available in the last few years since they may still be in circulation and their names may still be referred to in the literature and in practice. Such preparations that have been withdrawn from the market or are no longer being actively marketed may be identified by the symbol †. Readers should be aware that since Part 3 was prepared other preparations are likely to have been withdrawn or introduced; also ingredients may change, as may indications.

The manufacturer's full name and address can be found in the Directory of Manufacturers.

Each preparation title is also listed in the General Index. Where thought helpful, preparation titles have also been listed at the end of the relevant monograph.

217 Frosst, Canad.
Aspirin (p.16·1); caffeine citrate (p.749·3).
Fever; inflammation; pain.

222 Frosst, Canad.
Aspirin (p.16·1); caffeine citrate (p.749·3); codeine phosphate (p.26·1).
Fever; inflammation; pain.

282 Frosst, Canad.
Aspirin (p.16·1); caffeine citrate (p.749·3); codeine phosphate (p.26·1).
Fever; inflammation; pain.

292 Frosst, Canad.
Aspirin (p.16·1); caffeine citrate (p.749·3); codeine phosphate (p.26·1).
Fever; inflammation; pain.

642 Frosst, Canad.
Dextropropoxyphene hydrochloride (p.27·3).
Pain.

692 Frosst, Canad.
Dextropropoxyphene hydrochloride (p.27·3); aspirin (p.16·1); caffeine (p.749·3).
Pain.

A-200 Hogil, USA.
Pyrethrins; piperonyl butoxide (p.1409·3).
Pediculosis.

A 313 Pharmadeveloppement, Fr.
Capsules: Vitamin A (p.1358·1).
Vitamin A deficiency.
Ointment: Vitamin A (p.1358·1); tyrothricin (p.267·2).
Dermatitis; superficial wounds and burns.

A + B Balsam N Mickan, Ger.
Menthol (p.1600·2); camphor (p.1557·2); eucalyptus oil (p.1578·1).
Respiratory-tract disorders.

A C B Therapex, Canad.†
Barium sulphate (p.1003·1).
Radiographic contrast medium.

A + D + E-Vicotrat Heyl, Ger.
Retinol palmitate (p.1359·2); cholecalciferol (p.1366·3); alpha tocopheryl acetate (p.1369·2).
Deficiency of fat-soluble vitamins.

A and D Medicated Schering-Plough, USA.
Zinc oxide (p.1096·2); cod-liver oil (p.1337·3); vitamin A (p.1358·1); vitamin D (p.1366·3).
Nappy rash.

A & D Ointment Schering, Canad.
Vitamin A (p.1358·1); vitamin D (p.1366·3).
Minor skin disorders.

A + D_3-Vicotrat Heyl, Ger.
Vitamin A palmitate (p.1359·2); cholecalciferol (p.1366·3).
Vitamin A and D_3 deficiency.

A + E Thilo Alcon-Thilo, Ger.
Vitamin A acetate (p.1359·2); alpha tocopheryl acetate (p.1369·1).
Vitamin A and E deficiency.

A Vogel Capsules a l'ail Bioforce, Switz.
Garlic (p.1583·1).
Cerebrovascular disorders.

A Vogel Capsules polyvitaminees Bioforce, Switz.
Halibut-liver oil (p.1345·3); rose fruit (p.1365·2); red cherry (p.1001·1); dried yeast (p.1373·1); safflower oil (p.1353·3).
Tonic.

A to Z Centabs Hall, Canad.
Multivitamin and mineral preparation.

A to Z Plus 4 Hall, Canad.†
Multivitamin and mineral preparation.

AAA
Note. This name is used for preparations of different composition.
Rhone-Poulenc Rorer, Irl.
Benzocaine (p.1286·2); cetylpyridinium chloride (p.1106·2).
Mouth and throat disorders.
Roche, S.Afr.; Manx, UK.
Benzocaine (p.1286·2); cetalkonium chloride (p.1105·2).
Mouth and throat disorders.

Aacidexam Aaciphar, Belg.
Dexamethasone sodium phosphate (p.1037·2).
Corticosteroid.

Aacifemine Aaciphar, Belg.
Oestriol (p.1457·2).
Oestrogen deficiency.

AA-HC Otic Schein, USA.
Hydrocortisone (p.1043·3); glacial acetic acid (p.1541·2); propylene glycol diacetate (p.1328·2); benzethonium chloride (p.1102·3).
Ear infection.

Aarane
Schoeller, Aust.; Fisons, Ger.; Rhone-Poulenc Rorer, Ger.; Fisons, Switz.
Sodium cromoglycate (p.762·1); reproterol hydrochloride (p.758·1).
Obstructive airways disease.

AAS Sanofi Winthrop, Spain.
Aspirin (p.16·1).
Fever; inflammation; pain; thrombo-embolism prophylaxis.

AB FE Camps, Spain.
Aspirin (p.16·1); caffeine (p.749·3); phenazone (p.78·2).
Fever; pain.

Abacin Benedetti, Ital.
Co-trimoxazole (p.196·3).
Bacterial infections.

Abactrim Andreu, Spain.
Co-trimoxazole (p.196·3).
Bacterial infections; Pneumocystis carinii pneumonia.

Abactrim Balsamico Roche, Spain†.
Ammonium chloride (p.1055·2); guaiphenesin (p.1061·3); co-trimoxazole (p.196·3).
Respiratory-tract infections.

Abadox Lafar, Ital.†.
Doxycycline hydrochloride (p.202·3).
Bacterial infections.

Abaprim Gentili, Ital.
Trimethoprim (p.265·1).
Bacterial infections.

Abbemetic Abbott, S.Afr.†.
Metoclopramide hydrochloride (p.1200·3).
Gastro-intestinal disorders.

Abbenclamide Abbott, S.Afr.†.
Glibenclamide (p.319·3).
Diabetes mellitus.

Abbifen Abbott, S.Afr.†.
Ibuprofen (p.44·1).
Musculoskeletal and joint disorders.

Abbiofort Synpharma, Aust.
Caraway (p.1559·3); psyllium (p.1194·2).
Constipation; stool softener.

Abbocillin-V Abbott, Austral.
Benzathine phenoxymethylpenicillin (p.159·2).
Bacterial infections.

Abbocillin-VK Abbott, Austral.
Phenoxymethylpenicillin potassium (p.236·2).
Bacterial infections.

Abbodop Abbott, Swed.
Dopamine hydrochloride (p.861·1).
Shock.

Abbokinase
Abbott, Aust.; Abbott, Canad.; Abbott, Ger.†; Abbott, Spain; Abbott, Swed.; Abbott, USA.
Urokinase (p.959·3).
Intra-ocular haemorrhage; pulmonary embolism; thrombo-embolic disorders; to restore patency of intravenous shunts.

Abbolipid Abbott, Ger.
Safflower oil (p.1353·3); soya oil (p.1355·1).
Lipid infusion for parenteral nutrition.

Abbonidazole Abbott, S.Afr.†.
Metronidazole (p.585·1).
Anaerobic bacterial infections; protozoal infections.

Abbopen Abbott, Swed.†.
Phenoxymethylpenicillin potassium (p.236·2).
Bacterial infections.

Abboplegisol Abbott, Spain.
Electrolyte infusion (p.1147·1).
Adjunct to open-heart surgery.

Abboticin
Abbott, Norw.; Abbott, Swed.
Erythromycin (p.204·1), erythromycin ethyl succinate (p.204·2), or erythromycin lactobionate (p.204·2).
Bacterial infections.

Abboticine Abbott, Fr.
Erythromycin ethyl succinate (p.204·2).
Bacterial infections.

Abbottselsun Abbott, Spain.
Selenium sulphide (p.1091·1).
Skin disorders.

Abburic Quick-Med, S.Afr.†.
Allopurinol (p.390·2).
Gout; hyperuricaemia.

Abbutamol Norton, S.Afr.†.
Salbutamol (p.758·2).
Obstructive airways disease.

ABC Beiersdorf, Aust.
Capsicum (p.1559·2).
Muscle and joint pain.

ABC Warme-Pflaster N Beiersdorf, Ger.
Arnica flowers (p.1550·3); cayenne pepper.
Musculoskeletal and joint disorders.

ABC Warme-Pflaster Sensitive Beiersdorf, Ger.
Nonivamide (p.63·2).
Musculoskeletal, joint, peri-articular, and soft-tissue disorders.

ABC Warme-Salbe Beiersdorf, Ger.
Diethylamine salicylate (p.33·1); benzyl nicotinate (p.22·1); nonivamide (p.63·2).
Bruises; musculoskeletal and joint disorders; neuralgia; sprains.

ABC to Z Nature's Bounty, USA.
Ferrous fumarate (p.1339·3); folic acid (p.1340·3); multivitamins and minerals.
Iron-deficiency anaemias.

ABC-Bad Beiersdorf, Ger.†.
Salicylamide (p.82·3); benzyl nicotinate (p.22·1).
Bath additive; musculoskeletal and joint disorders; neuralgia; peripheral vascular disorders.

Abdijsiroop (Akker-Siroop) Chefaro, Neth.†.
Belladonna tincture (p.457·1); drosera (p.1574·1); ipecacuanha tincture (p.1062·2); primula tincture; ephedrine hydrochloride (p.1059·3).
Coughs.

Abdomilon Herchemie, Aust.†.
Absinthium (p.1541·1); angelica; calamus (p.1556·1); frangula bark (p.1193·2); gentian (p.1583·3); melissa (p.1600·1); rhubarb (p.1212·1).
Dyspepsia.

Abdomilon N Redel, Ger.
Absinthium (p.1541·1); angelica root; calamus root (p.1556·1); gentian root (p.1583·3); melissa leaves (p.1600·1).
Gastro-intestinal disorders.

Abdominol Medea, Spain.
Atropine methobromide (p.455·1); caffeine (p.749·3); propyphenazone (p.81·3).
Pain due to smooth muscle spasm.

Abdoscan
Nycomed, Ger.; Nycomed Imaging, Norw.; Nycomed, Swed.; Nycomed, Switz.; Nycomed, UK.
Ferristene (p.1004·2).
Contrast medium for magnetic resonance imaging.

Abelcet
Liposome Company, Irl.; Pensa, Spain; Liposome Company, Swed.; Liposome Company, UK.
Amphotericin (p.372·2).
Fungal infections.

Abenol SmithKline Beecham, Canad.
Paracetamol (p.72·2).
Fever; pain.

Aberel Janssen-Cilag, Fr.
Tretinoin (p.1093·3).
Acne; keratinisation disorders.

Aberela
Janssen-Cilag, Norw.; Janssen-Cilag, Swed.
Tretinoin (p.1093·3).
Acne.

Abesira Clariana, Spain.
Vitamin B substances and amino acids.
Anaemias; metabolic disorders; tonic.

Abetol CT, Ital.
Labetalol hydrochloride (p.896·1).
Hypertension.

Abflex Xeragen, S.Afr.
Paracetamol (p.72·2); doxylamine succinate (p.410·1); caffeine (p.749·3); codeine phosphate (p.26·1).
Pain with tension.

Abfuhrdragees Waldheim, Aust.
Aloes (p.1177·1); phenolphthalein (p.1208·2); hard soap (p.1468·2).
Constipation.

Abfuhrdragees mild Waldheim, Aust.
Aloes (p.1177·1); frangula bark (p.1193·2); hard soap (p.1468·2).
Bowel evacuation; constipation.

Abfuhrtee Waldheim, Aust.
Couch-grass (p.1567·3); chamomile (p.1561·2); centaurea cyanus; frangula bark (p.1193·2); rhubarb (p.1212·1); senna (p.1212·2).
Constipation.

Abfuhr-Tee Depuraflux Nattermann Tee-Arznei, Ger.†.
Plant tea: Senna (p.1212·2); aniseed (p.1549·3); caraway (p.1559·3); coriander (p.1567·3); fennel (p.1579·1); achillea (p.1542·2); viola tricolor; liquorice (p.1197·1); tartaric acid (p.1634·3).
Tea powder: Frangula bark (p.1193·2); aniseed (p.1549·3); caraway (p.1559·3); coriander (p.1567·3); fennel (p.1579·1); peppermint leaf (p.1208·1); senna (p.1212·2); centaury (p.1561·1); equisetum (p.1575·1); anise oil (p.1550·1); caraway oil (p.1559·3); coriander oil (p.1567·3); fennel oil (p.1579·2); peppermint oil (p.1208·1).
Constipation.

Abfuhrtee EF-EM-ES Smetana, Aust.
Achillea (p.1542·2); peppermint leaf (p.1208·1); senna (p.1212·2).
Formerly contained frangula bark, hypericum, peppermint leaf, and senna.
Bowel evacuation; constipation.

Abfuhrtee Solubilax N Heumann, Ger.†.
Senna leaf (p.1212·2); frangula bark (p.1193·2).
Constipation.

Abfuhr-Tee Stada Stada, Ger.†.
Mallow flower; calendula officinalis; fennel (p.1579·1); aniseed (p.1549·3); viola tricoloris; sambucus (p.1627·2); red sandalwood; convolvulus; ononis (p.1610·2); frangula bark (p.1193·2); senna (p.1212·2); liquorice (p.1197·1); phaseolus; anise oil (p.1550·1).
Constipation.

Abfuhrtropfen Ratiopharm, Ger.
Sodium picosulphate (p.1213·2).
Constipation.

Abi Medix, Fr.†.
Triethanolamine (p.1639·1); stearic acid (p.1632·3); cetyl palmitate.
Burns and wounds.

Abiadin Boehringer Ingelheim, Ger.†.
Orciprenaline sulphate (p.756·3); bromhexine hydrochloride (p.1055·3); doxylamine succinate (p.410·1).
Bronchitis; tracheobronchitis.

Abidec
Warner-Lambert, Irl.; Teofarma, Ital.; Parke, Davis, S.Afr.†; Parke, Davis, UK.
Multivitamin preparation.

Abiocef Nuovo, Ital.†.
Cephalexin monohydrate (p.178·2).
Bacterial infections.

Abiosan L'Arguenon, Fr.†.
Tetracycline hydrochloride (p.259·1); sodium aminobenzoate.
Bacterial infections.

Abiostil Deca, Ital.
Neomycin sulphate (p.229·2); cineole (p.1564·1); pumilio pine oil (p.1623·3); camphor (p.1557·2); menthol (p.1600·2).
Nasopharyngeal infections.

Abiplatin
Donau, Aust.; Abic, Neth.†; Intramed, S.Afr.
Cisplatin (p.513·3).
Malignant neoplasms.

Abiposid Donau, Aust.
Etoposide (p.532·3).
Malignant neoplasms.

Abitrexate
Donau, Aust.; Intramed, S.Afr.; International Pharmaceutical, USA.
Methotrexate sodium (p.547·1).
Malignant neoplasms; psoriasis.

Ablacton Schering, Ital.†.
Norethisterone acetate (p.1453·1); testosterone enanthate (p.1464·1); oestradiol valerate (p.1455·2); oestradiol benzoate (p.1455·1).
Inhibition of lactation.

Abnobaviscum Abnoba, Ger.
Mistletoe (p.1604·1).
Malignant neoplasms.

Abramen Mepha, Switz.†.
Ambroxol hydrochloride (p.1054·3).
Respiratory-tract disorders.

Abrasone Seid, Spain.
Fluocinolone acetonide (p.1041·1); framycetin sulphate (p.210·3).
Infected skin disorders.

Abrasone Rectal Seid, Spain.
Fluocinonide acetonide (p.1041·2); hexetidine (p.1116·1); ruscogenin (p.1627·1).
Anorectal disorders.

Abrinac Boots, Neth.†.
Pirenzepine hydrochloride (p.467·1).
Peptic ulcer; Zollinger-Ellison syndrome.

Absenor Orion, Swed.
Sodium valproate (p.361·2).
Epilepsy.

Absimed Synpharma, Aust.
Caraway (p.1559·3); melissa (p.1600·1); valerian (p.1643·1).
Gastro-intestinal disorders.

Absorbase Carolina, USA.
Vehicle for topical preparations.

Absorber HFV Artevo, Ger.
Simethicone (p.1213·1).
Reduction of gastro-intestinal gas.

Absorbine Analgesic Young, Canad.
Methyl salicylate (p.55·2); camphor (p.1557·2); menthol (p.1600·2); eucalyptus oil (p.1578·1).

Absorbine Antifungal
Young, Canad.; Young, USA†.
Tolnaftate (p.389·1).
Fungal skin infections.

Absorbine Antifungal Foot Powder Young, USA.
Miconazole nitrate (p.384·3).
Fungal skin infections.

Absorbine Athletes Foot Care Young, USA.
Tolnaftate (p.389·1); menthol (p.1600·2).
Fungal infections.

Absorbine Jr
Young, Canad.; Young, USA.
Menthol (p.1600·2).
Muscle, joint, and soft-tissue pain; neuralgia.

Absorbine Jr Antifungal Young, Canad.
Tolnaftate (p.389·1); menthol (p.1600·2).
Tinea pedis.

Absorbine Power Gel
Young, Canad.; Young, USA.
Menthol (p.1600·2).
Muscular aches.

Absorlent Esteve, Spain.
Oestradiol (p.1455·1).
Menopausal disorders.

Absorlent Plus Esteve, Spain.
Patch A, oestradiol (p.1455·1); patch B, oestradiol; norethisterone acetate (p.1453·1).
Menopausal disorders.

Abstem Wyeth, Irl.
Calcium carbimide (p.1556·2).
Alcoholism.

Abufene Doms-Adrian, Fr.
Beta-alanine (p.1333·3).
Menopausal disorders.

Abulen Searle, Swed.†.
Dimethicone 1000 (p.1213·1).
Flatulence.

AC & C WestCan, Canad.; Wampole, Canad.
Aspirin (p.16·1); caffeine (p.749·3); codeine phosphate (p.26·1).
Fever; inflammation; pain.

AC Crisina Syntex, Spain†.
Ascorbic acid (p.1365·2); vitamin A palmitate (p.1359·2).
Deficiency of vitamins A and C.

AC Vax SmithKline Beecham, UK.
A meningococcal vaccine (groups A and C) (p.1520·3).
Active immunisation.

Acacia Complex Blackmores, Austral.†.
Geranium maculatum; acacia catechu (p.1560·3); hamamelis virginiana (p.1587·1); agrimonia eupatoria; sodium ascorbate; vitamin B substances; folic acid.
Diarrhoea; dysentery; mucous colitis.

Acadione Cassenne, Fr.
Tiopronin (p.997·2).
Cystinuric lithiasis; polyarthritis.

A-Caine AVP, USA.
Diperodon hydrochloride (p.1292·3); mepyramine maleate (p.414·1); phenylephrine hydrochloride (p.1066·2); bismuth subcarbonate (p.1180·1); zinc oxide (p.1096·2).
Anorectal disorders.

Acalka Robert, Spain.
Potassium citrate (p.1153·1).
Alkalinisation of urine; renal calculi.

Acarcid Pierre Fabre, Fr.
Acetamide; crotamiton (p.1081·1); benzalkonium chloride (p.1101·3); thyme oil (p.1637·1); geranium oil (p.1584·1); myrtle oil.
Elimination of house dust mites.

Acardust
SCAT, Fr.; Geymonat, Ital.; SCAT, Switz.
Esdepallethrine (p.1406·1); piperonyl butoxide (p.1409·3).
Acaricide; house dust mite allergies (adjuvant).

Acaren Bio-Therabel, Belg.†.
Vitamin A acetate (p.1359·2).
Vitamin A deficiency.

Acarex
Allergopharma, Ger.; Crawford, UK†.
Potassium hydroxide (p.1621·1); methyl alcohol (p.1379·2).
Test for detection of house dust mite excretae.

Acarosan
Allergopharma, Ger.
Benzyl benzoate (p.1402·2).
Elimination of house dust mites.

Crawford, UK†.
Carbonic acid esters.
Elimination of house dust mites.

ACC
Hexal, Aust.; Hexal, Ger.
Acetylcysteine (p.1052·3) or acetylcysteine sodium (p.1053·1).
Respiratory-tract disorders with increased or viscous mucus.

ACC200 Hexal, S.Afr.
Acetylcysteine (p.1052·3).
Paracetamol overdosage; respiratory-tract disorders.

Accolate
Zeneca, Irl.; Zeneca, UK; Zeneca, USA.
Zafirlukast (p.774·2).
Asthma.

Accomin Whitehall, Austral.
Multivitamin and mineral preparation.

Accomin Centrum Whitehall, Austral.
Capsules: Multivitamin and mineral preparation with lysine.
Oral liquid: Multivitamin preparation with lysine and iron.

Accomin Vitamin Whitehall, Austral.
Amino-acid, vitamin, and iron preparation.

Accu-Check Advantage Boehringer Mannheim, USA.
Test for glucose in blood (p.1585·1).

Accu-Check III/Chemstrip bG Boehringer Mannheim, Canad.
Test for glucose in blood (p.1585·1).

Accu-Chek Boehringer Mannheim, Fr.
Test for glucose in blood (p.1585·1).

Accupaque Nycomed, Ger.
Iohexol (p.1006·3).
Radiographic contrast medium.

Accupep Sherwood, USA.
Preparation for enteral nutrition.
Gastro-intestinal disorders.

Accuprep Wyeth-Ayerst, Canad.†.
Preparation for enteral nutrition.

Accupril
Parke, Davis, Austral.; Parke, Davis, Belg.; Parke, Davis, Canad.; Parke, Davis, S.Afr.; Parke, Davis, USA.
Quinapril hydrochloride (p.938·1).
Heart failure; hypertension.

Accuprin Parke, Davis, Ital.
Quinapril hydrochloride (p.938·1).
Heart failure; hypertension.

Accupro
Parke, Davis, Aust.; Godecke, Ger.; Parke, Davis, Ger.; Parke, Davis, Irl.; Parke, Davis, Swed.; Warner-Lambert, Switz.; Parke, Davis, UK.
Quinapril hydrochloride (p.938·1) or quinaprilat (p.938·2).
Heart failure; hypertension.

Accupro Comp Parke, Davis, Swed.
Quinapril hydrochloride (p.938·1); hydrochlorothiazide (p.885·2).
Hypertension.

Accurbron Marion Merrell Dow, USA.
Theophylline (p.765·1).
Asthma; bronchospasm.

Accure Alphapharm, Austral.
Isotretinoin (p.1084·1).
Acne.

Accuretic
Parke, Davis, Belg.; Parke, Davis, Irl.; Parke, Davis, Ital.; Parke, Davis, S.Afr.; Warner-Lambert, Switz.; Parke, Davis, UK.
Quinapril hydrochloride (p.938·1); hydrochlorothiazide (p.885·2).
Hypertension.

AccuSite Matrix, UK†.
Fluorouracil (p.534·3).
Adrenaline (p.813·2) is included in this preparation as a vasoconstrictor to diminish absorption and localise the effect of the antineoplastic.
Genital warts.

Accutane
Roche, Canad.; Roche Dermatologics, USA.
Isotretinoin (p.1084·1).
Acne.

Accutrend Cholesterol
Boehringer Mannheim, Ital.; Boehringer Mannheim Diagnostics, UK.
Test for cholesterol in blood.

Accutrend GC Boehringer Mannheim, Canad.
Test for glucose and cholesterol in blood (p.1585·1).

Accutrend Glucose Boehringer Mannheim, Ital.
Test for glucose in blood (p.1585·1).

Accuzide
Parke, Davis, Aust.; Godecke, Ger.; Parke, Davis, Ger.
Quinapril hydrochloride (p.938·1); hydrochlorothiazide (p.885·2).
Hypertension.

Acdril Eurorga, Fr.†.
Arginine acetylasparaginate (p.1334·2).
Tonic.

ACE + Z Legere, USA†.
Vitamin and mineral preparation.

Acecol Sankyo, Jpn.
Temocapril hydrochloride (p.951·3).
Hypertension.

Acecomb Zeneca, Aust.
Hydrochlorothiazide (p.885·2); lisinopril (p.898·2).
Hypertension.

Acecor SPA, Ital.
Acebutolol hydrochloride (p.809·3).
Arrhythmias; heart failure; hypertension.

acecromol Wolff, Ger.
Sodium cromoglycate (p.762·1).
Asthma.

Acedicone Boehringer Ingelheim, Belg.
Thebacon hydrochloride (p.1070·3).
Coughs.

Acediur
Note. This name is used for preparations of different composition.
Menarini, Ital.
Captopril (p.836·3); hydrochlorothiazide (p.885·2).
Hypertension.

Sigma-Tau, Spain.
Enalapril maleate (p.863·2); hydrochlorothiazide (p.885·2).
Hypertension.

Acef Eurofarmaco, Ital.
Cephazolin sodium (p.181·1).
Bacterial infections.

ACE-Hemmer Ratiopharm, Ger.
Captopril (p.836·3).
Heart failure; hypertension.

Aceite Acalorico Ordesa, Spain.
Olive oil (p.1610·1); betacarotene (p.1335·2); liquid paraffin (p.1382·1).
Constipation; obesity.

Aceite Geve Concentrado Bama, Spain.
Cod-liver oil (p.1337·3).
Deficiency of vitamins A and D.

Acel-Imune
Lederle, Switz.; Lederle-Praxis, USA.
An adsorbed diphtheria, tetanus, and acellular pertussis vaccine (p.1509·1).
Active immunisation of infants and young children.

Acelluvax Biocine, Ital.
An acellular pertussis vaccine (p.1526·1).
Active immunisation.

Acel-P *Lederle, Ger.; Lederle, Switz.*
An adsorbed acellular pertussis vaccine (p.1526·1).
Active immunisation.

Acemin *Zeneca, Aust.*
Lisinopril (p.898·2).
Heart failure; hypertension; myocardial infarction.

Acemix *Bioprogress, Ital.*
Acemetacin (p.12·2).
Musculoskeletal and joint disorders.

Acemuc *Betapharm, Ger.*
Acetylcysteine (p.1052·3).
Respiratory-tract disorders with viscous mucus.

Acemucol *Streuli, Switz.*
Acetylcysteine (p.1052·3).
Respiratory-tract disorders associated with excess or viscous mucus.

Acenorm
Alphapharm, Austral.; Azupharma, Ger.
Captopril (p.836·3).
Diabetic nephropathy; heart failure; hypertension; myocardial infarction.

Acenterine *Christiaens, Belg.*
Aspirin (p.16·1).
Musculoskeletal and joint disorders.

Aceomel *Clonmel, Irl.*
Captopril (p.836·3).
Heart failure; hypertension.

Aceon *Ortho Pharmaceutical, USA.*
Perindopril erbumine (p.928·2).
Hypertension.

Acephen *G & W, USA.*
Paracetamol (p.72·2).
Pain.

Aceplus
Bristol-Myers Squibb, Ital.; Bristol-Myers Squibb, Neth.
Captopril (p.836·3); hydrochlorothiazide (p.885·2).
Hypertension.

Acepress *Bristol-Myers Squibb, Ital.*
Captopril (p.836·3).
Diabetic nephropathy; heart failure; hypertension; myocardial infarction.

Acepril *Squibb, UK.*
Captopril (p.836·3).
Diabetic nephropathy; heart failure; hypertension; myocardial infarction.

Acequide *Recordati, Ital.*
Quinapril hydrochloride (p.938·1); hydrochlorothiazide (p.885·2).
Hypertension.

Acequin *Recordati, Ital.*
Quinapril hydrochloride (p.938·1).
Heart failure; hypertension.

Acerbine
Note. This name is used for preparations of different composition.
Montavit, Aust.
Benzoic acid (p.1102·3); malic acid (p.1598·3); propylene glycol (p.1622·1); propylene glycol malate (p.1622·2); salicylic acid (p.1090·2).
Bruises; burns; sunburn; ulcers; wounds.

Lucchini, Switz.
Ointment: Benzoic acid (p.1102·3); malic acid (p.1598·3); salicylic acid (p.1090·2); propylene glycol (p.1622·1); propylene glycol malate (p.1622·2); hexachlorophane (p.1115·2).
Topical solution; topical gel: Benzoic acid (p.1102·3); malic acid (p.1598·3); salicylic acid (p.1090·2); propylene glycol (p.1622·1); propylene glycol malate (p.1622·2).
Burns; wounds.

Acerbiol *Vitafarma, Spain.*
Benzyl alcohol (p.1103·3); benzoic acid (p.1102·3); malic acid (p.1598·3); propylene glycol malate (p.1622·2); propylene glycol (p.1622·1); salicylic acid (p.1090·2).
Burns; wounds.

Acerbon *Zeneca, Ger.*
Lisinopril (p.898·2).
Heart failure; hypertension.

Acercomp *Zeneca, Ger.*
Lisinopril (p.898·2); hydrochlorothiazide (p.885·2).
Hypertension.

Acerola Complex *Suisse, Austral.†.*
Ascorbic acid (p.1365·2); hesperidin-rutin-buckwheat-citrus bioflavonoid complex (p.1580·1).
Vitamin C deficiency.

Acertol *Lacer, Spain.*
Paracetamol (p.72·2).
Fever; pain.

Acesal
OPW, Ger.; Roland, Ger.; Geymonat, Ital.
Aspirin (p.16·1).
Fever; musculoskeletal and joint disorders; pain.

Acesal Calcium *OPW, Ger.; Roland, Ger.*
Aspirin (p.16·1).
Calcium carbonate (p.1182·1) is included in this preparation in an attempt to limit adverse effects on the gastro-intestinal mucosa.
Fever; pain; rheumatism; thrombo-embolic disorders.

Acesistem *Sigma-Tau, Ital.*
Enalapril maleate (p.863·2); hydrochlorothiazide (p.885·2).
Hypertension.

Acet-2, Acet-3 *Pharmascience, Canad.*
Paracetamol (p.72·2); codeine phosphate (p.26·1); caffeine (p.749·3).
Fever; pain.

Acet Codeine *Pharmascience, Canad.*
Paracetamol (p.72·2); codeine phosphate (p.26·1).
Fever; pain.

Aceta *Century, USA.*
Paracetamol (p.72·2).
Fever; pain.

Aceta with Codeine *Century, USA.*
Paracetamol (p.72·2); codeine phosphate (p.26·1).
Pain.

Acetab *Romilo, Canad.*
Paracetamol (p.72·2).

Acetaco *Legere, USA†.*
Paracetamol (p.72·2); codeine phosphate (p.26·1).

Aceta-Gesic *Rugby, USA.*
Phenyltoloxamine citrate (p.416·1); paracetamol (p.72·2).
Upper respiratory-tract symptoms.

Acetalgine *Streuli, Switz.*
Paracetamol (p.72·2).
Fever; pain.

Acetaminophen with Codeine *Pharmascience, Canad.*
Paracetamol (p.72·2); caffeine (p.749·3); codeine phosphate (p.26·1).
Coughs; fever; pain.

Acetamol *Abiogen, Ital.*
Paracetamol (p.72·2).
Pain.

Acetapon *Pharmagen, S.Afr.†.*
Aspirin (p.16·1); paracetamol (p.72·2); codeine phosphate (p.26·1).
Fever; pain.

Acetard *Benzon, Swed.†.*
Aspirin (p.16·1).
Fever; inflammation; pain.

Acetasol *Barre-National, USA.*
Acetic acid (p.1541·2); propylene glycol acetate (p.1328·2); benzethonium chloride (p.1102·3).
Ear infection.

Acetasol HC *Barre-National, USA.*
Hydrocortisone (p.1043·3); acetic acid (p.1541·2); propylene glycol diacetate (p.1328·2); benzethonium chloride (p.1102·3).
Ear infection.

Acetat-Haemodialyse *Alte Kreis, Aust.*
Electrolytes with or without glucose (p.1151·1).
Haemodialysis solutions.

Acetazone Forte *Technilab, Canad.*
Chlorzoxazone (p.1313·1); paracetamol (p.72·2).
Pain; skeletal muscle spasm.

Acetazone Forte C8 *Technilab, Canad.*
Chlorzoxazone (p.1313·1); paracetamol (p.72·2); codeine phosphate (p.26·1).
Pain; skeletal muscle spasm.

Acetensil *Andromaco, Spain.*
Enalapril maleate (p.863·2).
Heart failure; hypertension.

Acetensil Plus *Andromaco, Spain.*
Enalapril maleate (p.863·2); hydrochlorothiazide (p.885·2).
Hypertension.

Acetest
Miles, Canad.†; Bayer Diagnostics, Fr.; Ames, Irl.; Bayer Diagnostics, UK; Bayer, USA.
Test for ketones in urine, plasma, or serum.
In the UK these are described in the Drug Tariff as Nitroprusside Reagent Tablets (Rothera's Tablets).

Acethropan *Hoechst, Ger.†.*
Corticotrophin (porcine) (p.1244·2).
Corticosteroid release stimulant; multiple sclerosis.

Acetocaustin *Asta Medica, Ger.*
Monochloroacetic acid.
Verrucas.

Acetocaustine *Asta Medica, Switz.*
Monochloroacetic acid.
Warts.

Acetolyt
Madaus, Aust.; Madaus, Ger.
Calcium-sodium-hydrogencitrate.
Metabolic acidosis.

Acetonal
Brady, Aust.
Aluminium acetotartrate (p.1547·3); trichlorisobutyl salicylate.
Anorectal disorders.

Athenstaedt, Ger.†.
Aluminium subacetate tartrate; (2,2,2-trichlor-1,1-dimethylethyl)-salicylate.
Anorectal disorders.

Acetonal Vaginale *Athenstaedt, Ger.†.*
Aluminium acetotartrate (p.1547·3); (2,2,2-trichlor-1,1-dimethylethyl)-salicylate; oestradiol benzoate (p.1455·1); sulphanilamide (p.256·3).
Vaginal infections; vaginitis.

Acetopt *Sigma, Austral.*
Sulphacetamide sodium (p.252·2).
Conjunctival infections.

Acetoxyl
Stiefel, Canad.; Stiefel, UK†.
Benzoyl peroxide (p.1079·2).
Acne.

Acetuber *ICN, Spain.*
Injection: Pituitary extract (p.1258·3).
Suppositories: Cocarboxylase (p.1361·2); dimenhydrinate (p.408·2); glucose (p.1343·3); pyridoxine (p.1363·1); potassium chloride (p.1161·1); dibasic sodium phosphate (p.1159·3).
Acetonaemia; vomiting in pregnancy.

Acetylcodone *Bios, Belg.*
Acetyldihydrocodeine hydrochloride (p.1054·2).
Coughs.

Acetylin *Bristol-Myers Squibb, Ger.*
Aspirin (p.16·1).
Fever; pain; rheumatism.

Acetyst *Yamanouchi, Ger.*
Acetylcysteine (p.1052·3).
Respiratory-tract disorders associated with increased or viscous mucus.

Acezide *Squibb, UK.*
Captopril (p.836·3); hydrochlorothiazide (p.885·2).
Hypertension.

Acfol *Italfarmaco, Spain.*
Folic acid (p.1340·3).
Folic acid deficiency; prevention of neural tube defects in pregnancy.

Aches-N-Pain *Lederle, USA†.*
Ibuprofen (p.44·1).
Fever; osteoarthritis; pain; rheumatoid arthritis.

Aches/Pains *Homeocan, Canad.*
Homoeopathic preparation.

Achisane Troubles du Sommeil *Dolisos, Fr.*
Crataegus (p.1568·2); tilia (p.1637·3); valerian (p.1643·1).
Insomnia.

Achrocidin *Wyeth-Ayerst, Canad.†.*
Tetracycline hydrochloride (p.259·1); caffeine (p.749·3); salicylamide (p.82·3); chloropyrilene citrate (p.405·1).
Bacterial infections.

Achromide *Propan, S.Afr.*
Mercurochrome (p.1119·2); acriflavine (p.1098·3); sulphanilamide (p.256·3); zinc oxide (p.1096·2); cod-liver oil (p.1337·3).
Burns; ulcers; wounds.

Achromycin
Cyanamid, Aust.; Lederle, Austral.; Wyeth-Ayerst, Canad.; Lederle, Ger.; Wyeth, Irl.; Lederle, S.Afr.; Wyeth Lederle, Swed.; Lederle, UK; Lederle, USA†; Storz, USA†.
Tetracycline hydrochloride (p.259·1).
Procaine hydrochloride (p.1299·2) is included in some intramuscular injections to alleviate the pain of injection.
Bacterial infections.

Achromycin V
Lederle, Austral.; Wyeth-Ayerst, Canad.; Lederle, USA†.
Tetracycline (p.259·1) or tetracycline hydrochloride (p.259·1).
Bacterial infections.

Achromycine *Lederle, Switz.*
Tetracycline hydrochloride (p.259·1).
Bacterial infections.

Aci Kestomal *Wasserman, Spain†.*
Aluminium-magnesium hydroxide co-dried gel (p.1198·1); dimethicone (p.1213·1); magnesium carbonate (p.1198·1); magnesium oxide (p.1198·3); metoclopramide hydrochloride (p.1200·3).
Gastro-intestinal disorders.

Acic *Hexal, Ger.*
Aciclovir (p.602·3) or aciclovir sodium (p.602·3).
Herpesvirus infections.

Aciclin *IFI, Ital.*
Aciclovir (p.602·3).
Herpesvirus infections.

Aciclobeta *Betapharm, Ger.*
Aciclovir (p.602·3).
Herpesvirus infections.

Acicloftal *Bruschettini, Ital.†.*
Aciclovir (p.602·3).
Herpes simplex keratitis.

Aciclostad *Stada, Ger.*
Aciclovir (p.602·3).
Herpesvirus infections.

Acic-Ophtal *Winzer, Ger.*
Aciclovir (p.602·3).
Herpes simplex eye infections.

Acid A Vit
Roche, Belg.†; Roche, Neth.†.
Tretinoin (p.1093·3).
Acne.

Acid Mantle
Note. This name is used for preparations of different composition.
Miles, Canad.†.
Aluminium acetate (p.1547·3).
Skin irritation.

Sandoz Consumer, USA.
An ointment base.

Acidac *Rovifarma, Spain.*
Aluminium hydroxide (p.1177·3); dimethicone (p.1213·1); magnesium carbonate (p.1198·1); magnesium hydroxide (p.1198·2).
Flatulence; hyperchlorhydria.

Acide acetylsalicylique comp. "Radix" *Streuli, Switz.*
Aspirin (p.16·1); paracetamol (p.72·2); codeine hydrochloride (p.26·1); lignocaine hydrochloride (p.1293·2).
Fever; pain.

Acid-Eze *Norton, UK.*
Cimetidine (p.1183·2).
Dyspepsia; heartburn.

Acidion *Inibsa, Spain.*
Oral solution†: Aluminium hydroxide (p.1177·3); dimethicone (p.1213·1); magnesium hydroxide (p.1198·2).
Gastro-intestinal disorders.
Tablets: Aluminium hydroxide (p.1177·3); dimethicone (p.1213·1); magnesium carbonate (p.1198·1); magnesium hydroxide (p.1198·2).
Flatulence; hyperacidity.

Acidodermil *Vifor, Switz.*
Bornyl salicylate (p.22·1); mint oil (p.1604·1); rosemary oil (p.1626·2).
Skin disorders.

Acidona *Vicente, Spain†.*
Ammonium fluoride; hydrochloric acid (p.1588·3); lactic-acid-producing organisms (p.1594·1); pepsin (p.1616·3).
Dyspepsia; hypochlorhydria.

Acidonorm *Searle, Ger.†.*
Aluminium hydroxide gel (p.1177·3); calcium carbonate (p.1182·1).
Gastro-intestinal disorders.

Acidophilus *Zyma, Ger.*
Lactobacillus acidophilus (p.1594·1).
Gastro-intestinal disorders.

Acidophilus Complex *Neo-Life, Austral.*
Lactobacillus acidophilus (p.1594·1); *Lactobacillus bulgaricus* (p.1594·1); *Bifidobacterium bifidum* (*Bacillus bifidus*) (p.1594·1).
Digestive disorders.

Acidophilus Plus *Quest, UK.*
Lactobacillus acidophilus (p.1594·1); *Lactobacillus rhamnosus* (p.1594·1); *Lactobacillus bifidus* (p.1594·1); *Streptococcus faecium* (p.1594·1).

Acidophilus Tablets *Vita Glow, Austral.*
Lactobacillus acidophilus (p.1594·1).
Formerly known as Vitaglow Acidophilus.
Vaginal and gastro-intestinal disorders.

Acidosis *Potter's, UK.*
Meadowsweet (p.1599·1); vegetable charcoal (p.972·3); rhubarb (p.1212·1).
Dyspepsia.

Acidovert *Klein, Ger.*
Calcium citrate (p.1155·1); magnesium citrate (p.1198·2).
Acid-base regulation; metabolic acidosis.

Acidown *Brunel, S.Afr.*
Cimetidine (p.1183·2).
Gastro-intestinal disorders.

Acidrina *Solvay, Spain.*
Aluminium hydroxide (p.1177·3); dimethicone (p.1213·1); magnesium hydroxide (p.1198·2).
Gastro-intestinal disorders.

Acidrine
Solvay, Aust.; Solvay, Belg.; Solvay, Fr.; Solvay, Ger.; Solvay, Ital.
Aluminium glycinate (p.1177·2); galactane sulphate; myrtecaine lauryl sulphate (p.1297·3).
Gastro-intestinal disorders.

Acidulin *Lilly, USA†.*
Glutamic acid hydrochloride (p.1344·3).
Gastric acidifier.

Acidum phosphoricum Med Complex *Dynamit, Aust.*
Homoeopathic preparation.

Acidum picrinicum Med Complex *Dynamit, Aust.*
Homoeopathic preparation.

Acid-X *BDI, USA.*
Paracetamol (p.72·2); calcium carbonate (p.1182·1).
Gastro-intestinal disorders.

Acidylina *Fermenti, Ital.*
Ascorbic acid (p.1365·2).

Aciflux *SmithKline Beecham, Neth.*
Cimetidine (p.1183·2); alginic acid (p.1470·3).
Gastro-oesophageal reflux.

Aciforin *Pharmonta, Aust.*
Formic acid (p.1581·3); methyl salicylate (p.55·2); turpentine oil (p.1641·1).
Musculoskeletal pain.

Acifugan
Henning, Ger.; Lacer, Spain; Henning, Switz.
Allopurinol (p.390·2); benzbromarone (p.392·3).
Gout; hyperuricaemia.

Aci-Jel
Note. This name is used for preparations of different composition.
Janssen-Cilag, Austral.; Ortho, Canad.†; Cilag, Swed.†; Ortho Pharmaceutical, USA.
Acetic acid (p.1541·2); hydroxyquinoline sulphate (p.1589·3); ricinoleic acid (p.1625·1); glycerol (p.1585·2).
Maintenance of vaginal acidity.

Janssen-Cilag, Irl.; Janssen-Cilag, UK.
Acetic acid (p.1541·2).
Maintenance of vaginal acidity.

Acilac *Technilab, Canad.*
Lactulose (p.1195·3).
Constipation; hepatic encephalopathy.

Acilen *IFI, Ital.*
Acetylcarnitine or acetylcarnitine hydrochloride (p.1542·1).
Cerebrovascular disorders; peripheral neuropathy.

Aciloc *Orion, Swed.*
Cimetidine (p.1183·2) or cimetidine hydrochloride (p.1185·3).
Gastro-oesophageal reflux; peptic ulcer; Zollinger-Ellison syndrome.

Aci-Med *Triomed, S.Afr.*
Cimetidine (p.1183·2).
Gastro-oesophageal reflux; peptic ulcer; upper gastro-intestinal haemorrhage; Zollinger-Ellison syndrome.

Acimethin
Madaus, Aust.; Gry, Ger.; Gry, Switz.
Methionine (p.984·2).
Adjunct in antibiotic therapy; paracetamol overdosage; renal calculi; urinary-tract disorders.

Acimetten *Pharmonta, Aust.*
Aspirin (p.16·1).
Fever; pain.

Acinil *GEA, Swed.*
Cimetidine (p.1183·2).
Gastro-oesophageal reflux; peptic ulcer; Zollinger-Ellison syndrome.

Acintor *Corvi, Ital.*
Klebsiella pneumoniae glycoprotein (p.1593·2).
Respiratory-tract infections.

Acipem *Caber, Ital.*
Pipemidic acid (p.237·2).
Urinary-tract infections.

Acipen *Yamanouchi, Neth.*
Phenoxymethylpenicillin potassium (p.236·2).
Bacterial infections.

Acipen-V *Yamanouchi, Neth.*
Phenoxymethylpenicillin (p.236·2).
Bacterial infections.

Aciril *Molteni, Ital.*
Ibuprofen lysine (p.44·3).
Musculoskeletal and joint disorders.

Acirufan *Madaus, Ger.*
Homoeopathic preparation.

Aci-Sanorania *Sanorania, Ger.*
Aciclovir (p.602·3).
Herpesvirus infections.

Aci-steril *Heyl, Ger.†.*
Hexamine orthophosphate (p.216·2).
Urinary-tract disorders.

Acistin *Medifood-Trufood, Ital.*
Infant feed.
Cystinosis.

Acitak *Opus, UK.*
Cimetidine (p.1183·2).
Aspiration syndrome; gastro-oesophageal reflux; peptic ulcer; Zollinger-Ellison syndrome.

Acivir *Curasan, Ger.*
Aciclovir sodium (p.602·3).
Herpes simplex infections.

Aciviran *Ripari-Gero, Ital.†.*
Aciclovir (p.602·3).
Herpesvirus infections.

Aclacin *Lundbeck, UK.*
Aclarubicin hydrochloride (p.502·1).
Acute non-lymphoblastic leukaemia.

Aclacinomycine *Bellon, Fr.†.*
Aclarubicin hydrochloride (p.502·1).
Leukaemias; lymphomas.

Aclaplastin
Ebewe, Aust.; Medac, Ger.
Aclarubicin hydrochloride (p.502·1).
Now known as Aclarubicin in *Aust.*
Acute myeloid leukaemia; thyroid cancer.

Aclin *Alphapharm, Austral.*
Sulindac (p.86·3).
Musculoskeletal and joint disorders; pain with inflammation.

Aclinda *Azupharma, Ger.*
Clindamycin hydrochloride (p.191·1) or clindamycin phosphate (p.191·1).
Bacterial infections.

Aclon Lievit *Geymonat, Ital.*
Dried yeast (p.1373·1); vitamins; echinacea (p.1574·2); betacarotene (p.1335·2).
Acne; seborrhoea.

Aclonium *SmithKline Beecham, Ital.*
Gabapentin (p.346·3).
Epilepsy.

Aclophen *Nutripharm, USA.*
Phenylephrine hydrochloride (p.1066·2); paracetamol (p.72·2); chlorpheniramine maleate (p.405·1).
Upper respiratory-tract symptoms.

Aclosone
Schering-Plough, Fr.; Schering-Plough, Neth.; Schering-Plough, S.Afr.
Alclometasone dipropionate (p.1031·3).
Skin disorders.

Aclovate *Glaxo Wellcome, USA.*
Alclometasone dipropionate (p.1031·3).
Skin disorders.

ACM 20 *Paraphar, Fr.*
Multivitamin, mineral, and amino-acid preparation.

ACN *Person & Covey, USA†.*
Vitamins A, B, and C.

Acnacyl *Parke, Davis, Austral.†.*
Benzoyl peroxide (p.1079·2).
Acne.

Acnaveen
Note. This name is used for preparations of different composition.
Rydelle, Fr.
Avena (p.1551·3); salicylic acid (p.1090·2); carbocisteine (p.1056·3).
Acne.

Rydelle, Ital.
Avena (p.1551·3); salicylic acid (p.1090·2).
Acne; seborrhoea.

Bioglan, UK.
Sulphur (p.1091·2); salicylic acid (p.1090·2).
Acne.

Acne Blemish Cream *Bonne Bell, Canad.*
Sulphur (p.1091·2).
Acne.

Acne Complex *Brauer, Austral.†.*
Homoeopathic preparation.

Acne Creme *Widmer, Switz.*
Salicylic acid (p.1090·2); colloidal sulphur (p.1091·2); colloidal silicon dioxide (p.1475·1); triclosan (p.1127·2).
Acne.

Acne Creme Plus *Widmer, Switz.*
Benzoyl peroxide (p.1079·2); miconazole nitrate (p.384·3).
Acne.

Acne Gel *Widmer, Switz.*
Colloidal sulphur (p.1091·2); pyridoxine hydrochloride (p.1362·3); triclosan (p.1127·2); urea (p.1095·2).
Acne.

Acne Lotion *Widmer, Switz.*
Salicylic acid (p.1090·2); lactic acid (p.1593·3); triclosan (p.1127·2); zinc sulphate (p.1373·2); magnesium sulphate dihydrate (p.1157·3).
Acne.

Acne Lotion 10 *C & M, USA.*
Sulphur (p.1091·2).
Acne.

Acne-Aid
Note. This name is used for preparations of different composition.
Stiefel, Austral.; Stiefel, Canad.; Stiefel, S.Afr.†; Stiefel, UK†; Stiefel, USA.
Soap.
Acne.

Stiefel, Canad.
Topical gel: Sulphur (p.1091·2); resorcinol (p.1090·1); chloroxylenol (p.1111·1).
Acne.

Cusi, Spain†.
Benzoyl peroxide (p.1079·2).
Acne.

Acne-Ban *Czarniak, Austral.†.*
Precipitated sulphur (p.1091·2); salicylic acid (p.1090·2); resorcinol (p.1090·1); chlorbutol (p.1106·3).
Acne.

Acnecide
Galderma, Irl.; Galderma, UK.
Benzoyl peroxide (p.1079·2).
Acne.

Acneclear *Janpharm, S.Afr.*
Miconazole nitrate (p.384·3); benzoyl peroxide (p.1079·2).
Acne.

Acnecolor *Spirig, Switz.*
Clotrimazole (p.376·3).
Acne.

Acnecure *Taxandria, Neth.*
Miconazole nitrate (p.384·3); benzoyl peroxide (p.1079·2).
Acne.

Acne-Cy-Clean *Brovar, S.Afr.†.*
Doxycycline hydrochloride (p.202·3).
Acne.

Acnederm *Ego, Austral.*
Sulphur (p.1091·2); ichthammol (p.1083·3); undecylenic alkanolamide (p.389·2); zinc oxide (p.1096·2).
Formerly contained alcloxa, sulphur, dimethicones, ichthammol, and undecylenic alkanolamide.
Acne.

Acnederm Wash *Ego, Austral.*
Cetrimide (p.1105·2); glycerol (p.1585·2).
Formerly contained cetrimide and chlorhexidine gluconate.
Acne.

Acnefuge *Spirig, Switz.*
Benzoyl peroxide (p.1079·2).
Acne.

Acnegel *Stiefel, UK†.*
Benzoyl peroxide (p.1079·2).
Acne.

Acne-Med *Max Ritter, Switz.†.*
Salicylic acid (p.1090·2); coal tar (p.1092·3).
Acne; seborrhoea.

Acne-Med Simplex *Max Ritter, Switz.†.*
Soap substitute.
Acne.

Acneryne *Galderma, Belg.*
Erythromycin (p.204·1).
Acne.

Acnesan *Novogaleno, Ital.*
Sulphur (p.1091·2); zinc sulphate (p.1373·2); glycolic acid (p.1083·1); enoxolone (p.35·2).
Seborrhoea.

Acnestrol *Poirier, Fr.*
Broparestrol (p.1439·1); pyridoxine (p.1363·1); hexachlorophane (p.1115·2).
Acne.

Acnex *Dermtek, Canad.*
Salicylic acid (p.1090·2).
Acne.

Acnidazil
Note. This name is used for preparations of different composition.
Janssen-Cilag, Aust.
Miconazole nitrate (p.384·3).
Formerly contained miconazole nitrate and benzoyl peroxide.
Acne.

Janssen-Cilag, Belg.; Janssen-Cilag, Ger.; Italchimici, Ital.; Janssen-Cilag, Neth.; Janssen-Cilag, S.Afr.; Janssen-Cilag, Switz.; Johnson & Johnson MSD Consumer, UK.
Miconazole nitrate (p.384·3); benzoyl peroxide (p.1079·2).
Acne.

Janssen-Cilag, Switz.†.
Topical lotion: Salicylic acid (p.1090·2); lactic acid (p.1593·3); magnesium sulphate dihydrate (p.1157·3); zinc sulphate (p.1373·2); triclosan (p.1127·2).
Acne.

Acnisal
Helsinn Birex, Irl.; Euroderma, UK.
Salicylic acid (p.1090·2).
Acne.

Acnisdin *Isdin, Spain.*
Sulphur (p.1091·2); calcium dobesilate (p.1556·3); resorcinol (p.1090·1).
Acne.

Acnisdin Retinoico *Isdin, Spain.*
Calcium dobesilate (p.1556·3); tretinoin (p.1093·3).
Acne; psoriasis.

Acno *Baker Cummins, USA.*
Sulphur (p.1091·2); salicylic acid (p.1090·2).
Acne.

Acno Cleanser *Baker Cummins, USA.*
Skin cleanser.

Acnomel
Note. This name is used for preparations of different composition.
Chattem, Canad.
Cream: Resorcinol (p.1090·1); sulphur (p.1091·2); isopropyl alcohol (p.1118·2).
Vanishing cream: Resorcinol (p.1090·1); sulphur (p.1091·2).
Acne.

Smith Kline & French, Spain†.
Resorcinol (p.1090·1); sulphur (p.1091·2).
Acne.

SmithKline Beecham Consumer, USA.
Resorcinol (p.1090·1); sulphur (p.1091·2); titanium dioxide (p.1093·3).
Acne.

Acnomel Acne Mask *Chattem, Canad.*
Salicylic acid (p.1090·2).
Acne.

Acnomel BP 5 *Chattem, Canad.*
Benzoyl peroxide (p.1079·2).
Acne.

Acnophill *Torch, USA†.*
Sulphur (p.1091·2); zinc oxide (p.1096·2).
Acne.

Acnosan *Bescansa, Spain.*
Camphor (p.1557·2); boric acid (p.1554·2); resorcinol (p.1090·1); salicylic acid (p.1090·2); undecenoic acid (p.389·2); zinc sulphate (p.1373·2); copper sulphate (p.1338·1).
Acne.

Acnotex *C & M, USA.*
Sulphur (p.1091·2); salicylic acid (p.1090·2); methylbenzethonium chloride (p.1119·3).
Acne.

ACNU
Asta Medica, Ger.; Asta Medica, Neth.; Asta Medica, Switz.
Nimustine hydrochloride (p.556·2).
Malignant neoplasms.

Acoband *Kabi Pharmacia, Austral.†.*
Zinc oxide (p.1096·2); white soft paraffin; liquid paraffin.
Venous leg ulcers.

Acoin *Combustin, Ger.*
Amethocaine hydrochloride (p.1285·2); laureth 9 (p.1325·2).
Local anaesthesia.

Acomin *ACO, Swed.†.*
A range of vitamin preparations.

Aconex *Agepha, Aust.*
Naphazoline hydrochloride (p.1064·2).
Eye irritation.

Aconitum *Truw, Ger.*
Homoeopathic preparation.

Aconitum Med Complex *Dynamit, Aust.*
Homoeopathic preparation.

Aconitysat *Ysatfabrik, Ger.†.*
Aconite tuber (p.1542·2).
Neuralgia.

Acordin
Note. This name is used for preparations of different composition.
Kwizda, Aust.
Isosorbide dinitrate (p.893·1); diazepam (p.661·1).
Angina pectoris.

Mepha, Switz.
Isosorbide dinitrate (p.893·1).
Angina pectoris; heart failure; myocardial infarction.

Acorus *Zeppenfeldt, Ger.*
Couch-grass (p.1567·3).
Urinary-tract disorders.

Acovil *Hoechst, Spain.*
Ramipril (p.941·1).
Heart failure following myocardial infarction; hypertension.

Acqua di Sirmione *Terme Sirmione, Ital.*
Sulphurous thermal water (p.1091·2).
Catarrh; cold symptoms; rhinitis; sinusitis.

Acqua Virginiana *Kelemata, Ital.*
Hamamelis virginiana (p.1587·1).
Skin irritation.

Acriflex *Seton, UK.*
Chlorhexidine gluconate (p.1107·2).
Burns; scalds; wounds.

Acrisuxin
Chemomedica, Aust.; Gewo, Ger.†; Geistlich, Switz.
Ethosuximide (p.344·3); mepacrine hydrochloride (p.584·2).
Absence seizures.

Acromicina *Cyanamid, Ital.*
Tetracycline hydrochloride (p.259·1).
Bacterial infections.

Acsacea *Chemomedica, Aust.*
Metronidazole (p.585·1).
Rosacea.

Acset *Bio-Transfusion, Fr.*
Activated factor VII (p.720·2).
Haemophilias A and B.

ACT *Johnson & Johnson Medical, USA.*
Sodium fluoride (p.742·1).
Dental caries prophylaxis.

ACT-3 *Whitehall, Austral.*
Ibuprofen (p.44·1).
Fever; inflammation; musculoskeletal and joint disorders; pain.

Actacode *Sigma, Austral.*
Codeine phosphate (p.26·1).
Coughs.

Actagen *Goldline, USA.*
Pseudoephedrine hydrochloride (p.1068·3); triprolidine hydrochloride (p.420·3).
Upper respiratory-tract symptoms.

Actagen-C Cough *Goldline, USA.*
Pseudoephedrine hydrochloride (p.1068·3); codeine phosphate (p.26·1); triprolidine hydrochloride (p.420·3).
Coughs and cold symptoms.

Actal
SmithKline Beecham, Irl.; Maggioni, Ital.†; Sterling Health, UK.
Alexitol sodium (p.1176·3).
Dyspepsia; gastric hyperacidity.

Actan *Restan, S.Afr.*
Alexitol sodium (p.1176·3).
Hyperchlorhydria; peptic ulcer; gastro-oesophageal reflux.

Actapulgite
Ipsen, Belg.; Beaufour, Fr.; Beaufour, Switz.
Attapulgite (p.1178·3).
Gastro-intestinal disorders.

Actebral
Menarini, Belg.; Biologiques de l'Ile-de-France, Fr.
Cyprodenate (p.1478·2) or cyprodenate maleate (p.1478·2).
Cerebral disorders.

Acthar
Rhone-Poulenc Rorer, Austral.†; Rorer, Irl.; Roche, S.Afr.; Rorer, UK; Rorer, USA.
Corticotrophin (p.1244·2).
Available on a named-patient basis only in the *UK.*
Corticosteroid release stimulant; diagnostic testing of adrenocortical function.

Actharn *Rhone-Poulenc Rorer, Canad.†.*
Corticotrophin (p.1244·2).
Corticosteroid release stimulant; diagnostic testing of adrenocortical function.

Act-HIB
Serotherapeutisches, Aust.; Pasteur Merieux, Austral.†; Pasteur Merieux, Belg.; Connaught, Canad.; Merieux, Fr.; Pasteur Merieux, Ger.; Pasteur Merieux, Ital.; Pasteur Merieux, Neth.; Pasteur Merieux, Norw.; Rhone-Poulenc Rorer, S.Afr.; Pasteur Merieux, Spain; Pasteur Merieux, Swed.; Pro Vaccine, Switz.; Pasteur Merieux, UK; Connaught, USA.
A haemophilus influenzae conjugate vaccine (tetanus toxoid conjugate) (p.1511·1).
Active immunisation.

Act-HIB DTP *Pasteur Merieux, UK.*
A diphtheria, tetanus, pertussis, and haemophilus influenzae vaccine (p.1509·3).
Active immunisation.

Act-HIB plus DPT *Serotherapeutisches, Aust.*
Haemophilus influenzae conjugate vaccine (tetanus toxoid conjugate) (p.1511·1); diphtheria, tetanus, and pertussis vaccine (p.1509·1).
Active immunisation.

Act-HIB Polio *Pasteur Merieux, Swed.*
A haemophilus influenzae conjugate vaccine (tetanus toxoid conjugate) and an injectable inactivated poliomyelitis vaccine (types I, II and III).
Active immunisation.

Acthrel *Ferring, USA.*
Corticorelin triflutate (p.1244·1).
Determination of ACTH production in Cushing's syndrome.

Acti 5 *Pierre Fabre, Fr.*
Oral liquid: Deanol glutamate; sodium ascorbate (p.1365·2); magnesium aminobenzoate; hesperidin methyl chalcone (p.1580·2).
Syrup: Deanol glutamate; lysine hydrochloride (p.1350·1); calcium gluconogluceptate; phosphoric acid (p.1618·1).
Tonic.

Acti-B$_{12}$ *Charton, Canad.*
Hydroxocobalamin (p.1363·3); amino acids.
Anaemia.

ActiBath *Jergens, USA.*
Avena (p.1551·3).
Dry skin; pruritus.

Actibil *Arkopharma, Fr.*
Cynara (p.1569·2); fumitory (p.1581·3).
Gastro-intestinal and urinary-tract disorders.

Actibrush *Colgate-Palmolive, UK.*
Triclosan (p.1127·2); gantrez.
Dental hygiene.

Acticarbine *Elerte, Fr.*
Papaverine hydrochloride (p.1614·2); activated charcoal (p.972·2).
Gastro-intestinal disorders.

Acticin *Alpharma, USA.*
Permethrin (p.1409·2).
Scabies.

Acticinco *Robapharm, Spain.*
Calcium gluceptate (p.1155·1); lysine hydrochloride (p.1350·1); deanol pyroglutamate (p.1478·2).
Tonic.

Acticolin *Upsamedica, Ital.*
Citicoline sodium (p.1564·3).
Cerebrovascular disorders; parkinsonism.

Acticort *Baker Cummins, USA.*
Hydrocortisone (p.1043·3).
Skin disorders.

Actidil
Glaxo Wellcome, Aust.; Wellcome, Irl.†; Warner-Lambert, Ital.
Triprolidine hydrochloride (p.420·3).
Hypersensitivity reactions.

Actidilon *Wellcome, Fr.†.*
Triprolidine hydrochloride (p.420·3).
Hypersensitivity reactions.

Actidilon Hydrocortisone *Wellcome, Fr.†.*
Triprolidine hydrochloride (p.420·3); hydrocortisone acetate (p.1043·3).
Local inflammatory reactions.

Actidose with Sorbitol *Paddock, USA.*
Activated charcoal (p.972·2); sorbitol (p.1354·2).
Emergency treatment of poisoning.

Actidose-Aqua *Paddock, USA.*
Activated charcoal (p.972·2).
Emergency treatment of poisoning.

Actifed
Note. This name is used for preparations of different composition.
Warner-Lambert, Austral.; Glaxo Wellcome, Belg.; Warner-Lambert, Canad.; Warner-Lambert, Ger.; Wellcome, Irl.; Warner-Lambert, Ital.; Glaxo Wellcome, S.Afr.; Warner-Lambert, UK; Wellcome, USA.
Triprolidine hydrochloride (p.420·3); pseudoephedrine hydrochloride (p.1068·3).
Upper respiratory-tract congestion.

Glaxo Wellcome, Belg.
Syrup: Triprolidine hydrochloride (p.420·3); codeine phosphate (p.26·1); pseudoephedrine hydrochloride (p.1068·3); guaiphenesin (p.1061·3).
Coughs.

Warner-Lambert, Fr.
Triprolidine hydrochloride (p.420·3); pseudoephedrine hydrochloride (p.1068·3); paracetamol (p.72·2).
Cold symptoms; upper respiratory-tract congestion.

Actifed Allergy *Wellcome, USA.*
White daytime caplets, pseudoephedrine (p.1068·3); blue night time caplets, pseudoephedrine; diphenhydramine hydrochloride (p.409·1).

Actifed Anaesthetic *Warner-Lambert, Austral.*
Lignocaine hydrochloride (p.1293·2); dichlorobenzyl alcohol (p.1112·2); cetylpyridinium chloride (p.1106·2).
Sore throat.

Actifed Antiseptic *Parke Davis-Wellcome, Austral.†.*
Cetylpyridinium chloride (p.1106·2).
Sore throat.

Actifed CC Chesty *Warner-Lambert, Austral.*
Capsules: Guaiphenesin (p.1061·3); pseudoephedrine hydrochloride (p.1068·3).
Elixir: Guaiphenesin (p.1061·3); pseudoephedrine hydrochloride (p.1068·3); triprolidine hydrochloride (p.420·3).
Upper respiratory-tract disorders.

Actifed CC Dry *Warner-Lambert, Austral.*
Capsules: Dextromethorphan hydrobromide (p.1057·3); pseudoephedrine hydrochloride (p.1068·3).
Syrup: Pseudoephedrine hydrochloride (p.1068·3); dextromethorphan hydrobromide (p.1057·3); triprolidine hydrochloride (p.420·3).
Upper respiratory-tract disorders.

Actifed CC Junior *Warner-Lambert, Austral.*
Dextromethorphan hydrobromide (p.1057·3); triprolidine hydrochloride (p.420·3).
Upper respiratory-tract disorders.

Actifed Co *Glaxo Wellcome, S.Afr.*
Triprolidine hydrochloride (p.420·3); pseudoephedrine hydrochloride (p.1068·3); codeine phosphate (p.26·1).
Coughs.

Actifed with Codeine *Glaxo Wellcome, USA†.*
Codeine phosphate (p.26·1); triprolidine hydrochloride (p.420·3); pseudoephedrine hydrochloride (p.1068·3).
Coughs and cold symptoms.

Actifed Composto *Warner-Lambert, Ital.*
Triprolidine hydrochloride (p.420·3); pseudoephedrine hydrochloride (p.1068·3); dextromethorphan hydrobromide (p.1057·3).
Coughs; respiratory tract congestion.

Actifed Compound
Wellcome, Irl.; Warner-Lambert, UK.
Triprolidine hydrochloride (p.420·3); pseudoephedrine hydrochloride (p.1068·3); dextromethorphan hydrobromide (p.1057·3).
Coughs; upper respiratory-tract congestion.

Actifed DM
Warner-Lambert, Canad.; Glaxo Wellcome, S.Afr.
Triprolidine hydrochloride (p.420·3); pseudoephedrine hydrochloride (p.1068·3); dextromethorphan hydrobromide (p.1057·3).
Upper respiratory-tract disorders.

Actifed Expectorant
Wellcome, Irl.; Warner-Lambert, UK.
Triprolidine hydrochloride (p.420·3); pseudoephedrine hydrochloride (p.1068·3); guaiphenesin (p.1061·3).
Coughs; upper respiratory-tract congestion.

Actifed 12 Hour *Wellcome, Canad.†.*
Triprolidine hydrochloride (p.420·3); pseudoephedrine hydrochloride (p.1068·3).
Upper respiratory-tract congestion.

Actifed jour et nuit *Warner-Lambert, Fr.*
Yellow tablets, paracetamol (p.72·2); phenylpropanolamine hydrochloride (p.1067·2); blue tablets, paracetamol; diphenhydramine hydrochloride (p.409·1).
Rhinitis.

Actifed Nasale *Warner-Lambert, Ital.*
Oxymetazoline hydrochloride (p.1065·3).
Nasal congestion.

Actifed Plus
Warner-Lambert, Canad.; Wellcome, USA.
Triprolidine hydrochloride (p.420·3); pseudoephedrine hydrochloride (p.1068·3); paracetamol (p.72·2).
Cold symptoms.

Actifed Sinus Daytime *Wellcome, USA.*
Pseudoephedrine hydrochloride (p.1068·3); paracetamol (p.72·2).
Upper respiratory-tract symptoms.

Actifed Sinus Nighttime *Wellcome, USA.*
Pseudoephedrine hydrochloride (p.1068·3); diphenhydramine hydrochloride (p.409·1); paracetamol (p.72·2).
Upper respiratory-tract symptoms.

Actifen *Sterling Health, Spain†.*
Ibuprofen (p.44·1).
Fever; pain.

Actiferrine *Mepha, Switz.*
Ferrous sulphate (p.1340·2); DL-serine.
Iron deficiency; iron-deficiency anaemia.

Actiferrine-F Nouvelle formule *Mepha, Switz.*
Ferrous sulphate (p.1340·2); DL-serine; folic acid (p.1340·3).
Pregnancy- or lactation-induced anaemia.

Actiferro *Lampugnani, Ital.*
Ferric sodium gluconate (p.1340·1).
Iron-deficiency disorders.

Actiflora *Brovar, S.Afr.†.*
Lactobacillus acidophilus (p.1594·1).
Restoration of a normal gastro-intestinal flora.

Actifral A + D3 Hidrosolub *Duphar, Spain†.*
Cholecalciferol (p.1366·3); vitamin A palmitate (p.1359·2).
Deficiency of vitamins A and D.

Actifral D3 *Duphar, Spain†.*
Cholecalciferol (p.1366·3).
Hypoparathyroidism; vitamin D deficiency.

Actigall *Novartis, USA.*
Ursodeoxycholic acid (p.1642·1).
Gallstones.

Actigesic *Glaxo Wellcome, S.Afr.*
Triprolidine hydrochloride (p.420·3); pseudoephedrine hydrochloride (p.1068·3); paracetamol (p.72·2).
Cold and influenza symptoms.

Actigrip *Warner-Lambert, Ital.*
Triprolidine hydrochloride (p.420·3); pseudoephedrine hydrochloride (p.1068·3); paracetamol (p.72·2).
Influenza symptoms; respiratory tract congestion.

Actihaemyl *Byk Gulden, Ger.*
Protein-free bovine blood extract.
Burns; ophthalmic disorders; peripheral and cerebral vascular disorders; wounds.

Actilax *Alphapharm, Austral.*
Lactulose (p.1195·3).
Constipation; hepatic encephalopathy.

Actilevol C *Wasserman, Spain†.*
Glycine (p.1345·2); ascorbic acid (p.1365·2); haematoporphyrin hydrochloride (p.1587·1); liver extract; yeast extract (p.1373·1).
Tonic.

Actilevol Orex *Wasserman, Spain.*
Vitamins; carnosine; cyproheptadine hydrochloride (p.407·2); haematoporphyrin hydrochloride (p.1587·1).
Tonic.

Actilife *Lifeplan, UK.*
Vitamins, minerals, fish oils, ginseng, and betacarotene.
Nutritional supplement.

Actilyse
Bender, Aust.; Boehringer Ingelheim, Austral.; Boehringer Ingelheim, Belg.; Boehringer Ingelheim, Fr.; Thomae, Ger.; Boehringer Ingelheim, Irl.; Boehringer Ingelheim, Ital.; Boehringer Ingelheim, Neth.; Boehringer Ingelheim, Norw.; Boehringer Ingelheim, S.Afr.; Boehringer Ingelheim, Spain; Boehringer Ingelheim, Swed.; Boehringer Ingelheim, Switz.; Boehringer Ingelheim, UK.
Alteplase (p.818·1).
Myocardial infarction; peripheral arterial thrombo-embolism; pulmonary embolism.

Actimag
Vita, Ital.; Iquinosa, Spain.
Magnesium pidolate (p.1157·3).
Magnesium depletion.

Actimidol *Sterling Health, Spain.*
Ibuprofen (p.44·1).
Fever; inflammation; musculoskeletal and joint disorders; pain.

Actimmune *Genentech, USA.*
Interferon gamma-1b (p.616·1).
Infections in chronic granulomatous disease.

Actimoxi *Clariana, Spain.*
Amoxycillin trihydrate (p.151·3).
Bacterial infections.

Actinac
Hoechst Marion Roussel, Canad.; Hoechst Marion Roussel, Irl.; Roussel, UK.
Chloramphenicol (p.182·1); hydrocortisone acetate (p.1043·3); nicoboxil (p.63·1); allantoin (p.1078·2); precipitated sulphur (p.1091·2).
Acne.

Actinex *Schwarz, USA.*
Masoprocol (p.544·3).
Solar keratoses.

Actino-Hermal *Hermal, Ger.*
Fluorouracil (p.534·3).
Skin cancer.

Actiol *SIT, Ital.†.*
Methyl cysteine hydrochloride (p.1064·1).
Respiratory-tract disorders.

Action
Note. This name is used for preparations of different composition.
Bayer, Austral.
Chlorpheniramine maleate (p.405·1); phenylephrine acid tartrate (p.1066·2); aspirin (p.16·1); ascorbic acid (p.1365·2).
Cold and influenza symptoms.

Upjohn, Austral.†.
Colloidal sulphur (p.1091·2); aluminium chlorohydrate (p.1078·3).
Acne.

Sante Naturelle, Canad.
Ascorbic acid (p.1365·2).

Action Chewable *Bayer, Austral.*
Chlorpheniramine maleate (p.405·1); phenylephrine tartrate (p.1066·2).
Cold symptoms; nasal congestion.

Actiphos *Theraplix, Fr.*
Phosphoric acid salts (p.1618·1).
Tonic.

Actiplas *Dompe Biotec, Ital.*
Alteplase (p.818·1).
Myocardial infarction.

Actiprofen
SmithKline Beecham, Austral.; Bayer, Canad.; SmithKline Beecham, Irl.
Ibuprofen (p.44·1).
Fever; inflammation; pain.

Actisane Constipation Occasionnelle *Dolisos, Fr.*
Senna (p.1212·2); tamarind (p.1217·3).
Constipation.

Actisane Digestion *Dolisos, Fr.*
Cynara (p.1569·2); boldo (p.1554·1); fumitory (p.1581·3).
Biliary-tract disorders.

Actisane Douleurs Articulaires *Dolisos, Fr.*
Harpagophytum procumbens (p.27·2); meadowsweet (p.1599·1).
Joint disorders.

Actisane Fatigue Passagere *Dolisos, Fr.*
Ginseng (p.1584·2); tea (p.1645·1).
Tonic.

Actisane Hemorroides, Jambes Lourdes *Dolisos, Fr.*
Aesculus (p.1543·3); melilotus officinalis; red vine.
Haemorrhoids; venous insufficiency.

Actisane Minceur *Dolisos, Fr.*
Bladderwrack (p.1554·1); orthosiphon (p.1592·2); meadowsweet (p.1599·1).
Obesity.

Actisane Nervosite *Dolisos, Fr.*
Crataegus (p.1568·2); red-poppy petal (p.1001·1); passion flower (p.1615·3).
Cardiac disorders.

Actisite
Willvonseder, Aust.; Dentaid, Spain.; Meda, Swed.; Alza, Switz.; Alza, USA.
Tetracycline hydrochloride (p.259·1).
Bacterial mouth infections.

Actisorb
Johnson & Johnson Medical, Fr.; Ethicon, Ital.†.
Activated charcoal (p.972·2).
Infected or malodorous wounds.

Actisorb Plus
Johnson & Johnson Medical, Fr.; Johnson & Johnson, Irl.; Ethicon, Ital.; Johnson & Johnson Medical, UK.
Activated charcoal (p.972·2); silver (p.1629·2).
Infected or malodorous wounds.

Actisoufre *Serozym, Fr.*
Sodium sulphate (p.1213·3); dried yeast (p.1373·1).
Upper respiratory-tract inflammation.

Actispirine *Millot-Solac, Fr.†.*
Aspirin (p.16·1).
Fever; pain.

Actisson *Urgo, Fr.*
Dietary fibre preparation.
Constipation.

Actithiol *Funk, Spain.*
Carbocisteine (p.1056·3).
Respiratory-tract disorders.

Actithiol Antihist *Funk, Spain.*
Carbocisteine (p.1056·3); promethazine hydrochloride (p.416·2).
Respiratory-tract disorders.

Actitonic *Amido, Fr.*
Solution for adults: Amino-acid and mineral preparation.
Solution for children: Amino-acid preparation.
Tonic.

Activadone
Cusi, Spain.
Eye drops: Chromocarb diethylamine (p.1562·3).
Adjunct in eye surgery; conjunctival capillary fragility.

Thea, Spain.
Capsules: Chromocarb diethylamine (p.1562·3).
Capillary haemorrhage; venous insufficiency.

Activante *Asta Medica, Belg.†.*
Allantoin (p.1078·2); retinol (p.1358·1); ergocalciferol (p.1367·1).
Corneal and conjunctival trauma.

Activarol
Note. This name is used for preparations of different composition.
Lipha, Belg.
Ascorbic acid; haematoporphyrin; glycine; vitamin B$_{12}$; dried yeast.
Tonic.

Monot, Fr.
Glycine (p.1345·2); arginine (p.1334·1).
Tonic.

Carlo Erba OTC, Ital.
Haematoporphyrin hydrochloride; glycine; cyanocobalamin; calcium gluconate.
Tonic.

Activarol C
Anphar-Rolland, Fr.†.
Haematoporphyrin hydrochloride; glycine; dried yeast; ascorbic acid.
Tonic.

Rolland, Switz.†.
Haematoporphyrin; glycine; liver extracts; yeast; ascorbic acid.
Tonic.

Activase
Roche, Canad.; Genentech, USA.
Alteplase (p.818·1).
Myocardial infarction; pulmonary embolism.

Active Dry Lotion *Norwood, Canad.*
SPF 15: Ethylhexyl *p*-methoxycinnamate (p.1487·1); oxybenzone (p.1487·3).
SPF 30: Ethylhexyl *p*-methoxycinnamate (p.1487·1); oxybenzone (p.1487·3); octyl salicylate (p.1487·3).
Sunscreen.

Activex 40 Plus *Mer-National, S.Afr.*
Ginseng (p.1584·2); muira puama; vitamins; minerals; kelp (p.1593·1); lysine hydrochloride.

Activir
Parke, Davis, Aust.; Warner-Lambert, Fr.; Glaxo Wellcome, S.Afr.
Aciclovir (p.602·3).
Herpes labialis.

Activital *ECR, Switz.*
Arginine aspartate (p.1334·2); calcium gluconate (p.1155·2); magnesium gluconate (p.1157·2).
Tonic.

Activox *Arkopharma, Fr.*
Erysimum; chamomile (p.1561·2).
Mouth and throat disorders.

Actizyme *Willvonseder, Aust.*
Subtilisin-A; poloxamer 338 (p.1326·3).
Cleaning of contact lenses.

Actocortina *Byk Elmu, Spain.*
Hydrocortisone sodium phosphate (p.1044·1).
Corticosteroid.

Actol
Mayrhofer, Aust.; Fournier, Ger.; Upsamedica, Spain†.
Niflumic acid (p.63·1) or morniflumate (p.56·1).
Inflammation; pain.

Actomin *Francia, Ital.*
Citicoline sodium (p.1564·3).
Cerebrovascular disorders; parkinsonism.

Actomite *Searle, UK.*
Bioallethrin (p.1402·3).
Elimination of house dust mite.

Acton prolongatum *Ferring, Swed.†.*
Corticotrophin (p.1244·2).
Corticosteroid release stimulant.

Actonel *Procter & Gamble, USA.*
Sodium risedronate (p.741·3).
Paget's disease of bone.

Actonorm *Wallace Mfg Chem., UK.*
Oral gel: Aluminium hydroxide (p.1177·3); magnesium hydroxide (p.1198·2); simethicone (p.1213·1).
Flatulence; hyperchlorhydria.
Oral powder: Magnesium carbonate (p.1198·1); aluminium hydroxide (p.1177·3); atropine sulphate (p.455·1); calcium carbonate (p.1182·1); magnesium trisilicate (p.1199·1); sodium bicarbonate (p.1153·2); peppermint oil (p.1208·1).
Gastro-intestinal spasm.

Actophlem *Covan, S.Afr.*
Theophylline (p.765·1); etofylline (p.753·1); diphenylpyraline hydrochloride (p.409·3); ammonium chloride (p.1055·2); sodium citrate (p.1153·2).
Coughs.

Actosolv
Hoechst, Aust.; Hoechst Marion Roussel, Belg.; Hoechst, Fr.; Hoechst, Ger.; Hoechst Marion Roussel, Ital.
Urokinase (p.959·3).
Thrombo-embolic disorders.

Actovegin
Hafslund Nycomed, Aust.; Nycomed, Ger.; Hafslund Nycomed, Switz.†.
Protein-free bovine blood extract.
Burns; cerebral circulatory and metabolic disorders; eye disorders; peripheral vascular disorders; ulcers; wounds.

Actraphane HM
CSL-Novo, Austral.†; Novo Nordisk, S.Afr.; Novo Nordisk, Switz.†.
Mixture of insulin injection (human, monocomponent) 30% and isophane insulin injection (human, monocomponent) 70% (p.322·1).
Diabetes mellitus.

Actraphane HM 10/90, 20/80, 30/70, 40/60, 50/50
Novo Nordisk, Ger.; Novo Nordisk, Ital.
Mixtures of neutral insulin injection (human, monocomponent) and isophane insulin injection (human, monocomponent) respectively in the proportions indicated (p.322·1).
Diabetes mellitus.

Actraphane MC *CSL-Novo, Austral.†.*
Mixture of neutral insulin injection (porcine, monocomponent) 30% and isophane insulin injection (porcine, monocomponent) 70% (p.322·1).
Diabetes mellitus.

Actrapid
Novo Nordisk, Austral.; Novo Nordisk, Irl.; Novo Nordisk, Neth.; Novo Nordisk, Norw.; Novo Nordisk, Spain; Novo Nordisk, Swed.
Neutral insulin injection (human, pyr, monocomponent) (p.322·1).
Formerly known as Human Actrapid in *Irl.*
Diabetes mellitus.

Actrapid HM
Novo Nordisk, Aust.; Novo Nordisk, Belg.; Novo Nordisk, Fr.; Novo Nordisk, Ger.; Novo Nordisk, Ital.; Novo Nordisk, S.Afr.; Novo Nordisk, Switz.
Neutral insulin injection (human, pyr, monocomponent) (p.322·1).
Diabetes mellitus.

Actrapid MC
CSL-Novo, Austral.†; Novo Nordisk, Switz.
Neutral insulin injection (porcine, monocomponent) (p.322·1).
Diabetes mellitus.

Actron
Note. This name is used for preparations of different composition.
Bayer, Aust.; Bayer, USA.
Ketoprofen (p.48·2).
Fever; pain.

Bayer, Fr.; Bayer, UK†.
Aspirin (p.16·1); paracetamol (p.72·2); caffeine (p.749·3).
Fever; pain.

Bayer, Spain.
Paracetamol (p.72·2).
Fever; pain.

Actron Compuesto *Bayer, Spain.*
Aspirin (p.16·1); caffeine (p.749·3); paracetamol (p.72·2).
Fever; pain.

Actuss *Sigma, Austral.*
Pholcodine (p.1068·1).
Coughs.

Acuatim *Otsuka, Jpn.*
Nadifloxacin (p.228·1).
Acne.

Acubiron *Bohm, Spain.*
Prunus africana.
Prostatic adenoma.

Acucil *Apotex, S.Afr.*
Amoxycillin trihydrate (p.151·3).
Bacterial infections.

Acuco *Apotex, S.Afr.*
Co-trimoxazole (p.196·3).
Bacterial infections.

ACU-dyne *Acme, USA.*
Povidone-iodine (p.1123·3).
Skin disinfection; vaginal disorders.

Acu-Erylate S *Apotex, S.Afr.*
Erythromycin estolate (p.204·1).
Bacterial infections.

Acuflex *Apotex, S.Afr.*
Indomethacin (p.45·2).
Gout; musculoskeletal and joint disorders.

Acuflu-P *Apotex, S.Afr.*
Triprolidine hydrochloride (p.420·3); pseudoephedrine hydrochloride (p.1068·3); paracetamol (p.72·2).
Cold and influenza symptoms.

Acugesil *Apotex, S.Afr.*
Paracetamol (p.72·2); codeine phosphate (p.26·1); caffeine (p.749·3); meprobamate (p.678·1).
Pain with tension.

Acugest *Apotex, S.Afr.*
Triprolidine hydrochloride (p.420·3); pseudoephedrine hydrochloride (p.1068·3).
Cold and influenza symptoms.

Acugest Co *Apotex, S.Afr.*
Triprolidine hydrochloride (p.420·3); pseudoephedrine hydrochloride (p.1068·3); codeine phosphate (p.26·1).
Coughs.

Acuilix *Parke, Davis, Fr.*
Hydrochlorothiazide (p.885·2); quinapril hydrochloride (p.938·1).
Hypertension.

Acuitel *Parke, Davis, Fr.*
Quinapril hydrochloride (p.938·1).
Heart failure; hypertension.

Acular
Allergan, Canad.; Allergan, Ger.; Allergan, Irl.; Allergan, Ital.; Allergan, Neth.†; Allergan, S.Afr.; Allergan, UK; Allergan, USA.
Ketorolac trometamol (p.49·1).
Allergic conjunctivitis; ocular inflammation following cataract surgery.

Aculare *Allergan, Belg.*
Ketorolac trometamol (p.49·1).
Ocular inflammation following cataract surgery.

Aculoid *Apotex, S.Afr.*
Cyclizine hydrochloride (p.407·1).
Nausea; vestibular disorders; vomiting.

Acumet *Apotex, S.Afr.*
Metoclopramide hydrochloride (p.1200·3).
Gastro-intestinal disorders.

Acumod *Apotex, S.Afr.*
Amiloride hydrochloride (p.819·2); hydrochlorothiazide (p.885·2).
Hypertension; oedema.

Acunaso *Apotex, S.Afr.*
Pseudoephedrine hydrochloride (p.1068·3).
Upper respiratory-tract congestion.

Acu-Oxytet *Apotex, S.Afr.*
Oxytetracycline hydrochloride (p.235·1).
Bacterial infections.

Acupan
3M, Belg.; Biocodex, Fr.; 3M, Irl.; Boehringer Mannheim, Ital.†; 3M, S.Afr.†; CEPA, Spain; 3M, Switz.; 3M, UK.
Nefopam hydrochloride (p.62·3).
Pain.

Acuphlem *Apotex, S.Afr.*
Carbocisteine (p.1056·3).
Respiratory-tract disorders with excess mucus.

Acupillin *Apotex, S.Afr.*
Ampicillin trihydrate (p.153·2).
Bacterial infections.

Acuprel *Parke, Davis, Spain.*
Quinapril hydrochloride (p.938·1).
Heart failure; hypertension.

Acupril *Parke, Davis, Neth.*
Quinapril hydrochloride (p.938·1).
Heart failure; hypertension.

Acurate *Acupharm, S.Afr.; Apotex, S.Afr.*
Paracetamol (p.72·2); doxylamine succinate (p.410·1); caffeine (p.749·3); codeine phosphate (p.26·1).
Pain with tension.

Acuretic *Parke, Davis, Spain.*
Quinapril hydrochloride (p.938·1); hydrochlorothiazide (p.885·2).
Hypertension.

Acusprain *Apotex, S.Afr.*
Naproxen (p.61·2).
Dysmenorrhoea; gout; musculoskeletal and joint disorders.

Acustop *Apotex, S.Afr.*
Paracetamol (p.72·2); codeine phosphate (p.26·1); promethazine hydrochloride (p.416·2).
Fever; pain.

Acutamine *Synthelabo, Belg.†.*
Amino-acid and vitamin preparation.

Acutil Fosforo *SmithKline Beecham, Ital.*
Aceglutamide or levoglutamide; L-asparagine; DL-phosphoserine; pyridoxine or pyridoxine hydrochloride.
Tonic.

Acutrim *Ciba, USA.*
Phenylpropanolamine hydrochloride (p.1067·2).
Obesity.

Acutussive *Apotex, S.Afr.*
Triprolidine hydrochloride (p.420·3); pseudoephedrine hydrochloride (p.1068·3); guaiphenesin (p.1061·3); codeine phosphate (p.26·1).
Coughs.

Acuzide *Parke, Davis, Neth.*
Quinapril hydrochloride (p.938·1); hydrochlorothiazide (p.885·2).
Hypertension.

Acuzole *Apotex, S.Afr.*
Metronidazole (p.585·1).
Anaerobic bacterial infections; protozoal infections.

Acyclo-V *Alphapharm, Austral.*
Aciclovir (p.602·3).
Herpesvirus infections.

Acyvir *Glaxo Allen, Ital.*
Aciclovir (p.602·3).
Herpes simplex infections.

AD7 *Medifood-Trufood, Ital.†.*
Sugar, fibre, protein, lipid, and mineral salts.
Diarrhoea; dyspepsia.

AD Pabyrn *Samil, Ital.*
Vitamin A palmitate (p.1359·2); cholecalciferol (p.1366·3).
Formerly contained vitamin A palmitate and ergocalciferol.
Vitamin A and D deficiency.

ADA *Estedi, Spain.*
Phenylephrine hydrochloride (p.1066·2).
Formerly contained phenylephrine hydrochloride, benzalkonium chloride and diphenhydramine hydrochloride.
Nasal congestion.

Adacol *Nelson, Austral.†.*
Cetylpyridinium chloride (p.1106·2); chlorhexidine hydrochloride (p.1107·2); benzocaine (p.1286·2).
Sore throat.

Adacor *Nelson, Austral.†.*
Hydrocortisone acetate (p.1043·3).
Skin disorders.

Adagen *Enzon, USA.*
Pegademase bovine (p.1616·1).
Adenosine deaminase deficiency.

Adalat
Bayer, Aust.; Bayer, Austral.; Bayer, Belg.; Bayer, Canad.; Bayer, Ger.; Bayer, Irl.; Bayer, Ital.; Bayer, Neth.; Bayer, Norw.; Bayer, S.Afr.; Bayer, Spain; Bayer, Swed.; Bayer, Switz.; Bayer, UK; Bayer, USA.
Nifedipine (p.916·2).
Angina pectoris; coronary spasm; hypertension; Raynaud's syndrome.

Adalate *Bayer, Fr.*
Nifedipine (p.916·2).
Angina pectoris; coronary spasm; hypertension; Raynaud's syndrome.

Adalgur *Roussel, Spain.*
Paracetamol (p.72·2); thiocolchicoside (p.1322·1).
Formerly contained glafenine and thiocolchicoside.
Painful skeletal muscle spasm.

Adalixin C *Nelson, Austral.†.*
Promethazine hydrochloride (p.416·2); codeine phosphate (p.26·1); ephedrine hydrochloride (p.1059·3); ammonium chloride (p.1055·2).
Coughs.

Adalixin (New Formula) *Nelson, Austral.†.*
Promethazine hydrochloride (p.416·2); dextromethorphan hydrobromide (p.1057·3); ephedrine hydrochloride (p.1059·3).
Coughs.

Adamucol *Ferrer, Spain†.*
Adamexine (p.1054·3).
Respiratory-tract disorders.

Adancor *Merck-Clevenot, Fr.*
Nicorandil (p.915·3).
Angina pectoris.

Adapettes *Alcon, USA.*
Range of solutions for contact lenses.

Adaphol *Nelson, Austral.†.*
Pholcodine (p.1068·1).

Adapin *Lotus, USA†.*
Doxepin hydrochloride (p.283·2).
Anxiety; depression.

Adapine *Amrad, Austral.*
Nifedipine (p.916·2).
Hypertension.

Adapress *Lagap, Switz.†.*
Nifedipine (p.916·2).
Angina pectoris; hypertension.

Adapt *Alcon, USA.*
Wetting solution for hard contact lenses.

Adapta *Wander Health Care, Switz.†.*
Preparation for enteral nutrition.

Adaquin *Nelson, Austral.†.*
Quinine sulphate (p.439·2).

Adasept *Odan, Canad.*
Cleanser: Triclosan (p.1127·2).
Skin cleanser.
Topical gel: Triclosan (p.1127·2); salicylic acid (p.1090·2); sodium thiosulphate (p.996·2).
Acne.

Adasone *Nelson, Austral.†.*
Prednisone (p.1049·2).
Corticosteroid.

Adavite *Hudson, USA.*
A range of vitamin preparations.

Adco-Dol *Adcock Ingram Generics, S.Afr.*
Paracetamol (p.72·2); codeine phosphate (p.26·1); caffeine (p.749·3); doxylamine succinate (p.410·1).
Fever; pain.

Adco-Flupain *Adcock Ingram Generics, S.Afr.*
Triprolidine hydrochloride (p.420·3); pseudoephedrine hydrochloride (p.1068·3); paracetamol (p.72·2).
Cold and influenza symptoms.

Adco-Linctopent *Adcock Ingram, S.Afr.*
Bromhexine hydrochloride (p.1055·3); orciprenaline sulphate (p.756·3).
Coughs.

Adco-Loten *Adcock Ingram Generics, S.Afr.*
Atenolol (p.825·3); chlorthalidone (p.839·3).
Hypertension.

Adco-Muco Expect *Adcock Ingram Generics, S.Afr.*
Triprolidine hydrochloride (p.420·3); pseudoephedrine hydrochloride (p.1068·3); guaiphenesin (p.1061·3).
Coughs.

Adco-Phenobarbitone Vitalet *Adcock Ingram, S.Afr.*
Phenobarbitone (p.350·2); vitamin B substances.
Epilepsy; insomnia; sedative.

Adco-Retic *Adcock Ingram Generics, S.Afr.*
Amiloride hydrochloride (p.819·2); hydrochlorothiazide (p.885·2).
Hypertension; oedema.

Adcortyl
Bristol-Myers Squibb, Irl.; Squibb, UK.
Triamcinolone acetonide (p.1050·2).
Musculoskeletal, joint, and peri-articular disorders; skin disorders.

Adcortyl with Graneodin *Squibb, UK.*
Triamcinolone acetonide (p.1050·2); neomycin sulphate (p.229·2); gramicidin (p.215·2).
Infected skin disorders.

Adcortyl in Orabase
Bristol-Myers Squibb, Irl.; Squibb, UK.
Triamcinolone acetonide (p.1050·2).
Inflammatory disorders of the mouth; lesions of the oral mucosa.

Adco-Sinal Co *Adcock Ingram Generics, S.Afr.*
Paracetamol (p.72·2); phenylpropanolamine hydrochloride (p.1067·2); phenyltoloxamine citrate (p.416·1); codeine phosphate (p.26·1).
Cold and influenza symptoms.

Adco-Sodasol *Adcock Ingram, S.Afr.*
Sodium citrate (p.1153·2); sodium bicarbonate (p.1153·2); anhydrous citric acid (p.1564·3); tartaric acid (p.1634·3).
Gastric hyperacidity; urinary alkalinisation.

Adco-Sufedrin *Adcock Ingram Generics, S.Afr.*
Pseudoephedrine hydrochloride (p.1068·3).
Upper respiratory-tract congestion.

Adco-Tussend *Adcock Ingram Generics, S.Afr.*
Triprolidine hydrochloride (p.420·3); pseudoephedrine hydrochloride (p.1068·3); codeine phosphate (p.26·1).
Coughs.

Addamel
Kabivitrum, Irl.†; Pharmacia, S.Afr.†; Kabi, Swed.†; KabiVitrum, UK†.
Electrolyte and trace element preparation (p.1147·1).
Parenteral nutrition.

Addamel N
Pharmacia Upjohn, Ital.; Pharmacia Upjohn, Neth.; Pharmacia Upjohn, Switz.
Electrolyte and trace element preparation (p.1147·1).
Parenteral nutrition.

Addamel Novum *Pharmacia Upjohn, Belg.*
Electrolyte and trace element preparation (p.1147·1).
Parenteral nutrition.

Addel N *Pharmacia Upjohn, Ger.*
Electrolyte and trace element preparation (p.1147·1).
Parenteral nutrition.

Adderall *Richwood, USA.*
Dexamphetamine sulphate (p.1478·2); dexamphetamine saccharate (p.1479·2); amphetamine sulphate (p.1477·3); amphetamine aspartate (p.1477·3).
Formerly known as Obetrol.
Attention deficit disorder with hyperactivity; narcoleptic syndrome; obesity.

Addergit *Klinge, Switz.†.*
Dihydroergotamine mesylate (p.444·2); etilefrine hydrochloride (p.867·2).
Hypotension.

Addex *Pharmacia Upjohn, Swed.*
A range of electrolyte preparations (p.1147·1).

Addiphos
Pharmacia Upjohn, Irl.; Pharmacia Upjohn, Neth.; Pharmacia Upjohn, Swed.; Kabi, Switz.†; Pharmacia Upjohn, UK.
Electrolyte preparation (p.1147·1).
Parenteral nutrition.

Additrace
Pharmacia Upjohn, Irl.; Pharmacia Upjohn, UK.
Trace-element preparation (p.1147·1).
Parenteral nutrition.

Adebilan *Schoning-Berlin, Ger.†.*
Glycerol (p.1585·2); wheat-germ oil; cod-liver oil (p.1337·3); allantoin (p.1078·2); chlorophyllin (p.1000·1); thymol (p.1127·1); yeast (p.1373·1); honey (p.1345·3).
Ulcers; wounds.

A+D+E+B_{12}-Vicotrat *Heyl, Ger.†.*
Multivitamin preparation.

Adecaps *Schoeller, Aust.*
Cod-liver oil (p.1337·3).
Vitamin A and D deficiency.

Adecut *Takeda, Jpn.*
Delapril hydrochloride (p.847·1).
Hypertension.

Adeflor M *Upjohn, USA.*
Multivitamin and mineral preparation with fluoride (p.742·1) and iron.
Dental caries prophylaxis; dietary supplement.

Adek *Falk, Ger.*
Multivitamin preparation.

Adeks
Jouveinal, Canad.; Scandipharm, USA.
Multivitamin and mineral preparation.

Adelfan
Ciba, Ital.†; Ciba-Geigy, Spain†.
Reserpine (p.942·1); dihydralazine sulphate (p.854·1).
Hypertension.

Adelfan-Esidrex
Ciba, Ital.†; Ciba-Geigy, Spain.
Reserpine (p.942·1); dihydralazine sulphate (p.854·1); hydrochlorothiazide (p.885·2).
Hypertension.

Adelheid-Jodquelle, Tolzer *Jodquellen, Ger.*
Sodium iodide (p.1493·2); potassium; sodium; ammonium; calcium; magnesium; iron; chloride; sodium bromide; bicarbonate.
Iodine-deficiency disorders.

Adelphan *Ciba, Ger.†; Ciba, Switz.†.*
Reserpine (p.942·1); dihydralazine sulphate (p.854·1).
Hypertension.

Adelphane-Esidrex *Ciba-Geigy, S.Afr.†.*
Reserpine (p.942·1); dihydralazine sulphate (p.854·1); hydrochlorothiazide (p.885·2).
Hypertension.

Adelphan-Esidrex *Ciba-Geigy, Aust.; Ciba, Switz.*
Reserpine (p.942·1); dihydralazine sulphate (p.854·1); hydrochlorothiazide (p.885·2).
Hypertension.

Adelphan-Esidrex-K *Ciba-Geigy, Aust.†; Ciba, Switz.†.*
Reserpine (p.942·1); dihydralazine sulphate (p.854·1); hydrochlorothiazide (p.885·2); potassium chloride (p.1161·1).
Hypertension.

Adelphan-Esidrix *Ciba, Ger.*
Reserpine (p.942·1); dihydralazine sulphate (p.854·1); hydrochlorothiazide (p.885·2).
Hypertension.

Adena C *Innothera, Fr.*
Pink tablets, deoxyribonucleic acid (p.1570·3); white tablets, ascorbic acid (p.1365·2).
Tonic.

Adenas *Eagle, Austral.*
Vitamins and minerals; ginger (p.1193·2); equisetum (p.1575·1).
Tonic.

Adeneurina *Panthox & Burck, Ital.†.*
Adenosine phosphate (p.1543·2); thiamine monophosphate chloride (p.1361·2); cyanocobalamin (p.1363·3).
Musculoskeletal and joint disorders; neuritis.

Adenobeta *Salus, Ital.*
Cocarboxylase chloride (p.1361·2); cyanocobalamin (p.1363·3).
Neuritis.

Adenocard *Fujisawa, Canad.; Fujisawa, USA.*
Adenosine (p.812·3).
Diagnosis of arrhythmias; paroxysmal supraventricular tachycardia.

Adenocor *Sanofi Winthrop, Austral.; Sanofi Winthrop, Belg.; Sanofi Winthrop, Irl.; Sanofi Winthrop, Neth.; Sanofi Winthrop, Norw.; Sanofi Omnimed, S.Afr.; Sanofi Winthrop, Spain; Sanofi, Swed.†; Sanofi Winthrop, UK.*
Adenosine (p.812·3).
Diagnosis of arrhythmias; paroxysmal supraventricular tachycardia.

Adenoplex *Marion Merrell Dow, Belg.†.*
Multivitamin preparation.

Adenoplex Forte *Lepetit, Ital.*
Cocarboxylase (p.1361·2); pyridoxine hydrochloride (p.1362·3); cyanocobalamin (p.1363·3).
Musculoskeletal and joint disorders; neuritis.

Adenoprostal *IBSA, Switz.*
Pollen extract.
Micturition disorders associated with benign prostatic hyperplasia.

Adenopurin *Herbrand, Ger.†.*
Injection: Adenosine (p.812·3); proxyphylline (p.757·3); ethaverine hydrochloride (p.1577·1).
Tablets: Adenosine (p.812·3); proxyphylline (p.757·3); ethaverine hydrochloride (p.1577·1); pentaerythritol tetranitrate (p.927·3); phenobarbitone (p.350·2).
Cardiac disorders.

Adenoscan *Sanofi Winthrop, Austral.; Sanofi Winthrop, Neth.; Sanofi Winthrop, UK; Fujisawa, USA.*
Adenosine (p.812·3).
Coronary vasodilator during radionuclide myocardial perfusion imaging.

Adenovasin *Pfleger, Ger.†.*
Glyceryl trinitrate (p.874·3); atropine sulphate (p.455·1); adenosine (p.812·3); ethaverine hydrochloride (p.1577·1); phenobarbitone (p.350·2); theophylline (p.765·1).
Cardiac disorders.

Adenovit *Nuovo, Ital.*
Cyanocobalamin (p.1363·3); cocarboxylase hydrochloride (p.1361·2); pyridoxine hydrochloride (p.1362·3).
Neuropathies.

Adenyl *Wyeth, Fr.*
Adenosine phosphate (p.1543·2).
Haemorrhoids; venous insufficiency.

Adenylocrat *Godecke, Ger.*
Crataegus (p.1568·2).
Cardiac disorders.

Adepal *Wyeth, Fr.*
Levonorgestrel (p.1454·1); ethinyloestradiol (p.1445·1).
Biphasic oral contraceptive; dysmenorrhoea.

Adepril *Lepetit, Ital.*
Amitriptyline hydrochloride (p.273·3).
Depression.

Adeptolon *Godecke, Ger.*
Prednisolone (p.1048·1); *N*-(4-bromobenzyl)-*N*′-ethyl-*N*′-methyl-*N*-(2-pyridyl)ethylenediamine maleate.
Hypersensitivity disorders; pruritus.

Aderman *Schulke & Mayr, Ger.†.*
Phenylmercuric acetate (p.1122·2).
Skin and mucous membrane disinfection.

Adermykon *Terramin, Aust.*
Chlorphenesin (p.376·2).
Fungal and bacterial infections.

Aderplus spezial Dr Hagedorn *Naturarzneimittel, Ger.*
Homoeopathic preparation.

Adesipress-TTS *Pharmacia Upjohn, Ital.*
Clonidine (p.842·2).
Hypertension.

Adesitrin *Pharmacia Upjohn, Ital.*
Glyceryl trinitrate (p.874·3).
Angina pectoris.

Adexolin *Seven Seas, UK.*
Multivitamin preparation.

Adfen *Adcock Ingram Self Medication, S.Afr.*
Ibuprofen (p.44·1).
Fever; inflammation; musculoskeletal and joint disorders; pain.

Adhaegon *Merckle, Aust.*
Dihydroergotamine mesylate (p.444·2).
Chronic venous insufficiency; hypotension; migraine; varicose veins.

Adiantine *Potter's, UK.*
Artemisia abrotanum; glycerol (p.1585·2); hamamelis (p.1587·1); rosemary oil (p.1626·2); bay oil (p.1552·2).
Seborrhoeic dermatitis.

Adiaril *Diepal, Fr.*
Glucose; sucrose; potassium gluconate; sodium bicarbonate; sodium chloride (p.1152·3).
Diarrhoea; oral rehydration therapy.

Adiazine *Doms-Adrian, Fr.*
Sulphadiazine (p.252·3).
Bacterial infections; Pneumocystis carinii pneumonia; toxoplasmosis.

Adiboran AD *Eurospital, Ital.*
Vitamin A palmitate (p.1359·2); cholecalciferol (p.1366·3).
Vitamin A and D deficiency.

Adical 12 Smit Forte *UCB, Ital.†.*
Multivitamin preparation with calcium laevulinate.

Adiclair *Ardeypharm, Ger.*
Nystatin (p.386·1).
Fungal infections.

Adifax *Servier, Austral.†; Servier, Irl.†; Servier, S.Afr.†; Servier, UK†.*
Dexfenfluramine hydrochloride (p.1479·2).
Obesity.

Adifteper *ISM, Ital.*
A diphtheria, tetanus, and pertussis vaccine (p.1509·1).
Active immunisation.

Adinepar *Lebens, Ital.†.*
Inosine (p.1591·1); cyanocobalamin (p.1363·3); calcium folinate (p.1342·2); suprarenal cortex (p.1050·1). Lignocaine hydrochloride (p.1293·2) is included in this preparation to alleviate the pain of injection.
Tonic.

Adiod *Bama, Spain.*
Cholecalciferol (p.1366·3); vitamin A (p.1358·1); iodine (p.1493·1).
Deficiency of vitamins A and D.

Adipex *Gerot, Aust.; Gerot, Switz.*
Phentermine polystyrene sulphonate (p.1484·3).
Obesity.

Adipex-P *Gate, USA.*
Phentermine hydrochloride (p.1484·3).
Obesity.

Adipine *Trinity, UK.*
Nifedipine (p.916·2).
Angina pectoris; hypertension.

Adipo Ro-Plex Arzneitee (Rowo-714) *Pharmakon, Ger.†.*
Sassafras; urtica; erica; achillea; viola tricolor; equisetum; senna; betula; juglandis; rosemary; phaseolus; rose fruit; juniper; frangula bark; liquorice; ebuli root; guaiacum wood.
Herbal preparation.

Adipomin *Streuli, Switz.†.*
Fenfluramine hydrochloride (p.1480·3).
Obesity.

Adiro *Bayer, Spain.*
Aspirin (p.16·1).
Fever; inflammation; pain; thrombo-embolism prophylaxis.

Adisole *Farmitalia Carlo Erba, Ital.†.*
Tuna-liver oil.
Vitamin A and D source.

Adisterolo *Abiogen, Ital.*
Vitamin A (p.1358·1); ergocalciferol (p.1367·1).
Vitamin A and D deficiency.

Adistop *Phyteia, Switz.*
Cathine hydrochloride (p.1478·1).
Obesity.

Adistop Lax *Phyteia, Switz.*
Frangula (p.1193·2); aloes (p.1177·1); senna (p.1212·2); peppermint leaf (p.1208·1); caraway (p.1559·3); fennel (p.1579·1).
Constipation.

Adiuvant *Manetti Roberts, Ital.*
Pirglutargine (p.1619·2).
Mental function disorders.

Adizem *Napp, Irl.; Napp, UK.*
Diltiazem hydrochloride (p.854·2).
Angina pectoris; hypertension.

Adizem-XL Plus *Napp, UK†.*
Diltiazem hydrochloride (p.854·2); hydrochlorothiazide (p.885·2).
Hypertension.

ADL *SmithKline Beecham, Ger.*
Allergen extracts (p.1545·1).
Hyposensitisation.

Adlone *UAD, USA.*
Methylprednisolone acetate (p.1046·1).

Admon *Esteve, Spain.*
Nimodipine (p.922·2).
Cerebrovascular disorders.

Ad-Muc *Merz, Ger.*
Chamomile (p.1561·2); myrrh (p.1606·1).
Inflammatory disorders of the mouth and gums.

Adnexol *Bama, Spain†.*
Ichthammol (p.1083·3).
Genital inflammatory conditions.

Adnisolone *Nelson, Austral.†.*
Prednisolone (p.1048·1).
Corticosteroid.

Ado C *Kwizda, Aust.*
Paracetamol (p.72·2); ascorbic acid (p.1365·2).
Fever; pain.

Adobiol *Menarini, Ital.†.*
Bufetolol hydrochloride (p.834·2).
Cardiovascular disorders.

Adocor *TAD, Ger.*
Captopril (p.836·3).
Heart failure; hypertension.

Adofen *Ferrer, Spain.*
Fluoxetine hydrochloride (p.284·1).
Bulimia nervosa; depression; obsessive-compulsive disorder.

Adolkin *Prodes, Spain.*
Metamizole magnesium (p.35·1).
Fever; pain.

Adolonta *Andromaco, Spain.*
Tramadol hydrochloride (p.90·1).
Pain.

Adolorin *Kwizda, Aust.*
Propyphenazone (p.81·3); paracetamol (p.72·2); caffeine (p.749·3).
Fever; pain.

Adolphs Salt Substitute *Adolphs, USA.*
Sodium-free dietary salt substitute.

Adoluron CC *Kwizda, Aust.*
Propyphenazone (p.81·3); paracetamol (p.72·2); codeine hydrochloride (p.26·1).
Fever; pain.

Adomal *Malesci, Ital.†.*
Diflunisal (p.33·2).
Pain.

Adomed *Kwizda, Aust.*
Bupranolol hydrochloride (p.835·2).
Hypertension.

Adona *SIT, Ital.; Tanabe, Jpn.*
Carbazochrome sodium sulphonate (p.714·2).
Haemorrhagic disorders.

Adphen *Ferndale, USA†.*
Phendimetrazine tartrate (p.1484·2).
Obesity.

Adprin-B *Pfeiffer, USA.*
Aspirin (p.16·1).
Calcium carbonate (p.1182·1), magnesium carbonate (p.1198·1), and magnesium oxide (p.1198·3) are included in this preparation in an attempt to limit adverse effects on the gastro-intestinal mucosa.
Pain.

Adrectal *Vifor, Switz.*
Ointment: Ephedrine hydrochloride (p.1059·3); lignocaine hydrochloride (p.1293·2); peppermint oil (p.1208·1); thymol (p.1127·1); zinc stearate (p.1469·3).
Suppositories: Ephedrine hydrochloride (p.1059·3); lignocaine hydrochloride (p.1293·2); amethocaine hydrochloride (p.1285·2); peppermint oil (p.1208·1); thymol (p.1127·1); zinc stearate (p.1469·3).
Anorectal disorders.

Adrekar *Sanofi Winthrop, Aust.; Sanofi Winthrop, Ger.*
Adenosine (p.812·3).
Arrhythmias.

Adrenam *NAM, Ger.*
Etilefrine hydrochloride (p.867·2).
Hypotension.

Adrenas *Eagle, Austral.†.*
Vitamins and minerals; equisetum (p.1575·1); ginger (p.1193·2).
Tonic.

Adrenor *Llorens, Spain.*
Noradrenaline acid tartrate (p.924·1).
Glaucoma.

Adrenosin Composto *Vis, Ital.†.*
Zinc sulphate (p.1373·2); boric acid (p.1554·2); lignocaine hydrochloride (p.1293·2); naphazoline nitrate (p.1064·2).
Eye disorders.

Adrenoxyl *Sanofi Winthrop, Belg.†; Labaz, Fr.†; Sanofi Winthrop, Ger.*
Carbazochrome (p.714·1).
Haemorrhagic disorders.

Adreson *Organon, Belg.; Organon, Neth.†.*
Cortisone acetate (p.1036·1).
Corticosteroid.

Adrevil *Zyma, Ger.*
Butalamine hydrochloride (p.835·2).
Peripheral and cerebral vascular disorders.

Adriblastin *Pharmacia Upjohn, Aust.; Pharmacia Upjohn, Ger.*
Doxorubicin hydrochloride (p.529·2).
Malignant neoplasms.

Adriblastina *Pharmacia Upjohn, Belg.; Pharmacia Upjohn, Ital.; Pharmacia Upjohn, Neth.; Pharmacia Upjohn, S.Afr.*
Doxorubicin hydrochloride (p.529·2).
Malignant neoplasms.

Adriblastine *Pharmacia Upjohn, Fr.; Pharmacia Upjohn, Switz.*
Doxorubicin hydrochloride (p.529·2).
Malignant neoplasms.

Adrigyl *Doms-Adrian, Fr.*
Cholecalciferol (p.1366·3).
Vitamin D deficiency.

Adrimedac *Medac, Ger.*
Doxorubicin hydrochloride (p.529·2).
Malignant neoplasms.

Adro-derm *Adroka, Switz.*
Propyl alcohol (p.1124·2); alcohol (p.1099·1); chlorhexidine gluconate (p.1107·2).
Skin disinfection.

Adro-med *Adroka, Switz.†.*
Soap substitute.
Skin disorders.

Adronat *Neopharmed, Ital.*
Alendronate sodium (p.733·2).
Osteoporosis.

Adroyd *Parke, Davis, Austral.†.*
Oxymetholone (p.1459·1).
Anaemias.

Adrucil *Pharmacia Upjohn, Canad.; Adria, USA.*
Fluorouracil (p.534·3).
Malignant neoplasms.

Ad-Sorb *Key, Austral.*
Activated charcoal (p.972·2).
Flatulence.

Adsorbocarpine *Alcon, USA.*
Pilocarpine hydrochloride (p.1396·3).
Glaucoma; raised intra-ocular pressure; reversal of mydriasis.

Adsorbonac *Alcon-Thilo, Ger.; Alcon, Ital.; Alcon, USA.*
Sodium chloride (p.1162·2).
Corneal oedema; eye irritation.

Adsorbotear *Alcon, USA.*
Hydroxyethylcellulose (p.1472·3); povidone (p.1474·2).
Dry eyes.

Adsorgan *Bristol-Myers Squibb, Ger.†.*
Colloidal silver chloride (p.1629·2); silicon dioxide (p.1474·3); colloidal silver; activated charcoal (p.972·2); dimethicone (p.1213·1); liquorice (p.1197·1).
Gastro-intestinal disorders.

ADT Vaccine *CSL, Austral.*
An adsorbed diphtheria and tetanus vaccine (p.1508·1).
Active immunisation.

A-D-Ton *Benvegna, Ital.†.*
Retinol; cholecalciferol.
Vitamin A and D supplement.

Adult Ideal Quota *Larkhall Laboratories, UK.*
Multivitamin and mineral preparation.

Adumbran *Bender, Aust.; Thomae, Ger.; Boehringer Ingelheim, Ital.†; Boehringer Ingelheim, Spain.*
Oxazepam (p.683·2).
Anxiety; hyperexcitability; insomnia.

Advance *Advanced Care, USA.*
Pregnancy test (p.1621·2).

Advanced Antioxidants Formula *Solgar, UK.*
Multivitamin and mineral preparation with superoxide dismutase inducers and proanthocyanidin complex.
Dietary supplement.

Advanced Formula Di-Gel *Schering-Plough, USA.*
Magnesium hydroxide (p.1198·2); calcium carbonate (p.1182·1); simethicone (p.1213·1).
Hyperacidity.

Advanced Formula Plax *Pfizer, USA.*
Sodium pyrophosphate.

Advanced Formula Tegrin *Block, USA.*
Coal tar (p.1092·3).
Scalp disorders.

Advanced Formula Zenate *Solvay, USA.*
Multivitamin and mineral preparation with iron and folic acid.
Formerly called Zenate.
Nutritional supplement in pregnancy and lactation.

Advantage
Note. This name is used for preparations of different composition.
Allergan, Austral.
Subtilisin.
Protein remover for soft and gas permeable contact lenses.

Boehringer Mannheim, Austral.
Test for glucose in blood (p.1585·1).

Advantage 24
Roberts, Canad.; Lake, USA.
Nonoxinol 9 (p.1326·1).
Contraceptive.

Advantan
Schering, Aust.; CSL, Austral.; Schering, Belg.; Schering, Ger.; Schering, Ital.; Schering, S.Afr.; Lederle, Switz.
Methylprednisolone aceponate (p.1046·2).
Skin disorders.

Adventan Schering, Spain.
Methylprednisolone aceponate (p.1046·2).
Skin disorders.

Advera
Abbott, Canad.; Abbott, Fr.; Abbott, Ital.; Ross, USA.
Preparation for enteral nutrition.
Nutritional supplement in HIV infection.

Adversuten Dresden, Ger.
Prazosin hydrochloride (p.932·3).
Heart failure; hypertension; Raynaud's syndrome.

Advil
Whitehall-Robins, Canad.; Whitehall, Fr.; Whitehall, Irl.; Whitehall, Neth.; Whitehall, UK; Wyeth-Ayerst, USA; Whitehall, USA.
Ibuprofen (p.44·1).
Fever; pain.

Advil Cold & Flu Whitehall, Irl.
Ibuprofen (p.44·1); pseudoephedrine (p.1068·3).
Cold and influenza symptoms.

Advil Cold & Sinus
Whitehall-Robins, Canad.; Whitehall, UK; Whitehall, USA.
Ibuprofen (p.44·1); pseudoephedrine hydrochloride (p.1068·3).
Formerly known as Coadvil in the *USA*.
Cold and influenza symptoms; sinusitis.

Advil CS Whitehall, S.Afr.
Ibuprofen (p.44·1); pseudoephedrine hydrochloride (p.1068·3).
Cold and influenza symptoms.

Advil NS Akromed, S.Afr.†.
Oxymetazoline hydrochloride (p.1065·3).
Nasal congestion.

Ad-Vitan Janssen-Cilag, Belg.
Vitamin A acetate (p.1359·2); cholecalciferol (p.1366·3).
Osteomalacia; rickets; vitamin A and D deficiency.

Adyston Krewel, Ger.
Pholedrine sulphate (p.930·2); norfenefrine hydrochloride (p.925·1).
Hypotension.

Aedolac Guieu, Fr.
Emollient.
Dry skin; eczema.

Aedurid Robugen, Ger.†.
Edoxudine (p.609·2).
Herpesvirus eye infections.

Aegrosan Opfermann, Ger.
Dimethicone (p.1213·1).
Gastro-intestinal disorders.

Aeine Gallier, Fr.†.
Phenobarbitone (p.350·2); crataegus (p.1568·2).
Nervous disorders; sleep disorders.

A-E-Mulsin
Mucos, Aust.; Mucos, Ger.
Vitamin A palmitate (p.1359·2); alpha tocopheryl acetate (p.1369·1).
Vitamin A and E deficiency.

Aequamen Promonta Lundbeck, Ger.
Betahistine mesylate (p.1553·1).
Ménière's syndrome; vestibular disorders.

Aequiseral Streuli, Switz.
Electrolyte and glucose solution (p.1147·1).
Dehydration.

Aequiton-P Sudmedica, Ger.
Phenazone (p.78·2).
Fever; pain.

A-E-R Birchwood, USA.
Hamamelis (p.1587·1).
Anorectal disorders; vaginal irritation.

Aero Plus Upsamedica, Spain.
Dimethicone (p.1213·1); metoclopramide hydrochloride (p.1200·3).
Formerly known as Aero Red Plus.
Gastro-intestinal disorders.

Aero Red Upsamedica, Spain.
Dimethicone (p.1213·1).
Flatulence.

Aero Red Eupeptico Upsamedica, Spain.
Dimethicone (p.1213·1); lipolytic enzymes; amylolytic enzymes; proteolytic enzymes; cellulolytic enzymes.
Formerly contained metoclopramide, dimethicone, lipolytic enzymes, amylolytic enzymes, proteolytic enzymes, and cellulolytic enzymes.
Gastro-intestinal disorders.

Aeroaid Health & Medical, USA; Graham-Field, USA.
Thiomersal (p.1126·3).
Skin disinfection; wounds.

AeroBec
3M, Ger.; Asta Medica, Ger.; 3M, Irl.; 3M, Neth.; 3M, S.Afr.; 3M, UK.
Beclomethasone dipropionate (p.1032·1).
Obstructive airways disease.

AeroBid Forest Pharmaceuticals, USA.
Flunisolide (p.1040·3).
Asthma.

Aerobin Farmasan, Ger.
Theophylline (p.765·1) or theophylline sodium glycinate (p.772·2).
Obstructive airways disease.

Aerocaine Aeroceuticals, USA.
Benzocaine (p.1286·2); benzethonium chloride (p.1102·3).
Skin disorders.

Aerocef Klinge, Aust.
Cefixime (p.165·3).
Bacterial infections.

Aerocid Aerocid, Fr.
Pancreas powder (porcine); simethicone (p.1213·1).
Formerly contained adrenaline, pancreatin, liver extract, and ergot.
Dyspepsia.

Aerocrom Castlemead, UK.
Sodium cromoglycate (p.762·1); salbutamol sulphate (p.758·2).
Asthma.

Aeroderm Seid, Spain.
Lignocaine hydrochloride (p.1293·2).
Skin irritation.

Aerodesin Lysoform, Ger.
Propyl alcohol (p.1124·2); alcohol (p.1099·1); glutaraldehyde (p.1114·3).
Surface disinfection.

Aerodine Graham-Field, USA.
Povidone-iodine (p.1123·3).
Skin disinfection.

Aerodur Stern, Ger.
Terbutaline sulphate (p.764·1).
Obstructive airways disease.

Aerodyne Klinge, Aust.
Theophylline (p.765·1) or theophylline sodium glycinate (p.772·2).
Obstructive airways disease.

Aerofagil Geymonat, Ital.
Sodium citrate (p.1153·2); dimethicone (p.1213·1).
Aerophagia; meteorism.

Aeroflat Biosarto, Spain.
Dimethicone (p.1213·1); metoclopramide (p.1202·1).
Gastro-intestinal disorders.

Aerofreeze Graham-Field, USA.
Dichlorodifluoromethane (p.1164·3); trichlorofluoromethane (p.1164·3).
Topical anaesthesia.

Aerogastol Sopar, Belg.†.
An antihistamine.

Aerolate Fleming, USA.
Theophylline (p.765·1).
Obstructive airways disease.

Aerolin
3M, Irl.; 3M, Neth.; 3M, UK.
Salbutamol sulphate (p.758·2).
Obstructive airways disease.

Aeromax Cascan, Ger.; Cascapharm, Ger.
Salmeterol xinafoate (p.761·2).
Obstructive airways disease.

Aeromuc Klinge, Aust.
Acetylcysteine (p.1052·3).
Otitis media; respiratory-tract disorders.

Aeropax
Ercopharm, Neth.†; Ercopharm, Switz.
Simethicone (p.1213·1).
Aid to gastroscopy; flatulence.

Aerophagyl Monal, Fr.†.
Hexamine (p.216·1); sodium bromide (p.1620·3); citric acid (p.1564·3); calcium carbonate (p.1182·1).
Dyspepsia.

Aeroseb-Dex Allergan Herbert, USA.
Dexamethasone (p.1037·1).
Skin disorders.

Aeroseb-HC Allergan Herbert, USA†.
Hydrocortisone (p.1043·3).
Skin disorders.

Aerosol Spitzner N Spitzner, Ger.
Oleum pini sylvestris; pumilio pine oil (p.1623·3); eucalyptus oil (p.1578·1); siberian fir oil; noble pine oil.
Respiratory-tract disorders.

Aerosoma Andreu, Spain†.
Beclomethasone dipropionate (p.1032·1); salbutamol (p.758·2).
Asthma.

Aerosporin
Glaxo Wellcome, Canad.; Wellcome, Irl.†; Calmic, UK†; Glaxo Wellcome, USA†.
Polymyxin B sulphate (p.239·1).
Gram-negative infections.

Aerospray Analgesico Alonga, Spain†.
Camphor (p.1557·2); methyl salicylate (p.55·2); menthol (p.1600·2).
Musculoskeletal and joint pain.

Aerospray Antialergico Alonga, Spain†.
Benzalkonium chloride (p.1101·3); diphenhydramine (p.409·1); menthol (p.1600·2).
Insect bites; pruritus.

Aerotec Synthelabo, Ital.
Salbutamol sulphate (p.758·2).
Obstructive airways disease.

Aerotherm Aeroceuticals, USA.
Benzocaine (p.1286·2); benzethonium chloride (p.1102·3).
Skin disorders.

Aerovacuna Nezel, Spain.
Lysates of *diplococcus*; *streptococcus*; *Micrococcus pyogenes*; *Gaffkya anaerobia*; *Neisseria*; *Haemophilus influenzae*; *Klebsiella pneumoniae*; *Moraxella*.
Respiratory-tract infections.

Aerozoin Graham-Field, USA.
Compound benzoin tincture.
Barrier preparation.

AErrane
ICI, Austral.; Pharmacia Upjohn, Belg.; Pharmacia Upjohn, Irl.; Pharmacia Upjohn, Ital.; Pharmacia Upjohn, Neth.; Pharmacia Upjohn, Spain; Pharmacia, UK.
Isoflurane (p.1225·1).
General anaesthesia.

Aescorin N Steigerwald, Ger.
Injection: Rutoside sodium sulphate (p.1580·2); esculoside (p.1543·3).
Haemorrhoids; vascular disorders.
Ointment: Aesculus (p.1543·3); hamamelis (p.1587·1).
Haemorrhoids; vascular disorders.
Tablets: Aesculus (p.1543·3).
Soft-tissue injury; venous insufficiency.

Aescosulf N Rorer, Ger.†.
Homoeopathic preparation.

Aesculaforce Bioforce, Switz.
Aesculus (p.1543·3).
Venous insufficiency.

Aesculaforce N Bioforce, Switz.
Homoeopathic preparation.

Aesculus Med Complex Dynamit, Aust.
Homoeopathic preparation.

Aescusan
Jenapharm, Ger.
Tablets; oral liquid: Aesculus (p.1543·3).
Soft-tissue inflammation; venous insufficiency.
LAW, Ger.
Cream: Aesculus (p.1543·3); hamamelis (p.1587·1).
Soft-tissue inflammation; venous insufficiency.

Aescuven Redel, Ger.
Aesculus (p.1543·3).
Soft-tissue inflammation; venous insufficiency.

Aesrutal S Steigerwald, Ger.
Convallaria (p.1567·2); crataegus (p.1568·2); ammi visnaga fruit (p.1593·2).
Circulatory insufficiency; heart failure.

Aesrutan Engelshof, Aust.
Rutin (p.1580·2); aesculus (p.1543·3).
Chronic venous insufficiency; haemorrhoids.

Aethone
Sopar, Belg.†; Biologiques de l'Ile-de-France, Fr.†.
Ethyl orthoformate (p.1061·1).
Coughs.

Aethoxysklerol
Provita, Aust.; Codali, Belg.; Kreussler, Ger.; Novartis, Neth.; Inverdia, Swed.; Kreussler, Switz.
Laureth 9 (p.1325·2).
Haemorrhoids; varices.

Aethroma
Merckle, Aust.; Mepha, Switz.
Vincamine (p.1644·1).
Cerebrovascular disorders; hearing disorders; tinnitus.

Aetoxisclerol Dexo, Fr.
Laureth 9 (p.1325·2).
Varices.

Aezodent Associated Dental, UK.
Chlorbutol (p.1106·3); methyl salicylate (p.55·2); benzocaine (p.1286·2); menthol (p.1600·2); eugenol (p.1578·2).
Denture irritation.

AF Lennon, S.Afr.
Zinc undecenoate (p.389·2); undecenoic acid (p.389·2); terpineol (p.1635·1).
Fungal skin infections.

222 AF Frosst, Canad.
Paracetamol (p.72·2).
Fever; pain.

AF Anacin Whitehall-Robins, Canad.
Paracetamol (p.72·2).
Fever; pain.

afdosa-duo Hefa, Ger.†.
Isoprenaline hydrochloride (p.892·1); atropine methonitrate (p.455·1).
Asthma; bronchitis; emphysema.

Afebrin Inkeysa, Spain.
Dipyrone (p.35·1).
Fever; pain.

Afebryl
SMB, Belg.; Galephar, Fr.
Aspirin (p.16·1); paracetamol (p.72·2); ascorbic acid (p.1365·2).
Fever; pain.

Aferadol Oberlin, Fr.
Paracetamol (p.72·2).
Fever; pain.

AFI-B$_6$ Nycomed, Norw.
Pyridoxine hydrochloride (p.1362·3).
Peripheral neuritis; pyridoxine deficiency; sideroblastic anaemia.

AFI-B-Total Nycomed, Norw.
Vitamin B substances.

AFI-C Nycomed, Norw.
Ascorbic acid (p.1365·2).
Vitamin C deficiency.

AFI-D$_2$ Nycomed, Norw.
Ergocalciferol (p.1367·1).
Hypoparathyroid tetany.

Afid Plus Fresenius, Ger.
Bis(3-aminopropyl)-dodecylamine; benzalkonium chloride (p.1101·3); cocospropylenediamineguanidinium diacetate.
Instrument disinfection.

AFI-E Nycomed, Norw.
Alpha tocopheryl acetate (p.1369·2).
Vitamin E deficiency.

A-Fil GenDerm, USA.
Methyl anthranilate; titanium dioxide (p.1093·3).
Sunscreen.

AFI-Nutrin Nycomed, Norw.†.
Multivitamin preparation.

Afipran AFI, Norw.
Metoclopramide (p.1202·1) or metoclopramide hydrochloride (p.1200·3).
Gastro-intestinal disorders.

Aflamin Hexal, S.Afr.
Indomethacin (p.45·2).
Gout; musculoskeletal and joint disorders.

Afloben Esseti, Ital.
Benzydamine hydrochloride (p.21·3).
Inflammation; pain.

Aflodac Biotekfarma, Ital.
Sulindac (p.86·3).
Gout; musculoskeletal and joint disorders.

Aflogine Deverge, Ital.
Cetrimonium tosylate (p.1106·1); allantoin (p.1078·2); lactic acid (p.1593·3); sodium adipate (p.1543·3).
Personal hygiene; vaginal douche.

Aflogos Biomedica, Ital.
Diflunisal arginine (p.33·3).
Pain.

Aflomin Ciba Vision, Spain†.
Trifluridine (p.627·3).
Herpes simplex infections of the eye.

Afloxan Rotta, Ital.
Proglumetacin dimaleate (p.81·2).
Inflammation; pain.

Afloyan Alter, Spain.
Etofibrate (p.1272·3).
Hyperlipidaemias.

Aflukin C IPS, Neth.
Quinine sulphate (p.439·2); ascorbic acid (p.1365·2).
Cold and influenza symptoms.

Afluon Asta Medica, Spain.
Azelastine hydrochloride (p.403·1).
Allergic rhinitis.

Afluvit IPS, Neth.
Paracetamol (p.72·2); ascorbic acid (p.1365·2).
Cold and influenza symptoms.

Afongan
Galderma, Ital.; Galderma, Spain.
Omoconazole nitrate (p.386·3).
Fungal skin and nail infections.

Afonilum
Ebewe, Aust.†.
Theophylline (p.765·1).
Obstructive airways disease.
Knoll, Ger.
Controlled-release capsules: Theophylline (p.765·1).
Injection: Aminophylline hydrate (p.748·1).
Obstructive airways disease.

Afonilum novo Knoll, Ger.
Theophylline sodium glycinate (p.772·2).
Obstructive airways disease.

Afos Salus, Ital.
Injection†: Fosfomycin sodium (p.210·2).
Tablets: Fosfomycin calcium (p.210·2).
Bacterial infections.

afpred-DEXA Hefa, Ger.
Dexamethasone sodium metasulphobenzoate (p.1037·2).
Formerly known as afpred-1.
Obstructive airways disease.

afpred-THEO Hefa, Ger.
Theophylline (p.765·1).
Formerly known as afpred-2.
Cor pulmonale; neonatal apnoea; obstructive airways disease.

Afrazine
Schering-Plough, Irl.†; Schering-Plough, UK.
Oxymetazoline hydrochloride (p.1065·3).
Nasal congestion.

African Gold Strickland, Canad.
Hydroquinone (p.1083·1).

Afrin
Note. This name is used for preparations of different composition.
Schering-Plough, S.Afr.†.
Oxymetazoline hydrochloride (p.1065·3).
Ocular vasoconstrictor.
Schering-Plough, USA.
Nasal drops; nasal spray: Oxymetazoline hydrochloride (p.1065·3).
Tablets: Pseudoephedrine sulphate (p.1068·3).
Nasal congestion.

Afrin Moisturizing Saline Mist Schering-Plough, USA.
Sodium chloride (p.1162·2).
Formerly called Afrin Saline Mist.
Inflammation and dryness of nasal membranes.

Afrodor Farco, Ger.
Quebracho; acetylcarbromal; vitamin E.
Tonic.

Afrolate Bayer, Spain.
Etofenamate (p.36·3).
Peri-articular disorders; soft-tissue disorders.

Afta Juventus, Spain.
Benzalkonium chloride (p.1101·3); hydrocortisone hemisuccinate (p.1044·1).
Stomatitis.

Aftab Rottapharm, Ital.
Triamcinolone acetonide (p.1050·2).
Aphthous ulcer; gingivitis; stomatitis.

Aftate Schering-Plough, USA.
Tolnaftate (p.389·1).
Fungal skin infections.

After Bite
Pensa, Spain; De Witt, UK.
Ammonia (p.1548·3).
Insect bites; stings.

After-Work Hamilton, Austral.
Emollient.
Dry skin.

Aftir Gel Biochimici, Ital.
Malathion (p.1407·3).
Pediculosis.

Aftir Shampoo Biochimici, Ital.
Hydroxyquinoline sulphate (p.1589·3).
For use after Aftir Gel; pediculosis.

AF-Tonic Blucher-Schering, Ger.†.
Formica rufa; formic acid; herb. urticae; apis mellifica; fol. et cort. hamamelidis; flor. arnicae; cort. salicis; sulfur; ol. betulae.
Circulatory disorders; neuralgia; rheumatism.

Agaffin Merck, Aust.
Sodium picosulphate (p.1213·2).
Bowel evacuation; constipation.

Agamadon Agamadon, Ger.
Aquilegia; sedi telephii; teucrii scor; equisetum (p.1575·1); sanicula; chamomile (p.1561·2); sage (p.1627·1); birch leaves (p.1553·3).
Gastro-intestinal disorders.

Agamadon N Agamadon, Ger.
Chamomile (p.1561·2); peppermint leaf (p.1208·1); caraway (p.1559·3).
Dyspepsia.

Agapurin Medphano, Ger.
Oxpentifylline (p.925·3).
Circulatory disorders.

Agarbil Ottolenghi, Ital.†.
Agar (p.1470·3); phenolphthalein (p.1208·2); sodium dehydrocholate (p.1570·3).
Constipation.

Agarol
Note. This name is used for preparations of different composition.
Parke, Davis, Austral.; Warner-Lambert, Ger.; Warner-Wellcome, Spain.
Liquid paraffin (p.1382·1); phenolphthalein (p.1208·2).
Constipation.

Warner-Lambert Consumer, Belg.; Warner-Lambert, Irl.; Warner-Lambert, Ital.†; Warner-Lambert, Neth.†; Parke, Davis, S.Afr.; Warner-Lambert Consumer, Switz.; Warner-Lambert, UK.
Liquid paraffin (p.1382·1); phenolphthalein (p.1208·2); agar (p.1470·3).
Constipation.

Warner-Lambert, Canad.
Oral emulsion: Liquid paraffin (p.1382·1); glycerol (p.1585·2); phenolphthalein (p.1208·2); agar (p.1470·3).
Tablets†: Aloin (p.1177·2); phenolphthalein (p.1208·2).
Constipation.

Agarol Plain Warner-Lambert, Canad.
Liquid paraffin (p.1382·1); glycerol (p.1585·2); agar (p.1470·3).
Constipation.

Agarol Rosa Parke, Davis, Ital.†.
Liquid paraffin (p.1382·1).
Constipation.

Agaroletten N Warner-Lambert, Ger.
Bisacodyl (p.1179·3).
Constipation.

Agastrin Rottapharm, Ital.
Trihydroxyaluminium magnesium carbonate.
Gastro-intestinal disorders associated with hyperacidity.

Agathol Iderne, Fr.
Zinc oxide (p.1096·2); titanium dioxide (p.1093·3); peru balsam (p.1617·2).
Formerly contained zinc oxide, titanium dioxide, peru balsam, and cresol.
Skin disorders.

Age Block Avon, Canad.
Avobenzone (p.1486·3); ethylhexyl *p*-methoxycinnamate (p.1487·1); oxybenzone (p.1487·3).
Sunscreen.

Agedin Plus GD, Ital.
Eicosapentaenoic acid (p.1276·1); ubidecarenone (p.1641·2); methionine (p.984·2); betacarotene (p.1335·2).
Nutritional supplement.

Agelan Antigen, Irl.
Indapamide (p.890·2).
Hypertension.

A-gen 53
Chemieprodukte, Aust.
Polysaccharide polysulphuric acid ester.
Contraceptive.

Herbrand, Ger.; Chefaro, Ger.
Cellulose poly(sulphuric acid ester), trisodium salt; nonoxinol 9 (p.1326·1).
Contraceptive.

Agena Lusofarmaco, Ital.
Vaginal gel: Benzalkonium chloride (p.1101·3); nonoxinol (p.1326·1); ethylene glycol monolaurate; carmellose sodium (p.1471·2).
Vaginal tablets: Benzalkonium chloride (p.1101·3); nonoxinol (p.1326·1); ethylene glycol monolaurate; macrogol (p.1597·3).
Contraceptive; vaginal disinfection.

Ageroplas
Serono, Ital.†; Farma Lepori, Spain.
Ditazole (p.859·3).
Thrombo-embolic disorders.

Agerpen CEPA, Spain.
Amoxycillin sodium (p.151·3) or amoxycillin trihydrate (p.151·3).
Bacterial infections.

Agerpen Mucolitico CEPA, Spain.
Amoxycillin trihydrate (p.151·3); bromhexine hydrochloride (p.1055·3).
Respiratory-tract infections.

Agevis Boehringer Ingelheim, Ger.†.
Ethoxyphenyl diethyl phenylbutylamine hydrochloride (p.1577·2); propyphenazone (p.81·3); caffeine (p.749·3).
Dysmenorrhoea.

Agevit Moreau, Fr.
A range of vitamin and mineral supplements.

Aggrastat Merck, USA.
Tirofiban hydrochloride (p.955·1).
Myocardial infarction.

Agilan Klinge, Aust.
Dihydroergotamine mesylate (p.444·2); etilefrine hydrochloride (p.867·2).
Hypotension.

Agiobulk Madaus, S.Afr.
Plantago ovata seeds (p.1194·2); ispaghula husk (p.1194·2).
Constipation.

Agiocur
Madaus, Aust.; Madaus, Ger.
Ispaghula (p.1194·2); ispaghula husk (p.1194·2).
Constipation; Crohn's disease; stool softener.

Agiofibe Knoll, Austral.
Ispaghula (p.1194·2); ispaghula husk (p.1194·2).
Dietary fibre supplement.

Agiolax
Note. This name is used for preparations of different composition.
Madaus, Aust.; Knoll, Austral.; Madaus, Ger.; Madaus, S.Afr.; Madaus, Spain; Madaus, Switz.
Ispaghula (p.1194·2); ispaghula husk (p.1194·2); senna (p.1212·2).
Bowel evacuation; constipation; stool softener.

Madaus, Fr.; Naturwaren, Ital.; Madaus, Neth.
Ispaghula (p.1194·2); senna (p.1212·2).
Constipation.

Madaus, Belg.
Ispaghula (p.1194·2); Tinnevelly senna (p.1212·2); guaiazulene (p.1586·3).
Constipation; stool softener.

Madaus, Ger.
Ispaghula (p.1194·2).
Constipation; stool softener.

Agiolax mite Madaus, Switz.
Ispaghula (p.1194·2); ispaghula husk (p.1194·2).
Constipation; irritable bowel syndrome; stool softener.

Agiolax Pico Madaus, Ger.
Sodium picosulphate (p.1213·2).
Constipation.

Agiolind
Note. This name is used for preparations of different composition.
Madaus, Aust.
Ispaghula (p.1194·2).
Constipation; stool softener.

Madaus, Ger.†.
Psyllium (p.1194·2).
Constipation.

Agipiu Candioli, Ital.
Silver carbonate (p.1629·2); alkylbenzyldimethylammonium saccharinate (p.1102·1).
Wound disinfection.

Agit Sanofi Winthrop, Ger.
Dihydroergotamine mesylate (p.444·2).
Hypotension; migraine and other vascular headaches; varices.

Agit plus Sanofi Winthrop, Ger.
Dihydroergotamine mesylate (p.444·2); etilefrine hydrochloride (p.867·2).
Hypotension.

Aglumin Eisai, Jpn†.
Ethamsylate (p.720·1).
Haemorrhagic disorders.

Aglutella
Distriborg, Fr.†; Gentili, Ital.; Ultrapharm, UK.
Low-protein, gluten-free food for special diets.

Aglycid IFI, Ital.†.
Tolbutamide (p.333·2).
Diabetes mellitus.

Agnolyt
Madaus, Ger.; Natural Touch, UK.
Vitex agnus castus (p.1544·2).
Mastalgia; menstrual disorders.

Agnucaston Bionorica, Ger.
Vitex agnus castus (p.1544·2).
Mastalgia; menstrual disorders.

Agnuchol Smetana, Aust.
Cynara (p.1569·2); taraxacum (p.1634·2); peppermint leaf (p.1208·1).
Digestive disorders; gallbladder disorders.

Agnufemil Steigerwald, Ger.
Agnus castus (p.1544·2).
Mastalgia; premenstrual syndrome.

Agnukliman Smetana, Aust.
Cimicifuga (p.1563·3).
Menopausal disorders.

Agnumens Smetana, Aust.
Agnus castus (p.1544·2).
Menstrual disorders; premenstrual syndrome.

Agnus castus Hevert, Ger.
Homoeopathic preparation.

Agofell Janssen-Cilag, S.Afr.
Di-isopromine hydrochloride (p.1189·1); sorbitol (p.1354·2).
Biliary-tract disorders.

Agolanid Sandoz, Spain†.
Acetyldigoxin (p.812·3).
Arrhythmias; heart failure.

Agon Hoechst Marion Roussel, Austral.
Felodipine (p.867·3).
Hypertension.

Agopton
Takeda, Aust.; Takeda, Ger.; Grunenthal, Switz.
Lansoprazole (p.1196·2).
Gastro-oesophageal reflux; peptic ulcer.

Agoral Warner-Lambert, USA.
Liquid paraffin (p.1382·1); phenolphthalein (p.1208·2); agar (p.1470·3).
Constipation.

Agoral Plain Warner-Lambert, USA†.
Liquid paraffin (p.1382·1).
Constipation.

A/G-Pro Miller, USA.
Multivitamin, mineral, and amino-acid preparation.

Agradil Synthelabo, Ital.
Veralipride (p.698·1).
Menopausal disorders.

A-Gram Inava, Fr.
Amoxycillin trihydrate (p.151·3) or amoxycillin sodium (p.151·3).
Bacterial infections.

Agreal
Synthelabo, Belg.; Synthelabo, Fr.; Delagrange, Spain.
Veralipride (p.698·1).
Menopausal disorders.

Agredamol Bio-Therabel, Belg.†.
Dipyridamole (p.857·1).
Angina pectoris; ischaemic heart disease; thrombo-embolic disorders.

Agre-Gola Vemedia, Neth.
Cetylpyridinium chloride (p.1106·2); phenol (p.1121·2); menthol (p.1600·2).
Sore throat.

Agrimonas N Niedermaier, Ger.
Taraxacum (p.1634·2); celandine; absinthium (p.1541·1).
Dyspepsia.

Agrippal
Chiron, Ital.; Biovac, S.Afr.
An inactivated influenza vaccine (p.1515·2).
Active immunisation.

Agrumina Also, Ital.
Ascorbic acid (p.1365·2).
Vitamin C deficiency; vitamin C supplement.

Agruton-C Sanofi Winthrop, Belg.†.
Citroflavonoids (p.1580·1); ascorbic acid (p.1365·2).
Capillary disorders.

Agruvit Hoechst Marion Roussel, Ital.
Ascorbic acid (p.1365·2); calcium ascorbate dihydrate (p.1365·2) or sodium ascorbate (p.1365·2).
Vitamin C deficiency; vitamin C supplement.

Agrylin Roberts, USA.
Anagrelide hydrochloride (p.1549·2).
Essential thrombocythaemia.

Agua del Carmen Fardi, Spain.
Coriander seeds (p.1567·3); matricaria (p.1561·2); melissa (p.1600·1); dried bitter-orange peel (p.1610·3); tilia platyphyllos flowers (p.1637·3); lippia citriodora; cinnamon (p.1564·2); angelica; nutmeg (p.1609·2); hyssopus officinalis.
Hyperactivity; nervous disorders; pain.

Agua Germana Liberman, Spain†.
Tartaric acid (p.1634·3); aluminium acetate (p.1547·3).
Aphthous ulcers; gum disorders; tonsillitis.

Agudil Sigma-Tau, Spain.
Levoglutamide (p.1344·3); asparagine; pyridoxine hydrochloride (p.1362·3); phosphoserine.
Tonic.

Agyrax
Note. This name is used for preparations of different composition.
Darci, Belg.
Buclizine hydrochloride (p.404·1); hydroxyzine hydrochloride (p.412·1); buphenine hydrochloride (p.1555·3).
Hearing disorders; tinnitus; vertigo.

Vedim, Fr.
Meclozine hydrochloride (p.413·3).
Formerly contained buphenine hydrochloride, meclozine hydrochloride, and hydroxyzine hydrochloride.
Vertigo.

AH 3 N Rodleben, Ger.
Hydroxyzine hydrochloride (p.412·1).
Pruritus.

AH-chew WE, USA.
Phenylephrine hydrochloride (p.1066·2); chlorpheniramine maleate (p.405·1); hyoscine methonitrate (p.463·1).
Upper respiratory-tract symptoms.

AH-chew D WE, USA.
Phenylephrine (p.1066·2).
Nasal congestion.

AHD 2000 Lysoform, Ger.
Alcohol (p.1099·1).
Hand disinfection; skin disinfection.

AHF CSL, Austral.
A factor VIII preparation (p.720·3).
Factor VIII deficiency; von Willebrand's disease.

AHP 200 Chephasaar, Ger.
Oxaceprol (p.1611·3).
Degenerative disorders of joints and connective tissue.

A-Hydrocort
Abbott, Canad.; Abbott, USA.
Hydrocortisone sodium succinate (p.1044·1).
Corticosteroid.

Aicamin Sanofi Winthrop, Belg.
Orazamide (p.1611·1).
Liver disorders.

Aicase FIRMA, Ital.†.
Urazamide (p.1641·3).
Liver disorders.

Aicorat Mack, Illert., Ger.†.
Orazamide (p.1611·1).
Liver disorders.

Aida Paraphar, Fr.
Hydroquinone (p.1083·1).
Hyperpigmentation.

Aidex Ovelle, Irl.†.
Aminacrine hydrochloride (p.1098·3); benzocaine (p.1286·2).
Burns; stings; sunburn; wounds.

Aid-Lax Nobel, Canad.
Aloin (p.1177·2); cascara (p.1183·1); phenolphthalein (p.1208·2); bile salts (p.1553·2).

Aigin Hevert, Ger.
Kava (p.1592·3).
Nervous disorders.

Aiglonyl Fumouze, Fr.
Sulpiride (p.692·3).
Neuroses.

Ailax Galen, UK.
Danthron (p.1188·2); poloxamer 188 (p.1326·3).
These ingredients can be described by the British Approved Name Co-danthramer.
Constipation.

Aima-Calcin ISI, Ital.
Elcatonin (p.735·3).
Hypercalcaemia; osteoporosis; Paget's disease of bone; reflex sympathetic dystrophy.

Aimafix ISI, Ital.
Factor IX (p.721·3).
Haemorrhagic disorders.

Ainscrid Gerda, Fr.
Indomethacin (p.45·2).
Fever; inflammation.

Airet Adams, USA.
Salbutamol sulphate (p.758·2).

Airol
Roche, Aust.; Roche, Austral.†; Roche, Ger.†; Roche, Ital.; Roche, Norw.†; Roche, S.Afr.†; Roche, Switz.
Tretinoin (p.1093·3).
Acne.

Airomir
3M, Belg.; 3M, Irl.; 3M, Neth.; 3M, Norw.; 3M, S.Afr.; 3M, Swed.; 3M, Switz.; 3M, UK.
Salbutamol (p.758·2) or salbutamol sulphate (p.758·2).
Obstructive airways disease.

Airtal
Rowex, Irl.; Prodes, Spain.
Aceclofenac (p.12·1).
Musculoskeletal, joint, and peri-articular disorders; pain.

Airtal Difucrem Prodes, Spain.
Aceclofenac (p.12·1).
Peri-articular and soft-tissue disorders.

Airvitess Farmasan, Ger.
Ketotifen fumarate (p.755·2).
Allergic disorders; asthma.

Ajaka Streuli, Switz.
Aloes (p.1177·1); aloin (p.1177·2); belladonna (p.457·1); caraway (p.1559·3); fennel (p.1579·1) juniper (p.1592·2); caraway oil (p.1559·3); fennel oil (p.1579·2); juniper oil (p.1592·3).
Constipation.

Ajan 3M, Ger.
Nefopam hydrochloride (p.62·3).
Pain.

Akamin Alphapharm, Austral.
Minocycline hydrochloride (p.226·2).
Bacterial infections.

Akarpine *Akorn, USA.*
Pilocarpine hydrochloride (p.1396·3).
Glaucoma; raised intra-ocular pressure; reversal of mydriasis.

Akatinol *Merz, Ger.*
Memantine hydrochloride (p.1142·2).
Mental function impairment; parkinsonism; spasticity.

Ak-Beta *Akorn, USA.*
Levobunolol hydrochloride (p.897·3).
Glaucoma; ocular hypertension.

Ak-Biocholine *Akorn, USA.*
Choline bitartrate (p.1337·1); citrus bioflavonoid complex (p.1580·1).

Ak-Chlor *Akorn, USA.*
Chloramphenicol (p.182·1).
Eye infections.

Ak-Cide *Akorn, USA.*
Prednisolone acetate (p.1048·1); sulphacetamide sodium (p.252·2).

Ak-Con
Akorn, Canad.; Akorn, USA.
Naphazoline hydrochloride (p.1064·2).
Minor eye irritation.

Ak-Con-A *Akorn, USA.*
Naphazoline hydrochloride (p.1064·2); pheniramine maleate (p.415·3).
Eye irritation.

Ak-Dex *Akorn, USA.*
Dexamethasone sodium phosphate (p.1037·2).
Eye inflammation.

Ak-Dilate *Akorn, USA.*
Phenylephrine hydrochloride (p.1066·2).
Funduscopy; open-angle glaucoma; ophthalmic examination; pupil dilatation during surgery; refraction without cycloplegia; uveitis.

AKE
Fresenius-Klinik, Ger.; Fresenius, Switz.
Amino-acid, carbohydrate, and electrolyte infusion.
Parenteral nutrition.

Akeral *Dermalife, Ital.†.*
Vitamin A acetate (p.1359·2).
Vitamin A deficiency disorders.

Akeson *Baer, Ger.†.*
Costae; glandulae thymi; hepar; spleen; medulla ossium; sanguis.
Neuromuscular and joint disorders.

Akfen *Wyeth, Irl.*
Guanfacine hydrochloride (p.879·1).
Hypertension.

Ak-Fluor *Akorn, USA.*
Fluorescein sodium (p.1581·1).
Ophthalmic diagnostic agent.

Akila mains et peau *Adam, Mon.*
Chlorhexidine gluconate (p.1107·2); hydrogen peroxide (p.1116·2); propyl alcohol (p.1124·2).
Skin disinfection.

Akila spray *Adam, Mon.*
Glutaraldehyde (p.1114·3); benzalkonium chloride (p.1101·3); bromonitrodioxan; alcohol (p.1099·1); propyl alcohol (p.1124·2).
Surface disinfection.

Akindex
Fournier, Belg.; Urgo, Fr.
Dextromethorphan hydrobromide (p.1057·3).
Coughs.

Akindol *Fournier, Spain.*
Paracetamol (p.72·2).
Fever; pain.

Akineton
Ebewe, Aust.; Knoll, Austral.; Knoll, Belg.; Knoll, Canad.; Knoll, Fr.; Knoll, Ger.; Knoll, Irl.; Ravizza, Ital.; Knoll, Neth.; Knoll, Norw.; Knoll, S.Afr.; Knoll, Spain; Meda, Swed.; Knoll, Switz.; Knoll, UK; Knoll, USA.
Biperiden (p.458·3), biperiden hydrochloride (p.458·3), or biperiden lactate (p.458·3).
Bronchospasm; drug-induced extrapyramidal disorders; nicotine poisoning; parkinsonism; phosphorus poisoning; spasticity; trigeminal neuralgia.

Akistin *Nycomed, Aust.†.*
Diethylamine salamidacetate (p.82·3).
Musculoskeletal and joint disorders; neuralgias.

Akkoclean *Akko, Ital.†.*
Soap substitute.

Aklonin *Wernigerode, Ger.*
Phenamazide hydrochloride (p.466·3).
Smooth muscle cramp; vomiting.

Ak-Mycin *Akorn, USA.*
Erythromycin (p.204·1).
Eye infections.

Ak-NaCl *Akorn, USA.*
Sodium chloride (p.1162·2).
Corneal oedema.

Akne *Ichthyol, Aust.*
Erythromycin (p.204·1).
Acne.

Akne Cordes *Ichthyol, Ger.*
Erythromycin (p.204·1).
Acne.

Akne-Aid-Creme *Stiefel, Ger.†.*
Chloroxylenol (p.1111·1); resorcinol (p.1090·1); sulphur (p.1091·2).
Acne.

Akne-Aid-Lotion mild *Stiefel, Ger.†.*
Benzoyl peroxide (p.1079·2).
Acne.

Akne-Aid-Seife *Stiefel, Ger.†.*
Sulphonated plant oils.
Acne; seborrhoea.

Aknederm *Rovi, Spain†.*
Sulphur (p.1091·2); ichthammol (p.1083·3); resorcinol (p.1090·1); zinc oxide (p.1096·2).
Acne.

Aknederm Ery *Gepepharm, Ger.*
Erythromycin (p.204·1).
Acne.

Aknederm N *Gepepharm, Ger.*
Salicylic acid (p.1090·2); lactic acid (p.1593·3).
Skin disorders.

Aknederm Neu *Gepepharm, Ger.*
Ictasol (p.1083·3); zinc oxide (p.1096·2).
Aknederm N ointment formerly contained sulphur, ichthammol, and zinc oxide.
Skin disorders.

Aknederm Oxid *Gepepharm, Ger.*
Benzoyl peroxide (p.1079·2).
Acne.

Aknedertim *Rovi, Spain†.*
Alcohol (p.1099·1); lactic acid (p.1593·3); lapyrium chloride; pyridoxine hydrochloride (p.1362·3); salicylic acid (p.1090·2); vitamin F.
Acne.

Ak-Nefrin *Akorn, USA.*
Phenylephrine hydrochloride (p.1066·2).
Minor eye irritation.

Aknefug simplex *Wolff, Ger.*
Hexachlorophane (p.1115·2).
Acne; rosacea.

Aknefug-EL *Wolff, Ger.*
Erythromycin (p.204·1).
Acne.

Aknefug-Emulsion N *Wolff, Ger.*
Oestradiol (p.1455·1); hexachlorophane (p.1115·2).
Acne.

Aknefug-liquid N *Wolff, Ger.*
Salicylic acid (p.1090·2); coal tar (p.1092·3).
Acne; seborrhoea.

Aknefug-oxid *Wolff, Ger.†.*
Benzoyl peroxide (p.1079·2).
Acne.

Aknelan Lotio *Beiersdorf, Ger.†.*
Salicylic acid (p.1090·2); colloidal sulphur (p.1091·2); dexpanthenol (p.1570·3).
Skin disorders.

Aknelan Milch *Beiersdorf, Ger.†.*
Benzalkonium chloride (p.1101·3); dexpanthenol (p.1570·3).
Skin disorders.

aknemago *Strathmann, Ger.*
Erythromycin (p.204·1).
Acne.

Akne-Medice Kombipackung *Medice, Ger.†.*
Topical powder, tannic acid (p.1634·2); hexylresorcinol (p.1116·1); sublimed sulphur (p.1091·2); lotion, salicylic acid (p.1090·2); camphor (p.1557·2); liquid phenol (p.1121·2); resorcinol (p.1090·1).
Acne.

Aknemin
E. Merck, Neth.; E. Merck, UK.
Minocycline hydrochloride (p.226·2).
Bacterial infections.

Aknemycin
Note. This name is used for preparations of different composition.
Merck, Aust.; Merck-Belgolabo, Belg.; Hermal, Ger.; Boots Healthcare, Neth.; Hermal, Switz.; Hermal, USA.
Erythromycin (p.204·1).
Acne.

Hermal, Ger.; Hermal, Switz.
Topical emulsion: Erythromycin (p.204·1); ichthammol (p.1083·3).
Acne.

Aknemycin compositum *Merck, Aust.*
Erythromycin (p.204·1); light ammonium bituminosulphonate (p.1083·3).
Acne.

Ak-Neo-Dex *Akorn, USA.*
Neomycin sulphate (p.229·2); dexamethasone sodium phosphate (p.1037·2).
Eye inflammation with bacterial infection.

Akne-Puren *Isis Puren, Ger.*
Minocycline hydrochloride (p.226·2).
Acne.

Akne-Pyodron Kur *Cassella-med, Ger.†.*
Lotion: Clorophene (p.1111·2).
Tablets: Tetracycline hydrochloride (p.259·1).
Topical gel: Aluminium magnesium silicate gel (p.1471·1).
Acne.

Akne-Pyodron lokal *Cassella-med, Ger.†.*
Lotion: Clorophene (p.1111·2).
Topical gel: Aluminium magnesium silicate gel (p.1471·1); glycerol (p.1585·2).
Acne.

Akne-Pyodron oral *Cassella-med, Ger.†.*
Tetracycline hydrochloride (p.259·1).
Acne.

Aknereduct *Azupharma, Ger.*
Minocycline hydrochloride (p.226·2).
Acne.

Akneroxid
Merck, Aust.; Merck-Belgolabo, Belg.; Hermal, Ger.; Boots Healthcare, Neth.; Hermal, Switz.
Benzoyl peroxide (p.1079·2).
Acne.

Aknex *Sanopharm, Switz.*
Benzoyl peroxide (p.1079·2).
Acne.

Aknichthol *Ichthyol, Aust.*
Ictasol (p.1083·3); salicylic acid (p.1090·2); colloidal sulphur (p.1091·2).
Acne.

Aknichthol Creme *Ichthyol, Ger.*
Ictasol (p.1083·3).
Acne.

Aknichthol Dexa *Ichthyol, Ger.†.*
Ictasol (p.1083·3); salicylic acid (p.1090·2); dexamethasone acetate (p.1037·1); colloidal sulphur (p.1091·2).
Acne.

Aknichthol N
Note. This name is used for preparations of different composition.
Ichthyol, Ger.
Ictasol (p.1083·3); salicylic acid (p.1090·2).
Acne; rosacea.

Ichthyol, Switz.
Sodium bituminosulphonate (Ichthyol sodium) (p.1083·3); salicylic acid (p.1090·2).
Acne.

Aknilox *Drossapharm, Switz.*
Erythromycin (p.204·1).
Acne.

Aknin
Note. This name is used for preparations of different composition.
Sanofi Winthrop, Ger.
Capsules†: Oxytetracycline hydrochloride (p.235·1).
Lotion: Erythromycin (p.204·1).
Ointment: Sulphur (p.1091·2); salicylic acid (p.1090·2).
Acne.

Winthrop, Switz.†.
Oxytetracycline hydrochloride (p.235·1).
Acne.

Aknin-Mino *Sanofi Winthrop, Ger.*
Minocycline hydrochloride (p.226·2).
Acne.

Aknin-N *Sodip, Switz.*
Minocycline hydrochloride (p.226·2).
Acne.

Aknoral *IBSA, Switz.*
Minocycline hydrochloride (p.226·2).
Acne.

Aknosan *Hermal, Ger.*
Minocycline hydrochloride (p.226·2).
Acne.

Akoline *Akorn, USA†.*
Vitamin B substances with vitamin C; methionine (p.984·2); lemon bioflavonoids (p.1580·1).

Ak-Pentolate *Akorn, USA.*
Cyclopentolate hydrochloride (p.459·3).
Production of mydriasis and cycloplegia.

Ak-Poly-Bac *Akorn, USA.*
Polymyxin B sulphate (p.239·1); bacitracin zinc (p.157·3).
Eye infections.

Ak-Pred *Akorn, USA.*
Prednisolone sodium phosphate (p.1048·1).
Eye inflammation.

AkPro *Akorn, USA.*
Dipivefrine hydrochloride (p.1572·3).
Glaucoma.

Akrinor
Note. This name is used for preparations of different composition.
Asta Medica, Aust.; Asta Medica, Ger.; Vesta, S.Afr.; Asta Medica, Switz.
Cafedrine hydrochloride (p.835·3); theodrenaline hydrochloride (p.1636·2).
Circulatory disorders; hypotension.

Asta Medica, Ital.†.
Cafedrine hydrochloride (p.835·3).
Hypotension; tachycardia.

Ak-Rinse *Akorn, USA.*
Electrolytes (p.1147·1).
Eye irrigation.

Ak-Rose *Akorn, Canad.*
Rose bengal sodium (p.1626·1).
Ophthalmic diagnostic agent.

Akrotherm *Gepepharm, Ger.*
Benzyl nicotinate (p.22·1); nonivamide (p.63·2).
Peripheral vascular disorders; soft-tissue injury.

Aksekapseln *Laves, Ger.†.*
Vitamin A (p.1358·1); wheat-germ oil and sunflower oil fatty-acid ethyl ester (p.1634·1); cholecalciferol (p.1366·3); alpha tocopheryl acetate (p.1369·1); calcium pantothenate (p.1352·3); sulphur (p.1091·2); iodine (p.1493·1); manganese sulphate monohydrate (p.1350·3).
Acne; seborrhoea.

Ak-Spore *Akorn, USA.*
Eye drops: Polymyxin B sulphate (p.239·1); neomycin sulphate (p.229·2); gramicidin (p.215·2).
Eye ointment: Polymyxin B sulphate (p.239·1); neomycin sulphate (p.229·2); bacitracin zinc (p.157·3).
Eye infections.

Ak-Spore HC *Akorn, USA.*
Ear drops: Hydrocortisone (p.1043·3); neomycin sulphate (p.229·2); polymyxin B (p.239·3).
Bacterial ear infections.
Eye drops; eye ointment: Polymyxin B sulphate (p.239·1); neomycin sulphate (p.229·2); hydrocortisone (p.1043·3).
Eye inflammation with bacterial infection.

Ak-Sulf *Akorn, USA.*
Sulphacetamide sodium (p.252·2).
Eye infections.

Ak-Taine
Akorn, Canad.; Akorn, USA.
Proxymetacaine hydrochloride (p.1300·1).
Local anaesthesia.

Ak-T-Caine *Akorn, USA.*
Amethocaine hydrochloride (p.1285·2).

Aktiferrin *Merckle, Aust.*
Ferrous sulphate (p.1340·2); DL-serine.
Iron deficiency; iron deficiency anaemia.

Aktiferrin compositum *Merckle, Aust.*
Ferrous sulphate (p.1340·2); DL-serine; folic acid (p.1340·3); cyanocobalamin (p.1363·3).
Iron deficiency anaemia with folic acid deficiency.

Aktiferrin E F *Merckle, Ger.†.*
Ferrous sulphate (p.1340·2); DL-serine; folic acid (p.1340·3).
Folic-acid deficiency; iron-deficiency; iron-deficiency anaemia.

Aktiferrin N *Merckle, Ger.*
Ferrous sulphate (p.1340·2).
Iron deficiency.

Aktiv Blasen- und Nierentee *Krug, Aust.*
Silver birch (p.1553·3); juniper (p.1592·2); ononis (p.1610·2); bearberry (p.1552·2); peppermint leaf (p.1208·1).
Renal and urinary-tract disorders.

Aktiv Husten- und Bronchialtee *Krug, Aust.*
Plantago lanceolata; aniseed (p.1549·3); thyme (p.1636·3); althaea (p.1546·3).
Catarrh; coughs.

Aktiv Leber- und Gallentee *Krug, Aust.*
Peppermint leaf (p.1208·1); achillea (p.1542·2); fennel (p.1579·1); turmeric (p.1001·3).
Liver and gallbladder disorders.

Aktiv milder Magen- und Darmtee *Krug, Aust.*
Aniseed (p.1549·3); fennel (p.1579·1); caraway (p.1559·3); chamomile (p.1561·2); achillea (p.1542·2).
Gastro-intestinal disorders.

Aktiv Nerven- und Schlaftee *Krug, Aust.*
Lupulus (p.1597·2); valerian (p.1643·1); melissa (p.1600·1); peppermint leaf (p.1208·1); orange flowers.
Nervous disorders; sleep disorders.

Aktivakid *Hoechst Marion Roussel, S.Afr.*
Liver extracts; vitamin B_{12}; yeast extract; ferric glycerophosphate; lysine.
Tonic.

Aktivanad
Ebewe, Aust.
Oral liquid: Liver extract; yeast; rose fruit; caffeine.
Syrup: Liver extract; yeast; rose fruit; ferric glycerophosphate; lysine.
Tonic.

Hoechst Marion Roussel, S.Afr.
Syrup: Haematoporphyrin; liver extracts; caffeine; yeast extract.
Tablets: Haematoporphyrin; liver extracts; amino acids; vitamins; caffeine; yeast extract; ferric glycerophosphate.
Tonic.

Knoll, Switz.†.
Caffeine; sodium acid phosphate; haematoporphyrin; liver extract; rose fruit; yeast.
Tonic.

Aktivanad-N *Knoll, Ger.*
Oral liquid: Liver extract; yeast extract; caffeine.
Tablets: Vitamins; caffeine.
Tonic.

Aktiv-Puder *Klosterfrau, Ger.*
Colloidal silicon dioxide (p.1475·1).
Burns; skin disorders.

AkTob *Akorn, USA.*
Tobramycin (p.264·1).

Akton *Exel, Belg.*
Cloxazolam (p.657·3).
Anxiety disorders; premedication.

Ak-Tracin *Akorn, USA.*
Bacitracin (p.157·3).
Eye infections.

Aktren *Bayer, Ger.*
Ibuprofen (p.44·1).
Fever; pain.

Ak-Trol *Akorn, USA.*
Dexamethasone (p.1037·1); neomycin sulphate (p.229·2); polymyxin B sulphate (p.239·1).
Eye inflammation with bacterial infection.

Ak-Vernacon *Akorn, Canad.*
Pheniramine maleate (p.415·3); phenylephrine hydrochloride (p.1066·2).
Antihistamine; decongestant.

Akwa Tears
Note. This name is used for preparations of different composition.
Akorn, Canad.; Akorn, USA.
Eye ointment: White soft paraffin (p.1382·3); liquid paraffin (p.1382·1); wool fat (p.1385·3).
Dry eyes.

Akorn, USA.
Eye drops: Polyvinyl alcohol (p.1474·2).
Dry eyes.

AKZ
Pfizer, Aust.; Howmedica, Switz.
Erythromycin gluceptate (p.204·2); colistin sulphomethate sodium (p.196·1); polymethylmethacrylate/methylmethacrylate copolymer (p.1603·2).
Bone cement for orthopaedic surgery.

Ak-Zol Akorn, USA†.
Acetazolamide (p.810·3).
Epilepsy; glaucoma; oedema; symptoms associated with acute mountain sickness.

al 110
Nestle, Fr.; Nestle, Ital.; Nestle, S.Afr.; Nestle, Switz.; Nestle, UK.
Food for special diets.
Lactose intolerance.

Alacetan N Palmicol, Ger.
Aspirin (p.16·1); paracetamol (p.72·2); caffeine (p.749·3).
Fever; inflammation; pain.

Ala-Cort Del-Ray, USA.
Hydrocortisone (p.1043·3).
Skin disorders.

Alamag Goldline, USA.
Aluminium hydroxide (p.1177·3); magnesium hydroxide (p.1198·2).
Hyperacidity.

Alamag Plus Goldline, USA.
Aluminium hydroxide (p.1177·3); magnesium hydroxide (p.1198·2); simethicone (p.1213·1).
Hyperacidity.

Alantomicina Cantabria, Spain.
Allantoin (p.1078·2); bacitracin (p.157·3); neomycin (p.229·2); zinc oxide (p.1096·2).
Skin infections.

Alantomicina Complex Cantabria, Spain.
Allantoin (p.1078·2); bacitracin (p.157·3); hydrocortisone acetate (p.1043·3); neomycin (p.229·2); zinc oxide (p.1096·2).
Infected skin disorders.

Alapril Mediolanum, Ital.
Lisinopril (p.898·2).
Heart failure; hypertension.

Alapryl Menarini, Spain.
Halazepam (p.673·2).
Anxiety.

Ala-Quin Del-Ray, USA.
Hydrocortisone (p.1043·3); clioquinol (p.193·2).
Skin disorders.

Alasenn Schworer, Ger.
Senna (p.1212·2); ononis (p.1610·2); achillea (p.1542·2); taraxacum (p.1634·2).
Constipation.

Alasulf Major, USA.
Sulphanilamide (p.256·3); aminacrine hydrochloride (p.1098·3); allantoin (p.1078·2).
Vaginal infections.

Alatone Major, USA.
Spironolactone (p.946·1).
Hyperaldosteronism; hypertension; hypokalaemia; oedema.

Alavac
SmithKline Beecham, Aust.†; Kallergen, Ital.†; Kalopharma, Ital.†.
Allergen extracts (p.1545·1).
Hyposensitisation.

Alavac-P Teomed, Switz.†.
Grass pollen extracts (p.1545·1).
Hyposensitisation.

Alavac-S
Artu, Neth.; Teomed, Switz.
Allergen extracts (p.1545·1).
Hyposensitisation.

Alaxa Angelini, Ital.
Bisacodyl (p.1179·3).
Constipation.

Alba-3 Alba, USA.
Eye drops: Polymyxin B sulphate (p.239·1); neomycin sulphate (p.229·2)l gramicidin (p.215·2).
Eye ointment: Polymyxin B sulphate (p.239·1); neomycin sulphate (p.229·2); bacitracin zinc (p.157·3).
Ointment: Polymyxin B sulphate (p.239·1); neomycin sulphate (p.229·2); bacitracin (p.157·3).

Alba CE Alba, USA.
Ascorbic acid (p.1365·2).

Alba Dex Alba, USA.
Dexamethasone sodium phosphate (p.1037·2).
Corticosteroid.

Alba Gyn Alba, USA.
Sulphathiazole (p.257·1); sulphacetamide (p.252·2); sulfabenzamide (p.251·1).

Alba Lybe Alba, USA.
Vitamin B substances with lysine.

Albacort Idrodispersibile Teknofarma, Ital.†.
Triamcinolone (p.1050·2).
Corticosteroid.

Albaform HC Alba, USA.
Hydrocortisone (p.1043·3); clioquinol (p.193·2).

Albafort Alba, USA.
Vitamin B substances with iron.

Albalon
Allergan, Austral.; Allergan, Belg.; Allergan, Irl.†; Allergan, S.Afr.; Allergan, Switz.; Allergan, USA.
Naphazoline hydrochloride (p.1064·2).
Eye irritation.

Albalon Liquifilm
Allergan, Canad.; Allergan, Neth.†.
Naphazoline hydrochloride (p.1064·2).
Conjunctival congestion; eye irritation.

Albalon Relief Allergan, Austral.
Phenylephrine hydrochloride (p.1066·2).
Eye irritation.

Albalon-A Allergan, S.Afr.
Naphazoline hydrochloride (p.1064·2); antazoline phosphate (p.401·3).
Eye irritation.

Albalon-A Liquifilm
Allergan, Austral.; Allergan, Canad.
Naphazoline hydrochloride (p.1064·2); antazoline phosphate (p.401·3).
Allergic inflammatory eye conditions; eye irritation; ocular congestion.

Albamycin Upjohn, USA.
Novobiocin sodium (p.233·3).
Bacterial infections.

AlbaTemp Alba, USA.
Paracetamol (p.72·2).
Fever; pain.

Albatran Beaufour, Fr.
Papaverine codecarboxylase derivative (p.1614·3).
Peripheral and cerebral vascular disorders.

Albatussin Alba, USA.
Guaiphenesin (p.1061·3); dextromethorphan hydrobromide (p.1057·3); phenylephrine hydrochloride (p.1066·2).
Coughs.

Albatussin NN Alba, USA.
Dextromethorphan hydrobromide (p.1057·3); mepyramine maleate (p.414·1); potassium guaiacolsulfonate (p.1068·3); phenylephrine hydrochloride (p.1066·2).
Coughs.

Albatussin Pediatric Alba, USA.
Dextromethorphan hydrobromide (p.1057·3); phenylephrine hydrochloride (p.1066·2).
Coughs.

Albaxin Pharmacia Upjohn, Ital.†.
Bacampicillin hydrochloride (p.157·2).
Bacterial infections.

Albay
Bayer, Austral.; Dome-Hollister-Stier, Fr.; Bayer, S.Afr.; Miles, USA.
Venoms of bee, wasp, hornet, yellow jacket, and mixed vespids (p.1545·1).
Diagnosis of hypersensitivity to insect stings; hyposensitisation to insect stings.

Albego
Simes, Ital.†; Daker Farmasimes, Spain; Inpharzam, Switz.†.
Camazepam (p.645·2).
Anxiety; insomnia; premedication.

Albenza SmithKline Beecham, USA.
Albendazole (p.96·2).
Cysticercosis; echinococcosis.

Albert Tiafen Albert, Canad.
Tiaprofenic acid (p.89·1).
Inflammation; pain.

Albicansan Sanum-Kehlbeck, Ger.
Homoeopathic preparation.

Albicort
Sanofi Winthrop, Belg.; Sanofi Winthrop, Neth.
Triamcinolone acetonide (p.1050·2).
Corticosteroid.

Albicort Compositum
Sanofi Winthrop, Belg.; Sanofi Winthrop, Neth.
Triamcinolone acetonide (p.1050·2); salicylic acid (p.1090·2).
Skin disorders.

Albicort Oticum Sanofi Winthrop, Belg.
Triamcinolone acetonide (p.1050·2); salicylic acid (p.1090·2).
Otitis externa.

Albiotic Pharmacia Upjohn, Ger.
Lincomycin hydrochloride (p.222·1).
Bacterial infections.

Albistat Janssen-Cilag, Belg.
Miconazole nitrate (p.384·3).
Vulvovaginal yeast infections.

Albital Sclavo, Ital.
Albumin (p.710·1).
Cerebral oedema; hyperbilirubinaemia; hypoproteinaemia; shock.

Albothyl
Byk, Aust.†; Byk Gulden, Ger.
Metacresolsulphonic acid-formaldehyde (p.725·1).
Gynaecological disorders; skin disorders.

Albraton Steigerwald, Ger.
Homoeopathic preparation.

Albucid
ankerpharm, Ger.; Schering-Plough, S.Afr.†; Nicholas, UK†.
Sulphacetamide sodium (p.252·2).
Chlamydial eye infections.

Albumaid Preparations Scientific Hospital Supplies, UK.
A range of amino-acid preparations for special diets.
Homocystinuria; phenylketonuria; protein malabsorption syndromes.

Albumaid XPhen, Tyr Scientific Hospital Supplies, Austral.†.
Food for special diets.
Tyrosinaemia.

Albuman
Berna, Belg.; Berna, Ital.; Berna, Switz.
Albumin (p.710·1).
Hypoalbuminaemia.

Albumarc American Red Cross, USA.
Albumin (p.710·1).

Albumer Pasteur Merieux, Swed.†.
Albumin (p.710·1).
Hypoalbuminaemia; hypovolaemia.

Albumex CSL, Austral.
Albumin (human) (p.710·1).
Adult respiratory distress syndrome; burns; cardiopulmonary bypass surgery; haemodialysis; hypoproteinaemia; hypovolaemia; plasma exchange; shock.

Albuminar
Centeon, Irl.; Rorer, Ital.†; Centeon, Swed.†; Centeon, UK; Armour, USA.
Albumin (p.710·1).
Burns; hypoproteinaemia; hypovolaemic shock; neonatal hyperbilirubinaemia; plasma volume expansion.

Albunex Mallinckrodt, USA.
Albumin (p.710·1).
Burns; hypoproteinaemia; shock.

Alburone
Clintec, Fr.; Roussel, S.Afr.†.
Food for special diets.
Protein supplement.

Albusol NBI, S.Afr.
Albumin (p.710·1).
Hypoproteinaemia; hypovolaemia.

Albustix
Bayer Diagnostics, Austral.; Miles, Canad.†; Bayer Diagnostics, Fr.; Ames, Irl.; Bayer Diagnostici, Ital.; Ames, S.Afr.; Bayer Diagnostics, UK; Bayer, USA.
Test for protein in urine.

Albutannin Berlin-Chemie, Ger.†.
Albumin tannate (p.1176·3).
Diarrhoea.

Albutein
Alpha Therapeutic, Ital.; Alpha Therapeutic, UK; Alpha Therapeutic, USA.
Albumin (p.710·1).
Dialysis solutions; hypoalbuminaemia; hypovolaemia; neonatal hyperbilirubinaemia.

Albyl minor Pharmacia Upjohn, Swed.
Aspirin (p.16·1).
Fever; pain.

Albyl-E Nycomed, Norw.
Aspirin (p.16·1).
Magnesium oxide (p.1198·3) is included in this preparation in an attempt to limit adverse effects on the gastro-intestinal mucosa.
Fever; pain; thrombosis prophylaxis.

Albyl-koffein Kabi, Swed.†.
Aspirin (p.16·1); caffeine (p.749·3).
Fever; inflammation; pain.

Albym-Test
Boehringer Mannheim Diagnostics, Irl.; Boehringer Mannheim Diagnostics, UK.
Test for protein in urine.

Alca-C Wander OTC, Switz.
Carbaspirin calcium (p.25·1); ascorbic acid (p.1365·2).
Cold symptoms.

Alcacyl Wander OTC, Switz.
Suppositories†: Carbaspirin calcium (p.25·1).
Tablets: Carbaspirin calcium (p.25·1).
Aluminium hydroxide (p.1177·3) is included in this preparation in an attempt to limit adverse effects on the gastro-intestinal mucosa.
Fever; inflammation; pain.

Alcacyl instant Wander OTC, Switz.
Lysine aspirin (p.50·3).
Fever; inflammation; pain.

Alcacyl-B$_1$ Wander OTC, Switz.†.
Carbaspirin calcium (p.25·1); thiamine mononitrate (p.1361·1).
Aluminium hydroxide (p.1177·3) is included in this preparation in an attempt to limit adverse effects on the gastro-intestinal mucosa.
Fever; inflammation; pain.

Alcaine
Alcon, Austral.; Alcon, Belg.†; Alcon, Canad.; Alcon, Norw.; Alcon, Switz.; Alcon, USA.
Proxymetacaine hydrochloride (p.1300·1).
Local anaesthesia.

Alcalinos Gelos Gelos, Spain.
Calcium carbonate (p.1182·1); magnesium hydroxide (p.1198·2); sodium bicarbonate (p.1153·2); dibasic sodium phosphate (p.1159·3).
Gastro-intestinal hyperacidity.

Alcalinos Vita Vita, Spain.
Aluminium hydroxide (p.1177·3); calcium carbonate (p.1182·1); magnesium hydroxide (p.1198·2).
Gastro-intestinal hyperacidity.

Alcalosio SIT, Ital.
Anhydrous glucose (p.1343·3); potassium citrate (p.1153·1); pyridoxine hydrochloride (p.1362·3); sodium bicarbonate (p.1153·2); sodium citrate (p.1153·2).
Electrolyte disorders; gastro-intestinal disorders.

Alcamen Menarini, Ital.†.
Vitamin B substances and electrolytes with fructose (p.1147·1).
Fluid and electrolyte disorders.

Alcaphor Theraplix, Fr.
Trometamol citrate (p.1640·1); sodium acid citrate (p.1153·2); dipotassium citrate.
Metabolic acidosis; renal calculi.

Alcare Calgon Vestal, USA.
Alcohol (p.1099·1).
Antiseptic.

Alcasedine
Note. This name is used for preparations of different composition.
Sopar, Belg.†.
Prepared belladonna herb (p.457·1); bismuth subcarbonate (p.1180·1); algeldrate (p.1177·3); magnesium trisilicate (p.1199·1); calcium carbonate (p.1182·1).
Gastro-intestinal disorders.

Sopar, Neth.
Algeldrate (p.1177·3); magnesium trisilicate (p.1199·1).
Dyspepsia; gastric hyperacidity.

Alcasol Asta Medica, Belg.
Sodium bicarbonate (p.1153·2); borax (p.1554·2); sodium chloride (p.1162·2).
Eye disorders.

Alclox Alphapharm, Austral.†.
Cloxacillin sodium (p.195·2).
Bacterial infections.

Alcobon
Roche, Irl.; Roche, S.Afr.†; ICN, UK.
Flucytosine (p.379·2).
Fungal infections.

Alcoderm
Note. This name is used for preparations of different composition.
Galderma, Irl.
Liquid paraffin (p.1382·1).
Dry skin.

Galderma, UK.
Moisturiser.
Dry skin.

Alcodin Alcon, Ital.
Myrtillus (p.1606·1).
Capillary fragility; eye disorders.

Alco-Gel Tweezerman, USA.
Alcohol (p.1099·1).
Disinfection of hands.

Alcohcan Marrero, Spain.
Alcohol (p.1099·1); benzalkonium chloride (p.1101·3).
Skin disinfection.

Alcohocel Calmante Vitaminado, Spain.
Alcohol (p.1099·1); cetylpyridinium chloride (p.1106·2).
Skin disinfection.

Alcohten Marrero, Spain.
Alcohol (p.1099·1).
Skin disinfection.

Alcojel Roberts, Canad.
Isopropyl alcohol (p.1118·2).
Antiseptic.

Alcomicin
Alcon, Belg.†; Alcon, Canad.
Gentamicin sulphate (p.212·1).
Eye infections.

Alcon Eye Gel Alcon, Belg.
Carbomer (p.1471·2); mannitol (p.900·3).
Dry eyes.

Alconefrin PolyMedica, USA.
Phenylephrine hydrochloride (p.1066·2).
Nasal congestion.

Alcopac Reforzado Agua del Carmen, Spain.
Alcohol (p.1099·1); benzalkonium chloride (p.1101·3).
Skin, wound, and surface disinfection.

Alcopar
Wellcome, Irl.†; Wellcome, UK†.
Bephenium hydroxynaphthoate (p.98·3).
Ascariasis; hookworm infections; trichostrongyliasis.

Alcophyllex Propan, S.Afr.
Theophylline (p.765·1); etofylline (p.753·1); diphenhydramine hydrochloride (p.409·1); ammonium chloride (p.1055·2); sodium citrate (p.1153·2).
Bronchospasm.

Alcophyllin Propan, S.Afr.
Theophylline (p.765·1).
Obstructive airways disease.

Alcorten Galderma, Spain†.
Triamcinolone benetonide (p.1050·3).
Skin disorders.

Alcos-Anal
Note. This name is used for preparations of different composition.
Norgine, Austral.†.
Sodium oleate (p.1469·1); laureth 9 (p.1325·2); chlorothymol (p.1111·1).
Haemorrhoids; pruritus ani.

Bristol-Myers Squibb, Ger.; Bristol-Myers Squibb, Norw.; Squibb, Switz.†.
Laureth 9 (p.1325·2); 5-chlorocarvacrol; sodium oleate (p.1469·1).
Anorectal disorders.

Meda, Swed.
Sodium oleate (p.1469·1); 2-hydroxy-5-chlorothymol.
Anorectal disorders.

Alcover CT, Ital.
Sodium oxybate (p.1232·2).
Alcohol withdrawal syndrome.

Alcowipe Seton, UK.
Isopropyl alcohol (p.1118·2).
Hard surface disinfection.

Alcusal Alcusal, Austral.
Copper (p.1337·3); salicylic acid (p.1090·2); alcohol (p.1099·1).
Inflammation; pain.

Alcusal Sport *Alcusal, Austral.*
Copper (p.1337·3); methyl salicylate (p.55·2); menthol (p.1600·2); camphor (p.1557·2); eucalyptus oil (p.1578·1); alcohol (p.1099·1).
Pain and inflammation due to sports injuries.

Aldace *Searle, Ger.†.*
Spironolactone (p.946·1).
Hyperaldosteronism; hypertension; liver cirrhosis with ascites; oedema.

Aldactacine *Searle, Spain.*
Althiazide (p.819·1); spironolactone (p.946·1).
Hypertension; oedema.

Aldactazide
Searle, Canad.; SPA, Ital.; Searle, USA.
Spironolactone (p.946·1); hydrochlorothiazide (p.885·2).
Heart failure; hypertension; liver cirrhosis with oedema or ascites; nephrotic syndrome.

Aldactazine
Searle, Belg.; Monsanto, Fr.
Althiazide (p.819·1); spironolactone (p.946·1).
Hypertension; oedema.

Aldactide
Searle, Irl.; Searle, UK.
Spironolactone (p.946·1); hydroflumethiazide (p.889·2).
These ingredients can be described by the British Approved Name Co-flumactone.
Heart failure; hypertension.

Aldactone
Boehringer Mannheim, Aust.; Searle, Austral.; Searle, Belg.; Searle, Canad.; Monsanto, Fr.; Boehringer Mannheim, Ger.; Searle, Irl.; Lepetit, Ital.; Searle, Neth.; Searle, Norw.; Searle, S.Afr.; Searle, Spain; Searle, Swed.; Searle, Switz.; Searle, UK; Searle, USA.
Canrenoate potassium (p.836·2) or spironolactone (p.946·1).
Cor pulmonale; heart failure; hirsutism in females; hyperaldosteronism; hypertension; hypokalaemia; liver cirrhosis with ascites and oedema; myasthenia gravis; nephrotic syndrome; oedema.

Aldactone Saltucin
Boehringer Mannheim, Aust.; Boehringer Mannheim, Ger.
Spironolactone (p.946·1); buthiazide (p.835·2).
Cor pulmonale; heart failure; hyperaldosteronism; hypertension; liver cirrhosis with ascites and oedema; nephrotic syndrome; oedema.

Aldalix *Monsanto, Fr.*
Spironolactone (p.946·1); frusemide (p.871·1).
Heart failure.

Aldara
3M, UK; 3M, USA.
Imiquimod (p.613·3).
Anogenital warts.

Aldazide *Searle, S.Afr.*
Spironolactone (p.946·1); buthiazide (p.835·2).
Glomerular kidney disease; hypertension; oedema.

Aldazine *Alphapharm, Austral.*
Thioridazine hydrochloride (p.695·1).
Psychoses.

Aldecin
Schering-Plough, Austral.; Byk, Belg.; Byk, Neth.†; Byk, Switz.
Beclomethasone dipropionate (p.1032·1).
Allergic rhinitis; obstructive airways disease.

Aldecine *Byk, Fr.†.*
Beclomethasone dipropionate (p.1032·1).
Allergic rhinitis; asthma; bronchospastic disorders; coughs.

Aldetex *Zeneca, Belg.†.*
Glutaraldehyde (p.1114·3).
Disinfection.

Aldipine *Helvepharm, Switz.*
Nifedipine (p.916·2).
Angina pectoris; hypertension; Raynaud's syndrome.

Aldira *Zyma, Spain†.*
Terfenadine (p.418·1).
Hypersensitivity reactions.

Aldo Asma *Aldo, Spain.*
Ascorbic acid; phenylephrine hydrochloride (p.1066·2); isoprenaline hydrochloride (p.892·1).
Obstructive airways disease.

Aldo Otico *Aldo, Spain.*
Framycetin sulphate (p.210·3); lignocaine hydrochloride (p.1293·2); triamcinolone acetonide (p.1050·2); choline salicylate (p.25·2).
External ear disorders.

Aldoacne *Aldo, Spain.*
Benzoyl peroxide (p.1079·2).
Acne.

Aldoclor *Merck Sharp & Dohme, USA.*
Methyldopa (p.904·2); chlorothiazide (p.839·1).
Hypertension.

Aldocorten *Ciba, Ger.†.*
Aldosterone (p.1031·3).
Adrenocortical insufficiency; salt deficiency syndrome; shock.

Aldocumar *Aldo, Spain.*
Warfarin sodium (p.964·2).
Thrombo-embolic disorders; thrombosis prophylaxis.

Aldoderma *Aldo, Spain.*
Framycetin sulphate (p.210·3); triamcinolone acetonide (p.1050·2).
Infected skin disorders.

Aldoleo *Byk Elmu, Spain.*
Chlorthalidone (p.839·3); spironolactone (p.946·1).
Hypertension; oedema.

Aldomet
Merck Sharp & Dohme, Austral.; Merck Sharp & Dohme, Belg.; Merck Sharp & Dohme, Canad.; Merck Sharp & Dohme-Chibret, Fr.; Merck Sharp & Dohme, Irl.; Merck Sharp & Dohme, Ital.; Merck Sharp & Dohme, Neth.; Merck Sharp & Dohme, Norw.; Merck Sharp & Dohme, S.Afr.; Merck Sharp & Dohme, Spain; Merck Sharp & Dohme, Swed.; Merck Sharp & Dohme, Switz.; Merck Sharp & Dohme, UK; Merck Sharp & Dohme, USA.
Methyldopa (p.904·2) or methyldopate hydrochloride (p.904·2).
Hypertension.

Aldometil *Merck Sharp & Dohme, Aust.*
Methyldopa (p.904·2).
Hypertension.

Aldopren *Amrad, Austral.*
Methyldopa (p.904·2).
Hypertension.

Aldopur
Kwizda, Aust.; Hormosan, Ger.
Spironolactone (p.946·1).
Cor pulmonale; heart failure; hyperaldosteronism; hypertension; liver cirrhosis with ascites and oedema; nephrotic syndrome.

Aldoretic
Merck Sharp & Dohme, Aust.; Merck Sharp & Dohme, S.Afr.; Merck Sharp & Dohme, Switz.
Amiloride hydrochloride (p.819·2); hydrochlorothiazide (p.885·2); methyldopa (p.904·2).
Hypertension.

Aldoril
Merck Sharp & Dohme, Canad.; Merck Sharp & Dohme, USA.
Methyldopa (p.904·2); hydrochlorothiazide (p.885·2).
Hypertension.

Aldospray Analgesico *Aldo, Spain.*
Ibuprofen aminoethanol (p.44·3).
Peri-articular and soft-tissue disorders.

Aldotride *Merck Sharp & Dohme, Ital.†.*
Hydrochlorothiazide (p.885·2); methyldopa (p.904·2).
Hypertension.

Aldozone *Searle, Switz.*
Spironolactone (p.946·1); buthiazide (p.835·2).
Heart failure; hypertension; liver cirrhosis with ascites; nephrotic syndrome; oedema.

Aldrisone *SIFI, Ital.†.*
Endrysone.
Eye disorders.

Aldrisone VC *SIFI, Ital.†.*
Endrysone; tetrahydrozoline hydrochloride (p.1070·2).
Eye disorders.

Aldrox
Note. This name is used for preparations of different composition.
Whitehall, Belg.†.
Algeldrate (p.1177·3).
Gastro-intestinal disorders associated with hyperacidity.

Wyeth, Ital.†.
Algeldrate (p.1177·3); magnesium hydroxide (p.1198·2).
Gastro-intestinal disorders associated with hyperacidity.

Alec *Britannia Pharmaceuticals, UK.*
Pumactant (p.1623·1).
Respiratory distress syndrome.

Aledin *Nestle, Switz.*
Preparation for enteral nutrition.
Coeliac disease; diarrhoea.

Aleevex *Pure Plant Products, UK.*
Eucalyptus oil (p.1578·1); camphor (p.1557·2); menthol (p.1600·2).
Cold symptoms.

Alegysal *Tokyo Tanabe, Jpn.*
Pemirolast potassium (p.757·2).
Allergic rhinitis; asthma.

Alembicol D *Alembic Products, UK.*
Fractionated coconut oil (p.1599·2).
Food for special diets; malabsorption syndromes.

Alendros *Abiogen, Ital.*
Alendronate sodium (p.733·2).
Osteoporosis.

Alene *Organon, Spain†.*
Epimestrol (p.1444·3).
Amenorrhoea; anovulatory infertility.

Alenic Alka *Rugby, USA.*
Oral liquid: Aluminium hydroxide (p.1177·3); magnesium carbonate (p.1198·1).
Tablets: Aluminium hydroxide (p.1177·3); magnesium trisilicate (p.1199·1); sodium bicarbonate (p.1153·2).
Hyperacidity.

Aleot *Apomedica, Aust.*
Chlorphenesin (p.376·2); diphenhydramine hydrochloride (p.409·1); chlorbutol (p.1106·3); benzalkonium chloride (p.1101·3); urea (p.1095·2).
Ear disorders.

Alepa *Duopharm, Ger.*
Silybum marianum (p.993·3).
Liver disorders.

Alepam *Alphapharm, Austral.*
Oxazepam (p.683·2).
Alcohol withdrawal syndrome; anxiety.

Alepsal *Genevrier, Fr.*
Phenobarbitone (p.350·2); caffeine (p.749·3).
Epilepsy; febrile convulsions.

Alercur *Schering, Spain†.*
Clemizole hydrochloride (p.406·3).
Hypersensitivity reactions.

Alerfrin *Allergan, Spain.*
Oxymetazoline hydrochloride (p.1065·3).
Ocular congestion and irritation.

Alergical
Iquinosa, Spain.
Cream: Betamethasone valerate (p.1033·3); fluocinolone acetonide (p.1041·1).
Skin disorders.

Llorente, Spain.
Syrup: Chlorpheniramine maleate (p.405·1); prednisolone sodium metasulphobenzoate (p.1048·1).
Tablets: Ascorbic acid (p.1365·2); chlorpheniramine maleate (p.405·1); prednisolone (p.1048·1).
Hypersensitivity reactions; skin disorders.

Alergical Expect *Llorente, Spain.*
Chlorpheniramine maleate (p.405·1); diprophylline (p.752·1); guaiphenesin (p.1061·3); paracetamol (p.72·2).
Catarrh; influenza.

Alergist *Prodes, Spain.*
Terfenadine (p.418·1).
Hypersensitivity reactions.

Alerglobulina *Rhone-Poulenc Rorer, Spain†.*
A normal immunoglobulin (p.1522·1).
Hypersensitivity reactions.

Alergoftal *Cusi, Spain.*
Antazoline phosphate (p.401·3); naphazoline hydrochloride (p.1064·2).
Eye irritation.

Alergogamma *Leti, Spain†.*
A normal immunoglobulin (p.1522·1).
Hypersensitivity reactions.

Alerion *Gerbiol, Fr.†.*
Sodium cromoglycate (p.762·1).
Allergic rhinitis.

Alerlisin *Prodes, Spain.*
Cetirizine hydrochloride (p.404·2).
Hypersensitivity reactions.

Alermizol *Septa, Spain.*
Astemizole (p.402·1).
Hypersensitivity reactions.

Alersule *Misemer, USA.*
Phenylephrine hydrochloride (p.1066·2); chlorpheniramine maleate (p.405·1).
Upper respiratory-tract symptoms.

Alertonic
Hoechst Marion Roussel, Austral.; Hoechst Marion Roussel, Canad.; Mer-National, S.Afr.
Pipradol hydrochloride (p.1485·1); vitamin B substances; minerals.
Tonic.

Alesion *Boehringer Ingelheim, Jpn.*
Epinastine hydrochloride (p.410·3).
Allergic rhinitis; asthma; pruritus.

Alesse *Wyeth-Ayerst, USA.*
Levonorgestrel (p.1454·1); ethinyloestradiol (p.1445·1).
28-Day packs also contain 7 inert tablets.
Combined oral contraceptive.

Aletor Compositum *Cantabria, Spain.*
Bromhexine (p.1055·3); codeine acephyllinate (p.27·1); diphenhydramine hydrochloride (p.409·1); papaverine teprosilate (p.1614·3); pyridofylline (p.757·3).
Upper-respiratory-tract disorders.

Aletris Oligoplex *Madaus, Ger.*
Homoeopathic preparation.

Aleudrina *Boehringer Ingelheim, Spain.*
Isoprenaline sulphate (p.892·1).
Bronchospasm; cardiac disorders; shock.

Alevaire *Sanofi Winthrop, Belg.†.*
Tyloxapol (p.1329·2).
Respiratory-tract congestion.

Aleve
Roche Nicholas, Neth.; Procter & Gamble, USA.
Naproxen sodium (p.61·2).
Fever; pain.

Aleviatin *Dainippon, Jpn.*
Phenytoin sodium (p.352·3).
Epilepsy.

Alexan
Pfizer, Aust.; Boots, Austral.†; Mack, Illert., Ger.; Byk Gulden, Ital.†; Mack, Neth.†; Intramed, S.Afr.; Nycomed, Swed.; Mack, Switz.; Pfizer, UK†.
Cytarabine (p.525·2).
Leukaemias; non-Hodgkin's lymphomas.

Alfa
Ravizza, Ital.†; Rovi, Spain.
Naphazoline nitrate (p.1064·2).
Eye disorders.

Alfa Acid *Erredici, Ital.*
Ammonium lactate (p.1079·1); salicylic acid (p.1090·2); dexpanthenol (p.1570·3).
Scalp disorders.

Alfa C *Bracco, Ital.*
Benzalkonium chloride (p.1101·3).
Eye irritation.

Alfa D *Du Pont Pharmaceuticals, UK.*
Alfacalcidol (p.1366·3).
Vitamin D deficiency.

Alfa Kappa *Biagini, Ital.*
Amino-acid preparation.
Nutritional supplement in renal failure.

Alfa Mirtillo *Ravizza, Ital.†.*
Myrtillus (p.1606·1); vitamin A palmitate (p.1359·2).
Eye disorders; vascular disorders.

Alfabetal *Mitim, Ital.*
Labetalol hydrochloride (p.896·1).
Hypertension.

Alfabios *Biotekfarma, Ital.*
Fluocinolone acetonide (p.1041·1).
Corticosteroid.

Alfacortone *Spirig, Switz.*
Hydrocortisone acetate (p.1043·3).
Skin disorders.

AlfaD *Du Pont Pharmaceuticals, UK.*
Alfacalcidol (p.1366·3).
Vitamin D deficiency.

Alfadelta *Ern, Spain.*
Alfacalcidol (p.1366·3).
Hypoparathyroidism; osteomalacia; renal osteodystrophy; vitamin D deficiency.

Alfadil *Pfizer, Swed.*
Doxazosin mesylate (p.862·3).
Benign prostatic hyperplasia; hypertension.

Alfaferone *Wassermann, Ital.*
Interferon alfa (p.615·3).
Malignant neoplasms; viral infections.

Alfaflor *INTES, Ital.*
Betamethasone sodium phosphate (p.1033·3); naphazoline nitrate (p.1064·2); tetracycline hydrochloride (p.259·1).
Inflammatory eye and ear disorders.

Alfa-Fluorone *New Farma, Ital.*
Lotion: Fluocinolone acetonide (p.1041·1).
Skin disorders.
Vaginal solution: Fluocinolone acetonide (p.1041·1); benzalkonium chloride (p.1101·3).
Vulvovaginal infections.

Alfagamma *Humana, Ital.*
Essential fatty acids; vitamin E; vitamin B_6.
Nutritional supplement.

Alfagen *Wassermann, Ital.*
Collagen (p.1566·3).
Ulcers; wounds.

Alfakinasi *Wassermann, Ital.*
Urokinase (p.959·3).
Thrombo-embolic disorders.

Alfalfa Tonic *Homeocan, Canad.*
Homoeopathic preparation.

Alfamox *Teofarma, Ital.*
Amoxycillin trihydrate (p.151·3).
Bacterial infections.

Alfare
Nestle, Austral.; Nestle, Fr.; Nestle, Ital.; Nestle, S.Afr.; Nestle, Switz.; Nestle, UK.
Preparation for enteral nutrition.
Diarrhoea; digestive disorders; food for low-birth-weight neonates; malabsorption; milk intolerance.

Alfarol *Chugai, Jpn.*
Alfacalcidol (p.1366·3).
Osteoporosis; vitamin D metabolic disorders.

Alfason *Yamanouchi, Ger.*
Hydrocortisone butyrate (p.1044·1).
Skin disorders.

Alfater *Sclavo, Ital.*
Interferon alfa (p.615·3).
Genital warts; hepatitis B; hepatitis non-A non-B; malignant neoplasms.

Alfatil *Lilly, Fr.*
Cefaclor (p.163·2).
Bacterial infections.

Alfa-Trofodermin *Pharmacia Upjohn, Ital.†.*
Clostebol acetate (p.1440·2).
Wounds.

Alfavit *Medgenix, Belg.*
Ephedrine tartrate (p.1060·1); vitamins.
Tonic.

Alfazina *Salus, Ital.*
Propyphenazone (p.81·3); caffeine (p.749·3).
Fever; pain.

Alfenta
Janssen-Ortho, Canad.; Janssen, USA.
Alfentanil hydrochloride (p.12·3).
Analgesia during anaesthesia.

Alferm *Schoning-Berlin, Ger.*
Ointment: Prednisolone (p.1048·1); thymol (p.1127·1); allantoin (p.1078·2).
Suppositories: Prednisolone (p.1048·1); thymol (p.1127·1); menthol (p.1600·2).
Anorectal disorders.

Alferon N *Purdue Frederick, USA.*
Interferon alfa-n3 (p.615·3).
Genital warts.

Alferos *Berenguer Infale, Spain.*
Azelastine hydrochloride (p.403·1).
Allergic rhinitis.

Alfetim *Morrith, Spain.*
Alfuzosin hydrochloride (p.817·2).
Benign prostatic hyperplasia.

Alformin *Merckle, Ger.†.*
Dequalinium chloride (p.1112·1); naphazoline hydrochloride (p.1064·2); eucalyptus oil (p.1578·1).
Inflammatory disorders and infections of the oropharynx.

Alfospas
Opfermann, Ger.; Rottapharm, Ital.
Tiropramide hydrochloride (p.1638·2).
Smooth muscle spasm.

Alganex *Roche, Swed.*
Tenoxicam (p.88·2).
Dysmenorrhoea; inflammation; musculoskeletal and joint disorders; postoperative pain.

Alganil *IBIS, Ital.†*
Naproxen piperazine (p.62·1).
Musculoskeletal and joint disorders.

Algefit *Solvay, Aust.*
Diclofenac sodium (p.31·2).
Soft-tissue and peri-articular disorders.

Algesal
Note. This name is used for preparations of different composition.
Solvay, Aust.; Solvay, Belg.; Solvay, Canad.; Latema, Fr.†; Solvay, Ital.; Vemedia, Neth.; Nycomed, Norw.; Solvay Duphar, Swed.; Solvay, UK.
Diethylamine salicylate (p.33·1).
Musculoskeletal, joint, soft-tissue, and peri-articular disorders.

Solvay, Belg.; Solvay, Ger.; Solvay, Spain; Solvay, Switz.
Diethylamine salicylate (p.33·1); myrtecaine (p.1297·3) or myrtecaine lauryl sulphate (p.1297·3).
Musculoskeletal, joint, peri-articular, and soft-tissue disorders; neuralgia.

Algesal Forte *Vemedia, Neth.*
Diethylamine salicylate (p.33·1); myrtecaine (p.1297·3).
Muscle and joint pain.

Algesal Suractive *Solvay, Fr.*
Diethylamine salicylate (p.33·1); myrtecaine (p.1297·3).
Soft-tissue disorders.

Algesalona
Solvay, Ger.; Solvay, Switz.
Diethylamine salicylate (p.33·1); myrtecaine (p.1297·3); flufenamic acid (p.41·3).
Musculoskeletal, joint, and soft-tissue disorders.

Algesalona E *Solvay, Ger.*
Etofenamate (p.36·3).
Musculoskeletal, joint, peri-articular, and soft-tissue disorders.

Algex *Sopar, Belg.†.*
Histamine chloride (p.1587·3); capsicum oleoresin; ethyl nicotinate (p.36·1); propylene glycol salicylate.
Musculoskeletal and joint disorders.

Algho *Rhone-Poulenc Rorer, Spain.*
Aspirin (p.16·1).
Fever; inflammation; pain; thrombo-embolism prophylaxis.

Algiasdin *Isdin, Spain.*
Ibuprofen (p.44·1).
Fever; inflammation; musculoskeletal and joint disorders; pain.

Algicon
Note. This name is used for preparations of different composition.
Rhone-Poulenc Rorer, Austral.; Rorer, Fr.†; Rhone-Poulenc Rorer, Irl.; Rhone-Poulenc Rorer, Neth.
Suspension: Magnesium alginate (p.1470·3); aluminium hydroxide-magnesium carbonate co-dried gel (p.1178·2); magnesium carbonate (p.1198·1); potassium bicarbonate (p.1153·1); calcium carbonate (p.1182·1).
Gastro-oesophageal reflux.

Rhone-Poulenc Rorer, Austral.; Rhone-Poulenc Rorer, Irl.; Rhone-Poulenc Rorer, Neth.; Rhone-Poulenc Rorer, Norw.; Rhone-Poulenc Rorer, Swed.†; Rhone-Poulenc Rorer, UK.
Suspension; tablets: Magnesium alginate (p.1470·3); aluminium hydroxide-magnesium carbonate co-dried gel (p.1178·2); magnesium carbonate (p.1198·1); potassium bicarbonate (p.1153·1).
Gastro-oesophageal reflux.

Rhone-Poulenc Rorer Consumer, Canad.†.
Magnesium alginate (p.1470·3); aluminium hydroxide-magnesium carbonate co-dried gel (p.1178·2); magnesium carbonate (p.1198·1).
Gastro-oesophageal reflux.

Algicortis *Vaillant, Ital.†.*
Hydrocortisone (p.1043·3).
Skin disorders.

Algidol
Sintesa, Belg.; Berenguer Infale, Spain.
Paracetamol (p.72·2); codeine phosphate (p.26·1); ascorbic acid (p.1365·2).
Fever; pain.

Algifene *Nicholas, Fr.*
Ibuprofen (p.44·1).
Fever; pain.

Algifor *Vifor, Switz.*
Ibuprofen (p.44·1).
Fever; pain.

Alginex *Sauter, Switz.†.*
Ethyl salicylate (p.36·1); camphor (p.1557·2); menthol (p.1600·2); turpentine oil (p.1641·1).
Musculoskeletal, joint, and tissue pain.

Alginina *Upsamedica, Spain†.*
Paracetamol (p.72·2).
Fever; pain.

Alginor *Boehringer Ingelheim, Ital.*
Cimetropium bromide (p.459·2).
Adjunct in gastro-intestinal examinations and surgical procedures; gastro-intestinal disorders.

Algiospray *Robert, Spain.*
Picolamine salicylate (p.80·1).
Peri-articular disorders; soft-tissue disorders.

Algipan
Note. This name is used for preparations of different composition.
SmithKline Beecham Consumer, Belg.
Methyl nicotinate (p.55·1); glycol salicylate (p.43·1); mephenesin (p.1315·3).
Musculoskeletal pain; skeletal muscle spasm.

Sterling Midy, Fr.†.
Mephenesin (p.1315·3); methyl nicotinate (p.55·1); glycol salicylate (p.43·1); histamine dihydrochloride (p.1587·3); capsicum oleoresin.
Cramp; muscle, tendon, and ligament pain.

Whitehall, Irl.
Cream: Methyl nicotinate (p.55·1); glycol salicylate (p.43·1); capsaicin (p.24·2).
Topical spray†: Methyl nicotinate (p.55·1); glycol salicylate (p.43·1).
Musculoskeletal and joint pain.

Whitehall, UK.
Cream: Methyl nicotinate (p.55·1); glycol salicylate (p.43·1); capsicum oleoresin.
Topical spray†: Methyl nicotinate (p.55·1); glycol salicylate (p.43·1).
Muscle and joint pain.

Algiquin *Berenguer Infale, Spain†.*
Hydroquinidine alginate (p.889·3).
Arrhythmias.

Algisan *Prodes, Spain.*
Ibuprofen (p.44·1).
Fever; inflammation; musculoskeletal and joint disorders; pain.

Algisedal *Asta Medica, Fr.*
Paracetamol (p.72·2); codeine phosphate (p.26·1).
Pain.

Algisin *Ram, USA†.*
Chlorzoxazone (p.1313·1); paracetamol (p.72·2).

Algispir *Soekami, Fr.†.*
Aspirin (p.16·1); codeine phosphate (p.26·1); ascorbic acid (p.1365·2).
Fever; pain.

Algist *Hoechst Marion Roussel, S.Afr.*
Paracetamol (p.72·2); caffeine (p.749·3); chlorpheniramine maleate (p.405·1); phenylephrine hydrochloride (p.1066·2).
Cold symptoms.

Algistat *ConvaTec, UK.*
Calcium alginate (p.714·1).
Haemostatic dressing.

Algitec
SmithKline Beecham, Irl.; SmithKline Beecham, UK.
Alginic acid (p.1470·3) or sodium alginate (p.1470·3); cimetidine (p.1183·2).
Gastro-oesophageal reflux.

Algobene *Merckle, Aust.*
Aspirin (p.16·1).
Fever; pain.

Algo-Buscopan *Delagrange, Fr.†.*
Hyoscine butylbromide (p.462·3); dipyrone (p.35·1).
Pain.

Algocetil *Francia, Ital.*
Sulindac sodium (p.87·2).
Gout; musculoskeletal, joint, and peri-articular disorders; neuritis.

Algocor *Ravizza, Ital.*
Gallopamil hydrochloride (p.874·2).
Ischaemic heart disease; myocardial infarction.

Algoderm
Note. This name is used for preparations of different composition.
Brothier, Fr.†.
Calcium alginate (p.714·1).
Wounds.

Inibsa, Spain.
Diethylamine salicylate (p.33·1).
Peri-articular and soft-tissue disorders.

Algofen *Blue Cross, Ital.*
Ibuprofen (p.44·1).
Pain.

Algoflex Same *Savoma, Ital.*
Diethylamine salicylate (p.33·1).
Musculoskeletal and joint disorders.

Algolider *Garant, Ital.*
Nimesulide (p.63·2).
Fever; inflammation; pain.

Algolisina *Celsius, Ital.*
Pridinol mesylate (p.1318·2); benzydamine hydrochloride (p.21·3); cinchocaine hydrochloride (p.1289·2); hyaluronidase (p.1588·1).
Musculoskeletal, joint, and soft-tissue disorders.

Algonerg *Eberth, Ger.†.*
Mofebutazone (p.56·1); glycol salicylate (p.43·1); benzyl nicotinate (p.22·1); histamine dihydrochloride (p.1587·3); rosemary oil (p.1626·2).
Arthroses; inflammation; neuralgia; neuritis; pain; rheumatism.

Algoneurina B12 *IBIS, Ital.†.*
Thiamine disulphide hydrochloride; cyanocobalamin.

Algo-Nevriton
Rhone-Poulenc Rorer, Belg.†; Sciencex, Fr.; Rhone-Poulenc Rorer, Switz.†.
Acetiamine hydrochloride (p.1360·3); aspirin (p.16·1).
Musculoskeletal and joint disorders; neuralgia; pain.

Algophytum *Herbaxt, Fr.*
Harpagophyton (p.27·2).
Joint pain.

Algoplaque HP *Urgo, Fr.*
A hydrocolloid dressing.
Ulcers.

Algopriv *Interdelta, Switz.*
Diproqualone camsylate (p.35·1); etenzamide (p.35·3).
Inflammation; pain.

Algo-Prolixan *Jacoby, Aust.*
Azapropazone (p.20·3); dextropropoxyphene hydrochloride (p.27·3).
Musculoskeletal and joint disorders.

Algostase *SMB, Belg.*
Paracetamol (p.72·2); caffeine (p.749·3).
Fever; pain.

Algosteril
Brothier, Fr.; Beiersdorf, UK.
Calcium alginate (p.714·1).
Haemostatic dressing.

Algotrex *CT, Ital.†.*
Nifenazone (p.63·1).
Musculoskeletal disorders; neuritis.

Algotropyl *Theraplix, Fr.*
Paracetamol (p.72·2); promethazine hydrochloride (p.416·2).
Allergy; fever; pain.

Alho Sedosan *Wiedemann, Ger.*
Homoeopathic preparation.

Alho-Arthrosan *Wiedemann, Ger.*
Homoeopathic preparation.

Alhydrate
Nestle, Fr.; Nestle, Ital.
Maltodextrin; sucrose; sodium chloride; citric acid; potassium citrate (p.1152·3).
Diarrhoea; oral rehydration therapy.

Ali Veg *SmithKline Beecham, Spain.*
Cimetidine (p.1183·2).
Gastro-intestinal disorders.

Alibron *Europharma, Spain†.*
Bromhexine hydrochloride (p.1055·3); erythromycin propionate (p.204·2).
Respiratory-tract infections.

Aligest *Schering-Plough, Spain.*
Aluminium hydroxide (p.1177·3); dimethicone (p.1213·1); magnesium hydroxide (p.1198·2).
Gastro-intestinal hyperacidity and flatulence.

Aligest Plus *Schering-Plough, Spain.*
Aluminium hydroxide (p.1177·3); calcium carbonate (p.1182·1); magnesium hydroxide (p.1198·2); simethicone (p.1213·1).
Gastro-intestinal hyperacidity and flatulence.

Alimentum
Ross, Canad.; Ross, USA.
Corn- and lactose-free infant feed.
Fat malabsorption; food hypersensitivity; protein maldigestion; protein sensitivity.

Alimix
SmithKline Beecham, Ger.; Cilag, Ital.; Janssen, UK†.
Cisapride (p.1187·1).
Gastric motility disorders; gastro-oesophageal reflux.

Alinam *Lucien, Fr.†.*
Chlormezanone (p.648·3).
Skeletal muscle spasm.

Alinamin-F *Takeda, Jpn.*
Fursultiamine hydrochloride.
Vitamin B_1 deficiency.

Alinda *Rorer, Ger.†.*
Glucose monohydrate (p.1343·3); fructose (p.1343·2); dilute phosphoric acid (p.1618·2).
Motion sickness; nausea; vomiting.

Alinor
Alpharma, Norw.; Dumex-Alpharma, Swed.†.
Atenolol (p.825·3).
Angina pectoris; arrhythmias; hypertension; hyperthyroidism; migraine; myocardial infarction.

Alipase *Janssen-Cilag, Fr.*
Pancrelipase (p.1613·3).
Pancreatic insufficiency.

Aliseum *Zoja, Ital.*
Diazepam (p.661·1).
Anxiety disorders; epilepsy.

Alitraq
Abbott, Austral.; Abbott, UK.
Preparation for enteral nutrition.

Alius *Roussel, Ital.†.*
Dimethothiazine mesylate (p.408·3).
Headache including migraine.

Aliviomas *Alacan, Spain.*
Naproxen (p.61·2).
Musculoskeletal and joint disorders; pain; peri-articular disorders.

Aliviosin *Alacan, Spain.*
Indomethacin (p.45·2).
Gout; musculoskeletal, joint, and peri-articular disorders; pain.

ALK *Epipharm, Aust.†.*
Range of allergen extracts (p.1545·1).
Hyposensitisation.

Alk *Scherax, Ger.*
A range of allergen extracts (p.1545·1).
Hyposensitisation.

Alka Butazolidin *Geigy, Canad.†.*
Phenylbutazone (p.79·2).
Dried aluminium hydroxide (p.1177·3) and magnesium trisilicate (p.1199·1) are included in this preparation in an attempt to limit adverse effects on the gastro-intestinal mucosa.
Ankylosing spondylitis; gout.

Alkaban *Quad, USA.*
Vinblastine sulphate (p.569·1).
Malignant neoplasms.

Alkafizz *Xeragen, S.Afr.*
Sodium citrate (p.1153·2); sodium bicarbonate (p.1153·2); anhydrous citric acid (p.1564·3); tartaric acid (p.1634·3).
Gastric hyperacidity; urinary alkalinisation.

Alkagin *Ganassini, Ital.*
Calendula officinalis; mallow; tilia (p.1637·3).
Personal hygiene.

Alkala N *Sanum-Kehlbeck, Ger.*
Sodium citrate dihydrate (p.1153·2); potassium bicarbonate (p.1153·1); sodium bicarbonate (p.1153·2).
Gastro-intestinal acidity.

Alkala T *Sanum-Kehlbeck, Ger.*
Sodium bicarbonate (p.1153·2).
Metabolic acidosis.

Alkalite D *Garec, S.Afr.*
Dicyclomine hydrochloride (p.460·1); dried aluminium hydroxide gel (p.1177·3); light magnesium oxide (p.1198·3).
Gastro-intestinal disorders.

Alkalovert *Klein, Ger.†.*
Phytic acid (p.995·3).
Alkalinising agent.

Alka-Mints *Bayer, USA.*
Calcium carbonate (p.1182·1).
Hyperacidity.

Alka-Seltzer
Note. This name is used for preparations of different composition.
Bayer, Aust.; Bayer, Austral.; Bayer, Canad.; Bayer, Fr.; Bayer, Ger.; Bayer, Ital.; Bayer, Neth.; Bayer, Swed.; Bayer Diagnostics, Switz.; Bayer, UK.
Aspirin (p.16·1); citric acid (p.1564·3); sodium bicarbonate (p.1153·2).
Fever; gastro-intestinal disorders; pain.

Bayer, Spain.
Aspirin (p.16·1); calcium phosphate (p.1155·3); citric acid (p.1564·3); sodium bicarbonate (p.1153·2).
Fever; musculoskeletal and joint disorders; pain.

Alka-Seltzer Advanced Formula *Miles Consumer Healthcare, USA†.*
Paracetamol (p.72·2).

Alka-Seltzer Antacid *Miles Consumer Healthcare, USA.*
Sodium bicarbonate (p.1153·2); citric acid (p.1564·3); potassium bicarbonate (p.1153·1).
Gastro-intestinal disorders.

Alka-Seltzer with Aspirin *Miles Consumer Healthcare, USA.*
Aspirin (p.16·1); citric acid (p.1564·3); sodium bicarbonate (p.1153·2).
Arthritis; fever; gastro-intestinal disorders; myocardial infarction; pain.

Alka-Seltzer Effervescent Tablets *Miles, USA.*
Sodium bicarbonate (p.1153·2); citric acid (p.1564·3); aspirin (p.16·1).
Hyperacidity.

Alka-Seltzer Plus Cold
Note. This name is used for preparations of different composition.
Bayer, Canad.; Miles Consumer Healthcare, USA.
Tablets: Phenylpropanolamine bitartrate (p.1067·3); chlorpheniramine maleate (p.405·1); aspirin (p.16·1).
Cold symptoms; nasal congestion.

Miles Consumer Healthcare, USA.
Capsules: Chlorpheniramine maleate (p.405·1); pseudoephedrine hydrochloride (p.1068·3); paracetamol (p.72·2).

Alka-Seltzer Plus Cold & Cough *Miles Consumer Healthcare, USA.*
Tablets: Phenylpropanolamine bitartrate (p.1067·3); chlorpheniramine maleate (p.405·1); dextromethorphan hydrobromide (p.1057·3); aspirin (p.16·1).
Capsules: Dextromethorphan (p.1057·3); pseudoephedrine hydrochloride (p.1068·3); chlorpheniramine maleate (p.405·1); paracetamol (p.72·2).
Coughs and cold symptoms.

Alka-Seltzer Plus Night-Time Cold *Miles Consumer Healthcare, USA.*
Capsules: Doxylamine succinate (p.410·1); dextromethorphan (p.1057·3); pseudoephedrine hydrochloride (p.1068·3); paracetamol (p.72·2).
Tablets: Phenylpropanolamine bitartrate (p.1067·3); brompheniramine maleate (p.403·2); dextromethorphan hydrobromide (p.1057·3); aspirin (p.16·1).
Coughs and cold symptoms.

Alka-Seltzer Plus Sinus *Bayer, USA.*
Phenylpropanolamine tartrate (p.1067·3); aspirin (p.16·1).
Upper-respiratory tract congestion.

Alka-Seltzer Plus Sinus Allergy *Miles, USA.*
Phenylpropanolamine bitartrate (p.1067·3); brompheniramine maleate (p.403·2); aspirin (p.16·1).
Upper respiratory-tract symptoms.

Alka-Seltzer XS *Bayer Consumer, UK.*
Aspirin (p.16·1); paracetamol (p.72·2); caffeine (p.749·3).
Headache.

Alkenide *Evans, Fr.*
Poloxamer 188 (p.1326·3).
Skin cleanser.

Alkeran
Glaxo Wellcome, Aust.; Glaxo Wellcome, Austral.; Glaxo Wellcome, Belg.; Glaxo Wellcome, Canad.; Glaxo Wellcome, Fr.; Glaxo Wellcome, Ger.; Wellcome, Irl.; Glaxo Wellcome, Ital.; Glaxo Wellcome, Neth.; Glaxo Wellcome, Norw.; Glaxo Wellcome, S.Afr.; Glaxo Wellcome, Swed.; Wellcome, Switz.; Wellcome, UK; Glaxo Wellcome, USA.
Melphalan (p.544·3) or melphalan hydrochloride (p.545·2).
Malignant neoplasms; polycythaemia vera.

Alkets Roberts, USA; Hauck, USA.
Calcium carbonate (p.1182·1).
Hyperacidity.

Alko Isol Marc-O, Canad.
Isopropyl alcohol (p.1118·2).

All In One Plus Grapefruit Solgar, UK.
Soya lecithin (p.1595·2); grapefruit powder concentrate; cider vinegar.
Dietary supplement.

Allbece Whitehall, Swed.†.
Vitamin B and C preparation.

Allbee Robins, USA.
A range of vitamin preparations.

Allbee with C
Whitehall, Austral.†; Whitehall-Robins, Canad.; Whitehall, Irl.; Whitehall, UK†.
Vitamin B substances with ascorbic acid.

Allbee C-550 Whitehall-Robins, Canad.
Vitamin B substances with ascorbic acid.

Allbee C-800 Whitehall-Robins, Canad.
Vitamin B substances, ascorbic acid, and vitamin E.

Allbee C-800 plus Iron Whitehall-Robins, Canad.
Vitamin B substances, ascorbic acid, vitamin E, folic acid, and iron.

Allcocks Plaster Allcock, Norw.†.
Cautchuc; burgundy pitch; olibanum; orris; capsicum (p.1559·2); camphor (p.1557·2); elemi; myrrh (p.1606·1).
Rheumatoid pain.

Allegra Hoechst Marion Roussel, USA.
Fexofenadine hydrochloride (p.410·3).
Allergic rhinitis.

Allegra-D Hoechst Marion Roussel, USA.
Fexofenadine (p.410·3); pseudoephedrine hydrochloride (p.1068·3).
Upper respiratory-tract disorders.

Allegron
Dista, Austral.; Dista, UK.
Nortriptyline hydrochloride (p.300·2).
Depression; nocturnal enuresis.

Allent Ascher, USA.
Brompheniramine maleate (p.403·2); pseudoephedrine hydrochloride (p.1068·3).
Allergic rhinitis; nasal congestion.

Aller-Aide Technilab, Canad.
Diphenhydramine hydrochloride (p.409·1).

Allerbiocid S Allerbio, Fr.
Benzyl benzoate (p.1402·2); tannic acid (p.1634·2).
Insecticide for bedding and upholstery.

Aller-Chlor Rugby, USA.
Chlorpheniramine maleate (p.405·1).
Hypersensitivity reactions.

Allercon Parmed, USA.
Pseudoephedrine hydrochloride (p.1068·3); triprolidine hydrochloride (p.420·3).
Upper respiratory-tract symptoms.

Allercreme Carme, USA.
Emollient and moisturiser.

Allercrom UCB, Aust.†.
Sodium cromoglycate (p.762·1).
Allergic conjunctivitis; allergic rhinitis.

Allerdryl
ICN, Canad.; Legere, USA†.
Diphenhydramine hydrochloride (p.409·1).
Hypersensitivity.

Allerest Fisons, USA.
Naphazoline hydrochloride (p.1064·2).
Minor eye irritation.

Allerest Headache Strength Ciba, USA.
Pseudoephedrine hydrochloride (p.1068·3); chlorpheniramine maleate (p.405·1); paracetamol (p.72·2).
Upper respiratory-tract symptoms.

Allerest 12 Hour Ciba, USA.
Phenylpropanolamine hydrochloride (p.1067·2); chlorpheniramine maleate (p.405·1).
Upper respiratory-tract symptoms.

Allerest 12 Hour Nasal Fisons, USA.
Oxymetazoline hydrochloride (p.1065·3).
Nasal congestion.

Allerest Maximum Strength Ciba, USA.
Pseudoephedrine hydrochloride (p.1068·3); chlorpheniramine maleate (p.405·1).
Upper respiratory-tract symptoms.

Allerest Sinus Pain Formula Ciba, USA.
Pseudoephedrine hydrochloride (p.1068·3); chlorpheniramine maleate (p.405·1); paracetamol (p.72·2).
Upper respiratory-tract symptoms.

Aller-eze Intercare, UK.
Cream: Diphenhydramine hydrochloride (p.409·1).
Hypersensitivity reactions of the skin; insect bites and stings.
Tablets: Clemastine hydrogen fumarate (p.406·2).
Hay fever; urticaria.

Aller-eze Clear Novartis Consumer, UK†.
Terfenadine (p.418·1).
Hay fever; urticaria.

Aller-eze Plus Intercare, UK.
Clemastine hydrogen fumarate (p.406·2); phenylpropanolamine hydrochloride (p.1067·2).
Hay fever.

Allerfen Sella, Ital.
Promethazine hydrochloride (p.416·2).
Hypersensitivity reactions; insomnia.

Allerfre Boots Healthcare, Neth.
Loratadine (p.413·1).
Hypersensitivity reactions.

Allerfrim Rugby, USA.
Pseudoephedrine hydrochloride (p.1068·3); triprolidine hydrochloride (p.420·3).
Upper respiratory-tract symptoms.

Allerfrin with Codeine Rugby, USA.
Pseudoephedrine hydrochloride (p.1068·3); codeine phosphate (p.26·1); triprolidine hydrochloride (p.420·3).
Coughs and cold symptoms.

Aller-G Hoechst, Austral.†.
Pheniramine maleate (p.415·3).
Hypersensitivity reactions.

Allerga Goupil, Fr.†.
Mefenidramium (p.413·3).
Hypersensitivity reactions; pruritic skin disorders.

Allergamma Association Nationale, Fr.†.
A normal immunoglobulin (p.1522·1).
Hypersensitivity reactions; hyposensitisation.

Allergan Bouty, Ital.
Diphenhydramine hydrochloride (p.409·1).
Insect bites; pruritus; sunburn.

Allergan Enzymatic Allergan, USA.
Papain (p.1614·1).
Cleansing solution for soft contact lenses.

Allergefon Lafon, Fr.
Carbinoxamine maleate (p.404·2).
Hypersensitivity reactions.

Allergen Goldline, USA.
Benzocaine (p.1286·2); phenazone (p.78·2); glycerol (p.1585·2).
Ear pain.

Allergenid Herbaline, Ital.
Agrimony; black currant (p.1365·2); echinacea (p.1574·2).
Hypersensitivity reactions.

Allergex
CP Protea, Austral.†; Propan, S.Afr.
Chlorpheniramine maleate (p.405·1).
Hypersensitivity reactions.

Allerg-Eze Rhone-Poulenc Rorer, Austral.†.
Pseudoephedrine hydrochloride (p.1068·3); vitamins and minerals; allium cepa; apis mel; natrum muriaticum.
Hay fever; nasal and bronchial congestion; sinusitis.

Allergie-Injektopas Pascoe, Ger.
Homoeopathic preparation.

Allergies Homeocan, Canad.
Homoeopathic preparation.

Allergin Propan, S.Afr.
Diphenhydramine hydrochloride (p.409·1); ammonium chloride (p.1055·2); sodium citrate (p.1153·2); menthol (p.1600·2).
Coughs.

Allergina De Angeli, Ital.†.
Diphenhydramine hydrochloride (p.409·1).
Hypersensitivity reactions.

Allergin-Coffein Nycomed, Norw.†.
Diphenhydramine hydrochloride (p.409·1); caffeine (p.749·3).
Hypersensitivity reactions; nausea and vomiting.

Allergipuran N Scheurich, Ger.
Bufexamac (p.22·2).
Inflammatory skin disorders.

Allergocrom Ursapharm, Ger.
Sodium cromoglycate (p.762·1).
Allergic conjunctivitis and rhinitis.

Allergodex ISM, Ital.†.
Plant allergen extracts (p.1545·1).
Hyposensitisation.

Allergodil
Asta Medica, Aust.; Asta Medica, Belg.; Asta Medica, Fr.; Asta Medica, Ger.; Asta Medica, Ital.; Asta Medica, Neth.; Asta Medica, Switz.
Azelastine hydrochloride (p.403·1).
Allergic rhinitis.

Allergopos N Ursapharm, Ger.
Antazoline phosphate (p.401·3); tetrahydrozoline hydrochloride (p.1070·2).
Eye disorders.

Allergospasmin
Asta Medica, Aust.; Asta Medica, Ger.
Sodium cromoglycate (p.762·1); reproterol hydrochloride (p.758·1).
Obstructive airways disease.

Allergospasmine Asta Medica, Switz.
Sodium cromoglycate (p.762·1); reproterol hydrochloride (p.758·1).
Obstructive airways disease.

Allergosyx Syxyl, Ger.
Homoeopathic preparation.

Allergovit
Allergopharma, Ger.; Allergopharma, Switz.
Allergen extracts (p.1545·1).
Hyposensitisation.

Allergy Parmed, USA.
Chlorpheniramine maleate (p.405·1).

Allergy Cold Geneva, USA.
Pseudoephedrine hydrochloride (p.1068·3); triprolidine hydrochloride (p.420·3).
Upper respiratory-tract symptoms.

Allergy Drops
Bausch & Lomb, Canad.; Bausch & Lomb, USA.
Naphazoline hydrochloride (p.1064·2).
Eye irritation.

Allergy Elixir Tanta, Canad.
Diphenhydramine hydrochloride (p.409·1).

Allergy Eyes Abbott, Austral.
Antazoline sulphate (p.402·1); xylometazoline hydrochloride (p.1071·2).
Eye irritation and inflammation.

Allergy Relief JCP, Canad.
Terfenadine (p.418·1).

Allergy Relief Medicine Rugby, USA.
Phenylpropanolamine hydrochloride (p.1067·2); chlorpheniramine maleate (p.405·1).
Upper respiratory-tract symptoms.

Allergy Sinus WestCan, Canad.
Pseudoephedrine hydrochloride (p.1068·3); chlorpheniramine maleate (p.405·1); paracetamol (p.72·2).

Allergy Symptoms Relief Brauer, Austral.
Homoeopathic preparation.

Allergy Tablets Tanta, Canad.
Diphenhydramine hydrochloride (p.409·1).

Allerhist
Note. This name is used for preparations of different composition.
Propan-Vernleigh, S.Afr.†.
Chlorpheniramine maleate (p.405·1).
Hypersensitivity reactions.
Warner Chilcott, USA†.
Brompheniramine maleate (p.403·2); phenylpropanolamine hydrochloride (p.1067·2).

AlleRid Murdock, USA†.
Pseudoephedrine hydrochloride (p.1068·3).

Allerkif Edmond Pharma, Ital.†.
Ketotifen fumarate (p.755·2).
Obstructive airways disease.

AllerMax Pfeiffer, USA.
Diphenhydramine hydrochloride (p.409·1).
Insomnia; motion sickness; parkinsonism.

Allermed Murdock, USA.
Pseudoephedrine hydrochloride (p.1068·3).
Nasal congestion.

Allernix Technilab, Canad.
Diphenhydramine hydrochloride (p.409·1).
Antihistamine.

Allerpant Lagap, Ital.†.
Clemizole hydrochloride (p.406·3).
Hypersensitivity reactions.

Allerphed Great Southern, USA.
Pseudoephedrine hydrochloride (p.1068·3); triprolidine hydrochloride (p.420·3).
Upper respiratory-tract symptoms.

Allerplus Astra, Ital.†.
Terfenadine (p.418·1).
Hypersensitivity reactions.

Allerset
Hal, Ger.†.
Allergen extracts of pollen, moulds, dust, mites, and skin (p.1545·1).
Hyposensitisation.
HAL, Neth.
Aqueous allergen extracts (p.1545·1).
Hyposensitisation.

Allersol Ocusoft, USA.
Naphazoline hydrochloride (p.1064·2).

Allertac Propan, S.Afr.
Atropine sulphate (p.455·1); hyoscine hydrobromide (p.462·3); hyoscyamine sulphate (p.464·2); phenylpropanolamine hydrochloride (p.1067·2); pheniramine maleate (p.415·3); chlorpheniramine maleate (p.405·1).
Congestion and hypersecretion of the nasal and paranasal sinuses.

Allevyn
Smith & Nephew, Irl.; Smith & Nephew, UK.
Hydrophilic polyurethane dressing.
Ulcers; wounds.

Allgauer Allga, Aust.
Pumilio pine oil (p.1623·3); eucalyptus oil (p.1578·1); peppermint oil (p.1208·1).
Cold and influenza symptoms.

Allium Plus Zeller, Switz.
Ginkgo biloba (p.1584·1); garlic (p.1583·1).
Cerebrovascular disorders; tonic.

All-Nite Cold Formula Major, USA.
Pseudoephedrine hydrochloride (p.1068·3); dextromethorphan hydrobromide (p.1057·3); doxylamine succinate (p.410·1); paracetamol (p.72·2).
Coughs and cold symptoms.

Allo CT, Ger.
Allopurinol (p.390·2).
Gout; hyperuricaemia; renal calculi.

allo-basan Schonenberger, Switz.
Allopurinol (p.390·2).
Gout; hyperuricaemia; renal calculi.

Allobenz Hofmann, Aust.
Allopurinol (p.390·2); benzbromarone (p.392·3).
Gout; hyperuricaemia; renal calculi.

Allobeta Betapharm, Ger.
Allopurinol (p.390·2).
Gout; hyperuricaemia; renal calculi.

Alloca Upjohn, Jpn†.
Ornoprostil (p.1420·3).

Allochrysine
Solvay, Belg.; Solvay, Fr.
Aurotioprol (p.20·2).
Rheumatoid arthritis.

allo.comp.-ratiopharm Ratiopharm, Ger.
Allopurinol (p.390·2); benzbromarone (p.392·3).
Gout; hyperuricaemia.

Allo-Efeka Brenner-Efeka, Ger.
Allopurinol (p.390·2).
Gout; hyperuricaemia.

Alloferin
Roche, Aust.; Roche, Austral.†; Roche, Ger.; Roche, Neth.†; Roche, S.Afr.; Roche, UK†.
Alcuronium chloride (p.1304·2).
Competitive neuromuscular blocker.

Alloferine Roche, Switz.†.
Alcuronium chloride (p.1304·2).
Competitive neuromuscular blocker.

Allohexal Hexal, Ger.
Allopurinol (p.390·2).
Hyperuricaemia.

Allomaron
Nattermann, Ger.; Rhone-Poulenc Rorer, S.Afr.
Allopurinol (p.390·2); benzbromarone (p.392·3).
Gout; hyperuricaemia.

Allop-Gry Gry, Ger.†.
Allopurinol (p.390·2).
Gout; hyperuricaemia.

Allopur
AFI, Norw.; Gea, Switz.
Allopurinol (p.390·2).
Gout; hyperuricaemia; renal calculi; uric acid nephropathy.

Allo-Puren Isis Puren, Ger.
Allopurinol (p.390·2).
Gout; hyperuricaemia; renal calculi.

Alloremed Rhone-Poulenc Rorer, Austral.†.
Allopurinol (p.390·2).
Gout; prevention of uric acid nephropathy in neoplastic conditions; urate stones.

Allorin Douglas, Austral.
Allopurinol (p.390·2).
Hyperuricaemia.

Allo-300-Tablinen
Sanorania, Ger.; Sanorania, Switz.†.
Allopurinol (p.390·2).
Gout; hyperuricaemia; renal calculi.

Allotropat Heyl, Ger.†.
Hydroxyapatite (p.1589·2).
Bone cement.

Allpargin Merz, Ger.
Allopurinol (p.390·2).
Gout; hyperuricaemia.

All-Pro Solgar, UK.
Amino-acid preparation.

Allpyral
Bayer, Austral.; Dome-Hollister-Stier, Fr.; Miles, USA.
A range of allergen extracts (p.1545·1).
Hyposensitisation.

Allpyral Pure Mite Bayer, S.Afr.
D. pteronyssinus extracts (p.1545·1).
Hyposensitisation.

Allpyral Special Grass Bayer, S.Afr.
Grass pollen extracts (p.1545·1).
Hyposensitisation.

Alltotal
Note. This name is used for preparations of different composition.
Allergan, Aust.
Cleaning, wetting, and storage solution for hard and gas permeable contact lenses.
Allergan, Ger.
Polyvinyl alcohol (p.1474·2).
Storage and wetting solution for contact lenses.

Alludex ISM, Ital.†.
Allergen extracts (p.1545·1).
Hyposensitisation.

All-Up Leppin, S.Afr.†.
Multivitamin and mineral preparation.

Allural Rovi, Spain†.
Allopurinol (p.390·2).
Gout; hyperuricaemia.

Allurit Rhone-Poulenc Rorer, Ital.
Allopurinol (p.390·2).
Gout; hyperuricaemia.

Allvoran TAD, Ger.
Diclofenac sodium (p.31·2).
Inflammation; pain; rheumatism.

Alma Restan, S.Afr.
Peppermint oil (p.1208·1); cardamom (p.1560·1).
Carminative.

Almacarb Boots, Austral.†.
Aluminium hydroxide-magnesium carbonate co-dried gel (p.1178·2).
Gastric hyperacidity.

Almacone Rugby, USA.
Aluminium hydroxide (p.1177·3); magnesium hydroxide (p.1198·2); simethicone (p.1213·1).
Hyperacidity.

Almag CT, Ger.
Algeldrate (p.1177·3); magnesium hydroxide (p.1198·2) or magnesium trisilicate (p.1199·1).
Gastric hyperacidity; phosphate binding.

Almagel Atlas, Canad.
Aluminium hydroxide (p.1177·3); magnesium hydroxide (p.1198·2).

Almaphar Pharma Plus, Switz.†.
Aluminium hydroxide (p.1177·3); magnesium trisilicate (p.1199·1).
Duodenal ulcer; gastric hyperacidity.

Almarl Sumitomo, Jpn.
Arotinolol hydrochloride (p.825·3).
Angina pectoris; hypertension; tachycardia; tremor.

Almarytm Synthelabo, Ital.
Flecainide acetate (p.868·3).
Arrhythmias.

Almax Almirall, Spain.
Almagate (p.1177·1).
Gastro-intestinal hyperacidity.

Almay Total Sunbloc Revlon, UK.
Cream: Padimate O (p.1488·1); oxybenzone (p.1487·3); titanium dioxide (p.1093·3).
Lip balm: Padimate O (p.1488·1); oxybenzone (p.1487·3).
Sunscreen.

Almebex Plus B_{12} Dayton, USA.
Vitamin B substances.

Almevax
Wellcome, Irl.; SBL, Swed.†; Medeva, UK.
A rubella vaccine (Wistar RA 27/3 strain) (p.1532·3).
Active immunisation.

Almide Alcon, Fr.
Lodoxamide trometamol (p.756·1).
Allergic eye disorders.

Almirid Desitin, Ger.
Dihydroergocryptine mesylate (p.1571·3).
Parkinsonism.

Almitil Almirall, Spain.
Enoxacin (p.203·3).
Urinary-tract infections.

Almodan
Berk, Irl.; Berk, UK.
Amoxycillin (p.151·3) or amoxycillin sodium (p.151·3).
Bacterial infections.

Almora Forest Pharmaceuticals, USA.
Magnesium gluconate (p.1157·2).
Dietary supplement.

Alna Boehringer Ingelheim, Ger.
Tamsulosin hydrochloride (p.951·2).
Benign prostatic hyperplasia.

Alnert Mitsubishi, Jpn.
Bifemelane hydrochloride.
Cerebrovascular disorders.

Alnide Cusi, UK†.
Cyclopentolate hydrochloride (p.459·3).
Production of cycloplegia and mydriasis.

Alodan Gerot, Aust.
Pethidine hydrochloride (p.76·1).
Pain.

Alodont Warner-Lambert, Fr.
Cetylpyridinium chloride (p.1106·2); chlorbutol (p.1106·3); eugenol (p.1578·2).
Mouth and throat infections.

Alodont nouvelle formule Parke, Davis, Switz.
Cetylpyridinium chloride (p.1106·2); chlorbutol (p.1106·3); eugenol (p.1578·2).
Mouth and throat disorders.

Alodorm Alphapharm, Austral.
Nitrazepam (p.682·2).
Insomnia.

Aloe Complex Dolisos, Canad.
Homoeopathic preparation.

Aloe Grande Gordon, USA.
Vitamin A (p.1358·1); vitamin E (p.1369·1); aloe vera (p.1177·1).
Skin disorders.

Aloe Vesta Calgon Vestal, USA.
Skin cleanser.

Alofedina Coll, Spain.
Aloin (p.1177·2); belladonna (p.457·1); phenolphthalein (p.1208·2); ipecacuanha (p.1062·2); nux vomica (p.1609·3); podophyllum (p.1089·1).
Constipation.

Aloinophen Streuli, Switz.
Aloes (p.1177·1); belladonna (p.457·1); bisacodyl (p.1179·3); ipecacuanha (p.1062·2).
Constipation.

Alol SIT, Ital.†.
Acebutolol hydrochloride (p.809·3).
Arrhythmias; hypertension.

Alomen Benedetti, Ital.
Ceftezole sodium (p.175·1).
Bacterial infections.

Alomide
Alcon, Belg.; Alcon, Canad.; Galen, Irl.; Alcon, Ital.; Alcon, S.Afr.; Alcon, UK; Alcon, USA.
Lodoxamide trometamol (p.756·1).
Allergic conjunctivitis.

Alongamicina Alonga, Spain†.
Ampicillin sodium (p.153·1); ampicillin benzathine (p.154·1).
Bacterial infections.

Alongamicina Balsa Alonga, Spain.
Ampicillin sodium (p.153·1); ampicillin benzathine (p.154·1); bromhexine hydrochloride (p.1055·3); guaiphenesin (p.1061·3).
Respiratory-tract infections.

Alopam
Alpharma, Norw.; Dumex-Alpharma, Swed.†.
Oxazepam (p.683·2).
Anxiety; insomnia; neuroses; restlessness.

Alopate Wolfs, Belg.
Zinc oxide (p.1096·2); titanium oxide (p.1093·3); kaolin (p.1195·1).
Skin disorders.

Alopexy
Pierre Fabre, Fr.; Pierre Fabre, Switz.
Minoxidil (p.910·3).
Alopecia androgenetica.

Alophen
Note. This name is used for preparations of different composition.
Parke, Davis, Austral.†.
Phenolphthalein (p.1208·2); aloin (p.1177·2); belladonna (p.457·1); ipecacuanha (p.1062·2).
Constipation.

Warner-Lambert, Canad.†.
Phenolphthalein (p.1208·2).
Constipation.

Warner-Lambert, Irl.; Warner-Lambert, UK.
Phenolphthalein (p.1208·2); aloin (p.1177·2).
Formerly contained phenolphthalein, aloin, belladonna, and ipecacuanha.
Constipation.

Alophen Pills Warner-Lambert, USA.
Phenolphthalein (p.1208·2).
Formerly called Alophen Pills No. 973.
Constipation.

Aloplastine
Wolfs, Belg.; Biologiques de l'Ile-de-France, Fr.
Zinc oxide (p.1096·2); purified talc (p.1092·1).
Skin disorders.

Aloplastine Acide
Note. This name is used for preparations of different composition.
Biologiques de l'Ile-de-France, Fr.†.
Glycerol (p.1585·2); purified talc (p.1092·1).
Skin disorders.

Sodip, Switz.†.
Magnesium silicate (p.1473·3); glycerol (p.1585·2); lactic acid (p.1593·3); citric acid (p.1564·3).
Infected skin disorders.

Aloplastine Ichthyolee Biologiques de l'Ile-de-France, Fr.†.
Ichthammol (p.1083·3); zinc oxide (p.1096·2); glycerol (p.1585·2); purified talc (p.1092·1).
Eczema.

Aloplastine poudre Sodip, Switz.†.
Barrier preparation.

Aloplastine simple Sodip, Switz.†.
Magnesium silicate (p.1473·3); zinc oxide (p.1096·2); glycerol (p.1585·2).
Skin disorders.

Alopon Resinag, Switz.
Aluminium chlorohydrate (p.1078·3).
Anorectal disorders.

Alopresin Alonga, Spain.
Captopril (p.836·3).
Diabetic nephropathy; heart failure; hypertension.

Alopresin Diu Alonga, Spain.
Hydrochlorothiazide (p.885·2); captopril (p.836·3).
Hypertension.

Aloquin Prosana, Austral.†.
Monobenzone (p.1088·3).
Hyperpigmentation.

Alor Atley, USA.
Hydrocodone tartrate (p.43·1); aspirin (p.16·1).
Pain.

Alora Procter & Gamble, USA.
Oestradiol (p.1455·1).
Menopausal disorders.

Aloral Lagap, UK.
Allopurinol (p.390·2).
Gout; hyperuricaemia.

Alorbat
Asta Medica, Ger.†; Asta Medica, Switz.†.
An influenza vaccine (p.1515·2).
Active immunisation.

Alostil Sanofi Winthrop, Fr.
Minoxidil (p.910·3).
Alopecia androgenetica.

Alovir Caber, Ital.
Aciclovir (p.602·3).
Herpesvirus infections.

Aloxidil IDI, Ital.
Minoxidil (p.910·3).
Alopecia androgenetica.

Alpagelle Pharmadeveloppement, Fr.
Miristalkonium chloride (p.1119·3).
Contraceptive.

1-Alpha Leo, Belg.
Alfacalcidol (p.1366·3).
Hypoparathyroidism; osteoporosis; renal osteodystrophy; rickets.

Alpha Keri
Note. This name is used for preparations of different composition.
Bristol-Myers, Austral.; Bristol-Myers Squibb, Canad.; Bristol-Myers Squibb, UK; Westwood, USA.
Bath oil; lotion: Liquid paraffin (p.1382·1); lanolin oil (p.1385·3).
Dermatitis; dry skin.

Bristol-Myers Squibb, Canad.
Soap: Glycerol (p.1585·2).

Westwood, USA†; Bristol-Myers Products, USA†.
Cleansing bar: Skin cleanser.

Alpha Keri Silky Smooth Bristol-Myers, Austral.
Vitamin E (p.1369·1).
Emollient.

Alpha Keri Tar Bristol-Myers, Austral.
Bath oil: Coal tar (p.1092·3); oil-soluble, dewaxed lanolin fraction (p.1385·3); liquid paraffin (p.1382·1).
Bath additive; skin disorders.
Gel: Coal tar (p.1092·3).
Skin disorders.
Shampoo: Coal tar (p.1092·3); salicylic acid (p.1090·2); sulphur (p.1091·2).
Scalp disorders.

Alpha Plus Tyson, USA†.
Amino acid preparation.

Alpha Renol Monin, Fr.†.
Equisetum (p.1575·1); maize; juniper (p.1592·2); couch-grass (p.1567·3).
Formerly contained chymotrypsin and trypsin.
Herbal preparation.

Alpha VIII
Alpha Therapeutic, Ger.†; Alpha Therapeutic, UK.
A factor VIII preparation (p.720·3).
Formerly known as Profilate HT and Profilate-SD in the *UK.*
Factor VIII deficiency.

Alpha-Apoplectal
Klinge, Aust.; Klinge, Ger.†.
Sodium aescinate (p.1543·3); etofylline (p.753·1).
Cerebrovascular disorders.

Alphacaine SPAD, Fr.
Carticaine hydrochloride (p.1289·1).
Adrenaline hydrochloride (p.813·3) is included in this preparation as a vasoconstrictor to diminish absorption and localise the effect of the local anaesthetic.
Local anaesthesia.

Alpha-Chymocutan Strathmann, Ger.
Chymotrypsin (p.1563·2).
Soft tissue inflammation and oedema.

Alpha-Chymotrase Strathmann, Ger.
Chymotrypsin (p.1563·2).
Respiratory-tract disorders; soft tissue inflammation and oedema.

Alphacin Alphapharm, Austral.
Ampicillin trihydrate (p.153·2).
Bacterial infections.

Alphacortison Procter & Gamble, Neth.
Hydrocortisone (p.1043·3); urea (p.1095·2).
Skin disorders.

Alphacutanee Leurquin, Fr.
Chymotrypsin (p.1563·2).
Oedema.

Alpha-Depressan OPW, Ger.
Urapidil (p.959·2).
Hypertension.

Alphaderm
Procter & Gamble, Belg.; Procter & Gamble, Irl.; Procter & Gamble, UK.
Hydrocortisone (p.1043·3); urea (p.1095·2).
Skin disorders.

Alphadrate Procter & Gamble, Neth.
Urea (p.1095·2).
Dry skin disorders.

Alphagan
Allergan, Austral.; Allergan, Swed.; Allergan, UK; Allergan, USA.
Brimonidine tartrate (p.834·1).
Glaucoma; ocular hypertension.

Alphaglobin
Alpha Therapeutic, Ger.; Alpha Therapeutic, Ital.; Alpha Therapeutic, UK.
A normal immunoglobulin (p.1522·1).
Chronic lymphocytic leukaemia; idiopathic thrombocytopenic purpura; immunodeficiencies; passive immunisation.

Alpha-Kadol Clin Midy, Fr.†.
Chymotrypsin (p.1563·2); phenylbutazone (p.79·2).
Musculoskeletal and joint disorders; soft tissue disorders; superficial phlebitis.

Alphakinase Alpha Therapeutic, Ger.
Urokinase (p.959·3).
Thrombo-embolic disorders.

Alpha-Lac Genpharm, Canad.†.
Lactulose (p.1195·3).
Constipation.

Alpha-Lipon Stada, Ger.
Thioctic acid (p.1636·2).
Diabetic polyneuropathy.

Alphamex Pharmagen, S.Afr.†.
Methyldopa (p.904·2).
Hypertension.

Alphamox Alphapharm, Austral.
Amoxycillin trihydrate (p.151·3).
Bacterial infections.

Alphanate
Alpha Therapeutic, Ital.; Alpha Therapeutic, UK; Alpha Therapeutic, USA.
A factor VIII preparation (p.720·3).
Haemorrhagic disorders.

Alphane Bailleul, Fr.
Zinc sulphate (p.1373·2); pyridoxine hydrochloride (p.1362·3).
Seborrhoea.

Alphanine
Alpha Therapeutic, Ger.; Alpha Therapeutic, Ital.; Alpha Therapeutic, UK; Alpha Therapeutic, USA.
Factor IX (p.721·3).
Factor IX deficiency.

Alphaparin Alpha Therapeutic, UK.
Certoparin sodium (p.839·1).
Venous thrombo-embolism prophylaxis.

Alphapress Alphapharm, Austral.
Hydralazine hydrochloride (p.883·2).
Hypertension.

Alpha-R Bayer, Fr.†.
A range of allergen extracts (p.1545·1).
Hyposensitisation.

Alphastria Inpharzam, Switz.
Sodium hyaluronate (p.1630·3); vitamin A palmitate (p.1358·1); alpha tocopheryl acetate (p.1369·2); dexpanthenol (p.1570·3); allantoin (p.1078·2); camphor (p.1557·2); menthol (p.1600·2).
Prevention of skin striae.

Alphatest Bayer, Fr.†.
A range of allergen extracts (p.1545·1).
Diagnosis of hypersensitivity.

Alphatrex Savage, USA.
Betamethasone dipropionate (p.1033·3).
Skin disorders.

Alphavase Ashbourne, UK.
Prazosin hydrochloride (p.932·3).

alpha-Vibolex Chephasaar, Ger.
Thioctic acid (p.1636·2).
Diabetic polyneuropathy.

Alphintern
Leurquin, Fr.; Hasenclever, Ger.†.
Chymotrypsin (p.1563·2); trypsin (p.1640·1).
Oedema; upper respiratory-tract inflammation.

Alphodith Stafford-Miller, UK†.
Dithranol (p.1082·1).
Psoriasis.

Alphosyl
Note. This name is used for preparations of different composition.
Salus, Aust.; Stafford-Miller, Austral.; Stafford-Miller Continental, Belg.; Reed & Carnrick, Canad.; Stafford-Miller, Fr.; Stafford-Miller, Irl.; Searle, S.Afr.; Stafford-Miller, Spain; Meda, Swed.; Stafford-Miller, Switz.; Stafford-Miller, UK.
Allantoin (p.1078·2); coal tar (p.1092·3).
Psoriasis; seborrhoeic dermatitis.

Stafford-Miller, Austral.
Shampoo: Coal tar (p.1092·3).
Dandruff; psoriasis; seborrhoeic dermatitis.

Alphosyl 2 in 1 Stafford-Miller, UK.
Coal tar (p.1092·3).
Scalp disorders.

Alphosyl HC
Stafford-Miller, Irl.; Stafford-Miller, UK.
Coal tar (p.1092·3); allantoin (p.1078·2); hydrocortisone (p.1043·3).
Psoriasis.

Alphosyle Poli, Ital.
Allantoin (p.1078·2); coal tar (p.1092·3).
Psoriasis.

Alpicort
Note. This name is used for preparations of different composition.
Montavit, Aust.†.
Prednisolone (p.1048·1); salicylic acid (p.1090·2); coal tar (p.1092·3); colloidal sulphur (p.1091·2); thymol (p.1127·1).
Scalp disorders.

Wolff, Ger.; Cimex, Switz.
Prednisolone (p.1048·1); salicylic acid (p.1090·2).
Formerly known as Alpicort-N in *Ger.*
Scalp disorders.

Alpicort F
Wolff, Ger.; Cimex, Switz.
Prednisolone (p.1048·1); salicylic acid (p.1090·2); oestradiol benzoate (p.1455·1).
Formerly known as Alpicort-F neu in *Ger.*
Scalp disorders.

Alpina Gel a la consoude Alpinamed, Switz.
Comfrey (p.1567·1); hypericum (p.1590·1); calendula officinalis; spearmint (p.1632·1); echinacea purpurea (p.1574·2).
Soft-tissue injury.

Alpina Gel a l'arnica avec spilanthes Alpinamed, Switz.
Arnica (p.1550·3); spilanthes oleracea.
Musculoskeletal and joint pain; soft-tissue disorders.

Alpina Pommade au souci Alpinamed, Switz.
Calendula officinalis; calendula oil.
Burns; wounds.

Alpoxen
Alpharma, Norw.; Dumex-Alpharma, Swed.
Naproxen (p.61·2).
Inflammation; musculoskeletal and joint disorders; pain.

Alpralid Dumex-Alpharma, Swed.†.
Alprazolam (p.640·3).
Anxiety.

Alpraz SMB, Belg.
Alprazolam (p.640·3).
Anxiety disorders; depression; nervous tension.

Alpress Pfizer, Fr.
Prazosin hydrochloride (p.932·3).
Hypertension.

Alprim Alphapharm, Austral.
Trimethoprim (p.265·1).
Bacterial infections of the urinary tract.

The symbol † denotes a preparation no longer actively marketed

Alprimol *Biochemie, Aust.†.*
Trimethoprim (p.265·1).
Bacterial infections.

Alprostar *Recordati, Ital.*
Alprostadil alfadex (p.1413·1).
Thromboangiitis obliterans.

Alprox *Orion, Irl.*
Alprazolam (p.640·3).
Anxiety.

Alquat *SCAM, Ital.†.*
Benzalkonium chloride (p.1101·3); didecyldimethylammonium chloride (p.1112·2); glutaraldehyde (p.1114·3); polyoxyethylene alkylarylether; sodium lauryl ether sulphate.
Skin disinfection.

Alquil Dermol *Zyma, Spain†.*
Citric acid (p.1564·3); lemon oil (p.1595·3); alkylsulphonate sodium.
Skin disinfection.

Alramucil *Alra, USA.*
Psyllium hydrophilic mucilloid (p.1194·2).
Constipation.

Alramucil Instant Mix *Alra, USA.*
Ispaghula husk (p.1194·2).

Alredase
John Wyeth, Irl.†; Wyeth, Ital.†.
Tolrestat (p.333·3).
Diabetic neuropathy.

Alrex *Bausch & Lomb, USA.*
Loteprednol etabonate (p.1045·3).
Allergic conjunctivitis.

Alrheumat
Bayer, Irl.†; Bayer, UK†.
Ketoprofen (p.48·2).
Musculoskeletal and joint disorders; pain.

Alrheumun *Bayer, Ger.*
Ketoprofen (p.48·2).
Gout; inflammation; musculoskeletal and joint disorders; pain.

Alsadorm *Woelm, Ger.†.*
Doxylamine succinate (p.410·1).
Sleep disorders.

Alsicur *Alsitan, Ger.*
Cucurbita (p.1569·1); cucurbita oil; pollen; centaury (p.1561·1); echinacea (p.1574·2); vitamin E (p.1369·1).
Urinary-tract disorders.

Alsidrine *Alsi, Canad.*
Ammonium chloride (p.1055·2); coccilana (p.1057·2).

Alsilax *Alsi, Canad.*
Magnesium sulphate (p.1157·3); cascara (p.1183·1); boldo (p.1554·1); pancreatin (p.1612·1); peptone.

Alsiline *Alsi, Canad.*
Aloin (p.1177·2); cascara (p.1183·1); phenolphthalein (p.1208·2); bile salts (p.1553·2).

Alsilon *DCG, Swed.†.*
Dried aluminium hydroxide (p.1177·3); magnesium oxide (p.1198·3); magnesium trisilicate (p.1199·1).

Alsimine with Vitamins A & D *Alsi, Canad.*
Multivitamins with calcium and iron.

Alsiphene *Alsi, Canad.*
Paracetamol (p.72·2).

Alsiroyal *Alsitan, Ger.*
Royal jelly (p.1626·3); vitamin E (p.1369·1); ginseng (p.1584·2).
Tonic.

Alsirub *Alsi, Canad.*
Methyl salicylate (p.55·2); menthol (p.1600·2); cineole (p.1564·1).

Alsogil *Also, Ital.*
Suppositories: Aspirin (p.16·1); paracetamol (p.72·2).
Tablets: Aspirin (p.16·1); paracetamol (p.72·2); caffeine (p.749·3).
Cold symptoms; pain.

Alsol
Note. This name is used for preparations of different composition.
Athenstaedt, Ger.
Ointment†: Basic aluminium acetotartrate (p.1547·3); chlorbutol (p.1106·3); corn oil; wheat oil.
Topical inflammatory conditions.
Topical solution: Basic aluminium acetotartrate (p.1547·3).
Astringent.
Also, Ital.
Cetylpyridinium chloride (p.1106·2).
Formerly contained bisdequalinium diacetate.
Mouth and throat infections.

Alsol N *Athenstaedt, Ger.*
Basic aluminium acetotartrate (p.1547·3).
Napkin rash; skin disorders; wounds.

Alsoy
Nestle, Canad.; Nestle, Ital.
Soya infant feed.
Cow's milk intolerance; lactose intolerance.

Altace
Hoechst Marion Roussel, Canad.; Hoechst Marion Roussel, USA.
Ramipril (p.941·1).
Heart failure following myocardial infarction; hypertension.

Altacet *Hoechst Marion Roussel, Swed.*
Hydrotalcite (p.1194·1).
Gastro-intestinal disorders.

Altacite
Hoechst Marion Roussel, Irl.; Hoechst Marion Roussel, S.Afr.; Roussel, UK.
Hydrotalcite (p.1194·1).
Gastro-intestinal hyperacidity.

Altacite Plus
Hoechst Marion Roussel, Irl.; Roussel, UK.
Hydrotalcite (p.1194·1); simethicone (p.1213·1).
These ingredients can be described by the British Approved Name Co-simalcite.
Gastro-intestinal disorders.

Altan *Rottapharm, Ital.*
Promelase (p.1621·3).
Respiratory-system disorders.

Altat *Teikoku, Jpn.*
Roxatidine acetate hydrochloride (p.1212·1).
Aspiration syndrome; gastritis; gastro-intestinal haemorrhage; gastro-oesophageal reflux; peptic ulcer; Zollinger-Ellison syndrome.

Altego *Goldschmidt, Ger.†.*
Isopropyl alcohol (p.1118·2); glutaraldehyde (p.1114·3); propyl alcohol (p.1124·2); alkylbenzyldimethylammonium chloride (p.1101·3).
Surface disinfection.

Alteporina *Alter, Spain.*
Cefminox sodium (p.167·1).
Bacterial infections.

ALternaGEL *J&J-Merck, USA.*
Dried aluminium hydroxide gel (p.1177·3).
Hyperacidity symptoms.

Altesona *Alter, Spain.*
Cortisone acetate (p.1036·1).
Corticosteroid.

Althaea Complex *Blackmores, Austral.*
Maize; althaea (p.1546·3); buchu (p.1555·2); bearberry (p.1552·2); *d*-alpha tocopheryl acid succinate (p.1369·2); vitamin A acetate (p.1359·2).
Urinary-tract disorders.

Altiazem *Lusofarmaco, Ital.*
Diltiazem hydrochloride (p.854·2).
Cardiovascular disorders.

Altim *Roussel, Fr.*
Cortivazol (p.1036·2).
Corticosteroid.

Altior *Pensa, Spain.*
Ibuprofen (p.44·1).
Fever; musculoskeletal, joint, and peri-articular disorders; pain.

Altocel *Irex, Fr.*
Loperamide hydrochloride (p.1197·2).
Diarrhoea.

Altodor *Synthelabo, Ger.†.*
Ethamsylate (p.720·1).
Haemorrhagic disorders.

Altosone *Purofarma, Ital.*
Mometasone furoate (p.1047·2).
Skin disorders.

Altracart II *Althin, Swed.*
Sodium bicarbonate (p.1151·1).
Haemodialysis.

Altramet *Dresden, Ger.*
Cimetidine (p.1183·2) or cimetidine hydrochloride (p.1185·3).
Aspiration syndromes; gastro-oesophageal reflux; hypersensitivity reactions; peptic ulcer; Zollinger-Ellison syndrome.

Altren *Rhone-Poulenc Rorer, Belg.†.*
Acemetacin (p.12·2).
Inflammation; musculoskeletal, joint, and peri-articular disorders; pain.

Altris *Isnardi, Ital.†.*
Aloglutamol (p.1177·2).
Gastro-intestinal disorders.

Alu-3 *Germania, Aust.*
Aluminium tyrosinate.
Gastro-intestinal disorders; hyperphosphataemia.

Alubifar *Rottapharm, Spain.*
Almasilate (p.1177·1).
Formerly contained almasilate, aluminium polygalacturonate, dimethicone, and magnesium oxide.
Gastro-intestinal hyperacidity.

Alubron-Saar *CPF, Ger.*
Aluminium chloride (p.1078·3).
Inflammatory disorders of the oropharynx.

Alu-Cap
3M, Ger.†; 3M, UK; 3M, USA.
Dried aluminium hydroxide gel (p.1177·3).
Gastro-intestinal hyperacidity; hyperphosphataemia.

Alucid *Labima, Belg.*
Aluminium glycinate (p.1177·2); calcium carbonate (p.1182·1); magnesium trisilicate (p.1199·1); sodium bicarbonate (p.1153·2).
Gastro-intestinal disorders.

Alucol
Note. This name is used for preparations of different composition.
Schoeller, Aust.; Wander OTC, Switz.
Dried aluminium hydroxide gel (p.1177·3); magnesium hydroxide (p.1198·2).
Gastric hyperacidity; gastric irritation; gastro-oesophageal reflux.
Sandoz, Ital.†.
Aluminium hydroxide (p.1177·3).
Gastric hyperacidity.

Alucol Silicona *Sandoz, Spain.*
Aluminium hydroxide (p.1177·3); dimethicone (p.1213·1); magnesium hydroxide (p.1198·2).
Gastro-intestinal hyperacidity and flatulence.

Alucol-S *Wander, Switz.†.*
Dried aluminium hydroxide gel (p.1177·3); magnesium hydroxide (p.1198·2); simethicone (p.1213·1).
Flatulence; hyperacidity.

Alucone *Drug Houses Austral., Austral.†.*
Aluminium hydroxide (p.1177·3); magnesium hydroxide (p.1198·2); simethicone (p.1213·1).
Flatulence; gastric acidity.

Aluctyl
Monal, Fr.; Yamanouchi, Ital.
Aluminium lactate (p.1548·1).
Mouth and throat disorders.

Aludrox
Note. This name is used for preparations of different composition.
Whitehall, Austral.†; Akromed, S.Afr.†.
Aluminium hydroxide (p.1177·3); magnesium hydroxide (p.1198·2).
Hyperchlorhydria; peptic ulcer.
Wyeth, Ger.; Charwell Pharmaceuticals, Irl.
Aluminium hydroxide (p.1177·3).
Gastric hyperacidity; hyperphosphataemia; peptic ulcer.
Pfizer Consumer, UK.
Oral liquid: Aluminium hydroxide (p.1177·3).
Tablets: Aluminium hydroxide-magnesium carbonate co-dried gel (p.1178·2); magnesium hydroxide (p.1198·2).
Dyspepsia; hyperphosphataemia.
Wyeth-Ayerst, USA.
Aluminium hydroxide (p.1177·3); magnesium hydroxide (p.1198·2); simethicone (p.1213·1).
Hyperacidity.

Aludyal *Sandoz, Ital.†.*
Algeldrate (p.1177·3).
Hyperphosphataemia.

Alufilm *Boots, Spain†.*
Almasilate (p.1177·1).
Gastro-intestinal hyperacidity.

Alugel *Atlas, Canad.*
Aluminium hydroxide (p.1177·3).

Alugelibys *Pharmacia Upjohn, Spain.*
Aluminium hydroxide (p.1177·3).
Gastro-intestinal hyperacidity.

Alugelibys Magn Susp *Pharmacia Upjohn, Spain.*
Aluminium hydroxide (p.1177·3); magnesium hydroxide (p.1198·2).
Gastro-intestinal hyperacidity.

Alugelibys Magnesiado *Pharmacia Upjohn, Spain.*
Aluminium hydroxide (p.1177·3); magnesium oxide (p.1198·3).
Formerly contained aluminium magnesium hydroxide.
Gastro-intestinal hyperacidity.

Aluhyde *Sinclair, UK†.*
Aluminium hydroxide (p.1177·3); magnesium trisilicate (p.1199·1); belladonna (p.457·1).
Gastro-intestinal spasm.

Alukon *Apotex, S.Afr.*
Aluminium hydroxide (p.1177·3).
Gastric hyperacidity.

Alumadrine *Fleming, USA.*
Phenylpropanolamine hydrochloride (p.1067·2); chlorpheniramine maleate (p.405·1); paracetamol (p.72·2).
Upper respiratory-tract symptoms.

Alumag *Trianon, Canad.*
Aluminium hydroxide (p.1177·3); magnesium hydroxide (p.1198·2).

Alumagall *Interdelta, Switz.*
Dried aluminium hydroxide gel (p.1177·3); magnesium hydroxide (p.1198·2); allantoin (p.1078·2).
Gastric hyperacidity.

Aluminium Free Indigestion *Larkhall Laboratories, UK.*
Calcium carbonate (p.1182·1); cinnamon (p.1564·2); nutmeg (p.1609·2); clove (p.1565·2); cardamom seed (p.1560·1).

Alumite *Xixia, S.Afr.*
Dicyclomine hydrochloride (p.460·1); aluminium hydroxide (p.1177·3); magnesium oxide (p.1198·3).
Gastro-intestinal disorders.

Alun Difter *Evans, Spain†.*
A diphtheria vaccine (p.1507·3).
Active immunisation.

Alupent
Bender, Aust.; Boehringer Ingelheim, Austral.; Boehringer Ingelheim, Belg.; Boehringer Ingelheim, Canad.; Boehringer Ingelheim, Fr.; Boehringer Ingelheim, Ger.; Boehringer Ingelheim, Irl.; Boehringer Ingelheim, Ital.; Boehringer Ingelheim, Neth.†; Boehringer Ingelheim, S.Afr.; Boehringer Ingelheim, Spain; Boehringer Ingelheim, Switz.; Boehringer Ingelheim, UK; Boehringer Ingelheim, USA.
Orciprenaline sulphate (p.756·3).
Arrhythmias; beta blocker overdosage; digitalis intoxication; obstructive airways disease; Stokes-Adams syndrome.

Alupent Expectorant *Boehringer Ingelheim, Irl.*
Orciprenaline sulphate (p.756·3); bromhexine hydrochloride (p.1055·3).
Obstructive airways disease.

Alu-Phar *Pharma Plus, Switz.†.*
Dried aluminium hydroxide gel (p.1177·3).
Duodenal ulcer; gastric hyperacidity.

Alupir *Farmacologico Milanese, Ital.†.*
Aluminium aspirin (p.15·1).
Cold symptoms; musculoskeletal disorders; neuritis.

Alurate *Roche, USA.*
Aprobarbital (p.642·2).
Insomnia; sedative.

Aluspastyl *Pharmatec, S.Afr.†.*
Dicyclomine hydrochloride (p.460·1); dried aluminium hydroxide (p.1177·3); light magnesium oxide (p.1198·3).
Gastro-intestinal disorders.

Alu-Tab
3M, Austral.; 3M, Canad.; 3M, USA.
Dried aluminium hydroxide gel (p.1177·3).
Gastric hyperacidity; hyperphosphataemia; peptic ulcer.

Alutard
Epipharm, Aust.†.
Range of allergen extracts (p.1545·1).
Hyposensitisation.
ALK, Norw.
Allergen extracts (p.1545·1) from timothy (*Phleum pratense*) or birch (*Betula verrucosa*).
Hyposensitisation.

Alutard SQ
ALK, Swed.; Trimedal, Switz.
Allergen extracts (p.1545·1).
Hyposensitisation.

Alutoxoide D T *Antibioticos, Spain†.*
A diphtheria and tetanus vaccine (p.1508·1).
Active immunisation of infants and young children.

Alutoxoide D T P *Antibioticos, Spain†.*
A diphtheria, tetanus, and pertussis vaccine (p.1509·1).
Active immunisation of infants and young children.

Alutoxoide T *Antibioticos, Spain†.*
A tetanus vaccine (p.1535·3).
Active immunisation.

Aluzime *Alter, Spain.*
Coenzyme A (p.1566·2).
Glomerular kidney disease; metabolic disorders.

Alvadermo Fuerte *Inexfa, Spain.*
Fluocinolone acetonide (p.1041·1).
Skin disorders.

Alvear *Whitehall, Ital.*
Royal jelly (p.1626·3).
Nutritional supplement.

Alvear Complex *Whitehall, Ital.*
Royal jelly (p.1626·3); pollen; dried yeast (p.1373·1); lactic-acid-producing organisms (p.1594·1).
Nutritional supplement.

Alvear Sport *Whitehall, Ital.*
Yellow capsules: royal jelly (p.1626·3); pollen; red capsules: ginkgo biloba (p.1584·1); myrtillus (p.1606·1); tablets: glucose (p.1343·3); royal jelly.
Nutritional supplement.

Alvedon
Astra, Norw.; Astra, Swed.; Novex Pharma, UK.
Paracetamol (p.72·2).
Fever; pain.

Alven *Wassermann, Ital.*
Diosmin (p.1580·1).
Peripheral vascular disorders.

Alveofact
Bender, Aust.; Thomae, Ger.; Boehringer Ingelheim, Ital.
Bovactant (p.1623·1).
Neonatal respiratory distress syndrome.

Alveolex *Klinge, Irl.*
Acetylcysteine (p.1052·3).
Cystic fibrosis; respiratory-tract disorders with excess or viscous mucus.

Alveoten *Ibi, Ital.*
Neltenexine (p.1065·1) or neltenexine hydrochloride (p.1065·1).
Respiratory-tract disorders.

Alvercol
Norgine, Austral.; Norgine, Irl.; Norgine, S.Afr.; Norgine, UK.
Sterculia (p.1214·1); alverine citrate (p.1548·1).
Formerly known as Normacol Antispasmodic in *S.Afr.* and *UK*.
Hypertonic colon; irritable bowel syndrome.

Alvesin *Berlin-Chemie, Ger.*
Amino-acid and electrolyte infusion.
Parenteral nutrition.

Alvinorm *Wolfer, Ger.†.*
Placentae deproteinisatum (p.1599·1).
Tonic.

Alvityl
Solvay, Belg.†; Solvay, Fr.
Multivitamin preparation.

Alvityl Plus *Solvay, Belg.†.*
Multivitamin, amino-acid, and mineral preparation.

Alvofact
Boehringer Ingelheim, Belg.; Boehringer Ingelheim, Neth.
Bovactant (p.1623·1).
Neonatal respiratory distress syndrome.

Alvogil *Prats, Spain.*
Butyl aminobenzoate (p.1289·1); eugenol (p.1578·2); iodoform (p.1118·2).

Alvogyl *Septodont, Switz.*
Butyl aminobenzoate (p.1289·1); iodoform (p.1118·2); eugenol (p.1578·2); spearmint oil (p.1632·1); penghawar djambi fibra.
Pain following tooth extraction.

Alvonal MR *Godecke, Ger.†.*
Cymarin (p.845·3).
Heart failure.

Alyma *Morrith, Spain†.*
Almasilate (p.1177·1).
Gastro-intestinal hyperacidity.

Alymphon *Iso, Ger.*
Homoeopathic preparation.

Alyostal *Stallergenes, Fr.; Stallergenes, Switz.*
A range of allergen extracts (p.1545·1).
Diagnosis of hypersensitivity; hyposensitisation.

Alyrane *ICI, Austral.; Pharmacia Upjohn, Belg.; Pharmacia Upjohn, Neth.; Pharmacia Upjohn, Swed.*
Enflurane (p.1222·1).
General anaesthesia.

Alzam *Parke-Med, S.Afr.*
Alprazolam (p.640·3).
Anxiety disorders.

AM 73 *Medici, Ital.†.*
Amoxycillin trihydrate (p.151·3).
Bacterial infections.

Am Lactin *Upsher-Smith, USA.*
Ammonium lactate (p.1079·1).
Dry skin.

Amacodone *Trimen, USA.*
Hydrocodone tartrate (p.43·1); paracetamol (p.72·2).
Pain.

Amadol *TAD, Ger.*
Tramadol hydrochloride (p.90·1).
Pain.

Amagesan *Yamanouchi, Ger.*
Amoxycillin trihydrate (p.151·3).
Bacterial infections.

Amalium *Janssen-Cilag, Aust.*
Flunarizine hydrochloride (p.411·1).
Ménière's disease; migraine; vertigo.

Amantan *Byk, Belg.*
Amantadine hydrochloride (p.1129·2).
Influenza A; parkinsonism.

Amaphen *Trimen, USA.*
Paracetamol (p.72·2); caffeine (p.749·3); butalbital (p.644·3).
Pain.

Amaphen with Codeine *Trimen, USA.*
Codeine phosphate (p.26·1); paracetamol (p.72·2); caffeine (p.749·3); butalbital (p.644·3).
Pain.

Amaphil *Be-Tabs, S.Afr.†.*
Aminophylline (p.748·1); ephedrine hydrochloride (p.1059·3); amylobarbitone (p.641·3).
Obstructive airways disease.

Amara *Koch, Aust.*
Gentian tincture (p.1583·3); cinchona bark tincture (p.1564·1); absinthium tincture (p.1541·1).
Gastro-intestinal disorders.

Amara-Tropfen-Pascoe *Pascoe, Ger.*
Gentian (p.1583·3); cinchona bark (p.1564·1); absinthium (p.1541·1); cinnamon bark (p.1564·2).
Gastro-intestinal disorders.

Amaro *Giuliani, Switz.†.*
Rhubarb (p.1212·1); cascara (p.1183·1); gentian (p.1583·3); boldo (p.1554·1).
Tonic.

Amaro Lassativo *Sofar, Ital.†.*
Rhubarb (p.1212·1); cascara (p.1183·1); boldo (p.1554·1); phenolphthalein (p.1208·2).
Constipation.

Amaro Maffioli *Sofar, Ital.†.*
Nux vomica (p.1609·3); kola (p.1645·1); rhubarb (p.1212·1); gentian (p.1583·3); calamus (p.1556·1); orange; cinchona (p.1564·1); calumba (p.1557·2); quassia (p.1624·1).
Dyspepsia.

Amaro Medicinale *Giuliani, Ital.*
Rhubarb (p.1212·1); cascara (p.1183·1); gentian (p.1583·3); boldo (p.1554·1).
Gastro-intestinal disorders.

Amaro Padil *Blue Cross, Ital.*
Cascara (p.1183·1); gentian (p.1583·3).
Constipation.

Amaryl
Hoechst, Ger.; Hoechst Marion Roussel, Irl.; Hoechst Marion Roussel, Neth.; Hoechst Marion Roussel, S.Afr.; Hoechst Marion Roussel, Swed.; Hoechst Marion Roussel, Switz.; Hoechst Marion Roussel, UK; Hoechst Marion Roussel, USA.
Glimepiride (p.320·2).
Diabetes mellitus.

Amasin *Heilit, Ger.†.*
Menthyl salicylate; benzyl nicotinate (p.22·1).
Circulatory disorders of the skin.

Amasulin *Takeda, Jpn.*
Carumonam sodium (p.163·2).
Mepivacaine hydrochloride (p.1297·2) is contained in the intramuscular injection to alleviate the pain of injection.
Bacterial infections.

Amatine *Knoll, Canad.*
Midodrine hydrochloride (p.910·1).
Idiopathic orthostatic hypotension.

Amazin *Pharmalab, S.Afr.†.*
Chlorpromazine hydrochloride (p.649·1).
Psychoses.

Amazyl *Christiaens, Belg.*
Bismuth subnitrate (p.1180·2); magnesium trisilicate (p.1199·1); borax (p.1554·2).
Cracked nipples.

Ambacamp *Pharmacia Upjohn, Ger.*
Bacampicillin hydrochloride (p.157·2).
Bacterial infections.

Ambatrol *SmithKline Beecham, Fr.*
Nifuroxazide (p.231·3).
Diarrhoea.

Ambaxin
Upjohn, Irl.†; Pharmacia Upjohn, UK†.
Bacampicillin hydrochloride (p.157·2).
Bacterial infections.

Ambaxino *Upjohn, Spain.*
Bacampicillin hydrochloride (p.157·2).
Bacterial infections.

Ambe 12 *Merckle, Ger.*
Cyanocobalamin (p.1363·3).
Vitamin B_{12} deficiency.

Ambenat *Merckle, Aust.*
Glycol salicylate (p.43·1); benzyl nicotinate (p.22·1); heparin sodium (p.879·3).
Muscle, nerve, and joint pain.

Ambene
Note. This name is used for preparations of different composition.
Merckle, Aust.
Ampoule A, phenylbutazone sodium (p.79·3); sodium salamidacetate (p.82·3); dexamethasone (p.1037·1); ampoule B, cyanocobalamin (p.1363·3).
Lignocaine hydrochloride (p.1293·2) is included in both ampoules to alleviate the pain of injection.
Arthritis; degenerative spinal disorders; neuralgias; neuritis.

Merckle, Ger.
Phenylbutazone (p.79·2) or phenylbutazone sodium (p.79·3).
Lignocaine hydrochloride (p.1293·2) is included in the injection to alleviate the pain of injection.
Gout; musculoskeletal and joint disorders.

Ambene Comp *Merckle, Ger.*
Ampoule 1, phenylbutazone sodium (p.79·3); ampoule 2, cyanocobalamin (p.1363·3).
Lignocaine hydrochloride (p.1293·2) is included in each ampoule to alleviate the pain of injection.
Gout; musculoskeletal and joint-disorders.

Ambene N
Note. This name is used for preparations of different composition.
Merckle, Aust.
Suppositories: Phenylbutazone (p.79·2); cyanocobalamin (p.1363·3).
Tablets: Phenylbutazone (p.79·2); thiamine hydrochloride (p.1361·1); cyanocobalamin (p.1363·3).
Aluminium glycinate (p.1177·2) is included in this preparation in an attempt to limit adverse effects on the gastro-intestinal mucosa.
Gout; musculoskeletal, joint, soft-tissue, and peri-articular disorders; neuritis; superficial thrombophlebitis.

Merckle, Ger.
Glycol salicylate (p.43·1); benzyl nicotinate (p.22·1).
Formerly contained glycol salicylate, benzyl nicotinate, and heparin sodium.
Bruising; musculoskeletal inflammatory disorders.

Ambenyl *Parke, Davis, Canad.*
Codeine phosphate (p.26·1); bromodiphenhydramine hydrochloride (p.403·2); diphenhydramine hydrochloride (p.409·1); ammonium chloride (p.1055·2); potassium guaiacolsulfonate (p.1068·3).
Coughs.

Ambenyl Cough Syrup *Forest Pharmaceuticals, USA.*
Codeine phosphate (p.26·1); bromodiphenhydramine hydrochloride (p.403·2).
Allergic upper respiratory symptoms; coughs and cold symptoms.

Ambenyl-D *Forest Pharmaceuticals, USA.*
Guaiphenesin (p.1061·3); pseudoephedrine hydrochloride (p.1068·3); dextromethorphan hydrobromide (p.1057·3).
Coughs; nasal congestion.

Amber Gold *Larkhall Laboratories, UK.*
Tea tree oil (p.1599·2).

Amberin *ACO, Swed.†.*
Hydrocortisone (p.1043·3).
Anogenital pruritus; eczema.

Ambi 10 *Kiwi, USA.*
Cream: Benzoyl peroxide (p.1079·2).
Acne.
Soap: Triclosan (p.1127·2).

Ambi Skin Tone *Kiwi, USA.*
Hydroquinone (p.1083·1); padimate O (p.1488·1).
Hyperpigmentation.

Ambien *Searle, USA.*
Zolpidem tartrate (p.698·3).
Insomnia.

Ambifon *Helvepharm, Switz.†.*
Lysine hydrochloride (p.1350·1).
Gastro-intestinal disorders.

Ambilhar *Ciba, Switz.†.*
Niridazole (p.106·2).
Worm infections.

AmBisome
Laevosan, Aust.; Nexstar, Belg.; Nexstar, Ital.; Nextar, Neth.; Nextar, Spain; Swedish Orphan, Swed.; Nexstar, UK; Fujisawa, USA.
Amphotericin (p.372·2).
Fungal infections; leishmaniasis.

Amblosin *Hoechst, Ger.†.*
Ampicillin sodium (p.153·1) or ampicillin trihydrate (p.153·2).
Bacterial infections.

Amboneural *Hofmann, Aust.*
Selegiline hydrochloride (p.1144·2).
Parkinsonism.

Ambra Med Complex *Dynamit, Aust.*
Homoeopathic preparation.

Ambral *Beige, S.Afr.†.*
Metronidazole (p.585·1).
Anaerobic bacterial infections; protozoal infections.

Ambramicina
Farmochimica, Ital.; Marion Merrell, Spain.
Tetracycline hydrochloride (p.259·1).
Bacterial infections.

Ambre Solaire *Garnier, UK.*
Avobenzone (p.1486·3); benzylidine camphor; phenylbenzimidazolesulphonic acid (p.1488·2); titanium dioxide (p.1093·3).
Sunscreen.

Ambredin *Chemieprodukte, Aust.*
Theophylline (p.765·1); aceverine hydrochloride; octodrine phosphate (p.925·1).
Obstructive airways disease.

Ambril *Cascan, Ger.; Cascapharm, Ger.*
Ambroxol hydrochloride (p.1054·3).
Respiratory-tract disorders associated with increased or viscous mucus.

Ambritan *Daker Farmasimes, Spain.*
Cobamamide (p.1364·2).
Tonic.

Ambrobene *Merckle, Aust.*
Ambroxol hydrochloride (p.1054·3).
Respiratory-tract disorders with viscous mucus.

Ambrobeta *Betapharm, Ger.*
Ambroxol hydrochloride (p.1054·3).
Respiratory-tract disorders with viscous mucus.

Ambrodoxy *Hexal, Ger.*
Doxycycline hydrochloride (p.202·3); ambroxol hydrochloride (p.1054·3).
Respiratory-tract infections with increased or viscous mucus.

Ambrohexal *Hexal, Ger.*
Ambroxol hydrochloride (p.1054·3).
Respiratory-tract disorders associated with increased or viscous mucus.

Ambrolan *Lannacher, Aust.†.*
Ambroxol hydrochloride (p.1054·3).
Respiratory-tract disorders.

Ambrolitic *Wasserman, Spain.*
Ambroxol hydrochloride (p.1054·3).
Respiratory-tract disorders.

Ambrolos *Hexal, Ger.*
Ambroxol hydrochloride (p.1054·3).
Respiratory-tract disorders.

Ambromucil *Malesci, Ital.*
Ambroxol acefyllinate (p.1054·3).
Obstructive airways disease.

Ambro-Puren *Isis Puren, Ger.*
Ambroxol hydrochloride (p.1054·3).
Respiratory-tract disorders with viscous mucus.

Ambroxol AL comp *Aliud, Ger.*
Ambroxol hydrochloride (p.1054·3); doxycycline hydrochloride (p.202·3).
Respiratory-tract infections.

Ambroxol comp *Ratiopharm, Ger.*
Ambroxol hydrochloride (p.1054·3); doxycycline hydrochloride (p.202·3).
Respiratory-tract infections.

Amcacid *Glaxo Allen, Ital.†.*
Tranexamic acid (p.728·2).
Haemorrhagic disorders.

Amchafibrin *Fides, Spain.*
Tranexamic acid (p.728·2).
Haemorrhage.

Amciderm *Hermal, Ger.*
Amcinonide (p.1032·1).
Skin disorders.

Amcinil *Crosara, Ital.*
Amcinonide (p.1032·1).
Skin disorders.

Amcoral *Meiji, Jpn.*
Amrinone (p.823·2).
Heart failure.

Amcort *Keene, USA.*
Triamcinolone diacetate (p.1050·2).
Corticosteroid.

Amc-Puren *Isis Puren, Ger.*
Amoxycillin trihydrate (p.151·3).
Bacterial infections.

Amdox-Puren *Isis Puren, Ger.*
Doxycycline hydrochloride (p.202·3); ambroxol hydrochloride (p.1054·3).
Respiratory-tract infections with increased or viscous mucus.

Amekrin
Warner-Lambert, Norw.; Parke, Davis, Swed.
Amsacrine (p.503·3).
Acute leukaemias.

Amen *Carnrick, USA.*
Medroxyprogesterone acetate (p.1448·3).
Abnormal uterine bleeding; secondary amenorrhoea.

Amerge *Glaxo Wellcome, USA.*
Naratriptan hydrochloride (p.448·3).
Migraine.

Americaine *Ciba, USA.*
Benzocaine (p.1286·2); benzethonium chloride (p.1102·3).
Anorectal disorders.

Americaine Anesthetic *Ciba, USA.*
Benzocaine (p.1286·2).
Local anaesthesia.

Americaine Anesthetic Lubricant *Fisons, USA.*
Benzocaine (p.1286·2).
Local anaesthesia; lubrication.

Americaine First Aid *Ciba, USA.*
Benzocaine (p.1286·2); benzethonium chloride (p.1102·3).
Skin disorders.

Americaine Otic *Fisons, USA.*
Benzocaine (p.1286·2); benzethonium chloride (p.1102·3); glycerol (p.1585·2).
Pain and pruritus in otitis.

Ameride *Du Pont, Spain.*
Amiloride hydrochloride (p.819·2); hydrochlorothiazide (p.885·2).
Hypertension; oedema.

Amersan *Austroplant, Aust.*
Agrimony herb; achillea (p.1542·2); peppermint oil (p.1208·1); rose fruit (p.1365·2); berberis; black currant (p.1365·2); myrtillus (p.1606·1).
Liver and biliary tract disorders.

Ames-BG *Bayer Diagnostics, Austral.†.*
Test for glucose in blood (p.1585·1).

Amesec
Lilly, Canad.†; Lilly, S.Afr.†.
Aminophylline (p.748·1); ephedrine hydrochloride (p.1059·3); amylobarbitone (p.641·3).
Asthma.

A-Methapred *Abbott, USA.*
Methylprednisolone sodium succinate (p.1046·1).
Corticosteroid.

Ametic *Garec, S.Afr.*
Metoclopramide hydrochloride (p.1200·3).
Gastro-intestinal disorders.

Ametionin *Medifood-Trufood, Ital.*
Food for special diets.
Homocystinuria.

Ametop *Smith & Nephew, UK.*
Amethocaine (p.1285·2).
Local anaesthesia.

Ametycine *Sanofi Winthrop, Fr.*
Mitomycin (p.552·2).
Malignant neoplasms.

Ameu *Pharmacal, Switz.*
Omega-3 triglycerides (p.1276·1).
Hyperlipidaemias.

Amfamox *Amrad, Austral.*
Famotidine (p.1192·1).
Gastro-oesophageal reflux; peptic ulcer; Zollinger-Ellison syndrome.

Amfed TD *Legere, USA†.*
Phenylpropanolamine (p.1067·2).

Amfipen
Yamanouchi, Irl.; Brocades, Neth.†; Brocades, UK†; Yamanouchi, UK.
Ampicillin (p.153·1) or ampicillin sodium (p.153·1).
Bacterial infections.

Amgenal Cough *Goldline, USA.*
Bromodiphenhydramine hydrochloride (p.403·2); codeine phosphate (p.26·1).
Coughs and cold symptoms.

Amias *Astra, UK.*
Candesartan cilexetil (p.836·1).
Hypertension.

Amicaliq *Tanabe, Jpn.*
Amino-acid, carbohydrate, and electrolyte infusion.
Parenteral nutrition.

Amicar
Lederle, Austral.; Wyeth-Ayerst, Canad.; Wyeth, S.Afr.; Immunex, USA.
Aminocaproic acid (p.711·1).
Fibrinolysis.

Amicasil *Lineamedica, Ital.*
Amikacin sulphate (p.150·2).
Bacterial infections.

Amicel *Salus, Ital.*
Econazole nitrate (p.377·2).
Fungal infections.

Amicic
Ciba Vision, Fr.; Ciba Vision, Switz.
Amino-acid preparation.
Corneal ulcers.

Amicla
Wyeth Lederle, Belg.; Lederle, Neth.†.
Amcinonide (p.1032·1).
Skin disorders.

Amiclair
Gelflex, Austral.†.
Protease; lipase; pronase.
Contact lens cleaner.

Abatron, UK.
Contact lens cleanser.

Amico *SIT, Ital.*
Amino-acid preparation with cobamamide.
Tonic.

Amicrobin *Hosbon, Spain.*
Norfloxacin (p.233·1).
Bacterial infections.

Amidal *Douglas, Austral.*
Amiloride hydrochloride (p.819·2).
Hepatic cirrhosis with ascites; hypertension; oedema.

Amidate *Abbott, USA.*
Etomidate (p.1223·2).
General anaesthesia.

Amidonal *PCR, Ger.*
Aprindine hydrochloride (p.825·1).
Arrhythmias.

Amidox *Approved Prescription Services, UK.*
Amiodarone hydrochloride (p.820·1).
Arrhythmias.

Amidoyina *Puerto Galiano, Spain†.*
Camphor (p.1557·2); boric acid (p.1554·2); cineole (p.1564·1); ephedrine (p.1059·3); niaouli oil (p.1607·1); menthol (p.1600·2).
Nasal congestion.

Amidral *Dicofarm, Ital.†.*
Sodium chloride; sodium bicarbonate; potassium chloride; rice starch (p.1152·3).
Diarrhoea; oral rehydration therapy.

Amidrin *Fardi, Spain.*
Ephedrine hydrochloride (p.1059·3); sulphanilamide (p.256·3).
Nasal congestion and infection.

Amidrin Bio *Fardi, Spain†.*
Chloramphenicol (p.182·1); ephedrine hydrochloride (p.1059·3); sulphacetamide sodium (p.252·2).
Nasal congestion and infection.

Ami-Drix *Amide, USA.*
Pseudoephedrine sulphate (p.1068·3); dexbrompheniramine maleate (p.403·2).
Upper respiratory-tract symptoms.

Amiduret *Trommsdorff, Ger.*
Amiloride hydrochloride (p.819·2); hydrochlorothiazide (p.885·2).
Ascites; hypertension; oedema.

Amigen *Baxter, Ital.†.*
Amino-acid, carbohydrate, and electrolyte infusion.
Parenteral nutrition.

Amigesic *Amide, USA.*
Salsalate (p.83·1).
Fever; inflammation; pain.

Amikal *Selena, Swed.†.*
Amiloride hydrochloride (p.819·2).
Hypertension; liver cirrhosis with ascites; oedema.

Amikan *SoSe, Ital.*
Amikacin sulphate (p.150·2).
Bacterial infections.

Amikin
Bristol-Myers Squibb, Austral.; Bristol, Canad.; Bristol-Myers Squibb, Irl.; Bristol-Myers Squibb, S.Afr.; Bristol-Myers Squibb, UK; Apothecon, USA.
Amikacin sulphate (p.150·2).
Bacterial infections.

Amikine *Bristol-Myers Squibb, Switz.*
Amikacin sulphate (p.150·2).
Bacterial infections.

Amiklin *Bristol-Myers Squibb, Fr.*
Amikacin sulphate (p.150·2).
Bacterial infections.

Amilamont *Rosemont, UK.*
Amiloride hydrochloride (p.819·2).
Heart failure; hepatic cirrhosis with ascites; hypertension.

Amilco *Norton, UK.*
Hydrochlorothiazide (p.885·2); amiloride hydrochloride (p.819·2).
These ingredients can be described by the British Approved Name Co-amilozide.
Ascites; heart failure; hepatic cirrhosis; hypertension.

Amilit-IFI *IFI, Ital.*
Amitriptyline hydrochloride (p.273·3).
Depression.

Amilmaxco *Ashbourne, UK.*
Amiloride hydrochloride (p.819·2); hydrochlorothiazide (p.885·2).
These ingredients can be described by the British Approved Name Co-amilozide.
Ascites; heart failure; hypertension.

Amilo-basan *Schonenberger, Switz.*
Amiloride hydrochloride (p.819·2); hydrochlorothiazide (p.885·2).
Hypertension; liver cirrhosis with ascites; oedema.

Amiloferm *Nordic, Swed.*
Amiloride hydrochloride (p.819·2); hydrochlorothiazide (p.885·2).
Hypertension; liver cirrhosis with ascites; oedema.

Amilo-OPT *Truw, Ger.†.*
Amiloride hydrochloride (p.819·2); hydrochlorothiazide (p.885·2).
Hypertension; oedema.

Amiloretic *Lennon, S.Afr.*
Amiloride hydrochloride (p.819·2); hydrochlorothiazide (p.885·2).
Hypertension; oedema.

Amiloretik
Hexal, Aust.; Hexal, Ger.
Amiloride hydrochloride (p.819·2); hydrochlorothiazide (p.885·2).
Hypertension; liver cirrhosis with ascites; oedema.

Amilorid comp
Genericon, Aust.; Heumann, Ger.; Ratiopharm, Ger.; Upsamedica, Switz.
Amiloride hydrochloride (p.819·2); hydrochlorothiazide (p.885·2).
Heart failure; hypertension; liver cirrhosis with ascites; oedema.

Amilospare *Ashbourne, UK.*
Amiloride hydrochloride (p.819·2).
Ascites; heart failure; hypertension.

Amilothiazid *Isis Puren, Ger.*
Amiloride hydrochloride (p.819·2); hydrochlorothiazide (p.885·2).
Hypertension; oedema.

Amilozid *CT, Ger.*
Amiloride hydrochloride (p.819·2); hydrochlorothiazide (p.885·2).
Hypertension; oedema.

Amilprats *Prats, Spain†.*
Metampicillin sodium (p.224·3).
Bacterial infections.

Amimox
Tika, Norw.; Tika, Swed.
Amoxycillin (p.151·3) or amoxycillin trihydrate (p.151·3).
Bacterial infections; peptic ulcer associated with Helicobacter pylori.

Amin-Aid
Baxter, Ital.†; McGaw, USA†.
Food for special diets.
Renal failure.

Amindan
Note. This name is used for preparations of different composition.
Desitin, Ger.
Selegiline hydrochloride (p.1144·2).
Parkinsonism.

Eberth, Ger.†.
Chloramphenicol (p.182·1); vitamin B substances.
Bacterial infections.

Aminess
Pharmacia Upjohn, Neth.; Clintec, USA.
Amino-acid infusion.
Parenteral nutrition in renal impairment.

Recip, Norw.; Pharmacia, Swed.
Amino-acid preparation.
Uraemia.

Aminess-N *Pharmacia, Neth.†.*
Amino-acid preparation.
Dietary supplement.

Amineurin *Hexal, Ger.*
Amitriptyline hydrochloride (p.273·3).
Depression; pain.

Amino 3 *Fiori, Ital.*
Amino-acid preparation.

Amino B Compound 240 *Medical Research, Austral.†.*
Vitamin B substances, mineral, and amino acid preparation.

Amino Essence Complex *Suisse, Austral.†.*
Amino acid and digestive enzyme preparation.
Nutritional supplement.

Amino Essence Figure Formula Day-time Use *Suisse, Austral.†.*
Amino acids; vitamins; minerals; royal jelly; bee pollen; natural digestive enzymes; dietary fibre; ginseng complex; fo-ti-tieng.
Nutritional supplement.

Amino Essence Figure Formula Night Time Use *Suisse, Austral.†.*
Amino acids; vitamins; minerals; natural digestive enzymes; dietary fibre; chamomile; passion flower; valerian; scullcap; lupulus.
Nutritional supplement.

Amino MS *Larkhall Laboratories, UK.*
L-Alanine (p.1333·3); L-lysine hydrochloride (p.1350·1); L-glutamic acid hydrochloride (p.1344·3); L-tyrosine (p.1357·3).

Amino PG *Cantassium Co., UK.*
Amino-acid and zinc preparation.

Aminoblastin *Pharmacia, S.Afr.†.*
Aminoglutethimide (p.502·3).
Adrenocortical adenoma; breast cancer; Cushing's syndrome.

Amino-Cerv
Milex, Canad.; Milex, USA.
Benzalkonium chloride (p.1101·3); cystine (p.1339·1); inositol (p.1591·1); methionine (p.984·2); sodium propionate (p.387·1); urea (p.1095·2).
Cervicitis; post cauterisation; post conisation; post cryosurgery; postpartum cervical tears.

Aminoflex *Vifor Medical, Switz.*
Amino-acid and electrolyte infusion.
Parenteral nutrition.

Aminoflor *Crosara, Ital.†.*
Amino-acid infusion.
Parenteral nutrition.

Aminofusin *Kabi, Switz.†.*
Amino-acid, electrolyte, and multivitamin infusion.
Parenteral nutrition.

Aminofusin 600 *Kabi Pharmacia, Ger.†.*
Amino-acid, carbohydrate, and electrolyte infusion.
Parenteral nutrition.

Aminofusin Hepar *Kabi Pharmacia, Ger.†.*
Amino-acid, carbohydrate, and electrolyte infusion.
Parenteral nutrition in liver disease.

Aminofusin Hepar sine *Pharmacia Upjohn, Ger.*
Amino-acid and electrolyte infusion.
Parenteral nutrition in liver disorders.

Aminofusin L *Kabi Pharmacia, Ger.†.*
Amino-acid, carbohydrate, electrolyte, and vitamin infusion.
Parenteral nutrition.

Aminofusin L Forte *E. Merck, UK†.*
Amino acid, vitamin, and electrolyte infusion.
Parenteral nutrition.

Aminofusin L kohlenhydratfrei
Pharmacia Upjohn, Aust.; Kabi Pharmacia, Ger.†.
Amino-acid, electrolyte, and vitamin infusion.
Parenteral nutrition.

Aminofusin N *Pharmacia Upjohn, Ger.*
Amino-acid, xylitol, and electrolyte infusion.
Parenteral nutrition.

Aminofusin 10% Plus *Pharmacia Upjohn, Ger.*
Amino-acid and electrolyte infusion.
Parenteral nutrition.

Aminogran
Faulding, Austral.; UCB, Irl.; Eurospital, Ital.; Glaxo Wellcome, S.Afr.†; UCB, Swed.; UCB, UK.
Food for special diets.
Phenylketonuria.

Aminogran Mineral Mixture
Faulding, Austral.; UCB, Irl.
Mineral preparation.

Aminohorm 5 G-E *Fresenius-Klinik, Ger.†.*
Amino-acid, carbohydrate, and electrolyte infusion.
Parenteral nutrition.

Aminohorm hepa *Schiwa, Ger.†; Hormonchemie, Ger.†.*
Amino-acid and electrolyte infusion.
Parenteral nutrition in liver disease.

Aminohorm PE *Schiwa, Ger.†; Hormonchemie, Ger.†.*
Amino-acid, carbohydrate, and electrolyte infusion.
Parenteral nutrition.

Aminohorm pur *Schiwa, Ger.†; Hormonchemie, Ger.†.*
Amino-acid infusion.
Parenteral nutrition.

Aminoleban *Otsuka, Jpn.*
Amino-acid infusion.
Hepatic encephalopathy.

Aminoleban EN *Otsuka, Jpn.*
Nutritional supplement.
Hepatic encephalopathy.

Aminolete *Tyson, USA.*
Amino acid preparation.

Aminomal *Malesci, Ital.*
Elixir: Theophylline (p.765·1).
Tablets; injection; suppositories: Aminophylline (p.748·1).
Lignocaine hydrochloride (p.1293·2) is included in the intramuscular injection to alleviate the pain of injection; lignocaine (p.1293·2) is also included in the suppositories.
Obstructive airways disease.

Aminomal con Antiasmatico *Malesci, Ital.†.*
Suppositories: Aminophylline (p.748·1); ephedrine hydrochloride (p.1059·3); lignocaine (p.1293·2).
Tablets: Aminophylline (p.748·1); ephedrine hydrochloride (p.1059·3).
Bronchospasm.

Aminomega *Larkhall Laboratories, UK.*
Amino-acid preparation.

Amino-Mel *Leopold, Aust.*
A range of amino-acid infusions with or without carbohydrate or electrolytes.
Parenteral nutrition.

Aminomel *Baxter, Ger.*
A range of amino-acid infusions with or without carbohydrate or electrolytes.
Parenteral nutrition.

Amino-Min-D *Tyson, USA.*
Calcium with vitamin D and minerals.
Calcium deficiency; dietary supplement.

Aminomine *Tyson, USA.*
Amino acid preparation.

Aminomix
Fresenius, Fr.; Fresenius-Klinik, Ger.; Meda, Swed.; Fresenius, Switz.
A range of amino-acid and carbohydrate infusions with or without electrolytes.
Parenteral nutrition.

Amino-Opti-C *Tyson, USA.*
Lemon bioflavonoids (p.1580·1); rutin (p.1580·2); hesperidin (p.1580·2); vitamin C (p.1365·2); rose hips (p.1365·2).
Capillary bleeding.

Amino-Opti-E *Tyson, USA.*
Vitamin E (p.1369·1).
Vitamin E deficiency.

Aminopad
Pharmacia Upjohn, Aust.; Pharmacia Upjohn, Ger.
Amino-acid infusion.
Parenteral nutrition.

Aminopan *UCB, Ger.*
Somatostatin acetate (p.1261·1).
Gastro-intestinal haemorrhage; postoperative pancreatic disorders.

Aminoplasmal
Braun, Aust.; Braun, Belg.†; Braun, Ger.; Braun, Irl.; SIFRA, Ital.; Braun, Norw.; Braun, Spain; Braun, Swed.; Braun, UK.
A range of amino-acid infusions with or without electrolytes.
Parenteral nutrition.

Aminoplex *Tyson, USA.*
Amino acid preparation.

Aminoplex *Geistlich, UK.*
A range of amino-acid infusions with or without carbohydrate or electrolytes.
Parenteral nutrition.

Aminopt *Sigma, Austral.*
Aminacrine hydrochloride (p.1098·3).
Eye infections.

Aminoram *Torre, Ital.*
Food for special diets.
Liver disorders.

Aminosine *Tyson, USA†.*
Amino acid preparation.

Aminostab *Pharmacia Upjohn, Fr.*
Amino-acid infusion.
Parenteral nutrition.

Aminostasis *Tyson, USA.*
Amino acid preparation.

Aminosteril
Leopold, Aust.; Fresenius, Ger.; Mein, Spain; Fresenius, Switz.; Fresenius, UK.
A range of amino-acid infusions with or without carbohydrate or electrolytes.
Parenteral nutrition.

Aminostress *Lafare, Ital.*
Nutritional supplement.

Aminosyn
Abbott, Canad.; Abbott, USA.
A range of amino-acid infusions with or without carbohydrate or electrolytes.
Parenteral nutrition.

Aminotate *Tyson, USA.*
Amino acid preparation.

Aminotool *Volchem, Ital.*
Amino-acid preparation.

Aminotril *Progest, Ital.*
Lotion: Triaminodil; vitamin A palmitate (p.1359·2).
Shampoo: Pyrithione zinc (p.1089·3); Triaminodil.
Hair loss; seborrhoeic dermatitis.

Aminotripa *Otsuka, Jpn.*
Amino-acid, carbohydrate, and electrolyte infusion.
Parenteral nutrition.

Aminoveinte *Madariaga, Spain.*
Multivitamin and amino-acid preparation.
Tonic.

Aminovenos Pad
Fresenius, Belg.; Fresenius-Klinik, Ger.; Fresenius, Switz.
Amino-acid infusion.
Parenteral nutrition.

Aminovit con Carnosina *FAMA, Ital.*
Carbohydrate, amino acids, minerals, and vitamins.
Nutritional supplement.

Aminoxin *Tyson, USA.*
Pyridoxal phosphate (p.1363·1).

Aminozim *Poli, Ital.*
Amino-acid preparation with cobamamide.
Tonic.

Aminsane *Dolisos, Fr.*
Bladderwrack (p.1554·1); orthosiphon (p.1592·2); meadowsweet (p.1599·1).
Obesity.

Aminsolut *Delta, Ger.*
Amino-acid, carbohydrate, and electrolyte infusion.
Parenteral nutrition.

Amiodar *Sanofi Winthrop, Ital.*
Amiodarone hydrochloride (p.820·1).
Angina pectoris; arrhythmias.

Amiopia *Medical, Spain.*
Vitamins, minerals, amino acids; isoniazid (p.218·1).
Eye disorders.

Amipaque
Winthrop, Austral.†; Sanofi Winthrop, Canad.†; Alter, Spain†; Winthrop, USA.
Metrizamide (p.1009·2).
Radiographic contrast medium.

Amiparen *Otsuka, Jpn.*
Amino-acid infusion.
Parenteral nutrition.

Amipress *Salus, Ital.*
Labetalol hydrochloride (p.896·1).
Hypertension.

Amirale *IDI, Ital.†.*
Vitamin A acetate (p.1359·2).
Vitamin-A deficiency.

Amitase *Schering-Plough, Swed.†.*
Dithranol (p.1082·1).
Psoriasis.

Ami-Tex LA *Amide, USA.*
Phenylpropanolamine hydrochloride (p.1067·2); guaiphenesin (p.1061·3).
Coughs.

Amitone *Menley & James, USA.*
Calcium carbonate (p.1182·1).
Hyperacidity.

Amitrol *Douglas, Austral.*
Amitriptyline hydrochloride (p.273·3).
Depression; nocturnal enuresis.

Amitron *Torlan, Spain.*
Amoxycillin trihydrate (p.151·3).
Bacterial infections.

Amix *Ashbourne, UK.*
Amoxycillin trihydrate (p.151·3).
Bacterial infections.

Amixx *Krewel, Ger.*
Amantadine hydrochloride (p.1129·2).
Drug-induced extrapyramidal disorders; parkinsonism.

Amizet 10 *Tanabe, Jpn.*
Amino-acid infusion.
Parenteral nutrition.

Amizet 10X *Tanabe, Jpn.*
Amino-acid and carbohydrate infusion.
Parenteral nutrition.

Amizide
Alphapharm, Austral.; Pinewood, Irl.†; Rolab, S.Afr.
Amiloride hydrochloride (p.819·2); hydrochlorothiazide (p.885·2).
Cardiac oedema; hepatic cirrhosis with ascites; hypertension.

AMK Plantes Tropicales, Fr.
Glucomannan (p.1584·3); bladderwrack (p.1554·1).
Slimming aid.

Amlodin Sumitomo, Jpn.
Amlodipine besylate (p.822·3).
Angina pectoris; hypertension.

Amlor
Roerig, Belg.; Pfizer, Fr.
Amlodipine besylate (p.822·3).
Angina pectoris; hypertension.

Amniex Mastelli, Ital.
Amniotic membrane (human) (p.1549·1).
Skin substitute.

Amniolina Reig Jofre, Spain.
Talc (p.1092·1); zinc oxide (p.1096·2).
Skin disorders.

Amnivent Ashbourne, UK.
Aminophylline (p.748·1).
Bronchospasm.

AMO Endosol
Allergan, Austral.; Allergan, USA.
Electrolytes (p.1147·1).
Eye irrigation; irrigation solution during surgery.

Amo Resan Alacan, Spain.
Amoxycillin trihydrate (p.151·3); bromhexine hydrochloride (p.1055·3).
Respiratory-tract infections.

AMO Vitrax
Allergan, Austral.; Allergan, Swed.; Allergan, Switz.; Allergan, USA.
Sodium hyaluronate (p.1630·3).
Aid to ocular surgery.

Amobronc Ist. Chim. Inter., Ital.
Ambroxol hydrochloride (p.1054·3).
Respiratory-system disorders.

Amocid Lysoform, Ger.
Orthophenylphenol (p.1120·3).
Surface disinfection.

Amocillin Caps, S.Afr.
Amoxycillin sodium (p.151·3).
Bacterial infections.

Amodex
Note. This name is used for preparations of different composition.
Bouchara, Fr.
Amoxycillin trihydrate (p.151·3) or amoxycillin sodium (p.151·3).
Bacterial infections.

Kabi, Swed.†.
Amino acid and electrolyte infusion.
Parenteral nutrition.

Amoflamisan Morrith, Spain.
Amoxycillin trihydrate (p.151·3).
Bacterial infections.

Amoflux Lampugnani, Ital.
Amoxycillin trihydrate (p.151·3).
Bacterial infections.

Amol Heilkrautergeist N Roland, Ger.
Melissa oil; clove oil (p.1565·2); cinnamon oil (p.1564·2); lemon oil (p.1595·3); peppermint oil (p.1208·1); lavender oil (p.1594·3); menthol (p.1600·2).
Colds; coughs; gastro-intestinal disorders; neuralgia; rheumatoid disorders; sore throat.

Amolin Helsinn Birex, Irl.
Atenolol (p.825·3).
Angina pectoris; arrhythmias; hypertension; myocardial infarction.

Amopen Yorkshire Pharmaceuticals, UK.
Amoxycillin (p.151·3).
Bacterial infections.

Amophar Dakota, Fr.
Amoxycillin trihydrate (p.151·3).
Bacterial infections.

Amoram Eastern Pharmaceuticals, UK.
Amoxycillin (p.151·3).
Bacterial infections.

Amorphan Heumann, Ger.†.
Cathine hydrochloride (p.1478·1).
Obesity.

Amosan
Note. This name is used for preparations of different composition.
Oral-B, Austral.
Sodium perborate (p.1125·2); sodium bitartrate.
Inflammation of the oral cavity.

Oral-B, Canad.; Oral-B, USA.
Sodium perborate (p.1125·2).
Oral disinfection; oral lesions.

Amosedil Roussel, Ital.†.
Quinalbital (p.938·1).
Arrhythmias.

Amosyt Abigo, Swed.
Dimenhydrinate (p.408·2).
Ménière's syndrome; nausea; vertigo.

Amotein Wasserman, Spain.
Metronidazole (p.585·1).
Amoebiasis; anaerobic bacterial infections; dracunculiasis; trichomoniasis.

Amox
Salus, Ital.; Berenguer Infale, Spain.
Amoxycillin trihydrate (p.151·3).
Bacterial infections.

Amoxaren Areu, Spain.
Amoxycillin trihydrate (p.151·3).
Bacterial infections.

Amoxi
SMB, Belg.†; CT, Ger.; BASF, Ger.; Schwarz, Ger.; Sanol, Ger.; Lichtenstein, Ger.; Sanorania, Ger.
Amoxycillin trihydrate (p.151·3).
Bacterial infections.

Amoxi Gobens Normon, Spain.
Amoxycillin sodium (p.151·3) or amoxycillin trihydrate (p.151·3).
Bacterial infections.

Amoxi Gobens Mucol Normon, Spain.
Amoxycillin trihydrate (p.151·3); bromhexine hydrochloride (p.1055·3).
Respiratory-tract infections.

Amoxibacter Rubio, Spain.
Amoxycillin trihydrate (p.151·3).
Bacterial infections.

amoxi-basan
Sagitta, Ger.†; Schonenberger, Switz.
Amoxycillin trihydrate (p.151·3).
Bacterial infections.

Amoxibeta Betapharm, Ger.
Amoxycillin trihydrate (p.151·3).
Bacterial infections.

Amoxibiocin Nycomed, Ger.†.
Amoxycillin (p.151·3) or amoxycillin trihydrate (p.151·3).
Bacterial infections.

Amoxibiotic Lagap, Ital.†.
Amoxycillin sodium (p.151·3) or amoxycillin trihydrate (p.151·3).
Bacterial infections.

Amoxid Kwizda, Aust.
Amoxycillin trihydrate (p.151·3).
Bacterial infections.

Amoxidel Synthelabo Delagrange, Spain.
Amoxycillin trihydrate (p.151·3).
Bacterial infections.

Amoxidel Bronquial Synthelabo Delagrange, Spain.
Amoxycillin trihydrate (p.151·3); brovanexine hydrochloride (p.1056·1).
Respiratory-tract infections.

Amoxi-Diolan Engelhard, Ger.
Amoxycillin trihydrate (p.151·3).
Bacterial infections.

Amoxiferm Fermenta, Swed.†.
Amoxycillin trihydrate (p.151·3).
Bacterial infections.

Amoxi-Hefa Hefa, Ger.
Amoxycillin trihydrate (p.151·3).
Bacterial infections.

Amoxihexal Hexal, Ger.
Amoxycillin trihydrate (p.151·3).
Bacterial infections.

Amoxil
SmithKline Beecham, Austral.; Wyeth-Ayerst, Canad.; SmithKline Beecham, Irl.; SmithKline Beecham, S.Afr.; Bencard, UK; SmithKline Beecham, USA.
Amoxycillin sodium (p.151·3) or amoxycillin trihydrate (p.151·3).
Bacterial infections.

Amoxilan Lannacher, Aust.
Amoxycillin trihydrate (p.151·3).
Bacterial infections.

Amoxillat Azupharma, Ger.
Amoxycillin trihydrate (p.151·3).
Bacterial infections.

Amoxillin
Esseti, Ital.; Alpharma, Norw.
Amoxycillin sodium (p.151·3) or amoxycillin trihydrate (p.151·3).
Bacterial infections.

Amoximedical Medical, Spain.
Amoxycillin trihydrate (p.151·3).
Bacterial infections.

Amoxi-Mepha Mepha, Switz.
Amoxycillin trihydrate (p.151·3).
Bacterial infections.

Amoximerck Merck, Ger.
Amoxycillin trihydrate (p.151·3).
Bacterial infections.

Amoximex Cimex, Switz.
Amoxycillin trihydrate (p.151·3).
Bacterial infections.

Amoxina Aesculapius, Ital.
Amoxycillin trihydrate (p.151·3).
Bacterial infections.

Amoxipen
Metapharma, Ital.; Hortel, Spain†.
Amoxycillin sodium (p.151·3) or amoxycillin trihydrate (p.151·3).
Bacterial infections.

Amoxi-Tablinen Sanorania, Ger.
Amoxycillin trihydrate (p.151·3).
Bacterial infections.

Amoxi-Wolff Wolff, Ger.
Injection†: Amoxycillin sodium (p.151·3).
Oral liquid; tablets: Amoxycillin trihydrate (p.151·3).
Bacterial infections.

Amoxtiol Daker Farmasimes, Spain.
Amoxycillin trihydrate (p.151·3); carbocisteine (p.1056·3).
Respiratory-tract infections.

Amoxycaps Wolfs, Belg.†.
Amoxycillin trihydrate (p.151·3).
Bacterial infections.

Amoxyfizz Schwulst, S.Afr.
Amoxycillin (p.151·3).
Bacterial infections.

Amoxymed Bradford Chemists Alliance, UK†.
Amoxycillin trihydrate (p.151·3).
Bacterial infections.

Amoxypen
Farmabel, Belg.†; Grunenthal, Ger.
Amoxycillin trihydrate (p.151·3).
Bacterial infections.

Amoxyplus Novag, Spain.
Amoxycillin trihydrate (p.151·3); potassium clavulanate (p.190·2).
Bacterial infections.

Amoxyvinco Mucolitico Reig Jofre, Spain.
Amoxycillin trihydrate (p.151·3); guaiphenesin (p.1061·3).
Respiratory-tract infections.

Ampamet Menarini, Ital.
Aniracetam (p.1549·3).
Mental function impairment.

Ampecyclal Sarget, Fr.; Asta Medica, Fr.
Heptaminol adenosine phosphate (p.1587·2).
Haemorrhoids; metrorrhagia; peripheral vascular disorders.

Ampen Medosan, Ital.†.
Ampicillin (p.153·1) or ampicillin sodium (p.153·1).
Bacterial infections.

Ampensaar Chephasaar, Ger.†.
Ampicillin trihydrate (p.153·2).
Bacterial infections.

Ampexin Amrad, Austral.
Amoxycillin trihydrate (p.151·3).
Bacterial infections.

Amphisept Goldschmidt, Switz.
Alcohol (p.1099·1).
Hand disinfection.

Amphisept E Bode, Ger.
Alcohol (p.1099·1).
Hand disinfection.

Amphocil
Zeneca, Aust.; Zeneca, Irl.; Zeneca, Ital.; Zeneca, Neth.; Zeneca, Swed.; Zeneca, UK.
Amphotericin (p.372·2).
Fungal infections.

Amphocycline
Bristol-Myers Squibb, Fr.; Squibb, Neth.†; Squibb, Switz.†.
Amphotericin (p.372·2); tetracycline (p.259·1) or tetracycline hydrochloride (p.259·1).
Bacterial and fungal infections.

Amphocycline Combipack Squibb, Switz.†.
Pessaries, Amphocycline; tablets, Ampho-Moronal; cream, Halciderm comp.
Bacterial or fungal infections of the vagina; balanitis; intestinal disinfection.

Amphodyn
Note. This name is used for preparations of different composition.
Klinge, Aust.
Etilefrine hydrochloride (p.867·2); aescin (p.1543·3).
Circulatory disorders; hypotension.

Klinge, Ger.
Etilefrine hydrochloride (p.867·2); aesculus (p.1543·3).
Circulatory disorders; hypotension.

Amphodyn mono Klinge, Aust.
Etilefrine hydrochloride (p.867·2).
Hypotension.

Amphodyn special Klinge Munich, Switz.†.
Etilefrine hydrochloride (p.867·2); aesculus (p.1543·3).
Circulatory disorders.

Amphojel
Whitehall, Austral.; Axcan, Canad.; Akromed, S.Afr.; Wyeth-Ayerst, USA.
Aluminium hydroxide (p.1177·3).
Hyperacidity; hyperphosphataemia.

Amphojel 500 Axcan, Canad.
Aluminium hydroxide (p.1177·3); magnesium hydroxide (p.1198·2).
Antacid.

Amphojel Plus Axcan, Canad.
Oral liquid: Aluminium hydroxide (p.1177·3); magnesium hydroxide (p.1198·2); simethicone (p.1213·1).
Tablets: Aluminium hydroxide-magnesium carbonate co-dried gel (p.1178·2); magnesium hydroxide (p.1198·2); simethicone (p.1213·1).
Antacid; flatulence.

Ampholysine Plus Peters, Fr.†.
Polyhexanide (p.1123·1); mixed amphoteric and quaternary ammonium salts.
Instrument disinfection.

Ampho-Moronal
Bristol-Myers Squibb, Aust.; Bristol-Myers Squibb, Ger.; Bristol-Myers Squibb, Switz.
Amphotericin (p.372·2).
Fungal infections.

Ampho-Moronal V Bristol-Myers Squibb, Ger.
Amphotericin (p.372·2); triamcinolone acetonide (p.1050·2).
Fungal skin infections.

Ampho-Moronal V N Bristol-Myers Squibb, Ger.†.
Amphotericin (p.372·2); triamcinolone acetonide (p.1050·2).
Skin disorders with fungal infection.

Amphosca a l'orchitine Lehning, Fr.
Homoeopathic preparation.

Amphosca a l'ovarine Lehning, Fr.
Homoeopathic preparation.

Amphosca Orchitine Homeocan, Canad.
Homoeopathic preparation.

Amphosca Ovarine Homeocan, Canad.
Homoeopathic preparation.

Amphosept BV Anios, Fr.
Didecyldimethylammonium chloride (p.1112·2); alkylbenzylammonium chloride; alkylethylbenzylammonium chloride; alylaminoalkyl glycine.
Instrument disinfection.

Amphotabs Whitehall, Austral.†.
Aluminium hydroxide (p.1177·3).
Hyperacidity.

Ampho-Vaccin intestinal Sanofi Winthrop, Fr.
Bifidobacterium bifidum (p.1594·1); *Escherichia coli*; *Streptococcus faecalis* (p.1594·1); *Proteus vulgaris*; *Pseudomonas aeruginosa*.
Diarrhoea.

Ampiciliber Bronquial Dimportex, Spain†.
Ampicillin sodium (p.153·1); ampicillin benzathine (p.154·1); bromhexine (p.1055·3).
Respiratory-tract infections.

Ampicillat Azuchemie, Ger.†.
Ampicillin trihydrate (p.153·2).
Bacterial infections.

Ampicin Bristol, Canad.
Ampicillin sodium (p.153·1).
Bacterial infections.

Ampiclox
SmithKline Beecham, Irl.; SmithKline Beecham, S.Afr.; Beecham Research, UK†.
Ampicillin sodium (p.153·1) or ampicillin trihydrate (p.153·2); cloxacillin sodium (p.195·2).
Bacterial infections.

Ampicyn
Note. This name is used for preparations of different composition.
Rhone-Poulenc Rorer, Austral.
Ampicillin sodium (p.153·1); ampicillin (p.153·1).
Bacterial infections.

Xixia, S.Afr.†.
Ampicillin trihydrate (p.153·2).
Bacterial infections.

Ampilan Ibirn, Ital.†.
Ampicillin (p.153·1).
Bacterial infections.

Ampilisa Lisapharma, Ital.
Ampicillin (p.153·1) or ampicillin sodium (p.153·1).
Bacterial infections.

Ampilux Allergan, Ital.
Ampicillin sodium (p.153·1).
Eye infections.

Ampimax Hexal, S.Afr.
Ampicillin trihydrate (p.153·2).
Bacterial infections.

Ampiorus Balsamico Llorente, Spain†.
Ampicillin trihydrate (p.153·2); carbocisteine (p.1056·3); guaiphenesin (p.1061·3).
Respiratory-tract infections.

Ampipen Caps, S.Afr.
Ampicillin (p.153·1).
Bacterial infections.

Ampiplus
Note. This name is used for preparations of different composition.
Menarini, Ital.
Ampicillin (p.153·1) or ampicillin sodium (p.153·1); dicloxacillin sodium (p.202·1).
Bacterial infections.

Menarini, Spain.
Ampicillin trihydrate (p.153·2).
Bacterial infections.

Ampiplus Simplex Menarini, Ital.
Ampicillin sodium (p.153·1).
Bacterial infections.

Ampi-Rol Rolab, S.Afr.
Ampicillin trihydrate (p.153·2).
Bacterial infections.

Ampisalt Propan, S.Afr.
Ampicillin trihydrate (p.153·2).
Bacterial infections.

Ampisint Proter, Ital.†.
Ampicillin (p.153·1) or ampicillin sodium (p.153·1).
Bacterial infections.

Ampi-Tablinen Sanorania, Ger.†.
Ampicillin trihydrate (p.153·2).
Bacterial infections.

Ampi-Zoja Zoja, Ital.†.
Ampicillin trihydrate (p.153·2).
Bacterial infections.

Amplibac Schwarz, Ital.†.
Bacampicillin hydrochloride (p.157·2).
Bacterial infections.

Amplidermis Medea, Spain.
Acedoben (p.1541·1); allantoin (p.1078·2); chlorquinaldol (p.185·1); dexamethasone (p.1037·1); mepyramine maleate (p.414·1); vitamin F.
Infected skin disorders.

Ampligen *HemispheRx, USA.*
Poly I.poly C (p.1619·3).
HIV infection; malignant neoplasms.

Amplipenyl *ISF, Ital.†.*
Ampicillin (p.153·1) or ampicillin sodium (p.153·1).
Bacterial infections.

Amplital *Pharmacia Upjohn, Ital.*
Ampicillin (p.153·1), ampicillin sodium (p.153·1), or ampicillin trihydrate (p.153·2).
Bacterial infections.

Amplium *Sigma-Tau, Ital.*
Ampicillin sodium (p.153·1) or ampicillin trihydrate (p.153·2); cloxacillin sodium (p.195·2).
Bacterial infections.

Amplizer *OFF, Ital.*
Ampicillin (p.153·1).
Bacterial infections.

Amprace *Amrad, Austral.*
Enalapril maleate (p.863·2).
Heart failure; hypertension.

Amrit *BHR, UK.*
Amoxycillin trihydrate (p.151·3).
Bacterial infections.

Amsa P-D *Parke, Davis, Canad.*
Amsacrine (p.503·3).
Acute leukaemias.

Amsidine
Parke, Davis, Belg.; Parke, Davis, Fr.; Parke, Davis, Irl.; Parke, Davis, Neth.; Goldshield, UK.
Amsacrine (p.503·3).
Acute leukaemias.

Amsidyl
Parke, Davis, Austral.; Godecke, Ger.; Warner-Lambert, Switz.
Amsacrine (p.503·3).
Acute leukaemias.

Amuchina *Sokosi, Switz.†.*
Sodium chloride (p.1162·2).
Hand, skin, and wound disinfection.

Amukin
Bristol-Myers Squibb, Belg.; Bristol-Myers Squibb, Neth.
Amikacin sulphate (p.150·2).
Bacterial infections.

Amukine *Gifrer Barbezat, Fr.*
Sodium hypochlorite (p.1124·3); sodium chloride (p.1162·2).
Skin, mucous membrane and wound cleansing.

A-Mulsin *Mucos, Ger.*
Retinol palmitate (p.1359·2).
Vitamin A deficiency.

A-Mulsion *Seroyal, Canad.*
Vitamin A palmitate (p.1359·2).

Amuno *Merck Sharp & Dohme, Ger.*
Indomethacin (p.45·2).
Gout; inflammation; musculoskeletal, joint, peri-articular, and soft-tissue disorders; pain.

Amuno M *Merck Sharp & Dohme, Ger.†.*
Indomethacin (p.45·2).
Magnesium hydroxide (p.1198·2) and aluminium hydroxide magnesium carbonate co-dried gel (p.1178·2) are included in this preparation in an attempt to limit adverse effects on the gastro-intestinal mucosa.
Inflammation; musculoskeletal and joint disorders; pain.

Amunovax *Pasteur Merieux, Spain.*
A measles vaccine (Schwarz strain) (p.1517·3).
Active immunisation.

Amvisc
Johnson & Johnson, Aust.; Iolab, Canad.†; Iolab, Norw.†; MCM, S.Afr.; Johnson & Johnson, Swed.; Iolab, USA.
Sodium hyaluronate (p.1630·3).
Aid in ophthalmic surgery.

AMX *Brovar, S.Afr.†.*
Amoxycillin trihydrate (p.151·3).
Bacterial infections.

Amycor *Lipha Sante, Fr.*
Bifonazole (p.375·3).
Fungal skin infections.

Amycor Onychoset *Lipha Sante, Fr.*
Bifonazole (p.375·3); urea (p.1095·2).
Fungal nail infections.

Amyderm S *Schulke & Mayr, Ger.†.*
Povidone-iodine (p.1123·3).
Pre-operative skin disinfection.

Amygdorectol
Merck-Clevenot, Fr.; Merck-Clevenot, Switz.
Bismuth camphocarbonate (p.1181·1).
Pharyngeal disorders.

Amygdospray *Merck-Clevenot, Fr.*
Hexamidine isethionate (p.1115·3); amethocaine hydrochloride (p.1285·2).
Mouth and throat disorders.

Amylatin *Synpharma, Aust.*
Angelica; centaury (p.1561·1); absinthium (p.1541·1).
Gastro-intestinal disorders.

Amyline *Antigen, Irl.†.*
Amitriptyline hydrochloride (p.273·3).
Depression.

Amylodiastase *Thepenier, Fr.*
Amylase (cereal extract) (p.1549·1).
Dyspepsia.

Amytal
Lilly, Austral.†; Lilly, Canad.; Lilly, UK; Lilly, USA.
Amylobarbitone (p.641·3) or amylobarbitone sodium (p.641·3).
Anxiety; convulsive disorders; insomnia; sedative.

AN 1 *Krugmann, Ger.*
Amphetaminil (p.1477·3).
Narcoleptic syndrome.

Anabact *Asta Medica, UK.*
Metronidazole (p.585·1).
Malodorous fungating tumours.

Anabasi *Zilliken, Ital.†.*
Cobamamide (p.1364·2).
Tonic.

Anabloc *IRBI, Ital.†.*
Phenyramidol hydrochloride (p.80·1).
Inflammation; pain.

Anabol-Hevert *Hevert, Ger.*
Homoeopathic preparation.

Anabolico Navarro *Navarro, Spain†.*
Calcium camsylate; vitamin B substances; carnitine hydrochloride; cyproheptadine hydrochloride.
Tonic.

Anabol-Injektopas *Pascoe, Ger.†.*
Homoeopathic preparation.

anabol-loges *Loges, Ger.*
Alpha tocopheryl acetate (p.1369·1); magnesium hydrogen phosphate; potassium chloride; terra silicea; hypericum (p.1590·1).
Bone and connective tissue disorders.

Anacal *Panpharma, UK.*
A heparinoid (p.882·3); laureth 9 (p.1325·2).
Formerly contained a heparinoid, prednisolone, laureth 9, and hexachlorophane.
Anorectal disorders.

Anacalcit *Belmac, Spain.*
Sodium cellulose phosphate (p.994·3).
Hypercalcaemia; hypercalciuria; osteopetrosis; vitamin D intoxication.

Anacervix *Farma Lepori, Spain.*
Piracetam (p.1619·1); vincamine (p.1644·1).
Cerebral trauma; cerebrovascular disorders.

Anacidase *Pharkos, Ital.†.*
Aluminium glycinate (p.1177·2); light magnesium carbonate (p.1198·1); sodium bicarbonate (p.1153·2); heavy kaolin (p.1195·1); belladonna (p.457·1).
Gastric hyperacidity; gastro-intestinal spasm.

Anacidol
Note. This name is used for preparations of different composition.
Menarini, Ital.
Aluminium hydroxide dried gel (p.1177·3); magnesium hydroxide (p.1198·2); dimethicone (p.1213·1); milk powder.
Gastro-intestinal disorders.

Spirig, Switz.
Calcium carbonate (p.1182·1); aluminium hydroxide-magnesium carbonate co-dried gel (p.1178·2).
Gastric disorders.

Anacin
Whitehall-Robins, Canad.; Robins, USA.
Aspirin (p.16·1); caffeine (p.749·3).
Fever; pain.

Anacin-3 *Whitehall, Canad.†.*
Paracetamol (p.72·2).
Fever; pain.

Anacin with Codeine *Whitehall-Robins, Canad.*
Aspirin (p.16·1); caffeine (p.749·3); codeine phosphate (p.26·1).
Fever; pain.

Anaclosil *Pharmacia Upjohn, Spain.*
Cloxacillin sodium (p.195·2).
Bacterial infections.

Anacufen *Difa, Ital.†.*
Vitamin A (p.1358·1); vitamin E (p.1369·1); papaverine hydrochloride (p.1614·2); methandriol propionate; xenbucin; niaouli oil (p.1607·1); eucalyptus oil (p.1578·1).
Ear disorders.

Anacyclin *Geigy, Ger.*
Lynoestrenol (p.1448·2); ethinyloestradiol (p.1445·1).
Combined oral contraceptive.

Anadermin *Ecobi, Ital.*
Chlorhexidine gluconate (p.1107·2); precipitated sulphur (p.1091·2).
Skin disinfection.

Anadin
Whitehall, Irl.; Whitehall, UK.
Aspirin (p.16·1); caffeine (p.749·3); quinine sulphate (p.439·2).
Fever; pain.

Anadin Extra
Whitehall, Irl.; Whitehall, UK.
Aspirin (p.16·1); paracetamol (p.72·2); caffeine (p.749·3).
Fever; pain.

Anadin Ibuprofen *Whitehall, UK†.*
Ibuprofen (p.44·1).
Fever; pain.

Anadin Maximum *Whitehall, UK.*
Aspirin (p.16·1); caffeine (p.749·3).
Fever; pain.

Anadin Paracetamol *Whitehall, UK.*
Paracetamol (p.72·2).
Fever; pain.

Anadin Soluble *Whitehall, UK†.*
Aspirin (p.16·1); caffeine citrate (p.749·3).
Fever; pain.

Anador *Pharmacia Upjohn, Fr.†.*
Nandrolone propionate (p.1452·2).
Anabolic; osteoporosis.

Anadrol *Syntex, USA.*
Oxymetholone (p.1459·1).
Anaemias.

Anadur
Pharmacia Upjohn, Aust.; Kabi Pharmacia, Belg.†; Pharmacia Upjohn, Ger.†; Kabi Pharmacia, Neth.†; Kabi, Swed.†; Kabi, Switz.†.
Nandrolone hexyloxyphenylpropionate (p.1452·2).
Anabolic; chronic renal and intestinal disorders; osteoporosis; radiation and chemotherapy induced myelosuppression.

Anaemodoron *Weleda, Aust.*
Fragaria vesca; urtica dioica (p.1642·3).
Iron-deficiency anaemia.

Anaerobex *Gerot, Aust.*
Metronidazole (p.585·1).
Anaerobic bacterial infections; Helicobacter pylori infections.

Anaerobyl *Searle, S.Afr.†.*
Metronidazole (p.585·1).
Anaerobic bacterial infections; protozoal infections.

Anaeromet *Glaxo Wellcome, Belg.*
Metronidazole (p.585·1).
Anaerobic bacterial infections; protozoal infections.

Anaestalgin *Streuli, Switz.*
Procaine hydrochloride (p.1299·2); caffeine (p.749·3).
Pain.

Anaesthecomp N *Ritsert, Ger.*
Lignocaine hydrochloride (p.1293·2); diphenhydramine hydrochloride (p.409·1).
Allergic rashes; insect stings; sunburn.

Anaestherit *Salus, Aust.*
Benzocaine (p.1286·2).
Anorectal disorders; skin disorders.

Anaesthesetten N *Ritsert, Ger.†.*
Butethamate citrate (p.1056·2); benzocaine (p.1286·2).
Coughs and associated throat disorders.

Anaesthesie *ankerpharm, Ger.†.*
Propipocaine (p.1300·1).
Surface anaesthesia.

Anaesthesierende Salbe *Lichtenstein, Ger.†.*
Benzocaine (p.1286·2).
Burns; haemorrhoids; insect stings; skin disorders.

Anaesthesin *Ritsert, Ger.*
Benzocaine (p.1286·2).
Coughs and associated throat disorders; haemorrhoids; skin disorders; wounds.

Anaesthesin N *Ritsert, Ger.*
Benzocaine (p.1286·2).
Anorectal disorders; skin disorders.

Anaesthesin-Rivanol *Ritsert, Ger.*
Benzocaine (p.1286·2); ethacridine lactate (p.1098·3).
Painful throat infections.

Anaesthesulf P *Ritsert, Ger.*
Laureth 9 (p.1325·2); zinc oxide (p.1096·2).
Pruritic skin disorders.

Anaesthol *Merz, Ger.*
Lignocaine hydrochloride (p.1293·2).
Adrenaline (p.813·2) and noradrenaline (p.924·1) are included in this preparation as vasoconstrictors to diminish absorption and localise the effect of the local anaesthetic.
Local anaesthesia.

Anafilaxol *Juventus, Spain†.*
Benzalkonium chloride (p.1101·3); diphenhydramine hydrochloride (p.409·1); prednisone (p.1049·2); zinc oxide (p.1096·2).
Infected skin disorders.

Anafilaxol B *Juventus, Spain†.*
Calcium chloride (p.1155·1); diphenhydramine hydrochloride (p.409·1); prednisolone (p.1048·1).
Hypersensitivity reactions; inflammatory eye disorders; skin disorders.

Anaflex
Chemomedica, Aust.; Geistlich, Switz.†; Geistlich, UK.
Polynoxylin (p.1123·1).
Infected skin disorders.

Anaflon *Sanofi Winthrop, Ger.†.*
Paracetamol (p.72·2).
Fever; pain.

Anafranil
Ciba-Geigy, Aust.; Novartis, Austral.; Ciba-Geigy, Belg.; Geigy, Canad.; Ciba-Geigy, Fr.; Geigy, Ger.; Geigy, Irl.; Ciba, Ital.; Novartis, Neth.; Geigy, Norw.; Novartis, S.Afr.; Ciba-Geigy, Spain; Novartis, Swed.; Geigy, Switz.; Geigy, UK; Novartis, USA.
Clomipramine hydrochloride (p.281·2).
Depression; narcoleptic syndrome; nocturnal enuresis; obsessive-compulsive disorder; pain syndromes; panic attacks; phobic states.

Anagastra *Madaus, Spain.*
Pantoprazole sodium (p.1207·3).
Gastro-oesophageal; peptic ulcer.

Anagen *Rydelle, Fr.*
Amino-acid, vitamin, and mineral preparation.
Hair and nail disorders.

Anagregal *Gentili, Ital.*
Ticlopidine hydrochloride (p.953·1).
Thrombosis prophylaxis.

Ana-Guard *Bayer, S.Afr.*
Adrenaline hydrochloride (p.813·3).
Anaphylaxis.

Anahelp *Stallergenes, Fr.*
Adrenaline (p.813·2).
Anaphylaxis.

Ana-Kit
Bayer, Canad.; Hollister-Stier, USA.
Combination pack: Injection, adrenaline (p.813·2) or adrenaline hydrochloride (p.813·3); 4 chewable tablets, chlorpheniramine maleate (p.405·1).
Anaphylaxis.

Anakit *Dome-Hollister-Stier, Fr.*
Adrenaline (p.813·2).
Anaphylaxis.

Analergyl *Qualiphar, Belg.†.*
Diphenhydramine hydrochloride (p.409·1); dimenhydrinate (p.408·2); caffeine hydrate (p.750·1).
Hypersensitivity reactions; motion sickness; vertigo.

Analexin *Biotrading, Ital.†.*
Phenyramidol hydrochloride (p.80·1).
Muscle and joint pain and spasms.

Analgen
Note. A similar name is used for preparations of different composition.
Noristan, S.Afr.†.
Ointment: Diethylamine salicylate (p.33·1); myrtecaine (p.1297·3).
Musculoskeletal pain.
Tablets: Aspirin (p.16·1); paracetamol (p.72·2); codeine phosphate (p.26·1); caffeine (p.749·3).
Fever; pain.

Anal-Gen
Note. A similar name is used for preparations of different composition.
BCL, Switz.
Hamamelis water (p.1587·1); melissa oil.
Anogenital skin disorders.

Analgen-SA *Noristan, S.Afr.*
Aluminium aspirin (p.15·1); paracetamol (p.72·2); codeine phosphate (p.26·1); caffeine (p.749·3); chlorphenoxamine (p.405·3); phenobarbitone (p.350·2); ascorbic acid (p.1365·2).
Fever; pain.

Analgesia Creme *Rugby, USA.*
Triethanolamine salicylate (p.1639·2).
Muscle, joint, and soft-tissue pain; neuralgia.

Analgesic Balm
Note. This name is used for preparations of different composition.
Parke, Davis, Austral.†; Warner-Lambert, Canad.; Goldline, USA; Major, USA; Schein, USA; URL, USA.
Menthol (p.1600·2); methyl salicylate (p.55·2).
Muscle, joint, and soft-tissue pain; neuralgia.

Drug Trading, Canad.
Methyl salicylate (p.55·2); menthol (p.1600·2); chloral hydrate (p.645·3).

Stanley, Canad.
Methyl salicylate (p.55·2); menthol (p.1600·2); eucalyptus oil (p.1578·1); guaiacol (p.1061·2).

Analgesic Otic Solution *Akorn, USA.*
Phenazone (p.78·2); benzocaine (p.1286·2); hydroxyquinoline sulphate (p.1589·3).

Analgesic Rub *McGloin, Austral.†.*
Menthol (p.1600·2); camphor (p.1557·2); eucalyptus oil (p.1578·1); methyl salicylate (p.55·2); pumilio pine oil (p.1623·3).
Muscle and joint pain.

Analgesic Rub (NCP) *Arjo, Canad.†.*
Menthol (p.1600·2); methyl salicylate (p.55·2).
Musculoskeletal and joint pain.

Analgesico Pyre *Salvat, Spain†.*
Aspirin (p.16·1); caffeine (p.749·3).
Fever; pain.

Analgesico Ut Asens Fn *Asens, Spain.*
Camphor (p.1557·2); alcohol (p.1099·1); ammonia (p.1548·3); menthol (p.1600·2).
Soft-tissue disorders.

Analgesico Viviar *Viviar, Spain†.*
Aspirin (p.16·1); caffeine (p.749·3).
Fever; pain.

Analgilasa *Lasa, Spain.*
Suppositories: Caffeine (p.749·3); codeine phosphate (p.26·1); papaverine hydrochloride (p.1614·2); paracetamol (p.72·2).
Tablets: Caffeine (p.749·3); codeine phosphate (p.26·1); paracetamol (p.72·2).
Pain.

Analgin *Medphano, Ger.*
Dipyrone (p.35·1).
Fever; pain.

Analgit *Krewel, Ger.*
Dipyrone (p.35·1).
Fever; pain.

Analgyl *Specia, Fr.†.*
Ibuprofen (p.44·1).
Fever; pain.

Analip
Iketon, Ital.†.
Pantethine (p.1276·3); fosforylcholine calcium tetrahydrate (p.1581·3).
Lipid metabolism disorders; liver disorders.

Iketon, Ital.
Pantethine (p.1276·3).
Hyperlipidaemias.

Analog MSUD *Scientific Hospital Supplies, UK.*
Food for special diets.
Maple syrup urine disease.

Analog RVHB
Scientific Hospital Supplies, Irl.; Scientific Hospital Supplies, UK.
Food for special diets.
Homocystinuria; hypermethioninaemia.

Analog Xmet, Thre, Val, Isoleu *Scientific Hospital Supplies, UK.*
Food for special diets.
Methylmalonic or propionic acidaemia.

Analog XP *Taranis, Fr.†; Scientific Hospital Supplies, Irl.; Scientific Hospital Supplies, UK.*
Food for special diets.
Phenylketonuria.

Analog Xphen, Tyr *Scientific Hospital Supplies, UK.*
Food for special diets.

Analpram-HC *Ferndale, USA.*
Hydrocortisone acetate (p.1043·3); pramoxine (p.1298·2).

Analter *Alter, Spain.*
Paracetamol (p.72·2).
Fever; pain.

Analux *Cusi, Spain.*
Phenylephrine hydrochloride (p.1066·2).
Eye irritation.

Anamine *Mayrand, USA.*
Pseudoephedrine hydrochloride (p.1068·3); chlorpheniramine maleate (p.405·1).
Cold symptoms.

Anamorph *Fawns & McAllan, Austral.*
Morphine sulphate (p.56·2).
Pain.

Ananase
Rhone-Poulenc Rorer, Irl.; Rottapharm, Ital.; Rhone-Poulenc Rorer, S.Afr.
Bromelains (p.1555·1).
Skin disorders; skin ulceration; soft-tissue inflammation and oedema.

Ananda *Glaxo Allen, Ital.†.*
Metoclopramide hydrochloride (p.1200·3).
Gastro-intestinal disorders.

Anandron
Hoechst Marion Roussel, Austral.; Hoechst Marion Roussel, Canad.; Cassenne, Fr.; Hoechst Marion Roussel, Neth.; Hoechst Marion Roussel, Norw.; Hoechst Marion Roussel, Swed.
Nilutamide (p.556·2).
Prostatic cancer.

Ananxyl *Synthelabo, Fr.†.*
Alpidem (p.640·3).
Anxiety disorders.

Anapen *CEPA, Spain.*
Benzylpenicillin sodium (p.159·3); clemizole penicillin (p.191·1).
Bacterial infections.

Anaphylaxie-Besteck *SmithKline Beecham, Ger.*
Adrenaline hydrochloride (p.813·3).
Anaphylactic shock.

Anaplex *Medi-Plex, USA.*
Pseudoephedrine hydrochloride (p.1068·3); chlorpheniramine maleate (p.405·1).
Cold symptoms.

Anaplex HD *Medi-Plex, USA.*
Hydrocodone tartrate (p.43·1); phenylephrine hydrochloride (p.1066·2); chlorpheniramine maleate (p.405·1).
Coughs and cold symptoms.

Anapolon
Syntex, Austral.†; Syntex, Canad.†; Roche, S.Afr.†; Syntex, UK.
Oxymetholone (p.1459·1).
Anaemias.

Anaprox
Syntex, Austral.; Syntex, USA.
Naproxen sodium (p.61·2).
Musculoskeletal and joint disorders; pain; peri-articular disorders.

Anartril *Farma Lepori, Spain.*
Glucosamine sulphate (p.1585·1); glucosamine hydriodide (p.1585·1).
Inflammation; osteomyelitis.

Anasclerol *Expharma, Ital.*
Vincamine hydrochloride (p.1644·1).
Cerebrovascular disorders.

Ana-Sed *Potter's, UK.*
Lupulus (p.1597·2); Jamaica dogwood; wild lettuce (p.1645·1); passion flower (p.1615·3); pulsatilla (p.1623·3).
Irritability; pain; tension.

Anasilpiel *Euroexim, Spain.*
Ointment: Dexpanthenol (p.1570·3); neomycin undecenoate (p.229·2); triamcinolone acetonide (p.1050·2).
Topical aerosol†: Neomycin undecenoate (p.229·2); triamcinolone acetonide (p.1041·1).
Infected skin disorders.

Anaspaz *Ascher, USA.*
Hyoscyamine sulphate (p.464·2).
Smooth muscle spasm.

Anastil *Eberth, Ger.*
Lozenges: Thyme (p.1636·3).
Bronchitis; catarrh.
Oral liquid†: Thyme (p.1636·3); guaiphenesin (p.1061·3); guaiacol (p.1061·2); potassium guaiacolsulfonate (p.1068·3); sodium salicylate (p.85·1); menthol (p.1600·2); chlorophyllin (p.1000·1); anise oil (p.1550·1).
Coughs and colds.
Suppositories; injection: Guaiacol (p.1061·2).
Bronchitis; pneumonia.
Tablets†: Thyme (p.1636·3); guaiphenesin (p.1061·3); guaiacol (p.1061·2); potassium guaiacolsulfonate (p.1068·3); sodium salicylate (p.85·1); menthol (p.1600·2); camphor (p.1557·2).
Coughs and colds.

Anastil N *Eberth, Ger.*
Thyme (p.1636·3); camphor (p.1557·2); guaiphenesin (p.1061·3).
Bronchitis; catarrh; coughs.

Anatac *UCB, Spain.*
Carbocisteine (p.1056·3).
Respiratory-tract disorders.

Anatensol
Bristol-Myers Squibb, Austral.; Bristol-Myers Squibb, Belg.†; Mead Johnson, Ital.; Bristol-Myers Squibb, Neth.
Fluphenazine decanoate (p.671·2) or fluphenazine hydrochloride (p.671·3).
Psychoses.

Anatetall *Biocine, Ital.*
An adsorbed tetanus vaccine (p.1535·3).
Active immunisation.

Anatopic *Martin, Spain.*
Fluocinolone acetonide (p.1041·1).
Skin disorders.

Anatox *Lagap, Ital.†.*
Cogalactoisomerase sodium (p.1566·2).
Liver disorders.

Anatoxal Di
Berna, Spain†; Berna, Switz.
An adsorbed diphtheria vaccine (p.1507·3).
Active immunisation.

Anatoxal Di Te
Kwizda, Aust.; Berna, Belg.; Berna, Ital.; Berna, Spain; Berna, Switz.
An adsorbed diphtheria and tetanus vaccine (p.1508·1). Separate preparations are available for infants and young children and for older children and adults.
Active immunisation.

Anatoxal Di Te Per
Kwizda, Aust.; Berna, Belg.; Berna, Ital.; Berna, Spain; Berna, Switz.
An adsorbed diphtheria, tetanus, and pertussis vaccine (p.1509·1).
Active immunisation of infants and young children.

Anatoxal Te
Berna, Belg.; Berna, Spain; Berna, Switz.
An adsorbed tetanus vaccine (p.1535·3).
Active immunisation.

Anatrast *Lafayette, USA.*
Barium sulphate (p.1003·1).
Contrast medium for gastro-intestinal radiography.

Anatuss *Mayrand, USA.*
Syrup: Phenylpropanolamine hydrochloride (p.1067·2); dextromethorphan hydrobromide (p.1057·3); guaiphenesin (p.1061·3).
Tablets: Phenylpropanolamine hydrochloride (p.1067·2); dextromethorphan hydrobromide (p.1057·3); guaiphenesin (p.1061·3); paracetamol (p.72·2).
Coughs.

Anatuss DM *Mayrand, USA.*
Guaiphenesin (p.1061·3); pseudoephedrine hydrochloride (p.1068·3); dextromethorphan hydrobromide (p.1057·3).

Anatuss LA *Mayrand, USA.*
Guaiphenesin (p.1061·3); pseudoephedrine hydrochloride (p.1067·2).
Coughs.

Anauran *Zambon, Ital.*
Polymyxin B sulphate (p.239·1); neomycin sulphate (p.229·2); lignocaine hydrochloride (p.1293·2).
Formerly contained polymyxin B sulphate, neomycin sulphate, lignocaine hydrochloride, betamethasone, and furaltadone hydrochloride.
External ear disorders.

Anaus *Molteni, Ital.†.*
Trimethobenzamide hydrochloride (p.420·1).
Nausea and vomiting.

Anausin *Asta Medica, Fr.*
Metoclopramide hydrochloride (p.1200·3).
Adjunct to gastro-intestinal procedures; dyspepsia; nausea and vomiting.

Anavir *Errekappa, Ital.†.*
Inosine pranobex (p.615·2).
Viral infections.

Anaxeryl *Bailly, Fr.*
Dithranol (p.1082·1); ichthammol (p.1083·3); salicylic acid (p.1090·2); resorcinol (p.1090·1); peru balsam (p.1617·2); birch tar oil (p.1092·2).
Alopecia; dry skin conditions; psoriasis.

Anbesol
Note. This name is used for preparations of different composition.
Whitehall-Robins, Canad.
Topical gel: Benzocaine (p.1286·2); phenol (p.1121·2).
Topical liquid: Benzocaine (p.1286·2); phenol (p.1121·2); camphor (p.1557·2); menthol (p.1600·2).
Minor skin abrasions; mouth pain.
Whitehall, Irl.; Seton, UK.
Lignocaine hydrochloride (p.1293·2); chlorocresol (p.1110·3); cetylpyridinium chloride (p.1106·2).
Aphthous stomatitis; gingival pain; teething.
Whitehall, USA.
Topical gel: Benzocaine (p.1286·2); phenol (p.1121·2).
Topical liquid: Benzocaine (p.1286·2); phenol (p.1121·2); menthol (p.1600·2); camphor (p.1557·2); povidone-iodine (p.1123·3).
Mouth and throat disorders.

Anbesol Baby *Whitehall-Robins, Canad.*
Benzocaine (p.1286·2).
Teething.

Ancatropine Gel *Sandoz, Canad.†.*
Aluminium oxide (p.1077·2); magnesium hydroxide (p.1198·2); methylphenobarbitone (p.349·2).
Gastro-intestinal hyperacidity and hypertonicity.

Ancatropine Infant Drops *Sandoz, Canad.†.*
Homatropine methobromide (p.462·2); butobarbitone (p.645·1).
Gastro-intestinal hyperacidity and hypertonicity.

Ancef
SmithKline Beecham, Canad.; SmithKline Beecham, USA.
Cephazolin sodium (p.181·1).
Bacterial infections.

Ancet *C & M, USA.*
Skin cleanser.

Ancid *Hexal, Ger.*
Hydrotalcite (p.1194·1).
Gastric hyperacidity; peptic ulcer.

Anco *Kanoldt, Ger.*
Ibuprofen (p.44·1).
Inflammation; pain; rheumatism.

Ancobon *Roche, USA.*
Flucytosine (p.379·2).
Candidiasis; cryptococcosis.

Ancolan *Boots, Austral.†.*
Meclozine hydrochloride (p.413·3).
Allergic rhinitis; allergy; eczema; Ménière's disease; nasal congestion; nausea and vomiting; urticaria.

Ancopir *Grossmann, Switz.*
Vitamin B substances.
Lignocaine hydrochloride (p.1293·2) is included in the intramuscular injection to alleviate the pain of injection.
Adjuvant in radiation therapy; alcoholism; lumbago; neuralgia; neuritis; sciatica; vitamin B deficiency.

Ancotil
Roche, Aust.; Roche, Austral.†; Roche, Canad.†; Roche, Fr.; Roche, Ger.†; Roche, Ital.; Roche, Neth.; Roche, Norw.; Roche, Swed.; Roche, Switz.
Flucytosine (p.379·2).
Fungal infections.

Andante *Boehringer Ingelheim, Ger.*
Bunazosin hydrochloride (p.835·2).
Hypertension.

Andantol
Asta Medica, Belg.; Rorer, Ital.†; Vesta, S.Afr.†.
Isothipendyl hydrochloride (p.412·2).
Skin disorders.

Andapsin *Orion, Swed.*
Sucralfate (p.1214·2).
Peptic ulcer.

Andergin *Poli, Ital.*
Miconazole (p.384·3) or miconazole nitrate (p.384·3).
Fungal infections.

Andolex
3M, S.Afr.; 3M, Swed.
Benzydamine hydrochloride (p.21·3).
Painful inflammation of the mouth and throat.

Andolex-C *3M, S.Afr.*
Benzydamine hydrochloride (p.21·3); chlorhexidine gluconate (p.1107·2).
Inflammation and infection of the mouth and throat.

Andractim
Piette, Belg.; Besins-Iscovesco, Fr.
Stanolone (p.1462·2).
Lichen; male hypogonadism.

Andrews
SmithKline Beecham Consumer, Belg.; SmithKline Beecham, Irl.†; Winthrop, Switz.†; Sterling Health, UK.
Citric acid (p.1564·3); magnesium sulphate (p.1157·3); sodium bicarbonate (p.1153·2).
Bile disorders; constipation; gastric hyperacidity.

Andrews Answer *Sterling Health, UK.*
Paracetamol (p.72·2); caffeine (p.749·3).
Dyspepsia; headache.

Andrews Antacid
SmithKline Beecham Consumer, Irl.; Sterling Health, UK.
Calcium carbonate (p.1182·1); magnesium carbonate (p.1198·1).
Dyspepsia.

Andrews Laxeerzout *Sterling, Neth.†.*
Magnesium sulphate (p.1157·3).
Constipation.

Andrews Tums Antacid *SmithKline Beecham Consumer, Austral.*
Calcium carbonate (p.1182·1).
Dyspepsia; heartburn.

Andriol
Organon, Aust.; Organon, Austral.; Organon, Canad.; Organon, Ger.; Organon, Ital.; Organon, Neth.; Organon, Switz.
Testosterone undecanoate (p.1464·2).
Delayed puberty; primary and hypogonadotrophic hypogonadism; testosterone deficiency.

Andro *Forest Pharmaceuticals, USA.*
Testosterone enanthate (p.1464·1).
Breast cancer; delayed puberty (males); male hypogonadism.

Androcur
Schering, Aust.; Schering, Austral.; Schering, Belg.; Berlex, Canad.; Schering, Fr.; Schering, Ger.; Schering, Irl.; Schering, Ital.; Schering, Neth.; Schering, Norw.; Schering, S.Afr.; Schering, Spain; Schering, Swed.; Schering, Switz.; Schering, UK.
Cyproterone acetate (p.1440·2).
Androgen-dependent hirsutism, alopecia, acne, and seborrhoea in females; male sexual deviation; male virilisation; precocious puberty; prostatic cancer.

Androderm *SmithKline Beecham, USA.*
Testosterone (p.1464·1).
Testosterone deficiency.

Andro-Diane *Schering, Aust.*
Cyproterone acetate (p.1440·2).
Androgen-dependent hirsutism, alopecia, acne, and seborrhoea in females.

Andro/Fem *Pasadena, USA†.*
Oestradiol cypionate (p.1455·1); testosterone cypionate (p.1464·1).
Menopausal vasomotor symptoms; prevention of postpartum breast engorgement.

Android *ICN, USA.*
Methyltestosterone (p.1450·3).
Androgen replacement therapy; breast cancer; male hypogonadism; postpartum breast engorgement; postpubertal cryptorchidism.

Androlone-D *Keene, USA.*
Nandrolone decanoate (p.1452·2).
Anaemia in renal disease.

Andropatch
SmithKline Beecham, Irl.; SmithKline Beecham, UK.
Testosterone (p.1464·1).
Hypogonadism.

Andropository *Rugby, USA.*
Testosterone enanthate (p.1464·1).
Breast cancer; delayed puberty (males); male hypogonadism.

Androskat
Byk, Aust.; Byk, Neth.
Papaverine hydrochloride (p.1614·2); phentolamine mesylate (p.930·1).
Impotence.

Androtardyl *Schering, Fr.*
Testosterone enanthate (p.1464·1).
Male hypogonadism.

Androvite *Optimox, USA.*
Multivitamin and mineral preparation with iron and folic acid.

Androxon
Organon, Norw.; Donmed, S.Afr.
Testosterone undecanoate (p.1464·2).
Male hypogonadism.

Andrumin *Janssen-Cilag, Austral.*
Dimenhydrinate (p.408·2).
Motion sickness; vestibular disorders.

Andursil
Note. This name is used for preparations of different composition.
Ciba-Geigy, Ger.†.
Magnesium hydroxide (p.1198·2); heavy magnesium carbonate (p.1198·1); dried aluminium hydroxide gel (p.1177·3); simethicone (p.1213·1).
Gastro-intestinal disorders.
CCP, Irl.†; Ciba-Geigy, Switz.†.
Oral suspension: Aluminium hydroxide gel (p.1177·3); magnesium hydroxide (p.1198·2); aluminium hydroxide-magnesium carbonate co-dried gel (p.1178·2); simethicone (p.1213·1).
Flatulence; hyperacidity.
CCP, Irl.†; Zyma, Switz.
Tablets: Aluminium hydroxide-magnesium carbonate co-dried gel (p.1178·2); simethicone (p.1213·1).
Flatulence; gastro-intestinal hyperacidity; gastro-oesophageal reflux.

Andursil N *Zyma, Ger.*
Heavy magnesium carbonate (p.1198·1); dried aluminium hydroxide gel (p.1177·3).
Gastro-intestinal disorders.

Anectine
Glaxo Wellcome, Canad.; Wellcome, Irl.; Wellcome, Spain; Wellcome, UK; Wellcome, USA.
Suxamethonium chloride (p.1319·1).
Depolarising neuromuscular blocker.

Anemial *Malesci, Ital.†.*
Ferritin (p.1580·1).
Iron-deficiency disorders.

Anemotron *Rovi, Spain†.*
Cyanocobalamin (p.1363·3); intrinsic factor; ferrous fumarate (p.1339·3); thiamine (p.1361·2).
Anaemias.

Anemul mono *Medopharm, Ger.*
Dexamethasone (p.1037·1).
Skin disorders.

Anergan *Forest Pharmaceuticals, USA.*
Promethazine hydrochloride (p.416·2).
Hypersensitivity reactions; motion sickness; nausea; postoperative pain (adjunct); sedative; vomiting.

Anervan
Recip, Norw.; Recip, Swed.
Ergotamine tartrate (p.445·3); chlorcyclizine hydrochloride (p.404·3); caffeine (p.749·3); meprobamate (p.678·1).
Migraine.

Anest Compuesto *Llorens, Spain.*
Amethocaine (p.1285·2).
Naphazoline nitrate (p.1064·2) is included in this preparation as a vasoconstrictor to diminish absorption and localise the effect of the local anaesthetic.
Local anaesthesia.

Anestacon *PolyMedica, USA.*
Lignocaine hydrochloride (p.1293·2).
Urethral pain.

Anestan *Seton, UK†.*
Ephedrine hydrochloride (p.1059·3); theophylline (p.765·1).
Respiratory-tract disorders.

Anestecidan Noradrenalin *Cidan, Spain†.*
Lignocaine hydrochloride (p.1293·2).
Noradrenaline acid tartrate (p.924·1) is included in this preparation as a vasoconstrictor to diminish absorption and localise the effect of the local anaesthetic.
Local anaesthesia.

Anestecidan Simple *Cidan, Spain†.*
Lignocaine hydrochloride (p.1293·2).
Local anaesthesia.

Anestesia Loc Braun C/A *Braun, Spain.*
Procaine hydrochloride (p.1299·2).
Adrenaline (p.813·2) is included in this preparation as a vasoconstrictor to diminish absorption and localise the effect of the local anaesthetic.
Formerly known as Anestesia Local Miro C/A.
Local anaesthesia.

Anestesia Loc Braun S/A *Braun, Spain.*
Cinchocaine (p.1289·2); procaine hydrochloride (p.1299·2).
Formerly known as Anestesia Local Miro S/A.
Local anaesthesia.

Anestesia Topi Braun C/A *Braun, Spain.*
Amethocaine hydrochloride (p.1285·2).
Adrenaline (p.813·2) is included in this preparation as a vasoconstrictor to diminish absorption and localise the effect of the local anaesthetic.
Formerly known as Anestesia Topi C/A and F.
Local anaesthesia.

Anestesia Topica And Far *Palex, Spain†.*
Amethocaine (p.1285·2).
Local anaesthesia.

Anestesico *Cusi, Spain.*
Amethocaine hydrochloride (p.1285·2).
Naphazoline hydrochloride (p.1064·2) is included in this preparation as a vasoconstrictor to diminish absorption and localise the effect of the local anaesthetic.
Local anaesthesia.

Anesthesique Double *Asta Medica, Belg.*
Oxybuprocaine hydrochloride (p.1298·1); amethocaine hydrochloride (p.1285·2).
Local anaesthesia.

Anesti Doble *Cusi, Spain.*
Oxybuprocaine hydrochloride (p.1298·1); amethocaine hydrochloride (p.1285·2).
Local anaesthesia.

Anestina Braun *Palex, Spain.*
Lignocaine hydrochloride (p.1293·2); procaine hydrochloride (p.1299·2); amethocaine hydrochloride (p.1285·2).
Formerly known as Anestina Miro.
Local anaesthesia.

Anethaine
Salusa, S.Afr.†; Torbet Laboratories, UK.
Amethocaine hydrochloride (p.1285·2).
Local anaesthesia.

Anetin *Ibirn, Ital.*
Carnitine (p.1336·2).
Carnitine deficiency; myocardial ischaemia.

Aneural *Wyeth, Ger.*
Maprotiline hydrochloride (p.296·2).
Depression.

Aneurin *A.S., Ger.*
Thiamine hydrochloride (p.1361·1).
Vitamin B deficiency.

Aneurol
Note. This name is used for preparations of different composition.
Sanico, Belg.
Thiamine hydrochloride (p.1361·1).
Neurogenic pain; rheumatic pain; vitamin B_1 deficiency.

Lacer, Spain.
Diazepam (p.661·1).
Contains pyridoxine hydrochloride.
Alcohol withdrawal syndrome; anxiety; febrile convulsions; insomnia; skeletal muscle spasm.

Anevrasi *Donini, Ital.*
Passion flower (p.1615·3); crataegus (p.1568·2); valerian (p.1643·1).
Insomnia.

Anexate
Roche, Aust.; Roche, Austral.; Roche, Belg.; Roche, Canad.; Roche, Fr.; Roche, Ger.; Roche, Irl.; Roche, Ital.; Roche, Neth.; Roche, Norw.; Roche, S.Afr.; Roche, Spain; Roche, Switz.; Roche, UK.
Flumazenil (p.981·1).
Benzodiazepine overdosage; reversal of benzodiazepine-induced sedation.

Anexsia *Mallinckrodt, USA.*
Hydrocodone tartrate (p.43·1); paracetamol (p.72·2).
Pain.

Anfenax *Xixia, S.Afr.†.*
Diclofenac sodium (p.31·2).
Inflammation; pain.

Anfocort *Bristol-Myers Squibb, Ital.*
Halcinonide (p.1043·2); neomycin sulphate (p.229·2); amphotericin (p.372·2).
Infected skin disorders.

Angass *Medice, Ger.*
Bismuth subnitrate (p.1180·2); bismuth aluminate (p.1180·1).
Peptic ulcer.

Angass S *Medice, Ger.*
Bismuth subnitrate (p.1180·2).
Peptic ulcer.

Angesil Plus *Drug Houses Austral., Austral.†.*
Paracetamol (p.72·2); thiamine hydrochloride (p.1361·1); pyridoxine hydrochloride (p.1362·3).
Pain.

Angettes *Bristol-Myers Squibb, UK.*
Aspirin (p.16·1).
Cardiovascular disorders.

Angeze *Opus, UK.*
Isosorbide mononitrate (p.893·3).
Angina pectoris.

Angi *Sterling Health, Spain†.*
Cineole (p.1564·1); enoxolone (p.35·2); menthol (p.1600·2); sodium cetylsulphate.
Upper-respiratory-tract inflammation.

Angi C *Trenker, Belg.†.*
Tablet A, formaldehyde (p.1113·2); tablet C, ascorbic acid (p.1365·2).
Mouth and throat infections.

Angi Truw N *Truw, Ger.†.*
Homoeopathic preparation.

Angichrome *Pharmethic, Belg.†.*
Sulphanilamide (p.256·3); mercurochrome (p.1119·2).
Disinfection of skin and mucous membranes.

Angicola *Sterling Health, Spain†.*
Lozenges: Chlorhexidine hydrochloride (p.1107·2); benzocaine (p.1286·2).
Throat spray: Chlorhexidine gluconate (p.1107·2); amethocaine hydrochloride (p.1285·2).
Mouth and throat disorders.

Angidil *Benedetti, Ital.*
Diltiazem hydrochloride (p.854·2).
Angina pectoris; hypertension.

Angidine *Vifor, Switz.*
Gramicidin (p.215·2); benzethonium chloride (p.1102·3); amethocaine hydrochloride (p.1285·2).
Mouth and throat disorders.

Angifebrine *Pharmacal, Switz.*
Propyphenazone (p.81·3); paracetamol (p.72·2).
Fever; pain.

Angifonil *Diviser Aquilea, Spain.*
Cetylpyridinium chloride (p.1106·2).
Bacterial mouth infections.

Angileptol *Sigma-Tau, Spain.*
Enoxolone (p.35·2); benzocaine (p.1286·2); sulphaguanidine (p.254·1).
Mouth and throat disorders.

Angilol *DDSA Pharmaceuticals, UK.*
Propranolol hydrochloride (p.937·1).
Angina pectoris; arrhythmias; essential tremor; hypertension; migraine; myocardial infarction.

Angimuth *Darci, Belg.†.*
Bismuth camphocarboxylate (p.1181·1).
Infections of the mouth and throat.

Angina MCC *Streuli, Switz.*
Cetylpyridinium chloride (p.1106·2); lignocaine hydrochloride (p.1293·2); menthol (p.1600·2).
Mouth and throat disorders.

Angina-Gastreu N R1 *Reckeweg, Ger.*
Homoeopathic preparation.

Anginamide *Medgenix, Belg.*
Sulphacetamide sodium (p.252·2).
Infections of the mouth and throat.

Anginasin N *Opfermann, Ger.*
Hexetidine (p.1116·1); camphor (p.1557·2); menthol (p.1600·2).
Inflammatory disorders and infections of the oropharynx.

Anginesin *Grossmann, Switz.*
Aluminium acetotartrate (p.1547·3); sage (p.1627·1).
Mouth and throat pain.

Anginetten *Divapharma, Ger.†.*
Cetylpyridinium chloride (p.1106·2); dequalinium chloride (p.1112·1); menthol (p.1600·2).
Infections of the oropharynx.

Anginin *Banyu, Jpn.*
Pyricarbate (p.1624·1).
Thrombo-embolic disorders; vascular disorders.

Anginine *Glaxo Wellcome, Austral.*
Glyceryl trinitrate (p.874·3).
Angina pectoris.

Anginol
Note. This name is used for preparations of different composition.
Labima, Belg.
Dequalinium chloride (p.1112·1).
Mouth and throat disorders.

Streuli, Switz.
Ethacridine lactate (p.1098·3); levomenthol (p.1600·2); camphor (p.1557·2); peru balsam (p.1617·2).
Mouth and throat disorders.

Anginomycin *Chephasaar, Ger.*
Tyrothricin (p.267·2); bacitracin (p.157·3).
Infections of the oropharynx.

Anginor *Vesta, S.Afr.*
Nifedipine (p.916·2).
Angina pectoris; hypertension.

Anginova Nouvelle formule *Medinova, Switz.*
Dequalinium chloride (p.1112·1); lignocaine hydrochloride (p.1293·2).
Mouth and throat disorders.

Anginovag *Novag, Spain.*
Dequalinium chloride (p.1112·1); enoxolone (p.35·2); hydrocortisone acetate (p.1043·3); lignocaine hydrochloride (p.1293·2); tyrothricin (p.267·2).
Mouth and throat disorders.

Anginovin H *Pfluger, Ger.*
Homoeopathic preparation.

Angiocardyl N *Rhenomed, Ger.*
Atropine sulphate (p.455·1); glyceryl trinitrate (p.874·3); theobromine and sodium salicylate (p.765·1).
Formerly contained atropine sulphate, glyceryl trinitrate, phenobarbitone, and theobromine and sodium salicylate.
Cardiac disorders.

Angiociclan *Organon, Ital.†.*
Bencyclane fumarate (p.827·3).
Circulatory disorders.

Angio-Conray
Bracco, Ital.; Mallinckrodt, USA.
Sodium iothalamate (p.1008·1).
Radiographic contrast medium.

Angiocontrast 370 *Juste, Spain†.*
Sodium metrizoate (p.1009·2); meglumine metrizoate (p.1009·2); calcium metrizoate (p.1009·2).
Radiographic contrast medium.

Angiodrox *Nezel, Spain.*
Diltiazem hydrochloride (p.854·2).
Angina pectoris; hypertension; myocardial infarction.

Angiofiline *Seid, Spain†.*
Ephedrine hydrochloride (p.1059·3); potassium iodide (p.1493·1); theophylline glycinate (p.772·2); thonzylamine hydrochloride (p.419·2); menthol (p.1600·2).
Respiratory-tract disorders.

Angioflux *Mitim, Ital.*
A heparinoid (p.882·3).
Thrombosis prophylaxis.

Angiografin
Schering, Aust.; Schering, Ger.; Schering, Ital.†; Schering, Neth.; Schering, S.Afr.
Meglumine diatrizoate (p.1003·2).
Radiographic contrast medium.

Angiografine *Schering, Fr.*
Meglumine diatrizoate (p.1003·2).
Radiographic contrast medium.

Angiolast *Manetti Roberts, Ital.†.*
Bamethan nicotinate (p.827·1).
Peripheral vascular disorders.

Angionorm *Farmasan, Ger.*
Dihydroergotamine mesylate (p.444·2).
Hypotension; migraine and other vascular headache; venous insufficiency.

Angiopac *UCB, Ger.†.*
Vincamine (p.1644·1).
Ménière's disease; mental function disorders; metabolic and circulatory disorders of the brain, retina, and inner ear.

Angiopan *Gentili, Ital.†.*
Injection: Rutin sodium sulphate (p.1580·2); sulmarin sodium; hesperidin methyl chalcone (p.1580·2); epicatechin; ascorbic acid (p.1365·2).
Tablets: Rutin (p.1580·2); sulmarin sodium; hesperidin (p.1580·2); epicatechin; ascorbic acid (p.1365·2).
Vascular disorders.

Angiopas *Pascoe, Ger.*
Homoeopathic preparation.

Angiophtal
Bournonville, Belg.; Merck Sharp & Dohme-Chibret, Fr.
Chromocarb diethylamine (p.1562·3).
Capillary fragility in the eye; subconjunctival haemorrhage.

Angiopine *Ashbourne, UK.*
Nifedipine (p.916·2).
Angina pectoris; hypertension; Raynaud's syndrome.

Angiorex *Lampugnani, Ital.*
Myrtillus (p.1606·1).
Capillary disorders.

Angiosedante *Unifarma, Spain.*
Aminophylline (p.748·1); papaverine hydrochloride (p.1614·2).
Biliary colic; cardiac stimulation; obstructive airways disease.

Angiospray *UCB, Ital.†.*
Glyceryl trinitrate (p.874·3).
Cardiovascular disorders.

Angioton *GD, Ital.*
Centella (p.1080·3); rubina; vitamins.
Venous disorders.

Angioton S *DHU, Ger.*
Homoeopathic preparation.

Angiovist 282 *Berlex, USA.*
Meglumine diatrizoate (p.1003·2).
Radiographic contrast medium.

Angiovist 292, Angiovist 370 *Berlex, USA.*
Meglumine diatrizoate (p.1003·2); sodium diatrizoate (p.1003·2).
Radiographic contrast medium.

Angioxil *FIRMA, Ital.†.*
Pyricarbate (p.1624·1).
Vascular disorders.

Angiozem *Ashbourne, UK.*
Diltiazem hydrochloride (p.854·2).
Angina pectoris.

Angiplex *Leiras, Swed.†.*
Glyceryl trinitrate (p.874·3).
Angina pectoris.

Angipress *Crinos, Ital.*
Diltiazem hydrochloride (p.854·2).
Hypertension; ischaemic heart disease.

Angisan *Sanabo, Aust.*
Chlorhexidine gluconate (p.1107·2).
Mouth disorders.

Angised
Wellcome, Irl.; Glaxo Wellcome, S.Afr.
Glyceryl trinitrate (p.874·3).
Angina pectoris.

Angiseptina *Hosbon, Spain†.*
Dichlorobenzyl alcohol (p.1112·2); amylmetacresol (p.1101·3).
Mouth and throat infections.

Angispray
Note. A similar name is used for preparations of different composition.
Monot, Fr.
Hexetidine (p.1116·1); propionic acid (p.387·1); chlorbutol (p.1106·3).
Mouth and throat disorders.

Angi-Spray
Note. A similar name is used for preparations of different composition.
Akromed, S.Afr.
Isosorbide dinitrate (p.893·1).
Angina pectoris; heart failure; myocardial infarction.

Angitil *Trinity, UK.*
Diltiazem hydrochloride (p.854·2).
Angina pectoris; hypertension.

Angitrate *Akromed, S.Afr.*
Isosorbide mononitrate (p.893·3).
Angina pectoris.

Angizem *Inverni della Beffa, Ital.*
Diltiazem hydrochloride (p.854·2).
Cardiovascular disorders.

Angocin Anti-Infekt N *Repha, Ger.*
Tropaeolum majus; armoracia.
Respiratory-tract infections; urinary-tract infections.

Angocin Bronchialtropfen *Repha, Ger.*
Marrubium vulgare (p.1063·3).
Respiratory-tract catarrh.

Angocin percutan *Repha, Ger.*
Camphor (p.1557·2); eucalyptus oil (p.1578·1); turpentine oil (p.1641·1).
Muscle and joint pain; respiratory-tract disorders.

Angonit *Cedona, Neth.†.*
Glyceryl trinitrate (p.874·3).
Angina pectoris.

Angstrom Anti-Acqua *Restiva, Ital.†.*
Ethylhexyl *p*-methoxycinnamate (p.1487·1); avobenzone (p.1486·3).
Sunscreen.

Angstrom Corpo *Restiva, Ital.*
Ethylhexyl *p*-methoxycinnamate (p.1487·1); avobenzone (p.1486·3).
Sunscreen.

Angstrom Viso/Labbra Alta Protezione
Restiva, Ital.
Cream: Ethylhexyl *p*-methoxycinnamate (p.1487·1); avobenzone (p.1486·3); vitamin E acetate (p.1369·1); dimethicone (p.1384·2); betacarotene (p.1335·2); allantoin (p.1078·2); sodium pidolate (p.1091·2); triclosan (p.1127·2).
Stick: Ethylhexyl *p*-methoxycinnamate (p.1487·1); avobenzone (p.1486·3); vitamin E acetate (p.1369·1); betacarotene (p.1335·2).
Barrier preparation; sunscreen.

Angurate Magentee *Alsitan, Ger.*
Mentzelia cordifolia.
Gastro-intestinal disorders.

Anhydrol Forte
Dermal Laboratories, Irl.; Dermal Laboratories, UK.
Aluminium chloride (p.1078·3).
Hyperhidrosis.

Anifed *Formenti, Ital.*
Nifedipine (p.916·2).
Hypertension; ischaemic heart disease.

Anifer Hustenbalsam *Anifer, Aust.*
Eucalyptus oil (p.1578·1); pumilio pine oil (p.1623·3); sage oil.
Respiratory-tract disorders.

Anifer Hustentee *Anifer, Aust.*
Althaea (p.1546·3); aniseed (p.1549·3); thyme (p.1636·3); plantago lanceolata leaf; mallow flowers.
Respiratory-tract disorders.

Anifer Hustentropfen *Anifer, Aust.*
Thyme (p.1636·3); primula rhizome.
Coughs.

Anifer Krauterol *Anifer, Aust.*
Eucalyptus oil (p.1578·1); oleum pini sylvestris; pumilio pine oil (p.1623·3).
Respiratory-tract disorders.

Aniflazym *Madaus, Ger.; Takeda, Ger.*
Serrapeptase (p.1628·3).
Treatment of inflammatory symptoms.

Animal Shapes *Major, USA.*
Multivitamin preparation.

Animal Shapes + Iron *Major, USA.*
Multivitamin preparation with iron.

Animbo-N *Trommsdorff, Ger.†.*
Hexylresorcinol (p.1116·1); bromchlorophane; salicylic acid (p.1090·2); isopropyl alcohol (p.1118·2); menthol (p.1600·2).
Acne.

Animbo-Tinktur *Trommsdorff, Ger.†.*
Sozoiodol sodium (p.1125·3); ammonium thiocyanate; thymol (p.1127·1); salicylic acid (p.1090·2); isopropyl alcohol (p.1118·2).
Acne.

Animine
Note. This name is used for preparations of different composition.
McGloin, Austral.
Cream: Benzocaine (p.1286·2); benzalkonium chloride (p.1101·3).
Lotion: Lignocaine hydrochloride (p.1293·2); benzalkonium chloride (p.1101·3); calamine (p.1080·1).
Bites; pruritus; stings.

Synthelabo, Belg.
Trimethylxanthine sodium alphanaphthylacetate.
Mental function impairment; tonic.

Anionen-Spurenelement Leopold, Aust.
Electrolytes for infusion (p.1147·1).
Parenteral nutrition.

Aniospray Anios, Fr.
Formaldehyde (p.1113·2); glyoxal (p.1115·1); glutaraldehyde (p.1114·3); didecyldimethylammonium chloride (p.1112·2).
Disinfection of instruments and surfaces.

Anisan Pascoe, Ger.
Menthol (p.1600·2); bismuth subgallate (p.1180·2); aluminium acetate tartrate (p.1547·3); hypericum oil (p.1590·1); aesculus (p.1543·3); chamomile (p.1561·2); hamamelis (p.1587·1); liver oil.
Anorectal disorders.

Anivy Roberts, Canad.
Chlorphenesin (p.376·2); benzocaine (p.1286·2).
Insect bites; poison ivy; skin irritation.

Annexine
Berna, Belg.†; Berna, Ital.†.
Neisseria gonorrhoeae; Streptococcus haemolyticus A; Staphylococcus aureus; Staphylococcus albus; Escherichia coli.
Immunotherapy of gynaecological inflammation.

Anningzochin Laves, Ger.
Mycobacterium chelonae subsp. *chelonae.*
Immunotherapy.

Anocaine Mallard, USA†.
Benzocaine (p.1286·2); zinc oxide (p.1096·2); bismuth subgallate (p.1180·2); peru balsam (p.1617·2).
Anorectal disorders.

Anoclor Rolab, S.Afr.
Chloroquine phosphate (p.426·3).
Malaria.

Anodan-HC Odan, Canad.
Hydrocortisone acetate (p.1043·3); zinc sulphate (p.1373·2).
Anorectal disorders.

Anodesyn Seton, UK.
Ephedrine hydrochloride (p.1059·3); lignocaine hydrochloride (p.1293·2); allantoin (p.1078·2).
Anorectal disorders.

Anodynos Buffington, USA.
Aspirin (p.16·1); salicylamide (p.82·3); caffeine (p.749·3).
Pain.

Anolan Goupil, Fr.†.
Enoxolone (p.35·2); amylocaine hydrochloride (p.1286·1).
Anorectal disorders.

Anoquan Roberts, USA.
Paracetamol (p.72·2); caffeine (p.749·3); butalbital (p.644·3).
Pain.

Anoran Labima, Belg.
Phendimetrazine hydrochloride (p.1484·2).
Obesity.

Anore Dolor Schwarzwalder, Ger.
Homoeopathic preparation.

Anore rheumatic N Schwarzwalder, Ger.
Homoeopathic preparation.

Anore X N Schwarzwalder, Ger.
Absinthium (p.1541·1); gentian (p.1583·3); angelica.
Appetite loss; dyspepsia.

Anoreine
Note. This name is used for preparations of different composition.
Germania, Aust.
Carrageenan (p.1471·3); titanium dioxide (p.1093·3); zinc oxide (p.1096·2).
Anorectal disorders.

Martin, Fr.
Carrageenan (p.1471·3); bismuth subgallate (p.1180·2); zinc oxide (p.1096·2).
Anorectal disorders.

Anoreine mit Lidocain Germania, Aust.
Carrageenan (p.1471·3); titanium dioxide (p.1093·3); zinc oxide (p.1096·2); lignocaine (p.1293·2).
Anorectal disorders.

Anorex
Note. This name is used for preparations of different composition.
Crinex, Fr.†.
Diethylpropion hydrochloride (p.1479·3).
Obesity.

Dunhall, USA.
Phendimetrazine tartrate (p.1484·2).
Obesity.

Anovlar Schering, Ital.†.
Norethisterone acetate (p.1453·1); ethinyloestradiol (p.1445·1).
Combined oral contraceptive; gynaecological disorders.

Anoxid Volchem, Ital.
Vitamins A, C, and E with selenium.
Nutritional supplement.

Anpec Alphapharm, Austral.
Verapamil hydrochloride (p.960·3).
Angina; arrhythmias; hypertension.

Anpine Alphapharm, Austral.†.
Nifedipine (p.916·2).
Angina pectoris.

Anplag Mitsubishi, Jpn.
Sarpogrelate hydrochloride (p.943·1).
Thrombo-embolic disorders.

Anquil
Janssen-Cilag, Irl.; Janssen, UK.
Benperidol (p.642·3).
Deviant sexual behaviour.

Ansaid
Pharmacia Upjohn, Canad.; Upjohn, USA.
Flurbiprofen (p.42·1).
Inflammation; musculoskeletal and joint disorders; pain.

Ansatipin
Kenfarma, Spain; Pharmacia Upjohn, Swed.
Rifabutin (p.242·2).
Opportunistic mycobacterial infections; tuberculosis.

Ansatipine Pharmacia Upjohn, Fr.
Rifabutin (p.242·2).
Mycobacterial infections; tuberculosis.

Anselol Douglas, Austral.
Atenolol (p.825·3).
Angina pectoris; arrhythmias; hypertension; myocardial infarction.

Ansene Nelson, Austral.†.
Cetrimide (p.1105·2); calamine (p.1080·1); vitamins A, D, & E.
Nappy rash.

Ansene L Nelson, Austral.†.
Cetrimide (p.1105·2); lignocaine hydrochloride (p.1293·2); chlorhexidine acetate (p.1107·2); vitamins A, D, & E.
Minor cuts; sunburn.

Anseren Ciba, Ital.
Ketazolam (p.675·2).
Anxiety disorders.

Ansial Vita, Spain†.
Buspirone hydrochloride (p.643·3).
Anxiety.

Ansimar ABC, Ital.
Doxofylline (p.752·2).
Obstructive airways disease.

Ansiolin Corvi, Ital.
Diazepam (p.661·1).
Anxiety; epilepsy; insomnia.

Ansiowas Wasserman, Spain†.
Meprobamate (p.678·1).
Anxiety; insomnia; skeletal muscle spasm.

Ansium Vita Elan, Spain.
Diazepam (p.661·1); sulpiride (p.692·3).
Neurosis.

Anso Lacer, Spain.
Hexetidine (p.1116·1); lignocaine hydrochloride (p.1293·2); triamcinolone acetonide (p.1050·2); pentosan polysulphate (p.928·1).
Anorectal disorders.

Ansopal Kabi, Swed.†.
Acetylglycinamide-chloral hydrate (p.640·2).
Insomnia; sedative.

Ansudor Basotherm, Ger.
Aluminium chlorohydrate (p.1078·3); triclocarban (p.1127·2).
Hyperhidrosis; intertrigo; wound exudate.

Ansudoral Basotherm, Ger.†.
Dihydroergotamine tartrate (p.444·3); atropine methonitrate (p.455·1); amylobarbitone (p.641·3); calcium pantothenate (p.1352·3).
Hyperhidrosis.

Answer Carter, USA.
Fertility test or pregnancy test (p.1621·2).

Answer Now Carter Horner, Canad.
Pregnancy test (p.1621·2).

Antabus
Chemomedica, Aust.; Tosse, Ger.; Dumex, Neth.†; Dumex, Norw.; Bohm, Spain; Dumex-Alpharma, Swed.; Dumex, Switz.
Disulfiram (p.1573·1).
Chronic alcoholism.

Antabuse
Orphan, Austral.; Synthelabo, Belg.; Wyeth-Ayerst, Canad.; Dumex, Irl.; Crinos, Ital.; Lagamed, S.Afr.; Dumex, UK; Wyeth-Ayerst, USA.
Disulfiram (p.1573·1).
Chronic alcoholism.

Antacal Errekappa, Ital.
Amlodipine besylate (p.822·3).
Angina pectoris; hypertension.

Antacid
Geneva, USA.
Oral suspension: Aluminium hydroxide (p.1177·3); magnesium hydroxide (p.1198·2).
Hyperacidity.

Goldline, USA.
Tablets: Calcium carbonate (p.1182·1).
Hyperacidity.

Antacid Liquid Shoppers Drug Mart, Canad.
Aluminium hydroxide (p.1177·3); magnesium hydroxide (p.1198·2); simethicone (p.1213·1).

Antacid Plus Antiflatulant Stanley, Canad.; Drug Trading, Canad.
Aluminium hydroxide (p.1177·3); magnesium hydroxide (p.1198·2); simethicone (p.1213·1).

Antacid Suspension Pharmel, Canad.
Aluminium hydroxide (p.1177·3); magnesium hydroxide (p.1198·2).

Antacid Tablet
Note. This name is used for preparations of different composition.
Stanley, Canad.
Aluminium hydroxide (p.1177·3); magnesium hydroxide (p.1198·2); simethicone (p.1213·1).

Swiss Herbal, Canad.
Magnesium hydroxide (p.1198·2); calcium carbonate (p.1182·1).

Antacide Suspension Therapex, Canad.
Aluminium hydroxide (p.1177·3); magnesium hydroxide (p.1198·2).

Antacide Suspension avec Antiflatulent Therapex, Canad.
Aluminium hydroxide (p.1177·3); magnesium hydroxide (p.1198·2); simethicone (p.1213·1).

Antacidum Pfizer, Aust.
Dihydroxyaluminium sodium carbonate (p.1188·3).
Dyspepsia; hyperacidity; peptic ulcer.

Antacidum OPT Optimed, Ger.
Aluminium hydroxide (p.1177·3).
Gastric hyperacidity; hyperphosphaturia.

Antacidum-Rennie Roche, Aust.
Calcium carbonate (p.1182·1); magnesium carbonate (p.1198·1).
Hyperacidity.

Antacin John Wyeth, Irl.†.
Magaldrate (p.1198·1).
Hyperacidity.

Antadine
Boots, Austral.†; Boots, S.Afr.†.
Amantadine hydrochloride (p.1129·2).
Drug-induced extrapyramidal disorders; influenza A; parkinsonism.

Antadys Theramex, Mon.
Flurbiprofen (p.42·1).
Dysmenorrhoea; musculoskeletal and joint disorders.

Antagonil Ciba, Ger.
Nicardipine hydrochloride (p.915·1).
Angina pectoris; hypertension.

Antagosan
Hoechst, Fr.; Hoechst, Ger.; Hoechst Marion Roussel, Ital.
Aprotinin (p.711·3).
Haemorrhagic disorders; shock.

Antalgic Caps, S.Afr.
Paracetamol (p.72·2).
Fever; pain.

Antalgil Janssen-Cilag, Ital.
Ibuprofen (p.44·1).
Pain.

Antalgin Syntex, Spain.
Naproxen sodium (p.61·2).
Fever; gout; musculoskeletal, joint, and peri-articular disorders; pain.

Antalgit Klinge, Switz.†.
Ibuprofen (p.44·1).
Fever; inflammation; pain.

Antalgola Janssen-Cilag, Ital.†.
Benzalkonium saccharinate (p.1102·1); menthol (p.1600·2); cineole (p.1564·1); pumilio pine oil (p.1623·3).
Mouth and throat disorders.

Antalgola Plus Janssen-Cilag, Ital.†.
Benzalkonium saccharinate (p.1102·1); enoxolone (p.35·2); pumilio pine oil (p.1623·3).
Mouth and throat disorders.

Antalon Dresden, Ger.
Pimozide (p.686·2).
Schizophrenia.

Antalvic Houde, Fr.
Dextropropoxyphene hydrochloride (p.27·3).
Pain.

Antalyre Boehringer Ingelheim, Fr.
Chlorhexidine gluconate (p.1107·2); oxedrine tartrate (p.925·3).
Conjunctival irritation.

Antamex Cimex, Switz.†.
Nifedipine (p.916·2).
Hypertension; ischaemic heart disease.

Antapentan
Byk, Belg.†; Gerot, Switz.†.
Phendimetrazine (p.1484·2) or phendimetrazine hydrochloride (p.1484·2).
Concentration loss; depression; fatigue; obesity.

Antares Krewel, Ger.
Kava (p.1592·3).
Nervous disorders.

Antarol Antigen, Irl.†.
Propranolol hydrochloride (p.937·1).
Angina pectoris; anxiety; arrhythmias; hypertension; hyperthyroidism; migraine; phaeochromocytoma.

Antasten-Privin Ciba Vision, Swed.
Antazoline sulphate (p.402·1); naphazoline nitrate (p.1064·2); boric acid (p.1554·2); borax (p.1554·2).
Allergic conjunctivitis.

Antaxone
Zambon, Ital.; Pharmazam, Spain.
Naltrexone hydrochloride (p.988·1).
Opioid intoxication.

Antazoline-V Rugby, USA.
Naphazoline hydrochloride (p.1064·2); antazoline phosphate (p.401·3).
Eye irritation.

Antebor
Wolfs, Belg.; Biologiques de l'Ile-de-France, Fr.; Sodip, Switz.†.
Sulphacetamide sodium (p.252·2).
Bacterial skin infections.

Antebor B$_6$
Biologiques de l'Ile-de-France, Fr.; Sodip, Switz.†.
Sulphacetamide sodium (p.252·2); pyridoxine hydrochloride (p.1362·3).
Bacterial skin infections.

Antebor N Sodip, Switz.
Chlorhexidine (p.1107·2); triclosan (p.1127·2).
Acne.

Antelepsin Dresden, Ger.
Clonazepam (p.343·3).
Epilepsy.

Antelmina Gerda, Fr.
Piperazine hydrate (p.107·2).
Intestinal nematode infections.

Antemesyl Molteni, Ital.
Injection: Mepyramine hydrochloride (p.414·1); pyridoxine hydrochloride (p.1362·3).
Suppositories: Mepyramine hydrochloride (p.414·1).
Nausea and vomiting.

Antemin Streuli, Switz.
Dimenhydrinate (p.408·2).
Nausea and vomiting.

Antemin compositum Streuli, Switz.
Dimenhydrinate (p.408·2); caffeine (p.749·3); pyridoxine hydrochloride (p.1362·3).
Nausea and vomiting.

Antenex Alphapharm, Austral.
Diazepam (p.661·1).
Alcohol withdrawal syndrome; anxiety; skeletal muscle spasm; spasticity.

Antepan
Mayrhofer, Aust.; Henning, Ger.
Protirelin (p.1259·1).
Assessment of pituitary and thyroid function.

Antepar Wellcome, Irl.†.
Piperazine hydrate (p.107·2); piperazine citrate (p.107·2).
Ascariasis; enterobiasis.

Antepsin
Wyeth, Irl.; Baldacci, Ital.; Orion, Norw.; Wyeth, UK.
Sucralfate (p.1214·2).
Gastritis; gastro-intestinal haemorrhage; gastro-oesophageal reflux; peptic ulcer.

Anthel Alphapharm, Austral.
Pyrantel embonate (p.109·3).
Worm infections.

Anthelios Cosmair, Canad.
Avobenzone (p.1486·3); 3-(4-methylbenzylidene)bornan-2-one (p.1487·2); terephthalylidene dicamphor sulphonic acid; titanium dioxide (p.1093·3).
Sunscreen.

Anthelios Stick Cosmair, Canad.
Avobenzone (p.1486·3); 3-(4-methylbenzylidene)bornan-2-one (p.1487·2).
Sunscreen.

Anthelox Lesourd, Fr.†.
Geraniol; niaouli oil (p.1607·1).
Worm infections.

Anthex Rolab, S.Afr.
Mebendazole (p.104·1).
Worm infections.

Anthiphen Rhone-Poulenc Rorer, S.Afr.†.
Dichlorophen (p.99·2).
Taeniasis.

Anthisan
Rhone-Poulenc Rorer, Austral.; Rhone-Poulenc Rorer, Irl.; Rhone-Poulenc Rorer, S.Afr.; Rhone-Poulenc Rorer, UK.
Mepyramine maleate (p.414·1).
Allergic skin disorders; insect bites and stings.

Anthisan Plus Rhone-Poulenc Rorer, UK.
Mepyramine maleate (p.414·1); benzocaine (p.1286·2).
Bites and stings.

Anthozym Petrasch, Aust.
Beta vulgaris extract; lactic acid (p.1593·3); ferrous lactate (p.1340·1); ascorbic acid (p.1365·2); calcium lactate (p.1155·2); potassium aspartate (p.1161·3); magnesium aspartate (p.1157·2); black currant juice (p.1365·2).
Tonic.

Anthozym N Reith & Petrasch, Ger.
Beetroot; lactic acid (p.1593·3).
Tonic.

Anthra-Derm
Note. This name is used for preparations of different composition.
Gerot, Aust.
Dithranol (p.1082·1); salicylic acid (p.1090·2).
Psoriasis.

Dermik, USA.
Dithranol (p.1082·1).
Psoriasis.

Anthraforte Stiefel, Canad.
Dithranol (p.1082·1).
Psoriasis.

Anthranol
Stiefel, Canad.; Stiefel, Fr.†; Stiefel, S.Afr.†; Stiefel, Spain; Stiefel, UK†.
Dithranol (p.1082·1).
Psoriasis.

Anthrascalp Stiefel, Canad.
Dithranol (p.1082·1).
Psoriasis.

Anthraxivore Picot, Fr.
Arctium lappa (p.1594·2).
Skin infections.

Anti Anorex Triple Lesvi, Spain.
Cyproheptadine hydrochloride (p.407·2); deanol aceglumate (p.1478·2); metoclopramide hydrochloride (p.1200·3).
Tonic.

Anti Itch Blistex, USA.
Pramoxine hydrochloride (p.1298·2).
Pruritus.

Anti-Ac Clement, Fr.
Pyrimiphos methyl; permethrin (p.1409·2); piperonyl butoxide (p.1409·3).
House dust mite acaricide.

Antiacide Marc-O, Canad.
Aluminium hydroxide (p.1177·3); magnesium hydroxide (p.1198·2).

Anti-Acido Giuliani, Ital.
Aluminium hydroxide dried gel (p.1177·3); magnesium hydroxide (p.1198·2); dimethicone (p.1213·1).
Aerophagia; gastric hyperacidity; meteorism.

Antiacido Eno SmithKline Beecham, Spain.
Calcium carbonate (p.1182·1); magnesium carbonate (p.1198·1).
Gastro-intestinal hyperacidity.

Antiacido Salud Boots Healthcare, Spain.
Aluminium hydroxide (p.1177·3); calcium carbonate (p.1182·1); magnesium hydroxide (p.1198·2).
Gastro-intestinal hyperacidity and flatulence.

Anti-Acne
Note. This name is used for preparations of different composition.
Samil, Ital.
Sublimed sulphur (p.1091·2); meclocycline sulphosalicylate (p.224·1); nicoboxil (p.63·1).
Formerly contained sulphur, nicoboxil, chloramphenicol, hydrocortisone acetate, and titanium dioxide.
Acne.

Byk Leo, Spain.
Alcohol; sulphur (p.1091·2); resorcinol (p.1090·1); triclosan (p.1127·2).
Acne.

Anti-Acne Control Formula Clinique, Canad.
Salicylic acid (p.1090·2).
Acne.

Anti-Acne Formula for Men Clinique, Canad.
Salicylic acid (p.1090·2); sulphur (p.1091·2).
Acne.

Anti-Acne Spot Treatment Clinique, Canad.
Salicylic acid (p.1090·2).
Acne.

Antiadipositum X-112
Hanseler, Ger.; Hanseler, Switz.
Cathine hydrochloride (p.1478·1).
Obesity.

Antiadiposo Teofarma, Ital.
Iodocasein; thiamine nitrate (p.1361·1).
Metabolic activator.

Anti-Ageing Kalmia Homeocan, Canad.
Homoeopathic preparation.

Antial Ellem, Ital.†.
Brompheniramine maleate (p.403·2).
Hypersensitivity reactions.

Anti-Algos Truw, Ger.
Paracetamol (p.72·2).
Fever; pain.

Antiallergicum Truw, Ger.†.
Homoeopathic preparation.

Antib Max Farma, Ital.†.
Inosine pranobex (p.615·2).
Herpesvirus infections.

Antibex Bristol, Ger.†.
Lichen islandicus; guaiphenesin (p.1061·3); butethamate citrate (p.1056·2); thyme (p.1636·3).
Catarrh; coughs.

Antibex cum Ephedrino Bristol, Ger.†.
Lichen islandicus; potassium guaiacolsulfonate (p.1068·3); ephedrine hydrochloride (p.1059·3); caffeine (p.749·3); peppermint oil (p.1208·1).
Asthma; bronchitis; emphysema; silicosis.

Antibio-Aberel Janssen-Cilag, Fr.
Tretinoin (p.1093·3); erythromycin (p.204·1).
Acne.

Antibiocin Nycomed, Ger.†.
Phenoxymethylpenicillin potassium (p.236·2).
Bacterial infections.

Antibiofilus Llorente, Spain.
Lactobacillus acidophilus (p.1594·1); choline orotate (p.1611·2); vitamins.
Gastro-intestinal disorders; restoration of the gastro-intestinal flora.

Antibiopen Antibioticos, Spain.
Ampicillin sodium (p.153·1) or ampicillin trihydrate (p.153·2).
Bacterial infections.

Antibiophilus
Germania, Aust.; Lyocentre, Fr.
Lactobacillus rhamnosus (p.1594·1).
Diarrhoea.

Antibioptal Farmila, Ital.
Chloramphenicol (p.182·1); neomycin sulphate (p.229·2).
Bacterial eye infections.

Antibio-Synalar Cassenne, Fr.
Fluocinolone acetonide (p.1041·1); polymyxin B sulphate (p.239·1); neomycin sulphate (p.229·2).
Otitis.

AntibiOtic Parnell, USA.
Hydrocortisone (p.1043·3); neomycin sulphate (p.229·2); polymyxin B (p.239·3).
Bacterial ear infections.

Antibiotic Ointment Stanley, Canad.; Technilab, Canad.
Bacitracin (p.157·3); polymyxin B sulphate (p.239·1).

Antibioticoedermin B Damor, Ital.†.
Betamethasone valerate (p.1033·3); neomycin sulphate (p.229·2); tyrothricin (p.267·2).
Infected skin disorders.

Antibiotique Onguent Prodemdis, Canad.
Bacitracin (p.157·3); polymyxin B sulphate (p.239·1).

Antibiotulle Lumiere
Solvay, Fr.; Hefa, Ger.
Neomycin sulphate (p.229·2); polymyxin B sulphate (p.239·1).
Infected leg ulcers; infected wounds and burns.

Antiblef Eczem Ciba Vision, Spain.
Clioquinol (p.193·2); hydrocortisone acetate (p.1043·3).
Infected eye disorders.

Antiblefarica Ciba Vision, Spain.
Bismuth loretinate; chlortetracycline hydrochloride (p.185·1); cortisone acetate (p.1036·1).
Eye disorders.

Antibron Potter's, UK.
Lobelia (p.1481·3); wild lettuce (p.1645·1); coltsfoot (p.1057·2); euphorbia; pleurisy root; senega (p.1069·3).
Coughs.

Anticatarral Alcala Farm Alcala, Spain.
Chlorpheniramine maleate (p.405·1); phenylephrine hydrochloride (p.1066·2); guaiazulene (p.1586·3); muramidase hydrochloride (p.1604·3); paracetamol (p.72·2).
Formerly known as Anticatarral Alesa.
Upper-respiratory-tract disorders.

Anticerumen Knoll, Spain.
Sodium lauryl sulphate (p.1468·3).
Removal of ear wax.

Antichloric Bio-Therabel, Belg.
Calcium carbonate (p.1182·1); heavy magnesium carbonate (p.1198·1).
Formerly contained light calcium carbonate, heavy magnesium carbonate, belladonna, and liquorice.
Peptic ulcer.

Anticholium
Kohler, Aust.; Kohler, Ger.
Physostigmine salicylate (p.1395·3).
Alcohol withdrawal syndrome; antimuscarinic poisoning; central anticholinergic syndrome.

Anticongestiva Cusi, Spain.
Zinc oxide (p.1096·2).
Skin disorders.

Anticorizza Ogna, Ital.
Paracetamol (p.72·2); salicylamide (p.82·3); caffeine (p.749·3); tripelennamine hydrochloride (p.420·2).
Cold and influenza symptoms.

Anticude UCB, Spain.
Edrophonium bromide (p.1392·2).
Diagnosis of myasthenia gravis; reversal of competitive neuromuscular blockade.

Anti-Dandruff Shampoo Avant Garde, Canad.
Pyrithione zinc (p.1089·3).

Anti-Dessechement Lierac, Fr.†.
Urea (p.1095·2).
Dry skin.

Anti-Diarrheal Stanley, Canad.
Loperamide hydrochloride (p.1197·2).

Antidol
Note. This name is used for preparations of different composition.
Gerbex, Canad.
Aspirin (p.16·1); caffeine (p.749·3).

Cinfa, Spain.
Paracetamol (p.72·2).
Fever; pain.

Antidoloroso Rudol Areu, Spain.
Aspirin (p.16·1); caffeine (p.749·3).
Fever; pain.

Antidot zu Arwin Knoll, Ger.
Ancrod antiserum.
Overdosage with or adverse effects of ancrod.

Antidote Anti-Digitale Boehringer Mannheim, Switz.
Digoxin-specific antibody fragments (p.979·1).
Digitalis poisoning.

Antidoto Arvin Knoll, Spain.
Ancrod antiserum.
Overdosage with ancrod.

Antidotum Thallii Heyl Heyl, Ger.
Prussian blue (p.993·3).
Thallium poisoning.

Antidrasi Pharmec, Ital.
Dichlorphenamide (p.848·2) or dichlorphenamide sodium (p.848·2).
Control of intra-ocular pressure during eye surgery; glaucoma.

Antidry Adroka, Switz.
Bath oil: Liquid paraffin (p.1382·1); almond oil (p.1546·2).
Shower oil: Liquid paraffin (p.1382·1); soya oil (p.1355·1); levomenol (p.1596·1).
Topical lotion: Sodium lactate (p.1153·2); almond oil (p.1546·2).
Skin disorders.

Antiedema Cusi, Spain.
Sodium chloride (p.1162·2).
Corneal oedema.

Antiemorroidale Milanfarma Milanfarma, Ital.†.
Hydrocortisone acetate (p.1043·3); benzocaine (p.1286·2).
Haemorrhoids.

Antiemorroidali Ogna, Ital.
Ichthammol (p.1083·3); zinc oxide (p.1096·2); bismuth subgallate (p.1180·2); belladonna (p.457·1).
Haemorrhoids.

Antifect
Note. This name is used for preparations of different composition.
Schulke & Mayr, Ger.
Alcohol (p.1099·1); propyl alcohol (p.1124·2); glyoxal (p.1115·1).
Surface disinfection.

Potter's, UK.
Garlic (p.1583·1); garlic oil; echinacea (p.1574·2).
Nasal congestion.

Anti-Flab Suisse, Austral.†.
Arginine (p.1334·1); ornithine (p.1352·3).
Nutritional supplement.

Antiflam Rolab, S.Afr.
Ibuprofen (p.44·1).
Musculoskeletal and joint disorders.

Antiflog FIRMA, Ital.
Piroxicam (p.80·2).
Rheumatic disorders.

Antifloxil Alter, Spain.
Nimesulide (p.63·2).
Fever; inflammation; pain.

Antiflu
Note. This name is used for preparations of different composition.
Byk Gulden, Ital.
Paracetamol (p.72·2); chlorpheniramine maleate (p.405·1); caffeine (p.749·3).
Cold and influenza symptoms.

Pharmco, S.Afr.
Paracetamol (p.72·2); mepyramine maleate (p.414·1); diphenhydramine hydrochloride (p.409·1); caffeine (p.749·3); codeine phosphate (p.26·1); phenylephrine hydrochloride (p.1066·2).
Cold and influenza symptoms.

AntiFocal Vitorgan, Ger.
Animal tissue extract: diencephalon; cerebellum (p.1599·1); cort. cerebri; cerebrum fet.; medulla spinal; hepar.; pancreas; lien; thyreoidea (p.1496·3); thymus juvenil.; placenta; mucosae misc.
Nervous system disorders.

AntiFocal N Vitorgan, Ger.
Methenolone acetate (p.1450·3); liothyronine hydrochloride (p.1495·2); chorionic gonadotrophin (p.1243·1); pyridoxine hydrochloride (p.1362·3); cyanocobalamin (p.1363·3).
Nervous system disorders.

Antifohnon-N Sudmedica, Ger.
Ephedrine hydrochloride (p.1059·3); etenzamide (p.35·3).
Circulatory disorders; pain.

Antifungal Foot Deodorant Or-Dov, Austral.
Tolnaftate (p.389·1).
Tinea pedis.

Antifungol Hexal, Ger.
Clotrimazole (p.376·3).
Fungal infections of skin and genito-urinary tract.

Anti-Gas Antacid Invamed, USA.
Calcium carbonate (p.1182·1); magnesium hydroxide (p.1198·2); simethicone (p.1213·1).

Antiglan Potter's, UK.
Kava (p.1592·3); saw palmetto (p.1462·1); equisetum (p.1575·1); hydrangea.
Bladder discomfort.

Antigoutteux Rezall Medecine Vegetale, Fr.
Lithium benzoate (p.1596·3); lithium salicylate (p.50·3); colchicum (p.394·2); maize; bitter-orange (p.1610·3).
Gout; rheumatism.

Antigreg Piam, Ital.
Ticlopidine hydrochloride (p.953·1).
Thrombosis prophylaxis.

Antigrietun Casen Fleet, Spain.
Allantoin (p.1078·2); aminacrine (p.1098·3); peru balsam (p.1617·2); prednisolone (p.1048·1).
Skin disorders.

Antigrip Warner-Lambert Consumer, Belg.†.
Pholcodine (p.1068·1); quinine sulphate (p.439·2); caffeine hydrate (p.750·1); salicylamide (p.82·3); ascorbic acid (p.1365·2).
Cold symptoms.

Antigrippalin Sanofi Winthrop, Ger.†.
Quinine sulphate (p.439·2); caffeine (p.749·3); ascorbic acid (p.1365·2); salicylamide (p.82·3); paracetamol (p.72·2).
Cold symptoms; fever; influenza.

Antigrippine
Note. This name is used for preparations of different composition.
Sanofi Winthrop, Switz.†.
Paracetamol (p.72·2); codeine phosphate (p.26·1).
Cold symptoms.

SmithKline Beecham Consumer, Switz.
Paracetamol (p.72·2); ascorbic acid (p.1365·2).
Fever; pain.

Antigrippine a l'Aspirine SmithKline Beecham Sante, Fr.
Aspirin (p.16·1); ascorbic acid (p.1365·2); caffeine hydrate (p.750·1).
Fever; pain.

Antigrippine C Sanofi Winthrop, Switz.†.
Paracetamol (p.72·2); codeine phosphate (p.26·1); ascorbic acid (p.1365·2).
Cold symptoms.

Antigrippine Comp. Sanofi Winthrop, Switz.†.
Paracetamol (p.72·2); cresotamide; codeine phosphate (p.26·1); ascorbic acid (p.1365·2).
Cold symptoms.

Antigrippine Hot Drink Sanofi Midy, Neth.†.
Paracetamol (p.72·2); ascorbic acid (p.1365·2).
Cold symptoms; pain.

Antigrippine Midy SmithKline Beecham Consumer, Belg.
Paracetamol (p.72·2); 3-methylsalicylamide; codeine phosphate (p.26·1); caffeine (p.749·3); ascorbic acid (p.1365·2).
Cold symptoms.

Antigrippine Midy a la Vitamine C Sterling Midy, Fr.†.
Aspirin (p.16·1); ascorbic acid (p.1365·2); caffeine (p.749·3).
Fever; pain.

Antigrippine Nieuwe Formule SmithKline Beecham Consumer, Neth.
Paracetamol (p.72·2); caffeine (p.749·3); ascorbic acid (p.1365·2).
Fever; pain.

Anti-H Amido, Fr.
Aluminium sodium silicate (p.1178·3); kaolin (p.1195·1); sodium bicarbonate (p.1153·2); calcium carbonate (p.1182·1).
Flatulence; gastro-intestinal pain.

Antihemorr Cinfa, Spain.
Benzocaine (p.1286·2); hydrocortisone acetate (p.1043·3); neomycin sulphate (p.229·2); tannic acid (p.1634·2).
Anorectal disorders.

Anti-Hemorroidaires Cassenne, Fr.
Rectal ointment: Hydrocortisone (p.1043·3); cinchocaine hydrochloride (p.1289·2).
Suppositories: Hydrocortisone acetate (p.1043·3); esculoside (p.1543·3); benzocaine (p.1286·2).
Formerly contained hydrocortisone acetate, benzocaine, esculoside, framycetin sulphate, heparin, and butyl amino benzoate.
Anorectal disorders.

Antihemorroidal
ICN, Spain.
Ointment: Hydrocortisone acetate (p.1043·3); neomycin sulphate (p.229·2); promethazine hydrochloride (p.416·2); retinol (p.1358·1).
Suppositories: Hydrocortisone acetate (p.1043·3); promethazine hydrochloride (p.416·2); retinol (p.1358·1).
Anorectal disorders.

Rovi, Spain†.
Ointment: Belladonna (p.457·1); adrenaline (p.813·2); phenol (p.1121·2); hamamelis (p.1587·1); ichthammol (p.1083·3); tannic acid (p.1634·2); peru balsam (p.1617·2).
Anorectal disorders.

Antihist
Clonmel, Irl.; Llorens, Spain.
Chlorpheniramine maleate (p.405·1).
Hypersensitivity reactions.

Antihist-1 Goldline, USA; Major, USA; Rugby, USA.
Clemastine fumarate (p.406·2).

Antihistamine Forte Unichem, UK.
Terfenadine (p.418·1).
Hay fever; hypersensitivity reactions.

Antihist-D Goldline, USA.
Clemastine fumarate (p.406·2); phenylpropanolamine hydrochloride (p.1067·2).
Upper-respiratory-tract disorders.

Antihydral
Schmidgall, Aust.†; Robugen, Ger.; Medipharm, Switz.
Hexamine (p.216·1).
Hyperhidrosis; skin infections; wounds.

Antihydral M
Schmidgall, Aust.†; Robugen, Ger.; Medipharm, Switz.
Hexamine (p.216·1); sulphur (p.1091·2).
Fungal skin infections.

Antihypertonicum Molitor, Ger.†.
Homoeopathic preparation.

Antihypertonicum S Schuck, Ger.
Betula (p.1553·3); crataegus (p.1568·2); mistletoe (p.1604·1); fol. oleae europ.; rhododendron leaf; rutin (p.1580·2); proxyphylline (p.757·3).
Arteriosclerosis; hypertension.

Antihypertonicum-Weliplex Weber & Weber, Ger.
Homoeopathic preparation.

Antihypertonikum-Tropfen N Schuck, Ger.
Homoeopathic preparation.

Anti-inhibitor Coagulant Complex Baxter, UK.
A factor VIII inhibitor bypassing fraction (p.721·3).
Haemorrhage in patients with inhibitors to factor VIII.

Anti-Kalium Medice, Ger.
Calcium polystyrene sulphonate (p.974·3).
Hyperkalaemia.

Antikataraktikum N Ursapharm, Ger.
Disodium inosinate (p.1573·1).
Visual disturbances.

Antikataraktikum N oral Ursapharm, Ger.
Disodium uridine 5′-monophosphate.
Cataracts.

Antilinfatico E Isnardi, Ital.†.
Multivitamin preparation.

Anti-Lipide-ratiopharm Ratiopharm, Ger.†.
Clofibrate (p.1271·1); inositol nicotinate (p.891·3).
Lipid disorders.

Antilirium Forest Pharmaceuticals, USA†.
Physostigmine salicylate (p.1395·3).
Reversal of drug-induced CNS antimuscarinic effects.

Antimast N Selz, Ger.
Homoeopathic preparation.

Antimast T Selz, Ger.
Homoeopathic preparation.

Antimet
Note. This name is used for preparations of different composition.
Antigen, Irl.
Metoclopramide hydrochloride (p.1200·3).
Gastro-intestinal disorders.

Rolab, S.Afr.
Cinnarizine (p.406·1).
Nausea; vertigo.

Antimicotico
Note. This name is used for preparations of different composition.
IFI, Ital.†.
Ear drops: Benzoxiquine; dexamethasone (p.1037·1); polyenacid; benzyl alcohol (p.1103·3).
Fungal ear infections.

IFI, Ital.
Ointment: Benzoxiquine; dexamethasone (p.1037·1); pyridoxine (p.1363·1); polyenacid.
Fungal skin infections.

Savoma, Ital.
Cream: Clotrimazole (p.376·3).
Fungal infections.

Antiminth Pfizer, USA.
Pyrantel embonate (p.109·3).
Worm infections.

Antimucose Promedica, Fr.
Ox bile extract (p.1553·2).
Bowel evacuation; constipation.

Antimycoticum Stulln, Ger.†.
Hydroxyquinoline silicofluoride (p.1589·3); hydroxyquinoline hexafluorosilicate.
Fungal infections.

Antimyk Pfleger, Ger.†.
Clotrimazole (p.376·3).
Fungal infections.

Antimyopikum Ursapharm, Ger.
Troxerutin (p.1580·2); alpha tocopheryl acetate (p.1369·1).
Progressive myopia.

Antinal
Roques, Fr.; Interdelta, Switz.†.
Nifuroxazide (p.231·3).
Diarrhoea.

Anti-Naus CP Protea, Austral.†.
Prochlorperazine maleate (p.687·3).
Mental and emotional disorders; nausea and vomiting; vertigo.

Antinephrin M Hanosan, Ger.
Homoeopathic preparation.

Antinerveux Lesourd Lesourd, Fr.
Lotus petal; melilot.
Insomnia; irritability.

Antineuralgica Alpharma, Norw.
Caffeine (p.749·3); phenazone (p.78·2).
Fever; pain.

Antineuralgicum (Rowo-633) Pharmakon, Ger.
Homoeopathic preparation.
Lignocaine hydrochloride (p.1293·2) is included in this preparation to alleviate the pain of injection.

Antineurina Mabo, Spain.
Cyanocobalamin (p.1363·3); pyridoxine hydrochloride (p.1362·3); thiamine hydrochloride (p.1361·1).
Lignocaine hydrochloride (p.1293·2) is included in this preparation to alleviate the pain of injection.
Neuralgia; neuritis; peripheral neuropathy.

Antinevralgico Dr Knapp Montefarmaco, Ital.
Paracetamol (p.72·2); aspirin (p.16·1); caffeine (p.749·3).
Fever; pain.

Antinevralgico Penegal FAMA, Ital.
Paracetamol (p.72·2); aspirin (p.16·1).
Fever; pain.

Antinicoticum sine (Rowo-100) Pharmakon, Ger.
Homoeopathic preparation.

Antiobes Zyma, Spain.
Fenproporex hydrochloride (p.1481·3).
Obesity.

Anti.opt Truw, Ger.†.
Codeine phosphate (p.26·1); paracetamol (p.72·2); salicylamide (p.82·3).
Coughs and cold symptoms; neuralgia; pain.

Antiotic Andreabal, Switz.
Amoxycillin trihydrate (p.151·3).
Bacterial infections.

Antiox Mayrand, USA.
Betacarotene (p.1335·2); ascorbic acid (p.1365·2).

Antioxidans E Hevert, Ger.
dl-Alpha tocopheryl acetate (p.1369·2).
Vitamin E deficiency.

Antioxidant Nutrients Solgar, UK.
Multivitamin preparation with amino acids and zinc.
Dietary supplement.

Antioxidant Tablets Cenovis, Austral.; Vitelle, Austral.
Ascorbic acid (p.1365·2); sodium ascorbate (p.1365·2); betacarotene (p.1335·2); *d*-alpha tocopheryl acid succinate (p.1369·2); zinc amino acid chelate (p.1373·3); riboflavine (p.1362·1).
Vitamin A, C, E, B_2, and zinc deficiencies.

Antipanin N Michallik, Ger.†.
Etenzamide (p.35·3); paracetamol (p.72·2).
Pain.

Antipark Mayrhofer, Aust.†.
Bromocriptine mesylate (p.1132·2).
Acromegaly; parkinsonism.

Antiparkin Asta Medica, Ger.
Selegiline hydrochloride (p.1144·2).
Formerly known as Movergan.
Parkinsonism.

Antipen Biochemie, Aust.
Clemizole penicillin (p.191·1); benzylpenicillin sodium (p.159·3).
Lignocaine hydrochloride (p.1293·2) is included in the highest strength injections to alleviate the pain of injection.
Bacterial infections.

Antipeol
Restan, S.Afr.
Zinc oxide (p.1096·2); ichthammol (p.1083·3); salicylic acid (p.1090·2).
Skin disorders.

Medico-Biological Laboratories, UK.
Zinc oxide (p.1096·2); ichthammol (p.1083·3); salicylic acid (p.1090·2); urea (p.1095·2).
Skin disorders.

Antiphlebin Sudmedica, Ger.
Quinine hydrochloride (p.439·2); lignocaine hydrochloride (p.1293·2).
Haemorrhoids.

Antiphlogistine
Note. This name is used for preparations of different composition.
Fumouze, Fr.
Kaolin (p.1195·1); salicylic acid (p.1090·2).
Muscle and connective tissue pain.

Carter-Wallace, Switz.
Salicylic acid (p.1090·2); methyl salicylate (p.55·2); eucalyptus oil (p.1578·1); peppermint oil (p.1208·1).
Inflammation; pain.

Antiphlogistine Rub A-535 Carter Horner, Canad.
Methyl salicylate (p.55·2); camphor (p.1557·2); menthol (p.1600·2); eucalyptus oil (p.1578·1).
Musculoskeletal pain.

Antiphlogistine Rub A-535 Ice Carter Horner, Canad.
Menthol (p.1600·2).
Musculoskeletal pain.

Antiphlogistine Rub A-535 No Odour Carter Horner, Canad.
Triethanolamine salicylate (p.1639·2).
Musculoskeletal pain.

Anti-Phosphat
Brady, Aust.; Gry, Ger.
Aluminium hydroxide (p.1177·3).
Hyperphosphataemia.

Anti-Phosphate Bichsel, Switz.
Dried aluminium hydroxide (p.1177·3).
Hyperphosphataemia.

Anti-Plaque Chewing Gum Or-Dov, Austral.
Chlorhexidine acetate (p.1107·2).
Dental plaque.

Antipressan
Berk, Irl.; Berk, UK.
Atenolol (p.825·3).
Angina pectoris; arrhythmias; hypertension; myocardial infarction.

Antiprurit
Note. This name is used for preparations of different composition.
Kade, Ger.
Cell-contents and metabolic products of *Staphylococcus aureus*; *Enterococcus faecalis* (p.1594·1); *Pseudomonas aeruginosa*; and *Escherichia coli*; hydrocortisone (p.1043·3).
Skin disorders.

Kade, Switz.†.
Hydrocortisone acetate (p.1043·3); chlorphenesin (p.376·2).
Skin disorders.

Antipulmina Lisapharma, Ital.†.
Peppermint oil (p.1208·1); pumilio pine oil (p.1623·3); eucalyptus oil (p.1578·1).
Respiratory-tract disorders.

Antipyn Garec, S.Afr.
Paracetamol (p.72·2); codeine phosphate (p.26·1); caffeine (p.749·3).
Fever; pain.

Antireumina ISI, Ital.
Aspirin (p.16·1); paracetamol (p.72·2); caffeine (p.749·3).
Fever; pain.

Anti-Rhinyl Pierre Fabre, Fr.†.
Framycetin sulphate (p.210·3); sodium propionate (p.387·1).
Upper respiratory-tract infections.

Antirrinum Bama, Spain.
Chlorhexidine gluconate (p.1107·2); oxymetazoline hydrochloride (p.1065·3).
Nasal congestion.

Antisacer Wander, Switz.†.
Phenytoin sodium (p.352·3).
Epilepsy.

Antisacer comp. Wander, Ger.†.
Phenytoin sodium (p.352·3); phenobarbitone (p.350·2); potassium bromide (p.1620·3); caffeine citrate (p.749·3); atropine sulphate (p.455·1).
Epilepsy.

Antiscabbia Candioli al DDT Terapeutico
Candioli, Ital.
Benzyl benzoate (p.1402·2); benzocaine (p.1286·2); dicophane (p.1404·3).
Scabies.

Antiscabiosum Strathmann, Ger.
Benzyl benzoate (p.1402·2).
Scabies.

Antiseptic Foot Balm Scholl, UK.
Menthol (p.1600·2); halquinol (p.215·3); methyl salicylate (p.55·2).
Sore feet.

Antiseptic Lozenges Mentholatum, UK.
Menthol (p.1600·2); eucalyptus oil (p.1578·1); amylmetacresol (p.1101·3).
Colds; coughs.

Antiseptic Mouthwash Scott, Canad.
Cineole (p.1564·1); menthol (p.1600·2); thymol (p.1127·1).

Antiseptic Ointment Arjo, Canad.
Chloroxylenol (p.1111·1); benzethonium chloride (p.1102·3).
Skin protection.

Antiseptic Skin Cream National Care, Canad.
Benzethonium chloride (p.1102·3); vitamin A (p.1358·1); vitamin D (p.1366·3).
Ostomy care; skin irritation.

Antiseptic Sore Throat Lozenges Sutton, Canad.
Hexylresorcinol (p.1116·1).

Antiseptic Throat Lozenges
Note. This name is used for preparations of different composition.
Ernest Jackson, UK.
Amylmetacresol (p.1101·3); dichlorobenzyl alcohol (p.1112·2).
Sore throat.

Unichem, UK.
Amylmetacresol (p.1101·3).
Sore throat.

Antiseptic Throat Pastilles Ernest Jackson, UK.
Menthol (p.1600·2); camphor (p.1557·2); benzoic acid (p.1102·3).
Sore throats.

Antiseptico Dent Donner Domenech Garcia, Spain†.
Emetine; formaldehyde (p.1113·2); sweet birch oil (p.55·3); resorcinol (p.1090·1); zinc phenolsulphonate (p.1096·3); menthol (p.1600·2); styrax tonkinensis; myrrh (p.1606·1).
Gingivitis; pyorrhoea; stomatitis.

Antiseptique Pastilles Prodemdis, Canad.
Domiphen bromide (p.1112·3).

Antiseptique-Calmante Chauvin, Fr.
Methylene blue (p.984·3); crystal violet (p.1111·2); boric acid (p.1554·2); procaine hydrochloride (p.1299·2).
Eye disorders.

Antisettico Astringente Sedativo Bruschettini, Ital.
Zinc phenolsulphonate (p.1096·3); sulphacetamide sodium (p.252·2); naphazoline hydrochloride (p.1064·2); lignocaine hydrochloride (p.1293·2).
Conjunctivitis.

Antisklerosin S Medopharm, Ger.
Crataegus (p.1568·2); mistletoe (p.1604·1); nicotinic acid (p.1351·2); magnesium orotate (p.1611·2); rutin (p.1580·2).
Arteriosclerosis and associated circulatory disorders; hyperlipidaemias.

Anti-Smoking Tablets Potter's, UK.
Lobelia (p.1481·3).
Aid to smoking withdrawal.

Antispas Keene, USA.
Dicyclomine hydrochloride (p.460·1).
Functional bowel syndrome; irritable bowel syndrome.

Antispasmina Colica Recordati, Ital.
Papaverine hydrochloride (p.1614·2); belladonna (p.457·1).
Gastro-intestinal spasm.

Antispasmina Colica B Recordati, Ital.†.
Belladonna (p.457·1); valerian (p.1643·1).
Smooth muscle spasm.

Antispasmodic Elixir Morton Grove, USA.
Phenobarbitone (p.350·2); hyoscyamine sulphate (p.464·2); atropine sulphate (p.455·1); hyoscine hydrobromide (p.462·3).

Antistax Pharmaton, Ger.
Red vine leaves.
Venous disorders.

Antistine-Privine Ciba Vision, Austral.
Antazoline sulphate (p.402·1); naphazoline nitrate (p.1064·2).
Allergic conjunctivitis; eye irritation.

Antistin-Privin
Ciba Vision, Ger.; Ciba Vision, Norw.†; Novartis, S.Afr.; Ciba Vision, Switz.
Antazoline sulphate (p.402·1); naphazoline nitrate (p.1064·2).
Allergic conjunctivitis.

Antistin-Privina Ciba Vision, Ital.
Antazoline sulphate (p.402·1); naphazoline nitrate (p.1064·2).
Allergic conjunctivitis.

Antitiroide Panthox & Burck, Ital.†.
Methimazole (p.1495·3).
Hyperthyroidism.

Antitis Potter's, UK.
Buchu leaf (p.1555·2); clivers (p.1565·2); couch-grass (p.1567·3); equisetum (p.1575·1); shepherds purse; uva ursi (p.1552·2).
Urinary or bladder discomfort.

Antituss
Note. A similar name is used for preparations of different composition.
Pharmco, S.Afr.
Promethazine hydrochloride (p.416·2); codeine phosphate (p.26·1); ephedrine hydrochloride (p.1059·3).
Cold symptoms; coughs.

Anti-Tuss
Note. A similar name is used for preparations of different composition.
Century, USA.
Guaiphenesin (p.1061·3).
Coughs.

Antitussive Decongestant Antihistamine Syrup Prodemdis, Canad.
Phenylpropanolamine hydrochloride (p.1067·2); pheniramine maleate (p.415·3); mepyramine maleate (p.414·1); dextromethorphan hydrobromide (p.1057·3).

Antitussivum Burger Ysatfabrik, Ger.
Dihydrocodeine tartrate (p.34·1); thyme oil (p.1637·1).
Coughs.

Antituxil-Z Ghimas, Ital.†.
Zipeprol hydrochloride (p.1071·3).
Coughs.

Antivenin Wyeth-Ayerst, Canad.
Crotalidae antiserum (p.1534·1).
Snake envenomation.

Antivenin (Latrodectus Mactans) Merck Sharp & Dohme, Canad.
Black widow spider antiserum (p.1534·3).
Black widow spider bite.

Antiverrugas Isdin, Spain.
Lactic acid (p.1593·3); salicylic acid (p.1090·2).
Warts.

Antivert
Note. This name is used for preparations of different composition.
Pfizer, Canad.
Meclozine hydrochloride (p.413·3); nicotinic acid (p.1351·2).
Radiation sickness; vascular headaches; vertigo.

Roerig, USA.
Meclozine hydrochloride (p.413·3).
Motion sickness; vertigo.

Antiviscosin-N-Schlankheitstee Hameln, Ger.†.
Senna; frangula bark; aniseed; fennel; achillea; couch-grass.
Herbal preparation.

Antizid Lilly, S.Afr.
Nizatidine (p.1203·2).
Heartburn; hyperacidity.

Antizol
Cambridge, UK; Orphan Medical, USA.
Fomepizole (p.982·1).
Available on a named patient basis only in the *UK*.
Ethylene glycol poisoning.

Antizona Alonga, Spain.
Idoxuridine (p.613·2) in dimethyl sulphoxide.
Cutaneous herpes infections.

Antocin Allergan, Ital.
Vaccinium myrtillus (p.1606·1).
Capillary disorders.

Antoderin Rosen, Ger.†.
Oxazepam (p.683·2).
Anxiety; nervous disorders; sleep disorders.

Antodrel Ciba Vision, Spain†.
Pilocarpine hydrochloride (p.1396·3).
Glaucoma; ocular hypertension; production of miosis.

Antomiopic Ciba Vision, Spain.
Vitamins and amino acids; myrtillus (p.1606·1).
Eye disorders.

Antopal Bama, Spain.
Binifibrate (p.1269·2).
Hyperlipidaemias.

Antoral Recordati, Ital.
Tibezonium iodide (p.1637·3).
Mouth and throat disinfection.

Antoxymega Larkhall Laboratories, UK.
Multivitamin and mineral preparation.

Antra
Recipe, Aust.; Astra, Ger.; Astra, Ital.; Astra, Switz.
Omeprazole (p.1204·2) or omeprazole sodium (p.1204·2).
Gastro-oesophageal reflux; peptic ulcer; Zollinger-Ellison syndrome.

Antrenyl
Ciba-Geigy, Belg.†.; Ciba, Neth.†.; Ciba, Switz.†.
Oxyphenonium bromide (p.466·3).
Smooth muscle spasm.

Antrima Doms-Adrian, Fr.
Co-trimazine (p.196·3).
Bacterial infections; Pneumocystis carinii pneumonia.

Antrimox Antigen, Irl.
Co-trimoxazole (p.196·3).
Bacterial infections.

Antrizine Major, USA.
Meclozine hydrochloride (p.413·3).
Motion sickness; vertigo.

Antrocol Poythress, USA.
Atropine sulphate (p.455·1); phenobarbitone (p.350·2).
Gastro-intestinal disorders.

Anturan
Ciba-Geigy, Aust.; Novartis, Austral.; Geigy, Canad.; Ciba-Geigy, Irl.†; Ciba-Geigy, S.Afr.†; Geigy, Switz.; Geigy, UK.
Sulphinpyrazone (p.395·2).
Gout; hyperuricaemia; myocardial infarction; thrombo-embolic disorders.

Anturane Novartis, USA.
Sulphinpyrazone (p.395·2).
Gouty arthritis.

Anturano Ciba, Ger.†.
Sulphinpyrazone (p.395·2).
Gout; hyperuricaemia; thrombo-embolic disorders.

Antussan *Dolorgiet, Ger.*
Oral drops; oral liquid: Thyme (p.1636·3).
Formerly contained menthol, camphor, benzoic acid, ephedrine hydrochloride, sodium dibunate, thyme, and primula rhizome.
Catarrh; coughs.
Tablets: Ambroxol hydrochloride (p.1054·3).
Respiratory-tract disorders with increased or viscous mucus.

Antussan "T" *Henk, Ger.†.*
Thyme (p.1636·3).
Respiratory-tract disorders.

Anucort-HC *G & W, USA.*
Hydrocortisone acetate (p.1043·3).

Anugesic *Parke, Davis, S.Afr.*
Ointment: Pramoxine hydrochloride (p.1298·2).
Suppositories: Bismuth subgallate (p.1180·2); bismuth oxide (p.1180·1); resorcinol (p.1090·1); bismuth oxyiodide (p.1181·1); peru balsam (p.1617·2); benzyl benzoate (p.1402·2); zinc oxide (p.1096·2); boric acid (p.1554·2); pramoxine hydrochloride (p.1298·2).
Anorectal disorders.

Anugesic-HC
Note. This name is used for preparations of different composition.
Parke, Davis, Canad.
Pramoxine hydrochloride (p.1298·2); hydrocortisone acetate (p.1043·3); zinc sulphate (p.1373·2).
Anorectal disorders.

Parke, Davis, Irl.
Cream: Pramoxine hydrochloride (p.1298·2); hydrocortisone acetate (p.1043·3); zinc oxide (p.1096·2); peru balsam (p.1617·2); benzyl benzoate (p.1402·2); bismuth oxide (p.1180·1); resorcinol (p.1090·1).
Suppositories: Pramoxine hydrochloride (p.1298·2); hydrocortisone acetate (p.1043·3); zinc oxide (p.1096·2); bismuth subgallate (p.1180·2); peru balsam (p.1617·2); benzyl benzoate (p.1402·2); bismuth oxide (p.1180·1).
Anorectal disorders.

Parke, Davis, UK.
Cream: Pramoxine hydrochloride (p.1298·2); hydrocortisone acetate (p.1043·3); bismuth oxide (p.1180·1); peru balsam (p.1617·2); zinc oxide (p.1096·2); benzyl benzoate (p.1402·2).
Suppositories: Pramoxine hydrochloride (p.1298·2); hydrocortisone acetate (p.1043·3); zinc oxide (p.1096·2); bismuth subgallate (p.1180·2); bismuth oxide (p.1180·1); Peru balsam (p.1617·2); benzyl benzoate (p.1402·2).
Anorectal disorders.

Anumed *Major, USA.*
Bismuth subgallate (p.1180·2); bismuth resorcinol compound (p.1181·1); benzyl benzoate (p.1402·2); zinc oxide (p.1096·2); peru balsam (p.1617·2).
Anorectal disorders.

Anumed HC *Major, USA.*
Hydrocortisone acetate (p.1043·3); bismuth subgallate (p.1180·2); bismuth resorcinol compound (p.1181·1); benzyl benzoate (p.1402·2); peru balsam (p.1617·2); zinc oxide (p.1096·2).
Anorectal disorders.

Anumedin *Kade, Ger.*
Prednisolone acetate (p.1048·1); cinchocaine hydrochloride (p.1289·2).
Anorectal disorders.

Anuprep HC *Great Southern, USA†.*
Hydrocortisone acetate (p.1043·3).

Anuprep Hemorrhoidal *Great Southern, USA†.*
Bismuth subgallate (p.1180·2); bismuth resorcinol compound (p.1181·1); benzyl benzoate (p.1402·2); peru balsam (p.1617·2); zinc oxide (p.1096·2).

Anusept *Lichtenstein, Ger.*
Bismuth subnitrate (p.1180·2); zinc oxide (p.1096·2); benzocaine (p.1286·2).
Anorectal disorders.

Anusol
Note. This name is used for preparations of different composition.
Parke, Davis, Austral.
Suppositories; ointment: Zinc oxide (p.1096·2); peru balsam (p.1617·2); benzyl benzoate (p.1402·2).
Anorectal disorders.

Warner-Lambert, Austral.
Wipes: Hamamelis water (p.1587·1); glycerol (p.1585·2).
Anorectal irritation.

Warner-Lambert, Canad.
Zinc sulphate (p.1373·2).
Anorectal disorders.

Warner-Lambert, Fr.
Bismuth oxide (p.1180·1); bismuth subgallate (p.1180·2); zinc oxide (p.1096·2).
Anorectal disorders.

Warner-Lambert, Ger.
Bismuth oxide-bismuthoxyiodide-1,3-bis-(ammoniumoxy)-benzol-4,5-(bismuthylsulphonate); zinc oxide (p.1096·2); peru balsam (p.1617·2).
Anorectal disorders.

Warner-Lambert, Irl.
Cream: Zinc oxide (p.1096·2); bismuth oxide (p.1180·1); peru balsam (p.1617·2).
Suppositories; ointment: Bismuth subgallate (p.1180·2); bismuth oxide (p.1180·1); peru balsam (p.1617·2); zinc oxide (p.1096·2).
Anorectal disorders.

Warner-Lambert, Ital.
Resorcinol (p.1090·1); yellow bismuth oxide (p.1180·1); bismuth subgallate (p.1180·2); bismuth oxyiodide (p.1181·1); peru balsam (p.1617·2); zinc oxide (p.1096·2).
Anorectal disorders.

Warner-Lambert, Neth.
Bismuth subgallate (p.1180·2); zinc oxide (p.1096·2).
Anorectal disorders.

Lundbeck, Norw.†.
Bismuth resorcinol compound (p.1181·1); zinc oxide (p.1096·2); peru balsam (p.1617·2).
Anorectal disorders.

Parke, Davis, S.Afr.
Ointment: Bismuth subgallate (p.1180·2); bismuth oxide (p.1180·1); zinc oxide (p.1096·2).
Formerly contained bismuth subgallate, bismuth oxide, resorcinol, bismuth oxyiodide, benzyl benzoate, Peru balsam, and zinc oxide.
Suppositories: Bismuth subgallate (p.1180·2); bismuth oxide (p.1180·1); zinc oxide (p.1096·2).
Formerly contained bismuth oxyiodide, bismuth subgallate, bismuth oxide, resorcinol, Peru balsam, benzyl benzoate, and zinc oxide.
Anorectal disorders.

Warner-Lambert, Spain†.
Ointment: Bismuth resorcinol compound (p.1181·1); bismuth oxyiodide (p.1181·1); bismuth subgallate (p.1180·2); peru balsam (p.1617·2).
Suppositories: Peru balsam (p.1617·2); bismuth iodoresorcinol sulphate (p.1181·1); zinc oxide (p.1096·2).
Anorectal disorders.

Lundbeck, Swed.
Bismuth oxyiodoresorcinsulphonate; zinc oxide (p.1096·2); peru balsam (p.1617·2).
Anorectal disorders.

Warner-Lambert Consumer, Switz.
Bismuth oxide (p.1180·1); bismuth subgallate (p.1180·2); bismuth oxyiodide (p.1181·1); peru balsam (p.1617·2); benzyl benzoate (p.1402·2); zinc oxide (p.1096·2).
Anorectal disorders.

Parke, Davis, UK.
Cream: Bismuth oxide (p.1180·1); peru balsam (p.1617·2); zinc oxide (p.1096·2).
Ointment; suppositories: Bismuth subgallate (p.1180·2); bismuth oxide (p.1180·1); peru balsam (p.1617·2); zinc oxide (p.1096·2).
Anorectal disorders.

Glaxo Wellcome, USA.
Suppositories: Starch (p.1356·2); benzyl alcohol (p.1103·3); soybean oil (p.1355·1); tocopheryl acetate (p.1369·1).
Formerly contained bismuth subgallate, bismuth resorcinol compound, benzyl benzoate, zinc oxide, and peru balsam.
Anorectal disorders.

Parke, Davis, USA.
Ointment: Zinc oxide (p.1096·2); pramoxine hydrochloride (p.1298·2); peru balsam (p.1617·2); benzyl benzoate (p.1402·2).
Anorectal disorders.

Anusol Antifungal Foot Powder *Young, USA.*
Miconazole nitrate (p.384·3).
Fungal infections.

Anusol + H *Godecke, Ger.†.*
Bismuth oxide-bismuth oxyiodide-1,3-bis-(ammonium oxy)benzol-4,6-bis-(bismuthylsulphonate) complex (pp.1180·1 and 1181·1); zinc oxide (p.1096·2); peru balsam (p.1617·2); hydrocortisone acetate (p.1043·3).
Anorectal disorders.

Anusol Plus *Warner-Lambert, Canad.*
Pramoxine hydrochloride (p.1298·2); zinc sulphate (p.1373·2).
Anorectal disorders.

Anusol-HC
Note. This name is used for preparations of different composition.
Warner-Lambert, Austral.†.
Hydrocortisone acetate (p.1043·3); bismuth subgallate (p.1180·2); bismuth resorcinol compound (p.1181·1); bismuth oxyiodide (p.1181·1); boric acid (p.1554·2); zinc oxide (p.1096·2); peru balsam (p.1617·2); benzyl benzoate (p.1402·2).
Anorectal disorders.

Parke, Davis, Canad.
Zinc sulphate (p.1373·2); hydrocortisone acetate (p.1043·3).
Anorectal disorders.

Parke, Davis, Irl.
Hydrocortisone acetate (p.1043·3); benzyl benzoate (p.1402·2); bismuth subgallate (p.1180·2); bismuth oxide (p.1180·1); peru balsam (p.1617·2); zinc oxide (p.1096·2).
Anorectal disorders.

Parke, Davis, S.Afr.
Bismuth subgallate (p.1180·2); bismuth oxide (p.1180·1); bismuth oxyiodide (p.1181·1); resorcinol (p.1090·1); peru balsam (p.1617·2); benzyl benzoate (p.1402·2); zinc oxide (p.1096·2); boric acid (p.1554·2); hydrocortisone acetate (p.1043·3).
Anorectal disorders.

Parke, Davis, USA.
Hydrocortisone acetate (p.1043·3).
Anorectal disorders; skin disorders.

Anusol-HC, Anusol Plus HC *Warner-Lambert, UK.*
Bismuth subgallate (p.1180·2); bismuth oxide (p.1180·1); peru balsam (p.1617·2); zinc oxide (p.1096·2); hydrocortisone acetate (p.1043·3); benzyl benzoate (p.1402·2).
Anusol HC formerly contained bismuth subgallate, bismuth oxide, peru balsam, zinc oxide, hydrocortisone acetate, benzyl benzoate, and resorcinol.
Anorectal disorders.

Anuzinc *Technilab, Canad.*
Zinc sulphate (p.1373·2).
Anorectal disorders.

Anvatrol *Nelson, Austral.†.*
Fructose (p.1343·2); anhydrous glucose (p.1343·3); phosphoric acid (p.1618·1).
Nausea and vomiting.

Anvitoff
Knoll, Ger.; Knoll, Switz.
Tranexamic acid (p.728·2).
Haemorrhagic disorders.

Anxanil *Econo Med, USA†.*
Hydroxyzine hydrochloride (p.412·1).
Anxiety; hypersensitivity reactions.

Anxicalm *Clonmel, Irl.*
Diazepam (p.661·1).
Anxiety; epilepsy; insomnia; premedication; skeletal muscle spasm.

Anxiocard *Gerot, Aust.†.*
Oxazepam (p.683·2); dipyridamole (p.857·1).
Cardiovascular disorders.

Anxiolit
Gerot, Aust.; Medichemie, Switz.
Oxazepam (p.683·2).
Anxiety; insomnia.

Anxiolit plus *Gerot, Aust.*
Oxazepam (p.683·2); methylbenactyzium bromide (p.465·2).
Anxiety disorders.

Anxoral *IPRAD, Fr.*
Phenobarbitone (p.350·2); crataegus (p.1568·2); passion flower (p.1615·3); valerian (p.1643·1).
Formerly contained crataegus, passion flower, valerian, sparteine sulphate, phenobarbitone, and papaverine hydrochloride.
Anxiety; insomnia.

Any *Homme de Fer, Fr.*
Mequinol (p.1086·2).
Hyperpigmentation.

Anzatax *Faulding, Austral.*
Paclitaxel (p.556·3).
Breast cancer; ovarian cancer.

Anzem *Rolab, S.Afr.*
Diltiazem hydrochloride (p.854·2).
Angina pectoris; hypertension.

Anzemet
Hoechst Marion Roussel, Austral.; Hoechst Marion Roussel, USA.
Dolasetron mesylate (p.1190·2).
Nausea and vomiting.

Aolept *Bayer, Ger.†.*
Pericyazine (p.685·2).
Pain; psychiatric disorders.

A-O-Q10 MaxiPower Formula *Solgar, UK.*
Multivitamin and mineral preparation with amino acids, coenzyme Q-10, and fibre.
Dietary supplement.

Aosept
Ciba Vision, Aust.; Ciba Vision, Austral.; Ciba Vision, Fr.†; Ciba Vision, USA.
Hydrogen peroxide (p.1116·2).
Disinfecting solution for soft contact lenses.

Aotal *Lipha Sante, Fr.*
Acamprosate calcium (p.640·1).
Alcoholism.

APA *Lannacher, Aust.*
Suppositories: Paracetamol (p.72·2); propyphenazone (p.81·3).
Fever; pain.
Tablets: Paracetamol (p.72·2); dextropropoxyphene hydrochloride (p.27·3).
Pain.

APAC Improved *Vortech, USA.*
Aspirin (p.16·1); caffeine (p.749·3).
Pain.

Apacef
Zeneca, Belg.; Zeneca, Fr.
Cefotetan disodium (p.170·1).
Lignocaine hydrochloride (p.1293·2) is included in the intramuscular injection to alleviate the pain of injection.
Bacterial infections.

Apacet
Merck, Aust.†.; Parmed, USA.
Paracetamol (p.72·2).
Fever; pain.

Apagen *Stomygen, Ital.*
Hydroxyapatite (p.1589·2).
Dental disorders.

Apaisance *Lierac, Fr.*
Tilia (p.1637·3); levomenol (p.1596·1).
Hypersensitive skin.

Apaisyl *Monot, Fr.*
Isothipendyl hydrochloride (p.412·2).
Hypersensitivity.

Apamid
Weifa, Norw.; Parke, Davis, Swed.
Glipizide (p.320·3).
Diabetes mellitus.

Apamox *Martin, Spain.*
Amoxycillin trihydrate (p.151·3).
Bacterial infections.

Apap *Alra, USA.*
Paracetamol (p.72·2).

A-Par
Note. This name is used for preparations of different composition.
SCAT, Fr.
Esdepallethrine (p.1406·1); piperonyl butoxide (p.1409·3).
Adjunct to treatment of scabies; destruction of scabies mite in textiles.

SCAT, Switz.
Pyrethrum (p.1410·1); piperonyl butoxide (p.1409·3).
Pediculosis.

Aparoxal *Veyron-Froment, Fr.*
Phenobarbitone (p.350·2).
Epilepsy; tremor.

Aparsonin N *Merckle, Ger.*
Bromhexine hydrochloride (p.1055·3).
Respiratory-tract disorders associated with increased mucus.

Apatate *Kenwood, USA.*
Vitamin B complex.

Apatate with Fluoride *Kenwood, USA.*
Vitamin B substances with sodium fluoride (p.742·1).

Apatef
Lederle, Austral.; Zeneca, Ger.†; Zeneca, Ital.
Cefotetan disodium (p.170·1).
Bacterial infections.

Apatite *Weleda, UK.*
Homoeopathic preparation.

Apegmone *Lipha Sante, Fr.*
Tioclomarol (p.954·3).
Thrombo-embolic disorders.

Apekumarol *Pharmacia Upjohn, Swed.*
Dicoumarol (p.848·2).
Thrombo-embolic disorders.

Apen *Xixia, S.Afr.*
Ampicillin (p.153·1); cloxacillin (p.195·2).
Bacterial infections.

Aperamid *Ardeypharm, Ger.*
Loperamide hydrochloride (p.1197·2).
Diarrhoea.

Aperdan *ABC, Ital.*
Naproxen cetrimonium (p.62·1).
Formerly contained dequalinium chloride, crotamiton, undecenoic acid diethanolamide, thymol, and phenoxyethanol.
Vulvovaginal disorders.

Apergan *Panzera, Ital.*
Royal jelly (p.1626·3); glucose (p.1343·3); ginseng (p.1584·2).
Nutritional supplement.

Aperisan *Dentinox, Ger.*
Sage (p.1627·1).
Mouth and throat inflammation.

Apernyl
Bayer, Ger.†; Bayer, Ital.†.
Aspirin (p.16·1).
Dental pain and inflammation.

Aperop *Pharmacobel, Belg.*
Nux vomica (p.1609·3); kola (p.1645·1); orange peel (p.1610·3); cinchona bark (p.1564·1); haemoglobin (p.723·3); iodine (p.1493·1); tannic acid (p.1634·2); calcium phosphate hydrochloride.
Tonic.

Apetil *Ram, USA.*
Multivitamin and mineral preparation.

Apetinil-Depo *Syntex, Switz.*
Ethylamphetamine hydrochloride.
Obesity.

Aphenylbarbit *Streuli, Switz.*
Phenobarbitone (p.350·2).
Epilepsy.

Aphilan *Darcy, Fr.*
Buclizine hydrochloride (p.404·1).
Allergic disorders; pruritic skin disorders.

Aphloine P *DB, Fr.*
Aphloia; hamamelis (p.1587·1); hydrastis (p.1588·2); piscidia; viburnum; esculoside (p.1543·3).
Haemorrhoids; peripheral vascular insufficiency.

Aphlomycine *Fumouze, Fr.†.*
Tetracycline hydrochloride (p.259·1); chymotrypsin (p.1563·2).
Bacterial infections.

Aphrodyne *Star, USA.*
Yohimbine hydrochloride (p.1645·3).

Aphthasol *Block, USA.*
Amlexanox (p.749·1).
Aphthous ulcers.

Aphtiria *Debat, Fr.*
Lindane (p.1407·2).
Disinfection of clothes and bedding; pediculosis.

Api Baby *Sanitalia, Ital.*
Pollen; royal jelly (p.1626·3); fructose; myrtillus (p.1606·1).
Nutritional supplement.

Apifor *Parke, Davis, Spain†.*
Thymoxamine hydrochloride (p.952·2).
Vascular disorders.

Apihepar *Asta Medica, Aust.*
Silybum marianum (p.993·3).
Liver disorders.

Apimid *Apogepha, Ger.*
Flutamide (p.537·1).
Prostatic cancer.

Apiocolina *Bruschettini, Ital.*
Escherichia coli lysate.
Anorectal inflammation.

Apir Clorurado *Pharmacia Upjohn, Spain.*
Sodium chloride (p.1162·2).
Fluid and electrolyte disorders.

Apir Cloruro Amonico *Pharmacia Upjohn, Spain.*
Ammonium chloride (p.1055·2).
Hypochloraemia; metabolic alkalosis.

Apir Glucoibys *Pharmacia Upjohn, Spain.*
Glucose (p.1343·3).
Carbohydrate source; fluid and electrolyte disorders.

Apir Glucopotasico *Pharmacia Upjohn, Spain.*
Glucose (p.1343·3); potassium chloride (p.1161·1).
Hypokalaemia.

Apir Glucosado *Pharmacia Upjohn, Spain.*
Glucose (p.1343·3).
Fluid and electrolyte disorders; parenteral nutrition.

Apir Glucosalino *Pharmacia Upjohn, Spain.*
Glucose (p.1343·3); sodium chloride (p.1162·2).
Fluid and electrolyte disorders.

Apir Ringer *Pharmacia Upjohn, Spain.*
Electrolyte infusion (p.1147·1).
Fluid and electrolyte depletion.

Apir Ringer Lactate *Pharmacia Upjohn, Spain.*
Electrolyte infusion with sodium lactate (p.1147·1).
Fluid and electrolyte depletion.

Apiretal *Ern, Spain.*
Paracetamol (p.72·2).
Fever; pain.

Apiroflex Clorurado Simp *Antibioticos, Spain†.*
Sodium chloride (p.1162·2).
Fluid and electrolyte disorders.

Apiroflex Glucosada *Pharmacia Upjohn, Spain.*
Glucose (p.1343·3).
Fluid and electrolyte disorders; parenteral nutrition.

Apis *Brauer, Austral.*
Homoeopathic preparation.

Apisate
John Wyeth, Irl.†; Wyeth, UK†.
Diethylpropion hydrochloride (p.1479·3); vitamin B substances.
Obesity.

Apiserum *DB, Fr.*
Royal jelly (p.1626·3).
Tonic.

Apiserum con Telergon I *Codit, Ital.*
Wine; acacia honey (p.1345·3); royal jelly (p.1626·3).
Nutritional supplement.

Apisgel *Dolisos, Canad.*
Homoeopathic preparation.

Apistress *Sanitalia, Ital.*
Royal jelly (p.1626·3); pollen; propolis (p.1621·3).
Nutritional supplement.

APL
Wyeth, Austral.; Wyeth-Ayerst, Canad.; Akromed, S.Afr.; Ayerst, USA.
Chorionic gonadotrophin (p.1243·1).
Cryptorchidism; infertility; habitual abortion; male hypogonadism; pituitary dwarfism.

Aplace *Kyorin, Jpn.*
Troxipide (p.1218·1).
Gastritis; peptic ulcer.

Aplactin *Mead Johnson, Ital.*
Pravastatin sodium (p.1277·1).
Arteriosclerosis; hyperlipidaemias.

Aplaket *Rottapharm, Ital.*
Ticlopidine hydrochloride (p.953·1).
Thrombotic disorders.

Aplakil *Aristegui, Spain†.*
Oxazepam (p.683·2).
Anxiety; insomnia.

Aplexil
Gerot, Aust.; Rhone-Poulenc, Ger.†.
Oxomemazine (p.415·2); guaiphenesin (p.1061·3); paracetamol (p.72·2); sodium benzoate (p.1102·3).
Respiratory-tract disorders.

Aplisol *Parke, Davis, USA.*
Tuberculin purified protein derivative (p.1640·2).
Diagnosis of tuberculosis.

Aplitest *Parke, Davis, USA.*
Tuberculin purified protein derivative (p.1640·2).
Diagnosis of tuberculosis.

Aplodan *Astra, Ital.*
Injection†: Creatinolfosfate sodium (p.1568·3).
Tablets; effervescent granules: Creatinolfosfate (p.1568·3).
Cardiac disorders.

Aplona *Gastropharm, Ger.*
Apple powder; colloidal silicon dioxide (p.1475·1).
Diarrhoea.

Apo-Amilzide *Apotex, Canad.*
Hydrochlorothiazide (p.885·2); amiloride hydrochloride (p.819·2).
Hypertension; oedema.

Apo-C *Apotex, Canad.*
Ascorbic acid (p.1365·2).
Vitamin supplement.

Apo-Cal *Apotex, Canad.*
Calcium carbonate (p.1182·1).
Calcium supplement.

Apocanda *Apogepha, Ger.*
Clotrimazole (p.376·3).
Fungal infections.

Apocard *Esteve, Spain.*
Flecainide acetate (p.868·3).
Arrhythmias.

Apo-Chlorax *Apotex, Canad.*
Chlordiazepoxide hydrochloride (p.646·3); clidinium bromide (p.459·2).
Anticholinergic; anxiolytic.

Apocillin *Alpharma, Norw.*
Phenoxymethylpenicillin potassium (p.236·2).
Bacterial infections.

Apo-Cloxi *Apotex, Canad.*
Cloxacillin sodium (p.195·2).
Bacterial infections.

Apocortal *Alpharma, Norw.*
Hydrocortisone acetate (p.1043·3).
Skin disorders.

Apodorm
Alpharma, Norw.; Dumex-Alpharma, Swed.
Nitrazepam (p.682·2).
Epilepsy; infantile spasm; insomnia.

Apo-Doxy *Apotex, Canad.*
Doxycycline hydrochloride (p.202·3).
Bacterial infections.

Apo-Gain *Apotex, Canad.*
Minoxidil (p.910·3).
Alopecia androgenetica.

Apo-Hepat *Pekana, Ger.*
Homoeopathic preparation.

Apo-Hexa *Apotex, Canad.*
Multivitamin preparation.

Apo-Hydro *Apotex, Canad.*
Hydrochlorothiazide (p.885·2).
Hypertension; oedema.

Apo-Infekt *Pekana, Ger.*
Homoeopathic preparation.

Apo-Ipravent *Apotex, Canad.*
Ipratropium bromide (p.754·2).
Bronchodilator.

Apo-ISDN *Apotex, Canad.*
Isosorbide dinitrate (p.893·1).
Angina pectoris.

Apo-K *Apotex, Canad.*
Potassium chloride (p.1161·1).
Potassium depletion.

Apo-Keto *Apotex, Canad.*
Ketoprofen (p.48·2).
Inflammation; pain.

Apokinon *Aguettant, Fr.*
Apomorphine hydrochloride (p.1131·1).
Parkinsonism.

Apolar
Alpharma, Norw.; Dumex-Alpharma, Swed.
Desonide (p.1036·3).
Skin disorders.

Apolar med dekvalon *Alpharma, Norw.*
Desonide (p.1036·3); dequalinium chloride (p.1112·1).
Infected skin disorders.

Apo-Levocarb *Apotex, Canad.*
Levodopa (p.1137·1); carbidopa (p.1136·1).
Parkinsonism.

Apo-Methazide *Apotex, Canad.*
Methyldopa (p.904·2); hydrochlorothiazide (p.885·2).
Hypertension.

Apomine *Faulding, Austral.*
Apomorphine hydrochloride (p.1131·1).
Parkinsonism.

Aponal *Boehringer Mannheim, Ger.; Dresden, Ger.*
Doxepin hydrochloride (p.283·2).
Anxiety; depression; insomnia; withdrawal syndromes.

Apo-Napro-Na *Apotex, Canad.*
Naproxen sodium (p.61·2).
Inflammation; pain.

Apo-Nifed *Apotex, Canad.*
Nifedipine (p.916·2).
Angina pectoris; hypertension.

Aponil *Glaxo Allen, Ital.*
Lacidipine (p.897·1).
Hypertension.

Apo-Pen-VK *Apotex, Canad.*
Phenoxymethylpenicillin potassium (p.236·2).
Bacterial infections.

Apoplectal *Klinge, Aust.*
Etofylline (p.753·1); aesculus extract (p.1543·3); buphenine hydrochloride (p.1555·3).
Cerebrovascular disorders.

Apoplectal N *Klinge, Ger.*
Aesculus (p.1543·3); buphenine hydrochloride (p.1555·3).
Formerly contained aesculus, buphenine hydrochloride, and etofylline.
Cerebrovascular disorders.

Apo-Prazo *Apotex, Canad.*
Prazosin hydrochloride (p.932·3).
Hypertension.

Apo-Pulm *Pekana, Ger.*
Homoeopathic preparation.

Aporex *Alpharma, Norw.*
Dextropropoxyphene hydrochloride (p.27·3); paracetamol (p.72·2).
Pain.

Aporil *Qualiphar, Belg.*
Salicylic acid (p.1090·2); acetic acid (p.1541·2); lactic acid (p.1593·3); thuja (p.1636·3); chelidonium.
Warts.

Apo-Salvent *Apotex, Canad.*
Salbutamol (p.758·2) or salbutamol sulphate (p.758·2).
Bronchoconstriction.

Apo-Sulfatrim *Apotex, Canad.*
Co-trimoxazole (p.196·3).
Bacterial infections; Pneumocystis carinii pneumonia.

Apo-Sulin *Apotex, Canad.*
Sulindac (p.86·3).
Inflammation; pain.

Apo-Tamox *Apotex, Canad.*
Tamoxifen citrate (p.563·3).
Malignant neoplasms.

Apo-Tetra *Apotex, Canad.*
Tetracycline hydrochloride (p.259·1).
Bacterial infections.

Apotheker Bauer's Blahungstee *Jauntal, Aust.*
Angelica; fennel (p.1579·1); chamomile (p.1561·2); coriander (p.1567·3); sage (p.1627·1).
Flatulence.

Apotheker Bauer's Brust- und Hustentee
Jauntal, Aust.
Fennel (p.1579·1); Iceland moss; primula flowers; thyme leaf (p.1636·3); verbascum flowers.
Catarrh.

Apotheker Bauer's Franzbranntwein-Gel
Jauntal, Aust.
Brandy (p.1099·1); concentrated ammonia (p.1548·3).
Insect bites; minor injuries.

Apotheker Bauer's Grippetee *Jauntal, Aust.*
Primula rhizome; pimpinella; sambucus (p.1627·2); tilia (p.1637·3); crataegus (p.1568·2).
Cold and influenza symptoms.

Apotheker Bauer's Harntreibender Tee
Jauntal, Aust.
Urtica (p.1642·3); orthosiphon leaves (p.1592·2); parsley root (p.1615·3); solidago virgaurea; juniper (p.1592·2).
Renal calculi.

Apotheker Bauer's Huhneraugentinktur
Jauntal, Aust.
Salicylic acid (p.1090·2); lactic acid (p.1593·3); resorcinol (p.1090·1); flexible collodion.
Corns and callouses.

Apotheker Bauer's Inhalationsmischung
Jauntal, Aust.
Eucalyptus oil (p.1578·1); juniper oil (p.1592·3); pumilio pine oil (p.1623·3).
Respiratory-tract disorders.

Apotheker Bauer's Kindertee *Jauntal, Aust.*
Orange flowers; fennel (p.1579·1); clove (p.1565·2); hibiscus flowers; pansy.
Gastro-intestinal disorders.

Apotheker Bauer's Magentee *Jauntal, Aust.*
Angelica; caraway (p.1559·3); mallow leaves; rosemary leaves; centaury (p.1561·1); calendula officinalis.
Gastro-intestinal disorders.

Apotheker Bauer's Misteltinktur *Jauntal, Aust.*
Mistletoe (p.1604·1).
Circulatory disorders.

Apotheker Bauer's Nieren- und Blasentee
Jauntal, Aust.
Silver birch leaves (p.1553·3); urtica (p.1642·3); orthosiphon leaves (p.1592·2); solidago virgaurea; bearberry (p.1552·2).
Kidney and bladder disorders.

Apo-Theo *Apotex, Canad.*
Theophylline (p.765·1).
Bronchospasm.

Apo-Timol *Apotex, Canad.*
Timolol maleate (p.953·3).
Angina pectoris; hypertension.

Apo-Timop *Apotex, Canad.*
Timolol maleate (p.953·3).
Glaucoma.

Apo-Triazide *Apotex, Canad.*
Triamterene (p.957·2); hydrochlorothiazide (p.885·2).
Hypertension; oedema.

Apo-Triazo *Apotex, Canad.*
Triazolam (p.696·3).
Insomnia.

Apo-Trihex *Apotex, Canad.*
Benzhexol hydrochloride (p.457·3).
Antispasmodic.

Apo-Trimip *Apotex, Canad.*
Trimipramine maleate (p.310·1).
Depression.

Apotrin *Ridupharm, Switz.*
Betacarotene (p.1335·2); canthaxanthin (p.999·3).
Photodermatoses; protoporphyria.

Apo-Tuss *Pekana, Ger.*
Homoeopathic preparation.

Apo-Verap *Apotex, Canad.*
Verapamil hydrochloride (p.960·3).
Angina; arrhythmias; hypertension.

Apozepam *Dumex-Alpharma, Swed.*
Diazepam (p.661·1).
Alcohol withdrawal syndrome; anxiety; insomnia; premedication; restlessness; sedative; skeletal muscle spasm; status epilepticus; tetanus.

APP Stomach Preparations *Chancellor, UK†.*
Magnesium carbonate (p.1198·1); magnesium trisilicate (p.1199·1); aluminium hydroxide (p.1177·3); bismuth carbonate (p.1181·1); calcium carbonate (p.1182·1); homatropine methobromide (p.462·2).
Formerly contained magnesium carbonate, magnesium trisilicate, aluminium hydroxide, bismuth carbonate, calcium carbonate, homatropine methobromide, and papaverine hydrochloride.
Gastro-intestinal disorders.

Appedrine
Note. This name is used for preparations of different composition.
Stella, Canad.
Benzocaine (p.1286·2); ferrous fumarate (p.1339·3); carmellose sodium (p.1471·2); vitamins.
Obesity.
Thompson, USA.
Phenylpropanolamine hydrochloride (p.1067·2); multivitamins and minerals.

Appetiser Mixture *Potter's, UK.*
Chamomile (p.1561·2); calumba (p.1557·2); compound gentian infusion (p.1583·3).
Flatulence; tonic.

Appetrol *Covan, S.Afr.*
Cathine hydrochloride (p.1478·1).
Obesity.

Applicaine *Carter-Wallace, Austral.*
Oral gel: Choline salicylate (p.25·2).
Topical liquid: Benzocaine (p.1286·2).
Mouth ulcers; teething.

Apracur *Schering, Aust.*
Paracetamol (p.72·2); clemizole hydrochloride (p.406·3); phenylephrine hydrochloride (p.1066·2).
Cold and influenza symptoms.

Apra-Gel *Roche, Belg.*
Naproxen (p.61·2).
Musculoskeletal, joint, and peri-articular disorders.

Apranax
Roche, Belg.; Roche, Fr.; Syntex, Ger.; Roche, Ger.; Roche, Switz.
Naproxen (p.61·2) or naproxen sodium (p.61·2).
Lignocaine (p.1293·2) is included in the intramuscular injection to alleviate the pain of injection.
Gout; inflammation; musculoskeletal, joint, and peri-articular disorders; pain.

Aprednislon *Merck, Aust.*
Prednisolone (p.1048·1).
Corticosteroid.

Apresazide *Novartis, USA.*
Hydralazine hydrochloride (p.883·2); hydrochlorothiazide (p.885·2).
Hypertension.

Apresolin
Ciba, Ital.†; Ciba, Norw.; Novartis, Swed.
Hydralazine hydrochloride (p.883·2).
Heart failure; hypertension.

Apresoline
Novartis, Austral.; Ciba, Canad.; Ciba-Geigy, Irl.; Novartis, Neth.; Novartis, S.Afr.; Alliance, UK; Novartis, USA.
Hydralazine hydrochloride (p.883·2).
Heart failure; hypertension.

Aprical *Rentschler, Ger.*
Nifedipine (p.916·2).
Angina pectoris; hypertension; Raynaud's syndrome.

Aprinox
Knoll, Austral.; Knoll, UK.
Bendrofluazide (p.827·3).
Hypertension; oedema; suppression of lactation.

Aprodine *Major, USA.*
Pseudoephedrine hydrochloride (p.1068·3); triprolidine hydrochloride (p.420·3).
Upper respiratory-tract symptoms.

Aprodine with Codeine *Major, USA.*
Pseudoephedrine hydrochloride (p.1068·3); codeine phosphate (p.26·1); triprolidine hydrochloride (p.420·3).
Coughs and cold symptoms.

Aprolis *Dietavigor, Ital.†.*
Propolis (p.1621·3); acerola (p.1001·1).
Nutritional supplement.

Aproten
Distriborg, Fr.†; Ultrapharm, UK.
Low-protein, gluten-free foods for special diets.

Aprovel
Sanofi Winthrop, Irl.; Bristol-Myers Squibb, Irl.; Sanofi Winthrop, Neth.; Bristol-Myers Squibb, Neth.; Sanofi, Swed.; Bristol-Myers Squibb, Swed.; Sanofi Winthrop, UK.
Irbesartan (p.891·3).
Hypertension.

Aprozide *Major, USA†.*
Hydrochlorothiazide (p.885·2); hydralazine hydrochloride (p.883·2).

APS Balneum *APS, Ger.*
Chamomile oil.
Bath additive; skin disorders.

Apsifen *Approved Prescription Services, UK.*
Ibuprofen (p.44·1).
Fever; inflammation; pain; rheumatoid arthritis.

Apsin VK *Approved Prescription Services, UK.*
Phenoxymethylpenicillin potassium (p.236·2).
Bacterial infections.

Apsolol *Approved Prescription Services, UK.*
Propranolol hydrochloride (p.937·1).
Angina pectoris; anxiety; arrhythmias; essential tremor; hypertension; hyperthyroidism; migraine; myocardial infarction.

Apsolox *Approved Prescription Services, UK†.*
Oxprenolol hydrochloride (p.926·2).
Angina pectoris; arrhythmias; hypertension; hypertrophic obstructive cardiomyopathy.

Apsomol *Farmasan, Ger.*
Salbutamol (p.758·2) or salbutamol sulphate (p.758·2).
Obstructive airways disease.

Apsor *IDI, Ital.*
Betamethasone valero-acetate (p.1034·1); tretinoin (p.1093·3); salicylic acid (p.1090·2).

Formerly contained betamethasone valero-acetate, tretinoin, precipitated sulphur, salicylic acid, camphor, and allantoin.
Psoriasis.

Apstil Approved Prescription Services, UK.
Stilboestrol (p.1462·3).
Breast cancer; prostatic cancer.

Aptamil HA con LCP Milupan Milupa, Ital.
Infant feed.
Milk intolerance.

Aptin
Astra, Austral.†; Astra, Ger.; Byk Gulden, Ital.†; Astra, Norw.; Hassle, Swed.
Alprenolol benzoate (p.817·3) or alprenolol hydrochloride (p.817·3).
Angina pectoris; arrhythmias; hypertension; hyperthyroidism; idiopathic hypertrophic sub-aortic stenosis; myocardial infarction.

Aptine
Astra, Belg.; Astra, Neth.
Alprenolol benzoate (p.817·3).
Angina pectoris; arrhythmias; hypertension; myocardial infarction.

Aptodin Plus GD, Ital.
Vitamin, mineral, and amino-acid preparation.

Apulonga Dorsch, Ger.†.
Allopurinol (p.390·2).
Gout; hyperuricaemia.

Apurin
Laevosan, Aust.; Gea, Neth.†.
Allopurinol (p.390·2) or allopurinol sodium (p.391·3).
Gout; hyperuricaemia; renal calculi.

Apurone
3M, Belg.; 3M, Fr.
Flumequine (p.210·1).
Bacterial infections of the urinary tract.

Aqium Active Defence Ego, Austral.
Barrier cream; emollient.

Aqsia
Opsia, Fr.†; Chauvin, UK.
Electrolyte solution (p.1147·1).
Eye irrigation.

Aqua Ban
Thompson, UK; Thompson, USA.
Ammonium chloride (p.1055·2); caffeine (p.749·3).
Premenstrual water retention.

Aqua Ban Plus Thompson, USA.
Ammonium chloride (p.1055·2); caffeine (p.749·3); ferrous sulphate (p.1340·2).
Premenstrual water retention.

Aqua Care Chattem, Canad.†.
Urea (p.1095·2).
Dry skin.

Aqua Emoform Byk Gulden, Ital.
Sodium monofluorophosphate (p.743·3); sodium fluoride (p.742·1).
Gingival inflammation; oral hygiene.

Aquabase
Note. This name is used for preparations of different composition.
Westbrook, UK.
A non ionic emulsifying wax (p.1383·2).
Paddock, USA.
Vehicle for topical preparations.

Aquacaps Muller Goppingen, Ger.
Orthosiphon (p.1592·2).
Urinary-tract disorders.

Aquacare
Allergan, Austral.†; Menley & James, USA.
Urea (p.1095·2).
Dry skin; hyperkeratosis.

Aquacare-HP Allergan, Austral.
Urea (p.1095·2).
Eczema; skin disorders.

Aquacel Convatec, Fr.
Carmellose sodium (p.1471·2).
Ulcers; wounds.

Aquachloral PolyMedica, USA.
Chloral hydrate (p.645·3).
Sedative.

Aquacort Draxis, Canad.
Hydrocortisone (p.1043·3).
Skin disorders.

Aquaderm
Note. This name is used for preparations of different composition.
Baker Cummins, Canad.
Emollient.
Baker Cummins, Canad.
SPF 15: Octyl salicylate (p.1487·3); avobenzone (p.1486·3); ethylhexyl *p*-methoxycinnamate (p.1487·1); titanium dioxide (p.1093·3).
SPF 30: Avobenzone (p.1486·3); octocrylene (p.1487·3); ethylhexyl *p*-methoxycinnamate (p.1487·1); titanium dioxide (p.1093·3).
Sunscreen.
Baker Cummins, USA.
SPF 15: Ethylhexyl *p*-methoxycinnamate (p.1487·1); oxybenzone (p.1487·3).
Sunscreen.

Aquadrate
Procter & Gamble, Austral.†; Procter & Gamble, Irl.; Procter & Gamble, UK.
Urea (p.1095·2).
Dry skin disorders; eczema; rosacea.

Aquadrex Parke-Med, S.Afr.†.
Amiloride (p.819·3); hydrochlorothiazide (p.885·2).
Hypertension; oedema.

Aquae Hamilton, Austral.
Carmellose sodium (p.1471·2); sorbitol (p.1354·2); electrolytes (p.1147·1).
Artificial saliva.

Aquaear Whitehall, Austral.
Glacial acetic acid (p.1541·2); isopropyl alcohol (p.1118·2).
Prevention of otitis externa.

Aquafor Asta Medica, Ital.
Xipamide (p.971·2).
Hypertension.

Aquaform Scimat, UK.
Hydrogel dressing.
Ulcers; wounds.

Aquagen SQ ALK, Swed.
Allergen extracts (p.1545·1).
Diagnosis of hypersensitivity; hyposensitisation.

Aqualcium Aqualab, Fr.
Mineral preparation.
Calcium deficiency.

Aqualette Lichtwer, UK.
Taraxacum (p.1634·2); equisetum (p.1575·1).

Aqualibra Medice, Ger.
Ononis (p.1610·2); orthosiphon (p.1592·2); solidago.
Urinary-tract disorders.

Aquamag Aqualab, Fr.
Mineral preparation.
Magnesium deficiency.

Aquamephyton Merck Sharp & Dohme, USA.
Phytomenadione (p.1371·1).
Coagulation disorders associated with vitamin K deficiency, due to faulty formation of factors II, VII, IX, and X.

Aquamox
Lederle, Austral.†; Cyanamid, Ital.†; Lederle, Neth.†.
Quinethazone (p.938·3).
Hypertension; oedema.

Aquamycetin Winzer, Ger.
Chloramphenicol (p.182·1).
Bacterial infections of the ear and eye.

Aquanil
Note. This name is used for preparations of different composition.
Gea, Norw.; GEA, Swed.
Timolol maleate (p.953·3).
Glaucoma; ocular hypertension.
Person & Covey, USA.
Emollient and moisturiser.

Aquanil HC Person & Covey, USA.
Hydrocortisone (p.1043·3).
Skin disorders.

Aquaphilic Medco, USA.
Vehicle for topical preparations.

Aquaphor
Note. This name is used for preparations of different composition.
Smith & Nephew, Canad.
White soft paraffin (p.1382·3).
Dry skin; ointment base.
Beiersdorf-Lilly, Ger.
Xipamide (p.971·2).
Hypertension; oedema.
Beiersdorf, USA.
Yellow soft paraffin; liquid paraffin; mineral wax; wool wax alcohol.
Barrier ointment; ointment base.

Aquaphor Antibiotic Beiersdorf, USA.
Polymyxin B sulphate (p.239·1); bacitracin zinc (p.157·3).

Aquaphoril Asta Medica, Aust.
Xipamide (p.971·2).
Oedema.

Aquaphyllin Ferndale, USA.
Theophylline (p.765·1).
Asthma; bronchospasm.

Aquapred Winzer, Ger.
Ear drops†: Dexamethasone (p.1037·1); naphazoline hydrochloride (p.1064·2); chloramphenicol (p.182·1).
Inflammatory disorders and infections of the ear.
Eye drops: Chloramphenicol hydrogen succinate (p.184·2); prednisolone hemisuccinate (p.1048·1).
Inflammatory disorders and infections of the eye.

Aquareduct Azupharma, Ger.
Spironolactone (p.946·1).
Ascites; hyperaldosteronism; oedema.

Aquaretic Azuchemie, Ger.
Amiloride hydrochloride (p.819·2); hydrochlorothiazide (p.885·2).
Ascites; hypertension; oedema.

Aquarid
Note. A similar name is used for preparations of different composition.
Schwulst, S.Afr.
Frusemide (p.871·1).
Oedema.

Aqua-Rid
Note. A similar name is used for preparations of different composition.
Goldline, USA.
Buchu (p.1555·2); couch grass (p.1567·3); corn silk; hydrangea.
Premenstrual water retention.

Aquasept Houghs Healthcare, UK.
Triclosan (p.1127·2).
Skin disinfection.

Aquasite
Ciba Vision, Canad.
Macrogol 400 (p.1598·2); dextran 70 (p.717·1).
Ciba Vision, USA.
Macrogol 400 (p.1598·2); dextran 70 (p.717·1); polycarbophil (p.1209·1).
Dry eyes.

Aquasol Seton, UK.
Purified water.

Aquasol A
Note. This name is used for preparations of different composition.
Dermik, Canad.
Cream: Vitamin A palmitate (p.1359·2); dexpanthenol (p.1570·3).
Skin disorders.
Rhone-Poulenc Rorer Consumer, Canad.†.
Capsules: Vitamin A (p.1358·1).
Vitamin A deficiency.
Astra, USA.
Vitamin A (p.1358·1).
Vitamin A deficiency.

Aquasol A & D Rhone-Poulenc Rorer Consumer, Canad.†.
Vitamin A (p.1358·1); vitamin D (p.1366·3).
Vitamin A and D deficiency.

Aquasol E
Novartis Consumer, Canad.; Astra, USA.
Vitamin E (p.1369·1).
Vitamin E deficiency.

Aquasport Also, Ital.
Mineral preparation.

Aquasun Blockout Roche, Austral.†.
A range of sunscreen preparations based on padimates and avobenzone.

Aquasun (SPF4/8/12) Roche, Austral.†.
A range of sunscreen preparations based on padimates.

Aquatabs Medentech, Irl.
Sodium dichloroisocyanurate (p.1124·3).
Water purification.

Aquatain
Whitehall, Austral.; Whitehall-Robins, Canad.
Emollient.

AquaTar Allergan Herbert, USA.
Coal tar (p.1092·3).
Skin disorders.

Aquatensen Wallace, USA.
Methyclothiazide (p.904·1).
Hypertension; oedema.

Aquavit-E Cypress, USA.
dl-Alpha tocopheryl acetate (p.1369·2).
Vitamin E deficiency.

Aqua-Vite Super Kelp Bio-Health, UK.
Multivitamins; ascophyllum nodosum.

Aqucilina Pharmacia Upjohn, Spain.
Procaine penicillin (p.240·2).
Bacterial infections.

Aqucilina D A Pharmacia Upjohn, Spain.
Benzylpenicillin potassium (p.159·2); procaine penicillin (p.240·2).
Bacterial infections.

Aquest Dunhall, USA.
Oestrone (p.1458·2).

Aquo-Cytobion Merck, Ger.
Hydroxocobalamin acetate (p.1364·2).
Vitamin B_{12} deficiency.

Aquo-Trinitrosan
Merck, Ger.; E. Merck, Switz.†.
Glyceryl trinitrate (p.874·3).
Cardiovascular disorders.

Aqupla Shionogi, Jpn.
Nedaplatin (p.556·2).
Malignant neoplasms.

Arabine Baxter, Swed.
Cytarabine (p.525·2).
Acute leukaemias.

ARA-cell Cell Pharm, Ger.
Cytarabine (p.525·2).
Malignant neoplasms.

Aracytin Pharmacia Upjohn, Ital.
Cytarabine (p.525·2).
Proliferative blood disorders.

Aracytine Pharmacia Upjohn, Fr.
Cytarabine (p.525·2).
Leukaemias; lymphomas.

Aralen
Sanofi Winthrop, Canad.; Sanofi Winthrop, USA.
Chloroquine hydrochloride (p.426·3) or chloroquine phosphate (p.426·3).
Amoebiasis; malaria.

Aralen with Primaquine Phosphate Sanofi Winthrop, USA†.
Chloroquine phosphate (p.426·3); primaquine phosphate (p.434·3).
Malaria prophylaxis.

Aralia Med Complex Dynamit, Aust.
Homoeopathic preparation.

Aramexe Merckle, Aust.
Co-dergocrine mesylate (p.1566·1).
Cerebrovascular disorders; cervical syndrome; hypertension; migraine; peripheral vascular disease.

Aramine
Merck Sharp & Dohme, Austral.; Merck Sharp & Dohme, Belg.; Merck Sharp & Dohme, Neth.†; Merck Sharp & Dohme, Norw.; Merck Sharp & Dohme, UK; Merck Sharp & Dohme, USA.
Metaraminol tartrate (p.903·1).
Hypotension.

Aran C Schiapparelli, Ital.†.
Ascorbic acid (p.1365·2).
Vitamin C deficiency.

Aranidorm-S Weber & Weber, Ger.
Centaury (p.1561·1); chamomile (p.1561·2); passion flower (p.1615·3); valerian (p.1643·1); lavender (p.1594·3); lupulus (p.1597·2); melissa (p.1600·1); atropa bellad.; avena sat.; coffeinum; datura stram.; eschscholtzia calif.; hyoscyamus nig.; lactuca vir.; papaver dub.; zincum isovalerianicum.
Hyperactivity; insomnia.

Araniforce-forte Weber & Weber, Ger.
Homoeopathic preparation.

Aranisan-N Weber & Weber, Ger.
Homoeopathic preparation.

Arantil P Hoechst, Ger.†.
Propyphenazone (p.81·3).
Fever; pain.

Arasena-A Mochida, Jpn.
Vidarabine (p.628·2).
Herpesvirus infections.

Aratac Alphapharm, Austral.
Amiodarone hydrochloride (p.820·1).
Arrhythmias.

Arava Hoechst Marion Roussel, USA.
Leflunomide (p.543·3).
Rheumatoid arthritis.

Arbid
Note. This name is used for preparations of different composition.
Kolassa, Aust.; Medichemie, Switz.
Buphenine hydrochloride (p.1555·3); diphenylpyraline hydrochloride (p.409·3).
Rhinitis; sinusitis.
Tropon, Ger.†.
Controlled-release tablets: Buphenine hydrochloride (p.1555·3); diphenylpyraline hydrochloride (p.409·3).
Oral drops: Buphenine hydrochloride (p.1555·3); diphenylpyraline hydrochloride (p.409·3); sodium salamidacetate (p.82·3).
Tablets: Buphenine hydrochloride (p.1555·3); diphenylpyraline hydrochloride (p.409·3); salicylamide (p.82·3).
Rhinitis.

Arbid N Bayer, Ger.
Diphenylpyraline hydrochloride (p.409·3).
Cold symptoms.

Arbid-top Medichemie, Switz.
Phenylephrine hydrochloride (p.1066·2); dequalinium chloride (p.1112·1); muramidase hydrochloride (p.1604·3).
Nasal congestion.

Arbralene Berk, UK.
Metoprolol tartrate (p.907·3).
Angina pectoris; arrhythmias; hypertension; hyperthyroidism; migraine; myocardial infarction.

Arbum Jaldes, Fr.
Lappa (p.1594·2); cystine (p.1339·1); zinc gluconate (p.1373·2); pyridoxine hydrochloride (p.1362·3); biotin (p.1336·1).
Seborrhoea.

Arca-Be Arcana, Aust.
Thiamine disulphide (p.1361·2); pyridoxine hydrochloride (p.1362·3); cyanocobalamin (p.1363·3).
Neuralgia; neuritis.

Arcablock Arcana, Aust.
Atenolol (p.825·3).
Angina pectoris; arrhythmias; hypertension; myocardial infarction.

Arcablock comp Arcana, Aust.
Atenolol (p.825·3); chlorthalidone (p.839·3).
Hypertension.

Arcadipin Merck, Aust.
Nilvadipine (p.922·1).
Hypertension.

Arca-Enzym Merck, Aust.
Pancreatin (p.1612·1); cellulase (p.1561·1); ox bile (p.1553·2); bromelains (p.1555·1).
Digestive disorders.

Arcalion
Therval, Fr.; Servier, Spain; Servier, Switz.
Sulbutiamine (p.1360·3).
Tonic.

Arcana Cough Linctus Arcana, S.Afr.†.
Triprolidine hydrochloride (p.420·3); pseudoephedrine hydrochloride (p.1068·3); codeine phosphate (p.26·1).
Coughs.

Arcana Expectorant Arcana, S.Afr.
Triprolidine hydrochloride (p.420·3); pseudoephedrine hydrochloride (p.1068·3); codeine phosphate (p.26·1); guaiphenesin (p.1061·3).
Coughs.

Arcanacillin Arcana, S.Afr.†.
Amoxycillin trihydrate (p.151·3).
Bacterial infections.

Arcanacycline Arcana, S.Afr.
Tetracycline hydrochloride (p.259·1).
Bacterial infections.

Arcanacysteine Arcana, S.Afr.
Carbocisteine (p.1056·3).
Respiratory-tract disorders with increased or viscous mucus.

Arcanadopa Arcana, S.Afr.†.
Methyldopa (p.904·2).
Hypertension.

Arcanafed *Arcana, S.Afr.*
Triprolidine hydrochloride (p.420·3); pseudoephedrine hydrochloride (p.1068·3).
Cold and influenza symptoms.

Arcanafenac *Arcana, S.Afr.*
Diclofenac sodium (p.31·2).
Gout; inflammation; musculoskeletal and joint disorders; pain.

Arcanaflex *Arcana, S.Afr.*
Paracetamol (p.72·2); chlormezanone (p.648·3).
Pain with tension.

Arcanaflu *Arcana, S.Afr.*
Capsules: Paracetamol (p.72·2); vitamin C (p.1365·2); phenylephrine hydrochloride (p.1066·2); chlorpheniramine maleate (p.405·1); caffeine (p.749·3).
Syrup: Paracetamol (p.72·2); phenylpropanolamine hydrochloride (p.1067·2); dextromethorphan hydrobromide (p.1057·3).
Cold and influenza symptoms.

Arcanagesic *Arcana, S.Afr.*
Syrup: Paracetamol (p.72·2).
Tablets: Paracetamol (p.72·2); codeine phosphate (p.26·1).
Fever; pain.

Arcanamide *Arcana, S.Afr.†.*
Frusemide (p.871·1).
Ascites; hypertension; oedema.

Arcanamycin *Arcana, S.Afr.*
Erythromycin estolate (p.204·1) or erythromycin stearate (p.204·2).
Bacterial infections.

Arcanaprim *Arcana, S.Afr.*
Co-trimoxazole (p.196·3).
Bacterial infections.

Arcanaretic *Arcana, S.Afr.†.*
Amiloride hydrochloride (p.819·2); hydrochlorothiazide (p.885·2).
Hypertension; oedema.

Arcanum *Strath-Labor, Ger.†.*
Fruct. avenae; herba basilici; herba calendulae; equisetum; hypericum; turiones pini; taraxacum; thyme.
Tonic.

Arcasin
Note. This name is used for preparations of different composition.
Engelhard, Ger.; Cimex, Switz.
Phenoxymethylpenicillin potassium (p.236·2).
Bacterial infections.

Esteve, Spain.
Cisapride (p.1187·1).
Gastro-oesophageal reflux.

Arcavit A *Merck, Aust.*
Vitamin A acetate (p.1359·2).
Vitamin A deficiency.

Arcavit A/E *Arcana, Aust.*
Vitamin A palmitate (p.1359·2); dl-alpha tocopheryl acetate (p.1369·2).
Vitamin A and E deficiency.

Arcental *Martin, Spain.*
Ketoprofen (p.48·2).
Fever; inflammation; pain.

Arcet *Econo Med, USA.*
Butalbital (p.644·3); paracetamol (p.72·2); caffeine (p.749·3).

Architex *Cooperation Pharmaceutique, Fr.*
Sodium monofluorophosphate (p.743·3); calcium carbonate (p.1182·1).
Osteoporosis.

Arco Pain *Romilo, Canad.*
Aspirin (p.16·1); caffeine citrate (p.749·3).

Arcobee with C *Nature's Bounty, USA.*
Vitamin B substances with vitamin C.

Arcocillin *Arcolab, Switz.†.*
Ampicillin (p.153·1).
Bacterial infections.

Arcoiran *Alter, Spain.*
Sumatriptan succinate (p.450·1).
Cluster headache; migraine.

Arco-Lase *Arco, USA.*
Amylolytic enzymes (p.1549·1); proteolytic enzymes; cellulolytic enzymes (p.1561·1); lipase.
Poor digestion.

Arco-Lase Plus *Arco, USA.*
Amylolytic enzymes (p.1549·1); proteolytic enzymes; cellulolytic enzymes (p.1561·1); lipase; hyoscyamine sulphate (p.464·2); atropine sulphate (p.455·1); phenobarbitone (p.350·2).
Gastro-intestinal disorders.

Arconeurine *Arcolab, Switz.†.*
Cyanocobalamin (p.1363·3); thiamine hydrochloride (p.1361·1).
Nephritis; pain.

Arcored *Arcolab, Switz.†.*
Cyanocobalamin (p.1363·3).
Lignocaine hydrochloride (p.1293·2) is included in this preparation to alleviate the pain of injection.
Vitamin B_{12} deficiency.

Arcotinic *Arco, USA†.*
Iron (p.1346·1); liver (desiccated).
Vitamin C (p.1365·2) is included in this preparation to increase the absorption and availability of iron.
Iron-deficiency anaemias.

Arctuvan N *Klinge, Ger.*
Bearberry leaves (p.1552·2).
Formerly contained hexamine, salol, and bearberry leaves.
Urinary-tract infections.

Ardey aktiv *Ardeypharm, Ger.*
Ginseng (p.1584·2).
Tonic.

Ardeyceryl *Ardeypharm, Ger.†.*
Cerebral cortex lipid extract (p.1599·1).
Central nervous system disorders.

Ardeyceryl P *Ardeypharm, Ger.*
Pyritinol hydrochloride (p.1624·1).
Mental function disorders.

Ardeycholan N *Ardeypharm, Ger.*
Chelidonium majus.
Smooth muscle spasm.

Ardeycordal N *Ardeypharm, Ger.*
Crataegus (p.1568·2); potassium aspartate (p.1161·3); magnesium aspartate (p.1157·2).
Formerly contained ethaverine, crataegus, valerian, potassium aspartate, magnesium aspartate, and sparteine sulphate.
Arrhythmias.

Ardeydystin *Ardeypharm, Ger.*
Kava (p.1592·3).
Formerly contained valerian root, kavain, and crataegus.
Nervous disorders.

Ardeyhepan N *Ardeypharm, Ger.*
Silybum marianum (p.993·3).
Liver disorders.

Ardeysedon N *Ardeypharm, Ger.*
Valerian root (p.1643·1); lupulus (p.1597·2).
Nervous disorders; sleep disorders.

Ardeytropin *Ardeypharm, Ger.*
Tryptophan (p.310·2).
Depression; sleep disorders.

Ardine *Antibioticos, Spain.*
Amoxycillin trihydrate (p.151·3).
Bacterial infections.

Ardine Bronquial *Antibioticos, Spain.*
Amoxycillin trihydrate (p.151·3); bromhexine hydrochloride (p.1055·3).
Respiratory-tract infections.

Ardinex *Astra, Swed.*
Ibuprofen (p.44·1); codeine phosphate (p.26·1).
Pain.

Arduan
Organon Teknika, Ital.; Organon, USA.
Pipecuronium bromide (p.1318·1).
Competitive neuromuscular blocker.

Aredia
Ciba-Geigy, Aust.; Novartis, Austral.; Ciba-Geigy, Belg.; Geigy, Canad.; Ciba-Geigy, Fr.; Ciba, Ger.; Ciba-Geigy, Irl.; Ciba, Ital.; Novartis, Neth.; Ciba, Norw.; Novartis, S.Afr.; Novartis, Swed.; Ciba, Switz.; Ciba, UK; Novartis, USA.
Disodium pamidronate (p.740·2).
Hypercalcaemia of malignancy; osteolytic lesions and bone pain in multiple myeloma and in bone metastases associated with breast cancer; Paget's disease of bone.

Arelcant *Bender, Aust.*
Fenoterol hydrobromide (p.753·2); ipratropium bromide (p.754·2).
Obstructive airways disease.

Arelix
Albert-Roussel, Aust.; Hoechst, Ger.; Hoechst Marion Roussel, Irl.; Bipharma, Neth.†; Hoechst Marion Roussel, S.Afr.; Hoechst Marion Roussel, Switz.; Hoechst Marion Roussel, UK†.
Piretanide (p.931·3) or piretanide sodium (p.931·3).
Forced diuresis; heart failure; hypertension; oedema; renal failure.

Arelix ACE *Hoechst, Ger.*
Piretanide (p.931·3); ramipril (p.941·1).
Hypertension.

Arem *Lennon, S.Afr.*
Nitrazepam (p.682·2).
Insomnia.

Aremin *Boniscontro & Gazzone, Ital.*
Heparan sulphate (p.879·2).
Thrombo-embolic disorders.

Aremis *Esteve, Spain.*
Sertraline hydrochloride (p.307·2).
Depression.

Arestal *Janssen-Cilag, Aust.*
Loperamide oxide (p.1197·3).
Diarrhoea.

Areuzolin *Areu, Spain.*
Cephazolin sodium (p.181·1).
Bacterial infections.

Arfen *Lisapharma, Ital.*
Ibuprofen lysine (p.44·3).
Arthritic disorders; gynaecological disorders; radiculitis.

Arfonad
Roche, Canad.†; Roche, Irl.†; Roche, Ital.†; Cambridge, UK; Roche, USA†.
Trimetaphan camsylate (p.958·3).
Now known as Trimetaphan Camsylate Ampoules in the UK.
Hypertensive crises; induction of controlled hypotension; pulmonary oedema.

Argenpal *Braun, Spain.*
Silver nitrate (p.1629·2).
Skin disorders; verrucas.

Argent-Eze *Lennon, S.Afr.*
Silver sulphadiazine (p.247·3).
Burns.

Argentocromo *Bucca, Spain.*
Mercurochrome (p.1119·2); silver (p.1629·2).
Gingivitis; mouth infection.

Argentofenol *Bucca, Spain.*
Phenol (p.1121·2); methylene blue (p.984·3); silver nitrate (p.1629·2).
Aphthous stomatitis; oral bleeding; tonsillitis.

Argentum Med Complex *Dynamit, Aust.*
Homoeopathic preparation.

Argesic *Econo Med, USA.*
Methyl salicylate (p.55·2).
Muscle, joint, and soft-tissue pain; neuralgia.

Argesic-SA *Econo Med, USA.*
Salsalate (p.83·1).
Fever; inflammation; pain.

Argicilline *Monot, Fr.*
Gramicidin (p.215·2).
Formerly contained methocidin and cetylpyridinium chloride.
Nose and throat infections.

Argin *Volchem, Ital.*
Protein supplement.
Arginine deficiency.

Arginil *SPA, Ital.†.*
Arginine glucose-1-phosphate.
Liver disorders.

Arginotri-B
Bouchara, Fr.; Bouchara, Switz.
Arginine hydrochloride (p.1334·1); thiamine hydrochloride (p.1361·1); pyridoxine hydrochloride (p.1362·3); hydroxocobalamin (p.1363·3).
Alcoholism; hepatic disorders; neuritis; nutritional supplement; pain.

Argirofedrina *Vaillant, Ital.*
Ephedrine sulphate (p.1059·3); anhydrous sodium sulphate (p.1213·3); mild silver protein.
Nasal congestion.

Argisone *Teofarma, Ital.*
Hydrocortisone acetate (p.1043·3); mild silver protein.
Bacterial eye infections.

Argobase *Westbrook, UK.*
A range of emulsifying product bases.

Argotone *Lipha, Ital.*
Ephedrine hydrochloride (p.1059·3); mild silver protein.
Nasal congestion.

Argun *Merckle, Ger.*
Lonazolac calcium (p.50·3).
Inflammation; musculoskeletal and joint disorders; pain.

Argyrol *Asta Medica, Belg.†.*
Mild silver protein.
Bacterial infections of the eye.

Argyrophedrine
Note. This name is used for preparations of different composition.
Lipha, Belg.; Lipha, Switz.†.
Ephedrine hydrochloride (p.1059·3) or ephedrine laevulinate; mild silver protein.
Nasal congestion.

Lipha Sante, Fr.
Ephedrine laevulinate; mild silver protein; sodium laevulinate; calcium laevulinate (p.1155·2).
Nasal congestion.

Arhemapectine Antihemorragique *Aerocid, Fr.*
Pectin (p.1474·1).
Haemorrhage.

Arial *Dompe, Ital.*
Salmeterol xinafoate (p.761·2).
Obstructive airways disease.

Aricept
Pfizer, Irl.; Pfizer, Swed.; Pfizer, UK; Pfizer, USA.
Donepezil hydrochloride (p.1391·2).
Alzheimer's disease.

Aricodil *Malesci, Ital.*
Dextromethorphan hydrobromide (p.1057·3).
Coughs.

Aridil *CP Pharmaceuticals, UK.*
Frusemide (p.871·1); amiloride hydrochloride (p.819·2).
These ingredients can be described by the British Approved Name Co-amilofruse.
Ascites; oedema.

Arilin
Wolff, Ger.; Cimex, Switz.
Metronidazole (p.585·1).
Amoebiasis; anaerobic bacterial infections; trichomoniasis.

Ariline *Montavit, Aust.*
Metronidazole (p.585·1).
Anaerobic bacterial infections; protozoal infections.

Arilvax
Wellcome, Belg.†; Evans Medical, Irl.; Evans, Neth.; Medpro, S.Afr.; SBL, Swed.; Wellcome, Switz.†; Medeva, UK.
A yellow fever vaccine (17D strain) (p.1539·1).
Active immunisation.

Arima *Alphapharm, Austral.*
Moclobemide (p.298·3).
Depression.

Arimidex
Zeneca, Aust.; ICI, Austral.; Zeneca, Canad.; Zeneca, Ger.; Zeneca, Irl.; Zeneca, Ital.; Zeneca, Neth.; Zeneca, Norw.; Zeneca, S.Afr.; Zeneca, Swed.; Zeneca, Switz.; Zeneca, UK; Zeneca, USA.
Anastrozole (p.504·1).
Breast cancer.

Aristamid
Ebewe, Aust.†; Nordmark, Ger.†.
Sulphasomidine sodium (p.257·1).
Burns; infected skin disorders; infected wounds.

Aristo L *Steiner, Ger.*
Aloes (p.1177·1).
Constipation.

Aristochol
Note. This name is used for preparations of different composition.
Linobion, Aust.
Chelidonium; curcuma zanthorrhiza; silybum marianum (p.993·3); aloes (p.1177·1); pancreatin (p.1612·1).

Steiner, Ger.
Capsules†: Chelidonium; Javanese curcuma (p.1001·3); cape aloe (p.1177·1).
Biliary disorders; digestive disorders; hepatitis.
Oral granules: Chelidonium; cape aloe (p.1177·1).
Constipation.

Steiner, Switz.†.
Chelidonium; cape aloe (p.1177·1).
Constipation.

Aristochol CC *Steiner, Ger.*
Chelidonium; turmeric (p.1001·3).
Gastro-intestinal spasm.

Aristochol N *Steiner, Ger.*
Chelidonium; achillea (p.1542·2); taraxacum (p.1634·2); gnaphalii flowers; absinthium (p.1541·1).
Biliary disorders.

Aristocomb *Lederle, Austral.*
Triamcinolone acetonide (p.1050·2); neomycin sulphate (p.229·2); gramicidin (p.215·2); nystatin (p.386·1).
Infected skin disorders.

Aristocor *Kwizda, Aust.*
Flecainide acetate (p.868·3).
Arrhythmias.

Aristocort
Lederle, Austral.; Stiefel, Canad.; Fujisawa, USA.
Triamcinolone (p.1050·2), triamcinolone acetonide (p.1050·2), or triamcinolone diacetate (p.1050·2).
Corticosteroid.

Aristoforat *Steiner, Ger.*
Hypericum (p.1590·1).
Depression; nervous disorders.

Aristoform *Stiefel, Canad.†.*
Triamcinolone acetonide (p.1050·2); clioquinol (p.193·2).
Skin disorders.

Aristospan
Stiefel, Canad.; Fujisawa, USA.
Triamcinolone hexacetonide (p.1050·2).
Musculoskeletal and joint disorders.

Aritmina *Solvay, Ital.*
Ajmaline (p.817·1).
Arrhythmias.

Ariven *Beiersdorf-Lilly, Ger.*
Topical gel: Heparin sodium (p.879·3).
Skin trauma.

Ariven SN *Beiersdorf, Ger.†.*
Propyphenazone (p.81·3); solidago.
Vascular disorders.

Arkin-Z *Otsuka, Jpn.*
Vesnarinone (p.964·2).
Heart failure.

Arkogelules *Arkopharma, Fr.*
A range of herbal preparations.

Arkonsol *Romilo, Canad.*
Benzalkonium chloride (p.1101·3).

Arkonutril MM *Arkopharma, Fr.*
Preparation for enteral nutrition.

Arkophytum *Arkopharma, Fr.*
Harpagophytum (p.27·2); black currant (p.1365·2); willow (p.82·3).
Painful joint disorders.

Arkotonic *Arkopharma, Fr.*
Pollen; carnitine (p.1336·2); vitamin E (p.1369·1); ascorbic acid (p.1365·2); royal jelly (p.1626·3); soya lecithin (p.1595·2).
Tonic.

Arkovital *Arkopharma, Fr.*
A range of vitamin, mineral, and trace element supplements.

Arkovital C *Arkopharma, Fr.*
Ascorbic acid (p.1365·2).
Cold symptoms; tonic; vitamin C deficiency.

Arlevert *Hennig, Ger.*
Cinnarizine (p.406·1); dimenhydrinate (p.408·2).
Vertigo.

Arlidin
Rhone-Poulenc Rorer, Canad.; Rhone-Poulenc Rorer, USA†.
Buphenine hydrochloride (p.1555·3).
Cerebrovascular disorders; circulatory disturbances of the inner ear; peripheral vascular disease.

Arlitene *Asta Medica, Ital.*
Thymoxamine hydrochloride (p.952·2).
Cardiovascular disorders.

ARM *Menley & James, USA.*
Phenylpropanolamine hydrochloride (p.1067·2); chlorpheniramine maleate (p.405·1).
Upper respiratory-tract symptoms.

Armaya *Centrum, Spain.*
Polypodium leucotomos.
Eczema; psoriasis.

Armil *Squibb, Spain.*
Benzalkonium chloride (p.1101·3).
Disinfection.

Arminol Krewel, Ger.
Sulpiride (p.692·3).
Depression; schizophrenia; vestibular disorders.

Armophylline Bellon, Fr.†.
Theophylline (p.765·1).
Asthma; bronchospastic disorders.

Arnica + Homeocan, Canad.
Homoeopathic preparation.

Arnica comp. DHU, Ger.
Homoeopathic preparation.

Arnica Kneipp Salbe Kneipp, Ger.
Arnica oil (p.1550·3); heparin (p.879·3).
Peripheral vascular disorders; skin trauma.

Arnica Komplex Richter, Aust.
Homoeopathic preparation.

Arnica Med Complex Dynamit, Aust.
Homoeopathic preparation.

Arnica Oligoplex Madaus, Ger.
Homoeopathic preparation.

Arnicadol Phytomedica, Fr.
Arnica (p.1550·3); menthol (p.1600·2).
Soft-tissue injury.

Arnicalm Boiron, Canad.
Homoeopathic preparation.

Arnican Cooperation Pharmaceutique, Fr.
Arnica (p.1550·3).
Soft-tissue disorders.

Arnicet Metochem, Aust.
Arnica (p.1550·3); hamamelis (p.1587·1).
Muscle pain; skin disorders.

Arnicon Cusi, Spain.
Arnica (p.1550·3); methyl salicylate (p.55·2); menthol (p.1600·2).
Musculoskeletal and joint pain.

Arniflor VSM, Neth.†.
Arnica (p.1550·3).
Bruising; haematoma; muscle pain; sprain.

Arniflor-N Spitzner, Ger.; Schwabe, Ger.
Arnica (p.1550·3).
Boils; insect bites; musculoskeletal and joint disorders; superficial phlebitis; wounds.

Arnika plus Ratiopharm, Ger.
Arnica (p.1550·3); heparin sodium (p.879·3); aesculus (p.1543·3).
Soft-tissue injury; venous disorders.

Arnika-Balsam Doerr, Ger.†.
Arnica (p.1550·3); rosemary oil (p.1626·2); camphor (p.1557·2).
Bruises; pain; rheumatic disorders; sprains.

Arnikamill Biomo, Ger.
Chamomile (p.1561·2); arnica flowers (p.1550·3).
Haemorrhoids; skin disorders; soft-tissue inflammation; wounds.

Arnilose AJC, Fr.
Arginine hydrochloride (p.1334·1); ornithine hydrochloride (p.1352·3); sorbitol (p.1354·2); fructose (p.1343·2).
Dyspepsia.

Arobon
Salus, Aust.; Nestle, Ital.; Nestle, Norw.; Nestle, Switz.†; Nestle, UK.
Ceratonia (p.1472·2).
Diarrhoea.

Arocin Modern Health Products, UK.
Betacarotene (p.1335·2).

Arofuto Tanabe, Jpn†.
Afloqualone (p.1304·2).
Muscle hypertonia; spastic paralysis.

Arola Rosebalm Pharmaceutical Enterprises, S.Afr.
Bismuth subnitrate (p.1180·2); dimethicone (p.1384·2); allantoin (p.1078·2); zinc oxide (p.1096·2).
Skin disorders.

Arolac IPRAD, Fr.
Lysuride maleate (p.1142·1).
Hyperprolactinaemia; lactation inhibition.

Aromabyl Plantes et Medecines, Fr.
Cynara (p.1569·2); lappa (p.1594·2); cascara (p.1183·1); juglans regia; sodium salicylate (p.85·1); sodium arsenate (p.1630·2); boldo (p.1554·1).
Constipation; dyspepsia.

Aromalgyl Plantes et Medecines, Fr.
Maize; hexamine (p.216·1); fleabane; orthosiphon (p.1592·2); ash.
Rheumatism.

Aromasol Plantes et Medecines, Fr.
Clove oil (p.1565·2); peppermint oil (p.1208·1); pine oil; lavender oil (p.1594·3); cinnamon oil (p.1564·2); rosemary oil (p.1626·2); wild thyme oil.
Respiratory-tract congestion.

Aropax
SmithKline Beecham, Austral.; Beecham, Belg.; SmithKline Beecham, S.Afr.; Morrith, Spain†.
Paroxetine hydrochloride (p.301·2).
Depression; obsessive-compulsive disorder; panic disorders.

Arovit
Roche Consumer, Belg.†; Bio-Sante, Canad.; Roche, Fr.; Roche, Ital.; Roche, S.Afr.; Roche, Spain†; Roche, Swed.; Roche, Switz.
Vitamin A (p.1359·2).
Atrophic rhinitis; neurosensory disorders; vitamin A deficiency.

Arpamyl LP Jouveinal, Fr.†.
Verapamil hydrochloride (p.960·3).
Hypertension.

Arpha
Note. This name is used for preparations of different composition.
Fournier, Fr.†.
Nasal spray: Benzododecinium bromide (p.1103·2); procaine hydrochloride (p.1299·2); phenylephrine hydrochloride (p.1066·2); ephedrine hydrochloride (p.1059·3).
Rhinitis; rhinopharyngitis; sinusitis.
Spray: Benzododecinium bromide (p.1103·2); acetarsol sodium (p.578·2); amylocaine hydrochloride (p.1286·1).
Mouth and throat disorders.

Urgo, Fr.
Capsules: Paracetamol (p.72·2); chlorpheniramine maleate (p.405·1).
Cold symptoms.

Arpha Hustensirup Fournier, Ger.†.
Dextromethorphan hydrobromide (p.1057·3).
Coughs.

Arphos Fournier, Fr.
Cyanocobalamin (p.1363·3); phosphoric acid (p.1618·1); calcium gluceptate (p.1155·1).
Tonic.

Arpicolin Rosemont, UK.
Procyclidine hydrochloride (p.467·3).
Drug-induced extrapyramidal disorders; parkinsonism.

Arpilon
Organon, Aust.; Organon Teknika, Ger.†; Organon Teknika, Neth.†; Organon, Switz.†.
Pipecuronium bromide (p.1318·1).
Competitive neuromuscular blocker.

Arpimycin Rosemont, UK.
Erythromycin ethyl succinate (p.204·2).
Bacterial infections.

Arrestin Vortech, USA.
Trimethobenzamide hydrochloride (p.420·1).
Nausea and vomiting.

Arret
Janssen-Cilag, Irl.; Johnson & Johnson MSD Consumer, UK.
Loperamide hydrochloride (p.1197·2).
Diarrhoea.

Arsacol Zambon, Fr.
Ursodeoxycholic acid (p.1642·1).
Gallstones.

Arscolloid SIT, Ital.
Dichlorobenzyl alcohol (p.1112·2); silver protein (p.1629·3).
Oral disinfection.

Arsiquinoforme Synthelabo, Fr.
Quinine acetarsolate (p.441·2); quinine formate (p.441·2).
Malaria.

Arsobal
Specia, Fr.†; Rhone-Poulenc Rorer, S.Afr.
Melarsoprol (p.583·3).
African trypanosomiasis.

Art Negma, Fr.
Diacerein (p.29·3).
Osteoarthritis.

Artamin Biochemie, Aust.
Penicillamine (p.988·3).
Benign purpura hyperglobulinaemia; chronic active hepatitis; cystinuria; heavy metal poisoning; primary biliary cirrhosis; rheumatoid arthritis; scleroderma; Wilson's disease.

Artane
Wyeth Lederle, Aust.; Lederle, Austral.; Wyeth Lederle, Belg.; Wyeth-Ayerst, Canad.; Specia, Fr.; Lederle, Ger.; Wyeth, Irl.; Cyanamid, Ital.; Lederle, Neth.; Wyeth, S.Afr.; Cyanamid, Spain; Lederle, Switz.; Wyeth, UK†; Lederle, USA.
Benzhexol hydrochloride (p.457·3).
Drug-induced extrapyramidal disorders; parkinsonism.

Artaxan SmithKline Beecham, Ital.
Nabumetone (p.60·1).
Musculoskeletal, joint, peri-articular, and soft-tissue disorders.

Arte Rautin forte S Maurer, Ger.
Rauwolfia serpentina (p.941·3).
Formerly contained rauwolfia serpentina, olive leaf, crataegus, mistletoe, juniper, valerian, rutin, and etofylline.
Anxiety disorders; hypertension.

Arte Rutin C Maurer, Ger.
Crataegus (p.1568·2).
Formerly contained rutin, crataegus, olive leaf, valerian, lupulus, and mistletoe.
Heart failure.

Artedil Wasserman, Spain†.
Co-dergocrine mesylate (p.1566·1).
Cerebrovascular insufficiency; migraine; peripheral vascular disorders.

Artelac
Riel, Aust.; Tramedico, Belg.; Mann, Ger.; Mann, Irl.
Hypromellose (p.1473·1).
Dry eyes.

Artensen Cusi, Spain†.
Vincamine (p.1644·1).
Cerebral trauma; cerebrovascular disorders.

Arteolol Lacer, Spain.
Carteolol hydrochloride (p.837·3).
Angina pectoris; arrhythmias; hypertension.

Arteoptic
Ciba Vision, Ger.; Ciba Vision, Spain†; Ciba Vision, Swed.; Novopharma, Switz.
Carteolol hydrochloride (p.837·3).
Glaucoma; ocular hypertension.

Arteparon
Luitpold, Ger.†; Swisspharm, S.Afr.†; Alfarma, Spain†.
A heparinoid (p.882·3).
Musculoskeletal and joint disorders.

Arterase Poutrat, Fr.
Equisetum (p.1575·1); garlic (p.1583·1); cypress; aesculus (p.1543·3).
Formerly contained equisetum, garlic, cypress, aesculus, mistletoe, magnesium thiosulphate, and sodium citrate.
Capillary fragility; venous insufficiency.

Arterenol Hoechst, Ger.
Noradrenaline hydrochloride (p.924·2).
Hypotension.

Arteria -cyl Ho-Len-Complex Liebermann, Ger.
Homoeopathic preparation.

Arteriobrate Farma Lepori, Spain.
Aluminium clofibrate (p.1271·1); vincamine (p.1644·1).
Exudative diabetic retinopathy; hyperlipidaemias.

Arterioflexin
Lannacher, Aust.; CP Protea, Austral.†.
Clofibrate (p.1271·1).
Hyperlipidaemias.

Arteriovinca Farma Lepori, Spain.
Vincamine (p.1644·1) or vincamine hydrochloride (p.1644·1).
Cerebral trauma; cerebrovascular disorders.

Arterium
Schwarz, Ital.†; Llorens, Spain.
Nicofibrate hydrochloride (p.1276·1).
Hyperlipidaemias.

Arterodiet Yves Ponroy, Fr.
Fish oil.
Nutritional supplement.

Arterosan Nordmark, Ger.†.
Garlic; Mexican valerian; hawthorn; melissa.
Tonic.

Arterosan Plus Galactina, Switz.
Crataegus (p.1568·2); melissa (p.1600·1); garlic oil; ginkgo biloba (p.1584·1).
Cerebrovascular disorders.

Artes Sumitomo, Jpn†.
Melinamide (p.1275·3).
Hypercholesterolaemia.

Artesunate Atlantic, Thai.
Artesunate (p.425·2).

Arteven Boehringer Ingelheim, Ital.
Heparan sulphate (p.879·2).
Thrombosis prophylaxis.

Artex
Servier, Belg.; Therval, Fr.; Servier, Neth.
Tertatolol hydrochloride (p.952·2).
Hypertension.

Artexal Servier, Irl.
Tertatolol hydrochloride (p.952·2).
Hypertension.

Arth-A Oligocan Homeocan, Canad.
Homoeopathic preparation.

Artha-G Williams, USA.
Salsalate (p.83·1).
Fever; inflammation; pain.

Arthaxan SmithKline Beecham, Ger.
Nabumetone (p.60·1).
Musculoskeletal and joint disorders.

Arth-B Oligocan Homeocan, Canad.
Homoeopathic preparation.

Arthotec Heumann, Ger.; Albert-Roussel, Ger.
Diclofenac sodium (p.31·2).
Misoprostol (p.1419·3) is included in this preparation in an attempt to limit adverse effects on the gastro-intestinal mucosa.
Musculoskeletal and joint disorders.

Arthrabas Tosse, Ger.
Chloroquine phosphate (p.426·3).
Arthritis; lupus erythematosus.

Arthrex BASF, Ger.
Diclofenac sodium (p.31·2).
Gout; inflammation; musculoskeletal, joint, and soft-tissue disorders; pain.

Arthrex Duo BASF, Ger.
Diclofenac sodium (p.31·2).
Gout; inflammation; musculoskeletal and joint disorders; pain.

Arthrexin
Alphapharm, Austral.; Lennon, S.Afr.
Indomethacin (p.45·2).
Dysmenorrhoea; gout; musculoskeletal and joint disorders; peri-articular disorders.

Arthribosan B 31 Bock, Ger.
Homoeopathic preparation.

Arthricare Double Ice Del, USA; Commerce, USA.
Menthol (p.1600·2); camphor (p.1557·2).
Muscle and joint pain.

Arthricare Odor Free
Del, Canad.; Del, USA; Commerce, USA.
Menthol (p.1600·2); methyl nicotinate (p.55·1); capsaicin (p.24·2).
Muscle and joint pain.

Arthricare Triple Medicated
Del, Canad.; Del, USA; Commerce, USA.
Methyl salicylate (p.55·2); menthol (p.1600·2); methyl nicotinate (p.55·1).
Muscle and joint pain.

Arthrifid S Fides, Ger.
Homoeopathic preparation.

Arthrisan Planta, Canad.
Capsules: Salix (p.82·3); juniper (p.1592·2).
Oral drops: Salix (p.82·3); juniper (p.1592·2); solidago canadensis.
Arthritis.

Arthrisel Ramon Sala, Spain†.
Lithium citrate (p.290·3); monosodium citrate; sodium acid citrate (p.1153·2); sodium sulphate (p.1213·3); sodium bitartrate.
Arthritis; constipation; diuresis; renal calculi; rheumatism.

Arthritic Pain Homeocan, Canad.
Homoeopathic preparation.

Arthritic Pain Herbal Formula 1 Vitelle, Austral.
Celery (p.1561·1); juniper (p.1592·2); harpagophytum procumbens (p.27·2); salix alba (p.82·3).
Arthritis; rheumatism.

Arthritic Pain L10 Homeocan, Canad.
Homoeopathic preparation.

Arthritis Foundation Ibuprofen McNeil Consumer, USA†.
Ibuprofen (p.44·1).
Fever; osteoarthritis; pain; rheumatoid arthritis.

Arthritis Foundation Nighttime McNeil Consumer, USA†.
Paracetamol (p.72·2); diphenhydramine hydrochloride (p.409·1).
Insomnia associated with pain.

Arthritis Foundation Pain Reliever McNeil Consumer, USA.
Aspirin (p.16·1).
Fever; musculoskeletal and joint disorders; myocardial infarction; pain; transient ischaemic attacks.

Arthritis Foundation Pain Reliever, Aspirin Free McNeil Consumer, USA†.
Paracetamol (p.72·2).
Fever; musculoskeletal and joint disorders; pain.

Arthritis Hot Creme Thompson, USA.
Methyl salicylate (p.55·2); menthol (p.1600·2).
Muscle, joint, and soft-tissue pain; neuralgia.

Arthritis Pain Formula Whitehall, USA.
Aspirin (p.16·1).
Aluminium hydroxide (p.1177·3) and magnesium hydroxide (p.1198·2) are included in this preparation in an attempt to limit adverse effects on the gastro-intestinal mucosa.
Arthritis; fever; pain.

Arthritis Pain Formula Aspirin Free Whitehall, USA.
Paracetamol (p.72·2).
Fever; pain.

Arthritis Pain Tablets Invamed, USA.
Aspirin (p.16·1).
Calcium carbonate (p.1182·1), magnesium carbonate (p.1198·1), and magnesium oxide (p.1198·3) are included in this preparation in an attempt to limit adverse effects on the gastro-intestinal mucosa.

Arthrixyl N Syxyl, Ger.
Homoeopathic preparation.

arthro akut Tosse, Ger.
Lonazolac calcium (p.50·3).
Inflammation; musculoskeletal and joint disorders; pain.

Arthrocine Merck Sharp & Dohme-Chibret, Fr.
Sulindac (p.86·3).
Musculoskeletal, joint, and peri-articular disorders.

Arthrodeformat P Ziethen, Ger.
Pituitary extract (p.1050·1); rosemary oil (p.1626·2).
Rheumatic disorders.

Arthrodestal N Krugmann, Ger.
Glycol salicylate (p.43·1); camphor (p.1557·2); benzyl nicotinate (p.22·1).
Nerve, joint, and muscle pain.

Arthrodont Veyron-Froment, Fr.
Enoxolone (p.35·2); formaldehyde (p.1113·2); sodium formaldehyde sulphoxylate (p.1124·3).
Gum disorders.

Arthrodynat N Ziethen, Ger.
Urtica (p.1642·3).
Rheumatic disorders.

Arthrodynat P Ziethen, Ger.
Rosemary oil (p.1626·2); camphor (p.1557·2); hypericum oil (p.1590·1).
Rheumatic disorders.

Arthrofen Ashbourne, UK.
Ibuprofen (p.44·1).
Inflammation; musculoskeletal and joint disorders; pain.

Arthrokehlan "A" Sanum-Kehlbeck, Ger.
Formoltoxoid from *Corynebacterium parvum* (p.516·1).
Musculoskeletal and joint disorders.

Arthrokehlan "U" Sanum-Kehlbeck, Ger.
Formol toxoid from Corynebacterium spp.
Tonic.

Arthro-Menthoneurin Tosse, Ger.†.
Diethylamine salicylate (p.33·1); methyl nicotinate (p.55·1); heparin (p.879·3).
Muscle and joint disorders.

Arthropan Purdue Frederick, USA.
Choline salicylate (p.25·2).
Fever; inflammation; pain.

Arthrorell Sanorell, Ger.
Homoeopathic preparation.

Arthrose-Echtroplex *Weber & Weber, Ger.*
Homoeopathic preparation.

Arthrose-Gastreu R73 *Reckeweg, Ger.*
Homoeopathic preparation.

Arthrosenex AR *Brenner-Efeka, Ger.; LAW, Ger.*
Arnica (p.1550·3).
Muscular and joint disorders.

Arthrosetten H *Brenner-Efeka, Ger.*
Harpagophytum procumbens (p.27·2).
Musculoskeletal disorders.

Arthrosin *Ashbourne, UK.*
Naproxen (p.61·2).
Dysmenorrhoea; gout; musculoskeletal and joint disorders.

Arthrotabs *Duopharm, Ger.*
Harpagophytum procumbens (p.27·2).
Musculoskeletal and joint disorders.

Arthrotec
Searle, Austral.; Searle, Canad.; Searle, Irl.; Searle, Neth.; Searle, Norw.; Searle, S.Afr.; Searle, Swed.; Searle, Switz.; Searle, UK; Searle, USA.
Diclofenac sodium (p.31·2).
Misoprostol (p.1419·3) is included in this preparation in an attempt to limit adverse effects on the gastro-intestinal mucosa.
Musculoskeletal and joint disorders.

Arthrotone *Pharmadass, UK.*
Harpagophytum procumbens (p.27·2); royal jelly (p.1626·3).

Arthroxen *CP Pharmaceuticals, UK.*
Naproxen (p.61·2).
Musculoskeletal and joint disorders.

Arthryl *Synlab, Fr.†.*
N-Acetyl glucosamine; sodium sulphate (p.1213·3).
Arthroses.

Articulen *Rolab, S.Afr.*
Indomethacin (p.45·2).
Gout; musculoskeletal and joint disorders.

Articulose-50 *Seatrace, USA.*
Prednisolone acetate (p.1048·1).
Corticosteroid.

Articulose LA *Seatrace, USA.*
Triamcinolone diacetate (p.1050·2).
Corticosteroid.

Artiflam *Hoechst Marion Roussel, Belg.*
Tiaprofenic acid (p.89·1) or tiaprofenic acid, trometamol salt (p.89·1).
Inflammation.

Artigel *SAN, Ital.†.*
Harpagophytum procumbens (p.27·2).

Artin *Schoeller, Aust.*
Aloes (p.1177·1); frangula bark (p.1193·2).
Constipation; stool softener.

Artisial
Jouveinal, Canad.; Jouveinal, Fr.; Cell Pharm, Ger.
Electrolytes (p.1147·1); carmellose sodium (p.1471·2); sorbitol (p.1354·2).
Saliva substitute.

Artival *Chefaro Ardeval, Fr.†.*
Black currant (p.1365·2); meadowsweet (p.1599·1).
Joint pain.

Artocoron *Knoll, Ger.*
Naftidrofuryl oxalate (p.914·2).
Peripheral vascular disorders.

Artoid *Artu, Neth.*
Pollen extracts (p.1545·1).
Hyposensitisation.

Artonil *GEA, Swed.*
Ranitidine hydrochloride (p.1209·3).
Gastro-oesophageal reflux; peptic ulcer; Zollinger-Ellison syndrome.

Artosin
Boehringer Mannheim, Ger.; Boehringer Mannheim, Neth.
Tolbutamide (p.333·2).
Diabetes mellitus.

Artoxan *Herbaline, Ital.*
Harpagophytum procumbens (p.27·2); silver birch (p.1553·3); fraxinus excelsior; meadowsweet (p.1599·1).
Musculoskeletal, joint, and peri-articular disorders; myalgia.

Artracin *Trinity, UK.*
Indomethacin (p.45·2).
Inflammation; musculoskeletal, joint, and peri-articular disorders; pain.

Artragel *Interdelta, Switz.*
Glycol salicylate (p.43·1); benzyl nicotinate (p.22·1); camphor (p.1557·2); levomenthol (p.1600·2); turpentine oil (p.1641·1).
Musculoskeletal and joint pain.

Artragil *Iquinosa, Spain.*
Piroxicam (p.80·2).
Dysmenorrhoea; gout; musculoskeletal and joint disorders.

Artralgon *Saunier-Daguin, Fr.*
Amylocaine hydrochloride (p.1286·1); glycol orthocresotinate; guaiacyl nicotinate.
Soft-tissue disorders.

Artrene *IRBI, Ital.†.*
Ibuprofen meglumine (p.44·3).
Musculoskeletal and joint disorders.

Artri *Medical, Spain.*
Adenosine phosphate (p.1543·2); indomethacin (p.45·2).
Fever; inflammation; pain.

Artri Ben *Benarth, Canad.†.*
Fir oil; cedar oil; pine oil.
Musculoskeletal and joint pain.

Artrinovo *Llorens, Spain.*
Indomethacin (p.45·2).
Gout; inflammation; musculoskeletal and joint disorders; pain; peri-articular disorders.

Artritol *Bio-Sante, Canad.*
Capsules: Paracetamol (p.72·2).
Cream: Methyl salicylate (p.55·2); menthol (p.1600·2).

Artriunic *Novag, Spain.*
Tenoxicam (p.88·2).
Musculoskeletal and joint disorders; peri-articular disorders.

Artrivia Prednisolona *Sabater, Spain†.*
Indomethacin (p.45·2); methylprednisolone (p.1046·1).
Musculoskeletal and joint disorders; peri-articular disorders.

Artrobetin *Lenza, Ital.†.*
Injection: Cocarboxylase (p.1361·2); cyanocobalamin (p.1363·3); pyridoxine hydrochloride (p.1362·3).
Tablets: Thiamine hydrochloride (p.1361·1); cyanocobalamin (p.1363·3); pyridoxine hydrochloride (p.1362·3).
Neuropathies.

Artrocaptin *Estedi, Spain.*
Tolmetin sodium (p.89·3).
Inflammation; musculoskeletal and joint disorders; pain.

Artrocur *IRBI, Ital.*
Injection†: A heparinoid (p.882·3); dipyrone (p.35·1).
Topical gel: A heparinoid (p.882·3); aminopropylone (p.15·2).
Pain.

Artrodar *Ecupharma, Ital.*
Diacerein (p.29·3).
Osteoarthritis.

Artrodesmol Extra *Reig Jofre, Spain.*
Dimethyl sulphoxide (p.1377·2); phenylbutazone (p.79·2); fluocinolone acetonide (p.1041·1); methyl salicylate (p.55·2).
Soft-tissue disorders.

Artrodif *Andreu, Spain†.*
Animal organ hydrolysates (p.1599·1).
Inflammation.

Artrodol *AGIPS, Ital.*
Diflunisal (p.33·2).
Pain.

Artroglobina *Tedec Meiji, Spain†.*
Immunoglobulins (p.1522·1).
Inflammation.

Artrogota *Parisis, Spain.*
Diethylamine salicylate (p.33·1).
Peri-articular and soft-tissue disorders.

Artrolasi *Lenza, Ital.†.*
Orgotein (p.87·3).
Inflammatory disorders.

Artromed *Medosan, Ital.*
Amtolmetin guacil (p.15·3).
Musculoskeletal and joint disorders; pain.

Artroreuma *Teofarma, Ital.*
Tiaprofenic acid (p.89·1).
Inflammation; pain.

Artrosal *OTC, Spain.*
Ethyl vanillin (p.1577·2); phenylpropanol salicylate.
Rheumatic and muscle pain.

Artrosan *Dolisos, Fr.*
Harpagophytum procumbens (p.27·2); meadowsweet (p.1599·1).
Joint disorders.

Artrosilene *Dompe, Ital.*
Ketoprofen lysine (p.48·3).
Musculoskeletal and joint disorders.

Artrosone *Belmac, Spain†.*
Dexamethasone (p.1037·1).
Corticosteroid.

Artrotec *Monsanto, Ital.*
Diclofenac sodium (p.31·2).
Misoprostol (p.1419·3) is included in this preparation in an attempt to limit adverse effects on the gastro-intestinal mucosa.
Inflammation; musculoskeletal and joint disorders; pain.

Artroxen *Errekappa, Ital.*
Naproxen (p.61·2).
Musculoskeletal and joint disorders.

Artroxicam *Coli, Ital.*
Piroxicam (p.80·2).
Musculoskeletal, joint, peri-articular, and soft-tissue disorders.

Arturic *Alpharma, Norw.*
Allopurinol (p.390·2).
Gout; hyperuricaemia; renal calculi; uric acid nephropathy.

Artz *Luitpold, Ital.*
Sodium hyaluronate (p.1630·3).
Osteoarthritis of the knee.

Artzal
Luitpold, Aust.; Astra, Swed.
Sodium hyaluronate (p.1630·3).
Arthrosis of the knee.

Aru C *ankerpharm, Ger.*
Clotrimazole (p.376·3).
Corynebacterium skin infections; fungal skin infections.

Arubendol
Note. This name is used for preparations of different composition.
Isis, Ger.
Terbutaline sulphate (p.764·1).
Obstructive airways disease.

Klinge, Ger.
Salbutamol (p.758·2).
Obstructive airways disease.

Aruclonin *ankerpharm, Ger.*
Clonidine hydrochloride (p.841·2).
Glaucoma; ocular hypertension.

Arufil *ankerpharm, Ger.*
Povidone (p.1474·2).
Dry eyes.

Arumalon *Robapharm, Ger.†; Tosse, Ger.†.*
Bovine cartilage extract; bone marrow extract.
Degenerative joint disorders.

Aru-Sept-Spray *ankerpharm, Ger.†.*
Chlorocresol (p.1110·3); clorophene (p.1111·2).
Fungal foot infections.

Aruterol *Klinge, Ger.†.*
Fenoterol hydrobromide (p.753·2).
Obstructive airways disease.

Arutimol *ankerpharm, Ger.*
Timolol maleate (p.953·3).
Glaucoma; ocular hypertension.

Aruto-Magenpulver *Hotz, Ger.†.*
Magnesium oxide (p.1198·3); calcium carbonate (p.1182·1); charcoal (p.972·3); kaolin (p.1195·1).
Gastro-intestinal disorders.

Aruto-Magenpulver-forte *Hotz, Ger.†.*
Kaolin (p.1195·1); magnesium oxide (p.1198·3); aluminium magnesium trisilicate; calcium carbonate (p.1182·1); bismuth subnitrate (p.1180·2); chamomile (p.1561·2); peppermint leaf (p.1208·1); achillea (p.1542·2); absinthium (p.1541·1); caraway (p.1559·3); fennel (p.1579·1); rhubarb (p.1212·1); gentian (p.1583·3).
Gastro-intestinal disorders.

Arutrin *ankerpharm, Ger.*
Triamcinolone acetonide (p.1050·2).
Skin disorders.

Arutropid *Klinge, Ger.†.*
Ipratropium bromide (p.754·2).
Obstructive airways disease.

Arvenum *Stroder, Ital.*
Diosmin (p.1580·1).
Peripheral vascular disorders.

Arvin
Knoll, Canad.; Knoll, Spain; Knoll, UK†.
Ancrod (p.823·3).
Peripheral vascular disorders; thrombo-embolic disorders.

Arvin Antidote
Knoll, Canad.†; Knoll, UK†.
Ancrod antiserum.
Overdosage with or adverse effects of ancrod.

Arwin
Ebewe, Aust.; Knoll, Ger.
Ancrod (p.823·3).
Peripheral vascular disorders.

Arythmol
Knoll, Irl.; Knoll, UK.
Propafenone hydrochloride (p.935·3).
Arrhythmias.

Arzimol *Daker Farmasimes, Spain.*
Cefprozil (p.172·3).
Bacterial infections.

AS 101 VA N *Staufen, Ger.*
Homoeopathic preparation.

ASA *Lilly, USA†.*
Aspirin (p.16·1).

ASA and Codeine Compound, No.3 *Lilly, USA†.*
Codeine phosphate (p.26·1); aspirin (p.16·1); caffeine (p.749·3).

Asa Right Powder *Eagle, Austral.*
Vitamin and mineral preparation.
Formerly known as Asma Right Powder.
Respiratory congestion.

ASA Tones *Eagle, Austral.*
Grindelia camporum; hedera helix; potassium iodide (p.1493·1); crataegus (p.1568·2); euphorbia hirta; liquorice (p.1197·1); polygala tenuifolia (p.1069·3); drosera longifolia (p.1574·1).
Upper respiratory-tract symptoms.

Asacol
Byk, Belg.; Procter & Gamble, Canad.; Giuliani, Ital.; Byk, Neth.; Leiras, Norw.; Hoechst Marion Roussel, S.Afr.; Leiras, Swed.; Giuliani, Switz.; SmithKline Beecham, UK; Procter & Gamble, USA.
Mesalazine (p.1199·2).
Anorectal disorders; inflammatory bowel disease.

Asacolitin *Henning, Ger.*
Mesalazine (p.1199·2).
Ulcerative colitis.

Asacolon *Evans Medical, Irl.*
Mesalazine (p.1199·2).
Proctitis; proctosigmoiditis; ulcerative colitis.

ASAD
Stallergenes, Fr.; Stallergenes, Switz.
A range of allergen extracts (p.1545·1).
Hyposensitisation.

Asaferm *Merckle, Swed.†.*
Aspirin (p.16·1).
Cardiovascular disorders; fever; inflammation; pain.

Asaflow *Sandipro, Belg.*
Aspirin (p.16·1).
Cardiovascular and cerebrovascular disorders.

Asalen *Covan, S.Afr.*
Phenylephrine hydrochloride (p.1066·2); chlorpheniramine maleate (p.405·1); paracetamol (p.72·2); caffeine (p.749·3).
Formerly contained phenylephrine hydrochloride, thenyldiamine hydrochloride, paracetamol, and caffeine.
Cold symptoms.

Asalen Cough Linctus *Saphar, S.Afr.†.*
Codeine phosphate (p.26·1); ammonium chloride (p.1055·2); potassium guaiacolsulfonate (p.1068·3); phenylephrine hydrochloride (p.1066·2).
Coughs.

Asalite *Kabi, Swed.†.*
Aspirin (p.16·1).
Cardiovascular disorders.

Asaphen *Pharmascience, Canad.*
Aspirin (p.16·1).
Fever; pain.

Asarid *Boehringer Ingelheim, Belg.*
Aspirin (p.16·1).
Cardiovascular disorders; fever; pain.

Asarum Med Complex *Dynamit, Aust.*
Homoeopathic preparation.

Asasantin
Thomae, Ger.; Boehringer Ingelheim, Spain; Boehringer Ingelheim, UK.
Dipyridamole (p.857·1); aspirin (p.16·1).
Thrombo-embolic disorders.

Asasantine
Boehringer Ingelheim, Canad.; Boehringer Ingelheim, Switz.†.
Dipyridamole (p.857·1); aspirin (p.16·1).
Thrombo-embolic disorders; vascular disorders.

ASAtard *Boehringer Ingelheim, S.Afr.*
Aspirin (p.16·1).
Thrombosis prophylaxis.

Asba *Medirel, Switz.*
Calcium carbonate (p.1182·1); camphor (p.1557·2); peppermint oil (p.1208·1).
Mouth and throat disorders.

Asboi *BOI, Spain†.*
Aspirin (p.16·1).
Fever; musculoskeletal and joint disorders; pain; thrombo-embolism prophylaxis.

Asbron G *Sandoz, USA†.*
Theophylline sodium glycinate (p.772·2); guaiphenesin (p.1061·3).
Obstructive airways disease.

Ascabiol
Note. This name is used for preparations of different composition.
Rhone-Poulenc Rorer, Austral.; Rhone-Poulenc Rorer, Irl.; Rhone-Poulenc Rorer, S.Afr.; May & Baker, UK.
Benzyl benzoate (p.1402·2).
Pediculosis; scabies.

Evans, Fr.
Benzyl benzoate (p.1402·2); monosulfiram (p.1408·2).
Scabies.

Ascal
Helsinn Birex, Irl.†; Asta Medica, Neth.
Carbaspirin calcium (p.25·1).
Fever; pain; thrombo-embolism prophylaxis.

Ascal 38 *Asta Medica, Spain.*
Carbaspirin calcium (p.25·1).
Thrombo-embolism prophylaxis.

Ascarient *Propan, S.Afr.†.*
Piperazine citrate (p.107·2).
Enterobiasis; roundworm infections.

Ascencyl *Theraplix, Fr.*
Adenosine phosphate; cyanocobalamin; magnesium aspartate; manganese gluconate.
Tonic.

Ascodyne *Chemedica, Switz.*
Multivitamin preparation with amino acids.
Tonic.

Ascofer
Desbergers, Canad.; Gerda, Fr.; Sodip, Switz.†.
Ferrous ascorbate (p.1339·2).
Iron-deficiency anaemias.

Ascold *Propan, S.Afr.*
Phenylephrine hydrochloride (p.1066·2); salicylamide (p.82·3); mepyramine maleate (p.414·1); caffeine (p.749·3); ascorbic acid (p.1365·2).
Cold and influenza symptoms.

Ascomed *Ripari-Gero, Ital.*
Ascorbic acid (p.1365·2).
Vitamin C deficiency.

Ascorb *CP Protea, Austral.†.*
Ascorbic acid (p.1365·2).

Ascorbamina 1500 *Rhone-Poulenc Rorer, Spain†.*
Ascorbic acid; cyanocobalamin; lysine hydrochloride; sarcosine ascorbate.
Tonic.

Ascorbamina Infantil *Rhone-Poulenc Rorer, Spain†.*
Ascorbic acid; carnitine hydrochloride; cyanocobalamin; lysine; sarcosine ascorbate.
Tonic.

Ascorbeta *Manetti Roberts, Ital.†.*
Betaine ascorbate (p.1553·2).
Vitamin C deficiency.

Ascorbex *Sante Naturelle, Canad.*
Ascorbic acid (p.1365·2).

Ascorbicap *ICN, USA.*
Ascorbic acid (p.1365·2).
Scurvy; vitamin C deficiency.

Ascorbin
Montavit, Aust.
Ascorbic acid (p.1365·2) or sodium ascorbate (p.1365·2).
Vitamin C deficiency.

Italfarmaco, Ital.†.
Calcium ascorbate (p.1365·2).
Calcium and vitamin C deficiency.

Ascorbin-Chinin-Dragees Michallik *Michallik, Ger.†.*
Quinine sulphate (p.439·2); ascorbic acid (p.1365·2); caffeine (p.749·3); etenzamide (p.35·3).
Cold symptoms; influenza.

Ascorbisal *Lannacher, Aust.*
Aspirin (p.16·1); ascorbic acid (p.1365·2).
Fever; musculoskeletal and joint disorders; pain.

Ascorell *Sanorell, Ger.*
Ascorbic acid (p.1365·2).
Vitamin C deficiency.

Ascorgil *Biomedica, Ital.†.*
Ascorbic acid (p.1365·2).
Vitamin C deficiency.

Ascortonyl *Gerda, Fr.*
Ascorbic acid (p.1365·2); magnesium potassium aspartate.
Formerly contained ascorbic acid, magnesium potassium aspartate, and cyanocobalamin.
Tonic.

Ascorvit *Jenapharm, Ger.*
Ascorbic acid (p.1365·2).
Vitamin C deficiency.

Ascotodin *Bruschettini, Ital.*
Mebechinium methylsulphate; thonzylamine hydrochloride (p.419·2).
Eye disorders.

Ascoxal
Astra, Austral.; Astra, Norw.; Astra, Swed.
Ascorbic acid (p.1365·2); sodium percarbonate; copper sulphate (p.1338·1).
Mouth and throat inflammation and infection.

Ascredar *Boehringer Mannheim, Aust.*
Disodium clodronate (p.737·3).
Hypercalcaemia of malignancy; osteolytic bone metastases; Paget's disease of bone.

Ascriptin
Rhone-Poulenc Rorer, Irl.; Rhone-Poulenc Rorer, Ital.
Aspirin (p.16·1).
Aluminium hydroxide (p.1177·3) and magnesium hydroxide (p.1198·2) are included in this preparation in an attempt to limit adverse effects on the gastro-intestinal mucosa.
Fever; inflammation; pain.

Rhone-Poulenc Rorer, USA.
Aspirin (p.16·1).
Aluminium hydroxide (p.1177·3), calcium carbonate (p.1182·1), and magnesium hydroxide (p.1198·2) are included in this preparation in an attempt to limit adverse effects on the gastro-intestinal mucosa.
Fever; inflammation; myocardial infarction; pain; transient ischaemic attacks.

Aselli *Weifa, Norw.*
Cream: Cetylpyridinium chloride (p.1106·2); zinc tannate.
Minor skin disorders; skin disinfection; sunburn.
Ointment: Zinc tannate; zinc oxide (p.1096·2); titanium dioxide (p.1093·3); cod-liver oil (p.1337·3).
Minor skin disorders.

Asendin
Wyeth-Ayerst, Canad.; Lederle, USA.
Amoxapine (p.279·2).
Depression.

Asendis
Wyeth, Irl.; Wyeth, UK.
Amoxapine (p.279·2).
Depression.

ASEP *Galen, UK.*
Glutaraldehyde (p.1114·3).
Instrument disinfection.

Asepsal *Magis, Ital.*
Ibuprofen isobutanolammonium (p.44·3).
Gynaecological disorders.

Aseptiderm *Pharmethic, Belg.*
Cetrimonium bromide (p.1106·1).
Disinfection of skin and instruments.

Aseptil *SmithKline Beecham, Ital.*
Copper usnate (p.1643·1); diazolidinyl urea; zinc oxide (p.1096·2); alcloxa (p.1078·2).
Skin and wound disinfection.

Aseptil Liquido *Maggioni, Ital.†.*
Chlorhexidine gluconate (p.1107·2).
Skin and wound disinfection.

Aseptisol *Bode, Ger.*
Glutaraldehyde (p.1114·3); formaldehyde (p.1113·2); didecylmethyloxethylammonium propionate.
Instrument disinfection.

Asepto 7 *Riom, Fr.*
Cetrimide (p.1105·2).
Burns; wounds.

Aseptoman *Geistlich, Switz.*
Isopropyl alcohol (p.1118·2); 1,3-butanediol.
Hand disinfection.

Aseptosyl *Synthelabo, Belg.*
Potassium hydroxyquinoline sulphate (p.1621·1); lignocaine hydrochloride (p.1293·2).
Mouth and throat disorders.

Aserbine
Bencard, Irl.†; SmithKline Beecham, S.Afr.; Forley, UK.
Benzoic acid (p.1102·3); malic acid (p.1598·3); salicylic acid (p.1090·2); propylene glycol (p.1622·1).
Burns; skin ulcers; wounds.

Asgocholan *Rhein-Pharma, Ger.†.*
Chelidonium; frangula bark (p.1193·2); peppermint leaf (p.1208·1); silybum marianum (p.993·3); absinthium (p.1541·1); carduus benedictus (p.1565·3); achillea (p.1542·2); taraxacum (p.1634·2).
Biliary disorders; liver disorders.

Asgoviscum N *Rhein-Pharma, Ger.*
Mistletoe (p.1604·1); crataegus (p.1568·2); garlic (p.1583·1).
Cardiac disorders.

Ashton & Parsons Infants Powders *SmithKline Beecham Consumer, UK.*
Matricaria tincture (p.1561·2).
Colic; teething.

Asic *Pharmaceutical Enterprises, S.Afr.*
Dicyclomine hydrochloride (p.460·1); doxylamine succinate (p.410·1); pyridoxine hydrochloride (p.1362·3).
Nausea and vomiting in pregnancy.

Asig *Sigma, Austral.*
Quinapril hydrochloride (p.938·1).
Heart failure; hypertension.

Asilone
Knoll, Irl.; Roche, S.Afr.; Seton, UK.
Oral suspension; oral gel: Aluminium hydroxide (p.1177·3); magnesium oxide (p.1198·3); simethicone (p.1213·1).
Dyspepsia; flatulence; gastritis; gastro-oesophageal reflux; hiatus hernia; peptic ulcer.

Knoll, Irl.; Roche, S.Afr.; Seton, UK.
Tablets: Aluminium hydroxide (p.1177·3); simethicone (p.1213·1).
Dyspepsia; flatulence; gastritis; gastro-oesophageal reflux; hiatus hernia; peptic ulcer.

Asilone Heartburn *Seton, UK.*
Alginic acid (p.1470·3); aluminium hydroxide (p.1177·3); magnesium hydroxide (p.1198·2); sodium bicarbonate (p.1153·2).
Dyspepsia; heartburn.

Asilone Windcheaters *Seton, UK.*
Simethicone (p.1213·1).
Flatulence.

Asimil B12 *Torlan, Spain.*
Mecobalamin (p.1364·2).
Vitamin B12 deficiency.

Askarutina *Gentili, Ital.†.*
Injection: Sodium ascorbate (p.1365·2); menadiol sodium sulphate (p.1371·3); sulmarin.
Syrup: Sodium ascorbate (p.1365·2); menadiol sodium sulphate (p.1371·3); sulmarin; rutin (p.1580·2).
Tablets: Ascorbic acid (p.1365·2); menadiol sodium sulphate (p.1371·3); sulmarin; rutin (p.1580·2).
Haemorrhagic disorders.

Askenzyme *Laleuf, Fr.†.*
Aspergillus aureus enzymes.
Dyspepsia.

Askina *Braun Biotrol, Fr.*
Carmellose (p.1471·2).
Wounds.

Askit *Askit, UK.*
Capsules: Aspirin (p.16·1); aloxiprin (p.15·1); caffeine (p.749·3).
Tablets; oral powders: Aspirin (p.16·1); aloxiprin (p.15·1); caffeine citrate (p.749·3).
Aluminium glycinate (p.1177·2) is included in this preparation in an attempt to limit adverse effects on the gastro-intestinal mucosa.
Fever; pain.

ASL *Normon, Spain.*
Lysine aspirin (p.50·3).
Fever; inflammation; pain; thrombo-embolism prophylaxis.

Aslavital *Schoeller, Aust.†.*
Injection: Procaine hydrochloride (p.1299·2); glutamic acid (p.1344·3).
Tablets: Procaine hydrochloride (p.1299·2); pyridoxine hydrochloride (p.1362·3); inositol (p.1591·1).
Tonic.

Asmabec *Medeva, UK.*
Beclomethasone dipropionate (p.1032·1).
Asthma.

Asmacortone *Nuovo, Ital.*
Methylprednisolone sodium hemisuccinate (p.1046·1).
Corticosteroid.

Asmalene *FIRMA, Ital.*
Bitolterol mesylate (p.749·2).
Obstructive airways disease.

Asmalix *Century, USA.*
Theophylline (p.765·1).
Obstructive airways disease.

Asmalline *Be-Tabs, S.Afr.†.*
Aminophylline (p.748·1).
Obstructive airways disease.

Asman-Valeas *Valeas, Ital.†.*
Adrenaline acid tartrate (p.813·3); atropine methobromide (p.455·1).
Asthma; hay fever.

Asmarectal *Serpero, Ital.†.*
Diphenhydramine methylbromide (p.409·2); aminophylline (p.748·1); lignocaine (p.1293·2).
Obstructive airways disease.

Asmasal *Medeva, UK.*
Salbutamol sulphate (p.758·2).
Obstructive airways disease.

Asmaven *Approved Prescription Services, UK.*
Salbutamol sulphate (p.758·2).
Obstructive airways disease; premature labour.

Asmavent *Technilab, Canad.*
Salbutamol sulphate (p.758·2).
Obstructive airways disease.

Asmaxen *Doetsch, Grether, Switz.†.*
Salbutamol (p.758·2).
Obstructive airways disease.

Asmetil *Benvegna, Ital.†.*
Protokylol hydrochloride.
Respiratory-system disorders.

Asmisul *Inibsa, Spain†.*
Eprozinol hydrochloride (p.1574·3).
Asthmatic and dyspnoeic disorders.

Asmo *ICN, Spain.*
Theophylline (p.765·1).
Heart failure; obstructive airways disease; paroxysmal dyspnoea.

Asmol *Alphapharm, Austral.*
Salbutamol (p.758·2) or salbutamol sulphate (p.758·2).
Obstructive airways disease.

Asocid *Volchem, Ital.*
Peptide, lipid, and carbohydrate preparation with vitamin C.
Nutritional supplement.

Asonacor *Ebewe, Aust.*
Propafenone hydrochloride (p.935·3).
Arrhythmias.

Asorec *Radiumfarma, Ital.†.*
Sulphaguanole.
Infective diarrhoea.

Aspac *Inexfa, Spain.*
Paracetamol (p.72·2).
Fever; pain.

Aspalgin *Fawns & McAllan, Austral.*
Aspirin (p.16·1); codeine phosphate (p.26·1).
Fever; inflammation; pain.

Aspalox *Rorer, Ger.†.*
Aspirin (p.16·1).
Arthritis; fever; pain; rheumatism; thrombo-embolic disorders.

Asparagin N (Rowo-119) *Pharmakon, Ger.†.*
Vitamin and electrolyte preparation.
Tonic.

Asparagus-P *Plantina, Ger.*
Asparagus; parsley (p.1615·3).
Oedema; renal calculi.

Aspartamins *Solgar, UK.*
Mineral aspartate preparation.

Aspartatol *Eagle, Austral.*
Potassium aspartate (p.1161·3); magnesium aspartate (p.1157·2); levoglutamide (p.1344·3).
Tonic.

Aspartina
Bouty, Ital.; Vick International, Ital.†.
Aspartame (p.1335·1).
Sugar substitute.

Aspartono *Medix, Spain.*
Adenosine triphosphate; glucose; magnesium aspartate; potassium aspartate.
Cardiopathies; liver disorders; muscular dystrophies; tonic.

A-Spas *Hyrex, USA.*
Hyoscyamine sulphate (p.464·2).
Gastro-intestinal disorders.

Aspaserine B6 Tranq *UCB, Spain.*
Diazepam (p.661·1).
Contains pyridoxine.
Alcohol withdrawal syndrome; anxiety; febrile convulsions; insomnia; skeletal muscle spasm.

Aspasmon N *Norgine, Ger.*
Peppermint oil (p.1208·1); anise oil (p.1550·1); caraway oil (p.1559·3).
Asthma; gastro-intestinal disorders.

Aspav *Roussel, UK.*
Aspirin (p.16·1); papaveretum (p.71·1).
Pain.

Aspecton *Krewel, Ger.*
Thyme (p.1636·3).
Catarrh; coughs.

Aspecton N *Krewel, Ger.*
Thyme (p.1636·3); gypsophila saponins.
Respiratory-tract disorders.

Aspecton-Balsam *Krewel, Ger.*
Camphor (p.1557·2); thyme oil (p.1637·1); eucalyptus oil (p.1578·1).
Cold symptoms; coughs.

Aspectonetten N *Krewel, Ger.*
Gypsophila saponins.
Formerly contained butethamate citrate.
Respiratory-tract catarrh.

Aspegic
Synthelabo, Belg.; Synthelabo, Fr.; Synthelabo, Ital.; Lorex Synthelabo, Neth.; Cantabria, Spain; Synthelabo, Switz.
Lysine aspirin (p.50·3).
Fever; musculoskeletal and joint disorders; pain; thrombo-embolism prophylaxis.

Aspellin *Fisons, UK.*
Methyl salicylate (p.55·2); ethyl salicylate (p.36·1); ammonium salicylate (p.15·2); menthol (p.1600·2); camphor (p.1557·2).
Pain.

Aspenil *Chemil, Ital.†.*
Amoxycillin (p.151·3).
Bacterial infections.

Asperal-B *Bio-Therabel, Belg.†.*
Theophylline (p.765·1); phenobarbitone (p.350·2); papaverine hydrochloride (p.1614·2); belladonna extract (p.457·1).
Asthma; dyspnoea.

Aspercreme
Note. This name is used for preparations of different composition.
Stella, Canad.; Thompson, USA.
Triethanolamine salicylate (p.1639·2).
Muscle, joint, and soft-tissue pain; neuralgia.

Roche, Ital.
Diethylamine salicylate (p.33·1); methyl nicotinate (p.55·1).
Musculoskeletal disorders.

Aspergum
Schering-Plough, Canad.; Farmades, Ital.†; Schering-Plough, USA.
Aspirin (p.16·1).
Fever; inflammation; myocardial infarction; pain; transient ischaemic attacks.

Asphaline *Galenica, Switz.*
Camphor (p.1557·2); thymol (p.1127·1); paraformaldehyde (p.1121·1); zinc oxide (p.1096·2).
Root canal infections.

Aspidol *Piam, Ital.*
Lysine aspirin (p.50·3).
Pain.

Aspidolce *Alonga, Spain†.*
Aspirin (p.16·1).
Fever; musculoskeletal and joint disorders; pain; periarticular disorders; thrombo-embolism prophylaxis.

Aspiglicina *Antonetto, Ital.*
Aspirin (p.16·1).
Glycine (p.1345·2) is included in this preparation in an attempt to limit adverse effects on the gastro-intestinal mucosa.
Neuralgia.

Aspinfantil *Diviser Aquilea, Spain.*
Aspirin (p.16·1).
Fever; musculoskeletal and joint disorders; pain; thrombo-embolism prophylaxis.

Aspirange *Schwarz, Fr.†.*
Aspirin (p.16·1); ascorbic acid (p.1365·2).
Fever; pain.

Aspiricor *Bayer, Aust.*
Aspirin (p.16·1).
Migraine; thrombo-embolism prophylaxis.

Aspirin Backache *Bayer, Canad.*
Aspirin (p.16·1); methocarbamol (p.1316·1).
Back pain.

Aspirin + C *Bayer, Aust.*
Aspirin (p.16·1); ascorbic acid (p.1365·2).
Fever; pain.

Aspirin forte *Bayer, Ger.*
Aspirin (p.16·1); caffeine (p.749·3).
Inflammation; pain.

Aspirin Free Anacin *Robins, USA.*
Paracetamol (p.72·2).
Formerly known as Anacin-3.

Aspirin Free Anacin PM *Whitehall, USA.*
Paracetamol (p.72·2); diphenhydramine hydrochloride (p.409·1).
Insomnia; pain.

Aspirin Free Excedrin *Bristol-Myers Squibb, USA.*
Paracetamol (p.72·2); caffeine (p.749·3).

Aspirin Free Excedrin Dual *Bristol-Myers Squibb, USA.*
Paracetamol (p.72·2); calcium carbonate (p.1182·1); magnesium carbonate (p.1198·1); magnesium oxide (p.1198·3).

Aspirin Free Pain Relief *Hudson, USA.*
Paracetamol (p.72·2).
Fever; pain.

Aspirin Plus *Invamed, USA.*
Paracetamol (p.72·2); aspirin (p.16·1); caffeine (p.749·3).

Aspirin plus C *Bayer, Ger.*
Aspirin (p.16·1); ascorbic acid (p.1365·2).
Cold symptoms; fever; pain.

Aspirin Plus Stomach Guard *Bayer, Canad.*
Aspirin (p.16·1).
Calcium carbonate (p.1182·1), magnesium carbonate (p.1198·1), and magnesium oxide (p.1198·3) are included in this preparation in an attempt to limit adverse effects on the gastro-intestinal mucosa.
Fever; inflammation; pain.

Aspirina
Bayer, Ital.; Bayer, Spain.
Aspirin (p.16·1).
Fever; musculoskeletal and joint disorders; pain; periarticular disorders; thrombo-embolism prophylaxis.

Aspirina 05 *Bayer, Ital.*
Chewable tablets: Aspirin (p.16·1).
Calcium carbonate (p.1182·1) is included in this preparation in an attempt to limit adverse effects on the gastro-intestinal mucosa.
Fever; pain.

Aspirina 03 and 05 *Bayer, Ital.*
Tablets: Aspirin (p.16·1).

Magnesium hydroxide (p.1198·2) and aluminium glycinate (p.1177·2) are included in this preparation in an attempt to limit adverse effects on the gastro-intestinal mucosa.
Fever; pain.

Aspirina C
Bayer, Ital.; Bayer, Spain.
Aspirin (p.16·1); ascorbic acid (p.1365·2).
Fever; musculoskeletal disorders; pain.

Aspirine *Bayer, Belg.*
Aspirin (p.16·1).
Cardiovascular and cerebrovascular disorders; fever; pain.

Aspirine C
Bayer, Belg.; Bayer, Neth.
Aspirin (p.16·1); ascorbic acid (p.1365·2).
Fever; pain.

Aspirinetta *Bayer, Ital.*
Aspirin (p.16·1).
Fever; inflammation; pain.

Aspirinetta C *Bayer, Ital.*
Aspirin (p.16·1); ascorbic acid (p.1365·2).
Fever; inflammation; pain.

Aspirin-Free Bayer Select Allergy Sinus *Sterling, USA.*
Pseudoephedrine hydrochloride (p.1068·3); chlorpheniramine maleate (p.405·1); paracetamol (p.72·2).

Aspirin-Free Bayer Select Head & Chest Cold *Sterling, USA.*
Pseudoephedrine hydrochloride (p.1068·3); dextromethorphan hydrobromide (p.1057·3); guaiphenesin (p.1061·3); paracetamol (p.72·2).

Aspirin-Free Bayer Select Headache *Sterling, USA.*
Paracetamol (p.72·2); caffeine (p.749·3).

Aspisol *Bayer, Ger.*
Lysine aspirin (p.50·3).
Fever; pain; rheumatism; thrombo-embolic disorders.

Asplin *Diafarm, Spain.*
Paracetamol (p.72·2).
Fever; pain.

Asporin 0.5 *MC, Ital.*
Sodium phenolate; glutaraldehyde (p.1114·3).
Instrument sterilisation.

Asporin 2 *MC, Ital.*
Glutaraldehyde (p.1114·3).
Instrument sterilisation.

Asprimox *Invamed, USA.*
Aspirin (p.16·1).
Aluminium hydroxide (p.1177·3), calcium carbonate (p.1182·1), and magnesium hydroxide (p.1198·2) are included in this preparation in an attempt to limit adverse effects on the gastro-intestinal mucosa.

Aspro
Roche, Aust.; Roche Consumer, Austral.; Roche, Belg.; Roche Nicholas, Fr.; Roche Nicholas, Ger.; Roche Consumer, Irl.; Roche, Ital.; Roche Nicholas, Neth.; Roche, S.Afr.; Roche Nicholas, Spain; Roche, Switz.; Roche Consumer, UK.
Aspirin (p.16·1).
Fever; musculoskeletal and joint disorders; pain; thrombo-embolism prophylaxis.

Aspro C
Roche, Aust.; Roche, Ital.; Roche, Switz.
Aspirin (p.16·1); ascorbic acid (p.1365·2).
Fever; pain.

Aspro + C *Roche, Belg.*
Aspirin (p.16·1); ascorbic acid (p.1365·2).
Fever; pain.

Aspro Paraclear *Roche Consumer, UK†.*
Paracetamol (p.72·2).

Aspro vitamine C *Roche Nicholas, Fr.*
Aspirin (p.16·1); ascorbic acid (p.1365·2).
Fever; pain.

ASS
Schoeller, Aust.; Aspro-Nicholas, Aust.; Hexal, Ger.; CT, Ger.; Durachemie, Ger.; Ratiopharm, Ger.; Stada, Ger.; Worwag, Ger.; Azupharma, Ger.
Aspirin (p.16·1).
Fever; inflammation; pain; rheumatism; thrombo-embolic disorders.

ASS + C *Ratiopharm, Ger.*
Aspirin (p.16·1); ascorbic acid (p.1365·2).
Cold symptoms; fever; pain.

ASS OPT *Optimed, Ger.*
Aspirin (p.1365·2).
Fever; musculoskeletal and joint disorders; pain; thrombo-embolic disorders.

Assagix *Plantes et Medecines, Fr.*
Tilia (p.1637·3); calcium bromolactobionate (p.645·1).
Insomnia.

Assan *Permamed, Switz.*
Flufenamic acid (p.41·3); glycol salicylate (p.43·1); heparin sodium (p.879·3).
Musculoskeletal and joint pain; peripheral vascular disorders; soft-tissue injury.

Assan-Thermo *Permamed, Switz.*
Flufenamic acid (p.41·3); glycol salicylate (p.43·1); benzyl nicotinate (p.22·1); heparin sodium (p.879·3).
Musculoskeletal and joint disorders.

Assist Energetico *Ledi, Ital.*
Vitamin preparation.

Assist Reintegratore *Ledi, Ital.*
Nutritional supplement.
Fluid and electrolyte imbalance.

ASS-Kombi *Ratiopharm, Ger.*
Paracetamol (p.72·2); aspirin (p.16·1); ascorbic acid (p.1365·2).
Pain.

ASS-Kreuz *RAN, Ger.*
Aspirin (p.1365·2).
Fever; musculoskeletal and joint disorders; pain; thrombo-embolic disorders.

Assocort *Bristol-Myers Squibb, Ital.*
Triamcinolone acetonide (p.1050·2); neomycin sulphate (p.229·2); gramicidin (p.215·2); nystatin (p.386·1).
Infected skin disorders.

Assogen *Metapharma, Ital.*
Cloricromen hydrochloride (p.845·1).
Thrombosis prophylaxis.

Assoral *Savio, Ital.*
Roxithromycin (p.247·1).
Bacterial infections.

Assur
Delagrange, Belg.†; Delagrange, Fr.†.
Moroxydine hydrochloride (p.623·1); aspirin (p.16·1).
Fever; pain; viral infections.

Astat *Tsumura, Jpn†.*
Lanoconazole (p.384·2).
Fungal skin infections.

Astec *Gebro, Aust.*
Salbutamol sulphate (p.758·2).
Obstructive airways disease.

Astelin *Wallace, USA.*
Azelastine hydrochloride (p.403·1).
Allergic rhinitis.

Astenile *Recordati, Ital.†.*
Prasterone sodium sulphate (p.1459·2).
Asthenia.

Astenolit *Byk Leo, Spain.*
Vitamin, mineral and amino-acid preparation.
Tonic.

Aster C *Corvi, Ital.†.*
Ascorbic acid (p.1365·2).
Vitamin C deficiency.

Asthavent *Cipla-Medpro, S.Afr.*
Salbutamol (p.758·2).
Obstructive airways disease.

Asthenal *Grossmann, Switz.*
Sodium dimethyl aminophenylphosphinate; glutamic acid; thiamine hydrochloride; ascorbic acid.
Tonic.

Asthenopin *Mann, Ger.*
Pilocarpine hydrochloride (p.1396·3).
Eye disorders.

Asthma *Disperga, Aust.*
Papaverine hydrochloride (p.1614·2); ephedrine hydrochloride (p.1059·3); propyphenazone (p.81·3); hyoscine hydrobromide (p.462·3).
Obstructive airways disease.

Asthma 23 D *Donau, Aust.*
Ephedrine hydrochloride (p.1059·3); belladonna (p.457·1); papaverine hydrochloride (p.1614·2); caffeine-naphthylacetic acid sodium; theophylline (p.765·1).
Obstructive airways disease.

Asthma Efeum *Apomedica, Aust.†.*
Proxyphylline (p.757·3); phenazone (p.78·2); ethaverine sulphamate (p.1577·1); ephedrine hydrochloride (p.1059·3); diphenhydramine hydrochloride (p.409·1).
Obstructive airways disease.

Asthma 6-N *Hobein, Ger.*
Ephedrine hydrochloride (p.1059·3); grindelia; senega root (p.1069·3).
Obstructive airways disease.

Asthma-Bisolvon
Bender, Aust.; Thomae, Ger.†.
Bromhexine hydrochloride (p.1055·3); ephedrine hydrochloride (p.1059·3); theophylline (p.765·1).
Obstructive airways disease.

Asthma-Bomin H *Pfluger, Ger.*
Homoeopathic preparation.

Asthmacolat *Galenika, Ger.†.*
Etofylline (p.753·1); ephedrine hydrochloride (p.1059·3); stramonium (p.468·2); adonis vernalis (p.1543·3); arnica (p.1550·3); belladonna (p.457·1).
Adjunct in pertussis; asthma; bronchitis.

Asthma-Frenon *Richter, Aust.*
Guaiphenesin (p.1061·3); caffeine (p.749·3); phenazone (p.78·2); potassium thiocyanate; ephedrine hydrochloride (p.1059·3); monobenzylphthalate; menthol (p.1600·2); cineole (p.1564·1); camphor (p.1557·2).

Asthma-Frenon-S *Hefa, Ger.†.*
Caffeine-guaiphenesin compound (pp.749·3 and 1061·3); ephedrine hydrochloride (p.1059·3); camphor (p.1557·2); cineole (p.1564·1); menthol (p.1600·2).
Asthma; bronchitis; emphysema.

AsthmaHaler Mist *Menley & James, USA.*
Adrenaline acid tartrate (p.813·3).
Bronchospasm.

Asthma-Hilfe *Agepha, Aust.*
Aminophylline (p.748·1); theobromine (p.765·1); ephedrine hydrochloride (p.1059·3); potassium guaiacolsulphonate (p.1068·3).
Obstructive airways disease.

Asthmakhell N *Steigerwald, Ger.*
Homoeopathic preparation.

Asthmalgine *Cochon, Fr.*
Sodium benzoate (p.1102·3); ephedrine hydrochloride (p.1059·3); caffeine (p.749·3); hyoscyamus (p.464·3).
The oral solution also contains Desessartz syrup.
Asthma.

Asthmalitan *3M, Ger.†.*
Isoetharine hydrochloride (p.755·1).
Obstructive airways disease.

Asthmalyticum-Ampullen N (Rowo-210)
Pharmakon, Ger.
Homoeopathic preparation.
Lignocaine hydrochloride (p.1293·2) is included in this preparation to alleviate the pain of injection.

AsthmaNefrin *Menley & James, USA.*
Racepinephrine hydrochloride (p.815·2).
Obstructive airways disease.

Asthmasedine *Soekami, Fr.†.*
Theophylline (p.765·1); sodium benzoate (p.1102·3); phenobarbitone sodium (p.350·2); ephedrine hydrochloride (p.1059·3); caffeine (p.749·3); potassium iodide (p.1493·1); belladonna herb (p.457·1); lobelia (p.1481·3).
Obstructive airways disease.

Asthma-Spray *CT, Ger.*
Salbutamol (p.758·2).
Obstructive airways disease.

Asthmatee *Smetana, Aust.*
Enulae root; marrubium vulgare (p.1063·3); origanum; aniseed (p.1549·3); arnica (p.1550·3); cacao husk (p.1636·2).
Obstructive airways disease.

Asthmavowen-N *Weber & Weber, Ger.*
Homoeopathic preparation.

Asthmocupin *Fisons, Ger.†.*
Sodium cromoglycate (p.762·1); reproterol hydrochloride (p.758·1).
Obstructive airways disease.

Asthmo-Kranit Mono *Krewel, Ger.*
Terbutaline sulphate (p.764·1).
Formerly contained ethaverine hydrochloride, ephedrine hydrochloride, phenobarbitone, and theophylline.
Obstructive airways disease.

Asthmoprotect *Azupharma, Ger.*
Terbutaline sulphate (p.764·1).
Obstructive airways disease.

Astho-Med *Schonenberger, Switz.*
Diphenhydramine hydrochloride (p.409·1); diprophylline (p.752·1); guaiphenesin (p.1061·3); phenylpropanolamine hydrochloride (p.1067·2).
Bronchitis; coughs.

Asticol *Clinced, Aust.*
Paracetamol nicotinate (p.74·2); propyphenazone (p.81·3); caffeine (p.749·3).

Astidin *Medifood-Trufood, Ital.*
Infant feed.
Histidinaemia.

Astifat *Fatol, Ger.*
Ketotifen fumarate (p.755·2).
Asthma; bronchitis; hypersensitivity reactions.

Astomin *Yamanouchi, Jpn.*
Dimemorfan phosphate (p.1058·3).
Coughs.

Astone *Ramelco, Canad.*
Aspirin (p.16·1); caffeine (p.749·3).

Astonin
Merck, Aust.; Merck, Ger.; Merck, Spain.
Fludrocortisone (p.1040·1).
Adrenocortical insufficiency; congenital adrenal hyperplasia; hypotension; peripheral perfusion disorders.

Astramorph PF *Astra, USA.*
Morphine sulphate (p.56·2).
Pain.

Astratonil *Astra, Swed.*
Multivitamin preparation.

Astreptine *Darci, Belg.*
Sulphanilamide (p.256·3).
Infected wounds.

Astressane *Dolisos, Fr.*
Crataegus (p.1568·2); red-poppy petal (p.1001·1); passion flower (p.1615·3).
Cardiac irritability.

Astring-O-Sol *Mentholatum, USA.*
Methyl salicylate (p.55·2); myrrh (p.1606·1); zinc chloride (p.1373·1).
Mouthwash.

Astrix *Faulding, Austral.*
Aspirin (p.16·1).
Thrombo-embolic disorders.

Astroderm *Lagap, Ital.†.*
Dichlorisone acetate (p.1039·2).
Skin disorders.

Astroglide
Lodim, Switz.†.
Glycerol (p.1585·2); propylene glycol (p.1622·1).
Lubricant.

Biofilm, USA.
Glycerol (p.1585·2); propylene glycol (p.1622·1); polyquaternium 5.
Vaginal lubricant.

Astronautal *Strallhofer, Aust.*
Diphenylpyraline hydrochloride (p.409·3); pyridoxine hydrochloride (p.1362·3).
Motion sickness; nausea; vertigo.

Astudal *Almirall, Spain.*
Amlodipine besylate (p.822·3).
Angina pectoris; hypertension.

Astyl *Lophal, Fr.*
Deanol bisorcate (p.1478·2).
Tonic.

Asvelik *Medinsa, Spain.*
Tipepidine hybenzate (p.1070·3).
Coughs.

Asverin *Tanabe, Jpn.*
Tipepidine hybenzate (p.1070·3).
Coughs.

AT 10
Merck, Aust.; Sanofi Winthrop, Austral.; Merck-Belgolabo, Belg.; Bayer, Ger.; Sanofi Winthrop, Irl.; Bayer, Ital.; Bayer, S.Afr.†; Bayer, Switz.; Sanofi Winthrop, UK.
Dihydrotachysterol (p.1366·3).
Hypoparathyroidism with hypocalcaemia; osteomalacia; renal osteodystrophy; tetany; vitamin D-resistant rickets.

Atabrine *Winthrop, USA†.*
Mepacrine hydrochloride (p.584·2).

Atacand
Hassle, Swed.; Astra Merck, USA.
Candesartan cilexetil (p.836·1).
Hypertension.

Ataclor *SoSe, Ital.*
Atenolol (p.825·3); chlorthalidone (p.839·3).
Hypertension.

Atarax
UCB, Aust.; Pfizer, Austral.; UCB, Belg.; Pfizer, Canad.; UCB, Fr.; UCB, Ger.; Rodleben, Ger.; Vedim, Ger.; Pfizer, Irl.; UCB, Ital.; UCB, Neth.; UCB, Norw.; UCB, Spain; UCB, Swed.; UCB, Switz.; Pfizer, UK; Roerig, USA.
Hydroxyzine (p.412·2), hydroxyzine embonate (p.411·3), or hydroxyzine hydrochloride (p.412·1).
Alcohol withdrawal syndrome; anxiety disorders; hypersensitivity reactions; insomnia; nausea and vomiting; premedication; pruritus; senile agitation; urticaria.

Atarone *Vinas, Spain.*
Pantethine (p.1276·3).
Hyperlipidaemias.

Atasol *Carter Horner, Canad.*
Paracetamol (p.72·2).
Fever; pain.

Atasol-8, -15, -30 *Carter Horner, Canad.*
Paracetamol (p.72·2); codeine phosphate (p.26·1); caffeine citrate (p.749·3).
Fever; pain.

Atazina *Panthox & Burck, Ital.†.*
Hydroxyzine hydrochloride (p.412·1).
Nervous system disorders.

Atebemyxine *Chauvin, Fr.*
Neomycin sulphate (p.229·2); polymyxin B sulphate (p.239·1).
Bacterial eye infections.

Atebeta *Betapharm, Ger.*
Atenolol (p.825·3).
Angina pectoris; arrhythmias; hypertension.

Atecor *Rowex, Irl.*
Atenolol (p.825·3).
Angina pectoris; arrhythmias; hypertension; myocardial infarction.

Atehexal
Hexal, Austral.; Hexal, Ger.
Atenolol (p.825·3).
Angina pectoris; arrhythmias; hypertension; myocardial infarction.

Atehexal comp *Hexal, Ger.*
Atenolol (p.825·3); chlorthalidone (p.839·3).
Hypertension.

Atem *Chiesi, Ital.*
Ipratropium bromide (p.754·2).
Obstructive airways disease.

Atemaron NR30 *Reckeweg, Ger.*
Homoeopathic preparation.

Atemur *Cascan, Ger.; Cascapharm, Ger.*
Fluticasone propionate (p.1042·3).
Asthma.

Atenativ
Pharmacia Upjohn, Aust.; Pharmacia Upjohn, Ger.; Pharmacia Upjohn, Neth.; Pharmacia Upjohn, Norw.; Pharmacia, Spain; Pharmacia Upjohn, Swed.; ZLB, Switz.
Antithrombin III (p.711·2).
Antithrombin III deficiency.

Atendol *Pohl, Ger.*
Atenolol (p.825·3).
Acute myocardial infarction; arrhythmias; hypertension; ischaemic heart disease.

Atenetic *Gerard, Irl.*
Atenolol (p.825·3); chlorthalidone (p.839·3).
Hypertension.

Ateni *Gerard, Irl.*
Atenolol (p.825·3).
Angina pectoris; arrhythmias; hypertension; myocardial infarction.

Atenigron *Mitim, Ital.*
Atenolol (p.825·3); chlorthalidone (p.839·3).
Hypertension.

Atenil *Ecosol, Switz.*
Atenolol (p.825·3).
Angina pectoris; arrhythmias; hypertension; myocardial infarction.

Atenix *Ashbourne, UK.*
Atenolol (p.825·3).
Angina pectoris; arrhythmias; hypertension.

AtenixCo *Ashbourne, UK.*
Atenolol (p.825·3); chlorthalidone (p.839·3).

These ingredients can be described by the British Approved Name Co-tenidone.
Hypertension.

Ateno Isis Puren, Ger.
Atenolol (p.825·3).
Angina pectoris; arrhythmias; hypertension.

Ateno comp Isis Puren, Ger.
Atenolol (p.825·3); chlorthalidone (p.839·3).
Hypertension.

ateno-basan comp. Schonenberger, Switz.
Atenolol (p.825·3); chlorthalidone (p.839·3).
Hypertension.

ateno-basan mite Schonenberger, Switz.
Atenolol (p.825·3).
Angina pectoris; arrhythmias; hypertension.

Atenobene Merckle, Aust.
Atenolol (p.825·3).
Angina pectoris; arrhythmias; hypertension; myocardial infarction.

Atenoblok Triomed, S.Afr.
Atenolol (p.825·3).
Angina pectoris; hypertension; myocardial infarction.

Atenogen Antigen, Irl.
Atenolol (p.825·3).
Angina pectoris; arrhythmias; hypertension; myocardial infarction.

Atenol CT, Ital.
Atenolol (p.825·3).
Angina pectoris; arrhythmias; hypertension.

Atenolan Lannacher, Aust.
Atenolol (p.825·3).
Angina pectoris; arrhythmias; hypertension; myocardial infarction.

Atenolan comp Lannacher, Aust.
Atenolol (p.825·3); chlorthalidone (p.839·3).
Hypertension.

Atenolol AL comp Aliud, Ger.
Atenolol (p.825·3); chlorthalidone (p.839·3).
Hypertension.

Atenolol comp
Genericon, Aust.; Ratiopharm, Ger.; CT, Ger.; Heumann, Ger.
Atenolol (p.825·3); chlorthalidone (p.839·3).
Hypertension.

Atenomel Clonmel, Irl.
Atenolol (p.825·3).
Angina pectoris; arrhythmias; hypertension; myocardial infarction.

Atenomerck Merck, Ger.
Atenolol (p.825·3).
Angina pectoris; arrhythmias; hypertension.

Atenomerck comp Merck, Ger.
Atenolol (p.825·3); chlorthalidone (p.839·3).
Hypertension.

Atenos UCB, Ger.
Tulobuterol hydrochloride (p.774·2).
Asthma; bronchitis; bronchospastic disorders.

Atensine
Berk, Irl.†; Berk, UK†.
Diazepam (p.661·1).
Alcohol withdrawal syndrome; anxiety; epilepsy; insomnia; premedication; skeletal muscle spasm.

Atepadene Mayoly-Spindler, Fr.
Adenosine triphosphate disodium (p.1543·2).
Pain.

Atepium Berenguer Infale, Spain†.
Nicofibrate hydrochloride (p.1276·1).
Hyperlipidaemias.

Atepodin Medix, Spain.
Adenosine triphosphate sodium (p.1543·2).
Arrhythmias; muscular dystrophies; prevention of anoxia.

Ateran Eurofarmaco, Ital.
A heparinoid (p.882·3).
Thrombosis prophylaxis.

Aterax UCB, S.Afr.
Hydroxyzine hydrochloride (p.412·1).
Anxiety; hypersensitivity reactions; premedication.

Atereal Realpharma, Ger.
Atenolol (p.825·3).
Angina pectoris; arrhythmias; hypertension; myocardial infarction.

Ateren Rolab, S.Afr.
Atenolol (p.825·3); chlorthalidone (p.839·3).
Hypertension.

Aterina Tedec Meiji, Spain.
Sulodexide (p.951·1).
Arteriosclerosis; hyperlipidaemias.

Ateroclar Mediolanum, Ital.
Heparin sodium (p.879·3).
Thrombo-embolic disorders.

Ateroid Crinos, Ital.
A heparinoid (p.882·3).
Thrombosis prophylaxis.

Aterol Rolab, S.Afr.
Atenolol (p.825·3).
Angina pectoris; hypertension.

Ateroxide Ripari-Gero, Ital.
A heparinoid (p.882·3).
Thrombosis prophylaxis.

Aterozot Boizot, Spain†.
Binifibrate (p.1269·2).
Hyperlipidaemias.

Atesifar Siphar, Switz.
Atenolol (p.825·3).
Angina pectoris; arrhythmias; hypertension.

Atezym Scharper, Ital.†.
Pancreatin (p.1612·1).
Pancreatic exocrine disorders.

ATG
Serotherapeutisches, Aust.; Hoechst Marion Roussel, Belg.; Fresenius, Switz.
Antilymphocyte immunoglobulin (p.504·2).
Transplant rejection.

Atgam
Pharmacia Upjohn, Austral.; Pharmacia Upjohn, Canad.; Upjohn, Neth.†; Upjohn, Spain; Pharmacia Upjohn, Switz.; Upjohn, USA.
Antithymocyte immunoglobulin (horse) (p.504·2).
Aplastic anaemia; renal transplant rejection.

Athensa-ferro-Saft Athenstaedt, Ger.†.
Ferrous gluconate (p.1340·1) with vitamins and amino acids.
Iron-deficiency anaemia.

Athera Modern Health Products, UK.
Parsley (p.1615·3); vervain; senna leaf (p.1212·2); clivers (p.1565·2).
Menopausal symptoms.

atherolipin Schwarz, Ger.†.
Aluminium clofibrate (p.1271·1).
Hyperlipidaemias.

Athimbin HS Centeon, Aust.
Antithrombin III (p.711·2).
Antithrombin III deficiency.

Athlete's Foot Scholl, UK.
Tolnaftate (p.389·1).
Tinea pedis.

Athletes Foot Antifungal Pedi-Pak, Canad.
Aluminium chlorohydrate (p.1078·3); undecenoic acid (p.389·2); zinc undecenoate (p.389·2).
Tinea pedis.

Athletes Foot Cream Wallis, UK.
Clotrimazole (p.376·3).
Tinea pedis.

Athymil Organon, Fr.
Mianserin hydrochloride (p.297·1).
Depression.

Atinorm Bioprogress, Ital.
Atenolol (p.825·3); indapamide (p.890·2).
Hypertension.

Atiramin Juste, Spain.
Azatadine maleate (p.402·3); pseudoephedrine sulphate (p.1068·3).
Allergic rhinitis.

Atirosin Medifood-Trufood, Ital.
Infant feed.
Tyrosinaemia.

Atisuril Kaliforma, Spain†.
Salsalate (p.83·1).
Fever; inflammation; pain.

Ativan
Wyeth, Austral.; Wyeth-Ayerst, Canad.; Wyeth, Irl.; Akromed, S.Afr.; Wyeth, UK; Wyeth-Ayerst, USA.
Lorazepam (p.675·3).
Anxiety; insomnia; mania; premedication; status epilepticus.

Atkinson & Barker's Gripe Mixture Torbet Laboratories, UK.
Light magnesium carbonate (p.1198·1); sodium bicarbonate (p.1153·2); fennel oil (p.1579·2); dill oil (p.1572·1).
Colic.

Atmocol Thackray, UK.
A deodorant spray for use with colostomies and ileostomies.

Atmos Astra, Swed.
Testosterone (p.1464·1).
Hypogonadism.

Atmulen E Fides, Ger.†.
Juniper (p.1592·2); liquorice (p.1197·1); thyme (p.1636·3); pumilio pine oil (p.1623·3); peppermint oil (p.1208·1); silicea (p.1474·3); drosera (p.1574·1); ephedrine hydrochloride (p.1059·3).
Coughs and associated upper respiratory-tract disorders.

Atmulen K Fides, Ger.†.
Eryngium; pulmonaria; althaea (p.1546·3); fennel (p.1579·1).
Coughs and associated upper respiratory-tract disorders.

ATnativ Hyland, USA.
Antithrombin III (p.711·2).
Antithrombin III deficiency.

Atock Yamanouchi, Jpn.
Eformoterol fumarate (p.752·3).
Obstructive airways disease.

Atolant SS, Jpn.
Neticonazole hydrochloride (p.386·1).
Fungal skin infections.

Atolone Major, USA.
Triamcinolone (p.1050·2).
Corticosteroid.

Atomolan Kyowa, Jpn.
Glutathione (p.983·1).
Corneal injury; drug and metal poisoning; liver disorders; radiation-induced inflammation of oral mucosa; radiation-induced leucopenia; skin disorders; vomiting.

Atosil
Bayer, Ger.
Tablets; syrup; oral solution; injection: Promethazine hydrochloride (p.416·2).
Gastro-intestinal disorders; hypersensitivity reactions; insomnia; motion sickness; nausea and vomiting; premedication; psychiatric disorders; respiratory disorders.

Tropon, Ger.†.
Suppositories: Promethazine (p.416·2).
Gastro-intestinal disorders; hypersensitivity reactions; premedication; psychiatric disorders; respiratory disorders.

Atossisclerol Kreussler Also, Ital.
Laureth 9 (p.1325·2).
Sclerotherapy of varices.

Atover Recordati, Ital.†.
Pyricarbate (p.1624·1).
Vascular disorders.

Atoxan
Note. This name is used for preparations of different composition.
Lagap, Ital.†.
Thioctic acid (p.1636·2); nicotinamide (p.1351·2).
Liver disorders.

Bicther, Spain†.
Oxatomide (p.415·1).
Hypersensitivity reactions.

Atoxepan Dukron, Ital.†.
Cogalactoisomerase sodium (p.1566·2).
Liver disorders.

ATP-Uvocal N Stroschein, Ger.†.
Adenosine triphosphate, disodium salt (p.1543·2).
Peripheral circulatory disorders.

Atrac-Tain Sween, USA.
Urea (p.1095·2).
Dry skin.

Atractil Trenker, Belg.
Diethylpropion (p.1479·3).
Obesity.

Atretol Athena Neurosciences, USA.
Carbamazepine (p.339·2).
Epilepsy; trigeminal neuralgia.

Atrican
Innotech, Fr.; Bouty, Ital.†.
Tenonitrozole (p.594·1).
Urogenital trichomoniasis and candidiasis.

Atrimycon Bioindustria, Ital.†.
Protiofate (p.387·1).
Trichomonal and fungal infections.

Atrium
Riom, Fr.; Roche, Switz.
Tetrabamate, a complex of febarbamate (p.670·1), difebarbamate (p.668·1), and phenobarbitone (p.350·2).
Alcohol withdrawal syndrome; anxiety; tremor.

Atrobel Fawns & McAllan, Austral.
Belladonna herb (p.457·1).
Peptic ulcer; reduction of secretions; smooth muscle spasm.

Atrofed Lennon, S.Afr.†.
Phenazone (p.78·2); theobromine (p.765·1); caffeine (p.749·3); belladonna (p.457·1); ephedrine hydrochloride (p.1059·3).
Asthma.

Atrohist Pediatric Adams, USA.
Phenylephrine tannate (p.1067·1); chlorpheniramine tannate (p.405·2); mepyramine tannate (p.414·1).
Allergic rhinitis; nasal congestion.

Atrohist Plus Adams, USA.
Phenylpropanolamine hydrochloride (p.1067·2); phenylephrine hydrochloride (p.1066·2); chlorpheniramine maleate (p.405·1); hyoscyamine sulphate (p.464·2); atropine sulphate (p.455·1); hyoscine hydrobromide (p.462·3).
Upper respiratory-tract symptoms.

Atrohist Sprinkle Adams, USA.
Pseudoephedrine hydrochloride (p.1068·3); chlorpheniramine maleate (p.405·1).
Formerly contained brompheniramine maleate, phenyltoloxamine citrate and phenylephrine hydrochloride.
Cold symptoms.

Atromidin
Zeneca, Belg.; ICI, Ital.†; Zeneca, Swed.
Clofibrate (p.1271·1).
Diabetic retinopathy; hyperlipidaemias; prophylaxis of ischaemic heart disease in high-risk patients; xanthoma.

Atromid-S
ICI, Austral.; Wyeth-Ayerst, Canad.; Zeneca, Irl.; Zeneca, S.Afr.; Zeneca, UK; Wyeth-Ayerst, USA.
Clofibrate (p.1271·1).
Diabetic retinopathy; hyperlipidaemias.

Atronase
Bender, Aust.; Boehringer Ingelheim, Belg.; Boehringer Ingelheim, S.Afr.†.
Ipratropium bromide (p.754·2).
Rhinitis.

AtroPen Survival Technology, USA.
Atropine sulphate (p.455·1).
Organophosphorus or carbamate pesticide poisoning.

Atropine and Demerol Sanofi Winthrop, USA.
Atropine sulphate (p.455·1); pethidine hydrochloride (p.76·1).
Sedative.

Atropinol Winzer, Ger.
Atropine (p.455·1).
Eye disorders.

Atropisol
Ciba Vision, Canad.; Iolab, USA.
Atropine sulphate (p.455·1).
Production of cycloplegia and mydriasis.

Atropt Sigma, Austral.
Atropine sulphate (p.455·1).
Production of cycloplegia and mydriasis.

Atrosept Geneva, USA.
Hexamine (p.216·1); salol (p.83·1); atropine sulphate (p.455·1); hyoscyamine sulphate (p.464·2); benzoic acid (p.1102·3); methylene blue (p.984·3).
Urinary-tract infections.

Atrovent
Bender, Aust.; Boehringer Ingelheim, Austral.; Boehringer Ingelheim, Belg.; Boehringer Ingelheim, Canad.; Boehringer Ingelheim, Fr.; Boehringer Ingelheim, Ger.; Boehringer Ingelheim, Irl.; Boehringer Ingelheim, Ital.; Boehringer Ingelheim, Neth.; Boehringer Ingelheim, Norw.; Boehringer Ingelheim, S.Afr.; Boehringer Ingelheim, Spain; Boehringer Ingelheim, Swed.; Boehringer Ingelheim, Switz.; Boehringer Ingelheim, UK; Boehringer Ingelheim, USA.
Ipratropium bromide (p.754·2).
Allergic rhinitis; obstructive airways disease; rhinorrhoea.

ATS
Note. This name is used for preparations of different composition.
Doms-Adrian, Fr.†.
Trichloroacetic acid (p.1639·1); salicylic acid (p.1090·2).
Mucosal infections of the mouth and throat; pruritus.

Hoechst Marion Roussel, USA.
Erythromycin (p.204·1).
Acne.

Attain
Wyeth-Ayerst, Canad.†; Sherwood, USA.
Lactose-free preparation for enteral nutrition.

Attentil Ravizza, Ital.†.
Fipexide hydrochloride.
Fatigue.

Attenuvax
Merck Sharp & Dohme, Aust.; CSL, Austral.†; Merck Sharp & Dohme, Belg.†; Pasteur Merieux, Ital.; Merck Sharp & Dohme, Neth.†; Pro Vaccine, Switz.; Merck Sharp & Dohme, USA.
A live measles vaccine (more attenuated Enders' Edmonston strain) (p.1517·3).
Active immunisation.

Aturgyl Synthelabo, Fr.
Oxymetazoline hydrochloride (p.1065·3).
Formerly contained fenoxazoline hydrochloride.
Rhinopharyngeal congestion.

Atus Metapharma, Ital.
Ambroxol hydrochloride (p.1054·3).
Respiratory-tract disorders.

Atuss DM Atley, USA.
Dextromethorphan hydrobromide (p.1057·3); phenylephrine hydrochloride (p.1066·2); chlorpheniramine maleate (p.405·1).
Coughs and associated respiratory-tract disorders.

Atuss EX Atley, USA.
Hydrocodone tartrate (p.43·1); guaiphenesin (p.1061·3).
Coughs and associated respiratory-tract disorders.

Atuss G Atley, USA.
Hydrocodone tartrate (p.43·1); phenylephrine hydrochloride (p.1066·2); guaiphenesin (p.1061·3).
Coughs and associated respiratory-tract disorders.

Atuss HD Atley, USA.
Hydrocodone tartrate (p.43·1); phenylephrine hydrochloride (p.1066·2); chlorpheniramine maleate (p.405·1).

Atussil Goupil, Fr.†.
Pentoxyverine hydrochloride (p.1066·2).
Coughs.

Atussil-Eucalyptol Goupil, Fr.†.
Pentoxyverine (p.1066·1); cineole (p.1564·1).
Coughs.

Atuxane Monot, Fr.
Dextromethorphan hydrobromide (p.1057·3).
Coughs.

AU 4 Regeneresen Dyckerhoff, Ger.
Ribonucleic acid (p.1624·3).
Ear disorders.

Aubeline Arkopharma, Fr.
Crataegus (p.1568·2).
Cardiac disorders; nervous disorders.

Audax
Mundipharma, Ger.; Seton, Irl.; Ethimed, S.Afr.†; Seton, UK.
Choline salicylate (p.25·2).
Aid to ear wax removal; earache.

Audazol Lesvi, Spain.
Omeprazole (p.1204·2) or omeprazole sodium (p.1204·2).
Gastro-oesophageal reflux; peptic ulcer; Zollinger-Ellison syndrome.

Audicort
Wyeth, Irl.; Lederle, UK.
Neomycin undecenoate (p.229·2); triamcinolone acetonide (p.1050·2).
The UK preparation formerly contained benzocaine, triamcinolone acetonide, and neomycin undecenoate.
Inflammatory ear disorders with bacterial infection.

Audinorme Carlton Laboratories, UK†.
Docusate sodium (p.1189·3); glycerol (p.1585·2).
Ear wax removal.

Audione Serra Pamies, Spain.
Vitamins; iodine (p.1493·1) or potassium iodide (p.1493·1).
Ear disorders; eye disorders.

Audispray Diepha, Fr.
Sea water.
External ear hygiene.

Augentonicum *Stulln, Switz.*
Digitalis (p.848·3); digitoxin (p.848·3); esculoside (p.1543·3).
Eye disorders.

Augentonikum *Stulln, Ger.*
Digitalin (p.1571·3); retinol palmitate (p.1359·2).
Eye disorders.

Augentropfen "Jso-Werk" *Iso, Ger.†.*
Homoeopathic preparation.

Augentropfen Mucokehl D5 *Sanum-Kehlbeck, Ger.*
Homoeopathic preparation.

Augentropfen Stulln *Salus, Aust.*
Digitalis (p.848·3); esculoside (p.1543·3).

Augentropfen Stulln Mono *Stulln, Ger.*
Digitalis leaf (p.848·3); esculoside (p.1543·3).
Eye disorders.

Augentropfen Thilo *Alcon-Thilo, Ger.†.*
Pilocarpine hydrochloride (p.1396·3); thiamine hydrochloride (p.1361·1).
Eye disorders.

Augmentan *SmithKline Beecham, Ger.*
Amoxycillin sodium (p.151·3) or amoxycillin trihydrate (p.151·3); potassium clavulanate (p.190·2).
Bacterial infections.

Augmentin
SmithKline Beecham, Aust.; SmithKline Beecham, Austral.; Beecham, Belg.; SmithKline Beecham, Fr.; SmithKline Beecham, Irl.; SmithKline Beecham, Ital.; SmithKline Beecham, Neth.; SmithKline Beecham, S.Afr.; SmithKline Beecham, Switz.; Beecham Research, UK; SmithKline Beecham, USA.
Amoxycillin sodium (p.151·3) or amoxycillin trihydrate (p.151·3); potassium clavulanate (p.190·2).
These ingredients can be described by the British Approved Name Co-amoxiclav.
Bacterial infections.

Augmentin-Duo *SmithKline Beecham, UK.*
Amoxycillin trihydrate (p.151·3); potassium clavulanate (p.190·2).
These ingredients can be described by the British Approved Name Co-amoxiclav.
Bacterial infections.

Augmentine *SmithKline Beecham, Spain.*
Amoxycillin sodium (p.151·3) or amoxycillin trihydrate (p.151·3); potassium clavulanate (p.190·2).
Bacterial infections.

Aulcer *Alacan, Spain.*
Omeprazole (p.1204·2).
Gastro-oesophageal reflux; peptic ulcers; Zollinger-Ellison syndrome.

Aulin
Helsinn Birex, Irl.; Boehringer Mannheim, Ital.; Boehringer Mannheim, Switz.
Nimesulide (p.63·2).
Fever; musculoskeletal, joint, peri-articular, and soft-tissue disorders; pain.

Aunativ
Pharmacia Upjohn, Aust.; Pharmacia Upjohn, Ger.; Pharmacia Upjohn, Norw.; Pharmacia Upjohn, Swed.
A hepatitis B immunoglobulin (p.1512·3).
Passive immunisation.

Aunative *Jorba, Spain†.*
A hepatitis B immunoglobulin (p.1512·3).
Passive immunisation.

Aurafair Otic *Pharmafair, USA†.*
Phenazone (p.78·2); benzocaine (p.1286·2).

Auralgan
Whitehall, Austral.; Whitehall-Robins, Canad.; Wyeth-Ayerst, USA.
Phenazone (p.78·2); benzocaine (p.1286·2); glycerol (p.1585·2).
Otitis media; removal of ear wax.

Auralgicin *Roche, S.Afr.*
Ephedrine hydrochloride (p.1059·3); phenazone (p.78·2); benzocaine (p.1286·2); potassium hydroxyquinoline sulphate (p.1621·1).
Otitis media.

Auraltone *Rhone-Poulenc Rorer, Irl.†.*
Phenazone (p.78·2); benzocaine (p.1286·2).
Otitis.

Aurantin *Parke, Davis, Ital.*
Phenytoin sodium (p.352·3).
Arrhythmias; epilepsy.

Aurasept *Restan, S.Afr.*
Benzocaine (p.1286·2); phenazone (p.78·2).
Otitis.

Aurasol *Optimax, USA.*
Colloidal gold (p.1586·2).

Auratek hCG *Organon Teknika, UK.*
Pregnancy test (p.1621·2).

Aureal *Syxyl, Ger.†.*
Cereus grandiflorus; crataegus (p.1568·2); cheiranthi cheiri; calamus (p.1556·1); motherwort (p.1604·2); passion flower (p.1615·3); avena (p.1551·3); scoparium (p.1628·1); valerian (p.1643·1); adonis; aurum natr. chlorat.; camphora; convallaria; digitalis; gelsemium; naja tripud.; strophantus; apocynum; arnica; lobelia.
Cardiac disorders.

Aureocort
Wyeth Lederle, Aust.; Stiefel, Canad.†; Wyeth, Irl.; Cyanamid, Ital.; Lederle, UK.
Chlortetracycline (p.185·1) or chlortetracycline hydrochloride (p.185·1); triamcinolone acetonide (p.1050·2).
Infected skin disorders.

Aureodelf *Lederle, Ger.*
Chlortetracycline hydrochloride (p.185·1); triamcinolone acetonide (p.1050·2).
Infected skin disorders.

Aureomicina
Cyanamid, Ital.; Cyanamid, Spain.
Chlortetracycline hydrochloride (p.185·1).
Bacterial infections.

Aureomix *SIT, Ital.*
Chlortetracycline hydrochloride (p.185·1); sulphacetamide sodium (p.252·2).
Ear, nose, throat, and eye infections.

Aureomycin
Wyeth Lederle, Aust.; Lederle, Austral.; Wyeth Lederle, Belg.; Wyeth-Ayerst, Canad.; Lederle, Ger.; Wyeth, Irl.; Lederle, Neth.; Wyeth, Norw.; Wyeth, S.Afr.; Wyeth Lederle, Swed.; Lederle, Switz.; Lederle, UK; Lederle, USA†; Storz, USA†.
Chlortetracycline (p.185·1) or chlortetracycline hydrochloride (p.185·1).
Bacterial infections.

Aureomycin N *Lederle, Ger.*
Chlortetracycline hydrochloride (p.185·1); nystatin (p.386·1).
Vaginal infections.

Aureomycine
Asta Medica, Belg.; Theraplix, Fr.
Chlortetracycline hydrochloride (p.185·1).
Eye and skin infections.

Aureotan *Tosse, Ger.*
Aurothioglucose (p.20·2).
Chronic polyarthritis; psoriatic arthritis.

Auricovit *Farmades, Ital.†.*
Vitamin A (p.1358·1); vitamin E (p.1369·1); pumilio pine oil (p.1623·3); niaouli oil (p.1607·1); guaiacol (p.1061·2).
Otosclerosis.

Auricularum *Serolam, Fr.*
Oxytetracycline hydrochloride (p.235·1); polymyxin B sulphate (p.239·1); dexamethasone sodium phosphate (p.1037·2); nystatin (p.386·1).
Otitis.

Auricum *Dolisos, Canad.*
Homoeopathic preparation.

Aurisan *Nadeau, Canad.*
Benzocaine (p.1286·2); camphor (p.1557·2); chlorbutol (p.1106·3).
Ear ache.

Auristan
Note. This name is used for preparations of different composition.
Monin, Fr.
Phenylephrine hydrochloride (p.1066·2).
Otitis externa.

Novopharma, Switz.†.
Chlorhexidine gluconate (p.1107·2); phenylephrine hydrochloride (p.1066·2).
Otitis externa.

Aurizone *SIFI, Ital.†.*
Dexamethasone (p.1037·1); polymyxin B sulphate (p.239·1); chloramphenicol (p.182·1); lignocaine hydrochloride (p.1293·2).
Ear disorders.

Auro *Del, USA.*
Urea hydrogen peroxide (p.1127·3).
Ear wax removal.

Auroanalin *Hevert, Ger.*
Glycol salicylate (p.43·1); benzyl nicotinate (p.22·1).
Inflammation; rheumatism.

Auro-Detoxin
Brady, Aust.†; SmithKline Beecham, Ger.†.
Gold keratinate (p.43·1).
Chronic polyarthritis.

Auro-Dri *Del, USA.*
Isopropyl alcohol (p.1118·2); boric acid (p.1554·2).
Ear disorders.

Aurolate *Pasadena, USA.*
Sodium aurothiomalate (p.83·2).

Auromyose *Nourypharma, Neth.*
Aurothioglucose (p.20·2).
Rheumatoid arthritis.

Aurone *Pharmacare Consumer, S.Afr.*
Phenazone (p.78·2).
Earache; otitis media.

Aurone Forte *Pharmacare Consumer, S.Afr.*
Phenazone (p.78·2); benzocaine (p.1286·2).
Earache; otitis media.

Auroplatin
Steigerwald, Ger.
Homoeopathic preparation.

Aurorix
Roche, Aust.; Roche, Austral.; Roche, Belg.; Roche, Ger.; Roche, Ital.; Roche, Neth.; Roche, Norw.; Roche, S.Afr.; Roche, Swed.; Roche, Switz.
Moclobemide (p.298·3).
Depression; phobias.

Aurosulfo *Geymonat, Ital.*
Colloidal gold sulphide.
Rheumatoid arthritis.

Aurosyx N *Syxyl, Ger.*
Homoeopathic preparation.

Auroto *Barre-National, USA.*
Benzocaine (p.1286·2); phenazone (p.78·2).
Earache.

Aurum-Gastreu NR2 *Reckeweg, Ger.*
Homoeopathic preparation.

Auscard *Sigma, Austral.*
Diltiazem hydrochloride (p.854·2).
Angina pectoris.

Ausgem *Sigma, Austral.*
Gemfibrozil (p.1273·3).
Hyperlipidaemias.

Ausobronc *Biotekfarma, Ital.*
Mesna (p.983·3).
Respiratory-tract disorders.

Ausomina *Biotekfarma, Ital.*
Vincamine (p.1644·1).
Cerebrovascular disorders.

Ausovit B Complesso *Pharkos, Ital.†.*
Vitamin B substances.

Aussie Tan
Or-Dov, Austral.
SPF 4: Ethylhexyl *p*-methoxycinnamate (p.1487·1); avobenzone (p.1486·3).
SPF 7: Ethylhexyl *p*-methoxycinnamate (p.1487·1); avobenzone (p.1486·3); oxybenzone (p.1487·3).
SPF 15 Lotion: Ethylhexyl *p*-methoxycinnamate (p.1487·1); avobenzone (p.1486·3); oxybenzone (p.1487·3).
SPF 15 Topical gel: Ethylhexyl *p*-methoxycinnamate (p.1487·1); avobenzone (p.1486·3).
Sunscreen.

Aussie Tan Pre-Tan *Or-Dov, Austral.*
Tyrosine (p.1357·3); tyrosinase.
To accelerate tanning.

Aussie Tan Skin Moisturiser *Or-Dov, Austral.*
Urea (p.1095·2); lactic acid (p.1593·3).

Aussie Tan Sunstick *Or-Dov, Austral.*
Salol (p.83·1).
Sunscreen.

Austrapen *CSL, Austral.*
Injection: Ampicillin sodium (p.153·1).
Syrup†; capsules†: Ampicillin trihydrate (p.153·2).
Bacterial infections.

Austrialens *Austroflex, Aust.*
Cleaning, wetting, and storage solutions for hard and gas-permeable contact lenses.

Austroflex *Austroflex, Aust.*
Range of contact lens solutions.

Austrophyllin *Petrasch, Aust.*
Diprophylline (p.752·1).

Austrorinse *Austroflex, Aust.*
Rinsing solution for contact lenses.

Austrosept *Austroflex, Aust.*
Hydrogen peroxide (p.1116·2).
Disinfecting solution for soft contact lenses.

Austyn *Faulding, Austral.*
Theophylline (p.765·1).
Obstructive airways disease.

Autan *Bayer, Ger.*
Diethyltoluamide (p.1405·1).
Insect repellent.

Autonic *Acusan, Ger.*
Caffeine (p.749·3).
Fatigue.

Autoplasme Vaillant *Chefaro Ardeval, Fr.*
Black mustard (p.1605·3).
Respiratory-tract congestion.

Autoplex
Baxter, Ger.; Baxter, Swed.; Travenol, UK.
A factor VIII inhibitor bypassing fraction (p.721·3).
Haemorrhage in patients with inhibitors to factor VIII.

Autoplex T
Baxter, Belg.; Baxter, Spain; Hyland, USA.
Factor VIII inhibitor bypassing fraction (p.721·3).
Haemorrhage in patients with inhibitors to factor VIII.

Autosterile *Allergan, Aust.*
Contact lens cleaner.

Autrin *Wyeth, S.Afr.*
Vitamin B_{12}; intrinsic factor; ferrous fumarate; vitamin C; folic acid.
Anaemias.

Auxergyl D₃ *Roussel, Fr.*
Vitamin A acetate (p.1359·2); cholecalciferol (p.1366·3).
Hypocalcaemic tetany; osteomalacia; rickets; vitamin D deficiency.

Auxibilina *Granata, Ital.†.*
Metochalcone (p.1603·2).
Biliary-tract disorders.

Auxidor *Fher, Spain†.*
Paracetamol (p.72·2).
Fever; pain.

Auxiloson *Thomae, Ger.*
Dexamethasone isonicotinate (p.1037·1).
Respiratory-tract disorders.

Auxina A + E *Alcala, Spain.*
Vitamin A palmitate (p.1359·2); tocopherol (p.1369·2).
Deficiency of vitamins A and E; eye disorders; habitual abortion; infertility; skin disorders.

Auxina A Masiva *Alcala, Spain.*
Vitamin A palmitate (p.1359·2).
Vitamin A deficiency.

Auxina Complejo B *Alcala, Spain.*
Vitamin B substances.

Auxina Complejo Total *Wellcome, Spain†.*
Multivitamin preparation.

Auxina E *Alcala, Spain.*
Tocopheryl acetate (p.1369·1).
Hypoproteinaemia; intermittent claudication; mastalgia; muscular dystrophies; prevention of intraventricular haemorrhage in premature neonates; vitamin E deficiency.

Auxisone *Boehringer Ingelheim, Fr.†.*
Dexamethasone isonicotinate (p.1037·1).
Obstructive airways disease.

Auxitrans *Jumer, Fr.*
Pentaerythritol (p.1208·1).
Constipation.

Avacan *Noristan, S.Afr.†.*
Camylofin hydrochloride (p.1558·2).
Gastro-intestinal spasm.

Avafortan *Therabel, Fr.*
Camylofin hydrochloride (p.1558·2) or camylofin noramidopyrine mesylate (p.1558·2); dipyrone (p.35·1).
Pain; smooth muscle spasm.

Avail *Menley & James, USA.*
Multivitamin and mineral preparation with iron and folic acid.

Avalin *Medifood-Trufood, Ital.*
Infant feed.
Maple syrup urine disease.

Avallone *Sanabo, Aust.*
Ibuprofen (p.44·1).
Inflammation; musculoskeletal and joint disorders; pain.

Avamigran *Asta Medica, Aust.*
Ergotamine tartrate (p.445·3); mecloxamine citrate (p.465·1); camylofin hydrochloride (p.1558·2); anhydrous caffeine (p.749·3); propyphenazone (p.81·3).
Cluster headache; migraine.

Avamigran N *Asta Medica, Ger.*
Ergotamine tartrate (p.445·3); propyphenazone (p.81·3).
Formerly contained ergotamine tartrate, propyphenazone, mecloxamine citrate, camylofin hydrochloride, and caffeine.
Cluster headache; migraine.

Avan *Takeda, Jpn.*
Idebenone (p.1590·2).
Cerebrovascular disorders.

Avancort *Farmades, Ital.*
Methylprednisolone aceponate (p.1046·2).
Skin disorders.

Avant Garde Shampoo *Avant Garde, Canad.*
Pyrithione zinc (p.1089·3).

Avantol *Hosbon, Spain†.*
Fenoterol hydrobromide (p.753·2).
Bronchospasm; premature labour.

Avantrin *UCB, Ital.*
Trapidil (p.957·2).
Ischaemic heart disease.

Avapro *Sanofi Winthrop, USA.*
Irbesartan (p.891·3).
Hypertension.

Avaxim
Pasteur Merieux, Neth.; Pasteur Merieux, Swed.; Pasteur Merieux, UK.
A hepatitis A vaccine (p.1512·2).
Active immunisation.

AVC
Hoechst Marion Roussel, Canad.; Hoechst Marion Roussel, USA.
Sulphanilamide (p.256·3).
Vulvovaginal candidiasis.

AVC/Dienestrol *Merrell Dow, Canad.†.*
Dienoestrol (p.1444·1); sulphanilamide (p.256·3); aminacrine hydrochloride (p.1098·3); allantoin (p.1078·2).
Atrophic vaginitis.

Avecyde *3M, Austral.*
Lactic acid (p.1593·3).
Nappy rash; skin irritation; soap substitute.

Avedorm *Eberth, Ger.*
Oral liquid: Valerian (p.1643·1); melissa (p.1600·1); passion flower (p.1615·3).
Tablets: Valerian (p.1643·1); lupulus (p.1597·2).
Agitation; sleep disorders.

Avedorm N *Eberth, Ger.*
Lupulus (p.1597·2); passiflora; zinc valerianic.
Nervous disorders.

Aveeno
Note. This name is used for preparations of different composition.
Bioglan, Irl.
Avena (p.1551·3).
Dry skin.

Rydelle, USA.
Soap-free skin cleanser; emollient and moisturiser.

Aveeno Acne Bar *Johnson, Canad.*
Avena (p.1551·3); salicylic acid (p.1090·2).
Acne.

Aveeno Anti-Itch
Note. This name is used for preparations of different composition.
Johnson, Canad.
Calamine (p.1080·1); pramoxine hydrochloride (p.1298·2).
Aveeno Anti-Itch cream formerly contained calamine, pramoxine hydrochloride, and camphor.
Skin disorders.

Rydelle, USA.
Calamine (p.1080·1); pramoxine hydrochloride (p.1298·2); camphor (p.1557·2).
Minor skin irritation.

Aveeno Cleansing Bar *Rydelle, USA.*
Sulphur (p.1091·2); salicylic acid (p.1090·2); colloidal oatmeal (p.1551·3).
Acne.

Aveeno Preparations Dermatech, Austral.†; Johnson, Canad.; Rydelle, Fr.; Rydelle, Ital.; Bioglan, UK.
A range of preparations containing avena (p.1551·3).
Dry skin; skin care; skin irritation.

Aveenobar (for acne) Dermatech, Austral.†.
Avena (p.1551·3); sulphur (p.1091·2); salicylic acid (p.1090·2).

Aveenoderm Rydelle, Fr.
Avena (p.1551·3); zinc oxide (p.1096·2); allantoin (p.1078·2).
Skin disorders.

Avena Complex Blackmores, Austral.
Rosemary; avena (p.1551·3); verbena officinalis; kola (p.1645·1); vitamin B substances.
Tonic.

Avena Med Complex Dynamit, Aust.
Homoeopathic preparation.

Avena Rihom Komplex Richter, Aust.
Homoeopathic preparation.

Avena sativa comp. Weleda, UK.
Avena (p.1551·3); lupulus (p.1597·2); passion flower (p.1615·3); valerian root (p.1643·1); coffea tosta.
To aid relaxation.

Avenaforce Bioforce, Switz.
Avena sativa (p.1551·3).
Insomnia; nervousness.

Avene Pierre Fabre, Fr.†.
Ruscus aculeatus; dextran sulphate (p.1571·1); melilot.
Skin redness.

Avenoc
Note. This name is used for preparations of different composition.
Boiron, Canad.
Ointment: Homoeopathic preparation.
Boiron, Canad.; Boiron, Fr.
Suppositories: Homoeopathic preparation.
Boiron, Fr.
Ointment: Ficaria verna; paeonia officinalis; adrenaline; amylocaine hydrochloride (p.1286·1).
Anorectal disorders; haemorrhoids.

Aventyl
Lilly, Canad.; Lilly, Irl.; Lilly, S.Afr.; Lilly, UK†; Lilly, USA.
Nortriptyline hydrochloride (p.300·2).
Depression; nocturnal enuresis.

Averuk Bruciaporri Boots Healthcare, Ital.
Trichloroacetic acid (p.1639·1).
Verrucas; warts.

Avibon Theraplix, Fr.
Vitamin A (p.1358·1).
Skin disorders; vitamin A deficiency.

A-Vicotrat Heyl, Ger.
Retinol palmitate (p.1359·2).
Vitamin A deficiency.

Avigilen
Note. This name is used for preparations of different composition.
Schoeller, Aust.
Alpha tocopheryl acetate (p.1369·2).
Intermittent claudication; muscle and connective tissue disorders.
Brenner-Efeka, Ger.
Piracetam (p.1619·1).
Mental function disorders.

Avil
Note. This name is used for preparations of different composition.
Albert-Roussel, Aust.; Hoechst Marion Roussel, Belg.; Albert-Roussel, Ger.; Hoechst, Ger.; Albert, S.Afr.†.
Pheniramine aminosalicylate (p.415·3) or pheniramine maleate (p.415·3).
Burns; eczema; hypersensitivity reactions; sunburn.
Hoechst Marion Roussel, Austral.
Nasal spray†: Phenylephrine hydrochloride (p.1066·2); pheniramine maleate (p.415·3).
Colds; hay fever; rhinitis.
Syrup; controlled-release tablets; tablets: Pheniramine maleate (p.415·3).
Hypersensitivity reactions; motion sickness; pruritus; rhinitis; vestibular disorders.

Avil Decongestant Hoechst Marion Roussel, Austral.
Pheniramine maleate (p.415·3); ammonium chloride (p.1055·2); menthol (p.1600·2).
Bronchial and nasal congestion; coughs.

Aviletten Albert-Roussel, Ger.†.
Pheniramine aminosalicylate (p.415·3).
Hypersensitivity reactions.

Avilettes Hoechst Marion Roussel, Austral.†.
Pheniramine aminosalicylate (p.415·3).
Hypersensitivity reactions; motion sickness; pruritus; rhinitis; vestibular disorders.

Aviral IBIS, Ital.†.
Inosine pranobex (p.615·2).
Viral infections.

Avirase Lampugnani, Ital.
Aciclovir (p.602·3).
Herpesvirus infections.

Avirax Fabrigen, Canad.
Aciclovir (p.602·3).
Herpesvirus infections.

Avirin Eurofarmaco, Ital.
Inosine pranobex (p.615·2).
Viral infections.

Avita DPT, USA.
Tretinoin (p.1093·3).
Acne.

Avitene
Agepha, Aust.; Shionogi, USA.
Microfibrillar collagen (p.1566·3).
Haemorrhage in surgical procedures.

Avitina CT, Ital.†.
Vitamin A palmitate (p.1359·2).

Avitol Lannacher, Aust.
Vitamin A acetate (p.1359·2).
Vitamin A deficiency.

Avix Ibirn, Ital.
Aciclovir (p.602·3).
Herpesvirus infections.

Avlocardyl Zeneca, Fr.
Propranolol hydrochloride (p.937·1).
Cardiovascular disorders; migraine; oesophageal varices; tremor.

Avloclor
Zeneca, Irl.; Zeneca, UK.
Chloroquine phosphate (p.426·3).
Hepatic amoebiasis; lupus erythematosus; malaria; rheumatoid arthritis.

Avlosulfon Wyeth-Ayerst, Canad.
Dapsone (p.199·2).
Actinomycotic mycetoma; dermatitis herpetiformis; leprosy.

AVOCA Robinson, UK.
Silver nitrate (p.1629·2); potassium nitrate (p.1123·1).
Warts.

Avocin Cyanamid, Ital.
Piperacillin sodium (p.237·2).
Lignocaine hydrochloride (p.1293·2) is included in this preparation to alleviate the pain of injection.
Bacterial infections.

Avomine
Rhone-Poulenc Rorer, Austral.; Rhone-Poulenc Rorer, Irl.; Manx, UK.
Promethazine theoclate (p.416·2).
Motion sickness; nausea; vertigo; vomiting.

Avonex
Dompe Biotec, Ital.; Biogen, Neth.; Astra, Swed.; Biogen, UK; Biogen, USA.
Interferon beta-1a (p.616·1).
Multiple sclerosis.

Avril Sterling Health, Spain.
Cod-liver oil (p.1337·3); aluminium acetotartrate (p.1547·3); benzalkonium chloride (p.1101·3); zinc oxide (p.1096·2).
Burns; wounds.

Avyclor Uno, Ital.
Aciclovir (p.602·3).
Herpesvirus infections.

Avyplus Epifarma, Ital.
Aciclovir (p.602·3).
Herpesvirus infections.

Axacef Tika, Swed.
Cefuroxime sodium (p.177·1).
Bacterial infections.

Axamin Lennon, S.Afr.†.
Chlorthalidone (p.839·3).
Hypertension; oedema.

Axeen
Hommel, Ger.†; Zyma, Switz.†.
Proxibarbal (p.689·3).
Headache including migraine.

Axepim Bristol-Myers Squibb, Fr.
Cefepime hydrochloride (p.165·1).
Bacterial infections.

Axer Wassermann, Ital.
Naproxen sodium (p.61·2).
Inflammation; pain.

Axerol Wander, Switz.†.
Vitamin A (p.1358·1).
Vitamin A deficiency.

Axid
Lilly, Aust.†; Lilly, Canad.; Lilly, Irl.; Dista, Neth.; Lilly, Neth.; Lilly, S.Afr.; Lilly, UK; Lilly, USA; Whitehall-Robins, USA.
Nizatidine (p.1203·2).
Dyspepsia; gastro-oesophageal reflux; heartburn; peptic ulcer.

Axil Boehringer Mannheim, Ital.†.
Pidotimod (p.1618·3).
Immunostimulant.

Axiten Zambon, Ital.†.
Mebutamate (p.901·3).
Hypertension.

Axiten Tre Zambon, Ital.†.
Mebutamate (p.901·3); reserpine (p.942·1); dihydralazine sulphate (p.854·1).
Arteriosclerosis; hypertension.

Axocet Savage, USA.
Butobarbitone (p.645·1); paracetamol (p.72·2).
Pain.

Axonyl Parke, Davis, Fr.
Piracetam (p.1619·1).
Cerebrovascular insufficiency; mental function disorders; vertigo.

Axoren Glaxo Wellcome, Ital.
Buspirone hydrochloride (p.643·3).
Anxiety.

Axotal Adria, USA†.
Butalbital (p.644·3); aspirin (p.16·1).
Tension headache.

Axotide Glaxo Wellcome, Switz.
Fluticasone propionate (p.1042·3).
Asthma.

Axsain
GenDerm, Canad.; Helsinn Birex, Irl.; Euroderma, UK.
Capsaicin (p.24·2).
Diabetic polyneuropathy; joint pain; neuralgia; post-surgical pain.

Axyol Richard, Fr.
Iodine (p.1493·1).
Burns; leg ulcers; wounds.

Aydolid Farma Lepori, Spain.
Fosfosal (p.42·3).
Pain.

Aydolid Codeina Farma Lepori, Spain.
Codeine phosphate (p.26·1); fosfosal (p.42·3).
Pain.

Ayercillin Wyeth-Ayerst, Canad.
Procaine penicillin (p.240·2).
Bacterial infections.

Aygestin Wyeth-Ayerst, USA.
Norethisterone acetate (p.1453·1).
Abnormal uterine bleeding; endometriosis; secondary amenorrhoea.

Ayr Saline Ascher, USA.
Sodium chloride (p.1162·2).
Nasal irritation.

Ayrton's Antiseptic McGloin, Austral.
Zinc oxide (p.1096·2); dichlorobenzyl alcohol (p.1112·2).
Superficial skin infections.

Ayrton's Chilblain McGloin, Austral.
Camphor (p.1557·2); benzocaine (p.1286·2); peru balsam (p.1617·2); phenol (p.1121·2).
Chilblains.

Ayrton's Iodised McGloin, Austral.†.
Iodine (p.1493·1); phenol (p.1121·2); menthol (p.1600·2).
Sore throat.

Aywet Willvonseder, Aust.
Wetting solution for hard and soft contact lenses.

AZ 15 Gengidentifricio Procter & Gamble, Ital.
Sodium chloride (p.1162·2); benzalkonium chloride (p.1101·3); azulene (p.1552·1).
Gum protection; oral hygiene.

AZ Junior Procter & Gamble, Ital.
Sodium fluoride (p.742·1); mica-titanium dioxide complex.
Dental caries prophylaxis.

Azacortid Lepetit, Ital.†.
Fluazacort.
Skin disorders.

Azactam
Laevosan, Aust.; Bristol-Myers Squibb, Austral.; Bristol-Myers Squibb, Belg.; Sanofi Winthrop, Fr.; Bristol-Myers Squibb, Ger.; Grunenthal, Ger.; Bristol-Myers Squibb, Irl.; Bristol-Myers Squibb, Ital.; Eisai, Jpn; Bristol-Myers Squibb, Neth.; Bristol-Myers Squibb, Norw.; Squibb, Spain; Bristol-Myers Squibb, Swed.; Bristol-Myers Squibb, Switz.; Squibb, UK; Squibb, USA.
Aztreonam (p.156·3).
Gram-negative bacterial infections.

Azamedac Medac, Ger.
Azathioprine sodium (p.506·2).
Auto-immune disorders; organ transplantation.

Azameno
Wyeth Lederle, Aust.; Wyeth, Switz.
Omoconazole nitrate (p.386·3).
Fungal and Gram-positive bacterial vaginal infections; fungal infections.

Azamune Penn, UK.
Azathioprine (p.505·3).
Auto-immune disorders; organ transplantation.

Azantac Glaxo Wellcome, Fr.
Ranitidine hydrochloride (p.1209·3).
Gastro-oesophageal reflux; peptic ulcers; Zollinger-Ellison syndrome.

Azapress Intramed, S.Afr.
Azathioprine (p.505·3).
Transplant rejection.

Azaron
Schoeller, Aust.; Chefaro, Ger.; Chefaro, Neth.†; Organon, Spain.
Tripelennamine hydrochloride (p.420·2).
Hypersensitivity reactions; insect bites.

Azdone Schwarz, USA†.
Hydrocodone tartrate (p.43·1); aspirin (p.16·1).
Pain.

Azedavit Whitehall, Fr.
Multivitamin and mineral preparation.

Azelex Allergan Herbert, USA.
Azelaic acid (p.1079·1).
Acne.

Azeptin Eisai, Jpn.
Azelastine hydrochloride (p.403·1).
Allergic rhinitis; asthma; pruritus.

Azerodol Edmond Pharma, Ital.
Salicylamide (p.82·3); propyphenazone (p.81·3); caffeine (p.749·3).
Pain.

Azilline Spirig, Switz.
Amoxycillin trihydrate (p.151·3).
Bacterial infections.

Azinc
Arkopharma, Fr.; Arkochim, Spain.
Multivitamin and mineral preparation.

Azinc Complex Arkopharma, UK.
Multivitamin and mineral preparation.

Azitrocin Roerig, Ital.
Azithromycin (p.155·2).
Bacterial infections.

Azitromax
Pfizer, Norw.; Pfizer, Swed.
Azithromycin (p.155·2).
Bacterial infections.

Azmacort
Rhone-Poulenc Rorer, Canad.; Rhone-Poulenc Rorer, USA.
Triamcinolone acetonide (p.1050·2).
Asthma.

AZM-Tab Alra, USA.
Acetazolamide (p.810·3).

Azo Gantanol Roche, USA†.
Phenazopyridine hydrochloride (p.78·3); sulphamethoxazole (p.254·3).
Bacterial infections of the urinary tract.

Azo Gantrisin
Roche, Canad.†; Roche, USA†.
Phenazopyridine hydrochloride (p.78·3); sulphafurazole (p.253·3).
Bacterial infections of the urinary tract.

Azodine Propan, S.Afr.
Phenazopyridine hydrochloride (p.78·3).
Urinary-tract pain.

Azol
Note. This name is used for preparations of different composition.
Alphapharm, Austral.
Danazol (p.1441·3).
Endometriosis; hereditary angioedema; mastalgia; menorrhagia.
Andreu, Spain†.
Ointment: Cholesterol; sulphanilamide (p.256·3); zinc oxide (p.1096·2).
Skin infections.
Roche Nicholas, Spain.
Topical powder: Sulphanilamide (p.256·3).
Skin infections.

Azolmen Menarini, Ital.
Bifonazole (p.375·3).
Fungal skin infections.

Azo-Mandelamine Parke, Davis, S.Afr.†.
Hexamine mandelate (p.216·1); phenazopyridine hydrochloride (p.78·3).
Urinary-tract infections.

Azonutril
Pharmacia Upjohn, Fr.; Rhone-Poulenc Rorer, Neth.†; Rhone-Poulenc Rorer, Spain.
Amino-acid infusion.
Parenteral nutrition.

Azopine Pinewood, Irl.
Azathioprine (p.505·3).
Auto-immune disorders; organ transplantation.

Azopt Alcon, USA.
Brinzolamide (p.834·1).
Glaucoma; ocular hypertension.

Azor Lennon, S.Afr.
Alprazolam (p.640·3).
Anxiety.

Azo-Standard PolyMedica, USA.
Phenazopyridine hydrochloride (p.78·3).
Urinary-tract pain.

Azostix
Bayer Diagnostics, Austral.; Miles, Canad.; Ames, Irl.; Bayer Diagnostici, Ital.†; Ames, S.Afr.; Bayer Diagnostics, UK; Bayer, USA.
Test for urea in blood.

Azosulfin Panto, Spain†.
Co-trimoxazole (p.196·3).
Bacterial infections; Pneumocystis carinii pneumonia.

Azuben Lasa, Spain.
Pefloxacin mesylate (p.236·1).
Bacterial infections.

Azubromaron Azupharma, Ger.†.
Benzbromarone (p.392·3).
Gout; hyperuricaemia.

Azubronchin Azupharma, Ger.
Acetylcysteine (p.1052·3).
Respiratory-tract disorders associated with increased or viscous mucus.

Azucalcit Azupharma, Ger.
Salcatonin (p.735·3).
Hypercalcaemia; osteoporosis; Paget's disease of bone; reflex sympathetic dystrophy.

Azucimet Azupharma, Ger.
Cimetidine (p.1183·2).
Aspiration syndromes; gastro-oesophageal reflux; peptic ulcer; Zollinger-Ellison syndrome.

Azudoxat Azupharma, Ger.
Doxycycline hydrochloride (p.202·3).
Bacterial infections.

Azudoxat comp Azupharma, Ger.
Doxycycline hydrochloride (p.202·3); ambroxol hydrochloride (p.1054·3).
Respiratory-tract infections.

Azudoxat-T Azuchemie, Ger.†.
Doxycycline (p.202·3).
Bacterial infections.

Azufibrat Azupharma, Ger.
Bezafibrate (p.1268·2).
Hyperlipidaemias.

Azuglucon Azupharma, Ger.
Glibenclamide (p.319·3).
Diabetes mellitus.

Azul Metile *Ciba Vision, Spain.*
Methylene blue (p.984·3).
Ophthalmic diagnostic agent.

Azulen *Provita, Aust.*
Guaiazulene (p.1586·3).
Hypersensitivity and inflammatory disorders.

Azulenal *Agepha, Aust.*
Guaiazulene (p.1586·3).
Hypersensitivity disorders; mucus membrane inflammation; skin disorders.

Azulene
Note. This name is used for preparations of different composition.
Allergan, Fr.†.
Guaiazulene (p.1586·3).
Conjunctival irritation.

Allergan, Switz.†.
Azulene (p.1552·1); benzododecinium (p.1103·2).
Conjunctival irritation.

Azulfidine
Pharmacia Upjohn, Ger.; Pharmacia Upjohn, USA.
Sulphasalazine (p.1215·2).
Inflammatory bowel diseases; rheumatoid arthritis.

Azulipont *Azupharma, Ger.*
Thioctic acid (p.1636·2).
Diabetic polyneuropathy.

Azulon *Asta Medica, Ger.*
Chamomile (p.1561·2).
Skin disorders.

Azulon compositum Homburg *Asta Medica, Ger.*†.
Sodium gualenate; butinoline phosphate (p.1555·3); aluminium hydroxide-magnesium carbonate gel (p.1178·2); colloidal silicon dioxide (p.1474·3).
Gastro-intestinal disorders.

Azulon liquidum Homburg *Asta Medica, Ger.*†.
Sodium gualenate; laureth 9 (p.1325·2).
Gastro-intestinal disorders.

Azumetop *Azupharma, Ger.*
Metoprolol tartrate (p.907·3).
Angina pectoris; arrhythmias; hypertension; migraine; myocardial infarction.

Azunaftil *Azupharma, Ger.*
Naftidrofuryl oxalate (p.914·2).
Peripheral vascular disorders.

Azupamil *Azupharma, Ger.*
Verapamil hydrochloride (p.960·3).
Angina pectoris; arrhythmias; hypertension.

Azupanthenol *Parke, Davis, Ger.*
Oral liquid: Guaiazulene (p.1586·3); sodium pantothenate (p.1353·1).
Tablets†: Ammonium salt of guaiazulene-3-sulphonic acid; calcium pantothenate (p.1352·3); bismuth aluminate (p.1180·1); dried aluminium hydroxide gel (p.1177·3); magnesium trisilicate (p.1199·1); light magnesium carbonate (p.1198·1); frangula bark (p.1193·2); calamus (p.1556·1); fennel oil (p.1579·2).
Gastro-intestinal disorders.

Azupentat *Azupharma, Ger.*
Oxpentifylline (p.925·3).
Peripheral vascular disorders.

Azuperamid *Azupharma, Ger.*
Loperamide hydrochloride (p.1197·2).
Diarrhoea.

Azuprostat M *Azupharma, Ger.*
Sitosterol (p.1279·3).
Prostatic disorders.

Azur *Steiner, Ger.*
Paracetamol (p.72·2); caffeine (p.749·3).
Pain.

Azur compositum *Steiner, Ger.*
Paracetamol (p.72·2); caffeine (p.749·3); codeine phosphate (p.26·1).
Pain.

Azuranit *Azupharma, Ger.*
Ranitidine hydrochloride (p.1209·3).
Aspiration syndromes; gastro-oesophageal reflux; peptic ulcer; Zollinger-Ellison syndrome.

Azutranquil *Azuchemie, Ger.*†.
Oxazepam (p.683·2).
Insomnia.

Azutrimazol *Azupharma, Ger.*
Clotrimazole (p.376·3).
Fungal skin and genito-urinary tract infections.

Azym *Laphal, Fr.*
Magnesium hydroxide (p.1198·2); magnesium carbonate (p.1198·1); anhydrous sodium sulphate (p.1213·3); dibasic sodium phosphate (p.1159·3); calcium carbonate (p.1182·1); sodium bicarbonate (p.1153·2).
Gastro-intestinal disorders.

B_{12} Ankermann *Worwag, Ger.*
Cyanocobalamin (p.1363·3).
Vitamin B_{12} deficiency.

B 15 APS *APS, Ger.*†.
Di-isopropylammonium dichloroacetate (p.854·1).
Circulatory disorders; liver disorders.

B Chabre *AJC, Fr.*
Vitamin B substances.

B Complex
Jamieson, Canad.; Sante Naturelle, Canad.; Shaklee, Canad.
Vitamin B substances.

Phillips Yeast, UK.
Yeast (p.1373·1); vitamin B substances.

B Complex 100 *Bioglan, Austral.*†.
Vitamin B preparation.

B Complex 500 *Nobel, Canad.*
Vitamin B substances and vitamin C.

B Complex with C *Everest, Canad.*
Vitamin B substances and vitamin C.

B Complex C 550 *Adams, Canad.*
Vitamin B substances and vitamin C.

B Complex Fosforilado *Alter, Spain.*
Vitamin B substances.

B Complex Plus *Vita Glow, Austral.*†.
B vitamins and vitamin C; methionine; pectin; lecithin; liver extract; calcium phosphate.
Vitamin B and C deficiencies.

B Complex plus C *Jamieson, Canad.*
Vitamin B substances and vitamin C.

B 12 compositum N *Siegfried, Ger.*†.
Cyanocobalamin (p.1363·3); folic acid (p.1340·3); iron(III)-saccharose complex.
Hypochromic and secondary anaemias; tonic.

B Compound *Swiss Herbal, Canad.*
Vitamin B substances.

B Forte *Bio-Health, UK.*
Vitamin B preparation.

B4 Hemosan *Zambon, Spain*†.
Adenine (p.1543·2) or adenine hydrochloride (p.1543·2).
Agranulocytosis; white blood cell disorders.

B 12-L 90 *Loges, Ger.*
Cyanocobalamin (p.1363·3).
Anaemias; tonic; vitamin B deficiency.

B12 Latino Depot *Syntex, Spain*†.
Cyanocobalamin tannate (p.1364·2).
Vitamin B12 deficiency.

B 12 Nervinfant *Josso-Arznei, Ger.*†.
Cyanocobalamin (p.1363·3); thiamine hydrochloride (p.1361·1); lupulus (p.1597·2); passion flower (p.1615·3); piscidia erythrina; mistletoe (p.1604·1); sodium phytate (p.995·3); guaiphenesin (p.1061·3); sodium glycerophosphate (p.1586·2).
Nervous disorders.

B & O Supprettes No. 15A *PolyMedica, USA.*
Prepared opium (p.70·3); powdered belladonna extract (p.457·1).
Ureteral spasm pain.

B & O Supprettes No. 16A *PolyMedica, USA.*
Prepared opium (p.70·3); powdered belladonna extract (p.457·1).
Ureteral spasm pain.

B plus C *Novopharm, Canad.*
Vitamin B substances and vitamin C.

B 10-Strath *Strath-Labor, Ger.*†.
Bryonia (p.1555·2); ephedra (p.1059·3); turiones pini; polygonum avicularis; valerian (p.1643·1).
Bronchitis; colds; influenza.

B Stress C plus Iron & Vitamins *Stanley, Canad.*
Vitamin preparation with iron.

B Stress Select *Sisu, Canad.*
Vitamin B substances.

B Totum *Desbergers, Canad.*
Vitamin B substances and vitamin C.

B Virol *Rolmex, Canad.*
Multivitamin preparation.

Babee *Pfeiffer, USA.*
Benzocaine (p.1286·2); cetalkonium chloride (p.1105·2); camphor (p.1557·2); menthol (p.1600·2); cineole (p.1564·1).
Oral lesions.

Babiforton *Sanofi Winthrop, Ger.*
Eucalyptus oil (p.1578·1); pine needle oil; peppermint oil (p.1208·1).
Respiratory-tract catarrh.

Babigoz Crema Protettiva *Guigoz, Ital.*
Zinc oxide (p.1096·2); magnesium silicate (p.1473·3); wheat-germ oil.
Nappy rash.

Babix *Madaus, Aust.*
Cajuput oil (p.1556·1); pumilio pine oil (p.1623·3); eucalyptus oil (p.1578·1).
Respiratory-tract disorders.

Babix-Inhalat N *Mickan, Ger.*
Eucalyptus oil (p.1578·1); Norway spruce oil.
Respiratory-tract disorders.

Babix-Wundsalbe N *Mickan, Ger.*
Zinc oxide (p.1096·2); lemon oil (p.1595·3); chamomile oil.
Skin disorders.

Baby Anbesol *Whitehall, USA.*
Benzocaine (p.1286·2).
Teething pain.

Baby Block *Estee Lauder, Canad.*
Titanium dioxide (p.1093·3).
Sunscreen.

Baby Chest Rub *Seton, UK*†.
Turpentine oil (p.1641·1); menthol (p.1600·2); eucalyptus oil (p.1578·1).
Bronchial congestion.

Baby Cough Syrup *Cupal, UK*†.
Acetic acid (p.1541·2).
Coughs.

Baby Liberol *Galactina, Switz.*
Hyoscyamus oil (p.464·3); eucalyptus oil (p.1578·1); pumilio pine oil (p.1623·3); star anise oil; juniper oil (p.1592·3); methyl salicylate (p.55·2).
Cold symptoms.

Baby Luuf *Apomedica, Aust.*
Camphor (p.1557·2); eucalyptus oil (p.1578·1); turpentine oil (p.1641·1); majoram oil.
Respiratory-tract disorders.

Baby Orajel
Del, Canad.; Del, USA.
Benzocaine (p.1286·2).
Teething pain.

Baby Orajel Tooth and Gum Cleanser *Del, USA.*
Poloxamer 407 (p.1326·3); simethicone (p.1213·1).
Dental hygiene.

Baby Rinol *Marion Merrell, Spain.*
Chlorpheniramine maleate (p.405·1); phenylpropanolamine hydrochloride (p.1067·2); paracetamol (p.72·2).
Upper-respiratory-tract disorders.

Babygella *Guieu, Ital.*
Cream: Calendula; chamomile (p.1561·2); zinc oxide (p.1096·2).
Topical paste: Squalane; sweet almond oil; lactic acid; zinc oxide (p.1096·2).
Topical powder†: Zinc oxide (p.1096·2); sage (p.1627·1).
Barrier preparation.

Babygencal *Qualiphar, Belg.*
Amylocaine hydrochloride (p.1286·1); potassium bromide (p.1620·3); chloral hydrate (p.645·3).
Teething pain.

Babylax
Byk, Aust.; Mann, Ger.; Mann, Irl.; Mann, S.Afr.†.
Glycerol (p.1585·2).
Bowel evacuation; constipation.

Baby-Rinolo *Lepetit, Ital.*
Phenylpropanolamine hydrochloride (p.1067·2); chlorpheniramine maleate (p.405·1); paracetamol (p.72·2).
Respiratory-tract disorders.

Babys Own Gripe Water *Block, Canad.*
Anise oil (p.1550·1); dill oil (p.1572·1); fennel oil (p.1579·2); sodium bicarbonate (p.1153·2).
Gastro-intestinal disorders.

Babys Own Infant Drops *Block, Canad.*
Simethicone (p.1213·1).
Infant colic, bloating, and flatulence.

Babys Own Ointment *Block, Canad.*
Zinc oxide (p.1096·2).
Nappy rash.

Babys Own Teething Gel *Block, Canad.*
Benzyl alcohol (p.1103·3).
Teething pain.

Babysiton *Faes, Spain.*
Cetylpyridinium chloride (p.1106·2); zinc oxide (p.1096·2).
Skin disorders.

Babysteril *Eurospital, Ital.*
Zinc oxide (p.1096·2); almond oil (p.1546·2); wheat-germ oil; vitamin A (p.1358·1); vitamin E (p.1369·1).
Formerly contained zinc oxide, silicon, and wool fat, and was known as Pastasil.
Napkin rash.

Baby-Transpulmin *Asta Medica, Ger.*
Eucalyptus oil (p.1578·1); pine needle oil.
Cold symptoms.

Bacacil
Roerig, Ital.; Mack, Switz.†.
Bacampicillin hydrochloride (p.157·2).
Bacterial infections.

Bacampicin
Pharmacia Upjohn, Belg.; Pharmacia Upjohn, Switz.
Bacampicillin hydrochloride (p.157·2).
Bacterial infections.

Bacampicine *Pharmacia Upjohn, Fr.*
Bacampicillin hydrochloride (p.157·2).
Bacterial infections.

Bacarate *Reid-Rowell, USA*†.
Phendimetrazine tartrate (p.1484·2).
Obesity.

Baccalin *Bode, Ger.*
Benzalkonium chloride (p.1101·3); didecyldimethylammonium chloride (p.1112·2).
Disinfection.

Baccidal
Kyorin, Jpn; Knoll, Spain.
Norfloxacin (p.233·1).
Bacterial infections.

Bach Rescue Remedy *Bach, UK.*
Homoeopathic preparation.

Bacicoline
Note. This name is used for preparations of different composition.
Merck Sharp & Dohme-Chibret, Fr.
Bacitracin (p.157·3); colistin sulphomethate (p.196·2); hydrocortisone acetate (p.1043·3).
Eye infections.

Merck Sharp & Dohme, Switz.†.
Colistin sulphomethate sodium (p.196·1); chloramphenicol (p.182·1); hydrocortisone acetate (p.1043·3).
Eye infections; otitis.

Bacicoline-B *Chibret, Neth.*
Colistin sulphomethate sodium (p.196·1); bacitracin (p.157·3); hydrocortisone acetate (p.1043·3).
Inflammatory ear infections.

Bacid
Rhone-Poulenc Rorer, Canad.; Ciba, USA.
Lactobacillus acidophilus (p.1594·1).
Diarrhoea; stomatitis.

Bacifurane
Rhone-Poulenc Rorer, Belg.; Meram, Fr.†.
Nifuroxazide (p.231·3).
Diarrhoea.

Baciguent
McNeil Consumer, Canad.; Upjohn, USA.
Bacitracin (p.157·3).
Bacterial skin infections.

Baciguent Plus Pain Reliever *McNeil Consumer, Canad.*
Bacitracin (p.157·3); lignocaine (p.1293·2).
Pain and infection in burns and wounds.

Baci-IM *Pharma Tek, USA.*
Bacitracin (p.157·3).
Bacterial infections.

Bacillocid rasant *Bode, Ger.*
Glutaraldehyde (p.1114·3); benzalkonium chloride (p.1101·3); didecyldimethylammonium chloride (p.1112·2).
Surface disinfection.

Bacillocid Spezial *Bode, Ger.*
1,6-Dihydroxy-2,5-dioxahexan; glutaraldehyde (p.1114·3); benzalkonium chloride (p.1101·3); cocos-guanidinium chloride.
Surface disinfection.

Bacillol *Bode, Ger.*
Propyl alcohol (p.1124·2); isopropyl alcohol (p.1118·2); alcohol (p.1099·1); 1,6-dihydroxy-2,5-dioxahexan; mecetronium ethylsulphate (p.1119·1).
Surface disinfection.

Bacillol plus *Bode, Ger.*
Propyl alcohol (p.1124·2); isopropyl alcohol (p.1118·2); glutaraldehyde (p.1114·3).
Surface disinfection.

Bacillotox *Bode, Ger.*
Chlorocresol (p.1110·3); orthophenylphenol (p.1120·3); chloroxylenol (p.1111·1); clorophene (p.1111·2).
Disinfection.

Bacimex *Alter, Spain.*
Injection†: Ampicillin sodium (p.153·1); sulbactam sodium (p.250·3).
Lignocaine hydrochloride (p.1293·2) is included in the intramuscular injection to alleviate the pain of injection.
Tablets; oral suspension: Sultamicillin tosylate (p.257·2).
Bacterial infections.

Bacimycin *Alpharma, Norw.*
Bacitracin zinc (p.157·3); chlorhexidine acetate (p.1107·2).
Bacterial infections of the skin.

Bacimycine *Grossmann, Switz.*
Bacitracin (p.157·3); neomycin sulphate (p.229·2).
Infected skin disorders.

Bacimyxin *Pharmascience, Canad.*
Polymyxin B sulphate (p.239·1); bacitracin (p.157·3).
Bacterial infections.

Bacisporin *Wellcome, Spain.*
Bacitracin zinc (p.157·3); hydrocortisone (p.1043·3); neomycin sulphate (p.229·2); polymyxin B sulphate (p.239·1).
Infected skin disorders.

Bacitin *Pharmascience, Canad.*
Bacitracin (p.157·3).
Bacterial infections of the skin.

Backache Ledum *Homeocan, Canad.*
Homoeopathic preparation.

Backache Maximum Strength Relief *Bristol-Myers Squibb, USA.*
Magnesium salicylate (p.51·1).

Backache Tablets *Potter's, UK.*
Eupatorium purpurea root; hydrangea root; buchu (p.1555·2); bearberry (p.1552·2); capsicum (p.1559·2).
Backache.

Back-Aid *Technilab, Canad.*
Paracetamol (p.72·2); chlorzoxazone (p.1313·1).

Back-Ese M *Dannorth, Canad.*
Magnesium salicylate (p.51·1).

Baclospas *Ashbourne, UK.*
Baclofen (p.1308·2).
Skeletal muscle spasm or spasticity.

Baclysar *Artu, Neth.*†.
Bacterial extracts for specific hyposensitisation (p.1545·1).

Bacmin *Marnel, USA.*
Multivitamin and mineral preparation with iron and folic acid.

Bacocil *Roerig, Belg.*
Bacampicillin hydrochloride (p.157·2).
Bacterial infections.

Bactekod *Biogalenique, Fr.*†.
Co-trimoxazole (p.196·3).
Bacterial infections; Pneumocystis carinii pneumonia; toxoplasmosis.

Bacteomycine *Monot, Fr.*
Bacitracin (p.157·3); neomycin sulphate (p.229·2).
Infected skin disorders.

Bacterial *CT, Ital.*
Co-trimoxazole (p.196·3).
Bacterial infections.

Bacterianos D *Anios, Fr.*
Formaldehyde (p.1113·2); glyoxal (p.1115·1); glutaraldehyde (p.1114·3); didecyldimethylammonium chloride (p.1112·2).
Disinfection of surfaces.

Bacti-Cleanse *Pedinol, USA.*
Benzalkonium chloride (p.1101·3).
Skin cleanser.

Bacticlens Seton, UK†.
Chlorhexidine gluconate (p.1107·2).
Bladder irrigation; skin disinfection.

Bacticort Rugby, USA.
Hydrocortisone (p.1043·3); neomycin sulphate (p.229·2); polymyxin B sulphate (p.239·1).
Eye inflammation with bacterial infection.

Bactidan Pierre Fabre, Ital.
Enoxacin (p.203·3).
Urinary-tract and respiratory-tract infections.

Bactident Oberlin, Fr.
Sodium perborate (p.1125·2); sodium carbonate (p.1630·2); sodium phosphate (p.1159·3); sodium lauryl sulphate (p.1468·3).
False teeth hygiene.

Bactidox TAD, Ger.
Doxycycline (p.202·3).
Bacterial infections.

Bactidron Hoechst Marion Roussel, S.Afr.
Enoxacin (p.203·3).
Cystitis.

Bactifor Andromaco, Spain.
Co-trimoxazole (p.196·3).
Bacterial infections; Pneumocystis carinii pneumonia.

Bactigras
Smith & Nephew, Austral.; Smith & Nephew, Canad.; Braun, Ger.; Smith & Nephew, S.Afr.; Smith & Nephew, UK.
Chlorhexidine acetate (p.1107·2).
Burns; skin infections; ulcers; wounds.

Bactine
Note. This name is used for preparations of different composition.
Bayer, Canad.
Benzalkonium chloride (p.1101·3); lignocaine hydrochloride (p.1293·2).
Skin disorders; wound cleansing.
Miles, USA.
Hydrocortisone (p.1043·3).
Skin disorders.

Bactine Antiseptic Miles, USA.
Lignocaine (p.1293·2); benzalkonium chloride (p.1101·3).
Skin disorders.

Bactine First Aid Antibiotic Plus Anesthetic
Miles Laboratories, USA.
Polymyxin B sulphate (p.239·1); bacitracin (p.157·3); neomycin sulphate (p.229·2); diperodon hydrochloride (p.1292·3).
Bacterial skin infections.

Bactisubtil
Hoechst Marion Roussel, Belg.; Marion Merrell, Fr.; Cassella-med, Ger.; Leti, Spain.
Bacillus cereus (strain IP 5832) or *Bacillus subtilis.*
Diarrhoea; restoration of the gastro-intestinal flora.

Bactocef Gerec, S.Afr.
Cephradine (p.181·3).
Bacterial infections.

Bactocill SmithKline Beecham, USA.
Oxacillin sodium (p.234·2).
Bacterial infections.

Bactofen Hoechst Marion Roussel, Ital.
Benzoxonium chloride (p.1103·3).
Instrument disinfection; skin and mucous membrane disinfection.

Bactopumon Cinfa, Spain.
Tolu balsam (p.1071·1); bromhexine hydrochloride (p.1055·3); co-trimoxazole (p.196·3).
Respiratory-tract infections.

Bactoreduct Azupharma, Ger.
Co-trimoxazole (p.196·3).
Bacterial infections; Pneumocystis carinii pneumonia.

BactoShield Amsco, USA.
Chlorhexidine gluconate (p.1107·2); isopropyl alcohol (p.1118·2).
Skin disinfection.

Bactosone Belmac, Spain†.
Ampicillin sodium (p.153·1); bromhexine hydrochloride (p.1055·3); guaiphenesin (p.1061·3).
Lignocaine hydrochloride (p.1293·2) is included in this preparation to alleviate the pain of injection.
Respiratory-tract infections.

Bactosone Retard Belmac, Spain.
Ampicillin sodium (p.153·1); ampicillin benzathine (p.154·1); bromhexine hydrochloride (p.1055·3) guaiphenesin (p.1061·3).
Lignocaine hydrochloride (p.1293·2) is included in this preparation to alleviate the pain of injection.
Respiratory-tract infections.

Bactox Innotech, Fr.
Amoxycillin sodium (p.151·3) or amoxycillin trihydrate (p.151·3).
Bacterial infections.

Bactrazine Smith & Nephew, S.Afr.
Silver sulphadiazine (p.247·3).
Infected ulcers and burns.

Bactrian Loveridge, UK.
Cetrimide (p.1105·2).
Skin infections.

Bactrim
Roche, Aust.; Roche, Austral.; Roche, Belg.; Roche, Canad.; Roche, Fr.; Roche, Ger.; Roche, Irl.; Roche, Ital.; Roche, Norw.; Roche, S.Afr.; Roche, Swed.; Roche, Switz.; Roche, UK†; Roche, USA.
Co-trimoxazole (p.196·3).
Bacterial infections; blastomycosis; mycetoma; Pneumocystis carinii pneumonia; toxoplasmosis.

Bactrimel Roche, Neth.
Co-trimoxazole (p.196·3).
Bacterial infections; Pneumocystis carinii pneumonia.

Bactroban
SmithKline Beecham, Aust.; SmithKline Beecham, Austral.; Bencard, Belg.; SmithKline Beecham, Canad.; SmithKline Beecham, Fr.; SmithKline Beecham, Irl.; SmithKline Beecham, Ital.; SmithKline Beecham, Neth.; SmithKline Beecham, S.Afr.; SmithKline Beecham, Spain; SmithKline Beecham, Swed.; SmithKline Beecham, Switz.; Beecham Research, UK; SmithKline Beecham, USA.
Mupirocin (p.227·2) or calcium mupirocin (p.227·3).
Bacterial skin infections; elimination of nasal staphylococci.

Bactylisine Peters, Fr.
Mixed quaternary ammonium salts; polyalkylamine.
Surface disinfection.

Bad Heilbrunner Abfuhrtee N extra Bad Heilbrunner, Ger.
Senna (p.1212·2).
Constipation.

Badeol Agepha, Aust.
Sulphur (p.1091·2); soya oil (p.1355·1).
Skin disorders.

Bafucin Pharmacia Upjohn, Swed.
Benzocaine (p.1286·2); gramicidin (p.215·2); cetylpyridinium chloride (p.1106·2); dichlorobenzyl alcohol (p.1112·2).
Mouth and throat disorders.

Bagnisan med Heilbad Klemenz, Ger.
Echinacea purpurea (p.1574·2); hamamelis (p.1587·1); chlorophyllin (p.1000·1).
Bath additive; circulatory disorders; deodorant; neuralgia; neuritis; skin disorders.

Bagnisan S med Rheumabad Klemenz, Ger.†.
Sodium sulphate (p.1213·3); echinacea purpurea (p.1574·2); hamamelis (p.1587·1); chlorophyllin (p.1000·1).
Bath additive; nervous disorders; rheumatic disorders.

Bagno Oculare Ogna, Ital.
Zinc sulphate (p.1373·2); boric acid (p.1554·2); borax (p.1554·2).
Eye irritation.

Bain de Bouche Bancaud Cooperation Pharmaceutique, Fr.†.
Phenol (p.1121·2); chloral hydrate (p.645·3); sodium salicylate (p.85·1).
Mouth disorders.

Bain de Bouche Lipha Lipha, Fr.†.
Veratrol; menthol (p.1600·2); resorcinol (p.1090·1) chloral hydrate (p.645·3).
Mouthwash.

Bain de Soleil
Charton, Canad.
SPF 4; SPF 8: Octocrylene (p.1487·3); ethylhexyl *p*-methoxycinnamate (p.1487·1); titanium dioxide (p.1093·3).
SPF 15; SPF 30: Octocrylene (p.1487·3); ethylhexyl *p*-methoxycinnamate (p.1487·1); oxybenzone (p.1487·3); titanium dioxide (p.1093·3).
Sunscreen.
Procter & Gamble, USA.
SPF 4: Ethylhexyl *p*-methoxycinnamate (p.1487·1); 2-ethylhexyl salicylate (p.1487·3).
Sunscreen.

Bain de Soleil All Day Procter & Gamble, USA.
SPF 4; SPF 8: Ethylhexyl *p*-methoxycinnamate (p.1487·1); octocrylene (p.1487·3); titanium dioxide (p.1093·3).
SPF 15; SPF 30: Ethylhexyl *p*-methoxycinnamate (p.1487·1); octocrylene (p.1487·3); oxybenzone (p.1487·3); titanium dioxide (p.1093·3).
Sunscreen.

Bain de Soleil Color Procter & Gamble, USA.
SPF 8+: Ethylhexyl *p*-methoxycinnamate (p.1487·1); octocrylene (p.1487·3).
SPF 15+; SPF 30+: Ethylhexyl *p*-methoxycinnamate (p.1487·1); octocrylene (p.1487·3); oxybenzone (p.1487·3).
Sunscreen.

Bain de Soleil Mega Tan Charton, Canad.
SPF 4: Octocrylene (p.1487·3); ethylhexyl *p*-methoxycinnamate (p.1487·1).
Sunscreen.

Bain de Soleil Sport Charton, Canad.
SPF 8: Octocrylene (p.1487·3); ethylhexyl *p*-methoxycinnamate (p.1487·1); titanium dioxide (p.1093·3).
SPF 15: Octocrylene (p.1487·3); ethylhexyl *p*-methoxycinnamate (p.1487·1); oxybenzone (p.1487·3); titanium dioxide (p.1093·3).
Sunscreen.

Bain extra-doux dermatologique Widmer, Switz.
Coal tar (p.1092·3); chamomile (p.1561·2).
Skin disorders.

Bain Soufre au Sulfuryl Aerocid, Fr.
Sulphurated aluminium sodium silicate (p.1178·3); precipitated sulphur (p.1091·2).
Arthroses; skin disorders.

Bakanasan Einschlaf Bregenzer, Aust.
Valerian (p.1643·1); lupulus (p.1597·2).
Anxiety; sleep disorders.

Bakanasan Entwasserungs Bregenzer, Aust.
Silver birch (p.1553·3).
Urinary-tract disorders.

Bakanasan Leber-Galle Bregenzer, Aust.
Silybum marianum (p.993·3); turmeric (p.1001·3).
Gastro-intestinal disorders; liver and gallbladder disorders.

Baktar Shionogi, Jpn†.
Co-trimoxazole (p.196·3).
Bacterial infections.

Bakteriostat "Herbrand" Herbrand, Ger.
Dequalinium chloride (p.1112·1); ascorbic acid (p.1365·2).
Mouth and throat disorders.

Baktobod Bode, Ger.
Glutaraldehyde (p.1114·3); glyoxal (p.1115·1); benzalkonium chloride (p.1101·3).
Surface disinfection.

Baktobod N Bode, Ger.
Glyoxal (p.1115·1); benzalkonium chloride (p.1101·3).
Surface disinfection.

Bakto-Diaront Rosen, Ger.†.
Colistin sulphate (p.195·3).
Bacterial infections of the gastro-intestinal tract.

Baktonium Bode, Ger.
Benzalkonium chloride (p.1101·3).
Hand and skin disinfection.

Baktozil Chephasaar, Ger.†.
Cephazolin sodium (p.181·1).
Bacterial infections.

Bal Tar Euroderm, Ital.
Castor oil (p.1560·2); ichthammol (p.1083·3).
Seborrhoeic dermatitis.

Balanced B Adams, Canad.; Hall, Canad.; Pharmavite, Canad.; Stanley, Canad.
Vitamin B substances.

Balanced B Complex plus Vitamins C & E
Pharmavite, Canad.
Vitamin B substances, vitamin C, and Vitamin E.

Balanced C Complex Jamieson, Canad.
Ascorbic acid (p.1365·2).

Balanced E Jamieson, Canad.
Vitamin C, vitamin E, and selenium.

Balanced Ratio Cal-Mag Quest, UK.
Calcium, magnesium, and vitamin D preparation.

Balanced Salt Solution
Abbott, Canad.; Alcon, UK; Abbott, USA; Bausch & Lomb, USA.
Electrolyte solution (p.1147·1).
Eye irrigation.

Balancid Astra, Norw.
Magnesium carbonate (p.1198·1) or magnesium hydroxide (p.1198·2); aluminium hydroxide (p.1177·3).
Gastro-intestinal disorders associated with hyperacidity.

Balans IBP, Ital.†.
Benfluorex hydrochloride (p.1268·2).
Lipid metabolism disorders.

Baldex Bausch & Lomb, USA†.
Dexamethasone sodium phosphate (p.1037·2).
Eye inflammation.

Baldracin Austroplant, Aust.
Valerian (p.1643·1); peppermint leaf (p.1208·1); melissa (p.1600·1); lupulus (p.1597·2).
Nervous disorders.

Baldrian AMA Kwizda, Aust.
Valerian (p.1643·1); lupulus (p.1597·2).
Nervous disorders; sleep disorders.

Baldrian Dispert Compositum Solvay, Aust.
Valerian (p.1643·1); lupulus (p.1597·2).
Nervous disorders; sleep disorders.

Baldrian-Dispert Solvay Duphar, Swed.
Valerian (p.1643·1).
Nervous disorders; sleep disorders.

Baldrian-Dispert Nacht Solvay, Ger.
Valerian (p.1643·1); lupulus (p.1597·2).
Insomnia.

Baldrian-Elixier Ehrmann, Aust.
Valerian (p.1643·1); lupulus (p.1597·2); melissa (p.1600·1).
Nervous disorders; sleep disorders.

Baldrianetten N Eu Rho, Ger.
Valerian (p.1643·1).
Anxiety disorders; sleep disorders.

Baldrian-Krautertonikum Bioflora, Aust.
Melissa (p.1600·1); valerian (p.1643·1); lupulus (p.1597·2); orange flowers; lavender flowers (p.1594·3).
Nervous disorders; sleep disorders.

Baldrianox S Hermes, Ger.
Valerian (p.1643·1); lupulus (p.1597·2).
Nervous and sleep disorders.

Baldrinetten Solvay, Aust.
Valerian (p.1643·1).
Sedative.

Baldriparan Whitehall-Robins, Switz.
Valerian (p.1643·1); melissa (p.1600·1); lupulus (p.1597·2).
Nervous disorders.

Baldriparan Beruhigungs Salus, Aust.
Valerian (p.1643·1); lupulus (p.1597·2); melissa (p.1600·1).
Nervous disorders; sleep disorders.

Baldriparan N Much, Ger.
Valerian (p.1643·1); lupulus (p.1597·2).
Formerly contained valerian, lupulus, crataegus, and mistletoe.
Nervous disorders; sleep disorders.

Baldriparan stark N Much, Ger.
Valerian (p.1643·1); lupulus (p.1597·2); melissa (p.1600·1).
Formerly contained valerian, lupulus, crataegus, mistletoe, and guaiphenesin.
Nervous disorders; sleep disorders.

Baldrisedon
Much, Ger.; Wild, Switz.
Valerian (p.1643·1).
Anxiety; sleep disorders.

Baldronit cum Nitro Redel, Ger.†.
Valerian (p.1643·1); adonis vernalis (p.1543·3); barbitone sodium (p.642·3); glyceryl trinitrate (p.874·3).
Cardiac disorders.

Baldronit forte N Redel, Ger.†.
Barbitone sodium (p.642·3); phenobarbitone sodium (p.350·2); valerian (p.1643·1); belladonna (p.457·1); adonis vernalis (p.1543·3); mistletoe (p.1604·1).
Nervous disorders; sleep disorders.

Baldronit N Redel, Ger.†.
Valerian (p.1643·1); adonis vernalis (p.1543·3).
Formerly contained valerian, adonis vernalis, and barbitone sodium.
Insomnia; nervous disorders.

Balgifen Berk, UK.
Baclofen (p.1308·2).
Skeletal muscle spasm or spasticity.

Balisa Zyma, Ger.†.
Urea (p.1095·2).
Hyperkeratotic skin disorders.

Balisa VAS Zyma, Ger.†.
Urea (p.1095·2); tretinoin (p.1093·3).
Hyperkeratotic skin disorders.

Balkis Dolorgiet, Ger.
Capsules: Phenylephrine hydrochloride (p.1066·2); chlorpheniramine maleate (p.405·1).
Formerly contained etilefrine polistirex and chlorpheniramine polistirex.
Colds; hay fever.
Nasal drops; nasal spray: Xylometazoline hydrochloride (p.1071·2).
Allergic rhinitis; rhinitis.

Balkis Spezial Dolorgiet, Ger.
Terfenadine (p.418·1).
Allergic rhinitis.

Balm of Gilead
Healthcrafts, UK.
Oral mixture; pastilles: Balm of Gilead (p.1620·1); squill (p.1070·1); lobelia (p.1481·3).
Catarrh; coughs.
Potter's, UK.
Oral mixture: Balm of Gilead (p.1620·1); squill (p.1070·1); lobelia (p.1481·3); lungwort.
Coughs.

Balmandol
Smith & Nephew, Irl.†; Spirig, Switz.; Goldshield, UK†.
Almond oil (p.1546·2); light liquid paraffin (p.1382·1).
Skin disorders.

Balmex Stafford-Miller, Fr.
Zinc oxide (p.1096·2); liquid paraffin (p.1382·1); beeswax (p.1383·1); silicone (p.1384·2).
Nappy rash.

Balmex Baby Macsil, USA.
Zinc oxide (p.1096·2); peru balsam (p.1617·2); corn starch (p.1356·2); calcium carbonate (p.1182·1).
Nappy rash.

Balmex Emollient Macsil, USA.
Emollient and moisturiser.

Balminil Decongestant Rougier, Canad.
Pseudoephedrine hydrochloride (p.1068·3).
Nasal and sinus congestion.

Balminil DM Rougier, Canad.
Dextromethorphan hydrobromide (p.1057·3).
Coughs.

Balminil DM D Rougier, Canad.
Pseudoephedrine hydrochloride (p.1068·3); dextromethorphan hydrobromide (p.1057·3).
Congestion; coughs.

Balminil Expectorant Rougier, Canad.
Guaiphenesin (p.1061·3).
Coughs.

Balminil Lozenges Rougier, Canad.
Cetylpyridinium chloride (p.1106·2); benzocaine (p.1286·2).
Mouth and throat disorders.

Balminil Nasal Ointment Rougier, Canad.
Camphor (p.1557·2); menthol (p.1600·2); cineole (p.1564·1); chlorbutol (p.1106·3); ephedrine hydrochloride (p.1059·3).
Nasal congestion.

Balminil Suppositoires Rougier, Canad.
Cineole (p.1564·1); niaouli oil (p.1607·1); menthol (p.1600·2); sodium dibunate (p.1070·1).
Coughs.

Balmosa Pharmax, UK.
Methyl salicylate (p.55·2); menthol (p.1600·2); camphor (p.1557·2); capsicum oleoresin.
Pain.

Balmox SmithKline Beecham, Switz.
Nabumetone (p.60·1).
Musculoskeletal and joint disorders.

Balneoconzen S & K, Ger.
Soya oil (p.1355·1); lecithin (p.1595·2).
Skin disorders.

Balneogel Merck, Spain.
Allantoin (p.1078·2); chlorophyllin (p.1000·1); guaiazulene (p.1586·3); lauryl polyoxyethylene sulphate; riboflavine sodium phosphate (p.1362·1); sorbitol.
Skin disorders.

Balneol Solvay, USA.
Skin cleanser.

Balneovit O *Jossa-Arznei, Ger.†.*
Wheat-germ oil; avocado oil; carotene; soya oil (p.1355·1); light liquid paraffin (p.1382·1).
Bath additive; skin disorders.

Balnetar
Westwood-Squibb, Canad.; Westwood-Squibb, USA.
Coal tar (p.1092·3).
Dermatitis; psoriasis.

Balneum
Hermal, Ger.; E. Merck, Irl.; Hermal, Switz.; E. Merck, UK.
Soya oil (p.1355·1).
Bath additive; dry skin.

Balneum F
Hermal, Ger.; Hermal, Switz.
Arachis oil (p.1550·2); light liquid paraffin (p.1382·1).
Bath additive; skin disorders.

Balneum Hermal *Merck, Aust.*
Soya oil (p.1355·1).
Skin disorders.

Balneum Hermal F *Merck, Aust.*
Arachis oil (p.1550·2); light liquid paraffin (p.1382·1).
Skin disorders.

Balneum Hermal mit Teer *Merck, Aust.*
Soya oil (p.1355·1); coal tar (p.1092·3).
Skin disorders.

Balneum Hermal Plus *Merck, Aust.*
Soya oil (p.1355·1); laureth 9 (p.1325·2).
Skin disorders.

Balneum mit Schwefel *Hermal, Ger.†.*
Soya oil (p.1355·1); sulphur (p.1091·2).
Bath additive; skin disorders.

Balneum mit Teer *Hermal, Ger.†.*
Soya oil (p.1355·1); coal tar (p.1092·3).
Bath additive; skin disorders.

Balneum normal *Merck-Clevenot, Fr.†.*
Soya oil (p.1355·1).
Bath additive; skin disorders.

Balneum Plus
Note. This name is used for preparations of different composition.
Hermal, Ger.; E. Merck, Irl.; Hermal, Switz.; E. Merck, UK.
Bath additive: Soya oil (p.1355·1); laureth compounds (p.1325·2).
Dry skin; pruritus.

E. Merck, UK.
Cream: Laureth compounds (p.1325·2); urea (p.1095·2).
Skin disorders.

Balneum surgras *Merck-Clevenot, Fr.*
Arachis oil (p.1550·2); liquid paraffin (p.1382·1).
Bath additive; skin disorders.

Balneum with Tar
E. Merck, Irl.; E. Merck, UK†.
Soya oil (p.1355·1); coal tar (p.1092·3).
Bath additive; skin disorders.

Balnostim Bad N *Hoernecke, Ger.*
Pine needle oil; rosemary oil (p.1626·2).
Musculoskeletal, joint, and soft-tissue disorders.

Balodin *Ferrer, Spain.*
Dirithromycin (p.202·2).
Bacterial infections.

Balsacetil *Biotekfarma, Ital.*
Guacetisal (p.1061·2).
Respiratory-tract disorders.

Balsafissan *Uhlmann-Eyraud, Switz.†.*
Casein hydrolysate (Labiline); colloidal silicon dioxide (p.1475·1); acid. polysilicicum fluorat.; bismuth subnitrate (p.1180·2); dichlorophen (p.99·2).
Breast and nipple care.

Balsamico F. di M. *Kelemata, Ital.†.*
Pine oil; bornyl acetate (p.1555·1); benzyl benzoate (p.1402·2); cineole (p.1564·1); niaouli (p.1607·1); camphor (p.1557·2); linalyl acetate; amber musk (p.1605·3); rosemary oil (p.1626·2); menthol (p.1600·2).
Respiratory-tract disorders.

Balsamicum *Weleda, UK.*
Calendula; mercurialis perennis; peru balsam (p.1617·2); stibium metallicum praeparatum.
Minor wounds; nappy rash.

Balsamina Kroner *Ceccarelli, Ital.*
Potassium guaiacolsulfonate (p.1068·3); mepyramine (p.414·1); hedera; cherry-laurel.
Coughs.

Balsamo Analgesic Karmel *Agua del Carmen, Spain.*
Camphor (p.1557·2); beleo; stramonium (p.468·2); amyl salicylate (p.15·3); menthol (p.1600·2).
Formerly known as Karmel Balsamo.
Rheumatic and muscle pain.

Balsamo BOI *BOI, Spain†.*
Benzoic acid; bismuth subnitrate (p.1180·2); calcium hydroxide solution (p.1556·3); kaolin (p.1195·1); chlorophyll (p.1000·1); zinc oxide (p.1096·2); rose essence.
Burns; ulcers; wounds.

Balsamo Germano *Ponto, Spain†.*
Camphor (p.1557·2); styrax tonkinensis; phenol (p.1121·2); glycerol; potassium iodide (p.1493·1); potash soap.
Chilblains.

Balsamo Italstadium *Falqui, Ital.*
Methyl salicylate (p.55·2); menthol (p.1600·2); camphor (p.1557·2).
Musculoskeletal and joint pain.

Balsamo Midalgan *Sanofi Winthrop, Spain.*
Capsicum (p.1559·2); methyl nicotinate (p.55·1); methyl salicylate (p.55·2).
Rheumatic and muscle pain.

Balsamo Sifcamina *Maggioni, Ital.*
Methyl nicotinate (p.55·1); glycol salicylate (p.43·1).
Musculoskeletal disorders.

Balsamorhinol *Etris, Fr.*
Chlorbutol (p.1106·3); menthol (p.1600·2); bergamot oil (p.1553·1); orange oil (p.1610·3); neroli oil (p.1606·3).
Nose and throat infections.

Balsatux *Edmond Pharma, Ital.*
Potassium guaiacolsulfonate (p.1068·3); dextromethorphan hydrobromide (p.1057·3).
Coughs.

Balseptol *Bouteille, Fr.†.*
Thymol (p.1127·1); cajuput oil (p.1556·1); origanum oil; niaouli oil (p.1607·1); cineole (p.1564·1).
Dermatitis.

Balsoclase
Note. This name is used for preparations of different composition.
Bios, Belg.
Oral drops: Pentoxyverine citrate (p.1066·1); guaiphenesin (p.1061·3); cineole (p.1564·1); terpin hydrate (p.1070·2); thymol (p.1127·1).
Oral solution: Pentoxyverine citrate (p.1066·1); terpin hydrate (p.1070·2).
Suppositories: Pentoxyverine (p.1066·1); guaiphenesin (p.1061·3); cineole (p.1564·1); terpineol (p.1635·1); terpin hydrate (p.1070·2).
Syrup: Pentoxyverine citrate (p.1066·1); cineole (p.1564·1); terpin hydrate (p.1070·2); thyme (p.1636·3).
Coughs.

UCB, Neth.
Pentoxyverine citrate (p.1066·1).
Coughs.

Balsoclase Compositum *UCB, Neth.*
Pentoxyverine citrate (p.1066·1); cineole (p.1564·1); sodium citrate (p.1153·2); terpin hydrate (p.1070·2); thyme (p.1636·3).
Coughs.

Balsoclase-E *UCB, Neth.*
Pentoxyverine (p.1066·1); cineole (p.1564·1).
Coughs.

Balsofletol *Pharmascience, Fr.†.*
Retinol (p.1358·1); eucalyptus oil (p.1578·1); pine oil; thyme oil (p.1637·1); rosemary oil (p.1626·2); lemon oil (p.1595·3); lavender oil (p.1594·3); camphor (p.1557·2); resorcinol (p.1090·1).
Nose and throat infections.

Balsofumine *Sanofi Winthrop, Fr.*
Peru balsam (p.1617·2); sumatra benzoin (p.1634·1); eucalyptus (p.1578·1); lavender oil (p.1594·3); thyme oil (p.1637·1).
Respiratory-tract congestion.

Balsofumine Mentholee *Sanofi Winthrop, Fr.*
Peru balsam (p.1617·2); sumatra benzoin (p.1634·1); eucalyptus (p.1578·1); lavender oil (p.1594·3); thyme oil (p.1637·1); menthol (p.1600·2).
Respiratory-tract congestion.

Balsolene *Cooperation Pharmaceutique, Fr.*
Eucalyptus oil (p.1578·1); niaouli oil (p.1607·1); menthol (p.1600·2); siam benzoin (p.1628·3).
Respiratory-tract congestion.

Balsoprim *Juste, Spain.*
Bromhexine hydrochloride (p.1055·3); co-trimoxazole (p.196·3).
Respiratory-tract infections.

Balta Intimo Soluzione *Lutsia, Ital.*
Menthol (p.1600·2); cineole (p.1564·1); Iceland moss; undecenoic acid (p.389·2).
Personal hygiene.

Balta-Crin Tar *Lutsia, Ital.*
Tar (p.1092·3); allantoin (p.1078·2).
Seborrhoeic dermatitis.

Baltar
E. Merck, Irl.; E. Merck, UK†.
Coal tar (p.1092·3).
Scalp disorders.

Balto Foot Balm *Lane, UK.*
Camphor (p.1557·2); menthol (p.1600·2); zinc oxide (p.1096·2); precipitated sulphur (p.1091·2).
Dry skin; excessive perspiration.

Bamalite *Tecnobio, Spain.*
Lansoprazole (p.1196·2).
Gastro-oesophageal reflux; peptic ulcer.

Bambec
Astra, Aust.; Stern, Ger.; Astra, Ger.; Astra, Ital.; Astra, Norw.; Astra, Spain; Draco, Swed.; Astra, Switz.; Astra, UK.
Bambuterol hydrochloride (p.749·1).
Obstructive airways disease.

Bamifix *Chiesi, Ital.*
Bamifylline hydrochloride (p.749·2).
Obstructive airways disease.

Bami-med *Permamed, Switz.†.*
Bamifylline hydrochloride (p.749·2).
Obstructive airways disease.

Bamycor
Astra, Norw.; Hassle, Swed.
Aspirin (p.16·1).
Cardiovascular and cerebrovascular disorders.

Bamyl *Hassle, Swed.*
Aspirin (p.16·1).
Fever; inflammation; pain.

Bamyl koffein *Hassle, Swed.*
Aspirin (p.16·1); caffeine (p.749·3).
Fever; pain.

Ban Pain *Triomed, S.Afr.*
Syrup: Paracetamol (p.72·2); codeine phosphate (p.26·1); promethazine hydrochloride (p.416·2).
Fever; pain.
Tablets: Paracetamol (p.72·2); codeine phosphate (p.26·1); caffeine (p.749·3); meprobamate (p.678·1).
Pain.

Banadyne-3 *Norstar, USA.*
Lignocaine (p.1293·2); menthol (p.1600·2); alcohol (p.1099·1).
Herpes labialis.

Banalg *Forest Pharmaceuticals, USA.*
Methyl salicylate (p.55·2); camphor (p.1557·2); menthol (p.1600·2).
Muscle, joint, and soft-tissue pain; neuralgia.

Banan *Sankyo, Jpn.*
Cefpodoxime proxetil (p.172·1).
Bacterial infections.

Banana Boat Active Kids *Banana Boat, Canad.*
SPF 30: Ethylhexyl *p*-methoxycinnamate (p.1487·1); octyl salicylate (p.1487·3); oxybenzone (p.1487·3); titanium dioxide (p.1093·3).
SPF 50: Octocrylene (p.1487·3); ethylhexyl *p*-methoxycinnamate (p.1487·1); octyl salicylate (p.1487·3); oxybenzone (p.1487·3).
Sunscreen.

Banana Boat Aloe Vera Lip Balm Sunblock
Banana Boat, Canad.
SPF 30: Padimate O (p.1488·1); ethylhexyl *p*-methoxycinnamate (p.1487·1); oxybenzone (p.1487·3).
SPF 30: Padimate O (p.1488·1); ethylhexyl *p*-methoxycinnamate (p.1487·1); oxybenzone (p.1487·3); homosalate (p.1487·2).
Sunscreen.

Banana Boat Baby Sunblock *Banana Boat, Canad.*
SPF 50: Octocrylene (p.1487·3); ethylhexyl *p*-methoxycinnamate (p.1487·1); octyl salicylate (p.1487·3); oxybenzone (p.1487·3).
Sunscreen.

Banana Boat Dark Tanning *Banana Boat, Canad.*
Lotion SPF 4: Padimate O (p.1488·1).
Oil SPF 4: Padimate O (p.1488·1); ethylhexyl *p*-methoxycinnamate (p.1487·1).
Sunscreen.

Banana Boat Faces Plus *Banana Boat, Canad.*
SPF 15; SPF 23: Ethylhexyl *p*-methoxycinnamate (p.1487·1); octyl salicylate (p.1487·3); oxybenzone (p.1487·3).
SPF 31: Ethylhexyl *p*-methoxycinnamate (p.1487·1); octyl salicylate (p.1487·3); oxybenzone (p.1487·3); titanium dioxide (p.1093·3).
Sunscreen.

Banana Boat Funky Fruit Lip Balm *Banana Boat, Canad.*
SPF 15: Padimate O (p.1488·1); homosalate (p.1487·2); ethylhexyl *p*-methoxycinnamate (p.1487·1); oxybenzone (p.1487·3).
Sunscreen.

Banana Boat Oil Free *Banana Boat, Canad.*
SPF 30: Ethylhexyl *p*-methoxycinnamate (p.1487·1); octyl salicylate (p.1487·3); oxybenzone (p.1487·3).
Sunscreen.

Banana Boat Sooth-A-Caine *Banana Boat, Canad.*
Menthol (p.1600·2); lignocaine (p.1293·2).

Banana Boat Sport *Banana Boat, Canad.*
SPF 15: Ethylhexyl *p*-methoxycinnamate (p.1487·1); octyl salicylate (p.1487·3); oxybenzone (p.1487·3).
SPF 30: Ethylhexyl *p*-methoxycinnamate (p.1487·1); octyl salicylate (p.1487·3); oxybenzone (p.1487·3); titanium dioxide (p.1093·3).
SPF 50: Ethylhexyl *p*-methoxycinnamate (p.1487·1); octyl salicylate (p.1487·3); oxybenzone (p.1487·3); octocrylene (p.1487·3).
Sunscreen.

Banana Boat Sunblock *Banana Boat, Canad.*
SPF 15: Ethylhexyl *p*-methoxycinnamate (p.1487·1); octyl salicylate (p.1487·3); oxybenzone (p.1487·3).
Sunscreen.

Banana Boat Sunscreen *Banana Boat, Canad.*
SPF 8: Padimate O (p.1488·1); oxybenzone (p.1487·3).
Sunscreen.

Banana Boat Ultra *Banana Boat, Canad.*
SPF 30: Ethylhexyl *p*-methoxycinnamate (p.1487·1); octyl salicylate (p.1487·3); oxybenzone (p.1487·3); titanium dioxide (p.1093·3).
Sunscreen.

Banana Boat Ultra Plus *Banana Boat, Canad.*
SPF 50: Ethylhexyl *p*-methoxycinnamate (p.1487·1); octyl salicylate (p.1487·3); oxybenzone (p.1487·3); octocrylene (p.1487·3).
Sunscreen.

Banana Boat Vitamin E Lip Balm Sunblock
Banana Boat, Canad.
SPF 30: Ethylhexyl *p*-methoxycinnamate (p.1487·1); octocrylene (p.1487·3); oxybenzone (p.1487·3); padimate O (p.1488·1).
Sunscreen.

Bancap HC *Forest Pharmaceuticals, USA.*
Hydrocodone tartrate (p.43·1); paracetamol (p.72·2).
Pain.

Banedif *Roche Nicholas, Spain.*
Bacitracin (p.157·3); neomycin sulphate (p.229·2); zinc oxide (p.1096·2).
Infected skin disorders.

Baneocin *Biochemie, Aust.*
Bacitracin (p.157·3) or bacitracin zinc (p.157·3); neomycin sulphate (p.229·2).
Bacterial infections.

Baneopol *Streuli, Switz.*
Bacitracin (p.157·3); polymyxin B sulphate (p.239·1); neomycin sulphate (p.229·2).
Infected eye and skin disorders.

Banex *Lu Chem, USA†.*
Phenylpropanolamine hydrochloride (p.1067·2); phenylephrine hydrochloride (p.1066·2); guaiphenesin (p.1061·3).

Banflex *Forest Pharmaceuticals, USA.*
Orphenadrine citrate (p.465·2).
Musculoskeletal pain.

Banikol Vitamine B_1 *Pharmy, Fr.†.*
Tetramethylammonium iodide (p.1635·2); thiamine hydrochloride (p.1361·1).
Neuralgia; neuritis.

Banimax *SmithKline Beecham, UK.*
Aspirin (p.16·1); paracetamol (p.72·2).

Banish II *Smith & Nephew, Austral.*
Zinc ricinoleate; dipropylene glycol.
Colostomy and ileostomy odour.

Banishing Cream *Avon, Canad.*
Hydroquinone (p.1083·1).

Banistyl *May & Baker, S.Afr.†.*
Dimethothiazine mesylate (p.408·3).
Hypersensitivity reactions.

Banlice *Pfizer, Austral.*
Pyrethrins; piperonyl butoxide (p.1409·3).
Pediculosis.

Banoftal *Cusi, Spain.*
Boric acid (p.1554·2); calendula officinalis; hamamelis (p.1587·1); borax (p.1554·2).
Formerly contained boric acid, borax, adrenaline, mercuric cyanide, and trinitrophenol.
Eye disorders.

Banophen *Major, USA.*
Diphenhydramine hydrochloride (p.409·1).
Hypersensitivity reactions; insomnia; motion sickness.

Banophen Decongestant *Major, USA.*
Diphenhydramine hydrochloride (p.409·1); pseudoephedrine hydrochloride (p.1068·3).
Hypersensitivity reactions; insomnia; motion sickness.

BanSmoke *Thompson, USA.*
Benzocaine (p.1286·2).
Aid to smoking withdrawal.

Bansor *Thornton & Ross, UK.*
Cetrimide (p.1105·2).
Sore gums.

Bansuk *Parke, Davis, Austral.†.*
Sucrose octa-acetate (p.1633·2); nonivamide (p.63·2).
Habitual nail biting.

Bantenol *Abello, Spain.*
Mebendazole (p.104·1).
Worm infections.

Banthine *Schiapparelli Searle, USA.*
Methantheline bromide (p.465·1).
Adjunct in peptic ulcer; neurogenic bladder.

Bantron *DEP, USA.*
Lobeline sulphate (p.1481·3).
Aid to smoking withdrawal.

Baokang *Hefa, Ger.†.*
Peppermint oil (p.1208·1); eucalyptus oil (p.1578·1).
Cold symptoms.

Baralgan *Albert, S.Afr.†.*
Dipyrone (p.35·1); pitofenone hydrochloride (p.1619·2); fenpiverinium bromide (p.1579·3).
Colic; genital-tract spasm.

Baralgin
Note. This name is used for preparations of different composition.
Albert-Roussel, Aust.†; Hoechst, Belg.†; Hoechst, Spain†.
Dipyrone (p.35·1); pitofenone hydrochloride (p.1619·2); fenpiverinium bromide (p.1579·3).
Biliary and renal colic; smooth muscle spasm.

Albert-Roussel, Ger.; Hoechst, Ger.
Dipyrone (p.35·1).
Colic; pain.

Baralgina *Hoechst Marion Roussel, Ital.†.*
Dipyrone (p.35·1); pitofenone hydrochloride (p.1619·2); fenpiverinium bromide (p.1579·3).
Painful smooth muscle spasm.

Baralgine
Hoechst, Fr.†; Hoechst Marion Roussel, Switz.†.
Dipyrone (p.35·1); pitofenone hydrochloride (p.1619·2); fenpiverinium bromide (p.1579·3).
Colic; pain.

Baran-mild N *Mickan, Ger.*
Benzocaine (p.1286·2); olive oil (p.1610·1); zinc oil (p.1373·1).
Skin ulcers; wounds.

Baratol
Monmouth, Irl.; Akromed, S.Afr.; Monmouth, UK.
Indoramin hydrochloride (p.891·1).
Hypertension.

Barazan *Dieckmann, Ger.*
Norfloxacin (p.233·1).
Bacterial infections of the urinary tract.

Barbamin *Streuli, Switz.*
Propyphenazone (p.81·3); diphenhydramine hydrochloride (p.409·1).
Fever; pain.

Barbidonna *Wallace, USA.*
Atropine sulphate (p.455·1); hyoscine hydrobromide (p.462·3); hyoscyamine hydrobromide (p.464·2) or hyoscyamine sulphate (p.464·2); phenobarbitone (p.350·2).
Gastro-intestinal disorders.

Barbloc *Alphapharm, Austral.*
Pindolol (p.931·1).
Angina pectoris; arrhythmias; hypertension.

Barc *Del, USA.*
Pyrethrins; piperonyl butoxide (p.1409·3).
Pediculosis.

Barcan *UCB, Swed.*
Aceclofenac (p.12·1).
Musculoskeletal and joint disorders.

Barclyd *Biogalenique, Fr.†.*
Clonidine hydrochloride (p.841·2).
Hypertension.

Bareon *Hokuriku, Jpn.*
Lomefloxacin hydrochloride (p.222·2).
Bacterial infections.

Barexal *Ipsen, Belg.*
Smectite; aluminium hydroxide-magnesium carbonate co-dried gel (p.1178·2).
Diarrhoea.

Baricon *Lafayette, USA.*
Barium sulphate (p.1003·1).
Contrast medium for gastro-intestinal radiography.

Baridium *Pfeiffer, USA.*
Phenazopyridine hydrochloride (p.78·3).
Irritation of the lower urinary tract.

Barigraf *Juste, Spain.*
Barium sulphate (p.1003·1).
Contrast medium for gastro-intestinal radiography.

Barigraf Tac *Juste, Spain.*
Barium sulphate (p.1003·1).
Simethicone (p.1213·1) is included in this preparation to eliminate gas from the gastro-intestinal tract before tomography.
Contrast medium for gastro-intestinal computerised axial tomography.

Bario Cidan *Cidan, Spain†.*
Barium sulphate (p.1003·1).
Contrast medium for gastro-intestinal radiography.

Bario Dif *Rovi, Spain.*
Barium sulphate (p.1003·1).
Dimethicone (p.1213·1) is included in this preparation to eliminate gas from the gastro-intestinal tract before radiography.
Contrast medium for gastro-intestinal radiography.

Bario Faes *Faes, Spain.*
Barium sulphate (p.1003·1).
Dimethicone (p.1213·1) is included in this preparation to eliminate gas from the gastro-intestinal tract before radiography.
Contrast medium for gastro-intestinal radiography.

Bario Faes Ultra *Faes, Spain.*
Barium sulphate (p.1003·1).
Contrast medium for gastro-intestinal radiography.

Bario Llorente *Llorente, Spain.*
Barium sulphate (p.1003·1).
Contrast medium for gastro-intestinal radiography.

Bariopacin *Serra Pamies, Spain.*
Barium sulphate (p.1003·1).
Contrast medium for gastro-intestinal radiography.

Baripril *Lesvi, Spain.*
Enalapril maleate (p.863·2).
Heart failure; hypertension.

Baripril Diu *Lesvi, Spain.*
Enalapril maleate (p.863·2); hydrochlorothiazide (p.885·2).
Hypertension.

Baritop *Bioglan, UK.*
Barium sulphate (p.1003·1).
Contrast medium for gastro-intestinal tract radiography.

Barium Med Complex *Dynamit, Aust.*
Homoeopathic preparation.

Barnes-Hind Cleaning and Soaking Solution *Allergan, Austral.*
Cleansing and storage solution for hard contact lenses .

Barnes-Hind Wetting and Soaking Solution *Barnes-Hind, Austral.†.*
Polyvinyl alcohol (p.1474·2); povidone (p.1474·2); hydroxyethylcellulose (p.1472·3).
Soaking solution for hard contact lenses.

Barnes-Hind Wetting Solution *Allergan, Austral.*
Polyvinyl alcohol (p.1474·2).
Wetting solution for hard contact lenses.

Barnetil
Synthelabo, Belg.; Synthelabo, Fr.
Sultopride hydrochloride (p.693·2).
Aggression; delirium; mania; schizophrenia.

Barnotil *Synthelabo, Ital.*
Sultopride hydrochloride (p.693·2).
Psychoses.

Barobag *Lafayette, USA†.*
Barium sulphate (p.1003·1).
Contrast medium for gastro-intestinal radiography.

Baro-cat *Lafayette, USA.*
Barium sulphate (p.1003·1).
Contrast medium for gastro-intestinal radiography.

Baroflave *Lannett, USA.*
Barium sulphate (p.1003·1).
Contrast medium for gastro-intestinal radiography.

Barokaton *Donau, Aust.†.*
Injection: 1-(β-Diethylaminoethyl)-theobromin-ethylbromide; 2-diethylaminoethanol hydrochloride (p.1479·3).
Tablets: 1-(β-Diethylaminoethyl)-theobromin-ethylbromide.
Asthma; cardiovascular disorders.

Baros *Lafayette, USA.*
Sodium bicarbonate (p.1153·2); tartaric acid (p.1634·3); simethicone (p.1213·1).
Adjunct in gastro-intestinal radiography.

Barosperse *Lafayette, USA.*
Barium sulphate (p.1003·1).
Contrast medium for gastro-intestinal radiography.

Barotonal *Brenner-Efeka, Ger.*
Hydrochlorothiazide (p.885·2); reserpine (p.942·1).
Hypertension.

Barrier Cream *National Care, Canad.*
Dimethicone (p.1384·2).
Skin disorders.

Barriere *Roberts, Canad.*
Dimethicone (p.1384·2).
Skin disorders.

Barriere-HC *Roberts, Canad.*
Hydrocortisone (p.1043·3).
Skin disorders.

Barrycidal *Barry, Ital.*
Alkylbenzyldimethylammonium chloride (p.1101·3); benzethonium chloride (p.1102·3); diisobutylcresoxyethoxyethylbenzyldimethylammonium chloride.
Instrument disinfection.

Bartal *Andreu, Spain†.*
Camphor (p.1557·2); methyl salicylate (p.55·2); turpentine oil (p.1641·1); menthol (p.1600·2).
Muscular and joint pain.

Bartelin N *OTW, Ger.*
Diethylamine salicylate (p.33·1); camphor (p.1557·2); turpentine oil (p.1641·1).
Musculoskeletal and joint disorders; neuralgia; neuritis.

Bartelin nico *OTW, Ger.*
Diethylamine salicylate (p.33·1); benzyl nicotinate (p.22·1); oleum pini sylvestris.
Musculoskeletal and joint disorders; neuralgia; neuritis.

Barytgen
Byk Gulden, Ital.†; Fuji, Swed.
Barium sulphate (p.1003·1).
Contrast medium for gastro-intestinal radiography.

B_{12}-AS *A.S., Ger.*
Cyanocobalamin (p.1363·3).
Vitamin B_{12} deficiency.

Basal-H-Insulin *Hoechst, Ger.*
Isophane insulin (human) (p.322·1).
Diabetes mellitus.

Basaljel
Note. This name is used for preparations of different composition.
Axcan, Canad.
Aluminium hydroxide (p.1177·3).
Phosphate binding in renal failure.
Wyeth-Ayerst, USA.
Dried basic aluminium carbonate gel (p.1177·2).
Hyperacidity; hyperphosphataemia.

Bascardial *Bastian, Ger.*
Potassium aspartate (p.1161·3); magnesium aspartate (p.1157·2).
Coronary circulation disorders with magnesium and potassium deficiency.

Basdene *Doms-Adrian, Fr.*
Benzylthiouracil (p.1491·2).
Hyperthyroidism.

Baseler Haussalbe *Sanico, Belg.*
Zinc oxide (p.1096·2); zinc stearate (p.1469·3); bismuth subnitrate (p.1180·2); titanium dioxide (p.1093·3); borax (p.1554·2); sodium salicylate (p.85·1); purified talc (p.1092·1).
Barrier cream; skin disorders.

Basen *Takeda, Jpn.*
Voglibose (p.334·3).
Diabetes mellitus.

Basic *Corvi, Ital.†.*
Colloidal aluminium hydroxide (p.1177·3); magnesium trisilicate (p.1199·1).
Dyspepsia.

Basiron
Nycomed, Norw.; Nycomed, Swed.; Basotherm, Switz.
Benzoyl peroxide (p.1079·2).
Acne.

Basis-Infusionslosung N *Stroschein, Ger.†.*
Electrolyte infusion (p.1147·1).
Fluid and electrolyte disorders.

Basiter *Basotherm, Ger.*
Coal tar (p.1092·3).
Eczema; psoriasis.

Basocef *Curasan, Ger.*
Cephazolin sodium (p.181·1).
Bacterial infections.

Basocin *Basotherm, Ger.*
Clindamycin phosphate (p.191·1).
Acne.

Basodexan
Procter & Gamble, Aust.; Hermal, Ger.; Max Ritter, Switz.†.
Urea (p.1095·2).
Skin disorders.

Basofer *Zwintscher, Ger.†.*
Oral granules: Caraway (p.1559·3); turmeric (p.1001·3); sodium potassium tartrate (p.1213·3); sodium citrate (p.1153·2); sodium bicarbonate (p.1153·2).
Tablets: Papain (p.1614·1); caraway (p.1559·3); sodium potassium tartrate (p.1213·3); sodium citrate (p.1153·2); sodium bicarbonate (p.1153·2).
Gastro-intestinal disorders.

Basofer forte *Zwintscher, Ger.†.*
Curcuma zanthorrhiza; caraway (p.1559·3); potassium citrate (p.1153·1); sodium potassium tartrate (p.1213·3); sodium bicarbonate (p.1153·2).
Gastro-intestinal disorders.

Basoplex *Palmicol, Ger.*
Paracetamol (p.72·2); phenylpropanolamine hydrochloride (p.1067·2); dextromethorphan hydrobromide (p.1057·3).
Coughs and cold symptoms.

Basotar *Nycomed, Swed.†.*
Coal tar (p.1092·3).
Psoriasis.

Bassado *Poli, Ital.*
Doxycycline hydrochloride (p.202·3).
Infections.

Basticrat *Bastian, Ger.*
Crataegus (p.1568·2).
Cardiac disorders.

Basti-Mag *Bastian, Ger.*
Magnesium aspartate (p.1157·2).
Magnesium deficiency.

Bastiverit *Bastian, Ger.*
Glibenclamide (p.319·3).
Diabetes mellitus.

Bastoncino *Whitehall, Ital.*
Eugenol (p.1578·2).
Oral hygiene; temporary dental filling.

Bat *Zeta, Ital.*
Cetylpyridinium chloride (p.1106·2).
Disinfection of wounds and burns.

Bath E45 *Crookes Healthcare, UK.*
Bath additive.
Dry skin.

Batkaletta *Reinecke, Ger.†.*
Senna (p.1212·2); chamomile (p.1561·2); frangula bark (p.1193·2).
Constipation.

Batmen *Menarini, Spain.*
Prednicarbate (p.1047·3).
Skin disorders.

Batrafen
Albert-Roussel, Aust.; Hoechst, Ger.; Hoechst Marion Roussel, Irl.; Hoechst Marion Roussel, Ital.; Hoechst, Spain; Knoll, Switz.
Ciclopirox (p.376·2) or ciclopirox olamine (p.376·2).
Fungal infections.

Batramycine *Geistlich, Switz.*
Nasal ointment: Bacitracin (p.157·3); neomycin sulphate (p.229·2); octacaine hydrochloride (p.1298·1).
Bacterial nasal infections.
Ointment; topical powder: Bacitracin (p.157·3); neomycin sulphate (p.229·2).
Infected wounds or burns.
Paste†: Bacitracin (p.157·3); neomycin sulphate (p.229·2).
Bacterial infections.
Pastilles†: Bacitracin (p.157·3); neomycin sulphate (p.229·2); clibucaine hydrochloride (p.1289·3).
Mouth and throat disorders.

Batrax *Gewo, Ger.*
Nasal ointment: Bacitracin (p.157·3); neomycin sulphate (p.229·2); octacaine hydrochloride (p.1298·1).
Nasal infections.
Ointment; topical powder: Bacitracin (p.157·3); neomycin sulphate (p.229·2).
Bacterial skin infections.

Batticon S *Trommsdorff, Ger.†.*
Povidone-iodine (p.1123·3).
Antiseptic; skin disinfection.

Baudry *Boiron, Canad.*
Homoeopathic preparation.

Baume
Note. This name is used for preparations of different composition.
Wild, Switz.†.
Ointment: Zinc oxide (p.1096·2); zinc peroxide (p.1127·3); laureth 9 (p.1325·2).
Skin disorders.
Zeller, Switz.†.
Oral drops: Achillea (p.1542·2); absinthium (p.1541·1); poppy flowers (p.1001·1); guaiacum wood; tormentil root (p.1638·3); cinnamon bark (p.1564·2); benzoin (p.1634·1); myrrh (p.1606·1); tolu balsam (p.1071·1).
Gastro-intestinal disorders.

Baume Analgesique *Multi-Pro, Canad.*
Methyl salicylate (p.55·2); camphor (p.1557·2).

Baume Analgesique Medicamente *Prodemdis, Canad.*
Methyl salicylate (p.55·2); camphor (p.1557·2); menthol (p.1600·2); eucalyptus oil (p.1578·1).

Baume Aroma *Mayoly-Spindler, Fr.*
Juniper oil (p.1592·3); clove oil (p.1565·2); capsicum oil; amyl salicylate (p.15·3); salicylic acid (p.1090·2).
Muscle and joint pain.

Baume Bengue *URPAC, Fr.*
Methyl salicylate (p.55·2); menthol (p.1600·2).
Muscle and joint pain.

Baume Dalet
Note. This name is used for preparations of different composition.
COB, Belg.
Menthol (p.1600·2); guaiacol (p.1061·2); chloroform (p.1220·3); methyl salicylate (p.55·2); belladonna (p.457·1).
Bunions.
Phygiene, Fr.
Hyoscyamus oil (p.464·3); amyl salicylate (p.15·3); guaiacol (p.1061·2); menthol (p.1600·2); chloroform (p.1220·3).
Calluses; corns.

Baume de Chine Temple of Heaven blanc *Panax, Switz.*
Menthol (p.1600·2); camphor (p.1557·2); peppermint oil (p.1208·1); eucalyptus oil (p.1578·1); clove oil (p.1565·2); cinnamon oil (p.1564·2).
Musculoskeletal and joint disorders; soft-tissue injury.

Baume Disalgyl *Monin, Fr.†.*
Methyl salicylate (p.55·2); borax (p.1554·2); capsicum oleoresin; camphor (p.1557·2).
Muscle and joint pain.

Baume du Chalet *Plan, Switz.*
Lavender oil (p.1594·3); melissa oil; spike lavender oil (p.1632·2); terebinthin (p.1641·1).
Skin disorders; wounds.

Baume du Tigre *Phytomedica, Fr.†.*
Camphor (p.1557·2); menthol (p.1600·2); clove oil (p.1565·2); eucalyptus oil (p.1578·1); peppermint oil (p.1208·1); cinnamon oil (p.1564·2).

Baume Esco *Streuli, Switz.*
Salicylic acid (p.1090·2); menthol (p.1600·2); methyl salicylate (p.55·2).
Musculoskeletal and joint pain.

Baume Esco Forte *Streuli, Switz.*
Salicylic acid (p.1090·2); menthol (p.1600·2); methyl salicylate (p.55·2); ethyl nicotinate (p.36·1).
Musculoskeletal and joint pain.

Baume Kytta *Whitehall-Robins, Switz.†.*
Comfrey (p.1567·1); methyl nicotinate (p.55·1); eucalyptus essence (p.1578·1); pine needle essence (p.1623·3); lavender essence (p.1594·3).
Musculoskeletal and joint disorders.

Baume Saint-Bernard *Monot, Fr.*
Salicylic acid (p.1090·2); menthol (p.1600·2); camphor (p.1557·2); amyl salicylate (p.15·3); capsicum (p.1559·2); benzylidene acetone.
Muscle and joint pain.

Bausch & Lomb Concentrated Cleaner *Bausch & Lomb, Austral.*
Cleansing solution for gas permeable and hard contact lenses.

Bausch & Lomb Conditioning Solution *Bausch & Lomb, Austral.*
Disinfecting and storage solution for gas permeable and hard contact lenses.

Bausch & Lomb ReNu Multipurpose *Bausch & Lomb, Austral.*
Cleansing and disinfecting solution for soft contact lenses.

Bausch & Lomb Saline Plus *Bausch & Lomb, Austral.*
Sodium chloride (p.1162·2).
Solution for soft contact lenses.

Bausch & Lomb Sensitive Eyes Daily Cleaner *Bausch & Lomb, Austral.*
Cleansing solution for soft contact lenses.

Bausch & Lomb Sensitive Eyes Lens Lubricant *Bausch & Lomb, Austral.*
Povidone (p.1474·2); hypromellose (p.1473·1).
Wetting solution for contact lenses.

Bausch & Lomb Sensitive Eyes Protein Removal *Bausch & Lomb, Austral.*
Proteolytic enzyme.
Cleanser for contact lenses.

Bausch & Lomb Sensitive Eyes Saline *Bausch & Lomb, Austral.*
Sodium chloride (p.1162·2).
Saline solution for soft contact lenses.

Bausch & Lomb Sensitive Eyes Thermal Protein Removal *Bausch & Lomb, Austral.†.*
Proteolytic enzyme.
Cleanser for soft contact lenses.

Baxacor
Sanus, Aust.†; Helopharm, Ger.†; Schering, Ital.†.
Etafenone hydrochloride (p.866·3).
Cardiac disorders.

Baxal *Ital Suisse, Ital.†.*
Latamoxef disodium (p.221·2).
Bacterial infections.

Baxan *Bristol-Myers Squibb, UK.*
Cefadroxil (p.163·3).
Bacterial infections.

Baxanitrat *Sanus, Aust.†.*
Isosorbide dinitrate (p.893·1); etafenone hydrochloride (p.866·3).
Angina pectoris.

Baxedin *Luvabec, Canad.*
Chlorhexidine gluconate (p.1107·2).
Disinfection and antisepsis.

Baxidin *Bergamon, Ital.*
Cetrimide (p.1105·2); chlorhexidine gluconate (p.1107·2).
Disinfection of wounds and burns.

Baycaron
Bayer, Ger.; Bayer, Irl.; Bayer, Neth.; Bayer, Norw.; Bayer, Swed.†; Bayer, UK.
Mefruside (p.902·2).
Hypertension; oedema.

Baycillin Bayer, Ger.
Propicillin potassium (p.240·3).
Bacterial infections.

Baycip Bayer, Spain.
Ciprofloxacin hydrochloride (p.185·3) or ciprofloxacin lactate (p.185·3).
Bacterial infections.

Baycol Bayer, USA.
Cerivastatin sodium (p.1269·3).
Hyperlipidaemia.

Baycuten Bayer, Ger.
Clotrimazole (p.376·3); dexamethasone acetate (p.1037·1).
Infected skin disorders.

Bayer Children's Cold Tablets Glenbrook, USA†.
Phenylpropanolamine hydrochloride (p.1067·2); aspirin (p.16·1).
Cold symptoms.

Bayer Children's Cough Syrup Glenbrook, USA†.
Phenylpropanolamine hydrochloride (p.1067·2); dextromethorphan hydrobromide (p.1057·3).
Coughs.

Bayer Low Adult Strength Sterling Health, USA.
Aspirin (p.16·1).

Bayer Select Chest Cold Sterling, USA.
Dextromethorphan hydrobromide (p.1057·3); paracetamol (p.72·2).

Bayer Select Flu Relief Sterling, USA.
Paracetamol (p.72·2); pseudoephedrine hydrochloride (p.1068·3); dextromethorphan hydrobromide (p.1057·3); chlorpheniramine maleate (p.405·1).

Bayer Select Head Cold Sterling, USA.
Pseudoephedrine hydrochloride (p.1068·3); paracetamol (p.72·2).

Bayer Select Maximum Strength Backache Sterling, USA.
Magnesium salicylate (p.51·1).

Bayer Select Maximum Strength Headache Sterling, USA.
Paracetamol (p.72·2); caffeine (p.749·3).

Bayer Select Maximum Strength Menstrual Sterling, USA.
Paracetamol (p.72·2); pamabrom (p.927·1).

Bayer Select Maximum Strength Night Time Pain Relief Sterling, USA.
Paracetamol (p.72·2); diphenhydramine hydrochloride (p.409·1).
Insomnia; pain.

Bayer Select Maximum Strength Sinus Pain Relief Sterling, USA.
Paracetamol (p.72·2); pseudoephedrine hydrochloride (p.1068·3).
Nasal congestion; pain.

Bayer Select Night Time Cold Sterling, USA.
Paracetamol (p.72·2); pseudoephedrine hydrochloride (p.1068·3); dextromethorphan hydrobromide (p.1057·3); triprolidine hydrochloride (p.420·3).

Bayer Select Pain Relief Formula Sterling, USA.
Ibuprofen (p.44·1).

Baygon N Bayer, Ital.
Propoxur (p.1410·1); tetramethrin (p.1410·3); piperonyl butoxide (p.1409·3).
Insecticide.

Baymycard Bayer, Ger.; Zeneca, Ger.
Nisoldipine (p.922·3).
Angina pectoris; hypertension.

Bayolin
Bayer, Aust.; Bayropharm, Ger.†; Bayer, Irl.†; Bayer, UK†.
A heparinoid (p.882·3); glycol salicylate (p.43·1); benzyl nicotinate (p.22·1).
Bruising; haematoma; muscle, joint, and nerve pain.

Bayoline
Bayer, Belg.†; Bayer, Fr.†.
A heparinoid (p.882·3); glycol salicylate (p.43·1); benzyl nicotinate (p.22·1).
Muscle and joint pain; neuralgia; neuritis.

Bayotensin Bayer, Ger.
Nitrendipine (p.923·1).
Angina pectoris; hypertension.

Baypen
Bayer, Aust.; Bayer, Fr.; Bayer, Ger.; Bayer, Ital.; Bayer, Spain.
Mezlocillin sodium (p.225·3).
Bacterial infections.

Baypresol Bayer, Spain.
Nitrendipine (p.923·1).
Angina pectoris; hypertension; Raynaud's syndrome.

Baypress
Bayer, Aust.; Bayer, Belg.; Bayer, Fr.; Bayer, Ital.; Bayer, Neth.; Bayer, Switz.
Nitrendipine (p.923·1).
Hypertension.

Bayro Bayer, Ital.
Etofenamate (p.36·3).
Musculoskeletal, joint, peri-articular, and soft-tissue disorders.

Baythion EC Bayer, Ital.
Phoxim (p.1409·3).
Insecticide.

Bazalin Yamanouchi, Spain.
Coal tar (p.1092·3); fluocinolone acetonide (p.1041·1); salicylic acid (p.1090·2).
Hyperkeratotic skin disorders; psoriasis.

Bazoton Kanoldt, Ger.
Urtica root (p.1642·3).
Prostatic disorders.

Bazuka Dendron, UK.
Salicylic acid (p.1090·2); lactic acid (p.1593·3).
Calluses; corns; verrucas; warts.

BB-K8 Bristol-Myers Squibb, Ital.
Amikacin sulphate (p.150·2).
Bacterial infections.

BC Block, USA.
Aspirin (p.16·1); salicylamide (p.82·3); caffeine (p.749·3).
Pain.

BC 500
Whitehall, Irl.; Whitehall, UK.
Vitamin B substances and vitamin C.
Vitamin supplement.

BC Cold-Sinus Block, USA.
Phenylpropanolamine hydrochloride (p.1067·2); aspirin (p.16·1).
Upper respiratory-tract symptoms.

BC 500 with Iron Whitehall, Irl.
Ferrous fumarate (p.1339·3); vitamin B and C substances.
Dietary supplement; vitamin B and C and iron deficiencies.

BC Multi Symptom Cold Powder Block, USA.
Phenylpropanolamine hydrochloride (p.1067·2); chlorpheniramine maleate (p.405·1); aspirin (p.16·1).
Upper respiratory-tract symptoms.

B-C-Bid Roberts, USA.
Vitamin B complex with vitamin C.

BCM G.P. Laboratories, Austral.
Vitamin and mineral preparation.

B-Complex Plus Vita Glow, Austral.†.
Vitamin B substances and vitamin C.

B-Complex Threshold Neo-Life, Austral.
Vitamin B substances; rutin (p.1580·2).

B_{12}N-Compositum Stada, Switz.
Cyanocobalamin (p.1363·3); saccharated iron oxide (p.1353·2); calcium glycerophosphate (p.1155·2).
Tonic.

B12-Depot-Hevert Hevert, Ger.
Hydroxocobalamin acetate (p.1364·2).
Vitamin B_{12} deficiency.

B_{12}-Depot-Vicotrat Heyl, Ger.
Hydroxocobalamin (p.1363·3).
Vitamin B_{12} deficiency.

Be-Ampicil Be-Tabs, S.Afr.
Ampicillin trihydrate (p.153·2).
Bacterial infections.

Beano
Jan, Canad.; AkPharma, USA.
α-D-Galactosidase.
Gas/bloating from ingestion of raffinose, stachyose, or verbascose.

Bear Essentials Hall, Canad.
Multivitamin preparation with glucose.

Bebedermis Abbott, Ital.
Glycerol; wool fat; vegetable oil; zinc oxide (p.1096·2).
Barrier cream.

Bebegel Sarget, Fr.
Glycerol (p.1585·2).
Bowel evacuation; constipation.

Beben
Parke, Davis, Canad.; Parke, Davis, Ital.
Betamethasone benzoate (p.1033·3).
Skin disorders.

Beben Clorossina Parke, Davis, Ital.
Betamethasone benzoate (p.1033·3); chloroxine (p.215·3).
Infected skin disorders.

Bebesales Pharmacia Upjohn, Spain.
Calcium lactate pentahydrate; citric acid monohydrate; magnesium sulphate; potassium chloride; sodium bicarbonate; sodium chloride; glucose (p.1152·3).
Oral rehydration therapy.

Bebesan N Sanopharm, Switz.†.
Paracetamol (p.72·2).
Fever; pain.

Bebia
Note. This name is used for preparations of different composition.
Stiefel, Canad.
Bath Oil†: Light liquid paraffin (p.1382·1).
Moisturiser; pruritus.
Cream: Zinc oxide (p.1096·2); kaolin (p.1195·1); talc (p.1092·1).
Skin disorders.
Stiefel, Fr.
Zinc oxide (p.1096·2); talc (p.1092·1); heavy kaolin (p.1195·1).
Skin disorders.

Bebia Antiseptic Soap Stiefel, Canad.†.
Trichlorban (p.1127·2); triclosan (p.1127·2).
Bacterial skin infections.

Bebiclean Stiefel, Canad.†.
Soap substitute.

Bebimix Sella, Ital.
Honey (p.1345·3); royal jelly (p.1626·3); myrtillus (p.1606·1).
Nutritional supplement.

Bebitar Stiefel, Canad.†.
Tars (p.1092·2).
Seborrhoea.

Bebulin Immuno, Canad.†.
Factor IX (p.721·3).
Factor IX deficiency.

Bebulin S-TIM 4 Immuno, Aust.
A factor IX preparation (p.721·3).
Factor IX deficiency.

Bebulin TIM 3 Immuno, Ital.
Factor IX (p.721·3).
Factor IX deficiency; haemophilia B.

Bebulin TIM 4
Omnimed, S.Afr.†; Immuno, Spain.
Factor IX (p.721·3).
Factor IX deficiency.

Bebuline S-TIM 4 Immuno, Switz.†.
Factor IX (p.721·3).
Factor IX deficiency.

Becalm Healthcrafts, UK.
Valerian (p.1643·1); lupulus (p.1597·2); passion flower (p.1615·3).
Stress.

Becantex
SmithKline Beecham Consumer, Belg.
Syrup: Sodium dibunate (p.1070·1); guaiphenesin (p.1061·3).
Coughs.
Sterling Health, Belg.†.
Tablets: Sodium dibunate (p.1070·1).
Coughs.

Because Schering, USA.
Nonoxinol 9 (p.1326·1).
Contraceptive.

Becenun
Bristol-Myers Squibb, Norw.; Bristol-Myers Squibb, Swed.
Carmustine (p.511·3).
Malignant neoplasms.

Beceze
Norton, S.Afr.; Norton, UK.
Beclomethasone dipropionate (p.1032·1).
Allergic rhinitis; asthma.

Bechicon Tosi, Ital.†.
Piperidione (p.1068·2); hedera helix.
Coughs.

Bechilar Montefarmaco, Ital.
Dextromethorphan hydrobromide (p.1057·3).
Coughs.

Bechisan Salus, Ital.†.
Sodium dibunate (p.1070·1).
Coughs.

Bechitus Recofarma, Ital.†.
Chlorcyclizine dibunate (p.404·3).
Coughs.

Bechizolo Tosi, Ital.†.
Zipeprol hydrochloride (p.1071·3).
Coughs.

Becholine D Medical Research, Austral.†.
Choline chloride (p.1337·1).
Liver cirrhosis.

Becilan Specia, Fr.
Pyridoxine hydrochloride (p.1362·3).
Drug-induced neuropathies; vitamin deficiency.

Beclate Cipla-Medpro, S.Afr.
Beclomethasone dipropionate (p.1032·1).
Allergic rhinitis; asthma.

Beclazone Norton, UK.
Beclomethasone dipropionate (p.1032·1).
Asthma.

Beclo Aqua Bartholomew Rhodes, UK.
Beclomethasone dipropionate (p.1032·1).

Beclo Asma Aldo, Spain.
Beclomethasone dipropionate (p.1032·1).
Asthma.

Beclo Rino Aldo, Spain.
Beclomethasone dipropionate (p.1032·1).
Nasal polyps; rhinitis.

Beclodisk Glaxo Wellcome, Canad.
Beclomethasone dipropionate (p.1032·1).
Asthma.

Becloforte
Allen & Hanburys, Austral.; Glaxo Wellcome, Canad.; Glaxo Wellcome, Neth.; Allen & Hanburys, S.Afr.; Allen, Spain; Glaxo Wellcome, Switz.; Allen & Hanburys, UK.
Beclomethasone dipropionate (p.1032·1).
Asthma.

Beclojet Promedica, Fr.
Beclomethasone dipropionate (p.1032·1).
Asthma.

Beclomet Orion, Ger.
Beclomethasone dipropionate (p.1032·1).
Obstructive airways disease; rhinitis.

Beclonarin Rappai, Switz.
Beclomethasone dipropionate (p.1032·1); chamomile (p.1561·2).
Allergic rhinitis; polyps.

Beclorhinol Fisons, Ger.
Beclomethasone dipropionate (p.1032·1).
Allergic rhinitis; nasal polyps.

Beclosona Spyfarma, Spain.
Beclomethasone dipropionate (p.1032·1).
Skin disorders.

Becloturmant Fisons, Ger.
Beclomethasone dipropionate (p.1032·1).
Obstructive airways disease.

Beclovent
Glaxo Wellcome, Canad.; Glaxo Wellcome, USA.
Beclomethasone dipropionate (p.1032·1).
Asthma.

Beco Mepha, Switz.
Vitamin B substances.
Alcoholism; liver disorders; neuropathies; vitamin B deficiency.

Becodisk Glaxo Wellcome, Switz.
Beclomethasone dipropionate (p.1032·1).
Asthma.

Becodisks
Allen & Hanburys, Irl.; Allen & Hanburys, S.Afr.; Allen & Hanburys, UK.
Beclomethasone dipropionate (p.1032·1).
Asthma.

Becof Compu, S.Afr.
Diphenhydramine hydrochloride (p.409·1); ammonium chloride (p.1055·2); sodium citrate (p.1153·2).
Coughs.

Becomject Mayrand, USA†.
Vitamin B substances.
Parenteral nutrition.

Beconase
Glaxo Wellcome, Aust.; Allen & Hanburys, Austral.†; Glaxo Wellcome, Belg.; Glaxo Wellcome, Canad.; Glaxo Wellcome, Fr.; Glaxo Wellcome, Ger.†; Allen & Hanburys, Irl.; Glaxo Wellcome, Neth.; Allen & Hanburys, S.Afr.; Allen, Spain; Glaxo Wellcome, Switz.†; Allen & Hanburys, UK; Glaxo Wellcome, USA.
Beclomethasone dipropionate (p.1032·1).
Nasal polyps; rhinitis.

Beconase AQ
Allen & Hanburys, Austral.; Glaxo Wellcome, USA.
Beclomethasone dipropionate (p.1032·1).
Nasal polyps; rhinitis.

Beconase Aquosum Glaxo Wellcome, Ger.
Beclomethasone dipropionate (p.1032·1).
Allergic rhinitis; nasal polyps.

Beconasol Glaxo Wellcome, Switz.
Beclomethasone dipropionate (p.1032·1).
Nasal polyps; rhinitis.

Becoplex Ido Novo Nordisk, S.Afr.
Vitamin B substances.

Becosym
Roche Consumer, Irl.; Roche, UK†.
Vitamin B substances.
Vitamin B deficiency.

Becotal Streuli, Switz.
Vitamin B substances.
Neuropathies; vitamin B deficiency.

Becotide
Glaxo Wellcome, Aust.; Glaxo Wellcome, Austral.; Glaxo Wellcome, Belg.; Glaxo Wellcome, Fr.; Allen & Hanburys, Irl.; Glaxo Wellcome, Ital.; Glaxo Wellcome, Neth.; Glaxo Wellcome, Norw.; Allen & Hanburys, S.Afr.; Glaxo Wellcome, Spain; Glaxo Wellcome, Swed.; Glaxo Wellcome, Switz.; Allen & Hanburys, UK.
Beclomethasone dipropionate (p.1032·1).
Asthma; nasal polyps; rhinitis.

Becotide A Glaxo Wellcome, Ital.
Beclomethasone dipropionate (p.1032·1).
Formerly known as Inalone A.
Nasal disorders; obstructive airways disease.

Becovitan Janssen-Cilag, Belg.
Vitamin B substances.
Dietary supplementation; digestive disorders; nervous disorders; skin disorders; vitamin B deficiency.

Becozym
Roche, Aust.; Roche, Ital.; Roche, Swed.
Vitamin B substances.
Alcoholism; neuropathies; vitamin B deficiency.

Becozyme
Roche, Belg.; Roche, Fr.; Roche Nicholas, Spain; Roche, Switz.
Vitamin B substances.
Alcoholism; liver disorders; neuralgia; neuropathies; vitamin B deficiency.

Becozyme C Forte Roche Nicholas, Spain.
Vitamin B substances and vitamin C.

Bed Wetting Brauer, Austral.
Homoeopathic preparation.

Bedelix Beaufour, Fr.
Montmorillonite beidellitique.
Gastro-intestinal disorders.

Bedermin Damor, Ital.†.
Betamethasone valerate (p.1033·3).
Skin disorders.

Bedorma Nouvelle formulation Singer, Switz.
Diphenhydramine hydrochloride (p.409·1).
Sleep disorders.

Bedoxine Meuse, Belg.
Pyridoxine hydrochloride (p.1362·3).
Vitamin B_6 deficiency.

Bedranol Lagap, Switz.†.
Propranolol hydrochloride (p.937·1).
Angina pectoris; arrhythmias; hypertension; migraine.

Bedranol SR Lagap, UK.
Propranolol hydrochloride (p.937·1).
Anxiety; cardiac disorders; essential tremor; hypertension; migraine.

Bedrenal *Lagap, Switz.*†.
Pindolol (p.931·1).
Angina pectoris; arrhythmias; hypertension.

Beech Nut Cough Drops *Lifesavers, Canad.*
Black: Menthol (p.1600·2); anise oil (p.1550·1).
Honey-Lemon; wild cherry: Menthol (p.1600·2); eucalyptus (p.1578·1).
Menthol: Menthol (p.1600·2); anethole (p.1549·3); eucalyptus oil (p.1578·1).

Beecham Lemon *SmithKline Beecham, Spain.*
Ascorbic acid (p.1365·2); phenylephrine hydrochloride (p.1066·2); paracetamol (p.72·2).
Cold symptoms.

Beecham Lemon Miel *SmithKline Beecham, Spain.*
Paracetamol (p.72·2); caffeine (p.749·3); ascorbic acid (p.1365·2).
Cold symptoms; fever; pain.

Beechams All-In-One *SmithKline Beecham Consumer, UK.*
Paracetamol (p.72·2); guaiphenesin (p.1061·3); phenylephrine (p.1066·2).
Cold symptoms.

Beechams Flu-Plus *SmithKline Beecham Consumer, UK.*
Paracetamol (p.72·2); phenylephrine (p.1066·2); caffeine (p.749·3); vitamin C (p.1365·2).
Influenza symptoms.

Beechams Hot Blackcurrant *SmithKline Beecham Consumer, UK.*
Paracetamol (p.72·2); phenylephrine hydrochloride (p.1066·2); ascorbic acid (p.1365·2).
Cold symptoms.

Beechams Hot Honey and Lemon *SmithKline Beecham Consumer, UK.*
Paracetamol (p.72·2); phenylephrine hydrochloride (p.1066·2); ascorbic acid (p.1365·2).
Cold symptoms.

Beechams Hot Lemon *SmithKline Beecham Consumer, UK.*
Paracetamol (p.72·2); phenylephrine hydrochloride (p.1066·2); ascorbic acid (p.1365·2).
Cold symptoms.

Beechams Lemon Tablets *SmithKline Beecham Consumer, UK.*
Aspirin (p.16·1).
Cold symptoms; pain.

Beechams Pills *SmithKline Beecham Consumer, UK*†.
Aloin (p.1177·2).
Constipation.

Beechams Powders *SmithKline Beecham Consumer, UK.*
Aspirin (p.16·1); caffeine (p.749·3).
Cold symptoms; fever; pain.

Beechams Powders Capsules *SmithKline Beecham Consumer, UK.*
Paracetamol (p.72·2); caffeine (p.749·3); phenylephrine hydrochloride (p.1066·2).
Cold symptoms; fever; pain.

Beechams Powders Tablets *SmithKline Beecham Consumer, UK*†.
Aspirin (p.16·1); caffeine (p.749·3).
Cold symptoms; fever; pain.

Beechams Throat-Plus *SmithKline Beecham Consumer, UK.*
Benzalkonium chloride (p.1101·3); hexylresorcinol (p.1116·1).

Beeline *Lifeplan, UK.*
Propolis (p.1621·3); pollen; royal jelly (p.1626·3).
Nutritional supplement.

Beelith *Beach, USA.*
Pyridoxine hydrochloride (p.1362·3); magnesium salts (p.1157·2).
Dietary supplement.

Beepen-VK *SmithKline Beecham, USA.*
Phenoxymethylpenicillin potassium (p.236·2).
Bacterial infections.

Beesix *SA Druggists, S.Afr.*†.
Pyridoxine hydrochloride (p.1362·3).
Vitamin B_6 deficiencies.

Beespan *Garec, S.Afr.*
Vitamin B substances.
Vitamin B deficiencies.

Bee-T-Vites *Rugby, USA*†.
Vitamin B substances with vitamin C.

Bee-Zee *Rugby, USA.*
Multivitamin and mineral preparation.

Befact *SMB, Belg.*
Vitamin B substances.
Neuralgia; neuritis; skin disorders; vitamin B deficiency.

Befelka Herz-Dragees *Befelka, Ger.*†.
Motherwort (p.1604·2); squill (p.1070·1); crataegus (p.1568·2).
Cardiac disorders.

Befelka-Asthma N *Befelka, Ger.*†.
Diphenhydramine hydrochloride (p.409·1); ephedrine hydrochloride (p.1059·3).
Asthma; hay fever.

Befelka-Oel *Befelka, Ger.*
Hypericum oil (p.1590·1); calendula oil; chamomile oil; olive oil (p.1610·1); viola tricoloris oil; liquid paraffin (p.1382·1).
Skin disorders.

Befelka-Tinktur *Befelka, Ger.*
Aloes (p.1177·1); achillea (p.1542·2); melissa (p.1600·1); juniper fruit (p.1592·2); ononis (p.1610·2); betula; urtica (p.1642·3); chamomile (p.1561·2); arnica (p.1550·3); pimpinella; turiones pini; liquorice (p.1197·1).
Circulatory disorders; metabolic disorders; skin disorders.

$B_{1/6}$-Effekton *Brenner-Efeka, Ger.*
Thiamine hydrochloride (p.1361·1); pyridoxine hydrochloride (p.1362·3).
Neurological disorders.

Befibrat *Hennig, Ger.*
Bezafibrate (p.1268·2).
Hyperlipidaemias.

Befizal *Boehringer Mannheim, Fr.*
Bezafibrate (p.1268·2).
Hyperlipidaemias.

Beflavina *Roche, Ital.*†.
Riboflavine (p.1362·1).
Vitamin B_2 deficiency.

Beflavine *Roche, Fr.*
Riboflavine (p.1362·1).
Vitamin B deficiency.

Beforplex *Bournonville, Belg.*
Vitamin B substances.
Digestive disorders; neuritis; skin disorders; vitamin B deficiency.

Beglan *Faes, Spain.*
Salmeterol xinafoate (p.761·2).
Asthma; bronchitis.

Beglunina *Llorens, Spain.*
Pyridoxine (p.1363·1).
Alcohol intoxication; vitamin B_6 deficiency.

Begrivac
Hoechst, Aust.; Chiron Behring, Ger.; Hoechst Marion Roussel, Swed.; Wyeth, UK.
An inactivated influenza vaccine (p.1515·2).
Active immunisation.

Begrivac-F *Hoechst Marion Roussel, Irl.*†.
An influenza vaccine (p.1515·2).
Active immunisation.

Begrocit *Grossmann, Switz.*
Vitamin and mineral preparation.

Behepan *Pharmacia Upjohn, Swed.*
Injection: Hydroxocobalamin acetate (p.1364·2).
Tablets: Cyanocobalamin (p.1363·3).
Megaloblastic anaemia; Schilling test; sprue; vitamin B_{12} deficiency.

B12-Ehrl *Hormosan, Ger.*
Cyanocobalamin (p.1363·3).
Vitamin B_{12} deficiency.

Bekunis
Note. This name is used for preparations of different composition.
Schulke & Mayr, Aust.; Roha, Irl.; Naturwaren, Ital.†.
Senna (p.1212·2).
Constipation.

Roha, Switz.
Senna (p.1212·2); bisacodyl (p.1179·3).
Constipation.

Bekunis Bisacodyl *Roha, Ger.*
Bisacodyl (p.1179·3).
Constipation.

Bekunis Chocolate *Polcopharma, Austral.*†.
Senna (p.1212·2).
Constipation.

Bekunis Complex *Sandoz Nutrition, Spain*†.
Bisacodyl (p.1179·3); senna (p.1212·2).
Constipation.

Bekunis Fine Herbal Blend *Polcopharma, Austral.*†.
Senna (p.1212·2); hibiscus blossoms; liquorice (p.1197·1); peppermint leaf (p.1208·1).
Constipation.

Bekunis Herbal Tea *Polcopharma, Austral.*
Senna (p.1212·2).
Constipation.

Bekunis Instant
Polcopharma, Austral.; Roha, Ger.
Senna (p.1212·2).
Constipation.

Bekunis Leicht *Roha, Ger.*
Ispaghula (p.1194·2).
Constipation.

Bekunis Plantago Granule *Roha, Switz.*
Ispaghula (p.1194·2).
Constipation; diarrhoea; irritable bowel; obesity; stool softener.

Bekunis-Krautertee *Roha, Ger.*
Senna (p.1212·2).
Constipation.

Belcomycine *Rhone-Poulenc Rorer, Neth.*
Colistin sulphate (p.195·3).
Bacterial infections.

Belidral *Sintesa, Belg.*
Amiloride hydrochloride (p.819·2); hydrochlorothiazide (p.885·2).
Ascites; heart failure; hypertension; oedema.

Belivon
Organon, Aust.; Organon, Ital.
Risperidone (p.690·3).
Psychoses.

Belix *Halsey, USA*†.
Diphenhydramine hydrochloride (p.409·1).
Insomnia; motion sickness; parkinsonism.

bella sanol *Sanol, Ger.*†.
Ergotamine tartrate (p.445·3); hyoscine hydrobromide (p.462·3); hyoscyamine (p.464·2); phenobarbitone (p.350·2).
Nervous disorders.

Bellacane *Treiner, USA.*
Hyoscyamine sulphate (p.464·2); phenobarbitone (p.350·2).
Gastro-intestinal disorders.

Bellacanfor *Inkeysa, Spain*†.
Camphor (p.1557·2); lavender oil (p.1594·3); methyl salicylate (p.55·2); mustard oil (p.1605·3); rosemary oil (p.1626·2); eucalyptus oil (p.1578·1); belladonna (p.457·1); capsicum (p.1559·2); menthol (p.1600·2).
Rheumatic and muscular pain.

BellaCarotin mono *3M, Ger.*
Betacarotene (p.1335·2).
Sunburn.

Belladenal *Wander, S.Afr.*†.
Belladonna alkaloids (p.457·1); phenobarbitone (p.350·2).
Gastro-intestinal disorders; smooth muscle spasm.

Belladol *Dolisos, Canad.*
Homoeopathic preparation.

Belladonna Med Complex *Dynamit, Aust.*
Homoeopathic preparation.

Belladonna-Strath *Strath-Labor, Ger.*†.
Belladonna (p.457·1); chelidonium; gratiola; valerian (p.1643·1).
Dystonias; gastro-intestinal disorders.

Belladonna-Valobonin *Hanseler, Ger.*†.
Belladonna (p.457·1); valerian (p.1643·1); crataegus (p.1568·2); passion flower (p.1615·3); lupulus (p.1597·2).
Colic; dysmenorrhoea.

Belladonnysat Burger *Ysatfabrik, Ger.*
Belladonna (p.457·1).
Smooth muscle spasms.

Bellafit N *Streuli, Switz.*
Atropine sulphate (p.455·1).
Colic; hyperhidrosis; sialorrhoea.

Bellafolin *Sandoz, Ger.*†.
Belladonna alkaloids (p.457·1).
Smooth muscle spasms.

Bellafolina *Sandoz, Ital.*†.
Belladonna alkaloids (p.457·1).
Smooth muscle spasm.

Bellafoline *Sandoz, USA*†.
Belladonna (p.457·1).
Asthma; dysmenorrhoea; gastro-intestinal disorders; motion sickness; nocturnal enuresis; parkinsonism; renal colic; vagal inhibition.

Bellagotin *Streuli, Switz.*
Belladonna (p.457·1); diphenhydramine hydrochloride (p.409·1); ergotamine tartrate (p.445·3).
Nervous disorders.

Bellanorm *Rosch & Handel, Aust.*
Belladonna (p.457·1).
Bronchospasm; gastro-intestinal disorders; motion sickness; night sweats.

Bellanox *Bios, Belg.*
Brallobarbital (p.643·1); amylobarbitone (p.641·3); quinalbarbitone (p.690·2).
Insomnia.

Bell/ans *Dent, USA.*
Sodium bicarbonate (p.1153·2).
Hyperacidity.

Bellaravil *Ravensberg, Ger.*†.
Ergot (p.1576·1); belladonna (p.457·1); phenobarbitone (p.350·2); procaine hydrochloride (p.1299·2).
Nervous disorders.

Bellaravil-retard *Ravensberg, Ger.*†.
Ergotamine tartrate (p.445·3); belladonna (p.457·1); phenobarbitone (p.350·2); procaine hydrochloride (p.1299·2).
Nervous disorders.

Bellasthman
Note. This name is used for preparations of different composition.
Petrasch, Aust.
Ephedrine hydrochloride (p.1059·3); belladonna (p.457·1); theophylline (p.765·1); caffeine (p.749·3); phenazone (p.78·2).

3M, Ger.†.
Isoprenaline sulphate (p.892·1).
Bronchospastic disorders.

Bellatal *Richwood, USA.*
Phenobarbitone (p.350·2); hyoscyamine sulphate (p.464·2); atropine sulphate (p.455·1); hyoscine hydrobromide (p.462·3).
Hypnotic; sedative.

Bellatard *Propan, S.Afr.*
Phenobarbitone (p.350·2); atropine sulphate (p.455·1); hyoscine hydrobromide (p.462·3); hyoscyamine sulphate (p.464·2).
Smooth muscle spasm.

BellaVal *Ysatfabrik, Ger.*†.
Homoeopathic preparation.

Bellavern *Propan-Vernleigh, S.Afr.*†.
Hyoscyamine sulphate (p.464·2); atropine sulphate (p.455·1); hyoscine hydrobromide (p.462·3); phenobarbitone (p.350·2).
Smooth muscle spasm.

Bellergal
Sandoz, Canad.; Sandoz, Ger.†*; Novartis, S.Afr.; Sandoz, Spain*†*; Sandoz, Switz.*
Belladonna alkaloids (p.457·1); ergotamine tartrate (p.445·3); phenobarbitone (p.350·2).
Gastro-intestinal disorders; insomnia; menopausal disorders; nervous disorders; premenstrual syndrome.

Bellergal-S *Sandoz, USA.*
Levorotatory alkaloids of belladonna (Bellafoline) (p.457·1); ergotamine tartrate (p.445·3); phenobarbitone (p.350·2).
Cardiovascular disorders; gastro-intestinal disorders; menopausal disorders; recurrent throbbing headache.

Bellergil *Sandoz, Ital.*
Belladonna alkaloids (p.457·1); ergotamine tartrate (p.445·3); phenobarbitone (p.350·2).
Dystonias.

Bellocarb *Sinclair, UK*†.
Belladonna (p.457·1); magnesium carbonate (p.1198·1); magnesium trisilicate (p.1199·1).
Gastro-intestinal disorders.

Belloform nouvelle formule *Tentan, Switz.*
Cathine hydrochloride (p.1478·1).
Obesity.

Belmacina *CEPA, Spain.*
Ciprofloxacin hydrochloride (p.185·3).
Bacterial infections.

Belmalax *Belmac, Spain.*
Lactulose (p.1195·3).
Constipation; hepatic encephalopathy; salmonella eradication.

Belmazol *Belmac, Spain.*
Omeprazole (p.1204·2).
Gastro-oesophageal reflux; peptic ulcer; Zollinger-Ellison syndrome.

Belnif *Promed, Ger.; Astra, Ger.*
Metoprolol tartrate (p.907·3); nifedipine (p.916·2).
Angina pectoris; hypertension.

Beloc
Astra, Aust.; Astra, Ger.
Metoprolol tartrate (p.907·3).
Angina pectoris; arrhythmias; hypertension; hyperthyroidism; migraine; myocardial infarction.

Beloc comp
Astra, Aust.; Astra, Ger.
Metoprolol tartrate (p.907·3); hydrochlorothiazide (p.885·2).
Hypertension.

Beloc-Zok
Astra, Ger.; Promed, Ger.; Astra, Switz.
Metoprolol succinate (p.908·2).
Arrhythmias; hypertension; migraine; myocardial infarction.

Beloc-Zok comp *Astra, Ger.; Promed, Ger.*
Metoprolol succinate (p.908·2); hydrochlorothiazide (p.885·2).
Hypertension.

Bel-Phen-Ergot S *Goldline, USA.*
Phenobarbitone (p.350·2); ergotamine tartrate (p.445·3); belladonna (p.457·1).

Belsar *Schering-Plough, Ital.*†.
Oral liquid: Dimethicone (p.1213·1); almasilate (p.1177·1); magnesium hydroxide (p.1198·2); aluminium hydroxide (p.1177·3).
Tablets: Dimethicone (p.1213·1); anhydrous colloidal silicon dioxide (p.1475·1); aluminium hydroxide-magnesium carbonate (p.1178·2); magnesium hydroxide (p.1198·2).
Gastro-intestinal disorders.

Beltop *Janssen-Cilag, Aust.*
Ketoconazole (p.383·1).
Dandruff.

Belustine
Bellon, Fr.; Rhone-Poulenc Rorer, Ital.; Rhone-Poulenc Rorer, Spain.
Lomustine (p.544·1).
Malignant neoplasms.

Bemetrazole *Be-Tabs, S.Afr.*
Metronidazole (p.585·1).
Anaerobic bacterial infections; protozoal infections.

Beminal
Whitehall-Robins, Canad.; Akromed, S.Afr.†*; Whitehall, USA.*
Vitamin B substances with vitamin C.
Alcoholism; stress; vitamin deficiencies.

Beminal C Fortis *Whitehall-Robins, Canad.*
Vitamin B substances with ascorbic acid.

Beminal Fortis *Whitehall-Robins, Canad.*
Vitamin B substances.

Beminal with Iron *Akromed, S.Afr.*†.
Vitamin B substances; vitamin C; ferrous fumarate.
Iron deficiency; vitamin deficiencies.

Beminal with Iron and Liver *Whitehall-Robins, Canad.*
Vitamin B substances with ferrous sulphate and liver.

Beminal Z *Whitehall-Robins, Canad.*
Multivitamins; zinc sulphate (p.1373·2).

Bemolan *Boehringer Mannheim, Spain.*
Magaldrate (p.1198·1).
Gastro-intestinal hyperacidity.

Bemote *Everett, USA*†.
Dicyclomine hydrochloride (p.460·1).
Functional bowel syndrome; irritable bowel syndrome.

Benacine *Parke, Davis, Austral.*†.
Diphenhydramine hydrochloride (p.409·1); hyoscine hydrobromide (p.462·3).
Motion sickness; parkinsonism.

Bena-D *Seatrace, USA*†.
Diphenhydramine hydrochloride (p.409·1).
Motion sickness; parkinsonism.

Benadon
Roche, Aust.; Roche, Ger.†; Roche Consumer, Irl.; Roche, Ital.; Roche Nicholas, Spain; Roche, Swed.; Roche, Switz.; Roche Consumer, UK.
Pyridoxine hydrochloride (p.1362·3).
Acute alcohol intoxication; hypoacousia; premenstrual syndrome; vitamin B_6 deficiency; vomiting.

Benadryl
Note. This name is used for preparations of different composition.
Parke, Davis, Aust.
Capsules: Diphenhydramine hydrochloride (p.409·1); codeine phosphate sesquihydrate (p.26·1).
Coughs.
Oral liquid; oral drops: Diphenhydramine hydrochloride (p.409·1); ammonium chloride (p.1055·2); menthol (p.1600·2); sodium citrate (p.1153·2).
Cold and influenza symptoms; coughs.
Parke, Davis, Austral.†; Warner-Lambert, Canad.; Warner-Lambert, Ital.; Warner-Lambert, Spain; Parke, Davis, Switz.†; Parke, Davis, USA; Glaxo Wellcome, USA.
Diphenhydramine hydrochloride (p.409·1) or diphenhydramine (p.409·1).
Hypersensitivity disorders; migraine; motion sickness; nausea and vomiting; parkinsonism; sedative.
Parke, Davis, Fr.†.
Paracetamol (p.72·2); phenylpropanolamine hydrochloride (p.1067·2).
Nasal congestion.
Parke, Davis, Ital.
Syrup: Diphenhydramine hydrochloride (p.409·1); ammonium chloride (p.1055·2); sodium citrate (p.1153·2); menthol (p.1600·2).
Coughs.
Warner-Lambert, UK.
Acrivastine (p.401·3).
Formerly contained diphenhydramine hydrochloride.
Hypersensitivity reactions.

Benadryl Allergy/Sinus Headache Warner-Wellcome, USA.
Diphenhydramine hydrochloride (p.409·1); pseudoephedrine hydrochloride (p.1068·3); paracetamol (p.72·2).

Benadryl Allergy/Sinus/Headache Warner-Lambert, Canad.
Diphenhydramine hydrochloride (p.409·1); pseudoephedrine hydrochloride (p.1068·3); paracetamol (p.72·2).
Eye irritation; headache; upper respiratory-tract disorders.

Benadryl Cold Nighttime Formula Parke, Davis, USA.
Pseudoephedrine hydrochloride (p.1068·3); diphenhydramine hydrochloride (p.409·1); paracetamol (p.72·2).
Upper respiratory-tract symptoms.

Benadryl Cold/Flu Parke, Davis, USA†.
Pseudoephedrine hydrochloride (p.1068·3); diphenhydramine hydrochloride (p.409·1); paracetamol (p.72·2).
Upper respiratory-tract symptoms.

Benadryl Complex Parke, Davis, Ital.
Diphenhydramine hydrochloride (p.409·1); dextromethorphan hydrobromide (p.1057·3); pseudoephedrine hydrochloride (p.1068·3); ammonium chloride (p.1055·2); sodium citrate (p.1153·2); menthol (p.1600·2).
Coughs.

Benadryl Cough Medicine Warner-Lambert, Austral.
Diphenhydramine hydrochloride (p.409·1); ammonium chloride (p.1055·2); sodium citrate (p.1153·2).
Allergic rhinitis; cough and cold symptoms.

Benadryl Cough Medicine for Chesty Coughs Warner-Lambert, Austral.
Guaiphenesin (p.1061·3); pseudoephedrine hydrochloride (p.1068·3).
Coughs.

Benadryl Cough Medicine for Children Parke, Davis, Austral.†.
Diphenhydramine hydrochloride (p.409·1); pseudoephedrine hydrochloride (p.1068·3).
Upper respiratory-tract symptoms.

Benadryl Decongestant
Warner-Lambert, Canad.; Parke, Davis, USA.
Diphenhydramine hydrochloride (p.409·1); pseudoephedrine hydrochloride (p.1068·3).
Cold symptoms; hay fever.

Benadryl Expectorante Warner-Lambert, Spain.
Ammonium chloride (p.1055·2); diphenhydramine hydrochloride (p.409·1); sodium citrate (p.1153·2); menthol (p.1600·2).
Respiratory-tract disorders.

Benadryl Itch Glaxo Wellcome, USA.
Diphenhydramine hydrochloride (p.409·1); zinc acetate (p.1646·2).
Hypersensitivity reactions.

Benadryl mit Codein
Note. This name is used for preparations of different composition.
Parke, Davis, Aust.
Oral drops: Codeine phosphate (p.26·1); diphenhydramine hydrochloride (p.409·1); ammonium chloride (p.1055·2).
Oral liquid: Codeine phosphate (p.26·1); diphenhydramine hydrochloride (p.409·1); ammonium chloride (p.1055·2); menthol (p.1600·2); sodium citrate (p.1153·2).
Coughs.
Warner-Wellcome, Ger.†.
Diphenhydramine hydrochloride (p.409·1); codeine phosphate (p.26·1).
Coughs.

Benadryl N Warner-Lambert, Ger.
Diphenhydramine hydrochloride (p.409·1).
Coughs, colds and associated respiratory-tract disorders.

Benadryl N mit Codein Warner-Wellcome, Ger.†.
Diphenhydramine hydrochloride (p.409·1); codeine phosphate (p.26·1).
Coughs, colds, and associated respiratory-tract disorders.

Benadryl Plus Parke, Davis, USA†.
Diphenhydramine hydrochloride (p.409·1); paracetamol (p.72·2); pseudoephedrine hydrochloride (p.1068·3).
Nasal congestion.

Benagol Boots Healthcare, Ital.
Dichlorobenzyl alcohol (p.1112·2); amylmetacresol (p.1101·3).
Oral hygiene.

Benagol Collutorio Boots Healthcare, Ital.
Amylmetacresol (p.1101·3).
Oral hygiene.

Benagol Mentolo-Eucaliptolo Boots Healthcare, Ital.
Dichlorobenzyl alcohol (p.1112·2); amylmetacresol (p.1101·3); menthol (p.1600·2).
Oral hygiene.

Benagol Vitamina C Boots Healthcare, Ital.
Dichlorobenzyl alcohol (p.1112·2); amylmetacresol (p.1101·3); sodium ascorbate (p.1365·2); ascorbic acid (p.1365·2).
Adjunct in cold symptoms; oral hygiene.

Benahist Keene, USA†.
Diphenhydramine hydrochloride (p.409·1).
Motion sickness; parkinsonism.

Ben-Allergin Dunhall, USA†.
Diphenhydramine hydrochloride (p.409·1).
Motion sickness; parkinsonism.

Ben-Aqua Syosset, USA.
Benzoyl peroxide (p.1079·2).
Acne.

Be-Natal Be-Tabs, S.Afr.
Multivitamin and mineral preparation.

Benatuss Parke, Davis, Austral.†.
Diphenhydramine hydrochloride (p.409·1); dextromethorphan hydrobromide (p.1057·3); phenylephrine hydrochloride (p.1066·2); ammonium chloride (p.1055·2); sodium citrate (p.1153·2).
Coughs; nasal congestion.

Bencard DP6 Kalopharma, Ital.†.
Allergen extracts of *Dermatophagoides pteronyssinus* (p.1545·1).
Hyposensitisation.

Bencard Skin Testing Solutions Bencard, UK.
Allergen extracts (single and mixed) (p.1545·1).
Diagnosis of hypersensitivity.

Bencef Benvegna, Ital.†.
Pivcephalexin hydrochloride (p.238·3).
Bacterial infections.

Benciclina Benvegna, Ital.†.
Methacycline hydrochloride (p.225·1).
Bacterial infections.

Bencole Propan, S.Afr.
Co-trimoxazole (p.196·3).
Bacterial infections.

Bendalina
Angelini, Ital.; Farma Lepori, Spain†.
Bendazac lysine (p.21·1).
Cataracts.

Bendigon Bayer, Aust.†.
Reserpine (p.942·1); mefruside (p.902·2); inositol nicotinate (p.891·3).
Hypertension.

Bendigon N Bayer, Ger.
Mefruside (p.902·2); reserpine (p.942·1).
Formerly contained inositol nicotinate, mefruside, and reserpine.
Hypertension.

Bendogen Lagap, UK†.
Bethanidine sulphate (p.832·2).
Hypertension.

Bendralan Antibioticos, Spain†.
Phenethicillin potassium (p.236·2).
Bacterial infections.

Benecut Salus, Aust.
Naftifine hydrochloride (p.385·3).
Fungal skin infections.

Benedar Benedetti, Ital.†.
Diacerein (p.29·3).
Osteoarthritis.

Benedorm Dresden, Ger.
Valerian (p.1643·1).
Anxiety disorders; insomnia.

Benefix Genetics Institute, USA.
A factor IX preparation (recombinant DNA) (p.721·3).
Factor IX deficiency.

Beneflur Schering, Spain.
Fludarabine phosphate (p.534·1).
Chronic lymphocytic leukaemia.

Benegyn Vortech, USA†.
Sulphanilamide (p.256·3); aminacrine hydrochloride (p.1098·3); allantoin (p.1078·2).
Vaginal infections.

Benemid
Merck Sharp & Dohme, Austral.; Merck Sharp & Dohme, Canad.; Merck Sharp & Dohme, Irl.; Merck Sharp & Dohme, Neth.†; Merck Sharp & Dohme, S.Afr.; Merck Sharp & Dohme, Switz.; Merck Sharp & Dohme, UK; Merck Sharp & Dohme, USA†.
Probenecid (p.394·3).
Adjunct to beta-lactam antibacterials; gout; hyperuricaemia.

Benemide Doms-Adrian, Fr.†.
Probenecid (p.394·3).
Adjunct to beta-lactam antibacterials; gout; hyperuricaemia.

Beneroc Roche, Aust.
Multivitamin and mineral preparation.

Benerva
Roche Consumer, Belg.; Roche, Fr.; Roche Consumer, Irl.; Roche, Ital.; Roche Nicholas, Spain; Roche, Swed.; Roche, Switz.; Roche Consumer, UK.
Thiamine hydrochloride (p.1361·1).
Alcoholism; beri beri; neuropathies; vitamin B_1 deficiency; Wernicke's encephalopathy.

Benerva Compound
Roche, Irl.†; Roche Consumer, UK†.
Vitamin B substances.
Vitamin B deficiencies.

Benestan
Vita, Ital.; Alonga, Spain.
Alfuzosin hydrochloride (p.817·2).
Benign prostatic hyperplasia.

Beneuran Hafslund Nycomed, Aust.
Thiamine hydrochloride (p.1361·1).
Vitamin B_1 deficiency.

Beneuran compositum Hafslund Nycomed, Aust.
Thiamine hydrochloride (p.1361·1); pyridoxine hydrochloride (p.1362·3); folic acid (p.1340·3); cyanocobalamin (p.1363·3).
Cervical syndrome; funicular myelosis; herpes zoster infection; nervous exhaustion; neuralgia; neuritis; pregnancy induced vomiting.

Beneuran Vit B-Komplex Hafslund Nycomed, Aust.
Riboflavine sodium phosphate (p.1362·1); pyridoxine hydrochloride (p.1362·3); dexpanthenol (p.1570·3); thiamine hydrochloride (p.1361·1); nicotinamide (p.1351·2).
Eye disorders; gastro-intestinal disorders; liver disorders; mouth and throat disorders; neurological disorders; obstetric disorders; skin disorders; vitamin deficiency.

Beneurol Meuse, Belg.
Thiamine hydrochloride (p.1361·1).
Beri-beri; dietary supplementation; digestive disorders; neuritis.

Benevit Salus, Ital.†.
Vitamin B substances.

Benexol Roche, Switz.
Vitamin B substances.
Alcoholism; neuropathies; vitamin B deficiency.

Benexol B12 Roche, Ital.
Injection: Cocarboxylase (p.1361·2); pyridoxine hydrochloride (p.1362·3); hydroxocobalamin (p.1363·3).
Tablets: Thiamine hydrochloride (p.1361·1); pyridoxine hydrochloride (p.1362·3); cyanocobalamin (p.1363·3).
Neuropathies; vitamin B_1, B_6, and B_{12} deficiency; vomiting.

Benexol B1 B6 B12 Roche Nicholas, Spain.
Cyanocobalamin (p.1363·3); pyridoxine hydrochloride (p.1362·3); thiamine hydrochloride (p.1361·1).
Vitamin B deficiency.

Benflogin Angelini, Ital.
Ibuprofen guaiacol ester (p.44·3).
Fever; inflammation; pain.

Benfofen Sanofi Winthrop, Ger.
Diclofenac sodium (p.31·2).
Gout; inflammation; musculoskeletal and joint disorders; pain.

Benfogamma Worwag, Ger.
Benfotiamine (p.1360·3).
Vitamin B_1 deficiency.

Ben-Gay Pfizer, USA.
Methyl salicylate (p.55·2); menthol (p.1600·2).
Muscle, joint, and soft-tissue pain; neuralgia.

Ben-Gay Ice Pfizer, Canad.
Menthol (p.1600·2).

Ben-Gay No Odor Pfizer, Canad.
Triethanolamine salicylate (p.1639·2).
Muscle and joint pain.

Ben-Gay Original, Ben-Gay Extra Strength
Pfizer, Canad.
Methyl salicylate (p.55·2); menthol (p.1600·2).
Muscle and joint pain.

Ben-Gay Ultra
Pfizer, Canad.; Pfizer, USA.
Methyl salicylate (p.55·2); menthol (p.1600·2); camphor (p.1557·2).
Muscle, joint, and soft-tissue pain; neuralgia.

Ben-Gay Vanishing Pfizer, USA.
Menthol (p.1600·2).
Muscle, joint, and soft-tissue pain; neuralgia.

Bengers Key, Austral.†.
Infant feed.

Benglau Angelini, Aust.
Dapiprazole hydrochloride (p.1570·2).
Reversal of mydriasis.

Bengue's Balsam
Bengue, Irl.; Pfizer, UK.
Menthol (p.1600·2); methyl salicylate (p.55·2).
Chilblains; cough and cold symptoms; rheumatic and muscular pain.

Benical Roche, Switz.
Dextromethorphan hydrobromide (p.1057·3); pseudoephedrine hydrochloride (p.1068·3); chlorpheniramine maleate (p.405·1).
Coughs.

Beni-cur Beni-med, Ger.
Garlic (p.1583·1).
Vascular disorders.

Benium Merckle, Ger.
Anise oil (p.1550·1); fennel oil (p.1579·2); caraway oil (p.1559·3).
Flatulence; gastro-intestinal cramp.

Benocten Medinova, Switz.
Diphenhydramine hydrochloride (p.409·1).
Sleep disorders.

Benoject Mayrand, USA†.
Diphenhydramine hydrochloride (p.409·1).
Motion sickness; parkinsonism.

Benoquin
ICN, Canad.; ICN, USA.
Monobenzone (p.1088·3).
Skin hyperpigmentation.

Benoral
Note. This name is used for preparations of different composition.
Sanofi Winthrop, Irl.; Sanofi Winthrop, UK.
Benorylate (p.21·2).
Fever; musculoskeletal and joint disorders; pain.
Reig Jofre, Spain.
Benzathine phenoxymethylpenicillin (p.159·2).
Bacterial infections.

Benortan
Sanofi Winthrop, Belg.†; Sanofi Winthrop, Ger.†; Winthrop, Neth.†; Winthrop, Switz.†.
Benorylate (p.21·2).
Fever; musculoskeletal and joint disorders; pain.

Benoxid Yamanouchi, Ital.
Benzoyl peroxide (p.1079·2).
Acne; skin disinfection.

Benoxinat SE Alcon-Thilo, Ger.
Oxybuprocaine hydrochloride (p.1298·1).
Local anaesthesia.

Benoxinato Cusi, Spain.
Oxybuprocaine hydrochloride (p.1298·1).
Local anaesthesia.

Benoxygel Stiefel, Spain.
Benzoyl peroxide (p.1079·2).
Acne.

Benoxyl
Stiefel, Canad.; Stiefel, Irl.; Stiefel, S.Afr.; Stiefel, UK; Stiefel, USA.
Benzoyl peroxide (p.1079·2).
Acne.

Benpen CSL, Austral.
Benzylpenicillin sodium (p.159·3).
Bacterial infections.

Benpon Tropon, Ger.†.
Flupenthixol hydrochloride (p.670·3); nortriptyline hydrochloride (p.300·2).
Psychiatric disorders.

Bensulfoid
Note. This name is used for preparations of different composition.
ECR, USA.
Cream: Colloidal sulphur (p.1091·2); resorcinol (p.1090·1).
Acne.
Poythress, USA†.
Tablets: Colloidal sulphur (p.1091·2).

Bentasil Carter Horner, Canad.
Green lozenges: Anethole (p.1549·3); cineole (p.1564·1); menthol (p.1600·2).
Nasal congestion.
Red lozenges; yellow lozenges: Anethole (p.1549·3); menthol (p.1600·2).
Coughs; sore throats.

Bentelan Glaxo Wellcome, Ital.
Depot injection†: Betamethasone disodium phosphate (p.1033·3); betamethasone (p.1033·2).
Effervescent tablets; injection: Betamethasone disodium phosphate (p.1033·3).
Corticosteroid.

Bentos
Ciba Vision, Fr.; Kaken, Jpn.
Befunolol hydrochloride (p.827·1).
Glaucoma; ocular hypertension.

Bentum Zambon, Ital.†.
Benorylate (p.21·2).
Musculoskeletal and joint disorders; pain.

Bentyl
Lepetit, Ital.†; Lakeside, USA.
Dicyclomine hydrochloride (p.460·1).
Functional bowel syndrome; irritable bowel syndrome.

Bentylol
Hoechst Marion Roussel, Canad.; Marion Merrell, Spain.
Dicyclomine hydrochloride (p.460·1).
Adjuvant in peptic ulcer; irritable bowel syndrome; smooth muscle spasm.

Benur Roerig, Ital.
Doxazosin mesylate (p.862·3).
Benign prostatic hyperplasia.

Benuride Roche, Switz.
Pheneturide (p.350·1).
Epilepsy.

Ben-u-ron
Bene, Ger.; Milupa, Switz.
Paracetamol (p.72·2).
Fever; pain.

Benuryl *ICN, Canad.*
Probenecid (p.394·3).
Hyperuricaemia.

Beny-Caps a la codeine *Warner-Lambert Consumer, Switz.*
Codeine phosphate (p.26·1); diphenhydramine hydrochloride (p.409·1).
Coughs.

Benylan *Parke, Davis, Swed.*
Diphenhydramine hydrochloride (p.409·1).
Formerly contained diphenhydramine hydrochloride, ammonium chloride and menthol.
Hypersensitivity reactions.

Benylin
Note. This name is used for preparations of different composition.
Parke, Davis, Fr.†.
Diphenhydramine hydrochloride (p.409·1).
Coughs.

Parke, Davis, S.Afr.
Diphenhydramine hydrochloride (p.409·1); ammonium chloride (p.1055·2); menthol (p.1600·2).
Coughs.

Warner-Lambert Consumer, Switz.
Diphenhydramine hydrochloride (p.409·1); ammonium chloride (p.1055·2).
Coughs.

Benylin a la codeine *Warner-Lambert Consumer, Switz.*
Diphenhydramine hydrochloride (p.409·1); codeine phosphate (p.26·1); ammonium chloride (p.1055·2).
Coughs.

Benylin Adult *Glaxo Wellcome, USA.*
Dextromethorphan hydrobromide (p.1057·3).
Formerly called Benylin Cough Syrup and contained diphenhydramine hydrochloride.
Coughs.

Benylin for Allergies *Warner-Lambert, Canad.†.*
Diphenhydramine hydrochloride (p.409·1); pseudoephedrine hydrochloride (p.1068·3).
Nasal congestion.

Benylin Antihistaminicum *Warner-Lambert Consumer, Belg.*
Diphenhydramine hydrochloride (p.409·1).
Coughs; respiratory-tract disorders.

Benylin Antitusivo *Warner-Lambert, Spain.*
Dextromethorphan hydrobromide (p.1057·3).
Coughs.

Benylin Antitussivum *Warner-Lambert Consumer, Belg.*
Dextromethorphan hydrobromide (p.1057·3).
Coughs.

Benylin (Benylin Original) *Warner-Lambert, Irl.*
Diphenhydramine hydrochloride (p.409·1); menthol (p.1600·2).
Coughs; hypersensitivity reactions.

Benylin Chesty Cough
Warner-Lambert, Irl.†; Warner-Lambert, UK.
Diphenhydramine hydrochloride (p.409·1); ammonium chloride (p.1055·2); sodium citrate (p.1153·2); menthol (p.1600·2).
Formerly known as Benylin Expectorant in the *UK.*
Coughs; respiratory-tract congestion.

Benylin Childrens Chesty Coughs *Warner-Lambert, UK.*
Guaiphenesin (p.1061·3).
Coughs.

Benylin Childrens Cough *Warner-Lambert, Irl.*
Diphenhydramine hydrochloride (p.409·1); sodium citrate (p.1153·2); menthol (p.1600·2).
Coughs.

Benylin Childrens Coughs & Colds *Warner-Lambert, UK.*
Dextromethorphan hydrobromide (p.1057·3); triprolidine hydrochloride (p.420·3).
Coughs and cold symptoms.

Benylin Childrens Dry Coughs *Warner-Lambert, UK.*
Pholcodine (p.1068·1).
Coughs.

Benylin Childrens Night Coughs *Warner-Lambert, UK.*
Diphenhydramine hydrochloride (p.409·1); menthol (p.1600·2).
Formerly known as Benylin Paediatric.
Coughs; respiratory-tract congestion.

Benylin Codeine *Warner-Lambert, Canad.*
Codeine phosphate (p.26·1); pseudoephedrine hydrochloride (p.1068·3); guaiphenesin (p.1061·3).
Coughs; nasal congestion.

Benylin with Codeine
Note. This name is used for preparations of different composition.
Warner-Lambert, Irl.
Diphenhydramine hydrochloride (p.409·1); codeine phosphate (p.26·1); menthol (p.1600·2).
Coughs.

Parke, Davis, S.Afr.
Diphenhydramine hydrochloride (p.409·1); codeine phosphate (p.26·1); ammonium chloride (p.1055·2); menthol (p.1600·2).
Coughs.

Warner-Lambert, UK.
Diphenhydramine hydrochloride (p.409·1); codeine phosphate (p.26·1); sodium citrate (p.1153·2); menthol (p.1600·2).
Coughs.

Benylin Cold *Warner-Lambert, Canad.†.*
Pseudoephedrine hydrochloride (p.1068·3); chlorpheniramine maleate (p.405·1).
Nasal congestion.

Benylin Cough & Congestion *Warner-Lambert, UK.*
Diphenhydramine hydrochloride (p.409·1); menthol (p.1600·2); dextromethorphan hydrobromide (p.1057·3); pseudoephedrine hydrochloride (p.1068·3).
Coughs and congestion.

Benylin Day & Night
Warner-Lambert, Ital.; Parke, Davis, S.Afr.; Warner-Lambert, UK.
Day tablets, paracetamol (p.72·2); phenylpropanolamine hydrochloride (p.1067·2); night tablets, paracetamol; diphenhydramine hydrochloride (p.409·1).
Cold and influenza symptoms; upper respiratory-tract congestion.

Benylin Decongestant
Note. This name is used for preparations of different composition.
Warner-Lambert, Canad.†.
Pseudoephedrine hydrochloride (p.1068·3).
Nasal congestion.

Warner-Lambert, Irl.†.
Diphenhydramine hydrochloride (p.409·1); pseudoephedrine hydrochloride (p.1068·3); sodium citrate (p.1153·2); menthol (p.1600·2).
Coughs; respiratory-tract congestion.

Parke, Davis, USA.
Diphenhydramine hydrochloride (p.409·1); pseudoephedrine hydrochloride (p.1068·3).
Upper respiratory-tract symptoms.

Benylin Decongestivo *Warner-Lambert, Spain.*
Dextromethorphan hydrobromide (p.1057·3); pseudoephedrine hydrochloride (p.1068·3).
Coughs; nasal congestion.

Benylin DM
Warner-Lambert, Canad.; Parke, Davis, S.Afr.; Parke, Davis, USA.
Dextromethorphan hydrobromide (p.1057·3).
Coughs.

Benylin DM-D
Warner-Lambert, Canad.; Parke, Davis, S.Afr.
Dextromethorphan hydrobromide (p.1057·3); pseudoephedrine hydrochloride (p.1068·3).
Coughs; nasal congestion.

Benylin DM-D-E *Warner-Lambert, Canad.*
Dextromethorphan hydrobromide (p.1057·3); pseudoephedrine hydrochloride (p.1068·3); guaiphenesin (p.1061·3).
Coughs; nasal congestion.

Benylin DM-E *Warner-Lambert, Canad.*
Dextromethorphan hydrobromide (p.1057·3); guaiphenesin (p.1061·3).
Coughs.

Benylin Dry Cough
Warner-Lambert, Irl.; Warner-Lambert, UK.
Diphenhydramine hydrochloride (p.409·1); dextromethorphan hydrobromide (p.1057·3); sodium citrate (p.1153·2); menthol (p.1600·2).
Formerly known as Benylin Fortified in the *UK.*
Coughs.

Benylin Expectorant *Glaxo Wellcome, USA.*
Dextromethorphan hydrobromide (p.1057·3); guaiphenesin (p.1061·3).
Coughs.

Benylin 4 Flu
Note. This name is used for preparations of different composition.
Warner-Wellcome, Canad.
Dextromethorphan hydrobromide (p.1057·3); pseudoephedrine hydrochloride (p.1068·3); guaiphenesin (p.1061·3); paracetamol (p.72·2).
Coughs and cold symptoms.

Warner-Lambert, UK.
Hot drink: Diphenhydramine (p.409·1); paracetamol (p.72·2); phenylephrine (p.1066·2).
Oral liquid; tablets: Diphenhydramine hydrochloride (p.409·1); paracetamol (p.72·2); pseudoephedrine hydrochloride (p.1068·3).
Influenza symptoms.

Benylin Mentholated Linctus *Warner-Lambert, UK.*
Diphenhydramine hydrochloride (p.409·1); dextromethorphan hydrobromide (p.1057·3); pseudoephedrine hydrochloride (p.1068·3); menthol (p.1600·2).
Coughs.

Benylin Multi-Symptom *Glaxo Wellcome, USA.*
Dextromethorphan hydrobromide (p.1057·3); pseudoephedrine hydrochloride (p.1068·3); guaiphenesin (p.1061·3).
Cough and cold symptoms.

Benylin Non-Drowsy *Warner-Lambert, UK.*
Guaiphenesin (p.1061·3); menthol (p.1600·2).
Coughs.

Benylin Non-Drowsy Chesty Coughs
Warner-Lambert, Irl.; Warner-Lambert, UK.
Guaiphenesin (p.1061·3); menthol (p.1600·2).
Coughs.

Benylin Non-Drowsy Dry Coughs
Warner-Lambert, Irl.; Warner-Lambert, UK.
Dextromethorphan hydrobromide (p.1057·3).
Coughs.

Benylin Paediatric *Warner-Lambert Consumer, Switz.*
Diphenhydramine hydrochloride (p.409·1).
Coughs.

Benylin Pediatric *Glaxo Wellcome, USA.*
Dextromethorphan hydrobromide (p.1057·3).
Coughs.

Benylin Solid *Parke, Davis, S.Afr.*
Dextromethorphan hydrobromide (p.1057·3).
Coughs.

Benylin Sore Throat Lozenges *Warner-Lambert, Canad.†.*
Cetylpyridinium chloride (p.1106·2).
Sore throat.

Benylin-Dextromethorfanhydrobromide *Warner-Lambert, Neth.*
Dextromethorphan hydrobromide (p.1057·3).
Coughs.

Benylin-Difenhydraminehydrochloride *Warner-Lambert, Neth.*
Diphenhydramine hydrochloride (p.409·1).
Coughs.

Benylin-E *Warner-Lambert, Canad.*
Guaiphenesin (p.1061·3).
Coughs.

Benyphed
Note. This name is used for preparations of different composition.
Parke, Davis, Austral.†.
Diphenhydramine hydrochloride (p.409·1); dextromethorphan hydrobromide (p.1057·3); phenylephrine hydrochloride (p.1066·2); ammonium chloride (p.1055·2); sodium citrate (p.1153·2).
Coughs; nasal congestion.

Parke, Davis, S.Afr.†.
Diphenhydramine hydrochloride (Benadryl) (p.409·1); dextromethorphan hydrobromide (p.1057·3); phenylephrine hydrochloride (p.1066·2).
Coughs.

Benza *Century, USA.*
Benzalkonium chloride (p.1101·3).
Eye, bladder, urethra, and body cavity irrigation; skin, mucous membrane, and wound disinfection; vaginal douching.

Benzac
Galderma, Austral.; Galderma, Belg.; Galderma, Canad.; Galderma, Ital.; Galderma, Neth.; Galderma, Switz.; Galderma, USA.
Benzoyl peroxide (p.1079·2).
Acne.

Benzac-AC *Galderma, S.Afr.*
Benzoyl peroxide (p.1079·2).
Acne.

Benzagel
Novartis Consumer, Canad.; Bioglan, UK†; Dermik, USA.
Benzoyl peroxide (p.1079·2).
Acne.

Benzaknen
AB-Consult, Aust.; Galderma, Ger.
Benzoyl peroxide (p.1079·2).
Acne.

Benzalc *Asens, Spain.*
Benzalkonium chloride (p.1101·3).
Skin and mucous membrane disinfection.

Benzaltex *Innothera, Switz.†.*
Benzalkonium chloride (p.1101·3).
Contraceptive; disinfectant.

Benzamycin
Trenker, Belg.; Bioglan, Irl.; Bioglan, UK; Dermik, USA.
Benzoyl peroxide (p.1079·2); erythromycin (p.204·1).
Acne.

Benzamycine *UCB, S.Afr.*
Benzoyl peroxide (p.1079·2); erythromycin (p.204·1).
Acne.

Benzashave *Medicis, USA.*
Benzoyl peroxide (p.1079·2).
Acne.

Benzatec *Caps, S.Afr.*
Benzylpenicillin sodium (p.159·3).
Bacterial infections.

Benzedrex *Menley & James, USA.*
Propylhexedrine (p.1485·1).
Nasal congestion.

Benzemul *McGloin, Austral.*
Benzyl benzoate (p.1402·2).
Pediculosis; scabies.

Benzet *Covan, S.Afr.*
Cetrimide (p.1105·2); benzocaine (p.1286·2).
Mouth and throat disorders.

Benzetacil *Pharmacia Upjohn, Spain.*
Benzathine penicillin (p.158·3).
Bacterial infections.

Benzetacil Compuesta *Pharmacia Upjohn, Spain.*
Benzylpenicillin potassium (p.159·2); procaine penicillin (p.240·2); benzathine penicillin (p.158·3).
Bacterial infections.

Benzibel *Lusofarmaco, Ital.*
Methylbenzethonium chloride (p.1119·3).
Barrier preparation; skin irritation and infection.

Benzide *CP Protea, Austral.†.*
Bendrofluazide (p.827·3).
Hypertension; oedema.

Benzirin *Fater, Ital.*
Benzydamine hydrochloride (p.21·3).
Inflammatory mouth disorders.

Benzocaine PD *Produits Dentaires, Switz.*
Benzocaine (p.1286·2); hydroxyquinoline sulphate (p.1589·3); eugenol (p.1578·2).
Dental pain.

Benzochloryl *Goupil, Fr.†.*
Dicophane (p.1404·3).
Lice infestation; scabies.

Benzocol *Hauck, USA†.*
Benzocaine (p.1286·2).
Local anaesthesia.

Benzodent *Procter & Gamble, USA.*
Benzocaine (p.1286·2).
Oral lesions.

Benzoderm *Athenstaedt, Ger.†.*
Cream; ointment: Undecenoic acid (p.389·2); zinc oxide (p.1096·2).
Medicated soap: Undecenoic acid (p.389·2).
Topical powder: Zinc undecenoate (p.389·2).
Topical solution: Undecenoic acid (p.389·2); salicylic acid (p.1090·2).
Fungal infections.

Benzoderm Myco *Athenstaedt, Ger.*
Clotrimazole (p.376·3).
Fungal skin infections.

Benzodiapin *Lisapharma, Ital.†.*
Chlordiazepoxide hydrochloride (p.646·3).
Nervous system disorders.

Benzogen Ferri *Cos Farma, Ital.*
Benzalkonium chloride (p.1101·3); sodium nitrite (p.995·2); acetone (p.1375·1).
Instrument disinfection.

Benzo-Gynoestryl *Roussel, Fr.*
Oestradiol benzoate (p.1455·1) or oestradiol hexahydrobenzoate (p.1455·2).
Lactation disorders; menopausal disorders; menorrhagia; menstrual disorders.

Benzomix *Savoma, Ital.*
Benzoyl peroxide (p.1079·2).
Acne; skin disinfection.

Benzopin *Schwulst, S.Afr.*
Diazepam (p.661·1).
Alcohol withdrawal syndrome; anxiety; premedication.

Benzotic *Alba, USA.*
Phenazone (p.78·2); benzocaine (p.1286·2).

Benzotol *Nelson, Austral.†.*
Benzocaine (p.1286·2); chlorbutol (p.1106·3).
Ear ache.

Benzotran *CP Protea, Austral.†.*
Oxazepam (p.683·2).
Anxiety; psychoses.

Benzoyt *Hexal, Ger.*
Benzoyl peroxide (p.1079·2).
Acne.

Benztrone *Amsa, Ital.*
Oestradiol benzoate (p.1455·1).
Now known as Estradiolo Amsa.
Labour induction; menstrual disorders.

Beocid Puroptal *Metochem, Aust.*
Sulphacetamide sodium (p.252·2).
Bacterial eye infections.

Beogaze *Hoechst Marion Roussel, Belg.*
Gauze impregnated with camphor (p.1557·2) and niaouli oil (p.1607·1).
Burns; wounds.

Be-Oxytet *Be-Tabs, S.Afr.*
Oxytetracycline hydrochloride (p.235·1).
Bacterial infections.

Bepanten *Roche, Ital.*
Dexpanthenol (p.1570·3).
Intestinal atony.

Bepanthen
Note. This name is used for preparations of different composition.
Roche, Aust.
Cream; ointment: Dexpanthenol (p.1570·3).
Skin damage; wounds.
Oral liquid; topical solution: Dexpanthenol (p.1570·3); domiphen bromide (p.1112·3).
Gastro-intestinal disorders; mouth and throat disorders; nasal disorders; respiratory tract disorders; skin damage.

Roche Consumer, Austral.
Panthenol (p.1571·1).
Burns; minor skin lesions; skin irritation.

Roche Nicholas, Ger.
Dexpanthenol (p.1570·3).
Conjunctivitis; dexpanthenol deficiency disorders; gastro-intestinal disorders; respiratory-tract disorders; skin disorders.

Roche, Swed.†.
Dexpanthenol (p.1570·3).
Pantothenic acid deficiency.

Bepanthen plus *Roche, Aust.*
Dexpanthenol (p.1570·3); chlorhexidine hydrochloride (p.1107·2).
Wounds.

Bepanthen V *Roche, Ger.†.*
Dexpanthenol (p.1570·3); lactic acid (p.1593·3); sodium lactate (p.1153·2).
Vaginitis.

Bepanthene
Note. This name is used for preparations of different composition.
Roche, Belg.
Panthenol (p.1571·1).
Hepatitis; intestinal atony; muscular cramps; respiratory-tract disorders; skin disorders.

Roche, Fr.; Roche Nicholas, Spain; Roche, Switz.
Dexpanthenol (p.1570·3).
Gastro-intestinal disorders; mouth and throat disorders; nasal disorders; respiratory-tract disorders; skin disorders.

Bepanthene Plus *Roche, Switz.*
Dexpanthenol (p.1570·3); chlorhexidine hydrochloride (p.1107·2).
Skin disorders; wounds.

Bepantol *Roche, S.Afr.*
Dexpanthenol (p.1570·3).
Skin disorders.

Beprolo *Lusofarmaco, Ital.†.*
Metoprolol tartrate (p.907·3).
Angina pectoris; hypertension.

Bequipecto *Llorens, Spain.*
Bromelains (p.1555·1); bromhexine (p.1055·3); oxolamine citrate (p.1065·3).
Respiratory-tract disorders.

Beracal *Noristan, S.Afr.†.*
Diphenhydramine hydrochloride (p.409·1); calamine (p.1080·1); benzocaine (p.1286·2).
Skin disorders.

Beramin *Hoechst Marion Roussel, S.Afr.*
Diphenhydramine hydrochloride (p.409·1); ammonium chloride (p.1055·2).
Coughs.

Berazole *Hoechst Marion Roussel, S.Afr.*
Metronidazole (p.585·1).
Anaerobic bacterial infections; protozoal infections.

Berberil N *Mann, Ger.*
Tetrahydrozoline hydrochloride (p.1070·2).
Formerly contained berberine hydrochloride and tetrahydrozoline hydrochloride.
Eye disorders.

Berberis Complex *Blackmores, Austral.*
Berberis vulgaris; taraxacum (p.1634·2); chelidonium majus; boldo (p.1554·1); lecithin (p.1595·2); methionine (p.984·2); thiamine hydrochloride (p.1361·1).
Constipation; dyspepsia; liver disorders.

Berberis Med Complex *Dynamit, Aust.*
Homoeopathic preparation.

Berberis Oligoplex *Madaus, Ger.*
Homoeopathic preparation.

Berberis-Tonikum *Pascoe, Ger.†.*
Homoeopathic preparation.

Bergacef *Bergamon, Ital.†.*
Cephamandole nafate sodium (p.180·1).
Bacterial infections.

Bergamon Sapone *Bergamon, Ital.*
Tribromsalan (p.1104·3).
Skin cleansing.

Bergasol *Bergaderm, Fr.†.*
A range of preparations containing various sunscreen agents including ethylhexyl cinnamate; dibenzoylmethane (p.1487·1); benzylidene-heptanone.
Sunscreen.

Bergauf *Huls, Ger.†.*
Hexylresorcinol (p.1116·1); eucalyptus oil (p.1578·1); sage oil; rosemary oil (p.1626·2).
Fungal skin infections of the hands and feet.

Berggeist *Kur und Stadtapotheke, Aust.*
Arnica tincture (p.1550·3); urtica tincture (p.1642·3); formic acid (p.1581·3); menthol (p.1600·2); methyl nicotinate (p.55·1); juniper oil (p.1592·3); lavender oil (p.1594·3); eucalyptus oil (p.1578·1); rosemary oil (p.1626·2); pumilio pine oil (p.1623·3).
Bruising; musculoskeletal and joint disorders; neuralgia.

Beriate
Centeon, Aust.; Centeon, Ger.; Centeon, Swed.
A factor VIII preparation (p.720·3).
Haemorrhagic disorders.

Beriate P *Centeon, Spain.*
Factor VIII (p.720·3).
Factor VIII deficiencies.

Beriglobin
Centeon, Aust.; Chiron Behring, Ger.; Centeon, Ger.; Hoechst Marion Roussel, S.Afr.; Centeon, Swed.
A normal immunoglobulin (p.1522·1).
Hypogammaglobulinaemia; passive immunisation.

Beriglobina *Centeon, Spain.*
A normal immunoglobulin (p.1522·1).
Passive immunisation.

Beriglobina Anti D-P *Centeon, Spain.*
An anti-D immunoglobulin (p.1503·2).
Formerly known as Beriglobina Anti Rho(D).
Prevention of rhesus sensitisation.

Berinert
Centeon, Aust.; Centeon, Ger.
C 1-inactivator (p.1567·2).
Hereditary angioedema.

Berinert HS *Centeon, Switz.*
C1-inactivator (p.1567·2).
Hereditary angioedema.

Berinert P *Centeon, UK.*
C1 inactivator (p.1567·2).
Hereditary angioedema.

Berinin *Centeon, Ger.*
Factor IX (p.721·3).
Factor IX deficiency; haemophilia B.

Beriplast
Centeon, Aust.
Combination pack: 1 ampoule: fibrinogen (p.722·3); factor XIII (p.722·2); aprotinin (p.711·3); 1 ampoule: thrombin (p.728·1); calcium chloride (p.1155·1).
Haemorrhage; wounds.

Centeon, Ger.
Combination pack: 1 ampoule: fibrinogen (p.722·3); factor XIII (p.722·2); 1 ampoule: aprotinin (p.711·3); 1 ampoule: thrombin (p.728·1); 1 ampoule: calcium chloride (p.1155·1)
On mixing this forms a fibrin glue (p.722·2).
Surgical bleeding.

Beriplex
Centeon, Aust.; Centeon, Ger.
A factor IX preparation (p.721·3).
Factor II, VII, IX, and X deficiency; haemorrhagic disorders.

Beriplex PN *Centeon, UK.*
A factor IX preparation (p.721·3).
Anticoagulant overdose; haemorrhagic disorders.

Berirab
Centeon, Aust.; Chiron Behring, Ger.; Centeon, Ger.
A rabies immunoglobulin (p.1530·2).
Passive immunisation.

Berirubin *Ebewe, Aust.*
Pirarubicin hydrochloride (p.558·1).
Now known as Pirarubicin.
Malignant neoplasms.

Berivine *Meuse, Belg.*
Riboflavine (p.1362·1).
Dietary supplement; nocturnal cramps; vitamin B_2 deficiency.

Berkamil
Berk, Irl.; Berk, UK.
Amiloride (p.819·3).
Heart failure; hepatic cirrhosis with ascites; hypertension.

Berkaprine *Berk, UK†.*
Azathioprine (p.505·3).
Auto-immune disorders; organ transplantation.

Berkatens
Berk, Irl.; Berk, UK.
Verapamil hydrochloride (p.960·3).
Angina; arrhythmias; hypertension.

Berkmycen
Berk, Irl.; Berk, UK.
Oxytetracycline (p.235·1).
Bacterial infections.

Berkolol
Berk, Irl.; Berk, UK.
Propranolol hydrochloride (p.937·1).
Angina pectoris; anxiety; arrhythmias; essential tremor; hypertension; hyperthyroidism; migraine; myocardial infarction.

Berkozide *Berk, UK.*
Bendrofluazide (p.827·3).
Heart failure; hypertension; oedema; suppression of lactation.

Berlicetin *Berlin-Chemie, Ger.*
Chloramphenicol (p.182·1), chloramphenicol palmitate (p.182·2), or chloramphenicol sodium succinate (p.182·2).
Bacterial infections.

Berlicetin-Augentropfen *ankerpharm, Ger.*
Azidamfenicol (p.155·2).
Bacterial eye infections.

Berlicetin-Ohrentropfen *Wernigerode, Ger.*
Chloramphenicol (p.182·1); prednisolone (p.1048·1).
Bacterial ear infections with inflammation.

Berlicort *Berlin-Chemie, Ger.*
Triamcinolone (p.1050·2).
Corticosteroid.

Berlinsulin H 10/90, 20/80, 30/70, 40/60, 50/50 *Berlin-Chemie, Ger.*
Mixtures of insulin injection (human, prb) and isophane insulin injection (human, prb) respectively in the proportions indicated (p.322·1).
Diabetes mellitus.

Berlinsulin H Basal *Berlin-Chemie, Ger.*
Isophane insulin injection (human, prb) (p.322·1).
Diabetes mellitus.

Berlinsulin H Normal *Berlin-Chemie, Ger.*
Insulin injection (human, prb) (p.322·1).
Diabetes mellitus.

Berlithion *Berlin-Chemie, Ger.*
Thioctic acid (p.1636·2) or ethylenediamine thioctate (p.1636·2).
Diabetic polyneuropathy.

Berlocid *Berlin-Chemie, Ger.*
Co-trimoxazole (p.196·3).
Bacterial infections; Pneumocystis carinii pneumonia.

Berlocombin *Berlin-Chemie, Ger.*
Trimethoprim (p.265·1); sulfamerazine (p.251·3).
Bacterial infections.

Berlopentin *Berlin-Chemie, Ger.†.*
Diacetylsplenopentin hydrochloride.
Immunodeficiency associated with HIV infection and AIDS.

Berlosin *Berlin-Chemie, Ger.*
Dipyrone (p.35·1).
Fever; pain.

Berlthyrox *Berlin-Chemie, Ger.*
Thyroxine sodium (p.1497·1).
Hypothyroidism.

Berniter *Basotherm, Ger.*
Coal tar (p.1092·3).
Scalp disorders.

Berocca
Roche Consumer, Austral.; Roche Nicholas, Fr.; Roche, Ital.; Roche, Switz.†; Roche Consumer, UK; Roche, USA.
Vitamin B substances with vitamin C.
Vitamin B and C deficiency.

Berocca C *Roche, Canad.†.*
Vitamin B substances with vitamin C.

Berocca Calcium
Roche, Aust.; Roche, Ital.†; Roche, S.Afr.
Vitamin B substances with vitamin C and calcium.

Berocca calcium et magnesium *Roche, Switz.*
Vitamin B substances with vitamin C, calcium, and magnesium.
Alcoholism; vitamin deficiency.

Berocca Calmag *Roche, S.Afr.*
Multivitamins with calcium and magnesium.

Berocca Parenteral Nutrition *Roche, USA†.*
Multivitamin preparation for parenteral nutrition.

Berocca Plus
Note. This name is used for preparations of different composition.
Roche, Aust.
Vitamin B substances with vitamin C, calcium, and magnesium.

Roche, USA.
Ferrous fumarate (p.1339·3); folic acid (p.1340·3); multivitamins and minerals.
Iron-deficiency anaemias.

Berodual
Bender, Aust.; Boehringer Ingelheim, Ger.; Boehringer Ingelheim, Neth.; Boehringer Ingelheim, Spain; Boehringer Ingelheim, Switz.
Fenoterol hydrobromide (p.753·2); ipratropium bromide (p.754·2).
Obstructive airways disease; respiratory-function tests.

Berodualin *Bender, Aust.*
Fenoterol hydrobromide (p.753·2); ipratropium bromide (p.754·2).
Obstructive airways disease.

Berofor
Bender, Aust.; Boehringer Ingelheim, Belg.†; Basotherm, Ger.†.
Interferon alfa-2c (p.615·3).
Anogenital warts; chronic active hepatitis; herpes infections; malignant neoplasms.

Berotec
Bender, Aust.; Boehringer Ingelheim, Austral.; Boehringer Ingelheim, Belg.; Boehringer Ingelheim, Canad.; Boehringer Ingelheim, Fr.; Boehringer Ingelheim, Ger.; Boehringer Ingelheim, Irl.; Boehringer Ingelheim, Neth.; Boehringer Ingelheim, Norw.; Boehringer Ingelheim, S.Afr.; Boehringer Ingelheim, Spain; Boehringer Ingelheim, Swed.; Boehringer Ingelheim, Switz.; Boehringer Ingelheim, UK.
Fenoterol hydrobromide (p.753·2).
Obstructive airways disease; premature labour; pulmonary-function tests; uterine hypertonia.

Berotec solvens *Boehringer Ingelheim, Ger.*
Fenoterol hydrobromide (p.753·2); bromhexine hydrochloride (p.1055·3).
Bronchiectasis; bronchitis; emphysema; interstitial lung disease.

Berplex *Schein, USA.*
Ferrous fumarate (p.1339·3); folic acid (p.1340·3); multivitamins and minerals.
Iron-deficiency anaemias.

Bersicaran N *Janssen-Cilag, Ger.†.*
Ambucetamide hydrochloride (p.1548·2); aspirin (p.16·1); paracetamol (p.72·2); codeine phosphate (p.26·1).
Dysmenorrhoea.

Bertabronc *Berta, Ital.†.*
Bromhexine hydrochloride (p.1055·3); potassium guaiacolsulfonate (p.1068·3).
Coughs.

Berubi *Redel, Ger.†.*
Cyanocobalamin (p.1363·3).
Vitamin B deficiency.

Berubi-compositum N *Redel, Ger.†.*
B vitamin preparation with iron.
Anaemia; tonic.

Berubi-long *Redel, Ger.†.*
Hydroxocobalamin (p.1363·3).
Vitamin B deficiency.

Beruhigungskapseln *Klosterfrau, Aust.*
Valerian (p.1643·1); lupulus (p.1597·2).
Nervous disorders; sleep disorders.

Beruhigungstee *Salus, Aust.*
Valerian (p.1643·1); melissa (p.1600·1); lupulus (p.1597·2); lavender flower (p.1594·3); orange flowers.
Anxiety; sleep disturbances.

Beruhigungs-Tee Nervoflux *Nattermann Tee-Arznei, Ger.†.*
Flor. aurantii; lavander (p.1594·3); melissa (p.1600·1); liquorice (p.1197·1); lupulus (p.1597·2); valerian (p.1643·1); glucose (p.1343·3); maltose (p.1350·2).
Nervous excitability; sleep disorders.

Besenol *Covan, S.Afr.*
Paracetamol (p.72·2); chlormezanone (p.648·3).
Fever; pain; skeletal muscle spasm.

Besinergial *Delagrange, Spain†.*
Ascorbic acid (p.1365·2); cyanocobalamin (p.1363·3); pyridoxine hydrochloride (p.1362·3); thiamine hydrochloride (p.1361·1).
Deficiency of vitamins B and C.

Besitran *Pfizer, Spain.*
Sertraline hydrochloride (p.307·2).
Depression.

Besopartin *Bender, Aust.*
Alteplase (p.818·1).
Myocardial infarction; peripheral arterial thromboembolism; pulmonary embolism.

Bespar *Bristol-Myers Squibb, Ger.*
Buspirone hydrochloride (p.643·3).
Anxiety.

Best EPA *Contassium Co., UK.*
Fish oil (eicosapentaenoic acid, and docosahexaenoic acid) (p.1276·1).

Bestatin *Kayaku, Jpn.*
Ubenimex (p.568·3).
Prophylaxis following the induction of remission against adult acute nonlymphoid leukaemias.

Bestcall *Takeda, Jpn.*
Cefmenoxime hydrochloride (p.166·2).
Mepivacaine hydrochloride (p.1297·2) is included in the intramuscular injection to alleviate the pain of injection.
Bacterial infections.

Bester Complex *Salvat, Spain.*
Benfotiamine (p.1360·3); hydroxocobalamin acetate (p.1364·2); pyridoxine hydrochloride (p.1362·3).
Vitamin B deficiency.

Beston *Solvay, Belg.†.*
Bisbentiamine (p.1360·3).
Muscular disorders; vitamin B_1 deficiency.

Beta-2 *Nephron, USA.*
Isoetharine hydrochloride (p.755·1).
Asthma; bronchospasm.

Beta 21 *IDI, Ital.*
Betamethasone valero-acetate (p.1034·1).
Skin disorders.

Beta A-C *Eagle, Austral.*
Ascorbic acid (p.1365·2); sodium ascorbate (p.1365·2); calcium ascorbate (p.1365·2); *dl*-alpha-tocopheryl acetate (p.1369·2); rutin (p.1580·2); zinc amino acid chelate (p.1373·3); betacarotene (p.1335·2).
Vitamin supplement.

Beta C E with Selenium *Stanley, Canad.*
Betacarotene, selenium, vitamin C, and vitamin E.

Beta Micoter *Farmacusi, Spain.*
Betamethasone dipropionate (p.1033·3); clotrimazole (p.376·3).
Fungal skin infections.

Beta plus Vitamins C, E & Selenium *Quest, Canad.*
Betacarotene, selenium, vitamin C, and vitamin E.

Beta-Ace Tablets *Vita Glow, Austral.*
Betacarotene; ascorbic acid; *d*-alpha tocopheryl acid succinate; zinc amino acid chelate.
Formerly known as Vitaglow Beta Ace.
Dietary supplement.

Beta-Acigoxin *Inverni della Beffa, Ital.†.*
β-Acetyldigoxin (p.812·3).
Arrhythmias; heart failure.

Beta-Adalat
Bayer, Aust.; Bayer, Belg.; Bayer, Irl.; Bayer, Neth.†; Bayer, Switz.; Bayer, UK.
Atenolol (p.825·3); nifedipine (p.916·2).
Angina pectoris; hypertension.

Beta-Adalate *Bayer, Fr.*
Atenolol (p.825·3); nifedipine (p.916·2).
Hypertension.

Betabactyl *SmithKline Beecham, Ger.*
Ticarcillin sodium (p.263·2); potassium clavulanate (p.190·2).
Bacterial infections.

Betabion
Merck, Ger.; Bracco, Ital.; Meda, Swed.
Thiamine hydrochloride (p.1361·1).
Vitamin B_1 deficiency.

Betabioptal *Farmila, Ital.*
Betamethasone (p.1033·2); chloramphenicol (p.182·1).
Infected eye disorders.

Betabiotic *Esseti, Ital.*
Flucloxacillin sodium (p.209·2).
Lignocaine hydrochloride (p.1293·2) is included in the intramuscular injection to alleviate the pain of injection.
Bacterial infections.

Betacap
Dermal Laboratories, Irl.; Dermal Laboratories, UK.
Betamethasone valerate (p.1033·3).
Scalp disorders.

Beta-Cardone *Medeva, UK.*
Sotalol hydrochloride (p.945·1).
Arrhythmias.

Betacarpin *Riel, Aust.*
Pilocarpine hydrochloride (p.1396·3); metipranolol hydrochloride (p.906·3).
Glaucoma.

Betacef
Note. This name is used for preparations of different composition.
FIRMA, Ital.
Cefoxitin sodium (p.170·3).
Bacterial infections.

Be-Tabs, S.Afr.
Cephalexin (p.178·2).
Bacterial infections.

Betacept *Wampole, Canad.*
Vitamin C, vitamin E, and betacarotene.

Betachron *Inwood, USA.*
Propranolol hydrochloride (p.937·1).

Betacillin *Be-Tabs, S.Afr.†.*
Phenoxymethylpenicillin potassium (p.236·2).
Bacterial infections.

Betacin *Be-Tabs, S.Afr.*
Indomethacin (p.45·2).
Gout; musculoskeletal and joint disorders.

Betaclar *Angelini, Ital.*
Befunolol hydrochloride (p.827·1).
Glaucoma.

Betaclomin *Be-Tabs, S.Afr.*
Dicyclomine hydrochloride (p.460·1); dried aluminium hydroxide gel (p.1177·3); light magnesium oxide (p.1198·3).
Gastro-intestinal disorders.

Betaclopramide *Be-Tabs, S.Afr.*
Metoclopramide hydrochloride (p.1200·3).
Gastro-intestinal disorders.

Betacod *Be-Tabs, S.Afr.†.*
Paracetamol (p.72·2); codeine phosphate (p.26·1).
Fever; pain.

The symbol † denotes a preparation no longer actively marketed

Betacomplesso *Medosan, Ital.*
Vitamin B substances.
Tonic; vitamin B deficiency.

Betacort
ICN, Canad.; Pharmagalen, Ger.†.
Betamethasone valerate (p.1033·3).
Scalp disorders.

Beta-Cortex B12 *Manetti Roberts, Ital.†.*
Cyanocobalamin (p.1363·3); betaine ascorbate (p.1553·2); suprarenal cortex (p.1050·1).
Tonic.

Betacortone *Spirig, Switz.*
Cream: Halcinonide (p.1043·2); urea (p.1095·2).
Topical solution: Halcinonide (p.1043·2).
Skin disorders.

Betacortone S *Spirig, Switz.*
Halcinonide (p.1043·2); salicylic acid (p.1090·2).
Skin disorders.

BetaCreme *Lichtenstein, Ger.*
Betamethasone valerate (p.1033·3).
Skin disorders.

Betacycline *Restan, S.Afr.†.*
Oxytetracycline hydrochloride (p.235·1).
Bacterial infections.

Betaderm
Note. This name is used for preparations of different composition.
Taro, Canad.
Betamethasone valerate (p.1033·3).
Scalp disorders; skin disorders.

Beta, Ital.
Salicylic acid (p.1090·2); aluminium acetate (p.1547·3); zinc oxide (p.1096·2).
Skin disinfection.

Betadermic *Hexal, Ger.*
Betamethasone dipropionate (p.1033·3); salicylic acid (p.1090·2).
Skin disorders.

Betadermyl
Chinoin, Ital.†; Dagra, Neth.†.
Povidone-iodine (p.1123·3).
Skin disinfection.

Betades *Farmades, Ital.*
Sotalol hydrochloride (p.945·1).
Angina pectoris; arrhythmias; hypertension.

Betadine
Faulding, Austral.; Purdue Frederick, Canad.; Asta Medica, Fr.; Intra Pharma, Irl.; Asta Medica, Ital.; Asta Medica, Neth.; Adcock Ingram Self Medication, S.Afr.; Restan, S.Afr.; Asta Medica, Spain; Mundipharma, Switz.; Seton, UK; Purdue Frederick, USA.
Povidone-iodine (p.1123·3).
Herpes labialis; infections of the skin, wounds, oropharynx, and vagina; skin, mucous membrane, and wound disinfection; viral sore throat.

Betadine First Aid Antibiotics + Moisturizer
Purdue Frederick, USA.
Polymyxin B sulphate (p.239·1); bacitracin zinc (p.157·3).
Skin infections.

Betadine Plus First Aid Antibiotics & Pain Reliever *Purdue Frederick, USA.*
Polymyxin B Sulphate (p.239·1); bacitracin zinc (p.157·3); pramoxine (p.1298·2).
Skin infections.

Betadipresan *Fides, Spain.*
Hydralazine hydrochloride (p.883·2); propranolol hydrochloride (p.937·1).
Hypertension.

Betadipresan Diu *Fides, Spain.*
Bendrofluazide (p.827·3); hydralazine hydrochloride (p.883·2); propranolol hydrochloride (p.937·1).
Hypertension.

Betadiur *Siphar, Switz.*
Amiloride hydrochloride (p.819·2); hydrochlorothiazide (p.885·2).
Hypertension; liver failure with ascites; oedema.

Betadorm *Woelm, Ger.†.*
Diphenhydramine hydrochloride (p.409·1); carbromal (p.645·2).
Sleep disorders.

Betadorm-A *Woelm, Ger.*
Diphenhydramine hydrochloride (p.409·1); 8-chlorotheophylline.
Sleep disorders.

Betadorm-N *Woelm, Ger.†.*
Diphenhydramine hydrochloride (p.409·1); valdetamide.
Sleep disorders.

Betadrenol
Schwarz, Ger.; Schwarz, Ital.†.
Bupranolol hydrochloride (p.835·2).
Cardiac disorders; hypertension.

Betadur CR *Monmouth, UK.*
Propranolol hydrochloride (p.937·1).
Angina pectoris; anxiety; essential tremor; hypertension; migraine; variceal haemorrhage.

Betaeffe Plus *Mavi, Ital.*
Betacarotene, vitamin E, and selenium preparation.
Nutritional supplement.

Betaferon
Schering, Austral.; Schering, Belg.; Schering, Fr.; Schering, Ger.; Schering, Irl.; Farmades, Ital.; Schering, Neth.; Schering, Norw.; Schering, S.Afr.; Schering, Spain; Schering, Switz.; Schering, UK.
Interferon beta-1b (p.616·1).
Multiple sclerosis.

Betaflex *Mer-National, S.Afr.*
Paracetamol (p.72·2); chlormezanone (p.648·3).
Pain and associated tension.

Betafolin B12 *Beta, Ital.†.*
Vitamin B substances; vitamin C.

Betaform Habitat *Cos Farma, Ital.*
Benzalkonium chloride (p.1101·3); a nonoxinol (p.1326·1).
Surface and room disinfection.

Betagalen *Pharmagalen, Ger.*
Betamethasone valerate (p.1033·3).
Skin disorders.

Betagan
Allergan, Austral.; Allergan, Belg.; Allergan, Canad.; Allergan, Fr.; Allergan, Irl.; Allergan, Neth.†; Allergan, S.Afr.; Allergan, Spain; Allergan, Swed.; Allergan, UK; Allergan, USA.
Levobunolol hydrochloride (p.897·3).
Glaucoma; ocular hypertension.

Betagard *Neo-Life, Austral.*
Vitamin, mineral, and amino-acid preparation.

Betagentam *Winzer, Ger.*
Betamethasone sodium phosphate (p.1033·3); gentamicin sulphate (p.212·1).
Infected eye disorders.

Betagesic *Restan, S.Afr.*
Ibuprofen (p.44·1).
Fever; musculoskeletal and joint disorders; pain.

Betagon *Schering, Ital.*
Mepindolol sulphate (p.902·3).
Angina pectoris; cardiac hyperkinesis; hypertension.

Betaimune *Pharmadass, UK.*
Vitamins A, C, and E; selenium; zinc.

Betaine Digestive Aid *Neo-Life, Austral.*
Betaine hydrochloride (p.1553·2); pepsin (p.1616·3); papain (p.1614·1); pectin (p.1474·1); natural dried beef; rhubarb (p.1212·1); liquorice (p.1197·1).
Digestive disorders.

Betaisodona
Mundipharma, Aust.; Mundipharma, Ger.
Povidone-iodine (p.1123·3).
Burns; mouth and throat disorders; skin and mucous membrane disinfection; skin disorders; vaginal infections; wounds.

Beta-Isoket
Gebro, Aust.†.
Bupranolol hydrochloride (p.835·2); isosorbide dinitrate (p.893·1).
Angina pectoris; myocardial infarction.

Schwarz, Ger.†.
Bupranolol hydrochloride (p.835·2); isosorbide dinitrate (p.893·1).
Cardiovascular disorders.

Betalactam *Bergamon, Ital.†.*
Latamoxef disodium (p.221·2).
Bacterial infections.

Betalevo *Simes, Ital.†.*
Levomoprolol hydrochloride (p.898·1); mebutizide (p.901·3).
Hypertension.

Betalin *Be-Tabs, S.Afr.*
Diphenhydramine hydrochloride (p.409·1); ammonium chloride (p.1055·2); sodium citrate (p.1153·2); menthol (p.1600·2).
Coughs.

Betalin Compound *Lilly, USA†.*
Vitamin B complex.

Betalix *Be-Tabs, S.Afr.*
Chlorpheniramine maleate (p.405·1); phenylpropanolamine hydrochloride (p.1067·2); phenylephrine hydrochloride (p.1066·2).
Nasal congestion.

Betaloc
Astra, Austral.; Astra, Canad.; Astra, Irl.; Astra, UK.
Metoprolol tartrate (p.907·3).
Angina pectoris; arrhythmias; hypertension; hyperthyroidism; migraine; myocardial infarction.

Betamann *Mann, Ger.*
Metipranolol hydrochloride (p.906·3).
Glaucoma.

Betamatil *Inibsa, Spain.*
Betamethasone valerate (p.1033·3).
Skin disorders.

Betamatil con Neomicina *Inibsa, Spain.*
Betamethasone valerate (p.1033·3); neomycin sulphate (p.229·2).
Infected skin disorders.

Betamaze *Pfizer, Fr.*
Sulbactam sodium (p.250·3).
Bacterial infections.

Betamed *Kwizda, Aust.*
Bupranolol hydrochloride (p.835·2); diazepam (p.661·1).
Anxiety disorders.

Betamethason Plus *Heumann, Ger.*
Betamethasone dipropionate (p.1033·3); salicylic acid (p.1090·2).
Skin disorders.

Betamican *Alter, Spain.*
Salmeterol xinafoate (p.761·2).
Obstructive airways disease.

Betamida *Cusi, Spain.*
Betamethasone sodium phosphate (p.1033·3); sulphacetamide sodium (p.252·2).
Eye disorders.

Betamin *Rhone-Poulenc Rorer, Austral.*
Thiamine hydrochloride (p.1361·1).
Vitamin B_1 deficiency.

Betamine *Wolfs, Belg.*
Thiamine hydrochloride (p.1361·1).
Alcoholic polyneuropathy; beri-beri; neuralgia.

Betam-Ophtal *Winzer, Ger.*
Betamethasone sodium phosphate (p.1033·3).
Eye disorders.

Betamox *Be-Tabs, S.Afr.*
Amoxycillin trihydrate (p.151·3).
Bacterial infections.

Betamycin *Be-Tabs, S.Afr.*
Erythromycin estolate (p.204·1).
Bacterial infections.

Beta-Nephral *Pfleger, Ger.*
Propranolol hydrochloride (p.937·1); triamterene (p.957·2); hydrochlorothiazide (p.885·2).
Hypertension.

Betanol *Allergan, Fr.†.*
Metipranolol (p.906·2).
Glaucoma; ocular hypertension.

Betantrone *Italfarmaco, Ital.*
Interferon beta (p.616·1).
Hepatitis; malignant neoplasms; viral infections.

Beta-Ophtiole
Riel, Aust.; Tramedico, Belg.; Mann, Neth.; Bausch & Lomb, S.Afr.
Metipranolol hydrochloride (p.906·3).
Glaucoma; ocular hypertension.

Betapace *Berlex, USA.*
Sotalol hydrochloride (p.945·1).
Arrhythmias.

Betapam *Be-Tabs, S.Afr.*
Diazepam (p.661·1).
Alcohol withdrawal syndrome; anxiety; premedication.

Betapen *Be-Tabs, S.Afr.*
Phenoxymethylpenicillin potassium (p.236·2).
Bacterial infections.

Betapen-VK *Apothecon, USA†.*
Phenoxymethylpenicillin potassium (p.236·2).
Bacterial infections.

Betaperamide *Restan, S.Afr.*
Loperamide hydrochloride (p.1197·2).
Diarrhoea.

Betaphlem *Be-Tabs, S.Afr.*
Carbocisteine (p.1056·3).
Respiratory-tract disorders.

Betapindol *Helvepharm, Switz.*
Pindolol (p.931·1).
Angina pectoris; arrhythmias; hypertension.

Betaplex B12 *Molteni, Ital.†.*
Vitamin B substances.

Betaplus *Sigma-Tau, Ital.†.*
Vitamin B substances; carnitine; glycocyamine.

Betapred *Glaxo Wellcome, Swed.*
Betamethasone sodium phosphate (p.1033·3).
Corticosteroid.

Betapressin
Hoechst, Aust.; Hoechst, Ger.; Hoechst Marion Roussel, Ital.†.
Penbutolol sulphate (p.927·2).
Angina pectoris; arrhythmias; hypertension; myocardial infarction.

Betapressine
Roussel, Fr.; Hoechst Marion Roussel, Switz.†.
Penbutolol sulphate (p.927·2).
Angina pectoris; hypertension.

Betaprofen *Be-Tabs, S.Afr.*
Ibuprofen (p.44·1).
Musculoskeletal and joint disorders.

Beta-Prograne *Tillomed, UK.*
Propranolol hydrochloride (p.937·1).
Angina pectoris; anxiety; essential tremor; hypertension; hyperthyroidism; migraine; prophylaxis of upper gastro-intestinal bleeding.

Betaprol *Helvepharm, Switz.*
Propranolol hydrochloride (p.937·1).
Angina pectoris; arrhythmias; hypertension; migraine; phaeochromocytoma.

Betapyn *Restan, S.Afr.*
Syrup†: Diphenhydramine hydrochloride (p.409·1); paracetamol (p.72·2); codeine phosphate (p.26·1).
Tablets: Paracetamol (p.72·2); codeine phosphate (p.26·1); doxylamine succinate (p.410·1); caffeine (p.749·3).
Fever; muscular tension; pain.

Betapyr *Wolfs, Belg.*
Thiamine hydrochloride (p.1361·1); pyridoxine hydrochloride (p.1362·3).
Alcoholic polyneuritis; prophylaxis during isoniazid therapy; vitamin B_1 and/or B_6 deficiency.

Betarelix *Hoechst, Ger.*
Penbutolol sulphate (p.927·2); piretanide (p.931·3).
Hypertension.

Betaretic *Be-Tabs, S.Afr.*
Amiloride hydrochloride (p.819·2); hydrochlorothiazide (p.885·2).
Hypertension; oedema.

Betartrinovo *Llorens, Spain.*
Betamethasone phosphate (p.1034·1); indomethacin (p.45·2).
Musculoskeletal and joint disorders; peri-articular disorders.

BetaSalbe *Lichtenstein, Ger.*
Betamethasone valerate (p.1033·3).
Skin disorders.

Betasan *Mundipharma, Aust.*
Povidone-iodine (p.1123·3).
Mouth and throat infections; wounds.

Betascor B12 *Manetti Roberts, Ital.*
Betaine ascorbate (p.1553·2); cyanocobalamin (p.1363·3).
Vitamin C deficiency.

Betaselen *Arkopharma, Fr.*
Multivitamin and mineral preparation.
Tonic.

Betasemid
Hoechst, Ger.; Hoechst Marion Roussel, Ital.†.
Penbutolol sulphate (p.927·2); frusemide (p.871·1).
Hypertension.

Betasept
Note. This name is used for preparations of different composition.
Napp, UK†.
Povidone-iodine (p.1123·3).
Acne; oro-pharyngeal infections; seborrhoeic scalp disorders.

Purdue Frederick, USA.
Chlorhexidine gluconate (p.1107·2).
Skin and wound disinfection.

Betaseptic
Note. This name is used for preparations of different composition.
Mundipharma, Aust.; Asta Medica, Ital.; Asta Medica, Spain†.
Povidone-iodine (p.1123·3).
Burns; skin disinfection; wounds.

Mundipharma, Ger.; Mundipharma, Switz.
Povidone-iodine (p.1123·3); isopropyl alcohol (p.1118·2); alcohol (p.1099·1).
Skin disinfection.

Betaserc
Solvay, Aust.; Solvay, Belg.; Solvay, Neth.; Solvay, Switz.
Betahistine hydrochloride (p.1553·1).
Ménière's disease; vestibular disorders.

Betaseron
Berlex, Canad.; Berlex, USA.
Interferon beta-1b (p.616·1).
Multiple sclerosis.

Betasit Plus *Ferrer, Spain.*
Chlorthalidone (p.839·3); atenolol (p.825·3).
Hypertension.

Betasleep *Restan, S.Afr.*
Diphenhydramine hydrochloride (p.409·1).
Insomnia.

Betasoda *Restan, S.Afr.*
Citric acid (p.1564·3); sodium bicarbonate (p.1153·2).
Urinary alkalinisation.

Beta-Sol *Fawns & McAllan, Austral.*
Thiamine hydrochloride (p.1361·1).
Symptoms of vitamin B_1 deficiency.

Beta-Stulln *Stulln, Ger.*
Betamethasone sodium phosphate (p.1033·3).
Eye disorders.

Betasyn *Jacoby, Aust.*
Atenolol (p.825·3).
Angina pectoris; arrhythmias; hypertension; myocardial infarction.

Beta-Tablinen *Sanorania, Ger.*
Propranolol hydrochloride (p.937·1).
Angina pectoris; anxiety; arrhythmias; essential tremor; hypertension; migraine.

Betathiazid *Henning, Ger.*
Propranolol hydrochloride (p.937·1); triamterene (p.957·2); hydrochlorothiazide (p.885·2).
Hypertension.

Betathiazid A *Henning, Ger.*
Propranolol hydrochloride (p.937·1); hydrochlorothiazide (p.885·2).
Hypertension.

Beta-Tim *Ciba Vision, Canad.*
Timolol maleate (p.953·3).
Glaucoma.

Beta-Timelets *Temmler, Ger.†.*
Propranolol hydrochloride (p.937·1).
Angina pectoris; hypertension.

Betatop *Marcofina, Fr.*
Atenolol (p.825·3).
Angina pectoris; hypertension.

Betatrex *Savage, USA.*
Betamethasone valerate (p.1033·3).
Skin disorders.

Betatul *Asta Medica, Spain.*
Povidone-iodine (p.1123·3).
Skin disinfection; skin infections.

Beta-Turfa *BASF, Ger.*
Propranolol hydrochloride (p.937·1); triamterene (p.957·2); hydrochlorothiazide (p.885·2).
Hypertension.

Beta-Val *Lemmon, USA.*
Betamethasone valerate (p.1033·3).
Skin disorders.

Betavit *Rivopharm, Switz.†.*
Vitamin preparation.

Betaxin *Sanofi Winthrop, Canad.*
Thiamine hydrochloride (p.1361·1).

Betaxina *Terapeutico, Ital.*
Nalidixic acid (p.228·2).
Gram-negative genito-urinary tract infections.

Betazok *Astra, Irl.*
Metoprolol succinate (p.908·2).
Angina pectoris; hypertension.

BETE *Laevosan, Aust.*
Benztropine hydrochloride (p.458·2).
Pain with spasmodic disorders.

Bethacil *Bioindustria, Ital.*
Injection: Sulbactam sodium (p.250·3); ampicillin sodium (p.153·1).
Lignocaine hydrochloride (p.1293·2) is included in the intramuscular injection to alleviate the pain of injection.
Oral suspension: Sultamicillin (p.257·2).
Tablets: Sultamicillin tosylate (p.257·2).
Bacterial infections.

Betim
Leo, Irl.†; Leo, Norw.; Leo, UK.
Timolol maleate (p.953·3).
Angina pectoris; hypertension; hyperthyroidism; migraine; myocardial infarction.

Betimol *Ciba Vision, USA.*
Timolol (p.954·1).
Raised intra-ocular pressure.

Betinex *Approved Prescription Services, UK.*
Bumetanide (p.834·3).
Oedema.

Betitotal *Propan, S.Afr.*
Multivitamin and mineral preparation.

Betnelan
Evans Medical, Irl.; Glaxo Wellcome, Neth.; Glaxo Wellcome, S.Afr.†; Medeva, UK.
Betamethasone (p.1033·2) or betamethasone valerate (p.1033·3).
Corticosteroid.

Betnelan Clioquinol *Glaxo Wellcome, Neth.†.*
Betamethasone valerate (p.1033·3); clioquinol (p.193·2).
Infected skin disorders.

Betnelan Neomycine *Glaxo Wellcome, Neth.†.*
Betamethasone valerate (p.1033·3); neomycin sulphate (p.229·2).
Infected skin disorders.

Betnelan-V *Glaxo Wellcome, Belg.*
Betamethasone valerate (p.1033·3).
Skin disorders.

Betnelan-VC *Glaxo Wellcome, Belg.*
Betamethasone valerate (p.1033·3); clioquinol (p.193·2).
Infected skin disorders.

Betnelan-VN *Glaxo Wellcome, Belg.*
Betamethasone valerate (p.1033·3); neomycin sulphate (p.229·2).
Infected skin disorders.

Betnesalic
Glaxo Wellcome, Fr.; Glaxo Wellcome, Ger.; Wolff, Ger.; Glaxo Wellcome, Switz.
Betamethasone valerate (p.1033·3); salicylic acid (p.1090·2).
Skin disorders.

Betnesol
Glaxo Wellcome, Aust.; Glaxo Wellcome, Belg.; Roberts, Canad.; Glaxo Wellcome, Fr.; Evans Medical, Irl.; Glaxo Wellcome, Neth.; Allen & Hanburys, S.Afr.; Glaxo Wellcome, Switz.; Medeva, UK.
Betamethasone (p.1033·2) or betamethasone sodium phosphate (p.1033·3).
Corticosteroid.

Glaxo Wellcome, Ger.†.
Depot injection†: Betamethasone (p.1033·2); betamethasone sodium phosphate (p.1033·3).
Parenteral corticosteroid.
Enema: Betamethasone sodium phosphate (p.1033·3).
Ulcerative colitis.
Pastilles†: Betamethasone (p.1033·2).
Hypersensitivity reactions; inflammation of oral mucous membranes; lichen; pemphigoid.

Betnesol-N
Glaxo Wellcome, Aust.; Evans Medical, Irl.; Allen & Hanburys, S.Afr.; Medeva, UK.
Betamethasone sodium phosphate (p.1033·3); neomycin sulphate (p.229·2).
Infected eye, ear, and nasal disorders.

Betnesol-V *Glaxo Wellcome, Ger.; Wolff, Ger.*
Betamethasone valerate (p.1033·3).
Scalp disorders; skin disorders.

Betnesol-VN *Glaxo Wellcome, Ger.†.*
Betamethasone valerate (p.1033·3); neomycin sulphate (p.229·2).
Skin disorders.

Betnesol-WL *Glaxo Wellcome, Ger.†.*
Betamethasone sodium phosphate (p.1033·3).
Corticosteroid.

Betneval *Glaxo Wellcome, Fr.*
Betamethasone valerate (p.1033·3).
Mouth disorders; skin disorders.

Betneval-Neomycine *Glaxo Wellcome, Fr.*
Betamethasone valerate (p.1033·3); neomycin sulphate (p.229·2).
Infected skin disorders.

Betnovat
Glaxo Wellcome, Norw.; Glaxo Wellcome, Swed.
Betamethasone valerate (p.1033·3).
Otitis externa; skin disorders.

Betnovat med Chinoform
Glaxo Wellcome, Norw.; Glaxo Wellcome, Swed.
Betamethasone valerate (p.1033·3); clioquinol (p.193·2).
Infected skin disorders.

Betnovat med neomycin *Glaxo Wellcome, Swed.*
Betamethasone valerate (p.1033·3); neomycin sulphate (p.229·2).
Infected skin disorders.

Betnovate
Glaxo Wellcome, Aust.; Glaxo Wellcome, Austral.; Roberts, Canad.; Glaxo Wellcome, Irl.; Allen & Hanburys, S.Afr.; Evans, Spain; Glaxo Wellcome, Switz.; Glaxo, UK.
Betamethasone valerate (p.1033·3).
Skin and scalp disorders.

Betnovate RD (Ready Diluted) *Glaxo, UK.*
Betamethasone valerate (p.1033·3).
Skin disorders.

Betnovate Rectal Ointment *Glaxo, UK.*
Betamethasone valerate (p.1033·3); lignocaine hydrochloride (p.1293·2); phenylephrine hydrochloride (p.1066·2).
Anorectal disorders.

Betnovate-C
Glaxo Wellcome, Aust.; Glaxo Wellcome, Irl.; Allen & Hanburys, S.Afr.; Glaxo Wellcome, Switz.; Glaxo, UK.
Betamethasone valerate (p.1033·3); clioquinol (p.193·2).
Infected skin disorders.

Betnovate-N
Glaxo Wellcome, Aust.; Glaxo Wellcome, Canad.†; Glaxo Wellcome, Irl.; Allen & Hanburys, S.Afr.†; Glaxo Wellcome, Switz.; Glaxo, UK.
Betamethasone valerate (p.1033·3); neomycin sulphate (p.229·2).
Infected skin disorders.

Betoid
Yamanouchi, Norw.; Yamanouchi, Swed.
Betamethasone valerate (p.1033·3).
Skin disorders.

Betolvex
Dumex, Neth.†; Dumex, Norw.; Lagamed, S.Afr.; Dumex-Alpharma, Swed.; Dumex, Switz.
Cyanocobalamin (p.1363·3) or cyanocobalamin tannate (p.1364·2).
Vitamin B_{12} deficiency.

Betoptic
Alcon, Aust.; Bayer, Austral.; Alcon, Belg.; Alcon, Canad.; Alcon, Fr.; Alcon, Irl.; Alcon, Ital.; Alcon, Neth.†; Alcon, Norw.; Alcon, S.Afr.; Alcon, Spain; Alcon, Swed.; Alcon, Switz.; Alcon, UK; Alcon, USA.
Betaxolol hydrochloride (p.832·1).
Glaucoma; ocular hypertension.

Betoptima *Alcon-Thilo, Ger.*
Betaxolol hydrochloride (p.832·1).
Glaucoma; ocular hypertension.

Betoquin *Ioquin, Austral.*
Betaxolol hydrochloride (p.832·1).
Glaucoma; ocular hypertension.

Be-Total *Pharmacia Upjohn, Ital.*
Vitamin B substances.
Vitamin B deficiency.

Betrimax
Anphar-Rolland, Fr.†; Lipha, Ger.†; Rolland, Switz.†.
Vitamin B substances.
Chronic alcoholism; neuropathies; pain; rheumatic disorders; vitamin B deficiency.

Betriphos-C *Schwarz, Fr.*
Adenosine triphosphate sodium (p.1543·2); vitamin B substances; ascorbic acid.
Tonic.

Betron R *Italfarmaco, Ital.*
Interferon beta (human, recombinant) (p.616·1).
Malignant neoplasms; viral infections.

Betsuril *Berenguer Infale, Spain.*
Beclomethasone dipropionate (p.1032·1).
Asthma.

Bettamousse *Medeva, UK.*
Betamethasone valerate (p.1033·3).
Scalp disorders.

Betulac *Meda, Swed.*
Lactulose (p.1195·3).
Constipation; hepatic encephalopathy.

Betuline *Ferndale, USA.*
Methyl salicylate (p.55·2); camphor (p.1557·2); menthol (p.1600·2).
Muscle, joint, and soft-tissue pain; neuralgia.

Betullosin *Vis, Ital.†.*
Betula (p.1553·3); resorcinol (p.1090·1); lignocaine hydrochloride (p.1293·2); hamamelis (p.1587·1).
Eye disorders.

Be-Uric *Be-Tabs, S.Afr.*
Allopurinol (p.390·2).
Gout; hyperuricaemia.

Beviplex *Meuse, Belg.*
Vitamin B substances.
Neuritis; vitamin B deficiency.

Beviplex forte *Abigo, Swed.*
Vitamin B substances.
Alcoholism; neuropathies; vitamin B deficiency.

Bevispas *Lennon, S.Afr.*
Mebeverine hydrochloride (p.1199·2).
Irritable bowel syndrome.

Bevit Forte *Biocur, Ger.*
Thiamine hydrochloride (p.1361·1) pyridoxine hydrochloride (p.1362·3).
Nervous system disorders.

Be-Vital *Be-Tabs, S.Afr.*
Multivitamin and mineral preparation.

Bevitin *Abbott, Ital.*
Vitamin B substances.
Vitamin B deficiency.

Bevitine *Specia, Fr.*
Thiamine hydrochloride (p.1361·1).
Beri beri; neuritis; vitamin B deficiency.

Bevitol *Lannacher, Aust.*
Thiamine hydrochloride (p.1361·1).
Vitamin B_1 deficiency.

Bevitotal comp. *Astra, Swed.*
Vitamin B substances with vitamin C.
Neuropathies; vitamin B and C deficiency.

Bevoren *Sintesa, Belg.*
Glibenclamide (p.319·3).
Diabetes mellitus.

Bewon *Charton, Canad.*
Thiamine hydrochloride (p.1361·1).

Bex
Note. This name is used for preparations of different composition.
Roche Consumer, Austral.
Aspirin (p.16·1).
Fever; pain.

Lalco, Canad.
Vitamin B substances and vitamin C.

Bexalin *Pinewood, Irl.†.*
Diphenhydramine hydrochloride (p.409·1); ammonium chloride (p.1055·2); sodium citrate (p.1153·2); menthol (p.1600·2).
Coughs; respiratory-tract congestion.

Bexedan *UCB, Ital.†.*
Chlorcyclizine dibunate (p.404·3).
Coughs.

Bexedyl *Sanofi Midy, Neth.†.*
Sodium dibunate (p.1070·1).
Coughs.

Bexedyl Expectorans *Sanofi Midy, Neth.†.*
Sodium dibunate (p.1070·1); guaiphenesin (p.1061·3).
Coughs.

Bexicortil *Isdin, Spain.*
Fluorometholone (p.1042·1); miconazole nitrate (p.384·3); neomycin sulphate (p.229·2).
Infected skin disorders.

Bexidermil *Isdin, Spain.*
Triethanolamine salicylate (p.1639·2).
Peri-articular disorders; soft-tissue disorders.

Bexilona *Isdin, Spain†.*
Diflorasone diacetate (p.1039·3).
Skin disorders.

Bexine *Spirig, Switz.*
Dextromethorphan hydrobromide (p.1057·3).
Coughs.

Beza *CT, Ger.*
Bezafibrate (p.1268·2).
Hyperlipidaemias.

Beza Lande *Synthelabo, Ger.*
Bezafibrate (p.1268·2).
Hyperlipidaemias.

Beza Puren *Isis Puren, Ger.*
Bezafibrate (p.1268·2).
Hyperlipidaemias.

Bezacur *Hexal, Ger.*
Bezafibrate (p.1268·2).
Hyperlipidaemias.

Bezalip
Boehringer Mannheim, Aust.; Boehringer Mannheim, Canad.; Boehringer Mannheim, Ital.; Boehringer Mannheim, Jpn; Boehringer Mannheim, Neth.; Boehringer Mannheim, S.Afr.; Boehringer Mannheim, Swed.; Boehringer Mannheim, UK.
Bezafibrate (p.1268·2).
Hyperlipidaemias.

Bezalip Mono *Boehringer Mannheim, UK.*
Bezafibrate (p.1268·2).
Hyperlipidaemias.

Bezamerck *Merck, Ger.*
Bezafibrate (p.1268·2).
Hyperlipidaemias.

BFI
Merck Sharp & Dohme, Austral.
Bismuth-formic-iodide (p.1181·1); magnesium carbonate (p.1198·1); zinc *p*-phenolsulphonate (p.1096·3); pentyloxyphenol; alum (p.1547·1); thymol (p.1127·1); menthol (p.1600·2); cineole (p.1564·1); bismuth subgallate (p.1180·2).
Damaged skin; pruritus.

Menley & James, USA.
Bismuth-formic-iodide (p.1181·1); zinc phenolsulphonate (p.1096·3); alum (p.1547·1); bismuth subgallate (p.1180·2); boric acid (p.1554·2); menthol (p.1600·2); cineole (p.1564·1); thymol (p.1127·1).
Antiseptic.

B_{12}-Fol-Vicotrat *Heyl, Ger.*
Cyanocobalamin (p.1363·3); folic acid (p.1340·3).
Vitamin B_{12} and folic acid deficiency.

Bgramin *Douglas, Austral.*
Amoxycillin trihydrate (p.151·3).
Bacterial infections.

B12-Horfervit *Arteva, Ger.*
Cyanocobalamin (p.1363·3).
Vitamin B_{12} deficiency.

Biactol Antibacterial Double Action Pads *Procter & Gamble (H&B Care), UK†.*
Salicylic acid (p.1090·2).

Biactol Antibacterial Facewash *Procter & Gamble, Irl.*
Phenoxypropanol (p.1122·2).
Acne.

Biactol Liquid *Procter & Gamble (H&B Care), UK.*
Phenoxypropanol (p.1122·2).
Acne.

Biaferone *Biagini, Ital.*
Interferon alfa (p.615·3).
Hepatitis; malignant neoplasms; viral infections.

Biafine *Medix, Fr.*
Soap substitute.
Burns.

Biaflu *Biagini, Ital.*
An adsorbed inactivated influenza vaccine (p.1515·2).
Active immunisation.

Biaflu-Zonale SU *Biagini, Ital.*
An influenza vaccine (p.1515·2).
Active immunisation.

Bi-Aglut
Distriborg, Fr.; Plasmon, Ital.; Ultrapharm, UK.
A range of gluten-free and lactose-reduced foods.
Gluten and lactose intolerance.

Bialcol *Zyma, Ital.*
Benzoxonium chloride (p.1103·3).
Disinfection of skin, wounds, burns, and surfaces.

Bianco Val *Edmond Pharma, Ital.*
Valerian (p.1643·1); crataegus (p.1568·2).
Hyperexcitability; insomnia.

Biarison
Biochemie, Aust.; Wander, Switz.†.
Proquazone (p.81·3).
Gout; musculoskeletal, joint, peri-articular, and soft tissue disorders.

Biartac *Merck Sharp & Dohme, Belg.*
Diflunisal (p.33·2).
Arthrosis; polyarthritis.

Biavax II *Merck Sharp & Dohme, USA.*
A rubella and mumps vaccine (Wistar RA 27/3 and Jeryl Lynn (B level) strains respectively) (p.1533·2).
Active immunisation.

Biaven *Biagini, Ital.*
A normal immunoglobulin (p.1522·1).
Hypogammaglobulinaemia; idiopathic thrombocytopenic purpura; immunodeficiency.

Biaxin
Note. This name is used for preparations of different composition.
Sigma, Austral.†.
Roxithromycin (p.247·1).
Bacterial infections.

Abbott, Canad.; Abbott, USA.
Clarithromycin (p.189·1).
Bacterial infections.

Biaxin HP *Abbott, Ger.*
Clarithromycin (p.189·1).
Helicobacter pylori infections.

Biaxsig *Sigma, Austral.*
Roxithromycin (p.247·1).
Bacterial infections.

Biazolina *Fermenti, Ital.*
Cephazolin sodium (p.181·1).
Bacterial infections.

Bibivit Light *Lampugnani, Ital.*
Multivitamin and carbohydrate preparation with fruit and plant extracts.
Nutritional supplement.

BiCart *Gambro, Swed.*
Concentrates for haemodialysis solutions: Sodium chloride; potassium chloride; magnesium chloride; calcium chloride glacial acetic acid (p.1151·1).
To be used with BiCart powder.
Powder for haemodialysis solutions: Sodium bicarbonate (p.1151·1).
To be used with BiCart concentrates.

Bicbag *Dicamed, Swed.*
Sodium bicarbonate (p.1151·1).
Haemodialysis.

Bicetil *Menarini, Spain.*
Quinapril hydrochloride (p.938·1); hydrochlorothiazide (p.885·2).
Hypertension.

Bi-Chinine *Rhone-Poulenc Rorer, Austral.†.*
Quinine bisulphate (p.439·1).
Malaria; night cramps.

Bicholate *Sabex, Canad.*
Bile salts (p.1553·2); cascara (p.1183·1); phenolphthalein (p.1208·2); aloin (p.1177·2).
Constipation.

Bicillin *Yamanouchi, UK.*
Procaine penicillin (p.240·2); benzylpenicillin sodium (p.159·3).
Bacterial infections.

Bicillin All Purpose *Wyeth, Austral.†.*
Benzathine penicillin (p.158·3); procaine penicillin (p.240·2); benzylpenicillin potassium (p.159·2).
Bacterial infections.

Bicillin A-P *Wyeth-Ayerst, Canad.*
Benzathine penicillin (p.158·3); procaine penicillin (p.240·2); benzylpenicillin potassium (p.159·2).
Bacterial infections.

Bicillin C-R *Wyeth-Ayerst, USA.*
Benzathine penicillin (p.158·3); procaine penicillin (p.240·2).
Bacterial infections.

Bicillin L-A
Lederle, Austral.; Wyeth-Ayerst, Canad.; Akromed, S.Afr.; Wyeth-Ayerst, USA.
Benzathine penicillin (p.158·3).
Bacterial infections.

Bicilline *Yamanouchi, Neth.*
Procaine penicillin (p.240·2); benzylpenicillin sodium (p.159·3).
Bacterial infections.

Biciron *Basotherm, Ger.*
Tramazoline hydrochloride (p.1071·1).
Eye disorders.

Bicitra *Willen, USA.*
Sodium citrate (p.1153·2); citric acid monohydrate (p.1564·3).
Chronic metabolic acidosis; urine alkalinising agent.

Bi-Citrol
Pharmethic, Belg.; Diepha, Fr.
Monosodium citrate; sodium citrate (p.1153·2).
Dyspepsia.

Biclar *Abbott, Belg.*
Clarithromycin (p.189·1).
Bacterial infections; toxoplasmosis.

Biclin *Bristol-Myers, Spain.*
Amikacin sulphate (p.150·2).
Bacterial infections.

Biclinocilline *Sanofi Winthrop, Fr.*
Benethamine penicillin (p.158·3); benzylpenicillin sodium (p.159·3).
Bacterial infections.

BiCNU
Bristol-Myers Squibb, Austral.; Bristol, Canad.; Bristol-Myers Squibb, Fr.; Bristol-Myers Squibb, Irl.; Bristol-Myers Squibb, S.Afr.; Bristol-Myers Squibb, UK; Bristol-Myers Oncology, USA.
Carmustine (p.511·3).
Malignant neoplasms.

Bicomplex *ABC, Ital.*
Vitamin B substances.
Vitamin B deficiency.

Bicozene *Sandoz, USA.*
Benzocaine (p.1286·2); resorcinol (p.1090·1).
Local anaesthesia.

Bidiabe *Sanofi Winthrop, Ital.*
Chlorpropamide (p.319·1); phenformin hydrochloride (p.330·3).
Diabetes mellitus.

Bidiamet *Guidotti, Ital.†.*
Chlorpropamide (p.319·1); metformin hydrochloride (p.330·1).
Diabetes mellitus.

Bidien *IDI, Ital.*
Budesonide (p.1034·3).
Skin disorders.

Bidocef *Bristol-Myers Squibb, Ger.*
Cefadroxil (p.163·3).
Bacterial infections.

Bidor *Weleda, UK.*
Ferrous sulphate (p.1340·2); silica (p.1474·3).
Headaches; migraine.

Bidramine *Nelson, Austral.†.*
Diphenhydramine hydrochloride (p.409·1); ammonium chloride (p.1055·2); sodium citrate (p.1153·2); menthol (p.1600·2).
Cough and cold symptoms.

Bidrolar *Spyfarma, Spain.*
Prunus africana.
Prostatic adenoma.

Bienfait Total *Lancome, Canad.*
SPF 15: Ethylhexyl *p*-methoxycinnamate (p.1487·1); 2-phenyl-1*H*-benzimidazole-5-sulphonic acid (p.1488·2).
Sunscreen.

Bietapres *Medix, Spain†.*
Bietaserpine (p.832·3); hydrochlorothiazide (p.885·2).
Hypertension.

Bietapres Complex *Medix, Spain†.*
Bietaserpine (p.832·3); dihydralazine hydrochloride (p.854·1); hydrochlorothiazide (p.885·2).
Hypertension.

Bi-Euglucon *Boehringer Mannheim, Ital.*
Glibenclamide (p.319·3); phenformin hydrochloride (p.330·3).
Diabetes mellitus.

Bi-Euglucon M *Boehringer Mannheim, Ital.*
Glibenclamide (p.319·3); metformin hydrochloride (p.330·1).
Diabetes mellitus.

Bifazol *Bayer, Ital.*
Bifonazole (p.375·3).
Fungal skin infections.

Bifenabid *Marion Merrell, Spain.*
Probucol (p.1277·3).
Hyperlipidaemias.

Bifilact *Fermenti, Ital.*
Lactobacillus acidophilus (p.1594·1); *Bifidobacterium bifidum* (p.1594·1).
Maintenance of normal gastro-intestinal flora.

Bifinorma *Merckle, Ger.*
Lactulose (p.1195·3).
Constipation; hepatic encephalopathy; salmonella enteritis.

Bifiteral
Solvay, Aust.; Solvay, Belg.; Solvay, Ger.
Lactulose (p.1195·3).
Constipation; hepatic encephalopathy; salmonella enteritis.

Bifokey *Inkeysa, Spain.*
Bifonazole (p.375·3).
Fungal skin and nail infections.

Bifomyk *Hexal, Ger.*
Bifonazole (p.375·3).
Fungal skin infections.

Bifort *Merck, Spain.*
Cafedrine hydrochloride (p.835·3); theodrenaline hydrochloride (p.1636·2).
Hypotension.

Big V *Tanning Research, Canad.*
SPF 15: Ethylhexyl *p*-methoxycinnamate (p.1487·1); oxybenzone (p.1487·3).
SPF 30: Homosalate (p.1487·2); ethylhexyl *p*-methoxycinnamate (p.1487·1); octyl salicylate (p.1487·3); oxybenzone (p.1487·3).
Sunscreen.

Big V Baby *Tanning Research, Canad.*
SPF 30: Homosalate (p.1487·2); ethylhexyl *p*-methoxycinnamate (p.1487·1); octyl salicylate (p.1487·3); oxybenzone (p.1487·3).
Sunscreen.

Big V Cough Lozenge *Sutton, Canad.*
Menthol (p.1600·2).

Big V Kids *Tanning Research, Canad.*
Ethylhexyl *p*-methoxycinnamate (p.1487·1); octocrylene (p.1487·3); octyl salicylate (p.1487·3); oxybenzone (p.1487·3).
Sunscreen.

Bigasan *Phyteia, Switz.*
Aluminium hydroxide (p.1177·3); magnesium hydroxide (p.1198·2); magnesium oxide (p.1198·3); magnesium silicate (p.1473·3); mannitol (p.900·3).
Gastric hyperacidity.

Bigonist *Cassenne, Fr.*
Buserelin acetate (p.1241·3).
Prostatic cancer.

Bigpen *Fides, Spain.*
Amoxycillin trihydrate (p.151·3); potassium clavulanate (p.190·2).
Bacterial infections.

Bikalm *Byk Gulden, Ger.*
Zolpidem tartrate (p.698·3).
Sleep disorders.

Biklin
Frika, Aust.; Bristol-Myers Squibb, Ger.; Bristol-Myers Squibb, Swed.
Amikacin sulphate (p.150·2).
Bacterial infections.

Bilagar *SIT, Ital.†.*
Phenolphthalein (p.1208·2); ox bile extract (p.1553·2).
Constipation.

Bilagit Mono *Temmler, Ger.*
Curcuma zanthorrhiza.
Dyspepsia.

Bilagol *Janssen-Cilag, Belg.*
Di-isopromine hydrochloride (p.1189·1); sorbitol (p.1354·2).
Constipation; hepatobiliary disorders.

Bilancen *Biomedica, Ital.†.*
Vincamine (p.1644·1); papaverine hydrochloride (p.1614·2).
Cerebrovascular disorders.

Bilarcil *Bayer, Ger.†.*
Metriphonate (p.105·1).
Schistosomiasis.

Bilarvis *Vis, Ital.†.*
Cynarine (p.1569·3); boldo (p.1554·1); gentian (p.1583·3); rhubarb (p.1212·1); cascara (p.1183·1); sorbitol (p.1354·2).
Biliary-tract disorders; liver disorders.

Bilatin *Stada, Aust.*
Lecithin (p.1595·2); liver extract.
Tonic.

Bilatin Fischol *Stada, Ger.*
Marine triglycerides (p.1276·1).
Hyperlipidaemias.

Bilberry Plus *Eagle, Austral.*
Bilberry (p.1606·1); euphrasia; fenugreek (p.1579·3); golden seal (p.1588·2).
Eye disorders.

Bilenor *Schwarz, Ital.*
Magnesium trihydrate salt of chenodeoxycholic and ursodeoxycholic acids (pp.1562·1 and 1642·1).
Biliary dyspepsia; gallstones.

Bilezyme *Geriatric Pharm. Corp., USA†.*
Standardised amylolytic enzyme (Gerilase) (p.1549·1); standardised proteolytic enzyme (Geriprotase); dehydrocholic acid (p.1570·2); deoxycholic acid.
Gastro-intestinal disorders.

Bilgast *Rorer, Ger.†.*
Ox bile (p.1553·2); turmeric (p.1001·3); silybum marianum (p.993·3); chelidonium; peppermint leaf (p.1208·1); frangula bark (p.1193·2).
Biliary disorders; digestive disorders of the liver and bile; meteorism.

Bilgast echinac *Bilgast, Ger.*
Echinacea purpurea (p.1574·2).
Respiratory- and urinary-tract infections.

Bilibyk *Byk Gulden, Ital.†.*
Iobenzamic acid.
Contrast medium for biliary-tract radiography.

Bilibyk/KM-Suspension *Byk Gulden, Ger.†.*
Combination pack: Tablets, iobenzamic acid; suspension, sorbitol (p.1354·2).
Contrast medium for biliary-tract radiography.

Bilicanta *Boehringer Mannheim, Spain.*
Hymecromone (p.1589·3).
Biliary-tract disorders.

Bilicante *Lipha, Switz.†.*
Hymecromone (p.1589·3).
Biliary disorders; dyspepsia.

Bilicombin sp *Brunnengraber, Ger.†.*
Atropine sulphate (p.455·1); bile acids (p.1553·2).
Formerly contained atropine sulphate, papaverine hydrochloride, and bile acids.
Biliary disorders; gallstones.

Bili-Combur-6 *Boehringer Mannheim, Austral.†.*
Test for urinary ketones, bilirubin, blood, pH, protein and glucose.

Bilicordan *Repha, Ger.†.*
Homoeopathic preparation.

Bilicura Forte *Muller Goppingen, Ger.*
Kava (p.1592·3); cynara (p.1569·2).
Biliary disorders; dyspepsia.

Biliepar *Ibirn, Ital.*
Ursodeoxycholic acid (p.1642·1).
Biliary dyspepsia; gallstones.

Bilifluine *Promedica, Fr.*
Depigmented and decholesterolised ox bile (p.1553·2); sodium oleate (p.1469·1).
Constipation; dyspepsia.

Bilifuge *Plan, Switz.*
Cynara (p.1569·2); berberis vulgaris; orthosiphon (p.1592·2); kinkeliba (p.1593·2).
Digestive disorders.

Bili-Labstix
Bayer Diagnostics, Austral.†; Ames, Irl.; Bayer Diagnostici, Ital.; Ames, S.Afr.; Bayer Diagnostics, UK; Bayer, USA.
Test for pH, protein, glucose, ketones, bilirubin, and blood in urine.

Bilimiro *Byk Gulden, Ger.†.*
Iopronic acid.
Contrast medium for biliary-tract radiography.

Bilina *Esteve, Spain.*
Levocabastine hydrochloride (p.412·3).
Allergic conjunctivitis; allergic rhinitis.

Biliopaco *Rovi, Spain†.*
Iopanoic acid (p.1007·1).
Contrast medium for biliary-tract radiography.

Bi-Lipanor *Sterling Winthrop, Fr.†.*
Ciprofibrate (p.1270·3).
Hyperlipidaemias.

Bilipax *Taphlan, Switz.*
Naphthylacetic acid (p.1606·2); methylphenylethyl nicotinate.
Adjuvant in cholangiography; digestive disorders.

Bilipeptal forte *Brunnengraber, Ger.†.*
Pancreatin (p.1612·1); pepsin (p.1616·3); bile acids (p.1553·2).
Digestive system disorders.

Bilipeptal Mono *Gastropharm, Ger.*
Pancreatin (p.1612·1).
Pancreatic disorders.

Bilisan C3 *Repha, Ger.*
Silybum marianum (p.993·3); chelidonium majus; curcuma zanthorrhiza.
Biliary disorders; gallstones; liver disorders.

Bilisan forte *Repha, Ger.†.*
Capsella bursa pastoris; peppermint leaf (p.1208·1); chelidonium; senna (p.1212·2); cichorium intybus; rubia tinctorum; turmeric (p.1001·3); cnicus benedictus (p.1565·3); calendula officinalis; frangula bark (p.1193·2); lycopodium; chamomile (p.1561·2); silybum marianum (p.993·3); cholesterol; fel tauri; magnesium sulphate (p.1157·3); sodium potassium tartrate (p.1213·3).
Liver and biliary-tract disorders.

Biliscopin
Schering, Aust.; Schering, Ger.; Schering, Neth.†; Schering, Swed.; Schering, Switz.; Schering, UK.
Meglumine iotroxate (p.1008·2).
Contrast medium for biliary-tract radiography.

Bilisegrol *Schering, Spain.*
Meglumine iotroxate (p.1008·2).
Contrast medium for biliary-tract radiography.

Biliton H *Berlin-Chemie, Ger.†.*
Hymecromone (p.1589·3).
Biliary-tract spasm.

Bilivist *Berlex, USA.*
Sodium iopodate (p.1007·3).
Radiographic contrast medium for cholecystography.

Bilkaby *Bailly, Fr.*
Menadione (p.1370·3); bile salts (p.1553·2).
Haemorrhagic disorders due to vitamin K deficiency.

Billerol *Lehning, Fr.*
Homoeopathic preparation.

Bilobene
Merckle, Aust.; Merckle, Ger.
Fumitory (p.1581·3).
Biliary-tract disorders.

Bilopaque *Nycomed, USA.*
Sodium tyropanoate (p.1009·3).
Radiographic contrast medium for cholecystography.

Biloptin
Schering, Aust.; Schering, Ger.; Schering, Ital.†; Schering, S.Afr.; Schering, Switz.; Schering, UK.
Sodium iopodate (p.1007·3).
Contrast medium for biliary-tract radiography.

Bilordyl *Fisons, Ger.†.*
Theophylline (p.765·1).
Obstructive airways disease.

Bilron
Lilly, S.Afr.; Lilly, USA†.
Iron bile salts (p.1553·2).
Bile salt deficiency.

Biltricide
Bayer, Austral.; Bayer, Fr.; Bayer, Ger.; Bayer, Neth.; Bayer, S.Afr.; Miles, USA.
Praziquantel (p.108·2).
Worm infections.

Bilugen
Boehringer Mannheim, Austral.; Boehringer Mannheim Diagnostics, UK.
Test for urobilinogen and bilirubin in urine.

Bilugen-Test *Boehringer Mannheim Diagnostics, Irl.*
Test for bilirubin and urobilinogen.

Bimixin *Sanofi Winthrop, Ital.*
Bacitracin (p.157·3); neomycin sulphate (p.229·2).
Enteric infections.

Bimoxi *Jorba, Spain†.*
Amoxycillin trihydrate (p.151·3).
Bacterial infections.

Bimoxi Mucolitico *Jorba, Spain†.*
Capsules: Amoxycillin trihydrate (p.151·3); bromhexine hydrochloride (p.1055·3); guaiphenesin (p.1061·3).
Oral suspension: Amoxycillin (p.151·3); bromhexine (p.1055·3); guaiacol cinnamate (p.1061·2).
Respiratory-tract infections.

Bi-Myconase *Yamanouchi, Neth.†.*
Glucamylase; invertase.
Diarrhoea due to amylase, isomaltase, or invertase deficiency.

Binaldan *Vifor, Switz.*
Loperamide hydrochloride (p.1197·2).
Diarrhoea.

Binevrilplus *Biagini, Ital.†.*
Hydroxocobalamin hydriodide; thiamine phosphate; di-isopropylammonium dichloroacetate (p.854·1); lignocaine hydrochloride (p.1293·2).
Neuropathies.

Biniwas *Wasserman, Spain.*
Binifibrate (p.1269·2).
Hyperlipidaemias.

Binordiol
Wyeth Lederle, Belg.; Wyeth, Ital.†; Wyeth, Neth.; Wyeth, Switz.
Levonorgestrel (p.1454·1); ethinyloestradiol (p.1445·1).
Biphasic oral contraceptive; menstrual disorders.

Binotal
Bayer, Aust.; Grunenthal, Ger.
Ampicillin sodium (p.153·1) or ampicillin trihydrate (p.153·2).
Bacterial infections.

Binovum
Janssen-Cilag, Irl.; Cilag, UK.
Norethisterone (p.1453·1); ethinyloestradiol (p.1445·1).
Biphasic oral contraceptive.

Bio² *Bio2, Fr.*
Protein, fibre, and vitamin preparation.
Low body weight.

Bio-200 *Dermofarma, Ital.*
Royal jelly (p.1626·3); pollen.
Nutritional supplement.

Bio Acidophilus *Bioceuticals, UK.*
Lactobacillus acidophilus (p.1594·1).

Bio E *Bio-Health, UK.*
Vitamin E (p.1369·1).

Bio Espectrum *Centrum, Spain.*
Ampicillin sodium (p.153·1); ampicillin benzathine (p.154·1); bromhexine (p.1055·3).
Lignocaine hydrochloride (p.1293·2) is included in this preparation to alleviate the pain of injection.
Respiratory-tract infections.

Bio Exazol *Leti, Spain.*
Erythromycin ethyl succinate (p.204·2) or erythromycin propionate (p.204·2).
Bacterial infections.

Bio Exazol Balsamico *Leti, Spain†.*
Erythromycin ethyl succinate (p.204·2); guaiphenesin (p.1061·3).
Respiratory-tract infections.

Bio Hubber *ICN, Spain.*
Streptomycin sulphate (p.249·3); neomycin sulphate (p.229·2); pectin (p.1474·1); sulphadiazine (p.252·3); menadione sodium bisulphite; nicotinamide.
Gastro-intestinal infections.

Bio Hubber Fuerte *ICN, Spain.*
Bacitracin zinc (p.157·3); streptomycin sulphate (p.249·3); menadione sodium bisulphite; neomycin sulphate (p.229·2); nicotinamide; pectin (p.1474·1); sulphadiazine (p.252·3).
Gastro-intestinal infections.

Bio Mineral Formula *Blackmores, Austral.*
Mineral preparation.

Bio Notte Baby *IBP, Ital.†.*
Lettuce (p.1645·1); passion flower (p.1615·3); matricaria flowers (p.1561·2).
Insomnia.

Bio Ritz *IBP, Ital.†.*
Fructose; yeast (p.1373·1); royal jelly (p.1626·3).
Nutritional supplement.

Bio Soufre *Luchon, Fr.†.*
Laminaria digitata (p.1594·2).
Sulphur deficiency.

Bio Star *Novag, Spain.*
Ginseng (p.1584·2).
Tonic.

Bio-Acerola C Complex
Solgar, UK.
Vitamin C with bioflavonoids.

Solgar, USA.
Vitamin C (p.1365·2); citrus bioflavonoids complex (p.1580·1); rutin (p.1580·2); acerola (p.1001·1); rose hips (p.1365·2).
Capillary bleeding.

Bioagil Eurodrug, Aust.
Ascorbic acid (p.1365·2).
Vitamin C deficiency.

Bioaminal Lenza, Ital.†.
Amino-acid and pantothenic acid preparation.

Bioarginina Damor, Ital.
Arginine hydrochloride (p.1334·1).
Asthenia; hyperammonaemia.

Bio-Arscolloid SIT, Ital.
Dichlorobenzyl alcohol (p.1112·2); silver protein (p.1629·3); tyrothricin (p.267·2).
Bacterial mouth infections.

Bio-Ascorbate Solgar, UK.
Vitamin C with bioflavonoids.

Biobalm Modern Health Products, UK.
Slippery elm bark (p.1630·1); marshmallow root (p.1546·3); irish moss (p.1471·3).
Gastro-intestinal disorders.

Biobase Odan, Canad.
Alcohol (p.1099·1); (+)-cetyl steryl ethylene oxide.
Disinfection of the skin.

Bio-Biol Searle, Ital.
Vitamin B substances; coenzyme A (p.1566·2).
Vitamin deficiency.

Bio-C Bioforce, Switz.
Vitamin C preparation.

Bio-C Complex Blackmores, Austral.
Ascorbic acid (p.1365·2); sodium ascorbate (p.1365·2); calcium ascorbate (p.1365·2); lemon bioflavonoids (p.1580·1); rutin (p.1580·2); hesperidin (p.1580·2); acerola (p.1001·1).
Vitamin C preparation.

Biocadmio Uriach, Spain.
Cadmium sulphide (p.1555·3).
Skin and scalp disorders.

Biocalcin Esseti, Ital.
Salcatonin (p.735·3).
Hypercalcaemia; osteoporosis; Paget's disease of bone; sympathetic pain syndrome.

Bio-Calcium + D$_3$ Pharma Nord, Irl.
Calcium (p.1155·1); magnesium (p.1157·2); cholecalciferol (p.1366·3).
Calcium deficiency.

Bio-Calcium + D$_3$ + K Pharma Nord, Irl.
Calcium (p.1155·1); cholecalciferol (p.1366·3); vitamin K (p.1370·3).

Biocalyptol Laphal, Fr.
Pholcodine (p.1068·1); cineole (p.1564·1); guaiacol (p.1061·2).
The syrup formerly contained pholcodine, cineole, guaiacol, belladonna, and sodium camsylate. The suppositories formerly contained pholcodine, cineole, guaiacol, and sodium camsylate.
Coughs.

Bio-Caps Bio-Health, UK.
Multivitamin and mineral preparation.

Biocarde Lehning, Fr.
Pulsatilla (p.1623·3); crataegus (p.1568·2); passion flower (p.1615·3); convallaria (p.1567·2); strophanthus (p.951·1); avena (p.1551·3); valerian (p.1643·1); cereus grandiflorus; camphor (p.1557·2); colloidal gold (p.1586·2).
Insomnia; nervous disorders.

Biocarn Medice, Ger.
Carnitine (p.1336·2).
Carnitine deficiency.

Biocarnil Abiogen, Ital.
Carnitine hydrochloride (p.1336·2); L-lysine hydrochloride (p.1350·1).
Nutritional supplement.

Biocarotine Bioceuticals, UK.
Betacarotene (p.1335·2).

Biocatalase Fournier SA, Spain.
Catalase (p.1560·3).
Burns; skin disorders; ulcers; wounds.

Biocatines C Fuerte Garcia Suarez, Spain†.
Ascorbic acid (p.1365·2).
Methaemoglobinaemia; vitamin C deficiency.

Bioceanat Plantes Tropicales, Fr.
Sea water; copper gluconate (p.1338·1).
Nasal irrigation.

Bioceane Martin, Fr.†.
Electrolyte and mineral preparation.
Cold symptoms; nutritional and digestive disorders.

Biocebe Nutergia, Fr.
Amino-acid, vitamin, and zinc preparation.

Biocef
Note. This name is used for preparations of different composition.
Biochemie, Aust.
Cefpodoxime proxetil (p.172·1).
Bacterial infections.
Pharmacia Upjohn, Spain.
Ceftibuten (p.175·1).
Bacterial infections.
International Ethical, USA.
Cephalexin (p.178·2).
Bacterial infections.

Biochetasi Sigma-Tau, Ital.
Injection; suppositories: Vitamin B substances and electrolytes.
Oral granules: Vitamin B substances, electrolytes, and carbohydrate.
Fluid and electrolyte disorders; liver disorders.

Bio-Chrome Herbaxt, Fr.
Chromium (p.1337·1) from *Saccharomyces cerevisiae*; nicotinamide (p.1351·2).
Nutritional supplement.

Bio-Chromium Blackmores, Austral.
Mineral preparation with nicotinamide.
Alcoholism; hyperglycaemia; hypoglycaemia; sugar cravings.

Bio-Ci Ceccarelli, Ital.
Ascorbic acid (p.1365·2).

Biociclin Del Saz & Filippini, Ital.
Cefuroxime sodium (p.177·1).
Bacterial infections.

Biocidan Menarini, Fr.
Eye drops: Cethexonium bromide (p.1105·2).
Minor eye infections.
Nasal spray: Cethexonium bromide (p.1105·2); phenyltoloxamine citrate (p.416·1).
Nose and throat disorders.

Biocil Ibirn, Ital.
Cefonicid sodium (p.167·2).
Lignocaine hydrochloride (p.1293·2) is included in this preparation to alleviate the pain of injection.
Formerly known as Cefid.
Bacterial infections.

Biocin Ibirn, Ital.
Fosfomycin calcium (p.210·2).
Bacterial infections.

Biocitrin International Research, Austral.†.
Vitamin P (p.1580·1); ascorbic acid (p.1365·2).
Capillary damage.

Bioclate
Centeon, Ger.; Centeon, Spain; Centeon, UK; Armour, USA.
A factor VIII preparation (p.720·3).
Haemophilia A.

Biocodone Bios, Belg.
Hydrocodone bitartrate (p.43·1).
Coughs.

Biocol Bio-Transfusion, Fr.
1 Vial, fibrinogen (p.722·3); fibronectin (p.1580·1); factor XIII (p.722·2); 1 syringe, aprotinin (p.711·3); 1 vial, thrombin (p.728·1); calcium chloride (p.1155·1)
On mixing this forms a fibrin glue (p.722·2).
Haemorrhage.

Biocomplexes Yves Ponroy, Fr.†.
A range of multivitamin preparations.

Bioconseils Yves Ponroy, Fr.
A range of herbal preparations.

Biocortex Lenza, Ital.†.
Vitamin B substances; inosine (p.1591·1); suprarenal cortex (p.1050·1).
Anaemias; asthenia; liver disorders.

Biocortison Nezel, Spain†.
Bismuth subgallate (p.1180·2); phthalylsulphathiazole (p.237·1); papaverine hydrochloride (p.1614·2); prednisone hemisuccinate (p.1049·3).
Rectitis; rectosigmoiditis; ulcerative colitis.

Biocortone Vit Gibipharma, Ital.†.
Suprarenal cortex (p.1050·1); pyridoxine hydrochloride (p.1362·3); ascorbic acid (p.1365·2).
Adrenocortical insufficiency.

Biocoryl Uriach, Spain.
Procainamide hydrochloride (p.934·1).
Arrhythmias.

BioCox Iatric, USA.
Coccidioidin (p.1566·1).
Skin test for coccidioidomycosis.

Biocream BritHealth, UK.
Tissue salts; terpineol (p.1635·1); germall.
Skin disorders.

Bio-Cuivre Herbaxt, Fr.
Copper and manganese conjugated with 5-oxo-proline.
Nutritional supplement.

Biocyclin Biochemie, Aust.
Doxycycline hydrochloride (p.202·3).
Bacterial and protozoal infections.

Bio-Delta Cortilen SIFI, Ital.
Prednisolone acetate (p.1048·1); neomycin sulphate (p.229·2).
Eye infections.

Bioderm Odan, Canad.
Polymyxin B sulphate (p.239·1); bacitracin (p.157·3).
Bacterial infections.

Biodermatin Lafare, Ital.
Biotin (p.1336·1).
Skin disorders.

Biodermin Biotekfarma, Ital.†.
Econazole nitrate (p.377·2).
Fungal infections.

Biodine Major, USA.
Povidone-iodine (p.1123·3).
Skin disinfection.

Bio-Disc Blackmores, Austral.
Minerals; vitamins; silicon dioxide (p.1474·3); bromelains (p.1555·1); papain (p.1614·1).
Delayed bone healing; muscular and joint pain.

Biodophilus Bioceuticals, UK.
Lactobacillus acidophilus (p.1594·1).

Biodramina Uriach, Spain.
Dimenhydrinate (p.408·2).
Motion sickness; vertigo.

Biodramina Cafeina Uriach, Spain.
Caffeine (p.749·3); dimenhydrinate (p.408·2); pyridoxine hydrochloride (p.1362·3).
Motion sickness; vertigo.

Biodroxil Biochemie, Aust.
Cefadroxil (p.163·3).
Bacterial infections.

Biodyn Proter, Ital.†.
Ascorbic acid (p.1365·2); bioflavonoids (rutin and quercetin) (p.1580·1).
Asthenia; vascular disorders.

Bioepar Ripari-Gero, Ital.†.
Vitamin B substances; suprarenal cortex (p.1050·1); lignocaine (p.1293·2).
Anaemias; asthenia.

Bioequiseto Ghimas, Ital.
Equisetum (p.1575·1).
Nutritional supplement.

Bioesse Mavi, Ital.
L-Cystine, L-methionine, zinc, and copper.
Nutritional supplement.

Biofanal Pfleger, Ger.
Nystatin (p.386·1).
Candidiasis.

Biofenac UCB, Belg.
Aceclofenac (p.12·1).
Inflammation; musculoskeletal, joint, and peri-articular disorders.

Biofenicol-N Dorsch, Ger.†.
Chloramphenicol (p.182·1); amethocaine hydrochloride (p.1285·2).
Inflammatory disorders and infections of the ear.

Bio-Fer Herbaxt, Fr.
Iron pidolate; folic acid; ascorbic acid.
Nutritional supplement.

Biofilm
Biotrol, Fr.†.; CliniMed, UK.
Hydrocolloid dressing.
Ulcers; wounds.

Bioflorin
Schoeller, Aust.; Bio-Therabel, Belg.†; Bracco, Ital.; Giuliani, Switz.
Lactic-acid-producing enterococci (p.1594·1).
Gastro-intestinal disorders.

Bioflutin-N Sudmedica, Ger.
Etilefrine hydrochloride (p.867·2).
Hypotension.

Biofolic Esseti, Ital.
Calcium methyltetrahydrofolate (p.1342·3).
Antidote to folic acid antagonists; folic acid deficiency; reduction of aminopterin and methotrexate toxicity.

Biofos Lebens, Ital.†.
Fosfomycin calcium (p.210·2).
Bacterial infections.

Bio-Frin IBP, Ital.†.
Hydroxyquinoline sulphate (p.1589·3).
Vaginal douche.

Biofurex KBR, Ital.
Cefuroxime sodium (p.177·1).
Bacterial infections.

Biogam Biogam, Switz.
Trace element preparations.

Biogardol Biophytarom, Fr.
Vitamin E; betacarotene; vitamin C.

Bio-Garten Entschlackungstee Bio-Garten, Aust.
Silver birch (p.1553·3); dandelion leaf (p.1634·2); prunus spinosa; rose fruit (p.1365·2); sambucus (p.1627·2); calendula officinalis.
Herbal preparation.

Bio-Garten Tee fur den Magen Bio-Garten, Aust.
Chamomile (p.1561·2); peppermint leaf (p.1208·1); caraway (p.1559·3); valerian (p.1643·1).
Gastro-intestinal disorders.

Bio-Garten Tee fur Leber und Galle Bio-Garten, Aust.
Absinthium (p.1541·1); calamus (p.1556·1); angelica; peppermint leaf (p.1208·1); bitter-orange leaf.
Liver and gallbladder disorders.

Bio-Garten Tee fur Niere und Blase Bio-Garten, Aust.
Bearberry (p.1552·2); equisetum (p.1575·1); sliver birch (p.1553·3).
Kidney and bladder disorders.

Bio-Garten Tee gegen Blahungen Bio-Garten, Aust.
Fennel (p.1579·1); chamomile (p.1561·2); caraway (p.1559·3); achillea (p.1542·2); peppermint leaf (p.1208·1).
Flatulence.

Bio-Garten Tee gegen Durchfall Bio-Garten, Aust.
Tormentil (p.1638·3); chamomile (p.1561·2); strawberry leaf; blackberry leaf; raspberry leaf (p.1624·2).
Diarrhoea.

Bio-Garten Tee gegen Erkaltung Bio-Garten, Aust.
Thyme (p.1636·3); althaea (p.1546·3); verbascum flowers; plantago lanceolata leaf.
Catarrh; cold symptoms.

Bio-Garten Tee gegen Verstopfung Bio-Garten, Aust.
Prunus spinosa; peppermint leaf (p.1208·1); chamomile (p.1561·2); fennel (p.1579·1).
Constipation.

Bio-Garten Tee zur Beruhigung Bio-Garten, Aust.
Valerian (p.1643·1); melissa (p.1600·1); lupulus (p.1597·2); lavender flowers (p.1594·3); orange flowers.
Anxiety; insomnia.

Bio-Garten Tee zur Erhohung der Harnmenge Bio-Garten, Aust.
Urtica (p.1642·3); silver birch (p.1553·3); taraxacum leaf (p.1634·2); prunus spinosa; ononis (p.1610·2).
Diuretic.

Bio-Garten Tee zur Starkung und Kraftigung Bio-Garten, Aust.
Achillea (p.1542·2); dried bitter-orange peel (p.1610·3); gentian (p.1583·3); rosemary leaf; rose fruit (p.1365·2).
Tonic.

Bio-Garten Tropfen fur Galle und Leber Bio-Garten, Aust.
Absinthium (p.1541·1); achillea (p.1542·2); taraxacum (p.1634·2).
Liver and gallbladder disorders.

Bio-Garten Tropfen fur Magen und Darm Bio-Garten, Aust.
Peppermint (p.1208·1); valerian (p.1643·1); chamomile (p.1561·2).
Gastro-intestinal disorders.

Bio-Garten Tropfen fur Niere und Blase Bio-Garten, Aust.
Silver birch (p.1553·3); equisetum (p.1575·1).
Kidney and bladder disorders.

Bio-Garten Tropfen gegen Blahungen Bio-Garten, Aust.
Caraway (p.1559·3); coriander (p.1567·3); peppermint (p.1208·1).
Flatulence.

Bio-Garten Tropfen gegen Husten Bio-Garten, Aust.
Thyme (p.1636·3); plantago lanceolata.
Catarrh; coughs.

Bio-Garten Tropfen zur Beruhigung Bio-Garten, Aust.
Lupulus (p.1597·2); melissa (p.1600·1).
Nervous disorders.

Biogastrone
Sanofi Winthrop, Irl.†; Sterling Winthrop, UK†.
Carbenoxolone sodium (p.1182·2).
Gastric ulcer.

Biogaze Evans, Fr.
Niaouli oil (p.1607·1); thyme oil (p.1637·1).
Burns.

Biogel Ghimas, Ital.
Royal jelly (p.1626·3).

Biogelat Erkaltungs & Grippe Metochem, Aust.
Salix (p.82·3).
Cold and flu symptoms; pain.

Biogelat Leberschutz Metochem, Aust.
Silybum marianum (p.993·3).
Liver disorders.

Biogelat Schlaf Metochem, Aust.
Valerian (p.1643·1); lupulus (p.1597·2).
Sleep disorders.

Biogen Cusi, Spain†.
Gentamicin sulphate (p.212·1).
Bacterial infections.

Biogena Baby Farmoderm, Ital.†.
Zinc oxide (p.1096·2).
Barrier preparation.

Biogena Dermo Biogena, Ital.
Soap substitute.

Biogenis Bayer, Ger.
dl-Alpha tocopheryl acetate (p.1369·2); magnesium oxide (p.1198·3).
Vitamin E or magnesium deficiency.

Bioget Michallik, Ger.
Tannic acid (p.1634·2); cetylpyridinium chloride (p.1106·2).
Burns; wounds.

Bioglan Acidophilus Bioglan, Austral.
Lactobacillus acidophilus (p.1594·1).
Restoration of gastro-intestinal flora.

Bioglan Active Enzyme Complex Rhone-Poulenc Rorer, Austral.†.
Maltase (p.1546·2); lipase AP6; protease M6; cellulase (p.1561·1); papain (p.1614·1).
Gastric or duodenal enzyme deficiency.

Bioglan Cal C Bioglan, Austral.
Calcium ascorbate (p.1365·2).
Vitamin C deficiency.

Bioglan Children's Micelle Rhone-Poulenc Rorer, Austral.†.
Multivitamin preparation.

Bioglan Daily Plus Bioglan, Austral.
Vitamin and mineral preparation.

Bioglan Digestive Zyme Rhone-Poulenc Rorer, Austral.†.
Betaine hydrochloride (p.1553·2); glutamic acid (p.1344·3); pepsin (p.1616·3).
Achlorhydria; hypochlorhydria.

Bioglan Discone Rhone-Poulenc Rorer, Austral.†.
Vitamin and mineral preparation with bromelain (p.1555·1) and papain (p.1614·1).
Soft tissue inflammation.

Bioglan Effervescent Granules Bioglan, UK.
Tartaric acid (p.1634·3); sodium bicarbonate (p.1153·2); dimethicone (p.1384·2).
Adjunct in gastro-intestinal radiography.

Bioglan Effervescent Tablets Bioglan, UK.
Sodium bicarbonate (p.1153·2); tartaric acid (p.1634·3); calcium carbonate (p.1182·1); dimethicone (p.1213·1).
Adjunct to gastro-intestinal radiography.

Bioglan E-Plus *Bioglan, Austral.*
d-Alpha tocopherol (p.1369·1); fish oil (p.1276·1); evening primrose oil (p.1582·1); rosemary oil (p.1626·2); lecithin (p.1595·2).
Aid in skin tissue repair; antoxidant.

Bioglan Fingers & Toes *Bioglan, Austral.*
Calcium ascorbate (p.1365·2); *d*-alpha tocopheryl acid succinate (p.1369·2); rutin (p.1580·2); bioflavonoids (p.1580·1); nicotinic acid (p.1351·2); aesculus (p.1543·3); hamamelis (p.1587·1); ginkgo biloba (p.1584·1); rosemary oil (p.1626·2).
Peripheral vascular disorders.

Bioglan Formula Four *Bioglan, Austral.*
Vitamin and mineral preparation.

Bioglan Hemo Factor *Bioglan, Austral.*
Vitamin preparation with iron and folic acid.
Anaemia.

Bioglan Junior Sesame Street Childrens Chewable Vitamin C *Bioglan, Austral.*
Vitamin C substances (p.1365·2).

Bioglan Junior Sesame Street Multivitamins with Calcium *Bioglan, Austral.*
Multivitamin and mineral preparation.

Bioglan Maxepa *Bioglan, Austral.*
Fish oil (p.1276·1); *d*-alpha tocopheryl acetate (p.1369·2).
Atherosclerosis; hypertriglyceridaemia.

Bioglan Micelle A plus E *Bioglan, Austral.*
Vitamin A (p.1358·1); *d*-alpha tocopheryl acetate (p.1369·2).
Fat malabsorption syndromes; vitamin A and E supplement.

Bioglan Micelle B *Rhone-Poulenc Rorer, Austral.†.*
Multivitamin preparation.

Bioglan Micelle E *Bioglan, Austral.*
d-Alpha tocopheryl acetate (p.1369·2).
Vitamin E supplement.

Bioglan Natural E *Bioglan, Austral.*
d-Alpha tocopherol (p.1369·1).
Vitamin E deficiency; vitamin E supplement.

Bioglan Neo Stress Formula *Bioglan, Austral.*
Multivitamin, mineral, and amino-acid preparation.

Bioglan Organic Mineral *Bioglan, Austral.*
Mineral supplement.

Bioglan Panazyme *Rhone-Poulenc Rorer, Austral.†.*
Pancreatin (p.1612·1).
Digestive enzyme supplement.

Bioglan Primrose Micelle *Bioglan, Austral.*
Evening primrose oil (p.1582·1).
Eczema; mastalgia.

Bioglan Primrose-E *Bioglan, Austral.*
Evening primrose oil (p.1582·1); *d*-alpha tocopherol (p.1369·1).
Premenstrual syndrome.

Bioglan Stress Formula *Rhone-Poulenc Rorer, Austral.†.*
Multivitamin, mineral, and nutritional preparation.

Bioglan Sucro Formula *Bioglan, Austral.*
Vitamin and mineral preparation.

Bioglan Super Cal C *Bioglan, Austral.*
Calcium ascorbate (p.1365·2); citrus bioflavonoids (p.1580·1); hesperidin (p.1580·2); rutin (p.1580·2); rose fruit (p.1365·2).
Vitamin C supplement.

Bioglan Superdophilus *Bioglan, Austral.*
Lactobacillus acidophilus (p.1594·1).
Restoration of the gastro-intestinal flora.

Bioglan Tri-B3 *Bioglan, Austral.†.*
Nicotinic acid (p.1351·2).
Chilblains; frostbite; pellagra.

Bioglan Vegetable Enzymes *Rhone-Poulenc Rorer, Austral.†.*
Amylase (p.1549·1); protease; lipase; cellulase (p.1561·1).
Digestive enzyme deficiency.

Bioglan Water Soluble E *Rhone-Poulenc Rorer, Austral.†.*
d-Alpha tocopherol (p.1369·1).
Vitamin E supplement.

Bioglan Zinc Chelate *Bioglan, Austral.*
Zinc amino acid chelate (p.1373·3).
Zinc deficiency.

Bioglan Zn-A-C *Bioglan, Austral.*
Ascorbic acid (p.1365·2); retinol (p.1358·1); zinc amino acid chelate (p.1373·3); calcium pantothenate (p.1352·3); rutin (p.1580·2).
Vitamin and mineral supplement.

Biogrisin *Biochemie, Aust.†.*
Griseofulvin (p.380·2).
Fungal skin infections.

Biohisdex DM *Everest, Canad.*
Dextromethorphan hydrobromide (p.1057·3); phenylephrine hydrochloride (p.1066·2); diphenylpyraline hydrochloride (p.409·3).
Coughs; respiratory congestion.

Biohisdine DM *Everest, Canad.*
Dextromethorphan hydrobromide (p.1057·3); phenylephrine hydrochloride (p.1066·2); diphenylpyraline hydrochloride (p.409·3).
Coughs; respiratory congestion.

Biohist *Propan, S.Afr.*
Diphenhydramine hydrochloride (p.409·1); zinc oxide (p.1096·2); calamine (p.1080·1); phenol (p.1121·2).
Skin disorders.

Biohist-LA *Wakefield, USA.*
Carbinoxamine maleate (p.404·2); pseudoephedrine hydrochloride (p.1068·3).
Cold symptoms.

BIO-H-TIN *Mauermann, Ger.*
Biotin (p.1336·1).
Biotin deficiency.

Bio-Insulin 10/90, 20/80, 30/70, 40/60, and 50/50 *Guidotti, Ital.*
Mixtures of insulin injection (human, biosynthetic) and isophane insulin injection (human, biosynthetic) respectively in the proportions indicated (p.322·1).
Diabetes mellitus.

Bio-Insulin I *Guidotti, Ital.*
Isophane insulin (human, biosynthetic) (p.322·1).
Diabetes mellitus.

Bio-Insulin L *Guidotti, Ital.*
Insulin zinc suspension (human, biosynthetic) (p.322·1).
Diabetes mellitus.

Bio-Insulin R *Guidotti, Ital.*
Insulin (human, biosynthetic) (p.322·1).
Diabetes mellitus.

Bio-Insulin U *Guidotti, Ital.*
Insulin zinc suspension (crystalline) (human, biosynthetic) (p.322·1).
Diabetes mellitus.

Bioiodine *Bioceuticals, UK.*
Potassium iodate (p.1495·3).

Biojad *Schieffer, Aust.*
Multivitamin and iron preparation.
Tonic.

Biolac EPS *Eurofarmaco, Ital.*
Lactulose (p.1195·3).
Hepatic cirrhosis; hepatic encephalopathy.

Biolactine *Sella, Ital.*
Vitamin B substances; lactic-acid-producing organisms (p.1594·1); myrtillus (p.1606·1).
Nutritional supplement.

Biolan Cad *Biopha, Fr.†.*
Cade oil (p.1092·2); salicylic acid (p.1090·2).
Seborrhoea.

Biolan Tar *Biopha, Fr.*
Coal tar (p.1092·3); piroctone olamine (p.1089·1); salicylic acid (p.1090·2).
Seborrhoeic dermatitis.

Biolau *Luchon, Fr.*
Linalol; geraniol; neroli; d-borneol; cinol; cineole (p.1564·1); sodium chloride (p.1162·2).
Nasal and oral hygiene.

Biolavan *Pharmaton, Ger.*
Equisetum (p.1575·1).
Oedema; urinary-tract disorders.

Biolecit *Nattermann, Ger.†.*
Plant phosphatide fraction.
Lipid disorders.

Biolecit H3 *Schieffer, Aust.*
Procaine hydrochloride (p.1299·2); essential phospholipids; *dl*-alpha tocopheryl acetate (p.1369·2).
Tonic.

Bioleine *Nutergia, Fr.*
Evening primrose oil (p.1582·1).
Nutritional supplement.

Biolens Nettoyage *Bausch & Lomb, Fr.†.*
Cleansing solution for soft and hard contact lenses.

Biolens Rincage *Bausch & Lomb, Fr.†.*
Rinsing solution for contact lenses.

Biolid *Belmac, Fr.†.*
Erythromycin ethyl succinate (p.204·2).
Bacterial infections.

Biolina *Bioceuticals, UK.*
Spirulina (p.1632·2).

Biologische Migrane-Tropfen *Rodler, Ger.†.*
Homoeopathic preparation.

Bio-Logos *Sigma-Tau, Switz.*
Hydroxocobalamin; amino acids.
Tonic.

Biolon
Ophtapharma, Canad.; SIFI, Ital.; Novopharma, Switz.
Sodium hyaluronate (p.1630·3).
Aid in eye surgery.

Biolucchini *Geymonat, Ital.*
Proteins (mol. wt 30-300 kD).
Tissue repair.

Biomag
Note. This name is used for preparations of different composition.
Homeocan, Canad.; Lehning, Fr.
Homoeopathic preparation.

Pulitzer, Ital.
Cimetidine (p.1183·2).
Gastro-intestinal disorders associated with hyperacidity.

Biomagnesin *Madaus, Ger.*
Dibasic magnesium phosphate; dibasic magnesium citrate.
Magnesium deficiency.

Bio-Magnesium *Phytomed, Switz.*
Homoeopathic preparation.

Biomax *Alonga, Spain†.*
Adenosine triphosphate sodium (p.1543·2); cyproheptadine acetylaspartate (p.407·3); cobamamide (p.1364·2).
Anorexia; tonic; weight loss.

Biometalle II-Heyl *Heyl, Ger.*
Mineral preparation.
Correction of metal balance following penicillamine therapy.

Biometalle III-Heyl *Heyl, Ger.*
Mineral preparation.
Correction of metal balance following penicillamine therapy.

Biomineral *Biochimici, Ital.*
Mineral preparation with cystine.
Nutritional supplement.

Biominol A *Alter, Spain.*
Vitamin A palmitate (p.1359·2).
Vitamin A deficiency.

Biominol A D *Alter, Spain.*
Vitamin A palmitate (p.1359·2); ergocalciferol (p.1367·1).
Deficiency of vitamins A and D.

Biomioran *Bioindustria, Ital.†.*
Chlorzoxazone (p.1313·1).
Skeletal muscle spasm.

Biomo-lipon *Biomo, Ger.*
Thioctic acid (p.1636·2).
Diabetic polyneuropathy.

Biomorphol *Winzer, Ger.†.*
Multivitamin preparation.
Arteriosclerosis; convalescence; diabetes mellitus; Ménière's disease; ophthalmic disorders.

Biomox *International Ethical, USA†.*
Amoxycillin trihydrate (p.151·3).
Bacterial infections.

Biomunil *Lusofarmaco, Ital.*
Klebsiella pneumoniae ribosomes and membrane fraction; *Diplococcus pneumoniae* ribosomes; *Streptococcus pyogenes* ribosomes; *Haemophilus influenzae* ribosomes.
Immunostimulant.

Biomunyl *Pierre Fabre, Ger.†.*
Ribosomes of *Klebsiella pneumoniae*; *Streptococcus pneumoniae*; *Haemophilus influenzae* (p.1593·2); proteoglycan of *Klebsiella pneumoniae*.
Respiratory-tract infections.

Bion Tears
Alcon, Canad.; Alcon, USA.
Dextran 70 (p.717·1); hypromellose (p.1473·1).
Dry eyes.

Bionagre plus E *Bio-Sante, Canad.*
Linoleic acid (p.1582·1); linolenic acid; vitamin E (p.1369·1).

Bionagrol *Biophytarom, Fr.*
Evening primrose oil (p.1582·1).
Nutritional supplement.

Bionagrol Plus *Biophytarom, Fr.*
Evening primrose oil (p.1582·1); omega-3 fatty acids (p.1276·1).
Nutritional supplement.

Bionect *Sinax, Ital.†.*
Sodium hyaluronate (Hyalastine) (p.1630·3).
Wounds.

Bionet *Carter Horner, Canad.*
Benzocaine (p.1286·2); cetalkonium chloride (p.1105·2).
Mouth disorders.

Bioneural (Rowo-634) *Pharmakon, Ger.†.*
Homoeopathic preparation.

Bionicard *Bioindustria, Ital.*
Nicardipine hydrochloride (p.915·1).
Angina pectoris; hypertension.

Bionocalcin *Kendall, Spain.*
Salcatonin (p.735·3).
Hypercalcaemia; metastatic bone pain; Paget's disease of bone; postmenopausal osteoporosis.

Biontop *Merck, Spain†.*
Aspirin (p.16·1).
Fever; pain.

Biopac *Svenska Dental, Swed.†.*
Aluminium chlorohydrate (p.1078·3).
Dental care.

Biopasal Fibra *Derly, Spain.*
Ispaghula husk (p.1194·2).
Constipation.

Biopatch *Johnson & Johnson Medical, USA.*
Chlorhexidine gluconate (p.1107·2).
Wound dressing.

Bioperazone *Biopharma, Ital.*
Cefoperazone sodium (p.167·3).
Bacterial infections.

Bioperidolo *FIRMA, Ital.*
Haloperidol (p.673·3).
Psychoses.

Biophenicol *Biochemie, Aust.*
Chloramphenicol (p.182·1) or chloramphenicol sodium succinate (p.182·2).
Bacterial infections.

Biophil *Kemiprogress, Ital.*
Vitamin B substances; myrtillus (p.1606·1).
Disturbances of the gastro-intestinal flora.

Biophylin *Gerard House, UK.*
Valerian (p.1643·1); scullcap; jamaican dogwood; black cohosh (p.1563·3).
Tenseness, restlessness, nervous irritability.

Biophyllin *Propan, S.Afr.*
Theophylline (p.765·1).
Obstructive airways disease.

Biophylline *Delandale, UK†.*
Theophylline sodium glycinate (p.772·2) or theophylline (p.765·1).
Obstructive airways disease.

Biopim *Kemyos, Ital.*
Pipemidic acid (p.237·2).
Urinary-tract infections.

Bioplak *Berenguer Infale, Spain.*
Aspirin (p.16·1).
Thrombo-embolism prophylaxis.

bioplant-Kamillenfluid *Serum-Werk Bernburg, Ger.*
Chamomile (p.1561·2); calendula.
Bedsores; inflammation of the oral cavity; skin inflammation.

bioplant-Kinderol *Serum-Werk Bernburg, Ger.†.*
Guaiazulene (p.1586·3); calendula; melissa (p.1600·1).
Skin care; skin inflammation.

Bioplasma FDP *NBI, S.Afr.*
Plasma protein fraction (p.726·3).
Fluid depletion; haemorrhagic disorders.

Bioplex
Note. This name is used for preparations of different composition.
Sante Naturelle, Canad.
Vitamin B substances.

Torre, Ital.
Amino-acid infusion.
Parenteral nutrition.

Thames, UK.
Carbenoxolone sodium (p.1182·2).
Mouth ulcers.

Bioplus *Mer-National, S.Afr.*
Caffeine; vitamin B substances; calcium citrate; calcium gluconate.
Tonic.

Biopto-E *Jenapharm, Ger.*
d-Alpha tocopherol (p.1369·1).
Tonic; vitamin E deficiency.

Biopulmin *Savoma, Ital.†.*
Benzyl cinnamate; niaouli oil (p.1607·1); guaiacol (p.1061·2).
Respiratory-tract disorders.

Biopyn *Laser, S.Afr.†.*
Paracetamol (p.72·2); codeine phosphate (p.26·1); caffeine (p.749·3).
Fever; pain.

Biopyr *Madaus, Ger.*
Homoeopathic preparation.

Bioral
Smith & Nephew, Austral.; SmithKline Beecham, Irl.; Roche, S.Afr.†; SmithKline Beecham, UK.
Carbenoxolone sodium (p.1182·2).
Mouth ulcers.

Bio-Real *Farmetrusca, Ital.*
Royal jelly (p.1626·3); yeast (p.1373·1).

Bio-Real Complex *Farmetrusca, Ital.*
Royal jelly (p.1626·3); ginseng (p.1584·2).

Bio-Real Plus *Farmetrusca, Ital.*
Royal jelly (p.1626·3); ginseng (p.1584·2).

Bio-Regenerat *Dibropharm, Ger.*
Adenosine phosphate disodium (p.1543·2).
Psoriasis.

Biorenal *Pharmalink, Swed.*
Anhydrous glucose; sodium chloride; sodium lactate; calcium chloride; magnesium chloride (p.1151·1).
Peritoneal dialysis.

Bio-Rex *Aandersen, Ital.†.*
Cobamamide (p.1364·2); calcium folinate (p.1342·2); suprarenal cortex (p.1050·1).
Anaemias; asthenia; liver disorders.

Biorganic Geri *Gisand, Switz.*
Vitamin, mineral, and amino-acid preparation with ginseng (p.1584·2).
Dietary supplement; tonic.

Biorinil *Farmila, Ital.*
Betamethasone (p.1033·2); tetrahydrozoline hydrochloride (p.1070·2).
Formerly contained betamethasone, chlorpheniramine maleate, kanamycin sulphate, and tetrahydrozoline hydrochloride.
Rhinitis; rhinopharyngitis; sinusitis.

Biormon *Amsa, Ital.*
Oestradiol benzoate (p.1455·1); progesterone (p.1459·3).
Amenorrhoea; oligomenorrhoea.

Biorphen *Bioglan, UK.*
Orphenadrine hydrochloride (p.465·2).
Drug-induced extrapyramidal disorders; parkinsonism.

Biortho *Nutergia, Fr.*
Vitamin, mineral, and triglyceride preparation.
Nutritional supplement.

Bios Ferro *Recordati, Ital.†.*
Ferritin (p.1580·1).
Iron-deficiency disorders.

Biosal *Yauyip, Austral.*
Methyl salicylate (p.55·2); menthol (p.1600·2); camphor (p.1557·2); eucalyptus oil (p.1578·1); pumilio pine oil (p.1623·3).
Arthritis pain.

Bioscefal *Unibios, Spain.*
Cephalexin (p.178·2).
Bacterial infections.

Biosedon S *Biocur, Ger.*
Valerian (p.1643·1); passion flower (p.1615·3); lupulus (p.1597·2).
Anxiety disorders; insomnia.

Bio-Selenium *Herbaxt, Fr.*
Selenium (p.1353·3) from *Saccharomyces cerevisiae*; alpha tocopheryl acetate (p.1369·1); wheat-germ oil.
Muscular disorders; skin disorders.

Bioselenium *Uriach, Spain.*
Selenium sulphide (p.1091·1).
Skin disorders.

Biosilit-Heilsalbe *Evers, Ger.†.*
Silicon dioxide (p.1474·3); tannic acid (p.1634·2).
Skin disorders.

Biosinax *Rorer, Ital.†.*
A mixture of the gangliosides G_{M1}, G_{D1a}, G_{D1b}, and G_{T1b} (p.1582·3).
Peripheral neurological disorders.

Biosol A *Pharmalink, Swed.*
Sodium chloride; potassium chloride; magnesium chloride; calcium chloride; acetic acid; with or without glucose (p.1151·1).
Haemodialysis.

Biosol B *Pharmalink, Swed.*
Sodium bicarbonate (p.1151·1).
Haemodialysis.

Biosorbin MCT *Pfrimmer Nutricia, Switz.†.*
Preparation for enteral nutrition.

Biosor-C *Hamilton, Austral.*
Hesperidin methyl chalcone (p.1580·2); hesperidin (p.1580·2); ascorbic acid (p.1365·2).
Gingivitis; herpes labialis.

Bio-Sprint *Poli, Switz.†.*
Cyanocobalamin; amino acids.
Tonic.

Biosteril *Biotest, Ger.†.*
Sodium chloride (p.1162·2).
Fluid replacement.

Biostim
Cassenne, Fr.; Hoechst Marion Roussel, Ital.; Roussel, S.Afr.†.
Klebsiella pneumoniae glycoprotein (p.1593·2).
Burns; prophylaxis of respiratory-tract infection; ulcers; wounds.

Bio-Strath *Lizofarm, Ital.*
Valerian (p.1643·1); passion flower (p.1615·3); peppermint leaf (p.1208·1).
Insomnia; sedative.

Biosun *Banana Boat, Canad.*
SPF 25; SPF 30: Ethylhexyl *p*-methoxycinnamate (p.1487·1); octyl salicylate (p.1487·3); oxybenzone (p.1487·3); titanium dioxide (p.1093·3).
SPF 45: Ethylhexyl *p*-methoxycinnamate (p.1487·1); octyl salicylate (p.1487·3); oxybenzone (p.1487·3); octocrylene (p.1487·3).
Sunscreen.

Biosym *Anatomia, UK†.*
Lactobacillus bulgaricus (p.1594·1); *Streptococcus thermophilus* (p.1594·1).
Dietary supplement.

Biotab
Note. A similar name is used for preparations of different composition.
Bioline, USA†.
Phenylpropanolamine hydrochloride (p.1067·2); phenyltoloxamine citrate (p.416·1); paracetamol (p.72·2).

Bio-Tab
Note. A similar name is used for preparations of different composition.
International Ethical, USA.
Doxycycline hydrochloride (p.202·3).

Biotamin *Sankyo, Jpn.*
Benfotiamine (p.1360·3).
Vitamin B_1 deficiency.

Biotassina *Teofarma, Ital.*
Amino acids; vitamin B substances; calcium gluconate (p.1155·2).
Lignocaine hydrochloride (p.1293·2) is included in the intramuscular injection to alleviate the pain of injection.
Asthenia.

Biotel diabetes *Biotel, USA.*
Test for glucose in urine (p.1585·1).

Biotel kidney *Biotel, USA.*
Test for haemoglobin, red blood cells, and albumin in urine.

Biotel uti *Biotel, USA†.*
Test for nitrite in urine.

Biotene *Biotene, Austral.†.*
Glucose oxidase (p.1585·1); lactoperoxidase.
Prevention of caries and gum disease in dry mouth.

Biotens *Kemyos, Ital.*
Labetalol hydrochloride (p.896·1); chlorthalidone (p.839·3).
Hypertension.

Bioterciclin *Lisapharma, Ital.†.*
Capsules: Demeclocycline hydrochloride (p.201·2).
Oral drops: Demeclocycline hydrochloride (p.201·2); vitamin B substances.
Bacterial infections.

Biotherm *Biotherm, Canad.*
SPF 15; SPF 25; SPF 30: Avobenzone (p.1486·3); 3-(4-methylbenzylidene)bornan-2-one (p.1487·2); terephthalylidene dicamphor sulphonic acid; titanium dioxide (p.1093·3).
Sunscreen.

Biotherm Gelee Bronzante *Biotherm, Canad.*
SPF 8: Ethylhexyl *p*-methoxycinnamate (p.1487·1); octyl salicylate (p.1487·3); oxybenzone (p.1487·3).
Sunscreen.

Biotherm Gelee Fraiche *Biotherm, Canad.*
SPF 8: Ethylhexyl *p*-methoxycinnamate (p.1487·1); 3-(4-methylbenzylidene)bornan-2-one (p.1487·2); terephthalylidene dicamphor sulphonic acid; titanium dioxide (p.1093·3).
Sunscreen.

Biotherm Lait Bronzant *Biotherm, Canad.*
SPF 8: Ethylhexyl *p*-methoxycinnamate (p.1487·1); terephthalylidene dicamphor sulphonic acid; titanium dioxide (p.1093·3).
Sunscreen.

Biotherm Lait Protecteur *Biotherm, Canad.*
SPF 15: Ethylhexyl *p*-methoxycinnamate (p.1487·1); terephthalylidene dicamphor sulphonic acid; titanium dioxide (p.1093·3).
Sunscreen.

Biotherm Soin des Levres *Biotherm, Canad.*
SPF 8: Ethylhexyl *p*-methoxycinnamate (p.1487·1).
Sunscreen.

Biotherm Soin Solaire *Biotherm, Canad.*
SPF 8: Ethylhexyl *p*-methoxycinnamate (p.1487·1); terephthalylidene dicamphor sulphonic acid; titanium dioxide (p.1093·3).
Sunscreen.

Biotherm Soin Solaire Autobronzant *Biotherm, Canad.*
SPF 8: Avobenzone (p.1486·3); 3-(4-methylbenzylidene)bornan-2-one (p.1487·2); terephthalylidene dicamphor sulphonic acid.
Sunscreen.

Biotherm Stick Ecran *Biotherm, Canad.*
SPF 20: Avobenzone (p.1486·3); octocrylene (p.1487·3); titanium dioxide (p.1093·3).
Sunscreen.

Biotinas *Eagle, Austral.†.*
Biotin (p.1336·1).
Inflammation; nutritional deficiency.

Bioton *Sella, Ital.*
Honey (p.1345·3); ginseng (p.1584·2); royal jelly (p.1626·3).
Nutritional supplement.

Biotone *Lophal, Fr.*
Kola (p.1645·1); phosphoric acid (p.1618·1); inositol calcium; manganese glycerophosphate (p.1586·2).
Tonic.

Biotrefon Plus *Whitehall, Ital.*
Pollen; royal jelly (p.1626·3); liver extract.

Biotrin *Galway, Irl.†.*
Neomycin sulphate (p.229·2); bacitracin zinc (p.157·3); L-cysteine; DL-threonine.
Abscesses; burns; skin ulcers; wounds.

Biotrixina *Benedetti, Ital.*
Cefatrizine (p.164·2).
Bacterial infections.

Biotron *Covan, S.Afr.*
Multivitamin and mineral preparation.

Biotropic *Madaus, Spain.*
Guar gum (p.321·3).
Diabetes mellitus.

Biotuss N *Spitzner, Ger.*
Thyme (p.1636·3); althaea (p.1546·3); drosera (p.1574·1).
Catarrh; coughs.

Biovaline *Gerda, Fr.†.*
DL-Valine; pyridoxine (p.1363·1); cyanocobalamin (p.1363·3).
Tonic.

Bioveinal *Fuca, Fr.†.*
Hamamelis (p.1587·1); viburnum; aesculus (p.1543·3); esculoside (p.1543·3).
Peripheral vascular disorders.

Biovelbin *Biogalenica, Spain.*
Vinorelbine tartrate (p.571·2).
Breast cancer; lung cancer.

Biovigor *Biotrading, Ital.*
Royal jelly (p.1626·3); honey (p.1345·3).
Nutritional supplement.

Biovigor Polline *Biotrading, Ital.†.*
Pollen; honey (p.1345·3).
Nutritional supplement.

Biovit-A *Bioceuticals, UK.*
Vitamin A (p.1358·1).

Biovital
Note. This name is used for preparations of different composition.
Polcopharma, Austral.†; Rhone-Poulenc Rorer, Irl.; Rhone-Poulenc Rorer, S.Afr.†; Roche, UK.
Multivitamin and mineral preparation.

Lampugnani, Ital.
Royal jelly (p.1626·3).
Nutritional supplement.

Biovital Forte N *Schieffer, Ger.*
Crataegus (p.1568·2); caffeine citrate (p.749·3); ferrous gluconate (p.1340·1); vitamins.
Tonic.

Biovital Ginseng *Schieffer, Switz.*
Ginseng (p.1584·2); caffeine (p.749·3); lecithin (p.1595·2); vitamins and minerals.
Tonic.

Biovital N *Schieffer, Ger.*
Oral liquid: Crataegus (p.1568·2); motherwort (p.1604·2); ferric sodium citrate; vitamins.
Tablets: Crataegus (p.1568·2); motherwort (p.1604·2); ferrous sulphate (p.1340·2); ferric sodium citrate; vitamins.
Tonic.

Bioxidona *Faes, Spain.*
Amoxycillin trihydrate (p.151·3).
Bacterial infections.

Bioxima *Kemyos, Ital.*
Cefuroxime sodium (p.177·1).
Bacterial infections.

Bioxyol *Richard, Fr.*
Zinc oxide (p.1096·2); zinc peroxide (p.1127·3); titanium dioxide (p.1093·3); diatom powder.
Burns; ulcers; wounds.

Bio-Zinc *Herbaxt, Fr.*
Zinc pidolate; vitamin A; vitamin B_6.
Nutritional supplement.

Biozolene *Bioindustria, Ital.*
Fluconazole (p.378·1).
Fungal infections.

Bipectinol *Propan, S.Afr.*
Kaolin (p.1195·1); pectin (p.1474·1); electrolytes (p.1147·1).
Diarrhoea.

Bipenicilline *Diamant, Fr.†.*
Benzylpenicillin sodium (p.159·3); procaine penicillin (p.240·2).
Bacterial infections.

Bipensaar *Rosen, Ger.*
Benzylpenicillin sodium (p.159·3); procaine penicillin (p.240·2).
Lignocaine hydrochloride (p.1293·2) is included in this preparation to alleviate the pain of injection.
Bacterial infections.

Biphasil
Wyeth, Austral.; Akromed, S.Afr.
Levonorgestrel (p.1454·1); ethinyloestradiol (p.1445·1).
28-Day packs also contain 7 inert tablets.
Biphasic oral contraceptive; menstrual disorders.

Biphedrine Aqueuse *Bouchara, Fr.†.*
Ephedrine hydrochloride (p.1059·3); amylocaine hydrochloride (p.1286·1); chlorbutol (p.1106·3).
Rhinitis; sinusitis.

Biphedrine Huileuse *Bouchara, Fr.†.*
Ephedrine (p.1059·3); camphor (p.1557·2); cineole (p.1564·1); mint oil (p.1208·1); lemon oil (p.1595·3); anise oil (p.1550·1).
Nasal congestion.

Biplatrix *Smith & Nephew, Fr.*
Dried calcium sulphate (p.1557·2).
External splinting.

Bi-Profenid *Specia, Fr.*
Ketoprofen (p.48·2).
Musculoskeletal and joint disorders.

Biquin
Note. This name is used for preparations of different composition.
Nelson, Austral.†.
Quinine bisulphate (p.439·1).

Astra, Canad.
Quinidine bisulphate (p.938·3).
Arrhythmias.

Biquinate *Rhone-Poulenc Rorer, Austral.*
Quinine bisulphate (p.439·1).
Diagnosis of myasthenia gravis; malaria; muscle cramps; myotonia congenita.

Bi-Qui-Nol *Monot, Fr.*
Cineole (p.1564·1); guaiacol (p.1061·2); camphor (p.1557·2); bismuth succinate (p.1181·1).
Formerly contained cineole, guaiacol, camphor, bismuth succinate, and quinine sulphate.
Mouth and throat disorders.

Biral
Madaus, Ger.; Madaus, S.Afr.
Valerian (p.1643·1); passion flower (p.1615·3).
Anxiety; minor nervous disorders.

Birley's *Torbet Laboratories, UK.*
Dried aluminium hydroxide (p.1177·3); magnesium trisilicate (p.1199·1); light magnesium carbonate (p.1198·1).
Gastro-intestinal hyperacidity.

Birobin *Sandoz, Aust.*
Metolazone (p.907·2).
Hypertension; oedema.

Birofenid *Rhone-Poulenc Rorer, Belg.*
Ketoprofen (p.48·2).
Inflammation; musculoskeletal, joint, and peri-articular disorders; oedema; pain.

Biroxol *Salus, Ital.*
Ciclopirox olamine (p.376·2).
Fungal infections.

Bisac-Evac *G & W, USA.*
Bisacodyl (p.1179·3).
Constipation.

Bisacolax *ICN, Canad.*
Bisacodyl (p.1179·3).
Constipation.

Bisalax *Rhone-Poulenc Rorer, Austral.*
Bisacodyl (p.1179·3).
Bowel evacuation; constipation.

Bisco-Lax *Raway, USA.*
Bisacodyl (p.1179·3).
Constipation.

Biscotto Plasmon *Plasmon, Ital.*
Protein, carbohydrate, and lipid preparation with minerals and vitamins.
Nutritional supplement.

Biscotto Polial *Plasmon, Ital.†.*
Food for special diets.
Milk and gluten intolerance.

Bisco-Zitron *Biscova, Ger.*
Bisacodyl (p.1179·3).
Constipation.

Biseko
Note. This name is used for preparations of different composition.
Biotest, Aust.; Biotest, Ger.
A plasma protein fraction (p.726·3).
Hypoproteinaemia; hypovolaemia; passive immunisation.

Biotest, Switz.†.
Albumin (p.710·1).
Hypoalbuminaemia.

Biseptidine *Pan Quimica, Spain†.*
Benzalkonium chloride (p.1101·3); chlorhexidine gluconate (p.1107·2).
Disinfection of skin, body cavities, and instruments.

Biseptine *Nicholas, Fr.*
Chlorhexidine gluconate (p.1107·2); benzalkonium chloride (p.1101·3); benzyl alcohol (p.1103·3).
Skin and wound disinfection.

Biseptol compositum *Winzer, Ger.†.*
Ethacridine (p.1098·3); cetalkonium chloride (p.1105·2); (+)-propyl-(*O*-benzoyl-pseudotropin-2-carboxylate).
Eye disorders.

Biseptol simplex *Winzer, Ger.*
Ethacridine (p.1098·3).
Antiseptic; eye infections.

Biserirte Magnesia *Whitehall, Norw.*
Magnesium subcarbonate (p.1198·1); sodium bicarbonate (p.1153·2); bismuth subcarbonate (p.1180·1).
Gastro-intestinal disorders associated with hyperacidity.

Biskapect *Propan, S.Afr.*
Light kaolin (p.1195·1); apple pectin (p.1474·1); bismuth subcarbonate (p.1180·1).
Diarrhoea.

Bismag *Whitehall, UK.*
Sodium bicarbonate (p.1153·2); heavy magnesium carbonate (p.1198·1); light magnesium carbonate.
Dyspepsia; flatulence.

Bisma-Rex *3M, UK.*
Bismuth subcarbonate (p.1180·1); calcium carbonate (p.1182·1); magnesium trisilicate (p.1199·1); magnesium carbonate (p.1198·1); peppermint oil (p.1208·1).
Dyspepsia; flatulence.

Bismatrol *Major, USA.*
Bismuth salicylate (p.1180·1).
Diarrhoea; dyspepsia; nausea.

Bismed *Technilab, Canad.*
Oral liquid: Bismuth salicylate (p.1180·1).
Tablets: Bismuth salicylate (p.1180·1); calcium carbonate (p.1182·1).
Diarrhoea; dyspepsia.

Bismofalk *Falk, Ger.*
Bismuth subgallate (p.1180·2); bismuth subnitrate (p.1180·2).
Gastro-intestinal disorders.

Bismolan *Gastropharm, Ger.*
Bismuth subnitrate (p.1180·2); butoxycaine hydrochloride (p.1289·1); zinc oxide (p.1096·2).
Formerly contained bismuth oxychloride, procaine hydrochloride, and peru balsam.
Anorectal disorders.

Bismolan H *Gastropharm, Ger.*
Prednisolone acetate (p.1048·1); bismuth oxychloride (p.1181·1); zinc oxide (p.1096·2).
Anorectal disorders.

Bismorectal *Vifor, Switz.*
Bismuth succinate (p.1181·1); bismuth hydroxyquinoline (p.1181·1); eucalyptus oil (p.1578·1).
Mouth and throat disorders.

Bismulcid *Azuchemie, Ger.†.*
Bismuth salicylate (p.1180·1); calcium carbonate (p.1182·1); magnesium peroxide (p.1119·1).
Gastro-intestinal disorders.

Bismurectol *Bouchara Sante, Fr.*
Bismuth succinate (p.1181·1); cineole (p.1564·1); camphor (p.1557·2).
Upper respiratory-tract congestion.

Bismuth Tulasne *Rhone-Poulenc Rorer, Switz.*
Bismuth subnitrate (p.1180·2).
Dyspepsia; peptic ulcer.

Bismylate *Stanley, Canad.*
Bismuth salicylate (p.1180·1).

Bisobloc
Azupharma, Ger.; Lederle, Neth.
Bisoprolol fumarate (p.833·1).
Angina pectoris; hypertension.

Bisodol
Whitehall, Irl.; Whitehall, UK.
Oral powder: Heavy magnesium carbonate (p.1198·1); light magnesium carbonate; sodium bicarbonate (p.1153·2).
Dyspepsia; flatulence.

Whitehall, Irl.; Whitehall, UK.
Tablets: Calcium carbonate (p.1182·1); light magnesium carbonate (p.1198·1); sodium bicarbonate (p.1153·2).
Dyspepsia; flatulence.

Bisodol Extra
Whitehall, Irl.†; Whitehall, UK.
Calcium carbonate (p.1182·1); light magnesium carbonate (p.1198·1); sodium bicarbonate (p.1153·2); simethicone (p.1213·1).
Dyspepsia; flatulence.

Bisodol Heartburn Whitehall, UK.
Alginic acid (p.1470·3); magaldrate (p.1198·1); sodium bicarbonate (p.1153·2).
Heartburn.

Bisolapid Boehringer Ingelheim, Switz.
Acetylcysteine (p.1052·3).
Excess respiratory mucus.

Bisolbruis Boehringer Ingelheim, Neth.
Acetylcysteine (p.1052·3).
Respiratory-tract disorders associated with increased mucus.

Bisolgrip Fher, Spain.
Chlorpheniramine maleate (p.405·1); phenylephrine hydrochloride (p.1066·2); paracetamol (p.72·2).
Cold symptoms.

Bisolnasal Boehringer Ingelheim, Neth.
Tramazoline hydrochloride (p.1071·1).
Nasal congestion.

Bisolpent
Boehringer Ingelheim, Ital.†; Boehringer Ingelheim, S.Afr.†.
Bromhexine hydrochloride (p.1055·3); orciprenaline sulphate (p.756·3).
Respiratory-tract disorders.

Bisoltus Fher, Spain.
Codeine hydrochloride (p.26·1).
Cough; diarrhoea; pain.

Bisolvex Boehringer Ingelheim, Switz.
Cineole (p.1564·1); camphor (p.1557·2); niaouli oil (p.1607·1).
Cold symptoms.

Bisolvit Nuovo, Ital.†.
Thiamine hydrochloride (p.1361·1).

Bisolvomed Thomae, Ger.†.
Oral drops: Bromhexine hydrochloride (p.1055·3); ephedrine hydrochloride (p.1059·3); menthol (p.1600·2); fennel oil (p.1579·2); anise oil (p.1550·1); thyme oil (p.1637·1); peppermint oil (p.1208·1); cineole (p.1564·1).
Oral liquid: Bromhexine hydrochloride (p.1055·3); ephedrine hydrochloride (p.1059·3).
Coughs and associated respiratory-tract disorders.

Bisolvomed mit Codein Thomae, Ger.†.
Bromhexine hydrochloride (p.1055·3); ephedrine hydrochloride (p.1059·3); menthol (p.1600·2); fennel oil (p.1579·2); anise oil (p.1550·1); thyme oil (p.1637·1); peppermint oil (p.1208·1); cineole (p.1564·1); codeine phosphate (p.26·1).
Coughs and associated respiratory-tract disorders.

Bisolvomicin Boehringer Ingelheim, Ital.†.
Bromhexine hydrochloride (p.1055·3); oxytetracycline hydrochloride (p.235·1).
Respiratory-tract disorders.

Bisolvomycin
Bender, Aust.; Thomae, Ger.; Boehringer Ingelheim, S.Afr.
Bromhexine hydrochloride (p.1055·3); oxytetracycline hydrochloride (p.235·1).
Bacterial infections of the respiratory tract.

Bisolvon
Bender, Aust.; Boehringer Ingelheim, Austral.; Boehringer Ingelheim, Belg.; Boehringer Ingelheim, Fr.; Thomae, Ger.; Boehringer Ingelheim, Irl.; Boehringer Ingelheim, Ital.; Boehringer Ingelheim, Neth.; Boehringer Ingelheim, Norw.; Boehringer Ingelheim, S.Afr.; Fher, Spain; Boehringer Ingelheim, Swed.; Boehringer Ingelheim, Switz.
Bromhexine hydrochloride (p.1055·3).
Respiratory-tract disorders.

Bisolvon AM Thomae, Ger.
Ambroxol hydrochloride (p.1054·3).
Respiratory-tract disorders associated with increased or viscous mucus.

Bisolvon Amoxycilina Fher, Spain.
Amoxycillin trihydrate (p.151·3); bromhexine hydrochloride (p.1055·3).
Respiratory-tract infections.

Bisolvon Ampicil Retard Fher, Spain†.
Ampicillin sodium (p.153·1); ampicillin benzathine (p.154·1); bromhexine hydrochloride (p.1055·3).
Respiratory-tract infections.

Bisolvon Ampicilina Fher, Spain†.
Ampicillin trihydrate (p.153·2); bromhexine hydrochloride (p.1055·3).
Respiratory-tract infections.

Bisolvon Ciclina Fher, Spain†.
Bromhexine hydrochloride (p.1055·3); oxytetracycline hydrochloride (p.235·1).
Formerly also available as an oral suspension which contained bromhexine and tetracycline.
Respiratory-tract infections.

Bisolvon Compositum Fher, Spain.
Bromhexine hydrochloride (p.1055·3); codeine hydrochloride (p.26·1); diphenhydramine hydrochloride (p.409·1); ephedrine hydrochloride (p.1059·3).
Formerly contained bromhexine hydrochloride, codeine hydrochloride, diphenhydramine hydrochloride, ephedrine hydrochloride, noscapine hydrochloride, and papaverine hydrochloride.
Respiratory-tract disorders.

Bisolvon F Thomae, Ger.†.
Bromhexine hydrochloride (p.1055·3).
Respiratory-tract disorders associated with increased or viscous mucus.

Bisolvon Gribletten Thomae, Ger.†.
Bromhexine hydrochloride (p.1055·3); codeine phosphate (p.26·1); aspirin (p.16·1).
Coughs and cold symptoms.

Bisolvon Linctus Boehringer Ingelheim, Switz.
Bromhexine hydrochloride (p.1055·3); ammonium chloride (p.1055·2).
Respiratory-tract disorders.

Bisolvon Linctus DA Boehringer Ingelheim, S.Afr.
Bromhexine hydrochloride (p.1055·3); orciprenaline sulphate (p.756·3).
Obstructive airways disease.

Bisolvon NAC Thomae, Ger.
Acetylcysteine (p.1052·3).
Bronchitis.

Bisolvon Pilules antigrippales Boehringer Ingelheim, Switz.†.
Bromhexine hydrochloride (p.1055·3); codeine phosphate (p.26·1); aspirin (p.16·1).
Bronchial catarrh; cold symptoms.

Bisolvonamid
Bender, Aust.; Thomae, Ger.†.
Bromhexine hydrochloride (p.1055·3); sulphadiazine (p.252·3).
Bacterial respiratory-tract infections.

Bisolvonat Thomae, Ger.
Bromhexine hydrochloride (p.1055·3); erythromycin ethyl succinate (p.204·2).
Bacterial respiratory-tract infections.

Bisolvonat Mono Thomae, Ger.
Erythromycin (p.204·1) or erythromycin ethyl succinate (p.204·2).
Bacterial infections.

Bisolvotin Bender, Aust.
Bromhexine hydrochloride (p.1055·3); ammonium chloride (p.1055·2); benzoic acid (p.1102·3).
Coughs.

Bisomerck Merck, Ger.
Bisoprolol fumarate (p.833·1).
Angina pectoris; hypertension.

Bispan Chinoin, Hung.
Isopropamide iodide (p.464·3); drotaverine hydrochloride (p.1574·2).
Peptic ulcer; smooth muscle spasm.

Bisrenin Winzer, Ger.
Bismuth subgallate (p.1180·2); naphazoline hydrochloride (p.1064·2).
Eye disorders.

Bitensil UCB, Spain.
Enalapril maleate (p.863·2).
Heart failure; hypertension.

Bitensil Diu UCB, Spain.
Enalapril maleate (p.863·2); hydrochlorothiazide (p.885·2).
Hypertension.

Bi-Tildiem Synthelabo, Fr.
Diltiazem hydrochloride (p.854·2).
Angina pectoris.

Bitteridina AFOM, Ital.
Cinchona calisaya (p.1564·1); calumba (p.1557·2); angelica; cascara (p.1183·1); valerian (p.1643·1).
Constipation.

Biuricowas Wasserman, Spain†.
Allopurinol (p.390·2); benziodarone (p.393·1).
Gout; hyperuricaemia; renal calculi.

Bivacyn Medphano, Ger.
Neomycin sulphate (p.229·2); bacitracin (p.157·3).
Ear inflammation; eye disorders; skin disorders; urinary-tract infections; wounds.

Bivaraten Swisspharm, S.Afr.
A measles and mumps vaccine (p.1519·2).
Active immunisation.

Bi-Vaspit Asche, Ger.
Fluocortin butyl (p.1041·3); isoconazole nitrate (p.381·2).
Nappy rash.

Biviol Nourypharma, Ger.
Desogestrel (p.1443·3); ethinyloestradiol (p.1445·1).
Biphasic oral contraceptive.

Biviraten Berna, Switz.
A measles and mumps vaccine (p.1519·2).
Active immunisation.

Bivitasi ISI, Ital.
Cocarboxylase (p.1361·2).
Vitamin B_1 deficiency.

Bivitox Terapeutico, Ital.
Cogalactoisomerase disodium (p.1566·2).
Liver disorders.

Bivlar Schering, Ital.†.
Levonorgestrel (p.1454·1); ethinyloestradiol (p.1445·1).
Biphasic oral contraceptive.

BJ6 Macarthys, UK†; Thornton & Ross, UK†.
Hypromellose (p.1473·1).
Dry eyes.

B-Ject Hyrex, USA.
Vitamin B substances.
2.
Parenteral nutrition.

B-kombin ACO, Swed.
Vitamin B substances.
Vitamin B deficiency.

Black Be-Tabs, S.Afr.†.
Nutritional supplement.

Black-Draught Chattem, USA.
Syrup: Casanthranol (p.1182·3); senna (p.1212·2); rhubarb (p.1212·1).
Tablets; oral granules: Senna (p.1212·2).
Constipation.

Blackoids du Docteur Meur SERP, Mon.
Menthol (p.1600·2); liquorice (p.1197·1).
Sore throat.

Blairex Lens Lubricant Blairex, USA.
Range of solutions for soft contact lenses.

Blandonal Falqui, Ital.
Passion flower (p.1615·3); crataegus (p.1568·2).
Insomnia.

Blapidon Vitaminado Perez Gimenez, Spain†.
Caffeine (p.749·3); chlorpheniramine maleate (p.405·1); ascorbic acid (p.1365·2); paracetamol (p.72·2).
Fever; nasal congestion; pain.

Blascorid Guidotti, Ital.†.
Benproperine embonate (p.1055·2).
Coughs.

Blasen- und Nierentee
Note. This name is used for preparations of different composition.
Salus, Aust.
Bearberry (p.1552·2); equisetum (p.1575·1); birch leaf (p.1553·3).
Kidney and bladder disorders.

Schoeller, Aust.
Bearberry (p.1552·2); equisetum (p.1575·1); birch leaf (p.1553·3); orthosiphon (p.1592·2); mate leaf (p.1645·1).
Kidney and bladder disorders.

Blasen-Nieren-Tee Stada Stada, Ger.
Couch-grass (p.1567·3); ononis (p.1610·2); solidago virgaurea; liquorice (p.1197·1); betulae (p.1553·3).
Urinary-tract infections.

Blasen-Nieren-Tee Uroflux Nattermann Tee-Arznei, Ger.†.
Betula (p.1553·3); juniper (p.1592·2); phaseolus vulgaris; equisetum (p.1575·1); ononis (p.1610·2); couch-grass (p.1567·3); bearberry (p.1552·2).
Urinary-tract infections.

Blasen-Nieren-Tee Uroflux S Nattermann Tee-Arznei, Ger.†.
Bearberry (p.1552·2); silver birch (p.1553·3); couch-grass (p.1567·3).
Urinary-tract disorders.

Blasen-Tee Mayrhofer, Aust.
Bearberry (p.1552·2); herniaria (p.1587·2); juniper (p.1592·2); ononis (p.1610·2); parsley root (p.1615·3); peppermint leaf (p.1208·1).
Kidney and bladder disorders.

Blasentee Smetana, Aust.
Birch leaf (p.1553·3); herniaria (p.1587·2); equisetum (p.1575·1); calluna vulgaris.
Kidney and bladder disorders.

Blastoestimulina Funk, Spain.
Injection; topical powder; eye drops: Centella asiatica (p.1080·3).
Burns; eye disorders; ulcers; wounds.
Ointment; medicated dressing: Centella asiatica (p.1080·3); neomycin sulphate (p.229·2).
Burns; skin infections; ulcers; wounds.
Pessaries: Centella asiatica (p.1080·3); chlordantoin (p.376·2); metronidazole (p.585·1); neomycin sulphate (p.229·2); polymyxin B sulphate (p.239·1).
Vulvovaginal infections.
Topical aerosol: Centella asiatica (p.1080·3); amethocaine (p.1285·2).
Burns; ulcers; wounds.

Blastoidin R.C. Giuliani, Switz.†.
Cyanocobalamin; liver extract; folic acid.
Tonic.

Blastoifer Giuliani, Switz.†.
Ferrous fumarate (p.1339·3); liver extract; manganese-sodium citrate.
Iron deficiency.

Blaston Tecnobio, Spain.
Cinitapride acid tartrate (p.1187·1).
Gastro-oesophageal reflux; gastroparesis.

Bled Poli, Ital.†.
Ciclonicate.
Vascular disorders.

Blefarida Cusi, Spain.
Chloramphenicol (p.182·1); cortisone acetate (p.1036·1).
Infected eye disorders.

Blefarolin Bruschettini, Ital.
Tannic acid (p.1634·2); resorcinol (p.1090·1); menthol (p.1600·2).
Eye disorders.

Blefcon
Note. This name is used for preparations of different composition.
Alcon-Thilo, Ger.
Sulphacetamide sodium (p.252·2); prednisolone acetate (p.1048·1).
Allergic and inflammatory disorders of the eye.

Allergan, Swed.
Sulphacetamide sodium (p.252·2); prednisolone acetate (p.1048·1); phenylephrine hydrochloride (p.1066·2).
Blepharitis.

Blemaren N Esparma, Ger.
Citric acid (p.1564·3); anhydrous sodium citrate (p.1153·2); potassium bicarbonate (p.1153·1).
Hyperuricaemia; porphyria cutanea tarda; renal calculi.

Blemerase Young, USA.
Benzoyl peroxide (p.1079·2).
Acne.

Bleminol Gepepharm, Ger.
Allopurinol (p.390·2).
Gout; hyperuricaemia; renal calculi.

Blemish Control Kay, Canad.
Salicylic acid (p.1090·2).
Acne.

Blemix Ashbourne, UK.
Minocycline (p.227·1).
Bacterial infections.

Blend-a-med Fluid Blend-a-med, Ger.†.
2,2′-Dihydroxy-3,3′-dibromo-5,5′-dichlorodiphenylmethane; guaiazulene (p.1586·3); arnica (p.1550·3); myrrh (p.1606·1).
Gingivitis; stomatitis.

Blenox Pharmacia Upjohn, Spain.
Amoxycillin (p.151·3).
Probenecid (p.394·3) is included in this preparation to reduce renal tubular excretion of amoxycillin.
Bacterial infections.

Blenoxane
Bristol-Myers Squibb, Austral.; Bristol, Canad.; Bristol-Myers Squibb, S.Afr.; Bristol-Myers Oncology, USA.
Bleomycin sulphate (p.507·3).
Malignant neoplasms.

Bleo
Kayaku, Jpn; Kyowa, UK.
Bleomycin hydrochloride (p.508·3) or bleomycin sulphate (p.507·3).
Malignant neoplasms.

Bleo-cell Cell Pharm, Ger.
Bleomycin sulphate (p.507·3).
Malignant neoplasms.

Bleo-S Kayaku, Jpn.
Bleomycin sulphate (p.507·3).
Skin cancer.

Bleph-10
Allergan, Austral.; Allergan, Irl.†; Allergan, S.Afr.; Allergan, USA.
Sulphacetamide sodium (p.252·2).
Eye infections.

Bleph-10 Liquifilm Allergan, Canad.
Sulphacetamide sodium (p.252·2).
Eye infections.

Blephamide
Note. This name is used for preparations of different composition.
Allergan, Aust.; Allergan, Austral.; Allergan, Irl.†; Allergan, S.Afr.
Sulphacetamide sodium (p.252·2); prednisolone acetate (p.1048·1); phenylephrine hydrochloride (p.1066·2).
Blepharitis; conjunctivitis.

Allergan, Canad.; Allergan, Ger.; Allergan, Switz.; Allergan, USA.
Sulphacetamide sodium (p.252·2); prednisolone acetate (p.1048·1).
Formerly contained sulphacetamide sodium, phenazone, sodium thiosulphate, prednisolone acetate, and phenylephrine hydrochloride in *Switz.*
Blepharitis; conjunctivitis.

Blephamide N Liquifilm Allergan, Ger.
Sulphacetamide sodium (p.252·2); prednisolone acetate (p.1048·1).
Blepharitis; conjunctivitis; eye infections.

Blephaseptyl
Chauvin, Fr.†; Novopharma, Switz.†.
Fludrocortisone acetate (p.1040·1); hexamidine diisethionate (p.1115·3); selenium sulphide (p.1091·1).
Blepharitis.

Blephasulf Allergan, Aust.†.
Sulphacetamide sodium (p.252·2).
Blepharitis; conjunctivitis; dacryocystitis.

Bleukawine Ern, Spain.
Homatropine methobromide (p.462·2); kava (p.1592·3); methylene blue (p.984·3).
Urinary-tract infections.

Blink-N-Clean Allergan, Austral.†.
Polyoxyl 40 stearate (p.1327·2); macrogol 300 (p.1598·2).
Hard contact lens cleanser.

Blinx
Note. This name is used for preparations of different composition.
Barnes-Hind, Austral.†.
Boric acid (p.1554·2); borax (p.1554·2).
Eye irrigation.

Pilkington Barnes-Hind, USA.
Electrolytes (p.1147·1).
Eye irrigation.

BlisterGard Medtech, USA.
Topical barrier preparation.

Blistex Blistex, USA.
Camphor (p.1557·2); phenol (p.1121·2); allantoin (p.1078·2).
Oral lesions.

Blistex Aloe & Vitamin E Key, Austral.†.
Padimate O (p.1488·1); vitamin E acetate (p.1369·1); aloe vera (p.1177·1).
Dry lips; sunscreen.

Blistex DCT Lip Balm Blistex, Canad.
SPF 15: Padimate O (p.1488·1); oxybenzone (p.1487·3); menthol (p.1600·2); phenol (p.1121·2); camphor (p.1557·2).
Chapped lips; sunscreen.

Blistex Faceblock Key, Austral.†.
SPF15+: Ethylhexyl *p*-methoxycinnamate (p.1487·1); menthyl anthranilate (p.1487·2); oxybenzone (p.1487·3).
Sunscreen.

Blistex Lip Balm
Note. This name is used for preparations of different composition.
Blistex, Canad.
SPF 10: Padimate O (p.1488·1); oxybenzone (p.1487·3); dimethicone (p.1384·2).
Chapped lips; sunscreen.

Blistex, USA.
SPF 10: Camphor (p.1557·2); phenol (p.1121·2); allantoin (p.1078·2); dimethicone (p.1384·2); padimate O (p.1488·1); oxybenzone (p.1487·3).
Chapped lips; sunscreen.

Blistex Lip Ointment *Blistex, Canad.*
Allantoin (p.1078·2); camphor (p.1557·2); phenol (p.1121·2).
Chapped lips; herpes labialis.

Blistex Lip Tone
Note. This name is used for preparations of different composition.
Key, Austral.
SPF15+: Ethylhexyl *p*-methoxycinnamate (p.1487·1); oxybenzone (p.1487·3).
Dry lips; sunscreen.

Blistex, Canad.
SPF 15: Padimate O (p.1488·1); menthyl anthranilate (p.1487·2); dimethicone (p.1384·2).
Chapped lips; sunscreen.

Blistex Medicated Lip Balm *Key, Austral.*
SPF15+: Padimate O (p.1488·1); oxybenzone (p.1487·3).
Dry lips; sunscreen.

Blistex Medicated Lip Conditioner *Key, Austral.*
SPF15+: Yellow soft paraffin (p.1382·3); padimate O (p.1488·1); oxybenzone (p.1487·3).
Dry lips; sunscreen.

Blistex Medicated Lip Conditioner Jar *Blistex, Canad.*
Camphor (p.1557·2); menthol (p.1600·2); menthyl anthranilate (p.1487·2); padimate O (p.1488·1); phenol (p.1121·2).
Chapped lips; herpes labialis.

Blistex Medicated Lip Conditioner Tube *Blistex, Canad.*
SPF 15: Padimate O (p.1488·1); oxybenzone (p.1487·3); camphor (p.1557·2).
Sunscreen.

Blistex Medicated Lip Ointment *Key, Austral.*
SPF15+: Padimate O (p.1488·1); oxybenzone (p.1487·3); allantoin (p.1078·2); camphor (p.1557·2).
Dry lips; sunscreen.

Blistex Sun Block Lip Balm *Key, Austral.†.*
SPF15+: Padimate O (p.1488·1); oxybenzone (p.1487·3); allantoin (p.1078·2).
Dry lips; sunscreen.

Blistex Sunblock *Blistex, Canad.†.*
SPF 15: Dimethicone (p.1384·2); padimate O (p.1488·1); oxybenzone (p.1487·3).
Sunscreen.

Blistex Ultra *Blistex, USA.*
SPF 30: Ethylhexyl *p*-methoxycinnamate (p.1487·1); oxybenzone (p.1487·3); octyl salicylate (p.1487·3); methyl anthranilate; homosalate (p.1487·2).
Sunscreen.

Blistex Ultra Lip Balm *Blistex, Canad.*
SPF 30: Ethylhexyl *p* methoxycinnamate (p.1487·1); oxybenzone (p.1487·3); octyl salicylate (p.1487·3); menthyl anthranilate (p.1487·2); homosalate (p.1487·2); dimethicone (p.1384·2).
Chapped lips; sunscreen.

Blisteze *DDD, UK.*
Strong ammonia solution (p.1548·3); ammonia solution aromatic; phenol (p.1121·2).
Chapped lips; herpes labialis.

Blistik *Key, Austral.†.*
Padimate O (p.1488·1); oxybenzone (p.1487·3); allantoin (p.1078·2).
Dry lips; sunscreen.

Blis-To-Sol *Chattem, USA.*
Topical liquid: Tolnaftate (p.389·1).
Topical powder: Zinc undecenoate (p.389·2).
Formerly contained benzoic acid and salicylic acid.
Fungal skin infections.

Blocadren
Merck Sharp & Dohme, Aust.; Frosst, Austral.; Merck Sharp & Dohme, Belg.; Frosst, Canad.; Merck Sharp & Dohme, Irl.; Merck Sharp & Dohme, Ital.; Merck Sharp & Dohme, Neth.; Merck Sharp & Dohme, Norw.; Merck Sharp & Dohme, S.Afr.; Merck Sharp & Dohme, Spain†; Merck Sharp & Dohme, Swed.; Merck Sharp & Dohme, Switz.; Merck Sharp & Dohme, UK; Merck, USA.
Timolol maleate (p.953·3).
Angina pectoris; arrhythmias; glaucoma; hypertension; migraine; myocardial infarction; ocular hypertension.

Block-Aid *ICN, Canad.†.*
Roxadimate (p.1488·2); oxybenzone (p.1487·3).
Sunscreen.

Blockel *Mochida, Jpn†.*
Carbazochrome sodium sulphonate (p.714·2).
Haemorrhage.

Blocotenol *Azupharma, Ger.*
Atenolol (p.825·3).
Angina pectoris; arrhythmias; hypertension.

Blocotenol comp *Azupharma, Ger.*
Atenolol (p.825·3); chlorthalidone (p.839·3).
Hypertension.

Blocotin *Hoechst, Spain†.*
Penbutolol sulphate (p.927·2).
Angina pectoris; arrhythmias; hypertension.

Blodex *Estedi, Spain.*
Vegetable oil (p.1643·3).
Adjunct in cholecystography and cholangiography.

Blokium *Prodes, Spain.*
Atenolol (p.825·3).
Angina pectoris; arrhythmias; hypertension; myocardial infarction.

Blokium Diu *Prodes, Spain.*
Chlorthalidone (p.839·3); atenolol (p.825·3).
Hypertension.

Blood Tone Organic Iron *Suisse, Austral.†.*
B vitamins, minerals and iron preparation.
Anaemias.

Blox *Biomedica, Ital.†.*
Loperamide hydrochloride (p.1197·2).
Diarrhoea.

Bluboro *Allergan Herbert, USA.*
Aluminium sulphate (p.1548·1); calcium acetate (p.1155·1).
Bruises; skin inflammation.

Blue *Ambix, USA; Moore, USA.*
Pyrethrins; piperonyl butoxide (p.1409·3).
Pediculosis.

Blue Collyrium *Sabex, Canad.*
Methylene blue (p.984·3); naphazoline hydrochloride (p.1064·2).
Eye irritation.

Blue Flag Root Compound *Gerard House, UK.*
Blue flag root (p.1591·3); burdock (p.1594·2); sarsaparilla (p.1627·2).
Minor skin disorders.

Blue Gel Muscular Pain Reliever *Rugby, USA.*
Menthol (p.1600·2).

Bluesteril *IMS, Ital.*
Benzalkonium chloride (p.1101·3).
Instrument disinfection.

Bluetest *Quidel, Fr.*
Pregnancy or fertility test (p.1621·2).

Blunorm *Pharma-Natura, Ital.*
Hesperidin (p.1580·2); diosmin (p.1580·1); vitamin C (p.1365·2).
Nutritional supplement in vascular disorders.

Blutal *Dainippon, Jpn.*
Chondroitin sulphate-iron colloid (p.1337·1).
Iron-deficiency anaemia.

Blutquick Forte *Duopharm, Ger.*
Ferrous gluconate (p.1340·1); vitamin B substances.
Iron deficiency; tonic.

Blutquick Forte S *Duopharm, Ger.*
Ferrous fumarate (p.1339·3); ferric sodium citrate; ferrous gluconate (p.1340·1).
Iron-deficiency anaemia.

Blutreinigungstee *Smetana, Aust.†.*
Senna leaf (p.1212·2); frangula bark (p.1193·2); equisetum (p.1575·1); sambucus (p.1627·2); cortex cacao (p.1636·2); flores calcatrippae.
Skin disorders; tonic.

Blutreinigungs-Tee *Kneipp, Ger.†.*
Juniper berries; peppermint leaves; birch leaves.
Herbal preparation.

BM-Accutest
Boehringer Mannheim Diagnostics, Irl.; Boehringer Mannheim Diagnostics, UK.
Test for glucose in blood (p.1585·1).

BM-Hopitest *Boehringer Mannheim Diagnostics, UK.*
Test for protein, glucose, ketones, and blood in urine.

BMS *Bio-Medical, UK†.*
Liquid paraffin (p.1382·1); wool alcohols (p.1385·2).

BM-Test 1-44
Boehringer Mannheim Diagnostics, Irl.; Boehringer Mannheim Diagnostics, UK.
Test for glucose in blood (p.1585·1).
Formerly known as BM-Test Glycemie 1-44 in the *UK.*

BM-Test 3
Boehringer Mannheim Diagnostics, Irl.; Boehringer Mannheim Diagnostics, UK.
Test for pH, protein, and glucose in urine.

BM-Test 4
Boehringer Mannheim Diagnostics, Irl.; Boehringer Mannheim Diagnostics, UK.
Test for nitrite, pH, protein, and glucose in urine.

BM-Test 7
Boehringer Mannheim Diagnostics, Irl.; Boehringer Mannheim Diagnostics, UK.
Test for pH, protein, glucose, ketones, urobilinogen, bilirubin, and blood in urine.

BM-Test 8
Boehringer Mannheim Diagnostics, Irl.; Boehringer Mannheim Diagnostics, UK.
Test for nitrite, pH, protein, glucose, ketones, urobilinogen, bilirubin, and blood in urine.

BM-Test BG
Boehringer Mannheim, Austral.; Boehringer Mannheim, Ital.; Boehringer Mannheim Diagnostics, UK†.
Test for glucose in blood (p.1585·1).

BM-Test Colon-Albumin *Boehringer Mannheim, S.Afr.*
Test for blood in faeces.

BM-Test Glycemie *Boehringer Mannheim, Fr.*
Test for glucose in blood (p.1585·1).

BM-Test Glycemie 20-800 *Boehringer Mannheim, Austral.*
Test for glucose in blood (p.1585·1).

BM-Test GP
Boehringer Mannheim, Austral.; Boehringer Mannheim Diagnostics, UK.
Test for glucose and protein in urine.

BM-Test Ketur *Boehringer Mannheim Diagnostics, Irl.*
Test for ketones in urine.

BM-Test 5L
Boehringer Mannheim Diagnostics, Irl.; Boehringer Mannheim Diagnostics, UK.
Test for pH, protein, glucose, ketones, and blood in urine.

BM-Test LN *Boehringer Mannheim, Fr.*
Test for leucocytes and nitrites in urine.

BM-Test Meconium *Boehringer Mannheim Diagnostics, UK.*
Test for cystic fibrosis by detection of albumin in the meconium.

BN *3M, UK.*
Turpentine oil (p.1641·1); strong ammonia (p.1548·3); ammonium chloride (p.1055·2).
Musculoskeletal and joint disorders; pain.

BN 53 *Staufen, Ger.*
Homoeopathic preparation.

B_1-Neurischian *Krewel, Ger.†.*
Procaine hydrochloride (p.1299·2); hyoscine methonitrate (p.463·1); homatropine hydrobromide (p.462·2); thiamine hydrochloride (p.1361·1).
Local anaesthesia with nervous system disorders.

Bo-Cal *Fibertone, USA.*
Calcium with vitamins B and D, and magnesium.

Bocasan
Oral-B, Irl.; Oral-B, UK.
Sodium perborate (p.1125·2).
Oral hygiene.

Bodaril *Byk Elmu, Spain.*
Inosine pranobex (p.615·2).
Viral infections.

Bodigarde *Lifeplan, UK.*
Vitamins, fish oils, borage oil, and garlic oil.
Nutritional supplement.

Body *Progest, Ital.*
Barrier gel.

Body Lotion *Hamilton, Austral.*
Chlorhexidine gluconate (p.1107·2).
Emollient.

Boestrol *Antigen, Irl.†.*
Stilboestrol (p.1462·3).
Breast cancer; prostatic cancer.

Bogil *Llorente, Spain.*
Aminohydroxybutyric acid (p.339·1).
Behaviour disorders; convulsions; emotional disorders.

Bo-Gum *Solvay, Ital.*
Cetylpyridinium chloride (p.1106·2); sorbic acid (p.1125·2); bioflavonoids (p.1580·1).
Oral hygiene.

Bogumil-tassenfertiger milder Abfurtee *Enzypharm, Aust.*
Sambucus (p.1627·2); equisetum (p.1575·1); urtica (p.1642·3); chamomile (p.1561·2); tilia (p.1637·3).
Constipation; dyspepsia; flatulence.

Boi K *BOI, Spain.*
Potassium ascorbate (p.1161·3).
Potassium depletion.

Boi K Aspartico *BOI, Spain.*
Potassium ascorbate (p.1161·3).
Potassium depletion.

Boifilina *BOI, Spain†.*
Etamiphylline camsylate (p.753·1).
Cardiorespiratory failure; obstructive airways disease.

Boil Ease
Note. This name is used for preparations of different composition.
Del, Canad.
Benzocaine (p.1286·2); ichthammol (p.1083·3); sulphur (p.1091·2); cade oil (p.1092·2); camphor (p.1557·2); phenol (p.1121·2); zinc oxide (p.1096·2); thymol (p.1127·1).

Del, USA; Commerce, USA.
Benzocaine (p.1286·2); ichthammol (p.1083·3); sulphur (p.1091·2); cade oil (p.1092·2); camphor (p.1557·2); phenol (p.1121·2); zinc oxide (p.1096·2); thymol (p.1127·1); menthol (p.1600·2); eucalyptus oil (p.1578·1).
Boils.

Bok-C-Lin *Brovar, S.Afr.†.*
Doxycycline hydrochloride (p.202·3).
Bacterial infections.

Bolchipen *Cruz, Spain.*
Amoxycillin trihydrate (p.151·3).
Bacterial infections.

Bolcitol *Lesourd, Fr.*
Fumitory (p.1581·3); boldo (p.1554·1); sage (p.1627·1); fennel (p.1579·1).
Biliary disorders; gastro-intestinal disorders; kidney disorders.

Boldina He *Teofarma, Ital.*
Boldine (p.1554·1); aloin (p.1177·2).
Constipation.

Boldo
Note. This name is used for preparations of different composition.
Larkhall Laboratories, UK.
Boldo (p.1554·1); clivers (p.1565·2); bearberry (p.1552·2); fucus vesiculosus (p.1554·1); taraxacum (p.1634·2).

Potter's, UK.
Taraxacum (p.1634·2); butternut bark; boldo (p.1554·1); fucus (p.1554·1).
Slimming aid.

Boldo "Dr. Eberth" *Eberth, Ger.†.*
Boldoglucin (p.1554·1); cynara (p.1569·2); aloin amorph. (p.1177·2).
Biliary disorders; hepatogenic constipation associated with cholecystectomy.

Boldo N "Hanosan" *Hanosan, Ger.*
Homoeopathic preparation.

Boldocynara N *Bioforce, Switz.*
Cynara (p.1569·2); silybum marianum (p.993·3); taraxacum (p.1634·2); boldo (p.1554·1); peppermint leaf (p.1208·1).
Digestive disorders.

Boldoflorine
Note. This name is used for preparations of different composition.
Exflora, Fr.†; Exflora, Switz.
Tablets: Boldine (p.1554·1); senna (p.1212·2); frangula bark (p.1193·2); rosemary.
Constipation.

Exflora, Switz.
Herbal tea: Senna (p.1212·2); boldo (p.1554·1); rosemary; peppermint leaf (p.1208·1); fraxinus excelsior; corylus avellana leaf; castanea vulgaris; frangula bark (p.1193·2); apple; coriander (p.1567·3); inula helenium (p.1059·2); liquorice (p.1197·1).
Constipation.

Boldolaxin *Diviser Aquilea, Spain.*
Belladonna (p.457·1); bisacodyl (p.1179·3); boldo leaves (p.1554·1); calcium phosphate (p.1155·3); docusate sodium (p.1189·3).
Bowel evacuation; constipation.

Boldolaxine *Bouchara, Fr.†.*
Phenolphthalein (p.1208·2); belladonna (p.457·1); boldo (p.1554·1); lichen.
Constipation.

Boldolaxine Aloes *Pharmethic, Belg.†.*
Phenolphthalein (p.1208·2); Iceland moss; aloes (p.1177·1); boldo (p.1554·1); belladonna (p.457·1).
Constipation.

Boldosal *Ern, Spain.*
Boldine (p.1554·1); inosine (p.1591·1); magnesium sulphate (p.1157·3); sodium bicarbonate (p.1153·2); dibasic sodium phosphate (p.1159·3); sodium sulphate (p.1213·3).
Constipation; hepatobiliary disorders.

Boldosten *Sofar, Ital.†.*
Boldo (p.1554·1); rhubarb (p.1212·1); artichoke (p.1569·2); kinkeliba (p.1593·2); taraxacum (p.1634·2); equisetum (p.1575·1); depigmented bile (p.1553·2); inositol (p.1591·1); nicotinamide (p.1351·2); cascara sagrada (p.1183·1).
Biliary-tract disorders; liver disorders.

Bolinan
Syntex, Fr.†; Syntex, Switz.†.
Povidone (p.1474·2).
Gastro-intestinal disorders.

Bolo *Eagle, Austral.*
Vitamin, mineral and amino-acid preparation with Siberian ginseng (p.1584·2).
Tonic.

Boltin *Organon, Spain.*
Tibolone (p.1466·3).
Menopausal disorders.

Bolus Eucalypti Comp
Note. This name is used for preparations of different composition.
Weleda, Aust.
Homoeopathic preparation.

Weleda, UK.
Apis mellifera (p.1550·2); belladonna (p.457·1); eucalyptus (p.1578·1); light kaolin (p.1195·1).
Sore throat.

Bolutol *ICN, Spain.*
Gemfibrozil (p.1273·3).
Hyperlipidaemias.

Bolvidon *Organon, UK†.*
Mianserin hydrochloride (p.297·1).
Depression.

B-OM *OM, Switz.*
Cyanocobalamin; sorbitol; yeast.
Tonic.

B-OM Forte *OM, Switz.*
Cyanocobalamin; nicotinamide; sorbitol; yeast.
Tonic.

Bomacorin *Hevert, Ger.*
Crataegus (p.1568·2).
Cardiac disorders.

Bomagall forte S *Hevert, Ger.*
Ammi visnaga; atropin sulf.; carduus marianus; taraxacum; burs. past.; cardui benedict. (p.1565·3); herb. chelidonii; echinacea; echinaceae pallidae (p.1574·2).
Painful and spastic biliary disorders.

Bomagall mono *Hevert, Ger.*
Fumitory (p.1581·3).
Smooth muscle spasm.

Bomaklim *Hevert, Ger.*
Homoeopathic preparation.

Bomapect *Hevert, Ger.*
Homoeopathic preparation.

Bom-Bon *Montefarmaco, Ital.†.*
Phenolphthalein (p.1208·2).
Constipation.

Bomix *Bode, Ger.*
Clorophene (p.1111·2); orthophenylphenol (p.1120·3); chlorocresol (p.1110·3).
Instrument disinfection.

Bonactin *Almed, Switz.*
Zinc sulphate (p.1373·2); heparin sodium (p.879·3).
Herpesvirus infections.

Bonakiddi *Weimer, Ger.†.*
Aspirin (p.16·1).
Fever; inflammation; pain.

Bonamine
Pfizer, Canad.; Pfizer, Ger.
Meclozine hydrochloride (p.413·3).
Nausea; vertigo; vomiting.

Bonasanit *Weimer, Ger.*
Pyridoxine hydrochloride (p.1362·3).
Vitamin B deficiency.

Bonased-L *Dolorgiet, Ger.*
Lupulus (p.1597·2).
Nervous disorders; sleep disorders.

Bonceur *Rolab, S.Afr.*
Verapamil hydrochloride (p.960·3).
Angina; arrhythmias.

Bonciclol *CEPA, Spain†.*
Papaverine hydrochloride (p.1614·2); paracetamol (p.72·2); salicylamide (p.82·3).
Dysmenorrhoea.

Bondiol *Gry, Ger.*
Alfacalcidol (p.1366·3).
Osteomalacia; osteoporosis; renal osteodystrophy.

Bondronat
Boehringer Mannheim, Ger.; Boehringer Mannheim, Swed.
Sodium ibandronate (p.739·3).
Hypercalcaemia of malignancy.

Bonefos
Laevosan, Aust.; Rhone-Poulenc Rorer, Austral.; UCB, Belg.; Rhone-Poulenc Rorer, Canad.; Astra, Ger.; Medac, Ger.; Boehringer Ingelheim, Irl.; Leiras, Norw.; Funk, Spain; Astra, Swed.; Astra, Switz.; Boehringer Ingelheim, UK.
Disodium clodronate (p.737·3).
Hypercalcaemia of malignancy; osteolysis.

Bonfal *Worwag, Ger.†.*
Aspirin (p.16·1).
Thrombosis prophylaxis.

Boniderma *Boniscontro & Gazzone, Ital.*
Fluocinolone acetonide (p.1041·1).
Skin disorders.

Bonidon *Mepha, Switz.*
Indomethacin (p.45·2).
Aluminium glycinate (p.1177·2) is included in the tablets in an attempt to limit adverse effects on the gastro-intestinal mucosa.
Inflammation; pain.

Bonifen *Merck, Spain†.*
Pyritinol hydrochloride (p.1624·1).
Cerebrovascular disorders; tonic.

Bonifen B6 *Merck, Spain†.*
Pyridoxine hydrochloride (p.1362·3); pyritinol hydrochloride (p.1624·1).
Alcoholism; cerebrovascular disorders; tonic.

Bonifen H *Merck, Spain†.*
Phenytoin sodium (p.352·3); pyritinol hydrochloride (p.1624·1).
Epilepsy; trigeminal neuralgia.

Bonine *Roerig, USA; Leeming, USA.*
Meclozine hydrochloride (p.413·3).
Motion sickness; vertigo.

Bonjela
Note. This name is used for preparations of different composition.
Reckitt & Colman, Austral.; Reckitts, Irl.
Choline salicylate (p.25·2); cetalkonium chloride (p.1105·2).
Oral and nasal pain and inflammation.

Reckitt & Colman, UK.
Oral gel: Choline salicylate (p.25·2); cetalkonium chloride (p.1105·2); menthol (p.1600·2).
Oral pain and irritation.
Pastilles: Lignocaine hydrochloride (p.1293·2); aminacrine hydrochloride (p.1098·3).
Mouth ulcers.

Bonlax *Synthelabo, Ital.*
Cascara (p.1183·1).
Constipation.

Bonnington's Irish Moss *SmithKline Beecham Consumer, Austral.*
Carrageenan (p.1471·3); camphor (p.1557·2); menthol (p.1600·2).
Coughs; sore throat.

Bonomint *Intercare, UK.*
Yellow phenolphthalein (p.1208·2).
Constipation.

Bontril *Carnrick, USA.*
Phendimetrazine tartrate (p.1484·2).
Obesity.

Boost
Mead Johnson, Canad.†; Mead Johnson Nutritionals, USA.
Preparation for enteral nutrition.

Boots Covering Cream *Boots, UK.*
A covering cream.
Concealment of birth marks, scars, and disfiguring skin disease.

Boots Hayfever Relief Antihistamine *Boots, UK.*
Terfenadine (p.418·1).
Formerly known as One-a-Day Antihistamine.
Hypersensitivity reactions.

Boots Vapour Rub *Boots, UK.*
Eucalyptus oil (p.1578·1); camphor (p.1557·2); turpentine oil (p.1641·1); menthol (p.1600·2); thymol (p.1127·1); pumilio pine oil (p.1623·3).

B.O.P. *Pautrat, Fr.*
Olive leaf; birch leaf (p.1553·3).
Oedema.

Boracelle
Swiss Herbal, Canad.; Bio-Oil Research, UK.
Borage oil (p.1582·1).
Dietary supplement.

Boradren *Ciba Vision, Spain.*
Boric acid (p.1554·2); phenylephrine hydrochloride (p.1066·2); borax (p.1554·2).
Eye disorders.

Boradrine
Note. This name is used for preparations of different composition.
Bournonville, Belg.
Borax (p.1554·2); boric acid (p.1554·2); phenylephrine hydrochloride (p.1066·2).
Eye irritation.

Bournonville, Neth.
Phenylephrine hydrochloride (p.1066·2).
Congestion.

Boraline *Abello, Spain.*
Phenylephrine hydrochloride (p.1066·2).
Eye disorders.

Borbalan *Spyfarma, Spain.*
Amoxycillin trihydrate (p.151·3).
Bacterial infections.

Bor-Cefazol *Proter, Ital.†.*
Cephazolin sodium (p.181·1).
Bacterial infections.

Borea *Boehringer Mannheim, Spain.*
Megestrol acetate (p.1449·3).
Breast cancer; endometrial cancer.

Bormelin *Fresenius, Ger.†.*
Menthol (p.1600·2); camphor (p.1557·2); mace oil (p.1597·3); cedar wood oil; thymol (p.1127·1); pumilio pine oil (p.1623·3).
Catarrh.

Bormelin N *Fresenius, Ger.†.*
Menthol (p.1600·2).
Colds; hay fever.

Bormelin N-Adrenalin *Fresenius, Ger.†.*
Menthol (p.1600·2); adrenaline (p.813·2).
Rhinitis.

Born
Jacoby, Aust.†; Lichtwer, Ger.
Crataegus (p.1568·2).
Cardiac disorders.

Bornamid *Farmades, Ital.†.*
Pentanobornamide (p.1616·3).
Digestive, biliary, and genito-urinary spasm.

Borocaina *Schiapparelli, Ital.*
Benzyl alcohol (p.1103·3); sodium benzoate (p.1102·3).
Mouth and throat disinfection.

Borocaina Gola *Schiapparelli, Ital.*
Cetylpyridinium chloride (p.1106·2).
Mouth disinfection.

Borocarpin *Winzer, Ger.†.*
Pilocarpine borate (p.1396·3); naphazoline hydrochloride (p.1064·2).
Glaucoma; production of miosis.

Borocarpin-N *Winzer, Ger.†.*
Pilocarpine borate (p.1396·3); pilocarpine hydrochloride (p.1396·3); naphazoline hydrochloride (p.1064·2).
Glaucoma; production of miosis.

Borocarpin-S *Winzer, Ger.*
Pilocarpine hydrochloride (p.1396·3).
Glaucoma; production of miosis.

Borocell *Neutron Technology, USA.*
Sodium monomercaptoundecahydro-closo-dodecaborate.
Glioblastoma multiforme.

Boroclarine *Ciba Vision, Fr.*
Borax (p.1554·2); boric acid (p.1554·2); phenylephrine hydrochloride (p.1066·2).
Conjunctivitis.

Borofair Otic *Major, USA.*
Acetic acid (p.1541·2); aluminium acetate (p.1547·3).

Borofax *Warner-Wellcome, USA.*
Zinc oxide (p.1096·2).
Formerly contained boric acid.
Skin irritation.

Boro-Hexamin *Winzer, Ger.†.*
Hexamine borate (p.1554·3); naphazoline hydrochloride (p.1064·2).
Inflammatory eye disorders.

Boropak
Glenwood, Canad.†; Glenwood, USA.
Aluminium sulphate (p.1548·1); calcium acetate (p.1155·1).
Inflammatory skin disorders.

Boro-Scopol *Winzer, Ger.*
Hyoscine borate (p.463·2).
Eye disorders.

Borossigeno Plus Stomatologico *Warner-Lambert, Ital.*
Sodium perborate (p.1125·2); benzethonium chloride (p.1102·3); borax (p.1554·2); boric acid (p.1554·2).
Oral hygiene.

Borostyrol
Note. This name is used for preparations of different composition.
ACP, Belg.
Ointment: Thymol (p.1127·1); benzophenol salicylate; menthol (p.1600·2); boric acid (p.1554·2).
Burns; skin disorders; wounds.
Topical solution: Thymol (p.1127·1); benzophenol salicylate; menthol (p.1600·2); boric acid (p.1554·2); benzoin (p.1634·1).
Insect stings; mouth disorders; skin disinfection.

Mayoly-Spindler, Fr.
Cream: Thymol (p.1127·1); salol (p.83·1); menthol (p.1600·2).
Minor skin disorders.
Topical Solution: Thymol (p.1127·1); salol (p.83·1); menthol (p.1600·2); boric acid (p.1554·2); siam benzoin (p.1628·3).
Minor skin and mouth disorders.

Borostyrol N *Uhlmann-Eyraud, Switz.*
Thymol (p.1127·1); salol (p.83·1); menthol (p.1600·2); Siam benzoin (p.1628·3).
Mouth disorders.

Borotropin *Winzer, Ger.†.*
Atropine borate (p.456·1).
Eye disorders.

Bosisto's Eucalyptus Inhalant *Felton, Austral.*
Eucalyptus oil (p.1578·1); menthol (p.1600·2).
Cold symptoms.

Bosisto's Eucalyptus Rub *Felton, Austral.*
Eucalyptus oil (p.1578·1); menthol (p.1600·2); methyl salicylate (p.55·2).
Muscular aches and pains.

Bosisto's Eucalyptus Spray *Felton, Austral.*
Eucalyptus oil (p.1578·1).
Muscular aches and pains.

Boston
Bausch & Lomb, Fr.; Polymer Technology, USA.
Range of solutions for contact lenses.

Boston Advance *Essilor, Aust.*
Storage solution for hard and gas permeable contact lens.

Boston Lens Cleaning Solution *Gelflex, Austral.†.*
Cleansing solution for hard contact lenses.

Boston Lens Conditioning Solution *Gelflex, Austral.†.*
Soaking and wetting solution for hard contact lenses.

Botox
Allergan, Austral.; Allergan, Canad.; Allergan, Fr.; Merz, Ger.; Allergan, Irl.; Allergan, Ital.; Allergan, Norw.; Allergan, Swed.; Allergan, Switz.; Allergan, UK; Allergan, USA.
Botulinum A toxin (p.1310·1).
Blepharospasm; foot spasticity associated with paediatric cerebral palsy; hemifacial spasm; spasmodic torticollis; strabismus.

Botropase *Ravizza, Ital.*
Batroxobin (p.712·3).
Haemorrhagic disorders.

Bottom Better *InnoVisions, USA.*
Yellow soft paraffin (p.1382·3); wool fat (p.1385·3).
Nappy rash.

Bouillet *Dietetique et Sante, Fr.*
Potassium chloride; calcium glutamate; adipic acid; glutamic acid; magnesium carbonate.
Dietary salt substitute.

Bounty Bears *Nature's Bounty, USA.*
A range of vitamin preparations.

Bourget N *Medipharma, Ger.*
Sodium citrate (p.1153·2); sodium bicarbonate (p.1153·2); tartaric acid (p.1634·3).
Gastro-intestinal tract disorders.

Boutycin *Bouty, Ital.†.*
Indomethacin (p.45·2).
Musculoskeletal disorders.

Bovisan D5 *Sanum-Kehlbeck, Ger.*
Homoeopathic preparation.

Boviserin *Behringwerke, Ger.†.*
Bovine serum.
Tonic.

Boxazin plus C *Thomae, Ger.*
Aspirin (p.16·1); ascorbic acid (p.1365·2).
Cold symptoms; fever; inflammation; pain.

Boxocalm *Boxo, Ger.*
Valerian (p.1643·1); lupulus (p.1597·2).
Anxiety; insomnia.

Boxol *Rovi, Spain.*
Dalteparin sodium (p.845·3).
Deep vein thrombosis; thrombosis prophylaxis.

Boxolip *Boxo, Ger.*
Loperamide hydrochloride (p.1197·2).
Diarrhoea.

Boydenex *Bama, Spain†.*
Glycerol (p.1585·2); egg yolk.
Adjunct in cholecystography.

Boyol Salve *Pfeiffer, USA.*
Ichthammol (p.1083·3); benzocaine (p.1286·2).
Skin disorders.

Boz *Prosana, Austral.†.*
Boric acid (p.1554·2); olive oil (p.1610·1); zinc oxide (p.1096·2).
Eczema; psoriasis.

B-Plex *Stanley, Canad.*
Vitamin B substances.

B-Plex C *Stanley, Canad.*
Vitamin B substances and vitamin C.

B-Plus *Volchem, Ital.*
Multivitamin and amino-acid preparation.
Nutritional supplement.

Bracen *Zyma, Ital.†.*
Xibornol (p.270·3).
Respiratory-tract infections.

Brachialin *Steigerwald, Switz.†.*
Camphor (p.1557·2); diethylamine salicylate (p.33·1); methyl salicylate (p.55·2); benzyl nicotinate (p.22·1); rosemary oil (p.1626·2).
Musculoskeletal and joint pain.

Brachialin percutan N *Steigerwald, Ger.*
Diethylamine salicylate (p.33·1); benzyl nicotinate (p.22·1); methyl salicylate (p.55·2).
Bruising; lumbago; neuralgia; rheumatism; sciatica; sports injuries.

Brachiapas S *Pascoe, Ger.*
Homoeopathic preparation.

Brachont *Azupharma, Ger.*
Glycol salicylate (p.43·1); benzyl nicotinate (p.22·1).
Bruising; muscle and joint disorders.

Bradilan
Napp, Irl.†; Napp, UK†.
Nicofuranose (p.915·2).
Hyperlipidaemias; peripheral and cerebral vascular disorders.

Bradimox *Yamanouchi, Ital.*
Amoxycillin trihydrate (p.151·3).
Bacterial infections.

Bradoral
Note. This name is used for preparations of different composition.
Zyma, Ital.
Domiphen bromide (p.1112·3).
Mouth and throat disinfection.

Zyma, Switz.†.
Domiphen bromide (p.1112·3); eucalyptus oil (p.1578·1); menthol (p.1600·2).
Mouth and throat disorders.

Bradosol
Note. This name is used for preparations of different composition.
Zyma, Aust.
Domiphen bromide (p.1112·3); peppermint oil (p.1208·1); eucalyptus oil (p.1578·1); anise oil (p.1550·1).
Sore throat.

Novartis Consumer, Canad.
Hexylresorcinol (p.1116·1).
Sore throat.

CCP, Irl.†.
Domiphen bromide (p.1112·3).
Mouth and throat infections.

Zyma, UK.
Benzalkonium chloride (p.1101·3).
Formerly contained domiphen bromide.
Sore throat.

Bradosol Plus *Zyma, UK.*
Domiphen bromide (p.1112·3); lignocaine hydrochloride (p.1293·2).
Sore throat.

Bradyl *Lafon, Fr.*
Nadoxolol hydrochloride (p.914·1).
Arrhythmias.

Brady's-Magentropfen *Brady, Aust.*
Cinchona bark (p.1564·1); cinnamon (p.1564·2); aniseed (p.1549·3); coriander (p.1567·3); fennel (p.1579·1); myrrh (p.1606·1); santalum album; gentian (p.1583·3); rhubarb (p.1212·1); zedoary.
Gastro-intestinal disorders.

Bragg's *Bragg, UK.*
Activated charcoal (p.972·2).
Dyspepsia; flatulence; heartburn.

Brain *Fidia, Ital.†.*
Phospholipids from cortical grey matter; pyridoxine hydrochloride (p.1362·3); cyanocobalamin (p.1363·3).
Tonic.

Brainal *Andromaco, Spain.*
Nimodipine (p.922·2).
Cerebral ischaemia; cerebral vasospasm due to subarachnoid haemorrhage.

Braintop *Exel, Belg.*
Piracetam (p.1619·1).
Alcohol withdrawal syndrome; mental function disorders.

Bramin-hepa *Merz, Ger.*
Isoleucine (p.1349·2); leucine (p.1350·1); valine (p.1358·1); pyridoxine hydrochloride (p.1362·3).
Hepatic encephalopathy.

Bramserene *Corvi, Ital.†.*
Red-poppy petal (p.1001·1); matricaria (p.1561·2); lime flowers (p.1637·3); valerian (p.1643·1).
Insomnia.

BranchAmin
Clintec, Canad.†; Clintec, USA.
Amino-acid infusion.
Parenteral nutrition in hepatic encephalopathy.

Brand- u. Wundgel-Medice N *Medice, Ger.*
Benzethonium chloride (p.1102·3); laureth 9 (p.1325·2); urea (p.1095·2).
Wounds, burns, and other skin disorders.

Brandiazin *Medphano, Ger.*
Silver sulphadiazine (p.247·3).
Burns.

Branigen *Glaxo Wellcome, Ital.*
Acetylcarnitine hydrochloride (p.1542·1).
Cerebrovascular disorders; diabetic neuropathy; peripheral nerve disorders.

Branolind *Perfecta, Switz.†.*
Peru balsam (p.1617·2).
Wounds.

Branolind L *Hartmann, Ger.†.*
Peru balsam (p.1617·2); butoxycaine (p.1289·1).
Wounds.

Branolind N *Hartmann, Ger.*
Peru balsam (p.1617·2).
Wounds.

Brasivil *Stiefel, Ger.*
Aluminium oxide (p.1077·2).
Acne.

Brasivol
Stiefel, Austral.; Stiefel, Canad.; Stiefel, Fr.†; Stiefel, S.Afr.†; Stiefel, UK; Stiefel, USA.
Aluminium oxide (p.1077·2).
Acne.

Brassel *Searle, Ital.*
Citicoline sodium (p.1564·3).
Cerebrovascular disorders; parkinsonism.

Bratenol *Byk Elmu, Spain.*
Pirifibrate (p.1277·1).
Arteriosclerosis; hyperlipidaemias.

Braunoderm
Note. This name is used for preparations of different composition.
Braun, Aust.; Braun, Belg.; Braun, Ger.; Braun, Irl.; Braun, Ital.; Braun, Switz.
Povidone-iodine (p.1123·3); isopropyl alcohol (p.1118·2).
Skin disinfection; wounds.

Braun, Spain.
Povidone-iodine (p.1123·3).
Catheter lubrication; skin and mucous membrane disinfection.

Braunol
Braun, Aust.; Braun, Belg.; Braun, Ger.; Braun, Irl.; Braun, Ital.; Braun, Spain; Braun, Switz.
Povidone-iodine (p.1123·3).
Skin, mucous membrane, and wound disinfection.

Braunosan
Braun, Irl.; Braun, Ital.†; Braun, Switz.
Povidone-iodine (p.1123·3).
Hand and wound disinfection.

Braunosan H Plus *Braun, Switz.*
Povidone-iodine (p.1123·3).
Hand and skin disinfection.

Braunovidon
Salus, Aust.; Braun, Ger.; Braun, Irl.; Braun, Ital.†; Braun, Switz.
Povidone-iodine (p.1123·3).
Infected skin disorders; infected wounds.

Brazepam *Lennon, S.Afr.*
Bromazepam (p.643·1).
Anxiety.

Breathe Free *Thompson, USA.*
Sodium chloride (p.1162·2).
Inflammation and dryness of nasal membranes.

Breatheze *Rolab, S.Afr.*
Salbutamol (p.758·2).
Bronchospasm.

Bredon *Organon, Austral.†.*
Oxolamine citrate (p.1065·3).
Coughs.

Breezee Mist Antifungal
Note. This name is used for preparations of different composition.
Pedinol, USA.
Tolnaftate (p.389·1).
Formerly contained aluminium chlorohydrate, menthol, and undecenoic acid.
Fungal skin infections.

Pedinol, USA.
Miconazole nitrate (p.384·3).
Fungal infections.

Brek *IRBI, Ital.†.*
Loperamide hydrochloride (p.1197·2).
Diarrhoea.

Brelomax
Abbott, Ger.; Abbott, UK†.
Tulobuterol hydrochloride (p.774·2).
Obstructive airways disease.

Bremax *Abbott, Aust.*
Tulobuterol hydrochloride (p.774·2).
Obstructive airways disease.

Bremide *Astra, Norw.*
Amoxycillin trihydrate (p.151·3); potassium clavulanate (p.190·2).
Otitis media.

Bremon *Pensa, Spain.*
Clarithromycin (p.189·1).
Bacterial infections.

Brenda-35 ED *Alphapharm, Austral.*
21 Tablets, cyproterone acetate (p.1440·2); ethinyloestradiol (p.1445·1); 7 inert tablets.
Androgenisation in females; combined oral contraceptive.

Brennesseltonikum *Bioflora, Aust.*
Urtica (p.1642·3); taraxacum (p.1634·2); silver birch (p.1553·3).
Diuretic.

Brentan *Esteve, Spain.*
Hydrocortisone (p.1043·3); miconazole nitrate (p.384·3).
Fungal infections with inflammation.

Breonesin *Sanofi Winthrop, USA.*
Guaiphenesin (p.1061·3).
Coughs.

Bres *Farmacologico Milanese, Ital.*
Bromelains (p.1555·1); aescin (p.1543·3).
Peripheral vascular disorders.

Bresben *Ciba, Ger.*
Atenolol (p.825·3); nifedipine (p.916·2).
Hypertension.

Brethaire *Novartis, USA.*
Terbutaline sulphate (p.764·1).
Asthma; bronchospasm.

Brethine *Novartis, USA.*
Terbutaline sulphate (p.764·1).
Asthma; bronchospasm.

Bretylate
Wellcome, Austral.†; Glaxo Wellcome, Belg.; Glaxo Wellcome, Canad.; Wellcome, Fr.†; Wellcome, Irl.; Glaxo Wellcome, Neth.†; Wellcome, UK.
Bretylium tosylate (p.833·2).
Ventricular arrhythmias.

Bretylol
Boots, S.Afr.†; Du Pont, USA†.
Bretylium tosylate (p.833·2).
Ventricular arrhythmias.

Breva *Valeas, Ital.*
Salbutamol (p.758·2); ipratropium bromide (p.754·2).
Obstructive airways disease.

Brevibloc
Torrex, Aust.; Boots, Austral.; Zeneca, Canad.; Isotec, Fr.; Gensia, Irl.; Boots, S.Afr.; Gensia, Switz.; Sanofi Winthrop, UK; Ohmeda, USA.
Esmolol hydrochloride (p.866·1).
Hypertension; tachycardia.

Brevicon
Searle, Canad.; Syntex, USA.
Norethisterone (p.1453·1); ethinyloestradiol (p.1445·1).
28-Day packs also contain 7 inert tablets.
Combined oral contraceptive.

Brevilax *Cassella-med, Ital.†.*
Cascara sagrada (p.1183·1).
Constipation.

Brevilon *Roche Nicholas, Spain.*
Passion flower (p.1615·3); valerian (p.1643·1).
Sedative.

Brevimytal *Lilly, Ger.*
Methohexitone sodium (p.1227·2).
General anaesthesia.

Brevinaze *Intramed, S.Afr.*
Ketamine hydrochloride (p.1226·2).
General anaesthesia.

Brevinor
Syntex, Austral.; Searle, Irl.; Searle, S.Afr.; Searle, UK.
Norethisterone (p.1453·1); ethinyloestradiol (p.1445·1).
28-Day packs also contain 7 inert tablets.
Combined oral contraceptive.

Brevital *Lilly, USA.*
Methohexitone sodium (p.1227·2).
General anaesthesia.

Brevoxyl
Stiefel, Austral.; Stiefel, USA.
Benzoyl peroxide (p.1079·2).
Acne.

Brewers Yeast
Jamieson, Canad.; Phillips Yeast, UK; Nature's Bounty, USA.
Vitamin B substances.

Brewers Yeast with Garlic *Phillips Yeast, UK.*
Yeast (p.1373·1); garlic (p.1583·1); vitamin B substances.

Brexecam *Mer-National, S.Afr.*
Piroxicam betadex (p.81·1).
Gout; musculoskeletal and joint disorders.

Brexidol
Pharmacia Upjohn, Ger.; Nycomed, Norw.; Nycomed, Swed.
Piroxicam betadex (p.81·1).
Gout; musculoskeletal and joint disorders; pain.

Brexin
Pharmacia Upjohn, Aust.; Robapharm, Fr.; Chiesi, Ital.
Piroxicam betadex (p.81·1).
Gout; inflammation; musculoskeletal, joint, and peri-articular disorders; pain.

Brexin LA *Savage, USA.*
Chlorpheniramine maleate (p.405·1); pseudoephedrine hydrochloride (p.1068·3).
Cold symptoms.

Brexine
Christiaens, Belg.; Christiaens, Neth.
Piroxicam betadex (p.81·1).
Gout; musculoskeletal and joint disorders; pain.

Brexinil *Andromaco, Spain.*
Piroxicam betadex (p.81·1).
Gout; musculoskeletal, joint, and peri-articular disorders; pain.

Brezal *Sandoz, Ital.*
Choline alfoscerate (p.1390·3).
Mental function impairment in the elderly.

Briantum *Sauter, Switz.†.*
Delorazepam (p.660·3).
Convulsions; non-psychotic mental disorders; premedication.

Briazide *Pierre Fabre, Fr.*
Benazepril hydrochloride (p.827·1); hydrochlorothiazide (p.885·2).
Hypertension.

Bricanyl
Astra, Aust.; Astra, Austral.; Astra, Belg.; Astra, Canad.; Astra, Fr.; Stern, Ger.; Astra, Irl.; Astra, Neth.; Astra, Norw.; Astra, S.Afr.; Draco, Swed.; Astra, Switz.; Astra, UK; Lakeside, USA.
Terbutaline sulphate (p.764·1).
Obstructive airways disease; premature labour.

Bricanyl comp
Astra, Aust.; Astra, Ger.
Terbutaline sulphate (p.764·1); guaiphenesin (p.1061·3).
Obstructive airways disease.

Bricanyl Expectorant *Astra, Irl.*
Terbutaline sulphate (p.764·1); guaiphenesin (p.1061·3).
Obstructive airways disease.

Bridotrim *Quimifar, Spain.*
Co-trimoxazole (p.196·3).
Bacterial infections; Pneumocystis carinii pneumonia.

Briem *Pierre Fabre, Fr.*
Benazepril hydrochloride (p.827·1).
Hypertension.

Brietal
Lilly, Aust.; Lilly, Austral.; Lilly, Belg.†; Lilly, Canad.; Lilly, Fr.†; Lilly, Irl.; Lilly, Neth.; Lilly, Norw.; Lilly, S.Afr.; Lilly, Swed.; Lilly, Switz.; Lilly, UK.
Methohexitone sodium (p.1227·2).
General anaesthesia.

Brimexate *Bristol-Myers Squibb, Ital.†.*
Methotrexate sodium (p.547·1).
Malignant neoplasms.

Brinaldix
Sandoz, Fr.†; Sandoz, Ger.; Sandoz, Ital.†; Sandoz, Neth.†; Sandoz, Swed.†.
Clopamide (p.844·2).
Heart failure; hypertension; oedema.

Brinerdin
Sandoz, Aust.; Wander, Neth.†; Novartis, S.Afr.
Clopamide (p.844·2); dihydroergocristine mesylate (p.1571·3); reserpine (p.942·1).
Hypertension.

Brinerdina
Sandoz, Ital.; Sandoz, Spain.
Clopamide (p.844·2); dihydroergocristine mesylate (p.1571·3); reserpine (p.942·1).
Hypertension.

Brinerdine *Sandoz, Switz.*
Clopamide (p.844·2); dihydroergocristine mesylate (p.1571·3); reserpine (p.942·1).
Hypertension.

Briocor *Upsamedica, Ital.*
Carnitine (p.1336·2).
Carnitine deficiency; myocardial ischaemia.

Briofil *Wassermann, Ital.*
Bamifylline hydrochloride (p.749·2).
Bronchospasm.

Briogen *ABC, Ital.*
Levoglutamide (p.1344·3); DL-phosphoserine; cyanocobalamin (p.1363·3).
Tonic.

Brionil *Vita, Spain.*
Nedocromil sodium (p.756·2).
Asthma.

Brioschi *Brioschi, Canad.*
Sodium bicarbonate (p.1153·2).

Briovitan *Monteformaco, Ital.*
Multivitamin and mineral preparation.
Nutritional supplement.

Brisantin *Lacer, Spain†.*
Amoxycillin trihydrate (p.151·3); bromhexine (p.1055·3).
Respiratory-tract infections.

Briscocough *Quatromed, S.Afr.*
Diphenhydramine hydrochloride (p.409·1); ammonium chloride (p.1055·2); sodium citrate (p.1153·2).
Coughs.

Briscopyn *Quatromed, S.Afr.*
Paracetamol (p.72·2); caffeine (p.749·3); meprobamate (p.678·1); codeine phosphate (p.26·1).
Formerly contained paracetamol, caffeine, and meprobamate.
Pain with tension.

Briscotrim *Brissenco, S.Afr.†.*
Co-trimoxazole (p.196·3).
Bacterial infections.

Briserin N *Sandoz, Ger.*
Clopamide (p.844·2); reserpine (p.942·1).
Formerly contained dihydroergocristine mesylate, clopamide, and reserpine.
Hypertension.

Brisfirina *Juste, Spain.*
Cefapirin sodium (p.164·1).
Lignocaine (p.1293·2) is included in the intramuscular injection to alleviate the pain of injection.
Bacterial infections.

Brisfirina Balsamica *Juste, Spain.*
Cefapirin (p.164·1); niaouli oil (p.1607·1); guaiphenesin (p.1061·3).
Respiratory-tract infections.

Brisoral *Bristol-Myers, Spain.*
Cefprozil (p.172·3).
Bacterial infections.

Bristaciclina *Pharmacia Upjohn, Spain.*
Tetracycline hydrochloride (p.259·1).
Bacterial infections.

Bristaciclina Dental *Pharmacia Upjohn, Spain.*
Benzydamine hydrochloride (p.21·3); chymotrypsin (p.1563·2); tetracycline hydrochloride (p.259·1); trypsin (p.1640·1).
Mouth and upper respiratory-tract infections.

Bristacol *Bristol-Myers, Spain.*
Pravastatin sodium (p.1277·1).
Hypercholesterolaemia; myocardial infarction.

Bristamox
Bristol-Myers Squibb, Fr.; Bristol-Myers Squibb, Swed.
Amoxycillin (p.151·3) or amoxycillin trihydrate (p.151·3).
Bacterial infections.

Bristopen *Bristol-Myers Squibb, Fr.*
Oxacillin sodium (p.234·2).
Bacterial infections.

Britaject *Britannia Pharmaceuticals, UK.*
Apomorphine hydrochloride (p.1131·1).
Parkinsonism.

Britane *Martin, Fr.*
Miconazole nitrate (p.384·3).
Fungal infections.

Britapen *SmithKline Beecham, Spain.*
Ampicillin sodium (p.153·1) or ampicillin trihydrate (p.153·2).
Bacterial infections.

Britiazim *Thames, UK†.*
Diltiazem hydrochloride (p.854·2).
Angina pectoris.

British Army Foot Powder *Regal, Canad.*
Boric acid (p.1554·2); formaldehyde (p.1113·2); salicylic acid (p.1090·2); zinc oxide (p.1096·2).
Tinea pedis.

Britlofex *Britannia Pharmaceuticals, UK.*
Lofexidine hydrochloride (p.1596·3).
Opioid withdrawal symptoms.

Brixilon *Cantabria, Spain†.*
Ampicillin sodium (p.153·1); ampicillin benzathine (p.154·1).
Bacterial infections.

Brizolina *Juste, Spain.*
Cephazolin sodium (p.181·1).
Lignocaine (p.1293·2) is included in the intramuscular injection to alleviate the pain of injection.
Bacterial infections.

Brocadopa *Brocades, UK†.*
Levodopa (p.1137·1).
Parkinsonism.

Brodiwas *Wasserman, Spain†.*
Procaterol hydrochloride (p.757·3).
Obstructive airways disease.

Brofed *Marnel, USA.*
Pseudoephedrine hydrochloride (p.1068·3); brompheniramine maleate (p.403·2).
Upper respiratory-tract symptoms.

Broflex *Bioglan, UK.*
Benzhexol hydrochloride (p.457·3).
Drug-induced extrapyramidal disorders; parkinsonism.

Brolene
Rhone-Poulenc Rorer, Austral.; Rhone-Poulenc Rorer, Irl.; May & Baker, UK.
Dibromopropamidine isethionate (p.1112·2) or propamidine isethionate (p.1124·1).
Eye infections.

Brol-eze *Rhone-Poulenc Rorer, UK.*
Sodium cromoglycate (p.762·1).
Allergic conjunctivitis.

Brolimine Antibiotico *Quimifar, Spain†.*
Amoxycillin (p.151·3); bromhexine hydrochloride (p.1055·3).
Respiratory-tract infections.

Brolin *UCB, Spain.*
Famotidine (p.1192·1).
Gastro-oesophageal reflux; peptic ulcers; Zollinger-Ellison syndrome.

Broluidan *Kenfarma, Spain.*
Letosteine (p.1063·2).
Respiratory-tract disorders.

Brolumin *ISI, Ital.†.*
Suppositories: Phenobarbitone (p.350·2); prolonium bromide (p.689·1); lignocaine (p.1293·2).
Tablets: Phenobarbitone (p.350·2); prolonium bromide (p.689·1).
Insomnia; sedative.

Bromadine-DM *Cypress, USA.*
Brompheniramine maleate (p.403·2); pseudoephedrine hydrochloride (p.1068·3); dextromethorphan hydrobromide (p.1057·3).
Coughs.

Bromaline *Rugby, USA.*
Phenylpropanolamine hydrochloride (p.1067·2); brompheniramine maleate (p.403·2).
Upper respiratory-tract symptoms.

Bromaline Plus *Rugby, USA.*
Phenylpropanolamine hydrochloride (p.1067·2); brompheniramine maleate (p.403·2); paracetamol (p.72·2).
Upper respiratory-tract symptoms.

Broman *Hofmann, Aust.*
Bromocriptine mesylate (p.1132·2).
Parkinsonism.

Bromanate *Barre-National, USA.*
Phenylpropanolamine hydrochloride (p.1067·2); brompheniramine maleate (p.403·2).
Upper respiratory-tract symptoms.

Bromapect forte *Hevert, Ger.†.*
Homoeopathic preparation.

Bromarest *Warner Chilcott, USA†.*
Brompheniramine maleate (p.403·2).

Bromarest DC *Warner Chilcott, USA†.*
Brompheniramine maleate (p.403·2); phenylpropanolamine hydrochloride (p.1067·2); codeine phosphate (p.26·1).

Bromarest DX *Warner Chilcott, USA.*
Brompheniramine maleate (p.403·2); pseudoephedrine hydrochloride (p.1068·3); dextromethorphan hydrobromide (p.1057·3).
Coughs and cold symptoms.

Bromatane DX *Goldline, USA.*
Pseudoephedrine hydrochloride (p.1068·3); brompheniramine maleate (p.403·2); dextromethorphan hydrobromide (p.1057·3).
Coughs.

Bromatapp *Copley, USA.*
Phenylpropanolamine hydrochloride (p.1067·2); brompheniramine maleate (p.403·2).
Upper respiratory-tract symptoms.

Bromazanil *Hexal, Ger.*
Bromazepam (p.643·1).
Anxiety; insomnia; tension.

Bromaze *Hexal, S.Afr.*
Bromazepam (p.643·1).
Anxiety.

Bromazep *CT, Ger.*
Bromazepam (p.643·1).
Anxiety; insomnia.

Bromazolo *Baldacci, Ital.*
Methimazole (p.1495·3); dibromotyrosine (p.1493·1).
Hyperthyroidism.

Bromed *Schoeller, Aust.*
Bromocriptine mesylate (p.1132·2).
Acromegaly; parkinsonism.

Bromex *Qualiphar, Belg.*
Bromhexine hydrochloride (p.1055·3).
Bronchiectasis; obstructive bronchopneumonopathies; respiratory-tract disorders associated with increased mucus; sinusitis; Sjögren's syndrome.

Bromfed *Muro, USA.*
Brompheniramine maleate (p.403·2); pseudoephedrine hydrochloride (p.1068·3).
Allergic rhinitis; nasal congestion.

Bromfed-DM *Muro, USA.*
Brompheniramine maleate (p.403·2); pseudoephedrine hydrochloride (p.1068·3); dextromethorphan hydrobromide (p.1057·3).
Allergic rhinitis; coughs; vasomotor rhinitis.

Bromfed-PD *Muro, USA.*
Brompheniramine maleate (p.403·2); pseudoephedrine hydrochloride (p.1068·3).
Symptoms of seasonal and perennial allergic rhinitis and vasomotor rhinitis.

Bromfenex *Ethex, USA.*
Brompheniramine maleate (p.403·2); pseudoephedrine hydrochloride (p.1068·3).
Respiratory-tract disorders.

Bromidem *Sandipro, Belg.*
Bromazepam (p.643·1).
Anxiety; insomnia.

Bromo Madelon *St Laurent, Canad.*
Sodium bicarbonate (p.1153·2); citric acid (p.1564·3).

Bromo Seltzer
Note. This name is used for preparations of different composition.
Warner-Lambert, Canad.†.
Sodium citrate (p.1153·2).
Dyspepsia; gastric hyperacidity.
Warner-Lambert, USA.
Paracetamol (p.72·2).
Fever; pain.

Bromo Seltzer Effervescent Granules *Warner-Lambert, USA.*
Sodium bicarbonate (p.1153·2); paracetamol (p.72·2); citric acid (p.1564·3).
Hyperacidity.

Bromocod N *Streuli, Switz.*
Codeine phosphate (p.26·1); belladonna (p.457·1); drosera (p.1574·1); ipecacuanha (p.1062·2); opium (p.70·3); terpin hydrate (p.1070·2).
Coughs.

Bromocodeina *Menarini, Ital.†.*
Bromoform (p.1620·3); codeine phosphate (p.26·1); tolu balsam (p.1071·1).
Respiratory-tract disorders.

Bromofotyl *Centrapharm, Belg.†.*
Pholcodine (p.1068·1); bromoform (p.1620·3); aconite (p.1542·2); cherry-laurel water; ipecacuanha (p.1062·2); tolu (p.1071·1).
Respiratory-tract disorders.

Bromo-Kin *Irex, Fr.*
Bromocriptine mesylate (p.1132·2).
Hyperprolactinaemia; parkinsonism.

Bromolactin *Sigma, Austral.*
Bromocriptine mesylate (p.1132·2).
Acromegaly; hyperprolactinaemia; lactation inhibition; parkinsonism.

Bromophen TD *Rugby, USA.*
Phenylpropanolamine hydrochloride (p.1067·2); phenylephrine hydrochloride (p.1066·2); brompheniramine maleate (p.403·2).
Upper respiratory-tract symptoms.

Bromoterpina *Panthox & Burck, Ital.†.*
Terpin monohydrate (p.1070·2); ephedrine hydrochloride (p.1059·3); tolu balsam (p.1071·1).
Respiratory-tract disorders.

Bromotiren *Baldacci, Ital.*
Dibromotyrosine (p.1493·1).
Hyperthyroidism.

Bromotuss with Codeine *Rugby, USA.*
Bromodiphenhydramine hydrochloride (p.403·2); codeine phosphate (p.26·1).
Coughs and cold symptoms.

Bromphen *Schein, USA†.*
Phenylpropanolamine hydrochloride (p.1067·2); brompheniramine maleate (p.403·2).
Upper respiratory-tract symptoms.

Bromphen DX Cough *Muro, USA.*
Pseudoephedrine hydrochloride (p.1068·3); brompheniramine maleate (p.403·2); dextromethorphan hydrobromide (p.1057·3).
Coughs and cold symptoms.

Brompheniramine Cough *Geneva, USA.*
Pseudoephedrine hydrochloride (p.1068·3); brompheniramine maleate (p.403·2); dextromethorphan hydrobromide (p.1057·3).
Coughs and cold symptoms.

Brompheniramine DC Cough *Geneva, USA.*
Phenylpropanolamine hydrochloride (p.1067·2); codeine phosphate (p.26·1); brompheniramine maleate (p.403·2).
Coughs and cold symptoms.

Bromselon *Tecnobio, Spain.*
Ebastine (p.410·2).
Hypersensitivity reactions.

Bromuc *Klinge, Ger.*
Acetylcysteine (p.1052·3).
Respiratory-tract disorders associated with increased or viscous mucus.

Bron *Roussel, Ital.†.*
Potassium guaiacolsulfonate (p.1068·3).
Respiratory-tract disorders.

Bronal *Cupal, UK†.*
Dextromethorphan hydrobromide (p.1057·3); glycerol (p.1585·2).
Coughs.

Bronalide *Boehringer Ingelheim, Canad.*
Flunisolide (p.1040·3).
Asthma.

Bronalin Decongestant *Seton, UK.*
Pseudoephedrine (p.1068·3).
Cough and cold symptoms.

Bronalin Dry Cough *Seton, UK.*
Dextromethorphan hydrobromide (p.1057·3); pseudoephedrine hydrochloride (p.1068·3).
Coughs.

Bronalin Expectorant *Seton, UK.*
Diphenhydramine hydrochloride (p.409·1); sodium citrate (p.1153·2); ammonium chloride (p.1055·2).
Coughs.

Bronalin Junior *Seton, UK.*
Diphenhydramine hydrochloride (p.409·1); sodium citrate (p.1153·2).
Formerly known as Bronalin Paediatric.
Coughs.

Bronas *Swisspharm, S.Afr.†.*
Pneumococci; streptococci; staphylococci; *M. (Branhamella) catarrhalis*; *M. tetragenes*; *B. pyocyaneus*; *Klebsiella pneumoniae*; *Haemophilus influenzae*.
Active immunisation against bronchitis.

Broncal
Note. This name is used for preparations of different composition.
Pharmacobel, Belg.
Pholcodine (p.1068·1); ephedrine hydrochloride (p.1059·3); chlorpheniramine maleate (p.405·1); potassium guaiacolsulfonate (p.1068·3).
Coughs.
SmithKline Beecham, Ital.
Dextromethorphan hydrobromide (p.1057·3); potassium guaiacolsulfonate (p.1068·3).
Coughs.

Broncasma
Berna, Belg.; Berna, Switz.
Pneumococcus I, II, III; *Streptococcus*; *Staphylococcus*; *Neisseria catarrhalis*; *Gaffkya tetragena*; *Pseudomonas aeruginosa*; *Klebsiella pneumoniae*; *Haemophilus influenzae*.
Obstructive airways disease.

Broncaspin *Bayer, Ital.*
Guacetisal (p.1061·2).
Respiratory-tract disorders.

Bronch Eze *Pharmavite, Canad.*
Ephedrine hydrochloride (p.1059·3); ammonium chloride (p.1055·2).

Bronchalene
Note. This name is used for preparations of different composition.
Rhone-Poulenc Rorer, Belg.
Syrup for adults and children: Pholcodine (p.1068·1); chlorpheniramine maleate (p.405·1).
Syrup for infants: Chlorpheniramine maleate (p.405·1).
Coughs.
Martin, Fr.
Pholcodine (p.1068·1); chlorpheniramine maleate (p.405·1); sodium benzoate (p.1102·3).
Coughs.

Bronchalene Nourisson *Martin, Fr.*
Chlorpheniramine maleate (p.405·1); sodium benzoate (p.1102·3); tolu balsam (p.1071·1).
Coughs.

Bronchalin *Gubler, Switz.*
Ephedrine hydrochloride (p.1059·3); guaiphenesin (p.1061·3); hyoscyamine sulphate (p.464·2); castanea vulgaris; drosera (p.1574·1); liquorice (p.1197·1); psyllium (p.1194·2); thyme (p.1636·3); belladonna (p.457·1); ipecacuanha (p.1062·2); sodium benzoate (p.1102·3).
Respiratory-tract disorders.

Bronchangin *Bionorica, Ger.†.*
Althaea (p.1546·3); coltsfoot leaf (p.1057·2); galeopsis ochroleuca; phellandri; pulmonaria; scabiosa columbaria; comfrey (p.1567·1).
Coughs and associated respiratory-tract disorders.

Bronchathiol
Rhone-Poulenc Rorer, Belg.; Martin, Fr.
Carbocisteine (p.1056·3).
Respiratory-tract congestion.

Bronchenolo
Note. This name is used for preparations of different composition.
Maggioni, Ital.
Syrup: Dextromethorphan hydrobromide (p.1057·3); potassium guaiacolsulfonate (p.1068·3); ammonium acetate (p.1055·1).
Tablets: Dextromethorphan hydrobromide (adsorbed onto magnesium trisilicate) (p.1057·3).
Coughs.
Midy, Ital.
Oral drops†: Dextromethorphan hydrobromide (p.1057·3).
Coughs.
Pastilles: Cetylpyridinium chloride (p.1106·2).
Mouth and throat disinfection.

Bronchenolo Antiflu *SmithKline Beecham, Ital.*
Paracetamol (p.72·2); ascorbic acid (p.1365·2).
Fever; pain.

Bronchenolo Balsamo *Midy, Ital.†.*
Cineole (p.1564·1); camphor (p.1557·2); menthol (p.1600·2).
Cold symptoms.

Bronchette *Lennon, S.Afr.†.*
Carbocisteine (p.1056·3).
Respiratory-tract disorders.

Bronchex *Hilarys, Canad.*
Ammonium chloride (p.1055·2); ammonia (p.1548·3); ammonium carbonate (p.1055·1); glycerol (p.1585·2); liquorice (p.1197·1); menthol (p.1600·2); siberian fir oil; white pine compound.

Bronchial *Theralab, Canad.*
Ammonium chloride (p.1055·2); senega (p.1069·3); white pine compound.

Bronchialtee *TAD, Ger.†.*
Fennel (p.1579·1); lichen islandicus; thyme (p.1636·3); althaea (p.1546·3); sage (p.1627·1); tilia (p.1637·3).
Bronchitis; colds.

Bronchiase *Lafare, Ital.*
Dextromethorphan hydrobromide (p.1057·3); potassium guaiacolsulfonate (p.1068·3).
Coughs.

Bronchicough *Rhone-Poulenc Rorer, S.Afr.*
Cimicifuga (p.1563·3); grindelia; pimpinella; primula; quebracho; thyme (p.1636·3); ephedrine hydrochloride (p.1059·3); menthol (p.1600·2); eucalyptus oil (p.1578·1); saponin.
Coughs.

Bronchicum
Note. This name is used for preparations of different composition.
Nattermann, Ger.
Thyme oil (p.1637·1).
Bath additive; respiratory-tract disorders.
Nattermann, Neth.
Thyme (p.1636·3); primula root; grindelia; pimpinella root; anise oil (p.1550·1); eucalyptus oil (p.1578·1); menthol (p.1600·2); saponin.
Formerly marketed as Bronchicum Hoestsiroop.
Coughs.
Rhone-Poulenc Rorer, S.Afr.
Cimicifuga (p.1563·3); grindelia; pimpinella; primula; quebracho; thyme (p.1636·3); ephedrine hydrochloride (p.1059·3); menthol (p.1600·2); sodium bromide (p.1620·3); eucalyptus oil (p.1578·1); saponin.
Bronchitis.

Bronchicum Balsam mit Eukalyptusol *Nattermann, Ger.*
Eucalyptus oil (p.1578·1); camphor (p.1557·2); oleum pini sylvestris.
Catarrh; cold symptoms.

Bronchicum Elixir N *Nattermann, Ger.*
Grindelia; pimpinella; primula root; quebracho; thyme (p.1636·3).
Coughs and associated respiratory-tract disorders.

Bronchicum Elixir Plus *Nattermann, Ger.*
Thyme (p.1636·3); plantago lanceolata; primula root.
Bronchial congestion; coughs.

Bronchicum Extra Sterk *Nattermann, Neth.*
Ephedrine hydrochloride (p.1059·3); codeine phosphate (p.26·1); vegetable extracts.
Coughs.

Bronchicum Husten-Pastillen *Nattermann, Ger.†.*
Thyme (p.1636·3).
Mouth and throat catarrh and inflammation.

Bronchicum Hustentee *Nattermann, Ger.*
Thyme (p.1636·3); fennel oil (p.1579·2); anise oil (p.1550·1); saponaria; liquorice (p.1197·1).
Coughs and cold symptoms; sore throat.

Bronchicum Inhalat *Nattermann, Ger.†.*
Cineole (p.1564·1); pine needle oil; thyme oil (p.1637·1); rosemary oil (p.1626·2); α-terpineol (p.1635·1).
Respiratory-tract disorders.

Bronchicum Mono Codein *Nattermann, Ger.*
Codeine phosphate (p.26·1).
Coughs.

Bronchicum Pflanzlicher *Nattermann, Ger.*
Thyme (p.1636·3); drosera (p.1574·1).
Coughs.

Bronchicum SB *Nattermann, S.Afr.†.*
Cimicifuga (p.1563·3); grindelia; pimpinella; primula; quebracho; thyme (p.1636·3); ephedrine hydrochloride (p.1059·3); menthol (p.1600·2); eucalyptus oil (p.1578·1); saponin.
Coughs.

Bronchicum Sekret-Loser *Nattermann, Ger.*
Eucalyptus oil (p.1578·1); primula root; thyme (p.1636·3).
Upper respiratory-tract disorders with thickened secretions.

Bronchicum Thymian *Nattermann, Ger.*
Primula root; thyme (p.1636·3).
Bronchitis; coughs.

Bronchicum Tropfen mit Codein *Nattermann, Ger.†.*
Codeine phosphate (p.26·1); quebracho; saponaria; thyme (p.1636·3); menthol (p.1600·2).
Coughs and associated respiratory-tract disorders.

Bronchicum Tropfen N *Nattermann, Ger.*
Quebracho; saponaria; thyme (p.1636·3).
Bronchitis.

Bronchi-Do *Grasler, Ger.*
Homoeopathic preparation.

Bronchiflu *Rhone-Poulenc Rorer, S.Afr.*
Mepyramine maleate (p.414·1); menthol (p.1600·2); ammonium chloride (p.1055·2); paracetamol (p.72·2); phenylpropanolamine hydrochloride (p.1067·2).
Cold symptoms; coughs.

Bronchilate *Nattermann, S.Afr.†.*
Pholcodine (p.1068·1); ephedrine hydrochloride (p.1059·3); cetrimide (p.1105·2); mepyramine maleate (p.414·1); menthol (p.1600·2).
Coughs.

Bronchi-Pertu *Pekana, Ger.*
Homoeopathic preparation.

Bronchiplant *Apotheke Heiligen Josef, Aust.*
Balsam: Eucalyptus oil (p.1578·1); rosemary oil (p.1626·2); camphor (p.1557·2).
Coughs and cold symptoms.
Oral liquid; syrup: Thyme (p.1636·3); iceland moss; senega root (p.1069·3); bitter-orange peel (p.1610·3).
Catarrh; coughs.

Bronchiplant light *Apotheke Heiligen Josef, Aust.*
Iceland moss; senega root (p.1069·3); thyme (p.1636·3); bitter-orange peel (p.1610·3).
Catarrh; coughs.

Bronchipret *Bionorica, Ger.*
Oral drops; oral liquid: Thyme (p.1636·3); hedera helix.
Tablets: Primula root; thyme (p.1636·3).
Bronchitis.

Bronchisaft *Hilarys, Canad.*
Ammonia (p.1548·3); glycerol (p.1585·2); ipecacuanha (p.1062·2); menthol (p.1600·2); sodium citrate (p.1153·2).

Bronchisan *Disperga, Aust.*
Theophylline (p.765·1); ephedrine hydrochloride (p.1059·3).
Obstructive airways disease.

Bronchised *Corvi, Ital.†.*
Calcium chloride (p.1155·1); sodium benzoate (p.1102·3); potassium guaiacolsulfonate (p.1068·3); ephedrine hydrochloride (p.1059·3); bromoform (p.1620·3).
Respiratory-tract disorders.

Bronchiselect *Dreluso, Ger.*
Homoeopathic preparation.

Bronchistop *Rhone-Poulenc Rorer, S.Afr.*
Pholcodine (p.1068·1); ephedrine hydrochloride (p.1059·3); mepyramine maleate (p.414·1); menthol (p.1600·2); cetrimide (p.1105·2).
Coughs.

Bronchitten *Medopharm, Ger.*
Thyme (p.1636·3).
Bronchial catarrh; bronchitis; coughs.

Bronchitten forte K *Medopharm, Ger.*
Thyme (p.1636·3); primula root.
Upper respiratory-tract disorders with thickened secretions.

Bronchitussin *Schuck, Ger.†.*
Primula officinalis.
Bronchial catarrh.

Bronchitussin SC *Schuck, Ger.†.*
Orris; plantago lanceolata; primula root; thyme (p.1636·3); viola tricolor; althaea (p.1546·3); liquorice (p.1197·1); ammonium chloride (p.1055·2); sodium benzoate (p.1102·3); saponin.
Coughs and associated respiratory-tract disorders.

Broncho Inhalat *Klinge, Ger.*
Salbutamol sulphate (p.758·2).
Atelectasia; obstructive airways disease.

Broncho Munal
OM, Ger.; Abiogen, Ital.
Lysates of *Haemophilus infuenzae*; *Diplococcus pneumoniae*; *Klebsiella pneumoniae*; *Klebsiella ozaenae*; *Staphylococcus aureus*; *Streptococcus pyogenese*; *Streptococcus viridans*; *Branhamella catarrhalis*.
Respiratory-tract infections.

Broncho Rub *Mathieu, Canad.*
Camphor (p.1557·2); menthol (p.1600·2); cajuput oil (p.1556·1); turpentine.

Broncho Saline *Blairex, USA.*
Sodium chloride (p.1162·2).
Diluent for bronchodilator solutions for inhalation.

Broncho Sanol *Sanol, Ger.†.*
Polysorbate 20 (p.1327·3); thyme oil (p.1637·1); anise oil (p.1550·1); fennel oil (p.1579·2).
Respiratory-tract disorders.

Broncho Spray *Klinge, Ger.*
Salbutamol (p.758·2).
Atelectasia; obstructive airways disease.

Bronchobactan *Klinge, Ger.*
Lysate of *Staphylococcus aureus*; *Streptococcus mitis*; *Streptococcus pyogenes*; *Streptococcus pneumoniae*; *Klebsiella pneumoniae*; *Branhamella catarrhalis*; *Haemophilus influenzae*.
Respiratory-tract infections.

Bronchobel *Pharmethic, Belg.*
Codeine (p.26·1); ephedrine hydrochloride (p.1059·3); potassium guaiacolsulfonate (p.1068·3); sodium benzoate (p.1102·3).
Coughs.

Bronchobest *CT, Ger.*
Spike lavender oil (p.1632·2).
Bronchitis.

Broncho-Binotal *Bayer, Ger.†.*
Ampicillin trihydrate (p.153·2); theophylline (p.765·1); papaverine hydrochloride (p.1614·2); guaiphenesin (p.1061·3).
Bacterial infections of the respiratory tract.

Bronchocedin *Wolfer, Ger.†.*
Pimpinella; thyme (p.1636·3); eucalyptus oil (p.1578·1).
Respiratory-tract disorders.

Bronchocedin N *Strathmann, Ger.*
Anise oil (p.1550·1); eucalyptus oil (p.1578·1); peppermint oil (p.1208·1).
Catarrh.

Bronchocodin *Grossmann, Switz.*
Codeine phosphate (p.26·1); sodium benzoate (p.1102·3); tolu balsam (p.1071·1); senega root (p.1069·3); menthol (p.1600·2); star anise (p.1549·3); peppermint oil (p.1208·1); liquorice (p.1197·1).
Coughs.

Bronchocort *Klinge, Ger.*
Beclomethasone dipropionate (p.1032·1).
Respiratory-tract disorders.

Bronchocyst *SmithKline Beecham, Fr.*
Carbocisteine (p.1056·3).
Respiratory-tract disorders associated with increased or viscous mucus.

Bronchodermine
Note. This name is used for preparations of different composition.
Tissot, Fr.
Ointment: Cineole (p.1564·1); guaiacol (p.1061·2); pine oil; terpin hydrate (p.1070·2); terpineol (p.1635·1).
Suppositories: Amylocaine hydrochloride (p.1286·1); cineole (p.1564·1); guaiacol (p.1061·2); pine oil; terpin hydrate (p.1070·2).
Respiratory disorders.
Tissot, Switz.†.
Cineole (p.1564·1); guaiacol (p.1061·2); pine oil; terpin hydrate (p.1070·2).
Respiratory-tract infections.

Bronchodex D *Prodemdis, Canad.*
Phenylpropanolamine hydrochloride (p.1067·2); chlorpheniramine maleate (p.405·1); pheniramine maleate (p.415·3).

Bronchodex DM *Prodemdis, Canad.*
Mepyramine maleate (p.414·1); dextromethorphan hydrobromide (p.1057·3); ammonium chloride (p.1055·2); menthol (p.1600·2); sodium citrate (p.1153·2).

Bronchodex Pastilles *Prodemdis, Canad.*
Domiphen bromide (p.1112·3).

Bronchodex Pastilles Antiseptiques *Prodemdis, Canad.*
Hexylresorcinol (p.1116·1).

Bronchodex Pediatrique *Therapex, Canad.*
Pseudoephedrine hydrochloride (p.1068·3); pheniramine maleate (p.415·3); dextromethorphan hydrobromide (p.1057·3); guaiphenesin (p.1061·3).

Bronchodex Vapo *Theralab, Canad.*
Camphor (p.1557·2); eucalyptus oil (p.1578·1); menthol (p.1600·2).

Bronchodil *Asta Medica, UK.*
Reproterol hydrochloride (p.758·1).
Bronchospasm.

Bronchodine *Pharmethic, Belg.*
Codeine phosphate (p.26·1).
Coughs.

Bronchodual *Boehringer Ingelheim, Fr.*
Fenoterol hydrobromide (p.753·2); ipratropium bromide (p.754·2).
Obstructive airways disease.

Bronchodurat *Pohl, Ger.*
Eucalyptus oil (p.1578·1); menthol (p.1600·2).
Bronchitis; cold symptoms.

Bronchodurat Eucalyptusol *Pohl, Ger.*
Eucalyptus oil (p.1578·1).
Respiratory-tract disorders.

Broncho-Euphyllin *Byk Gulden, Ger.*
Theophylline (p.765·1); ambroxol hydrochloride (p.1054·3).
Formerly contained theophylline and guaiphenesin.
Obstructive airways disease.

Broncho-Fips *Lichtenstein, Ger.*
Acetylcysteine (p.1052·3).
Respiratory-tract disorders with viscous mucus.

Bronchofluid *DP-Medica, Switz.*
Baby: Codeine phosphate (p.26·1); ephedrine hydrochloride (p.1059·3); guaiphenesin (p.1061·3); belladonna (p.457·1); drosera (p.1574·1); hedera helix; plantago lanceolata; senega root (p.1069·3); thyme (p.1636·3).
Infant; Adult: Codeine phosphate (p.26·1); ephedrine hydrochloride (p.1059·3); guaiphenesin (p.1061·3); belladonna (p.457·1); ipecacuanha (p.1062·2); drosera (p.1574·1); hedera helix; plantago lanceolata; senega root (p.1069·3); thyme (p.1636·3); cherry-laurel.
Coughs; laryngitis; sore throat.

Bronchoforton
Note. This name is used for preparations of different composition.
Kwizda, Aust.
Eucalyptus oil (p.1578·1); oleum pini sylvestris; peppermint oil (p.1208·1).
Cold and influenza symptoms.
Sanofi Winthrop, Ger.
Capsules: Eucalyptus oil (p.1578·1); anise oil (p.1550·1); peppermint oil (p.1208·1).
Bronchitis; sinusitis.
Ointment: Eucalyptus oil (p.1578·1); pine needle oil; peppermint oil (p.1208·1).
Catarrh; cold symptoms.
Oral liquid; oral drops: Hedera helix.
Bronchitis; sinusitis.
Plantorgan, Neth.†.
Eucalyptus oil (p.1578·1); pumilio pine oil (p.1623·3); camphor (p.1557·2); menthol (p.1600·2).
Cold symptoms.
Sodip, Switz.
Eucalyptus oil (p.1578·1); pine oil; peppermint oil (p.1208·1).
Respiratory-tract disorders.

Bronchoforton Infant *Plantorgan, Ger.†.*
Eucalyptus oil (p.1578·1); pine needle oil; rosemary oil (p.1626·2).
Coughs and associated respiratory-tract disorders.

Bronchoforton Kinderbalsam *Sanofi Winthrop, Ger.*
Eucalyptus oil (p.1578·1); pine needle oil.
Respiratory-tract disorders.

Bronchoforton Kodeinsaft *Plantorgan, Ger.†.*
Codeine phosphate (p.26·1).
Coughs.

Bronchoforton N *Plantorgan, Ger.†.*
Eucalyptus oil (p.1578·1); pine needle oil menthol (p.1600·2).
Bronchitis; sinusitis.

Bronchoforton-Solinat *Sanofi Winthrop, Ger.*
Cations: sodium, potassium, magnesium, calcium; anions: chloride, sulphate, bicarbonate.
Respiratory-tract disorders.

Broncho-Grippol-DM *Charton, Canad.*
Dextromethorphan hydrobromide (p.1057·3).
Coughs.

Bronchokod *Biogalenique, Fr.*
Carbocisteine (p.1056·3).
Respiratory-tract disorders associated with increased or viscous mucus.

Bronchol *Streuli, Switz.*
Guaiphenesin (p.1061·3).
Upper-respiratory-tract disorders.

Bronchol N *DP-Medica, Switz.*
Guaiphenesin (p.1061·3); ephedrine hydrochloride (p.1059·3); codeine phosphate (p.26·1); camphor (p.1557·2); cineole (p.1564·1); anise oil (p.1550·1).
Coughs.

Broncholate *Sanofi Winthrop, USA.*
Ephedrine hydrochloride (p.1059·3); guaiphenesin (p.1061·3).
Coughs.

Broncholate CS *Bock, USA†.*
Codeine phosphate (p.26·1); ephedrine hydrochloride (p.1059·3); guaiphenesin (p.1061·3).

Broncholind *Divapharma, Ger.†.*
Aniseed (p.1549·3); eucalyptus leaf (p.1578·1); fennel (p.1579·1); matricaria flowers (p.1561·2); peppermint leaf (p.1208·1); sage leaf (p.1627·1); thyme (p.1636·3).
Coughs and associated respiratory-tract disorders.

Broncholind Balsam *Divapharma, Ger.†.*
Camphor (p.1557·2); menthol (p.1600·2); eucalyptus oil (p.1578·1).
Formerly contained camphor, menthol, eucalyptus oil, turpentine oil, pumilio pine oil, rosemary oil, sage oil, and thyme oil.
Cold symptoms; respiratory-tract catarrh.

Bronchomed *Pohl, Ger.*
Eucalyptus oil (p.1578·1).
Bronchitis; cold symptoms.

Broncho-Noleptan *Thomae, Ger.†.*
Bromhexine hydrochloride (p.1055·3); fominoben hydrochloride (p.1061·2).
Respiratory-tract disorders associated with increased or viscous mucus.

Bronchopan DM *Atlas, Canad.*
Dextromethorphan hydrobromide (p.1057·3).

Bronchoparat *Klinge, Ger.*
Theophylline sodium glycinate (p.772·2).
Cor pulmonale; obstructive airways disease.

Broncho-pectoralis *Medgenix, Belg.*
Pholcodine (p.1068·1); diphenhydramine hydrochloride (p.409·1); ephedrine sulphate (p.1059·3); potassium guaiacolsulfonate (p.1068·3); Desessartz fluidextract; red-poppy petal fluidextract.
Coughs and nasal congestion.

Bronchoped *Adcock Ingram, S.Afr.*
Terbutaline sulphate (p.764·1); ammonium chloride (p.1055·2); sodium citrate (p.1153·2).
Coughs with bronchospasm.

Bronchophen *Rolab, S.Afr.*
Theophylline (p.765·1).
Obstructive airways disease.

Bronchopront *Mack, Illert., Ger.*
Ambroxol hydrochloride (p.1054·3).
Respiratory-tract disorders associated with increased or viscous mucus.

Bronchorectine *Mayoly-Spindler, Switz.†.*
Adult preparation: Citralum; guaiacol (p.1061·2); terpin hydrate (p.1070·2); pine oil; wild thyme.
Infant preparation: Citralum; terpin hydrate (p.1070·2); pine oil; wild thyme.
Respiratory-tract infections.

Bronchorectine au Citral *Mayoly-Spindler, Fr.*
Citral; benzyl cinnamate; guaiacol (p.1061·2); terpin hydrate (p.1070·2); oleum pini sylvestris; thyme oil (p.1637·1).
Respiratory disorders.

Bronchoretard *Klinge, Ger.*
Theophylline (p.765·1).
Obstructive airways disease.

Broncho-Rivo *Rivopharm, Switz.*
Adult: Diphenhydramine hydrochloride (p.409·1); ammonium chloride (p.1055·2); sodium citrate (p.1153·2); menthol (p.1600·2).
Paediatric: Diphenhydramine hydrochloride (p.409·1); sodium citrate (p.1153·2); menthol (p.1600·2).
Coughs.

Bronchosan *Bioforce, Switz.*
Hedera helix; thyme (p.1636·3); anise oil (p.1550·1); horehound (p.1063·3); liquorice (p.1197·1).
Bronchitis; coughs; influenza.

Bronchosedal *Janssen-Cilag, Belg.*
Oral liquid: Dextromethorphan hydrobromide (p.1057·3).
Syrup: Cherry-laurel water; aconite tincture (p.1542·2); codeine phosphate (p.26·1); sodium benzoate (p.1102·3).
Coughs.

Broncho-Sern *Serturner, Ger.*
Plantago major (p.1208·3).
Coughs; inflammation of mouth and throat; respiratory catarrh.

Bronchosirum *Bronchosirum, Canad.*
Phenylpropanolamine hydrochloride (p.1067·2); pheniramine maleate (p.415·3); mepyramine maleate (p.414·1); dextromethorphan hydrobromide (p.1057·3).

Bronchospasmin
Asta Medica, Aust.; Asta Medica, Ger.
Reproterol hydrochloride (p.758·1).
Obstructive airways disease.

Bronchospasmine *Asta Medica, Switz.*
Reproterol hydrochloride (p.758·1).
Obstructive airways disease.

Bronchospray
Note. This name is used for preparations of different composition.
Tissot, Fr.
Guethol nicotinate (p.1062·1); guaiphenesin (p.1061·3); terpineol (p.1635·1); cineole (p.1564·1); pine oil; lavender oil (p.1594·3).
Respiratory disorders.
Parke-Med, S.Afr.
Salbutamol (p.758·2).
Obstructive airways disease.

Bronchostad *Stada, Ger.†.*
Plantago; althaeae root (p.1546·3); liquorice root (p.1197·1); pulmonaria; coltsfoot leaf (p.1057·2).
Bronchitis; tracheitis.

Bronchostop *Metochem, Aust.*
Capsules: Mentholum valerianicum; guaiphenesin (p.1061·3); eucalyptus oil (p.1578·1); camphor (p.1557·2).
Formerly known as Nicogelat.
Coughs.
Ointment: Camphor (p.1557·2); menthol (p.1600·2); eucalyptus oil (p.1578·1); turpentine oil (p.1641·1); pumilio pine oil (p.1623·3); thyme oil (p.1637·1).
Catarrh; colds; cough; sore throat.
Oral drops: Guaiphenesin (p.1061·3); thyme (p.1636·3); chamomile (p.1561·2); anise oil (p.1550·1).
Coughs.
Oral liquid: Ascorbic acid (p.1365·2); thyme extract (p.1636·3); althaea syrup (p.1546·3).
Catarrh; colds; cough; sore throat.
Spray: Sage tincture (p.1627·1); thyme tincture (p.1636·3); peppermint leaf tincture (p.1208·1).
Mouth and throat inflammation.

Bronchosyl *Pharmalab, Canad.*
Ammonium chloride (p.1055·2); cocillana (p.1057·2).

Bronchosyx N *Syxyl, Ger.*
Liquorice (p.1197·1); thyme (p.1636·3).
Cold symptoms.

Broncho-Tulisan Eucalyptol *Logeais, Fr.*
Noscapine camsylate (p.1065·2); aspirin (p.16·1); cineole (p.1564·1).
Coughs.

Bronchotussine *Medichemie, Switz.*
Butethamate citrate (p.1056·2); codeine phosphate (p.26·1).
Coughs.

Broncho-Tyrosolvetten *Tosse, Ger.*
Cetylpyridinium chloride (p.1106·2); ammonium chloride (p.1055·2); liquorice (p.1197·1).
Infections of the oropharynx; respiratory-tract catarrh.

Broncho-Vaxom
Byk, Aust.; Fournier, Belg.; Byk Gulden, Ger.; Byk Gulden, Ital.; OM, Switz.
Lysate of: *Haemophilus influenzae*; *Diplococcus pneumoniae*; *Klebsiella pneumoniae*; *Klebsiella ozaenae*; *Staphylococcus aureus*; *Streptococcus pyogenes*; *Streptococcus viridans*; *Branhamella catarrhalis*.
Respiratory-tract infections.

Bronchovydrin *Searle, Ger.†.*
Adrenaline (p.813·2); atropine methonitrate (p.455·1); papaverine hydrochloride (p.1614·2); amethocaine hydrochloride (p.1285·2).
Asthma; bronchitis; interstitial lung disease; silicosis.

Bronchowern *Wernigerode, Ger.*
Ambroxol hydrochloride (p.1054·3).
Respiratory-tract disorders with viscous mucus.

Bronchozone *Drug Trading, Canad.*
Ammonium chloride (p.1055·2); ammonium carbonate (p.1055·1); liquorice (p.1197·1); menthol (p.1600·2); senega (p.1069·3).

Broncivent *Boehringer Ingelheim, Spain.*
Beclomethasone dipropionate (p.1032·1).
Asthma.

Broncleer *Mer-National, S.Afr.*
Diphenhydramine hydrochloride (p.409·1); ammonium chloride (p.1055·2); sodium citrate (p.1153·2).
Coughs.

Broncleer with Codeine *Mer-National, S.Afr.; Propan, S.Afr.*
Codeine phosphate (p.26·1); diphenhydramine hydrochloride (p.409·1); ammonium chloride (p.1055·2); sodium citrate (p.1153·2).
Coughs.

Bronco Aseptilex *Wasserman, Spain.*
Sulphadiazine (p.252·3); guaiacol cinnamate (p.1061·2).
Respiratory-tract infections.

Bronco Aseptilex Fuerte *Wasserman, Spain.*
Bromhexine hydrochloride (p.1055·3); co-trimoxazole (p.196·3); guaiacol cinnamate (p.1061·2).
Respiratory-tract infections.

Bronco Asmol *Herbes Universelles, Canad.*
Ammonium bicarbonate (p.1055·1); anethole (p.1549·3); tolu balsam (p.1071·1); camphor (p.1557·2); squill (p.1070·1).

Bronco Bactifor *Andromaco, Spain.*
Bromhexine (p.1055·3); co-trimoxazole (p.196·3).
Respiratory-tract infections.

Bronco Lizom *Pensa, Spain.*
Haemophilus influenzae; *Klebsiella pneumoniae*; *Staphylococcus aureus*; *Streptococcus pyogenes*; *Streptococcus pneumoniae*; *Branhamella catarrhalis*.
Respiratory-tract infections.

Bronco Medical *Medical, Spain.*
Potassium guaiacolsulfonate (p.1068·3); dextromethorphan hydrobromide (p.1057·3).
Coughs.

Bronco Pensusan *Wasserman, Spain.*
Ampicillin sodium (p.153·1); ampicillin benzathine (p.154·1); bromhexine hydrochloride (p.1055·3).
Lignocaine hydrochloride (p.1293·2) is included in this preparation to alleviate the pain of injection.
Respiratory-tract infections.

Bronco Sergo *Inexfa, Spain.*
Tolu balsam (p.1071·1); bromhexine hydrochloride (p.1055·3); sodium benzoate (p.1102·3); co-trimoxazole (p.196·3).
Respiratory-tract infections.

Bronco Tonic N F *Vir, Spain.*
Amoxycillin trihydrate (p.151·3); bromhexine (p.1055·3).
Respiratory-tract infections.

Bronco Valda *Valda, Ital.†.*
Diiodhydrin (p.1572·1); camphor (p.1557·2); menthol (p.1600·2); guaiacol (p.1061·2); pumilio pine oil (p.1623·3).
Bronchial hypersecretion.

Broncobacter *Rubio, Spain†.*
Ampicillin trihydrate (p.153·2); bromhexine hydrochloride (p.1055·3).
Respiratory-tract infections.

Broncobeta *Beta, Ital.†.*
Dextromethorphan hydrobromide (p.1057·3); oxedrine tartrate (p.925·3); potassium guaiacolsulfonate (p.1068·3); sodium benzoate (p.1102·3).
Coughs.

Broncoclar *Oberlin, Fr.*
Oral solution: Acetylcysteine (p.1052·3).
Syrup: Carbocisteine (p.1056·3).
Respiratory-tract disorders associated with increased or viscous mucus.

Bronco-Dex *Pastor Farina, Ital.*
Dextromethorphan hydrobromide (p.1057·3); potassium guaiacolsulfonate (p.1068·3).
Coughs.

Broncodil
Note. This name is used for preparations of different composition.
Epifarma, Ital.
Clenbuterol hydrochloride (p.752·1).
Asthma.

Lagap, Switz.†.
Bromhexine hydrochloride (p.1055·3).
Respiratory-tract infections.

Broncofenil Forte *Almirall, Spain†.*
Potassium guaiacolsulfonate (p.1068·3); tetracycline edetate (p.261·1); thenoate sodium (p.262·2).
Respiratory-tract infections.

Broncofluid *Pharmarecord, Ital.*
Prenoxdiazine hybenzate (p.1068·3); carbocisteine (p.1056·3).
Coughs.

Broncoformo Muco Dexa *Ale, Spain.*
Dexamethasone (p.1037·1); dextromethorphan hydrobromide (p.1057·3); guaiphenesin (p.1061·3); sodium benzoate (p.1102·3).
Respiratory-tract disorders.

Broncokin *Geymonat, Ital.*
Bromhexine hydrochloride (p.1055·3).
Respiratory-tract disorders.

Broncol *Crown, S.Afr.*
Dextromethorphan hydrobromide (p.1057·3); ammonium chloride (p.1055·2); panthenol (p.1571·1).
Coughs.

Broncolitic *Wasserman, Spain†.*
Bromhexine hydrochloride (p.1055·3); erythromycin estolate (p.204·1); guaiacol cinnamate (p.1061·2).
Respiratory-tract infections.

Broncometil *Herdel, Ital.†.*
Guaiphenesin (p.1061·3); methyl cysteine hydrochloride (p.1064·1).
Respiratory-tract disorders.

Broncomicin Bals *Alcala, Spain.*
Tolu balsam (p.1071·1); sodium benzoate (p.1102·3); ammoniacal aniseed (p.1549·3); sulphadiazine (p.252·3).
Respiratory-tract infections.

Broncomnes *Bracco, Ital.*
Ambroxol acefyllinate (p.1054·3).
Bronchospasm.

Broncomucil *SmithKline Beecham, Ital.*
Carbocisteine (p.1056·3).
Respiratory-tract disorders associated with excess or viscous mucus.

Bronconovag *Novag, Spain.*
Amoxycillin trihydrate (p.151·3); bromhexine (p.1055·3).
Respiratory-tract infections.

Broncopiam *Piam, Ital.†.*
Oxolamine phosphate (p.1065·3); ephedrine hydrochloride (p.1059·3).
Bronchitis; coughs.

Broncoplus *Sigma-Tau, Ital.*
Stepronin sodium (p.1070·1).
Respiratory-tract disorders.

Broncopulmin *Ecobi, Ital.*
Camphor (p.1557·2); niaouli oil (p.1607·1); cineole (p.1564·1); menthol (p.1600·2).
Respiratory-tract disorders.

Broncorema *Septa, Spain.*
Guaiphenesin (p.1061·3); co-trimoxazole (p.196·3).
Respiratory-tract infections.

Broncorinol etats grippaux *Roche Nicholas, Fr.*
Paracetamol (p.72·2); pseudoephedrine hydrochloride (p.1068·3); chlorpheniramine maleate (p.405·1).
Cold symptoms.

Broncorinol Expectorant *Roche Nicholas, Fr.*
Carbocisteine (p.1056·3).
Viscous bronchial secretions.

Broncorinol maux de gorge *Roche Nicholas, Fr.*
Cetylpyridinium chloride (p.1106·2); amethocaine hydrochloride (p.1285·2); ascorbic acid (p.1365·2).
Sore throat.

Broncorinol rhinites *Roche Nicholas, Fr.*
Paracetamol (p.72·2); pseudoephedrine hydrochloride (p.1068·3).
Rhinitis.

Broncorinol toux seches *Roche Nicholas, Fr.*
Pholcodine (p.1068·1); sodium benzoate (p.1102·3); aconite (p.1542·2); hyoscyamus (p.464·3); lobelia (p.1481·3); polygala (p.1069·3); eucalyptus (p.1578·1).
Coughs.

Broncort
Boehringer Ingelheim, Belg.; Boehringer Ingelheim, Switz.
Flunisolide (p.1040·3).
Obstructive airways disease.

Broncosedina *FAMA, Ital.*
Cocillana (p.1057·2); eriodictyon (p.1060·3); marrubium (p.1063·3); grindelia; juniper (p.1592·2); compound thyme (p.1636·3); pumilio pine oil (p.1623·3); mint oil (p.1604·1).
Respiratory-tract disorders.

Broncosolvente EP *Ifidesa Aristegui, Spain†.*
Benzylpenicillin sodium (p.159·3); procaine penicillin (p.240·2); cineole (p.1564·1); niaouli oil (p.1607·1).
Respiratory-tract infections.

Broncospasmin *Merck, Spain.*
Reproterol hydrochloride (p.758·1).
Obstructive airways disease.

Broncospasmine *Asta Medica, Ital.*
Reproterol hydrochloride (p.758·1).
Asthma.

Broncostat *Rhone-Poulenc Rorer, Austral.†.*
Haemophilus influenzae killed cells.
Oral prophylaxis against bronchitis.

Broncostyl *Robert, Spain.*
Adamexine (p.1054·3).
Respiratory-tract disorders.

Broncosyl *Homberger, Switz.*
Homoeopathic preparation.

Bronco-Turbinal *Valeas, Ital.*
Beclomethasone dipropionate (p.1032·1).
Bronchospasm.

Broncotyfen *Cantabria, Spain†.*
Ampicillin sodium (p.153·1); ampicillin benzathine (p.154·1); bromhexine hydrochloride (p.1055·3); guaiphenesin (p.1061·3).
Respiratory-tract infections.

Broncovaleas *Valeas, Ital.*
Salbutamol (p.758·2).
Bronchospasm.

Broncovanil *Celafar, Ital.*
Guaiphenesin (p.1061·3).
Respiratory-tract disorders.

Broncovir NF *Vir, Spain.*
Co-trimoxazole (p.196·3); potassium guaiacolsulfonate (p.1068·3).
Bacterial infections of the respiratory tract.

Broncovital *Puerto Galiano, Spain.*
Cineole (p.1564·1); codeine phosphate (p.26·1); ephedrine hydrochloride (p.1059·3); niaouli oil (p.1607·1); sodium benzoate (p.1102·3); potassium guaiacolsulfonate (p.1068·3); belladonna (p.457·1); drosera (p.1574·1); quebracho; polygala (p.1069·3).
Respiratory-tract disorders.

Broncozina *Mendelejeff, Ital.†.*
Zipeprol hydrochloride (p.1071·3).
Coughs.

Brondecon *Parke, Davis, USA†.*
Choline theophyllinate (p.751·3); guaiphenesin (p.1061·3).

Brondecon Expectorant *Parke, Davis, Austral.*
Choline theophyllinate (p.751·3); guaiphenesin (p.1061·3).
Obstructive airways disease.

Brondecon-PD *Parke, Davis, Austral.*
Choline theophyllinate (p.751·3).
Obstructive airways disease.

Brondix *Pentafarm, Spain.*
Amoxycillin trihydrate (p.151·3).
Bacterial infections.

Brongenit *Elfar, Spain.*
Co-trimoxazole (p.196·3).
Bacterial infections; Pneumocystis carinii pneumonia.

Bronica *Takeda, Jpn.*
Seratrodast (p.762·1).
Asthma.

Bronilide
Cassenne, Fr.; Syntex, Switz.†.
Flunisolide (p.1040·3).
Asthma.

Bronitin Mist *Whitehall, USA.*
Adrenaline acid tartrate (p.813·3).
Bronchospasm.

Bronkaid
Note. This name is used for preparations of different composition.
Sanofi Winthrop, Canad.
Adrenaline (p.813·2).
Asthma.

Sterling Health, USA†.
Ephedrine sulphate (p.1059·3); guaiphenesin (p.1061·3); theophylline (p.765·1).
Bronchial asthma; bronchial congestion.

Bronkaid Dual Action *Sterling, USA.*
Ephedrine sulphate (p.1059·3); guaiphenesin (p.1061·3).

Bronkaid Mist *Sterling Health, USA.*
Adrenaline nitrate (p.815·2); adrenaline hydrochloride (p.813·3).
Bronchial asthma.

Bronkaid Mist Suspension *Winthrop Consumer, USA†.*
Adrenaline acid tartrate (p.813·3).
Bronchial asthma.

Bronkephrine *Winthrop, USA†.*
Ethylnoradrenaline hydrochloride (p.753·1).
Bronchial asthma; reversible bronchospasm.

Bronkese *Pharmacare Consumer, S.Afr.*
Bromhexine hydrochloride (p.1055·3).
Respiratory-tract disorders.

Bronkese Compound *Pharmacare Consumer, S.Afr.*
Bromhexine hydrochloride (p.1055·3); orciprenaline sulphate (p.756·3).
Respiratory-tract disorders.

Bronkodyl *Winthrop, USA†.*
Theophylline (p.765·1).
Asthma; bronchospasm.

Bronkolixir *Sterling, USA†.*
Theophylline (p.765·1); ephedrine sulphate (p.1059·3); guaiphenesin (p.1061·3); phenobarbitone (p.350·2).
Bronchospasm.

Bronkometer *Sanofi Winthrop, USA.*
Isoetharine mesylate (p.755·1).
Bronchial asthma; reversible bronchospasm.

Bronkosol *Sanofi Winthrop, USA.*
Isoetharine hydrochloride (p.755·1).

Bronkotabs *Sterling, USA†.*
Theophylline (p.765·1); ephedrine sulphate (p.1059·3); guaiphenesin (p.1061·3); phenobarbitone (p.350·2).
Bronchospasm.

Bronkotuss Expectorant *Hyrex, USA.*
Ephedrine sulphate (p.1059·3); chlorpheniramine maleate (p.405·1); guaiphenesin (p.1061·3).
Coughs.

Bronkyl *Weifa, Norw.*
Acetylcysteine (p.1052·3).
Chronic bronchitis; cystic fibrosis.

Bro-N-Pain *Brovar, S.Afr.†.*
Paracetamol (p.72·2); codeine phosphate (p.26·1).
Fever; pain.

Bronpax *Biocodex, Fr.*
Paediatric syrup: Potassium guaiacolsulfonate (p.1068·3); sodium benzoate (p.1102·3); piscidia; aconite (p.1542·2); belladonna (p.457·1); pine buds; frangula (p.1193·2); tolu balsam (p.1071·1); terpin hydrate (p.1070·2); liquorice (p.1197·1).
Respiratory disorders.
Pastilles: Tyrothricin (p.267·2); ethylmorphine hydrochloride (p.36·1); sodium benzoate (p.1102·3); menthol (p.1600·2); glycyrrhizinic acid; potassium guaiacolsulfonate (p.1068·3); terpin hydrate (p.1070·2).
Coughs.
Syrup: Codeine (p.26·1); potassium guaiacolsulfonate (p.1068·3); sodium benzoate (p.1102·3); piscidia; aconite (p.1542·2); belladonna (p.457·1); pine buds; Dessessartz syrup; tolu balsam (p.1071·1); terpin hydrate (p.1070·2); liquorice (p.1197·1).
Coughs.

Bronquiasmol *Berenguer Infale, Spain†.*
Aminophylline (p.748·1); lobelia inflata (p.1481·3); mepyramine maleate (p.414·1); pangamic acid (p.1614·1); polygala (p.1069·3); prednisolone (p.1048·1); ephedrine hydrochloride (p.1059·3); sodium iodide (p.1493·2); potassium iodide (p.1493·1); caffeine (p.749·3); sodium benzoate (p.1102·3); adenosine triphosphate (p.1543·2).
Respiratory-tract disorders.

Bronquicisteina *Iquinosa, Spain.*
Carbocisteine (p.1056·3); co-trimoxazole (p.196·3).
Respiratory-tract infections.

Bronquidiazina CR *Faes, Spain.*
Tolu balsam (p.1071·1); bromhexine (p.1055·3); sodium benzoate (p.1102·3); co-trimoxazole (p.196·3).
Respiratory-tract infections.

Bronquimar *Cruz, Spain.*
Oral suspension: Guaiphenesin (p.1061·3); sodium benzoate (p.1102·3); co-trimoxazole (p.196·3).
Respiratory-tract infections.
Suppositories: Camphor (p.1557·2); cineole (p.1564·1); niaouli oil (p.1607·1); guaiacol (p.1061·2); propyphenazone (p.81·3); menthol (p.1600·2).
Upper-respiratory-tract disorders.

Bronquimar Vit A *Cruz, Spain.*
Camphor (p.1557·2); cineole (p.1564·1); niaouli oil (p.1607·1); guaiacol (p.1061·2); vitamin A (p.1358·1); menthol (p.1600·2).
Respiratory-tract disorders.

Bronquimucil *Uriach, Spain.*
Brovanexine hydrochloride (p.1056·1); co-trimoxazole (p.196·3).
Respiratory-tract infections.

Bronquinflamatoria *Faes, Spain.*
Injection†: Bromhexine hydrochloride (p.1055·3); oxytetracycline (p.235·1).
Lignocaine hydrochloride (p.1293·2) is included in this preparation to alleviate the pain of injection.
Oral suspension: Bromhexine hydrochloride (p.1055·3); tetracycline phosphate (p.259·1); ammoniacal aniseed (p.1549·3).
Respiratory-tract infections.

Bronquium *Ferrer, Spain.*
Bromhexine hydrochloride (p.1055·3); co-trimoxazole (p.196·3).
Respiratory-tract infections.

Bronquium Amoxicilina *Ferrer, Spain.*
Amoxycillin trihydrate (p.151·3); bromhexine hydrochloride (p.1055·3).
Respiratory-tract infections.

Bronsal *UCB, Spain.*
Betamethasone sodium phosphate (p.1033·3); diprophylline (p.752·1); guaiphenesin (p.1061·3).
Respiratory-tract disorders.

Bronsecur *Parke, Davis, Ital.†.*
Carbuterol hydrochloride (p.751·3).
Bronchospasm.

Bronsema *Leti, Spain.*
Erythromycin ethyl succinate (p.204·2).
Bacterial infections.

Bronsema Balsamico *Leti, Spain.*
Erythromycin ethyl succinate (p.204·2); guaiphenesin (p.1061·3).
Respiratory-tract infections.

Bronteril *Manetti Roberts, Ital.*
Guaimesal (p.1061·3).
Respiratory-tract disorders.

Brontex *Procter & Gamble, USA.*
Codeine phosphate (p.26·1); guaiphenesin (p.1061·3).
Coughs.

Brontheo *Thomae, Ger.†.*
Choline theophyllinate (p.751·3).
Obstructive airways disease.

Brontin *Formenti, Ital.*
Deptropine citrate (p.408·1).
Respiratory-tract disorders.

Bronx *Lisapharma, Ital.*
Carbocisteine (p.1056·3).
Formerly contained zipeprol hydrochloride.
Respiratory-tract disorders.

Bronz *Nelson, Austral.†.*
Calamine (p.1080·1); zinc oxide (p.1096·2).
Sunscreen.

Bronze 8882 *Juvex, Fr.*
Ethylhexyl *p*-methoxycinnamate (p.1487·1); oxybenzone (p.1487·3); avobenzone (p.1486·3); mica-titanium dioxide complex (p.1093·3).
Sunscreen.

Brooklax *Intercare, UK.*
Yellow phenolphthalein (p.1208·2).
Constipation.

Bros *Fidia, Ital.†.*
Phosphatidylserine (p.1618·1).
Cerebrovascular disorders.

Brosol *Mepha, Switz.*
Codeine phosphate (p.26·1); diprophylline (p.752·1); atropine methobromide (p.455·1); thyme oil (p.1637·1).
Coughs.

Brosoline-Rectocaps *Mepha, Switz.*
Noscapine hydrochloride (p.1065·2); guaiphenesin (p.1061·3).
Bronchial disorders.

Brostalin *Synpharma, Aust.*
Urtica root and leaves (p.1642·3); couch-grass (p.1567·3).
Urinary-tract disorders.

Brota Rectal Bals *Escaned, Spain.*
Camphor (p.1557·2); cineole (p.1564·1); ephedrine hydrochloride (p.1059·3); niaouli oil (p.1607·1); quinine sulphate (p.439·2); potassium guaiacolsulfonate (p.1068·3).
Respiratory-tract disorders.

Brotane DX *Bioline, USA†.*
Pseudoephedrine hydrochloride (p.1068·3); brompheniramine maleate (p.403·2); dextromethorphan hydrobromide (p.1057·3).

Brotazona *Escaned, Spain.*
Feprazone (p.41·2).
Gout; musculoskeletal and joint disorders.

B12-Rotexmedica *Rotexmedica, Ger.*
Cyanocobalamin (p.1363·3) or hydroxocobalamin acetate (p.1364·2).
Vitamin B_{12} deficiency.

Brovaflamp *Brovar, S.Afr.†.*
Diclofenac sodium (p.31·2).
Gout; inflammation; musculoskeletal and joint disorders.

Brovel *Lepetit, Ital.†.*
Eprozinol hydrochloride (p.1574·3).
Respiratory-tract disorders.

Brox-Aerosol N *Redel, Ger.†.*
Adrenaline (p.813·2); atropine methonitrate (p.455·1); hyoscine hydrobromide (p.462·3); papaverine hydrochloride (p.1614·2); amethocaine hydrochloride (p.1285·2); ascorbic acid (p.1365·2).
Asthma.

Broxamox *UCB, Spain†.*
Amoxycillin trihydrate (p.151·3); bromhexine hydrochloride (p.1055·3).
Respiratory-tract infections.

Broxil *SmithKline Beecham, Neth.*
Phenethicillin potassium (p.236·2).
Bacterial infections.

Broxo al Fluoro *Cabon, Ital.*
Levomenol (p.1596·1); sodium fluoride (p.742·1); sodium monofluorophosphate (p.743·3).
Gum disorders; halitosis.

Broxodin *Cabon, Ital.*
Chlorhexidine gluconate (p.1107·2).
Oral hygiene.

Broxol
Mundipharma, Aust.; Pulitzer, Ital.
Ambroxol hydrochloride (p.1054·3).
Respiratory-tract disorders.

Brozam *Rolab, S.Afr.†.*
Bromazepam (p.643·1).
Anxiety.

Bruciaporri *Giovanardi, Ital.*
Salicylic acid (p.1090·2); lactic acid (p.1593·3).
Verrucas; warts.

Brufen
Ebewe, Aust.; Knoll, Austral.; Knoll, Belg.; Knoll, Fr.; Kanoldt, Ger.; Knoll, Irl.; Nordmark, Ital.; Knoll, Neth.; Knoll, Norw.; Knoll, S.Afr.; Meda, Swed.; Knoll, Switz.; Knoll, UK.
Ibuprofen (p.44·1) or ibuprofen sodium (p.44·3).
Fever; gout; musculoskeletal, joint, peri-articular, and soft-tissue disorders; pain.

Brufort *Lampugnani, Ital.*
Ibuprofen (p.44·1).
Inflammation; musculoskeletal and joint disorders; pain.

Brugesic *Garec, S.Afr.*
Ibuprofen (p.44·1).
Fever; muscle pain; pain.

Brulamycin
Torrex, Aust.; Medphano, Ger.
Tobramycin sulphate (p.264·1).
Bacterial infections.

Brulex *Bailly, Fr.*
Phenazone (p.78·2); zinc oxide (p.1096·2); peru balsam (p.1617·2); phenosalyl.
Formerly contained phenazone, zinc oxide, peru balsam, phenosalyl, and bismuth subgallate.
Burns; sunburn.

Brulidine
Rhone-Poulenc Rorer, Austral.; Rhone-Poulenc Rorer, Irl.; Rhone-Poulenc Rorer, Norw.; Manx, UK.
Dibromopropamidine isethionate (p.1112·2).
Burns; skin abrasions; skin infections.

Brulstop Tecnodif, Fr.
Hydrocolloid dressing.
Burns.

Brumetidina Bruschettini, Ital.
Cimetidine (p.1183·2).
Gastro-intestinal disorders associated with hyperacidity.

Brumeton Colloidale S Bruschettini, Ital.
Betamethasone (p.1033·2); sulphacetamide sodium (p.252·2).
Eye and ear disorders.

Brumixol Bruschettini, Ital.
Ciclopirox olamine (p.376·2).
Fungal skin and vulvovaginal infections.

Brunac Bruschettini, Ital.
Acetylcysteine (p.1052·3).
Eye disorders.

Brunacod Brunel, S.Afr.
Promethazine hydrochloride (p.416·2); ephedrine hydrochloride (p.1059·3); codeine phosphate (p.26·1).
Coughs.

Brunazine Brunel, S.Afr.
Promethazine hydrochloride (p.416·2).
Hypersensitivity reactions; motion sickness; nausea; vomiting.

Brunocilline Mepha, Switz.
Phenoxymethylpenicillin potassium (p.236·2).
Bacterial infections.

Brunomol Brunel, S.Afr.
Paracetamol (p.72·2).
Fever; pain.

Brush Off Seton, UK.
Povidone-iodine (p.1123·3).
Herpes labialis.

Brushtox Dentox, UK.
Denatured alcohol (p.1099·1).
Disinfection of toothbrushes.

Brust- und Hustentee Smetana, Aust.
Castaneae vulgaris; plantago lanceolata; verbascum leaf; thyme (p.1636·3); rad. enulae.
Respiratory-tract disorders.

Brust- und Husten-Tee Stada N Stada, Ger.
Spitzwegerichkraut thyme (p.1636·3); fennel (p.1579·1); liquorice (p.1197·1).
Bronchitis; tracheitis.

Brustol Vifor, Switz.
Dextromethorphan hydrobromide (p.1057·3); phenylephrine hydrochloride (p.1066·2); chlorpheniramine maleate (p.405·1).
Coughs.

Bruxicam Bruschettini, Ital.
Piroxicam (p.80·2).
Musculoskeletal, joint, peri-articular, and soft-tissue disorders.

Bryonia-Strath Strath-Labor, Ger.†.
Ointment: Hamamelis (p.1587·1); conii; aesculus (p.1543·3); echinacea (p.1574·2); bryonia (p.1555·2).
Circulatory disorders; haemorrhoids; inflammation; varicose veins.
Oral drops: Aconite (p.1542·2); conii; arnica (p.1550·3); bryonia (p.1555·2).
Inflammatory disorders and infections of the oropharynx.

Bryonon B-Komplex Protina, Ger.
Vitamin B substances.
Vitamin B deficiency.

Bryonon N Protina, Ger.
Vitamin B substances.
Vitamin B deficiency.

Bryorheum DHU, Ger.
Homoeopathic preparation.

B-Scorbic Pharmics, USA.
Vitamin C and vitamin B substances.

BSD 1800 Kabi, Switz.†.
Amino-acid, multivitamin, and mineral preparation.
Nutritional disorders.

B-S-P Legere, USA†.
Betamethasone sodium phosphate (p.1033·3).

BS-ratiopharm Ratiopharm, Ger.
Hyoscine butylbromide (p.462·3).
Smooth muscle cramp.

BSS
Alcon, Aust.; Alcon, Austral.; Alcon, Belg.; Alcon, Canad.; Alcon, Fr.; Alcon-Thilo, Ger.; Alcon, Irl.; Alcon, Neth.†; Alcon, S.Afr.; Alcon, Spain; Alcon, Switz.; Alcon, USA.
Electrolyte solution (p.1147·1).
Eye irrigation; otorhinolaryngeal irrigation.

BSS Compose Alcon, Fr.
Electrolytes (p.1147·1); glucose (p.1343·3); oxiglutatione.
Eye irrigation.

BSS Plus
Alcon, Aust.; Alcon, Austral.; Alcon, Belg.; Alcon, Canad.; Alcon, Ger.; Alcon, Neth.†; Alcon, Switz.; Alcon, UK.
Electrolytes (p.1147·1); glucose (p.1343·3); oxiglutatione.
Eye irrigation.

B12-Steigerwald Steigerwald, Ger.
Cyanocobalamin (p.1363·3).
Vitamin B_{12} deficiency.

BTE Verla, Ger.†.
Tropine benzilate hydrochloride (p.469·3).
Smooth muscle spasms.

B-Tene Vita Glow, Austral.
Betacarotene (p.1335·2).
Photosensitivity reactions in patients with erythropoietic protoporphyria.

BTH-N Broncho-Tetra-Holz Fournier, Ger.†.
Capsules: Oxytetracycline hydrochloride (p.235·1); guaiphenesin (p.1061·3).
Syrup: Oxytetracycline (p.235·1); guaiphenesin (p.1061·3); papaverine hydrochloride (p.1614·2).
Bacterial infections of the respiratory tract.

BTH-S (Broncho-Tetra-Holz) Fournier, Ger.†.
Oxytetracycline hydrochloride (p.235·1).
Bacterial infections.

B-Tonin Nycomed, Norw.
Vitamin B substances; caffeine (p.749·3).
Tonic; vitamin B deficiency.

Bucain Curasan, Ger.
Bupivacaine hydrochloride (p.1286·3).
Local anaesthesia.

Buccalin
Note. This name is used for preparations of different composition.
Kwizda, Aust.
Haemophilus influenzae; pneumococci; streptococci; staphylococci; ox bile extract (p.1553·2).
Prophylaxis of bacterial infections in patients with colds.
Berna, Ital.
Diplococcus pneumoniae I, II, and III; *Streptococcus haemolyticus*; *Staphylococcus aureus*; *Haemophilus influenzae*.
Prophylaxis of bacterial infections in patients with influenza.

Buccalin Complet Berna, Spain.
Pneumococcus; streptococcus; staphylococcus; *Haemophilus influenzae*.
Respiratory-tract infections.

Buccaline
Berna, Belg.; Berna, Switz.
Pneumococci; streptococci; staphylococci; *Haemophilus influenzae*; ox bile (p.1553·2).
Prophylaxis against colds.

Buccalsone
Will-Pharma, Belg.; Will-Pharma, Neth.
Hydrocortisone sodium succinate (p.1044·1).
Aphthous stomatitis.

Buccapol Kwizda, Aust.†.
An oral poliomyelitis vaccine (p.1528·2).
Active immunisation.

Buccastem
Reckitts, Irl.; Reckitt & Colman, UK.
Prochlorperazine maleate (p.687·3).
Migraine; nausea; vertigo; vomiting.

Buccawalter SmithKline Beecham, Fr.
Amylocaine hydrochloride (p.1286·1); chloral hydrate (p.645·3); phenosalyl; borax (p.1554·2).
Mouth and throat disorders.

Buccosan Warner-Lambert Consumer, Belg.
Dequalinium chloride (p.1112·1); lignocaine hydrochloride (p.1293·2).
Mouth and throat disorders.

Bucco-Spray Warner-Lambert Consumer, Belg.
Dequalinium chloride (p.1112·1); lignocaine hydrochloride (p.1293·2).
Mouth and throat disorders.

Bucco-Tantum Roche, Switz.
Benzydamine hydrochloride (p.21·3).
Mouth and throat inflammation.

Buccotean Labopharma, Ger.†.
Theobroma (p.1636·2); stoechados; betula leaf (p.1553·3); buchu (p.1555·2); jaborandi leaf; peppermint leaf (p.1208·1); orthosiphon (p.1592·2); raspberry leaf (p.1624·2); phaseolus vulgaris; rose fruit (p.1365·2); equisetum (p.1575·1); herniaria (p.1587·2); parietaria officinalis; juniper wood (p.1592·2); pterocarpus santalinus; liquorice (p.1197·1); ononis (p.1610·2); couch-grass (p.1567·3).
Urinary-tract infections.

Buccotean TF Labopharma, Ger.†.
Theobroma (p.1636·2); betula leaf (p.1553·3); orthosiphon (p.1592·2); equisetum (p.1575·1); herniaria (p.1587·2); parietaria officinalis; couch-grass (p.1567·3); buchu (p.1555·2); liquorice (p.1197·1); rose fruit (p.1365·2); peppermint oil (p.1208·1); juniper oil (p.1592·3).
Urinary-tract infections.

Bucet UAD, USA.
Butalbital (p.644·3); paracetamol (p.72·2).

Buchol Palmicol, Ger.
Sage oil.
Hyperhidrosis.

Buchu Compound Gerard House, UK.
Taraxacum (p.1634·2); buchu (p.1555·2); bearberry (p.1552·2); clivers (p.1565·2).
Fluid retention.

Buckley's DM Buckley, Canad.
Dextromethorphan hydrobromide (p.1057·3).
Dry cough.

Buckley's DM Decongestant Buckley, Canad.
Pseudoephedrine hydrochloride (p.1068·3); dextromethorphan hydrobromide (p.1057·3).
Coughs and cold symptoms.

Buckley's Mixture Buckley, Canad.
Ammonium carbonate (p.1055·1); potassium bicarbonate (p.1153·1); menthol (p.1600·2); camphor (p.1557·2).
Cough.

Buckleys Pain Relief Buckley, Canad.
Methyl salicylate (p.55·2); menthol (p.1600·2).

Buckley's White Rub Buckley, Canad.
Menthol (p.1600·2); camphor (p.1557·2); methyl salicylate (p.55·2); thymol (p.1127·1).
Cold symptoms; muscle and joint pain.

Bucladin-S Softab Stuart, USA.
Buclizine hydrochloride (p.404·1).
Motion sickness.

Buco Regis Ramon Sala, Spain.
Ipecacuanha (p.1062·2); methyl salicylate (p.55·2); myrrh (p.1606·1); sulphanilamide (p.256·3); zinc chloride (p.1373·1); menthol (p.1600·2).
Mouth and throat inflammation; pyorrhoea.

Bucodrin Fardi, Spain.
Ephedrine ricinoleate; ethacridine lactate (p.1098·3); sulphathiazole (p.257·1).
Mouth and throat inflammation.

Bucometasona Solvay, Spain.
Chlorhexidine hydrochloride (p.1107·2); benzocaine (p.1286·2); tyrothricin (p.267·2).
Formerly contained cetrimonium bromide, benzocaine, muramidase hydrochloride, tyrothricin, and triamcinolone acetonide.
Mouth and throat disorders.

Buconif Nycomed, Aust.†.
Nifedipine (p.916·2).
Hypertension; ischaemic heart disease; Raynaud's syndrome.

Bucospray Solvay, Spain.
Chlorhexidine gluconate (p.1107·2); benzocaine (p.1286·2).
Formerly known as Bucometasona. Formerly contained cetrimonium bromide, prednisolone phosphate, benzocaine, and tyrothricin.
Mouth and throat disorders.

Bucovacuna Nezel, Spain.
Diplococcus pneumoniae; *Micrococcus pyogenes*; *Haemophilus influenzae*; *Gaffkya tetragena*; *Moraxella (Branhamella) catarrhalis*; *Klebsiella pneumoniae*; *Moraxella*.
Prophylaxis of respiratory-tract infections.

Budamax PMC, Austral.
Budesonide (p.1034·3).
Allergic rhinitis.

Budeflam Cipla-Medpro, S.Afr.
Budesonide (p.1034·3).
Asthma.

Budirol Fher, Spain†.
Propyphenazone (p.81·3).
Fever; pain.

Budodouze Cambridge Laboratories, Austral.†.
B vitamins.
Lignocaine hydrochloride (p.1293·2) is included in the intramuscular injection to alleviate the pain of injection.

Buenoson Zilly, Ger.
Hypericum oil; wheatgerm oil; avocado oil; birch tar oil; neatsfoot oil; thiamine hydrochloride; dilute formic acid; garlic juice; birch leaf; juniper berry; gentian root; lupulus; clove; male fern leaf.
Herbal preparation.

Buer Vitamin E + Magnesium Roland, Ger.
α-Tocopheryl acetate (p.1369·2); magnesium oxide (p.1198·3).
Muscle weakness.

Buerlecithin
Schmidgall, Aust.
Lecithin (p.1595·2) with or without vitamins.
Tonic.
Polcopharma, Austral.; Roland, Ger.
Lecithin (p.1595·2).
Tonic.

Buerlecithin Compact Schmidgall, Aust.
Soya lecithin (p.1595·2).
Tonic.

Buerlecithine Compact Byk Roland, Switz.†.
Lecithin (p.1595·2).
Tonic.

Bufal Pierre Fabre, Fr.
Bufexamac (p.22·2).
Inflammatory skin disorders.

Buf-Bar 3M, USA†.
Sulphur (p.1091·2); titanium dioxide (p.1093·3).
Acne.

Bufederm Yamanouchi, Ger.
Bufexamac (p.22·2).
Skin disorders.

Bufedil Abbott, Ger.
Buflomedil hydrochloride (p.834·2).
Peripheral vascular disorders.

Bufedon Byk, Belg.
Ibuprofen (p.44·1).
Gout; musculoskeletal, joint, and peri-articular disorders; pain.

Bufene Ist. Chim. Inter., Ital.
Buflomedil hydrochloride (p.834·2).
Vascular disorders.

Bufeno Helvepharm, Switz.
Ibuprofen (p.44·1).
Musculoskeletal and joint disorders.

Bufeproct Hexal, Ger.
Bufexamac (p.22·2); lignocaine hydrochloride (p.1293·2); bismuth subgallate (p.1180·2); titanium dioxide (p.1093·3).
Haemorrhoids.

Bufexan Lannacher, Aust.
Bufexamac (p.22·2).
Inflammatory skin disorders.

Bufexine Belphar, Belg.
Bufexamac (p.22·2).
Arthritis; peri-articular inflammation.

Buffered C Quest, UK.
Calcium ascorbate (p.1365·2).

Buffered C 500 Bio-Health, UK.
Calcium ascorbate (p.1365·2).

Bufferin
Bristol-Myers, Austral.†; Bristol-Myers Squibb, Canad.
Aspirin (p.16·1).
Aluminium glycinate (p.1177·2) and magnesium carbonate (p.1198·1) are included in this preparation in an attempt to limit adverse effects on the gastro-intestinal mucosa.
Fever; pain; rheumatoid arthritis.
Bristol-Myers Squibb, Ital.; Bristol-Myers Products, USA.
Aspirin (p.16·1).
Calcium carbonate (p.1182·1), magnesium carbonate (p.1198·1), and magnesium oxide (p.1198·3) are included in this preparation in an attempt to limit adverse effects on the gastro-intestinal mucosa.
Fever; inflammation; myocardial infarction; pain; transient ischaemic attacks.

Bufferin AF Nite Time Bristol-Myers Squibb, USA.
Diphenhydramine citrate (p.409·1); paracetamol (p.72·2).
Insomnia.

Buffets II JMI, USA.
Paracetamol (p.72·2); aspirin (p.16·1); caffeine (p.749·3).
Aluminium hydroxide (p.1177·3) is included in this preparation in an attempt to limit adverse effects on the gastro-intestinal mucosa.
Pain.

Buffex Roberts, USA.
Aspirin (p.16·1).
Aluminium glycinate (p.1177·2) and magnesium carbonate (p.1198·1) are included in this preparation in an attempt to limit adverse effects on the gastro-intestinal mucosa.
Fever; inflammation; myocardial infarction; pain; transient ischaemic attacks.

Bufigen Antigen, Irl.
Ibuprofen (p.44·1).
Musculoskeletal, joint, and peri-articular disorders; pain; soft-tissue injuries.

Buflan Fournier, Ital.
Buflomedil hydrochloride (p.834·2).
Vascular disorders.

Buflocit CT, Ital.
Buflomedil hydrochloride (p.834·2).
Cerebral and peripheral vascular disorders.

Buflofar Upsamedica, Ital.
Buflomedil hydrochloride (p.834·2).
Cerebral and peripheral vascular disorders.

Buflohexal Hexal, Ger.
Buflomedil hydrochloride (p.834·2).
Peripheral vascular disorders.

Buflo-Puren Isis Puren, Ger.
Buflomedil hydrochloride (p.834·2).
Peripheral vascular disorders.

Buflo-Reu Reusch, Ger.
Buflomedil hydrochloride (p.834·2).
Peripheral vascular disorders.

Buf-Oxal 3M, USA†.
Benzoyl peroxide (p.1079·2).
Acne.

Bufoxin Fulton, Ital.
Buflomedil pyridoxal phosphate compound (p.834·2).
Cerebral and peripheral vascular disorders.

Bug Guards Go Travel, UK.
Diethyltoluamide (p.1405·1).
Insect repellent.

Bugs Bunny
Miles, Canad.; Miles, USA.
A range of vitamin preparations.

Build-Up Nestle, S.Afr.
Preparation for enteral nutrition.

Bulboid Wander OTC, Switz.
Glycerol (p.1585·2).
Bowel evacuation; constipation.

Bulboshap Farmagan, Ital.
Shampoo containing achillea, chamomile, cinchona, cornflower, gentian, lilly, and almond.
Seborrhoeic dermatitis.

Bulbotruw Truw, Ger.†.
Homoeopathic preparation.

Bulbotruw S Truw, Ger.†.
Homoeopathic preparation.

Bulk Agepha, Aust.
Methylcellulose (p.1473·3).
Constipation.

Bullfrog
Note. This name is used for preparations of different composition.
Parke, Davis, Austral.†.
Octocrylene (p.1487·3); roxadimate (p.1488·2); avobenzone (p.1486·3).
Sunscreen.
Chattem, USA.
Gel SPF 18: Oxybenzone (p.1487·3); octocrylene (p.1487·3); ethylhexyl *p*-methoxycinnamate (p.1487·1).
Stick SPF 18: Oxybenzone (p.1487·3); ethylhexyl *p*-methoxycinnamate (p.1487·1).

SPF 36: Oxybenzone (p.1487·3); octocrylene (p.1487·3); ethylhexyl *p*-methoxycinnamate (p.1487·1).
Sunscreen.

Bullfrog for Kids Chattem, USA.
SPF 18: Octocrylene (p.1487·3); ethylhexyl *p*-methoxycinnamate (p.1487·1) octyl salicylate (p.1487·3).
Sunscreen.

Bullfrog Sport Chattem, USA.
SPF 18: Oxybenzone (p.1487·3); octocrylene (p.1487·3); ethylhexyl *p*-methoxycinnamate (p.1487·1) octyl salicylate (p.1487·3); titanium dioxide (p.1093·3).
Sunscreen.

Bullrich Salz Mundipharma, Aust.
Sodium bicarbonate (p.1153·2).
Dyspepsia.

Bumex Roche, USA.
Bumetanide (p.834·3).
Oedema.

Buminate
Baxter, UK†; Hyland, USA.
Albumin (p.710·1).
Hypoalbuminaemia; hypovolaemia; neonatal hyperbilirubinaemia.

Bumps 'n Falls Dermamend, UK.
Benzalkonium chloride (p.1101·3); oxyesterified triglycerides.
Cuts; soft-tissue injury.

Bunetten Woelm, Ger.†.
Valerian (p.1643·1); crataegus (p.1568·2); passion flower (p.1615·3); lupulus (p.1597·2).
Nervous disorders; sleep disorders.

Bunion Salve Cress, Canad.
Camphor (p.1557·2); menthol (p.1600·2); phenol (p.1121·2); tannic acid (p.1634·2).

BUP-4 Taiho, Jpn†.
Propiverine hydrochloride (p.468·2).
Urinary frequency; urinary incontinence.

Bupap ECR, USA.
Butalbital (p.644·3); paracetamol (p.72·2).
Pain.

Buphenyl Ucyclyd, USA.
Sodium phenylbutyrate (p.1631·3).
Urea cycle disorders.

Bupiforan Bieffe, Ital.
Bupivacaine hydrochloride (p.1286·3).
Adrenaline acid tartrate (p.813·3) is included in some injections as a vasoconstrictor to diminish absorption and localise the effect of the local anaesthetic.
Local anaesthesia.

Buprenex Reckitt & Colman, USA.
Buprenorphine hydrochloride (p.22·2).
Pain.

Buprex Esteve, Spain.
Buprenorphine hydrochloride (p.22·2).
Pain.

Buram Leo, Irl.
Bumetanide (p.834·3); amiloride hydrochloride (p.819·2).
Oedema.

Buraton Schulke & Mayr, Ger.†.
Isopropyl alcohol (p.1118·2); formaldehyde (p.1113·2); glyoxal (p.1115·1); glyoxylic acid.
Instrument disinfection.

Buraton 25 Schulke & Mayr, Ger.†.
Formaldehyde (p.1113·2); glyoxal (p.1115·1); glyoxylic acid; benzalkonium chloride (p.1101·3).
Fungal skin infections; surface disinfection.

Buraton 10 F Schulke & Mayr, Ger.
Glyoxal (p.1115·1); formaldehyde (p.1113·2); glutaraldehyde (p.1114·3); 2-ethyl-1-hexanol.
Surface disinfection.

Burgerstein Geriatrikum Antistress, Switz.
Multivitamin and mineral preparation.
Tonic.

Burgerstein S Antistress, Switz.
Vitamin and mineral preparation.
Liver disorders.

Burgodin
Janssen-Cilag, Belg.; Janssen, Neth.†.
Bezitramide (p.22·1).
Pain.

Burinex
Merck, Aust.; Astra, Austral.; Leo, Belg.; Leo, Canad.; Leo, Fr.; Leo, Ger.; Leo, Irl.; Sigma-Tau, Ital.†; Leo, Neth.; Leo, Norw.; Adcock Ingram, S.Afr.; Lovens, Swed.; Leo, Switz.; Leo, UK.
Bumetanide (p.834·3).
Forced diuresis; heart failure; hypertension; oedema; renal failure; sodium retention.

Burinex A Leo, UK.
Bumetanide (p.834·3); amiloride hydrochloride (p.819·2).
Oedema.

Burinex K
Leo, Irl.; Leo, Norw.; Leo, S.Afr.†; Leo, UK.
Bumetanide (p.834·3); potassium chloride (p.1161·1).
Oedema.

Burmicin I Farmacologia, Spain.
Amoxycillin trihydrate (p.151·3); potassium clavulanate (p.190·2).
Bacterial infections.

Burn Healing Cream Brauer, Austral.
Homoeopathic preparation.

Burn-aid Seton, UK†.
Aminacrine hydrochloride (p.1098·3).
Minor burns or wounds.

Burneze Seton, UK.
Benzocaine (p.1286·2).
Burns; scalds.

Burns Ointment Nelson, UK.
Homoeopathic preparation.

Buro Derm Trans Canaderm, Canad.
Aluminium acetate (p.1547·3); benzethonium chloride (p.1102·3).

Buronil
Lundbeck, Aust.; Lundbeck, Belg.; Lundbeck, Norw.; Lundbeck, Swed.
Melperone hydrochloride (p.677·3).
Anxiety disorders; dementia; drug and alcohol withdrawal syndromes; pain; psychoses; sleep disorders.

Buro-Sol
Note. This name is used for preparations of different composition.
Trans Canaderm, Canad.
Aluminium acetate (p.1547·3); benzethonium chloride (p.1102·3).
Ear disorders; skin disorders.

Doak, USA.
Aluminium acetate (p.1547·3).
Skin inflammation.

Burow's Rugby, USA.
Acetic acid (p.1541·2); aluminium acetate (p.1547·3).
Ear infections.

Busala Selz, Ger.
Dimethicone (p.1213·1).
Gastro-intestinal disorders.

Buscapina Boehringer Ingelheim, Spain.
Hyoscine butylbromide (p.462·3).
Smooth muscle spasm.

Buscapina Compositum Boehringer Ingelheim, Spain.
Hyoscine butylbromide (p.462·3); dipyrone (p.35·1).
Pain.

Buscolysin Medphano, Ger.
Hyoscine butylbromide (p.462·3).
Smooth muscle spasm.

Buscopamol Bender, Aust.
Hyoscine butylbromide (p.462·3); paracetamol (p.72·2).
Cramp; pain.

Buscopan
Bender, Aust.; Boehringer Ingelheim, Austral.; Boehringer Ingelheim, Belg.; Boehringer Ingelheim, Canad.; Delagrange, Fr.†; Thomae, Ger.; Boehringer Ingelheim, Irl.; Boehringer Ingelheim, Ital.; Boehringer Ingelheim, Neth.; Boehringer Ingelheim, Norw.; Boehringer Ingelheim, S.Afr.; Boehringer Ingelheim, Swed.; Boehringer Ingelheim, Switz.; Boehringer Ingelheim, UK.
Hyoscine butylbromide (p.462·3).
Diagnostic aid in radiology or endoscopy; smooth muscle spasm.

Buscopan Compositum
Bender, Aust.; Boehringer Ingelheim, Belg.; Boehringer Ingelheim, Ital.; Boehringer Ingelheim, S.Afr.; Boehringer Ingelheim, Switz.†.
Hyoscine butylbromide (p.462·3); dipyrone (p.35·1).
Smooth muscle spasm.

Buscopan Plus Boehringer Ingelheim, Ger.
Hyoscine butylbromide (p.462·3); paracetamol (p.72·2).
Smooth muscle spasm.

Buscopax Boehringer Ingelheim, Spain†.
Hyoscine butylbromide (p.462·3); oxazepam (p.683·2).
Extrapyramidal disorders; gastro-intestinal disorders; smooth muscle spasm.

Bush Formula Or-Dov, Austral.
Chlorhexidine gluconate (p.1107·2).
Acne; skin rashes.

Buspar
Bristol-Myers Squibb, Aust.; Bristol-Myers Squibb, Austral.; Bristol-Myers Squibb, Belg.; Bristol, Canad.; Bristol-Myers Squibb, Fr.; Bristol-Myers Squibb, Irl.; Mead Johnson, Ital.; Bristol-Myers Squibb, Neth.; Bristol-Myers Squibb, Norw.; Bristol-Myers Squibb, S.Afr.; Bristol-Myers, Spain; Bristol-Myers Squibb, Swed.; Bristol-Myers Squibb, Switz.; Bristol-Myers Squibb, UK; Mead Johnson Pharmaceutical, USA.
Buspirone hydrochloride (p.643·3).
Anxiety.

Buspimen Menarini, Ital.
Buspirone hydrochloride (p.643·3).
Anxiety.

Buspisal Lesvi, Spain.
Buspirone hydrochloride (p.643·3).
Anxiety.

Butacote
Ciba-Geigy, Irl.†; Geigy, UK.
Phenylbutazone (p.79·2).
Ankylosing spondylitis; osteoarthritis; rheumatoid arthritis.

Butadion Streuli, Switz.
Phenylbutazone (p.79·2) or phenylbutazone sodium (p.79·3).
Lignocaine hydrochloride (p.1293·2) is included in the intramuscular injection to alleviate the pain of injection.
Gout; musculoskeletal and joint disorders; phlebitis; soft-tissue disorders.

Butadiona Miquel Otsuka, Spain†.
Phenylbutazone (p.79·2).
Musculoskeletal and joint disorders.

Butaliret Fatol, Ger.
Terbutaline sulphate (p.764·1).
Obstructive airways disease.

Butalitab Fatol, Ger.
Terbutaline sulphate (p.764·1).
Obstructive airways disease.

Butaparin Streuli, Switz.
Heparin sodium (p.879·3); phenylbutazone (p.79·2); thymol (p.1127·1).
Peripheral vascular disorders.

Butatensin Benvegna, Ital.†.
Mebutamate (p.901·3).
Hypertension.

Butazina Vis, Ital.†.
Phenylbutazone (p.79·2).
Pain; rheumatic disorders.

Butazolidin
Ciba-Geigy, Aust.; Novartis, Austral.; Ciba-Geigy, Belg.; Geigy, Canad.†; Geigy, Ger.; Ciba-Geigy, Irl.†; Novartis, Neth.; Ciba-Geigy, Swed.†; Geigy, USA†.
Phenylbutazone (p.79·2) or phenylbutazone sodium (p.79·3).
Cinchocaine (p.1289·2) or lignocaine (p.1293·2) may be included in the injection to alleviate the pain of injection.
Ankylosing spondylitis; degenerative joint disease; gouty arthritis; rheumatoid arthritis.

Butazolidina
Ciba, Ital.†; Padro, Spain.
Phenylbutazone (p.79·2).
Ankylosing spondylitis; arthrosis; gout; rheumatism.

Butazolidine
Ciba-Geigy, Fr.; Geigy, Switz.
Phenylbutazone (p.79·2) or phenylbutazone sodium (p.79·3).
Cinchocaine (p.1289·2) is included in the intramuscular injection to alleviate the pain of injection.
Ankylosing spondylitis; arthrosis; gout; rheumatoid arthritis.

Butazolidine Alca Geigy, Switz.†.
Phenylbutazone (p.79·2).
Colloidal aluminium hydroxide (p.1177·3) and magnesium trisilicate (p.1199·1) are included in this preparation in an attempt to limit adverse effects on the gastro-intestinal mucosa.
Ankylosing spondylitis; arthrosis; gout; rheumatoid arthritis.

Butazone DDSA Pharmaceuticals, UK.
Phenylbutazone (p.79·2).

Buteridol Promonta Lundbeck, Ger.
Haloperidol (p.673·3).
Anxiety; movement disorders; pain; psychoses; stuttering; vomiting.

Butesin Picrate
Note. This name is used for preparations of different composition.
Abbott, Austral.
Butyl aminobenzoate picrate (p.1289·1); nitromersol (p.1120·1).
Burns; skin abrasions.

Abbott, USA.
Butyl aminobenzoate picrate (p.1289·1).
Burns.

Butibel Wallace, USA.
Belladonna (p.457·1); secbutobarbitone sodium (p.692·1).
Gastro-intestinal disorders.

Butidil Iquinosa, Spain†.
Indomethacin (p.45·2).
Gout; inflammation; musculoskeletal, joint, and periarticular disorders; pain.

Butinat Mabo, Spain†.
Bumetanide (p.834·3).
Oedema.

Butiran Ecobi, Ital.
Butamyrate citrate (p.1056·2).
Coughs.

Butisol
Carter Horner, Canad.; Wallace, USA.
Secbutobarbitone sodium (p.692·1).
Anxiety; insomnia; sedative.

Butix Pierre Fabre, Fr.
Tablets: Mequitazine (p.414·2).
Hypersensitivity disorders; skin disorders.
Topical gel: Diphenhydramine hydrochloride (p.409·1).
Pruritus; urticaria.

Buto Asma Aldo, Spain.
Salbutamol (p.758·2) or salbutamol sulphate (p.758·2).
Obstructive airways disease.

Butohaler Chiesi, Switz.
Salbutamol (p.758·2).
Bronchospasm.

Butosol Aldo, Spain.
Beclomethasone dipropionate (p.1032·1); salbutamol (p.758·2).
Obstructive airways disease.

Butovent Siphar, Switz.
Salbutamol (p.758·2).
Bronchospasm.

Butrex Pharmalab, S.Afr.†.
Phenylbutazone (p.79·2).
Lignocaine (p.1293·2) is included in the injection to alleviate the pain of injection.
Ankylosing spondylitis.

Buttercup Lozenges LRC Products, UK.
Bee propolis (p.1621·3).
Coughs.

Buttercup Pol'N'Count LRC Products, UK.
Echinacea (p.1574·2); garlic (p.1583·1).
Hay fever.

Buttercup Syrup LRC Products, UK.
Squill liquid (p.1070·1); capsicum tincture (p.1559·2).
Coughs.

Buttercup Syrup (Blackcurrant flavour) LRC Products, UK.
Ipecacuanha (p.1062·2); glucose (p.1343·3); menthol (p.1600·2).
Coughs.

Buttercup Syrup (Honey and Lemon flavour) LRC Products, UK.
Ipecacuanha (p.1062·2); glucose (p.1343·3); menthol (p.1600·2); honey (p.1345·3).
Coughs.

Buventol Orion, Swed.
Salbutamol sulphate (p.758·2).
Obstructive airways disease.

Buzpel Torbet Laboratories, UK.
Pyrethrins; piperonyl butoxide (p.1409·3).
Insect repellent.

B-Vasc Garec, S.Afr.
Atenolol (p.825·3).
Angina pectoris; hypertension.

B_1-Vicotrat Heyl, Ger.
Thiamine nitrate (p.1361·1).
Vitamin B deficiency.

B_6-Vicotrat Heyl, Ger.
Pyridoxine hydrochloride (p.1362·3).
Premenstrual syndrome; vitamin B deficiency.

B_{12}-Vicotrat Heyl, Ger.
Cyanocobalamin (p.1363·3).
Vitamin B deficiency.

BVK Roche A Roche, Ger.†.
Vitamin B substances.
Vitamin B deficiency.

BVK Roche plus C Roche Nicholas, Ger.
Vitamin B substances with ascorbic acid.
Vitamin B and C deficiency.

B-Voltaren Geigy, Ger.†.
Diclofenac sodium (p.31·2); vitamin B substances.
Inflammation; pain; rheumatic and nerve disorders.

Byclomine Major, USA.
Dicyclomine hydrochloride (p.460·1).
Functional bowel/irritable bowel syndrome.

Byclomine with Phenobarbital Major, USA†.
Dicyclomine hydrochloride (p.460·1); phenobarbitone (p.350·2).

Bydramine Cough Major, USA†.
Diphenhydramine hydrochloride (p.409·1).
Coughs.

Bye Bye Bite Daniels, Canad.
Diphenhydramine hydrochloride (p.409·1); menthol (p.1600·2); benzocaine (p.1286·2).
Bites and stings.

Bye Bye Burn Daniels, Canad.
Benzocaine (p.1286·2); cetrimonium bromide (p.1106·1); allantoin (p.1078·2); vitamin E (p.1369·1).
Burns.

Bykomycetin Byk Gulden, Ital.†.
Spiramycin (p.249·2).
Infections.

Bykomycin
Byk, Aust.; Byk Gulden, Ger.
Neomycin sulphate (p.229·2).
Hepatic coma.

Bykomycin F Byk Gulden, Ger.†.
Neomycin sulphate (p.229·2); hydrocortisone acetate (p.1043·3).
Eye disorders.

Byodin Lucchini, Ital.
Proteins (mol. wt 30-300 kD).
Tissue repair.

C2 Wampole, Canad.†.
Aspirin (p.16·1); caffeine (p.749·3).
Cardiovascular disorders; fever; inflammation; pain.

C-1000 Seroyal, Canad.
Ascorbic acid (p.1365·2).

C-3000 Seroyal, Canad.
Ascorbic acid (p.1365·2).

C2 with Codeine Wampole, Canad.
Aspirin (p.16·1); caffeine (p.749·3); codeine phosphate (p.26·1).
Aluminium hydroxide (p.1177·3) and magnesium hydroxide (p.1198·2) are included in this preparation in an attempt to limit adverse effects on the gastro-intestinal mucosa.
Cardiovascular disorders; fever; inflammation; pain.

C Factors "1000" Plus Solgar, USA.
Vitamin C (p.1365·2); rose hips (p.1365·2); citrus bioflavonoids complex (p.1580·1); rutin (p.1580·2); hesperidin (p.1580·2).
Capillary bleeding.

C Forte Frega, Canad.
Ascorbic acid (p.1365·2).

C1 Inattivatore Umano Immuno, Ital.
Complement C_1 esterase inhibitor (p.1567·2).
Hereditary angioedema.

C Monovit Esseti, Ital.
Sodium ascorbate (p.1365·2).
Vitamin C deficiency.

C P P A Humain Bio-Transfusion, Fr.†.
Factor IX complex (p.721·3).
Haemophilia A.

C Pal
Eagle, Austral.†.
Vitamin and mineral preparation.

Eagle, Austral.
Vitamin and mineral preparation with lysine.

C Plus E Natural Larkhall Laboratories, UK.
Vitamin C and E preparation.

C Speridin Marlyn, USA.
Hesperidin (p.1580·2); lemon bioflavonoids (p.1580·1); ascorbic acid (p.1365·2).
Capillary bleeding.

C 34-Strath Strath-Labor, Ger.†.
Leontopodium alpinum; maize; rhus toxocodendron (p.1624·3); taraxacum (p.1634·2); urtica (p.1642·3).
Musculoskeletal and joint disorders; prostate disorders; ulcers.

C Supa + Bioflavonoids Vitaplex, Austral.
Calcium ascorbate (p.1365·2); citrus bioflavonoids (p.1580·1); hesperidin (p.1580·2); rutin (p.1580·2); rose fruit (p.1365·2).
Vitamin C deficiency.

Cabaser
Pharmacia Upjohn, Swed.; Pharmacia Upjohn, UK.
Cabergoline (p.1135·2).
Parkinsonism.

Cabdrivers Adult Linctus Seven Seas, UK.
Dextromethorphan hydrobromide (p.1057·3); menthol (p.1600·2); terpin hydrate (p.1070·2); pumilio pine oil (p.1623·3); eucalyptus oil (p.1578·1).
Coughs.

Cabdrivers Sugar-Free Linctus Seven Seas, UK.
Ephedrine hydrochloride (p.1059·3); dextromethorphan hydrobromide (p.1057·3).
Coughs.

Caberdelta M Caber, Ital.†.
Methylprednisolone (p.1046·1).
Oral corticosteroid.

Cabermox Caber, Ital.†.
Amoxycillin trihydrate (p.151·3).
Bacterial infections.

Cabral Solvay, Ger.†.
Phenyramidol hydrochloride (p.80·1).
Muscle relaxant.

Ca-C
Note. This name is used for preparations of different composition.
Wander, Belg.; Sandoz, Neth.†; Novartis Consumer, S.Afr.; Sandoz OTC, Switz.
Ascorbic acid (p.1365·2); calcium carbonate (p.1182·1); calcium lactate gluconate (p.1155·2).
Adjunct in colds and influenza; calcium deficiency; vitamin C deficiency.

Sandoz, Fr.
Ascorbic acid (p.1365·2); calcium lactate gluconate (p.1155·2).
Asthenia; vitamin C deficiency.

Cachexon Telluride, USA.
Glutathione (p.983·1).
AIDS-associated cachexia.

Cacit
Procter & Gamble, Belg.; Procter & Gamble, Fr.; Procter & Gamble, Irl.; Procter & Gamble, Ital.; Procter & Gamble, Neth.; Procter & Gamble, UK.
Calcium carbonate (p.1182·1).
Calcium deficiency; osteoporosis; tetany.

Cacit D3 Procter & Gamble, UK.
Calcium carbonate (p.1182·1); cholecalciferol (p.1366·3).
Calcium and vitamin D deficiency; osteoporosis.

Cacit Vitamine D_3
Procter & Gamble, Belg.; Procter & Gamble, Fr.
Calcium carbonate (p.1182·1); cholecalciferol (p.1366·3).
Calcium and vitamin D deficiency; osteoporosis.

Cacital Parke, Davis, Spain.
Papain (p.1614·1).
Hypersensitivity reactions; tissue injury.

Cactus compositum Peithner, Aust.
Homoeopathic preparation.

Cadexi Ale, Spain†.
Emollient.

Ca-Di IBP, Ital.†.
Calcium gluceptate (p.1155·1); ergocalciferol (p.1367·1).
Calcium and vitamin D deficiency.

Caditar IPRAD, Fr.
Cade oil (p.1092·2).
Skin disorders.

Cadmiofrine Novopharma, Switz.†.
Cadmium sulphate (p.1555·3); zinc sulphate (p.1373·2); phenylephrine hydrochloride (p.1066·2).
Eye irritation.

Cadraten SmithKline Beecham, Ital.
Cadralazine (p.835·3).
Hypertension.

Cadrilan Ciba, Ital.
Cadralazine (p.835·3).
Hypertension.

C-A-E Seroyal, Canad.
Vitamins A, C, and E.

Caedex Aesca, Aust.
Ceftibuten (p.175·1).
Bacterial infections.

Caelyx
Sequus, Aust.; Schering-Plough, Neth.; Schering-Plough, Swed.; Schering-Plough, UK.
Doxorubicin hydrochloride (p.529·2).
Kaposi's sarcoma.

Cafadol Typharm, UK.
Paracetamol (p.72·2); caffeine (p.749·3).
Fever; pain.

Cafatine Major, USA.
Ergotamine tartrate (p.445·3); caffeine (p.749·3).
Migraine.

Cafatine-PB Major, USA.
Ergotamine tartrate (p.445·3); caffeine (p.749·3); belladonna (p.457·1); pentobarbitone sodium (p.685·1).
Migraine.

Cafergot
Sandoz, Aust.; Novartis, Austral.; Wander, Belg.; Sandoz, Canad.; Sandoz, Irl.; Sandoz, Ital.; Novartis, Neth.; Sandoz, Norw.; Novartis, S.Afr.; Sandoz, Spain; Novartis, Swed.; Sandoz, Switz.; Alliance, UK; Sandoz, USA.
Ergotamine tartrate (p.445·3); caffeine (p.749·3).
Migraine and related vascular headache.

Cafergot Comp Sandoz, Norw.
Ergotamine tartrate (p.445·3); caffeine (p.749·3); belladonna alkaloids (p.457·1); butalbital (p.644·3).
Migraine and related vascular headache.

Cafergot N Sandoz, Ger.
Ergotamine tartrate (p.445·3); caffeine (p.749·3).
Headache including migraine.

Cafergot-PB
Note. This name is used for preparations of different composition.
Wander, Belg.†; Novartis, S.Afr.; Sandoz, Spain; Sandoz, Switz.
Ergotamine tartrate (p.445·3); caffeine (p.749·3); belladonna alkaloids (p.457·1); butalbital (p.644·3).
Migraine and related vascular headache.

Sandoz, Canad.
Ergotamine tartrate (p.445·3); caffeine (p.749·3); laevorotatory alkaloids of belladonna (p.457·1); pentobarbitone (p.684·3).
Migraine and related vascular headache.

Cafersona Labaz, Spain†.
Caffeine (p.749·3); paracetamol (p.72·2).
Fever; pain.

Cafetrate Schein, USA.
Ergotamine tartrate (p.445·3); caffeine (p.749·3).
Migraine.

Caffalgina Home, Ital.
Propyphenazone (p.81·3); caffeine (p.749·3).
Pain.

Caffedrine Thompson, USA.
Caffeine (p.749·3).
Fatigue.

Caffeine Withdrawal Support Homeocan, Canad.
Homoeopathic preparation.

Cafiaspirina
Bayer, Ital.; Bayer, Spain.
Aspirin (p.16·1); caffeine (p.749·3).
Fever; pain.

Cafinitrina Berenguer Infale, Spain.
Caffeine citrate (p.749·3); glyceryl trinitrate (p.874·3).
Angina pectoris; myocardial infarction.

Cal-500 Pro Doc, Canad.
Calcium carbonate (p.1182·1).

Cal Carb-HD Konsyl, USA.
Calcium carbonate (p.1182·1).
Calcium deficiency; dietary supplement.

Cal D Pro Doc, Canad.
Calcium carbonate (p.1182·1); vitamin D (p.1366·3).

Cal de Ce Sandoz, Spain†.
Ascorbic acid (p.1365·2); calcium gluceptate (p.1155·1); cholecalciferol (p.1366·3).
Bone and dental disorders; calcium deficiency; osteomalacia; rickets.

Cal Gel Lalco, Canad.
Calcium phosphate (p.1155·3).

Cal Mag plus Vitamin D Quest, Canad.
Calcium, magnesium, and vitamin D.

Cal Mo Dol Herbes Universelles, Canad.
Methyl salicylate (p.55·2); camphor (p.1557·2); menthol (p.1600·2); cineole (p.1564·1); turpentine oil (p.1641·1); peppermint oil (p.1208·1).

Calaband
Boots, Austral.; Seton, UK.
Calamine (p.1080·1); zinc oxide (p.1096·2).
Medicated bandage.

Calabren Berk, UK.
Glibenclamide (p.319·3).
Diabetes mellitus.

Cal-A-Cool Seton, UK†.
Calamine (p.1080·1); silicone (p.1384·2); zinc oxide (p.1096·2).
Skin disorders.

Caladryl
Note. This name is used for preparations of different composition.
Parke, Davis, Aust.; Warner-Lambert Consumer, Switz.
Diphenhydramine hydrochloride (p.409·1); camphor (p.1557·2); zinc oxide (p.1096·2).
Skin irritation and pain.

Warner-Lambert, Austral.
Lignocaine (p.1293·2) or lignocaine hydrochloride (p.1293·2); calamine (p.1080·1); camphor (p.1557·2).
Pruritus; skin irritation.

Warner-Lambert, Canad.; Warner-Lambert, Neth.
Diphenhydramine hydrochloride (p.409·1); calamine (p.1080·1).
Pruritus.

Warner-Lambert, Irl.; Parke, Davis, S.Afr.; Warner-Wellcome, Spain; Warner-Lambert, UK.
Diphenhydramine hydrochloride (p.409·1); calamine (p.1080·1); camphor (p.1557·2).
Pruritus; urticaria.

Parke, Davis, USA.
Pramoxine hydrochloride (p.1298·2); calamine (p.1080·1).

Caladryl Clear Parke, Davis, USA.
Pramoxine hydrochloride (p.1298·2); zinc acetate (p.1646·2).

Cala-gen Goldline, USA.
Diphenhydramine hydrochloride (p.409·1); camphor (p.1557·2).
Pruritus.

Calais Mead Johnson, Canad.
Calcium glycerophosphate hydroxide (p.1155·2).

Cal-Alkyline Eagle, Austral.
Calcium carbonate (p.1182·1); slippery elm (p.1630·1); glycine (p.1345·2); equisetum (p.1575·1); dibasic sodium phosphate (p.1159·3); spirulina (p.1632·2); magnesium carbonate (p.1198·1); ginger (p.1193·2).
Gastric hyperacidity.

Calamatum Blair, USA.
Calamine (p.1080·1); zinc oxide (p.1096·2); menthol (p.1600·2); camphor (p.1557·2); benzocaine (p.1286·2).
Minor skin irritation.

Calamine Antihistamine Stanley, Canad.
Calamine (p.1080·1); diphenhydramine hydrochloride (p.409·1).
Pruritus.

Calamox Hauck, USA.
Calamine (p.1080·1).
Minor skin irritation.

Calamycin Pfeiffer, USA.
Zinc oxide (p.1096·2); calamine (p.1080·1); benzocaine (p.1286·2); chloroxylenol (p.1111·1); mepyramine maleate (p.414·1).
Pruritus.

Calan
Note. This name is used for preparations of different composition.
Takeda, Jpn.
Vinpocetine (p.1644·2).
Cerebrovascular disorders.

Searle, USA.
Verapamil hydrochloride (p.960·3).
Angina; arrhythmias; hypertension.

Calanif Berk, UK.
Nifedipine (p.916·2).
Angina pectoris; hypertension; Raynaud's syndrome.

Calas Gewo, Ger.†.
Calcium laevulinate (p.1155·2); ascorbic acid (p.1365·2).
Allergy; asthma; influenza.

Calasept Scania, Swed.†.
Calcium hydroxide (p.1556·3); sodium chloride; potassium chloride; calcium chloride; sodium bicarbonate.
Dental cavities.

Calasthetic Restan, S.Afr.
Calamine (p.1080·1); benzocaine (p.1286·2); pheniramine maleate (p.415·3); phenol (p.1121·2).
Skin disorders.

Calax Odan, Canad.
Docusate calcium (p.1189·3).
Constipation.

Calazem Berk, UK.
Diltiazem hydrochloride (p.854·2).
Angina pectoris.

Calbion Merck, Spain.
Calcium pidolate (p.1155·3).
Hypocalcaemia; osteoporosis.

Calcascorbin Pharmonta, Aust.
Calcium ascorbate (p.1365·2).
Vitamin C deficiency.

Calced Therica, Fr.†.
Ampoule 1, ascorbic acid (p.1365·2); ampoule 2, ergocalciferol (p.1367·1); calcium hypophosphite; calcium pantothenate (p.1352·3).
Vitamin D deficiency.

Calcedon Worwag, Ger.
Injection†: Calcium gluconate (p.1155·2).
Tablets: Calcium carbonate (p.1182·1).
Calcium deficiency.

Calcefor Vifor, Switz.†.
Ascorbic acid (p.1365·2); calcium glycerophosphate (p.1155·2).
Adjunct in colds and influenza; calcium deficiency; vitamin C deficiency.

Calceos Thames, UK.
Calcium carbonate (p.1182·1); cholecalciferol (p.1366·3).
Calcium and vitamin D deficiency.

Calcet Mission Pharmacal, USA.
Calcium lactate (p.1155·2); calcium gluconate (p.1155·2); calcium carbonate (p.1182·1); vitamin D (p.1366·3).
Calcium supplement.

Calcet Plus Mission Pharmacal, USA.
Multivitamin and mineral preparation with iron and folic acid.
Low-calcium leg cramping; nursing mothers; osteoporosis; patients with milk allergies; pre- and postoperative patients.

Calcevita
Roche Nicholas, Neth.; Roche, Swed.
Multivitamin preparation with calcium.

Calcevitone Roche, Austral.†.
Multivitamin preparation with calcium carbonate (p.1182·1).
Vitamin and calcium deficiency.

Calci Hexal, Ger.
Salcatonin (p.735·3).
Hypercalcaemia; osteolysis; osteoporosis; Paget's disease of bone; reflex sympathetic dystrophy.

Calcia English Grains, UK.
Calcium carbonate (p.1182·1) with vitamins and iron.

Calciben FIRMA, Ital.
Salcatonin (p.735·3).
Hypercalcaemia; osteoporosis; Paget's disease of bone; prevention of fracture in osteoporosis; reflex sympathetic dystrophy.

Calcibind Mission Pharmacal, USA.
Sodium cellulose phosphate (p.994·3).
Ion exchange resin binding calcium.

Calcibronat
Sandoz, Fr.; Sandoz, Ital.
Calcium bromolactobionate (p.645·1).
Insomnia; nervous disorders; skin disorders; tetany.

CalciCaps Nion, USA.
Calcium with vitamin D and phosphorus.
Calcium deficiency; dietary supplement.

CalciCaps with iron Nion, USA.
Calcium with vitamin D, phosphorus, and iron.
Calcium deficiency; dietary supplement.

CalciCaps M-Z Nion, USA.
Calcium with vitamins A and D, and minerals.

Calcicard
Note. This name is used for preparations of different composition.
Parke-Med, S.Afr.
Verapamil hydrochloride (p.960·3).
Angina pectoris; arrhythmias; hypertension.

Norton, UK.
Diltiazem hydrochloride (p.854·2).
Angina pectoris; hypertension.

Calci-Chew
Piette, Belg.; Christiaens, Neth.; R&D, USA.
Calcium carbonate (p.1182·1).
Calcium deficiency; dietary supplement.

Calcichew
Shire, Irl.; Shire, UK.
Calcium carbonate (p.1182·1).
Calcium deficiency; phosphate binder for renal dialysis patients.

Calcichew D_3
Shire, Irl.; Nycomed, Swed.; Shire, UK.
Calcium carbonate (p.1182·1); cholecalciferol (p.1366·3).
Calcium and vitamin D deficiency; osteomalacia; osteoporosis.

Calciday Nature's Bounty, USA.
Calcium carbonate (p.1182·1).
Calcium deficiency; dietary supplement.

Calcidia Nicholas, Fr.
Calcium carbonate (p.1182·1).
Hypocalcaemia and hyperphosphoraemia related to kidney disorders; renal osteodystrophy.

Calcidon Roche, Ital.
Calcium carbonate (p.1182·1); cholecalciferol (p.1366·3).
Calcium and vitamin D deficiency.

Calcidose Opocalcium, Fr.
Calcium carbonate (p.1182·1).
Calcium deficiency; osteoporosis.

Calcidose Vitamine D Opocalcium, Fr.
Calcium carbonate (p.1182·1); cholecalciferol (p.1366·3).
Calcium and vitamin D deficiency; osteoporosis.

Calcidrine Abbott, USA.
Codeine (p.26·1); calcium iodide (p.1056·2).
Coughs.

Calcidrink Shire, UK.
Calcium carbonate (p.1182·1).
Calcium deficiency.

Calciferol
Richmond, Canad.†; Schwarz, USA.
Ergocalciferol (p.1367·1).
Familial hypophosphataemia; gastro-intestinal, liver, or biliary disease associated with malabsorption of vitamin D; hypoparathyroidism; refractory rickets.

Calcifolin Ibirn, Ital.
Calcium folinate (p.1342·2).
Antidote to folic acid antagonists; folic acid deficiency.

Calciforte Serozym, Fr.
Oral liquid: Calcium gluconate (p.1155·2); calcium lactate (p.1155·2); calcium gluceptate (p.1155·1); calcium chloride (p.1155·1); yeast (*Saccharomyces cerevisiae*) (p.1373·1).
Powder for oral solution: Calcium gluconate (p.1155·2); calcium lactate (p.1155·2); calcium gluceptate (p.1155·1); calcium chloride (p.1155·1); calcium carbonate (p.1182·1); yeast (*Saccharomyces cerevisiae*) (p.1373·1).
Calcium deficiency; osteoporosis.

Calcigenol Simple Darci, Belg.†.
Calcium triphosphate (p.1155·3); sodium methylarsinate (p.1631·2); sodium fluoride (p.742·1).
Dietary supplement.

Calcigenol Vitamine Darci, Belg.†.
Calcium triphosphate (p.1155·3); ergocalciferol (p.1367·1); sodium fluoride (p.742·1).
Dietary supplement.

Calcigran Nycomed, Norw.
Oral granules: Calcium carbonate (p.1182·1); ascorbic acid (p.1365·2); cholecalciferol (p.1366·3).
Tablets: Calcium carbonate (p.1182·1); cholecalciferol (p.1366·3).
Calcium supplement; osteoporosis.

Calcihep *Rhone-Poulenc Rorer, Austral.*
Heparin calcium (p.879·3).

Calciject
Note. This name is used for preparations of different composition.
Omega, Canad.†.
Calcium chloride (p.1155·1).
Calcium supplement.

GN, Ger.†.
Calcium gluconate (p.1155·2); calcium saccharate (p.1557·1); calcium laevulinate (p.1155·2).
Calcium deficiency.

Calcijex
Abbott, Aust.; Abbott, Austral.; Abbott, Canad.; Abbott, Irl.; Abbott, Ital.; Abbott, Norw.; Abbott, Spain; Abbott, Swed.; Abbott, Switz.; Abbott, UK; Abbott, USA.
Calcitriol (p.1366·3).
Hyperparathyroidism; hypocalcaemia in chronic renal dialysis; hypoparathyroidism; osteodystrophy; osteomalacia; rickets.

Calcilat *Eastern Pharmaceuticals, UK.*
Nifedipine (p.916·2).
Angina pectoris; hypertension; Raynaud's syndrome.

Calcilean *Organon Teknika, Canad.*
Heparin calcium (p.879·3).
Thrombo-embolic disorders; thrombosis prophylaxis.

Calcilin *Laevosan, Aust.*
Calcium laevulinate (p.1155·2).
Allergic and anaphylactic conditions; calcium deficiency; haemorrhage; inflammation.

Calcilin compositum *Laevosan, Aust.*
Chlorphenoxamine hydrochloride (p.405·3); calcium laevulinate (p.1155·2); calcium gluconate (p.1155·2).
Allergic disorders.

Calcilos *TAD, Ger.*
Calcium carbonate (p.1182·1).
Calcium deficiency.

Calcimagon *Nycomed, Ger.*
Calcium carbonate (p.1182·1).
Calcium deficiency.

Calcimar
Rhone-Poulenc Rorer, Canad.; Rhone-Poulenc Rorer, USA.
Salcatonin (p.735·3).
Hypercalcaemia; Paget's disease of bone; postmenopausal osteoporosis.

Calcimax
Note. This name is used for preparations of different composition.
Parke, Davis, Austral.†.
Calcium carbonate (p.1182·1).
Calcium deficiency; osteoporosis.

Carmaran, Canad.
Calcium lactate (p.1155·2).

Wallace Mfg Chem., UK.
Calcium laevulinate (p.1155·2); calcium chloride (p.1155·1); vitamins.
Calcium deficiency.

Calcimega *Larkhall Laboratories, UK.*
Calcium with vitamins and minerals.

Calci-Mix *R&D, USA.*
Calcium carbonate (p.1182·1).
Calcium deficiency; dietary supplement.

Calcimonta *Tosse, Ger.*
Salcatonin (p.735·3).
Algodystrophy; hypercalcaemia; osteolysis; osteoporosis; Paget's disease of bone.

Calcinatal *Warner-Lambert, Spain.*
Multivitamin and mineral preparation.

Calcinatal-MK *Propan-Vernleigh, S.Afr.*†.
Multivitamin and mineral preparation.

Calcinil *Sclavo, Ital.*
Elcatonin (p.735·3).
Hypercalcaemia; osteoporosis; Paget's disease of bone; reflex sympathetic dystrophy.

Calcio Colloidale con Ostelin con Vit *Glaxo Wellcome, Ital.*†.
Ergocalciferol (p.1367·1); cyanocobalamin (p.1363·3); calcium oleate.

Calcio 20 Complex *Madariaga, Spain.*
Ascorbic acid (p.1365·2); calcium phosphate (p.1155·3); calcium pantothenate (p.1352·3); cyanocobalamin (p.1363·3); cholecalciferol (p.1366·3); vitamin A palmitate (p.1358·1).
Calcium deficiency; osteoporosis.

Calcio Dobetin *Angelini, Ital.*
Cyanocobalamin (p.1363·3); calcium gluconate (p.1155·2); calcium gluceptate (p.1155·1).
Calcium and vitamin B_{12} deficiency.

Calcio 20 Emulsion *Madariaga, Spain.*
Calcium phosphate (p.1155·3).
Calcium deficiency.

Calcio Faes DYC *Faes, Spain.*
Ascorbic acid (p.1365·2); calcium carbonate (p.1182·1); calcium fluoride (p.1556·3); calcium phosphate (p.1155·3); cholecalciferol (p.1366·3).
Bone and dental disorders; calcium deficiency; osteomalacia.

Calcio 20 Fuerte *Madariaga, Spain.*
Calcium phosphate (p.1155·3); cholecalciferol (p.1366·3).
Calcium deficiency; osteoporosis.

Calcio Geve DYC *Bama, Spain.*
Ascorbic acid (p.1365·2); calcium gluceptate (p.1155·1); calcium hypophosphite; calcium laevulinolactogluconate; cholecalciferol (p.1366·3).
Calcium deficiency; vitamin C and D deficiency.

Calcio Geve Liquido *Bama, Spain*†.
Calcium phosphate (p.1155·3); cholecalciferol (p.1366·3).
Calcium deficiency.

Calcio Jodico *Allergan, Ital.*†.
Rubidium iodide (p.1626·3); calcium chloride (p.1155·1); sodium iodide (p.1493·2).
Cataract.

Calcio Vitam D3 *Berenguer Infale, Spain.*
Calcium hydrogen phosphate (p.1155·3); cholecalciferol (p.1366·3).
Bone and dental disorders; calcium deficiency; osteomalacia.

Calciofix *Damor, Ital.*
L-Arginine (p.1334·1); L-lysine (p.1350·1); glycerophosphoric acid (p.1586·2).
Tonic.

Calciopen *Astra, Swed.*
Phenoxymethylpenicillin potassium (p.236·2).
Bacterial infections.

Calciopor *Chiesi, Ital.*†.
Calcium pidolate (p.1155·3).
Calcium deficiency.

Calcioretard *Farmapros, Spain.*
Calcium ascorbate (p.1365·2); lysine hydrochloride (p.1350·1); tryptophan (p.310·2).
Bone and dental disorders; calcium deficiency; osteomalacia; rickets.

Calciosint *Pulitzer, Ital.*
Salcatonin (p.735·3).
Hypercalcaemia; osteoporosis; Paget's disease of bone; reflex sympathetic dystrophy.

Calci-ostelin B12 *Glaxo Wellcome, Ital.*†.
Calcium phosphate (p.1155·3); ergocalciferol (p.1367·1); cyanocobalamin (p.1363·3).

Calcioton *San Carlo, Ital.*
Salcatonin (p.735·3).
Hypercalcaemia; osteoporosis; Paget's disease of bone; reflex sympathetic dystrophy.

Calciovit Urto *Lafare, Ital.*
Calcium oleate; ergocalciferol (p.1367·1).
Vitamin deficiency.

Calciozim *Poli, Ital.*
Vitamin and mineral preparation.

Calciparin
Sanofi Winthrop, Aust.; Sanofi Winthrop, Ger.
Heparin calcium (p.879·3).
Thrombo-embolic disorders.

Calciparina
Italfarmaco, Ital.; Sanofi Winthrop, Spain.
Heparin calcium (p.879·3).
Thrombo-embolic disorders.

Calciparine
Sanofi Winthrop, Austral.; Sanofi Winthrop, Fr.; Sanofi Winthrop, Irl.; Mer-National, S.Afr.; Sanofi Winthrop, Switz.; Sanofi Winthrop, UK; Du Pont, USA†.
Heparin calcium (p.879·3).
Thrombo-embolic disorders.

Calcipen *Leo, Norw.*
Phenoxymethylpenicillin calcium (p.236·2).
Bacterial infections.

Calciplex *Vitaplex, Austral.*
Mineral and vitamin D preparation.
Calcium deficiency.

Calcipot *3M, Ger.*
Effervescent tablets: Calcium gluconate (p.1155·2).
Tablets: Calcium citrate (p.1155·1); calcium hydrogen phosphate (p.1155·3).
Calcium deficiency.

Calcipot C *Kolassa, Aust.*
Vitamin C (p.1365·2); rutin (p.1580·2); calcium citrate (p.1155·1); calcium glycerophosphate (p.1155·2).
Calcium and vitamin C deficiency.

Calcipot D_3
Kolassa, Aust.
Cholecalciferol (p.1366·3); calcium citrate (p.1155·1); calcium glycerophosphate (p.1155·2).
Calcium and vitamin D deficiency.

3M, Ger.†.
Cholecalciferol (p.1366·3); calcium citrate (p.1155·1); calcium hydrogen phosphate (p.1155·3).
Rickets.

Calcipot F *3M, Ger.*†.
Calcium citrate (p.1155·1); calcium fluoride (p.1556·3); calcium hydrogen phosphate (p.1155·3); magnesium fluoride; sodium fluoride (p.742·1); sodium hexafluoroferrate.
Dental caries prophylaxis.

Calcipot Plus C *3M, Ger.*†.
Calcium citrate (p.1155·1); calcium hydrogen phosphate (p.1155·3); ascorbic acid (p.1365·2).
Calcium and vitamin C deficiency.

Calciprat *IPRAD, Fr.*
Calcium carbonate (p.1182·1).
Calcium deficiency; osteoporosis.

Calcipulpe *Septodont, Switz.*
Barium sulphate (p.1003·1); calcium hydroxide (p.1556·3).
Covering for dental pulp.

Calciretard *Kohler-Pharma, Ger.*
Calcium aspartate.
Hypocalcaemia.

Calcisan *Petrasch, Aust.*
Calcium hydrogen phosphate (p.1155·3); calcium carbonate (p.1182·1).
Calcium deficiency.

Calcisan B + C *Petrasch, Aust.*
Calcium hydrogen phosphate (p.1155·3); calcium carbonate (p.1182·1); ascorbic acid (p.1365·2); thiamine hydrochloride (p.1361·1).
Calcium, vitamin B_1, and vitamin C deficiency.

Calcisan C *Petrasch, Aust.*
Calcium hydrogen phosphate (p.1155·3); calcium carbonate (p.1182·1); ascorbic acid (p.1365·2).
Calcium and vitamin C deficiency.

Calcisan D *Petrasch, Aust.*
Calcium hydrogen phosphate (p.1155·3); calcium carbonate (p.1182·1); ergocalciferol (p.1367·1).
Calcium and vitamin D deficiency.

Calcisorb
3M, Austral.; 3M, Belg.; 3M, Ger.†*; 3M, Neth.; 3M, S.Afr.*†*; 3M, UK.*
Sodium cellulose phosphate (p.994·3).
Hypercalcaemia; hypercalciuria; osteopetrosis; vitamin D intoxication.

Calcitar
Specia, Fr.; Rhone-Poulenc Rorer, Ital.
Calcitonin (pork) (p.735·3).
Hypercalcaemia; hyperphosphatasia; osteoporosis; Paget's disease of bone.

Calcitare
Rhone-Poulenc Rorer, Austral.; Rhone-Poulenc Rorer, Irl.; Rhone-Poulenc Rorer, Norw.†*; Rorer, UK.*
Calcitonin (pork) (p.735·3).
Hypercalcaemia; Paget's disease of bone.

Calcite *Riva, Canad.*
Calcium carbonate (p.1182·1).
Calcium supplement.

Calcite D *Riva, Canad.*
Calcium carbonate (p.1182·1); vitamin D (p.1366·3).
Dietary supplement.

Calcitol *Frega, Canad.*
Vitamin A, vitamin D, and calcium.

Calcitonin L *Rorer, Ger.*†.
Salcatonin (p.735·3).
Bone pain in malignancy; hypercalcaemia; osteoporosis; Paget's disease of bone; reflex sympathetic dystrophy.

Calcitonin S *Rorer, Ger.*†.
Calcitonin (pork) (p.735·3).
Bone pain in malignancy; hypercalcaemia; osteoporosis; Paget's disease of bone; reflex sympathetic dystrophy.

Calcitonina-Sandoz *Novartis, Ital.*
Salcatonin (p.735·3).
Hypercalcaemia; osteoporosis; Paget's disease of bone; reflex sympathetic dystrophy.

Calcitoran *Teikoku, Jpn.*
Salcatonin (p.735·3).
Osteoporosis.

Calcitrans *Fresenius-Praxis, Ger.*
Effervescent tablets†*:* Calcium gluconate (p.1155·2).
Oral granules†*:* Calcium chloride-lysine-citric acid complex (p.1155·1).
Injection: Calcium gluconate (p.1155·2); calcium gluceptate (p.1155·1); calcium saccharate (p.1557·1).
Calcium deficiency.

Calcitridin *Opfermann, Ger.*
Calcium carbonate (p.1182·1).
Calcium deficiency; osteoporosis.

Calcitugg *Nycomed, Swed.*
Calcium carbonate (p.1182·1).
Calcium deficiency; hyperphosphataemia; osteoporosis.

Calcium 600 *Solgar, USA*†.
Calcium carbonate (p.1182·1); vitamin D (p.1366·3).

Calcium Braun *Braun, Ger.*
Calcium gluconate (p.1155·2); calcium saccharate (p.1557·1).
Calcium deficiency.

Calcium Clear *Nutraceuticals, UK.*
Calcium lactate (p.1155·2); magnesium carbonate (p.1198·1).
Calcium supplement.

Calcium Corbiere *Sanofi Winthrop, Fr.*
Calcium glucoheptogluconate (p.1155·1).
Hypocalcaemia.

Calcium Corbiere vitamine CDPP *Sanofi Winthrop, Fr.*
Anhydrous calcium gluceptate (p.1155·1) or calcium glucoheptogluconate with vitamins.
Asthenia.

Calcium cum... *Worwag, Ger.*†.
Mineral preparation.
Calcium deficiency.

Calcium D Sauter *Roche, Switz.*
Calcium hydrogen phosphate (p.1155·3); calcium gluconate (p.1155·2); calcium lactate pentahydrate (p.1155·2); ergocalciferol (p.1367·1); ascorbic acid (p.1365·2).
Calcium supplement; disorders of calcium and phosphorus metabolism; vitamin C and D deficiencies.

Calcium Dago *Steiner, Ger.*
Calcium carbonate (p.1182·1).
Calcium deficiency.

Calcium Disodium Versenate *3M, USA.*
Sodium calciumedetate (p.994·1).
Lead poisoning.

Calcium Docuphen *Pharmascience, Canad.*
Docusate calcium (p.1189·3); yellow phenolphthalein (p.1208·2).
Constipation.

Calcium and Ergocalciferol Tablets *Cox, UK.*
Calcium lactate 300 mg (p.1155·2); calcium phosphate 150 mg (p.1155·3); ergocalciferol 10 µg (p.1367·1).
Each tablet contains 400 units of vitamin-D activity. They should be crushed or chewed before administration.
Distinguish from Calcium with Vitamin D Tablets (BPC 1973).

Calcium gluconicum *Eifelfango, Ger.*
Calcium gluconate (p.1155·2); calcium laevulinate (p.1155·2).
Calcium deficiency.

Calcium 600mg *Pharmadass, UK.*
Calcium carbonate (p.1182·1); vitamins A and D.

Calcium Resonium
Sanofi Winthrop, Austral.; Sanofi Winthrop, Ger.; Sanofi Winthrop, Irl.; Sanofi Winthrop, Neth.†*; Sanofi Winthrop, UK.*
Calcium polystyrene sulphonate (p.974·3).
Hyperkalaemia.

Calcium Rich Rolaids *Warner-Lambert, USA.*
Magnesium hydroxide (p.1198·2); calcium carbonate (p.1182·1).
Hyperacidity.

Calcium Stanley *Stanley, Canad.*
Calcium gluceptate (p.1155·1); calcium gluconate (p.1155·2).
Calcium deficiency; calcium supplement.

Calcium Truw *Truw, Ger.*
Calcium gluconate (p.1155·2); calcium saccharate (p.1557·1).
Calcium deficiency.

Calcium Verla *Verla, Ger.*
Effervescent tablets: Calcium carbonate (p.1182·1).
Calcium deficiency.
Injection: Calcium gluconate (p.1155·2); calcium saccharate (p.1557·1).
Allergic disorders; calcium deficiency; lead poisoning; tetany.
Tablets: Calcium phosphate (p.1155·3); calcium citrate (p.1155·1).
Allergic reactions; calcium deficiency; osteomalacia; osteoporosis; tetany.

Calcium-dura *Durachemie, Ger.*
Calcium carbonate (p.1182·1).
Osteoporosis.

Calcium-EAP *Kohler-Pharma, Ger.*
Phosphorylcolamine calcium.
Calcium deficiency; hypersensitivity reactions.

Calciumedetat-Heyl *Heyl, Ger.*†.
Sodium calciumedetate (p.994·1).
Metal poisoning.

Calcium-Gluconicum-Losung Phytopharma
OTW, Ger.†.
Calcium gluconate (p.1155·2); calcium laevulinate (p.1155·2); calcium saccharate (p.1557·1).
Calcium deficiency.

Calcium-Rotexmedica *Rotexmedica, Ger.*†.
Calcium gluconate (p.1155·2); calcium laevulinate (p.1155·2).
Calcium deficiency.

Calcium-Rutinion *Biomo, Ger.*
Rutin (p.1580·2); calcium gluconate (p.1155·2).
Capillary disorders; epistaxis; retinopathy; skin disorders.

Calcium-Sandoz
Note. This name is used for preparations of different composition.
Sandoz, Austral.†.
Tablets (Sandocal): Calcium lactate gluconate (p.1155·2); calcium carbonate (p.1182·1).
Calcium deficiency; calcium supplement.

Sandoz, Belg.
Effervescent tablets; oral powder: Calcium lactate gluconate (p.1155·2); calcium carbonate (p.1182·1).
Bone demineralisation; calcium supplement; osteoporosis; tetany.
Injection: Calcium glubionate (p.1155·1).
Hypocalcaemia; potassium poisoning; rickets; tetany.

Novartis Consumer, Canad.
Syrup: Calcium lactobionate (p.1155·2); calcium glubionate (p.1155·1).
Tablets: Calcium lactate gluconate (p.1155·2); calcium carbonate (p.1182·1).
Calcium deficiency; calcium supplement.

Sandoz, Fr.
Injection: Calcium glubionate (p.1155·1).
Hypersensitivity reactions; hypocalcaemia.
Syrup: Calcium gluconate (p.1155·2); calcium lactobionate (p.1155·2).
Calcium deficiency; normocalcaemic tetany; prevention of bone loss in immobilisation; rickets.
Tablets: Calcium lactate gluconate (p.1155·2); calcium carbonate (p.1182·1).
Calcium deficiency; osteoporosis.

Sandoz, Ger.
Effervescent tablets: Calcium lactate gluconate (p.1155·2); calcium carbonate (p.1182·1).
Calcium deficiency; osteoporosis.
Injection: Calcium gluconate (p.1155·2); calcium lactobionate (p.1155·2).
Calcium deficiency.

Sandoz, Irl.
Injection†*:* Calcium glubionate (p.1155·1).
Calcium deficiencies.
Syrup: Calcium glubionate (p.1155·1); calcium lactobionate (p.1155·2).
Calcium deficiencies; osteoporosis.

Sandoz, Ital.
Calcium lactate gluconate (p.1155·2); calcium carbonate (p.1182·1).
Calcium deficiency.

Novartis, Neth.
Injection: Calcium glubionate (p.1155·1).
Calcium deficiency; lead or tetrachloromethane poisoning.
Tablets; oral powder: Calcium lactate gluconate (p.1155·2); calcium carbonate (p.1182·1).
Calcium deficiency; osteoporosis; tetany.

Novartis, Norw.
Effervescent tablets; oral powder: Calcium lactate gluconate (p.1155·2); calcium carbonate (p.1182·1).
Calcium supplement; osteoporosis.
Injection: Calcium glubionate (p.1155·1).
Lead, fluoride, carbon tetrachloride, phosphate, or potassium poisoning; skin disorders.

Novartis, S.Afr.
Effervescent tablets: Calcium carbonate (p.1182·1); calcium lactate gluconate (p.1155·2).
Injection: Calcium glubionate (p.1155·1).
Syrup†: Calcium glubionate (p.1155·1); calcium lactobionate (p.1155·2).
Calcium deficiencies; osteoporosis; tetany.

Sandoz, Spain.
Calcium glubionate (p.1155·1).
Calcium deficiency.

Novartis, Swed.
Effervescent tablets: Calcium lactate gluconate (p.1155·2); calcium carbonate (p.1182·1).
Injection: Calcium glubionate (p.1155·1).
Calcium deficiency.

Sandoz, Switz.
Effervescent tablets; powder for oral solution: Calcium lactate gluconate (p.1155·2); calcium carbonate (p.1182·1).
Calcium deficiency; calcium supplement; osteoporosis.
Injection: Calcium glubionate (p.1155·1).
Adjuvant in hyperkalaemia; calcium deficiency; osteoporosis; poisoning with lead, fluorides, or magnesium.
Syrup†: Calcium glubionate (p.1155·1); calcium lactobionate (p.1155·2).
Calcium deficiency; calcium supplement.

Alliance, UK.
Syrup: Calcium glubionate (p.1155·1); calcium lactobionate (p.1155·2).
Hypocalcaemia; osteoporosis.

Sandoz, UK.
Injection: Calcium glubionate (p.1155·1).
Fluoride poisoning; hypocalcaemia; lead poisoning; neonatal tetany.

Calcium-Sandoz C *Sandoz, Spain.*
Ascorbic acid (p.1365·2); calcium glubionate (p.1155·1).
Calcium deficiency; vitamin C deficiency.

Calcium-Sandoz Forte *Sandoz, Spain.*
Calcium carbonate (p.1182·1); calcium glubionate (p.1155·1).
Calcium deficiency; hypoparathyroidism; osteomalacia; osteoporosis; rickets.

Calcium-Sandoz Forte D *Sandoz, Spain.*
Calcium gluceptate (p.1155·1); cholecalciferol(p.1366·3); calcium carbonate (p.1182·1).
Deficiencies of calcium and vitamin D; osteoporosis.

Calcium-Sandoz + Vitamine C *Sandoz, Switz.†.*
Calcium glubionate (p.1155·1); ascorbic acid (p.1365·2).
Calcium and vitamin C deficiencies; calcium and vitamin C supplement.

Calcium-Sorbisterit *Fresenius, Fr.*
Calcium polystyrene sulphonate (p.974·3).
Hyperkalaemia related to renal insufficiency.

Calcivit *UB Interpharm, Switz.*
Calcium hydrogen phosphate (p.1155·3); cholecalciferol (p.1366·3).
Hypocalcaemia.

Calcivita *Roche, Ital.†.*
Ascorbic acid (p.1365·2); ergocalciferol (p.1367·1); calcium carbonate (p.1182·1).
Vitamin and calcium deficiency.

calcivitase *GN, Ger.*
Calcium citrate (p.1155·1); calcium gluconate (p.1155·2); calcium glycerophosphate (p.1155·2); calcium silicate (p.1182·2); cholecalciferol (p.1366·3).
Calcium deficiency.

Calco *Lisapharma, Ital.*
Salcatonin (p.735·3).
Hypercalcaemia; osteoporosis; Paget's disease of bone; reflex sympathetic dystrophy.

Calcort
Albert-Roussel, Ger.; Hoechst, Ger.; Hoechst Marion Roussel, Switz.; Shire, UK.
Deflazacort (p.1036·2).
Corticosteroid.

Calcufel Aqua *Hevert, Ger.*
Solidago virgaurea.
Renal calculi; urinary-tract disorders.

Calculi H *Pfluger, Ger.*
Homoeopathic preparation.

Cal-C-Vita
Roche, Aust.; Roche, Ger.†; Roche, S.Afr.; Roche, Switz.
Calcium carbonate (p.1182·1); vitamins.
Calcium supplement; tonic.

Caldease *Roche Consumer, Irl.*
Zinc oxide (p.1096·2); cod-liver oil (p.1337·3).
Burns; nappy rash; skin irritation; wounds.

Cal-De-Ce *Sanabo, Aust.*
Calcium hydrogen phosphate (p.1155·3); cholecalciferol (p.1366·3); ascorbic acid (p.1365·2).
Calcium and vitamin deficiency.

CaldeCort *Fisons, USA†.*
Hydrocortisone (p.1043·3) or hydrocortisone acetate (p.1043·3).
Skin disorders.

Calderol *Organon, USA.*
Calcifediol (p.1366·3).
Hypocalcaemia associated with renal dialysis; metabolic bone disease.

Caldesene
Note. This name is used for preparations of different composition.
Novartis Consumer, Canad.; Fisons, USA.
Ointment: Cod-liver oil (p.1337·3); zinc oxide (p.1096·2).
Skin disorders.

Novartis Consumer, Canad.; Roche Consumer, Irl.; Fisons, USA.
Topical powder: Calcium undecenoate (p.389·2).
Bromhidrosis; fungal skin infections; hyperhidrosis; minor skin irritation; nappy rash.

Caldine *Boehringer Ingelheim, Fr.*
Lacidipine (p.897·1).
Hypertension.

Caldomine-DH *Technilab, Canad.*
Hydrocodone tartrate (p.43·1); phenylpropanolamine hydrochloride (p.1067·2); mepyramine maleate (p.414·1); pheniramine maleate (p.415·3).
Coughs.

Cal-D-Vita *Roche, Swed.*
Calcium carbonate (p.1182·1); cholecalciferol (p.1366·3).
Osteoporosis; vitamin D and calcium deficiencies.

Calel-D *Rhone-Poulenc Rorer, USA.*
Calcium carbonate (p.1182·1); cholecalciferol (p.1366·3).
Nutritional supplement.

Calendolon *Weleda, UK.*
Calendula officinalis.
Minor wounds and abrasions.

Calendula + *Homeocan, Canad.*
Homoeopathic preparation.

Calendulene
Allergan, Fr.; Allergan, Switz.†.
Calendula officinalis.
Contact lens care; eye irritation.

Calendumed *DHU, Ger.*
Homoeopathic preparation.

Calfolex *Crinos, Ital.*
Calcium folinate (p.1342·2).
Antidote to folic acid antagonists; folic acid deficiency; reduction of aminopterin and methotrexate toxicity.

Calgel *Warner-Lambert, UK.*
Lignocaine hydrochloride (p.1293·2); cetylpyridinium chloride (p.1106·2).
Teething pain.

Calglycine Antacid *Rugby, USA.*
Calcium carbonate (p.1182·1); glycine (p.1345·2).
Gastro-intestinal hyperacidity.

Cal-Guard *Rugby, USA.*
Calcium carbonate (p.1182·1).

Califig *Sterling Health, UK.*
Senna (p.1212·2); fig (p.1193·2).
Constipation.

California Syrup of Figs *SmithKline Beecham, Irl.*
Senna leaf (p.1212·2).

Californit *Merckle, Ger.†.*
Oxyphenbutazone (p.72·1).
Acute ankylosing spondylitis; rheumatism.

Calimal *Sussex, UK.*
Chlorpheniramine maleate (p.405·1).
Hypersensitivity reactions.

Calinat *Aesculapius, Ital.*
Calcium folinate (p.1342·2).
Folate deficiency; reduction of aminopterin and methotrexate toxicity.

Calispan D3 *Septa, Spain†.*
Mineral, vitamin, and amino-acid preparation.
Mineral deficiency.

Calistaflex *Boots, Austral.†.*
Aminacrine hydrochloride (p.1098·3); lignocaine (p.1293·2); calamine (p.1080·1).
Burns; insect bites and stings; sunburn.

Calisvit *Menarini, Ital.*
Cholecalciferol (p.1366·3); tribasic calcium phosphate (p.1155·3).
Calcium and vitamin D deficiency; osteoporosis.

Callicida Brujo *Calmante Vitaminado, Spain.*
Flexible collodion; lactic acid (p.1593·3); salicylic acid (p.1090·2).
Callosities.

Callicida Brum *Brum, Spain.*
Flexible collodion; salicylic acid (p.1090·2); trichloroacetic acid (p.1639·1).
Callosities.

Callicida Cor Pik *Boehringer Mannheim, Spain.*
Acetic acid (p.1541·2); flexible collodion; lactic acid (p.1593·3); castor oil; salicylic acid (p.1090·2).
Callosities.

Callicida Cor Pik Stick *Boehringer Mannheim, Spain†.*
Acetic acid (p.1541·2); salicylic acid (p.1090·2).
Callosities.

Callicida Durcall *Llorens, Spain.*
Acetic acid (p.1541·2); flexible collodion; lactic acid (p.1593·3); salicylic acid (p.1090·2).
Callosities.

Callicida Globodermis *Weinco, Spain.*
Salicylic acid (p.1090·2).
Callosities.

Callicida Gras *Quimifar, Spain.*
Salicylic acid (p.1090·2).
Calluses.

Callicida Rojo *Escaned, Spain.*
Acetic acid (p.1541·2); flexible collodion; benzocaine (p.1286·2); salicylic acid (p.1090·2); iodine tincture (p.1493·1).
Callosities.

Callicida Salve *Cederroth, Spain.*
Salicylic acid (p.1090·2).
Calluses; corns.

Callimon *Grossmann, Switz.*
Calcium carbonate (p.1182·1); calcium lactate (p.1155·2); ascorbic acid (p.1365·2).
Vitamin C and calcium deficiency.

Callivoro Marthand *Martinez Llenas, Spain.*
Salicylic acid (p.1090·2); benzocaine (p.1286·2).
Calluses; corns.

Callix D *Calmante Vitaminado, Spain.*
Flexible collodion; benzocaine (p.1286·2); lactic acid (p.1593·3); salicylic acid (p.1090·2).
Callosities.

Callofin *Alcor, Spain.*
Salicylic acid (p.1090·2).
Callosities.

Callous Removers *Scholl, UK.*
Salicylic acid (p.1090·2).
Calluses.

Calloverk *Verkos, Spain†.*
Salicylic acid (p.1090·2); lactic acid (p.1593·3); acetic acid (p.1541·2).
Callosities.

Callus Salve *Cress, Canad.*
Salicylic acid (p.1090·2).

Callusolve *Dermal Laboratories, UK†.*
Benzalkonium chloride-bromine (pp.1101·3 and 1555·1).
Warts.

Calmactiv *Schiapparelli, Ital.†.*
Valerian (p.1643·1); passion flower (p.1615·3).
Insomnia.

Calmaderm *Whitehall, Fr.*
Bufexamac (p.22·2).
Pruritus.

Cal-Mag
Note. This name is used for preparations of different composition.
Seroyal, Canad.
Calcium carbonate (p.1182·1); magnesium oxide (p.1198·3).

Swiss Herbal, Canad.
Calcium carbonate (p.1182·1); magnesium carbonate (p.1198·1).

Quest, UK.
Calcium, magnesium, and vitamin D.

Calmag D *Gerbex, Canad.*
Calcium, magnesium, and vitamin D.

Cal/Mag & D *Seroyal, Canad.*
Calcium, magnesium, and vitamin D.

Calmant Martou *Sanico, Belg.*
Belladonna extract (p.457·1); mint oil (p.1604·1); cinnamon oil (p.1564·2); orange-peel oil; melissa oil; eugenol (p.1578·2); anethole (p.1549·3); saffron (p.1001·1).
Gastro-intestinal disorders.

Calmante Murri *Bracco, Ital.†.*
Aspirin (p.16·1); paracetamol (p.72·2); caffeine (p.749·3).
Pain.

Calmante Vitaminado Infant *Perez Gimenez, Spain†.*
Aspirin (p.16·1); thiamine (p.1361·2).
Fever; pain.

Calmante Vitaminado P G *Calmante Vitaminado, Spain.*
Aspirin (p.16·1); caffeine (p.749·3); thiamine (p.1361·2).
Fever; pain.

Calmante Vitaminado PG Efervescente *Calmante Vitaminado, Spain.*
Aspirin (p.16·1); caffeine (p.749·3); thiamine mononitrate (p.1361·1); ascorbic acid (p.1365·2).
Fever; pain.

Calmante Vitaminado Rinver *Monik, Spain.*
Aspirin (p.16·1); thiamine (p.1361·2).
Formerly known as Calmante Vitaminado Rinver.
Fever; pain.

Calmanticold *Calmante Vitaminado, Spain.*
Paracetamol (p.72·2).
Fever; pain.

Calmanticold Vit C *Calmante Vitaminado, Spain.*
Ascorbic acid (p.1365·2); paracetamol (p.72·2).
Fever; pain.

Calmantina *Inexfa, Spain.*
Aspirin (p.16·1).
Fever; inflammation; pain; thrombo-embolism prophylaxis.

Calmapica *Calmante Vitaminado, Spain.*
Ammonia (p.1548·3).
Insect bites; stings.

Calmasol *Ethipharm, Canad.†.*
Diphenhydramine hydrochloride (p.409·1); calamine (p.1080·1); benzocaine (p.1286·2); zinc oxide (p.1096·2).
Pruritus; topical analgesic, antihistamine, anti-allergic, and antiseptic.

Calmatel *Almirall, Spain.*
Piketoprofen hydrochloride (p.80·1).
Inflammation; pain; peri-articular disorders.

Calmaven *Alter, Spain.*
Diazepam (p.661·1).
Alcohol withdrawal syndrome; anxiety; epilepsy; febrile convulsions; insomnia; premedication; skeletal muscle spasm.

Calmaverine *Tophlan, Switz.*
Caroverine (p.1560·1).
Smooth muscle spasm.

Calmaxid
Bios, Belg.†; Lilly, Switz.
Nizatidine (p.1203·2).
Gastric hyperacidity; gastro-oesophageal reflux; peptic ulcer.

Calmday
Will-Pharma, Belg.; Ravizza, Neth.
Nordazepam (p.682·3).
Anxiety; epilepsy.

Calmerphan-L *Doetsch, Grether, Switz.*
Dextromethorphan resin (p.1057·3).
Bronchitis; coughs.

Calmesine *Mepha, Switz.*
Dextromethorphan resin (p.1058·2).
Coughs.

Calmex *Novopharm, Canad.*
Diphenhydramine hydrochloride (p.409·1).
Insomnia.

Calmigen *Antigen, Irl.†.*
Diazepam (p.661·1).
Anxiety; cerebral palsy; skeletal muscle spasm; tension.

Calmine *Bouty, Ital.*
Ibuprofen (p.44·1).
Pain.

Calmixene *Sandoz, Fr.*
Pimethixene (p.416·1).
Coughs.

Calmo *Eagle, Austral.*
Mistletoe (p.1604·1); valerian (p.1643·1); verbena officinalis; gentian (p.1583·3); avena (p.1551·3); passion flower (p.1615·3); scutellaria; tansy; pulsatilla (p.1623·3).
Hypnotic; tension; tension headache.

Calmo Yer Cafeina *Yer, Spain†.*
Aspirin (p.16·1); caffeine (p.749·3).
Fever; inflammation; pain.

Calmogel *Rhone-Poulenc Rorer, Ital.*
Isothipendyl hydrochloride (p.412·2).
Insect bites; pruritus; sunburn.

Calmol *Mentholatum, USA.*
Zinc oxide (p.1096·2); bismuth subgallate (p.1180·2).
Anorectal disorders.

Calmomusc *Cardinaux, Canad.*
Methyl salicylate (p.55·2); menthol (p.1600·2); cineole (p.1564·1).

Calmonal *Bristol-Myers Squibb, Ger.†.*
Meclozine hydrochloride (p.413·3).
Nervous disorders; sleep disorders.

Calmophytum *Holistica, Fr.*
Tilia (p.1637·3); orange buds; chamomile (p.1561·2); verbena; hibiscus.
Insomnia.

Calmoplex *Knoll, Spain.*
Codeine phosphate (p.26·1); hydroxyzine hydrochloride (p.412·1); propyphenazone (p.81·3).
Coughs; fever; pain.

Calmoroide *Phygiene, Fr.*
Ruscogenin (p.1627·1); vitamin A palmitate (p.1359·2).
Haemorrhoids.

Calmoserpin *Roland, Ger.†.*
Triamterene (p.957·2); hydrochlorothiazide (p.885·2); reserpine (p.942·1).
Hypertension.

Calms *Hylands, Canad.*
Homoeopathic preparation.

Calms Forte *Hylands, Canad.*
Homoeopathic preparation.

Calmurid
AB-Consult, Aust.; Galderma, Austral.; Galderma, Belg.; Galderma, Canad.; Galderma, Ger.; Galderma, Irl.; Galderma, Neth.; Galderma, Switz.; Galderma, UK.
Urea (p.1095·2); lactic acid (p.1593·3).
Dry skin; hyperkeratosis.

Calmurid HC
Note. This name is used for preparations of different composition.
AB-Consult, Aust.; Galderma, Canad.; Galderma, Ger.; Galderma, Irl.; Galderma, Switz.; Galderma, UK.
Urea (p.1095·2); lactic acid (p.1593·3); hydrocortisone (p.1043·3).
Skin disorders.

Galderma, Neth.
Urea (p.1095·2); hydrocortisone (p.1043·3).
Skin disorders.

Calmuril *Pharmacia Upjohn, Swed.*
Urea (p.1095·2); lactic acid (p.1593·3).
Dry skin; eczema; hyperkeratosis.

Calmuril-Hydrokortison *Pharmacia Upjohn, Swed.*
Urea (p.1095·2); hydrocortisone (p.1043·3).
Skin disorders.

Calm-X *Republic, USA.*
Dimenhydrinate (p.408·2).
Motion sickness.

Calmydone *Technilab, Canad.*
Hydrocodone tartrate (p.43·1); etafedrine hydrochloride (p.1061·1); sodium citrate (p.1153·2); doxylamine succinate (p.410·1).
Coughs.

Calmylin #1 *Technilab, Canad.*
Dextromethorphan hydrobromide (p.1057·3).
Coughs.

Calmylin #2 *Technilab, Canad.*
Dextromethorphan hydrobromide (p.1057·3); pseudoephedrine hydrochloride (p.1068·3).
Formerly known as Calmylin-DM-D.
Coughs.

Calmylin #3 *Technilab, Canad.*
Dextromethorphan hydrobromide (p.1057·3); pseudoephedrine hydrochloride (p.1068·3); guaiphenesin (p.1061·3).
Formerly known as Calmylin-DM-D-E.
Coughs.

Calmylin #4 *Technilab, Canad.*
Diphenhydramine hydrochloride (p.409·1); ammonium chloride (p.1055·2); dextromethorphan hydrobromide (p.1057·3).
Formerly known as Calmylin-DM.
Coughs.

Calmylin Ace *Technilab, Canad.*
Guaiphenesin (p.1061·3); pheniramine maleate (p.415·3); codeine phosphate (p.26·1).
Coughs.

Calmylin Codeine D-E *Technilab, Canad.*
Pseudoephedrine hydrochloride (p.1068·3); codeine phosphate (p.26·1); guaiphenesin (p.1061·3).

Calmylin Cough & Flu *Technilab, Canad.*
Dextromethorphan hydrobromide (p.1057·3); pseudoephedrine hydrochloride (p.1068·3); guaiphenesin (p.1061·3); paracetamol (p.72·2).
Coughs and cold symptoms.

Calmylin Expectorant *Technilab, Canad.*
Guaiphenesin (p.1061·3).
Coughs.

Calmylin Original with Codeine *Technilab, Canad.†.*
Diphenhydramine hydrochloride (p.409·1); ammonium chloride (p.1055·2); codeine phosphate (p.26·1).
Coughs.

Calmylin Pediatric *Technilab, Canad.*
Dextromethorphan hydrobromide (p.1057·3); pseudoephedrine hydrochloride (p.1068·3).
Coughs and cold symptoms.

Calnit *Vita Elan, Spain.*
Nimodipine (p.922·2).
Cerebral ischaemia; cerebral vasospasm due to subarachnoid haemorrhage.

Calociclina *ISI, Ital.*
Tetracycline hydrochloride (p.259·1).
Bacterial infections.

Calogen
Note. This name is used for preparations of different composition.
Scientific Hospital Supplies, Austral.; Scientific Hospital Supplies, Irl.; Scientific Hospital Supplies, UK.
Arachis oil (p.1550·2).
Carbohydrate malabsorption; dietary supplement; disorders of amino acid metabolism; ketogenic diet in epilepsy.

Prodes, Spain.
Salcatonin (p.735·3).
Hypercalcaemia; metastatic bone pain; osteoporosis; Paget's disease of bone.

Calomide-S *Yamanouchi, Jpn.*
Cobamamide (p.1364·2).
Anaemias; vitamin B_{12} deficiency.

Calonat *Pharmacal, Switz.*
Carbaspirin calcium (p.25·1); ascorbic acid (p.1365·2).
Fever; pain.

Caloreen
Hoechst Marion Roussel, Canad.†; Clintec, Fr.; Clintec, Irl.; Roussel, S.Afr.; Nestle, UK.
Dextrin (p.1339·1).
Food for special diets.

Calox *Qualiphar, Belg.*
Sterculia (p.1214·1).
Formerly known as Fixobel.
Denture fixative.

Calpan *ICN, Canad.*
Calcium pantothenate (p.1352·3).

Calparine
Sanofi Winthrop, Belg.; Sanofi Winthrop, Neth.
Heparin calcium (p.879·3).
Thrombo-embolic disorders.

Calperos *Doms-Adrian, Fr.*
Calcium carbonate (p.1182·1).
Calcium deficiency; osteoporosis.

Calperos D_3 *Doms-Adrian, Fr.*
Calcium carbonate (p.1182·1); cholecalciferol (p.1366·3).
Calcium and vitamin D deficiency; osteoporosis.

Calphosan *Glenwood, USA.*
Calcium glycerophosphate (p.1155·2); calcium lactate (p.1155·2).
Calcium deficiency.

Calphron *Nephro-Tech, USA.*
Calcium acetate (p.1155·1).
Hyperphosphataemia.

Cal-Plus *Geriatric Pharm. Corp., USA.*
Calcium carbonate (p.1182·1).
High-potency calcium supplement.

Calpol
Warner-Lambert, Irl.; Wellcome, Ital.†; Glaxo Wellcome, S.Afr.; Warner-Lambert, UK.
Paracetamol (p.72·2).
Fever; pain.

Calpol Extra *Warner-Lambert, UK.*
Paracetamol (p.72·2); codeine phosphate (p.26·1); caffeine (p.749·3).
Fever; pain.

Calporo *Eagle, Austral.*
Multivitamin and mineral supplement with herbs and bone powder.

Calpred *Grossmann, Switz.*
Prednisolone acetate (p.1048·1); mepyramine maleate (p.414·1); calcium laevulinate (p.1155·2).
Skin disorders.

Calsalettes *Torbet Laboratories, UK.*
Aloin (p.1177·2).
Constipation.

Calsan *Sandoz, Canad.*
Calcium carbonate (p.1182·1).
Calcium supplement.

Calscorbat *Aerocid, Fr.†.*
Asphocalcium.
Asthenia.

Calsip *Rowa, Irl.*
Food for special diets.

Calslot *Takeda, Jpn.*
Manidipine dihydrochloride (p.900·2).
Hypertension.

Cal-Sup *3M, Austral.*
Calcium carbonate (p.1182·1).
Calcium deficiency; calcium supplement.

Calsyn *Specia, Fr.*
Salcatonin (p.735·3).
Algodystrophies; hypercalcaemia; hyperphosphatasia; osteoporosis; Paget's disease of bone; prevention of bone loss in immobilisation.

Calsynar
Rhone-Poulenc Rorer, Austral.; Rhone-Poulenc Rorer, Belg.; Rhone-Poulenc Rorer, Ger.; Rhone-Poulenc Rorer, Irl.; Rhone-Poulenc Rorer, Neth.†; Rhone-Poulenc Rorer, Spain; Rorer, UK.
Salcatonin (p.735·3) or salcatonin acetate (p.736·3).
Bone pain in malignancy; hypercalcaemia; osteoporosis; Paget's disease of bone; reflex sympathetic dystrophy.

Calsynar Lyo *Rhone-Poulenc Rorer, Ger.*
Salcatonin (p.735·3).
Bone pain in malignancy; hypercalcaemia; osteoporosis; Paget's disease of bone; reflex sympathetic dystrophy.

Calsynar Lyo S *Rorer, Ger.†.*
Calcitonin (pork) (p.735·3).
Hypercalcaemia; osteoporosis; Paget's disease of bone.

Caltabs *Lifeplan, UK.*
Vitamin and mineral preparation.

Caltheon *Chephasaar, Ger.*
Tetrahydrozoline hydrochloride (p.1070·2).
Formerly contained naphazoline nitrate and phenylephrine hydrochloride.
Nasal congestion.

Caltine *Ferring, Canad.*
Salcatonin (p.735·3).
Hypercalcaemia; Paget's disease of bone.

Caltoson Balsamico *Rottapharm, Spain.*
Cineole (p.1564·1); benzocaine (p.1286·2); pholcodine (p.1068·1); cherry-laurel; terpineol (p.1635·1); menthol (p.1600·2).
Respiratory-tract disorders.

Caltrate
Whitehall, Austral.; Whitehall-Robins, Canad.; Whitehall, Fr.; Whitehall, S.Afr.; Lederle, USA.
Calcium carbonate (p.1182·1).
Calcium deficiency; calcium supplement; osteomalacia; osteoporosis.

Caltrate + D *Whitehall, Austral.*
Calcium carbonate (p.1182·1); cholecalciferol (p.1366·3).
Calcium and vitamin D deficiency; calcium supplement; osteomalacia; osteoporosis.

Caltrate + Iron & Vitamin D
Whitehall-Robins, Canad.; Lederle, USA.
Calcium carbonate (p.1182·1); ferrous fumarate (p.1339·3); vitamin D (p.1366·3).
Calcium and iron deficiency.

Caltrate Jr. *Lederle, USA.*
Calcium carbonate (p.1182·1).
Formerly contained calcium carbonate and vitamin D.
Calcium deficiency.

Caltrate Plus *Lederle, USA.*
Vitamin D with minerals.

Caltrate + Vitamin D
Whitehall-Robins, Canad.; Lederle, USA.
Calcium carbonate (p.1182·1); vitamin D (p.1366·3).
Calcium deficiency.

Caltro *Geneva, USA.*
Calcium with vitamin D.
Calcium deficiency; dietary supplement.

Calvakehl *Sanum-Kehlbeck, Ger.*
Homoeopathic preparation.

Calvepen *Leo, Irl.*
Phenoxymethylpenicillin calcium (p.236·2).
Bacterial infections.

Calvita *Roche Consumer, Austral.*
Calcium phosphate (p.1155·3); vitamins and iron.
Calcium supplement; dietary supplement.

Calvita Osti *Roche Consumer, Austral.*
Calcium carbonate (p.1182·1); cholecalciferol (p.1366·3).
Calcium and vitamin D deficiency; calcium and vitamin D supplement; osteomalacia; osteoporosis.

Calyptol
Bellon, Belg.†; Rhone-Poulenc Rorer, Ital.; Techni-Pharma, Mon.
Cineole (p.1564·1); terpineol (p.1635·1); pine oil; thyme oil (p.1637·1); rosemary oil (p.1626·2).
Respiratory-tract congestion.

Calyptol Inhalante *Rhone-Poulenc Rorer, Spain.*
Pinus sylvestris oil; rosemary oil (p.1626·2); terpineol (p.1635·1); thyme oil (p.1637·1); eucalyptus (p.1578·1).
Respiratory-tract congestion.

CAM
Note. This name is used for preparations of different composition.
Rybar, Irl.
Butethamate citrate (p.1056·2).
Formerly contained butethamate citrate and ephedrine hydrochloride.
Bronchospasm.

Shire, UK.
Ephedrine hydrochloride (p.1059·3).
Formerly contained butethamate citrate and ephedrine hydrochloride.
Bronchospasm; cough.

CAM Bronchodilator Mixture *Rybar, UK.*
Ephedrine hydrochloride (p.1059·3).
Bronchospasm.

Cama Arthritis Pain Reliever *Sandoz, USA.*
Aspirin (p.16·1).
Aluminium hydroxide (p.1177·3) and magnesium oxide (p.1198·3) are included in this preparation in an attempt to limit adverse effects on the gastro-intestinal mucosa.
Arthritis; pain.

Camalox
Rorer, Irl.†; Rorer, Ital.†; Rhone-Poulenc Rorer, Swed.
Aluminium hydroxide (p.1177·3); magnesium hydroxide (p.1198·2); calcium carbonate (p.1182·1).
Heartburn; peptic ulcer.

Cam-ap-es *Camall, USA†.*
Hydrochlorothiazide (p.885·2); reserpine (p.942·1); hydralazine hydrochloride (p.883·2).
Hypertension.

Camcolit
Norgine, Belg.†; Norgine, Irl.; Norgine, S.Afr.; Norgine, UK.
Lithium carbonate (p.290·3).
Bipolar disorder; depression; mania.

Camegel *Bonomelli, Ital.*
Carrot; honey (p.1345·3).
Diarrhoea.

Cameo *Medco, USA.*
Emollient.

Camil *Martin, Spain†.*
Cephazolin sodium (p.181·1).
Bacterial infections.

Camiline *Arkopharma, Fr.*
Green tea (p.1645·1).
Slimming aid.

Campanyl *Temmler, Ger.*
Potassium polystyrene sulphonate (p.992·2).
Hypercalciuria.

Campel *Promedica, Fr.*
Chromocarb diethylamine (p.1562·3).
Circulatory disorders; haemorrhoids.

Camphoderm N *Li-il, Ger.*
Camphor (p.1557·2).
Catarrh; musculoskeletal, joint, and soft-tissue disorders.

Camphodionyl *Distri B3, Fr.*
Sodium camsylate; potassium guaiacolsulfonate (p.1068·3); codeine (p.26·1); ethylmorphine hydrochloride (p.36·1); aconite root (p.1542·2); Desessartz syrup; benzoic acid (p.1102·3).
Coughs.

Campholinct *Rhone-Poulenc Rorer, Austral.†.*
Camphor (p.1557·2).

Campho-Phenique *Winthrop Consumer, USA; Sterling, USA.*
Phenol (p.1121·2); camphor (p.1557·2).
Burns; cuts; herpes labialis; infections; insect bites; pain.

Campho-Phenique Antibiotic Plus Pain Reliever Ointment *Winthrop Consumer, USA.*
Bacitracin (p.157·3); neomycin sulphate (p.229·2); polymyxin B sulphate (p.239·1); lignocaine (p.1293·2).
Formerly contained diperodon hydrochloride in place of lignocaine.
Infection prophylaxis and pain relief in minor skin lesions.

Campho-Phenique Sting Relief Formula *Winthrop Consumer, USA†.*
Benzocaine (p.1286·2); menthol (p.1600·2).
Insect stings and bites.

Camphopin *Schoning-Berlin, Ger.*
Methyl salicylate (p.55·2); benzyl nicotinate (p.22·1); camphor (p.1557·2).
Frostbite; neuralgia; rheumatic disorders; sciatica; tendinitis.

Campho-Pneumine
Note. This name is used for preparations of different composition.
Marion Merrell Dow, Belg.†.
Sodium guaiacolate; cineole (p.1564·1); camphor (p.1557·2).
Respiratory-tract disorders.

Marion Merrell, Fr.
Adult suppositories: Camphor (p.1557·2); guaiacol (p.1061·2); cineole (p.1564·1); guaiphenesin (p.1061·3); amylocaine hydrochloride (p.1286·1).
Suppositories child: Camphor (p.1557·2); guaiacol (p.1061·2); cineole (p.1564·1); guaiphenesin (p.1061·3).
Suppositories infant: Cineole (p.1564·1); guaiphenesin (p.1061·3).
Syrup†: Sodium camsylate; sodium benzoate (p.1102·3); sodium bromide (p.1620·3); potassium guaiacolsulfonate (p.1068·3); thiamine dicamsylate (p.1361·2); maidenhair fern; tolu balsam (p.1071·1).
Respiratory-system disorders.

Campho-Pneumine Aminophylline
Marion Merrell, Fr.†.
Adult syrup: Codeine (p.26·1); belladonna (p.457·1); aconite (p.1542·2); bromoform (p.1620·3); sodium camsylate; sodium benzoate (p.1102·3); potassium guaiacolsulfonate (p.1068·3); thiamine dicamsylate (p.1361·2); aminophylline (p.748·1); potion de Todd; eucalyptus (p.1578·1); fumitory (p.1581·3); Desessartz syrup; tolu balsam (p.1071·1).
Paediatric syrup: Codeine (p.26·1); belladonna (p.457·1); grindelia; gelsemium (p.1583·2); sodium camsylate; sodium benzoate (p.1102·3); potassium guaiacolsulfonate (p.1068·3); thiamine dicamsylate (p.1361·2); aminophylline (p.748·1); fumitory (p.1581·3); Desessartz syrup; tolu balsam (p.1071·1).
Respiratory-system disorders.

Camphor Linctus Compound *McGloin, Austral.*
Camphor (p.1557·2); tolu balsam (p.1071·1).
Coughs.

Camphre Compose *Valmo, Canad.*
Camphor (p.1557·2); menthol (p.1600·2); cineole (p.1564·1).

Camphrice Du Canada *Homme de Fer, Fr.*
Camphor (p.1557·2).
Skin disorders.

Campral
Merck, Aust.; Lipha, Ger.; Lipha, Irl.; E. Merck, Neth.; Merck, Spain; E. Merck, Swed.; Lipha, Switz.; Lipha, UK.
Acamprosate calcium (p.640·1).
Alcoholism.

Campto
Bellon, Fr.; Rhone-Poulenc Rorer, Ital.; Rhone-Poulenc Rorer, S.Afr.; Rhone-Poulenc Rorer, UK.
Irinotecan hydrochloride (p.543·2).
Colorectal cancer.

Camptosar
Pharmacia Upjohn, Austral.; Pharmacia Upjohn, USA.
Irinotecan hydrochloride (p.543·2).
Colon cancer; rectal cancer.

Campylotec *Pfizer, Ger.†.*
Bismuth aluminate (p.1180·1).
Gastritis; peptic ulcer.

Camsilon *Cambridge, UK.*
Edrophonium chloride (p.1392·2).
Formerly known as Tensilon.
Now known as Edrophonium Chloride Ampoules.
Diagnosis of myasthenia gravis or phase-II block; reversal of competitive neuromuscular blockade.

Camyna *Nycomed, Swed.†.*
Thioxolone (p.1093·3).
Acne; seborrhoea.

Canadiol *Esteve, Spain.*
Itraconazole (p.381·3).
Fungal infections.

Canalba *Compu, S.Afr.*
Clotrimazole (p.376·3).
Fungal skin and vulvovaginal infections.

Candalba *Brauer, Austral.*
Homoeopathic preparation.

Candaspor *Be-Tabs, S.Afr.*
Clotrimazole (p.376·3).
Fungal skin and vulvovaginal infections.

Candermyl
Galderma, Austral.; Galderma, UK†.
Emollient.
Dry skin.

Candibene *Merckle, Aust.*
Clotrimazole (p.376·3).
Fungal infections; trichomoniasis.

Candi-Biffidus *Eagle, Austral.†.*
Lactobacillus spp. (p.1594·1).
Antibiotic-induced suppression of intestinal flora; candidiasis; constipation; digestive disorders; intestinal infection.

Candida Yeast *Homeocan, Canad.*
Homoeopathic preparation.

Candidal *IBSA, Switz.†.*
Mepartricin (p.384·2) or mepartricin sodium lauryl sulphate (p.384·2).
Fungal infections of the vagina.

Candida-Lokalicid *Dorsch, Ger.†.*
Nystatin (p.386·1).
Fungal infections.

Candidine *Stallergenes, Fr.*
Candida albicans antigen (p.1545·1).
Diagnosis of hypersensitivity to Candida albicans; hyposensitisation to Candida albicans.

Candio
Merck, Aust.; Hermal, Ger.; Hermal, Switz.
Nystatin (p.386·1).
Fungal infections.

Candio E *Hermal, Switz.†.*
Nystatin (p.386·1); fluprednidene acetate (p.1042·2); chlorquinaldol (p.185·1).
Fungal infections.

Candio E comp N *Hermal, Ger.*
Nystatin (p.386·1); fluprednidene acetate (p.1042·2).
Inflammatory skin disorders with fungal infection.

Candistatin *Westwood-Squibb, Canad.*
Nystatin (p.386·1).
Fungal infections.

Candizole *Lennon, S.Afr.*
Clotrimazole (p.376·3).
Fungal skin and vulvovaginal infections.

Candyl *Douglas, Austral.*
Piroxicam (p.80·2).
Musculoskeletal and joint disorders.

Canef
Astra, Neth.; Astra, Norw.; Hassle, Swed.
Fluvastatin sodium (p.1273·2).
Hyperlipidaemias.

Canephron N *Bionorica, Ger.*
Centaury (p.1561·1); levisticum (p.1597·2); rosemary.
Urinary-tract disorders.

Canephron novo *Bionorica, Ger.*
Birch leaves; orthosiphon (p.1592·2); solidago virgaurea.
Renal calculi; urinary-tract disorders.

Canesten
Bayer, Aust.; Bayer, Austral.; Bayer, Canad.; Bayer, Ger.; Bayer, Irl.; Bayer, Ital.; Bayer, Neth.; Bayer, Norw.; Bayer, S.Afr.; Bayer, Spain; Bayer, Swed.; Bayer, UK.
Clotrimazole (p.376·3).
Fungal and bacterial infections; trichomoniasis.

Canesten Combi *Bayer, UK.*
Combination pack containing Canesten Cream and Canesten 1 pessary: Clotrimazole (p.376·3).
Vulvovaginal candidiasis.

Canesten HC
Bayer, Ger.; Bayer, Irl.; Bayer, UK.
Clotrimazole (p.376·3); hydrocortisone (p.1043·3).
Fungal skin infections with inflammation.

Canestene
Bayer, Belg.; Bayer, Switz.
Clotrimazole (p.376·3).
Fungal and bacterial infections; trichomoniasis.

Canex *Schwulst, S.Afr.*
Clotrimazole (p.376·3).
Fungal skin infections; fungal vulvo-vaginitis.

Canfodion *Gentili, Ital.†.*
Dextromethorphan hydrobromide (p.1057·3).
Coughs.

Canifug *Wolff, Ger.*
Clotrimazole (p.376·3).
Fungal and bacterial infections; trichomoniasis.

Cankerol *Coradol, Ger.*
Homoeopathic preparation.

Canol *Jolly-Jatel, Fr.*
Cynara (p.1569·2); chimaphylla; aphloia.
Dyspepsia.

Canrenol *Prospa, Belg.*
Canrenoate potassium (p.836·2).
Cirrhosis; electrolyte disturbances; heart failure; hyperaldosteronism; hypertension; nephrotic syndrome.

Canscreen *Tican, Canad.*
Avobenzone (p.1486·3); ethylhexyl *p*-methoxycinnamate (p.1487·1); oxybenzone (p.1487·3).
Sunscreen.

Canstat *Wyeth, S.Afr.*
Nystatin (p.386·1).
Candidiasis.

Cantabilin *Formenti, Ital.*
Hymecromone (p.1589·3).
Biliary-tract disorders.

Cantabiline
Lipha, Belg.; Lipha Sante, Fr.
Hymecromone (p.1589·3).
Biliary-tract disorders; dyspepsia.

Cantalene *Cooperation Pharmaceutique, Fr.*
Muramidase hydrochloride (p.1604·3); chlorhexidine acetate (p.1107·2); amethocaine hydrochloride (p.1285·2).
Mouth and throat disorders.

Cantamac *Cantassium Co., UK.*
Multivitamin and mineral preparation.

Cantamega *Larkhall Laboratories, UK.*
Multivitamin and mineral preparation.

Cantan *Cassella-med, Ital.†.*
Ascorbic acid (p.1365·2).
Vitamin C deficiency.

Cantanidin *Bender, Aust.†.*
Clonidine hydrochloride (p.841·2).
Hypertension.

Cantapollen *Cantassium Co., UK.*
Dolomite; bee pollen.

Cantassium Discs *Cantassium Co., UK.*
Mineral preparation.

Cantavite with FF *Cantassium Co., UK.*
Multivitamin and mineral preparation.

Canteine Bouteille *Bouteille, Fr.†.*
Oral liquid: Crataegus (p.1568·2); hamamelis (p.1587·1); passion flower (p.1615·3); salix alba (p.82·3).
Tablets: Hamamelis (p.1587·1); crataegus (p.1568·2); passion flower (p.1615·3); salix alba (p.82·3); strophanthus (p.951·1); phenobarbitone (p.350·2).
Cardiovascular disorders; haemorrhoids; varicose veins.

Canthacur *Pharmascience, Canad.*
Cantharidin (p.1559·2).
Molluscum contagiosum; warts.

Canthacur-PS *Pharmascience, Canad.*
Cantharidin (p.1559·2); podophyllum resin (p.1089·1); salicylic acid (p.1090·2).
Molluscum contagiosum; warts.

Cantharis Med Complex *Dynamit, Aust.*
Homoeopathic preparation.

Cantharone
Dormer, Canad.; Seres, USA†.
Cantharidin (p.1559·2).
Molluscum contagiosum; warts.

Cantharone Plus
Dormer, Canad.; Seres, USA†.
Cantharidin (p.1559·2); podophyllum resin (p.1089·1); salicylic acid (p.1090·2).
Molluscum contagiosum; warts.

Cantil
Marion Merrell Dow, Belg.†; Tika, Swed.; Boehringer Mannheim, UK†; Hoechst Marion Roussel, USA.
Mepenzolate bromide (p.465·1).
Adjunctive therapy in peptic ulcer; lower gastro-intestinal tract motility disorders.

Cantopal *Larkhall Laboratories, UK.*
Calcium pantothenate (p.1352·3).

Cantor
Clin Midy, Fr.†; Midy, Ital.†.
Minaprine hydrochloride (p.298·1).
Depression.

Cantricin *Corvi, Ital.†.*
Pentamycin (p.386·3).
Vaginitis.

Canulase *Wander, Ital.†.*
Methixene hydrochloride (p.465·1); dimethicone (p.1213·1); cellulase (p.1561·1); glutamic acid hydrochloride (p.1344·3); pepsin (p.1616·3); pancreatin (p.1612·1); sodium dehydrocholate (p.1570·3).
Gastro-intestinal disorders.

Canusal *CP Pharmaceuticals, UK.*
Heparin sodium (p.879·3).
To maintain patency of in-dwelling intravascular lines.

Caolax *Labima, Belg.*
Phenolphthalein (p.1208·2).
Bowel evacuation; constipation.

Caomet *Astra, Ital.*
Ubidecarenone (p.1641·2).
Cardiac disorders.

Caosina *Ern, Spain.*
Calcium carbonate (p.1182·1).
Hypocalcaemia; osteoporosis.

Capace
Amrad, Austral.; Garec, S.Afr.
Captopril (p.836·3).
Diabetic nephropathy; heart failure; hypertension; myocardial infarction.

Capadex *Fawns & McAllan, Austral.*
Dextropropoxyphene hydrochloride (p.27·3); paracetamol (p.72·2).
Fever; pain.

Capasal
Dermal Laboratories, Irl.; Dermal Laboratories, UK.
Salicylic acid (p.1090·2); coal tar (p.1092·3).
Skin disorders of the scalp.

Capastat
Lilly, Aust.; Lilly, Austral.; Lilly, Canad.; Dista, Spain; Dista, UK; Dura, USA.
Capreomycin sulphate (p.162·1).
Pulmonary tuberculosis.

CAPD *Fresenius, Spain.*
Calcium chloride; magnesium chloride; sodium chloride; sodium lactate; glucose (p.1151·1).
Peritoneal dialysis.

Capergyl *Therica, Fr.*
Co-dergocrine mesylate (p.1566·1).
Mental function disorders.

Capilarema *Zambon, Spain.*
Aminaphthone (p.710·3).
Capillary disorders; haemorrhage.

Capillarema *Baldacci, Ital.*
Aminaphthone (p.710·3).
Capillary disorders.

Capillaron *Madaus, Ger.*
Homoeopathic preparation.

Capistan *Sanofi Winthrop, Fr.*
Saw palmetto (p.1462·1).
Benign prostatic hyperplasia.

Capital with Codeine Suspension *Carnrick, USA.*
Paracetamol (p.72·2); codeine phosphate (p.26·1).
Pain.

Capitol *Dermal Laboratories, UK†.*
Benzalkonium chloride (p.1101·3).
Seborrhoeic scalp conditions.

Capitrol *Westwood-Squibb, USA.*
Chloroxine (p.215·3).
Seborrhoeic dermatitis.

Caplenal
Berk, Irl.; Berk, UK.
Allopurinol (p.390·2).
Gout; hyperuricaemia; renal calculi.

Capolax *Propan-Vernleigh, S.Afr.†.*
Bisacodyl (p.1179·3).
Bowel evacuation; constipation.

Caposan *Adler, Switz.*
Propyphenazone (p.81·3); paracetamol (p.72·2); caffeine (p.749·3).
Fever; pain.

Capota *Faes, Spain.*
Cetylpyridinium chloride (p.1106·2); benzocaine (p.1286·2).
Skin and wound disinfection.

Capoten
Bristol-Myers Squibb, Austral.; Bristol-Myers Squibb, Belg.; Squibb, Canad.; Bristol-Myers Squibb, Irl.; Mead Johnson, Ital.; Bristol-Myers Squibb, Neth.; Bristol-Myers Squibb, Norw.; Bristol-Myers Squibb, S.Afr.; Squibb, Spain; Bristol-Myers Squibb, Swed.; Squibb, UK; Bristol-Myers Squibb, USA.
Captopril (p.836·3).
Diabetic nephropathy; heart failure; hypertension; myocardial infarction.

Capozid *Bristol-Myers Squibb, Swed.*
Captopril (p.836·3); hydrochlorothiazide (p.885·2).
Hypertension.

Capozide
Bristol-Myers Squibb, Aust.; Bristol-Myers Squibb, Ger.; Bristol-Myers Squibb, Irl.; Bristol-Myers Squibb, Neth.; Bristol-Myers Squibb, S.Afr.; Bristol-Myers Squibb, Switz.; Squibb, UK; Bristol-Myers Squibb, USA.
Captopril (p.836·3); hydrochlorothiazide (p.885·2).
Hypertension.

Capracid *Glaxo Allen, Ital.†.*
Aminocaproic acid (p.711·1).
Haemorrhagic disorders.

Capramin *Glaxo Wellcome, Aust.*
Aspirin (p.16·1); carbinoxamine maleate (p.404·2); phenylephrine hydrochloride (p.1066·2); caffeine (p.749·3).
Colds; influenza.

Capricin *Sisu, Canad.*
Caprylic acid (p.1609·3).
Elimination of intestinal Candida albicans.

Caprilate *Eagle, Austral.*
Sodium caprylate (p.1609·3); berberis vulgaris; magnesium chloride (p.1157·2); zinc gluconate (p.1373·2); lithium chloride (p.295·1); sorbic acid (p.1125·2).
Inhibition of gastro-intestinal yeast growth.

Caprilon
Cow & Gate, Irl.; Cow & Gate, UK.
Medium-chain triglycerides.
Formerly known as MCT(1) in the *UK*.
Malabsorption syndromes.

Caprin
Note. This name is used for preparations of different composition.
CSL, Austral.†.
Heparin calcium (p.879·3).
Cardiovascular procedures; disseminated intravascular coagulation; thrombo-embolic disorders.

Sinclair, Irl.; Sinclair, UK.
Aspirin (p.16·1).
Fever; pain; secondary prevention of myocardial infarction.

Caprinol *Bayer, Ger.†.*
Reserpine (p.942·1); methyldopa (p.904·2); mefruside (p.902·2).

Caprisana *Sidroga, Switz.*
Camphor (p.1557·2); juniper oil (p.1592·3); rosemary oil (p.1626·2); turpentine oil (p.1641·1); thyme oil (p.1637·1); larch oil.
Musculoskeletal and joint pain.

Caproamin *Fides, Spain.*
Aminocaproic acid (p.711·1).
Haemorrhage.

Caprofides Hemostatico *Fides, Spain.*
Injection†: Esculoside (p.1543·3); hesperidin methyl chalcone (p.1580·2); menadione sodium phosphate (p.1370·3); creatinine sulphate; tranexamic acid (p.728·2).
Oral solution: Aminocaproic acid (p.711·1); esculoside (p.1543·3); hesperidin methyl chalcone (p.1580·2); menadione (p.1370·3); creatinine sulphate.
Haemorrhage.

Caprolisin *Malesci, Ital.*
Aminocaproic acid (p.711·1).
Haemorrhagic disorders.

Capros *Rhone-Poulenc Rorer, Ger.; Medac, Ger.*
Morphine sulphate (p.56·2).
Pain.

Capsamol *Worwag, Ger.*
Ointment: Capsicum (p.1559·2).
Musculoskeletal and joint pain.
Topical application: Camphor (p.1557·2); benzyl nicotinate (p.22·1); capsaicin (p.24·2).
Rheumatic disorders.

Capsic *Pierre Fabre, Fr.*
Dressing: Capsicum (p.1559·2); methyl salicylate (p.55·2); camphor (p.1557·2).
Ointment: Capsaicin (p.24·2); methyl nicotinate (p.55·1).
Muscle cramp.

Capsicum + Arthri-Cream *Homeocan, Canad.*
Homoeopathic preparation.

Capsidol *Vinas, Spain.*
Capsaicin (p.24·2).
Pain.

Capsig *Schering, Austral.†.*
Capsaicin (p.24·2).
Postherpetic neuralgia.

Capsin *Fleming, USA.*
Capsaicin (p.24·2).
Neuralgia; pain.

Capsina *Astra, Swed.*
Capsaicin (p.24·2).
Postherpetic neuralgia.

Capsiplast *Beiersdorf, Aust.*
Capsaicin (p.24·2).
Musculoskeletal and joint disorders.

Capsoid *Caps, S.Afr.*
Prednisolone (p.1048·1).
Corticosteroid.

Capsolin
Note. This name is used for preparations of different composition.
Parke, Davis, Austral.†; Warner-Lambert, Canad.†.
Capsicum oleoresin; camphor (p.1557·2); turpentine oil (p.1641·1); cajuput oil (p.1556·1).
Joint and muscle pain.

Warner-Lambert, Ital.; Parke, Davis, Switz.
Capsicum oleoresin; camphor (p.1557·2); turpentine oil (p.1641·1); eucalyptus oil (p.1578·1).
Joint and muscle pain.

Capsules laxatives Nattermann Nr. 13 *Piraud, Switz.*
Senna (p.1212·2); caraway oil (p.1559·3); anise oil (p.1550·1).
Bowel evacuation; constipation.

Capsuvac *Galen, UK.*
Danthron (p.1188·2); docusate sodium (p.1189·3).
These ingredients can be described by the British Approved Name Co-danthrusate.
Constipation.

Capsyl *Sandoz, Fr.*
Dextromethorphan hydrobromide (p.1057·3).
Coughs.

Captagon
Asta Medica, Belg.; Asta Medica, Ger.
Fenethylline hydrochloride (p.1480·3).
Hyperactivity disorders.

Captea *Bellon, Fr.*
Captopril (p.836·3); hydrochlorothiazide (p.885·2).
Hypertension.

Captimer *Fresenius, Ger.*
Tiopronin (p.997·2).
Cystinuria; heavy metal poisoning; liver disorders.

Captin *Krewel, Ger.*
Paracetamol (p.72·2).
Fever; pain.

Capto *CT, Ger.; BASF, Ger.; corax, Ger.; Eu Rho, Ger.; Sanorania, Ger.*
Captopril (p.836·3).
Heart failure; hypertension.

Captobeta *Betapharm, Ger.*
Captopril (p.836·3).
Heart failure; hypertension.

Captocomp *Ebewe, Aust.*
Verapamil hydrochloride (p.960·3); captopril (p.836·3).
Hypertension.

Capto-dura Cor *Durachemie, Ger.*
Captopril (p.836·3).
Heart failure; hypertension.

Captoflux *Hennig, Ger.*
Captopril (p.836·3).
Heart failure; hypertension.

Captogamma *Worwag, Ger.*
Captopril (p.836·3).
Heart failure; hypertension.

Captohexal
Hexal, Austral.; Hexal, Ger.
Captopril (p.836·3).
Diabetic nephropathy; heart failure; hypertension; myocardial infarction.

Capto-ISIS *Isis Puren, Ger.*
Captopril (p.836·3).
Diabetic nephropathy; heart failure; hypertension; myocardial infarction.

Captol *Sanico, Belg.†.*
Bromoform (p.1620·3); codeine (p.26·1); aconite (p.1542·2); belladonna (p.457·1); potassium guaiacolsulfonate (p.1068·3); cineole (p.1564·1); sodium camsylate.
Bronchopulmonary disorders.

Captolane *Bellon, Fr.*
Captopril (p.836·3).
Heart failure; hypertension; myocardial infarction.

Captomerck *Merck, Ger.*
Captopril (p.836·3).
Heart failure; hypertension.

Captopress *Bayer, Ger.*
Captopril (p.836·3).
Heart failure; hypertension.

Captopril Compositum *Mayrhofer, Aust.*
Captopril (p.836·3); hydrochlorothiazide (p.885·2).
Hypertension.

Capto-Puren Cor *Isis Puren, Ger.*
Captopril (p.836·3).
Heart failure; hypertension.

Captor *Rowex, Irl.*
Captopril (p.836·3).
Heart failure; hypertension.

Captoreal *Realpharma, Ger.*
Captopril (p.836·3).
Heart failure; hypertension.

Capurate *Sigma, Austral.*
Allopurinol (p.390·2).
Hyperuricaemia.

Capval *Dreluso, Ger.*
Oral drops; oral liquid; tablets: Noscapine (p.1065·2) or noscapine hydrochloride (p.1065·2).
Coughs and associated respiratory-tract disorders.

Capzasin-P
Stella, Canad.; Thompson, USA.
Capsaicin (p.24·2).
Pain.

Carace
Du Pont, Irl.; Du Pont Pharmaceuticals, UK.
Lisinopril (p.898·2).
Heart failure; hypertension; myocardial infarction.

Carace Plus
Du Pont, Irl.; Du Pont Pharmaceuticals, UK.
Lisinopril (p.898·2); hydrochlorothiazide (p.885·2).
Hypertension.

Caradrin
Laevosan, Aust.; Boehringer Mannheim, Ital.†.
Proscillaridin (p.938·1).
Cardiac disorders.

Carafate
Hoechst Marion Roussel, Austral.; Marion Merrell Dow, USA.
Sucralfate (p.1214·2).
Peptic ulcer.

Caramelle alle Erbe Digestive *Giuliani, Ital.*
Gentian (p.1583·3); rhubarb (p.1212·1); boldo (p.1554·1).
Aid to digestion.

Caramelos Agua del Carmen *Fardi, Spain.*
Cineole (p.1564·1); melissa (p.1600·1); menthol (p.1600·2).
Nasal congestion.

Caramelos Balsam *Alcala, Spain.*
Cineole (p.1564·1); oleum pinus sylvestris; menthol (p.1600·2).
Throat irritation.

Caramelos Vit C *Alcala, Spain.*
Ascorbic acid (p.1365·2).
Deficiency of vitamin C.

Carasel *Almirall, Spain.*
Ramipril (p.941·1).
Heart failure; hypertension.

Carba *CT, Ger.*
Carbamazepine (p.339·2).
Alcohol withdrawal syndrome; diabetic neuropathy; epilepsy; neuralgias.

Carbagamma *Worwag, Ger.*
Carbamazepine (p.339·2).
Diabetic neuropathy; epilepsy; neuralgia.

Carbaica *Synthelabo, Ital.*
Urazamide (p.1641·3).
Liver disorders.

Carbalax *Pharmax, UK.*
Monobasic sodium phosphate (p.1159·3); sodium bicarbonate (p.1153·2).
Formerly known as Beogex.
Bowel evacuation; constipation.

Carbamann *Mann, Ger.*
Carbachol (p.1390·1).
Glaucoma.

Carbamid + VAS *Widmer, Ger.*
Tretinoin (p.1093·3); urea (p.1095·2).
Skin disorders.

Carbapen *CSL, Austral.†.*
Carbenicillin sodium (p.162·3).
Bacterial infections.

Carbastat *Ciba Vision, USA.*
Carbachol (p.1390·1).
Production of miosis in eye surgery.

Carbellon *Torbet Laboratories, UK.*
Activated charcoal (p.972·2); magnesium hydroxide (p.1198·2); peppermint oil (p.1208·1).
Formerly contained activated charcoal, belladonna dry extract, magnesium hydroxide, and peppermint oil.
Gastro-intestinal disorders.

Carbem *Lilly, Ital.*
Loracarbef (p.222·3).
Bacterial infections.

Carbenin *Sankyo, Jpn.*
Panipenem (p.235·3); betamipron (p.161·3).
Bacterial infections.

Carbex
Note. This name is used for preparations of different composition.
Nordic, UK.
Oral granules, sodium bicarbonate (p.1153·2); simethicone (p.1213·1); solution, anhydrous citric acid (p.1564·3).
Adjunct to contrast media for gastro-intestinal radiography.

Du Pont, USA.
Selegiline hydrochloride (p.1144·2).
Parkinsonism.

Carbicalcin
Procter & Gamble, Ital.; Smith Kline & French, Spain.
Elcatonin (p.735·3).
Hypercalcaemia; metastatic bone pain; osteoporosis; Paget's disease of bone; reflex sympathetic dystrophy.

Carbicarb *IMS, Canad.†.*
Sodium bicarbonate (p.1153·2); sodium carbonate anhydrous (p.1630·2).
Metabolic acidosis.

Carbilev *Lennon, S.Afr.*
Levodopa (p.1137·1); carbidopa (p.1136·1).
Parkinsonism.

Carbinoxamine Compound *Morton Grove, USA.*
Carbinoxamine maleate (p.404·2); pseudoephedrine hydrochloride (p.1068·3); dextromethorphan hydrobromide (p.1057·3).
Coughs and cold symptoms.

Carbiset *Nutripharm, USA.*
Pseudoephedrine hydrochloride (p.1068·3); carbinoxamine maleate (p.404·2).
Upper respiratory-tract symptoms.

Carbium *Hexal, Ger.*
Carbamazepine (p.339·2).
Alcohol withdrawal syndrome; diabetic neuropathy; epilepsy; neuralgias.

Carbo Konigsfeld *Muller Goppingen, Ger.*
Carbo coffea (p.1645·1).
Digestive system disorders.

Carbo Veg *Brauer, Austral.*
Homoeopathic preparation.

Carbobel *Medgenix, Belg.*
Activated charcoal (p.972·2); hexamine (p.216·1); magnesium citrate (p.1198·2).
Diarrhoea; dyspepsia; poisoning.

Carbocain
Astra, Norw.; Astra, Swed.
Mepivacaine hydrochloride (p.1297·2).
Adrenaline acid tartrate (p.813·3) is included in some injections as a vasoconstrictor to diminish absorption and localise the effect of the local anaesthetic.
Local anaesthesia.

Carbocaina
Note. This name is used for preparations of different composition.
Astra, Ital.
Mepivacaine hydrochloride (p.1297·2).
Adrenaline acid tartrate (p.813·3) is included in some injections as a vasoconstrictor to diminish absorption and localise the effect of the local anaesthetic.
Local anaesthesia.

Bucca, Spain.
Phenol (p.1121·2); methyl salicylate (p.55·2); amethocaine hydrochloride (p.1285·2).
Local anaesthesia.

Carbocaine
Astra, Austral.; Sanofi Winthrop, Canad.; Adcock Ingram, S.Afr.; Sanofi Winthrop, USA; Cook-Waite, USA.
Mepivacaine hydrochloride (p.1297·2).
Levonordefrin (p.1596·2) is included in some injections as a vasoconstrictor to diminish absorption and localise the effect of the local anaesthetic.
Local anaesthesia.

Carbocaine with Neo-Cobefrin *Cook-Waite, USA.*
Mepivacaine hydrochloride (p.1297·2).
Levonordefrin (p.1596·2) is included in this preparation as a vasoconstrictor to diminish absorption and localise the effect of the local anaesthetic.
Local anaesthesia.

Carbocal *Madariaga, Spain.*
Calcium carbonate (p.1182·1).
Hypocalcaemia; osteoporosis.

Carbocit *CT, Ital.*
Carbocisteine (p.1056·3).
Respiratory-tract disorders.

Carbo-Cort *Lagap, UK†.*
Coal tar (p.1092·3); hydrocortisone (p.1043·3).
Eczema; psoriasis.

Carbodec *Rugby, USA.*
Carbinoxamine maleate (p.404·2); pseudoephedrine hydrochloride (p.1068·3).
Allergic rhinitis; nasal congestion.

Carbodec DM *Rugby, USA.*
Pseudoephedrine hydrochloride (p.1068·3); dextromethorphan hydrobromide (p.1057·3); carbinoxamine maleate (p.404·2).
Coughs and cold symptoms.

Carbo-Dome
Dome-Hollister-Stier, Fr.†; Lagap, UK.
Coal tar (p.1092·3).
Psoriasis.

Carboguan *Aesca, Aust.†.*
Carbo medicinalis (p.972·2); sulphaguanidine (p.254·1).

Carbolactanose *Sopar, Belg.†.*
Streptococcus lactis; activated charcoal (p.972·2).
Diarrhoea; enterocolitis; meteorism; re-establishment of gastro-intestinal flora.

Carbolevure
Vedim, Fr.; UCB, Switz.
Saccharomyces cerevisiae (p.1373·1); activated charcoal (p.972·2).
Gastro-intestinal disorders.

Carbolith *ICN, Canad.*
Lithium carbonate (p.290·3).
Bipolar disorder.

Carbolithium *IFI, Ital.*
Lithium carbonate (p.290·3).
Adjunct in drug-induced leucopenia; cluster headache; psychiatric disorders.

Carbomix
SCAT, Fr.; Penn, Irl.; Selena, Swed.; Penn, UK.
Activated charcoal (p.972·2).
Acute poisoning; diarrhoea.

Carbomucil *Norgine, Ger.†.*
Activated charcoal (p.972·2); sterculia (p.1214·1); heavy magnesium carbonate (p.1198·1).

Carbonaphtine Pectinee *Giffer Barbezat, Fr.†.*
Benzonaphtol (p.98·3); aluminium salicylate; vegetable charcoal (p.972·3); pectin (p.1474·1); kaolin (p.1195·1); salicaire; raspberry leaf (p.1624·2).
Gastro-intestinal disorders.

Carbonesia *Geymonat, Ital.*
Activated charcoal (p.972·2); magnesium oxide (p.1198·3); calcium carbonate (p.1182·1); magnesium peroxide (p.1119·1).
Gastro-intestinal disorders.

Carbonet
Smith & Nephew, Fr.; Smith & Nephew, Irl.; Smith & Nephew, Ital.†; Smith & Nephew, UK.
Activated charcoal (p.972·2).
Malodorous wounds.

Carboneural *Recipe, Aust.*
Bupivacaine hydrochloride (p.1286·3).
Local anaesthesia.

Carbonex *Aerocid, Fr.*
Sublimed sulphur (p.1091·2); magnesium hydroxide (p.1198·2).
Gastro-intestinal disorders.

Carbophagix *Darcy, Fr.*
Activated charcoal (p.972·2); *Saccharomyces cerevisiae* (p.1373·1).
Gastro-intestinal disorders.

Carbophos *UPSA, Fr.*
Vegetable charcoal (p.972·3); calcium carbonate (p.1182·1); calcium phosphate (p.1155·3).
Gastro-intestinal disorders.

Carboplat *Bristol-Myers Squibb, Ger.*
Carboplatin (p.510·3).
Malignant neoplasms.

Carbosan *Rowa, Irl.*
Carbenoxolone sodium (p.1182·2).
Aphthous stomatitis; herpes labialis; lip sores.

Carboseptol *Herbes Universelles, Canad.*
Menthol (p.1600·2); cineole (p.1564·1); methyl salicylate (p.55·2); thymol (p.1127·1); zinc oxide (p.1096·2).

Carbosin
Nycomed, Norw.; Pharmachemie, S.Afr.
Carboplatin (p.510·3).
Malignant neoplasms.

Carbosol *Donau, Aust.*
Carboplatin (p.510·3).
Malignant neoplasms.

Carbosorb
Delta, Austral.; Seton, UK†.
Activated charcoal (p.972·2).
Malodorous wounds; poisoning.

Carbosorb S *Delta, Austral.*
Activated charcoal (p.972·2); sorbitol (p.1354·2).
Drug overdose; poisoning.

Carbospect *Mer-National, S.Afr.*
Carbocisteine (p.1056·3).
Respiratory-tract disorders.

Carbostesin
Astra, Aust.; Astra, Ger.; Astra, Switz.
Bupivacaine hydrochloride (p.1286·3).
Adrenaline acid tartrate (p.813·3) is included in some injections as a vasoconstrictor to diminish absorption and localise the effect of the local anaesthetic.
Local anaesthesia.

Carbosylane *Serolam, Fr.*
Activated charcoal (p.972·2); dimethicone (p.1213·1).
Gastro-intestinal disorders.

Carbosylane Bi-Attivo *Giuliani, Ital.†.*
Activated charcoal (p.972·2); simethicone (p.1213·1).
Gastro-intestinal disorders.

Carbo-Syrup *Brovar, S.Afr.†.*
Carbocisteine (p.1056·3).
Respiratory-tract disorders.

Carboticon
Note. This name is used for preparations of different composition.
Byk, Neth.†.
Simethicone (p.1213·1).
Flatulence.

Interdelta, Switz.
Activated charcoal (p.972·2); simethicone (p.1213·1).
Digestive disorders; flatulence.

Carbotiol *Bouty, Ital.*
Killed bacteria: *Escherichia coli*; *Streptococcus ovalis*; *Micrococcus pyogenes* var. *aureus*; *Proteus vulgaris*; vegetable charcoal (p.972·3); kaolin (p.1195·1); sodium sulphate (p.1213·3); sodium bicarbonate (p.1153·2).
Gastro-intestinal disorders.

Carboyoghurt *Ilex, Ital.*
Vegetable charcoal (p.972·3); simethicone (p.1213·1).
Gastro-intestinal disorders.

Carbrital *Parke, Davis, Austral.†.*
Pentobarbitone sodium (p.685·1).
Insomnia; mental disorders; nervous disorders; premedication.

Carcinil *Abbott, Ger.*
Leuprorelin acetate (p.1253·1).
Prostatic cancer.

Cardalept
Note. This name is used for preparations of different composition.
Synpharma, Aust.
Crataegus (p.1568·2); melissa (p.1600·1); rosemary.
Cardiac disorders.

Keimdiat, Ger.†.
Rosemary; convallaria (p.1567·2); adonis (p.1543·3); crataegus (p.1568·2); melissa (p.1600·1); peppermint leaf (p.1208·1).
Hypotension.

Cardaminol *Reinecke, Ger.†.*
Oral drops: Homoeopathic preparation.
Tablets: Crataegus (p.1568·2); scoparium (p.1628·1); adonis vernalis (p.1543·3); ammi visnaga (p.1593·2); ephedra (p.1059·3); passion flower (p.1615·3); cereus grandiflorus; nicotinamide (p.1351·2); pentetrazol (p.1484·2); camphor (p.1557·2).
Hypotension.

Cardanat *Temmler, Ger.*
Etilefrine hydrochloride (p.867·2).
Formerly contained dimepropion hydrochloride and crataegus.
Hypotension.

Cardaxen *Spirig, Switz.*
Atenolol (p.825·3).
Angina pectoris; arrhythmias; hypertension; myocardial infarction.

Cardaxen plus *Spirig, Switz.*
Atenolol (p.825·3); chlorthalidone (p.839·3).
Hypertension.

Cardcal *Amrad, Austral.*
Diltiazem hydrochloride (p.854·2).
Angina pectoris.

Card-Dusodril *Lipha, Ger.†.*
Digoxin (p.849·3); naftidrofuryl oxalate (p.914·2).
Cardiovascular disorders.

Cardec DM Pediatric *Schein, USA.*
Pseudoephedrine hydrochloride (p.1068·3); dextromethorphan hydrobromide (p.1057·3); carbinoxamine maleate (p.404·2).
Coughs and cold symptoms.

Cardec-S *Barre-National, USA.*
Pseudoephedrine hydrochloride (p.1068·3); carbinoxamine maleate (p.404·2).
Upper respiratory-tract symptoms.

Cardegic *Synthelabo, Belg.*
Lysine aspirin (p.50·3).
Thrombo-embolic disorders.

Cardem *Rhone-Poulenc Rorer, Spain.*
Celiprolol hydrochloride (p.838·3).
Angina pectoris; hypertension.

Cardene
Roche, Canad.; Roche, Irl.; Yamanouchi, Neth.; Roche, UK; Syntex, USA.
Nicardipine hydrochloride (p.915·1).
Angina pectoris; hypertension.

Cardeymin *Cantassium Co., UK.*
Magnesium orotate (p.1611·2); bromelain (p.1555·1); potassium orotate (p.1611·2).

Card-Floe II *Sisu, Canad.*
Multivitamin and mineral preparation.

Card-Fludilat *Thiemann, Ger.†.*
Bencyclane fumarate (p.827·3); digoxin (p.849·3).
Cardiovascular disorders.

Cardiacton *Byk, Aust.*
Diltiazem hydrochloride (p.854·2).
Angina pectoris; hypertension.

Cardiacum I S *Pascoe, Ger.†.*
Crataegus flowers (p.1568·2); convallaria (p.1567·2).
Cardiac disorders.

Cardiacum II S *Pascoe, Ger.†.*
Crataegus flowers (p.1568·2); quebracho bark; convallaria (p.1567·2); kalmia latifolia; santakraut.
Cardiac disorders.

Cardiacum PMD *Plantamed, Ger.*
Homoeopathic preparation.

Cardiaforce *Bioforce, Switz.*
Crataegus (p.1568·2); melissa (p.1600·1); wine.
Sleep disorders; tachycardia.

Cardiagen *APS, Ger.*
Crataegus (p.1568·2); camphor (p.1557·2).
Cardiovascular disorders.

Cardiagutt *Engelhard, Ger.†.*
Verapamil hydrochloride (p.960·3).
Cardiac disorders; hypertension.

Cardialgine *Rosen, Ger.*
Etilefrine hydrochloride (p.867·2).
Hypotension.

Cardiavis C *Truw, Ger.†.*
Herbal and homoeopathic preparation.

Cardiazol-Paracodina *Knoll, Ital.*
Pentetrazol (p.1484·2); dihydrocodeine thiocyanate (p.34·2).
Coughs.

cardibeltin *Schwarz, Ger.†.*
Verapamil hydrochloride (p.960·3).
Angina pectoris; arrhythmias; hypertension.

Cardibisana *Hotz, Ger.*
Crataegus (p.1568·2); cinchona bark (p.1564·1); cola (p.1645·1); convallaria (p.1567·2); cereus grandiflorus; ephedra (p.1059·3); ginseng (p.1584·2); camphora; thi-

amine hydrochloride; veratrum; strophanthus; phosphorus; glonoinum; arsenicum album.
Cardiovascular disorders.

Cardiblok *Xixia, S.Afr.*
Propranolol hydrochloride (p.937·1).
Angina pectoris; anxiety; arrhythmias; hypertension; hyperthyroidism; phaeochromocytoma.

Cardifen *SA Druggists, S.Afr.*
Nifedipine (p.916·2).
Angina pectoris.

Cardilate
Note. A similar name is used for preparations of different composition.
Glaxo Wellcome, Ital.; Wellcome, USA†.
Erythrityl tetranitrate (p.866·1).
Angina pectoris.

Cardilate MR
Note. A similar name is used for preparations of different composition.
Norton, UK.
Nifedipine (p.916·2).
Angina pectoris; hypertension.

Cardimax *Garec, S.Afr.*
Propranolol (p.937·2).
Angina pectoris; arrhythmias; hypertension; hyperthyroidism; phaeochromocytoma.

Cardimet *Errekappa, Ital.*
Carnitine (p.1336·2).
Carnitine deficiency; myocardial ischaemia.

Cardinol *CP Pharmaceuticals, UK.*
Propranolol hydrochloride (p.937·1).
Angina pectoris; anxiety; arrhythmias; essential tremor; hypertension; hyperthyroidism; migraine; myocardial infarction; phaeochromocytoma.

Cardinorma *Pekana, Ger.*
Homoeopathic preparation.

Card-Instenon *Byk Gulden, Ger.†.*
Hexobendine hydrochloride (p.883·1); ethamivan (p.1480·3); etofylline (p.753·1); digoxin (p.849·3).
Cardiovascular disorders.

Cardioaspirin *Bayer, Ital.*
Aspirin (p.16·1).
Thrombo-embolic disorders.

Cardiocalm *Pharmastra, Fr.*
Crataegus (p.1568·2); phenobarbitone (p.350·2).
Insomnia; nervous disorders.

Cardiocap *Miba, Ital.*
Chromonar hydrochloride (p.840·1).
Ischaemic heart disease.

Cardio-Conray *May & Baker, Austral.†.*
Meglumine iothalamate (p.1008·1); sodium iothalamate (p.1008·1).
Contrast medium for urography and angiography.

Cardiodest *Biotrading, Ital.†.*
Suxamidofylline.
Respiratory-tract disorders.

Cardiodisco *Juste, Spain.*
Glyceryl trinitrate (p.874·3).
Angina pectoris.

Cardiodoron
Weleda, Aust.; Weleda, Ger.
Hyoscyamus herba; onopordon flower; primula flower.
Cardiac disorders.

Cardiofrik *Frika, Aust.*
Convallaria (p.1567·2); crataegus (p.1568·2); valerian (p.1643·1).
Cardiac disorders.

Cardiogen *Chemil, Ital.*
Carnitine (p.1336·2).
Carnitine deficiency; myocardial ischaemia.

CardioGen 82 *Squibb Diagnostics, USA.*
Rubidium-82 (p.1424·3).

Cardio-Green
Becton, Dickinson, Canad.†; Paesel, Ger.; Becton Dickinson, USA.
Indocyanine green (p.1590·3).
Diagnostic aid.

Cardiolan *Tosi, Ital.*
Medigoxin (p.902·1).
Heart failure.

Cardiolite
Du Pont, Aust.; Du Pont, Fr.
Technetium-99m sestamibi (p.1425·1).
Diagnosis and location of myocardial infarction; diagnosis of myocardial ischaemia and ventricular dysfunction.

Cardio-Longoral *Artesan, Ger.; Cassella-med, Ger.*
Potassium aspartate (p.1161·3); magnesium aspartate (p.1157·2); crataegus (p.1568·2).
Cardiac disorders.

Cardi-Omega 3 *Thompson, USA.*
Omega-3 marine triglycerides (p.1276·1).
Dietary supplement.

Cardio-Plantina *Plantina, Ger.*
Homoeopathic preparation.

Cardioplegia A *Baxter, Austral.*
Sodium chloride (p.1162·2); potassium chloride (p.1161·1); magnesium chloride (p.1157·2); calcium chloride (p.1155·1).
Induction of cardiac arrest during heart surgery.

Cardioplegia Solution *DBL, Austral.*
Magnesium chloride (p.1157·2); potassium chloride (p.1161·1); procaine hydrochloride (p.1299·2).
Induction of ischaemic cardiac arrest in heart surgery.

Cardioplegin N *Kohler, Ger.*
Magnesium aspartate (p.1157·2); procaine hydrochloride (p.1299·2); xylitol (p.1372·3).
Cardioplegia in open-heart surgery.

Cardiopril *Schwarz, Switz.*
Spirapril hydrochloride (p.946·1).
Hypertension.

Cardioprotect *Kytta, Ger.*
Verapamil hydrochloride (p.960·3).
Arrhythmias; hypertension; ischaemic heart disease.

Cardioquin
Purdue Frederick, Canad.; Asta Medica, Neth.; Purdue Frederick, USA.
Quinidine polygalacturonate (p.938·3).
Arrhythmias.

Cardioquine
Asta Medica, Belg.†; Asta Medica, Fr.; Berenguer Infale, Spain.
Quinidine polygalacturonate (p.938·3).
Arrhythmias.

Cardiorapide *Rapide, Spain†.*
Pentetrazol (p.1484·2).
Respiratory failure.

Cardiorapide Efed *Rapide, Spain†.*
Ephedrine (p.1059·3); pentetrazol (p.1484·2).
Circulatory disorders; respiratory disorders.

Cardioreg *Rhone-Poulenc, Ital.*
Injection†: Digoxin (p.849·3).
Cardiac disorders.
Tablets: β-Acetyldigoxin (p.812·3).
Heart failure.

Cardioselect *Dreluso, Ger.*
Homoeopathic preparation.

Cardiosimpal *Inibsa, Spain†.*
Diethylphenylephrine hydrochloride.
Hypotension.

Cardiostenol *Molteni, Ital.*
Morphine hydrochloride (p.56·1); atropine sulphate (p.455·1).
Adjuvant in anaesthesia; pain.

Cardiosteril *Fresenius, Ger.†.*
Dopamine hydrochloride (p.861·1).
Heart failure; hypotension; shock.

CardioTec *Squibb Diagnostics, USA.*
Technetium-99m teboroxime (p.1425·1).
Assessment of myocardial function.

Cardioten *OFF, Ital.*
Nicardipine hydrochloride (p.915·1).
Angina pectoris; heart failure; hypertension.

cardiotensin *Schwarz, Ger.†.*
Bemetizide (p.827·1); triamterene (p.957·2); bupranolol hydrochloride (p.835·2).
Hypertension.

Cardioton *NCSN, Ital.*
Ubidecarenone (p.1641·2).
Cardiopathy; coenzyme Q10 deficiency.

Cardiotonicum (Rowo-15) *Pharmakon, Ger.*
Homoeopathic preparation.
Lignocaine hydrochloride (p.1293·2) is included in this preparation to alleviate the pain of injection.

Cardiotonique "S" *Hanseler, Switz.†.*
Homoeopathic preparation.

Cardiovas *Knoll, Spain.*
Isosorbide mononitrate (p.893·3).
Angina pectoris; heart failure.

Cardioxane
Chiron, Fr.; Chiron, Ital.
Dexrazoxane hydrochloride (p.978·3).
Prevention of doxorubicin cardiotoxicity.

Cardip *Francia, Ital.*
Nicardipine hydrochloride (p.915·1).
Angina pectoris; heart failure; hypertension.

Cardiphyt *Austroplant, Aust.*
Crataegus (p.1568·2).
Cardiac disorders.

Cardiplant
Also, Ital.†; Schwabe, Switz.
Crataegus (p.1568·2).
Cardiac disorders.

Cardiprin *Reckitt & Colman, Austral.*
Aspirin (p.16·1).
Prevention of deep-vein thrombosis; prevention of stroke; prevention of vascular occlusion; secondary prevention of myocardial infarction; transient ischaemia.

Cardirene *Synthelabo, Ital.*
Lysine aspirin (p.50·3).
Myocardial infarction.

Cardiser *Merck, Spain.*
Diltiazem hydrochloride (p.854·2).
Angina pectoris; hypertension.

Cardisetten *Brenner-Efeka, Ger.†.*
Crataegus (p.1568·2); motherwort (p.1604·2); ammi visnaga (p.1593·2); valerian (p.1643·1); cereus grandiflorus; camphor (p.1557·2).
Cardiac disorders.

Cardispare *Rolab, S.Afr.*
Propranolol hydrochloride (p.937·1).
Hypertension.

Cardizem
ICI, Austral.; Hoechst Marion Roussel, Canad.; Pharmacia Upjohn, Norw.; Pharmacia Upjohn, Swed.; Marion Merrell Dow, USA.
Diltiazem hydrochloride (p.854·2).
Angina pectoris; arrhythmias; hypertension.

Card-Lamuran
Boehringer Mannheim, Aust.†; Boehringer Mannheim, Ger.†.
Raubasine (p.941·3); digoxin (p.849·3).
Cardiovascular disorders.

Cardol *Alphapharm, Austral.*
Sotalol hydrochloride (p.945·1).
Arrhythmias.

Card-Ompin S *Heumann, Ger.†.*
Convallaria (p.1567·2); adonis vernalis (p.1543·3); crataegus (p.1568·2); valerian (p.1643·1).
Cardiac disorders.

Cardopax *Orion, Swed.†.*
Isosorbide dinitrate (p.893·1).
Vasodilator.

Cardophyllin *Hamilton, Austral.†.*
Aminophylline (p.748·1).
Obstructive airways disease.

Cardovar BD *Bristol, Ger.†.*
Trimazosin hydrochloride (p.958·3).
Hypertension.

Carduben *Madaus, Ger.*
Ammi visnaga fruit (p.1593·2).
Cardiac disorders.

Cardular *Pfizer, Ger.*
Doxazosin mesylate (p.862·3).
Benign prostatic hyperplasia; hypertension.

Cardura
Astra, Canad.; Invicta, Irl.; Roerig, Ital.; Pfizer, Neth.; Pfizer, S.Afr.; Pfizer, UK; Roerig, USA.
Doxazosin mesylate (p.862·3).
Benign prostatic hyperplasia; hypertension.

Carduran
Pfizer, Austral.; Pfizer, Norw.; Pfizer, Spain.
Doxazosin mesylate (p.862·3).
Benign prostatic hyperplasia; hypertension.

Carduus-monoplant *Weber & Weber, Ger.*
Silybum marianum (p.993·3).
Liver disorders.

Carefluor *Beta, Ital.†.*
Cetylpyridinium chloride (p.1106·2); sodium fluoride (p.742·1); sodium monofluorophosphate (p.743·3).
Oral disinfection.

Carencyl *Riom, Fr.*
Multivitamin, amino-acid, and mineral preparation.
Tonic.

Carentil *Funk, Spain.*
Conjugated oestrogens (p.1457·3).
Female hypogonadism; menopausal disorders; osteoporosis.

Caress *Schering-Plough, Swed.*
Urea (p.1095·2).
Dry skin.

Carfenil *Chugai, Jpn.*
Lobenzarit sodium (p.1596·3).
Rheumatoid arthritis.

Cargutt *Hanosan, Ger.†.*
Homoeopathic preparation.

Cariamyl *Delalande, Switz.†.*
Heptaminol acephyllinate (p.754·1).
Cardio-pulmonary insufficiency; hypotension.

Cariban *Inibsa, Spain.*
Doxylamine succinate (p.410·1); pyridoxine hydrochloride (p.1362·3).
Nausea; vomiting.

Caricef *Pharmacia Upjohn, Spain.*
Cephazolin sodium (p.181·1).
Lignocaine hydrochloride (p.1293·2) is included in the intramuscular injection to alleviate the pain of injection.
Bacterial infections.

Caril *Nutricia, Fr.*
Carrots, rice, dextrin-maltose, glucose, and electrolytes (p.1152·3).
Diarrhoea.

Carilax *Strallhofer, Aust.*
Senna (p.1212·2).
Bowel evacuation; constipation.

Carin *Corvi, Ital.†.*
Aspirin (p.16·1); ascorbic acid (p.1365·2).
Flu symptoms; pain.

Carin all'Arancia *Corvi, Ital.†.*
Aspirin (p.16·1); ascorbic acid (p.1365·2).
Flu symptoms; pain.

Carin 300 all'Arancia *Corvi, Ital.†.*
Ascorbic acid (p.1365·2); calcium ascorbate (p.1365·2); aspirin (p.16·1).
Flu symptoms; pain.

Carindapen *Pfizer, Ger.†.*
Carindacillin sodium (p.163·1).
Bacterial infections of the urinary tract.

Cariomix *INTES, Ital.*
Xanthopterin; human placenta extract.
Corneal ulcers, burns, and wounds; herpetic keratitis.

Carisano *Bilgast, Ger.*
Garlic (p.1583·1).
Lipid disorders.

Carisoma *Pharmax, UK.*
Carisoprodol (p.1312·3).
Skeletal muscle spasm.

Cari-Tab *Jones, USA†.*
Sodium fluoride (p.742·1) with multivitamins.

Carito *Hoyer, Ger.†.*
Onion (p.1610·2); echinacea purpururea (p.1574·2); cucurbita (p.1569·1); poplar buds (p.1620·1); damiana (p.1570·2); chondodendron tomentosum; aescin (p.1543·3).
Urinary-tract infections.

Carito mono
Europharm, Aust.; Hoyer, Ger.
Orthosiphon leaves (p.1592·2).
Urinary-tract disorders.

Carl Baders Divinal *Apotheke Heiligen Rupertus, Aust.*
Camphor and camphor spirit (p.1557·2); methyl salicylate (p.55·2); salicylic acid (p.1090·2); salol (p.83·1); turpentine oil (p.1641·1); rosemary oil (p.1626·2); menthol (p.1600·2).
Musculoskeletal and joint disorders.

Carlytene *Asta Medica, Fr.*
Thymoxamine hydrochloride (p.952·2).
Circulatory disorders.

Carmatis *Carmaran, Canad.*
Methyl salicylate (p.55·2); camphor (p.1557·2); menthol (p.1600·2).

Carmian *Teofarma, Ital.*
Atenolol (p.825·3); chlorthalidone (p.839·3).
Hypertension.

Carminagal N *Galenika, Ger.*
Cynara (p.1569·2).
Formerly contained cynara, pancreatin, and dimethicone.
Dyspepsia.

Carminat *Molitor, Ger.†.*
Peppermint leaf (p.1208·1); coriander (p.1567·3); caraway (p.1559·3); valerian (p.1643·1); cardamom (p.1560·1).
Gastro-intestinal disorders.

Carminative *Schoeller, Aust.*
Caraway tincture (p.1559·3); coriander tincture (p.1567·3); spearmint tincture (p.1632·1).
Flatulence.

Carminative Tea *Weleda, UK.*
Fennel seed (p.1579·1); aniseed (p.1549·3); caraway seed (p.1559·3); yarrow (p.1542·2); chamomile flowers (p.1561·2).
Flatulence.

Carminativo Ibys *Pharmacia Upjohn, Spain.*
Anise oil (p.1550·1); sodium bicarbonate (p.1153·2).
Aerophagia.

Carminativo Juventus *Juventus, Spain.*
Anise oil (p.1550·1); belladonna tincture (p.457·1); sodium bicarbonate (p.1153·2).
Aerophagia; flatulence; vomiting.

Carminativum Babynos
Byk, Aust.; Dentinox, Ger.
Fennel (p.1579·1); coriander (p.1567·3); matricaria flowers (p.1561·2).
Gastro-intestinal disorders.

Carminativum-Hetterich N *Galenika, Ger.*
Matricaria flowers (p.1561·2); peppermint leaf (p.1208·1); caraway (p.1559·3); fennel (p.1579·1); dried bitter-orange peel (p.1610·3).
Gastro-intestinal disorders.

Carminativum-Pascoe *Pascoe, Ger.*
Peppermint leaf (p.1208·1); chamomile (p.1561·2); caraway (p.1559·3).
Gastro-intestinal disorders.

Carminex *Propan, S.Afr.*
Magnesium carbonate (p.1198·1); sodium bicarbonate (p.1153·2); tinct. cardamom co. (p.1560·1); sodium citrate (p.1153·2).
Constipation; hyperchlorhydria.

Carmol
Note. This name is used for preparations of different composition.
Iromedica, Switz.†.
Drops for oral administration, topical administration, or inhalation: Anise oil (p.1550·1); clove oil (p.1565·2); cinnamon oil (p.1564·2); lemon oil (p.1595·3); lavender oil (p.1594·3); nutmeg oil (p.1609·3); lemon grass oil (p.1595·3); sage oil; thyme oil (p.1637·1); melissa (p.1600·1); mint.
Oil: Clove oil (p.1565·2); cinnamon oil (p.1564·2); lavender oil (p.1594·3); spike lavender oil (p.1632·2); nutmeg oil (p.1609·3); melissa oil; anise oil (p.1550·1); lemon oil (p.1595·3); thyme oil (p.1637·1); sage oil; mint oil (p.1604·1).
Gastro-intestinal disorders; musculoskeletal and joint pain; respiratory-tract disorders.
Topical gel: Menthol (p.1600·2); camphor (p.1557·2); anise oil (p.1550·1); clove oil (p.1565·2); lavender oil (p.1594·3); mace oil (p.1597·3); lemon grass oil (p.1595·3); sage oil; thyme oil (p.1637·1); eucalyptus oil (p.1578·1); turpentine oil (p.1641·1); oleum pini sylvestris; rosemary oil (p.1626·2); lignocaine hydrochloride (p.1293·2); methyl salicylate (p.55·2).
Musculoskeletal and joint disorders; soft-tissue disorders.

Doak, USA.
Urea (p.1095·2).
Dry skin; hyperkeratosis.

Carmol "blanche" *Iromedica, Switz.†.*
Menthol (p.1600·2); camphor (p.1557·2); methyl salicylate (p.55·2); guaiacol (p.1061·2); anise oil (p.1550·1); clove oil (p.1565·2); eucalyptus oil (p.1578·1); mace oil (p.1597·3); melissa oil; sage oil; thyme oil (p.1637·1); turpentine oil (p.1641·1).
Musculoskeletal and joint pain; respiratory-tract disorders; soft-tissue disorders.

Carmol HC *Doak, USA.*
Hydrocortisone acetate (p.1043·3).
Corticosteroid.

Carmol "thermogene" *Iromedica, Switz.†.*
Menthol (p.1600·2); camphor (p.1557·2); methyl salicylate (p.55·2); anise oil (p.1550·1); clove oil (p.1565·2); eucalyptus oil (p.1578·1); nutmeg oil (p.1609·3); melissa oil; rosemary oil (p.1626·2); sage

oil; thyme oil (p.1637·1); cayenne pepper; citral; allantoin (p.1078·2).
Musculoskeletal and joint pain; respiratory-tract disorders.

Carmubris *Bristol-Myers Squibb, Ger.*
Carmustine (p.511·3).
Malignant neoplasms.

Carnation
Note. This name is used for preparations of different composition.
Clintec, Canad.
A range of preparations for enteral nutrition.
Cuxson, Gerrard, UK.
Salicylic acid (p.1090·2).
Calluses; corns; verrucas.

Carnicor *Max Farma, Ital.; Sigma-Tau, Spain.*
Carnitine (p.1336·2).
Carnitine deficiency; myocardial ischaemia.

Carnidex *Farmades, Ital.†.*
Carnitine (p.1336·2).
Cardiac disorders.

Carnigen *Albert-Roussel, Aust.; Albert-Roussel, Ger.; Hoechst, Ger.*
Oxilofrine hydrochloride (p.925·3).
Circulatory disorders; orthostatic hypotension.

Carnitolo *Pharmarecord, Ital.*
Carnitine hydrochloride (p.1336·2).
Carnitine deficiency; myocardial ischaemia.

Carnitop *Virginia, Ital.*
Carnitine (p.1336·2).
Carnitine deficiency; myocardial ischaemia.

Carnitor *Sigma-Tau, Canad.; Shire, UK; Sigma-Tau, USA.*
Carnitine (p.1336·2).
Carnitine deficiency.

Carnovis *Duncan, Ital.*
Carnitine (p.1336·2) or carnitine hydrochloride (p.1336·2).
Carnitine deficiency; myocardial ischaemia.

Carnum *FIRMA, Ital.*
Carnitine (p.1336·2).
Carnitine deficiency.

Carobel *Baxter, Austral.†; Cow & Gate, Irl.; Cow & Gate, UK.*
Ceratonia (p.1472·2).
Feed thickener to control vomiting.

Carogil *Diepal, Fr.*
Carrots, rice, dextrin-maltose, and electrolytes (p.1152·3).
Diarrhoea.

Caroid *Mentholatum, Canad.*
Cascara (p.1183·1); phenolphthalein (p.1208·2); ox bile (p.1553·2).

Carominthe *Lehning, Fr.*
Homoeopathic preparation.

Carotaben *Merck, Aust.; Hermal, Ger.; Boots Healthcare, Neth.; Hermal, Switz.*
Betacarotene (p.1335·2).
Erythropoietic protoporphyria; photodermatitis; skin pigmentation disorders.

Carotin *Twardy, Ger.*
Betacarotene (p.1335·2); biotin (p.1336·1); calcium D-pantothenate (p.1352·3).
Sunburn.

Carovit *Biochimici, Ital.*
Betacarotene with vitamin E.
Nutritional supplement.

Carovit Forte *Biochimici, Ital.*
Betacarotene with vitamins E and C.
Nutritional supplement.

Carpantin *Sanofi Winthrop, Ital.*
Pantethine (p.1276·3); carnitine chloride (p.1336·2); cyproheptadine hydrochloride (p.407·2).
Tonic.

Carpaz *Rolab, S.Afr.*
Carbamazepine (p.339·2).
Epilepsy; trigeminal neuralgia.

Carpilo *Chauvin, Fr.*
Pilocarpine nitrate (p.1396·3); carteolol hydrochloride (p.837·3).
Glaucoma; ocular hypertension.

Carpinplast *Llorens, Spain†.*
Pilocarpine hydrochloride (p.1396·3).
Glaucoma; production of miosis.

Carreldon *Bama, Spain.*
Diltiazem hydrochloride (p.854·2).
Angina pectoris; hypertension; myocardial infarction.

Carrier *Chiesi, Ital.*
Carnitine (p.1336·2).
Carnitine deficiency; myocardial ischaemia.

Carteol *Asta Medica, Belg.; Chauvin, Fr.; SIFI, Ital.*
Carteolol hydrochloride (p.837·3).
Ocular hypertension; open-angle glaucoma.

Carter Petites Pilules *Carter-Wallace, Switz.*
Aloin (p.1177·2); phenolphthalein (p.1208·2); liquorice (p.1197·1).
Constipation.

Carters
Note. This name is used for preparations of different composition.
Therabel Pharma, Belg.
Aloes (p.1177·1); podophyllum resin (p.1089·1).
Constipation.
Carter-Wallace, UK.
Aloin (p.1177·2); phenolphthalein (p.1208·2).
Constipation.

Carters Little Pills *Carter Horner, Canad.*
Aloin (p.1177·2); phenolphthalein (p.1208·2).
Constipation.

Carthamex *Rolmex, Canad.*
Vitamin B_6 (p.1362·3) in safflower oil.

Cartia *SmithKline Beecham, Austral.*
Aspirin (p.16·1).
Anti-platelet agent; vascular disorders.

Cartrol *Sanofi, UK†; Abbott, USA.*
Carteolol hydrochloride (p.837·3).
Angina pectoris; hypertension.

Carudol
Note. This name is used for preparations of different composition.
Boehringer Ingelheim, Fr.
Phenylbutazone piperazine (p.79·3); methyl nicotinate (p.55·1); piperazine hydrate (p.107·2).
Musculoskeletal and joint disorders.
Boehringer Ingelheim, Ital.†; Fher, Spain.
Phenylbutazone piperazine (p.79·3).
Gout; musculoskeletal and joint disorders.
Wild, Switz.
Phenylbutazone piperazine (p.79·3); piperazine hydrate (p.107·2).
Musculoskeletal, joint, and peri-articular pain; soft-tissue disorders.

Carvasin *Wyeth, Ital.*
Isosorbide dinitrate (p.893·1).
Ischaemic heart disease.

Carvipress *Gentili, Ital.*
Carvedilol (p.838·1).
Angina pectoris; hypertension.

Carvis *Volchem, Ital.*
Carnitine (p.1336·2).
Tonic.

Carvit *AGIPS, Ital.*
Carnitine (p.1336·2).
Carnitine deficiency; myocardial ischaemia.

Carvomin *Wernigerode, Ger.*
Angelica; carduus benedictus (p.1565·3); peppermint leaf (p.1208·1).
Gastro-intestinal disorders.

Carvomin Magentropfen mit Pomeranze *Madaus, Ger.*
Bitter-orange peel (p.1610·3).
Dyspepsia.

Carylderm *Seton, Irl.; Seton, UK.*
Carbaryl (p.1403·1).
Carylderm Liquid was formerly known as Derbac-C in the *UK*.
Pediculosis.

Caryolysine *Synthelabo, Fr.*
Mustine hydrochloride (p.555·1).
Leukaemias; lymphomas; mycosis fungoides; psoriasis.

Carzem *Rottapharm, Ital.*
Diltiazem hydrochloride (p.854·2).
Hypertension; ischaemic heart disease.

Carzodelan *Gaschler, Ger.*
Pancreatin (p.1612·1).
Inflammatory disorders.

Casacol *Helsinn Birex, Irl.*
Methoxyphenamine hydrochloride (p.1063·3); guaiphenesin (p.1061·3); sodium citrate (p.1153·2).
Coughs.

Casalm *Pharmacia Upjohn, Aust.; Pharmacia Upjohn, Ger.*
Salcatonin (p.735·3).
Hypercalcaemia; osteolysis; osteoporosis; Paget's disease of bone; reflex sympathetic dystrophy.

Cascade *Modern Health Products, UK.*
Bearberry (p.1552·2); clivers (p.1565·2); burdock root (p.1594·2).
Water retention.

Cascalax *Will-Pharma, Belg.*
Casanthranol (p.1182·3).
Constipation.

Cascapride *Merck, Ger.*
Capsules: Bromopride (p.1181·3).
Oral drops†: Bromopride hydrochloride (p.1181·3).
Gastro-intestinal disorders.

Cascara-Salax *Ferring, Ger.; Ferring, Switz.*
Powder for oral solution, dried magnesium sulphate (p.1158·2); tablets, cascara (p.1183·1).
Bowel evacuation.

Casec *Mead Johnson, Canad.†; Mead Johnson Nutritionals, USA.*
Calcium caseinate.
Protein supplement.

Casilan *Crookes, Irl.†; Crookes Healthcare, UK†.*
Protein preparation.
Hypoproteinaemia.

Casodex *Zeneca, Canad.; Zeneca, Ger.; Zeneca, Irl.; Zeneca, Ital.; Zeneca, Neth.; Zeneca, Norw.; Zeneca, S.Afr.; Zeneca, Spain; Zeneca, Swed.; Zeneca, Switz.; Zeneca, UK; Zeneca, USA.*
Bicalutamide (p.507·2).
Prostatic cancer.

Caspiselenio *Kin, Spain.*
Selenium sulphide (p.1091·1).
Skin disorders.

Cassadan *Dresden, Ger.*
Alprazolam (p.640·3).
Anxiety.

Castaderm *Lannett, USA.*
Resorcinol (p.1090·1); boric acid (p.1554·2); phenol (p.1121·2).
Fungal skin infections.

Castel *Syosset, USA.*
Resorcinol (p.1090·1).
Fungal skin infections.

Castellani Neu *Hollborn, Ger.*
Miconazole (p.384·3).
Fungal and bacterial skin infections.

Ca-sterogyl *Roussel, Ital.†.*
Multivitamins and calcium.

Castindia *Vaillant, Ital.*
Aesculus (p.1543·3); silybum marianum (p.993·3); hamamelis (p.1587·1).
Peripheral vascular disorders.

Castoria *Mentholatum, Canad.*
Sennoside A and B (p.1212·3).

Castrophan *Repha, Ger.†.*
Convallaria (p.1567·2); melissa (p.1600·1); adonis vernalis (p.1543·3); mistletoe (p.1604·1); cinchona bark (p.1564·1); peppermint leaf (p.1208·1); arnica (p.1550·3); levisticum officinale (p.1597·2); hypericum (p.1590·1); valerian (p.1643·1); cactus; camphora; crataegus; scilla; oleander; aurum coll.; spigelia.
Cardiac disease.

Castufemin N *Ardeypharm, Ger.*
Agnus castus (p.1544·2).
Mastalgia; menstrual disorders.

Catabex
Note. This name is used for preparations of different composition.
Darci, Belg.
Dropropizine (p.1059·2).
Coughs.
Darcy, Fr.
Dropropizine (p.1059·2); guaiphenesin (p.1061·3).
Coughs.

Catabex Expectorans *Darci, Belg.*
Dropropizine (p.1059·2); guaiphenesin (p.1061·3).
Coughs.

Cataclot *Ono, Jpn.*
Ozagrel sodium (p.1612·1).
Cerebrovascular disorders.

Catacol *Alcon, Fr.; Alcon, Switz.*
Disodium inosinate (p.1573·1).
Eye disorders.

Cataflam *Ciba-Geigy, Belg.; Geigy, Irl.; Ciba, Ital.; Novartis, Neth.; Novartis, S.Afr.; Novartis, USA.*
Diclofenac potassium (p.31·2).
Gout; musculoskeletal, joint, and peri-articular disorders; pain.

Catalgine *Schwarz, Fr.*
Sodium aspirin (p.18·2).
Fever; musculoskeletal and joint disorders; myocardial infarction; pain.

Catalgine a la vitamine C *Pharmacia Upjohn, Fr.†.*
Sodium aspirin (p.18·2); ascorbic acid (p.1365·2).
Fever; influenza.

Catalgix *Rhone-Poulenc Rorer, Belg.*
Aspirin (p.16·1).
Fever; migraine; rheumatic disorders.

Catalgix C *Rhone-Poulenc Rorer, Belg.*
Aspirin (p.16·1); ascorbic acid (p.1365·2).
Fever; migraine; rheumatic disorders.

Catanidin *Bender, Aust.*
Clonidine hydrochloride (p.841·2) or clonidine tosylate (p.842·2).
Hypertension.

Catapres *Boehringer Ingelheim, Austral.; Boehringer Ingelheim, Canad.; Boehringer Ingelheim, Irl.; Boehringer Ingelheim, S.Afr.; Boehringer Ingelheim, UK; Boehringer Ingelheim, USA.*
Clonidine hydrochloride (p.841·2).
Hypertension; menopausal flushing; migraine.

Catapresan *Bender, Aust.; Boehringer Ingelheim, Ger.; Boehringer Ingelheim, Ital.; Boehringer Ingelheim, Neth.; Boehringer Ingelheim, Norw.; Boehringer Ingelheim, Spain; Boehringer Ingelheim, Swed.; Boehringer Ingelheim, Switz.*
Clonidine (p.842·2) or clonidine hydrochloride (p.841·2).
Hypertension; menopausal disorders; migraine; opioid withdrawal.

Catapressan *Boehringer Ingelheim, Belg.; Boehringer Ingelheim, Fr.*
Clonidine hydrochloride (p.841·2).
Hypertension.

Catarase *Iolab, Canad.†.*
Chymotrypsin (p.1563·2).
Adjunct in cataract surgery.

Cataridol *Ciba Vision, Fr.*
Sodium iodide (p.1493·2); calcium chloride (p.1155·1).
Eye disorders.

Catarrh *Larkhall Laboratories, UK.*
Yarrow (p.1542·2); vervain; horehound (p.1063·3); salvia (p.1627·1).

Catarrh Cream *Weleda, UK.*
Esculoside (p.1543·3); berberis fruit; prunus spinosa fruit; bryonia alba; camphor (p.1557·2); echinacea purp. (p.1574·2); mercurius sulph.; eucalyptus oil (p.1578·1); peppermint oil (p.1208·1); thyme oil (p.1637·1).
Nasal congestion.

Catarrh Mixture *Potter's, UK.*
Boneset; blue flag (p.1591·3); burdock root (p.1594·2); hyssop; capsicum (p.1559·2).
Catarrh.

Catarrh Pastilles
Note. This name is used for preparations of different composition.
Healthcrafts, UK.
Squill vinegar (p.1070·1); menthol (p.1600·2); pumilio pine oil (p.1623·3); eucalyptus oil (p.1578·1).
Cough and cold symptoms.
Unichem, UK.
Menthol (p.1600·2); siberian fir oil; oleum pini sylvestris; creosote (p.1057·3).
Catarrh; coughs.

Catarrh Tablets *Healthcrafts, UK.*
Horehound (p.1063·3); squill (p.1070·1).
Catarrh; coughs.

Catarrh-eeze *English Grains, UK.*
Marrubium (p.1063·3); achillea (p.1542·2); inula (p.1059·2).
Catarrh.

Catarrh-Ex *Thompson, UK.*
Pseudoephedrine hydrochloride (p.1068·3); paracetamol (p.72·2).
Cold symptoms.

Catarstat *Chauvin, Fr.*
Pyridoxine hydrochloride (p.1362·3); glycine (p.1345·2); aspartic acid (p.1335·1); glutamic acid (p.1344·3).
Cataracts.

Catarstat Nouvelle formule *Novopharma, Switz.*
Pyridoxine hydrochloride (p.1362·3); amino acids.
Cataracts.

CAT-Barium (E-Z-CAT) *Bracco, Switz.*
Barium sulphate (p.1003·1).
Contrast medium for gastro-intestinal radiography.

Catemine *Tyson, USA.*
Tyrosine (p.1357·3); pyridoxal phosphate (p.1363·1).

Catex *Cantabria, Spain.*
Ciprofloxacin hydrochloride (p.185·3).
Bacterial infections.

Cathejell *Montavit, Aust.; Sodip, Switz.†.*
Diphenhydramine hydrochloride (p.409·1); chlorhexidine hydrochloride (p.1107·2).
Cystoscopy; endoscopy; lubrication for catheter insertion.

Cathejell mit Lidocain *Montavit, Aust.*
Lignocaine hydrochloride (p.1293·2); chlorhexidine hydrochloride (p.1107·2).
Catheterisation; instrument insertion.

Cathejell-N *Geistlich, Switz.*
Lignocaine hydrochloride (p.1293·2); chlorhexidine hydrochloride (p.1107·2).
Catheterisation.

Catheter Preparation *Delta, Austral.*
Chlorhexidine gluconate (p.1107·2).
Skin disinfection prior to bladder catheterisation.

Catonin *Magis, Ital.*
Salcatonin (p.735·3).
Hypercalcaemia; osteoporosis; Paget's disease of bone; reflex sympathetic dystrophy.

Catorid *Boehringer Ingelheim, Belg.*
Prolintane hydrochloride (p.1485·1).
Narcoleptic syndrome.

Catovit *Boehringer Ingelheim, Austral.†; Boehringer Ingelheim, S.Afr.*
Prolintane hydrochloride (p.1485·1); multivitamins.
Tonic.

Catrix *Donell DerMedex, USA.*
Emollient and moisturiser.

Catrix Correction *Donell DerMedex, USA.*
SPF 15: Ethylhexyl *p*-methoxycinnamate (p.1487·1); methyl anthranilate; oxybenzone (p.1487·3); titanium dioxide (p.1093·3).
Sunscreen.

Catrix Lip *Donell DerMedex, USA.*
SPF 15: Ethylhexyl *p*-methoxycinnamate (p.1487·1); oxybenzone (p.1487·3).
Sunscreen.

Causat *Sanofi Winthrop, Aust.*
Procaine hydrochloride (p.1299·2); atropine sulphate (p.455·1).
Migraine; neuralgia; neuritis.

Causat B12 N *Sanofi Winthrop, Ger.*
Procaine hydrochloride (p.1299·2); atropine sulphate (p.455·1); hydroxocobalamin hydrochloride (p.1364·2).
Arthrosis; migraine; neuralgia; neuritis.

Causat N *Sanofi Winthrop, Ger.*
Procaine hydrochloride (p.1299·2); atropine sulphate (p.455·1).
Migraine; neuralgia; neuritis; postherpetic neuralgia; trigeminal neuralgia.

Caustinerf forte *Septodont, Switz.*
Lignocaine (p.1293·2); phenol (p.1121·2); paraformaldehyde (p.1121·1).
Dental pain.

Causyth *Inverni della Beffa, Ital.†.*
Propyphenazone (p.81·3).
Fever; pain.

Cavedess *Astra, Swed.†.*
Deglycyrrhizinised liquorice (p.1197·1); bismuth subnitrate (p.1180·2); colloidal aluminium hydroxide (p.1177·3); sodium bicarbonate (p.1153·2); magnesium subcarbonate (p.1198·1); fennel (p.1579·1).
Peptic ulcer.

Caved-S
Note. This name is used for preparations of different composition.
Byk, Aust.
Deglycyrrhizinised liquorice (p.1197·1); magnesium carbonate (p.1198·1); aluminium hydroxide (p.1177·3); sodium bicarbonate (p.1153·2); fennel (p.1579·1).
Hyperacidity; peptic ulcer.

Sarget, Fr.†.
Deglycyrrhizinised liquorice (p.1197·1); aluminium hydroxide (p.1177·3); magnesium carbonate (p.1198·1); calamus (p.1556·1).
Gastritis; peptic ulcer.

Recordati, Ital.†.
Deglycyrrhizinised liquorice (p.1197·1); aluminium hydroxide (p.1177·3); magnesium carbonate (p.1198·1); sodium bicarbonate (p.1153·2); frangula bark (p.1193·2).
Gastritis; hyperchlorhydria; peptic ulcer.

Byk, Neth.†; Byk Gulden, S.Afr.†; Pharmacia Upjohn, UK†.
Deglycyrrhizinised liquorice (p.1197·1); aluminium hydroxide (p.1177·3); magnesium carbonate (p.1198·1); sodium bicarbonate (p.1153·2); bismuth subnitrate (p.1180·2).
Gastritis; gastro-intestinal hyperacidity; peptic ulcer.

Casen Fisons, Spain.
Deglycyrrhizinised liquorice (p.1197·1); colloidal aluminium hydroxide (p.1177·3); magnesium carbonate (p.1198·1); sodium bicarbonate (p.1153·2); calamus (p.1556·1); frangula bark (p.1193·2).
Gastro-intestinal hyperacidity.

Pharmakon, Switz.
Deglycyrrhizinised liquorice (p.1197·1); dried aluminium hydroxide gel (p.1177·3); magnesium carbonate (p.1198·1); sodium bicarbonate (p.1153·2); frangula (p.1193·2); calamus (p.1556·1); fennel (p.1579·2).
Gastro-intestinal disorders.

Caved-S N *Promonta, Ger.†.*
Deglycyrrhizinised liquorice (p.1197·1); aluminium hydroxide gel (p.1177·3); light magnesium carbonate (p.1198·1).
Gastroduodenitis; peptic ulcer.

Caverject
Pharmacia Upjohn, Aust.; Pharmacia Upjohn, Austral.; Pharmacia Upjohn, Belg.; Pharmacia Upjohn, Canad.; Pharmacia Upjohn, Fr.; Pharmacia Upjohn, Irl.; Pharmacia Upjohn, Ital.; Pharmacia Upjohn, Neth.; Pharmacia Upjohn, Norw.; Pharmacia Upjohn, S.Afr.; Upjohn, Spain; Pharmacia Upjohn, Swed.; Pharmacia Upjohn, Switz.; Pharmacia Upjohn, UK.
Alprostadil (p.1412·2).
Impotence.

Cavinton
Kwizda, Aust.†; Thiemann, Ger.
Vinpocetine (p.1644·2).
Cerebrovascular disorders.

Cavum Pediatrico *Boots, Spain†.*
Chlorhexidine acetate (p.1107·2); tyrothricin (p.267·2); trypsin (p.1640·1).
Upper-respiratory-tract infection.

Cav-X *Palisades, USA†.*
Stannous fluoride (p.1632·2).

Caye Balsam *Medopharm, Ger.*
Glycol salicylate (p.43·1); sodium salamidacetate (p.82·3); benzyl nicotinate (p.22·1); capsicum (p.1559·2); coumarin (p.1568·1).
Muscular, neuromuscular, and joint disorders; sports injuries.

C-Calcium *Streuli, Switz.*
Calcium gluconate (p.1155·2); ascorbic acid (p.1365·2); calcium saccharate (p.1557·1).
Vitamin C and calcium deficiency.

CCNU
Almirall, Spain†; Lundbeck, UK.
Lomustine (p.544·1).
Malignant neoplasms.

C-Destrosio *Roussel, Ital.†.*
Ascorbic acid (p.1365·2); glucose (p.1343·3).
Vitamin C deficiency.

C-Dose *Medgenix, Belg.*
Ascorbic acid (p.1365·2).
Scurvy; vitamin C deficiency.

CDT Vaccine *CSL, Austral.*
An adsorbed diphtheria and tetanus vaccine (p.1508·1).
Active immunisation of infants and young children.

Ceanel
Quinoderm, Irl.; Hoechst Marion Roussel, S.Afr.; Quinoderm, UK.
Cetrimide (p.1105·2); undecenoic acid (p.389·2); phenethyl alcohol (p.1121·1).
Dandruff; psoriasis; seborrhoeic dermatitis.

CEA-Scan
Byk Gulden, Ital.; Immunomedics, USA.
Technetium-99m arcitumomab (p.1425·1).
Detection of colorectal cancer.

Cebedex *Chauvin, Fr.*
Dexamethasone sodium phosphate (p.1037·2).
Eye disorders.

Cebedexacol *Chauvin, Fr.*
Chloramphenicol (p.182·1); dexamethasone sodium phosphate (p.1037·2).
Eye infections.

Cebemyxine *Chauvin, Fr.*
Neomycin sulphate (p.229·2); polymyxin B sulphate (p.239·1).
The eye ointment formerly contained neomycin sulphate, polymyxin B sulphate, and bacitracin zinc.
Eye infections.

Cebenicol *Chauvin, Fr.*
Chloramphenicol (p.182·1).
Eye infections.

Cebera *Irex, Fr.*
Alibendol (p.1545·1).
Dyspepsia.

Cebesine *Chauvin, Fr.*
Oxybuprocaine hydrochloride (p.1298·1).
Local anaesthesia.

Cebid *Hauck, USA.*
Ascorbic acid (p.1365·2).
Scurvy; vitamin C deficiency.

Cebion
Merck, Aust.; Merck, Ger.; Bracco, Ital.; Merck, S.Afr.†; Merck, Spain.
Ascorbic acid (p.1365·2).
Gingivitis; methaemoglobinaemia; stomatitis; vitamin C deficiency.

Cebion Erkaltungs *Merck, Ger.*
Aspirin (p.16·1); ascorbic acid (p.1365·2).
Cold symptoms; fever; pain.

Cebion N *Merck, Ger.*
Sodium ascorbate (p.1365·2).
Methaemoglobinaemia; vitamin C deficiency.

Cebion-Calcium N *Merck, S.Afr.*
Calcium carbonate (p.1182·1); ascorbic acid (p.1365·2).
Calcium supplement.

Cebiopirina *Bracco, Ital.*
Ascorbic acid (p.1365·2); aspirin (p.16·1).
Cold symptoms; pain.

Cebran
Note. This name is used for preparations of different composition.
Garant, Ital.
Nicergoline (p.1607·1).
Cerebral and peripheral vascular disorders.

Ripari-Gero, Ital.†.
Suprarenal cortex (p.1050·1); cyanocobalamin (p.1363·3); inositol (p.1591·1); nicotinamide (p.1351·2).
Anaemias; asthenia.

Cebroton *San Carlo, Ital.*
Citicoline sodium (p.1564·3).
Cerebrovascular disorders; mental function impairment; parkinsonism.

Cebutid *Knoll, Fr.*
Flurbiprofen (p.42·1).
Inflammation; pain; prevention of vascular re-occlusion; secondary prevention of myocardial infarction.

Cec
Hexal, Ger.; Hexal, S.Afr.
Cefaclor (p.163·2).
Bacterial infections.

Ce-ca-bion N *Merck, Ger.†.*
Ascorbic acid (p.1365·2); calcium carbonate (p.1182·1).
Calcium and vitamin C deficiency.

Cecenu
Rhone-Poulenc Rorer, Belg.; Medac, Ger.
Lomustine (p.544·1).
Malignant neoplasms.

Ceclor
Lilly, Aust.; Lilly, Austral.; Lilly, Belg.; Lilly, Canad.; Lilly, Neth.; Lilly, S.Afr.; Lilly, Spain; Lilly, Switz.; Lilly, USA.
Cefaclor (p.163·2).
Bacterial infections.

Ceclorbeta *Betapharm, Ger.*
Cefaclor (p.163·2).
Bacterial infections.

Cecon
Note. This name is used for preparations of different composition.
Abbott, Austral.; Abbott, USA.
Ascorbic acid (p.1365·2).
Scurvy; vitamin C deficiency.

Abbott, Ital.
Oral drops; oral powder: Ascorbic acid (p.1365·2).
Tablets: Sodium ascorbate (p.1365·2); ascorbic acid (p.1365·2).
Vitamin C deficiency.

Cecrisina *Syntex, Spain†.*
Ascorbic acid (p.1365·2).
Methaemoglobinaemia; vitamin C deficiency.

Cedanon *Sanabo, Aust.*
Propyphenazone (p.81·3); dihydroergotamine mesylate (p.444·2); caffeine (p.749·3).
Migraine and related vascular headache.

Cedax
Schering-Plough, Irl.; Schering-Plough, Ital.; Schering-Plough, Neth.; Schering-Plough, S.Afr.; Schering-Plough, Spain; Schering-Plough, Swed.; Essex, Switz.; Schering-Plough, UK; Schering, USA.
Ceftibuten (p.175·1).
Bacterial infections.

Cedigocine *Sandoz, Switz.†.*
Acetyldigoxin (p.812·3).
Heart failure.

Cedigossina *Sandoz, Ital.†.*
Acetyldigoxin (p.812·3).
Cardiac disorders.

Cedilanid
Note. This name is used for preparations of different composition.
Sandoz, Aust.
Injection: Deslanoside (p.847·2).
Tablets: Lanatoside C (p.897·2).
Arrhythmias; heart failure.

Sandoz, Ger.†; Sandoz, Irl.†; Sandoz, Ital.†; Sandoz, S.Afr.†.
Lanatoside C (p.897·2).
Cardiac disorders.

Cedilanide *Sandoz, Fr.*
Deslanoside (p.847·2).
Pulmonary oedema; supraventricular arrhythmias.

Cedine *Rowex, Irl.*
Cimetidine (p.1183·2).
Gastric hyperacidity; peptic ulcer; Zollinger-Ellison syndrome.

Cedium *Qualiphar, Belg.*
Benzalkonium chloride (p.1101·3).
Disinfection of the skin, wounds, and hands.

Cedixen *Hoechst, Aust.*
Cefpirome sulphate (p.171·3).
Bacterial infections.

Cedocard
Byk, Aust.; Byk, Belg.; Pharmascience, Canad.; Pharmacia Upjohn, Irl.; Byk, Neth.; Byk, Switz.†; Tillotts, UK.
Isosorbide dinitrate (p.893·1).
Angina pectoris; heart failure; myocardial infarction; pulmonary hypertension.

Cedol *Euroformaco, Ital.*
Cephamandole nafate (p.180·1).
Bacterial infections.

Cedoxon *Roche, Ger.†.*
Ascorbic acid (p.1365·2) or sodium ascorbate (p.1365·2).
Vitamin C deficiency.

Cedril *MC, Ital.*
Benzalkonium chloride (p.1101·3); benzethonium chloride (p.1102·3); didecyldimethylammonium chloride (p.1112·2).
Disinfection of ulcers, burns, and wounds.

Cedril Strumenti *MC, Ital.*
Benzalkonium chloride (p.1101·3); benzethonium chloride (p.1102·3); didecyldimethylammonium chloride (p.1112·2); ethyl alcohol (p.1099·1).
Instrument disinfection.

Cedril Tintura *MC, Ital.†.*
Benzalkonium chloride (p.1101·3); benzethonium chloride (p.1102·3); didecyldimethylammonium chloride (p.1112·2); ethyl alcohol (p.1099·1).
Pre-operative skin disinfection.

Cedrol *Astra, Spain.*
Zolpidem tartrate (p.698·3).
Insomnia.

Cedrox *Hexal, Ger.*
Cefadroxil (p.163·3).
Bacterial infections.

Cedur
Boehringer Mannheim, Belg.; Boehringer Mannheim, Ger.; Boehringer Mannheim, Switz.
Bezafibrate (p.1268·2).
Hyperlipidaemias.

Cee-500 *Legere, USA†.*
Ascorbic acid (p.1365·2).

Cee-1000 TD *Legere, USA†.*
Ascorbic acid (p.1365·2).

CeeNU
Bristol-Myers Squibb, Austral.; Bristol, Canad.; Bristol-Myers Squibb, S.Afr.; Bristol-Myers Oncology, USA.
Lomustine (p.544·1).
Malignant neoplasms.

Ceetamol *CP Protea, Austral.†.*
Paracetamol (p.72·2).
Fever; pain.

Ceezinc *Lifeplan, UK.*
Zinc (p.1373·1); vitamin C (p.1365·2).

Cefa Resan *Alacan, Spain.*
Cephazolin sodium (p.181·1).
Lignocaine hydrochloride (p.1293·2) is included in this preparation to alleviate the pain of injection.
Bacterial infections.

Cefabene *Cefak, Ger.*
Stipites dulcamarae (p.1574·2).
Eczema.

Cefabiocin *Nycomed, Ger.†.*
Cefaclor (p.163·2).
Bacterial infections.

Cefabiot *Reig Jofre, Spain.*
Cephazolin sodium (p.181·1).
Lignocaine hydrochloride (p.1293·2) is included in this preparation to alleviate the pain of injection.
Bacterial infections.

Cefabiozim *IPA, Ital.*
Cephazolin sodium (p.181·1).
Lignocaine hydrochloride (p.1293·2) is included in this preparation to alleviate the pain of injection.
Bacterial infections.

Cefabol *Robert, Spain.*
Sodium cytidine monophosphate; gamma-aminobutyric acid (p.1582·1); aminohydroxybutyric acid (p.339·1); magnesium glutamate hydrobromide (p.1598·3); trisodium uridine triphosphate; pyridoxine hydrochloride (p.1362·3).
Mental function impairment; tonic.

Cefabronchin N *Cefak, Ger.*
Thyme (p.1636·3); Iceland moss; saponaria; pimpinella; eucalyptus (p.1578·1); fennel (p.1579·1); star anise.
Respiratory-tract inflammation.

Cefacene *Centrum, Spain.*
Cephazolin sodium (p.181·1).
Lignocaine (p.1293·2) is included in this preparation to alleviate the pain of injection.
Bacterial infections.

Cefacet *Norgine, Fr.*
Cephalexin (p.178·2).
Bacterial infections.

Cefachol N *Cefak, Ger.*
Chelidonium; taraxacum (p.1634·2); silybum marianum (p.993·3).
Biliary disorders; liver disorders.

Cefacidal
Bristol-Myers Squibb, Belg.; Bristol-Myers Squibb, Fr.; Bristol-Myers Squibb, Neth.; Bristol-Myers Squibb, S.Afr.
Cephazolin sodium (p.181·1).
Lignocaine (p.1293·2) is included in the intramuscular injection to alleviate the pain of injection.
Bacterial infections.

Cefacron *Faes, Spain.*
Cefotaxime sodium (p.168·2).
Bacterial infections.

Cefacutan *Cefak, Ger.†.*
Calendula; arnica (p.1550·3).
Skin disorders; wounds.

Cefadel *Del Saz & Filippini, Ital.*
Cefmetazole sodium (p.166·2).
Lignocaine hydrochloride (p.1293·2) is included in this preparation to alleviate the pain of injection.
Bacterial infections.

Cefadian *Cefak, Ger.*
Potentilla anserina.
Dysmenorrhoea.

Cefadiarrhon *Cefak, Ger.†.*
Tormentil (p.1638·3); chamomile (p.1561·2).
Diarrhoea.

Cefadina *Antibioticos, Spain†.*
Cephalexin (p.178·2).
Bacterial infections.

Cefadolor *Cefak, Ger.*
Guaiacum wood.
Rheumatic disorders.

Cefadrex *Vir, Spain.*
Cephazolin sodium (p.181·1).
Lignocaine (p.1293·2) is included in the injection to alleviate the pain of injection.
Bacterial infections.

Cefadril *AGIPS, Ital.*
Cefadroxil (p.163·3).
Bacterial infections.

Cefadros *Proter, Ital.†.*
Cephalexin (p.178·2).
Bacterial infections.

Cefadrox *Adcock Ingram, S.Afr.*
Cefadroxil (p.163·3).
Bacterial infections.

Cefadyl *Apothecon, USA†.*
Cefapirin sodium (p.164·1).
Bacterial infections.

Cefadysbasin *Cefak, Ger.*
Secale corn.; aesculus (p.1543·3); potentilla anserina.
Peripheral, coronary, and central circulatory disorders.

Cefagastrin *Cefak, Ger.*
Chamomile (p.1561·2); calendula officinalis; peppermint leaf (p.1208·1); centaury (p.1561·1); absinthium (p.1541·1); arnica (p.1550·3); fennel (p.1579·1).
Gastro-intestinal disorders.

Cefakava *Cefak, Ger.*
Kava (p.1592·3).
Anxiety; nervousness; tension.

Cefakes *Inexfa, Spain.*
Cephazolin sodium (p.181·1).
Bacterial infections.

Cefakliman *Cefak, Ger.*
Homoeopathic preparation.

Cefakliman mono *Cefak, Ger.*
Cimicifuga (p.1563·3).
Menopausal and menstrual disorders.

Cefakliman N *Cefak, Ger.*
Homoeopathic preparation.

Cefaktivon "novum" *Cefak, Ger.*
Injection: Protein-free extract of bovine blood; cerium chloride III; echinacea (p.1574·2); hypericum (p.1590·1); menyanthes (p.1601·2); calendula.
Adjuvant to cancer therapy; circulatory disorders.
Oral drops: Cerium (III)-chloride; echinacea (p.1574·2); hypericum (p.1590·1); menyanthes (p.1601·2); calendula.
Tonic.

Cefalen *Lenza, Ital.†.*
Pivcephalexin hydrochloride (p.238·3).
Bacterial infections.

Cefalexgobens *Normon, Spain.*
Cephalexin (p.178·2).
Bacterial infections.

Cefaline Hauth *Homme de Fer, Fr.*
Paracetamol (p.72·2); caffeine (p.749·3).
Fever; pain.

Cefaline-Pyrazole *Homme de Fer, Fr.*
Dipyrone (p.35·1); caffeine (p.749·3).
Pain.

Cefallone Azupharma, Ger.
Cefaclor (p.163·2).
Bacterial infections.

Cefaloject Bristol-Myers Squibb, Fr.
Cefapirin sodium (p.164·1).
Lignocaine hydrochloride (p.1293·2) is included in the intramuscular injection to alleviate the pain of injection.
Bacterial infections.

Cefalorex Inibsa, Spain†.
Cephalexin (p.178·2).
Bacterial infections.

Cefaluffa Cefak, Ger.
Homoeopathic preparation.

Cefalymphat N Cefak, Ger.
Homoeopathic preparation.

Cefam Magis, Ital.
Cephamandole nafate (p.180·1).
Lignocaine hydrochloride (p.1293·2) is included in this preparation to alleviate the pain of injection.
Bacterial infections.

Cefamadar Cefak, Ger.
Homoeopathic preparation.

Cefamar FIRMA, Ital.
Cefuroxime sodium (p.177·1).
Bacterial infections.

Cefamen Menarini, Ital.†.
Cephamandole nafate (p.180·1).
Bacterial infections.

Cefamezin
Sigma, Austral.; Pharmacia Upjohn, Ital.; Fujisawa, Jpn; Knoll, Spain.
Cephazolin sodium (p.181·1).
Lignocaine hydrochloride (p.1293·2) is included in the intramuscular injection to alleviate the pain of injection.
Bacterial infections.

Cefamid Gibipharma, Ital.†.
Cephradine (p.181·3).
Bacterial infections.

Cefamiso Inexfa, Spain.
Cephalexin (p.178·2).
Bacterial infections.

Cefamox Bristol-Myers Squibb, Swed.
Cefadroxil (p.163·3).
Bacterial infections.

Cefamusel Cruz, Spain.
Cephazolin sodium (p.181·1).
Lignocaine (p.1293·2) is included in the intramuscular injection to alleviate the pain of injection.
Bacterial infections.

Cefanalgin Cefak, Ger.
Homoeopathic preparation.

Cefanephrin N Cefak, Ger.
Solidago virgaurea; bearberry (p.1552·2).
Urinary-tract disorders.

Cefanex Apothecon, USA.
Cephalexin (p.178·2).
Bacterial infections.

Cefangipect N Cefak, Ger.
Homoeopathic preparation.

Cefanorm Cefak, Ger.
Agnus castus (p.1544·2).
Mastalgia; menstrual disorders.

Cefaperos
Bristol-Myers Squibb, Belg.; Bristol-Myers Squibb, Fr.
Propylene glycol cefatrizine (p.164·2).
Bacterial infections.

Cefapulmon mono Cefak, Ger.
Hedera helix.
Bronchial catarrh.

Cefarheumin Cefak, Ger.
Homoeopathic preparation.

Cefarheumin N Cefak, Ger.
Pumilio pine oil (p.1623·3); rosemary oil (p.1626·2); camphor (p.1557·2).
Muscle, joint, and nerve pain; neuritis.

Cefarheumin S Cefak, Ger.
Homoeopathic preparation.

Cefasabal Cefak, Ger.
Saw palmetto (p.1462·1); solidago virgaurea; aesculus (p.1543·3).
Prostatic disorders.

Cefascillan N Cefak, Ger.
Squill (p.1070·1); convallaria (p.1567·2).
Cardiac disorders; oedema.

Cefasedativ Cefak, Ger.
Valerian (p.1643·1); lupulus (p.1597·2); crataegus (p.1568·2).
Anxiety disorders; insomnia.

Cefasel Cefak, Ger.
Sodium selenite (p.1354·1).
Selenium deficiency.

Cefak, Ger.
Homoeopathic preparation.

Cefasept
Note. This name is used for preparations of different composition.
Cefak, Ger.
Injection; oral drops: Homoeopathic preparation.
Tablets: Echinacea angustifolia (p.1574·2).
Infections.

Medica, Neth.†.
Chlorhexidine gluconate (p.1107·2).
Hand disinfection.

Cefasept mono Cefak, Ger.
Echinacea purpura (p.1574·2).
Immunostimulant.

Cefaseptolo Miba, Ital.†.
Cephamandole nafate (p.180·1).
Lignocaine hydrochloride (p.1293·2) is included in this preparation to alleviate the pain of injection.
Bacterial infections.

Cefasliymarin Cefak, Ger.
Silybum marianum (p.993·3).
Liver disorders.

Cefaspasmon N Cefak, Ger.
Homoeopathic preparation.

Cefasulfon N Cefak, Ger.
Homoeopathic preparation.

Cefatrix Biotekfarma, Ital.
Propylene glycol cefatrizine (p.164·2).
Bacterial infections.

Cefavale Cefak, Ger.
Lycopus europaeus.
Thyroid disorders.

Cefavora Cefak, Ger.
Homoeopathic preparation.

Cefa-Wolff Wolff, Ger.
Cefaclor (p.163·2).
Bacterial infections.

Cefaxicina CEPA, Spain.
Cefoxitin sodium (p.170·3).
Lignocaine hydrochloride (p.1293·2) is included in the intramuscular injection to alleviate the pain of injection.
Bacterial infections.

Cefazil Italfarmaco, Ital.
Cephazolin sodium (p.181·1).
Lignocaine hydrochloride (p.1293·2) is included in this preparation to alleviate the pain of injection.
Bacterial infections.

Cefazina Chemil, Ital.†.
Cephazolin sodium (p.181·1).
Bacterial infections.

Cefazone Locatelli, Ital.
Cefoperazone sodium (p.167·3).
Lignocaine hydrochloride (p.1293·2) is included in this preparation to alleviate the pain of injection.
Bacterial infections.

Cef-Diolan Engelhard, Ger.
Cefaclor (p.163·2).
Bacterial infections.

Cefedrin N Cefak, Ger.
Ephedra (p.1059·3); thyme (p.1636·3); ammi visnaga (p.1593·2).
Asthma; coughs.

Ceferro Knoll, Ger.
Ferrous sulphate (p.1340·2).
Iron-deficiency; iron-deficiency anaemias.

Cefibacter Rubio, Spain†.
Cephalexin (p.178·2).
Bacterial infections.

Cefiran Poli, Ital.
Cephamandole nafate (p.180·1).
Lignocaine hydrochloride (p.1293·2) is included in this preparation to alleviate the pain of injection.
Bacterial infections.

Cefixoral Menarini, Ital.
Cefixime (p.165·3).
Bacterial infections.

Cefizox
Boehringer Mannheim, Aust.; SmithKline Beecham, Canad.; Bellon, Fr.; Wellcome, Irl.; Yamanouchi, Neth.; Smith Kline & French, Spain; Glaxo Wellcome, UK†; Fujisawa, USA.
Ceftizoxime sodium (p.175·2).
Lignocaine hydrochloride (p.1293·2) is included in the intramuscular injection to alleviate the pain of injection.
Bacterial infections.

Cefmetazon Sankyo, Jpn.
Cefmetazole sodium (p.166·2).
Bacterial infections.

Cefobid
Pfizer, Aust.; Pfizer, Canad.†; Pfizer, Ital.†; Pfizer, Spain; Roerig, USA.
Cefoperazone sodium (p.167·3).
Bacterial infections.

Cefobis
Pfizer, Fr.; Pfizer, Ger.; Pfizer, Switz.†.
Cefoperazone sodium (p.167·3).
Bacterial infections.

Cefociclin Francia, Ital.
Cefoxitin sodium (p.170·3).
Lignocaine hydrochloride (p.1293·2) is included in this preparation to alleviate the pain of injection.
Bacterial infections.

Cefodie SmithKline Beecham, Ital.
Cefonicid sodium (p.167·2).
Lignocaine hydrochloride (p.1293·2) is included in the intramuscular injections to alleviate the pain of injection.
Bacterial infections.

Cefodox
Roussel, Fr.†; Hoechst Marion Roussel, Irl.; Farmochimica, Ital.
Cefpodoxime proxetil (p.172·1).
Bacterial infections.

Cefogram Metapharma, Ital.
Cefoperazone sodium (p.167·3).
Lignocaine hydrochloride (p.1293·2) is included in this preparation to alleviate the pain of injection.
Bacterial infections.

Cefol Abbott, USA.
Multivitamin preparation.

Cefoneg Tosi, Ital.
Cefoperazone sodium (p.167·3).
Lignocaine hydrochloride (p.1293·2) is included in the intramuscular injection to alleviate the pain of injection.
Bacterial infections.

Cefoper Menarini, Ital.
Cefoperazone sodium (p.167·3).
Lignocaine hydrochloride (p.1293·2) is included in the intramuscular injection to alleviate the pain of injection.
Bacterial infections.

Cefoprim Esseti, Ital.
Cefuroxime sodium (p.177·1).
Lignocaine hydrochloride (p.1293·2) is included in this preparation to alleviate the pain of injection.
Bacterial infections.

Ceforcal Pensa, Spain†.
Piperazine sultamate (p.108·1).
Hyperlipidaemias.

Cefosint Crosara, Ital.
Cefoperazone sodium (p.167·3).
Lignocaine hydrochloride (p.1293·2) is included in this preparation to alleviate the pain of injection.
Bacterial infections.

Cefosporin Esseti, Ital.
Cefonicid sodium (p.167·2).
Lignocaine hydrochloride (p.1293·2) is included in the intramuscular injection to alleviate the pain of injection.
Bacterial infections.

Cefossin H Cefak, Ger.
Symphoricarpus; euphorbium cypariss.; gold in form of tetrachlorogold acid (p.1586·2).
Joint disorders.

Cefossin N Cefak, Ger.
Homoeopathic preparation.

Cefotan
Wyeth-Ayerst, Canad.; Zeneca, USA.
Cefotetan disodium (p.170·1).
Bacterial infections.

Cefotrizin FIRMA, Ital.
Propylene glycol cefatrizine (p.164·2).
Bacterial infections.

Cefrabiotic Prospa, Ital.
Cephradine (p.181·3).
Bacterial infections.

Cefral Juventus, Spain†.
Cephradine (p.181·3).
Bacterial infections.

Cefrasol Radiumfarma, Ital.†.
Cephradine (p.181·3).
Bacterial infections.

Cefril Bristol-Myers Squibb, S.Afr.
Cephradine (p.181·3).
Bacterial infections.

Cefrom
Albert-Roussel, Aust.; Hoechst Marion Roussel, Austral.; Hoechst Marion Roussel, Belg.; Roussel, Fr.; Hoechst Marion Roussel, Neth.; Hoechst Marion Roussel, Swed.; Hoechst Marion Roussel, Switz.; Roussel, UK.
Cefpirome sulphate (p.171·3).
Bacterial infections.

Cefroxil Bristol-Myers, Spain†.
Cefadroxil (p.163·3).
Bacterial infections.

Cefspan Fujisawa, Jpn.
Cefixime (p.165·3).
Bacterial infections.

Ceftenon Biochemie, Aust.
Cefotetan disodium (p.170·1).
Bacterial infections.

Ceftim Glaxo Allen, Ital.
Ceftazidime (p.173·3).
Bacterial infections.

Ceftin
Glaxo Wellcome, Canad.; Glaxo Wellcome, USA.
Cefuroxime axetil (p.177·1).
Bacterial infections.

Ceftix Boehringer Mannheim, Ger.
Ceftizoxime sodium (p.175·2).
Bacterial infections.

Cefumax SoSe, Ital.
Cefuroxime sodium (p.177·1).
Lignocaine hydrochloride (p.1293·2) is included in this preparation to alleviate the pain of injection.
Bacterial infections.

Cefur Eurofarmaco, Ital.
Cefuroxime sodium (p.177·1).
Bacterial infections.

Cefurex Salus, Ital.
Cefuroxime sodium (p.177·1).
Bacterial infections.

Cefurin Magis, Ital.
Cefuroxime sodium (p.177·1).
Bacterial infections.

Cefzil
Bristol-Myers Squibb, Canad.; Bristol-Myers Squibb, UK; Bristol, USA.
Cefprozil (p.172·3).
Bacterial infections.

Cefzon Fujisawa, Jpn.
Cefdinir (p.164·3).
Bacterial infections.

Ceglycon Braun, Ger.†.
Ascorbic acid (p.1365·2).
Vitamin C deficiency.

Cegrovit Grossmann, Switz.
Ascorbic acid (p.1365·2).
Vitamin C deficiency.

Cehafolin Donau, Aust.
Calcium folinate (p.1342·2).
Enhancement of fluorouracil activity; methotrexate toxicity.

Cehapark Schoeller, Aust.
Bromocriptine mesylate (p.1132·2).
Acromegaly; parkinsonism.

Cehaposid Donau, Aust.
Etoposide (p.532·3).
Malignant neoplasms.

Cehasol
Note. This name is used for preparations of different composition.
Donau, Aust.
Ointment: Sulphur-rich shale oil (Cehasol); vitamin F-glycerinester.
Skin disorders.

Schoeller, Aust.
Bath additive: Eucalyptus oil (p.1578·1); camphor (p.1557·2); menthol (p.1600·2).
Cold symptoms.

Celadigal Beiersdorf, Ger.†.
Lanatoside C (p.897·2).
Cardiac disorders.

Celanate Streuli, Switz.†.
Lanatoside C (p.897·2).
Cardiac disorders.

Celance
Lilly, Irl.; Lilly, UK.
Pergolide mesylate (p.1142·3).
Parkinsonism.

Celbenin Beecham Research, UK†.
Methicillin sodium (p.225·1).
Staphylococcal infections.

Celectol
Bellon, Fr.; Pantheon, UK.
Celiprolol hydrochloride (p.838·3).
Angina pectoris; hypertension.

Celefer Smith Kline & French, Spain†.
Mupirocin (p.227·2).
Bacterial skin infections.

Celesemine Schering-Plough, Spain.
Betamethasone (p.1033·2); dexchlorpheniramine maleate (p.405·1).
Formerly contained betamethasone, dexchlorpheniramine maleate, and fluphenazine hydrochloride.
Hypersensitivity reactions.

Celestamin Aesca, Aust.
Betamethasone (p.1033·2); dexchlorpheniramine maleate (p.405·1).
Hypersensitivity disorders.

Celestamine
Schering-Plough, Fr.; Essex, Ger.; Schering-Plough, S.Afr.; Essex, Switz.
Betamethasone (p.1033·2); dexchlorpheniramine maleate (p.405·1).
Hypersensitivity reactions.

Celestamine N Essex, Ger.
Betamethasone (p.1033·2).
Corticosteroid.

Celestamine-F Schering-Plough, Belg.†.
Betamethasone (p.1033·2); dexchlorpheniramine maleate (p.405·1); fluphenazine (p.672·1).
Allergic and inflammatory disorders.

Celestan
Aesca, Aust.; Essex, Ger.†.
Betamethasone (p.1033·2) or betamethasone sodium phosphate (p.1033·3) and betamethasone acetate (p.1033·2).
Corticosteroid.

Celestan Depot Essex, Ger.
Betamethasone sodium phosphate (p.1033·3); betamethasone acetate (p.1033·2).
Corticosteroid.

Celestan solubile Essex, Ger.
Betamethasone sodium phosphate (p.1033·3).
Corticosteroid.

Celestan-V Essex, Ger.
Betamethasone valerate (p.1033·3).
Scalp disorders; skin disorders.

Celestene Schering-Plough, Fr.
Betamethasone (p.1033·2) or betamethasone sodium phosphate (p.1033·3).
Corticosteroid.

Celestene Chronodose Schering-Plough, Fr.
Betamethasone sodium phosphate (p.1033·3); betamethasone acetate (p.1033·2).
Corticosteroid.

Celestoderm
Schering, Canad.; Schering-Plough, Fr.; Schering-Plough, Neth.; Schering-Plough, Spain.
Betamethasone valerate (p.1033·3).
Skin disorders.

Celestoderm Gentamicina Schering-Plough, Spain.
Betamethasone valerate (p.1033·3); gentamicin sulphate (p.212·1).
Infected skin disorders.

Celestoderm met Garamycin Schering-Plough, Neth.†.
Betamethasone valerate (p.1033·3); gentamicin sulphate (p.212·1).
Infected skin disorders.

Celestoderm met Neomycine *Schering-Plough, Neth.*
Betamethasone valerate (p.1033·3); neomycin sulphate (p.229·2).
Infected skin disorders.

Celestoderm-V
Schering-Plough, Ital.; Schering-Plough, S.Afr.; Schering-Plough, Spain; Essex, Switz.
Betamethasone valerate (p.1033·3).
Skin disorders.

Celestoderm-V with Garamycin *Schering-Plough, S.Afr.*
Betamethasone valerate (p.1033·3); gentamicin sulphate (p.212·1).
Infected skin disorders.

Celestoform *Schering-Plough, Neth.*
Betamethasone valerate (p.1033·3); clioquinol (p.193·2).
Infected skin disorders.

Celeston
Schering-Plough, Norw.
Injection: Betamethasone acetate (p.1033·2); betamethasone sodium phosphate (p.1033·3).
Corticosteroid.
Schering-Plough, Norw.†; Schering-Plough, Swed.†.
Tablets: Betamethasone (p.1033·2).
Corticosteroid.
Schering-Plough, Swed.
Injection: Betamethasone sodium phosphate (p.1033·3).
Corticosteroid.

Celeston bifas *Schering-Plough, Swed.*
Betamethasone acetate (p.1033·2); betamethasone sodium phosphate (p.1033·3).
Corticosteroid.

Celeston valerat *Schering-Plough, Swed.*
Betamethasone valerate (p.1033·3).
Otitis externa; skin disorders.

Celeston valerat comp. *Schering-Plough, Swed.*
Betamethasone valerate (p.1033·3); neomycin sulphate (p.229·2).
Infected skin disorders.

Celeston valerat med chinoform *Schering-Plough, Swed.*
Betamethasone valerate (p.1033·3); clioquinol (p.193·2).
Infected skin disorders; otitis externa.

Celeston valerat med gentamicin *Schering-Plough, Swed.*
Betamethasone valerate (p.1033·3); gentamicin sulphate (p.212·1).
Infected skin disorders.

Celestone
Schering-Plough, Austral.†; Schering-Plough, Belg.; Schering, Canad.; Schering-Plough, Ital.; Schering-Plough, Neth.; Schering-Plough, S.Afr.; Schering-Plough, Spain; Essex, Switz.; Schering, USA.
Betamethasone (p.1033·2) or betamethasone sodium phosphate (p.1033·3).
Corticosteroid.

Celestone Chronodose
Schering-Plough, Austral.; Schering-Plough, Belg.; Schering-Plough, Neth.; Essex, Switz.
Betamethasone sodium phosphate (p.1033·3); betamethasone acetate (p.1033·2).
Corticosteroid.

Celestone Cronodose
Schering-Plough, Ital.; Schering-Plough, Spain.
Betamethasone acetate (p.1033·2); betamethasone sodium phosphate (p.1033·3).
Corticosteroid.

Celestone M *Schering-Plough, Austral.*
Betamethasone valerate (p.1033·3).
Skin disorders.

Celestone S
Schering, Canad.†; Schering-Plough, Spain.
Betamethasone (p.1033·2) or betamethasone sodium phosphate (p.1033·3); sulphacetamide sodium (p.252·2).
Infected eye and ear disorders.

Celestone Soluspan
Schering, Canad.; Schering-Plough, S.Afr.; Schering, USA.
Betamethasone sodium phosphate (p.1033·3); betamethasone acetate (p.1033·2).
Corticosteroid.

Celestone V *Schering-Plough, Austral.*
Betamethasone valerate (p.1033·3).
Skin disorders.

Celestone VG *Schering-Plough, Austral.*
Betamethasone valerate (p.1033·3); gentamicin sulphate (p.212·1).
Infected skin disorders.

Celetil *Schering, Ger.†.*
Ergotamine tartrate (p.445·3); caffeine (p.749·3).
Headache including migraine.

Celevac
Monmouth, Irl.; Monmouth, UK.
Methylcellulose (p.1473·3).
Colostomy and ileostomy management; constipation; diarrhoea; diverticular disease; obesity.

Celex *Lagap, Ital.†.*
Cephradine (p.181·3).
Bacterial infections.

Celexa *Forest Pharmaceuticals, USA.*
Citalopram hydrobromide (p.281·1).
Depression.

Ce-Limo *Asta Medica, Aust.*
Ascorbic acid (p.1365·2).
Vitamin C deficiency.

Ce-Limo plus 10 Vitamine *Asta Medica, Aust.*
Multivitamin preparation.

Ce-Limo-Calcium *Asta Medica, Aust.*
Ascorbic acid (p.1365·2); calcium carbonate (p.1182·1).
Calcium and vitamin C deficiency.

Celipro *Sanorania, Ger.*
Celiprolol hydrochloride (p.838·3).
Angina pectoris; hypertension.

Cellaforte *Polcopharma, Austral.†.*
Procaine hydrochloride (p.1299·2); multivitamins and trace elements.
Tonic.

Cellblastin *Cell Pharm, Ger.*
Vinblastine sulphate (p.569·1).
Malignant neoplasms.

Cellbloc *Larkhall Laboratories, UK†.*
Potassium gluconate (p.1161·1); kelp (p.1593·1); magnesium carbonate (p.1198·1); bromelain (p.1555·1); vitamin E (p.1369·1); vitamin B_6 (p.1362·3).

CellCept
Roche, Aust.; Roche, Austral.; Roche, Belg.; Roche, Canad.; Roche, Fr.; Roche, Ger.; Roche, Irl.; Roche, Ital.; Roche, Neth.; Roche, Norw.; Roche, Spain; Roche, Swed.; Roche, Switz.; Roche, UK; Roche, USA.
Mycophenolate mofetil (p.555·3).
Renal or cardiac transplant rejection.

Cellcristin *Cell Pharm, Ger.*
Vincristine sulphate (p.570·1).
Malignant neoplasms.

Cellferon *Cell Pharm, Ger.*
Interferon alpha-1 (p.615·3).
Hairy-cell leukaemia.

Cellidrin *Hennig, Ger.*
Allopurinol (p.390·2).
Gout; hyperuricaemia; renal calculi.

Cellidrine *Sodip, Switz.*
Allopurinol (p.390·2).
Hyperuricaemia.

cellmustin *Cell Pharm, Ger.*
Estramustine sodium phosphate (p.532·2) or estramustine meglumine phosphate.
Prostatic cancer.

Cellobexon *Agepha, Aust.*
Methylcellulose (p.1473·3); vitamin B_1 (p.1361·2); vitamin C (p.1365·2).

Celloid Compounds Magcal Plus *Blackmores, Austral.*
Dibasic sodium phosphate (p.1159·3); magnesium phosphate (p.1157·3); calcium phosphate (p.1155·3); dibasic potassium phosphate (p.1159·2); iron phosphate.

Celloid Compounds Sodical Plus *Blackmores, Austral.*
Dibasic sodium phosphate (p.1159·3); calcium phosphate (p.1155·3); iron phosphate.

Celloids CF 43 *Blackmores, Austral.*
Homoeopathic preparation.

Celloids CP 57 *Blackmores, Austral.*
Calcium phosphate (p.1155·3).

Celloids CS 36 *Blackmores, Austral.*
Calcium sulphate (p.1557·1).

Celloids IP 82 *Blackmores, Austral.*
Iron phosphate.

Celloids MP 65 *Blackmores, Austral.*
Magnesium phosphate (p.1157·3).

Celloids PC 73 *Blackmores, Austral.*
Potassium chloride (p.1161·1).

Celloids PP 85 *Blackmores, Austral.*
Potassium phosphate (p.1159·3).

Celloids PS 29 *Blackmores, Austral.*
Potassium sulphate (p.1161·2).

Celloids S 79 *Blackmores, Austral.*
Silicon dioxide (p.1474·3).

Celloids SP 96 *Blackmores, Austral.*
Dibasic sodium phosphate (p.1159·3).

Celloids SS 69 *Blackmores, Austral.*
Anhydrous sodium sulphate (p.1213·3).

Celltop *Asta Medica, Fr.*
Etoposide (p.532·3).
Malignant neoplasms.

Cellucor *Magis, Ital.†.*
Cardiac phospholipids.
Lipid disorders.

Cellufresh
Allergan, Austral.; Allergan, Canad.; Allergan, USA.
Carmellose sodium (p.1471·2).
Dry eyes.

Cellulin Retinale *INTES, Ital.*
Retina extract.
Eye disorders.

Cellulone *Alphapharm, Austral.*
Methylcellulose (p.1473·3).
Bowel disorders; constipation; diarrhoea.

Celluson *Saunier-Daguin, Fr.*
Bran (p.1181·2).
Dietary fibre supplement.

Celluvisc
Allergan, Austral.; Allergan, Canad.; Allergan, Fr.; Allergan, Ger.; Allergan, Ital.; Allergan, S.Afr.; Allergan, Spain; Allergan, Swed.; Allergan, Switz.; Allergan, USA.
Carmellose sodium (p.1471·2).
Dry eyes.

Celnium *Sanofi Winthrop, Fr.*
Selenium (p.1353·3) from *Saccharomyces cerevisiae.*
Skin and muscular disorders.

Celocurin *Pharmacia Upjohn, Swed.*
Suxamethonium chloride (p.1319·1).
Depolarising neuromuscular blocker.

Celocurine *Pharmacia Upjohn, Fr.*
Suxamethonium iodide (p.1321·3).
Depolarising neuromuscular blocker.

Celontin
Parke, Davis, Austral.†; Parke, Davis, Belg.†; Parke, Davis, Canad.; Parke, Davis, Neth.; Parke, Davis, S.Afr.†; Parke, Davis, USA.
Methsuximide (p.349·1).
Absence seizures.

Celospor
Ciba, Ital.†; Ciba, Switz.†.
Cephacetrile sodium (p.178·1).
Lignocaine hydrochloride (p.1293·2) is included in this preparation to alleviate the pain of injection.
Bacterial infections.

Cel-U-Jec *Hauck, USA.*
Betamethasone sodium phosphate (p.1033·3).
Corticosteroid.

Celupan *Lacer, Spain.*
Naltrexone hydrochloride (p.988·1).
Opioid withdrawal.

Cemac B12 *Larkhall Laboratories, UK.*
Vitamin B_{12} (p.1363·3).

Cemado *Francia, Ital.*
Cephamandole nafate (p.180·1).
Lignocaine hydrochloride (p.1293·2) is included in this preparation to alleviate the pain of injection.
Bacterial infections.

Cemaflavone *Therica, Fr.*
Citroflavonoids (p.1580·1); magnesium ascorbate (p.1157·2).
Circulatory disorders; haemorrhoids.

Cemalyt *Madaus, Spain.*
Human placenta extract; triamcinolone acetonide (p.1050·2); calendula officinalis.
Bruising; skin disorders.

Cemaquin *Cimex, Switz.†.*
Benzethonium chloride (p.1102·3); ascorbic acid (p.1365·2).
Mouth and throat infections.

Cemetol *Pharmacia Upjohn, Spain.*
Cefmetazole sodium (p.166·2).
Lignocaine hydrochloride (p.1293·2) is included in the intramuscular injection to alleviate the pain of injection.
Bacterial infections.

Cemidon *Alcala, Spain.*
Isoniazid (p.218·1).
Opportunistic mycobacterial infections; tuberculosis.

Cemidon B6 *Alcala, Spain.*
Isoniazid (p.218·1).
Pyridoxine hydrochloride (p.1362·3) is included in this preparation for the prophylaxis of peripheral neuropathy.
Opportunistic mycobacterial infections; tuberculosis.

Cemirit *Bayer, Ital.*
Aspirin (p.16·1).
Fever; inflammation; influenza symptoms; pain.

Cenafed *Century, USA.*
Pseudoephedrine hydrochloride (p.1068·3).
Nasal congestion.

Cenafed Plus *Century, USA.*
Pseudoephedrine hydrochloride (p.1068·3); triprolidine hydrochloride (p.420·3).
Upper respiratory-tract symptoms.

Cena-K *Century, USA.*
Potassium chloride (p.1161·1).
Hypokalaemia; potassium depletion.

Cenat *Madaus, Spain.*
Ispaghula (p.1194·2); ispaghula husk (p.1194·2).
Constipation; functional diarrhoeas.

Ceneo *Pensa, Spain.*
Hydrocortisone butyrate (p.1044·1) or hydrocortisone propionate (p.1044·2).
Skin disorders.

Cennlacs *Westward, Canad.*
Senna (p.1212·2); liquorice (p.1197·1).

Cenol *Solvay, Belg.*
Ascorbic acid (p.1365·2).
Dietary supplement; methaemoglobinaemia; scurvy.

Cenolate *Abbott, USA.*
Sodium ascorbate (p.1365·2).
Scurvy; vitamin C deficiency.

Centellase *Corvi, Ital.*
Centella asiatica (p.1080·3).
Burns; skin ulceration; venous insufficiency; wounds.

Center-Al *Center Laboratories, USA.*
Range of allergen extracts (p.1545·1).
Hyposensitisation.

Centilux *Cusi, Spain.*
Methylene blue (p.984·3); naphazoline hydrochloride (p.1064·2).
Eye disorders.

Centoxin
Centocor, Fr.†; Centocor, Neth.†; Centocor, UK†.
Nebacumab (p.1510·2).
Septic shock.

Centra Acid *Therapex, Canad.*
Aluminium hydroxide (p.1177·3); magnesium hydroxide (p.1198·2).

Centra Acid Plus *Therapex, Canad.*
Aluminium hydroxide (p.1177·3); magnesium hydroxide (p.1198·2); simethicone (p.1213·1).

Centracol *Therapex, Canad.*
Phenylephrine hydrochloride (p.1066·2); phenylpropanolamine hydrochloride (p.1067·2); brompheniramine maleate (p.403·2).

Centracol DM *Therapex, Canad.*
Phenylpropanolamine hydrochloride (p.1067·2); pheniramine maleate (p.415·3); mepyramine maleate (p.414·1); dextromethorphan hydrobromide (p.1057·3).

Centracol Pediatrique *Therapex, Canad.*
Pseudoephedrine hydrochloride (p.1068·3); pheniramine maleate (p.415·3); dextromethorphan hydrobromide (p.1057·3); guaiphenesin (p.1061·3).

Centralgine *Amino, Switz.*
Pethidine hydrochloride (p.76·1).
Pain; smooth muscle spasm.

Centralgol *Zyma, Fr.*
Proxibarbal (p.689·3).
Anxiety; menopausal symptoms.

Centramin *Rosch & Handel, Aust.*
Glycine (p.1345·2); magnesium chloride hexahydrate (p.1157·2); calcium chloride dihydrate (p.1155·1); potassium chloride (p.1161·1).
Pruritus; tetany.

Centramina *Miquel Otsuka, Spain.*
Amphetamine sulphate (p.1477·3).
Hyperactivity; narcoleptic syndrome.

Centrapryl *Opus, UK.*
Selegiline hydrochloride (p.1144·2).
Parkinsonism.

Centratuss DM *Therapex, Canad.*
Dextromethorphan hydrobromide (p.1057·3).

Centratuss DM Expectorant *Therapex, Canad.*
Dextromethorphan hydrobromide (p.1057·3); guaiphenesin (p.1061·3).

Centratuss DM-D *Therapex, Canad.*
Dextromethorphan hydrobromide (p.1057·3); pseudoephedrine hydrochloride (p.1068·3).

Centrax
Parke, Davis, Irl.; Parke, Davis, USA†.
Prazepam (p.687·2).
Anxiety.

Centren *Esteve, Spain†.*
Etoperidone hydrochloride (p.284·1).
Depression.

Centrovite *Rugby, USA.*
A range of multivitamin and mineral preparations with iron and folic acid.

Centrum
Note. This name is used for preparations of different composition.
Whitehall-Robins, Canad.; Whitehall, Irl.; Lederle, Switz.†; Whitehall, UK; Lederle, USA.
A range of multivitamin and mineral preparations.
Polifarma, Ital.
Cytidine; uridine (p.1641·3).
Mental function impairment.

Centurion A–Z *Mission Pharmacal, USA.*
Iron (p.1346·1); folic acid (p.1340·3); multivitamins and minerals.
Iron-deficiency anaemias.

Century B-100 Complex *Suisse, Austral.†.*
Vitamin B substances with nutrients and enzymes.

Centyl
Leo, Irl.; Leo, Norw.; Leo, UK†.
Bendrofluazide (p.827·3).
Diabetes insipidus; hypertension; oedema; renal calcium stones.

Centyl K
Leo, Irl.; Leo, UK†.
Bendrofluazide (p.827·3); potassium chloride (p.1161·1).
Hypertension; oedema; renal calculi.

Centyl med Kaliumklorid *Leo, Norw.*
Bendrofluazide (p.827·3); potassium chloride (p.1161·1).
Diabetes insipidus; hypertension; oedema; renal calcium stones.

Ceolat
Solvay, Ger.; Solvay, Neth.; Solvay, Norw.; Solvay Duphar, Swed.
Dimethicone (p.1213·1).
Adjunct to gastroscopy and gastro-intestinal radiography; flatulence.

Ceolat Compositum *Lannacher, Aust.*
Dimethicone (p.1384·2); metoclopramide (p.1202·1).
Gastro-intestinal disorders.

Ceo-Two *Beutlich, USA.*
Sodium bicarbonate (p.1153·2); potassium acid tartrate (p.1209·1).
Constipation.

Ceoxil *Magis, Ital.*
Cefadroxil (p.163·3).
Bacterial infections.

Cepa Med Complex *Dynamit, Aust.*
Homoeopathic preparation.

Cepacaine
Note. This name is used for preparations of different composition.
Hoechst Marion Roussel, Austral.
Mouthwash: Benzocaine (p.1286·2); cetylpyridinium chloride (p.1106·2).
Mouth and throat disorders.
Mer-National, S.Afr.
Lozenges: Benzocaine (p.1286·2); cetylpyridinium chloride (p.1106·2).

Mouthwash: Benzocaine (p.1286·2); cinchocaine hydrochloride (p.1289·2); cetylpyridinium chloride (p.1106·2).
Mouth and throat disorders.

Cepacilina
Note. This name is used for preparations of different composition.
I Farmacologia, Spain.
Benzathine penicillin (p.158·3).
Bacterial infections; rheumatic fever.

CEPA, Spain.
Benzylpenicillin sodium (p.159·3); procaine penicillin (p.240·2); benzathine penicillin (p.158·3).
Bacterial infections; rheumatic fever.

Cepacol
Note. This name is used for preparations of different composition.
Hoechst Marion Roussel, Canad.
Cetylpyridinium chloride (p.1106·2).
Mouth and throat disorders; oral hygiene.

Lepetit, Ital.
Alkylbenzyldimethylammonium saccharinate (p.1102·1); sodium monofluorophosphate (p.743·3); calcium hydrogen phosphate (p.1155·3).
Oral disinfection; oral hygiene.

Mer-National, S.Afr.
Linctus: Dextromethorphan hydrobromide (p.1057·3); doxylamine succinate (p.410·1); sodium citrate (p.1153·2); cetylpyridinium chloride (p.1106·2).
Coughs.
Lozenges; mouthwash: Cetylpyridinium chloride (p.1106·2).
Mouth and throat disorders.

JB Williams, USA.
Cetylpyridinium chloride (p.1106·2).
Minor mouth or throat disorders.

Cepacol Anaesthetic Hoechst Marion Roussel, Austral.
Benzocaine (p.1286·2); cetylpyridinium chloride (p.1106·2).
Mouth and throat disorders.

Cepacol Anesthetic
Hoechst Marion Roussel, Canad.; JB Williams, USA.
Benzocaine (p.1286·2); cetylpyridinium chloride (p.1106·2).
Mouth and throat disorders.

Cepacol Antibacterial Hoechst Marion Roussel, Austral.
Cetylpyridinium chloride (p.1106·2).
Infective disorders of the mouth and throat; prevention of dental plaque.

Cepacol Cough Discs Mer-National, S.Afr.
Dextromethorphan (p.1057·3); cetylpyridinium chloride (p.1106·2); benzocaine (p.1286·2).
Coughs; sore throat.

Cepacol Cough and Sore Throat Hoechst Marion Roussel, Austral.
Dextromethorphan hydrobromide (p.1057·3); cetylpyridinium chloride (p.1106·2); benzocaine (p.1286·2); menthol (p.1600·2).
Coughs; sore throat.

Cepacol with Fluoride Hoechst Marion Roussel, Canad.
Cetylpyridinium chloride (p.1106·2); sodium fluoride (p.742·1).

Cepacol Maximum Strength JB Williams, USA.
Benzocaine (p.1286·2); menthol (p.1600·2); cetylpyridinium chloride (p.1106·2).
Sore throat.

Cepacol Maximum Strength Sore Throat JB Williams, USA.
Dyclocaine hydrochloride (p.1292·3); cetylpyridinium chloride (p.1106·2).
Sore throat.

Cepacol Mint Hoechst Marion Roussel, Austral.
Cetylpyridinium chloride (p.1106·2).
Reduction in plaque accumulation; sore throat; throat irritation.

Cepacol Regular Hoechst Marion Roussel, Austral.
Cetylpyridinium chloride (p.1106·2).
Minor mouth and throat infections.

Cepacol Regular Strength JB Williams, USA.
Menthol (p.1600·2); cetylpyridinium chloride (p.1106·2).
Sore throat.

Cepacol Throat JB Williams, USA.
Benzyl alcohol (p.1103·3); cetylpyridinium chloride (p.1106·2).
Sore throat.

Cepalorin Glaxo, Belg.†.
Cephaloridine (p.179·1).
Bacterial infections.

Cepan Ibi, Ital.†.
Cefotetan disodium (p.170·1).
Bacterial infections.

Cepasium Cortunon, Canad.
Magnesium carbonate (p.1198·1).

Cepastat
Hoechst Marion Roussel, Canad.; SmithKline Beecham Consumer, USA.
Phenol (p.1121·2); menthol (p.1600·2); eucalyptus oil (p.1578·1).
Sore throat.

Cepastat Cherry SmithKline Beecham Consumer, USA.
Phenol (p.1121·2); menthol (p.1600·2).
Sore throat.

Cepazine Sanofi Winthrop, Fr.
Cefuroxime axetil (p.177·1).
Bacterial infections.

Cepevit Darcy, Fr.
Ascorbic acid (p.1365·2); hesperidin methyl chalcone (p.1580·2); hesperidin (p.1580·2); esculoside (p.1543·3).
Capillary fragility.

Cepexin Glaxo Wellcome, Aust.
Cephalexin (p.178·2).
Bacterial infections.

Cephalex CT, Ger.
Cephalexin (p.178·2).
Bacterial infections.

Cephalgan UPSA, Fr.
Carbaspirin calcium (p.25·1); metoclopramide hydrochloride (p.1200·3).
Migraine.

Cephalo Plantina, Ger.
Homoeopathic preparation.

Cephalobene Merckle, Aust.
Cephalexin monohydrate (p.178·2).
Bacterial infections.

Cephanol Riva, Canad.
Paracetamol (p.72·2).

Cephoral
Merck, Ger.; E. Merck, Switz.
Cefixime (p.165·3).
Bacterial infections.

Cephos CT, Ital.
Cefadroxil (p.163·3).
Bacterial infections.

Cephulac
Hoechst Marion Roussel, Canad.; Hoechst Marion Roussel, USA.
Lactulose (p.1195·3).
Hepatic encephalopathy.

Cephyl Boiron, Fr.
Aspirin (p.16·1); etenzamide (p.35·3); caffeine hydrate (p.750·1); belladonna; iris versicolor; nux vomica; spigelia; gelsemium.
Pain.

Cepifran Juste, Spain.
Ceftibuten (p.175·1).
Bacterial infections.

Cepim Upsamedica, Ital.
Cefepime hydrochloride (p.165·1).
Bacterial infections.

Cepimex Mead Johnson, Ital.
Cefepime hydrochloride (p.165·1).
Bacterial infections.

Ceplac Rhone-Poulenc Rorer, UK.
Erythrosine (p.1000·2).
Disclosing agent for plaque.

Cepo Glaxo Wellcome, Ital.†.
Cephalexin sodium (p.178·3).
Bacterial infections.

Ceporacin
Bioniche, Canad.; Glaxo Wellcome, Neth.†.
Cephalothin sodium (p.179·1).
Bacterial infections.

Ceporex
Duncan, Flockhart, Austral.†; Glaxo Wellcome, Belg.; Glaxo Wellcome, Irl.; Glaxo Wellcome, Ital.; Glaxo Wellcome, Neth.†; Glaxo Wellcome, S.Afr.†; Glaxo Wellcome, Switz.†; Glaxo, UK.
Cephalexin (p.178·2).
Bacterial infections.

Ceporexin Hoechst, Ger.; Glaxo Wellcome, Ger.
Cephalexin (p.178·2).
Bacterial infections.

Ceporexine Glaxo Wellcome, Fr.
Cephalexin (p.178·2).
Bacterial infections.

Ceporin Glaxo Wellcome, Ital.†.
Cephaloridine (p.179·1).
Bacterial infections.

Ceporine Glaxo, Fr.†.
Cephaloridine (p.179·1).
Bacterial infections.

Cepovenin Hoechst, Ger.†; Glaxo Wellcome, Ger.†.
Cephalothin sodium (p.179·1).
Bacterial infections.

Cepral Kemyos, Ital.
Aluminium sulphate (p.1548·1); cetylpyridinium chloride (p.1106·2).
Mouth and throat disorders.

Ceprandal Sigma-Tau, Spain.
Omeprazole (p.1204·2).
Gastro-oesophageal reflux; peptic ulcer; Zollinger-Ellison syndrome.

Ceprimax Fides, Spain.
Ciprofloxacin hydrochloride (p.185·3).
Bacterial infections.

Ceprin Dolisos, Canad.
Homoeopathic preparation.

Ceprovit Wider, Ger.
Lemon oil (p.1595·3); chamomile oil; arnica (p.1550·3).
Healing of amputations.

Ceptaz
Glaxo Wellcome, Canad.; Glaxo Wellcome, USA.
Ceftazidime (p.173·3).
Bacterial infections.

Cepticol Banyu, Jpn.
Propylene glycol cefatrizine (p.164·2).
Bacterial infections.

Cepton Zyma, UK.
Chlorhexidine gluconate (p.1107·2).
Acne.

Cequinyl SmithKline Beecham, Fr.
Paracetamol (p.72·2); ascorbic acid (p.1365·2); quinine hydrochloride (p.439·2).
Formerly contained phenacetin, ascorbic acid, and quinine hydrochloride.
Fever; pain.

Ceralba Wild, Switz.†.
Wool alcohols (p.1385·2); white beeswax (p.1383·1); liquid paraffin (p.1382·1); almond oil (p.1546·2).
Dry skin.

Cerasorb Curasan, Ger.
Calcium phosphate (p.1155·3).
Artificial bone and dental enamel.

Cerat Inalterable Roche-Posay, Fr.
Titanium dioxide (p.1093·3); aluminium silicate (p.1178·3); white beeswax (p.1383·1); light liquid paraffin (p.1382·1).
Barrier ointment.

Cere Kolassa, Aust.
Ornithine aspartate (p.1352·3).
Hepatic encephalopathy.

Cerebral-Uvocal Mulli, Ger.†.
Protein-free brain extract (p.1599·1).
Mental function disorders; migraine.

Cerebramina Benvegna, Ital.†.
Vincamine (p.1644·1).
Cerebrovascular disorders.

Cerebrino Mandri, Spain.
Aspirin (p.16·1); paracetamol (p.72·2); caffeine (p.749·3).
Influenza symptoms; pain.

Cerebrix Roussel, Ital.†.
Cobamamide (p.1364·2); L-lysine hydrochloride (p.1350·1); levoglutamide (p.1344·3); DL-carnitine chloride (p.1336·2).
Tonic.

Cerebroforte Azupharma, Ger.
Piracetam (p.1619·1).
Mental function disorders.

Cerebrol
Note. This name is used for preparations of different composition.
Boehringer Ingelheim, Fr.
Diethylaminoethanol malate (p.1479·3).
Asthenia.

Actipharm, Switz.
Codeine phosphate (p.26·1); caffeine (p.749·3); paracetamol (p.72·2); propyphenazone (p.81·3).
Pain.

Cerebrol sans codeine Actipharm, Switz.
Caffeine (p.749·3); paracetamol (p.72·2).
Pain.

Cerebrolysin
Ebewe, Aust.; Knoll, Ger.
Porcine brain extract (p.1599·1).
Alzheimer's disease; cerebral disorders.

Cerebropan ISM, Ital.
Piracetam (p.1619·1).
Mental function impairment.

Cerebrosteril Fresenius, Ger.†.
Piracetam (p.1619·1).
Mental function disorders.

Cerebrotrofina Nuovo, Ital.†.
Pyritinol hydrochloride (p.1624·1).
Mental function impairment.

Cerebrovase Ashbourne, UK.
Dipyridamole (p.857·1).
Thrombo-embolism prophylaxis.

Cerebroxine Therabel Pharma, Belg.
Vincamine (p.1644·1).
Cerebrovascular disorders.

Cerebryl Kwizda, Aust.
Piracetam (p.1619·1).
Cerebral disorders.

Cerebyx Parke, Davis, USA.
Fosphenytoin sodium (p.346·2).
Epilepsy.

Ceredase
Genzyme, Ger.; Genzyme, Ital.; Genzyme, Spain; Genzyme, UK; Genzyme, USA.
Alglucerase (p.1544·2).
Gaucher disease.

Ceredilan Martin, Spain†.
Vincamine (p.1644·1).
Cerebral trauma; cerebrovascular disorders.

Ceredopa Merckle, Aust.
Levodopa (p.1137·1).
Parkinsonism.

Ceredor IRBI, Ital.†.
Acetylcarnitine hydrochloride (p.1542·1).
Cerebrovascular disorders; diabetic neuropathy; peripheral nerve disorders.

Cereen Rolab, S.Afr.
Haloperidol (p.673·3).
Psychoses.

Cereginkgo Pfluger, Ger.
Homoeopathic preparation.

Cerekinon Tanabe, Jpn.
Trimebutine maleate (p.1639·3).
Chronic gastritis; irritable bowel syndrome.

Ceremente Perez Gimenez, Spain†.
Calcium glycerophosphate (p.1155·2); levoglutamide (p.1344·3); pyridoxine (p.1363·1).
Mental function impairment.

Ceremin Madaus, Aust.
Gingko biloba (p.1584·1).
Cerebral and peripheral vascular disorders.

Cerepar
Merckle, Ger.†; Mepha, Switz.
Cinnarizine (p.406·1).
Cerebral and peripheral circulatory disorders; vestibular disorders.

Cerepar N Merckle, Ger.
Piracetam (p.1619·1).
Mental function impairment.

Cerespan Rorer, USA†.
Papaverine hydrochloride (p.1614·2).
Cerebral and peripheral ischaemia; smooth muscle spasm.

Ceretec
Amersham, Fr.; Sorin, Ital.; Amersham International, UK.
Technetium-99m exametazime (p.1425·1).
Cerebral blood flow scintigraphy; leucocyte labelling.

Cerevon Wellcome, Canad.
Ferrous succinate (p.1340·2).
Iron-deficiency anaemias.

Cerexin Rolab, S.Afr.
Cephalexin (p.178·2).
Bacterial infections.

Cerezyme
Genzyme, UK; Genzyme, USA.
Imiglucerase (p.1544·3).
Gaucher disease.

Cergem Nourypharma, Ger.
Gemeprost (p.1418·3).
Cervical dilatation.

Ceridal Rhone-Poulenc Rorer, Irl.
A range of emollient preparations.
Dry skin and scalp disorders.

Cerivikehl Sanum-Kehlbeck, Ger.
Homoeopathic preparation.

Cernevit
Clintec, Fr.; Baxter, Ger.; Clintec, Irl.; Clintec, Ital.; Clintec, Spain; Baxter, UK.
Multivitamin preparation.
Parenteral nutrition.

Cernilton
Strathmann, Ger.; Cernitin, Switz.
Pollen extracts.
Micturation disorders; prostatitis.

Cerose DM Wyeth-Ayerst, USA.
Dextromethorphan hydrobromide (p.1057·3); chlorpheniramine maleate (p.405·1); phenylephrine hydrochloride (p.1066·2).
Coughs and cold symptoms.

Cerotto Bertelli Arnikos Kelemata, Ital.
Capsicum oleoresin.
Musculoskeletal disorders.

Cerovite Rugby, USA.
Multivitamin and mineral preparation with iron and folic acid.

Ceroxmed Steril Bouty, Ital.
Benzalkonium chloride (p.1101·3).
Instrument and surface disinfection; skin, wound, and hand disinfection.

Cerson LAW, Ger.
Flumethasone pivalate (p.1040·3).
Skin disorders.

Certagen Goldline, USA.
Oral liquid: Multivitamin and mineral preparation.
Tablets: Ferrous fumarate (p.1339·3); folic acid (p.1340·3); multivitamins and minerals.
Iron-deficiency anaemias.

Certagen Senior Goldline, USA.
Multivitamin and mineral preparation with iron and folic acid.

Certain Dri Numark, USA.
Aluminium chloride (p.1078·3).
Hyperhidrosis.

Certa-Vite Major, USA.
Multivitamin and mineral preparation.

Certified Decongestant Prodemdis, Canad.
Xylometazoline hydrochloride (p.1071·2).

Certiva Ross, USA.
A diphtheria, tetanus, and pertussis vaccine (p.1509·1).
Active immunisation.

Certobil Metapharma, Ital.
Dehydrocholic acid (p.1570·2); rhubarb (p.1212·1); cascara (p.1183·1); boldo (p.1554·1); manna (p.1199·1).
Constipation.

Certomycin
Aesca, Aust.; Essex, Ger.
Netilmicin sulphate (p.231·1).
Bacterial infections.

Certonal Serturner, Ger.
Moxaverine hydrochloride (p.1604·3).
Circulatory disorders.

Certostat Jenapharm, Ger.†.
Ethinyloestradiol (p.1445·1); dienogest (p.1444·1).
Combined oral contraceptive.

Ceru Spray Ghimas, Ital.
Chamomile (p.1561·2).
Aural hygiene.

Cerubidin
Rhone-Poulenc Rorer, Austral.†; Rhone-Poulenc Rorer, Norw.; Rhone-

Poulenc Rorer, S.Afr.; Rhone-Poulenc Rorer, Swed.; Rhone-Poulenc Rorer, UK.
Daunorubicin hydrochloride (p.528·1).
Leukaemias.

Cerubidine
Rhone-Poulenc Rorer, Belg.; Rhone-Poulenc Rorer, Canad.; Bellon, Fr.; Rhone-Poulenc Rorer, Neth.; Rhone-Poulenc Rorer, Switz.; Chiron, USA†.
Daunorubicin hydrochloride (p.528·1).
Malignant neoplasms.

Cerucal Dresden, Ger.
Metoclopramide hydrochloride (p.1200·3).
Gastro-intestinal disorders.

Cerulex Farmitalia Carlo Erba, Fr.†.
Ceruletide diethylamine (p.1561·2).
Test for pancreatic function.

Cerulisina Bouty, Ital.
Xylene (p.1381·3).
Ear wax removal.

Cerulyse Chauvin, Fr.
Xylene (p.1381·3).
Ear wax removal.

Cerumenex
Purdue Frederick, Canad.; Mundipharma, Ger.; Asta Medica, Ital.; Hoechst Marion Roussel, S.Afr.; Mundipharma, Switz.; Purdue Frederick, USA.
Triethanolamine polypeptide oleate-condensate (p.1639·2).
Ear wax removal.

Cerumenol
Note. This name is used for preparations of different composition.
Martin, Fr.
Polysorbate 80 (p.1327·3).
Ear wax removal.

Berna, Spain.
Potassium hydroxide (p.1621·1).
Ear wax removal.

LAB, Switz.
Paradichlorobenzene (p.1615·2); chlorbutol hemihydrate (p.1106·3); turpentine oil (p.1641·1); orthodichlorobenzene (p.1611·2).
Ear wax removal.

Cerumol
Note. This name is used for preparations of different composition.
Culver, Austral.
Paradichlorobenzene (p.1615·2); chlorbutol (p.1106·3); turpentine oil (p.1641·1); arachis oil (p.1550·2).
Ear wax removal.

Solvay, Canad.; Laboratories for Applied Biology, Irl.
Paradichlorobenzene (p.1615·2); chlorbutol (p.1106·3); turpentine oil (p.1641·1).
Ear wax removal.

Pharmafrica, S.Afr.; Laboratories for Applied Biology, UK.
Paradichlorobenzene (p.1615·2); arachis oil (p.1550·2); chlorbutol (p.1106·3).
The name Cerumenol has also been used for this preparation in the *UK*.
Ear wax removal.

Cerutil Isis, Ger.
Meclofenoxate hydrochloride (p.1599·1).
Cerebral circulatory disorders; mental function impairment.

Cervagem
Rhone-Poulenc Rorer, Austral.; Rhone-Poulenc Rorer, Neth.†; Rhone-Poulenc Rorer, Norw.; Rhone-Poulenc Rorer, Swed.; May & Baker, UK†.
Gemeprost (p.1418·3).
Cervical dilatation; termination of pregnancy.

Cervageme Bellon, Fr.
Gemeprost (p.1418·3).
Cervical dilatation prior to uterine procedures; termination of pregnancy.

Cervicaletten Prospa, Switz.†.
Tetracycline hydrochloride (p.259·1); nystatin (p.386·1).
Vaginal infections.

Cervidil
Note. This name is used for preparations of different composition.
Serono, Ital.
Gemeprost (p.1418·3).
Cervical dilatation.

Forest Pharmaceuticals, USA.
Dinoprostone (p.1414·3).
Labour induction.

Cervilane Cassenne, Fr.
Lomifylline; dihydroergocristine mesylate (p.1571·3).
Cerebral circulatory disorders.

Cerviprost
Organon, Aust.; Nourypharma, Ger.; Organon, Neth.†; Organon, Norw.†; Organon, Swed.†; Organon, Switz.
Dinoprostone (p.1414·3).
Cervical dilatation; labour induction; termination of pregnancy.

Cervitalin Savoma, Ital.†.
Pyritinol hydrochloride (p.1624·1).
Mental function impairment.

Cervitec DAB, Swed.
Chlorhexidine acetate (p.1107·2).
Dental hygiene.

Cervoxan
SmithKline Beecham, Fr.; Mabo, Spain.
Vinburnine (p.1644·1).
Cerebrovascular disorders; retinal disorders.

CES ICN, Canad.
Conjugated oestrogens (p.1457·3).
Oestrogen deficiency.

Cesamet
Lilly, Canad.; Lilly, Irl.; Lilly, UK; Lilly, USA†.
Nabilone (p.1203·1).
Nausea and vomiting associated with cancer chemotherapy.

Cesol Merck, Ger.
Praziquantel (p.108·2).
Cestode infections.

Cesplon Esteve, Spain.
Captopril (p.836·3).
Diabetic nephropathy; heart failure; hypertension; myocardial infarction.

Cesplon Plus Esteve, Spain.
Hydrochlorothiazide (p.885·2); captopril (p.836·3).
Hypertension.

Cesporan Caber, Ital.†.
Cephradine (p.181·3).
Bacterial infections.

Cesra Redel, Ger.
Ibuprofen (p.44·1).
Fever; gout; inflammation; musculoskeletal and joint disorders; pain.

Cesradyston Redel, Ger.
Hypericum (p.1590·1).
Formerly contained belladonna, phenobarbitone, secalia corn., gelsemium, atropine sulphate, and hamamelis.
Nervous disorders.

Cesralax N Redel, Ger.†.
Rhubarb (p.1212·1); senna leaves (p.1212·2); cape aloe (p.1177·1).
Constipation.

Cesrasanol Redel, Ger.
Chamomile; hamamelis; calendula; arnica; achillea; centaury.
Inflammation; spasms.

Ceta C & M, USA.
Skin cleanser.

Ceta Plus Seatrace, USA.
Hydrocodone tartrate (p.43·1); paracetamol (p.72·2).
Pain.

Cetacaine Cetylite, USA.
Benzocaine (p.1286·2); butyl aminobenzoate (p.1289·1); amethocaine hydrochloride (p.1285·2).
Local anaesthesia.

Cetacort Galderma, USA.
Hydrocortisone (p.1043·3).
Skin disorders.

Cetal
Note. This name is used for preparations of different composition.
Parke, Davis, Aust.; Parke, Davis, Ger.; Warner-Lambert, Switz.
Slow-release capsules: Vincamine (p.1644·1).
Ménière's disease; mental function disorders; metabolic and circulatory disorders of the brain, retina, and ear.

Parke, Davis, Ger.†.
Injection: Vincamine hydrochloride (p.1644·1).
Ménière's disease; mental function disorders; metabolic and circulatory disorders of the brain, retina, and ear.

Cetal Concentrate
Note. A similar name is used for preparations of different composition.
Colgate Oral Care, Austral.
Benzalkonium chloride (p.1101·3).
Instrument and surface disinfection.

Cetal Instrument Disinfectant
Note. A similar name is used for preparations of different composition.
Colgate Oral Care, Austral.
Chlorhexidine gluconate (p.1107·2); cetrimide (p.1105·2).
Disinfection of instruments, linen, and furniture.

Cetam Formenti, Ital.†.
Piracetam (p.1619·1).
Mental function impairment.

Cetamide
Alcon, Canad.; Alcon, USA.
Sulphacetamide sodium (p.252·2).
Bacterial eye infections.

Cetamine
Note. This name is used for preparations of different composition.
Wolfs, Belg.
Ascorbic acid (p.1365·2).
Vitamin C deficiency; vitamin C supplement.

Covan, S.Afr.
Syrup: Paracetamol (p.72·2); mepyramine maleate (p.414·1); phenylephrine hydrochloride (p.1066·2); caffeine (p.749·3).
Tablets: Quinine sulphate (p.439·2); ascorbic acid (p.1365·2); paracetamol (p.72·2); mepyramine maleate (p.414·1); phenylephrine hydrochloride (p.1066·2).
Cold and influenza symptoms.

Cetamol Antigen, Irl.†.
Paracetamol (p.72·2).
Pain.

Cetanorm Norma, UK.
Benzalkonium chloride (p.1101·3); aldioxa (p.1078·2); chlorbutol (p.1106·3); cetrimide (p.1105·2).

Cetanovo Llorens, Spain†.
Cinmetacin (p.25·3).
Musculoskeletal and joint disorders.

Cetaphil
Galderma, Austral.; Galderma, Canad.; Alcon, S.Afr.†; Galderma, UK; Galderma, USA; Owen, USA.
Skin cleanser.

Cetapon Pharmagen, S.Afr.†.
Paracetamol (p.72·2).
Fever; pain.

Cetapred
Alcon, Belg.†; Alcon, Switz.†; Alcon, USA.
Prednisolone acetate (p.1048·1); sulphacetamide sodium (p.252·2).
Bacterial eye infections with inflammation.

Cetapril Dainippon, Jpn.
Alacepril (p.817·2).
Hypertension.

Cetavlex
Note. This name is used for preparations of different composition.
Zeneca, Belg.
Cetrimonium bromide (p.1106·1); chlorhexidine gluconate (p.1107·2).
Disinfection of wounds, skin, and hands; skin disorders.

Zeneca, Irl.; Bioglan, UK.
Cetrimide (p.1105·2).
Minor wounds, burns, and abrasions; napkin rash; skin disinfection; skin disorders.

Boots Healthcare, Neth.†.
Cetrimide (p.1105·2); chlorhexidine hydrochloride (p.1107·2).
Burns; skin disinfection; wounds.

Cetavlon
ICI, Austral.†; Zeneca, Fr.; Zeneca, Irl.†; ICI, Ital.†; Zeneca, Neth.; Zeneca, S.Afr.; Zeneca, Spain; ICI, UK†.
Cetrimide (p.1105·2).
Burns; skin disinfection; skin disorders; wounds.

Cetazin Sigmapharm, Aust.
Sulphacetamide sodium (p.252·2).
Bacterial eye infections.

Cetebe Fink, Ger.
Ascorbic acid (p.1365·2).
Vitamin C deficiency.

Cetilsan Sella, Ital.
Cetylpyridinium chloride (p.1106·2).
Oral hygiene; skin and wound disinfection.

Cetimil Lesvi, Spain.
Nedocromil sodium (p.756·2).
Asthma.

Cetiprin
Pharmacia Upjohn, Aust.; Pharmacia Upjohn, Irl.; Pharmacia Upjohn, Neth.; Pharmacia Upjohn, Norw.; Kabi, S.Afr.†; Pharmacia Upjohn, Swed.; Pharmacia Upjohn, Switz.
Emepronium bromide (p.461·1) or emepronium carrageenate (p.461·1).
Pancreatitis; smooth muscle spasm; tenesmus; urinary frequency; urinary incontinence.

Cetoderm Nelson, Austral.†.
Cetrimide (p.1105·2).
Seborrhoeic dermatitis.

Cetoglutaran Soekami, Fr.†.
Calcium di-oxoglurate.
Asthenia.

Cetolog Clintec, Fr.†.
Amino-acid preparation.
Prevention of uraemia in patients with renal failure.

Cetona Demopharm, Switz.
Aluminium acetate (p.1547·3); arnica (p.1550·3); chamomile (p.1561·2); calendula officinalis; hypericum (p.1590·1); comfrey (p.1567·1); dexpanthenol (p.1570·3); lignocaine hydrochloride (p.1293·2).
Skin swelling.

Cetornan Logeais, Fr.
Ornithine oxoglurate (p.1352·3).
Nutritional supplement.

Cetovinca Byk Elmu, Spain.
Vincamine oxoglurate (p.1644·1).
Cerebral trauma; cerebrovascular disorders.

Cetoxol Pharmacare Consumer, S.Afr.
Benzocaine (p.1286·2); cetylpyridinium chloride (p.1106·2).
Sore throat.

Cetraben Pharma Health, UK.
White soft paraffin (p.1382·3); liquid paraffin (p.1382·1).
Dry skin.

Cetraben Bath Oil Pharma Health, UK.
Light liquid paraffin (p.1382·1).
Dry skin.

Cetraphylline Schering-Plough, Fr.†.
Theophylline (p.765·1).
Asthma.

Cetraxal Salvat, Spain.
Ciprofloxacin (p.185·3) or ciprofloxacin hydrochloride (p.185·3).
Bacterial infections.

Cetrazil Virginia, Ital.
Propylene glycol cefatrizine (p.164·2).
Bacterial infections.

Cetriclens Seton, UK†.
Cetrimide (p.1105·2); chlorhexidine gluconate (p.1107·2).
Bladder irrigation; skin disinfection.

Cetrinox Magis, Ital.
Propylene glycol cefatrizine (p.164·2).
Bacterial infections.

Cetrisan Gedis, Ital.
Chlorhexidine gluconate (p.1107·2); cetrimide (p.1105·2).
Surface disinfection.

Cetrispect Propan, S.Afr.
Mepyramine maleate (p.414·1); ammonium chloride (p.1055·2); sodium citrate (p.1153·2); ephedrine hydrochloride (p.1059·3).
Coughs.

Cetylcide Cetylite, USA†.
Cetyldimethylethylammonium bromide (p.1106·2); benzalkonium chloride (p.1101·3); isopropyl alcohol (p.1118·2).
Instrument and hard surface disinfection.

Cevalin Lilly, USA.
Ascorbic acid (p.1365·2).
Vitamin C deficiency.

Cevi-Bid Geriatric Pharm. Corp., USA.
Ascorbic acid (p.1365·2).
Vitamin C deficiency.

Cevi-drops Centrapharm, Belg.†.
Ascorbic acid (p.1365·2).
Vitamin C supplement.

Cevi-Fer Geriatric Pharm. Corp., USA.
Ferrous fumarate (p.1339·3); folic acid (p.1340·3).
Ascorbic acid (p.1365·2) is included in this preparation to increase the absorption and availability of iron.
Iron and folic acid deficiency.

Cevigen Gentili, Ital.†.
Sodium ascorbate (p.1365·2).
Vitamin C deficiency.

Cevirin Esseti, Ital.
Aciclovir (p.602·3).
Herpesvirus infections.

Ce-Vi-Sol
Mead Johnson, Canad.†; Mead Johnson Nutritionals, USA.
Ascorbic acid (p.1365·2).
Scurvy; vitamin C deficiency.

Cevit Italfarmaco, Ital.†.
Ascorbic acid (p.1365·2).
Vitamin C deficiency.

Cevitan Sopar, Belg.†.
Ascorbic acid (p.1365·2).
Dietary supplement.

Cevitine Warner-Lambert Consumer, Belg.
Ascorbic acid (p.1365·2); calcium ascorbate (p.1365·2).
Vitamin C deficiency; vitamin C supplement.

Cevitol Lannacher, Aust.
Ascorbic acid (p.1365·2).
Vitamin C deficiency.

Cezin UAD, USA.
Multivitamin and mineral preparation.

C-Film
Geymonat, Ital.; Abello, Spain†; Lucchini, Switz.; Arun, UK.
Nonoxinol 9 (p.1326·1).
Contraceptive.

Cha-mill Ritsert, Ger.†.
Chamomile flowers (p.1561·2); achillea (p.1542·2).
Inflammation.

Chamo Ysatfabrik, Ger.
Chamomile flowers (p.1561·2).
Gastro-intestinal disorders; mouth and throat inflammation; skin disorders; wounds.

Chamoca Hanosan, Ger.†.
Homoeopathic preparation.

Championyl Synthelabo, Ital.
Sulpiride (p.692·3).
Dysthymia; psychoses.

Chantaline Madaus, Spain.
Theophylline (p.765·1).
Asthma; bronchospasm; heart failure; paroxysmal dyspnoea.

Chapstick
Note. This name is used for preparations of different composition.
Whitehall, Austral.
Padimate O (p.1488·1).
SPF 15: Padimate O (p.1488·1); oxybenzone (p.1487·3).
Dry or chapped lips; sunscreen for lips.

Whitehall-Robins, Canad.
SPF 15: Padimate O (p.1488·1); oxybenzone (p.1487·3).
Sunscreen.

Robins, USA.
Lip balm SPF 15: Padimate O (p.1488·1); oxybenzone (p.1487·3); titanium dioxide (p.1093·3).
Ointment SPF 15: Padimate O (p.1488·1); oxybenzone (p.1487·3).
Sunscreen.

Chapstick Medicated Lip Balm
Whitehall-Robins, Canad.; Robins, USA.
Yellow soft paraffin (p.1382·3); camphor (p.1557·2); menthol (p.1600·2); phenol (p.1121·2).

Chapstick Petroleum Jelly Plus - With Sunblock Robins, Austral.†.
SPF 15: Padimate O (p.1488·1); oxybenzone (p.1487·3).
Dry or chapped lips; sunscreen for lips.

Charabs Lane, UK.
Caffeine (p.749·3); vitamin B substances.
Tonic.

Charac Valtec, Canad.†.
Activated charcoal (p.972·2).
Poison antidote.

Charbon de Belloc Chefaro Ardeval, Fr.
Activated charcoal (p.972·2).
Gastro-intestinal disorders.

Charcoaid Requa, USA.
Activated charcoal (p.972·2).
Emergency treatment of poisoning.

Charcoal Plus Kramer, USA.
Simethicone (p.1213·1); activated charcoal (p.972·2).
Flatulence.

CharcoCaps
Key, Austral.; Requa, USA.
Activated charcoal (p.972·2).
Diarrhoea; flatulence; poisoning.

Charcodote *Pharmascience, Canad.*
Activated charcoal (p.972·2); sorbitol (p.1354·2).
Poison antidote.

Charcodote Aqueous *Pharmascience, Canad.*
Activated charcoal (p.972·2).
Poison antidote.

Charcotabs *Key, Austral.*
Activated charcoal (p.972·2).
Diarrhoea; drug poisoning; excess gastro-intestinal gas.

Chardonna-2 *Schwarz, USA.*
Belladonna (p.457·1); phenobarbitone (p.350·2).
Gastro-intestinal disorders.

Charlieu Anti-Poux *Mayoly-Spindler, Fr.*
Permethrin (p.1409·2); piperonyl butoxide (p.1409·3).
Lice infestation.

Chase Kolik Gripe Water *Stella, Canad.*
Alcohol (p.1099·1); ginger (p.1193·2); dill oil (p.1572·1); sodium bicarbonate (p.1153·2).

Chase Kolik Gripe Water Alcohol-Free *Stella, Canad.*
Fennel oil (p.1579·2); sodium bicarbonate (p.1153·2).

Chefarine 4 *Chefaro, Neth.†.*
Aspirin (p.16·1); paracetamol (p.72·2).
Fever; pain.

Chefir *Drug Research, Ital.*
Cefonicid sodium (p.167·2).
Lignocaine hydrochloride (p.1293·2) is included in this preparation to alleviate the pain of injection.
Bacterial infections.

Cheihepar *Steigerwald, Ger.†.*
Cheiranthus cheiri; iberis amara; angelica; peppermint leaf (p.1208·1); chelidonium; absinthium (p.1541·1); achillea (p.1542·2); hypericum (p.1590·1); thiamine hydrochloride (p.1361·1); pyridoxine hydrochloride (p.1362·3); cysteine hydrochloride (p.1338·3).
Biliary disorders; liver disorders.

Cheiranthol *Klein, Ger.*
Cheiranthus cheiri; silybum marianum (p.993·3); cnicus benedictus (p.1565·3); achillea (p.1542·2); hypericum (p.1590·1).
Liver disorders.

Chek-Stix *Bayer, Austral.*
Positive and negative controls for tests for glucose, bilirubin, ketones, specific gravity, blood, pH, protein, urobilinogen, nitrite, and leucocytes in urine.

Chelante *IPIT, Ital.†.*
Sodium calciumedetate (p.994·1).
Chelation therapy.

Chelated Cal-Mag *Neo-Life, Austral.*
Calcium glycinate; magnesium glycinate; fish-liver oil.
Calcium and magnesium deficiency.

Chelated Solamins *Solgar, UK.*
Minerals as amino-acid chelates.

Chelatran *L'Arguenon, Fr.*
Disodium edetate (p.980·1).
Digitalis intoxication.

Cheliboldo *Terapeutico, Ital.†.*
Boldo (p.1554·1); frangula bark (p.1193·2); lappa (p.1594·2); taraxacum (p.1634·2); chelidonium; combretum (p.1593·2); bile salts (p.1553·2); dehydrocholic acid (p.1570·2).
Constipation.

Chelidonium Compose *Boiron, Fr.*
Homoeopathic preparation.

Chelidonium-Strath *Strath-Labor, Ger.†.*
Chelidonium; agrimony; sage (p.1627·1); hypericum (p.1590·1).
Liver disorders.

Chelidophyt *Galenika, Ger.*
Chelidonium major.
Formerly contained chelidonium, achillea, peppermint leaf, and scopolia root.
Biliary and gastro-intestinal spasm.

Chelintox *Hausmann, Switz.†.*
Sodium calciumedetate (p.994·1).
Heavy-metal poisoning.

Chelobil *Inexfa, Spain†.*
Chenodeoxycholic acid (p.1562·1).
Cholesterol gallstones.

Chemacin *CT, Ital.*
Amikacin sulphate (p.150·2).
Bacterial infections.

Chemet
Janssen-Cilag, Aust.; Sanofi Winthrop, USA.
Succimer (p.997·1).
Lead poisoning.

Chemicetina
Fournier, Ital.; Astra, Spain.
Chloramphenicol (p.182·1), chloramphenicol palmitate (p.182·2), chloramphenicol sodium succinate (p.182·2), or chloramphenicol stearate (p.184·2).
Bacterial infections.

Chemiofurin *Torlan, Spain.*
Nitrofurantoin (p.231·3).
Urinary-tract infections.

Chemionazolo *NCSN, Ital.*
Econazole nitrate (p.377·2).
Fungal and bacterial skin and vulvovaginal infections.

Chemiosalfa *Salfa, Ital.†.*
Sulphadimethoxine (p.253·2).
Bacterial infections.

Chemiovis *SIT, Ital.†.*
Sulphathiazole (p.257·1); sulphadiazine (p.252·3); sulphanilamide (p.256·3); vitamin A (p.1358·1); ergocalciferol (p.1367·1).
Vaginitis.

Chemitrim *Biomedica, Ital.*
Co-trimoxazole (p.196·3).
Bacterial infections.

Chemotrim *Rosemont, UK.*
Co-trimoxazole (p.196·3).
Bacterial infections.

Chemstrip 6 *Boehringer Mannheim, USA.*
Test for glucose, protein, blood, ketones, leukocytes, and pH in urine.

Chemstrip 7 *Boehringer Mannheim, USA.*
Test for glucose, protein, blood, ketones, bilirubin, leukocytes, and pH in urine.

Chemstrip 8 *Boehringer Mannheim, USA.*
Test for glucose, protein, blood, ketones, bilirubin, urobilinogen, leukocytes, and pH in urine.

Chemstrip 9 *Boehringer Mannheim, USA.*
Test for glucose, protein, blood, ketones, bilirubin, urobilinogen, nitrite, leukocytes, and pH in urine.

Chemstrip bG
Boehringer Mannheim, Canad.; Boehringer Mannheim Diagnostics, USA.
Test for glucose in blood (p.1585·1).

Chemstrip 2 GP *Boehringer Mannheim, USA.*
Test for glucose and protein in urine.

Chemstrip K
Boehringer Mannheim, Canad.; Boehringer Mannheim, USA.
Test for ketones in urine.

Chemstrip 2 LN *Boehringer Mannheim, USA.*
Test for nitrite and leukocytes in urine.

Chemstrip Micral *Boehringer Mannheim, USA.*
Test for albumin in urine.

Chemstrip 4 the OB *Boehringer Mannheim, USA.*
Test for glucose, protein, blood, and leukocytes in urine.

Chemstrip 10 with SG *Boehringer Mannheim, USA.*
Test for nitrite, pH, protein, glucose, ketones, urobilinogen, bilirubin, blood, leucocytes, and specific gravity in urine.

Chemstrip uG
Boehringer Mannheim, Canad.; Boehringer Mannheim, USA.
Test for glucose in urine (p.1585·1).

Chemstrip uG 5000K *Boehringer Mannheim, Canad.*
Test for glucose and ketones in urine.

Chemstrip uGK *Boehringer Mannheim, USA.*
Test for glucose and ketones in urine.

Chemyparin *SIT, Ital.*
Heparin sodium (p.879·3).
Eye disorders.

Chemyterral *SIT, Ital.†.*
Oxytetracycline hydrochloride (p.235·1); chloramphenicol (p.182·1); sulphacetamide sodium (p.252·2).
Bacterial infections of the eye.

Chendol
Fisons, Austral.†; CP Pharmaceuticals, Irl.; CP Pharmaceuticals, UK†.
Chenodeoxycholic acid (p.1562·1).
Cholesterol gallstones.

Chenix *Solvay, USA†.*
Chenodeoxycholic acid (p.1562·1).
Cholesterol gallstones.

Chenocol *Caber, Ital.†.*
Chenodeoxycholic acid (p.1562·1).
Cholesterol gallstones.

Chenodex *Houde, Fr.*
Chenodeoxycholic acid (p.1562·1).
Cholesterol gallstones.

Chenofalk
Merck, Aust.; Codali, Belg.; Falk, Ger.; Antigen, Irl.; Also, Ital.†; Falk, Neth.; Falk, Switz.; Thames, UK.
Chenodeoxycholic acid (p.1562·1).
Cholesterol gallstones.

Chenossil *Midy, Ital.†.*
Chenodeoxycholic acid (p.1562·1).
Cholesterol gallstones.

Chephapyrin N *Chephasaar, Ger.*
Aspirin (p.16·1); paracetamol (p.72·2); caffeine (p.749·3).
Cold symptoms; pain.

Cheracol *Roberts, Canad.*
Codeine phosphate (p.26·1); guaiphenesin (p.1061·3); ammonium chloride (p.1055·2).
Coughs.

Cheracol Cough *Roberts, USA.*
Codeine phosphate (p.26·1); guaiphenesin (p.1061·3).
Coughs.

Cheracol D Cough *Roberts, USA.*
Dextromethorphan hydrobromide (p.1057·3); guaiphenesin (p.1061·3).
Coughs.

Cheracol Nasal *Roberts, USA.*
Oxymetazoline hydrochloride (p.1065·3).

Cheracol Plus *Roberts, USA.*
Phenylpropanolamine hydrochloride (p.1067·2); chlorpheniramine maleate (p.405·1); dextromethorphan hydrobromide (p.1057·3).
Coughs and cold symptoms.

Cheracol Sinus *Roberts, USA†.*
Pseudoephedrine sulphate (p.1068·3); dexbrompheniramine maleate (p.403·2).
Allergic rhinitis; nasal congestion.

Cheracol Sore Throat *Roberts, USA.*
Phenol (p.1121·2).
Sore throat.

Cheratil *Francia, Ital.†.*
Idoxuridine (p.613·2).
Herpes keratitis.

Cherry Chest Rub *Mentholatum, Canad.*
Camphor (p.1557·2); eucalyptus oil (p.1578·1); menthol (p.1600·2).

Chest Cold Relief *Brauer, Austral.*
Homoeopathic preparation.
Formerly known as Chest Cold Complex.

Chest Mixture *Potter's, UK.*
Horehound (p.1063·3); pleurisy root; senega (p.1069·3); lobelia (p.1481·3); acetum scillae (p.1070·1).
Catarrh; coughs.

Chetopir *Sarm, Ital.†.*
Kebuzone (p.48·1).
Musculoskeletal and joint disorders.

Chetotest *SPA, Ital.*
Test for acetone in urine.

Chew-E *Eagle, Austral.*
d-Alpha tocopheryl acid succinate (p.1369·2).
Vitamin E supplement.

Chibro B12 *Chibret, Ger.†.*
Cyanocobalamin (p.1363·3).
Eye disorders.

Chibro-Amuno 3 *Chibret, Ger.*
Indomethacin (p.45·2).
Macular oedema following cataract surgery.

Chibro-Atropine *Merck Sharp & Dohme-Chibret, Fr.*
Atropine sulphate (p.455·1).
Eye disorders.

Chibro-Boraline
Merck Sharp & Dohme-Chibret, Fr.†; Merck Sharp & Dohme, Switz.
Oxedrine tartrate (p.925·3); borax (p.1554·2); boric acid (p.1554·2).
Eye irritation.

Chibro-Cadron
Merck Sharp & Dohme-Chibret, Fr.; Chibret, Ger.
Dexamethasone sodium phosphate (p.1037·2); neomycin sulphate (p.229·2).
Eye and nose disorders.

Chibro-Kerakain *Chibret, Ger.*
Proxymetacaine hydrochloride (p.1300·1).
Local anaesthesia.

Chibro-Pilocarpin *Chibret, Ger.†.*
Pilocarpine nitrate (p.1396·3).
Glaucoma.

Chibro-Pilocarpine *Merck Sharp & Dohme-Chibret, Fr.*
Pilocarpine nitrate (p.1396·3).
Glaucoma; reversal of mydriasis.

Chibro-Proscar *Merck Sharp & Dohme-Chibret, Fr.*
Finasteride (p.1446·1).
Benign prostatic hyperplasia.

Chibro-Rifamycin *Chibret, Ger.†.*
Rifamycin sodium (p.246·2).
Bacterial eye infections.

Chibro-Timoptol *Chibret, Ger.*
Timolol maleate (p.953·3).
Glaucoma.

Chibro-Uvelin *Chibret, Ger.†.*
Methylhydroxyquinoline methylsulphate (p.1603·2).
Light- and radiation-induced ocular damage.

Chibro-Uvelina *Merck Sharp & Dohme, Spain.*
Methylhydroxyquinoline methylsulphate (p.1603·2).
Eye irritation.

Chibroxin
Chibret, Ger.; Merck Sharp & Dohme, Spain; Merck Sharp & Dohme, USA.
Norfloxacin (p.233·1).
Bacterial eye infections.

Chibroxine *Merck Sharp & Dohme-Chibret, Fr.*
Norfloxacin (p.233·1).
Bacterial eye infections.

Chibroxol
Merck Sharp & Dohme, Belg.; Merck Sharp & Dohme, Neth.; Merck Sharp & Dohme, Switz.
Norfloxacin (p.233·1).
Bacterial eye infections.

Chiclida *Torrens, Spain.*
Meclozine hydrochloride (p.413·3).
Motion sickness.

Chiggerex *Scherer, USA.*
Benzocaine (p.1286·2); camphor (p.1557·2); menthol (p.1600·2).
Skin disorders.

Chigger-Tox *Scherer, USA.*
Benzocaine (p.1286·2).
Local anaesthesia.

Chilblain Formula *Vitaplex, Austral.*
Nicotinamide (p.1351·2); acetomenaphthone (p.1370·3).
Chilblains; poor peripheral circulation.

Chilblains Ointment *Nelson, UK.*
Homoeopathic preparation.

Child Formula *Avon, Canad.*
Multivitamin and mineral preparation.

Children's Allerest *Ciba, USA.*
Phenylpropanolamine hydrochloride (p.1067·2); chlorpheniramine maleate (p.405·1).
Upper respiratory-tract symptoms.

Children's Benylin DM-D *Warner-Lambert, Canad.*
Dextromethorphan hydrobromide (p.1057·3) pseudoephedrine hydrochloride (p.1068·3).
Coughs; nasal congestion.

Children's Calcium With Minerals *Cenovis, Austral.; Vitelle, Austral.*
Calcium ascorbate (p.1365·2); cholecalciferol (p.1366·3); ferrous fumarate (p.1339·3); folic acid (p.1340·3); zinc amino acid chelate (p.1373·3).
Dietary supplement.

Childrens Cepacol *JB Williams, USA.*
Paracetamol (p.72·2); pseudoephedrine hydrochloride (p.1068·3).
Upper respiratory-tract disorders.

Childrens Chesty Cough Syrup *Boots, UK.*
Guaiphenesin (p.1061·3).
Formerly known as Nirolex for Children.
Coughs.

Childrens Chewable
Quest, Canad.; Quest, UK.
Multivitamin and mineral preparation.

Childrens Chewables *Sisu, Canad.*
Multivitamin and mineral preparation.

Children's CoTylenol *McNeil Consumer, USA†.*
Paracetamol (p.72·2); chlorpheniramine maleate (p.405·1); pseudoephedrine hydrochloride (p.1068·3).
Cold symptoms.

Childrens Diarrhoea Mixture *Unichem, UK.*
Kaolin (p.1195·1).
Diarrhoea.

Childrens Dynafed Jr *BDI, USA.*
Paracetamol (p.72·2).
Fever; pain.

Children's Formula Cough *Pharmakon, USA.*
Dextromethorphan hydrobromide (p.1057·3); guaiphenesin (p.1061·3).
Coughs.

Children's Hold *Menley & James, USA†.*
Dextromethorphan hydrobromide (p.1057·3).
Coughs.

Children's Kaopectate *Upjohn, USA.*
Attapulgite (p.1178·3).
Diarrhoea.

Childrens Mapap *Major, USA.*
Paracetamol (p.72·2).
Fever; pain.

Childrens Motion Sickness Liquid *Tanta, Canad.*
Dimenhydrinate (p.408·2).

Childrens Multi *Vitaplex, Austral.*
Multivitamin and mineral preparation with lysine hydrochloride.

Children's Multivitamins *Cenovis, Austral.; Vitelle, Austral.*
Multivitamin and mineral preparation.

Children's Nostril *Ciba, USA.*
Phenylephrine hydrochloride (p.1066·2).
Nasal congestion.

Childrens Nyquil *Procter & Gamble, Canad.*
Pseudoephedrine hydrochloride (p.1068·3); chlorpheniramine maleate (p.405·1); dextromethorphan hydrobromide (p.1057·3).
Coughs and cold symptoms.

Children's SunKist Multivitamins Complete
Ciba, USA.
Multivitamin and mineral preparation.

Children's SunKist Multivitamins + Extra C
Ciba, USA.
Multivitamin preparation.

Children's SunKist Multivitamins + Iron *Ciba, USA.*
Multivitamin preparation with iron.

Children's Tylenol Cold Multi-Symptom *McNeil Consumer, USA.*
Pseudoephedrine hydrochloride (p.1068·3); chlorpheniramine maleate (p.405·1); paracetamol (p.72·2).
Upper respiratory-tract symptoms.

Children's Tylenol Cold Multi-Symptom Plus Cough *McNeil Consumer, USA.*
Paracetamol (p.72·2); dextromethorphan hydrobromide (p.1057·3); chlorpheniramine maleate (p.405·1); pseudoephedrine hydrochloride (p.1068·3).
Coughs and cold symptoms.

Childrevit *Diviser Aquilea, Spain.*
Cyproheptadine hydrochloride (p.407·2); amino acids and vitamins.
Tonic.

Chimax *Chiron, UK.*
Flutamide (p.537·1).
Prostatic cancer.

Chimodil *Yamanouchi, Ital.*
Aluminium hydroxide (p.1177·3); magnesium hydroxide (p.1198·2).
Dyspepsia associated with gastric hyperacidity.

Chimono *Lusofarmaco, Ital.*
Lomefloxacin hydrochloride (p.222·2).
Bacterial infections.

Chimotetra *Serono, Ital.†.*
Tetracycline hydrochloride (p.259·1); chymotrypsin (p.1563·2); trypsin (p.1640·1).
Bacterial infections.

China *Sanamed, Aust.*
Camphor (p.1557·2); clove oil (p.1565·2); menthol (p.1600·2).
Musculoskeletal and joint disorders; neuralgia; respiratory-tract disorders.

China Diarrhea L107 Homeocan, Canad.
Homoeopathic preparation.

China Eisenwein Ungar, Aust.
Ferrous citrate; tinct. cinchona comp (p.1564·1).
Iron deficiency; tonic.

China Med Complex Dynamit, Aust.
Homoeopathic preparation.

China Minze Serturner, Ger.†.
Peppermint oil (p.1208·1).
Cold symptoms.

China-Eisenwein Mayrhofer, Aust.
Mace flowers; gentian (p.1583·3); bitter-orange peel (p.1610·3); centaury (p.1561·1); ceratonia (p.1472·2); cinchona bark (p.1564·1); cinnamon (p.1564·2); ferrous citrate; ferrous ascorbate (p.1339·2).
Tonic.

Chinavit Nattermann, Ger.†.
Salicylamide (p.82·3); cinchona bark (p.1564·1); ascorbic acid (p.1365·2).
Cold symptoms; influenza.

Chinine Rhone-Poulenc Rorer, Austral.†.
Quinine sulphate (p.439·2).
Malaria; night cramps.

Chinoidina Giovanardi, Ital.
Cinchona calisaya (p.1564·1); gentian (p.1583·3); kola (p.1645·1).
Dyspepsia.

Chinomint Plus Chinosolfabrik, Ger.†.
Hydroxyquinoline sulphate (p.1589·3); potassium sulphate (p.1161·2); cetylpyridinium chloride (p.1106·2).
Bacterial and fungal infections of the oropharynx.

Chinosol Chinosolfabrik, Ger.
Hydroxyquinoline sulphate (p.1589·3); potassium sulphate (p.1161·2).
Skin disinfection.

Chinosol S Vaseline Chinosolfabrik, Ger.
Hydroxyquinoline sulphate (p.1589·3); potassium sulphate (p.1161·2).
Formerly contained hydroxyquinoline and methyl salicylate.
Infective skin disorders.

Chinson Corvi, Ital.†.
Ambroxol acefyllinate (p.1054·3).
Bronchospasm.

Chinteina Lafare, Ital.
Quinidine sulphate (p.939·1).
Arrhythmias.

Chirofossat N Dreluso, Ger.
Homoeopathic preparation.

Chiron Barrier Cream Simcare, UK.
Aluminium chlorohydrate (p.1078·3).

Chironair Odour Control Liquid Simcare, UK.
A deodorant for use with colostomies and ileostomies.

Chiroplexan H Pfluger, Ger.
Homoeopathic preparation.

Chisi Propan, S.Afr.
Turpentine oil (p.1641·1); rectified camphor oil; capsicum oleoresin; methyl salicylate (p.55·2).
Musculoskeletal and joint disorders.

Chlo-Amine Hollister-Stier, USA.
Chlorpheniramine maleate (p.405·1).
Hypersensitivity reactions.

Chlor Vortech, USA.
Chlorpheniramine maleate (p.405·1).
Hypersensitivity reactions.

Chlor-3 Fleming, USA.
Sodium chloride (p.1162·2); potassium chloride (p.1161·1); magnesium chloride (p.1157·2).
Medical condiment; table salt substitute.

Chloractil DDSA Pharmaceuticals, UK.
Chlorpromazine hydrochloride (p.649·1).
Anxiety; intractable hiccup; premedication; psychoses; vomiting.

Chloraethyl "Dr Henning" Henning Walldorf, Ger.
Ethyl chloride (p.1292·3).
Local anaesthesia.

Chlorafed Roberts, USA.
Chlorpheniramine maleate (p.405·1); pseudoephedrine hydrochloride (p.1068·3).
Cold symptoms.

Chloraldurat
Salus, Aust.; Pohl, Ger.; Pohl, Neth.; Pohl, Switz.
Chloral hydrate (p.645·3).
Insomnia; sedative; tetany.

Chloralix Riker, Austral.†.
Chloral hydrate (p.645·3).
Insomnia.

Chloramex Lagamed, S.Afr.
Chloramphenicol (p.182·1).
Eye infections.

Chloramex H Lagamed, S.Afr.†.
Chloramphenicol (p.182·1); hydrocortisone acetate (p.1043·3).
Inflammatory bacterial infections.

Chloraminophene Techni-Pharma, Mon.
Chlorambucil (p.512·3).
Glomerulonephritis; leukaemia; lymphoma.

Chlorammonic Promedica, Fr.
Ammonium chloride (p.1055·2).
Alkalosis; sodium and water retention; urinary-tract disorders.

Chloramon Streuli, Switz.
Ammonium chloride (p.1055·2).
Bronchitis; metabolic alkalosis.

Chloramsaar N Chephasaar, Ger.
Chloramphenicol (p.182·1).
Bacterial infections.

Chlorasept Baxter, UK.
Chlorhexidine acetate (p.1107·2).
Bladder irrigation; skin disinfection.

Chloraseptic
Note. This name is used for preparations of different composition.
Procter & Gamble, Canad.
Lozenges: Benzocaine (p.1286·2); menthol (p.1600·2).

Procter & Gamble, Canad.; Pharmatec, S.Afr.†.
Throat spray: Phenol (p.1121·2).
Sore throat.

Procter & Gamble (H&B Care), UK†.
Phenol (p.1121·2); sodium phenolate; menthol (p.1600·2); thymol (p.1127·1); glycerol.
Oral hygiene.

Chlorasol Seton, UK.
Sodium hypochlorite (p.1124·3).
Skin disinfection.

Chlorate Major, USA†.
Chlorpheniramine maleate (p.405·1).
Hypersensitivity reactions.

Chlor-Athrombon Berlin-Chemie, Ger.†.
Clorindione.
Thrombo-embolic disorders.

Chlorazin Streuli, Switz.
Chlorpromazine hydrochloride (p.649·1).
Nausea; pain; pruritus; psychoses; vertigo; vomiting.

Chlorazol Qualiphar, Belg.
Chloramine (p.1106·3).
Disinfection.

Chlorcol Propan, S.Afr.
Chloramphenicol (p.182·1).
Bacterial infections.

Chlordrine Rugby, USA.
Pseudoephedrine hydrochloride (p.1068·3); chlorpheniramine maleate (p.405·1).
Upper respiratory-tract symptoms.

Chloresium Rystan, USA.
Chlorophyllin copper complex (p.1000·1).
Relief of pain, malodour, and inflammation of wounds, burns, surface ulcers, cuts, abrasions and skin irritations; wound healing.

Chlorethyl Adroka, Switz.
Ethyl chloride (p.1292·3).
Local anaesthesia.

Chlorgest-HD Great Southern, USA†.
Phenylephrine hydrochloride (p.1066·2); chlorpheniramine maleate (p.405·1); hydrocodone tartrate (p.43·1).
Coughs and cold symptoms.

Chlorhexamed
Procter & Gamble, Aust.; Procter & Gamble, Belg.†; Blend-a-med, Ger.; Procter & Gamble, Switz.
Chlorhexidine gluconate (p.1107·2).
Mouth infections; oral hygiene.

Chlorhex-a-myl Blend-a-pharm, Fr.†.
Chlorhexidine gluconate (p.1107·2).
Mouth infections.

Chlorhexseptic Pharmascience, Canad.
Chlorhexidine gluconate (p.1107·2).
Disinfection.

Chlorhist Propan, S.Afr.
Chlorpheniramine maleate (p.405·1).
Hypersensitivity reactions.

Chloridia Aerocid, Fr.†.
Hydrochloric acid (p.1588·3); pepsin (p.1616·3); amylocaine hydrochloride (p.1286·1); chloroform (p.1220·3).
Achlorhydria.

Chlorisept N Chinosolfabrik, Ger.†.
Tolnaftate (p.389·1).
Powder and ointment formerly contained cloxyquin. Topical solution formerly contained cloxyquin, salicylic acid, and benzoic acid.
Fungal infections.

Chlorispray Anios, Fr.
Chlorhexidine gluconate (p.1107·2); formaldehyde (p.1113·2); glutaraldehyde (p.1114·3); didecyldimethylammonium chloride (p.1112·2); alcohol (p.1099·1).
Surface disinfection.

Chlorochin Streuli, Switz.
Chloroquine phosphate (p.426·3).
Lupus erythematosus; malaria; polyarthritis.

Chlorocort Parke, Davis, Austral.
Chloramphenicol (p.182·1); hydrocortisone acetate (p.1043·3).
Eye infections.

Chlorohex
Note. This name is used for preparations of different composition.
Colgate Oral Care, Austral.; Colgate-Palmolive, UK.
Chlorhexidine gluconate (p.1107·2).
Mouth infections; oral hygiene.

Geistlich, Switz.
Chlorhexidine gluconate (p.1107·2) and/or chlorhexidine hydrochloride (p.1107·2).
Skin and hand disinfection.

Chlorohex-U Geistlich, Switz.†.
Chlorhexidine gluconate (p.1107·2).
Cystoscopic investigations.

Chloro-Magnesion Pautrat, Fr.
Magnesium chloride (p.1157·2); calcium chloride (p.1155·1).
Magnesium deficiency.

Chloromycetin
Parke, Davis, Austral.; Parke, Davis, Belg.†; Parke, Davis, Canad.; Parke, Davis, Irl.; Parke, Davis, Ital.; Parke, Davis, S.Afr.; Parke, Davis, Spain; Parke, Davis, Swed.; Parke, Davis, Switz.; Forley, UK; Parke, Davis, UK†; Parke, Davis, USA.
Chloramphenicol (p.182·1), chloramphenicol palmitate (p.182·2), or chloramphenicol sodium succinate (p.182·2).
Bacterial infections.

Chloromycetin Hydrocortison Parke, Davis, Swed.†.
Chloramphenicol (p.182·1); hydrocortisone acetate (p.1043·3).
Eye inflammation with bacterial infection.

Chloromycetin Hydrocortisone
Parke, Davis, UK.; Parke, Davis, USA.
Chloramphenicol (p.182·1); hydrocortisone acetate (p.1043·3).
Eye inflammation with bacterial infection.

Chloromyxin Parke, Davis, Austral.†.
Chloramphenicol (p.182·1); polymyxin B sulphate (p.239·1).
Bacterial eye infections.

Chloropect Laser, S.Afr.
Kaolin (p.1195·1); pectin (p.1474·1); bismuth subcarbonate (p.1180·1); chloroform and morphine tincture (p.56·1).
Diarrhoea.

Chlorophyll Potter's, UK.
Kola nut (p.1645·1); chlorophyllin (p.1000·1).
Tonic.

Chlorophyllin Salbe "Schuh" Coradol, Ger.
Chlorophyllin (p.1000·1); chamomilla; arnica; hamamelis (p.1587·1).
Wounds.

Chloropotassuril Rhone-Poulenc Rorer, Belg.
Potassium chloride (p.1161·1).
Potassium depletion.

Chloroptic
Allergan, Austral.†; Allergan, Canad.; Allergan, Ger.†; Allergan, Irl.; Allergan, S.Afr.; Allergan, USA.
Chloramphenicol (p.182·1).
Eye infections.

Chloroserpine Rugby, USA†.
Chlorothiazide (p.839·1); reserpine (p.942·1).
Hypertension.

Chlorphed-LA Roberts, USA; Hauck, USA.
Oxymetazoline hydrochloride (p.1065·3).
Nasal congestion.

Chlorphedrine SR Goldline, USA.
Pseudoephedrine hydrochloride (p.1068·3); chlorpheniramine maleate (p.405·1).
Upper respiratory-tract symptoms.

Chlorphen Caps, S.Afr.
Chloramphenicol (p.182·1).
Bacterial infections.

Chlor-Pro Schein, USA.
Chlorpheniramine maleate (p.405·1).
Hypersensitivity reactions.

Chlorpromanyl Technilab, Canad.
Chlorpromazine hydrochloride (p.649·1).
Nausea and vomiting; psychoses.

Chlorquin Rhone-Poulenc Rorer, Austral.
Chloroquine phosphate (p.426·3).
Amoebic hepatitis; lupus erythematosus; malaria; rheumatoid arthritis and related collagen disease.

Chlor-Rest Rugby, USA.
Phenylpropanolamine hydrochloride (p.1067·2); chlorpheniramine maleate (p.405·1).
Upper respiratory-tract symptoms.

Chlorsig Sigma, Austral.
Chloramphenicol (p.182·1).
Bacterial eye infections.

Chlorspan Vortech, USA.
Chlorpheniramine maleate (p.405·1).
Hypersensitivity reactions.

Chlortab Vortech, USA†.
Chlorpheniramine maleate (p.405·1).
Hypersensitivity reactions.

Chlortesin-N Atzinger, Ger.†.
Allantoin (p.1078·2); glucose; hamamelis water (p.1587·1); cod-liver oil (p.1337·3).
Ulcers.

Chlor-Trimeton
Schering-Plough, S.Afr.; Schering-Plough, USA.
Chlorpheniramine maleate (p.405·1).
Hypersensitivity reactions.

Chlor-Trimeton Allergy Sinus Schering-Plough, USA.
Phenylpropanolamine hydrochloride (p.1067·2); chlorpheniramine maleate (p.405·1); paracetamol (p.72·2).
Upper respiratory-tract symptoms.

Chlor-Trimeton 4 Hour Relief Schering-Plough, USA.
Pseudoephedrine sulphate (p.1068·3); chlorpheniramine maleate (p.405·1).
Upper respiratory-tract symptoms.

Chlor-Trimeton 12 Hour Relief Schering-Plough, USA.
Pseudoephedrine sulphate (p.1068·3); chlorpheniramine maleate (p.405·1).
Upper respiratory-tract symptoms.

Chlor-Tripolon Schering, Canad.
Chlorpheniramine maleate (p.405·1).
Hypersensitivity disorders; pruritus.

Chlor-Tripolon Decongestant Schering, Canad.
Syrup: Chlorpheniramine maleate (p.405·1); phenylpropanolamine hydrochloride (p.1067·2).
Tablets: Chlorpheniramine maleate (p.405·1); pseudoephedrine sulphate (p.1068·3).
Respiratory congestion.

Chlor-Tripolon ND Schering, Canad.
Loratadine (p.413·1); pseudoephedrine sulphate (p.1068·3).
Upper respiratory-tract congestion.

Chlorumagene
Thepenier, Fr.; Thepenier, Switz.
Magnesium hydroxide (p.1198·2).
Constipation.

Chlorvescent Rhone-Poulenc Rorer, Austral.
Potassium chloride (p.1161·1); potassium bicarbonate (p.1153·1).
Potassium deficiency.

Chlotride
Amrad, Austral.; Merck Sharp & Dohme, Neth.
Chlorothiazide (p.839·1).
Hypertension; oedema.

Choanol Hanosan, Ger.†.
Chelidonium; silybum marianum (p.993·3); turmeric (p.1001·3); berberis; echinacea angustifolia (p.1574·2); quassia amara; leptandra; nux vomica; lycopodium.
Liver and biliary disorders.

Chocaton Mirren, S.Afr.
Multivitamin preparation.

Chocovite
Torbet, Irl.; Torbet Laboratories, UK.
Calcium gluconate (p.1155·2); ergocalciferol (p.1367·1).
Calcium and vitamin D deficiency.

Choice dm Mead Johnson Nutritionals, USA.
Preparation for enteral nutrition.
Abnormal glucose tolerance.

Chol 4000 Lichtenstein, Ger.
Chelidonium.
Biliary and gastro-intestinal spasm.

Cholac Alra, USA.
Lactulose (p.1195·3).
Constipation; hepatic encephalopathy.

Cholacid Madaus, Ger.
Ursodeoxycholic acid (p.1642·1).
Biliary-tract disorders.

Cholaflux Nattermann Tee-Arznei, Ger.†.
Powder for tea: Spinacia oleracea; silybum marianum (p.993·3); potentilla anserina; chelidonium; achillea (p.1542·2); liquorice (p.1197·1); rhubarb (p.1212·1); taraxacum (p.1634·2); turmeric (p.1001·3); aloes (p.1177·1); curcuma oil.
Tea: Peppermint leaf (p.1208·1); senna (p.1212·2); caraway (p.1559·3); centaury (p.1561·1); chelidonium; achillea (p.1542·2); liquorice (p.1197·1); taraxacum (p.1634·2); turmeric (p.1001·3); spinacia oleracea; urtica (p.1642·3).
Herbal tea.

Cholaflux N Nattermann Tee-Arznei, Ger.†.
Piscidia erythrina; peppermint leaf (p.1208·1); spinacia oleracea; aniseed (p.1549·3); silybum marianum (p.993·3); caraway (p.1559·3); fennel (p.1579·1); potentilla anserina; chelidonium; achillea (p.1542·2); liquorice (p.1197·1); taraxacum (p.1634·2); turmeric (p.1001·3); rhubarb (p.1212·1); aloes (p.1177·1).
Herbal tea.

Cholagogum Polcopharma, Austral.†.
Carum carvi (p.1559·3); chelidonium majus; curcumis sativus; glycyrrhiza glabra (p.1197·1); achillea millefolium (p.1542·2); spinacea oleracea; taraxacum officinale (p.1634·2).
Biliary disorders.

Cholagogum F Nattermann, Ger.
Turmeric (p.1001·3); chelidonium.
Biliary-tract disorders.

Cholagogum N Nattermann, Ger.
Chelidonium; turmeric (p.1001·3); peppermint oil (p.1208·1).
Biliary disorders; gallstones.

Cholagutt-N Albert-Roussel, Ger.; Hoechst, Ger.
Chelidonium majus; lavandula latifolia; peppermint leaf (p.1208·1).
Biliary disorders.

Cholaktol forte Medopharm, Ger.
Peppermint oil (p.1208·1).
Biliary-tract spasm.

Cholaktol TR Medopharm, Ger.†.
Taraxacum (p.1634·2).
Biliary-tract disorders.

Cholaktol-L Pharmasal, Ger.†.
Peppermint oil (p.1208·1); caraway oil (p.1559·3); rhubarb (p.1212·1); aloes (p.1177·1); cascara (p.1183·1); magnesium oxide (p.1198·3).
Biliary disorders; constipation associated with liver or biliary disorders.

Cholan-HMB Ciba Consumer, USA.
Dehydrocholic acid (p.1570·2).
Biliary stasis; constipation.

Cholapret Bionorica, Ger.
Boldo (p.1554·1); chelidonium; curcuma zanthorrhiza.
Biliary disorders; gastro-intestinal disorders.

Cholarist Steiner, Ger.
Chelidonium.
Smooth muscle spasm.

Cholasitrol Lifeplan, UK.
Sitosterol (p.1279·3); vitamins; minerals.
Nutritional supplement.

Cholasyn Rolmex, Canad.
Cascara (p.1183·1); phenolphthalein (p.1208·2).

Cholasyn II Rolmex, Canad.
Cascara (p.1183·1); senna (p.1212·2).

Choldestal
Krugmann, Ger.
Capsules: Turmeric (p.1001·3).
Dyspepsia.
Oral drops†: Curcuma zanthorrhiza; gentian (p.1583·3); fumitory (p.1581·3); berberis; rhubarb (p.1212·1); zedoary; agaricus albus; aloes (p.1177·1).
Tablets†: Papain (p.1614·1); cysteine hydrochloride (p.1338·3); caraway oil (p.1559·3); cineole (p.1564·1); curcuma zanthorrhiza; gentian (p.1583·3); fumitory (p.1581·3); berberis; rhubarb (p.1212·1); zedoary; agaricus albus; aloes (p.1177·1).
Gastro-intestinal disorders.

Chol-Do Grasler, Ger.
Homoeopathic preparation.

Cholebrin Nycomed, Swed.
Iocetamic acid (p.1005·2).
Contrast medium for cholecystography.

Cholebrine
Mundipharma, Ger.†; Asta Medica, Neth.; Mallinckrodt, USA.
Iocetamic acid (p.1005·2).
Contrast medium for cholecystography.

Cholebrine-Reizmahlzeit Mundipharma, Ger.†.
Theobroma seed (p.1636·2); theobroma oil (p.1385·2); milk powder; sorbitol (p.1354·2).
Adjuvant to biliary-tract radiography.

Chole-cyl Ho-Len-Complex Liebermann, Ger.
Homoeopathic preparation.

Cholecysmon Dresden, Ger.
Ox bile extract (p.1553·2).
Liver, bile, and pancreas disorders.

Choledyl
Warner-Lambert, Austral.†; Parke, Davis, Canad.; Parke, Davis, Irl.; Parke, Davis, S.Afr.; Parke, Davis, Spain†; Parke, Davis, UK†; Parke, Davis, USA.
Choline theophyllinate (p.751·3).
Obstructive airways disease.

Choledyl Expectorant Parke, Davis, Canad.
Choline theophyllinate (p.751·3); guaiphenesin (p.1061·3).
Obstructive airways disease.

Cholegerol Holistica, Fr.
Soya lecithin (p.1595·2); wheat germ; shiitake; herbs.
Cholesterol reduction.

Cholemin Berk, UK.
Cholestyramine (p.1269·3).
Hyperlipidaemias.

Choleodoron
Note. This name is used for preparations of different composition.
Weleda, Aust.; Weleda, Ger.; Weleda, UK.
Chelidonium; turmeric (p.1001·3).
Liver and biliary disorders.
Weleda, Fr.
Homoeopathic preparation.

Cholesolvin
Cyanamid, Ital.; Yoshitomi, Jpn.
Simfibrate (p.1278·2).
Hyperlipidaemias.

Cholestabyl Fournier, Ger.
Colestipol hydrochloride (p.1272·1).
Hypercholesterolaemia.

Cholest-X L112 Homeocan, Canad.
Homoeopathic preparation.

Choletec
Squibb Diagnostics, Canad.; Squibb Diagnostics, USA.
Technetium-99m mebrofenin (p.1425·1).
Hepatobiliary imaging.

Chol-Grandelat Synpharma, Aust.
Chamomile (p.1561·2); peppermint oil (p.1208·1); achillea (p.1542·2).
Gallbladder disorders.

Cholhepan N Schuck, Ger.
Silybum marianum (p.993·3); chelidonium majus; aloes (p.1177·1).
Biliary disorders; constipation; flatulence.

Cholidase Freeda, USA.
Vitamin B substances with vitamin E.

Cholinoid Goldline, USA.
Vitamin B substances with vitamin C; lemon bioflavonoids (p.1580·1).

Cholipin
Boehringer Ingelheim, Belg.†; Boehringer Ingelheim, Spain†.
Fenipentol (p.1579·1); octibenzonium bromide.
Biliary-tract disorders.

Cholit-Chenosan Fresenius, Ger.†.
Chenodeoxycholic acid (p.1562·1).
Gallstones.

Cholit-Ursan Fresenius, Ger.
Ursodeoxycholic acid (p.1642·1).
Cholesterol gallstones.

Chol-Kugeletten Neu Dolorgiet, Ger.
Chelidonium; aloes (p.1177·1).
Biliary disorders.

Cholofalk Falk, Ger.
Ursodeoxycholic acid (p.1642·1).
Primary biliary cirrhosis.

Cholografin
Squibb Diagnostics, Canad.; Squibb Diagnostics, USA.
Meglumine iodipamide (p.1005·3).
Contrast medium for biliary-tract radiography.

Chologram Schering, Ital.†.
Meglumine iotroxate (p.1008·2).
Contrast medium for biliary-tract radiography.

Cholonerton
Schoeller, Aust.†; Dolorgiet, Ger.†.
Hymecromone (p.1589·3).
Liver and gallbladder disorders.

Cholongal Molitor, Ger.†.
Oral liquid: Castor; valerian (p.1643·1); rhubarb (p.1212·1); cardamom (p.1560·1); peppermint leaf (p.1208·1); chelidonium; rorippa nasturtium aquaticum; taraxacum (p.1634·2); fumitory (p.1581·3).
Tablets: Pancreatin (p.1612·1); rhubarb (p.1212·1); valerian (p.1643·1); silybum marianum (p.993·3); castor; cardamom (p.1560·1).
Biliary disorders; gallstones.

Cholongal plus Molitor, Ger.†.
Castor; valerian (p.1643·1); silybum marianum (p.993·3); rhubarb (p.1212·1); cardamom (p.1560·1); peppermint leaf (p.1208·1); fumitory (p.1581·3); chelidonium; herba nasturtii; taraxacum (p.1634·2).
Biliary disorders; gallstones.

Cholosan Spreewald, Ger.
Raphanus sativus var nigra.
Dyspepsia.

Cholosolm Phyto Hevert, Ger.
Chelidonium; turmeric (p.1001·3); taraxacum (p.1634·2).
Liver and bile disorders.

Cholosom Hevert, Ger.†.
Acriflavine (p.1098·3); aloes (p.1177·1); chelidonium; turmeric (p.1001·3); rhubarb (p.1212·1); taraxacum (p.1634·2); ox bile (p.1553·2); caraway oil (p.1559·3); peppermint oil (p.1208·1).
Gastro-intestinal disorders.

Cholosom SL Hevert, Ger.
Chelidonium; curcuma zanthorrhiza; taraxacum (p.1634·2).
Liver and bile disorders.

Cholosom-Tee Hevert, Ger.
Caraway (p.1559·3); curcuma zanthorrhiza; taraxacum (p.1634·2); silybum marianum (p.993·3) peppermint leaf (p.1208·1).
Biliary-tract disorders; gastro-intestinal disorders.

Cholosum N Hevert, Ger.†.
Cascara (p.1183·1); chelidonium; curcuma zanthorrhiza; rhubarb (p.1212·1); taraxacum (p.1634·2); caraway oil (p.1559·3); peppermint oil (p.1208·1).
Biliary disorders; gastro-intestinal disorders.

Choloxin
Knoll, Canad.; Boots-Flint, USA.
Dextrothyroxine sodium (p.1272·2).
Hyperlipidaemias.

Cholsoy L Giuliani, Ital.†.
Lecithin (p.1595·2).
Hypercholesterolaemia.

Cholspasmin Lipha, Ger.
Hymecromone (p.1589·3) or hymecromone sodium (p.1589·3).
Biliary-tract disorders.

Cholspasminase Lipha, Ger.†.
Hymecromone (p.1589·3); pancreatin (p.1612·1); cellulase (p.1561·1).
Digestive system disorders.

Cholspasminase N Lipha, Ger.
Pancreatin (p.1612·1).
Pancreatic disorders.

Chol-Spasmoletten Dolorgiet, Ger.
Hymecromone (p.1589·3).
Biliary disorders.

Chol-Truw S Truw, Ger.
Oral drops: Homoeopathic preparation.
Tablets: Curcuma zanthorrhiza; chelidonium; acetic acid (p.1541·2); absinthium (p.1541·1).
Biliary disorders.

Chomelanum
Brady, Aust.; Schur, Ger.
Choline stearate.
Skin disorders; soft-tissue disorders.

Chondrosulf Genevrier, Fr.
Sodium chondroitin sulphate A (p.1562·2).
Osteoarthritis.

Chooz Schering-Plough, USA.
Calcium carbonate (p.1182·1).
Hyperacidity.

Chophytol
Rosa-Phytopharma, Fr.; Rosa-Phytopharma, Switz.
Cynara (p.1569·2).
Gastro-intestinal disorders; kidney disorders.

Choragon
Ferring, Ger.; Ferring, UK.
Chorionic gonadotrophin (p.1243·1).
Delayed puberty; female infertility; oligospermia; undescended testes.

Chorex Hyrex, USA.
Chorionic gonadotrophin (p.1243·1).
Male and female infertility; male hypogonadism; prepubertal cryptorchidism.

Chorigon Dunhall, USA†.
Chorionic gonadotrophin (p.1243·1).
Male and female infertility; male hypogonadism; prepubertal cryptorchidism.

Choron Forest Pharmaceuticals, USA.
Chorionic gonadotrophin (p.1243·1).
Male and female infertility; male hypogonadism; prepubertal cryptorchidism.

Chromagen Savage, USA.
Ferrous fumarate (p.1339·3); vitamin B_{12} substances (p.1363·3); intrinsic factor (stomach preparation).
Vitamin C (p.1365·2) is included in this preparation to increase the absorption and availability of iron.
Anaemias.

Chromagen FA Savage, USA.
Ferrous fumarate (p.1339·3); cyanocobalamin (p.1363·3); folic acid (p.1340·3).
Vitamin C (p.1365·2) is included in this preparation to increase the absorption and availability of iron.
Anaemias.

Chromagen Forte Savage, USA.
Ferrous fumarate (p.1339·3); cyanocobalamin (p.1363·3); folic acid (p.1340·3).
Vitamin C (p.1365·2) is included in this preparation to increase the absorption and availability of iron.
Anaemias.

Chroma-Pak Smith & Nephew SoloPak, USA.
Chromium trichloride (p.1337·1).
Additive for intravenous total parenteral nutrition solutions.

Chromargon Richard, Fr.
Hydroxyquinoline sulphate (p.1589·3); acriflavine (p.1098·3).
Skin infections.

Chrome Eagle, Austral.
Chromium chelate.
Dietary supplement.

Chromelin Complexion Blender Summers, USA.
Dihydroxyacetone (p.1081·2).
Hypopigmentation; vitiligo.

Chrometrace Rorer, Austral.†.
Chromium trichloride (p.1337·1).
Additive for intravenous total parenteral nutrition solutions.

Chromitope Squibb Diagnostics, USA.
Chromium-51 (p.1423·2) as sodium chromate.

Chronadalate Bayer, Fr.
Nifedipine (p.916·2).
Angina pectoris; hypertension.

Chronexan Asta Medica, Fr.
Xipamide (p.971·2).
Hypertension; oedema.

Chronocard Redel, Ger.
Crataegus (p.1568·2).
Cardiac disorders.

Chronocorte Streuli, Switz.
Dexamethasone (p.1037·1); dexamethasone sodium phosphate (p.1037·2).
Corticosteroid.

Chrono-Indocid Merck Sharp & Dohme-Chibret, Fr.
Indomethacin (p.45·2).
Musculoskeletal and joint disorders.

Chronophyllin Byk Madaus, S.Afr.
Theophylline (p.765·1).
Obstructive airways disease.

Chronulac
Hoechst Marion Roussel, Canad.; Merrell Dow, USA.
Lactulose (p.1195·3).
Constipation.

Chrysocor Sanum-Kehlbeck, Ger.
Placenta extracts (human).
Sexual disorders.

Chymalgyl Rhone-Poulenc Rorer, Belg.†.
Aspirin (p.16·1); pancreatic proteolytic enzymes.
Fever; muscle and tissue damage; pain.

Chymar
Note. This name is used for preparations of different composition.
Rorer, Irl.†.
Chymotrypsin (p.1563·2).
Inflammation; oedema.
Semar, Spain†.
Chymotrypsin (p.1563·2); trypsin (p.1640·1).
Inflammation; oedema.

Chymex Adria, USA.
Bentiromide (p.1552·2).
Diagnosis of pancreatic insufficiency.

Chymocyclar
Note. This name is used for preparations of different composition.
Rorer, Irl.†.
Tetracycline (p.259·1); purified pancreatic concentrate.
Bacterial infections.
Semar, Spain†.
Tetracycline hydrochloride (p.259·1); trypsin (p.1640·1); chymotrypsin (p.1563·2).
Bacterial infections.

Chymocycline Rhone-Poulenc Rorer, Switz.†.
Tetracycline hydrochloride (p.259·1); pancreatin (p.1612·1).
Bacterial infections.

Chymodiactin
Knoll, Austral.; Knoll, Canad.; Knoll, Irl.; Knoll, Spain; Knoll, UK; Boots-Flint, USA.
Chymopapain (p.1562·3).
Herniated lumbar intervertebral disc.

Chymodiactine Knoll, Fr.
Chymopapain (p.1562·3).
Sciatica secondary to herniated disc.

Chymol Emollient Balm Waterhouse, UK.
Eucalyptus oil (p.1578·1); terpineol (p.1635·1); methyl salicylate (p.55·2); phenol (p.1121·2).
Bruises; chapped skin; chilblains; sprains.

Chymoral
Rorer, Irl.†; Rorer, Ital.†.
Chymotrypsin (p.1563·2); trypsin (p.1640·1).
Inflammation; oedema.

Chymoser Serono, Ital.†.
Chymotrypsin (p.1563·2); trypsin (p.1640·1).
Inflammation.

Chymoser Balsamico Serono, Ital.†.
Chymotrypsin (p.1563·2); trypsin (p.1640·1); potassium guaiacolsulfonate (p.1068·3); terpin hydrate (p.1070·2); guaiphenesin (p.1061·3); sodium benzoate (p.1102·3).
Respiratory-tract disorders.

Ciarbiot Vir, Spain.
Ampicillin trihydrate (p.153·2).
Bacterial infections.

Ciatyl Tropon, Ger.
Zuclopenthixol acetate (p.700·2), zuclopenthixol decanoate (p.700·2), or zuclopenthixol hydrochloride (p.700·2).
Psychoses.

Ciba Vision Cleaner For Sensitive Eyes Ciba Vision, USA.
Cleaning solution for soft contact lenses.

Cibacalcin
Ciba-Geigy, Aust.; Novartis, Austral.; Geigy, Ger.; Ciba, Ital.; Novartis, Neth.; Novartis, Swed.; Ciba, USA†.
Calcitonin (human) (p.735·3).
Hypercalcaemia; osteolysis; osteoporosis; Paget's disease of bone; reflex sympathetic dystrophy.

Cibacalcina Ciba-Geigy, Spain.
Calcitonin (human) (p.735·3).
Hypercalcaemia; metastatic bone pain; osteoporosis; Paget's disease of bone.

Cibacalcine
Ciba-Geigy, Belg.; Ciba-Geigy, Fr.; Ciba, Switz.
Calcitonin (human) (p.735·3).
Algodystrophy; hypercalcaemia; hyperphosphatasia; osteoporosis; Paget's disease of bone; prevention of bone loss in immobilisation.

Cibace Novartis, S.Afr.
Benazepril hydrochloride (p.827·1).
Hypertension.

Cibacen
Ciba-Geigy, Aust.; Ciba-Geigy, Belg.; Ciba, Ger.; Ciba-Geigy, Irl.; Ciba, Ital.; Novartis, Neth.; Ciba-Geigy, Spain; Ciba, Switz.
Benazepril hydrochloride (p.827·1).
Heart failure; hypertension.

Cibacene Ciba-Geigy, Fr.
Benazepril hydrochloride (p.827·1).
Hypertension.

Cibadrex
Ciba-Geigy, Aust.; Ciba-Geigy, Fr.; Ciba, Ger.; Ciba, Ital.; Novartis, Neth.; Novartis, S.Afr.; Ciba-Geigy, Swed.†; Ciba, Switz.
Benazepril hydrochloride (p.827·1); hydrochlorothiazide (p.885·2).
Hypertension.

Cibalen Geigy, Ger.†.
Propyphenazone (p.81·3); drofenine hydrochloride (p.460·3); codeine phosphate (p.26·1).
Cramp; fever; pain.

Cibalgina
Zyma, Ital.†; Ciba-Geigy, Spain.
Propyphenazone (p.81·3).
Formerly contained propyphenazone and allobarbitone in *Ital.*
Fever; pain.

Cibalgina Compuesta Ciba-Geigy, Spain.
Codeine phosphate (p.26·1); propyphenazone (p.81·3).
Fever; pain.

Cibalgina Due Fast Novartis Consumer, Ital.
Ibuprofen (p.44·1).
Fever; influenza symptoms; pain.

Cibalgine Zyma, Belg.†.
Propyphenazone (p.81·3).
Fever; pain.

Cibalith-S Ciba, USA†.
Lithium citrate (p.290·3).
Bipolar disorder.

Ciblor Inava, Fr.
Amoxycillin trihydrate (p.151·3); potassium clavulanate (p.190·2).
Bacterial infections.

Cica-Care
Smith & Nephew, Fr.; Smith & Nephew Healthcare, UK.
Silicone (p.1384·2).
Hypertrophic scars; keloids.

Cicaderma Boiron, Fr.
Calendula officinalis; hypericum perforatum (p.1590·1); achillea millefolium (p.1542·2); ledum palustre; anemone pulsatilla (p.1623·3).
Superficial burns and wounds.

Cicafissan Uhlmann-Eyraud, Switz.
Casein hydrolysate; kaolin (p.1195·1); colloidal silicon dioxide (p.1475·1); bismuth subnitrate (p.1180·2); zinc oxide (p.1096·2).
Burns; skin disorders; wounds.

Cicamosa Lutsia, Fr.
Mimosa tenuiflora.

Cicatral Diviser Aquilea, Spain.
Peru balsam (p.1617·2); ergocalciferol (p.1367·1); oestrone (p.1458·2); benzocaine (p.1286·2); retinol (p.1358·1); tyrothricin (p.267·2).
Skin disorders.

Cicatrene Warner-Lambert, Ital.
Neomycin sulphate (p.229·2); bacitracin zinc (p.157·3).
Skin infections.

Cicatrex Glaxo Wellcome, Aust.; Glaxo Wellcome, Ger.; Wellcome, Switz.
Bacitracin zinc (p.157·3); neomycin sulphate (p.229·2); cysteine; glycine; DL-threonine.
Bacterial skin infections; infected wounds and burns.

Cicatrin Glaxo Wellcome, Austral.; Glaxo Wellcome, Canad.; Wellcome, Irl.; Glaxo Wellcome, S.Afr.; Wellcome, UK.
Bacitracin zinc (p.157·3); neomycin sulphate (p.229·2); L-cysteine; glycine DL-threonine.
Bacterial skin infections; burns; wounds.

Cicatryl Darcy, Fr.
Allantoin (p.1078·2); guaiazulene (p.1586·3); chlorocresol (p.1110·3); alpha tocopheryl acetate (p.1369·1).
Superficial burns and wounds.

Cicladol Master Pharma, Ital.
Piroxicam betadex (p.81·1).
Musculoskeletal and joint disorders; pain.

Cicladol L Master Pharma, Ital.†.
Piroxicam (p.80·2).
Musculoskeletal and joint disorders.

Ciclafast Master Pharma, Ital.
Piroxicam pivalate (p.81·1).
Musculoskeletal and joint disorders.

Ciclochem Novag, Spain.
Ciclopirox olamine (p.376·2).
Cutaneous and mucosal fungal infections.

Ciclofalina Almirall, Spain.
Piracetam (p.1619·1).
Alcoholism; cerebrovascular disorders; mental function impairment; vertigo.

Ciclolux Allergan, Ital.
Cyclopentolate hydrochloride (p.459·3).
Production of mydriasis and cycloplegia.

Ciclople Llorens, Spain.
Cyclopentolate hydrochloride (p.459·3).
Eye disorders; production of mydriasis.

Cicloplejic Ciba Vision, Spain.
Cyclopentolate hydrochloride (p.459·3).
Eye disorders; production of mydriasis.

Cicloplejico Cusi, Spain.
Cyclopentolate hydrochloride (p.459·3).
Production of mydriasis.

Ciclospasmol Yamanouchi, Ital.
Cyclandelate (p.845·2).
Vascular disorders.

Ciclotres Pierre Fabre, Spain†.
Ascorbic acid (p.1365·2); hesperidin methyl chalcone (p.1580·2); ruscus aculeatus; troxerutin (p.1580·2).
Capillary disorders.

Cicloven AGIPS, Ital.
Pyricarbate (p.1624·1).
Vascular disorders.

Cicloxal Prodes, Spain.
Cyclophosphamide (p.516·2).
Malignant neoplasms.

Cidalgon Ecobi, Ital.†.
Indomethacin (p.45·2).
Ankylosing spondylitis; arthritis; osteoarthritis.

Cidan Est Cidan, Spain†.
Streptomycin sulphate (p.249·3).
Bacterial infections.

Cidanamox Cidan, Spain†.
Amoxycillin (p.151·3).
Bacterial infections.

Cidanbutol Cidan, Spain†.
Ethambutol hydrochloride (p.207·2).
Tuberculosis.

Cidancaina Cidan, Spain†.
Lignocaine hydrochloride (p.1293·2).
Noradrenaline acid tartrate (p.924·1) is included in some injections as a vasoconstrictor to diminish absorption and localise the effect of the local anaesthetic.
Local anaesthesia.

Cidanchin Cidan, Spain†.
Chloroquine phosphate (p.426·3).
Amoebiasis; malaria; rheumatoid arthritis; systemic lupus erythematosus.

Cidantos Cidan, Spain†.
Codeine (p.26·1) or codeine camsylate (p.27·1); ethylmorphine (p.36·1) or ethylmorphine camsylate (p.36·1).
Coughs.

Cidegol C Hofmann & Sommer, Ger.
Chlorhexidine gluconate (p.1107·2).
Mouth and throat infections and inflammation.

Cidermex Evans, Fr.
Triamcinolone acetonide (p.1050·2); neomycin sulphate (p.229·2).
Skin and eye disorders.

Cidex Johnson & Johnson Medical, Fr.; Johnson & Johnson, Ger.; Ethicon, Ital.; Johnson & Johnson Medical, UK; Johnson & Johnson Medical, USA.
Glutaraldehyde (p.1114·3).
Instrument disinfection.

Cidifos Neopharmed, Ital.†.
Citicoline sodium (p.1564·3).
Cerebrovascular disorders.

Cidilin Errekappa, Ital.
Citicoline sodium (p.1564·3).
Cerebrovascular disorders.

Cidine Almirall, Spain.
Cinitapride acid tartrate (p.1187·1).
Gastro-oesophageal reflux; gastroparesis.

Cidomel Clonmel, Irl.
Indomethacin (p.45·2).
Gout; musculoskeletal and joint disorders; pain.

Cidomycin Roussel, Austral.†; Hoechst Marion Roussel, Canad.; Hoechst Marion Roussel, Irl.; Hoechst Marion Roussel, S.Afr.; Roussel, UK.
Gentamicin sulphate (p.212·1).
Bacterial infections.

Ciella Cooperation Pharmaceutique, Fr.
Chlorbutol (p.1106·3); zinc sulphate (p.1373·2).
Eye disorders.

Ciergin Rorer, Ital.†.
Ascorbic acid (p.1365·2).
Vitamin C deficiency.

Ciergin Calcium Rorer, Ital.†.
Ascorbic acid (p.1365·2); calcium gluconate (p.1155·2).
Vitamin C and calcium deficiency.

Ciflox Bayer, Fr.; Bayropharm, Ital.†.
Ciprofloxacin (p.185·3) or ciprofloxacin hydrochloride (p.185·3).
Bacterial infections.

Cigarettes Anti-asthmatiques Denolin, Belg.†.
Belladonna herb (p.457·1); stramonium leaf (p.468·2); sage (p.1627·1); lavender flower (p.1594·3).
Asthma; bronchitis; coughs; respiratory depression.

Cigarettes Berthiot Monal, Fr.†.
Lobelia inflata (p.1481·3); coltsfoot leaf; rose petals; cinnamon oil; glycerol; honey; catechu; citric acid; potassium nitrate; peppermint oil.
Aid to smoking withdrawal.

Cig-Ridettes Or-Dov, Austral.
Lobeline hydrochloride (p.1481·3).
Aid to smoking withdrawal.

Cilamox Sigma, Austral.
Amoxycillin trihydrate (p.151·3).
Bacterial infections.

Cilest Janssen-Cilag, Belg.; Janssen-Cilag, Fr.; Janssen-Cilag, Ger.; Janssen-Cilag, Irl.; Janssen-Cilag, Ital.†; Janssen-Cilag, Neth.; Janssen-Cilag, Switz.; Cilag, UK.
Norgestimate (p.1453·3); ethinyloestradiol (p.1445·1).
Combined oral contraceptive.

Cileste Janssen-Cilag, Aust.
Norgestimate (p.1453·3); ethinyloestradiol (p.1445·1).
Combined oral contraceptive.

Cilferon-A Janssen-Cilag, Ital.
Interferon alfa (p.615·3).
Malignant neoplasms; viral infections.

Ciliar Crinos, Ital.
Timonacic methyl hydrochloride (p.1638·1).
Respiratory-tract disorders associated with viscous mucus.

Cilicaine Syringe Sigma, Austral.
Procaine penicillin (p.240·2).
Bacterial infections.

Cilicaine V Sigma, Austral.
Benzathine phenoxymethylpenicillin (p.159·2).
Bacterial infections.

Cilicaine VK Sigma, Austral.
Phenoxymethylpenicillin potassium (p.236·2).
Bacterial infections.

Cilicef Hortel, Spain†.
Capsules; oral powder: Cephalexin (p.178·2).
Bacterial infections.

Cilina Cidan, Spain†.
Benzylpenicillin sodium (p.159·3).
Bacterial infections.

Cilina 400 Cidan, Spain†.
Benzylpenicillin sodium (p.159·3); procaine penicillin (p.240·2).
Bacterial infections; rheumatic fever.

Cilinafosal Medical, Spain.
Ephedrine hydrochloride (p.1059·3); sulphanilamide sodium mesylate (p.256·3).
Nasal congestion and infection.

Cilinafosal DHD Estrep Medical, Spain.
Dihydrostreptomycin sulphate (p.202·2); ephedrine hydrochloride (p.1059·3); sulphanilamide sodium mesylate (p.256·3).
Nasal congestion and infection.

Cilinafosal Hidrocort Medical, Spain.
Ephedrine hydrochloride (p.1059·3); hydrocortisone acetate (p.1043·3); neomycin sulphate (p.229·2); sulphanilamide sodium mesylate (p.256·3).
Nasal congestion and infection.

Cilinafosal Neomicina Medical, Spain.
Ephedrine hydrochloride (p.1059·3); neomycin sulphate (p.229·2).
Nasal congestion and infection.

Cilinavagin Neomicina Medical, Spain.
Stilboestrol dipropionate (p.1462·3); neomycin sulphate (p.229·2); sulphanilamide sodium mesylate (p.256·3); zinc sulphate (p.1373·2).
Vulvovaginal infections.

Cilinvita Bronquial Vita, Spain†.
Amoxycillin trihydrate (p.151·3); bromhexine hydrochloride (p.1055·3).
Respiratory-tract infections.

Cilipen Hortel, Spain†.
Benzylpenicillin sodium (p.159·3).
Bacterial infections.

Cillimicina Hoechst Marion Roussel, Ital.†; Normon, Spain.
Lincomycin hydrochloride (p.222·1).
Bacterial infections.

Cilopen VK Douglas, Austral.
Phenoxymethylpenicillin potassium (p.236·2).
Bacterial infections.

Ciloprin Janssen-Cilag, Swed.
Acediasulfone sodium (p.150·1); oxymethurea.
Ear infections.

Ciloprin cum Anaesthetico Janssen-Cilag, Aust.
Acediasulfone (p.150·1); cinchocaine (p.1289·2).
Ear disorders.

Ciloprine ca Janssen-Cilag, Switz.
Acediasulfone sodium (p.150·1); cinchocaine (p.1289·2); oxymethurea.
Otitis.

Cilox Alcon, Norw.
Ciprofloxacin hydrochloride (p.185·3).
Bacterial keratitis.

Ciloxan Alcon, Aust.; Alcon, Austral.; Alcon, Belg.; Alcon, Canad.; Alcon-Thilo, Ger.; Alcon, S.Afr.; Alcon, Swed.; Alcon, Switz.; Alcon, UK; Alcon, USA.
Ciprofloxacin hydrochloride (p.185·3).
Bacterial eye infections.

Cimagen Antigen, Irl.
Cimetidine (p.1183·2).
Gastric hyperacidity; peptic ulcer; Zollinger-Ellison syndrome.

Cimal Alpharma, Norw.; Dumex-Alpharma, Swed.†.
Cimetidine (p.1183·2).
Aspiration syndrome; gastro-oesophageal reflux; peptic ulcer; Zollinger-Ellison syndrome.

Cime Eu Rho, Ger.; Sanorania, Ger.
Cimetidine (p.1183·2).
Aspiration syndromes; gastro-oesophageal reflux; peptic ulcer; Zollinger-Ellison syndrome.

Cimebeta Betapharm, Ger.
Cimetidine (p.1183·2).
Aspiration syndromes; gastro-intestinal haemorrhage; gastro-oesophageal reflux; peptic ulcer; Zollinger-Ellison syndrome.

Cimehexal Hexal, Ger.
Cimetidine (p.1183·2) or cimetidine hydrochloride (p.1185·3).
Aspiration syndromes; gastro-intestinal haemorrhage; gastro-oesophageal reflux; peptic ulcer; Zollinger-Ellison syndrome.

Cimeldine Clonmel, Irl.
Cimetidine (p.1183·2).
Gastric hyperacidity; peptic ulcer; Zollinger-Ellison syndrome.

Cimelin Donau, Aust.
Acetylcysteine (p.1052·3).
Respiratory-tract disorders with viscous mucus.

Cimemerck Merck, Ger.
Cimetidine (p.1183·2).
Aspiration syndromes; gastro-intestinal haemorrhage; gastro-oesophageal reflux; peptic ulcer; Zollinger-Ellison syndrome.

Cimephil Philopharm, Ger.
Cimetidine (p.1183·2).
Aspiration syndrome; gastro-oesophageal reflux; peptic ulcer; Zollinger-Ellison syndrome.

Cime-Puren Isis Puren, Ger.
Cimetidine (p.1183·2).
Aspiration syndromes; gastro-oesophageal reflux; peptic ulcer; Zollinger-Ellison syndrome.

Cimet Thiemann, Ger.
Cimetidine (p.1183·2).
Gastro-oesophageal reflux; peptic ulcer; Zollinger-Ellison syndrome.

Cimetag SmithKline Beecham, Aust.
Cimetidine (p.1183·2) or cimetidine hydrochloride (p.1185·3).
Anaphylactoid reactions; gastro-intestinal disorders associated with hyperacidity.

Cimetalgin SmithKline Beecham, Aust.
Oral suspension: Cimetidine (p.1183·2); sodium alginate (p.1470·3).
Tablets: Cimetidine (p.1183·2); alginic acid (p.1470·3); sodium bicarbonate (p.1153·2).
Gastro-oesophageal reflux.

Cimetimax PMC, Austral.
Cimetidine (p.1183·2).
Gastro-oesophageal reflux; peptic ulcer; scleroderma oesophagus; Zollinger-Ellison syndrome.

Cimetrin Cimex, Switz.
Erythromycin ethyl succinate (p.204·2) or erythromycin stearate (p.204·2).
Bacterial infections.

Cimex Sirop contre la toux Cimex, Switz.
Codeine phosphate (p.26·1); ephedrine hydrochloride (p.1059·3); ipecacuanha (p.1062·2); tolu balsam (p.1071·1); cherry-laurel.
Coughs.

Cimexillin Cimex, Switz.†.
Ampicillin trihydrate (p.153·2).
Bacterial infections.

Cimexon Cimex, Switz.†.
Multivitamin and mineral preparation.

Cimexon G Cimex, Switz.†.
Multivitamin and mineral preparation with ginseng (p.1584·2).
Tonic.

Cimexyl Schoeller, Aust.
Acetylcysteine (p.1052·3).
Mucolytic in asthma and bronchitis.

Cimicifuga Med Complex Dynamit, Aust.
Homoeopathic preparation.

Cimicifuga Oligoplex Madaus, Ger.
Homoeopathic preparation.

Cimisan APS, Ger.
Cimicifuga (p.1563·3).
Menstrual and menopausal disorders.

CimLich Lichtenstein, Ger.
Cimetidine (p.1183·2).
Aspiration syndrome; gastro-oesophageal reflux; peptic ulcer; Zollinger-Ellison syndrome.

Cimporhin Thomae, Ger.†.
Tramazoline hydrochloride (p.1071·1); chlorpheniramine maleate (p.405·1); chlorthenoxazin.
Rhinitis.

Cin Vis, Ital.†.
Isoniazid (p.218·1).
Tuberculosis.

Cinadine Garec, S.Afr.
Cimetidine (p.1183·2).
Gastro-oesophageal reflux; peptic ulcer; upper gastro-intestinal haemorrhage; Zollinger-Ellison syndrome.

Cinalone 40 Legere, USA†.
Triamcinolone diacetate (p.1050·2).

Cinarbile Benvegna, Ital.†.
Sodium dehydrocholate (p.1570·3); hexamine (p.216·1); cynara (p.1569·2); rhubarb (p.1212·1); frangula bark (p.1193·2); nicotinamide (p.1351·2).
Gastro-intestinal disorders.

Cinaro Bilina Semar, Spain.
Cynara scolymus (p.1569·2); aloes (p.1177·1).
Constipation; hepatobiliary disorders.

Cinaziere Ashbourne, UK.
Cinnarizine (p.406·1).

Cinazyn Italchimici, Ital.
Cinnarizine (p.406·1).
Vascular disorders; vestibular disorders.

Cincain Ipex, Swed.
Cinchocaine (p.1289·2).
Eye disorders.

Cincofarm Farma Lepori, Spain.
Oxitriptan (p.301·2).
Depression; epilepsy.

Cincopal Cyanamid, Spain.
Fenbufen (p.37·1).
Gout; musculoskeletal disorders; pain; peri-articular disorders.

Cinetic IRBI, Ital.
Thyroid (p.1496·3).
Hypothyroidism.

Cinfacromin Cinfa, Spain.
Mercurochrome (p.1119·2).
Skin disinfection.

Cinfamar Cinfa, Spain.
Dimenhydrinate (p.408·2).
Motion sickness; vertigo.

Cinfamar Cafeina Cinfa, Spain.
Caffeine (p.749·3); dimenhydrinate (p.408·2).
Motion sickness; vertigo.

Cinfatos Cinfa, Spain.
Dextromethorphan hydrobromide (p.1057·3).
Cough.

Cinnabene Merckle, Aust.
Cinnarizine (p.406·1).
Cerebral and peripheral vascular disease.

Cinnacet Sanofi Winthrop, Ger.
Cinnarizine (p.406·1).
Cerebral and peripheral circulatory disorders; vestibular disorders.

Cinnaforte Winthrop, Switz.†.
Cinnarizine (p.406·1).
Motion sickness; vertigo; vestibular disorders.

Cinnageron Streuli, Switz.
Cinnarizine (p.406·1).
Cochlear disorders; motion sickness; vestibular disorders.

Cinnarplus Gerot, Aust.
Cinnarizine (p.406·1); ethamivan (p.1480·3).
Cerebral and peripheral vascular disease.

Cinnipirine Artu, Neth.
Cinnarizine (p.406·1).
Hypersensitivity reactions; motion sickness; vertigo; vestibular disorders.

Cinobac Lilly, Aust.; Lilly, Belg.; Lilly, Ital.; Lilly, Neth.†; Lilly, UK; Oclassen, USA.
Cinoxacin (p.185·2).
Urinary-tract infections.

Cinobactin Lilly, Ger.; Lilly, S.Afr.; Lilly, Swed.†.
Cinoxacin (p.185·2).
Urinary-tract infections.

Cinonide 40 Legere, USA†.
Triamcinolone acetonide (p.1050·2).

Cinopal Novalis, Fr.; Cyanamid, Ital.; Wyeth, S.Afr.
Fenbufen (p.37·1).
Musculoskeletal, joint, and peri-articular disorders.

CiNU Bristol-Myers Squibb, Switz.†.
Lomustine (p.544·1).
Malignant neoplasms.

Cinulcus Wasserman, Spain†.
Cimetidine (p.1183·2).
Gastro-intestinal disorders.

Cional
Provita, Aust.; Kreussler, Switz.†.
Aluminium formate; arnica (p.1550·3); chamomile (p.1561·2); sage (p.1627·1).
Mouth and throat disorders.

Cional S Kreussler, Ger.
Aluminium formate.
Inflammatory disorders of the oropharynx.

Cipadur Cipla-Medpro, S.Afr.
Cefadroxil (p.163·3).
Bacterial infections.

Cipex Cipla-Medpro, S.Afr.
Mebendazole (p.104·1).
Worm infections.

Cipobacter Rubio, Spain.
Ciprofloxacin hydrochloride (p.185·3) or ciprofloxacin lactate (p.185·3).
Bacterial infections.

Cipralan
Searle, Belg.; UPSA, Fr.
Tablets: Cibenzoline succinate (p.840·2).
Arrhythmias.

UPSA, Fr.
Injection: Cibenzoline succinate (p.840·2); cibenzoline (p.840·1).
Arrhythmias.

Cipramil
Lundbeck, Austral.; Lundbeck, Belg.; Promonta Lundbeck, Ger.; Lundbeck, Irl.; Lundbeck, Neth.; Lundbeck, Norw.; Lundbeck, S.Afr.; Lundbeck, Swed.; Lundbeck, UK.
Citalopram hydrobromide (p.281·1) or citalopram hydrochloride (p.281·1).
Depression; panic attacks.

Cipril Italchimici, Ital.
Cisapride (p.1187·1).
Gastro-intestinal disorders.

Cipro
Miles, Canad.; Bayer, USA.
Ciprofloxacin (p.185·3) or ciprofloxacin hydrochloride (p.185·3).
Bacterial infections.

Cipro HC Otic Bayer, USA.
Ciprofloxacin (p.185·3); hydrocortisone (p.1043·3).
Infected ear disorders.

Ciprobay
Bayer, Ger.; Bayer, S.Afr.
Ciprofloxacin (p.185·3), ciprofloxacin hydrochloride (p.185·3), or ciprofloxacin lactate (p.185·3).
Bacterial infections.

Ciprok Alonga, Spain.
Ciprofloxacin hydrochloride (p.185·3).
Bacterial infections.

Ciproxin
Bayer, Aust.; Bayer, Austral.; Bayer, Irl.; Bayer, Ital.; Bayer, Neth.; Bayer, Norw.; Bayer, Swed.; Bayer, UK.
Ciprofloxacin (p.185·3), ciprofloxacin hydrochloride (p.185·3), or ciprofloxacin lactate (p.185·3).
Bacterial infections.

Ciproxine
Bayer, Belg.; Bayer, Switz.
Ciprofloxacin (p.185·3), ciprofloxacin hydrochloride (p.185·3), or ciprofloxacin lactate (p.185·3).
Bacterial infections.

Circanol 3M, Ger.
Co-dergocrine mesylate (p.1566·1).
Adjuvant in mental function disorders; cervical disc syndrome; hypertension.

Circavite-T Circle, USA.
Multivitamin and mineral preparation with iron.

Circolene Inverni della Beffa, Ital.†.
Raubasine (p.941·3).
Vascular disorders.

Circo-Maren Krewel, Ger.
Nicergoline (p.1607·1).
Mental function disorders.

Circonyl N Medidom, Switz.
Quinine sulphate (p.439·2).
Nocturnal leg cramps.

Circovegetalin Verla, Ger.†.
Ergotoxine phosphate (p.1576·1); quinine sulphate (p.439·2); quinidine sulphate (p.939·1); theobromine (p.765·1); magnesium glutamate; magnesium dehydrocholate; magnesium nicotinate.
Cardiovascular disorders.

Circovegetalin compositum Verla, Ger.†.
Pink tablets, ergotoxine phosphate (p.1576·1); quinine sulphate (p.439·2); quinidine sulphate (p.939·1); theobromine (p.765·1); magnesium glutamate; magnesium dehydrocholate; magnesium nicotinate; brown tablets, ergotamine tartrate (p.445·3); ergotoxine phosphate; hyoscyamine (p.464·2); hyoscine hydrobromide (p.462·3); phenobarbitone (p.350·2).
Cardiovascular disorders.

Circovenil Wyeth, Spain.
Buphenine hydrochloride (p.1555·3); aescin (p.1543·3); sodium polygalacturonate sulphonate.
Peripheral vascular disorders.

Circovenil Fuerte Wyeth, Spain.
Buphenine hydrochloride (p.1555·3); aescin (p.1543·3); esculoside (p.1543·3); hesperidin (p.1580·2).
Circulatory disorders.

Circularine Negma, Fr.
Alpha tocopheryl acetate (p.1369·1); troxerutin (p.1580·2); esculoside (p.1543·3).
Peripheral vascular disorders.

Circulation Homeocan, Canad.
Homoeopathic preparation.

Circulatonic Phytomedica, Fr.
Menthol (p.1600·2); camphor (p.1557·2); cypress oil; equisetum (p.1575·1).
Circulatory disorders.

Circupon
Kolassa, Aust.; Gepepharm, Ger.; Medichemie, Switz.
Etilefrine hydrochloride (p.867·2).
Hypotension.

Circuvit E Wernigerode, Ger.
Etilefrine hydrochloride (p.867·2).
Hypotension.

Cirflo Rhone-Poulenc Rorer, Austral.†.
Oxerutins (p.1580·2); nicotinic acid (p.1351·2); bioflavonoids (p.1580·1); calcium ascorbate (p.1365·2); calcium gluconate (p.1155·2); calcium fluoride (p.1556·3); ruscus aculeatus; aesculus (p.1543·3); hamamelis (p.1587·1); pulsatilla (p.1623·3).
Circulatory disorders.

Cirkan Sinbio, Fr.
Pancreatic enzymes (expressed as chymotrypsin and trypsin activities); ruscosides; ascorbic acid (p.1365·2); hesperidin methyl chalcone (p.1580·2); metesculetol sodium (p.1602·3).
Haemorrhoids; peripheral vascular disorders.

Cirkan a la Prednacinolone Sinbio, Fr.
Desonide (p.1036·3); lignocaine hydrochloride (p.1293·2); vitamin A palmitate (p.1359·2); ruscosides; tocopheryl acetate (p.1369·1); heparin sodium (p.879·3).
Anorectal disorders.

Cirkufemal Roha, Ger.
Cimicifuga (p.1563·3).
Menopausal disorders.

Cirkulin
Polcopharma, Austral.†; Cedar Health, UK†.
Garlic (p.1583·1).

Cirkuprostan Roha, Ger.
Urtica root (p.1642·3).
Prostatic hyperplasia.

Cirrus Bios, Belg.
Cetirizine hydrochloride (p.404·2); pseudoephedrine hydrochloride (p.1068·3).
Nasal congestion; rhinitis.

Cirumycin Novo Nordisk, Swed.†.
Roxithromycin (p.247·1).
Bacterial infections.

Cisday Kytta, Ger.
Nifedipine (p.916·2).
Angina pectoris; hypertension.

Cisordinol
Lundbeck, Aust.; Lundbeck, Belg.; Lundbeck, Neth.; Lundbeck, Norw.; Duphar, Spain; Lundbeck, Swed.
Zuclopenthixol (p.700·2), zuclopenthixol acetate (p.700·2), zuclopenthixol decanoate (p.700·2), or zuclopenthixol hydrochloride (p.700·2).
Psychoses.

Cisplatyl Bellon, Fr.
Cisplatin (p.513·3).
Malignant neoplasms.

Cistalgan Recordati, Ital.
Flavoxate hydrochloride (p.461·2); propyphenazone (p.81·3).
Spasm of the female genital tract; urinary-tract disorders.

Cistidil IDI, Ital.
L-Cystine (p.1339·1).
Skin disorders.

Cistobil
Bracco, Ital.; Bracco, Switz.
Iopanoic acid (p.1007·1).
Contrast medium for biliary-tract radiography.

Cistofuran Crosara, Ital.
Nitrofurantoin (p.231·3).
Urinary-tract infections.

Cistomid Biotekfarma, Ital.
Pipemidic acid (p.237·2).
Urinary-tract infections.

Cistus canadensis Oligoplex Madaus, Ger.
Homoeopathic preparation.

Citaethol Medopharm, Ger.†.
Peppermint oil (p.1208·1).
Biliary-tract disorders.

Cital Bichsel, Switz.
Mannitol (p.900·3); sorbitol (p.1354·2).
Irrigation solution.

Citanest
Note. This name is used for preparations of different composition.
Astra, Austral.; Astra, Belg.; Astra, Canad.; Astra, Irl.; Astra, Neth.; Inibsa, Spain; Astra, Swed.; Astra, UK; Astra, USA.
Prilocaine hydrochloride (p.1298·3).
Adrenaline (p.813·2) or adrenaline acid tartrate (p.813·3) is included in some injections as a vasoconstrictor to diminish absorption and localise the effect of the local anaesthetic.
Local anaesthesia.

Astra, Norw.
Prilocaine hydrochloride (p.1298·3); chlorhexidine gluconate (p.1107·2).
Cystitis; cystoscopy; local anaesthesia.

Citanest con Octapressin Astra, Ital.
Prilocaine hydrochloride (p.1298·3).
Felypressin (p.1246·3) is included in this preparation as a vasoconstrictor to diminish absorption and localise the effect of the local anaesthetic.
Local anaesthesia.

Citanest Dental Astra, Austral.
Prilocaine hydrochloride (p.1298·3).
Felypressin (p.1246·3) is included in this preparation as a vasoconstrictor to diminish absorption and localise the effect of the local anaesthetic.
Formerly known as Citanest with Octapressin.
Local anaesthesia.

Citanest with Octapressin
Astra, Irl.; Astra, UK.
Prilocaine hydrochloride (p.1298·3).
Felypressin (p.1246·3) is included in this preparation as a vasoconstrictor to diminish absorption and localise the effect of the local anaesthetic.
Local anaesthesia in dentistry.

Citanest Octapressin
Astra, Norw.; Inibsa, Spain; Astra, Swed.
Prilocaine hydrochloride (p.1298·3).
Felypressin (p.1246·3) is included in this preparation as a vasoconstrictor to diminish absorption and localise the effect of the local anaesthetic.
Local anaesthesia.

Citanest Octapressine Astra, Neth.
Prilocaine hydrochloride (p.1298·3).
Felypressin (p.1246·3) is included in this preparation as a vasoconstrictor to diminish absorption and localise the effect of the local anaesthetic.
Local anaesthesia.

Citanest Octopressin Adcock Ingram, S.Afr.†.
Prilocaine (p.1299·1).
Felypressin (p.1246·3) is included in this preparation as a vasoconstrictor to diminish absorption and localise the effect of the local anaesthetic.
Local anaesthesia in dentistry.

Citanest Plain Astra, Austral.
Prilocaine hydrochloride (p.1298·3).
Local anaesthesia.

Citemul S Medopharm, Ger.
Mesulphen (p.1086·3).
Scabies; skin disorders.

Citicef CT, Ital.
Cephradine (p.181·3).
Bacterial infections.

Citicil CT, Ital.
Ampicillin (p.153·1) or ampicillin sodium (p.153·1).
Bacterial infections.

Citicortex CT, Ital.†.
Suprarenal cortex (p.1050·1); cyanocobalamin (p.1363·3); adenosine triphosphate sodium (p.1543·2); cytidine; uridine (p.1641·3); guanosine; betaine ascorbate (p.1553·2).
Lignocaine (p.1293·2) is included in this preparation to alleviate the pain of injection.
Tonic.

Citidel Del Saz & Filippini, Ital.
Citicoline sodium (p.1564·3).
Cerebrovascular disorders; parkinsonism.

Citidol CT, Ital.†.
Diflunisal (p.33·2).
Inflammation; pain.

Citifar Lafare, Ital.
Citicoline (p.1564·3).
Cerebrovascular disorders.

Citilat CT, Ital.
Nifedipine (p.916·2).
Hypertension; ischaemic heart disease.

Citimid CT, Ital.
Cimetidine (p.1183·2).
Gastro-intestinal haemorrhage; gastro-oesophageal reflux; peptic ulcer; Zollinger-Ellison syndrome.

Citinoides Serra Pamies, Spain.
Lithium carbonate (p.290·3); sodium bicarbonate (p.1153·2).
Hyperacidity.

Citiolase Hoechst Marion Roussel, Ital.
Citiolone (p.1564·3).
Liver disorders.

Citireuma CT, Ital.
Sulindac (p.86·3).
Musculoskeletal and joint disorders.

Citivir CT, Ital.
Aciclovir (p.602·3).
Herpesvirus infections.

Citizem CT, Ital.
Diltiazem hydrochloride (p.854·2).
Hypertension; ischaemic heart disease.

Citoburol Richter, Aust.
Calcium acetate (p.1155·1); aluminium sulphate (p.1548·1).
Bruises; inflammation.

Citocartin Molteni, Ital.
Carticaine hydrochloride (p.1289·1).
Adrenaline acid tartrate (p.813·3) is included in this preparation as a vasoconstrictor to diminish absorption and localise the effect of the local anaesthetic.
Local anaesthesia in dentistry.

Citochol Strallhofer, Aust.
Taraxacum (p.1634·2); achillea (p.1542·2); peppermint oil (p.1208·1).
Biliary disorders; gastro-intestinal disorders.

Citodon Astra, Swed.
Paracetamol (p.72·2); codeine phosphate (p.26·1).
Pain.

Citofolin Bracco, Ital.
Calcium folinate (p.1342·2).
Antidote to folic acid antagonists; folic acid deficiency; reduction of aminopterin and methotrexate toxicity.

Citofur Lusofarmaco, Ital.
Tegafur (p.565·2).
Malignant neoplasms.

Citogel Novartis Consumer, Ital.
Sucralfate (p.1214·2).
Gastro-intestinal disorders associated with hyperacidity.

Citoglutar Bruco, Ital.†.
Pyridoxine hydrochloride (p.1362·3); cyanocobalamin (p.1363·3); uridine (p.1641·3); cytidine.
Tonic.

Cito-Guakalin Stada, Ger.†.
Sodium dibunate (p.1070·1); guaiphenesin (p.1061·3); thyme (p.1636·3).
Coughs and associated respiratory-tract disorders.

Citokrebiol Locatelli, Ital.†.
Uridine (p.1641·3); cytidine; arginine malate.
Tonic.

Citoplatino Rhone-Poulenc Rorer, Ital.
Cisplatin (p.513·3).
Malignant neoplasms.

Citotal Muller Goppingen, Ger.†.
Combination pack: Tablets, lobeline sulphate (p.1481·3); with additional multivitamin tablets.
Aid to smoking withdrawal.

Citovirax Roche, Ital.
Ganciclovir sodium (p.611·3).
Cytomegalovirus infections.

Citra pH ValMed, USA.
Sodium citrate (p.1153·2).
Hyperacidity.

Citracal Mission Pharmacal, USA.
Calcium citrate (p.1155·1).
Aluminium-free phosphate binder in renal disease; calcium supplement.

Citracal + D Mission Pharmacal, USA.
Calcium citrate (p.1155·1); ergocalciferol (p.1367·1).

Citralite Rhone-Poulenc Rorer, Austral.
Sodium bicarbonate (p.1153·2); citric acid (p.1564·3).
Urinary alkalinisation.

Citralka Parke, Davis, Austral.†.
Sodium acid citrate (p.1153·2).
Urinary alkalinisation.

Citramag Bioglan, UK.
Magnesium citrate (p.1198·2).
Bowel evacuation.

Citrarginine Laphal, Fr.
Neutral arginine citrate (p.1334·2); betaine (p.1553·2); betaine hydrochloride (p.1553·2).
Liver disorders.

Citrato Espresso Gabbiani Montefarmaco, Ital.
Magnesium oxide (p.1198·3); magnesium carbonate (p.1198·1).
Gastro-intestinal disorders.

Citrato Espresso S. Pellegrino Synthelabo, Ital.
Magnesium hydroxide (p.1198·2).
Constipation.

Citravescent Rhone-Poulenc Rorer, Austral.
Sodium bicarbonate (p.1153·2); citric acid (p.1564·3).
Urinary alkalinisation.

Citrazine Antigen, Irl.
Piperazine citrate (p.107·2).
Ascariasis; enterobiasis.

Citrec Orion, Swed.
Calcium folinate (p.1342·2).
Methotrexate antagonist.

Citrical Shire, UK†.
Calcium carbonate (p.1182·1).
Calcium deficiency.

Citrisource Sandoz Nutrition, Canad.
Preparation for enteral nutrition.

Citrizan IDI, Ital.
Catalase (equine) (p.1560·3).
Burns; skin ulceration.

Citrizan Antibiotico IDI, Ital.
Catalase (equine) (p.1560·3); gentamicin sulphate (p.212·1).
Infected burns and skin ulcers.

Citro-B_6 Plantier, Fr.†.
Monopyridoxine citrate (p.1363·1); anhydrous betaine (p.1553·2); citric acid (p.1564·3).
Steatosis, particularly associated with alcohol withdrawal.

Citrocarbonate
Note. This name is used for preparations of different composition.
Roberts, Canad.
Sodium bicarbonate (p.1153·2); sodium citrate (p.1153·2); anhydrous citric acid (p.1564·3); calcium lactate pentahydrate (p.1155·2); sodium chloride (p.1162·2); anhydrous monobasic sodium phosphate (p.1159·3); magnesium sulphate (p.1157·3).
Antacid; urinary alkaliniser.

Roberts, USA; Hauck, USA.
Sodium bicarbonate (p.1153·2); anhydrous sodium citrate (p.1153·2).
Hyperacidity.

Citrocholine Therica, Fr.
Granules for oral solution: Sodium citrate (p.1153·2); magnesium citrate (p.1198·2); choline citrate (p.1337·1).

Oral Solution: Choline citrate (p.1337·1); sodium acid citrate (p.1153·2); citric acid monohydrate (p.1564·3); light magnesium carbonate (p.1198·1).
Dyspepsia.

Citrocholine vit. C 250 *Therica, Fr.†.*
Monosodium citrate; dibasic magnesium citrate; choline dihydrogen citrate (p.1337·1); ascorbic acid (p.1365·2).
Gastro-intestinal disorders.

Citrocil *I Farmacologia, Spain.*
Dihydrostreptomycin sulphate (p.202·2); sodium citrate (p.1153·2).
Gastro-intestinal infections.

Citrocit *Propan, S.Afr.*
Citric acid (p.1564·3); sodium bicarbonate (p.1153·2).
Urinary alkalinisation.

Citroen Action 2 Collutorio *Iketon, Ital.†.*
Cetylpyridinium chloride (p.1106·2); guaiazulene (p.1586·3).
Oral disinfection; oral hygiene.

Citroen Action 2 Dentrificio *Iketon, Ital.†.*
Cetylpyridinium chloride (p.1106·2); sodium chloride (p.1162·2); guaiazulene (p.1586·3); calcium carbonate (p.1182·1).
Oral disinfection; oral hygiene.

Citroen Alcolico *Iketon, Ital.†.*
Cetrimide (p.1105·2); isopropyl alcohol (p.1118·2); propyl alcohol (p.1124·2).
Skin and wound disinfection.

Citroen Alcolico Strumenti *Iketon, Ital.†.*
Cetrimide (p.1105·2); isopropyl alcohol (p.1118·2); propyl alcohol (p.1124·2); sodium nitrite.
Instrument disinfection.

Citroen Disinfettante *Iketon, Ital.†.*
Cetylpyridinium chloride (p.1106·2).
Skin and wound disinfection; surface disinfection.

Citroen Towel *Iketon, Ital.†.*
Cetylpyridinium chloride (p.1106·2).
Skin and wound disinfection; surface disinfection.

Citroepatina *Roussel, Ital.*
Betaine monocitrate (p.1553·2); sorbitol (p.1354·2); sodium bicarbonate (p.1153·2); anhydrous citric acid (p.1564·3).
Digestive disorders.

Citro-Flav *Goldline, USA.*
Citrus bioflavonoids complex (p.1580·1).
Capillary bleeding.

Citroflavona *Funk, Spain.*
Ascorbic acid (p.1365·2); bioflavonoids (p.1580·1).
Capillary disorders.

Citroflavona Mag *Funk, Spain.*
Ascorbic acid (p.1365·2); bioflavonoids (p.1580·1); hydroxyflavone.
Capillary disorders.

Citroflavona Solu *Funk, Spain†.*
Ascorbic acid (p.1365·2); bioflavonoids (p.1580·1); menadione (p.1370·3).
Capillary disorders.

Citroftalmina *SIFI, Ital.*
Zinc phenolsulphonate (p.1096·3); procaine hydrochloride (p.1299·2).
Eye irritation and congestion.

Citroftalmina VC *SIFI, Ital.*
Naphazoline nitrate (p.1064·2); zinc phenolsulphonate (p.1096·3); procaine hydrochloride (p.1299·2).
Eye irritation and congestion.

Citrokehl *Sanum-Kehlbeck, Ger.*
Homoeopathic preparation.

Citrolider *Farmalider, Spain.*
Ascorbic acid (p.1365·2).
Vitamin C deficiency.

Citrolith *Beach, USA.*
Anhydrous potassium citrate (p.1153·1); anhydrous sodium citrate (p.1153·2).
Urinary alkalinising agent.

Citro-Mag *Rougier, Canad.*
Anhydrous magnesium citrate (p.1198·2).
Bowel evacuation; constipation.

Citron Chaud *Prodemdis, Canad.*
Phenylephrine hydrochloride (p.1066·2); pheniramine maleate (p.415·3); paracetamol (p.72·2); ascorbic acid (p.1365·2).

Citron Chaud DM *Prodemdis, Canad.*
Phenylephrine hydrochloride (p.1066·2); pheniramine maleate (p.415·3); dextromethorphan hydrobromide (p.1057·3); ascorbic acid (p.1365·2).

Citropepsin *Byk Gulden, Ger.*
Pepsin (p.1616·3); citric acid (p.1564·3).
Gastro-intestinal disorders.

Citropiperazina *Rhone-Poulenc Rorer, Ital.*
Piperazine (p.107·2).
Urinary alkalinisation.

Citroplus *IRBI, Ital.*
Metoclopramide hydrochloride (p.1200·3).
Gastro-intestinal disorders.

Citrosan *Boots Healthcare, Neth.*
Paracetamol (p.72·2); ascorbic acid (p.1365·2); sodium citrate (p.1153·2).
Cold and influenza symptoms; fever; pain.

Citrosil
Note. This name is used for preparations of different composition.
Plantes et Medecines, Fr.
Thyme oil (p.1637·1); lemon oil (p.1595·3); lavender oil (p.1594·3).
House dust mite acaricide.

Manetti Roberts, Ital.
Benzalkonium chloride (p.1101·3).
Skin and wound disinfection.

Citrosil Alcolico Azzuro *Manetti Roberts, Ital.*
Benzalkonium chloride (p.1101·3); alcohol (p.1099·1); sodium nitrite (p.995·2).
Instrument disinfection.

Citrosil Alcolico Bruno *Manetti Roberts, Ital.*
Benzalkonium chloride (p.1101·3); alcohol (p.1099·1).
Skin and wound disinfection.

Citrosil Alcolico Incolore *Manetti Roberts, Ital.*
Benzalkonium chloride (p.1101·3); alcohol (p.1099·1).
Skin and wound disinfection.

Citrosil Nubesan *Manetti Roberts, Ital.*
Benzalkonium chloride (p.1101·3); benzoin resin (p.1634·1).
Surface disinfection.

Citrosil Sapone *Manetti Roberts, Ital.*
Triclocarban (p.1127·2).
Skin cleansing.

Citrosil Sapoplus *Manetti Roberts, Ital.*
Benzalkonium chloride (p.1101·3).
Skin and wound disinfection.

Citrosil Spray *Manetti Roberts, Ital.*
Benzalkonium chloride (p.1101·3).
Skin and wound disinfection.

Citro-Soda *Abbott, S.Afr.*
Sodium citrate (p.1153·2); sodium bicarbonate (p.1153·2); tartaric acid (p.1634·3); citric acid (p.1564·3).
Antacid; urinary alkalinisation.

Citrosodina *Roche, Ital.*
Sodium citrate (p.1153·2).
Gastric hyperacidity.

Citrosorbina B6 *Granata, Ital.†.*
Pyridoxine hydrochloride (p.1362·3); choline chloride (p.1337·1); trisodium citrate (p.1153·2); D-sorbitol (p.1354·2).
Liver disorders.

Citrosteril *Fresenius, Ger.*
Citric acid monohydrate (p.1564·3).
Instrument disinfection.

Citrosystem *Antipiol, Ital.*
Citronella oil (p.1565·1); basil oil; lavender oil (p.1594·3).
Insect repellent.

Citrotein
Sandoz Nutrition, Canad.; Sandoz Nutrition, USA.
Lactose-, cholesterol-, and gluten-free preparation for enteral nutrition.

Citrovescent *Lagamed, S.Afr.†.*
Sodium bicarbonate (p.1153·2); citric acid (p.1564·3); tartaric acid (p.1634·3).
Urinary alkalinisation.

Citrovit *Abello, Spain.*
Ascorbic acid (p.1365·2).
Vitamin C deficiency.

Citrucel
Merrell Dow, Canad.†.
Methylcellulose (p.1473·3).
Constipation.

SmithKline Beecham Consumer, USA.
Methylcellulose (p.1473·3).
Bowel evacuation; constipation.

Citruplexina *Synthelabo, Ital.†.*
L-Citrulline (p.1337·2); L-ornithine hydrochloride (p.1352·3); L-arginine hydrochloride (p.1334·1).
Liver disorders.

Citrus-flav C *Fibertone, USA.*
Citrus bioflavonoids complex (p.1580·1); vitamin C (p.1365·2); hesperidin (p.1580·2); acerola (p.1001·1); rutin (p.1580·2).
Capillary bleeding.

Citsav *Savio, Ital.*
Citicoline sodium (p.1564·3).
Cerebrovascular disorders.

Cituridina *Zambon, Ital.*
Cytidine; uridine (p.1641·3).
Hepatic encephalopathy.

Ciuk *BASF, Ger.*
Cimetidine (p.1183·2).
Aspiration syndrome; gastro-intestinal haemorrhage; gastro-oesophageal reflux; peptic ulcer; Zollinger-Ellison syndrome.

Civeran *Lesvi, Spain.*
Loratadine (p.413·1).
Hypersensitivity reactions.

CL 3 Bruciaporri *Nova Argentia, Ital.*
Trichloroacetic acid (p.1639·1).
Warts.

Clabin
Sagitta, Ger.†; Schonenberger, Switz.
Salicylic acid (p.1090·2); lactic acid (p.1593·3); resorcinol (p.1090·1).
Calluses; corns; verrucas; warts.

Claforan
Albert-Roussel, Aust.; Hoechst Marion Roussel, Austral.; Hoechst Marion Roussel, Belg.; Hoechst Marion Roussel, Canad.; Roussel, Fr.; Hoechst, Ger.; Hoechst Marion Roussel, Irl.; Corvi, Ital.; Hoechst Marion Roussel, Neth.; Hoechst Marion Roussel, Norw.; Hoechst Marion Roussel, S.Afr.; Roussel, Spain; Hoechst Marion Roussel, Swed.; Hoechst Marion Roussel, Switz.; Hoechst Marion Roussel, UK; Hoechst Marion Roussel, USA.
Cefotaxime sodium (p.168·2).
Lignocaine hydrochloride (p.1293·2) is included in some intramuscular injections to alleviate the pain of injection.
Bacterial infections.

Claim *Apomedica, Aust.*
Curcumae oleosum extract (p.1001·3); tolynol (p.1638·2); peppermint oil (p.1208·1); eucalyptus oil (p.1578·1); camphor (p.1557·2); menthol (p.1600·2).
Gastro-intestinal disorders.

Clairo Tea *Weleda, UK.*
Senna leaf (p.1212·2); peppermint leaf (p.1208·1); aniseed (p.1549·3); clove (p.1565·2).
Constipation.

Clairodermyl *BCS, Fr.*
Mequinol (p.1086·2).
Hyperpigmentation.

Clairvan *Sinclair, UK†.*
Ethamivan (p.1480·3).
Respiratory failure.

Clamarvit *Clariana, Spain.*
Ascorbic acid (p.1365·2); vitamin B substances; ferrous gluconate (p.1340·1); ferrous gluceptate (p.1339·3).
Anaemias; tonic.

Clamoxyl
Note. This name is used for preparations of different composition.
SmithKline Beecham, Aust.; Beecham, Belg.; SmithKline Beecham, Fr.; SmithKline Beecham, Ger.; SmithKline Beecham, Neth.; SmithKline Beecham, Spain; SmithKline Beecham, Switz.
Amoxycillin sodium (p.151·3) or amoxycillin trihydrate (p.151·3).
Bacterial infections.

Alphapharm, Austral.
Amoxycillin trihydrate (p.151·3); potassium clavulanate (p.190·2).
Bacterial infections.

Clamoxyl Mucolitico *SmithKline Beecham, Spain.*
Amoxycillin trihydrate (p.151·3); bromhexine hydrochloride (p.1055·3).
Respiratory-tract infections.

Clanzoflat *Wyeth, Spain.*
Dimethicone (p.1213·1); clebopride (p.1188·2).
Gastro-intestinal disorders.

Clanzol *Wyeth, Spain.*
Clebopride malate (p.1188·2).
Gastro-intestinal disorders; nausea and vomiting.

Claradin *Nicholas, Irl.†.*
Aspirin (p.16·1).
Fever; pain.

Claradol *Nicholas, Fr.*
Paracetamol (p.72·2).
Fever; pain.

Claradol Cafeine *Nicholas, Fr.*
Paracetamol (p.72·2); caffeine (p.749·3).
Fever; pain.

Claradol Codeine *Nicholas, Fr.*
Paracetamol (p.72·2); codeine phosphate (p.26·1).
Pain.

Claragine *Nicholas, Fr.*
Aspirin (p.16·1).
Fever; pain.

Claral *Schering, Spain.*
Diflucortolone valerate (p.1039·3).
Skin disorders.

Claral Plus *Schering, Spain.*
Chlorquinaldol (p.185·1); diflucortolone valerate (p.1039·3).
Infected skin disorders.

Claramid
Zambon, Belg.; Jouveinal, Fr.
Roxithromycin (p.247·1).
Bacterial infections.

Claratyne *Schering-Plough, Austral.*
Loratadine (p.413·1).
Allergic rhinitis; urticaria.

Clarema *Damor, Ital.*
Heparan sulphate (p.879·2).
Thrombosis prophylaxis.

Clarens *Upsamedica, Ital.*
Sulodexide (p.951·1).
Thrombosis prophylaxis.

Clarinase
Aesca, Aust.; Schering-Plough, Austral.; Schering-Plough, Belg.; Schering-Plough, Fr.; Essex, Spain.
Loratadine (p.413·1); pseudoephedrine sulphate (p.1068·3).
Allergic rhinitis; coughs and colds.

Clarisco *Schwarz, Ital.*
Heparin sodium (p.879·3).
Vascular disorders.

Clariteyes *Schering-Plough, UK.*
Sodium cromoglycate (p.762·1).
Allergic conjunctivitis.

Claritin
Schering, Canad.; Schering-Plough, USA.
Loratadine (p.413·1).
Allergic rhinitis; hypersensitivity reactions of the skin.

Claritin Extra *Schering, Canad.*
Loratadine (p.413·1); pseudoephedrine sulphate (p.1068·3).
Upper respiratory-tract congestion.

Claritin-D *Schering, USA.*
Loratadine (p.413·1); pseudoephedrine (p.1068·3) or pseudoephedrine sulphate (p.1068·3).
Upper respiratory-tract symptoms.

Claritine
Schering-Plough, Belg.; Schering-Plough, Neth.; Essex, Switz.
Loratadine (p.413·1).
Allergic rhinitis; urticaria.

Clarityn
Aesca, Aust.; Schering-Plough, Irl.; Schering-Plough, Ital.; Schering-Plough, Norw.; Schering-Plough, Swed.; Schering-Plough, UK.
Loratadine (p.413·1).
Allergic conjunctivitis; allergic rhinitis; hypersensitivity reactions of the skin.

Clarityne
Schering-Plough, Fr.; Schering-Plough, S.Afr.; Schering-Plough, Spain.
Loratadine (p.413·1).
Allergic rhinitis; hypersensitivity reactions of the skin.

Clarityne D *Schering-Plough, S.Afr.*
Loratadine (p.413·1); pseudoephedrine hydrochloride (p.1068·3).
Upper respiratory-tract congestion.

Clarix *Cooperation Pharmaceutique, Fr.*
Ephedrine hydrochloride (p.1059·3); pholcodine (p.1068·1); aconite root (p.1542·2); belladonna (p.457·1); sodium camsylate; potassium guaiacolsulfonate (p.1068·3).
Coughs; throat disorders.

Clarmyl *Roussel, Spain.*
Clobazam (p.656·3).
Anxiety; insomnia.

Clarograf *Juste, Spain.*
Iopromide (p.1007·3).
Radiographic contrast medium.

Clarvisan
Allergan, Ital.; Cusi, Spain.
Pirenoxine sodium (p.1619·1).
Cataracts.

Clarvisor *Alcon-Thilo, Ger.*
Pirenoxine sodium (p.1619·1).
Cataracts.

Clast *Meiji, Jpn†.*
Clebopride malate (p.1188·2).
Gastric ulcer.

Clasteon *Abiogen, Ital.*
Disodium clodronate (p.737·3).
Hyperparathyroidism; multiple myeloma; osteolytic tumours; osteoporosis.

Clastoban *Bellon, Fr.*
Disodium clodronate (p.737·3).
Hypercalcaemia of malignancy; osteolytic tumours.

Claudemor *Luitpold, Ger.†.*
Thromboplastin (p.728·1); benzocaine (p.1286·2); procaine (p.1299·2); zinc oxide (p.1096·2); bismuth subgallate (p.1180·2); peru balsam (p.1617·2).
Anorectal disorders.

Claudicat *Promonta, Ger.*
Oxpentifylline (p.925·3).
Peripheral vascular disorders; vascular eye disorders.

Clauparest *Pekana, Ger.*
Homoeopathic preparation.

Clavamox *SmithKline Beecham, Aust.*
Amoxycillin sodium (p.151·3) or amoxycillin trihydrate (p.151·3); potassium clavulanate (p.190·2).
Bacterial infections.

Claventin *SmithKline Beecham, Fr.*
Ticarcillin sodium (p.263·2); potassium clavulanate (p.190·2).
Bacterial infections.

Clavepen *Prodes, Spain.*
Amoxycillin trihydrate (p.151·3); potassium clavulanate (p.190·2).
Bacterial infections.

Claversal
SmithKline Beecham, Aust.; SK-RIT, Belg.; SmithKline Beecham, Ger.; Merckle, Ger.; Parke, Davis, Ital.; Smith Kline & French, Spain.
Mesalazine (p.1199·2).
Inflammatory bowel disease.

Clavigrenin *Hormosan, Ger.*
Dihydroergotamine mesylate (p.444·2).
Hypotension; migraine and related vascular headaches.

Clavigrenin akut *Hormosan, Ger.†.*
Ergotamine tartrate (p.445·3).
Migraine.

Clavius *IBYS, Spain†.*
Amoxycillin trihydrate (p.151·3); potassium clavulanate (p.190·2).
Bacterial infections.

Clavucar *Procter & Gamble, Ital.*
Ticarcillin sodium (p.263·2); potassium clavulanate (p.190·2).
Lignocaine hydrochloride (p.1293·2) is included in the intramuscular injection to alleviate the pain of injection.
Bacterial infections.

Clavucid
Bencard, Belg.; Recordati Elmu, Spain.
Amoxycillin trihydrate (p.151·3); potassium clavulanate (p.190·2).
Bacterial infections.

Clavulin
CSL, Austral.; SmithKline Beecham, Canad.; Fournier, Ital.
Amoxycillin trihydrate (p.151·3); potassium clavulanate (p.190·2).
Bacterial infections.

Clavumox *Pharmacia Upjohn, Spain.*
Amoxycillin trihydrate (p.151·3); potassium clavulanate (p.190·2).
Bacterial infections.

Clean & Clear Antibacterial Foam Cleanser *Johnson & Johnson, Canad.*
Triclosan (p.1127·2).
Acne.

Clean & Clear Deep Cleaning Astringent *Johnson & Johnson, Canad.*
Salicylic acid (p.1090·2).
Acne.

Clean & Clear Invsible Blemish *Johnson & Johnson, Canad.*
Salicylic acid (p.1090·2).
Acne.

Clean Skin Anti Acne *Mentholatum, Austral.*
Tea tree oil (p.1599·2).
Acne.

Clean Skin Face Wash *Mentholatum, Austral.*
Tea tree oil (p.1599·2); benzalkonium chloride (p.1101·3).
Acne.

Clean-N-Soak *Allergan, Austral.*
Hard and gas permeable contact lens cleaning and soaking solution.

Cleanomed *Agepha, Aust.*
Alcohol (p.1099·1); isopropyl alcohol (p.1118·2); benzalkonium chloride (p.1101·3).
Skin and hand disinfection.

Cleansing Herb Tablets *Potter's, UK.*
Tinnevelly senna leaves (p.1212·2); aloes (p.1177·1); cascara (p.1183·1); taraxacum (p.1634·2); fennel seed (p.1579·1).
Constipation.

Cleansing Lotion *Hamilton, Austral.*
Glycerol (p.1585·2); liquid paraffin (p.1382·1); chlorhexidine gluconate (p.1107·2).
Skin cleansing; skin disorders.

Clear Away
Schering-Plough, Austral.; Schering-Plough, Canad.
Salicylic acid (p.1090·2).
Warts.

Clear By Design *SmithKline Beecham Consumer, USA.*
Benzoyl peroxide (p.1079·2).
Acne.

Clear Caladryl Spray *Warner-Lambert, Canad.†.*
Diphenhydramine hydrochloride (p.409·1).
Pain; pruritus.

Clear Cough *Be-Tabs, S.Afr.*
Diphenhydramine hydrochloride (p.409·1); ammonium chloride (p.1055·2); sodium citrate (p.1153·2).
Coughs.

Clear Eyes
Abbott, Austral.; Abbott, Canad.; Ross, USA.
Naphazoline hydrochloride (p.1064·2).
Eye irritation.

Clear Eyes ACR *Ross, USA.*
Naphazoline hydrochloride (p.1064·2); zinc sulphate (p.1373·2).
Eye irritation.

Clear Pore Treatment *Professional Health, Canad.*
Salicylic acid (p.1090·2).
Acne.

Clear Total Lice Elimination System *Care, USA.*
Shampoo, pyrethrum extract (p.1410·1); piperonyl butoxide (p.1409·3); enzymic lice egg remover; comb.
Pediculosis.

Clear Tussin 30 *Goldline, USA.*
Guaiphenesin (p.1061·3); dextromethorphan hydrobromide (p.1057·3).
Coughs.

Clearamed
Procter & Gamble, Spain; Procter & Gamble, Swed.†.
Benzoyl peroxide (p.1079·2).
Acne.

Clearasil
Note. This name is used for preparations of different composition.
Procter & Gamble, Switz.†.
Sulphur (p.1091·2); triclosan (p.1127·2).
Acne.

Richardson-Vicks Personal Care, USA.
Benzoyl peroxide (p.1079·2).
Acne.

Clearasil Acne Cream *Procter & Gamble, Canad.*
Sulphur (p.1091·2); resorcinol (p.1090·1); triclosan (p.1127·2).
Acne.

Clearasil Acne Treatment Cream *Procter & Gamble, Austral.*
Sulphur (p.1091·2); triclosan (p.1127·2).
Formerly known as Clearasil Cream Medication and contained sulphur, resorcinol, triclosan, and aluminium hydroxide.
Acne.

Clearasil Antibacterial *Richardson-Vicks Personal Care, USA.*
Triclosan (p.1127·2); glycerol (p.1585·2); titanium dioxide (p.1093·3).
Acne.

Clearasil B.P. Plus *Procter & Gamble, Canad.*
Benzoyl peroxide (p.1079·2).
Acne.

Clearasil Clearstick
Procter & Gamble, Canad.; Procter & Gamble, USA.
Salicylic acid (p.1090·2).
Acne.

Clearasil Cream
Note. This name is used for preparations of different composition.
Lachartre, Fr.†.
Sulphur (p.1091·2); alcohol (p.1099·1); triclosan (p.1127·2).
Acne.

Procter & Gamble (H&B Care), UK†.
Salicylic acid (p.1090·2); sulphur (p.1091·2).
Acne.

Clearasil Daily Face Wash
Note. This name is used for preparations of different composition.
Procter & Gamble, Austral.
Phenoxyisopropanol.
Formerly contained triclosan.
Acne.

Procter & Gamble, USA.
Triclosan (p.1127·2).

Clearasil Disques *Lachartre, Fr.†.*
Salicylic acid (p.1090·2); alcohol (p.1099·1).
Acne.

Clearasil Double Clear *Richardson-Vicks, USA.*
Salicylic acid (p.1090·2); alcohol (p.1099·1); hamamelis (p.1587·1).

Clearasil Double Textured Pads *Procter & Gamble, USA.*
Salicylic acid (p.1090·2); alcohol (p.1099·1).

Clearasil Dual Action Pads *Procter & Gamble (H&B Care), UK.*
Salicylic acid (p.1090·2).
Acne.

Clearasil Extra Strength *Procter & Gamble, Austral.†.*
Benzoyl peroxide (p.1079·2); aluminium hydroxide (p.1177·3).
Acne.

Clearasil Face Wash
Procter & Gamble, Canad.; Lachartre, Fr.†.
Phenoxypropanol (p.1122·2).
Acne.

Clearasil Gel de soin invisible *Lachartre, Fr.†.*
Salicylic acid (p.1090·2); alcohol (p.1099·1).
Acne.

Clearasil Gel soin de nuit *Lachartre, Fr.†.*
Salicylic acid (p.1090·2).
Acne.

Clearasil Lotion *Lachartre, Fr.†.*
Alcohol (p.1099·1); allantoin (p.1078·2); chlorhexidine gluconate (p.1107·2).
Acne.

Clearasil Max 10 *Procter & Gamble, UK.*
Benzoyl peroxide (p.1079·2).
Acne.

Clearasil Medicated Astringent *Richardson-Vicks Personal Care, USA†.*
Salicylic acid (p.1090·2).
Acne.

Clearasil Medicated Cleanser *Procter & Gamble, Canad.*
Salicylic acid (p.1090·2); alcohol (p.1099·1).
Acne.

Clearasil Medicated Face Wash *Procter & Gamble (H&B Care), UK.*
Phenoxypropanol (p.1122·2).
Acne.

Clearasil Medicated Foam *Procter & Gamble, Austral.†.*
Triclosan (p.1127·2); salicylic acid (p.1090·2).
Acne.

Clearasil Medicated Lotion *Procter & Gamble (H&B Care), UK.*
Chlorhexidine gluconate (p.1107·2); alcohol (p.1099·1).
Acne.

Clearasil Medicated Moisturiser *Procter & Gamble (H&B Care), UK.*
Triclosan (p.1127·2).
Acne.

Clearasil Medicated Wipes *Procter & Gamble, Austral.*
Salicylic acid (p.1090·2).
Acne.

Clearasil Milk *Procter & Gamble (H&B Care), UK†.*
Alcohol (p.1099·1); ergosan.
Acne.

Clearasil Nightclear *Procter & Gamble (H&B Care), UK.*
Salicylic acid (p.1090·2).
Acne.

Clearasil Pads *Procter & Gamble, Canad.*
Salicylic acid (p.1090·2).
Acne.

Clearasil Sensitive Skin Cleanser *Procter & Gamble, Canad.*
Cetrimonium bromide (p.1106·1); chlorhexidine gluconate (p.1107·2); alcohol (p.1099·1).
Acne.

Clearasil Soap *Procter & Gamble (H&B Care), UK.*
Triclosan (p.1127·2).
Acne.

Clearasil Treatment Cream *Procter & Gamble (H&B Care), UK.*
Triclosan (p.1127·2); sulphur (p.1091·2).
Acne.

Clearasil Ultra *Procter & Gamble, Ital.*
Benzoyl peroxide (p.1079·2).
Acne; skin disinfection.

Clearasil Ultra Medication *Procter & Gamble, Austral.*
Benzoyl peroxide (p.1079·2).
Acne.

Clearblue
Fisons Consumer, Austral.†; Warner-Lambert, Austral.; Novartis Consumer, Canad.; Polive, Fr.; Farmades, Ital.; Unipath, UK; Whitehall, USA.
Pregnancy test (p.1621·2).

Clear-Flex Formula 13, 15, 55, 62, 91, AA, AB, AC *Bieffe, Switz.*
A range of glucose and electrolyte solutions for peritoneal dialysis (p.1151·1).

Clearly Cala-gel *Tec, USA.*
Diphenhydramine hydrochloride (p.409·1); zinc acetate (p.1646·2).

Clearon *Semar, Spain.*
Binifibrate (p.1269·2).
Hyperlipidaemias.

Clearplan
Warner-Lambert, Austral.; Novartis Consumer, Canad.; Polive, Fr.; Farmades, Ital.; Unipath, UK; Whitehall, USA.
Fertility test (p.1621·2).

Clearskin Acne Defense Stick *Avon, Canad.*
Salicylic acid (p.1090·2); alcohol (p.1099·1).
Acne.

Clearskin 2 Overnight Acne Treatment *Avon, Canad.*
Salicylic acid (p.1090·2); alcohol (p.1099·1).
Acne.

Clearskin 2 Tinted Blemish *Avon, Canad.*
Sulphur (p.1091·2); resorcinol (p.1090·1).
Acne.

Clearsol *Coventry, UK.*
Tar acids (p.1126·2).

Clearstick *Lachartre, Fr.†.*
Salicylic acid (p.1090·2); alcohol (p.1099·1).
Acne.

Clearview
Note. A similar name is used for preparations of different composition.
Colgate Oral Care, Austral.
Demisting solution for dental mirrors and spectacles.

Clearview HCG
Note. A similar name is used for preparations of different composition.
Warner-Lambert, Austral.; Unipath, UK; Wampole, USA†.
Pregnancy test (p.1621·2).

Cleboril *Almirall, Spain.*
Clebopride malate (p.1188·2).
Gastro-intestinal disorders; nausea and vomiting.

Cledial *Lipha Sante, Fr.*
Medifoxamine (p.296·3).
Depression.

Cleensheen *Florafaun, Austral.*
Malathion (Maldison) (p.1407·3).
Pediculosis.

Cleer *Mack, Illert., Ger.†.*
Tetrahydrozoline hydrochloride (p.1070·2).
Conjunctivitis.

Clements Iron *Felton, Austral.*
Multivitamin, mineral, and glucose preparation with iron (p.1346·1).
Iron deficiency; nutritional anaemia.

Clements Tonic *Felton, Austral.*
Vitamin and mineral preparation with malt, honey, and yeast.
Dietary supplement.

Clemenzil *Medopharm, Ger.†.*
Aesculus (p.1543·3); 3',4',7-tris(*O*-hydroxymethyl) rutoside.
Vascular disorders.

Clemenzil ST *Medopharm, Ger.*
Melilotus officinalis.
Chronic venous insufficiency; haemorrhoids; thrombophlebitis.

Clemipen *Biochemie, Aust.*
Clemizole penicillin (p.191·1).
Syphilis.

Clenasma *Biomedica, Ital.*
Clenbuterol hydrochloride (p.752·1).
Obstructive airways disease.

Clenbutol *Scharper, Ital.†.*
Clenbuterol hydrochloride (p.752·1).
Respiratory-tract disorders.

Cleniderm *Chiesi, Ital.*
Beclomethasone dipropionate (p.1032·1).
Skin disorders.

Clenil
Chiesi, Ital.; Chiesi, Neth.†; Rolab, S.Afr.
Beclomethasone dipropionate (p.1032·1).
Asthma; rhinitis.

Clenil Compositum *Chiesi, Ital.*
Beclomethasone dipropionate (p.1032·1); salbutamol (p.758·2) or salbutamol sulphate (p.758·2).
Obstructive airways disease.

Clens
Alcon, Austral.†; Alcon, USA.
Cleansing solution for hard contact lenses.

Clen-Zym *Alcon, UK.*
Pancreatin (p.1612·1).
Soft contact lens cleanser.

Cleocin
Pharmacia Upjohn, Aust.; Kenral, Austral.; Pharmacia Upjohn, Ital.; Upjohn, USA.
Clindamycin hydrochloride (p.191·1), clindamycin palmitate hydrochloride (p.191·1), or clindamycin phosphate (p.191·1).
Bacterial infections.

Cleocin T *Upjohn, USA.*
Clindamycin phosphate (p.191·1).
Acne.

Clepríd *Recordati, Ital.†.*
Clebopride malate (p.1188·2).
Gastro-intestinal disorders.

Cleregil *Merck-Clevenot, Fr.*
Deanol aceglumate (p.1478·2).
Asthenia.

Cleridium *Marcofina, Fr.*
Dipyridamole (p.857·1).
Cardiovascular disorders; diagnostic aid.

Clerz
Note. This name is used for preparations of different composition.
Ciba Vision, Austral.
Poloxamer 407 (p.1326·3).
Lubricating, cleansing, and hydrating eye drops for use with soft contact lenses.

Alcon, USA.
Range of solutions for contact lenses.

Clerz Moisturising Drops *Ciba Vision, Austral.*
Povidone (p.1474·2).
Formerly contained hydroxyethylcellulose and poloxamer 407.
Dry eyes.

Clesidren *Farmochimica, Ital.*
Epomediol (p.1574·3).
Liver disorders.

Cletan *Intersan, Ger.*
Urtica (p.1642·3).
Benign prostatic hyperplasia.

Cletanol *Corvi, Ital.†.*
Paracetamol (p.72·2); ephedrine sulphate (p.1059·3); caffeine (p.749·3); mepyramine maleate (p.414·1); phenylpropanolamine hydrochloride (p.1067·2).
Respiratory-tract symptoms.

Cletanol C *Corvi, Ital.†.*
Paracetamol (p.72·2); ephedrine sulphate (p.1059·3); caffeine (p.749·3); mepyramine maleate (p.414·1); phenylpropanolamine hydrochloride (p.1067·2); calcium ascorbate (p.1365·2).
Respiratory-tract symptoms.

Cleveral *Aesculapius, Ital.*
Piracetam (p.1619·1).
Mental function impairment.

Clevian *Aesculapius, Ital.*
Piroxicam (p.80·2).
Musculoskeletal and joint disorders.

Clexane
Rhone-Poulenc Rorer, Austral.; Rhone-Poulenc Rorer, Belg.; Rhone-Poulenc Rorer, Ger.; Rhone-Poulenc Rorer, Irl.; Rhone-Poulenc Rorer, Ital.; Rhone-Poulenc Rorer, Neth.; Rhone-Poulenc Rorer, S.Afr.; Rhone-Poulenc Rorer, Spain; Rhone-Poulenc Rorer, Switz.; Rhone-Poulenc Rorer, UK.
Enoxaparin sodium (p.864·2).
Angina pectoris; deep vein thrombosis; myocardial infarction; thrombo-embolism prophylaxis.

Cliacil
Hoechst, Aust.; Hoechst Marion Roussel, Switz.†.
Phenoxymethylpenicillin potassium (p.236·2).
Bacterial infections.

Clift *Knoll, Ger.†.*
Meproscillarin (p.902·3).
Heart failure.

Climacteron *Sabex, Canad.*
Testosterone enanthate benzilic acid hydrazone; oestradiol dienanthate (p.1455·2); oestradiol benzoate (p.1455·1).
Hormone replacement therapy.

Climagest *Sandoz, UK.*
Grey-blue tablets, oestradiol valerate (p.1455·2); white tablets, oestradiol valerate; norethisterone (p.1453·1).
Menopausal disorders.

Climara
Schering, Aust.; Schering, Austral.; Schering, Irl.; Schering, Ital.; Schering, Neth.; Schering, S.Afr.; Schering, Swed.; Schering, Switz.; Berlex, USA.
Oestradiol (p.1455·1).
Menopausal disorders; osteoporosis.

Climarest *LAW, Ger.; Brenner-Efeka, Ger.*
Conjugated oestrogens (p.1457·3).
Menopausal disorders.

Climaval *Sandoz, UK.*
Oestradiol valerate (p.1455·2).
Menopausal disorders.

Climaxol *Lehning, Fr.*
Hamamelis (p.1587·1); viburnum; fragon epineux; hydrastis (p.1588·2); aesculus (p.1543·3).
Peripheral vascular disorders.

Climen
Schering, Aust.; Schering, Austral.; Schering, Belg.; Schering, Ger.; Schering, Ital.; Schering, S.Afr.; Schering, Switz.†.
11 tablets, oestradiol valerate (p.1455·2); 10 tablets, oestradiol valerate; cyproterone acetate (p.1440·2).
28-Day packs also contain 7 inert tablets.
Menopausal disorders; osteoporosis.

Climene Schering, Fr.
11 Tablets, oestradiol valerate (p.1455·2); 10 tablets, oestradiol valerate; cyproterone acetate (p.1440·2).
Menopausal disorders.
Schering, Neth.
16 Tablets, oestradiol valerate (p.1455·2); 12 tablets, cyproterone acetate (p.1440·2); oestradiol valerate.
Menopausal disorders; osteoporosis.

Climesse Sandoz, UK.
Oestradiol valerate (p.1455·2); norethisterone (p.1453·1).
Menopausal disorders.

Clinadil Andromaco, Spain.
Cinnarizine (p.406·1); dihydroergocristine mesylate (p.1571·3).
Cerebrovascular disorders.

Clinadil Compositum Andromaco, Spain.
Cinnarizine (p.406·1); co-dergocrine mesylate (p.1566·1); heptaminol acephyllinate (p.754·1).
Cerebrovascular disorders.

Clinamide Norton, S.Afr.†.
Metoclopramide hydrochloride (p.1200·3).
Gastro-intestinal disorders.

Clinasol Gambar, Ital.
Sodium tetrachloroiodite.
Infections; water purification.

Clinaten Norton, S.Afr.†.
Atenolol (p.825·3).
Angina pectoris; hypertension; myocardial infarction.

Clinazole Norton, S.Afr.†.
Metronidazole (p.585·1).
Anaerobic bacterial infections; protozoal infections.

Clinda Reusch, Ger.
Clindamycin phosphate (p.191·1).
Bacterial infections.

Clindac Intramed, S.Afr.
Clindamycin.
Bacterial infections.

Clinda-Derm Paddock, USA.
Clindamycin phosphate (p.191·1).
Acne.

Clindahexal Hexal, Ger.
Clindamycin hydrochloride (p.191·1).
Bacterial infections.

Clinda-saar Rosen, Ger.
Clindamycin hydrochloride (p.191·1) or clindamycin phosphate (p.191·1).
Bacterial infections.

Clindastad Stada, Ger.
Clindamycin hydrochloride (p.191·1).
Bacterial infections.

Clindatech Dermatech, Austral.
Clindamycin hydrochloride (p.191·1).
Acne.

Clindets Stiefel, USA.
Clindamycin.
Acne.

Clindex Chelsea, USA.
Clidinium bromide (p.459·2); chlordiazepoxide hydrochloride (p.646·3).
Gastro-intestinal disorders.

Clinesfar Essex, Ger.
Erythromycin (p.204·1); tretinoin (p.1093·3).
Acne.

Cliniben Norton, S.Afr.†.
Glibenclamide (p.319·3).
Diabetes mellitus.

Clinicide De Witt, UK†.
Carbaryl (p.1403·1).
Pediculosis.

Cliniclens Cleansing Bar Johnson & Johnson, Austral.†.
Soap substitute.

Cliniclens Cream Johnson & Johnson, Austral.†.
Moisturiser.

Cliniclens Glycerine Cream Johnson & Johnson, Austral.†.
Emollient.

Cliniclens Liquid Cleanser Johnson & Johnson, Austral.†.
Soap substitute.

Cliniclens Shampoo Johnson & Johnson, Austral.†.
Soap-free shampoo.

Cliniclens Skin Lotion Johnson & Johnson, Austral.†.
Moisturiser.

Cliniderm Max Ritter, Switz.
Cream: Polyethylene granules (abrasive) (p.1077·2); salicylic acid (p.1090·2).
Topical solution: Triclosan (p.1127·2).
Acne; seborrhoea.

Clinifeed
Clintec, Irl.; Nestle, UK.
Preparation for enteral nutrition.

Cliniflam Norton, S.Afr.†.
Diclofenac sodium (p.31·2).
Gout; inflammation; musculoskeletal and joint disorders; pain.

Clinigel Delta, Austral.
Lubricating gel.

Clinimix
Laevosan, Aust.; Baxter, Ger.; Clintec, Ital.; Baxter, UK.
Amino-acid and carbohydrate infusion with or without electrolytes.
Parenteral nutrition.

Clinimycin Galen, Irl.
Oxytetracycline (p.235·1).
Bacterial infections.

Cliniretic Norton, S.Afr.†.
Amiloride hydrochloride (p.819·2); hydrochlorothiazide (p.885·2).
Hypertension; oedema.

Clinisorb CliniMed, UK.
Activated charcoal (p.972·2).
Formerly known as Cliniflex.
Malodorous wounds.

Clinispas Norton, S.Afr.†.
Baclofen (p.1308·2).
Skeletal muscle spasm or spasticity.

Clinispon Swissphar, Neth.†.
Gelatin (p.723·2).
Wounds.

Clinistix
Bayer Diagnostics, Austral.; Miles, Canad.; Bayer Diagnostics, Fr.; Ames, Irl.; Bayer Diagnostici, Ital.; Ames, S.Afr.; Bayer Diagnostics, UK; Bayer, USA.
Test for glucose in urine (p.1585·1).

Clinit
Note. This name is used for preparations of different composition.
Kwizda, Aust.
Ampoule 1, mofebutazone sodium (p.56·1); lignocaine (p.1293·2); ampoule 2, dexamethasone (p.1037·1); cyanocobalamin (p.1363·3); lignocaine (p.1293·2).
Musculoskeletal and joint disorders.
Kwizda, Switz.†.
Solution A, mofebutazone sodium (p.56·1); amidopyrine (p.15·2); dexamethasone (p.1037·1); lignocaine (p.1293·2); solution B, cyanocobalamin (p.1363·3).
Rheumatic disorders.

Clinit N Hormosan, Ger.
Injection: Sodium salamidacetate (p.82·3).
Lignocaine (p.1293·2) is included in this preparation to alleviate the pain of injection.
Formerly consisted of 2 ampoules: ampoule 1, sodium salamidacetate and ampoule 2, cyanocobalamin.
Joint disorders; severe pain.
Ointment†: Nonivamide (p.63·2); methyl salicylate (p.55·2).
Neuralgia; rheumatism.
Tablets†: Mofebutazone (p.56·1); propyphenazone (p.81·3).
Rheumatic disorders.

Clinitar
Shire, Irl.; Shire, UK.
Coal tar (Stantar) (p.1092·3).
Dandruff; eczema; psoriasis; seborrhoeic dermatitis.

Clinitest
Bayer Diagnostics, Austral.; Miles, Canad.; Bayer Diagnostics, Fr.; Ames, Irl.; Bayer Diagnostici, Ital.; Ames, S.Afr.; Bayer Diagnostics, UK; Bayer, USA.
Test for reducing substances in urine (p.1585·1).
In the *UK* these are described in the Drug Tariff as Copper Solution Reagent Tablets.

Clinium Janssen-Cilag, Ger.†.
Lidoflazine (p.898·1).
Angina pectoris; myocardial infarction.

Clinofem Pharmacia Upjohn, Ger.
Medroxyprogesterone acetate (p.1448·3).
Progestogenic; test of ovarian function.

Clinofen Norton, S.Afr.†.
Ibuprofen (p.44·1).
Inflammation; musculoskeletal and joint disorders; pain.

Clinofug D Wolff, Ger.
Doxycycline hydrochloride (p.202·3).
Acne.

Clinofug Gel Wolff, Ger.
Erythromycin (p.204·1).
Acne.

Clinolat Norton, S.Afr.†.
Nifedipine (p.916·2).
Angina pectoris.

Clinoleic Clintec, Fr.
Soya oil (p.1355·1); olive oil (p.1610·1).
Contains egg lecithin.
Lipid infusion for parenteral nutrition.

Clinomel Baxter, UK.
Amino-acid, electrolyte, glucose, and lipid (from soya oil (p.1355·1)) infusion.
Contains egg phosphatides.
Parenteral nutrition.

Clinoril
Merck Sharp & Dohme, Aust.; Frosst, Austral.; Merck Sharp & Dohme, Belg.; Merck Frosst, Canad.; Merck Sharp & Dohme, Irl.; Neopharmed, Ital.; Merck Sharp & Dohme, Neth.; Merck Sharp & Dohme, Norw.; Merck Sharp & Dohme, S.Afr.; Merck Sharp & Dohme, Swed.; Merck Sharp & Dohme, Switz.; Merck Sharp & Dohme, UK; Merck Sharp & Dohme, USA.
Sulindac (p.86·3).
Gout; musculoskeletal, joint, and peri-articular disorders.

Clinosyn Norton, S.Afr.†.
Naproxen (p.61·2).
Dysmenorrhoea; gout; musculoskeletal and joint disorders.

Clinovir Pharmacia Upjohn, Ger.
Medroxyprogesterone acetate (p.1448·3).
Breast cancer; endometrial cancer.

Clinoxide Geneva, USA†.
Clidinium (p.459·2); chlordiazepoxide hydrochloride (p.646·3).
Gastro-intestinal disorders.

Clin-Sanorania Sanorania, Ger.
Clindamycin hydrochloride (p.191·1) or clindamycin palmitate hydrochloride (p.191·1).
Bacterial infections.

Clinstan Norton, S.Afr.†.
Mefenamic acid (p.51·2).
Fever; pain.

Clinutren Clintec, UK†.
Preparation for enteral nutrition.

Clinvit Plants, Ital.
Royal jelly (p.1626·3).
Nutritional supplement.

Clinwas Wasserman, Spain.
Clindamycin hydrochloride (p.191·1) or clindamycin phosphate (p.191·1).
Bacterial infections.

Clipoxide Schein, USA†.
Clidinium (p.459·2); chlordiazepoxide hydrochloride (p.646·3).
Gastro-intestinal disorders.

Clipto Quimifar, Spain.
Enalapril maleate (p.863·2).
Heart failure; hypertension.

C-Lisa Lisapharma, Ital.
Ascorbic acid (p.1365·2) or sodium ascorbate (p.1365·2).
Vitamin C deficiency; vitamin C supplement.

Clisemina Juventus, Spain.
Doxycycline hydrochloride (p.202·3).
Bacterial infections.

Clisflex Sella, Ital.
Monobasic sodium phosphate (p.1159·3); dibasic sodium phosphate (p.1159·3).
Bowel evacuation; constipation.

Clisma Bieffe Medital Bieffe, Ital.†.
Monobasic sodium phosphate (p.1159·3); dibasic sodium phosphate (p.1159·3).
Bowel evacuation; constipation.

Clisma Evacuante Sofar, Ital.
Monobasic sodium phosphate monohydrate (p.1159·3); dibasic sodium phosphate heptahydrate (p.1159·3).
Bowel evacuation.

Clisma Fleet
Bergamon, Ital.; Fresenius, Switz.†.
Dibasic sodium phosphate (p.1159·3); monobasic sodium phosphate (p.1159·3).
Bowel evacuation; constipation.

Clisma-Lax Sofar, Ital.
Monobasic sodium phosphate monohydrate (p.1159·3); hydrated dibasic sodium phosphate (p.1159·3).
Bowel evacuation; constipation.

Clistere Evacuativo Carminativo Interfarma, Ital.†.
Sodium oleate-stearate; sodium palmitate.
Bowel evacuation.

Clisundac Lagap, Ital.†.
Sulindac (p.86·3).
Musculoskeletal and joint disorders.

Clivarin
Knoll, Ger.; Immuno, Ger.; Meda, Swed.
Reviparin sodium (p.943·1).
Thrombosis prophylaxis.

Clivarine Knoll, Fr.
Reviparin sodium (p.943·1).
Thrombo-embolic disorders.

Clivoten Italfarmaco, Ital.
Isradipine (p.894·2).
Hypertension.

Clo Zinc Llorens, Spain.
Chloramphenicol (p.182·1); naphazoline hydrochloride (p.1064·2); zinc sulphate (p.1373·2).
Eye disorders; eye infections.

Clobendian Efarmes, Spain.
Diltiazem hydrochloride (p.854·2).
Angina pectoris; hypertension; myocardial infarction.

Clobesol Glaxo Wellcome, Ital.
Clobetasol propionate (p.1035·2).
Skin disorders.

Clobet Angelini, Ital.
Clobetasone butyrate (p.1035·3).
Eye disorders.

Cloburate Dominion, UK.
Clobetasone butyrate (p.1035·3).
Formerly known as Eumovate Eye Drops.
Eye disorders.

Cloburate-N Dominion, UK†.
Clobetasone butyrate (p.1035·3); neomycin sulphate (p.229·2).
Formerly known as Eumovate-N Eye Drops.
Infected eye disorders.

Clocillin Rolab, S.Afr.
Cloxacillin sodium (p.195·2).
Staphylococcal infections.

Clocim Cimex, Switz.
Clotrimazole (p.376·3).
Fungal skin and vaginal infections.

Clocream Roberts, USA.
Cod-liver oil (p.1337·3); cholecalciferol (p.1366·3); vitamin A palmitate (p.1359·2).
Skin disorders.

Cloderm Hermal, USA.
Clocortolone pivalate (p.1035·3).
Skin disorders.

Cloel Aesculapius, Ital.
Cloperastine fendizoate (p.1057·2).
Coughs.

Clofen Alphapharm, Austral.
Baclofen (p.1308·2).
Skeletal muscle spasm or spasticity.

Clofend Fidia, Ital.
Cloperastine fendizoate (p.1057·2).
Coughs.

Clofi ICN, Neth.†.
Clofibrate (p.1271·1).
Hyperlipidaemias.

Clofinit Gentili, Ital.†.
Clofibrate (p.1271·1).
Hyperlipidaemias.

Clomaderm Parke-Med, S.Afr.
Clotrimazole (p.376·3).
Fungal skin infections.

Clomhexal Hexal, Ger.
Clomiphene citrate (p.1439·2).
Female infertility.

Clomid
Hoechst, Aust.; Hoechst Marion Roussel, Austral.; Hoechst Marion Roussel, Belg.; Nordic, Canad.; Marion Merrell, Fr.; Hoechst Marion Roussel, Irl.; Bruno, Ital.; Hoechst Marion Roussel, Neth.; Mer-National, S.Afr.; Hoechst Marion Roussel, Switz.; Hoechst Marion Roussel, UK; Merrell Dow, USA.
Clomiphene citrate (p.1439·2).
Anovulatory infertility.

Clomifen Casen Fleet, Spain.
Clomiphene citrate (p.1439·2).
Anovulatory infertility; male infertility.

Clomin Noristan, S.Afr.†.
Dicyclomine hydrochloride (p.460·1).
Smooth muscle spasm.

Clomivid
Astra, Norw.; Tika, Swed.
Clomiphene citrate (p.1439·2).
Anovulatory infertility.

Clomycin Roberts, USA.
Bacitracin (p.157·3); neomycin sulphate (p.229·2); polymyxin B sulphate (p.239·1); lignocaine (p.1293·2).
Skin infections.

Clonalin Clonmel, Irl.
Diphenhydramine hydrochloride (p.409·1); sodium citrate (p.1153·2); ammonium chloride (p.1055·2); menthol (p.1600·2).
Coughs; respiratory-tract congestion.

Clonamox Clonmel, Irl.
Amoxycillin trihydrate (p.151·3).
Bacterial infections.

Clonamp Clonmel, Irl.
Ampicillin trihydrate (p.153·2).
Bacterial infections.

Clonazine Clonmel, Irl.
Chlorpromazine hydrochloride (p.649·1).
Hypothermia induction; premedication; schizophrenia; sedative; vomiting.

Clondepryl Clonmel, Irl.
Selegiline hydrochloride (p.1144·2).
Parkinsonism.

Clonea Alphapharm, Austral.
Clotrimazole (p.376·3).
Fungal skin infections.

Clonfolic Clonmel, Irl.
Folic acid (p.1340·3).
Prevention of fetal neural tube defects.

Clonilix Clonmel, Irl.
Indapamide (p.890·2).
Hypertension.

Clonistada Stada, Ger.
Clonidine hydrochloride (p.841·2).
Hypertension.

Clonofilin Clonmel, Irl.
Aminophylline (p.748·1).
Obstructive airways disease.

Clonorax Clonmel, Irl.
Aciclovir (p.602·3).
Herpes simplex infections of the lips and face.

Clonoxifen Clonmel, Irl.
Tamoxifen citrate (p.563·3).
Breast cancer; endometrial cancer.

Clont Bayer, Ger.
Metronidazole (p.585·1).
Anaerobic bacterial infections; trichomoniasis.

Clonteric Clonmel, Irl.
Aspirin (p.16·1).
Fever; inflammation; pain; thrombosis prophylaxis.

Clonuretic Clonmel, Irl.
Amiloride hydrochloride (p.819·2); hydrochlorothiazide (p.885·2).
Heart failure; hepatic cirrhosis; hypertension; oedema.

Clopamon Intramed, S.Afr.
Metoclopramide hydrochloride (p.1200·3).
Gastro-intestinal disorders.

Clopan FIRMA, Ital.
Metoclopramide hydrochloride (p.1200·3).
Gastro-intestinal disorders.

Clopax Funk, Spain†.
Clobazam (p.656·3).
Anxiety; insomnia.

Clopir IRBI, Ital.†.
Clofibrate (p.1271·1); pyricarbate (p.1624·1).
Hyperlipidaemias.

Clopixol
Lundbeck, Austral.; Lundbeck, Belg.; Hoechst Marion Roussel, Canad.; Lundbeck, Fr.; Lundbeck, Irl.; Lundbeck, Ital.; Lundbeck, S.Afr.; Lundbeck, Spain; Lundbeck, Switz.; Lundbeck, UK.
Zuclopenthixol acetate (p.700·2), zuclopenthixol decanoate (p.700·2), or zuclopenthixol hydrochloride (p.700·2).
Psychoses.

Clopra Quantum, USA.
Metoclopramide hydrochloride (p.1200·3).
Nausea and vomiting.

Cloprane Luitpold, Ital.
Ronifibrate (p.1278·1).
Hyperlipidaemias.

Cloptison
Merck Sharp & Dohme, Norw.; Merck Sharp & Dohme, Switz.
Clobetasone butyrate (p.1035·3).
Eye disorders.

Cloptison-N Merck Sharp & Dohme, Switz.
Clobetasone butyrate (p.1035·3); neomycin sulphate (p.229·2).
Infected eye disorders.

Clor Hemi Llorens, Spain.
Boric acid (p.1554·2); chloramphenicol (p.182·1); dexamethasone hemisuccinate (p.1037·3).
Infected eye disorders.

Cloradryn Recordati, Ital.
Cloprednol (p.1035·3).
Corticosteroid.

Cloraethyl "Dr. Henning" Henning Walldorf, Ger.†.
Ethyl chloride (p.1292·3).
Topical anaesthesia.

Cloramfen Sclavo, Ital.
Chloramphenicol (p.182·1).
Bacterial eye infections.

Cloramplast Llorens, Spain†.
Chloramphenicol (p.182·1).
Skin infections.

Cloranfe Llorens, Spain.
Chloramphenicol (p.182·1).
Bacterial eye infections.

Cloranfenic Ciba Vision, Spain.
Chloramphenicol (p.182·1).
Bacterial eye infections.

Cloraseptic Prodes, Spain.
Chlorhexidine gluconate (p.1107·2); chlorbutol (p.1106·3).
Mouth and throat infections.

Clorazecaps Martec, USA†.
Potassium clorazepate (p.657·1).

Clorazetabs Martec, USA†.
Potassium clorazepate (p.657·1).

Clordispenser Molteni, Ital.
Halazone (p.1115·1).
Waste disinfection.

Cloretilo Chemirosa Ern, Spain.
Ethyl chloride (p.1292·3).
Local anaesthesia.

Clorexan IMS, Ital.
Chlorhexidine gluconate (p.1107·2); isopropyl alcohol (p.1118·2).
Wound disinfection.

Clorexident Warner-Lambert, Ital.
Chlorhexidine gluconate (p.1107·2).
Mouth disorders; oral disinfection.

Clorexident Ortodontico Warner-Lambert, Ital.
Chlorhexidine gluconate (p.1107·2); sodium fluoride (p.742·1).
Oral disinfection; prophylaxis of dental caries and gingivitis.

Clorhexitulle
Hoechst Marion Roussel, Austral.; Roussel, UK.
Chlorhexidine acetate (p.1107·2).
Wounds.

Clorina
Lysoform, Ger.; Squibb, Spain.
Chloramine (p.1106·3).
Hand disinfection; instrument and surface disinfection; vaginal irrigation; water purification.

Cloristamina Procemsa, Ital.†.
Diethylamine salicylate (p.33·1); methyl nicotinate (p.55·1); natural camphor (p.1557·2).
Musculoskeletal disorders.

Cloritines Torlan, Spain.
Halazone (p.1115·1); sodium carbonate (p.1630·2); sodium chloride (p.1162·2).
Disinfection of drinking water.

Clormetadone Nuovo, Ital.†.
Chlormezanone (p.648·3); amidopyrine (p.15·2).
Musculoskeletal disorders.

Cloroboral Inexfa, Spain.
Alum (p.1547·1); boric acid (p.1554·2); potassium chlorate (p.1620·3); thymol (p.1127·1); menthol (p.1600·2).
Gingivitis; mouth and throat irritation; pyorrhoea; stomatitis.

Clorofenicina Antibioticos, Spain†.
Chloramphenicol sodium succinate (p.182·2).
Bacterial infections.

Cloromi-T Formenti, Ital.
Chloramine (p.1106·3).
Disinfection of minor wounds.

Clorosan Lachifarma, Ital.
Chlorhexidine gluconate (p.1107·2).
Disinfection of skin, wounds, and burns.

Clorpactin Guardian, Canad.
Sodium oxychlorosene (p.1120·3).
Antiseptic.

Clorpactin WCS-90 Guardian, USA.
Sodium oxychlorosene (p.1120·3).
Disinfection; skin infections.

Clorpactin XCB Guardian, USA†.
Oxychlorosene (p.1120·3).
Irrigation and disinfection of skin, wounds, and mucous membranes; skin infections.

Clortanol CT, Ital.
Atenolol (p.825·3); chlorthalidone (p.839·3).
Hypertension.

Clorten Panthox & Burck, Ital.†.
Chlorpheniramine maleate (p.405·1).
Hypersensitivity reactions.

Clortetrin Medosan, Ital.†.
Demeclocycline hydrochloride (p.201·2).
Bacterial infections.

Closcript Searle, S.Afr.†.
Clotrimazole (p.376·3).
Fungal skin and vulvovaginal infections.

Closina Lilly, Austral.
Cycloserine (p.198·3).
Tuberculosis; urinary-tract infections.

Clostene SIFI, Ital.†.
Clostebol acetate (p.1440·2).
Eye disorders.

Clostet Medeva, UK.
An adsorbed tetanus vaccine (p.1535·3).
Active immunisation.

Clostilbegyt Medphano, Ger.
Clomiphene citrate (p.1439·2).
Female infertility.

Clotam
Salus, Aust.; Gea, Switz.; Thames, UK.
Tolfenamic acid (p.89·3).
Dysmenorrhoea; migraine; musculoskeletal and joint pain.

clot-basan Schonenberger, Switz.†.
Clotrimazole (p.376·3).
Fungal skin infections.

Clotest
Delta, Austral.; Bripharm, Irl.
Test for presence of *Helicobacter pylori* in gastric mucosal biopsy samples.

Clotrasone Schering-Plough, Spain.
Betamethasone dipropionate (p.1033·3); clotrimazole (p.376·3).
Fungal skin infections.

Clotri OPT Optimed, Ger.
Clotrimazole (p.376·3).
Fungal skin infections.

Clotriferm Fermenta, Swed.†.
Clotrimazole (p.376·3).
Fungal infections.

Clotrifug Wolff, Ger.
Clotrimazole (p.376·3).
Fungal and bacterial vaginal infections.

Clotrigalen Pharmagalen, Ger.
Clotrimazole (p.376·3).
Fungal skin infections.

Clotrimaderm Taro, Canad.
Clotrimazole (p.376·3).
Fungal infections.

Clovate Evans, Spain.
Clobetasol propionate (p.1035·2).
Skin disorders.

Clovix Valeas, Ital.†.
Aciclovir (p.602·3).
Herpesvirus infections.

Clox Caber, Ital.
Ticlopidine hydrochloride (p.953·1).
Thrombosis prophylaxis.

Cloxam Lennon, S.Afr.
Ampicillin (p.153·1); cloxacillin (p.195·2).
Bacterial infections.

Cloxapen SmithKline Beecham, USA.
Cloxacillin sodium (p.195·2).
Bacterial infections.

Cloxin Intramed, S.Afr.
Cloxacillin sodium (p.195·2).
Staphylococcal infections.

Clozan Roerig, Belg.
Clotiazepam (p.657·2).
Anxiety disorders.

Clozaril
Novartis, Austral.; Sandoz, Canad.; Sandoz, Irl.; Novartis, UK; Sandoz, USA.
Clozapine (p.657·3).
Schizophrenia.

Clusinol Amrad, Austral.
Sulindac (p.86·3).
Musculoskeletal and joint disorders; pain with inflammation.

Clusivol
Akromed, S.Afr.†.
Chewable tablets: Multivitamin preparation.
Pharmacare Consumer, S.Afr.
Syrup: Multivitamin and mineral preparation.

Clym-Depositum Poli, Ital.†.
Testosterone cypionate (p.1464·1); oestradiol cypionate (p.1455·1).
Androgenic/oestrogenic.

Clysmol Pharmacia Upjohn, Aust.
Monobasic sodium phosphate (p.1159·3); dibasic sodium phosphate (p.1159·3).
Bowel evacuation; constipation.

Clysodrast Rhone-Poulenc Rorer, USA.
Bisacodyl tannex (p.1179·3).
Constipation.

C-Max Bio-Tech, USA.
Vitamin C and mineral preparation.

C-Mox Columbia, S.Afr.
Amoxycillin trihydrate (p.151·3).
Bacterial infections.

CMV Immunoglobulin CSL, Austral.
A cytomegalovirus immunoglobulin (human) (p.1507·1).
Passive immunisation.

CMV Iveegam Immuno, Canad.
A cytomegalovirus immunoglobulin (p.1507·1).
Passive immunisation.

C-Naryl Homberger, Switz.
Ascorbic acid (p.1365·2).
Vitamin C supplement.

Co Amoxin Smaller, Spain.
Amoxycillin trihydrate (p.151·3).
Bacterial infections.

Co Bucal Smaller, Spain.
Alum (p.1547·1); procaine hydrochloride (p.1299·2); salicylic acid (p.1090·2); sodium chlorate (p.1630·3); thymol (p.1127·1); cherry laurel water; peppermint oil.
Gingivitis; pyorrhoea; stomatitis.

Co Fluocin Fuerte Smaller, Spain.
Fluocinolone acetonide (p.1041·1).
Skin disorders.

CO_2 Granulat
Salus, Aust.; Guerbet, Ger.
Betaine hydrochloride (p.1553·2); sodium bicarbonate (p.1153·2); simethicone (p.1213·1); colloidal silicone dioxide (p.1475·1).
Adjunct in double contrast radiography.

Co Hepa B12 Smaller, Spain.
Vitamin B substances; liver extract.
Tonic; vitamin B deficiency.

Co-A Millot-Solac, Fr.†.
Coenzyme A (p.1566·2); calcium gluconate (p.1155·2); cysteine hydrochloride (p.1338·3).
Myocardial infarction.

CoActifed Glaxo Wellcome, Canad.
Expectorant: Triprolidine hydrochloride (p.420·3); pseudoephedrine hydrochloride (p.1068·3); guaiphenesin (p.1061·3); codeine phosphate (p.26·1).
Syrup; tablets: Triprolidine hydrochloride (p.420·3); pseudoephedrine hydrochloride (p.1068·3); codeine phosphate (p.26·1).
Coughs.

Coalgan Brothier, Fr.
Calcium alginate (p.714·1).
Haemorrhage.

Coalgel Ducray, Fr.†.
Coal tar (p.1092·3); salicylic acid (p.1090·2).
Seborrhoeic dermatitis.

Coalip SmithKline Beecham, Ital.
Coenzyme A (p.1566·2).
Hypertriglyceridaemia.

Coaltar Saponine le Beuf Gerda, Fr.
Coal tar (p.1092·3); quillaia (p.1328·2).
Gingivitis; skin disorders; stomatitis.

Co-Apap Rugby, USA.
Chlorpheniramine maleate (p.405·1); dextromethorphan hydrobromide (p.1057·3); paracetamol (p.72·2); pseudoephedrine hydrochloride (p.1068·3).
Coughs and cold symptoms.

CO-B1 Bruco, Ital.†.
Cocarboxylase (p.1361·2).
Metabolic disorders.

CO-B12 (Cobidodici) Bruco, Ital.†.
Cocarboxylase (p.1361·2); thiamine monophosphate (p.1361·2); cyanocobalamin (p.1363·3).
Neuralgia symptoms.

Coba-12 Nordic, Canad.†.
Vitamin B substances; lysine hydrochloride (p.1350·1); lignocaine hydrochloride (p.1293·2).
Vitamin B deficiency.

Cobadex Cox, UK.
Hydrocortisone (p.1043·3); dimethicones (p.1384·2).
Skin disorders.

Cobaforte Hoechst Marion Roussel, Ital.
Cobamamide (p.1364·2).
Tonic; vitamin B_{12} deficiency.

Cobalatec Caps, S.Afr.
Cyanocobalamin (p.1363·3).
Vitamin B_{12} deficiency.

Cobaldocemetil Clariana, Spain†.
Mecobalamin (p.1364·2).
Vitamin B_{12} deficiency.

Cobalin-H Link, UK.
Hydroxocobalamin (p.1363·3).
Anaemia due to B_{12} deficiency; Leber's atrophy; tobacco amblyopia.

Cobalton Lagap, Ital.†.
Cocarboxylase (p.1361·2); cyanocobalamin (p.1363·3); sodium glycerophosphate (p.1586·2).
Neuralgia.

Cobamas Tafir, Spain†.
Cyproheptadine hydrochloride (p.407·2); amino acids and vitamins.
Tonic.

Cobamide UCB, Ital.†.
Hydroxocobalamin (p.1363·3).
Anaemias; neurological symptoms.

Cobantril Pfizer, Switz.
Pyrantel embonate (p.109·3).
Nematode infections.

Cobanzyme L'Arguenon, Fr.
Cobamamide (p.1364·2).
Debilitated states.

Cobazymase Bouchara, Switz.†.
Cobamamide (p.1364·2).
Vitamin B_{12} deficiency.

Cobed Marion Merrell Dow, Ger.†.
Drops; syrup: Guaiphenesin (p.1061·3); sodium camsylate.
Gel: Camphor (p.1557·2); guaiacol ethylglycolate (p.1061·2); turpentine oil (p.1641·1); peppermint oil (p.1208·1); menthol (p.1600·2); rosemary oil (p.1626·2); thymol (p.1127·1); methyl nicotinate (p.55·1).
Bronchitis; bronchopneumonia.

Cobergon Mendelejeff, Ital.†.
Cobamamide (p.1364·2).
Tonic.

Co-Betaloc
Astra, Irl.; Astra, UK.
Metoprolol tartrate (p.907·3); hydrochlorothiazide (p.885·2).
Hypertension.

Cobeton Propan, S.Afr.†.
Vitamin B substances.

cobidec n Warner-Lambert, Ger.
Multivitamin and mineral preparation.

Cobiona Esteve, Spain.
Oxatomide (p.415·1).
Hypersensitivity reactions.

Cobolin-M Legere, USA†.
Cyanocobalamin (p.1363·3).

Cobratope Squibb Diagnostics, USA.
Cobalt-57 (p.1423·2) as cobalt chloride.

Co-Carnetina B12 Sigma-Tau, Ital.
Cobamamide (p.1364·2); carnitine (p.1336·2).
Tonic.

Cocarvit CT, Ital.†.
Cocarboxylase (p.1361·2).

Cocculine
Boiron, Canad.; Boiron, Fr.
Homoeopathic preparation.

Cocculus Oligoplex Madaus, Ger.
Homoeopathic preparation.

Cocilix Vernleigh, S.Afr.†.
Cocillana (p.1057·2); senega (p.1069·3); squill (p.1070·1); guaiacol (p.1061·2); terpin hydrate (p.1070·2); menthol (p.1600·2); codeine phosphate (p.26·1).
Coughs.

Cocillana Co Propan, S.Afr.
Cocillana (p.1057·2); squill (p.1070·1); menthol (p.1600·2).
Coughs.

Cocillana-Etyfin Pharmacia Upjohn, Swed.
Ethylmorphine hydrochloride (p.36·1); senega (p.1069·3); cocillana (p.1057·2).
Coughs.

Co-Cillin Docmed, S.Afr.
Ampicillin trihydrate (p.153·2).
Bacterial infections.

Cocktail Reale Sella, Ital.
Honey (p.1345·3); pollen; ginseng (p.1584·2); royal jelly (p.1626·3); propolis (p.1621·3).
Nutritional supplement.

Cocois
Bioglan, Irl.; Bioglan, UK.
Coal tar (p.1092·3); salicylic acid (p.1090·2); precipitated sulphur (p.1091·2).
Dry scalp conditions.

Cocresol Areu, Spain†.
Feprazone (p.41·2).
Fever; inflammation; pain.

Cocydal Xixia, S.Afr.
Co-trimoxazole (p.196·3).
Bacterial infections.

Cocyntal Boiron, Canad.
Homoeopathic preparation.

Cod Efferalgan Upsamedica, Spain.
Paracetamol (p.72·2); codeine phosphate (p.26·1).
Pain.

COD N 70 Torre, Ital.
Amino-acid infusion.
Parenteral nutrition.

Codacetyl A.L., Norw.†.
Codeine phosphate (p.26·1); aspirin (p.16·1).
Pain.

Co-Dafalgan Upsamedica, Switz.
Paracetamol (p.72·2); codeine phosphate (p.26·1).
Pain.

Codafen Continus
Napp, Irl.; Napp, UK.
Ibuprofen (p.44·1); codeine phosphate (p.26·1).
Inflammation; pain.

Codagest Expectorant *Great Southern, USA.*
Phenylpropanolamine hydrochloride (p.1067·2); guaiphenesin (p.1061·3); codeine phosphate (p.26·1).
Coughs.

Codalax
Napp, Irl.; Napp, UK.
Danthron (p.1188·2); poloxamer 188 (p.1326·3).
These ingredients can be described by the British Approved Name Co-danthramer.
Constipation.

Codalgin
Note. This name is used for preparations of different composition.
Fawns & McAllan, Austral.
Paracetamol (p.72·2); codeine phosphate (p.26·1).
Fever; pain.

Nycomed, Norw.
Codeine phosphate (p.26·1); phenazone (p.78·2).
Pain.

Coda-Med *Broad, UK.*
Paracetamol (p.72·2); codeine phosphate (p.26·1); caffeine citrate (p.749·3).

Codamine *Barre-National, USA.*
Phenylpropanolamine hydrochloride (p.1067·2); hydrocodone tartrate (p.43·1).
Coughs and cold symptoms.

Codan *Warner Chilcott, USA†.*
Hydrocodone tartrate (p.43·1); homatropine methobromide (p.462·2).

Codanin *Whitehall, UK†.*
Codeine phosphate (p.26·1); paracetamol (p.72·2).
These ingredients can be described by the British Approved Name Co-codamol.
Fever; pain.

Codant *Antigen, Irl.*
Codeine phosphate (p.26·1).
Coughs; pain.

Codapane *Alphapharm, Austral.*
Paracetamol (p.72·2); codeine phosphate (p.26·1).
Fever; pain.

Codate *Rhone-Poulenc Rorer, Austral.†.*
Codeine phosphate (p.26·1).
Coughs; diarrhoea; pain.

Codef *Be-Tabs, S.Afr.*
Codeine phosphate (p.26·1); mepyramine maleate (p.414·1); ephedrine hydrochloride (p.1059·3).
Coughs.

Codefilona *Lasa, Spain†.*
Aminophylline (p.748·1); codeine (p.26·1).
Bronchospasm; coughs.

Codegest Expectorant *Great Southern, USA.*
Phenylpropanolamine hydrochloride (p.1067·2); codeine phosphate (p.26·1); guaiphenesin (p.1061·3).
Coughs.

Codehist DH *Geneva, USA.*
Pseudoephedrine hydrochloride (p.1068·3); chlorpheniramine maleate (p.405·1); codeine phosphate (p.26·1).
Coughs and cold symptoms.

Codeinol *Saba, Ital.*
Codeine hydrochloride (p.26·1); ephedrine hydrochloride (p.1059·3).
Respiratory-tract symptoms with cough.

Codeisan *Abello, Spain.*
Codeine phosphate (p.26·1).
The syrup formerly contained codeine phosphate, ephedrine hydrochloride, primula veris, and sodium benzoate.
Coughs; diarrhoea; pain.

Codelasa *Lasa, Spain†.*
Codeine (p.26·1); ephedrine hydrochloride (p.1059·3); potassium guaiacolsulfonate (p.1068·3).
Respiratory-tract disorders.

Codelix *Rhone-Poulenc Rorer, Austral.†.*
Codeine phosphate (p.26·1).
Coughs; diarrhoea; pain.

Codella *Napp, UK.*
Glycerol (p.1585·2); kaolin (p.1195·1); povidone-iodine (p.1123·3).
Dry skin.

Codelum *Schoeller, Aust.*
Thyme extract (p.1636·3); codeine phosphate (p.26·1).
Coughs.

Coderma *Biotrading, Ital.†.*
Fluocinolone acetonide (p.1041·1).
Skin disorders.

Codethyline *Hoechst Marion Roussel, Belg.*
Ethylmorphine hydrochloride (p.36·1).
Coughs.

Codetilina-Eucaliptolo He *Teofarma, Ital.*
Ethylmorphine hydrochloride (p.36·1); cineole (p.1564·1).
Coughs.

Codetricine *Roche Nicholas, Fr.*
Tyrothricin (p.267·2).
Mouth and throat disorders.

Codetricine vitamine C *Roche Nicholas, Fr.*
Tyrothricin (p.267·2); amethocaine hydrochloride (p.1285·2); ascorbic acid (p.1365·2).
Mouth and throat disorders.

Codex *SmithKline Beecham, Ital.*
Saccharomyces boulardii (p.1594·1).
Gastro-intestinal disorders.

codi OPT *Optimed, Ger.*
Codeine phosphate (p.26·1).
Pain.

Codicaps *Thiemann, Ger.*
Codeine (p.26·1) or codeine polistirex (p.27·1); chlorpheniramine maleate (p.405·1) or chlorpheniramine polistirex (p.405·2).
Coughs and associated respiratory-tract disorders.

Codicaps B *Thiemann, Ger.†.*
Codeine (p.26·1); chlorpheniramine maleate (p.405·1); bromhexine hydrochloride (p.1055·3).
Coughs and associated respiratory-tract disorders.

Codicaps mono *Thiemann, Ger.*
Codeine (p.26·1).
Coughs.

Codicept *Sanol, Ger.†.*
Codeine (p.26·1).
Coughs.

Codiclear DH *Schwarz, USA.*
Hydrocodone tartrate (p.43·1); guaiphenesin (p.1061·3).
Coughs.

Codicompren *Cascan, Ger.; Cascapharm, Ger.*
Codeine phosphate (p.26·1).
Coughs.

Codicontin
Asta Medica, Belg.; Mundipharma, Switz.
Dihydrocodeine tartrate (p.34·1).
Pain.

Codidol *Mundipharma, Aust.*
Dihydrocodeine tartrate (p.34·1).
Pain.

Codidoxal *Mack, Illert., Ger.†.*
Doxycycline hydrochloride (p.202·3); codeine polistirex (p.27·1).
Coughs associated with infections of the respiratory-tract.

Codiforton *Sanofi Winthrop, Ger.*
Codeine phosphate (p.26·1).
Coughs.

Codimal *Schwarz, USA.*
Chlorpheniramine maleate (p.405·1); pseudoephedrine hydrochloride (p.1068·3); paracetamol (p.72·2).
Upper respiratory-tract symptoms.

Codimal DH *Schwarz, USA.*
Hydrocodone tartrate (p.43·1); phenylephrine hydrochloride (p.1066·2); mepyramine maleate (p.414·1).
Coughs and cold symptoms.

Codimal DM *Schwarz, USA.*
Dextromethorphan hydrobromide (p.1057·3); phenylephrine hydrochloride (p.1066·2); mepyramine maleate (p.414·1).
Coughs.

Codimal Expectorant *Central Pharmaceuticals, USA†.*
Phenylpropanolamine hydrochloride (p.1067·2); guaiphenesin (p.1061·3).
Coughs.

Codimal LA *Schwarz, USA.*
Chlorpheniramine maleate (p.405·1); pseudoephedrine hydrochloride (p.1068·3).
Cold symptoms.

Codimal PH *Schwarz, USA.*
Codeine phosphate (p.26·1); phenylephrine hydrochloride (p.1066·2); mepyramine maleate (p.414·1).
Coughs and cold symptoms.

Codinol *Prosana, Austral.†.*
Paracetamol (p.72·2); codeine phosphate (p.26·1).
Pain.

Codipar *Rolab, S.Afr.†.*
Paracetamol (p.72·2); codeine phosphate (p.26·1); diphenhydramine hydrochloride (p.409·1); caffeine (p.749·3).
Pain.

Codipertussin
Klinge, Aust.; SmithKline Beecham, Ger.†.
Codeine polistirex (p.27·1).
Bronchitis; coughs.

Codiphen *G.P. Laboratories, Austral.*
Codeine phosphate (p.26·1); aspirin (p.16·1).
Fever; pain.

Codipront
Pfizer, Aust.; Mack, Illert., Ger.; Bracco, Ital.; Pfizer, Spain; Mack, Switz.
Codeine phosphate (p.26·1) or codeine polistirex (p.27·1); phenyltoloxamine citrate (p.416·1) or phenyltoloxamine polistirex (p.416·1).
Coughs.

Codipront cum Expectorans
Pfizer, Aust.; Mack, Illert., Ger.†; Mack, Switz.
Capsules: Codeine polistirex (p.27·1); phenyltoloxamine polistirex (p.416·1); guaiphenesin (p.1061·3).
Coughs.

Pfizer, Aust.; Mack, Illert., Ger.†; Mack, Switz.
Oral liquid: Codeine polistirex (p.27·1); phenyltoloxamine polistirex (p.416·1); guaiphenesin (p.1061·3); thyme (p.1636·3).
Coughs.

Codipront mono *Mack, Illert., Ger.*
Codeine polistirex (p.27·1).
Coughs.

Codis
Reckitt & Colman, Austral.; Reckitt & Colman, Belg.; Reckitts, Irl.; Reckitt & Colman, S.Afr.; Reckitt & Colman, UK.
Aspirin (p.16·1); codeine phosphate (p.26·1).
Fever; pain.

Codlin *Nelson, Austral.†.*
Codeine phosphate (p.26·1).
Coughs; pain.

Codocalyptol *Qualiphar, Belg.*
Codeine (p.26·1).
Coughs.

Codol *Mundipharma, Switz.*
Paracetamol (p.72·2); codeine phosphate (p.26·1).
Fever; pain.

Codoliprane *Theraplix, Fr.*
Paracetamol (p.72·2); codeine phosphate (p.26·1).
Pain.

Codomill *Brunel, S.Afr.*
Mepyramine maleate (p.414·1); ephedrine hydrochloride (p.1059·3); codeine phosphate (p.26·1).
Coughs.

Codotussyl
Lederle, Fr.†.
Pastilles: Pholcodine (p.1068·1); aconite (p.1542·2); belladonna (p.457·1); sodium benzoate (p.1102·3); terpin (p.1070·2).
Coughs.

Whitehall, Fr.
Syrup: Pholcodine (p.1068·1); sodium benzoate (p.1102·3); potassium guaiacolsulfonate (p.1068·3); aconite (p.1542·2); belladonna (p.457·1); cherry-laurel water; tolu syrup (p.1071·1); Desessartz syrup.
Coughs.

Codotussyl Expectorant *Whitehall, Fr.*
Oral solution: Acetylcysteine (p.1052·3).
Syrup: Carbocisteine (p.1056·3).
Respiratory-tract congestion.

Codox *Boots, Austral.*
Aspirin (p.16·1); dihydrocodeine tartrate (p.34·1).
Coughs; fever; pain.

Codral Blue Label *Wellcome, Austral.†.*
Aspirin (p.16·1); codeine phosphate (p.26·1).
Fever; pain.

Codral Cold and Flu Tablets *Warner-Lambert, Austral.*
Paracetamol (p.72·2); pseudoephedrine hydrochloride (p.1068·3); codeine phosphate (p.26·1).
Cold and influenza symptoms.

Codral Daytime/Nightime *Warner-Lambert, Austral.*
White tablets, paracetamol (p.72·2); pseudoephedrine hydrochloride (p.1068·3); codeine phosphate (p.26·1); blue tablets, paracetamol; pseudoephedrine hydrochloride; triprolidine hydrochloride (p.420·3).
Cold and influenza symptoms.

Codral Forte *Glaxo Wellcome, Austral.*
Aspirin (p.16·1); codeine phosphate (p.26·1).
Coughs; pain.

Codral Linctus *Warner-Lambert, Austral.*
Pseudoephedrine hydrochloride (p.1068·3); codeine phosphate (p.26·1).
Cold symptoms; coughs.

Codral Pain Relief *Warner-Lambert, Austral.*
Paracetamol (p.72·2); codeine phosphate (p.26·1).
Pain.

Codral Period Pain *Parke Davis-Wellcome, Austral.†.*
Ibuprofen (p.44·1).
Dysmenorrhoea.

Codral Tension Headache *Parke Davis-Wellcome, Austral.†.*
Paracetamol (p.72·2); codeine phosphate (p.26·1); doxylamine succinate (p.410·1).
Tension headache.

Codyl *Kabi, Swed.†.*
Aspirin (p.16·1); codeine phosphate (p.26·1).
Pain.

Coedieci *Mitim, Ital.*
Ubidecarenone (p.1641·2).
Cardiopathy; coenzyme Q10 deficiency.

Co-Efferalagan *Upsamedica, Ital.*
Paracetamol (p.72·2); codeine phosphate (p.26·1).
Pain.

Coffalon *Stark, Ger.*
Paracetamol (p.72·2); salicylamide (p.82·3); caffeine (p.749·3); tiemonium iodide (p.468·3).
Pain.

Coffee Break *Columbia, USA†.*
Caffeine (p.749·3).
Fatigue.

Coffeemed N *Passauer, Ger.*
Caffeine (p.749·3); phenazone (p.78·2).
Influenza; migraine; neuralgia; pain.

Coffein-Enervit *Pfleger, Ger.†.*
Caffeine (p.749·3); ascorbic acid (p.1365·2).
Tonic.

Coffetylin *Bristol-Myers Squibb, Ger.*
Aspirin (p.16·1); caffeine (p.749·3).
Fever; pain.

Coffo Selt *Rosch & Handel, Aust.*
Phenazone (p.78·2); caffeine (p.749·3).
Pain.

Coff-Rest *Garec, S.Afr.*
Triprolidine hydrochloride (p.420·3); pseudoephedrine hydrochloride (p.1068·3); dextromethorphan hydrobromide (p.1057·3).
Coughs.

Coff-Up *Universal, S.Afr.*
Pheniramine maleate (p.415·3); menthol (p.1600·2); ammonium chloride (p.1055·2); sodium citrate (p.1153·2).
Respiratory-tract congestion.

Co-Flem *Compu, S.Afr.*
Carbocisteine (p.1056·3).
Respiratory-tract disorders.

Co-Gel *Compu, S.Afr.*
Dicyclomine hydrochloride (p.460·1); compressed aluminium hydroxide gel (p.1177·3); light magnesium oxide (p.1198·3).
Gastro-intestinal disorders.

Cogentin
Merck Sharp & Dohme, Aust.; Merck Sharp & Dohme, Austral.; Merck Sharp & Dohme, Canad.; Merck Sharp & Dohme, Irl.; Merck Sharp & Dohme, Norw.; Merck Sharp & Dohme, Swed.; Merck Sharp & Dohme, UK; Merck Sharp & Dohme, USA.
Benztropine mesylate (p.458·2).
Drug-induced extrapyramidal disorders; parkinsonism.

Cogentinol *Astra, Ger.*
Benztropine mesylate (p.458·2).
Parkinsonism.

Co-Gesic
Note. This name is used for preparations of different composition.
Docmed, S.Afr.
Paracetamol (p.72·2); codeine phosphate (p.26·1).
Fever; pain.

Schwarz, USA.
Hydrocodone tartrate (p.43·1); paracetamol (p.72·2).
Pain.

Cogitum *SmithKline Beecham, Fr.*
Bipotassium *N*-acetylaspartate.
Asthenia.

Cognex
Parke, Davis, Aust.; Parke, Davis, Austral.; Parke, Davis, Belg.; Parke, Davis, Fr.; Parke, Davis, Ger.; Parke, Davis, Spain; Parke, Davis, Swed.; Parke, Davis, Switz.; Parke, Davis, USA.
Tacrine hydrochloride (p.1399·1).
Alzheimer's disease.

Cognitiv *Ebewe, Aust.*
Selegiline hydrochloride (p.1144·2).
Parkinsonism.

Cognito *Health Perception, UK.*
Phosphatidyl serine (p.1618·1).
Memory impairment.

Co-Hist *Roberts, USA.*
Pseudoephedrine hydrochloride (p.1068·3); chlorpheniramine (p.405·2); paracetamol (p.72·2).
Upper respiratory-tract symptoms.

Cohortan *Fher, Spain.*
Cream: Benzoxonium chloride (p.1103·3); hydrocortisone acetate (p.1043·3).
Infected skin disorders.
Suppositories; rectal ointment: Hydrocortisone (p.1043·3); tyrothricin (p.267·2); isopropyl benztropine mesylate.
Anorectal disorders.

Cohortan Antibiotico *Fher, Spain.*
Hydrocortisone (p.1043·3); tyrothricin (p.267·2); benzoxonium chloride (p.1103·3).
Infected skin disorders.

Co-Hypert *Pekana, Ger.*
Homoeopathic preparation.

Co-Inhibace *Roche, Belg.*
Cilazapril (p.840·3); hydrochlorothiazide (p.885·2).
Hypertension.

Cojene *Roche Consumer, UK†.*
Aspirin (p.16·1); codeine phosphate (p.26·1); caffeine citrate (p.749·3).
Fever; pain.

Col *Alphapharm, Austral.†.*
Clofibrate (p.1271·1).
Hyperlipidaemia.

Cola Tonic *Fiori, Ital.*
Fructose; kola; ginseng; fieno greco; guarana.
Nutritional supplement.

Colace
Roberts, Canad.; Bristol-Myers Squibb, Irl.†; Apothecon, USA.
Docusate sodium (p.1189·3).
Constipation.

Coladren *Coop. Farm., Ital.*
Cascara (p.1183·1); boldo (p.1554·1).
Constipation.

Colagain *Metochem, Aust.*
Kola extract (p.1645·1); soya lecithin (p.1595·2); vitamin E (p.1369·1).
Tonic.

Colambil *Madaus, Spain.*
Fumitory (p.1581·3).
Biliary-tract disorders.

Colamin *Solvay, Ital.*
Cascara (p.1183·1).
Constipation.

Colarine *Sterling Midy, Fr.†.*
Belladonna (p.457·1); hyoscyamus (p.464·3); liquid paraffin (p.1382·1).
Gastro-intestinal disorders.

Co-Lav *Copley, USA.*
Macrogol 3350 (p.1598·2); electrolytes (p.1147·1).
Bowel evacuation.

Colax
Note. This name is used for preparations of different composition.
OFF, Ital.
Senna (p.1212·2); rhubarb (p.1212·1); cynara (p.1569·2); boldo (p.1554·1).
Constipation; digestive disorders; loss of appetite.

Rugby, USA.
Docusate sodium (p.1189·3); phenolphthalein (p.1208·2).
Constipation.

Colax-C *Metapharma, Canad.*
Docusate calcium (p.1189·3).
Constipation.

Colax-S *Metapharma, Canad.*
Docusate sodium (p.1189·3).
Constipation.

Colazide *Astra, UK.*
Balsalazide sodium (p.1179·1).
Ulcerative colitis.

ColBenemid *Merck Sharp & Dohme, USA†.*
Probenecid (p.394·3); colchicine (p.393·1).
Chronic gouty arthritis.

Colbiocin *SIFI, Ital.*
Eye drops: Rolitetracycline (p.247·1); chloramphenicol (p.182·1); colistin sulphomethate sodium (p.196·1).
Eye ointment: Tetracycline (p.259·1); chloramphenicol (p.182·1); colistin sulphomethate sodium (p.196·1).
Eye infections.

Colcaps *Covan, S.Afr.*
Capsules: Phenylpropanolamine hydrochloride (p.1067·2); phenylephrine hydrochloride (p.1066·2); mepyramine maleate (p.414·1); caffeine (p.749·3); salicylamide (p.82·3); chlorpheniramine maleate (p.405·1).
Syrup: Paracetamol (p.72·2); codeine phosphate (p.26·1); promethazine hydrochloride (p.416·2); pseudoephedrine hydrochloride (p.1068·3).
Cold symptoms; nasal congestion; rhinitis.

Colchicum Med Complex *Dynamit, Aust.*
Homoeopathic preparation.

Colchicum-Strath *Strath-Labor, Ger.†.*
Colchicum (p.394·2); rhus toxicodendron (p.1624·3); urtica (p.1642·3); leontopodium alpinum; taraxacum (p.1634·2).
Joint disorders.

Colchimax
Note. This name is used for preparations of different composition.
Houde, Fr.
Colchicine (p.393·1); tiemonium methylsulphate (p.468·3); opium powder (p.70·3).
Formerly contained phenobarbitone, colchicine, tiemonium iodide, and opium.
Gout; inflammatory disorders.

Seid, Spain.
Colchicine (p.393·1); dicyclomine hydrochloride (p.460·1).
Gout.

Colchysat *Ysatfabrik, Ger.*
Colchicum autumnale (p.394·2).
Acute gout.

Colcleer *Propan, S.Afr.*
Chlorpheniramine maleate (p.405·1); ephedrine hydrochloride (p.1059·3); paracetamol (p.72·2); caffeine (p.749·3).
Cold symptoms.

Cold & Allergy Relief *Stanley, Canad.*
Phenylpropanolamine hydrochloride (p.1067·2); phenylephrine hydrochloride (p.1066·2); brompheniramine maleate (p.403·2).

Cold Cream Naturel *Roche-Posay, Fr.*
Cetyl palmitate; white beeswax (p.1383·1); light liquid paraffin (p.1382·1).
Skin dryness and irritation.

Cold Cream Salicyle *Roche-Posay, Fr.*
Salicylic acid (p.1090·2); titanium dioxide (p.1093·3).
Skin disorders.

Cold Decongestant *Novopharm, Canad.*
Phenylpropanolamine hydrochloride (p.1067·2); chlorpheniramine maleate (p.405·1); pheniramine maleate (p.415·3).

Cold and Flu Symptoms Relief *Brauer, Austral.*
Ascorbic acid (p.1365·2); echinacea angustifolia (p.1574·2); zinc gluconate (p.1373·2); aurum met.; arsen. alb.; belladonna; merc. sol.; baptisia tinct.; apis mel.; bryonia; ferrum phos.
Cold and influenza symptoms.

Cold & Flu Tablets
Note. This name is used for preparations of different composition.
Hamilton, Austral.
Paracetamol (p.72·2); pseudoephedrine hydrochloride (p.1068·3); codeine phosphate (p.26·1).
Cold and influenza symptoms.

Or-Dov, Austral.
Pseudoephedrine hydrochloride (p.1068·3); paracetamol (p.72·2); phenylephrine hydrochloride (p.1066·2); bioflavonoids (p.1580·1); ascorbic acid (p.1365·2).
Cold and flu symptoms; hay fever.

Prosana, Austral.†.
Paracetamol (p.72·2); codeine phosphate (p.26·1); ephedrine hydrochloride (p.1059·3); chlorpheniramine maleate (p.405·1); belladonna (p.457·1).
Cold and flu symptoms; hay fever.

Cold Medication D *Prodemdis, Canad.*
Pseudoephedrine hydrochloride (p.1068·3); dextromethorphan hydrobromide (p.1057·3); paracetamol (p.72·2).

Cold Medication Daytime Relief *Stanley, Canad.; WestCan, Canad.*
Pseudoephedrine hydrochloride (p.1068·3); dextromethorphan hydrobromide (p.1057·3); paracetamol (p.72·2).

Cold Medication N *Prodemdis, Canad.*
Pseudoephedrine hydrochloride (p.1068·3); chlorpheniramine maleate (p.405·1); dextromethorphan hydrobromide (p.1057·3); paracetamol (p.72·2).

Cold Medication Nighttime Relief *WestCan, Canad.*
Pseudoephedrine hydrochloride (p.1068·3); chlorpheniramine maleate (p.405·1); dextromethorphan hydrobromide (p.1057·3); paracetamol (p.72·2).

Cold Relief
Note. This name is used for preparations of different composition.
Sussex, UK.
Caffeine (p.749·3); paracetamol (p.72·2); phenylephrine hydrochloride (p.1066·2).
Cold symptoms.

Unichem, UK.
Capsules: Paracetamol (p.72·2); caffeine (p.749·3); phenylephrine hydrochloride (p.1066·2).
Oral powders: Paracetamol (p.72·2); ascorbic acid (p.1365·2).
Cold and influenza symptoms.

Rugby, USA.
Chlorpheniramine maleate (p.405·1); dextromethorphan hydrobromide (p.1057·3); paracetamol (p.72·2); phenylpropanolamine hydrochloride (p.1067·2).
Coughs and cold symptoms.

Cold Relief Daytime *Unichem, UK.*
Paracetamol (p.72·2); pholcodine (p.1068·1); pseudoephedrine hydrochloride (p.1068·3).
Cold and influenza symptoms.

Cold Relief Night-Time *Unichem, UK.*
Paracetamol (p.72·2); pholcodine (p.1068·1); pseudoephedrine hydrochloride (p.1068·3); diphenhydramine hydrochloride (p.409·1).
Cold and influenza symptoms.

Cold Sore Balm *Abbott, Austral.†.*
Lignocaine (p.1293·2); nitromersol (p.1120·1).
Herpes labialis.

Cold Sore Cream *Nyal, Austral.†.*
Menthol (p.1600·2); camphor (p.1557·2).
Cracked lips; herpes labialis.

Cold Sore Lotion
Note. This name is used for preparations of different composition.
Nyal, Austral.†.
Menthol (p.1600·2); camphor (p.1557·2); benzoin (p.1634·1).
Herpes labialis.

Drug Trading, Canad.
Benzocaine (p.1286·2); benzoin (p.1634·1); camphor (p.1557·2); menthol (p.1600·2); myrrh (p.1606·1).

Sabex, Canad.
Menthol (p.1600·2); myrrh (p.1606·1); benzoin (p.1634·1 and p.1628·3); camphor (p.1557·2); alcohol (p.1099·1).
Herpes labialis.

Stanley, Canad.
Benzoin (p.1634·1); camphor (p.1557·2); menthol (p.1600·2).

Numark, UK†.
Povidone-iodine (p.1123·3).

Cold Sore Ointment *Seton, UK†.*
Diperodon (p.1292·3); camphor (p.1557·2); zinc oxide (p.1096·2); allantoin (p.1078·2).

Cold Sore Relief *Vitaplex, Austral.*
Lysine hydrochloride (p.1350·1); ascorbic acid (p.1365·2); zinc amino acid chelate (p.1373·3).
Herpes labialis.

Cold Sore Tablets
Note. This name is used for preparations of different composition.
Rhone-Poulenc Rorer, Austral.†.
L-Lysine; zinc oxide (p.1096·2).
Herpes genitalis; herpes labialis.

Vita Glow, Austral.
Lysine hydrochloride (p.1350·1); ascorbic acid (p.1365·2); betacarotene (p.1335·2); zinc amino acid chelate (p.1373·3).
Herpes labialis.

Cold Tablets *Invamed, USA.*
Paracetamol (p.72·2); chlorpheniramine maleate (p.405·1).

Cold Tablets-D *Invamed, USA.*
Paracetamol (p.72·2); chlorpheniramine maleate (p.405·1); phenylpropanolamine hydrochloride (p.1067·2).

Colda *Sigmapharm, Aust.*
Sage oil; thuja oil; pumilio pine oil (p.1623·3); camphor (p.1557·2); oleum pini sylvestris (p.1570·3); dexpanthenol (p.1570·3); eucalyptus oil (p.1578·1).
Respiratory-tract disorders.

Coldadolin *Sigmapharm, Aust.*
Etenzamide (p.35·3); paracetamol (p.72·2); caffeine (p.749·3); butethamate citrate (p.1056·2).
Pain.

Coldagrippin *Sigmapharm, Aust.*
Paracetamol (p.72·2); propyphenazone (p.81·3); anhydrous caffeine (p.749·3).
Fever; pain.

Coldan *Sigmapharm, Aust.*
Naphazoline hydrochloride (p.1064·2).
Adjunct in rhinoscopy; conjunctivitis; hay fever; rhinitis; sinusitis; sore throat.

Coldangin *Sigmapharm, Aust.*
Dichlorobenzyl alcohol (p.1112·2); amylmetacresol (p.1101·3).
Mouth and throat disorders.

Coldargan
Sigmapharm, Aust.; Desitin, Ger.†.
Silver protein (p.1629·3); ephedrine laevulinate; calcium laevulinate (p.1155·2); sodium laevulinate.
Mouth and throat disorders; rhinitis; sinusitis.

Coldastop *Desitin, Ger.*
Vitamin A palmitate (p.1359·2); alpha tocopheryl acetate (p.1369·1).
Rhinitis.

Cold-eeze *English Grains, UK.*
Garlic (p.1583·1); echinacea (p.1574·2).
Cold symptoms.

Coldenza *Nelson, UK.*
Homoeopathic preparation.

Cold-Gard *Weider, UK.*
Zinc acetate (p.1646·2).
Cold symptoms.

Coldil *Dolisos, Canad.*
Homoeopathic preparation.

Coldistan *Sigmapharm, Aust.*
Eye drops; nasal drops: Diphenhydramine hydrochloride (p.409·1); naphazoline hydrochloride (p.1064·2).
Allergic eye disorders; eye irritation; rhinitis; sinusitis.
Nasal ointment: Diphenhydramine hydrochloride (p.409·1); phenylephrine hydrochloride (p.1066·2); calcium laevulinate (p.1155·2); cetylpyridinium chloride (p.1106·2); dexpanthenol (p.1570·3); sage oil.
Hay fever; rhinitis; sinusitis.

Coldistop
Sigmapharm, Aust.; Sigmapharm, Switz.
Vitamin A palmitate (p.1359·2); alpha tocopheryl acetate (p.1369·1).
Nasal and sinus disorders.

Coldloc *Fleming, USA.*
Guaiphenesin (p.1061·3); phenylpropanolamine hydrochloride (p.1067·2); phenylephrine hydrochloride (p.1066·2).
Upper respiratory-tract symptoms.

Coldloc-LA *Fleming, USA.*
Phenylpropanolamine hydrochloride (p.1067·2); guaiphenesin (p.1061·3).
Upper respiratory-tract symptoms.

Coldophthal *Sigmapharm, Aust.*
Naphazoline hydrochloride (p.1064·2); mercuric oxycyanide (p.1602·2); boric acid (p.1554·2).
Conjunctivitis; eye irritation.

Coldrex
Note. This name is used for preparations of different composition.
Sterling Health, Belg.†; Sterling, Neth.†.
Aspirin (p.16·1); phenylephrine hydrochloride (p.1066·2) ascorbic acid (p.1365·2).
Cold symptoms.

SmithKline Beecham, Irl.; Sterling Health, UK.
Paracetamol (p.72·2); phenylephrine hydrochloride (p.1066·2); caffeine (p.749·3); terpin hydrate (p.1070·2); ascorbic acid (p.1365·2).
Cold symptoms.

Coldrex C *SmithKline Beecham Consumer, Neth.*
Aspirin (p.16·1); ascorbic acid (p.1365·2).
Cold and influenza symptoms.

Coldrex Cold and Flu Capsules *Nyal, Austral.†.*
Paracetamol (p.72·2); dextromethorphan hydrobromide (p.1057·3); pseudoephedrine hydrochloride (p.1068·3); chlorpheniramine maleate (p.405·1).
Cold and flu symptoms.

Coldrex Nasal Spray *Nyal, Austral.†.*
Oxymetazoline hydrochloride (p.1065·3).
Nasal congestion.

Coldrine *Roberts, USA; Hauck, USA.*
Pseudoephedrine hydrochloride (p.1068·3); paracetamol (p.72·2).
Upper respiratory-tract symptoms.

Coldvac *Swisspharm, S.Afr.*
Pneumococci; streptococci; staphylococci; *Haemophilus influenzae*.
Active oral immunisation against colds.

Coldvico *Merck, S.Afr.*
Paracetamol (p.72·2); ascorbic acid (p.1365·2); phenylephrine hydrochloride (p.1066·2); chlorpheniramine maleate (p.405·1); caffeine (p.749·3).
Cold and influenza symptoms.

Coleb *Promed, Ger.; Astra, Ger.*
Isosorbide mononitrate (p.893·3).
Angina pectoris; heart failure; pulmonary hypertension.

Colebrin *Schering, Ital.†.*
Iocetamic acid (p.1005·2).
Contrast medium for biliary-tract radiography.

Colebrina *Asta Medica, Spain†.*
Iocetamic acid (p.1005·2).
Contrast medium for biliary-tract radiography.

Colegraf *Estedi, Spain.*
Iopanoic acid (p.1007·1).
Contrast medium for biliary-tract radiography.

Colemin *Biohorm, Spain.*
Simvastatin (p.1278·2).
Hyperlipidaemias.

Coleminal *Mitsui, Jpn†.*
Flutazolam.

Colenitral *Seid, Spain.*
Glyceryl trinitrate (p.874·3).
Angina pectoris.

Colese *Alphapharm, Austral.*
Mebeverine hydrochloride (p.1199·2).
Irritable bowel syndrome.

Colesterinex *Prodes, Spain.*
Pyricarbate (p.1624·1).
Hyperlipidaemias.

Colestid
Pharmacia Upjohn, Austral.; Pharmacia Upjohn, Belg.; Pharmacia Upjohn, Canad.; Pharmacia Upjohn, Ger.; Pharmacia Upjohn, Irl.; Pharmacia Upjohn, Neth.; Pharmacia Upjohn, S.Afr.†; Upjohn, Spain; Pharmacia Upjohn, Switz.; Upjohn, UK; Upjohn, USA.
Colestipol hydrochloride (p.1272·1).
Hypercholesterolaemia.

Colestrol *Formenti, Ital.*
Cholestyramine (p.1269·3).
Hyperlipidaemias.

Colestyr *CT, Ger.*
Cholestyramine (p.1269·3).
Hyperlipidaemias.

Colex *Tramedico, Neth.*
Dibasic sodium phosphate (p.1159·3); monobasic sodium phosphate (p.1159·3).
Bowel evacuation; constipation.

Colfarit
Bayer, Aust.; Bayer, Ger.†; Bayer, Switz.†.
Aspirin (p.16·1).
Thrombo-embolic disorders.

Colfed-A *Parmed, USA.*
Pseudoephedrine hydrochloride (p.1068·3); chlorpheniramine maleate (p.405·1).
Upper respiratory-tract symptoms.

Colgen *Bournonville, Belg.*
Collagen (bovine, non-denatured) (p.1566·3).
Haemorrhage.

Colgout *Rhone-Poulenc Rorer, Austral.*
Colchicine (p.393·1).
Gout; leukaemia; polyarthritis associated with sarcoidosis.

Coliacron *Enzypharm, Neth.†.*
Glutamine synthetase; acetylcoenzyme A kinase; oxidative phosphorylating enzymes.
Psychosomatic and neurovegetative disorders.

Colibiogen *Laves, Ger.*
Peptide extract from *Escherichia coli*.
Gastro-intestinal disorders; hypersensitivity; musculoskeletal and joint disorders.

Colic Relief *Brauer, Austral.*
Homoeopathic preparation.

Coliceflor *Coli, Ital.†.*
Cephalexin (p.178·2).
Bacterial infections.

Colicitina *Panthox & Burck, Ital.†.*
Phthalylsulphathiazole (p.237·1).

Colicort *Merck Sharp & Dohme-Chibret, Fr.*
Colistin sulphomethate sodium (p.196·1); tetracycline hydrochloride (p.259·1); prednisolone sodium phosphate (p.1048·1).
Infections of the ear and nose.

Coli-Fagina S *ABC, Ital.*
Lysate of *Escherichia coli*; *Bacillus pumilus*; *Morganella morgani*; *Alcaligenes faecalis*; *Shigella flexneri*; *Enterococcus faecalis* (p.1594·1); *Bacillus subtilis*; *Proteus vulgaris*.
Gastro-intestinal infections; genito-urinary infections.

Colifoam
Salus, Aust.; Stafford-Miller, Austral.; Stafford-Miller Continental, Belg.; Trommsdorff, Ger.; Stafford-Miller, Irl.; Stafford-Miller, Ital.; Stafford-Miller, Norw.; Searle, S.Afr.; Meda, Swed.; Stafford-Miller, Switz.; Stafford-Miller, UK.
Hydrocortisone acetate (p.1043·3).
Inflammatory bowel disorders.

Colifossim *Day, Ital.*
Cefuroxime sodium (p.177·1).
Bacterial infections.

Colimax *Qualiphar, Belg.*
Ephedrine hydrochloride (p.1059·3); sodium benzoate (p.1102·3); aconite (p.1542·2); belladonna (p.457·1); thyme (p.1636·3); wild thyme; maidenhair fern.
Coughs.

Colimicina
Note. This name is used for preparations of different composition.
UCB, Ital.
Injection: Colistin sulphomethate sodium (p.196·1).
Bacterial infections.
Ointment†: Colistin sulphate (p.195·3); tyrothricin (p.267·2).
Skin disorders.
Tablets; oral drops: Colistin sulphate (p.195·3).
Bacterial infections of the gastro-intestinal tract.

Syntex, Spain.
Colistin sulphate (p.195·3).
Bacterial infections.

Colimune *Fisons, Ger.*
Sodium cromoglycate (p.762·1).
Food hypersensitivity; ulcerative colitis; ulcerative proctitis.

Colimycin *Lundbeck, Norw.*
Colistin sulphomethate sodium (p.196·1).
Gram-negative bacterial infections.

Colimycine
Glaxo Wellcome, Belg.; Bellon, Fr.; Rhone-Poulenc Rorer, Neth.
Colistin sulphate (p.195·3) or colistin sulphomethate sodium (p.196·1).
Bacterial infections.

Colina *Intersan, Ger.*
Smectite.
Diarrhoea; gastro-intestinal disorders.

Colina Spezial *Intersan, Ger.*
Smectite; aluminium hydroxide-magnesium carbonate gel (p.1178·2).
Formerly known as Skilpin.
Diarrhoea; gastro-intestinal disorders.

Coliopan *Eisai, Jpn.*
Butropium bromide (p.459·1).
Painful gastro-intestinal spasm.

Coliquifilm *Allergan, Ger.; Allergan, Switz.*
White soft paraffin (p.1382·3); wool alcohols (p.1385·2); light liquid paraffin (p.1382·1).
Eye disorders.

Coliriocilina *Medical, Spain.*
Benzylpenicillin potassium (p.159·2).
Eye infections.

Coliriocilina Adren Astr *Medical, Spain.*
Boric acid (p.1554·2); adrenaline hydrochloride (p.813·3); naphazoline hydrochloride (p.1064·2); procaine hydrochloride (p.1299·2); zinc sulphate (p.1373·2).
Eye disorders.

Coliriocilina Espectro *Medical, Spain.*
Neomycin sulphate (p.229·2); oxytetracycline (p.235·1).
Eye infections.

Coliriocilina Gentam *Medical, Spain.*
Gentamicin sulphate (p.212·1).
Eye infections.

Coliriocilina Homatrop *Medical, Spain.*
Homatropine hydrobromide (p.462·2).
Production of mydriasis and cycloplegia.

Coliriocilina Prednisona *Medical, Spain.*
Neomycin sulphate (p.229·2); prednisone (p.1049·2).
Eye disorders.

Colitique *Lacteol du Dr Boucard, Fr.*
Whole and lysed coliform bacteria.
Infections with coliform bacteria.

Colitofalk *Codali, Belg.*
Mesalazine (p.1199·2).
Inflammatory bowel disease.

Collafilm *Immuno, Fr.*
Collagen (p.1566·3).
Ulcers; wounds.

Collaven *Kolassa, Aust.*
Centella (p.1080·3).
Chronic venous insufficiency.

Collazin *Selmag, Switz.*
Zinc sulphate (p.1373·2).
Zinc deficiency.

Collett Spesialdiett *Nycomed, Norw.*†.
Preparation for enteral nutrition.

Colli *Gricar, Ital.*
Benzalkonium chloride (p.1101·3); hamamelis; chamomile.
Eye disinfection; eye irritation.

Collins Elixir *Collins Elixir, UK.*
Ethylmorphine hydrochloride (p.36·1).
Coughs.

Collins Elixir Pastilles *Collins Elixir, UK.*
Citric acid (p.1564·3); lemon oil (p.1595·3); squill vinegar (p.1070·1); glycerol (p.1585·2).
Coughs; sore throats.

Collirio Alfa *Bracco, Ital.*
Naphazoline nitrate (p.1064·2).
Eye irritation.

Collirio Alfa Antistaminico *Bracco, Ital.*
Thonzylamine hydrochloride (p.419·2); naphazoline nitrate (p.1064·2).
Conjunctival disorders.

Collirium Geymonat *Geymonat, Ital.*
Boric acid (p.1554·2); agrimonia eupatoria.
Eye infections.

Collis Browne's *Seton, UK.*
Oral mixture: Morphine (p.56·1); peppermint oil (p.1208·1).
Tablets: Light kaolin (p.1195·1); morphine hydrochloride (p.56·1); heavy calcium carbonate (p.1182·1).
Diarrhoea.

Collodyne *Universal, S.Afr.*
Light kaolin (p.1195·1); pectin (p.1474·1); bismuth subcarbonate (p.1180·1); chloroform and morphine tincture (p.56·1).
Diarrhoea.

Collomack *Polcopharma, Austral.*†*; Mack, Illert., Ger.*
Salicylic acid (p.1090·2); lactic acid (p.1593·3); laureth 9 (p.1325·2).
Skin disorders.

Collu-Blache *Gallier, Fr.*†*; Novopharma, Switz.*
Chlorhexidine gluconate (p.1107·2); oxybuprocaine hydrochloride (p.1298·1).
Mouth and throat disorders.

Collucalmyl *Sterling Midy, Fr.*†.
Hexamidine isethionate (p.1115·3); amethocaine hydrochloride (p.1285·2).
Mouth and throat disorders.

Colludol *Rhone-Poulenc Rorer, Belg.; Lipha, Fr.*†.
Hexamidine isethionate (p.1115·3); lignocaine hydrochloride (p.1293·2).
Mouth and throat disorders.

Collu-Hextril *Warner-Lambert Consumer, Belg.*†*; Warner-Lambert, Fr.*
Hexetidine (p.1116·1).
Mouth and throat infections.

Collunosol *Sodip, Switz.*†.
2,4,5-Trichlorophenol; amethocaine hydrochloride (p.1285·2).
Mouth and throat infections.

Collunosol-N *Sodip, Switz.*
Chlorhexidine gluconate (p.1107·2); lignocaine hydrochloride (p.1293·2).
Mouth and throat disorders.

Collunovar
Note. This name is used for preparations of different composition.
Dexo, Fr.
Mouthwash; throat spray: Chlorhexidine gluconate (p.1107·2).
Formerly contained neoarsphenamine.
Pastilles: Bacitracin zinc (p.157·3); tyrothricin (p.267·2).
Formerly contained neoarsphenamine, bacitracin zinc, and amethocaine hydrochloride.
Mouth and throat infections.
Dexo, Switz.
Chlorhexidine gluconate (p.1107·2).
Mouth and throat disorders.

Collupressine *Synthelabo, Fr.*
Felypressin (p.1246·3); chlorhexidine gluconate (p.1107·2).
Mouth and throat disorders.

Colluspir *Soekami, Fr.*†.
Hexamidine isethionate (p.1115·3); amethocaine hydrochloride (p.1285·2).
Mouth and throat disorders.

Collustan *Oberlin, Fr.*
Chlorhexidine gluconate (p.1107·2); amylocaine hydrochloride (p.1286·1); menthol.
Mouth and throat disorders.

Collylarm *Vifor, Switz.*
Povidone (p.1474·2); polyvinyl alcohol (p.1474·2).
Dry eyes.

Collypan *Vifor, Switz.*
Tetrahydrozoline hydrochloride (p.1070·2); zinc sulphate (p.1373·2); digitalis (p.848·3); hamamelis (p.1587·1); euphrasia.
Eye irritation.

Collyre Alpha *Bracco, Switz.*
Naphazoline nitrate (p.1064·2); camphor (p.1557·2).
Eye irritation.

Collyre Bleu *Sabex, Canad.; Leurquin, Fr.*
Methylene blue (p.984·3); naphazoline hydrochloride (p.1064·2) or naphazoline nitrate (p.1064·2).
Eye disorders.

Collyre Bleu Laiter *Opocalcium, Switz.*
Methylene blue (p.984·3); naphazoline nitrate (p.1064·2).
Eye irritation.

Collyrex *SmithKline Beecham, Fr.*
Thiomersal (p.1126·3); phenylephrine hydrochloride (p.1066·2); pentosan polysulphate (p.928·1).
Eye disorders.

Collyria *Nova Argentia, Ital.*
Benzalkonium chloride (p.1101·3); guaiazulene (p.1586·3); polyvinyl alcohol (p.1474·2).
Eye hygiene; eye irritation.

Collyrium *Charton, Canad.*
Tetrahydrozoline hydrochloride (p.1070·2); glycerol (p.1585·2).
Eye irritation.

Collyrium Fresh *Wyeth-Ayerst, USA.*
Tetrahydrozoline hydrochloride (p.1070·2); glycerol (p.1585·2).
Eye irritation.

Collyrium for Fresh Eyes *Wyeth-Ayerst, USA.*
Borax (p.1554·2); boric acid (p.1554·2).
Eye irrigation.

Colme *Croma, Aust.; Lasa, Spain.*
Calcium carbimide (p.1556·2).
Alcoholism.

ColoCare *Helena, USA.*
Test for occult blood in faeces.

Colocler *Rice Steele, Irl.*†.
Macrogol (p.1597·3); electrolytes (p.1147·1).
Bowel evacuation.

Colofac *Solvay, Aust.; Solvay, Austral.; Solvay, Irl.; Solvay, S.Afr.; Solvay, UK.*
Mebeverine embonate (p.1199·2) or mebeverine hydrochloride (p.1199·2).
Gastro-intestinal spasm; irritable bowel syndrome.

Colofiber *Madaus, Belg.*
Ispaghula (p.1194·2).
Colopathy; constipation.

Colofoam *Norgine, Fr.*
Hydrocortisone acetate (p.1043·3).
Inflammatory bowel disease.

Cololyt *Spirig, Switz.*
Macrogol 4000 (p.1598·2); electrolytes (p.1147·1).
Bowel evacuation.

Colomba N *Mauermann, Ger.*†.
Ephedrine hydrochloride (p.1059·3); calcium gluconate (p.1155·2); grindelia; theobromine and sodium salicylate (p.765·1); lobelia; menthol (p.1600·2).
Asthma; bronchitis; catarrh; silicosis.

Colomba spezial *Mauermann, Ger.*
Homoeopathic preparation.

Colominthe *Arkopharma, Fr.*
Peppermint leaf (p.1208·1); fennel (p.1579·1); melissa (p.1600·1).
Gastro-intestinal disorders.

Colomycin *Pharmax, Irl.; Pharmax, UK.*
Colistin sulphate (p.195·3) or colistin sulphomethate sodium (p.196·1).
Bacterial infections.

Colonlytely *Dendy, Austral.*
Macrogol 3350 (p.1598·2); electrolytes (p.1147·1).
Bowel evacuation.

Colonorm *Mundipharma, Aust.; Mundipharma, Ger.*†.
Senna (p.1212·2).
Constipation.

Colopeg *Roche, Belg.; Nicholas, Fr.; Sodip, Switz.*†.
Electrolytes (p.1147·1); macrogol 3350 (p.1598·2) or macrogol 4000 (p.1598·2).
Bowel evacuation.

Colo-Pleon *Mayrhofer, Aust.*†*; Henning, Ger.*
Sulphasalazine (p.1215·2).
Inflammatory bowel diseases.

Colopriv *Biotherapie, Fr.*
Mebeverine hydrochloride (p.1199·2).
Gastro-intestinal and biliary-tract disorders.

Colopten *Debat, Fr.; Hoechst Marion Roussel, Ital.; Fournier SA, Spain.*
Antigenic extracts of: *Staphylococcus aureus*; *Escherichia coli*; *Klebsiella pneumoniae*; *Proteus vulgaris*.
Diarrhoea.

Colo-Rectal Test *Roche, Canad.*
Test for occult blood in stools.

Colosan *Medichemie, Switz.*
Sterculia (p.1214·1); frangula (p.1193·2).
Constipation.

Colosan mite *Medichemie, Switz.*
Sterculia (p.1214·1).
Constipation; obesity.

Coloscreen *Helena, USA.*
Test for faecal occult blood.

Colosoft *Medichemie, Switz.*
Psyllium (p.1194·2).
Constipation.

Colovage *Dynapharm, USA.*
Macrogol 3350 (p.1598·2); electrolytes (p.1147·1).
Bowel evacuation; constipation.

Coloxyl *Fawns & McAllan, Austral.*
Enema; tablets: Docusate sodium (p.1189·3).
Bowel evacuation (enema); constipation.
Oral drops: Poloxamer 188 (p.1326·3).
Faecal softener.
Suppositories: Docusate sodium (p.1189·3); bisacodyl (p.1179·3).
Bowel evacuation; constipation.

Coloxyl with Senna *Fawns & McAllan, Austral.*
Docusate sodium (p.1189·3); sennosides (p.1212·3).
Constipation.

Colpermin *Germania, Aust.; Pharmascience, Canad.; Pharmacia Upjohn, Irl.; Gebro, Switz.; Pharmacia Upjohn, UK.*
Peppermint oil (p.1208·1).
Irritable bowel syndrome.

Colphen *Propan, S.Afr.*
Codeine phosphate (p.26·1); chlorpheniramine maleate (p.405·1); sodium salicylate (p.85·1); guaiphenesin (p.1061·3); phenylephrine hydrochloride (p.1066·2); caffeine (p.749·3); cetylpyridinium chloride (p.1106·2).
Coughs.

Colpogyn *Angelini, Ital.*
Oestriol (p.1457·2).
Cervical erosion; menopausal disorders.

Colpormon *Lipha Sante, Fr.*
Hydroxyestrone diacetate (p.1448·1).
Infertility caused by cervical mucus deficiency; vaginal and cervical oestrogen deficiency.

Colposeptina *Rhone-Poulenc Rorer, Spain*†.
Chlorquinaldol (p.185·1); promestriene (p.1461·2).
Leucorrhoea.

Colposeptine *Theramex, Mon.*
Chlorquinaldol (p.185·1); promestriene (p.1461·2).
Vaginal atrophy.

Colpotrofin *Andromaco, Spain.*
Promestriene (p.1461·2).
Vulvovaginitis.

Colpotrophine *Schering, Ital.; Theramex, Mon.; Golaz, Switz.*
Promestriene (p.1461·2).
Vulvovaginal disorders.

Colpovis *SIT, Ital.*
Quinestradol (p.1461·3).
Vulvovaginal disorders.

Colpro *Wyeth Lederle, Belg.; Wyeth, Neth.; Akromed, S.Afr.; Wyeth, Spain; Wyeth, Switz.*
Medrogestone (p.1448·2).
Benign breast disorders; endometriosis; infertility; menopausal disorders; menorrhagia; menstrual disorders; prostatic hyperplasia.

Colpron *Wyeth Lederle, Aust.*
Medrogestone (p.1448·2).
Hormone replacement therapy; menorrhagia; secondary amenorrhoea.

Colprone *Wyeth-Ayerst, Canad.; Wyeth, Fr.; Wyeth, Ital.*
Medrogestone (p.1448·2).
Endometriosis; fibroids; functional uterine bleeding; habitual abortion; infertility; menopausal disorders; menstrual disorders; threatened abortion.

Colsor *Pickles, UK.*
Phenol (p.1121·2); menthol (p.1600·2); tannic acid (p.1634·2).
Herpes labialis.

Colstat *Reston, S.Afr.*
Paracetamol (p.72·2); ascorbic acid (p.1365·2); caffeine (p.749·3); phenylephrine hydrochloride (p.1066·2); chlorpheniramine maleate (p.405·1); atropine sulphate (p.455·1).
Cold and influenza symptoms.

Coltapaste
Note. This name is used for preparations of different composition.
Smith & Nephew, Irl.
Zinc oxide (p.1096·2).
Medicated bandage.
Smith & Nephew, Ital.†*; Smith & Nephew, UK.*
Zinc oxide (p.1096·2); coal tar (p.1092·3).
Medicated bandage.

Coltec *Approved Prescription Services, UK*†.
Mesalazine (p.1199·2).
Ulcerative colitis.

Coltramyl *Roussel, Fr.*
Thiocolchicoside (p.1322·1).
Skeletal muscle spasm.

Coly-Mycin *Warner-Lambert, Austral.*†.
Colistin sulphate (p.195·3); neomycin sulphate (p.229·2); thonzonium bromide.
Otitis externa associated with bacterial infections.

Coly-Mycin M *Parke, Davis, Austral.; Parke, Davis, Canad.; Parke, Davis, USA.*
Colistin sulphomethate sodium (p.196·1).
Bacterial infections.

Coly-Mycin Otic *Parke, Davis, Canad.*†.
Colistin sulphate (p.195·3); neomycin sulphate (p.229·2); hydrocortisone acetate (p.1043·3); thonzonium bromide (p.1636·3).
Otitis externa associated with bacterial infections.

Coly-Mycin S Otic *Parke, Davis, USA.*
Colistin sulphate (p.195·3); neomycin sulphate (p.229·2); hydrocortisone acetate (p.1043·3); thonzonium bromide (p.1636·3).
Bacterial ear infections.

CoLyte *Reed & Carnrick, Canad.; Schwarz, USA.*
Macrogol 3350 (p.1598·2); electrolytes (p.1147·1).
Bowel evacuation.

Comafusin Hepar *Pharmacia Upjohn, Ger.*
Amino-acid, vitamin, and electrolyte infusion with xylitol.
Hepatic coma.

Comalose-R *Rougier, Canad.*
Lactulose (p.1195·3).
Hepatic encephalopathy.

Combacid *Streuli, Switz.*
Aluminium hydroxide-magnesium carbonate co-dried gel (p.1178·2); simethicone (p.1213·1).
Gastric hyperacidity.

Combactam *Pfizer, Aust.; Pfizer, Ger.*
Sulbactam sodium (p.250·3).
Adjunct to beta-lactam antibiotics.

Comba-Gripp *Doetsch, Grether, Switz.*
Aspirin (p.16·1); salicylamide (p.82·3); caffeine (p.749·3).
Cold symptoms.

Combantrin *Pfizer, Aust.; G.P. Laboratories, Austral.; Pfizer, Canad.; Pfizer, Fr.; Pfizer, Ital.; Pfizer, S.Afr.; Pfizer, UK*†.
Pyrantel embonate (p.109·3).
Worm infections.

Combaren *Ciba Cancer Care, Ger.*
Diclofenac sodium (p.31·2); codeine phosphate (p.26·1).
Pain.

Combetasi *ISI, Ital.*
Vitamin B substances.
Tonic.

Combevit *Sanico, Belg.*†.
Vitamin B substances.
Dietary supplement; megaloblastic anaemia; vitamin B deficiency.

Combeylax *Thera, Fr.*†.
Pentaerythritol (p.1208·1).
Constipation.

Combi 4A Medi-Test *Macherey Nagel Duren, S.Afr.*
Test for protein, pH, blood, ascorbic acid, and nitrite in urine.

Combi 6A Medi-Test *Macherey Nagel Duren, S.Afr.*
Test for glucose, protein, pH, blood, ascorbic acid and ketones in urine.

Combi 3 Medi-Test *Macherey Nagel Duren, S.Afr.*
Test for glucose, protein, and pH in urine.

Combi 5 Medi-Test *Macherey Nagel Duren, S.Afr.*
Test for glucose, protein, pH, blood, and ascorbic acid in urine.

Combi 7 Medi-Test *Macherey Nagel Duren, S.Afr.*
Test for glucose, protein, pH, blood, ascorbic acid, ketones, and nitrite in urine.

Combi 9 Medi-Test *Macherey Nagel Duren, S.Afr.*
Test for glucose, protein, pH, blood, ascorbic acid, ketones, nitrite, bilirubin, and urobilinogen in urine.

Combiamid *Winzer, Ger.*
Sulphacetamide sodium (p.252·2); mafenide hydrochloride (p.223·2); naphazoline hydrochloride (p.1064·2).
Formerly contained sulphacetamide sodium, mafenide hydrochloride, naphazoline hydrochloride, and antazoline hydrochloride.
Eye infections.

Combicilline *Wolfs, Belg.†.*
Benzylpenicillin sodium (p.159·3); procaine penicillin (p.240·2).
Bacterial infections.

Combiderm *Recordati, Ital.†.*
Fluocinonide (p.1041·2); neomycin sulphate (p.229·2); gramicidin (p.215·2); nystatin (p.386·1).
Skin disorders.

Combidol *CP Pharmaceuticals, UK†.*
Chenodeoxycholic acid (p.1562·1); ursodeoxycholic acid (p.1642·1).
Gallstones.

Combiflexona *Miquel Otsuka, Spain†.*
Isamfazone (p.48·1); prednisone (p.1049·2); indoarginine (p.46·3).
Inflammation; pain.

Combifusin *Pharmacia Upjohn, Ger.*
Amino-acid, carbohydrate, and electrolyte infusion.
Parenteral nutrition.

Combilosung *Agepha, Aust.*
Disinfection and storage solution for contact lens.

Combionta N *Merck, Ger.†.*
Multivitamin and mineral preparation.

Combiplasmal *Braun, Ger.*
Amino-acid, carbohydrate, and electrolyte infusion.
Parenteral nutrition.

Combipres
Boehringer Ingelheim, Canad.; Boehringer Ingelheim, USA.
Clonidine hydrochloride (p.841·2); chlorthalidone (p.839·3).
Hypertension.

Combipresan
Bender, Aust.; Boehringer Ingelheim, Ger.; Boehringer Ingelheim, Ital.†.
Clonidine hydrochloride (p.841·2); chlorthalidone (p.839·3).
Hypertension.

Combiprotect *Brenner-Efeka, Ger.†.*
Amiloride hydrochloride (p.819·2); hydrochlorothiazide (p.885·2).
Hypertension; oedema.

Combisan Plus *Esoform, Ital.†.*
Benzalkonium chloride (p.1101·3); glutaraldehyde (p.1114·3); alkylphenoxypolyglycol ether.
Surface disinfection.

Combisteril *Fresenius, Ger.†.*
Carbohydrate infusion with or without electrolytes.
Parenteral nutrition.

Combistix
Bayer Diagnostics, Austral.; Bayer, USA.
Test for pH, protein, and glucose in urine.

Combitard Humana 15/85 *Novo Nordisk, Spain†.*
Mixture of insulin injection (human) 15% and isophane insulin injection (human) 85% (p.322·1).
Diabetes mellitus.

Combithyrex *Sanabo, Aust.*
Thyroxine sodium (p.1497·1); liothyronine sodium (p.1495·1).
Hypothyroidism.

Combitorax *Nezel, Spain.*
Capsules: Amoxycillin trihydrate (p.151·3); bromhexine hydrochloride (p.1055·3).
Oral suspension: Amoxycillin trihydrate (p.151·3); bromhexine (p.1055·3); guaiphenesin (p.1061·3); polygala (p.1069·3); liquorice (p.1197·1).
Respiratory-tract infections.

Combitorax Ampicilina *Nezel, Spain†.*
Ampicillin sodium (p.153·1); ampicillin benzathine (p.154·1); cineole (p.1564·1); niaouli oil (p.1607·1).
Lignocaine hydrochloride (p.1293·2) is included in this preparation to alleviate the pain of injection.
Respiratory-tract infections.

Combivax *SK-RIT, Belg.*
An adsorbed diphtheria, tetanus, and pertussis vaccine (p.1509·1).
Active immunisation.

Combivent
Bender, Aust.; Boehringer Ingelheim, Canad.; Boehringer Ingelheim, Fr.; Boehringer Ingelheim, Irl.; Boehringer Ingelheim, S.Afr.; Boehringer Ingelheim, UK; Boehringer Ingelheim, USA.
Ipratropium bromide (p.754·2); salbutamol sulphate (p.758·2).
Obstructive airways disease.

Combivir
Glaxo Wellcome, UK; Glaxo Wellcome, USA.
Lamivudine (p.622·1); zidovudine (p.630·2).
HIV infection.

Combivit *Biomedica, Ital.†.*
Dicalcium fructose-1,6-diphosphate; L-lysine monohydrochloride (p.1350·1); multivitamins and minerals.

Combivite *SA Druggists Self Med, S.Afr.†.*
Multivitamin preparation.

Combivitol *Lannacher, Aust.*
Multivitamin preparation.

Combizym
Kwizda, Aust.; Luitpold, Austral.†; Luitpold, Belg.; Luitpold, Ger.; Luitpold, Ital.; Luitpold, Neth.; Luitpold, Norw.; Selena, Swed.; Luitpold, Switz.
Pancreatin (p.1612·1); enzymes from *Aspergillus oryzae*.
Cystic fibrosis; digestive disorders; pancreatic insufficiency.

Combizym Co *Luitpold, Austral.†.*
Pancreatin (p.1612·1); enzymes from *Aspergillus oryzae*; ox bile extract (p.1553·2).
Gastro-intestinal disorders.

Combizym Compositum
Kwizda, Aust.; Luitpold, Ger.; Luitpold, Ital.†; Luitpold, Neth.; Selena, Swed.; Luitpold, Switz.†.
Pancreatin (p.1612·1); enzymes from *Aspergillus oryzae*; ox bile (p.1553·2).
Digestive disorders; pancreatic insufficiency.

Combudoron
Note. This name is used for preparations of different composition.
Weleda, Ger.
Arnica (p.1550·3); urtica (p.1642·3).
Skin disorders.

Weleda, UK.
Homoeopathic preparation.

Combur 6 + Leuco *Boehringer Mannheim, Ital.†.*
Test for leucocytes, pH, protein, glucose, ketones, urobilinogen, and blood.

Combur Test *Boehringer Mannheim, Austral.*
Test for pH, protein, and glucose in urine.

Combur 7 Test *Boehringer Mannheim, Austral.*
Test for pH, protein, glucose, ketones, bilirubin, urobilinogen, and blood in urine.

Combur 8 Test *Boehringer Mannheim, Austral.*
Test for ketones, urobilinogen, bilirubin, blood, nitrite, pH, protein, and glucose in urine.

Combur 9 Test
Boehringer Mannheim, Austral.; Boehringer Mannheim, Ital.†; Boehringer Mannheim, S.Afr.
Test for leucocytes, nitrite, pH, protein, glucose, ketones, urobilinogen, bilirubin, and blood in urine.

Combur 10 Test
Boehringer Mannheim, Austral.; Boehringer Mannheim, Ital.†; Boehringer Mannheim, S.Afr.
Test for specific gravity, leucocytes, nitrite, pH, protein, glucose, ketones, urobilinogen, bilirubin, and blood in urine.

Combur 5 Test & Leucocytes *Boehringer Mannheim, S.Afr.*
Test for leucocytes, nitrites, glucose, protein, urobilinogen, and blood in urine.

Comburic *Bio-Therabel, Belg.*
Allopurinol (p.390·2); benzbromarone (p.392·3).
Gout; hyperuricaemia.

Combustin Heilsalbe *Combustin, Ger.*
Bismuth subgallate (p.1180·2); zinc oxide (p.1096·2); benzocaine (p.1286·2).
Skin disorders.

Cometamin *Yamanouchi, Jpn.*
Cycotiamine (p.1360·3).
Vitamin B_1 deficiency.

Cometon *Metapharma, Ital.*
Vitamin B substances.
Vitamin B deficiency.

Comfeel
Coloplast, Fr.; Coloplast, Switz.; Coloplast, UK.
Medicated dressing: Carmellose sodium (p.1471·2).
Wounds.

Coloplast, UK.
Barrier cream.
Peristomal care.

Comfeel Plus *Coloplast, UK.*
Carmellose sodium (p.1471·2); calcium alginate (p.714·1).
Wounds.

Comfeel Seasorb *Coloplast, UK.*
Calcium sodium alginate (p.714·1 and p.1470·3).
Exudating wounds.

Comfort Eye Drops *Pilkington Barnes-Hind, USA.*
Naphazoline hydrochloride (p.1064·2).
Minor eye irritation.

Comfort Tears *Pilkington Barnes-Hind, USA.*
Hydroxyethylcellulose (p.1472·3).
Dry eyes.

Comfortcare GP *Pilkington Barnes-Hind, USA.*
Disinfecting, wetting, and soaking solution for gas permeable contact lenses.

Comfortcare GP Comfort Drops *Barnes-Hind, Austral.†.*
Hydroxyethylcellulose (p.1472·3).
Lubricating solution for hard and gas permeable contact lenses.

Comfortcare GP Dual Action *Allergan, Austral.*
Subtilisin; poloxamer 338 (p.1326·3).
Cleanser for gas permeable contact lenses.

Comfortcare GP Wetting and Soaking *Allergan, Austral.*
Wetting and soaking solution for hard gas permeable contact lenses.

Comforte *3M, Ger.†.*
Bamethan; aescin (p.1543·3).
Vascular disorders.

Comfortine *Dermik, USA.*
Vitamin A (p.1358·1); vitamin E (p.1369·1); zinc oxide (p.1096·2); chloroxylenol (p.1111·1).
Skin disorders.

Comhist LA *Procter & Gamble, USA.*
Chlorpheniramine maleate (p.405·1); phenyltoloxamine citrate (p.416·1); phenylephrine hydrochloride (p.1066·2).
Nasal congestion; rhinorrhoea.

Comilorid *Mepha, Switz.*
Amiloride hydrochloride (p.819·2); hydrochlorothiazide (p.885·2).
Hypertension; liver cirrhosis with ascites; oedema.

Comital L *Bayer, Spain.*
Phenytoin (p.352·3); methylphenobarbitone (p.349·2); phenobarbitone (p.350·2).
Epilepsy; Sydenham's chorea.

Comixco *Ashbourne, UK.*
Co-trimoxazole (p.196·3).
Bacterial infections.

Comizial *Ogna, Ital.*
Phenobarbitone (p.350·2).
Sedative.

Commotional S *Declimed, Ger.†.*
Caffeine (p.749·3); propyphenazone (p.81·3).
Formerly contained papaverine hydrochloride, caffeine, and propyphenazone.
Migraine; pain; premedication for myelography.

Comox *Norton, UK†.*
Co-trimoxazole (p.196·3).
Bacterial infections.

Compagel *Derly, Spain.*
Aluminium hydroxide (p.1177·3); magnesium hydroxide (p.1198·2); magaldrate (p.1198·1).
Gastro-intestinal hyperacidity.

Companion 2 *MediSense, Canad.*
Test for glucose in blood (p.1585·1).

Compazine *SmithKline Beecham, USA.*
Prochlorperazine (p.687·3), prochlorperazine edisylate (p.687·3), or prochlorperazine maleate (p.687·3).
Behaviour disorders in mental retardation; non-psychotic anxiety; psychoses; severe nausea and vomiting.

Compendium *Poliforma, Ital.*
Bromazepam (p.643·1).
Anxiety disorders.

Compete *Mission Pharmacal, USA.*
Ferrous gluconate (p.1340·1); folic acid (p.1340·3); multivitamins and minerals.
Iron-deficiency anaemias.

Complamin
SmithKline Beecham, Aust.; Beecham, Belg.; SmithKline Beecham, Canad.; SmithKline Beecham, Ger.; Italchimici, Ital.; SmithKline Beecham, Neth.; Tika, Swed.; SmithKline Beecham, Switz.
Xanthinol nicotinate (p.971·1).
Cerebral circulatory and metabolic disorders; hearing disorders; hypercholesterolaemia; Ménière's disease; peripheral arterial disorders; retinal vascular disorders.

Complamin spezial *SmithKline Beecham, Ger.*
Xanthinol nicotinate (p.971·1).
Lipid disorders.

Complan
Boots, Austral.†; Crookes, Irl.†; Crookes Healthcare, UK.
Preparation for enteral nutrition.

Compleat
Sandoz Nutrition, Canad.; Sandoz Nutrition, USA.
A range of preparations for enteral nutrition.

Complegil *Diepal, Fr.*
Nutritional supplement.
Convalescence.

Complenatal FF *Pharmaceutical Enterprises, S.Afr.*
Multivitamin and mineral preparation.

Complesso B Antitossico Jamco *SIT, Ital.*
Capsules: Dried yeast (p.1373·1); vitamin B substances.
Injection; syrup: Vitamin B substances.
Tonic.

Complete *Allergan, Ger.*
Polyhexanide (p.1123·1); tyloxapol (p.1329·2); trometamol (p.1639·3); disodium edetate (p.980·1).
Disinfectant, storage, and rinsing solution for soft contact lenses.

Completovit *Biotherax, Ger.†.*
Multivitamin preparation.

Complex 15
Schering, Canad.
Dimethicone (p.1384·2); lecithin (p.1595·2).
Emollient.

Schering-Plough, USA.
Emollient and moisturiser.

Complex 75 *Frega, Canad.*
Vitamin B substances.

Complex B *Pharmalab, Canad.*
Vitamin B substances.

Complex-CHO *Tyson, USA†.*
Complex carbohydrate formulation from rice with minerals and fibre.

Complexe B Compose *Bio-Sante, Canad.*
Vitamin B substances.

Complexobiotico Bals *Roger, Spain†.*
Ampicillin sodium (p.153·1); ampicillin benzathine (p.154·1); bromhexine hydrochloride (p.1055·3); cineole (p.1564·1); niaouli oil (p.1607·1); guaiphenesin (p.1061·3).
Respiratory-tract infections.

Complexol *Sanico, Belg.†.*
Vitamin A (p.1358·1); cholecalciferol (p.1366·3).
Vitamin A and D deficiency.

Complidermol *Medea, Spain.*
Multivitamins and amino acids; inositol (p.1591·1).
Skin disorders.

Comploment Continus
Seton, Irl.; Mundipharma, Switz.; Seton, UK.
Pyridoxine hydrochloride (p.1362·3).
Premenstrual syndrome; vitamin B_6 deficiency.

Complutine *Zyma, Spain.*
Diazepam (p.661·1).
Contains pyridoxine hydrochloride.
Alcohol withdrawal syndrome; anxiety; febrile convulsions; insomnia; skeletal muscle spasm.

Comply
Wyeth-Ayerst, Canad.†.
Preparation for enteral nutrition.

Sherwood, USA.
Lactose-free preparation for enteral nutrition.

Compound V *Whitehall, UK.*
Salicylic acid (p.1090·2).
Verrucas.

Compound W
Whitehall-Robins, Canad.; Whitehall, Irl.; Seton, UK; Whitehall, USA.
Salicylic acid (p.1090·2).
Hyperkeratosis; verrucas; warts.

Compound W Plus *Whitehall-Robins, Canad.*
Salicylic acid (p.1090·2).
Warts.

Compoz Night-time Sleep Aid *Medtech, USA.*
Diphenhydramine hydrochloride (p.409·1).
Insomnia.

Compralgyl *Gifrer Barbezat, Fr.*
Aspirin (p.16·1); codeine phosphate (p.26·1).
Fever; pain.

Comprecin *Parke, Davis, UK†.*
Enoxacin (p.203·3).
Bacterial infections.

Comprimes analgesiques no 534 *Renapharm, Switz.*
Paracetamol (p.72·2).
Fever; pain.

Comprimes analgesiques "S" *Synpharma, Switz.*
Paracetamol (p.72·2); caffeine (p.749·3); propyphenazone (p.81·3).
Fever; pain.

Comprimes contre la toux *Zeller, Switz.*
Hedera helix.
Bronchial disorders with viscous mucus.

Comprimes Gynecologiques Pharmatex *Innothera, Fr.*
Benzalkonium chloride (p.1101·3).
Contraceptive.

Comprimes laxatifs de Worishofen *Hogapharm, Switz.†.*
Aloes (p.1177·1); fennel (p.1579·1); cuminum; frangula bark (p.1193·2).
Constipation; stool softener.

Comprimes pour l'estomac *Zeller, Switz.*
Calcium carbonate (p.1182·1); magnesium trisilicate (p.1199·1).
Gastric hyperacidity.

Comprimes somniferes no 533 nouvelle formule *Renapharm, Switz.*
Diphenhydramine hydrochloride (p.409·1).
Insomnia.

Comprimes somniferes "S" *Synpharma, Switz.*
Diphenhydramine (p.409·1).
Agitation; insomnia; nervousness.

Compu-Gel *Docmed, S.Afr.*
Aluminium hydroxide (p.1177·3); magnesium oxide (p.1198·3).
Gastric hyperacidity.

Compu-Pain *Compu, S.Afr.†.*
Paracetamol (p.72·2).
Fever; pain.

Comtess *Orion, UK.*
Entacapone (p.1136·2).
Parkinsonism.

Comtrex *Bristol-Myers Products, USA.*
Paracetamol (p.72·2); pseudoephedrine hydrochloride (p.1068·3); chlorpheniramine maleate (p.405·1); dextromethorphan hydrobromide (p.1057·3).
Coughs and cold symptoms.

Comtrex Allergy-Sinus *Bristol-Myers Products, USA.*
Paracetamol (p.72·2); pseudoephedrine hydrochloride (p.1068·3); chlorpheniramine maleate (p.405·1).
Upper respiratory-tract symptoms.

Comtrex Day & Night Maximum Strength
Bristol-Myers Products, USA.
Orange caplets, dextromethorphan hydrobromide (p.1057·3); paracetamol (p.72·2); pseudoephedrine hydrochloride (p.1068·3); blue tablets, dextromethorphan hydrobromide (p.1057·3); paracetamol (p.72·2); pseudoephedrine hydrochloride (p.1068·3); chlorpheniramine maleate (p.405·1).
Coughs and cold symptoms.

Comtrex Day & Night Multi-Symptom *Bristol-Myers Products, USA.*
Orange caplets, dextromethorphan hydrobromide (p.1057·3); paracetamol (p.72·2); pseudoephedrine hydrochloride (p.1068·3); yellow tablets, dextromethorphan hydrobromide (p.1057·3); paracetamol (p.72·2); pseudoephedrine hydrochloride (p.1068·3); chlorpheniramine maleate (p.405·1).
Coughs and cold symptoms.

Comtrex Hot Flu Relief *Bristol-Myers Products, USA.*
Chlorpheniramine maleate (p.405·1); dextromethorphan hydrobromide (p.1057·3); paracetamol (p.72·2); pseudoephedrine hydrochloride (p.1068·3).
Coughs and cold symptoms.

Comtrex Liqui-Gels *Bristol-Myers Products, USA.*
Chlorpheniramine maleate (p.405·1); dextromethorphan hydrobromide (p.1057·3); paracetamol (p.72·2); phenylpropanolamine hydrochloride (p.1067·2).
Coughs and cold symptoms.

Comvax *Merck, USA.*
A haemophilus influenzae and hepatitis B vaccine (p.1512·1).
Active immunisation in infants.

Concardisett *Brenner-Efeka, Ger.†.*
Convallaria (p.1567·2); crataegus (p.1568·2); cereus grandiflorus; valerian (p.1643·1); motherwort (p.1604·2); camphor (p.1557·2).
Cardiac disorders.

Concavit *Wallace Mfg Chem., UK.*
Multivitamin preparation.

Conceive *Pharmascience, Canad.*
Fertility test or pregnancy test (p.1621·2).

Conceive Ovulation Predictor *Quidel, USA.*
Fertility test (p.1621·2).

Conceive Pregnancy *Quidel, USA.*
Pregnancy test (p.1621·2).

Concentraid *Ferring, USA†.*
Desmopressin acetate (p.1245·2).
Renal concentration capacity testing.

Concentrated Milk of Magnesia-Cascara *Roxane, USA.*
Magnesium hydroxide (p.1198·2); cascara (p.1183·1).

Concentrin *CT, Ger.*
Aesculus (p.1543·3).
Soft-tissue disorders; venous disorders.

Conceplan M *Grunenthal, Ger.*
Ethinyloestradiol (p.1445·1); norethisterone (p.1453·1).
Combined oral contraceptive.

Concept Blue *Invitech, UK.*
Pregnancy test (p.1621·2).

Conchae comp. *Weleda, UK.*
Conchae; quercus cortex (p.1609·3).
Aid to enhance calcium absorption.

Conchivit *Ghimas, Ital.*
Multivitamin preparation.
Vitamin supplement.

Concise *BHR, UK.*
Pregnancy test (p.1621·2).

Concor
Merck, Aust.; Merck, Ger.; Bracco, Ital.; Continental Ethicals, S.Afr.; E. Merck, Switz.
Bisoprolol fumarate (p.833·1).
Angina pectoris; hypertension.

Concor Plus
Merck, Aust.; Merck, Ger.; E. Merck, Switz.
Bisoprolol fumarate (p.833·1); hydrochlorothiazide (p.885·2).
Hypertension.

Concordin
Merck Sharp & Dohme, Irl.; Merck Sharp & Dohme, Swed.; Merck Sharp & Dohme, UK.
Protriptyline hydrochloride (p.306·3).
Depression.

Condelone *Lacer, Spain.*
Podophyllotoxin (p.1089·1).
Anogenital warts.

Condilan *Pharmacia Upjohn, Ger.†.*
Hydrocortisone (p.1043·3); urea (p.1095·2); sodium chloride (p.1162·2).
Skin disorders.

Condiuren *Gentili, Ital.*
Enalapril maleate (p.863·2); hydrochlorothiazide (p.885·2).
Hypertension.

Condol *Maggioni, Ital.†.*
Dipyrone (p.35·1); chlormezanone (p.648·3).
Pain.

CondomMate *Upsher-Smith, USA†.*
Vaginal lubricant.

Condossan *Roland, Ger.†.*
Multivitamin and mineral preparation.
Calcium deficiency.

Condral *SPA, Ital.*
A heparinoid (p.882·3).
Osteoarthritis; pain.

Condress *Gentili, Ital.*
Collagen (p.1566·3).
Cicatrisation of wounds and skin ulcers.

Condrin-LA *Roberts, USA; Hauck, USA.*
Phenylpropanolamine hydrochloride (p.1067·2); chlorpheniramine maleate (p.405·1).
Upper respiratory-tract symptoms.

Condrofer *UCB, Ital.*
Chondroitin sulphate A-iron complex (p.1337·1).
Iron deficiency; iron deficiency anaemias.

Condrosulf
Salus, Aust.; IBSA, Switz.
Sodium chondroitin sulphate A (p.1562·2).
Joint disorders.

Condrotec *Searle, UK.*
Naproxen (p.61·2).
Misoprostol (p.1419·3) is included in this preparation in an attempt to limit adverse effects on the gastro-intestinal mucosa.
Ankylosing spondylitis; osteoarthritis; rheumatoid arthritis.

Conductasa *Bioresearch, Spain.*
Pyridoxine oxoglurate (p.1363·1).
Vitamin B6 deficiency.

Conducton
Klinge, Aust.; Klinge, Ger.
Carazolol (p.837·3).
Cardiac disorders; hypertension.

Condyline
Hamilton, Austral.; Yamanouchi, Belg.; Canderm, Canad.; Yamanouchi, Fr.; Yamanouchi, Ital.; Yamanouchi, Neth.; Nycomed, Norw.; Nycomed, Swed.; Nycomed, Switz.; Nycomed, UK.
Podophyllotoxin (p.1089·1).
Anogenital warts.

Condylox
Gerot, Aust.; Wolff, Ger.; Oclassen, USA.
Podophyllotoxin (p.1089·1).
Anogenital warts.

Coneurase *Alter, Spain†.*
Diclofenac sodium (p.31·2); vitamin B substances.
Formerly contained glafenine and vitamin B substances.
Pain.

Conex *Forest Pharmaceuticals, USA.*
Phenylpropanolamine hydrochloride (p.1067·2); guaiphenesin (p.1061·3).
Coughs.

Conex with Codeine *Forest Pharmaceuticals, USA.*
Phenylpropanolamine hydrochloride (p.1067·2); guaiphenesin (p.1061·3); codeine phosphate (p.26·1).
Coughs.

Confetti Lassativi *Giuliani, Ital.†.*
Rhubarb (p.1212·1); cascara (p.1183·1); boldo (p.1554·1); phenolphthalein (p.1208·2).
Constipation.

Confetto *Falqui, Ital.†.*
Phenolphthalein (p.1208·2).
Constipation.

Confetto Complex *Falqui, Ital.†.*
Phenolphthalein (p.1208·2); rhubarb (p.1212·1); boldo (p.1554·1).
Constipation.

Confiance *Wassen, UK.*
Multivitamin and mineral preparation.

Confiance Donna *Wassen, Ital.*
Multivitamin and mineral preparation.
Nutritional supplement.

Confidan *Bouty, Ital.†.*
Sulpiride (p.692·3).
Adjunct in peptic ulcer; psychiatric disorders.

Confidelle *Carter Horner, Canad.*
Pregnancy test (p.1621·2).

Confidelle Progress *Bouty, Ital.*
Pregnancy test (p.1621·2).

Confidol *Medopharm, Ger.*
Etilefrine hydrochloride (p.867·2).
Circulatory disorders; hypotension.

Confirm
Schmid, Canad.; Chefaro, UK†.
Pregnancy test (p.1621·2).

Confit *Procter & Gamble, Aust.*
Verapamil hydrochloride (p.960·3); triamterene (p.957·2); hydrochlorothiazide (p.885·2).
Hypertension.

Conflictan *Solvay, Fr.*
Oxaflozane hydrochloride (p.301·1).
Depression.

Confludin N *Bilgast, Ger.*
Homoeopathic preparation.

Confobos *Smaller, Spain.*
Famotidine (p.1192·1).
Gastro-oesophageal reflux; peptic ulcer; Zollinger-Ellison syndrome.

Confortid
Dumex, Ger.; Dumex, Norw.; Dumex-Alpharma, Swed.; Dumex, Switz.†.
Indomethacin (p.45·2) or indomethacin sodium (p.45·2).
Gout; inflammation; musculoskeletal, joint, and periarticular disorders; pain; renal and biliary colic.

Congespirin *Bristol-Myers Squibb, USA.*
Chewable tablets: Paracetamol (p.72·2); phenylephrine hydrochloride (p.1066·2).
Cold symptoms.
Oral liquid†: Paracetamol (p.72·2); phenylpropanolamine hydrochloride (p.1067·2).
Cold symptoms.
Syrup†: Dextromethorphan hydrobromide (p.1057·3).
Coughs.

Congess *Fleming, USA.*
Guaiphenesin (p.1061·3); pseudoephedrine hydrochloride (p.1068·3).
Asthma; coughs and cold symptoms; nasal congestion.

Congest *Trianon, Canad.*
Conjugated oestrogens (p.1457·3).
Oestrogen therapy.

Congest Aid *Zee, Canad.*
Pseudoephedrine hydrochloride (p.1068·3).

Congestac *Menley & James, USA.*
Pseudoephedrine hydrochloride (p.1068·3); guaiphenesin (p.1061·3).
Coughs.

Congestan *Schering-Plough, Neth.†.*
Azatadine maleate (p.402·3); pseudoephedrine sulphate (p.1068·3).
Allergic rhinitis.

Congestant *Rugby, USA.*
Paracetamol (p.72·2); chlorpheniramine maleate (p.405·1).
Upper respiratory-tract symptoms.

Congestant D *Rugby, USA.*
Phenylpropanolamine hydrochloride (p.1067·2); chlorpheniramine maleate (p.405·1); paracetamol (p.72·2).
Upper respiratory-tract symptoms.

Congest-Eze *Stanley, Canad.*
Pseudoephedrine hydrochloride (p.1068·3).

Congestion Relief *Schein, USA.*
Pseudoephedrine hydrochloride (p.1068·3).
Nasal congestion.

Coniel *Kyowa, Jpn.*
Benidipine hydrochloride (p.828·1).
Hypertension.

Conjonctyl *Sedifa, Mon.*
Sodium methylsilanetriol salicylate.
Arteritis; mastalgia; osteoporosis.

Conjugen
Klinge, Aust.; Klinge, Ger.; Klinge Munich, Switz.
Conjugated oestrogens (p.1457·3).
Menopausal disorders.

Conjuncain-EDO *Mann, Ger.*
Oxybuprocaine hydrochloride (p.1298·1).
Local anaesthesia.

Conjunctin
Allergan, Aust.†; Allergan, Belg.†.
Neomycin sulphate (p.229·2); polymyxin B sulphate (p.239·1).
Bacterial eye infections.

Conjunctin-S *Allergan, Aust.†.*
Prednisolone acetate (p.1048·1); neomycin sulphate (p.229·2); polymyxin B sulphate (p.239·1).
Bacterial eye infections.

Conjunctisan-A *Vitorgan, Ger.*
Bulb. oc. fet.; lens; vasa fet.; placenta; retina; nerv. opt.; chorioidea; corp. vitr.; cort. cerebri (p.1599·1); diencephalon; deslanoside (p.847·2); esculoside (p.1543·3).
Eye disorders.

Conjunctisan-B *Vitorgan, Ger.*
Cornea; conjunctiva; mucosa nasopharyng.; thymus fet.; lien fet.; lymphonodi; gland. supraren. (p.1050·1); placenta mat.; retina; nerv. opt.; lens; corp. vitr.; chorioidea; cort. cerebri (p.1599·1); diencephalon; esculoside (p.1543·3).
Eye disorders.

Conjuvac *SmithKline Beecham, Ger.†.*
Allergen extracts of *Dermatophagoides pteronyssinus*, grass pollens, or tree pollens (p.1545·1).
Hyposensitisation.

Conludag *Searle, Norw.*
Norethisterone (p.1453·1).
Progestogen-only oral contraceptive.

Connettivina
Kolassa, Aust.; Fidia, Ital.
Sodium hyaluronate (p.1630·3).
Burns; skin disorders; ulcers; wounds.

Connettivina Plus *Fidia, Ital.*
Sodium hyaluronate (p.1630·3); silver sulphadiazine (p.247·3).
Burns; skin ulceration; wound.

Conotrane
Boehringer Ingelheim, Irl.; Yamanouchi, UK.
Benzalkonium chloride (p.1101·3); dimethicone (p.1384·2).
Formerly contained hydrargaphen and dimethicone.
Barrier cream.

Conova
Searle, Belg.; Searle, Irl.†; Gold Cross, UK†.
Ethynodiol diacetate (p.1445·3); ethinyloestradiol (p.1445·1).
Combined oral contraceptive; menstrual disorders.

Conpec *Teral, USA.*
Pseudoephedrine hydrochloride (p.1068·3); guaiphenesin (p.1061·3).
Coughs.

Conpin *TAD, Ger.*
Isosorbide mononitrate (p.893·3).
Cardiac disorders.

Conray
Mallinckrodt, Austral.; May & Baker, Austral.†; Mallinckrodt, Canad.; Bracco, Ital.; May & Baker, UK.; Mallinckrodt, USA.
Meglumine iothalamate (p.1008·1) or sodium iothalamate (p.1008·1).
Radiographic contrast medium.

Conray 30 *Mallinckrodt, Ger.†.*
Meglumine iothalamate (p.1008·1).
Radiographic contrast medium.

Conray 60 *Mallinckrodt, Ger.†.*
Meglumine iothalamate (p.1008·1).
Radiographic contrast medium.

Conray 70 *Mallinckrodt, Ger.†.*
Meglumine iothalamate (p.1008·1); sodium iothalamate (p.1008·1).
Radiographic contrast medium.

Conray 80 *Mallinckrodt, Ger.†.*
Sodium iothalamate (p.1008·1).
Radiographic contrast medium.

Conray EV *Mallinckrodt, Ger.†.*
Meglumine iothalamate (p.1008·1); sodium iothalamate (p.1008·1).
Radiographic contrast medium.

Conray FL *Mallinckrodt, Ger.†.*
Meglumine iothalamate (p.1008·1).
Contrast medium for urography.

Consablitz *Agil, Ger.†.*
Salicylic acid (p.1090·2); benzocaine (p.1286·2); castor oil (p.1560·2); lactic acid (p.1593·3); solvent ether (p.1378·2).
Skin disorders.

Constant-T *Geigy, USA†.*
Theophylline (p.765·1).
Asthma; bronchospasm.

Constilac *Alra, USA.*
Lactulose (p.1195·3).
Constipation.

Constipation *Homeocan, Canad.*
Homoeopathic preparation.

Constrilia
Alcon, Fr.; Alcon, Neth.†; Alcon, Switz.†.
Tetrahydrozoline hydrochloride (p.1070·2).
Eye irritation.

Constulose *Barre-National, USA.*
Lactulose (p.1195·3).
Constipation.

Contac
Note. This name is used for preparations of different composition.
Schoeller, Aust.; Fink, Ger.; SmithKline Beecham Consumer, Irl.
Chlorpheniramine maleate (p.405·1); phenylpropanolamine hydrochloride (p.1067·2).
Cold symptoms; hay fever; sinusitis.

SmithKline Beecham Consumer, Austral.
Atropine sulphate (p.455·1); hyoscine hydrobromide (p.462·3); hyoscyamine sulphate (p.464·2); pseudoephedrine hydrochloride (p.1068·3).
Cold symptoms.

Contac 400 *SmithKline Beecham Consumer, UK.*
Chlorpheniramine maleate (p.405·1); phenylpropanolamine hydrochloride (p.1067·2).
Cold symptoms.

Contac Allergy Formula *SmithKline Beecham Consumer, Canad.*
Terfenadine (p.418·1).
Hypersensitivity disorders.

Contac C *SmithKline Beecham Consumer, Canad.*
Chlorpheniramine maleate (p.405·1); phenylpropanolamine hydrochloride (p.1067·2).
Respiratory congestion.

Contac C Nighttime *SmithKline Beecham Consumer, Canad.*
Pseudoephedrine hydrochloride (p.1068·3); diphenhydramine hydrochloride (p.409·1); paracetamol (p.72·2).

Contac C Nondrowsy *SmithKline Beecham Consumer, Canad.*
Pseudoephedrine hydrochloride (p.1068·3).

Contac Cough & Chest Cold *SmithKline Beecham Consumer, USA†.*
Pseudoephedrine hydrochloride (p.1068·3); dextromethorphan hydrobromide (p.1057·3); guaiphenesin (p.1061·3).
Coughs and cold symptoms.

Contac Cough Cold and Flu *SmithKline Beecham Consumer, Canad.*
Paracetamol (p.72·2); chlorpheniramine maleate (p.405·1); dextromethorphan hydrobromide (p.1057·3); phenylpropanolamine hydrochloride (p.1067·2).
Formerly known as Contac C Cold Care Formula.
Coughs and cold symptoms.

Contac Cough & Sore Throat *SmithKline Beecham Consumer, USA†.*
Dextromethorphan hydrobromide (p.1057·3); paracetamol (p.72·2).
Coughs.

Contac Coughcaps
SmithKline Beecham Consumer, Canad.†; SmithKline Beecham Consumer, UK.
Dextromethorphan hydrobromide (p.1057·3).
Coughs.

Contac Day & Night Allergy Sinus *SmithKline Beecham Consumer, USA.*
Paracetamol (p.72·2); pseudoephedrine hydrochloride (p.1068·3); diphenhydramine hydrochloride (p.409·1).

Contac Day & Night Cold and Flu *SmithKline Beecham Consumer, Canad.*
Yellow caplets, pseudoephedrine hydrochloride (p.1068·3); dextromethorphan hydrobromide (p.1057·3); paracetamol (p.72·2); blue caplets, diphenhydramine hydrochloride (p.409·1); pseudoephedrine hydrochloride; paracetamol.
Cold symptoms.

Contac Day and Night Cold & Flu Caplets *SmithKline Beecham Consumer, USA.*
Pseudoephedrine hydrochloride (p.1068·3); dextromethorphan hydrobromide (p.1057·3); paracetamol (p.72·2).
Coughs and cold symptoms.

Contac Day & Night Sinus/Allergy *SmithKline Beecham Consumer, Canad.*
Paracetamol (p.72·2); pseudoephedrine hydrochloride (p.1068·3); diphenhydramine hydrochloride (p.409·1).
Cold symptoms; coughs.

Contac Erkaltungs-Trunk *Fink, Ger.*
Paracetamol (p.72·2).
Cold symptoms; fever; pain.

Contac Erkaltungs-Trunk Forte *Fink, Ger.*
Paracetamol (p.72·2); phenylephrine hydrochloride (p.1066·2); dextromethorphan hydrobromide (p.1057·3).
Cold symptoms; influenza symptoms.

Contac H *Fink, Ger.*
Chlorpheniramine maleate (p.405·1); dextromethorphan hydrobromide (p.1057·3); phenylpropanolamine hydrochloride (p.1067·2).
Cold symptoms; coughs.

Contac 12 Hour *SmithKline Beecham Consumer, USA.*
Chlorpheniramine maleate (p.405·1); phenylpropanolamine hydrochloride (p.1067·2).
Upper respiratory-tract symptoms.

Contac 12 Hour Allergy *SmithKline Beecham Consumer, USA.*
Clemastine fumarate (p.406·2).

Contac Husten-Trunk *Fink, Ger.*
Ambroxol hydrochloride (p.1054·3).
Respiratory disorders associated with viscid or excessive mucus.

Contac Maximum Strength 12 Hour *SmithKline Beecham Consumer, USA†.*
Chlorpheniramine maleate (p.405·1); phenylpropanolamine hydrochloride (p.1067·2).
Upper respiratory-tract symptoms.

Contac Night Cold & Flu Caplets *SmithKline Beecham Consumer, USA†.*
Diphenhydramine hydrochloride (p.409·1); pseudoephedrine hydrochloride (p.1068·3); dextromethorphan hydrobromide (p.1057·3); paracetamol (p.72·2).
Coughs and cold symptoms.

Contac Night-Time Hot Drink *SmithKline Beecham Consumer, Canad.†.*
Paracetamol (p.72·2); ascorbic acid (p.1365·2); pheniramine maleate (p.415·3); phenylephrine hydrochloride (p.1066·2).
Cold symptoms.

Contac Rhume *SmithKline Beecham Consumer, Switz.*
Chlorpheniramine maleate (p.405·1); phenylpropanolamine hydrochloride (p.1067·2).
Allergic rhinitis; cold symptoms.

Contac Severe Cold and Flu Formula *SmithKline Beecham Consumer, USA.*
Chlorpheniramine maleate (p.405·1); dextromethorphan hydrobromide (p.1057·3); paracetamol (p.72·2); phenylpropanolamine hydrochloride (p.1067·2).
Coughs and cold symptoms.

Contac Severe Cold & Flu Hot Medicine *SmithKline Beecham Consumer, USA†.*
Chlorpheniramine maleate (p.405·1); dextromethorphan hydrobromide (p.1057·3); paracetamol (p.72·2); pseudoephedrine hydrochloride (p.1068·3).
Coughs and cold symptoms.

Contac Severe Cold & Flu Nighttime *SmithKline Beecham Consumer, USA†.*
Chlorpheniramine maleate (p.405·1); dextromethorphan hydrobromide (p.1057·3); paracetamol (p.72·2); pseudoephedrine hydrochloride (p.1068·3).
Coughs and cold symptoms.

Contac Severe Cold & Flu Non-Drowsy *SmithKline Beecham Consumer, USA.*
Pseudoephedrine hydrochloride (p.1068·3); paracetamol (p.72·2); dextromethorphan hydrobromide (p.1057·3).

Contac Sinus *SmithKline Beecham Consumer, Canad.*
Paracetamol (p.72·2); pseudoephedrine hydrochloride (p.1068·3).
Sinus pain and congestion.

Contac Sinus Formula *SmithKline Beecham Consumer, USA.*
Pseudoephedrine hydrochloride (p.1068·3); paracetamol (p.72·2).
Upper respiratory-tract symptoms.

Contac Toux *SmithKline Beecham Consumer, Switz.*
Chlorpheniramine maleate (p.405·1); phenylpropanolamine hydrochloride (p.1067·2); dextromethorphan hydrobromide (p.1057·3).
Coughs.

Contaclair *Akripan, Aust.*
Rinsing, disinfecting and storage solution for contact lens.

Contact *VAAS, Ital.*
Chlorhexidine hydrochloride (p.1107·2).
Skin disinfection; wounds.

Contactol *Merck Sharp & Dohme-Chibret, Fr.*
Hypromellose 4000 (p.1473·1).
Contact lens and ocular prostheses; dry eye disorders.

Contafilm *Allergan, Ger.*
Polyvinyl alcohol (p.1474·2).
Dry eye disorders.

Contalax *3M, Fr.*
Bisacodyl (p.1179·3).
Constipation.

Conta-Lens Wetting *Baif, Ital.*
Benzalkonium chloride (p.1101·3); edetic acid (p.980·3); methylcellulose (p.1473·3).
Wetting solution for hard contact lens.

Contamex *SmithKline Beecham, Ger.†.*
Ketazolam (p.675·2).
Head injuries; multiple sclerosis; myelitis; psychiatric disorders.

Contaren *Sintesa, Belg.*
Canrenone (p.836·2).
Hypertension; oedema.

Contenton *SmithKline Beecham, Ger.†.*
Amantadine sulphate (p.1129·2).
Influenza A; parkinsonism.

ConTE-PAK *SoloPak, USA.*
Trace element preparation.
Additive for intravenous total parenteral nutrition solutions.

Contigen *Bard, UK.*
Bovine dermal collagen (p.1566·3).
Urinary incontinence.

Contimit *Lindopharm, Ger.*
Terbutaline sulphate (p.764·1).
Obstructive airways disease.

Continucor *Parke, Davis, Aust.*
Quinapril hydrochloride (p.938·1).
Heart failure; hypertension.

Contiphyllin *Lindopharm, Ger.*
Theophylline (p.765·1).
Obstructive airways disease.

Contop *Rohm, Ger.†.*
Paracetamol (p.72·2); phenylpropanolamine hydrochloride (p.1067·2); caffeine (p.749·3).
Cold symptoms.

Contopharma *Silhouette, Aust.*
Wetting, disinfecting, and storage solutions for contact lenses.

Contra Infekt *Rentschler, Ger.†.*
Echinacea purpurea (p.1574·2).
Respiratory-tract infections; urinary-tract infections.

Contraceptivum *Donau, Aust.†.*
Nonoxinol 9 (p.1326·1).
Contraceptive.

Contracid *Thiemann, Ger.*
Cimetidine (p.1183·2).
Gastro-oesophageal reflux; peptic ulcer; Zollinger-Ellison syndrome.

Contracide *Norgine, Fr.*
Aluminium hydroxide (p.1177·3); magnesium trisilicate (p.1199·1); dimethicone (p.1213·1).
Gastro-intestinal disorders.

Contra-Coff *Universal, S.Afr.*
Pholcodine (p.1068·1); squill (p.1070·1).
Coughs.

Contractubex
Kolassa, Aust.; Merz, Ger.; Merz, Switz.
Onion (p.1610·2); heparin (p.879·3) or heparin sodium (p.879·3); allantoin (p.1078·2).
Keloids; scars.

Contradol *Merz, Ger.†.*
Aspirin (p.16·1).
Cold symptoms; fever; pain.

Contraflam *Berk, UK.*
Mefenamic acid (p.51·2).
Inflammation; menorrhagia; pain.

Contraforte *Waldheim, Aust.*
Propyphenazone (p.81·3); dextropropoxyphene (p.27·3); caffeine (p.749·3).
Pain.

Contrafungin *Pharmagalen, Ger.†.*
Clotrimazole (p.376·3).
Fungal skin infections.

Contragrippine *Sterling Midy, Fr.†.*
Paracetamol (p.72·2); ascorbic acid (p.1365·2).
Fever; pain.

Contralorin *Waldheim, Aust.*
Propyphenazone (p.81·3); paracetamol (p.72·2); anhydrous caffeine (p.749·3).
Fever; pain.

Contralum *Hermal, Ger.†.*
Benzophenone-6 (p.1487·1); sodium 3,4-dimethoxyphenylglyoxylate (p.1488·3).
Photosensitive skin disorders; sunscreen.

Contralum Ultra
Note. This name is used for preparations of different composition.
Hermal, Ger.†.
3-(4-Methylbenzylidene)bornan-2-one (p.1487·2); isopropyldibenzoylmethane (p.1487·2); 2-phenyl-1*H*-benzimidazole-5-sulphonic acid (p.1488·2).
Photosensitive skin disorders; sunscreen.
Boots Healthcare, Neth.
3-(4-Methylbenzylidene)bornan-2-one (p.1487·2); avobenzone (p.1486·3); sodium 2-phenyl-1*H*-benzimidazole-5-sulphonate (p.1488·2).
Photosensitive skin disorders; sunscreen.
Hermal, Switz.
3-(4-Methylbenzylidene) bornan-2-one (p.1487·2); avobenzone (p.1486·3); 2-phenyl-1*H*-benzimidazole-5-sulphonic acid (p.1488·2).
Sunscreen.

Contramal
Searle, Belg.; Formenti, Ital.
Tramadol hydrochloride (p.90·1).
Pain.

Contramareo *Orravan, Spain.*
Dimenhydrinate (p.408·2).
Motion sickness; vertigo.

Contramutan *Nattermann, Ger.*
Homoeopathic preparation.

Contraneural *Pfleger, Ger.*
Ibuprofen (p.44·1).
Fever; inflammation; musculoskeletal and joint disorders; pain.

Contraneural Forte *Pfleger, Ger.*
Paracetamol (p.72·2); codeine phosphate (p.26·1).
Pain.

Contraneural N *Pfleger, Ger.†.*
Aspirin (p.16·1); paracetamol (p.72·2); codeine phosphate (p.26·1).
Coughs and cold symptoms; neuralgia; pain.

Contrapect *Krewel, Ger.†.*
Codeine phosphate (p.26·1).
Formerly contained dioxethedrin hydrochloride, promethazine hydrochloride, and codeine phosphate.
Coughs.

Contrapect infant N *Krewel, Ger.†.*
Codeine phosphate (p.26·1).
Formerly contained dioxethadrin hydrochloride, promethazine hydrochloride, pholcodine, and potassium guaiacolsulfonate.
Coughs and associated respiratory-tract disorders.

Contrasmina *Falqui, Ital.*
Clenbuterol hydrochloride (p.752·1).
Obstructive airways disease.

Contraspasmin *Dresden, Ger.*
Clenbuterol hydrochloride (p.752·1).
Obstructive airways disease.

Contrasthenyl
Eumedis, Belg.†; Doms, Switz.
Vitamin B_6 preparation with minerals.
Asthenia.

Contrathion
SERB, Fr.; Rhone-Poulenc Rorer, Ital.
Pralidoxime methylsulphate (p.992·2).
Organophosphorus poisoning.

Contravenenum M *Fides, Ger.†.*
Rad. paeoniae; sarsaparilla; rad. cichorii; arnica; couch-grass; urtica; echinacea angustifolia; sulfur; ginseng; acid. phosphor.; tinctura amara; tinctura aromatica.
Herbal preparation.

Contravert B_6 *Waldheim, Aust.*
Meclozine hydrochloride (p.413·3); pyridoxine hydrochloride (p.1362·3).
Motion sickness; vertigo; vomiting.

Contre-Douleurs *Wild, Switz.*
Aspirin (p.16·1); paracetamol (p.72·2); caffeine (p.749·3).
Colloidal aluminium hydroxide (p.1177·3) is included in the tablets in an attempt to limit adverse effects on the gastro-intestinal mucosa.
Fever; pain.

Contre-Douleurs P *Wild, Switz.*
Paracetamol (p.72·2).
Fever; pain.

Contre-Douleurs-C *Wild, Switz.*
Aspirin (p.16·1); paracetamol (p.72·2); caffeine (p.749·3); ascorbic acid (p.1365·2).
Cold symptoms; fever.

Contrheuma *Spitzner, Ger.*
Sustained-release tablets†: Aspirin (p.16·1).
Arthritis; pain; rheumatism; thrombosis.
Topical gel: Glycol salicylate (p.43·1); benzyl nicotinate (p.22·1).
Circulatory disorders; inflammatory disorders; muscle and nerve pain; rheumatism.

Contrheuma Bad L *Spitzner, Ger.*
Salicylic acid (p.1090·2); sodium humate.
Bath additive; neuromuscular, musculoskeletal, and joint disorders.

Contrheuma flussig *Spitzner, Ger.†.*
Glycol salicylate (p.43·1); methyl nicotinate (p.55·1); Norway spruce oil; orange oil (p.1610·3).
Cervical syndrome; circulatory disorders; muscle pain; neuralgia; rheumatism.

Contrheuma V + T Bad N *Spitzner, Ger.*
Glycol salicylate (p.43·1); diethylamine salicylate (p.33·1); oleum pini sylvestris.
Bath additive; cold symptoms; musculoskeletal and joint disorders; neuralgia; peripheral circulatory disorders.

Contrheuma-Gel forte N *Spitzner, Ger.*
Bornyl salicylate (p.22·1); ethyl salicylate (p.36·1); methyl nicotinate (p.55·1).
Neuralgia; neuritis; rheumatism; sports injuries.

Contrin *Geneva, USA.*
Ferrous fumarate (p.1339·3); folic acid (p.1340·3); intrinsic factor; vitamin B_{12} substances (p.1363·3).
Vitamin C (p.1365·2) is included in this preparation to increase the absorption and availability of iron.
Anaemias.

Contrix
Codali, Belg.; Guerbet, Fr.†.
Meglumine iothalamate (p.1008·1).
Radiographic contrast medium.

Control
Note. This name is used for preparations of different composition.
Bio-Sante, Canad.
Cascara (p.1183·1); sennosides A and B (p.1212·3).
Bayer, Ital.
Lorazepam (p.675·3).
Convulsions; nervous disorders; sedative.
OM, Switz.
Mephenoxalone (p.678·1).
Anxiety; muscle tension.
Thompson, USA.
Phenylpropanolamine hydrochloride (p.1067·2).
Obesity.

Control-L *Schein, USA†.*
Pyrethrins; piperonyl butoxide technical (p.1409·3).
Pediculosis.

Controloc *Bayer, S.Afr.*
Pantoprazole (p.1207·3).
Gastro-oesophageal reflux; peptic ulcer.

Controlvas *Belmac, Spain.*
Enalapril maleate (p.863·2).
Heart failure; hypertension.

Contromet *Propan, S.Afr.*
Metoclopramide hydrochloride (p.1200·3).
Gastro-intestinal disorders.

Contugel *Klinge, Switz.†.*
Heparin sodium (p.879·3); glycol salicylate (p.43·1); menthol (p.1600·2).
Musculoskeletal, joint, and peri-articular disorders; soft-tissue disorders.

Contugesic *Asta Medica, Spain.*
Dihydrocodeine tartrate (p.34·1).
Pain.

Contumax *Casen Fisons, Spain.*
Sodium picosulphate (p.1213·2).
Constipation.

Contusin *Herbamed, Switz.*
Homoeopathic preparation.

Contuss *Parmed, USA.*
Phenylpropanolamine hydrochloride (p.1067·2); guaiphenesin (p.1061·3); phenylephrine hydrochloride (p.1066·2).
Coughs.

Convacard *Madaus, Ger.*
Convallaria glycosides (p.1567·2).
Heart failure.

Conva-cyl Ho-Len-Complex *Liebermann, Ger.*
Homoeopathic preparation.

Convallocor *Hevert, Ger.*
Homoeopathic preparation.

Convallocor-SL *Hevert, Ger.*
Crataegus (p.1568·2); convallaria (p.1567·2).
Cardiac disorders.

Convallysan *Hanosan, Ger.†.*
Homoeopathic preparation.

Convastabil *Klein, Ger.*
Convallaria (p.1567·2); crataegus (p.1568·2).
Cardiac disorders.

Convectal *Vita Elan, Spain.*
Diltiazem hydrochloride (p.854·2).
Angina pectoris; hypertension; myocardial infarction.

Conveen Protact *Coloplast, Fr.*
Barrier cream.

Converten *Gentili, Ital.*
Enalapril maleate (p.863·2).
Heart failure; hypertension; ischaemic heart disease.

Convivial *Malesci, Ital.†.*
Pepsin (p.1616·3); pancreatin (p.1612·1); bromelains (p.1555·1); cellulase (p.1561·1).
Digestive disorders.

Convulex
Gerot, Aust.; Byk, Belg.; Promonta Lundbeck, Ger.; Byk, Neth.; Byk Madaus, S.Afr.; Gerot, Switz.; Farmitalia Carlo Erba, UK.
Valproic acid (p.361·2) or sodium valproate (p.361·2).
Epilepsy.

Convulsofin *Dresden, Ger.; Boehringer Mannheim, Ger.; Wernigerode, Ger.*
Calcium valproate (p.363·3) or sodium valproate (p.361·2).
Epilepsy.

Cool-Mint Listerine *Warner-Lambert, USA.*
Thymol (p.1127·1); cineole (p.1564·1); methyl salicylate (p.55·2); menthol (p.1600·2).

Cooper AR *Coopervision, Canad.*
Antazoline phosphate (p.401·3); naphazoline hydrochloride (p.1064·2).

Cooper Tears *Coopervision, Canad.*
Polyvinyl alcohol (p.1474·2).

Copaltra *Plantes Tropicales, Fr.*
Coutarea; centaury (p.1561·1).
Diabetes.

Coparvax
Wellcome, Ital.†; Calmic, UK†.
Corynebacterium parvum (p.516·1).
Malignant ascites; malignant pleural effusion.

Copavin *Lilly, USA†.*
Codeine sulphate (p.26·2); papaverine hydrochloride (p.1614·2).

Copaxone *Teva, USA.*
Glatiramer acetate (p.1584·3).
Multiple sclerosis.

Cope *Mentholatum, USA.*
Aspirin (p.16·1); caffeine (p.749·3).
Aluminium hydroxide (p.1177·3) and magnesium hydroxide (p.1198·2) are included in this preparation in an attempt to limit adverse effects on the gastro-intestinal mucosa.
Pain.

Copen *Covan, S.Afr.†.*
Phenoxymethylpenicillin potassium (p.236·2).
Bacterial infections.

Cophene No. 2 *Dunhall, USA.*
Pseudoephedrine hydrochloride (p.1068·3); chlorpheniramine maleate (p.405·1).
Upper respiratory-tract symptoms.

Cophene XP *Dunhall, USA.*
Pseudoephedrine hydrochloride (p.1068·3); guaiphenesin (p.1061·3); hydrocodone tartrate (p.43·1).
Coughs.

Cophene-B *Dunhall, USA†.*
Brompheniramine maleate (p.403·2).
Hypersensitivity reactions.

Cophene-X *Dunhall, USA.*
Phenylephrine hydrochloride (p.1066·2); phenylpropanolamine hydrochloride (p.1067·2); pentoxyverine cit-

rate (p.1066·1); potassium guaiacolsulfonate (p.1068·3).
Coughs.

Cophenylcaine Paedpharm, Austral.
Phenylephrine hydrochloride (p.1066·2); lignocaine hydrochloride (p.1293·2).
Preparation of nasal mucosa for surgical procedures.

Copholco Roche Consumer, UK†.
Pholcodine (p.1068·1); terpin hydrate (p.1070·2); menthol (p.1600·2); cineole (p.1564·1).
Coughs.

Copholcoids Roche Consumer, UK†.
Pholcodine (p.1068·1); terpin hydrate (p.1070·2); menthol (p.1600·2); cineole (p.1564·1); chloroform (p.1220·3).
Coughs.

Cophylac Hoechst Marion Roussel, Canad.
Expectorant: Normethadone hydrochloride (p.1065·2); oxilofrine hydrochloride (p.925·3); emetine hydrochloride (p.582·2).
Oral solution: Normethadone hydrochloride (p.1065·2); oxilofrine hydrochloride (p.925·3).
Coughs.

Copinal Vinas, Spain.
Zinc acexamate (p.1542·1).
Peptic ulcer.

Copper T Schering, Ital.†.
Copper-wound plastic (p.1337·3).
Intra-uterine contraceptive device.

Coppertone Bug & Sunblock Schering-Plough, Canad.
Homosalate (p.1487·2); ethylhexyl *p*-methoxycinnamate (p.1487·1); octyl salicylate (p.1487·3); oxybenzone (p.1487·3).
Sunscreen.

Coppertone Kids
Note. This name is used for preparations of different composition.
Schering-Plough, Canad.
SPF 15; SPF 30; SPF 40: Homosalate (p.1487·2); ethylhexyl *p*-methoxycinnamate (p.1487·1); octyl salicylate (p.1487·3); oxybenzone (p.1487·3).
Sunscreen.

Schering-Plough, USA.
SPF 15: Ethylhexyl *p*-methoxycinnamate (p.1487·1); 2-ethylhexyl salicylate (p.1487·3); homosalate (p.1487·2); oxybenzone (p.1487·3).
SPF 30: Ethylhexyl *p*-methoxycinnamate (p.1487·1); 2-ethylhexyl salicylate (p.1487·3); oxybenzone (p.1487·3); octocrylene (p.1487·3).
Sunscreen.

Coppertone Lipkote
Schering-Plough, Canad.; Schering-Plough, USA.
SPF 15: Ethylhexyl *p*-methoxycinnamate (p.1487·1); oxybenzone (p.1487·3).
Sunscreen.

Coppertone Moisturizing Schering-Plough, USA.
SPF 2: Homosalate (p.1487·2).
SPF 4; SPF 6; SPF 8; SPF 15: Ethylhexyl *p*-methoxycinnamate (p.1487·1); oxybenzone (p.1487·3).
SPF 25; SPF 30: Ethylhexyl *p*-methoxycinnamate (p.1487·1); 2-ethylhexyl salicylate (p.1487·3); homosalate (p.1487·2); oxybenzone (p.1487·3).
SPF 45: Ethylhexyl *p*-methoxycinnamate (p.1487·1); 2-ethylhexyl salicylate (p.1487·3); octocrylene (p.1487·3); oxybenzone (p.1487·3).
Sunscreen.

Coppertone Noskote Schering-Plough, Canad.
SPF 15: Ethylhexyl *p*-methoxycinnamate (p.1487·1); octyl salicylate (p.1487·3); oxybenzone (p.1487·3).
Sunscreen.

Coppertone Oil-Free Schering-Plough, Canad.
SPF 8; SPF 15: Ethylhexyl *p*-methoxycinnamate (p.1487·1); oxybenzone (p.1487·3).
SPF 30: Homosalate (p.1487·2); ethylhexyl *p*-methoxycinnamate (p.1487·1); octyl salicylate (p.1487·3); oxybenzone (p.1487·3).
Sunscreen.

Coppertone Skin Selects Schering-Plough, Canad.
SPF 15: Ethylhexyl *p*-methoxycinnamate (p.1487·1); oxybenzone (p.1487·3).
Sunscreen.

Coppertone Skin Selects Sensitive Schering-Plough, Canad.
SPF 15: Ethylhexyl *p*-methoxycinnamate (p.1487·1); titanium dioxide (p.1093·3).
Sunscreen.

Coppertone Sport
Schering-Plough, Canad.; Schering-Plough, USA.
SPF 30: Ethylhexyl *p*-methoxycinnamate (p.1487·1); octyl salicylate (p.1487·3); oxybenzone (p.1487·3).
Sunscreen.

Schering-Plough, Canad.; Schering-Plough, USA.
SPF 4; SPF 8; SPF 15: Ethylhexyl *p*-methoxycinnamate (p.1487·1); oxybenzone (p.1487·3).
Sunscreen.

Coppertone Sunblock Schering-Plough, Canad.
SPF 45: Homosalate (p.1487·2); ethylhexyl *p*-methoxycinnamate (p.1487·1); octyl salicylate (p.1487·3); oxybenzone (p.1487·3).
Sunscreen.

Coppertone Sunscreen Schering-Plough, Canad.
SPF 4; SPF 8: Ethylhexyl *p*-methoxycinnamate (p.1487·1); oxybenzone (p.1487·3).
Sunscreen.

Coppertone Sunstick Cheshire, UK.
SPF 15: Titanium dioxide (p.1093·3).
Sunscreen.

Coppertone Supershade Cheshire, UK.
SPF 15: Oxybenzone (p.1487·3); padimate O (p.1488·1).
Sunscreen.

Coppertone Tan Magnifier Schering-Plough, USA.
SPF 2: Triethanolamine salicylate (p.1639·2).
Gel SPF 4: 2-Phenyl-1*H*-benzimidazole-5-sulphonic acid (p.1488·2).
Lotion SPF 4: Ethylhexyl *p*-methoxycinnamate (p.1487·1).
Sunscreen.

Coppertone Ultrashade Cheshire, UK.
SPF 23: Ethylhexyl *p*-methoxycinnamate (p.1487·1); oxybenzone (p.1487·3); padimate O (p.1488·1).
Sunscreen.

Coppertone UVGuard Schering-Plough, Canad.
SPF 15: Avobenzone (p.1486·3); ethylhexyl *p*-methoxycinnamate (p.1487·1); oxybenzone (p.1487·3).
SPF 30: Avobenzone (p.1486·3); ethylhexyl *p*-methoxycinnamate (p.1487·1); oxybenzone (p.1487·3); octyl salicylate (p.1487·3).
Sunscreen.

Coppertone Waterproof Sunblock Schering-Plough, Canad.
SPF 15: Ethylhexyl *p*-methoxycinnamate (p.1487·1); oxybenzone (p.1487·3).
SPF 30; SPF 45: Ethylhexyl *p*-methoxycinnamate (p.1487·1); homosalate (p.1487·2); octyl salicylate (p.1487·3); oxybenzone (p.1487·3).
Sunscreen.

Coppertrace Rorer, Austral.†.
Copper chloride (p.1337·3).
Additive for total parenteral nutrition solutions.

Coptin Jouveinal, Canad.
Sulphadiazine (p.252·3); trimethoprim (p.265·1).
Bacterial infections of the urinary tract.

Copyrkal N Berlin-Chemie, Ger.†.
Propyphenazone (p.81·3); caffeine (p.749·3).
Fever; pain.

Co-Pyronil 2 Dista, USA.
Pseudoephedrine hydrochloride (p.1068·3); chlorpheniramine maleate (p.405·1).
Upper respiratory-tract symptoms.

Co-Q-10
Larkhall Laboratories, UK; Solgar, USA†.
Ubidecarenone (p.1641·2).

Coquelusedal Elerte, Fr.
Niaouli oil (p.1607·1); camphor (p.1557·2); grindelia; gelsemium (p.1583·2); phenobarbitone (p.350·2).
Coughs.

Coquelusedal Paracetamol Elerte, Fr.
Paracetamol (p.72·2); niaouli oil (p.1607·1); grindelia; gelsemium (p.1583·2).
Respiratory-tract disorders.

cor tensobon Schwarz, Ger.
Captopril (p.836·3).
Diabetic nephropathy; heart failure; hypertension.

Coracin Roberts, USA; Hauck, USA.
Hydrocortisone acetate (p.1043·3); neomycin sulphate (p.229·2); bacitracin zinc (p.157·3); polymyxin B sulphate (p.239·1).
Infected eye disorders.

Coracten Medeva, UK.
Nifedipine (p.916·2).
Angina pectoris; hypertension.

Coradol Coradol, Ger.
Homoeopathic preparation.

Coradur Glaxo Wellcome, Canad.
Isosorbide dinitrate (p.893·1).
Angina pectoris.

Corafusin Kabi Pharmacia, Ger.†.
Lignocaine hydrochloride (p.1293·2).
Arrhythmias.

Coral Drug Research, Ital.
Nifedipine (p.916·2).
Hypertension; ischaemic heart disease.

Coralen Alter, Spain.
Ranitidine hydrochloride (p.1209·3).
Acid aspiration; gastro-intestinal haemorrhage; gastro-oesophageal reflux; peptic ulcer; Zollinger-Ellison syndrome.

Coralgesic Vesta, S.Afr.
Paracetamol (p.72·2); codeine phosphate (p.26·1); vitamin B substances.
Fever; pain.

Corallium I/ 02 B Phonix, Ger.†.
Homoeopathic preparation.

Coramedan Medice, Ger.
Digitoxin (p.848·3).
Arrhythmias; heart failure.

Coramil Tika, Swed.
Diltiazem hydrochloride (p.854·2).
Angina pectoris; hypertension.

Coramina Ciba-Geigy, Spain†.
Nikethamide (p.1483·3).
Circulatory disorders; respiratory depression.

Coramine Glucose Zyma, Fr.
Nikethamide (p.1483·3); glucose monohydrate (p.1343·3).
Asthenia; fainting.

Corangin
Ciba-Geigy, Aust.; Ciba, Ger.
Isosorbide mononitrate (p.893·3).
Chronic heart failure; ischaemic heart disease; pulmonary hypertension.

Corangin Nitrokapseln and Nitrospray Ciba, Ger.
Glyceryl trinitrate (p.874·3).
Cardiac disorders.

Corangine Ciba, Switz.
Isosorbide mononitrate (p.893·3).
Heart failure; ischaemic heart disease.

Corangor Berenguer Infale, Spain†.
Molsidomine (p.912·2).
Angina pectoris.

Coras Alphapharm, Austral.
Diltiazem hydrochloride (p.854·2).
Angina pectoris.

Corase Medac, Ger.
Urokinase (p.959·3).
Thrombo-embolic disorders.

Coratol Weifa, Norw.
Atenolol (p.825·3).
Angina pectoris; arrhythmias; hypertension; hyperthyroidism; migraine; myocardial infarction.

Coratoline Prodes, Spain†.
Dilazep hydrochloride (p.854·1).
Cardiac disorders.

Coraunol (Rowo-16) Pharmakon, Ger.†.
Homoeopathic preparation.

Corazem Mundipharma, Aust.
Diltiazem hydrochloride (p.854·2).
Angina pectoris; hypertension.

Corazet Mundipharma, Ger.
Diltiazem hydrochloride (p.854·2).
Angina pectoris; hypertension.

Corbar Covan, S.Afr.
Guaiphenesin (p.1061·3); ephedrine hydrochloride (p.1059·3); codeine phosphate (p.26·1); chlorpheniramine maleate (p.405·1); co. cocillana syrup (p.1057·2).
Coughs.

Corbar M Covan, S.Afr.
Carbocisteine (p.1056·3).
Respiratory-tract disorders.

Corbar S Covan, S.Afr.
Fedrilate (p.1061·1).
Coughs.

Corbeton Alphapharm, Austral.
Oxprenolol hydrochloride (p.926·2).
Angina pectoris; arrhythmias; hypertension.

Corbionax Dakota, Fr.
Amiodarone hydrochloride (p.820·1).
Arrhythmias.

Corbiovin Kattwiga, Ger.†.
Herba leonuri card.; sarothamni scop.; cactus; arnica; haematoporphyrin; adenosine triphosphate disodium salt; pentetrazol; thiamine chloride; riboflavine; cyanocobalamin; pangamic acid; calcium glycerophosphate; sodium phosphate; vinum malaga.
Cardiotonic.

Cordalin Dresden, Ger.
Bisoprolol fumarate (p.833·1).
A preparation of this name formerly contained etofylline and theophylline hydrate.
Angina pectoris; hypertension.

Cordalin-Strophanthin Asta Medica, Ger.†.
Etofylline (p.753·1); theophylline hydrate (p.765·1); strophanthin-K (p.951·1).
Cardiac disorders.

Cordan Ibi, Ital.†.
Fendiline hydrochloride (p.868·1).
Cardiac disorders.

Cordanum Dresden, Ger.
Talinolol (p.951·2).
Arrhythmias; hypertension; ischaemic heart disease; myocardial infarction.

Cordapur APS, Ger.
Crataegus (p.1568·2).
Cardiac disorders.

Cordarex Sanofi Winthrop, Ger.
Amiodarone hydrochloride (p.820·1).
Arrhythmias.

Cordarone
Sanofi Winthrop, Belg.; Wyeth-Ayerst, Canad.; Sanofi Winthrop, Fr.; Sigma-Tau, Ital.; Sanofi Winthrop, Neth.; Sanofi Winthrop, Norw.; Sanofi, Swed.; Sanofi Winthrop, Switz.; Wyeth-Ayerst, USA.
Amiodarone hydrochloride (p.820·1).
Arrhythmias.

Cordarone X
Sanofi Winthrop, Austral.; Sanofi Winthrop, Irl.; Sanofi Omnimed, S.Afr.; Sanofi Winthrop, UK.
Amiodarone hydrochloride (p.820·1).
Arrhythmias.

Cordema Charton, Canad.†.
Sodium chloride (p.1162·2).
Corneal oedema.

Cordes Beta Ichthyol, Ger.
Betamethasone valerate (p.1033·3).
Skin disorders.

Cordes BPO Ichthyol, Ger.
Benzoyl peroxide (p.1079·2).
Acne.

Cordes Estriol Ichthyol, Ger.
Oestriol (p.1457·2).
Vaginal disorders.

Cordes Granulat Ichthyol, Ger.†.
Acetylcysteine (p.1052·3).
Respiratory-tract disorders associated with increased or viscous mucus.

Cordes H Ichthyol, Ger.†.
Hydrocortisone acetate (p.1043·3).
Skin disorders.

Cordes Nystatin Soft Ichthyol, Ger.
Nystatin (p.386·1).
Fungal skin infections.

Cordes VAS Ichthyol, Ger.
Tretinoin (p.1093·3).
Acne.

Cordesin Serag-Wiessner, Ger.
Potassium aspartate (p.1161·3); magnesium aspartate (p.1157·2).
Heart failure; myocardial infarction; potassium and magnesium deficiency.

Cordicant Mundipharma, Ger.
Nifedipine (p.916·2).
Hypertension; ischaemic heart disease; Raynaud's syndrome.

Cordichin Knoll, Ger.
Verapamil hydrochloride (p.960·3); quinidine (p.938·3).
Arrhythmias.

Cordilan Andreu, Spain.
Nifedipine (p.916·2).
Angina pectoris; hypertension.

Cordilox
Schering, Austral.; Baker Norton, UK.
Verapamil hydrochloride (p.960·3).
Angina pectoris; arrhythmias; hypertension.

Cordipatch Schwarz, Fr.
Glyceryl trinitrate (p.874·3).
Angina pectoris.

Cordipina IBP, Ital.
Nicardipine hydrochloride (p.915·1).
Angina pectoris; heart failure; hypertension.

Cordiplast Bayer, Spain.
Glyceryl trinitrate (p.874·3).
Angina pectoris; heart failure.

Corditrine Specia, Fr.
Glyceryl trinitrate (p.874·3).
Angina pectoris; heart failure.

Cordium
Aaciphar, Belg.; Riom, Fr.
Bepridil hydrochloride (p.828·2).
Angina pectoris.

Cordran Oclassen, USA.
Flurandrenolone (p.1042·2).
Skin disorders.

Coreg SmithKline Beecham, USA.
Carvedilol (p.838·1).
Hypertension.

Coreine
Germania, Aust.; Martin, Fr.†.
Carrageenan (p.1471·3).
Constipation; obesity.

Coremax Zyma, Spain†.
Imolamine hydrochloride (p.890·2).
Cardiac disorders.

Co-Renitec
Merck Sharp & Dohme, Aust.; Merck Sharp & Dohme, Belg.; Merck Sharp & Dohme-Chibret, Fr.; Merck Sharp & Dohme, Neth.; Merck Sharp & Dohme, S.Afr.; Merck Sharp & Dohme, Spain.
Enalapril maleate (p.863·2); hydrochlorothiazide (p.885·2).
Hypertension.

Co-Reniten Merck Sharp & Dohme, Switz.
Enalapril maleate (p.863·2); hydrochlorothiazide (p.885·2).
Hypertension.

Corenza C Restan, S.Afr.
Aspirin (p.16·1); ascorbic acid (p.1365·2); chlorpheniramine maleate (p.405·1); phenylephrine hydrochloride (p.1066·2); moroxydine hydrochloride (p.623·1).
Cold and influenza symptoms.

Coreptil Synthelabo, Ital.
Heptaminol hydrochloride (p.1587·2).
Adjunct in overdosage with neuroleptics and barbiturates; cardiac disorders.

Corethium Johnson & Johnson Medical, UK.
Porcine skin (p.1630·1).
Skin grafts.

Corflene Rubio, Spain†.
Flecainide acetate (p.868·3).
Ventricular arrhythmias.

Corgard
Bristol-Myers Squibb, Belg.; Squibb, Canad.; Sanofi Winthrop, Fr.; Bristol-Myers Squibb, Irl.; Bristol-Myers Squibb, Ital.; Bristol-Myers Squibb, S.Afr.; Squibb, Spain; Bristol-Myers Squibb, Switz.; Sanofi Winthrop, UK; Bristol-Myers Squibb, USA.
Nadolol (p.913·2).
Angina pectoris; arrhythmias; hypertension; hyperthyroidism; migraine.

Corgaretic
Bristol-Myers Squibb, Irl.; Bristol-Myers Squibb, S.Afr.; Bristol-Myers Squibb, Switz.; Sanofi Winthrop, UK.
Nadolol (p.913·2); bendrofluazide (p.827·3).
Hypertension.

Corguttin Roland, Ger.†.
Convallaria (p.1567·2); adonis vernalis (p.1543·3); valerian (p.1643·1); crataegus (p.1568·2); primula; camphor.
Cardiovascular disorders.

Corguttin + Magnesium Roland, Ger.†.
Convallaria (p.1567·2); adonis vernalis (p.1543·3); magnesium aspartate (p.1157·2).
Cardiac disorders; magnesium deficiency.

Corguttin N plus *Roland, Ger.*
Adonis vernalis (p.1543·3); convallaria (p.1567·2); crataegus (p.1568·2).
Cardiovascular disorders.

Coribon *Radiumfarma, Ital.†.*
Dipyridamole (p.857·1).
Vascular disorders.

Coric *Du Pont, Ger.; Dresden, Ger.*
Lisinopril (p.898·2).
Heart failure; hypertension.

Coric plus *Du Pont, Ger.; Dresden, Ger.*
Lisinopril (p.898·2); hydrochlorothiazide (p.885·2).
Hypertension.

Coricide le Diable *Sodia, Fr.*
Salicylic acid (p.1090·2).
Callosities; corns; verrucae.

Coricide Rodell *Parke, Davis, Fr.†.*
Sodium hydroxide (p.1631·1); triethanolamine (p.1639·1).
Callosities; corns.

Coricides feuille de saule *Gilbert, Fr.†.*
Salicylic acid (p.1090·2).
Calluses; corns.

Coricidin
Note. This name is used for preparations of different composition.
Schering-Plough, Spain.
Ascorbic acid (p.1365·2); caffeine (p.749·3); chlorpheniramine maleate (p.405·1); salicylamide (p.82·3).
Influenza and cold symptoms.

Schering-Plough, USA.
Paracetamol (p.72·2); chlorpheniramine maleate (p.405·1).
Upper respiratory-tract symptoms.

Coricidin Cold *Schering, Canad.*
Chlorpheniramine maleate (p.405·1); aspirin (p.16·1).
Cold symptoms.

Coricidin D
Note. This name is used for preparations of different composition.
Schering-Plough, Belg.†.
Chlorpheniramine maleate (p.405·1); aspirin (p.16·1); caffeine (p.749·3); phenylephrine hydrochloride (p.1066·2).
Rhinitis; sinusitis.

Schering, Canad.
Long-acting tablets: Chlorpheniramine maleate (p.405·1); phenylpropanolamine hydrochloride (p.1067·2).
Tablets: Chlorpheniramine maleate (p.405·1); aspirin (p.16·1); phenylpropanolamine (p.1067·2).
Cold symptoms; respiratory congestion.

Schering-Plough, USA.
Phenylpropanolamine hydrochloride (p.1067·2); chlorpheniramine maleate (p.405·1); paracetamol (p.72·2).
Upper respiratory-tract symptoms.

Coricidin Fuerte *Schering-Plough, Spain.*
Chlorpheniramine maleate (p.405·1); phenylpropanolamine hydrochloride (p.1067·2); paracetamol (p.72·2).
Influenza and cold symptoms.

Coricidin Maximum Strength Sinus Headache *Schering-Plough, USA.*
Phenylpropanolamine hydrochloride (p.1067·2); chlorpheniramine maleate (p.405·1); paracetamol (p.72·2).
Upper respiratory-tract symptoms.

Coricidin Non-Drowsy *Schering, Canad.*
Phenylpropanolamine hydrochloride (p.1067·2); aspirin (p.16·1).
Sinus pain and congestion.

Coricidin Sinus Headache *Schering, Canad.*
Paracetamol (p.72·2); phenylpropanolamine hydrochloride (p.1067·2); chlorpheniramine maleate (p.405·1).
Cold symptoms; nasal congestion; sinus headache.

Coridil *Ecosol, Switz.*
Diltiazem hydrochloride (p.854·2).
Hypertension; ischaemic heart disease.

Corilisina *Pensa, Spain.*
Nasal spray: Benzalkonium chloride (p.1101·3); oxymetazoline hydrochloride (p.1065·3).
Nasal congestion.

Corindocomb
Schering, Aust.; Schering, Ger.
Mepindolol sulphate (p.902·3); hydrochlorothiazide (p.885·2).
Hypertension.

Corindolan
Schering, Aust.; Schering, Ger.
Mepindolol sulphate (p.902·3).
Angina pectoris; cardiac hyperkinetic syndrome; hypertension.

Corinfar *Dresden, Ger.*
Nifedipine (p.916·2).
Hypertension; ischaemic heart disease; Raynaud's syndrome.

Coristex-DH *Technilab, Canad.*
Phenylephrine hydrochloride (p.1066·2); hydrocodone tartrate (p.43·1).
Coughs.

Coristin *San Carlo, Ital.†.*
Co-dergocrine mesylate (p.1566·1).
Vascular disorders.

Coristine-DH *Technilab, Canad.*
Hydrocodone tartrate (p.43·1); phenylephrine hydrochloride (p.1066·2).
Coughs.

Coritrat *Nordmark, Ger.†.*
Procainamide hydrochloride (p.934·1); ajmaline monoethanolate (p.817·2); quinidine (p.938·3); meprobamate (p.678·1); phenobarbitone (p.350·2); theophylline (p.765·1).
Arrhythmias.

Corium *ICN, Canad.*
Chlordiazepoxide hydrochloride (p.646·3); clidinium bromide (p.459·2).
Gastro-intestinal disorders with associated anxiety.

Corizzina *SIT, Ital.*
Amethocaine hydrochloride (p.1285·2); naphazoline nitrate (p.1064·2).
Nasal congestion.

cor-L 90 N *Loges, Ger.*
Homoeopathic preparation.

Corlan
Boots, Austral.†; Evans Medical, Irl.; Medeva, UK.
Hydrocortisone sodium succinate (p.1044·1).
Aphthous stomatitis.

Corliprol
Upjohn, Ger.†; Upjohn, Switz.†.
Celiprolol hydrochloride (p.838·3).
Angina pectoris; hypertension.

Cor-loges *Loges, Ger.*
Squill (p.1070·1); convallaria (p.1567·2).
Cardiac disorders; oedema.

Corlopam *Neurex, USA.*
Fenoldopam mesylate (p.868·1).
Hypertension.

Cormagnesin
Asta Medica, Aust.; Worwag, Ger.
Magnesium sulphate (p.1157·3).
Arrhythmias; eclampsia; magnesium deficiency; premature labour.

Cormax *Oclassen, USA.*
Clobetasol propionate (p.1035·2).
Skin disorders.

Cormelian
Asta Medica, Ger.†; Schering, Ital.
Dilazep hydrochloride (p.854·1).
Cardiac disorders.

Cormelian-Digotab *Asta Medica, Ger.†.*
β-Acetyldigoxin (p.812·3); dilazep hydrochloride (p.854·1).
Heart failure.

Cor-myocrat *Schwabe, Ger.†.*
Convallaria (p.1567·2); adonis vernalis (p.1543·3); crataegus (p.1568·2).
Cardiac disorders.

Corn & Callous Removal Liquid *Scholl, UK.*
Salicylic acid (p.1090·2); camphor (p.1557·2).
Calluses; corns.

Corn Huskers *Warner-Lambert, USA.*
Emollient and moisturiser.

Corn Removers *Scholl, UK.*
Salicylic acid (p.1090·2).
Corns.

Corn Salve *Cress, Canad.*
Methyl salicylate (p.55·2); salicylic acid (p.1090·2).

Corn Solvent *Seton, UK†.*
Salicylic acid (p.1090·2).

Cornel *Berenguer Infale, Spain.*
Nisoldipine (p.922·3).
Angina pectoris; hypertension.

Cor-Neo-Nervacit-S *Herbert, Ger.†.*
Oral liquid: Phenazone (p.78·2); ouabain (p.925·2); diprophylline (p.752·1); chlorophyllin.
Tablets: Phenazone (p.78·2); ouabain (p.925·2); diprophylline (p.752·1).
Cardiac disorders.

Corneregel *Mann, Ger.*
Dexpanthenol (p.1570·3).
Eye disorders.

Corneregen N *Mann, Ger.†.*
Cyanocobalamin (p.1363·3); riboflavine sodium phosphate (p.1362·1); panthenol (p.1570·3).
Eye disorders.

Cornina Hornhaut *Beiersdorf, Ger.*
Salicylic acid (p.1090·2).
Calluses; corns.

Cornina Huhneraugen *Beiersdorf, Ger.*
Salicylic acid (p.1090·2).
Corns.

Cornkil *Norgine, Austral.*
Benzocaine (p.1286·2); salicylic acid (p.1090·2); lactic acid (p.1593·3).
Corns.

Corocrat *Biomo, Ger.*
Crataegus (p.1568·2).
Heart failure.

Coroday *Generics, UK.*
Nifedipine (p.916·2).
Angina pectoris; hypertension.

Corodoc S *Fides, Ger.†.*
Homoeopathic preparation.

Corodyn *Schmidgall, Aust.*
Crataegus tincture (p.1568·2); camphor (p.1557·2); menthol (p.1600·2).
Cardiovascular disorders.

Coro-Lanitop *Boehringer Mannheim, Aust.*
Chromonar hydrochloride (p.840·1); medigoxin (p.902·1).
Heart failure.

Corolater *Vita Elan, Spain.*
Diltiazem hydrochloride (p.854·2).
Angina pectoris; hypertension; myocardial infarction.

Coronarine *Negma, Fr.*
Dipyridamole (p.857·1).
Thrombo-embolic disorders.

Coronator *Roland, Ger.*
Crataegus (p.1568·2).
Heart failure.

Coronex *Wyeth-Ayerst, Canad.†.*
Isosorbide dinitrate (p.893·1).
Ischaemic heart disease.

Coro-Nitro
3M, Ger.; Boehringer Mannheim, UK.
Glyceryl trinitrate (p.874·3).
Angina pectoris; heart failure; myocardial infarction.

Coronorm *Wolff, Ger.*
Captopril (p.836·3).
Heart failure; hypertension.

Coronur *Boehringer Mannheim, Spain.*
Isosorbide mononitrate (p.893·3).
Angina pectoris; heart failure.

Coropar *Redel, Ger.†.*
Diprophylline (p.752·1); khellin (p.1593·1); ethaverine hydrochloride (p.1577·1); phenobarbitone (p.350·2); rutin (p.1580·2).
Asthma; cardiovascular disorders; migraine.

Corophylline *Gerda, Fr.†.*
Heptaminol acephyllinate (p.754·1).
Dyspnoea.

Coropres *Boehringer Mannheim, Spain.*
Carvedilol (p.838·1).
Hypertension; ischaemic heart disease.

Corosan *Farmacologico Milanese, Ital.*
Dipyridamole (p.857·1).
Vascular disorders.

Corotal *Rosch & Handel, Aust.*
β-Acetyldigoxin (p.812·3).
Arrhythmias; heart failure.

Corotrend
Kytta, Ger.; Siegfried, Switz.
Nifedipine (p.916·2).
Hypertension; ischaemic heart disease; Raynaud's syndrome.

Corotrop
Sanofi Winthrop, Aust.; Sanofi Winthrop, Ger.; Sanofi, Swed.; Sanofi Winthrop, Switz.
Milrinone (p.910·2) or milrinone lactate (p.910·2).
Heart failure.

Corotrope
Sanofi Winthrop, Belg.; Sanofi Winthrop, Fr.; Sanofi Winthrop, Neth.; Sanofi Winthrop, Spain.
Milrinone (p.910·2) or milrinone lactate (p.910·2).
Heart failure.

Coroverlan
Mayrhofer, Aust.; Verla, Ger.
Magnesium aspartate (p.1157·2); potassium aspartate (p.1161·3); etofylline (p.753·1); crataegus (p.1568·2).
Cardiac disorders.

Coroverlan-Digoxin *Verla, Ger.†.*
Magnesium aspartate (p.1157·2); potassium aspartate (p.1161·3); etofylline (p.753·1); digoxin (p.849·3); crataegus (p.1568·2).
Cardiac disorders.

Corovliss *Boehringer Mannheim, Ger.*
Isosorbide dinitrate (p.893·1).
Cardiac disorders.

Coroxin *Malesci, Ital.†.*
Dipyridamole (p.857·1).
Vascular disorders.

Corpamil *Helvepharm, Switz.*
Verapamil hydrochloride (p.960·3).
Angina; arrhythmias; hypertension.

Corpea *Normon, Spain.*
Molsidomine (p.912·2).
Angina pectoris.

Corprilor *Rubio, Spain.*
Enalapril maleate (p.863·2).
Heart failure; hypertension.

Corque *Geneva, USA.*
Hydrocortisone (p.1043·3); clioquinol (p.193·2).
Skin disorders.

Correctol
Note. This name is used for preparations of different composition.
Schering-Plough, Canad.
Bisacodyl (p.1179·3).
Constipation.

Alcon, Fr.
Disodium inosinate (p.1573·1).
Visual disturbances.

Schering-Plough, UK†.
Docusate sodium (p.1189·3); yellow phenolphthalein (p.1208·2).
Constipation.

Schering-Plough, USA.
Bisacodyl (p.1179·3).
Formerly contained docusate sodium and phenolphthalein.
Constipation.

Correctol Extra Gentle *Schering-Plough, USA.*
Docusate sodium (p.1189·3).

Correctol Stool Softener *Schering-Plough, Canad.*
Docusate sodium (p.1189·3).
Formerly contained docusate sodium and phenolphthalein.
Constipation.

Corrigast *Searle, Ger.†.*
Propantheline bromide (p.468·1).
Gastro-intestinal disorders.

Corsalbene *Merckle, Aust.*
Aspirin (p.16·1).
Migraine; myocardial infarction; thrombosis prophylaxis.

Cor-Select *Dreluso, Ger.*
Ointment: Crataegus (p.1568·2); valerian (p.1643·1); camphor (p.1557·2); ol. sinapis (p.1605·3); benzyl nicotinate (p.22·1); peppermint oil (p.1208·1); melissa oil.
Cardiovascular disorders.
Oral drops: Homoeopathic preparation.

Corsodyl
SmithKline Beecham Consumer, Belg.; SmithKline Beecham Sante, Fr.; Fink, Ger.; SmithKline Beecham Consumer, Irl.; SmithKline Beecham, Ital.; SmithKline Beecham Consumer, Neth.; SmithKline Beecham, Norw.; SmithKline Beecham, Swed.; SmithKline Beecham Consumer, Switz.; SmithKline Beecham Consumer, UK.
Chlorhexidine gluconate (p.1107·2).
Formerly known as Hibitane Dental in *Swed.*
Mouth infections; oral hygiene.

CorSotalol *Durachemie, Ger.*
Sotalol hydrochloride (p.945·1).
Arrhythmias.

Corsym *Novartis Consumer, Canad.*
Phenylpropanolamine polistirex (p.1067·3); chlorpheniramine polistirex (p.405·2).
Nasal congestion.

Cort 2000 *IPA, Ital.†.*
Suprarenal cortex (p.1050·1).
Steroid deficiency.

Cortacet *Whitehall-Robins, Canad.*
Hydrocortisone acetate (p.1043·3).
Skin disorders.

Cortafriol C *Derly, Spain.*
Paracetamol (p.72·2); pseudoephedrine sulphate (p.1068·3); ascorbic acid (p.1365·2).
Fever; influenza and cold symptoms; pain.

Cortafriol Complex *Derly, Spain.*
Paracetamol (p.72·2); pseudoephedrine sulphate (p.1068·3); chlorpheniramine maleate (p.405·1).
Fever; nasal congestion; pain.

CortaGel *Norstar, USA†.*
Hydrocortisone (p.1043·3).
Skin disorders.

Cortaid
Pharmacia Upjohn, Austral.†; Carlo Erba OTC, Ital.; Pharmacia Upjohn, USA.
Hydrocortisone (p.1043·3) or hydrocortisone acetate (p.1043·3).
Skin disorders.

Cortal *Organon, Swed.*
Cortisone acetate (p.1036·1).
Corticosteroid.

Cortalar *Bergamon, Ital.†.*
Fluocinolone acetonide (p.1041·1).
Skin disorders.

Cortamed *Sabex, Canad.*
Hydrocortisone acetate (p.1043·3).
Eye and ear disorders.

Cortamide *Ottolenghi, Ital.*
Fluocinolone acetonide (p.1041·1).
Skin disorders.

Cortancyl *Roussel, Fr.*
Prednisone (p.1049·2).
Corticosteroid.

Cortanest *Piam, Ital.*
Hydrocortamate hydrochloride (p.1043·3); lignocaine hydrochloride (p.1293·2).
Burns; skin disorders; wounds.

Cortanest Plus *Piam, Ital.*
Fluocinolone acetonide (p.1041·1); lignocaine hydrochloride (p.1293·2).
Anogenital disorders; burns; skin disorders.

Cortate
Note. This name is used for preparations of different composition.
Rhone-Poulenc Rorer, Austral.
Cortisone acetate (p.1036·1).
Oral corticosteroid.

Schering, Canad.
Hydrocortisone (p.1043·3).
Skin disorders.

Cortatrigen *Goldline, USA.*
Hydrocortisone (p.1043·3); neomycin sulphate (p.229·2); polymyxin B (p.239·3).
Bacterial ear infections.

Cort-Dome *Miles, USA.*
Hydrocortisone (p.1043·3) or hydrocortisone acetate (p.1043·3).
Anorectal disorders; skin disorders.

Cortef
Pharmacia Upjohn, Austral.; Pharmacia Upjohn, Canad.; Upjohn, USA.
Hydrocortisone (p.1043·3) or hydrocortisone cypionate (p.1044·1).
Corticosteroid.

Cortef Feminine Itch *Upjohn, USA.*
Hydrocortisone acetate (p.1043·3).
Pruritus.

Cortelan
Note. This name is used for preparations of different composition.
Aandersen, Ital.†.
Suprarenal cortex (p.1050·1).
Steroid deficiency.

Glaxo, UK†.
Cortisone acetate (p.1036·1).
Corticosteroid.

Cortenema
Note. This name is used for preparations of different composition.
Axcan, Canad.; Solvay, USA.
Hydrocortisone (p.1043·3).
Inflammatory bowel disease.

Casen Fisons, Spain.
Allantoin (p.1078·2); hydrocortisone hemisuccinate (p.1044·1); homatropine methobromide (p.462·2); zinc oxide (p.1096·2).
Anorectal disorders.

Cortepacitina Salus, Ital.†.
Suprarenal cortex (p.1050·1).
Steroid deficiency.

Cortepar B12 Ripari-Gero, Ital.†.
Suprarenal cortex (p.1050·1); cyanocobalamin (p.1363·3).
Anaemias; tonic.

Cortevit 100 Dukron, Ital.†.
Vitamin B substances; suprarenal cortex (p.1050·1); lignocaine hydrochloride (p.1293·2).

Cortexyl Soekami, Fr.†.
Calcium di-oxoglutarate.
Asthenia.

Corti Biciron N S & K, Ger.
Dexamethasone isonicotinate (p.1037·1); oxytetracycline hydrochloride (p.235·1).
Infected eye disorders.

Corti Jaikal S & K, Ger.
Hydrocortisone acetate (p.1043·3); sodium thiosulphate (p.996·2); salicylic acid (p.1090·2).
Acne.

Corti-Arscolloid SIT, Ital.
Dichlorobenzyl alcohol (p.1112·2); silver protein (p.1629·3); dexamethasone sodium phosphate (p.1037·2).
Stomatitis.

Cortic
Note. This name is used for preparations of different composition.
Sigma, Austral.
Hydrocortisone acetate (p.1043·3).
Anogenital pruritus; skin disorders.

Everett, USA.
Hydrocortisone (p.1043·3); pramoxine hydrochloride (p.1298·2); chloroxylenol (p.1111·1).
Inflammatory ear disorders.

Corticaine
Note. This name is used for preparations of different composition.
Glaxo, USA.
Rectal cream: Hydrocortisone acetate (p.1043·3); cinchocaine (p.1289·2).
Anorectal disorders.

UCB, USA.
Cream: Hydrocortisone acetate (p.1043·3).
Skin disorders.

Cortical Caber, Ital.
Diflucortolone valerate (p.1039·3).
Formerly contained suprarenal cortex.
Skin disorders.

Corticetine
Chauvin, Fr.; Novopharma, Switz.
Framycetin sulphate (p.210·3); dexamethasone sodium phosphate (p.1037·2).
Ear disorders.

Corti-Clyss Vifor Medical, Switz.
Prednisolone sodium metasulphobenzoate (p.1048·1).
Crohn's disease; ulcerative colitis.

Corticobiss Bissendorf, Neth.†.
Corticorelin triflutate (p.1244·1).
Diagnosis of Cushing's syndrome.

Corticoderm
Hermal, Norw.; Meda, Swed.
Fluprednidene acetate (p.1042·2).
Skin disorders.

Corticoderm comp Meda, Swed.†.
Fluprednidene acetate (p.1042·2); gentamicin sulphate (p.212·1).
Infected eczema.

Corticotherapique Mepha, Switz.†.
Triamcinolone acetonide (p.1050·2).
Skin disorders.

Corticotulle Lumiere
Solvay, Fr.; Hefa, Ger.
Neomycin sulphate (p.229·2); polymyxin B sulphate (p.239·1); triamcinolone acetonide (p.1050·2).
Burns; wounds.

Corticreme Rougier, Canad.
Hydrocortisone acetate (p.1043·3).
Skin disorders.

Corticyklin Nycomed, Norw.†.
Hydrocortisone acetate (p.1043·3); oxytetracycline hydrochloride (p.235·1).
Infected skin disorders.

Cortidene Berna, Spain.
Paramethasone acetate (p.1047·3).
Corticosteroid.

Cortidexason Dermapharm, Ger.
Dexamethasone (p.1037·1).
Skin and scalp disorders.

Cortidexason comp Dermapharm, Ger.
Dexamethasone (p.1037·1); neomycin sulphate (p.229·2).
Infected skin disorders.

Cortidexason-S Dorsch, Ger.†.
Dexamethasone (p.1037·1); salicylic acid (p.1090·2).
Skin disorders.

Cortidin Crinos, Ital.†.
Suprarenal cortex (p.1050·1).
Steroid deficiency.

Cortidro Salus, Ital.
Hydrocortisone acetate (p.1043·3).
Burns; skin disorders; wounds.

Corti-Dynexan Kreussler, Ger.
Prednisolone acetate (p.1048·1); laureth 9 (p.1325·2); dequalinium chloride (p.1112·1).
Inflammatory disorders of the mouth.

Cortiespec Centrum, Spain.
Fluocinolone acetonide (p.1041·1).
Skin disorders.

Cortifair Pharmafair, USA†.
Hydrocortisone (p.1043·3).

Corti-Flexiole
Mann, Ger.; Restan, S.Afr.†.
Hydrocortisone (p.1043·3); chloramphenicol (p.182·1); vitamin A palmitate (p.1359·2).
Eye, ear, and skin disorders.

Cortifluid N Streuli, Switz.
Calcium pantothenate (p.1352·3); hydrocortisone acetate (p.1043·3); neomycin sulphate (p.229·2).
Infected skin disorders.

Corti-Fluoral Schering, Ital.
Chloramphenicol (p.182·1); diflucortolone valerate (p.1039·3).
Mouth disorders.

Cortifoam
Reed & Carnrick, Canad.; Schwarz, USA.
Hydrocortisone acetate (p.1043·3).
Colitis; proctitis.

Cortifra Bouchara, Fr.†.
Prednisolone sodium metasulphobenzoate (p.1048·1); framycetin sulphate (p.210·3).
Nose disorders.

Cortigen B6 Lepetit, Ital.†.
Suprarenal cortex (p.1050·1); pyridoxine hydrochloride (p.1362·3).
Tonic; vomiting.

Cortiglanden Disperga, Aust.
Suprarenal cortex (p.1050·1).
Adrenocortical insufficiency; congenital adrenal hyperplasia.

Cortikinol Nycomed, Norw.†.
Hydrocortisone acetate (p.1043·3); chlorquinaldol (p.185·1).
Infected skin disorders.

Cortilen TC SIFI, Ital.†.
Hydrocortisone acetate (p.1043·3); tetracycline hydrochloride (p.259·1).
Eye disorders.

Cortiment Hoechst Marion Roussel, Canad.
Hydrocortisone acetate (p.1043·3).
Anorectal inflammatory disorders.

Cortimycine Syntex, Switz.
Cream: Hydrocortisone acetate (p.1043·3); neomycin sulphate (p.229·2); dexpanthenol (p.1570·3).
Infected skin disorders.
Ear drops; nose drops; eye drops; eye ointment; ointment: Hydrocortisone acetate (p.1043·3); neomycin sulphate (p.229·2).
Infected inflammatory disorders.

Cortimyk CCS, Swed.
Miconazole nitrate (p.384·3); hydrocortisone (p.1043·3).
Fungal skin infections with inflammation.

Cort-Inal Teofarma, Ital.
Hydrocortisone acetate (p.1043·3); diprophylline (p.752·1); sodium benzoate (p.1102·3).
Bronchial catarrh.

Cortine Naturelle Roche Nicholas, Fr.
Suprarenal cortex (porcine) (p.1050·1).
Asthenia.

Cortinorex Spyfarma, Spain.
Cyanocobalamin; suprarenal cortex; glutathione; liver extract; inosine.
Tonic.

Cortiphenol H Ciba Vision, Switz.†.
Chloramphenicol (p.182·1); hydrocortisone acetate (p.1043·3).
Infected eye disorders.

Cortiplastol Medici Domus, Ital.†.
Fluocinolone acetonide (p.1041·1).
Skin disorders.

Cortiplex Forte Lepetit, Ital.†.
Vitamin B substances; suprarenal cortex (p.1050·1); lignocaine (p.1293·2).

Corti-Refobacin Hermal, Ger.†.
Gentamicin sulphate (p.212·1); hydrocortisone (p.1043·3).
Burns; skin disorders.

Cortiron
Schering, Aust.; Schering, Ital.
Deoxycortone acetate (p.1036·2) or deoxycortone enanthate (p.1036·3).
Adrenocortical insufficiency; hypotension.

Cortisal Monin, Fr.
Propylene glycol mono- and disalicylate; prednisolone (p.1048·1).
Musculoskeletal and joint disorders; superficial thrombophlebitis.

Cortisdin Urea Isdin, Spain.
Fluorometholone (p.1042·1); urea (p.1095·2).
Skin disorders.

Cortisolone SIT, Ital.†.
Prednisolone (p.1048·1).
Oral corticosteroid.

Cortison Chemicet Topica Astra, Spain.
Chloramphenicol (p.182·1); hydrocortisone acetate (p.1043·3).
Infected skin disorders.

Cortison Chemicetina
Note. This name is used for preparations of different composition.
Fournier, Ital.
Chloramphenicol (p.182·1); hydrocortisone acetate (p.1043·3).
Infected eye or skin disorders.

Astra, Spain†.
Chloramphenicol (p.182·1); dexamethasone (p.1037·1); amethocaine hydrochloride (p.1285·2).
Infected external ear disorders.

Cortison Kemicetin Pharmacia Upjohn, Aust.
Chloramphenicol (p.182·1); hydrocortisone acetate (p.1043·3).
Bacterial eye infections; inflammation.

Cortisporin
Glaxo Wellcome, Canad.; Glaxo Wellcome, USA.
Ophthalmic suspension; otic solution; otic suspension: Polymyxin B sulphate (p.239·1); neomycin sulphate (p.229·2); hydrocortisone (p.1043·3).
Inflammatory conditions of the eye or ear with associated bacterial infection.

Glaxo Wellcome, Canad.; Glaxo Wellcome, USA.
Ointment; eye ointment: Polymyxin B sulphate (p.239·1); bacitracin zinc (p.157·3); neomycin sulphate (p.229·2); hydrocortisone (p.1043·3).
Inflammation with secondary bacterial infection.

Glaxo Wellcome, USA.
Cream: Polymyxin B sulphate (p.239·1); neomycin sulphate (p.229·2); hydrocortisone acetate (p.1043·3).
Infected skin disorders.

Cortisporin-TC Monarch, USA.
Colistin sulphate (p.195·3); neomycin sulphate (p.229·2); hydrocortisone acetate (p.1043·3); thonzonium bromide (p.1636·3).
Infected ear disorders.

Cortistab Knoll, UK†.
Cortisone acetate (p.1036·1).
Corticosteroid.

Cortisteron Streuli, Switz.
Deoxycortone acetate (p.1036·2).
Lignocaine hydrochloride (p.1293·2) is included in some injections to alleviate the pain of injection.
Adrenocortical insufficiency.

Cortisumman Winzer, Ger.
Dexamethasone (p.1037·1).
Eye disorders.

Cortisyl
Roussel, Irl.†; Roussel, UK.
Cortisone acetate (p.1036·1).
Corticosteroid.

Cortivel Ern, Spain.
Chloramphenicol (p.182·1); prednisolone sodium metasulphobenzoate (p.1048·1).
External ear or nasal disorders.

Cortizone Thompson, USA.
Hydrocortisone (p.1043·3).
Skin disorders.

Cortneo Ciba Vision, Fr.†.
Neomycin sulphate (p.229·2); hydrocortisone acetate (p.1043·3).
Eye disorders.

Cortoderm
Note. This name is used for preparations of different composition.
Taro, Canad.
Hydrocortisone (p.1043·3).
Skin disorders.

Lennon, S.Afr.
Fluocinolone acetonide (p.1041·1).
Skin disorders.

Cortoftal Cusi, Spain.
Clobetasone butyrate (p.1035·3).
Inflammatory eye disorders.

Cortogen Schering-Plough, S.Afr.
Cortisone acetate (p.1036·1).
Corticosteroid.

Cortone
Merck Sharp & Dohme, Aust.; Merck Sharp & Dohme, Canad.; Merck Sharp & Dohme, Ital.; Merck Sharp & Dohme, Norw.; Merck Sharp & Dohme, Swed.; Merck Sharp & Dohme, USA.
Cortisone acetate (p.1036·1).
Corticosteroid.

Cortopin Pinewood, Irl.
Hydrocortisone (p.1043·3).
Insect bites; skin disorders.

cortotact Feldhoff, Ger.†.
Calf heart extract; bovine testes extract (p.1464·1); bovine placenta extract.
Cardiac disorders.

Corto-Tavegil Sandoz, Ger.
Tablets: Clemastine fumarate (p.406·2); dexamethasone (p.1037·1).
Hypersensitivity reactions.
Topical gel: Clemastine fumarate (p.406·2); clocortolone pivalate (p.1035·3).
Insect stings; skin disorders; sunburn.

Cortril Pfizer, Belg.
Hydrocortisone (p.1043·3) or hydrocortisone acetate (p.1043·3).
Eye disorders; skin disorders.

Cortrosyn
Organon, Belg.†; Organon, Canad.; Organon, Ital.; Organon, Neth.†; Organon, USA.
Tetracosactrin (p.1261·3) or tetracosactrin hexa-acetate (p.1261·3).
Adrenocorticotrophic hormone; diagnosis of adrenocortical insufficiency.

Cortucid Nicholas, Irl.†.
Sulphacetamide sodium (p.252·2); hydrocortisone acetate (p.1043·3).
Eye inflammation.

Cor-Uvocal Stroschein, Ger.†.
Injection: Heart extract.
Cardiac disorders.
Tablets: Heart extract; potassium aspartate (p.1161·3); magnesium aspartate (p.1157·2).
Cardiac disorders; potassium and magnesium deficiency.

Corvasal
Note. This name is used for preparations of different composition.
Hoechst, Fr.
Injection: Linsidomine hydrochloride (p.898·2).
Angina pectoris; cardiac investigations; coronary arterial spasm.
Tablets: Molsidomine (p.912·2).
Angina pectoris.

Plantorgan, Ger.†.
Isosorbide mononitrate (p.893·3).
Cardiac disorders.

Corvaton
Therabel Pharma, Belg.; Hoechst, Ger.; Hoechst Marion Roussel, Switz.
Molsidomine (p.912·2).
Cardiac disorders.

Cor-Vel Truw, Ger.
Camphor (p.1557·2); menthol (p.1600·2); Norway spruce oil; rosemary oil (p.1626·2).
Cardiac disorders.

Cor-Vel N Truw, Ger.
Oral drops: Convallaria (p.1567·2); squill (p.1070·1).
Tablets: Convallaria (p.1567·2); crataegus (p.1568·2).
Heart failure.

Corvert
Pharmacia Upjohn, Neth.; Pharmacia Upjohn, Swed.; Pharmacia Upjohn, USA.
Ibutilide fumarate (p.890·1).
Arrhythmias.

Corvipas Pascoe, Ger.
Homoeopathic preparation.

Corwil Zeneca, Aust.
Xamoterol fumarate (p.970·1).
Heart failure.

Corwin
Zeneca, Belg.; Zeneca, UK.
Xamoterol fumarate (p.970·1).
Heart failure.

Coryfin C SIT, Ital.
Menglytate (p.1063·3); ascorbic acid (p.1365·2).
Coughs; hoarseness.

Coryphen Rougier, Canad.
Aspirin (p.16·1).

Coryretard-C Madaus, S.Afr.†.
Carbinoxamine maleate (p.404·2); phenylephrine hydrochloride (p.1066·2).
Allergic rhinitis.

Coryretard-S Ethimed, S.Afr.†.
Carbinoxamine (p.404·2); phenylpropanolamine (p.1067·2).
Cold symptoms.

Coryx Mirren, S.Afr.
Chlorpheniramine maleate (p.405·1); pseudoephedrine hydrochloride (p.1068·3); aspirin (p.16·1); ascorbic acid (p.1365·2).
Cold and influenza symptoms.

Coryzalia
Boiron, Canad.; Boiron, Fr.
Homoeopathic preparation.

Corzide
Squibb, Canad.; Bristol, USA.
Nadolol (p.913·2); bendrofluazide (p.827·3).
Hypertension.

Cosaar
Merck Sharp & Dohme, Aust.; Merck Sharp & Dohme, Switz.
Losartan potassium (p.899·1).
Hypertension.

Cosadon Hoechst, Fr.†.
Pentifylline (p.927·3); nicotinic acid (p.1351·2).
Mental function disorders in the elderly.

Cosaldon
Note. This name is used for preparations of different composition.
Albert-Roussel, Aust.; Hoechst Marion Roussel, S.Afr.
Pentifylline (p.927·3); nicotinic acid (p.1351·2).
Vascular disorders.

Albert-Roussel, Ger.; Hoechst, Ger.
Pentifylline (p.927·3).
Cerebrovascular insufficiency; vascular eye disorders; vestibular disorders.

Cosaldon A Albert-Roussel, Ger.; Hoechst, Ger.
Pentifylline (p.927·3); retinol palmitate (p.1359·2).
Vascular eye disorders; vestibular disorders.

Cosalgesic
Cox, Irl.; Cox, UK.
Dextropropoxyphene hydrochloride (p.27·3); paracetamol (p.72·2).
These ingredients can be described by the British Approved Name Co-proxamol.
Pain.

Cosavil Chinosolfabrik, Ger.†.
Phenazone salicylate (p.78·2); pheniramine maleate (p.415·3); caffeine (p.749·3).
Cold symptoms.

Coslan Parke, Davis, Spain.
Mefenamic acid (p.51·2).
Musculoskeletal, joint, and peri-articular disorders; pain.

Cosmegen
Merck Sharp & Dohme, Aust.; Merck Sharp & Dohme, Austral.; Merck Sharp & Dohme, Canad.; Merck Sharp & Dohme, Irl.; Merck Sharp & Dohme, Ital.; Merck Sharp & Dohme, Norw.; Merck Sharp & Dohme, S.Afr.; Merck Sharp & Dohme, Swed.; Merck Sharp & Dohme, Switz.; Merck Sharp & Dohme, UK; Merck Sharp & Dohme, USA.
Dactinomycin (p.527·2).
Malignant neoplasms.

Cosmetar-S Promedica, Fr.
Coal tar (Stantar) (p.1092·3).
Seborrhoeic dermatitis.

Cosmiciclina INTES, Ital.
Oxytetracycline hydrochloride (p.235·1); chloramphenicol (p.182·1); sulphacetamide sodium (p.252·2).
Bacterial infections of the eye or ear.

Cosmosin Lederle, Jpn†.
Cefuzonam sodium (p.178·1).
Bacterial infections.

Coso McGloin, Austral.
Menthol (p.1600·2); camphor (p.1557·2); benzyl alcohol (p.1103·3).
Herpes labialis.

Cosopt
Merck Sharp & Dohme, UK; Merck, USA.
Dorzolamide hydrochloride (p.862·3); timolol maleate (p.953·3).
Glaucoma; ocular hypertension.

Cospanon Eisai, Jpn.
Flopropione (p.1580·3).
Smooth muscle spasm.

CoSudafed Wellcome, Canad.†.
Pseudoephedrine hydrochloride (p.1068·3); codeine phosphate (p.26·1).
Coughs; nasal congestion.

CoSudafed Expectorant Wellcome, Canad.†.
Pseudoephedrine hydrochloride (p.1068·3); codeine phosphate (p.26·1); guaiphenesin (p.1061·3).
Coughs; nasal congestion.

Cosudex ICI, Austral.
Bicalutamide (p.507·2).
Prostatic cancer.

Cosuric DDSA Pharmaceuticals, UK.
Allopurinol (p.390·2).
Gout; hyperuricaemia.

Cosylan
Warner-Lambert, Norw.; Parke, Davis, Swed.
Ethylmorphine hydrochloride (p.36·1); cascara (p.1183·1); menthol (p.1600·2).
Coughs; respiratory-tract irritation.

Cotazym
Note. This name is used for preparations of different composition.
Organon, Canad.; Organon, USA.
Pancrelipase (p.1613·3).
Pancreatic enzyme deficiency.

Thiemann, Ger.
Pancreatin (p.1612·1).
Pancreatic enzyme deficiency.

Cotazym Forte Organon, Neth.†.
Pancreas; ox bile (p.1553·2).
Digestive disorders.

Cotazym S Forte Organon, Austral.
Pancrelipase (p.1613·3).
Pancreatic enzyme deficiency.

Cotenolol Mepha, Switz.
Atenolol (p.825·3); chlorthalidone (p.839·3).
Hypertension.

Cotenomel Clonmel, Irl.
Atenolol (p.825·3); chlorthalidone (p.839·3).
Hypertension.

Cotet Covan, S.Afr.
Capsules: Oxytetracycline hydrochloride (p.235·1); vitamin B substances.
Bacterial infections; protozoal infections.
Oral suspension†: Dioxytetracycline calcium (p.235·1).
Bacterial infections.

Cothera Wyeth, Ital.†.
Dimethoxanate hydrochloride (p.1058·3).
Coughs.

Cothera Compound Akromed, S.Afr.†.
Dimethoxanate hydrochloride (p.1058·3); isothipendyl hydrochloride (p.412·2); phenylephrine hydrochloride (p.1066·2); paracetamol (p.72·2); ammonium chloride (p.1055·2); sodium citrate (p.1153·2).
Coughs.

Cothilyne Haemacure, Canad.
Centella (p.1080·3).
Wounds.

Cotim Eu Rho, Ger.
Co-trimoxazole (p.196·3).
Bacterial infections.

Cotone Emostatico Boots Healthcare, Ital.; Farmatre, Ital.; Iema, Ital.; Morigi, Ital.; Nova Argentia, Ital.
Ferrous chloride (p.1339·3).
Haemorrhagic disorders.

Cotrane Sanofi Winthrop, Belg.
Dimethoxanate hydrochloride (p.1058·3).
Coughs.

Cotribene Merckle, Aust.
Co-trimoxazole (p.196·3).
Bacterial infections.

Cotridin Technilab, Canad.
Triprolidine hydrochloride (p.420·3); pseudoephedrine hydrochloride (p.1068·3); codeine phosphate (p.26·1).
Coughs.

Cotridin Expectorant Technilab, Canad.
Triprolidine hydrochloride (p.420·3); pseudoephedrine hydrochloride (p.1068·3); guaiphenesin (p.1061·3); codeine phosphate (p.26·1).
Coughs.

Cotrim
BASF, Ger.; Heumann, Ger.; CT, Ger.; Ratiopharm, Ger.; Spirig, Switz.; Lemmon, USA.
Co-trimoxazole (p.196·3).
Bacterial infections; Pneumocystis carinii pneumonia.

Cotrim Holsten Holsten, Ger.
Co-trimoxazole (p.196·3).
Bacterial infections.

Cotrimazol Lafon-Ratiopharm, Fr.
Co-trimoxazole (p.196·3).
Bacterial infections; Pneumocystis carinii pneumonia; toxoplasmosis.

Cotrim-basan Sagitta, Ger.†.
Co-trimoxazole (p.196·3).
Bacterial infections.

Cotrim-Diolan Engelhard, Ger.
Co-trimoxazole (p.196·3).
Bacterial infections; fungal mycetoma; paracoccidioidomycosis.

Cotrimel Clonmel, Irl.
Co-trimoxazole (p.196·3).
Bacterial infections.

Cotrim-Hefa Hefa, Ger.
Co-trimoxazole (p.196·3).
Bacterial and protozoal infections.

Cotrimhexal Hexal, Ger.
Co-trimoxazole (p.196·3).
Bacterial infections; protozoal infections.

Cotrimox-Wolff Wolff, Ger.
Co-trimoxazole (p.196·3).
Bacterial infections.

Cotrim-Puren Isis Puren, Ger.
Co-trimoxazole (p.196·3).
Bacterial infections; Pneumocystis carinii pneumonia.

Cotrim-Riker 3M, Ger.†.
Co-trimoxazole (p.196·3).
Bacterial infections.

Cotrimstada Stada, Ger.
Co-trimoxazole (p.196·3).
Bacterial infections.

Co-trim-Tablinen Sanorania, Ger.
Co-trimoxazole (p.196·3).
Bacterial infections; fungal mycetoma; paracoccidioidomycosis; Pneumocystis carinii pneumonia.

Cotrivan Zurich, S.Afr.†.
Co-trimoxazole (p.196·3).
Bacterial infections.

Co-Tuss V Rugby, USA.
Hydrocodone tartrate (p.43·1); guaiphenesin (p.1061·3).
Coughs.

Cotylbutazone Truxton, USA†.
Phenylbutazone (p.79·2).

Co-Tylenol
Johnson & Johnson, Aust.; Johnson & Johnson, Switz.†.
Paracetamol (p.72·2); carbinoxamine maleate (p.404·2); phenylephrine hydrochloride (p.1066·2).
Cold symptoms; sinusitis.

Cough & Cold Homeocan, Canad.
Homoeopathic preparation.

Cough & Cold L52 Homeocan, Canad.
Homoeopathic preparation.

Cough Drops
Note. This name is used for preparations of different composition.
Zee, Canad.
Menthol (p.1600·2).

Weleda, UK.
Archangelica root; cinnamon (p.1564·2); clove (p.1565·2); coriander (p.1567·3); lemon oil (p.1595·3); melissa leaf (p.1600·1); nutmeg (p.1609·2); cherry-laurel water.
Coughs.

Cough Elixir Weleda, UK.
Aniseed (p.1549·3); horehound (p.1063·3); marshmallow root (p.1546·3); thyme (p.1636·3); drosera; ipecacuanha root; pulsatilla.
Coughs.

Cough & Flu Syrup Technilab, Canad.
Pseudoephedrine hydrochloride (p.1068·3); dextromethorphan hydrobromide (p.1057·3); guaiphenesin (p.1061·3); paracetamol (p.72·2).

Cough Formula Comtrex Bristol-Myers Products, USA.
Paracetamol (p.72·2); pseudoephedrine hydrochloride (p.1068·3); guaiphenesin (p.1061·3); dextromethorphan hydrobromide (p.1057·3).
Coughs and cold symptoms.

Cough L64 Homeocan, Canad.
Homoeopathic preparation.

Cough N Cold Syrup Golden Pride, Canad.; Rawleigh, Canad.
Ephedrine hydrochloride (p.1059·3); guaiphenesin (p.1061·3); sodium citrate (p.1153·2).

Cough Relief Brauer, Austral.
Oral liquid: Anise oil (p.1550·1); althaea officinalis (p.1546·3); bryonia alba (p.1555·2); Iceland moss; echinacea angustifolia (p.1574·2); matricaria recutita (p.1561·2); thymus vulgaris (p.1636·3); urtica dioica (p.1642·3); aconitum nap.; coccus cacti; corallium rub.; drosera; ipecacuanha; kali bich.; kreosotum; spongia tosta; sticta pulm.
Coughs.
Oral spray: Homoeopathic preparation.

Cough Suppressant Syrup DM Drug Trading, Canad.
Dextromethorphan hydrobromide (p.1057·3).

Cough Syrup
Note. This name is used for preparations of different composition.
Marc-O, Canad.
Dextromethorphan hydrobromide (p.1057·3).

Stanley, Canad.
Pseudoephedrine hydrochloride (p.1068·3); codeine phosphate (p.26·1); guaiphenesin (p.1061·3).

Technilab, Canad.
Diphenhydramine hydrochloride (p.409·1); codeine phosphate (p.26·1); ammonium chloride (p.1055·2).

Goldline, USA.
Phenylephrine hydrochloride (p.1066·2); dextromethorphan hydrobromide (p.1057·3); guaiphenesin (p.1061·3).
Coughs.

Cough Syrup with Codeine Stanley, Canad.
Diphenhydramine hydrochloride (p.409·1); codeine phosphate (p.26·1); ammonium chloride (p.1055·2).

Cough Syrup DM Stanley, Canad.; WestCan, Canad.
Dextromethorphan hydrobromide (p.1057·3).

Cough Syrup DM Decongestant WestCan, Canad.
Dextromethorphan hydrobromide (p.1057·3); pseudoephedrine hydrochloride (p.1068·3).

Cough Syrup DM Decongestant for Children Stanley, Canad.
Dextromethorphan hydrobromide (p.1057·3); pseudoephedrine hydrochloride (p.1068·3).

Cough Syrup DM Decongestant Expectorant Stanley, Canad.
Dextromethorphan hydrobromide (p.1057·3); pseudoephedrine hydrochloride (p.1068·3); guaiphenesin (p.1061·3).

Cough Syrup DM Expectorant Stanley, Canad.
Dextromethorphan hydrobromide (p.1057·3); guaiphenesin (p.1061·3).

Cough Syrup DM-D-E WestCan, Canad.
Dextromethorphan hydrobromide (p.1057·3); pseudoephedrine hydrochloride (p.1068·3); guaiphenesin (p.1061·3).

Cough Syrup DM-E WestCan, Canad.
Dextromethorphan hydrobromide (p.1057·3); guaiphenesin (p.1061·3).

Cough Syrup Expectorant Stanley, Canad.
Guaiphenesin (p.1061·3).

Cough Syrup with Guaifenesin Tanta, Canad.
Dextromethorphan hydrobromide (p.1057·3); guaiphenesin (p.1061·3).

Cough Syrup with Honey Hylands, Canad.
Homoeopathic preparation.

Coughcod Compu, S.Afr.
Ephedrine hydrochloride (p.1059·3); ammonium chloride (p.1055·2); sodium citrate (p.1153·2); codeine phosphate (p.26·1); mepyramine maleate (p.414·1).
Coughs.

Cough-eeze English Grains, UK.
Ipecacuanha (p.1062·2); marrubium (p.1063·3); inula (p.1059·2).
Coughs.

Cough-X Ascher, USA.
Dextromethorphan hydrobromide (p.1057·3); benzocaine (p.1286·2).
Coughs.

Couldina Alter, Spain.
Aspirin (p.16·1); chlorpheniramine maleate (p.405·1); phenylephrine hydrochloride (p.1066·2).
Formerly contained aspirin, ascorbic acid, chlorpheniramine maleate, phenylephrine hydrochloride, and moroxydine hydrochloride.
Influenza and cold symptoms.

Couldina C Alter, Spain.
Aspirin (p.16·1); ascorbic acid (p.1365·2); chlorpheniramine maleate (p.405·1); phenylephrine hydrochloride (p.1066·2).
Fever; influenza and cold symptoms; pain.

Couldina Instant Alter, Spain.
Aspirin (p.16·1); chlorpheniramine maleate (p.405·1); ascorbic acid (p.1365·2).
Fever; influenza and cold symptoms; pain.

Coumadin
Boots, Austral.; Du Pont, Canad.; Du Pont, Ger.; Du Pont, Ital.; Boots, S.Afr.†; Du Pont, USA.
Warfarin sodium (p.964·2).
Thrombo-embolic disorders.

Coumadine Du Pont, Fr.
Warfarin sodium (p.964·2).
Thrombo-embolic disorders.

Counterpain Bristol-Myers Squibb, S.Afr.
Eugenol (p.1578·2); menthol (p.1600·2); methyl salicylate (p.55·2).
Musculoskeletal pain.

Covamet Covan, S.Afr.
Cyclizine hydrochloride (p.407·1).
Nausea; vestibular disorders; vomiting.

Covancaine Covan, S.Afr.
Phenazone (p.78·2); urea (p.1095·2); sulphacetamide sodium (p.252·2); benzocaine (p.1286·2).
Ear pain; otitis media.

Covangesic Wallace, USA.
Phenylpropanolamine hydrochloride (p.1067·2); phenylephrine hydrochloride (p.1066·2); chlorpheniramine maleate (p.405·1); mepyramine maleate (p.414·1); paracetamol (p.72·2).
Upper respiratory-tract symptoms.

Covatine Bailly, Fr.
Captodiame hydrochloride (p.645·2).
Anxiety.

Covera Searle, USA.
Verapamil hydrochloride (p.960·3).
Hypertension.

Covermark Cupharma, UK.
A covering cream.
Concealment of birth marks, scars, and disfiguring skin disease.

Coversum
Servier, Aust.; Servier, Ger.; Servier, Switz.
Perindopril erbumine (p.928·2).
Heart failure; hypertension.

Coversyl
Servier, Austral.; Servier, Belg.; Servier, Canad.; Servier, Fr.; Servier, Irl.; Servier, Ital.; Servier, Neth.; Servier, S.Afr.; Servier, Spain; Servier, UK.
Perindopril erbumine (p.928·2).
Heart failure; hypertension.

Covitasa B12 Seid, Spain.
Cyproheptadine hydrochloride (p.407·2); cobamamide (p.1364·2).
Tonic.

Covite Covan, S.Afr.
Haematoporphyrin; liver extracts; caffeine; yeast.
Tonic.

Covitol Drug Houses Austral., Austral.†.
Cod-liver oil (p.1337·3); zinc oxide (p.1096·2).
Burns; chilblains; skin disorders; wounds.

Covochol Covan, S.Afr.
Acetylcholine chloride (p.1389·1).
Production of miosis in eye surgery.

Covocort Covan, S.Afr.
Hydrocortisone (p.1043·3).
Corticosteroid.

Covomycin Covan, S.Afr.
Chloramphenicol (p.182·1); neomycin sulphate (p.229·2); naphazoline hydrochloride (p.1064·2).
Eye, ear, and nose infections.

Covomycin-D Covan, S.Afr.
Chloramphenicol (p.182·1); neomycin sulphate (p.229·2); dexamethasone sodium phosphate (p.1037·2).
Inflammatory eye and ear infections.

Covonia Bronchial Balsam Thornton & Ross, UK.
Dextromethorphan hydrobromide (p.1057·3); menthol (p.1600·2); cineole (p.1564·1).
Formerly contained dextromethorphan hydrobromide, guaiphenesin, menthol, and cineole.
Coughs.

Covonia for Children Thornton & Ross, UK.
Dextromethorphan hydrobromide (p.1057·3).
Coughs.

Covosan Covan, S.Afr.
Naphazoline hydrochloride (p.1064·2); antazoline phosphate (p.401·3); sulphacetamide sodium (p.252·2).
Conjunctivitis.

Covospor Covan, S.Afr.
Clotrimazole (p.376·3).
Fungal infections.

Covostet Covan, S.Afr.
Amethocaine hydrochloride (p.1285·2).
Local anaesthesia.

Covosulf Covan, S.Afr.
Sulphacetamide sodium (p.252·2).
Eye infections.

Covotop Covan, S.Afr.
Chloramphenicol (p.182·1); benzocaine (p.1286·2).
Ear infections.

Coxa -cyl Ho-Len-Complex Liebermann, Ger.
Homoeopathic preparation.

Coxanturenasi Teofarma, Ital.
Pyridoxine hydrochloride (p.1362·3); pyridoxal phosphate (p.1363·1).
Lignocaine hydrochloride (p.1293·2) is included in the intramuscular injection to alleviate the pain of injection.
Vitamin B_6 and its co-enzyme deficiency.

Cozaar
Merck Sharp & Dohme, Austral.; Merck Sharp & Dohme, Belg.; Merck Sharp & Dohme, Canad.; Merck Sharp & Dohme-Chibret, Fr.; Merck Sharp & Dohme, Irl.; Merck Sharp & Dohme, Neth.; Merck Sharp & Dohme, Norw.; Merck Sharp & Dohme, S.Afr.; Merck Sharp & Dohme, Spain; Merck Sharp & Dohme, Swed.; Merck Sharp & Dohme, UK; Merck, USA.
Losartan potassium (p.899·1).
Hypertension.

Cozaar Comp *Merck Sharp & Dohme, Norw.; Merck Sharp & Dohme, S.Afr.; Merck Sharp & Dohme, UK.*
Losartan potassium (p.899·1); hydrochlorothiazide (p.885·2).
Hypertension.

Cozole *Be-Tabs, S.Afr.*
Co-trimoxazole (p.196·3).
Bacterial infections.

C-Plus *Gentili, Ital.†.*
Ascorbic acid (p.1365·2); troxerutin (p.1580·2); calcium carbonate (p.1182·1).
Vitamin C deficiency.

CPS Pulver *Gry, Ger.*
Calcium polystyrene sulphonate (p.974·3).
Hyperkalaemia.

Cracoa B *Neusc, Spain.*
Aluminium hydroxide (p.1177·3); calcium carbonate (p.1182·1); magnesium carbonate (p.1198·1); magnesium trisilicate (p.1199·1).
Gastro-intestinal hyperacidity.

Cradocap
Napp, Irl.†; Napp, UK.
Cetrimide (p.1105·2).
Cradle cap.

Craegium *Biocur, Ger.*
Crataegus (p.1568·2).
Bradycardia; heart failure.

Crafilm *Francia, Ital.*
Sucralfate (p.1214·2).
Gastro-intestinal disorders associated with hyperacidity.

Cralonin *Heel, Ger.*
Homoeopathic preparation.

Cralsanic *Hexal, S.Afr.*
Sucralfate (p.1214·2).
Peptic ulcer.

Cramp End *Ohm, USA†.*
Ibuprofen (p.44·1).

Crampex *Seton, UK.*
Calcium gluconate (p.1155·2); nicotinic acid (p.1351·2); ergocalciferol (p.1367·1).
Night cramps.

Cranio -cyl Ho-Len-Complex *Liebermann, Ger.*
Homoeopathic preparation.

Cranoc *Astra, Ger.; Promed, Ger.*
Fluvastatin sodium (p.1273·2).
Hyperlipidaemias.

Crasnitin
Bayer, Ger.†; Bayer, Ital.; Bayer, Neth.†.
Asparaginase (p.504·3).
Leukaemias; non-Hodgkin's lymphoma.

Crasnitine *Bayer, Switz.†.*
Asparaginase (p.504·3).
Leukaemias; non-Hodgkin's lymphoma.

Crataegan *Asta Medica, Aust.*
Crataegus (p.1568·2).
Cardiac disorders.

Crataegisan N *Bioforce, Switz.*
Crataegus (p.1568·2).
Cardiac disorders.

Crataegitan *Amino, Switz.*
Crataegus (p.1568·2).
Cardiac disorders.

Crataegol *LDM, Fr.*
Crataegus (p.1568·2).
Insomnia; nervous disorders.

Crataegus Complex *Blackmores, Austral.*
Tilia platyphyllos (p.1637·3); achillea (p.1542·2); crataegus (p.1568·2); garlic (p.1583·1); ascorbic acid (p.1365·2); hesperidin (p.1580·2); rutin (p.1580·2).
Cardiovascular disorders.

Crataegus Med Complex *Dynamit, Aust.*
Homoeopathic preparation.

Crataegutt
Austroplant, Aust.; Schwabe, Ger.; Schwabe, Neth.†; Semar, Spain.
Crataegus (p.1568·2).
Cardiac disorders.

Crataegutt-Strophanthin *Schwabe, Ger.†.*
Ouabain (p.925·2); crataegus (p.1568·2).

Crataegysat *Ysatfabrik, Ger.*
Crataegus (p.1568·2).
Cardiac disorders.

Crataelanat *Schwabe, Ger.*
Digoxin (p.849·3); crataegus (p.1568·2).
Heart failure.

Crataepas *Pascoe, Ger.*
Crataegus (p.1568·2).
Cardiac disorders.

Crataesan *Henk, Ger.†.*
Crataegus (p.1568·2).
Cardiac disorders.

Crataezyma *Zyma, Ger.*
Crataegus (p.1568·2).
Cardiac disorders.

Crataezyma N *Zyma, Ger.†.*
Crataegus (p.1568·2); leonurus cardiaca (p.1604·2).
Cardiac disorders.

Cratamed novo *Redel, Ger.*
Crataegus (p.1568·2).
Cardiac disorders.

Cratecor *Bionorica, Ger.*
Crataegus (p.1568·2).
Heart failure.

Cratylen *Madaus, Ger.†.*
Crataegus (p.1568·2); rutin sodium sulphate (p.1580·2); potassium fluoride; copper chloride; manganese sulphate monohydrate; cobalt chloride.
Cardiac disorders.

Craviscum *CPF, Ger.†.*
Crataegus (p.1568·2); mistletoe (p.1604·1).
Cardiovascular disorders.

Craviscum mono *CPF, Ger.*
Crataegus (p.1568·2).
Cardiac disorders.

Cravit *Daiichi, Jpn.*
Levofloxacin (p.221·2).
Bacterial infections.

Creacal *Prodes, Spain.*
Calcium phosphate (p.1155·3); cholecalciferol (p.1366·3).
Calcium deficiency.

Creamy Tar *C & M, USA.*
Coal tar (p.1092·3).
Scalp disorders.

Creanol *Helsinn Birex, Irl.†.*
Propranolol (p.937·2).
Angina pectoris; anxiety; arrhythmias; hypertension; myocardial infarction.

Creanolona *Bohm, Spain.*
Fluocinolone acetonide (p.1041·1); neomycin (p.229·2); polymyxin B (p.239·3).
Skin infections with inflammation.

Creatergyl *Midy, Ital.†.*
Fosfocreatinine sodium (p.1581·3).
Striated muscle disorders.

Creatile *New Farma, Ital.*
Creatine (p.1568·3).
Nutritional supplement.

Creatyl *Volchem, Ital.*
Amino-acid preparation or amino-acid and carbohydrate preparation.
Nutritional supplement.

Creci Baby *Wasserman, Spain†.*
Vitamin B substances; muramidase; amino acids.
Tonic.

Crecisan *Fides, Spain†.*
Minoxidil (p.910·3).
Alopecia.

Crema Anitallergica Antipruriginosa *Dynacren, Ital.†.*
Promethazine (p.416·2).
Hypersensitivity reactions; insect bites; skin irritation.

Crema Antisolar Evanesce *Perez Gimenez, Spain†.*
Almond oil (p.1546·2); phenazone (p.78·2); glycerol.
Skin disorders.

Crema Contracepti Lanzas *Lanzas, Spain.*
Benzalkonium chloride (p.1101·3).
Contraceptive.

Crema de Magnesia *Cinfa, Spain.*
Magnesium hydroxide (p.1198·2).
Constipation; gastro-intestinal hyperacidity.

Crema Glaan *Madaus, Spain†.*
Human placental extract.
Burns; skin disorders; wounds.

Crema Glaan Corticoide *Madaus, Spain†.*
Human placental extract; triamcinolone acetonide (p.1050·2); calendula.
Skin disorders.

Crema Grasa *Genove, Spain†.*
Cholesterol; salicylic acid (p.1090·2); borax.
Skin disorders.

Crema Neutra *Genove, Spain†.*
Stearylsulfamide (p.249·2); cetyl alcohol; cholesterol; spermaceti; glycerol; salicylic acid (p.1090·2).
Skin disorders.

Crema Protettiva *Guigoz, Ital.†.*
Wheat-germ oil; zinc oxide (p.1096·2); magnesium silicate (p.1473·3).
Barrier preparation.

Crema Transcutan Astier *Semar, Spain†.*
Hydrocortisone acetate (p.1043·3).
Skin disorders.

Cremalgin
Berk, Irl.†; Co-Pharma, UK.
Methyl nicotinate (p.55·1); glycol salicylate (p.43·1); capsicum oleoresin.
Muscle and joint pain.

Creme antikeloides *Widmer, Switz.*
Dexamethasone (p.1037·1); urea (p.1095·2); vitamin A palmitate (p.1359·2).
Scars.

Creme Anti-Rides Auto-Bronzante *Clarins, Canad.*
SPF 15: Ethylhexyl *p*-methoxycinnamate (p.1487·1); oxybenzone (p.1487·3); titanium dioxide (p.1093·3).
Sunscreen.

Creme Autobronzante Visage *Lancome, Canad.*
Avobenzone (p.1486·3); 3-(4-methylbenzylidene)bornan-2-one (p.1487·2).
Sunscreen.

Creme bij Wondjes *SAN, Neth.†.*
Pramoxine hydrochloride (p.1298·2); hydroxyquinoline (p.1589·3); lauryldimethyl benzylammoniumbromide.
Skin disorders.

Creme Carbamide *Widmer, Switz.*
Urea (p.1095·2); vitamin A palmitate (p.1359·2); dexpanthenol (p.1570·3).
Skin disorders.

Creme Carbamide + VAS *Widmer, Switz.*
Tretinoin (p.1093·3); urea (p.1095·2); dexpanthenol (p.1570·3).
Skin disorders.

Creme de base *Glaxo Wellcome, Switz.*
Emollient.
Skin disorders.

Creme des 3 Fleurs d'Orient *Creme d'Orient, Fr.*
Cream: Hydroquinone (p.1083·1).
Ointment: Mequinol (p.1086·2).
Hyperpigmentation.

Creme Domistan a la vitamine F *Therval, Fr.†.*
Histapyrrodine (p.411·3); ethyl isolinoleate.
Pruritic skin disorders.

Creme Ecran Total *Lancome, Canad.*
SPF 25: Avobenzone (p.1486·3); 3-(4-methylbenzylidene)bornan-2-one (p.1487·2); terephthalylidene dicamphor sulphonic acid; titanium dioxide (p.1093·3).
Sunscreen.

Creme Haute Protection *Vichy, Canad.*
SPF 15: Avobenzone (p.1486·3); 3-(4-methylbenzylidene)bornan-2-one (p.1487·2); terephthalylidene dicamphor sulphonic acid; titanium dioxide (p.1093·3).
Sunscreen.

Creme Protectrice *Lancome, Canad.*
SPF 15: Avobenzone (p.1486·3); 3-(4-methylbenzylidene)bornan-2-one (p.1487·2); terephthalylidene dicamphor sulphonic acid; titanium dioxide (p.1093·3).
Sunscreen.

Creme Rap *Monal, Fr.*
Scoparium (p.1628·1); arnica (p.1550·3); aconite root (p.1542·2); aesculus (p.1543·3); cigue; hyoscyamus (p.464·3); nux vomica (p.1609·3).
Circulatory disorders; musculoskeletal and joint disorders.

Creme Solaire Anti-Rides *Clarins, Canad.*
SPF 10: Ethylhexyl *p*-methoxycinnamate (p.1487·1); oxybenzone (p.1487·3); titanium dioxide (p.1093·3).
Sunscreen.

Creme Solaire Bronzage *Clarins, Canad.*
SPF 15: Ethylhexyl *p*-methoxycinnamate (p.1487·1); oxybenzone (p.1487·3); titanium dioxide (p.1093·3).
Sunscreen.

Cremes Tegen Spierpijn *SAN, Neth.†.*
Methyl nicotinate (p.55·1); histamine dihydrochloride (p.1587·3); glycol salicylate (p.43·1); capsaicin (p.24·2).
Muscle and joint pain.

Cremicort-H *Chefaro, Belg.*
Hydrocortisone (p.1043·3).
Skin disorders.

Cremol *Max Ritter, Switz.*
Bath additive.
Lotion: Emollient.
Soap substitute.
Skin disorders.

Cremol-P *Max Ritter, Switz.*
Evening primrose oil (p.1582·1).
Dry skin.

Cremor Menthol *Prosana, Austral.†.*
Methyl salicylate (p.55·2); menthol (p.1600·2); camphor (p.1557·2); eucalyptus oil (p.1578·1).
Pruritus; topical analgesic.

Cremsol *Quimifar, Spain.*
Linseed oil; calcium hydroxide (p.1556·3); benzocaine (p.1286·2); sulphathiazole (p.257·1); triamcinolone acetonide (p.1050·2); zinc oxide (p.1096·2).
Infected skin disorders.

Crenodyn *Francia, Ital.*
Cefadroxil (p.163·3).
Bacterial infections.

Creo Grippe *Marc-O, Canad.*
Camphor (p.1557·2); cineole (p.1564·1); guaiphenesin (p.1061·3).

Creolina *Pearson, Ital.*
Cresol (p.1111·2).
Surface disinfection.

Creon
Solvay, Belg.; Solvay, Canad.; Solvay, Fr.; Solvay, Irl.; Solvay, Ital.; Solvay, Neth.; Solvay, S.Afr.; Solvay, Switz.; Solvay, UK; Solvay, USA.
Pancreatin (p.1612·1).
Cystic fibrosis; pancreatic insufficiency.

Creo-Rectal *Nadeau, Canad.*
Diphenylpyraline hydrochloride (p.409·3); guaiacol carbonate (p.1061·2); camphor (p.1557·2).
Coughs.

Creosolactol Adulti *Sempio, Ital.†.*
Calcium glycerophosphate (p.1155·2); lactic acid (p.1593·3); codeine phosphate (p.26·1); aconite (p.1542·2); creosote (p.1057·3); cherry-laurel.
Coughs.

Creosolactol Bambini *Sempio, Ital.†.*
Calcium glycerophosphate (p.1155·2); lactic acid (p.1593·3); sodium benzoate (p.1102·3); sodium salicylate (p.85·1); potassium guaiacolsulfonate (p.1068·3); cherry-laurel; tolu balsam (p.1071·1); creosote carbonate (p.1057·3).
Coughs.

Creo-Terpin *Lee, USA.*
Dextromethorphan hydrobromide (p.1057·3).

Crescom *Esoform, Ital.*
Sodium *o*-phenylphenol (p.1120·3).
Surface disinfection.

Cresolox *Coventry, UK.*
Tar acids (p.1126·2).

Cresophene
Note. This name is used for preparations of different composition.
Prats, Spain.
Dexamethasone (p.1037·1); hexachlorophane (p.1115·2); prajmalium bitartrate (p.932·2); parachlorophenol (p.1120·3).
Dental caries; oral disinfection.

Septodont, Switz.
Dexamethasone acetate (p.1037·1); thymol (p.1127·1); parachlorophenol (p.1120·3); camphor (p.1557·2).
Root canal infections.

Cresylate *Recsei, USA.*
m-Cresyl acetate (p.1111·2); isopropyl alcohol (p.1118·2).
Ear infection.

CRH
Ferring, Ger.; Ferring, Neth.
Corticorelin (p.1244·1) or corticorelin trifluoroacetate (p.1244·1).
Diagnosis of adrenal disorders.

Crimanex *Drossapharm, Switz.*
Scalp application†: Dipyrithione (p.1081·3); undecenoic acid polyethanolamide (p.389·2).
Shampoo: Dipyrithione (p.1081·3); undecenoic acid diethanolamide (p.389·2).
Scalp disorders.

Crinex *Crinex, Fr.†.*
Ovarian extract (porcine) (p.1458·2).
Menopausal disorders; menstrual disorders.

Criniton
Richter, Aust.; Atzinger, Ger.
Thymol (p.1127·1); salicylic acid (p.1090·2); rosemary oil (p.1626·2).
Scalp disorders.

Crino Cordes *Ichthyol, Aust.*
Sodium bituminosulphonate (p.1083·3); sodium sulphosuccinated undecenoic acid monoethanolamide (p.389·2).
Scalp disorders.

Crino Cordes N *Ichthyol, Ger.*
Ictasol (p.1083·3).
Scalp disorders; skin disorders.

Crinocedin *Wolfer, Ger.†.*
Urtica (p.1642·3); rosemary oil (p.1626·2); calcium pantothenate (p.1352·3).
Hair tonic.

Crinohermal
Hermal, Ger.†.
Salicylic acid (p.1090·2); resorcinol (p.1090·1); light ammonium bituminosulphonate (p.1083·3).
Scalp disorders.

Hermal, Switz.†.
Salicylic acid (p.1090·2); resorcinol (p.1090·1); ichthammol (p.1083·3).
Alopecia; scalp disorders.

Crinohermal FEM *Hermal, Switz.†.*
Fluprednidene acetate (p.1042·2); dienoestrol diacetate (p.1444·1); ichthammol (p.1083·3).
Alopecia; scalp disorders.

Crinohermal fem neu *Hermal, Ger.*
Fluprednidene acetate (p.1042·2); oestradiol (p.1455·1).
Female hair loss.

Crinohermal P
Hermal, Ger.†.
Salicylic acid (p.1090·2); resorcinol (p.1090·1); light ammonium bituminosulphonate (p.1083·3); prednisolone (p.1048·1).
Scalp disorders.

Hermal, Switz.†.
Salicylic acid (p.1090·2); resorcinol (p.1090·1); ichthammol (p.1083·3); prednisolone (p.1048·1).
Alopecia; scalp disorders.

Crino-Kaban N *Asche, Ger.*
Clocortolone pivalate (p.1035·3); salicylic acid (p.1090·2).
Scalp disorders.

Crinone
Wyeth, UK; Wyeth-Ayerst, USA.
Progesterone (p.1459·3).
Female infertility; menopausal disorders.

Crinopex *Schering-Plough, Swed.*
Pyrethrin (p.1410·1); piperonyl butoxide (p.1409·3).
Pediculosis.

Crinopex-N *Boehringer Ingelheim, Neth.*
Pyrethrum (p.1410·1); piperonyl butoxide (p.1409·3).
Pediculosis.

Crinoren *Uriach, Spain.*
Enalapril maleate (p.863·2).
Heart failure; hypertension.

Crinoretic *Uriach, Spain.*
Enalapril maleate (p.863·2); hydrochlorothiazide (p.885·2).
Hypertension.

Crinotar *Agpharm, Switz.*
Pyrithione zinc (p.1089·3); coal tar (p.1092·3).
Scalp disorders.

Criostat SD 2 *Grifols, Spain.*
Factor VIII (p.720·3).
Factor VIII deficiency.

Crisinor *Rubio, Spain.*
Auranofin (p.19·3).
Rheumatoid arthritis.

Crislaxo *Quimifar, Spain.*
Aloes (p.1177·1); aniseed (p.1549·3); cascara (p.1183·1); senna (p.1212·2); fennel (p.1579·1); rhu-

barb (p.1212·1); sulphur (p.1091·2); belladonna (p.457·1).
Constipation.

Crismol Funk, Spain.
Fenoterol hydrobromide (p.753·2); ipratropium bromide (p.754·2).
Obstructive airways disease.

Crisofin Allergan, Ital.†.
Auranofin (p.19·3).
Rheumatoid arthritis.

Crisolax Italfarmaco, Ital.†.
Phenolphthalein (p.1208·2); rhubarb (p.1212·1); cascara (p.1183·1); cinchona bark (p.1564·1); frangula (p.1193·2); aloes (p.1177·1).
Constipation; gastro-intestinal disorders.

Cristal
Note. This name is used for preparations of different composition.
Pfizer, Ital.
Multivitamin preparation.

Vifor, Switz.
Glycerol (p.1585·2).
Constipation.

Cristalcrom Cinfa, Spain.
Chlorhexidine gluconate (p.1107·2).
Skin and wound disinfection.

Cristalmina Salvat, Spain.
Chlorhexidine gluconate (p.1107·2).
Skin disinfection.

Cristanyl Biogalenique, Fr.†.
Raubasine (p.941·3); dihydroergocristine mesylate (p.1571·3).
Cerebrovascular disorders.

Cristopal Alcon, Fr.
Calcium chloride (p.1155·1); sodium iodide (p.1493·2); glycine (p.1345·2).
Lens opacities.

Criticare HN
Mead Johnson, Austral.; Mead Johnson, Canad.†; Mead Johnson Nutritionals, USA.
Lactose-free preparation for enteral nutrition.

Critichol Angelini, Ital.
Fenipentol hemisuccinate (p.1579·1); cascara (p.1183·1); boldo (p.1554·1); rhubarb (p.1212·1).
Constipation.

Critifib Boots, Austral.†.
Bretylium tosylate (p.833·2).
Arrhythmias.

Crixivan
Merck Sharp & Dohme, Austral.; Merck Sharp & Dohme, Belg.; Merck Frosst, Canad.; Merck Sharp & Dohme, Ger.; Merck Sharp & Dohme, Irl.; Merck Sharp & Dohme, Ital.; Merck Sharp & Dohme, Neth.; Merck Sharp & Dohme, S.Afr.; Merck Sharp & Dohme, Spain; Merck Sharp & Dohme, Swed.; Merck Sharp & Dohme, Switz.; Merck Sharp & Dohme, UK; Merck, USA.
Indinavir sulphate (p.614·1).
HIV infection.

Crodamols Croda, UK.
A range of emollient esters.

Crolom Bausch & Lomb, USA.
Sodium cromoglycate (p.762·1).
Inflammatory disorders of the eye.

Cromacort Medosan, Ital.†.
Vitamin B substances; suprarenal cortex (p.1050·1); lignocaine hydrochloride (p.1293·2).
Tonic.

Cromal Mundipharma, Aust.
Sodium cromoglycate (p.762·1).
Obstructive airways disease.

Cromantal NCSN, Ital.
Disodium cromoglycate (p.762·1).
Hypersensitivity reactions.

Cro-Man-Zin Freeda, USA.
Chromium, manganese, and zinc preparation.
Mineral supplement.

Cromaton Menarini, Belg.
Liver extract; suprarenal cortex extract (p.1050·1).
Tonic.

Cromaton Cortex Menarini, Spain†.
Cyanocobalamin (p.1363·3); suprarenal cortex extract (p.1050·1); liver extract.
Lignocaine hydrochloride (p.1293·2) is included in this preparation to alleviate the pain of injection.
Hepatic insufficiency; tonic; vitamin B_{12} deficiency.

Cromatonbic 5000 Menarini, Spain†.
Calcium folinate (p.1342·2); cyanocobalamin (p.1363·3).
Anaemias; tonic.

Cromatonbic B12 Menarini, Spain.
Cyanocobalamin (p.1363·3).
Vitamin B12 deficiency.

Cromatonbic Ferro Menarini, Spain.
Ferrous lactate (p.1340·1).
Formerly contained calcium folinate, ferric ammonium citrate and cyanocobalamin.
Anaemias.

Cromatonbic 5000 Ferro Menarini, Spain†.
Ferrocholinate (p.1339·2); calcium folinate (p.1342·2); cyanocobalamin (p.1363·3).
Anaemias.

Cromatonbic Folinico Menarini, Spain.
Calcium folinate (p.1342·2).
Folic acid deficiency; megaloblastic anaemia.

Cromatonferro Menarini, Ital.
Ferrous gluconate (p.1340·1).
Anaemias; iron deficiency.

Cromedil Europhta, Mon.
Sodium cromoglycate (p.762·1).
Allergic eye disorders.

Cromene Scharper, Ital.†.
Chromonar hydrochloride (p.840·1).
Cardiac disorders.

Cromer Orto Normon, Spain.
Mercurochrome (p.1119·2).
Skin disinfection.

Cromex Herdel, Ital.†.
Cobamamide (p.1364·2); suprarenal cortex (p.1050·1).
Tonic.

Cromeze Pharmacia Upjohn, Austral.
Sodium cromoglycate (p.762·1).
Asthma.

Cromezin SoSe, Ital.
Cephazolin sodium (p.181·1).
Bacterial infections.

Cromo Ratiopharm, Ger.; CT, Ger.
Sodium cromoglycate (p.762·1).
Allergic rhinitis; asthma; eye disorders; food hypersensitivity; hay fever.

Cromo Asma Aldo, Spain.
Sodium cromoglycate (p.762·1).
Allergic rhinitis; asthma.

Cromo Pur CT, Ger.
Sodium cromoglycate (p.762·1).
Allergic rhinitis.

Cromocur Tipomark, Ital.†.
Mercurochrome (p.1119·2).
Wound disinfection.

Cromodyn Rappai, Switz.
Sodium cromoglycate (p.762·1).
Allergic rhinitis.

Cromoftol Merck Sharp & Dohme, Spain.
Chlorpheniramine maleate (p.405·1); sodium cromoglycate (p.762·1).
Eye disorders.

Cromogen
Norton Waterford, Irl.; Norton, S.Afr.; Norton, UK.
Sodium cromoglycate (p.762·1).
Asthma.

Cromoglicin Heumann, Ger.
Sodium cromoglycate (p.762·1).
Allergic conjunctivitis; allergic rhinitis; asthma.

Cromoglicin-ratiopharm Ratiopharm, Ger.†.
Sodium cromoglycate (p.762·1).
Allergic rhinitis; asthma.

Cromoglin Merckle, Aust.
Sodium cromoglycate (p.762·1).
Allergic eye disorders; obstructive airways disease; rhinitis.

Cromohexal
Hexal, Ger.; Hexal, S.Afr.
Sodium cromoglycate (p.762·1).
Allergic conjunctivitis; allergic rhinitis; asthma.

Cromol Betapharm, Ger.
Sodium cromoglycate (p.762·1).
Hay fever.

Cromolind Lindopharm, Ger.
Sodium cromoglycate (p.762·1).
Asthma.

Cromolyn Fatol, Ger.; Orion, Ger.
Sodium cromoglycate (p.762·1).
Asthma.

Crom-Ophtal Winzer, Ger.
Sodium cromoglycate (p.762·1).
Allergic conjunctivitis; allergic rhinitis.

Cromoptic Chauvin, Fr.
Sodium cromoglycate (p.762·1).
Allergic eye disorders.

Cromosan Medici, Ital.
Sodium cromoglycate (p.762·1).
Food hypersensitivity.

Cromosol Ophta Ecosol, Switz.
Sodium cromoglycate (p.762·1).
Conjunctivitis.

Cromovist Fisons, Neth.†.
Sodium cromoglycate (p.762·1); hypromellose (p.1473·1).
Allergic conjunctivitis.

Cromoxin Rius, Spain†.
Carbazochrome (p.714·1).
Haemorrhage.

Cromoxin K Rius, Spain.
Carbazochrome (p.714·1); phytomenadione (p.1371·1).
Haemorrhage.

Cromoxin Perfus Fortific Rius, Spain†.
Carbazochrome (p.714·1); multivitamins.
Haemorrhage; muscle atony.

Cromozil Allergan, Ital.
Tetrahydrozoline hydrochloride (p.1070·2); sodium cromoglycate (p.762·1).
Conjunctivitis.

Cronacol Biotekfarma, Ital.
Sodium cromoglycate (p.762·1).
Food hypersensitivity.

Cronasma Orion, Ger.
Theophylline (p.765·1).
Asthma; bronchitis; emphysema.

Cronassial Fidia, Ital.†.
Gangliosides (p.1582·3).
Peripheral neuropathies.

Cronauzan Chinoin, Ital.†.
Metoclopramide hydrochloride (p.1200·3).
Nausea and vomiting.

Croneparina Chemil, Ital.
Heparin calcium (p.879·3).
Atherosclerosis; thrombo-embolic disorders.

Cronizat Pharmacia Upjohn, Ital.
Nizatidine (p.1203·2).
Peptic ulcers.

Cronodine Reig Jofre, Spain.
Diltiazem hydrochloride (p.854·2).
Angina pectoris; hypertension; myocardial infarction.

Cronol Solvay, Spain.
Famotidine (p.1192·1).
Gastro-oesophageal reflux; peptic ulcer; Zollinger-Ellison syndrome.

Cross Prep Colgate Oral Care, Austral.
Chlorhexidine gluconate (p.1107·2); cetrimide (p.1105·2).
Surface disinfection.

Crotamitex Gepepharm, Ger.
Crotamiton (p.1081·1).
Pruritic skin disorders.

Cruex
Novartis Consumer, Canad.; Ciba Consumer, USA.
Aerosol; cream: Undecenoic acid (p.389·2); zinc undecenoate (p.389·2).
Bromhidrosis; fungal skin infections; hyperhidrosis; minor skin irritation; nappy rash.

Novartis Consumer, Canad.; Ciba Consumer, USA.
Topical powder: Calcium undecenoate (p.389·2).
Bromhidrosis; fungal skin infections; hyperhidrosis; minor skin irritation; nappy rash.

Cruscaprugna Dietetica Recordati, Ital.†.
Dietary fibre supplement with prune and minerals (p.1209·2).
Gastro-intestinal disorders; weight reduction.

Cruscasohn Antonetto, Ital.
Cereal fibre; guar gum (p.321·3); pectin (p.1474·1).
Constipation.

Crusken
Maggioni, Ital.; Sterling Midy, Ital.
A range of dietary fibre supplements (p.1181·2).
Delayed gastro-intestinal transit.

Cruzzy SIT, Ital.
Lotion: Pyrethrum (p.1410·1); piperonyl butoxide (p.1409·3); diethyltoluamide (p.1405·1).
Shampoo: Phenothrin (p.1409·2).
Pediculosis.

Cruzzy Antiparassitario SIT, Ital.
Pyrethrum (p.1410·1); piperonyl butoxide (p.1409·3).
Pediculosis.

Cryptocur
Hoechst Marion Roussel, Irl.†; Hoechst Marion Roussel, Neth.
Gonadorelin (p.1247·2).
Cryptorchidism.

Crystacide
Evans Medical, Irl.; Medeva, UK.
Hydrogen peroxide (p.1116·2).
Skin infections.

Crystamine Dunhall, USA.
Cyanocobalamin (p.1363·3).
Schilling test; vitamin B_{12} deficiency.

Crystapen
Duncan, Flockhart, Austral.†; Bioniche, Canad.; Britannia Pharmaceuticals, Irl.; Britannia Pharmaceuticals, UK.
Benzylpenicillin sodium (p.159·3).
Bacterial infections.

Crysti 1000 Roberts, USA; Hauck, USA.
Cyanocobalamin (p.1363·3).
Schilling test; vitamin B_{12} deficiency.

Crysticillin Apothecon, USA.
Procaine penicillin (p.240·2).
Bacterial infections.

Crystodigin Lilly, USA.
Digitoxin (p.848·3).
Atrial flutter and fibrillation; heart failure; supraventricular tachycardia.

C-Soft Austroflex, Aust.
Rinsing and storage solution for soft contact lenses.

C-Solve Syosset, USA.
Vehicle for topical preparations.

C-Tard Whitehall, Ital.
Ascorbic acid (p.1365·2).
Vitamin C deficiency.

C-Tol Rhone-Poulenc Rorer, Austral.†.
Ascorbic acid (p.1365·2); sodium ascorbate (p.1365·2).
Vitamin C deficiency.

C-Tron Calcium Sauter, Switz.†.
Vitamin C and D preparation with calcium.
Cold symptoms; tonic.

C/T/S Hoechst Roussel, USA.
Clindamycin phosphate (p.191·1).
Acne.

Cu-7 Searle, USA†.
Copper-wound plastic (p.1337·3).
Intra-uterine contraceptive device.

Cuantin Mabo, Spain†.
Famotidine (p.1192·1).
Gastro-oesophageal reflux; peptic ulcer; Zollinger-Ellison syndrome.

Cuatroderm Schering-Plough, Spain.
Betamethasone valerate (p.1033·3); clioquinol (p.193·2); gentamicin sulphate (p.212·1); tolnaftate (p.389·1).
Infected skin disorders.

Culat Boehringer Mannheim, Aust.
Epoetin beta (p.718·3).
Anaemia of prematurity, chronic renal failure or malignant disease; autologous blood transfusions.

Cullens Headache Powders Cullen & Davison, UK.
Aspirin (p.16·1); caffeine (p.749·3).

Cumulit Giuliani, Switz.†.
Ursodeoxycholic acid (p.1642·1); chenodeoxycholic acid (p.1562·1).
Gallstones.

Cunesin Elmu, Spain.
Ciprofloxacin hydrochloride (p.185·3).
Bacterial infections.

Cunil Helsinn Birex, Irl.
Ibuprofen (p.44·1).
Musculoskeletal, joint, and peri-articular disorders; pain; soft-tissue injuries.

Cunticina Rovi, Spain.
Albumin tannate (p.1176·3).
Diarrhoea.

Cunticina Adultos Rovi, Spain†.
Albumin tannate (p.1176·3); dihydrostreptomycin sulphate (p.202·2); phthalylsulphathiazole (p.237·1); powdered opium (p.70·3).
Infectious diarrhoea.

Cunticina Infantil Rovi, Spain†.
Albumin tannate (p.1176·3); dihydrostreptomycin sulphate (p.202·2); phthalylsulphathiazole (p.237·1).
Infectious diarrhoea.

Cupanol Inibsa, Spain.
Paracetamol (p.72·2).
Fever; pain.

Cuplex
Trans Canaderm, Canad.; Smith & Nephew, Irl.; Smith & Nephew Pharmaceuticals, UK.
Salicylic acid (p.1090·2); lactic acid (p.1593·3); copper acetate.
Calluses; corns; warts.

Cuprenase GN, Ger.†.
Copper gluconate (p.1338·1).
Copper deficiency.

Cuprex Merck, Ger.†.
Copper oleate (p.1403·3).
Pediculosis.

Cupridium DHU, Ger.
Homoeopathic preparation.

Cuprimine
Merck Sharp & Dohme, Canad.; Merck Sharp & Dohme, Neth.; Merck Sharp & Dohme, Norw.; Merck Sharp & Dohme, Swed.; Merck Sharp & Dohme, USA.
Penicillamine (p.988·3).
Chronic lead poisoning; cystinuria; rheumatoid arthritis; Wilson's disease.

Cupripen Rubio, Spain.
Penicillamine (p.988·3).
Biliary cirrhosis; cystinuria; heavy-metal poisoning; rheumatoid arthritis; Wilson's disease.

Cuprocept CCL Cuprocept, S.Afr.
Copper-wound plastic (p.1337·3).
Intra-uterine contraceptive device.

Cuprofen Seton, UK.
Ibuprofen (p.44·1).
Inflammation; pain.

Cuprum Ro-Plex (Rowo-392) Pharmakon, Ger.†.
Homoeopathic preparation.

Cuprum Ro-Plex (Rowo-1000) Pharmakon, Ger.†.
Homoeopathic preparation.

Cura Arnaldi-Uscio, Ital.
Tablets (500 mg): Aloes (p.1177·1); senna (p.1212·2); althaea (p.1546·3); liquorice (p.1197·1); ferrous sulphate (p.1340·2); vegetable charcoal (p.972·3).
Tablets (1 g); oral powder: Melissa (p.1600·1); cascarilla; quassia (p.1624·1); senna (p.1212·2); ginger (p.1193·2); aloes (p.1177·1); althaea (p.1546·3); laurel; myrtle; bergamot oil (p.1553·1).
Constipation.

Curacallos Pedykur Domenech Garcia, Spain†.
Alcohol; chloral hydrate (p.645·3); ethyl ether; pyroxylin (p.1090·1); salicylic acid (p.1090·2).
Callosities.

Curacit Nycomed, Norw.
Suxamethonium chloride (p.1319·1).
Depolarising neuromuscular blocker.

Curadent Leti, Spain.
Lignocaine hydrochloride (p.1293·2).
Local anaesthesia in dentistry.

Curadon Tika, Swed.
Paracetamol (p.72·2).
Fever; pain.

Curafil Betafar, Spain.
Chlorhexidine gluconate (p.1107·2).
Skin and wound disinfection.

Curantyl Berlin-Chemie, Ger.
Dipyridamole (p.857·1).
Ischaemic heart disease.

Curapic Leti, Spain.
Diphenhydramine hydrochloride (p.409·1); lignocaine hydrochloride (p.1293·2).
Insect stings; pruritus.

Curarina Miro *Palex, Spain.*
Tubocurarine chloride (p.1322·3).
Competitive neuromuscular blocker.

Curash Anti-Rash *Carter-Wallace, Austral.*
Zinc oxide (p.1096·2).
Hyperhidrosis; nappy rash; skin irritation.

Curash Baby Wipes *Carter-Wallace, Austral.*
Vitamin E (p.1369·1); sorbolene.
Moisturiser.

Curastain *Young, USA.*
Triethanolamine (p.1639·1).
Reduction of dithranol-induced staining.

Curastatin *Austroplant, Aust.*
Somatostatin acetate (p.1261·1).
Gastro-intestinal haemorrhage; prevention of postoperative complications following pancreatic surgery.

Curasten *Therabel, Fr.*
Lysine hydrochloride (p.1350·1); calcium gluceptate (p.1155·1).
Asthenia.

Curatin *Carter-Wallace, Austral.*
Cream: Tolnaftate (p.389·1); chlorocresol (p.1110·3).
Powder: Tolnaftate (p.389·1).
Fungal skin infections.

Curatoderm
Hermal, Ger.; Hermal, Switz.; Crookes Healthcare, UK.
Tacalcitol (p.1092·1).
Psoriasis.

Curaven *Biomedica, Ital.*
Aesculus (p.1543·3).
Peripheral vascular disorders.

Curcumen *Temmler, Ger.*
Curcuma zanthorrhiza.
Dyspepsia.

Curel *Bausch & Lomb, USA.*
Emollient and moisturiser.

Curethyl *AJC, Fr.*
Alcohol (p.1099·1).
Alcohol withdrawal syndromes.

Curibronches *Splenodex, Fr.†.*
Adult syrup: Bromoform (p.1620·3); potassium guaiacolsulfonate (p.1068·3); aconite (p.1542·2); belladonna (p.457·1); codeine (p.26·1); ethylmorphine hydrochloride (p.36·1); cherry-laurel; tolu balsam (p.1071·1); eucalyptus (p.1578·1).
Infant syrup: Sodium benzoate (p.1102·3); potassium guaiacolsulfonate (p.1068·3); sodium bromide (p.1620·3); belladonna (p.457·1); tolu balsam (p.1071·1); eucalyptus (p.1578·1).
Paediatric syrup: Sodium benzoate (p.1102·3); potassium guaiacolsulfonate (p.1068·3); sodium bromide (p.1620·3); belladonna (p.457·1); codeine (p.26·1); tolu balsam (p.1071·1); Desessartz syrup; eucalyptus (p.1578·1).
Respiratory system disorders.

Curine *Leti, Spain.*
Benzalkonium chloride (p.1101·3); lignocaine hydrochloride (p.1293·2).
Pain; pruritus.

Curocef *Glaxo Wellcome, Aust.*
Cefuroxime sodium (p.177·1).
Bacterial infections.

Curon-B *Intramed, S.Afr.*
Pancuronium bromide (p.1317·2).
Competitive neuromuscular blocker.

Curosurf
Serono, Aust.; Serono, Fr.; Serono, Ger.; Serono, Irl.; Chiesi, Ital.; Serono, Neth.; Serono, Norw.; Serono, Spain; Serono, Swed.; Serono, Switz.; Serono, UK.
Poractant alfa (p.1623·1).
Neonatal respiratory distress syndrome.

Curoveinyl *Pharmygiene, Fr.*
Aesculus (p.1543·3); hamamelis (p.1587·1); hydrastis (p.1588·2); cupressus sempervirens; scoparium (p.1628·1); nux vomica (p.1609·3).
Peripheral vascular disorders.

Curoxim *Glaxo Wellcome, Ital.*
Cefuroxime sodium (p.177·1).
Bacterial infections.

Curoxima *Glaxo Wellcome, Spain.*
Cefuroxime sodium (p.177·1).
Bacterial infections.

Curpol *Warner-Lambert Consumer, Belg.*
Paracetamol (p.72·2).
Fever; pain.

Curretab *Solvay, USA.*
Medroxyprogesterone acetate (p.1448·3).
Abnormal uterine bleeding; secondary amenorrhoea.

Curzon *Gerard House, UK.*
Damiana (p.1570·2).
Tonic.

Cuscutine *Geymonat, Ital.*
Senna (p.1212·2); aloin (p.1177·2).
Constipation.

Cusialgil *Cusi, Spain†.*
Ibuprofen (p.44·1).
Fever; pain.

Cusicrom *Cusi, Spain; Farmacusi, Spain.*
Sodium cromoglycate (p.762·1).
Allergic rhinitis; eye disorders.

Cusigel *Farmacusi, Spain.*
Fluocinonide (p.1041·2).
Skin disorders.

Cusilyn *Cusi, UK†.*
Sodium cromoglycate (p.762·1).

Cusimolol *Cusi, Spain.*
Timolol maleate (p.953·3).
Glaucoma; ocular hypertension.

Cusispray *Cusi, Spain†.*
Dexamethasone phosphate (p.1037·2); framycetin sulphate (p.210·3); lignocaine hydrochloride (p.1293·2).
Mouth and throat infections.

Cusiter *Cusi, Spain.*
Lactic acid (p.1593·3); triclocarban (p.1127·2).
Skin disinfection.

Cusiviral *Cusi, Spain; Britisfarma, Spain.*
Aciclovir (p.602·3) or aciclovir sodium (p.602·3).
Herpesvirus infections.

Custodiol
Raith, Aust.; Kohler, Ger.
Electrolytes, amino acids, and mannitol.
Organ perfusion solution.

Customed *Chefaro, Ger.*
Bromhexine hydrochloride (p.1055·3); thymol (p.1127·1).
Coughs; respiratory-tract disorders; sinusitis.

Cutacnyl *Galderma, Fr.*
Benzoyl peroxide (p.1079·2).
Acne.

Cutaderm *Schering-Plough, S.Afr.*
Hydrocortisone (p.1043·3).
Skin disorders.

Cutanit *Yamanouchi, Spain.*
Fluclorolone acetonide (p.1040·1).
Skin disorders.

Cutar *Summers, USA.*
Coal tar (p.1092·3).
Skin disorders.

Cutasept
Beiersdorf, Aust.; Bode, Ger.
Isopropyl alcohol (p.1118·2); benzalkonium chloride (p.1101·3).
Skin disinfection.

Cutemol *Summers, USA.*
Emollient and moisturiser.

Cutemul *Medopharm, Ger.*
Dexpanthenol (p.1570·3).
Burns; inflammatory skin disorders; wounds.

Cuterpes *Chauvin, Fr.*
Ibacitabine (p.613·2).
Herpes infections.

Cuticura *DEP, USA.*
Cream†: Benzoyl peroxide (p.1079·2).
Ointment†: Sulphur (p.1091·2); phenol (p.1121·2); hydroxyquinoline (p.1589·3).
Acne.
Soap: Triclocarban (p.1127·2).
Skin cleanser.

Cutifitol *Llorente, Spain.*
Progesterone (p.1459·3).
Hair, scalp, and skin disorders.

Cutimix *Metochem, Aust.*
Zinc oxide (p.1096·2); talc (p.1092·1).
Skin disorders.

Cutinea *Cupal, UK†.*
Chlorphenesin (p.376·2); zinc oxide (p.1096·2).
Fungal skin infections.

Cutinova *Beiersdorf, UK.*
Polyurethane foam dressing.
Burns; ulcers; wounds.

Cutisan *Boots Healthcare, Fr.*
Triclocarban (p.1127·2).
Skin disorders.

Cutisan a l'Hydrocortisone *Boots, Fr.†.*
Triclocarban (p.1127·2); hydrocortisone acetate (p.1043·3).
Skin disorders.

cutistad
Stada, Ger.; Helvepharm, Switz.
Clotrimazole (p.376·3).
Fungal skin infections.

Cutivate
Glaxo Wellcome, Aust.; Glaxo Wellcome, Neth.; Allen & Hanburys, S.Afr.; Glaxo Wellcome, Switz.; Glaxo, UK; Glaxo Wellcome, USA.
Fluticasone propionate (p.1042·3).
Skin disorders.

Cutterglobin *Tropon-Cutter, Ger.†.*
A normal immunoglobulin (p.1522·1).
Hypogammaglobulinaemia; passive immunisation.

Cuvalit
Schering, Ger.; Schering, Ital.†.
Lysuride maleate (p.1142·1).
Migraine.

Cuvefilm *Calmante Vitaminado, Spain.*
Chlorhexidine gluconate (p.1107·2).
Skin and wound disinfection.

Cuxabrain *TAD, Ger.*
Piracetam (p.1619·1).
Mental function disorders.

Cuxacillin *TAD, Ger.*
Amoxycillin trihydrate (p.151·3).
Bacterial infections.

Cuxaflex N *TAD, Ger.*
Ointment: Methyl salicylate (p.55·2); benzyl nicotinate (p.22·1); turpentine oil (p.1641·1).
Cold damage; musculoskeletal and joint disorders; neuralgia.
Topical gel: Glycol salicylate (p.43·1); benzyl nicotinate (p.22·1).
Musculoskeletal, joint, and soft-tissue disorders; neuralgia.

Cuxaflex Thermo *TAD, Ger.*
Glycol salicylate (p.43·1); benzyl nicotinate (p.22·1).
Musculoskeletal, joint, and soft-tissue disorders.

Cuxanorm *TAD, Ger.*
Atenolol (p.825·3).
Arrhythmias; hypertension; ischaemic heart disease.

C-vimin *Astra, Swed.*
Ascorbic acid (p.1365·2).
Vitamin C deficiency.

C-Vit *Sanabo, Aust.*
Ascorbic acid (p.1365·2).
Vitamin C deficiency.

CVP *Rhone-Poulenc Rorer, Ital.*
Bioflavonoids (p.1580·1); ascorbic acid (p.1365·2).
Gingivitis; stomatitis; vitamin C deficiency.

C-Will
Will-Pharma, Belg.; Will-Pharma, Neth.
Ascorbic acid (p.1365·2).
Vitamin C deficiency.

CX Powder *Adams, UK.*
Chlorhexidine acetate (p.1107·2).
Skin disinfection.

Cyanide Antidote Package *Lilly, USA.*
Combination pack: 2 Ampoules, sodium nitrite (p.995·2); 2 ampoules, sodium thiosulphate (p.996·2); 12 aspirols, amyl nitrite (p.974·2).
Cyanide poisoning.

Cyanoject *Mayrand, USA.*
Cyanocobalamin (p.1363·3).
Schilling test; vitamin B_{12} deficiency.

Cyanokit *Lipha Sante, Fr.*
Hydroxocobalamin (p.1363·3).
Cyanide poisoning.

Cyater *Sigma-Tau, Spain.*
Terfenadine (p.418·1).
Hypersensitivity reactions.

Cyclabil
Schering, Norw.; Schering, Swed.
11 Tablets, oestradiol valerate (p.1455·2); 10 tablets, oestradiol valerate; levonorgestrel (p.1454·1).
Menopausal disorders; osteoporosis.

Cyclacur
Schering, Aust.; Schering, Ital.†; Schering, Switz.
11 Tablets, oestradiol valerate (p.1455·2); 10 tablets, oestradiol valerate; norgestrel (p.1454·1).
Menopausal disorders; menstrual disorders.

Cycladol
Promedica, Fr.; Wasserman, Spain.
Piroxicam betadex (p.81·1).
Gout; musculoskeletal, joint, and peri-articular disorders; pain.

Cyclan *Major, USA†.*
Cyclandelate (p.845·2).
Cerebrovascular and peripheral vascular disorders.

Cycleane *Monsanto, Fr.*
Desogestrel (p.1443·3); ethinyloestradiol (p.1445·1).
Combined oral contraceptive.

Cyclen *Janssen-Ortho, Canad.*
Norgestimate (p.1453·3); ethinyloestradiol (p.1445·1).
28-Day packs also contain 7 inert tablets.
Combined oral contraceptive.

Cyclergine *Poirier, Fr.*
Cyclandelate (p.845·2).
Peripheral vascular disorders.

Cyclidox *Triomed, S.Afr.*
Doxycycline hydrochloride (p.202·3).
Bacterial infections.

Cyclimorph
Wellcome, Irl.; Glaxo Wellcome, S.Afr.; Wellcome, UK.
Morphine tartrate (p.56·3); cyclizine tartrate (p.407·1).
Pain.

Cyclimycin *Lennon, S.Afr.*
Minocycline (p.227·1).
Bacterial infections.

Cyclinex *Ross, USA.*
A range of preparations for enteral nutrition including an infant feed.
Gyrate atrophy; urea cycle disorder.

Cyclivex *Lennon, S.Afr.*
Aciclovir (p.602·3).
Herpesvirus infections.

Cyclo 3 *Pierre Fabre, Fr.*
Cream: Sterol heterosides from Ruscus aculeatus; melilot.
Circulatory disorders.

Cyclo 3 Fort *Pierre Fabre, Fr.*
Ruscus aculeatus; hesperidin methyl chalcone (p.1580·2); ascorbic acid (p.1365·2).
Circulatory disorders.

Cycloarthrin *Schaper & Brummer, Ger.†.*
Coumarin (p.1568·1); benzyl nicotinate (p.22·1); glycol salicylate (p.43·1); heparin (p.879·3).
Musculoskeletal and joint disorders; neuralgia; neuritis.

Cyclobiol *Yves Ponroy, Fr.*
Nutritional supplement.
Premenstrual syndrome.

Cycloblastin
Pharmacia Upjohn, Austral.; Pharmacia Upjohn, S.Afr.
Cyclophosphamide (p.516·2).
Auto-immune diseases; malignant neoplasms; transplant rejection.

Cycloblastine
Pharmacia Upjohn, Belg.; Pharmacia, Neth.†.
Cyclophosphamide (p.516·2).
Malignant neoplasms.

Cyclobral *Norgine, UK†.*
Cyclandelate (p.845·2).
Peripheral and cerebral vascular disorders.

Cyclocaps *Goldshield, UK†.*
Salbutamol (p.758·2).
Asthma.

Cyclo-cell *Cell Pharm, Ger.*
Cyclophosphamide (p.516·2).
Malignant neoplasms.

Cyclocort
Stiefel, Canad.; Fujisawa, USA.
Amcinonide (p.1032·1).
Skin disorders.

Cyclocur
Schering, Belg.; Schering, Neth.
11 Tablets, oestradiol valerate (p.1455·2); 10 tablets, oestradiol valerate; norgestrel (p.1454·1).
Menopausal disorders; menstrual disorders.

Cycloderm
Note. This name is used for preparations of different composition.
Belphar, Belg.†.
Amcinonide (p.1032·1).
Skin disorders.
Rottapharm, Ital.†.
Ciclomethasone.
Skin disorders.

Cyclodox *Berk, UK.*
Doxycycline (p.202·3).
Bacterial infections.

Cyclogest
Hoechst Marion Roussel, S.Afr.; Shire, UK.
Progesterone (p.1459·3).
Fertility disorders; premenstrual syndrome; puerperal depression.

Cyclogyl
Alcon, Austral.; Alcon, Canad.; Alcon, Neth.†; Alcon, S.Afr.; Alcon, Swed.; Alcon, Switz.; Alcon, USA.
Cyclopentolate hydrochloride (p.459·3).
Production of cycloplegia and mydriasis.

Cyclomandol *Yamanouchi, Swed.*
Cyclandelate (p.845·2).
Vascular disorders.

Cyclomen *Sanofi Winthrop, Canad.*
Danazol (p.1441·3).
Endometriosis; mastalgia; primary menorrhagia.

Cyclo-Menorette *Wyeth, Ger.*
11 Tablets, oestradiol valerate (p.1455·2); oestriol (p.1457·2); 10 tablets, oestradiol valerate; oestriol; levonorgestrel (p.1454·1).
Menopausal disorders.

Cyclomin *Berk, UK.*
Minocycline (p.227·1).
Bacterial infections.

Cyclomydri *Thilo, Neth.†.*
Cyclopentolate hydrochloride (p.459·3).
Production of cycloplegia and mydriasis.

Cyclomydril
Alcon, S.Afr.; Alcon, USA.
Cyclopentolate hydrochloride (p.459·3); phenylephrine hydrochloride (p.1066·2).
Production of mydriasis.

CycloOstrogynal *Asche, Ger.*
11 Tablets, oestradiol valerate (p.1455·2); oestriol (p.1457·2); 10 tablets, oestradiol valerate; oestriol; levonorgestrel (p.1454·1).
Menopausal disorders.

Cyclopent *ankerpharm, Ger.†.*
Cyclodrine hydrochloride (p.459·2).
Production of mydriasis and cycloplegia.

Cyclopentol *Asta Medica, Belg.*
Cyclopentolate hydrochloride (p.459·3).
Prevention of iridocrystalline adherences; prevention of synechiae; production of cycloplegia and mydriasis.

Cyclo-Premarin-MPA *Wyeth Lederle, Aust.*
Redbrown tablets, conjugated oestrogens (p.1457·3); blue tablets, conjugated oestrogens; medroxyprogesterone acetate (p.1448·3).
Menopausal disorders.

Cyclo-Premella
Wyeth Lederle, Aust.
14 Tablets, conjugated oestrogens (p.1457·3); 14 tablets, conjugated oestrogens; medroxyprogesterone acetate (p.1448·3).
Menopausal disorders.
Wyeth, Switz.
28 Tablets, conjugated oestrogens (p.1457·3); 14 tablets medroxyprogesterone acetate (p.1448·3).
Menopausal disorders; oestrogen deficiency.

Cyclo-Progynova
Schering, Ger.; Schering, Irl.†.
11 Tablets, oestradiol valerate (p.1455·2); 10 tablets, oestradiol valerate; norgestrel (p.1454·1).
Menopausal disorders; menstrual disorders.

Cyclo-Progynova 1 mg *Asta Medica, UK.*
11 Tablets, oestradiol valerate (p.1455·2); 10 tablets, oestradiol valerate; levonorgestrel (p.1454·1).
Menopausal disorders.

Cyclo-Progynova 2 mg *Asta Medica, UK.*
11 Tablets, oestradiol valerate (p.1455·2); 10 tablets, oestradiol valerate; norgestrel (p.1454·1).
Menopausal disorders.

Cyclorel *Thera, Fr.*
Naringin sodium.
Circulatory disorders.

Cyclosa *Nourypharma, Ger.*
7 Tablets, ethinyloestradiol (p.1445·1); 15 tablets, ethinyloestradiol; desogestrel (p.1443·3).
Menstrual disorders.

Cycloserine *Lilly, UK.*
Cycloserine (p.198·3).
Tuberculosis; urinary-tract infections.

Cyclospasmol
Byk, Aust.†; Yamanouchi, Belg.; Wyeth-Ayerst, Canad.; Yamanouchi, Fr.; Yamanouchi, Neth.†; Wyeth-Ayerst, USA†.
Cyclandelate (p.845·2).
Peripheral and cerebral vascular disorders.

Cyclostin *Pharmacia Upjohn, Ger.*
Cyclophosphamide (p.516·2).
Malignant neoplasms.

Cycloteriam *Roussel, Fr.*
Triamterene (p.957·2); cyclothiazide (p.845·3).
Hypertension; oedema.

Cycloven Forte N *CT, Ger.*
Aesculus (p.1543·3); esculoside (p.1543·3); rutin (p.1580·2).
Peripheral vascular disorders.

Cycloviran *Sigma-Tau, Ital.*
Aciclovir (p.602·3).
Herpesvirus infections.

Cycofed *Cypress, USA.*
Codeine phosphate (p.26·1); pseudoephedrine hydrochloride (p.1068·3); guaiphenesin (p.1061·3).
Coughs.

Cycrin *ESI, USA.*
Medroxyprogesterone acetate (p.1448·3).
Abnormal uterine bleeding; secondary amenorrhoea.

Cyfol *Shire, Irl.†.*
Ferrous gluconate (p.1340·1); folic acid (p.1340·3); cyanocobalamin (p.1363·3).
Anaemias.

Cyklo-F *Pharmacia Upjohn, Swed.*
Tranexamic acid (p.728·2).
Menorrhagia.

Cyklokapron
Pharmacia Upjohn, Aust.; Pharmacia Upjohn, Austral.; Pharmacia Upjohn, Canad.; Pharmacia Upjohn, Ger.; Pharmacia Upjohn, Irl.; Pharmacia Upjohn, Neth.; Pharmacia Upjohn, Norw.; Pharmacia Upjohn, S.Afr.; Pharmacia Upjohn, Swed.; Pharmacia Upjohn, Switz.; Kabivitrum, UK; Kabivitrum, USA.
Tranexamic acid (p.728·2).
Hereditary angioedema; hyphaemia; local and general fibrinolysis; menorrhagia; surgical procedures in those with coagulopathies.

Cykrina *Wyeth Lederle, Swed.*
Medroxyprogesterone acetate (p.1448·3).
Endometriosis; menstrual disorders.

Cylate *Ocusoft, USA.*
Cyclopentolate hydrochloride (p.459·3).

Cylert
Abbott, Canad.; Abbott, USA.
Pemoline (p.1484·1).
Attention deficit disorders; hyperactivity.

Cylex *Pharmakon, USA.*
Benzocaine (p.1286·2); cetylpyridinium chloride (p.1106·2).
Sore throat.

Cyllind *Abbott, Ger.*
Clarithromycin (p.189·1).
Bacterial infections.

Cymalon
Note. This name is used for preparations of different composition.
Seton, Irl.
Sodium citrate (p.1153·2); anhydrous citric acid (p.1564·3); sodium bicarbonate (p.1153·2); sodium carbonate (p.1630·2).
Cystitis.
Sterling Health, UK.
Sodium citrate (p.1153·2).
Cystitis.

Cymerin *Tokyo Tanabe, Jpn.*
Ranimustine (p.560·2).
Blood disorders; malignant neoplasms.

Cymevan *Roche, Fr.*
Ganciclovir (p.612·3) or ganciclovir sodium (p.611·3).
Cytomegalovirus infections.

Cymeven *Syntex, Ger.; Roche, Ger.*
Ganciclovir sodium (p.611·3).
Cytomegalovirus infections.

Cymevene
Roche, Aust.; Roche, Austral.; Roche, Belg.; Roche, Irl.; Recordati, Ital.; Roche, Neth.; Roche, Norw.; Roche, S.Afr.; Roche, Spain; Roche, Swed.; Roche, Switz.; Roche, UK.
Ganciclovir (p.612·3) or ganciclovir sodium (p.611·3).
Cytomegalovirus infections.

Cymex *De Witt, UK.*
Urea (p.1095·2); dimethicone (p.1384·2); cetrimide (p.1105·2); chlorocresol (p.1110·3).
Cracked lips; herpes labialis.

Cymi *Lennon, S.Afr.†.*
Cimetidine (p.1183·2).
Gastric hyperacidity; peptic ulcer; Zollinger-Ellison syndrome.

Cyna Bilisan *Repha, Ger.*
Cynara (p.1569·2).
Dyspepsia.

Cynacur *Biocur, Ger.*
Cynara (p.1569·2).
Dyspepsia.

Cynafol *Kanoldt, Ger.*
Cynara (p.1569·2).
Dyspepsia.

Cynarix
Montavit, Aust.; Sagitta, Ger.†.
Cynara (p.1569·2); rhubarb (p.1212·1).
Biliary disorders; hepatogenic digestive disorders; liver disorders; repletion.

Cynarix comp *Montavit, Aust.*
Cynara (p.1569·2); rhubarb (p.1212·1) salverine hydrochloride (p.1627·2).
Biliary disorders.

Cynarol *Pharmethic, Belg.*
Cynara (p.1569·2).
Biliary disorders; promotion of diuresis.

Cynarzym N *Roland, Ger.*
Cynara (p.1569·2); boldo (p.1554·1); chelidonium.
Digestive disorders; liver disorders.

Cynomel *Marion Merrell, Fr.*
Liothyronine sodium (p.1495·1).
Hypothyroidism.

Cynt *Beiersdorf-Lilly, Ger.*
Moxonidine (p.913·1).
Hypertension.

Cyomin *Forest Pharmaceuticals, USA.*
Cyanocobalamin (p.1363·3).
Schilling test; vitamin B_{12} deficiency.

Cyprid *Janssen-Cilag, Belg.*
Cisapride (p.1187·1).
Digestive disorders.

Cyprone *Alphapharm, Austral.*
Cyproterone acetate (p.1440·2).
Androgenisation; deviant sexual behaviour; prostatic cancer.

Cyprostat *Schering, UK.*
Cyproterone acetate (p.1440·2).
Prostatic cancer.

Cyprostol *Salus, Aust.*
Misoprostol (p.1419·3).
Peptic ulcer.

Cyral *Gerot, Aust.*
Primidone (p.358·3).
Epilepsy.

Cyrpon *Kolassa, Aust.*
Meprobamate (p.678·1).
Anxiety.

Cystadane *Orphan, Austral.*
Betaine (p.1553·2).
Homocystinuria.

Cystagon
Orphan, Austral.; Swedish Orphan, Swed.; Orphan Europe, UK.
Cysteamine bitartrate (p.1569·3).
Nephropathic cystinosis.

Cystelle Antipelliculaire *Bailleul, Fr.*
Piroctone olamine (p.1089·1).
Formerly contained soluble pyrithione.
Seborrhoeic dermatitis.

Cystelle Shampooing Cheveux Gras *Bailleul, Fr.*
Cade oil (p.1092·2); zinc gluconate (p.1373·2); pyridoxine hydrochloride (p.1362·3).
Seborrhoea.

Cystemme *Abbott, UK.*
Sodium citrate (p.1153·2).
Cystitis.

Cystex *Numark, USA.*
Hexamine (p.216·1); sodium salicylate (p.85·1); benzoic acid (p.1102·3).
Urinary-tract infections.

Cystibosin B 48 *Bock, Ger.*
Homoeopathic preparation.

Cystichol *Bailleul, Fr.*
Cystine (p.1339·1); choline bitartrate (p.1337·1).
Liver disorders.

Cysticide
Merck, Ger.; Merck, S.Afr.
Praziquantel (p.108·2).
Neurocysticercosis.

Cystinol *Schaper & Brummer, Ger.*
Betula; equisetum (p.1575·1); solidago virgaurea; bearberry (p.1552·2).
Urinary-tract disorders.

Cystinol Akut *Schaper & Brummer, Ger.*
Bearberry (p.1552·2).
Urinary-tract inflammation.

Cystinol Long *Schaper & Brummer, Ger.*
Solidago virgaurea.
Renal calculi.

Cystinol N *Asta Medica, Switz.†.*
Silver birch (p.1553·3); equisetum (p.1575·1); juniper (p.1592·2); solidago virgaurea; bearberry (p.1552·2).
Urinary-tract disorders.

Cystiselect N *Dreluso, Ger.*
Homoeopathic preparation.

Cystistat *Bioniche, Canad.*
Sodium hyaluronate (p.1630·3).
Replacement of bladder glycosaminoglycan.

Cystit *Bristol-Myers Squibb, Ger.*
Nitrofurantoin (p.231·3).
Urinary-tract infections.

Cystitis Juniperus *Homeocan, Canad.*
Homoeopathic preparation.

Cystitis Treatment *Numark, UK†.*
Sodium citrate (p.1153·2).

Cystium *Wernigerode, Ger.*
Fennel oil (p.1579·2); camphor oil.
Renal calculi.

Cysti-Z *Bailleul, Fr.*
DL-Methionine (p.984·2); zinc sulphate (p.1373·2); pyridoxine hydrochloride (p.1362·3).
Alopecia; seborrhoea.

Cysto -cyl Ho-Len-Complex *Liebermann, Ger.*
Homoeopathic preparation.

Cysto Fink
Kade, Ger.; Fink, Ger.; SmithKline Beecham Consumer, Switz.
Bearberry (p.1552·2); cucurbita oil; kava (p.1592·3); lupulus (p.1597·2); rhus aromatica.
Bladder disorders.

Cystocalm *Galpharm, UK.*
Sodium citrate (p.1153·2).
Cystitis.

Cysto-Caps Chassot *Ebi, Switz.*
Bearberry (p.1552·2); cucurbita (p.1569·1); kava (p.1592·3); lupulus (p.1597·2); rhus aromatica.
Bladder disorders.

Cysto-Conray
Mallinckrodt, Canad.; Mallinckrodt, USA.
Meglumine iothalamate (p.1008·1).
Radiographic contrast medium.

Cystoforce *Bioforce, Canad.†.*
Bearberry (p.1552·2); echinacea (p.1574·2); hypericum (p.1590·1); rhus aromatica; achillea (p.1542·2); avena (p.1551·3); belladonna (p.457·1); aspen.
Urinary-tract disorders.

Cysto-Gastreu N R18 *Reckeweg, Ger.*
Homoeopathic preparation.

Cystografin *Squibb Diagnostics, USA.*
Meglumine diatrizoate (p.1003·2).
Radiographic contrast medium.

Cystoleve *Seton, UK.*
Sodium citrate (p.1153·2).
Cystitis.

Cysto-Myacyne N *Schur, Ger.*
Neomycin sulphate (p.229·2).
Urinary-tract infections.

Cystopurin
Roche, Irl.; Roche Consumer, UK.
Potassium citrate (p.1153·1).
Cystitis.

Cystorenol *Homberger, Switz.†.*
Homoeopathic preparation.

Cystosol *Baxter, Swed.*
Sorbitol (p.1354·2).
Bladder irrigation.

Cystospaz *PolyMedica, USA.*
Hyoscyamine (p.464·2).
Urinary-tract spasm.

Cystospaz-M *PolyMedica, USA.*
Hyoscyamine sulphate (p.464·2).
Urinary-tract spasm.

Cysto-Urgenin *Madaus, Ger.*
Cucurbita oil.
Bladder irritability.

Cystrin
Lorex Synthelabo, Irl.; Lorex, UK.
Oxybutynin hydrochloride (p.466·1).
Neurogenic bladder disorders; nocturnal enuresis; urinary incontinence.

Cytacon
Goldshield, Irl.; Glaxo Wellcome, S.Afr.†; Goldshield, UK.
Cyanocobalamin (p.1363·3).
Megaloblastic anaemia; tropical sprue; vitamin B_{12} deficiency.

Cytadren
Novartis, Austral.; Ciba, Canad.; Ciba, USA.
Aminoglutethimide (p.502·3).
Breast cancer; Cushing's syndrome.

Cytamen
DBL, Austral.; Evans Medical, Irl.; Glaxo Wellcome, S.Afr.†; Medeva, UK.
Cyanocobalamin (p.1363·3).
Megaloblastic anaemia; Schilling test; vitamin B_{12} deficiency.

Cytarbel *Bellon, Fr.*
Cytarabine (p.525·2).
Malignant neoplasms.

Cyteal
Note. This name is used for preparations of different composition.
Sinbio, Fr.
Chlorhexidine gluconate (p.1107·2); chlorocresol (p.1110·3); hexamidine isethionate (p.1115·3).
Disinfection of skin and mucous membranes.
Pierre Fabre, Ital.†.
Chlorhexidine (p.1107·2).

Cyto-Biffidus *Eagle, Austral.*
Lactobacillus acidophilus (p.1594·1); *Lactobacillus bulgaricus* (p.1594·1); with seven other *Lactobacillus* species.
Gastro-intestinal disorders.

Cytobion *Merck, Ger.*
Cyanocobalamin (p.1363·3).
Vitamin B_{12} deficiency.

Cytochrom C-Uvocal *Strathmann, Ger.†.*
Cytochrome C (p.1570·1).
Angina pectoris; heart failure; oxygen deficiency states; peripheral and cerebral circulatory disorders.

CytoGam *Medimmune, USA.*
A cytomegalovirus immunoglobulin (p.1507·1).
Passive immunisation.

Cytoglobin *Bayer, Ger.*
A cytomegalovirus immunoglobulin (p.1507·1).
Passive immunisation.

Cytomel
SK-RIT, Belg.; SmithKline Beecham, Canad.; SmithKline Beecham, Neth.; SmithKline Beecham, USA.
Liothyronine sodium (p.1495·1).
Evaluation of thyroid function; goitre; hypothyroidism.

Cytorest *Mochida, Jpn†.*
Cytochrome C (p.1570·1).
Leucopenia.

Cytosafe *Biosyn, Ger.†.*
Fluorouracil (p.534·3).
Malignant neoplasms.

Cytosar
Pharmacia Upjohn, Aust.; Pharmacia Upjohn, Belg.; Pharmacia Upjohn, Canad.; Pharmacia Upjohn, Irl.; Pharmacia Upjohn, Neth.; Pharmacia Upjohn, Norw.; Pharmacia Upjohn, S.Afr.; Pharmacia Upjohn, Swed.; Pharmacia Upjohn, Switz.; Pharmacia Upjohn, UK.
Cytarabine (p.525·2).
Leukaemias; non-Hodgkin's lymphoma.

Cytosar-U
Pharmacia Upjohn, Austral.; Upjohn, USA.
Cytarabine (p.525·2).
Leukaemias; non-Hodgkin's lymphoma.

Cytosol *Cytosol Ophthalmics, USA.*
Electrolytes (p.1147·1).
Ocular irrigation.

Cytospray *ICN, Canad.†.*
Macrogols (p.1597·3); isopropyl alcohol (p.1118·2).
Diagnostic aid.

Cytotec
Searle, Austral.; Searle, Belg.; Searle, Canad.; Monsanto, Fr.; Heumann, Ger.; Searle, Irl.; Searle, Ital.; Searle, Neth.; Searle, Norw.; Searle, S.Afr.; Searle, Spain; Searle, Swed.; Searle, Switz.; Searle, UK; Searle, USA.
Misoprostol (p.1419·3).
Peptic ulcer.

Cytotect
Biotest, Aust.; Biotest, Ger.; Biotest, Ital.; Biotest, Switz.
A cytomegalovirus immunoglobulin (p.1507·1).
Passive immunisation.

Cytovene
Roche, Canad.; Roche, USA.
Ganciclovir sodium (p.611·3).
Cytomegalovirus infections.

Cytoxan
Bristol, Canad.; Bristol-Myers Oncology, USA.
Cyclophosphamide (p.516·2).
Glomerular kidney disease in children; malignant neoplasms.

Cytra-2 *Cypress, USA.*
Citric acid monohydrate (p.1564·3); sodium citrate (p.1153·2).
Metabolic acidosis; urinary alkalinisation.

Cytra-3 *Cypress, USA.*
Citric acid monohydrate (p.1564·3); potassium citrate (p.1153·1); sodium citrate (p.1153·2).
Metabolic acidosis; urinary alkalinisation.

Cytra-K *Cypress, USA.*
Citric acid monohydrate (p.1564·3); potassium citrate (p.1153·1).
Metabolic acidosis; urinary alkalinisation.

Cytra-LC *Cypress, USA.*
Citric acid monohydrate (p.1564·3); potassium citrate (p.1153·1); sodium citrate (p.1153·2).
Metabolic acidosis; urinary alkalinisation.

Cytur Test *Boehringer Mannheim, Austral.*
Test for leucocytes in urine.

d Epifrin *Allergan, Ger.*
Dipivefrine hydrochloride (p.1572·3).
Glaucoma.

D1 Handedesinfektion *Beiersdorf, Ger.†.*
Isopropyl alcohol (p.1118·2); propyl alcohol (p.1124·2); mecetronium ethylsulphate (p.1119·1).
Skin disinfection.

D Sucril *Pierre Fabre, Fr.*
Aspartame (p.1335·1).
Sugar substitute.

3D Tipo P-Disinfettante *Eurochimica, Ital.†.*
Benzalkonium chloride (p.1101·3).
Surface disinfection.

DA Chewable *Dura, USA.*
Chlorpheniramine maleate (p.405·1); phenylephrine hydrochloride (p.1066·2); hyoscine methonitrate (p.463·1).
Allergic rhinitis; cold symptoms; sinusitis.

DA II *Dura, USA.*
Chlorpheniramine maleate (p.405·1); phenylephrine hydrochloride (p.1066·2); hyoscine methonitrate (p.463·1).
Upper respiratory-tract symptoms.

Dabonal *Vita, Spain.*
Enalapril maleate (p.863·2).
Heart failure; hypertension.

Dabonal Plus *Vita, Spain.*
Hydrochlorothiazide (p.885·2); enalapril maleate (p.863·2).
Hypertension.

Dabroson *Hoyer, Ger.†.*
Allopurinol (p.390·2).
Gout; hyperuricaemia.

Dacala *Tafir, Spain†.*
Amoxycillin (p.151·3).
Bacterial infections.

Dacef *Lennon, S.Afr.*
Cefadroxil (p.163·3).
Bacterial infections.

Dacoren *Nattermann, Ger.*
Co-dergocrine mesylate (p.1566·1).
Hypertension; mental function disorders.

Dacortilen *Meda, Swed.†.*
Prednylidene (p.1049·3).
Corticosteroid.

Dacortin *Merck, Spain.*
Prednisone (p.1049·2).
Corticosteroid.

Dacortin H *Merck, Spain.*
Prednisolone (p.1048·1).
Corticosteroid.

Dacovo *Tafir, Spain†.*
Cephazolin sodium (p.181·1).
Bacterial infections.

Dacrin
Merck Sharp & Dohme, Aust.; Chibret, Ger.
Hydrastinine hydrochloride; oxedrine tartrate (p.925·3).
Conjunctivitis.

Dacrine
Merck Sharp & Dohme-Chibret, Fr.†; Merck Sharp & Dohme, Switz.
Hydrastinine hydrochloride; oxedrine tartrate (p.925·3).
Eye irritation.

Dacriogel *Alcon, Ital.*
Carbomer (p.1471·2).
Dry eyes.

Dacriose *Iolab, USA.*
Electrolytes (p.1147·1).
Eye irrigation.

Dacriosol *Alcon, Ital.*
Eye drops: Dextran 70 (p.717·1); hypromellose (p.1473·1).
Eye ointment†: Liquid paraffin (p.1382·1); wool fat (p.1385·3); white soft paraffin (p.1382·3).
Dry eyes.

Dacrolux *Cusi, Spain.*
Dextran 70 (p.717·1); hypromellose (p.1473·1).
Dry eyes.

Dacryne *Martin, Fr.*
Hydrastinine hydrochloride; oxedrine tartrate (p.925·3); chlorhexidine gluconate (p.1107·2).
Conjunctivitis; eye irritation.

Dacryoboraline *Martin, Fr.*
Oxedrine tartrate (p.925·3); borax (p.1554·2); boric acid (p.1554·2).
Eye irritation.

Dacryolarmes *Martin, Fr.*
Methylcellulose 4000 (p.1473·3).
Dry eyes; protection during eye examinations.

Dacryoserum *Martin, Fr.*
Boric acid (p.1554·2); borax (p.1554·2); sodium chloride (p.1162·2).
Minor eye disorders.

Dactil *Marion Merrell Dow, Belg.†.*
Piperidolate hydrochloride (p.467·1); phenobarbitone (p.350·2).
Gastro-intestinal spasm.

Dafalgan
Upsamedica, Belg.; UPSA, Fr.; Upsamedica, Switz.
Paracetamol (p.72·2).
Fever; pain.

Dafalgan Codeine
Upsamedica, Belg.; UPSA, Fr.
Paracetamol (p.72·2); codeine phosphate (p.26·1).
Pain.

Daflon
Note. This name is used for preparations of different composition.
Bender, Aust.; Eutherapie, Belg.
Diosmin (p.1580·1); hesperidin (p.1580·2).
Haemorrhoids; peripheral vascular disorders.

Servier, Fr.
Bioflavonoids (p.1580·1).
Vascular disorders.

Servier, Ger.†.
Diosmin (p.1580·1); hesperidin (p.1580·2); flavonoids derived from orange peel.
Vascular disorders.

Servier, Ital.†; Servier, Spain; Servier, Switz.
Diosmin (p.1580·1).
Haemorrhoids; vascular disorders.

Daflon 500
Servier, Ital.; Servier, Spain; Servier, Switz.
Diosmin (p.1580·1); hesperidin (p.1580·2).
Haemorrhoids; venous insufficiency.

Dafnegil *Poli, Switz.*
Nifuratel (p.589·1); nystatin (p.386·1).
Balanitis; skin infections; vulvovaginal infections.

Dafnegin *Poli, Ital.*
Ciclopirox olamine (p.376·2).
Vulvovaginal and peri-anal candidiasis.

Dagan *Tedec Meiji, Spain.*
Nicardipine hydrochloride (p.915·1).
Angina pectoris; cerebrovascular disorders; hypertension.

Dagenan *Rhone-Poulenc Rorer, Canad.*
Sulphapyridine (p.256·3).
Bacterial infections.

Dagra Fluor *Asta Medica, Neth.*
Sodium fluoride (p.742·1).
Dental caries prophylaxis.

Dagracycline *Asta Medica, Neth.*
Doxycycline fosfatex (p.202·3).
Bacterial infections.

Dagramycine *Asta Medica, Belg.*
Doxycycline polyphosphate sodium (p.202·3).
Bacterial infections.

Dagravit A *Asta Medica, Belg.*
Vitamin A acetate (p.1359·2).
Vitamin A deficiency.

Dagravit A Forte *Asta Medica, Neth.*
Vitamin A acetate (p.1359·2).
Vitamin A deficiency.

Dagravit A-E *Asta Medica, Belg.*
Vitamin A palmitate (p.1359·2); *dl*-alpha tocopheryl acetate (p.1369·2).
Vitamin A and E deficiency.

Dagravit A-E Forte *Asta Medica, Neth.*
Vitamin A palmitate (p.1359·2); *dl*-alpha-tocopheryl acetate (p.1369·2).
Vitamin A and E deficiency.

Dagravit B-Complex
Asta Medica, Belg.; Dagra, Neth.†.
Vitamin B substances.
Vitamin B deficiency.

Dagravit B-Complex Forte *Asta Medica, Neth.*
Vitamin B substances; intrinsic factor.
Vitamin B deficiency.

Dagravit Becoforte *Dagra, Neth.†.*
Vitamin B substances.
Vitamin B deficiency.

Dagravit C *Asta Medica, Neth.†.*
Vitamin C (p.1365·2).
Vitamin C deficiency.

Dagravit D-Kalk *Dagra, Neth.†.*
Cholecalciferol (p.1366·3); calcium carbonate (p.1182·1).
Calcium or vitamin D deficiency.

Dagravit Totaal 8 *Asta Medica, Neth.*
Multivitamin preparation.

Dagravit Totaal 30 *Dagra, Neth.†.*
Multivitamin and mineral preparation.

Dagravit Total *Asta Medica, Belg.*
Multivitamin preparation with iron.

Dagravit Total 8 *Asta Medica, Belg.*
Multivitamin preparation.

Dagynil *Asta Medica, Neth.*
Conjugated oestrogens (p.1457·3).
Menopausal disorders; osteoporosis; prostatic cancer.

Daiet B *Humana, Ital.*
Fatty-acid, lipid, and vitamin preparation.
Nutritional supplement.

Daily Balance *Pharmavite, Canad.*
Multivitamin preparation.

Daily Care *Pfizer, USA.*
Zinc oxide (p.1096·2).

Daily Conditioning *Blistex, USA.*
SPF 15†: Padimate O (p.1488·1); oxybenzone (p.1487·3).
SPF 20: Ethylhexyl *p*-methoxycinnamate (p.1487·1); oxybenzone (p.1487·3).
Sunscreen.

Daily Gold Pack *Solgar, UK.*
Multivitamin and mineral preparation.

Daily Lip Protector *Retsews, USA.*
SPF 15: Padimate O (p.1488·1); oxybenzone (p.1487·3).
Sunscreen.

Daily Multi *Vitaplex, Austral.*
Multivitamin, mineral, and amino-acid preparation.

Daily-Vite *Rugby, USA.*
Multivitamin and mineral preparation with iron and folic acid.

Dairy Ease *Sterling, USA.*
Tilactase (p.1637·3).
Lactase insufficiency.

Dairyaid *Tanta, Canad.*
Tilactase (p.1637·3).
Lactase insufficiency.

Daisy *Advanced Care, USA.*
Pregnancy test (p.1621·2).

Daital *Alter, Spain†.*
Etersalate (p.35·3).
Fever; inflammation; pain; thrombo-embolism prophylaxis.

Daivonex
CSL, Austral.; Leo, Belg.; Leo, Fr.; Leo, Ger.; Formenti, Ital.; Leo, Neth.; Leo, Norw.; Farmacusi, Spain; Lovens, Swed.; Leo, Switz.
Calcipotriol (p.1080·2).
Psoriasis.

Dakar *Hoechst Marion Roussel, Belg.*
Lansoprazole (p.1196·2).
Gastro-oesophageal reflux; peptic ulcer.

Dakin *Cooperation Pharmaceutique, Fr.*
Sodium hypochlorite (p.1124·3).
Skin and mucous membrane disinfection.

Dakincooper *Rhone-Poulenc Rorer, Belg.*
Sodium hypochlorite (p.1124·3).
Skin and mucous membrane disinfection.

Dakryo Biciron *Basotherm, Ger.†.*
Bromhexine hydrochloride (p.1055·3).
Dry eye disorders.

Daktacort
Janssen-Cilag, Aust.; Janssen-Cilag, Belg.; Janssen-Cilag, Fr.; Janssen-Cilag, Irl.; Janssen-Cilag, Ital.†; Janssen-Cilag, Neth.; Janssen-Cilag, Norw.; Janssen-Cilag, S.Afr.; Janssen-Cilag, Swed.; Janssen-Cilag, Switz.; Janssen, UK.
Miconazole nitrate (p.384·3); hydrocortisone (p.1043·3).
Fungal and Gram-positive bacterial skin infections.

Daktar
Janssen-Cilag, Ger.; Janssen-Cilag, Norw.; Janssen-Cilag, Swed.; Janssen-Cilag, Switz.†.
Miconazole (p.384·3) or miconazole nitrate (p.384·3).
Fungal infections.

Daktar Duo *Janssen, Belg.†.*
Miconazole nitrate (p.384·3).
Fungal skin infections.

Daktar-Hydrocortison *Janssen-Cilag, Ger.†.*
Miconazole nitrate (p.384·3); hydrocortisone (p.1043·3).
Fungal infections with inflammation.

Daktarin
Janssen-Cilag, Aust.; Janssen-Cilag, Austral.; Janssen-Cilag, Belg.; Janssen-Cilag, Fr.; Janssen-Cilag, Irl.; Janssen-Cilag, Ital.; Janssen-Cilag, Neth.; Janssen-Cilag, S.Afr.; Esteve, Spain; Janssen-Cilag, Switz.; Janssen-Cilag, UK.
Miconazole (p.384·3) or miconazole nitrate (p.384·3).
Fungal and Gram-positive bacterial infections.

Daktozin
Janssen-Cilag, Austral.; Janssen-Cilag, Belg.
Miconazole nitrate (p.384·3); zinc oxide (p.1096·2).
Fungal skin infections.

Dalacin
Pharmacia Upjohn, Aust.; Pharmacia Upjohn, Irl.; Pharmacia Upjohn, Norw.; Upjohn, Spain; Pharmacia Upjohn, Swed.; Upjohn, UK.
Clindamycin hydrochloride (p.191·1), clindamycin palmitate hydrochloride (p.191·1), or clindamycin phosphate (p.191·1).
Bacterial infections.

Dalacin C
Pharmacia Upjohn, Austral.; Pharmacia Upjohn, Belg.; Pharmacia Upjohn, Canad.; Pharmacia Upjohn, Irl.; Pharmacia Upjohn, Ital.; Pharmacia Upjohn, Neth.; Pharmacia Upjohn, S.Afr.; Pharmacia Upjohn, Switz.; Upjohn, UK.
Clindamycin hydrochloride (p.191·1), clindamycin palmitate hydrochloride (p.191·1), or clindamycin phosphate (p.191·1).
Bacterial infections.

Dalacin T
Pharmacia Upjohn, Belg.; Pharmacia Upjohn, Canad.; Pharmacia Upjohn, Irl.; Pharmacia Upjohn, Ital.; Pharmacia Upjohn, Neth.; Pharmacia Upjohn, S.Afr.; Pharmacia Upjohn, Switz.; Upjohn, UK.
Clindamycin phosphate (p.191·1).
Acne.

Dalacin V
Pharmacia Upjohn, Austral.; Pharmacia Upjohn, Switz.
Clindamycin phosphate (p.191·1).
Bacterial vaginitis.

Dalacin Vaginal
Pharmacia Upjohn, Belg.; Pharmacia Upjohn, Canad.
Clindamycin phosphate (p.191·1).
Bacterial vaginosis.

Dalacin VC *Pharmacia Upjohn, S.Afr.*
Clindamycin phosphate (p.191·1).
Bacterial vaginosis.

Dalacine *Pharmacia Upjohn, Fr.*
Clindamycin hydrochloride (p.191·1) or clindamycin phosphate (p.191·1).
Bacterial infections.

Dalacine T *Pharmacia Upjohn, Fr.*
Clindamycin phosphate (p.191·1).
Acne.

Dalalone *Forest Pharmaceuticals, USA.*
Dexamethasone acetate (p.1037·1) or dexamethasone sodium phosphate (p.1037·2).
Corticosteroid.

Dalamon *Alter, Spain.*
Capsules: Cobamamide (p.1364·2); pyridoxine phosphate (p.1363·1); thiamine phosphate (p.1361·2).
Injection: Cyanocobalamin (p.1363·3); dexamethasone sodium diacid phosphate (p.1037·2); pyridoxine hydrochloride (p.1362·3); thiamine hydrochloride (p.1361·1).
Lignocaine hydrochloride (p.1293·2) is included in this preparation to alleviate the pain of injection.
Neuralgia; neuritis.

Dalcept *Cuprocept, S.Afr.*
Copper-wound plastic (p.1337·3).
Intra-uterine contraceptive device.

Dal-E *Dal-Vita, Austral.*
d-Alpha tocopheryl acetate (p.1369·2).
Burns; minor wounds; skin irritation.

Dalet-Balsam *Mauermann, Ger.*
Guaiacol (p.1061·2); methyl salicylate (p.55·2); belladonna (p.457·1); menthol (p.1600·2).
Hallux valgus; inflammation of big toe joint.

Dalfaz *Synthelabo Delagrange, Spain.*
Alfuzosin hydrochloride (p.817·2).
Benign prostatic hyperplasia.

Dalgan *Astra, USA.*
Dezocine (p.29·2).
Pain.

Dalgen *Recordati Elmu, Spain.*
Fepradinol hydrochloride (p.41·2).
Peri-articular disorders; soft-tissue disorders.

Dalinar *Essex, Spain.*
Netilmicin sulphate (p.231·1).
Bacterial infections.

Dalivit
Note. This name is used for preparations of different composition.
Samil, Ital.†.
Vitamin B substances; levoglutamide (p.1344·3); magnesium fructose-1,6-diphosphate.
Tonic.

Eastern Pharmaceuticals, UK.
Multivitamin preparation.

Dallergy *Laser, USA.*
Chlorpheniramine maleate (p.405·1); phenylephrine hydrochloride (p.1066·2); hyoscine methonitrate (p.463·1).
Upper respiratory-tract symptoms.

Dallergy-D *Laser, USA.*
Capsules: Pseudoephedrine hydrochloride (p.1068·3); chlorpheniramine maleate (p.405·1).
Syrup: Phenylephrine hydrochloride (p.1066·2); chlorpheniramine maleate (p.405·1).
Upper respiratory-tract symptoms.

Dallergy-JR *Laser, USA.*
Brompheniramine maleate (p.403·2); pseudoephedrine hydrochloride (p.1068·3).
Allergic rhinitis; nasal congestion.

Dalmadorm
Roche, Ger.; Roche, Ital.; Roche, Neth.; Roche, S.Afr.; Roche, Switz.
Flurazepam hydrochloride (p.672·2) or flurazepam monohydrochloride (p.672·2).
Insomnia.

Dalmane
Roche, Austral.†; Roche, Canad.; Roche, Irl.; Roche, UK; Roche, USA.
Flurazepam hydrochloride (p.672·2) or flurazepam monohydrochloride (p.672·2).
Insomnia.

Dalparan *Farma Lepori, Spain.*
Zolpidem tartrate (p.698·3).
Insomnia.

Dalsy *Knoll, Spain.*
Ibuprofen (p.44·1).
Fever; musculoskeletal, joint, and peri-articular disorders; pain.

Daluwal *Cascan, Ger.†.*
Rhubarb (p.1212·1); aloes (p.1177·1); cascara (p.1183·1); peppermint oil.
Constipation.

Daluwal Forte *Cascan, Ger.†.*
Rhubarb (p.1212·1); aloes (p.1177·1); cascara (p.1183·1); bisacodyl (p.1179·3); peppermint oil (p.1208·1).
Constipation.

Dam *Terapeutico, Ital.*
Damiana (p.1570·2); muira puama; santoreggia; kola (p.1645·1); cinnamon (p.1564·2).
Asthenia; impotence.

Damalax *Schering-Plough, Spain.*
Docusate sodium (p.1189·3); phenolphthalein (p.1208·2).
Constipation.

Damason-P *Mason, USA.*
Hydrocodone tartrate (p.43·1); aspirin (p.16·1).
Pain.

Damide *Benedetti, Ital.*
Indapamide (p.890·2).
Hypertension.

Damira *Wander Health Care, Switz.*
Preparation for enteral nutrition.
Cow's milk intolerance.

Damoxicil *Byk Elmu, Spain.*
Amoxycillin trihydrate (p.151·3).
Bacterial infections.

Damoxicil Mucolitico *Byk Elmu, Spain.*
Amoxycillin trihydrate (p.151·3); bromhexine hydrochloride (p.1055·3).
Respiratory-tract infections.

D-Amp *Dunhall, USA†.*
Ampicillin trihydrate (p.153·2).
Bacterial infections.

Dampo *Roche Nicholas, Neth.*
Nasal spray: Oxymetazoline hydrochloride (p.1065·3).
Nasal congestion.
Ointment for inhalation: Camphor (p.1557·2); menthol (p.1600·2); eucalyptus oil (p.1578·1).
Cold symptoms.

Dampo bij droge hoest *Roche Nicholas, Neth.*
Dextromethorphan hydrobromide (p.1057·3).
Coughs.

Dampo Mucopect *Roche Nicholas, Neth.*
Acetylcysteine (p.1052·3).
Respiratory-tract congestion.

Dampo "Solvopect" *Roche Nicholas, Neth.*
Carbocisteine (p.1056·3).
Respiratory-tract congestion.

Danatrol
Sanofi Winthrop, Belg.; Sanofi Winthrop, Fr.; Sanofi Winthrop, Ital.; Sanofi Winthrop, Neth.; Sanofi Winthrop, Spain; Sanofi Winthrop, Switz.
Danazol (p.1441·3).
Benign breast disorders; endometriosis; female infertility; hereditary angioedema; menorrhagia.

Danazant *Antigen, Irl.*
Danazol (p.1441·3).
Benign breast disorders; dysfunctional uterine bleeding; endometriosis; gynaecomastia.

Dancor Merck, Aust.; E. Merck, Neth.†; E. Merck, Switz.
Nicorandil (p.915·3).
Angina pectoris.

Dandruff Control Pert 2 in 1 Procter & Gamble, Austral.
Pyrithione zinc (p.1089·3).
Dandruff.

Dandruff Treatment Shampoo Sutton, Canad.
Pyrithione zinc (p.1089·3).

Daneral
Hoechst Marion Roussel, Irl.; Hoechst, UK†.
Pheniramine maleate (p.415·3).
Hypersensitivity reactions.

Dan-Gard
Faulding, Austral.; Stiefel, Canad.
Pyrithione zinc (p.1089·3).
Dandruff; seborrhoeic dermatitis.

Danilon Esteve, Spain.
Suxibuzone (p.88·2).
Musculoskeletal, joint, and peri-articular disorders.

Danka Angelini, Ital.
Levodropropizine (p.1059·2).
Coughs.

Danlene SIT, Ital.†.
Dantrolene sodium (p.1313·3).
Spastic disorders.

Danocrine
Sanofi Winthrop, Austral.; Sanofi Winthrop, Norw.; Sanofi, Swed.; Sanofi Winthrop, USA.
Danazol (p.1441·3).
Endometriosis; hereditary angioedema; mastalgia; menorrhagia.

Danokrin Sanofi Winthrop, Aust.
Danazol (p.1441·3).
Endometriosis; gynaecomastia; hereditary angioedema; precocious puberty.

Danol
Sanofi Winthrop, Irl.; Sanofi Winthrop, UK.
Danazol (p.1441·3).
Endometriosis; gynaecomastia; mastalgia; menstrual disorders; precocious puberty.

Dantamacrin
Procter & Gamble, Aust.; Procter & Gamble, Ger.; Procter & Gamble, Switz.
Dantrolene sodium (p.1313·3).
Skeletal muscle spasm; spasticity.

Dan-Tar Plus Stiefel, Canad.
Polytar (a blend of wood and mineral tars) (p.1092·2); pyrithione disulphide (p.1089·3).
Seborrhoeic dermatitis.

Dantrium
Pharmacia Upjohn, Austral.; Procter & Gamble, Belg.; Procter & Gamble, Canad.; Lipha Sante, Fr.; Procter & Gamble, Irl.; Formenti, Ital.; Procter & Gamble, Neth.; SmithKline Beecham, S.Afr.; Procter & Gamble, UK; Procter & Gamble, USA.
Dantrolene sodium (p.1313·3).
Malignant hyperthermia; skeletal muscle spasm; spasticity.

Danzen Takeda, Ital.
Serrapeptase (p.1628·3).
Inflammation; oedema.

Daonil
Hoechst Marion Roussel, Austral.; Hoechst Marion Roussel, Belg.; Hoechst, Fr.; Hoechst Marion Roussel, Irl.; Hoechst Marion Roussel, Ital.; Hoechst Marion Roussel, Neth.; Hoechst Marion Roussel, Norw.; Hoechst Marion Roussel, S.Afr.; Hoechst, Spain; Hoechst Marion Roussel, Swed.; Hoechst Marion Roussel, Switz.; Hoechst Marion Roussel, UK.
Glibenclamide (p.319·3).
Diabetes mellitus.

Dapa Ferndale, USA.
Paracetamol (p.72·2).
Fever; pain.

Dapacin Cold Ferndale, USA.
Phenylpropanolamine hydrochloride (p.1067·2); chlorpheniramine maleate (p.405·1); paracetamol (p.72·2).
Upper respiratory-tract symptoms.

Dapamax Parke-Med, S.Afr.
Indapamide (p.890·2).
Hypertension; oedema.

Dapa-tabs Alphapharm, Austral.
Indapamide (p.890·2).
Hypertension.

Dapaz Alter, Spain.
Meprobamate (p.678·1).
Anxiety; insomnia; skeletal muscle spasm.

Dapotum
Bristol-Myers Squibb, Aust.; Bristol-Myers Squibb, Ger.; Sanofi Winthrop, Ger.; Bristol-Myers Squibb, Switz.
Fluphenazine hydrochloride (p.671·3) or fluphenazine decanoate (p.671·2).
Psychoses.

Daptazile Roche, Ger.†.
Amiphenazole hydrochloride (p.1477·3).
Respiratory insufficiency.

Daptazole Aspro-Nicholas, Aust.†.
Amiphenazole hydrochloride (p.1477·3).
Respiratory disorders.

Daptril Xeragen, S.Afr.
Indapamide (p.890·2).
Hypertension.

Daraclor Glaxo Wellcome, S.Afr.†.
Pyrimethamine (p.436·3); chloroquine sulphate (p.426·3).
Malaria.

Daral Noristan Generica, S.Afr.†.
Aminophylline (p.748·1); ephedrine hydrochloride (p.1059·3); amylobarbitone (p.641·3).
Asthma; bronchitis; bronchopneumonia.

Daralix Hoechst Marion Roussel, S.Afr.
Promethazine hydrochloride (p.416·2).
Hypersensitivity reactions; nausea; vomiting.

Daramal Glaxo Wellcome, S.Afr.
Chloroquine sulphate (p.426·3).
Discoid lupus erythematosus; malaria; rheumatoid arthritis.

Daranide
Sigma, Austral.; Merck Sharp & Dohme, Irl.; Merck Sharp & Dohme, UK†; Merck Sharp & Dohme, USA.
Dichlorphenamide (p.848·2).
Glaucoma.

Daraprim
Glaxo Wellcome, Aust.; Glaxo Wellcome, Austral.; Glaxo Wellcome, Belg.; Glaxo Wellcome, Canad.; Glaxo Wellcome, Ger.; Wellcome, Irl.; Glaxo Wellcome, Neth.; Glaxo Wellcome, S.Afr.; Wellcome, Spain; Glaxo Wellcome, Swed.†; Wellcome, Switz.; Wellcome, UK; Glaxo Wellcome, USA.
Pyrimethamine (p.436·3).
Malaria; toxoplasmosis.

Dardex Llorente, Spain.
Captopril (p.836·3).
Diabetic nephropathy; heart failure; hypertension; myocardial infarction.

Dardum Lisapharma, Ital.
Cefoperazone sodium (p.167·3).
Lignocaine hydrochloride (p.1293·2) is included in the intramuscular injection to alleviate the pain of injection.
Bacterial infections.

Darebon
Ciba-Geigy, Aust.; Ciba, Ger.
Chlorthalidone (p.839·3); reserpine (p.942·1).
Hypertension.

Daren Antibioticos, Spain†.
Cephazolin sodium (p.181·1); cephazolin dibenzylamine (p.181·2).
Lignocaine hydrochloride (p.1293·2) is included in this preparation to alleviate the pain of injection.
Bacterial infections.

Dari Vita Elan, Spain.
Nifedipine (p.916·2).
Angina pectoris; hypertension.

Daricol Pfizer, Swed.†.
Oxyphencyclimine hydrochloride (p.466·3).
Gastro-intestinal disorders.

Daricon
Roerig, Belg.†; Pfizer, Neth.†.
Oxyphencyclimine hydrochloride (p.466·3).
Irritable bowel syndrome; peptic ulcer.

Darkene Bayer, Ital.
Flunitrazepam (p.670·1).
Insomnia.

Darlin Sandipro, Belg.
Senna fruit (p.1212·2).
Constipation.

Darmen Salt Ern, Spain.
Magnesium sulphate (p.1157·3); sodium bicarbonate (p.1153·2); dibasic sodium phosphate (p.1159·3); sodium sulphate (p.1213·3).
Constipation; dyspepsia.

Darmol
Note. This name is used for preparations of different composition.
Schmidgall, Aust.; Iromedica, Switz.
Senna (p.1212·2).
Bowel evacuation; constipation.

Omegin, Ger.
Phenolphthalein (p.1208·2).
Constipation.

Darmol Bisacodyl Omegin, Ger.
Bisacodyl (p.1179·3).
Constipation.

Daro SmithKline Beecham Consumer, Neth.†.
Paracetamol (p.72·2).
Fever; pain.

Daro Hoofdpijnpoeders SmithKline Beecham Consumer, Neth.
Paracetamol (p.72·2); propyphenazone (p.81·3); caffeine (p.749·3).
Headache.

Daro Thijm SmithKline Beecham Consumer, Neth.
Thyme (p.1636·3).
Coughs.

Darob
Knoll, Ger.; Meda, Swed.
Sotalol hydrochloride (p.945·1).
Arrhythmias.

Darocet SmithKline Beecham Consumer, Neth.†.
Paracetamol (p.72·2).
Fever; pain.

Darocillin Hoechst Marion Roussel, S.Afr.
Phenoxymethylpenicillin potassium (p.236·2).
Bacterial infections.

Darolan Hoestprikkeldempende SmithKline Beecham Consumer, Neth.
Dextromethorphan hydrobromide (p.1057·3).
Coughs.

Darolan Slijmplossende SmithKline Beecham Consumer, Neth.
Bromhexine hydrochloride (p.1055·3).
Respiratory-tract disorders with viscous mucus.

Daromide Noristan Generica, S.Afr.†.
Mercurochrome (p.1119·2); sulphanilamide (p.256·3); acriflavine (p.1098·3); cod-liver oil (p.1337·3).
Skin infections; wounds.

Daronvite Pharmalab, S.Afr.†.
Vitamin B substances.

Darosed Hoechst Marion Roussel, S.Afr.
Promethazine hydrochloride (p.416·2); codeine phosphate (p.26·1); ephedrine hydrochloride (p.1059·3).
Coughs.

Darrow-Liq Brunel, S.Afr.
Sodium chloride; potassium chloride; sodium citrate dihydrate; glucose (p.1152·3).
Oral rehydration therapy.

Darrowped Pharmacare Consumer, S.Afr.
Potassium chloride; sodium chloride; sodium citrate; glucose (p.1152·3).
Diarrhoea; oral rehydration therapy.

Daruma Cyanamid, Ital.
Idebenone (p.1590·2).
Mental and movement disturbances associated with cerebrovascular disorders.

Darvilen Schering, Ital.†.
Cefotetan disodium (p.170·1).
Bacterial infections.

Darvocet-N Lilly, USA.
Dextropropoxyphene napsylate (p.27·3); paracetamol (p.72·2).
Fever; pain.

Darvon
Lilly, Spain; Lilly, USA.
Dextropropoxyphene hydrochloride (p.27·3).
Pain.

Darvon Compound Lilly, USA.
Dextropropoxyphene hydrochloride (p.27·3); aspirin (p.16·1); caffeine (p.749·3).
Fever; pain.

Darvon-N
Lilly, Canad.; Lilly, USA.
Dextropropoxyphene napsylate (p.27·3).
Fever; pain.

Darvon-N with ASA Lilly, Canad.†.
Dextropropoxyphene napsylate (p.27·3); aspirin (p.16·1).
Fever; pain.

Darvon-N Compound Lilly, Canad.†.
Dextropropoxyphene napsylate (p.27·3); aspirin (p.16·1); caffeine (p.749·3).
Fever; pain.

Dasen Takeda, Jpn.
Serrapeptase (p.1628·3).
Inflammation; respiratory-tract congestion.

Dasin SmithKline Beecham Consumer, USA†.
Aspirin (p.16·1); caffeine (p.749·3); atropine sulphate (p.455·1); ipecacuanha (p.1062·2); camphor (p.1557·2).
Pain.

Daskil
Sandoz, Aust.; LPB, Ital.
Terbinafine hydrochloride (p.387·3).
Fungal skin and nail infections.

Dasovas Pharmacia Upjohn, Ital.†.
Defibrotide (p.847·1).
Thrombo-embolic disorders.

Dastosin Yamanouchi, Spain.
Dimemorfan phosphate (p.1058·3).
Coughs.

Dasuen Knoll, Spain†.
Temazepam (p.693·3).
Anxiety; insomnia.

Datolan Faes, Spain.
Zopiclone (p.699·2).
Insomnia.

Datron Allen, Spain†.
Ondansetron hydrochloride (p.1206·2).
Nausea and vomiting induced by cytotoxics or radiotherapy.

Daunoblastin
Pharmacia Upjohn, Aust.; Pharmacia Upjohn, Ger.; Pharmacia Upjohn, S.Afr.
Daunorubicin hydrochloride (p.528·1).
Acute leukaemias.

Daunoblastina
Pharmacia Upjohn, Ital.; Kenfarma, Spain.
Daunorubicin hydrochloride (p.528·1).
Leukaemias; non-Hodgkins lymphomas.

DaunoXome
Laevosan, Aust.; Nexstar, Belg.; Nexstar, Ital.; Nextar, Neth.; Swedish Orphan, Swed.; Nexstar, UK; Nexstar, USA.
Daunorubicin (p.528·2), daunorubicin citrate (p.528·2), or daunorubicin hydrochloride (p.528·1).
HIV-related Kaposi's sarcoma.

Davasal Sandoz, Ital.†.
Sodium-free dietary salt substitute.

Davenol Whitehall, UK†.
Carbinoxamine maleate (p.404·2); ephedrine hydrochloride (p.1059·3); pholcodine (p.1068·1).
Coughs.

Daverium Poli, Ital.
α-Dihydroergocryptine mesylate (p.1571·3).
Age-related mental and movement disorders; headache; hyperprolactinaemia; lactation inhibition; migraine; parkinsonism.

David Morton's Quintessential Lifeplan, UK.
A range of multivitamin and mineral supplements.

Davitamon AD Chefaro, Neth.†.
Retinol palmitate (p.1359·2); cholecalciferol (p.1366·3).

Davitamon AD Fluor Chefaro, Neth.†.
Retinol palmitate (p.1359·2); cholecalciferol (p.1366·3); sodium fluoride (p.742·1).
Dental caries prophylaxis; rickets.

Davitamon C Chefaro, Neth.†.
Ascorbic acid (p.1365·2).

Davurmicin Belmac, Spain†.
Benzylpenicillin sodium (p.159·3); procaine penicillin (p.240·2); benzathine penicillin (p.158·3).
Bacterial infections.

Day Cold Comfort Boots, UK.
Paracetamol (p.72·2); pseudoephedrine hydrochloride (p.1068·3); pholcodine (p.1068·1).
Cold symptoms.

Day & Night Warner-Lambert, Irl.
15 Tablets, paracetamol (p.72·2); phenylpropanolamine hydrochloride (p.1067·2); 5 tablets, paracetamol; diphenhydramine hydrochloride (p.409·1).
Cold and influenza symptoms.

Day and Night Cold and Flu Warner-Lambert, Austral.
White/green capsules, paracetamol (p.72·2); pseudoephedrine hydrochloride (p.1068·3); dextromethorphan hydrobromide (p.1057·3); white/red capsules, paracetamol; dextromethorphan hydrobromide; chlorpheniramine maleate (p.405·1).
Cold and influenza symptoms.

Day Nurse
Note. This name is used for preparations of different composition.
SmithKline Beecham Consumer, Irl.; SmithKline Beecham Consumer, UK.
Capsules: Paracetamol (p.72·2); dextromethorphan hydrobromide (p.1057·3); phenylpropanolamine hydrochloride (p.1067·2).
Cold symptoms.

SmithKline Beecham Consumer, UK.
Oral liquid: Paracetamol (p.72·2); dextromethorphan hydrobromide (p.1057·3); phenylpropanolamine hydrochloride (p.1067·2); ascorbic acid (p.1365·2).
Cold symptoms.

Dayalets Abbott, USA.
Multivitamin preparation.

Dayalets + Iron Abbott, USA.
Multivitamin preparation with iron and folic acid.

Dayamineral Abbott, Spain.
Multivitamin and mineral preparation.

Daypro Searle, USA.
Oxaprozin (p.71·2).
Osteoarthritis; rheumatoid arthritis.

Dayquil Procter & Gamble, Canad.
Pseudoephedrine hydrochloride (p.1068·3); dextromethorphan hydrobromide (p.1057·3); paracetamol (p.72·2).
Cold and influenza symptoms.

Dayquil Sinus with Pain Relief Procter & Gamble, Canad.
Pseudoephedrine hydrochloride (p.1068·3); ibuprofen (p.44·1).

Daytime Cold & Flu Stanley, Canad.
Pseudoephedrine hydrochloride (p.1068·3); dextromethorphan hydrobromide (p.1057·3); guaiphenesin (p.1061·3); paracetamol (p.72·2).

Dayto Himbin Dayton, USA.
Yohimbine hydrochloride (p.1645·3).

Dayto Sulf Dayton, USA.
Sulphathiazole (p.257·1); sulphacetamide (p.252·2); sulfabenzamide (p.251·1); urea (p.1095·2).
Vaginitis due to Gardnerella vaginalis.

Dayto-Anase Dayton, USA.
Bromelains (p.1555·1).

Daywear Estee Lauder, Canad.
SPF 15: Ethylhexyl *p*-methoxycinnamate (p.1487·1); titanium dioxide (p.1093·3).
Sunscreen.

Dazamide Major, USA.
Acetazolamide (p.810·3).
Epilepsy; glaucoma; oedema; symptoms associated with acute mountain sickness.

Dazen Takeda, Fr.
Serrapeptase (p.1628·3).
Oedema; respiratory-tract congestion.

DC Softgels Goldline, USA.
Docusate calcium (p.1189·3).
Constipation.

DCCK Rentschler, Ger.
Co-dergocrine mesylate (p.1566·1).
Cerebral and peripheral vascular disorders; cervical disc syndrome; hypertension; migraine; shock.

DCP 340 Parke, Davis, Austral.†.
Calcium hydrogen phosphate (p.1155·3).
Calcium and phosphorus deficiency disorders.

D-Cure SMB, Belg.
Cholecalciferol (p.1366·3).
Dietary supplement; hypoparathyroidism; pseudohypoparathyroidism; vitamin D deficiency.

DDAVP
Ferring, Canad.; Ferring, Ger.; Akromed, S.Afr.†; Ferring, UK; Rhone-Poulenc Rorer, USA.
Desmopressin (p.1245·1) or desmopressin acetate (p.1245·2).
Diabetes insipidus; haemophilia; headache resulting from lumbar puncture; nocturnal enuresis; polyuria; test of fibrinolytic response; test of renal concentrating capacity; von Willebrand's disease.

DDD
Note. This name is used for preparations of different composition.
Austroplant, Aust.
Lotion: Salicylic acid (p.1090·2); chlorbutol (p.1106·3); methyl salicylate (p.55·2); thymol (p.1127·1); with or without phenol (p.1121·2).
Lotion, extra strong: Salicylic acid (p.1090·2); chlorbutol (p.1106·3); methyl salicylate (p.55·2); thymol (p.1127·1); phenol (p.1121·2).
Ointment: Salicylic acid (p.1090·2); chlorbutol (p.1106·3); methyl salicylate (p.55·2); thymol (p.1127·1); camphor (p.1557·2).
Skin disorders.
delta pronatura, Ger.
Thymol (p.1127·1); salicylic acid (p.1090·2); methyl salicylate (p.55·2).
Skin disorders.
DDD, UK.
Cream: Thymol (p.1127·1); menthol (p.1600·2); methyl salicylate (p.55·2); chlorbutol (p.1106·3); titanium dioxide (p.1093·3).
Lotion: Thymol (p.1127·1); menthol (p.1600·2); salicylic acid (p.1090·2); chlorbutol (p.1106·3); methyl salicylate (p.55·2).
Skin disorders.

De Icin *Asta Medica, Belg.*
Dexamethasone sodium metasulphobenzoate (p.1037·2); neomycin sulphate (p.229·2); polymyxin B sulphate (p.239·1).
Infected eye disorders.

De Icol *Asta Medica, Belg.*
Dexamethasone sodium phosphate (p.1037·2); chloramphenicol (p.182·1).
Infected eye disorders.

De Oxin *Berenguer Infale, Spain†.*
Etofylline nicotinate (p.753·1).
Dyspnoea.

de STAT *Sherman, USA.*
Range of solutions for contact lenses.

De Witt's Analgesic *De Witt, UK.*
Paracetamol (p.72·2); caffeine (p.749·3).
Fever; pain.

De Witt's Antacid
Note. This name is used for preparations of different composition.
Fleet, Austral.
Oral powder: Magnesium trisilicate (p.1199·1); magnesium carbonate (p.1198·1); calcium carbonate (p.1182·1); sodium bicarbonate (p.1153·2); kaolin (p.1195·1); aluminium hydroxide (p.1177·3).
Tablets: Magnesium trisilicate (p.1199·1); magnesium carbonate (p.1198·1); calcium carbonate (p.1182·1); sodium bicarbonate (p.1153·2); aluminium hydroxide (p.1177·3).
Gastro-intestinal hyperacidity.
De Witt, UK.
Oral powder: Magnesium trisilicate (p.1199·1); light magnesium carbonate (p.1198·1); calcium carbonate (p.1182·1); sodium bicarbonate (p.1153·2); light kaolin (p.1195·1); peppermint oil (p.1208·1).
Tablets: Calcium carbonate (p.1182·1); magnesium carbonate (p.1198·1); magnesium trisilicate (p.1199·1); peppermint oil (p.1208·1).
Gastro-intestinal hyperacidity.

De Witt's Lozenges *De Witt, UK.*
Benzocaine (p.1286·2); cetylpyridinium chloride (p.1106·2).
Formerly contained tyrothricin, benzocaine, and cetylpyridinium chloride.
Sore throat.

De Witt's Pills *Fleet, Austral.*
Bearberry (p.1552·2); buchu (p.1555·2); caffeine (p.749·3); methylene blue (p.984·3).
Fluid retention.

Deacura *Dermapharm, Ger.*
Biotin (p.1336·1).
Biotin deficiency.

Deadyn *Boehringer Ingelheim, Ital.†.*
Pemoline (p.1484·1); levoglutamide (p.1344·3).
Tonic.

Deaftol avec lidocaine *Roche, Switz.*
Aluminium lactate (p.1548·1); lignocaine hydrochloride (p.1293·2).
Mouth and throat disorders.

Dealgic *Poli, Ital.*
Diclofenac sodium (p.31·2).
Inflammation; musculoskeletal and joint disorders; pain.

Dealyd *Rosch & Handel, Aust.*
Polyphloroglucinol phosphate (p.1089·3).
Skin disorders.

Deanxit
Lundbeck, Aust.; Lundbeck, Belg.; Lundbeck, Ital.; Lundbeck, Spain; Lundbeck, Switz.
Flupenthixol hydrochloride (p.670·3); melitracen hydrochloride (p.296·3).
Anxiety; depression.

Debax *Gebro, Aust.*
Captopril (p.836·3).
Diabetic nephropathy; heart failure; hypertension; myocardial infarction.

Debekacyl *Bellon, Fr.*
Dibekacin sulphate (p.201·3).
Bacterial infections.

Debizima *Miba, Ital.†.*
Muramidase (p.1604·3).
Viral infections.

Deblaston
Madaus, Aust.; Madaus, Ger.; Byk Madaus, S.Afr.; Madaus, Switz.
Pipemidic acid (p.237·2).
Bacterial infections of the urinary tract.

Debridat
Croma, Aust.; Jouveinal, Fr.; Sigma-Tau, Ital.; Uhlmann-Eyraud, Switz.
Trimebutine (p.1639·3) or trimebutine maleate (p.1639·3).
Gastro-intestinal disorders.

Debridat Enzimatico *Sigma-Tau, Ital.†.*
Trimebutine maleate (p.1639·3); dehydrocholic acid (p.1570·2); pancreatin (p.1612·1); bromelains (p.1555·1); dimethicone (p.1213·1).
Gastro-intestinal disorders.

Debripad *Pharmacia, Neth.†.*
Dextranomer (p.1081·1).
Infected wounds.

Debrisan
Johnson & Johnson, Austral.†; Pharmacia Upjohn, Belg.; Pharmacia Upjohn, Canad.; Pharmacia Upjohn, Fr.; Pharmacia Upjohn, Irl.; Pharmacia Upjohn, Ital.; Pharmacia Upjohn, Neth.; Pharmacia Upjohn, S.Afr.; Pharmacia Upjohn, Swed.; Pharmacia Upjohn, Switz.; Pharmacia, UK; Johnson & Johnson, USA.
Beads: Dextranomer (p.1081·1).
Burns; skin ulcers; wounds.
Pharmacia, UK.
Topical paste; dressing: Dextranomer (p.1081·1); polyethylene glycol.
Wounds.

Debrisorb
Pharmacia Upjohn, Aust.; Pharmacia Upjohn, Ger.
Dextranomer (p.1081·1).
Wounds.

Debrox
Farmila, Ital.; Marion Merrell Dow, USA.
Urea hydrogen peroxide (p.1127·3).
Ear wax removal.

Debrum *Sigma-Tau, Ital.*
Trimebutine maleate (p.1639·3); medazepam (p.677·3).
Gastro-intestinal spasm with a component of anxiety.

Debrumyl *Pierre Fabre, Fr.*
Deanol pidolate (p.1478·2); heptaminol hydrochloride (p.1587·2).
Tonic.

Deca *Medinova, Switz.*
Aluminium chloride (p.1078·3); lignocaine hydrochloride (p.1293·2); cetalkonium chloride (p.1105·2); menthol (p.1600·2).
Mouth and throat disorders.

Decabis *Gazzoni, Ital.†.*
Dequalinium chloride (p.1112·1).
Oral infections.

Decacef *Boniscontro & Gazzone, Ital.*
Cefmetazole sodium (p.166·2).
Lignocaine hydrochloride (p.1293·2) is included in this preparation to alleviate the pain of injection.
Bacterial infections.

Decaderm in Estergel *Merck Sharp & Dohme, USA†.*
Dexamethasone (p.1037·1).
Skin disorders.

Decadran *Merck Sharp & Dohme, Spain.*
Dexamethasone (p.1037·1), dexamethasone phosphate (p.1037·2), or dexamethasone sodium phosphate (p.1037·2).
Corticosteroid.

Decadran Neomicina *Merck Sharp & Dohme, Spain.*
Dexamethasone phosphate (p.1037·2); neomycin sulphate (p.229·2).
Eye or ear disorders.

Decadron
Merck Sharp & Dohme, Aust.†; Merck Sharp & Dohme, Austral.; Merck Sharp & Dohme, Belg.; Merck Sharp & Dohme, Canad.; Merck Sharp & Dohme-Chibret, Fr.; Chibret, Ger.†; Merck Sharp & Dohme, Irl.; Merck Sharp & Dohme, Ital.; Merck Sharp & Dohme, Neth.; Merck Sharp & Dohme, Norw.; Merck Sharp & Dohme, S.Afr.; Merck Sharp & Dohme, Swed.; Merck Sharp & Dohme, Switz.; Merck Sharp & Dohme, UK.
Dexamethasone (p.1037·1) or dexamethasone sodium phosphate (p.1037·2).
Corticosteroid.

Decadron a la neomycine *Merck Sharp & Dohme, Switz.†.*
Dexamethasone sodium phosphate (p.1037·2); neomycin sulphate (p.229·2).
Infected eye and ear disorders.

Decadron avec Neomycine *Merck Sharp & Dohme, Belg.*
Dexamethasone sodium phosphate (p.1037·2); neomycin sulphate (p.229·2).
Infected eye and external ear disorders.

Decadron cum neomycin *Merck Sharp & Dohme, Swed.*
Dexamethasone sodium phosphate (p.1037·2); neomycin sulphate (p.229·2).
Infected eye and ear disorders.

Decadron Depot *Merck Sharp & Dohme, Neth.†.*
Dexamethasone acetate (p.1037·1).
Corticosteroid.

Decadron met neomycine *Chibret, Neth.*
Dexamethasone sodium phosphate (p.1037·2); neomycin sulphate (p.229·2).
Infected eye and ear disorders.

Decadron mit Neomycin *Merck Sharp & Dohme, Aust.†.*
Dexamethasone sodium phosphate (p.1037·2); neomycin sulphate (p.229·2).

Decadron Phosphat *Merck Sharp & Dohme, Ger.*
Dexamethasone phosphate (p.1037·2).
Corticosteroid.

Deca-Durabol *Organon, Swed.*
Nandrolone decanoate (p.1452·2).
Anabolic.

Deca-Durabolin
Organon, Aust.; Organon, Austral.; Organon, Belg.; Organon, Canad.; Organon, Fr.†; Organon, Ger.; Organon, Irl.; Organon, Ital.; Organon, Neth.; Organon, Norw.; Donmed, S.Afr.; Organon, Spain; Organon, Switz.; Organon, UK; Organon, USA.
Nandrolone decanoate (p.1452·2).
Anabolic; anaemia; breast cancer; osteoporosis; renal failure.

Decafar *Lafare, Ital.*
Ubidecarenone (p.1641·2).
Cardiac disorders.

Decafen *Rolab, S.Afr.*
Fluphenazine decanoate (p.671·2).
Psychoses.

Decagen *Goldline, USA.*
Multivitamin and mineral preparation with iron and folic acid.

Decaject *Mayrand, USA.*
Dexamethasone acetate (p.1037·1) or dexamethasone sodium phosphate (p.1037·2).
Corticosteroid.

Decal *Rice Steele, Irl.*
Calcium lactate (p.1155·2); calcium gluconate (p.1155·2); calcium phosphate (p.1155·3); ergocalciferol (p.1367·1).
Calcium deficiencies; calcium supplement.

Decalcit *Geistlich, Switz.*
Ergocalciferol (p.1367·1); calcium hydrogen phosphate (p.1155·3).
Calcium and vitamin D deficiencies.

Decapeptyl
Sigmapharm, Aust.; Ipsen, Belg.; IPSEN Biotech, Fr.; Ferring, Ger.; Tosse, Ger.; Ipsen, Irl.; Ipsen, Ital.; Ferring, Neth.; Adcock Ingram, S.Afr.; Lasa, Spain; Ferring, Swed.; Ferring, Switz.; Speywood, UK.
Triptorelin (p.1262·2), triptorelin acetate (p.1262·2), or triptorelin embonate (p.1262·2).
Breast cancer; endometriosis; female infertility; ovarian cancer; precocious puberty; prostatic cancer; uterine fibroids.

Decaprednil *Nycomed, Ger.*
Prednisolone (p.1048·1) or prednisolone acetate (p.1048·1).
Parenteral corticosteroid.

Decarene *Recordati, Ital.†.*
Ubidecarenone (p.1641·2).
Cardiac disorders.

Decasept *Streuli, Switz.*
Dequalinium chloride (p.1112·1); calcium pantothenate (p.1352·3); ammonium gualenate; laureth 9 (p.1325·2).
Mouth and throat disorders.

Decasona *Alter, Spain.*
Beclomethasone dipropionate (p.1032·1).
Asthma.

Decasone *Intramed, S.Afr.*
Dexamethasone phosphate (p.1037·2).
Corticosteroid.

Decaspir *Pulitzer, Ital.†.*
Fenspiride hydrochloride (p.1579·3).
Respiratory-tract disorders.

Decaspray *Merck Sharp & Dohme, USA†.*
Dexamethasone (p.1037·1).
Skin disorders.

Decatylene *Mepha, Switz.*
Dequalinium chloride (p.1112·1).
Mouth and throat disorders.

Decatylene Neo *Mepha, Switz.*
Dequalinium chloride (p.1112·1); cinchocaine hydrochloride (p.1289·2).
Mouth and throat disorders.

Decavit *Rowa, Irl.*
Multivitamin preparation.

Decazate *Berk, UK†.*
Fluphenazine decanoate (p.671·2).

Decentan
Merck, Aust.; Merck, Ger.; Merck, Spain.
Perphenazine (p.685·2) or perphenazine enanthate (p.685·3).
Anxiety disorders; depression; nausea; psychoses; vomiting.

Decholin *Miles, USA.*
Dehydrocholic acid (p.1570·2).
Constipation.

Deciclina *Farmades, Ital.†.*
Demeclocycline (p.201·2); multivitamins.
Bacterial infections; protozoal infections; rickettsial infections.

Decima Nil *ICN, Spain†.*
Magnesium aminobutyrate; paracetamol (p.72·2); passion flower (p.1615·3).
Fever; pain.

Decipar *Italfarmaco, Spain.*
Enoxaparin sodium (p.864·2).
Thrombo-embolism prophylaxis.

Declinax
Roche, Irl.†; Cambridge, UK.
Debrisoquine sulphate (p.846·2).
Now known as Debrisoquine Tablets in the *UK.*
Hypertension.

Decloban *Farmacusi, Spain.*
Clobetasol propionate (p.1035·2).
Skin disorders.

Declomycin
Wyeth-Ayerst, Canad.; Lederle, USA.
Demeclocycline hydrochloride (p.201·2).
Bacterial infections; intestinal amoebiasis.

Decme *Zyma, Ger.†.*
Dihydroergocristine mesylate (p.1571·3).
Cerebrovascular disorders.

Decoderm
Merck, Aust.; Merck-Belgolabo, Belg.; Hermal, Ger.; Boots Healthcare, Neth.; Merck, Spain; Hermal, Switz.
Fluprednidene acetate (p.1042·2).
Skin disorders.

Decoderm Base *Hermal, Switz.*
Emollient.
Skin disorders.

Decoderm Basiscreme *Hermal, Ger.*
Emollient.
Skin disorders.

Decoderm bivalent *Hermal, Switz.*
Fluprednidene acetate (p.1042·2); miconazole nitrate (p.384·3).
Infected skin disorders.

Decoderm Comp
Merck-Belgolabo, Belg.; Hermal, Ger.
Fluprednidene acetate (p.1042·2); gentamicin sulphate (p.212·1).
Infected skin disorders.

Decoderm compositum
Merck, Aust.; Hermal, Switz.†.
Fluprednidene acetate (p.1042·2); gentamicin sulphate (p.212·1).
Infected skin disorders.

Decoderm tri *Hermal, Ger.*
Fluprednidene acetate (p.1042·2); miconazole nitrate (p.384·3).
Infected skin disorders.

Decoderm trivalent
Merck, Aust.; Hermal, Ger.†; E. Merck, Switz.†.
Fluprednidene acetate (p.1042·2); gentamicin sulphate (p.212·1); cloxyquin (p.215·3).
Infected skin disorders.

Decoderm Trivalente *Merck, Spain.*
Fluprednidene acetate (p.1042·2); neomycin sulphate (p.229·2); cloxyquin (p.215·3).
Infected skin disorders.

Decofed *Barre-National, USA; Major, USA.*
Pseudoephedrine hydrochloride (p.1068·3).
Nasal congestion.

Decofluor *Salfa, Ital.†.*
Dexamethasone (p.1037·1).
Oral corticosteroid.

Decohistine DH *Morton Grove, USA.*
Pseudoephedrine hydrochloride (p.1068·3); chlorpheniramine maleate (p.405·1); codeine phosphate (p.26·1).
Coughs and cold symptoms.

Decohistine Expectorant *Morton Grove, USA.*
Guaiphenesin (p.1061·3); pseudoephedrine hydrochloride (p.1068·3); codeine phosphate (p.26·1).

Decon *Noristan Generica, S.Afr.†.*
Paracetamol (p.72·2); phenylephrine hydrochloride (p.1066·2); phenyltoloxamine citrate (p.416·1); caffeine (p.749·3); chlorpheniramine maleate (p.405·1).
Upper respiratory-tract disorders.

Deconamine *Kenwood, USA.*
Chlorpheniramine maleate (p.405·1); pseudoephedrine hydrochloride (p.1068·3).
Nasal congestion.

Deconamine CX *Bradley, USA.*
Guaiphenesin (p.1061·3); hydrocodone tartrate (p.43·1); pseudoephedrine hydrochloride (p.1068·3).
Coughs.

Decongene *Ravasini, Ital.†.*
Paracetamol (p.72·2); mepyramine maleate (p.414·1); phenylpropanolamine hydrochloride (p.1067·2); caffeine (p.749·3).
Nasal congestion.

Decongestabs *Parmed, USA.*
Phenylpropanolamine hydrochloride (p.1067·2); phenylephrine hydrochloride (p.1066·2); chlorpheniramine maleate (p.405·1); phenyltoloxamine citrate (p.416·1).
Upper respiratory-tract symptoms.

Decongestant
Note. This name is used for preparations of different composition.
Moore, USA.
Phenylpropanolamine hydrochloride (p.1067·2); phenylephrine hydrochloride (p.1066·2); chlorpheniramine maleate (p.405·1); phenyltoloxamine citrate (p.416·1).
Upper respiratory-tract symptoms.
Rugby, USA.
Phenylephrine hydrochloride (p.1066·2); paracetamol (p.72·2); chlorpheniramine maleate (p.405·1).
Upper respiratory-tract symptoms.

Decongestant Antihistaminic Syrup *Pharmascience, Canad.*
Brompheniramine maleate (p.403·2); phenylephrine hydrochloride (p.1066·2); phenylpropanolamine hydrochloride (p.1067·2).
Antihistamine; decongestant.

Decongestant Cough Elixir *Nyal, Austral.†.*
Pseudoephedrine hydrochloride (p.1068·3); codeine phosphate (p.26·1); potassium guaiacolsulfonate

(p.1068·3); ammonium chloride; creosote; squill; eucalyptus oil; menthol; honey; glycerol.
Coughs and cold symptoms.

Decongestant Cough Elixir Junior *Nyal, Austral.†.*
Pseudoephedrine hydrochloride (p.1068·3); pholcodine (p.1068·1); potassium guaiacolsulfonate (p.1068·3); ammonium chloride; creosote; squill; eucalyptus oil; menthol; glycerol.
Coughs and cold symptoms.

Decongestant Expectorant *Schein, USA.*
Pseudoephedrine hydrochloride (p.1068·3); guaiphenesin (p.1061·3); codeine phosphate (p.26·1).
Coughs.

Decongestant Eye Drops *Nyal, Austral.†.*
Phenylephrine hydrochloride (p.1066·2).
Conjunctival congestion.

Decongestant Nasal Spray
Note. This name is used for preparations of different composition.
Nyal, Austral.†.
Phenylephrine hydrochloride (p.1066·2).
Nasal congestion.

Prodemdis, Canad.; Technilab, Canad.; Stanley, Canad.
Xylometazoline hydrochloride (p.1071·2).

Decongestant Nose Drops *Prodemdis, Canad.*
Xylometazoline hydrochloride (p.1071·2).

Decongestant SR *Geneva, USA.*
Phenylpropanolamine hydrochloride (p.1067·2); phenylephrine hydrochloride (p.1066·2); chlorpheniramine maleate (p.405·1); phenyltoloxamine citrate (p.416·1).
Upper respiratory-tract symptoms.

Decongestant Tablets
Stanley, Canad.; Unichem, UK.
Pseudoephedrine hydrochloride (p.1068·3).

Decongestine *Sauter, Switz.†.*
Kaolin (p.1195·1); glycerol (p.1585·2); zinc oxide (p.1096·2); salicylic acid (p.1090·2); methyl salicylate (p.55·2).
Musculoskeletal disorders.

Deconhist LA *Goldline, USA.*
Phenylephrine hydrochloride (p.1066·2); phenylpropanolamine hydrochloride (p.1067·2); chlorpheniramine maleate (p.405·1); hyoscyamine sulphate (p.464·2); atropine sulphate (p.455·1); hyoscine hydrobromide (p.462·3).
Upper respiratory-tract symptoms.

Deconsal II *Adams, USA.*
Pseudoephedrine hydrochloride (p.1068·3); guaiphenesin (p.1061·3).
Coughs.

Deconsal Pediatric *Adams, USA.*
Codeine phosphate (p.26·1); pseudoephedrine hydrochloride (p.1068·3); guaiphenesin (p.1061·3).

Deconsal Sprinkle *Adams, USA.*
Phenylephrine hydrochloride (p.1066·2); guaiphenesin (p.1061·3).
Coughs; nasal congestion.

Decontractyl
Note. This name is used for preparations of different composition.
Synthelabo, Belg.; Robert & Carriere, Canad.; Synthelabo, Fr.
Ointment: Mephenesin (p.1315·3); methyl nicotinate (p.55·1).
Painful muscular disorders.

Synthelabo, Belg.†; Synthelabo, Fr.
Tablets: Mephenesin (p.1315·3).
Painful muscular disorders.

Decorenone *Italfarmaco, Ital.*
Ubidecarenone (p.1641·2).
Cardiac disorders; co-enzyme Q deficiency.

Decorin *Invamed, USA.*
Pseudoephedrine hydrochloride (p.1068·3).

Decorpa
Norgine, Fr.†; Norgine, Ger.
Sterculia (p.1214·1).
Obesity.

Decortilen *Merck, Ger.*
Prednylidene (p.1049·3) or prednylidene diethylaminoacetate hydrochloride.
Corticosteroid.

Decortin *Merck, Ger.*
Prednisone (p.1049·2).
Oral corticosteroid.

Decortin H *Merck, Ger.*
Prednisolone (p.1048·1).
Oral corticosteroid.

Decortin-H-KS *Merck, Ger.†.*
Prednisolone acetate (p.1048·1).
Parenteral corticosteroid.

Decortisyl
Roussel, Irl.†; Roussel, UK†.
Prednisone (p.1049·2).
Hypersensitivity reactions; inflammatory disorders.

Decorton *Salfa, Ital.†.*
Prednisone (p.1049·2).
Oral corticosteroid.

Decrelip *Ferrer, Spain.*
Gemfibrozil (p.1273·3).
Hyperlipidaemias.

Decresco *Searle, Spain.*
Captopril (p.836·3); hydrochlorothiazide (p.885·2).
Hypertension.

Decreten *Dumex, Norw.†.*
Pindolol (p.931·1).
Angina pectoris; arrhythmias; hypertension.

Decrin *Roche Consumer, Austral.*
Aspirin (p.16·1); codeine phosphate (p.26·1).
Fever; pain.

Dectancyl *Roussel, Fr.*
Dexamethasone acetate (p.1037·1).
Corticosteroid.

Decylenes *Rugby, USA.*
Undecenoic acid (p.389·2); zinc undecenoate (p.389·2).
Bromhidrosis; fungal skin infections; hyperhidrosis; minor skin irritation; nappy rash.

Dediol *Rhone-Poulenc Rorer, Ital.*
Alfacalcidol (p.1366·3).
Vitamin D deficiency.

Dedolor *Klinge, Aust.*
Diclofenac sodium (p.31·2).
Inflammation; musculoskeletal and joint disorders; pain.

Dedralen *Italfarmaco, Ital.*
Doxazosin mesylate (p.862·3).
Hypertension.

Dedrogyl
Hoechst Marion Roussel, Belg.; Roussel, Fr.; Albert-Roussel, Ger.; Hoechst, Ger.
Calcifediol (p.1366·3).
Hypocalcaemia; hypoparathyroidism; osteomalacia; renal osteodystrophy; rickets.

Deep Cold *Mentholatum, Canad.*
Menthol (p.1600·2).

Deep Freeze *Mentholatum, UK.*
Trichlorofluoromethane (p.1164·3); dichlorodifluoromethane (p.1164·3).
Painful muscular spasm.

Deep Freeze Cold Gel *Mentholatum, UK†.*
Menthol (p.1600·2).
Musculoskeletal and joint disorders; pain.

Deep Heat *Mentholatum, Austral.*
Cream: Methyl salicylate (p.55·2); menthol (p.1600·2).
Topical spray: Methyl salicylate (p.55·2); ethyl salicylate (p.36·1); glycol salicylate (p.43·1); methyl nicotinate (p.55·1).
Muscular aches and pains.

Deep Heat Massage *Mentholatum, UK.*
Menthol (p.1600·2); methyl salicylate (p.55·2).
Rheumatic and muscular pain.

Deep Heat Maximum Strength *Mentholatum, UK.*
Menthol (p.1600·2); methyl salicylate (p.55·2).
Formerly known as Deep Heat Extra Strength.
Rheumatic and muscular pain.

Deep Heat Rub *Mentholatum, UK.*
Menthol (p.1600·2); eucalyptus oil (p.1578·1); methyl salicylate (p.55·2); turpentine oil (p.1641·1).
Rheumatic and muscular pain.

Deep Heat Spray *Mentholatum, UK.*
Methyl nicotinate (p.55·1); glycol salicylate (p.43·1); methyl salicylate (p.55·2); ethyl salicylate (p.36·1).
Rheumatic and muscular pain.

Deep Heating *Mentholatum, Canad.*
Methyl salicylate (p.55·2); menthol (p.1600·2).

Deep Heating Lotion *Mentholatum, USA.*
Methyl salicylate (p.55·2); menthol (p.1600·2).
Musculoskeletal, joint, and soft-tissue pain; neuralgia.

Deep Heating Rub *Mentholatum, USA.*
Methyl salicylate (p.55·2); menthol (p.1600·2).
Arthritis; musculoskeletal, joint, and soft-tissue pain; neuralgia.

Deep Relief *Mentholatum, UK.*
Ibuprofen (p.44·1); menthol (p.1600·2).
Musculoskeletal disorders.

Deep-Down Rub *SmithKline Beecham, USA.*
Methyl salicylate (p.55·2); menthol (p.1600·2); camphor (p.1557·2).
Muscle, joint, and soft-tissue pain; neuralgia.

Defanyl *Novalis, Fr.*
Amoxapine (p.279·2).
Depression.

Defaxina *Smaller, Spain.*
Cephalexin (p.178·2).
Bacterial infections.

DeFed *Ferndale, USA.*
Pseudoephedrine hydrochloride (p.1068·3).
Nasal congestion.

Defencid *Duopharm, Ger.*
Harpagophytum (p.27·2).
Musculoskeletal and joint disorders.

Defen-LA *Horizon, USA.*
Pseudoephedrine hydrochloride (p.1068·3); guaiphenesin (p.1061·3).

Defesto C *Boileau & Boyd, Irl.†.*
Carbaryl (p.1403·1).
Pediculosis.

Defibrase
Gerot, Aust.; Serono, Ger.†; Pentapharm, Switz.†.
Batroxobin (p.712·3).
Peripheral arterial disorders; thrombo-embolic disorders.

Defiltran *Jumer, Fr.*
Acetazolamide (p.810·3).
Soft tissue injury.

Deflam *Akromed, S.Afr.*
Oxaprozin (p.71·2).
Musculoskeletal and joint disorders.

Deflamat
Klinge, Aust.; Luitpold, Ital.
Diclofenac sodium (p.31·2).
Inflammation; musculoskeletal and joint disorders; pain.

Deflamol *Fumouze, Fr.*
Titanium dioxide (p.1093·3); zinc oxide (p.1096·2).
Dermatitis.

Deflamon *SPA, Ital.*
Metronidazole (p.585·1).
Anaerobic bacterial infections; trichomoniasis.

Deflan *Guidotti, Ital.*
Deflazacort (p.1036·2).
Oral corticosteroid.

Deflogon *Damor, Ital.†.*
Ibuproxam (p.45·2).
Musculoskeletal disorders.

Deflox *Abbott, Spain.*
Terazosin hydrochloride (p.952·1).
Benign prostatic hyperplasia; hypertension.

Defluina
Note. This name is used for preparations of different composition.
Ebewe, Aust.
Raubasine (p.941·3) or raubasine hydrochloride (p.941·3); dihydroergocristine mesylate (p.1571·3); dihydroergotamine mesylate (p.444·2).
Cerebral and peripheral vascular disease.

Nattermann, Ger.
Buflomedil hydrochloride (p.834·2).
Peripheral vascular disorders.

Teofarma, Ital.
Dihydroergocristine mesylate (p.1571·3).
Vascular disorders.

Defluina N *Nattermann, Ger.*
Co-dergocrine mesylate (p.1566·1).
Mental function disorders.

Defonamid *Blucher-Schering, Ger.†.*
Sulphanilamide (p.256·3).
Vaginal infections; vaginitis.

Deftan *Merck, Spain.*
Lofepramine hydrochloride (p.296·1).
Depression.

Defy *Akorn, USA.*
Tobramycin (p.264·1).
Eye infections.

Degas
Note. This name is used for preparations of different composition.
Whitehall, Austral.
Simethicone (p.1213·1); calcium carbonate (p.1182·1); light magnesium carbonate (p.1198·1); sodium bicarbonate (p.1153·2).
Formerly contained only simethicone.
Flatulence.

Invamed, USA.
Simethicone (p.1213·1).

Degest *Akorn, USA.*
Naphazoline hydrochloride (p.1064·2).
Minor eye irritation.

Degoran
Note. This name is used for preparations of different composition.
Novartis Consumer, S.Afr.
Effervescent tablets: Phenylephrine hydrochloride (p.1066·2); paracetamol (p.72·2); pheniramine maleate (p.415·3).
Formerly contained phenylpropanolamine hydrochloride, paracetamol, and pheniramine maleate.
Tablets; oral liquid: Chlorpheniramine maleate (p.405·1); phenylpropanolamine hydrochloride (p.1067·2); dextromethorphan hydrobromide (p.1057·3); paracetamol (p.72·2).
Cold symptoms.

Wander, S.Afr.†.
Phenylpropanolamine hydrochloride (p.1067·2); pheniramine maleate (p.415·3); mepyramine maleate (p.414·1); noscapine (p.1065·2); terpin hydrochloride (p.1070·2); paracetamol (p.72·2).
Cold symptoms; coughs.

Degranol *Lennon, S.Afr.*
Carbamazepine (p.339·2).
Epilepsy; trigeminal neuralgia.

Dehidrobenzperidol *Syntex, Spain.*
Droperidol (p.668·2).
General anaesthesia; neuroleptanalgesia; premedication.

Dehist *Forest Pharmaceuticals, USA†.*
Phenylpropanolamine hydrochloride (p.1067·2); chlorpheniramine maleate (p.405·1).
Upper respiratory-tract symptoms.

Dehydral *Trans Canaderm, Canad.*
Hexamine (p.216·1).
Bacterial infections; hyperhidrosis.

dehydro sanol *Sanol, Ger.†.*
Bemetizide (p.827·1); hesperidin complex (p.1580·2); thiamine nitrate; potassium chloride (p.1161·1).
Oedema associated with venous insufficiency.

dehydro sanol tri *Sanol, Ger.*
Bemetizide (p.827·1); triamterene (p.957·2).
Leg pain associated with venous insufficiency.

dehydro tri mite *Sanol, Ger.*
Bemetizide (p.827·1); triamterene (p.957·2).
Leg pain associated with venous insufficiency.

Dehydrobenzperidol
Janssen-Cilag, Aust.; Janssen-Cilag, Belg.; Janssen-Cilag, Ger.; Janssen-Cilag, Neth.; Janssen-Cilag, Switz.
Droperidol (p.668·2) or droperidol tartrate (p.668·3).
Agitation; neuroleptanalgesia; pain; postoperative medication; premedication; vomiting.

Dehydrosin *Mayrhofer, Aust.*
Bemetizide (p.827·1); triamterene (p.957·2).
Oedema.

Deidroepar *Iema, Ital.†.*
Sodium dehydrocholate (p.1570·3).
Biliary disorders.

Deiron *Iquinosa, Spain†.*
Etofenamate (p.36·3).
Peri-articular disorders; soft-tissue disorders.

Deiten *ABC, Ital.*
Nitrendipine (p.923·1).
Hypertension.

Dekamega *Omega, Spain.*
Piroxicam choline (p.81·1).
Gout; musculoskeletal, joint, and peri-articular disorders; pain.

Dekamin *Monico, Ital.*
Amino-acid infusion.
Parenteral nutrition.

Dekristol *Jenapharm, Ger.*
Cholecalciferol (p.1366·3).
Hypoparathyroidism; osteomalacia; osteoporosis; pseudohypoparathyroidism; rickets; vitamin D deficiency.

Del Aqua *Del-Ray, USA.*
Benzoyl peroxide (p.1079·2).
Acne.

Delabarre *Fumouze, Fr.*
Tamarind (p.1217·3); saffron (p.1001·1).
Teething pain.

De-Lact *Sharpe, Austral.*
Infant feed.
Lactose intolerance.

Deladiol *Steris, USA†.*
Oestradiol valerate (p.1455·2).
Female castration; female hypogonadism; menopausal vasomotor symptoms; prevention of breast engorgement; primary ovarian failure; prostatic cancer; vulval and vaginal atrophy.

Deladumone *Bristol-Myers Squibb, USA†.*
Oestradiol valerate (p.1455·2); testosterone enanthate (p.1464·1).
Menopausal vasomotor symptoms; prevention of postpartum breast engorgement.

Delagil *Dermapharm, Ger.*
Phenol-formaldehyde-urea polycondensate sodium sulphate.
Skin disorders.

Delaket *Chiesi, Ital.*
Delapril (p.847·1).
Hypertension.

Delakmin *Albert-Roussel, Ger.; Hoechst, Ger.*
(5*E*,7*E*)-9,10-Secocholesta-5,7,10(19)-triene-3β,25-diol.
Renal osteopathy.

Delapride *Chiesi, Ital.*
Delapril hydrochloride (p.847·1); indapamide (p.890·2).
Hypertension.

Delatestryl
Squibb, Canad.; BTG, USA.
Testosterone enanthate (p.1464·1).
Breast cancer; delayed puberty (males); male hypogonadism.

Delbiase *Promedica, Fr.*
Magnesium chloride (p.1157·2); magnesium bromide hydrate.
Magnesium deficiency.

Delcoprep *Delta, Ger.*
Macrogol 4000 (p.1598·2); electrolytes (p.1147·1).
Bowel evacuation.

Delcort *Roberts, USA.*
Hydrocortisone (p.1043·3).
Corticosteroid.

Delecit *LPB, Ital.*
Choline alfoscerate (p.1390·3).
Mental function impairment.

Delegol *Bayer, Ital.†.*
Partially chlorinated benzylphenol.
Surface disinfection.

Delestrogen
Squibb, Canad.; Mead Johnson Laboratories, USA.
Oestradiol valerate (p.1455·2).
Hypoestrogenism due to hypogonadism, castration, or primary ovarian failure; menopausal vasomotor symptoms; prostatic cancer; vulval and vaginal atrophy.

Delfen
Janssen-Cilag, Aust.; Janssen-Cilag, Austral.; Cilag, Belg.†; Johnson & Johnson, Canad.; Janssen-Cilag, Irl.; Cilag, Neth.†; Janssen-Cilag, S.Afr.; Janssen-Cilag, Switz.; Cilag, UK; Ortho Pharmaceutical, USA.
Nonoxinol 9 (p.1326·1).
Contraceptive.

Delgamer *Marion Merrell, Spain.*
Diethylpropion hydrochloride (p.1479·3).
Obesity.

Delgian *Sanofi Winthrop, Ger.†.*
Maprotiline hydrochloride (p.296·2).
Depression.

Delica-Sol *Medichemie, Switz.†.*
Dequalinium chloride (p.1112·1); lactic acid (p.1593·3); mint oil; fennel oil (p.1579·2); anise oil (p.1550·1); origanum oil.
Mouth and throat disorders.

delimmun *Synthelabo, Ger.*
Inosine pranobex (p.615·2).
Viral infections.

Delipid *Coop. Farm., Ital.†.*
Tiadenol (p.1279·3).
Hyperlipidaemias.

Delipoderm
Theramex, Mon.; Reig Jofre, Spain.
Promestriene (p.1461·2).
Acne; seborrhoea.

Deliproct *Schering, Fr.*
Prednisolone hexanoate (p.1048·1); cinchocaine hydrochloride (p.1289·2).
Formerly contained prednisolone hexanoate, cinchocaine hydrochloride, and clemizole undecanoate.
Anorectal disorders.

Deliver *Mead Johnson, Austral.*
Preparation for enteral nutrition.
Fluid or volume restriction; hypermetabolic states.

Delix *Hoechst, Ger.*
Ramipril (p.941·1).
Heart failure; hypertension.

Delix plus *Hoechst, Ger.*
Ramipril (p.941·1); hydrochlorothiazide (p.885·2).
Hypertension.

Delixir *Hamilton, Austral.*
Diphenhydramine hydrochloride (p.409·1); ammonium chloride (p.1055·2); sodium citrate (p.1153·2).
Coughs and cold symptoms.

Dellova *Poutrat, Fr.*
Bladderwrack (p.1554·1); orthosiphon (p.1592·2).
Formerly contained ovary extracts, thyroid, digitalis purpurea, and phenolphthalein (.
Obesity.

Delmofulvina *Coli, Ital.†.*
Griseofulvin (p.380·2).
Fungal infections.

Del-Mycin *Del-Ray, USA.*
Erythromycin (p.204·1).

Delonal
Essex, Ger.; Essex, Switz.
Alclometasone dipropionate (p.1031·3).
Skin disorders.

Delphi
Wyeth Lederle, Belg.; Lederle, Neth.
Triamcinolone acetonide (p.1050·2).
Skin disorders.

Delphicort
Cyanamid, Aust.; Lederle, Ger.
Triamcinolone (p.1050·2), triamcinolone acetonide (p.1050·2), or triamcinolone diacetate (p.1050·2).
Corticosteroid.

Delphimix *Lederle, Ger.*
Triamcinolone diacetate (p.1050·2).
Musculoskeletal and joint disorders.

Delphinac *Lederle, Ger.*
Diclofenac sodium (p.31·2).
Inflammation; musculoskeletal and joint disorders; pain.

Delpral *Synthelabo, Aust.*
Tiapride hydrochloride (p.696·1).
Alcohol withdrawal syndrome; movement disorders; pain.

Delsacid *Selvi, Ital.*
Cefonicid sodium (p.167·2).
Lignocaine hydrochloride (p.1293·2) is included in this preparation to alleviate the pain of injection.
Bacterial infections.

Delsym
Novartis Consumer, Canad.; Roche Consumer, Irl.; Fisons Consumer, USA.
Dextromethorphan polistirex (p.1058·2).
Coughs.

Delta 80 *IDI, Ital.*
Benzoyl peroxide (p.1079·2).
Acne; skin disinfection.

Delta 80 Plus *IDI, Ital.*
Benzoyl peroxide (p.1079·2); cetylpyridinium chloride (p.1106·2).
Acne; skin disinfection.

Deltacef *Pulitzer, Ital.*
Cefuroxime sodium (p.177·1).
Bacterial infections.

Deltacillin *Lagamed, S.Afr.†.*
Phenoxymethylpenicillin potassium (p.236·2).
Bacterial infections.

Deltacina *Upsamedica, Spain.*
Neomycin sulphate (p.229·2); thiomersal (p.1126·3).
Skin infections.

Delta-Cortef
Upjohn, Austral.†; Upjohn, USA.
Prednisolone (p.1048·1).
Corticosteroid.

Deltacortene *Lepetit, Ital.*
Prednisone (p.1049·2).
Oral corticosteroid.

Deltacortilen *SIFI, Ital.†.*
Prednisolone acetate (p.1048·1).
Inflammatory eye disorders.

Deltacortril
Pfizer, Belg.; Pfizer, Ger.†; Pfizer, Irl.; Pfizer, UK.
Prednisolone (p.1048·1) or prednisolone acetate (p.1048·1).
Corticosteroid.

Delta-D *Freeda, USA.*
Cholecalciferol (p.1366·3).
Dietary supplement; vitamin D deficiency.

Delta-Hadensa *Kolassa, Aust.*
Prednisolone sodium metasulphobenzoate (p.1048·1); chlorcarvacrol; ichthammol (p.1083·3); menthol (p.1600·2); with or without chamomile oil.
Anorectal disorders.

Deltalipid *Delta, Ger.*
Soya oil (p.1355·1).
Contains egg phospholipids.
Lipid infusion for parenteral nutrition.

Deltamidrina *Allergan, Ital.*
Prednisolone acetate (p.1048·1); atropine sulphate (p.455·1); phenylephrine hydrochloride (p.1066·2).
Inflammatory eye disorders.

Deltarhinol *Hoechst Marion Roussel, Belg.*
Isoflupredone acetate (p.1045·3); ephedrine hydrochloride (p.1059·3); naphazoline nitrate (p.1064·2).
Rhinitis.

Deltarinolo *Hoechst Marion Roussel, Ital.*
Ephedrine hydrochloride (p.1059·3); naphazoline nitrate (p.1064·2).
Nasal congestion.

Deltasiton *Faes, Spain.*
Coal tar (p.1092·3); cloxyquin (p.215·3); gramicidin (p.215·2); neomycin sulphate (p.229·2); nystatin (p.386·1); triamcinolone acetate (p.1050·2); keratinase (p.1593·1); titanium dioxide (p.1093·3).
Infected skin disorders.

Deltasolone *Rhone-Poulenc Rorer, Austral.†.*
Prednisolone (p.1048·1).
Corticosteroid.

Deltasone
Rhone-Poulenc Rorer, Austral.†; Pharmacia Upjohn, Canad.; Upjohn, USA.
Prednisone (p.1049·2).
Corticosteroid.

Deltasoralen *Delta Laboratories, Irl.*
Methoxsalen (p.1086·3).
Leucoderma; psoriasis; vitiligo.

Deltastab *Knoll, UK.*
Prednisolone acetate (p.1048·1).
Corticosteroid.

Delta-Tomanol *Byk, Aust.*
Ramifenazone (p.82·1); phenylbutazone (p.79·3); prednisolone sodium phosphate (p.1048·1); hydroxocobalamin acetate (p.1364·2).
Cinchocaine (p.1289·2) is included in this preparation to alleviate the pain of injection.
Musculoskeletal and joint disorders; neuralgia.

Delta-Tritex *Dermol, USA.*
Triamcinolone acetonide (p.1050·2).
Skin disorders.

Deltavac *Trimen, USA.*
Sulphanilamide (p.256·3); aminacrine hydrochloride (p.1098·3); allantoin (p.1078·2).
Vaginal infections.

Deltavagin *Biagini, Ital.*
Betamethasone (p.1033·2); tyrothricin (p.267·2); norvaline.
Formerly contained betamethasone, sulphamethoxypyridazine, tyrothricin, and norvaline.
Vaginitis.

Deltazen *Pharmacia Upjohn, Fr.*
Diltiazem hydrochloride (p.854·2).
Hypertension.

Deltidrosol *Poli, Ital.†.*
Prednisolone (p.1048·1).
Parenteral corticosteroid.

Deltin *IFI, Ital.†.*
Sulphadimethoxine (p.253·2).
Prostate infections.

Deltison *Recip, Swed.*
Prednisone (p.1049·2).
Magnesium trisilicate (p.1199·1) and calcium hydrogen phosphate (p.1155·3) are included in this preparation in an attempt to limit adverse effects on the gastro-intestinal mucosa.
Corticosteroid.

Delto-cyl Ho-Len-Complex *Liebermann, Ger.*
Homoeopathic preparation.

Delursan *Houde, Fr.*
Ursodeoxycholic acid (p.1642·1).
Gallstones; liver and biliary disorders.

Delvas *Berk, UK.*
Amiloride hydrochloride (p.819·2); hydrochlorothiazide (p.885·2).
These ingredients can be described by the British Approved Name Co-amilozide.
Cirrhosis with ascites; heart failure; hypertension.

Del-Vi-A *Del-Ray, USA.*
Vitamin A (p.1358·1).
Vitamin A deficiency.

Demadex
Boehringer Mannheim, Canad.; Jouveinal, Canad.; Boehringer Mannheim, USA.
Torasemide (p.956·3).
Hypertension; oedema.

Demalit *Baldacci, Ital.†.*
Lithium glutamate (p.295·1).
Formerly known as Lithium Bruco.
Psychoses.

Demazin
Note. This name is used for preparations of different composition.
Schering-Plough, Austral.
Delayed-release tablets: Dexchlorpheniramine maleate (p.405·1); pseudoephedrine sulphate (p.1068·3).
Syrup: Chlorpheniramine maleate (p.405·1); phenylephrine hydrochloride (p.1066·2).
Tablets: Chlorpheniramine maleate (p.405·1); pseudoephedrine sulphate (p.1068·3).
Upper respiratory tract symptoms.
Schering-Plough, S.Afr.
Sustained-release capsules: Dexchlorpheniramine maleate (p.405·1); pseudoephedrine sulphate (p.1068·3).
Syrup: Chlorpheniramine maleate (p.405·1); phenylephrine hydrochloride (p.1066·2).
Upper respiratory-tract symptoms.
Schering-Plough, USA.
Chlorpheniramine maleate (p.405·1); phenylpropanolamine hydrochloride (p.1067·2).
Upper respiratory-tract symptoms.

Demazin Anti-Tussive *Schering-Plough, S.Afr.*
Chlorpheniramine maleate (p.405·1); dextromethorphan hydrobromide (p.1057·3); phenylpropanolamine hydrochloride (p.1067·2).
Coughs.

Demazin Cold & Flu *Schering-Plough, Austral.*
Chlorpheniramine maleate (p.405·1); pseudoephedrine sulphate (p.1068·3); paracetamol (p.72·2).
Cold and influenza symptoms; sinusitis.

Demazin Expectorant *Schering-Plough, S.Afr.*
Dexchlorpheniramine maleate (p.405·1) pseudoephedrine sulphate (p.1068·3) guaiphenesin (p.1061·3).
Respiratory-tract disorders.

Demazin NS *Schering-Plough, S.Afr.*
Loratadine (p.413·1); pseudoephedrine sulphate (p.1068·3).
Rhinitis.

Demazin Sinus *Schering-Plough, Austral.*
Pseudoephedrine sulphate (p.1068·3).
Upper respiratory-tract congestion.

Demdec *Rougier, Canad.*
Pseudoephedrine hydrochloride (p.1068·3); dextromethorphan hydrobromide (p.1057·3).
Coughs; respiratory-tract congestion.

Demebronc *Cyanamid, Ital.†.*
Demeclocycline (p.201·2); dextromethorphan hydrobromide (p.1057·3); potassium guaiacolsulfonate (p.1068·3).
Respiratory-tract infections.

De-menthasin *Scheurich, Ger.*
Dequalinium salicylate (p.1112·1); hexetidine (p.1116·1).
Mouth and throat inflammation.

Dementrin *Parke, Davis, Aust.*
Prazepam (p.687·2).
Anxiety; skeletal muscle spasm.

Demerol
Sanofi Winthrop, Canad.; Sanofi Winthrop, USA.
Pethidine hydrochloride (p.76·1).
Pain.

Demetil *Farmila, Ital.*
Tetrahydrozoline hydrochloride (p.1070·2).
Eye congestion.

Demetrin
Godecke, Ger.; Parke, Davis, Ger.; Parke, Davis, S.Afr.; Parke, Davis, Spain†; Parke, Davis, Switz.
Prazepam (p.687·2).
Anxiety; insomnia; neuroses.

Demex *Berlin-Chemie, Ger.*
Propyphenazone (p.81·3).
Pain.

Demiax *Merck, Spain.*
Xipamide (p.971·2).
Hypertension; oedema.

Demicina *Medosan, Ital.†.*
Neomycin sulphate (p.229·2); prednisone (p.1049·2); ephedrine hydrochloride (p.1059·3).
Otitis; rhinitis; sinusitis.

Demi-Regroton *Rhone-Poulenc Rorer, USA.*
Chlorthalidone (p.839·3); reserpine (p.942·1).
Hypertension.

Demix *Ashbourne, UK.*
Doxycycline hydrochloride (p.202·3).

Demo baume *Demopharm, Switz.*
Chlorbutol (p.1106·3); ephedrine hydrochloride (p.1059·3); lignocaine hydrochloride (p.1293·2); camphor (p.1557·2); menthol (p.1600·2); lavender oil (p.1594·3); niaouli oil (p.1607·1).
Rhinitis.

Demo collyre No 2 *Demopharm, Switz.†.*
Tetrahydrozoline hydrochloride (p.1070·2).
Eye irritation.

Demo elixir pectoral *Demopharm, Switz.*
Codeine phosphate (p.26·1); ephedrine hydrochloride (p.1059·3); guaiphenesin (p.1061·3); belladonna (p.457·1); drosera (p.1574·1); hedera helix; ipecacuanha (p.1062·2).
Bronchitis; catarrh; coughs.

Demo gouttes bronchiques *Demopharm, Switz.*
Thyme (p.1636·3); lierre; liquorice (p.1197·1).
Coughs with viscous mucus.

Demo gouttes contre la toux *Demopharm, Switz.*
Codeine phosphate (p.26·1); ephedrine hydrochloride (p.1059·3); guaiphenesin (p.1061·3); drosera (p.1574·1); hedera helix; ipecacuanha (p.1062·2); thyme oil (p.1637·1).
Coughs; respiratory-tract disorders with increased or viscous mucus.

Demo gouttes pour les yeux No 1 *Demopharm, Switz.†.*
Hamamelis (p.1587·1); euphrasia; dexpanthenol (p.1570·3).
Eye irritation.

Demo pates pectorales *Demopharm, Switz.*
Codeine phosphate (p.26·1); benzoic acid (p.1102·3); ipecacuanha (p.1062·2); tolu balsam (p.1071·1); drosera (p.1574·1); hedera helix; plantaginis; menthol (p.1600·2); anise oil (p.1550·1); bitter orange oil; eucalyptus oil (p.1578·1); peppermint oil (p.1208·1).
Bronchitis; coughs.

Demo pommade contre les refroidissements *Demopharm, Switz.*
Eucalyptus oil (p.1578·1); pine needle oil (p.1623·3); peru balsam (p.1617·2); camphor (p.1557·2); thyme oil (p.1637·1).
Cold symptoms.

Demo pommade contre les refroidissements pour bebes *Demopharm, Switz.*
Eucalyptus oil (p.1578·1); pine needle oil (p.1623·3); sage oil; thyme oil (p.1637·1); juniper oil (p.1592·3); peru balsam (p.1617·2).
Respiratory-tract disorders.

Demo sirop bronchique N *Demopharm, Switz.*
Thyme (p.1636·3); primula rhizome; hedera helix.
Coughs.

Demo sirop contre la toux *Demopharm, Switz.*
Ephedrine hydrochloride (p.1059·3); guaiphenesin (p.1061·3); tolu balsam (p.1071·1); drosera (p.1574·1); ipecacuanha (p.1062·2); thyme (p.1636·3); belladonna (p.457·1); liquorice (p.1197·1).
Bronchitis; catarrh; coughs.

DemoAngina *Demopharm, Switz.†.*
Dichlorobenzyl alcohol (p.1112·2); cetylpyridinium chloride (p.1106·2); althaea (p.1546·3).
Sore throat.

Demo-Cineol *Sabex, Canad.*
Cineole (p.1564·1); guaiacol (p.1061·2); camphor (p.1557·2).
Cough; rheumatic pain.

Democyl *Demopharm, Switz.*
Paracetamol (p.72·2).
Fever; pain.

Demodenal *Demopharm, Switz.*
Dimenhydrinate (p.408·2).
Motion sickness.

Demodenal compositum *Demopharm, Switz.*
Dimenhydrinate (p.408·2); pyridoxine hydrochloride (p.1362·3); caffeine (p.749·3).
Motion sickness.

Demoderhin *Demopharm, Switz.*
Diphenhydramine hydrochloride (p.409·1); mepyramine maleate (p.414·1); caffeine (p.749·3).
Nasal congestion; rhinitis.

Demodon *Demopharm, Switz.†.*
Aloes (p.1177·1); frangula bark (p.1193·2); turmeric (p.1001·3); taraxacum (p.1634·2); belladonna alkaloids (p.457·1).
Constipation.

Demodon N *Demopharm, Switz.*
Senna (p.1212·2).
Constipation.

Demogripal *Demopharm, Switz.*
Paracetamol (p.72·2).
Fever; pain.

Demogripal C *Demopharm, Switz.*
Paracetamol (p.72·2); ascorbic acid (p.1365·2).
Cold symptoms.

Demogripp *Demopharm, Switz.†.*
Salicylamide (p.82·3); paracetamol (p.72·2).
Cold and influenza symptoms.

Demolaxin *Demopharm, Switz.*
Bisacodyl (p.1179·3).
Constipation.

Demolox *Cyanamid, Spain.*
Amoxapine (p.279·2).
Depression.

Demonatur Capsules ail-aubepine *Demopharm, Switz.†.*
Crataegus (p.1568·2); garlic oil; leonura cardiaca (p.1604·2); cactus flower; tocopherol acetate (p.1369·1).
Atherosclerosis.

Demonatur Capsules contre les refroidissements *Demopharm, Switz.*
Brown capsules, thyme oil (p.1637·1); origanum oil; savory oil; green capsules, echinacea purpurea (p.1574·2).
Influenza symptoms.

Demonatur Dragees calmantes *Demopharm, Switz.†.*
Valerian (p.1643·1); lupulus (p.1597·2); melissa (p.1600·1).
Anxiety; nervousness.

Demonatur Dragees pour les reins et la vessie *Demopharm, Switz.*
Bearberry (p.1552·2); solidago virgaurea; ononis (p.1610·2); echinacea (p.1574·2); Java tea (p.1592·2).
Urinary-tract disorders.

Demonatur Gouttes pour le foie et la bile *Demopharm, Switz.*
Vial no 1: gentian (p.1583·3); taraxacum (p.1634·2); cynara (p.1569·2); vial no 2: silybum marianum (p.993·3); celandine; berberis.
Gastro-intestinal disorders.

Demoplas *Godecke, Ger.*
Injection: Phenylbutazone sodium (p.79·3).
Lignocaine hydrochloride (p.1293·2) is included in this preparation to alleviate the pain of injection.
Acute ankylosing spondylitis; rheumatism.

Demoprin nouvelle formule *Demopharm, Switz.*
Aspirin (p.16·1).
Fever; pain.

Demo-Rhinil *Demopharm, Switz.†.*
Oxedrine tartrate (p.925·3); ephedrine hydrochloride (p.1059·3); allantoin (p.1078·2); lignocaine hydrochloride (p.1293·2); dexpanthenol (p.1570·3).
Nasal congestion.

Demosept *Demopharm, Switz.*
Chlorhexidine gluconate (p.1107·2); dichlorobenzyl alcohol (p.1112·2); allantoin (p.1078·2); vitamin A (p.1358·1); cholecalciferol (p.1366·3).
Skin abrasions; skin irritation.

Demosept Jod *Demopharm, Switz.†.*
Povidone-iodine (p.1123·3).
Wound disinfection.

Demostan *Demopharm, Switz.*
Ointment: Diphenhydramine hydrochloride (p.409·1); lignocaine hydrochloride (p.1293·2); menthol (p.1600·2).
Topical gel: Diphenhydramine hydrochloride (p.409·1); lignocaine hydrochloride (p.1293·2).
Burns; insect bites; skin irritation.

Demosvelte N *Demopharm, Switz.*
Agar (p.1470·3); guar gum (p.321·3); sodium alginate (p.1470·3); pectin (p.1474·1); soya (p.1355·1).
Obesity.

Demotest *Pierre Fabre, Spain.*
Budesonide (p.1034·3).
Skin disorders.

Demotherm Pommade contre le rhumatisme *Demopharm, Switz.*
Benzyl nicotinate (p.22·1); glycol salicylate (p.43·1).
Musculoskeletal and joint pain.

Demotussil *Demopharm, Switz.*
Codeine phosphate (p.26·1); ephedrine hydrochloride (p.1059·3); ipecacuanha (p.1062·2); guaiphenesin (p.1061·3); cineole (p.1564·1).
Coughs.

Demovarin *Demopharm, Switz.*
Heparin sodium (p.879·3); thymol (p.1127·1).
Superficial vascular disorders.

Demoven N *Demopharm, Switz.*
Troxerutin (p.1580·2); aesculus (p.1543·3).
Venous insufficiency.

Demovit *Demopharm, Switz.*
A range of multivitamin and mineral preparations.
Dietary supplementation.

Demozem *Evers, Ger.†.*
Palm kernel oil (p.1384·2); bay-laurel oil.
Psoriasis.

Dempol *Esoform, Ital.*
Chlorhexidine gluconate (p.1107·2).
Hand disinfection.

Demser
Merck Sharp & Dohme, Neth.†; Merck Sharp & Dohme, UK; Merck Sharp & Dohme, USA.
Metirosine (p.906·3).
Phaeochromocytoma.

Demulen
Searle, Canad.; Searle, S.Afr.†; Searle, USA.
Ethynodiol diacetate (p.1445·3); ethinyloestradiol (p.1445·1).
28-Day packs also contain 7 inert tablets.
Combined oral contraceptive.

Demusin *Bama, Spain.*
Albumin tannate (p.1176·3); amylase (p.1549·1); ethylmorphine hydrochloride (p.36·1).
Diarrhoea.

Demykosan *Bayrol, Ger.†.*
Benzalkonium chloride (p.1101·3); didecyldimethylammonium chloride (p.1112·2); formaldehyde (p.1113·2); glyoxal (p.1115·1); glutaraldehyde (p.1114·3).
Fungal skin infection prophylaxis; surface disinfection.

Demykosan S *Bayrol, Ger.†.*
Benzalkonium chloride (p.1101·3); didecyldimethylammonium chloride (p.1112·2); glyoxal (p.1115·1); glutaraldehyde (p.1114·3).
Disinfection.

Denan *Thomae, Ger.*
Simvastatin (p.1278·2).
Hypercholesterolaemia.

Denaxpren *Smaller, Spain.*
Naproxen (p.61·2).
Fever; gout; musculoskeletal, joint, and peri-articular disorders; pain.

Denco *Horner, Canad.†.*
Pregnancy test (p.1621·2).

Dencoccult *Carter-Wallace, Austral.†.*
Test for occult blood in faeces.

Dencorub *Carter-Wallace, Austral.*
Camphor (p.1557·2); menthol (p.1600·2); eucalyptus oil (p.1578·1); methyl salicylate (p.55·2).
Musculoskeletal pain.

Dencorub Arthritis *Carter-Wallace, Austral.*
Triethanolamine salicylate (p.1639·2).
Arthritis; muscle pain.

Dencorub Extra Strength *Carter-Wallace, Austral.*
Methyl salicylate (p.55·2); menthol (p.1600·2).
Muscle pain.

Dencorub Ice *Carter-Wallace, Austral.*
Menthol (p.1600·2).
Musculoskeletal pain.

Dencyl *SmithKline Beecham, UK.*
Dried ferrous sulphate (p.1340·2); zinc sulphate (p.1373·2); folic acid (p.1340·3).
Prophylaxis of iron and folic acid deficiency in pregnancy.

Deniban
Bender, Aust.; Synthelabo, Ital.
Amisulpride (p.641·2).
Dysthymia.

Denisoline *Aerocid, Fr.*
Talc (p.1092·1); precipitated sulphur (p.1091·2); glycerol (p.1585·2); alum (p.1547·1).
Acne.

De-Nol
Parke, Davis, Austral.; Yamanouchi, Belg.; Yamanouchi, Irl.; Yamanouchi, Ital.; Yamanouchi, Neth.; Yamanouchi, Norw.; Pharmaplan, S.Afr.; Yamanouchi, Switz.; Yamanouchi, UK.
Tripotassium dicitratobismuthate (p.1180·2).
Dyspepsia; gastritis; peptic ulcer.

De-Noltab
Yamanouchi, Irl.; Yamanouchi, UK.
Tripotassium dicitratobismuthate (p.1180·2).
Dyspepsia; gastritis; peptic ulcer.

Denoral
Note. This name is used for preparations of different composition.
Rhone-Poulenc Rorer, Belg.; Theraplix, Fr.; Rhone-Poulenc Rorer, Ital.
Tablets: Buzepide metiodide (p.459·2); clocinizine hydrochloride (p.406·3); phenylpropanolamine hydrochloride (p.1067·2).
Upper respiratory-tract congestion.
Theraplix, Fr.
Syrup: Buzepide metiodide (p.459·2); clocinizine hydrochloride (p.406·3); pholcodine (p.1068·1).
Coughs; upper respiratory-tract congestion.

Denorex
Whitehall-Robins, Canad.; Whitehall, Irl.; Whitehall, Neth.; Whitehall, UK; Whitehall, USA.
Coal tar (p.1092·3); menthol (p.1600·2).
Dandruff; psoriasis; seborrhoeic dermatitis.

Denosol *Doerenkamp, Ger.*
Cineole (p.1564·1); menthol (p.1600·2); camphor (p.1557·2); thymol (p.1127·1).
Colds; influenza.

Denquel *Procter & Gamble, USA.*
Potassium nitrate (p.1123·1).
Sensitive teeth.

Dentafijal *Navarro, Spain†.*
Pagliari water; resorcinol (p.1090·1).
Gingivitis; mouthwash in oral surgery; pyorrhoea.

Dental Ointment *Abbott, Austral.†.*
Lignocaine (p.1293·2); nitromersol (p.1120·1).
Denture pain; pain of dry socket and pyorrhoea.

Dentalgar *Marc-O, Canad.*
Benzocaine (p.1286·2); camphor (p.1557·2); guaiacol (p.1061·2); menthol (p.1600·2); clove oil (p.1565·2).

Dental-Phenjoca *Worndli, Switz.*
Iodine (p.1493·1); camphor (p.1557·2); thymol (p.1127·1); anethole (p.1549·3); safrole; eugenol (p.1578·2); chlorbutol (p.1106·3); phenol (p.1121·2).
Dental extraction pain.

Denta-Mint Mouth Rinse *Colgate Oral Care, Austral.*
Detergent mouthwash.
Oral hygiene.

Denta-Mint Topical Fluoride Solution *Colgate Oral Care, Austral.*
Sodium fluoride (p.742·1).
Fluoridation of tooth enamel.

Dentan *Ipex, Swed.*
Sodium fluoride (p.742·1).
Dental caries prophylaxis.

Dentaton Antisettico *Ghimas, Ital.*
Chlorhexidine gluconate (p.1107·2); benzalkonium chloride (p.1101·3).
Oral disinfection.

Dentese *McGloin, Austral.†.*
Phenol (p.1121·2); camphor (p.1557·2); eucalyptus oil (p.1578·1); clove oil (p.1565·2).
Toothache.

Denti Gum C *Brovar, S.Afr.†.*
Cetylpyridinium chloride (p.1106·2).
Mouth and throat infections.

Denti Gum CF *Brovar, S.Afr.†.*
Sodium fluoride (p.742·1); cetylpyridinium chloride (p.1106·2).
Dental caries prophylaxis; plaque removal.

Denti Gum F *Brovar, S.Afr.†.*
Sodium fluoride (p.742·1).
Dental caries prophylaxis; fluoride supplement.

Dentiform *Roche Nicholas, Neth.†.*
Lignocaine hydrochloride (p.1293·2).
Mouth irritation.

Dentigoa *Scheurich, Ger.*
Ibuprofen (p.44·1).
Fever; pain.

Dentikrisos *Quimifar, Spain.*
Creosote (p.1057·3); benzocaine (p.1286·2); amethocaine hydrochloride (p.1285·2); menthol (p.1600·2).
Toothache.

Dentinale *Montefarmaco, Ital.*
Amylocaine hydrochloride (p.1286·1); sodium benzoate (p.1102·3).
Teething pain.

Dentinox
Note. This name is used for preparations of different composition.
Byk, Aust.
Chamomile tincture (p.1561·2); myrrh tincture (p.1606·1); cetylpyridinium chloride (p.1106·2); laureth 9 (p.1325·2).
Teething pain.
Roche Nicholas, Neth.
Lignocaine hydrochloride (p.1293·2).
Teething pain.
Dentinox, Switz.
Chamomile (p.1561·2); lignocaine hydrochloride (p.1293·2); laureth 9 (p.1325·2).
Dental pain.

Dentinox Colic Drops *DDD, UK.*
Activated dimethicone (p.1213·1).
Colic.

Dentinox Cradle Cap *DDD, UK.*
Sodium lauryl ether sulphosuccinate; sodium lauryl ether sulphate (p.1468·3).
Cradle cap.

Dentinox N *Dentinox, Ger.*
Chamomile (p.1561·2); lignocaine hydrochloride (p.1293·2); laureth 9 (p.1325·2).
Gingivitis.

Dentinox Teething Gel *DDD, UK.*
Lignocaine hydrochloride (p.1293·2); cetylpyridinium chloride (p.1106·2).
Teething pain.

Dentipatch *Noven, USA.*
Lignocaine (p.1293·2).
Local anaesthesia.

Dentispray *Vinas, Spain.*
Benzocaine (p.1286·2).
Local anaesthesia.

Dentogen *Dental Health Products, UK.*
Clove oil (p.1565·2).
Toothache.

Dentohexine *Streuli, Switz.*
Chlorhexidine gluconate (p.1107·2).
Mouth and throat disorders.

Dentol Topico *Calmante Vitaminado, Spain.*
Camphor (p.1557·2); clove oil (p.1565·2); chloral hydrate (p.645·3); procaine hydrochloride (p.1299·2); menthol (p.1600·2).
Toothache.

Dentomicin *Seid, Spain.*
Saffron (p.1001·1); tamarind (p.1217·3).
Toothache.

Dentomycin
Wyeth, Irl.; Lederle, UK.
Minocycline hydrochloride (p.226·2).
Bacterial mouth infections.

Dentomycine *Lederle, Switz.*
Minocycline hydrochloride (p.226·2).
Bacterial mouth infections.

Dentophar *Qualiphar, Belg.*
Amylocaine hydrochloride (p.1286·1); chloral hydrate (p.645·3); chloroform (p.1220·3); menthol (p.1600·2); thymol (p.1127·1); eugenol (p.1578·2).
Dental pain.

Dentosan Mese *Pagni, Ital.†.*
Peppermint oil (p.1208·1); geranium oil (p.1584·1); melissa oil; clove oil (p.1565·2); spearmint oil (p.1632·1); chlorhexidine gluconate (p.1107·2).
Oral hygiene.

Dentosan Ortodontico Collutorio *Parke, Davis, Ital.*
Chlorhexidine gluconate (p.1107·2); sodium fluoride (p.742·1); xylitol (p.1372·3); peppermint oil (p.1208·1).
Oral hygiene.

Dentosan "Pagni" Collutorio *Parke, Davis, Ital.†.*
Chlorhexidine gluconate (p.1107·2); xylitol (p.1372·3); peppermint oil (p.1208·1); geranium oil (p.1584·1); melissa oil; clove oil (p.1565·2); spearmint oil (p.1632·1).
Oral hygiene.

Dentosan Parodontale *Warner-Lambert, Ital.*
Chlorhexidine gluconate (p.1107·2).
Bacterial mouth infections; dental plaque prevention.

Dentosedina *Teofarma, Ital.*
Procaine (p.1299·2); procaine hydrochloride (p.1299·2); benzocaine hydrochloride (p.1286·2); ephedrine hydrochloride (p.1059·3).
Dental pain.

Dentovax *Bouty, Ital.*
Inactivated cells of: *Escherichia coli*; *Streptococcus ovalis*; *Staphylococcus pyog. aur.*; *Proteus vulgaris*; chlorophyll (p.1000·1).
Gingivitis.

Dent's Extra Strength Toothache Gum *Dent, USA.*
Benzocaine (p.1286·2).

Dent's Lotion-Jel *Dent, USA.*
Benzocaine (p.1286·2).

Dent's Maximum Strength Toothache Drops *Dent, USA.*
Benzocaine (p.1286·2).

Dentyl pH *Grafton, UK.*
Triclosan (p.1127·2); fluoride (p.742·1).
Oral hygiene.

Denubil *Pierre Fabre, Spain.*
Heptaminol hydrochloride (p.1587·2); deanol pidolate (p.1478·2).
Mental function impairment.

Denvar *Merck, Spain.*
Cefixime (p.165·3).
Bacterial infections.

Deopens *Brunel, S.Afr.*
Magnesium hydroxide (p.1198·2).
Gastro-oesophageal reflux.

Depa *Alra, USA†.*
Valproic acid (p.361·2).
Epilepsy.

Depacon *Abbott, USA.*
Sodium valproate (p.361·2).
Epilepsy.

Depade *Mallinckrodt, USA.*
Naltrexone hydrochloride (p.988·1).
Alcohol withdrawal syndrome; opioid withdrawal.

Depain *Laser, S.Afr.†.*
Paracetamol (p.72·2); codeine phosphate (p.26·1); caffeine (p.749·3).
Pain.

Depain Plus *Vesta, S.Afr.*
Paracetamol (p.72·2); codeine phosphate (p.26·1); phenobarbitone (p.350·2).
Pain and associated tension.

Depakene
Abbott, Canad.; Kyowa, Jpn; Abbott, USA.
Sodium valproate (p.361·2) or valproic acid (p.361·2).
Epilepsy.

Depakin *Sanofi Winthrop, Ital.*
Sodium valproate (p.361·2).
Epilepsy.

Depakine
Sanofi Winthrop, Aust.; Sanofi Winthrop, Belg.; Sanofi Winthrop, Fr.; Sanofi Winthrop, Neth.; Sanofi Winthrop, Spain; Sanofi Winthrop, Switz.
Sodium valproate (p.361·2).
Epilepsy; febrile convulsions; infantile convulsions.

Depakine Chrono
Sanofi Winthrop, Aust.; Sanofi Winthrop, Fr.; Sanofi Winthrop, Neth.; Sanofi Winthrop, Switz.
Sodium valproate (p.361·2); valproic acid (p.361·2).
Epilepsy.

Depakote *Abbott, USA.*
Semisodium valproate (p.361·2).
Epilepsy.

Depamag *Sigma-Tau, Ital.*
Magnesium valproate (p.363·3).
Epilepsy.

Depamide
Sanofi Winthrop, Fr.; Sigma-Tau, Ital.; Sanofi Winthrop, Spain.
Valpromide (p.361·2).
Depression; epilepsy; psychoses.

depAndro *Forest Pharmaceuticals, USA.*
Testosterone cypionate (p.1464·1).
Breast cancer; delayed puberty (males); male hypogonadism.

depAndrogyn *Forest Pharmaceuticals, USA.*
Oestradiol cypionate (p.1455·1); testosterone cypionate (p.1464·1).
Menopausal vasomotor symptoms; prevention of post-partum breast engorgement.

Depas
Fournier, Ital.; Yoshitomi, Jpn.
Etizolam (p.669·3).
Anxiety; sleep disorders.

Depasan *Giulini, Ger.†.*
Sparteine sulphate (p.1632·1).
Arrhythmias.

Depen
Carter Horner, Canad.; Wallace, USA.
Penicillamine (p.988·3).
Cystinuria; rheumatoid arthritis; Wilson's disease.

Depex *Rolab, S.Afr.*
Sulpiride (p.692·3).
Behaviour disorders; depression; peptic ulcer; psychoses; vertigo.

depGynogen *Forest Pharmaceuticals, USA.*
Oestradiol cypionate (p.1455·1).
Female hypogonadism; menopausal vasomotor symptoms.

Depigman *Hermal, Ger.†.*
Monobenzone (p.1088·3).
Hyperpigmentation disorders.

Depixol
Lundbeck, Irl.; Lundbeck, UK.
Flupenthixol decanoate (p.670·3) or flupenthixol hydrochloride (p.670·3).
Psychoses.

depMedalone *Forest Pharmaceuticals, USA.*
Methylprednisolone acetate (p.1046·1).
Corticosteroid.

Depo Moderin *Upjohn, Spain.*
Methylprednisolone acetate (p.1046·1).
Corticosteroid.

Depo-Clinovir *Pharmacia Upjohn, Ger.*
Medroxyprogesterone acetate (p.1448·3).
Progestogen-only injectable contraceptive.

Depocon *Pharmacia Upjohn, Aust.*
Medroxyprogesterone acetate (p.1448·3).
Endometriosis.

Depodillar
Syntex, Belg.†; Syntex, Neth.†.
Paramethasone acetate (p.1047·3).
Corticosteroid.

Depogamma *Worwag, Ger.†.*
Hydroxocobalamin acetate (p.1364·2).
Vitamin B deficiency.

Depogen *Hyrex, USA.*
Oestradiol cypionate (p.1455·1).
Female hypogonadism; menopausal vasomotor symptoms.

Depoject *Mayrand, USA.*
Methylprednisolone acetate (p.1046·1).
Corticosteroid.

Depo-Medrate *Pharmacia Upjohn, Ger.*
Methylprednisolone acetate (p.1046·1).
Parenteral corticosteroid.

Depo-Medrol
Pharmacia Upjohn, Aust.; Pharmacia Upjohn, Austral.; Pharmacia Upjohn, Belg.; Pharmacia Upjohn, Canad.; Pharmacia Upjohn, Fr.; Pharmacia Upjohn, Ital.; Pharmacia Upjohn, Neth.; Pharmacia Upjohn, Norw.; Pharmacia Upjohn, S.Afr.; Pharmacia Upjohn, Swed.; Pharmacia Upjohn, Switz.; Upjohn, USA.
Methylprednisolone acetate (p.1046·1).
Corticosteroid.

Depo-Medrol cum Lidocain *Pharmacia Upjohn, Norw.*
Methylprednisolone acetate (p.1046·1); lignocaine hydrochloride (p.1293·2).
Musculoskeletal and joint disorders.

Depo-Medrol cum Lidokain *Pharmacia Upjohn, Swed.*
Methylprednisolone acetate (p.1046·1); lignocaine hydrochloride (p.1293·2).
Musculoskeletal, joint, and peri-articular disorders.

Depo-Medrol + Lidocaina *Pharmacia Upjohn, Ital.*
Methylprednisolone acetate (p.1046·1); lignocaine hydrochloride (p.1293·2).
Musculoskeletal, joint, and peri-articular disorders.

Depo-Medrol with Lidocaine
Pharmacia Upjohn, Canad.; Pharmacia Upjohn, S.Afr.
Methylprednisolone acetate (p.1046·1); lignocaine hydrochloride (p.1293·2).
Musculoskeletal, joint, and peri-articular disorders.

Depo-Medrol Lidocaine *Pharmacia Upjohn, Switz.*
Methylprednisolone acetate (p.1046·1); lignocaine hydrochloride (p.1293·2).
Musculoskeletal, joint, and peri-articular disorders.

Depo-Medrol + Lidocaine
Pharmacia Upjohn, Belg.; Pharmacia Upjohn, Neth.
Methylprednisolone acetate (p.1046·1); lignocaine hydrochloride (p.1293·2).
Musculoskeletal, joint, and peri-articular disorders.

Depo-Medrol mit Lidocain *Pharmacia Upjohn, Aust.*
Methylprednisolone acetate (p.1046·1); lignocaine hydrochloride (p.1293·2).
Musculoskeletal and joint disorders.

Depo-Medrone
Pharmacia Upjohn, Irl.; Upjohn, Swed.†; Upjohn, UK.
Methylprednisolone acetate (p.1046·1).
Corticosteroid.

Depo-Medrone with Lidocaine
Pharmacia Upjohn, Irl.; Upjohn, UK.
Methylprednisolone acetate (p.1046·1); lignocaine hydrochloride (p.1293·2).
Musculoskeletal, joint, and peri-articular disorders.

Depo-Medrone med lidokain *Upjohn, Swed.†.*
Methylprednisolone acetate (p.1046·1); lignocaine hydrochloride (p.1293·2).
Inflammatory joint disorders.

Deponit
Gebro, Aust.; Byk, Belg.; Schwarz, Ger.; Schwarz, Irl.; Schwarz, Ital.; Byk, Neth.; Schwarz, Switz.; Schwarz, UK; Schwarz, USA.
Glyceryl trinitrate (p.874·3).
Angina pectoris; heart failure; prophylaxis of phlebitis and extravasation.

Depopred *Hyrex, USA.*
Methylprednisolone acetate (p.1046·1).
Corticosteroid.

Depo-Predate *Legere, USA†.*
Methylprednisolone acetate (p.1046·1).

Depo-Prodasone *Pharmacia Upjohn, Fr.*
Medroxyprogesterone acetate (p.1448·3).
Endometriosis; malignant neoplasms; precocious puberty.

Depo-Progevera *Upjohn, Spain.*
Medroxyprogesterone acetate (p.1448·3).
Endometrial cancer; progestogen-only injectable contraceptive.

Depo-Provera
Pharmacia Upjohn, Aust.; Pharmacia Upjohn, Austral.; Pharmacia Upjohn, Belg.; Pharmacia Upjohn, Canad.; Pharmacia Upjohn, Fr.; Pharmacia Upjohn, Irl.; Pharmacia Upjohn, Ital.; Pharmacia Upjohn, Neth.; Pharmacia Upjohn, Norw.; Pharmacia Upjohn, S.Afr.; Pharmacia Upjohn, Swed.; Pharmacia Upjohn, Switz.; Pharmacia Upjohn, UK; Upjohn, USA.
Medroxyprogesterone acetate (p.1448·3).
Endometriosis; malignant neoplasms; menopausal disorders; progestogen-only injectable contraceptive.

Depo-Ralovera *Kenral, Austral.*
Medroxyprogesterone acetate (p.1448·3).
Breast cancer; endometrial cancer; endometriosis; progestogen-only injectable contraceptive; renal cancer.

Deposal *Benvegna, Ital.†.*
Morpholine salicylate (p.60·1).
Musculoskeletal disorders.

Depositon *Jenapharm, Ger.†.*
3 Tablets, ethinyloestradiol propane sulphonate (p.1445·1); 2 tablets, norethisterone acetate (p.1453·1).
Growth disorders in young girls; sequential-type oral contraceptive.

Depostat
Schering, Aust.; Schering, Belg.†; Schering, Ger.; Schering, Ital.; Schering, Neth.†; Schering, Spain; Schering, Switz.; Cambridge, UK.
Gestronol hexanoate (p.1448·1).
Now known as Gestronol Hexanoate Ampoules in the UK.
Benign prostatic hyperplasia; breast cancer; endometrial cancer.

Depotest *Hyrex, USA.*
Testosterone cypionate (p.1464·1).
Breast cancer; delayed puberty (males); male hypogonadism.

Depo-Testadiol *Upjohn, USA.*
Oestradiol cypionate (p.1455·1); testosterone cypionate (p.1464·1).
Menopausal vasomotor symptoms; prevention of postpartum breast engorgement.

Depotestogen *Hyrex, USA.*
Oestradiol cypionate (p.1455·1); testosterone cypionate (p.1464·1).
Menopausal vasomotor symptoms; prevention of postpartum breast engorgement.

Depot-Hal
Delta, Aust.†.
Allergen extracts (p.1545·1).
Hyposensitisation.

Hal, Ger.
Allergen extracts of pollen, fungi, house dust, mites, and skin (p.1545·1).
Hyposensitisation.

HAL, Neth.
Allergen extracts (p.1545·1).
Hyposensitisation.

Depot-H-Insulin *Hoechst, Ger.*
Neutral insulin suspension (human, highly-purified) (75% crystalline) (p.322·1).
Diabetes mellitus.

Depot-H15-Insulin *Hoechst, Ger.*
Neutral insulin suspension (human, highly-purified) (85% crystalline) (p.322·1).
Diabetes mellitus.

Depot-Insulin
Hoechst, Aust.; Hoechst, Ger.
Insulin injection (bovine) (p.322·1).
Diabetes mellitus.

Depot-Insulin Horm *Hormonchemie, Ger.†.*
Insulin injection (crystalline, bovine) with zinc chloride and protamine sulphate (p.322·1).
Diabetes mellitus.

Depot-Insulin S *Hoechst, Ger.*
Insulin injection (porcine) (p.322·1).
Diabetes mellitus.

Depot-Padutin *Bayropharm, Ger.†.*
Kallidinogenase (Kallikrein) (p.1592·3).
Male fertility disorders; peripheral and cerebral vascular disorders.

Depotpen *SmithKline Beecham, Ger.†.*
Benzathine penicillin (p.158·3); procaine penicillin (p.240·2).
Bacterial infections.

Depotrone *Propan, S.Afr.*
Testosterone cypionate (p.1464·1).
Gynaecomastia; lactation suppression; male hypogonadism; mastitis; menstrual disorders.

Depot-Thrombophob-N *Knoll, Ger.; Immuno, Ger.*
Heparin sodium (p.879·3).
Formerly contained heparin sodium and ephedrine hydrochloride.
Thrombo-embolic disorders.

Deprakine *Sanofi Winthrop, Norw.*
Sodium valproate (p.361·2).
Epilepsy.

Deprancol *Parke, Davis, Spain.*
Dextropropoxyphene hydrochloride (p.27·3).
Pain.

Depraser *Farma Lepori, Spain.*
Etoperidone or etoperidone hydrochloride (p.284·1).
Depression.

Deprax *Farma Lepori, Spain.*
Trazodone hydrochloride (p.308·3).
Depression; premedication.

Deprece *Tecnobio, Spain.*
Almagate (p.1177·1).
Gastric hyperacidity.

Deprelio *Estedi, Spain.*
Amitriptyline hydrochloride (p.273·3); perphenazine (p.685·2).
Bipolar disorder; depression.

Deprenyl
Schering-Plough, Fr.; Sanofi Winthrop, Ger.
Selegiline hydrochloride (p.1144·2).
Parkinsonism.

Depressan *OPW, Ger.*
Dihydralazine sulphate (p.854·1).
Hypertension.

Depressase *Azuchemie, Ger.†.*
Maprotiline hydrochloride (p.296·2).
Depression.

Deprilept *Promonta Lundbeck, Ger.*
Maprotiline hydrochloride (p.296·2).
Depression.

Deproic *Reid-Rowell, USA†.*
Valproic acid (p.361·2).

Deproist Expectorant with Codeine *Geneva, USA.*
Pseudoephedrine hydrochloride (p.1068·3); guaiphenesin (p.1061·3); codeine phosphate (p.26·1).
Coughs.

Deprol *Wallace, USA†.*
Meprobamate (p.678·1); benactyzine hydrochloride (p.280·1).
Depression.

Depronal
Parke, Davis, Belg.; Parke, Davis, Neth.; Warner-Lambert, Switz.
Dextropropoxyphene hydrochloride (p.27·3).
Pain.

Deptran *Alphapharm, Austral.*
Doxepin hydrochloride (p.283·2).
Depression.

Depuran
Woelm, Ger.; Rhone-Poulenc, Ital.†; Rhone-Poulenc Rorer, S.Afr.; Nattermann, Spain.
Senna (p.1212·2).
Constipation.

Depuratif des Alpes *Sodia, Fr.*
Senna (p.1212·2); frangula bark (p.1193·2); liquorice (p.1197·1); magnesium chloride (p.1157·2).
Constipation.

Depuratif Parnel *Medecine Vegetale, Fr.*
Lappa (p.1594·2); viola tricolor; saponaria; fumitory (p.1581·3); sarsaparilla (p.1627·2); senna (p.1212·2).
Constipation.

Depuratif Richelet *Richelet, Fr.*
Walnut leaves; cresson leaves; cochlearia armoracia root; cochlearia officinalis leaves; menyanthes leaves; cinnamon bark; bitter orange; gentian; tannic acid; magnesium chloride; magnesium bromide; nicotinamide.
Tonic.

Depurativo *IDI, Ital.*
Sarsaparilla (p.1627·2); fumitory (p.1581·3); borrana; saponaria; viola; walnut leaves; clover; rhubarb (p.1212·1); senna (p.1212·2); cascara (p.1183·1); lappa (p.1594·2); chicory; dulcamara (p.1574·2); couch-grass (p.1567·3); bitter-orange (p.1610·3); gentian (p.1583·3); willow (p.82·3).
Constipation.

Depurativo Richelet *Vitafarma, Spain.*
Gentian (p.1583·3); potassium iodide (p.1493·1); salicylic acid (p.1090·2); tannic acid (p.1634·2); iodine (p.1493·1); cinnamon oil (p.1564·2); magnesium chloride (p.1157·2); magnesium bromide; nicotinamide (p.1351·2).
Detoxification.

Depuratum *Lehning, Fr.*
Ononis (p.1610·2); birch; calamus rhizome (p.1556·1); rosemary leaves; juniper fruit (p.1592·2); rhapontic root (p.1212·1); fumitory (p.1581·3); aloes (p.1177·1); senna (p.1212·2); frangula bark (p.1193·2); thyme (p.1636·3).
Constipation; dyspepsia.

Depurfat *Herbaline, Ital.*
Rosemary; silver birch (p.1553·3); taraxacum (p.1634·2); cupressus sempervirens; juniper (p.1592·2).
Adjuvant in obesity; biliary disorders; liver disorders; venous disorders; water retention.

Dequacaine
Boots Healthcare, Irl.; Crookes Healthcare, UK.
Benzocaine (p.1286·2); dequalinium chloride (p.1112·1).
Sore throat.

Dequadin
Glaxo Wellcome, Aust.; Boots, Austral.†; Roberts, Canad.; Boots Healthcare, Irl.; Eurospital, Ital.; Salusa, S.Afr.†; Inibsa, Spain; Crookes Healthcare, UK.
Dequalinium chloride (p.1112·1).
Mouth and throat infections.

Dequadin Mouth Paint *Rhone-Poulenc Rorer, S.Afr.*
Dequalinium chloride (p.1112·1); lignocaine (p.1293·2).
Mouth disorders.

Dequadin Mouth Ulcer Paint *Boots, Austral.†.*
Dequalinium chloride (p.1112·1); lignocaine (p.1293·2).
Mouth ulcers.

Dequafungan *Provita, Aust.*
Dequalinium chloride (p.1112·1); undecenoic acid (p.389·2).
Skin infections.

Dequalinetten *Provita, Aust.*
Dequalinium chloride (p.1112·1); benzocaine (p.1286·2).
Mouth and throat disorders.

Dequalinium *Wolfs, Belg.*
Dequalinium chloride (p.1112·1); amylocaine (p.1286·1).
Mouth and throat disorders.

Dequamed *Salusa, S.Afr.†.*
Dequalinium chloride (p.1112·1); lignocaine hydrochloride (p.1293·2).
Sore throat.

Dequasine *Miller, USA.*
Vitamin C with minerals and amino-acids.

Dequavagyn *Provita, Aust.*
Dequalinium chloride (p.1112·1).

Dequin *Inibsa, Spain†.*
Dequalinium chloride (p.1112·1).
Mouth and throat infections.

Dequonal
Provita, Aust.; Kreussler, Ger.; Kreussler, Switz.
Dequalinium chloride (p.1112·1); benzalkonium chloride (p.1101·3).
Mouth and throat infections.

Dequosangola *Eurospital, Ital.*
Dequalinium chloride (p.1112·1).
Mouth disinfection.

Dera *Ingram & Bell, Canad.*
Zinc oxide (p.1096·2); peru balsam (p.1617·2).
Napkin rash.

Deralin *Alphapharm, Austral.*
Propranolol hydrochloride (p.937·1).
Angina pectoris; arrhythmias; hypertension; hypertrophic subaortic stenosis; migraine; myocardial infarction; phaeochromocytoma; tremor.

Deratin *Normon, Spain.*
Chlorhexidine gluconate (p.1107·2).
Mouth and throat infections; skin and wound disinfection.

Derbac-C *Seton, Irl.*
Carbaryl (p.1403·1).
Pediculosis.

Derbac-M
Seton, Irl.; Seton, UK.
Malathion (p.1407·3).
Pediculosis; scabies.

Derbitan Antibiotico *Normon, Spain.*
Atropine methobromide (p.455·1); streptomycin sulphate (p.249·3); phthalylsulphathiazole (p.237·1); neomycin sulphate (p.229·2).
Gastro-intestinal infections.

Dercusan *Asta Medica, Belg.*
Chloramine (p.1106·3).
Superficial wounds.

Dercut *Pekana, Ger.*
Homoeopathic preparation.

Dereme *Menarini, Spain.*
Beclomethasone salicylate (p.1032·3).
Skin disorders.

Dergiflux *Gallier, Fr.†.*
Dihydroergotamine mesylate (p.444·2).
Circulatory insufficiency; migraine and vascular headache; orthostatic hypotension.

Dergotamine *Abbott, Fr.†.*
Dihydroergotamine mesylate (p.444·2).
Migraine and vascular headache; orthostatic hypotension.

Derifil
Iketon, Ital.†; Rystan, USA.
Chlorophyllin copper complex (p.1000·1).
Ostomy deodorant; reduction of faecal or urinary odour in incontinence.

Derilate *Hosbon, Spain.*
Tiaprofenic acid (p.89·1).
Inflammation; musculoskeletal, joint, and peri-articular disorders; pain.

Derinase Plus *Bioindustria, Ital.*
Deoxyribonuclease (p.1059·1); bromelains (p.1555·1).
Inflammatory disorders.

Derinox
Therabel, Fr.; Sodip, Switz.
Prednisolone (p.1048·1); phenylephrine hydrochloride (p.1066·2); naphazoline nitrate (p.1064·2).
Inflammatory and allergic disorders of upper respiratory tract.

Deripil *Galderma, Spain.*
Erythromycin (p.204·1).
Acne.

Derivatio H *Pfluger, Ger.*
Homoeopathic preparation.

Derivon *Gerot, Aust.*
Cream: Benzyl nicotinate (p.22·1); diethylamine salicylate (p.33·1); heparin (p.879·3).
Liniment: Benzyl nicotinate (p.22·1); camphor (p.1557·2); methyl salicylate (p.55·2).
Neuralgia; soft-tissue, peri-articular, musculoskeletal, and joint disorders.

Derma Bad *Lichtenstein, Ger.†.*
Wheat-germ oil; avocado oil; light liquid paraffin (p.1382·1); soya oil (p.1355·1).
Bath additive; skin disorders.

Derma Care *Nelson, Austral.†.*
Chlorhexidine (p.1107·2); dimethicone (p.1384·2).
Dry skin and minor abrasions.

Derma Viva *Rugby, USA.*
Emollient and moisturiser.

Dermabase *Paddock, USA.*
Vehicle for topical preparations.

Dermablend *DDC, UK.*
A covering cream.
Concealment of birth marks, scars, and disfiguring skin disease.

Dermacalm *Sauter, Switz.†.*
Hydrocortisone (p.1043·3) or hydrocortisone acetate (p.1043·3).
Skin disorders.

Dermacalm-d *Roche, Switz.*
Hydrocortisone acetate (p.1043·3); dexpanthenol (p.1570·3).
Skin disorders.

Dermachrome *Synthelabo, Fr.*
Thiomersal (p.1126·3); lignocaine hydrochloride (p.1293·2); phenylephrine hydrochloride (p.1066·2).
Skin disinfection.

Dermacide
Note. This name is used for preparations of different composition.
Sterling Health, Belg.†.
Sodium lauryl sulphate (p.1468·3); benzoic acid (p.1102·3); salicylic acid (p.1090·2).
Cleansing of skin and mucous membranes.
CS, Fr.
Soap: Tartaric acid (p.1634·3); salicylic acid (p.1090·2); benzoic acid (p.1102·3).
Cleansing of skin.
Topical solution: Hydroxyquinoline sulphate (p.1589·3); sodium propionate (p.387·1); salicylic acid (p.1090·2); tartaric acid (p.1634·3).
Skin disinfection.

Dermacne *Bio-Sante, Canad.*
Benzoyl peroxide (p.1079·2).
Acne.

Dermacoat *Century, USA.*
Benzocaine (p.1286·2); chloroxylenol (p.1111·1); menthol (p.1600·2).
Skin disorders.

Dermacolor *Fox, UK.*
A covering cream.
Concealment of birth marks, scars, and disfiguring skin disease.

Dermacort
Parke, Davis, Austral.†; Panpharma, UK; Solvay, USA.
Hydrocortisone (p.1043·3) or hydrocortisone acetate (p.1043·3).
Skin disorders.

Dermacreme *Potter's, UK.*
Menthol (p.1600·2); methyl salicylate (p.55·2); liquefied phenol (p.1121·2).
Antiseptic for minor skin injuries.

Dermacure *Taxandria, Neth.*
Miconazole nitrate (p.384·3).
Fungal skin and nail infections.

Dermadex *Teofarma, Ital.*
Dexamethasone valerate (p.1037·3).
Skin disorders.

Dermadex Chinolinico *SmithKline Beecham, Ital.†.*
Dexamethasone valerate (p.1037·3); clioquinol (p.193·2).
Skin disorders.

Dermadex Neomicina *SmithKline Beecham, Ital.†.*
Dexamethasone valerate (p.1037·3); neomycin sulphate (p.229·2).
Skin disorders.

Dermadine *Medpro, S.Afr.*
Povidone-iodine (p.1123·3).
Mouth and throat disorders; skin disinfection.

Dermadrate *Dermatech, Austral.*
Lactic acid (p.1593·3); urea (p.1095·2); sodium pidolate (p.1091·2).
Dry skin.

Dermaethyl *Medice, Ger.†.*
Coal tar (p.1092·3); laureth 9 (p.1325·2); undecenoic acid (p.389·2); hexylresorcinol (p.1116·1).
Skin disorders.

Dermaethyl-H *Medice, Ger.†.*
Coal tar (p.1092·3); laureth 9 (p.1325·2); undecenoic acid (p.389·2); hexylresorcinol (p.1116·1); hydrocortisone (p.1043·3).
Skin disorders.

Dermafilm *Parke, Davis, Austral.†.*
Dimethicone (p.1384·2).
Barrier cream.

Dermaflex
Note. This name is used for preparations of different composition.
Neolab, Canad.
Urea (p.1095·2).
Emollient; moisturiser.
Zila, USA.
Lignocaine (p.1293·2).

Dermaflogil *NCSN, Ital.*
Diflucortolone valerate (p.1039·3); kanamycin sulphate (p.220·3).
Skin disorders.

Dermaflor *NCSN, Ital.*
Diflorasone diacetate (p.1039·3).
Skin disorders.

Dermagor *Coryne de Bruynes, Mon.*
Aluminium chlorohydrate (p.1078·3).
Hyperhidrosis.

Dermagraft *Smith & Nephew, UK.*
Human dermal tissue.
Diabetic foot ulcers.

Derm-Aid *Ego, Austral.*
Hydrocortisone (p.1043·3).
Skin disorders.

Dermaide *Dermaide, USA.*
Aloe vera (p.1177·1).
Superficial burns, infections, cuts, abrasions, and irritation of the skin.

Dermairol *Roche, Swed.†.*
Tretinoin (p.1093·3).
Acne.

Dermaisom *Teofarma, Ital.†.*
Fluocinolone acetonide (p.1041·1).
Skin disorders.

Dermaknin *Winthrop, Switz.†.*
Salicylic acid (p.1090·2); sulphur (p.1091·2).
Acne.

Dermalex *Sanofi Winthrop, UK.*
Hexachlorophane (p.1115·2) in an emollient base.
Bed sores; rashes; skin disinfection.

Dermalibour *Ducray, Fr.*
Avena (p.1551·3); zinc oxide (p.1096·2); copper sulphate (p.1338·1); zinc sulphate (p.1373·2).
Skin disorders.

Dermalid *Blucher-Schering, Ger.†.*
Camphor (p.1557·2); methyl salicylate (p.55·2).
Circulatory disorders of the skin; frostbite; rheumatic disorders; skin damage.

Dermalife *Delta, Austral.*
Vitamin A palmitate (p.1359·2).
Burns; minor skin lesions; nappy rash.

Dermalife Plus *Delta, Austral.*
Calamine (p.1080·1); vitamin A palmitate (p.1359·2); dimethicone (p.1384·2).
Burns; cradle cap; minor skin lesions; nappy rash; pruritus.

derma-loges N *Loges, Ger.*
Peru balsam (p.1617·2); arnica tincture (p.1550·3); hamamelis water (p.1587·1); matricaria (p.1561·2); sunflower oil (p.1634·1).
Burns; haemorrhoids; skin disorders; wounds.

Dermal-Rub *Hauck, USA.*
Methyl salicylate (p.55·2); camphor (p.1557·2); menthol (p.1600·2); cajuput oil (p.1556·1).
Muscle, joint, and soft-tissue pain; neuralgia.

Dermamist *Yamanouchi, UK.*
White soft paraffin (p.1382·3).
Dry skin disorders.

Dermamycin *Pfeiffer, USA.*
Diphenhydramine hydrochloride (p.409·1).

Derma-Mykotral *Rosen, Ger.*
Miconazole nitrate (p.384·3).
Fungal infections of the skin and mucous membranes.

Dermana *Humana, Ital.*
Zinc oxide (p.1096·2); gamolenic acid (p.1582·1); omega-3 triglyceride (p.1276·1); vitamin E (p.1369·1); vitamin A (p.1358·1).
Nappy rash; skin irritation.

Derma-Oil *Hamilton, Austral.†.*
Light liquid paraffin (p.1382·1).
Dry skin.

Derma-Pax *Recsei, USA.*
Mepyramine maleate (p.414·1); chlorpheniramine (p.405·2).
Pruritus.

Dermaplus *Ripari-Gero, Ital.†.*
Fluocinolone acetonide (p.1041·1).
Skin disorders.

Dermaren *Areu, Spain.*
Dichlorisone acetate (p.1039·2).
Skin disorders.

Dermarest *Del, USA.*
Diphenhydramine hydrochloride (p.409·1); resorcinol (p.1090·1).
Pruritus.

Dermarest Dri-Cort *Del, USA.*
Hydrocortisone acetate (p.1043·3).
Skin disorders.

Dermarest Plus *Del, USA.*
Diphenhydramine hydrochloride (p.409·1); menthol (p.1600·2).
Pruritus.

DermaSept *Sauter, Switz.†.*
Chlorhexidine gluconate (p.1107·2); isopropyl alcohol (p.1118·2).
Skin disinfection.

Dermasept Antifungal *Pharmakon, USA.*
Tannic acid (p.1634·2); zinc chloride (p.1373·1); benzocaine (p.1286·2); methylbenzethonium chloride (p.1119·3); tolnaftate (p.389·1); undecenoic acid (p.389·2).
Fungal skin infections.

DermaSept-d *Sauter, Switz.†.*
Chlorhexidine hydrochloride (p.1107·2); dexpanthenol (p.1570·3).
Wounds.

Dermasil *Chesebrough-Pond's, USA.*
Glycerol (p.1585·2); dimethicone (p.1384·2).

Derma-Smoothe *Camcos, Canad.†.*
Fluocinolone acetonide (p.1041·1).
Skin disorders.

Derma-Smoothe/FS *Hill, USA.*
Fluocinolone acetonide (p.1041·1).
Skin disorders.

Dermasone *Technilab, Canad.*
Clobetasol propionate (p.1035·2).
Skin disorders.

Dermaspray
Roche, Aust.; Roche, Belg.; Roche Nicholas, Fr.†; Nicholas, Neth.†.
Chlorhexidine gluconate (p.1107·2); benzalkonium chloride (p.1101·3); benzyl alcohol (p.1103·3).
Wound disinfection.

Dermastine Solaire *Bergaderm, Fr.†.*
A range of sunscreen preparations containing: ethylhexyl *p*-methoxycinnamate (p.1487·1); 3-(4-methylbenzylidene)bornan-2-one (p.1487·2).

Dermatar
Note. This name is used for preparations of different composition.
Hamilton, Austral.
Tar (p.1092·3).
Skin inflammation and pruritus.
IDI, Ital.
Betamethasone valero-acetate (p.1034·1); salicylic acid (p.1090·2); ichthammol (p.1083·3).
Skin disorders.

Dermatech Liquid *Dermatech, Austral.*
Alcohol (p.1099·1); propylene glycol (p.1622·1).
Vehicle for topical drugs.

Dermatech Wart Treatment *Dermatech, Austral.*
Lactic acid (p.1593·3); salicylic acid (p.1090·2).
Warts.

Dermatodoron
Weleda, Aust.; Weleda, UK.
Dulcamara flowers (p.1574·2); lysimachia nummularia.
Eczema.

Dermatol *Chinosolfabrik, Ger.*
Bismuth subgallate (p.1180·2).
Burns; excoriations.

Dermatop
Hoechst, Ger.; Hoechst Marion Roussel, Ital.; Hoechst Marion Roussel, USA.
Prednicarbate (p.1047·3).
Burns; skin disorders.

Dermatophytin O (Oidiomycin) *Miles, USA†.*
Oidiomycin.
Assessment of cell-mediated immunity; detection of delayed hypersensitivity.

Dermatophytin (Trichophytin) *Miles, USA†.*
Trichophyton antigen.
Assessment of cell-mediated immunity; detection of delayed hypersensitivity.

Dermaval *FIRMA, Ital.*
Diflucortolone valerate (p.1039·3).
Skin disorders.

DermaVeen Acne *Dermatech, Austral.*
Colloidal oatmeal (p.1551·3); salicylic acid (p.1090·2).
Acne; soap-free cleanser.

DermaVeen Bath *Dermatech, Austral.*
Colloidal oatmeal (p.1551·3).
Dry skin; pruritus.

DermaVeen Dry Skin *Dermatech, Austral.*
Colloidal oatmeal (p.1551·3).
Soap-free cleanser.

DermaVeen Moisturising *Dermatech, Austral.*
Colloidal oatmeal (p.1551·3); sodium pidolate (p.1091·2); white soft paraffin (p.1382·3).
Dry skin; pruritus.

DermaVeen Shower and Bath *Dermatech, Austral.*
Colloidal oatmeal (p.1551·3); sodium pidolate (p.1091·2); liquid paraffin (p.1382·1).
Dry skin; pruritus; soap-free cleanser.

Dermazellon *Kohler, Ger.*
Silver salt of 2-aminoethyldihydrogen phosphate.
Burns; skin disorders; wounds.

Dermazin *Pharmascience, Canad.*
Silver sulphadiazine (p.247·3).
Bacterial skin infections.

Dermazol
Bailleul, Fr.; CT, Ital.†.
Econazole nitrate (p.377·2).
Fungal infections.

Dermazole *Ego, Austral.*
Econazole nitrate (p.377·2).
Fungal infections.

Der-med *Permamed, Switz.*
Soap substitute.
Skin disorders.

Dermedal *Farmec, Ital.*
Chloramine (p.1106·3).
Disinfection of wounds and surfaces; genital hygiene.

Dermestril
Sanofi Winthrop, Austral.; Sanofi Winthrop, Belg.; Opfermann, Ger.; Rottapharm, Ital.; Sanofi Winthrop, Neth.; Sanofi Winthrop, UK.
Oestradiol (p.1455·1).
Menopausal disorders; osteoporosis.

Dermex *Hamilton, Austral.*
Range of barrier creams.

Derm-Freeze *Eagle, Austral.*
Trichlorofluoromethane (p.1164·3); dichlorodifluoromethane (p.1164·3).
Local anaesthesia; pain.

Dermichthol *Ichthyol, Ger.*
Ictasol (p.1083·3).
Skin disorders.

Dermiclone *Soekami, Fr.†.*
Phenylbutazone (p.79·2); hydrocortisone acetate (p.1043·3); lignocaine (p.1293·2).
Inflammation; pain.

Dermico *Dermon, Ital.†.*
Triclosan (p.1127·2).
Skin cleansing; skin disorders.

Dermi-cyl *Liebermann, Ger.*
Calcium hydroxide solution (p.1556·3).
Burns; skin disorders.

Dermidex *Seton, UK.*
Lignocaine (p.1293·2); alcloxa (p.1078·2); chlorbutol (p.1106·3); cetrimide (p.1105·2).
Skin irritation.

Dermido *Tosse, Ger.†.*
Metacresolsulphonic acid-formaldehyde (p.725·1).
Infected skin disorders.

Dermiflex *Johnson & Johnson, UK†.*
Hydrocolloid dressing.
Wounds.

Dermijabon Acido *Sterling Health, Spain†.*
Amino acids; lactic acid (p.1593·3); lecithin; lanolin; mineral salts.
Skin disinfection; skin disorders.

Dermijabon Antiseborreic *Sterling Health, Spain†.*
Ammonium lauryl polyethylenesulphonate; sulphur (p.1091·2); docusate sodium (p.1189·3); salicylic acid (p.1090·2); sodium lauryl sulphate; sodium lauryl besylate.
Eczema; seborrhoea.

Dermilon
Herchemie, Aust.†; Redel, Ger.
Zinc oxide (p.1096·2); cod-liver oil (p.1337·3).
Skin disorders.

Derminovag *Novag, Spain.*
Hydrocortisone acetate (p.1043·3).
Formerly contained dexamethasone, hydrocortisone acetate, and neomycin sulphate.
Skin disorders.

Dermintact *Dietavigor, Ital.†.*
Propolis (p.1621·3).

Dermisdin *Isdin, Spain.*
Sulphur (p.1091·2); fenticlor (p.377·3); miconazole nitrate (p.384·3); salicylic acid (p.1090·2).
Acne; scalp disorders; seborrhoea.

Dermisone Beclo *Zyma, Spain.*
Beclomethasone dipropionate (p.1032·1).
Skin disorders.

Dermisone Epitelizante *Zyma, Spain†.*
Amino acids; chloramphenicol (p.182·1); vitamin A palmitate; vitamin F.
Wound healing.

Dermisone Fentiazaco *Zyma, Spain†.*
Fentiazac (p.41·1).
Peri-articular disorders; soft-tissue disorders.

Dermisone Hidroc Neomic *Zyma, Spain†.*
Hydrocortisone (p.1043·3); neomycin sulphate (p.229·2).
Formerly known as Dermisone Hidrocorti Neomicina.
Infected skin disorders.

Dermisone Tri Antibiotic *Zyma, Spain.*
Bacitracin (p.157·3); neomycin sulphate (p.229·2); polymyxin B sulphate (p.239·1).
Skin infections.

Dermitina *Donini, Ital.*
Hamamelis (p.1587·1); sodium glutamate; fatty acids.
Soap substitute.

Dermo 6 *Pharmadeveloppement, Fr.*
Pyridoxine hydrochloride (p.1362·3).
Seborrhoea.

Dermo Base Grassa *Restiva, Ital.*
Product basis.

Dermo Base Magra *Restiva, Ital.*
Product basis.

Dermo Chabre B6 *Reig Jofre, Spain†.*
Pyridoxine hydrochloride (p.1362·3).
Hair, scalp, and skin disorders.

Dermo H Infantil *Zyma, Spain.*
Dimethicone (p.1384·2); benzalkonium chloride (p.1101·3); retinol (p.1358·1); zinc oxide (p.1096·2).
Skin disorders.

Dermo Hubber *ICN, Spain.*
Bacitracin zinc (p.157·3); hydrocortisone acetate (p.1043·3); neomycin sulphate (p.229·2).
Infected skin disorders.

Dermo Posterisan *Kade, Ger.*
Hydrocortisone (p.1043·3).
Skin disorders.

Dermo WAS *Montavit, Aust.*
Lecithin (p.1595·2).
Skin disorders.

Dermoangiopan *Abiogen, Ital.*
Troxerutin (p.1580·2); sulodexide (p.951·1).
Soft-tissue disorders; vascular disorders.

DermoAntage *Antonetto, Ital.†.*
Multivitamin and mineral preparation with collagen and lysine.

Dermobaby *Wintec, Fr.†.*
Titanium dioxide (p.1093·3); vitamin E acetate (p.1369·2).
Nappy rash.

Dermobeta *Terapeutico, Ital.*
Fluocinolone acetonide (p.1041·1).
Skin disorders.

Dermobios *Biotekfarma, Ital.*
Diflucortolone valerate (p.1039·3); tetracycline (p.259·1); polymyxin B sulphate (p.239·1).
Infected skin disorders.

Dermobios Oto *Biotekfarma, Ital.†.*
Diflucortolone valerate (p.1039·3); tetracycline hydrochloride (p.259·1); polymyxin B sulphate (p.239·1).
Skin disorders.

Dermocaine *Ego, Austral.*
Lignocaine hydrochloride (p.1293·2); menthol (p.1600·2); phenoxypropanol (p.1122·2); cetrimide (p.1105·2).
Pain and pruritus.

Dermocalm *Pharmadeveloppement, Fr.*
Vitamin A (p.1358·1); lignocaine (p.1293·2); framycetin sulphate (p.210·3); hydrocortisone acetate (p.1043·3).
Burns.

Dermochinona *Chinoin, Ital.†.*
Monobenzone (p.1088·3).
Hyperpigmentation.

Dermocinetic *Geymonat, Ital.*
Thyroxine sodium (p.1497·1); aescin (p.1543·3).
Cellulite; local build up of adipose tissue.

Dermocortal *Blue Cross, Ital.*
Hydrocortisone (p.1043·3).
Skin disorders.

Dermocreme *Chauvin, Fr.*
Zinc oxide (p.1096·2); copper sulphate (p.1338·1).
Skin irritation.

Dermocuivre *Chauvin, Fr.*
Copper sulphate (p.1338·1); zinc oxide (p.1096·2).
Skin disorders.

Dermocur *Schering, Ital.*†.
Fluocortolone (p.1041·3); fluocortolone hexanoate (p.1041·3); neomycin sulphate (p.229·2).
Skin disorders.

Dermodis *Farmades, Ital.*
Rifaximin (p.246·3).
Bacterial skin infections.

Dermodrin *Montavit, Aust.*
Diphenhydramine hydrochloride (p.409·1).
Skin disorders.

Dermofil *Nuovo, Ital.*†.
Fluocinolone acetonide (p.1041·1).
Skin disorders.

Dermofix *Ferrer, Spain.*
Sertaconazole nitrate (p.387·2).
Fungal infections.

Dermofug *Wolff, Ger.*
Dodecylbenzolsulphonic acid triethanolamine; ammonium lauryl sulphate (p.1468·3).
Acne; fungal infections; seborrhoeic dermatitis.

Dermogamma *IPFI, Ital.*†.
Precipitated sulphur (p.1091·2); resorcinol (p.1090·1); irgasan DP 300 (p.1127·2); allantoin (p.1078·2).
Skin disinfection.

Dermojuventus *Juventus, Spain.*
Tretinoin (p.1093·3).
Acne.

Dermokey *Inkeysa, Spain*†.
Bifonazole (p.375·3).
Fungal skin infections.

Dermol
Note. This name is used for preparations of different composition.
Schwulst, S.Afr.†.
Emollient.
Dry skin.

Dermal Laboratories, UK.
Benzalkonium chloride (p.1101·3); chlorhexidine hydrochloride (p.1107·2); liquid paraffin (p.1382·1); isopropyl myristate (p.1384·1).
Dry and pruritic skin disorders.

Dermol HC *Dermol, USA.*
Hydrocortisone (p.1043·3).

Dermolan *Organon, Canad.*†.
Wool fat (as hypoallergenic fraction) (p.1385·3) allantoin (p.1078·2); triclosan (Irgasan DP 300) (p.1127·2); menthol (p.1600·2).
Antiseptic emollient.

Dermolate *Schering-Plough, USA.*
Hydrocortisone (p.1043·3).
Skin disorders.

Dermolin
Note. This name is used for preparations of different composition.
Lafare, Ital.
Fluocinolone acetonide (p.1041·1).
Skin disorders.

Roberts, USA.
Methyl salicylate (p.55·2); camphor (p.1557·2); menthol (p.1600·2); mustard oil (p.1605·3).
Muscle, joint, and soft-tissue pain; neuralgia.

Dermomycose *Reig Jofre, Spain.*
Boric acid (p.1554·2); phenol (p.1121·2); rosaniline; resorcinol (p.1090·1).
Fungal infections.

Dermomycose Talco *Reig Jofre, Spain.*
Neomycin undecenoate (p.229·2); menthol (p.1600·2).
Skin infections.

Dermophil Indien
Note. This name is used for preparations of different composition.
Couvreur, Belg.†.
Chloral hydrate (p.645·3); peru balsam (p.1617·2); benzophenol salicylate.
Burns; stings; wounds.

Dermophil Indien, Switz.
Peru balsam (p.1617·2); levomenol (p.1596·1); salol (p.83·1).
Emollient.

Dermoplast
Note. This name is used for preparations of different composition.
Wyeth-Ayerst, Canad.
Benzocaine (p.1286·2); benzethonium chloride (p.1102·3); menthol (p.1600·2); hydroxyquinoline benzoate (p.1589·3).
Local anaesthesia.

Akromed, S.Afr.†.
Benzocaine (p.1286·2); benzethonium chloride (p.1102·3); menthol (p.1600·2); hydroxyquinoline (p.1589·3).
Painful conditions of the skin and perineum.

Whitehall, USA.
Benzocaine (p.1286·2).
Painful conditions of the skin and perineum.

Dermoprolyn *Virginia, Ital.*
Aescin (p.1543·3); hamamelis (p.1587·1); ruscus aculeatus; hedera helix.
Skin disorders.

Dermosa Aureomicina *Farmacusi, Spain.*
Chlortetracycline hydrochloride (p.185·1).
Skin infections.

Dermosa Cusi Anticongest *Cusi, Spain*†.
Starch; zinc oxide (p.1096·2).
Skin disorders.

Dermosa Hidrocortisona *Farmacusi, Spain.*
Hydrocortisone acetate (p.1043·3).
Skin disorders.

Dermoseptic *SmithKline Beecham, Spain.*
Sertaconazole nitrate (p.387·2).
Fungal skin and nail infections.

Dermo-Steril
Note. A similar name is used for preparations of different composition.
Ghimas, Ital.
Triclosan (p.1127·2).
Acne.

Dermosteril
Note. A similar name is used for preparations of different composition.
Vis, Ital.†.
Cod-liver oil (p.1337·3); ascorbic acid (p.1365·2).
Vascular disorders.

Dermo-Sulfuryl *Aerocid, Fr.*
Precipitated sulphur (p.1091·2); copper sulphate (p.1338·1); zinc sulphate (p.1373·2).
Skin disorders.

Dermoswab *Schwulst, S.Afr.*†.
Chlorhexidine (p.1107·2); isopropyl alcohol (p.1118·2).
Skin disinfection.

Dermotherma N *Luitpold, Ger.*†.
Benzyl nicotinate (p.22·1).
Peripheral circulatory disorders.

Dermoval *Glaxo Wellcome, Fr.*
Clobetasol propionate (p.1035·2).
Skin disorders.

Dermovan *Owen, USA; Galderma, USA.*
Vehicle for topical preparations.

Dermovat
Glaxo Wellcome, Norw.; Glaxo Wellcome, Swed.
Clobetasol propionate (p.1035·2).
Skin disorders.

Dermovate
Glaxo Wellcome, Aust.; Glaxo Wellcome, Belg.; Glaxo Wellcome, Canad.; Glaxo Wellcome, Irl.; Glaxo Wellcome, Neth.; Allen & Hanburys, S.Afr.; Glaxo Wellcome, Switz.; Glaxo, UK.
Clobetasol propionate (p.1035·2).
Skin and scalp disorders.

Dermovate-NN
Glaxo Wellcome, Switz.; Glaxo, UK.
Clobetasol propionate (p.1035·2); neomycin sulphate (p.229·2); nystatin (p.386·1).
Skin disorders with bacterial or fungal infection.

Dermovit *Kemiprogress, Ital.*
Vitamin, selenium, yeast, and coenzyme Q10.
Nutritional supplement.

Dermovitamina *Difer, Ital.*
Cod-liver oil (p.1337·3).
Skin disorders.

Dermowas N *Wolff, Ger.*
Dodecylbenzolsulphonic acid triethanolamine.
Skin disorders.

Dermowund *Adler, Aust.*
Acriflavine (p.1098·3); diacetylaminoazotoluene; cod-liver oil (p.1337·3); linseed oil (p.1596·2); sodium propionate (p.387·1); zinc oxide (p.1096·2).
Wounds.

Dermoxin *Glaxo Wellcome, Ger.; Wolff, Ger.*
Clobetasol propionate (p.1035·2).
Skin disorders.

Dermoxinale *Glaxo Wellcome, Ger.; Wolff, Ger.*
Clobetasol propionate (p.1035·2).
Scalp disorders.

Dermoxyl
Note. This name is used for preparations of different composition.
ICN, Canad.; ICN, USA†.
Benzoyl peroxide (p.1079·2).
Acne.

RDC, Ital.
Urea hydrogen peroxide (p.1127·3).
Skin disinfection and cleansing.

Dermster *Oberlin, Fr.*†.
Hexamidine isethionate (p.1115·3); hydroxyquinoline sulphate (p.1589·3).
Skin disinfection for skin infections, wounds, and burns.

Dermtex HC with Aloe *Pfeiffer, USA.*
Hydrocortisone (p.1043·3); aloe vera (p.1177·1).
Skin disorders.

Dermuspray *Warner Chilcott, USA.*
Trypsin (p.1640·1); peru balsam (p.1617·2); castor oil (p.1560·2).
Wounds.

Deronga Heilpaste *Basotherm, Ger.*
Natamycin (p.385·3).
Fungal skin infections.

Deroxat
SmithKline Beecham, Fr.; SmithKline Beecham, Switz.; Ciba-Geigy, Switz.
Paroxetine hydrochloride (p.301·2).
Anxiety disorders; depression.

Dertrase *UCB, Spain.*
Carbamoylglutamic acid; inositol (p.1591·1); methionine (p.984·2); chymotrypsin (p.1563·2); ribonucleic acid (p.1624·3); trypsin (p.1640·1); nitrofurazone (p.232·3).
Burns; skin disorders; ulcers; wounds.

Dervin *Boniscontro & Gazzone, Ital.*
Diflucortolone valerate (p.1039·3).
Skin disorders.

Desaci *Simes, Ital.*†.
Deslanoside (p.847·2).
Cardiac disorders.

Desagamma K *IBP, Ital.*†.
Dexamethasone sodium phosphate (p.1037·2); kanamycin sulphate (p.220·3).
Skin disorders.

Desalark *Farmacologico Milanese, Ital.*
Eye/ear drops: Dexamethasone sodium phosphate (p.1037·2).
Eye/ear disorders.
Tablets†*:* Dexamethasone (p.1037·1).
Corticosteroid.

Desalfa *INTES, Ital.*
Cream; ointment: Dexamethasone isonicotinate (p.1037·1); lignocaine hydrochloride (p.1293·2).
Haemorrhoids; skin disorders.
Eye drops; eye ointment: Dexamethasone isonicotinate (p.1037·1); phenylephrine hydrochloride (p.1066·2); neomycin (p.229·2).
Eye disorders.
Inhalation†*:* Dexamethasone isonicotinate (p.1037·1); bromhexine hydrochloride (p.1055·3).
Respiratory-tract disorders.
Lotion: Dexamethasone isonicotinate (p.1037·1); neomycin (p.229·2); nystatin (p.386·1).
Skin disorders.
Topical solution: Dexamethasone isonicotinate (p.1037·1); neomycin (p.229·2); lignocaine hydrochloride (p.1293·2); phenylephrine hydrochloride (p.1066·2); nystatin (p.386·1).
Nasal/ear disorders.

Desamin Same *Savoma, Ital.*
Naphazoline hydrochloride (p.1064·2).
Nasal congestion.

Desamix Effe *Savoma, Ital.*
Dexamethasone (p.1037·1); clotrimazole (p.376·3).
Infected skin disorders.

Desamix-Neomicina *Savoma, Ital.*
Dexamethasone (p.1037·1); neomycin sulphate (p.229·2).
Skin disorders.

Desamon *Streuli, Switz.*
Didecyldiammonium chloride isopropyl alcohol (p.1118·2).
Disinfection of instruments, clothing, hands, skin, and mucous membranes.

Desanden *Nycomed, Switz.*
Benzoyl peroxide (p.1079·2).
Acne.

Desarell *Sanorell, Ger.*
Homoeopathic preparation.

Desarrol *Iquinosa, Spain.*
Cyproheptadine hydrochloride (p.407·2); amino acids.
Tonic.

Desaten *Martin, Spain*†.
Adenosine triphosphate; glutathione; vitamin B substances; pyritinol dihydrochloride; amino acids; betaine.
Tonic.

Desatura *Sanofi Winthrop, Fr.*
Allopurinol (p.390·2); benzbromarone (p.392·3).
Hyperuricaemia.

Desbly *Cooperation Pharmaceutique, Fr.*†.
Drosera (p.1574·1); grindelia; sodium bromide (p.1620·3); sodium benzoate (p.1102·3); magnesium sulphate (p.1157·3); wild thyme.
Respiratory-tract disorders.

Desclidium *Nattermann, Ger.*
Viquidil hydrochloride (p.1644·2).
Circulatory and metabolic disorders of the brain, eyes, and inner ear.

Desconasal *Warner-Lambert, Spain.*
Xylometazoline hydrochloride (p.1071·2).
Nasal congestion.

Desconex *Reig Jofre, Spain.*
Loxapine hydrochloride (p.677·1) or loxapine succinate (p.677·1).
Psychoses.

Descongestan *Merck, Spain.*
Oxymetazoline hydrochloride (p.1065·3).
Nasal congestion.

Descongestivo Cuve Nasal *Perez Gimenez, Spain*†.
Phenylephrine hydrochloride (p.1066·2); menthol (p.1600·2).
Nasal congestion.

Descutan *Pharmacia Upjohn, Swed.*
Chlorhexidine gluconate (p.1107·2).
Skin disinfection.

Desderman
Winthrop, Belg.†.
Tetrabromocresol (p.1126·3); isopropyl alcohol (p.1118·2); alcohol (p.1099·1).
Hand disinfection.

Schulke & Mayr, Ger.
Tetrabromocresol (p.1126·3); alcohol (p.1099·1).
Hand disinfection.

Desenex
Note. This name is used for preparations of different composition.
Novartis Consumer, Canad.; Roche Consumer, Irl.; Ciba, USA.
Ointment; cream; foam; soap; spray powder; powder: Undecenoic acid (p.389·2) and/or zinc undecenoate (p.389·2).
Fungal skin infections; minor skin disorders.

Fisons, USA†.
Topical spray: Tolnaftate (p.389·1).
Fungal skin infections.

Desenfriol *Schering-Plough, Spain.*
Aspirin (p.16·1); caffeine (p.749·3); chlorpheniramine maleate (p.405·1).
Influenza and cold symptoms.

Desenfriol C *Schering-Plough, Spain.*
Aspirin (p.16·1); ascorbic acid (p.1365·2); caffeine (p.749·3); chlorpheniramine maleate (p.405·1).
Influenza and cold symptoms.

Desenfriol D *Schering-Plough, Spain.*
Aspirin (p.16·1); caffeine (p.749·3); chlorpheniramine maleate (p.405·1); phenylephrine hydrochloride (p.1066·2).
Influenza and cold symptoms.

Desenfriol Infantil *Schering-Plough, Spain.*
Aspirin (p.16·1); chlorpheniramine maleate (p.405·1); phenylephrine hydrochloride (p.1066·2).
Influenza and cold symptoms.

Desensib *Wiedemann, Ger.*
Homoeopathic preparation.

Desentol *Pharmacia Upjohn, Swed.*
Diphenhydramine hydrochloride (p.409·1).
Hypersensitivity reactions.

Deseril
Novartis, Austral.; Wander, Belg.; Sandoz, Ger.; Sandoz, Irl.; Novartis, Neth.; Sandoz, Norw.†*; Novartis, S.Afr.; Sandoz, Spain*†*; Sandoz, Switz.; Alliance, UK.*
Methysergide maleate (p.448·1).
Diarrhoea associated with carcinoid disease; migraine and other vascular headaches.

Desernil *Sandoz, Fr.*
Methysergide maleate (p.448·1).
Migraine.

Deseronil *Essex, Ital.*†.
Dexamethasone (p.1037·1).
Oral corticosteroid.

Deserril *Sandoz, Ital.*
Methysergide maleate (p.448·1).
Migraine.

Desert Pure Calcium *Cal-White, USA.*
Calcium carbonate (p.1182·1); vitamin D (p.1366·3).

Desfebre *Lasa, Spain*†.
Paracetamol (p.72·2).
Fever; pain.

Desferal
Ciba-Geigy, Aust.; Novartis, Austral.; Ciba-Geigy, Belg.; Ciba, Canad.; Ciba-Geigy, Fr.; Ciba Cancer Care, Ger.; Ciba-Geigy, Irl.; Ciba, Ital.; Novartis, Neth.; Ciba, Norw.; Novartis, S.Afr.; Novartis, Swed.; Ciba, Switz.; Ciba, UK; Ciba, USA.
Desferrioxamine mesylate (p.975·2).
Aluminium overload; iron overload.

Desferin *Padro, Spain.*
Desferrioxamine mesylate (p.975·2).
Iron overload.

Deshisan *LAW, Ger.*†.
Cellulose (p.1472·1).
Burns; skin disorders; wounds.

Desidox *Desitin, Ger.*
Doxepin hydrochloride (p.283·2).
Anxiety; depression.

Desintex *Richard, Fr.*
Sodium thiosulphate (p.996·2); magnesium thiosulphate (p.996·3).
Dyspepsia; rhinitis; rhinopharyngitis.

Desintex Infantile *Richard, Fr.*
Sodium thiosulphate (p.996·2); magnesium thiosulphate (p.996·3); calcium gluconate (p.1155·2); calcium carbonate (p.1182·1).
Dyspepsia; rhinitis; rhinopharyngitis.

Desintex-Choline *Richard, Fr.*
Sodium thiosulphate (p.996·2); magnesium thiosulphate (p.996·3); choline chloride (p.1337·1).
Dyspepsia.

Desinto *Alter, Spain*†.
Crataegus (p.1568·2); quinine ascorbate (p.1624·2); vitamins.
Aid to smoking withdrawal.

Desinvag *Casen Fisons, Spain.*
Benzalkonium chloride (p.1101·3); furazolidone (p.583·1).
Vaginal antiseptic; vulvovaginal trichomoniasis.

Desiperiden *Desitin, Ger.*
Biperiden hydrochloride (p.458·3) or biperiden lactate (p.458·3).
Drug-induced extrapyramidal disorders; nicotine poisoning; parkinsonism.

Desisulpid *Desitin, Ger.*
Sulpiride (p.692·3).
Depression; schizophrenia; vestibular disorders.

Desitin
Note. This name is used for preparations of different composition.
Sigmapharm, Aust.; Pfizer, Canad.; Desitin, Ger.; Leeming, USA.
Ointment; topical spray: Cod-liver oil (p.1337·3); zinc oxide (p.1096·2).
Burns; skin disorders; wounds.

Desitin, Ger.
Topical powder: Zinc oxide (p.1096·2).
Burns; skin disorders.

Desitin Creamy *Pfizer, USA.*
Zinc oxide (p.1096·2); liquid paraffin (p.1382·1); white soft paraffin (p.1382·3).
Formerly known as Daily Care.
Nappy rash.

Desitin with Zinc Oxide *Pfizer, USA.*
Corn starch (p.1356·2); zinc oxide (p.1096·2).

Desitur *Turimed, Switz.*
Alcohol (p.1099·1); cetrimonium bromide (p.1106·1).
Hand disinfection.

Deskoval N *Sanol, Ger.†.*
Aluminium aspirin (p.15·1); aspirin (p.16·1).
Back pain; rheumatism; spondylosis.

Desmanol *Schulke & Mayr, Ger.*
Chlorhexidine gluconate (p.1107·2); propyl alcohol (p.1124·2); isopropyl alcohol (p.1118·2).
Hand disinfection.

Desmoidpillen *Pohl, Ger.†.*
Methylene blue (p.984·3).
Diagnostic agent.

Desmospray
Ferring, Irl.; Ferring, UK.
Desmopressin (p.1245·1) or desmopressin acetate (p.1245·2).
Diabetes insipidus; nocturnal enuresis; test of renal concentrating capacity.

Desmotabs
Ferring, Irl.; Ferring, UK.
Desmopressin acetate (p.1245·2).
Diabetes insipidus; nocturnal enuresis; post-hypophysectomy polyuria/polydipsia.

Desocol *Lampugnani, Ital.*
Ursodeoxycholic acid (p.1642·1).
Biliary dyspepsia; cholesterol gallstones.

Desocort
Note. This name is used for preparations of different composition.
Galderma, Canad.
Desonide (p.1036·3).
Skin disorders.

Chauvin, Fr.; Novopharma, Switz.†.
Prednisolone sodium metasulphobenzoate (p.1048·1); chlorhexidine gluconate (p.1107·2).
Ear and eye disorders.

Desoform *Lysoform, Ger.*
Glyoxal (p.1115·1); formaldehyde (p.1113·2); glutaraldehyde (p.1114·3); didecyldimethylammonium chloride (p.1112·2).
Instrument disinfection.

Desogen
Note. This name is used for preparations of different composition.
Hoechst Marion Roussel, Ital.
Toloconium methylsulphate (p.1127·2).
Skin, burn, and wound disinfection.

Organon, USA.
21 Tablets, desogestrel (p.1443·3); ethinyloestradiol (p.1445·1); 7 tablets, inert.
Combined oral contraceptive.

Desogene *Ciba-Geigy, Switz.†.*
Toloconium methylsulphate (p.1127·2).
Disinfection of skin and instruments; mouth and throat infections; vaginal infections.

Desolett *Organon, Swed.*
Desogestrel (p.1443·3); ethinyloestradiol (p.1445·1).
28-Day packs also contain 7 inert tablets.
Combined oral contraceptive.

Desomedine
Chauvin, Fr.; Novopharma, Switz.
Hexamidine isethionate (p.1115·3).
Infections of the eye or nose.

Desonix *Difa, Ital.†.*
Desonide (p.1036·3); tetracycline (p.259·1); tetrahydrozoline hydrochloride (p.1070·2).
Eye disorders.

Desopan *Mochida, Jpn†.*
Trilostane (p.1639·2).
Adrenocortical suppressant.

DesOwen *Galderma, USA.*
Desonide (p.1036·3).
Skin disorders.

Desoxil *Boniscontro & Gazzone, Ital.*
Ursodeoxycholic acid (p.1642·1).
Biliary disorders.

Desoxyn *Abbott, USA.*
Methylamphetamine hydrochloride (p.1482·2).
Attention deficit hyperactivity disorder; obesity.

Desquam *Westwood-Squibb, USA.*
Benzoyl peroxide (p.1079·2).
Acne.

Desquaman
Merck, Aust.; Hermal, Switz.†.
Pyrithione zinc (p.1089·3).
Scalp infections; seborrhoeic dermatitis.

Desquaman N *Hermal, Ger.*
Pyrithione zinc (p.1089·3).
Scalp disorders.

Desquam-X *Westwood-Squibb, Canad.*
Benzoyl peroxide (p.1079·2).
Acne.

Dessertase *Inpharzam, Switz.†.*
Fentonium bromide (p.461·2); pancreatin (p.1612·1); dehydrocholic acid (p.1570·2); lactulose (p.1195·3).
Gastro-intestinal disorders.

deSTAT 3 *Sherman, USA.*
Cleaning, disinfectant, and storage solution for gas permeable contact lenses.

Destolit
Marion Merrell, Fr.; Norgine, UK.
Ursodeoxycholic acid (p.1642·1).
Cholesterol gallstones.

Destrobac
Hoechst Marion Roussel, Ital.; Max Ritter, Switz.
Povidone-iodine (p.1123·3).
Skin disinfection; wounds.

Desuric
Sanofi Winthrop, Belg.; Sanofi Winthrop, Fr.; Sanofi Winthrop, Neth.; Sanofi Winthrop, Switz.
Benzbromarone (p.392·3).
Gout; hyperuricaemia.

Desyrel
Bristol, Canad.; Apothecon, USA.
Trazodone hydrochloride (p.308·3).
Depression.

DET MS *Rentschler, Ger.*
Dihydroergotamine mesylate (p.444·2).
Hypotension; migraine and other vascular headaches.

DET MS spezial *Rentschler, Ger.*
Dihydroergotamine (p.445·1).
Chronic venous insufficiency; hypotension; migraine and other vascular headaches.

Detane *Del, USA.*
Benzocaine (p.1286·2).
Genital desensitising lubricant.

Detantol *Eisai, Jpn.*
Bunazosin hydrochloride (p.835·2).
Hypertension.

Deteclo
Wyeth, Irl.; Lederle, UK.
Tetracycline hydrochloride (p.259·1); chlortetracycline hydrochloride (p.185·1); demeclocycline hydrochloride (p.201·2).
Bacterial infections.

Detemes *Procter & Gamble, Aust.*
Dihydroergotamine mesylate (p.444·2).
Hypotension; migraine and related vascular headaches; vascular disorders.

Detensiel *Merck-Clevenot, Fr.*
Bisoprolol fumarate (p.833·1).
Angina pectoris; hypertension.

Detensor *Sandoz OTC, Switz.*
Diphenhydramine hydrochloride (p.409·1); 8-chlorotheophylline.
Sleep disorders.

Detergente Cusi Acido *Cusi, Spain†.*
Boric acid (p.1554·2); citric acid; sodium lauryl sulphate.
Skin disorders.

Detergil
Citrosil, Ital.; Manetti Roberts, Ital.
Benzalkonium chloride (p.1101·3).
Wound disinfection.

Deterzyme
Thylmer, Belg.†; Fournier, Fr.†.
Proteolytic and amylolytic fraction of *Aspergillus oryzae*.
Wound cleanser.

Deticene
Bellon, Fr.; Medac, Ger.†; Rhone-Poulenc Rorer, Ital.; Rhone-Poulenc Rorer, Neth.
Dacarbazine (p.526·3).
Malignant neoplasms.

Detimedac *Medac, Ger.*
Dacarbazine (p.526·3).
Malignant neoplasms.

Detox Thuja *Homeocan, Canad.*
Homoeopathic preparation.

Detoxalgine *Lyocentre, Fr.*
Glucuronamide; aspirin (p.16·1); ascorbic acid (p.1365·2).
Fever; musculoskeletal and joint disorders; pain.

Detoxasi *Miba, Ital.†.*
Cogalactoisomerase sodium (p.1566·2).
Liver disorders.

Detoxepa *Wyeth, Ital.†.*
Timonacic (p.1638·1).
Liver disorders.

Detoxergon *Baldacci, Ital.*
Injection†: Pirglutargine (p.1619·2); pyridoxine hydrochloride (p.1362·3); taurine (p.1635·1); potassium pidolate; magnesium pidolate (p.1157·3); calcium pidolate (p.1155·3); sodium pidolate (p.1091·2).
Hyperammonaemia.
Oral powder: Pidolic acid; pirglutargine (p.1619·2); taurine (p.1635·1); pyridoxine hydrochloride (p.1362·3); sodium citrate (p.1153·2); potassium chloride (p.1161·1); magnesium chloride (p.1157·2); calcium chloride (p.1155·1).
Gastro-intestinal disorders.

Detoxicon
Note. This name is used for preparations of different composition.
Schering, Ital.†.
Tablets; injection: Glutathione (p.983·1); glucurolactone; glycine (p.1345·2); inositol (p.1591·1); ascorbic acid (p.1365·2); methionine (p.984·2).
Liver disorders.

SIT, Ital.
Tablets: Glycine (p.1345·2); acetylmethionine.
Formerly contained glucurolactone, glycine, and acetylmethionine.
Tonic.

Detraine *Seid, Spain.*
Hydrocortisone (p.1043·3); propanocaine hydrochloride (p.1299·3).
Skin disorders.

Detravis *Vis, Ital.†.*
Demeclocycline hydrochloride (p.201·2).
Bacterial infections.

Detrixin *Astra, Swed.*
Cholecalciferol (p.1366·3).
Osteoporosis; vitamin D deficiency.

Detrol *Pharmacia Upjohn, USA.*
Tolterodine tartrate (p.469·1).
Urinary incontinence.

Detrulisin *Glaxo Allen, Ital.†.*
Emepronium bromide (p.461·1).
Muscle spasms.

Detrunorm *Schering-Plough, UK.*
Propiverine hydrochloride (p.468·2).
Bladder instability; neurogenic bladder.

Detrusitol
Pharmacia Upjohn, Swed.; Pharmacia Upjohn, UK.
Tolterodine tartrate (p.469·1).
Bladder instability.

Dettol
Note. This name is used for preparations of different composition.
Reckitt & Colman, Austral.; Reckitts, Irl.; Reckitt & Colman, UK.
Cream; soap: Chloroxylenol (p.1111·1); triclosan (p.1127·2).
Skin disinfection.

Reckitt & Colman, Belg.; Reckitt & Colman, UK.
Topical solution: Chloroxylenol (p.1111·1).
Skin disinfection.

Reckitt & Colman, UK.
Mouthwash†: Cetylpyridinium chloride (p.1106·2).
Formerly contained chloroxylenol.
Oral hygiene.
Topical spray: Benzalkonium chloride (p.1101·3); lignocaine (p.1293·2).
Bites and stings; minor burns; minor wounds.
Topical wipe†: Triclosan (p.1127·2).
Skin disinfection.

Dettol Classic *Reckitt & Colman, Austral.*
Chloroxylenol (p.1111·1).
Disinfection.

Dettol Fresh
Reckitt & Colman, Austral.; Reckitt & Colman, UK.
Benzalkonium chloride (p.1101·3).
Skin disinfection.

Dettol Liquid Wash *Reckitt & Colman, Austral.*
Triclosan (p.1127·2).
Skin disinfection.

Detulin *Woelm, Ger.*
dl-Alpha tocopheryl acetate (p.1369·2).
Vitamin E deficiency.

Deturgylone *Synthelabo, Fr.*
Prednazoline (p.1068·3).
Congestion and inflammation of the upper respiratory tract.

Deursil
Sanofi Winthrop, Ital.; Giuliani, Switz.
Ursodeoxycholic acid (p.1642·1).
Gallstones.

Devaron *Solvay, Neth.*
Cholecalciferol (p.1366·3).
Vitamin D deficiency.

Develin *Godecke, Ger.*
Dextropropoxyphene hydrochloride (p.27·3).
Pain.

Deverol *Waldheim, Aust.*
Spironolactone (p.946·1).
Hyperaldosteronism; hypertension; liver cirrhosis with ascites; nephrotic syndrome; oedema.

Deverol mit Thiazid *Waldheim, Aust.*
Spironolactone (p.946·1); hydrochlorothiazide (p.885·2).
Ascites; heart failure; nephrotic syndrome; oedema.

Devian *Farmacologico Milanese, Ital.†.*
Metformin hydrochloride (p.330·1).
Diabetes mellitus.

Devigen *Stomygen, Ital.†.*
Paraformaldehyde (p.1121·1); lignocaine hydrochloride (p.1293·2).
Toothache.

Devils Claw Plus *Eagle, Austral.*
Harpagophytum procumbens (p.27·2); murraya; celery (p.1561·1) hesperidin (p.1580·2).
Arthritis; rheumatism.

Devincal *Prodes, Spain.*
Piracetam (p.1619·1); vincamine (p.1644·1).
Cerebrovascular disorders.

Devitre *Nycomed, Swed.*
Cholecalciferol (p.1366·3).
Osteoporosis; vitamin D deficiency.

Devorfungi *Combe, Spain.*
Tolnaftate (p.389·1).
Fungal skin infections.

Devrom *Parthenon, USA.*
Bismuth subgallate (p.1180·2).
Ostomy deodorant.

Dex4 Glucose *Can-Am Care, USA.*
Glucose (p.1343·3).
Hypoglycaemia.

Dexa Biciron *Basotherm, Ger.*
Dexamethasone isonicotinate (p.1037·1); tramazoline hydrochloride (p.1071·1).
Allergic and inflammatory disorders of the eye.

Dexa in der Ophtiole *Mann, Ger.*
Dexamethasone sodium phosphate (p.1037·2).
Eye disorders.

Dexa Fenic *Ciba Vision, Spain.*
Chloramphenicol (p.182·1); dexamethasone (p.1037·1).
Infected eye disorders.

Dexa Loscon
Note. This name is used for preparations of different composition.
Basotherm, Ger.†.
Dexamethasone isonicotinate (p.1037·1); thioxolone (p.1093·3); benzoxonium chloride (p.1103·3).
Scalp disorders.

Basotherm, Switz.†.
Dexamethasone isonicotinate (p.1037·1); thioxolone (p.1093·3); dexpanthenol (p.1570·3).
Scalp disorders.

Dexa Loscon mono *Basotherm, Ger.*
Dexamethasone isonicotinate (p.1037·1).
Scalp disorders.

Dexa Polyspectran N *Alcon-Thilo, Ger.*
Polymyxin B sulphate (p.239·1); neomycin sulphate (p.229·2); dexamethasone sodium phosphate (p.1037·2).
Infected eye and ear disorders.

Dexa Tavegil *Sandoz, Spain.*
Clemastine fumarate (p.406·2); dexamethasone (p.1037·1).
Hypersensitivity reactions; inflammatory eye disorders; skin disorders.

Dexa Vasoc *Ciba Vision, Spain.*
Dexamethasone (p.1037·1); naphazoline hydrochloride (p.1064·2); zinc sulphate (p.1373·2).
Eye congestion; inflammatory eye disorders.

Dexa-Allvoran *TAD, Ger.*
Dexamethasone sodium phosphate (p.1037·2).
Corticosteroid.

Dexabene
Merckle, Aust.; Merckle, Ger.
Dexamethasone sodium phosphate (p.1037·2).
Parenteral corticosteroid.

Dexa-Biofenicol-N *Dorsch, Ger.†.*
Dexamethasone (p.1037·1); chloramphenicol (p.182·1); amethocaine hydrochloride (p.1285·2).
Ear disorders.

Dexabiotan in der Ophtiole *Mann, Ger.†.*
Dexamethasone sodium phosphate (p.1037·2); polymyxin B sulphate (p.239·1); framycetin sulphate (p.210·3); sulphacetamide (p.252·2); phenylephrine hydrochloride (p.1066·2); dexpanthenol (p.1570·3).
Eye disorders.

Dexa-Brachialin N *Steigerwald, Ger.*
Dexamethasone sodium phosphate (p.1037·2).
Acute inflammatory rheumatic disorders.

Dexabronchisan *Boehringer Mannheim, Spain†.*
Calcium lactate (p.1155·2); dexamethasone (p.1037·1); diphenhydramine hydrochloride (p.409·1); ephedrine hydrochloride (p.1059·3); theophylline (p.765·1).
Obstructive airways disease.

Dexacidin *Iolab, USA.*
Dexamethasone (p.1037·1); neomycin sulphate (p.229·2); polymyxin B sulphate (p.239·1).
Eye inflammation with bacterial infection.

dexa-clinit *Hormosan, Ger.*
Dexamethasone sodium phosphate (p.1037·2).
Parenteral corticosteroid.

Dexacort *Adams, USA.*
Dexamethasone (p.1037·1), dexamethasone acetate (p.1037·1), or dexamethasone sodium phosphate (p.1037·2).
Lignocaine hydrochloride (p.1293·2) is included in some injections to alleviate the pain of injection.
Formerly known as Decadron.
Corticosteroid.

Dexacortal *Organon, Swed.*
Dexamethasone (p.1037·1).
Corticosteroid.

Dexacrinin *Pharmagalen, Ger.*
Dexamethasone (p.1037·1); salicylic acid (p.1090·2); coal tar (p.1092·3).
Scalp disorders.

Dexaderme Kefrane *RoC, Fr.†.*
Copper sulphate (p.1338·1); zinc sulphate (p.1373·2); dexamethasone sodium phosphate (p.1037·2).
Skin disorders.

Dexa-Effekton *Brenner-Efeka, Ger.; LAW, Ger.*
Dexamethasone sodium phosphate (p.1037·2).
Rheumatic disorders.

Dexafed Cough *Mallard, USA.*
Phenylephrine hydrochloride (p.1066·2); dextromethorphan hydrobromide (p.1057·3); guaiphenesin (p.1061·3).
Coughs.

Dexafenicol *Ciba Vision, Spain.*
Chloramphenicol (p.182·1); dexamethasone (p.1037·1).
Infected eye disorders.

Dexaflam N *Lichtenstein, Ger.*
Dexamethasone sodium phosphate (p.1037·2).
Musculoskeletal, joint, and peri-articular disorders.

Dexa-Gentamicin *Ursapharm, Ger.*
Dexamethasone (p.1037·1) or dexamethasone sodium phosphate (p.1037·2); gentamicin sulphate (p.212·1).
Infected eye disorders.

Dexagrane *Leurquin, Fr.*
Dexamethasone sodium phosphate (p.1037·2); neomycin sulphate (p.229·2).
Infected eye disorders.

Dexahexal *Hexal, Ger.*
Dexamethasone sodium phosphate (p.1037·2).
Corticosteroid.

Dexal *Pulitzer, Ital.†.*
Ketoprofen (p.48·2).
Musculoskeletal disorders.

Dexalocal *Medinova, Switz.*
Dexamethasone (p.1037·1).
Skin and scalp disorders.

Dexalocal-F *Medinova, Switz.*
Dexamethasone (p.1037·1); framycetin sulphate (p.210·3).
Infected skin disorders.

Dexam Constric *Cusi, Spain.*
Chloramphenicol succinate (p.184·2); dexamethasone sodium phosphate (p.1037·2); tetrahydrozoline hydrochloride (p.1070·2).
Eye disorders.

Dexambutol *L'Arguenon, Fr.*
Ethambutol hydrochloride (p.207·2).
Opportunistic mycobacterial infections; tuberculosis.

Dexambutol-INH *L'Arguenon, Fr.*
Ethambutol hydrochloride (p.207·2); isoniazid (p.218·1).
Opportunistic mycobacterial infections; tuberculosis.

Dexamed *Medice, Ger.†.*
Injection: Dexamethasone sodium phosphate (p.1037·2).
Parenteral corticosteroid.
Topical spray: Dexamethasone (p.1037·1); hexylresorcinol (p.1116·1); cetylpyridinium chloride (p.1106·2); benzethonium chloride (p.1102·3); laureth 9 (p.1325·2).
Anogenital pruritus; skin disorders.

Dexameth *Major, USA.*
Dexamethasone (p.1037·1).
Corticosteroid.

Dexamethason-mp *Medphano, Ger.*
Dexamethasone (p.1037·1) or dexamethasone phosphate (p.1037·2).
Corticosteroid.

Dexamin
Note. This name is used for preparations of different composition.
Nycomed, Norw.†.
Amphetamine sulphate (p.1477·3).
Hyperactivity; narcoleptic syndrome.
Streuli, Switz.
Dexamphetamine sulphate (p.1478·2).
Obesity.

Dexamonozon *Medice, Ger.*
Dexamethasone (p.1037·1).
Oral corticosteroid.

Dexamonozon N *Medice, Ger.*
Dexamethasone (p.1037·1).
Lignocaine hydrochloride (p.1293·2) is included in the intramuscular injection to alleviate the pain of injection.
Musculoskeletal and joint disorders.

Dexamytrex
Mann, Ger.; Mann, Neth.
Gentamicin sulphate (p.212·1); dexamethasone (p.1037·1) or dexamethasone sodium phosphate (p.1037·2).
Inflammatory eye infections.

Dexaphen-SA *Major, USA.*
Pseudoephedrine sulphate (p.1068·3); dexbrompheniramine maleate (p.403·2).
Upper respiratory-tract symptoms.

Dexa-Phlogont L *Azupharma, Ger.*
Prednisolone (p.1048·1); dexamethasone (p.1037·1); lignocaine hydrochloride (p.1293·2).
Musculoskeletal and joint disorders.

Dexaplast *Llorens, Spain†.*
Dexamethasone (p.1037·1).
Skin disorders.

Dexapolyfra *Poirier, Fr.†.*
Dexamethasone sodium phosphate (p.1037·2); framycetin sulphate (p.210·3); polymyxin B sulphate (p.239·1).
Ear and nose infections.

Dexapos *Ursapharm, Ger.*
Dexamethasone sodium metasulphobenzoate (p.1037·2).
Allergic and inflammatory disorders of the eye.

Dexa-ratiopharm *Ratiopharm, Ger.*
Dexamethasone sodium phosphate (p.1037·2).
Corticosteroid.

Dexa-Rhinaspray
Boehringer Ingelheim, Irl.; Boehringer Ingelheim, UK†.
Tramazoline hydrochloride (p.1071·1); dexamethasone isonicotinate (p.1037·1); neomycin sulphate (p.229·2).
Allergic rhinitis.

Dexa-Rhinaspray Duo *Boehringer Ingelheim, UK.*
Tramazoline hydrochloride (p.1071·1); dexamethasone isonicotinate (p.1037·1).
Allergic rhinitis.

Dexa-Rhinospray
Bender, Aust.; Boehringer Ingelheim, Belg.; Boehringer Ingelheim, Switz.†.
Tramazoline hydrochloride (p.1071·1); dexamethasone isonicotinate (p.1037·1); neomycin sulphate (p.229·2).
Nasal oedema; rhinitis.

Dexa-Rhinospray N *Thomae, Ger.*
Tramazoline hydrochloride (p.1071·1); dexamethasone isonicotinate (p.1037·1).
Rhinitis.

Dexasalyl
Mayrhofer, Aust.†; Nourypharma, Ger.; Medinova, Switz.
Dexamethasone (p.1037·1) or dexamethasone acetate (p.1037·1); salicylic acid (p.1090·2).
Skin and scalp disorders.

Dexa-sine *Alcon-Thilo, Ger.*
Dexamethasone sodium phosphate (p.1037·2).
Eye disorders.

Dexa-Siozwo N *Febena, Ger.*
Dexamethasone acetate (p.1037·1); naphazoline hydrochloride (p.1064·2); peppermint oil (p.1208·1).
Catarrh; rhinitis; sinusitis.

Dexa-Sol *Hoechst Marion Roussel, Belg.†.*
Dexamethasone sodium metasulphobenzoate (p.1037·2).
Eye disorders.

Dexa-Sol Soframycine *Hoechst Marion Roussel, Belg.†.*
Dexamethasone sodium metasulphobenzoate (p.1037·2); framycetin sulphate (p.210·3); gramicidin (p.215·2).
Infected eye disorders.

Dexasone
ICN, Canad.; Hauck, USA.
Dexamethasone (p.1037·1), dexamethasone acetate (p.1037·1), or dexamethasone sodium phosphate (p.1037·2).
Corticosteroid.

Dexasporin *Moore, USA; Rugby, USA; URL, USA.*
Dexamethasone (p.1037·1); neomycin sulphate (p.229·2); polymyxin B sulphate (p.239·1).
Eye inflammation with bacterial infection.

Dexatopic
Organon, Ger.†; Ravasini, Ital.†; Organon, Neth.; Organon, Spain†.
Dexamethasone (p.1037·1); nandrolone decanoate (p.1452·2); chlorhexidine hydrochloride (p.1107·2).
Skin disorders.

Dexatrim
Note. This name is used for preparations of different composition.
Stella, Canad.
Benzocaine (p.1286·2); ferrous fumarate (p.1339·3); carmellose sodium (p.1471·2).
Obesity.
Roche, Switz.; Thompson, USA.
Phenylpropanolamine hydrochloride (p.1067·2).
Obesity.

Dexatrim Plus Vitamin C *Thompson, USA.*
Phenylpropanolamine hydrochloride (p.1067·2); ascorbic acid (p.1365·2).
Obesity.

Dexatrim Plus Vitamins
Note. This name is used for preparations of different composition.
Thompson, USA.
Caplets: Multivitamin and mineral preparation.
Thompson, USA.
Controlled release caplets: Phenylpropanolamine (p.1067·2); vitamin C (p.1365·2).
Obesity.

Dexchlor *Schein, USA†.*
Dexchlorpheniramine maleate (p.405·1).
Hypersensitivity reactions.

Dexedrine
SmithKline Beecham, Canad.; Medeva, UK; SmithKline Beecham, USA.
Dexamphetamine sulphate (p.1478·2).
Attention deficit disorder with hyperactivity; epilepsy; narcoleptic syndrome; parkinsonism.

DexFerrum *American Regent, USA.*
Iron dextran (p.1348·1).
Iron deficiency.

Dexicam *OFF, Ital.*
Piroxicam (p.80·2).
Musculoskeletal and joint disorders.

Dexide
Synthelabo, Ital.; Rottapharm, Spain.
Colextran hydrochloride (p.1272·2).
Hyperlipidaemias.

Dexir
Upsamedica, Belg.; Oberlin, Fr.
Dextromethorphan hydrobromide (p.1057·3).
Coughs.

Dexium *Synthelabo, Ger.*
Calcium dobesilate (p.1556·3).
Vascular disorders.

Dexkaf *Key, Austral.†.*
Caffeine (p.749·3); vitamin B substances.
Stimulant.

Dexmethsone *Rhone-Poulenc Rorer, Austral.*
Dexamethasone (p.1037·1).
Corticosteroid.

Dexnon *Allen, Spain.*
Thyroxine sodium (p.1497·1).
Hypothyroidism.

Dexodon *Tika, Swed.*
Dextropropoxyphene hydrochloride (p.27·3); paracetamol (p.72·2).
Pain.

Dexofen *Astra, Swed.*
Dextropropoxyphene napsylate (p.27·3).
Pain.

Dexol 250 *Legere, USA†.*
Dexpanthenol (p.1570·3).

Dexol TD *Legere, USA†.*
Pantothenic acid (p.1352·3).

Dexolan *Streuli, Switz.*
Dexamethasone (p.1037·1); zinc oxide (p.1096·2).
Skin disorders.

Dexoline *Ciba Vision, Ital.*
Chloramphenicol (p.182·1); dexamethasone sodium phosphate (p.1037·2); tetrahydrozoline hydrochloride (p.1070·2).
Eye disorders.

Dexomon *Hillcross, UK.*
Diclofenac sodium (p.31·2).
Gout; inflammation; musculoskeletal, joint, peri-articular, and soft-tissue disorders; pain.

Dexone *Solvay, USA.*
Dexamethasone (p.1037·1), dexamethasone acetate (p.1037·1), or dexamethasone sodium phosphate (p.1037·2).
Corticosteroid.

Dexsal *Reckitt & Colman, Austral.*
Oral granules: Sodium citrotartrate; tartaric acid (p.1634·3); glucose; sodium bicarbonate (p.1153·2).
Oral liquid: Calcium carbonate (p.1182·1); simethicone (p.1213·1).
Dyspepsia; flatulence.

Dextin *Rolab, S.Afr.*
Metformin hydrochloride (p.330·1).
Diabetes mellitus.

Dextoma *Arkomedika, Fr.*
Aluminium hydroxide (p.1177·3); aluminium carbonate (p.1177·2); magnesium hydroxide (p.1198·2); magnesium carbonate (p.1198·1).
Gastro-intestinal disorders.

Dextrarine Phenylbutazone *Synthelabo, Fr.*
Dextran sulphate (p.1571·1); phenylbutazone (p.79·2).
Musculoskeletal and joint disorders; superficial phlebitis.

Dextraven *CP Pharmaceuticals, UK†.*
Dextran 110 (p.717·3) in sodium chloride.
Hypovolaemia.

Dextricea *Durban, Spain.*
Rice; gelatin tannate; pectin (p.1474·1); wheat germ.
Diarrhoea.

Dextro med *Maizena, Ger.†.*
Glucose monohydrate (p.1343·3).
Fluid depletion.

Dextro OG-T *Boehringer Mannheim, Ger.*
Mono- and oligosaccharide mixture.
Glucose tolerance test.

Dextrocalmine *Pharmacal, Switz.*
Dextromethorphan hydrobromide (p.1057·3).
Coughs.

Dextrolag *Lagap, Switz.†.*
Dextromethorphan hydrobromide (p.1057·3); guaiphenesin (p.1061·3); chlorpheniramine maleate (p.405·1); ammonium chloride (p.1055·2).
Coughs.

Dextromon *Maizena, Ger.†.*
Glucose monohydrate (p.1343·3).
Prophylaxis of mastitis.

Dextrostat *Richwood, USA.*
Dexamphetamine sulphate (p.1478·2).
Attention deficit disorder; narcoleptic syndrome; obesity.

Dextrostix
Bayer Diagnostics, Fr.; Ames, Irl.; Bayer, Ital.; Ames, S.Afr.; Bayer Diagnostics, UK†; Bayer, USA.
Test for glucose in blood (p.1585·1).

Dezacor *Marion Merrell, Spain.*
Deflazacort (p.1036·2).
Corticosteroid.

DF 118
Galen, Irl.; Glaxo Wellcome, S.Afr.; Napp, UK.
Dihydrocodeine tartrate (p.34·1).
Pain.

D-Fluoretten *Albert-Roussel, Ger.; Hoechst, Ger.*
Cholecalciferol (p.1366·3); sodium fluoride (p.742·1).
Dental caries prophylaxis; rickets prophylaxis.

DH 112 *Holzinger, Aust.†.*
Procaine hydrochloride (p.1299·2); royal jelly (p.1626·3).

DHC *Mundipharma, Ger.*
Dihydrocodeine tartrate (p.34·1).
Pain.

DHC Continus
Napp, Irl.; Napp, UK.
Dihydrocodeine tartrate (p.34·1).
Pain.

DHC Plus *Purdue Frederick, USA.*
Dihydrocodeine tartrate (p.34·1); paracetamol (p.72·2); caffeine (p.749·3).

DHE 45 *Sandoz, USA.*
Dihydroergotamine mesylate (p.444·2).
Vascular headache.

DHS Sal *Person & Covey, USA.*
Salicylic acid (p.1090·2).
Psoriasis; seborrhoeic dermatitis.

DHS Tar *Person & Covey, USA.*
Coal tar (p.1092·3).
Scalp disorders; seborrhoea.

DHS Zinc *Person & Covey, USA.*
Pyrithione zinc (p.1089·3).
Scalp disorders.

DHT *Roxane, USA.*
Dihydrotachysterol (p.1366·3).
Hypoparathyroidism; postoperative and idiopathic tetany.

DH-Tox *Sanorania, Ger.†.*
Co-dergocrine mesylate (p.1566·1).
Vascular headache including migraine.

Di Retard *Llorens, Spain.*
Diclofenac sodium (p.31·2).
Gout; inflammation; musculoskeletal, joint, and periarticular disorders; pain; renal colic.

Dia-Aktivanad-N *Knoll, Ger.*
Bovine liver extract; yeast extract; caffeine.
Tonic.

Diabacil *Hosbon, Spain†.*
Rifampicin (p.243·2).
Asymptomatic carriers of Neisseria meningitidis; opportunistic mycobacterial infections; tuberculosis.

dia-basan *Sagitta, Ger.†.*
Glibenclamide (p.319·3).
Diabetes mellitus.

Dia-BASF *BASF, Ger.*
Glibenclamide (p.319·3).
Diabetes mellitus.

Diabe Strip *Midy, Ital.†.*
Test for glucose in blood (p.1585·1).

Diabemide *Guidotti, Ital.*
Chlorpropamide (p.319·1).
Diabetes mellitus.

Diabene *Lehning, Fr.*
Homoeopathic preparation.

Diabenor *IFI, Ital.*
Glisolamide (p.321·2).
Diabetes mellitus.

Diabenyl *ankerpharm, Ger.†.*
Diphenhydramine hydrochloride (p.409·1); naphazoline hydrochloride (p.1064·2).
Allergic conjunctivitis.

Diabenyl T *ankerpharm, Ger.*
Tetrahydrozoline hydrochloride (p.1070·2).
Eye irritation.

Diabenyl-Rhinex *Wernigerode, Ger.*
Diphenhydramine hydrochloride (p.409·1); naphazoline hydrochloride (p.1064·2).
Allergic rhinitis.

Diaberit *IFI, Ital.†.*
Metformin hydrochloride (p.330·1).
Diabetes mellitus.

DiaBeta
Hoechst Marion Roussel, Canad.; Hoechst, USA.
Glibenclamide (p.319·3).
Diabetes mellitus.

Diabetamide *Ashbourne, UK.*
Glibenclamide (p.319·3).
Diabetes mellitus.

Diabetan S *Schuck, Ger.*
Homoeopathic preparation.

Diabetase *Azupharma, Ger.*
Metformin hydrochloride (p.330·1).
Diabetes mellitus.

Diabetes-Entoxin N *Klein & Steube, Ger.†.*
Homoeopathic preparation.

Diabetes-Gastreu N R40 *Reckeweg, Ger.*
Homoeopathic preparation.

Diabetex *Germania, Aust.*
Metformin hydrochloride (p.330·1).
Diabetes mellitus.

Diabetic Tussin *Roberts, USA.*
Dextromethorphan hydrobromide (p.1057·3); guaiphenesin (p.1061·3); phenylephrine (p.1066·2).
Coughs.

Diabetic Tussin Allergy Relief *Health Care Products, USA.*
Chlorpheniramine maleate (p.405·1).
Upper respiratory-tract symptoms.

Diabetic Tussin DM *Roberts, USA.*
Dextromethorphan hydrobromide (p.1057·3); guaiphenesin (p.1061·3).
Coughs.

Diabetic Tussin EX *Health Care Products, USA.*
Guaiphenesin (p.1061·3).
Coughs.

Diabeton Metilato *Teknofarma, Ital.†.*
Tolbutamide (p.333·2).
Diabetes mellitus.

Diabetosan
Note. This name is used for preparations of different composition.
Brocchieri, Ital.†.
Metformin hydrochloride (p.330·1).
Diabetes mellitus.
Pharmacal, Switz.†.
Lignocaine hydrochloride (p.1293·2); dequalinium chloride (p.1112·1); amethocaine hydrochloride (p.1285·2); menthol (p.1600·2).
Sore throat.

diabetoSome (Revitorgan) *Vitorgan, Ger.†.*
Pancreatic extract; zinc sulphate (p.1373·2); manganese sulphate (p.1350·3); magnesium chloride (p.1157·2); potassium chloride (p.1161·1); calcium chloride (p.1155·1).
Angiopathies; diabetes mellitus; neuropathies.

Diabetylin N *Diabetylin, Ger.†.*
Faex medicinalis (p.1373·1); sulphur (p.1091·2); galega officinale; phaseolus vulgaris.
Diabetes mellitus (adjuvant).

Diabewas *IFI, Ital.†.*
Tolazamide (p.333·2).
Diabetes mellitus.

Diabex *Alphapharm, Austral.*
Metformin hydrochloride (p.330·1).
Diabetes mellitus.

Diabexan *Crosara, Ital.*
Chlorpropamide (p.319·1).
Diabetes mellitus.

Diabiformine *Pfizer, Switz.*
Chlorpropamide (p.319·1); metformin hydrochloride (p.330·1).
Diabetes mellitus.

Diabines *Pfizer, Swed.*
Chlorpropamide (p.319·1).
Diabetes mellitus.

Diabinese
Pfizer, Austral.; Roerig, Belg.; Pfizer, Canad.; Pfizer, Fr.†; Pfizer, Irl.; Pfizer, Ital.†; Pfizer, Norw.; Pfizer, S.Afr.; Pfizer, Spain; Pfizer, Switz.; Pfizer, UK†; Pfizer, USA.
Chlorpropamide (p.319·1).
Diabetes insipidus; diabetes mellitus.

Diabis Activado *Funk, Spain†.*
Aminoglucosidase; phenformin hydrochloride (p.330·3).
Diabetes mellitus.

Diabitex *Salters, S.Afr.†.*
Chlorpropamide (p.319·1).
Diabetes mellitus.

Diabomet *Carlo Erba, Ital.†.*
Metformin (p.330·2); glycyclamide (p.321·2).
Diabetes mellitus.

Diaborale *Pharmacia Upjohn, Ital.*
Glycyclamide (p.321·2).
Diabetes mellitus.

Diabrezide *Molteni, Ital.*
Gliclazide (p.320·1).
Diabetes mellitus.

Diabur-Test 5000
Boehringer Mannheim, Austral.; Boehringer Mannheim Diagnostics, Irl.; Boehringer Mannheim, Ital.; Boehringer Mannheim Diagnostics, UK.
Test for glucose in urine (p.1585·1).

Diacard *Madaus, Ger.*
Homoeopathic preparation.

Diaceplex *Salvat, Spain.*
Diazepam (p.661·1).
Diaceplax capsules also contain pyridoxine hydrochloride.
Alcohol withdrawal syndrome; anxiety; epilepsy; febrile convulsions; general anaesthesia; insomnia; skeletal muscle spasm.

Diaceplex Simple *Salvat, Spain.*
Diazepam (p.661·1).
Alcohol withdrawal syndrome; anxiety; epilepsy; febrile convulsions; general anaesthesia; insomnia; skeletal muscle spasm.

Dia-Chek *Searle, Austral.*
Codeine phosphate (p.26·1); aluminium hydroxide (p.1177·3).
Diarrhoea.

Diachlor *Major, USA.*
Chlorothiazide (p.839·1).
Hypertension; oedema.

Dia-Colon *Piam, Ital.*
Lactulose (p.1195·3).
Gastro-intestinal disorders; liver disorders.

Diacor *Houde, Fr.*
Diltiazem hydrochloride (p.854·2).
Angina pectoris.

Di-Actane *Menarini, Fr.*
Naftidrofuryl oxalate (p.914·2).
Cerebral and peripheral vascular disorders; mental function impairment in the elderly.

Diacure
Note. This name is used for preparations of different composition.
Lehning, Fr.
Taraxacum (p.1634·2); berberis; juglans; millefolium; myrtillus (p.1606·1); centaury (p.1561·1); natrum phosphoricum.
Metabolic disorders.

Taxandria, Neth.
Loperamide hydrochloride (p.1197·2).
Diarrhoea.

Diadar *Prophin, Ital.†.*
Diacerein (p.29·3).
Osteoarthritis.

Diadin M *Diadin, Ger.*
Mofebutazone (p.56·1).
Musculoskeletal and joint disorders.

Di-Adreson-F *Organon, Neth.*
Prednisolone acetate (p.1048·1) or prednisolone sodium succinate (p.1048·2).
Corticosteroid.

Dia-Eptal *Montavit, Aust.*
Glibenclamide (p.319·3).
Diabetes mellitus.

Diafen *MC, Ital.†.*
Povidone-iodine (p.1123·3); isopropyl alcohol (p.1118·2).
Skin and wound disinfection.

Diaformin *Alphapharm, Austral.*
Metformin hydrochloride (p.330·1).
Diabetes mellitus.

Diafusor
Schering-Plough, Belg.; Pierre Fabre, Fr.; Pierre Fabre, Spain.
Glyceryl trinitrate (p.874·3).
Angina pectoris.

Diagesil *Berk, UK.*
Diamorphine hydrochloride (p.29·3).
Pain.

Diaglyk *Generics, UK.*
Gliclazide (p.320·1).
Diabetes mellitus.

Diagnosis *Boehringer Mannheim, Ital.*
Pregnancy test (p.1621·2).

Diagnostic Skin Testing Kit *Bayer, S.Afr.*
Allergen extracts (p.1545·1).
Diagnostic agent.

Diagran *Bristol-Myers Squibb, Ital.*
Multivitamin preparation.

Diagran Minerale *Bristol-Myers Squibb, Ital.*
Multivitamin and mineral preparation.

Diaguard *Nelson, Austral.†.*
Mixture: Kaolin (p.1195·1); pectin (p.1474·1); simethicone (p.1213·1).
Tablets: Aluminium hydroxide (p.1177·3); activated attapulgite (p.1178·3); pectin (p.1474·1); benzalkonium chloride (p.1101·3).
Diarrhoea.

Diaguard Forte *Nelson, Austral.†.*
Codeine phosphate (p.26·1); kaolin (p.1195·1); pectin (p.1474·1); simethicone (p.1213·1).
Diarrhoea.

Diah-Limit *Wallis, UK.*
Loperamide hydrochloride (p.1197·2).
Diarrhoea.

Dialaflex Solutions *Kendall, UK†.*
Electrolytes; anhydrous glucose (p.1151·1).
Peritoneal dialysis.

Dialamine
Scientific Hospital Supplies, Austral.; Scientific Hospital Supplies, Irl.; Scientific Hospital Supplies, UK.
Amino acid, carbohydrate, ascorbic acid, and mineral preparation.
Enteral nutrition.

Dialar *Lagap, UK.*
Diazepam (p.661·1).

Dialax *Brady, Aust.†.*
Rhubarb extract (p.1212·1); cascara extract (p.1183·1); aloes extract (p.1177·1); Kissingen salts.

Dialens
Specia, Fr.; Novopharma, Switz.
Dextran 60-85 (p.716·3).
Dry eyes; wetting agent for contact lenses.

Dialgine forte N *Intermedica, Switz.*
Paracetamol (p.72·2); propyphenazone (p.81·3); caffeine (p.749·3).
Fever; pain.

Dialibra *Dieterba, Ital.*
Dietary fibre supplement (p.1181·2).
Disorders of glucose and lipid metabolism.

Dialicor *Guidotti, Ital.†.*
Etafenone hydrochloride (p.866·3).
Cardiac disorders.

Dialisol *Pharmacia Upjohn, Spain.*
A peritoneal dialysis solution (p.1151·1).

Dialose *J&J-Merck, USA.*
Docusate potassium (p.1189·3) or docusate sodium (p.1189·3).
Constipation; hard stools.

Dialose Plus *J&J-Merck, USA.*
Docusate sodium (p.1189·3); yellow phenolphthalein (p.1208·2).
Constipation; hard stools.

Dialster *Esoform, Ital.*
Sodium dichloroisocyanurate (p.1124·3).
Disinfection of surfaces, water, food, and feeding bottles.

Dialume
Rorer, Spain†; Rhone-Poulenc Rorer, USA.
Aluminium hydroxide (p.1177·3).
Hyperacidity; hyperphosphataemia.

Dialycare *Abbott, Ital.*
Preparation for enteral nutrition.
Renal dialysis.

Dialysol Acide *Soludia, Fr.*
Sodium chloride; potassium chloride; calcium chloride; magnesium chloride; acetic acid (p.1151·1).
Haemodialysis solution.

Dialysol Bicarbonate *Soludia, Fr.*
Sodium bicarbonate; sodium chloride (p.1151·1).
Haemodialysis solution.

Dialytan H *Aguettant, Fr.*
Haemodialysis solution (p.1151·1).

Dialyte *Gambro, USA.*
Glucose; electrolytes (p.1151·1).
Peritoneal dialysis solution.

Diamantil *IBIS, Ital.†.*
Heart and lymph gland extract (p.1599·1).
Male infertility.

Diambulate Solutions *Kendall, UK†.*
Electrolytes; anhydrous glucose (p.1151·1).
Peritoneal dialysis.

Diamicron
Servier, Aust.; Servier, Austral.; Servier, Belg.; Servier, Canad.; Servier, Fr.; Servier, Ger.; Servier, Irl.; Servier, Ital.; Servier, Neth.; Servier, S.Afr.; Servier, Spain; Servier, Switz.; Servier, UK.
Gliclazide (p.320·1).
Diabetes mellitus.

Diamine TD *Major, USA†.*
Brompheniramine maleate (p.403·2).
Hypersensitivity reactions.

Diaminocillina *Fournier, Ital.*
Benzathine penicillin (p.158·3).
Bacterial infections.

Diamoril *Roques, Fr.*
Benzquercin (p.1580·1).
Peripheral vascular disorders.

Diamox
Cyanamid, Aust.; Storz, Austral.; Storz, Belg.; Storz, Canad.; Theraplix, Fr.; Lederle, Ger.; Storz, Irl.; Cyanamid, Ital.; Lederle, Neth.; Wyeth, Norw.; Wyeth, S.Afr.; Cyanamid, Spain; Wyeth Lederle, Swed.; Lederle, Switz.; Wyeth, UK; Lederle, USA.
Acetazolamide (p.810·3) or acetazolamide sodium (p.810·3).
Acute mountain sickness; cerebral oedema; epilepsy; glaucoma; hypercapnia; Ménière's disease; ocular hypertension; oedema; pancreatic disorders; respiratory insufficiency.

Diamplicil *Pharmacia Upjohn, Ital.*
Ampicillin (p.153·1); dicloxacillin (p.201·3).
Bacterial infections.

Diane
Schering, Aust.; Schering, Austral.; Schering, Belg.; Schering, Fr.; Schering, Ger.; Schering, Ital.; Schering, Neth.; Schering, Norw.; Schering, S.Afr.; Schering, Spain; Schering, Switz.
Cyproterone acetate (p.1440·2); ethinyloestradiol (p.1445·1).
28-Day packs contain 7 inert tablets.
Androgen-dependent acne, seborrhoea, alopecia, and hirsutism in females; oral contraceptive in women with androgenic symptoms.

Dianeal
Baxter, Aust.; Baxter, Austral.; Baxter, Spain; Baxter, Swed.; Baxter, Switz.; Baxter, UK; Travenol, USA†.
Glucose; sodium chloride; sodium lactate; calcium chloride; magnesium chloride (p.1151·1).
Peritoneal dialysis.

Dianette
Schering, Irl.; Schering, UK.
Cyproterone acetate (p.1440·2); ethinyloestradiol (p.1445·1).
Acne and hirsutism in females.

Di-Antalvic *Houde, Fr.*
Dextropropoxyphene hydrochloride (p.27·3); paracetamol (p.72·2).
Pain.

Diaparene *Lehn & Fink, USA†.*
Methylbenzethonium chloride (p.1119·3).
Skin irritation or chafing.

Diaparene Baby *Lehn & Fink, USA†.*
Emollient barrier cream.
Nappy rash.

Diaparene Corn Starch *Personal Care, USA.*
Corn starch (p.1356·2); aloes (p.1177·1).
Nappy rash.

Diaparene Cradol *Lehn & Fink, USA†.*
Methylbenzethonium chloride (p.1119·3).
Cradle cap and scalp infections in infants.

Diaparene Diaper Rash *Personal Care, USA.*
Zinc oxide (p.1096·2).
Nappy rash.

Diaparene Peri-Anal *Glenbrook, USA†.*
Methylbenzethonium chloride (p.1119·3); cod-liver oil (p.1337·3); zinc oxide (p.1096·2).
Nappy rash; skin irritation or chafing.

Diapatol *Teofarma, Ital.*
Amitriptyline hydrochloride (p.273·3); chlordiazepoxide hydrochloride (p.646·3).
Anxiety disorders; depression; insomnia.

Diaper Guard
Note. This name is used for preparations of different composition.
Del, Canad.
Dimethicone (p.1384·2); soft paraffin (p.1382·3); zinc oxide (p.1096·2).

Del, USA.
Dimethicone (p.1384·2); white soft paraffin (p.1382·3); vitamin A (p.1358·1); vitamin D_3 (p.1366·3); vitamin E (p.1369·1).
Nappy rash.

Diaper Rash
Note. This name is used for preparations of different composition.
Drug Trading, Canad.
Zinc oxide (p.1096·2).

Goldline, USA; Rugby, USA; Schein, USA.
Zinc oxide (p.1096·2); cod-liver oil (p.1337·3).
Nappy rash.

Diaphal *Pierre Fabre, Ger.*
Frusemide (p.871·1); amiloride hydrochloride (p.819·2).
Ascites; hypertension; oedema.

Diapid
Sandoz, Fr.; Sandoz, USA.
Lypressin (p.1263·2).
Diabetes insipidus.

Diaporin *Merckle-Diadin, Ger.†.*
Iodine (p.1493·1); aconite (p.1542·2).
Antiseptic; skin disinfection.

Diaqua *Hauck, USA.*
Hydrochlorothiazide (p.885·2).
Hypertension; oedema.

Diaquel *Rolab, S.Afr.*
Diazepam (p.661·1).
Alcohol withdrawal syndrome; anxiety; premedication.

Diar-Aid *Thompson, USA†.*
Loperamide hydrochloride (p.1197·2).

Diarcalm *McGloin, Austral.*
Oral liquid: Light kaolin (p.1195·1); pectin (p.1474·1); catechu (p.1560·3); aluminium hydroxide (p.1177·3).
Tablets†: Codeine phosphate (p.26·1); attapulgite (p.1178·3); pectin (p.1474·1).
Diarrhoea; stomach pain.

Diarconal *Recordati, Ital.†.*
Conalbumin.
Gastro-intestinal disorders.

Diarex *Pharmavite, Canad.*
Kaolin (p.1195·1); pectin (p.1474·1).

Diareze
Note. This name is used for preparations of different composition.
Key, Austral.
Oral suspension: Attapulgite (p.1178·3); pectin (p.1474·1); simethicone (p.1213·1).
Tablets: Attapulgite (p.1178·3); pectin (p.1474·1); aluminium hydroxide (p.1177·3).
Diarrhoea.

Boots, UK.
Loperamide hydrochloride (p.1197·2).
Diarrhoea.

Diargal
Diepal, Fr.; Bonomelli, Ital.†.
Infant feed; food for special diets.
Coeliac disease; diarrhoea; irritable bowel syndrome; lactose intolerance; sucrose intolerance.

Diaril *MC, Ital.*
Glutaraldehyde (p.1114·3); sodium phenate.
Instrument disinfection.

Diarlac *Urgo, Fr.*
Lactobacillus acidophilus (p.1594·1).
Diarrhoea.

Diaront mono *Chephasaar, Ger.*
Colistin sulphate (p.195·3).
Selective gastro-intestinal tract decontamination.

Diaront NN *Chephasaar, Ger.†.*
Capsules: Bismuth subcarbonate (p.1180·1); phthalylsulphathiazole (p.237·1); chloroxine (p.215·3).
Formerly contained bismuth subcarbonate, belladonna, phthalylsulphathiazole, sulphaguanidine, and chloroxine.
Oral liquid: Bismuth subcarbonate (p.1180·1); albumin tannate (p.1176·3); formosulphathiazole (p.210·1); phthalylsulphathiazole (p.237·1); chloroxine (p.215·3).
Formerly contained bismuth subcarbonate, albumin tannate, formosulphathiazole, phthalylsulphathiazole, sulphaguanidine, chloroxine, tinct. catechu, and tinct. belladonnae.
Diarrhoea.

Diarphen *Mepra-Pharm, UK.*
Diphenoxylate hydrochloride (p.1189·1).
Atropine sulphate (p.455·1) is included in this preparation to discourage abuse.
These ingredients can be described by the British Approved Name Co-phenotrope.
Diarrhoea.

Diarrest
Galen, Irl.; Galen, UK.
Codeine phosphate (p.26·1); dicyclomine hydrochloride (p.460·1); sodium chloride; potassium chloride; sodium citrate.
Diarrhoea.

Diarret *Geymonat, Ital.*
Nifuroxazide (p.231·3).
Acute infective diarrhoea.

Diarrex *Hylands, Canad.*
Homoeopathic preparation.

Diarrhea Relief *Stanley, Canad.*
Loperamide hydrochloride (p.1197·2).

Diarrheel S *Heel, Ger.*
Homoeopathic preparation.

Diarrhoea Complex *Brauer, Austral.*
Homoeopathic preparation.

Diarrhoea Tablets *Brauer, Austral.*
Homoeopathic preparation.

Diarrhoesan
Salvator, Aust.; Loges, Ger.
Apple pectin (p.1474·1); chamomile (p.1561·2).
Diarrhoea.

Diarsed *Sanofi Winthrop, Fr.*
Diphenoxylate hydrochloride (p.1189·1).
Atropine sulphate (p.455·1) is included in this preparation to discourage abuse.
Diarrhoea.

Diarstop
Note. This name is used for preparations of different composition.
Giuliani, Ital.
Loperamide hydrochloride (p.1197·2).
Diarrhoea.

Schering, Ital.†.
Fenalamide (p.1578·3); dihydrostreptomycin sulphate (p.202·2).
Gastro-intestinal disorders.

Diarstop L *Henk, Ger.†.*
Loperamide hydrochloride (p.1197·2).
Diarrhoea.

Diascan *Home Diagnostics, USA.*
Test for glucose in blood (p.1585·1).

Diasol *Baxter, Swed.†.*
Electrolytes (p.1151·1).
Haemodialysis solution.

Diasorb
Note. This name is used for preparations of different composition.
Norton, UK.
Loperamide (p.1197·3).
Diarrhoea.

Columbia, USA.
Activated attapulgite (p.1178·3).
Diarrhoea.

Diastat *Mer-National, S.Afr.*†.
Streptomycin (p.249·3); phthalylsulphathiazole (p.237·1); belladonna tincture (p.457·1); chloroform and morphine tincture (p.56·1); kaolin (p.1195·1); pectin (p.1474·1); tinct. card. co.
Diarrhoea.

Diastix
Bayer Diagnostics, Austral.; Bayer, Canad.; Ames, Irl.; Bayer Diagnostici, Ital.; Bayer Diagnostics, UK; Bayer, USA.
Test for glucose in urine (p.1585·1).

Diathynil *Dermolife, Ital.*†.
Biotin (p.1336·1).
Skin disorders.

Diatin *Ferrer, Spain.*
Elcatonin (p.735·3).
Metastatic bone pain; osteoporosis; Paget's disease of bone.

Diatolil *Fardi, Spain.*
Buphenine hydrochloride (p.1555·3).
Circulatory disorders; dysmenorrhoea.

Diatracin *Dista, Spain.*
Vancomycin hydrochloride (p.267·2).
Bacterial infections.

Di-Atro *Legere, USA*†.
Diphenoxylate hydrochloride (p.1189·1).
Atropine sulphate (p.455·1) is included in this preparation to discourage abuse.

Diatrum *Romilo, Canad.*
Multivitamin and mineral preparation.

Diatussin *Propan, S.Afr.*
Diphenhydramine hydrochloride (p.409·1); sodium citrate (p.1153·2); menthol (p.1600·2); ammonium chloride (p.1055·2); theophylline (p.765·1).
Coughs.

Dia-Vite *Landmark, Canad.*†.
Vitamin B substances with ascorbic acid.

Diawern *Wernigerode, Ger.*
Crataegus (p.1568·2); valerian (p.1643·1).
Heart failure.

Diazemuls
Pharmacia Upjohn, Austral.; Pharmacia Upjohn, Canad.; Dumex, Ger.†; Dumex, Irl.; Pharmacia Upjohn, Ital.; Dumex, Neth.†; Dumex, UK.
Diazepam (p.661·1).
Alcohol withdrawal syndrome; anxiety; convulsions; premedication; skeletal muscle spasm; status epilepticus; tetanus.

Diazep *CT, Ger.*
Diazepam (p.661·1).
Anxiety; premedication; skeletal muscle spasm.

Diba *Manetti Roberts, Ital.*
Glutaraldehyde (p.1114·3).
Instrument disinfection; surface disinfection.

Diban *Wyeth-Ayerst, Canad.*
Activated attapulgite (p.1178·3); pectin (p.1474·1); prepared opium (p.70·3); hyoscyamine sulphate (p.464·2); atropine sulphate (p.455·1); hyoscine hydrobromide (p.462·3).
Diarrhoea.

Diben-amid *Heumann, Ger.*†.
Sulphadiazine (p.252·3); guaiphenesin (p.1061·3); oxilofrine hydrochloride (p.925·3).
Bacterial infections of the respiratory tract.

Dibencozan *Houde, Fr.*†.
Cobamamide (p.1364·2).
Neuralgias; neuritis.

Dibent *Hauck, USA.*
Dicyclomine hydrochloride (p.460·1).
Functional bowel/irritable bowel syndrome.

Dibenyline
SmithKline Beecham, Austral.; SK-RIT, Belg.; Smith Kline & French, Irl.†; SmithKline Beecham, Neth.; SmithKline Beecham, S.Afr.†; Forley, UK.
Phenoxybenzamine hydrochloride (p.929·1).
Phaeochromocytoma; shock; urinary retention due to neurogenic bladder.

Dibenzyline *SmithKline Beecham, USA.*
Phenoxybenzamine hydrochloride (p.929·1).
Phaeochromocytoma.

Dibenzyran
Procter & Gamble, Aust.; Procter & Gamble, Ger.
Phenoxybenzamine hydrochloride (p.929·1).
Neurogenic bladder; phaeochromocytoma.

Dibertil *Christiaens, Belg.*
Metoclopramide hydrochloride (p.1200·3).
Adjunct in gastro-intestinal examination; gastro-intestinal motility disorders; nausea and vomiting.

Diblocin *Astra, Ger.*
Doxazosin mesylate (p.862·3).
Benign prostatic hyperplasia; hypertension.

Dibondrin *Montavit, Aust.*
Diphenhydramine hydrochloride (p.409·1).
Hypersensitivity disorders; prophylaxis against anaphylactic shock.

Dibro-Be Mono *Dibropharm, Ger.*
Potassium bromide (p.1620·3).
Epilepsy.

Dibromol *Trommsdorff, Ger.*
Sodium 3,5-dibromo-4-hydroxybenzenesulphonate; bromchlorophen (p.1104·2); isopropyl alcohol (p.1118·2).
Burns; skin disinfection; wounds.

Dical *Abbott, USA.*
Calcium with vitamin D and phosphorus.
Calcium deficiency; dietary supplement.

Dicalcium *Abiogen, Ital.*
Vitamin A palmitate (p.1359·2); cholecalciferol (p.1366·3); calcium carbonate (p.1182·1).
Formerly contained vitamin A palmitate, ergocalciferol, and calcium carbonate.
Vitamin or mineral deficiency.

Dicalm *Schieffer, Switz.*†.
Valerian (p.1643·1); lupulus (p.1597·2); hyoscyamus (p.464·3); ballota; passion flower (p.1615·3).
Anxiety; nervousness.

Dicalmir *Dicofarm, Ital.*
Fennel (p.1579·1); chamomile (p.1561·2); aniseed (p.1549·3); liquorice (p.1197·1); cumin; coriander (p.1567·3).
Colic; meteorism.

Dicalys 11 *Dicamed, Swed.*
Sodium chloride; potassium chloride; calcium chloride; magnesium chloride; sodium lactate; glucose (p.1151·1).
Haemofiltration.

Dicapen *Leo, UK*†.
Sulbactam (p.250·3); ampicillin (p.153·1).
Bacterial infections.

Dicarbosil *Bira, USA.*
Calcium carbonate (p.1182·1).
Hyperacidity.

Dicel *Lasa, Spain.*
Fenproporex hydrochloride (p.1481·3).
Obesity.

Dicepin B6 *Lasa, Spain.*
Diazepam (p.661·1).
Contains pyridoxine hydrochloride.
Alcohol withdrawal syndrome; anxiety; febrile convulsions; insomnia; skeletal muscle spasm.

Dicetel
Solvay, Aust.; Solvay, Belg.; Solvay, Canad.; Solvay, Fr.; Solvay, Ital.; Solvay, Neth.; Solvay, Switz.
Pinaverium bromide (p.1618·3).
Gastro-intestinal and biliary-tract spasm; irritable bowel syndrome; preparation of gastro-intestinal tract for radiography.

Dichinalex *Recordati, Ital.*†.
Chloroquine phosphate (p.426·3).
Malaria.

Dichlor-Stapenor *Bayer, Ger.*
Dicloxacillin sodium (p.202·1).
Benzylpenicillin-resistant staphylococcal infections.

Dichlotride
Merck Sharp & Dohme, Austral.; Merck Sharp & Dohme, Belg.; Merck Sharp & Dohme, Neth.; Merck Sharp & Dohme, Norw.; Merck Sharp & Dohme, S.Afr.; Merck Sharp & Dohme, Swed.
Hydrochlorothiazide (p.885·2).
Hypertension; oedema; premenstrual syndrome.

dichronase *GN, Ger.*†.
Pepsin (p.1616·3); pancreatin (p.1612·1); trypsin (p.1640·1); amylase (p.1549·1); caraway oil (p.1559·3).
Gastro-intestinal disorders.

Dicil *Chemil, Ital.*†.
Amoxycillin (p.151·3); dicloxacillin sodium (p.202·1).
Bacterial infections.

Dicinone *Pensa, Spain.*
Ethamsylate (p.720·1).
Haemorrhage.

Diclac
Hexal, Ger.; Rowex, Irl.
Diclofenac sodium (p.31·2).
Gout; inflammation; musculoskeletal and joint disorders; pain.

Diclamina *Esteve, Spain.*
Cinnarizine (p.406·1); heptaminol acephyllinate (p.754·1).
Vascular headache; vertigo.

Diclectin *Duchesnay, Canad.*
Doxylamine succinate (p.410·1); pyridoxine hydrochloride (p.1362·3).
Nausea and vomiting of pregnancy.

Diclo
Note. This name is used for preparations of different composition.
Kade, Ger.; CT, Ger.; Betapharm, Ger.; Isis Puren, Ger.; Ratiopharm, Ger.; Pinewood, Irl.
Diclofenac sodium (p.31·2).
Gout; musculoskeletal and joint disorders; pain; soft-tissue disorders.

FIRMA, Ital.
Dicloxacillin sodium (p.202·1).
Bacterial infections.

diclo-basan *Schonenberger, Switz.*
Diclofenac sodium (p.31·2).
Gout; inflammation; musculoskeletal and joint disorders; pain; soft-tissue injuries.

Diclobene *Merckle, Aust.*
Diclofenac sodium (p.31·2).
Gout; inflammation; pain; peri-articular, musculoskeletal, and joint disorders.

Dicloberl *Berlin-Chemie, Ger.*†.
Diclofenac sodium (p.31·2).
Inflammation; musculoskeletal and joint disorders; pain.

Diclocil
Bristol-Myers Squibb, Austral.; Bristol-Myers Squibb, Belg.†; Bristol-Myers Squibb, Fr.†; Bristol-Myers Squibb, Neth.†; Bristol-Myers Squibb, Norw.; Bristol-Myers Squibb, Swed.
Dicloxacillin sodium (p.202·1).
Bacterial infections.

Diclocillin *Lagap, Ital.*†.
Dicloxacillin sodium (p.202·1).
Bacterial infections.

Diclocular *Angelini, Ital.*
Diclofenac sodium (p.31·2).
Adjunct in eye surgery; corneal ulcers; pain and inflammation of the eye.

Dicloderm Forte *Cruz, Spain.*
Dichlorisone acetate (p.1039·2).
Skin disorders.

Diclofam *Garec, S.Afr.*
Diclofenac sodium (p.31·2).
Inflammation; musculoskeletal and joint disorders; pain.

Diclofenbeta *Betapharm, Ger.*
Diclofenac sodium (p.31·2).
Gout; inflammation; musculoskeletal and joint disorders; pain.

Dicloflex *Dexcel, UK.*
Diclofenac sodium (p.31·2).
Gout; inflammation; musculoskeletal, joint, peri-articular, and soft-tissue disorders; pain.

Dicloftil *Farmigea, Ital.*
Diclofenac sodium (p.31·2).
Inflammatory eye disorders.

Diclohexal *Hexal, Austral.*
Diclofenac sodium (p.31·2).
Inflammation; musculoskeletal and joint disorders; pain.

Diclomax Retard *Parke, Davis, UK.*
Diclofenac sodium (p.31·2).
Inflammation; musculoskeletal and joint disorders; pain.

Diclomel *Clonmel, Irl.*
Diclofenac sodium (p.31·2).
Gout; inflammation; musculoskeletal, joint, and periarticular disorders; pain.

Diclomelan *Lannacher, Aust.*
Diclofenac sodium (p.31·2).
Inflammation; musculoskeletal and joint disorders; pain.

Diclomerck *Merck, Ger.*
Diclofenac sodium (p.31·2).
Gout; inflammation; musculoskeletal and joint disorders; pain.

Diclo-OPT *Truw, Ger.*†.
Diclofenac sodium (p.31·2).
Inflammation; rheumatism.

Diclophlogont *Azupharma, Ger.*
Diclofenac sodium (p.31·2).
Gout; inflammation; musculoskeletal, joint, peri-articular, and soft-tissue disorders; pain.

Diclo-Puren *Isis Puren, Ger.*
Diclofenac sodium (p.31·2).
Inflammation; musculoskeletal, joint, peri-articular, and soft-tissue disorders; pain.

Diclorektal *Sanorania, Ger.*
Diclofenac sodium (p.31·2).
Gout; inflammation; musculoskeletal and joint disorders.

Dicloreum *Wassermann, Ital.*
Diclofenac epolamine (p.32·3) or diclofenac sodium (p.31·2).
Inflammation; musculoskeletal, joint, and peri-articular disorders; pain.

Diclo-saar *Chephasaar, Ger.*
Diclofenac sodium (p.31·2).
Gout; inflammation; musculoskeletal and joint disorders; pain.

Diclosifar *Siphar, Switz.*
Diclofenac sodium (p.31·2).
Gout; inflammation; musculoskeletal and joint disorders; oedema; pain.

Diclo-Spondyril *Nycomed, Ger.*†.
Diclofenac sodium (p.31·2).
Acute gout; inflammation; neuralgia; neuritis; rheumatism.

Diclosyl *Solvay, Aust.*
Diclofenac sodium (p.31·2).
Musculoskeletal, joint, peri-articular, and soft-tissue disorders.

Diclo-Tablinen *Sanorania, Ger.*
Diclofenac sodium (p.31·2).
Gout; inflammation; musculoskeletal and joint disorders.

Diclotard *Bartholomew Rhodes, UK.*
Diclofenac sodium (p.31·2).
Inflammation; musculoskeletal, joint, peri-articular, and soft-tissue disorders; pain.

Diclovol *CP Pharmaceuticals, UK.*
Diclofenac sodium (p.31·2).

Diclo-Wolff *Wolff, Ger.*
Diclofenac sodium (p.31·2).
Gout; inflammation; musculoskeletal and joint disorders; neuralgia; neuritis.

Dicloxan *Ibi, Ital.*†.
Dicloxacillin sodium (p.202·1).
Bacterial infections.

Diclozip *Ashbourne, UK.*
Diclofenac sodium (p.31·2).
Inflammation; pain.

Dicodid
Knoll, Ger.; Knoll, Switz.
Hydrocodone hydrochloride (p.43·1) or hydrocodone tartrate (p.43·1).
Coughs; pain.

Dicodin *Asta Medica, Fr.*
Dihydrocodeine tartrate (p.34·1).
Pain.

Dicodral *Dicofarm, Ital.*
Sodium chloride; potassium chloride; sodium bicarbonate; glucose (p.1152·3).
Diarrhoea; oral rehydration therapy.

Dicoflor *Dicofarm, Ital.*
Food containing lactic-acid-producing organisms (p.1594·1).
Disturbances of the gastro-intestinal flora.

Dicoman *Dicofarm, Ital.*
Dietary fibre supplement.

Diconal
Wellcome, Irl.; Wellcome, UK.
Dipipanone hydrochloride (p.34·3); cyclizine hydrochloride (p.407·1).
Pain.

Dicopac *Amersham International, UK.*
1 capsule, cyanocobalamin (cobalt-57) (p.1423·2); 1 capsule, cyanocobalamin (cobalt-58) (p.1423·2); 1 ampoule, cyanocobalamin (p.1363·3).

Dicoplus *Dicofarm, Ital.*
Glucomannan (p.1584·3).
Disorders of lipid metabolism.

Dicortal *Medici, Ital.*†.
Diflucortolone valerate (p.1039·3).
Skin disorders.

Dicorvin *ICN, Spain.*
Acetylspiramycin (p.249·2).
Bacterial infections.

Dicorynan *Roussel, Spain.*
Disopyramide (p.858·1).
Arrhythmias.

Dicton *Dolorgiet, Ger.*
Codeine polistirex (p.27·1).
Coughs.

Dicynene
Delandale, Irl.; Delandale, UK.
Ethamsylate (p.720·1).
Small-vessel haemorrhage.

Dicynone
Synthelabo, Belg.; Synthelabo, Fr.; Synthelabo, Ital.; OM, Switz.
Ethamsylate (p.720·1).
Haemorrhage; menorrhagia.

Didamega *Larkhall Laboratories, UK.*
Multivitamin and mineral preparation.

Didamol *Byk, Belg.*
Dipyridamole (p.857·1).
Angina pectoris; thrombo-embolism prophylaxis.

Di-Delamine *Del, USA; Commerce, USA.*
Diphenhydramine hydrochloride (p.409·1); tripelennamine hydrochloride (p.420·2).
Pruritus.

Didrex *Upjohn, USA.*
Benzphetamine hydrochloride (p.1478·1).
Obesity.

Didrica *Pensa, Spain.*
Calcium chloride; potassium chloride; sodium chloride; sodium lactate; glucose (p.1152·3).
Oral rehydration therapy.

Didrocal
Pharmacia Upjohn, Austral.; Procter & Gamble, Canad.
White tablets, disodium etidronate (p.738·3); blue tablets, calcium carbonate (p.1182·1).
Osteoporosis.

Didrocolo *Recofarma, Ital.*†.
Dehydrocholic acid (p.1570·2).
Biliary-tract disorders.

Didrogyl *Bruno, Ital.*
Calcifediol (p.1366·3).
Vitamin D deficiency.

Didro-Kit *Procter & Gamble, Ital.*
White tablets, disodium etidronate (p.738·3); blue tablets, calcium carbonate (p.1182·1).
Osteoporosis.

Didrokit *Procter & Gamble, Neth.*
Didronel tablets, disodium etidronate (p.738·3); Cacit tablets, calcium carbonate (p.1182·1).
Osteoporosis.

Didronate
Procter & Gamble, Norw.; Roche, Swed.
Disodium etidronate (p.738·3).
Paget's disease of bone; postmenopausal osteoporosis.

Didronel
Procter & Gamble, Aust.; Pharmacia Upjohn, Austral.; Procter & Gamble, Belg.; Procter & Gamble, Canad.; Knoll, Canad.; Procter & Gamble, Fr.; Procter & Gamble, Ger.; Procter & Gamble, Irl.; Procter & Gamble, Neth.†; Boehringer Mannheim, S.Afr.; Procter & Gamble, Switz.; Procter & Gamble, UK; Procter & Gamble, USA.
Disodium etidronate (p.738·3).
Ectopic ossification; hypercalcaemia of malignancy; osteoporosis; Paget's disease of bone.

Didronel PMO *Procter & Gamble, UK.*
Didronel tablets, disodium etidronate (p.738·3); Cacit tablets, calcium carbonate (p.1182·1).
Osteoporosis.

Diele *Diele, Fr.*
Food for special diets.
A range of foods for patients with amino acid metabolic disorders.

Diemil *Almirall, Spain.*
Dihydroergocristine mesylate (p.1571·3); piracetam (p.1619·1).
Cerebral trauma; cerebrovascular disorders.

Dienol *Doms-Adrian, Fr.*†.
Iron oxides; manganese oxides (p.1351·1).
Hyperthermia.

Diergo *Wander, Belg.; Sandoz, Fr.*
Dihydroergotamine mesylate (p.444·2); caffeine (p.749·3).
Migraine.

Diertina *Mundipharma, Aust.; Poli, Ital.; Poli, Switz.*
Dihydroergocristine mesylate (p.1571·3).
Dopamine deficiency; headache; hypertension; metabolic or vascular cerebral disorders; migraine; peripheral vascular disease; tinnitus; vertigo.

Diertina Ipotensiva *Poli, Ital.†.*
Dihydroergocristine mesylate (p.1571·3); reserpine (p.942·1); hydrochlorothiazide (p.885·2).
Hypertension.

Diertine *Morrith, Spain.*
Dihydroergocristine mesylate (p.1571·3).
Cerebrovascular disorders.

Diet Ayds *DEP, USA.*
Benzocaine (p.1286·2).
Obesity.

Diet Fibre Complex 1500 *Suisse, Austral.†.*
Soy bran (p.1181·2); ispaghula husk (p.1194·2); apple pectin (p.1474·1); citrus pectin; guar gum (p.321·3); ceratonia (p.1472·2); rice bran; wheat bran; agar (p.1470·3); sea vegetable.
Constipation and other gastro-intestinal disorders; obesity.

Diet Plan with Diadax *O'Connor, USA†.*
Phenylpropanolamine hydrochloride (p.1067·2).
Also contains grapefruit extract.
Obesity.

Diet Sucaryl *Abbott, Ital.*
Sodium cyclamate (p.1338·3); saccharin (p.1353·2).
Sugar substitute.

Dietaid *Mer-National, S.Afr.†.*
Caffeine (p.749·3); ephedrine hydrochloride (p.1059·3); phenolphthalein (p.1208·2).
Obesity.

Diet-Aid *O'Connor, USA†.*
Phenylpropanolamine hydrochloride (p.1067·2).

Dietason *Formenti, Ital.†.*
Aspartame (p.1335·1).
Sugar substitute.

Dietene *Restan, S.Afr.*
Cathine hydrochloride (p.1478·1).
Obesity.

Dietil *Trenker, Belg.*
Diethylpropion hydrochloride (p.1479·3).
Obesity.

Dietoglucid *Nutricia, Ital.†.*
Preparation for enteral nutrition.

Dietolipid *Nutricia, Ital.†.*
Lipid preparation for enteral nutrition.

Dietoman *Teofarma, Ital.*
Glucomannan (p.1584·3).
Diabetes; lipid disorders; obesity.

Dietosal *Nutricia, Ital.†.*
Mineral preparation for enteral nutrition.

Diet-Trim *Marpa, Austral.†.*
Carmellose sodium (p.1471·2); spirulina (p.1632·2); apple pectin (p.1474·1) ascorbic acid; vitamin B substances.
Obesity.

Dieutrim *Legere, USA.*
Phenylpropanolamine hydrochloride (p.1067·2); benzocaine (p.1286·2); carmellose sodium (p.1471·2).
Obesity.

Dievril *FIRMA, Ital.*
Vitamin B preparation.
Lignocaine hydrochloride (p.1293·2) is included in the intramuscular injection to alleviate the pain of injection.
Neuralgia; neuritis.

Diezime *Recordati, Ital.*
Cefodizime sodium (p.167·1).
Lignocaine hydrochloride (p.1293·2) is included in this preparation to alleviate the pain of injection.
Bacterial infections.

Dif Vitamin A Masivo *Roche Nicholas, Spain.*
Vitamin A acetate (p.1359·2).
Vitamin A deficiency.

Difaterol *Andreu, Spain.*
Bezafibrate (p.1268·2).
Hyperlipidaemias.

Difco *Lagamed, S.Afr.†.*
Diphenhydramine hydrochloride (p.409·1); ammonium chloride (p.1055·2); sodium citrate (p.1153·2); menthol (p.1600·2).
Coughs.

Difenac *Rolab, S.Afr.*
Diclofenac sodium (p.31·2).
Inflammation; musculoskeletal and joint disorders; pain.

Difenax *SmithKline Beecham, Ital.†.*
Difenpiramide (p.33·2).
Musculoskeletal disorders.

Difene *Klinge, Irl.*
Diclofenac sodium (p.31·2).
Gout; inflammation; musculoskeletal, joint, peri-articular, and soft-tissue disorders; pain; renal colic.

Differin
AB-Consult, Aust.; Galderma, Austral.; Galderma, Canad.; Galderma, Ger.; Galderma, Irl.; Galderma, Ital.; Galderma, S.Afr.; Meda, Swed.; Galderma, Switz.; Galderma, UK; Galderma, USA.
Adapalene (p.1078·1).
Acne.

Differine
Galderma, Fr.; Galderma, Spain.
Adapalene (p.1078·1).
Acne.

Difflam
3M, Austral.; 3M, Irl.; 3M, UK.
Benzydamine hydrochloride (p.21·3).
Inflammation; musculoskeletal, joint, and soft-tissue disorders; pain.

Difflam Anti-inflammatory Antiseptic Mouth Gel *3M, Austral.*
Benzydamine hydrochloride (p.21·3); cetylpyridinium chloride (p.1106·2).
Painful inflammatory mouth disorders.

Difflam Anti-Inflammatory Cough Lozenges *3M, Austral.*
Benzydamine hydrochloride (p.21·3); cetylpyridinium chloride (p.1106·2); pholcodine (p.1068·1).
Coughs; sore throat.

Difflam Anti-inflammatory Lozenges *3M, Austral.*
Benzydamine hydrochloride (p.21·3); cetylpyridinium chloride (p.1106·2).
Mouth and throat pain.

Difflam Anti-inflammatory Solution *3M, Austral.*
Benzydamine hydrochloride (p.21·3).
Mouth and throat pain.

Difflam Anti-inflammatory Throat Spray *3M, Austral.*
Benzydamine hydrochloride (p.21·3).
Mouth and throat pain.

Difflam Dental *3M, Austral.†.*
Benzydamine hydrochloride (p.21·3); chlorhexidine gluconate (p.1107·2).
Mouth and throat pain.

Difflam-C *3M, Austral.*
Benzydamine hydrochloride (p.21·3); chlorhexidine gluconate (p.1107·2).
Mouth and throat pain.

Diffu-K *UCB, Fr.*
Potassium chloride (p.1161·1).
Hypokalaemia.

Diffumal *Malesci, Ital.*
Theophylline (p.765·1).
Respiratory-tract disorders.

Diffusyl *Farmasan, Ger.*
Sodium cromoglycate (p.762·1).
Asthma.

Difilina Asmorax *Liade, Spain.*
Diprophylline (p.752·1); ephedrine hydrochloride (p.1059·3); hydroxyzine hydrochloride (p.412·1).
Obstructive airways disease.

Difillin *Lisapharma, Ital.†.*
Diprophylline (p.752·1).
Respiratory-tract disorders.

Difix *Chiesi, Ital.*
Calcitriol (p.1366·3).
Hypoparathyroidism; osteoporosis; pseudohypoparathyroidism; renal osteodystrophy; rickets.

Diflamil *Belmac, Spain.*
Oxyphenbutazone piperazine (p.72·1).
Gout; musculoskeletal and joint disorders.

Diflonid
Dumex, Norw.; Dumex-Alpharma, Swed.†.
Diflunisal (p.33·2).
Musculoskeletal and joint disorders; pain.

Diflor *Coli, Ital.†.*
Dicloxacillin sodium (p.202·1).
Bacterial infections.

Diflucan
Pfizer, Aust.; Pfizer, Austral.; Pfizer, Belg.; Pfizer, Canad.; Pfizer, Ger.; Pfizer, Irl.; Roerig, Ital.; Pfizer, Neth.; Pfizer, Norw.; Pfizer, S.Afr.; Pfizer, Spain; Pfizer, Swed.; Pfizer, Switz.; Pfizer, UK; Roerig, USA.
Fluconazole (p.378·1).
Fungal infections.

Difludol *Edmond Pharma, Ital.*
Diflunisal (p.33·2).
Musculoskeletal disorders; pain.

Difluid *Bioprogress, Ital.*
Dihydroergocristine mesylate (p.1571·3).
Cerebral and peripheral disorders; headache; hypertension; migraine.

Diflunil *Schwarz, Ital.†.*
Diflunisal (p.33·2).
Musculoskeletal disorders; pain.

Diflusal *Merck Sharp & Dohme, Belg.*
Diflunisal (p.33·2).
Pain.

Diflusan *Lebens, Ital.†.*
Diflunisal (p.33·2).
Musculoskeletal disorders; pain.

Difmecor *Solvay, Ital.*
Fendiline hydrochloride (p.868·1).
Cardiac disorders.

Difmedol *UCM-Difme, Ital.†.*
Oxyphenbutazone piperazine (p.72·1); methyl nicotinate (p.55·1).
Musculoskeletal disorders.

Difmetre *Solvay, Ital.*
Indomethacin (p.45·2); caffeine (p.749·3); prochlorperazine maleate (p.687·3).
Headache; migraine.

Difmetus *UCM-Difme, Ital.†.*
Noscapine embonate (p.1065·2); noscapine (p.1065·2).
Coughs.

Difmetus Compositum *Solvay, Ital.*
Noscapine embonate (p.1065·2); noscapine (p.1065·2); promethazine embonate (p.417·1).
Coughs.

Diformil *Faes, Spain.*
Formaldehyde (p.1113·2).
Mouth infections.

Diformiltricina *Faes, Spain.*
Cetrimonium bromide (p.1106·1); benzocaine (p.1286·2); formaldehyde (p.1113·2); tyrothricin (p.267·2).
Mouth and throat disorders.

Difosfen *Rubio, Spain.*
Disodium etidronate (p.738·3).
Ectopic ossification; osteoporosis; Paget's disease of bone.

Difosfocin *Magis, Ital.*
Citicoline (p.1564·3).
Cerebrovascular disorders; parkinsonism.

Difosfonal *SPA, Ital.*
Disodium clodronate (p.737·3).
Hyperparathyroidism; multiple myeloma; osteolytic tumours; osteoporosis.

Dif-Per-Tet-All *Biocine, Ital.†.*
An adsorbed diphtheria, tetanus, and pertussis vaccine (p.1509·1).
Active immunisation.

Difrarel
Note. This name is used for preparations of different composition.
Leurquin, Fr.; Sigma-Tau, Switz.†.
Myrtillus (p.1606·1); betacarotene (p.1335·2).
Peripheral vascular disorders.

Basotherm, Ger.; Sigma-Tau, Spain.
Myrtillus (p.1606·1).
Eye disorders; peripheral vascular disorders.

Difrarel E
Leurquin, Fr.; Sigma-Tau, Spain.
Myrtillus (p.1606·1); tocopherol (p.1369·1).
Myopias; vascular disorders.

Difravit *Difa, Ital.†.*
Myrtillus (p.1606·1); vitamin A palmitate (p.1359·2); tocopheryl acetate (p.1369·1).
Eye disorders.

Diftavax
Pasteur Merieux, Irl.; Pasteur Merieux, Spain; Pasteur Merieux, UK.
An adsorbed diphtheria and tetanus vaccine (p.1508·1).
Active immunisation of older children and adults.

Dif-Tet-All *Biocine, Ital.*
An adsorbed diphtheria and tetanus vaccine (p.1508·1).
Active immunisation.

Difur *Cantabria, Spain.*
Polypodium leucotomos.
Skin disorders.

Difusor *Kendall, UK†.*
Electrolytes; anhydrous glucose (p.1151·1).
Peritoneal dialysis.

Digacin *Beiersdorf-Lilly, Ger.*
Digoxin (p.849·3).
Arrhythmias; heart failure.

Digaloid *Molimin, Ger.†.*
Convallaria (p.1567·2); adonis vernalis (p.1543·3); crataegus fruit (p.1568·2); valerian root (p.1643·1); cereus grandiflorus.
Cardiovascular disorders.

Digaol *Leurquin, Fr.*
Timolol maleate (p.953·3).
Glaucoma; ocular hypertension.

Digedryl *Cooperation Pharmaceutique, Fr.*
Anhydrous sodium sulphate (p.1213·3); monobasic sodium phosphate (p.1159·3).
Dyspepsia.

Digeflash *Boehringer Ingelheim, Fr.*
Pancreas.
Dyspepsia.

Di-Gel
Note. This name is used for preparations of different composition.
Schering-Plough, Canad.†; Schering-Plough, USA.
Oral suspension: Aluminium hydroxide (p.1177·3); magnesium hydroxide (p.1198·2); simethicone (p.1213·1).
Flatulence; gastric hyperacidity.

Schering-Plough, Canad.†.
Tablets: Magnesium hydroxide (p.1198·2); calcium carbonate (p.1182·1); simethicone (p.1213·1).
Flatulence; gastric hyperacidity.

Digenac *Ethical Generics, UK.*
Diclofenac sodium (p.31·2).

Digepepsin *Kenwood, USA.*
Pepsin (p.1616·3); pancreatin (p.1612·1); bile salts (p.1553·2).

Digerall *Falqui, Ital.*
Alginic acid (p.1470·3); aluminium hydroxide (p.1177·3); magnesium trisilicate (p.1199·1); sodium bicarbonate (p.1153·2).
Gastro-intestinal disorders.

Digerent *Polifarma, Ital.*
Trimebutine maleate (p.1639·3).
Gastro-intestinal disorders.

Digeron *Piraud, Switz.†.*
Garlic; garlic oil; ginseng; crataegus; troxerutin; PCF-lecithin; orotic acid.
Tonic.

Digervin *Alacan, Spain.*
Famotidine (p.1192·1).
Gastro-oesophageal reflux; peptic ulcer; Zollinger-Ellison syndrome.

Di-Gesic *Dista, Austral.*
Dextropropoxyphene hydrochloride (p.27·3); paracetamol (p.72·2).
Fever; pain.

Digess *Axcan, Canad.*
Pancrelipase (p.1613·3).
Pancreatic insufficiency.

Digest *Modern Health Products, UK.*
Parsley (p.1615·3); centaury (p.1561·1); marshmallow root (p.1546·3).
Dyspepsia; flatulence.

Digest Merz *Merz, Ger.†.*
Porcine pancreatin (p.1612·1); Javanese turmeric; dimethicone (p.1213·1).
Digestive system disorders.

Digest Merz forte *Merz, Ger.†.*
Pancreatin (p.1612·1).
Gastro-intestinal disorders.

Digestaid *Eagle, Austral.*
Betaine hydrochloride (p.1553·2); pepsin (p.1616·3); pancreatin (p.1612·1); ox bile salt (p.1553·2); bromelain (p.1555·1); papain (p.1614·1); maltase (p.1546·2); potassium chloride (p.1161·1); gentian (p.1583·3); fennel (p.1579·1); peppermint oil (p.1208·1); chromium chelate (p.1337·1).
Gastro-intestinal disorders.

Digestelact *Sharpe, Austral.*
Food for special diets.
Lactose intolerance.

Digest-eze *Medinat, Austral.†.*
Alginic acid (p.1470·3); glycine (p.1345·2); pancreatin (p.1612·1); magnesium hydroxide (p.1198·2); magnesium trisilicate (p.1199·1); calcium carbonate (p.1182·1); sodium bicarbonate (p.1153·2); peppermint oil (p.1208·1); gentian (p.1583·3); chamaemelum (p.1561·2); taraxacum (p.1634·2).
Gastro-intestinal disorders.

Digestibys *IBYS, Spain†.*
Amylase (p.1549·1); pancreatin (p.1612·1); pepsin (p.1616·3).
Digestive enzyme deficiency; dyspepsia.

Digestif Marga *Cooperation Pharmaceutique, Fr.*
Magnesium hydroxide (p.1198·2); dried aluminium hydroxide (p.1177·3); calcium carbonate (p.1182·1).
Gastro-intestinal disorders.

Digestif Rennie
Note. This name is used for preparations of different composition.
Roche, Aust.
Papain (p.1614·1); pancreatin (p.1612·1); calcium carbonate (p.1182·1); magnesium carbonate (p.1198·1).
Dyspepsia.

Roche Consumer, Irl.; Roche, S.Afr.
Calcium carbonate (p.1182·1); magnesium carbonate (p.1198·1).
Dyspepsia.

Digestinas *Geminis, Spain†.*
Aluminium hydroxide (p.1177·3); aluminium glycinate (p.1177·2).
Gastro-intestinal disorders.

Digestinas Super *Geminis, Spain.*
Aluminium glycinate (p.1177·2); aluminium hydroxide (p.1177·3).
Formerly contained aluminium hydroxide, magnesium hydroxide, and magaldrate.
Gastro-intestinal hyperacidity.

Digestion L114 *Homeocan, Canad.*
Homoeopathic preparation.

Digestive Aid *Blackmores, Austral.*
Slippery elm (p.1630·1); fennel (p.1579·1); ginger (p.1193·2); gentian (p.1583·3); papain (p.1614·1); bromelains (p.1555·1); peppermint (p.1208·1); anise oil (p.1550·1).
Digestive disorders.

Digestive Rennie *Roche Consumer, Austral.*
Calcium carbonate (p.1182·1); heavy magnesium carbonate (p.1198·1).
Dyspepsia; flatulence.

Digestivo Antonetto *Antonetto, Ital.*
Anionic resin; glycine (p.1345·2); calcium carbonate (p.1182·1).
Gastric hyperacidity.

Digestivo Dr. Ragionieri *Ragionieri, Ital.†.*
Calcium carbonate (p.1182·1); magnesium carbonate (p.1198·1); dibasic sodium phosphate (p.1159·3); calcium phosphate (p.1155·3); magnesium hydroxide (p.1198·2); sodium citrate (p.1153·2); sodium bicarbonate (p.1153·2).
Digestive disorders.

Digestivo Giuliani *Giuliani, Ital.*
Domperidone (p.1190·3).
Dyspepsia.

Digestivo Rennie *Roche Nicholas, Spain.*
Calcium carbonate (p.1182·1); magnesium carbonate (p.1198·1); peppermint oil (p.1208·1).
Flatulence; gastro-intestinal hyperacidity.

Digestivum-Hetterich S *Galenika, Ger.*
Gentian (p.1583·3).
Gastro-intestinal disorders.

Digestobiase
Note. This name is used for preparations of different composition.
Couvreur, Belg.†.
Erepsin; kinase; pancreatin (p.1612·1); nux vomica (p.1609·3); pepsin (p.1616·3).
Digestive enzyme deficiency.

Wyeth, Fr.†.
Pepsin (p.1616·3); pancreatin (p.1612·1); papain (p.1614·1); enterokinase; activated charcoal (p.972·2); nux vomica (p.1609·3).
Dyspepsia.

Digestodoron Weleda, Aust.; Weleda, Fr.; Weleda, UK.
Male fern (p.104·1); polypodium; scolopendrium; salix alba (p.82·3); salix purpurea (p.82·3); salix viminalis; salix vitellina.
Dyspepsia; flatulence.

Digestofluid Amino, Switz.†.
Ox bile extract (p.1553·2); turmeric (p.1001·3); caraway (p.1559·3); fennel (p.1579·1); citrus sinensis; peppermint leaf (p.1208·1); chamomile (p.1561·2).
Digestive disorders.

Digestol Richter, Aust.
Gentian (p.1583·3); bitter-orange peel (p.1610·3); taraxacum (p.1634·2).
Gastro-intestinal disorders.

Digestol Sanatorium Santiveri, Spain.
Aniseed (p.1549·3); centaurium erythraea (p.1561·1); gentian (p.1583·3); chamomile (p.1561·2); melissa (p.1600·1); peppermint (p.1208·1).
Gastro-intestinal disorders.

Digestomen Menarini, Belg.
Betaine hydrochloride (p.1553·2); pepsin (p.1616·3); papain (p.1614·1); amylase (p.1549·1); pancreatin (p.1612·1); pancrelipase (p.1613·3); cellulase (p.1561·1).
Digestive disorders due to pancreatic insufficiency.

Digestomen Complex Menarini, Spain.
Betaine hydrochloride (p.1553·2); amylase (p.1549·1); lipase; pancreatin (p.1612·1); papain (p.1614·1); pepsin (p.1616·3); bile (p.1553·2); cellulase (p.1561·1); hemicellulase (p.1561·1).
Digestive enzyme deficiency; dyspepsia; flatulence.

Digestonico Vicente, Spain†.
Aluminium hydroxide (p.1177·3); bismuth citrate (p.1180·1); calcium carbonate (p.1182·1); magnesium carbonate (p.1198·1); pepsin (p.1616·3).
Gastritis; gastro-intestinal hyperacidity; peptic ulcer.

Digestonico Solucion Vicente, Spain†.
Ammonium fluoride; bismuth subnitrate (p.1180·2); inula helenium (p.1059·2); sodium citrate (p.1153·2).
Gastritis; gastro-intestinal hyperacidity; peptic ulcer.

Digestopan Menarini, Ital.
Pepsin (p.1616·3); papain (p.1614·1); amylase (p.1549·1); pancreatin (p.1612·1); pancreatic lipase; cellulase (p.1561·1).
Digestive disorders.

Digestosan Laevosan, Aust.
Ranitidine hydrochloride (p.1209·3).
Acid aspiration; gastro-intestinal haemorrhage; gastro-oesophageal reflux; peptic ulcer; Zollinger-Ellison syndrome.

Digestovital Puerto Galiano, Spain.
Belladonna (p.457·1); opium (p.70·3); sodium bicarbonate (p.1153·2); sodium citrate (p.1153·2); sodium sulphate (p.1213·3); star anise; aniseed (p.1549·3) cardamom (p.1560·1).
Gastritis; gastro-intestinal hyperacidity; peptic ulcer.

Digestozim Guidotti, Ital.†.
Pepsin (p.1616·3); papain (p.1614·1); amylase (p.1549·1); pancreatin (p.1612·1); pancreatic lipase; cellulase (p.1561·1).
Digestive disorders.

Digestozym Amino, Switz.†.
Ox bile extract (p.1553·2); aloes (p.1177·1); turmeric (p.1001·3); papain (p.1614·1); pancreatin (p.1612·1); caraway oil (p.1559·3); fennel oil (p.1579·2); bitter orange oil; peppermint oil (p.1208·1); chamomile oil.
Digestive disorders.

Digestum Rhone-Poulenc, Ital.†.
Pepsin (p.1616·3); simethicone (p.1213·1); pancreatin (p.1612·1).
Digestive disorders.

Digest-X Yucca L110 Homeocan, Canad.
Homoeopathic preparation.

Digezyme Cantassium Co., UK.
Betaine hydrochloride (p.1553·2); ox bile (p.1553·2); pepsin (p.1616·3); pancrelipase (p.1613·3); bromelain (p.1555·1).

Digi-Aldopur Kwizda, Aust.
Spironolactone (p.946·1); β-acetyldigoxin (p.812·3).
Arrhythmias; heart failure.

Digibind
Glaxo Wellcome, Austral.; Glaxo Wellcome, Canad.; Wellcome, UK; Wellcome, USA.
Digoxin-specific antibody fragments (p.979·1).
Digoxin or digitoxin toxicity.

Digicor Hennig, Ger.†.
Digitoxin (p.848·3).
Arrhythmias; heart failure.

Digifar Farmila, Ital.
Digitalin (p.1571·3); vitamin P (p.1580·1).
Eye disorders.

Digilateral Ursapharm, Ger.†.
β-Acetyldigoxin (p.812·3).
Arrhythmias; heart failure.

Digimed Gepepharm, Ger.
Digitoxin (p.848·3).
Heart failure.

Digimerck
Merck, Aust.; Merck, Ger.
Digitoxin (p.848·3).
Arrhythmias; heart failure.

Digi-Nitronal Pohl, Ger.†.
Glyceryl trinitrate (p.874·3); digoxin (p.849·3).
Cardiovascular disorders.

Digi-Pulsnorma Giulini, Ger.†.
Digoxin (p.849·3); ajmaline hydrochloride (p.817·2); sparteine sulphate (p.1632·1); antazoline hydrochloride (p.401·3); phenobarbitone (p.350·2).
Cardiac disorders.

Digipural Schaper & Brummer, Ger.†.
Digitoxin (p.848·3).
Cardiac disorders.

Digitaline
Procter & Gamble, Belg.; Welcker-Lyster, Canad.; Procter & Gamble, Fr.; Pan Quimica, Spain†; Nativelle, Switz.†.
Digitoxin (p.848·3).
Arrhythmias; heart failure.

Digitalis Antidot
Boehringer Mannheim, Aust.; Boehringer Mannheim, Belg.; Boehringer Mannheim, Ger.; Boehringer Mannheim, Swed.
Digoxin-specific antibody fragments (p.979·1).
Digitalis poisoning.

Digitalysat Ysatfabrik, Ger.†.
Digitalis purpurea leaf (p.848·3).
Cardiac disorders.

Digitalysat Scilla-Digitaloid Ysatfabrik, Ger.
Squill (p.1070·1).
Cardiac disorders.

Digitasid Sopar, Belg.†.
Digitoxin (p.848·3).
Arrhythmias; cardiac decompensation.

Digitrin
Astra, Norw.; Tika, Swed.
Digitoxin (p.848·3).
Arrhythmias; heart failure.

Digi-Tromcardin Trommsdorff, Ger.†.
Digoxin (p.849·3); potassium aspartate (p.1161·3); magnesium aspartate (p.1157·2).
Cardiac disorders.

Dignoamoxicillin Luitpold, Ger.†.
Amoxycillin trihydrate (p.151·3).
Bacterial infections.

Dignobeta Luitpold, Ger.
Atenolol (p.825·3).
Arrhythmias; hypertension; ischaemic heart disease.

Dignobroxol Luitpold, Ger.
Ambroxol hydrochloride (p.1054·3).
Respiratory-tract disorders associated with increased or viscous mucus.

Dignocetamol Luitpold, Ger.†.
Paracetamol (p.72·2).
Fever; pain.

Dignodenum Luitpold, Ger.†.
Bismuth subcarbonate (p.1180·1).
Gastritis; peptic ulcer.

Dignodolin Luitpold, Ger.
Flufenamic acid (p.41·3).
Musculoskeletal and joint disorders.

Dignofenac Dignos, Ger.†.
Diclofenac sodium (p.31·2).
Inflammation; musculoskeletal and joint disorders; pain.

Dignoflex Luitpold, Ger.
Ibuprofen (p.44·1).
Gout; inflammation; musculoskeletal and joint disorders; pain.

Dignokonstant Luitpold, Ger.
Nifedipine (p.916·2).
Angina pectoris; hypertension; myocardial infarction; Raynaud's syndrome.

Dignometoprol Luitpold, Ger.
Metoprolol tartrate (p.907·3).
Angina pectoris; arrhythmias; hypertension; migraine; myocardial infarction.

Dignonitrat Luitpold, Ger.
Isosorbide dinitrate (p.893·1).
Angina pectoris; heart failure; pulmonary hypertension.

Dignopenicillin Luitpold, Ger.†.
Phenoxymethylpenicillin potassium (p.236·2).
Bacterial infections.

Dignoquine Luitpold, Ger.†.
Chloroxine (p.215·3); chlorquinaldol (p.185·1).
Amoebic dysentery; diarrhoea.

Dignoretik Luitpold, Ger.
Amiloride hydrochloride (p.819·2); hydrochlorothiazide (p.885·2).
Ascites; hypertension; oedema.

Dignotamoxi Luitpold, Ger.†.
Tamoxifen citrate (p.563·3).
Breast cancer.

Dignotrimazol Luitpold, Ger.
Clotrimazole (p.376·3).
Fungal skin infections.

Dignover Luitpold, Ger.
Verapamil hydrochloride (p.960·3).
Angina pectoris; arrhythmias; hypertension.

Dignowell Luitpold, Ger.
Phenylephrine hydrochloride (p.1066·2); a heparinoid (p.882·3).
Venous insufficiency.

Digomal Malesci, Ital.
Digoxin (p.849·3).
Cardiac disorders.

Digophton ankerpharm, Ger.
Digitalis (p.848·3).
Eye strain.

Digo-Sensit Thiemann, Ger.†.
Fendiline hydrochloride (p.868·1); β-acetyldigoxin (p.812·3).
Heart failure.

Digostada Stada, Ger.
β-Acetyldigoxin (p.812·3).
Arrhythmias; heart failure.

Digotab Asta Medica, Ger.
β-Acetyldigoxin (p.812·3).
Heart failure.

Digox CT, Ger.
β-Acetyldigoxin (p.812·3).
Arrhythmias; heart failure.

Digoxin "Didier" Hormosan, Ger.
β-Acetyldigoxin (p.812·3).
Heart failure.

Digton Areu, Spain.
Sulpiride (p.692·3).
Psychoses; vertigo.

Di-Hydan
Synthelabo, Belg.; Synthelabo, Fr.
Phenytoin (p.352·3).
Arrhythmias; epilepsy; facial neuralgias.

Dihydergot
Note. This name is used for preparations of different composition.
Sandoz, Aust.; Novartis, Austral.; Wander, Belg.; Sandoz, Ger.; Novartis, Neth.; Novartis, S.Afr.; Sandoz, Spain; Sandoz, Switz.; Sandoz, UK†.
Injection; tablets; oral drops: Dihydroergotamine mesylate (p.444·2).
Chronic functional constipation; gastro-intestinal disorders; hypotension; migraine and related vascular headache; thrombosis prophylaxis; urinary retention; venous disorders of the legs.

Sandoz, Aust.; Sandoz, Norw.; Sandoz, Switz.
Nasal spray: Dihydroergotamine mesylate (p.444·2); caffeine (p.749·3).
Migraine and other vascular headaches.

Dihydergot plus
Sandoz, Ger.; Sandoz, Switz.
Dihydroergotamine mesylate (p.444·2); etilefrine hydrochloride (p.867·2).
Hypotension.

Dihydral
Note. This name is used for preparations of different composition.
Solvay, Belg.; Solvay, Neth.
Dihydrotachysterol (p.1366·3).
Hypoparathyroidism; renal osteodystrophy; rickets.

Pharmalab, S.Afr.†.
Diphenhydramine hydrochloride (p.409·1).
Hypersensitivity reactions.

Dihydrex Kay, USA.
Diphenhydramine hydrochloride (p.409·1).
Motion sickness; parkinsonism.

Dihytamin Dresden, Ger.; Wernigerode, Ger.
Dihydroergotamine mesylate (p.444·2).
Hypotension; migraine and other vascular headaches.

Dihyzin Henning, Ger.
Dihydralazine sulphate (p.854·1).
Hypertension.

Diidergot Sandoz, Ital.
Dihydroergotamine mesylate (p.444·2).
Headache; vascular disorders.

Dijene Boots, Austral.†.
Aluminium hydroxide-magnesium carbonate co-dried gel (p.1178·2).
Dyspepsia; peptic ulcer.

Dijex
Note. This name is used for preparations of different composition.
Boots Healthcare, Irl.†; Seton, UK.
Oral liquid: Aluminium hydroxide (p.1177·3); magnesium hydroxide (p.1198·2).
These ingredients can be described by the British Approved Name Co-magaldrox.
Dyspepsia.

Seton, UK.
Tablets: Aluminium hydroxide-magnesium carbonate co-dried gel (p.1178·2).
Dyspepsia.

Dikacine Belphar, Belg.
Dibekacin sulphate (p.201·3).
Gram-negative bacterial infections; staphylococcal infections.

Dilabar Vita, Spain.
Captopril (p.836·3).
Diabetic nephropathy; heart failure; hypertension; myocardial infarction.

Dilabar Diu Vita, Spain.
Hydrochlorothiazide (p.885·2); captopril (p.836·3).
Hypertension.

Dilaclan CEPA, Spain.
Diltiazem hydrochloride (p.854·2).
Angina pectoris; hypertension; myocardial infarction.

Dilacor XR Rhone-Poulenc Rorer, USA.
Diltiazem hydrochloride (p.854·2).
Hypertension.

Diladel Synthelabo, Ital.
Diltiazem hydrochloride (p.854·2).
Hypertension; ischaemic heart disease.

Dilaescol Kolassa, Aust.
Buphenine hydrochloride (p.1555·3); thiamine hydrochloride (p.1361·1); aesculus extract (p.1543·3).
Migraine; peripheral vascular disease; premenstrual syndrome; reflex sympathetic dystrophy.

Dilafurane Sanofi Winthrop, Spain.
Benziodarone (p.393·1).
Hyperuricaemia.

Dilanacin Dresden, Ger.
Digoxin (p.849·3).
Arrhythmias; heart failure.

Dilangio Compositum Fournier SA, Spain.
Bencyclane acephyllinate (p.827·3); bencyclane fumarate (p.827·3).
Cardiac disorders; vascular disorders.

Dilanid Rolab, S.Afr.
Isosorbide dinitrate (p.893·1).
Angina pectoris.

Dilanorm Rhone-Poulenc Rorer, Neth.
Celiprolol hydrochloride (p.838·3).
Angina pectoris; hypertension.

Dilantin
Parke, Davis, Austral.; Parke, Davis, Canad.; Parke, Davis, USA.
Phenytoin (p.352·3) or phenytoin sodium (p.352·3).
Arrhythmias; epilepsy.

Dilantin with Phenobarbital Parke, Davis, Canad.
Phenytoin sodium (p.352·3); phenobarbitone (p.350·2).
Epilepsy.

Dilaphylline Streuli, Switz.†.
Injection; oral drops: Etofylline (p.753·1); theophylline hydrate (p.765·1).
Tablets: Etofylline (p.753·1).
Obstructive airways disease.

Dilapres Quimifar, Spain.
Bencyclane fumarate (p.827·3); clonidine hydrochloride (p.841·2); hydrochlorothiazide (p.885·2).
Hypertension.

Dilar
Note. This name is used for preparations of different composition.
Cassenne, Fr.
Paramethasone acetate (p.1047·3).
Corticosteroid.

Teofarma, Ital.†.
Vincamine (p.1644·1).
Vascular disorders.

Dilarterial Llorente, Spain.
Vincamine (p.1644·1).
Cerebral trauma; cerebrovascular disorders.

Dilatam Lennon, S.Afr.
Diltiazem hydrochloride (p.854·2).
Angina pectoris; hypertension.

Dilatame Donau, Aust.
Diltiazem hydrochloride (p.854·2).
Angina pectoris; hypertension.

Dilatan Kore Lenza, Ital.†.
Efloxate (p.863·1).
Cardiac disorders.

Dilatol
Kolassa, Aust.; Tropon, Ger.†; Vesta, S.Afr.†.
Buphenine hydrochloride (p.1555·3).
Inhibition of labour; peripheral vascular disease; uterine relaxant; vascular headache.

Dilatol-Chinin Kolassa, Aust.
Buphenine hydrochloride (p.1555·3); quinine sulphate (p.439·2).
Cramp.

Dilatrane Labomed, Fr.
Theophylline (p.765·1) or theophylline sodium acetate (p.772·2).
Obstructive airways disease.

Dilatrate Schwarz, USA.
Isosorbide dinitrate (p.893·1).
Angina pectoris.

Dilatrend
Boehringer Mannheim, Aust.; Boehringer Mannheim, Ger.; Boehringer Mannheim, Ital.; Boehringer Mannheim, Norw.; Boehringer Mannheim, S.Afr.; Boehringer Mannheim, Switz.
Carvedilol (p.838·1).
Angina pectoris; heart failure; hypertension.

Dilaudid
Knoll, Canad.; Knoll, Ger.; Knoll, Irl.†; Knoll, USA.
Hydromorphone hydrochloride (p.43·2).
Pain.

Dilaudid Cough Knoll, USA.
Hydromorphone hydrochloride (p.43·2); guaiphenesin (p.1061·3).
Coughs.

Dilaudid-Atropin
Knoll, Ger.; Meda, Swed.; Knoll, Switz.
Hydromorphone hydrochloride (p.43·2); atropine sulphate (p.455·1).
Pain; smooth muscle spasm.

Dilcardia Generics, UK.
Diltiazem hydrochloride (p.854·2).

Dilcor BOI, Spain.
Nifedipine (p.916·2).
Angina pectoris; hypertension; Raynaud's syndrome.

Dilcoran
Parke, Davis, Aust.; Godecke, Ger.
Pentaerythritol tetranitrate (p.927·3).
Ischaemic heart disease.

Dilcovit OFF, Ital.†.
Bufylline ethiodide (p.749·3).
Asthma; cardiac disorders; hypertension; vascular disorders.

Dilem *Ist. Chim. Inter., Ital.*
Diltiazem hydrochloride (p.854·2).
Hypertension; ischaemic heart disease.

Dilena *Organon, Aust.†.*
Combination pack: White tablets, oestradiol valerate (p.1455·2); blue tablets, oestradiol valerate (p.1455·2); medroxyprogesterone acetate (p.1448·3).
Hormone replacement therapy.

Diligan
Note. This name is used for preparations of different composition.
UCB, Aust.; UCB, Belg.†; UCB, S.Afr.†.
Hydroxyzine (p.412·2); meclozine (p.413·3); nicotinic acid (p.1351·2).
Ménière's disease; vertigo.
Rodleben, Ger.; Vedim, Ger.
Hydroxyzine hydrochloride (p.412·1); meclozine hydrochloride (p.413·3).
Ménière's disease; vertigo.

Dilinct *Restan, S.Afr.*
Etofylline (p.753·1); diphenhydramine hydrochloride (p.409·1); ammonium chloride (p.1055·2); polysorbate 20 (p.1327·3).
Bronchodilator; coughs.

Diliter *Pulitzer, Ital.*
Diltiazem hydrochloride (p.854·2).
Angina pectoris; heart failure; hypertension.

Dillar *Syntex, Belg.†.*
Paramethasone acetate (p.1047·3).
Corticosteroid.

Diloc *Tramedico, Neth.*
Diltiazem hydrochloride (p.854·2).
Angina pectoris; hypertension.

Dilocaine *Hauck, USA.*
Lignocaine hydrochloride (p.1293·2).
Local anaesthesia.

Dilomine *Kay, USA.*
Dicyclomine hydrochloride (p.460·1).
Functional bowel/irritable bowel syndrome.

Dilor *Savage, USA.*
Diprophylline (p.752·1).
Acute bronchial asthma; reversible bronchospasm.

Dilor-G *Savage, USA.*
Diprophylline (p.752·1); guaiphenesin (p.1061·3).
Bronchospasm.

Dilosyn *Sigma, Austral.*
Methdilazine hydrochloride (p.414·2).
Hypersensitivity reactions; migraine; pruritus.

Dilotab *Zee, Canad.*
Phenylpropanolamine hydrochloride (p.1067·2); paracetamol (p.72·2).

Dilpavan *Biogalenique, Fr.†.*
Hesperidin methyl chalcone (p.1580·2); ascorbic acid (p.1365·2); pyridoxine hydrochloride (p.1362·3); papaverine hydrochloride (p.1614·2).
Peripheral vascular disorders.

Dilrene *Dakota, Fr.*
Diltiazem hydrochloride (p.854·2).
Angina pectoris; hypertension.

Dilsana *Milupa, Switz.*
Preparation for enteral nutrition.

Dil-Sanorania *Sanorania, Ger.*
Diltiazem hydrochloride (p.854·2).
Angina pectoris; hypertension.

Diltahexal
Hexal, Austral.; Hexal, Ger.
Diltiazem hydrochloride (p.854·2).
Angina pectoris; hypertension.

Diltam *Rowex, Irl.*
Diltiazem hydrochloride (p.854·2).
Angina pectoris; hypertension.

Diltaretard *Betapharm, Ger.*
Diltiazem hydrochloride (p.854·2).
Angina pectoris; hypertension.

Dilti *CT, Ger.; BASF, Ger.; Wolff, Ger.*
Diltiazem hydrochloride (p.854·2).
Angina pectoris; hypertension.

Diltiamax *PMC, Austral.*
Diltiazem hydrochloride (p.854·2).
Angina pectoris.

Diltiamerck *Merck, Ger.*
Diltiazem hydrochloride (p.854·2).
Angina pectoris; hypertension.

Dilti-Essex *Essex, Ger.†.*
Diltiazem hydrochloride (p.854·2).
Hypertension; ischaemic heart disease.

Diltiuc *Durachemie, Ger.*
Diltiazem hydrochloride (p.854·2).
Angina pectoris; hypertension.

Diltiwas *Wasserman, Spain.*
Diltiazem hydrochloride (p.854·2).
Angina pectoris; hypertension; myocardial infarction.

Dilucort *Triomed, S.Afr.*
Hydrocortisone acetate (p.1043·3).
Skin disorders.

Dilusol *Dermtek, Canad.*
Alcohol (p.1099·1); isopropyl alcohol; propylene glycol; laureth-4.
Topical vehicle.

Dilutol *Boehringer Mannheim, Spain.*
Torasemide (p.956·3) or torasemide sodium (p.956·3).
Hypertension; oedema.

Dilydrin *Willvonseder, Aust.*
Buphenine hydrochloride (p.1555·3).
Dysmenorrhoea; premature labour.

Dilydrine Retard *Medichemie, Switz.*
Buphenine hydrochloride (p.1555·3).
Peripheral vascular disorders.

Dilzem
Parke, Davis, Aust.; Douglas, Austral.; Godecke, Ger.; Elan, Irl.; Warner-Lambert, Switz.; Elan, UK.
Diltiazem hydrochloride (p.854·2).
Adjunct in transluminal coronary angioplasty or bypass surgery; angina pectoris; arrhythmias; hypertension; myocardial infarction; prevention of kidney transplant rejection; reduction of cyclosporin nephrotoxicity.

Dilzene *Sigma-Tau, Ital.*
Diltiazem hydrochloride (p.854·2).
Arrhythmias; hypertension; ischaemic heart disease.

Dilzereal *Realpharma, Ger.*
Diltiazem hydrochloride (p.854·2).
Angina pectoris; hypertension.

Dilzicardin *Azupharma, Ger.*
Diltiazem hydrochloride (p.854·2).
Angina pectoris; hypertension.

Dimac *Lilly, Aust.*
Dirithromycin (p.202·2).
Bacterial infections.

Dimacol *Robins, USA.*
Guaiphenesin (p.1061·3); pseudoephedrine hydrochloride (p.1068·3); dextromethorphan hydrobromide (p.1057·3).
Coughs.

Dimaestad *Stada, Ger.†.*
Deanol hydrogen tartrate (p.1478·2); adenosine phosphate sodium (p.1543·2); B vitamins; methionine (p.984·2).
Circulatory disorders; migraine; psychiatric and nervous system disorders.

Dima-Fen *Stroder, Ital.†.*
Fenfluramine hydrochloride (p.1480·3).
Obesity.

Dimalan *Parke, Davis, Fr.†.*
Algeldrate (p.1177·3); magnesium hydroxide (p.1198·2); dimethicone (p.1213·1).
Gastro-intestinal disorders.

Dim-Antos *Pharmonta, Aust.*
Propyphenazone (p.81·3).
Fever; pain.

Dimaphen *Major, USA.*
Phenylpropanolamine hydrochloride (p.1067·2); brompheniramine maleate (p.403·2).
Upper respiratory-tract symptoms.

Dimatab Cold Tablets *Whitehall, Austral.†.*
Paracetamol (p.72·2); pseudoephedrine hydrochloride (p.1068·3).
Cold symptoms.

Dimaval *Heyl, Ger.*
Unithiol (p.998·2).
Heavy metal poisoning.

Dimayon *Sabater, Spain.*
Camphor (p.1557·2); cineole (p.1564·1); niaouli oil (p.1607·1); oxolamine citrate (p.1065·3); paracetamol (p.72·2); choline theophyllinate (p.751·3); vitamin A (p.1358·1).
Influenza and cold symptoms.

Dimegan
Dexo, Fr.; Kreussler, Ger.
Brompheniramine maleate (p.403·2).
Hypersensitivity reactions of skin or mucous membranes.

Dimelor
Lilly, Canad.; Lilly, Ital.†; Lilly, S.Afr.
Acetohexamide (p.318·1).
Diabetes mellitus.

Dimen *Heumann, Ger.*
Dimenhydrinate (p.408·2).
Dizziness; nausea; vomiting.

Dimenformon
Note. This name is used for preparations of different composition.
Organon, Belg.
Oestradiol benzoate (p.1455·1); oestradiol phenylpropionate (p.1455·2).
Menstrual disorders; oestrogen replacement therapy.
Organon, Neth.†.
Oestradiol (p.1455·1).
Menopausal disorders.

Dimenhydrinat comp *Ratiopharm, Ger.†.*
Dimenhydrinate (p.408·2); pyridoxine hydrochloride (p.1362·3); caffeine (p.749·3).
Motion sickness; nausea; postoperative vomiting.

Dimenhydrinat retard *Ratiopharm, Ger.†.*
Dimenhydrinate (p.408·2); pyridoxine hydrochloride (p.1362·3).
Motion sickness; nausea; postoperative vomiting.

Dimetabs *Jones, USA.*
Dimenhydrinate (p.408·2).
Motion sickness.

Dimetane
Note. This name is used for preparations of different composition.
Whitehall, Austral.†; Whitehall-Robins, Canad.; Robins, Swed.†; Robins, USA.
Brompheniramine maleate (p.403·2).
Hypersensitivity reactions.
Wyeth, Fr.
Paediatric syrup: Brompheniramine maleate (p.403·2); guaiphenesin (p.1061·3); sodium benzoate (p.1102·3).
Upper respiratory-tract congestion.
Syrup: Brompheniramine maleate (p.403·2); pholcodine (p.1068·1); phenylephrine hydrochloride (p.1066·2); guaiphenesin (p.1061·3); sodium benzoate (p.1102·3).
Coughs.
Wyeth, Switz.
Codeine phosphate (p.26·1); phenylephrine hydrochloride (p.1066·2); phenylpropanolamine hydrochloride (p.1067·2); guaiphenesin (p.1061·3).
Coughs and associated respiratory-tract disorders.

Dimetane Decongestant *Robins, USA.*
Brompheniramine maleate (p.403·2); phenylephrine hydrochloride (p.1066·2).
Upper respiratory-tract symptoms.

Dimetane Expectorant *Whitehall-Robins, Canad.*
Brompheniramine maleate (p.403·2); guaiphenesin (p.1061·3); phenylephrine hydrochloride (p.1066·2); phenylpropanolamine hydrochloride (p.1067·2).
Upper respiratory-tract disorders.

Dimetane Expectorant-C *Whitehall-Robins, Canad.*
Brompheniramine maleate (p.403·2); phenylephrine hydrochloride (p.1066·2); phenylpropanolamine hydrochloride (p.1067·2); guaiphenesin (p.1061·3); codeine phosphate (p.26·1).
Upper respiratory-tract disorders.

Dimetane Expectorant-DC *Whitehall-Robins, Canad.*
Brompheniramine maleate (p.403·2); hydrocodone tartrate (p.43·1); guaiphenesin (p.1061·3); phenylephrine hydrochloride (p.1066·2); phenylpropanolamine hydrochloride (p.1067·2).
Upper respiratory-tract disorders.

Dimetane-DC *Robins, USA.*
Brompheniramine maleate (p.403·2); phenylpropanolamine hydrochloride (p.1067·2); codeine phosphate (p.26·1).
Coughs.

Dimetane-DX *Robins, USA.*
Brompheniramine maleate (p.403·2); pseudoephedrine hydrochloride (p.1068·3); dextromethorphan hydrobromide (p.1057·3).
Coughs.

Dimetapp
Note. This name is used for preparations of different composition.
Whitehall, Austral.
Brompheniramine maleate (p.403·2); phenylephrine hydrochloride (p.1066·2).
Upper respiratory-tract symptoms.
Whitehall-Robins, Canad.; Pharmacare Consumer, S.Afr.; Wyeth, Switz.
Brompheniramine maleate (p.403·2); phenylephrine hydrochloride (p.1066·2); phenylpropanolamine hydrochloride (p.1067·2).
Hypersensitivity reactions; upper respiratory-tract disorders.
Robins, USA.
Brompheniramine maleate (p.403·2); phenylpropanolamine hydrochloride (p.1067·2).
Allergic rhinitis; nasal congestion.

Dimetapp Chewables *Whitehall-Robins, Canad.*
Brompheniramine maleate (p.403·2); phenylpropanolamine hydrochloride (p.1067·2).
Upper respiratory-tract disorders.

Dimetapp Clear *Whitehall-Robins, Canad.*
Brompheniramine maleate (p.403·2); phenylpropanolamine hydrochloride (p.1067·2).

Dimetapp Cold & Allergy Chewable *Robins, USA.*
Brompheniramine maleate (p.403·2); phenylpropanolamine hydrochloride (p.1067·2).
Upper respiratory-tract symptoms.

Dimetapp Cold, Cough & Flu *Whitehall, Austral.*
Day capsules, dextromethorphan hydrobromide (p.1057·3); pseudoephedrine hydrochloride (p.1068·3); paracetamol (p.72·2); night capsules, dextromethorphan hydrobromide; pseudoephedrine hydrochloride; doxylamine succinate (p.410·1); paracetamol.
Cold and influenza symptoms.

Dimetapp Cold, Cough & Sinus *Whitehall, Austral.*
Dextromethorphan hydrobromide (p.1057·3); pseudoephedrine hydrochloride (p.1068·3); guaiphenesin (p.1061·3).
Coughs; nasal congestion.

Dimetapp Cold & Flu *Robins, USA.*
Brompheniramine maleate (p.403·2); phenylpropanolamine hydrochloride (p.1067·2); paracetamol (p.72·2).
Upper respiratory-tract symptoms.

Dimetapp Cough & Cold Liqui-Gels *Whitehall-Robins, Canad.*
Brompheniramine maleate (p.403·2); phenylpropanolamine hydrochloride (p.1067·2); dextromethorphan hydrobromide (p.1057·3).
Coughs and cold symptoms.

Dimetapp Cough Expectorant *SA Druggists Self Med, S.Afr.†.*
Guaiphenesin (p.1061·3).
Coughs.

Dimetapp Daytime *Whitehall, Austral.†.*
Pseudoephedrine hydrochloride (p.1068·3).
Cold symptoms.

Dimetapp DM
Note. This name is used for preparations of different composition.
Whitehall, Austral.
Brompheniramine maleate (p.403·2); phenylephrine hydrochloride (p.1066·2); dextromethorphan hydrobromide (p.1057·3).
Upper respiratory-tract symptoms.
Whitehall-Robins, Canad.
Brompheniramine maleate (p.403·2); phenylephrine hydrochloride (p.1066·2); phenylpropanolamine hydrochloride (p.1067·2); dextromethorphan hydrobromide (p.1057·3).
Cold symptoms; upper respiratory-tract disorders.
Robins, USA.
Brompheniramine maleate (p.403·2); phenylpropanolamine hydrochloride (p.1067·2); dextromethorphan hydrobromide (p.1057·3).
Coughs and cold symptoms.

Dimetapp Elixir-Plus *Whitehall, Austral.†.*
Brompheniramine maleate (p.403·2); phenylephrine hydrochloride (p.1066·2); phenylpropanolamine hydrochloride (p.1067·2); paracetamol (p.72·2).
Coughs and cold symptoms.

Dimetapp 12 Hour Nasal *Whitehall, Austral.*
Oxymetazoline hydrochloride (p.1065·3).
Nasal congestion.

Dimetapp LA *Whitehall, Austral.†.*
Brompheniramine maleate (p.403·2); phenylephrine hydrochloride (p.1066·2); phenylpropanolamine hydrochloride (p.1067·2).
Upper respiratory tract symptoms.

Dimetapp Liqui-Gels *Whitehall-Robins, Canad.*
Brompheniramine maleate (p.403·2); phenylpropanolamine hydrochloride (p.1067·2).
Upper respiratory-tract disorders.

Dimetapp Oral Infant Drops *Whitehall-Robins, Canad.*
Brompheniramine maleate (p.403·2); phenylephrine hydrochloride (p.1066·2); phenylpropanolamine hydrochloride (p.1067·2).
Cold symptoms; hypersensitivity reactions.

Dimetapp Sinus Caplets *Robins, USA.*
Pseudoephedrine hydrochloride (p.1068·3); ibuprofen (p.44·1).
Nasal congestion.

Dimetapp Sinus Relief *Whitehall, Austral.†.*
Paracetamol (p.72·2); pseudoephedrine hydrochloride (p.1068·3).
Sinus pain and congestion.

Dimetapp-A Sinus *Whitehall-Robins, Canad.*
Phenylephrine hydrochloride (p.1066·2); phenylpropanolamine hydrochloride (p.1067·2); paracetamol (p.72·2).
Cold symptoms.

Dimetapp-C *Whitehall-Robins, Canad.*
Brompheniramine maleate (p.403·2); phenylpropanolamine hydrochloride (p.1067·2); phenylephrine hydrochloride (p.1066·2); codeine phosphate (p.26·1).
Cold symptoms; upper respiratory-tract disorders.

Dimethicream *Hamilton, Austral.*
Dimethicone (p.1384·2); cetrimide (p.1105·2).
Emollient barrier cream.

Dimetriose
Hoechst Marion Roussel, Austral.; Roussel, Irl.†; Florizel, UK.
Gestrinone (p.1447·3).
Endometriosis.

Dimetrose
Piette, Belg.; Poli, Ital.
Gestrinone (p.1447·3).
Endometriosis.

Dimidon *Hexal, Ger.†.*
Ibuprofen (p.44·1).
Pain.

Di-Mill *SIT, Ital.*
Benzalkonium chloride (p.1101·3).
Eye disinfection; eye irritation.

Diminex Antitusigeno *Vinas, Spain.*
Cineole (p.1564·1); chlorcyclizine hydrochloride (p.404·3); codeine phosphate (p.26·1); guaiphenesin (p.1061·3).
Respiratory-tract disorders.

Diminex Balsamico *Vinas, Spain.*
Cineole (p.1564·1); chlorcyclizine hydrochloride (p.404·3); chlorpromazine hydrochloride (p.649·1); dextromethorphan hydrobromide (p.1057·3); niaouli oil (p.1607·1); guaiphenesin (p.1061·3).
Respiratory-tract disorders.

Dimiprol
Note. This name is used for preparations of different composition.
Propan, S.Afr.
Tablets: Paracetamol (p.72·2); codeine phosphate (p.26·1); caffeine (p.749·3); meprobamate (p.678·1).
Pain; tension.
Zurich, S.Afr.†.
Syrup: Paracetamol (p.72·2); codeine phosphate (p.26·1); promethazine hydrochloride (p.416·2).
Pain; tension.

Dimitone *Boehringer Mannheim, Belg.*
Carvedilol (p.838·1).
Hypertension.

Dimor *Nordic, Swed.*
Loperamide hydrochloride (p.1197·2).
Diarrhoea.

Dimotane
Wyeth, Irl.; Wyeth, UK.
Brompheniramine maleate (p.403·2).
Allergic rhinitis; urticaria.

Dimotane Co
Whitehall, Irl.; Whitehall, UK.
Brompheniramine maleate (p.403·2); codeine phosphate (p.26·1); pseudoephedrine hydrochloride (p.1068·3).
Formerly contained codeine phosphate, guaiphenesin, phenylephrine hydrochloride, phenylpropanolamine hydrochloride, and brompheniramine maleate in *Irl.*
Coughs.

Dimotane Expectorant *Whitehall, Irl.; Whitehall, UK.*
Brompheniramine maleate (p.403·2); guaiphenesin (p.1061·3); pseudoephedrine hydrochloride (p.1068·3).
Formerly contained phenylephrine hydrochloride, phenylpropanolamine hydrochloride, brompheniramine maleate, and guaiphenesin.
Upper respiratory-tract disorders.

Dimotane Plus *Robins, Irl.†; Wyeth, UK.*
Brompheniramine maleate (p.403·2); pseudoephedrine hydrochloride (p.1068·3).
Allergic rhinitis.

Dimotapp *Whitehall, Irl.; Whitehall, UK.*
Phenylephrine hydrochloride (p.1066·2); phenylpropanolamine hydrochloride (p.1067·2); brompheniramine maleate (p.403·2).
Rhinitis; sinusitis.

Dimyril *Fisons, UK†.*
Isoaminile citrate (p.1063·2).
Coughs.

Dina *San Carlo, Ital.*
Cimetidine (p.1183·2).
Gastro-intestinal disorders associated with hyperacidity.

Dinabac *Lilly, Ital.*
Dirithromycin (p.202·2).
Bacterial infections.

Dinacode *Picot, Fr.*
Cream: Turpentine oil (p.1641·1); pine oil; rosemary oil (p.1626·2); wild thyme oil; white thyme oil; niaouli oil (p.1607·1); cineole (p.1564·1); quinine sulphate (p.439·2).
Respiratory congestion.
Paediatric suppositories: Potassium borotartrate (p.1620·2); sodium benzoate (p.1102·3); sodium bromide (p.1620·3); phenobarbitone (p.350·2).
Coughs.
Paediatric syrup: Sodium bromide (p.1620·3); sodium benzoate (p.1102·3); grindelia; senega (p.1069·3); tolu balsam (p.1071·1).
Coughs.

Dinacode avec codeine *Picot, Fr.*
Paediatric syrup: Sodium benzoate (p.1102·3); potassium guaiacolsulfonate (p.1068·3); belladonna (p.457·1); grindelia; senega (p.1069·3); tolu balsam (p.1071·1); codeine (p.26·1).
Syrup; suppositories; tablets: Codeine (p.26·1); belladonna (p.457·1); stramonium (p.468·2); sodium benzoate (p.1102·3).
Coughs.

Dinacode N *Picot, Switz.*
Syrup: Codeine (p.26·1); sodium benzoate (p.1102·3); thyme (p.1636·3); tolu balsam (p.1071·1).
Tablets: Codeine (p.26·1); sodium benzoate (p.1102·3).
Coughs.

Dinamozim *San Carlo, Ital.†.*
Uridine triphosphate (p.1641·3); cyanocobalamin (p.1363·3).
Muscular disorders.

Dinapres *Master Pharma, Ital.*
Delapril (p.847·1); indapamide (p.890·2).
Hypertension.

Dinasint *Proter, Ital.†.*
Cephaloridine (p.179·1).
Bacterial infections.

Dinate *Seatrace, USA.*
Dimenhydrinate (p.408·2).
Motion sickness.

Dinatrofon *Rhone-Poulenc Rorer, Spain†.*
Oestradiol propionate nicotinate (p.1456·1); nandrolone undecanoate (p.1452·2); progesterone enanthate (p.1460·3).
Atherosclerosis; cerebrovascular disorders; diabetes; metabolic bone disorders.

Dindevan *Boots, Austral.; Goldshield, UK.*
Phenindione (p.928·3).
Thrombo-embolic disorders.

Diniket *Schwarz, Ital.*
Isosorbide dinitrate (p.893·1).
Angina pectoris; heart failure.

Dinintel *Diamant, Fr.*
Clobenzorex hydrochloride (p.1478·2).
Obesity.

Dinisor *Parke, Davis, Spain.*
Diltiazem hydrochloride (p.854·2).
Angina pectoris; hypertension.

Dinneford's *SmithKline Beecham Consumer, UK†.*
Heavy magnesium carbonate (p.1198·1); citric acid monohydrate (p.1564·3); sodium bicarbonate (p.1153·2).

Dinnefords Teejel *Seton, UK.*
Choline salicylate (p.25·2).
Oral lesions.

Dinobroxol *Alfarma, Spain.*
Ambroxol hydrochloride (p.1054·3).
Respiratory-tract disorders.

Dinoldin *Lacer, Spain†.*
Rifampicin (p.243·2).
Meningitis; opportunistic mycobacterial infections; tuberculosis.

Dinosan *SCAM, Ital.†.*
Alkylaminoethylglycine (p.1112·3).
Surface disinfection.

Dinostral *Helvepharm, Switz.*
Oxpentifylline (p.925·3).
Vascular disorders.

Dinoven *Alfarma, Spain.*
A heparinoid (p.882·3).
Superficial thrombophlebitis; varices.

Dintoina *Recordati, Ital.*
Phenytoin sodium (p.352·3).
Arrhythmias; epilepsy; trigeminal neuralgia.

Dintoinale *Recordati, Ital.*
Phenytoin sodium (p.352·3); methylphenobarbitone (p.349·2).
Epilepsy.

Dintospina *Recordati, Ital.†.*
Phenytoin sodium (p.352·3); methylphenobarbitone (p.349·2); amphetamine sulphate (p.1477·3).
Epilepsy.

Dio *Sciencex, Fr.*
Diosmin (p.1580·1).
Capillary fragility; haemorrhoids; venous insufficiency.

Diocaine *Dioptic, Canad.*
Proxymetacaine hydrochloride (p.1300·1).
Local anaesthesia.

Diocalm *SmithKline Beecham Consumer, Irl.*
Morphine hydrochloride (p.56·1); attapulgite (p.1178·3); activated attapulgite.
Diarrhoea.

Diocalm Dual Action *Seton, UK.*
Morphine hydrochloride (p.56·1); attapulgite (p.1178·3).
Formerly known as Diocalm.
Diarrhoea.

Diocalm Replenish *Seton, UK.*
Anhydrous glucose; sodium chloride; sodium citrate; potassium chloride (p.1152·3).
Formerly known as Diocalm Junior.
Diarrhoea; oral rehydration therapy.

Diocalm Ultra *Seton, UK.*
Loperamide hydrochloride (p.1197·2).
Diarrhoea.

Diocaps *Berk, UK.*
Loperamide hydrochloride (p.1197·2).
Diarrhoea.

Diocarpine *Dioptic, Canad.*
Pilocarpine hydrochloride (p.1396·3).
Cholinergic; production of miosis.

Diochloram *Dioptic, Canad.*
Chloramphenicol (p.182·1).
Bacterial eye infections.

Diocimex *Cimex, Switz.*
Doxycycline hydrochloride (p.202·3).
Bacterial infections.

Dioctin *Abbott, S.Afr.†.*
Difenoxin hydrochloride (p.1188·3).
Atropine sulphate (p.455·1) is included in this preparation to discourage abuse.
Diarrhoea.

Diocto-K *Rugby, USA.*
Docusate potassium (p.1189·3).
Constipation.

Diocto-K Plus *Rugby, USA.*
Docusate potassium (p.1189·3); casanthranol (p.1182·3).
Constipation.

Dioctolose Plus *Goldline, USA.*
Docusate potassium (p.1189·3); casanthranol (p.1182·3).
Constipation.

Dioctyl *Everest, Canad.; Schwarz, UK.*
Docusate sodium (p.1189·3).
Constipation.

Dioderm *Dermal Laboratories, Irl.; Dermal Laboratories, UK.*
Hydrocortisone (p.1043·3).
Dermatitis; eczema.

Diodex *Dioptic, Canad.*
Dexamethasone sodium phosphate (p.1037·2).
Corticosteroid.

Diodine *Marc-O, Canad.*
Iodine (p.1493·1); isopropyl alcohol (p.1118·2); potassium iodide (p.1493·1).

Diodoquin *Glenwood, Canad.*
Di-iodohydroxyquinoline (p.581·1).
Amoebiasis.

Dioeze *Century, USA.*
Docusate sodium (p.1189·3).
Constipation.

Diofluor *Dioptic, Canad.*
Fluorescein sodium (p.1581·1).
Aid to ophthalmic examination.

Dioflur-P *Dioptic, Canad.†.*
Fluorescein sodium (p.1581·1); proxymetacaine hydrochloride (p.1300·1).
Aid to eye examination.

Diogent *Dioptic, Canad.*
Gentamicin sulphate (p.212·1).
Bacterial eye infections.

Diolaxil *Derly, Spain.*
Sennosides A and B (p.1212·3).
Constipation.

Diomycin *Dioptic, Canad.*
Erythromycin (p.204·1).
Bacterial eye infections.

Diondel *Sanofi Winthrop, Spain†.*
Metolazone (p.907·2).
Hypertension; oedema.

Dionephrine *Dioptic, Canad.*
Phenylephrine hydrochloride (p.1066·2).

Dionosil *Glaxo Wellcome, Swed.†.*
Propyliodone (p.1009·3).
Radiographic contrast medium for bronchography.

Dionosil Oily *Allen & Hanburys, USA.*
Propyliodone (p.1009·3) in arachis oil.
Radiographic contrast medium for bronchography.

Dioparine *Thea, Fr.; Ciba Vision, Switz.*
Sodium iodoheparinate (p.1631·2).
Burns to the eye; corneal damage.

Diopentolate *Dioptic, Canad.*
Cyclopentolate hydrochloride (p.459·3).
Production of mydriasis and cycloplegia.

Diophenyl-T *Dioptic, Canad.*
Phenylephrine hydrochloride (p.1066·2); tropicamide (p.469·2).
Production of mydriasis and cycloplegia.

Diopine *Allergan, Neth.†; Allergan, Spain; Allergan, Switz.*
Dipivefrine hydrochloride (p.1572·3).
Glaucoma; raised intra-ocular pressure.

Diopred *Dioptic, Canad.*
Prednisolone acetate (p.1048·1).
Eye inflammation.

Diopticon *Dioptic, Canad.*
Naphazoline hydrochloride (p.1064·2).

Diopticon A *Dioptic, Canad.*
Naphazoline hydrochloride (p.1064·2); pheniramine maleate (p.415·3).

Dioptimyd *Dioptic, Canad.*
Sulphacetamide sodium (p.252·2); prednisolone acetate (p.1048·1).
Eye disorders.

Dioptrol *Dioptic, Canad.*
Neomycin sulphate (p.229·2); polymyxin B sulphate (p.239·1); dexamethasone (p.1037·1).
Eye disorders.

Dioralyte *Rhone-Poulenc Rorer, Irl.; Nattermann, Neth.; Rhone-Poulenc Rorer, UK.*
Sodium chloride; potassium chloride; disodium hydrogen citrate; glucose (p.1152·3).
Diarrhoea; oral rehydration therapy.

Dioralyte Relief *Rhone-Poulenc Rorer, UK.*
Rice powder; sodium citrate; sodium chloride; potassium chloride (p.1152·3).
Diarrhoea; oral rehydration therapy.

Dioron *Marion Merrell Dow, Belg.†.*
Potassium orotate (p.1611·2).
Hepatobiliary insufficiency.

Diorouge *Dioptic, Canad.†.*
Pheniramine maleate (p.415·3); phenylephrine hydrochloride (p.1066·2).

Diosmectal *Malesci, Ital.*
Diosmectite.
Gastro-intestinal disorders.

Diosmil *Theraplix, Fr.*
Diosmin (p.1580·1).
Peripheral vascular disorders.

Diosminil *Faes, Spain.*
Diosmin (p.1580·1).
Haemorrhoids; vascular disorders.

Diospor HC *Dioptic, Canad.*
Neomycin sulphate (p.229·2); polymyxin B sulphate (p.239·1); hydrocortisone (p.1043·3).
Eye disorders.

Diosporin *Dioptic, Canad.*
Neomycin sulphate (p.229·2); polymyxin B sulphate (p.239·1); gramicidin (p.215·2).
Bacterial eye infections.

Diostate *Roberts, USA.*
Calcium with vitamin D and phosphorus.
Calcium deficiency; dietary supplement.

Diosulf *Dioptic, Canad.*
Sulphacetamide sodium (p.252·2).
Bacterial eye infections.

Diosven *CT, Ital.*
Diosmin (p.1580·1).
Peripheral vascular disorders.

Diotrope *Dioptic, Canad.*
Tropicamide (p.469·2).
Production of mydriasis and cycloplegia.

Diotroxin *Glaxo Wellcome, S.Afr.*
Thyroxine sodium (p.1497·1); liothyronine sodium (p.1495·1).
Hypothyroidism.

Dioval *Keene, USA.*
Oestradiol valerate (p.1455·2).
Female castration; female hypogonadism; menopausal vasomotor symptoms; prevention of breast engorgement; primary ovarian failure; prostatic cancer; vulval and vaginal atrophy.

Diovan *Ciba, Ger.; Novartis, Irl.; Novartis, Neth.; Novartis, S.Afr.; Novartis, Swed.; Ciba, Switz.; Ciba, UK; Ciba-Geigy, USA.*
Valsartan (p.960·2).
Hypertension.

Diovenor *Innothera, Fr.*
Diosmin (p.1580·1).
Peripheral vascular disorders.

Diovol
Note. This name is used for preparations of different composition.
Carter Horner, Canad.
Oral suspension; caplets: Aluminium hydroxide (p.1177·3); magnesium hydroxide (p.1198·2).
Tablets: Aluminium hydroxide-magnesium carbonate co-dried gel (p.1178·2); magnesium hydroxide (p.1198·2).
Dyspepsia; heartburn.
Pharmax, UK.
Aluminium hydroxide (p.1177·3); magnesium hydroxide (p.1198·2); simethicone (p.1213·1).
Flatulence; gastro-intestinal hyperacidity.

Diovol EX *Carter Horner, Canad.*
Aluminium hydroxide (p.1177·3); magnesium hydroxide (p.1198·2).
Dyspepsia; gastro-oesophageal reflux; heartburn.

Diovol Plus *Carter Horner, Canad.*
Oral suspension: Aluminium hydroxide (p.1177·3); magnesium hydroxide (p.1198·2); simethicone (p.1213·1).
Tablets: Aluminium hydroxide-magnesium carbonate co-dried gel (p.1178·2); magnesium hydroxide (p.1198·2); simethicone (p.1213·1).
Dyspepsia; flatulence; heartburn.

Diovol Plus AF *Carter Horner, Canad.*
Calcium carbonate (p.1182·1); magnesium hydroxide (p.1198·2); simethicone (p.1213·1).
Dyspepsia; flatulence; heartburn.

Di-Paralene *Abbott, Swed.†.*
Chlorcyclizine chloride (p.404·3).
Hypersensitivity reactions.

Diparene *Bios, Belg.†.*
Naproxen (p.61·2).
Gout; inflammation; musculoskeletal and joint disorders; pain.

Dipasic *Gewo, Ger.†; Inibsa, Spain†.*
Isoniazid aminosalicylate (p.220·1).
Tuberculosis.

Dipect *Schieffer, Switz.†.*
Capsules (day): Guaiphenesin (p.1061·3); ephedrine hydrochloride (p.1059·3); ipecacuanha (p.1062·2); hedera helix; drosera (p.1574·1); liquorice (p.1197·1); primula rhizome; eucalyptus (p.1578·1).
Capsules (night): Codeine phosphate (p.26·1); belladonna (p.457·1); hedera helix; drosera (p.1574·1); passion flower (p.1615·3); thyme (p.1636·3); grindelia; piscidia.
Syrup (day): Guaiphenesin (p.1061·3); ephedrine hydrochloride (p.1059·3); althaea (p.1546·3); ipecacuanha (p.1062·2); hedera helix; drosera (p.1574·1); liquorice (p.1197·1); primula; eucalyptus (p.1578·1).
Syrup (night): Codeine phosphate (p.26·1); belladonna (p.457·1); hedera helix; drosera (p.1574·1); passion flower (p.1615·3); thyme (p.1636·3); grindelia; piscidia; althaea (p.1546·3).
Coughs.

Dipentum *Pharmacia Upjohn, Aust.; Pharmacia Upjohn, Austral.; Pharmacia Upjohn, Canad.; Pharmacia Upjohn, Fr.; Pharmacia Upjohn, Ger.; Pharmacia Upjohn, Irl.; Pharmacia Upjohn, Ital.; Pharmacia Upjohn, Neth.; Pharmacia Upjohn, Norw.; Pharmacia Upjohn, S.Afr.; Pharmacia Upjohn, Swed.; Pharmacia Upjohn, Switz.; Pharmacia, UK; Pharmacia, USA.*
Olsalazine sodium (p.1204·1).
Ulcerative colitis.

Dipeptamin *Fresenius-Klinik, Ger.*
L-Alanyl-L-glutamine (p.1344·3).
Parenteral nutrition.

Dipeptiven *Leopold, Aust.; SIFRA, Ital.; Meda, Swed.; Fresenius, UK.*
L-alanyl-L-glutamine (p.1344·3).
Parenteral nutrition.

Diperpen *Francia, Ital.*
Pipemidic acid (p.237·2).
Bacterial infections of the urinary tract.

Dipervina *Farma Lepori, Spain.*
Dihydroergocristine mesylate (p.1571·3); vincamine (p.1644·1) or vincamine hydrochloride (p.1644·1).
Cerebral trauma; cerebrovascular disorders.

Diphamine *Medgenix, Belg.*
Diphenhydramine hydrochloride (p.409·1).
Hypersensitivity reactions; insect stings; pruritus; sunburn; urticaria.

Diphantoine *Wolfs, Belg.*
Phenytoin sodium (p.352·3).
Arrhythmias; epilepsy.

Diphar *Pharbiol, Fr.†.*
Dipyridamole (p.857·1).
Thrombo-embolic disorders.

Diphemin *Alcon, Switz.*
Dipivefrine hydrochloride (p.1572·3).
Glaucoma.

Diphen AF *Morton Grove, USA.*
Diphenhydramine hydrochloride (p.409·1).

Diphen Cough *Morton Grove, USA.*
Diphenhydramine hydrochloride (p.409·1).
Coughs.

Diphenamill *Brunel, S.Afr.*
Aminophylline (p.748·1); diphenhydramine hydrochloride (p.409·1); ammonium chloride (p.1055·2); sodium citrate (p.1153·2).
Coughs.

Diphenhist *Rugby, USA.*
Diphenhydramine hydrochloride (p.409·1).

Diphenhydramine Constrictor *Asta Medica, Belg.*
Diphenhydramine hydrochloride (p.409·1); naphazoline hydrochloride (p.1064·2).
Hypersensitivity reactions.

Diphenylan *Lannett, USA†.*
Phenytoin sodium (p.352·3).
Epilepsy.

Diphlogen *Zyma, Aust.*
Methyl salicylate (p.55·2); eucalyptus oil (p.1578·1); menthol (p.1600·2).
Musculoskeletal, joint, peri-articular, and soft-tissue disorders.

Diphos *Procter & Gamble, Ger.*
Disodium etidronate (p.738·3).
Ectopic ossification; Paget's disease of bone.

Diphuman *Berna, Switz.*
A diphtheria immunoglobulin (p.1507·3).
Passive immunisation.

Dipidolor
Janssen-Cilag, Aust.; Janssen-Cilag, Belg.; Janssen-Cilag, Ger.; Janssen-Cilag, Neth.
Piritramide (p.80·2).
Pain.

Dipiperon
Janssen-Cilag, Belg.; Janssen-Cilag, Fr.; Janssen-Cilag, Ger.; Janssen-Cilag, Neth.; Janssen-Cilag, Switz.
Pipamperone hydrochloride (p.687·1).
Mood disturbances; psychoses; sleep disorders.

Diplogel *Ircafarm, Ital.*
Aluminium hydroxide (p.1177·3).
Gastro-intestinal disorders associated with hyperacidity.

Diplovax *Biovac, S.Afr.*
A measles vaccine (Edmonston-Zagreb strain) (p.1517·3).
Active immunisation.

Dipondal *Servier, Spain†.*
Dexfenfluramine hydrochloride (p.1479·2).
Obesity.

Dipramid *Valeas, Ital.†.*
Isopropamide iodide (p.464·3).
Gastro-intestinal disorders.

Diprin *Alcon, Swed.*
Dipivefrine hydrochloride (p.1572·3).
Glaucoma.

Diprivan
Zeneca, Aust.; ICI, Austral.; Zeneca, Belg.; Zeneca, Canad.; Zeneca, Fr.; Zeneca, Irl.; Zeneca, Ital.; Zeneca, Neth.; Zeneca, Norw.; Zeneca, S.Afr.; Zeneca, Spain; Zeneca, Swed.; Zeneca, UK; Zeneca, USA.
Propofol (p.1229·3).
General anaesthesia; sedative.

Diprobase
Schering-Plough, Irl.; Schering-Plough, UK.
Emollient.
Dry skin conditions; topical vehicle.

Diprobath
Schering-Plough, Irl.; Schering-Plough, UK.
Light liquid paraffin (p.1382·1); isopropyl myristate (p.1384·1); laureth 4.
Bath additive; dry skin disorders; hyperkeratoses.

Diproderm
Aesca, Aust.; Schering-Plough, Spain; Schering-Plough, Swed.
Betamethasone dipropionate (p.1033·3).
Otitis externa; skin disorders.

Diproform *Schering-Plough, Ital.*
Betamethasone dipropionate (p.1033·3); clioquinol (p.193·2).
Skin disorders.

Diproforte *Aesca, Aust.*
Betamethasone dipropionate (p.1033·3).
Skin disorders.

Diprogen *Schering, Canad.*
Betamethasone dipropionate (p.1033·3); gentamicin sulphate (p.212·1).
Infected skin disorders.

Diprogenta
Aesca, Aust.; Essex, Ger.; Essex, Ital.; Schering-Plough, S.Afr.; Schering-Plough, Spain; Essex, Switz.
Betamethasone dipropionate (p.1033·3); gentamicin sulphate (p.212·1).
Infected skin disorders.

Diprolene
Schering-Plough, Belg.; Schering-Plough, Fr.; Schering-Plough, Neth.; Schering-Plough, S.Afr.; Essex, Switz.; Schering, USA.
Betamethasone dipropionate (p.1033·3).
Skin disorders.

Diprolene Glycol *Schering, Canad.*
Betamethasone dipropionate (p.1033·3).
Skin disorders.

Di-Promal *Mundipharma, Aust.*
Ipratropium bromide (p.754·2); salbutamol (p.758·2).
Obstructive airways disease.

Diprophos
Aesca, Aust.; Schering-Plough, Belg.; Essex, Switz.
Betamethasone dipropionate (p.1033·3); betamethasone sodium phosphate (p.1033·3).
Corticosteroid.

Diprorecto *Schering-Plough, Ital.†.*
Betamethasone dipropionate (p.1033·3); phenylephrine hydrochloride (p.1066·2); lignocaine hydrochloride (p.1293·2).
Anorectal disorders.

Diprosalic
Aesca, Aust.; Schering-Plough, Belg.; Schering, Canad.; Schering-Plough, Fr.; Essex, Ger.; Schering-Plough, Irl.; Schering-Plough, Ital.; Schering-Plough, Neth.; Schering-Plough, Norw.; Schering-Plough, S.Afr.; Schering-Plough, Spain; Schering-Plough, Swed.; Essex, Switz.; Schering-Plough, UK.
Betamethasone dipropionate (p.1033·3); salicylic acid (p.1090·2).
Skin and scalp disorders.

Diprosept *Schering-Plough, Fr.*
Betamethasone dipropionate (p.1033·3); clioquinol (p.193·2).
Infected skin disorders.

Diprosis *Essex, Ger.*
Betamethasone dipropionate (p.1033·3).
Skin disorders.

Diprosone
Schering-Plough, Austral.; Schering-Plough, Belg.; Schering, Canad.; Schering-Plough, Fr.; Essex, Ger.; Schering-Plough, Irl.; Schering-Plough, Ital.; Schering-Plough, Neth.; Schering-Plough, S.Afr.; Essex, Switz.; Schering-Plough, UK; Schering, USA.
Betamethasone dipropionate (p.1033·3).
Skin and scalp disorders.

Diprosone Depot *Essex, Ger.*
Betamethasone dipropionate (p.1033·3); betamethasone sodium phosphate (p.1033·3).
Parenteral corticosteroid.

Diprosone Duopack *Schering-Plough, Irl.†.*
Combination preparation: Ointment or cream, betamethasone dipropionate (p.1033·3); ointment or cream, Diprobase emollient.
Skin disorders.

Diprosone Neomycine *Schering-Plough, Fr.*
Betamethasone dipropionate (p.1033·3); neomycin sulphate (p.229·2).
Infected skin disorders.

Diprostene *Schering-Plough, Fr.*
Betamethasone dipropionate (p.1033·3); betamethasone sodium phosphate (p.1033·3).
Corticosteroid.

Dipsan
Lederle, Austral.†; Lederle, Neth.†; Lederle, S.Afr.†; Wyeth Lederle, Swed.†.
Calcium carbimide (p.1556·2).
Alcoholism.

Diptol Antihist *Navarro, Spain†.*
Oral drops: Diphenhydramine hydrochloride (p.409·1); mepyramine maleate (p.414·1).
Hypersensitivity reactions.
Syrup: Diphenhydramine hydrochloride (p.409·1); ephedrine hydrochloride (p.1059·3); ethylmorphine hydrochloride (p.36·1); bitter orange; potassium iodide (p.1493·1); sodium benzoate (p.1102·3).
Upper respiratory-tract disorders.

Dipulmin *Daker Farmasimes, Spain.*
Salbutamol sulphate (p.758·2).
Obstructive airways disease; premature labour; status asthmaticus.

Dipyridan *Rhone-Poulenc Rorer, Belg.*
Dipyridamole (p.857·1).
Angina pectoris; thrombo-embolism prophylaxis.

Dipyrol *Rolab, S.Afr.*
Dipyridamole (p.857·1).
Thrombo-embolic disorders.

Dirahist *Cyanamid, Ital.*
Triamcinolone (p.1050·2); chlorpheniramine maleate (p.405·1).
Hypersensitivity reactions.

Direct Formulary Cough Lozenges *Sutton, Canad.*
Menthol (p.1600·2).

Directaclone CG *Alpha Laboratories, UK†.*
Pregnancy test (p.1621·2).

Direktan *Gerot, Aust.*
Sodium nicotinate.
Decubitus ulcer; peripheral vascular disease; sports massage.

Direxiode *Delalande, Fr.†.*
Di-iodohydroxyquinoline (p.581·1).
Infectious diarrhoea; intestinal amoebiasis.

Diribiotine CK *Lipha, Switz.†.*
Lysate of: *Escherichia coli*; *Klebsiella pneumoniae.*
Bacterial infections.

Dirythmin
Astra, Irl.†; Astra, UK.
Disopyramide phosphate (p.858·1).
Arrhythmias.

Dirytmin
Astra, Belg.; Astra, Neth.; Hassle, Norw.†; Hassle, Swed.
Disopyramide phosphate (p.858·1).
Arrhythmias.

Disadine DP *Zeneca, Irl.†.*
Povidone-iodine (p.1123·3).
Bed sores; burns; varicose ulcers; wounds.

Disalcid
3M, Canad.; Riker, UK†; 3M, USA.
Salsalate (p.83·1).
Fever; musculoskeletal and joint disorders; pain.

Disalgesic *3M, Ger.†.*
Salsalate (p.83·1).
Musculoskeletal and joint disorders.

Disalgil *Also, Ital.*
Glycol salicylate (p.43·1); camphor (p.1557·2); capsaicin (p.24·2).
Musculoskeletal, joint, and soft-tissue disorders.

Disalgyl *Monin, Fr.*
Methyl salicylate (p.55·2); capsicum oleoresin; camphor (p.1557·2).
Musculoskeletal and joint pain.

Disalpin *Dresden, Ger.*
Hydrochlorothiazide (p.885·2); reserpine (p.942·1).
Hypertension.

Disalunil *Berlin-Chemie, Ger.*
Hydrochlorothiazide (p.885·2).
Diabetes insipidus; heart failure; hypertension; oedema.

Disanal *Humana, Ital.*
Gluten-free food.

Disanthrol *Lannett, USA.*
Docusate sodium (p.1189·3); casanthranol (p.1182·3).
Constipation.

Discase *Knoll, Belg.*
Chymopapain (p.1562·3).
Herniated lumbar intervertebral disc.

Disci Bamb *Pfluger, Ger.†.*
Homoeopathic preparation.

Dis-Cinil Complex *Menarini, Ital.*
Dihydroxydibutylether (p.1571·3); cascara (p.1183·1); rhubarb (p.1212·1); boldo (p.1554·1).
Constipation.

Dis-Cinil Ilfi *Menarini, Ital.*
Dihydroxydibutylether (p.1571·3).
Constipation with digestive disorders.

Disclar *Casen Fleet, Spain.*
Tocopheryl nicotinate (p.1280·1).
Hyperlipidaemias.

Disclo-Gel *Colgate Oral Care, Austral.*
Erythrosine (p.1000·2).
Disclosing agent for dental plaque.

Disclo-Plaque *Colgate Oral Care, Austral.*
Fluorescein (p.1581·1).
Disclosing agent for dental plaque.

Disclo-Tabs *Colgate Oral Care, Austral.*
Erythrosine (p.1000·2).
Disclosing agent for dental plaque.

Discmigon *Zilly, Ger.*
Hypericum oil (p.1590·1); wheat-germ oil; avocado oil; birch tar oil (p.1092·2); beef hoof oil; thiamine hydrochloride (p.1361·1); formic acid (p.1581·3); garlic juice (p.1583·1); birch leaf (p.1553·3); juniper berry (p.1592·2); gentian root (p.1583·3); lupulus (p.1597·2); clove (p.1565·2); male fern leaf (p.104·1).
Joint disorders; keloid scars; rheumatism.

Disco-cyl Ho-Len-Complex *Liebermann, Ger.*
Homoeopathic preparation.

Discotrine *3M, Fr.*
Glyceryl trinitrate (p.874·3).
Angina pectoris.

Discover *Carter-Wallace, UK.*
Pregnancy test (p.1621·2).

Discover-2 *Carter-Wallace, Austral.†.*
Pregnancy test (p.1621·2).

Discover Onestep *Carter-Wallace, Austral.*
Pregnancy test (p.1621·2).

Discretest
Chefaro, Fr.†; Angelini, Ital.†; Chefaro, UK†.
Fertility test (p.1621·2).

Discromil *Pergam, Ital.*
Hydroquinone (p.1083·1).
Skin hyperpigmentation.

Discus compositum *Heel, Ger.*
Homoeopathic preparation.

Disdolen *Uriach, Spain.*
Fosfosal (p.42·3).
Pain.

Disdolen Codeina *Uriach, Spain.*
Codeine phosphate (p.26·1); fosfosal (p.42·3).
Pain.

Disebrin *Allergan, Ital.*
Heparin sodium (p.879·3).
Eye disorders.

Diseon *Prosintex, Ital.*
Alfacalcidol (p.1366·3).
Vitamin D deficiency.

Diseptil *Gedis, Ital.*
Benzalkonium chloride (p.1101·3).
Skin disinfection.

Disfil *Llorente, Spain.*
Ectylurea; phenytoin (p.352·3); phenobarbitone (p.350·2); aminohydroxybutyric acid (p.339·1).
Epilepsy.

Disflatyl *Solco, Switz.*
Simethicone (p.1213·1).
Flatulence; preparation for gastro-intestinal investigations.

Disgren
Poli, Ital.; Uriach, Spain.
Triflusal (p.958·3).
Thrombo-embolic disorders.

Disinclor *Tipomark, Ital.*
Chloramine (p.1106·3).
Disinfection of wounds and external genitals.

Disintox *IRBI, Ital.†.*
Calcium folinate (p.1342·2).
Anaemias; antidote to folic acid antagonists.

Disintox Cortex *IRBI, Ital.†.*
Cyanocobalamin (p.1363·3); suprarenal cortex (p.1050·1); calcium folinate (p.1342·2).
Tonic.

Disintyl *Zeta, Ital.*
Benzalkonium chloride (p.1101·3).
Disinfection of wounds, burns, and external genitals.

Disipal
3M, Austral.; Yamanouchi, Belg.; 3M, Canad.; Yamanouchi, Fr.†; Yamanouchi, Irl.; Yamanouchi, Ital.; Brocades, Neth.†; Yamanouchi, Norw.; Yamanouchi, S.Afr.; Yamanouchi, Swed.; Yamanouchi, Switz.†; Yamanouchi, UK.
Orphenadrine hydrochloride (p.465·2).
Akinesia; drug-induced extrapyramidal disorders; parkinsonism; senile depression; skeletal muscle spasm; vertigo.

Disipaletten *Brocades, Neth.†.*
Orphenadrine hydrochloride (p.465·2).
Akinesia; parkinsonism; vertigo.

Diskin *Benedetti, Ital.*
Dihydroxydibutylether (p.1571·3).
Constipation with digestive disorders.

Dismenol *Agpharm, Switz.†.*
Carzenide (p.1560·2); propyphenazone (p.81·3).
Dysmenorrhoea; smooth muscle spasm.

Dismenol N
Simons, Ger.; Agpharm, Switz.
Ibuprofen (p.44·1).
Formerly contained propyphenazone and carzenide in *Ger.*
Pain.

Dismenol neu *Salus, Aust.*
Ibuprofen (p.44·1).
Pain.

Dismozon pur *Bode, Ger.*
Magnesium monoperoxyphthalate.
Surface disinfection.

Disne Asmol *Berenguer Infale, Spain.*
Ipratropium bromide (p.754·2).
Obstructive airways disease.

Disneumon Pernasal *Solvay, Spain.*
Phenylephrine hydrochloride (p.1066·2).
Formerly contained cineole, dexamethasone phosphate, muramidase hydrochloride, phenylephrine hydrochloride, and menthol.
Nasal and sinus congestion.

D-Iso *Ratiopharm, Ger.*
Sodium chloride; sodium citrate; potassium chloride; glucose (p.1152·3).
Diarrhoea; oral rehydration therapy.

Disobrom *Geneva, USA.*
Pseudoephedrine sulphate (p.1068·3); dexbrompheniramine maleate (p.403·2).
Upper respiratory-tract symptoms.

Diso-Duriles *Astra, Ger.*
Disopyramide phosphate (p.858·1).
Arrhythmias.

Disofrol
Schering-Plough, Spain; Schering-Plough, Swed.; Essex, Switz.
Pseudoephedrine sulphate (p.1068·3); dexbrompheniramine maleate (p.403·2).
Upper respiratory-tract disorders.

Disolan *Lannett, USA.*
Docusate sodium (p.1189·3); phenolphthalein (p.1208·2).
Constipation.

Disolan Forte *Lannett, USA.*
Docusate sodium (p.1189·3); carmellose sodium (p.1471·2); casanthranol (p.1182·3).
Constipation.

Disonate *Lannett, USA.*
Docusate sodium (p.1189·3).
Constipation.

Disonorm *Solvay, Ger.*
Disopyramide (p.858·1) or disopyramide phosphate (p.858·1).
Arrhythmias.

Disophrol
Aesca, Aust.; Schering-Plough, USA.
Dexbrompheniramine maleate (p.403·2); pseudoephedrine sulphate (p.1068·3).
Eustachian tube congestion; rhinitis; sinusitis.

Disoplex *Lannett, USA.*
Docusate sodium (p.1189·3); carmellose sodium (p.1471·2).
Constipation.

Disoprivan
Zeneca, Ger.; Glaxo Wellcome, Ger.; Zeneca, Switz.
Propofol (p.1229·3).
General anaesthesia; sedative.

Disorat *Boehringer Mannheim, Ger.†.*
Metipranolol (p.906·2).
Cardiac disorders; hypertension.

Disorlon *Riom, Fr.*
Isosorbide dinitrate (p.893·1).
Angina pectoris; heart failure.

Disotat *Isis, Ger.*
Di-isopropylammonium dichloroacetate (p.854·1) or di-isopropylammonium hydrochloride (p.854·1).
Hypertension.

Disotate *Forest Pharmaceuticals, USA.*
Disodium edetate (p.980·1).
Digitalis-induced cardiac arrhythmias; hypercalcaemia.

Dispaclonidin *Ciba Vision, Ger.*
Clonidine hydrochloride (p.841·2).
Glaucoma; ocular hypertension.

Dispacromil *Ciba Vision, Ger.*
Sodium cromoglycate (p.762·1).
Allergic conjunctivitis.

Dispadex comp *Ciba Vision, Ger.*
Dexamethasone sodium phosphate (p.1037·2); neomycin sulphate (p.229·2).
Bacterial infections and inflammation of the eye.

Dispagent *Ciba Vision, Ger.*
Gentamicin sulphate (p.212·1).
Bacterial eye infections.

Dispaphenicol *Ciba Vision, Ger.†.*
Chloramphenicol (p.182·1).
Bacterial eye infections.

Dispasan *Ciba Vision, Ger.*
Sodium hyaluronate (p.1630·3).
Adjunct in ocular surgery.

Dispatenol *Ciba Vision, Ger.*
Dexpanthenol (p.1570·3); polyvinyl alcohol (p.1474·2).
Dry eyes.

Dispatetrin *Ciba Vision, Ger.*
Tetracycline hydrochloride (p.259·1).
Bacterial eye infections.

Dispatim *Ciba Vision, Ger.*
Timolol maleate (p.953·3).
Glaucoma; ocular hypertension.

Di-Spaz *Vortech, USA.*
Dicyclomine hydrochloride (p.460·1).
Functional bowel/irritable bowel syndrome.

Disperbarium *Rovi, Spain.*
Barium sulphate (p.1003·1).
Contrast medium for gastro-intestinal radiography.

Display *Solea, Ital.*
Benzalkonium chloride (p.1101·3).
Eye disinfection; eye irritation.

Dispon *Poli, Ital.*
Liothyronine (p.1495·2).
Cellulite; local accumulation of adipose tissue.

Dispril
Reckitt & Colman, Belg.; Reckitt & Colman, Norw.; Meda, Swed.
Aspirin (p.16·1).
Fever; inflammation; pain.

Disprin
Reckitt & Colman, Austral.; Reckitts, Irl.; Reckitt & Colman, S.Afr.; Reckitt & Colman, UK.
Aspirin (p.16·1).
Fever; inflammation; pain; thrombo-embolic disorders.

Disprin Direct
Reckitt & Colman, Austral.
Aspirin (p.16·1).
Glycine (p.1345·2) is included in this preparation in an attempt to limit adverse effects on the gastro-intestinal mucosa.
Fever; inflammation; pain.
Reckitt & Colman, UK.
Aspirin (p.16·1).
Formerly known as Solmin and Disprin Solmin.
Fever; pain.

Disprin Extra
Reckitts, Irl.; Reckitt & Colman, UK.
Aspirin (p.16·1); paracetamol (p.72·2).
Cold symptoms; pain; rheumatism.

Disprin Forte *Reckitt & Colman, Austral.*
Aspirin (p.16·1); codeine phosphate (p.26·1).
Fever; inflammation; pain.

Disprol
Reckitts, Irl.; Reckitt & Colman, UK.
Paracetamol (p.72·2).
Fever; pain.

Dispromil *Diviser Aquilea, Spain.*
Famotidine (p.1192·1).
Gastro-oesophageal reflux; peptic ulcers; Zollinger-Ellison syndrome.

Dissenten *SPA, Ital.*
Loperamide hydrochloride (p.1197·2).
Diarrhoea.

Dissolvurol *Dissolvurol, Mon.*
Oral drops: Colloidal silicon dioxide (p.1475·1).
Musculoskeletal and joint disorders.

Distaclor
Dista, Irl.; Lilly, Irl.; Dista, UK.
Cefaclor (p.163·2).
Bacterial infections.

Distalgesic
Napp, Irl.; Lilly, S.Afr.; Lilly, Swed.; Dista, Switz.; Dista, UK.
Dextropropoxyphene hydrochloride (p.27·3) or dextropropoxyphene napsylate (p.27·3); paracetamol (p.72·2).
These ingredients can be described by the British Approved Name Co-proxamol.
Pain.

Distalgic *Dista, Belg.*
Dextropropoxyphene hydrochloride (p.27·3); paracetamol (p.72·2).
Fever; pain.

Distamine
Lilly, Aust.; Dista, Irl.; Lilly, Neth.; Dista, UK.
Penicillamine (p.988·3).
Cystinuria; hepatitis; lead poisoning; rheumatoid arthritis; Wilson's disease.

Distaph *Alphapharm, Austral.*
Dicloxacillin sodium (p.202·1).
Gram-positive bacterial infections.

Distaquaine V-K *Dista, UK.*
Phenoxymethylpenicillin potassium (p.236·2).
Bacterial infections.

Distasil *Milana, Ital.*
Benzalkonium chloride (p.1101·3).
Skin disinfection.

Distaxid *Dista, Spain.*
Nizatidine (p.1203·2).
Gastro-oesophageal reflux; peptic ulcer.

Distensan *Esteve, Spain.*
Clotiazepam (p.657·2).
Anxiety; insomnia; neuroleptanalgesia.

Disteril *Lachifarma, Ital.*
Benzalkonium chloride (p.1101·3).
Genital hygiene; skin, wound, and burn disinfection.

Distilbene *Gerda, Fr.*
Stilboestrol (p.1462·3).
Prostatic cancer.

Distonium *Zilliken, Ital.†.*
Meprobamate (p.678·1); homatropine methobromide (p.462·2); ergotamine tartrate (p.445·3).
Gastro-intestinal disorders.

Distovagal *Tedec Meiji, Spain.*
Belladonna alkaloids (p.457·1); ergotamine tartrate (p.445·3); phenobarbitone (p.350·2).
Cardiovascular disorders; gastro-intestinal disorders; genito-urinary disorders; menopausal disorders; premenstrual syndrome; vascular headaches.

Distra-cid *Astra, Ger.†.*
Aluminium hydroxide gel (p.1177·3); magnesium oxide (p.1198·3); aluminium hydroxide-magnesium carbonate gel (p.1178·2).
Gastro-intestinal disorders.

Distraneurin
Astra, Aust.; Astra, Ger.; Astra, Switz.
Chlormethiazole (p.647·2) or chlormethiazole edisylate (p.647·2).
Alcohol withdrawal syndromes; pre-eclampsia and eclampsia; psychiatric disorders; sleep disorders; status epilepticus.

Distraneurine
Astra, Belg.; Astra, Neth.; Astra, Spain.
Chlormethiazole (p.647·2) or chlormethiazole edisylate (p.647·2).
Alcohol withdrawal syndrome; eclampsia; sedative; status epilepticus.

Disulone *Specia, Fr.*
Dapsone (p.199·2); ferrous oxalate (p.1340·1).
Dermatitis herpetiformis; leprosy; polychondritis.

Diswart *Dermatech, Austral.*
Glutaraldehyde (p.1114·3).
Common warts.

DIT I-2 *Dunhall, USA.*
Sulphanilamide (p.256·3); aminacrine hydrochloride (p.1098·3); allantoin (p.1078·2).
Vaginal infections.

Dital *UAD, USA†.*
Phendimetrazine tartrate (p.1484·2).

Ditanrix
SmithKline Beecham, Aust.; SmithKline Beecham, Ital.; Smith Kline & French, Spain.
An adsorbed diphtheria and tetanus vaccine (p.1508·1). Separate preparations are available for infants and young children and for children and adults.
Active immunisation.

Ditaven
Merck, Aust.; Merck, Ger.
Digitoxin (p.848·3).
Haematomas; leg oedema; peripheral vascular disease; varicose ulcers; venous insufficiency.

Ditaven comp *Merck, Aust.*
Digitoxin (p.848·3); heparin sodium (p.879·3).
Leg oedema; soft-tissue injuries; varicose ulcers; venous insufficiency.

Ditavene *Pharmadeveloppement, Fr.*
Digitoxin (p.848·3); heparin sodium (p.879·3).
Capillary disorders; erythrosis; rosacea.

Di-Te Kik *Meda, Swed.*
A diphtheria, tetanus, and pertussis vaccine (p.1509·1).
Active immunisation.

Ditec
Bender, Aust.; Thomae, Ger.
Fenoterol hydrobromide (p.753·2); sodium cromoglycate (p.762·1).
Obstructive airways disease.

Ditemer *Pasteur Merieux, Belg.*
An adsorbed diphtheria and tetanus vaccine (p.1508·1).
Active immunisation.

Ditemic *SmithKline Beecham, UK.*
Dried ferrous sulphate (p.1340·2); zinc sulphate (p.1373·2); vitamin B substances; ascorbic acid (p.1365·2).

Ditenate *Marion Merrell Dow, Ger.†.*
Controlled-release tablets; syrup: Bufylline (p.749·3); etafedrine hydrochloride (p.1061·1); doxylamine succinate (p.410·1).
Suppositories: Theophylline (p.765·1); etafedrine hydrochloride (p.1061·1); doxylamine succinate (p.410·1); ephedrine hydrochloride (p.1059·3).
Allergic respiratory disorders; bronchospastic disorders.

Ditenate N *Marion Merrell Dow, Ger.†.*
Theophylline (p.765·1).
Asthma; bronchitis; emphysema.

Ditenside *Funk, Spain.*
Enalapril maleate (p.863·2); hydrochlorothiazide (p.885·2).
Hypertension.

Ditensor *Funk, Spain.*
Enalapril maleate (p.863·2).
Heart failure; hypertension.

DiTePerPol Vaccin *Berna, Switz.†.*
A diphtheria, tetanus, pertussis, and polio vaccine (p.1509·3).
Formerly known as Vaccin Di Te Per Pol.
Active immunisation.

Dithiazid *Merck, Aust.†.*
Hydrochlorothiazide (p.885·2).
Hypertension; oedema.

Dithrasal *Dermatech, Austral.*
Dithranol (p.1082·1); salicylic acid (p.1090·2).
Psoriasis.

Dithrasis *Galderma, Fr.†.*
Dithranol (p.1082·1).
Psoriasis.

Dithrocream
Hamilton, Austral.; Dermal Laboratories, Irl.; Dermal Laboratories, UK.
Dithranol (p.1082·1).
Psoriasis.

Dithrolan *Dermal Laboratories, UK†.*
Dithranol (p.1082·1); salicylic acid (p.1090·2).
Psoriasis.

Ditonal *Athenstaedt, Ger.†.*
Suppositories: Trichlor-dimethylethyl-salicylate; paracetamol (p.72·2).
Cold symptoms; fever; pain; sedative.
Tablets: Trichlor-dimethylethyl-salicylate; paracetamol (p.72·2); caffeine (p.749·3); calcium ascorbate.
Neuralgia; pain.

Ditonal N *Athenstaedt, Ger.*
Paracetamol (p.72·2); caffeine (p.749·3).
Pain.

Ditripentat-Heyl *Heyl, Ger.*
Calcium trisodium pentetate (p.975·1).
Poisoning with heavy or radioactive metals.

Ditropan
Pharmacia Upjohn, Aust.; Rhone-Poulenc Rorer, Austral.; Synthelabo, Belg.; Procter & Gamble, Canad.; Synthelabo, Fr.; Lorex, Irl.; Synthelabo, Ital.; Hoechst Marion Roussel, S.Afr.; Alonga, Spain; Pharmacia Upjohn, Swed.; Hoechst Marion Roussel, Switz.; Lorex, UK; Hoechst Marion Roussel, USA.
Oxybutynin hydrochloride (p.466·1).
Neurogenic bladder; urinary incontinence.

Diu Rauwiplus *Lacer, Spain.*
Ajmaline (p.817·1); hydrochlorothiazide (p.885·2); methylrauhimbine; sarpagine (p.941·3); rescinnamide (p.942·1); reserpine hydrochloride (p.942·2).
Hypertension.

Diu Venostasin *Klinge, Ger.*
Tablets, triamterene (p.957·2); hydrochlorothiazide (p.885·2); controlled-release capsules, aesculus (p.1543·3).
Venous insufficiency.

Diu-Atenolol *Verla, Ger.*
Atenolol (p.825·3); chlorthalidone (p.839·3).
Hypertension.

Diube *SIT, Ital.*
Atenolol (p.825·3); chlorthalidone (p.839·3).
Hypertension.

Diucardin *Wyeth-Ayerst, USA.*
Hydroflumethiazide (p.889·2).
Hypertension; oedema.

Diuciclin *Benvegna, Ital.†.*
Demeclocycline magnesium (p.201·2).
Bacterial infections.

Diucomb
Gebro, Aust.; Byk, Belg.; Synthelabo, Ger.; Schwarz, Switz.
Bemetizide (p.827·1); triamterene (p.957·2).
Hypertension; oedema.

Diulo
Searle, Austral.†; Schiapparelli Searle, USA.
Metolazone (p.907·2).
Ascites; hypertension; oedema.

diu-melusin *Schwarz, Ger.*
Hydrochlorothiazide (p.885·2).
Hypertension; oedema.

Diumide-K Continus
Napp, Irl.; Asta Medica, UK.
Frusemide (p.871·1); potassium chloride (p.1161·1).
Hypertension; oedema.

Diumid+K *Mundipharma, Switz.†.*
Frusemide (p.871·1); potassium chloride (p.1161·1).
Hypertension; oedema.

Diupres *Merck Sharp & Dohme, USA†.*
Reserpine (p.942·1); chlorothiazide (p.839·1).
Hypertension.

Diural
Alpharma, Norw.; Dumex-Alpharma, Swed.†.
Frusemide (p.871·1).
Forced diuresis; hypertension; oedema; renal failure.

Diuramid *Medphano, Ger.*
Acetazolamide (p.810·3).
Glaucoma.

Diurapid *Jenapharm, Ger.*
Frusemide (p.871·1).
Oedema; oliguria.

Diuraupur *Giulini, Ger.†.*
Benzylhydrochlorothiazide; reserpine hydrochloride (p.942·2); rescinnamine (p.942·1); sarpagine (p.941·3); ajmaline (p.817·1); yohimbine (p.1645·3); potassium chloride (p.1161·1).
Hypertension.

Diuraupur sine *Giulini, Ger.†.*
Benzylhydrochlorothiazide; rescinnamine (p.942·1); sarpagine (p.941·3); ajmaline (p.817·1); yohimbine (p.1645·3); potassium chloride (p.1161·1).
Hypertension.

Diuremid *Guidotti, Ital.*
Torasemide (p.956·3) or torasemide sodium (p.956·3).
Ascites; heart failure; oedema; renal failure.

Diuresal *Lagap, Switz.†.*
Frusemide (p.871·1).
Hypertension; oedema; renal failure.

Diurese *American Urologicals, USA.*
Trichlormethiazide (p.958·2).
Hypertension; oedema.

Diuresix *Menarini, Ital.*
Torasemide sodium.
Ascites; heart failure; kidney disorders; oedema.

Diuretabs *Potter's, UK.*
Buchu leaf (p.1555·2); juniper berry oil (p.1592·3); parsley piert; bearberry (p.1552·2).
Fluid retention.

Diureticum *Holzinger, Aust.†.*
Acetazolamide (p.810·3).

Diureticum Truw *Truw, Ger.†.*
Homoeopathic preparation.

Diureticum-Medice *Medice, Ger.†.*
Crataegus (p.1568·2); inula helenium (p.1059·2); herniaria (p.1587·2); ononis (p.1610·2); orthosiphon (p.1592·2); phaseolus vulgaris; solidago virgaurea; squill (p.1070·1); dill; parsley (p.1615·3); chelidonium; rubia tinctorum.
Renal and cardiac disorders.

Diuretikum Verla *Verla, Ger.*
Triamterene (p.957·2); hydrochlorothiazide (p.885·2).
Hypertension; oedema.

Diurex *Lacer, Spain.*
Xipamide (p.971·2).
Hypertension; oedema.

Diurexan
Asta Medica, Belg.; E. Merck, Irl.; Vesta, S.Afr.; Asta Medica, UK.
Xipamide (p.971·2).
Hypertension; oedema.

Diurid *Laevosan, Aust.*
Triamterene (p.957·2); hydrochlorothiazide (p.885·2).
Heart failure; hypertension; oedema.

Diurigen *Goldline, USA.*
Chlorothiazide (p.839·1).
Hypertension; oedema.

Diuril *Merck Sharp & Dohme, USA.*
Chlorothiazide (p.839·1) or chlorothiazide sodium (p.839·2).
Hypertension; oedema.

Diurin *Pharmalab, S.Afr.†.*
Benzthiazide (p.828·1).
Hypertension; oedema; premenstrual syndrome.

Diuritens *Biotrading, Ital.†.*
Hydroflumethiazide (p.889·2); reserpine (p.942·1).
Hypertension.

Diurix *Helvepharm, Switz.*
Frusemide (p.871·1).
Forced diuresis; hypertension; oedema.

Diurolab *Lebens, Ital.†.*
Labetalol hydrochloride (p.896·1); chlorthalidone (p.839·3).
Hypertension.

Diurolasa *Lasa, Spain†.*
Frusemide (p.871·1).
Hypertension; oedema.

Diursan *TAD, Ger.*
Hydrochlorothiazide (p.885·2); amiloride hydrochloride (p.819·2).
Hypertension; oedema.

Diutec *Garec, S.Afr.*
Amiloride hydrochloride (p.819·2); hydrochlorothiazide (p.885·2).
Hypertension; oedema.

Diutensat *Azupharma, Ger.*
Triamterene (p.957·2); hydrochlorothiazide (p.885·2).
Hypertension; oedema.

Diutensat comp *Azupharma, Ger.*
Triamterene (p.957·2); hydrochlorothiazide (p.885·2); propranolol hydrochloride (p.937·1).
Hypertension.

Diutensen-R *Wallace, USA.*
Methyclothiazide (p.904·1); reserpine (p.942·1).
Hypertension.

Diu-Tonolytril *Dorsch, Ger.†.*
Triamterene (p.957·2); hydrochlorothiazide (p.885·2).
Hypertension; oedema.

Diuzine *CEPA, Spain.*
Amiloride hydrochloride (p.819·2); hydrochlorothiazide (p.885·2).
Hypertension; oedema.

Diuzolin *Llorente, Spain†.*
Etozolin (p.867·2).
Hypertension; oedema.

Divacuna TD *Leti, Spain.*
A diphtheria and tetanus vaccine (p.1508·1).
Active immunisation of infants and young children.

Divalol W *Wernigerode, Ger.*
Curcuma zanthorrhiza; peppermint oil (p.1208·1).
Biliary disorders.

Divane *Monin, Fr.†.*
Crataegus (p.1568·2).
Nervous disorders.

Divascan *Berlin-Chemie, Ger.*
Iprazochrome.
Diabetic retinopathy; headache; migraine.

Divegal *Waldheim, Aust.*
Dihydroergotamine tartrate (p.444·3).
Migraine and related vascular headaches.

Divial *Merck, Spain.*
Lorazepam pivalate (p.676·3).
Alcohol withdrawal syndrome; anxiety; chemotherapy-induced nausea and vomiting; epilepsy; insomnia.

Divical *Zilliken, Ital.*
Calcium folinate (p.1342·2).
Folate deficiency.

Dividol *Zambon, Ital.*
Viminol hydroxybenzoate (p.91·2).
Pain.

Divigel
Orion, Irl.; Orion, Swed.
Oestradiol (p.1455·1).
Menopausal disorders; osteoporosis.

Divina
Organon, Austral.; Innothera, Fr.; Byk, Neth.; Continental Ethicals, S.Afr.; Orion, Swed.
11 Tablets, oestradiol valerate (p.1455·2); 10 tablets, oestradiol valerate; medroxyprogesterone acetate (p.1448·3).
Menopausal disorders; osteoporosis.

Divinal Galle *Divinal, Ger.*
Cynara (p.1569·2).
Dyspepsia.

Divinal Gastro *Divinal, Ger.*
Caraway (p.1559·3); peppermint leaf (p.1208·1); fennel (p.1579·1).
Dyspepsia; flatulence.

Divinal Rheuma *Divinal, Ger.*
Camphor (p.1557·2).
Rheumatism.

Divinal Seda *Divinal, Ger.*
Hypericum (p.1590·1).
Anxiety; depression; psychovegetative states.

Divinal-Bohnen *Divinal, Ger.†.*
Agrimony; boldo (p.1554·1); chelidonium; frangula bark (p.1193·2); gentian (p.1583·3); hedera helix; senna (p.1212·2); peppermint oil (p.1208·1); fennel oil (p.1579·2); caraway oil (p.1559·3); guaiazulene (p.1586·3); papain (p.1614·1); dried yogurt powder; pancreatin (p.1612·1); ox bile (p.1553·2); cholic acid; docusate sodium (p.1189·3); anhydrous orotic acid (p.1611·2); cysteine hydrochloride; benzyl mandelate.
Digestive system disorders.

Divinal-Broncho-Balsam *Divinal, Ger.*
Camphor (p.1557·2); eucalyptus oil (p.1578·1); turpentine oil (p.1641·1).
Respiratory-tract disorders.

Divinal-Hepa *Divinal, Ger.*
Silybum marianum (p.993·3).
Liver disorders.

Diviva *Pharmacia Upjohn, Belg.*
11 Tablets, oestradiol valerate (p.1455·2); 10 tablets, oestradiol valerate; medroxyprogesterone acetate (p.1448·3).
Menopausal disorders; oestrogen replacement therapy.

Dixarit
Boehringer Ingelheim, Austral.†; Boehringer Ingelheim, Belg.; Boehringer Ingelheim, Canad.; Boehringer Ingelheim, Ger.; Boehringer Ingelheim, Irl.; Boehringer Ingelheim, Neth.; Boehringer Ingelheim, S.Afr.; Boehringer Ingelheim, UK.
Clonidine hydrochloride (p.841·2).
Menopausal flushing; migraine or vascular headache.

Dixeran
Lundbeck, Aust.; Lundbeck, Belg.; Lundbeck, Switz.
Melitracen hydrochloride (p.296·3).
Depression.

Dixibon *Sandoz, Spain†.*
Sulpiride (p.692·3).
Psychoses; vertigo.

Dizac *Ohmeda, USA.*
Diazepam (p.661·1).
Anxiety; epilepsy; skeletal muscle relaxant.

Dizmiss *JMI, USA.*
Meclozine hydrochloride (p.413·3).
Motion sickness; vertigo.

DLPA *Contassium Co., UK.*
DL-Phenylalanine.

DM Cough Syrup
Note. This name is used for preparations of different composition.
Prodemdis, Canad.
Diphenhydramine hydrochloride (p.409·1); dextromethorphan hydrobromide (p.1057·3); ammonium chloride (p.1055·2).
Technilab, Canad.
Dextromethorphan hydrobromide (p.1057·3).

DM E Suppressant Expectorant *Drug Trading, Canad.*
Dextromethorphan hydrobromide (p.1057·3); guaiphenesin (p.1061·3).

DM Plus Decongestant *Technilab, Canad.*
Dextromethorphan hydrobromide (p.1057·3); pseudoephedrine hydrochloride (p.1068·3).

DM Plus Decongestant Expectorant *Technilab, Canad.*
Dextromethorphan hydrobromide (p.1057·3); pseudoephedrine hydrochloride (p.1068·3); guaiphenesin (p.1061·3).

DM Plus Expectorant *Technilab, Canad.*
Dextromethorphan hydrobromide (p.1057·3); guaiphenesin (p.1061·3).

DM Sans Sucre *Trianon, Canad.*
Dextromethorphan hydrobromide (p.1057·3).
Coughs.

DM Syrup *Technilab, Canad.*
Dextromethorphan hydrobromide (p.1057·3); diphenhydramine hydrochloride (p.409·1); ammonium chloride (p.1055·2).

4-DMAP
Kohler, Ger.; Kohler, Neth.
4-Dimethylaminophenol hydrochloride (p.980·1).
Cyanide, hydrocyanic acid, nitrile, or hydrogen sulphide poisoning.

D-Med *Ortega, USA.*
Methylprednisolone acetate (p.1046·1).
Corticosteroid.

DMG-B15 *Contassium Co., UK.*
Calcium gluconate (p.1155·2); NN-dimethylglycine hydrochloride.

DMH *Alra, USA.*
Dimenhydrinate (p.408·2).

DML *Person & Covey, USA.*
A range of moisturisers.

D-Mulsin *Mucos, Ger.*
Cholecalciferol (p.1366·3).
Vitamin D deficiency.

DNCG *Mundipharma, Ger.; Stada, Ger.; Trommsdorff, Ger.*
Sodium cromoglycate (p.762·1).
Asthma; conjunctivitis; rhinitis.

Doak-Oil *Trans Canaderm, Canad.*
Liquid paraffin (p.1382·1); isopropyl palmitate (p.1384·1); coal tar (p.1092·3).
Skin disorders.

Doans
Note. This name is used for preparations of different composition.
Zyma, UK†.
Paracetamol (p.72·2); sodium salicylate (p.85·1).
Backache.
Ciba Consumer, USA.
Magnesium salicylate (p.51·1).
Fever; inflammation; pain.

Doans Backache Pills *Novartis Consumer, Canad.*
Magnesium salicylate (p.51·1).
Muscular back pain.

Dobacen *Brandt, Switz.*
Diphenhydramine hydrochloride (p.409·1).
Insomnia.

Dobacen plus *Brandt, Switz.†.*
Diphenhydramine hydrochloride (p.409·1); promethazine hydrochloride (p.416·2).
Insomnia.

Dobenam *Angelini, Ital.†.*
Droxicam (p.35·2).
Rheumatic disorders.

Dobendan
Hoechst, Aust.; Cassella-med, Ger.
Cetylpyridinium chloride (p.1106·2).
Mouth and throat disorders.

Dobendan X *Cassella-med, Ger.*
Cetylpyridinium chloride (p.1106·2).
Mouth and throat disorders.

Dobesifar *Farmila, Ital.†.*
Calcium dobesilate (p.1556·3).
Haemorrhagic disorders.

Dobetin *Angelini, Ital.*
Cyanocobalamin (p.1363·3).
Tonic; vitamin B_{12} deficiency.

Dobetin con Vitamina B1 *Angelini, Ital.*
Vitamin B preparation.
Neuralgia; neuritis.

Dobetin Totale *Angelini, Ital.*
Vitamin B preparation.
Neuralgia.

Dobica *OPW, Ger.*
Calcium dobesilate (p.1556·3).
Capillary fragility and leakage; venous insufficiency.

Doblexan *Quimifar, Spain.*
Piroxicam (p.80·2).
Dysmenorrhoea; gout; musculoskeletal and joint disorders.

Dobo 600 *Wolfer, Ger.†.*
Calcium gluconate (p.1155·2).
Calcium deficiency.

Dobren *Ravizza, Ital.*
Sulpiride (p.692·3).
Dysthymia; psychoses.

Dobriciclin *Quimifar, Spain.*
Amoxycillin trihydrate (p.151·3).
Bacterial infections.

Dobuject *Leiras, Swed.*
Dobutamine hydrochloride (p.860·1).
Heart failure.

Dobupal *Almirall, Spain.*
Venlafaxine hydrochloride (p.311·2).
Depression.

Dobutrex
Lilly, Aust.; Lilly, Austral.; Lilly, Belg.; Lilly, Canad.; Lilly, Fr.; Lilly, Ger.; Lilly, Irl.; Lilly, Ital.; Lilly, Neth.; Lilly, Norw.; Lilly, S.Afr.; Lilly, Spain; Lilly, Swed.; Lilly, Switz.; Lilly, UK; Lilly, USA.
Dobutamine hydrochloride (p.860·1).
Cardiac stress testing; heart failure.

Docabolin *Nourypharma, Ger.†.*
Deoxycortone phenylpropionate (p.1036·3); nandrolone phenylpropionate (p.1452·2).
Hypotension.

Docabolina *Organon, Spain†.*
Deoxycortone phenylpropionate (p.1036·3); nandrolone phenylpropionate (p.1452·2).
Asthenia; hypotension.

Docatone *Wyeth, Spain.*
Doxapram (p.1480·2).
CNS depression; respiratory depression.

Docdol *Mer-National, S.Afr.*
Paracetamol (p.72·2); codeine phosphate (p.26·1); caffeine (p.749·3).
Pain.

Docgel *Docmed, S.Afr.*
Dried aluminium hydroxide gel (p.1177·3); magnesium oxide (p.1198·3); simethicone (p.1213·1).
Dyspepsia; gastritis; gastro-oesophageal reflux; peptic ulcer.

Docidrazin *Zeneca, Ger.; Rhein-Pharma, Ger.*
Propranolol hydrochloride (p.937·1); hydralazine hydrochloride (p.883·2); bendrofluazide (p.827·3).
Hypertension.

Dociretic *Thiemann, Ger.*
Propranolol hydrochloride (p.937·1); bendrofluazide (p.827·3).
Hypertension.

Dociteren *Procter & Gamble, Ger.; Rhein-Pharma, Ger.*
Propranolol hydrochloride (p.937·1); triamterene (p.957·2); hydrochlorothiazide (p.885·2).
Hypertension.

Dociton *Zeneca, Ger.; Rhein-Pharma, Ger.*
Propranolol hydrochloride (p.937·1).
Anxiety; cardiac disorders; essential tremor; hypertension; hyperthyroidism; migraine.

Dociton Dytide H *Rhein-Pharma, Ger.†; Rohm, Ger.†.*
Combination pack: Dociton: propranolol hydrochloride (p.937·1) Dytide H: triamterene (p.957·2); hydrochlorothiazide (p.885·2).
Hypertension.

Doclis *Boehringer Mannheim, Spain.*
Diltiazem hydrochloride (p.854·2).
Angina pectoris; hypertension; myocardial infarction.

Docostyl *Pentafarm, Spain.*
Doxycycline hydrochloride (p.202·3).
Bacterial infections.

Docrub *Docmed, S.Afr.*
Camphor (p.1557·2); menthol (p.1600·2); methyl salicylate (p.55·2); eucalyptus oil (p.1578·1); buchu oil (p.1555·2).
Cold symptoms; coughs; soft-tissue disorders.

Docsed *Docmed, S.Afr.*
Mepyramine maleate (p.414·1); codeine phosphate (p.26·1); pholcodine (p.1068·1); ephedrine hydrochloride (p.1059·3).
Coughs.

Doctar *Savage, USA.*
Coal tar (p.1092·3).
Scalp disorders.

Doctodermis *Medea, Spain.*
Biotin; methyl hydroxybenzoate (p.1117·2); triethanolamine lauryl sulphate.
Skin cleansing.

Doctofril Antiinflamat *Medea, Spain.*
Phenylbutazone (p.79·2); lignocaine (p.1293·2); methyl nicotinate (p.55·1); vitamin F.
Chilblains; rheumatic and muscle pain.

Doctogaster *Medea, Spain.*
Aluminium silicate (p.1178·3); frangula bark (p.1193·2); magnesium carbonate (p.1198·1); magnesium polygalacturonate; liquorice (p.1197·1); sodium bicarbonate (p.1153·2).
Gastritis; hyperacidity; peptic ulcer.

Doctomitil *Medea, Spain.*
Cineole (p.1564·1); diethylamine salicylate (p.33·1); methyl nicotinate (p.55·1).
Soft-tissue disorders.

Doctril *Abello, Spain.*
Ibuprofen lysine (p.44·3).
Fever; inflammation; musculoskeletal, joint, and periarticular disorders; pain.

Doctrim *Docmed, S.Afr.*
Co-trimoxazole (p.196·3).
Bacterial infections.

Docucal-P *Parmed, USA.*
Docusate calcium (p.1189·3); phenolphthalein (p.1208·2).
Constipation.

Docusoft Plus *G & W, USA.*
Docusate sodium (p.1189·3); casanthranol (p.1182·3).
Constipation.

Docusoft S *G & W, USA.*
Docusate sodium (p.1189·3).
Constipation.

Docusol *Typharm, UK.*
Docusate sodium (p.1189·3).
Bowel evacuation; constipation.

Docutrix *Lilly, Spain†.*
Fluoxetine hydrochloride (p.284·1).
Depression.

Dodds *Dannorth, Canad.*
Sodium salicylate (p.85·1).
Musculoskeletal pain.

Dodecan *Vernleigh, S.Afr.†.*
Multivitamin and mineral preparation.

Dodecatol N *Heyl, Ger.*
Procaine hydrochloride (p.1299·2); cyanocobalamin (p.1363·3).
Inflammation; pain.

Dodecavit *L'Arguenon, Fr.*
Hydroxocobalamin acetate (p.1364·2).
Neuralgias.

Dodemox *Epifarma, Ital.*
Amoxycillin trihydrate (p.151·3).
Bacterial infections.

Doderlein Med *Zyma, Ger.*
Lactobacillus gasseri.
Vaginal disorders.

Do-Do
Note. This name is used for preparations of different composition.
COB, Belg.†.
Ephedrine hydrochloride (p.1059·3); caffeine (p.749·3); amidopyrine (p.15·2); theobromine and calcium salicylate (p.765·1); grindelia.
Asthma; coughs.
Zyma, UK.
Theophylline (p.765·1); ephedrine hydrochloride (p.1059·3); caffeine (p.749·3).
Bronchial coughs; wheezing.

Do-Do Expectorant Linctus *Zyma, UK.*
Guaiphenesin (p.1061·3).
Coughs.

Doederlein *Zyma, Aust.*
Lactobacillus acidophilus (p.1594·1).
Vaginal candidiasis.

Dogmagel *Delagrange, Spain†.*
Aluminium hydroxide (p.1177·3); sulpiride (p.692·3).
Psychosomatic gastroduodenal disorders.

Dogmatil
Synthelabo, Aust.; Synthelabo, Belg.; Synthelabo, Fr.; Synthelabo, Ger.; Lorex Synthelabo, Neth.; Delagrange, Spain; Synthelabo, Switz.
Sulpiride (p.692·3).
Depression; Ménière's disease; neuroses; peptic ulcer; psychoses; vertigo.

Dohyfral Vitamine AD3 *Solvay, Neth.*
Retinol (p.1358·1); cholecalciferol (p.1366·3).
Vitamin A and vitamin D deficiency.

DOK *Major, USA.*
Docusate sodium (p.1189·3).
Constipation.

Doktacillin
Astra, Aust.; Astra, Norw.; Astra, Swed.
Ampicillin sodium (p.153·1).
Bacterial infections.

Dolacet *Roberts, USA.*
Hydrocodone tartrate (p.43·1); paracetamol (p.72·2).
Pain.

Dolak *Bama, Spain.*
Isosorbide mononitrate (p.893·3).
Angina pectoris.

Dolal
Biocodex, Fr.; Biocodex, Switz.†.
Ethylmethoxy salicylate; phenylpropyl salicylate.
Musculoskeletal and joint pain.

Dolalgial *Sanofi Winthrop, Spain.*
Clonixin lysine (p.26·1).
Pain; peri-articular disorders.

Dolanal *Exel, Belg.†.*
Lignocaine hydrochloride (p.1293·2); hydrocortisone acetate (p.1043·3).
Haemorrhoids.

Dolanex *Lannett, USA.*
Paracetamol (p.72·2).
Fever; pain.

Dolantin *Hoechst, Ger.*
Pethidine hydrochloride (p.76·1).
Pain.

Dolantina *Bayer, Spain.*
Pethidine hydrochloride (p.76·1).
Pain; premedication.

Dolantine
Hoechst Marion Roussel, Belg.; Hoechst Marion Roussel, Switz.†.
Pethidine hydrochloride (p.76·1).
Pain; premedication; sedative.

Dolarist *Steiner, Ger.†.*
Paracetamol (p.72·2).
Fever; pain.

Dolarist comp *Steiner, Ger.†.*
Paracetamol (p.72·2); codeine phosphate (p.26·1).
Pain.

Dolazol *Galephar, Neth.†.*
Indomethacin (p.45·2).
Musculoskeletal and joint disorders; pain.

Dolcidium *SMB, Belg.†.*
Indomethacin (p.45·2).
Musculoskeletal and joint disorders.

Dolcol *Dainippon, Jpn.*
Pipemidic acid (p.237·2).
Bacterial infections.

Dolcontin
Pharmacia Upjohn, Norw.; Pharmacia Upjohn, Swed.
Morphine sulphate (p.56·2).
Pain.

Dolcopin *Rottapharm, Spain.*
Magnesium trisilicate (p.1199·1); sodium bicarbonate (p.1153·2); almasilate (p.1177·1).
Formerly contained alginic acid, magnesium trisilicate, sodium bicarbonate, almasilate.
Gastro-oesophageal reflux.

Dolcor *Gazzoni, Ital.*
Aspartame (p.1335·1).
Sugar substitute.

Dolcymene *Semar, Spain†.*
Cymene (p.27·2).
Rheumatic and muscle pain.

Doldieta *Ottolenghi, Ital.*
Maltodextrin (p.1350·2); aspartame (p.1335·1).
Sugar substitute.

Dolean *3M, Belg.†.*
Aspirin (p.16·1).
Musculoskeletal and joint inflammation.

Dolean pH 8 *3M, Switz.†.*
Aspirin (p.16·1).
Fever; inflammation; pain.

Dolefin Paracetamol *Pharmacia, Spain.*
Paracetamol (p.72·2).
Fever; pain.

Dolemicin *Alcala, Spain.*
Dipyrone (p.35·1).
Fever; pain.

Dolene *Lederle, USA.*
Dextropropoxyphene hydrochloride (p.27·3).
Pain.

Dolenon *Strathmann, Ger.*
Cayenne pepper.
Muscle pain; nerve pain.

Dolerax *Propan, S.Afr.*
Paracetamol (p.72·2); doxylamine succinate (p.410·1); caffeine (p.749·3); codeine phosphate (p.26·1).
Pain associated with tension.

Doleron *Astra, Swed.*
Aspirin (p.16·1); dextropropoxyphene napsylate (p.27·3); phenazone (p.78·2).
Pain.

Dolestan *Much, Ger.*
Diphenhydramine hydrochloride (p.409·1).
Sleep disorders.

Dolestan forte comp *Much, Ger.*
Diphenhydramine hydrochloride (p.409·1); guaiphenesin (p.1061·3).
Sleep disorders.

Dolex
Note. This name is used for preparations of different composition.
Terramin, Aust.
Glycol salicylate (p.43·1); salicylic acid (p.1090·2); camphor (p.1557·2); turpentine oil (p.1641·1).
Rheumatic and muscle pain.

IFI, Ital.
Furprofen (p.42·3).
Pain.

Dolexaderm H *Strathmann, Ger.*
Dulcamara (p.1574·2).
Eczema.

Dolexamed N *Strathmann, Ger.*
Eucalyptus oil (p.1578·1); peppermint oil (p.1208·1); rosemary oil (p.1626·2).
Myalgia; neuralgia; rheumatism.

Dolgesic *Novag, Spain.*
Paracetamol (p.72·2).
Fever; pain.

Dolgesic Codeina *Novag, Spain.*
Codeine phosphate (p.26·1); paracetamol (p.72·2).
Pain.

Dolgit
Schoeller, Aust.; Merck-Belgolabo, Belg.†; Merck-Clevenot, Fr.; Dolorgiet, Ger.; Dolorgiet, Switz.
Ibuprofen (p.44·1).
Fever; inflammation; musculoskeletal, joint, and peri-articular disorders; pain; soft-tissue injury.

Dolgit-Diclo *Dolorgiet, Ger.*
Diclofenac sodium (p.31·2).
Gout; inflammation; musculoskeletal and joint disorders; pain.

Dolibu *Klinge, Aust.*
Ibuprofen (p.44·1).
Fever; musculoskeletal and joint disorders; pain.

Dolicoccil *Dolisos, Canad.*
Homoeopathic preparation.

Dolinac
Durachemie, Ger.; IRBI, Ital.; Whitehall, S.Afr.
Felbinac (p.37·1) or diisopropanolamine felbinac (p.37·1).
Inflammation; pain; soft-tissue disorders.

Doline *Ferrer, Spain.*
Benorylate (p.21·2).
Fever; musculoskeletal and joint disorders; pain.

Dolipol *Hoechst, Fr.*
Tolbutamide (p.333·2).
Diabetes mellitus.

Doliprane *Theraplix, Fr.*
Paracetamol (p.72·2).
Fever; pain.

Dolisal *Guidotti, Ital.†.*
Diflunisal (p.33·2).
Pain.

Dolko *Therabel, Fr.*
Paracetamol (p.72·2).
Fever; pain.

Dolmatil
Delandale, Irl.; Delandale, UK.
Sulpiride (p.692·3).
Schizophrenia.

Dolmen
Note. This name is used for preparations of different composition.
Sigma-Tau, Ital.
Tenoxicam (p.88·2).
Musculoskeletal disorders.

Uriach, Spain.
Aspirin (p.16·1); ascorbic acid (p.1365·2); codeine phosphate (p.26·1).
Fever; influenza symptoms; pain.

Dolmitin *Medea, Spain.*
Cineole (p.1564·1); diethylamine salicylate (p.33·1).
Soft-tissue disorders.

Dolmix *Apomedica, Aust.†.*
Etenzamide (p.35·3); paracetamol (p.72·2); caffeine (p.749·3).
Fever; pain.

Dolo Buscopan *Boehringer Ingelheim, Spain†.*
Dipyrone (p.35·1).
Fever; pain.

Dolo Coneurase *Tedec Meiji, Spain†.*
Lysine aspirin (p.50·3); vitamin B substances.
Lignocaine hydrochloride (p.1293·2) is included in this preparation to alleviate the pain of injection.
Pain.

Dolo Demotherm *Demopharm, Switz.*
Dimethyl sulphoxide (p.1377·2); benzyl nicotinate (p.22·1); glycol salicylate (p.43·1).
Musculoskeletal and joint pain.

Dolo Mobilat *Luitpold, Ger.*
Phenylephrine hydrochloride (p.1066·2); a heparinoid (p.882·3); glycol salicylate (p.43·1).
Joint, peri-articular, and soft-tissue disorders.

Dolo neos *Optimed, Ger.*
Ibuprofen (p.44·1).
Fever; inflammation; musculoskeletal and joint disorders; pain.

Dolo Nervobion *Merck, Spain.*
Diclofenac sodium (p.31·2); vitamin B substances.
Rheumatism, neuritis.

Doloana *Quimifar, Spain.*
Aspirin (p.16·1); salicylamide (p.82·3).
Fever; pain.

Dolo-Arthrodynat *Ziethen, Ger.*
Harpagophytum procumbens (p.27·2).
Musculoskeletal and joint disorders.

Dolo-Arthrosenex *Whitehall-Robins, Switz.*
Glycol salicylate (p.43·1); heparin sodium (p.879·3); camphor (p.1557·2).
Musculoskeletal, joint, peri-articular, and soft-tissue disorders.

Dolo-Arthrosenex N *Brenner-Efeka, Ger.*
Glycol salicylate (p.43·1).
Formerly marketed as Dolo-Arthrosenex which contained glycol salicylate, heparin sodium, and camphor.
Muscle, joint, and soft-tissue injuries and disorders.

Dolo-Arthrosetten *Brenner-Efeka, Ger.†.*
Paracetamol (p.72·2); kava (p.1592·3); tropaeolum majus; rhododendron ferrugineum; taraxacum (p.1634·2); bryonia (p.1555·2).
Painful joint, muscle and nerve disorders.

Dolo-Arthrosetten H *Brenner-Efeka, Ger.*
Harpagophytum procumbens (p.27·2).
Musculoskeletal and joint disorders.

dolobasan *Sagitta, Ger.†.*
Diclofenac sodium (p.31·2).
Inflammation; rheumatism.

Dolobene
Merckle, Ger.; Mepha, Switz.
Dimethyl sulphoxide (p.1377·2); heparin sodium (p.879·3); dexpanthenol (p.1570·3).
Neuralgia; peri-articular and soft-tissue disorders.

Dolobid
Merck Sharp & Dohme, Austral.; Frosst, Canad.; Morson, Irl.; Merck Sharp & Dohme, Ital.; Merck Sharp & Dohme, S.Afr.; Merck Sharp & Dohme, Spain; Morson, UK; Merck Sharp & Dohme, USA.
Diflunisal (p.33·2).
Inflammation; musculoskeletal, joint, and peri-articular disorders; pain.

Dolobis *Merck Sharp & Dohme-Chibret, Fr.*
Diflunisal (p.33·2).
Pain.

Dolocid *Merck Sharp & Dohme, Neth.*
Diflunisal (p.33·2).
Musculoskeletal and joint disorders; pain.

Dolocod *Klinge, Aust.*
Aspirin (p.16·1); paracetamol (p.72·2); codeine phosphate (p.26·1).
Fever; pain.

Dolo-cyl
Note. A similar name is used for preparations of different composition.
Liebermann, Ger.
Arnica oil (p.1550·3); eucalyptus oil (p.1578·1); hypericum oil (p.1590·1); juniper oil (p.1592·3); lavender oil (p.1594·3); pumilio pine oil (p.1623·3); rosemary oil (p.1626·2).
Musculoskeletal and joint disorders; sports injuries.

Dolocyl
Note. A similar name is used for preparations of different composition.
Novartis, Ital.; Sandoz, Spain.; Wander OTC, Switz.
Ibuprofen (p.44·1).
Fever; musculoskeletal, joint, and peri-articular disorders; pain.

Dolodens *Knoll, Spain.*
Codeine phosphate (p.26·1); hydroxyzine hydrochloride (p.412·1); propyphenazone (p.81·3).
Pain.

Dolodent *Theranol-Deglaude, Fr.*
Amylocaine hydrochloride (p.1286·1); chloral hydrate (p.645·3).
Aphthous ulcers; teething pain.

Doloderm
Theraplix, Fr.; Rhone-Poulenc Rorer, Ital.
Methyl butetisalicylate (p.55·1).
Musculoskeletal and joint pain.

Dolo-Dobendan *Cassella-med, Ger.*
Cetylpyridinium chloride (p.1106·2); benzocaine (p.1286·2).
Mouth and throat disorders.

Dolo-Dolgit *Dolorgiet, Ger.†.*
Ibuprofen (p.44·1).
Inflammation; rheumatism.

Dolo-Exhirud *Plantorgan, Ger.†.*
Hirudin (p.883·1); glycol salicylate (p.43·1); benzyl nicotinate (p.22·1).
Muscle and joint disorders; pain.

Dolofarma *Maxfarma, Spain.*
Aspirin (p.16·1); caffeine (p.749·3); paracetamol (p.72·2).
Fever; pain.

Dolofin *Farmabel, Belg.†.*
Ibuprofen (p.44·1).
Fever; inflammation; musculoskeletal, joint, and peri-articular disorders; pain.

Doloflex *Byk Gulden, Ital.*
Paracetamol (p.72·2); aspirin (p.16·1).
Pain.

Dolofort *Klinge, Aust.*
Ibuprofen (p.44·1).
Pain.

Dolofugin *Sanol, Ger.†.*
Paracetamol (p.72·2).
Fever; pain.

Dologastrine *Gifrer Barbezat, Fr.†.*
Codeine (p.26·1); magnesium hydroxide (p.1198·2); sodium bicarbonate (p.1153·2); anhydrous dibasic sodium phosphate (p.1159·3); anhydrous sodium sulphate (p.1213·3).
Gastro-intestinal disorders.

Dologel *Wander OTC, Switz.*
Ibuprofen (p.44·1).
Musculoskeletal, joint, and soft-tissue disorders.

Dologyne *Arkopharma, Fr.*
Artemisia vulgaris; chamomile (p.1561·2).
Pain.

Doloject *Syxyl, Ger.*
Homoeopathic preparation.

Dolokapton *Strallhofer, Aust.*
Paracetamol (p.72·2); codeine phosphate (p.26·1).
Coughs; fever; pain.

Dolokey *Inkeysa, Spain.*
Camphor (p.1557·2); lavender oil (p.1594·3); methyl salicylate (p.55·2); expressed mustard oil (p.1605·3); rosemary oil (p.1626·2); eucalyptus oil (p.1578·1); belladonna (p.457·1); capsicum (p.1559·2); menthol (p.1600·2).
Musculoskeletal and joint disorders.

Dolomedil *Daker Farmasimes, Spain.*
Codeine phosphate (p.26·1); paracetamol (p.72·2).
Pain.

Dolo-Menthoneurin
Byk, Aust.; Tosse, Ger.; Byk, Switz.†.
Diethylamine salicylate (p.33·1); heparin sodium (p.879·3); menthol (p.1600·2).
Muscle, joint, peri-articular, and soft-tissue disorders; neuralgia.

Dolo-Menthoneurin CreSa *Tosse, Ger.*
Glycol salicylate (p.43·1); benzyl nicotinate (p.22·1); camphor (p.1557·2).
Muscle, joint, and peri-articular disorders.

Dolomine *Frega, Canad.*
Aspirin (p.16·1); caffeine (p.749·3).

Dolomite *Nature's Bounty, USA.*
Calcium salts (p.1155·1); magnesium salts (p.1157·2).
Dietary supplement.

Dolomo *Klinge, Aust.*
Aspirin (p.16·1); paracetamol (p.72·2); caffeine (p.749·3).
Fever; pain.

Dolomo Nacht *Klinge, Aust.†.*
Aspirin (p.16·1); paracetamol (p.72·2); codeine phosphate (p.26·1).
Fever; pain.

Dolomo TN *Klinge, Ger.*
White tablets, aspirin (p.16·1); paracetamol (p.72·2); caffeine (p.749·3); blue tablets, aspirin; paracetamol; codeine phosphate (p.26·1).
Pain.

Dolonerv *Gerot, Aust.*
Paracetamol (p.72·2); vitamin B substances.
Pain.

Doloneuro *Merck, Ger.*
Diethylamine salicylate (p.33·1); glycol salicylate (p.43·1); methyl nicotinate (p.55·1).
Muscle, nerve, and joint pain.

Dolo-Neurobion
Note. This name is used for preparations of different composition.
Merck, Aust.
Diclofenac sodium (p.31·2); vitamin B substances.
Musculoskeletal and joint disorders; pain.

E. Merck, Switz.†.
Vitamin B substances; dipyrone (p.35·1).
Procaine hydrochloride (p.1299·2) is included in the injection to alleviate the pain of injection.
Muscle, nerve, and joint pain.

Dolo-Neurobion forte *Merck, Ger.*
Vitamin B substances; paracetamol (p.72·2).
Arthritis; back pain; neuralgia.

Dolo-Neurobion N *Merck, Ger.*
Vitamin B substances; paracetamol (p.72·2).
Formerly contained vitamin B substances, paracetamol, and etenzamide.
Joint disorders; lumbago; neuralgia; neuritis; sciatica.

Dolo-Neurotrat *Nordmark, Ger.†.*
Dextropropoxyphene hydrochloride (p.27·3); vitamins.
Pain.

Dolonevran *Synthelabo, Fr.†.*
Cobamamide (p.1364·2).
Neuralgias.

Dolophine *Lilly, USA.*
Methadone hydrochloride (p.53·2).
Detoxification and treatment of opioid addiction; pain.

Dolo-Phlogase *Godecke, Ger.†.*
Oxyphenbutazone (p.72·1); propyphenazone (p.81·3).
Acute ankylosing spondylitis; rheumatism.

DoloPosterine N *Kade, Ger.*
Cinchocaine hydrochloride (p.1289·2).
Formerly contained allantoin, cinchocaine hydrochloride, and diphenylpyraline hydrochloride and was known as DoloPosterine.
Anorectal disorders.

Doloproct *Schering, Ger.*
Fluocortolone pivalate (p.1041·3); lignocaine hydrochloride (p.1293·2).
Anorectal disorders.

Dolo-Prolixan
Siegfried, Ger.†; Siegfried, Switz.
Yellow tablets, azapropazone (p.20·3); dextropropoxyphene hydrochloride (p.27·3); blue tablets, azapropazone; phenprobamate (p.686·1).
Musculoskeletal, joint, and peri-articular pain.

Dolo-Puren *Isis, Ger.*
Ibuprofen (p.44·1).
Gout; inflammation; musculoskeletal and joint disorders; pain; soft-tissue disorders.

Dolopyrine *Streuli, Switz.*
Propyphenazone (p.81·3); atropine methobromide (p.455·1); papaverine hydrochloride (p.1614·2); diphenhydramine hydrochloride (p.409·1); codeine phosphate (p.26·1).
Pain.

Dolorac *GenDerm, USA.*
Capsaicin (p.24·2).
Pain.

Doloreduct *Azupharma, Ger.*
Paracetamol (p.72·2).
Fever; pain.

Doloren *Merckle, Aust.*
Ibuprofen (p.44·1).
Fever; musculoskeletal and joint disorders; pain.

Dolorex *Whitehall-Robins, Switz.*
Glycol salicylate (p.43·1); camphor (p.1557·2); lavender oil (p.1594·3); thyme oil (p.1637·1); siberian fir oil; isopropyl alcohol (p.1118·2).
Musculoskeletal, joint, peri-articular, and soft-tissue disorders.

Dolorex Neo *Whitehall-Robins, Switz.*
Glycol salicylate (p.43·1); allantoin (p.1078·2).
Musculoskeletal and joint disorders; superficial circulatory disorders.

Dolorfug *Wolff, Ger.†.*
Paracetamol (p.72·2).
Fever; pain.

Dolorgiet *Dolorgiet, Ger.*
Glycol salicylate (p.43·1); benzyl nicotinate (p.22·1).
Musculoskeletal and joint disorders.

Dolor-loges *Loges, Ger.*
Homoeopathic preparation.

Dolormin *Woelm, Ger.*
Ibuprofen lysine (p.44·3).
Fever; pain.

Dolorol *Lennon, S.Afr.*
Paracetamol (p.72·2).
Fever; pain.

Dolorol Forte *Lennon, S.Afr.*
Paracetamol (p.72·2); codeine phosphate (p.26·1).
Fever; pain.

Dolorsan-Balsam *Opfermann, Ger.*
Methyl salicylate (p.55·2); menthol (p.1600·2); camphor (p.1557·2).
Catarrh; musculoskeletal and joint disorders; neuralgia; sports injuries.

Dolo-Rubriment *Knoll, Ger.*
Glycol salicylate (p.43·1); benzyl nicotinate (p.22·1); heparin sodium (p.879·3).
Muscle, nerve, joint, and soft-tissue disorders.

Dolosal *Specia, Fr.*
Pethidine hydrochloride (p.76·1).
Adjunct in anaesthesia; pain.

Dolosarto *Biosarto, Spain.*
Aspirin (p.16·1); benzydamine hydrochloride (p.21·3).
Fever; inflammation; musculoskeletal and joint disorders; pain.

Dolostop
Note. This name is used for preparations of different composition.
Bayer, Spain.
Paracetamol (p.72·2).
Fever; pain.

Zeller, Switz.
Propyphenazone (p.81·3); paracetamol (p.72·2); caffeine (p.749·3).
Fever; pain.

Dolotard *Nycomed, Swed.*
Dextropropoxyphene chloride (p.27·3).
Pain.

Dolotec *Innothera, Fr.*
Paracetamol (p.72·2).
Fever; pain.

Doloteffin *Ardeypharm, Ger.*
Harpagophytum procumbens (p.27·2).
Musculoskeletal and joint disorders.

DoloTendin *Divinal, Ger.*
Dexamethasone (p.1037·1); lignocaine hydrochloride (p.1293·2).
Musculoskeletal, joint, and peri-articular disorders.

Dolothricin *Provita, Aust.*
Tyrothricin (p.267·2); neomycin sulphate (p.229·2); benzocaine (p.1286·2); camphor (p.1557·2); chloroxylenol (p.1111·1).
Bacterial ear infections.

Dolotren *Faes, Spain.*
Diclofenac diethylamine (p.31·2) or diclofenac sodium (p.31·2).
Dysmenorrhoea; gout; musculoskeletal, joint, peri-articular, and soft-tissue disorders.

Dolo-Veniten *Whitehall-Robins, Switz.*
Glycol salicylate (p.43·1); a heparinoid (p.882·3); aescin (p.1543·3).
Vascular disorders.

DoloVisano Diclo *Kade, Ger.†.*
Diclofenac sodium (p.31·2).
Inflammation; musculoskeletal and joint disorders.

DoloVisano M *Kade, Ger.*
Mephenesin (p.1315·3).
Cervical syndrome; lumbago; muscle pain; skeletal muscle spasm.

DoloVisano Salbe *Kade, Ger.*
Glycol salicylate (p.43·1); benzyl nicotinate (p.22·1).
Circulatory disorders of the skin; muscle and joint pain; soft-tissue disorders.

Doloxene
Lilly, Austral.; Lilly, Irl.; Lilly, S.Afr.; Lilly, Swed.; Lilly, UK.
Dextropropoxyphene hydrochloride (p.27·3) or dextropropoxyphene napsylate (p.27·3).
Pain.

Doloxene Co
Note. This name is used for preparations of different composition.
Lilly, Austral.†.
Dextropropoxyphene napsylate (p.27·3); aspirin (p.16·1).
Pain.

Lilly, S.Afr.
Dextropropoxyphene hydrochloride (p.27·3); aspirin (p.16·1); caffeine (p.749·3).
Pain.

Doloxene Compound
Lilly, Irl.; Lilly, UK†.
Dextropropoxyphene napsylate (p.27·3); aspirin (p.16·1); caffeine (p.749·3).
Pain.

Dolpasse *Leopold, Aust.†.*
Dipyrone (p.35·1); orphenadrine citrate (p.465·2).
Back pain; headache.

Dolprone
Hoechst Marion Roussel, Belg.; Rhone-Poulenc Rorer, Switz.
Paracetamol (p.72·2).
Fever; pain.

Dolpyc
Note. This name is used for preparations of different composition.
Bournonville, Belg.; Warner-Lambert, Fr.
Capsicum oleoresin; chloroform (p.1220·3).
Muscle and joint pain.

Teofarma, Ital.
Capsicum oleoresin.
Musculoskeletal and joint pain.

Dol.S Regaliz *Cinfa, Spain†.*
Liquorice (p.1197·1); menthol (p.1600·2).
Coughs; throat irritation.

Dolsed *American Urologicals, USA.*
Hexamine (p.216·1); salol (p.83·1); atropine sulphate (p.455·1); hyoscyamine sulphate (p.464·2); benzoic acid (p.1102·3); methylene blue (p.984·3).
Urinary-tract infections.

Dolsinal *Ferrer, Spain.*
Nabumetone (p.60·1).
Musculoskeletal and joint disorders.

Dol-Stop *Warner-Lambert Consumer, Belg.*
Paracetamol (p.72·2); codeine phosphate (p.26·1).
Fever; pain.

Dolviran
Bayer, Belg.; Bayer, Ger.†; Bayer, Spain.
Aspirin (p.16·1); codeine phosphate (p.26·1); caffeine (p.749·3).
Fever; influenza symptoms; pain.

Dolviran N
Note. This name is used for preparations of different composition.
Bayer, Ger.
Aspirin (p.16·1); codeine phosphate (p.26·1).
Pain.

Bayer, Neth.
Aspirin (p.16·1); codeine phosphate (p.26·1); caffeine (p.749·3).
Fever; pain.

Dolvis *Bayer, Ital.†.*
Aspirin (p.16·1); paracetamol (p.72·2); caffeine (p.749·3).
Fever; pain.

Dolzam *Zambon, Belg.*
Tramadol hydrochloride (p.90·1).
Pain.

Domar *Teofarma, Ital.*
Pinazepam (p.687·1).
Nervous disorders.

Domeboro *Miles, USA.*
Aluminium sulphate (p.1548·1); calcium acetate (p.1155·1).
Inflammatory skin conditions.

Domenan *Kissei, Jpn.*
Ozagrel hydrochloride (p.1612·1).
Asthma.

Domeni *Tafir, Spain†.*
Vincamine (p.1644·1).
Cerebral trauma; cerebrovascular disorders.

Dome-Paste *Miles, USA.*
Zinc oxide (p.1096·2); calamine (p.1080·1); gelatin (p.723·2).
Conditions of the extremities requiring protection and support.

Dometin *Nycomed, Neth.†.*
Indomethacin (p.45·2).
Musculoskeletal, joint, and peri-articular disorders.

Domex *Sante Naturelle, Canad.*
Calcium and magnesium.

Domical
Berk, Irl.; Berk, UK.
Amitriptyline hydrochloride (p.273·3).
Depression.

Domidorm *Asta Medica, Belg.*
Prothipendyl hydrochloride (p.689·2); cyclobarbitone calcium (p.660·2).
Agitation; insomnia; premedication.

Dominal
Asta Medica, Aust.; Asta Medica, Belg.; Asta Medica, Ger.
Prothipendyl hydrochloride (p.689·2).
Atopic dermatitis; eclampsia; pruritus; psychiatric disorders; sedative.

Dominans *Lundbeck, Ital.*
Nortriptyline hydrochloride (p.300·2); fluphenazine hydrochloride (p.671·3).
Mixed anxiety depressive states.

Domistan *Therval, Fr.†.*
Histapyrrodine hydrochloride (p.411·3).
Hypersensitivity reactions.

Domol
Miles, Canad.†; Miles, USA.
Bath additive.
Lubrication of the skin; pruritus.

Domperamol *Servier, UK.*
Paracetamol (p.72·2); domperidone maleate (p.1191·1).
Migraine.

Dompil *Spyfarma, Spain.*
Metampicillin sodium (p.224·3).
Bacterial infections.

Dompil Balsamico *Spyfarma, Spain†.*
Guaiphenesin (p.1061·3); metampicillin sodium (p.224·3).
Respiratory-tract infections.

Domucef *Medici Domus, Ital.†.*
Cephalexin (p.178·2).
Bacterial infections.

Domupirina *Medici Domus, Ital.†.*
Aspirin (p.16·1).
Flu symptoms; pain.

Domureuma *Medici Domus, Ital.†.*
Fentiazac (p.41·1) or fentiazac calcium (p.41·1).
Fever; inflammation; pain.

Domutussina *Medici Domus, Ital.†.*
Dropropizine (p.1059·2).
Coughs.

Domuvar *Bioprogress, Ital.*
Spores of *Bacillus subtilis*.
Gastro-intestinal disorders.

Dona *Rottapharm, Ital.*
Glucosamine sulphate (p.1585·1).
Arthroses.

Dona 200-S *Opfermann, Ger.*
Tablets: Glucosamine sulphate (p.1585·1).
Degenerative joint disorders.

Donalg *Dynacren, Ital.*
Amethocaine hydrochloride (p.1285·2); potassium guaiacolsulfonate (p.1068·3); salicylic acid (p.1090·2); menthol (p.1600·2); sage (p.1627·1); chamomile (p.1561·2); willow (p.82·3); ginger (p.1193·2).
Dental pain.

Donamet *Ravizza, Ital.*
Ademetionine (p.1543·1).
Hepatic cholestasis.

Donatiol *AGIPS, Ital.*
Methyl cysteine hydrochloride (p.1064·1); guaiphenesin (p.1061·3); camphor (p.1557·2).
Respiratory-tract disorders.

Donatussin *Laser, USA.*
Oral drops: Chlorpheniramine maleate (p.405·1); phenylephrine hydrochloride (p.1066·2); guaiphenesin (p.1061·3).
Syrup: Chlorpheniramine maleate (p.405·1); phenylephrine hydrochloride (p.1066·2); dextromethorphan hydrobromide (p.1057·3); guaiphenesin (p.1061·3).
Coughs.

Donatussin DC *Laser, USA.*
Hydrocodone tartrate (p.43·1); phenylephrine hydrochloride (p.1066·2); guaiphenesin (p.1061·3).
Coughs.

Doncef *Pharma 2000, Fr.*
Cephradine (p.181·3).
Bacterial infections.

Doneka *Vita, Spain.*
Lisinopril (p.898·2).
Heart failure; hypertension; myocardial infarction.

Doneka Plus *Vita, Spain.*
Lisinopril (p.898·2); hydrochlorothiazide (p.885·2).
Hypertension.

Doneurin *Hexal, Ger.*
Doxepin hydrochloride (p.283·2).
Anxiety; depression; withdrawal syndromes.

Doneurina *Delagrange, Spain†.*
Cyanocobalamin (p.1363·3); thiamine hydrochloride (p.1361·1).
Vitamin B deficiency.

Dong Quai Complex *Blackmores, Austral.*
Angelica sinensis; avena (p.1551·3); cimicifuga (p.1563·3); vitex agnus castus (p.1544·2); vitamins and minerals.
Menopausal disorders; premenstrual syndrome; uterine cramping.

Donicer *Novag, Spain.*
Amiloride hydrochloride (p.819·2); hydrochlorothiazide (p.885·2).
Hypertension; oedema.

Donix *Llorens, Spain.*
Lorazepam (p.675·3).
Alcohol withdrawal syndrome; anxiety; chemotherapy-induced nausea and vomiting; epilepsy; insomnia.

Donnagel
Note. This name is used for preparations of different composition.
Whitehall, Austral.; Wyeth-Ayerst, Canad.†.
Hyoscyamine sulphate (p.464·2); atropine sulphate (p.455·1); hyoscine hydrobromide (p.462·3); kaolin (p.1195·1); pectin (p.1474·1).
Gastro-intestinal disorders.

Wyeth-Ayerst, USA.
Attapulgite (p.1178·3).
Diarrhoea.

Donnagel-MB *Wyeth-Ayerst, Canad.†.*
Kaolin (p.1195·1); pectin (p.1474·1).
Diarrhoea.

Donnagel-PG
Note. This name is used for preparations of different composition.
Wyeth-Ayerst, Canad.
Capsules: Activated attapulgite (p.1178·3); pectin (p.1474·1); prepared opium (p.70·3).
Oral suspension: Kaolin (p.1195·1); pectin (p.1474·1); prepared opium (p.70·3).
Diarrhoea.

Robins, USA†.
Hyoscyamine sulphate (p.464·2); atropine sulphate (p.455·1); hyoscine hydrobromide (p.462·3); kaolin (p.1195·1); pectin (p.1474·1); prepared opium (p.70·3).
Diarrhoea.

Donnalix *Whitehall, Austral.*
Hyoscyamine sulphate (p.464·2); atropine sulphate (p.455·1); hyoscine hydrobromide (p.462·3).
Gastro-intestinal disorders.

Donnamar *Marnel, USA.*
Hyoscyamine sulphate (p.464·2).

Donnamor *Moore, USA.*
Atropine sulphate (p.455·1); hyoscine hydrobromide (p.462·3); hyoscyamine hydrobromide (p.464·2) or hyoscyamine sulphate (p.464·2); phenobarbitone (p.350·2).
Gastro-intestinal disorders.

Donnapine *Major, USA†.*
Atropine sulphate (p.455·1); hyoscine hydrobromide (p.462·3); hyoscyamine hydrobromide (p.464·2) or hyoscyamine sulphate (p.464·2); phenobarbitone (p.350·2).
Gastro-intestinal disorders.

Donna-Sed *Vortech, USA.*
Atropine sulphate (p.455·1); hyoscine hydrobromide (p.462·3); hyoscyamine hydrobromide (p.464·2) or hyoscyamine sulphate (p.464·2); phenobarbitone (p.350·2).
Gastro-intestinal disorders.

Donnatab *Whitehall, Austral.*
Hyoscyamine sulphate (p.464·2); atropine sulphate (p.455·1); hyoscine hydrobromide (p.462·3).
Gastro-intestinal disorders.

Donnatal
Wyeth-Ayerst, Canad.; Continental Ethicals, S.Afr.; Robins, USA.
Hyoscyamine sulphate (p.464·2); atropine sulphate (p.455·1); hyoscine hydrobromide (p.462·3); phenobarbitone (p.350·2).
Biliary-tract disorders; gastro-intestinal disorders; genitourinary-tract disorders; motion sickness.

Donnazyme *Robins, USA.*
Pancreatin (p.1612·1).
Decreased digestive enzyme secretory activity; dyspepsia.

Donobid
Merck Sharp & Dohme, Norw.; Merck Sharp & Dohme, Swed.
Diflunisal (p.33·2).
Inflammation; musculoskeletal and joint disorders; pain.

Donorest *Wyeth, Spain.*
Fentiazac (p.41·1).
Fever; musculoskeletal, joint, and peri-articular disorders; pain.

Donormyl
Oberlin, Fr.; Upsamedica, Spain.
Doxylamine succinate (p.410·1).
Insomnia.

Don't *Del, USA.*
Sucrose octa-acetate (p.1633·2); isopropyl alcohol (p.1118·2).
Nail biting deterrent.

Dontisolon D *Hoechst, Ger.*
Prednisolone (p.1048·1) or prednisolone acetate (p.1048·1).
Inflammatory disorders of the mouth.

Dontisolon M *Hoechst Marion Roussel, Switz.†.*
Prednisolone (p.1048·1) or prednisolone acetate (p.1048·1); neomycin hydrochloride (p.230·1); aminoquinuride hydrochloride (p.1101·2).
Inflammatory disorders of the mouth.

Dontisolon M Mundheilpaste *Hoechst, Ger.†.*
Prednisolone acetate (p.1048·1); neomycin hydrochloride (p.230·1); aminoquinuride hydrochloride (p.1101·2).
Inflammatory disorders of the mouth.

Dontisolon M Zylinderampullen *Hoechst, Ger.†.*
Prednisolone (p.1048·1); neomycin hydrochloride (p.230·1); aminoquinuride hydrochloride (p.1101·2).
Dental dressing; inflammatory disorders of the mouth.

Dontopivalone *Jouveinal, Fr.*
Tixocortol pivalate (p.1050·1); chlorhexidine acetate (p.1107·2).
Mouth disorders.

Dopacard
IPSEN Biotech, Fr.; Ipsen, Irl.; Fisons, Neth.†; Speywood, Swed.; Galenica, Switz.; Speywood, UK.
Dopexamine hydrochloride (p.862·1).
Heart failure.

Dopaflex *Medphano, Ger.*
Levodopa (p.1137·1).
Parkinsonism.

Dopagen *Antigen, Irl.†.*
Methyldopa (p.904·2).
Hypertension.

Dopamed *SMP, S.Afr.†.*
Dopamine hydrochloride (p.861·1).
Heart failure; shock.

Dopamet
Berk, Irl.; Dumex, Norw.; Dumex-Alpharma, Swed.†; Dumex, Switz.; Berk, UK†.
Methyldopa (p.904·2).
Hypertension.

Dopar *Procter & Gamble, USA.*
Levodopa (p.1137·1).
Parkinsonism.

Dopatox *Angelini, Ital.†.*
Cyanocobalamin (p.1363·3); calcium folinate (p.1342·2).
Tonic.

Dopegyt *Thiemann, Ger.*
Methyldopa (p.904·2).
Hypertension.

Dopergin
Schering, Aust.; Schering, Ger.; Schering, Ital.; Schering, Neth.; Schering, Spain; Schering, Switz.
Lysuride maleate (p.1142·1).
Acromegaly; amenorrhoea; hyperprolactinaemia; infertility; lactation inhibition; male hypogonadism; parkinsonism; premenstrual syndrome; prolactinoma.

Dopergine
Schering, Belg.†; Schering, Fr.
Lysuride maleate (p.1142·1).
Galactorrhoea; gynaecomastia and impotence in males; infertility; menstrual disorders; parkinsonism.

Dopo Pik *Tipomark, Ital.*
Triclosan (Irgasan 300) (p.1127·2); triethanolamine (p.1639·1); propylene glycol (p.1622·1).
Skin disinfection.

Doppelherz Energie-Tonikum N *Queisser, Ger.*
Vitamin B substances; honey; invert sugar; crataegus; valerian; lupulus.
Tonic.

Doppelherz Ginseng Aktiv *Queisser, Ger.*
Ginseng; pyridoxine hydrochloride; nicotinamide; caffeine.
Tonic.

Doppelherz Magenstarkung *Queisser, Ger.*
Peppermint leaf (p.1208·1); absinthium (p.1541·1); silybum marianum (p.993·3).
Gastro-intestinal disorders.

Doppelherz Melissengeist *Queisser, Ger.*
Melissa (p.1600·1); angelica; cinnamon (p.1564·2); nutmeg (p.1609·2); bitter-orange peel (p.1610·3); clove (p.1565·2); lemon peel.
Cold symptoms; insomnia; musculoskeletal and joint pain; nervous disorders.

Doppelherz Tonikum *Pharmonta, Aust.*
Crataegus (p.1568·2); melissa (p.1600·1); lupulus (p.1597·2).
Tonic.

Doppel-Spalt Compact *Much, Ger.*
Aspirin (p.16·1); caffeine (p.749·3).
Fever; inflammation; pain.

Dopram
Salus, Aust.; Wyeth, Austral.; Wyeth Lederle, Belg.; Wyeth-Ayerst, Canad.; Brenner-Efeka, Ger.†; Antigen, Irl.; Wyeth, Neth.; Wyeth, Norw.; Intramed, S.Afr.; Wyeth, Switz.; Anpharm, UK; Robins, USA.
Doxapram hydrochloride (p.1480·1).
Respiratory depression.

Dops
Note. This name is used for preparations of different composition.
Fuca, Fr.
Sodium bicarbonate (p.1153·2); calcium carbonate (p.1182·1); calcium phosphate (p.1155·3); magnesium

hydroxide (p.1198·2); titanium dioxide (p.1093·3); magnesium carbonate (p.1198·1).
Gastric hyperacidity.

Sumitomo, Jpn.
Droxidopa (p.1136·2).
Familial amyloid polyneuropathy; parkinsonism.

Doral Wallace, USA.
Quazepam (p.689·3).
Insomnia.

Doralese
SmithKline Beecham, Irl.; Bencard, UK.
Indoramin (p.891·2).
Benign prostatic hyperplasia.

Doranol Antibioticos, Spain†.
Erythromycin stearate (p.204·2).
Bacterial infections.

Dorant Laboratories for Applied Biology, UK†.
Hydroxybenzoates (p.1117·2).
Oral hygiene.

Dorcol Children's Cold Formula Sandoz, USA.
Pseudoephedrine hydrochloride (p.1068·3); chlorpheniramine maleate (p.405·1).
Cold symptoms.

Dorcol Children's Cough Syrup Sandoz, USA.
Pseudoephedrine hydrochloride (p.1068·3); guaiphenesin (p.1061·3); dextromethorphan hydrobromide (p.1057·3).
Coughs.

Dorcol Children's Decongestant Sandoz, USA.
Pseudoephedrine hydrochloride (p.1068·3).
Nasal congestion.

Dorcol Children's Fever & Pain Reducer Sandoz, USA.
Paracetamol (p.72·2).
Fever; pain.

Dorcol DM Sandoz, Canad.†.
Dextromethorphan hydrobromide (p.1057·3); phenylpropanolamine hydrochloride (p.1067·2); guaiphenesin (p.1061·3).
Coughs; nasal congestion.

Doregrippin Rentschler, Ger.
Paracetamol (p.72·2); phenylephrine hydrochloride (p.1066·2).
Cold and influenza symptoms.

Doregrippin S Rentschler, Ger.†.
Etenzamide (p.35·3); diphenylpyraline hydrochloride (p.409·3).
Catarrh; influenza.

Dorehydrin Procter & Gamble, Aust.
Co-dergocrine mesylate (p.1566·1).
Cervical syndrome; hypertension; mental function impairment; migraine and related vascular headache; peripheral vascular disease.

Dorenasin Rentschler, Ger.
Xylometazoline hydrochloride (p.1071·2).
Nasal congestion.

Doreperol N Rentschler, Ger.
Hexetidine (p.1116·1).
Inflammatory disorders of the oropharynx; oral hygiene.

Doretonsin Rentschler, Ger.†.
Chlorhexidine hydrochloride (p.1107·2); benzocaine (p.1286·2).
Mouth and throat disorders.

Dorex Woelm, Ger.†.
Benzocaine (p.1286·2); ephedrine hydrochloride (p.1059·3); liquorice juice (p.1197·1); saponin; ammonium chloride (p.1055·2); eucalyptus oil (p.1578·1); menthol (p.1600·2).
Coughs.

Dorex Hustensaft N mit Oxeladin Woelm, Ger.†.
Oral drops: Oxeladin citrate (p.1065·3); ephedrine hydrochloride (p.1059·3); thyme (p.1636·3); ammonium chloride (p.1055·2); eucalyptus oil (p.1578·1); anise oil (p.1550·1); sage oil; camphor (p.1557·2).
Oral liquid: Oxeladin citrate (p.1065·3); ephedrine hydrochloride (p.1059·3); thyme (p.1636·3); wild thyme leaf; ammoniacal extract of liquorice root (p.1197·1); saponin; thyme oil (p.1637·1); anise oil (p.1550·1); sage oil; ammonium chloride (p.1055·2).
Coughs.

Dorex-retard Woelm, Ger.†.
Oxeladin citrate (p.1065·3).
Coughs.

Dori Rentschler, Ger.
Benzocaine (p.1286·2); cetylpyridinium chloride (p.1106·2); tyrothricin (p.267·2).
Mouth and throat inflammation.

Doricum Farmila, Ital.
Fluocinolone acetonide (p.1041·1); neomycin sulphate (p.229·2).
Eye, ear, and nose disorders.

Doricum Semplice Farmila, Ital.†.
Fluocinolone acetonide (p.1041·1).
Skin disorders.

Doridamina Angelini, Ital.
Lonidamine (p.544·2).
Malignant neoplasms.

Dorithricin
Note. This name is used for preparations of different composition.
Provita, Aust.
Tyrothricin (p.267·2); neomycin sulphate (p.229·2).

Rentschler, Ger.
Tyrothricin (p.267·2); benzalkonium chloride (p.1101·3); benzocaine (p.1286·2).
Mouth and throat disorders.

Dorival Bayer, Spain.
Ibuprofen (p.44·1).
Fever; musculoskeletal and joint disorders; pain; peri-articular disorders.

Dorken UCB, Spain.
Potassium clorazepate (p.657·1); aminohydroxybutyric acid (p.339·1); pyridoxine (p.1363·1).
Anxiety; behaviour disorders.

Dormacil Vinas, Spain†.
Doxylamine succinate (p.410·1).
Insomnia.

Dormarex 2 Republic, USA†.
Diphenhydramine hydrochloride (p.409·1).
Insomnia; motion sickness; parkinsonism.

Dormarist Steiner, Ger.
Valerian (p.1643·1); melissa (p.1600·1).
Sleep disorders.

Dorme Hoechst Marion Roussel, S.Afr.
Quazepam (p.689·3).
Insomnia.

Dormeasan
Note. This name is used for preparations of different composition.
Bioforce, Ger.
Valerian (p.1643·1); lupulus (p.1597·2).
Agitation; insomnia.

Bioforce, Switz.†.
Melissa (p.1600·1); avena (p.1551·3); passion flower (p.1615·3); lupulus (p.1597·2); valerian (p.1643·1); lupulin.
Insomnia; nervous disorders.

Dormeasan N Bioforce, Switz.
Lupulus (p.1597·2); valerian (p.1643·1).
Agitation; insomnia; irritability.

Dormel Rhone-Poulenc Rorer, Austral.†.
Chloral hydrate (p.645·3).
Anxiety; insomnia.

Dormen Labima, Belg.
Pyrithyldione (p.689·3); diphenhydramine hydrochloride (p.409·1).
Insomnia.

Dormer 211 Dormer, Canad.
Emollient.
Dry skin.

Dormex Nobel, Canad.
Diphenhydramine hydrochloride (p.409·1).
Insomnia.

Dormicum
Roche, Aust.; Roche, Belg.; Roche, Ger.; Roche, Neth.; Roche, Norw.; Roche, S.Afr.; Roche, Spain; Roche, Swed.; Roche, Switz.
Midazolam (p.679·3), midazolam hydrochloride (p.679·3), or midazolam maleate (p.680·1).
General anaesthesia; premedication; sedative; sleep disorders; status epilepticus.

Dormidina Pensa, Spain.
Doxylamine succinate (p.410·1).
Insomnia.

Dormi-Gastreu N R14 Reckeweg, Ger.
Homoeopathic preparation.

Dormigen Antigen, Irl.†.
Nitrazepam (p.682·2).
Insomnia.

Dormigoa N Scheurich, Ger.
Diphenhydramine hydrochloride (p.409·1).
Dormigoa formerly contained diphenhydramine hydrochloride and guaiphenesin.
Sleep disorders.

Dormilfo N Redel, Ger.†.
Secbutobarbitone sodium (p.692·1); meprobamate (p.678·1).
Sleep disorders.

Dormin Randob, USA.
Diphenhydramine hydrochloride (p.409·1).
Insomnia.

Dormiphen Lalco, Canad.
Diphenhydramine hydrochloride (p.409·1).
Insomnia.

Dormiplant Schwabe, Switz.
Valerian (p.1643·1); melissa (p.1600·1).
Sleep disorders.

Dormodor Andreu, Spain.
Flurazepam hydrochloride (p.672·2).
Insomnia.

Dormonoct
Hoechst Marion Roussel, Belg.; Hoechst Marion Roussel, Irl.; Hoechst Marion Roussel, Neth.; Hoechst Marion Roussel, S.Afr.; Roussel, UK†.
Loprazolam mesylate (p.675·3).
Insomnia; premedication.

Dormo-Puren Isis Puren, Ger.
Nitrazepam (p.682·2).
Sleep disorders.

Dormo-Sern Serturner, Ger.
Valerian (p.1643·1); passion flower (p.1615·3).
Nervous disorders; sleep disorders.

Dormoverlan Verla, Ger.
Valerian (p.1643·1); lupulus (p.1597·2); passion flower (p.1615·3).
Agitation; insomnia.

Dormplus Pensa, Spain.
Diphenhydramine hydrochloride (p.409·1).
Insomnia.

Dormutil N Isis, Ger.
Diphenhydramine hydrochloride (p.409·1).
Sleep disorders.

Dorner Toray, Jpn.
Beraprost sodium (p.1413·3).
Thrombo-embolic disorders.

Dorocoff-ASS plus Hevert, Ger.
Aspirin (p.16·1); caffeine (p.749·3).
Pain.

Dorocoff-Paracetamol Hevert, Ger.
Paracetamol (p.72·2).
Fever; pain.

Dorsec Quimifar, Spain†.
Bismuth subgallate (p.1180·2); chloramphenicol (p.182·1); sulphamethizole (p.254·2); sulphanilamide (p.256·3).
Skin infections.

Dorsiflex Medial, Neth.
Mephenoxalone (p.678·1).
Muscle pain.

Dorsilon Drossapharm, Switz.
Mephenoxalone (p.678·1); paracetamol (p.72·2).
Musculoskeletal pain.

Doryl
Merck, Ger.; E. Merck, Switz.
Carbachol (p.1390·1).
Gastro-intestinal motility disorders; urinary retention.

Doryx
Faulding, Austral.; Parke, Davis, Canad.; Parke-Med, S.Afr.; Scand Pharm, Swed.; Parke, Davis, USA.
Doxycycline hydrochloride (p.202·3).
Bacterial infections.

DOS Softgel Goldline, USA.
Docusate sodium (p.1189·3).
Constipation.

Dosaflex Richwood, USA.
Senna (p.1212·2).
Constipation.

Dosalax Richwood, USA.
Senna (p.1212·2).
Constipation.

Dosberotec Boehringer Ingelheim, Ital.
Fenoterol hydrobromide (p.753·2).
Respiratory-tract disorders.

Doscafis Llorens, Spain.
Aspirin (p.16·1); caffeine (p.749·3); paracetamol (p.72·2).
Fever; inflammation; musculoskeletal and joint disorders; pain.

Dose Iketon, Ital.†.
Lactic acid (p.1593·3); alkylamidobetaine.
Vaginal douche.

Doses-O-Son Realdyme, Fr.
Bran (p.1181·2).
Dietary fibre supplement.

Dosil Llorens, Spain.
Doxycycline hydrochloride (p.202·3).
Bacterial infections.

Dosil Enzimatico Llorens, Spain.
Doxycycline hydrochloride (p.202·3); chymotrypsin (p.1563·2); trypsin (p.1640·1).
Bacterial infections.

Dospir Boehringer Ingelheim, Switz.
Ipratropium bromide (p.754·2); salbutamol sulphate (p.758·2).
Obstructive airways disease.

Doss
Note. This name is used for preparations of different composition.
SmithKline Beecham, Canad.
Danthron (p.1188·2); docusate sodium (p.1189·3).
Constipation.

Tosse, Ger.
Alfacalcidol (p.1366·3).
Bone disorders; hypoparathyroidism.

Dossifil Therica, Fr.
Ergocalciferol (p.1367·1); calcium hypophosphite; calcium pantothenate (p.1352·3).
Vitamin D deficiency.

Dostil Triomed, S.Afr.
Capsules†: Aspirin (p.16·1); codeine phosphate (p.26·1).
Syrup: Paracetamol (p.72·2); codeine phosphate (p.26·1).
Fever; pain.

Dostinex
Pharmacia Upjohn, Aust.; Pharmacia Upjohn, Austral.; Pharmacia Upjohn, Belg.; Pharmacia Upjohn, Ger.; Pharmacia Upjohn, Irl.; Pharmacia Upjohn, Ital.; Pharmacia Upjohn, Neth.; Pharmacia Upjohn, Norw.; Kenfarma, Spain; Pharmacia Upjohn, Swed.; Pharmacia Upjohn, Switz.; Farmitalia Carlo Erba, UK; Pharmacia Upjohn, USA.
Cabergoline (p.1135·2).
Hyperprolactinaemia; lactation inhibition; prolactinomas.

Dotarem
Codali, Belg.; Guerbet, Fr.; Farmades, Ital.; Guerbet, Neth.; Gothia, Swed.; Guerbet, Switz.
Meglumine gadoterate (p.1005·1).
Contrast medium for magnetic resonance imaging.

Dothep Alphapharm, Austral.
Dothiepin hydrochloride (p.283·1).
Depression.

Dotur Sanabo, Aust.
Doxycycline hydrochloride (p.202·3).
Bacterial infections; protozoal infections.

Double Check Family Planning Sales, UK.
Nonoxinol 9 (p.1326·1).
Contraceptive.

Double-Action Toothache Kit Dent, USA.
Liquid, benzocaine (p.1286·2); tablets, paracetamol (p.72·2) (Maranox).

Doudol Monot, Fr.†.
Emetine hydrochloride (p.582·2); ethylmorphine hydrochloride (p.36·1); ammonium chloride (p.1055·2).
Respiratory-tract disorders.

Doulax
Note. This name is used for preparations of different composition.
Bio-Sante, Canad.
Cascara (p.1183·1); senna (p.1212·2).

Bio-Sante, Canad.
Cascara (p.1183·1); phenolphthalein (p.1208·2).

Doval Pharmaceutical Enterprises, S.Afr.
Diazepam (p.661·1).
Alcohol withdrawal syndrome; anxiety; depression; premedication.

Dovate Lennon, S.Afr.
Clobetasol propionate (p.1035·2).
Skin disorders.

Doven Eurofarmaco, Ital.
Diosmin (p.1580·1).
Vascular disorders.

Dovida Tedec Meiji, Spain†.
Dimetofrine hydrochloride (p.857·1).
Circulatory disorders; hypotension.

Dovonex
Leo, Canad.; Leo, Irl.; Adcock Ingram, S.Afr.; Leo, UK; Westwood-Squibb, USA.
Calcipotriol (p.1080·2).
Psoriasis.

Doxakne Hexal, Ger.
Doxycycline (p.202·3).
Acne.

Doxam TAD, Ger.
Doxycycline hydrochloride (p.202·3); ambroxol hydrochloride (p.1054·3).
Respiratory-tract infections.

Doxans Schiapparelli Searle, Ital.†.
Doxefazepam.
Insomnia.

Doxapril Carlo Erba, Ital.†.
Doxapram hydrochloride (p.1480·1).
Respiratory depression.

Doxate-C Richmond, Canad.
Docusate calcium (p.1189·3).
Constipation.

Doxate-S Richmond, Canad.
Docusate sodium (p.1189·3).
Constipation.

Doxergan
Rhone-Poulenc Rorer, Belg.; Rhone-Poulenc Rorer, Neth.†.
Oxomemazine (p.415·2).
Coughs; gastritis; hypersensitivity reactions; insomnia.

Doxi Crisol Quimifar, Spain.
Doxycycline hydrochloride (p.202·3).
Bacterial infections.

Doxi Sergo Inexfa, Spain.
Doxycycline hydrochloride (p.202·3).
Bacterial infections.

Doxicento Recordati, Ital.†.
Doxycycline hydrochloride (p.202·3).
Bacterial infections.

Doxiclat Inkeysa, Spain.
Doxycycline hydrochloride (p.202·3).
Bacterial infections.

Doxidan
Hoechst Marion Roussel, Canad.; Upjohn, USA.
Docusate calcium (p.1189·3); phenolphthalein (p.1208·2).
Constipation.

Doxifin IFI, Ital.†.
Doxycycline hydrochloride (p.202·3).
Bacterial infections.

Doxil Sequus, USA.
Doxorubicin hydrochloride (p.529·2).
AIDS-related Kaposi's sarcoma.

Doxilen Lenza, Ital.†.
Doxycycline hydrochloride (p.202·3).
Bacterial infections.

Doximucol Sanorania, Ger.
Doxycycline hydrochloride (p.202·3); ambroxol hydrochloride (p.1054·3).
Bacterial infections of the respiratory tract associated with increased or viscous mucus.

Doxina IPFI, Ital.
Doxycycline hydrochloride (p.202·3).
Bacterial infections.

Doxinate Torlan, Spain.
Doxycycline hydrochloride (p.202·3).
Bacterial infections.

Doxiproct
Ebewe, Aust.†; Delalande, Ital.†; OM, Switz.
Calcium dobesilate (p.1556·3); lignocaine hydrochloride (p.1293·2).
Anorectal disorders.

Doxiproct mit Dexamethason Ebewe, Aust.†.
Calcium dobesilate (p.1556·3); lignocaine hydrochloride (p.1293·2); dexamethasone acetate (p.1037·1).
Anorectal disorders.

Doxiproct Plus *Synthelabo, Ital.; OM, Switz.*
Calcium dobesilate (p.1556·3); lignocaine hydrochloride (p.1293·2); dexamethasone acetate (p.1037·1).
Anorectal disorders.

Doxised *Corvi, Ital.†.*
Doxylamine succinate (p.410·1).
Hypersensitivity reactions.

Doxitab Cold Tablets *Nelson, Austral.†.*
Pseudoephedrine hydrochloride (p.1068·3); phenylpropanolamine hydrochloride (p.1067·2); paracetamol (p.72·2); chlorpheniramine maleate (p.405·1).
Cold symptoms.

Doxiten *Zyma, Spain.*
Doxycycline hydrochloride (p.202·3).
Bacterial infections.

Doxiten Bio *Zyma, Spain.*
Doxycycline hydrochloride (p.202·3).
Bacterial infections.

Doxiten Enzimatico *Zyma, Spain.*
Doxycycline hydrochloride (p.202·3); chymotrypsin (p.1563·2); trypsin (p.1640·1).
Bacterial infections.

Doxium
Ebewe, Aust.; Synthelabo, Belg.; Synthelabo, Fr.; Synthelabo, Ital.; Esteve, Spain; OM, Switz.
Calcium dobesilate (p.1556·3).
Chronic venous insufficiency; microcirculatory disorders.

Doxivenil
Delalande, Ital.†; OM, Switz.
Calcium dobesilate (p.1556·3); dextran sulphate potassium (p.1571·1).
Peripheral vascular disorders.

Doxivis *Vis, Ital.†.*
Doxycycline hydrochloride (p.202·3).
Bacterial infections.

DOXO-cell *Cell Pharm, Ger.*
Doxorubicin hydrochloride (p.529·2).
Malignant neoplasms.

Doxsig *Sigma, Austral.*
Doxycycline hydrochloride (p.202·3).
Amoebiasis; bacterial infections.

Doxy
Douglas, Austral.; Elerte, Fr.; Engelhard, Ger.; CT, Ger.; BASF, Ger.; Eu Rho, Ger.; Edwards, USA.
Doxycycline (p.202·3) or doxycycline hydrochloride (p.202·3).
Amoebiasis; bacterial infections; malaria.

Doxy Comp *CT, Ger.*
Doxycycline hydrochloride (p.202·3); ambroxol hydrochloride (p.1054·3).
Respiratory-tract infections.

Doxy Komb *Engelhard, Ger.*
Doxycycline hydrochloride (p.202·3).
Bacterial infections.

Doxy Lindoxyl *Lindopharm, Ger.*
Doxycycline hydrochloride (p.202·3); ambroxol hydrochloride (p.1054·3).
Bacterial infections of the respiratory-tract associated with increased or viscous mucus.

Doxy M *CT, Ger.; Ratiopharm, Ger.*
Doxycycline (p.202·3).
Bacterial infections.

Doxy Plus *Stada, Ger.*
Doxycycline hydrochloride (p.202·3); ambroxol hydrochloride (p.1054·3).
Respiratory-tract infections.

Doxy Pohl *Pohl, Ger.†.*
Doxycycline (p.202·3).
Bacterial infections.

Doxy S+K *S & K, Ger.*
Doxycycline hydrochloride (p.202·3).
Bacterial infections.

Doxy-basan
Sagitta, Ger.†; Schonenberger, Switz.
Doxycycline hydrochloride (p.202·3).
Bacterial infections.

Doxybene *Merckle, Aust.*
Doxycycline (p.202·3) or doxycycline hydrochloride (p.202·3).
Bacterial infections; protozoal infections.

Doxybiocin *Nycomed, Ger.†.*
Doxycycline hydrochloride (p.202·3).
Bacterial infections.

Doxychel *Rachelle, USA.*
Doxycycline hydrochloride (p.202·3).
Bacterial infections.

Doxycin *Riva, Canad.*
Doxycycline hydrochloride (p.202·3).
Bacterial infections.

Doxyclin *Pharmador, S.Afr.†.*
Doxycycline hydrochloride (p.202·3).
Bacterial infections.

Doxycline *Spirig, Switz.*
Doxycycline hydrochloride (p.202·3).
Bacterial infections.

Doxycyl *Lennon, S.Afr.*
Doxycycline hydrochloride (p.202·3).
Bacterial infections.

Doxy-Dagra *Asta Medica, Neth.*
Doxycycline fosfatex (p.202·3).
Bacterial infections.

Doxyderm *Klinge, Aust.*
Doxycycline hydrochloride (p.202·3).
Acne.

Doxyderma *Dermapharm, Ger.*
Doxycycline (p.202·3).
Bacterial infections.

Doxy-Diolan *Engelhard, Ger.*
Doxycycline hydrochloride (p.202·3).
Bacterial infections.

Doxy-duramucal *Durachemie, Ger.*
Doxycycline hydrochloride (p.202·3); ambroxol hydrochloride (p.1054·3).
Bacterial infections of the respiratory-tract associated with increased or viscous mucus.

Doxydyn *Klinge, Aust.*
Doxycycline hydrochloride (p.202·3).
Bacterial infections.

Doxyfene *Covan, S.Afr.*
Dextropropoxyphene hydrochloride (p.27·3); paracetamol (p.72·2).
Fever; pain.

Doxyferm *Nordic, Swed.*
Doxycycline (p.202·3) or doxycycline hydrochloride (p.202·3).
Bacterial infections.

Doxyfim *Wolfs, Belg.*
Doxycycline hydrochloride (p.202·3).
Bacterial infections.

Doxygram *Pharma 2000, Fr.*
Doxycycline hydrochloride (p.202·3).
Bacterial infections.

Doxyhexal *Hexal, Ger.*
Doxycycline (p.202·3) or doxycycline hydrochloride (p.202·3).
Bacterial infections.

Doxy-HP *Hefa, Ger.*
Doxycycline (p.202·3).
Bacterial infections.

Doxylag *Lagap, Switz.†.*
Doxycycline hydrochloride (p.202·3).
Bacterial infections.

Doxylan *Lannacher, Aust.*
Doxycycline (p.202·3) or doxycycline hydrochloride (p.202·3).
Bacterial infections.

Doxylar *Lagap, UK.*
Doxycycline hydrochloride (p.202·3).
Bacterial infections.

Doxylets
SMB, Belg.; Galephar, Fr.; Brovar, S.Afr.†.
Doxycycline hydrochloride (p.202·3).
Bacterial infections.

Doxylin
Alphapharm, Austral.; Alpharma, Norw.
Doxycycline (p.202·3) or doxycycline hydrochloride (p.202·3).
Amoebiasis; bacterial infections; trachoma.

Doxymono *Betapharm, Ger.*
Doxycycline (p.202·3).
Bacterial infections.

Doxymycin
Rhone-Poulenc Rorer, Neth.†; SA Druggists, S.Afr.†.
Doxycycline (p.202·3) or doxycycline hydrochloride (p.202·3).
Bacterial infections.

Doxymycine *Rhone-Poulenc Rorer, Belg.†.*
Doxycycline hydrochloride (p.202·3).
Bacterial infections.

Doxy-N-Tablinen *Sanorania, Ger.*
Doxycycline (p.202·3).
Bacterial infections.

Doxy-P *Ratiopharm, Ger.*
Doxycycline hydrochloride (p.202·3).
Bacterial infections.

Doxypol *Beige, S.Afr.†.*
Dextropropoxyphene hydrochloride (p.27·3); paracetamol (p.72·2); caffeine (p.749·3).
Pain.

Doxy-Puren *Isis Puren, Ger.*
Doxycycline hydrochloride (p.202·3).
Bacterial infections.

Doxyremed *Lichtenstein, Ger.†.*
Doxycycline (p.202·3) or doxycycline hydrochloride (p.202·3).
Bacterial infections.

Doxysol *Ecosol, Switz.*
Doxycycline (p.202·3).
Bacterial infections.

Doxysolvat *Betapharm, Ger.*
Doxycycline hydrochloride (p.202·3); ambroxol hydrochloride (p.1054·3).
Respiratory-tract infections.

Doxysom *Quantum, USA†.*
Doxylamine succinate (p.410·1).

Doxytab *Farmabel, Belg.†.*
Doxycycline (p.202·3) or doxycycline hydrochloride (p.202·3).
Bacterial infections.

Doxy-Tablinen *Sanorania, Ger.*
Doxycycline hydrochloride (p.202·3).
Bacterial infections.

Doxy-Tabs *Barr, USA†.*
Doxycycline (p.202·3).

Doxytec *Technilab, Canad.*
Doxycycline hydrochloride (p.202·3).
Bacterial infections.

Doxytem *Temmler, Ger.*
Doxycycline hydrochloride (p.202·3).
Bacterial infections.

Doxy-Wolff *Wolff, Ger.*
Doxycycline (p.202·3) or doxycycline hydrochloride (p.202·3).
Bacterial infections.

Doxy-Wolff Mucolyt *Wolff, Ger.*
Doxycycline hydrochloride (p.202·3); ambroxol hydrochloride (p.1054·3).
Respiratory-tract infections associated with increased or viscous mucus.

Doyle *Tanabe, Jpn.*
Aspoxicillin (p.155·1).
Bacterial infections.

Dozic *Rosemont, UK.*
Haloperidol (p.673·3).
Anxiety; intractable hiccup; motor tics; nausea and vomiting; psychoses.

Dozile *Sunspot, Austral.*
Doxylamine succinate (p.410·1).
Insomnia.

Dozol *Rice Steele, Irl.*
Paracetamol (p.72·2); diphenhydramine hydrochloride (p.409·1).
Fever; pain.

dp *Scientific Hospital Supplies, UK.*
Low-protein food for special diets.

DPCA
Grifols, Spain†; Fresenius, Switz.
Electrolytes; glucose (p.1151·1).
Peritoneal dialysis.

DPCA 2 *Fresenius, Fr.*
Sodium chloride; sodium lactate; calcium chloride; magnesium chloride; glucose monohydrate (p.1151·1).
Peritoneal dialysis.

D-Penamine *Disto, Austral.*
Penicillamine (p.988·3).
Cystinuria; heavy-metal poisoning; rheumatoid arthritis; Wilson's disease.

DPH
Note. This name is used for preparations of different composition.
Propan, S.Afr.
Diphenhydramine hydrochloride (p.409·1); ammonium chloride (p.1055·2); sodium citrate (p.1153·2).
Coughs.

Alra, USA†.
Diphenhydramine hydrochloride (p.409·1).

DPN *Alclin, S.Afr.*
Nadide (p.1606·1).
Alcoholism; drug addiction.

D-Pronto-Disinfettante Analcolico *Eurochimica, Ital.†.*
Benzalkonium chloride (p.1101·3).
Skin and wound disinfection.

DPT Merieux *Pasteur Merieux, Ger.*
An adsorbed diphtheria, tetanus, and pertussis vaccine (p.1509·1).
Active immunisation of infants and young children.

DPT-Impfstoff *Chiron Behring, Ger.*
An adsorbed diphtheria, tetanus, and pertussis vaccine (p.1509·1).
Active immunisation of infants and young children.

DPT-Vaccinol *Procter & Gamble, Ger.*
An adsorbed diphtheria, tetanus, and pertussis vaccine (p.1509·1).
Active immunisation of infants and young children.

Dr. Boether Bronchial Tropfen *Medopharm, Ger.†.*
Thyme (p.1636·3).
Bronchitis; catarrh; coughs.

Dr. Boether Bronchitten forte N *Medopharm, Ger.†.*
Proxyphylline (p.757·3); ephedrine hydrochloride (p.1059·3); thyme (p.1636·3); primula root.
Acute attacks of asthma, bronchitis, and coughing spasm.

Dr. Boether Bronchitten S *Medopharm, Ger.†.*
Polygonum; equisetum (p.1575·1); plantago lanceolata; thyme (p.1636·3).
Coughs and associated respiratory-tract disorders.

Dr Caldwell Senna Laxative *Gebauer, USA.*
Senna (p.1212·2).
Constipation.

Dr Dermi-Heal *Quality Formulations, USA.*
Allantoin (p.1078·2); zinc oxide (p.1096·2); peru balsam (p.1617·2); castor oil (p.1560·2).
Skin disorders.

Dr Ernst Richter's Abfuhrtee *Salus, Aust.*
Senna (p.1212·2); frangula bark (p.1193·2).
Constipation.

Dr Ernst Richter's Abfuhrtee-tassen-fertig *Salus, Aust.*
Senna (p.1212·2); frangula bark (p.1193·2); peppermint oil (p.1208·1); liquorice (p.1197·1).
Constipation.

Dr Fischers Melissengeist *Pharmonta, Aust.*
Nutmeg oil (p.1609·3); clove oil (p.1565·2); cinnamon oil (p.1564·2); citronella oil (p.1565·1).
Gastro-intestinal disorders; musculoskeletal and joint disorders; nervous disorders.

Dr Fischer's Minzol *Pharmonta, Aust.*
Menthae arvensis oil (p.1208·1).
Gastro-intestinal disorders; headache; musculoskeletal and joint disorders; respiratory-tract disorders.

Dr. Grandel Brennessel Vital Tonikum *Grandel-Synpharma, Ger.†.*
Urtica (p.1642·3).
Tonic.

Dr. Grandel Granobil *Grandel-Synpharma, Ger.*
Usnea barbata (p.1643·1).
Bacterial infections of the oropharynx.

Dr. Grandel Weizenkeim-Vollextract-Kapseln *Grandel-Synpharma, Ger.†.*
Germinum tritici; vitamins; wheat-germ oil.
Tonic.

Dr. Hotz Vollbad *Hotz, Ger.*
Whey; sorbitol (p.1354·2); lactic acid (p.1593·3); alum (p.1547·1); gentian (p.1583·3); achillea (p.1542·2); crataegus (p.1568·2); olive oil (p.1610·1); arachis oil (p.1550·2); sage oil; rosemary oil (p.1626·2); chamomile oil; alpha tocopheryl acetate (p.1369·1).
Bath additive; skin disorders.

Dr. Janssens Teebohnen *Dr Janssen, Ger.*
Aloes (p.1177·1).
Constipation.

Dr. Kleinschrod's Cor-Insuffin *Dronania, Ger.†.*
Crataegus (p.1568·2); convallaria (p.1567·2); cereus grandiflorus; kalmia latifolia; scoparium (p.1628·1); mistletoe (p.1604·1); valerian (p.1643·1); potentilla anserina; achillea (p.1542·2); arnica (p.1550·3); levisticum officinale (p.1597·2); peppermint leaf (p.1208·1); melissa (p.1600·1); rosemary; rue.
Cardiovascular disorders.

Dr. Kleinschrod's Spasmi Tropfen *Dronania, Ger.†.*
Potentilla anserina; artemisia; valerian (p.1643·1); cardamine pratensis; melissa (p.1600·1); chamomile (p.1561·2); fennel (p.1579·1); dictamus albus; achillea (p.1542·2); gomphocarpus fructicosus; paeonia officinalis; caraway (p.1559·3).
Smooth muscle spasms.

Dr. Klinger's Bergischer Krautertee, Abfuhr- und Verdauungstee *Mack, Illert., Ger.†.*
Senna (p.1212·2); frangula bark (p.1193·2); prunus spinosa; juglans regia; phaseolus vulgaris; urtica (p.1642·3); fennel (p.1579·1); ononis (p.1610·2); sarsaparilla (p.1627·2).
Constipation.

Dr. Klinger's Bergischer Krautertee, Blasen- u. Nierentee *Mack, Illert., Ger.†.*
Orthosiphon (p.1592·2); equisetum (p.1575·1); betula leaf; ononis (p.1610·2); calendula officinalis; fennel oil (p.1579·2).
Urinary-tract disorders.

Dr. Klinger's Bergischer Krautertee, Blutreinigungs- und Stoffwechselkrautertee *Mack, Illert., Ger.†.*
Taraxacum; achillea; juniper; urtica; couch-grass; fennel; betula leaf.
Herbal preparation.

Dr. Klinger's Bergischer Krautertee, Herz- und Kreislauftee *Mack, Illert., Ger.†.*
Crataegus (p.1568·2); motherwort (p.1604·2); melissa (p.1600·1); angelica; achillea (p.1542·2); potentilla anserina; solidago virgaurea.
Heart and nerve tonic.

Dr. Klinger's Bergischer Krautertee, Husten- u. Bronchial-tee *Mack, Illert., Ger.†.*
Mallow flower; verbascum flowers; coltsfoot leaf (p.1057·2); thyme (p.1636·3); pulmonaria; lichen islandicus; liquorice (p.1197·1); tilia (p.1637·3); althaea (p.1546·3); primula root; ascorbic acid (p.1365·2).
Colds; coughs.

Dr. Klinger's Bergischer Krautertee, Leber- und Gallentee *Mack, Illert., Ger.†.*
Taraxacum (p.1634·2); curcuma zanthorrhiza; rhubarb (p.1212·1); frangula bark (p.1193·2); chamomile (p.1561·2); calendula officinalis; boldo (p.1554·1); absinthium (p.1541·1); capsella bursa pastoris; liquorice (p.1197·1).
Liver disorders.

Dr. Klinger's Bergischer Krautertee, Magentee *Mack, Illert., Ger.†.*
Condurango (p.1567·2); arnica (p.1550·3); gentian (p.1583·3); angelica; liquorice (p.1197·1); fennel (p.1579·1); chamomile (p.1561·2).
Gastro-intestinal disorders.

Dr. Klinger's Bergischer Krautertee, Nerven- und Beruhigungstee *Mack, Illert., Ger.†.*
Peppermint leaf (p.1208·1); melissa (p.1600·1); liquorice (p.1197·1); fennel (p.1579·1); aniseed (p.1549·3); lupulus (p.1597·2); lavender (p.1594·3); flor. aurantii.
Nervousness; sleep disorders.

Dr. Maurers Magen-Apotheke *Herzpunkt, Ger.†.*
Cinchona bark (p.1564·1); dried bitter-orange peel (p.1610·3); cardamom (p.1560·1); aniseed (p.1549·3); clove (p.1565·2); sandalwood; cinnamon (p.1564·2); galanga; ginger (p.1193·2); harongarinde; pepsin (p.1616·3); liquorice (p.1197·1); silybum marianum (p.993·3); cynara (p.1569·2); chamomile (p.1561·2); sorbitol.
Gastro-intestinal disorders.

Dr Schmidgall Halsweh *Schmidgall, Aust.†.*
dl-Alpha tocopheryl acetate (p.1369·2); benzalkonium chloride (p.1101·3).
Mouth and throat inflammation.

Dr Scholl's Athlete's Foot *Schering-Plough, USA.*
Tolnaftate (p.389·1).
Tinea pedis.

Dr Scholl's Callus Removers *Schering-Plough, USA.*
Salicylic acid (p.1090·2).

Dr Scholl's Clear Away *Schering-Plough, USA.*
Salicylic acid (p.1090·2).
Hyperkeratosis.

Dr Scholl's Corn Removers *Schering-Plough, USA.*
Salicylic acid (p.1090·2).

Dr Scholl's Corn/Callus Remover *Schering-Plough, USA.*
Salicylic acid (p.1090·2).
Hyperkeratosis.

Dr Scholl's Cracked Heel Relief *Schering-Plough, USA.*
Lignocaine (p.1293·2).

Dr Scholl's Smooth Touch Deep Moisturizing Cream *Scholl, USA†.*
Urea (p.1095·2).
Dry skin.

Dr Scholl's Super Deodorant Foot Powder *Scholl, USA†.*
Aluminium chlorohydrate (p.1078·3).
Bromhidrosis.

Dr Scholl's Tritin Antifungal Powder *Scholl, USA.*
Tolnaftate (p.389·1).
Tinea pedis.

Dr Scholl's Wart Remover *Schering-Plough, USA.*
Salicylic acid (p.1090·2).

Dracodermalin
Richter, Aust.; Atzinger, Ger.†.
Camphor (p.1557·2); rosemary oil (p.1626·2); turpentine oil (p.1641·1).
Coughs and colds; soft tissue and muscle disorders.

Draganon *Roche, Ital.*
Aniracetam (p.1549·3).
Mental function disorders.

Dragees 19 *Berlin-Chemie, Ger.†.*
Phenolphthalein (p.1208·2); rhubarb (p.1212·1).
A preparation of the same name manufactured by Much, *Ger.* formerly contained aloes, cascara, frangula bark, and bile extract.
Constipation.

Dragees antirhumatismales fortes *Zeller, Switz.*
Salix (p.82·3); passion flower (p.1615·3).
Musculoskeletal and joint disorders.

Dragees aux figues avec du sene *Zeller, Switz.*
Fig (p.1193·2); senna (p.1212·2); petasites officinalis.
Constipation.

Dragees contre la toux no 536 *Renapharm, Switz.*
Butethamate citrate (p.1056·2); codeine phosphate (p.26·1); thyme (p.1636·3).
Coughs.

Dragees contre les maux de tete *Zeller, Switz.*
Salix (p.82·3); kola (p.1645·1).
Headache.

Dragees contre les maux de voyage no 537 *Renapharm, Switz.*
Dimenhydrinate (p.408·2); caffeine (p.749·3).
Motion sickness.

Dragees Fuca *Fuca, Fr.*
Frangula bark (p.1193·2); cascara (p.1183·1); bladderwrack (p.1554·1).
Constipation.

Dragees laxatives no 510 *Renapharm, Switz.*
Aloes (p.1177·1); belladonna (p.457·1); rhubarb (p.1212·1).
Constipation.

Dragees Neunzehn *Salus, Aust.*
Aloes (p.1177·1); frangula (p.1193·2); cascara (p.1183·1); fel suis (p.1553·2).
Constipation.

Dragees Neunzehn Senna *Salus, Aust.*
Senna (p.1212·2).
Constipation.

Dragees pour la detente nerveuse *Zeller, Switz.*
Petasites officinalis; valerian (p.1643·1); passion flower (p.1615·3); melissa (p.1600·1).
Nervous disorders.

Dragees pour le coeur et les nerfs *Zeller, Switz.*
Crataegus (p.1568·2); passion flower (p.1615·3); lupulus (p.1597·2); valerian (p.1643·1).
Nervous disorders.

Dragees pour le sommeil nouvelle formule *Zeller, Switz.*
Valerian (p.1643·1); lupulus (p.1597·2).
Sleep disorders.

Dragees pour reins et vessie S *Synpharma, Switz.*
Orthosiphon (p.1592·2); solidago virgaurea; ononis (p.1610·2); bearberry (p.1552·2); boldo (p.1554·1).
Urinary-tract disorders.

Dragees relaxantes et tranquillisantes *Piraud, Switz.†.*
Valerian (p.1643·1); lupulus (p.1597·2); bois ivrant; passion flower (p.1615·3).
Agitation; sleep disorders; tension.

Dragees Vegetales Rex *Lehning, Fr.*
Frangula bark (p.1193·2); cascara (p.1183·1).
Formerly contained euonymine, bladderwrack, agar, belladonna, bile, cascara, hyoscyamus, star anise, frangula, and aloes.
Constipation.

Dragon Balm *Gerard House, UK.*
Camphor (p.1557·2); menthol (p.1600·2); turpentine oil (p.1641·1); nutmeg oil (p.1609·3); eucalyptus oil (p.1578·1); cassia oil (p.1560·2); pine oil; thymol (p.1127·1); guaiacol (p.1061·2); peru balsam (p.1617·2).
Muscular aches.

Dragosil *Daker Farmasimes, Spain.*
Creatinolfosfate (p.1568·3) or creatinolfosfate sodium (p.1568·3).
Cardiac disorders.

Drainactil *IPRAD, Fr.*
Boldo (p.1554·1); birch leaf (p.1553·3); black currant leaf (p.1365·2).
Gastro-intestinal disorders; kidney disorders.

Dralinsa *Duopharm, Ger.*
Linseed (p.1596·2); senna leaf (p.1212·2).
Constipation.

Dramamine
Searle, Austral.; Searle, Belg.; Monsanto, Fr.; Searle, Irl.; Searle, Neth.; Searle, S.Afr.†; Searle, Switz.; Searle, UK; Upjohn, USA.
Dimenhydrinate (p.408·2).
Motion sickness; nausea and vomiting; vestibular disorders.

Dramamine Cafeina *Searle, Spain†.*
Dimenhydrinate (p.408·2); caffeine (p.749·3).
Motion sickness.

Dramamine II *Upjohn, USA.*
Meclozine hydrochloride (p.413·3).
Motion sickness.

Dramamine-compositum *Searle, Switz.*
Dimenhydrinate (p.408·2); caffeine (p.749·3).
Motion sickness.

Dramanate *Pasadena, USA.*
Dimenhydrinate (p.408·2).
Motion sickness.

Dramigel *Drug Research, Ital.*
Amikacin sulphate (p.150·2).
Gram-negative bacterial infections.

Dramilin *Kay, USA.*
Dimenhydrinate (p.408·2).
Motion sickness.

Dramine *Uriach, Spain.*
Meclozine hydrochloride (p.413·3).
Motion sickness.

Dramoject *Mayrand, USA†.*
Dimenhydrinate (p.408·2).
Motion sickness.

Drapolene
Wellcome, Irl.; Warner-Lambert, UK.
Benzalkonium chloride (p.1101·3); cetrimide (p.1105·2).
Minor burns and wounds; napkin rash.

Drapolex *Wellcome, Austral.†.*
Benzalkonium chloride (p.1101·3); cetrimide (p.1105·2).
Antiseptic barrier cream.

Dravyr *Drug Research, Ital.*
Aciclovir (p.602·3).
Herpesvirus infections.

Drazin *Wellcome, Spain†.*
Paracetamol (p.72·2).
Fever; pain.

Drazoic *Lambda, USA.*
Benzoic acid (p.1102·3).
Fungal infections.

Dreamtrim *Cantassium Co., UK†.*
Amino-acid, vitamin, and mineral preparation.

Dregan *drepharm, Ger.†.*
Activated charcoal (p.972·2).
Diarrhoea; gastro-enteritis.

Dreimal *Rhone-Poulenc, Ital.†.*
Aspirin (p.16·1).
Cold and flu symptoms; pain.

Dreisacal *Gry, Ger.†.*
Calcium gluconate (p.1155·2).
Calcium deficiency.

Dreisacarb *Gry, Ger.*
Calcium carbonate (p.1182·1).
Hyperphosphataemia.

Dreisafer *Gry, Ger.*
Ferrous sulphate (p.1340·2).
Iron-deficiency.

Dreisalan *Gry, Ger.†.*
Ichthammol (p.1083·3); zinc oxide (p.1096·2).
Wounds.

Dreisalind *Gry, Ger.†.*
Inosine (p.1591·1); dexpanthenol (p.1570·3).
Skin disorders.

Dreisavit *Brady, Aust.*
Multivitamin preparation.

Dreisavit N
Gry, Ger.; Bichsel, Switz.
Multivitamin preparation.
Dietary supplement; renal failure.

Dremisan *drepharm, Ger.†.*
Simethicone (p.1213·1).
Defoaming agent in gastro-intestinal radiography or endoscopy; disorders associated with excessive intestinal gas.

Drenian *Ern, Spain.*
Diazepam (p.661·1).
Alcohol withdrawal syndrome; anxiety; epilepsy; insomnia; premedication; skeletal muscle spasm; status epilepticus.

Drenison
Lilly, Canad.; Lilly, Ital.†; Derly, Spain.
Flurandrenolone (p.1042·2).
Skin disorders.

Drenison con Neomicina *Lilly, Ital.†.*
Flurandrenolone (p.1042·2); neomycin sulphate (p.229·2).
Skin disorders.

Drenison Neomicina *Derly, Spain.*
Flurandrenolone (p.1042·2); neomycin sulphate (p.229·2).
Infected skin disorders.

Drenusil *Pfizer, Ger.†.*
Polythiazide (p.932·1).
Hypertension; oedema.

Drenusil-R *Pfizer, Ger.†.*
Polythiazide (p.932·1); reserpine (p.942·1).
Hypertension.

Driclor
Stiefel, Austral.; Stiefel, Fr.; Stiefel, UK.
Aluminium chloride (p.1078·3).
Hyperhidrosis.

Dridase
Pharmacia Upjohn, Ger.; Byk, Neth.
Oxybutynin hydrochloride (p.466·1).
Bladder disorders.

Dridol
Janssen-Cilag, Norw.; Janssen-Cilag, Swed.
Droperidol (p.668·2).
Nausea; neuroleptanalgesia; premedication; vomiting.

Dri/Ear *Pfeiffer, USA.*
Boric acid (p.1554·2); isopropyl alcohol (p.1118·2).
Ear disorders.

Drilix *Be-Tabs, S.Afr.*
Pseudoephedrine hydrochloride (p.1068·3).
Upper respiratory-tract congestion.

Drill
Note. This name is used for preparations of different composition.
Pierre Fabre, Fr.
Chlorhexidine gluconate (p.1107·2); amethocaine hydrochloride (p.1285·2).
Sore throat.

Pierre Fabre, Spain.
Chlorhexidine gluconate (p.1107·2); benzocaine (p.1286·2).
Mouth and throat infections.

Drill Expectorant *Pierre Fabre Sante, Fr.*
Carbocisteine (p.1056·3).
Respiratory-tract congestion.

Drill rhinites *Pierre Fabre Sante, Fr.*
Pseudoephedrine hydrochloride (p.1068·3).
Nasal congestion.

Drill toux seche *Pierre Fabre Sante, Fr.*
Dextromethorphan hydrobromide (p.1057·3).
Coughs.

Drin *Schiapparelli, Ital.*
Aspirin (p.16·1); paracetamol (p.72·2); caffeine (p.749·3).
Fever; pain.

Driol *Bournonville, Belg.*
Osalmid (p.1611·2).
Biliary disorders.

Driptane
Fournier, Belg.; Debat, Fr.
Oxybutynin hydrochloride (p.466·1).
Enuresis; neurogenic bladder.

Drisdol
Sanofi Winthrop, Canad.; Sanofi Winthrop, USA.
Ergocalciferol (p.1367·1).
Familial hypophosphataemia; hypoparathyroidism; rickets.

Drisi-gast *Serturner, Ger.†.*
Liquorice (p.1197·1); bismuth subnitrate (p.1180·2).
Gastritis; peptic ulcer.

Drisi-Ven *Serturner, Ger.*
Troxerutin (p.1580·2).
Vascular disorders.

Dristan
Note. This name is used for preparations of different composition.
Whitehall-Robins, Canad.
Caplets; tablets: Paracetamol (p.72·2); phenylephrine hydrochloride (p.1066·2); chlorpheniramine maleate (p.405·1).
Cold symptoms.
Capsules: Phenylpropanolamine hydrochloride (p.1067·2); chlorpheniramine maleate (p.405·1); aspirin (p.16·1); caffeine (p.749·3).
Cold symptoms; fever; headache; pain; upper respiratory-tract disorders.
Long-acting nasal spray: Oxymetazoline hydrochloride (p.1065·3).
Nasal congestion.
Nasal spray: Phenylephrine hydrochloride (p.1066·2); pheniramine maleate (p.415·3).
Nasal congestion.
Sustained release capsules†: Chlorpheniramine maleate (p.405·1); phenylpropanolamine hydrochloride (p.1067·2).
Cold symptoms; upper respiratory-tract congestion.

Whitehall, Irl.; Whitehall, UK.
Nasal spray: Oxymetazoline hydrochloride (p.1065·3).
Nasal congestion.
Tablets: Aspirin (p.16·1); caffeine (p.749·3); phenylephrine hydrochloride (p.1066·2); chlorpheniramine maleate (p.405·1).
Cold symptoms.

Dristan Allergy *Whitehall, USA.*
Pseudoephedrine hydrochloride (p.1068·3); brompheniramine maleate (p.403·2).
Hypersensitivity reactions.

Dristan Cold *Whitehall, USA.*
Chlorpheniramine maleate (p.405·1); phenylephrine hydrochloride (p.1066·2); paracetamol (p.72·2).
Formerly known as Advanced Formula Dristan.
Cold symptoms.

Dristan Cold Caplets *Whitehall, USA.*
Pseudoephedrine hydrochloride (p.1068·3); paracetamol (p.72·2).
Upper respiratory-tract symptoms.

Dristan Cold & Flu *Whitehall, USA.*
Chlorpheniramine maleate (p.405·1); dextromethorphan hydrobromide (p.1057·3); paracetamol (p.72·2); pseudoephedrine hydrochloride (p.1068·3).
Coughs and cold symptoms.

Dristan Cold Maximum Strength Multi-symptom Formula *Whitehall, USA.*
Paracetamol (p.72·2); pseudoephedrine hydrochloride (p.1068·3); brompheniramine maleate (p.403·2).
Cold symptoms; hypersensitivity reactions.

Dristan Cold Maximum Strength No Drowsiness Formula *Whitehall, USA.*
Paracetamol (p.72·2); pseudoephedrine hydrochloride (p.1068·3).
Cold symptoms.

Dristan Cold Multi-Symptom Formula *Whitehall, USA.*
Phenylephrine hydrochloride (p.1066·2); paracetamol (p.72·2); chlorpheniramine maleate (p.405·1).
Upper respiratory-tract symptoms.

Dristan Formula P *Whitehall-Robins, Canad.†.*
Phenylephrine hydrochloride (p.1066·2); mepyramine maleate (p.414·1); aspirin (p.16·1); caffeine (p.749·3).
Cold symptoms; fever; headache; pain; upper respiratory-tract disorders.

Dristan 12-hr Nasal Decongestant Spray *Whitehall, USA.*
Oxymetazoline hydrochloride (p.1065·3).
Formerly known as Dristan Long Lasting.
Nasal congestion.

Dristan Juice Mix-in *Whitehall, USA.*
Paracetamol (p.72·2); pseudoephedrine hydrochloride (p.1068·3); dextromethorphan hydrobromide (p.1057·3).
Coughs and cold symptoms.

Dristan Long Lasting *Whitehall, USA.*
Oxymetazoline hydrochloride (p.1065·3).
Nasal congestion.

Dristan Nasal Spray *Whitehall, USA.*
Phenylephrine hydrochloride (p.1066·2); pheniramine maleate (p.415·3).
Nasal congestion.

Dristan Non Drowsy *Whitehall-Robins, Canad.*
Pseudoephedrine hydrochloride (p.1068·3); paracetamol (p.72·2).
Cold symptoms; fever; headache; pain; upper respiratory-tract disorders.

Dristan Saline Spray *Whitehall, USA.*
Sodium chloride (p.1162·2).
Inflammation and dryness of nasal membranes.

Dristan Sinus
Whitehall-Robins, Canad.; Whitehall, USA.
Ibuprofen (p.44·1); pseudoephedrine hydrochloride (p.1068·3).
Cold and influenza symptoms.

Drithocreme *Dermik, USA.*
Dithranol (p.1082·1).
Psoriasis.

Dritho-Scalp *Dermik, USA.*
Dithranol (p.1082·1).
Psoriasis.

Drix *Pharmacal, Switz.*
Bisacodyl (p.1179·3); frangula bark (p.1193·2); senna (p.1212·2); sodium sulphate (p.1213·3).
Constipation.

Drix Abfuhr-Dragees *Hermes, Ger.*
Senna leaf (p.1212·2).
Constipation.

Drix N *Hermes, Ger.*
Bisacodyl (p.1179·3).
Constipation.

Drix Richter's Krautertee *Hermes, Ger.†.*
Tea: Senna leaf (p.1212·2); frangula bark (p.1193·2); birch leaf; taraxacum (p.1634·2); viola tricoloris; crataegus (p.1568·2); blackberry leaf; coriander (p.1567·3); sunflower; larkspur flowers; delphinium consolida; centaurea cyanus.
Tea in filter-bag: Senna leaf (p.1212·2); frangula bark (p.1193·2); birch leaf; taraxacum (p.1634·2); viola tricolor; crataegus (p.1568·2); blackberry leaf; coriander (p.1567·3).
Tea powder: Senna leaf (p.1212·2); frangula bark (p.1193·2); birch leaf; crataegus (p.1568·2).
Constipation.

Drixine *Schering-Plough, S.Afr.*
Oxymetazoline hydrochloride (p.1065·3).
Nasal congestion.

Drixine Cough Expectorant *Schering-Plough, Austral.†.*
Dexchlorpheniramine maleate (p.405·1); phenylephrine hydrochloride (p.1066·2); ammonium chloride (p.1055·2); guaiphenesin (p.1061·3).
Coughs and cold symptoms.

Drixine Cough Suppressant *Schering-Plough, Austral.†.*
Dexchlorpheniramine maleate (p.405·1); dextromethorphan hydrobromide (p.1057·3); caffeine (p.749·3); sodium salicylate (p.85·1).
Coughs and cold symptoms.

Drixine Nasal *Schering-Plough, Austral.*
Oxymetazoline hydrochloride (p.1065·3).
Nasal congestion.

Drixomed *Iomed, USA.*
Dexbrompheniramine maleate (p.403·2); pseudoephedrine sulphate (p.1068·3).
Respiratory-tract disorders.

Drixora
Schering-Plough, Austral.†; Schering-Plough, S.Afr.
Pseudoephedrine sulphate (p.1068·3).
Aid for correcting habitual use of nasal vasoconstrictors; upper respiratory mucosal congestion.

Drixoral
Note. This name is used for preparations of different composition.
Schering, Canad.
Capsules: Dextromethorphan hydrobromide (p.1057·3).
Coughs.
Nasal spray: Oxymetazoline hydrochloride (p.1065·3).
Upper respiratory-tract congestion.
Sustained release capsules; sustained release tablets; syrup: Dexbrompheniramine maleate (p.403·2); pseudoephedrine sulphate (p.1068·3).
Upper respiratory-tract congestion.
Schering-Plough, USA.
Pseudoephedrine sulphate (p.1068·3); brompheniramine maleate (p.403·2).
Upper respiratory-tract symptoms.

Drixoral Cold & Allergy *Schering-Plough, USA.*
Pseudoephedrine sulphate (p.1068·3); dexbrompheniramine maleate (p.403·2).
Upper respiratory-tract symptoms.

Drixoral Cold & Flu *Schering-Plough, USA.*
Pseudoephedrine sulphate (p.1068·3); paracetamol (p.72·2); dexbrompheniramine maleate (p.403·2).
Upper respiratory-tract symptoms.

Drixoral Cough
Schering, Canad.; Schering-Plough, USA.
Dextromethorphan hydrobromide (p.1057·3).
Coughs.

Drixoral Cough & Congestion *Schering-Plough, USA.*
Pseudoephedrine hydrochloride (p.1068·3); dextromethorphan hydrobromide (p.1057·3).

Drixoral Cough & Sore Throat *Schering-Plough, USA.*
Dextromethorphan hydrobromide (p.1057·3); paracetamol (p.72·2).

Drixoral Day/Night *Schering, Canad.*
Yellow tablets, pseudoephedrine sulphate (p.1068·3); white tablets, dexbrompheniramine maleate (p.403·2); pseudoephedrine sulphate.
Ear disorders; upper respiratory-tract congestion.

Drixoral ND *Schering, Canad.*
Pseudoephedrine sulphate (p.1068·3).
Ear disorders; upper respiratory-tract congestion.

Drixoral Non-Drowsy Formula *Schering, USA.*
Pseudoephedrine sulphate (p.1068·3).
Nasal congestion.

Drixoral Plus *Schering-Plough, USA.*
Pseudoephedrine sulphate (p.1068·3); paracetamol (p.72·2); dexbrompheniramine maleate (p.403·2).
Formerly known as Drixoral Allergy Sinus.
Upper respiratory-tract symptoms.

Drixtab *Schering, Canad.*
Dexbrompheniramine maleate (p.403·2); pseudoephedrine sulphate (p.1068·3).
Upper respiratory-tract congestion.

Drize *Jones, USA.*
Chlorpheniramine maleate (p.405·1); phenylpropanolamine hydrochloride (p.1067·2).
Cold symptoms.

Droal *Vita, Spain.*
Ketorolac trometamol (p.49·1).
Pain.

Drocorcina *Bama, Spain†.*
Thyme (p.1636·3).
Immunotherapy.

Droctil *Ciba, Ital.†.*
Exiproben sodium (p.1578·3).
Hepato-biliary disorders.

Drofaron *Demopharm, Switz.*
Aluminium hydroxide (p.1177·3); magnesium trisilicate (p.1199·1); dimethicone (p.1213·1).
Flatulence; gastric hyperacidity; gastritis.

Drogelon *Farma Lepori, Spain†.*
Droxicam (p.35·2).
Musculoskeletal and joint disorders; peri-articular disorders.

Drogenil
Schering-Plough, Irl.; Essex, Ital.; Schering-Plough, Neth.; Schering-Plough, UK.
Flutamide (p.537·1).
Prostatic cancer.

Drogimed *Synpharma, Aust.*
Silver birch (p.1553·3); equisetum (p.1575·1).
Urinary-tract disorders.

Droleptan
Janssen-Cilag, Austral.; Janssen-Cilag, Fr.; Janssen-Cilag, Irl.; Janssen, UK.
Droperidol (p.668·2).
Adjunct in neuroleptanalgesia; nausea and vomiting; premedication; psychoses.

Dronal *Sigma-Tau, Ital.*
Alendronate sodium (p.733·2).
Postmenopausal osteoporosis.

Dropilton *Bruschettini, Ital.*
Pilocarpine hydrochloride (p.1396·3).
Glaucoma.

Dropstar *Farmigea, Ital.*
Sodium hyaluronate (p.1630·3).
Dry eyes.

Droptimol *Farmigea, Ital.*
Timolol maleate (p.953·3).
Glaucoma; ocular hypertension.

Dropyal *Bruschettini, Ital.*
Sodium hyaluronate (p.1630·3); carbomer 941 (p.1471·2); glycerol (p.1585·2).
Dry eyes.

Drosera Komplex *Richter, Aust.*
Homoeopathic preparation.

Droserapect-N *Weber & Weber, Ger.*
Homoeopathic preparation.

Drosetux
Dolisos, Canad.; Dolisos, Fr.
Homoeopathic preparation.

Drosinula N *Bioforce, Switz.*
Norway spruce buds; drosera (p.1574·1); hedera helix; pear.
Respiratory-tract disorders.

Drosithym-N *Ysatfabrik, Ger.*
Primula rhizome; thyme (p.1636·3); drosera (p.1574·1).
Catarrh; coughs.

Drossadin *Drossapharm, Switz.*
Hexetidine (p.1116·1).
Mouth and throat disorders.

Drossa-Nose *Drossapharm, Switz.†.*
Sea salt (p.1162·2).
Nasal dryness.

Drotic *Ascher, USA†.*
Hydrocortisone (p.1043·3); neomycin sulphate (p.229·2); polymyxin B (p.239·3).
Bacterial ear infections.

Drovitol *Synpharma, Aust.*
Myrrh (p.1606·1); clove (p.1565·2); tormentil (p.1638·3).
Mouth and throat disorders.

Droxar *Pharmacia Upjohn, Ital.†.*
Droxicam (p.35·2).
Rheumatic disorders.

Droxaryl
Salus, Aust.; Continental Pharma, Belg.; Sanofi Winthrop, Neth.†.
Bufexamac (p.22·2).
Skin disorders.

Droxicef *Alfa Farmaceutici, Ital.†.*
Cefadroxil (p.163·3).
Bacterial infections.

Droxitop *Synpharma, Aust.*
Orthosiphon (p.1592·2); solidago virgaurea; equisetum (p.1575·1).
Kidney and urinary-tract disorders.

Drufusan N *Syxyl, Ger.*
Homoeopathic preparation.

Dry Cough Complex *Brauer, Austral.†.*
Homoeopathic preparation.

Dry Eye Gel *Alcon, Neth.†.*
Carbomer (p.1471·2).
Dry eyes.

Dry Eye Therapy *Bausch & Lomb, USA.*
Glycerol (p.1585·2).
Dry eyes.

Dry Eyes *Bausch & Lomb, USA.*
Eye drops: Polyvinyl alcohol (p.1474·2).
Eye ointment: White soft paraffin (p.1382·3); liquid paraffin (p.1382·1); wool fat (p.1385·3).
Dry eyes.

Drylin *Merckle, Ger.*
Co-trimoxazole (p.196·3).
Bacterial infections; Pneumocystis carinii pneumonia.

Dryptal
Berk, Irl.; Berk, UK†.
Frusemide (p.871·1).
Eclampsia; hypertension; oedema.

Drysol *Person & Covey, USA.*
Aluminium chloride (p.1078·3).
Hyperhidrosis.

Dry-Tar *Restiva, Ital.†.*
Willow oleoresin; sulphur (p.1091·2); dexpanthenol (p.1570·3).
Seborrhoeic dermatitis.

Drytergent *C & M, USA.*
Skin cleanser.

Drytex *C & M, USA.*
Salicylic acid (p.1090·2); methylbenzethonium chloride (p.1119·3).
Acne.

D-Seb *Rydelle, Ital.*
Chlorhexidine gluconate (p.1107·2).
Acne; seborrhoea.

DSMC Plus *Geneva, USA.*
Docusate potassium (p.1189·3); casanthranol (p.1182·3).
Constipation.

D-S-S *Warner Chilcott, USA.*
Docusate sodium (p.1189·3).
Constipation.

D-S-S Plus *Warner Chilcott, USA†.*
Docusate sodium (p.1189·3); casanthranol (p.1182·3).
Constipation.

D-Stop *Ratiopharm, Ger.*
Loperamide hydrochloride (p.1197·2).
Diarrhoea.

DT Bis *Merieux, Fr.*
A diphtheria and tetanus vaccine (p.1508·1).
Active immunisation of older children and adults.

DT Coq *Merieux, Fr.*
An adsorbed diphtheria, tetanus, and pertussis vaccine (p.1509·1).
Active immunisation.

DT Polio *Merieux, Fr.*
A diphtheria, tetanus, and poliomyelitis vaccine (p.1510·1).
Active immunisation.

DT Vax *Merieux, Fr.*
An adsorbed diphtheria and tetanus vaccine (p.1508·1).
Active immunisation.

D-Tabs *Riva, Canad.*
Cholecalciferol (p.1366·3).
Vitamin D supplement.

DT-HIB *SBL, Swed.†.*
A diphtheria, tetanus, and Haemophilus influenzae vaccine (p.1509·3).
Active immunisation.

DTIC
Bayer, Canad.; Rhone-Poulenc Rorer, Ger.; Bayer, Swed.; Dome, Switz.
Dacarbazine (p.526·3) or dacarbazine citrate (p.527·1).
Malignant neoplasms.

DTIC-Dome
Bayer, Aust.; Bayer, Belg.; Bayer, Irl.; Bayer, S.Afr.; Bayer, Spain; Bayer, UK; Miles, USA.
Dacarbazine (p.526·3).
Malignant neoplasms.

DT-Impfstoff *Pasteur Merieux, Ger.; Chiron Behring, Ger.*
An adsorbed diphtheria and tetanus vaccine (p.1508·1).
Active immunisation of infants and young children.

DTP-Merieux *Rhone-Poulenc Rorer, S.Afr.*
An adsorbed diphtheria, tetanus, and pertussis vaccine (p.1509·1).
Active immunisation.

DTP-Rix *SmithKline Beecham, Ger.*
An adsorbed diphtheria, tetanus, and pertussis vaccine (p.1509·1).
Active immunisation.

D-Tracetten *Albert-Roussel, Ger.; Hoechst, Ger.*
Cholecalciferol (p.1366·3).
Vitamin D deficiency.

DT-reduct *Serotherapeutisches, Aust.*
An adsorbed diphtheria and tetanus vaccine (p.1508·1).
Active immunisation.

DT-Rix *SmithKline Beecham, Ger.*
An adsorbed diphtheria and tetanus vaccine (p.1508·1).
Active immunisation of infants and young children.

D-Tussin *Pharmco, S.Afr.*
Etofylline (p.753·1); diphenhydramine hydrochloride (p.409·1); ammonium chloride (p.1055·2); sodium citrate (p.1153·2).
Coughs; obstructive airways disease.

DT-Vaccinol *Procter & Gamble, Ger.*
An adsorbed diphtheria and tetanus vaccine (p.1508·1).
Active immunisation of infants and young children.

DT-Wellcovax *Wellcopharm, Ger.†.*
An adsorbed diphtheria and tetanus vaccine (p.1508·1).
Active immunisation of infants and young children.

Duact *Glaxo Wellcome, Aust.*
Acrivastine (p.401·3); pseudoephedrine hydrochloride (p.1068·3).
Allergic rhinitis.

Duadacin *Kenwood, USA.*
Paracetamol (p.72·2); chlorpheniramine maleate (p.405·1); phenylpropanolamine hydrochloride (p.1067·2).
Upper respiratory-tract symptoms.

Duafen *Pharmed, Aust.*
Ibuprofen (p.44·1).
Fever; pain.

Dual-Lax Extra Strong *Lane, UK.*
Senna (p.1212·2); aloin (p.1177·2); cascara sagrada (p.1183·1).
Constipation.

Dual-Lax Normal Strength *Lane, UK.*
Senna (p.1212·2); cape aloes (p.1177·1); cascara sagrada (p.1183·1).
Constipation.

Duan *Pharmed, Aust.*
Aspirin (p.16·1); paracetamol (p.72·2); caffeine (p.749·3).
Fever; pain.

Duaneo *Pharmed, Aust.*
Paracetamol (p.72·2).
Fever; pain.

Duaneo mit Codein *Pharmed, Aust.*
Aspirin (p.16·1) paracetamol (p.72·2); codeine hydrochloride (p.26·1).
Pain.

Dubam *Norma, UK.*
Cream: Methyl salicylate (p.55·2); menthol (p.1600·2); cineole (p.1564·1).
Chilblains; muscle stiffness; soft-tissue injuries.
Topical spray: Methyl salicylate (p.55·2); ethyl salicylate (p.36·1); glycol salicylate (p.43·1); methyl nicotinate (p.55·1).
Pain.

Duboisine *Ciba Vision, Fr.†.*
Hyoscyamine sulphate (p.464·2).
Eye examination; uveitis.

Ducase *Medecine Vegetale, Fr.*
Calumba (p.1557·2); quassia (p.1624·1); cascara (p.1183·1); liquorice (p.1197·1); gentian (p.1583·3); ferrous oxalate (p.1340·1).
Tonic.

Ducene *Sauter, Austral.*
Diazepam (p.661·1).
Alcohol withdrawal syndrome; anxiety disorders; skeletal muscle spasm and spasticity.

Duebien *PQS, Spain.*
Doxylamine succinate (p.410·1).
Insomnia.

Dufaston *Solvay, Ital.*
Dydrogesterone (p.1444·2).
Progestogenic.

Dukoral *SBL, Swed.*
A cholera vaccine (p.1506·2).
Active immunisation.

Dulax *Antigen, Irl.*
Lactulose (p.1195·3).
Constipation; hepatic encephalopathy.

Dulcagen *Goldline, USA.*
Bisacodyl (p.1179·3).
Constipation.

Dulcargan *Winzer, Ger.†.*
Silver borate (p.1629·2).
Antiseptic; inflammatory eye disorders.

Dulcex *Blue Cross, Ital.†.*
Aspartame (p.1335·1); acesulfame (p.1333·3).
Sugar substitute.

Dulcibleu *Allergan, Fr.†.*
Methylthioninium (p.984·3); phenylephrine hydrochloride (p.1066·2).
Eye disorders.

Dulcicortine *Allergan, Fr.†.*
Neomycin sulphate (p.229·2); hydrocortisone acetate (p.1043·3).
Infected eye disorders.

Dulcidrine *Allergan, Fr.†.*
Oxedrine tartrate (p.925·3); chlorhexidine gluconate (p.1107·2).
Conjunctivitis.

Dulcilarmes
Allergan, Fr.; Allergan, Switz.†.
Povidone (p.1474·2).
Dry eyes; eye examinations.

Dulcimyxine *Allergan, Fr.†.*
Framycetin sulphate (p.210·3); polymyxin B sulphate (p.239·1).
Bacterial eye infections.

Dulcion *Allergan, Fr.†.*
Co-dergocrine mesylate (p.1566·1).
Mental function disorders in the elderly; peripheral vascular disorders.

Dulciphak *Allergan, Fr.*
Sodium monomethyltrisilanol orthohydroxybenzoate; parahydroxycinnamic acid.
Eye lens disorders.

Dulcipirina *SmithKline Beecham, Spain†.*
Aspirin (p.16·1).
Glycine (p.1345·2) is included in this preparation in an attempt to limit adverse effects on the gastro-intestinal mucosa.
Fever; musculoskeletal and joint disorders; pain; thrombo-embolism prophylaxis.

Dulcivit *Abigo, Swed.*
Multivitamin preparation.

Dulco Laxo *Fher, Spain.*
Bisacodyl (p.1179·3).
Bowel evacuation; constipation.

Dulcodruppels *Boehringer Ingelheim, Neth.*
Sodium picosulphate (p.1213·2).
Constipation.

Dulcolax
Bender, Aust.; Boehringer Ingelheim, Belg.; Boehringer Ingelheim, Canad.; Boehringer Ingelheim, Fr.; Thomae, Ger.; Windsor, Irl.; Boehringer Ingelheim, Ital.; Boehringer Ingelheim, Neth.; Boehringer Ingelheim, Norw.; Boehringer Ingelheim, S.Afr.; Boehringer Ingelheim, Swed.; Boehringer Ingelheim, Switz.; Windsor, UK; Ciba Consumer, USA.
Bisacodyl (p.1179·3).
Bowel evacuation; constipation.

Dulcolax Bowel Prep Kit *Ciba, USA.*
Combination pack: 4 Dulcolax tablets (p.1179·3); 1 Dulcolax suppository.
Pre-operative bowel preparation.

Dulcolax Liquid *Windsor, UK.*
Sodium picosulphate (p.1213·2).
Constipation.

Dulcolax NP *Thomae, Ger.*
Sodium picosulphate (p.1213·2).
Constipation.

Dulconatur *Boehringer Ingelheim, Switz.*
Psyllium (p.1194·2).
Constipation; gastro-intestinal disorders.

Dull-C *Freeda, USA.*
Ascorbic acid (p.1365·2).
Scurvy; vitamin C deficiency.

Dumicoat
Dumex, Ger.; Dumex, Norw.; Dumex-Alpharma, Swed.; Dumex, Switz.; Dumex, UK.
Miconazole (p.384·3).
Fungal mouth infections.

Dumirox
Pharmacia Upjohn, Ital.; Duphar, Spain.
Fluvoxamine maleate (p.288·3).
Depression; obsessive-compulsive disorder.

Dumoxin *Dumex, Neth.†; Dumex, Norw.; Lagamed, S.Afr.*
Doxycycline (p.202·3) or doxycycline hydrochloride (p.202·3).
Bacterial infections.

Dumozolam *Dumex-Alpharma, Swed.†.*
Triazolam (p.696·3).
Sleep disorders.

Duna *Tedec Meiji, Spain.*
Pinazepam (p.687·1).
Anxiety; insomnia.

Duo Celloid CSIP *Blackmores, Austral.†.*
Calcium sulphate (p.1557·1); iron phosphate.

Duo Celloids CPIP *Blackmores, Austral.*
Calcium phosphate (p.1155·3); iron phosphate.

Duo Celloids CPMP *Blackmores, Austral.*
Calcium phosphate (p.1155·3); magnesium phosphate (p.1157·3).

Duo Celloids PCCP *Blackmores, Austral.*
Potassium chloride (p.1161·1); calcium phosphate (p.1155·3).

Duo Celloids PCIP *Blackmores, Austral.*
Potassium chloride (p.1161·1); iron phosphate.

Duo Celloids PCMP *Blackmores, Austral.*
Potassium chloride (p.1161·1); magnesium phosphate (p.1157·3).

Duo Celloids PPIP *Blackmores, Austral.*
Potassium phosphate (p.1159·3); iron phosphate.

Duo Celloids PPMP *Blackmores, Austral.*
Potassium phosphate (p.1159·3); magnesium phosphate (p.1157·3).

Duo Celloids PSMP *Blackmores, Austral.*
Potassium sulphate (p.1161·2); magnesium phosphate (p.1157·3).

Duo Celloids PSPC *Blackmores, Austral.*
Potassium sulphate (p.1161·2); potassium chloride (p.1161·1).

Duo Celloids SCF *Blackmores, Austral.*
Silicon dioxide (p.1474·3); calcium fluoride.

Duo Celloids SPCF *Blackmores, Austral.*
Dibasic sodium phosphate (p.1159·3); calcium fluoride.

Duo Celloids SPCP *Blackmores, Austral.*
Dibasic sodium phosphate (p.1159·3); calcium phosphate (p.1155·3).

Duo Celloids SPIP *Blackmores, Austral.*
Dibasic sodium phosphate (p.1159·3); iron phosphate.

Duo Celloids SPMP *Blackmores, Austral.*
Dibasic sodium phosphate (p.1159·3); magnesium phosphate (p.1157·3).

Duo Celloids SPPC *Blackmores, Austral.*
Dibasic sodium phosphate (p.1159·3); potassium chloride (p.1161·1).

Duo Celloids SPPP *Blackmores, Austral.*
Dibasic sodium phosphate (p.1159·3); potassium phosphate (p.1159·3).

Duo Celloids SPPS *Blackmores, Austral.*
Dibasic sodium phosphate (p.1159·3); potassium sulphate (p.1161·2).

Duo Celloids SPS *Blackmores, Austral.*
Dibasic sodium phosphate (p.1159·3); silicon dioxide (p.1474·3).

Duo Celloids SPSS *Blackmores, Austral.*
Dibasic sodium phosphate (p.1159·3); sodium sulphate (p.1213·3).

Duo Celloids SSMP *Blackmores, Austral.*
Sodium sulphate (p.1213·3); magnesium phosphate (p.1157·3).

Duo Celloids SSPC *Blackmores, Austral.*
Sodium sulphate (p.1213·3); potassium chloride (p.1161·1).

Duo Celloids SSS *Blackmores, Austral.*
Sodium sulphate (p.1213·3); silicon dioxide (p.1474·3).

Duo Gobens *Normon, Spain.*
Doxycycline hydrochloride (p.202·3); chymotrypsin (p.1563·2); trypsin (p.1640·1).
Bacterial infections.

Duobact *Orion, Irl.*
Co-trimoxazole (p.196·3).
Bacterial infections.

Duobar
Scientific Hospital Supplies, Austral.; Scientific Hospital Supplies, Irl.; Medifood-Trufood, Ital.; Scientific Hospital Supplies, UK.
Food for special diets.
Liver disorders; phenylketonuria; renal disorders.

Duobiocin *Nycomed, Ger.†.*
Co-trimoxazole (p.196·3).
Bacterial infections.

Duobrus *Searle, Swed.*
Ibuprofen (p.44·1).
Fever; pain.

Duo-C *Geymonat, Ital.*
Ascorbic acid (p.1365·2).
Vitamin C deficiency; vitamin C supplement.

Duocal
Note. This name is used for preparations of different composition.
Scientific Hospital Supplies, Austral.; Scientific Hospital Supplies, Irl.; Medifood-Trufood, Ital.; Scientific Hospital Supplies, UK.
Low-electrolyte, protein-free carbohydrate preparation for special diets.

Serag-Wiessner, Ger.†.
Glucose monohydrate (p.1343·3); xylitol (p.1372·3).
Parenteral nutrition.

Duocet *Mason, USA.*
Hydrocodone tartrate (p.43·1); paracetamol (p.72·2).
Pain.

Duo-CVP *Rhone-Poulenc Rorer, Canad.*
Bioflavonoids (p.1580·1); ascorbic acid (p.1365·2).
Capillary bleeding.

Duo-CVP with Vitamin K *Rhone-Poulenc Rorer, Canad.†.*
Bioflavonoids (p.1580·1); ascorbic acid (p.1365·2); menadione (p.1370·3).
Capillary bleeding.

Duo-Cyp *Keene, USA.*
Oestradiol cypionate (p.1455·1); testosterone cypionate (p.1464·1).
Menopausal vasomotor symptoms; prevention of postpartum breast engorgement.

Duoderm
Note. This name is used for preparations of different composition.
Convatec, Austral.; Bristol-Myers Squibb, Belg.; Convatec, Fr.
A range of hydrocolloid dressings.
Burns; ulcers; wounds.

Scherag, S.Afr.†.
Tolnaftate (p.389·1); nystatin (p.386·1).
Fungal skin infections.

Duodexa N *Kade, Ger.*
Dexamethasone (p.1037·1); dexamethasone sodium metasulphobenzoate (p.1037·2).
Skin disorders.

Duofer *Andreabal, Switz.*
Ferrous fumarate (p.1339·3); ferrous gluconate (p.1340·1).
Ascorbic acid (p.1365·2) is included in this preparation to increase the absorption and availability of iron.
Iron deficiency.

Duofer Fol *Andreabal, Switz.*
Ferrous fumarate (p.1339·3); ferrous gluconate (p.1340·1); folic acid (p.1340·3).
Ascorbic acid (p.1365·2) is included in this preparation to increase the absorption and availability of iron.
Iron and folic acid deficiency.

Duofilm
Note. This name is used for preparations of different composition.
Salus, Aust.; Stiefel, Austral.; Stiefel, Canad.; Stiefel, Fr.; Stiefel, Ger.; Stiefel, Irl.; Stiefel, S.Afr.; Stiefel, Switz.; Stiefel, UK.
Salicylic acid (p.1090·2); lactic acid (p.1593·3).
Warts.

Schering-Plough, USA.
Salicylic acid (p.1090·2).
Benign epithelial tumours; hyperkeratosis.

Duoform *Mauermann, Ger.†.*
Sedum acre; silybum marianum (p.993·3); aesculus (p.1543·3); capsella bursa pastoris; frangula bark (p.1193·2); nux vomica; acid. nitricum; carbo vegetabilis.
Anorectal disorders.

Duoform Med *Mauermann, Ger.†.*
Ruscus aculeatus.
Haemorrhoids.

Duoform Novo *Mauermann, Ger.*
Mouse thorn root.
Haemorrhoids.

Duoform-Balsam *Mauermann, Ger.†.*
Benzocaine (p.1286·2); peru balsam (p.1617·2); glycerol (p.1585·2); calendula officinalis; hamamelis (p.1587·1); tormentil (p.1638·3); cydonia; phytohormon.
Anorectal disorders.

Duoforte *Stiefel, Canad.*
Salicylic acid (p.1090·2).
Warts.

Duogas *Bracco, Ital.*
Sodium bicarbonate (p.1153·2); anhydrous citric acid (p.1564·3); dimethicone (p.1213·1).
Double-contrast radiography of the oesophagus and stomach.

Duogastral *ISM, Ital.*
Pirenzepine hydrochloride (p.467·1).
Gastroduodenitis; peptic ulcer.

Duogastril *Hosbon, Spain†.*
Cimetidine (p.1183·2).
Acid aspiration; gastro-intestinal haemorrhage; gastro-oesophageal reflux; peptic ulcer; Zollinger-Ellison syndrome.

Duogastrone *Sanofi Winthrop, Irl.†.*
Carbenoxolone sodium (p.1182·2).
Duodenal ulcers.

Duogink *Duopharm, Ger.*
Ginkgo biloba (p.1584·1).
Cerebrovascular disorders.

Duokapton *Strallhofer, Aust.*
Aspirin (p.16·1); paracetamol (p.72·2).
Fever; pain.

Duolax *Almirall, Spain.*
Lactulose (p.1195·3).
Constipation; hepatic encephalopathy; salmonella enteritis.

Duolip
Merckle, Aust.; Merckle, Ger.; Mepha, Switz.
Theofibrate (p.1279·3).
Hyperlipidaemias.

Duolube *Bausch & Lomb, Canad.*
White soft paraffin (p.1382·3); liquid paraffin (p.1382·1).
Corneal dryness.

Duoluton *Schering, Ger.†.*
Norgestrel (p.1454·1); ethinyloestradiol (p.1445·1).
Endometriosis; menstrual disorders.

Duolys A *Dicamed, Swed.*
A range of haemodialysis solutions (p.1151·1).

Duolys B *Dicamed, Swed.*
Sodium bicarbonate; disodium edetate (p.1151·1).
Haemodialysis solution.

Duo-Medihaler
3M, Ger.†; 3M, USA†.
Isoprenaline hydrochloride (p.892·1); phenylephrine acid tartrate (p.1066·2).
Asthma; bronchitis; bronchospastic disorders; emphysema; postoperative atelectasis.

Duomet *Propan, S.Afr.*
Cimetidine (p.1183·2).
Gastric hyperacidity; gastro-oesophageal reflux; peptic ulcer; Zollinger-Ellison syndrome.

Duonalc *ICN, Canad.*
Isopropyl alcohol (p.1118·2).
Skin cleanser.

Duonalc-E *ICN, Canad.*
Alcohol (p.1099·1); isopropyl alcohol (p.1118·2).
Skin cleanser.

Duonasa *Normon, Spain.*
Amoxycillin trihydrate (p.151·3); potassium clavulanate (p.190·2).
Bacterial infections.

Duo-Norgesic N *3M, Ger.†.*
Dipyrone (p.35·1); lignocaine hydrochloride (p.1293·2).
Pain.

Duo-Ormogyn *Amsa, Ital.*
Oestradiol benzoate (p.1455·1); progesterone (p.1459·3).
Menstrual disorders.

Duoplant
Note. This name is used for preparations of different composition.
Stiefel, Canad.
Salicylic acid (p.1090·2); lactic acid (p.1593·3); formaldehyde (p.1113·2).
Plantar warts.

Schering-Plough, USA.
Salicylic acid (p.1090·2).
Warts.

Duorol *Pharmacia Upjohn, Spain.*
Paracetamol (p.72·2).
Fever; pain.

Duospirel *Gebro, Aust.*
Salbutamol (p.758·2); beclomethasone dipropionate (p.1032·1).
Obstructive airways disease.

Duotal *Bristol-Myers Squibb, Ger.†.*
Tetracycline hydrochloride (p.259·1); fedrilate maleate (p.1061·1).
Bronchitis; broncho-pneumonia; pneumonia.

Duo-Trach Kit *Astra, USA.*
Lignocaine hydrochloride (p.1293·2).
Local anaesthesia.

Duotrate *Jones, USA†.*
Pentaerythritol tetranitrate (p.927·3).
Angina pectoris.

Duotrim *Genpharm, S.Afr.†.*
Co-trimoxazole (p.196·3).
Bacterial infections.

Duovax *Merck Sharp & Dohme, Belg.*
A live measles and mumps vaccine (Enders' attenuated Edmonston strain and Jeryl Lynn B strain, respectively) (p.1519·2).
Active immunisation.

Duovent
Boehringer Ingelheim, Belg.; Boehringer Ingelheim, Canad.; Boehringer Ingelheim, Irl.; Boehringer Ingelheim, Ital.; Boehringer Ingelheim, S.Afr.; Boehringer Ingelheim, UK.
Fenoterol hydrobromide (p.753·2); ipratropium bromide (p.754·2).
Obstructive airways disease.

Duoventrin *Schwörer, Ger.*
Bismuth subnitrate (p.1180·2); linseed (p.1596·2); lactose.
Gastro-intestinal disorders.

Duoventrinetten N *Schwörer, Ger.*
Aluminium hydroxide-magnesium carbonate gel, dried (p.1178·2); magnesium trisilicate (p.1199·1); magnesium hydroxide (p.1198·2).
Gastro-intestinal disorders.

Duovisc
Alcon, Austral.; Alcon-Thilo, Ger.
1 Syringe, sodium hyaluronate (p.1630·3); sodium chondroitin sulphate (p.1562·2) (Viscoat); one syringe, sodium hyaluronate (Provisc).
Adjunct in ocular surgery.

Duovitan *Asta Medica, Aust.*
Allopurinol (p.390·2); benzbromarone (p.392·3).
Gout; hyperuricaemia.

Duphalac
Solvay, Aust.; Solvay, Austral.; Solvay, Belg.; Solvay, Canad.; Solvay, Fr.; Solvay, Irl.; Solvay, Ital.; Solvay, Neth.; Solvay, Norw.; Solvay, S.Afr.; Duphar, Spain; Meda, Swed.; Solvay, Switz.; Solvay, UK; Solvay, USA.
Lactulose (p.1195·3).
Constipation; hepatic encephalopathy; salmonella enteritis.

Duphaston
Solvay, Aust.; Solvay, Austral.; Solvay, Belg.; Solvay, Fr.; Solvay, Ger.; Solvay, Irl.; Solvay, Neth.; Solvay, S.Afr.; Duphar, Spain; Solvay Duphar, Swed.; Solvay, Switz.; Solvay, UK.
Dydrogesterone (p.1444·2).
Endometriosis; female infertility; hormone replacement therapy; menorrhagia; menstrual disorders; threatened and habitual abortion.

Duplamin *Bruschettini, Ital.*
Promethazine hydrochloride (p.416·2).
Skin irritation.

Duplamox *ISF, Ital.†.*
Injection: Amoxycillin sodium (p.151·3); dicloxacillin sodium (p.202·1).
Tablets; oral powder; oral suspension: Amoxycillin trihydrate (p.151·3); dicloxacillin (p.201·3).
Bacterial infections.

Duplamox Mucolitico *ISF, Ital.†.*
Amoxycillin trihydrate (p.151·3); carbocisteine (p.1056·3).
Bacterial infections of the respiratory tract.

Duplex
Note. This name is used for preparations of different composition.
SBL, Swed.
A diphtheria and tetanus vaccine (p.1508·1).
Active immunisation.

C & M, USA.
Skin cleanser.

Duplex T *C & M, USA.*
Coal tar (p.1092·3).
Scalp disorders.

Duplexcillina *Metapharma, Ital.*
Ampicillin (p.153·1); dicloxacillin (p.201·3).
Bacterial infections.

Duplexil *Eurofarmaco, Ital.*
Capsules: Ampicillin trihydrate (p.153·2); dicloxacillin sodium (p.202·1).
Injection†: Ampicillin sodium (p.153·1); dicloxacillin sodium (p.202·1).
Bacterial infections.

Duplicalcio *Medical, Spain.*
Calcium laevulinate (p.1155·2); vitamin B substances; ergocalciferol (p.1367·1); liver extract; isoniazid (p.218·1).
Anaemias; bone and dental disorders; calcium deficiency; osteomalacia; rickets; tonic.

Duplicalcio 150 *Medical, Spain.*
Isoniazid (p.218·1); pyridoxine (p.1363·1).
Also contains calcium gluconate.
Tuberculosis.

Duplicalcio B12 *Medical, Spain.*
Calcium gluconate (p.1155·2); calcium laevulinate (p.1155·2); cyanocobalamin (p.1363·3); isoniazid (p.218·1).
Anaemias; tonic; tuberculosis.

Duplicalcio Hidraz *Medical, Spain.*
Calcium gluconate (p.1155·2); calcium laevulinate (p.1155·2); isoniazid (p.218·1).
Tonic; tuberculosis.

Duplinal *Hexal, Aust.*
Dipyridamole (p.857·1); aspirin (p.16·1).
Membranous proliferative glomerulonephritis; thrombosis prophylaxis.

Duplotrast *Gerot, Aust.*
Sodium carbonate (p.1153·2); simethicone (p.1213·1).
Adjunct in double contrast radiography.

Duplotrast Z *Gerot, Aust.*
Citric acid (p.1564·3); sodium bicarbonate (p.1153·2); simethicone (p.1213·1).
Adjunct in double contrast radiography.

Duplovac
Berna, Ital.†; Berna, Spain†.
A staphylococcal vaccine (p.1535·1).
Adjunct in prophylaxis of staphylococcal infections.

Duponil *Inkeysa, Spain.*
Ammonium chloride (p.1055·2); codeine phosphate (p.26·1); diphenhydramine hydrochloride (p.409·1); ephedrine hydrochloride (p.1059·3).
Respiratory-tract disorders.

dura AL *Durachemie, Ger.*
Allopurinol (p.390·2).
Adenine-phosphoribosyl-transferase deficiency; gout; hyperuricaemia; Lesch-Nyhan syndrome.

dura AX *Durachemie, Ger.*
Amoxycillin trihydrate (p.151·3).
Bacterial infections.

duraampicillin *Durachemie, Ger.*
Ampicillin trihydrate (p.153·2).
Bacterial infections.

durabetagent *Durachemie, Ger.†.*
Betamethasone sodium phosphate (p.1033·3); gentamicin sulphate (p.212·1).
Eye disorders.

durabetason *Durachemie, Ger.†.*
Betamethasone sodium phosphate (p.1033·3).
Eye disorders.

Durabezur *Durachemie, Ger.*
Bezafibrate (p.1268·2).
Hyperlipidaemias.

Durabolin
Organon, Austral.†; Organon, Belg.†; Organon, Canad.†; Organon, Fr.†; Ravasini, Ital.†; Organon, Neth.†; Donmed, S.Afr.†; Organon, Spain†; Organon, UK†; Organon, USA.
Nandrolone phenylpropionate (p.1452·2).
Anabolic; breast cancer; osteoporosis.

Durabronchal *Durachemie, Ger.*
Acetylcysteine (p.1052·3).
Respiratory-tract disorders associated with increased or viscous mucus.

Duracare
Note. This name is used for preparations of different composition.
Allergan, Aust.; Allergan, Austral.; Allergan, Ger.
Polyvinyl alcohol (p.1474·2); disodium edetate (p.980·1).
Disinfection and storage solution for gas-permeable hard contact lenses.
Blairex, USA.
Cleansing solution for soft contact lenses.

duracebrol Durachemie, Ger.
Nicergoline (p.1607·1).
Mental function disorders.

Duracef
Frika, Aust.; Bristol-Myers Squibb, Belg.; Bristol-Myers Squibb, S.Afr.; Juste, Spain; Bristol-Myers Squibb, Switz.
Cefadroxil (p.163·3).
Bacterial infections.

duracetamol Durachemie, Ger.
Paracetamol (p.72·2).
Fever; pain.

Duracid Fielding, USA†.
Calcium carbonate (p.1182·1); aluminium hydroxide-magnesium carbonate co-dried gel (p.1178·2).
Hyperacidity.

duraclamid Durachemie, Ger.†.
Metoclopramide hydrochloride (p.1200·3).
Gastro-intestinal disorders.

Duraclean Allergan, Austral.
Cleansing solution for gas permeable contact lenses.

Duracoll Schering-Plough, Belg.
Gentamicin sulphate (p.212·1); collagen (bovine) (p.1566·3).
Bone infections.

duracoron Durachemie, Ger.
Molsidomine (p.912·2).
Angina pectoris.

duracralfat Durachemie, Ger.†.
Sucralfate (p.1214·2).
Peptic ulcer.

Duracreme LRC Products, UK.
Nonoxinol 9 (p.1326·1).
Contraceptive.

duracroman Durachemie, Ger.
Sodium cromoglycate (p.762·1).
Allergic conjunctivitis; allergic rhinitis; asthma.

Duract Wyeth-Ayerst, USA†.
Bromfenac sodium (p.22·2).
Pain.

duradermal Durachemie, Ger.
Bufexamac (p.22·2).
Skin disorders.

duradiazepam Durachemie, Ger.†.
Diazepam (p.661·1).
Anxiety disorders; sleep disorders.

duradiuret Durachemie, Ger.
Triamterene (p.957·2); hydrochlorothiazide (p.885·2).
Hypertension; oedema.

duradoxal Durachemie, Ger.
Doxycycline (p.202·3) or doxycycline hydrochloride (p.202·3).
Bacterial infections.

duraerythromycin Durachemie, Ger.
Erythromycin ethyl succinate (p.204·2) or erythromycin stearate (p.204·2).
Bacterial infections.

Dura-Estrin Roberts, USA†; Hauck, USA†.
Oestradiol cypionate (p.1455·1).
Female hypogonadism; menopausal vasomotor symptoms.

Durafedrin Ciba Self Medication, Canad.†.
Pseudoephedrine polistirex (p.1069·2).
Nasal congestion.

durafenat Durachemie, Ger.
Fenofibrate (p.1273·1).
Hyperlipidaemias.

Duraflor Pharmascience, Canad.
Sodium fluoride (p.742·1).

duraforte Durachemie, Ger.†.
Naphazoline nitrate (p.1064·2); phenylephrine hydrochloride (p.1066·2); antazoline sulphate (p.402·1).
Eye disorders.

durafungol Durachemie, Ger.
Clotrimazole (p.376·3).
Fungal infections; vaginal infections.

durafurid Durachemie, Ger.
Frusemide (p.871·1) or frusemide sodium (p.872·3).
Hypertension; oedema; venous insufficiency.

Duragel LRC Products, UK.
Nonoxinol 9 (p.1326·1).
Contraceptive.

Duragen Roberts, USA†; Hauck, USA†.
Oestradiol valerate (p.1455·2).
Female castration; female hypogonadism; menopausal vasomotor symptoms; prevention of breast engorgement; primary ovarian failure; prostatic cancer; vulval and vaginal atrophy.

duragentam Durachemie, Ger.†.
Gentamicin sulphate (p.212·1).
Bacterial eye infections.

duragentamicin Durachemie, Ger.
Gentamicin sulphate (p.212·1).
Bacterial infections.

Duragesic
Janssen-Ortho, Canad.; Janssen, USA.
Fentanyl (p.38·1).
Pain.

Dura-Gest Dura, USA.
Phenylephrine hydrochloride (p.1066·2); phenylpropanolamine hydrochloride (p.1067·2); guaiphenesin (p.1061·3).
Coughs and cold symptoms; nasal congestion.

duraglucon N Durachemie, Ger.
Glibenclamide (p.319·3).
Diabetes mellitus.

duraH2 Durachemie, Ger.
Cimetidine (p.1183·2).
Aspiration syndrome; gastro-oesophageal reflux; peptic ulcer; Zollinger-Ellison syndrome.

dura-Ibu Durachemie, Ger.
Ibuprofen (p.44·1).
Inflammation; musculoskeletal, joint, and soft-tissue disorders; pain.

duraibuprofen Durachemie, Ger.
Ibuprofen (p.44·1).
Gout; inflammation; musculoskeletal and joint disorders.

durajod Durachemie, Ger.†.
Digitalin (p.1571·3); calcium iodide (p.1056·2); rubidium iodide (p.1626·3).
Eye disorders.

durakne Durachemie, Ger.
Minocycline hydrochloride (p.226·2).
Acne.

Duralex American Urologicals, USA.
Pseudoephedrine hydrochloride (p.1068·3); chlorpheniramine maleate (p.405·1).
Upper respiratory-tract symptoms.

duralipon Durachemie, Ger.
Thioctic acid (p.1636·2).
Diabetic polyneuropathy.

Duralith Janssen-Ortho, Canad.
Lithium carbonate (p.290·3).
Bipolar disorder.

Duralone Hauck, USA.
Methylprednisolone acetate (p.1046·1).
Corticosteroid.

duralopid Durachemie, Ger.
Loperamide hydrochloride (p.1197·2).
Diarrhoea.

duralozam Durachemie, Ger.
Lorazepam (p.675·3).
Sleep disorders.

Duralutin Roberts, USA†; Hauck, USA†.
Hydroxyprogesterone hexanoate (p.1448·1).
Abnormal uterine bleeding; amenorrhoea; metrorrhagia.

duraMCP Durachemie, Ger.
Metoclopramide hydrochloride (p.1200·3).
Gastro-intestinal disorders.

durametacin Durachemie, Ger.†.
Indomethacin (p.45·2).
Gout; inflammation; rheumatism.

duramipress Durachemie, Ger.
Prazosin hydrochloride (p.932·3).
Heart failure; hypertension; Raynaud's syndrome.

Duramist Plus Pfeiffer, USA.
Oxymetazoline hydrochloride (p.1065·3).
Nasal congestion.

duramonitat Durachemie, Ger.
Isosorbide mononitrate (p.893·3).
Heart failure; ischaemic heart disease.

Duramorph Elkins-Sinn, USA.
Morphine sulphate (p.56·2).
Pain.

duramucal Durachemie, Ger.
Ambroxol hydrochloride (p.1054·3).
Respiratory-tract disorders associated with increased or viscous mucus.

Duranest
Astra, Aust.; Astra, Austral.†; Astra, Fr.; Astra, Ger.; Astra, Swed.†; Astra, USA.
Etidocaine hydrochloride (p.1293·1).
Adrenaline (p.813·2) or adrenaline acid tartrate (p.813·3) is included in some injections as a vasoconstrictor to diminish absorption and localise the effect of the local anaesthetic.
Local anaesthesia.

duranifin Durachemie, Ger.
Nifedipine (p.916·2).
Hypertension; ischaemic heart disease; Raynaud's syndrome.

duranifin Sali Durachemie, Ger.
Nifedipine (p.916·2); mefruside (p.902·2).
Hypertension.

duranitrat Durachemie, Ger.
Isosorbide dinitrate (p.893·1).
Cardiac disorders; pulmonary hypertension.

Duranol Parke, Davis, Irl.†.
Propranolol hydrochloride (p.937·1).
Angina pectoris; anxiety; hypertension; migraine.

durapaediat Durachemie, Ger.
Erythromycin ethyl succinate (p.204·2).
Bacterial infections.

durapenicillin Durachemie, Ger.
Phenoxymethylpenicillin potassium (p.236·2).
Bacterial infections.

durapental Durachemie, Ger.
Oxpentifylline (p.925·3).
Peripheral vascular disorders.

duraperidol Durachemie, Ger.†.
Haloperidol (p.673·3).
Psychoses.

Duraphat
Austrodent, Aust.; Rhone-Poulenc Rorer, Ger.; Rorer, Norw.; Inpharma, Swed.
Sodium fluoride (p.742·1).
Dental caries prophylaxis; sensitive teeth.

Duraphyl Forest Pharmaceuticals, USA†.
Theophylline (p.765·1).

duraphyllin Durachemie, Ger.
Controlled-release capsules: Theophylline (p.765·1).
Injection†: Aminophylline monohydrate (p.748·1).
Obstructive airways disease.

durapindol Durachemie, Ger.
Pindolol (p.931·1).
Cardiac hyperkinesis; hypertension; ischaemic heart disease.

durapirenz Durachemie, Ger.
Pirenzepine hydrochloride (p.467·1).
Gastro-intestinal disorders.

durapirox Durachemie, Ger.
Piroxicam (p.80·2).
Gout; musculoskeletal and joint disorders.

durapitrop Durachemie, Ger.
Piracetam (p.1619·1).
Mental function disorders.

duraprednisolon Durachemie, Ger.
Prednisolone (p.1048·1) or prednisolone acetate (p.1048·1).
Corticosteroid.

Duraquin Warner Chilcott, USA†.
Quinidine gluconate (p.938·3).

durarese Durachemie, Ger.
Amiloride hydrochloride (p.819·2); hydrochlorothiazide (p.885·2).
Hypertension; oedema.

Durascreen
Note. This name is used for preparations of different composition.
Pharmascience, Canad.
SPF 15: Ethylhexyl *p*-methoxycinnamate (p.1487·1); octyl salicylate (p.1487·3); oxybenzone (p.1487·3); titanium dioxide (p.1093·3).
SPF 30: Ethylhexyl *p*-methoxycinnamate (p.1487·1); octyl salicylate (p.1487·3); oxybenzone (p.1487·3); titanium dioxide (p.1093·3); 2-phenyl-1*H*-benzimidazole-5-sulphonic acid (p.1488·2).
Sunscreen.
Schwarz, USA.
SPF 15: Ethylhexyl *p*-methoxycinnamate (p.1487·1); 2-ethylhexyl salicylate (p.1487·3); oxybenzone (p.1487·3).
SPF 30: Ethylhexyl *p*-methoxycinnamate (p.1487·1); octyl salicylate (p.1487·3); oxybenzone (p.1487·3); 2-phenylbenzimidazole-5-sulphonic acid (p.1488·2); titanium dioxide (p.1093·3).
Sunscreen.

durasilymarin Durachemie, Ger.
Silymarin (p.993·3).
Liver disorders.

Durasina SmithKline Beecham, Spain.
Chlorpheniramine maleate (p.405·1); phenylpropanolamine hydrochloride (p.1067·2).
Cold symptoms; nasal congestion.

duraskleral Durachemie, Ger.†.
Inositol nicotinate (p.891·3); vitamin A palmitate (p.1359·2); *dl*-alpha tocopheryl acid succinate (p.1369·2); diprophylline (p.752·1).
Coronary, cerebral, and peripheral vascular disorders.

Durasol-Badesalz Plantorgan, Ger.†.
Sodium chloride (p.1162·2); calcium sulphate dihydrate (p.1557·1); calcium chloride hexahydrate (p.1155·1); magnesium chloride (p.1157·2).
Anorexia; atopy; bath additive; catarrh; gynaecological disorders; musculoskeletal and joint disorders.

durasoptin Durachemie, Ger.
Verapamil hydrochloride (p.960·3).
Cardiac disorders; hypertension.

duraspiron Durachemie, Ger.
Spironolactone (p.946·1).
Hyperaldosteronism; hypertension; liver cirrhosis with ascites; oedema.

duraspiron-comp. Durachemie, Ger.
Spironolactone (p.946·1); frusemide (p.871·1).
Ascites; hyperaldosteronism; hypertension; oedema.

duratamoxifen Durachemie, Ger.
Tamoxifen citrate (p.563·3).
Breast cancer.

Dura-Tap/PD Dura, USA.
Chlorpheniramine maleate (p.405·1); pseudoephedrine hydrochloride (p.1068·3).
Allergic rhinitis; nasal congestion.

Duratears
Note. This name is used for preparations of different composition.
Alcon, Austral.; Alcon, Belg.; Alcon, Canad.
Liquid paraffin (p.1382·1); wool fat (p.1385·3); white soft paraffin (p.1382·3).
Dry eyes.
Alcon, Neth.†.
Electrolytes (p.1147·1); hypromellose (p.1473·1); dextran 70 (p.717·1).
Dry eyes.
Alcon, S.Afr.
Anhydrous liquid lanolin (p.1385·3).
Dry eyes.
Alcon, Switz.
Liquid paraffin (p.1382·1); wool fat (p.1385·3).
Dry eyes.

Duratears Free Alcon, Neth.†.
Povidone (p.1474·2).
Dry eyes.

Duratears Naturale Alcon, USA.
Liquid paraffin (p.1382·1); wool fat (p.1385·3); white soft paraffin (p.1382·3).
Dry eyes.

Duratears Z Alcon, Neth.†.
Liquid paraffin (p.1382·1); hydrous wool fat (p.1385·3); white soft paraffin (p.1382·3).
Dry eyes.

duratenol Durachemie, Ger.
Atenolol (p.825·3).
Angina pectoris; arrhythmias; hypertension.

duratenol comp Durachemie, Ger.
Atenolol (p.825·3); chlorthalidone (p.839·3).
Hypertension.

Duratest Roberts, USA; Hauck, USA.
Testosterone cypionate (p.1464·1).
Breast cancer; delayed puberty (males); male hypogonadism.

Duratestrin Hauck, USA.
Oestradiol cypionate (p.1455·1); testosterone cypionate (p.1464·1).
Menopausal vasomotor symptoms; prevention of post-partum breast engorgement.

duratetracyclin Durachemie, Ger.†.
Oxytetracycline hydrochloride (p.235·1).
Bacterial infections; infections with large viruses.

Durathate Roberts, USA; Hauck, USA.
Testosterone enanthate (p.1464·1).
Breast cancer; delayed puberty (males); male hypogonadism.

duratimol Durachemie, Ger.
Timolol maleate (p.953·3).
Glaucoma; ocular hypertension.

Duration
Schering-Plough, Canad.†; Schering-Plough, USA.
Oxymetazoline hydrochloride (p.1065·3).
Nasal congestion.

Duratirs Alcon, Ital.
Liquid paraffin (p.1382·1).
Dry eyes.

duratrimet Durachemie, Ger.†.
Co-trimoxazole (p.196·3).
Bacterial infections.

Duratuss UCB, USA.
Pseudoephedrine hydrochloride (p.1068·3); guaiphenesin (p.1061·3).
Nasal congestion.

Duratuss HD UCB, USA.
Pseudoephedrine hydrochloride (p.1068·3); guaiphenesin (p.1061·3); hydrocodone tartrate (p.43·1).
Coughs; nasal congestion.

Duratuss-G UCB, USA.
Guaiphenesin (p.1061·3).
Coughs.

duraultra Durachemie, Ger.
Retinol (p.1358·1); actinoquinol sodium (p.1543·1); naphazoline nitrate (p.1064·2).
Eye disorders.

duraultra forte Durachemie, Ger.†.
Retinol (p.1358·1); actinoquinol sodium (p.1543·1); naphazoline nitrate (p.1064·2); oxybuprocaine hydrochloride (p.1298·1).
Eye disorders.

Dura-Vent Dura, USA.
Phenylpropanolamine hydrochloride (p.1067·2); guaiphenesin (p.1061·3).
Coughs and cold symptoms.

Dura-Vent/A Dura, USA.
Phenylpropanolamine hydrochloride (p.1067·2); chlorpheniramine maleate (p.405·1).
Upper respiratory-tract symptoms.

Dura-Vent/DA Dura, USA.
Chlorpheniramine maleate (p.405·1); phenylephrine hydrochloride (p.1066·2); hyoscine methonitrate (p.463·1).
Upper respiratory-tract symptoms.

duravolten Durachemie, Ger.
Diclofenac sodium (p.31·2).
Inflammation; rheumatism.

durazanil Durachemie, Ger.
Bromazepam (p.643·1).
Anxiety disorders; insomnia.

durazepam Durachemie, Ger.
Oxazepam (p.683·2).
Anxiety disorders; sleep disorders.

durazidum Durachemie, Ger.
Magnesium hydroxide gel (p.1198·2); aluminium hydroxide gel (p.1177·3).
Gastro-intestinal disorders.

Durazina Maggioni, Ital.
Chlorpheniramine maleate (p.405·1); phenylpropanolamine hydrochloride (p.1067·2).
Nasal congestion.

Durbis
Hoechst Marion Roussel, Norw.; Hoechst Marion Roussel, Swed.
Disopyramide (p.858·1) or disopyramide phosphate (p.858·1).
Arrhythmias.

Dur-Elix 3M, Austral.
Bromhexine hydrochloride (p.1055·3).
Expectoration of excess mucus.

Dur-Elix Plus 3M, Austral.
Bromhexine hydrochloride (p.1055·3); pseudoephedrine hydrochloride (p.1068·3).
Expectoration of excess mucus; nasal congestion.

Duremesan Streuli, Switz.
Suppositories: Meclozine hydrochloride (p.413·3).
Tablets: Meclozine hydrochloride (p.413·3); caffeine (p.749·3).
Nausea and vomiting.

Duretic Abbott, Canad.†.
Methyclothiazide (p.904·1).
Hypertension; oedema.

Dureticyl Abbott, Canad.†.
Methyclothiazide (p.904·1); deserpidine (p.847·2).
Hypertension.

Duricef
Bristol, Canad.; Princeton, USA.
Cefadroxil (p.163·3).
Bacterial infections.

Duride Alphapharm, Austral.
Isosorbide mononitrate (p.893·3).
Angina pectoris.

Durobac Pharmaceutical Enterprises, S.Afr.
Co-trimoxazole (p.196·3).
Bacterial infections.

Duroferon
Astra, Norw.; Hassle, Swed.
Ferrous sulphate (p.1340·2).
Iron deficiency; iron-deficiency anaemia.

Duroferon vitamin Hassle, Swed.
Multivitamin preparation with iron.
Iron-deficiency anaemia of pregnancy.

Durogesic
Janssen-Cilag, Aust.; Janssen-Cilag, Ger.; Janssen-Cilag, Irl.; Janssen-Cilag, Ital.; Janssen-Cilag, Neth.; Janssen-Cilag, Norw.; Janssen-Cilag, S.Afr.; Janssen-Cilag, Swed.; Janssen, UK.
Fentanyl (p.38·1).
Pain.

Durolax Boehringer Ingelheim, Austral.
Bisacodyl (p.1179·3).
Bowel evacuation; constipation.

Durolax X-Pack Boehringer Ingelheim, Austral.
Combination pack: 3 Tablets, bisacodyl (p.1179·3); 1 suppository, bisacodyl; 1 sachet, citric acid (p.1564·3); heavy magnesium carbonate (p.1198·1).
Bowel evacuation.

Duromine
3M, Austral.; 3M, S.Afr.; 3M, UK.
Phentermine (as an ion-exchange resin complex) (p.1484·3).
Obesity.

Duronitrin Astra, Ital.
Isosorbide mononitrate (p.893·3).
Cardiac disorders.

Durotan Beiersdorf-Lilly, Ger.
Xipamide (p.971·2); reserpine (p.942·1).
Hypertension.

Duro-Tuss 3M, Austral.
Pholcodine (p.1068·1).
Coughs.

Duro-Tuss Cough Lozenges 3M, Austral.
Pholcodine (p.1068·1); cetylpyridinium chloride (p.1106·2).
Coughs; sore throat.

Duro-Tuss Decongestant 3M, Austral.
Pholcodine (p.1068·1); pseudoephedrine hydrochloride (p.1068·3).
Coughs; nasal congestion.

Duro-Tuss Expectorant 3M, Austral.
Pholcodine (p.1068·1); bromhexine hydrochloride (p.1055·3).
Coughs.

Durvitan Seid, Spain.
Caffeine (p.749·3).
Fatigue.

Dusk Seton, UK.
Diethyltoluamide (p.1405·1).
Insect repellent.

Dusodril
Merck, Aust.; Lipha, Ger.
Naftidrofuryl oxalate (p.914·2).
Peripheral circulatory disorders; vascular disorders of the brain, ears, and eyes.

Duspatal
Solvay, Ger.; Solvay, Ital.; Solvay, Neth.
Mebeverine embonate (p.1199·2) or mebeverine hydrochloride (p.1199·2).
Gastro-intestinal spasm; irritable bowel syndrome.

Duspatalin
Solvay, Belg.; Solvay, Fr.; Duphar, Spain; Solvay, Switz.
Mebeverine embonate (p.1199·2) or mebeverine hydrochloride (p.1199·2).
Gastro-intestinal and biliary tract disorders.

Dustinex HAL, Neth.
House-dust mite extracts.
Hyposensitisation.

Dutimelan Hoechst Marion Roussel, Ital.
Ten tablets, prednisolone acetate (p.1048·1); prednisolone (p.1048·1); ten tablets, prednisolone; cortisone acetate (p.1036·1).
Oral corticosteroid.

Dutonin
Bristol-Myers Squibb, Irl.; Bristol-Myers Squibb, Neth.; Bristol-Myers Squibb, UK.
Nefazodone hydrochloride (p.299·3).
Depression.

Duvadilan
Solvay, Austral.; Solvay, Belg.; Solvay, Fr.; Duphar, Ger.†; Solvay, Irl.; Solvay, Ital.; Solvay, Neth.; Duphar, Spain; Duphar, UK†.
Isoxsuprine hydrochloride (p.1592·1) or isoxsuprine resinate (p.1592·1).
Cerebral and peripheral vascular disorders; premature labour.

Duvaline Almirall, Spain†.
Pyricarbate (p.1624·1).
Arteriosclerosis; peripheral vascular disorders.

Duvaline Compositum Almirall, Spain†.
A heparinoid (p.882·3); inosine (p.1591·1); pyricarbate (p.1624·1); pyridoxine aceglutamate (p.1363·1); xanthinol nicotinate (p.971·1).
Arteriosclerosis; cerebrovascular insufficiency; hyperlipidaemias.

Duvaline Flebo Almirall, Spain†.
Pyricarbate (p.1624·1); troxerutin (p.1580·2).
Vascular disorders.

Duvium
Zambon, Belg.; Inpharzam, Switz.
Benorylate (p.21·2).
Fever; musculoskeletal and joint disorders; pain.

Duvoid
Roberts, Canad.; Roberts, USA.
Bethanechol chloride (p.1389·3).
Urinary retention.

Duxil Therval, Fr.
Almitrine (p.1477·2) or almitrine dimesylate (p.1477·2); raubasine (p.941·3).
Mental function impairment in the elderly.

Duxima Ecobi, Ital.
Cefuroxime sodium (p.177·1).
Bacterial infections.

Duxor Servier, Spain.
Raubasine (p.941·3); almitrine dimesylate (p.1477·2).
Cerebrovascular disorders; vestibular disorders.

DV Marion Merrell Dow, USA.
Dienoestrol (p.1444·1).
Menopausal vulval and vaginal atrophy.

D_3-Vicotrat Heyl, Ger.
Cholecalciferol (p.1366·3).
Vitamin D deficiency.

D-Vi-Sol Mead Johnson, Canad.
Vitamin D (p.1366·3).
Vitamin supplement.

D-Worm Triomed, S.Afr.
Mebendazole (p.104·1).
Worm infections.

Dyazide
SmithKline Beecham, Austral.; SmithKline Beecham, Canad.; SmithKline Beecham, Irl.; SmithKline Beecham, S.Afr.; SmithKline Beecham, Switz.; SmithKline Beecham, UK; SmithKline Beecham, USA.
Hydrochlorothiazide (p.885·2); triamterene (p.957·2).
These ingredients can be described by the British Approved Name Co-triamterzide.
Hypertension; oedema.

Dycholium Ciba Self Medication, Canad.
Dehydrocholic acid (p.1570·2).
Biliary-tract disorders.

Dycill SmithKline Beecham, USA.
Dicloxacillin sodium (p.202·1).
Bacterial infections.

Dyclone Astra, USA.
Dyclocaine hydrochloride (p.1292·3).
Local anaesthesia.

Dycol Delandale, UK†.
Sodium chloride; potassium chloride; sodium citrate; glucose (p.1152·3).
Diarrhoea; oral rehydration therapy.

Dyflex Econo Med, USA†.
Diprophylline (p.752·1).
Asthma; bronchospasm.

Dyflex-G Econo Med, USA.
Diprophylline (p.752·1); guaiphenesin (p.1061·3).
Bronchospasm.

Dygratyl Solvay Duphar, Swed.
Dihydrotachysterol (p.1366·3).
Hypocalcaemia; osteomalacia; rickets; secondary hyperparathyroidism.

Dyka-D Vesta, S.Afr.
Chlorpheniramine maleate (p.405·1); phenylephrine hydrochloride (p.1066·2); hyoscine methonitrate (p.463·1).
Hypersensitivity reactions; nasal congestion.

Dykatuss Vesta, S.Afr.†.
Chlorpheniramine maleate (p.405·1); phenylephrine hydrochloride (p.1066·2); hyoscine methonitrate (p.463·1).
Hypersensitivity reactions; nasal congestion.

Dykatuss Co Vesta, S.Afr.
Mepyramine maleate (p.414·1); ephedrine hydrochloride (p.1059·3); codeine phosphate (p.26·1).
Cold symptoms; coughs.

Dykatuss Expectorant Vesta, S.Afr.†.
Pentoxyverine citrate (p.1066·1); terpin hydrate (p.1070·2); sodium citrate (p.1153·2).
Coughs.

Dykatuss "S" Vesta, S.Afr.†.
Fedrilate (p.1061·1).
Coughs.

Dyline GG Seatrace, USA.
Diprophylline (p.752·1); guaiphenesin (p.1061·3).
Bronchospasm.

Dymadon Warner-Lambert, Austral.
Paracetamol (p.72·2).
Fever; pain.

Dymadon Co Warner-Lambert, Austral.
Paracetamol (p.72·2); codeine phosphate (p.26·1).
Pain.

Dymadon Forte Glaxo Wellcome, Austral.
Paracetamol (p.72·2); codeine phosphate (p.26·1).
Pain.

Dymelor Lilly, USA.
Acetohexamide (p.318·1).
Diabetes mellitus.

Dymenate Keene, USA.
Dimenhydrinate (p.408·2).
Motion sickness.

Dymion Pulitzer, Ital.
Ubidecarenone (p.1641·2).
Cardiac disorders; co-enzyme Q deficiency.

Dyn IBIS, Ital.†.
Food for special diets.
Hyperlipidaemias; weight reduction.

Dyna Jets Roche, S.Afr.
Multivitamin preparation.

Dyna Paks Suisse, Austral.†.
Bee pollen; royal jelly; pollen extract; chlorophyll; siberian ginseng; ginseng; sarsaparilla; calcium ascorbate; sodium ascorbate; bioflavonoids; pantothenic acid; *d*-alpha tocopheryl acid succinate; potassium aspartate; lecithin; liquorice; eleutherococcus; bladderwrack; fo-ti-tieng; gotu cola; kola nut; liver extracts.
Tonic.

Dyna-Ampcil Salters, S.Afr.
Ampicillin trihydrate (p.153·2).
Bacterial infections.

Dynabac
Lilly, Fr.; Bock, USA; Sanofi Winthrop, USA.
Dirithromycin (p.202·2).
Bacterial infections.

Dynablok Dynamed, S.Afr.†.
Propranolol hydrochloride (p.937·1).
Angina pectoris; arrhythmias; hypertension; hyperthyroidism; phaeochromocytoma; tremor.

Dynabolon
Fournier, Ital.; Theramex, Mon.
Nandrolone undecanoate (p.1452·2).
Anabolic; osteoporosis.

Dynacil Schwarz, Ger.; Sanol, Ger.
Fosinopril sodium (p.870·3).
Hypertension.

Dynacin Medicis, USA.
Minocycline hydrochloride (p.226·2).

Dynacirc
Sandoz, Canad.†; Novartis, S.Afr.; Novartis, USA.
Isradipine (p.894·2).
Hypertension.

Dynacold Thuasne, Fr.
Dichlorodifluoromethane (p.1164·3); trichlorofluoromethane (p.1164·3).
Joint and muscle pain.

Dynadol Salters, S.Afr.
Paracetamol (p.72·2).
Pain.

Dynafed Asthma Relief BDI, USA.
Ephedrine hydrochloride (p.1059·3); guaiphenesin (p.1061·3).
Coughs.

Dynafed IB BDI, USA.
Ibuprofen (p.44·1).
Fever; musculoskeletal and joint disorders; pain.

Dynafed Pseudo BDI, USA.
Pseudoephedrine hydrochloride (p.1068·3).
Nasal congestion.

Dynafemme Diepha, Fr.
Vitamin, mineral, and fish oil preparation.
Nutritional supplement.

Dynagastrin Salters, S.Afr.
Dicyclomine hydrochloride (p.460·1); dried aluminium hydroxide gel (p.1177·3); light magnesium oxide (p.1198·3).
Gastric hyperacidity.

Dyna-Hex Western Medical, USA.
Chlorhexidine gluconate (p.1107·2).
Skin disinfection.

Dynalert Restan, S.Afr.
Pemoline (p.1484·1).
Fatigue; stimulant.

Dynalin Dynamed, S.Afr.†.
Diphenhydramine hydrochloride (p.409·1); ammonium chloride (p.1055·2); sodium citrate (p.1153·2).
Coughs.

Dynametcin Dynamed, S.Afr.†.
Indomethacin (p.45·2).
Gout; musculoskeletal and joint disorders.

Dynametron Salters, S.Afr.
Metronidazole (p.585·1).
Anaerobic bacterial infections; protozoal infections.

Dynamide Dynamed, S.Afr.†.
Metoclopramide hydrochloride (p.1200·3).
Gastro-intestinal disorders.

Dynamin
Note. This name is used for preparations of different composition.
Ern, Spain.
Vitamin B substances; haematoporphyrin; amino acids; glutathione; nucleosides; procaine hydrochloride; orotic acid; magnesium molybdate; pemoline magnesium.
Tonic.

Berk, UK.
Isosorbide mononitrate (p.893·3).
Angina pectoris; heart failure.

Dynamisan
Wander, Belg.; Sandoz, Fr.; Novartis, Ital.; Sandoz OTC, Switz.
Arginine aspartate (p.1334·2) or arginine glutamate (p.1334·1).
Tonic.

Dynamo Key, Austral.
Caffeine (p.749·3); glucose (p.1343·3); thiamine hydrochloride (p.1361·1); nicotinic acid (p.1351·2).
Drowsiness; mental fatigue.

Dynamogen Faes, Spain.
Arginine aspartate (p.1334·2); glutodina.
Anorexia; tonic; weight loss.

Dynamol Eberth, Ger.†.
Garlic (p.1583·1); theobromine (p.765·1); chlorophyllin (p.1000·1); activated charcoal (p.972·2).
Arteriosclerosis; gastro-intestinal disorders; hypertension; menopausal disorders.

Dynamucil Siphar, Switz.
Acetylcysteine (p.1052·3).
Respiratory-tract disorders with viscous mucus.

Dynapam Dynamed, S.Afr.†.
Diazepam (p.661·1).
Alcohol withdrawal syndrome; anxiety; premedication.

Dynapayne Salters, S.Afr.
Paracetamol (p.72·2); codeine phosphate (p.26·1); promethazine (p.416·2).
Fever; pain.

Dynapen
Note. This name is used for preparations of different composition.
Merck, Aust.†.
Sultamicillin (p.257·2) or sultamicillin tosylate (p.257·2).
Bacterial infections.

Dynamed, S.Afr.
Phenoxymethylpenicillin potassium (p.236·2).
Bacterial infections.

Apothecon, USA.
Dicloxacillin sodium (p.202·1).
Bacterial infections.

Dynaphlem Dynamed, S.Afr.†.
Carbocisteine (p.1056·3).
Respiratory-tract disorders.

Dynaphos-C Sofar, Ital.
Ascorbic acid (p.1365·2).
Gingivitis; stomatitis; vitamin C deficiency.

Dynaplex Chemedica, Switz.
Multivitamin and amino-acid preparation.

Dynaspor Salters, S.Afr.
Clotrimazole (p.376·3).
Fungal infections.

Dynatra
Sintesa, Belg.; Zambon, Neth.
Dopamine hydrochloride (p.861·1).
Hypotension; shock.

Dynavent Piam, Ital.†.
Carbuterol hydrochloride (p.751·3).
Respiratory-tract disorders.

Dynavital Monal, Fr.
A range of trace element preparations.

Dynazole Salters, S.Afr.
Co-trimoxazole (p.196·3).
Bacterial infections.

Dynef Basotherm, Ger.
Anthocyanins from myrtillus; alpha tocopheryl acetate (p.1369·1).
Eye disorders.

Dyneric Henning, Ger.
Clomiphene citrate (p.1439·2).
Anovulatory infertility.

Dynese Galen, UK.
Magaldrate (p.1198·1).
Dyspepsia.

Dynexan
Note. This name is used for preparations of different composition.
Provita, Aust.; Kreussler, Ger.†; Mer-National, S.Afr.; Kreussler, Switz.
Ointment: Amethocaine hydrochloride (p.1285·2); chamomile (p.1561·2); arnica (p.1550·3); sage (p.1627·1); aluminium formate.
Mouth and throat disorders.

Vernleigh, S.Afr.†.
Oral powder: Amethocaine hydrochloride (p.1285·2); chlorophyllin (p.1000·1); chamomile (p.1561·2); arnica (p.1550·3); sage (p.1627·1); aluminium formate.
Mouth and throat disorders.

Dynexan A Kreussler, Ger.
Lignocaine hydrochloride (p.1293·2); benzalkonium chloride (p.1101·3).
Painful inflammatory disorders of the mouth.

Dynexan MHP *Kreussler, Ger.†.*
Laureth 9 (p.1325·2); dequalinium chloride (p.1112·1).
Bacterial and fungal infections associated with dentures.

Dynofen *Salters, S.Afr.*
Ibuprofen (p.44·1).
Musculoskeletal and joint disorders.

Dynorm *Merck, Ger.; Roche, Ger.*
Cilazapril (p.840·3).
Hypertension.

Dynorm Plus *Merck, Ger.; Roche, Ger.*
Cilazapril (p.840·3); hydrochlorothiazide (p.885·2).
Hypertension.

Dynos *Intramed, S.Afr.*
Dopamine hydrochloride (p.861·1).
Heart failure; shock.

Dynothel *Henning, Ger.*
Dextrothyroxine sodium (p.1272·2).
Hyperlipidaemias.

Dynoxytet *Salters, S.Afr.*
Oxytetracycline hydrochloride (p.235·1).
Bacterial infections.

Dyphylline-GG *Silarx, USA.*
Diprophylline (p.752·1); guaiphenesin (p.1061·3).
Asthma with associated cough.

Dyprotex
Note. This name is used for preparations of different composition.
Blistex, Canad.†.
Dimethicone (p.1384·2); zinc oxide (p.1096·2).
Nappy rash.

Blistex, USA.
Dimethicone (p.1384·2); zinc oxide (p.1096·2); cod-liver oil (p.1337·3).
Nappy rash.

Dyrenium
SmithKline Beecham, Canad.; SmithKline Beecham, Switz.; SmithKline Beecham, USA.
Triamterene (p.957·2).
Heart failure; oedema.

Dyrenium compositum *SmithKline Beecham, Switz.*
Triamterene (p.957·2); benzthiazide (p.828·1).
Hypertension; oedema.

Dyrexan-OD *Trimen, USA.*
Phendimetrazine tartrate (p.1484·2).
Obesity.

Dyrosol *Vesta, S.Afr.*
Bismuth salicylate (p.1180·1); codeine phosphate (p.26·1); atropine sulphate (p.455·1).
Diarrhoea.

Dyscornut-N *Weber & Weber, Ger.*
Homoeopathic preparation.

Dysdolen *Wander, Ger.†.*
Ibuprofen (p.44·1).
Inflammation; musculoskeletal and joint disorders.

Dyskinebyl *Zyma, Fr.*
Dihydroxydibutylether (p.1571·3).
Dyspepsia.

Dysman *Ashbourne, UK.*
Mefenamic acid (p.51·2).
Dysfunctional menorrhagia; pain.

Dysmenalgit *Krewel, Ger.*
Naproxen (p.61·2).
Pain.

Dysmenosyx *Syxyl, Ger.†.*
Homoeopathic preparation.

Dyspagon *Pierre Fabre, Fr.*
Loperamide hydrochloride (p.1197·2).
Diarrhoea.

Dyspamet
SmithKline Beecham, Irl.; SmithKline Beecham, UK.
Cimetidine (p.1183·2).
Gastric hyperacidity; gastro-oesophageal reflux; peptic ulcer; Zollinger-Ellison syndrome.

Dyspne-Inhal *Augot, Fr.*
Adrenaline (p.813·2).
Asthma; glottal oedema.

Dysport
IPSEN Biotech, Fr.; Ipsen, Irl.; Ipsen, Ital.; Speywood, UK.
Botulinum A toxin (p.1310·1).
Blepharospasm; hemifacial spasm; spasmodic torticollis.

dysto-L 90 N *Loges, Ger.*
Homoeopathic preparation.

dysto-loges *Loges, Ger.*
Homoeopathic preparation.

Dystomin E *Redel, Ger.†.*
Magnesium peroxide (p.1119·1); sal carol. fact.; light magnesium carbonate (p.1198·1); bismuth subnitrate (p.1180·2); kaolin (p.1195·1); tannin; vegetable charcoal (p.972·3); sodium bicarbonate (p.1153·2).
Gastro-intestinal disorders.

Dystomin forte *Redel, Ger.†.*
Heavy magnesium carbonate (p.1198·1); bismuth subnitrate (p.1180·2); calcium carbonate (p.1182·1); sodium bicarbonate (p.1153·2); belladonna (p.457·1); gelsemium (p.1583·2).
Gastro-intestinal disorders.

Dystomin M *Redel, Ger.*
Heavy magnesium oxide (p.1198·3).
Gastric hyperacidity.

Dystonal *Pharmethic, Belg.*
Belladonna extract (p.457·1); ergotamine tartrate (p.445·3); phenobarbitone (p.350·2).
Agitation; anxiety; dyspepsia; dystonia; fatigue; insomnia; irritability; Ménière's disease; migraine; motion sickness; urinary incontinence; urticaria.

Dystophan *Kattwiga, Ger.*
Homoeopathic preparation.

Dystoselect *Dreluso, Ger.†.*
Homoeopathic preparation.

Dysurgal *Disperga, Aust.*
Atropine sulphate (p.455·1); ephedrine hydrochloride (p.1059·3); strychnine nitrate (p.1633·1).
Urinary-tract disorders.

Dysurgal N *Galenika, Ger.*
Atropine sulphate (p.455·1).
Dysurgal formerly contained atropine sulphate, ephedrine hydrochloride, and strychnine nitrate.
Dysmenorrhoea; urinary-tract disorders.

Dytac
SmithKline Beecham, Austral.†; SK-RIT, Belg.†; Smith Kline & French, Irl.†; SmithKline Beecham, Neth.; Pharmark, UK.
Triamterene (p.957·2).
Hypertension; oedema.

Dyta-Urese
SMB, Belg.; SmithKline Beecham, Neth.
Triamterene (p.957·2); epithiazide (p.865·3).
Hypertension; oedema.

Dytenzide
SK-RIT, Belg.; SmithKline Beecham, Neth.
Triamterene (p.957·2); hydrochlorothiazide (p.885·2).
Hypertension; oedema.

Dytide
Smith Kline & French, Irl.†; Pharmark, UK.
Triamterene (p.957·2); benzthiazide (p.828·1).
Oedema.

Dytide H
Procter & Gamble, Aust.; Procter & Gamble, Ger.
Triamterene (p.957·2); hydrochlorothiazide (p.885·2).
Heart failure; hypertension; oedema.

Dytuss *Lunsco, USA.*
Diphenhydramine hydrochloride (p.409·1).

E45
Boots, Austral.; Boots Healthcare, Irl.; Boots, S.Afr.; Crookes Healthcare, UK.
Emollient.
Dry skin disorders.

E Perle *Scherer, Ital.†.*
d-Alpha tocopheryl acetate (p.1369·2).
Vitamin E deficiency.

EAP-61 *Hanosan, Ger.*
Homoeopathic preparation.

Ear Clear *Key, Austral.*
Urea hydrogen peroxide (p.1127·3).
Ear wax removal.

Ear Clear for Swimmer's Ear *Key, Austral.*
Acetic acid (p.1541·2); isopropyl alcohol (p.1118·2).
Otitis externa.

Earache Pain *Homeocan, Canad.*
Homoeopathic preparation.

Ear-Dry *Scherer, USA.*
Boric acid (p.1554·2); isopropyl alcohol (p.1118·2).
Ear disorders.

Earex *Seton, UK.*
Arachis oil (p.1550·2); almond oil (p.1546·2); rectified camphor oil.
Ear wax removal.

Earex Plus *Seton, UK.*
Choline salicylate (p.25·2); glycerol (p.1585·2).
Ear wax removal; earache.

Ear-Eze *Hyrex, USA.*
Hydrocortisone (p.1043·3); neomycin sulphate (p.229·2); polymyxin B (p.239·3).
Bacterial ear infections.

Early Bird
Note. This name is used for preparations of different composition.
Mentholatum, Austral.
Pyrantel embonate (p.109·3).
Enterobiasis.

Kent, UK†.
Fertility test (p.1621·2).

Kent, UK.
Pregnancy test (p.1621·2).

Early Detector *Warner-Lambert, USA†.*
Test for occult blood in faeces.

EarSol *Parnell, USA.*
Alcohol (p.1099·1).
Ear disorders.

EarSol-HC *Parnell, USA.*
Hydrocortisone (p.1043·3); alcohol (p.1099·1).
Ear inflammation.

EAS *Fresenius, Switz.*
Amino-acid preparation.
Nutritional supplement in renal failure.

Ease Pain Away *RMC, Canad.*
Menthol (p.1600·2); triethanolamine salicylate (p.1639·2).

Easistix BG *Eastern Pharmaceuticals, UK.*
Test for glucose in blood (p.1585·1).

Easistix UG *Eastern Pharmaceuticals, UK.*
Test for glucose in urine (p.1585·1).

Easprin *Parke, Davis, USA.*
Aspirin (p.16·1).
Fever; inflammation; pain.

Easy Check *Solent, UK†.*
Pregnancy test kit (p.1621·2).

Easy hCG *Carter-Wallace, Austral.†.*
Pregnancy test (p.1621·2).

Easy Strip *Boehringer Mannheim, Canad.*
Test for glucose in blood (p.1585·1).

Eatan N *Desitin, Ger.*
Nitrazepam (p.682·2).
Sleep disorders.

Eau Precieuse Depensier *Phygiene, Fr.*
Boric acid (p.1554·2); resorcinol (p.1090·1); salicylic acid (p.1090·2); tannic acid (p.1634·2); lysol (p.1111·2); phenol (p.1121·2); menthol (p.1600·2).
Skin disorders.

Eau-de-vie de France avec huile de pin nain du Tirol *Luond, Switz.*
Menthol (p.1600·2); pumilio pine oil (p.1623·3).
Muscular pain and fatigue.

Eavit *Terapeutico, Ital.*
Gelatin; wheat-germ oil; carrot oil; soya lecithin; royal jelly; beeswax.
Nutritional supplement.

E-Base *Barr, USA.*
Erythromycin (p.204·1).
Bacterial infections.

Ebastel *Almirall, Spain.*
Ebastine (p.410·2).
Hypersensitivity reactions.

Ebenol *Strathmann, Ger.*
Hydrocortisone acetate (p.1043·3).
Skin disorders.

Ebexol *Lyssia, Belg.†.*
Sodium dibunate (p.1070·1); guaiphenesin (p.1061·3); bergamot oil (p.1553·1); niaouli oil (p.1607·1); camphor (p.1557·2); guaiacol (p.1061·2).
Coughs; throat disorders.

Eblimon *Guidotti, Ital.†.*
Chlormezanone (p.648·3); dipyrone (p.35·1); codeine phosphate (p.26·1); caffeine (p.749·3).
Pain.

Ebrantil
Byk, Aust.; Byk, Belg.; Byk Gulden, Ger.; Byk Gulden, Ital.; Byk, Neth.; Byk, Switz.
Urapidil (p.959·2), urapidil fumarate (p.959·2), or urapidil hydrochloride (p.959·2).
Hypertension.

Ebrocit *Robert, Spain.*
Ebrotidine (p.1191·3).
Peptic ulcer.

Ebufac *DDSA Pharmaceuticals, UK.*
Ibuprofen (p.44·1).

Eburdent F *Acro, Ital.*
Miristalkonium saccharinate (p.1119·3); sodium fluoride (p.742·1).
Dental caries prophylaxis; oral hygiene.

Eburnal *Chiesi, Ital.*
Vinburnine phosphate (p.1644·1).
Cerebrovascular disorders.

Eburnoxin *Astra, Spain.*
Vinburnine (p.1644·1).
Cerebrovascular disorders; retinopathies.

Eburos *Acro, Ital.*
Chlorhexidine gluconate (p.1107·2).
Oral hygiene.

Ecabil *Biologici Italia, Ital.*
Heparin calcium (p.879·3).
Thrombo-embolic disorders.

Ecadiu *Vita Elan, Spain.*
Hydrochlorothiazide (p.885·2); captopril (p.836·3).
Hypertension.

Ecafast *Crinos, Ital.*
Heparin calcium (p.879·3).
Thrombo-embolic disorders.

Ecamannan *CaDiGroup, Ital.*
Glucomannan (p.1584·3); vitamin E (p.1369·1); vitamin C (p.1365·2); betacarotene (p.1335·2).
Arteriosclerosis; cellular ageing.

Ecasolv *Lepetit, Ital.*
Heparin calcium (p.879·3).
Thrombo-embolic disorders.

Ecazide
Bristol-Myers Squibb, Fr.; Squibb, Spain.
Captopril (p.836·3); hydrochlorothiazide (p.885·2).
Hypertension.

Eccarvit *CaDiGroup, Ital.*
Vitamin C (p.1365·2); vitamin E (p.1369·1); betacarotene (p.1335·2).
Antoxidant nutritional supplement.

Eccelium *Manetti Roberts, Ital.*
Econazole sulfosalicylate (p.377·2).
Fungal infections; Gram-positive bacterial superinfections.

Ecdylin *De Witt, UK.*
Diphenhydramine (p.409·1); ammonium chloride (p.1055·2).
Coughs.

Ecee Plus *Edwards, USA.*
Vitamins C and E with minerals.

Echan *Biocur, Ger.*
Echinacea purpura (p.1574·2).
Respiratory- and urinary-tract infections.

Echiherb *Duopharm, Ger.*
Echinacea purpurea (p.1574·2).
Infections of the respiratory and urinary tracts.

Echina Pro *Planta, Canad.*
Echinacea (p.1574·2).
Cold and influenza symptoms.

Echinacea *Pfluger, Ger.†.*
Homoeopathic preparation.

Echinacea ACE Plus Zinc *Blackmores, Austral.*
Echinacea angustifolia (p.1574·2); vitamins; zinc amino acid chelate (p.1373·3); garlic (p.1583·1).
Tonic.

Echinacea akut *Hevert, Ger.*
Homoeopathic preparation.

Echinacea & Antioxidants *Vitaplex, Austral.*
Ascorbic acid (p.1365·2); *d*-alpha tocopheryl acid succinate (p.1369·2); zinc gluconate (p.1373·2); echinacea (p.1574·2); garlic (p.1583·1).
Upper respiratory-tract disorders.

Echinacea comp
Hevert, Ger.†; Steigerwald, Ger.
Homoeopathic preparation.

Echinacea Herbal Plus Formula *Vitelle, Austral.*
Multivitamins with echinacea and zinc amino acid chelate (p.1574·2 and p.1373·3).
Minor upper respiratory-tract disorders; skin disorders.

Echinacea Hevert purp. forte *Hevert, Ger.*
Echinacea purpurea (p.1574·2).
Immunomodulator.

Echinacea L40 *Homeocan, Canad.*
Homoeopathic preparation.

Echinacea Med Complex *Dynamit, Aust.*
Homoeopathic preparation.

Echinacea Oligoplex *Madaus, Ger.*
Homoeopathic preparation.

Echinacea Plus *Eagle, Austral.*
Echinacea (p.1574·2); astragalus membranaceus; schizandra chinensis; tabebuia avellanedae.
Minor infections; tonic.

Echinacea Rodler *Rodler, Ger.†.*
Homoeopathic preparation.

Echinacea Ro-Plex (Rowo-298) *Pharmakon, Ger.†.*
Homoeopathic preparation.

Echinacea Ro-Plex (Rowo-415) *Pharmakon, Ger.†.*
Homoeopathic preparation.

Echinacea Ro-Plex (Rowo-849) *Pharmakon, Ger.†.*
Homoeopathic preparation.

Echinacea Urtinktur *Hevert, Ger.*
Homoeopathic preparation.

Echinacea-Complex *Weber & Weber, Ger.*
Homoeopathic preparation.

Echinacin
Polcopharma, Austral.; Madaus, Ger.
Echinacea purpurea (p.1574·2).
Infections of the respiratory and urinary tracts; wounds.

Echinaforce
Bio-Garten, Aust.; Bioforce, Ger.; Bioforce, Switz.
Echinacea purpurea (p.1574·2).
Cold symptoms; fever; mild infections.

Echinapur *Lappe, Ger.*
Echinacea purpura (p.1574·2).
Respiratory- and urinary-tract infections.

Echinarell *Sanorell, Ger.*
Homoeopathic preparation.

Echinasyx *Syxyl, Ger.*
Homoeopathic preparation.

Echinatruw *Truw, Ger.†.*
Echinacea purpurea (p.1574·2).
Infections of the respiratory and urinary tracts.

Echine *Eagle, Austral.*
Herbal and homoeopathic antiseptic.

Echnatol *Gerot, Aust.*
Cyclizine hydrochloride (p.407·1).
Motion sickness; nausea and vomiting.

Echnatol B_6 *Gerot, Aust.*
Cyclizine hydrochloride (p.407·1); pyridoxine hydrochloride (p.1362·3).
Inner ear disorders; Ménière's disease; motion sickness; nausea and vomiting; vertigo.

Echovist
Schering, Aust.; Schering, Fr.; Schering, Ger.; Schering, Neth.; Schering, Norw.; Schering, S.Afr.; Schering, Swed.; Schering, Switz.; Schering, UK.
Galactose (p.1005·2).
Ultrasound contrast medium.

Echtroferment-N *Weber & Weber, Ger.*
Aniseed (p.1549·3); caraway (p.1559·3); fennel (p.1579·1); potentilla anserina.
Gastro-intestinal disorders.

Echtromint *Weber & Weber, Ger.†.*
Peppermint oil (p.1208·1); echinacea purpurea (p.1574·2); hypericum oil (p.1590·1); melissa oil.
Angina pectoris; gastro-intestinal disorders; insect bites; migraine; neuralgia; respiratory-tract disorders; rheumatism.

Echtronephrin-N *Weber & Weber, Ger.†.*
Homoeopathic preparation.

Echtronerval-N *Weber & Weber, Ger.*
Homoeopathic preparation.

Echtrosept-GT *Weber & Weber, Ger.†.*
Lactic acid (p.1593·3); peppermint leaf (p.1208·1); echinacea purpurea (p.1574·2); tropaeolum majus; arnica (p.1550·3); clove (p.1565·2); chamomile

(p.1561·2); myrrh (p.1606·1); rhatany root (p.1624·3); sage (p.1627·1).
Inflammatory disorders of the oropharynx.

Echtrosept-N *Weber & Weber, Ger.*
Homoeopathic preparation.

Echtrovit-K *Weber & Weber, Ger.*
Procaine hydrochloride (p.1299·2); vitamins; rutin (p.1580·2).
Tonic.

Eclaran *Pierre Fabre, Fr.*
Benzoyl peroxide (p.1079·2).
Acne.

Eclipse Lip and Face *Triangle, USA.*
SPF 15: Padimate O (p.1488·1); oxybenzone (p.1487·3).
Sunscreen.

Eco Mi *Geymonat, Ital.*
Econazole nitrate (p.377·2).
Fungal skin or vulvovaginal infections.

Ecocain *Molteni, Ital.*
Lignocaine hydrochloride (p.1293·2).
Adrenaline acid tartrate (p.813·3) is included in some injections as a vasoconstrictor to diminish absorption and localise the effect of the local anaesthetic.
Local anaesthesia.

Ecodergin *Von Boch, Ital.†.*
Econazole nitrate (p.377·2).
Vulvo-vaginal or dermatological fungal infections.

Ecodipine *Ecosol, Switz.*
Nifedipine (p.916·2).
Hypertension; ischaemic heart disease; Raynaud's syndrome.

Ecodurex *Ecosol, Switz.*
Hydrochlorothiazide (p.885·2); amiloride hydrochloride (p.819·2).
Hypertension; oedema.

Ecoendocilli Testimonia *Istoria, Ital.*
Lactic-acid-producing organisms (p.1594·1); vitamins.
Disturbances of the gastro-intestinal flora; nutritional supplement.

Ecofenac *Ecosol, Switz.*
Diclofenac sodium (p.31·2).
Gout; inflammation; musculoskeletal, joint, and peri-articular disorders; pain.

Ecofermenti *Echo, Ital.*
Lactic-acid-producing organisms (p.1594·1); vitamins.
Disturbances of the gastro-intestinal flora.

Ecofibra *Echo, Ital.*
Dietary fibre supplement (p.1181·2).
Delayed gastro-intestinal transit; obesity.

Ecoflorina *Ecobi, Ital.*
Lactic-acid-producing organisms (p.1594·1).
Nutritional supplement.

Ecofol *Ecobi, Ital.*
Calcium folinate (p.1342·2).
Anaemias; antidote to overdosage with folic acid antagonists; folic acid deficiency.

Ecogel *Ecobi, Ital.†.*
Royal jelly (p.1626·3).

Ecolicin *ankerpharm, Ger.*
Erythromycin lactobionate (p.204·2); colistin sulphomethate sodium (p.196·1).
Bacterial eye infections.

Ecomitrin *Syntex, Spain†.*
Amphomycin calcium (p.153·1); hydrocortisone (p.1043·3); neomycin hydrochloride (p.230·1).
Infected skin disorders.

Ecomucyl *Ecosol, Switz.*
Acetylcysteine (p.1052·3).
Paracetamol overdosage; respiratory-tract disorders.

Ecomytrin
Lundbeck, Aust.; Lundbeck, Swed.†.
Amphomycin calcium (p.153·1); neomycin hydrochloride (p.230·1).
Infected skin disorders.

Ecomytrin-Hydrocortison
Lundbeck, Aust.; Lundbeck, Norw.†; Lundbeck, Swed.†; Lundbeck, Switz.†.
Amphomycin calcium (p.153·1); neomycin hydrochloride (p.230·1); hydrocortisone (p.1043·3).
Eye infections; infected skin disorders; otitis externa.

Econacort *Squibb, UK.*
Econazole nitrate (p.377·2); hydrocortisone (p.1043·3).
Infected skin disorders.

Economycin *DDSA Pharmaceuticals, UK.*
Tetracycline hydrochloride (p.259·1).

Econopred *Alcon, USA.*
Prednisolone acetate (p.1048·1).
Eye disorders.

Ecopan *Ecosol, Switz.†.*
Mefenamic acid (p.51·2).
Fever; inflammation; pain.

Ecoprofen *Ecosol, Switz.*
Ibuprofen (p.44·1).
Inflammation; musculoskeletal, joint, and peri-articular disorders; pain.

Ecorex *Tosi, Ital.*
Econazole nitrate (p.377·2).
Fungal or bacterial skin or vulvovaginal infections.

Ecoro *Eu Rho, Ger.*
d-Alpha tocopherol (p.1369·1).
Vitamin E deficiency.

Ecosporina *Ecobi, Ital.*
Cephradine (p.181·3).
Bacterial infections.

Ecostatin
Bristol-Myers Squibb, Austral.; Westwood-Squibb, Canad.; Bristol-Myers Squibb, Irl.; Squibb, UK.
Econazole nitrate (p.377·2).
Fungal infections.

Ecotam *Alacan, Spain.*
Econazole nitrate (p.377·2).
Fungal infections.

Ecotrin
SmithKline Beecham Consumer, Austral.; SmithKline Beecham Consumer, Canad.†; SmithKline Beecham, S.Afr.; SmithKline Beecham Consumer, USA.
Aspirin (p.16·1).
Fever; inflammation; myocardial infarction; pain; recurrent transient ischaemic attacks.

Ecoval *Glaxo Wellcome, Ital.*
Betamethasone valerate (p.1033·3).
Skin and scalp disorders.

Ecoval con Neomicina *Glaxo Wellcome, Ital.*
Betamethasone valerate (p.1033·3); neomycin sulphate (p.229·2).
Infected skin disorders.

Ecovent *Ecosol, Switz.*
Salbutamol (p.758·2).
Obstructive airways disease.

Ecran Anti-Solaire *Clarins, Canad.*
SPF 25: Ethylhexyl *p*-methoxycinnamate (p.1487·1); oxybenzone (p.1487·3); 2-phenyl-1*H*-benzimidazole-5-sulphonic acid (p.1488·2); titanium dioxide (p.1093·3).
Sunscreen.

Ecran Total *Vichy, Canad.*
SPF 15; SPF 25; SPF 30: Avobenzone (p.1486·3); 3-(4-methylbenzylidene)bornan-2-one (p.1487·2); terephthalylidene dicamphor sulphonic acid; titanium dioxide (p.1093·3).
Sunscreen.

Ectodyne *Wigglesworth, UK.*
Piperazine citrate (p.107·2).
Ascariasis; enterobiasis.

Ectosone *Technilab, Canad.*
Betamethasone valerate (p.1033·3).
Skin disorders.

Ectren *Menarini, Spain.*
Quinapril hydrochloride (p.938·1).
Heart failure; hypertension.

Ecur Test *Boehringer Mannheim, Austral.*
Test for glucose, protein, and blood in urine.

Ecur 4-Test *Boehringer Mannheim, S.Afr.*
Test for leucocytes, glucose, protein, and blood in urine.

Ecur Test and Leucocytes *Boehringer Mannheim, Austral.*
Test for protein, glucose, blood, and leucocytes in urine.

Ecural *Essex, Ger.*
Mometasone furoate (p.1047·2).
Scalp disorders; skin disorders.

E-Cypionate *Legere, USA†.*
Oestradiol cypionate (p.1455·1).

Eczecur *Schering, Ital.†.*
Fluocortolone hexanoate (p.1041·3); fluocortolone pivalate (p.1041·3); chlorquinaldol (p.185·1).
Infected eczema.

Eczederm *Quinoderm, UK†.*
Calamine (p.1080·1); arachis oil (p.1550·2).
Skin disorders.

Eczema Cream *Hamilton, Austral.*
Coal tar (p.1092·3); silicone fluid (p.1384·2); zinc oxide (p.1096·2).
Dermatitis; eczema.

Eczema Ointment
Note. This name is used for preparations of different composition.
Stanley, Canad.
Bismuth subcarbonate (p.1180·1); salicylic acid (p.1090·2); zinc oxide (p.1096·2).

Potter's, UK.
Zinc oxide (p.1096·2); salicylic acid (p.1090·2); benzoic acid (p.1102·3); chickweed.
Eczema.

Ed A-Hist *Edwards, USA.*
Phenylephrine hydrochloride (p.1066·2); chlorpheniramine maleate (p.405·1).
Allergic rhinitis; nasal congestion.

ED Tuss HC *Edwards, USA.*
Phenylephrine hydrochloride (p.1066·2); chlorpheniramine maleate (p.405·1); hydrocodone tartrate (p.43·1).
Coughs and cold symptoms.

Ede *Teofarma, Ital.*
Metoclopramide (p.1202·1); simethicone (p.1213·1).
Gastro-intestinal disorders.

Ede 6 *Teofarma, Ital.*
Dimethicone (p.1213·1); pancreatin (p.1612·1).
Formerly contained bromelains, alpha-amylase, metoclopramide hydrochloride, dimethicone, pancreatin, and sodium dehydrocholate.
Digestive insufficiency.

Edecril *Merck Sharp & Dohme, Austral.*
Ethacrynic acid (p.866·3).
Oedema.

Edecrin
Merck Sharp & Dohme, Aust.; Merck Sharp & Dohme, Canad.; Merck Sharp & Dohme, Irl.; Merck Sharp & Dohme, Ital.; Merck Sharp & Dohme, Neth.; Merck Sharp & Dohme, Norw.†; Merck Sharp & Dohme, UK; Merck Sharp & Dohme, USA.
Ethacrynic acid (p.866·3) or sodium ethacrynate (p.866·3).
Oedema.

Edecrina *Merck Sharp & Dohme, Swed.*
Ethacrynic acid (p.866·3) or sodium ethacrynate (p.866·3).
Oedema.

Edemox *Wasserman, Spain.*
Acetazolamide (p.810·3).
Epilepsy; glaucoma; high-altitude disorders; oedema.

Ederal *Esteve, Spain.*
Cinnarizine (p.406·1); calcium dobesilate (p.1556·3).
Cerebrovascular disorders; vestibular disorders.

Edex
Schwarz, Fr.; Schwarz, USA.
Alprostadil (p.1412·2).
Impotence.

Ediluna *Vinas, Spain.*
Ibuprofen (p.44·1).
Fever; musculoskeletal and joint disorders; pain; peri-articular disorders.

Edirel *Inava, Fr.*
Erdosteine (p.1060·3).
Respiratory-tract congestion.

Edistol *Pierre Fabre, Spain†.*
Isosorbide mononitrate (p.893·1).
Angina pectoris; heart failure.

Ediwal *Schering, Ger.†.*
Levonorgestrel (p.1454·1); ethinyloestradiol (p.1445·1).
Combined oral contraceptive.

Edmilla *Hanseler, Switz.*
Chamomile (p.1561·2).
Inflammatory disorders of the skin and mouth.

Edolan *Lepetit, Ital.†.*
Etodolac (p.36·2).
Osteoarthritis; rheumatoid arthritis.

Edoxil *ICN, Spain.*
Amoxycillin trihydrate (p.151·3).
Bacterial infections.

Edoxil Mucolitico *ICN, Spain.*
Amoxycillin trihydrate (p.151·3); bromhexine hydrochloride (p.1055·3).
Respiratory-tract infections.

EDP-Evans Dermal Powder *Boots, Austral.*
Povidone-iodine (p.1123·3).
Formerly contained thymol iodide, bismuth oxyiodide, chlorbutol, magnesium carbonate, magnesium borate, and magnesium stearate.
Burns; chafing; tinea pedis; ulcers; wounds.

Edronax
Pharmacia Upjohn, Swed.; Pharmacia Upjohn, UK.
Reboxetine mesylate (p.307·1).
Depression.

ED-SPAZ *Edwards, USA.*
Hyoscyamine sulphate (p.464·2).

ED-TLC *Edwards, USA.*
Phenylephrine hydrochloride (p.1066·2); chlorpheniramine maleate (p.405·1); hydrocodone tartrate (p.43·1).
Coughs and cold symptoms.

Eductyl *Techni-Pharma, Mon.*
Potassium acid tartrate (p.1209·1); sodium bicarbonate (p.1153·2).
Bowel evacuation; constipation.

Edulcor codeine, tolu, laurier-cerise *Pierre Fabre, Fr.†.*
Codeine phosphate (p.26·1); cherry laurel; tolu balsam (p.1071·1).
Coughs.

Edulcor eucalyptus *Pierre Fabre, Fr.†.*
Eucalyptus oil (p.1578·1).
Sore throat.

Edulcor eucalyptus et menthol *Pierre Fabre, Fr.†.*
Eucalyptus oil (p.1578·1); menthol (p.1600·2).
Sore throat.

Edulcor sans sucre *Pierre Fabre, Fr.†.*
Pastilles acidulees: Acacia (p.1470·2); glycerol (p.1585·2).
Pastilles reglisse: Liquorice (p.1197·1); acacia (p.1470·2); glycerol (p.1585·2).
Sore throat.

Eduprim *FS Profas, Spain.*
Co-trimoxazole (p.196·3).
Bacterial infections; Pneumocystis carinii pneumonia.

Eduprim Mucolitico *FS Profas, Spain.*
Carbocisteine (p.1056·3); guaiphenesin (p.1061·3); co-trimoxazole (p.196·3).
Respiratory-tract infections.

Edurid *Medipharm, Switz.*
Edoxudine (p.609·2).
Herpes simplex infections.

Edusan Fte Rectal *Casen Fleet, Spain.*
Camphor (p.1557·2); cineole (p.1564·1); niaouli oil (p.1607·1); guaiacol (p.1061·2).
Respiratory-tract disorders.

Edym Sedante *Vita, Spain.*
Diazepam (p.661·1); dimethicone (p.1213·1); metoclopramide hydrochloride (p.1200·3); pancreatin (p.1612·1).
Gastro-intestinal disorders.

EES
Abbott, Austral.; Abbott, Canad.; Abbott, USA.
Erythromycin ethyl succinate (p.204·2).
Bacterial infections.

Eetless *Mer-National, S.Afr.*
Cathine hydrochloride (p.1478·1).
Obesity.

EFA Plus *Tyson, USA†.*
Omega 3, 6, and essential fatty acids (p.1276·1).

EFA Steri *Pharmavite, Canad.*
Sodium chloride (p.1162·2).

Efacal *Efamol, UK.*
Evening primrose oil (p.1582·1); fish oil (p.1276·1); calcium (p.1155·1).
Calcium supplement.

Efadermin *Galderma, Ger.*
Lithium succinate (p.1086·2); zinc sulphate (p.1373·2).
Seborrhoeic dermatitis.

Efagel *Mavi, Ital.*
Gamolenic acid (p.1582·1); vitamin E (p.1369·1).
Nutritional supplement.

Efalex *Novartis, UK.*
Marine fatty acids (p.1276·1); evening primrose oil (p.1582·1); thyme oil (p.1637·1).

Efalith
Searle, Irl.; Widmer, Switz.; Searle, UK.
Lithium succinate (p.1086·2); zinc sulphate (p.1373·2).
Seborrhoeic dermatitis.

Efamarine *Efamol, UK.*
Evening primrose oil (p.1582·1); marine fish oil (p.1276·1).
Formerly known as Efamol Marine.

Efamast *Searle, UK.*
Evening primrose oil (p.1582·1).
Mastalgia.

Efamol
Vita Glow, Austral.†; Efamol, Canad.; Serono OTC, Ital.†; Sidroga, Switz.; Efamol, UK.
Evening primrose oil (p.1582·1).
Nutritional supplement.

Efamol G *Efamed, S.Afr.*
Gamolenic acid (p.1582·1); linoleic acid (p.1582·1).
Nutritional supplement.

Efamol Marine Capsules *Vita Glow, Austral.†.*
Evening primrose oil (p.1582·1); marine fish oil (p.1276·1).
Prostaglandin modulator.

Efamol Plus Coenzyme Q10 *Efamol, UK.*
Evening primrose oil (p.1582·1); ubidecarenone (p.1641·2).
Tonic.

Efamol PMP *Efamol, UK.*
Evening primrose oil (p.1582·1); vitamins; minerals.
Premenstrual syndrome.

Efamol PMS *Murdock, USA†.*
Evening primrose oil (p.1582·1); omega-3 marine triglycerides (p.1276·1); vitamins and minerals.

Efamol Safflower & Linseed *Efamol, UK.*
Evening primrose oil (p.1582·1); linseed oil (p.1596·2); safflower oil (p.1353·3).

Efanatal *Efamol, UK.*
Fatty acids (p.1276·1); evening primrose oil (p.1582·1).
Nutritional supplement in pregnancy and lactation.

Efargen *Teofarma, Ital.*
Cyanocobalamin (p.1363·3); folic acid (p.1340·3); nicotinamide (p.1351·2); pyridoxine hydrochloride (p.1362·3).
Vitamin deficiency.

Efasit N *Togal, Ger.*
Plaster: Salicylic acid (p.1090·2).
Tincture: Salicylic acid (p.1090·2); lactic acid (p.1593·3).
Calluses; corns; hard skin.

Efatime *Efamol, UK.*
Fatty acids (p.1276·1); vitamin E (p.1369·1); red thyme oil.

Efavite *Efamol, UK.*
Multivitamin and mineral preparation.

Efcod *Covan, S.Afr.†.*
Aminophylline (p.748·1); mepyramine maleate (p.414·1); codeine phosphate (p.26·1); ephedrine hydrochloride (p.1059·3); ipecacuanha (p.1062·2).
Coughs; obstructive airways disease.

Efcortelan
Duncan, Flockhart, Austral.†.
Hydrocortisone sodium succinate (p.1044·1).
Corticosteroid.

Glaxo, UK.
Hydrocortisone (p.1043·3).
Skin disorders.

Efcortelan Soluble
Glaxo Wellcome, Irl.†; Glaxo, UK†.
Hydrocortisone sodium succinate (p.1044·1).
Corticosteroid.

Efcortesol *Glaxo, UK.*
Hydrocortisone sodium phosphate (p.1044·1).
Corticosteroid.

Efcospect *Covan, S.Afr.†.*
Potassium iodide (p.1493·1); ephedrine hydrochloride (p.1059·3); ipecacuanha (p.1062·2).
Respiratory-tract disorders.

Efedrocanfine Vis, Ital.†.
Ephedrine hydrochloride (p.1059·3); menthol (p.1600·2); camphor (p.1557·2); cineole (p.1564·1).
Respiratory congestion.

Efektolol Brenner-Efeka, Ger.
Propranolol hydrochloride (p.937·1).
Angina pectoris; arrhythmias; essential tremor; hypertension; hyperthyroidism; migraine.

Efemida Llorens, Spain.
Cephalexin (p.178·2).
Bacterial infections.

Efemolin Ciba Vision, Ger.
Fluorometholone (p.1042·1); tetrahydrozoline hydrochloride (p.1070·2).
Allergic and inflammatory disorders of the eye.

Efemoline
Ciba Vision, Ital.; Restan, S.Afr.; Ciba Vision, Switz.
Fluorometholone (p.1042·1); tetrahydrozoline hydrochloride (p.1070·2).
Allergic and inflammatory disorders of the eye.

Efensol Lasa, Spain.
Filicol.
Diarrhoea associated with malabsorption of bile acids; hypercholesterolaemia; pruritus associated with partial biliary obstruction.

Eferox Wyeth, Ger.
Thyroxine sodium (p.1497·1).
Hypothyroidism.

Efexor
Wyeth Lederle, Aust.; Wyeth, Austral.; Wyeth, Ital.; Wyeth, Neth.; Wyeth, S.Afr.; Wyeth Lederle, Swed.; Wyeth, Switz.; Wyeth, UK.
Venlafaxine hydrochloride (p.311·2).
Depression.

Effacne
Roche-Posay, Fr.; Roche Posay, Switz.
Benzoyl peroxide (p.1079·2).
Acne.

Effective Strength Cough Formula Barre-National, USA.
Chlorpheniramine maleate (p.405·1); dextromethorphan hydrobromide (p.1057·3).
Coughs and cold symptoms.

Effective Strength Cough Formula Liquid With Decongestant Barre-National, USA.
Dextromethorphan hydrobromide (p.1057·3); pseudoephedrine hydrochloride (p.1068·3).
Coughs and cold symptoms.

Effederm CS, Fr.
Tretinoin (p.1093·3).
Acne.

Effee Propan, S.Afr.
Ferrous sulphate (p.1340·2); folic acid (p.1340·3).
Iron-deficiency anaemia.

Effekton Brenner-Efeka, Ger.; LAW, Ger.
Diclofenac sodium (p.31·2).
Gout; inflammation; musculoskeletal, joint, and soft-tissue disorders; pain.

Efferalgan
Upsamedica, Belg.; UPSA, Fr.; Upsamedica, Ital.; Upsamedica, Spain.
Paracetamol (p.72·2).
Fever; pain.

Efferalgan C
Upsamedica, Belg.; Upsamedica, Ital.; Upsamedica, Switz.
Paracetamol (p.72·2); ascorbic acid (p.1365·2).
Fever; pain.

Efferalgan Codeine UPSA, Fr.
Paracetamol (p.72·2); codeine phosphate (p.26·1).
Pain.

Efferalgan Vit C Upsamedica, Spain.
Paracetamol (p.72·2); ascorbic acid (p.1365·2).
Fever; pain.

Efferalgan Vitamine C UPSA, Fr.
Paracetamol (p.72·2); ascorbic acid (p.1365·2).
Fever; pain.

Effercal Akromed, S.Afr.
Vitamin B_6 and mineral preparation.

Effercal-600 Hamilton, Austral.†.
Calcium carbonate (p.1182·1).
Calcium supplement.

Effercitrate Typharm, UK.
Potassium citrate (p.1153·1); citric acid (p.1564·3).
Cystitis.

Effer-K Nomax, USA.
Potassium bicarbonate (p.1153·1); potassium citrate (p.1153·1).
Hypokalaemia; potassium depletion.

Effersol Pharmacare Consumer, S.Afr.
Sodium bicarbonate (p.1153·2); citric acid (p.1564·3); tartaric acid (p.1634·3).
Acidosis; urinary alkalinisation.

Effersyllium Johnson & Johnson, Aust.
Ispaghula husk (p.1194·2).
Constipation.

Effer-Syllium J&J-Merck, USA.
Psyllium hydrocolloid (p.1194·2).
Anorectal disorders; constipation; irritable bowel syndrome.

Effetre Farmatre, Ital.
Chlorhexidine gluconate (p.1107·2).
Disinfection of skin, wounds, burns, hands, and surgical materials; skin irritation.

Effexor
Wyeth-Ayerst, Canad.; Wyeth-Ayerst, USA.
Venlafaxine hydrochloride (p.311·2).
Depression.

Efficlean Bausch & Lomb, Fr.
Subtilisin-A.
Protein remover for contact lenses.

Effico
Pharmax, Irl.
Thiamine hydrochloride; nicotinamide; caffeine.
Tonic.

Pharmax, UK.
Nicotinamide; thiamine hydrochloride; caffeine; compound gentian infusion.
Tonic.

Efficort Galderma, Fr.
Hydrocortisone aceponate (p.1044·2).
Skin disorders.

Effidigest Yves Ponroy, Fr.
Nutritional supplement.
Gastro-intestinal disorders.

Effidose Chefaro Ardeval, Fr.
A range of herbal preparations.

Effiplen Effik, Spain.
Buspirone hydrochloride (p.643·3).
Anxiety.

Effiprev Effik, Fr.
Norgestimate (p.1453·3); ethinyloestradiol (p.1445·1).
Combined oral contraceptive.

Efflumidex Allergan, Ger.
Fluorometholone (p.1042·1).
Allergic and inflammatory disorders of the eye.

Efflumycin Allergan, Ger.
Fluorometholone (p.1042·1); neomycin sulphate (p.229·2).
Infected eye disorders.

Effortil
Bender, Aust.; Boehringer Ingelheim, Belg.; Boehringer Ingelheim, Fr.; Boehringer Ingelheim, Ger.; Boehringer Ingelheim, Ital.; Boehringer Ingelheim, Norw.; Boehringer Ingelheim, S.Afr.; Boehringer Ingelheim, Swed.; Boehringer Ingelheim, Switz.
Etilefrine hydrochloride (p.867·2).
Hypotension.

Effortil comp Bender, Aust.
Etilefrine hydrochloride (p.867·2); dihydroergotamine mesylate (p.444·2).
Hypotension.

Effortil plus
Boehringer Ingelheim, Ger.; Boehringer Ingelheim, Switz.
Etilefrine hydrochloride (p.867·2); dihydroergotamine mesylate (p.444·2).
Hypotension.

Efical Sanofi Winthrop, Fr.
Calcium pidolate (p.1155·3); calcium carbonate (p.1182·1).
Calcium deficiency; osteoporosis.

Efidac Ciba, USA.
Pseudoephedrine hydrochloride (p.1068·3).

Efidac 24-Chlorpheniramine Ciba, USA.
Chlorpheniramine maleate (p.405·1).
Hypersensitivity reactions.

Efimag Fornet, Fr.
Magnesium pidolate (p.1157·3).
Magnesium deficiency.

Efisalin N Woelm, Ger.†.
Ephedrine hydrochloride (p.1059·3); quebracho; phenazone (p.78·2); menthol (p.1600·2); gypsophila saponin.
Asthma; bronchitis; emphysema.

Efisol S Roland, Ger.
Dequalinium chloride (p.1112·1).
Inflammatory disorders of the oropharynx.

Efisol-H Roland, Ger.†.
Dequalinium chloride (p.1112·1); hydrocortisone (p.1043·3).
Skin disorders.

Efodine Fougera, USA.
Povidone-iodine (p.1123·3).
Skin disinfection.

Efortil Fher, Spain.
Etilefrine hydrochloride (p.867·2).
Hypotension.

Efralen Italfarmaco, Spain†.
Trimeprazine tartrate (p.419·3); ammonium acetate (p.1055·1); magnesium sulphate (p.1157·3); sodium benzoate (p.1102·3).
Upper-respiratory-tract disorders.

Efrane
Abbott, Norw.; Abbott, Swed.
Enflurane (p.1222·1).
General anaesthesia.

Efrarel Mediolanum, Ital.
L-α-Glycerophosphorylethanolamine monohydrate.
Nervous disorders.

Efriviral Aesculapius, Ital.
Aciclovir (p.602·3).
Formerly known as Efrivir.
Herpesvirus infections.

Eftab Thornton & Ross, UK.
Peppermint oil (p.1208·1); clove oil (p.1565·2); spearmint oil (p.1632·1); menthol (p.1600·2); thymol (p.1127·1); methyl salicylate (p.55·2).
Oral hygiene.

Eftapan
Merckle, Aust.; Merckle, Ger.
Eprazinone hydrochloride (p.1060·3).
Respiratory-tract disorders.

Eftapan Doxy Merckle, Ger.†.
Eprazinone hydrochloride (p.1060·3); doxycycline hydrochloride (p.202·3).
Bacterial infections of the respiratory tract.

Eftapan Tetra
Merckle, Aust.; Merckle, Ger.†.
Eprazinone hydrochloride (p.1060·3); tetracycline hydrochloride (p.259·1).
Bacterial infections of the respiratory tract.

Efudex
Roche, Canad.; Roche, USA.
Fluorouracil (p.534·3).
Skin cancer; solar keratoses.

Efudix
Roche, Austral.†; Roche, Belg.; Roche, Fr.; Roche, Ger.; Roche, Irl.; Roche, Ital.; Roche, Neth.; Roche, S.Afr.; Andreu, Spain; Roche, Switz.; ICN, UK.
Fluorouracil (p.534·3).
Anogenital warts; premalignant skin lesions; skin cancer; solar and senile keratoses.

Egacene Durettes Astra, Neth.
Hyoscyamine sulphate (p.464·2).
Bradycardia; gastro-intestinal spasm; hyperhidrosis.

Egarone Alcala, Spain.
Allantoin (p.1078·2); benzalkonium chloride (p.1101·3); muramidase hydrochloride (p.1604·3); oxymetazoline (p.1066·1).
Nasal congestion.

Egarone Oximetazolina Alcala, Spain.
Oxymetazoline hydrochloride (p.1065·3).
Nasal congestion; sinus congestion.

Egazil
Astra, Norw.; Hassle, Swed.
Hyoscyamine sulphate (p.464·2).
Biliary colic; bladder tenesmus; hypersecretion; irritable bowel syndrome.

E/Gel Fulton, USA.
Erythromycin (p.204·1).

Egery Biorga, Fr.
Erythromycin (p.204·1).
Bacterial infections.

Egibren Chiesi, Ital.
Selegiline hydrochloride (p.1144·2).
Psychiatric disorders.

Eglonyl Hoechst Marion Roussel, S.Afr.
Sulpiride (p.692·3).
Depression; peptic ulcer; psychoses; vertigo.

Egmovit Iromedica, Switz.†.
Multivitamin and mineral preparation.

Ego Prickly Heat Powder Ego, Austral.†.
Light liquid paraffin (p.1382·1); salicylic acid (p.1090·2); zinc oxide (p.1096·2).
Prickly heat rash.

Ego Skin Cream Ego, Austral.
Emollient.

Egocappol Ego, Austral.†.
Salicylic acid (p.1090·2).
Cradle cap.

Egocort Cream Ego, Austral.
Hydrocortisone (p.1043·3).
Skin disorders.

Egoderm Cream Ego, Austral.
Ammoniumsulfobitol (p.1083·3).
Formerly contained ammoniumsulfobitol and allantoin.
Skin disorders.

Egoderm Ointment Ego, Austral.
Ammoniumsulfobitol (p.1083·3); zinc oxide (p.1096·2).
Skin disorders.

Egogyn 30 Schering, Ital.
Levonorgestrel (p.1454·1); ethinyloestradiol (p.1445·1).
Combined oral contraceptive.

Egomycol Ego, Austral.
Undecylenic alkanolamide (p.389·2); chlorhexidine gluconate (p.1107·2); salicylic acid (p.1090·2); benzoic acid (p.1102·3); resorcinol (p.1090·1).
Fungal and bacterial skin and nail infections.

Egopsoryl TA Ego, Austral.
Sulphur (p.1091·2); phenol (p.1121·2); coal tar (p.1092·3).
Formerly contained allantoin, sulphur, phenol, coal tar, menthol, and glycerol.
Psoriasis.

Egozite Baby Cream Ego, Austral.
Zinc oxide (p.1096·2); dimethicone (p.1384·2); light liquid paraffin (p.1382·1).
Skin disorders.

Egozite Cradle Cap Ego, Austral.
Salicylic acid (p.1090·2); olive oil (p.1610·1); castor oil (p.1560·2).
Cradle cap.

Egozite Cream Ego, Austral.†.
Olive oil (p.1610·1); glycerol (p.1585·2); zinc oxide (p.1096·2).
Eczema; skin irritation; vulval inflammation.

Egozite Protective Baby Lotion Ego, Austral.
Dimethicone (p.1384·2).
Barrier preparation; nappy rash.

Ehrenhofer-Salbe Ehrenhofer, Aust.
Colophony (p.1567·1); levisticum root (p.1597·2).
Bronchitis; skin disorders; soft-tissue, peri-articular, musculoskeletal, and joint disorders.

Ehrmann's Entschlackungstee Ehrmann, Aust.
Prunus spinosa; equisetum (p.1575·1); silver birch (p.1553·3); urtica (p.1642·3); taraxacum (p.1634·2); peppermint leaf (p.1208·1); chamomile (p.1561·2).
Urinary disorders.

Eicosapen
Nefro, Aust.; Nycomed, Ger.; Byk, Switz.
Marine fish oil (p.1276·1).
Hyperlipidaemias.

Eicovis NBF-Lanes, Ital.
Omega-3 triglycerides, vitamins, and minerals.
Eye disorders; nutritional supplement.

Eifelfango-Neuenahr Eifelfango, Ger.
Medicinal mud.
Gastro-intestinal disorders; musculoskeletal and joint disorders.

Einalat Bayer, Aust.
Nifedipine (p.916·2).
Hypertension.

EinsAlpha Leo, Ger.
Alfacalcidol (p.1366·3).
Vitamin D deficiency.

Einschlafkapseln Twardy, Aust.
Valerian extract (p.1643·1); lupulus extract (p.1597·2).
Nervous disorders; sleep disorders.

Einschlaf-Kapseln biologisch Twardy, Ger.
Valerian (p.1643·1); lupulus (p.1597·2).
Nervous disorders; sleep disorders.

Eisen-Diasporal Protina, Ger.
Ferrous sulphate (p.1340·2).
Iron deficiency.

Eisendragees-ratiopharm Ratiopharm, Ger.
Ferrous sulphate (p.1340·2).
Iron deficiency; iron-deficiency anaemia.

Eismycin SmithKline Beecham, Ger.†.
Mupirocin (p.227·2).
Bacterial skin infections.

EK Burger Ysatfabrik, Ger.
Dried bovine parathyroid gland.
Disorders of calcium metabolism; hypoparathyroidism; hypoparathyroidism with tetany.

Eksalb Kade, S.Afr.†.
Cell contents and metabolites of *Escherichia coli; Staphylococcus aureus; Enterococcus faecalis* (p.1594·1); *Pseudomonas aeruginosa*.
Skin disorders.

Eksplorasjonskrem Nycomed, Norw.†.
Chlorhexidine acetate (p.1107·2).
Aid in vaginal examination.

ektebin Hefa, Ger.
Prothionamide (p.241·1).
Tuberculosis.

Ektogan
Hoechst, Fr.; Teofarma, Ital.
Zinc peroxide (p.1127·3); zinc oxide (p.1096·2); magnesium peroxide (p.1119·1).
Skin disorders; wound disinfection.

Ektoselene Robapharm, Switz.
Selenium disulphide (p.1091·1); sulphur (p.1091·2).
Scalp disorders.

Ekuba
Note. This name is used for preparations of different composition.
Solvay, Ital.†.
Toothpaste; chewing gum: Chlorhexidine acetate (p.1107·2); sodium fluoride (p.742·1); aminocaproic acid (p.711·1).
Oral disinfection; oral hygiene.

Teofarma, Ital.
Vaginal douche: Chlorhexidine gluconate (p.1107·2).
Personal hygiene.

UCM-Difme, Ital.†.
Cream: Chlorhexidine hydrochloride (p.1107·2).
Skin disinfection.

Ekvacillin
Astra, Norw.; Astra, Swed.
Cloxacillin sodium (p.195·2).
Bacterial infections.

Ekzemase Azupharma, Ger.
Bufexamac (p.22·2).
Eczema.

Ekzemex Serturner, Ger.†.
Hydrocortisone acetate (p.1043·3); tyrothricin (p.267·2); cetylpyridinium chloride (p.1106·2).
Skin disorders with bacterial or fungal infection.

Ekzemsalbe Agepha, Aust.
Hydrocortisone acetate (p.1043·3).
Eczema.

Ekzesin Mago, Ger.†.
Hydrocortisone acetate (p.1043·3).
Skin disorders.

Ekzevowen Weber & Weber, Ger.
Acid. arsenicosum; calendula offic.; centella asiat.; lytta ves.; mahonia aquifolium; peru balsam (p.1617·2); semecarpus anacard.; viola tric.; zinc oxide (p.1096·2).
Eczema; pruritus ani; pruritus vulvae.

Elacur LAW, Ger.
Propyl nicotinate (p.81·3).
Musculoskeletal and joint disorders; neuralgia.

Elacur NO LAW, Ger.†.
Nonivamide (p.63·2); propyl nicotinate (p.81·3).
Musculoskeletal and joint disorders; pain.

Elacutan LAW, Ger.
Urea (p.1095·2).
Skin disorders.

Elagen Eladon, UK.
Eleutherococcus senticosus (p.1584·2).
Tonic.

Elan Schwarz, Ital.
Isosorbide mononitrate (p.893·3).
Cardiac disorders.

Elana OTW, Ger.
Homoeopathic preparation.

Elanpres Parke, Davis, Irl.†.
Methyldopa (p.904·2).
Hypertension.

Elanpress Recordati, Ital.†.
Methyldopa (p.904·2).
Hypertension.

Elantan
Gebro, Aust.; Synthelabo, Ger.; Schwarz, Irl.; Sanofi Omnimed, S.Afr.; Schwarz, Switz.; Schwarz, UK.
Isosorbide mononitrate (p.893·3).
Heart failure; ischaemic heart disease; pulmonary hypertension.

Elase
Parke, Davis, Austral.; Parke, Davis, Canad.; Parke, Davis, Fr.; Parke, Davis, Ital.; Parke, Davis, Neth.; Fujisawa, USA.
Plasmin (p.932·1); deoxyribonuclease (p.1059·1).
Cervicitis; debridement of wounds; vaginitis.

Elase-Chloromycetin
Parke, Davis, Canad.; Fujisawa, USA.
Plasmin (p.932·1); deoxyribonuclease (p.1059·1); chloramphenicol (p.182·1).
Debridement of infected lesions.

Elastocapsil Smith & Nephew, Fr.†.
Capsicum (p.1559·2); belladonna (p.457·1); arnica (p.1550·3).
Joint and muscle pain.

Elasven Euroexim, Spain†.
Fluocinolone acetonide (p.1041·1).
Skin disorders.

Elaubat Desitin, Ger.†.
Haloperidol (p.673·3).
Psychiatric disorders.

Elavil
Merck Sharp & Dohme, Canad.; Merck Sharp & Dohme-Chibret, Fr.; DDSA Pharmaceuticals, UK; Zeneca, USA.
Amitriptyline embonate (p.273·3) or amitriptyline hydrochloride (p.273·3).
Depression; nocturnal enuresis.

Elavil Plus Merck Sharp & Dohme, Canad.
Amitriptyline hydrochloride (p.273·3); perphenazine (p.685·2).
Depression.

Elazor Sigma-Tau, Ital.
Fluconazole (p.378·1).
Fungal infections.

Elbozon Merckle-Diadin, Ger.†.
Zinc oxide (p.1096·2); cod-liver oil (p.1337·3); allantoin (p.1078·2); levomenol (p.1596·1); retinol palmitate (p.1359·2); cholecalciferol (p.1366·3).
Skin disorders.

Elbrol Pfleger, Ger.
Propranolol hydrochloride (p.937·1).
Arrhythmias; essential tremor; hypertension; hyperthyroidism; ischaemic heart disease; migraine.

Elcarn Co-Pharma, UK.
Carnitine (p.1336·2).
Carnitine deficiency.

Elcarnitol Genera, Switz.†.
Carnitine tartrate (p.1336·2).
Dietary supplement.

Elcimen Hafslund Nycomed, Aust.
Elcatonin (p.735·3).
Hypercalcaemia; osteoporosis; Paget's disease of bone; reflex sympathetic dystrophy.

Elcitonin Asahi, Jpn.
Elcatonin (p.735·3).
Hypercalcaemia; osteoporosis; Paget's disease of bone.

Eldepryl
Reckitt & Colman, Austral.; Asta Medica, Belg.; Draxis, Canad.; Orion, Irl.; Asta Medica, Neth.; Orion, Norw.; Reckitt & Colman, S.Afr.; Orion, Swed.; Britannia Pharmaceuticals, UK; Somerset, USA.
Selegiline hydrochloride (p.1144·2).
Parkinsonism.

Elder Flowers with Peppermint and Composition Essence Potter's, UK.
Bayberry bark; hemlock spruce; elder flowers (p.1627·2); peppermint oil (p.1208·1).
Colds; sore throat.

Eldercaps Mayrand, USA.
Multivitamin and mineral preparation.

Eldertonic Mayrand, USA.
Vitamin B substances with minerals.

Eldicet Solvay, Spain.
Pinaverium bromide (p.1618·3).
Gastro-intestinal spasm; irritable bowel syndrome.

Eldisin Lilly, Aust.
Vindesine sulphate (p.571·1).
Malignant neoplasms.

Eldisine
Lilly, Austral.; Lilly, Belg.; Lilly, Canad.; Lilly, Fr.; Lilly, Ger.; Lilly, Ital.; Lilly, Neth.; Lilly, S.Afr.; Lilly, Swed.; Lilly, Switz.; Lilly, UK.
Vindesine sulphate (p.571·1).
Malignant neoplasms.

Eldopal Yamanouchi, Neth.†.
Levodopa (p.1137·1).
Parkinsonism.

Eldopaque
ICN, Canad.; ICN, USA.
Hydroquinone (p.1083·1) in a sunblocking basis.
Hyperpigmented skin conditions.

Eldoquin
ICN, Canad.; ICN, USA.
Hydroquinone (p.1083·1).
Hyperpigmented skin conditions.

Eldox Lennon, S.Afr.
Diphenoxylate hydrochloride (p.1189·1).
Atropine sulphate (p.455·1) is included in this preparation to discourage abuse.
Diarrhoea.

Elebloc Cusi, Spain.
Carteolol hydrochloride (p.837·3).
Glaucoma; ocular hypertension.

Electopen Alter, Spain.
Ampicillin sodium (p.153·1) or ampicillin trihydrate (p.153·2).
Bacterial infections.

Electopen Balsam Alter, Spain†.
Ampicillin trihydrate (p.153·2); carbocisteine (p.1056·3); guaiphenesin (p.1061·3).
Respiratory-tract infections.

Electopen Balsam Retard Alter, Spain.
Ampicillin sodium (p.153·1); ampicillin benzathine (p.154·1); niaouli oil (p.1607·1); guaiphenesin (p.1061·3).
Respiratory-tract infections.

Electopen Retard Alter, Spain.
Ampicillin sodium (p.153·1); ampicillin benzathine (p.154·1).
Bacterial infections.

Electro C-1000 Quest, Canad.†.
Vitamin and mineral preparation.

Electrolactil Sol Electrolactil, Spain†.
Lactic-acid-producing organisms (p.1594·1).
Restoration of the gastro-intestinal flora; skin disorders.

Electrolade
Nicholas, Irl.†; Eastern Pharmaceuticals, UK.
Sodium chloride; potassium chloride; sodium bicarbonate; glucose (p.1152·3).
Diarrhoea; oral rehydration therapy.

Electrona Lagamed, S.Afr.
Potassium chloride; sodium chloride; sodium bicarbonate; calcium lactate; sodium acid phosphate; magnesium sulphate; magnesium carbonate; glucose (p.1152·3).
Diarrhoea; oral rehydration therapy.

Electropak Mirren, S.Afr.
Potassium chloride; sodium chloride; sodium bicarbonate; glucose (p.1152·3).
Diarrhoea; oral rehydration therapy.

Elemental 028
Scientific Hospital Supplies, Austral.; Scientific Hospital Supplies, UK.
Preparation for enteral nutrition.

Elen Yamanouchi, Jpn.
Indeloxazine hydrochloride (p.1590·2).
Cerebrovascular disorders.

Elenol Gerda, Fr.
Lindane (p.1407·2); amylocaine hydrochloride (p.1286·1).
Scabies.

Elentol Gerda, Fr.
Lindane (p.1407·2).
Disinfection of clothing and bedding; pediculosis.

Eleu-Kokk Pharmaton, Ger.
Eleutherococcus senticosus root (p.1584·2).
Tonic.

Eleutheroforce Bioforce, Ger.
Eleutherococcus senticosis root (p.1584·2).
Tonic.

Eleutherokokk-Aktiv-Kapseln SenticoMega
Twardy, Ger.
Eleutherococcus senticosus root (p.1584·2).
Tonic.

Elevat Lagamed, S.Afr.
Dronabinol (p.1191·2).
Anorexia with weight loss in AIDS; nausea and vomiting.

Elevit
Roche, Aust.; Roche, Switz.
Range of multivitamin or multivitamin and mineral preparations.

Elevit Pronatal
Roche, Aust.; Roche Consumer, Belg.†.
Multivitamin and mineral preparation.

Elevit RDI Roche, Austral.†.
Multivitamin and mineral preparation.

Elevit Vitamine B$_9$ Nicholas, Fr.
Multivitamin and mineral preparation.

Elex Verla, Ger.
dl-Alpha tocopheryl acetate (p.1369·2); magnesium oxide (p.1198·3).
Vitamin E and magnesium deficiency.

Elfanex
Ciba-Geigy, Aust.; Ciba, Ger.†.
Reserpine (p.942·1); dihydralazine sulphate (p.854·1); hydrochlorothiazide (p.885·2); potassium chloride (p.1161·1).
Hypertension.

Elgadil Byk Elmu, Spain.
Urapidil hydrochloride (p.959·2).
Hypertension.

Elgam Alfarma, Spain.
Omeprazole (p.1204·2).
Gastro-oesophageal reflux; peptic ulcer; Zollinger-Ellison syndrome.

Elgydium
Pierre Fabre, Fr.; Pierre Fabre, Spain†; Chefaro, UK.
Chlorhexidine gluconate (p.1107·2).
Dental caries prophylaxis; mouth disorders.

Elialconio Eliovit, Ital.†.
Benzalkonium chloride (p.1101·3).
Skin and wound disinfection.

Elica Schering-Plough, Spain.
Mometasone furoate (p.1047·2).
Skin disorders.

Elicodil Menarini, Ital.
Ranitidine bismutrex (p.1211·2).
Peptic ulcer.

Elidiur Bristol-Myers Squibb, Ital.
Fosinopril sodium (p.870·3); hydrochlorothiazide (p.885·2).
Hypertension.

Elimin Cantabria, Spain.
Sodium picosulphate (p.1213·2).
Constipation.

Elimite Allergan Herbert, USA.
Permethrin (p.1409·2).
Scabies.

Elimitona Brauer, Austral.
Homoeopathic preparation.

Elingrip Wasserman, Spain.
Aspirin (p.16·1); ascorbic acid (p.1365·2); chlorpheniramine maleate (p.405·1); kola (p.1645·1).
Cold and influenza symptoms.

Elios Rydelle, Fr.
Amino-acid, fatty-acid, and vitamin preparation.
UV-induced skin damage.

Elisir Depurativo Ambrosiano Alckamed, Ital.
Aesculus hippocastanum (p.1543·3); hypericum perforatum (p.1590·1); arnica montana (p.1550·3); polygonum avicolare; hamamelis virginiana (p.1587·1); gentiana lutea (p.1583·3).
Circulatory disorders.

Elisir Terpina Teofarma, Ital.
Terpin hydrate (p.1070·2); dropropizine (p.1059·2).
Coughs.

Elisor Bristol-Myers Squibb, Fr.
Pravastatin sodium (p.1277·1).
Hypercholesterolaemia.

Eliten Bristol-Myers Squibb, Ital.
Fosinopril sodium (p.870·3).
Heart failure; hypertension.

Elixifilin Morrith, Spain.
Potassium iodide (p.1493·1); theophylline (p.765·1).
Obstructive airways disease.

Elixir Bonjean Thepenier, Fr.
Melissa (p.1600·1); bitter-orange peel (p.1610·3); aniseed (p.1549·3); cumin seed; catechu (p.1560·3); mint oil (p.1208·1).
Digestive disorders.

Elixir Contre La Toux Weleda Weleda, Fr.
Aniseed (p.1549·3); dulcamara (p.1574·2); drosera; althaea (p.1546·3); ipecacuanha (p.1062·2); malt (p.1350·1); white marrubium (p.1063·3); pulsatilla; thyme (p.1636·3).
Coughs.

Elixir Dental Formahina Domenech Garcia, Spain†.
Formaldehyde (p.1113·2); peppermint oil; methyl salicylate (p.55·2); thymic acid; menthol (p.1600·2); cinnamon oil; clove oil (p.1565·2); borax (p.1554·2); boric acid (p.1554·2).
Mouth infection and inflammation.

Elixir Grez Monin, Fr.
Bitter-orange (p.1610·3); gentian (p.1583·3); cinnamon (p.1564·2); citric acid monohydrate (p.1564·3).
Digestive disorders.

Elixir Grez Chlorhydropepsique Monin, Fr.†.
Pepsin (p.1616·3); hydrochloric acid (p.1588·3); nux vomica (p.1609·3); gentian (p.1583·3); bitter-orange peel (p.1610·3).
Gastro-intestinal disorders.

Elixir Rebleuten Pharmacal, Switz.
Aloes (p.1177·1).
Constipation.

Elixir Spark Medecine Vegetale, Fr.
Boldo (p.1554·1); cynara (p.1569·2).
Formerly contained cascara, senna, boldo, cynara, lupulus, bitter orange, gentian, sage, chamomile, absinthium, quassia, chicory, calumba, and centaury.
Constipation; dyspepsia.

Elixirol Lennon, S.Afr.†.
Diphenhydramine hydrochloride (p.409·1); ammonium chloride (p.1055·2); sodium citrate (p.1153·2); menthol (p.1600·2).
Coughs.

Elix-Nocte Nelson, Austral.†.
Chloral hydrate (p.645·3).
Insomnia.

Elixomin Cenci, USA.
Theophylline (p.765·1).
Obstructive airways disease.

Elixophyllin
Schering, Austral.†; Forest Pharmaceuticals, USA.
Theophylline (p.765·1).
Obstructive airways disease.

Elixophyllin-GG Forest Pharmaceuticals, USA.
Theophylline (p.765·1); guaiphenesin (p.1061·3).
Obstructive airways disease.

Elixophyllin-KI
Schering, Austral.†; Forest Pharmaceuticals, USA.
Theophylline (p.765·1); potassium iodide (p.1493·1).
Tenacious mucus in asthma and bronchitis.

Elkamol Kendon, UK.
Paracetamol (p.72·2).

Elkapin
Parke, Davis, Aust.; Godecke, Ger.; Parke, Davis, Ital.; Parke, Davis, Spain.
Etozolin (p.867·2).
Hypertension; oedema.

Elkin Byk, Neth.
Frusemide (p.871·1); amiloride hydrochloride (p.819·2).
Hypertension; oedema.

Ellatun Basotherm, Ger.
Tramazoline hydrochloride (p.1071·1).
Nasal congestion.

Ell-Cranell Basotherm, Ger.
Oestradiol (p.1455·1); dexamethasone (p.1037·1); salicylic acid (p.1090·2).
Hair loss; scalp disorders.

Elle-care Geistlich, Switz.
Lactic acid (p.1593·3); sodium lactate (p.1153·2); docusate sodium (p.1189·3).
Vaginal disorders.

Elleci Lampugnani, Ital.
Carnitine (p.1336·2).
Carnitine deficiency; myocardial ischaemia.

Ellemger Ellem, Ital.†.
Clofibrate (p.1271·1); pyricarbate (p.1624·1).
Hyperlipidaemias.

Elleste Duet Conti Shire, UK.
Oestradiol (p.1455·1); norethisterone acetate (p.1453·1).
Menopausal disorders.

Elleste-Duet Searle, UK.
16 Tablets, oestradiol (p.1455·1); 12 tablets, oestradiol; norethisterone acetate (p.1453·1).
Menopausal disorders.

Elleste-Solo Searle, UK.
Oestradiol (p.1455·1).
Menopausal disorders.

Elle-Test Beta Theranol-Deglaude, Fr.†.
Pregnancy test (p.1621·2).

Ellimans Seton, UK.
Turpentine oil (p.1641·1); acetic acid (p.1541·2).
Musculoskeletal and joint disorders; pain.

Ellsurex Basotherm, Ger.
Selenium sulphide (p.1091·1); colloidal sulphur (p.1091·2); allantoin (p.1078·2).
Scalp disorders.

Elmetacin
Luitpold, Ger.; Byk Madaus, S.Afr.; Luitpold, Switz.
Indomethacin (p.45·2).
Musculoskeletal, joint, peri-articular, and soft-tissue pain and inflammation.

Elmex
Note. This name is used for preparations of different composition.
Gebro, Aust.; Wybert, Ger.; GABA, Switz.
Topical solution: Olaflur (p.1610·1); dectaflur (p.1570·2).
Dental caries prophylaxis; sensitive teeth.
Wybert, Ger.; Crinos, Ital.; GABA, Switz.
Topical gel: Olaflur (p.1610·1); dectaflur (p.1570·2); sodium fluoride (p.742·1).
Dental caries prophylaxis; sensitive teeth.

Elmiron Baker Cummins, Canad.
Pentosan polysulphate sodium (p.928·1).
Interstitial cystitis.

Elmuten Byk Elmu, Spain.
Aceglutamide; acetylaspartic acid; cyanocobalamin; citrulline; inositol; thiamine nitrate; magnesium potassium aspartate; pyridoxal phosphate; serine phosphate. Lignocaine hydrochloride (p.1293·2) is included in this preparation to alleviate the pain of injection.
Tonic.

Elo-admix Leopold, Aust.
Electrolyte infusion (p.1147·1).
Fluid and electrolyte disorders.

Eloamin Leopold, Aust.
Amino-acid and electrolyte infusion.
Parenteral nutrition.

Elobact Cascan, Ger.; Cascapharm, Ger.
Cefuroxime axetil (p.177·1).
Bacterial infections.

Elocom
Schering-Plough, Belg.; Schering, Canad.; Schering-Plough, Spain; Essex, Switz.
Mometasone furoate (p.1047·2).
Skin disorders.

Elocon
Aesca, Aust.; Schering-Plough, Austral.; Schering-Plough, Irl.; Schering-Plough, Ital.; Schering-Plough, Neth.; Schering-Plough, Norw.; Schering-Plough, S.Afr.; Schering-Plough, Swed.; Schering-Plough, UK; Schering, USA.
Mometasone furoate (p.1047·2).
Skin disorders.

Elodrink Leopold, Aust.†.
Sodium chloride; potassium chloride; sodium bicarbonate; glucose monohydrate (p.1152·3).
Diarrhoea; oral rehydration therapy.

Eloglucose Leopold, Aust.
Electrolyte infusion with glucose (p.1147·1).
Carbohydrate source; fluid and electrolyte disorders.

Elohaes
Fresenius, Belg.; Fresenius, UK.
Hexastarch (p.724·2) in sodium chloride.
Extracorporeal circulation; hypovolaemic shock; leucopheresis.

Elohast
Leopold, Aust.; Schiwa, Ger.†; Hormonchemie, Ger.†; Fresenius, Switz.
A hydroxyethyl ether starch (p.724·2) in electrolytes.
Hypovolaemia; shock.

Elohes
Biosedra, Fr.; Oxford Nutrition, UK.
A hydroxyethyl ether starch (p.724·2) in sodium chloride.
Extracorporeal circulation; leucopheresis; plasma volume expansion.

Eloisin Cusi, Spain.
Eledoisin trifluoroacetate (p.1574·3).
Dry eyes.

Elolipid Leopold, Aust.
Soya oil (p.1355·1).
Contains egg lecithin.
Lipid infusion for parenteral nutrition.

elomel Boehringer Mannheim, Ger.†.
A range of electrolyte infusions with or without carbohydrate (p.1147·1).
Carbohydrate source; fluid and electrolyte disorders.

ELO-MEL Leopold, Aust.
A range of electrolyte infusions with or without glucose (p.1147·1).
Carbohydrate source; fluid and electrolyte disorders.

ELO-oral Leopold, Aust.
Electrolytes (p.1147·1).
Fluid and electrolyte disorders.

Elopram Recordati, Ital.
Citalopram hydrobromide (p.281·1).
Depression.

E-Lor UAD, USA†.
Dextropropoxyphene hydrochloride (p.27·3); paracetamol (p.72·2).
Pain.

Elorgan Hoechst, Spain.
Oxpentifylline (p.925·3).
Vascular disorders.

Elorheo Leopold, Aust.
Dextran 40 (p.716·2) in electrolytes.
Fluid and electrolyte disorders.

Elotrace Leopold, Aust.
Electrolyte infusion with trace elements (p.1147·1).
Parenteral nutrition; trace element deficiency.

Elotrans
Leopold, Aust.; Fresenius-Praxis, Ger.; Rowa, Irl.†; Fresenius, Switz.
Glucose; sodium chloride; sodium citrate; potassium chloride (p.1152·3).
Diarrhoea; oral rehydration therapy.

Eloverlan Mayrhofer, Aust.†.
Anhydrous glucose; sodium chloride; potassium chloride; sodium bicarbonate (p.1152·3).
Diarrhoea; oral rehydration therapy.

Elovol Leopold, Aust.
Electrolyte infusion (p.1147·1).
Fluid and electrolyte disorders.

Eloxatine Sanofi Winthrop, Fr.
Oxaliplatin (p.556·3).
Colorectal cancer.

Elozell Leopold, Aust.
Magnesium aspartate (p.1157·2); potassium aspartate (p.1161·3).
Cardiac disorders; digitalis toxicity; potassium and magnesium deficiency.

Elpimed Stada, Ger.†.
Blood extract free of albumin and neutral lipids.
Immunotherapy.

Elroquil N Rodleben, Ger.
Hydroxyzine hydrochloride (p.412·1).
Anxiety disorders; premedication; pruritus; sleep disorders.

Elspar Merck Sharp & Dohme, USA.
Asparaginase (p.504·3).
Acute lymphocytic leukaemia.

Elteans Jaldes, Fr.
Salmon oil (p.1276·1); borage oil (p.1582·1); carrot and soya oils.
Nutritional fatty acid supplement.

Elthon Knoll, Ger.†.
Verapamil hydrochloride (p.960·3); diazepam (p.661·1).
Ischaemic heart disease; tachycardia.

Elthyrone Knoll, Belg.
Thyroxine sodium (p.1497·1).
Hypothyroidism.

Eltor Hoechst Marion Roussel, Canad.
Pseudoephedrine hydrochloride (p.1068·3).
Nasal and sinus congestion.

Eltroxin
Glaxo Wellcome, Canad.; Goldshield, Irl.; Glaxo Wellcome, Neth.; Glaxo Wellcome, S.Afr.; Goldshield, UK; Roberts, USA.
Thyroxine sodium (p.1497·1).
Hypothyroidism.

Eltroxine Sigma-Tau, Switz.
Thyroxine sodium (p.1497·1).
Hypothyroidism.

Eludril
Note. This name is used for preparations of different composition.
Inava, Fr.; Pierre Fabre, Switz.; Chefaro, UK.
Throat spray: Chlorhexidine gluconate (p.1107·2); amethocaine hydrochloride (p.1285·2).
Mouth and throat disorders.

Inava, Fr.
Mouthwash: Chlorhexidine gluconate (p.1107·2); chlorbutol (p.1106·3); chloroform (p.1220·3).
Tablets: Chlorhexidine gluconate (p.1107·2); amethocaine hydrochloride (p.1285·2); ascorbic acid (p.1365·2).
Mouth disorders.

Pierre Fabre, Spain; Chefaro, UK.
Mouthwash: Chlorhexidine gluconate (p.1107·2); chlorbutol (p.1106·3).
Mouth and throat disorders.

Pierre Fabre, Switz.
Mouthwash: Chlorhexidine gluconate (p.1107·2); chlorbutol (p.1106·3); laureth 9 (p.1325·2).
Mouth and throat disorders.

Elugan Menadier, Ger.
Simethicone (p.1213·1).
Elugan chewable tablets formerly contained simethicone, pancreatin, and beta-amylase.
Gastro-intestinal disorders.

Elugan N Menadier, Ger.
Simethicone (p.1213·1).
Gastro-intestinal disorders.

Elugel Inava, Fr.
Chlorhexidine gluconate (p.1107·2).
Gum disorders; mouth hygiene.

Elusanes Plantes et Medecines, Fr.
A range of herbal preparations.

Elutit-Calcium Felgentrager, Ger.
Calcium polystyrene sulphonate (p.974·3).
Hyperkalaemia.

Elutit-Natrium Felgentrager, Ger.
Sodium polystyrene sulphonate (p.995·3).
Hyperkalaemia.

Elvorine
Wyeth Lederle, Belg.; Lederle, Fr.
Calcium levofolinate (p.1342·3).
Adjuvant to fluorouracil therapy; drug-induced megaloblastic anaemia; folic acid deficiency; prevention of methotrexate-induced toxicity.

Elyzol
Chemomedica, Aust.; Dumex, Ger.; Dumex, Irl.; Dumex, Neth.†; Dumex, Norw.; Dumex-Alpharma, Swed.; Dumex, Switz.; Dumex, UK.
Metronidazole (p.585·1) or metronidazole benzoate (p.585·1).
Anaerobic bacterial infections; Crohn's disease; protozoal infections; rosacea.

Elzogram Lilly, Ger.
Cephazolin sodium (p.181·1).
Bacterial infections.

Elzym Luitpold, Switz.
Simethicone (p.1213·1); dried extract from *Aspergillus oryzae*; ethaverine hydrochloride (p.1577·1).
Gastro-intestinal disorders with excess gas; preparation of gastro-intestinal tract for radiological examination.

Elzym N Luitpold, Ger.†.
Simethicone (p.1213·1); dried extract from *Aspergillus oryzae*.
Elzym formerly contained simethicone, dried extract from *A. oryzae*, and ethaverine hydrochloride.
Gastro-intestinal disorders.

EM Eukal Sohan, Canad.
Eucalyptus oil (p.1578·1); menthol (p.1600·2).

Emadine Alcon, USA.
Emedastine fumarate (p.410·2).
Allergic conjunctivitis.

Emagel Hoechst Marion Roussel, Ital.
Polygeline (p.727·1).
Plasma volume expansion.

emagnesit Worwag, Ger.†.
dl-Alpha tocopheryl acetate (p.1369·2); magnesium orotate (p.1611·2); racemic magnesium aspartate (p.1157·2).
Neuromuscular disorders; vitamin E deficiency.

Emaseril Geymonat, Ital.†.
Deproteinised blood extract.
Peptic ulcer; varicose ulcer.

Emasex A Eurim, Ger.
Bamethan sulphate (p.827·1).
Impotence.

Emasex-N Eurim, Ger.
Bamethan sulphate (p.827·1); benzyl nicotinate (p.22·1).
Impotence; tonic.

Emazian B12 Bioindustria, Ital.
Injection: Thiamine hydrochloride (p.1361·1); riboflavine (p.1362·1); panthenol (p.1571·1); nicotinamide (p.1351·2); calcium folinate (p.1342·2); cyanocobalamin (p.1363·3).
Oral liquid†; syrup†: Thiamine hydrochloride (p.1361·1); riboflavine (p.1362·1); nicotinamide (p.1351·2); pyridoxine hydrochloride (p.1362·3); panthenol (p.1571·1); cyanocobalamin (p.1363·3); calcium folinate (p.1342·2).
Deficiency states; macrocytic anaemia.

Emazian Cortex Bioindustria, Ital.†.
Suprarenal cortex (p.1050·1); disodium inosinate heptahydrate (p.1573·1); disodium guanylate (p.1573·1); disodium uridine monophosphate dihydrate; disodium cytidine phosphate; calcium folinate (p.1342·2); cyanocobalamin (p.1363·3); pyridoxine hydrochloride (p.1362·3).
Anaemias; deficiency states.

EMB Fatol, Ger.
Ethambutol hydrochloride (p.207·2).
Tuberculosis.

Embarin Merckle, Ger.†.
Allopurinol (p.390·2).
Gout; hyperuricaemia.

Embial Merck, Ger.
dl-Alpha tocopheryl acetate (p.1369·2).
Vitamin E deficiency.

EMB-INH Fatol, Ger.
Ethambutol hydrochloride (p.207·2); isoniazid (p.218·1).
Tuberculosis.

Emblon Berk, UK.
Tamoxifen citrate (p.563·3).
Anovulatory infertility; breast cancer.

Embolex Sandoz, Aust.
Certoparin sodium (p.839·1) dihydroergotamine mesylate (p.444·2).
Lignocaine hydrochloride (p.1293·2) is included in this preparation to alleviate the pain of injection.
Thrombo-embolic disorders.

Embolex LM Sandoz, Switz.†.
Certoparin sodium (p.839·1); dihydroergotamine mesylate (p.444·2).
Lignocaine hydrochloride (p.1293·2) is included in this preparation to alleviate the pain of injection.
Thrombo-embolic disorders.

Embolex NM Sandoz, Ger.
Certoparin sodium (p.839·1); dihydroergotamine mesylate (p.444·2).
Lignocaine hydrochloride (p.1293·2) is included in this preparation to alleviate the pain of injection.
Thrombo-embolic disorders.

Embran Sudmedica, Ger.†.
Nucleoside (p.1609·2).
Circulatory insufficiency.

Embrocacion Gras Quimifar, Spain.
Alcohol (p.1099·1); capsicum oleoresin; methyl salicylate (p.55·2); turpentine oil (p.1641·1).
Rheumatic and muscle pain.

Embrocation Synpharma, Aust.
Menthol (p.1600·2); peppermint oil (p.1208·1); methyl salicylate (p.55·2); eucalyptus oil (p.1578·1); rosemary oil (p.1626·2); anise oil (p.1550·1); citronella oil (p.1565·1); arnica (p.1550·3).
Musculoskeletal and joint disorders.

Embropax Taphlan, Switz.
Methyl salicylate (p.55·2); isopropyl nicotinate; capsicum (p.1559·2); camphor (p.1557·2); turpentine oil (p.1641·1); eucalyptus oil (p.1578·1); lavender oil (p.1594·3).
Peri-articular and soft-tissue disorders.

Emconcor
Merck-Belgolabo, Belg.; Merck, Spain; Meda, Swed.
Bisoprolol fumarate (p.833·1).
Angina pectoris; arrhythmias; hypertension.

Emcor
E. Merck, Irl.; E. Merck, Neth.; E. Merck, UK.
Bisoprolol fumarate (p.833·1).
Angina pectoris; hypertension.

Emcoretic
Merck-Belgolabo, Belg.; E. Merck, Neth.; Merck, Spain.
Bisoprolol fumarate (p.833·1); hydrochlorothiazide (p.885·2).
Hypertension.

Emcyt
Pharmacia Upjohn, Canad.; Pharmacia, USA.
Estramustine sodium phosphate (p.532·2).
Prostatic cancer.

Emdalen Merck, S.Afr.
Lofepramine hydrochloride (p.296·1).
Depression.

Emdecassol Nattermann, Ger.†.
Asiaticoside; centella (p.1080·3).
Skin disorders.

Emecheck Savage, USA†.
Phosphoric acid (p.1618·1); glucose (p.1343·3); fructose (p.1343·2).
Nausea and vomiting.

Emedyl Montavit, Aust.
Dimenhydrinate (p.408·2).
Nausea and vomiting; vestibular disorders.

Emelis
Clintec, Fr.; Clintec, Irl.
High-protein semi-solid dietary supplement.
Chewing or swallowing disorders.

Emeproton Cantabria, Spain.
Omeprazole (p.1204·2).
Gastro-oesophageal reflux; peptic ulcer; Zollinger-Ellison syndrome.

Emercol Pharmavite, Canad.
Benzocaine (p.1286·2); cetalkonium chloride (p.1105·2); cetylpyridinium chloride (p.1106·2).

Emercreme No 4 Pharmavite, Canad.
Cetylpyridinium chloride (p.1106·2); bacitracin (p.157·3); tyrothricin (p.267·2); diphenylpyraline hydrochloride (p.409·3); benzocaine (p.1286·2).

Emereze Plus Pharmavite, Canad.
Cetylpyridinium chloride (p.1106·2).

Emergent-Ez Healthfirst, USA.
Combination pack: 2 Ampoules, adrenaline (p.813·2); 1 ampoule, aminophylline (p.748·1); 3 inhalants, ammonia (p.1548·3); 2 inhalants, amyl nitrite (p.974·2); 2 ampoules, atropine (p.455·1); 2 ampoules, diphenhydramine hydrochloride (Benadryl) (p.409·1); tablets, glyceryl trinitrate (p.874·3); 1 vial, hydrocortisone sodium succinate (Solu-Cortef) (p.1044·1); 1 ampoule, pentazocine lactate (Talwin) (p.75·1); 1 ampoule, trimethobenzamide hydrochloride (Tigan) (p.420·1); 2 ampoules, diazepam (Valium) (p.661·1); 2 ampoules, mephentermine sulphate (Wyamine) (p.902·2).
Emergency treatment.

Emersal Medco, USA.
Ammoniated mercury (p.1086·3); salicylic acid (p.1090·2).
Psoriasis.

Emesafene Asta Medica, Neth.
Meclozine hydrochloride (p.413·3); pyridoxine hydrochloride (p.1362·3).
Nausea; vomiting.

Emesan Lindopharm, Ger.
Diphenhydramine hydrochloride (p.409·1).
Formerly contained diphenhydramine hydrochloride and belladonna.
Nausea; vertigo; vomiting.

Emeside Laboratories for Applied Biology, UK.
Ethosuximide (p.344·3).
Absence seizures; myoclonic seizures.

Emete-con Roerig, USA†.
Benzquinamide hydrochloride (p.1179·2).
Nausea and vomiting following anaesthesia and surgery.

Emetrol
Note. This name is used for preparations of different composition.
Rhone-Poulenc Rorer, Austral.; Sanofi Winthrop, USA.
Fructose (p.1343·2); glucose (p.1343·3); phosphoric acid (p.1618·1).
Nausea; vomiting.

Rhone-Poulenc Rorer, S.Afr.
Sucrose (p.1357·1); phosphoric acid (p.1618·1).
Nausea; vomiting.

Emex Mirren, S.Afr.
Invert sugar (p.1357·3); phosphoric acid (p.1618·1).
Nausea.

Emfib Berk, UK.
Gemfibrozil (p.1273·3).
Hyperlipidaemias.

Emflex E. Merck, UK.
Acemetacin (p.12·2).
Inflammation; pain; rheumatoid arthritis.

Emgecard Mayrhofer, Aust.
Magnesium aspartate hydrochloride trihydrate (p.1158·2).
Magnesium deficiency.

Emgel Glaxo Wellcome, USA.
Erythromycin (p.204·1).
Acne.

Emgesan Pharmacia Upjohn, Swed.
Magnesium hydroxide (p.1198·2).
Magnesium deficiency; renal calculi.

Emican Alter, Spain.
Salbutamol sulphate (p.758·2).
Obstructive airways disease; premature labour; status asthmaticus.

Emidote APF Prosana, Austral.†.
Ipecacuanha (p.1062·2); dilute acetic acid (p.1541·2); glycerol (p.1585·2).
Induction of vomiting.

Emilace Yamanouchi, Jpn.
Nemonapride (p.682·1).
Schizophrenia.

Eminase
SmithKline Beecham, Aust.; Therabel Pharma, Belg.; SmithKline Beecham, Fr.; Reusch, Ger.; Beecham, Irl.†; SmithKline Beecham, Ital.†; Tramedico, Neth.; SmithKline Beecham, Switz.; Monmouth, UK; Roberts, USA.
Anistreplase (p.824·2).
Myocardial infarction.

Emitex Garec, S.Afr.
Cyclizine hydrochloride (p.407·1).
Motion sickness; nausea; vestibular disorders; vomiting.

Emko
Schering, Canad.†; Schering-Plough, S.Afr.†; Schering, USA.
Nonoxinol 9 (p.1326·1).
Contraceptive.

Emla
Astra, Aust.; Astra, Austral.; Astra, Belg.; Astra, Canad.; Astra, Fr.; Astra, Ger.; Astra, Irl.; Astra, Ital.; Astra, Neth.; Astra, Norw.; Astra, S.Afr.; Astra, Swed.; Astra, Switz.; Astra, UK; Astra, USA.
Lignocaine (p.1293·2); prilocaine (p.1299·1).
Local anaesthesia.

Emmetipi Sicor, Ital.
Methylprednisolone sodium succinate (p.1046·1).
Parenteral corticosteroid.

Emmolate Bio-Medical, UK.
Liquid paraffin (p.1382·1); acetylated wool alcohols (p.1385·2).
Dry skin.

Emoantitossina Piam, Ital.
Calcium folinate (p.1342·2); cyanocobalamin (p.1363·3); thiamine monophosphate chloride (p.1361·2); riboflavine sodium phosphate (p.1362·1); pyridoxine hydrochloride (p.1362·3); nicotinamide (p.1351·2); panthenol (p.1571·1).
Anaemias; deficiency states.

Emocicatrol Bouty, Ital.†.
Tannic acid (p.1634·2); hamamelis (p.1587·1); phenazone (p.78·2).
Epistaxis.

Emoclot DI *ISI, Ital.*
A factor VIII preparation (p.720·3).
Haemophilia A; von Willebrand's disease.

Emo-Cort *Trans Canaderm, Canad.*
Hydrocortisone (p.1043·3).
Skin disorders.

Emocrat forte *Hevert, Ger.*
Crataegus; rutin sodium sulphate (p.1580·2).
Arrhythmias; ischaemic heart disease.

Emodella *GABA, Switz.*
Frangula bark (p.1193·2).
Constipation.

Emodisintox *IRBI, Ital.†.*
Ferritin (p.1580·1).
Anaemias.

Emofer *Salus, Ital.†.*
Ferrocholinate (p.1339·2).
Anaemias.

Emoferrina *Piam, Ital.*
Ferric sodium gluconate (p.1340·1).
Iron deficiency; iron-deficiency anaemias.

Emoflux *Metapharma, Ital.*
Buflomedil hydrochloride (p.834·2).
Vascular disorders.

Emofol *Simes, Ital.†.*
Thiamine hydrochloride (p.1361·1); nicotinamide (p.1351·2); choline chloride (p.1337·1); cyanocobalamin (p.1363·3); folic acid (p.1340·3).
Folate deficiency; megaloblastic anaemia.

Emoform
Note. This name is used for preparations of different composition.
Warner-Lambert, Fr.
Formaldehyde (p.1113·2); electrolytes (p.1147·1).
Bleeding gums; hypersensitive teeth.

Wild, Switz.†.
Lignocaine hydrochloride (p.1293·2); chlorbutol (p.1106·3); formaldehyde (p.1113·2); sodium fluoride (p.742·1); electrolytes (p.1147·1).
Mouth pain; oral hygiene; sensitive teeth.

Norgine, UK†.
Formaldehyde (p.1113·2).
Hypersensitive teeth.

Emoform nouvelle formule *Wild, Switz.*
Electrolytes (p.1147·1).
Oral hygiene; sensitive teeth.

Emoform-F au fluor *Wild, Switz.*
Electrolytes (p.1147·1); sodium monofluorophosphate (p.743·3).
Dental caries prophylaxis; oral hygiene; sensitive teeth.

Emoklar *Savio, Ital.*
Heparin calcium (p.879·3).
Thrombo-embolic disorders.

Emollia *Gordon, USA.*
Emollient and moisturiser.

Emolytar *Stiefel, Spain.*
Tar (p.1092·3); juniper oil (p.1592·3); coal tar (p.1092·3).
Skin disorders.

Emonucleosina Cortex *Piam, Ital.†.*
Suprarenal cortex (p.1050·1); hydroxocobalamin (p.1363·3); cytidine; uridine (p.1641·3); inosine (p.1591·1); calcium folinate (p.1342·2).
Anaemias; deficiency states.

Emoplast *Schiapparelli, Ital.*
Benzalkonium chloride (p.1101·3); alum (p.1547·1).
Skin and wound disinfection.

Emopon *Terapeutico, Ital.*
Calcium folinate (p.1342·2); cyanocobalamin (p.1363·3); ferric ammonium citrate (p.1339·2); thiamine hydrochloride (p.1361·1); nicotinamide (p.1351·2).
Macrocytic anaemia.

Emopremarin *Wyeth, Ital.*
Conjugated oestrogens (p.1457·3).
Haemorrhage.

Emoren *IFI, Ital.*
Oxethazaine hydrochloride (p.1298·1).
Haemorrhoids.

Emorril *Poli, Ital.*
Troxerutin (p.1580·2); hydrocortisone acetate (p.1043·3); nifuratel (p.589·1); lignocaine (p.1293·2) or lignocaine hydrochloride (p.1293·2).
Adjunct in anorectal surgery; haemorrhoids.

Emosint *Sclavo, Ital.*
Desmopressin acetate (p.1245·2).
Haemorrhagic disorders.

Emoton *Rentsch, Switz.*
Agnus castus (p.1544·2).
Premenstrual disorders.

Emovat *Glaxo Wellcome, Swed.*
Clobetasone butyrate (p.1035·3).
Skin disorders.

Emovate
Glaxo Wellcome, Aust.; Glaxo Wellcome, Ger.; Wolff, Ger.; Glaxo Wellcome, Neth.; Evans, Spain; Glaxo Wellcome, Switz.
Clobetasone butyrate (p.1035·3).
Skin disorders.

Emovis *Boniscontro & Gazzone, Ital.*
Calcium folinate (p.1342·2).
Anaemias; antidote to overdosage with folic acid antagonists; folate deficiency; reduction of aminopterin and methotrexate toxicity.

Emozide B6 *Piam, Ital.†.*
Isoniazid (p.218·1); pyridoxine hydrochloride (p.1362·3).
Tuberculosis.

Empacod *Byk Madaus, S.Afr.*
Paracetamol (p.72·2); codeine phosphate (p.26·1).
Fever; pain.

Empaped *Byk Madaus, S.Afr.*
Paracetamol (p.72·2).
Fever; pain.

Empapol *Vilardell, Spain.*
Terpineol (p.1635·1); cresol (p.1111·2); pinus sylvestris resin (p.1567·1).
Formerly contained olive oil, cineole, cresol, pinus sylvestris resin, and sodium hydroxide.
Wounds.

Empicols *Albright & Wilson, UK.*
A range of sodium lauryl sulphates (p.1468·3).

Empirin *Wellcome, USA.*
Aspirin (p.16·1).
Fever; inflammation; myocardial infarction; pain; transient ischaemic attacks.

Empirin with Codeine *Wellcome, USA.*
Aspirin (p.16·1); codeine phosphate (p.26·1).
Pain.

Emplatre Croix D *Demopharm, Switz.*
Cayenne pepper; methyl salicylate (p.55·2); venice turpentine.
Musculoskeletal and joint pain.

Emportal *Zyma, Spain.*
Lactitol (p.1195·2).
Constipation; hepatic encephalopathy.

Empracet *Glaxo Wellcome, Canad.*
Paracetamol (p.72·2); codeine phosphate (p.26·1).
Pain.

Emprazil-A *Glaxo Wellcome, S.Afr.*
Syrup†: Triprolidine hydrochloride (p.420·3); pseudoephedrine hydrochloride (p.1068·3); paracetamol (p.72·2).
Tablets: Triprolidine hydrochloride (p.420·3); pseudoephedrine hydrochloride (p.1068·3); caffeine (p.749·3); paracetamol (p.72·2).
Cold and influenza symptoms.

Empynase *Kaken, Jpn.*
Pronase.
Inflammation; respiratory-tract congestion.

Emser Balsam echt *Siemens, Ger.†.*
Emser salz; azulene (p.1552·1); nutmeg oil (p.1609·3); pine needle oil; pumilio pine oil (p.1623·3); eucalyptus oil (p.1578·1); cedar leaf oil; camphor (p.1557·2); turpentine oil (p.1641·1).
Respiratory-tract disorders.

Emser Erkaltungsgel *Siemens, Ger.*
Pumilio pine oil (p.1623·3); eucalyptus oil (p.1578·1); camphor (p.1557·2).
Cold symptoms.

Emser Nasensalbe *Hochstetter, Aust.*
Natural emser salt; azulene (p.1552·1); nutmeg oil (p.1609·3); oleum pini sylvestris; pumilio pine oil (p.1623·3); eucalyptus oil (p.1578·1); cedar wood oil; turpentine oil (p.1641·1); camphor (p.1557·2).
Colds; hay fever.

Emser Nasensalbe N *Siemens, Ger.*
Emser salz; azulene (p.1552·1); nutmeg oil (p.1609·3); pumilio pine oil (p.1623·3); eucalyptus oil (p.1578·1); cedar wood oil; camphor (p.1557·2); turpentine oil (p.1641·1).
Colds; hay fever.

Emser Pastillen *Hochstetter, Aust.*
Natural emser salt.
Respiratory-tract disorders.

Emser Pastillen echt "Stark" *Siemens, Ger.†.*
Emser salz; menthol (p.1600·2); cetylpyridinium chloride (p.1106·2).
Mouth and throat disorders.

Emser Pastillen mit Menthol *Hochstetter, Aust.*
Natural emser salt; menthol (p.1600·2); peppermint oil (p.1208·1); eucalyptus oil (p.1578·1).
Respiratory-tract disorders.

Emser Pastillen mit Menthol N *Siemens, Ger.*
Natural emser salt (see Emser Salz); menthol (p.1600·2).
Throat disorders.

Emser Pastillen ohne Menthol *Siemens, Ger.*
Natural emser salt (see Emser Salz).
Throat disorders.

Emser Pastillen zuckerfrei *Siemens, Ger.*
Natural emser salt (see Emser Salz).
Throat disorders.

Emser Salz *Siemens, Ger.*
Natural emser salt (containing sodium, potassium, chloride, sulphate, and bicarbonate ions).
Dyspepsia; respiratory-tract disorders.

Emser Sole *Siemens, Ger.*
Cations: sodium, potassium; anions: chloride, sulphate, bicarbonate.
Respiratory-tract disorders.

Emsilat *Siemens, Ger.*
Eucalyptus oil (p.1578·1); pine needle oil.
Cold symptoms.

Emsogen *Scientific Hospital Supplies, Irl.*
Preparation for enteral nutrition.

Emtec-30 *Technilab, Canad.*
Paracetamol (p.72·2); codeine phosphate (p.26·1).
Cold symptoms; pain; upper respiratory-tract disorders.

Emthexat
Nycomed, Norw.; Nycomed, Swed.
Methotrexate (p.547·1).
Malignant neoplasms; psoriasis; rheumatoid arthritis.

Emthexate
Pharmachemie, S.Afr.; Pras, Spain.
Methotrexate (p.547·1) or methotrexate sodium (p.547·1).
Graft-versus-host disease; malignant neoplasms; psoriasis; rheumatoid arthritis.

Emtobil *Astra, Austral.†.*
Sorbitol (p.1354·2); arachis oil (p.1550·2); sorbimacrogol oleate.
Examination of gallbladder evacuation.

Emuclens *Ovelle, Irl.*
Cleanser in an emollient base.
Water-free cleansing.

Emucream *Ovelle, Irl.*
Emollient.
Dry skin.

Emu-K *Pharmacia Upjohn, S.Afr.†.*
Erythromycin estolate (p.204·1).
Bacterial infections.

Emulave
Note. This name is used for preparations of different composition.
Rydelle, Fr.; Rydelle, Ital.
Avena (p.1551·3).
Dry skin disorders; soap substitute.

Ovelle, Irl.
Soap substitute.

Emulax *Hassle, Swed.*
Cascara (p.1183·1); docusate sodium (p.1189·3).
Constipation.

Emuliquen Antiespasmodic *Lainco, Spain†.*
Belladonna (p.457·1); carrageenan mucilage (p.1471·3); paraffin (p.1382·1).
Constipation with muscle spasm.

Emuliquen Laxante *Lainco, Spain.*
Phenolphthalein (p.1208·2); paraffin (p.1382·1).
Formerly contained carrageenan mucilage, phenolphthalein, and paraffin.
Constipation.

Emuliquen Simple *Lainco, Spain.*
Paraffin (p.1382·1).
Constipation.

Emulsan *Leiras, Swed.†.*
Fractionated soya oil (p.1355·1).
Contains fractionated egg lecithin.
Lipid infusion for parenteral nutrition.

Emulsiderm
Dermal Laboratories, Irl.; Dermal Laboratories, UK.
Isopropyl myristate (p.1384·1); liquid paraffin (p.1382·1); benzalkonium chloride (p.1101·3).
Dry skin conditions.

E-Mulsin *Mucos, Ger.*
Alpha tocopheryl acetate (p.1369·1).
Vitamin E deficiency.

Emulsione Lassativa *FAMA, Ital.†.*
Liquid paraffin (p.1382·1); phenolphthalein (p.1208·2); agar (p.1470·3).
Constipation.

Emulsoil *Paddock, USA.*
Castor oil (p.1560·2).
Constipation.

Emu-V
Pharmacia Upjohn, Austral.; Pharmacia Upjohn, S.Afr.
Erythromycin (p.204·1).
Bacterial infections.

Emuvin *Pharmacia Upjohn, Aust.*
Erythromycin (p.204·1).
Bacterial infections.

Emvit *Madaus, S.Afr.†.*
Multivitamin and mineral preparation.

Emvit Pedia *Madaus, S.Afr.†.*
Multivitamin and mineral preparation.

E-Mycin
Alphapharm, Austral.; Pharmacia Upjohn, Canad.; Docmed, S.Afr.; Boots, USA.
Erythromycin (p.204·1), erythromycin estolate (p.204·1), or erythromycin ethyl succinate (p.204·2).
Bacterial infections.

En *Ravizza, Ital.*
Delorazepam (p.660·3).
Anxiety disorders; epilepsy; premedication; sleep disorders.

Enanton
Orion, Norw.; Orion, Swed.
Leuprorelin acetate (p.1253·1).
Prostatic cancer.

Enantone
Takeda, Aust.; Takeda, Fr.; Takeda, Ger.; Takeda, Ital.
Leuprorelin acetate (p.1253·1).
Breast cancer; endometriosis; fibromyoma; precocious puberty; prostatic cancer.

Enantone-Gyn *Takeda, Ger.*
Leuprorelin acetate (p.1253·1).
Breast cancer; endometriosis.

Enantyum *Menarini, Spain.*
Dexketoprofen trometamol.
Pain.

Enapren *Merck Sharp & Dohme, Ital.*
Enalapril maleate (p.863·2).
Heart failure; hypertension; ischaemic heart disease.

Enarax *UCB, S.Afr.†.*
Hydroxyzine hydrochloride (p.412·1); oxyphencyclimine hydrochloride (p.466·3).
Gastro-intestinal disorders.

Encare
Stella, Canad.; Thompson, USA.
Nonoxinol 9 (p.1326·1).
Contraceptive.

En-Cebrin *Lilly, USA†.*
Multivitamin and mineral preparation.

Encebrovit *Herdel, Ital.†.*
Pyritinol hydrochloride (p.1624·1).
Organic brain disorders.

Encefabol *Bracco, Ital.*
Pyritinol or pyritinol hydrochloride (p.1624·1).
Organic brain disorders.

Encegam *Centeon, Ger.; Chiron Behring, Ger.*
A tick-borne encephalitis immunoglobulin (p.1510·2).
Passive immunisation.

Encelin *Crosara, Ital.*
Citicoline sodium (p.1564·3).
Cerebrovascular disorders; parkinsonism.

Encephabol
Merck, Aust.; Merck-Belgolabo, Belg.†; Merck-Clevenot, Fr.†; Merck, Ger.; Merck, S.Afr.; E. Merck, Switz.†.
Pyritinol or pyritinol hydrochloride (p.1624·1).
Migraine; organic brain disorders; trigeminal neuralgia.

Encepur *Chiron Behring, Ger.*
An inactivated tick-borne encephalitis vaccine (p.1510·2).
Separate preparations are available for infants and children and for older children and adults.
Active immunisation.

Encerebron *Pulitzer, Ital.†.*
Pyritinol hydrochloride (p.1624·1).
Organic brain disorders.

Encetrop *Kytta, Ger.*
Piracetam (p.1619·1).
Mental function disorders.

Encevin *Savio, Ital.†.*
Vincamine (p.1644·1).
Cerebrovascular disorders.

Encialina *Bucca, Spain.*
Aconite (p.1542·2); arnica (p.1550·3); ipecacuanha (p.1062·2); matricaria (p.1561·2); rhatany (p.1624·3); iodine (p.1493·1).
Mouth inflammation; pyorrhoea.

End Lice *Thompson, USA.*
Pyrethrins; piperonyl butoxide (p.1409·3).
Pediculosis.

End Pain *Brovar, S.Afr.†.*
Syrup: Paracetamol (p.72·2); codeine phosphate (p.26·1); promethazine hydrochloride (p.416·2).
Fever; pain.
Tablets: Paracetamol (p.72·2); codeine phosphate (p.26·1); caffeine (p.749·3); meprobamate (p.678·1).
Pain and associated tension.

Endafed *UAD, USA.*
Pseudoephedrine hydrochloride (p.1068·3); brompheniramine maleate (p.403·2).
Allergic rhinitis; nasal congestion.

Endagen-HD *Abana, USA.*
Phenylephrine hydrochloride (p.1066·2); chlorpheniramine maleate (p.405·1); hydrocodone tartrate (p.43·1).
Coughs and cold symptoms.

Endak
Madaus, Aust.; Madaus, Ger.
Carteolol hydrochloride (p.837·3).
Angina pectoris; arrhythmias; hypertension; myocardial infarction.

Endal *UAD, USA.*
Phenylephrine hydrochloride (p.1066·2); guaiphenesin (p.1061·3).
Coughs.

Endal Expectorant *UAD, USA.*
Phenylpropanolamine hydrochloride (p.1067·2); guaiphenesin (p.1061·3); codeine phosphate (p.26·1).
Coughs.

Endalbumin *Alfa Biotech, Ital.*
Albumin (p.710·1).
Hypoalbuminaemia.

Endal-HD *UAD, USA.*
Chlorpheniramine maleate (p.405·1); phenylephrine hydrochloride (p.1066·2); hydrocodone tartrate (p.43·1).
Coughs and cold symptoms.

Endal-HD Plus *UAD, USA.*
Chlorpheniramine maleate (p.405·1); phenylephrine hydrochloride (p.1066·2); hydrocodone tartrate (p.43·1).
Coughs and cold symptoms.

Endantadine *Endo, Canad.*
Amantadine hydrochloride (p.1129·2).
Influenza A; parkinsonism.

Endcol *SA Druggists Self Med, S.Afr.†.*
Paracetamol (p.72·2); ascorbic acid (p.1365·2); phenylephrine hydrochloride (p.1066·2); chlorpheniramine maleate (p.405·1); caffeine (p.749·3).
Cold symptoms.

Endcol Cough Linctus *SA Druggists Self Med, S.Afr.†.*
Triprolidine hydrochloride (p.420·3); pseudoephedrine hydrochloride (p.1068·3); codeine phosphate (p.26·1).
Coughs.

Endcol Decongestant *SA Druggists Self Med, S.Afr.†.*
Triprolidine hydrochloride (p.420·3); pseudoephedrine hydrochloride (p.1068·3).
Cold symptoms.

Endcol Expectorant *Lennon, S.Afr.†.*
Triprolidine hydrochloride (p.420·3); pseudoephedrine hydrochloride (p.1068·3); codeine phosphate (p.26·1); guaiphenesin (p.1061·3).
Coughs.

En-De-Kay *Manx, UK.*
Sodium fluoride (p.742·1).
Dental caries prophylaxis.

Endep
Alphapharm, Austral.; Rolab, S.Afr.; Roche, USA†.
Amitriptyline hydrochloride (p.273·3).
Depression; nocturnal enuresis.

Endermyl *Galderma, Canad.*
Emollient.
Dry skin.

Endiaron *Medphano, Ger.*
Loperamide hydrochloride (p.1197·2).
Diarrhoea.

Endium *Europhta, Mon.*
Diosmin (p.1580·1).
Haemorrhoids; peripheral vascular disorders.

Endobil
Gerot, Aust.; E. Merck, Irl.; Bracco, Ital.†; Dagra, Neth.†; Bracco, Switz.†; E. Merck, UK†.
Meglumine iodoxamate (p.1006·2).
Contrast medium for biliary-tract radiography.

Endobulin
Immuno, Aust.; Immuno, Ger.; Immuno, Ital.; Omnimed, S.Afr.; Immuno, Spain; Baxter, Swed.; Immuno, Switz.; Immuno, UK†.
A normal immunoglobulin (p.1522·1).
Auto-immune and immune complex disorders; idiopathic thrombocytopenic purpura; immunoglobulin deficiency; Kawasaki disease; passive immunisation.

Endocet *Endo, Canad.*
Oxycodone hydrochloride (p.71·2); paracetamol (p.72·2).
Fever; pain.

Endociclina *Del Saz & Filippini, Ital.†.*
Fosfomycin calcium (p.210·2) or fosfomycin disodium (p.210·2).
Bacterial infections.

Endodan *Endo, Canad.*
Oxycodone hydrochloride (p.71·2); aspirin (p.16·1).
Fever; inflammation; pain.

Endoepacort B12 *Nuovo, Ital.†.*
Cyanocobalamin (p.1363·3); suprarenal cortex (p.1050·1).
Anaemias; asthenia.

Endofren *Bamo, Spain†.*
Diiodotyrosine (p.1493·1); reserpine (p.942·1).
Hyperthyroidism.

Endogen HS 15 *Panthox & Burck, Ital.†.*
Acidic enterococci.
Gastro-intestinal disorders.

Endol *Cruz, Spain.*
Tiadenol (p.1279·3).
Hyperlipidaemias.

Endolipide *Braun, Fr.*
Soya oil (p.1355·1).
Contains egg lecithin.
Lipid infusion for parenteral nutrition.

Endolor *Keene, USA.*
Paracetamol (p.72·2); caffeine (p.749·3); butalbital (p.644·3).
Pain.

Endomethasone *Septodont, Switz.*
Powder, hydrocortisone acetate (p.1043·3); thymol iodide (p.1127·1); barium sulphate (p.1003·1); liquid, eugenol (p.1578·2); peppermint oil (p.1208·1); anise oil (p.1550·1).
Root canal sealant.

Endomethazone *Rinnerthaler, Aust.*
Dexamethasone (p.1037·1); hydrocortisone acetate (p.1043·3).

Endomirabil *Byk Gulden, Ger.†.*
Meglumine iodoxamate (p.1006·2).
Contrast medium for biliary-tract radiography.

Endomixin *Lusofarmaco, Ital.†.*
Neomycin sulphate (p.229·2).
Hyperammonaemia associated with liver failure; intestinal infections.

Endone *Boots, Austral.*
Oxycodone hydrochloride (p.71·2).
Pain.

Endoneutralio *Crosara, Ital.*
Sodium citrate (p.1153·2); potassium citrate (p.1153·1).
Gastric hyperacidity.

Endopancrine 40 *Organon, Fr.*
Insulin injection (crystalline) (porcine, highly purified) (p.322·1).
Diabetes mellitus.

Endopancrine 100 *Organon, Fr.*
Insulin zinc suspension (porcine, highly purified) (p.322·1).
Diabetes mellitus.

Endopancrine Protamine *Organon, Fr.*
Isophane insulin injection (crystalline) (porcine, highly purified) (p.322·1).
Diabetes mellitus.

Endopancrine Zinc Protamine *Organon, Fr.*
A protamine zinc insulin suspension (porcine, highly purified) (p.322·1).
Diabetes mellitus.

Endo-Paractol *Asta Medica, Ger.*
Simethicone (p.1213·1).
Adjuvant for endoscopy and double contrast radiography.

Endophleban *Rentschler, Ger.*
Dihydroergotamine mesylate (p.444·2).
Chronic venous insufficiency; hypotension; migraine and related vascular headache.

Endoprost *Italfarmaco, Ital.*
Iloprost trometamol (p.1419·1).
Buerger's disease.

Endorem
Guerbet, Fr.; Guerbet, Ger.; Farmades, Ital.; Guerbet, Neth.; Rovi, Spain; Gothia, Swed.; Guerbet, Switz.
Ferumoxides (p.1004·2).
Contrast medium for magnetic resonance imaging.

Endorphan *Tyson, USA†.*
Amino acid preparation.

Endorphenyl *Tyson, USA.*
Phenylalanine (p.1353·1).

Endosgel
Chemieprodukte, Aust.; Melisana, Belg.†; Farco, Ger.; Almed, Switz.
Chlorhexidine gluconate (p.1107·2); sodium lactate (p.1153·2).
Aid to endoscopy and catheterisation.

Endosporine *Peters, Fr.†.*
Glutaraldehyde (p.1114·3).
Instrument disinfection.

Endotelon
Sanofi Winthrop, Fr.; Sanofi Winthrop, Switz.†.
Grape seeds.
Lymphoedema; peripheral vascular disorders.

Endoxan
Asta Medica, Aust.; Asta Medica, Austral.; Asta Medica, Belg.; Asta Medica, Fr.; Asta Medica, Ger.; Asta Medica, Ital.; Asta Medica, Neth.; Hoechst Marion Roussel, S.Afr.; Asta Medica, Switz.
Cyclophosphamide (p.516·2).
Auto-immune disorders; malignant neoplasms.

Endoxana *Asta Medica, UK.*
Cyclophosphamide (p.516·2).
Malignant neoplasms.

Endrate *Abbott, USA.*
Disodium edetate (p.980·1).
Digitalis-induced cardiac arrhythmias; hypercalcaemia.

Endrine
Note. This name is used for preparations of different composition.
Kwizda, Aust.†.
Ephedrine (p.1059·3); camphor (p.1557·2); menthol (p.1600·2); castor oil (p.1560·2); cineole (p.1564·1).
Catarrh; rhinitis.

Christiaens, Belg.
Ephedrine (p.1059·3); camphor (p.1557·2); menthol (p.1600·2); cineole (p.1564·1).
Cold symptoms.

Asche, Ger.†.
Nasal drops: Ephedrine (p.1059·3).
Allergic rhinitis; nasal congestion.
Nasal gel: Ephedrine (p.1059·3); camphor (p.1557·2); menthol (p.1600·2); eucalyptus oil (p.1578·1).
Catarrh; colds; hay fever.

Endrine Doux *Christiaens, Belg.*
Ephedrine (p.1059·3); camphor (p.1557·2); cineole (p.1564·1).
Cold symptoms.

Endrine mild
Kwizda, Aust.†.
Ephedrine (p.1059·3); camphor (p.1557·2); castor oil (p.1560·2); cineole (p.1564·1).
Catarrh; rhinitis.

Asche, Ger.†.
Nasal drops: Ephedrine (p.1059·3).
Allergic rhinitis; nasal congestion.
Nasal gel: Ephedrine (p.1059·3); camphor (p.1557·2); eucalyptus oil (p.1578·1).
Catarrh; colds; hay fever.

Endur-acin *Innovite, USA†.*
Nicotinic acid (p.1351·2).
Vitamin deficiency.

Enduron
Abbott, Austral.; Abbott, UK†; Abbott, USA.
Methyclothiazide (p.904·1).
Hypertension; oedema.

Endurona *Abbott, Swed.†.*
Methyclothiazide (p.904·1).
Hypertension; oedema.

Enduronil *Abbott, Ital.*
Methyclothiazide (p.904·1); deserpidine (p.847·2).
Hypertension.

Enduronyl *Abbott, USA.*
Methyclothiazide (p.904·1); deserpidine (p.847·2).
Hypertension.

Endydol *Guidotti, Ital.†.*
Aspirin (p.16·1).
Cold symptoms; pain.

Enecat *Lafayette, USA.*
Barium sulphate (p.1003·1).
Contrast medium for gastro-intestinal radiography.

Enelbin-Paste N *Cassella-med, Ger.*
Zinc oxide (p.1096·2); salicylic acid (p.1090·2); aluminium silicate (p.1178·3).
Inflammation.

Enelbin-Salbe forte *Cassella-med, Ger.†.*
Glycol salicylate (p.43·1); nonivamide (p.63·2); heparin sodium (p.879·3).
Rheumatic disorders.

Enelbin-Salbe N *Cassella-med, Ger.*
Heparin sodium (p.879·3); salicylic acid (p.1090·2).
Bruising; muscle and joint disorders.

Enelbin-Venen Salbe *Cassella-med, Ger.*
Heparin sodium (p.879·3).
Soft-tissue injury; superficial vascular disorders.

Enelfa
Schoeller, Aust.†; Dolorgiet, Ger.
Paracetamol (p.72·2).
Fever; pain.

Enema Casen *Casen Fleet, Spain.*
Dibasic sodium phosphate (p.1159·3); monobasic sodium phosphate (p.1159·3).
Bowel evacuation.

Enemac *Eurospital, Ital.*
Monobasic sodium phosphate (p.1159·3); dibasic sodium phosphate (p.1159·3).
Bowel evacuation; constipation.

Enemol *Pharmascience, Canad.*
Dibasic sodium phosphate (p.1159·3); monobasic sodium phosphate (p.1159·3).
Laxative.

Ener-B *Nature's Bounty, USA.*
Vitamin B_{12} (p.1363·3).
Dietary supplement.

Enercal *Wyeth-Ayerst, Canad.†.*
Preparation for enteral nutrition.

Ener-E *Wassen, Ital.*
Vitamin E (p.1369·1); ubidecarenone (p.1641·2).
Nutritional supplement.

Ener-G *General Dietary, UK.*
Gluten-free bread, rice bran, and pasta.
Gluten-sensitive enteropathies.

Energeia *Sanitalia, Ital.*
Ginseng; ginkgo biloba; eleutherococcus; minerals.
Nutritional supplement.

Energen *Volchem, Ital.*
Glucose (p.1343·3).
Energy loss; hypoglycaemia.

Energetic B-Aspart *Plan, Switz.†.*
Multivitamin and mineral preparation.

Energex Fort *Frega, Canad.*
Multivitamin and mineral preparation.

Energitum *SmithKline Beecham Sante, Fr.*
Arginine glutamate (p.1334·1).
Tonic.

Energon Rende *Ist. Chim. Inter., Ital.†.*
Disodium glucose-1-phosphate; cobamamide (p.1364·2); citrulline (p.1337·2); magnesium aspartate (p.1157·2); phosphothreonine; levoglutamide (p.1344·3).
Tonic.

Energona *Maurer, Ger.*
Norfenefrine hydrochloride (p.925·1).
Hypotension.

Energy Alfa *Dolisos, Canad.*
Homoeopathic preparation.

Ener-Mix *Also, Ital.*
Multivitamin and mineral preparation.

Enertonic *Bifarma, Ital.*
Eleutherococcus senticosis (p.1584·2); ginkgo biloba (p.1584·1); guarana (p.1645·1); echinacea (p.1574·2).
Dietary supplement.

Enervit *Also, Ital.*
A range nutritional supplements.

Enfalac Lactose Free *Mead Johnson, Canad.*
Lactose-free infant feed.
Lactose intolerance.

Enfalac Nutramigen *Mead Johnson, Canad.*
Gluten-free, lactose-free casein hydrolysate preparation for special diets.
Galactosaemia; protein sensitivity.

Enfalac Pregestimil *Mead Johnson, Canad.*
Infant feed.
Malabsorption syndromes.

Enfalac Soy *Mead Johnson, Canad.*
Soy based infant feed.
Hypersensitivity to cow's milk.

Enfamil AR *Mead Johnson Nutritionals, UK.*
Infant feed.
Gastro-oesophageal reflux.

Engerix-B
SmithKline Beecham, Aust.; SmithKline Beecham, Austral.; SK-RIT, Belg.; SmithKline Beecham, Canad.; SmithKline Beecham, Fr.; SmithKline Beecham, Ger.; SSW, Ger.; SmithKline Beecham, Irl.; SmithKline Beecham, Ital.; SmithKline Beecham, Neth.; SmithKline Beecham, Norw.; SmithKline Beecham, S.Afr.; Smith Kline & French, Spain; SmithKline Beecham, Swed.; SmithKline Beecham, Switz.; SmithKline Beecham, UK; SmithKline Beecham, USA.
A hepatitis B vaccine (recombinant DNA) (p.1513·1).
Active immunisation.

Engran-HP *Bristol-Myers Squibb, Irl.†.*
Multivitamin and mineral preparation.

Engystol *Heel, Ger.*
Homoeopathic preparation.

Engystol N *Heel, Ger.*
Homoeopathic preparation.

Enicul *Apomedica, Aust.†.*
Magnesium trisilicate (p.1199·1); algeldrate (p.1177·3); ammonium glycyrrhizinate (p.1055·2).
Gastro-intestinal disorders.

Enirant *Gepepharm, Ger.*
Co-dergocrine mesylate (p.1566·1).
Cerebral circulatory disorders; hypertension.

Enison *Lilly, Spain.*
Vindesine sulphate (p.571·1).
Malignant neoplasms.

Enisyl *Person & Covey, USA†.*
Lysine (p.1350·1).
Dietary supplement.

Enlive *Ross, UK.*
A range of products for enteral nutrition.

Enlon
Zeneca, Canad.; Ohmeda, USA.
Edrophonium chloride (p.1392·2).
Differential diagnosis of myasthenia gravis; reversal of competitive neuromuscular blockade.

Enlon-Plus *Ohmeda, USA.*
Edrophonium chloride (p.1392·2).
Atropine sulphate (p.455·1) is included in this preparation to protect against the muscarinic actions.
Curare antagonist; reversal of competitive neuromuscular blockade.

Ennagesic *Vernleigh, S.Afr.†.*
Paracetamol (p.72·2).
Fever; pain.

Eno
Note. This name is used for preparations of different composition.
Reckitt & Colman, Austral.; SmithKline Beecham, Ital.; SmithKline Beecham, Spain†.
Citric acid (p.1564·3); sodium bicarbonate (p.1153·2); sodium carbonate (p.1630·2).
Dyspepsia.

SmithKline Beecham Consumer, Canad.
Sodium citrate (p.1153·2).
Dyspepsia.

SmithKline Beecham, Fr.†.
Tartaric acid (p.1634·3); sodium bicarbonate (p.1153·2); sodium carbonate (p.1630·2).
Dyspepsia.

SmithKline Beecham Consumer, UK.
Citric acid (p.1564·3); tartaric acid (p.1634·3); sodium bicarbonate (p.1153·2).
Dyspepsia; flatulence.

Enofosforina Vigor *Serra Pamies, Spain.*
Calcium lactophosphate; magnesium glycerophosphate; kola; pyridoxine; sodium glycerophosphate; potassium glycerophosphate; nicotinamide.
Tonic.

Enomdan *Pharmacia Upjohn, Swed.*
Multivitamin preparation.

Enomine *Major, USA.*
Phenylpropanolamine hydrochloride (p.1067·2); guaiphenesin (p.1061·3); phenylephrine hydrochloride (p.1066·2).
Coughs.

Enoton *Pensa, Spain.*
Cyproheptadine aspartate (p.407·3); mecobalamin (p.1364·2).
Anorexia; tonic; weight loss.

Enovid *Searle, USA†.*
Norethynodrel (p.1453·3); mestranol (p.1450·2).
Endometriosis; hypermenorrhoea; production of cyclical withdrawal bleeding.

Enovil *Hauck, USA†.*
Amitriptyline hydrochloride (p.273·3).
Depression.

Enoxen *SmithKline Beecham, Ital.*
Enoxacin (p.203·3).
Bacterial infections.

Enoxin *Faulding, Austral.*
Enoxacin (p.203·3).
Bacterial infections.

Enoxor
Sinbio, Fr.; Pierre Fabre, Ger.
Enoxacin (p.203·3).
Bacterial infections.

Enpac *Brovar, S.Afr.†.*
Lactobacillus acidophilus (p.1594·1).
Replacement of intestinal flora.

Enpovax HDC *CSL, Austral.*
An inactivated poliomyelitis vaccine (p.1528·2).
Active immunisation.

Enprin *Galpharm, UK.*
Aspirin (p.16·1).
Cardiovascular disease.

Enrich
Abbott, Austral.†; Abbott, Fr.; Abbott, Irl.; Abbott, Ital.; Abbott, S.Afr.; Abbott, Switz.; Abbott, UK; Ross, USA†.
Preparation for enteral nutrition.

Enrich with Fibre *Ross, Canad.†.*
Preparation for enteral nutrition.

Ensidon *Ciba-Geigy, Swed.†.*
Opipramol hydrochloride (p.301·1).
Nonpsychotic mental disorders.

Ensure
Abbott, Austral.; Ross, Canad.†; Abbott, Irl.; Abbott, Ital.; Abbott, S.Afr.; Abbott, Switz.; Abbott, UK; Ross, USA.
Preparation for enteral nutrition.

Ensure Plus
Abbott, Irl.; Abbott, Ital.; Abbott, Switz.; Abbott, UK.
High calorie preparation for enteral nutrition.

ENT
Note. This name is used for preparations of different composition.
Mer-National, S.Afr.
Phenylephrine hydrochloride (p.1066·2); naphazoline nitrate (p.1064·2).
Nasal congestion.

Ion, USA†.
Phenylpropanolamine hydrochloride (p.1067·2); brompheniramine maleate (p.403·2).
Upper respiratory-tract symptoms.

Entacyl Roberts, Canad.
Piperazine adipate (p.107·2).
Ascariasis; enterobiasis.

Entalgic Salters, S.Afr.
Paracetamol (p.72·2).
Fever; pain.

Entamizole Boots, UK†.
Diloxanide furoate (p.581·2); metronidazole (p.585·1).
Amoebiasis.

Entecet Irex, Fr.
Barley germ; enzymes derived from aspergillus including amylase and protease; lipase derived from rhizopus.
Dyspepsia.

Entera Rowa, Irl.
Preparation for enteral nutrition.
Formerly known as Fresium High Energy.

Enteral 400 Scientific Hospital Supplies, UK.
Preparation for enteral nutrition.

Entercine Biogalenique, Fr.†.
Dihydrostreptomycin sulphate (p.202·2); sulphaguanidine (p.254·1); broxyquinoline; homatropine methobromide (p.462·2).
Diarrhoea.

entero sanol Sanol, Ger.†.
Oak bark (p.1609·3); salix (p.82·3); juglans regia; sage (p.1627·1); absinthium (p.1541·1); chelidonium.
Gastro-intestinal disorders.

Enterobene Merckle, Aust.
Loperamide hydrochloride (p.1197·2).
Diarrhoea.

Enterocantril Rhone-Poulenc, Ital.†.
Mepenzolate bromide (p.465·1); neomycin sulphate (p.229·2); dimethicone (p.1213·1); potassium gluconate (p.1161·1).
Gastro-intestinal disorders.

Enterocura
Nordmark, Ger.†; De Angeli, Ital.†.
Sulphaguanole.
Diarrhoea.

Enterodrip Diepal, Fr.
Preparation for enteral nutrition.

Enterodyne Mer-National, S.Afr.
Bismuth carbonate (p.1180·1); calcium carbonate (p.1182·1); chloroform and morphine tincture (p.56·1); aromatic ammonia liquid (p.1548·3); nutmeg oil (p.1609·3); clove oil (p.1565·2); cardamom tincture (p.1560·1); catechu tincture (p.1560·3); conc. cinnamon water; cinnamon oil (p.1564·2).
Gastro-intestinal disorders.

Enterogermina Sanofi Winthrop, Ital.
Spores of *Bacillus subtilis*.
Gastro-intestinal disorders.

Enterogil Diepal, Fr.
Preparation for enteral nutrition.

Enterol Lenza, Ital.†.
Piromidic acid (p.238·2).
Bacterial infections.

Enterolyte Propan, S.Afr.
Kaolin (p.1195·1); pectin (p.1474·1); sodium lactate; potassium chloride; sodium chloride (p.1152·3).
Diarrhoea.

Enteromix Bioprogress, Ital.
Piromidic acid (p.238·2).
Bacterial infections of the gastro-intestinal tract.

Enteromucilage Bayer, Fr.
Sterculia (p.1214·1).
Constipation.

Enteroplant Schwabe, Ger.; Spitzner, Ger.
Peppermint oil (p.1208·1); caraway oil (p.1559·3).
Dyspepsia.

Enterosan Windsor, UK.
Light kaolin (p.1195·1); morphine hydrochloride (p.56·1); belladonna (p.457·1).
Diarrhoea.

Enterosarine Synthelabo, Switz.†.
Aspirin (p.16·1).
Circulatory disorders; fever; inflammation; pain.

Enterosil Vis, Ital.†.
Metoclopramide hydrochloride (p.1200·3).
Gastro-intestinal disorders.

Enterosilicona Estedi, Spain.
Dimethicone (p.1213·1).
Flatulence.

Enterospasmyl N Interdelta, Switz.†.
Sterculia (p.1214·1); frangula bark (p.1193·2).
Constipation.

Enterostop Teofarma, Ital.
Bacitracin (p.157·3); neomycin sulphate (p.229·2).
Gastro-intestinal infections.

Entero-Teknosal Taco, Ger.
Colloidal silicon dioxide (p.1475·1).
Diarrhoea.

Enteroton Digestivo Panthox & Burck, Ital.†.
Papain (p.1614·1); pancreatin (p.1612·1); cascara (p.1183·1); cape aloes (p.1177·1); belladonna (p.457·1); pepsin (p.1616·3); kola (p.1645·1); boldo (p.1554·1); rhubarb (p.1212·1); nux vomica (p.1609·3).
Digestive disorders.

Enteroton Lassativo Panthox & Burck, Ital.†.
Inositol (p.1591·1); sodium taurocholate; bile extract (p.1553·2); boldo (p.1554·1); rhubarb (p.1212·1); aloin (p.1177·2); orthosiphon stamineus (p.1592·2); cascara (p.1183·1); belladonna (p.457·1).
Constipation; liver disorders.

Enterotropin Laves, Ger.†.
Metabolic product of *Escherichia coli*; choline bitartrate (p.1337·1); pancreatin (p.1612·1); fel tauri (p.1553·2); magnesium orotate (p.1611·2).
Digestive system disorders.

Entero-V Milanfarma, Ital.†.
Belladonna (p.457·1); papaverine hydrochloride (p.1614·2); valerian (p.1643·1); rhubarb (p.1212·1).
Gastro-intestinal spasms.

Enterovaccino ISI (Antitifico) ISI, Ital.
A killed oral typhoid vaccine (p.1536·3).
Active immunisation.

Enterovaccino Nuovo ISM ISM, Ital.
A killed oral typhoid vaccine (p.1536·3).
Active immunisation.

Enterowas Wasserman, Spain†.
Oral suspension: Dihydrostreptomycin (p.202·2); phthalylsulphathiazole (p.237·1); phthalylsulphathiazole-neomycin (p.229·2); povidone tannate.
Tablets: Dihydrostreptomycin (p.202·2); phthalylsulphathiazole (p.237·1); phthalylsulphathiazole-neomycin (p.229·2); homatropine methobromide (p.462·2); povidone tannate.
Gastro-intestinal infections.

Entertainer's Secret KLI, USA.
Artificial saliva.
Formerly known as Moi-Stir 10.
Throat discomfort.

Entex
Note. This name is used for preparations of different composition.
Procter & Gamble, Canad.
Phenylpropanolamine hydrochloride (p.1067·2); guaiphenesin (p.1061·3).
Upper respiratory-tract congestion.

Procter & Gamble, USA.
Phenylephrine hydrochloride (p.1066·2); phenylpropanolamine hydrochloride (p.1067·2); guaiphenesin (p.1061·3).
Coughs and cold symptoms; nasal congestion.

Entex LA Procter & Gamble, USA.
Phenylpropanolamine hydrochloride (p.1067·2); guaiphenesin (p.1061·3).
Coughs and cold symptoms; nasal congestion.

Entex PSE Procter & Gamble, USA.
Pseudoephedrine hydrochloride (p.1068·3); guaiphenesin (p.1061·3).
Coughs and cold symptoms.

Entocord Astra, S.Afr.
Budesonide (p.1034·3).
Ulcerative colitis.

Entocort
Astra, Aust.; Astra, Austral.; Astra, Canad.; Astra, Irl.; Astra, Neth.; Astra, Norw.; Tika, Swed.; Astra, Switz.; Astra, UK.
Budesonide (p.1034·3).
Inflammatory bowel disease.

Entolase Robins, USA†.
Pancrelipase (p.1613·3).
Exocrine pancreatic insufficiency.

Entom Dynacren, Ital.
Diethyltoluamide (p.1405·1); piperonyl butoxide (p.1409·3); pyrethrum (p.1410·1).
Insect repellent.

Entom Nature Dynacren, Ital.
Geranium oil (p.1584·1).
Insect repellent.

Entonox BOC, UK.
Nitrous oxide (p.1228·3); oxygen (p.1165·3).
Pain.

Entosorbine-N Roche Nicholas, Neth.
Albumin tannate (p.1176·3).
Diarrhoea.

Entoxin pur N Klein & Steube, Ger.†.
Homoeopathic preparation.

Entozyme
Note. This name is used for preparations of different composition.
Wyeth-Ayerst, Canad.†.
Pancreatin (p.1612·1).
Exocrine pancreatic insufficiency.

Robins, USA†.
Pancreatin (p.1612·1); pepsin (p.1616·3); bile salts (p.1553·2).
Deficiency of digestive enzymes.

Entrin Acidophilus Murdock, USA.
Lactobacillus rhamnosus (p.1594·1); *Lactobacillus acidophilus* (p.1594·1).

Entrin Bifidus Murdock, USA.
Bifidobacterium longum; *Bifidobacterium breve*; *Lactobacillus rhamnosus*; *Lactobacillus acidophilus* (p.1594·1).

Entrition Clintec, USA.
A range of lactose-free preparations for enteral nutrition.

Entrobar Lafayette, USA.
Barium sulphate (p.1003·1).
Contrast medium for gastro-intestinal radiography.

Entrocalm Galpharm, UK.
Kaolin (p.1195·1); calcium carbonate (p.1182·1).
Diarrhoea.

Entrodyn Ravensberg, Ger.
Phenylephrine (p.1066·2); caffeine (p.749·3).
Hypotension.

Entrophen Frosst, Canad.
Aspirin (p.16·1).
Fever; musculoskeletal and joint disorders; myocardial infarction; pain; transient ischaemic attacks.

Entrydil Orion, Irl.
Diltiazem hydrochloride (p.854·2).
Angina pectoris; hypertension.

Entschlackungstee
Note. This name is used for preparations of different composition.
Salus, Aust.
Silver birch (p.1553·3); taraxacum (p.1634·2); prunus spinosa; rose fruit (p.1365·2).
Herbal preparation.

Smetana, Aust.
Senna (p.1212·2); equisetum (p.1575·1); sambucus (p.1627·2); calcatrippae flowers.
Skin disorders.

Entumin Novartis, Ital.
Clothiapine (p.657·2).
Anxiety disorders; psychoses.

Entumine Sandoz, Switz.
Clothiapine (p.657·2).
Alcohol withdrawal syndrome; anxiety disorders; hyperactivity; psychoses; sleep disorders.

Enturen Ciba Vision, Ital.
Sulphinpyrazone (p.395·2).
Thrombo-embolic disorders.

Entuss Expectorant Roberts, USA; Hauck, USA.
Oral liquid: Hydrocodone tartrate (p.43·1); potassium guaiacolsulfonate (p.1068·3).
Tablets: Hydrocodone tartrate (p.43·1); guaiphenesin (p.1061·3).
Coughs.

Entuss Pediatric Roberts, USA†.
Hydrocodone tartrate (p.43·1); pseudoephedrine hydrochloride (p.1068·3); guaiphenesin (p.1061·3).
Coughs.

Entuss-D Roberts, USA.
Liquid: Hydrocodone tartrate (p.43·1); pseudoephedrine hydrochloride (p.1068·3).
Tablets: Hydrocodone tartrate (p.43·1); pseudoephedrine hydrochloride (p.1068·3); guaiphenesin (p.1061·3).
Coughs.

Entuss-D Jr Roberts, USA.
Hydrocodone tartrate (p.43·1); pseudoephedrine hydrochloride (p.1068·3); guaiphenesin (p.1061·3).
Coughs.

Entwasserungs-Tee Hevert, Ger.†.
Pterocarpus santalinus; rosemary; juniper (p.1592·2); asparagus; levisticum officinale (p.1597·2); ononis (p.1610·2); taraxacum (p.1634·2); rose fruit (p.1365·2); calendula officinalis; squill (p.1070·1); birch leaf (p.1553·3); buchu (p.1555·2); centaurea cyanus.
Oedema; renal disorders.

Enuclen N Alcon-Thilo, Ger.
Tyloxapol (p.1329·2).
Cleansing and lubrication of eye prostheses.

Enuclene
Alcon, Canad.; Alcon, USA.
Tyloxapol (p.1329·2).
Lubrication, cleaning, and wetting of artificial eyes.

Enulose Barre-National, USA.
Lactulose (p.1195·3).
Hepatic encephalopathy.

Enuretine Le Marchand, Fr.
Isopropamide iodide (p.464·3); vitamin E (p.1369·1); thiamine (p.1361·2); ephedrine hydrochloride (p.1059·3); phenobarbitone (p.350·2).
Urinary incontinence.

Enuroplant DHU, Ger.
Homoeopathic preparation.

Enveloppements ECR ECR, Switz.
Hay flowers; chamomile (p.1561·2); achillea (p.1542·2); linseed (p.1596·2); equisetum (p.1575·1).
Cold symptoms.

Enviro-Stress Vitaline, USA.
Vitamin B substances with vitamin C and minerals.

Envisan Marion Merrell Dow, USA†.
Dextranomer (p.1081·1).
Cleansing of wet wounds.

Enzace Sigma, Austral.
Captopril (p.836·3).
Diabetic nephropathy; heart failure; hypertension; myocardial infarction.

Enziagil Magenplus Serturner, Ger.
Gentian (p.1583·3).
Digestive system disorders.

Enzimepar Nuovo, Ital.†.
Ornicarbase (p.1611·1).
Liver disorders.

Enzipan Ravizza, Ital.
Pancreatin (p.1612·1).
Pancreatic disorders.

Enzone UAD, USA.
Hydrocortisone acetate (p.1043·3); pramoxine (p.1298·2).

Enzyflat Solvay, Aust.
Pancreatin (p.1612·1); dimethicone (p.1213·1).
Flatulence; meteorism; preparation for gastro-intestinal radiography and ultrasound.

Enzygaster Benvegna, Ital.†.
Gallbladder wall extract; bile salts (p.1553·2); gastric mucin (p.1472·3); pepsin (p.1616·3); papain (p.1614·1); pancreatin (p.1612·1); amylase (p.1549·1); invertase; protease; cellulase (p.1561·1); yeast (p.1373·1).
Digestive disorders.

enzym gallo sanol N Sanol, Ger.†.
Pancreatin (p.1612·1); enzyme concentrate from Aspergillus; fel tauri (p.1553·2).
Digestive system disorders.

Enzymatic Cleaner Alcon, USA.
Pancreatin (p.1612·1).
Cleansing solution for soft contact lenses.

Enzyme
Note. This name is used for preparations of different composition.
Neo-Life, Austral.
Pancreatin (p.1612·1); pepsin (p.1616·3); ox bile (p.1553·2); papain (p.1614·1); amylase (p.1549·1).
Digestive disorders.

Nature's Bounty, USA.
Amylase (p.1549·1); cellulase (p.1561·1); lipase; protease.
Gastro-intestinal disorders.

Enzyme Digest Quest, UK.
Betaine hydrochloride (p.1553·2); papain (p.1614·1); bromelain (p.1555·1); amylase (p.1549·1).

Enzymed Medice, Ger.†.
Sodium dehydrocholate (p.1570·3); pancreatin (p.1612·1); trypsin (p.1640·1); pepsin (p.1616·3); ascorbic acid; thiamine nitrate; riboflavine sodium phosphate; folic acid; syzygii.
Digestive system disorders.

Enzymed N Medice, Ger.†.
Pancreatin (p.1612·1).
Digestive system disorders.

Enzym-Harongan Schwabe, Ger.
Harongae; curcuma zanthorrhiza; pancreas powder.
Digestive system disorders.

Enzym-Hepaduran Zwintscher, Ger.†.
Bromelains (p.1555·1); pancreatin (p.1612·1); trypsin (p.1640·1); curcuma zanthorrhiza; berberis vulgaris; silybum marianum (p.993·3); ox bile (p.1553·2); vitamins.
Digestive disorders.

Enzym-Lefax Asche, Ger.
Pancreatin (p.1612·1); simethicone (p.1213·1).
Digestive system disorders.

Enzym-Lefax forte Asche, Ger.
Pancreatin (p.1612·1); dimethicone (p.1213·1).
Digestive system disorders.

Enzym-Paractol Asta Medica, Ger.†.
Enzyme concentrate from *Rhizopus arrhizus*; enzyme concentrate from *Aspergillus oryzae*; simethicone (p.1213·1); aluminium hydroxide gel (p.1177·3).
Digestive system disorders.

Enzym-Tyrosolvetten Tosse, Ger.†.
Tyrothricin (p.267·2); cetylpyridinium chloride (p.1106·2); muramidase (p.1604·3); papain (p.1614·1).
Inflammatory disorders and infections of the oropharynx.

Enzym-Wied Wiedemann, Ger.
Pancreatin (p.1612·1); bromelains (p.1555·1); papain (p.1614·1); triacylglycerollipase; amylase (p.1549·1); trypsin (p.1640·1); chymotrypsin (p.1563·2); rutin (p.1580·2).
Arteriosclerosis; soft-tissue injury; thrombosis; venous inflammation.

Enzynorm
Ebewe, Aust.; Nordmark, Ger.†; Hoechst Marion Roussel, S.Afr.
Stomach extract.
Anaemia; digestive disorders.

Enzynorm forte Knoll, Ger.
Gastric mucous membrane extract; amino acids.
Gastro-intestinal disorders; hypochromic anaemias.

eoden Rorer, Ger.†.
Heptaminol hydrochloride (p.1587·2).
Cardiac disorders.

Eogran Sympharma, Aust.
Chamomile (p.1561·2); peppermint leaf (p.1208·1); tormentil (p.1638·3).
Diarrhoea.

Eolarix SmithKline Beecham, UK†.
A measles and rubella vaccine (p.1519·2).
Active immunisation.

Eolene Fisons, Fr.†.
Salbutamol (p.758·2).
Asthma; obstructive airways disease.

Eoline Pfizer, Belg.
Hydrocortisone (p.1043·3); nystatin (p.386·1); di-oxytetracycline calcium (p.235·1).
Infected skin disorders.

Eolus Sigma-Tau, Ital.
Eformoterol fumarate (p.752·3).
Obstructive airways disease.

E.P. Pharmax, UK.
Paracetamol (p.72·2); caffeine (p.749·3); codeine phosphate (p.26·1).
Pain.

EPA Vitaplex, Austral.†.
Omega-3 marine triglycerides (p.1276·1).
Essential fatty acid deficiencies.

Epabetina OFF, Ital.
Betaine glucuronate (p.1553·2); trigonelline.
Liver disorders.

Epa-Bon Siforma, Ital.
Cyclobutyrol sodium (p.1569·2).
Biliary disorders.

Epacaps Byk Roland, Switz.
Marine fish oil (p.1276·1).
Hyperlipidaemias; nutritional supplement.

Epadel Mochida, Jpn†.
Ethyl icosapentate.
Arteriosclerosis obliterans.

Epaderm Bioglan, UK.
Yellow soft paraffin (p.1382·3); emulsifying wax (p.1383·3); liquid paraffin (p.1382·1).
Dry skin.

Epadora Herdel, Ital.†.
Ferritin (p.1580·1).
Anaemias.

Epaglifer Lagap, Ital.†.
Ferrous glycine sulphate (p.1340·1); cyanocobalamin (p.1363·3).
Anaemias; deficiency states.

Epaglutone Milanfarma, Ital.†.
Gentian (p.1583·3); cynara (p.1569·2); boldo (p.1554·1).
Digestive disorders.

Epalat EPS OFF, Ital.
Lactulose (p.1195·3).
Liver disorders.

Epalfen Zambon, Ital.
Lactulose (p.1195·3).
Bacterial gastro-intestinal infections; constipation; digestive disorders; hepatic encephalopathy.

Epanal Bouchara, Fr.†.
Tablets: Phenobarbitone (p.350·2); crataegus (p.1568·2).
Anxiety; epilepsy; insomnia; tremor.

Epanutin
Parke, Davis, Aust.; Parke, Davis, Belg.; Parke, Davis, Ger.; Parke, Davis, Irl.; Parke, Davis, Neth.; Parke, Davis, S.Afr.; Parke, Davis, Spain; Parke, Davis, Swed.; Parke, Davis, Switz.; Parke, Davis, UK.
Phenytoin (p.352·3) or phenytoin sodium (p.352·3).
Arrhythmias; epilepsy; migraine; parkinsonism; psychoses; Sydenham's chorea; trigeminal neuralgia.

Epanutin Fenobarbitona Parke, Davis, Spain†.
Phenytoin sodium (p.352·3); phenobarbitone (p.350·2).
Epilepsy.

Epaplex Aandersen, Ital.†.
Ferritin (p.1580·1); cyanocobalamin (p.1363·3); thioctic acid (p.1636·2).
Hypochromic anaemia.

Epaplex 40 Uno, Ital.
Ferric sodium gluconate (p.1340·1).
Sideropenic anaemia.

Epaq
Kolassa, Aust.; 3M, Ger.; Asta Medica, Ger.
Salbutamol sulphate (p.758·2).
Obstructive airways disease.

Epar Euchessina Antonetto, Ital.†.
Fencibutirol (p.1578·3); belladonna (p.457·1); boldo (p.1554·1); rhubarb (p.1212·1); cascara (p.1183·1).
Constipation.

Eparema SIT, Ital.
Cascara (p.1183·1); boldo (p.1554·1); rhubarb (p.1212·1).
Constipation.

Eparema-Levul SIT, Ital.
Cascara (p.1183·1); boldo (p.1554·1); rhubarb (p.1212·1); fructose (p.1343·2).
Constipation.

Epargriseovit Pharmacia Upjohn, Ital.
Cyanocobalamin (p.1363·3); folic acid (p.1340·3); nicotinamide (p.1351·2); ascorbic acid (p.1365·2).
Anaemias; peripheral neuropathies; tonic.

Eparical Rhone-Poulenc Rorer, Ital.
Heparin calcium (p.879·3).
Thrombo-embolic disorders.

Eparinlider Pharmaland, Ital.
Heparin calcium (p.879·3).
Thrombo-embolic disorders.

Eparinovis INTES, Ital.
Heparin sodium (p.879·3).
Eye disorders.

Eparmefolin Bracco, Ital.
Cyanocobalamin (p.1363·3); calcium folinate (p.1342·2).
Anaemias; deficiency states.

Eparsil Pulitzer, Ital.
Silymarin (p.993·3).
Liver disorders.

Epartisone Bouty, Ital.†.
Heparin sodium (p.879·3); hydrocortisone acetate (p.1043·3).
Anorectal disorders; varicose disorders.

Epartonno Benvegna, Ital.†.
Calcium folinate (p.1342·2); cyanocobalamin (p.1363·3); ascorbic acid (p.1365·2).
Anaemias.

Epaspes Nuovo, Ital.†.
Fosforylcholine calcium (p.1581·3).
Liver disorders.

Epatiol Medici, Ital.†.
Tiopronin (p.997·2).
Liver disorders.

Epatoxil Tosi, Ital.
Cogalactoisomerase sodium (p.1566·2).
Liver disorders.

Epa-Treis Ecobi, Ital.
Calcium oxoglurate; choline orotate (p.1611·2).
Liver disorders.

Epaxal
Cortec, Swed.; Berna, Switz.
An inactivated hepatitis A vaccine (p.1512·2).
Active immunisation.

Epha-retard Woelm, Ger.†.
Dimenhydrinate (p.408·2).
Motion sickness.

Ephecuan Staufen, Ger.†.
Homoeopathic preparation.

Ephedrine and Amytal Lilly, USA†.
Ephedrine sulphate (p.1059·3); amylobarbitone (p.641·3).

Ephepect Bolder, Ger.
Ephedrine hydrochloride (p.1059·3); ammonium chloride (p.1055·2); thyme (p.1636·3); primula rhizome; anise oil (p.1550·1); fennel oil (p.1579·2); peppermint oil (p.1208·1); eucalyptus oil (p.1578·1).
Bronchitis; catarrh.

Ephepect-Blocker-Pastillen N Bolder, Ger.
Sodium dibunate (p.1070·1); dequalinium chloride (p.1112·1).
Coughs and associated respiratory-tract disorders.

Ephex Teral, USA.
Guaiphenesin (p.1061·3); ephedrine hydrochloride (p.1059·3).

Ephydion Aerocid, Fr.
Syrup: Ethylmorphine hydrochloride (p.36·1); potassium guaiacolsulfonate (p.1068·3); grindelia.
Formerly contained ephedrine hydrochloride, ethylmorphine hydrochloride, potassium guaiacolsulfonate, belladonna, grindelia, and drosera.
Tablets; oral drops: Ethylmorphine hydrochloride (p.36·1); sodium benzoate (p.1102·3); grindelia.
Formerly contained ephedrine hydrochloride, ethylmorphine hydrochloride, sodium benzoate, belladonna, grindelia, and drosera.
Coughs.

Ephydrol Saunier-Daguin, Fr.
Cream: Fioravanti oil; lavender oil (p.1594·3); bergamot oil (p.1553·1); lemon oil (p.1595·3); camphor (p.1557·2); menthol (p.1600·2); saligenin; formaldehyde solution (p.1113·2).
Topical solution: Sanicle; fioravanti; camphor (p.1557·2); lavender oil (p.1594·3); bergamot oil (p.1553·1); lemon oil (p.1595·3); menthol (p.1600·2); saligenin; formaldehyde solution (p.1113·2).
Hyperhidrosis.

Ephynal
Roche, Aust.; Roche, Belg.; Roche, Fr.; Roche Nicholas, Ger.; Roche Consumer, Irl.; Roche, Ital.; Roche, S.Afr.; Roche Nicholas, Spain; Roche, Swed.†; Roche, Switz.; Roche Consumer, UK.
Alpha tocopheryl acetate (p.1369·2).
Benign mammary dysplasias; habitual abortion; haemolytic anaemia; haemorrhagic disease of the newborn; lipid malabsorption; male infertility; myopia; myotonic dystrophy; Peyronie's disease; urinary incontinence; vascular disorders; vitamin E deficiency.

Epi EZ Allerex, Canad.
Adrenaline (p.813·2).
Anaphylactic shock.

Epi-Aberel Janssen-Cilag, Ger.
Tretinoin (p.1093·3).
Acne.

Epianal Will-Pharma, Neth.
Sodium oleate (p.1469·1); oxypolyethoxydodecanum; chlorocarvacrol.
Haemorrhoids.

Epi-C Lafayette, USA.
Barium sulphate (p.1003·1).
Contrast medium for gastro-intestinal radiography.

Epicon Valeas, Ital.†.
Sodium valproate (p.361·2).
Epilepsy.

Epicordin
Note. This name is used for preparations of different composition.
Solvay, Aust.
Isosorbide mononitrate (p.893·3).
Angina pectoris; heart failure; pulmonary hypertension.

Solvay, Ger.
Captopril (p.836·3).
Heart failure; hypertension.

Epicrin Gebro, Switz.†.
Vitamin A palmitate; biotin; dexpanthenol; zinc amino acid chelate; millet extract; cystine; wheat-germ oil.
Hair and nail disorders.

Epidosin Solvay, Ger.
Valethamate bromide (p.469·3).
Smooth muscle spasms.

Epidropal Fresenius, Ger.†.
Allopurinol (p.390·2).
Gout; hyperuricaemia.

Epiestrol Roerig, Ital.
Oestradiol (p.1455·1).
Menopausal disorders.

Epiferol Juventus, Spain†.
Reproterol hydrochloride (p.758·1).
Obstructive airways disease.

Epifoam
Stafford-Miller, UK†; Schwarz, USA.
Hydrocortisone acetate (p.1043·3); pramoxine hydrochloride (p.1298·2).
Perineal injury.

Epifrin
Allergan, Austral.†; Allergan, Belg.†; Allergan, Canad.; Allergan, Irl.†; Allergan, S.Afr.†; Allergan, Switz.†; Allergan, USA.
Adrenaline (p.813·2) or adrenaline hydrochloride (p.813·3).
Open-angle glaucoma.

Epiglaufrin Allergan, Ger.†.
Adrenaline (p.813·2).
Glaucoma.

Epikur Agepha, Aust.
Meprobamate (p.678·1).
Anxiety; sleep disturbances.

Epilan Gerot, Aust.
Methoin (p.349·1).
Epilepsy.

Epilan-D Gerot, Aust.
Phenytoin (p.352·3).
Epilepsy.

Epilantin Miquel Otsuka, Spain.
Phenytoin (p.352·3); phenobarbitone (p.350·2).
Epilepsy.

Epilantine Streuli, Switz.
Phenytoin sodium (p.352·3).
Epilepsy.

Epilim
Reckitt & Colman, Austral.; Sanofi Winthrop, Irl.; Reckitt & Colman, S.Afr.; Sanofi Winthrop, UK.
Sodium valproate (p.361·2).
Epilepsy.

Epilim Chrono
Sanofi Winthrop, Irl.; Sanofi Winthrop, UK.
Sodium valproate (p.361·2); valproic acid (p.361·2).
Epilepsy.

E-Pilo
Ciba Vision, Canad.; Iolab, USA.
Adrenaline acid tartrate (p.813·3); pilocarpine hydrochloride (p.1396·3).
Glaucoma; raised intra-ocular pressure.

Epi-Lyt
Stiefel, Canad.; Stiefel, USA.
Glycerol (p.1585·2); lactic acid (p.1593·3).
Dry skin.

Epimaz Norton, UK.
Carbamazepine (p.339·2).

Epi-Monistat Janssen-Cilag, Ger.
Miconazole nitrate (p.384·3).
Fungal infections.

Epimorph Wyeth-Ayerst, Canad.†.
Morphine sulphate (p.56·2).
Pain.

Epinal Alcon, USA.
Adrenaline borate complex (p.815·2).
Open-angle glaucoma.

Epinat AFI, Norw.
Phenytoin (p.352·3) or phenytoin sodium (p.352·3).
Arrhythmias; epilepsy.

Epipak Espe, Ger.
Aluminium chlorohydrate (p.1078·3); polyethyleneimine hydrochloride.
Mouth disorders.

Epipen
CSL, Austral.; Allerex, Canad.; Merck, S.Afr.; ALK, Swed.; ALK, UK; Center Laboratories, USA.
Adrenaline (p.813·2) or adrenaline hydrochloride (p.813·3).
Anaphylaxis.

Epi-Pevaryl Janssen-Cilag, Ger.
Econazole nitrate (p.377·2).
Fungal skin and nail infections.

Epi-Pevaryl Heilpaste Janssen-Cilag, Ger.
Econazole nitrate (p.377·2); zinc oxide (p.1096·2).
Fungal skin infections.

Epi-Pevaryl Pv Janssen-Cilag, Ger.
Econazole (p.377·2).
Pityriasis versicolor.

Epipevisone Janssen-Cilag, Ger.
Econazole nitrate (p.377·2); triamcinolone acetonide (p.1050·2).
Fungal skin infections.

Epiphane Biorga, Fr.
Gelatin (p.723·2).
Fragile nails and hair.

Epiphysan Disperga, Aust.
Bovine pineal gland extract (p.1599·1).
Hypersexuality; psychoses.

Epipropane Medgenix, Belg.
Phenobarbitone magnesium (p.351·3); amphetamine sulphate (p.1477·3).
Agitation; epilepsy; hypertension.

Episcorit Sanum-Kehlbeck, Ger.
Echinacea purpura (p.1574·2).
Respiratory- and urinary-tract infections.

Episeal Richelin, S.Afr.†.
Trypsin (p.1640·1); peru balsam (p.1617·2); castor oil (p.1560·2).
Sunburn; wounds.

Episec Odan, Canad.
Liquid paraffin (p.1382·1); propylene glycol (p.1622·1); triethanolamine stearate.

Epistaxol Medical, Spain.
Adrenaline (p.813·2); phenazone (p.78·2); naphazoline hydrochloride (p.1064·2); rutin (p.1580·2).
Epistaxis; mucous membrane haemorrhage.

Epiteliplast Llorens, Spain†.
Sodium aminobenzoate.
Herpes simplex infections.

Epitelizante Ciba Vision, Spain.
Amino acids; chloramphenicol (p.182·1); retinol palmitate (p.1359·2).
Corneal damage.

Epithelial Wiedenmann, Switz.†.
Ichthammol (p.1083·3); linseed oil (p.1596·2); titanium dioxide (p.1093·3); zinc oxide (p.1096·2).
Wounds.

Epitheliale Ducray, Fr.
Avena (p.1551·3); vitamins A and E.
Skin disorders.

Epitol Lemmon, USA.
Carbamazepine (p.339·2).
Epilepsy; trigeminal neuralgia.

Epitopic Gerda, Fr.
Difluprednate (p.1039·3).
Skin disorders.

Epival Abbott, Canad.
Semisodium valproate (p.361·2).
Epilepsy; mania.

Epivir
Glaxo Wellcome, Fr.; Glaxo Wellcome, Ger.; Glaxo Wellcome, Ital.; Glaxo Wellcome, Neth.; Glaxo Wellcome, Spain; Glaxo Wellcome, Swed.; Glaxo Wellcome, UK.
Lamivudine (p.622·1).
HIV infection.

Epixian UCB, Spain.
Cocarboxylase (p.1361·2); magnesium phosphate (p.1157·3); magnesium succinate; pyridoxal phosphate (p.1363·1); chymotrypsin (p.1563·2); trypsin (p.1640·1).
Renal calculi.

Epixine Wolfs, Belg.†.
Lauroyldiacetylpyridoxine.
Seborrhoeic skin disorders.

Epizon Mepha, Switz.†.
Paracetamol (p.72·2); propyphenazone (p.81·3); guaiphenesin (p.1061·3); valerian (p.1643·1); passion flower (p.1615·3).
Fever; pain.

Eplonat Nattermann, Ger.†.
d-Alpha tocopherol (p.1369·1).
Vitamin E deficiency.

E.P.O. & E Quest, UK.
Evening primrose oil (p.1582·1); vitamin E.

Epo + Maxepa + Vitamin E Herbal Plus Formula 8 Vitelle, Austral.
d-Alpha tocopherol (p.1369·1); evening primrose oil (p.1582·1); marine fish oil (p.1276·1).
Nutritional supplement.

EPOC Evening Primrose Oil Co., UK.
Evening primrose oil (p.1582·1).

EPOC Marine Evening Primrose Oil Co., UK.
Evening primrose oil (p.1582·1); marine fish oil (p.1276·1).

Epocelin
Fujisawa, Jpn; CEPA, Spain.
Ceftizoxime sodium (p.175·2).
Lignocaine (p.1293·2) or lignocaine hydrochloride (p.1293·2) is included in the intramuscular injection to alleviate the pain of injection.
Bacterial infections.

Epocler Whitehall, Ital.
Hydroquinone (p.1083·1).
Skin hyperpigmentation.

Epodyl Zeneca, Aust.†.
Ethoglucid.
Bladder cancer.

Epogam
Note. This name is used for preparations of different composition.
Searle, Austral.; Beiersdorf, Ger.; Searle, Irl.; Whitehall, Ital.; Searle, UK.
Evening primrose oil (p.1582·1).
Eczema.

Scotia, S.Afr.; Leti, Spain.
Gamolenic acid (p.1582·1).
Eczema.

Epogen Amgen, USA.
Epoetin alfa (p.718·3).
Anaemia in cancer patients on chemotherapy; anaemia in zidovudine-treated HIV-infected patients; anaemia of chronic renal failure.

Epogin Chugai, Jpn.
Epoetin beta (p.718·3).
Anaemia in renal dialysis patients; autologous blood transfusion.

Epopa Vitalia, UK.
Safflower oil (p.1353·3); salmon oil (p.1276·1); evening primrose oil (p.1582·1); borage oil (p.1582·1); nicotinic acid (p.1351·2).

Epopen Pensa, Spain.
Epoetin alfa (p.718·3).
Anaemia of chronic renal failure; cisplatin-induced anaemia.

Eposerin Pharmacia Upjohn, Ital.
Ceftizoxime sodium (p.175·2).
Lignocaine hydrochloride (p.1293·2) is included in the intramuscular injection to alleviate the pain of injection.
Bacterial infections.

Eposin Nycomed, Norw.; Nycomed, Swed.
Etoposide (p.532·3).
Malignant neoplasms.

Epoxitin Cilag, Ital.
Epoetin alfa (p.718·3).
Anaemia of renal failure.

Eppy
Allergan, Fr.; Chauvin, Irl.; Pharmec, Ital.; Kabi Pharmacia, Neth.†; Smith & Nephew, S.Afr.; Abigo, Swed.; Chauvin, UK.
Adrenaline (p.813·2).
Open-angle glaucoma.

Eppy/N
Barnes-Hind, Austral.†; Barnes-Hind, Switz.†; Pilkington Barnes-Hind, USA.
Adrenaline borate complex (p.815·2).
Open-angle glaucoma.

Eppystabil Pharmacia Upjohn, Aust.
Adrenaline (p.813·2).
Open-angle glaucoma.

Eprex
Janssen-Cilag, Austral.; Janssen-Cilag, Belg.; Janssen-Ortho, Canad.; Janssen-Cilag, Fr.; Janssen-Cilag, Irl.; Janssen-Cilag, Ital.; Janssen-Cilag, Neth.; Janssen-Cilag, Norw.; Janssen-Cilag, S.Afr.; Janssen-Cilag, Spain; Janssen-Cilag, Swed.; Janssen-Cilag, Switz.; Janssen-Cilag, UK.
Epoetin alfa (p.718·3).
Anaemia; autologous blood transfusions.

Epromate Major, USA.
Aspirin (p.16·1); meprobamate (p.678·1).
Pain.

Epsoclar Biologici Italia, Ital.
Heparin sodium (p.879·3).
Thrombo-embolic disorders.

ept Stick Test Warner-Lambert, USA.
Pregnancy test (p.1621·2).

Eptacalcin Sigma-Tau, Ital.†.
Salcatonin (p.735·3).
Osteoporosis; Paget's disease of bone.

Eptadone Zambon, Ital.
Methadone hydrochloride (p.53·2).
Opioid withdrawal; pain.

Eptico Watsons, Canad.
Camphor (p.1557·2); zinc oxide (p.1096·2).

Epuram Pharmafarm, Fr.
Citrulline (p.1337·2); arginine hydrochloride (p.1334·1); ornithine hydrochloride (p.1352·3).
Liver disorders.

Equagesic
Note. This name is used for preparations of different composition.
Wyeth-Ayerst, Canad.; John Wyeth, Irl.†; Akromed, S.Afr.; Wyeth, UK.
Aspirin (p.16·1); meprobamate (p.678·1); ethoheptazine citrate (p.36·1).
Musculoskeletal pain; skeletal muscle spasm.
Wyeth-Ayerst, USA.
Aspirin (p.16·1); meprobamate (p.678·1).
Musculoskeletal pain.

Equalactin Numark, USA.
Polycarbophil calcium (p.1209·1).
Constipation; diarrhoea.

Equanil
Wyeth, Austral.; Wyeth-Ayerst, Canad.; Sanofi Winthrop, Fr.; John Wyeth, Irl.†; Akromed, S.Afr.; Wyeth, UK; Wyeth-Ayerst, USA.
Meprobamate (p.678·1).
Alcohol withdrawal syndrome; anxiety; premedication; skeletal muscle spasm.

Equation Pierre Fabre, Fr.†.
Chlorhexidine gluconate (p.1107·2).
Skin cleanser.

Equazine M Rugby, USA.
Aspirin (p.16·1); meprobamate (p.678·1).
Pain.

Equibar Biogalenique, Fr.†.
Methyldopa (p.904·2).
Hypertension.

Equidan Miquel Otsuka, Spain†.
Belladonna alkaloids (p.457·1); phenytoin (p.352·3); phenobarbitone (p.350·2).
Anxiety; infantile spasms; insomnia; menopausal disorders; migraine.

Equiday E Solvay, Ger.
d-Alpha tocopherol (p.1369·1).
Vitamin E deficiency.

Equidral Scherer, Ital.
Maltodextrin; electrolytes (p.1147·1).
Electrolyte depletion in hyperhidrosis.

Equilet Mission Pharmacal, USA.
Calcium carbonate (p.1182·1).
Hyperacidity.

Equilibrin Rhone-Poulenc Rorer, Ger.
Amitriptylinoxide (p.278·1).
Depression.

Equilid Bruno, Ital.
Sulpiride (p.692·3).
Adjuvant in gastric ulcer; depression; nausea and vomiting; nervous disorders; psychoses.

Equilium Fumouze, Fr.
Tiapride (p.696·2).
Aggressive states; agitation; choreiform movements; neuralgias.

Equilon Chefaro, UK.
Mebeverine hydrochloride (p.1199·2).
Irritable bowel syndrome.

Equin Aldo, Spain.
Conjugated oestrogens (p.1457·3).
Menopausal disorders.

Equipar Lampugnani, Ital.†.
Phosphorylcolaminecholine; betaine (p.1553·2); nicotinamide (p.1351·2); inositol (p.1591·1).
Liver and biliary disorders.

Equipur Medipharma, Ger.
Vincamine (p.1644·1).
Ménière's disease; mental function disorders; metabolic and circulatory disorders of the brain, retina, and inner ear.

Equisil Klein, Ger.
Equisetum (p.1575·1); plantago lanceolata; castanea vulgaris; primula rhizome; verbascum flowers; thyme (p.1636·3); ephedrine hydrochloride (p.1059·3); colloidal silicon dioxide (p.1475·1).
Coughs and associated respiratory-tract disorders.

Equiton Bruschettini, Ital.
Timolol maleate (p.953·3); pilocarpine hydrochloride (p.1396·3).
Glaucoma; ocular hypertension.

Eracine Sanofi Winthrop, Fr.
Acrosoxacin (p.150·1).
Bacterial infections.

Eradacil Sanofi Winthrop, Spain†.
Acrosoxacin (p.150·1).
Gonorrhoea.

Eradacin
Sanofi Winthrop, Irl.†; Sterling Winthrop, UK†.
Acrosoxacin (p.150·1).
Gonorrhoea.

Eramycin Wesley, USA.
Erythromycin stearate (p.204·2).
Bacterial infections.

Erantin Boehringer Mannheim, Spain.
Epoetin beta (p.718·3).
Anaemia of chronic renal failure; cisplatin-induced anaemia.

Erasol McGloin, Austral.
Phenazone (p.78·2).
Ear ache.

Ercaf Geneva, USA.
Ergotamine tartrate (p.445·3); caffeine (p.749·3).
Migraine and related vascular headache.

Ercar Almirall, Spain.
Carboplatin (p.510·3).
Bladder cancer; head and neck cancer; ovarian cancer; small-cell lung cancer.

Ercefuril Promesa, Spain†.
Nifuroxazide (p.231·3).
Diarrhoea.

Ercefuryl
Synthelabo, Belg.; Synthelabo, Fr.; Luitpold, Ital.
Nifuroxazide (p.231·3).
Acute infective diarrhoea.

Ercevit Synthelabo, Fr.
Rutin (p.1580·2); rutin propylsulphonate sodium.
Peripheral vascular disorders.

Erco-Fer Orion, Swed.
Ferrous fumarate (p.1339·3).
Iron deficiency; iron-deficiency anaemia.

Erco-Fer vitamin Orion, Swed.
Multivitamin preparation with ferrous fumarate (p.1339·3).
Iron deficiency; iron-deficiency anaemia.

Ercolax Ercopharm, Switz.
Bisacodyl (p.1179·3).
Bowel evacuation; constipation.

Ercoquin Nycomed, Norw.
Hydroxychloroquine sulphate (p.431·2).
Lupus erythematosus; malaria; photosensitivity; rheumatoid arthritis; Sjögren's syndrome.

Ercorax Roll-on Ercopharm, Switz.
Propantheline bromide (p.468·1).
Hyperhidrosis.

Ercotina Orion, Swed.
Propantheline bromide (p.468·1).
Gastro-intestinal disorders.

Ereclase Pharmethic, Belg.†.
Phenobarbitone sparteine (p.351·3).
Arrhythmias.

Erecnos Fournier, UK.
Thymoxamine hydrochloride (p.952·2).
Impotence.

Eremfat
Kolassa, Aust.; Fatol, Ger.
Rifampicin (p.243·2) or rifampicin sodium (p.245·3).
Brucellosis; leprosy; meningococcal meningitis prophylaxis; staphylococcal infections; tuberculosis.

Eres N Muller Goppingen, Ger.
Verbascum flowers.
Bronchial catarrh.

Erevan Fournier, Ital.
A heparinoid (p.882·3).
Thrombosis prophylaxis; vascular disorders.

Erfolgan Boehringer Mannheim, Spain.
Ibopamine hydrochloride (p.889·3).
Heart failure.

Ergadyl RP-LABO, Fr.†.
Fosfocreatinine disodium (p.1581·3); potassium fumarate; methylcolamine succinate.
Tonic.

Ergamisol
Janssen-Cilag, Austral.; Janssen-Cilag, Belg.; Janssen-Ortho, Canad.; Janssen-Cilag, Ger.; Janssen-Cilag, Ital.; Janssen-Cilag, Neth.; Janssen-Cilag, S.Afr.; Janssen, USA.
Levamisole hydrochloride (p.102·3).
Adjunct to fluorouracil therapy in colonic cancer; nephrotic syndrome.

Ergate Propan-Vernleigh, S.Afr.†.
Ergotamine tartrate (p.445·3).
Migraine.

Ergenyl
Kwizda, Aust.†; Sanofi Winthrop, Ger.; Sanofi, Swed.
Sodium valproate (p.361·2).
Epilepsy.

Ergenyl Chrono Sanofi Winthrop, Ger.
Sodium valproate (p.361·2); valproic acid (p.361·2).
Epilepsy.

Ergix Monot, Fr.
Ibuprofen (p.44·1).
Fever; pain.

Ergo Foletto, Ital.†.
Dihydroergocristine mesylate (p.1571·3).
Cerebral and peripheral vascular disorders; dopaminergic deficiency syndromes; hypertension; migraine.

ergo sanol Sanol, Ger.†.
Ergotamine tartrate (p.445·3); etenzamide (p.35·3).
Formerly contained ergotamine tartrate, thiamine nitrate, caffeine or caffeine and caffeine-citric acid, and etenzamide.
Headache; migraine.

ergo sanol SL Sanol, Ger.†.
Ergotamine tartrate (p.445·3).
Formerly contained ergotamine tartrate and caffeine.
Headache; migraine.

ergo sanol spezial Sanol, Ger.†.
Ergotamine tartrate (p.445·3); phenyltoloxamine citrate (p.416·1); etenzamide (p.35·3).
Formerly contained ergotamine tartrate, thiamine nitrate, phenyltoloxamine citrate, caffeine or caffeine and caffeine-citric acid, and etenzamide.
Migraine and other vascular headaches.

ergo sanol spezial N Sanol, Ger.
Ergotamine tartrate (p.445·3).
Migraine and other vascular headache.

ergobel Hormosan, Ger.
Nicergoline (p.1607·1).
Mental function disorders.

Ergocalm
Note. This name is used for preparations of different composition.
Mayrhofer, Aust.
Lorazepam (p.675·3).
Anxiety disorders; premedication; sleep disorders.
Brenner-Efeka, Ger.
Lormetazepam (p.677·1).
Premedication; sleep disorders.

Ergocris Magis, Ital.
Dihydroergocristine mesylate (p.1571·3).
Cerebral and peripheral vascular disorders; dopaminergic deficiency; headache; hypertension; migraine.

Ergodavur Belmac, Spain.
Dihydroergocristine mesylate (p.1571·3).
Cerebrovascular disorders; vestibular disorders.

Ergodesit Desitin, Ger.
Co-dergocrine mesylate (p.1566·1).
Hypertension; mental function disorders.

Ergodilat Diviser Aquilea, Spain.
Co-dergocrine mesylate (p.1566·1).
Cerebrovascular disorders; circulatory disorders.

Ergodose Murat, Fr.
Co-dergocrine mesylate (p.1566·1).
Mental function impairment in the elderly.

Ergodryl
Parke, Davis, Austral.; Parke, Davis, Canad.
Ergotamine tartrate (p.445·3); caffeine citrate (p.749·3); diphenhydramine hydrochloride (p.409·1).
Migraine and other vascular headaches.

Ergodryl Mono Parke, Davis, Austral.
Ergotamine tartrate (p.445·3).
Migraine and other vascular headaches.

Ergodystan Krewel, Ger.†.
Dihydroergotamine tartrate (p.444·3); caffeine (p.749·3).
Dysmenorrhoea; headache; migraine.

Ergoffin Dresden, Ger.
Ergotamine tartrate (p.445·3); caffeine (p.749·3).
Headache; migraine.

Ergofit Bonomelli, Ital.
Vitamin C (p.1365·2).
Nutritional supplement.

Ergohydrine Streuli, Switz.
Co-dergocrine mesylate (p.1566·1).
Cerebrovascular disorders.

Ergokapton Strallhofer, Aust.
Ergotamine tartrate (p.445·3).
Migraine and related vascular headaches.

Ergokod Biogalenique, Fr.†.
Co-dergocrine mesylate (p.1566·1).
Mental function impairment in the elderly; vascular disorders.

Ergo-Kranit Krewel, Ger.
Ergotamine tartrate (p.445·3); propyphenazone (p.81·3); paracetamol (p.72·2).
Headache including migraine.

Ergo-Kranit mono Krewel, Ger.
Ergotamine tartrate (p.445·3).
Migraine and other vascular headaches.

Ergolefrin Gepepharm, Ger.
Dihydroergotamine mesylate (p.444·2); etilefrine hydrochloride (p.867·2).
Hypotension.

Ergo-Lonarid Boehringer Ingelheim, Ger.†.
Dihydroergotamine tartrate (p.444·3); paracetamol (p.72·2); codeine phosphate (p.26·1); caffeine (p.749·3).
Headache including migraine.

Ergo-Lonarid PD Boehringer Ingelheim, Ger.
Dihydroergotamine tartrate (p.444·3); paracetamol (p.72·2).
Headache; migraine.

Ergomar
Rhone-Poulenc Rorer, Canad.; Lotus, USA.
Ergotamine tartrate (p.445·3).
Migraine and other vascular headaches.

Ergomed Kwizda, Aust.
Co-dergocrine mesylate (p.1566·1).
Cerebral insufficiency; hypertension; migraine and related vascular headache.

Ergometron Vernleigh, S.Afr.†.
Ergometrine maleate (p.1575·1).
Migraine; postpartum or postabortal haemorrhage.

Ergomimet Klinge, Ger.
Dihydroergotamine mesylate (p.444·2).
Hypotension; migraine and other vascular headaches; vascular disorders.

Ergomimet plus Klinge, Ger.
Dihydroergotamine mesylate (p.444·2); etilefrine hydrochloride (p.867·2).
Hypotension.

Ergon Biotrading, Ital.†.
Pollen.
Nutritional supplement.

Ergon 1000 Biotrading, Ital.†.
Royal jelly (p.1626·3).
Nutritional supplement.

Ergont
Sigmapharm, Aust.; Desitin, Ger.; Cimex, Switz.†.
Dihydroergotamine mesylate (p.444·2).
Chronic venous insufficiency; hypotension; migraine and related vascular headache.

Ergoplex Kwizda, Aust.
Co-dergocrine mesylate (p.1566·1).
Cerebral insufficiency; hypertension; migraine and related vascular headache.

Ergoplus Hormosan, Ger.
Co-dergocrine mesylate (p.1566·1).
Cervical disc syndrome; hypertension; mental function disorders.

Ergoram Bonomelli, Ital.
Amino-acid preparation.
Nutritional supplement.

Ergosanol Schwarz, Switz.
Ergotamine tartrate (p.445·3); etenzamide (p.35·3); caffeine (p.749·3).
Cluster headache; migraine and related vascular headache.

Ergosanol a la cafeine Schwarz, Switz.
Ergotamine tartrate (p.445·3); etenzamide (p.35·3); caffeine (p.749·3); caffeine citrate (p.749·3).
Cluster headache; migraine and other vascular headaches.

Ergosanol SL Schwarz, Switz.†.
Ergotamine tartrate (p.445·3).
Migraine and related vascular headache.

Ergosanol special Schwarz, Switz.
Ergotamine tartrate (p.445·3); phenyltoloxamine citrate (p.416·1); etenzamide (p.35·3); caffeine (p.749·3).
Cluster headache; migraine and related vascular headache.

Ergosanol special a la cafeine Schwarz, Switz.
Ergotamine tartrate (p.445·3); etenzamide (p.35·3); caffeine (p.749·3); caffeine citrate (p.749·3); phenyltoloxamine citrate (p.416·1).
Cluster headache; migraine and other vascular headaches.

Ergostat Parke, Davis, USA†.
Ergotamine tartrate (p.445·3).
Migraine.

Ergotam CT, Ger.
Dihydroergotamine mesylate (p.444·2).
Hypotension; migraine and other vascular headaches.

Ergotan Salf, Ital.
Ergotamine tartrate (p.445·3).
Migraine and related vascular headache.

Ergotartrat Rosch & Handel, Aust.†.
Ergotamine tartrate (p.445·3).
Migraine and related vascular headache.

Ergotina Ist. Chim. Inter., Ital.†.
Dihydroergocristine mesylate (p.1571·3).
Cerebral and peripheral vascular disorders; dopaminergic deficiency syndromes; hypertension; migraine.

Ergotonine Streuli, Switz.
Dihydroergotamine mesylate (p.444·2).
Fatigue; hypotension; migraine.

Ergotop Kwizda, Aust.
Nicergoline (p.1607·1).
Peripheral and cerebral vascular disorders.

Ergotox CT, Ger.
Co-dergocrine mesylate (p.1566·1).
Dementia.

Ergotrate
Lilly, Canad.; Lilly, S.Afr.†; Lilly, USA.
Ergometrine maleate (p.1575·1).
Postpartum atony and haemorrhage.

Ergovasan Klinge, Aust.
Dihydroergotamine mesylate (p.444·2).
Circulatory disorders; hypotension; migraine and related vascular headaches.

Ergozim Lactis Corvi, Ital.†.
Lactobacillus acidophilus (p.1594·1); *Streptococcus lactis*.
Gastro-intestinal disorders.

Ergybiol Nutergia, Fr.
Mineral preparation.

Ergymag Nutergia, Fr.
Vitamin B and mineral preparation.

Ergyphilus Nutergia, Fr.
Lactobacillus species, fibre, and mineral preparation.
Maintenance of normal gastro-intestinal flora.

Eridan SIT, Ital.
Diazepam (p.661·1).
Adjuvant in epilepsy; anxiety disorders.

Eridium Roberts, USA†.
Phenazopyridine hydrochloride (p.78·3).
Irritation of the lower urinary tract.

Eridosis Stiefel, Spain.
Erythromycin (p.204·1).
Acne.

Erifoscin I Farmacologia, Spain.
Erythromycin estolate (p.204·1); fosfomycin calcium (p.210·2).
Bacterial infections.

Eril Savio, Ital.
Piperacillin sodium (p.237·2).
Lignocaine hydrochloride (p.1293·2) is included in this preparation to alleviate the pain of injection.
Bacterial infections.

Erimin Sumitomo, Jpn.
Nimetazepam (p.682·2).
Insomnia.

Erios Mepha, Switz.
Erythromycin ethyl succinate (p.204·2) or erythromycin stearate (p.204·2).
Bacterial infections.

Eriprodin Prodes, Spain†.
Erythromycin (p.204·1).
Bacterial infections.

Erisidoron 1 Weleda, UK.
Homoeopathic preparation.

Erispan Sumitomo, Jpn.
Fludiazepam (p.670·1).
Autonomic imbalance; psychosomatic disorders.

Eritrobios Nuovo, Ital.†.
Erythromycin estolate (p.204·1).
Bacterial infections.

Eritrocina Abbott, Ital.
Erythromycin ethyl succinate (p.204·2) or erythromycin stearate (p.204·2).
Bacterial infections.

Eritrocist Edmond Pharma, Ital.
Erythromycin stinoprate (p.206·2).
Bacterial infections.

Eritrogen Boehringer Mannheim, Ital.
Epoetin beta (p.718·3).
Anaemia associated with renal impairment; autologous blood transfusion.

Eritrogobens Normon, Spain.
Erythromycin ethyl succinate (p.204·2).
Bacterial infections.

Eritrolag Lagap, Switz.†.
Erythromycin ethyl succinate (p.204·2) or erythromycin stearate (p.204·2).
Bacterial infections.

Eritroveinte Madariaga, Spain.
Erythromycin estolate (p.204·1).
Bacterial infections.

Eritrovit B12 Lisapharma, Ital.
Cyanocobalamin (p.1363·3).
Anaemia; neuritis.

Erkaltungsbad Agepha, Aust.
Eucalyptus oil (p.1578·1); pumilio pine oil (p.1623·3); menthol (p.1600·2).
Catarrh.

Erkaltungsbalsam
Note. This name is used for preparations of different composition.
Agepha, Aust.
Peppermint oil (p.1208·1); camphor (p.1557·2); menthol (p.1600·2).
Catarrh.
Kwizda, Aust.
Eucalyptus oil (p.1578·1); pumilio pine oil (p.1623·3); oleum pini sylvestris; camphor (p.1557·2); menthol (p.1600·2).
Cold symptoms.
Doerr, Ger.†.
Thyme oil (p.1637·1); eucalyptus oil (p.1578·1); menthol (p.1600·2).
Bronchitis; cold symptoms.

Erkaltungsbalsam-ratiopharm E Ratiopharm, Ger.
Eucalyptus oil (p.1578·1); camphor (p.1557·2); turpentine oil (p.1641·1).
Cold symptoms.

Erkaltungstee
Note. This name is used for preparations of different composition.
Salus, Aust.
Thyme leaf (p.1636·3); althaea (p.1546·3); verbascum flowers; plantago lanceolata leaf.
Mouth and throat disorders; respiratory-tract disorders.
Schoeller, Aust.
Thyme leaf (p.1636·3); althaea (p.1546·3); verbascum flowers; drosera (p.1574·1); plantago lanceolata leaf.
Mouth and throat disorders; respiratory-tract disorders.

Ermsech Heumann, Ger.
Calcium lactate (p.1155·2); echinacea (p.1574·2).
Hypersensitivity disorders; increase of immune capacity.

Ernodasa Ern, Spain.
Streptodornase (p.1632·3); streptokinase (p.948·2).
Inflammation; soft-tissue damage; ulcers.

ERO Scherer, USA.
Urea hydrogen peroxide (p.1127·3).
Ear wax removal.

Erocap Douglas, Austral.
Fluoxetine hydrochloride (p.284·1).
Depression.

Eromel Lagamed, S.Afr.
Erythromycin stearate (p.204·2).
Bacterial infections.

Eromel-S Lagamed, S.Afr.
Erythromycin ethyl succinate (p.204·2).
Bacterial infections.

Erpalfa INTES, Ital.
Cytarabine (p.525·2).
Viral keratitis.

Errevit Combi Erredici, Ital.
Vitamin E; betacarotene; selenium.
Nutritional supplement.

Ervasil Warner-Wellcome, Spain†.
Aluminium hydroxide (p.1177·3); calcium phosphate (p.1155·3); magnesium trisilicate (p.1199·1).
Gastro-intestinal hyperacidity.

Ervasil Lac Warner-Wellcome, Spain†.
Aluminium hydroxide (p.1177·3); skimmed milk; magnesium trisilicate (p.1199·1).
Gastro-intestinal hyperacidity.

Ervevax
SmithKline Beecham, Aust.; SmithKline Beecham, Austral.; SK-RIT, Belg.; SmithKline Beecham, Ger.; Dresden, Ger.; SmithKline Beecham, Irl.; SmithKline Beecham, Ital.; SmithKline Beecham, Neth.†; SmithKline Beecham, Switz.; SmithKline Beecham, UK.
A rubella vaccine (Wistar RA 27/3 or Cendehill strain) (p.1532·3).
Active immunisation.

Erwinase
Meda, Swed.; Speywood, UK.
Crisantaspase (asparaginase) (p.504·3).
Malignant neoplasms.

Ery
Bouchara, Fr.; Bouchara, Switz.
Erythromycin ethyl succinate (p.204·2) or erythromycin propionate (p.204·2).
Bacterial infections.

Eryacne
Galderma, Austral.; Galderma, Neth.; Galderma, UK.
Erythromycin (p.204·1).
Acne.

Eryaknen
AB-Consult, Aust.; Galderma, Ger.; Galderma, Switz.
Erythromycin (p.204·1).
Acne.

Erybesan Biochemie, Aust.
Erythromycin ethyl succinate (p.204·2) or erythromycin stearate (p.204·2).
Bacterial infections.

Erybeta Betapharm, Ger.
Erythromycin ethyl succinate (p.204·2) or erythromycin stearate (p.204·2).
Bacterial infections.

Erybid Abbott, Canad.
Erythromycin (p.204·1).
Bacterial infections.

Eryc
Faulding, Austral.; Parke, Davis, Canad.; Parke, Davis, Neth.; Parke, Davis, USA.
Erythromycin (p.204·1).
Bacterial infections.

Erycen
Berk, Irl.†; Berk, UK.
Erythromycin (p.204·1) or erythromycin ethyl succinate (p.204·2).
Bacterial infections.

Erycette
Janssen-Cilag, S.Afr.; Ortho Dermatological, USA.
Erythromycin (p.204·1).
Acne.

Erycinum
Schering, Aust.; CytoChemia, Ger.
Erythromycin (p.204·1), erythromycin ethyl succinate (p.204·2), erythromycin lactobionate (p.204·2), or erythromycin stearate (p.204·2).
Erycinum injection formerly contained erythromycin gluceptate.
Bacterial infections.

Erycocci Pharmafarm, Fr.
Erythromycin ethyl succinate (p.204·2).
Bacterial infections.

Erycytol Lannacher, Aust.
Hydroxocobalamin (p.1363·3).
Herpes zoster infections; liver disorders; macrocytic anaemias; neuralgia; neuritis; tobacco amblyopia; vitamin B_{12} deficiency.

Eryderm
Abbott, Belg.; Abbott, Neth.; Abbott, S.Afr.; Abbott, Switz.; Abbott, USA.
Erythromycin (p.204·1).
Acne.

Erydermec Hexal, Ger.
Erythromycin (p.204·1).
Acne.

Ery-Diolan Engelhard, Ger.
Erythromycin ethyl succinate (p.204·2) or erythromycin stearate (p.204·2).
Bacterial infections.

Eryfer
Cassella-med, Ger.; Hoechst Marion Roussel, Ital.†; Hoechst, Neth.†.
Ferrous sulphate (p.1340·2).
Iron-deficiency; iron-deficiency anaemias.

Eryfer comp. Cassella-med, Ger.
Ferrous sulphate (p.1340·2); cyanocobalamin (p.1363·3); folic acid (p.1340·3).
Iron and vitamin deficiency.

Eryfluid Pierre Fabre, Fr.
Erythromycin (p.204·1).
Acne.

Erygel Allergan Herbert, USA.
Erythromycin (p.204·1).
Acne; skin infections.

Eryhexal Hexal, Ger.
Erythromycin (p.204·1), erythromycin ethyl succinate (p.204·2), or erythromycin stearate (p.204·2).
Bacterial infections.

Ery-Max
Astra, Norw.; CEPA, Spain; Astra, Swed.
Erythromycin (p.204·1), erythromycin ethyl succinate (p.204·2), or erythromycin lactobionate (p.204·2).
Bacterial infections.

Erymax
Elan, Irl.; Parke-Med, S.Afr.; Helsinn, Switz.†; Parke, Davis, UK; Allergan Herbert, USA.
Erythromycin (p.204·1).
Acne.

Ery-Maxin Astra, Aust.
Erythromycin (p.204·1) or erythromycin ethyl succinate (p.204·2).
Bacterial infections.

Erymin Elan, UK.
Erythromycin ethyl succinate (p.204·2).
Bacterial infections.

Erymin S Parke-Med, S.Afr.†.
Erythromycin estolate (p.204·1).
Bacterial infections.

Erymycin Triomed, S.Afr.
Erythromycin estolate (p.204·1) or erythromycin stearate (p.204·2).
Bacterial infections.

Eryped
Abbott, Canad.†; Abbott, USA.
Erythromycin ethyl succinate (p.204·2).
Bacterial infections.

Eryphar Diophar, Fr.†.
Erythromycin ethyl succinate (p.204·2).
Bacterial infections.

Erypo
Janssen-Cilag, Aust.; Janssen-Cilag, Ger.
Epoetin alfa (p.718·3).
Anaemia; autologous blood transfusion.

Ery-Reu Reusch, Ger.
Erythromycin lactobionate (p.204·2).
Bacterial infections.

Erysec Lindopharm, Ger.
Erythromycin stinoprate (p.206·2).
Bacterial infections.

Erysidoron
Weleda, Aust.
Homoeopathic preparation.
Weleda, UK.
Birch (p.1553·3); sulphur.
Boils; tonsillitis.

Erysol
Stiefel, Canad.; Dermol, USA†.
Erythromycin (p.204·1).
Acne.

Erysolvan Laevosan, Aust.
Erythromycin stinoprate (p.206·2).
Bacterial infections.

Erystat Medpro, S.Afr.
Erythromycin estolate (p.204·1).
Bacterial infections.

Ery-Tab Abbott, USA.
Erythromycin (p.204·1).
Bacterial infections.

Eryteal Pierre Fabre, Fr.
Cod-liver oil (p.1337·3); halibut-liver oil (p.1345·3); zinc oxide (p.1096·2); cetrimonium bromide (p.1106·1).
Burns; nappy rash.

Erythra-Derm Paddock, USA.
Erythromycin (p.204·1).
Formerly known as ETS-2%.
Acne.

Erythro CT, Ger.
Erythromycin ethyl succinate (p.204·2).
Bacterial infections.

erythro-basan Sagitta, Ger.†.
Erythromycin ethyl succinate (p.204·2).
Bacterial infections.

Erythrocin
Abbott, Aust.; Abbott, Austral.; Abbott, Canad.; Abbott, Ger.; Abbott, Irl.; Abbott, S.Afr.; Abbott, UK; Abbott, USA.
Erythromycin ethyl succinate (p.204·2), erythromycin lactobionate (p.204·2), or erythromycin stearate (p.204·2).
Bacterial infections.

Erythrocin Neo Abbott, Ger.
Erythromycin ethyl succinate (p.204·2).
Bacterial infections.

Erythrocine
Abbott, Belg.; Abbott, Fr.; Abbott, Neth.; Abbott, Switz.
Erythromycin ethyl succinate (p.204·2), erythromycin lactobionate (p.204·2), or erythromycin stearate (p.204·2).
Bacterial infections.

Erythroforte Abbott, Belg.
Erythromycin ethyl succinate (p.204·2).
Bacterial infections.

Erythrogel Biorga, Fr.
Erythromycin (p.204·1).
Acne.

Erythrogenat Azupharma, Ger.
Erythromycin ethyl succinate (p.204·2) or erythromycin stearate (p.204·2).
Bacterial infections.

Erythrogram Pharma 2000, Fr.
Erythromycin ethyl succinate (p.204·2).
Bacterial infections.

Erythro-Hefa Hefa, Ger.
Erythromycin ethyl succinate (p.204·2) or erythromycin stearate (p.204·2).
Bacterial infections.

Erythromid
Abbott, Canad.†; Abbott, Irl.; Abbott, S.Afr.; Abbott, UK.
Erythromycin (p.204·1).
Bacterial infections.

Erythroped
Abbott, Irl.; Abbott, S.Afr.; Abbott, UK.
Erythromycin (p.204·1) or erythromycin ethyl succinate (p.204·2).
Bacterial infections.

Erythroton Anphar-Rolland, Fr.†.
Ferrous betainate hydrochloride.
Formerly contained ferrous betainate hydrochloride, cyanocobalamin, intrinsic factor, and liver.
Anaemias.

Erytop Stada, Ger.
Erythromycin (p.204·1).
Acne.

Erytran Spirig, Switz.
Erythromycin ethyl succinate (p.204·2) or erythromycin stearate (p.204·2).
Bacterial infections.

Erytrociclin Lisapharma, Ital.
Erythromycin stearate (p.204·2).
Bacterial infections.

Eryval Smetana, Aust.
Absinthium (p.1541·1); centaury (p.1561·1); hypericum (p.1590·1); menthol (p.1600·2); valerian (p.1643·1).
Gastro-intestinal disorders.

Eryzole Alra, USA.
Erythromycin ethyl succinate (p.204·2); acetyl sulphafurazole (p.253·3).
Otitis media.

ES Bronchial Mixture Torbet Laboratories, UK.
Squill (p.1070·1); ipecacuanha tincture (p.1062·2); senna (p.1212·2); ammonium bicarbonate (p.1055·1).
Coughs.

Esacinone Lisapharma, Ital.
Fluocinolone acetonide (p.1041·1).
Skin disorders.

Esadoxi Benvegna, Ital.†.
Doxycycline hydrochloride (p.202·3).
Bacterial infections.

Esafosfina Biomedica, Ital.
Sodium fructose-1,6-diphosphate hydrate.
Cardiac disorders; phosphate deficiency.

Esaglut Biomedica, Ital.
Levoglutamide (p.1344·3); dicalcium fructose-1,6-diphosphate; thiamine nitrate (p.1361·1); pyridoxine hydrochloride (p.1362·3); calcium pantothenate (p.1352·3).
Asthenia; mental function impairment; tonic.

Esametone Lisapharma, Ital.
Methylprednisolone (p.1046·1).
Oral corticosteroid.

Esapent Pharmacia Upjohn, Ital.
Omega-3 triglycerides (p.1276·1).
Hypertriglyceridaemia.

Esarondil Terapeutico, Ital.
Methacycline hydrochloride (p.225·1).
Bacterial infections.

Esavir Boniscontro & Gazzone, Ital.
Aciclovir (p.602·3).
Herpesvirus infections.

Esbatal Wellcome, Irl.†.
Bethanidine sulphate (p.832·2).
Hypertension.

Esbericard
Provita, Aust.; Schaper & Brummer, Ger.; Asta Medica, Switz.
Crataegus (p.1568·2).
Cardiac disorders.

Esbericid *Schaper & Brummer, Ger.†.*
Bendrofluazide (p.827·3).
Diabetes insipidus; hypertension; oedema; renal calculi.

Esbericum *Schaper & Brummer, Ger.*
Hypericum (p.1590·1).
Psychiatric disorders.

Esberidin *Schaper & Brummer, Ger.†.*
Vincamine hydrochloride (p.1644·1).
Metabolic and circulatory disorders of the brain, retina, and inner ear.

Esberigal N *Schaper & Brummer, Ger.*
Cnicus benedictus (p.1565·3); silybum marianum (p.993·3); chelidonium majus; chamomile (p.1561·2).
Biliary disorders.

Esberilan *Schaper & Brummer, Ger.†.*
β-Acetyldigoxin (p.812·3); potassium aspartate (p.1161·3); magnesium aspartate (p.1157·2).
Cardiac disorders.

Esberi-Nervin *Laves, Ger.†.*
Peppermint leaf (p.1208·1); potentilla anserina; valerian (p.1643·1); avena sativa (p.1551·3); melissa (p.1600·1).
Nervous disorders; sleeplessness.

Esberitox mono *Schaper & Brummer, Ger.*
Echinacea purpurea (p.1574·2).
Respiratory-tract infections.

Esberitox N
Schaper & Brummer, Ger.; Asta Medica, Switz.
Thuja (p.1636·3); baptisia tinctoria; echinacea purpurea (p.1574·2).
Cold symptoms.

Esberiven
Note. This name is used for preparations of different composition.
Knoll, Fr.
Melilot; heparin sodium (p.879·3).
Peripheral vascular disorders.

Iquinosa, Spain.
Melilot; troxerutin (p.1580·2).
Peripheral vascular disorders.

Esberiven Forte *Knoll, Fr.*
Melilot; rutin (p.1580·2).
Peripheral vascular disorders.

Esberizym N *Schaper & Brummer, Ger.*
Porcine pancreatin (p.1612·1); bromelains (p.1555·1); dimethicone (p.1213·1).
Digestive system disorders.

Esbuphon *Schaper & Brummer, Ger.†.*
Norfenefrine hydrochloride (p.925·1).
Hypotension.

Escalgin sans codeine *Streuli, Switz.*
Salicylamide (p.82·3); propyphenazone (p.81·3); caffeine (p.749·3).
Fever; pain.

Escandine
Strallhofer, Aust.; Pharmazam, Spain.
Ibopamine hydrochloride (p.889·3).
Heart failure.

Escarol *Muller Goppingen, Ger.*
Asarabacca (p.1551·2).
Respiratory-tract disorders.

Escatitona *Madaus, Aust.*
Homoeopathic preparation.

Escinogel *Doms-Adrian, Fr.*
Bamethan sulphate (p.827·1); aescin (p.1543·3).
Formerly contained bamethan sulphate, buphenine hydrochloride, and aescin.
Peripheral vascular disorders.

Esclama *Pharmacia Upjohn, Ger.*
Nimorazole (p.589·3).
Protozoal infections.

Esclebin *Wasserman, Spain.*
Norfloxacin (p.233·1).
Bacterial infections.

Esclerobion *Merck, Spain†.*
Pyricarbate (p.1624·1); pyritinol hydrochloride (p.1624·1); tocopheryl nicotinate (p.1280·1).
Arteriosclerosis; diabetic vascular complications; thrombo-embolic disorders.

Esclim *Serono, USA.*
Oestradiol (p.1455·1).
Menopausal disorders; osteoporosis.

Escoflex *Streuli, Switz.†.*
Chlorzoxazone (p.1313·1).
Musculoskeletal pain with spasm.

Escoflex Compositum *Streuli, Switz.†.*
Chlorzoxazone (p.1313·1); propyphenazone (p.81·3).
Musculoskeletal pain with spasm.

Escogripp *Streuli, Switz.†.*
Caffeine (p.749·3); propyphenazone (p.81·3); codeine phosphate (p.26·1); ipecacuanha (p.1062·2); ascorbic acid (p.1365·2); mepyramine maleate (p.414·1); salicylamide (p.82·3).
Cold symptoms.

Escogripp sans codeine *Streuli, Switz.*
Propyphenazone (p.81·3); salicylamide (p.82·3); caffeine (p.749·3); ascorbic acid (p.1365·2); mepyramine maleate (p.414·1).
Cold and influenza symptoms.

Escophylline *Streuli, Switz.*
Aminophylline (p.748·1) or theophylline (p.765·1).
Obstructive airways disease.

Escopon *Streuli, Switz.†.*
Mixed opium alkaloids (p.71·1).
Pain with smooth muscle spasm; premedication.

Escoprim *Streuli, Switz.*
Co-trimoxazole (p.196·3).
Bacterial infections.

Escor *Merck, Ger.*
Nilvadipine (p.922·1).
Hypertension.

Escothyol *Streuli, Switz.†.*
Ichthammol (p.1083·3); ammoniumsulfobitol (p.1083·3); hamamelis (p.1587·1); peru balsam (p.1617·2); lavender oil (p.1594·3); zinc oxide (p.1096·2).
Skin disorders.

Escotussin *Streuli, Switz.*
Dihydrocodeine thiocyanate (p.34·2); belladonna (p.457·1); drosera (p.1574·1); guaiphenesin (p.1061·3).
Coughs.

Escouflaire *Denolin, Belg.*
Belladonna leaf (p.457·1); stramonium leaf (p.468·2); hyoscyamus leaf (p.464·3); peppermint leaf (p.1208·1); potassium nitrate (p.1123·1).
Respiratory disorders.

Esedril *Lipha, Ital.*
Naftidrofuryl oxalate (p.914·2).
Cerebral and peripheral vascular disorders.

Eselin *Ravizza, Ital.*
Ethamsylate (p.720·1).
Haemorrhage; vascular disorders.

Esencial Nattermann *Nattermann, Spain†.*
Multivitamin and phospholipid preparation.
Liver disorders.

Esgic-Plus *Forest Pharmaceuticals, USA.*
Butalbital (p.644·3); paracetamol (p.72·2); caffeine (p.749·3).
Tension headache.

Esiclene *LPB, Ital.†.*
Formebolone (p.1447·1).
Osteoporosis.

Esidrex
Ciba-Geigy, Aust.; Ciba-Geigy, Belg.; Ciba-Geigy, Fr.; Ciba, Ital.; Novartis, Neth.; Ciba, Norw.; Ciba-Geigy, Spain; Novartis, Swed.; Ciba, Switz.; Ciba, UK†.
Hydrochlorothiazide (p.885·2).
Diabetes insipidus; heart failure; hypercalciuria; hypertension; Ménière's disease; oedema; renal calculi.

Esidrex-K
Ciba-Geigy, Belg.†; Ciba-Geigy, Swed.†; Ciba, Switz.†.
Hydrochlorothiazide (p.885·2); potassium chloride (p.1161·1).
Diabetes insipidus; hypercalciuria; hypertension; Ménière's disease; oedema.

Esidrix
Ciba, Ger.; Ciba, USA.
Hydrochlorothiazide (p.885·2).
Ascites; hypertension; oedema.

Esilgan *Takeda, Ital.*
Estazolam (p.669·2).
Insomnia.

Esilon *SIT, Ital.†.*
Fluocinolone acetonide (p.1041·1).
Skin disorders.

Esimil
Ciba-Geigy, Fr.†; Ciba, Ger.; Ciba, USA.
Guanethidine monosulphate (p.878·1); hydrochlorothiazide (p.885·2).
Hypertension.

Esirhinol *Desitin, Ger.†.*
Sodium cromoglycate (p.762·1).
Allergic rhinitis.

Esiteren *Ciba, Ger.*
Hydrochlorothiazide (p.885·2); triamterene (p.957·2).
Hypertension; oedema.

Eskalith *SmithKline Beecham, USA.*
Lithium carbonate (p.290·3).
Bipolar disorder.

Eskamel
SmithKline Beecham Consumer, Austral.; Smith Kline & French, Irl.†; SmithKline Beecham, S.Afr.†; Goldshield, UK.
Resorcinol (p.1090·1); sulphur (p.1091·2).
Acne.

Eskazine *SmithKline Beecham, Spain.*
Trifluoperazine hydrochloride (p.697·3).
Anxiety; psychoses.

Eskazole
SmithKline Beecham, Aust.; SmithKline Beecham, Austral.; SmithKline Beecham, Ger.; SmithKline Beecham, Neth.; Smith Kline & French, Spain; SmithKline Beecham, UK.
Albendazole (p.96·2).
Capillariasis; cysticercosis; echinococcosis; strongyloidiasis; trichinosis.

Eskim *Prospa, Ital.*
Omega-3 triglycerides (p.1276·1).
Hypertriglyceridaemia.

Eskornade
Smith Kline & French, Irl.†; SmithKline Beecham, S.Afr.; Goldshield, UK.
Phenylpropanolamine hydrochloride (p.1067·2); diphenylpyraline hydrochloride (p.409·3).
Formerly contained isopropamide, phenylpropanolamine hydrochloride, and diphenylpyraline hydrochloride in *S.Afr.*
Upper respiratory-tract disorders.

Esmacen *Smaller, Spain.*
Astemizole (p.402·1).
Hypersensitivity reactions.

Esmalorid *Merck, Ger.*
Trichlormethiazide (p.958·2); amiloride hydrochloride (p.819·2).
Hypertension; oedema.

Esmaloride *E. Merck, Switz.†.*
Trichlormethiazide (p.958·2); amiloride hydrochloride (p.819·2).
Hypertension; oedema.

Esmarin *Merck, Ger.†.*
Trichlormethiazide (p.958·2).
Hypertension; oedema.

Esmeron
Organon Teknika, Belg.; Organon Teknika, Fr.; Organon Teknika, Ger.; Organon Teknika, Irl.; Organon Teknika, Ital.; Organon Teknika, Neth.; Organon Teknika, Norw.; Sanofi Omnimed, S.Afr.; Organon, Spain; Organon Teknika, Swed.; Organon Teknika, Switz.; Organon Teknika, UK.
Rocuronium bromide (p.1318·2).
Competitive neuromuscular blocker.

Eso Cem *Esoform, Ital.*
Glutaraldehyde (p.1114·3).
Instrument disinfection.

Eso Deterferri *Esoform, Ital.*
Benzalkonium chloride (p.1101·3).
Instrument disinfection.

Eso Din *Esoform, Ital.*
Glutaraldehyde (p.1114·3); phenol (p.1121·2).
Instrument disinfection.

Eso Ferri *Esoform, Ital.*
Benzalkonium chloride (p.1101·3).
Instrument disinfection.

Eso Ferri Alcolico *Esoform, Ital.*
Benzalkonium chloride (p.1101·3); alcohol (p.1099·1).
Instrument disinfection.

Eso Ferri Alcolico Plus *Esoform, Ital.*
Benzalkonium chloride (p.1101·3); isopropyl alcohol (p.1118·2).
Instrument disinfection.

Eso Ferri Plus *Esoform, Ital.*
Chlorhexidine gluconate (p.1107·2); isopropyl alcohol (p.1118·2).
Instrument disinfection and storage.

Eso H1, HP, and HP1 *Esoform, Ital.*
Glutaraldehyde (p.1114·3).
Instrument disinfection.

Eso S 80 *Esoform, Ital.*
Benzalkonium chloride (p.1101·3); chlorhexidine gluconate (p.1107·2).
Instrument disinfection.

Esoalcolico Incolore *Esoform, Ital.*
Benzalkonium chloride (p.1101·3); alcohol (p.1099·1).
Skin, hand, and wound disinfection.

Esobar *Therapex, Canad.†.*
Barium sulphate (p.1003·1).
Radiographic contrast medium.

Esochlor 20 EC *Esoform, Ital.†.*
Propoxur (p.1410·1).
Insecticide.

Esofenol 60 *Esoform, Ital.*
Sodium *o*-phenylphenol (p.1120·3).
Waste disinfection.

Esofenol Ferri *Esoform, Ital.*
Orthobenzyl parachlorophenol (p.1120·3); orthophenylphenol (p.1120·3).
Instrument disinfection.

Esoform 92 *Esoform, Ital.*
Benzalkonium chloride (p.1101·3); glutaraldehyde (p.1114·3); alkylphenoxypolyglycol ether.
Surface disinfection.

Esoform Alcolico *Esoform, Ital.*
Benzalkonium chloride (p.1101·3); methyl salicylate; camphor; thyme oil; alcohol (p.1099·1); acetone; chloroform.
Skin disinfection.

Esoform Deterferri *Esoform, Ital.*
Benzalkonium chloride (p.1101·3).
Instrument disinfection.

Esoform Ferri *Esoform, Ital.*
Benzalkonium chloride (p.1101·3); sodium nitrite (p.995·2); methylene blue.
Instrument disinfection.

Esoform Ferri Alcolico *Esoform, Ital.*
Benzalkonium chloride (p.1101·3); alcohol (p.1099·1); sodium nitrite (p.995·2); acetone; chloroform.
Instrument disinfection.

Esoform HP *Esoform, Ital.†.*
Glutaraldehyde (p.1114·3).
Instrument disinfection.

Esoform Jod 10, 35, 75, 100, and 500 *Esoform, Ital.*
Povidone-iodine (p.1123·3).
Skin, wound, and hand disinfection.

Esoform Jod 20 and 50 *Esoform, Ital.*
Iodine (p.1493·1); potassium iodide (p.1493·1); alcohol; chloroform; isopropyl alcohol.
Skin and hand disinfection.

Esoform Jod 25 *Esoform, Ital.*
Alkylphenoxypolyglycol-iodine-ether complex.
Room and surface disinfection.

Esoform Mani *Esoform, Ital.*
Chlorhexidine gluconate (p.1107·2); isopropyl alcohol; chloroform; alcohol.
Skin and hand disinfection.

Esoform Maniferri *Esoform, Ital.*
Chlorhexidine gluconate (p.1107·2); isopropyl alcohol (p.1118·2).
Skin, hand, and instrument disinfection.

Esoform 7 mc *Esoform, Ital.*
Paraformaldehyde (p.1121·1); hydrogen peroxide (40-45 volume) (p.1116·2).
Surface and room disinfection.

Esoform 70 mc *Esoform, Ital.*
Paraformaldehyde (p.1121·1); hydrogen peroxide (40-45 volume) (p.1116·2).
Room disinfection.

Esoform Sanacasa *Esoform, Ital.†.*
Benzalkonium chloride (p.1101·3).
Surface disinfection.

Esolut *Angelini, Ital.*
Progesterone (p.1459·3).
Luteal insufficiency.

E-Solve *Syosset, USA.*
Vehicle for topical preparations.

Espho-Cat *Therapex, Canad.†.*
Barium sulphate (p.1003·1).
Contrast medium for computerised axial tomography.

Esosan *Esoform, Ital.*
Benzalkonium chloride (p.1101·3).
Skin and surface disinfection.

Esoterica
Note. This name is used for preparations of different composition.
Nasmark, Canad.
Hydroquinone (p.1083·1); oxybenzone (p.1487·3); padimate O (p.1488·1).
Skin pigmentation disorders.

Lentheric Morny, UK.
Hydroquinone (p.1083·1).

SmithKline Beecham Consumer, USA†.
Emollient and moisturiser.

Esoterica Facial and Sunscreen *Medicis, USA.*
Hydroquinone (p.1083·1); padimate O (p.1488·1); oxybenzone (p.1487·3).
Hyperpigmentation.

Esoterica Regular *Nasmark, Canad.*
Hydroquinone (p.1083·1).
Skin pigmentation disorders.

Esoterica Sensitive Skin and Regular *Medicis, USA.*
Hydroquinone (p.1083·1).
Hyperpigmentation.

Esotran *Almirall, Spain.*
Oestradiol (p.1455·1).
Menopausal disorders; osteoporosis.

Esoxid *Esoform, Ital.*
Glutaraldehyde (p.1114·3).
Instrument disinfection.

ESP *Barr, USA†.*
Erythromycin ethyl succinate (p.204·2); acetyl sulphafurazole (p.253·3).

espa-butyl *Esparma, Ger.*
Hyoscine butylbromide (p.462·3).
Smooth muscle spasm.

espa-lipon *Esparma, Ger.*
Thioctic acid (p.1636·2) or ethylenediamine thioctate (p.1636·2).
Diabetic polyneuropathy.

Esparil *Esparma, Ger.*
Captopril (p.836·3).
Heart failure; hypertension.

Esparon *Orion, Ger.*
Alprazolam (p.640·3).
Anxiety.

Espasmo Canulasa *Sandoz, Spain.*
Cellulase (p.1561·1); dimethicone (p.1213·1); glutamic acid hydrochloride (p.1344·3); methixene hydrochloride (p.465·1); pancreatin (p.1612·1); pepsin (p.1616·3); dehydrocholic acid (p.1570·2).
Digestive system insufficiency; meteorism.

Espasmo Cibalgina *Ciba-Geigy, Spain†.*
Drofenine hydrochloride (p.460·3); propyphenazone (p.81·3).
Pain.

Espasmo Digestomen *Menarini, Spain.*
Amylase (p.1549·1); methionine phenylbutyrate; nicotinic acid (p.1351·2); papain (p.1614·1); pepsin (p.1616·3); flopropione (p.1580·3); betaine hydrochloride (p.1553·2); pancreatin (p.1612·1); lipase; bile extract (p.1553·2); cellulase (p.1561·1); hemicellulase (p.1561·1).
Biliary-tract disorders; digestive system insufficiency; dyspepsia; meteorism.

Espectona Compositum *Fournier SA, Spain†.*
Bromhexine hydrochloride (p.1055·3); dextromethorphan hydrobromide (p.1057·3); diprophylline (p.752·1); pentetrazol (p.1484·2).
Obstructive airways disease.

Espectral *Centrum, Spain.*
Ampicillin trihydrate (p.153·2); muramidase hydrochloride (p.1604·3).
Bacterial infections.

Espectral Balsamico *Centrum, Spain.*
Ampicillin trihydrate (p.153·2); guaiphenesin (p.1061·3); muramidase hydrochloride (p.1604·3).
Respiratory-tract infections.

Espectrosira *Clariana, Spain.*
Ampicillin sodium (p.153·1); ampicillin benzathine (p.154·1); bromhexine hydrochloride (p.1055·3); guaiphenesin (p.1061·3).

Lignocaine hydrochloride (p.1293·2) is included in this preparation to alleviate the pain of injection.
Respiratory-tract infections.

Espeden *Vita, Spain.*
Norfloxacin (p.233·1).
Bacterial infections.

Esperal
Exel, Belg.†; Sanofi Winthrop, Fr.
Disulfiram (p.1573·1).
Chronic alcoholism.

Espidifen *Zambon, Spain.*
Ibuprofen arginine (p.44·3).
Fever; musculoskeletal, joint, and peri-articular disorders; pain.

Espiran *ICT, Ital.*
Fenspiride hydrochloride (p.1579·3).
Respiratory-tract disorders.

Espiride *Lennon, S.Afr.*
Sulpiride (p.692·3).
Behaviour disorders; depression; peptic ulcer; psychoses; vertigo.

Espledol *Fher, Spain.*
Acemetacin (p.12·2).
Musculoskeletal and joint disorders; peri-articular disorders.

Espo *Kirin, Jpn.*
Epoetin alfa (p.718·3).
Anaemia; autologous blood transfusion.

Espongostan *Byk Leo, Spain.*
Gelatin (p.723·2).
Mucous membrane haemorrhage.

Espotabs
Combe, Canad.; Combe, USA.
Yellow phenolphthalein (p.1208·2).
Constipation.

Esprenit *Hennig, Ger.*
Ibuprofen (p.44·1) or ibuprofen sodium (p.44·3).
Fever; musculoskeletal and joint disorders; pain.

Esprit *Bayer, Austral.*
Test for glucose in blood (p.1585·1).

Espritin *Petrasch, Aust.*
Lactic acid (p.1593·3).
Psoriasis.

Espumisan *Berlin-Chemie, Ger.*
Simethicone (p.1213·1).
Defoaming agent in radiography and endoscopy of the gastro-intestinal tract.

Esquinon *Sankyo, Jpn.*
Carboquone (p.511·3).
Malignant neoplasms.

Esradin *Sigma-Tau, Ital.*
Isradipine (p.894·2).
Hypertension.

Essamin *Torre, Ital.*
Amino-acid preparation.
Renal failure.

Essaproct *Rhone-Poulenc, Ital.†.*
Ointment: Ichthammol (p.1083·3); menthol (p.1600·2); chlorocarvacrol.
Suppositories: Ichthammol (p.1083·3); menthol (p.1600·2); matricaria oil; chlorocarvacrol.
Haemorrhoids.

Essasorb *Nattermann, Ger.†.*
Cadexomer-iodine (p.1105·1).
Infected wounds.

Essaven
Note. This name is used for preparations of different composition.
Nattermann, Ger.; Rhone-Poulenc Rorer, S.Afr.
Topical gel: Aescin (p.1543·3); heparin sodium (p.879·3); essential phospholipids.
Soft-tissue trauma; vascular disorders.

Rhone-Poulenc Rorer, Ital.
Capsules: Aescin (p.1543·3); rutin (p.1580·2); phosphatidylcholine (p.1618·1).
Topical gel: Aescin (p.1543·3); heparin sodium (p.879·3); phosphatidylcholine (p.1618·1).
Peripheral vascular disorders.

Rhone-Poulenc Rorer, S.Afr.
Capsules: Aescin (p.1543·3); rutin (p.1580·2); essential phospholipids.
Vascular disorders.

Essaven 50 000 *Nattermann, Ger.†.*
Heparin sodium (p.879·3); arnica (p.1550·3); aesculus (p.1543·3).
Skin trauma.

Essaven 60 000 *Nattermann, Ger.*
Heparin sodium (p.879·3).
Soft-tissue disorders; superficial vascular disorders.

Essaven Mono *Nattermann, Ger.*
Aesculus (p.1543·3).
Chronic venous insufficiency.

Essaven N *Nattermann, Ger.*
Aesculus (p.1543·3); trimethylhesperidin chalcone (p.1580·2).
Soft-tissue disorders; vascular disorders.

Essaven Sportgel *Nattermann, Ger.*
Glycol salicylate (p.43·1); arnica tincture (p.1550·3).
Sports injuries.

Essaven Tri-Complex *Nattermann, Ger.*
Heparin sodium (p.879·3); allantoin (p.1078·2); dexpanthenol (p.1570·3).
Soft-tissue disorders; superficial vascular disorders.

Essaven ultra *Nattermann, Ger.*
Aesculus (p.1543·3); trimethylhesperidin chalcone (p.1580·2); essential phospholipids.
Soft-tissue injury; vascular disorders.

Essavenon *Nattermann, Spain.*
Capsules†: Aesculus (p.1543·3); phospholipids; rutin (p.1580·2).
Topical gel: Aescin (p.1543·3); phospholipids; heparin sodium (p.879·3).
Peripheral vascular disorders; soft-tissue disorders.

Essen *Scharper, Ital.†.*
Metoclopramide hydrochloride (p.1200·3); pepsin (p.1616·3); dimethicone (p.1213·1); amylase (p.1549·1); lipase; trypsin (p.1640·1); chymotrypsin (p.1563·2); cellulase (p.1561·1).
Gastro-intestinal disorders.

Essen Enzimatico *Farmochimica, Ital.*
Pepsin (p.1616·3); amylase (p.1549·1); lipase; trypsin (p.1640·1); chymotrypsin (p.1563·2); cellulase (p.1561·1).
Dyspepsia.

Essence Algerienne *Toulade, Fr.*
Cineole (p.1564·1); menthol (p.1600·2); guaiacol (p.1061·2).
Upper respiratory-tract congestion.

Essential Balance *Pharmavite, Canad.*
Multivitamin and mineral preparation.

Essentiale
Note. This name is used for preparations of different composition.
Gerot, Aust.; Rhone-Poulenc Rorer, S.Afr.
Essential phospholipids and multivitamins.
Liver disorders.

Rhone-Poulenc Rorer, Ital.
Phosphatidyl choline (p.1618·1).
Liver disorders.

Essentiale N *Nattermann, Ger.*
Essential phospholipids.
Gallstones; liver disorders; psoriasis; radiation trauma.

Essentials *Ross, Canad.†.*
Preparation for enteral nutrition.

Essentielle Aminosauren *Fresenius-Praxis, Ger.*
Amino-acid preparation.
Dietary supplement in renal failure.

Essex
Essex, Ger.†; Essex, Switz.
Emollient.
Skin disorders.

Essigsaure Tonerde-Salbe *Michallik, Ger.*
Aluminium acetotartrate (p.1547·3).
Soft-tissue disorders.

Essitol *Athenstaedt, Ger.*
Aluminium acetotartrate (p.1547·3).
Insect stings; soft-tissue injury.

EST *Rosch & Handel, Aust.*
Alum (p.1547·1); calcium acetate (p.1155·1); calcium carbonate (p.1182·1).
Bruises; insect bites; sprains; swelling.

Estandron
Organon, Aust.; Ravasini, Ital.†.
Oestradiol benzoate (p.1455·1); oestradiol phenylpropionate (p.1455·2); testosterone propionate (p.1464·2); testosterone phenylpropionate (p.1464·2); testosterone isocaproate (p.1464·2).
Menopausal disorders.

Estandron Prolongado *Organon, Spain†.*
Oestradiol benzoate (p.1455·1); oestradiol phenylpropionate (p.1455·2); testosterone propionate (p.1464·2); testosterone phenylpropionate (p.1464·2); testosterone isocaproate (p.1464·2).
Menopausal disorders.

Estandron Prolongatum *Organon, Switz.†.*
Oestradiol benzoate (p.1455·1); oestradiol phenylpropionate (p.1455·2); testosterone propionate (p.1464·2); testosterone phenylpropionate (p.1464·2); testosterone isocaproate (p.1464·2).
Menopausal disorders.

Estar
Westwood-Squibb, Canad.; Westwood-Squibb, USA.
Coal tar (p.1092·3).
Psoriasis.

Estecina *Normon, Spain.*
Ciprofloxacin hydrochloride (p.185·3) or ciprofloxacin lactate (p.185·3).
Bacterial infections.

Esten *Rhone-Poulenc Rorer, Austral.†.*
Vitamins and minerals; arizona garlic (p.1583·1); lecithin (p.1595·2); cimicifuga (p.1563·3); viburnum opulus; passion flower (p.1615·3); smilax (p.1627·2).
Menopausal disorders.

Ester Aces *Sisu, Canad.*
Betacarotene, selenium, vitamin C, and vitamin E.

Esterbiol *Inexfa, Spain.*
Pyricarbate (p.1624·1).
Arteriosclerosis; peripheral vascular disorders.

Ester-C
Note. This name is used for preparations of different composition.
Quest, Canad.; Sisu, Canad.
Calcium ascorbate (p.1365·2).

Solgar, UK.
Vitamin C with bioflavonoids.

Ester-C Plus *Solgar, USA.*
Vitamin C (p.1365·2); citrus bioflavonoids complex (p.1580·1); acerola (p.1001·1); rose hips (p.1365·2); rutin (p.1580·2); calcium (p.1155·1).
Capillary bleeding.

Ester-C Plus Multi-Mineral *Solgar, USA.*
Vitamin C (p.1365·2); citrus bioflavonoids complex (p.1580·1); acerola (p.1001·1); rose hips (p.1365·2); rutin (p.1580·2); calcium (p.1155·1); magnesium (p.1157·2); potassium (p.1161·1); zinc (p.1373·1).
Capillary bleeding.

Estericlean *Braun, Spain.*
Sodium chloride (p.1162·2).
Fluid and electrolyte replacement; hypovolaemia.

Esterofundina P G Braun *Braun, Spain†.*
Electrolyte infusion with glucose (p.1147·1).
Fluid and electrolyte depletion.

Esterofundina Poliel Lev *Braun, Spain†.*
Electrolyte infusion with fructose (p.1147·1).
Carbohydrate source; fluid and electrolyte depletion.

Estiamen *UCM-Difme, Ital.†.*
Oestrone (p.1458·2); oestradiol (p.1455·1); oestriol (p.1457·2).
Oestrogen deficiency.

Estiamen B *UCM-Difme, Ital.†.*
Oestrone (p.1458·2); oestradiol (p.1455·1); oestriol (p.1457·2).
Menopausal disorders.

Estigyn *Glaxo Wellcome, Austral.*
Ethinyloestradiol (p.1445·1).
Amenorrhoea; menopausal disorders.

Estilsona *Astra, Spain.*
Prednisolone steaglate (p.1048·2).
Corticosteroid.

Estimulocel *Alonga, Spain.*
Procodazole ethyl ester (p.1621·3).
Immunotherapy.

Estinyl
Schering, Canad.; Schering-Plough, S.Afr.; Schering, USA.
Ethinyloestradiol (p.1445·1).
Breast cancer; functional uterine bleeding; hypogonadism; menopausal disorders; prostatic cancer.

Estivin *Alcon, USA.*
Naphazoline hydrochloride (p.1064·2); hypromellose (p.1473·1).
Minor eye irritation.

Esto *Angelini, Ital.*
Alfoscerate olamine.
Anxiety disorders.

Estomycin *Columbia, S.Afr.*
Erythromycin estolate (p.204·1).
Bacterial infections.

Estrace
Roberts, Canad.; Mead Johnson Laboratories, USA.
Oestradiol (p.1455·1).
Breast cancer; female castration; female hypogonadism; menopausal vasomotor symptoms; osteoporosis; primary ovarian failure; prostatic cancer; vulval and vaginal atrophy.

Estracomb
Ciba-Geigy, Aust.; Ciba, Canad.; Geigy, Ger.; Novartis, Ital.; Novartis, Neth.; Ciba, Norw.; Ciba-Geigy, Spain; Novartis, Swed.; Ciba, Switz.
4 Patches, oestradiol (p.1455·1) (Estraderm); 4 patches, oestradiol; norethisterone acetate (p.1453·1) (Estragest).
Menopausal disorders; oestrogen deficiency; osteoporosis.

Estracombi
Novartis, Austral.; Ciba-Geigy, Belg.; Ciba-Geigy, Irl.; Novartis, S.Afr.; Ciba, UK.
4 Patches, oestradiol (p.1455·1) (Estraderm TTS); 4 patches, oestradiol; norethisterone acetate (p.1453·1) (Estragest TTS).
Menopausal disorders; osteoporosis.

Estracyt
Pharmacia Upjohn, Aust.; Pharmacia Upjohn, Austral.; Pharmacia Upjohn, Belg.; Pharmacia Upjohn, Fr.; Pharmacia Upjohn, Ger.; Pharmacia Upjohn, Irl.; Pharmacia Upjohn, Ital.; Pharmacia Upjohn, Neth.; Pharmacia Upjohn, Norw.; Pharmacia Upjohn, S.Afr.; Pharmacia Upjohn, Spain; Pharmacia Upjohn, Swed.; Pharmacia Upjohn, Switz.; Pharmacia, UK.
Estramustine meglumine phosphate, estramustine phosphate, or estramustine sodium phosphate (p.532·2).
Prostatic cancer.

Estra-D *Seatrace, USA†.*
Oestradiol cypionate (p.1455·1).
Female hypogonadism; menopausal vasomotor symptoms.

Estraderm
Ciba-Geigy, Aust.; Novartis, Austral.; Ciba-Geigy, Belg.; Ciba, Canad.; Ciba-Geigy, Fr.; Geigy, Ger.; Ciba-Geigy, Irl.; Novartis, Ital.; Novartis, Neth.; Ciba, Norw.; Novartis, S.Afr.; Ciba-Geigy, Spain; Novartis, Swed.; Ciba, Switz.; Ciba, UK; Ciba, USA.
Oestradiol (p.1455·1).
Female castration; female hypogonadism; menopausal disorders; osteoporosis; primary ovarian failure; vulval and vaginal atrophy.

Estradurin
Pharmacia Upjohn, Aust.; Pharmacia Upjohn, Ger.; Parke, Davis, Ital.†; Pharmacia Upjohn, Neth.; Pharmacia Upjohn, Norw.; Pharmacia Upjohn, Spain; Pharmacia Upjohn, Swed.; Pharmacia Upjohn, Switz.; Pharmacia Upjohn, UK†; Wyeth-Ayerst, USA†.
Polyestradiol phosphate (p.1459·2).
Mepivacaine hydrochloride (p.1297·2) is included in this preparation to alleviate the pain of injection.
Amenorrhoea; breast cancer; functional uterine bleeding; menopausal disorders; osteoporosis; prostatic cancer.

Estradurine *Pharmacia Upjohn, Belg.*
Polyestradiol phosphate (p.1459·2).
Prostatic cancer.

Estragest *Ciba-Geigy, Aust.*
Oestradiol (p.1455·1); norethisterone acetate (p.1453·1).
Menopausal disorders; osteoporosis.

Estra-L *Pasadena, USA.*
Oestradiol valerate (p.1455·2).
Female castration; female hypogonadism; menopausal vasomotor symptoms; prevention of breast engorgement; primary ovarian failure; prostatic cancer; vulval and vaginal atrophy.

Estrapak
Note. This name is used for preparations of different composition.
Novartis, Austral.
8 Patches, oestradiol (p.1455·1); 14 tablets, medroxyprogesterone acetate (p.1448·3).
Menopausal disorders; osteoporosis.

Ciba-Geigy, Irl.; Ciba, UK.
Transdermal patches, oestradiol (p.1455·1); tablets, norethisterone acetate (p.1453·1).
Menopausal disorders; osteoporosis.

Estratab *Solvay, USA.*
Esterified oestrogens (p.1458·1).
Breast cancer; female castration; female hypogonadism; menopausal vasomotor symptoms; primary ovarian failure; prostatic cancer; vulval and vaginal atrophy.

Estratest *Solvay, USA.*
Esterified oestrogens (p.1458·1); methyltestosterone (p.1450·3).
Menopausal disorders.

Estra-Testrin *Pasadena, USA†.*
Oestradiol valerate (p.1455·2); testosterone enanthate (p.1464·1).
Menopausal vasomotor symptoms; prevention of postpartum breast engorgement.

Estrepto P H *Wasserman, Spain†.*
Streptomycin pantoheptagluconate calcium (p.250·1); streptomycin sulphate (p.249·3).
Bacterial infections.

Estreptoenterol *Juste, Spain.*
Dihydrostreptomycin sulphate (p.202·2); phthalylsulphathiazole (p.237·1); pectin (p.1474·1).
Gastro-intestinal infections.

Estreptosirup *Durban, Spain†.*
Dihydrostreptomycin sulphate (p.202·2); formosulphathiazole (p.210·1); neomycin sulphate (p.229·2); pectin (p.1474·1).
Gastro-intestinal infections.

Estreva *Theramex, Mon.*
Oestradiol (p.1455·1).
Oestrogen deficiency.

Estriel *Mochida, Jpn†.*
Oestriol (p.1457·2).
Menopausal disorders; osteoporosis.

Estrifam *Novo Nordisk, Ger.*
Oestradiol (p.1455·1).
Formerly contained oestradiol and oestriol.
Oestrogen replacement therapy.

Estring
Pharmacia Upjohn, Aust.; Pharmacia Upjohn, Austral.; Pharmacia Upjohn, Canad.; Pharmacia Upjohn, Ger.; Pharmacia Upjohn, Neth.; Pharmacia Upjohn, Norw.; Pharmacia Upjohn, S.Afr.; Pharmacia Upjohn, Switz.; Pharmacia, UK; Pharmacia Upjohn, USA.
Oestradiol (p.1455·1).
Postmenopausal atrophy of the vagina or lower urinary-tract.

Estroclim *Sigma-Tau, Ital.*
Oestradiol (p.1455·1).
Menopausal disorders; osteoporosis.

Estro-Cyp *Keene, USA.*
Oestradiol cypionate (p.1455·1).
Female hypogonadism; menopausal vasomotor symptoms.

Estrofem
Novo Nordisk, Aust.; Novo Nordisk, Belg.; Novo Nordisk, Fr.; Novo Nordisk, Irl.; Novo Nordisk, Neth.; Novo Nordisk, S.Afr.
Oestradiol (p.1455·1).
Formerly contained oestradiol and oestriol in *Fr.* and *S.Afr.*
Menopausal disorders; oestrogen deficiency; osteoporosis.

Estrofem N *Novo Nordisk, Switz.*
Oestradiol (p.1455·1).
Estrofem formerly contained oestradiol and oestriol.
Oestrogen deficiency.

Estroject *Mayrand, USA†.*
Oestradiol cypionate (p.1455·1).
Female hypogonadism; menopausal vasomotor symptoms.

Estro-Pause *Adcock Ingram, S.Afr.*
Oestradiol valerate (p.1455·2).
Menopausal disorders.

Estro-Primolut *Schering, Ital.†.*
Norethisterone acetate (p.1453·1); ethinyloestradiol (p.1445·1).
Secondary amenorrhoea.

Estrostep *Parke, Davis, USA.*
Norethisterone acetate (p.1453·1); ethinyloestradiol (p.1445·1).
Triphasic oral contraceptive.

Estrostep Fe *Parke, Davis, USA.*
21 Tablets, norethisterone acetate (p.1453·1); ethinyloestradiol (p.1445·1); 7 tablets, ferrous fumarate (p.1339·3).
Triphasic oral contraceptive.

Estrovis
Godecke, Ger.†; Parke, Davis, USA†.
Quinestrol (p.1461·3).
Female castration; female hypogonadism; menopausal vasomotor symptoms; primary ovarian failure; vulval and vaginal atrophy.

Estroxyn *Pharmacia Upjohn, Austral.*
Tamoxifen citrate (p.563·3).
Breast cancer.

Estulic
Wander, Belg.; Sandoz, Fr.; Wander, Ger.; Mochida, Jpn†; Asta Medica, Neth.; Sandoz, Spain†; Sandoz, Switz.†.
Guanfacine hydrochloride (p.879·1).
Hypertension.

Esucos
UCB, Aust.; UCB, Belg.; Rodleben, Ger.†; SIT, Ital.; UCB, Norw.; UCB, S.Afr.†; UCB, Swed.
Dixyrazine (p.668·2).
Alcohol withdrawal syndrome; anxiety; confusion; depression; nausea; nervous disorders; neuroleptanalgesia; premedication; vomiting.

Eta Biocortilen *SIFI, Ital.*
Dexamethasone sodium phosphate (p.1037·2); neomycin sulphate (p.229·2).
Formerly contained dexamethasone sodium phosphate, neomycin sulphate, and gramicidin.
Infected eye disorders.

Eta Biocortilen VC *SIFI, Ital.*
Dexamethasone sodium phosphate (p.1037·2); neomycin sulphate (p.229·2); gramicidin (p.215·2); tetrahydrozoline hydrochloride (p.1070·2).
Infected eye disorders.

Eta Cortilen *SIFI, Ital.*
Dexamethasone sodium phosphate (p.1037·2).
Eye disorders.

Etaciland *Landerlan, Spain†.*
Hetacillin (p.216·1).
Bacterial infections.

Etafillina *Delalande, Ital.†.*
Acepifylline.
Respiratory disorders.

Etalontin
Parke, Davis, Aust.; Parke, Davis, Ger.†.
Ethinyloestradiol (p.1445·1); norethisterone acetate (p.1453·1).
Combined oral contraceptive.

Etalpha
Merck, Aust.; Leo, Neth.; Leo, Norw.; Farmacusi, Spain; Lovens, Swed.
Alfacalcidol (p.1366·3).
Hypoparathyroidism; osteomalacia; renal osteodystrophy; osteoporosis; rickets; vitamin-D deficiency states.

Etamicina *Pharkos, Ital.†.*
Hydrocortamate hydrochloride (p.1043·3); neomycin sulphate (p.229·2); diphenhydramine hydrochloride (p.409·1).
Skin disorders.

Etamucin *Schoeller, Aust.†.*
Sodium hyaluronate (p.1630·3).
Adjunct in ophthalmic surgery.

Etanicozid B6 *Piam, Ital.*
Ethambutol hydrochloride (p.207·2); isoniazid (p.218·1).
Pyridoxine hydrochloride (p.1362·3) is included in this preparation for the prophylaxis of peripheral neuropathy.
Tuberculosis.

Etaphylline *Delalande, Switz.†.*
Acepifylline.
Obstructive airways disease.

Etapiam *Piam, Ital.*
Ethambutol hydrochloride (p.207·2).
Tuberculosis.

Etaproctene *Angelini, Ital.†.*
Prednisolamate hydrochloride (p.1047·3); tetrahydrozoline hydrochloride (p.1070·2); lignocaine (p.1293·2).
Anorectal disorders.

Etaretin *Etapharm, Aust.*
Retinal phosphatides; sodium bicarbonate (p.1153·2).
Eye disorders.

Etaxene *Wassermann, Ital.*
Somatostatin acetate (p.1261·1).
Gastro-intestinal haemorrhage.

Etermol *Quimpe, Spain.*
Aconite (p.1542·2); calcium lactophosphate; ephedrine hydrochloride (p.1059·3); beech; lemon; potassium guaiacolsulfonate (p.1068·3).
Upper-respiratory-tract disorders.

Etermol Antitusivo *Quimpe, Spain.*
Benzydamine hydrochloride (p.21·3); dextromethorphan hydrobromide (p.1057·3); guaiphenesin (p.1061·3); sodium benzoate (p.1102·3).
Coughs.

Ethamolin
DBL, Austral.†; Reed & Carnrick, Canad.; Schwarz, USA.
Ethanolamine oleate (p.1576·2).
Haemorrhoids; oesophageal varices; varicose veins.

Ethaquin *Ascher, USA†.*
Ethaverine hydrochloride (p.1577·1).
Cerebral and peripheral ischaemia; smooth muscle spasm.

Ethatab *Whitby, USA†.*
Ethaverine hydrochloride (p.1577·1).
Peripheral and cerebral vascular insufficiency.

Ethatyl *Hoechst Marion Roussel, S.Afr.*
Ethionamide (p.208·2).
Tuberculosis.

Ethavex *Econo Med, USA†.*
Ethaverine hydrochloride (p.1577·1).
Cerebral and peripheral ischaemia; smooth muscle spasm.

Etheophyl *Lindopharm, Ger.*
Theophylline (p.765·1).
Obstructive airways disease.

Ethibloc *Johnson & Johnson, Switz.*
Sodium diatrizoate (p.1003·2).
Packing of pancreatic duct following partial pancreatic resection; pre-operative vascular embolisation for renal tumours.

Ethibloc Okklusions-Emulsion *Ethicon, Ger.*
Sodium diatrizoate (p.1003·2).
Packing the residual pancreatic duct after partial resection of the pancreas; pre-operative vascular embolisation for renal tumours.

Ethicod *Pharmalab, S.Afr.†.*
Aspirin (p.16·1); codeine phosphate (p.26·1).
Fever; inflammation; pain.

Ethimil *Dexcel, UK.*
Verapamil hydrochloride (p.960·3).
Angina pectoris; hypertension.

Ethimycin *Noristan Generica, S.Afr.†.*
Erythromycin stearate (p.204·2).
Bacterial infections.

Ethiodol *Savage, USA.*
Iodised oil (p.1006·1).
Contrast medium for hysterosalpingography and lymphography.

Ethipam *Noristan Generica, S.Afr.†.*
Diazepam (p.661·1).
Alcohol withdrawal syndrome; anxiety; premedication.

Ethipramine *Noristan Generica, S.Afr.†.*
Imipramine hydrochloride (p.289·2).
Alcohol withdrawal syndrome; behaviour disorders; depression; parkinsonism.

Ethipurinol *Noristan Generica, S.Afr.†.*
Allopurinol (p.390·2).
Gout; hyperuricaemia.

Ethivite *Pharmalab, S.Afr.†.*
Multivitamin preparation.

Ethmozine
Monmouth, Irl.; Monmouth, UK; Roberts, USA.
Moracizine hydrochloride (p.912·3).
Ventricular arrhythmias.

Ethrane
Abbott, Aust.; Abbott, Austral.; Abbott, Belg.; Zeneca, Canad.; Abbott, Ger.; Abbott, Irl.; Abbott, Ital.†; Abbott, Neth.; Abbott, S.Afr.; Abbott, Spain†; Abbott, Switz.; Ohmeda, USA.
Enflurane (p.1222·1).
Anaesthesia and analgesia in obstetrics; general anaesthesia.

Ethyol
Schering-Plough, Austral.; Lilly, Canad.; Schering-Plough, Fr.; Essex, Ger.; Schering-Plough, Neth.; Schering-Plough, S.Afr.; Schering-Plough, Spain; Schering-Plough, UK; Alza, USA; US Bioscience, USA.
Amifostine (p.973·3).
Reduction of neutropenia and nephrotoxicity due to chemotherapy.

Etiaxil
Note. This name is used for preparations of different composition.
RP-LABO, Fr.†.
Aluminium chloride (p.1078·3) aluminium lactate (p.1548·1).
Hyperhidrosis.

Interdelta, Switz.
Aluminium chloride (p.1078·3).
Hyperhidrosis.

Etibi
Gerot, Aust.; ICN, Canad.; Zoja, Ital.
Ethambutol hydrochloride (p.207·2).
Tuberculosis.

Etibi-INH *Zoja, Ital.*
Ethambutol hydrochloride (p.207·2); isoniazid (p.218·1).
Tuberculosis.

Etidron *Abiogen, Ital.*
Disodium etidronate (p.738·3).
Paget's disease of bone.

Etifollin *Nycomed, Norw.*
Ethinyloestradiol (p.1445·1).
Menopausal disorders; prostatic cancer.

Etil *CT, Ger.*
Etilefrine hydrochloride (p.867·2).
Hypotension.

Etiltox *AFOM, Ital.*
Disulfiram (p.1573·1).
Alcoholism.

Etimonis *Ecosol, Switz.*
Isosorbide mononitrate (p.893·3).
Heart failure; ischaemic heart disease.

Etioven *Cassenne, Fr.*
Naftazone (p.725·2).
Peripheral vascular disorders.

Eti-Puren *Isis Puren, Ger.*
Etilefrine hydrochloride (p.867·2).
Hypotension.

Etmocard *Evers, Ger.†.*
Wheat-germ oil; dried yeast (p.1373·1); belladonna.
Cardiovascular disorders.

Etmoren *Evers, Ger.*
Silver birch (p.1553·3); orthosiphon leaves (p.1592·2); solidago virgaurea.
Diuretic.

Etocil Caffeina *Biomedica, Ital.†.*
Etenzamide (p.35·3); caffeine (p.749·3).
Fever; pain.

Etocil Pirina *Biomedica, Ital.†.*
Etenzamide (p.35·3); propyphenazone (p.81·3).
Fever; pain.

Etocovit *Richter, Aust.*
d-Alpha-tocopherol (p.1369·1).
Vitamin E deficiency.

Etofen *Ecosol, Switz.*
Etofenamate (p.36·3).
Musculoskeletal, joint, and soft-tissue disorders.

Etomine *Novartis, S.Afr.*
Clothiapine (p.657·2).
Agitation; anxiety; depression; psychoses.

Etopofos *Bristol-Myers Squibb, Swed.*
Etoposide phosphate (p.533·2).
Malignant neoplasms.

Etopophos
Bristol-Myers Squibb, Austral.; Bristol-Myers Squibb, Fr.; Bristol-Myers Squibb, Neth.; Bristol-Myers Squibb, UK; Bristol-Myers Oncology, USA.
Etoposide phosphate (p.533·2).
Malignant neoplasms.

Etoscol *Byk Gulden, Ger.†.*
Hexoprenaline sulphate (p.754·1).
Obstructive airways disease.

Etoxisclerol *Bama, Spain.*
Laureth 9 (p.1325·2).
Varices.

Etrafon
Schering, Canad.; Schering-Plough, S.Afr.; Schering, USA.
Perphenazine (p.685·2); amitriptyline hydrochloride (p.273·3).
Mixed anxiety depressive states.

Etramon *Janssen-Cilag, Spain.*
Econazole nitrate (p.377·2).
Fungal infections.

Etrat *Klinge, Aust.*
Heparin sodium (p.879·3); menthol (p.1600·2); glycol salicylate (p.43·1).
Post-traumatic oedema and haematoma.

Etrat Sportgel *Klinge, Ger.*
Heparin sodium (p.879·3); menthol (p.1600·2); glycol salicylate (p.43·1).
Sports injuries.

Etrat Sportsalbe *Schwab, Ger.†.*
Heparin sodium (p.879·3); benzyl nicotinate (p.22·1).
Sports injuries.

Etrat Sportsalbe MPS *Klinge, Ger.*
A heparinoid (p.882·3).
Soft-tissue injury; superficial vascular disorders.

Etro *Inexfa, Spain.*
Ampicillin sodium (p.153·1); ampicillin benzathine (p.154·1).
Lignocaine hydrochloride (p.1293·2) is included in this preparation to alleviate the pain of injection.
Bacterial infections.

Etro Balsamico *Inexfa, Spain.*
Ampicillin sodium (p.153·1); ampicillin benzathine (p.154·1); cineole (p.1564·1); niaouli oil (p.1607·1); guaiphenesin (p.1061·3).
Lignocaine hydrochloride (p.1293·2) is included in this preparation to alleviate the pain of injection.
Respiratory-tract infections.

Etrynit *Inibsa, Spain†.*
Propatylnitrate (p.936·3).
Angina pectoris; heart failure; myocardial infarction.

ETS *Paddock, USA†.*
Erythromycin (p.204·1).
Acne.

Etumina *Sandoz, Spain.*
Clothiapine (p.657·2).
Anxiety; psychoses.

Etumine *Wander, Belg.*
Clothiapine (p.657·2).
Agitation; alcohol withdrawal syndrome; anxiety; psychoses.

Etyzem *Caber, Ital.*
Diltiazem hydrochloride (p.854·2).
Angina pectoris; heart failure; hypertension.

Eubetal *SIFI, Ital.*
Betamethasone sodium phosphate (p.1033·3); antazoline phosphate (p.401·3).
Eye disorders.

Eubetal Antibiotico *SIFI, Ital.*
Eye drops: Betamethasone sodium phosphate (p.1033·3); rolitetracycline (p.247·1); chloramphenicol (p.182·1); colistin sulphomethate sodium (p.196·1).
Eye ointment: Betamethasone sodium phosphate (p.1033·3); tetracycline (p.259·1); chloramphenicol (p.182·1); colistin sulphomethate sodium (p.196·1).
Eye disorders.

Eubine *Promedica, Fr.*
Oxycodone hydrochloride (p.71·2).
Pain.

Eubiol *Chephasaar, Ger.*
Arginine aspartate (p.1334·2).
Liver disorders.

Eubispasme Codethyline *Promedica, Fr.*
Suppositories†: Opium (p.70·3); ethylmorphine camphorate (p.36·1); anisohydrocinnamol oleate.
Smooth muscle spasm.
Tablets: Opium (p.70·3); ethylmorphine (p.36·1); camphoric acid; anisohydrocinnamol hydrochloride.
Coughs.

Euboral *Bama, Spain.*
Naphazoline hydrochloride (p.1064·2); borax (p.1554·2).
Eye irritation.

Eubran *ICT-Lodi, Ital.†.*
Vinburnine phosphate (p.1644·1).
Cerebrovascular disorders.

Eubucal *Priorin, Switz.†.*
Chlorhexidine gluconate (p.1107·2); myrrh (p.1606·1); chamomile (p.1561·2); arnica (p.1550·3); rhatany (p.1624·3); menthol (p.1600·2).
Mouth disorders.

Eucabal *Esparma, Ger.*
Plantago lanceolata; thyme (p.1636·3).
Catarrh.

Eucabal-Balsam S *Esparma, Ger.*
Eucalyptus oil (p.1578·1); scotch pine needle oil.
Respiratory-tract disorders.

Eucafluid N *Steigerwald, Ger.*
Eucalyptus oil (p.1578·1); scotch pine needle oil; peppermint oil (p.1208·1); rosemary oil (p.1626·2).
Musculoskeletal and joint disorders; neuralgia.

Eucalcic *Byk, Fr.*
Calcium carbonate (p.1182·1).
Renal osteodystrophy.

Eucaliptina *Blue Cross, Ital.*
Cineole (p.1564·1); guaiacol (p.1061·2).
Respiratory disorders.

Eucalipto Composto *Dynacren, Ital.*
Eucalyptus oil (p.1578·1); camphor (p.1557·2); levomenthol (p.1600·2); thymol (p.1127·1).
Nasal congestion.

Eucalyptamint
Ciba Self Medication, Canad.†; Ciba, USA.
Menthol (p.1600·2); eucalyptus oil (p.1578·1).
Muscle pain and stiffness.

Eucalyptine Le Brun
Note. This name is used for preparations of different composition.
Medgenix, Belg.
Capsules: Cineole (p.1564·1); guaiacol (p.1061·2); phenol (p.1121·2); codeine (p.26·1); camphor (p.1557·2); bromoform (p.1620·3).
Suppositories for adults and children: Camphor (p.1557·2); phenol (p.1121·2); cineole (p.1564·1); guaiacol (p.1061·2).
Suppositories for infants: Camphor (p.1557·2); cineole (p.1564·1); guaiacol (p.1061·2).
Syrup: Potassium guaiacolsulfonate (p.1068·3); sodium phenolsulphonate; sodium camsylate; codeine (p.26·1); belladonna (p.457·1); aconite (p.1542·2); bromoform (p.1620·3); cineole (p.1564·1).
Respiratory disorders.

Martin, Fr.
Capsules: Cineole (p.1564·1); guaiacol (p.1061·2); phenol (p.1121·2); camphor (p.1557·2); bromoform (p.1620·3); codeine (p.26·1).
Neonatal suppositories: Cineole (p.1564·1); potassium guaiacolsulfonate (p.1068·3); sodium camsylate.
Suppositories: Cineole (p.1564·1); guaiacol (p.1061·2); phenol (p.1121·2); camphor (p.1557·2); codeine phosphate (p.26·1).
Syrup: Cineole (p.1564·1); codeine (p.26·1).
Formerly contained eucalyptus oil, sodium phenolsulphonate, sodium camsylate, potassium guaiacolsulfonate, bromoform, codeine, belladonna, and aconite.
Coughs.

Eucalyptine Pholcodine *Martin, Fr.*
Cineole (p.1564·1); guaiacol (p.1061·2); phenol (p.1121·2); camphor (p.1557·2); pholcodine (p.1068·1).
Coughs.

Eucalyptine Pholcodine Le Brun *Medgenix, Belg.*
Suppositories for adults and children: Cineole (p.1564·1); camphor (p.1557·2); phenol (p.1121·2); guaiacol (p.1061·2); pholcodine (p.1068·1).
Suppositories for infants: Cineole (p.1564·1); camphor (p.1557·2); guaiacol (p.1061·2); pholcodine (p.1068·1).
Syrup: Potassium guaiacolsulfonate (p.1068·3); sodium camsylate; sodium phenolsulphonate; pholcodine (p.1068·1); belladonna (p.457·1); aconite (p.1542·2); bromoform (p.1620·3); cineole (p.1564·1).
Respiratory disorders.

Eucalyptospirine *Rovi, Spain.*
Aspirin (p.16·1); amylocaine hydrochloride (p.1286·1); cineole (p.1564·1); ethylmorphine (p.36·1); guaiacol (p.1061·2); sodium camsylate.
Influenza and cold symptoms.

Eucalyptospirine Lact *Rovi, Spain.*
Aspirin (p.16·1); amylocaine hydrochloride (p.1286·1); cineole (p.1564·1); guaiacol (p.1061·2); sodium camsylate.
Influenza and cold symptoms.

Eucalyptrol L *Medopharm, Ger.*
Eucalyptus oil (p.1578·1).
Cold symptoms.

Eucamenth *Planta, Canad.*
Camphor oil; eucalyptus oil (p.1578·1); menthol (p.1600·2).
Coughs; nasal and sinus congestion.

Eucar *Salus, Ital.*
Levocarnitine hydrochloride (p.1336·2).
Carnitine deficiency; myocardial ischaemia.

Eucarbon
Note. This name is used for preparations of different composition.
Schmidgall, Aust.; Trenker, Belg.
Senna (p.1212·2); rhubarb (p.1212·1); vegetable charcoal (p.972·3); sulphur (p.1091·2); peppermint oil (p.1208·1); fennel oil (p.1579·2).
Constipation; dyspepsia; flatulence.

Difer, Ital.
Senna (p.1212·2); rhubarb (p.1212·1); vegetable charcoal (p.972·3); sublimed sulphur (p.1091·2).
Constipation.

Trenka, Switz.
Senna (p.1212·2); rhubarb (p.1212·1); vegetable charcoal (p.972·3); peppermint oil (p.1208·1); fennel oil (p.1579·2).
Constipation; flatulence.

Eucard *Sudmedica, Ger.†.*
Etofylline (p.753·1); quinidine (p.938·3).
Arrhythmias; heart failure.

Eucardic
Boehringer Mannheim, Neth.; Boehringer Mannheim, Swed.; SmithKline Beecham, UK.
Carvedilol (p.838·1).
Formerly known as Dilatrend in *Neth.*
Angina pectoris; heart failure; hypertension.

Eucardion *Dompe Biotec, Ital.*
Dexrazoxane hydrochloride (p.978·3).
Prevention of doxorubicin cardiotoxicity.

Eucarnil *Pulitzer, Ital.*
Levocarnitine (p.1336·2).
Carnitine deficiency; myocardial ischaemia.

Eucebral-N *Sudmedica, Ger.*
Etofylline (p.753·1); cyclandelate (p.845·2).
Cerebral and peripheral vascular disorders.

Eucerin
Smith & Nephew, Canad.; Beiersdorf, Irl.; Beiersdorf, UK; Beiersdorf, USA.
Emollient.
Dry skin.

Eucerin (Anhydrous) *Beiersdorf, Austral.*
Wool alcohols (p.1385·2).
Minor skin disorders; ointment basis; skin cleanser.

Eucerin Dry Skin Care Daily Facial *Beiersdorf, USA.*
SPF 20: Ethylhexyl *p*-methoxycinnamate (p.1487·1); titanium dioxide (p.1093·3); 2-phenyl-1*H*-benzimidazole-5-sulphonic acid (p.1488·2); 2-ethylhexyl salicylate (p.1487·3).
Sunscreen.

Euceta
Sandoz, Ital.; Wander, Neth.†; Wander OTC, Switz.
Aluminium acetotartrate (p.1547·3).
Skin disorders.

Euceta avec camomille et arnica *Wander, Switz.*
Aluminium acetotartrate (p.1547·3); chamomile (p.1561·2); arnica (p.1550·3).
Skin disorders.

Euceta mit Kamille *Sanabo, Aust.*
Aluminium acetotartrate (p.1547·3); chamomile.
Skin disorders.

Euceta Pic *Wander, Switz.†.*
Aluminium acetotartrate (p.1547·3); mepyramine maleate (p.414·1); lignocaine hydrochloride (p.1293·2).
Insect bites.

Euchessina *Antonetto, Ital.†.*
Phenolphthalein (p.1208·2).
Constipation.

Euchon *Steiner, Ger.†.*
Propranolol hydrochloride (p.937·1); valerian root (p.1643·1).
Hyperthyroidism; nervous disorders with cardiac symptoms; tremor.

Euci *Falqui, Ital.*
Paracetamol (p.72·2); ascorbic acid (p.1365·2); pseudoephedrine hydrochloride (p.1068·3); dextromethorphan hydrobromide (p.1057·3).
Cold symptoms.

Eucillin *Petrasch, Aust.*
Bacitracin (p.157·3); dequalinium chloride (p.1112·1); diphenylpyraline hydrochloride (p.409·3).
Infected skin disorders.

Euclean Eucalyptus Hand Cleaner *Felton, Austral.†.*
Coconut soap; eucalyptus oil (p.1578·1).
Skin cleanser.

Euclorina *SmithKline Beecham, Ital.*
Chloramine (p.1106·3).
Skin, wound, and genital disinfection.

Eucol *Soekami, Fr.†.*
Arginine oxoglurate (p.1334·2).
Hepatic encephalopathy; tonic.

Euctan *Synthelabo, Fr.†.*
Tolonidine nitrate (p.956·3).
Hypertension.

Eudal-SR *UAD, USA.*
Pseudoephedrine hydrochloride (p.1068·3); guaiphenesin (p.1061·3).
Coughs.

Eudemine
Allen & Hanburys, Irl.†; Goldshield, UK; Medeva, UK.
Diazoxide (p.847·2).
Hypertensive crises; hypoglycaemia.

Eudent con Glysan *Kemiprogress, Ital.*
Glysan (enoxolone (p.35·2); sanguinaria (p.1627·2)); sodium monofluorophosphate (p.743·3) or sodium fluoride (p.742·1).
Gum disorders; oral hygiene.

Eudermal Pasta *Pentaderm, Ital.*
Barrier cream.

Eudermal Sapone Allo Zolfo pH 5 *Pentaderm, Ital.*
Sulphur (p.1091·2).
Skin cleansing.

Eudextran *Bieffe, Ital.*
Dextran 40 (p.716·2) in sodium chloride or glucose.
Plasma volume expansion; thrombo-embolic disorders.

Eudigestio *Ogna, Ital.*
Pancreatin (p.1612·1); pepsin (p.1616·3).
Dyspepsia.

Eudigox *Astra, Ital.*
Digoxin (p.849·3).
Arrhythmias; heart failure.

Eudolene *Savio, Ital.*
Nimesulide (p.63·2).
Fever; inflammation; pain.

Eudorlin *Berlin-Chemie, Ger.†.*
Propyphenazone (p.81·3); paracetamol (p.72·2) caffeine (p.749·3).
Pain.

Eudur
Recipe, Aust.; Astra, Ger.; Astra, Switz.†.
Terbutaline sulphate (p.764·1); theophylline (p.765·1).
Obstructive airways disease.

Eudyna
Ebewe, Aust.; Knoll, Ger.
Tretinoin (p.1093·3).
Acne.

Eufans *Sigma-Tau, Ital.*
Amtolmetin guacil (p.15·3).
Musculoskeletal and joint disorders; pain.

Euffekt *OTW, Ger.†.*
Etenzamide (p.35·3).
Fever; pain.

Eufibron *Berlin-Chemie, Ger.*
Propyphenazone (p.81·3).
Fever; pain.

Eufilina *Byk Elmu, Spain.*
Aminophylline (p.748·1).
Neonatal dyspnoea; obstructive airways disease.

Eufimenth N mild *Lichtenstein, Ger.*
Eucalyptus oil (p.1578·1); Norway spruce oil.
Respiratory-tract disorders.

Eufimenth-Balsam N *Lichtenstein, Ger.*
Cineole (p.1564·1); Norway spruce oil; menthol (p.1600·2).
Respiratory-tract disorders.

Eufipulmo *Elmu, Spain†.*
Aminophylline (p.748·1); cineole (p.1564·1); niaouli oil (p.1607·1).
Respiratory-tract disorders.

Euflat *Solus, Aust.*
Pancreatin (p.1612·1); papaverine hydrochloride (p.1614·2); angelica; aloes (p.1177·1); fel tauri (p.1553·2); carbo coffea (p.1645·1).
Gastro-intestinal disorders.

Euflat I *SSW, Ger.*
Dimethicone (p.1213·1); caraway oil (p.1559·3); fennel oil (p.1579·2).
Digestive system disorders.

Euflat-E *Sudmedica, Ger.*
Pancreatin (p.1612·1).
Digestive system disorders.

Euflat-N *Sudmedica, Ger.†.*
Porcine pancreatin (p.1612·1); papaverine hydrochloride (p.1614·2); carbo coffea (p.1645·1).
Gastro-intestinal disorders.

Euflex *Schering, Canad.*
Flutamide (p.537·1).
Prostatic cancer.

Euflux-N *Sudmedica, Ger.*
Pumilio pine oil (p.1623·3); camphor (p.1557·2).
Cardiac disorders; respiratory disorders.

Eufosyl *Sterling Midy, Fr.†.*
Dequalinium chloride (p.1112·1); amethocaine hydrochloride (p.1285·2); muramidase chloride (p.1604·3).
Mouth disorders.

Eufusin *Bieffe, Ital.*
Succinylated gelatin (p.723·2).
Hypovolaemia.

Eufusol *Hormonchemie, Ger.†; Schiwa, Ger.†.*
A range of electrolyte infusions with or without carbohydrate (p.1147·1).
Fluid and electrolyte disorders.

Eufusol M 20 *Hormonchemie, Ger.†; Schiwa, Ger.†.*
Mannitol (p.900·3).
Fluid retention; renal failure.

Eufusol OP-S 5 *Hormonchemie, Ger.†.*
Electrolyte infusion with sorbitol (p.1147·1).
Carbohydrate source; fluid and electrolyte disorders.

Eugalac
Chepharin, Aust.; Topfer, Ger.
Lactulose (p.1195·3).
Constipation; liver disorders; salmonella enteritis.

Eugalan Topfer forte *Topfer, Ger.*
Bifidum bacteria; albumin; lactose (p.1349·3); lactulose (p.1195·3); minerals.
Cirrhosis; gastro-intestinal disorders.

Eugalan Topfer forte LC *Topfer, Ger.*
Bifidobacteria; lactulose (p.1195·3); albumin; lactose (p.1349·3); galactose; minerals.
Constipation; hepatic encephalopathy.

Eugastran *Piam, Ital.†.*
Metoclopramide (p.1202·1); dihydroxyaluminum sodium carbonate (p.1188·3); dimethicone (p.1213·1).
Gastro-intestinal disorders.

Eugiron *Denolin, Belg.*
Clove flower (p.1565·2); althaea root and leaf (p.1546·3); raspberry leaf (p.1624·2); tilia flower (p.1637·3); eucalyptus leaf (p.1578·1); aniseed fruit (p.1549·3); fennel fruit (p.1579·1).
Mouth and throat disorders.

Euglucan *Boehringer Mannheim, Fr.*
Glibenclamide (p.319·3).
Diabetes mellitus.

Euglucon
Boehringer Mannheim, Aust.; Hoechst, Aust.; Boehringer Mannheim, Austral.; Boehringer Mannheim, Belg.; Boehringer Mannheim, Canad.; Roussel, Irl.†; Boehringer Mannheim, Ital.; Boehringer Mannheim, Jpn; Boehringer Mannheim, Neth.; Boehringer Mannheim, Norw.; Boehringer Mannheim, S.Afr.; Boehringer Mannheim, Spain; Boehringer Mannheim, Swed.; Boehringer Mannheim, Switz.; Hoechst Marion Roussel, UK.
Glibenclamide (p.319·3).
Diabetes mellitus.

Euglucon N *Boehringer Mannheim, Ger.; Hoechst, Ger.*
Glibenclamide (p.319·3).
Diabetes mellitus.

Eugrippine *Synthelabo, Belg.*
Diphenhydramine hydrochloride (p.409·1); caffeine (p.749·3); quinine sulphate (p.439·2); ascorbic acid (p.1365·2).
Fever associated with influenza.

Eugynon
Schering, Ger.†; Schering, Ital.; Schering, Norw.; Schering, Spain.
Norgestrel (p.1454·1); ethinyloestradiol (p.1445·1).
28-Day packs also contain 7 inert tablets.
Combined oral contraceptive; endometriosis; menstrual disorders.

Eugynon 30
Schering, Irl.†; Schering, UK.
Levonorgestrel (p.1454·1); ethinyloestradiol (p.1445·1).
Combined oral contraceptive.

Euhypnos
Sigma, Austral.; Pharmacia Upjohn, Belg.; Pharmacia Upjohn, Irl.; Pharmacia, S.Afr.†; Farmitalia Carlo Erba, UK.
Temazepam (p.693·3).

Euipnos *Pharmacia Upjohn, Ital.*
Temazepam (p.693·3).
Insomnia.

Euka *Pharmonta, Aust.*
Fennel (p.1579·1); aniseed (p.1549·3); rosemary; eucalyptus (p.1578·1); lavender flowers (p.1594·3); laurel leaves; camphor (p.1557·2); peppermint oil (p.1208·1); spearmint oil (p.1632·1).
Gastro-intestinal disorders.

Eukalisan forte *Steigerwald, Ger.*
Cyanocobalamin (p.1363·3); nicotinamide (p.1351·2); rutin sodium sulphate (p.1580·2).
Lignocaine hydrochloride (p.1293·2) is included in this preparation to alleviate the pain of injection.
Liver disorders.

Eukalisan N *Steigerwald, Ger.*
Cyanocobalamin (p.1363·3); nicotinamide (p.1351·2); rutin sodium sulphate (p.1580·2).
Procaine hydrochloride (p.1299·2) is included in this preparation to alleviate the pain of injection.
Liver disorders; neuralgia; peripheral vascular disorders; tonic.

Eukamillat *Biocur, Ger.*
Chamomile (p.1561·2).
Gastro-intestinal, anogenital, dental, respiratory-tract, and skin disorders.

Eukavan *Duopharm, Ger.*
Kava (p.1592·3).
Anxiety disorders.

Eukliman *Albert-Roussel, Ger.†.*
Belladonna (p.457·1); glyceryl trinitrate (p.874·3); phenobarbitone (p.350·2); sage oil; menthyl isovalerate.
Autonomic dystonia; hyperhidrosis; menopausal disorders; nocturnal enuresis.

Euky Bear Cough Syrup *Felton, Austral.*
Chlorpheniramine (p.405·2); dextromethorphan (p.1057·3); sodium citrate (p.1153·2).
Coughs and cold symptoms.

Euky Bear Eu-Clear Inhalant *Felton, Austral.*
Eucalyptus oil (p.1578·1); menthol (p.1600·2).
Cold symptoms; respiratory-tract congestion.

Euky Bear Limberub *Felton, Austral.†.*
Eucalyptus oil (p.1578·1); menthol (p.1600·2); glycol salicylate (p.43·1); capsicum oleoresin.
Musculoskeletal and joint pain.

Euky Bear Nasex *Felton, Austral.*
Oxymetazoline hydrochloride (p.1065·3); cineole (p.1564·1); menthol (p.1600·2).
Nasal congestion.

Euky Bearub *Felton, Austral.*
Eucalyptus oil (p.1578·1); cineole (p.1564·1); menthol (p.1600·2); camphor (p.1557·2); rosemary oil (p.1626·2).
Cold and influenza symptoms; insect bites; muscular aches and pains; nasal congestion.

Eulactol *Eulactol, S.Afr.†.*
Urea (p.1095·2).
Dry skin.

Eulatin N *Lichtwer, Ger.*
Lignocaine (p.1293·2); bismuth subgallate (p.1180·2).
Anorectal disorders.

Eulatin NN *Lichtwer, Ger.*
Hamamelis (p.1587·1); bismuth subgallate (p.1180·2); benzocaine (p.1286·2).
Anorectal disorders.

Eulexin
Schering-Plough, Austral.; Schering-Plough, Belg.; Schering-Plough, Ital.; Schering-Plough, Neth.; Schering-Plough, Norw.; Schering-Plough, S.Afr.; Schering-Plough, Spain; Schering-Plough, Swed.; Schering, USA.
Flutamide (p.537·1).
Prostatic cancer.

Eulexine *Schering-Plough, Fr.*
Flutamide (p.537·1).
Prostatic cancer.

Eulip *SIT, Ital.*
Tiadenol (p.1279·3).
Hyperlipidaemias.

Eulipos *Boehringer Mannheim, Ger.†.*
Dextrothyroxine sodium (p.1272·2).
Hyperlipidaemias.

Eulitop
Boehringer Mannheim, Belg.; Boehringer Mannheim, Spain.
Bezafibrate (p.1268·2).
Hyperlipidaemias.

Eu-Med
Note. This name is used for preparations of different composition.
Zyma, Aust.
Paracetamol (p.72·2); caffeine (p.749·3); propyphenazone (p.81·3).
Formerly contained salacetamide, caffeine, propyphenazone, and phenazone.
Fever; pain.

Zyma, Ger.
Phenazone (p.78·2).
Fever; pain.

Eu-Med S *Zyma, Ger.†.*
Aspirin (p.16·1); etenzamide (p.35·3); caffeine (p.749·3).
Arthritis; cold symptoms; fever; inflammation; pain; postoperative thrombo-embolic disorders; rheumatism.

Eu-Med SC *Med Fabrik, Ger.†.*
Phenazone (p.78·2); propyphenazone (p.81·3); salacetamide (p.82·3).
Fever; pain.

Eu-Med Schmerzzapfschen *Zyma, Ger.†.*
Paracetamol (p.72·2).
Fever; pain.

Euminex *Asta Medica, Spain†.*
Glucametacin (p.42·3).
Inflammation; musculoskeletal and joint disorders; peri-articular disorders.

Euminz N *Lichtwer, Ger.*
Peppermint oil (p.1208·1).
Myalgia; neuralgia.

Eumotol *Byk Gulden, S.Afr.†.*
Bumadizone calcium (p.22·2).
Ankylosing spondylitis.

Eumovate
Glaxo Wellcome, Belg.; Glaxo Wellcome, Canad.; Glaxo Wellcome, Irl.; Glaxo Wellcome, Ital.; Allen & Hanburys, S.Afr.; Glaxo, UK.
Clobetasone butyrate (p.1035·3).
Skin disorders.

Eunasin *Bracco, Ital.*
Metyzoline hydrochloride (p.1064·2).
Upper respiratory-tract disorders.

Eunerpan *Knoll, Ger.*
Melperone hydrochloride (p.677·3).
Psychiatric disorders; sleep disorders.

Eunomin *Grunenthal, Ger.†.*
White tablets, mestranol (p.1450·2); green tablets, mestranol; chlormadinone acetate (p.1439·1).
Sequential-type oral contraceptive.

Eunova *Fink, Ger.*
Multivitamin and mineral preparation.

Eupantol *Byk, Fr.*
Pantoprazole sodium (p.1207·3).
Gastro-oesophageal reflux; peptic ulcer.

Eupasal Sodico *Bieffe, Ital.†.*
Sodium aminosalicylate (p.151·1).
Tuberculosis.

Eupatal *Madaus, Ger.*
Thyme (p.1636·3); star anise oil.
Cold symptoms.

Eupatol *Donini, Ital.*
Cascara (p.1183·1); boldo (p.1554·1); rhubarb (p.1212·1).
Constipation.

Eupatorium Oligoplex *Madaus, Ger.*
Homoeopathic preparation.

Eupaverin *E. Merck, Swed.†.*
Moxaverine (p.1604·3).
Vascular spasm.

Eupaverina *Bracco, Ital.†.*
Moxaverine hydrochloride (p.1604·3).
Peripheral vascular spasm.

Eupeclanic *Uriach, Spain.*
Amoxycillin trihydrate (p.151·3); potassium clavulanate (p.190·2).
Bacterial infections.

Eupen *Uriach, Spain.*
Amoxycillin trihydrate (p.151·3).
Bacterial infections.

Eupen Bronquial *Uriach, Spain.*
Amoxycillin trihydrate (p.151·3); brovanexine hydrochloride (p.1056·1).
Respiratory-tract infections.

Eupeptina *Diviser Aquilea, Spain.*
Dibasic sodium phosphate (p.1159·3); magnesium carbonate (p.1198·1); magnesium phosphate (p.1157·3); magnesium oxide (p.1198·3); pepsin carbonate.
Constipation; dyspepsia.

Eupeptique Tisy *Laphal, Fr.†.*
Pancreas; gastro-intestinal mucous membrane extract (porcine); barley.
Dyspepsia.

Euphidra G2 Radical *Zeta, Ital.*
Multivitamin and mineral preparation.
Nutritional supplement.

Euphon
Note. This name is used for preparations of different composition.
ACP, Belg.
Codeine (p.26·1); aconite (p.1542·2); sodium formate (p.1581·3); erysimin; inula (p.1059·2).
Throat disorders.

Mayoly-Spindler, Fr.
Oral solution: Codeine (p.26·1); aconite (p.1542·2); sodium formate (p.1581·3); erysimin.
Coughs.
Pastilles: Erysimin.
Sore throat.
Syrup: Erysimin; codeine (p.26·1).
Coughs.

Euphon N *Mayoly-Spindler, Switz.*
Codeine (p.26·1); tolu balsam (p.1071·1).
Coughs and associated respiratory-tract disorders.

Euphorbia Complex *Blackmores, Austral.*
Passion flower (p.1615·3); thyme (p.1636·3); grindelia; euphorbia; vitamins.
Respiratory tract disorders.

Euphorbium compositum-Nasentropfen S *Heel, Ger.*
Homoeopathic preparation.

Euphyllin
Byk, Aust.; Byk, Belg.; Byk Gulden, Ger.; Byk, Neth.; Byk Gulden, Norw.; Byk Madaus, S.Afr.; Byk, Switz.
Aminophylline (p.748·1), aminophylline hydrate (p.748·1), or theophylline (p.765·1).
Central respiratory disorders; cor pulmonale; heart failure; obstructive airways disease.

Euphyllina *Byk Gulden, Ital.*
Aminophylline (p.748·1).
Obstructive airways disease.

Euphyllina Rilcon *Byk Gulden, Ital.*
Theophylline (p.765·1).
Obstructive airways disease.

Euphyllina Ritardo *Byk Gulden, Ital.*
Theophylline (p.765·1).
Obstructive airways disease.

Euphyllin-Calcium *Byk, Aust.*
Aminophylline (p.748·1); calcium gluconate (p.1155·2).

Euphylline *Byk, Fr.*
Theophylline (p.765·1).
Obstructive airways disease.

Euphylong
Byk Gulden, Ger.; Byk, Neth.; Swedish Orphan, Swed.; Byk, Switz.
Theophylline (p.765·1).
Central respiratory disorders; obstructive airways disease.

Euphytose *Nicholas, Fr.*
Crataegus (p.1568·2); passion flower (p.1615·3); guarana (p.1645·1); kola (p.1645·1); valerian (p.1643·1); ballota.
Nervous disorders.

Euplit *Desitin, Ger.†.*
Amitriptyline hydrochloride (p.273·3).
Depression.

Eupneron *Lyocentre, Fr.*
Eprozinol hydrochloride (p.1574·3).
Obstructive airways disease.

Eupnol *Rottapharm, Spain.*
Benzethonium chloride (p.1102·3); cineole (p.1564·1); cherry-laurel; procaine hydrochloride (p.1299·2); terpineol (p.1635·1); menthol (p.1600·2).
Formerly called Eupnol Desinfectante.
Mouth and throat inflammation.

Eupond *Sudmedica, Ger.*
Theobromine (p.765·1); dehydrocholic acid (p.1570·2); ox bile (p.1553·2); atropine sulphate (p.455·1); aloes (p.1177·1); frangula bark (p.1193·2); cichorium; ononis (p.1610·2); parsley (p.1615·3); birch leaf (p.1553·3).
Heart conditions; obesity.

Eupond-F *Sudmedica, Ger.*
Frangula bark (p.1193·2).
Constipation.

Eupragin *Alcon-Thilo, Ger.*
Erythromycin estolate (p.204·1).
Bacterial eye infections.

Eupres *Searle, Ital.*
Atenolol (p.825·3); chlorthalidone (p.839·3).
Hypertension.

Eupressyl *Byk, Fr.*
Urapidil (p.959·2) or urapidil hydrochloride (p.959·2).
Hypertension.

Euproctol *Sanopharm, Switz.*
Ointment: Resorcinol (p.1090·1); ephedrine hydrochloride (p.1059·3); lignocaine hydrochloride (p.1293·2); menthol (p.1600·2).
Suppositories: Sozoiodol zinc (p.1125·3); resorcinol (p.1090·1); zinc oxide (p.1096·2).
Anorectal disorders.

Eupronerv *Roland, Ger.†.*
Tinct. aurantii (p.1610·3); valerian (p.1643·1); melissa (p.1600·1); crataegus (p.1568·2); passion flower (p.1615·3); avena (p.1551·3); dibasic potassium phosphate (p.1159·2); sodium glycerophosphate (p.1586·2); menthyl isovalerate.
Nervousness; sedative.

Euprotin *Almirall, Spain.*
Lenograstim (p.724·3).
Reduction of neutropenia associated with cancer chemotherapy.

Euradal *Lacer, Spain.*
Bisoprolol fumarate (p.833·1).
Angina pectoris; hypertension.

Eurax
Zyma, Aust.; Novartis, Austral.; Zyma, Belg.; Novartis Consumer, Canad.; Zyma, Fr.; Zyma, Irl.; Zyma, Ital.; Novartis, Norw.; Novartis Consumer, S.Afr.; Ciba-Geigy, Swed.†; Zyma, Switz.; Zyma, UK; Westwood-Squibb, USA.
Crotamiton (p.1081·1).
Pediculosis; pruritus; scabies.

Eurax-Hydrocortisone
Zyma, Irl.; Zyma, Switz.†; Zyma, UK.
Crotamiton (p.1081·1); hydrocortisone (p.1043·3).
Skin disorders.

Euraxil
Zyma, Ger.; Padro, Spain.
Crotamiton (p.1081·1).
Pruritus.

Euraxil Hidrocort *Padro, Spain.*
Crotamiton (p.1081·1); hydrocortisone (p.1043·3).
Skin disorders.

Eureceptor *Zambon, Ital.*
Cimetidine (p.1183·2).
Gastro-intestinal disorders.

EureCor *Kade, Ger.†.*
Isosorbide dinitrate (p.893·1).
Cardiac disorders.

Eurelix *Hoechst, Fr.*
Piretanide (p.931·3).
Hypertension.

Eurex *Sanofi Winthrop, Ger.*
Prazosin hydrochloride (p.932·3).
Heart failure; hypertension.

Eurhyton *Adima, Switz.*
Crataegus (p.1568·2).
Cardiac disorders.

Eurixor
Richter, Aust.; Medisculab, Ger.
Mistletoe (p.1604·1).
Joint disorders; malignant neoplasms.

Eurobiol
Eurorga, Fr.; Interdelta, Switz.
Pancreas extract.
Digestive disorders; pancreatic insufficiency.

Eurodin *Takeda, Jpn.*
Estazolam (p.669·2).
Insomnia; premedication.

Eurogel *Cielle, Ital.*
Royal jelly (p.1626·3); dried yeast (p.1373·1); wheat germ.
Nutritional supplement.

Euroiod-Disinfettante Iodoforo Analcolico *Eurochimica, Ital.†.*
Povidone-iodine (p.1123·3).
Skin and wound disinfection.

Euronac *Europhta, Mon.*
Acetylcysteine (p.1052·3).
Eye ulceration.

Euronormol-Disinfettante Concentrato Profumato *Eurochimica, Ital.†.*
Benzalkonium chloride (p.1101·3).
Surface disinfection.

europan *Hormosan, Ger.†.*
Ketoprofen (p.48·2) or ketoprofen sodium (p.48·3).
Inflammation; musculoskeletal and joint disorders.

Eurosan *Mepha, Switz.*
Clotrimazole (p.376·3).
Fungal skin and nail infections.

Eurosan-Antisettico Battericida *Eurochimica, Ital.†.*
Chlorhexidine gluconate (p.1107·2).
Hand disinfection.

Eusaprim
Glaxo Wellcome, Aust.; Glaxo Wellcome, Belg.; Glaxo Wellcome, Fr.; Glaxo Wellcome, Ger.; Glaxo Wellcome, Ital.; Glaxo Wellcome, Neth.; Wellcome, Norw.†; Glaxo Wellcome, Swed.; Wellcome, Switz.
Co-trimoxazole (p.196·3).
Bacterial infections; Pneumocystis carinii pneumonia; toxoplasmosis.

Eusedon mono *Krewel, Ger.*
Promethazine hydrochloride (p.416·2).
Hypersensitivity reactions; nervous disorders; sleep disorders.

eusept *Sagitta, Ger.†.*
Dequalinium chloride (p.1112·1); benzocaine (p.1286·2).
Mouth and throat disorders.

Euskin *Alfarma, Spain.*
Erythromycin (p.204·1).
Acne.

Eusovit *Strathmann, Ger.*
dl-Alpha tocopheryl acetate (p.1369·2).
Vitamin E deficiency.

Euspirax *Asche, Ger.*
Choline theophyllinate (p.751·3).
Asthma; bronchitis; emphysema.

Euspirax comp *Asche, Ger.†.*
Choline theophyllinate (p.751·3); guaiphenesin (p.1061·3).
Asthma; bronchitic disorders; emphysema.

Euspirol *AFOM, Ital.†.*
Methoxyphenamine hydrochloride (p.1063·3).
Allergic rhinitis; asthma; urticaria.

Eustoporin *Wellcopharm, Ger.†.*
Polymyxin B sulphate (p.239·1); neomycin sulphate (p.229·2).
Eye disorders.

Eusulpid *CT, Ital.†.*
Sulpiride (p.692·3).
Psychiatric disorders.

Eutalgic *Pierre Fabre, Fr.*
Menthol (p.1600·2); methyl salicylate (p.55·2); camphor (p.1557·2).
Soft-tissue injury.

Euthyral *Merck-Clevenot, Fr.*
Liothyronine sodium (p.1495·1); thyroxine sodium (p.1497·1).
Hypothyroidism.

Euthyrox
Merck, Aust.; Merck-Belgolabo, Belg.; Merck, Ger.; E. Merck, Neth.
Thyroxine sodium (p.1497·1).
Goitre; hypothyroidism; thyroid cancer.

Eutiman *Bristol-Myers, Spain†.*
Hydrochlorothiazide (p.885·2); captopril (p.836·3).
Hypertension.

Eutirox *Bracco, Ital.*
Thyroxine sodium (p.1497·1).
Hypothyroidism.

Eutuxal *Synlab, Fr.†.*
Cloroqualone (p.1057·2); guaiphenesin (p.1061·3).
Coughs.

Euvaderm *Parke, Davis, Ger.*
Cream: Betamethasone benzoate (p.1033·3).
Ointment: Betamethasone benzoate (p.1033·3); salicylic acid (p.1090·2).
Skin disorders.

Euvaderm N *Parke, Davis, Ger.*
Betamethasone benzoate (p.1033·3); salicylic acid (p.1090·2).
Skin disorders.

Euvalon *Hotz, Ger.*
Crataegus (p.1568·2); valerian (p.1643·1).
Cardiac disorders.

Euvanol *Monot, Fr.*
Geranium oil (p.1584·1); niaouli oil (p.1607·1); camphor (p.1557·2); benzalkonium bromide (p.1102·1).
Rhinopharyngeal infections.

Euvegal forte *Spitzner, Ger.*
Valerian (p.1643·1); melissa (p.1600·1).
Insomnia; nervous disorders.

Euvegal N *Spitzner, Ger.*
Oral drops: Valerian (p.1643·1); melissa (p.1600·1); passion flower (p.1615·3).
Neurosedative.
Oral liquid†; tablets†: Valerian (p.1643·1); lupulus (p.1597·2).
Nervous disorders.

Euvitan *Baer, Ger.*
Caffeine and sodium benzoate; rutin sodium sulphate (p.1580·2); tinct. amara; angelica; erica; juglandis; valerian (p.1643·1).
Dystonias; reduced appetite.

Euviterin *Sudmedica, Ger.*
Caffeine (p.749·3); nucleoside-nucleotide; melissa (p.1600·1); lavender flower (p.1594·3).
Hypotension.

Euvitil *Eumedis, Fr.†.*
Dihydroxyacetone (p.1081·2).
Vitiligo.

Euvitol *Bracco, Ital.*
Vitamin A palmitate (p.1359·2).
Skin disorders.

Euzymina I Bambini *Menarini, Ital.†.*
Pepsin (p.1616·3); nicotinic acid (p.1351·2); lactic acid (p.1593·3).
Gastro-intestinal disorders.

Euzymina II Adulti *Menarini, Ital.†.*
Pepsin (p.1616·3); nicotinic acid (p.1351·2).
Gastro-intestinal disorders.

Euzymina Lisina *Menarini, Spain.*
Lysine hydrochloride (p.1350·1); nicotinic acid (p.1351·2); pepsin (p.1616·3).
Formerly contained calcium chloride, hydrochloric acid, nicotinic acid, pepsin, lysine orotate, and sodium glycerophosphate.
Dyspepsia; gastric hyposecretion; hypochlorhydria.

Evacode *Norton, UK.*
Codeine phosphate (p.26·1).

Evac-Q-Kit *Adria, USA.*
Combination pack: Evac-Q-Mag; Evac-Q-Tabs, 2 tablets; Evac-Q-Sert, 2 suppositories.
Colon preparation prior to radiology.

Evac-Q-Kwik
Pharmacia Upjohn, Canad.; Adria, USA.
Combination preparation: Solution, magnesium citrate (p.1198·2); tablets, phenolphthalein (p.1208·2); suppository, bisacodyl (p.1179·3).
Bowel evacuation.

Evac-Q-Kwik Suppository *Adria, USA.*
Bisacodyl (p.1179·3).

Evac-Q-Mag *Adria, USA.*
Magnesium Citrate Oral Solution (USP) (p.1198·2).

Evac-Q-Sert *Adria, USA.*
Potassium acid tartrate (p.1209·1); sodium bicarbonate (p.1153·2).

Evac-Q-Tabs *Adria, USA.*
Phenolphthalein (p.1208·2).

Evacuante *Bohm, Spain.*
Macrogol (p.1597·3); electrolytes (p.1147·1).
Bowel evacuation.

Evac-U-Gen *Walker Pharmacal, USA.*
Yellow phenolphthalein (p.1208·2).
Constipation.

Evac-U-Lax *Hauck, USA.*
Phenolphthalein (p.1208·2).
Constipation.

Evacuol *Almirall, Spain.*
Sodium picosulphate (p.1213·2).
Constipation.

Evadene *Wyeth, Ital.*
Butriptyline hydrochloride (p.280·3).
Depression.

Evadermin *Gambar, Ital.*
Povidone-iodine (p.1123·3).
Genital hygiene.

Evadyne
Ayerst, Belg.†; John Wyeth, Irl.†; Wyeth, UK†.
Butriptyline hydrochloride (p.280·3).
Depression.

Evagrip *Evans, Spain.*
An influenza vaccine (p.1515·2).
Active immunisation.

Evalgan
Pharmacia Upjohn, Aust.; Pharmacia Upjohn, Ger.†.
Dimethicones (p.1384·2); zinc oxide (p.1096·2).
Skin disorders.

Evalose *Copley, USA.*
Lactulose (p.1195·3).

Evanor-D *Wyeth, Ital.*
Levonorgestrel (p.1454·1); ethinyloestradiol (p.1445·1).
Combined oral contraceptive.

Evans Blue Dye *New World Trading Corporation, USA.*
Aid for plasma volume measurement.

Evaphol *Norton, UK.*
Pholcodine (p.1068·1).

Evaplan *Boehringer Mannheim, Austral.*
Fertility test (p.1621·2).

Evasen Crema *Evapharm, Ital.*
Vitamin E (p.1369·1).
Cracked nipples.

Evasen Dischetti *Evapharm, Ital.*
Potassium sorbate (p.1125·2); glycerol (p.1585·2).
Cracked nipples.

Evasidol *Wyeth Lederle, Aust.*
Butriptyline hydrochloride (p.280·3).
Anxiety; depression.

Evasprin *Cantabria, Spain†.*
Ibuprofen (p.44·1).
Fever; pain.

Evatest One Step *Boehringer Mannheim, Austral.*
Pregnancy test (p.1621·2).

Evazol
Petrasch, Aust.; Ravensberg, Ger.
Dequalinium chloride (p.1112·1).
Skin infections.

EVC *Sisu, Canad.*
Vitamin and mineral preparation.

Eve *Grunenthal, Ger.*
Ethinyloestradiol (p.1445·1); norethisterone (p.1453·1).
Combined oral contraceptive.

Evening Gold *Larkhall Laboratories, UK.*
Evening primrose oil (p.1582·1).

Event Test Strip HCG *Boehringer Mannheim, S.Afr.*
Pregnancy test (p.1621·2).

Eventin
Note. This name is used for preparations of different composition.
Schering, Austral.†.
Propylhexedrine hydrochloride (p.1485·2).
Obesity.

Knoll, Ger.†.
Levopropylhexedrine hydrochloride (p.1485·2).
Obesity.

Everon *Weleda, Aust.*
Pepsin (p.1616·3); lemon juice; menthol (p.1600·2).
Colds.

Everone *Hyrex, USA.*
Testosterone enanthate (p.1464·1).
Breast cancer; delayed puberty (males); male hypogonadism.

Eversun *Pantene, Austral.†.*
SPF 4; SPF 8; SPF 12: Padimate O (p.1488·1).
Sunscreen.

Eversun Blockout *Pantene, Austral.†.*
SPF 15+: Padimate O (p.1488·1); 2-phenyl-1*H*-benzimidazole-5-sulphonic acid (p.1488·2); avobenzone (p.1486·3).
Sunscreen.

Eversun Facesaver Cream *Pantene, Austral.†.*
SPF 15+: Padimate O (p.1488·1); 2-phenyl-1*H*-benzimidazole-5-sulphonic acid (p.1488·2); avobenzone (p.1486·3).
Sunscreen.

Eversun Fair Skin Cream *Pantene, Austral.†.*
SPF 12: Padimate O (p.1488·1); 3-(4-methylbenzylidene)bornan-2-one (p.1487·2).
Sunscreen.

Eversun Sunstick *Pantene, Austral.†.*
Padimate O (p.1488·1).
Sunscreen.

E-Vicotrat *Heyl, Ger.*
Alpha tocopheryl acetate (p.1369·1).
Vitamin E deficiency.

E-Vicotrat + Magnesium *Heyl, Ger.*
dl-Alpha tocopheryl acetate (p.1369·2); magnesium oxide (p.1198·3).
Vitamin E and magnesium deficiency.

Evident *FIRMA, Ital.†.*
Cogalactoisomerase sodium (p.1566·2).
Liver disorders.

Eviletten N *Evers, Ger.*
Modified keratin.
Haemorrhoids; varicose veins.

E-vimin *Astra, Swed.*
Alpha-tocopheryl acetate (p.1369·1).
Vitamin E deficiency.

Evina *Nattermann, Ger.†.*
d-Alpha tocopherol with ascorbic acid.
Vitamin E and C deficiency.

Evion
Merck, Ger.; Bracco, Ital.
dl-Alpha tocopheryl acetate (p.1369·2).
Haemolytic anaemia; intermittent claudication; retrolenticular fibroplasia; vitamin E deficiency.

Eviprim *Key, Austral.†.*
Evening primrose oil (p.1582·1).
Dietary supplement.

Eviprostat *Interdelta, Switz.*
Wheat-germ oil; chimaphila umbellata; populus tremula (p.1620·1); pulsatilla (p.1623·3); equisetum (p.1575·1).
Prostatic disorders.

Eviprostat N *Evers, Ger.*
Chimaphila umbellata; populus tremula (p.1620·1); pulsatilla (p.1623·3); equisetum (p.1575·1).
Prostatic hyperplasia.

Eviprostat-S *Evers, Ger.*
Saw palmetto (p.1462·1).
Micturition disorders associated with benign prostatic hyperplasia.

Evista
Note. A similar name is used for preparations of different composition.
Lilly, UK; Lilly, USA.
Raloxifene hydrochloride (p.1461·3).
Osteoporosis.

E-Vista
Note. A similar name is used for preparations of different composition.
Seatrace, USA†.
Hydroxyzine hydrochloride (p.412·1).
Anxiety; hypersensitivity reactions.

Evit
Europharm, Aust.; Chefaro, Ger.; IBP, Ital.†.
Alpha tocopheryl acetate (p.1369·1).
Vitamin E deficiency.

Evitex *Alcon, Ital.*
Vitamin A (p.1358·1); tocopheryl nicotinate (p.1280·1).
Vitamin A and E deficiency.

Evitex A E Fuerte *Alcon, Spain.*
Vitamin A palmitate (p.1359·2); tocopheryl nicotinate (p.1280·1).
Deficiency of vitamins A and E; eye disorders; habitual abortion; infertility; skin disorders.

Evitina *CT, Ital.*
dl-Alpha tocopheryl acetate (p.1369·2).

Evitocor *Apogepha, Ger.*
Atenolol (p.825·3).
Angina pectoris; arrhythmias; cardiovascular disorders; hypertension.

Evitocor plus *Apogepha, Ger.*
Atenolol (p.825·3); chlorthalidone (p.839·3).
Hypertension.

Evitol *Lannacher, Aust.*
Vitamin E (p.1369·1).
Vitamin E deficiency.

E-Vitum *Lipha, Ital.*
d-Alpha tocopheryl acetate (p.1369·2).
Haemolytic anaemia; intermittent claudication; vitamin E deficiency.

Evopad *Janssen-Cilag, Spain.*
Oestradiol (p.1455·1).
Menopausal disorders; osteoporosis.

Evoprim *Bioceuticals, UK.*
Evening primrose oil (p.1582·1).

Evorel
Janssen-Cilag, Ger.; Janssen-Cilag, Irl.; Janssen-Cilag, Norw.; Janssen-Cilag, S.Afr.; Janssen-Cilag, Swed.; Janssen-Cilag, UK.
Oestradiol (p.1455·1).
Menopausal disorders; oestrogen deficiency; osteoporosis.

Evorel Conti *Janssen-Cilag, UK.*
Oestradiol (p.1455·1); norethisterone acetate (p.1453·1).
Menopausal disorders.

Evorel Sequi *Janssen-Cilag, UK.*
4 Patches, oestradiol (Evorel) (p.1455·1); 4 patches, oestradiol; norethisterone acetate (Evorel Conti) (p.1453·1).
Menopausal disorders.

Evorel.Pak *Ortho-Cilag, UK.*
Transdermal patches, oestradiol (p.1455·1); tablets, norethisterone (p.1453·1).
Menopausal disorders.

Exacor *Monsanto, Fr.*
Cibenzoline succinate (p.840·2).
Arrhythmias.

Exact *Premier, USA.*
Benzoyl peroxide (p.1079·2).
Acne.

Exactech *Medisense, UK.*
Test for glucose in blood (p.1585·1).

Exacyl
Bournonville, Belg.; Sanofi Winthrop, Fr.
Tranexamic acid (p.728·2).
Haemorrhagic disorders.

Ex'ail
Solvay, Belg.
Garlic (p.1583·1); rutin (p.1580·2); copper chlorophyll (p.1000·1).
Peripheral vascular disorders.

Phygiene, Fr.
Garlic (p.1583·1); rutin (p.1580·2); copper chlorophyll (p.1000·1).
Circulatory disorders.

Exangina N *Muller Goppingen, Ger.*
Homoeopathic preparation.

Exapenil Mucolitico *Hosbon, Spain†.*
Ampicillin sodium (p.153·1); ampicillin benzathine (p.154·1); citiolone (p.1564·3); niaouli oil (p.1607·1); guaiphenesin (p.1061·3); cineole (p.1564·1). Lignocaine hydrochloride (p.1293·2) is included in this preparation to alleviate the pain of injection.
Respiratory-tract infections.

Excedrin
Note. This name is used for preparations of different composition.
Bristol-Myers Squibb, Canad.
Paracetamol (p.72·2); caffeine (p.749·3).
Fever; pain.

Bristol-Myers Squibb, USA.
Paracetamol (p.72·2); aspirin (p.16·1); caffeine (p.749·3).
Pain.

Excedrin IB *Bristol-Myers Products, USA†.*
Ibuprofen (p.44·1).
Fever; osteoarthritis; pain; rheumatoid arthritis.

Excedrin PM *Bristol-Myers Squibb, USA.*
Paracetamol (p.72·2); diphenhydramine citrate (p.409·1) or diphenhydramine hydrochloride (p.409·1).
Pain and fever associated with sleeplessness.

Excegran *Dainippon, Jpn.*
Zonisamide (p.366·1).
Epilepsy.

Excillin *Propan, S.Afr.*
Ampicillin trihydrate (p.153·2).
Bacterial infections.

Excipial
Mayrhofer, Aust.; Spirig, Switz.
Emollient.
Skin disorders.

Excipial U
Mayrhofer, Aust.; Spirig, Switz.
Urea (p.1095·2).
Skin disorders.

Excita *Schmid, USA.*
Nonoxinol 9 (p.1326·1).
Contraceptive.

Excitans (Rowo-216) *Pharmakon, Ger.†.*
Homoeopathic preparation.

Excithol (Rowo-215) *Pharmakon, Ger.†.*
Homoeopathic preparation.

Exdol *Frosst, Canad.*
Paracetamol (p.72·2); caffeine citrate (p.749·3); codeine phosphate (p.26·1).
Fever; pain.

Executive B *Cenovis, Austral.; Vitelle, Austral.*
Vitamins and minerals; scutellaria; valerian (p.1643·1); passion flower (p.1615·3).
Stress; vitamin and mineral deficiencies.

Exelderm
Zeneca, Irl.; Schwarz, Ital.; Bioglan, UK; Westwood-Squibb, USA.
Sulconazole nitrate (p.387·2).
Fungal skin infections.

Exelon *Novartis, UK.*
Rivastigmine hydrogen tartrate (p.1398·3).
Alzheimers disease.

Exepin Cortex *SmithKline Beecham, Ital.†.*
Cyanocobalamin (p.1363·3); suprarenal cortex (p.1050·1); calcium folinate (p.1342·2); glycine (p.1345·2); lignocaine hydrochloride (p.1293·2).
Anaemias; asthenia; liver disorders.

Exgest LA *Carnrick, USA.*
Phenylpropanolamine hydrochloride (p.1067·2); guaiphenesin (p.1061·3).
Coughs.

Exhirud
Kwizda, Aust.; Sanofi Winthrop, Ger.
Leech extract (p.897·2).
Frostbite; haematoma; inflammation; insect bites; scar pain; superficial phlebitis; superficial thrombosis.

Ex-Histine *WE, USA.*
Phenylephrine (p.1066·2); chlorpheniramine (p.405·2); hyoscine (p.462·3).
Upper respiratory-tract disorders.

Exidine *Baxter, USA.*
Chlorhexidine gluconate (p.1107·2).
Skin disinfection.

Exidol *Sopar, Belg.†.*
Ibuprofen (p.44·1).
Fever; pain.

Exil *Esoform, Ital.*
Cetylpyridinium chloride (p.1106·2).
Genital hygiene.

Exirel
Byk, Aust.; 3M, UK†.
Pirbuterol acetate (p.757·2) or pirbuterol hydrochloride (p.757·2).
Obstructive airways disease.

Exit *Bracco, Ital.†.*
Salicylamide (p.82·3); propyphenazone (p.81·3); caffeine (p.749·3); brompheniramine maleate (p.403·2).
Cold symptoms; fever; pain.

Exitop
Asta Medica, Aust.; Asta Medica, Swed.; Pharmacia Upjohn, Switz.†.
Etoposide (p.532·3).
Malignant neoplasms.

Ex-Lax
Sandoz, Canad.; Intercare, UK; Novartis, USA.
Yellow phenolphthalein (p.1208·2).
Constipation.

Ex-Lax Extra Gentle Pills *Novartis, USA.*
Docusate sodium (p.1189·3); phenolphthalein (p.1208·2).
Constipation.

Ex-Lax Gentle Nature *Novartis, USA.*
Calcium sennoside A (p.1212·3); calcium sennoside B (p.1212·3).
Constipation.

Ex-Lax Light *Sandoz, Canad.*
Yellow phenolphthalein (p.1208·2); docusate sodium (p.1189·3).

Ex-Lax Maximum Relief *Novartis, USA.*
Yellow phenolphthalein (p.1208·2).

Exlutena *Organon, Swed.*
Lynoestrenol (p.1448·2).
Progestogen-only oral contraceptive.

Exluton
Organon, Belg.; Organon, Fr.; Organon, Neth.; Donmed, S.Afr.†.
Lynoestrenol (p.1448·2).
Progestogen-only oral contraceptive.

Exlutona
Organon, Ger.; Organon, Norw.; Organon, Switz.
Lynoestrenol (p.1448·2).
Progestogen-only oral contraceptive.

Exmykehl *Sanum-Kehlbeck, Ger.*
Homoeopathic preparation.

Exna *Robins, USA.*
Benzthiazide (p.828·1).
Hypertension; oedema.

Exneural *BASF, Ger.*
Ibuprofen (p.44·1).
Fever; inflammation; musculoskeletal and joint disorders; pain.

Exocaine *Del, USA; Commerce, USA.*
Methyl salicylate (p.55·2).
Muscle and joint pain.

Exocaine Odor Free *Commerce, USA†.*
Triethanolamine salicylate (p.1639·2).
Muscle, joint, and soft-tissue pain; neuralgia.

Exocin
Allergan, Irl.; Allergan, Ital.; Allergan, S.Afr.; Allergan, UK.
Ofloxacin (p.233·3).
Bacterial eye infections.

Exocine *Allergan, Fr.*
Ofloxacin (p.233·3).
Bacterial eye infections.

Exoderil
Sanabo, Aust.; Rentschler, Ger.; Sandoz, Switz.†.
Naftifine hydrochloride (p.385·3).
Fungal skin infections.

Exoderil Zinkpaste *Sanabo, Aust.*
Naftifine hydrochloride (p.385·3); zinc oxide (p.1096·2).
Fungal skin infections.

Exodor grun *Rorer, Ger.†.*
Copper-chlorophyllin complex (p.1000·1).
Catarrh; halitosis; inflammation of the mouth.

Exolan *Dermal Laboratories, UK†.*
Dithranol triacetate (p.1082·1).
Psoriasis.

Exolyt *Abigo, Swed.*
Chlorcyclizine hydrochloride (p.404·3); guaiphenesin (p.1061·3); ammonium chloride (p.1055·2).
Coughs.

Exomega *Ducray, Fr.*
Avena (p.1551·3); omega-6 fatty acids (p.1582·1).
Skin disorders.

Exomuc *Bouchara, Fr.*
Acetylcysteine (p.1052·3).
Respiratory-tract congestion.

Exorex *Vital Health, UK.*
Coal tar (p.1092·3).
Eczema; psoriasis.

Exoseptoplix *Diepha, Fr.*
Sulphanilamide (p.256·3).
Bacterial skin infections.

Exosurf
Glaxo Wellcome, Aust.; Glaxo Wellcome, Austral.; Glaxo Wellcome, Belg.; Glaxo Wellcome, Canad.; Glaxo Wellcome, Ger.; Wellcome, Irl.; Glaxo Wellcome, Ital.; Glaxo Wellcome, Neth.; Wellcome, Norw.†; Glaxo Wellcome, S.Afr.; Wellcome, Spain; Glaxo Wellcome, Swed.; Wellcome, Switz.; Wellcome, UK; Wellcome, USA†.
Colfosceril palmitate (p.1623·1).
Neonatal respiratory distress syndrome.

Expafusin
Pharmacia Upjohn, Aust.; Pharmacia Upjohn, Ger.; Pharmacia, Spain.
A hydroxyethyl ether starch (p.724·2) with electrolytes.
Plasma volume expansion.

Expahes
Laevosan, Aust.; Laevosan, Switz.
Hetastarch (p.724·1) with or without sodium chloride.
Blood-volume expansion.

Expectal Balsam *Tropon, Ger.†.*
Camphor (p.1557·2); pumilio pine oil (p.1623·3); nutmeg oil (p.1609·3) eucalyptus oil (p.1578·1); thyme oil (p.1637·1); benzyl nicotinate (p.22·1).
Respiratory-tract disorders.

Expectal N *Bayer, Ger.*
Thyme (p.1636·3).
Catarrh; coughs.

Expectal S *Tropon, Ger.†.*
Codeine (p.26·1); potassium guaiacolsulfonate (p.1068·3); thyme (p.1636·3).
Catarrh; coughs.

Expectal-Balsam *Kolassa, Aust.*
Pumilio pine oil (p.1623·3); camphor (p.1557·2); eucalyptus oil (p.1578·1); nutmeg oil (p.1609·3); thyme oil (p.1637·1); benzyl nicotinate (p.22·1).
Respiratory-tract disorders.

Expectalin *Parke-Med, S.Afr.*
Diphenhydramine hydrochloride (p.409·1); ammonium chloride (p.1055·2).
Coughs.

Expectalin with codeine *Parke-Med, S.Afr.*
Diphenhydramine hydrochloride (p.409·1); ammonium chloride (p.1055·2); codeine phosphate (p.26·1).
Coughs.

Expectal-Tropfen *Kolassa, Aust.*
Codeine (p.26·1); thyme extract (p.1636·3); orange extract; anise oil (p.1550·1).
Respiratory-tract disorders.

Expectco *Covan, S.Afr.†.*
Pseudoephedrine hydrochloride (p.1068·3); mepyramine maleate (p.414·1); ipecacuanha (p.1062·2).
Coughs.

Expectoran *Wiedenmann, Switz.†.*
Thyme (p.1636·3); primula; senega (p.1069·3); quillaia (p.1328·2); star anise oil.
Coughs and associated respiratory-tract disorders.

Expectoran avec codeine *Wiedenmann, Switz.†.*
Thyme (p.1636·3); primula; senega (p.1069·3); quillaia (p.1328·2); star anise oil; codeine phosphate (p.26·1).
Coughs and associated respiratory-tract disorders.

Expectoran Codein *Grossmann, Switz.*
Codeine phosphate (p.26·1); thyme (p.1636·3); senega (p.1069·3); quillaia (p.1328·2).
Adjuvant in bronchitis; coughs.

Expectorans Solucampher *Delalande, Ger.†.*
Ethylmorphine camsylate (p.36·1); codeine camsylate (p.27·1); ephedrine camsylate (p.1060·1); senna (p.1212·2); ipecacuanha (p.1062·2); aconite (p.1542·2); belladonna (p.457·1).
Catarrh.

Expectorant Cough Formula *Tanta, Canad.*
Guaiphenesin (p.1061·3).

Expectorant Cough Syrup
Note. This name is used for preparations of different composition.
Drug Trading, Canad.; Technilab, Canad.
Guaiphenesin (p.1061·3).

Kamfarma, Switz.†.
Diphenhydramine hydrochloride (p.409·1); ammonium chloride (p.1055·2); sodium citrate (p.1153·2); menthol (p.1600·2).
Coughs.

Expectorant Syrup *Marc-O, Canad.*
Guaiphenesin (p.1061·3).

Expectoryn *Pharma Plus, Switz.†.*
Diphenhydramine hydrochloride (p.409·1); ammonium chloride (p.1055·2); sodium citrate (p.1153·2); menthol (p.1600·2).
Coughs.

Expectoryn Paediatric *Pharma Plus, Switz.†.*
Diphenhydramine hydrochloride (p.409·1); sodium citrate (p.1153·2); menthol (p.1600·2).
Coughs.

Expectotussin "C" Propan, S.Afr.
Mepyramine maleate (p.414·1); ammonium chloride (p.1055·2); sodium citrate (p.1153·2); phenylephrine hydrochloride (p.1066·2); ascorbic acid (p.1365·2).
Coughs.

Expectysat Ysatfabrik, Ger.†.
Primula root; viola tricoloris; thyme (p.1636·3); potassium guaiacolsulfonate (p.1068·3).
Catarrh.

Expectysat-N Ysatfabrik, Ger.
Primula root; thyme (p.1636·3).
Cold symptoms.

Expelix Seton, UK†.
Piperazine citrate (p.107·2).
Intestinal nematode infections.

Exphobin N Lappe, Ger.†.
Meprobamate (p.678·1).
Menopausal disorders; muscular disorders; nervous system disorders; skin disorders.

Expigen
Note. This name is used for preparations of different composition.
Schoeller, Aust.
Polysorbate 20 (p.1327·3); ammonium chloride (p.1055·2); sodium benzoate (p.1102·3); anise oil (p.1550·1); niaouli oil (p.1607·1); thyme oil (p.1637·1); menglytate (p.1063·3).
Coughs; respiratory congestion.
Pharmacia Upjohn, Norw.; Adcock Ingram, S.Afr.
Polysorbate 20 (p.1327·3); ammonium chloride (p.1055·2).
Coughs; respiratory congestion.

Expit Yamanouchi, Ger.
Ambroxol hydrochloride (p.1054·3).
Respiratory-tract disorders associated with increased or viscous mucus.

Exponcit N Salutas, Ger.†.
Cathine hydrochloride (p.1478·1).
Obesity.

Expulin
Monmouth, Irl.; Monmouth, UK.
Pholcodine (p.1068·1); pseudoephedrine hydrochloride (p.1068·3); chlorpheniramine maleate (p.405·1); menthol (p.1600·2).
Coughs; respiratory-tract congestion.

Expulin Chesty Cough Monmouth, UK.
Guaiphenesin (p.1061·3).
Coughs.

Expulin Childrens Cough Monmouth, Irl.
Pholcodine (p.1068·1); chlorpheniramine maleate (p.405·1).
Coughs.

Expulin Dry Cough
Monmouth, Irl.; Monmouth, UK.
Pholcodine (p.1068·1).
Coughs.

Expulin Paediatric Monmouth, UK.
Pholcodine (p.1068·1); chlorpheniramine maleate (p.405·1); menthol (p.1600·2).
Coughs.

Expurhin Galen, UK†.
Ephedrine hydrochloride (p.1059·3); chlorpheniramine maleate (p.405·1); menthol (p.1600·2).
Upper respiratory-tract congestion.

Exputex Monmouth, Irl.
Carbocisteine (p.1056·3).
Respiratory-tract disorders with excessive or viscous mucus.

exrheudon OPT Optimed, Ger.
Ointment: Glycol salicylate (p.43·1); benzyl nicotinate (p.22·1).
Frostbite; inflammatory disorders; soft-tissue, nerve, and joint disorders; sports injuries.
Tablets: Phenylbutazone (p.79·2).
Acute ankylosing spondylitis; gout; rheumatism.

Exrhinin Wernigerode, Ger.
Tetrahydrozoline hydrochloride (p.1070·2).
Nasal congestion.

Exsel Allergan Herbert, USA.
Selenium sulphide (p.1091·1).
Dandruff; pityriasis versicolor; seborrhoeic dermatitis.

Extencilline Specia, Fr.
Benzathine penicillin (p.158·3).
Bacterial infections.

Extendryl Fleming, USA.
Phenylephrine hydrochloride (p.1066·2); hyoscine methonitrate (p.463·1); chlorpheniramine maleate (p.405·1).
Allergic rhinitis; respiratory congestion; urticaria and angioedema.

Exterol
Dermal Laboratories, Irl.; Dermal Laboratories, UK.
Urea hydrogen peroxide (p.1127·3).
Ear wax removal.

Extin Opfermann, Ger.
Adipic acid (p.1543·3); ammonium chloride (p.1055·2).
Urinary-tract infections.

Extovyl Marion Merrell, Fr.
Betahistine mesylate (p.1553·1).
Vertigo.

Extra Action Cough Rugby, USA.
Dextromethorphan hydrobromide (p.1057·3); guaiphenesin (p.1061·3).
Coughs.

Extra C 1000 Non Acid with Bioflavonoids Suisse, Austral.†.
Calcium ascorbate (p.1365·2); vitamin P (p.1580·1).
Vitamin-C deficiency.

Extra Strength Acetaminophen with Codeine WestCan, Canad.
Paracetamol (p.72·2); caffeine (p.749·3); codeine phosphate (p.26·1).
Fever; pain.

Extra Strength Alenic Alka Rugby, USA.
Aluminium hydroxide (p.1177·3); magnesium carbonate (p.1198·1).
Hyperacidity.

Extra Strength Alka-Seltzer Effervescent Tablets Bayer, USA.
Sodium bicarbonate (p.1153·2); citric acid (p.1564·3); aspirin (p.16·1).
Hyperacidity.

Extra Strength Bayer Plus Sterling Health, USA.
Aspirin (p.16·1).
Calcium carbonate (p.1182·1), magnesium carbonate (p.1198·1), and magnesium oxide (p.1198·3) are included in this preparation in an attempt to limit adverse effects on the gastro-intestinal mucosa.

Extra Strength Biotin Forte Vitaline, USA†.
Multivitamin preparation.

Extra Strength Datril Bristol-Myers Products, USA†.
Paracetamol (p.72·2).
Fever; pain.

Extra Strength Doans PM Ciba, USA.
Magnesium salicylate (p.51·1); diphenhydramine hydrochloride (p.409·1).

Extra Strength Dynafed EX BDI, USA.
Paracetamol (p.72·2).
Fever; pain.

Extra Strength Genaton Goldline, USA.
Aluminium hydroxide (p.1177·3); magnesium carbonate (p.1198·1).
Hyperacidity.

Extra Strength Maalox Rhone-Poulenc Rorer, USA.
Aluminium hydroxide (p.1177·3); magnesium hydroxide (p.1198·2); simethicone (p.1213·1).
Hyperacidity.

Extra Strength Mintox Plus Major, USA.
Simethicone (p.1213·1).

Extra Strength Pyrroxate Roberts, USA.
Phenylpropanolamine hydrochloride (p.1067·2); chlorpheniramine maleate (p.405·1); paracetamol (p.72·2).
Upper respiratory-tract symptoms.

Extra Strength Tri-Buffered Bufferin Bristol-Myers Products, USA†.
Aspirin (p.16·1).
Analgesic; anti-inflammatory.

Extra Strength Tylenol Headache Plus McNeil Consumer, USA.
Paracetamol (p.72·2); calcium carbonate (p.1182·1).
Gastro-intestinal pain associated with hyperacidity.

Extra Strength Tylenol PM McNeil Consumer, USA.
Diphenhydramine hydrochloride (p.409·1); paracetamol (p.72·2).
Insomnia.

Extra Strength Vicks Cough Drops Procter & Gamble, USA.
Menthol (p.1600·2).

Extracort Basotherm, Ger.
Triamcinolone acetonide (p.1050·2).
Skin disorders.

Extracort N Basotherm, Ger.
Triamcinolone acetonide (p.1050·2).
Formerly contained triamcinolone acetonide, neomycin sulphate, and gramicidin.
Skin disorders.

Extracort Rhin sine Basotherm, Ger.
Triamcinolone acetonide (p.1050·2); phenylephrine hydrochloride (p.1066·2).
Allergic nasal disorders.

Extracort Tinktur N Basotherm, Ger.
Triamcinolone acetonide (p.1050·2); salicylic acid (p.1090·2).
Skin disorders.

Extrafer SoSe, Ital.
Ferric sodium gluconate (p.1340·1).
Anaemias.

Extralin Lilly, USA†.
Liver-stomach concentrate.

Extranase
Rhone-Poulenc Rorer, Belg.†; Rottapharm, Fr.
Bromelains (p.1555·1).
Post-traumatic and postoperative oedema.

Extraneal Baxter, Swed.
Icodextrin; sodium chloride; sodium lactate; calcium chloride; magnesium chloride (p.1151·1).
Peritoneal dialysis.

Extraphytols Arkopharma, Fr.†.
A range of liquid herbal extracts.

Extraplus Pierre Fabre, Spain.
Ketoprofen (p.48·2).
Fever; gout; musculoskeletal and joint disorders; pain; peri-articular disorders.

Extravite Vitalia, UK.
Multivitamin and mineral preparation.

Extravits Lifeplan, UK.
Multivitamin and mineral preparation.

Extropin Bastian, Ger.†.
α-Terpineol (p.1635·1); eucalyptus oil (p.1578·1); borneol; anisaldehyde; turpentine oil (p.1641·1); siberian fir oil; camphor (p.1557·2).
Bath additive; nervous disorders.

Extur Normon, Spain.
Indapamide (p.890·2).
Hypertension; oedema.

Exuracid Rosch & Handel, Aust.
Tisopurine (p.396·3).
Gout; hyperuricaemia; urinary calculi.

Exzem Oil Pharmadass, UK.
Vitamin E oil (p.1369·1); evening primrose oil (p.1582·1); castor oil (p.1560·2); olive oil (p.1610·1); safflower oil (p.1353·3); grapeseed oil; chamomile oil.

Eye Drops Rivex, Canad.; Zee, Canad.
Tetrahydrozoline hydrochloride (p.1070·2).

Eye Drops Extra Ocusoft, USA.
Phenylephrine hydrochloride (p.1066·2).

Eye Eze Pharmavite, Canad.
Boric acid (p.1554·2); borax (p.1554·2).

Eye Formula Euphr Homeocan, Canad.
Homoeopathic preparation.

Eye Health Herbal Plus Formula 4 Vitelle, Austral.
Euphrasia; ginkgo biloba (p.1584·1); betacarotene (p.1335·2); *d*-alpha tocopheryl acid succinate (p.1369·2); ascorbic acid (p.1365·2); rutin (p.1580·2); hesperidin (p.1580·2).
Eye strain.

Eyebel Pharmacal, Switz.†.
Muramidase hydrochloride (p.1604·3).
Conjunctivitis; keratoconjunctivitis.

Eyelube Sabex, Canad.
Hypromellose (p.1473·1).
Dry eyes.

Eye-Lube-A Optopics, USA.
Glycerol (p.1585·2).
Dry eyes.

Eye-Sed Scherer, USA.
Zinc sulphate (p.1373·2).
Minor eye irritation.

Eyesine Akorn, USA.
Tetrahydrozoline hydrochloride (p.1070·2).
Minor eye irritation.

Eyestil Ophtapharma, Canad.
Sodium hyaluronate (p.1630·3).
Dry eyes.

Eye-Stream
Alcon, Austral.; Alcon, Canad.; Alcon, Spain; Alcon, USA.
Electrolyte preparation (p.1147·1).
Eye irrigation.

Eye-vit Pharmadass, UK.
Multivitamin, mineral, and trace element preparation.

Eyevite Allergan, Austral.
Vitamin and mineral preparation.
Eye disorders.

Eyewash Rivex, Canad.
Electrolyte solution (p.1147·1).
Eye irrigation.

EZ Detect Biomerica, USA.
Test for occult blood in faeces or urine.

EZ Paque-HD Codali, Belg.†.
Barium sulphate (p.1003·1).
Contrast medium for gastro-intestinal radiography.

E-Z-Cat
Therapex, Canad.; E-Z-EM, UK.
Barium sulphate (p.1003·1).
Contrast medium for computerised axial tomography of the gastro-intestinal tract.

E-Z-Gas II
Note. This name is used for preparations of different composition.
Therapex, Canad.
Sodium bicarbonate (p.1153·2); tartaric acid (p.1634·3); simethicone (p.1213·1).
Production of CO_2 in double contrast radiography of the gastro-intestinal tract.
Bracco, Switz.
Sodium bicarbonate (p.1153·2); citric acid (p.1564·3); simethicone (p.1213·1).
Production of CO_2 in double contrast radiography of the gastro-intestinal tract.

E-Z-HD
Therapex, Canad.†; E-Z-EM, Neth.†; E-Z-EM, UK.
Barium sulphate (p.1003·1).
Contrast medium for gastro-intestinal radiography.

E-Z-Jug Therapex, Canad.†.
Barium sulphate (p.1003·1).
Contrast medium for gastro-intestinal radiography.

E-Z-Paque
Therapex, Canad.†; E-Z-EM, UK.
Barium sulphate (p.1003·1).
Contrast medium for gastro-intestinal radiography.

I + I-F Dunhall, USA.
Hydrocortisone (p.1043·3); clioquinol (p.193·2); pramoxine (p.1298·2).
Skin disorders.

F080 Clintec, Ital.
Amino-acid infusion for parenteral nutrition.
Liver disorders.

F 99 Sulgan N Divapharma, Ger.
Hamamelis (p.1587·1).
Formerly contained aluminium chlorohydrex, benzocaine, camphor, dichlorobenzyl alcohol, ethyl linoleate, hamamelis, triclosan, menthol, and zinc oxide.
Anorectal disorders.

FAB Medical Research, Austral.
Iron and vitamin B substances.

FAB Co Medical Research, Austral.
Iron, vitamin B substances, and vitamin C.

FAB Tri-Cal Medical Research, Austral.
Calcium hydrogen phosphate (p.1155·3); calcium carbonate (p.1182·1); calcium gluconate (p.1155·2); zinc oxide (p.1096·2); magnesium oxide (p.1198·3); cholecalciferol (p.1366·3).
Nutritional supplement.

Fabahistin
Bayer, Austral.†; Bayer, Irl.†; Bayer, S.Afr.†; Bayer, UK†.
Mebhydrolin (p.413·2) or mebhydrolin napadisylate (p.413·2).
Hypersensitivity reactions.

Fabasma Propan, S.Afr.
Amylobarbitone (p.641·3); ephedrine hydrochloride (p.1059·3); aminophylline (p.748·1).
Asthma.

Fabrol
Zyma, Irl.†; Ciba-Geigy, Swed.†; Zyma, UK†.
Acetylcysteine (p.1052·3).
Bronchitis; cystic fibrosis; mucus hypersecretion.

Fabroven Pierre Fabre, Spain.
Capsules: Ascorbic acid (p.1365·2); hesperidin methyl chalcone (p.1580·2); ruscus aculeatus.
Cream: Dextran sulphate (p.1571·1); melilotus; ruscus aculeatus.
Peripheral vascular disorders.

Fabubac Brunel, S.Afr.
Co-trimoxazole (p.196·3).
Bacterial infections.

Face Foundation Avon, Canad.
SPF 15: Ethylhexyl *p*-methoxycinnamate (p.1487·1); titanium dioxide (p.1093·3).
Sunscreen.

Faces Only
Schering-Plough, Canad.†; Schering-Plough, USA.
Ethylhexyl *p*-methoxycinnamate (p.1487·1); oxybenzone (p.1487·3).
Sunscreen.

Facilit Fides, Spain.
Allopurinol (p.390·2); benzbromarone (p.392·3).
Gout; hyperuricaemia.

Facocinerin Difa, Ital.†.
Juglans cineraria; heparin sodium (p.879·3); hamamelis (p.1587·1).
Postoperative treatment of cataract.

Facogen NBF-Lanes, Ital.
Lipid, protein, carbohydrate, multivitamin, and trace-element preparation.
Nutritional supplement.

Facovit Teofarma, Ital.
Testosterone propionate (p.1464·2); rubidium iodide (p.1626·3); potassium iodide (p.1493·1); riboflavine (p.1362·1).
Cataract.

Fact Plus
Johnson & Johnson, Canad.; Johnson & Johnson, UK†; Advanced Care, USA.
Pregnancy test (p.1621·2).

Factor AF2 Biosyn, Ger.
Liver and spleen extract.
Supportive tumour therapy.

Factrel
Wyeth-Ayerst, Canad.; Wyeth-Ayerst, USA.
Gonadorelin hydrochloride (p.1248·1).
Diagnostic evaluation of anterior pituitary function.

Faderma Fader, Spain†.
Alum (p.1547·1); citric acid; sulphanilamide (p.256·3); tannic acid (p.1634·2); zinc chloride (p.1373·1).
Skin disorders.

Fadiamone CS, Fr.
Oestrone (p.1458·2); oestradiol (p.1455·1); testosterone propionate (p.1464·2); pregnenolone acetate; allantoin (p.1078·2).
Skin ageing.

Fado Caber, Ital.†.
Cephamandole nafate (p.180·1).
Bacterial infections.

Faexojodan Kanoldt, Ger.
Saccharomyces cerevisiae (non-fermentable) (p.1373·1).
Skin disorders.

Fagastril Quimifar, Spain.
Famotidine (p.1192·1).
Gastro-oesophageal reflux; peptic ulcer; Zollinger-Ellison syndrome.

Fagolitos Renal Falofi, Spain†.
Aloe (p.1177·1); arctostaphilus uva-ursi (p.1552·2); buchu (p.1555·2); glycerol (p.1585·2); maize; saw palmetto (p.1462·1).
Renal disorders.

Fagorutin Buchweizen Fink, Ger.
Tablets: Fagopyrum esculentum; troxerutin (p.1580·2).
Tea: Fagopyrum esculentum.
Capillary disorders; peripheral vascular disorders.

Fagorutin Ruscus Fink, Ger.
Ruscus aculeatus.
Chronic venous insufficiency; haemorrhoids.

Fagusan N Spreewald, Ger.
Guaiphenesin (p.1061·3).
Bronchitis.

Faktu
Tosse, Ger.; Byk, Switz.
Policresulen; cinchocaine hydrochloride (p.1289·2).
Anorectal disorders.

Falagan *Nattermann, Spain†.*
Fenproporex (p.1481·3).
Obesity.

Falcol *Bayer, Spain.*
Aceclofenac (p.12·1).
Musculoskeletal, joint, and peri-articular disorders; pain.

Falibaryt *Goldham, Ger.*
Barium sulphate (p.1003·1).
Radiographic contrast medium.

Falicard *Dresden, Ger.*
Verapamil hydrochloride (p.960·3).
Arrhythmias; hypertension; ischaemic heart disease.

Falimint *Berlin-Chemie, Ger.†.*
Acetylaminopropoxybenzene.
Mouth and throat disorders.

Falithrom *Hexal, Ger.*
Phenprocoumon (p.929·3).
Thrombo-embolism prophylaxis.

Falitonsin *Dresden, Ger.*
Atenolol (p.825·3).
Arrhythmias; hypertension; ischaemic heart disease.

Falizal *Ciba-Geigy, Spain†.*
Sulphinpyrazone (p.395·2).
Gout; hyperuricaemia; thrombo-embolic disorders.

Falkamin
Falk, Ger.; Knoll, Ital.
Leucine (p.1350·1); valine (p.1358·1); isoleucine (p.1349·2).
Liver disorders.

Falqui *Unipharma, Switz.*
Phenolphthalein (p.1208·2); liquid paraffin (p.1382·1); agar (p.1470·3); prune (p.1209·2).
Constipation.

Falquigut *Falqui, Ital.*
Sodium picosulphate (p.1213·2).
Constipation.

Falquilax *Falqui, Ital.*
Senna (p.1212·2).
Constipation.

Faltium *Prodes, Spain.*
Veralipride (p.698·1).
Menopausal disorders.

Falvin *Farmades, Ital.*
Fenticonazole nitrate (p.377·3).
Dermatological and gynaecological fungal infections.

Famcod *Salters, S.Afr.*
Paracetamol (p.72·2); codeine phosphate (p.26·1).
Pain.

Famel
Note. This name is used for preparations of different composition.
Boots, Ital.
Lactocreosote (p.1057·3); calcium lactophosphate; ephedrine hydrochloride (p.1059·3).
Bronchial catarrh.
Boots Healthcare, Neth.
Creosote (p.1057·3); ephedrine hydrochloride (p.1059·3).
Coughs.
Cassella-med, Switz.
Lactocreosote (p.1057·3); calcium lactophosphate; codeine (p.26·1); drosera (p.1574·1); grindelia.
Bronchitis; coughs; sore throat.

Famel Broomhexine *Boots Healthcare, Neth.*
Bromhexine hydrochloride (p.1055·3).
Coughs.

Famel Catarrh & Throat Pastilles *Seton, UK.*
Creosote (p.1057·3); cinnamon-leaf oil; lemon oil (p.1595·3); menthol (p.1600·2).
Coughs; sore throat.

Famel cum Codein *Brady, Aust.*
Lactocreosote (p.1057·3); calcium lactophosphate; codeine hydrochloride (p.26·1).
Asthma; bronchitis; catarrh; cold symptoms.

Famel cum Ephedrin *Brady, Aust.*
Lactocreosote (p.1057·3); calcium lactophosphate; ephedrine hydrochloride (p.1059·3).
Asthma; bronchitis; catarrh; cold symptoms.

Famel Expectorant *Seton, UK.*
Guaiphenesin (p.1061·3).
Coughs.

Famel Honey & Lemon Cough Pastilles *Seton, UK†.*
Guaiphenesin (p.1061·3).
Coughs; sore throat.

Famel Linctus *Seton, UK†.*
Pholcodine (p.1068·1).
Coughs.

Famel Original *Seton, UK.*
Creosote (p.1057·3); codeine phosphate (p.26·1).
Coughs.

Famethacin *Be-Tabs, S.Afr.*
Indomethacin (p.45·2).
Gout; musculoskeletal and joint disorders.

Family *Schein, USA†.*
Multivitamin preparation.

Family Medicated First Aid Treatment *Tender, Canad.*
Benzalkonium chloride (p.1101·3); lignocaine hydrochloride (p.1293·2).

Family Medicated Sunburn Relief *Tender, Canad.*
Lignocaine (p.1293·2).

Fam-Lax *Torbet Laboratories, UK.*
Yellow phenolphthalein (p.1208·2); rhubarb (p.1212·1).
Constipation.

Famodil *Sigma-Tau, Ital.*
Famotidine (p.1192·1).
Gastro-intestinal disorders.

Famotal *Alpharma, Norw.*
Famotidine (p.1192·1).
Gastro-oesophageal reflux; peptic ulcer; Zollinger-Ellison syndrome.

Famstim *Genpharm, S.Afr.*
Ammonium bicarbonate (p.1055·1); aromatic ammonium spirit (p.1548·3); spirit of ether (p.1378·2).
Coughs.

Famtuss *Genpharm, S.Afr.*
Diphenhydramine hydrochloride (p.409·1); ammonium chloride (p.1055·2); sodium citrate (p.1153·2).
Coughs.

Famucaps *Brunel, S.Afr.*
Phenylephrine hydrochloride (p.1066·2); chlorpheniramine maleate (p.405·1); ascorbic acid (p.1365·2); caffeine (p.749·3); paracetamol (p.72·2); atropine sulphate (p.455·1).
Upper respiratory-tract disorders.

Famulcer *Inkeysa, Spain.*
Famotidine (p.1192·1).
Gastro-oesophageal reflux; peptic ulcer; Zollinger-Ellison syndrome.

Famvir
Note. This name is used for preparations of different composition.
SmithKline Beecham, Aust.; SmithKline Beecham, Austral.; Beecham, Belg.; SmithKline Beecham, Canad.; SmithKline Beecham, Ger.; SmithKline Beecham, Irl.; SmithKline Beecham, Neth.; SmithKline Beecham, S.Afr.; SmithKline Beecham, Spain; SmithKline Beecham, Swed.; SmithKline Beecham, Switz.; SmithKline Beecham, UK; SmithKline Beecham, USA.
Famciclovir (p.609·3).
Herpesvirus infections.
SmithKline Beecham, Neth.
Cream: Penciclovir (p.624·1).
Herpes labialis.

Fanalgic *Mitchell, UK.*
Paracetamol (p.72·2).
Fever; pain.

Fanalgin *Weifa, Norw.*
Phenazone (p.78·2); caffeine (p.749·3).
Fever; pain.

Fanasil *Roche, Ital.*
Sulfadoxine (p.251·1).
Bacterial infections.

Fanaxal *Esteve, Spain.*
Alfentanil hydrochloride (p.12·3).
General anaesthesia.

Fangopress *Geistlich, Switz.*
Compress.
Musculoskeletal and joint disorders.

Fango-Rubriment *Knoll, Ger.*
Medicinal mud; sulphur (p.1091·2).
Musculoskeletal and joint disorders.

Fangotherm
Eifelfango, Ger.; Eifelfango, Switz.
Medicinal mud.
Gastro-intestinal, liver, and kidney disorders; gout; musculoskeletal and joint disorders; neuralgia.

Fangyol-Med-Bad *Eifelfango, Ger.†.*
Humic acid; sodium salicylate (p.85·1).
Bath additive; musculoskeletal and joint disorders; nervous disorders; peripheral circulatory disorders.

Fanhdi *Grifols, Spain.*
Factor VIII (p.720·3).
Factor VIII deficiency.

Fanosin *Abello, Spain.*
Famotidine (p.1192·1).
Gastro-oesophageal reflux; peptic ulcer; Zollinger-Ellison syndrome.

Fanox *Lesvi, Spain.*
Famotidine (p.1192·1).
Gastro-oesophageal reflux; peptic ulcer; Zollinger-Ellison syndrome.

Fansidar
Roche, Aust.; Roche, Austral.; Roche, Belg.; Roche, Canad.; Roche, Fr.; Roche, Ger.†; Roche, Irl.; Roche, Neth.†; Roche, Norw.†; Roche, S.Afr.; Roche, Swed.; Roche, Switz.; Roche, UK; Roche, USA.
Sulfadoxine (p.251·1); pyrimethamine (p.436·3).
Malaria; Pneumocystis carinii pneumonia; toxoplasmosis.

Fansidol *NCSN, Ital.*
Nimesulide (p.63·2).
Fever; inflammation; pain.

Fansimef *Roche, Switz.*
Mefloquine hydrochloride (p.432·2); sulfadoxine (p.251·1); pyrimethamine (p.436·3).
Malaria.

Fantomalt *Nutricia, Ital.*
Maltodextrin (p.1350·2).
Preparation for enteral nutrition.

Fapack *Hartmann, Ger.†.*
Medicinal mud.
Musculoskeletal and joint disorders; wounds.

Farbee with Vitamin C *Major, USA.*
Vitamin B substances with vitamin C.

Farco-Oxicyanid-Tupfer *Farco, Ger.*
Mercuric oxycyanide (p.1602·2).
Disinfection of skin and mucous membranes.

Farco-Uromycin *Farco, Ger.*
Neomycin sulphate (p.229·2); lignocaine hydrochloride (p.1293·2).
Urinary-tract infections.

Farecef *Lafare, Ital.*
Cefoperazone sodium (p.167·3).
Bacterial infections.

Faredina *Lafare, Ital.†.*
Cephaloridine (p.179·1).
Bacterial infections.

Faremicin *Lafare, Ital.*
Fosfomycin calcium (p.210·2).
Bacterial infections.

Faremid *Lafare, Ital.*
Pipemidic acid (p.237·2).
Bacterial infections.

Fareston
Ercopharm, Aust.; Orion, Irl.; Schering-Plough, Ital.; Asta Medica, Neth.; Orion, Swed.; Orion, UK; Schering-Plough, USA.
Toremifene citrate (p.567·3).
Breast cancer.

Faretrizin *Lafare, Ital.*
Propylene glycol cefatrizine (p.164·2).
Bacterial infections.

Fargan *Carlo Erba OTC, Ital.*
Promethazine (p.416·2).
Skin irritation.

Farganesse *Pharmacia Upjohn, Ital.*
Promethazine hydrochloride (p.416·2).
Hypersensitivity reactions; premedication.

Fargepirina *Upsamedica, Ital.†.*
Oxolamine citrate (p.1065·3); propyphenazone (p.81·3).
Influenza; respiratory-tract inflammation.

Fargo *Elexsam, Austral.†.*
Lignocaine (p.1293·2).
Bites and stings; muscle pain; pain; pruritus; skin irritation.

Farial *Knoll, Ger.*
Indanazoline hydrochloride (p.1062·1).
Colds.

Faril *Edmond Pharma, Ital.†.*
Nalidixic acid (p.228·2).
Urinary-tract infections.

Farin Gola *Montefarmaco, Ital.*
Cetylpyridinium chloride (p.1106·2).
Mouth and throat disinfection.

Faringesic *Diafarm, Spain.*
Chlorhexidine hydrochloride (p.1107·2); benzocaine (p.1286·2).
Formerly contained amylocaine hydrochloride, framycetin sulphate, and prednisolone.
Mouth and throat disorders.

Faringina *SIT, Ital.*
Dequalinium chloride (p.1112·1).
Mouth disinfection.

Faringotricina *SIT, Ital.*
Tyrothricin (p.267·2).
Stomatitis.

Farlutal
Pharmacia Upjohn, Aust.; Pharmacia, Austral.†; Pharmacia Upjohn, Belg.; Pharmacia Upjohn, Fr.; Pharmacia Upjohn, Ger.; Carlo Erba OTC, Ital.; Pharmacia Upjohn, Neth.; Pharmacia Upjohn, Norw.; Pharmacia Upjohn, S.Afr.; Kenfarma, Spain; Pharmacia Upjohn, Swed.; Pharmacia Upjohn, Switz.; Pharmacia Upjohn, UK.
Medroxyprogesterone acetate (p.1448·3).
Malignant neoplasms; metrorrhagia; secondary amenorrhoea.

Farmabroxol *Farmasan, Ger.*
Ambroxol hydrochloride (p.1054·3).
Respiratory disorders associated with viscid or excessive mucus.

Farmacetamol *Docmed, S.Afr.*
Paracetamol (p.72·2).
Fever; pain.

Farmacola *Roche Nicholas, Spain.*
Ginseng (p.1584·2); multivitamins and minerals; caffeine (p.749·3).
Tonic.

Farmadiuril *Farmacusi, Spain.*
Bumetanide (p.834·3).
Oedema, hypertension.

Farmagripine *Pensa, Spain.*
Chlorpheniramine maleate (p.405·1); phenylpropanolamine hydrochloride (p.1067·2); paracetamol (p.72·2).
Fever; influenza and cold symptoms; pain.

Farmaproina *I Farmacologia, Spain.*
Procaine penicillin (p.240·2).
Bacterial infections.

Farmiblastina *Kenfarma, Spain.*
Doxorubicin hydrochloride (p.529·2).
Malignant neoplasms.

Farmidone *Pharmacia Upjohn, Ital.†.*
Amidopyrine (p.15·2).
Fever; inflammation; pain.

Farmitrexat *Pharmacia Upjohn, Ger.*
Methotrexate sodium (p.547·1).
Malignant neoplasms; psoriasis.

Farmodoxi *Lifepharma, Ital.†.*
Doxycycline hydrochloride (p.202·3).
Bacterial infections.

Farmorubicin
Pharmacia Upjohn, Aust.; Pharmacia Upjohn, Ger.; Pharmacia Upjohn, Norw.; Pharmacia Upjohn, S.Afr.; Pharmacia Upjohn, Swed.
Epirubicin hydrochloride (p.532·1).
Malignant neoplasms.

Farmorubicina
Pharmacia Upjohn, Ital.; Kenfarma, Spain.
Epirubicin hydrochloride (p.532·1).
Malignant neoplasms.

Farmorubicine
Pharmacia Upjohn, Belg.; Pharmacia Upjohn, Fr.; Pharmacia Upjohn, Neth.; Pharmacia Upjohn, Switz.
Epirubicin hydrochloride (p.532·1).
Malignant neoplasms.

Farmospasmina Colica *Lifepharma, Ital.†.*
Papaverine hydrochloride (p.1614·2); belladonna (p.457·1).
Gastro-intestinal spasm.

Farmotal *Pharmacia Upjohn, Ital.*
Thiopentone sodium (p.1233·1).
General anaesthesia.

Farnesil *AGIPS, Ital.†.*
Gefarnate (p.1193·2).
Gastro-intestinal inflammation; peptic ulcer.

Farnic *Farge, Ital.†.*
Nicardipine hydrochloride (p.915·1).
Angina pectoris; heart failure; hypertension.

Farnisol *FIRMA, Ital.†.*
Gefarnate (p.1193·2).
Gastro-intestinal inflammation; peptic ulcer.

Farnitin *Lafare, Ital.*
Carnitine (p.1336·2).
Carnitine deficiency; myocardial ischaemia.

Farnolith *Almed, Switz.†.*
Potassium tartrate (p.1161·2); magnesium oxide (p.1198·3); ferrous fumarate (p.1339·3); zinc oxide (p.1096·2).
Renal calculi.

Faros *Lichtwer, Ger.*
Crataegus (p.1568·2).
Cardiac disorders.

Farvicett *Farmec, Ital.*
Chlorhexidine gluconate (p.1107·2); cetrimide (p.1105·2).
Skin, wound, burn, and mucous membrane disinfection.

Farviran *Farmigea, Ital.*
Inosine pranobex (p.615·2).
Viral gynaecological infections.

Fasax *BASF, Ger.*
Piroxicam (p.80·2).
Gout; musculoskeletal and joint disorders.

Fase *Schwarz, Ital.*
Aprotinin (p.711·3).
Oedema; pancreatic disorders; prevention of post-surgical adhesions; pulmonary embolism; shock.

Fasigin *Pfizer, Ital.*
Tinidazole (p.594·1).
Trichomoniasis.

Fasigin N *Pfizer, Ital.*
Tinidazole (p.594·1); nystatin (p.386·1).
Vulvovaginal trichomoniasis and candidiasis.

Fasigyn
Pfizer, Aust.; Pfizer, Austral.; Pfizer, Belg.; Pfizer, Neth.; Pfizer, Norw.†; Pfizer, S.Afr.; Pfizer, Swed.; Pfizer, UK.
Tinidazole (p.594·1).
Anaerobic bacterial infections; protozoal infections.

Fasigyne
Pfizer, Fr.; Pfizer, Switz.
Tinidazole (p.594·1).
Anaerobic bacterial infections; protozoal infections.

Faspic
Zambon, Ital.; Robapharm, Spain.
Ibuprofen (p.44·1).
Fever; gout; musculoskeletal, joint, and peri-articular disorders; pain.

Fastin
SmithKline Beecham, Canad.; SmithKline Beecham, USA.
Phentermine hydrochloride (p.1484·3).
Obesity.

Fastjekt
Allergopharma, Ger.; Bracco, Ital.
Adrenaline (p.813·2) or adrenaline hydrochloride (p.813·3).
Anaphylactic shock.

Fastum
Menarini, Belg.; Menarini, Ital.; Restan, S.Afr.; Menarini, Spain; Sokosi, Switz.
Ketoprofen (p.48·2).
Fever; gout; musculoskeletal, joint, peri-articular and soft-tissue disorders; pain; thrombophlebitis.

Fasupond *Eu Rho, Ger.*
Phenylpropanolamine hydrochloride (p.1067·2).
Obesity.

Father John's Medicine Plus *Oakhurst, USA.*
Phenylephrine hydrochloride (p.1066·2); dextromethorphan hydrobromide (p.1057·3); chlorpheniramine maleate (p.405·1); ammonium chloride (p.1055·2); guaiphenesin (p.1061·3).
Coughs.

Fatigue *Homeocan, Canad.*
Homoeopathic preparation.

Fat-Solv *Cantassium Co., UK.*
Inositol (p.1591·1); choline bitartrate (p.1337·1); methionine (p.984·2); betaine hydrochloride (p.1553·2); alfalfa (p.1544·2); kelp (p.1593·1); glutamic acid hydrochloride (p.1344·3); vitamin B_6 (p.1362·3).

Faustan *Dresden, Ger.*
Diazepam (p.661·1).
Anxiety disorders; premedication; skeletal muscle spasm; status epilepticus.

Fave di Fuca *Roche, Ital.*
Fucus vesiculus (p.1554·1); cascara (p.1183·1); frangula (p.1193·2).
Constipation.

Faverin
Solvay, Irl.; Solvay, UK.
Fluvoxamine maleate (p.288·3).
Depression; obsessive-compulsive disorder.

Favistan
Asta Medica, Aust.; Asta Medica, Ger.
Methimazole (p.1495·3).
Hyperthyroidism.

Fazadon *Glaxo Wellcome, Ital.†.*
Fazadinium bromide (p.1315·2).
Competitive neuromuscular blocker.

Fazol *Schering-Plough, Fr.*
Isoconazole nitrate (p.381·2).
Fungal skin infections.

Fazol G *Schering-Plough, Fr.*
Isoconazole nitrate (p.381·2).
Vaginal candidiasis.

Fazoplex *Inkeysa, Spain.*
Cephazolin sodium (p.181·1).
Bacterial infections.

Fe^{50} *Northampton Medical, USA.*
Dried ferrous sulphate (p.1340·2).
Iron-deficiency anaemia.

Febichol *Medphano, Ger.*
Fenipentol (p.1579·1).
Biliary disorders.

Febracyl *Vifor, Switz.*
Propyphenazone (p.81·3); paracetamol (p.72·2).
Fever; pain.

Febradolor sans codeine *Demopharm, Switz.†.*
Aspirin (p.16·1); paracetamol (p.72·2).
Colloidal aluminium phosphate (p.1178·3) is included in this preparation in an attempt to limit the adverse effects of aspirin on the gastro-intestinal mucosa.
Fever; inflammation; pain.

Febranine *Roche Nicholas, Spain.*
Paracetamol (p.72·2).
Fever; pain.

Febrectal *Funk, Spain.*
Mucopolysaccharidases; paracetamol (p.72·2); oleum pini sylvestris.
Fever; pain.

Febrectal Simple *Funk, Spain.*
Paracetamol (p.72·2).
Fever; pain.

Febrectol *Sanofi Winthrop, Fr.*
Adult suppositories: Paracetamol (p.72·2); pine needle oil (p.1623·3).
Paediatric and infant suppositories: Paracetamol (p.72·2); pine needle oil (p.1623·3); phenobarbitone (p.350·2).
Tablets: Paracetamol (p.72·2); alpha amylase (p.1549·1).
Fever; pain.

Febrinal *Singer, Switz.*
Paracetamol (p.72·2); dextromethorphan hydrobromide (p.1057·3); phenylephrine hydrochloride (p.1066·2).
Cold and influenza symptoms.

Febrispir *Soekami, Fr.†.*
Pheniramine maleate (p.415·3); paracetamol (p.72·2); ascorbic acid (p.1365·2).
Otorhinopharyngeal disorders.

Fectrim *DDSA Pharmaceuticals, UK.*
Co-trimoxazole (p.196·3).

Fedahist *Schwarz, USA.*
Pseudoephedrine hydrochloride (p.1068·3); chlorpheniramine maleate (p.405·1).
Cold symptoms; hay fever; other upper respiratory tract allergies; sinusitis.

Fedahist Decongestant *Schwarz, USA†.*
Pseudoephedrine hydrochloride (p.1068·3); chlorpheniramine maleate (p.405·1).
Cold symptoms; hay fever; other upper respiratory tract allergies; sinusitis.

Fedahist Expectorant *Schwarz, USA.*
Guaiphenesin (p.1061·3); pseudoephedrine hydrochloride (p.1068·3).
Coughs and cold symptoms.

Fedip
Gebro, Aust.; Gebro, Switz.
Nifedipine (p.916·2).
Angina pectoris; hypertension; Raynaud's syndrome.

Fedra *Schering, Ital.*
Gestodene (p.1447·2); ethinyloestradiol (p.1445·1).
Combined oral contraceptive.

Feel Perfecte *L'Oreal, Canad.*
SPF 15: Ethylhexyl *p*-methoxycinnamate (p.1487·1).
Sunscreen.

Feen-A-Mint
Schering-Plough, Canad.; Schering-Plough, USA.
Bisacodyl (p.1179·3).
Formerly contained phenolphthalein.
Constipation.

Feen-a-mint Pills *Schering-Plough, USA.*
Docusate sodium (p.1189·3); phenolphthalein (p.1208·2).
Constipation.

Fefol
SmithKline Beecham Consumer, Austral.; Evans Medical, Irl.; Xixia, S.Afr.; Medeva, UK.
Dried ferrous sulphate (p.1340·2); folic acid (p.1340·3).
Iron and folic acid deficiency in pregnancy.

Fefol Z *Medeva, UK†.*
Dried ferrous sulphate (p.1340·2); zinc sulphate (p.1373·2); folic acid (p.1340·3).
Iron and folic acid deficiency in pregnancy.

Fefol-Vit
Smith Kline & French, Irl.†; Xixia, S.Afr.†; Medeva, UK†.
Dried ferrous sulphate (p.1340·2); folic acid (p.1340·3); vitamin B and C substances.
Iron and vitamin deficiency in pregnancy.

FegaCoren *Vitorgan, Ger.*
Protein extracts from hepar, pancreas, thymus juv., lien, cor, ren, aorta, gland. suprarenal., mucosa intest., amnion, testes juvenil., gland thyreoidea, diencephalon.
Cardiovascular and liver disorders.

FegaCoren N *Vitorgan, Ger.*
Protein extracts from hepar, pancreas, thymus juv., lien, cor, ren, aorta, gland. suprarenal., mucosa intest., amnion, testes juvenil., gland. thyreoidea, diencephalon; methenolone acetate; prednisolone acetate; liothyronine hydrochloride; deslanoside; alpha-tocopheryl acetate; cyanocobalamin; pyridoxine hydrochloride.
Cardiovascular and liver disorders.

Fegacorten *Pulitzer, Ital.†.*
Suprarenal cortex (p.1050·1); cyanocobalamin (p.1363·3).
Anaemia; deficiency states; liver disorders.

Fegatex *Vifor, Switz.*
Vegetable extracts.
Digestive disorders.

Fegato *Lucchini, Ital.†.*
Fish-liver extract; cyanocobalamin (p.1363·3).
Anaemia; liver disorders.

Feiba
Immuno, Canad.; Immuno, Ital.; Baxter, Swed.; Immuno, Switz.; Immuno, UK; Immuno, USA.
A factor VIII inhibitor bypassing fraction (p.721·3).
Haemorrhagic disorders.

Feiba S-TIM 4
Immuno, Aust.; Immuno, Belg.; Immuno, Ger.
A factor VIII inhibitor bypassing fraction (p.721·3).
Haemorrhagic disorders.

Feiba TIM 4 *Immuno, Spain.*
A factor VIII inhibitor bypassing fraction (p.721·3).
Haemophilia.

Felbatol *Wallace, USA.*
Felbamate (p.345·3).
Epilepsy.

Felden
Pfizer, Aust.; Mack, Illert., Ger.; Pfizer, Ger.; ;Pfizer, Norw.; Pfizer, Swed.; Pfizer, Switz.
Piroxicam (p.80·2).
Gout; inflammation; musculoskeletal, joint, peri-articular, and soft-tissue disorders; pain.

Feldene
Pfizer, Austral.; Pfizer, Belg.; Pfizer, Canad.; Pfizer, Fr.; Pfizer, Irl.; Pfizer, Ital.; Pfizer, Neth.; Pfizer, S.Afr.; Pfizer, Spain; Pfizer, UK; Pfizer, USA.
Piroxicam (p.80·2).
Gout; musculoskeletal, joint, peri-articular, and soft-tissue disorders; pain.

Felidon neu *Schoeller, Aust.*
Absinthium (p.1541·1); achillea (p.1542·2); taraxacum (p.1634·2).
Hepatobiliary disorders.

Felis *Biocur, Ger.*
Hypericum (p.1590·1).
Anxiety; depression.

Felisedine *Monal, Fr.†.*
Phenobarbitone (p.350·2); crataegus (p.1568·2); valerian (p.1643·1).
Formerly contained papaverine hydrochloride, phenobarbitone, quinine hydrobromide, boldo, crataegus, anemone, and valerian.
Anxiety; insomnia.

Felison *Bayer, Ital.*
Flurazepam monohydrochloride (p.672·2).
Insomnia.

Felix *Apotheke Heiligen Josef, Aust.*
Hamamelis (p.1587·1); panthenol (p.1571·1); zinc oxide (p.1096·2).
Haemorrhoids; pruritus ani.

Fellesan *Recip, Swed.*
Cholic acid; dehydrocholic acid (p.1570·2).
Biliary-tract disorders.

Feloday *Ciba, Ital.*
Felodipine (p.867·3).
Angina pectoris; hypertension.

Felodur *PMC, Austral.*
Felodipine (p.867·3).
Hypertension.

Feloflux *Sauter, Switz.†.*
Dehydrocholic acid (p.1570·2); dehydrodesoxycholic acid.
Biliary-tract disorders.

Feloflux compose *Sauter, Switz.†.*
Dehydrocholic acid (p.1570·2); papaverine hydrochloride (p.1614·2).
Biliary-tract disorders.

Felsol Neo *Roland, Ger.*
Phenazone (p.78·2); nikethamide calcium thiocyanate (p.1483·3); ephedrine hydrochloride (p.1059·3).
Asthma; bronchitis; dyspnoea; emphysema; silicosis.

Felsolyn N *Roland, Ger.†.*
Hyoscine hydrochloride (p.463·2); paracetamol (p.72·2).
Cold symptoms; influenza; spasms.

Fem-1 *BDI, USA.*
Paracetamol (p.72·2); pamabrom (p.927·1).
Pain.

Femafen *Nicholas, UK†.*
Ibuprofen (p.44·1).

Femanest *Tika, Swed.*
Oestradiol (p.1455·1).
Oestrogen deficiency; osteoporosis.

Femanor *Tika, Swed.*
Oestradiol (p.1455·1); norethisterone acetate (p.1453·1).
Oestrogen deficiency; osteoporosis.

Femapak *Solvay, UK.*
Combination pack: Patches, oestradiol (p.1455·1) (Fematrix); tablets, dydrogesterone (p.1444·2) (Duphaston).
Menopausal disorders.

Femapirin *Chefaro, Neth.†.*
Ibuprofen (p.44·1).
Dysmenorrhoea.

Femaplus Spezial Dr Hagedorn *Naturarzneimittel, Ger.*
Homoeopathic preparation.

Femaprim *Organon, Spain.*
Ibuprofen (p.44·1).
Fever; musculoskeletal, joint, and peri-articular disorders; pain.

Femar *Novartis, Swed.*
Letrozole (p.543·3).
Breast cancer.

Femara
Novartis, Austral.; Novartis, Ital.; Novartis, S.Afr.; Ciba, UK; Novartis, USA.
Letrozole (p.543·3).
Breast cancer.

Femasekvens *Tika, Swed.*
16 tablets, oestradiol (p.1455·1); 12 tablets, oestradiol; norethisterone acetate (p.1453·1).
Oestrogen deficiency; osteoporosis.

Fematab *Solvay, Irl.*
Oestradiol (p.1455·1).
Menopausal disorders.

Fematrix
Solvay, Irl.; Solvay, UK.
Oestradiol (p.1455·1).
Menopausal disorders; osteoporosis.

Femavit *Pharmacia Upjohn, Ger.*
21 Tablets, conjugated oestrogens (p.1457·3); 7 tablets, inert.
Oestrogen replacement therapy.

FemCal *Freeda, USA.*
Calcium carbonate (p.1182·1); cholecalciferol (p.1366·3); vitamin B; minerals.

Femcare *Schering-Plough, USA†.*
Clotrimazole (p.376·3).
Vulvovaginal candidiasis.

Femcet *Russ, USA.*
Paracetamol (p.72·2); caffeine (p.749·3); butalbital (p.644·3).
Pain.

Femepen *AFI, Norw.*
Phenoxymethylpenicillin potassium (p.236·2).
Bacterial infections.

Femerital *Asta Medica, Neth.*
Ambucetamide (p.1548·2); paracetamol (p.72·2); caffeine hydrate (p.750·1).
Dysmenorrhoea.

Femeron *Johnson & Johnson MSD Consumer, UK.*
Miconazole nitrate (p.384·3).
Vaginal candidiasis.

Fem-Etts *Roberts, USA†.*
Paracetamol (p.72·2); pamabrom (p.927·1).
Pain.

Femex *Roche, Neth.*
Naproxen sodium (p.61·2).
Fever; inflammation; musculoskeletal and joint disorders; pain.

Femicine *Lake, USA†.*
Pulsatilla; mercurius vivus; sulphur.
Vaginal irritation.

Femidine *AVP, USA.*
Povidone-iodine (p.1123·3).
Vaginal disorders.

Femidol
Note. This name is used for preparations of different composition.
Lepetit, Ital.†.
Dextropropoxyphene hydrochloride (p.27·3); paracetamol (p.72·2); aspirin (p.16·1); caffeine (p.749·3); chlorpheniramine maleate (p.405·1).
Pain.

Merck, Spain.
Ibuprofen (p.44·1).
Fever; musculoskeletal, joint, and peri-articular disorders; pain.

Femigel *Scientific, S.Afr.*
Oestradiol (p.1455·1).
Menopausal disorders.

Femigoa *LAW, Ger.*
Levonorgestrel (p.1454·1); ethinyloestradiol (p.1445·1).
Combined oral contraceptive.

Femigraine *Roche Consumer, UK†.*
Aspirin (p.16·1); cyclizine hydrochloride (p.407·1).
Migraine.

Femilax *G & W, USA.*
Docusate sodium (p.1189·3); phenolphthalein (p.1208·2).
Constipation.

Femilla N *Steigerwald, Ger.*
Cimicifuga (p.1563·3).
Dysmenorrhoea.

Feminax
Roche Consumer, Irl.; Roche Consumer, UK.
Paracetamol (p.72·2); codeine phosphate (p.26·1); caffeine (p.749·3); hyoscine hydrobromide (p.462·3).
Dysmenorrhoea.

Femin-Do *Grasler, Ger.*
Homoeopathic preparation.

Feminesse *Unipath, UK.*
Sorbic acid; glycerol; liquid paraffin; polycarbophil.
Vaginal odour.

Feminex *Sante Naturelle, Canad.*
Multivitamin and mineral preparation.

Femininum Ro-Plex (Rowo-405) *Pharmakon, Ger.†.*
Homoeopathic preparation.

Feminique
Note. This name is used for preparations of different composition.
QHP, USA.
Sodium benzoate (p.1102·3); sorbic acid (p.1125·2); lactic acid (p.1593·3); octoxinol 9 (p.1326·2).
Vaginal disorders.

QHP, USA.
Vinegar (p.1541·2).
Vaginal disorders.

Feminique with Iron and Calcium *Stanley, Canad.*
Multivitamin preparation with calcium and iron.

Feminon N *Redel, Ger.*
Homoeopathic preparation.

Femiplexe *Lehning, Fr.*
Copper gluconate (p.1338·1); zinc gluconate (p.1373·2).
Menopausal disorders; menstrual disorders.

Femipres *Schwarz, Ital.*
Moexipril hydrochloride (p.912·1).
Hypertension.

Femiron *Menley & James, USA.*
Ferrous fumarate (p.1339·3).
Iron-deficiency anaemias.

Femiron Multi-Vitamins and Iron *Menley & James, USA.*
Multivitamin preparation with iron and folic acid.

Femisana N *Hotz, Ger.*
Agnus castus (p.1544·2); chelidonium; cimicifuga (p.1563·3); phosphorus.
Gynaecological disorders.

Femizol-M *Lake, USA.*
Miconazole nitrate (p.384·3).
Fungal vaginal infections.

Fem-Mono *Scand Pharm, Swed.*
Isosorbide mononitrate (p.893·3).
Angina pectoris.

Femodeen *Schering, Neth.*
Ethinyloestradiol (p.1445·1); gestodene (p.1447·2).
Combined oral contraceptive.

Femoden ED *Schering, Austral.*
21 Tablets, ethinyloestradiol (p.1445·1); gestodene (p.1447·2); 7 tablets, inert.
Combined oral contraceptive.

Femodene
Schering, Belg.; Schering, Irl.; Schering, S.Afr.; Schering, UK.
Ethinyloestradiol (p.1445·1); gestodene (p.1447·2).
28-Day packs also contain 7 inert tablets.
Combined oral contraceptive.

Femogex *Germiphene, Canad.*
Oestradiol valerate (p.1455·2).
Oestrogenic.

Femoston
Solvay, Austral.; Solvay, Belg.; Solvay, Neth.; Solvay, UK.
14 Tablets, oestradiol (p.1455·1); 14 tablets, oestradiol; dydrogesterone (p.1444·2).
Menopausal disorders; osteoporosis.

Femovan *Schering, Ger.*
Ethinyloestradiol (p.1445·1); gestodene (p.1447·2).
Combined oral contraceptive.

FemPatch *Parke, Davis, USA.*
Oestradiol (p.1455·1).
Menopausal disorders; oestrogen deficiency.

Femranette mikro *Brenner-Efeka, Ger.*
Ethinyloestradiol (p.1445·1); levonorgestrel (p.1454·1).
Combined oral contraceptive.

FemSeven
E. Merck, Swed.; E. Merck, UK.
Oestradiol (p.1455·1).
Menopausal disorders; osteoporosis.

Femstat
Syntex, Switz.†; Syntex, USA.
Butoconazole nitrate (p.376·1).
Vulvovaginal candidiasis.

Femtran *3M, Austral.*
Oestradiol (p.1455·1).
Menopausal disorders; osteoporosis.

Femulen
Searle, S.Afr.†; Searle, UK.
Ethynodiol diacetate (p.1445·3).
Progestogen-only oral contraceptive.

Fenac *Alphapharm, Austral.*
Diclofenac sodium (p.31·2).
Inflammation; musculoskeletal and joint disorders; pain.

Fenadol *Proge, Ital.*
Diclofenac sodium (p.31·2).
Inflammation; musculoskeletal and joint disorders; pain.

Fenalgic *Specia, Fr.†.*
Ibuprofen (p.44·1).
Dysmenorrhoea; musculoskeletal and joint disorders.

Fenalgin *Geminis, Spain.*
Caffeine (p.749·3); paracetamol (p.72·2); propyphenazone (p.81·3).
Pain.

Fenam *Solvay, Ital.*
Isoxsuprine resinate (polistirex) (p.1592·1).
Cerebrovascular disorders.

Fenamide *Farmigea, Ital.*
Dichlorphenamide (p.848·2).
Glaucoma.

Fenamin *Lennon, S.Afr.*
Mefenamic acid (p.51·2).
Musculoskeletal, joint, and soft-tissue disorders; pain.

Fenamine *Fawns & McAllan, Austral.*
Pheniramine maleate (p.415·3).
Hypersensitivity reactions; motion sickness; vestibular disorders.

Fenantoin *NM, Swed.*
Phenytoin (p.352·3).
Epilepsy.

Fenaren *Mundipharma, Aust.*
Diclofenac sodium (p.31·2).
Gout; inflammation; musculoskeletal, joint, and peri-articular disorders; pain; renal and biliary colic.

Fenazil *Sella, Ital.*
Promethazine hydrochloride (p.416·2).
Hypersensitivity reactions.

Fenazol *Hokuriku, Jpn.*
Ufenamate (p.91·2).
Skin disorders.

Fenazox *Meiji, Jpn†.*
Amfenac sodium (p.15·2).
Inflammation; pain.

Fenbid *Goldshield, UK.*
Ibuprofen (p.44·1).
Musculoskeletal and joint disorders; pain.

Fendilar *SPA, Ital.†.*
Fendiline hydrochloride (p.868·1).
Cardiac disorders.

Fendin *Ranbaxy, S.Afr.*
Terfenadine (p.418·1).
Hypersensitivity reactions.

Fenemal
AFI, Norw.; NM, Swed.
Phenobarbitone (p.350·2).
Epilepsy.

Fenergan Expectorante *Rhone-Poulenc Rorer, Spain.*
Ipecacuanha (p.1062·2); promethazine hydrochloride (p.416·2); potassium guaiacolsulfonate (p.1068·3).
Upper-respiratory-tract disorders.

Fenergan Topico *Rhone-Poulenc Rorer, Spain.*
Promethazine (p.416·2).
Cutaneous hypersensitivity reactions.

Fenesin *Dura, USA.*
Guaiphenesin (p.1061·3).
Coughs.

Fenesin DM *Dura, USA.*
Dextromethorphan hydrobromide (p.1057·3); guaiphenesin (p.1061·3).
Coughs.

Fengel *Zyma, Ital.†.*
Dimethindene maleate (p.408·3).
Pruritic skin disorders.

Fenicol
Alcon, Belg.†; Rolab, S.Afr.
Chloramphenicol (p.182·1).
Bacterial infections.

Fenigal *Sofar, Ital.†.*
Propoxur (p.1410·1).
Insecticide.

Fenilen *Nestle, Ital.†.*
Food for special diets.
Phenylketonuria.

Fenint *Pharmacia Upjohn, Ger.*
Thioctic acid (p.1636·2).
Diabetic polyneuropathy.

Fenipectum *Zyma, Ger.†.*
Dimethindene maleate (p.408·3); potassium guaiacolsulfonate (p.1068·3); phenylephrine (p.1066·2); codeine phosphate (p.26·1).
Coughs and associated respiratory-tract disorders.

Fenistil
Zyma, Aust.; Zyma, Belg.; Zyma, Ger.; Zyma, Ital.; Novartis Consumer, Neth.; Novartis, Norw.; Zyma, Spain; Zyma, Swed.†; Zyma, Switz.
Dimethindene maleate (p.408·3).
Hypersensitivity reactions; pruritic skin disorders.

Fenistil Plus *Zyma, Ger.†.*
Yellow and white capsules, betamethasone (p.1033·2); dimethindene maleate (p.408·3); white capsules, dimethindene maleate.
Hypersensitivity reactions.

Fenizolan
Organon, Aust.; Nourypharma, Ger.
Fenticonazole nitrate (p.377·3).
Genital candidiasis; vulvovaginal Gram-positive bacterial infections.

Fennings Children's Powders *Waterhouse, UK.*
Paracetamol (p.72·2).
Fever; pain.

Fennings Little Healers *Waterhouse, UK.*
Ipecacuanha (p.1062·2).
Coughs and colds.

Fennings Mixture *Fennings, UK†.*
Sodium salicylate (p.85·1).
Fever; pain.

Fenoket *Opus, UK.*
Ketoprofen (p.48·2).
Gout; musculoskeletal, joint, and peri-articular disorders; pain.

Fenolip *Lannacher, Aust.*
Fenofibrate (p.1273·1).
Hyperlipidaemias.

Fenomel *Clonmel, Irl.*
Flurbiprofen (p.42·1).
Musculoskeletal and joint disorders.

Fenopron
Dista, Irl.; Lilly, S.Afr.; Dista, UK.
Fenoprofen calcium (p.37·2).
Fever; gout; musculoskeletal and joint disorders; pain.

Fenospen *Pharmacia Upjohn, Ital.*
Phenoxymethylpenicillin (p.236·2).
Bacterial infections.

Fenostil
Zyma, Irl.†; Zyma, UK†.
Dimethindene maleate (p.408·3).
Hypersensitivity reactions; pruritic skin disorders.

Fenox
Note. This name is used for preparations of different composition.
Boots Healthcare, Irl.†; Boots, S.Afr.†; Seton, UK.
Phenylephrine hydrochloride (p.1066·2).
Nasal congestion; rhinitis; sinusitis.

Boots Healthcare, Ital.; Boots, S.Afr.
Phenylephrine hydrochloride (p.1066·2); naphazoline nitrate (p.1064·2).
Nasal congestion; sinusitis.

Fenoxypen
Novo Nordisk, Swed.†; Novo Nordisk, Switz.
Phenoxymethylpenicillin potassium (p.236·2).
Bacterial infections.

Fensaid *Amrad, Austral.*
Piroxicam (p.80·2).
Ankylosing spondylitis; osteoarthritis; rheumatoid arthritis.

Fensel *Pharmacia Upjohn, Spain.*
Felodipine (p.867·3).
Hypertension.

Fensol *Rolab, S.Afr.†.*
Fenoterol hydrobromide (p.753·2).
Obstructive airways disease.

Fenspir *Ibirn, Ital.*
Fenspiride hydrochloride (p.1579·3).
Respiratory disorders.

Fensum *Merckle, Ger.*
Paracetamol (p.72·2).
Formerly contained aspirin, paracetamol, and codeine phosphate.
Fever; pain.

Fensum N *Merckle, Ger.†.*
Aspirin (p.16·1); caffeine (p.749·3); ascorbic acid (p.1365·2).
Aluminium glycinate (p.1177·2) is included in this preparation in an attempt to limit adverse effects on the gastro-intestinal mucosa.
Cold symptoms; fever; inflammation; pain.

Fentac *Sarget, Fr.†.*
Fentiazac (p.41·1).
Musculoskeletal and joint disorders.

Fentalim *Angelini, Ital.*
Alfentanil hydrochloride (p.12·3).
General anaesthesia; neuroleptanalgesia.

Fentamox *Opus, UK.*
Tamoxifen citrate (p.563·3).
Anovulatory infertility; breast cancer.

Fentanest
Pharmacia Upjohn, Ital.; Syntex, Spain.
Fentanyl (p.38·1) or fentanyl citrate (p.38·1).
Analgesia during anaesthesia.

Fentatienil *Angelini, Ital.*
Sufentanil citrate (p.85·2).
General anaesthesia; neuroleptanalgesia.

Fentazin
Goldshield, Irl.; Forley, UK.
Perphenazine (p.685·2).
Anxiety; nausea; psychoses; vomiting.

Fentiderm *Zyma, Ital.*
Fenticonazole nitrate (p.377·3).
Fungal skin and anogenital infections.

Fentigyn *Ciba, Ital.*
Fenticonazole nitrate (p.377·3).
Fungal vulvovaginal infections.

Fentrate *Servier, Belg.†.*
Fenfluramine hydrochloride (p.1480·3).
Obesity.

Fentrinol *Frika, Aust.*
Amidephrine mesylate (p.1055·1).
Rhinitis.

Fenugrene *Aerocid, Fr.*
Fenugreek (p.1579·3).
Appetite stimulant.

Fenulin *Gerard House, UK.*
Fenugreek (p.1579·3); slippery elm (p.1630·1); hydrastis (p.1588·2).
Gastro-intestinal disorders.

Fenured *Technicon, S.Afr.†.*
Fenfluramine hydrochloride (p.1480·3).
Obesity.

Fenuril *Pharmacia Upjohn, Swed.*
Urea (p.1095·2).
Dry skin.

Fenuril-Hydrokortison *Pharmacia Upjohn, Swed.*
Urea (p.1095·2); hydrocortisone (p.1043·3).
Eczema.

Feocyte *Dunhall, USA.*
Iron (p.1346·1); liver extracts; folic acid (p.1340·3); vitamin B substances; copper.
Vitamin C (p.1365·2) is included in this preparation to increase the absorption and availability of iron.
Iron-deficiency anaemias.

Feosol *SmithKline Beecham Consumer, USA.*
Ferrous sulphate (as dried or hydrate) (p.1340·2).
Iron deficiency; iron-deficiency anaemia.

Feospan
Evans Medical, Irl.; Medeva, UK.
Dried ferrous sulphate (p.1340·2).
Iron deficiency; iron-deficiency anaemia.

Feospan Z *Medeva, UK†.*
Dried ferrous sulphate (p.1340·2); zinc sulphate (p.1373·2).
Iron deficiency.

Feostat *Forest Pharmaceuticals, USA.*
Ferrous fumarate (p.1339·3).
Iron-deficiency anaemias.

Feparil *Madaus, Spain.*
Tablets: Aescin (p.1543·3).
Oedema; peripheral vascular disorders.
Topical gel: Diethylamine salicylate (p.33·1); aescin (p.1543·3); sodium aescin polysulphate (p.1543·3).
Peripheral vascular disorders.

Fepramol *Schwarz, Ital.†.*
Feprazone (p.41·2); paracetamol (p.72·2); guaiphenesin (p.1061·3).
Coughs and cold symptoms.

Fepron
Dista, Belg.†; Lilly, Ital.; Lilly, Neth.†.
Fenoprofen calcium (p.37·2).
Inflammation; musculoskeletal, joint, and peri-articular disorders.

Fer UCB *UCB, Fr.*
Ferrous chloride (p.1339·3).
Ascorbic acid (p.1365·2) is included in this preparation to increase the absorption and availability of iron.
Anaemias.

Ferancee *J&J-Merck, USA.*
Ferrous fumarate (p.1339·3).
Ascorbic acid (p.1365·2) is included in this preparation to increase the absorption and availability of iron.
Iron-deficiency anaemias.

Feraplex *Lambda, USA.*
Vitamin B substance and iron.

Feratab *Upsher-Smith, USA.*
Ferrous sulphate (p.1340·2).
Iron-deficiency anaemias.

Feravol *Carlton Laboratories, UK†.*
Ferrous sulphate (p.1340·2); vitamin B and C substances.
Iron deficiency.

Feravol-F *Carlton Laboratories, UK†.*
Ferrous gluconate (p.1340·1); folic acid (p.1340·3).
Iron and folic acid deficiency.

Feravol-G *Carlton Laboratories, UK†.*
Syrup: Ferrous gluconate (p.1340·1); thiamine hydrochloride (p.1361·1).
Tablets: Ferrous gluconate (p.1340·1); vitamins and minerals.
Iron deficiency.

Ferfolic SV *Sinclair, UK.*
Ferrous gluconate (p.1340·1); folic acid (p.1340·3).
Iron and folic acid deficiency; neural tube defect prophylaxis.

Fer-gen-sol *Goldline, USA.*
Ferrous sulphate (p.1340·2).
Iron deficiency anaemia.

Fergon
Sanofi Winthrop, Austral.; Sanofi Winthrop, Irl.; Sterling Winthrop, UK†; Winthrop Consumer, USA.
Ferrous gluconate (p.1340·1).
Iron-deficiency anaemias.

Fergon Iron Plus Calcium *Winthrop Consumer, USA†.*
Ferrous fumarate (p.1339·3); calcium carbonate (p.1182·1); vitamin D (p.1366·3).
Iron and calcium deficiency.

Fergon Plus *Sanofi Winthrop, USA†.*
Ferrous gluconate (p.1340·1); intrinsic factor; vitamin B substances.
Vitamin C (p.1365·2) is included in this preparation to increase the absorption and availability of iron.
Anaemias.

Feridex *Berlex, USA.*
Ferumoxides (p.1004·2).
Contrast medium for magnetic resonance imaging of the liver.

Fer-In-Sol
Bristol-Myers Squibb, Belg.†; Mead Johnson, Canad.; Bristol-Myers Squibb, Irl.; Mead Johnson, Ital.; Mead Johnson Nutritionals, USA.
Ferrous sulphate (p.1340·2).
Iron-deficiency anaemias.

Fer-Iron *Rugby, USA.*
Ferrous sulphate (p.1340·2).
Iron-deficiency anaemias.

Ferlactis *AGIPS, Ital.*
Streptococcus lactis.
Gastro-intestinal disorders.

Ferlasin *Martin, Spain.*
Multivitamin, mineral, and amino-acid preparation.
Tonic.

Ferlatum *Zilliken, Ital.*
Iron succinyl-protein complex (p.1349·2).
Anaemias; iron deficiency.

Ferlixir *Rhone-Poulenc Rorer, S.Afr.*
Multivitamin and mineral preparation.

Ferlixir N *Nattermann, Ger.†.*
B vitamin preparation with iron and folic acid.
Iron-deficiency; iron-deficiency anaemias.

Ferlixir N triplex *Nattermann, Ger.†.*
B vitamin preparation with iron and folic acid.
Iron-deficiency; iron-deficiency anaemias.

Ferlixit *Rhone-Poulenc Rorer, Ital.*
Ferric sodium gluconate (p.1340·1).
Anaemias; iron deficiency.

Ferlucon *Allen & Hanburys, S.Afr.†.*
Ferrous gluconate (p.1340·1); vitamin B_1.
Iron deficiency.

Fermalac *Rougier, Canad.*
Lactobacillus acidophilus (p.1594·1); *Lactobacillus bulgaricus* (p.1594·1); *Streptococcus lactis.*
Diarrhoea.

Fermalac Vaginal *Rougier, Canad.*
Lactobacillus acidophilus (p.1594·1); *Lactobacillus bulgaricus* (p.1594·1); *Streptococcus lactis.*
Adjunct in treatment of vaginal infections.

Fermentmycin *Intramed, S.Afr.*
Gentamicin sulphate (p.212·1).
Bacterial infections.

Fermento duodenal
Sanol, Ger.; Schwarz, Switz.
Pancreatin (p.1612·1); dimethicone (p.1213·1).
Digestive disorders.

Fermentol *Carter Horner, Canad.*
Pepsin (p.1616·3).
Dyspepsia without hyperacidity; oral vehicle.

Fermenturto *Teknofarma, Ital.†.*
Lactic-acid-producing organisms (p.1594·1).
Gastro-intestinal disorders.

Fermenturto-Lio *Teknofarma, Ital.*
Lactic-acid-producing organisms (p.1594·1).
Gastro-intestinal disorders.

Ferocyl *Hudson, USA.*
Ferrous fumarate (p.1339·3).
Docusate sodium (p.1189·3) is included in this preparation to reduce the constipating effects of iron.
Iron-deficiency anaemias.

Ferodan *Odan, Canad.*
Ferrous sulphate (p.1340·2).
Anaemias.

Fero-Folic
Abbott, S.Afr.; Abbott, Switz.; Abbott, USA.
Ferrous sulphate (p.1340·2); folic acid (p.1340·3).
Vitamin C (p.1365·2) is included in this preparation to increase the absorption and availability of iron.
Folic acid deficiency; iron deficiency.

Feroglobin *Vitabiotics, UK.*
Iron, vitamin B, and mineral preparation.

Fero-Grad
Abbott, Belg.; Abbott, Canad.; Abbott, S.Afr.; Abbott, USA.
Ferrous sulphate (p.1340·2).
Vitamin C (p.1365·2) is included in this preparation to increase the absorption and availability of iron.
Iron-deficiency anaemias.

Fero-Grad vitamine C *Abbott, Fr.*
Ferrous sulphate (p.1340·2).
Ascorbic acid (p.1365·2) is included in this preparation to increase the absorption and availability of iron.
Anaemias.

Fero-Gradumet
Abbott, Belg.; Abbott, Neth.; Abbott, Spain; Abbott, USA.
Ferrous sulphate (p.1340·2).
Iron deficiency.

Ferolactan *Bioindustria, Ital.†.*
Prolactin (p.1259·1).
Lactation insufficiency; menstrual disorders; threatened abortion.

Feron *Toray, Jpn.*
Interferon beta (p.616·1).
Hepatitis; malignant neoplasms.

Ferospace *Hudson, USA.*
Ferrous sulphate (p.1340·2).
Iron-deficiency anaemias.

Ferotrinsic *Rugby, USA.*
Ferrous fumarate (p.1339·3); folic acid (p.1340·3); intrinsic factor; vitamin B_{12} substances (p.1363·3).
Vitamin C (p.1365·2) is included in this preparation to increase the absorption and availability of iron.
Anaemias.

Ferpan *Berenguer Infale, Spain†.*
Droxicam (p.35·2).
Musculoskeletal and joint disorders.

Ferplex
Italfarmaco, Ital.; Italfarmaco, Spain.
Iron succinyl-protein complex (p.1349·2).
Iron-deficiency anaemia.

Ferplex Fol *Lifepharma, Ital.†.*
Iron succinyl-protein complex (p.1349·2); calcium folinate (p.1342·2).
Anaemias; folate deficiency; iron-deficiency.

Ferralet *Mission Pharmacal, USA†.*
Ferrous gluconate (p.1340·1).
Iron-deficiency anaemias.

Ferralet Plus *Mission Pharmacal, USA.*
Ferrous gluconate (p.1340·1); folic acid (p.1340·3); vitamin B_{12} substances (p.1363·3).
Vitamin C (p.1365·2) is included in this preparation to increase the absorption and availability of iron.
Iron-deficiency anaemias.

Ferralyn *Lannett, USA†.*
Dried ferrous sulphate (p.1340·2).
Iron-deficiency anaemias.

Ferrascorbin *Streuli, Switz.*
Oral drops: Ferrous chloride (p.1339·3).
Ascorbic acid (p.1365·2) is included in this preparation to increase the absorption and availability of iron.
Tablets: Ferrous chloride (p.1339·3); ferrous gluconate (p.1340·1).
Ascorbic acid (p.1365·2) is included in this preparation to increase the absorption and availability of iron.
Iron deficiency; iron-deficiency anaemia.

Ferra-TD *Goldline, USA†.*
Dried ferrous sulphate (p.1340·2).
Iron-deficiency anaemias.

Ferrematos *Boniscontro & Gazzone, Ital.*
Ferrous gluconate (p.1340·1).
Iron deficiency; iron-deficiency anaemias.

Ferremon *Medici, Ital.*
Iron succinyl-protein complex (p.1349·2).
Anaemias; iron deficiency.

Ferretab *Lannacher, Aust.*
Ferrous fumarate (p.1339·3).
Iron deficiency anaemias.

Ferretab comp *Lannacher, Aust.*
Ferrous fumarate (p.1339·3); sodium folate (p.1341·2).
Iron and folic acid deficiency.

Ferretts *Pharmics, USA†.*
Ferrous fumarate (p.1339·3).

Ferricure *Trenker, Belg.*
Polysaccharide-iron complex (p.1353·2).
Iron-deficiency anaemia.

Ferri-Emina *Lafare, Ital.*
Ferric sodium gluconate (p.1340·1).
Anaemias; iron deficiency.

Ferrifol B12 *Sanico, Belg.*
Ferric ammonium citrate (p.1339·2); folic acid (p.1340·3); vitamin B_{12} (p.1363·3).
Anaemias; growth disorders.

Ferrimed *Byk Madaus, S.Afr.*
Capsules: Iron polymaltose (p.1349·1); folic acid (p.1340·3).
Injection; syrup: Iron polymaltose (p.1349·1).
Anaemias.

Ferrimed DS *Byk Madaus, S.Afr.*
Iron polymaltose (p.1349·1).
Iron-deficiency anaemias.

Ferriseltz *Bracco, Ital.*
Ferric ammonium citrate (p.1339·2).
Radiographic contrast medium.

Ferrisept *Pagni, Ital.†.*
Chlorhexidine gluconate (p.1107·2); dequalinium chloride (p.1112·1).
Instrument disinfection.

Ferriseptil *Gedis, Ital.*
Glutaraldehyde (p.1114·3).
Disinfection.

Ferritamin *Abigo, Swed.*
Multivitamin preparation with iron.

Ferritin Complex *ABC, Ital.*
Ferric sodium gluconate (p.1340·1); calcium folinate (p.1342·2).
Anaemias.

Ferritin Oti *ABC, Ital.*
Ferric sodium gluconate (p.1340·1).
Anaemias; iron deficiency.

Ferrivenin *Laevosan, Aust.*
Saccharated iron oxide (p.1353·2).
Hypochromic anaemias.

Ferriwas B12 Fuerte *Wasserman, Spain†.*
Cyanocobalamin (p.1363·3); folic acid (p.1340·3); ferrous sulphate (p.1340·2).
Anaemias.

Ferrlecit
Note. This name is used for preparations of different composition.
Nattermann, Ger.
Ferric sodium gluconate (p.1340·1).
Iron-deficiency; iron-deficiency anaemias.
Rhone-Poulenc, Ital.†.
Ferric sodium citrate; cobalt acetate (p.1565·3); copper sodium citrate; manganese citrate (p.1351·1).
Anaemia.

Ferrlecit 2 *Nattermann, Ger.*
Ferrous succinate (p.1340·2).
Iron-deficiency; iron-deficiency anaemias.

Ferro-12 *Wassen, Ital.*
Ferrous fumarate (p.1339·3).
Vitamin C (p.1365·2) is included in this preparation to increase the absorption and availability of iron.
Iron supplement.

Ferro 66 *Byk Gulden, Ger.*
Ferrous chloride (p.1339·3).
Iron-deficiency; iron-deficiency anaemias.

Ferro Angelini *Angelini, Ital.†.*
Ferric pyrophosphate (p.1339·2).
Anaemias.

Ferro Complex *Celafar, Ital.*
Sodium ironedetate (p.1354·2).
Anaemias.

Ferro Cytofol *Mead Johnson, Ger.†.*
Ferrous sulphate (p.1340·2); folic acid (p.1340·3).
Anaemias.

Ferro 66 DL *Promonta, Ger.†.*
Ferrous sulphate (p.1340·2).
Iron-deficiency; iron-deficiency anaemias.

Ferro Drops L *Parke, Davis, S.Afr.*
Ferrous lactate (p.1340·1).
Iron-deficiency anaemias.

Ferro Morgens *Llorente, Spain†.*
Ferritin (p.1580·1).
Anaemias.

Ferro sanol *Sanol, Ger.*
Ferrous glycine sulphate (p.1340·1).
Iron-deficiency; iron-deficiency anaemias.

Ferro sanol B N *Sanol, Ger.†.*
Vitamin B preparation with iron.
Iron and vitamin B deficiency.

Ferro sanol comp *Sanol, Ger.*
Ferrous glycine sulphate (p.1340·2); folic acid (p.1340·3); cyanocobalamin (p.1363·3).
Iron and vitamin B deficiency; iron-deficiency anaemias.

Ferro sanol duodenal *Sanol, Ger.*
Ferrous glycine sulphate (p.1340·1).
Iron-deficiency; iron-deficiency anaemias.

Ferro Semar *Semar, Spain.*
Ferrous ascorbate (p.1339·2).
Anaemias.

Ferro-Agepha *Agepha, Aust.*
Ferrous gluconate (p.1340·1).

Ferro-B 12 Ehrl *Hormosan, Ger.†.*
Ferrous gluconate (p.1340·1); cyanocobalamin (p.1363·3); folic acid (p.1340·3).
Iron-deficiency; iron-deficiency anaemias.

Ferrobet *Montavit, Aust.*
Ferrous fumarate (p.1339·3).
Iron deficiency anaemias.

Ferrocap *Consolidated Chemicals, UK†.*
Ferrous fumarate (p.1339·3).
Iron deficiency.

Ferrocap F *Consolidated Chemicals, Irl.*
Ferrous fumarate (p.1339·3); folic acid (p.1340·3).
Anaemia during pregnancy.

Ferrocap F 350 *Consolidated Chemicals, UK†.*
Ferrous fumarate (p.1339·3); folic acid (p.1340·3).
Iron and folic acid deficiency.

Ferro-C-Calcium *Hotz, Ger.*
Ferrous gluconate (p.1340·1); calcium gluconate (p.1155·2); ascorbic acid (p.1365·2).
Iron deficiency, especially with elevated calcium and vitamin C requirements.

Ferroce *Byk Elmu, Spain†.*
Copper sulphate (p.1338·1); ferrous sulphate (p.1340·2).
Ascorbic acid (p.1365·2) is included in this preparation to increase the absorption and availability of iron.
Anaemias.

Ferrocebrin *Lilly, S.Afr.†.*
Vitamin B substances with vitamin C and iron.
Anaemias; vitamin deficiencies.

Ferrocontin Continus
Napp, Irl.†; Asta Medica, UK†.
Ferrous glycine sulphate (p.1340·1).
Iron-deficiency anaemia.

Ferrocontin Folic Continus
Napp, Irl.†; Asta Medica, UK†.
Ferrous glycine sulphate (p.1340·1); folic acid (p.1340·3).
Iron and folic acid deficiency in pregnancy.

Ferrocur *Schering, Spain.*
Iron succinyl-protein complex (p.1349·2).
Iron-deficiency anaemia.

Ferro-Dok *Major, USA.*
Ferrous fumarate (p.1339·3).
Docusate sodium (p.1189·3) is included in this preparation to reduce the constipating effects of iron.
Iron-deficiency anaemias.

Ferro-Folgamma *Worwag, Ger.*
Ferrous sulphate (p.1340·2); folic acid (p.1340·3); cyanocobalamin (p.1363·3).
Iron and vitamin deficiency.

Ferrofolin *Farmades, Ital.*
Iron succinyl-protein complex (p.1349·2); calcium folinate (p.1342·2).
Anaemias; folic acid deficiency; iron deficiency.

Ferrofolin Simplex *Farmades, Ital.*
Iron succinyl-protein complex (p.1349·2).
Anaemias; iron deficiency.

Ferrofolin Venti *Farmades, Ital.†.*
Calcium folinate (p.1342·2); cobamamide (p.1364·2); ferritin (p.1580·1).
Anaemias.

Ferrofolin Venti Simplex *Farmades, Ital.†.*
Ferritin (p.1580·1).
Anaemias.

Ferro-Folsan *Solvay, Ger.*
Ferrous sulphate (p.1340·2); folic acid (p.1340·3).
Iron-deficiency anaemia.

Ferro-Folsan plus *Kali-Chemie, Ger.†.*
Ferrous sulphate (p.1340·2); folic acid (p.1340·3).
Succinic acid is included in this preparation to increase the absorption and availability of iron.
Anaemias.

Ferro-Folsaure-Vicotrat *Heyl, Ger.†.*
Ferrous sulphate (p.1340·2); folic acid (p.1340·3).
Anaemias; prevention of side-effects of folic acid antagonists.

Ferrograd
Abbott, Irl.; Abbott, Ital.; Abbott, UK.
Ferrous sulphate (p.1340·2).
Iron-deficiency anaemia.

Ferrograd C
Abbott, Aust.; Abbott, Irl.; Abbott, Ital.; Abbott, UK.
Ferrous sulphate (p.1340·2).
Sodium ascorbate (p.1365·2) is included in this preparation to increase the absorption and availability of iron.
Iron-deficiency anaemia.

Ferrograd Folic
Abbott, Irl.; Abbott, Ital.; Abbott, UK.
Ferrous sulphate (p.1340·2); folic acid (p.1340·3).
Sodium ascorbate (p.1365·2) may be included in this preparation to increase the absorption and availability of iron.
Iron and folic acid deficiency in pregnancy.

Ferrograd-Fol *Abbott, Aust.*
Ferrous sulphate (p.1340·2); folic acid (p.1340·3).
Iron and folic acid deficiency.

Ferro-Gradumet
Abbott, Aust.; Abbott, Austral.; Abbott, Switz.
Ferrous sulphate (p.1340·2).
Iron deficiency; iron-deficiency anaemia.

Ferroinfant *Jossa-Arznei, Ger.†.*
Vitamin B preparation with iron and minerals.
Iron deficiency.

Ferroinfant N *Jossa-Arznei, Ger.†.*
Vitamin B preparation with iron and minerals.
Iron deficiency.

Ferrokapsul *Strathmann, Ger.*
Ferrous fumarate (p.1339·3).
Iron-deficiency.

Ferro-Kobalt *Montavit, Aust.†.*
Ferrous gluconate (p.1340·1); cobalt gluconate.
Anaemias.

Ferro-Kombun N *Merckle, Ger.†.*
Iron (p.1346·1); ascorbic acid (p.1365·2); dried metabolic products of symbiotic gut bacteria (*Escherichia coli*, *Enterococcus faecalis* (p.1594·1), *Lactobacillus acidophilus* (p.1594·1)).
Primary and secondary anaemias.

Ferrol *Chemil, Ital.*
Chondroitin sulphate-iron complex (p.1337·1).
Iron deficiency; iron-deficiency anaemias.

Ferrolande *Synthelabo, Ger.†.*
Ferrous fumarate (p.1339·3).
Iron-deficiency anaemias.

Ferromar *Marnel, USA.*
Ferrous fumarate (p.1339·3).
Ascorbic acid (p.1365·2) is included in this preparation to increase the absorption and availability of iron.

Ferromax *Weifa, Norw.*
Ferrous sulphate (p.1340·2).
Iron deficiency; iron-deficiency anaemia.

Ferromia *Eisai, Jpn.*
Ferrous sodium citrate.
Iron-deficiency anaemia.

Ferrominerase *GN, Ger.†.*
Ferrous gluconate (p.1340·1).
Iron-deficiency anaemia.

Ferromyn
Wellcome, Irl.†; Calmic, UK†.
Ferrous succinate (p.1340·2).
Iron-deficiency anaemia.

Ferromyn S *Hassle, Swed.*
Ferrous succinate (p.1340·2).
Iron deficiency; iron-deficiency anaemia.

Ferronovin *Hommel, Ger.†.*
Vitamin preparation with iron, liver extract, and folic acid.
Iron deficiency.

Ferrophor *TAD, Ger.†.*
Ferrous sulphate (p.1340·2); liver extract.
Iron deficiency anaemias.

Ferroprotina *Faes, Spain.*
Ferritin (p.1580·1).
Anaemias.

Ferro-Retard *Nycomed, Norw.*
Ferrous sulphate (p.1340·2).
Iron deficiency; iron-deficiency anaemia.

Ferrosanol duodenal *Schwarz, Switz.*
Ferrous glycine sulphate (p.1340·1).
Iron deficiency; iron-deficiency anaemia.

Ferro-Sequels *Lederle, USA.*
Ferrous fumarate (p.1339·3).
Docusate sodium (p.1189·3) is included in this preparation to reduce the constipating effects of iron.
Iron deficiency; iron deficiency anaemias.

Ferrosprint *Poli, Ital.*
Ferric sodium gluconate (p.1340·1).
Anaemias.

Ferrostar *Mediolanum, Ital.†.*
Ferritin (p.1580·1).
Anaemias.

Ferrostrane *Parke, Davis, Fr.*
Sodium ironedetate (p.1354·2).
Anaemias.

Ferrostrene *Parke, Davis, Switz.†.*
Sodium ironedetate (p.1354·2).
Iron deficiency.

Ferrotab *Antigen, Irl.*
Dried ferrous sulphate (p.1340·2); copper sulphate (p.1338·1); manganese sulphate (p.1350·3).
Iron-deficiency anaemias.

Ferro-Tre *Mediolanum, Ital.*
Ferritin (p.1580·1); folic acid (p.1340·3).
Iron-deficiency anaemias.

Ferroven *Geymonat, Ital.*
Saccharated iron oxide (p.1353·2).
Iron-deficiency anaemias.

Ferrovin-Chinaeisenwein *Pharmonta, Aust.*
Ferric ammonium citrate (p.1339·2); manganese hypophosphite; cinchona bark (p.1564·1); citrus aurantium.
Anaemias; iron deficiency; tonic.

Ferrovin-Eisenelixier *Pharmonta, Aust.*
Saccharated iron oxide (p.1353·2); aromatic tincture; bitter orange tincture (p.1610·3).
Iron deficiency; tonic.

Ferrum *Hausmann, Irl.*
Iron polymaltose (p.1349·1).
Iron-deficiency anaemia.

Ferrum Fol B Hausmann *Vifor International, Switz.†.*
Ferrous fumarate (p.1339·3); folic acid (p.1340·3); cyanocobalamin (p.1363·3).
Iron and folic acid deficiency.

Ferrum H *Sigma, Austral.*
Iron polymaltose (p.1349·1).
Iron-deficiency anaemias.

Ferrum Hausmann
Richter, Aust.; Bio-Therabel, Belg.; Yamanouchi, Ger.; Geymonat, Ital.; Vifor International, Switz.
Ferrous fumarate (p.1339·3), iron polymaltose (p.1349·1), or saccharated iron oxide (p.1353·2).
Iron-deficiency; iron-deficiency anaemias.

Ferrum Klinge *Klinge, Ger.†.*
Ferrous fumarate (p.1339·3).
Iron-deficiency; iron-deficiency anaemias.

Ferrum Verla *Verla, Ger.*
Ferrous gluconate (p.1340·1).
Iron deficiency.

Ferrum-Quarz *Weleda, Aust.*
Ferrous sulphate (p.1340·2); quartz.
Migraine and related vascular headaches; tonic.

Ferrum-Strath *Strath-Labor, Ger.†.*
Calendula; echinacea angustifolia (p.1574·2); rue; reduced iron (p.1346·1).
Iron-deficiency anaemia.

Fersaday
Duncan, Flockhart, Irl.†; Goldshield, UK.
Ferrous fumarate (p.1339·3).
Iron deficiency.

Fersamal
Salusa, S.Afr.†; Forley, UK.
Ferrous fumarate (p.1339·3).
Iron deficiency.

Fertiline *Pharmagyne, Fr.*
Urofollitrophin (p.1263·1).
Female infertility.

Fertility Score *FertiPro, Irl.*
Test for male fertility (p.1621·2).

Fertilvit *Lafare, Ital.†.*
Vitamin E (p.1369·1).

Fertinex *Serono, USA.*
Urofollitrophin (p.1263·1).
Female infertility.

Fertinic *Desbergers, Canad.*
Ferrous gluconate (p.1340·1).
Iron-deficiency anaemias.

Fertinorm
Serono, Aust.; Serono, Canad.; Serono, Ger.; Serono, Norw.†; Serono, Spain†; Serono, Swed.†.
Urofollitrophin (p.1263·1).
Anovulatory infertility.

Fertiral
Hoechst Marion Roussel, Irl.†; Hoechst Marion Roussel, UK.
Gonadorelin (p.1247·2).
Amenorrhoea; male and female infertility.

Fertodur
Schering, Ger.†; Schering, Ital.†; Schering, Switz.†.
Cyclofenil (p.1440·2).
Anovulatory infertility.

Fertomcidina-U *Martini, Ital.†.*
Magnesium glycerophosphate (p.1157·2); salicylic acid (p.1090·2); sodium iodide (p.1493·2); ammonium bromide (p.1620·3).
Disinfection.

Ferumat
Continental Pharma, Belg.; Searle, Neth.†.
Ferrous fumarate (p.1339·3).
Iron-deficiency anaemia.

Ferus-B12 *Vitabiotics, UK†.*
Iron, vitamin B, and mineral preparation.

Fervex *Oberlin, Fr.*
Pheniramine maleate (p.415·3); paracetamol (p.72·2); ascorbic acid (p.1365·2).
Upper respiratory-tract disorders.

Ferybar *Pinewood, Irl.*
Liver extract; vitamin B substances; minerals.
Vitamin and mineral supplement.

Fesofor *Xixia, S.Afr.†.*
Ferrous sulphate (p.1340·2).
Iron-deficiency anaemias.

Fesovit
Evans Medical, Irl.; SmithKline Beecham, UK†.
Ferrous sulphate (p.1340·2); vitamin B and C substances.
Iron deficiency.

Fesovit Z *Medeva, UK.*
Ferrous sulphate (p.1340·2); zinc sulphate (p.1373·2); vitamin B and C substances.
Iron deficiency.

Fespan *SmithKline Beecham, Austral.†.*
Ferrous sulphate (p.1340·2).
Iron deficiency.

Festal
Note. This name is used for preparations of different composition.
Hoechst, Aust.; Hoechst, Canad.†; Hoechst, Swed.†.
Pancreas extract; hemicellulase (p.1561·1); ox bile (p.1553·2).
Pancreatic insufficiency; pancreatitis.

Cassella-med, Switz.†.
Pancreatin (p.1612·1); ox bile (p.1553·2).
Pancreatic insufficiency.

Festal N
Cassella-med, Ger.†; Hoechst Marion Roussel, Ital.
Pancreatin (p.1612·1).
Digestive system disorders.

Festalan *Hoechst, USA†.*
Lipase; amylase (p.1549·1); protease; atropine methonitrate (p.455·1).
Digestive enzyme deficiency; functional gastro-intestinal disorders.

Festale *Hoechst, Fr.†.*
Pancreas; beef bile (p.1553·2); hemicellulase (p.1561·1).
Dyspepsia.

Festamoxin *Shionogi, Ger.†.*
Latamoxef disodium (p.221·2).
Bacterial infections.

Feto-Longoral *Artesan, Ger.; Cassella-med, Ger.*
Multivitamin and mineral preparation.

Fetrin *Lunsco, USA.*
Ferrous fumarate (p.1339·3); cyanocobalamin (p.1363·3); intrinsic factor.
Ascorbic acid (p.1365·2) is included in this preparation to increase the absorption and availability of iron.

Feuille de Saule *Gilbert, Fr.*
Salicylic acid (p.1090·2).
Callus; corns; verrucas.

Fevamol *Garec, S.Afr.*
Paracetamol (p.72·2).
Fever; pain.

Fevarin
Solvay, Ger.; Solvay, Ital.; Solvay, Neth.; Solvay, Norw.; Solvay Duphar, Swed.
Fluvoxamine maleate (p.288·3).
Depression; obsessive-compulsive disorder.

Fever & Inflammation Complex *Brauer, Austral.†.*
Homoeopathic preparation.

Feverall *Upsher-Smith, USA.*
Paracetamol (p.72·2).
Fever; pain.

Feves De Fuca *Melisana, Belg.†.*
Frangula bark (p.1193·2); cascara (p.1183·1); fucus vesiculosus (p.1554·1).
Obesity.

Fevital *SPA, Ital.†.*
Ferritin (p.1580·1); cyanocobalamin (p.1363·3); thiamine hydrochloride (p.1361·1); riboflavine sodium phosphate (p.1362·1); pyridoxine hydrochloride (p.1362·3); nicotinamide (p.1351·2); sodium pantothenate (p.1353·1).
Anaemias.

Fevital Simplex *Prospa, Ital.*
Ferric sodium gluconate (p.1340·1).
Iron deficiency; iron-deficiency anaemias.

Fexin *Apotex, S.Afr.*
Cephalexin (p.178·2).
Bacterial infections.

FGF Tabs *Abbott, Austral.*
Dried ferrous sulphate (p.1340·2); folic acid (p.1340·3).
Folate deficiency; iron-deficiency anaemia; megaloblastic anaemia.

Fhbc *Clintec, Ital.*
Amino-acid infusion.
Parenteral nutrition.

Fherbolico *Fher, Spain†.*
Nandrolone cyclohexylpropionate (p.1452·2).
Anabolic; osteoporosis.

Fiacin *Biosarto, Spain.*
Indomethacin (p.45·2); prednisone (p.1049·2).
Musculoskeletal and joint disorders; peri-articular disorders.

Fialetta Odontalgica Dr Knapp *Montefarmaco, Ital.*
Benzocaine (p.1286·2); chlorbutol (p.1106·3); clove oil (p.1565·2); colophony (p.1567·1).
Toothache.

Fiber Rich *O'Connor, USA†.*
Phenylpropanolamine hydrochloride (p.1067·2); grain; citrus fruit fibre.

Fiberall *Ciba Consumer, USA.*
Chewable tablets: Polycarbophil calcium (p.1209·1).
Constipation; diarrhoea; stool softener in haemorrhoids.
Oral powder; wafers: Psyllium hydrophilic mucilloid (p.1194·2).
Constipation; stool softener in haemorrhoids.

Fibercon *Lederle, USA.*
Polycarbophil calcium (p.1209·1).
Bowel disorders; constipation.

Fiberform
Boehringer Ingelheim, Fr.†; Solvay, Neth.; Cederroth, Norw.†; Boehringer Ingelheim, Swed.
Wheat germ.
Constipation.

Fiberform Mix *Boehringer Ingelheim, Swed.*
Wheat germ.
Constipation.

Fiberlan *Elan, USA.*
Lactose-free, gluten-free preparation for enteral nutrition.

Fiber-Lax *Rugby, USA.*
Polycarbophil calcium (p.1209·1).
Constipation; diarrhoea.

FiberNorm *G & W, USA.*
Polycarbophil calcium (p.1209·1).
Constipation.

Fibertabletter *Kabi, Swed.†.*
Oat fibre (p.1181·2).
Dietary supplement.

Fibion *Asta Medica, Switz.*
Soya bran (p.1181·2).
Constipation.

Fiblaferon *Rentschler, Ger.*
Interferon beta (human) (p.616·1).
Viral infections.

Fiblet *Agpharm, Switz.†.*
Apple and potato fibre; cellulose (p.1472·2); pectin (p.1474·1).
Constipation; dietary supplement.

Fiboran
Christiaens, Belg.; Nycomed, Fr.; Nycomed, Spain.
Aprindine hydrochloride (p.825·1).
Arrhythmias.

Fibracol *Johnson & Johnson Medical, UK.*
Collagen alginate (p.1566·3).
Wounds.

Fibrad *Ross, USA†.*
Dietary fibre preparation.
Derived from pea, oat, and sugar-beet fibre.

Fibraflex *Nycomed, Ger.†.*
Lotion; ointment; cream: Heparin sodium (p.879·3); glycol salicylate (p.43·1); benzyl nicotinate (p.22·1).
Musculoskeletal, joint, and nerve disorders; sports injuries.
Tablets: Ibuprofen (p.44·1).
Formerly contained meprobamate and propyphenazone.
Fever; musculoskeletal, joint, and soft-tissue disorders; pain.
Topical emulsion: Diethylamine salicylate (p.33·1); turpentine oil (p.1641·1); benzyl nicotinate (p.22·1).
Musculoskeletal and joint disorders; sports injuries.
Topical gel: Heparin sodium (p.879·3); glycol salicylate (p.43·1); menthol (p.1600·2).
Musculoskeletal and joint disorders; sports injuries.

Fibraflex N *Dorsch, Ger.†.*
Glycol salicylate (p.43·1); benzyl nicotinate (p.22·1); menthol (p.1600·2).
Formerly contained heparin sodium, glycol salicylate, benzyl nicotinate, and menthol.
Neuralgia; rheumatism.

Fibraflex-W-Creme N *Dorsch, Ger.†.*
Glycol salicylate (p.43·1); benzyl nicotinate (p.22·1).
Formerly contained heparin, glycol salicylate, and benzyl nicotinate.
Neuralgia; rheumatism.

Fibraguar
Boehringer Ingelheim, Belg.†; Fardi, Spain.
Guar gum (p.321·3).
Diabetes mellitus; hyperlipidaemias.

Fibralax *Hosbon, Spain†.*
Wheat bran (p.1181·2).
Constipation.

Fibramucil *Procter & Gamble, Spain.*
Ispaghula husk (p.1194·2).
Constipation.

Fibrase *Teofarma, Ital.*
Pentosan polysulphate sodium (p.928·1).
Peripheral vascular disorders; soft-tissue disorders; thrombosis prophylaxis.

Fibrax *Whitehall-Robins, Canad.*
Grain and citrus fibre.
Constipation.

Fibrazeta *SmithKline Beecham, Ital.†.*
Dietary fibre supplement.
Delayed intestinal transit; weight reduction.

Fibre Dophilus *Pharmadass, UK.*
Acidophilus; bifidophilus.

Fibre Plus *Pharmadass, UK.*
Ispaghula husk (p.1194·2).
Formerly known as Fibrelax.

Fibrepur *Hoechst Marion Roussel, Canad.*
Ispaghula husk (p.1194·2).
Constipation.

Fibretime *Cenovis, Austral.†.*
Dietary fibre preparation.

Fibretrim *Cassella-med, Ital.†.*
Dietary fibre supplement.

Fibre-Vit *Vitalia, UK.*
Multivitamin, mineral, and fibre preparation.

Fibrex *Maggioni, Ital.†.*
Dietary fibre supplement with minerals.
Delayed intestinal transit; weight reduction.

Fibrex Hot Drink *Berlin-Chemie, Ger.†.*
Aspirin (p.16·1); ascorbic acid (p.1365·2).
Fever; inflammation; pain.

Fibrex Tabletten *Berlin-Chemie, Ger.†.*
Aspirin (p.16·1); paracetamol (p.72·2).
Fever; pain.

Fibrezym *Bene, Ger.*
Pentosan polysulphate sodium (p.928·1).
Thrombo-embolism prophylaxis.

Fibrinomer *ISI, Ital.*
Fibrinogen (p.722·3).
Haemorrhagic disorders; hypofibrinogenaemia.

Fibrocard *SMB, Belg.†.*
Verapamil hydrochloride (p.960·3).
Hypertension.

Fibrocid *Lacer, Spain.*
Pentosan polysulphate sodium (p.928·1).
Hyperlipidaemias; thrombo-embolic disorders.

Fibrocit *CT, Ital.*
Gemfibrozil (p.1273·3).
Hyperlipidaemias.

Fibroderm *Torlan, Spain.*
Acedoben potassium (p.1541·1); magnesium stearate.
Skin disorders.

Fibrogammin
Centeon, Aust.; Centeon, Ger.; Centeon, UK.
A factor XIII preparation (p.722·2).
Factor XIII deficiency.

Fibrolan
Parke, Davis, Aust.; Parke, Davis, Ger.; Parke, Davis, Switz.
Plasmin (p.932·1); deoxyribonuclease (p.1059·1).
Wounds.

Fibrolan mit Chloromycetin *Parke, Davis, Ger.†.*
Plasmin (bovine) (p.932·1); deoxyribonuclease (p.1059·1); chloramphenicol (p.182·1).
Wounds.

Fibrolax *Giuliani, Ital.*
Ispaghula husk (p.1194·2).
Constipation.

Fibrolax Complex *Giuliani, Ital.*
Ispaghula husk (p.1194·2); senna (p.1212·2).
Constipation.

Fibronevrina *Ceccarelli, Ital.*
Thiamine hydrochloride (p.1361·1); cyanocobalamin (p.1363·3).
Formerly contained d-isopropylammonium dichloroacetate, thiamine, and cyanocobalamin.
Peripheral neuralgia and neuritis.

Fibroral *Sodietal, Fr.*
Preparation for enteral nutrition.

Fibrosine *Whitehall, Irl.*
Maltodextrin (p.1350·2).
Constipation.

Fibro-Vein
STD, Irl.; STD Pharmaceutical Products, UK.
Sodium tetradecyl sulphate (p.1469·2).
Formerly known as STD Injection in the *UK.*
Varicose veins.

Fibyrax
Rhone-Poulenc Rorer, Austral.; Whitehall-Robins, Canad.
Grain and citrus fibres (p.1181·2).
Constipation; dietary fibre supplement.

Fichtensirup N *Jukunda, Ger.*
Spruce needles; thyme (p.1636·3); sage (p.1627·1); liquorice (p.1197·1); thyme oil (p.1637·1); sage oil.
Respiratory-tract disorders; tonic.

Ficortril
Pfizer, Ger.; Pfizer, Swed.
Hydrocortisone (p.1043·3) or hydrocortisone acetate (p.1043·3).
Anogenital pruritus; eczema; inflammatory eye disorders.

Ficortril Lotio m. Neomycin *Pfizer, Ger.†.*
Hydrocortisone (p.1043·3); neomycin sulphate (p.229·2).
Skin disorders.

Fidium *Fides, Spain.*
Betahistine hydrochloride (p.1553·1).
Ménière's disease; vestibular disorders.

Fidocin *Mendelejeff, Ital.†.*
Demeclocycline (p.201·2).
Bacterial infections.

Fidozon *Fides, Ger.†.*
Magnesium peroxide (p.1119·1); magnesium oxide (p.1198·3); dried magnesium sulphate (p.1158·2).
Gastro-intestinal disorders.

Fienamina *Recordati, Ital.*
Chlorpheniramine maleate (p.405·1); ephedrine hydrochloride (p.1059·3).
Hypersensitivity reactions.

Fiery Jack *Pickles, UK.*
Cream: Glycol salicylate (p.43·1); diethylamine salicylate (p.33·1); capsicum oleoresin; methyl nicotinate (p.55·1).
Ointment: Capsicum oleoresin.
Musculoskeletal and joint disorders; pain.

Figsen *Carter-Wallace, Austral.*
Phenolphthalein (p.1208·2).
Constipation.

FIII Hc *Clintec, Ital.*
Amino-acid infusion.
Parenteral nutrition.

Filair *3M, UK.*
Beclomethasone dipropionate (p.1032·1).
Obstructive airways disease.

Filarcidan *Cidan, Spain†.*
Diethylcarbamazine citrate (p.99·2).
Filariasis; loiasis; onchocerciasis.

Filena
Organon, Aust.; Organon, Ital.
11 White tablets, oestradiol valerate (p.1455·2); 10 blue tablets, oestradiol valerate; medroxyprogesterone acetate (p.1448·3).
Menopausal disorders; osteoporosis.

Filibon
Wyeth, S.Afr.; Lederle, USA†.
Multivitamin and mineral preparation with iron and folic acid.
Supplement for pregnant or lactating women.

Filmogen Same *Savoma, Ital.*
Barrier cream.

Filoklin *Sabater, Spain.*
Cephazolin sodium (p.181·1).
Lignocaine hydrochloride (p.1293·2) is included in this preparation to alleviate the pain of injection.
Bacterial infections.

Filteray Broad Spectrum *Wellcome, USA†.*
Avobenzone (p.1486·3); padimate O (p.1488·1).
Sunscreen.

Filtrax *Ipso, Ital.*
Pipemidic acid (p.237·2).
Bacterial urinary-tract infections.

Finac *C & M, USA.*
Sulphur (p.1091·2); methylbenzethonium chloride (p.1119·3).
Acne.

Finalgon
Bender, Aust.; Boehringer Ingelheim, Austral.; Boehringer Ingelheim, Canad.; Thomae, Ger.; Fher, Spain.
Nonivamide (p.63·2); nicoboxil (p.63·1).
Musculoskeletal, joint, and soft-tissue disorders; peripheral vascular disorders.

Finalgon N Schmerzpflaster *Thomae, Ger.*
Cayenne pepper; methyl salicylate (p.55·2).
Musculoskeletal and joint disorders; sprains.

Finalin *Yamanouchi, Jpn†.*
Methylbenactyzium bromide (p.465·2).
Gastro-intestinal spasm; nocturnal enuresis.

Finastid *Neopharmed, Ital.*
Finasteride (p.1446·1).
Benign prostatic hyperplasia.

Fincoid
Scientific, S.Afr.†; Orion, Switz.
Copper-wound polyethylene (p.1337·3).
Intra-uterine contraceptive device.

Finedal *Llorente, Spain.*
Clobenzorex hydrochloride (p.1478·2).
Obesity.

Finegosan *Merck, Spain†.*
Muramidase (p.1604·3); tetracycline hydrochloride (p.259·1).
Bacterial infections.

Fineural N *Molimin, Ger.*
Aspirin (p.16·1); paracetamol (p.72·2); caffeine (p.749·3).
Cold symptoms; fever; neuralgia; pain.

Finibron *Midy, Ital.†.*
Buprenorphine hydrochloride (p.22·2).
Pain.

Finidol *Sandoz, Fr.*
Aspirin (p.16·1); caffeine (p.749·3).
Colloidal aluminium hydroxide (p.1177·3) is included in this preparation in an attempt to limit adverse effects on the gastro-intestinal mucosa.
Fever; pain.

Finil *Coradol, Ger.*
Homoeopathic preparation.

Finimal
Roche, Belg.; Roche Nicholas, Neth.; Nicholas, Switz.†.
Paracetamol (p.72·2); caffeine (p.749·3).
Fever; pain.

Finipect *Roche Nicholas, Neth.*
Noscapine (p.1065·2).
Coughs.

Finiweh *Dentinox, Ger.*
Paracetamol (p.72·2).
Fever; pain.

Finlepsin *Dresden, Ger.; Boehringer Mannheim, Ger.*
Carbamazepine (p.339·2).
Alcohol withdrawal syndrome; epilepsy; neurogenic pain; psychoses.

Fiogesic *Sandoz, USA†.*
Aspirin (p.16·1); phenylpropanolamine hydrochloride (p.1067·2); pheniramine maleate (p.415·3); mepyramine maleate (p.414·1).
Cold symptoms; hay fever.

Fiorgen PF *Goldline, USA†.*
Aspirin (p.16·1); caffeine (p.749·3); butalbital (p.644·3).
Pain.

Fioricet *Sandoz, USA.*
Butalbital (p.644·3); paracetamol (p.72·2); caffeine (p.749·3).
Tension headache.

Fioricet with Codeine *Sandoz, USA.*
Codeine phosphate (p.26·1); butalbital (p.644·3); paracetamol (p.72·2); caffeine (p.749·3).
Pain.

Fiorinal
Note. This name is used for preparations of different composition.
Novartis, Austral.
Codeine phosphate (p.26·1); doxylamine succinate (p.410·1); paracetamol (p.72·2).
Pain.

Sandoz, Canad.; Sandoz, USA.
Aspirin (p.16·1); butalbital (p.644·3); caffeine (p.749·3).
Pain; vascular or tension headaches.

Sandoz, Spain.
Capsules: Aspirin (p.16·1); caffeine (p.749·3); paracetamol (p.72·2).
Suppositories†: Codeine phosphate (p.26·1); paracetamol (p.72·2); salicylamide (p.82·3).
Pain.

Fiorinal C *Sandoz, Canad.*
Butalbital (p.644·3); caffeine (p.749·3); aspirin (p.16·1); codeine phosphate (p.26·1).
Anxiety; pain; tension.

Fiorinal Codeina *Sandoz, Spain.*
Capsules: Aspirin (p.16·1); caffeine (p.749·3); codeine phosphate (p.26·1); paracetamol (p.72·2).
Suppositories†: Codeine phosphate (p.26·1); paracetamol (p.72·2); salicylamide (p.82·3).
Pain.

Fiorinal with Codeine *Sandoz, USA.*
Aspirin (p.16·1); butalbital (p.644·3); caffeine (p.749·3); codeine phosphate (p.26·1).
Pain.

Fiorinal Lact or Adul *Sandoz, Spain†.*
Paracetamol (p.72·2); salicylamide (p.82·3).
Fever; pain.

Fiorlin *IBP, Ital.†.*
Crataegus (p.1568·2); passion flower (p.1615·3).
Sedative.

Fiormil *Inpharzam, Switz.*
Enterococcus faecium (p.1594·1).
Restoration of normal gastro-intestinal flora.

Fiorpap *Creighton, USA.*
Butalbital (p.644·3); paracetamol (p.72·2); caffeine (p.749·3).
Pain.

Fiortal *Geneva, USA.*
Aspirin (p.16·1); caffeine (p.749·3); butalbital (p.644·3).
Pain.

Firmacef *FIRMA, Ital.*
Cephazolin sodium (p.181·1).
Lignocaine hydrochloride (p.1293·2) is included in the intramuscular injection to alleviate the pain of injection.
Bacterial infections.

Firmacort *FIRMA, Ital.*
Methylprednisolone (p.1046·1) or methylprednisolone sodium succinate (p.1046·1).
Corticosteroid.

Firmalone *FIRMA, Ital.†.*
Dexamethasone (p.1037·1).
Oral corticosteroid.

Firmavit *FIRMA, Ital.*
Cobamamide (p.1364·2); pyridoxal phosphate (p.1363·1); thiamine diphosphate (p.1361·2).
Neuritis.

First Aid Antiseptic Powder *Nelson, Austral.†.*
Chlorhexidine hydrochloride (p.1107·2); clioquinol (p.193·2); allantoin (p.1078·2).
Minor abrasions and wounds.

First Choice *Polymer Technology, USA.*
Test for glucose in blood (p.1585·1).

First Response
Carter-Wallace, Austral.; Carter Horner, Canad.; Carter-Wallace, UK; Carter, USA.
Fertility test or pregnancy test (p.1621·2).

Fisamox *Rhone-Poulenc Rorer, Austral.*
Amoxycillin sodium (p.151·3) or amoxycillin trihydrate (p.151·3).
Bacterial infections.

Fish Factor *Farmila, Ital.*
Omega-3 marine triglycerides (p.1276·1).
Arteriosclerosis; disorders of lipid metabolism.

Fishaphos *Felton, Austral.*
Omega-3 marine triglycerides (p.1276·1).
Dietary supplement.

Fisherman's Friend *Lofthouse of Fleetwood, Canad.*
Menthol (p.1600·2).
Coughs; sore throat.

Fisherman's Friend Honey Cough Syrup *Lofthouse of Fleetwood, UK†.*
Honey (p.1345·3); squill vinegar (p.1070·1); citric acid (p.1564·3); anise oil (p.1550·1); peppermint oil (p.1208·1); menthol (p.1600·2); cineole (p.1564·1).
Coughs.

Fisherman's Friend Original *Lofthouse of Fleetwood, Canad.*
Menthol (p.1600·2); eucalyptus oil (p.1578·1).
Cold symptoms.

Fisher's Phospherine *Felton, Austral.*
Vitamins and electrolytes; alstonia constricta; quassia (p.1624·1).
Tonic.

Fisifax *Septa, Spain.*
Nicergoline (p.1607·1).
Cerebral and peripheral vascular disorders; vascular headache.

Fisiobil *Salvat, Spain.*
Dimecrotic acid, magnesium salt.
Hepatobiliary disorders.

Fisiodar *Abiogen, Ital.*
Diacerein (p.29·3).
Osteoarthritis.

Fisiodex 40 *Grifols, Spain†.*
Dextran 40 (p.716·2) in sodium chloride.
Plasma volume expansion.

Fisiodex 70 *Grifols, Spain†.*
Dextran 70 (p.717·1) in sodium chloride.
Plasma volume expansion.

Fisiofer *Molteni, Ital.*
Ferric sodium gluconate (p.1340·1).
Iron deficiency; iron-deficiency anaemias.

Fisiogastrol *Salvat, Spain.*
Cisapride (p.1187·1).
Gastro-oesophageal reflux; gastroparesis.

Fisiolax *Manetti Roberts, Ital.†.*
Bisacodyl (p.1179·3); docusate sodium (p.1189·3); calcium pantothenate (p.1352·3).
Constipation.

Fisiologica *Farmasur, Spain; Fardi, Spain.*
Sodium chloride (p.1162·2).
Nasal congestion.

Fisiologico Betafar *Betafar, Spain; Cinfa, Spain; Neusc, Spain; Orravan, Spain; Calmante Vitaminado, Spain.*
Sodium chloride (p.1162·2).
Nasal congestion.

Fisiologico Bieffe M *Bieffe, Spain.*
Sodium chloride (p.1162·2).
Fluid and electrolyte depletion; hypovolaemia.

Fisiologico Braun *Braun, Spain.*
Sodium chloride (p.1162·2).
Fluid and electrolyte depletion; hypovolaemia.

Fisiologico Mein *Mein, Spain.*
Sodium chloride (p.1162·2).
Fluid and electrolyte depletion; hypovolaemia.

Fisiologico Vitulia *Ern, Spain.*
Sodium chloride (p.1162·2).
Fluid and electrolyte depletion; hypovolaemia.

Fisiozima *SIT, Ital.†.*
Muramidase hydrochloride (p.1604·3).
Viral infections.

Fissan *Uhlmann-Eyraud, Switz.*
Casein hydrolysate (Labiline); colloidal silicon dioxide (p.1475·1); polysilic acid fluoride; bismuth subnitrate (p.1180·2); kaolin (p.1195·1); silica clay (p.1474·3); titanium dioxide (p.1093·3); zinc oxide (p.1096·2).
Skin irritation.

Fissan-Azulenpaste *Fink, Ger.†.*
Guaiazulene (p.1586·3); zinc oxide (p.1096·2); bismuth subnitrate (p.1180·2).
Skin disorders.

Fissan-Brustwarzensalbe *Fink, Ger.†.*
Oestradiol (p.1455·1); dichlorophen (p.99·2); bismuth subnitrate (p.1180·2).
Breast or nipple tenderness.

Fissan-Silberpuder *Fink, Ger.†.*
Hexamine silver nitrate compound.
Umbilical cord care; wounds.

Fissan-Zinkol *Fink, Ger.†.*
Zinc oxide (p.1096·2); bismuth subnitrate (p.1180·2).
Skin disorders.

Fissan-Zinkschuttelmixtur *Fink, Ger.†.*
Zinc oxide (p.1096·2).
Skin disorders.

Fitacnol *Arkopharma, Fr.*
Lappa (p.1594·2); pensee sauvage; ortie dioique.
Acne.

Fitaxal *Phygiene, Fr.*
Lactulose (p.1195·3).
Constipation.

Fitepar Cortex *Biotekfarma, Ital.†.*
Inosine (p.1591·1); cyanocobalamin (p.1363·3); suprarenal cortex (p.1050·1).
Anaemias; asthenia.

Fitex E *Belmac, Spain†.*
Borogallic acid; salicylic acid (p.1090·2).
Fungal skin infections.

Fitocrem *Andromaco, Spain.*
Paraffin; wheat germ; phenoxyethanol.
Burns; ulcers; wounds.

Fitodorf Alghe Marine *Fitodorfarma, Ital.*
Quercia marine extract; frangula (p.1193·2); rhubarb (p.1212·1).
Constipation; dietary supplement.

Fitodorf Rabarbaro *Fitodorfarma, Ital.*
Boldo (p.1554·1); rhubarb (p.1212·1).
Digestive disorders; reduced intestinal motility.

Fitokey Harpagophytum *Inkeysa, Spain†.*
Harpagophytum procumbens (p.27·2).
Musculoskeletal and joint disorders.

Fitolinea *Ulrich, Ital.*
Bladderwrack (p.1554·1); senna (p.1212·2).
Constipation; obesity.

Fitosonno *Ulrich, Ital.*
Eschscholtzia californica; passion flower (p.1615·3); valerian (p.1643·1).
Insomnia.

Fitostimoline *Damor, Ital.*
Cream; medicated dressing; pessaries; vaginal wash: Wheat germ; phenoxyethanol (p.1122·2).
Burns; skin disorders; vaginal disorders; vascular disorders; wounds.
Injection: Wheat germ.
Burns; skin disorders; vascular disorders; wounds.

Fitostress *Ulrich, Ital.*
Ginseng (p.1584·2); kola (p.1645·1).
Tonic.

Fitsovelt *Arkochim, Spain.*
Black currant (p.1365·2); tea (p.1645·1).
Oedema.

Fittydent *Hoveler, Aust.*
Eucalyptus oil (p.1578·1); sage oil; clove oil (p.1565·2).
Mouth and throat inflammation; toothache.

Fixateur phospho-calcique *Bichsel, Switz.*
Calcium carbonate (p.1182·1).
Hyperphosphataemia.

Fixca *Lesvi, Spain.*
Ondansetron hydrochloride (p.1206·2).
Nausea and vomiting.

Fixim *Yamanouchi, Neth.*
Cefixime (p.165·3).
Bacterial infections.

Fixime *Merck, S.Afr.*
Cefixime (p.165·3).
Bacterial infections.

Fizz *Stanley, Canad.*
Multivitamin preparation.

Flacar *Schwabe, Ger.*
Betaine dihydrogen citrate (p.1553·2); sorbitol (p.1354·2).
Liver disorders.

Flagentyl *Specia, Fr.*
Secnidazole (p.592·3).
Protozoal infections.

Flagyl
Gerot, Aust.; Rhone-Poulenc Rorer, Austral.; Rhone-Poulenc Rorer, Belg.; Rhone-Poulenc Rorer, Canad.; Baxter, Canad.; Specia, Fr.; Rhone-Poulenc Rorer, Ger.; Rhone-Poulenc Rorer, Irl.; Pharmacia Upjohn, Ital.; Rhone-Poulenc Rorer, Neth.; Rhone-Poulenc Rorer, Norw.; Rhone-Poulenc Rorer, S.Afr.; Rhone-Poulenc Rorer, Spain; Rhone-Poulenc Rorer, Swed.; Rhone-Poulenc Rorer, Switz.; May & Baker, UK; Searle, USA.
Metronidazole (p.585·1), metronidazole benzoate (p.585·1), or metronidazole hydrochloride (p.585·1).
Anaerobic bacterial infections; protozoal infections.

Flagyl Compak
Rhone-Poulenc Rorer, Irl.; May & Baker, UK.
Combination preparation: Tablets, metronidazole (p.585·1); pessaries, nystatin (p.386·1).
Vaginitis.

Flagystatin *Rhone-Poulenc Rorer, Canad.*
Metronidazole (p.585·1); nystatin (p.386·1).
Vaginal trichomoniasis and candidiasis.

Flamaret *Xixia, S.Afr.*
Indomethacin (p.45·2).
Dysmenorrhoea; musculoskeletal and joint disorders.

Flamatak *Cox, UK.*
Diclofenac sodium (p.31·2).
Gout; inflammation; musculoskeletal, joint, peri-articular, and soft-tissue disorders; pain.

Flamatrol *Berk, UK.*
Piroxicam (p.80·2).
Inflammation; pain.

Flamazine
Smith & Nephew, Canad.; Smith & Nephew, Irl.; Smith & Nephew, Norw.; Smith & Nephew, S.Afr.; Smith & Nephew Pharmaceuticals, UK.
Silver sulphadiazine (p.247·3).
Infected wounds.

Flamazine C *Smith & Nephew, Canad.*
Silver sulphadiazine (p.247·3); chlorhexidine gluconate (p.1107·2).
Burns; ulcers; wounds.

Flamecid *Propan, S.Afr.*
Indomethacin (p.45·2).
Gout; musculoskeletal and joint disorders.

Flamilon *OM, Switz.†.*
Suxibuzone (p.88·2).
Inflammation.

Flaminase *Formenti, Ital.*
Promelase (p.1621·3).
Respiratory-tract disorders.

Flamlax *AGIPS, Ital.†.*
Carmellose (p.1471·2); phenolphthalein (p.1208·2).
Constipation.

Flammacerium
Solvay, Belg.; Solvay, Fr.; Solvay, Neth.
Silver sulphadiazine (p.247·3); cerous nitrate (p.1080·3).
Infected burns.

Flammazine
Solvay, Aust.; Solvay, Belg.; Solvay, Fr.; Solvay, Ger.; Solvay, Neth.; Duphar, Spain; Solvay, Switz.
Silver sulphadiazine (p.247·3).
Burns; infected wounds.

Flamon *Mepha, Switz.*
Verapamil hydrochloride (p.960·3).
Arrhythmias; hypertension; ischaemic heart disease.

Flamrase *Berk, UK.*
Diclofenac sodium (p.31·2).
Musculoskeletal, joint, peri-articular, and soft-tissue disorders; pain.

Flanamox
Wolff, Ger.; Proter, Ital.†.
Amoxycillin trihydrate (p.151·3); flucloxacillin sodium (p.209·2).
Bacterial infections.

Flanders Buttocks *Flanders, USA.*
Zinc oxide (p.1096·2); peru balsam (p.1617·2).
Nappy rash.

Flantadin *Lepetit, Ital.*
Deflazacort (p.1036·2).
Oral corticosteroid.

Flar *ISM, Ital.*
Streptococcus lactis; Lactobacillus acidophilus (p.1594·1); nicotinamide (p.1351·2).
Gastro-intestinal disorders.

Flarex
Alcon, Aust.; Alcon, Austral.; Alcon, Canad.; Alcon, Ital.; Alcon, Neth.†; Alcon, Switz.; Alcon, USA.
Fluorometholone acetate (p.1042·1).
Inflammatory eye disorders.

Flatoril *Almirall, Spain.*
Clebopride malate (p.1188·2); simethicone (p.1213·1).
Dyspepsia; gastro-oesophageal reflux; hiatus hernia.

Flatulex
Note. This name is used for preparations of different composition.
Globopharm, Switz.
Chewable tablets: Simethicone (p.1213·1); caraway oil (p.1559·3); fennel oil (p.1579·2); peppermint oil (p.1208·1).
Adjunct prior to gastro-intestinal examination; flatulence.

Globopharm, Switz.; Dayton, USA.
Oral drops: Simethicone (p.1213·1).
Adjunct prior to gastro-intestinal examination; flatulence.

Dayton, USA.
Tablets: Simethicone (p.1213·1); activated charcoal (p.972·2).
Flatulence.

Flatus-Pillen N Andreae *Kanoldt, Ger.†.*
Rhubarb (p.1212·1); aloes (p.1177·1); caraway oil (p.1559·3); fennel oil (p.1579·2); peppermint oil (p.1208·1).
Gastro-intestinal disorders.

Flavamed Halstabletten *Berlin-Chemie, Ger.*
Benzocaine (p.1286·2).
Hoarseness; sore throat.

Flavamed Hustentabletten, Husten-Heissgetrank, Hustensaft, Hustentropfen, and Husten-Retardkapseln *Berlin-Chemie, Ger.†.*
Ambroxol hydrochloride (p.1054·3).
Bronchopulmonary disorders associated with thickened secretions.

Flavan *Pharmafarm, Fr.*
Leucocianidol (p.1580·2).
Peripheral vascular disorders.

Flavangin *Streuli, Switz.*
Ethacridine lactate (p.1098·3); cetylpyridinium chloride (p.1106·2); lignocaine hydrochloride (p.1293·2); menthol (p.1600·2).
Mouth and throat disorders.

Flavettes *Parke, Davis, Austral.†.*
Ascorbic acid (p.1365·2).

Flaviastase *Iphym, Fr.*
Enzymes derived from Aspergillus.
Digestive disorders.

Flavigel *Solvay, Spain†.*
Dried aluminium hydroxide (p.1177·3); magnesium hydroxide (p.1198·2); simethicone (p.1213·1).
Gastro-intestinal hyperacidity and flatulence.

Flavis *Pulitzer, Ital.*
Piracetam (p.1619·1).
Mental function impairment.

Flavobetasi *Bruco, Ital.†.*
Cocarboxylase (p.1361·2); riboflavine (p.1362·1); nicotinamide (p.1351·2); sodium citrate (p.1153·2).

Flavone 500 *Ecobi, Ital.*
Ascorbic acid (p.1365·2); hesperidin (p.1580·2).

Flavonoid C *Vita Glow, Austral.†.*
Calcium ascorbate (p.1365·2); bioflavonoids (p.1580·1); hesperidin (p.1580·2); rutin (p.1580·2).
Cold symptoms; hypersensitivity reactions; peripheral vascular disorders; vitamin C deficiency.

Flavonoid Complex *Neo-Life, Austral.*
Cranberry; kale; green tea; red beetroot; mixed berry; oregon grape; grape; orange extract; lemon extract; grapefruit (p.1580·1).
Flavonoid supplement.

Flavons
Note. This name is used for preparations of different composition.
Eagle, Austral.
Ascorbic acid (p.1365·2); sodium ascorbate (p.1365·2); calcium ascorbate (p.1365·2); hesperidin (p.1580·2); bioflavonoids (p.1580·1); rutin (p.1580·2); rose hips (p.1365·2); boneset; echinacea (p.1574·2); yarrow (p.1542·2).
Minor wounds; tonic.
Freeda, USA.
Citrus bioflavonoids complex (p.1580·1); hesperidin (p.1580·2).
Capillary bleeding.

Flavoquine *Roussel, Fr.*
Amodiaquine hydrochloride (p.424·3).
Malaria.

Flavorcee *Hudson, USA.*
Ascorbic acid (p.1365·2).
Scurvy; vitamin C deficiency.

Flavorola C *Lifeplan, UK.*
Vitamin C (p.1365·2); bioflavonoids (p.1580·1).
Nutritional supplement.

Flavovenyl *Plan, Switz.*
Capsules; oral drops: Bioflavonoids (p.1580·1); hesperidin methyl chalcone (p.1580·2); esculoside (p.1543·3).
Ointment: Bioflavonoids (p.1580·1); hesperidin methyl chalcone (p.1580·2); esculoside (p.1543·3); menthol (p.1600·2).
Peripheral vascular disorders.

Flavovite *Covan, S.Afr.†.*
Multivitamin and mineral preparation.
Hepatic disorders; Ménière's disease.

Flavo-Zinc *Solgar, UK.*
Zinc gluconate (p.1373·2); zinc citrate.
Dietary supplement.

Flavozym *Lagap, Ital.†.*
Enzymes from *Aspergillus flavus.*
Dyspepsia; hepatic and pancreatic insufficiency.

Flaxedil
Rhone-Poulenc Rorer, Austral.; Rhone-Poulenc Rorer, Belg.†; Rhone-Poulenc Rorer, Canad.; Specia, Fr.†; Rhone-Poulenc Rorer, Neth.; Rhone-Poulenc Rorer, S.Afr.†; Concord, UK; Davis & Geck, USA†.
Gallamine triethiodide (p.1315·2).
Competitive neuromuscular blocker.

Flebeparoid *Bruco, Ital.†.*
A heparinoid (p.882·3).
Phlebitis; thrombophlebitis.

Flebeside *Jorba, Spain.*
Carbazochrome (p.714·1); troxerutin (p.1580·2).
Vascular disorders.

Flebil *Molteni, Ital.*
Troxerutin (p.1580·2).
Peripheral vascular disorders.

Flebo Stop *Inexfa, Spain.*
Bromelains (p.1555·1); esculoside (p.1543·3); etofylline (p.753·1); hydrochlorothiazide (p.885·2).
Oedema; vascular disorders.

Flebobag Fisio *Grifols, Spain.*
Sodium chloride infusion (p.1162·2).
Fluid and electrolyte depletion; hypovolaemia.

Flebobag Glucosal *Grifols, Spain.*
Sodium chloride infusion (p.1162·2) with glucose (p.1343·3).
Fluid and electrolyte depletion; hypovolaemia.

Flebocortid *Lepetit, Ital.*
Hydrocortisone sodium succinate (p.1044·1).
Parenteral corticosteroid.

Flebogamma
Note. This name is used for preparations of different composition.
IBP, Ital.†.
Heparin sodium (p.879·3); allantoin (p.1078·2).
Phlebitis; thrombophlebitis.
Grifols, Spain.
A normal immunoglobulin (p.1522·1).
Hypogammaglobulinaemia; idiopathic thrombocytopenic purpura.

Fleboplast Fisio *Grifols, Spain.*
Sodium chloride infusion (p.1162·2).
Fluid and electrolyte depletion; hypovolaemia.

Fleboplast Glucosal *Grifols, Spain.*
Sodium chloride infusion (p.1162·2) with glucose (p.1343·3).
Fluid and electrolyte depletion; hypovolaemia.

Fleboplast Plurisal *Grifols, Spain.*
Electrolyte infusion (p.1147·1) with sodium lactate (p.1153·2).
Fluid and electrolyte depletion; hypovolaemia.

Flebosan *Dukron, Ital.†.*
Tribenoside (p.1638·3).
Haemorrhoids; thrombophlebitis.

Fleboside *Synthelabo, Ital.*
Troxerutin (p.1580·2); carbazochrome (p.714·1).
Capillary fragility.

Flebosmil *Socopharm, Fr.*
Diosmin (p.1580·1).
Peripheral vascular disorders.

Flebostasin
Note. This name is used for preparations of different composition.
Luitpold, Ital.
Aesculus (p.1543·3).
Chronic venous insufficiency.
Alfarma, Spain.
Aescin (p.1543·3).
Oedema; peripheral vascular disorders.

Flebs *Pierre Fabre, Ital.*
Heparin sodium (p.879·3); a heparinoid (p.882·3).
Haemorrhoids; phlebitis; soft-tissue injury; thrombophlebitis.

Flecaine *3M, Fr.*
Flecainide acetate (p.868·3).
Arrhythmias.

Flectadol *Sanofi Winthrop, Ital.*
Lysine aspirin (p.50·3).
Cold symptoms; fever; musculoskeletal and joint disorders; pain.

Flectomas *Benvegna, Ital.†.*
Carisoprodol (p.1312·3); isophthalolic acid.
Musculoskeletal and joint disorders.

Flector
Genevrier, Fr.; IBSA, Ital.; IBSA, Switz.
Diclofenac epolamine (p.32·3) or diclofenac sodium (p.31·2).
Inflammation; musculoskeletal, joint, peri-articular, and soft-tissue disorders; pain.

Fleet *De Witt, Irl.*
Monobasic sodium phosphate (p.1159·3); dibasic sodium phosphate (p.1159·3).
Bowel evacuation; constipation.

Fleet Babylax *Fleet, USA.*
Glycerol (p.1585·2).
Constipation in children.

Fleet Bagenema *Fleet, USA.*
Liquid castile soap (p.1468·2).

Fleet Bisacodyl *Fleet, USA.*
Bisacodyl (p.1179·3).
Bowel evacuation; constipation.

Fleet Castor Oil Emulsion *Fleet, USA†.*
Castor oil (p.1560·2).
Constipation.

Fleet Enema
Wolfs, Belg.; Frosst, Canad.; Fleet, USA.
Dibasic sodium phosphate (p.1159·3); monobasic sodium phosphate (p.1159·3).
Bowel evacuation; constipation.

Fleet Enema Mineral Oil *Frosst, Canad.*
Liquid paraffin (p.1382·1).
Bowel evacuation; constipation.

Fleet Klysma *Fleet, Neth.†.*
Monobasic sodium phosphate (p.1159·3).
Bowel evacuation.

Fleet Laxative
Fleet, Austral.; Fleet, USA.
Bisacodyl (p.1179·3).
Bowel evacuation; constipation.

Fleet Medicated Pads *Fleet, USA.*
Hamamelis water (p.1587·1); alcohol; glycerol.
Anorectal disorders.

Fleet Micro *Ferring, Swed.*
Sodium citrate (p.1153·2); sodium lauryl sulphoacetate (p.1468·3).
Constipation.

Fleet Micro-Enema *De Witt, UK.*
Sodium citrate (p.1153·2); sodium lauryl sulphoacetate (p.1468·3).
Bowel evacuation; constipation.

Fleet Pain Relief *Fleet, USA.*
Pramoxine hydrochloride (p.1298·2).
Anorectal disorders.

Fleet Phospho-Soda
Fleet, Austral.; Wolfs, Belg.; Frosst, Canad.; De Witt, UK; Fleet, USA.
Monobasic sodium phosphate (p.1159·3); dibasic sodium phosphate (p.1159·3).
Bowel evacuation; constipation.

Fleet Prep Kit No. 1 *Fleet, USA.*
Combination pack: Fleet Phospho-Soda; Fleet Bisacodyl Tablets, 4 tablets; Fleet Bisacodyl Suppositories, 1 suppository.
Bowel evacuation.

Fleet Prep Kit No. 2 *Fleet, USA.*
Combination pack: Fleet Phospho-Soda; Fleet Bisacodyl Tablets, 4 tablets; Fleet Bagenema, 1 enema.
Bowel evacuation.

Fleet Prep Kit No. 3 *Fleet, USA.*
Combination pack: Fleet Phospho-Soda; Fleet Bisacodyl Tablets, 4 tablets; Fleet Bisacodyl Enema.
Bowel evacuation.

Fleet Prep Kit No. 4 *Fleet, USA.*
Combination pack: Fleet Magnesium Citrate (p.1198·2); Fleet Bisacodyl Tablets, 4 tablets; Fleet Bisacodyl Suppositories, 1 suppository.
Bowel evacuation.

Fleet Prep Kit No. 5 *Fleet, USA.*
Combination pack: Fleet Magnesium Citrate (p.1198·2); Fleet Bisacodyl Tablets, 4 tablets; Fleet Bagenema, 1 enema.
Bowel evacuation.

Fleet Prep Kit No. 6 *Fleet, USA.*
Combination pack: Fleet Magnesium Citrate (p.1198·2); Fleet Bisacodyl Tablets, 4 tablets; Fleet Bisacodyl Enema.
Bowel evacuation.

Fleet Ready-to-Use
Fleet, Austral.; De Witt, UK.
Monobasic sodium phosphate (p.1159·3); dibasic sodium phosphate (p.1159·3).
Bowel evacuation; constipation.

Fleet Relief *Fleet, USA†.*
Pramoxine hydrochloride (p.1298·2).
Anorectal pain and pruritus; haemorrhoids.

Flemex *Parke, Davis, S.Afr.*
Carbocisteine (p.1056·3).
Respiratory-tract disorders.

Flemeze *Parke, Davis, S.Afr.*
Orciprenaline sulphate (p.756·3); bromhexine hydrochloride (p.1055·3).
Coughs.

Flemgo *Schwulst, S.Afr.*
Carbocisteine (p.1056·3).
Respiratory-tract disorders.

Flemlite *Garec, S.Afr.*
Carbocisteine (p.1056·3).
Respiratory-tract disorders.

Flemoxin
Yamanouchi, Belg.; Yamanouchi, Neth.; Yamanouchi, Swed.; Yamanouchi, Switz.; Yamanouchi, UK†.
Amoxycillin (p.151·3), amoxycillin sodium (p.151·3), or amoxycillin trihydrate (p.151·3).
Bacterial infections.

Flemoxine *Yamanouchi, Fr.*
Amoxycillin trihydrate (p.151·3).
Bacterial infections.

Flemun *Intermuti, Ger.*
Sitosterol (p.1279·3).
Rheumatic disorders.

Flenin *Schuck, Ger.*
Homoeopathic preparation.

Flerudin *Janssen-Cilag, Spain.*
Flunarizine hydrochloride (p.411·1).
Ménière's disease; migraine; motion sickness; vestibular disorders.

Fletagex *Sterling Midy, Fr.†.*
Cod-liver oil (p.1337·3); vitamin A (p.1358·1).
Skin disorders.

Fletanol *Sante Naturelle, Canad.*
Vitamin A and vitamin D.

Fletchers Arachis Oil Retention Enema *Pharmax, UK.*
Arachis oil (p.1550·2).
Constipation.

Fletchers Castoria *Mentholatum, USA.*
Senna (p.1212·2).
Constipation.

Fletchers Childrens Laxative *Mentholatum, USA.*
Yellow phenolphthalein (p.1208·2).
Constipation.

Fletchers Enemette
Pharmax, Irl.; Pharmax, UK.
Docusate sodium (p.1189·3).
Bowel evacuation; constipation.

Fletchers Phosphate Enema
Pharmax, Irl.; Pharmax, UK.
Monobasic sodium phosphate (p.1159·3); dibasic sodium phosphate (p.1159·3).
Bowel evacuation; constipation.

Fletchers Sore Mouth Medicine *Nasmark, Canad.*
Alum (p.1547·1); potassium chlorate (p.1620·3).
Canker sores; denture irritation; herpes labialis.

Flexagen *Lennon, S.Afr.*
Diclofenac sodium (p.31·2).
Inflammation; musculoskeletal and joint disorders; pain.

Flexagil *Berenguer Infale, Spain.*
Carisoprodol (p.1312·3); propyphenazone (p.81·3).
Musculoskeletal spasms.

Flex-All *Chattem, Canad.*
Menthol (p.1600·2).
Muscle and joint pain.

Flex-all 454 *Chattem, USA.*
Menthol (p.1600·2); methyl salicylate (p.55·2).
Musculoskeletal pain and stiffness.

Flexaphen *Trimen, USA.*
Chlorzoxazone (p.1313·1); paracetamol (p.72·2).
Musculoskeletal pain.

Flexase *TAD, Ger.*
Piroxicam (p.80·2).
Gout; musculoskeletal and joint disorders.

Flex-Care
Alcon, Austral.†; Alcon, USA.
Range of solutions for contact lenses.

Flexen *Italfarmaco, Ital.*
Ketoprofen (p.48·2) or ketoprofen sodium (p.48·3).
Musculoskeletal, joint, and soft-tissue disorders.

Flexeril
Frosst, Canad.; Merck Sharp & Dohme, USA.
Cyclobenzaprine hydrochloride (p.1313·2).
Skeletal muscle spasm.

Flexfree *Whitehall, Belg.*
Felbinac (p.37·1).
Soft-tissue, peri-articular, and joint pain and inflammation.

Flexiban *Neopharmed, Ital.*
Cyclobenzaprine hydrochloride (p.1313·2).
Skeletal muscle spasm.

Flexical *Mead Johnson Nutritionals, UK†.*
Lactose- and gluten-free preparation for enteral nutrition.

Flexidin *Mundipharma, Aust.*
Indomethacin (p.45·2).
Gout; inflammation; musculoskeletal, joint, and periarticular disorders; oedema; pain.

Flexidol *Funk, Spain.*
Fepradinol hydrochloride (p.41·2).
Peri-articular disorders; soft-tissue disorders.

Flexidone *Poli, Ital.*
Carisoprodol (p.1312·3); propyphenazone (p.81·3).
Musculoskeletal and joint disorders.

Flexilat *Europharm, S.Afr.†.*
A heparinoid (p.882·3); flufenamic acid (p.41·3); glycol monosalicylate (p.43·1).
Musculoskeletal and joint disorders.

Flexin Continus
Napp, Irl.; Napp, UK.
Indomethacin (p.45·2).
Gout; inflammation; musculoskeletal, joint, and periarticular disorders; pain.

Flexinutryl *Clintec-Sopharga, Fr.†.*
Preparation for enteral nutrition.

Flexipyrin *Edmond Pharma, Ital.†.*
Suppositories: Amidopyrine (p.15·2); chlormezanone (p.648·3).
Tablets: Propyphenazone (p.81·3); chlormezanone (p.648·3).
Musculoskeletal and joint disorders.

Flexium *Rhone-Poulenc Rorer, Belg.*
Etofenamate (p.36·3).
Lumbar spondylosis; peri-articular disorders; soft-tissue injury.

Flexocutan N *Nycomed, Ger.†.*
Flufenamic acid (p.41·3); glycol salicylate (p.43·1); benzyl nicotinate (p.22·1).
Bruising; muscle and joint disorders; neuralgia.

Flexoject *Mayrand, USA.*
Orphenadrine citrate (p.465·2).
Musculoskeletal pain.

Flexon *Keene, USA.*
Orphenadrine citrate (p.465·2).
Musculoskeletal pain.

Flexotard *Dexcel, UK.*
Diclofenac sodium (p.31·2).
Gout; inflammation; musculoskeletal, joint, peri-articular, and soft-tissue disorders; pain.

Flextra *Poly, USA.*
Paracetamol (p.72·2); phenyltoloxamine citrate (p.416·1).
Pain.

Flexurat
Note. This name is used for preparations of different composition.
Nycomed, Aust.
Suprarenal cortex (p.1050·1); pentosan polysulphate sodium (p.928·1).
Peri-articular, and soft-tissue disorders.
Truw, Ger.
Bovine suprarenal cortex (p.1050·1); diethylamine salamidacetate (p.82·3); pentosan polysulphate sodium (p.928·1).
Joint and soft tissue disorders.

Flicum *Esteve, Spain.*
Flubendazole (p.100·3).
Ascariasis; enterobiasis; hookworm infections; trichuriasis.

Flint *Togal, Ger.*
Poly(butylmethacrylate, methylmethacrylate) (p.1603·2).
Wounds.

Flintstones
Bayer, Canad.; Miles Consumer Healthcare, USA.
A range of vitamin preparations.

Flixonase
Glaxo Wellcome, Aust.; Allen & Hanburys, Irl.; Glaxo Wellcome, Ital.; Glaxo Wellcome, Neth.; Allen & Hanburys, S.Afr.; Allen & Hanburys, UK.
Fluticasone propionate (p.1042·3).
Allergic rhinitis.

Flixotide
Glaxo Wellcome, Aust.; Allen & Hanburys, Austral.; Glaxo Wellcome, Belg.; Allen & Hanburys, Irl.; Glaxo Wellcome, Ital.; Glaxo Wellcome, Neth.; Allen & Hanburys, S.Afr.; Allen & Hanburys, UK.
Fluticasone propionate (p.1042·3).
Asthma.

Flobacin *Sigma-Tau, Ital.*
Ofloxacin (p.233·3).
Bacterial infections.

Flociprin *Ibi, Ital.*
Ciprofloxacin hydrochloride (p.185·3) or ciprofloxacin lactate (p.185·3).
Bacterial infections.

Flo-Coat *Lafayette, USA.*
Barium sulphate (p.1003·1).
Contrast medium for gastro-intestinal radiography.

Flodermol *Juventus, Spain.*
Fluocinolone acetonide (p.1041·1) gramicidin (p.215·2); neomycin sulphate (p.229·2).
Infected skin disorders.

Flodil *Astra, Fr.*
Felodipine (p.867·3).
Angina pectoris; hypertension.

Flodol *Uno, Ital.*
Piroxicam (p.80·2).
Musculoskeletal and joint disorders.

Flogaton *Radiumfarma, Ital.†.*
Benzydamine hydrochloride (p.21·3).
Fever; inflammation; pain.

Flogecyl *Wild, Switz.*
Aescin beta (p.1543·3); carrageenan (p.1471·3).
Mouth disorders.

Flogencyl *Parke, Davis, Fr.*
Aescin (p.1543·3).
Mouth ulcers.

Flogene *Polifarma, Ital.*
Fentiazac (p.41·1) or fentiazac calcium (p.41·1).
Fever; inflammation; pain.

Floginax *Teofarma, Ital.*
Naproxen (p.61·2).
Musculoskeletal and joint disorders; pain.

Flogobene *Upsamedica, Ital.*
Piroxicam (p.80·2).
Musculoskeletal and joint disorders.

Flogocid
Note. This name is used for preparations of different composition.
Salus, Aust.†; Continental Pharma, Switz.
Bufexamac (p.22·2).
Skin disorders.

Continental Pharma, Belg.
Bufexamac (p.22·2); neomycin sulphate (p.229·2); nystatin (p.386·1).
Infected skin disorders.

Flogocid NN *Continental Pharma, Switz.*
Bufexamac (p.22·2); nystatin (p.386·1); neomycin sulphate (p.229·2).
Infected skin disorders.

Flogofenac *Ecobi, Ital.*
Diclofenac diethylamine (p.31·2) or diclofenac sodium (p.31·2).
Musculoskeletal, joint, and soft-tissue disorders.

Flogogin *Tosi, Ital.*
Tablets; injection; suppositories: Naproxen sodium (p.61·2).
Lignocaine hydrochloride (p.1293·2) and lignocaine (p.1293·2) are included in the intramuscular injection to alleviate the pain of injection.
Topical gel: Naproxen sodium (p.61·2); a heparinoid (p.882·3).
Inflammation; musculoskeletal and joint disorders; pain.

Flogoprofen *Wasserman, Spain.*
Etofenamate (p.36·3).
Pain; peri-articular disorders.

Flogosone *Difa, Ital.†.*
Hydrocortisone acetate (p.1043·3); aminobenzoic acid (p.1486·3).
Inflammatory eye disorders.

Flogoter *Estedi, Spain.*
Indomethacin (p.45·2).
Gout; inflammation; musculoskeletal and joint disorders; pain; peri-articular disorders.

Flogotisol *Zambon, Ital.*
Thiamphenicol sodium glycinate isophthalolate (p.263·1).
Bacterial infections.

Flogozen *Valeas, Ital.*
Imidazole salicylate (p.45·2).
Fever; otorhinolaryngeal inflammation.

Flogozym *SPA, Ital.†.*
Trypsin (p.1640·1); chymotrypsin (p.1563·2).
Inflammation.

Flolan
Glaxo Wellcome, Aust.; Wellcome, Irl.; Glaxo Wellcome, Ital.; Glaxo Wellcome, Neth.; Wellcome, Spain; Wellcome, UK.
Epoprostenol sodium (p.1417·1).
Thrombosis prophylaxis during renal dialysis.

Flolid *CT, Ital.*
Nimesulide (p.63·2).
Fever; inflammation; pain.

Flomax
Note. This name is used for preparations of different composition.
Chiesi, Ital.
Morniflumate (p.56·1).
Fever; inflammation; pain.

Yamanouchi, UK; Boehringer Ingelheim, USA.
Tamsulosin hydrochloride (p.951·2).
Benign prostatic hyperplasia.

Flomed *Pulitzer, Ital.*
Buflomedil hydrochloride (p.834·2).
Cerebral and peripheral vascular disorders.

Flonase
Glaxo Wellcome, Canad.; Glaxo Wellcome, USA.
Fluticasone propionate (p.1042·3).
Allergic rhinitis.

Flopen *CSL, Austral.*
Flucloxacillin magnesium (p.209·1) or flucloxacillin sodium (p.209·2).
Gram-positive coccal infections.

Flora *Terme di Salsomaggiore, Ital.†.*
Sodium bicarbonate; sodium borate; sodium bromide; sodium iodide; sodium chloride; lithium chloride; thymol.
Feminine hygiene.

Floracit-Gummetten *Laves, Ger.†.*
Sweet whey concentrate.
Halitosis; inflammatory disorders of the oropharynx.

Floradix Krauterblut *Salushaus, Ger.*
Urtica; couch-grass; thall. rhodophyceae; crataegus; centaury; rose fruit; dried yeast; ferrous gluconate; vitamins.
Tonic.

Floradix Krauterblut-S-Saft *Salushaus, Ger.*
Thall. macrocystis pyrifera; urtica; couch-grass; achillea; fennel; rad. dauc. carot.; wheat-germ; dried bitter-orange peel; angelica; equisetum; juniper; ferrous gluconate; vitamins; rose fruit.
Tonic.

Floradix Maskam *Duopharm, Ger.*
Frangula bark (p.1193·2); rhubarb (p.1212·1); senna (p.1212·2); fennel (p.1579·1).
Constipation.

Floradix Multipretten *Salushaus, Ger.*
Caraway (p.1559·3); caraway oil (p.1559·3); fennel (p.1579·1); fennel oil (p.1579·2); anise oil (p.1550·1); coriander (p.1567·3); coriander oil (p.1567·3); peppermint leaf (p.1208·1); peppermint oil (p.1208·1); absinthium (p.1541·1); achillea (p.1542·2); imperatoria root; bromelains (p.1555·1); enzymes from *Aspergillus oryzae*.
Gastro-intestinal disorders.

Floralac *Laevosan, Aust.*
Lactitol monohydrate (p.1195·2).
Constipation; hepatic encephalopathy.

Floralax *Flora, Canad.*
Ispaghula husk (p.1194·2).

Floralaxative *Lalco, Canad.*
Buckthorn (p.1182·1); senna (p.1212·2).

Floran Effervescent *McGloin, Austral.†.*
Sodium fluoride (p.742·1).
Dental caries prophylaxis.

Floraquin
Note. This name is used for preparations of different composition.
Searle, Austral.
Di-iodohydroxyquinoline (p.581·1); boric acid (p.1554·2); phosphoric acid (p.1618·2).
Vaginal infections.

Searle, S.Afr.†.
Di-iodohydroxyquinoline (p.581·1).
Vaginal infections.

Searle, Spain†.
Di-iodohydroxyquinoline (p.581·1); boric acid (p.1554·2).
Vulvovaginal candidiasis; vulvovaginal trichomoniasis.

Florelax *Sanofi Winthrop, Ital.*
Dried yeast (p.1373·1); lactic-acid-producing organisms (p.1594·1); chamomile (p.1561·2); angelica; valerian (p.1643·1); peppermint leaf (p.1208·1); caraway (p.1559·3); vitamin B substances.
Gastro-intestinal disorders.

Florerbe Balsamica *Bonomelli, Ital.†.*
Thyme (p.1636·3); eucalyptus (p.1578·1); liquorice (p.1197·1); peppermint leaf (p.1208·1).
Respiratory-tract disorders.

Florerbe Calmante *Bonomelli, Ital.†.*
Valerian (p.1643·1); crataegus (p.1568·2); passion flower (p.1615·3); peppermint leaf (p.1208·1); liquorice (p.1197·1).
Sedative.

Florerbe Digestiva *Bonomelli, Ital.†.*
Boldo (p.1554·1); chamomile (p.1561·2); rhubarb (p.1212·1); gentian (p.1583·3); rosemary.
Digestive-system disorders.

Florerbe Lassativa *Bonomelli, Ital.*
Senna (p.1212·2); boldo (p.1554·1); cynara (p.1569·2); aniseed (p.1549·3); liquorice (p.1197·1).
Constipation.

Floresse *Roche Consumer, UK.*
Borage oil (p.1582·1) with or without vitamins.

Floria "Vitamin F"-Salbe *Cefak, Ger.†.*
Ethyl linoleate.
Skin disorders.

Floriabene *Cefak, Ger.*
Ethyl linoleate.
Skin disorders.

Florical *Mericon, USA.*
Calcium carbonate (p.1182·1); sodium fluoride (p.742·1).
Dietary supplement.

Florida Sunburn Relief *Pharmacel, USA.*
Benzyl alcohol (p.1103·3); phenol (p.1121·2); camphor (p.1557·2); menthol (p.1600·2).

Florid-F *Mochida, Jpn†.*
Miconazole (p.384·3).
Fungal infections.

Floridin *Coli, Ital.†.*
Cephaloridine (p.179·1).
Bacterial infections.

Florigien *Schering, Ital.*
Nonoxinol 9 (p.1326·1); phenoxyethanol (p.1122·2); sodium lauryl sulphate (p.1468·3); thymol (p.1127·1).
Vaginal infections.

Florigoz *Guigoz, Ital.†.*
A range of gluten-free foods.

Florinef
Bristol-Myers Squibb, Austral.; Roberts, Canad.; Bristol-Myers Squibb, Irl.; Bristol-Myers Squibb, Neth.; Bristol-Myers Squibb, Norw.; Bristol-Myers Squibb, S.Afr.; Bristol-Myers Squibb, Swed.; Bristol-Myers Squibb, Switz.; Squibb, UK; Apothecon, USA.
Fludrocortisone acetate (p.1040·1).
Adrenocortical insufficiency; congenital adrenal hyperplasia.

Florisan N *Boehringer Ingelheim, Ger.*
Bisacodyl (p.1179·3).
Constipation.

Florocycline *SmithKline Beecham, Fr.*
Tetracycline hydrochloride (p.259·1).
Bacterial infections.

Florone
Pharmacia Upjohn, Canad.; Basotherm, Ger.; Dermik, USA.
Diflorasone diacetate (p.1039·3).
Skin disorders.

Floropryl *Merck Sharp & Dohme, USA.*
Dyflos (p.1391·3).
Open-angle glaucoma; strabismus.

Florvite *Everett, USA.*
A range of vitamin and fluoride (p.742·1) preparations with or without minerals.
Dental caries prophylaxis; dietary supplement.

Flosa *Merckle, Ger.*
Ispaghula husk (p.1194·2).
Constipation; stool softener.

Flosine *Gastropharm, Ger.*
Ispaghula husk (p.1194·2).
Constipation; stool softener.

Flossac *Caber, Ital.*
Norfloxacin (p.233·1).
Bacterial urinary-tract infections.

Flotrin *Abbott, Ger.*
Terazosin hydrochloride (p.952·1).
Benign prostatic hyperplasia.

Flovent
Glaxo Wellcome, Canad.; Glaxo Wellcome, USA.
Fluticasone propionate (p.1042·3).
Asthma.

Flowmega *Lifeplan, UK.*
Omega-3 marine triglycerides (p.1276·1).

Floxal
Riel, Aust.; Mann, Ger.; Novopharma, Switz.
Ofloxacin (p.233·3).
Bacterial eye infections.

Floxalin *Salus, Ital.*
Naproxen sodium (p.61·2).
Musculoskeletal and joint disorders; pain.

Floxapen
SmithKline Beecham, Aust.; SmithKline Beecham, Austral.; Bencard, Belg.; SmithKline Beecham, Irl.; SmithKline Beecham, Neth.; SmithKline Beecham, S.Afr.; SmithKline Beecham, Switz.; Beecham Research, UK.
Flucloxacillin magnesium (p.209·1) or flucloxacillin sodium (p.209·2).
Bacterial infections.

Floxin
Janssen-Ortho, Canad.; McNeil Pharmaceutical, USA; Daiichi, USA.
Ofloxacin (p.233·3).
Bacterial infections.

Floxyfral
Solvay, Aust.; Solvay, Belg.; Solvay, Fr.; Solvay, Switz.
Fluvoxamine maleate (p.288·3).
Depression; obsessive-compulsive disorder.

Flu-21 *Uno, Ital.*
Fluocinonide (p.1041·2).
Skin disorders.

Flu, Cold & Cough Medicine *Major, USA.*
Chlorpheniramine maleate (p.405·1); dextromethorphan hydrobromide (p.1057·3); paracetamol (p.72·2); pseudoephedrine hydrochloride (p.1068·3).
Coughs and cold symptoms.

Flu & Fever Relief *Brauer, Austral.*
Homoeopathic preparation.

Fluad *Chiron, Ital.*
An influenza vaccine (p.1515·2).
Active immunisation.

Flu-Amp *Generics, UK.*
Ampicillin trihydrate (p.153·2); flucloxacillin sodium (p.209·2).
These ingredients can be described by the British Approved Name Co-fluampicil.
Bacterial infections.

Fluanxol
Lundbeck, Aust.; Fisons, Austral.; Lundbeck, Belg.; Lundbeck, Canad.; Lundbeck, Fr.; Bayer, Ger.; Lundbeck, Irl.; Lundbeck, Neth.; Lundbeck, Norw.; Lundbeck, S.Afr.; Lundbeck, Swed.; Lundbeck, Switz.; Lundbeck, UK.
Flupenthixol (p.671·1), flupenthixol decanoate (p.670·3), or flupenthixol hydrochloride (p.670·3).
Alcohol or opioid withdrawal syndromes; depression; neuroses; psychoses.

Fluarix
SmithKline Beecham, Fr.; SmithKline Beecham, Irl.; SmithKline Beecham, Ital.; SmithKline Beecham, Neth.; SmithKline Beecham, Norw.; Smith Kline & French, Spain; SmithKline Beecham, Swed.; SmithKline Beecham, Switz.; SmithKline Beecham, UK.
An inactivated influenza vaccine (split virion) (p.1515·2).
Active immunisation.

Fluaton *Allergan, Ital.*
Fluorometholone (p.1042·1).
Inflammatory eye disorders.

Flubason
Hoechst Marion Roussel, Ital.; Hoechst, Spain.
Desoxymethasone (p.1037·1).
Skin disorders.

Flubenil *Formenti, Ital.*
Ibuprofen guaiacol (p.44·3).
Cold symptoms; fever; pain.

Flubilar *Byk, Fr.*
Sodium methylcamphorate.
Constipation; digestive disorders.

Flubiotic *Pharmazam, Spain.*
Acetylcysteine (p.1052·3); amoxycillin trihydrate (p.151·3).
Respiratory-tract infections.

Flucil *Rhone-Poulenc Rorer, Austral.*
Flucloxacillin sodium (p.209·2).
Gram-positive coccal infections.

Flucillin
Pinewood, Irl.; Rolab, S.Afr.
Flucloxacillin sodium (p.209·2).
Bacterial infections.

Flucinar *Medphano, Ger.*
Fluocinolone acetonide (p.1041·1).
Skin disorders.

Flucinome *Essex, Switz.*
Flutamide (p.537·1).
Prostatic cancer.

Fluclomix *Ashbourne, UK.*
Flucloxacillin sodium (p.209·2).
Bacterial infections.

Fluclon *Clonmel, Irl.*
Flucloxacillin sodium (p.209·2).
Gram-positive bacterial infections.

Fluclox *Wyeth-Ayerst, Canad.†.*
Flucloxacillin sodium (p.209·2).
Staphylococcal infections.

Flucloxin *Rivopharm, Switz.*
Flucloxacillin sodium (p.209·2).
Gram-positive bacterial infections.

Flucol *Apotex, S.Afr.; Garec, S.Afr.*
Paracetamol (p.72·2); codeine phosphate (p.26·1); caffeine (p.749·3); mepyramine maleate (p.414·1); phenylephrine hydrochloride (p.1066·2).
Cold and influenza symptoms; sinusitis.

Flucon
Alcon, Austral.; Alcon, Belg.; Alcon, Fr.; Alcon, Neth.†; Alcon, S.Afr.; Alcon, Switz.†.
Fluorometholone (p.1042·1).
Inflammatory eye disorders.

Flu-Cortanest *Piam, Ital.*
Diflucortolone valerate (p.1039·3).
Burns; insect stings; skin disorders.

Fluctin *Lilly, Ger.*
Fluoxetine hydrochloride (p.284·1).
Bulimia; depression.

Fluctine
Lilly, Aust.; Lilly, Switz.
Fluoxetine hydrochloride (p.284·1).
Bulimia nervosa; depression; obsessive-compulsive disorder.

Fludactil *Garec, S.Afr.*
Triprolidine hydrochloride (p.420·3); pseudoephedrine hydrochloride (p.1068·3).
Cold and influenza symptoms.

Fludactil Co *Garec, S.Afr.*
Triprolidine hydrochloride (p.420·3); pseudoephedrine hydrochloride (p.1068·3); codeine phosphate (p.26·1).
Coughs.

Fludactil Expectorant *Garec, S.Afr.*
Triprolidine hydrochloride (p.420·3); pseudoephedrine hydrochloride (p.1068·3); guaiphenesin (p.1061·3).
Coughs.

Fludara
Schering, Austral.; Schering, Belg.; Berlex, Canad.; Schering, Fr.; Schering, Ital.; Schering, Neth.; Schering, Swed.; Schering, Switz.; Schering, UK; Berlex, USA.
Fludarabine phosphate (p.534·1) or fludarabine phosphate sodium (p.534·2).
Chronic lymphocytic leukaemia.

Fludarene *Merck Sharp & Dohme, Ital.*
Chromocarb diethylamine (p.1562·3).
Capillary fragility.

Fludecate *Intramed, S.Afr.*
Fluphenazine decanoate (p.671·2).
Psychoses.

Fludent *Dumex-Alpharma, Swed.*
Sodium fluoride (p.742·1).
Dental caries prophylaxis.

Fludestrin *Bristol-Myers Squibb, Ger.*
Testolactone (p.566·1).
Breast cancer.

Fludeten *Alter, Spain.*
Paracetamol (p.72·2); codeine phosphate (p.26·1).
Pain.

Fludex
Servier, Aust.; Servier, Belg.; Eutherapie, Fr.; Servier, Neth.; Servier, Switz.
Indapamide (p.890·2).
Hypertension.

Fludilat
Thiemann, Ger.; Organon, Switz.
Bencyclane fumarate (p.827·3).
Vascular disorders.

Fluditec *Innotech, Fr.*
Carbocisteine (p.1056·3).
Respiratory-tract congestion.

Fludixan *Doms-Adrian, Fr.†.*
Ethyl cysteine hydrochloride (p.1061·1).
Viscous bronchial secretions.

Fludren *Diafarm, Spain.*
Dextromethorphan hydrobromide (p.1057·3); ephedrine hydrochloride (p.1059·3); chlorpheniramine maleate (p.405·1).
Coughs.

Fludronef *Iquinosa, Spain.*
Fludrocortisone acetate (p.1040·1); gramicidin (p.215·2); neomycin sulphate (p.229·2).
Eye disorders; infected skin disorders.

Fluend
Note. This name is used for preparations of different composition.
Herbaline, Ital.
Silver birch (p.1553·3); salix (p.82·3); thyme (p.1636·3); tilia (p.1637·3); cynara (p.1569·2); rose fruit (p.1365·2); citrus aurantium.
Cold and influenza symptoms.

Genpharm, S.Afr.†.
Diphenhydramine hydrochloride (p.409·1); paracetamol (p.72·2); phenylephrine hydrochloride (p.1066·2); ascorbic acid (p.1365·2).
Cold symptoms.

Fluental Corvi, Ital.
Sobrerol (p.1069·3); paracetamol (p.72·2).
Respiratory disorders.

Fluenzen Ecupharma, Ital.
Imidazole salicylate (p.45·2).
Fever; otorhinolaryngeal inflammation.

Flugeral Italfarmaco, Ital.
Flunarizine hydrochloride (p.411·1).
Migraine; vertigo.

Flui-Amoxicillin Zambon, Ger.
Amoxycillin trihydrate (p.151·3).
Bacterial infections.

Fluibil Zambon, Ital.†.
Chenodeoxycholic acid (p.1562·1).
Gallstones.

Fluibron
Chiesi, Ital.; Chiesi, Switz.
Ambroxol hydrochloride (p.1054·3).
Respiratory-tract disorders.

Fluid Loss
Note. This name is used for preparations of different composition.
Vita Glow, Austral.
Celery (p.1561·1); juniper (p.1592·2); bearberry (p.1552·2); parsley (p.1615·3); potassium chloride (p.1161·1).
Fluid retention.

Vitaplex, Austral.
Celery (p.1561·1); buchu (p.1555·2); taraxacum (p.1634·2); bearberry (p.1552·2).
Fluid retention.

Fluidasa Knoll, Spain.
Mepifylline (p.414·1).
Obstructive airways disease.

Fluide Hydratant Matifiant Vichy, Canad.
SPF 13: Ethylhexyl *p*-methoxycinnamate (p.1487·1); 2-phenyl-1*H*-benzimidazole-5-sulphonic acid (p.1488·2).
Sunscreen.

Fluide Multi-Confort Clarins, Canad.
SPF 15: Ethylhexyl *p*-methoxycinnamate (p.1487·1); oxybenzone (p.1487·3); titanium dioxide (p.1093·3).
Sunscreen.

Fluiden Legon, Ital.
Fenspiride hydrochloride (p.1579·3).
Respiratory-tract disorders.

Fluidex O'Connor, USA.
Buchu (p.1555·2); couch grass (p.1567·3); corn silk; hydrangea.
Oedema.

Fluidex with Pamabrom O'Connor, USA.
Pamabrom (p.927·1).
Oedema associated with premenstrual syndrome.

Fluidin Lasa, Spain.
Guaiphenesin (p.1061·3).
Cough.

Fluidin Codeina Lasa, Spain†.
Codeine (p.26·1); guaiphenesin (p.1061·3); pseudoephedrine (p.1068·3).
Respiratory-tract disorders.

Fluidin Mucolitico Lasa, Spain.
Butethamate citrate (p.1056·2); carbocisteine (p.1056·3); diprophylline (p.752·1); guaiphenesin (p.1061·3).
Respiratory-tract disorders.

Flui-DNCG Zambon, Ger.
Sodium cromoglycate (p.762·1).
Allergic eye disorders; allergic rhinitis; asthma.

Fluidobil Lifepharma, Ital.†.
Dihydroxydibutylether (p.1571·3); frangula (p.1193·2); cascara (p.1183·1); rhubarb (p.1212·1).
Biliary disorders; constipation.

Fluifort Dompe, Ital.
Carbocisteine lysine (p.1056·3).
Respiratory disorders associated with excessive or viscous mucus.

Fluilast Boniscontro & Gazzone, Ital.
Ticlopidine hydrochloride (p.953·1).
Thrombosis prophylaxis.

Fluimucil
Strallhofer, Aust.; Zambon, Fr.; Zambon, Ger.; Zambon, Ital.; Zambon, Neth.; Zambon, Spain; Inpharzam, Switz.
Acetylcysteine (p.1052·3).
Paracetamol poisoning; respiratory-tract disorders; urotoxicity caused by ifosfamide and cyclophosphamide.

Fluimucil Antibiotic
Zambon, Belg.; Zambon, Fr.; Inpharzam, Switz.†.
Thiamphenicol acetylcysteinate (p.263·1) or thiamphenicol glycine acetylcysteinate (p.263·1).
Respiratory-tract infections.

Fluimucil Antibiotico
Zambon, Ital.; Zambon, Spain.
Thiamphenicol glycine acetylcysteinate (p.263·1).
Respiratory-tract infections.

Flu-Imune Lederle-Praxis, USA.
An influenza vaccine (p.1515·2).

Fluisedal Elerte, Fr.
Meglumine benzoate; polysorbate 20 (p.1327·3); promethazine hydrochloride (p.416·2).
Respiratory-tract congestion.

Fluisedal sans promethazine Elerte, Fr.
Meglumine benzoate; polysorbate 20 (p.1327·3).
Respiratory-tract congestion.

Flui-Theophylline Zambon, Ger.
Theophylline (p.765·1).
Obstructive airways disease.

Fluitran
Essex, Ital.†; Schering-Plough, Norw.†.
Trichlormethiazide (p.958·2).
Hypertension; oedema.

Fluiven Herbaline, Ital.
Achillea (p.1542·2); centella (p.1080·3); hamamelis (p.1587·1); myrtillus (p.1606·1).
Peripheral vascular disorders.

Fluixol Ripari-Gero, Ital.
Ambroxol hydrochloride (p.1054·3).
Respiratory-tract disorders.

Flumach Mayoly-Spindler, Fr.
Spironolactone (p.946·1).
Hyperaldosteronism; hypertension; myasthenia gravis.

Flumadine Forest Pharmaceuticals, USA.
Rimantadine hydrochloride (p.624·2).
Influenza A.

Flumarin Shionogi, Jpn.
Flomoxef sodium (p.209·1).
Bacterial infections.

Flumark Dainippon, Jpn.
Enoxacin (p.203·3).
Bacterial infections.

Flumetol Farmila, Ital.
Fluorometholone (p.1042·1); tetrahydrozoline hydrochloride (p.1070·2).
Inflammatory eye disorders.

Flumetol Antibiotico Farmila, Ital.
Fluorometholone (p.1042·1); tetracycline (p.259·1).
Infected eye disorders.

Flumetol Semplice Farmila, Ital.
Fluorometholone (p.1042·1).
Inflammatory eye disorders.

Flumox Rolab, S.Afr.
Amoxycillin (p.151·3); flucloxacillin (p.209·1).
Bacterial infections.

Flumural SPA, Ital.
Flumequine (p.210·1).
Urinary-tract infections.

Flunagen Gentili, Ital.
Flunarizine hydrochloride (p.411·1).
Migraine; vertigo.

Fluniget
Merck Sharp & Dohme, Aust.; Merck Sharp & Dohme, Ger.
Diflunisal (p.33·2).
Musculoskeletal and joint disorders; pain.

Flunimerck Merck, Ger.
Flunitrazepam (p.670·1).
Insomnia.

Fluninoc Hexal, Ger.
Flunitrazepam (p.670·1).
Insomnia.

Flunipam Alpharma, Norw.
Flunitrazepam (p.670·1).
Insomnia; premedication.

Flunir Oberlin, Fr.
Niflumic acid (p.63·1).
Sprains.

Flunitec Boehringer Ingelheim, Norw.
Flunisolide (p.1040·3).
Asthma.

Flunox Boehringer Mannheim, Ital.
Flurazepam monohydrochloride (p.672·2).
Insomnia.

Fluo Fenic Ciba Vision, Spain.
Chloramphenicol (p.182·1); fluocinolone acetonide (p.1041·1).
Infected eye disorders.

Fluo Vasoc Ciba Vision, Spain.
Fluocinolone acetonide (p.1041·1); naphazoline hydrochloride (p.1064·2); neomycin sulphate (p.229·2); zinc sulphate (p.1373·2).
Infected eye disorders.

Fluo-calc Searle, Switz.
Sodium monofluorophosphate (p.743·3); calcium carbonate (p.1182·1).
Osteoporosis.

Fluocalcic
Asta Medica, Aust.; Yamanouchi, Belg.; Yamanouchi, Fr.
Sodium monofluorophosphate (p.743·3); calcium carbonate (p.1182·1).
Osteoporosis.

Fluocaril Synthelabo, Belg.†.
Sodium fluoride (p.742·1); sodium monofluorophosphate (p.743·3).
Dental caries prophylaxis; dental hygiene.

Fluocaril Bi-Fluore
Synthelabo, Fr.; Goupil, Ital.
Sodium monofluorophosphate (p.743·3); sodium fluoride (p.742·1).
Dental caries prophylaxis.

Fluocid Forte Inkeysa, Spain.
Fluocinolone acetonide (p.1041·1).
Skin disorders.

Fluocinil Coli, Ital.†.
Fluocinolone acetonide (p.1041·1).
Skin disorders.

Fluocit CT, Ital.†.
Fluocinolone acetonide (p.1041·1).
Skin disorders.

Fluocortan Centrum, Spain.
Fluocinolone acetonide (p.1041·1).
Skin disorders.

Fluodent Scherer, Ital.
Sodium fluoride (p.742·1).
Dietary-fluoride deficiency.

Fluoderm
Taro, Canad.; Lennon, S.Afr.†.
Fluocinolone acetonide (p.1041·1).
Skin disorders.

Fluodermo Fuerte Septa, Spain.
Fluocinolone acetonide (p.1041·1).
Skin disorders.

Fluodermol Medosan, Ital.†.
Fluocinolone acetonide (p.1041·1).
Skin disorders.

Fluodonil Biologici Italia, Ital.
Diflunisal (p.33·2).
Musculoskeletal and joint disorders; pain.

Fluodont Gebro, Aust.
Sodium fluoride (p.742·1).
Dental caries prophylaxis.

Fluodontyl
Synthelabo, Belg.†; Synthelabo, Fr.; Goupil, Spain.
Sodium fluoride (p.742·1).
Formerly contained sodium fluoride and formaldehyde in *Fr.*
Dental caries prophylaxis; dental hygiene; dental hypersensitivity.

Fluoftal Agepha, Aust.
Fluorescein sodium (p.1581·1).
Diagnosis of corneal disorders.

Fluogel
Note. This name is used for preparations of different composition.
Synthelabo, Belg.†.
Sodium fluoride (p.742·1).
Dental caries prophylaxis following radiotherapy.

Dentoria, Fr.
Sodium fluoride (p.742·1); ammonium difluoride.
Dental caries prophylaxis following radiotherapy.

Fluogen Parke, Davis, USA.
An influenza vaccine (p.1515·2).
Active immunisation.

Fluogum Synthelabo, Fr.
Sodium fluoride (p.742·1).
Dental caries prophylaxis.

Fluomicetina Zoja, Ital.
Fluocinolone acetonide (p.1041·1); kanamycin sulphate (p.220·3).
Anogenital pruritus; skin disorders.

Fluomint Lysoform, Ger.
Potassium fluoride; myrrh tincture (p.1606·1); peppermint oil (p.1208·1).
Inflammatory disorders and infections of the oropharynx.

Fluomix Same Savoma, Ital.
Fluocinolone acetonide (p.1041·1).
Skin disorders.

Fluomycin N Nourypharma, Ger.
Dequalinium chloride (p.1112·1).
Fluomycin formerly contained phthalylsulphathiazole, neomycin sulphate, and dequalinium chloride.
Vaginal infections.

Fluon Rabi & Solabo, Fr.
Metesculetol sodium (p.1602·3); hamamelis (p.1587·1); aesculus (p.1543·3); senecio (p.1628·1); valerian (p.1643·1); viburnum.
Haemorrhoids; oedema; peripheral vascular disorders.

Fluonex ICN, USA.
Fluocinonide (p.1041·2).
Skin disorders.

Fluonid Allergan Herbert, USA.
Fluocinolone acetonide (p.1041·1).
Skin disorders.

Fluonilid Ascot, Austral.†.
Loflucarban (p.384·2).
Skin infections.

Fluopate Laphal, Fr.
Sodium fluoride (p.742·1); calcium fluoride (p.1556·3).
Dental caries prophylaxis.

Fluoplexe Lehning, Fr.
Sodium fluoride (p.742·1).
Peri-articular disorders.

Fluor
Or-Dov, Austral.; Lacer, Spain.
Sodium fluoride (p.742·1).
Dental caries prophylaxis.

Fluoracaine
Dioptic, Canad.; Akorn, USA.
Fluorescein sodium (p.1581·1); proxymetacaine hydrochloride (p.1300·1).
Aid to eye examination; local anaesthesia.

Fluor-A-Day
Pharmascience, Canad.; Dental Health Products, UK.
Sodium fluoride (p.742·1).
Dental caries prophylaxis.

Fluoralfa INTES, Ital.
Fluorescein sodium (p.1581·1).
Diagnosis of eye disorders.

Fluoran Inibsa, Spain†.
Sodium fluoride (p.742·1).
Dental caries prophylaxis.

Fluordent Warner-Lambert, Ital.
Sodium fluoride (p.742·1).
Dental caries prophylaxis.

Fluores Covan, S.Afr.†.
Fluorescein sodium (p.1581·1).
Ophthalmic diagnostic agent.

Fluorescite
Alcon, Austral.; Alcon, Canad.; Alcon, S.Afr.; Alcon, USA.
Fluorescein sodium (p.1581·1).
Aid to eye examination.

Fluorets
Smith & Nephew, Austral.; Ophtapharma, Canad.; Chauvin, Irl.; Smith & Nephew, S.Afr.; Chauvin, UK; Akorn, USA.
Fluorescein sodium (p.1581·1).
Aid to eye examination.

Fluorette
Fertin, Norw.; Meda, Swed.
Sodium fluoride (p.742·1).
Dental caries prophylaxis.

Fluoretten Albert-Roussel, Ger.; Hoechst, Ger.
Sodium fluoride (p.742·1).
Dental caries prophylaxis.

Fluorex Crinex, Fr.
Sodium fluoride (p.742·1).
Dental caries prophylaxis.

Fluorex Plus Gerot, Aust.
Tetracycline hydrochloride (p.259·1); dequalinium chloride (p.1112·1); prednisone (p.1049·2).
Colpitis.

Fluor-Gel Blend-a-med, Ger.†.
Sodium fluoride (p.742·1); dibasic sodium phosphate (p.1159·3).
Dental caries prophylaxis; sensitive teeth.

Fluorigard
Colgate-Palmolive, Ital.; Colgate-Palmolive, UK; Colgate-Palmolive, USA.
Sodium fluoride (p.742·1).
Dental caries prophylaxis.

Fluorigard Gel-Kam Colgate-Palmolive, UK.
Stannous fluoride (p.1632·2).
Dental caries prophylaxis.

Fluori-Methane Gebauer, USA.
Dichlorodifluoromethane (p.1164·3); trichlorofluoromethane (p.1164·3).
Local anaesthesia.

Fluor-In Goupil, Fr.†.
Sodium fluoride (p.742·1).
Dental caries prophylaxis.

Fluorinse
Oral-B, Canad.; Oral-B, USA.
Sodium fluoride (p.742·1).
Dental caries prophylaxis.

Fluor-I-Strip Wyeth-Ayerst, USA.
Fluorescein sodium (p.1581·1).
Aid to eye examination.

Fluor-I-Strip AT Storz, Canad.
Fluorescein sodium (p.1581·1).
Aid to eye examination.

Fluoritab Fluoritab, USA.
Sodium fluoride (p.742·1).
Dental caries prophylaxis.

Fluoritabs WestCan, Canad.
Sodium fluoride (p.742·1).

Fluorite 200 Galway, Irl.†.
Sodium fluoride (p.742·1).
Dental caries prophylaxis.

Fluor-Kin Kin, Spain.
Sodium fluoride (p.742·1).
Dental caries prophylaxis.

Fluorobioptal Farmila, Ital.
Dexamethasone (p.1037·1); chloramphenicol (p.182·1).
Formerly contained dexamethasone, chloramphenicol, nitrofurazone, and phenylephrine hydrochloride.
Inflammatory eye disorders.

Fluorocalciforte Serozym, Fr.
Calcium chloride (p.1155·1); calcium gluceptate (p.1155·1); calcium gluconate (p.1155·2); calcium lactate (p.1155·2); calcium carbonate (p.1182·1); sodium monofluorophosphate (p.743·3); yeast (p.1373·1).
Osteoporosis.

Fluorocortisol K Vis, Ital.†.
Kanamycin sulphate (p.220·3); dexamethasone phosphate (p.1037·2); phenylephrine hydrochloride (p.1066·2).
Inflammatory eye, nose, and ear, disorders.

Fluorogum Schwulst, S.Afr.†.
Sodium fluoride (p.742·1).
Fluoride supplement.

Fluor-Op Iolab, USA.
Fluorometholone (p.1042·1).
Inflammatory eye disorders.

Fluoroplex
Allergan, Austral.; Allergan, Canad.; Allergan Herbert, USA.
Fluorouracil (p.534·3).
Solar keratosis.

Fluororinil Farmila, Ital.
Betamethasone (p.1033·2); chlorpheniramine maleate (p.405·1).
Rhinitis.

Fluorosol WestCan, Canad.
Sodium fluoride (p.742·1).

Fluor-Retard Nycomed, Norw.†.
Sodium fluoride (p.742·1).
Osteoporosis.

Fluortabletjes SAN, Neth.†.
Sodium fluoride (p.742·1).
Dental caries prophylaxis.

Fluorthyrin Agepha, Aust.
Fluorotyrosine (p.1493·1).
Hyperthyroidism.

Fluortop GABA, Switz.
Sodium fluoride (p.742·1).
Dental caries prophylaxis.

Fluor-Vigantoletten Merck, Ger.
Cholecalciferol (p.1366·3); sodium fluoride (p.742·1).
Dental caries prophylaxis; vitamin D deficiency.

Fluorvitburck Fermenti, Ital.†.
Vitamin A (p.1358·1); ergocalciferol (p.1367·1); sodium fluoride (p.742·1); minerals.
Bone disorders.

Fluorvitin IPFI, Ital.
Sodium fluoride (p.742·1).
Dental caries prophylaxis.

Fluoselgine Zyma, Fr.
Domiphen bromide (p.1112·3); sodium fluoride (p.742·1).
Dental hygiene; gingivitis.

Fluosept Inava, Fr.
Ammonium difluoride; benzyl salicylate.
Dental caries prophylaxis.

Fluosol
Alpha Therapeutic, UK†; Alpha Therapeutic, USA†.
Perflunafene (p.1617·1); perfluamine (p.1617·1).
Adjunct in coronary angioplasty.

Fluotest Cusi, Spain.
Fluorescein sodium (p.1581·1); oxybuprocaine hydrochloride (p.1298·1).
Aid to eye examination.

Fluothane
Zeneca, Aust.; ICI, Austral.; Zeneca, Belg.; Wyeth-Ayerst, Canad.†; Zeneca, Fr.; Zeneca, Ger.; Zeneca, Irl.; Zeneca, Ital.; Zeneca, Neth.; Zeneca, Norw.; Zeneca, S.Afr.; Zeneca, Spain; Zeneca, Swed.; Zeneca, Switz.; Zeneca, UK; Wyeth-Ayerst, USA.
Halothane (p.1224·1).
General anaesthesia.

Fluotic Hoechst Marion Roussel, Canad.
Sodium fluoride (p.742·1).
Otospongiosis.

Fluovitef Teofarma, Ital.
Fluocinolone acetonide (p.1041·1).
Skin disorders.

Fluoxeren Menarini, Ital.
Fluoxetine hydrochloride (p.284·1).
Bulimia nervosa; depression; obsessive-compulsive disorder.

Flu-Oxinate Pasadena, USA.
Fluorescein sodium (p.1581·1); oxybuprocaine hydrochloride (p.1298·1).

Flupam Tika, Swed.
Flunitrazepam (p.670·1).
Premedication; sleep disorders.

Flupress Drug Research, Ital.
Buflomedil pyridoxal phosphate compound (p.834·2).
Cerebral and peripheral vascular disorders.

Fluprim Tosse Roche, Ital.
Dextromethorphan hydrobromide (p.1057·3).
Coughs.

Fluprim-Gola Roche, Ital.†.
Cetylpyridinium chloride (p.1106·2).
Oral hygiene.

Flura Kirkman, USA.
Sodium fluoride (p.742·1).
Dental caries prophylaxis.

Flurablastin
Pharmacia Upjohn, Norw.; Pharmacia Upjohn, Swed.
Fluorouracil (p.534·3) or fluorouracil sodium (p.536·1).
Malignant neoplasms.

Fluracedyl
Nycomed, Norw.; Nycomed, Swed.
Fluorouracil (p.534·3) or fluorouracil sodium (p.536·1).
Malignant neoplasms.

Flurate Bausch & Lomb, USA.
Fluorescein sodium (p.1581·1); oxybuprocaine hydrochloride (p.1298·1).
Local anaesthesia.

Flurekain Croma, Aust.
Oxybuprocaine hydrochloride (p.1298·1).
Local anaesthesia.

Fluress
Allergan, Austral.; Allergan, Canad.; Abigo, Swed.; Pilkington Barnes-Hind, USA.
Oxybuprocaine hydrochloride (p.1298·1); fluorescein sodium (p.1581·1).
Aid to eye examination; local anaesthesia.

Flurets Oral-B, Austral.
Sodium fluoride (p.742·1).
Prevention of tooth decay.

Flurex Seton, UK†.
Capsules: Paracetamol (p.72·2); phenylephrine hydrochloride (p.1066·2); dextromethorphan (p.1057·3).
Tablets: Paracetamol (p.72·2); phenylephrine hydrochloride (p.1066·2); caffeine (p.749·3).
Cold symptoms.

Flurex Bedtime Seton, UK†.
Paracetamol (p.72·2); diphenhydramine hydrochloride (p.409·1); pseudoephedrine (p.1068·3).
Cold symptoms.

Flurex Hot Lemon Seton, UK†.
Codeine phosphate (p.26·1); ephedrine hydrochloride (p.1059·3); diphenhydramine hydrochloride (p.409·1).
Cold symptoms.

Flurex Inhalant Seton, UK†.
Menthol (p.1600·2); camphor (p.1557·2); turpentine oil (p.1641·1); eucalyptus oil (p.1578·1).
Cold symptoms.

Flurexal Zyma, Switz.†.
Sodium fluoride (p.742·1).
Osteoporosis; otospongiosis.

Flurizic Pharmacia Upjohn, Ital.
Flurithromycin ethyl succinate (p.210·1).
Bacterial infections.

Fluroblastin
Pharmacia Upjohn, Ger.; Pharmacia Upjohn, S.Afr.
Fluorouracil (p.534·3).
Malignant neoplasms.

Fluroblastine
Pharmacia Upjohn, Belg.; Pharmacia Upjohn, Switz.†.
Fluorouracil (p.534·3) or fluorouracil sodium (p.536·1).
Malignant neoplasms.

Fluro-Ethyl Gebauer, USA.
Ethyl chloride (p.1292·3); dichlorotetrafluoroethane (p.1164·3).
Topical anaesthesia.

Flurosyn Rugby, USA.
Fluocinolone acetonide (p.1041·1).
Skin disorders.

Flurox Ocusoft, USA.
Fluorescein sodium (p.1581·1); oxybuprocaine hydrochloride (p.1298·1).

Flurpax Hosbon, Spain.
Flunarizine hydrochloride (p.411·1).
Ménière's disease; migraine; motion sickness; vestibular disorders.

Fluscand Enapharm, Swed.
Flunitrazepam (p.670·1).
Premedication; sleep disorders.

Flusemide UCB, Spain.
Nicardipine hydrochloride (p.915·1).
Angina pectoris; cerebral vasospasm; hypertension.

Flu-Shield Wyeth-Ayerst, USA.
An influenza vaccine (p.1515·2).
Active immunisation.

Flusin Columbia, S.Afr.
Chlorpheniramine maleate (p.405·1); ephedrine hydrochloride (p.1059·3); paracetamol (p.72·2); caffeine (p.749·3).
Cold and influenza symptoms.

Flusin DM Columbia, S.Afr.
Chlorpheniramine maleate (p.405·1); pseudoephedrine hydrochloride (p.1068·3); dextromethorphan hydrobromide (p.1057·3); ascorbic acid (p.1365·2).
Coughs; upper respiratory-tract congestion.

Fluspiral Menarini, Ital.
Fluticasone propionate (p.1042·3).
Obstructive airways disease.

Flusporan Menarini, Spain.
Flutrimazole (p.380·2).
Fungal infections.

Fluss 40 Hoechst Marion Roussel, Ital.
Frusemide (p.871·1); triamterene (p.957·2).
Ascites; hypertension; oedema.

Flussorex Lampugnani, Ital.
Citicoline sodium (p.1564·3).
Cerebrovascular disorders; mental function disorders; parkinsonism.

Flustar FIRMA, Ital.†.
Diflunisal (p.33·2).
Inflammation; pain.

Flu-Stat Be-Tabs, S.Afr.
Capsules: Paracetamol (p.72·2); ascorbic acid (p.1365·2); phenylephrine hydrochloride (p.1066·2); chlorpheniramine maleate (p.405·1); caffeine (p.749·3).
Syrup: Paracetamol (p.72·2); phenylpropanolamine hydrochloride (p.1067·2); dextromethorphan hydrobromide (p.1057·3).
Cold and influenza symptoms.

Flutacan Ferring, Swed.
Flutamide (p.537·1).
Prostatic cancer.

Fluta-Gry Gry, Ger.
Flutamide (p.537·1).
Prostatic cancer.

Flutamex Sanofi Winthrop, Ger.
Flutamide (p.537·1).
Prostatic cancer.

Flutenal Uriach, Spain.
Flupamesone (p.1050·3).
Skin disorders.

Flutenal Gentamicina Uriach, Spain.
Flupamesone (p.1050·3); gentamicin sulphate (p.212·1).
Infected skin disorders.

Flutenal Sali Uriach, Spain.
Flupamesone (p.1050·3); salicylic acid (p.1090·2).
Skin disorders.

Flutex
Note. This name is used for preparations of different composition.
Lennon, S.Afr.
Capsules: Ascorbic acid (p.1365·2); salicylamide (p.82·3); paracetamol (p.72·2); caffeine (p.749·3); phenylephrine hydrochloride (p.1066·2); chlorpheniramine maleate (p.405·1).
Syrup: Paracetamol (p.72·2); phenylephrine hydrochloride (p.1066·2).
Cold and influenza symptoms.

Syosset, USA.
Triamcinolone acetonide (p.1050·2).
Skin disorders.

Flutex Cough Linctus Lennon, S.Afr.
Diphenhydramine hydrochloride (p.409·1); codeine phosphate (p.26·1); ammonium chloride (p.1055·2).
Coughs.

Flutide
Glaxo Wellcome, Ger.; Glaxo Wellcome, Norw.; Glaxo Wellcome, Swed.
Fluticasone propionate (p.1042·3).
Allergic rhinitis; asthma.

Flutinase Glaxo Wellcome, Switz.
Fluticasone propionate (p.1042·3).
Rhinitis.

Flutivate
Glaxo Wellcome, Ger.; Wolff, Ger.; Glaxo Wellcome, Norw.; Glaxo Wellcome, Swed.
Fluticasone propionate (p.1042·3).
Skin disorders.

Flutox Pharmazam, Spain.
Cloperastine fendizoate (p.1057·2) or cloperastine hydrochloride (p.1057·2).
Coughs.

Flutraz Tika, Norw.
Flunitrazepam (p.670·1).
Insomnia.

Fluvaccin SBL, Swed.†.
An influenza vaccine (p.1515·2).
Active immunisation.

Fluvaleas Valeas, Ital.
Isopropamide iodide (p.464·3); paracetamol (p.72·2); diphenhydramine hydrochloride (p.409·1); caffeine (p.749·3).
Fever; inflammation; pain.

Fluvax CSL, Austral.
An influenza vaccine (p.1515·2).
Active immunisation.

Fluvermal Janssen-Cilag, Fr.
Flubendazole (p.100·3).
Veterinary names include Flubenol.
Intestinal nematode infections.

Fluvic Pierre Fabre Sante, Fr.
Carbocisteine (p.1056·3).
Respiratory-tract congestion.

Fluviral IAF Biovac, Canad.
An inactivated influenza vaccine (whole and split virion) (p.1515·2).
Active immunisation.

Fluvirin
Evans Medical, Irl.; Farmarekord, Ital.; Evans Medical, Norw.; Medpro, S.Afr.; SBL, Swed.; Medeva, UK; Adams, USA.
An inactivated influenza vaccine (surface antigen) (p.1515·2).
Active immunisation.

Fluvirine Evans, Fr.
An influenza vaccine (p.1515·2).
Active immunisation.

Flux Alpharma, Norw.
Sodium fluoride (p.742·1).
Dental caries prophylaxis.

Fluxal Rovi, Spain.
Lysine aspirin (p.50·3); calcium ascorbate (p.1365·2); chlorpheniramine maleate (p.405·1); phenylephrine hydrochloride (p.1066·2).
Influenza and cold symptoms.

Fluxapril
Wyeth Lederle, Aust.; Lederle, Ger.
Piperacillin sodium (p.237·2); flucloxacillin sodium (p.209·2).
Bacterial infections.

Fluxarten SmithKline Beecham, Ital.
Flunarizine hydrochloride (p.411·1).
Migraine; vertigo.

Fluxival Chefaro Ardeval, Fr.†.
Aesculus (p.1543·3); melilot.
Circulatory disorders.

Fluxoten Herbaline, Ital.
Melissa (p.1600·1); centaury (p.1561·1); calendula officinalis; artemisia vulgaris; saffron (p.1001·1).
Menstrual disorders.

Fluxum Wassermann, Ital.
Parnaparin sodium (p.927·1).
Thrombosis prophylaxis; vascular disorders.

Fluzone
Connaught, Canad.; Pasteur Merieux, Irl.; Connaught, Norw.; Meda, Swed.†; Pasteur Merieux, UK; Connaught, USA.
An inactivated influenza vaccine (split virion) (p.1515·2).
Active immunisation.

FML
Allergan, Austral.; Allergan, Belg.; Allergan, Canad.; Allergan, Irl.; Allergan, S.Afr.; Allergan, Spain; Allergan, Switz.; Allergan, USA.
Fluorometholone (p.1042·1).
Inflammatory eye disorders.

FML Liquifilm
Allergan, Canad.; Allergan, Neth.†; Allergan, UK.
Fluorometholone (p.1042·1).
Inflammatory eye disorders.

FML Neo
Allergan, Irl.†; Allergan, S.Afr.; Allergan, Spain; Allergan, Switz.
Fluorometholone (p.1042·1); neomycin sulphate (p.229·2).
Inflammatory eye infections.

FML Neo Liquifilm
Allergan, Canad.†; Allergan, UK.
Fluorometholone (p.1042·1); neomycin sulphate (p.229·2).
Inflammatory eye infections.

FML-S Allergan, USA.
Fluorometholone (p.1042·1); sulphacetamide sodium (p.252·2).
Inflammatory eye infections.

Foamicon Invamed, USA.
Aluminium hydroxide (p.1177·3); magnesium trisilicate (p.1199·1); sodium bicarbonate (p.1153·2); alginic acid (p.1470·3).
Hyperacidity.

Fobidon Biomedica, Ital.
Domperidone (p.1190·3).
Gastric discomfort; nausea; vomiting.

Foce Medici, Ital.†.
Fosfomycin (p.210·1); cephalexin (p.178·2).
Bacterial infections.

Focus Angelini, Ital.†.
Ibuprofen (p.44·1).
Musculoskeletal and joint disorders.

Focusan
Lundbeck, Aust.; Lundbeck, Neth.†; Lundbeck, Norw.†; Lundbeck, Switz.†.
Tolnaftate (p.389·1); cetylpyridinium chloride (p.1106·2).
Fungal skin infections.

Fohnetten N Ziethen, Ger.
Benzyl mandelate; caffeine (p.749·3); paracetamol (p.72·2).
Migraine; pain.

Foille
Note. This name is used for preparations of different composition.
Blistex, Canad.
Benzocaine (p.1286·2); benzyl alcohol (p.1103·3).
Burns; insect bites; wounds.

Synthelabo, Ital.
Benzocaine (p.1286·2); benzyl alcohol (p.1103·3); hydroxyquinoline (p.1589·3); colloidal sulphur (p.1091·2).
Burns; skin irritation; wounds.

Blistex, USA.
Benzocaine (p.1286·2); chloroxylenol (p.1111·1).
Local anaesthesia.

Foille Insetti Synthelabo, Ital.
Hydrocortisone (p.1043·3).
Insect stings; skin irritation.

Foille Sole Synthelabo, Ital.
Benzocaine (p.1286·2); benzyl alcohol (p.1103·3); chloroxylenol (p.1111·1).
Formerly known as Foille Plus.
Skin irritation; wounds.

Foipan Ono, Jpn.
Camostat mesylate (p.1557·2).
Gastro-oesophageal reflux; pancreatitis.

Fokalepsin Promonta Lundbeck, Ger.
Carbamazepine (p.339·2).
Diabetic neuropathy; epilepsy; trigeminal neuralgia.

Folacin Pharmacia Upjohn, Swed.
Folic acid (p.1340·3).
Folate deficiency; megaloblastic anaemia.

Folacin 12 Quest, Canad.
Vitamin B_{12} (p.1363·3); folic acid (p.1340·3).

Folamin Becker, Aust.†.
Folic acid (p.1340·3).

Folarell Sanorell, Ger.
Folic acid (p.1340·3).
Folate deficiency; megaloblastic anaemia.

Folaren Ist. Chim. Inter., Ital.
Calcium folinate (p.1342·2).
Antidote to folic acid antagonists; folate deficiency; reduction of aminopterin and methotrexate toxicity.

Folasic Nelson, Austral.†.
Folic acid (p.1340·3).

Folatine Lifeplan, UK.
Folic acid (p.1340·3).
Nutritional supplement.

Folavit Wolfs, Belg.†.
Folic acid (p.1340·3).
Prevention of neural tube defects in pregnancy.

Folaxin Zambon, Spain.
Calcium folinate (p.1342·2).
Folic acid deficiency; megaloblastic anaemia.

Folcodex Sanico, Belg.
Pholcodine (p.1068·1); ephedrine hydrochloride (p.1059·3); belladonna (p.457·1); aconite (p.1542·2); potassium guaiacolsulfonate (p.1068·3); ipecacuanha (p.1062·2); tolu balsam (p.1071·1).
Bronchopulmonary disorders.

Folcofen *Schwulst, S.Afr.*
Diphenhydramine hydrochloride (p.409·1); pholcodine (p.1068·1); guaiphenesin (p.1061·3).
Coughs.

Folepar B12 *Lisapharma, Ital.*
Folic acid (p.1340·3); nicotinamide (p.1351·2); thiamine hydrochloride (p.1361·1); cyanocobalamin (p.1363·3).
Deficiency states; macrocytic anaemia.

Folergot-DF *Marnel, USA.*
Phenobarbitone (p.350·2); ergotamine tartrate (p.445·3); belladonna (p.457·1).
Gastro-intestinal disorders.

Folex
Note. This name is used for preparations of different composition.
Qualiphar, Belg.
Pholcodine (p.1068·1); ephedrine hydrochloride (p.1059·3); sodium citrate (p.1153·2).
Bronchitis; coughs; laryngitis.
Rybar, Irl.
Ferrous fumarate (p.1339·3); folic acid (p.1340·3).
Iron and folic acid deficiency during pregnancy.
Adria, USA.
Methotrexate sodium (p.547·1).
Malignant neoplasms.

Folex-350 *Shire, UK.*
Ferrous fumarate (p.1339·3); folic acid (p.1340·3).
Iron and folic acid deficiency in pregnancy.

Folferite *Glaxo Wellcome, Irl.†.*
Ferrous sulphate (p.1340·2); folic acid (p.1340·3).
Iron and folic acid deficiency during pregnancy.

Folgamma *Worwag, Ger.*
Cyanocobalamin (p.1363·3); folic acid (p.1340·3).
Vitamin B_{12} and folic acid deficiency.

Foliben *FIRMA, Ital.*
Calcium folinate (p.1342·2).
Antidote to folic acid antagonists; folate deficiency; reduction of aminopterin and methotrexate toxicity.

Folic Acid Plus *Cenovis, Austral.; Vitelle, Austral.*
Vitamin and mineral preparation with iron and folic acid.

Folic Plus *English Grains, UK.*
Folic acid (p.1340·3); calcium (p.1155·1); vitamin D (p.1366·3).

Folicare *Rosemont, UK.*
Folic acid (p.1340·3).

FOLI-cell *Cell Pharm, Ger.*
Calcium folinate (p.1342·2).
Antidote to treatment with folic acid antagonists; folate deficiency.

Folicid *Rhone-Poulenc Rorer, Austral.†.*
Folic acid (p.1340·3).

Folicin *Paines & Byrne, UK†.*
Ferrous sulphate (p.1340·2); copper sulphate (p.1338·1); folic acid (p.1340·3); manganese sulphate (p.1350·3).
Anaemia of pregnancy.

Folico *Ecobi, Ital.†.*
Folic acid (p.1340·3).

Folicombin *Jenapharm, Ger.*
Ammonium iron sulphate; folic acid (p.1340·3).
Iron and folate deficiency.

Folidan *Almirall, Spain.*
Calcium folinate (p.1342·2).
Enhancement of fluorouracil; megaloblastic anaemia; methotrexate poisoning.

Folidar *Italfarmaco, Ital.*
Calcium folinate (p.1342·2).
Folate deficiency; reduction of aminopterin and methotrexate toxicity.

Foliferron *Wyeth, Spain.*
Folic acid (p.1340·3); ferrous fumarate (p.1339·3).
Iron and folic acid deficiency.

Foligan
Henning, Ger.; Henning, Switz.
Allopurinol (p.390·2).
Gout; hyperuricaemia; renal calculi.

Foliglobin *Pharmaceutical Enterprises, S.Afr.*
Ferrous sulphate (p.1340·2); folic acid (p.1340·3); vitamin B_{12} (p.1363·3).
Ascorbic acid (p.1365·2) is included in this preparation to increase the absorption and availability of iron.
Anaemias; iron deficiency.

Folina *Schwarz, Ital.*
Folic acid (p.1340·3) or sodium folinate.
Folate deficiency.

Folinac *Bioprogress, Ital.*
Calcium folinate (p.1342·2).
Antidote to overdosage with folic acid antagonists; folate deficiency; reduction of aminopterin and methotrexate toxicity.

Folincortex *Errekappa, Ital.†.*
Multivitamin and amino-acid preparation with suprarenal cortex (p.1050·1) and lignocaine hydrochloride (p.1293·2).
Anaemias; asthenia.

Folindor *Schaper & Brummer, Ger.†.*
Orthosiphon leaves (p.1592·2).
Urinary-tract infections.

Folinemic *FIRMA, Ital.†.*
Calcium folinate (p.1342·2); cyanocobalamin (p.1363·3).
Lignocaine hydrochloride (p.1293·2) is included in this preparation to alleviate the pain of injection.
Anaemias; asthenia.

Folinemic Cortex *FIRMA, Ital.†.*
Suprarenal cortex (p.1050·1); calcium folinate (p.1342·2); cyanocobalamin (p.1363·3).
Lignocaine hydrochloride (p.1293·2) is included in this preparation to alleviate the pain of injection.
Anaemias; asthenia.

Folinemic Ferro *FIRMA, Ital.*
Iron succinyl-protein complex (p.1349·2).
Iron deficiency; iron-deficiency anaemias.

Folinoral *Therabel, Fr.*
Calcium folinate (p.1342·2).
Drug-induced megaloblastic anaemia; methotrexate toxicity.

Folinvit *Garant, Ital.*
Calcium folinate (p.1342·2).
Anaemias; folate deficiency; reduction of aminopterin and methotrexate toxicity.

Foliplus *Sanofi Winthrop, Ital.*
Calcium folinate (p.1342·2).
Anaemias; folate deficiency; reduction of aminopterin and methotrexate toxicity.

Foli-Rivo *Rivopharm, Switz.*
Folic acid (p.1340·3).
Megaloblastic anaemias.

Folix *Caber, Ital.*
Calcium folinate (p.1342·2).
Antidote to overdosage with folic acid antagonists; folate deficiency; reduction of aminopterin and methotrexate toxicity.

Follegon *Organon, Neth.*
Urofollitrophin (p.1263·1).
Male and female infertility.

Follimin
Wyeth, Norw.; Wyeth Lederle, Swed.
Levonorgestrel (p.1454·1); ethinyloestradiol (p.1445·1).
28-Day packs also contain 7 inert tablets.
Combined oral contraceptive.

Follinett *Wyeth Lederle, Swed.*
Levonorgestrel (p.1454·1); ethinyloestradiol (p.1445·1).
Combined oral contraceptive.

Follistim *Organon, USA.*
Follitropin beta (p.1247·1).
Female infertility.

Follistrel *Wyeth Lederle, Swed.*
Levonorgestrel (p.1454·1).
Progestogen-only oral contraceptive.

Follutein *Squibb, USA†.*
Chorionic gonadotrophin (p.1243·1).
Male and female infertility; male hypogonadism; prepubertal cryptorchidism.

Folsan
Solvay, Aust.; Solvay, Ger.
Folic acid (p.1340·3).
Folic acid deficiency.

Folsana *Hotz, Ger.*
Ferrous gluconate (p.1340·1); folic acid (p.1340·3).
Formerly known as Ferro-Folsan.
Iron-deficiency anaemia.

Folvite
Wyeth-Ayerst, Canad.; Lederle, Switz.; Lederle, USA.
Folic acid (p.1340·3) or sodium folate (p.1341·2).
Folate deficiency; megaloblastic anaemia.

Fomac *Berk, UK.*
Mebeverine (p.1199·2).
Colonic spasm; irritable bowel syndrome.

Fomagrippin N *Michallik, Ger.*
Propyphenazone (p.81·3); ephedrine hydrochloride (p.1059·3); ascorbic acid (p.1365·2).
Cold symptoms.

Fomene *Funk, Spain.*
Tetrydamine maleate (p.88·3).
Vaginitis.

Fomentil *SIT, Ital.*
Eucalyptus oil (p.1578·1); menthol (p.1600·2); thyme oil (p.1637·1); peru balsam (p.1617·2); benzoin (p.1634·1).
Laryngitis; respiratory congestion; rhinitis; sore throat.

Fomos *Luitpold, Ger.*
Terfenadine (p.418·1).
Hypersensitivity reactions.

Fon Wan Eleuthero *Giuliani, Ital.*
Honey (p.1345·3); eleutherococcus senticosis (p.1584·2).
Nervous tension.

Fon Wan Ginsenergy *Giuliani, Ital.*
Honey (p.1345·3); royal jelly (p.1626·3); ginseng (p.1584·2).
Nutritional supplement.

Fon Wan Pocket Energy *Giuliani, Ital.*
Ginseng (p.1584·2); honey (p.1345·3).
Nutritional supplement.

Fon Wan Pollen *Giuliani, Ital.*
Pollen; honey (p.1345·3); royal jelly (p.1626·3); ginseng (p.1584·2).
Nutritional supplement.

Fonal N *Merckle, Ger.†.*
Aspirin (p.16·1); caffeine (p.749·3); codeine phosphate (p.26·1).
Coughs and cold symptoms; pain.

Foncitril *Lafon, Fr.*
Trimethylphloroglucinol (p.1618·1); citric acid monohydrate (p.1564·3); monobasic potassium citrate; monosodium citrate.
Urinary-tract disorders.

Fondril *Procter & Gamble, Ger.*
Bisoprolol fumarate (p.833·1).
Angina pectoris; hypertension.

Fondril-5 HCT *Procter & Gamble, Ger.*
Bisoprolol fumarate (p.833·1); hydrochlorothiazide (p.885·2).
Hypertension.

Fongamil
Biorga, Fr.; Juste, Spain.
Omoconazole nitrate (p.386·3).
Fungal infections.

Fongarex
Piette, Belg.; Besins-Iscovesco, Fr.
Omoconazole nitrate (p.386·3).
Fungal skin and vulvovaginal infections.

Fongeryl *L'Arguenon, Fr.*
Laurcetium bromide; lemoxinol.
Fungal skin infections.

Fongitar
Note. This name is used for preparations of different composition.
Stiefel, Austral.; Stiefel, Fr.†.
Pyrithione zinc (p.1089·3); tar (p.1092·3); cade oil (p.1092·2); coal tar (p.1092·3).
Scalp disorders.
Stiefel, Ital.
Pyrithione zinc (p.1089·3); tar (p.1092·3).
Seborrhoeic dermatitis.

Fonicef *RKG, Ital.*
Cefonicid sodium (p.167·2).
Lignocaine hydrochloride (p.1293·2) is included in this preparation to alleviate the pain of injection.
Bacterial infections.

Fonlipol
Lafon, Fr.; Recordati, Ital.†.
Tiadenol (p.1279·3).
Hyperlipidaemias.

Fonofos *Pulitzer, Ital.*
Fosfomycin calcium (p.210·2).
Bacterial infections.

Fontego *Polifarma, Ital.*
Bumetanide (p.834·3).
Oedema.

Fontex
Lilly, Norw.; Lilly, Swed.
Fluoxetine hydrochloride (p.284·1).
Anxiety disorders; bulimia; depression.

Fonx *Yamanouchi, Fr.*
Oxiconazole nitrate (p.386·3).
Fungal skin infections.

Fonzylane *Lafon, Fr.*
Buflomedil hydrochloride (p.834·2).
Intermittent claudication; Raynaud's syndrome.

For Liver *Tosi, Ital.*
Injection: Uridine (p.1641·3); inosine (p.1591·1); guanosine; cytidine; cyanocobalamin (p.1363·3); riboflavine sodium phosphate (p.1362·1); pyridoxine hydrochloride (p.1362·3); nicotinamide (p.1351·2); calcium folinate (p.1342·2).
Oral liquid: Uridine (p.1641·3); inosine (p.1591·1); guanosine; cytidine; cyanocobalamin (p.1363·3); thiamine hydrochloride (p.1361·1); riboflavine sodium phosphate (p.1362·1); pyridoxine hydrochloride (p.1362·3); nicotinamide (p.1351·2); calcium folinate (p.1342·2).
Anaemias; liver disorders.

For Men *Jamieson, Canad.*
Multivitamin and mineral preparation.

For Peripheral Circulation Herbal Plus Formula 5 *Vitelle, Austral.*
Ginkgo biloba (p.1584·1); crataegus (p.1568·2); zanthoxylum (p.1645·3); capsicum (p.1559·2); rutin (p.1580·2); hesperidin (p.1580·2).
Peripheral vascular disorders.

For the Post-Menopausal Years *Jamieson, Canad.*
Multivitamin and mineral preparation.

Foradil
Ciba-Geigy, Aust.; Ciba-Geigy, Fr.; Geigy, Irl.; Novartis, Ital.; Novartis, Neth.; Novartis, S.Afr.; Ciba-Geigy, Spain; Novartis, Swed.; Ciba, Switz.; Geigy, UK.
Eformoterol fumarate (p.752·3).
Obstructive airways disease.

Foradile *Novartis, Austral.*
Eformoterol fumarate (p.752·3).
Asthma.

Foral *Grossmann, Switz.*
Codeine phosphate (p.26·1); ephedrine hydrochloride (p.1059·3); sodium benzoate (p.1102·3); hedera helix; polygala (p.1069·3); liquorice (p.1197·1); star anise oil.
Coughs.

Forane
Abbott, Aust.; Zeneca, Canad.; Abbott, Irl.; Abbott, Ital.; Abbott, S.Afr.; Abbott, Spain; Anaquest, USA.
Isoflurane (p.1225·1).
General anaesthesia.

Forapin
Note. This name is used for preparations of different composition.
Pfizer, Aust.; Mack, Switz.†.
Liniment: Bee venom; benzyl nicotinate (p.22·1); bornyl salicylate (p.22·1); camphor (p.1557·2); methyl nicotinate (p.55·1).
Frostbite; musculoskeletal, joint, and peri-articular disorders; neuralgias.
Pfizer, Aust.; Mack, Belg.; Ethimed, S.Afr.†; Mack, Switz.
Ointment: Bee venom; benzyl nicotinate (p.22·1); bornyl salicylate (p.22·1); nonivamide (p.63·2).
Frostbite; musculoskeletal, joint, and peri-articular disorders; neuralgias; sports injuries.

Forapin E *Mack, Illert., Ger.*
Liniment: Bee venom; bornyl salicylate (p.22·1); methyl nicotinate (p.55·1).
Ointment: Bee venom; benzyl nicotinate (p.22·1); bornyl salicylate (p.22·1).
Cold damage; musculoskeletal and joint disorders; sports injuries.

Forcapil *Arkopharma, Fr.*
Calcium pantothenate (p.1352·3); biotin (p.1336·1); pyridoxine (p.1363·1); zinc pidolate; cystine (p.1339·1); methionine (p.984·2).
Hair and nail tonic.

Force S *Arik, Fr.†.*
Nutritional supplement.
Tonic.

Forcemil *Normon, Spain.*
Multivitamin and mineral preparation with ginseng.

Forceval
Unigreg, Irl.; Unigreg, UK.
Multivitamin and mineral preparation.

Forceval Protein
Unigreg, Irl.; Unigreg, UK.
Lactose- and gluten-free preparation for enteral nutrition.

Ford Pills *BML, Austral.*
Aloin (p.1177·2); phenolphthalein (p.1208·2).
Constipation.

Fordiuran
Thomae, Ger.†; Boehringer Ingelheim, Spain.
Bumetanide (p.834·3).
Hypertension; oedema.

Fordtran *Hanseler, Switz.; Streuli, Switz.*
Macrogol 4000 (p.1598·2) with electrolytes.
Bowel evacuation.

Forehead-C *Lina, UK.*
Aloe vera (p.1177·1).
Fever.

Forene
Abbott, Belg.; Abbott, Ger.; Abbott, Neth.; Abbott, Norw.; Abbott, Swed.; Abbott, Switz.
Isoflurane (p.1225·1).
General anaesthesia.

Foresight *Cantassium Co., UK.*
Multivitamin preparation.

Foresight Iron Formula *Cantassium Co., UK.*
Ferrous gluconate (p.1340·1); copper gluconate (p.1338·1).

Forgenac *Zoja, Ital.*
Diclofenac sodium (p.31·2).
Inflammation; musculoskeletal and joint disorders; oedema.

Forit *Sanofi Winthrop, Ger.†.*
Oxypertine (p.684·1).
Psychiatric disorders.

Forlax *Beaufour, Fr.*
Macrogol 4000 (p.1598·2).
Constipation.

Formamint *Beecham, Spain†.*
Cetylpyridinium chloride (p.1106·2).
Mouth infections.

Formamint N *Fink, Ger.†.*
Cetylpyridinium chloride (p.1106·2).
Inflammatory disorders and infections of the oropharynx.

Formasan *Sanum-Kehlbeck, Ger.*
Homoeopathic preparation.

Formicain *DHU, Ger.*
Homoeopathic preparation.

Formicare Bath *Hamilton, Austral.†.*
Tar (p.1092·3).
Inflammation; pruritus; skin irritation.

Formicare Shower *Hamilton, Austral.†.*
Tar (p.1092·3).
Inflammation; pruritus; skin irritation.

Formicare Skin Gel *Hamilton, Austral.†.*
Tar (p.1092·3).
Inflammation; pruritus; skin irritation.

Formicare Skin Relief *Hamilton, Austral.†.*
Menthol (p.1600·2); cetrimide (p.1105·2); dimethicone (p.1384·2); tar (p.1092·3).
Dermatitis; dry skin; eczema.

Formicare Skin Wash *Hamilton, Austral.†.*
Tar (p.1092·3).
Dermatitis; dry skin; eczema; soap substitute.

Formidium *DHU, Ger.*
Homoeopathic preparation.

Formisocard *Staufen, Ger.†.*
Homoeopathic preparation.

Formisoton *Staufen, Ger.*
Homoeopathic preparation.

Formistin *Vedim, Ital.*
Cetirizine hydrochloride (p.404·2).
Hypersensitivity reactions.

Formitrol *Novartis, Ital.*
Dextromethorphan hydrobromide (p.1057·3).
Coughs.

Formix *Milanfarma, Ital.†.*
Antimony potassium tartrate (p.98·1).
Insecticide.

Formocarbine *SmithKline Beecham Sante, Fr.*
Activated charcoal (p.972·2).
Gastro-intestinal disorders.

Formocillina al Dequalinium *Zyma, Ital.†.*
Dequalinium chloride (p.1112·1).
Mouth infections.

Formo-Cresol Mitis *Colgate Oral Care, Austral.*
Formaldehyde (p.1113·2); cresol (p.1111·2).
Endodontics.

Formoftil *Farmigea, Ital.*
Formocortal (p.1043·2).
Inflammatory eye disorders.

Formomicin *Farmigea, Ital.*
Formocortal (p.1043·2); gentamicin sulphate (p.212·1).
Infected inflammatory eye disorders.

Formula I *Vitaplex, Austral.†.*
Slippery elm bark (p.1630·1); propolis (p.1621·3); liquorice root (p.1197·1); tincture myrrh (p.1606·1).
Oral inflammation.

Formula 44
Note. This name is used for preparations of different composition.
Richardson-Vicks, Austral.†.
Dextromethorphan hydrobromide (p.1057·3); pseudoephedrine hydrochloride (p.1068·3); guaiphenesin (p.1061·3).
Cough and cold symptoms.
Procter & Gamble, Canad.
Dextromethorphan hydrobromide (p.1057·3).
Coughs.

Formula 405 *Doak, USA.*
Skin cleanser.

Formula B-50 *Solgar, USA†.*
High potency vitamin B complex.

Formula B Plus *Major, USA.*
Ferrous fumarate (p.1339·3); folic acid (p.1340·3); multivitamins and minerals.
Iron-deficiency anaemias.

Formula CDC *Seroyal, Canad.*
Vitamin C, manganese, and zinc.

Formula CI *Seroyal, Canad.*
Chromium proteinate (p.1337·1); inositol nicotinate (p.891·3).

Formula 44D *Procter & Gamble, Canad.*
Dextromethorphan hydrobromide (p.1057·3); pseudoephedrine hydrochloride (p.1068·3).
Coughs and cold symptoms.

Formula 44E *Procter & Gamble, Canad.*
Dextromethorphan hydrobromide (p.1057·3); guaiphenesin (p.1061·3).
Coughs.

Formula Forte Senior *Hall, Canad.*
Multivitamin and mineral preparation.

Formula Gln *Seroyal, Canad.*
Vitamin B_6 (p.1362·3); magnesium proteinate (p.1157·2).

Formula Gly *Seroyal, Canad.*
Multivitamin and mineral preparation.

Formula III *Sisu, Canad.*
Multivitamin and mineral preparation.

Formula IV *Neo-Life, Austral.*
Nutritional supplement with vitamins and minerals.

Formula 44M *Procter & Gamble, Canad.*
Dextromethorphan hydrobromide (p.1057·3); pseudoephedrine hydrochloride (p.1068·3); chlorpheniramine maleate (p.405·1); paracetamol (p.72·2).
Coughs and cold symptoms.

Formula 44M Pediatric *Procter & Gamble, Canad.*
Dextromethorphan hydrobromide (p.1057·3); pseudoephedrine hydrochloride (p.1068·3); chlorpheniramine maleate (p.405·1).
Cold symptoms.

Formula OSG *Seroyal, Canad.*
Vitamin A, vitamin C, and minerals.

Formula OSX *Seroyal, Canad.*
Mineral preparation.

Formula Q *Major, USA†.*
Quinine sulphate (p.439·2).
Nocturnal leg cramps.

Formula Three *Vita Glow, Austral.†.*
Pyridoxine hydrochloride (p.1362·3); magnesium oxide (p.1198·3); zinc amino acid chelate (p.1373·3).
Nutritional supplement.

Formula Three Triple Strength *Vita Glow, Austral.†.*
Pyridoxine hydrochloride (p.1362·3); magnesium oxide (p.1198·3); zinc amino acid chelate (p.1373·3); manganese amino acid chelate.
Nutritional supplement.

Formula VM *Solgar, USA.*
A range of vitamin preparations.

Formula VM-75 *Solgar, UK.*
Multivitamin and mineral preparation.

Formulaexpec *Procter & Gamble, Spain.*
Guaiphenesin (p.1061·3).
Coughs.

Formulatus *Procter & Gamble, Spain.*
Dextromethorphan hydrobromide (p.1057·3).
Coughs.

Formule de l'Abbe Chaupitre *Homeopathie Complexe, Fr.*
A range of homoeopathic preparations.

Formule 115 DM *Frega, Canad.*
Pseudoephedrine hydrochloride (p.1068·3); chlorpheniramine maleate (p.405·1); dextromethorphan hydrobromide (p.1057·3).

Formule No 203 Profil *Pharmalab, Canad.*
Multivitamin and mineral preparation.

Formule No 204 Profil *Pharmalab, Canad.*
Vitamin C, iron, and potassium.

Formule W *Whitehall, Neth.*
Salicylic acid (p.1090·2).
Corns; warts.

Formulex *ICN, Canad.*
Dicyclomine hydrochloride (p.460·1).
Antispasmodic.

Formulix *Ortho, UK.*
Paracetamol (p.72·2); codeine phosphate (p.26·1). These ingredients can be described by the British Approved Name Co-codamol.
Pain.

Forpyn *Rolab, S.Afr.*
Paracetamol (p.72·2); codeine phosphate (p.26·1); caffeine (p.749·3); doxylamine succinate (p.410·1).
Pain and associated tension.

Forta *Ross, USA.*
A range of preparations for enteral nutrition.

Forta B *Continental Pharma, Belg.*
Hydroxocobalamin acetate (p.1364·2).
Megaloblastic anaemia; neuralgia; vitamin B_{12} deficiency.

Fortagesic *Sanofi Winthrop, Irl.*
Pentazocine hydrochloride (p.75·1); paracetamol (p.72·2).
Musculoskeletal pain.

Fortakehl *Sanum-Kehlbeck, Ger.*
Homoeopathic preparation.

Fortal
Sanofi Winthrop, Belg.; Sanofi Winthrop, Fr.
Pentazocine (p.75·1).
Adjunct in anaesthesia; pain.

Fortalgesic
Sanofi, Swed.; Sanofi Winthrop, Switz.
Pentazocine (p.75·1), pentazocine hydrochloride (p.75·1), or pentazocine lactate (p.75·1).
Neuroleptanalgesia; pain; premedication.

Fortalidon *Sandoz, Switz.†.*
Propyphenazone (p.81·3); aspirin (p.16·1); caffeine (p.749·3); codeine phosphate (p.26·1).
Fever; inflammation; pain.

Fortalidon P *Sandoz OTC, Switz.*
Paracetamol (p.72·2).
Fever; pain.

Fortalidon S *Wander, Ger.†.*
Propyphenazone (p.81·3); codeine phosphate (p.26·1). Formerly contained propyphenazone, aspirin, caffeine, and codeine phosphate.
Pain.

Fortalidon sans codeine *Sandoz OTC, Switz.†.*
Propyphenazone (p.81·3); caffeine (p.749·3); aspirin (p.16·1).
Influenza symptoms; pain.

Fortalis *Interdelta, Switz.*
Methyl salicylate (p.55·2); salicylic acid (p.1090·2); formic acid (p.1581·3); camphor (p.1557·2).
Musculoskeletal and joint pain.

Fortam
Glaxo Wellcome, Spain; Glaxo Wellcome, Switz.
Ceftazidime (p.173·3).
Bacterial infections.

Fortamines 10 *Rougier, Canad.*
Multivitamin preparation.

Fortaneurin *Continental Pharma, Belg.*
Vitamin B substances.
Megaloblastic anaemia; neuralgia; polyneuritis; vitamin B_1 and/or B_{12} deficiency.

Fortasec *Esteve, Spain.*
Loperamide hydrochloride (p.1197·2).
Diarrhoea.

Fortasept *Wander, Aust.*
Oxybuprocaine hydrochloride (p.1298·1).

Fortaz
Glaxo Wellcome, Canad.; Glaxo Wellcome, USA.
Ceftazidime (p.173·3).
Bacterial infections.

Fortecortin
Merck, Aust.; Merck, Ger.; Merck, Spain; E. Merck, Switz.
Dexamethasone (p.1037·1), dexamethasone phosphate (p.1037·2), or dexamethasone sodium phosphate (p.1037·2).
Corticosteroid.

Fortefog *Agropharm, UK.*
Cypermethrin (Fortemethrin) (p.1404·1); piperonyl butoxide (p.1409·3); bioallethrin (p.1402·3); *N*-octylbicycloheptenedicarboximide.
Insecticide and repellent.

Fortel *Biomerica, USA.*
Fertility test or pregnancy test (p.1621·2).

Fortepen *Biochemie, Aust.*
Procaine penicillin (p.240·2); benzylpenicillin sodium (p.159·3).
Bacterial infections.

Fortespan *SmithKline Beecham, UK.*
Ferrous sulphate (p.1340·2); folic acid (p.1340·3).
Iron and folic acid deficiency in pregnancy.

Fortfen *Compu, S.Afr.*
Diclofenac sodium (p.31·2).
Gout; inflammation; musculoskeletal and joint disorders; pain.

Forthane *Abbott, Austral.*
Isoflurane (p.1225·1).
General anaesthesia.

Fortical *Rubio, Spain.*
Calcium carbonate (p.1182·1).
Hypocalcaemia; osteoporosis.

Forticine *Wolfs, Belg.*
Nutritional supplement.

Forticrin *Panzera, Ital.*
Vitamin B substances; vitamin E (p.1369·1); achillea (p.1542·2); ginkgo biloba (p.1584·1); ginseng (p.1584·2).
Hair loss.

Fortifresh
Nutricia, Fr.; Nutricia, Ital.
Preparation for enteral nutrition.

Fortijuice
Nutricia, Irl.; Nutricia, UK.
Preparation for enteral nutrition.

Fortimel
Nutricia, Fr.†; Nutricia, Irl.; Nutricia, Ital.; Nutricia, UK.
High-protein nutritional supplement.

Fortimicin *Kyowa, Jpn.*
Astromicin sulphate (p.155·1).
Bacterial infections.

Fortinic *Lambda, USA.*
Vitamin B substances and iron.

Fortipine *Goldshield, UK.*
Nifedipine (p.916·2).
Angina pectoris; hypertension; Raynaud's syndrome.

Fortiplex *Sante Naturelle, Canad.*
Vitamin B_{12} (p.1363·3); ferrous fumarate (p.1339·3).

Fortipudding
Nutricia, Fr.; Nutricia, Irl.; Nutricia, Ital.; Nutricia, UK.
High-protein nutritional supplement.

Fortisip
Nutricia, Irl.; Nutricia, UK.
Low-lactose and gluten-free, preparation for enteral nutrition.

Fortistress *Sante Naturelle, Canad.*
Vitamin B substances and vitamin C.

Fortovase *Roche, USA.*
Saquinavir (p.625·3).
HIV infection.

Fortradol *Bayer, Ital.*
Tramadol hydrochloride (p.90·1).
Pain.

Fortral
Sanofi Winthrop, Aust.; Sanofi Winthrop, Austral.; Sanofi Winthrop, Ger.; Sanofi Winthrop, Irl.; Sanofi Winthrop, Neth.; Sterling Research, UK†.
Pentazocine (p.75·1), pentazocine hydrochloride (p.75·1), or pentazocine lactate (p.75·1).
Pain.

Fortralin *Sanofi Winthrop, Norw.*
Pentazocine (p.75·1), pentazocine hydrochloride (p.75·1), or pentazocine lactate (p.75·1).
Pain.

Fortrans *Beaufour, Fr.*
Macrogol 4000 (p.1598·2); anhydrous sodium sulphate (p.1213·3); sodium bicarbonate; sodium chloride; potassium chloride.
Bowel evacuation.

Fortravel *Asta Medica, Aust.*
Cyclizine hydrochloride (p.407·1).
Motion sickness.

Fortum
Glaxo Wellcome, Aust.; Glaxo Wellcome, Austral.; Glaxo Wellcome, Fr.; Cascan, Ger.; Glaxo Wellcome, Ger.; Glaxo Wellcome, Irl.; Glaxo Wellcome, Neth.; Glaxo Wellcome, Norw.; Glaxo Wellcome, S.Afr.; Glaxo Wellcome, Swed.; Glaxo, UK.
Ceftazidime (p.173·3).
Bacterial infections.

Fortyplan *Lifeplan, UK.*
Vitamin, mineral, and nutritional preparation.

Forunculone *Labaz, Spain†.*
Tyrothricin (p.267·2); trypsin (p.1640·1).
Skin infections.

Forvital *Whitehall, Fr.*
Multivitamin and iron preparation.

Forvite *Lennon, S.Afr.†.*
Vitamin B substances.
Tonic.

Fosamax
Merck Sharp & Dohme, Aust.; Merck Sharp & Dohme, Austral.; Merck Sharp & Dohme, Belg.; Merck Sharp & Dohme, Canad.; Merck Sharp & Dohme, Ger.; Merck Sharp & Dohme, Irl.; Merck Sharp & Dohme, Ital.; Merck Sharp & Dohme, Neth.; Merck Sharp & Dohme, Norw.; Merck Sharp & Dohme, S.Afr.; Merck Sharp & Dohme, Spain; Merck Sharp & Dohme, Swed.; Merck Sharp & Dohme, Switz.; Merck Sharp & Dohme, UK.
Alendronate sodium (p.733·2).
Paget's disease of bone; osteoporosis.

Foscavir
Astra, Aust.; Astra, Austral.; Astra, Belg.; Astra, Fr.; Astra, Ger.; Astra, Ital.; Astra, Neth.; Astra, Norw.; Astra, Spain; Astra, Swed.; Astra, Switz.; Astra, UK; Astra, USA.
Foscarnet sodium (p.610·2).
Cytomegalovirus retinitis; herpes simplex infections.

Fosenema *Sabax, S.Afr.†.*
Monobasic sodium phosphate (p.1159·3); dibasic sodium phosphate (p.1159·3).
Bowel evacuation.

Fosfalugel *Yamanouchi, Ital.*
Aluminium phosphate (p.1178·3).
Gastric hyperacidity.

Fosfalumina *Schering-Plough, Spain.*
Aluminium phosphate (p.1178·3).
Gastro-intestinal hyperacidity; phosphate deficiency.

Fosfarginil *Wasserman, Spain†.*
Arginine glucose-1-phosphate.
Hyperammonaemia; liver disorders.

Fosfarsile Forte *Fitobucaneve, Ital.*
Oral liquid: Royal jelly (p.1626·3); propolis (p.1621·3); selenium (p.1353·3); ginseng (p.1584·2).
Tablets: Glucose (p.1343·3); royal jelly (p.1626·3); ginseng (p.1584·2).
Nutritional supplement.

Fosfarsile Yunior *Fitobucaneve, Ital.*
Royal jelly (p.1626·3); vitamins; phosphorus proteinate; cod-liver oil (p.1337·3).
Nutritional supplement.

Fosfidral *Angelini, Ital.†.*
Aluminium phosphate (p.1178·3).
Gastric hyperacidity; peptic ulcer.

Fosfo Plus *FAMA, Ital.*
Levoglutamide (p.1344·3); DL-phosphoserine; cyanocobalamin (p.1363·3).
Tonic.

Fosfoalugel *IBYS, Spain†.*
Aluminium phosphate (p.1178·3).
Gastro-intestinal disorders; phosphate deficiency.

Fosfobiotic *Bergamon, Ital.†.*
Fosfomycin calcium (p.210·2) or fosfomycin disodium (p.210·2).
Bacterial infections.

Fosfocin
Sanofi Winthrop, Belg.†; Boehringer Mannheim, Ger.; Crinos, Ital.; Dumex-Alpharma, Swed.†; Boehringer Mannheim, Switz.
Fosfomycin calcium (p.210·2) or fosfomycin disodium (p.210·2).
Bacterial infections.

Fosfocina *I Farmacologia, Spain.*
Fosfomycin calcium (p.210·2) or fosfomycin disodium (p.210·2).
Lignocaine hydrochloride (p.1293·2) is included in the intramuscular injection to alleviate the pain of injection.
Bacterial infections.

Fosfocine *Sanofi Winthrop, Fr.*
Fosfomycin sodium (p.210·2).
Bacterial infections.

Fosfocrisolo *Zambon, Ital.*
Sodium aurothiosulphate (p.85·1).
Rheumatoid arthritis.

Fosfodexa *Llorens, Spain†.*
Dexamethasone phosphate (p.1037·2).
Inflammatory eye disorders.

Fosfoglutil *Beta, Ital.†.*
Aceglutamide (p.1541·2) or levoglutamide (p.1344·3); asparagine; DL-phosphoserine; pyridoxine hydrochloride (p.1362·3).
Mental function impairment.

Fosfogram *FIRMA, Ital.†.*
Fosfomycin calcium (p.210·2) or fosfomycin disodium (p.210·2).
Bacterial infections.

Fosfoguaiacol *Ogna, Ital.*
Guaiacol (p.1061·2); eucalyptus (p.1578·1).
Respiratory congestion.

Fosfolexin *Lifepharma, Ital.†.*
Fosfomycin (p.210·1); cephalexin (p.178·2).
Bacterial infections.

Fosfolip *ISF, Ital.†.*
Pantethine (p.1276·3); fosforylcholine (p.1581·3).
Liver disorders.

Fosfor
Consolidated Chemicals, Irl.; Chancellor, UK.
Phosphorylcolamine.
Tonic.

Fosforal *Fournier, Ital.*
Fosfomycin calcium (p.210·2).
Bacterial infections.

Fosforil Calcium *SPA, Ital.*
Calcium glucose-1-phosphate; pyridoxine hydrochloride (p.1362·3); ergocalciferol (p.1367·1).
Calcium and vitamin deficiency.

Fosforilasi *Polifarma, Ital.*
Injection: Cocarboxylase (p.1361·2); riboflavine sodium phosphate (p.1362·1); pyridoxal phosphate (p.1363·1); nicotinamide (p.1351·2).
Lignocaine hydrochloride (p.1293·2) is included in this preparation to alleviate the pain of injection.
Neuritis; toxicosis.
Oral sachets†: Cocarboxylase hydrochloride (p.1361·2); riboflavine sodium phosphate (p.1362·1); pyridoxine hydrochloride (p.1362·3); nicotinamide (p.1351·2).

Fosfo-Soda Fleet *Bergamon, Ital.*
Monobasic sodium phosphate (p.1159·3); dibasic sodium phosphate (p.1159·3).
Constipation.

Fosfoutipi Vitaminico *Terapeutico, Ital.*
Uridine triphosphate (p.1641·3); cyanocobalamin (p.1363·3); thiamine hydrochloride (p.1361·1).
Peripheral neuropathies.

Fosfozimin *Medosan, Ital.†.*
Cyanocobalamin (p.1363·3); cocarboxylase (p.1361·2); lignocaine (p.1293·2).
Peripheral neuropathies.

Fosfree *Mission Pharmacal, USA.*
Multivitamin preparation with iron and calcium.
Calcium supplement; nocturnal leg cramping.

Fosglutamina B6 *Baldacci, Ital.†.*
Calcium pidolate (p.1155·3); tetraethylammonium phosphate; pyridoxine hydrochloride (p.1362·3); levoglutamide (p.1344·3).
Mental function impairment.

Fosgluten Reforzado *Alter, Spain.*
Calcium magnesium phytate; vitamin B substances; glutamine.
Tonic.

Fosicombi *Menarini, Ital.*
Fosinopril sodium (p.870·3); hydrochlorothiazide (p.885·2).
Hypertension.

Fosicomp *Bristol-Myers Squibb, Switz.*
Fosinopril sodium (p.870·3); hydrochlorothiazide (p.885·2).
Hypertension.

Fosinil *Solvay, Belg.*
Fosinopril sodium (p.870·3).
Hypertension.

Fosinorm *Bristol-Myers Squibb, Ger.*
Fosinopril sodium (p.870·3).
Hypertension.

Fosipres *Menarini, Ital.*
Fosinopril sodium (p.870·3).
Heart failure; hypertension.

Fositen *Bristol-Myers Squibb, Switz.*
Fosinopril sodium (p.870·3).
Heart failure; hypertension.

Fositens
Bristol-Myers Squibb, Aust.; Squibb, Spain.
Fosinopril sodium (p.870·3).
Heart failure; hypertension.

Foslymar *Bellon, Fr.†.*
Glycerol phosphate; monobasic magnesium phosphate.
Hypercalcaemia; hypercalciuria; magnesium deficiency; osteomalacia; osteoporosis; rickets; tetany.

Fosmicin *Meiji, Jpn†.*
Fosfomycin calcium (p.210·2).
Bacterial infections.

Fosmicin-S *Meiji, Jpn.*
Fosfomycin sodium (p.210·2).
Bacterial infections.

Fossyol *Merckle, Ger.*
Metronidazole (p.585·1).
Trichomoniasis.

Fostex *Westwood, USA.*
Benzoyl peroxide (p.1079·2).
Acne.

Fostex Acne Medication Cleansing *Bristol-Myers Products, USA.*
Salicylic acid (p.1090·2).
Acne; hyperkeratosis.

Fostex CM *Bristol-Myers Squibb, Canad.†.*
Sulphur (p.1091·2); laureth 4 (p.1325·2).
Acne.

Fostex Medicated *Westwood-Squibb, USA.*
Salicylic acid (p.1090·2); sulphur (p.1091·2).
Acne.

Fostex Medicated Cleansing *Bristol-Myers Squibb, Canad.*
Salicylic acid (p.1090·2).
Acne; oily skin.

Fostex Medicated Cleansing Bar *Westwood, USA†.*
Salicylic acid (p.1090·2); sulphur (p.1091·2); boric acid (p.1554·2); docusate sodium (p.1189·3); urea (p.1095·2).
Acne.

Fostril *Westwood, USA.*
Sulphur (p.1091·2); zinc oxide (p.1096·2).
Acne.

Fotil
Leiras, Norw.; Santen, Swed.
Pilocarpine hydrochloride (p.1396·3); timolol maleate (p.953·3).
Glaucoma; ocular hypertension.

Fotofil *INTES, Ital.*
Sodium aminobenzoate; actinoquinol (p.1543·1); naphazoline nitrate (p.1064·2); borax (p.1554·2).
Blepharitis; conjunctivitis; corneal damage.

Fotoretin *Farmila, Ital.†.*
Myrtillus (p.1606·1); betacarotene (p.1335·2).
Eye disorders.

Fototar *ICN, USA.*
Coal tar (Eldotar) (p.1092·3).
Chronic skin disorders such as psoriasis, eczema, or seborrhoea.

Four-Ton *Body Spring, Ital.*
Guarana (p.1645·1); damiana (p.1570·2); ginseng (p.1584·2); royal jelly (p.1626·3).
Nutritional supplement.

Fovysat *Ysatfabrik, Ger.†.*
Crataegus (p.1568·2); ginger (p.1193·2).
Dystonias; neuroses.

Fovysatum *Ysatfabrik, Ger.†.*
Ephedrine hydrochloride (p.1059·3); mistletoe (p.1604·1); crataegus (p.1568·2); ginger (p.1193·2).
Circulatory disorders; hypotension.

Fowlers Diarrhea Tablet *Sandoz, Canad.*
Attapulgite (p.1178·3).

Foximin *Caber, Ital.†.*
Fosfomycin calcium (p.210·2).
Bacterial infections.

Foy
Lepetit, Ital.; Ono, Jpn.
Gabexate mesylate (p.1582·1).
Disseminated intravascular coagulation; pancreatitis.

Fozitec *Lipha Sante, Fr.*
Fosinopril sodium (p.870·3).
Heart failure; hypertension.

Fractal *Sinbio, Fr.*
Fluvastatin sodium (p.1273·2).
Hyperlipidaemias.

Fradicilina *Reig Jofre, Spain.*
Procaine penicillin (p.240·2).
Bacterial infections.

Frador *Fenton, UK.*
Menthol (p.1600·2); chlorbutol (p.1106·3); storax (p.1632·3); benzoin (p.1634·1).
Mouth ulcers.

Fradyl *Christiaens, Belg.†.*
Neomycin sulphate (p.229·2).
Rhinitis; sinusitis.

Fragador *Weleda, UK.*
Cochlearia offic.; conchae; fragaria vesca fruit; glycogen; levisticum root (p.1597·2); mel; natrium carb.; pimpinella anisum fruit; sage leaves (p.1627·1); wheat germ; urtica leaves (p.1642·3); ferrum phos.
Stress.

Fragiprel *Biogalenique, Fr.†.*
Hesperidin methyl chalcone (p.1580·2); troxerutin (p.1580·2); ruscus; ascorbic acid (p.1365·2).
Peripheral vascular disorders.

Fragivix
Sanofi Winthrop, Belg.†; Sanol, Ger.†.
Benzarone (p.1552·3).
Vascular disorders.

Fragmin
Pharmacia Upjohn, Aust.; Pharmacia Upjohn, Austral.; Pharmacia Upjohn, Belg.; Pharmacia Upjohn, Canad.; Pharmacia Upjohn, Ger.; Pharmacia Upjohn, Ital.; Pharmacia Upjohn, Neth.; Pharmacia Upjohn, Norw.; Pharmacia Upjohn, S.Afr.; Pharmacia Upjohn, Spain; Pharmacia Upjohn, Swed.; Pharmacia Upjohn, Switz.; Pharmacia Upjohn, UK; Pharmacia Upjohn, USA.
Dalteparin sodium (p.845·3).
Deep vein thrombosis; prevention of clotting during haemodialysis and haemofiltration; thrombo-embolic disorders.

Fragmine *Pharmacia Upjohn, Fr.*
Dalteparin sodium (p.845·3).
Prevention of clotting during haemodialysis; thrombo-embolic disorders.

Fragonal *Phygiene, Fr.*
Ruscus aculeatus; esculoside (p.1543·3).
Circulatory disorders; haemorrhoids.

Frakidex
Chauvin, Fr.; Novopharma, Switz.
Dexamethasone sodium phosphate (p.1037·2); framycetin sulphate (p.210·3).
Infected eye disorders.

Frakitacine *Novopharma, Switz.*
Framycetin sulphate (p.210·3).
Bacterial eye infections.

Framil *Francia, Ital.*
Bicarnitine chloride (p.1336·2).
Anorexia; dyspepsia.

Framin *SIFRA, Ital.*
Amino-acid infusion.
Parenteral nutrition.

Framitulle *Cassenne, Fr.†.*
Framycetin sulphate (p.210·3).
Burns; wounds.

Framol *Saphar, S.Afr.†.*
Ephedrine sulphate (p.1059·3); theophylline (p.765·1); phenobarbitone (p.350·2).
Asthma; bronchospasm.

Framybiotal *Martin, Fr.*
Framycetin sulphate (p.210·3).
Rhinopharyngeal infections.

Francetin *Mochida, Jpn†.*
Neomycin sulphate (p.229·2).
Bacterial infections.

Franciclina *Francia, Ital.†.*
Methacycline hydrochloride (p.225·1).
Bacterial infections.

Francital *Francia, Ital.*
Capsules; tablets: Fosfomycin calcium (p.210·2).
Injection†: Fosfomycin disodium (p.210·2).
Bacterial infections.

Francomicina *Nuovo, Ital.†.*
Methacycline hydrochloride (p.225·1).
Bacterial infections.

Frangulina *Bruschettini, Ital.*
Frangula (p.1193·2); boldo (p.1554·1).
Constipation.

Franol
Sanofi Winthrop, Irl.; Sanofi Winthrop, UK.
Ephedrine hydrochloride (p.1059·3); theophylline (p.765·1).
Formerly contained phenobarbitone, ephedrine hydrochloride, and theophylline in the *UK*.
Bronchospasm.

Franol Expectorant *Sanofi Winthrop, Irl.*
Theophylline hydrate (p.765·1); guaiphenesin (p.1061·3).
Formerly contained ephedrine, theophylline hydrate, and guaiphenesin.
Obstructive airways disease.

Franol Plus *Sanofi Winthrop, UK.*
Ephedrine sulphate (p.1059·3); theophylline (p.765·1).
Formerly contained phenobarbitone, thenyldiamine hydrochloride, ephedrine sulphate, and theophylline.
Bronchospasm.

Franolyn Expectorant *Johnson & Johnson MSD Consumer, UK.*
Ephedrine (p.1059·3); guaiphenesin (p.1061·3); theophylline (p.765·1).
Formerly known as Strong Franolyn.
Coughs.

Franolyn Sedative *Johnson & Johnson MSD Consumer, UK.*
Dextromethorphan hydrobromide (p.1057·3).
Formerly known as Soothing Franolyn.
Coughs.

Franovul *Francia, Ital.†.*
Lynoestrenol (p.1448·2); mestranol (p.1450·2).
Menstrual disorders.

Franzbragil "F" *Agil, Ger.†.*
Oleum pini sylvestris; isobornyl acetate; terpinyl acetate; cineole (p.1564·1); cumin aldehyde; laurin aldehyde.
Pain; peripheral vascular disease.

Franzbragil "M" *Agil, Ger.†.*
Menthol (p.1600·2).
Back pain; bruising; lumbago; nerve disorders; rheumatism; sciatica.

Franzbranns *Hilarys, Canad.*
Menthol (p.1600·2); alcohol (p.1099·1); eucalyptus oil (p.1578·1); salol (p.83·1).

Franzbranntwein *Klosterfrau, Ger.*
Menthol (p.1600·2); camphor (p.1557·2); alcohol (p.1099·1).
Muscle and joint pain; soft-tissue disorders.

Fraurs *Francia, Ital.*
Ursodeoxycholic acid (p.1642·1).
Biliary disorders; gallstones.

Fravit B12 *Francia, Ital.†.*
Hydroxocobalamin (p.1363·3).
Anaemias; liver disorders; peripheral neuropathies.

Fraxiparin *Sanofi Winthrop, Ger.*
Nadroparin calcium (p.914·1).
Thrombosis prophylaxis.

Fraxiparina
Sanofi Winthrop, Ital.; Sanofi, Spain.
Nadroparin calcium (p.914·1).
Thrombo-embolic disorders.

Fraxiparine
Sanofi Winthrop, Austral.; Sanofi Winthrop, Belg.; Sanofi Winthrop, Fr.; Sanofi Winthrop, Neth.; Sanofi, Swed.; Sanofi Winthrop, Switz.
Nadroparin calcium (p.914·1).
Prevention of clotting during haemodialysis; thrombo-embolic disorders.

Fraxipos N *Ursapharm, Ger.†.*
Oxedrine hydrochloride (p.925·3).
Eye disorders.

Frazim *Francia, Ital.*
Pirenzepine hydrochloride (p.467·1).
Peptic ulcer.

Frazoline *Bouchara, Fr.*
Framycetin sulphate (p.210·3); naphazoline nitrate (p.1064·2); amylocaine hydrochloride (p.1286·1).
Nasal infection and congestion.

FreAmine
Kendall McGaw, Canad.†; Fresenius, UK.
Amino-acid and electrolyte infusions.
Parenteral nutrition.

FreAmine HBC *McGaw, USA.*
Amino-acid infusion.
Parenteral nutrition in hepatic encephalopathy.

FreAmine Hepatico *Pharmacia, Spain.*
Amino acid infusion.
Parenteral nutrition.

FreAmine III
Clintec, Ital.; Pharmacia, Spain†; McGaw, USA.
A range of amino-acid infusions with or without electrolytes.
Parenteral nutrition.

Free & Clear *Pharmaceutical Specialties, USA.*
Skin cleanser.

Freedavite *Freeda, USA.*
Multivitamin and mineral preparation with iron.

Freedox
Willvonseder, Aust.; Pharmacia Upjohn, Austral.; Pharmacia Upjohn, Norw.; Pharmacia Upjohn, S.Afr.; Pharmacia Upjohn, Swed.; Pharmacia Upjohn, Switz.
Tirilazad mesylate (p.954·3).
Subarachnoid haemorrhage.

Freezone
Whitehall-Robins, Canad.; Whitehall, Irl.; Whitehall, UK; Whitehall, USA.
Salicylic acid (p.1090·2).
Hyperkeratosis.

Freka nol *Fresenius, Ger.†.*
Alcohol (p.1099·1); glyoxal (p.1115·1); didecyldimethylammonium chloride (p.1112·2).
Surface disinfection.

Freka-cetamol *Fresenius, Ger.†.*
Paracetamol (p.72·2).
Fever; pain.

Freka-cid *Fresenius-Praxis, Ger.*
Povidone-iodine (p.1123·3).
Skin disinfection.

Freka-Clyss *Fresenius, Switz.*
Dibasic sodium phosphate (p.1159·3); monobasic sodium phosphate (p.1159·3).
Bowel evacuation; constipation.

Frekaderm
Fresenius, Fr.; Fresenius, Ger.; Fresenius, Switz.
Alcohol (p.1099·1); benzalkonium chloride (p.1101·3); orthophenylphenol (p.1120·3); clorophene (p.1111·2).
Skin disinfection.

Freka-Drainjet *Fresenius, Ger.*
Sodium chloride (p.1162·2).
Irrigation fluid.

Freka-Feindesinfektion *Fresenius, Ger.†.*
Dodecyl-1,4,7-triazaoctan-8-carbonic acid hydrochloride.
Disinfectant.

Freka-Sept 80 *Fresenius, Ger.*
Alcohol (p.1099·1); orthophenylphenol (p.1120·3); clorophene (p.1111·2); benzalkonium chloride (p.1101·3).
Hand disinfection.

Freka-Steril *Fresenius, Ger.*
Propyl alcohol (p.1124·2); isopropyl alcohol (p.1118·2).
Hand disinfection; skin disinfection.

Frekatuss *Fresenius-Praxis, Ger.†.*
Acetylcysteine (p.1052·3).
Ear and respiratory-tract disorders associated with increased or viscous mucus.

Fremet *Recordati Elmu, Spain.*
Cimetidine (p.1183·2).
Acid aspiration; gastro-oesophageal reflux; peptic ulcer; Zollinger-Ellison syndrome.

Frenactil
Janssen-Cilag, Belg.; Janssen-Cilag, Neth.
Benperidol (p.642·3).
Agitation; delirium; hallucinations; nausea and vomiting; sexually deviant behaviour.

Frenadol *Abello, Spain.*
Paracetamol (p.72·2); chlorpheniramine maleate (p.405·1); dextromethorphan hydrobromide (p.1057·3).
Formerly contained ascorbic acid, caffeine citrate, chlorpheniramine maleate, codeine phosphate, paracetamol, and salicylamide.
Coughs; fever; influenza and cold symptoms; pain.

Frenadol Complex *Abello, Spain.*
Ascorbic acid (p.1365·2); caffeine citrate (p.749·3); chlorpheniramine maleate (p.405·1); dextromethorphan hydrobromide (p.1057·3); paracetamol (p.72·2).
Cold and influenza symptoms; coughs; fever; pain.

Frenadol PS *Abello, Spain.*
Paracetamol (p.72·2); pseudoephedrine hydrochloride (p.1068·3); dextromethorphan hydrobromide (p.1057·3); chlorpheniramine maleate (p.405·1).
Cold and influenza symptoms; coughs; fever; pain.

Frenal
Searle, Ital.; Sigma-Tau, Spain.
Sodium cromoglycate (p.762·1).
Allergic rhinitis; asthma.

Frenal Compositum
Schiapparelli Searle, Ital.†; Sigma-Tau, Spain.
Sodium cromoglycate (p.762·1); isoprenaline sulphate (p.892·1).
Allergic bronchitis; asthma.

Frenal Rinologico *Searle, Ital.*
Sodium cromoglycate (p.762·1).
Allergic rhinitis.

Frenespan *Miquel Otsuka, Spain†.*
Isamfazone (p.48·1); metoclopramide piperazine-*n*-oxide; hyoscine butylbromide (p.462·3).
Smooth muscle spasm.

Frenolon *Thiemann, Ger.†.*
Metofenazate fumarate.
Psychoses.

frenopect *Hefa, Ger.*
Ambroxol hydrochloride (p.1054·3).
Respiratory-tract disorders associated with increased or viscous mucus.

Frerichs Maldifassi *Procemsa, Ital.*
Aloes (p.1177·1); rhubarb (p.1212·1); calamus (p.1556·1); gentian (p.1583·3).
Constipation.

Fresenius OPD *Rowa, Irl.*
Preparation for enteral nutrition.
Inflammatory bowel disease.

FreshBurst Listerine *Warner-Wellcome, USA.*
Thymol (p.1127·1); cineole (p.1564·1); methyl salicylate (p.55·2); menthol (p.1600·2).
Mouth disorders.

Fresubin
Rowa, Irl.; Fresenius, Switz.; Fresenius, UK.
Preparations for enteral nutrition.

Frezan *Drug Houses Austral., Austral.†.*
Dichlorotetrafluoroethane (p.1164·3); ethyl chloride (p.1292·3).
Topical anaesthesia.

Frialgina *Prodes, Spain.*
Aspirin (p.16·1); ascorbic acid (p.1365·2); caffeine (p.749·3).
Fever; pain.

Fribagyl *Vifor, Switz.†.*
Aspirin (p.16·1); paracetamol (p.72·2); codeine phosphate (p.26·1); caffeine (p.749·3).
Fever; pain.

Fribagyl sans codeine *Vifor, Switz.†.*
Aspirin (p.16·1); paracetamol (p.72·2); caffeine (p.749·3).
Fever; pain.

Friction Rub *Mathieu, Canad.*
Isopropyl alcohol (p.1118·2).

Fridol *Pharkos, Ital.†.*
Aspirin (p.16·1); caffeine (p.749·3).
Influenza; pain.

Frigol *Brady, Aust.*
Xanthinol nicotinate (p.971·1).
Cerebral and peripheral vascular disorders.

Frigoplasma *Kropf, Switz.*
Aluminium acetotartrate (p.1547·3); chamomile (p.1561·2); hamamelis (p.1587·1); camphor (p.1557·2); cajuput oil (p.1556·1); rosemary oil (p.1626·2); thyme oil (p.1637·1).
Phlebitis; soft-tissue and peri-articular disorders.

Frikton *Fader, Spain†.*
Cantharides (p.1559·1); pilocarpine (p.1396·3); quinine hydrochloride (p.439·2); resorcinol (p.1090·1); rum essence; sulphanilamide (p.256·3).
Hair loss; pityriasis.

Friliver *Bracco, Ital.*
Amino-acid preparations.
Hepatic failure; tonic.

Frinova *Rhone-Poulenc Rorer, Spain.*
Promethazine (p.416·2).
Hypersensitivity reactions; insomnia; nausea and vomiting; vertigo.

Frio Augentropfen "B" *Michallik, Ger.†.*
Panthenol (p.1571·1).
Eye irritation.

Friosmin *Michallik, Ger.†.*
Ointment: Liquefied phenol (p.1121·2); bismuth subgallate (p.1180·2); emplastrum lithargyri.
Burns; wounds.
Oral drops: Coriander (p.1567·3); caraway (p.1559·3); fennel (p.1579·1); aniseed (p.1549·3); cnicus benedictus (p.1565·3); thyme (p.1636·3); peppermint leaf (p.1208·1); cinchona bark (p.1564·1); angelica; rhubarb (p.1212·1); calamus (p.1556·1).
Gastro-intestinal disorders.

Friosmin N *Michallik, Ger.*
Bismuth subgallate (p.1180·2); emplastrum lithargyri.
Burns; wounds.

Fripouille *Dermophil Indien, Fr.†.*
Ethylpropoxyl aminobenzoate.
Sunscreen.

Frisium
Hoechst, Aust.; Hoechst Marion Roussel, Austral.; Hoechst Marion Roussel, Belg.; Hoechst Marion Roussel, Canad.; Hoechst, Ger.; Hoechst Marion Roussel, Irl.; Hoechst Marion Roussel, Ital.; Hoechst Marion Roussel, Neth.; Hoechst, UK.
Clobazam (p.656·3).
Anxiety; epilepsy; insomnia.

Fristamin *Italfarmaco, Ital.*
Loratadine (p.413·1).
Allergic rhinitis; hypersensitivity reactions.

Froben
Ebewe, Aust.; Knoll, Belg.; Knoll, Canad.; Kanoldt, Ger.; Knoll, Irl.; Nordmark, Ital.; Knoll, Neth.; Knoll, S.Afr.; Knoll, Spain; Knoll, Switz.; Knoll, UK.
Flurbiprofen (p.42·1).
Inflammation; musculoskeletal, joint, peri-articular, and soft-tissue disorders; pain.

Frone
Serono, Ital.; Serono, Spain.
Interferon beta (p.616·1).
Anogenital warts; malignant neoplasms; viral infections.

Frontal *Solvay, Ital.*
Alprazolam (p.640·3).
Anxiety disorders.

Froop *Ashbourne, UK.*
Frusemide (p.871·1).
Oedema; oliguria.

Froop Co *Ashbourne, UK.*
Frusemide (p.871·1); amiloride hydrochloride (p.819·2).
These ingredients can be described by the British Approved Name Co-amilofruse.
Ascites with cirrhosis; oedema.

Frosinor *Ciba-Geigy, Spain.*
Paroxetine hydrochloride (p.301·2).
Depression.

Frost Cream *Weleda, UK.*
Abrotanum; arnica (p.1550·3); peru balsam (p.1617·2); rosemary oil (p.1626·2); stibium metallicum.
Chilblains.

Frostsalbe *Weleda, Aust.*
Homoeopathic preparation.

Frubiase *Boehringer Ingelheim, Belg.†.*
Calcium gluconate (p.1155·2); calcium lactate (p.1155·2); phosphoric acid (p.1618·1); ergocalciferol (p.1367·1); ascorbic acid (p.1365·2).
Hypersensitivity disorders; osteomalacia; osteoporosis; rickets; spasmophilia.

Frubiase Calcium *Boehringer Ingelheim, Ger.*
Calcium carbonate (p.1182·1).
Calcium deficiency.

Frubiase Calcium forte *Boehringer Ingelheim, Ger.†.*
Calcium carbonate (p.1182·1); cholecalciferol (p.1366·3).
Osteomalacia; osteoporosis.

Frubiase Calcium forte 500 *Boehringer Ingelheim, Ger.*
Calcium gluconate (p.1155·2); calcium lactate (p.1155·2); ergocalciferol (p.1367·1).
Osteomalacia; osteoporosis.

Frubiase Calcium T *Boehringer Ingelheim, Ger.*
Calcium gluconate (p.1155·2); calcium lactate (p.1155·2).
Calcium deficiency.

Frubibalsam *Biotherax, Ger.†.*
Eucalyptus oil (p.1578·1); siberian fir oil; pumilio pine oil (p.1623·3); anise oil (p.1550·1).
Respiratory-tract disorders.

Frubienzym *Boehringer Ingelheim, Ger.*
Muramidase (p.1604·3); cetylpyridinium chloride (p.1106·2).
Inflammatory disorders and infections of the oropharynx.

Frubilurgyl *Boehringer Ingelheim, Ger.*
Chlorhexidine gluconate (p.1107·2).
Inflammatory disorders and infections of the oropharynx.

Frubiose Calcique *Boehringer Ingelheim, Fr.*
Ergocalciferol (p.1367·1); calcium gluconate (p.1155·2); calcium lactate (p.1155·2).
Hypocalcaemia; osteomalacia; rickets; vitamin D and calcium deficiency.

Frubiose Calcium *Wild, Switz.*
Calcium gluconate (p.1155·2); calcium lactate (p.1155·2); ergocalciferol (p.1367·1); phosphoric acid (p.1618·1).
Calcium deficiency.

Frubizin *Boehringer Ingelheim, Ger.*
Cetylpyridinium chloride (p.1106·2).
Mouth and throat infection and inflammation.

Frubizin Forte *Boehringer Ingelheim, Ger.*
Cetylpyridinium chloride (p.1106·2); benzocaine (p.1286·2).
Mouth and throat infection and inflammation.

Fru-Co
Norton Waterford, Irl.; Norton, UK.
Amiloride hydrochloride (p.819·2); frusemide (p.871·1).
These ingredients can be described by the British Approved Name Co-amilofruse.
Ascites; heart failure; nephrotic syndrome; oedema.

Frucol *Boehringer Ingelheim, Fr.†.*
Magnesium ferulate (p.1598·3).
Dyspepsia.

Fructal *Bieffe, Ital.*
Fructose (p.1343·2).

Fructan *Boehringer Mannheim, Ital.*
Fructose (p.1343·2).
Sugar substitute.

Fructines
Pharmethic, Belg.; DB, Fr.
Sodium picosulphate (p.1213·2).
Constipation.

Fructines nouvelle formule *DB, Switz.*
Sodium picosulphate (p.1213·2).
Constipation.

Fructine-Vichy *Lirca, Ital.†.*
Phenolphthalein (p.1208·2).
Constipation.

Fructoglucina *SPA, Ital.†.*
Disodium glucose-1-phosphate; disodium glucose-6-phosphate; trisodium fructose-1,6-diphosphate.
Glucose deficiency.

Fructopiran *Monico, Ital.*
Fructose (p.1343·2).

Fructosil *Volchem, Ital.*
Fructose (p.1343·2).
Supplementation of glycogen reserves.

Frugelletten *Bregenzer, Aust.*
Fig (p.1193·2); senna (p.1212·2); tamarind (p.1217·3).
Constipation.

Fruhjahrs-Elixier ohne Alkohol *Ehrmann, Aust.*
Urtica (p.1642·3); silver birch (p.1553·3); taraxacum (p.1634·2).
Diuretic.

Fruit of the Earth Moisturizing Aloe *Fruit of the Earth, Canad.*
SPF 8; SPF 15: Ethylhexyl *p*-methoxycinnamate (p.1487·1); oxybenzone (p.1487·3).
SPF 30; SPF 45: Ethylhexyl *p*-methoxycinnamate (p.1487·1); octocrylene (p.1487·3); octyl salicylate (p.1487·3); oxybenzone (p.1487·3); titanium dioxide (p.1093·3).
Sunscreen.

Fruit of the Earth Moisturizing Aloe Baby *Fruit of the Earth, Canad.*
SPF 45: Ethylhexyl *p*-methoxycinnamate (p.1487·1); octocrylene (p.1487·3); octyl salicylate (p.1487·3); oxybenzone (p.1487·3); titanium dioxide (p.1093·3).
Sunscreen.

Fruit of the Earth Moisturizing Aloe Kids *Fruit of the Earth, Canad.*
Topical liquid SPF 30: Ethylhexyl *p*-methoxycinnamate (p.1487·1); octocrylene (p.1487·3); octyl salicylate (p.1487·3); oxybenzone (p.1487·3); titanium dioxide (p.1093·3).
Topical spray SPF 30: Ethylhexyl *p*-methoxycinnamate (p.1487·1); octocrylene (p.1487·3); octyl salicylate (p.1487·3); oxybenzone (p.1487·3); DEA-methoxycinnamate.
Sunscreen.

Fruit of the Earth Moisturizing Aloe Sport *Fruit of the Earth, Canad.*
SPF 8; SPF 15: Ethylhexyl *p*-methoxycinnamate (p.1487·1); oxybenzone (p.1487·3).
SPF 30: Ethylhexyl *p*-methoxycinnamate (p.1487·1); octyl salicylate (p.1487·3); oxybenzone (p.1487·3).
Sunscreen.

Fruitatives *Rogers, Canad.*
Bisacodyl (p.1179·3); docusate sodium (p.1189·3); prune (p.1209·2).

Fruity Chews *Goldline, USA.*
A range of vitamin preparations.

Frumax *Ashbourne, UK.*
Frusemide (p.871·1).
Oedema.

Frumil
Rhone-Poulenc Rorer, Irl.; Rhone-Poulenc Rorer, Switz.; Rorer, UK.
Frusemide (p.871·1); amiloride hydrochloride (p.819·2).
These ingredients can be described by the British Approved Name Co-amilofruse.
Ascites; heart failure; oedema.

Frusamil
Rhone-Poulenc Rorer, Belg.; Rhone-Poulenc Rorer, Spain†.
Frusemide (p.871·1); amiloride hydrochloride (p.819·2).
Hypertension; oedema.

Frusemek *Berk, UK.*
Frusemide (p.871·1); amiloride hydrochloride (p.819·2).
These ingredients can be described by the British Approved Name Co-amilofruse.
Ascites; fluid retention; heart failure.

Frusene
Rhone-Poulenc Rorer, Irl.; Fisons, UK.
Frusemide (p.871·1); triamterene (p.957·2).
Oedema.

Frusid *DDSA Pharmaceuticals, UK.*
Frusemide (p.871·1).

Frusol *Rosemont, UK.*
Frusemide (p.871·1).
Hypertension; oedema.

Frutosel *Sterling Health, Spain†.*
Sodium bicarbonate (p.1153·2); sodium carbonate (p.1630·2); tartaric acid (p.1634·3).
Constipation; gastric hyperacidity.

Fruttidasi *Biomedica, Ital.†.*
Trisodium fructose-1,6-diphosphate; betaine (p.1553·2); thiamine mononitrate (p.1361·1); riboflavine sodium phosphate (p.1362·1); pyridoxine hydrochloride (p.1362·3); nicotinamide (p.1351·2); sodium pantothenate (p.1353·1); calcium folinate (p.1342·2); cyanocobalamin (p.1363·3).
Anaemias; deficiency states.

Fruttocal *Tosi, Ital.*
Ergocalciferol (p.1367·1); calcium ascorbate (p.1365·2); calcium gluconate (p.1155·2); inosine (p.1591·1).
Dental caries prophylaxis; osteoporosis; rickets.

Fruver *Bonomelli, Ital.*
Multivitamin preparation.

Frux *Pharmasal, Ger.†.*
Aloes (p.1177·1); frangula bark (p.1193·2).
Constipation.

Fruxucre *Etajesa, Fr.*
Fructose (p.1343·2).
Sugar substitute.

FS *Hill, USA.*
Fluocinolone acetonide (p.1041·1).
Scalp disorders.

FSME-Bulin
Immuno, Aust.; Immuno, Ger.; Immuno, Switz.
A tick-borne encephalitis immunoglobulin (p.1510·2).
Passive immunisation.

FSME-Immun
Note. This name is used for preparations of different composition.
Immuno, Aust.; Immuno, Belg.; Immuno, Ger.; Immuno, Switz.
A tick-borne encephalitis vaccine (p.1510·2).
Active immunisation.
Immuno, Canad.†.
A tick-borne encephalitis immunoglobulin (p.1510·2).
Passive immunisation.

FSME-Immunoglobulin *Behringwerke, Ger.†.*
A tick-borne encephalitis immunoglobulin (p.1510·2).
Passive immunisation.

Ftalazone *Terapeutico, Ital.†.*
Amidopyrine monohydroxyisophthalate (p.15·2).
Musculoskeletal and joint disorders.

Ftoralon *Donau, Aust.*
Tegafur (p.565·2).
Malignant neoplasms.

Fuca *Cassella-med, Switz.*
Frangula bark (p.1193·2); cascara (p.1183·1).
Constipation.

Fucafibres *Fuca, Fr.*
Fruit and cereal fibres; lactitol (p.1195·2).
Gastro-intestinal disorders.

Fucibet
Leo, Irl.; Farmacusi, Spain.; Leo, UK.
Betamethasone valerate (p.1033·3); fusidic acid (p.211·1).
Infected skin disorders.

Fucicort
Leo, Belg.; Leo, Ger.; Leo, Switz.
Betamethasone valerate (p.1033·3); fusidic acid (p.211·1).
Infected skin disorders.

Fucidin
Merck, Aust.; CSL, Austral.; Leo, Belg.; Leo, Canad.; Leo, Irl.; Sigma-Tau, Ital.†; Leo, Neth.; Leo, Norw.; Adcock Ingram, S.Afr.; Lovens, Swed.; Leo, UK.
Fusidic acid (p.211·1) or sodium fusidate (p.211·1).
Gram-positive bacterial infections.

Fucidin H
Leo, Irl.; Adcock Ingram, S.Afr.; Leo, UK.
Fusidic acid (p.211·1) or sodium fusidate (p.211·1); hydrocortisone acetate (p.1043·3).
Infected skin disorders.

Fucidine
Leo, Fr.; Thomae, Ger.; Farmacusi, Spain; Leo, Switz.
Fusidic acid (p.211·1) or sodium fusidate (p.211·1).
Bacterial infections.

Fucidine H *Thomae, Ger.†.*
Sodium fusidate (p.211·1); hydrocortisone acetate (p.1043·3).
Skin disorders.

Fucidine plus *Thomae, Ger.*
Sodium fusidate (p.211·1); hydrocortisone butyrate (p.1044·1).
Infected skin disorders.

Fucidin-Hydrocortison *Lovens, Swed.*
Fusidic acid (p.211·1); hydrocortisone (p.1043·3).
Infected skin disorders.

Fucithalmic
Merck, Aust.; Leo, Belg.; Leo, Fr.; Basotherm, Ger.; Thomae, Ger.; Leo, Irl.; Formenti, Ital.; Leo, Neth.; Leo, Norw.; Adcock Ingram, S.Afr.; Cusi, Spain; Lovens, Swed.; Leo, Switz.; Leo, UK.
Fusidic acid (p.211·1).
Bacterial eye infections.

Fucovesin *Berlin-Chemie, Ger.†.*
Frangula bark (p.1193·2); rhubarb (p.1212·1).
Constipation.

Fucus *Homeocan, Canad.*
Homoeopathic preparation.

Fudimun *Kanoldt, Ger.*
Echinacea purpura (p.1574·2).
Respiratory- and urinary-tract infections.

FUDR *Roche, USA.*
Floxuridine (p.534·1).
Gastro-intestinal adenocarcinoma metastatic to the liver.

Fugantil *Ghimas, Ital.†.*
Amidopyrine (p.15·2).
Fever; pain.

Fugaten *Lysoform, Ger.*
Alcohol (p.1099·1).
Surface disinfection.

Fugerel
Aesca, Aust.; Schering-Plough, Austral.; Essex, Ger.
Flutamide (p.537·1).
Anti-androgenic; prostatic cancer.

Fugisept *Lysoform, Ger.*
Didecyldimethylammonium chloride (p.1112·2); glyoxal (p.1115·1).
Fungal and bacterial skin infections.

Fugoa N *Robins, Switz.†.*
Phenylpropanolamine hydrochloride (p.1067·2).
Obesity.

Fulcin
Zeneca, Aust.†; ICI, Austral.; Zeneca, Irl.; SIT, Ital.; ICI, Neth.†; Zeneca, Norw.; Zeneca, S.Afr.; Zeneca, Spain; Zeneca, Swed.; Zeneca, Switz.; Zeneca, UK.
Griseofulvin (p.380·2).
Fungal skin, hair, and nail infections.

Fulcin S *Zeneca, Ger.*
Griseofulvin (microfine) (p.380·2).
Fungal infections.

Fulcine *Zeneca, Fr.*
Griseofulvin (p.380·2).
Fungal infections.

Fulcro *Fournier, Ital.*
Fenofibrate (p.1273·1).
Hyperlipidaemias.

Fulgium *Knoll, Spain.*
Benzydamine salicylate (p.21·3).
Musculoskeletal disorders.

Ful-Glo
Allergan, Austral.; Pilkington Barnes-Hind, USA.
Fluorescein sodium (p.1581·1).
Aid to eye examination.

Fulgram *ABC, Ital.*
Norfloxacin (p.233·1).
Urinary-tract infections.

Fulixan *Esteve, Spain†.*
Diflorasone diacetate (p.1039·3).
Skin disorders.

Full Marks *Seton, UK.*
Phenothrin (p.1409·2).
Pediculosis.

Full Service Sunblock *Clinique, Canad.*
SPF 15; SPF 20: Ethylhexyl *p*-methoxycinnamate (p.1487·1); octyl salicylate (p.1487·3); oxybenzone (p.1487·3).
Sunscreen.

Fultrexin *Zambon, Ital.†.*
Thiamphenicol (p.262·3); nifurtoinol (p.231·3); sulphafurazole (p.253·3).
Urinary-tract infections.

Fulvicin *Schering, Canad.*
Griseofulvin (p.380·2).
Fungal infections.

Fulvicin P/G *Schering, USA.*
Griseofulvin (as ultramicrosize crystals) (p.380·2).
Fungal infections of the skin, hair, and nails.

Fulvicin U/F *Schering, USA.*
Griseofulvin (as microsize crystals) (p.380·2).
Fungal infections of the skin, hair, and nails.

Fulvicina *Interpharma, Spain†.*
Griseofulvin (p.380·2).
Fungal skin infections.

Fumaderm *Fumedica, Ger.*
Dimethyl fumarate; calcium monoethyl fumarate (p.1083·1); magnesium monoethyl fumarate (p.1083·1); zinc monoethyl fumarate (p.1083·1).
Psoriasis.

Fumafer *Sanofi Winthrop, Fr.*
Ferrous fumarate (p.1339·3).
Anaemias.

Fumarenid *Brenner-Efeka, Ger.†.*
Frusemide (p.871·1).
Hypertension; oedema.

Fumasorb *Milance, USA†.*
Ferrous fumarate (p.1339·3).
Iron-deficiency anaemias.

Fumatinic *Laser, USA.*
Ferrous fumarate (p.1339·3); folic acid (p.1340·3); vitamin B_{12} substances (p.1363·3).
Vitamin C (p.1365·2) is included in this preparation to increase the absorption and availability of iron.
Iron-deficiency anaemias.

Fumerin *Laser, USA†.*
Ferrous fumarate (p.1339·3).
Iron-deficiency anaemias.

Fumidil *Sanofi Animal Health, UK.*
Bicyclohexyl ammonium fumagillin (p.582·3).
For veterinary use.
Nosema disease in bees.

Funcenal *Farma Lepori, Spain.*
Flutrimazole (p.380·2).
Fungal infections.

Funduscein
Ciba Vision, Canad.; Iolab, USA.
Fluorescein sodium (p.1581·1).
Aid to eye examination.

Funganiline *Squibb, Spain.*
Amphotericin (p.372·2).
Oropharyngeal candidiasis.

Fungarest *Janssen-Cilag, Spain.*
Ketoconazole (p.383·1).
Fungal infections.

Fungata
Pfizer, Aust.; Mack, Illert., Ger.
Fluconazole (p.378·1).
Vaginal candidiasis.

Fungederm *Nucare, UK.*
Clotrimazole (p.376·3).

Fungex *Streuli, Switz.*
Ointment: Undecenoic acid (p.389·2); zinc undecenoate (p.389·2).
Topical powder: Undecenoic acid (p.389·2); zinc undecenoate (p.389·2); aluminium acetotartrate (p.1547·3); calcium lactate (p.1155·2).
Fungal skin infections.

Fungibacid *Asche, Ger.*
Tioconazole (p.388·3).
Fungal infections.

Fungiderm
Note. This name is used for preparations of different composition.
Nycomed, Aust.
Bifonazole (p.375·3).
Fungal skin infections.

Janssen-Cilag, Ital.
Miconazole nitrate (p.384·3).
Fungal infections.

Fungiderm N *Terra-Bio, Ger.†.*
Salicylic acid (p.1090·2); undecenoic acid (p.389·2).
Fungal infections.

Fungidermo *Cinfa, Spain.*
Clotrimazole (p.376·3).
Fungal skin infections.

Fungidexan *Hermal, Ger.*
Clotrimazole (p.376·3); urea (p.1095·2).
Fungal skin infections.

Fungifos *Combustin, Ger.*
Tolciclate (p.388·3).
Fungal skin infections.

Fungilin
Bristol-Myers Squibb, Austral.; Bristol-Myers Squibb, Ital.; Squibb, UK.
Amphotericin (p.372·2).
Fungal infections.

Fungi-Nail *Kramer, USA.*
Resorcinol (p.1090·1); salicylic acid (p.1090·2); chloroxylenol (p.1111·1); benzocaine (p.1286·2); isopropyl alcohol (p.1118·2).
Fungal and bacterial skin infections; fungal nail infections.

Funginazol *Galderma, Spain†.*
Miconazole nitrate (p.384·3).
Fungal skin infections.

Fungiplex *Hermal, Ger.†.*
Sulbentine (p.387·2).
Fungal infections.

Fungireduct *Azupharma, Ger.*
Nystatin (p.386·1).
Candidiasis.

Fungisan *Galderma, Ger.*
Omoconazole nitrate (p.386·3).
Fungal skin infections.

Fungisdin *Isdin, Spain.*
Miconazole (p.384·3) or miconazole nitrate (p.384·3).
Candidiasis; fungal skin infections.

Fungispec *Bristol-Myers Squibb, Belg.†.*
Fludrocortisone acetate (p.1040·1); amphotericin (p.372·2); neomycin sulphate (p.229·2); gramicidin (p.215·2).
Infected skin disorders.

Fungisten *Weifa, Norw.*
Clotrimazole (p.376·3).
Fungal infections.

Fungivin *AFI, Norw.†.*
Griseofulvin (p.380·2).
Fungal infections.

Fungizid *Ratiopharm, Ger.*
Clotrimazole (p.376·3).
Fungal infections.

Fungizona *Squibb, Spain.*
Amphotericin (p.372·2).
Fungal infections.

Fungizone
Bristol-Myers Squibb, Austral.; Bristol-Myers Squibb, Belg.; Squibb, Canad.; Bristol-Myers Squibb, Fr.; Bristol-Myers Squibb, Irl.; Bristol-Myers Squibb, Ital.; Bristol-Myers Squibb, Neth.; Bristol-Myers Squibb, Norw.; Bristol-Myers Squibb, S.Afr.; Bristol-Myers Squibb, Swed.; Bristol-Myers Squibb, Switz.; Squibb, UK; Bristol-Myers Squibb, USA.
Amphotericin (p.372·2).
Fungal infections; leishmaniasis.

Fungo *Ego, Austral.*
Balm: Miconazole nitrate (p.384·3); bufexamac (p.22·2).
Cream; vaginal cream; topical powder: Miconazole nitrate (p.384·3).
Topical solution: Miconazole (p.384·3).
Fungal infections.

Fungo-Hubber *ICN, Spain.*
Ketoconazole (p.383·1).
Fungal infections.

Fungoid *Pedinol, USA.*
Cream; topical solution: Clotrimazole (p.376·3).
Topical tincture: Miconazole nitrate (p.384·3).
Fungal infections.

Fungoid AF *Pedinol, USA.*
Undecenoic acid (p.389·2).
Fungal skin infections.

Fungoid HC *Pedinol, USA.*
Miconazole nitrate (p.384·3); hydrocortisone (p.1043·3).
Bacterial and fungal skin infections.

Fungoral
Janssen-Cilag, Norw.; Janssen-Cilag, Swed.
Ketoconazole (p.383·1).
Fungal infections; seborrhoeic dermatitis.

Fungotox *Mepha, Switz.*
Clotrimazole (p.376·3).
Fungal skin and vaginal infections.

Fungowas *Wasserman, Spain.*
Ciclopirox olamine (p.376·2).
Cutaneous, mucosal and nail fungal infections.

Fungur M *Hexal, Ger.*
Miconazole nitrate (p.384·3).
Fungal skin and vaginal infections.

Fungusol *Roche Nicholas, Spain.*
Boric acid (p.1554·2); chlorocresol (p.1110·3); zinc oxide (p.1096·2).
Formerly contained boric acid, chlorocresol, zinc oxide, and silicic acid.
Fungal skin infections; intertrigo.

Fungusol Prednisona *Andreu, Spain†.*
Chlorocresol (p.1110·3); cholesterol; nicotinamide (p.1351·2); prednisolone (p.1048·1); zinc oxide (p.1096·2).
Infected skin disorders.

Furabid *Procter & Gamble, Neth.*
Nitrofurantoin (p.231·3).
Urinary-tract infections.

Furacin
Formenti, Ital.; SmithKline Beecham, S.Afr.; Seid, Spain; Procter & Gamble, USA; Roberts, USA.
Nitrofurazone (p.232·3).
Bacterial infections.

Furacine
Norgine, Belg.; Norgine, Neth.†.
Nitrofurazone (p.232·3).
Infected skin disorders.

Furacin-Otalgicum *Rohm, Ger.†.*
Nitrofurazone (p.232·3); amethocaine hydrochloride (p.1285·2); phenazone (p.78·2); glycerol.
Inflammatory disorders and bacterial infections of the ear.

Furacin-Sol *Procter & Gamble, Ger.*
Nitrofurazone (p.232·3).
Skin disinfection.

Furadantin
Boehringer Mannheim, Aust.; Pharmacia Upjohn, Austral.; Procter & Gamble, Ger.; Procter & Gamble, Irl.; Formenti, Ital.; Pharmacia Upjohn, Norw.; SmithKline Beecham, S.Afr.; Recip, Swed.; Procter & Gamble, UK; Dura, USA.
Nitrofurantoin (p.231·3).
Urinary-tract infections.

Furadantine
Procter & Gamble, Belg.; Lipha Sante, Fr.; Procter & Gamble, Neth.; Procter & Gamble, Switz.
Nitrofurantoin (p.231·3).
Urinary-tract infections.

Furadoine *Lipha Sante, Fr.*
Nitrofurantoin (p.231·3).
Urinary-tract infections.

Furamid *Knoll, Switz.*
Diloxanide furoate (p.581·2).
Amoebiasis.

Furamide
Boots, Austral.†; Knoll, Irl.; Knoll, UK.
Diloxanide furoate (p.581·2).
Amoebiasis.

Furanthril *Medphano, Ger.*
Frusemide (p.871·1) or frusemide sodium (p.872·3).
Forced diuresis; hypertension; oedema; oliguria.

Furantoina *Uriach, Spain.*
Nitrofurantoin (p.231·3).
Urinary-tract infections.

Furantoina Sedante *Uriach, Spain†.*
Phenazopyridine (p.79·1); nitrofurantoin (p.231·3); hyoscine methobromide (p.463·1).
Urinary-tract infections; urinary-tract spasm.

Furanvit *SIFI, Ital.*
Nitrofurazone (p.232·3); pyridoxine hydrochloride (p.1362·3).
Bacterial eye infections.

Furasept *Beige, S.Afr.*
Nitrofurazone (p.232·3).
Burns; skin infections; ulcers; wounds.

Furazanol *Monot, Fr.*
Econazole nitrate (p.377·2).
Fungal skin infections.

Furedan *Hoechst Marion Roussel, Ital.*
Nitrofurantoin (p.231·3).
Urinary-tract infections.

Furesis comp *Bristol-Myers Squibb, Ger.*
Frusemide (p.871·1); triamterene (p.957·2).
Hypertension; oedema.

Furex *Lennon, S.Afr.*
Nitrofurazone (p.232·3).
Burns; skin infections; ulcers; wounds.

Furil *OFF, Ital.*
Nitrofurantoin (p.231·3).
Urinary-tract infections.

Furix
AFI, Norw.; Nycomed, Swed.
Frusemide (p.871·1).
Forced diuresis; hypertension; nephrotic syndrome; oedema; renal insufficiency.

Furo
CT, Ger.; Ratiopharm, Ger.
Frusemide (p.871·1) or frusemide sodium (p.872·3).
Forced diuresis; heart failure; hypertension; oedema; oliguria.

Furo-Aldopur
Kwizda, Aust.; Hormosan, Ger.
Frusemide (p.871·1); spironolactone (p.946·1).
Ascites; oedema.

Furobactina *Dexter, Spain.*
Nitrofurantoin (p.231·3).
Urinary-tract infections.

furo-basan *Schonenberger, Switz.*
Frusemide (p.871·1).
Hypertension; oedema.

Furobeta *Betapharm, Ger.*
Frusemide (p.871·1).
Oedema; oliguria.

Furodermal *Streuli, Switz.*
Camphor (p.1557·2); ichthammol (p.1083·3); bismuth oxyiodogallate (p.1181·1); thymol (p.1127·1).
Skin infections.

Furodermil *Vifor, Switz.*
Ichthammol (p.1083·3); salicylic acid (p.1090·2); bismuth hydroxyquinoline (p.1181·1); peru balsam (p.1617·2).
Skin disorders.

Furodrix *Streuli, Switz.*
Frusemide sodium (p.872·3).
Heart failure; hypertension; oedema; oliguria in pregnancy; renal failure.

Furoic *Poli, Ital.*
Calcium mefolinate (p.1342·3).
Antidote in overdosage with folic acid antagonists; folate deficiency; reduction of aminopterin and methotrexate toxicity.

Furolacton *Lannacher, Aust.*
Spironolactone (p.946·1); frusemide (p.871·1).
Oedema.

Furomed *Wolff, Ger.*
Frusemide (p.871·1).
Hypertension; oedema; oliguria.

Furon *Merckle, Aust.*
Frusemide (p.871·1) or frusemide sodium (p.872·3).
Forced diuresis; hypercalcaemic crises; hypertension; oedema; renal failure.

Furo-Puren *Isis Puren, Ger.*
Frusemide (p.871·1).
Heart failure; hypertension; oedema.

Furorese *Hexal, Ger.*
Frusemide (p.871·1) or frusemide sodium (p.872·3).
Forced diuresis; hypertension; oedema; oliguria.

Furorese Comp *Hexal, Ger.*
Frusemide (p.871·1); spironolactone (p.946·1).
Ascites; oedema.

Furoscand *Enapharm, Swed.*
Frusemide (p.871·1).
Hypertension; oedema.

Furosemid comp *Upsamedica, Switz.*
Frusemide (p.871·1); spironolactone (p.946·1).
Ascites; oedema.

Furosemix *Biogalenique, Fr.†.*
Frusemide (p.871·1).
Hypertension; oedema; vertigo.

Furosifar *Siphar, Switz.*
Frusemide (p.871·1).
Hypertension; oedema; renal failure.

Furospir *Mepha, Switz.*
Frusemide (p.871·1); spironolactone (p.946·1).
Oedema.

Furotricina *Biomedica, Ital.*
Tyrothricin (p.267·2); nitrofurazone (p.232·3).
Gynaecological infections.

Furoxone
Formenti, Ital.; Xixia, S.Afr.†; Procter & Gamble, USA.
Furazolidone (p.583·1).
Gastro-intestinal infections.

Fursol *Ecosol, Switz.*
Frusemide (p.871·1).
Hypertension; oedema.

Furtulon *Roche, Jpn.*
Doxifluridine (p.529·2).
Malignant neoplasms.

Furunkulosin *Merckle, Ger.*
Yeast (p.1373·1).
Furunculosis.

Fusaloyos *Danval, Spain.*
Fusafungine (p.210·3).
Upper respiratory-tract infections and inflammation.

Fusid
Gry, Ger.; ICN, Neth.†.
Frusemide (p.871·1) or frusemide sodium (p.872·3).
Forced diuresis; heart failure; hypertension; oedema; oliguria.

Futraful *Taiho, Jpn.*
Tegafur (p.565·2).
Malignant neoplasms.

Futura *Marano, Ital.*
Aspartame (p.1335·1).
Sugar substitute.

FX Passage
Hestag, Aust.; Worwag, Ger.
Magnesium sulphate (p.1157·3).
Constipation; stool softener.

Fybogel
Reckitt & Colman, Austral.; Reckitt & Colman, Belg.†; Reckitts, Irl.; Reckitt & Colman, S.Afr.; Reckitt & Colman, Spain; Reckitt & Colman, UK.
Ispaghula husk (p.1194·2).
Constipation; dietary fibre supplement.

Fybogel Mebeverine
Reckitts, Irl.; Reckitt & Colman, UK.
Ispaghula husk (p.1194·2); mebeverine hydrochloride (p.1199·2).
Formerly known as Colven.
Gastro-intestinal disorders.

Fybozest *Reckitt & Colman, UK.*
Ispaghula husk (p.1194·2).
Hypercholesterolaemia.

Fybranta *Norgine, UK†.*
Bran (p.1181·2).
Constipation.

Fynnon Calcium Aspirin *Seton, UK.*
Aspirin (p.16·1).
Calcium carbonate (p.1182·1) is included in this preparation in an attempt to limit adverse effects on the gastro-intestinal mucosa.
Fever; pain.

Fynnon Salt *Seton, UK.*
Sodium sulphate (p.1213·3).
Constipation.

Fysioquens
Aacipharm, Belg.; Nourypharma, Neth.
7 Tablets, ethinyloestradiol (p.1445·1); 15 tablets, ethinyloestradiol; lynoestrenol (p.1448·2).
Sequential-type oral contraceptive.

G 1000 Record *Pierrel, Ital.†.*
Carbohydrate, multivitamin, and mineral preparation.

G Tril *Vinas, Spain.*
Febarbamate (p.670·1).
Alcohol withdrawal syndrome; insomnia; tremor.

Gabacet *Synthelabo, Fr.*
Piracetam (p.1619·1).
Cerebrovascular disorders; vertigo.

Gabakalm *Cantassium Co., UK†.*
Gamma aminobutyric acid; vitamins; minerals.

Gabbroral
Pharmacia Upjohn, Belg.; Pharmacia Upjohn, Ital.
Paromomycin sulphate (p.235·3).
Amoebiasis; bacterial intestinal infections; giardiasis.

Gabitril
Sanofi Winthrop, Austral.; Novo Nordisk, Irl.; Sanofi Winthrop, UK; Abbott, USA.
Tiagabine hydrochloride (p.360·1).
Epilepsy.

Gaboril Complex *Sigma-Tau, Spain†.*
Phenytoin (p.352·3); phenobarbitone (p.350·2); aminohydroxybutyric acid (p.339·1).
Epilepsy.

Gabrene *Synthelabo, Fr.*
Progabide (p.359·2).
Epilepsy.

Gabrilen *Kreussler, Ger.*
Ketoprofen (p.48·2).
Inflammation; musculoskeletal, joint, peri-articular, and soft-tissue disorders.

Gabroral *Farmitalia, Spain†.*
Paromomycin sulphate (p.235·3).
Gastro-intestinal amoebiasis; gastro-intestinal bacterial infections; taeniasis.

Gabunat *Strathmann, Ger.*
Biotin (p.1336·1).
Biotin deficiency.

Gafir *Mediolanum, Ital.†.*
Niperotidine hydrochloride (p.1203·2).
Gastro-intestinal disorders.

Gaiarsol *Monin, Fr.*
Methylarsenic acid; guaiacol (p.1061·2); aconite root (p.1542·2); codeine (p.26·1); tolu balsam (p.1071·1).
Coughs.

Galacordin *Biomo, Ger.*
Potassium aspartate (p.1161·3); magnesium aspartate (p.1157·2).
Potassium and magnesium deficiency.

Galactogil *Nutripharm Elgi, Fr.*
Galega; calcium phosphate (p.1155·3); malt extract (p.1350·1).
Insufficient milk production.

Galactomin
Cow & Gate, Irl.; Medifood-Trufood, Ital.; Cow & Gate, UK.
Food for special diets.
Lactose, glucose, or galactose intolerance.

Galactoquin
Mundipharma, Aust.; Mundipharma, Ger.†.
Quinidine polygalacturonate (p.938·3).
Arrhythmias.

Galake *Galen, UK.*
Dihydrocodeine tartrate (p.34·1); paracetamol (p.72·2).
These ingredients can be described by the British Approved Name Co-dydramol.
Pain.

Galama *Pharmonta, Aust.*
Silver birch (p.1553·3).
Kidney disorders.

Galamila *Galactina, Switz.*
Dexpanthenol (p.1570·3); chlorhexidine gluconate (p.1107·2) or chlorhexidine hydrochloride (p.1107·2).
Nipple care during breastfeeding.

Galanol GLX *Lifeplan, UK.*
Evening primrose oil (p.1582·1).
Nutritional supplement.

Galanol Gold *Lifeplan, UK.*
Evening primrose oil (p.1582·1); borage oil (p.1582·1).
Nutritional supplement.

Galantase
Tokyo Tanabe, Jpn; Hoechst Marion Roussel, S.Afr.
Tilactase (p.1637·3).
Lactose intolerance.

Galcodine *Galen, UK.*
Codeine phosphate (p.26·1).
Dry coughs.

Galenamet
Galen, Irl.; Galen, UK.
Cimetidine (p.1183·2).
Gastric hyperacidity; peptic ulcer; Zollinger-Ellison syndrome.

Galenamox
Galen, Irl.; Galen, UK.
Amoxycillin trihydrate (p.151·3).
Bacterial infections.

Galenavowen-N *Weber & Weber, Ger.*
Homoeopathic preparation.

Galenphol *Galen, UK.*
Pholcodine (p.1068·1).
Formerly known as Galphol.
Coughs.

Galfer
Galen, Irl.; Galen, UK.
Ferrous fumarate (p.1339·3).
Iron-deficiency anaemia.

Galfer FA
Galen, Irl.; Galen, UK.
Ferrous fumarate (p.1339·3); folic acid (p.1340·3).
Iron and folic acid deficiency in pregnancy.

Galfer-Vit *Galen, UK†.*
Ferrous fumarate (p.1339·3); vitamin B and C substances.
Iron deficiency.

Galfloxin *Galen, UK.*
Flucloxacillin sodium (p.209·2).
Bacterial infections.

Galirene *Jumer, Fr.*
Calcium bromide (p.1620·3); calcium lactate (p.1155·2).
Insomnia; nervous disorders.

Galium Complex *Blackmores, Austral.*
Galium aparine (p.1565·2); echinacea angustifolia (p.1574·2); calendula officinalis; baptisia tinctoria; vitamins; zinc amino acid chelate (p.1373·3).
Tonic.

Galivert *Luhr-Lehrs, Ger.*
Homoeopathic preparation.

Gallcusan (Rowo-29) *Pharmakon, Ger.†.*
Homoeopathic preparation.

Galleb *Hoyer, Ger.†.*
Chelidonium; curcuma zanthorrhiza; rubia tinctorum; silybum marianum (p.993·3); peppermint leaf (p.1208·1); taraxacum (p.1634·2); echinacea purpurea (p.1574·2); frangula bark (p.1193·2).
Biliary disorders; post-hepatitis syndrome.

Galleb S *Hoyer, Ger.*
Taraxacum (p.1634·2).
Biliary-tract disorders; dyspepsia.

Galle-Donau *Donau, Aust.*
Tolynol nicotinate (p.1638·3); α-naphthylacetic acid (p.1606·2).
Biliary-tract disorders.

Gallemolan forte *Redel, Ger.*
Chelidonium; absinthium (p.1541·1); taraxacum (p.1634·2).
Biliary-tract disorders; dyspepsia.

Gallemolan G *Redel, Ger.*
Absinthium (p.1541·1); boldo leaves (p.1554·1); chamomile flowers (p.1561·2); chelidonium; taraxacum (p.1634·2).
Biliary-tract disorders; dyspepsia.

Gallemolan N *Redel, Ger.†.*
Chelidonium; absinthium (p.1541·1); boldo (p.1554·1); taraxacum (p.1634·2); rhubarb (p.1212·1); chamomile (p.1561·2); ox bile (p.1553·2).
Biliary disorders; gallstones; liver disorders.

Gallen- und Lebertee *Smetana, Aust.*
Agrimony herb; marrubium vulgare (p.1063·3); peppermint leaf (p.1208·1); achillea (p.1542·2); taraxacum (p.1634·2).
Biliary-tract disorders.

Gallenja *OTW, Ger.*
Homoeopathic preparation.

Gallen-Leber-Tee Stada *Stada, Ger.†.*
Calendula; delphinium consolida; gentian (p.1583·3); fennel (p.1579·1); caraway (p.1559·3); chamomile (p.1561·2); ononis (p.1610·2); frangula bark (p.1193·2); chelidonium; peppermint leaf (p.1208·1); taraxacum (p.1634·2); caraway oil (p.1559·3).
Herbal tea.

Gallenperlen *Agepha, Aust.*
Phenylpropanol (p.1617·3).
Biliary-tract disorders.

Gallensteinkapseln *Evers, Ger.†.*
Glechoma hederaceum.
Gallstones.

Gallen-Tee Cholaflux S *Nattermann, Ger.†.*
Taraxacum (p.1634·2); peppermint leaves (p.1208·1); javanese turmeric; achillea (p.1542·2).
Biliary-tract disorders.

Gallesyn *Wenig, Aust.*
Oral drops: Frangula (p.1193·2); herba teucrii; peppermint oil (p.1208·1).
Tablets: Frangula (p.1193·2); herba teucrii; menthol (p.1600·2).
Biliary-tract disorders.

Gallexier *Salushaus, Ger.*
Oral liquid: Cynara (p.1569·2); taraxacum (p.1634·2); curcuma zanthorrhiza; silybum marianum (p.993·3); cnicus benedictus (p.1565·3); menyanthes (p.1601·2); achillea (p.1542·2); gentian (p.1583·3); absinthium (p.1541·1); calamus (p.1556·1); chamomile (p.1561·2); fennel (p.1579·1); fructose (p.1343·2).
Digestive system disorders.
Tablets: Curcuma zanthorrhiza; cynara (p.1569·2); silybum marianum (p.993·3); taraxacum (p.1634·2); chamomile (p.1561·2); peppermint leaf (p.1208·1).
Biliary disorders.

Gallia Lactofidus *Diepal, Fr.*
Infant feed.
Gastro-intestinal disorders.

Galliagene *Diepal, Fr.*
Infant feed; food for special diets.
Diarrhoea; malabsorption syndromes; milk-protein intolerance.

Gallialite *Gallia, Fr.†.*
Glucose; maltodextrin; potassium gluconate; sodium chloride; sodium sulphate (p.1152·3).
Diarrhoea; oral rehydration therapy.

Gallieva *Gallia, Fr.†.*
Infant feed; food for special diets.

Gallith *Evers, Ger.*
Hedera helix.
Cholesterol gallstones.

Gallitophen *Reinecke, Ger.†.*
Capsella bursa pastoris; frangula bark (p.1193·2); senna (p.1212·2); birch leaf (p.1553·3); chelidonium; equisetum (p.1575·1); cnicus benedictus (p.1565·3); silybum marianum (p.993·3); chamomile (p.1561·2); rorippa nasturtium aquaticum; taraxacum (p.1634·2); eschscholtzia californica; ox bile (p.1553·2); berberis; card. mar.; peppermint oil (p.1208·1).
Biliary disorders; liver disorders.

Gallo Merz *Kolassa, Aust.*
Dehydrocholic acid (p.1570·2); pancreatin (p.1612·1); cellulase (p.1561·1); dimethicone (p.1213·1); turmeric (p.1001·3).
Biliary-tract and pancreatic disorders.

Gallo Merz N *Merz, Ger.*
Dimethicone (p.1213·1); turmeric (p.1001·3).
Biliary-tract disorders.

Gallo Merz Spasmo *Merz, Ger.*
Hymecromone (p.1589·3).
Biliary-tract spasm.

Gallo sanol N *Sanol, Ger.†.*
Ox bile (p.1553·2); frangula bark (p.1193·2); aloes (p.1177·1).
Biliary disorders; post-hepatitis convalescence.

Gallogran *Synpharma, Aust.*
Taraxacum (p.1634·2); achillea (p.1542·2); absinthium (p.1541·1).
Biliary- and gastro-intestinal tract disorders.

Gallolingual *Pohl, Ger.†.*
Ethaverine hydrochloride (p.1577·1); glyceryl trinitrate (p.874·3).
Smooth muscle spasms.

Gallopas *Pascoe, Ger.*
Chelidonium majus.
Gastro-intestinal and biliary-tract spasm.

Galloselect *Dreluso, Ger.*
Homoeopathic preparation.

Galloselect M *Dreluso, Ger.*
Chelidonium; taraxacum (p.1634·2); silybum marianum (p.993·3); cynara (p.1569·2); chamomile (p.1561·2); peppermint oil (p.1208·1); caraway oil (p.1559·3).
Biliary-tract disorders.

Galloway's Cough Syrup *LRC Products, UK.*
Ipecacuanha liquid extract (p.1062·2); squill vinegar (p.1070·1); acetic acid (p.1541·2); chloroform (p.1220·3); ether.
Coughs.

Galmarin *Lifeplan, UK.*
Evening primrose oil (p.1582·1); borage oil (p.1582·1); omega 3 marine triglycerides (p.1276·1).
Nutritional supplement.

Galmax *Max Farma, Ital.*
Sodium succinate ursodeoxycholate (p.1642·1).
Biliary disorders; gallstones.

Galotam *Normon, Spain.*
Ampicillin sodium (p.153·1); sulbactam sodium (p.250·3).
Bacterial infections.

Galprofen *Galpharm, UK.*
Ibuprofen (p.44·1).
Pain.

Galpseud
Galen, Irl.; Galen, UK.
Pseudoephedrine hydrochloride (p.1068·3).
Upper respiratory-tract congestion.

Galpseud Plus *Galen, UK.*
Pseudoephedrine hydrochloride (p.1068·3); chlorpheniramine maleate (p.405·1).
Allergic rhinitis.

Galusan *Almirall, Spain.*
Pipemidic acid (p.237·2).
Urinary-tract infections.

Gamalate B6 *Novag, Spain.*
Gamma-aminobutyric acid (p.1582·1); aminohydroxybutyric acid (p.339·1); magnesium glutamate hydrobromide (p.1598·3); pyridoxine (p.1363·1).
Mental function impairment; senility.

Gamanil
E. Merck, Irl.; E. Merck, UK.
Lofepramine hydrochloride (p.296·1).
Depression.

Gamastan *Cutter, USA†.*
A normal immunoglobulin (p.1522·1).
Immunoglobulin deficiency; passive immunisation.

Gamatol *LED, Fr.*
Borage oil (p.1582·1).

Gambex *Pharmacare Consumer, S.Afr.*
Lindane (p.1407·2).
Pediculosis.

Gambrolys *Gambro, Swed.*
Sodium chloride; sodium hydroxide; potassium chloride; magnesium chloride; calcium chloride; acetic acid (p.1151·1).
Haemodialysis solution.

Gambrosol
Gambro, Swed.; Bichsel, Switz.
Glucose; sodium chloride; sodium lactate; calcium chloride; magnesium chloride (p.1151·1).
Peritoneal dialysis solution.

Gameval *Alter, Spain†.*
Cocarboxylase; coenzyme A; flavine adenine dinucleotide; nadide; nadide phosphate; thioctic acid; guanosine diphosphate.
Tonic.

Gamibetal *SIT, Ital.*
Aminohydroxybutyric acid (p.339·1).
Epilepsy.

Gamibetal Complex *SIT, Ital.*
Aminohydroxybutyric acid (p.339·1); phenobarbitone (p.350·2); phenytoin sodium (p.352·3).
Epilepsy.

Gamibetal Plus *SIT, Ital.*
Aminohydroxybutyric acid (p.339·1); diazepam (p.661·1).
Epilepsy.

Gamimune N
Bayer, Canad.; Cutter, UK†; Bayer, USA.
A normal immunoglobulin (p.1522·1).
Idiopathic thrombocytopenic purpura; immunodeficiency; passive immunisation.

Gamma 16
Merieux, Belg.†; Pasteur Merieux, Neth.†.
A normal immunoglobulin (p.1522·1).
Agammaglobulinaemia; hypogammaglobulinaemia; passive immunisation.

Gamma Coq *Association Nationale, Fr.†.*
A pertussis immunoglobulin (p.1525·3).
Passive immunisation.

Gamma EPA *Quest, UK.*
Concentrated fish oil (p.1276·1).

Gamma Glob *Grifols, Spain; ICN, Spain.*
A normal immunoglobulin (p.1522·1).
Passive immunisation.

Gamma Glob Anti D *Grifols, Spain.*
An anti-D immunoglobulin (p.1503·2).
Prevention of rhesus sensitisation.

Gamma Glob Anti Rh *ICN, Spain.*
An anti-D immunoglobulin (p.1503·2).
Prevention of rhesus sensitisation.

Gamma Glob Antial *ICN, Spain†.*
A normal immunoglobulin (p.1522·1).
Hypersensitivity reactions.

Gamma Glob Antihepa B *Alonga, Spain.*
A hepatitis B immunoglobulin (p.1512·3).
Passive immunisation.

Gamma Glob Antiparot *ICN, Spain†.*
A mumps immunoglobulin (p.1521·2).
Passive immunisation.

Gamma Glob Antiper *ICN, Spain†.*
A pertussis immunoglobulin (p.1525·3).
Passive immunisation.

Gamma Glob Antirub *ICN, Spain†.*
A rubella immunoglobulin (p.1532·3).
Passive immunisation.

Gamma Glob Antite *Alonga, Spain; Grifols, Spain.*
A tetanus immunoglobulin (p.1535·2).
Passive immunisation.

Gamma Marine *Quest, UK.*
Evening primrose oil (p.1582·1); borage oil (p.1582·1); fish oil (p.1276·1).

Gamma Oil
Quest, Canad.; Quest, UK.
Evening primrose oil (p.1582·1).
Nutritional supplement.

Gamma Oil Marine *Quest, Canad.*
Gamolenic acid (p.1582·1); linoleic acid (p.1582·1); vitamins.

Gamma Tetanos *Association Nationale, Fr.†.*
A tetanus immunoglobulin (p.1535·2).
Passive immunisation.

Gammabion *Sabater, Spain†.*
A normal immunoglobulin (p.1522·1).
Hypogammaglobulinaemia; passive immunisation.

Gammabulin
Immuno, Aust.; Immuno, Canad.†; Immuno, Ger.; Immuno, Irl.; Immuno, Ital.; Immuno, Swed.†; Immuno, UK.
A normal immunoglobulin (p.1522·1).
Agammaglobulinaemia; hypogammaglobulinaemia; passive immunisation.

Gammabulin A *Immuno, Ger.*
A hepatitis A immunoglobulin (p.1512·1).
Passive immunisation.

Gammabuline *Immuno, Switz.†.*
A normal immunoglobulin (p.1522·1).
Hypogammaglobulinaemia; passive immunisation.

Gammacur *Biocur, Ger.*
Evening primrose oil (p.1582·1).
Eczema.

Gammadin *OFF, Ital.*
Povidone-iodine (p.1123·3).
Skin and mucous membrane disinfection.

Gammagard
Baxter, Belg.; Baxter, Ger.; Baxter, Spain; Baxter, Swed.; Baxter, Switz.; Baxter, USA.
A normal immunoglobulin (p.1522·1).
B-cell chronic lymphocytic leukaemia; Guillain-Barré syndrome; hypogammaglobulinaemia; idiopathic thrombocytopenic purpura; Kawasaki disease; passive immunisation.

Gammaglob Antihep B *Grifols, Spain.*
A hepatitis B immunoglobulin (p.1512·3).
Passive immunisation.

Gammaglobulin *Pharmacia Upjohn, Norw.*
A normal immunoglobulin (p.1522·1).
Passive immunisation.

Gamma-Globuline *SRK, Switz.†.*
A normal immunoglobulin (p.1522·1).
Passive immunisation.

Gammakine *Dompe, Ital.*
Interferon gamma-1b (p.616·1).
Chronic granulomatous disease.

Gammalonga Varicela-Zona *Alonga, Spain†.*
A varicella-zoster immunoglobulin (p.1538·1).
Passive immunisation.

Gamma-Men *Nuovo ISM, Ital.*
An anti-D immunoglobulin (p.1503·2).
Prevention of rhesus sensitisation.

Gammamida Complex *Laproquifar, Spain.*
Cyanocobalamin (p.1363·3); glutamic acid (p.1344·3); pyridoxine (p.1363·1); thiamine (p.1361·2).
Alcoholism; muscular dystrophies; nausea and vomiting in pregnancy; vitamin B deficiency.

Gammanorm
Pharmacia Upjohn, Norw.; Pharmacia Upjohn, Swed.
A normal immunoglobulin (p.1522·1).
Hypogammaglobulinaemia.

Gamma-OH Clintec, Fr.
Sodium oxybate (p.1232·2).
General anaesthesia.

GammaOil Premium Quest, UK.
Evening primrose oil (p.1582·1).

Gammaprotect Biotest, Ger.†.
A hepatitis B immunoglobulin (p.1512·3).
Passive immunisation.

Gammaprotect Varizellen Biotest, Ger.†.
A varicella-zoster immunoglobulin (p.1538·1).
Passive immunisation.

Gammar-P Centeon, USA.
A normal immunoglobulin (p.1522·1).
Immunoglobulin deficiency; passive immunisation.

Gammatet Propan, S.Afr.
Tetracycline hydrochloride (p.259·1).
Bacterial infections.

Gamma-Tet P Centeon, Ital.
A tetanus immunoglobulin (p.1535·2).
Passive immunisation.

Gamma-Veinine Hoechst Marion Roussel, S.Afr.†.
A normal immunoglobulin (p.1522·1).
Passive immunisation.

Gamma-Venin
Centeon, Aust.; Centeon, Ger.; Centeon, Ital.; Hoechst, Spain†.
A normal immunoglobulin (p.1522·1).
Hypogammaglobulinaemia; passive immunisation.

Gammistin IBP, Ital.†.
Brompheniramine maleate (p.403·2).
Hypersensitivity reactions.

Gammonativ
Pharmacia Upjohn, Aust.; Pharmacia Upjohn, Ger.; Pharmacia Upjohn, Norw.; Pharmacia Upjohn, Swed.
A normal immunoglobulin (p.1522·1).
Hypogammaglobulinaemia; idiopathic thrombocytopenic purpura.

Gamonil
Merck, Ger.; E. Merck, Switz.
Lofepramine hydrochloride (p.296·1).
Depression.

Gamophen
Johnson & Johnson, Austral.; Johnson & Johnson Medical, UK.
Triclosan (p.1127·2).
Acne; soap substitute.

Gamulin Rh Armour, USA.
An anti-D immunoglobulin (p.1503·2).
Prevention of rhesus sensitisation.

Ganaton Hokuriku, Jpn.
Itopride hydrochloride (p.1195·1).
Gastro-intestinal symptoms of chronic gastritis.

Ganda
Chauvin, Irl.; Smith & Nephew, S.Afr.†; Chauvin, UK.
Guanethidine monosulphate (p.878·1); adrenaline (p.813·2).
Glaucoma.

Ganidan Specia, Fr.†.
Sulphaguanidine (p.254·1).
Bacterial infections.

Ganite Fujisawa, USA.
Gallium nitrate (p.739·3).
Hypercalcaemia of malignancy.

Ganor Thomae, Ger.
Famotidine (p.1192·1).
Gastro-intestinal haemorrhage; peptic ulcer; Zollinger-Ellison syndrome.

Gantanol Roche, USA.
Sulphamethoxazole (p.254·3).
Adjunct in falciparum malaria; bacterial infections.

Gantaprim Lenza, Ital.†.
Co-trimoxazole (p.196·3).
Bacterial infections.

Gantrim Geymonat, Ital.
Co-trimoxazole (p.196·3).
Bacterial infections.

Gantrimex Geymonat, Ital.
Oxolamine citrate (p.1065·3) or oxolamine phosphate (p.1065·3).
Respiratory-tract disorders.

Gantrisin Roche, USA†.
Sulphafurazole (p.253·3), acetyl sulphafurazole (p.253·3), or sulphafurazole diethanolamine (p.253·3).
Adjunct in falciparum malaria; bacterial infections.

Gaoptal Europhta, Mon.
Timolol maleate (p.953·3).
Glaucoma; ocular hypertension.

Gaosucryl Pharminter, Fr.†.
Saccharin sodium (p.1353·3).
Sugar substitute.

Garacol Schering-Plough, Neth.
Gentamicin sulphate (p.212·1).
Bacterial infections.

Garamycin
Schering-Plough, Austral.; Schering, Canad.; Schering-Plough, Neth.; Schering-Plough, Norw.; Schering-Plough, S.Afr.; Schering-Plough, Swed.; Essex, Switz.; Schering-Plough, UK; Schering, USA.
Gentamicin sulphate (p.212·1).
Bacterial infections.

Garanil Zambon, Spain.
Captopril (p.836·3).
Diabetic nephropathy; heart failure; hypertension; myocardial infarction.

Garasone
Schering-Plough, Belg.; Schering, Canad.; Schering-Plough, S.Afr.†.
Gentamicin sulphate (p.212·1); betamethasone sodium phosphate (p.1033·3).
Inflammatory eye infections; otitis externa.

Garaspirine IPRAD, Fr.†.
Infant suppositories: Aspirin (p.16·1); phenobarbitone (p.350·2).
Paediatric suppositories; adult suppositories; tablets: Aspirin (p.16·1); phenobarbitone (p.350·2); papaverine hydrochloride (p.1614·2).
Fever; pain.

Garatec Technilab, Canad.
Gentamicin sulphate (p.212·1).
Bacterial infections.

Gardenal
Rhone-Poulenc Rorer, Belg.; Specia, Fr.; Rhone-Poulenc Rorer, S.Afr.; Rhone-Poulenc Rorer, Spain; Concord, UK.
Phenobarbitone (p.350·2) or phenobarbitone sodium (p.350·2).
Epilepsy; febrile convulsions.

Gardenale Rhone-Poulenc Rorer, Ital.
Phenobarbitone (p.350·2) or phenobarbitone sodium (p.350·2).
Epilepsy; insomnia; sedative.

GA-301-Redskin 301 Madaus, Ger.
Histamine dihydrochloride (p.1587·3); clove oil (p.1565·2); juniper oil (p.1592·3).
Migraine; musculoskeletal and joint disorders; neuritis; respiratory-tract disorders.

Garfield
Whitehall-Robins, Canad.; Menley & James, USA.
A range of multivitamin and mineral preparations.

Gargaril Puerto Galiano, Spain†.
Formaldehyde (p.1113·2); menthol (p.1600·2).
Mouth and throat inflammation.

Gargaril Sulfamida Puerto Galiano, Spain†.
Formaldehyde (p.1113·2); sulphanilamide (p.256·3); menthol (p.1600·2).
Mouth and throat inflammation.

Gargarisma ankerpharm, Ger.
Aluminium chloride (p.1078·3); potassium chlorate (p.1620·3).
Mouth and throat inflammation.

Gargarol Boiron, Canad.
Homoeopathic preparation.

Gargilon Solvay, Neth.
Dequalinium chloride (p.1112·1).
Sore throat.

Garlic Allium Complex Neo-Life, Austral.
Garlic (p.1583·1); onion (p.1610·2); chive; leek; rosemary.
Upper respiratory-tract congestion.

Garlic Breathless Capsules Vitaplex, Austral.†.
Garlic oil.
Upper respiratory-tract disorders.

Garlic, Horseradish, A & C Capsules Vitaplex, Austral.
Garlic oil; horseradish root; ascorbic acid (p.1365·2); vitamin A palmitate (p.1359·2).
Excess body fluids; excess mucus formation.

Garlic and Horseradish + C Complex Cenovis, Austral.; Vitelle, Austral.
Cochlearia armoracia; garlic (p.1583·1); sodium ascorbate (p.1365·2); ascorbic acid (p.1365·2); fenugreek (p.1579·3); althaea (p.1546·3).
Upper respiratory-tract symptoms.

Garlic and Horseradish Complex 1000 Suisse, Austral.†.
Horseradish; garlic (p.1583·1); althaea (p.1546·3); parsley (p.1615·3); fenugreek (p.1579·3).
Hay fever; sinusitis.

Garlimega Cantassium Co., UK.
Garlic (p.1583·1).

Garlodex Modern Health Products, UK.
Marshmallow root (p.1546·3); parsley (p.1615·3); garlic oil.
Catarrh; colds.

Garmastan
Nycomed, Aust.; Protina, Ger.
Guaiazulene (p.1586·3).
Mastitis prophylaxis.

Garoin Rhone-Poulenc Rorer, S.Afr.
Phenytoin sodium (p.352·3); phenobarbitone sodium (p.350·2).
Epilepsy.

Gartech Eagle, Austral.
Astragalus; echinacea pallida (p.1574·2); garlic (p.1583·1); berberis vulgaris; paraformaldehyde (p.1121·1); garlic oil; anise oil (p.1550·1); thymol (p.1127·1); savory oil.
Cold and influenza symptoms.

Gartricin Cantabria, Spain.
Benzocaine (p.1286·2); niaouli oil (p.1607·1); menthol (p.1600·2); eucalyptus oil (p.1578·1).
Mouth and throat disorders.

Garze Disinfettanti alla Pomata Betadine Asta Medica, Ital.
Povidone-iodine (p.1123·3).
Medicated dressing.

Gas Ban Roberts, USA.
Calcium carbonate (p.1182·1); simethicone (p.1213·1).
Flatulence.

Gas Ban DS Roberts, USA.
Aluminium hydroxide (p.1177·3); magnesium hydroxide (p.1198·2); simethicone (p.1213·1).
Flatulence.

Gas Permeable Daily Cleaner Allergan, Austral.
Cleansing solution for hard and gas permeable contact lenses.

Gas Permeable Wetting and Soaking Solution Barnes-Hind, Austral.†.
Wetting and soaking solution for hard and gas permeable contact lenses.

Gas Relief Rugby, USA.
Simethicone (p.1213·1).
Flatulence.

Gasbrand-Antitoxin Chiron Behring, Ger.
A gas-gangrene antitoxin (p.1511·1).
Gas gangrene.

Gaslon N Shinyaku, Jpn.
Irsogladine maleate (p.1194·2).
Gastric ulcer.

Gas-Mag Valtec, Canad.†.
Magnesium hydroxide (p.1198·2); cascara (p.1183·1).
Constipation.

Gasmol Hilarys, Canad.
Magnesium carbonate (p.1198·1); magnesium hydroxide (p.1198·2); magnesium trisilicate (p.1199·1); calcium carbonate (p.1182·1); rhubarb (p.1212·1).

Gaster
Note. This name is used for preparations of different composition.
SoSe, Ital.
Sodium cromoglycate (p.762·1).
Food hypersensitivity; proctitis; ulcerative colitis.

Yamanouchi, Jpn.
Famotidine (p.1192·1).
Gastro-intestinal haemorrhage; gastro-oesophageal reflux; peptic ulcer; premedication; Zollinger-Ellison syndrome.

Gasteril Ripari-Gero, Ital.†.
Pirenzepine hydrochloride (p.467·1).
Gastritis; peptic ulcer.

Gasterine Bouchara, Fr.†.
Sodium bicarbonate (p.1153·2); calcium carbonate (p.1182·1); magnesium hydroxide (p.1198·2).
Gastro-intestinal pain.

Gastracol Streuli, Switz.
Aluminium hydroxide (p.1177·3).
Gastric hyperacidity.

Gastral Novag, Spain.
Sucralfate (p.1214·2).
Gastro-intestinal haemorrhage; peptic ulcer.

Gastralgin De Angeli, Ital.
Roxatidine acetate hydrochloride (p.1212·1).
Gastro-intestinal disorders associated with hyperacidity.

Gastralgine UPSA, Fr.
Aluminium hydroxide (p.1177·3); aluminium glycinate (p.1177·2); magnesium trisilicate (p.1199·1); simethicone (p.1213·1).
Gastro-intestinal disorders.

Gastralka GS, S.Afr.†.
Magnesium hydroxide (p.1198·2); aluminium hydroxide gel (p.1177·3).
Gastro-intestinal disorders.

Gastralon N Redel, Ger.
Chamomile (p.1561·2); gentian (p.1583·3); absinthium (p.1541·1).
Gastro-intestinal disorders.

Gastralsan
Note. This name is used for preparations of different composition.
Dolisos, Canad.
Homoeopathic preparation.

Dolisos, Fr.
Cynara (p.1569·2); boldo (p.1554·1); fumitory (p.1581·3).
Biliary-tract disorders.

Gastralugel Biogalenique, Fr.†.
Amorphous hydrated silica (p.1474·3); colloidal aluminium hydroxide (p.1177·3).
Gastro-intestinal disorders.

Gastrarctin N Serum-Werk Bernburg, Ger.
Colloidal silver; chamomile flowers (p.1561·2); peppermint leaf (p.1208·1).
Gastro-intestinal disorders.

Gastrausil Schiapparelli Searle, Ital.†.
Carbenoxolone sodium (p.1182·2).
Duodenitis; gastritis; peptic ulcer.

Gastrausil Complex Schiapparelli Searle, Ital.†.
Carbenoxolone sodium (p.1182·2); magnesium hydroxide (p.1198·2); aluminium hydroxide (p.1177·3).
Duodenitis; gastritis; peptic ulcer.

Gastrausil D Schiapparelli Searle, Ital.†.
Carbenoxolone sodium (p.1182·2); diazepam (p.661·1).
Duodenitis; gastritis; peptic ulcer.

Gastrax Asche, Ger.
Nizatidine (p.1203·2).
Peptic ulcer.

Gastregan Synpharma, Aust.
Chamomile flower (p.1561·2); melissa leaf (p.1600·1); peppermint leaf (p.1208·1).
Gastro-intestinal pain and inflammation.

Gastrex Boehringer Ingelheim, Fr.
Dihydroxyaluminium monohistidinate magnesium hydroxide (p.1198·2).
Gastro-intestinal disorders.

Gastribien Cinfa, Spain.
Aluminium hydroxide (p.1177·3); magnesium trisilicate (p.1199·1).
Gastro-intestinal hyperacidity.

Gastricalm Whitehall, Belg.
Magaldrate (p.1198·1).
Gastro-intestinal disorders associated with hyperacidity.

Gastricard N Cassella-med, Ger.
Oral drops: Gentian (p.1583·3); ginger oil; crataegus (p.1568·2); fennel oil (p.1579·2); peppermint oil (p.1208·1); caraway oil (p.1559·3); coriander oil (p.1567·3).
Tablets: Crataegus (p.1568·2); peppermint oil (p.1208·1); caraway oil (p.1559·3); fennel oil (p.1579·2); coriander oil (p.1567·3).
Gastro-intestinal disorders.

Gastricholan-L Sudmedica, Ger.
Matricaria flowers (p.1561·2); peppermint leaf (p.1208·1); fennel (p.1579·1).
Gastro-intestinal disorders.

Gastricum Truw, Ger.†.
Homoeopathic preparation.

Gastricur Heumann, Ger.
Pirenzepine hydrochloride (p.467·1).
Gastro-intestinal disorders.

Gastricure Bio-Familia, Switz.
Ceratonia (p.1472·2); marine algae; magnesium trisilicate (p.1199·1).
Bloating; gastric hyperacidity; gastric irritation.

Gastridin Merck Sharp & Dohme, Ital.
Famotidine (p.1192·1).
Gastro-intestinal disorders.

Gastrifom Tanta, Canad.
Aluminium hydroxide (p.1177·3); alginic acid (p.1470·3).

gastri-L 90 N Loges, Ger.
Homoeopathic preparation.

Gastrilax Saunier-Daguin, Fr.
Anhydrous sodium sulphate (p.1213·3); dibasic sodium phosphate (p.1159·3); citric acid monohydrate (p.1564·3).
Gastro-intestinal disorders.

Gastrils Ernest Jackson, UK.
Aluminium hydroxide-magnesium carbonate co-dried gel (p.1178·2).
Dyspepsia.

Gastrimagal Azupharma, Ger.
Magaldrate (p.1198·1).
Gastro-intestinal disorders associated with hyperacidity.

Gastrimut Normon, Spain.
Omeprazole (p.1204·2).
Gastro-oesophageal reflux; peptic ulcer; Zollinger-Ellison syndrome.

Gastrin-Do Grasler, Ger.
Homoeopathic preparation.

Gastrinol Frega, Canad.
Magnesium hydroxide (p.1198·2); aluminium hydroxide-magnesium carbonate co-dried gel (p.1178·2); simethicone (p.1213·1).

Gastrion Vita, Spain.
Famotidine (p.1192·1).
Gastro-oesophageal reflux; peptic ulcer; Zollinger-Ellison syndrome.

Gastri-P Sanorania, Ger.
Pirenzepine hydrochloride (p.467·1).
Gastro-intestinal disorders.

Gastripan
Note. This name is used for preparations of different composition.
Merckle, Aust.
Aluminium glycinate (p.1177·2); almasilate (p.1177·1); liquorice (p.1197·1); ethaverine hydrochloride (p.1577·1).
Gastro-intestinal disorders.

Merckle, Ger.
Magaldrate (p.1198·1).
Gastric hyperacidity; heartburn; peptic ulcer.

Gastripan M Merckle, Ger.†.
Bismuth subnitrate (p.1180·2).
Gastritis; peptic ulcer.

Gastrised Benvegna, Ital.†.
Oxyphencyclimine hydrochloride (p.466·3); meprobamate (p.678·1).
Gastro-intestinal disorders.

Gastriselect Dreluso, Ger.
Homoeopathic preparation.

Gastritol Klein, Ger.
Potentilla anserina; absinthium (p.1541·1); cnicus benedictus (p.1565·3); liquorice (p.1197·1); angelica; chamomile (p.1561·2); hypericum (p.1590·1).
Gastro-intestinal disorders.

Gastro Gobens Normon, Spain.
Aluminium hydroxide (p.1177·3); dimethicone (p.1213·1); levoglutamide (p.1344·3); metoclopramide hydrochloride (p.1200·3).
Dyspepsia; gastritis; meteorism; nausea; oesophagitis; peptic ulcer.

Gastro H2 Lesvi, Spain.
Cimetidine (p.1183·2).
Acid aspiration; gastro-oesophageal reflux; peptic ulcer; Zollinger-Ellison syndrome.

Gastroalgine Novag, Spain.
Aluminium hydroxide (p.1177·3); dimethicone (p.1213·1); enoxolone aluminium (p.1191·3); magnesium hydroxide (p.1198·2); sorbitol (p.1354·2).
Gastro-intestinal hyperacidity; meteorism; peptic ulcer.

Gastrobid Continus *Napp, Irl.; Napp, UK.*
Metoclopramide hydrochloride (p.1200·3).
Gastro-intestinal disorders; nausea and vomiting.

Gastrobin *Divapharma, Ger.†.*
Magnesium trisilicate (p.1199·1).
Gastro-intestinal disorders.

Gastrobitan *Gea, Norw.*
Cimetidine (p.1183·2).
Aspiration syndrome; gastro-oesophageal reflux; peptic ulcer; Zollinger-Ellison syndrome.

Gastrobon *Byk Madaus, S.Afr.*
Magaldrate (p.1198·1).
Dyspepsia; gastritis; gastro-oesophageal reflux disease; peptic ulcer.

Gastrobrom *Fawns & McAllan, Austral.†.*
Powdered milk; glucose; magnesium trisilicate (p.1199·1); magnesium hydroxide (p.1198·2); magnesium carbonate (p.1198·1); calcium carbonate (p.1182·1).
Dyspepsia.

Gastrobul
Codali, Belg.†; Guerbet, Fr.
Betaine hydrochloride (p.1553·2); sodium bicarbonate (p.1153·2); dimethicone (p.1213·1).
Gas production for double-contrast radiography.

Gastrocalm *Bio-Sante, Canad.*
Aluminium hydroxide-magnesium carbonate co-dried gel (p.1178·2); simethicone (p.1213·1).

Gastrocaps *Bouhon, Ger.†.*
Liquorice (p.1197·1); bismuth aluminate (p.1180·1); aluminium hydroxide gel (p.1177·3); sodium bicarbonate (p.1153·2); fennel oil (p.1579·2); condurango (p.1567·2); frangula bark (p.1193·2); valerian (p.1643·1); ox bile (p.1553·2); scopolia carniolica.
Gastro-intestinal disorders.

Gastrocaps A *Palmicol, Ger.*
Aluminium hydroxide (p.1177·3).
Gastro-intestinal disorders associated with hyperacidity; hyperphosphaturia.

Gastroccult *SmithKline Diagnostics, USA.*
Test for occult blood in gastric contents.

Gastrocolon *Pharmagen, S.Afr.†.*
Metoclopramide hydrochloride (p.1200·3).
Gastro-intestinal disorders.

Gastro-Conray *May & Baker, Austral.†.*
Sodium iothalamate (p.1008·1).
Contrast medium for gastro-enterography.

Gastrocote
Stanley, Canad.; SA Druggists, S.Afr.†; Seton, UK.
Alginic acid (p.1470·3) or sodium alginate (p.1470·3); aluminium hydroxide (p.1177·3); magnesium trisilicate (p.1199·1); sodium bicarbonate (p.1153·2).
Gastro-oesophageal reflux.

Gastrocrom *Fisons, USA.*
Sodium cromoglycate (p.762·1).
Mastocytosis.

Gastrocure *Taxandria, Neth.*
Domperidone maleate (p.1191·1).
Gastro-intestinal disorders.

Gastrocynesine *Boiron, Fr.*
Homoeopathic preparation.

Gastrodenol *Yamanouchi, Spain.*
Tripotassium dicitratobismuthate (p.1180·2).
Gastritis; peptic ulcer.

Gastrodiagnost *Merck, Ger.†.*
Pentagastrin (p.1616·3).
Diagnostic agent.

Gastrodomina *Berenguer Infale, Spain.*
Famotidine (p.1192·1).
Gastro-oesophageal reflux; peptic ulcer; Zollinger-Ellison syndrome.

Gastrofilm *Will-Pharma, Belg.*
Algeldrate (p.1177·3); magnesium carbonate (p.1198·1); calcium carbonate (p.1182·1); magnesium trisilicate (p.1199·1); bismuth subnitrate (p.1180·2); belladonna (p.457·1).
Dyspepsia; gastric hyperacidity.

Gastroflux *Ashbourne, UK.*
Metoclopramide hydrochloride (p.1200·3).
Gastro-intestinal disorders.

Gastrofrenal
Searle, Ital.; Sigma-Tau, Spain.
Sodium cromoglycate (p.762·1).
Food hypersensitivity; inflammatory bowel disease.

Gastrogel
Note. This name is used for preparations of different composition.
Fawns & McAllan, Austral.
Oral liquid: Aluminium hydroxide (p.1177·3); magnesium trisilicate (p.1199·1); magnesium hydroxide (p.1198·2).
Tablets: Aluminium hydroxide (p.1177·3); magnesium trisilicate (p.1199·1); magnesium hydroxide (p.1198·2); simethicone (p.1213·1).
Dyspepsia.
Giuliani, Ital.; Giuliani, Switz.
Sucralfate (p.1214·2).
Gastro-intestinal disorders.

Gastroglutal *Tedec Meiji, Spain.*
Magnesium oxide (p.1198·3); levoglutamide (p.1344·3); aluminium glycinate (p.1177·2).
Gastro-intestinal hyperacidity.

Gastrografin
Schering, Aust.; Squibb Diagnostics, Canad.; Schering, Ger.; Schering, Ital.; Schering, Neth.; Schering, Norw.; Schering, S.Afr.; Schering, Spain; Schering, Swed.; Schering, Switz.; Schering, UK; Squibb Diagnostics, USA.
Meglumine diatrizoate (p.1003·2); sodium diatrizoate (p.1003·2).
Contrast medium for gastro-intestinal radiography; meconium ileus.

Gastrografine *Schering, Fr.*
Meglumine diatrizoate (p.1003·2); sodium diatrizoate (p.1003·2).
Contrast medium for gastro-intestinal radiography.

Gastrol *Salus, Ital.*
Pirenzepine hydrochloride (p.467·1).
Gastroduodenitis; peptic ulcer.

Gastrol S *Fides, Ger.*
Gentian (p.1583·3); chamomile (p.1561·2); melissa (p.1600·1); caraway (p.1559·3); fennel (p.1579·1); coriander (p.1567·3); sweet basil; absinthium (p.1541·1); hypericum (p.1590·1); cinchona bark (p.1564·1); juniper (p.1592·2); calamus (p.1556·1); turmeric (p.1001·3).
Gastro-intestinal disorders.

Gastroloc *Stern, Ger.*
Capsules: Omeprazole (p.1204·2).
Injection†: Omeprazole sodium (p.1204·2).
Gastro-oesophageal reflux; peptic ulcer; Zollinger-Ellison syndrome.

Gastroluft
Fuji, Swed.; Nycomed, Switz.
Sodium bicarbonate (p.1153·2); tartaric acid (p.1634·3); dimethicone (p.1213·1).
Adjunct in gastro-intestinal double-contrast radiography.

Gastrolux *Goldham, Ger.*
Sodium diatrizoate (p.1003·2); meglumine diatrizoate (p.1003·2).
Contrast medium for gastro-intestinal radiography.

Gastrolyte
Rhone-Poulenc Rorer, Austral.; Rhone-Poulenc Rorer, Canad.
Sodium chloride; sodium acid citrate; potassium chloride; glucose (p.1152·3).
Diarrhoea; oral rehydration therapy.

Gastrolyte-R *Rhone-Poulenc Rorer, Austral.*
Rice powder; sodium chloride; sodium citrate; potassium chloride (p.1152·3).
Diarrhoea; oral rehydration therapy.

Gastrom *Tanabe, Jpn.*
Ecabet sodium (p.1191·3).
Gastric ulcer; gastritis.

Gastromax *Pfizer, UK.*
Metoclopramide hydrochloride (p.1200·3).
Gastro-intestinal disorders; nausea and vomiting.

Gastromet *Bayer, Ital.*
Cimetidine (p.1183·2) or cimetidine hydrochloride (p.1185·3).
Gastro-intestinal disorders.

Gastromiro
Gerot, Aust.; E. Merck, Irl.; Bracco, Ital.
Iopamidol (p.1007·1).
Contrast medium for gastro-intestinal radiography.

Gastromol *Byk Elmu, Spain.*
Magaldrate (p.1198·1).
Hyperacidity.

Gastron
Note. This name is used for preparations of different composition.
Lennon, S.Afr.
Loperamide hydrochloride (p.1197·2).
Colostomies; diarrhoea; ileostomies.
Sterling Winthrop, UK†.
Aluminium hydroxide (p.1177·3); sodium bicarbonate (p.1153·2); magnesium trisilicate (p.1199·1); alginic acid (p.1470·3).
Gastro-oesophageal reflux.

Gastronerton
Schoeller, Aust.†; Dolorgiet, Ger.
Metoclopramide (p.1202·1) or metoclopramide hydrochloride (p.1200·3).
Gastro-intestinal motility disorders; nausea and vomiting.

Gastronol *Bioforce, Switz.*
Homoeopathic preparation.

Gastronorm *Janssen-Cilag, Ital.*
Domperidone (p.1190·3).
Dyspepsia.

Gastro-Pasc *Pascoe, Ger.*
Homoeopathic preparation.

Gastropax *Lehning, Fr.*
Belladonna (p.457·1); star anise; kaolin (p.1195·1); calcium carbonate (p.1182·1); magnesium trisilicate (p.1199·1); magnesium carbonate (p.1198·1); vegetable charcoal (p.972·3); thyme (p.1636·3); calcium phosphate (p.1155·3); liquorice (p.1197·1); sodium bicarbonate (p.1153·2); sodium sulphate (p.1213·3); magnesium hydroxide (p.1198·2).
Gastro-intestinal disorders.

Gastropeache Susp *Italfarmaco, Spain.*
Aluminium hydroxide (p.1177·3); magnesium hydroxide (p.1198·2).
Hyperacidity.

Gastropect *Lennon, S.Afr.*
Kaolin (p.1195·1); pectin (p.1474·1).
Diarrhoea.

Gastropen *I Farmacologia, Spain.*
Famotidine (p.1192·1).
Gastro-oesophageal reflux; peptic ulcer; Zollinger-Ellison syndrome.

Gastro-Pepsin *Ceccarelli, Ital.*
Pepsin (p.1616·3); gastric mucosa; hydrochloric acid (p.1588·3); lactic acid (p.1593·3); bitter orange.
Formerly contained pepsin, gastric mucosa, hydrochloric acid, lactic acid, nux vomica, kola, gentian, condurango, cascarilla, and bitter orange.
Dyspepsia; hypoacidity.

Gastropiren *AGIPS, Ital.*
Pirenzepine hydrochloride (p.467·1).
Gastro-intestinal disorders.

Gastroplant *DHU, Ger.*
Homoeopathic preparation.

Gastroprotect *Brenner-Efeka, Ger.; LAW, Ger.*
Cimetidine (p.1183·2).
Aspiration syndrome; gastro-oesophageal reflux; peptic ulcer; Zollinger-Ellison syndrome.

Gastropulgit *Spitzner, Ger.*
Attapulgite (p.1178·3); aluminium hydroxide-magnesium carbonate dried gel (p.1178·2).
Gastro-intestinal disorders.

Gastropulgite
Ipsen, Belg.; Beaufour, Fr.; Beaufour, Switz.
Attapulgite (p.1178·3); aluminium hydroxide-magnesium carbonate co-dried gel (p.1178·2).
Gastro-intestinal disorders.

Gastrosan
Note. This name is used for preparations of different composition.
Inkeysa, Spain.
Aluminium hydroxide (p.1177·3); magnesium hydroxide (p.1198·2).
Gastro-intestinal hyperacidity.
Bioforce, Switz.
Achillea (p.1542·2); taraxacum (p.1634·2); melissa (p.1600·1); gentian (p.1583·3); cnicus benedictus (p.1565·3); angelica; centaury (p.1561·1).
Digestive disorders.

Gastrosanol *Lampugnani, Ital.†.*
Calcium carbonate (p.1182·1); bismuth subcarbonate (p.1180·1); light magnesium carbonate (p.1198·1); sodium bicarbonate (p.1153·2); procaine hydrochloride (p.1299·2); belladonna (p.457·1); heavy kaolin (p.1195·1).
Antacid.

Gastrosecur *Duopharm, Ger.*
Chirata; gentian (p.1583·3); ginger (p.1193·2); cinnamon (p.1564·2); dried bitter-orange peel (p.1610·3); caraway (p.1559·3).
Gastro-intestinal disorders.

Gastrosed
Note. This name is used for preparations of different composition.
Amsa, Ital.
Pirenzepine hydrochloride (p.467·1).
Gastritis; peptic ulcer.
Roberts, USA.
Hyoscyamine sulphate (p.464·2).

Gastrosedyl *Monin, Fr.*
Belladonna (p.457·1); hyoscyamus (p.464·3).
Gastro-intestinal and biliary-tract disorders.

Gastrosil
Salus, Aust.; Heumann, Ger.; Heumann, Switz.
Metoclopramide (p.1202·1) or metoclopramide hydrochloride (p.1200·3).
Adjunct in gastro-intestinal examination; gastro-intestinal disorders.

Gastrosindrom *Llorens, Spain†.*
Amylase (p.1549·1); dimethicone (p.1213·1); metoclopramide (p.1202·1); papain (p.1614·1); papaverine hydrochloride (p.1614·2); pepsin (p.1616·3); dehydrocholic acid (p.1570·2).
Digestive-system disorders.

Gastrosine *Boiron, Canad.*
Homoeopathic preparation.

Gastrostad *Stada, Ger.*
Magaldrate (p.1198·1).
Gastro-intestinal disorders associated with hyperacidity.

Gastro-Stop
Note. A similar name is used for preparations of different composition.
Rhone-Poulenc Rorer, Austral.
Loperamide hydrochloride (p.1197·2).
Diarrhoea.

Gastrostop
Note. A similar name is used for preparations of different composition.
Biomedica, Ital.
Aluminium glycinate (p.1177·2); magnesium hydroxide (p.1198·2).
Hyperchlorhydria.

Gastro-Tablinen *Sanorania, Ger.†.*
Metoclopramide hydrochloride (p.1200·3).
Gastro-intestinal disorders.

Gastrotat *Noristan Generica, S.Afr.†.*
Metoclopramide hydrochloride (p.1200·3).
Gastro-intestinal disorders.

Gastro-Teknosal *Taco, Ger.†.*
Magnesium trisilicate (p.1199·1); aluminium hydroxide gel (p.1177·3); calcium carbonate (p.1182·1).
Gastro-intestinal disorders.

Gastrotem *Temmler, Ger.†.*
Metoclopramide hydrochloride (p.1200·3).
Gastro-intestinal disorders.

Gastrotest *Waldheim, Aust.*
2 White tablets, caffeine and sodium benzoate; 3 yellow tablets, phenazopyridine (p.79·1).
Test for gastric acid production.

Gastro-Timelets
Salus, Aust.; Temmler, Ger.; Asta Medica, Switz.
Metoclopramide hydrochloride (p.1200·3).
Gastro-intestinal disorders.

Gastrotranquil *Azupharma, Ger.*
Metoclopramide hydrochloride (p.1200·3).
Gastro-intestinal disorders.

Gastrotrop *Sanol, Ger.†.*
Metoclopramide hydrochloride (p.1200·3).
Gastro-intestinal disorders.

Gastrovegetalin *Verla, Ger.*
Melissa (p.1600·1).
Gastro-intestinal disorders; sleep disorders.

Gastro-Vial *Klever, Ger.†.*
Sodium bicarbonate (p.1153·2); calcium carbonate (p.1182·1); sepia (p.1628·2); tubera salep; sal maris; sal bad vichy; angelica; marrubium vulgare (p.1063·3); potentilla anserina; centaury (p.1561·1); chamomile (p.1561·2); rue.
Gastro-intestinal disorders.

Gastrovison
Schering, Ger.†; Schering, Ital.
Sodium bicarbonate (p.1153·2); citric acid (p.1564·3); simethicone (p.1213·1); silicon dioxide (p.1474·3).
Gas production for double-contrast radiography.

Gastrozepin
Bender, Aust.; Boehringer Ingelheim, Canad.†; Thomae, Ger.; Knoll, Irl.†; Boehringer Ingelheim, Ital.; Boehringer Ingelheim, S.Afr.†; Boehringer Ingelheim, Spain†; Boots, UK†.
Pirenzepine hydrochloride (p.467·1).
Gastritis; peptic ulcer; Zollinger-Ellison syndrome.

Gastrozepine *Boehringer Ingelheim, Switz.*
Pirenzepine hydrochloride (p.467·1).
Gastroduodenitis; peptic ulcer.

Gasulsol *Herbes Universelles, Canad.*
Aluminium hydroxide (p.1177·3); magnesium trisilicate (p.1199·1).

Gasva *Gerbex, Canad.*
Aluminium hydroxide (p.1177·3); magnesium trisilicate (p.1199·1).

Gas-X
Sandoz, Canad.; Sandoz, USA.
Simethicone (p.1213·1).
Flatulence.

Gatinar
Sandoz, Spain; Wander OTC, Switz.
Lactulose (p.1195·3).
Constipation; hepatic encephalopathy; salmonella enteritis.

Gaurit *Merckle, Aust.*
Indomethacin (p.45·2).
Aluminium glycinate (p.1177·2) is included in this preparation in an attempt to limit adverse effects on the gastro-intestinal mucosa.
Gout; inflammation; musculoskeletal, joint, peri-articular, and soft-tissue disorders; pain.

Gavigrans *Reckitt & Colman, Austral.†.*
Alginic acid (p.1470·3); magnesium trisilicate (p.1199·1); aluminium hydroxide (p.1177·3); sodium bicarbonate (p.1153·2).
Gastro-oesophageal reflux.

Gaviscon
Note. This name is used for preparations of different composition.
Reckitt & Colman, Austral.; Reckitt & Colman, Belg.; SmithKline Beecham, Fr.; Reckitts, Irl.; Boehringer Mannheim, Ital.; Schering-Plough, Neth.; Reckitt & Colman, S.Afr.; Reckitt & Colman, UK.
Oral suspension: Sodium alginate (p.1470·3); calcium carbonate (p.1182·1); sodium bicarbonate (p.1153·2).
Gastro-oesophageal reflux; heartburn.
Reckitt & Colman, Austral.; Reckitt & Colman, Belg.; SmithKline Beecham, Fr.; Thomae, Ger.†; Reckitts, Irl.; Boehringer Mannheim, Ital.; Schering-Plough, Neth.; Reckitt & Colman, S.Afr.; Reckitt & Colman, UK; SmithKline Beecham Consumer, USA.
Chewable tablets; oral powder: Alginic acid (p.1470·3); aluminium hydroxide (p.1177·3); magnesium trisilicate (p.1199·1); sodium bicarbonate (p.1153·2).
Gastro-oesophageal reflux; heartburn.
Thomae, Ger.; Ferring, Norw.; Ferring, Swed.; Reckitt & Colman, Switz.
Oral suspension: Sodium alginate (p.1470·3); aluminium hydroxide (p.1177·3); sodium bicarbonate (p.1153·2); calcium carbonate (p.1182·1).
Abdominal distension; gastric hyperacidity; gastro-oesophageal reflux; heartburn.
Thomae, Ger.; Ferring, Norw.; Ferring, Swed.; Reckitt & Colman, Switz.
Chewable tablets: Alginic acid (p.1470·3); sodium bicarbonate (p.1153·2); aluminium hydroxide (p.1177·3).
Abdominal distension; gastric hyperacidity; gastro-oesophageal reflux; heartburn.
Reckitt & Colman, Spain.
Alginic acid (p.1470·3); sodium bicarbonate (p.1153·2).
Formerly contained alginic acid, aluminium hydroxide, magnesium trisilicate (tablets only), and sodium bicarbonate.
Gastro-oesophageal reflux.
SmithKline Beecham Consumer, USA.
Oral liquid: Aluminium hydroxide (p.1177·3); magnesium carbonate (p.1198·1); sodium alginate (p.1470·3).
Dyspepsia.

Gaviscon Acid *SmithKline Beecham Consumer, Canad.*
Magnesium hydroxide (p.1198·2); calcium carbonate (p.1182·1).

Gaviscon Advance *Reckitt & Colman, UK.*
Sodium alginate (p.1470·3); potassium bicarbonate (p.1153·1).
Dyspepsia; gastro-oesophageal reflux; heartburn.

Gaviscon Extra Strength *SmithKline Beecham Consumer, USA.*
Aluminium hydroxide (p.1177·3); magnesium carbonate (p.1198·1).
Dyspepsia.

Gaviscon Extra Strength Relief Formula *SmithKline Beecham Consumer, USA.*
Aluminium hydroxide (p.1177·3); magnesium carbonate (p.1198·1); simethicone (p.1213·1).
Hyperacidity.

Gaviscon Heartburn Relief *SmithKline Beecham Consumer, Canad.*
Alginic acid (p.1470·3) or sodium alginate (p.1470·3); aluminium hydroxide (p.1177·3).
Gastro-oesophageal reflux; heartburn.

Gaviscon Heartburn Relief Aluminium-Free *SmithKline Beecham Consumer, Canad.*
Alginic acid (p.1470·3); magnesium carbonate (p.1198·1).
Gastro-oesophageal reflux; heartburn.

Gaviscon Infant *Reckitt & Colman, UK.*
Magnesium alginate (p.1470·3); sodium alginate (p.1470·3).
Formerly known as Infant Gaviscon and contained aluminium hydroxide, magnesium alginate, and sodium alginate.
NOTE. In view of its high sodium content this preparation should not be used in premature infants or in situations where excess water-loss is likely, such as fever or high room-temperature; some sources have recommended that it should be avoided altogether in children less than 6 months of age.
Gastro-oesophageal reflux.

GB Tablets *Potter's, UK.*
Black-root; euonymus (p.1192·1); kava root (p.1592·3); burdock root (p.1594·2).
Formerly known as Gall Bladder Tablets.
Dyspepsia.

GBH *Rorer, Canad.†.*
Lindane (p.1407·2).
Pediculosis.

Geangin
Gea, Neth.†; Gea, Norw.; Cusi, UK†.
Verapamil hydrochloride (p.960·3).
Angina; arrhythmias; hypertension.

Geavir
Gea, Norw.; GEA, Swed.
Aciclovir (p.602·3) or aciclovir sodium (p.602·3).
Herpesvirus infections.

Gebauer "114" Spray *Gebauer, USA.*
Dichlorotetrafluoroethane (p.1164·3).
Topical anaesthetic.

Gee-Gee *Jones, USA.*
Guaiphenesin (p.1061·3).
Coughs.

Gefanil *Sumitomo, Jpn.*
Gefarnate (p.1193·2).
Gastritis; peptic ulcer.

Gefarnax *De Angeli, Ital.†.*
Gefarnate (p.1193·2); diazepam (p.661·1).
Gastro-intestinal disorders.

Gefarnil *De Angeli, Ital.†.*
Gefarnate (p.1193·2).
Gastro-intestinal disorders.

Gefarnil Compositum *De Angeli, Ital.†.*
Gefarnate (p.1193·2); nafiverine hydrochloride (p.1606·2); aluminium glycinate (p.1177·2); magnesium trisilicate (p.1199·1); aluminium hydroxide (p.1177·3).
Gastro-intestinal disorders.

Geffer *Boehringer Mannheim, Ital.*
Metoclopramide hydrochloride (p.1200·3); dimethicone (p.1213·1); potassium citrate (p.1153·1); citric acid (p.1564·3); tartaric acid (p.1634·3); sodium bicarbonate (p.1153·2).
Gastro-intestinal disorders associated with hyperacidity.

Gehwol Fungizid *Gerlach, Ger.*
Topical liquid: Undecenoic acid monoethanolamide (p.389·2); chloroxylenol (p.1111·1); 3,4,5,6-tetrabromo-*o*-cresol (p.1126·3); copper-triethanolamine complex.
Topical powder: Bromosalicylic acid (p.1090·3); undecenoic acid monoethanolamide (p.389·2); chloroxylenol (p.1111·1); 3,4,5,6-tetrabromo-*o*-cresol (p.1126·3).
Fungal infections.

Gehwol Fungizid Creme N *Gerlach, Ger.*
Undecenoic acid monoethanolamide (p.389·2); chloroxylenol (p.1111·1); 3,4,5,6-tetrabromo-*o*-cresol (p.1126·3).
Fungal infections.

Gehwol Huhneraugen Tinktur *Gerlach, Ger.*
Salicylic acid (p.1090·2); glacial acetic acid (p.1541·2).
Callouses; corns.

Gehwol Huhneraugenpflaster N *Gerlach, Ger.*
Salicylic acid (p.1090·2); lactic acid (p.1593·3).
Callouses; corns.

Gehwol Nagelpilz *Gerlach, Ger.*
Zinc chloride (p.1373·1); bromosalicylic acid (p.1090·3); salicylic acid (p.1090·2); undecenoic acid monoethanolamide (p.389·2).
Fungal nail infections.

Gehwol Schalpaste *Gerlach, Ger.*
Salicylic acid (p.1090·2).
Callouses; corns.

Gel "7" *Germiphene, Canad.†.*
Neutral sodium fluoride (p.742·1).
Dental caries prophylaxis.

Gel a l'Acetotartrate d'Alumine Defresne *Goupil, Fr.†.*
Methylcitrine; aluminium acetotartrate (p.1547·3).
Circulatory disorders; muscle pain.

Gel Kam *Scherer, USA.*
Stannous fluoride (p.1632·2).
Dental caries prophylaxis.

Gel Solaire Bronzage *Clarins, Canad.*
SPF 3: 2-phenyl-1*H*-benzimidazole-5-sulphonic acid (p.1488·2).
Sunscreen.

Gel Tar *Restiva, Ital.†.*
Willow oleoresin; sulphur (p.1091·2); urea (p.1095·2).
Skin disorders.

Gelacet
Merck, Aust.; Hermal, Ger.; Hermal, Switz.
Vitamin A acetate (p.1359·2); L-cystine (p.1339·1); gelatin (p.723·2).
Hair and nail disorders.

Gelafundin *Braun, Ger.*
Gelatin polysuccinate (p.723·2) with electrolytes.
Hypovolaemia.

Gelafusal-N in Ringeracetat *Serum-Werk Bernburg, Ger.*
Gelatin polysuccinate (p.723·2) in electrolytes.
Hypovolaemia; thrombosis prophylaxis.

Gelamel *Morado, Ital.*
Royal jelly (p.1626·3).
Nutritional supplement.

Gelaspon *ankerpharm, Ger.*
Gelatin (p.723·2).
Haemorrhage; haemostatic.

Gelastypt D *Hoechst, Ger.*
Gelatine (p.723·2).
Wounds.

Gelastypt M *Hoechst, Ger.†.*
Ethacridine lactate (p.1098·3).
Dental dressing.

Gelatine Medicinale *Geistlich, Switz.†.*
Amino-acid preparation.
Hair and nail disorders.

Gel-Caps *Nyal, Austral.†.*
Gelatin (p.723·2).
Nail defects.

Gelcen *Centrum, Spain.*
Capsaicin (p.24·2).
Pain.

Gelcosal *Quinoderm, UK.*
Coal tar (p.1092·3); tar (p.1092·3); salicylic acid (p.1090·2).
Dermatitis; psoriasis.

Gelcotar
Quinoderm, Irl.; Quinoderm, UK.
Shampoo: Coal tar (p.1092·3); cade oil (p.1092·2).
Dandruff; psoriasis of the scalp; seborrhoeic dermatitis.

Quinoderm, Irl.; Quinoderm, UK.
Topical gel: Coal tar (p.1092·3); tar (p.1092·3).
Dermatitis; psoriasis.

Geldene *Pfizer, Fr.*
Piroxicam (p.80·2).
Sprains; tendinitis.

Gelee lubrifiante simple *Bichsel, Switz.*
Chlorhexidine gluconate (p.1107·2); macrogol 400 (p.1598·2).
Lubrication for catheters and endoscopes.

Gelenk- und Rheumatropfen *Molitor, Ger.†.*
Homoeopathic preparation.

Gelenta *Warner-Lambert Consumer, Belg.†.*
Magnesium hydroxide (p.1198·2); aluminium hydroxide (p.1177·3).
Peptic ulcer.

Gelfilm
Pharmacia Upjohn, Austral.; Pharmacia Upjohn, Canad.; Pharmacia Upjohn, Neth.; Upjohn, USA.
Gelatin (p.723·2).
Haemorrhage.

Gelfoam
Pharmacia Upjohn, Austral.; Pharmacia Upjohn, Belg.; Pharmacia Upjohn, Canad.; Pharmacia Upjohn, Neth.; Pharmacia Upjohn, S.Afr.†; Pharmacia Upjohn, Switz.; Upjohn, USA.
Gelatin (p.723·2).
Haemostatic.

Gelictar de Charlieu *Nigy, Fr.†.*
A complex derived from ichthammol (p.1083·3) and coal tar (Ictar) (p.1092·3).
Seborrhoeic dermatitis.

Gelidina *Yamanouchi, Spain.*
Fluocinolone acetonide (p.1041·1).
Skin disorders.

Gelifundol
Biotest, Aust.; Biotest, Ger.; Mednostica, S.Afr.; Biotest, Switz.
Oxypolygelatin (p.725·2) with electrolytes.
Hypovolaemia; resuspension of concentrated erythrocytes.

Geliperm
Yamanouchi, Ger.; Geistlich, Switz.; Geistlich, UK.
Hydrogel dressing.
Burns; ulcers; wounds.

Geli-Stop *Schieffer, Switz.†.*
Magnesium peroxide (p.1119·1); pectin (p.1474·1); albumin tannate (p.1176·3).
Diarrhoea.

Gel-Larmes *Thea, Fr.*
Carbomer 934 P (p.1471·2).
Dry eyes.

Geloalumin *Gelos, Spain.*
Dried aluminium hydroxide (p.1177·3); dimethicone (p.1213·1); magnesium hydroxide (p.1198·2).
Gastro-intestinal hyperacidity and flatulence.

Gelocast *Beiersdorf, Ital.*
Zinc oxide (p.1096·2).
Medicated dressing.

Gelocatil *Gelos, Spain.*
Paracetamol (p.72·2).
Fever; pain.

Gelodiet *DHN, Fr.*
Gelatin (p.723·2); sucrose (p.1357·1).
Dehydration.

Gelodrox *Gelos, Spain.*
Dried aluminium hydroxide (p.1177·3); calcium carbonate (p.1182·1); magnesium carbonate (p.1198·1); magnesium trisilicate (p.1199·1).
Gastro-intestinal hyperacidity.

Gelodual *Gelos, Spain.*
Dried aluminium hydroxide (p.1177·3); magnesium hydroxide (p.1198·2); magnesium trisilicate (p.1199·1).
Gastro-intestinal hyperacidity.

Gelodurat *Pohl, Ger.†.*
Eucalyptus oil (p.1578·1).
Respiratory-tract disorders.

Gelofalk *Falk, Ger.*
Smectite; aluminium hydroxide gel (p.1177·3); magnesium hydroxide (p.1198·2).
Gastro-intestinal disorders.

Geloflex *Braun, UK.*
Succinylated gelatin (p.723·2) in sodium chloride.
Hypovolaemia.

Gelofusin *Braun, Aust.*
Gelatin (p.723·2).
Haemodilution; hypovolaemia.

Gelofusine
Braun, Belg.; Braun, Fr.; Braun, UK.
Succinylated gelatin (p.723·2) in sodium chloride.
Hypovolaemic shock.

Gelomyrtol
Salus, Aust.; Pohl, Ger.
Myrtol.
Bronchitis; sinusitis.

Gelonasal *Pohl, Ger.*
Xylometazoline hydrochloride (p.1071·2).
Nasal congestion.

Gelonida
Note. This name is used for preparations of different composition.
Godecke, Ger.
Paracetamol (p.72·2); codeine phosphate (p.26·1).
Pain.

Warner-Lambert, Switz.†.
Aspirin (p.16·1); paracetamol (p.72·2); codeine phosphate (p.26·1).
Fever; pain.

Gelonida NA *Godecke, Ger.*
Oral liquid: Sodium salicylate (p.85·1); paracetamol (p.72·2); codeine phosphate (p.26·1).
Cold symptoms; fever; neuralgia; neuritis; pain.
Suppositories: Aspirin (p.16·1); paracetamol (p.72·2); codeine phosphate (p.26·1).
Coughs and cold symptoms; pain.

Gelopectose *Nutripharm Elgi, Fr.*
Pectin (p.1474·1); microcrystalline cellulose (p.1472·1); hydrated colloidal silicon dioxide (p.1475·1).
Diarrhoea; regurgitation in infants.

Geloplasma
Pasteur Merieux, Belg.; Rhone-Poulenc Rorer, Neth.†; Rhone-Poulenc Rorer, Spain.
Gelatin (p.723·2) with electrolytes.
Blood-volume expansion.

Gelopol *Pohl, Ger.†.*
Ambroxol hydrochloride (p.1054·3).
Respiratory-tract disorders associated with increased or viscous mucus.

Gelosantal *Pohl, Ger.†.*
Sandalwood oil.
Disinfectant in chronic urinary-tract infections.

Gel-Ose *Jouveinal, Canad.†.*
Lactulose (p.1195·3).
Constipation.

Gelosedine *Bayer, Fr.†.*
Dimethicone (p.1213·1); sorbitol.
Formerly contained phencarbamide napadisylate, promethazine embonate, and dimethicone.
Gastro-intestinal disorders.

Gelotricar *Gelos, Spain.*
Calcium carbonate (p.1182·1); magnesium carbonate (p.1198·1); sodium bicarbonate (p.1153·2).
Gastro-intestinal hyperacidity; peptic ulcer.

Gelotrisin *Gelos, Spain.*
Aluminium hydroxide (p.1177·3); magnesium trisilicate (p.1199·1).
Gastro-intestinal hyperacidity.

Gelovit *Berenguer Infale, Spain.*
Stanolone (p.1462·2).
Atrophic vaginitis; gynaecomastia; male hypogonadism and androgen deficiency.

Gelovitall *Pohl, Ger.†.*
Garlic (p.1583·1); cod-liver oil (p.1337·3).
Tonic.

Gelox *Beaufour, Fr.*
Montmorillonite; aluminium hydroxide (p.1177·3); magnesium hydroxide (p.1198·2).
Gastro-intestinal disorders.

Gelparine *Streuli, Switz.*
Heparin sodium (p.879·3).
Soft-tissue injury; superficial inflammation and thrombosis.

Gel-Phan *Pierre Fabre, Fr.*
Gelatin (p.723·2).
Fragile hair or nails.

Gelpirin *Alra, USA.*
Paracetamol (p.72·2); aspirin (p.16·1); caffeine (p.749·3).

Gelpirin-CCF *Alra, USA.*
Paracetamol (p.72·2); guaiphenesin (p.1061·3); phenylpropanolamine hydrochloride (p.1067·2); chlorpheniramine maleate (p.405·1).
Coughs and cold symptoms.

Gelplex *SIFRA, Ital.*
Polygeline (p.727·1) with electrolytes.
Plasma volume expansion.

Gel-S *Propan, S.Afr.†.*
Dicyclomine hydrochloride (p.460·1); aluminium hydroxide (p.1177·3); magnesium oxide (p.1198·3); simethicone (p.1213·1).
Gastro-intestinal disorders.

Gelsadon *Jossa-Arznei, Ger.†.*
Oral drops: Sparteine sulphate (p.1632·1); squill (p.1070·1); adonis vernalis (p.1543·3); cereus grandiflorus; peppermint oil; citronella oil; caraway oil; fennel oil; gelsemium (p.1583·2).
Tablets: Gelsemium (p.1583·2); squill (p.1070·1); adonis vernalis (p.1543·3); cereus grandiflorus; sparteine sulphate (p.1632·1); peppermint oil; melissa oil; caraway oil; fennel oil.
Cardiac disorders; hyperthyroidism; migraine; sedative.

Gelsemium Oligoplex *Madaus, Ger.*
Homoeopathic preparation.

Gelsica *Resinag, Switz.*
Aluminium chlorohydrate (p.1078·3).
Wounds.

Geltears
Chauvin, Irl.; Chauvin, UK.
Carbomer 940 (p.1471·2).
Dry eyes.

Gel-Tin *Young, USA.*
Stannous fluoride (p.1632·2).
Dental caries prophylaxis.

Gelucystine *Parke, Davis, Fr.*
Cystine (p.1339·1).
Fragile nails and hair.

Gelufene *Cooperation Pharmaceutique, Fr.*
Ibuprofen (p.44·1).
Fever; pain; sprains.

Gelum *Medicopharm, Aust.*
Potassium iron phosphate-citrate complex.

Gelum oral-rd *Dreluso, Ger.†.*
Diferric potassium triphosphate-ferric dipotassium citrate complex; lactic acid; vitamin B substances.
Tonic.

Gelumaline *Solvay, Fr.*
Belladonna (p.457·1); codeine (p.26·1); caffeine (p.749·3); paracetamol (p.72·2).
Fever; pain.

Gelumen *Medpro, S.Afr.*
Dicyclomine hydrochloride (p.460·1); dried aluminium hydroxide gel (p.1177·3); light magnesium oxide (p.1198·3).
Gastric hyperacidity.

Gelum-Gel *Dreluso, Ger.*
Potassium-iron (III)-citrate-phosphate complex-poly citric acid glycerol ester.
Inflammatory disorders; soft tissue injuries.

Gelum-L *Dreluso, Ger.†.*
Ferric potassium triphosphate-ferric dipotassium citrate complex-poly citric acid glycerol ester.
Skin disorders.

Gelum-Supp *Dreluso, Ger.*
Potassium-iron (III)-citrate-phosphate complex; benzocaine (p.1286·2).
Anorectal disorders.

Gelum-Tropfen *Dreluso, Ger.*
Potassium-iron(III)-citrate-phosphate complex; lactic acid (p.1593·3).
Liver disorders; oxygen deficiency; sclerosis.

Geluprane *Theraplix, Fr.*
Paracetamol (p.72·2).
Fever; pain.

Gelusil
Note. This name is used for preparations of different composition.
Parke, Davis, Aust.; Warner-Lambert, Ger.; Warner-Lambert Consumer, Switz.
Almasilate (p.1177·1).
Gastro-intestinal disorders.

Parke, Davis, Austral.; Parke, Davis, USA.
Aluminium hydroxide (p.1177·3); magnesium hydroxide (p.1198·2); simethicone (p.1213·1).
Dyspepsia; gastro-oesophageal reflux.

Warner-Lambert Consumer, Belg.; Warner-Lambert, Canad.; Warner-Lambert, Fr.; Warner-Lambert, Irl.†; Warner-Lambert, Neth.†; Parke, Davis, S.Afr.; Parke, Davis, UK.
Aluminium hydroxide (p.1177·3); magnesium hydroxide (p.1198·2) or magnesium trisilicate (p.1199·1).
Gastro-intestinal disorders.

Gelusil ML *Warner-Lambert Consumer, Belg.†.*
Aluminium hydroxide (p.1177·3); magnesium hydroxide (p.1198·2); simethicone (p.1213·1).
Gastro-intestinal disorders.

Gelusil Simethicone *Warner-Lambert Consumer, Belg.*
Aluminium hydroxide (p.1177·3); magnesium hydroxide (p.1198·2); simethicone (p.1213·1).
Flatulence; gastro-intestinal disorders associated with hyperacidity.

Gelusil-Lac
Warner-Lambert, Ger.; Warner-Lambert Consumer, Switz.
Almasilate (p.1177·1); milk powder.
Gastro-intestinal disorders.

Gelusil-LacQuick *Warner-Wellcome, Ger.†.*
Almasilate (p.1177·1); fat-free milk powder.
Gastro-intestinal disorders.

Gelusil-Lact *Warner-Lambert Consumer, Belg.†.*
Aluminium hydroxide (p.1177·3); magnesium trisilicate (p.1199·1); debutyrated milk powder.
Gastro-intestinal disorders.

Gelusil-S *Parke, Davis, S.Afr.*
Aluminium hydroxide dried gel (p.1177·3); magnesium hydroxide (p.1198·2); simethicone (p.1213·1).
Bloating; gastric hyperacidity; peptic ulcer.

Gely *Lanzas, Spain.*
Emollient.

Gem
Note. A similar name is used for preparations of different composition.
Nycomed, Norw.
Sodium chloride; potassium chloride; sodium citrate; glucose (p.1152·3).
Diarrhoea; oral rehydration therapy.

GEM
Note. A similar name is used for preparations of different composition.
Piraud, Switz.†.
Pastilles: Codeine phosphate (p.26·1); benzoic acid (p.1102·3); anise oil (p.1550·1); star anise oil; eucalyptus oil (p.1578·1); polygala (p.1069·3); menthol (p.1600·2); liquorice (p.1197·1).
Coughs; throat disorders.
Tablets: Lignocaine hydrochloride (p.1293·2); tyrothricin (p.267·2); muramidase (p.1604·3); cetrimide (p.1105·2).
Mouth and throat disorders.

Gemalt *Pharmavite, Canad.*
Multivitamin preparation with iron.

Gemcor *Upsher-Smith, USA.*
Gemfibrozil (p.1273·3).

Gemfibromax *PMC, Austral.*
Gemfibrozil (p.1273·3).
Hyperlipidaemias.

Gemini *Mer-National, S.Afr.*
Antazoline hydrochloride (p.401·3); tetrahydrozoline hydrochloride (p.1070·2).
Eye irritation; inflammatory eye disorders.

Gemlipid *FIRMA, Ital.*
Gemfibrozil (p.1273·3).
Hyperlipidaemias.

Gemvites *Pharmavite, Canad.*
Multivitamin preparation.

Gemzar
Lilly, Aust.; Lilly, Austral.; Lilly, Fr.; Lilly, Ger.; Lilly, Ital.; Lilly, Neth.; Lilly, Norw.; Lilly, S.Afr.; Lilly, Spain; Lilly, Swed.; Lilly, UK; Lilly, USA.
Gemcitabine hydrochloride (p.538·1).
Non-small cell lung cancer; pancreatic cancer.

Gen H-B-Vax
Merck Sharp & Dohme, Aust.; Chiron Behring, Ger.; Pasteur Merieux, Ger.; Pro Vaccine, Switz.
A hepatitis B vaccine (recombinant DNA) (p.1513·1).
Separate preparations are available for children, adults, and adult dialysis patients.
Active immunisation.

Genabid *Goldline, USA†.*
Papaverine hydrochloride (p.1614·2).
Cerebral and peripheral ischaemia; smooth muscle spasm.

Genac
Note. This name is used for preparations of different composition.
Genevrier, Fr.
Acetylcysteine (p.1052·3).
Corneal ulceration.

Goldline, USA.
Pseudoephedrine hydrochloride (p.1068·3); triprolidine hydrochloride (p.420·3).
Upper respiratory-tract symptoms.

Genacol *Goldline, USA.*
Chlorpheniramine maleate (p.405·1); dextromethorphan hydrobromide (p.1057·3); paracetamol (p.72·2); pseudoephedrine hydrochloride (p.1068·3).
Coughs and cold symptoms.

Genagesic *Goldline, USA.*
Dextropropoxyphene hydrochloride (p.27·3); paracetamol (p.72·2).
Pain.

Genahist *Goldline, USA.*
Diphenhydramine hydrochloride (p.409·1).
Insomnia; motion sickness; parkinsonism.

Genalfa *INTES, Ital.*
Gentamicin sulphate (p.212·1); naphazoline nitrate (p.1064·2).
Eye infections.

Gen-Allerate *Goldline, USA.*
Chlorpheniramine maleate (p.405·1).

Genamin *Goldline, USA.*
Phenylpropanolamine hydrochloride (p.1067·2); chlorpheniramine maleate (p.405·1).
Upper respiratory-tract symptoms.

Genapap *Goldline, USA.*
Paracetamol (p.72·2).
Fever; pain.

Genapax *Key, USA†.*
Crystal violet (p.1111·2).
Vaginal candidiasis.

Genaphed *Goldline, USA.*
Pseudoephedrine hydrochloride (p.1068·3).
Nasal congestion.

Genasal *Goldline, USA.*
Oxymetazoline hydrochloride (p.1065·3).
Nasal congestion.

Genasoft Plus Softgels *Goldline, USA.*
Docusate sodium (p.1189·3); casanthranol (p.1182·3).
Constipation.

Genaspor *Goldline, USA.*
Tolnaftate (p.389·1).
Fungal skin infections.

Genaton *Goldline, USA.*
Oral liquid: Aluminium hydroxide (p.1177·3); magnesium carbonate (p.1198·1).
Tablets: Aluminium hydroxide (p.1177·3); magnesium trisilicate (p.1199·1); sodium bicarbonate (p.1153·2); alginic acid (p.1470·3).
Hyperacidity.

Genatrop *INTES, Ital.*
Gentamicin sulphate (p.212·1); atropine sulphate (p.455·1).
Bacterial eye infections.

Genatropine *Amido, Fr.*
Atropine oxide hydrochloride (p.456·1).
Biliary tract disorders; gastro-intestinal disorders.

Genatuss *Goldline, USA.*
Guaiphenesin (p.1061·3).
Coughs.

Genatuss DM *Goldline, USA.*
Dextromethorphan hydrobromide (p.1057·3); guaiphenesin (p.1061·3).
Coughs.

Gen-Beclo *Genpharm, Canad.*
Beclomethasone dipropionate (p.1032·1).
Corticosteroid.

Gen-bee with C *Goldline, USA.*
Vitamin B substances with vitamin C.

Gencalc *Goldline, USA.*
Calcium carbonate (p.1182·1).
Calcium deficiency; dietary supplement.

Gencefal *Llorente, Spain.*
Cephazolin sodium (p.181·1).
Bacterial infections.

GenCept 10/11 *Gencon, USA.*
Norethisterone (p.1453·1); ethinyloestradiol (p.1445·1).
Biphasic oral contraceptive.

GenCept 0.5/35 and 1/35 *Gencon, USA.*
Norethisterone (p.1453·1); ethinyloestradiol (p.1445·1).
28-Day packs also contain 7 inert tablets.
Combined oral contraceptive.

Gencifrice Baume 1re Dents *Goupil, Fr.†.*
Casein hydrolysate.
Dental antisepsis; teething pain.

Gencin
Curasan, Ger.; Rolab, S.Afr.
Gentamicin sulphate (p.212·1).
Bacterial infections.

Gencold *Goldline, USA.*
Phenylpropanolamine hydrochloride (p.1067·2); chlorpheniramine maleate (p.405·1).
Upper respiratory-tract symptoms.

Gencydo
Weleda, Aust.; Weleda, Ger.; Weleda, UK.
Lemon juice; cydonia seeds.
Hay fever.

Gendecon *Goldline, USA.*
Phenylephrine hydrochloride (p.1066·2); paracetamol (p.72·2); chlorpheniramine maleate (p.405·1).
Upper respiratory-tract symptoms.

Genebilina *Vitafarma, Spain†.*
Tolynol nicotinate (p.1638·3); naphthylacetic acid (p.1606·2).
Biliary-tract disorders.

Genebs *Goldline, USA.*
Paracetamol (p.72·2).
Fever; pain.

Generaid
Scientific Hospital Supplies, Austral.; Scientific Hospital Supplies, Irl.; Scientific Hospital Supplies, UK.
Amino-acid and protein preparation.
Chronic liver disease; porto-hepatic encephalopathy.

Generet *Goldline, USA.*
Ferrous sulphate (p.1340·2); vitamin B substances with vitamin C.
Iron-deficiency anaemias.

Generix-T *Goldline, USA.*
Multivitamin and mineral preparation with iron.

Generman *Byk Gulden, Ital.*
Multivitamin preparation with calcium glycerophosphate and sodium fluoride.
Bone and dental weakness.

Genesa
Gensia, Swed.; Gensia, USA.
Arbutamine hydrochloride (p.825·2).
Pharmacological cardiac stress test.

Geneserine *Amido, Fr.*
Eseridine salicylate (p.1393·1).
Dyspepsia.

Genesis *Wassen, UK.*
Multivitamin and mineral preparation.

Geneye AC Allergy *Goldline, USA†.*
Tetrahydrozoline hydrochloride (p.1070·2); zinc sulphate (p.1373·2).
Eye irritation.

Geneye Extra *Goldline, USA.*
Tetrahydrozoline hydrochloride (p.1070·2).
Eye irritation.

Gengivario *Farmatre, Ital.; Iema, Ital.*
Myrrh (p.1606·1); rhatany root (p.1624·3).
Astringent.

Gengivarium *Kemyos, Ital.*
Benzocaine (p.1286·2).
Mouth disorders.

Gen-Glybe *Genpharm, Canad.*
Glibenclamide (p.319·3).
Diabetes mellitus.

GenHevac B *Pasteur Vaccins, Fr.*
A hepatitis B vaccine (recombinant DNA) (p.1513·1).
Active immunisation.

Genisol
Fisons, Irl.; Teofarma, Ital.; Roche Consumer, UK†.
Coal tar (p.1092·3); sodium sulphosuccinated undecenoic acid monoethanolamide (p.389·2).
Dandruff; scalp psoriasis.

Genite *Goldline, USA.*
Pseudoephedrine hydrochloride (p.1068·3); dextromethorphan hydrobromide (p.1057·3); doxylamine succinate (p.410·1); paracetamol (p.72·2).
Coughs and cold symptoms.

Gen-K *Goldline, USA.*
Potassium chloride (p.1161·1).
Hypokalaemia; potassium depletion.

Gen-Lac *Genpharm, Canad.*
Lactulose (p.1195·3).
Constipation.

Genlip *Lusofarmaco, Ital.*
Gemfibrozil (p.1273·3).
Hyperlipidaemias.

Genoface *Genove, Spain†.*
Triclocarban (p.1127·2).
Skin infections.

Genogris *Vita, Spain.*
Piracetam (p.1619·1).
Alcoholism; cerebrovascular disorders; mental function impairment; vertigo.

Genola *CCD, Fr.*
Hexylresorcinol (p.1116·1); benzododecinium bromide (p.1103·2); allantoin (p.1078·2); boric acid (p.1554·2).
Spermicide.

Genoptic
Allergan, Austral.; Allergan, Belg.†; Allergan, S.Afr.; Allergan, Spain†; Allergan, USA.
Gentamicin sulphate (p.212·1).
Eye infections.

Genora 1/50 *Rugby, USA.*
Mestranol (p.1450·2); norethisterone (p.1453·1).
28-Day packs also contain 7 inert tablets.
Combined oral contraceptive.

Genora 0.5/35 and 1/35 *Rugby, USA.*
Ethinyloestradiol (p.1445·1); norethisterone (p.1453·1).
28-Day packs also contain 7 inert tablets.
Combined oral contraceptive.

Genoral *Kenral, Austral.*
Estropipate (p.1444·3).
Menopausal disorders; oestrogen deficiency.

Genoscopolamine *Amido, Fr.*
Hyoscine oxide hydrobromide (p.463·2).
Parkinsonism.

Genotonorm
Pharmacia Upjohn, Belg.; Pharmacia Upjohn, Fr.; Pharmacia Upjohn, Spain.
Somatropin (p.1249·3).
Growth hormone deficiency; Turner's syndrome.

Genotropin
Pharmacia Upjohn, Aust.; Pharmacia Upjohn, Austral.; Pharmacia Upjohn, Ger.; Pharmacia Upjohn, Irl.; Pharmacia Upjohn, Ital.; Pharmacia Upjohn, Neth.; Pharmacia Upjohn, Norw.; Pharmacia Upjohn, S.Afr.; Pharmacia Upjohn, Swed.; Pharmacia Upjohn, Switz.; Pharmacia Upjohn, UK; Pharmacia, USA.
Somatropin (p.1249·3).
Chronic renal insufficiency; growth hormone deficiency; Turner's syndrome.

Genox *Alphapharm, Austral.*
Tamoxifen citrate (p.563·3).
Breast cancer.

Genoxal *Pras, Spain.*
Cyclophosphamide (p.516·2).
Malignant neoplasms.

Genoxal Trofosfamida *Pras, Spain.*
Trofosfamide (p.568·2).
Malignant neoplasms.

Genoxen *Antigen, Irl.*
Naproxen (p.61·2).
Gout; musculoskeletal and joint disorders.

Genpril *Goldline, USA.*
Ibuprofen (p.44·1).
Fever; osteoarthritis; pain; rheumatoid arthritis.

Genprin *Goldline, USA.*
Aspirin (p.16·1).
Fever; inflammation; myocardial infarction; pain; transient ischaemic attacks.

Gensan *Goldline, USA.*
Aspirin (p.16·1); caffeine (p.749·3).

Gensasmol *Llorente, Spain†.*
Reproterol hydrochloride (p.758·1).
Obstructive airways disease.

Gensumycin
Hoechst Marion Roussel, Norw.; Hoechst Marion Roussel, Swed.
Gentamicin sulphate (p.212·1).
Bacterial infections.

Genta *CT, Ger.*
Gentamicin sulphate (p.212·1).
Bacterial infections.

Genta Gobens *Normon, Spain.*
Gentamicin sulphate (p.212·1).
Bacterial infections.

Gentabilles *Schering-Plough, Fr.*
Gentamicin sulphate (p.212·1).
Bacterial infections.

Gentacidin
Ciba Vision, Canad.; Iolab, USA.
Gentamicin sulphate (p.212·1).
Bacterial eye infections.

Gentacort *Ciba Vision, Ital.*
Fluorometholone (p.1042·1); gentamicin sulphate (p.212·1).
Infected eye disorders.

Gentafair *Pharmafair, USA†.*
Gentamicin sulphate (p.212·1).

Gentak *Akorn, USA.*
Gentamicin sulphate (p.212·1).
Bacterial infections.

Gentalline *Schering-Plough, Fr.*
Gentamicin sulphate (p.212·1).
Bacterial infections.

Gentallorens *Llorens, Spain†.*
Gentamicin sulphate (p.212·1).
Eye infections.

Gentalodina *Rhone-Poulenc Rorer, Spain.*
Gentamicin sulphate (p.212·1).
Bacterial infections.

Gentalyn *Schering-Plough, Ital.*
Gentamicin sulphate (p.212·1).
Bacterial infections.

Gentalyn Beta *Schering-Plough, Ital.*
Gentamicin sulphate (p.212·1); betamethasone valerate (p.1033·3).
Infected skin disorders.

Gentamedical *Medical, Spain.*
Gentamicin sulphate (p.212·1).
Bacterial infections.

Gentamen *Fournier, Ital.*
Gentamicin sulphate (p.212·1).
Bacterial infections.

Gentamin *Medix, Spain†.*
Gentamicin sulphate (p.212·1).
Bacterial infections.

Gentamival *Rovi, Spain.*
Gentamicin sulphate (p.212·1).
Bacterial infections.

Gentamix *Baxter, Ger.†.*
Gentamicin sulphate (p.212·1).
Bacterial infections.

Gentamorgens *Oykol, Spain†.*
Gentamicin sulphate (p.212·1).
Bacterial infections.

Gentamytrex
Tramedico, Belg.; Mann, Ger.; Mann, Neth.
Gentamicin sulphate (p.212·1).
Bacterial eye infections.

Gentarol N *UCB, Ger.†.*
Paracetamol (p.72·2); salicylamide (p.82·3); codeine phosphate (p.26·1); caffeine (p.749·3).
Migraine; pain.

Gentasol *Ocusoft, USA.*
Gentamicin sulphate (p.212·1).
Bacterial eye infections.

Gentasone *Schering-Plough, Fr.*
Gentamicin sulphate (p.212·1); betamethasone sodium phosphate (p.1033·3).
Bacterial eye infections with inflammation.

Gentax *Agepha, Aust.*
Gentamicin sulphate (p.212·1).
Bacterial eye infections.

Gentel *Inpharzam, Switz.†.*
Urogastrone (p.1218·1).
Eye wounds.

Gentibioptal *Farmila, Ital.*
Gentamicin sulphate (p.212·1).
Bacterial eye infections.

Genticin
Roche, Irl.; Roche, UK.
Gentamicin sulphate (p.212·1).
Bacterial infections.

Genticin HC
Nicholas, Irl.†; Nicholas, UK†.
Gentamicin sulphate (p.212·1); hydrocortisone acetate (p.1043·3).
Infected skin disorders.

Genticina *Pharmacia Upjohn, Spain.*
Gentamicin sulphate (p.212·1).
Bacterial infections.

Genticol *SIFI, Ital.*
Gentamicin sulphate (p.212·1).
Eye infections.

Gentil Spitzner, Ger.†.
Paracetamol (p.72·2); salicylamide (p.82·3); propyphenazone (p.81·3); ethaverine (p.1577·1); caffeine (p.749·3).
Cold symptoms; migraine; neuralgia; pain; rheumatism.

Gentisone HC
Roche, Irl.; Roche, UK.
Gentamicin sulphate (p.212·1); hydrocortisone acetate (p.1043·3).
Bacterial ear infections.

Gentisum Hortel, Spain†.
Gentamicin sulphate (p.212·1).
Bacterial infections.

Gentlax Blair, USA.
Senna (p.1212·2).
Constipation.

Gentlax S Blair, USA.
Docusate sodium (p.1189·3); senna (p.1212·2).
Constipation.

Gentlees Delamac, Austral.
Hamamelis water (p.1587·1); glycerol; cetylpyridinium chloride (p.1106·2).
Antiseptic astringent wipes.

Gent-L-Tip Baxter, Canad.
Monobasic sodium phosphate (p.1159·3); dibasic sodium phosphate (p.1159·3).
Bowel evacuation.

Gentogram E. Merck, Neth.†.
Gentamicin sulphate (p.212·1).
Bacterial infections.

Gentomil Biologici Italia, Ital.
Gentamicin sulphate (p.212·1).
Bacterial infections.

Gent-Ophtal Winzer, Ger.
Gentamicin sulphate (p.212·1).
Bacterial eye infections.

Gentos Llorente, Spain.
Chlophedianol hydrochloride (p.1057·1).
Coughs.

Gentralay Plevifarma, Spain.
Gentamicin sulphate (p.212·1).
Bacterial infections.

Gentran 40
Baxter, Canad.; Baxter, UK; Baxter, USA.
Dextran 40 (p.716·2) in glucose or sodium chloride.
Extracorporeal circulation; plasma volume expansion; thrombo-embolism prophylaxis.

Gentran 70
Baxter, Canad.; Baxter, UK; Baxter, USA.
Dextran 70 (p.717·1) in glucose or sodium chloride.
Plasma volume expansion.

Gentran 75 Baxter, USA.
Dextran 75 (p.717·3) in sodium chloride.
Plasma volume expansion.

Gentrasul Bausch & Lomb, USA†.
Gentamicin sulphate (p.212·1).
Eye infections.

Gentus Gentili, Ital.
Dimemorfan phosphate (p.1058·3).
Coughs.

Gentz Roxane, USA†.
Pramoxine hydrochloride (p.1298·2); alcloxa (p.1078·2); hamamelis (p.1587·1).
Perianal cleansing.

Genu-cyl Ho-Len-Complex Liebermann, Ger.
Homoeopathic preparation.

Genuine Australian Eucalyptus Drops Felton, Austral.
Eucalyptus oil (p.1578·1); menthol (p.1600·2); lemon oil (p.1595·3).
Cough; nasal congestion; sore throat.

Genurin Recordati, Ital.
Flavoxate hydrochloride (p.461·2).
Genito-urinary spasms.

Gen-Xene Alra, USA.
Potassium clorazepate (p.657·1).
Alcohol withdrawal syndrome; anxiety; epilepsy.

Geocillin Roerig, USA.
Carindacillin sodium (p.163·1).
Bacterial infections.

Geo-magnit Biomo, Ger.
Magnesium glutamate; dibasic magnesium phosphate.
Magnesium deficiency.

Geomix Difa, Ital.†.
Oxytetracycline (p.235·1); chloramphenicol (p.182·1); sulphadiazine (p.252·3).

Geomycine Schering-Plough, Belg.
Gentamicin sulphate (p.212·1).
Bacterial infections.

Geopen
Note. This name is used for preparations of different composition.
Pfizer, Canad.†.
Carindacillin sodium (p.163·1).
Bacterial infections of the urinary tract.
Pfizer, Ital.; Pfizer, Spain.
Carbenicillin sodium (p.162·3).
Bacterial infections.

Gepan Pohl, Ger.†.
Aspirin (p.16·1).
Fever; inflammation; pain; rheumatism; thrombosis prophylaxis.

Gepan CN Pohl, Ger.†.
Aspirin (p.16·1); caffeine (p.749·3); ascorbic acid (p.1365·2).
Influenza.

Ger N in der Ophtiole Mann, Ger.†.
Thiamine hydrochloride (p.1361·1); riboflavine sodium phosphate (p.1362·1); esculoside (p.1543·3); sodium iodide (p.1493·2).
Eye disorders.

Geralen Gerot, Aust.
Methoxsalen (p.1086·3).
Psoriasis.

Geram Vedim, Fr.
Piracetam (p.1619·1).
Cerebrovascular disorders; improvement of mental function in the elderly; vertigo.

Geramox Gerard, Irl.
Amoxycillin (p.151·3) or amoxycillin trihydrate (p.151·3).
Infections.

Gerard 99 Gerard House, UK.
Lupulus (p.1597·2); passion flower (p.1615·3); valerian (p.1643·1).
Irritability; tenseness.

Geratam Bios, Belg.
Piracetam (p.1619·1).
Mental function impairment.

Geratar UCB, S.Afr.
Inositol nicotinate (p.891·3); multivitamins; meclozine (p.413·3); hydroxyzine hydrochloride (p.412·1).
Vascular disorders; vertigo.

Geravim Major, USA.
Vitamin B substances with minerals.

Geravite Roberts, USA†; Hauck, USA†.
Vitamin B substances with lysine.

Gerax Gerard, Irl.
Alprazolam (p.640·3).
Alcohol withdrawal syndrome; anxiety disorders; depression; mixed anxiety-depression; panic attacks; phobias.

Gerbin Sanofi Winthrop, Spain.
Aceclofenac (p.12·1).
Inflammation; musculoskeletal, joint, peri-articular, and soft-tissue disorders; pain.

Gercid Goldschmidt, Ger.†.
Mixture of alkyloligoamines and alkyloligoamine carbonic acids; didecyldimethylammonium chloride (p.1112·2).
Surface disinfection.

Gercid forte Goldschmidt, Ger.†.
Didecyldimethylammonium chloride (p.1112·2).
Disinfection.

Geref
Serono, Aust.; Serono, Belg.†; Serono, Canad.; Serono, Ger.†; Serono, Irl.; Serono, Ital.; Serono, Norw.; Research Labs, S.Afr.; Serono, Spain; Serono, Swed.; Serono, Switz.; Serono, UK; Serono, USA.
Sermorelin (p.1260·3) or sermorelin acetate (p.1260·3).
Test for growth hormone secretion.

Gerel Serono, Fr.†.
Sermorelin acetate (p.1260·3).
Test for growth hormone secretion.

Gerelax Gerard, Irl.
Lactulose (p.1195·3).
Constipation; hepatic encephalopathy.

Geriaforce
Bioforce, Ger.; Bioforce, Switz.
Ginkgo biloba (p.1584·1).
Arteriosclerosis.

Geriakneipp N Kneipp, Ger.†.
Multivitamin preparation.
Tonic.

Geriaplasma Ardeypharm, Ger.
Bovine heart extract; bovine liver extract; bovine spleen extract.
Tonic.

Geriatric Stanley, Canad.; Herbes Universelles, Canad.
Multivitamin and mineral preparation.

Geriatric Pharmaton
Bender, Aust.; Thomae, Ger.; IBP, Ital.†.
Deanol tartrate; ginseng; vitamins; minerals; rutin.
Tonic.

Geriatricum-Pascoe Pascoe, Ger.†.
Vitamins; procaine hydrochloride; testes siccata; ovaria siccata; corpus luteum; arnica; barium carbonic.; convallaria maj.; crataegus; latrodectus mact.; lycopodium; rauwolfia.
Tonic.

Geriatrie-Mulsin Mucos, Ger.
Multivitamin preparation.

Geriavit
Note. This name is used for preparations of different composition.
Bergamon, Ital.†.
A heparinoid (p.882·3); homonicotinic acid (p.1274·3); pancreatic lipase; vitamins.
Hyperlipidaemias.
Pharmaton, Switz.
Ginseng; deanol bitartrate; multivitamins; minerals; rutin (p.1580·2); lecithin (p.1595·2).
Tonic.

Gericaps Pharmadass, UK.
Multivitamin and mineral preparation.

Gericarb Gerard, Irl.
Carbamazepine (p.339·2).
Alcohol withdrawal syndrome; epilepsy; pain.

Gericin Seid, Spain.
Nitrendipine (p.923·1).
Angina pectoris; hypertension; Raynaud's syndrome.

Gericomplex Boehringer Ingelheim, S.Afr.
Multivitamins; minerals; dimethylaminoethanol bitartrate; ginseng.
Tonic.

Geridium Goldline, USA†.
Phenazopyridine hydrochloride (p.78·3).
Irritation of the lower urinary tract.

Geriflox Gerard, Irl.
Flucloxacillin sodium (p.209·2).
Gram-positive bacterial infections.

Gerigoa Salus, Aust.
Procaine resinate; procaine hydrochloride; buphenine resinate; haematoporphyrin; orotic acid; vitamins.
Tonic.

Gerimal Rugby, USA.
Co-dergocrine mesylate (p.1566·1).
Senile dementia.

Gerimax Vitalia, UK.
Multivitamin and mineral preparation with ginseng.

Gerimax adultes Richelet, Fr.
Multivitamin and mineral preparation with ginseng.

Gerimax enfants Richelet, Fr.
Multivitamin and mineral preparation.

Gerimed Fielding, USA.
Multivitamin and mineral preparation.
Osteoporosis.

Gerinap Gerard, Irl.
Naproxen (p.61·2).
Gout; musculoskeletal and joint disorders.

Geriot Goldline, USA.
Ferrous fumarate (p.1339·3); folic acid (p.1340·3); multivitamins and minerals.
Iron-deficiency anaemias.

Geriplex
Parke, Davis, Austral.†.
Multivitamin preparation.
Warner-Lambert, Canad.†.
Multivitamin and mineral preparation.
Warner-Wellcome, Spain†.
Multivitamins and minerals; amylase; rutin.
Tonic.

Geriplex FS Parke, Davis, USA.
Multivitamin and mineral preparation.

Geri-Plus Herbes Universelles, Canad.
Betacarotene, selenium, vitamin C, and vitamin E.

Geritol
Note. This name is used for preparations of different composition.
SmithKline Beecham Consumer, Canad.
Multivitamins with iron.
SmithKline Beecham Consumer, USA.
Ferric ammonium citrate (p.1339·2); vitamin B substances with methionine.
Iron-deficiency anaemias.

Geritol Complete SmithKline Beecham Consumer, USA.
Iron (p.1346·1); folic acid (p.1340·3); multivitamins and minerals.
Iron-deficiency anaemias.

Geritol Extend SmithKline Beecham Consumer, USA.
Multivitamin and mineral preparation with iron and folic acid.

Geriton Gerbex, Canad.
Vitamin B substances, calcium, and iron.

Geritonic Geriatric Pharm. Corp., USA.
Ferric ammonium citrate (p.1339·2); liver fraction; vitamin B substances and minerals.
Iron-deficiency anaemias.

Gerivent Gerard, Irl.
Salbutamol (p.758·2).
Obstructive airways disease.

Gerivit Sanoreform, Ger.
Ginseng (p.1584·2).
Tonic.

Gerivite Goldline, USA.
Multivitamin and mineral preparation.

Gerivites Rugby, USA.
Ferrous sulphate (p.1340·2); vitamin B substances with vitamin C.
Iron-deficiency anaemias.

Gerlecit Piraud, Switz.†.
Vitamin and mineral preparation with pollen extracts and lecithin.
Tonic.

Germalyne Septfons, Fr.†.
Wheat germ.
Nutritional supplement.

Germanin Bayer, Ger.
Suramin (p.593·1).
Trypanosomiasis.

Germapect UCB, Ger.†.
Pentoxyverine citrate (p.1066·1).
Coughs.

Germex SA Druggists Self Med, S.Afr.†.
Nitrofurazone (p.232·3).
Bacterial infections; burns; wounds.

Germiciclin Mendelejeff, Ital.†.
Doxycycline hydrochloride (p.202·3).
Bacterial infections.

Germicidin IMS, Ital.
Benzalkonium chloride (p.1101·3).
Surface and instrument disinfection.

Germolene SmithKline Beecham Consumer, UK.
Cream: Chlorhexidine gluconate (p.1107·2); phenol (p.1121·2).
Ointment: Zinc oxide (p.1096·2); methyl salicylate (p.55·2); octaphonium chloride (p.1120·2); phenol (p.1121·2).
Topical spray: Triclosan (p.1127·2); dichlorophen (p.99·2).
Topical wipes: Benzalkonium chloride (p.1101·3); chlorhexidine gluconate (p.1107·2).
Skin disinfection.

Germoloids SmithKline Beecham Consumer, UK.
Cream; ointment; suppositories: Lignocaine hydrochloride (p.1293·2); zinc oxide (p.1096·2).
Topical wipes: Chlorhexidine gluconate (p.1107·2); benzalkonium chloride (p.1101·3); menthol (p.1600·2).
Haemorrhoids.

Germose Besins-Iscovesco, Fr.
Sodium benzoate (p.1102·3); potassium guaiacolsulfonate (p.1068·3); grindelia; crataegus (p.1568·2); peppermint (p.1208·1); thyme (p.1636·3).
Respiratory-tract congestion.

Germozero Carlo Erba OTC, Ital.
Chloramine (p.1106·3).
Skin disinfection.

Germozero Hospital Carlo Erba OTC, Ital.
Chlorhexidine gluconate (p.1107·2); cetrimide (p.1105·2).
Disinfection of wounds, external genitalia, surfaces, and instruments.

Germozero Plus Carlo Erba OTC, Ital.
Benzalkonium chloride (p.1101·3); orthophenylphenol (p.1120·3).
Wounds disinfection.

Gernebcin Lilly, Ger.
Tobramycin sulphate (p.264·1).
Bacterial infections.

Gernel Gerbex, Canad.
Cresol (p.1111·2); zinc oxide (p.1096·2).

Gero URPAC, Fr.†.
Procaine hydrochloride (p.1299·2).
Functional symptoms of old age.

Geroaslan H3 Schoeller, Aust.
Procaine hydrochloride (p.1299·2).
Tonic.

Gerobion Bracco, Ital.†.
Multivitamin preparation.

Geroderm
Note. This name is used for preparations of different composition.
Avantgarde, Ital.
Triclosan (p.1127·2).
Skin cleansing.
Maxwell, S.Afr.†.
Soap substitute.

Geroderm Zolfo Avantgarde, Ital.
Sulphur (p.1091·2); lactic acid (p.1593·3); triclosan (p.1127·2).
Skin cleansing in acne.

Gerodorm Gerot, Aust.
Cinolazepam (p.656·2).
Sleep disorders.

Gerodyl Gea, Neth.†.
Penicillamine (p.988·3).
Cystinuria; heavy-metal poisoning; rheumatoid arthritis; Wilson's disease.

Gerogelat Metochem, Aust.
Vitamin A palmitate (p.1359·2); tocopheryl acetate (p.1369·2).
Hearing loss; mucous membrane disorders; tinnitus; vitamin A and E deficiency.

Gero-H^3-Aslan Chefaro, Ger.
Procaine hydrochloride; benzoic acid; potassium disulphite; sodium phosphate.
Tonic.

Gerolin CT, Ital.
Citicoline sodium (p.1564·3).
Cerebrovascular disorders; parkinsonism.

Geromid Zoja, Ital.†.
Clofibrate (p.1271·1).
Hyperlipidaemias.

Gerontamin Pierre Fabre, Ger.
Gelatin (p.723·2); cystine (p.1339·1).
Joint disorders.

Gerontin Pharmonta, Aust.
Procaine hydrochloride (p.1299·2); anhydrous caffeine (p.749·3).
Tonic.

Geroten Gerard, Irl.
Captopril (p.836·3).
Heart failure; hypertension.

Geroton Forte Bradley, USA.
Multivitamin and mineral preparation.

Gerovital H3 Schoeller, Aust.
Procaine hydrochloride (p.1299·2).
Tonic.

Geroxalen
Sanofi Winthrop, Neth.; Nycomed, Norw.
Methoxsalen (p.1086·3).
Psoriasis.

Geroxicam Gerard, Irl.
Piroxicam (p.80·2).
Dysmenorrhoea; gout; musculoskeletal and joint disorders.

Gertac Gerard, Irl.
Ranitidine hydrochloride (p.1209·3).
Gastro-oesophageal reflux; peptic ulcer; Zollinger-Ellison syndrome.

Gerviton Andreabal, Switz.
Multivitamin and mineral preparation.

GES 45
Milupa, Fr.; Milupa, Switz.
Glucose; sucrose; potassium citrate; sodium bicarbonate; sodium chloride (p.1152·3).
Diarrhoea; oral rehydration therapy.

Gestafortin Merck, Ger.
Chlormadinone acetate (p.1439·1).
Endometriosis; menstrual disorders.

Gestakadin Kade, Ger.
Norethisterone acetate (p.1453·1).
Menopausal disorders; menstrual disorders.

Gestamater Cyanamid, Spain.
Multivitamin and mineral preparation.

Gestamestrol N Hermal, Ger.
Chlormadinone acetate (p.1439·1); mestranol (p.1450·2).
Androgen-dependent alopecia, acne, and seborrhoea; hirsutism.

Gestamine Nadeau, Canad.
Multivitamin preparation with calcium and iron.

Gestanin
Donmed, S.Afr.†; Organon, UK†.
Allyloestrenol (p.1439·1).
Threatened and habitual abortion.

Gestanon
Organon, Aust.; Organon, Belg.†; Organon, Ger.†; Organon, Ital.†; Organon, Spain†; Organon, Switz.†.
Allyloestrenol (p.1439·1).
Threatened and habitual abortion.

Gestantyl UCM-Difme, Ital.†.
Amino-acid, multivitamin, and mineral preparation.

Gestapuran Lovens, Swed.
Medroxyprogesterone acetate (p.1448·3).
Endometriosis; menopausal disorders; menstrual disorders.

Gesterol Germiphene, Canad.
Progesterone (p.1459·3).
Progestogenic.

Gestiferrol Wolfs, Belg.
Ferrous fumarate (p.1339·3); folic acid (p.1340·3).
Anaemias; dietary supplement during pregnancy.

Gestone Ferring, UK.
Progesterone (p.1459·3).
Adjunct in infertility disorders; menorrhagia.

Gestoral Ciba-Geigy, Fr.
Medroxyprogesterone acetate (p.1448·3).
Menopausal disorders.

Getderm Sepsi Geymonat, Ital.†.
Cetylpyridinium chloride (p.1106·2).
Skin disinfection.

Gets-It Oakhurst, USA.
Salicylic acid (p.1090·2); zinc chloride (p.1373·1).
Hyperkeratosis.

Gevatran Lipha Sante, Fr.
Naftidrofuryl oxalate (p.914·2).
Peripheral and cerebral vascular disorders.

Gevilon
Parke, Davis, Aust.; Parke, Davis, Ger.; Warner-Lambert, Switz.
Gemfibrozil (p.1273·3).
Hyperlipidaemias.

Gevirol Gerbex, Canad.
Multivitamin and mineral preparation.

Gevisol Maggioni, Ital.†.
Chlorocresol (p.1110·3); sodium hydroxide (p.1631·1).
Surface disinfection.

Gevrabon Lederle, USA.
Vitamin B substances with minerals.

Gevral
Cyanamid, Ital.; Whitehall, S.Afr.; Lederle, UK†; Lederle, USA.
Multivitamin and mineral preparation.

Gevral Instant Protein
Whitehall, Irl.; Whitehall-Robins, Switz.
Multivitamin, mineral, and protein preparation.
Tonic.

Gevral Protein
Lederle, UK†; Lederle, USA.
Multivitamin, mineral, and protein preparation.

Gevral Proteina Cyanamid, Spain.
Protein, vitamin, and mineral preparation.

Gevral T Lederle, USA.
Ferrous fumarate (p.1339·3); folic acid (p.1340·3); multivitamins and minerals.
Iron-deficiency anaemias.

Gevral Tablets Whitehall, Irl.
Multivitamin and mineral preparation.

Gevramycin Schering-Plough, Spain.
Gentamicin sulphate (p.212·1).
Bacterial infections.

Gevramycina Topica Schering-Plough, Spain.
Gentamicin sulphate (p.212·1).
Bacterial skin infections.

Gewacalm Nycomed, Aust.
Diazepam (p.661·1).
Anxiety disorders; eclampsia; neuroses; panic attacks; phobias; premedication; skeletal muscle spasm; sleep disorders; status epilepticus.

Gewacyclin Nycomed, Aust.†.
Doxycycline hydrochloride (p.202·3).
Bacterial infections.

Gewadal Nycomed, Aust.
Paracetamol (p.72·2); propyphenazone (p.81·3); caffeine (p.749·3).
Fever; pain.

Gewadilat Bayer, Aust.
Nifedipine (p.916·2).
Angina pectoris; hypertension; Raynaud's syndrome.

Gewaglucon Nycomed, Aust.
Glibenclamide (p.319·3).
Diabetes mellitus.

Gewapurol Nycomed, Aust.
Allopurinol (p.390·2).
Gout; hyperuricaemia; renal calculi.

Gewazem Nycomed, Aust.
Diltiazem hydrochloride (p.854·2).
Angina pectoris.

Gewodin Gewo, Ger.
Famprofazone (p.37·1); paracetamol (p.72·2); propyphenazone (p.81·3); caffeine (p.749·3).
Pain.

Gewodine Geistlich, Switz.
Paracetamol (p.72·2); caffeine (p.749·3); propyphenazone (p.81·3).
Fever; pain.

Gewusst wie Beruhigungs Metochem, Aust.
Valerian (p.1643·1).
Anxiety disorders.

Geyderm Geymonat, Ital.
Benzalkonium chloride (p.1101·3).
Disinfection of mucous membranes, wounds, burns, surfaces, and instruments.

Geyderm Sepsi Geymonat, Ital.
Cetylpyridinium chloride (p.1106·2).
Disinfection of wounds and burns.

Geyfritz Geymonat, Ital.
Aspirin (p.16·1); caffeine (p.749·3).
Glycine (p.1345·2) is included in this preparation in an attempt to limit adverse effects on the gastro-intestinal mucosa.
Cold symptoms; pain.

G-Farlutal Pharmacia Upjohn, Ger.
Medroxyprogesterone acetate (p.1448·3).
Menstrual disorders; test of ovarian function.

GG-Cen Schwarz, USA.
Guaiphenesin (p.1061·3).
Coughs.

Ghimadox Ghimas, Ital.†.
Doxycycline hydrochloride (p.202·3).
Bacterial infections.

GHRH Sanofi Winthrop, Neth.; Ferring, Neth.
Somatorelin acetate (p.1260·3).
Diagnosis of growth hormone deficiency.

Gibicef Metapharma, Ital.
Cefuroxime sodium (p.177·1).
Bacterial infections.

Gibifer Metapharma, Ital.
Ferric sodium gluconate (p.1340·1).
Iron-deficiency anaemias.

Gibiflu Metapharma, Ital.
Flunisolide (p.1040·3).
Rhinitis.

Gibinap Metapharma, Ital.
Naproxen sodium (p.61·2).
Lignocaine hydrochloride (p.1293·2) is included in the intramuscular injection to alleviate the pain of injection.
Musculoskeletal and joint disorders; pain.

Gibixen Metapharma, Ital.
Naproxen (p.61·2).
Musculoskeletal and joint disorders; pain.

Gichtex Gerot, Aust.
Allopurinol (p.390·2).
Gout; hyperuricaemia; renal calculi.

Gichtex plus Gerot, Aust.
Allopurinol (p.390·2); benzbromarone (p.392·3).
Gout; hyperuricaemia.

Giganten Tropon, Ger.†.
Cinnarizine (p.406·1).
Cerebral and peripheral circulatory disorders; vestibular disorders.

Gigasept Schulke & Mayr, Ger.
Succinic dialdehyde (p.1114·1); dimethoxytetrahydrofuran; formaldehyde (p.1113·2).
Instrument disinfection.

Gigasept FF Schulke & Mayr, Ger.
Succinic dialdehyde (p.1114·1); dimethoxytetrahydrofuran.
Instrument disinfection.

Gilemal Enzypharm, Aust.
Glibenclamide (p.319·3).
Diabetes mellitus.

Gillazyme Sandoz OTC, Switz.
Pancreatin (p.1612·1); dehydrocholic acid (p.1570·2); dimethicone (p.1213·1).
Digestive-system disorders.

Gillazyme plus Sandoz OTC, Switz.
Pancreatin (p.1612·1); dehydrocholic acid (p.1570·2); dimethicone (p.1213·1); methixene hydrochloride (p.465·1).
Digestive-system disorders.

Gilt Solvay, Ger.
Clotrimazole (p.376·3).
Fungal skin infections.

Gilucor Solvay, Ger.
Sotalol hydrochloride (p.945·1).
Formerly contained ajmaline, reserpine hydrochloride, belladonna, and pentaerythritol tetranitrate.
Arrhythmias.

Giludop Solvay Duphar, Swed.
Dopamine hydrochloride (p.861·1).
Shock.

Gilurytmal
Kali, Aust.; Solvay, Belg.†; Solvay, Ger.; Lacer, Spain.
Ajmaline (p.817·1) or ajmaline monoethanolate (p.817·2).
Arrhythmias.

Gilustenon Solvay, Ger.
Glyceryl trinitrate (p.874·3).
Angina pectoris; heart failure.

Ginatren LPB, Ital.
A trichomonal vaccine containing *Lactobacillus acidophilus* (p.1536·3).
Vaginitis.

Gincola Biocontrolfarm, Ital.
Ginseng (p.1584·2); kola (p.1645·1).

Gincosan Pharmaton, Switz.
Ginkgo biloba (p.1584·1); ginseng (p.1584·2).
Mental function impairment.

Gine Heyden Squibb, Spain.
Amphotericin (p.372·2); tetracycline hydrochloride (p.259·1).
Vulvovaginal infections.

Ginecofuran Crosara, Ital.
Nifuroxime (p.386·1); furazolidone (p.583·1).
Vaginitis.

Ginecrin Abbott, Spain.
Leuprorelin acetate (p.1253·1).
Endometriosis; prostatic cancer; uterine fibroma.

Gineflavir Crosara, Ital.†.
Metronidazole (p.585·1).
Giardiasis; trichomoniasis.

Gineflor Mitim, Ital.
Ibuprofen isobutanolammonium (p.44·3).
Gynaecological disorders.

Ginejuvent Juventus, Spain.
Benzalkonium chloride (p.1101·3); calcium lactate (p.1155·2); lactic acid (p.1593·3); chamomile (p.1561·2).
Vulvovaginal candidiasis; vulvovaginal trichomoniasis.

Ginenorm Aesculapius, Ital.
Ibuprofen isobutanolammonium (p.44·3).
Gynaecological inflammatory disorders.

Gineosepta Corvi, Ital.†.
Sodium perborate (p.1125·2); alum (p.1547·1); boric acid (p.1554·2).
Vaginal douche.

Ginesal Farmigea, Ital.
Benzydamine hydrochloride (p.21·3).
Gynaecological disorders; vaginal hygiene.

Ginesona Alonga, Spain†.
Chloramphenicol (p.182·1); benzocaine (p.1286·2); hydrocortisone acetate (p.1043·3).
Vulvovaginal infections.

Gingicaine D Hoechst, Ger.
Amethocaine (p.1285·2); benzalkonium chloride.
Local anaesthesia.

Gingiloba Biocur, Ger.
Ginkgo biloba (p.1584·1).
Dizziness; mental function disorders; peripheral vascular disorders; tinnitus.

Gingilone Zyma, Spain.
Ascorbic acid (p.1365·2); cortisone acetate (p.1036·1); neomycin sulphate (p.229·2); rutin (p.1580·2).
Bleeding gums; mouth ulcers; stomatitis.

Gingilone Comp Zyma, Spain†.
Ascorbic acid (p.1365·2); benzocaine (p.1286·2); hydrocortisone acetate (p.1043·3); neomycin sulphate (p.229·2); rutin (p.1580·2); menthol (p.1600·2).
Bleeding gums; mouth ulcers; stomatitis.

Gingi-Pak Gingi-Pak, Switz.
A range of threads and tampons impregnated with adrenaline hydrochloride (p.813·3).
Dental haemorrhage.

Gingium Hexal, Ger.
Ginkgo biloba (p.1584·1).
Dizziness; intermittent claudication; mental function disorders; tinnitus.

Gingivitol Sodip, Switz.†.
Dexpanthenol (p.1570·3); hydrastis (p.1588·2); tannic acid (p.1634·2).
Mouth and throat disorders.

Gingivitol N Hennig, Ger.
Hydrastis(p.1588·2).
Inflammatory disorders of the oropharynx.

Gingivyl Zyma, Fr.†.
Sodium saccharinate; sodium chloride (p.1162·2); sodium cyclamate.
Teeth and gum disorders.

Gingo A Eagle, Austral.
Ginkgo biloba (p.1584·1); crataegus (p.1568·2); eleutherococcus senticosis (p.1584·2); liquorice (p.1197·1); choline bitartrate (p.1337·1); cayenne; nicotinic acid (p.1351·2); potassium phosphate (p.1159·2).

Gingobeta Betapharm, Ger.
Ginkgo biloba (p.1584·1).
Dizziness; headache; mental function disorders; tinnitus.

Gingopret Bionorica, Ger.
Ginkgo biloba (p.1584·1).
Mental function disorders; peripheral vascular disorders; tinnitus; vertigo.

Ginkgo ACE Vita Glow, Austral.†.
Ginkgo biloba (p.1584·1); betacarotene (p.1335·2); ascorbic acid (p.1365·2); alpha tocopheryl succinate (p.1369·1); zinc amino acid chelate (p.1373·3); cysteine hydrochloride (p.1338·3); bioflavonoids (p.1580·1); choline bitartrate (p.1337·1); inositol (p.1591·1); calcium phosphate (p.1155·3).
Free radical scavenger.

Ginkgo biloba comp. Hevert, Ger.
Homoeopathic preparation.

Ginkgo Complex Blackmores, Austral.
Ginkgo biloba (p.1584·1); crataegus (p.1568·2); panax ginseng (p.1584·2); *d*-alpha tocopheryl acid succinate (p.1369·2).
Cerebral and peripheral vascular disorders.

Ginkgo Plus Biohorma, Ital.
Hamamelis (p.1587·1); aesculus (p.1543·3); ginkgo biloba (p.1584·1); cupressus sempervirens.
Peripheral vascular disorders.

Ginkgo Plus Herbal Plus Formula 10 Vitelle, Austral.
Ginkgo biloba (p.1584·1); ginger (p.1193·2); dibasic potassium phosphate (p.1159·2); magnesium oxide (p.1198·3).
Peripheral vascular disorders.

Ginkgobakehl Sanum-Kehlbeck, Ger.
Homoeopathic preparation.

Ginkgoforce Weber & Weber, Ger.
Homoeopathic preparation.

Ginkgorell Sanorell, Ger.
Homoeopathic preparation.

Ginkobil N Ratiopharm, Ger.
Ginkgo biloba (p.1584·1).
Cerebral and peripheral vascular disorders.

Ginkodilat Azupharma, Ger.
Ginkgo biloba (p.1584·1).
Mental function disorders; peripheral vascular disorders.

Ginkogink URPAC, Fr.
Ginkgo biloba (p.1584·1).
Mental function impairment in the elderly; peripheral and cerebral vascular disorders; vertigo.

Ginkopur Isis Puren, Ger.
Ginkgo biloba (p.1584·1).
Dizziness; headache; mental function disorders; peripheral vascular disorders; tinnitus.

Ginkor Beaufour, Fr.
Ginkgo biloba (p.1584·1); troxerutin (p.1580·2).
Peripheral vascular disorders.

Ginkor Fort Beaufour, Fr.
Ginkgo biloba (p.1584·1); heptaminol hydrochloride (p.1587·2); troxerutin (p.1580·2).
Peripheral vascular disorders.

Ginkor Procto Beaufour, Fr.
Ginkgo biloba (p.1584·1); butyl aminobenzoate (p.1289·1).
Haemorrhoids.

Ginkovit Roche, Switz.†.
Garlic (p.1583·1); glutamic acid (p.1344·3); crataegus (p.1568·2); ginseng (p.1584·2); ginkgo biloba (p.1584·1); magnesium orotate (p.1611·2); yeast (p.1373·1).
Mental function impairment.

Ginkovital Pharmadass, UK.
Ginkgo biloba (p.1584·1).

Ginocap Biocontrolfarm, Ital.
Bearberry (p.1552·2).

Ginoday Biocontrolfarm, Ital.
Birch (p.1553·3); alga clorella.

Ginoden Schering, Ital.
Gestodene (p.1447·2); ethinyloestradiol (p.1445·1).
Combined oral contraceptive.

Ginolax Biocontrolfarm, Ital.
Psyllium (p.1194·2); frangula (p.1193·2).

Ginomineral Biocontrolfarm, Ital.
Mineral preparation.
Nutritional supplement.

Ginopil Biocontrolfarm, Ital.
Pilosella.

Ginotricina UCB, Ital.†.
Tyrothricin (p.267·2).

Ginoven Biocontrolfarm, Ital.
Aesculus (p.1543·3).

Ginoxil RDC, Ital.
Urea hydrogen peroxide (p.1127·3).
Vaginal disorders; vaginal hygiene.

Ginroy Medisculab, Ger.
Ginseng (p.1584·2).
Tonic.

Ginsana
Bender, Aust.; Boehringer Ingelheim, Fr.; Pharmaton, Ger.; Swisspharm, S.Afr.†; Fher, Spain; GPL, Switz.
Ginseng (p.1584·2).
Tonic.

Ginsatonic Arkopharma, Fr.
Ginseng (p.1584·2).
Tonic.

Ginseng Komplex Truw, Ger.†.
Homoeopathic preparation.

Ginseng Med Complex *Dynamit, Aust.*
Homoeopathic preparation.

Ginseng-Biovital *Schieffer, Switz.†.*
Vitamins and minerals with ginseng, caffeine, and lecithin.
Tonic.

Ginseng-Complex "Schuh" *Coradol, Ger.*
Panax ginseng (p.1584·2); chlorophyllin (p.1000·1); crataegus (p.1568·2).
Tonic.

Ginvapast *Wild, Switz.*
Calcium gluconate (p.1155·2); procaine (p.1299·2); vitamins A and D.
Gum disorders.

Ginzinc *Nutergia, Fr.†.*
Red ginseng (p.1584·2); soya lecithin (p.1595·2); magnesium glycerophosphate (p.1157·2); zinc oxide (p.1096·2).

Ginzing *Vita Glow, Austral.*
Ginseng (p.1584·2).
Tonic.

Ginzing E *Vita Glow, Austral.*
Ginseng (p.1584·2); *d*-alpha tocopherol (p.1369·1).
Tonic.

Ginzing G *Vita Glow, Austral.*
Ginseng (p.1584·2); ginkgo biloba (p.1584·1).
Tonic.

Gipron *Serpero, Ital.†.*
Creatinolfosfate monosodium (p.1568·3).
Cardiac disorders.

Girha "Schuh" *Coradol, Ger.*
Homoeopathic preparation.

Girheulit H *Pflüger, Ger.*
Homoeopathic preparation.

Gittalun *Thomae, Ger.*
Doxylamine succinate (p.410·1).
Sleep disorders.

Gityl 6 *Krewel, Ger.*
Bromazepam (p.643·1).
Anxiety; sleep disorders.

Givalex
Norgine, Belg.; Norgine, Fr.; Norgine, Ger.
Hexetidine (p.1116·1); choline salicylate (p.25·2); chlorbutol (p.1106·3).
Mouth and throat infections.

Givitol
Galen, Irl.; Galen, UK.
Ferrous fumarate (p.1339·3); folic acid (p.1340·3); vitamin B and C substances.
Iron and folic acid deficiency in pregnancy.

Gladem
Bender, Aust.; Boehringer Ingelheim, Switz.
Sertraline hydrochloride (p.307·2).
Depression; obsessive-compulsive disorder.

Gladixol *Kolassa, Aust.*
β-Acetyldigoxin (p.812·3); potassium aspartate (p.1161·3); magnesium aspartate (p.1157·2).
Arrhythmias; heart failure.

Gladixol N *Gepepharm, Ger.*
β-Acetyldigoxin (p.812·3).
Heart failure.

Gladlax *Gerard House, UK.*
Aloes (p.1177·1); fennel (p.1579·1); valerian (p.1643·1); holy thistle (p.1565·3).
Constipation.

Glakay *Eisai, Jpn.*
Menatetrenone (p.1371·3).
Osteoporosis.

Glamidolo *Angelini, Ital.*
Dapiprazole hydrochloride (p.1570·2).
Glaucoma.

Glamin
Pharmacia Upjohn, Ger.; Pharmacia Upjohn, Irl.; Pharmacia Upjohn, Ital.; Pharmacia Upjohn, Neth.; Pharmacia Upjohn, Switz.; Pharmacia Upjohn, UK.
Amino-acid infusion.
Parenteral nutrition.

Glandosane
Leopold, Aust.; Fresenius, Ger.; Fresenius, Switz.; Fresenius, UK; Kenwood, USA.
Carmellose sodium (p.1471·2); sorbitol (p.1354·2); electrolytes (p.1147·1).
Dry mouth.

Glandulae-F-Gastreu R20 *Reckeweg, Ger.*
Homoeopathic preparation.

Glandulae-M-Gastreu R19 *Reckeweg, Ger.*
Homoeopathic preparation.

Glandulatherm *Feldhoff, Ger.†.*
Testicular extract (p.1464·1); placental extract.
Bath additive; circulatory disorders; pain syndromes.

Glanil *Janssen, Swed.†.*
Cinnarizine (p.406·1).
Motion sickness.

Glanoide *Hormosan, Ger.†.*
Animal ovarian extract (p.1458·2).
Lignocaine (p.1293·2) is included in this preparation to alleviate the pain of injection.
Gynaecological disorders.

Glanoide cerebrale *Hormosan, Ger.†.*
Albumin-free extract of calf brain (p.1599·1).
Lignocaine (p.1293·2) is included in this preparation to alleviate the pain of injection.
Cerebrovascular disorders.

Glanoide coreale *Hormosan, Ger.†.*
Animal heart extract.
Lignocaine (p.1293·2) is included in this preparation to alleviate the pain of injection.
Cardiovascular disorders.

Glanoide diencephale *Hormosan, Ger.†.*
Hormone- and protein-free brain lipid extract (p.1599·1).
Lignocaine (p.1293·2) is included in this preparation to alleviate the pain of injection.
Head injuries; psychiatric disorders.

Glanoide pancreale *Hormosan, Ger.†.*
Pancreatic extract, hormone-free.
Lignocaine (p.1293·2) is included in this preparation to alleviate the pain of injection.
Pancreatic insufficiency.

Glanoide renale *Hormosan, Ger.†.*
Albumin-free extract of animal kidneys.
Lignocaine (p.1293·2) is included in this preparation to alleviate the pain of injection.
Renal vascular disorders.

Glanoide retinale *Dispersa, Ger.†.*
Lipid extract of porcine retina.
Lignocaine (p.1293·2) is included in this preparation to alleviate the pain of injection.
Eye disorders.

Glanoide testoidale *Hormosan, Ger.†.*
Hormone-free testicular extract (p.1464·1).
Lignocaine (p.1293·2) is included in this preparation to alleviate the pain of injection.
Male impotence; male menopausal disorders.

GLA-Plus Vitamin E *Shaklee, Canad.*
Essential fatty acids with vitamin E.
Nutritional supplement.

Glassatan *Krewel, Ger.†.*
Amoxycillin trihydrate (p.151·3).
Bacterial infections.

Glaucadrin *Chibret, Ger.†.*
Aceclidine hydrochloride (p.1389·1); adrenaline (p.813·2).
Glaucoma.

Glaucadrine
Merck Sharp & Dohme-Chibret, Fr.; Merck Sharp & Dohme, Switz.
Aceclidine hydrochloride (p.1389·1); adrenaline (p.813·2).
Glaucoma.

Glaucocare
Bournonville, Belg.; Bournonville, Neth.
Aceclidine (p.1389·1) or aceclidine hydrochloride (p.1389·1).
Glaucoma; raised intra-ocular pressure.

Glaucofrin
Bournonville, Belg.; Bournonville, Neth.
Aceclidine (p.1389·1) or aceclidine hydrochloride (p.1389·1); adrenaline (p.813·2).
Glaucoma; raised intra-ocular pressure.

Glaucol
Note. This name is used for preparations of different composition.
Croma, Aust.
Dichlorphenamide (p.848·2).
Glaucoma.

Norton, UK.
Timolol maleate (p.953·3).
Ocular hypertension.

Glaucon *Alcon, USA.*
Adrenaline hydrochloride (p.813·3).
Open-angle glaucoma.

Glauconex
Agepha, Aust.; Bournonville, Belg.; Alcon-Thilo, Ger.; Thilo, Neth.†.
Befunolol hydrochloride (p.827·1).
Glaucoma; ocular hypertension.

Glauconide *Llorens, Spain.*
Dichlorphenamide (p.848·2).
Glaucoma; raised intra-ocular pressure.

Glaucosan *Hexal, S.Afr.*
Timolol maleate (p.953·3).
Raised intra-ocular pressure.

Glaucostat
Merck Sharp & Dohme-Chibret, Fr.; Merck Sharp & Dohme, Spain; Merck Sharp & Dohme, Switz.
Aceclidine hydrochloride (p.1389·1).
Glaucoma.

Glauco-Stulln *Stulln, Ger.*
Pindolol (p.931·1).
Glaucoma.

Glaucotat *Chibret, Ger.*
Aceclidine hydrochloride (p.1389·1).
Glaucoma.

Glaucothil
Agepha, Aust.; Alcon-Thilo, Ger.
Dipivefrine hydrochloride (p.1572·3).
Glaucoma.

GlaucTabs *Akorn, USA.*
Methazolamide (p.903·2).
Glaucoma.

Glaudrops *Cusi, Spain.*
Dipivefrine hydrochloride (p.1572·3).
Glaucoma; raised intra-ocular pressure.

Glaufrin *Allergan, Swed.*
Adrenaline hydrochloride (p.813·3).
Open-angle glaucoma.

Glauko Biciron *S & K, Ger.*
Pilocarpine hydrochloride (p.1396·3); phenylephrine hydrochloride (p.1066·2).
Glaucoma.

Glaumid *SIFI, Ital.*
Dichlorphenamide (p.848·2).
Glaucoma.

Glaunorm *Farmigea, Ital.*
Aceclidine hydrochloride (p.1389·1).
Glaucoma.

Glau-opt *Trinity, UK.*
Timolol maleate (p.953·3).
Glaucoma; ocular hypertension.

Glaupax
Ciba Vision, Ger.; Orion, Irl.; Ciba Vision, Neth.; Erco, Norw.; Orion, Swed.†; Ciba Vision, Switz.
Acetazolamide (p.810·3).
Epilepsy; glaucoma; Ménière's disease; oedema.

Glauposine *Alcon, Fr.†.*
Adrenaline (p.813·2).
Glaucoma; ocular hypertension.

Glautarakt *Pekana, Ger.*
Homoeopathic preparation.

Glavamin
Pharmacia Upjohn, Aust.; Pharmacia Upjohn, Norw.; Pharmacia Upjohn, Swed.
Amino-acid infusion.
Parenteral nutrition.

Glaxal Base *Roberts, Canad.*
Moisturiser.
Dermatological base.

Glazidim
Glaxo Wellcome, Belg.; Glaxo Wellcome, Ital.
Ceftazidime (p.173·3).
Bacterial infections.

Gleitgelen *Wolff, Ger.*
Liquid paraffin (p.1382·1); medium-chain triglycerides.
Vaginal dryness.

Gleitmittel *Bichsel, Switz.*
Chlorhexidine gluconate (p.1107·2).
Lubrication before catheterisation or endoscopy.

Gliadel *Rhone-Poulenc Rorer, USA.*
Carmustine (p.511·3).
Glioblastoma multiforme.

Glianimon *Bayer, Ger.*
Benperidol (p.642·3).
Psychoses.

Gliatilin *Italfarmaco, Ital.*
Choline alfoscerate (p.1390·3).
Mental function impairment.

gli-basan *Schonenberger, Switz.*
Glibenclamide (p.319·3).
Diabetes mellitus.

Gliben
CT, Ger.; Abiogen, Ital.
Glibenclamide (p.319·3).
Diabetes mellitus.

Gliben F *Abiogen, Ital.*
Glibenclamide (p.319·3); phenformin hydrochloride (p.330·3).
Diabetes mellitus.

Glibenese
Pfizer, Aust.; Pfizer, Fr.; Pfizer, Ger.; Pfizer, Irl.; Pfizer, Neth.; Pfizer, Spain; Pfizer, Swed.†; Mack, Switz.; Pfizer, UK.
Glipizide (p.320·3).
Diabetes mellitus.

Glibenhexal *Hexal, Ger.*
Glibenclamide (p.319·3).
Diabetes mellitus.

Gliben-Puren N *Isis Puren, Ger.*
Glibenclamide (p.319·3).
Diabetes mellitus.

Glibesifar *Siphar, Switz.*
Glibenclamide (p.319·3).
Diabetes mellitus.

Glibinese *Roerig, Belg.*
Glipizide (p.320·3).
Diabetes mellitus.

Glibomet *Guidotti, Ital.*
Glibenclamide (p.319·3); metformin hydrochloride (p.330·1).
Diabetes mellitus.

Gliboral *Guidotti, Ital.*
Glibenclamide (p.319·3).
Diabetes mellitus.

Glicacil *Bioprogress, Ital.*
Sodium cromoglycate (p.762·1).
Asthma; chronic intestinal inflammatory disease; food hypersensitivity.

Glicamin *Lafare, Ital.*
A heparinoid (p.882·3).
Thrombosis prophylaxis.

Glicermina *Bescansa, Spain.*
Stearic acid; glycerol.
Formerly contained potassium hydroxide, stearic acid, and glycerol.
Skin disorders.

Glicerolax *Dynacren, Ital.*
Glycerol (p.1585·2); mallow.
Constipation.

Glicerotens *Llorens, Spain.*
Glycerol (p.1585·2).
Glaucoma; ocular hypertension; ocular surgery.

Glicero-Valerovit *Teofarma, Ital.*
Sodium glycerophosphate (p.1586·2); valerian (p.1643·1).
Lignocaine hydrochloride (p.1293·2) is included in the intramuscular injection to alleviate the pain of injection.
Hyperexcitability; tonic.

Glico Test *Callegari, Ital.*
Test for glucose in blood (p.1585·1).

Glico Urine B *Callegari, Ital.*
Test for glucose in urine (p.1585·1).

Glicobase *Formenti, Ital.*
Acarbose (p.317·2).
Diabetes mellitus.

Glicocinnamina *Menarini, Ital.†.*
Guaiacol (p.1061·2); terpin hydrate (p.1070·2); codeine phosphate (p.26·1).
Catarrh; coughs.

Gliconorm *Gentili, Ital.†.*
Chlorpropamide (p.319·1).
Diabetes mellitus.

Glifan *Roussel, Ital.†.*
Glafenine hydrochloride (p.42·3).
Pain.

Glifanan *Roussel, Switz.†.*
Glafenine (p.42·3).
Pain.

Gliformin *Guidotti, Ital.*
Glibenclamide (p.319·3); phenformin hydrochloride (p.330·3).
Diabetes mellitus.

Glimbal *Angelini, Aust.*
Clocortolone pivalate (p.1035·3).
Skin disorders.

Glimel *Alphapharm, Austral.*
Glibenclamide (p.319·3).
Diabetes mellitus.

Glimidstada *Stada, Ger.*
Glibenclamide (p.319·3).
Diabetes mellitus.

Glios *Pharmacia Upjohn, Ital.*
Serine alfoscerate.
Cerebrovascular disorders; mental function impairment.

Glipressina *Ferring, Ital.*
Terlipressin acetate hydrate (p.1261·2).
Haemorrhage from oesophageal varices.

Gliptide *Crinos, Ital.*
Sulglycotide (p.1215·1).
Gastro-intestinal disorders; peptic ulcer.

Glissitol *Schwabe, Ger.†.*
Rhubarb (p.1212·1); ox bile (p.1553·2).
Biliary disorders; liver disorders.

Glitisol *Zambon, Ital.*
Thiamphenicol glycinate hydrochloride (p.262·3).
Bacterial infections.

Gliviton *SIFI, Ital.†.*
Elixir: Manganese glycerophosphate (p.1586·2); nicotinamide (p.1351·2); dexpanthenol (p.1570·3); lysine hydrochloride (p.1350·1); levoglutamide (p.1344·3); cyanocobalamin (p.1363·3).
Tablets: Levoglutamide (p.1344·3); cyanocobalamin (p.1363·3); manganese glycerophosphate (p.1586·2); lysine hydrochloride (p.1350·1); calcium pantothenate (p.1352·3); nicotinamide (p.1351·2).
Tonic.

Globase *Amino, Switz.†.*
Pancreatin (p.1612·1); bromelains (p.1555·1); papain (p.1614·1); colloidal silicon dioxide (p.1475·1); dimethicone (p.1213·1); ox bile (p.1553·2); turmeric (p.1001·3); caraway oil (p.1559·3); fennel oil (p.1579·2); orange-peel oil (p.1610·3); peppermint oil (p.1208·1); chamomile oil.
Digestive system disorders.

Globenicol *Yamanouchi, Neth.*
Chloramphenicol (p.182·1).
Bacterial eye infections.

Globentyl *Nycomed, Norw.*
Aspirin (p.16·1).
Fever; pain; rheumatic disorders.

Globocef
Roche, Aust.; Biochemie, Aust.; Roche, Ger.; Roche, Ital.; Roche, Switz.
Cefetamet pivoxil hydrochloride (p.165·2).
Bacterial infections.

Globofil *Chemdorf, Spain†.*
Ketotifen fumarate (p.755·2).
Allergic rhinitis; asthma.

Globoid *Nycomed, Norw.*
Aspirin (p.16·1).
Fever; pain; rheumatic disorders.

Globuce *Sigma-Tau, Spain.*
Ciprofloxacin hydrochloride (p.185·3).
Bacterial infections.

Globuleno *Polifarma, Ital.†.*
Thiamine mononitrate (p.1361·1); riboflavine sodium phosphate (p.1362·1); pyridoxine hydrochloride (p.1362·3); nicotinamide (p.1351·2); panthenol (p.1571·1); cyanocobalamin (p.1363·3); calcium folinate (p.1342·2).
Vitamin deficiency.

Globuli *Jacoby, Aust.*
Homoeopathic preparation.

Globulina Lloren Anti RH *Llorente, Spain.*
An anti-D immunoglobulin (p.1503·2).
Prevention of rhesus sensitivity.

Globuman
Note. This name is used for preparations of different composition.
Kwizda, Aust.
A hepatitis A immunoglobulin (p.1512·1).
Passive immunisation.

Berna, Belg.; Berna, Ital.; Swisspharm, S.Afr.; Berna, Spain; Berna, Switz.
A normal immunoglobulin (p.1522·1).
Idiopathic thrombocytopenic purpura; immune deficiency; passive immunisation.

Globuman Hepatite A Berna, Belg.; Berna, Switz.
A hepatitis A immunoglobulin (p.1512·1).
Passive immunisation.

Globuman Hepatitis A Swisspharm, S.Afr.
A hepatitis A immunoglobulin (p.1512·1).
Passive immunisation.

Globuman iv Anti-CMV Berna, Switz.
A cytomegalovirus immunoglobulin (p.1507·1).
Passive immunisation.

Globuren Dompe Biotec, Ital.
Epoetin alfa (p.718·3).
Anaemia in chronic renal failure.

Gloceda Medgenix, Belg.
Erysimin; aconite (p.1542·2); belladonna (p.457·1); euphorbia; drosera (p.1574·1); cherry-laurel; codeine phosphate (p.26·1).
Coughs.

Glogama Evans, Spain†.
A normal immunoglobulin (p.1522·1).
Hypogammaglobulinaemia; passive immunisation.

Glogama Antialergica Llorente, Spain†.
A normal immunoglobulin (p.1522·1).
Hypersensitivity reactions.

Glogama Antihepatitis B Evans, Spain.
A hepatitis B immunoglobulin (p.1512·3).
Passive immunisation.

Glogama Antiparotiditis Llorente, Spain†.
A mumps immunoglobulin (p.1521·2).
Passive immunisation.

Glogama Antipertusis Llorente, Spain†.
A pertussis immunoglobulin (p.1525·3).
Passive immunisation.

Glogama Antirubeola Llorente, Spain†.
A rubella immunoglobulin (p.1532·3).
Passive immunisation.

Glogama Antisarampion Llorente, Spain†.
A measles immunoglobulin (p.1517·3).
Passive immunisation.

Glogama Antitetanica Evans, Spain†.
A tetanus immunoglobulin (p.1535·2).
Passive immunisation.

Gloinar Rhone-Poulenc Rorer, Spain†.
A normal immunoglobulin (p.1522·1).
Hypogammaglobulinaemia.

Glonoin Coradol, Ger.
Herbal and homoeopathic preparation.

Glonoinum Hevert, Ger.
Homoeopathic preparation.

Gloquat C Rhone Poulenc Chemicals, UK.
Alkylaryltrimethylammonium chloride (p.1101·2).
Disinfection.

Glossithiase Jolly-Jatel, Fr.
Thenoate ethanolamine (p.262·2); muramidase hydrochloride (p.1604·3).
Infections of the mouth and throat.

Glotone Vita, Spain.
Cyproheptadine hydrochloride (p.407·2); embryo extract; gastric mucosa extract; muscle extract.
Tonic.

Glottyl
Note. This name is used for preparations of different composition.
Asta Medica, Belg.
Oral drops†: Amylocaine (p.1286·1); aconite (p.1542·2); belladonna (p.457·1); drosera (p.1574·1); erysimin; euphorbia.
Respiratory-system disorders.
Syrup: Codeine phosphate (p.26·1).
Formerly contained aconite, codeine phosphate, cherry-laurel, belladonna, drosera, erysimin, and euphorbia.
Coughs.
Tablets†: Amylocaine (p.1286·1); aconite (p.1542·2); belladonna (p.457·1); drosera (p.1574·1); erysimin; euphorbia; tyrothricin (p.267·2).
Respiratory-system disorders.
Marion Merrell, Fr.
Amylocaine hydrochloride (p.1286·1); erysimum; grindelia.
Sore throat.

Gluborid
Waldheim, Aust.; Grunenthal, Ger.; Grunenthal, Switz.
Glibornuride (p.320·1).
Diabetes mellitus.

GlucaGen
Novo Nordisk, Austral.; Novo Nordisk, Belg.; Novo Nordisk, Ger.; Novo Nordisk, Irl.; Novo Nordisk, Ital.; Novo Nordisk, S.Afr.; Novo Nordisk, Switz.; Novo Nordisk, UK.
Glucagon hydrochloride (p.982·2).
Adjunct in gastro-intestinal endoscopy and radiography; hypoglycaemia.

Glucagon Lilly, UK.
Glucagon hydrochloride (p.982·2).
Aid in gastro-intestinal radiography; hypoglycaemia.

Glucal Lennon, S.Afr.†.
Calcium gluconate (p.1155·2).
Calcium deficiencies.

Glucamet Opus, UK.
Metformin hydrochloride (p.330·1).
Diabetes mellitus.

Glucantim Rhone-Poulenc Rorer, Ital.
Meglumine antimonate (p.578·3).
Leishmaniasis.

Glucantime
Specia, Fr.; Rhone-Poulenc Rorer, Spain.
Meglumine antimonate (p.578·3).
Leishmaniasis.

Glucerna
Abbott, Austral.; Abbott, Canad.; Abbott, Irl.; Ross, USA.
Preparation for enteral nutrition.
Glucose intolerance.

Glucidoral Servier, Fr.
Carbutamide (p.319·1).
Diabetes mellitus.

Glucinan Lipha Sante, Fr.
Metformin chlorophenoxyacetate (p.330·2).
Diabetes mellitus.

Glucobay
Bayer, Aust.; Bayer, Austral.; Bayer, Belg.; Bayer, Ger.; Bayer, Irl.; Bayer, Ital.; Bayer, Neth.; Bayer, Norw.; Bayer, S.Afr.; Bayer, Spain; Bayer, Swed.; Bayer, Switz.; Bayer, UK.
Acarbose (p.317·2).
Diabetes mellitus.

Glucoben Farmades, Ital.†.
Glisoxepide (p.321·2).
Diabetes mellitus.

Glucobene Merckle, Aust.
Glibenclamide (p.319·3).
Diabetes mellitus.

Glucocalcium Streuli, Switz.
Calcium gluconate (p.1155·2); calcium sucrate.
Hypocalcaemia; poisoning.

Glucochaux Darci, Belg.
Calcium gluconate (p.1155·2); calcium hydrogen phosphate (p.1155·3).
Calcium deficiency; calcium supplement.

Glucodex Rougier, Canad.
Glucose (p.1343·3).
Oral glucose tolerance test.

Glucodin
Note. This name is used for preparations of different composition.
Boots Healthcare, Irl.
Glucose (p.1343·3); vitamin C (p.1365·2).
Crookes Laboratories, UK.
Glucose (p.1343·3).

Glucodulco Faes, Spain†.
Calcium phosphate; calcium gluconate; ergocalciferol; glucose.
Tonic.

Glucoferon Waldheim, Ger.†.
Interferon alfa (p.615·3).
Hairy-cell leukaemia.

Glucoferro Guidotti, Ital.
Ferrous gluconate (p.1340·1).
Iron deficiency; iron-deficiency anaemias.

Glucofilm
Bayer Diagnostics, Austral.; Miles, Canad.; Bayer Diagnostics, Fr.; Bayer Diagnostici, Ital.; Bayer, USA.
Test for glucose in blood (p.1585·1).

Glucolon Sabater, Spain.
Glibenclamide (p.319·3).
Diabetes mellitus.

Gluco-lyte Seton, UK†.
Sodium chloride; potassium chloride; sodium bicarbonate; glucose (p.1152·3).
Diarrhoea; oral rehydration therapy.

Glucomagma Drug Houses Austral., Austral.†.
Kaolin (p.1195·1); aluminium hydroxide (p.1177·3); glucose; codeine phosphate (p.26·1); pectin (p.1474·1).
Diarrhoea.

Glucoman Volchem, Ital.
Dietary fibre supplement containing glucomannan (p.1584·3), galactomannan, and minerals.
Disorders of carbohydrate and lipid metabolism; gastro-intestinal disorders; obesity.

Glucometer
Bayer, Austral.; Bayer Diagnostici, Ital.
Test for glucose in blood (p.1585·1).
For use with Glucometer Elite blood glucose meter.

Glucomide Lipha, Ital.
Metformin hydrochloride (p.330·1); glibenclamide (p.319·3).
Diabetes mellitus.

Gluconorm Wolff, Ger.
Glibenclamide (p.319·3).
Diabetes mellitus.

Glucophage
Merck, Aust.; 3M, Austral.; Lipha, Belg.; Hoechst Marion Roussel, Canad.; Lipha Sante, Fr.; Lipha, Ger.; Lipha, Irl.; Lipha, Ital.; E. Merck, Neth.; Lipha, Norw.; Mer-National, S.Afr.; Boehringer Mannheim, Spain; Meda, Swed.; Lipha, Switz.; Lipha, UK; Bristol-Myers Squibb, USA.
Metformin hydrochloride (p.330·1).
Diabetes mellitus.

Glucoplasmal
Braun, Aust.†.
Amino-acid and electrolyte infusion.
Parenteral nutrition.
Braun, Ger.; Braun, Spain.
Amino-acid, glucose, and electrolyte infusion.
Parenteral nutrition.

Glucoplex Geistlich, UK.
Carbohydrate, electrolyte, and trace element infusion.
Parenteral nutrition.

Glucoplurisalina Mein, Spain.
Electrolyte infusion with glucose (p.1147·1).
Fluid and electrolyte depletion.

Glucopolielectrol Baxter, Spain.
Electrolyte infusion with glucose.
Fluid and electrolyte depletion.

Glucopotasica Braun, Spain; Mein, Spain.
Potassium chloride infusion (p.1161·1) with glucose (p.1343·3).
Fluid and electrolyte depletion.

Glucopotasico Bieffe, Spain; Rapide, Spain; Ern, Spain.
Potassium chloride infusion (p.1161·1) with glucose (p.1343·3).
Fluid and electrolyte depletion.

Glucor Bayer, Fr.
Acarbose (p.317·2).
Diabetes mellitus.

Glucoremed Lichtenstein, Ger.
Glibenclamide (p.319·3).
Diabetes mellitus.

Glucosa CLNA CLK Baxter, Spain†.
Sodium chloride (p.1162·2) and potassium chloride infusion (p.1161·1) with glucose (p.1343·3).
Fluid and electrolyte depletion.

Glucosalin Baxter, Switz.
Anhydrous glucose (p.1343·3); sodium chloride (p.1162·2).
Carbohydrate source; fluid and electrolyte disorders.

Glucosalina Grifols, Spain; Instituto Farmacologico, Spain; Mein, Spain; Navarro, Spain; Braun, Spain.
Sodium chloride infusion (p.1162·2) with glucose (p.1343·3).
Fluid and electrolyte depletion.

Glucosalina Modific Mein, Spain.
Sodium chloride (p.1162·2) and sodium lactate (p.1153·2) infusion with glucose (p.1343·3).
Fluid and electrolyte depletion.

Glucosalino Bieffe, Spain; Ern, Spain; Braun, Spain; Pharmacia Upjohn, Spain.
Sodium chloride (p.1162·2) infusion with glucose (p.1343·3).
Fluid and electrolyte depletion.

Glucosan
Note. This name is used for preparations of different composition.
Laevosan, Aust.
Anhydrous glucose (p.1343·3).
Carbohydrate source; fluid depletion.
Ortho, Ital.
Test for glucose in blood (p.1585·1).

Glucose Medi-Test Macherey Nagel Duren, S.Afr.
Test for glucose in urine (p.1585·1).

Glucose 2 Medi-Test Macherey Nagel Duren, S.Afr.
Test for glucose and ascorbic acid in urine.

Glucose 3 Medi-Test Macherey Nagel Duren, S.Afr.
Test for glucose, ascorbic acid, and ketones in urine.

Glucoseral Streuli, Switz.
Electrolyte infusion with glucose (p.1147·1).
Fluid and electrolyte disorders; parenteral nutrition.

Glucosmon Byk Elmu, Spain.
Glucose (p.1343·3).
Carbohydrate source; hypoglycaemia.

Glucosteril Fresenius, Ger.
Glucose monohydrate (p.1343·3).
Carbohydrate source; fluid depletion.

Glucostix
Bayer Diagnostics, Austral.; Bayer, Canad.; Bayer Diagnostics, Fr.; Ames, Irl.; Bayer Diagnostici, Ital.; Ames, S.Afr.; Bayer Diagnostics, UK; Bayer, USA.
Test for glucose in blood (p.1585·1).

Glucosulfa Lipha, Ital.
Metformin (p.330·2); tolbutamide (p.333·2).
Diabetes mellitus.

Gluco-Tablinen
Sanorania, Ger.; Sanorania, Switz.†.
Glibenclamide (p.319·3).
Diabetes mellitus.

Glucotard
Boehringer Mannheim, Ger.; Boehringer Mannheim, Switz.†.
Guar gum (p.321·3).
Diabetes mellitus; hyperlipidaemias.

Glucotide
Bayer Diagnostics, Fr.; Ames, Irl.; Bayer Diagnostics, UK.
Test for glucose in blood (p.1585·1).

Glucotrol Pfizer, USA.
Glipizide (p.320·3).
Diabetes mellitus.

Glucovenos pad Fresenius, Ger.
Carbohydrate and electrolyte infusion.
Parenteral nutrition.

Glukacel Braun, Norw.
Electrolyte infusion with glucose (p.1147·1).
Carbohydrate source; fluid and electrolyte disorders.

Gluketurtest Boehringer Mannheim, Ital.
Test for glucose and ketone bodies in urine.

Gluko Savio, Ital.
Glutathione sodium (p.983·1).
Alcohol and drug poisoning; radiation trauma.

Glukor Hyrex, USA†.
Chorionic gonadotrophin (p.1243·1).
Male and female infertility; male hypogonadism; prepubertal cryptorchidism.

Glukoreduct Sanofi Winthrop, Ger.
Glibenclamide (p.319·3).
Diabetes mellitus.

Glukos-El Braun, Swed.
Carbohydrate and electrolyte infusion.
Parenteral nutrition.

Glukovital Wolff, Ger.
Glibenclamide (p.319·3).
Diabetes mellitus.

Glukurtest Boehringer Mannheim, Ital.
Test for glucose in urine (p.1585·1).

Glumal
Kyowa, Jpn; Knoll, Spain.
Aceglutamide aluminium (p.1176·2).
Gastro-intestinal hyperacidity; peptic ulcer.

Glumida Pensa, Spain.
Acarbose (p.317·2).
Diabetes mellitus.

Gluparin Locatelli, Ital.
A heparinoid (p.882·3).
Hyperlipidaemias; peripheral vascular disorders; thrombosis prophylaxis.

Glu-Phos SPA, Ital.
Disodium glucose-1-phosphate.
Glucose deficiency.

Glurenor
Guidotti, Ital.; Yamanouchi, Spain.
Gliquidone (p.321·1).
Diabetes mellitus.

Glurenorm
Bender, Aust.; Menarini, Belg.; Yamanouchi, Ger.; Sanofi Winthrop, UK.
Gliquidone (p.321·1).
Diabetes mellitus.

Gluronazid Hormonchemie, Ger.†.
Isoniazid sodium glucuronate (p.220·1).
Tuberculosis.

Gluserin B12 Montefarmaco, Ital.†.
Levoglutamide (p.1344·3); DL-phosphoserine; cyanocobalamin (p.1363·3).
Tonic.

Gluta Complex UCB, Ital.
Cobamamide (p.1364·2); amino acids.
Tonic.

Glutacerebro AFOM, Ital.
Levoglutamide (p.1344·3).
Mental function impairment.

Glutacid Nycomed, Norw.
Glutamic acid (p.1344·3).
Achlorhydria; hypochlorhydria.

Glutacide Germiphene, Canad.†.
Glutaraldehyde (p.1114·3).
Disinfection.

Glutacortin IBP, Ital.†.
Pyridoxal phosphate (p.1363·1); suprarenal cortex (p.1050·1); ascorbic acid (p.1365·2); cyanocobalamin (p.1363·3); lignocaine hydrochloride (p.1293·2).
Asthenia.

Glutadouze Bouchara, Switz.†.
Liver extract; pylorus extract; cerebral medulla extract (p.1599·1); sodium glycerophosphate (p.1586·2); monosodium glutamate (p.1351·2).
Tonic.

Glutaferro Medix, Spain.
Ferrous gluconate (p.1340·1) or ferrous glycine sulphate (p.1340·1).
Ascorbic acid (p.1365·2) is included in the capsules to increase absorption and availability of iron and docusate sodium (p.1189·3) is included to reduce the constipating effects of iron.
Anaemias.

Glutafin
Nutricia, Fr.†; Nutricia, Irl.; Nutricia, UK.
Gluten-free food for special diets.

Glutamag Trivit B
Aerocid, Fr.†; Sodip, Switz.†.
Magnesium glutamate; vitamin B substances.
Tonic.

Glutamag Vitamine Aerocid, Fr.
Magnesium glutamate; riboflavine (p.1362·1); nicotinamide (p.1351·2).
Tonic.

Glutamed Boehringer Mannheim, Ital.
Glutathione sodium (p.983·1).
Alcohol and drug poisoning; protection against toxicity induced by cytotoxic chemotherapy; radiation trauma.

Glutamin Fosforo SIT, Ital.
Levoglutamide (p.1344·3); DL-phosphoserine; cyanocobalamin (p.1363·3).
Mental function impairment.

Glutaminol B$_6$ Syntex, Fr.†.
Glutamic acid (p.1344·3); pyridoxine hydrochloride (p.1362·3).
Tonic.

Glutamin-Verla Verla, Ger.
Glutamic acid (p.1344·3).
Tonic.

Glutaneurina B6 Fte Zyma, Spain†.
Glutamic acid (p.1344·3); pyridoxine (p.1363·1); thiamine (p.1361·2); tocopheryl acetate (p.1369·1).
Motion sickness; neurological disorders.

Glutanil Bioprogress, Ital.
Reduced glutathione sodium (p.983·1).
Alcohol and drug poisoning; radiation trauma.

Glutarall Colgate Oral Care, Austral.
Glutaraldehyde (p.1114·3).
Disinfection.

Glutarase *Lusofarmaco, Ital.†.*
Pyridoxine oxoglurate (p.1363·1).
Liver disorders.

Glutarex *Ross, USA.*
A range of lysine- and tryptophan-free preparations for enteral nutrition including an infant feed.
Glutaric aciduria type I.

Glutargin *Terapeutico, Ital.*
Arginine glutamate (p.1334·1); arginine aspartate (p.1334·2).
Liver disorders.

Glutarol
Dermal Laboratories, Irl.; Vifor, Switz.; Dermal Laboratories, UK.
Glutaraldehyde (p.1114·3).
Warts.

Glutarsin E *Berlin-Chemie, Ger.*
Glutamic acid (p.1344·3); arginine hydrochloride (p.1334·1); potassium hydroxide (p.1621·1); sodium hydroxide (p.1631·1).
Hyperammonaemia.

Glutasan *San Carlo, Ital.*
Glutathione sodium (p.983·1).
Alcohol and drug poisoning; radiation trauma.

Glutathin *Mochida, Jpn†.*
Glutathione (p.983·1).
Liver disorders.

Glutatox *Ist. Chim. Inter., Ital.†.*
Glutathione sodium (p.983·1).
Alcohol and drug poisoning; radiation trauma.

Glutaven *Teofarma, Ital.*
Levoglutamide (p.1344·3).
Mental function impairment.

Glutergen + H 3 *Verla, Ger.†.*
Magnesium hydrogen glutamate; potassium chloride; ethyl linolate; ethyl octadecadienoate; ethyl linolenate; maize oil; cholic acid; lecithin; procaine hydrochloride; haematoporphyrin; troxerutin; vitamins.
Tonic.

Glutestere B-Complesso *Maggioni, Ital.†.*
Capsules: Acetylmethionine; inositol (p.1591·1); ethyl glutamate; potassium aspartate (p.1161·3); magnesium aspartate (p.1157·2); pantethine (p.1276·3); betaine hydrochloride (p.1553·2); thiamine nitrate (p.1361·1); riboflavine (p.1362·1); pyridoxine hydrochloride (p.1362·3); cyanocobalamin (p.1363·3); nicotinamide (p.1351·2); sodium ascorbate (p.1365·2).
Injection: Acetylmethionine; inositol (p.1591·1); choline bitartrate (p.1337·1); ethyl glutamate; potassium aspartate (p.1161·3); magnesium aspartate (p.1157·2); pantethine (p.1276·3); riboflavine sodium phosphate (p.1362·1); pyridoxine hydrochloride (p.1362·3); nicotinamide (p.1351·2); ascorbic acid (p.1365·2); cyanocobalamin (p.1363·3).
Liver disorders.

Gluthion *CT, Ital.*
Reduced glutathione sodium (p.983·1).
Alcohol and drug poisoning; radiation trauma.

Gluti-Agil *Serturner, Ger.*
Glutamic acid (p.1344·3).
Mental function stimulant.

Glutisal *Ravensberg, Ger.*
Ointment†: Procaine hydrochloride (p.1299·2); salicylamide (p.82·3); benzyl nicotinate (p.22·1).
Myalgia; neuralgia; peripheral vascular disorders; rheumatic disorders.
Tablets: Salicylamide (p.82·3); etenzamide (p.35·3).
Fever; gout; neuralgia; pain.

Glutisal-buton *Ravensberg, Ger.†.*
Phenylbutazone (p.79·2); salicylamide (p.82·3).
Acute ankylosing spondylitis; gout; rheumatism.

Glutisal-buton-Salbe *Ravensberg, Ger.†.*
Mofebutazone (p.56·1); sodium salamidacetate (p.82·3); benzyl nicotinate (p.22·1); menthol (p.1600·2); camphor (p.1557·2).
Rheumatism; sports injuries.

Glutofac *Kenwood, USA.*
A range of vitamin preparations.

Glutose *Paddock, USA.*
Glucose (p.1343·3).
Hypoglycaemia.

Glutoxil *Rottapharm, Ital.*
Glutathione sodium (p.983·1).
Alcohol and drug poisoning; radiation trauma.

Glutril
Roche, Austr.; Roche, Fr.; Roche, Ger.†; Roche, Ital.†; Roche, Switz.
Glibornuride (p.320·1).
Diabetes mellitus.

Glyate *Geneva, USA.*
Guaiphenesin (p.1061·3).
Coughs.

Glyben *Rolab, S.Afr.*
Glibenclamide (p.319·3).
Diabetes mellitus.

Glycaemie Medi-Test *Macherey Nagel Duren, S.Afr.*
Test for glucose in blood (p.1585·1).

Glycalis *Clintec-Sopharga, Fr.†.*
Preparation for enteral nutrition.

Glyceol *Chugai, Jpn.*
Glycerol concentrated (p.1585·2).
Cerebral oedema; ocular hypertension; raised intracranial pressure.

Glycerosteril *Fresenius, Ger.*
Glycerol (p.1585·2).
Cerebral oedema.

Glycerotone *Ciba Vision, Fr.*
Glycerol (p.1585·2).
Ocular hypertension; raised intracranial pressure.

Glyceryl-T *Rugby, USA.*
Theophylline (p.765·1); guaiphenesin (p.1061·3).
Bronchospasm.

Glycilax *Engelhard, Ger.*
Glycerol (p.1585·2).
Constipation.

Glycirenan *Disperga, Aust.*
Adrenaline hydrochloride (p.813·3).
Bronchospasm.

Glycobal *Nadeau, Canad.*
Multivitamin and mineral preparation.

Glycocortison *Ciba Vision, Ger.*
Hydrocortisone acetate (p.1043·3).
Eye disorders.

Glycocortisone H *Ciba Vision, Switz.*
Hydrocortisone acetate (p.1043·3) in glucose.
Corneal disorders.

Glycofed *Pal-Pak, USA.*
Pseudoephedrine hydrochloride (p.1068·3); guaiphenesin (p.1061·3).
Coughs.

glycolande N *Synthelabo, Ger.*
Glibenclamide (p.319·3).
Diabetes mellitus.

Glycomin *Lennon, S.Afr.*
Glibenclamide (p.319·3).
Diabetes mellitus.

Glycomycin *Dispersa, Ger.†.*
Neomycin sulphate (p.229·2) in glucose.
Eye disorders.

Glyconon *DDSA Pharmaceuticals, UK.*
Tolbutamide (p.333·2).
Diabetes mellitus.

Glycophos
Pharmacia Upjohn, Aust.; Pharmacia, Neth.†; Pharmacia Upjohn, Swed.†; Pharmacia Upjohn, Switz.
Sodium glycerophosphate (p.1586·2).
Phosphate supplement for parenteral nutrition.

Glycoplex *Vitaplex, Austral.*
Vitamins, minerals, and amino acids; liquorice (p.1197·1); taraxacum (p.1634·2).
Dietary supplement.

Gly-Coramin *Zyma, Switz.*
Nikethamide (p.1483·3); glucose and other reduced sugars (p.1343·3).
Tonic.

Glyco-Thymoline *Labomed, Fr.*
Sodium benzoate (p.1102·3); sodium bicarbonate (p.1153·2); borax (p.1554·2); sodium salicylate (p.85·1); thymol (p.1127·1); cineole (p.1564·1); pine oil; birch tar oil (p.1092·2); menthol (p.1600·2); glycerol (p.1585·2).
Skin and mucous membrane disinfection.

Glycotuss *Pal-Pak, USA.*
Guaiphenesin (p.1061·3).
Coughs.

Glycotuss-dM *Pal-Pak, USA.*
Dextromethorphan hydrobromide (p.1057·3); guaiphenesin (p.1061·3).
Coughs.

Glycovit *Alifarma, Ital.*
Amino-acid, multivitamin, and mineral preparation.
Nutritional supplement.

Glycylpressin
Sigmapharm, Aust.; Ferring, Ger.
Terlipressin acetate (p.1261·2).
Haemorrhagic gastritis; variceal haemorrhage.

Glycyron *Minophagen, Jpn.*
Ammonium glycyrrhizinate (p.1055·2).
Liver disorders; skin disorders; stomatitis.

Glycyrrhiza Complex *Blackmores, Austral.*
Liquorice (p.1197·1); avena sativa (p.1551·3); rose fruit (p.1365·2); vitamins; ginseng (p.1584·2).
Tonic.

Glymese *DDSA Pharmaceuticals, UK.*
Chlorpropamide (p.319·1).
Diabetes mellitus.

Glynase *Upjohn, USA.*
Glibenclamide (p.319·3).
Diabetes mellitus.

Gly-Oxide *SmithKline Beecham Consumer, USA.*
Urea hydrogen peroxide (p.1127·3).
Oral hygiene; oral inflammation.

Glypolix *Stroder, Ital.†.*
Dexfenfluramine hydrochloride (p.1479·2).
Obesity.

Glypressin
Ferring, Belg.; Ferring, Irl.; Ferring, Neth.; Ferring, UK.
Terlipressin (p.1261·2) or terlipressin acetate (p.1261·2).
Variceal haemorrhage.

Glypressine
Ferring, Fr.; Ferring, Switz.
Terlipressin acetate (p.1261·2).
Variceal haemorrhage.

Gly-Rectal *Valmo, Canad.*
Glycerol (p.1585·2).

Glyrol *Iolab, USA.*
Glycerol (p.1585·2).
Glaucoma; raised intra-ocular pressure before ophthalmic surgery.

Glysan *Brenner-Efeka, Ger.; LAW, Ger.*
Magaldrate (p.1198·1).
Gastric hyperacidity; heartburn; peptic ulcer.

Glysennid *Novartis Consumer, Canad.*
Sennosides (p.1212·3).
Constipation.

Glyset *Bayer, USA.*
Miglitol (p.330·3).
Diabetes mellitus.

Glytrin
Sanofi Winthrop, Irl.; Sanofi, UK†.
Glyceryl trinitrate (p.874·3).
Angina pectoris.

Glytuss *Mayrand, USA.*
Guaiphenesin (p.1061·3).
Coughs.

Glyvenol
Note. This name is used for preparations of different composition.
Ciba-Geigy, Aust.; Ciba-Geigy, Belg.; Ciba-Geigy, Fr.†; Ciba, Ger.†; Ciba, Ital.†; Padro, Spain†; Ciba, Switz.
Tribenoside (p.1638·3).
Peripheral vascular disorders.

Ciba-Geigy, Fr.†.
Suppositories: Tribenoside (p.1638·3); lignocaine (p.1293·2).
Haemorrhoids.

G-Myticin *Pedinol, USA.*
Gentamicin sulphate (p.212·1).
Bacterial infections.

G-Nol *Germiphene, Canad.†.*
Orthophenylphenol (p.1120·3); *o*-benzol-*p*-chlorophenol.
Disinfection.

GnRH *Serono, Ger.†.*
Gonadorelin acetate (p.1248·1).
Diagnosis of hypothalamic-pituitary-gonadal dysfunction.

Gobanal *Normon, Spain.*
Diazepam (p.661·1).
Contains pyridoxine.
Alcohol withdrawal syndrome; anxiety; febrile convulsions; insomnia; skeletal muscle spasm.

Gobemicina *Normon, Spain.*
Ampicillin trihydrate (p.153·2) or ampicillin sodium (p.153·1).
Bacterial infections.

Gobemicina Retard *Normon, Spain.*
Ampicillin sodium (p.153·1); ampicillin benzathine (p.154·1).
Lignocaine hydrochloride (p.1293·2) is included in this preparation to alleviate the pain of injection.
Bacterial infections.

Gobens Trim *Normon, Spain.*
Co-trimoxazole (p.196·3).
Bacterial infections.

Gocce Antonetto *Antonetto, Ital.*
Sodium picosulphate (p.1213·2).
Constipation.

Gocce D'Erbe *Kelemata, Ital.†.*
Hamamelis virginiana water (p.1587·1); rose water (p.1001·1); orange flower water; matricaria water (p.1561·2).
Eye irritation.

Gocce Lassative Aicardi *SIT, Ital.*
Sodium picosulphate (p.1213·2).
Constipation.

Gocce Sedative Della Tosse *Giovanardi, Ital.†.*
Dextromethorphan hydrobromide (p.1057·3).
Coughs.

Goccemed *Iodosan, Ital.*
Iodine (p.1493·1).
Oral hygiene.

Godabion B6 *Merck, Spain.*
Pyridoxine hydrochloride (p.1362·3).
Vitamin B6 deficiency.

Godafilin *Merck, Spain†.*
Theophylline (p.765·1).
Heart failure; obstructive airways disease; paroxysmal dyspnoea.

Godal *Merck, Spain.*
Bisoprolol fumarate (p.833·1).
Angina pectoris; hypertension.

Godamed *Pfleger, Ger.*
Aspirin (p.16·1).
Glycine (p.1345·2) is included in this preparation in an attempt to limit adverse effects on the gastro-intestinal mucosa.
Fever; pain; thrombo-embolic disorders.

Goddards White Oil Embrocation *LRC Products, UK.*
Turpentine oil (p.1641·1); dilute acetic acid (p.1541·2); dilute ammonia solution (p.1548·3).
Muscular aches and pains.

Go-Evac *Copley, USA.*
Macrogol 3350 (p.1598·2); electrolytes (p.1147·1).
Bowel evacuation.

Gofreely *Promedical, Ital.*
Macrogol 3350 (p.1598·2); electrolytes (p.1147·1).
Bowel evacuation.

Gola *Pierrel, Ital.†.*
Benzalkonium saccharinate (p.1102·1).
Oro-pharyngeal inflammation.

Gola Sel *Sella, Ital.†.*
Cetylpyridinium chloride (p.1106·2).
Oral hygiene.

Golacetin *Vaillant, Ital.*
Cetylpyridinium chloride (p.1106·2).
Oral disinfection.

Golamed Due *Iodosan, Ital.*
Cicliomenol; hexylresorcinol (p.1116·1).
Mouth and throat disinfection; sore throat.

Golamed Oral *Iodosan, Ital.*
Iodinated glycerol (p.1062·2); domiphen bromide (p.1112·3).
Oropharyngeal disinfection.

Golamixin *Fournier, Ital.*
Tyrothricin (p.267·2); cetrimonium bromide (p.1106·1); benzocaine (p.1286·2).
Bacterial stomatitis.

Golasan *Dynacren, Ital.*
Chlorhexidine gluconate (p.1107·2) or chlorhexidine hydrochloride (p.1107·2).
Mouth and throat disinfection; oral hygiene.

Golasept *Zeta, Ital.*
Povidone-iodine (p.1123·3).
Oral disinfection.

Golaseptine *SMB, Belg.†.*
Chlorhexidine hydrochloride (p.1107·2).
Mouth and throat disorders.

Golasol *Gambar, Ital.*
Chlorhexidine gluconate (p.1107·2).
Mouth and throat disinfection; oral hygiene.

Golaval *Carlo Erba OTC, Ital.*
Cetrimonium tosylate (p.1106·1).
Mouth and throat disinfection.

Gold-50 *Schering-Plough, Austral.*
Aurothioglucose (p.20·2).
Rheumatoid arthritis.

Gold Alka-Seltzer *Bayer, USA.*
Sodium bicarbonate (p.1153·2); citric acid (p.1564·3); potassium bicarbonate (p.1153·1).
Hyperacidity.

Gold Bond *Chattem, Canad.*
Menthol (p.1600·2); zinc oxide (p.1096·2).
Pruritus.

Golden Eye Drops *Typharm, UK.*
Propamidine isethionate (p.1124·1).
Eye infections.

Golden Eye Ointment
Note. This name is used for preparations of different composition.
Sigma, Austral.
Yellow mercuric oxide (p.1601·3).
Bacterial eye infections.

Typharm, UK.
Dibromopropamidine isethionate (p.1112·2).
Eye infections.

Golden Seal Compound *Gerard House, UK.*
Marshmallow root (p.1546·3); golden seal (p.1588·2); geum maculatum; taraxacum (p.1634·2).
Gastro-intestinal disorders.

Goldgeist *Gerlach, Ger.*
Pyrethrum (p.1410·1); piperonyl butoxide (p.1409·3).
Pediculosis.

Goldgesic *Searle, S.Afr.†.*
Paracetamol (p.72·2); codeine phosphate (p.26·1); promethazine hydrochloride (p.416·2).
Fever; pain.

Goldgestant *Searle, S.Afr.†.*
Chlorpheniramine maleate (p.405·1); phenylpropanolamine hydrochloride (p.1067·2); phenylephrine hydrochloride (p.1066·2).
Cold symptoms.

Gold-Komplex *Steigerwald, Ger.*
Homoeopathic preparation.

Goldtropfen N *DHU, Ger.*
Homoeopathic preparation.

Goldtropfen-Hetterich *Galenika, Ger.*
Crataegus (p.1568·2); valerian (p.1643·1); convallaria (p.1567·2); scoparium (p.1628·1); camphor (p.1557·2); gold chloride.
Cardiac disorders.

Golosan *Lifepharma, Ital.†.*
Dequalinium chloride (p.1112·1); menthol (p.1600·2); thymol (p.1127·1).
Mouth and throat inflammation.

GoLytely
Stafford-Miller, Austral.; Baxter, Canad.; Westermans, S.Afr.; Braintree, USA.
Macrogol 3350 (p.1598·2); electrolytes (p.1147·1).
Bowel evacuation.

Gomenol *Gomenol, Fr.*
Niaouli oil (p.1607·1).
Respiratory-tract disorders.

Gomenoleo *Gomenol, Fr.*
Niaouli oil (p.1607·1).
Burns; infections; ulcers; wounds.

Gomenol-Syner-Penicilline *Gomenol, Fr.*
Benzylpenicillin sodium (p.159·3); niaouli oil (p.1607·1).
Bacterial infections.

Gonacard *Mochida, Jpn†.*
Pregnancy test (p.1621·2).

Gonadoryl *Mochida, Jpn†.*
Menotrophin (p.1252·1).

Gonadotraphon LH
Paines & Byrne, Irl.; Ferring, UK†.
Chorionic gonadotrophin (p.1243·1).
Anovulatory infertility; delayed puberty, cryptorchidism, and oligospermia in the male.

Gonak *Akorn, USA.*
Hypromellose (p.1473·1).
Gonioscopic examination.

Gonal-F
Serono, Austr.; Serono, Fr.; Serono, Ger.; Serono, Irl.; Serono, Ital.; Serono, Neth.; Serono, Norw.; Serono, Swed.; Serono, Switz.; Serono, UK; Serono, USA.
Follitropin alfa (p.1247·1).
Anovulatory infertility; stimulation of ovulation.

Gonasi HP Amsa, Ital.
Chorionic gonadotrophin (p.1243·1).
Formerly known as Gonadotrafon LH.
Amenorrhoea; cryptorchidism; habitual abortion; hypogonadism; infertility; threatened abortion.

Gonavis Mochida, Jpn†.
Pregnancy test (p.1621·2).

Gonavislide
Sigma, Austral.†; Ames, S.Afr.
Pregnancy test (p.1621·2).

Gonic Hauck, USA.
Chorionic gonadotrophin (p.1243·1).
Male and female infertility; male hypogonadism; prepubertal cryptorchidism.

Gonioscopic Alcon, USA.
Hydroxyethylcellulose (p.1472·3).
Gonioscopic examination.

Goniosoft Ocusoft, USA.
Hypromellose (p.1473·1).

Goniosol Iolab, USA.
Hypromellose (p.1473·1).
Gonioscopic examination.

Gonne Balm Lane, UK.
Camphor (p.1557·2); menthol (p.1600·2); eucalyptus oil (p.1578·1); methyl salicylate (p.55·2); turpentine oil (p.1641·1).
Joint and muscular pain.

Gonoform Merckle, Aust.
Amoxycillin trihydrate (p.151·3).
Bacterial infections.

Goodnight Formula Vitaplex, Austral.
Valerian (p.1643·1); chamomile (p.1561·2); passion flower (p.1615·3); scutellaria; vitamin B substances; zinc sulphate (p.1373·2).
Insomnia.

Goody's Headache Powders Goodys, USA.
Aspirin (p.16·1); paracetamol (p.72·2); caffeine (p.749·3).

Go-Pain PD Pharm, S.Afr.
Syrup: Paracetamol (p.72·2); codeine phosphate (p.26·1); promethazine hydrochloride (p.416·2).
Fever; pain.
Tablets: Paracetamol (p.72·2); codeine phosphate (p.26·1); caffeine (p.749·3); meprobamate (p.678·1).
Pain with tension.

Goppilax Muller Goppingen, Ger.†.
Aloes (p.1177·1); cascara bark (p.1183·1); frangula bark (p.1193·2); senna leaves (p.1212·2).
Bowel evacuation; constipation.

Gopten
Knoll, Austral.; Knoll, Fr.; Knoll, Ger.; Knoll, Irl.; Knoll, Ital.; Knoll, Neth.; Knoll, S.Afr.; Knoll, Spain; Meda, Swed.; Knoll, Switz.; Knoll, UK.
Trandolapril (p.957·1).
Heart failure following myocardial infarction; hypertension.

Gordobalm Gordon, USA.
Methyl salicylate (p.55·2); menthol (p.1600·2); camphor (p.1557·2).
Muscle, joint, and soft-tissue pain; neuralgia.

Gordochom Gordon, USA.
Undecenoic acid (p.389·2); chloroxylenol (p.1111·1).
Fungal skin infections.

Gordofilm Gordon, USA.
Salicylic acid (p.1090·2).
Verrucas.

Gordogesic Gordon, USA.
Methyl salicylate (p.55·2).
Muscle, joint, and soft-tissue pain; neuralgia.

Gorgonium Drossapharm, Switz.
Heparin (p.879·3); allantoin (p.1078·2); dexpanthenol (p.1570·3); collagen (p.1566·3).
Scars.

Gormel Gordon, USA.
Urea (p.1095·2).
Dry skin; hyperkeratosis.

Gota Cebrina Derly, Spain.
Multivitamin preparation.

Gouttes aux Essences Plantes et Medecines, Fr.
Peppermint oil (p.1208·1); clove oil (p.1565·2); thyme oil (p.1637·1); cinnamon oil (p.1564·2); lavender oil (p.1594·3).
Respiratory-tract disorders.

Gouttes bile Wiedenmann, Switz.†.
Chelidonium; artichoke (p.1569·2); turmeric (p.1001·3).
Digestive system disorders.

Gouttes contre la toux "S" Synpharma, Switz.
Codeine phosphate (p.26·1); aromatic tincture; hyoscyamus (p.464·3); ipecacuanha (p.1062·2); drosera (p.1574·1); plantago lanceolata.
Coughs.

Gouttes Dentaires Valmo, Canad.
Benzocaine (p.1286·2); camphor (p.1557·2); guaiacol (p.1061·2); menthol (p.1600·2); clove oil (p.1565·2).

Gouttes homeopathiques contre le rhume des foins Phytomed, Switz.
Homoeopathic preparation.

Gouttes nasales Spirig, Switz.
Phenylephrine (p.1066·2).
Nasal congestion; rhinitis; sinusitis.

Gouttes nasales N Spirig, Switz.
Naphazoline nitrate (p.1064·2); phenylephrine (p.1066·2).
Nasal congestion; rhinitis; sinusitis.

Gouttes pour le coeur et les nerfs Concentrees Zeller, Switz.
Crataegus (p.1568·2); passion flower (p.1615·3).
Cardiac disorders; nervous disorders.

Gouttes pour Mal d'Orreilles Valmo, Canad.
Benzocaine (p.1286·2); camphor (p.1557·2); chlorbutol (p.1106·3).

Govil Stada, Ger.†.
Glyceryl trinitrate (p.874·3); pentaerythritol tetranitrate (p.927·3); nicotinic acid (p.1351·2); benzyl mandelate; phenobarbitone (p.350·2).
Cardiac disorders.

Goxil Pharmacia Upjohn, Spain.
Azithromycin (p.155·2).
Bacterial infections.

GP-500 Marnel, USA.
Pseudoephedrine hydrochloride (p.1068·3); guaiphenesin (p.1061·3).
Coughs.

Gracial
Organon, Aust.; Organon, Belg.; Organon, Switz.
Desogestrel (p.1443·3); ethinyloestradiol (p.1445·1).
Biphasic oral contraceptive.

Gradient Polifarma, Ital.
Flunarizine hydrochloride (p.411·1).
Migraine; vertigo.

Gradin Del D Andreu Roche Nicholas, Spain.
Benzalkonium chloride (p.1101·3); benzocaine (p.1286·2); tyrothricin (p.267·2).
Mouth and throat disorders.

Gradulon Ebewe, Aust.
Digoxin (p.849·3); verapamil hydrochloride (p.960·3).
Arrhythmias; heart failure; myocardial infarction.

Gradulon s. T. Minden, Ger.†.
Digoxin (p.849·3); verapamil hydrochloride (p.960·3).
Cardiovascular disorders.

Grafco VFZ, Switz.†.
Silver protein (p.1629·2); potassium nitrate (p.1123·1).
Verrucas; wounds.

Gragenil Reig Jofre, Spain.
Codeine phosphate (p.26·1); diphenhydramine hydrochloride (p.409·1); ephedrine hydrochloride (p.1059·3).
Cough; respiratory-tract disorders.

Grains de Vals
Note. This name is used for preparations of different composition.
Qualiphar, Belg.
Aloes (p.1177·1); belladonna (p.457·1); cascara (p.1183·1); frangula bark (p.1193·2); intestinal mucosa extract; ox bile extract (p.1553·2); phenolphthalein (p.1208·2).
Constipation.

Nogues, Fr.
Aloes (p.1177·1); belladonna (p.457·1); cascara (p.1183·1); frangula bark (p.1193·2); ox bile extract (p.1553·2).
Constipation.

Nogues, Switz.
Boldo (p.1554·1); cascara (p.1183·1); senna (p.1212·2).
Constipation.

Gral Boniscontro & Gazzone, Ital.
Dihydroergocristine mesylate (p.1571·3).
Cerebrovascular disorders; dopaminergic deficiency; headache; hypertension; migraine; peripheral vascular disorders.

Gram 2 Bergamon, Ital.†.
Didecyldimethylammonium chloride (p.1112·2).
Skin disinfection.

Gramaxin
Boehringer Mannheim, Aust.†; Boehringer Mannheim, Ger.
Cephazolin sodium (p.181·1).
Lignocaine hydrochloride (p.1293·2) is included in the intramuscular preparation to alleviate the pain of injection.
Bacterial infections.

Gramcal Sandoz, Canad.
Calcium lactate gluconate (p.1155·2); calcium carbonate (p.1182·1).
Calcium supplement; osteoporosis.

Gramcillina Caber, Ital.†.
Ampicillin (p.153·1).
Bacterial infections.

Gramicidin Andreu, Spain†.
Benzalkonium chloride (p.1101·3); benzocaine (p.1286·2); neomycin sulphate (p.229·2); tyrothricin (p.267·2).
Mouth and throat disorders.

Gramidil Leurquin, Fr.
Amoxycillin trihydrate (p.151·3).
Bacterial infections.

Graminflor
Adroka, Switz.
Bath additive: Hay flower.
Musculoskeletal and joint disorders.

Wolo, Switz.†.
Ointment: Hay flower; rosemary oil (p.1626·2); spike lavender oil (p.1632·2); thyme oil (p.1637·1); anise oil (p.1550·1).
Musculoskeletal disorders.

Gramipan Mayoly-Spindler, Switz.
Dequalinium chloride (p.1112·1); ascorbic acid (p.1365·2).
Mouth and throat infections.

Gram-Micina Lagap, Ital.†.
Fosfomycin calcium (p.210·2).
Bacterial infections.

Gramoce A Vir, Spain.
Ascorbic acid (p.1365·2); vitamin A (p.1358·1).
Deficiency of vitamins A and C.

Gramplus Chiesi, Ital.
Clofoctol (p.195·1).
Bacterial infections.

Gram-Val Polifarma, Ital.
Doxycycline hydrochloride (p.202·3).
Bacterial infections.

Gran Kirin, Jpn.
Filgrastim (p.723·1).
Neutropenia.

Granamon Norgine, Ger.
Sterculia (p.1214·1).
Constipation.

Grandaxin
EGIS, Hung.; Mochida, Jpn†.
Tofisopam (p.696·3).
Anxiety.

Grandelat eisen Grandel-Synpharma, Ger.†.
Ferrous aspartate (p.1339·2).
Iron-deficiency; iron-deficiency anaemias.

Grandelat magnesium Grandel-Synpharma, Ger.†.
Magnesium-amino acid chelate.
Magnesium deficiency.

Grandelat multimineral Grandel-Synpharma, Ger.†.
Mineral preparation.

Graneodin
Bristol-Myers Squibb, Austral.†; Bristol-Myers Squibb, Irl.; Squibb, UK.
Neomycin sulphate (p.229·2); gramicidin (p.215·2).
Bacterial infections of the skin and ear.

Graneodine Bristol-Myers Squibb, Belg.
Neomycin sulphate (p.229·2); gramicidin (p.215·2).
Skin infections.

Grani di Vals Geymonat, Ital.
Cascara (p.1183·1); aloes (p.1177·1); aloin (p.1177·2).
Constipation.

Granions Granions, Mon.
A range of mineral supplements.

Granobil Synpharma, Aust.
Fennel (p.1579·1); primula root; thyme leaf (p.1636·3).
Catarrh; coughs.

Granocol Schering, Austral.
Sterculia (p.1214·1); frangula bark (p.1193·2).
Constipation.

Granocyte
Rhone-Poulenc Rorer, Aust.; Amrad, Austral.; Rhone-Poulenc Rorer, Belg.; Bellon, Fr.; Rhone-Poulenc Rorer, Ger.; Rhone-Poulenc Rorer, Irl.; Rhone-Poulenc Rorer, Ital.; Rhone-Poulenc Rorer, Neth.; Rhone-Poulenc Rorer, Norw.; Rhone-Poulenc Rorer, Spain; Rhone-Poulenc Rorer, Swed.; Rhone-Poulenc Rorer, Switz.; Chugai, UK.
Lenograstim (p.724·3).
Mobilisation of autologous peripheral blood progenitor cells; reduction of neutropenia associated with cytotoxic therapy or bone marrow transplantation.

Granoleina SIFI, Ital.
dl-Alpha tocopheryl acetate (p.1369·2); linoleic acid (p.1582·1); vitamin A palmitate (p.1359·2); ergocalciferol (p.1367·1).
Vitamin deficiencies.

Granoton Grandel-Synpharma, Ger.
Tocopherol; tritici sativi e embryo; ethanol.
Tonic.

Granudoxy Pierre Fabre, Fr.
Doxycycline hydrochloride (p.202·3).
Bacterial infections.

Granufink Kurbiskern Fink, Ger.
Cucurbita (p.1569·1).
Urinary-tract disorders.

Granufink N Fink, Ger.
Cucurbita (p.1569·1); cucurbita oil.
Urinary-tract disorders.

Granuflex
Bristol-Myers Squibb, S.Afr.; ConvaTec, UK.
Hydrocolloid dressing.
Ulcers; wounds.

Granugen
Note. This name is used for preparations of different composition.
Knoll, Austral.
Paraffin oil (p.1382·1); zinc oxide (p.1096·2); titanium dioxide (p.1093·3); paraffin viscous; soft paraffin.
Minor wounds and ulcers.

Knoll, Ger.†.
Zinc oxide (p.1096·2); talc (p.1092·1); liquid paraffin (p.1382·1).
Skin disorders.

Granugenol Knoll, Ger.†.
Liquid paraffin (p.1382·1).
Skin disorders; vaginitis.

Granulderm Copley, USA.
Trypsin (p.1640·1); peru balsam (p.1617·2); castor oil (p.1560·2).
Wounds.

Granules Boribel Homeopathie Boribel, Fr.
A range of homoeopathic preparations.

Granulex Hickam, USA.
Trypsin (p.1640·1); peru balsam (p.1617·2); castor oil (p.1560·2).
Wound dressing.

Granulokine
Roche, Ital.; Pensa, Spain.
Filgrastim (p.723·1).
Neutropenia.

GranuMed Rugby, USA.
Trypsin (p.1640·1); peru balsam (p.1617·2); castor oil (p.1560·2).
Wounds.

Granvit Plants, Ital.
Royal jelly (p.1626·3) with wheat-germ oil, carrot oil, and soya lecithin.
Nutritional supplement.

Grasmin Berenguer Infale, Spain.
Fenproporex resinate (p.1481·3).
Obesity.

Gratusminal Daker Farmasimes, Spain.
Phenobarbitone diethylamine (p.351·3).
Epilepsy.

Gravergol Carter Horner, Canad.
Ergotamine tartrate (p.445·3); caffeine (p.749·3); dimenhydrinate (p.408·2).
Migraine and other vascular headaches.

Gravibinan
Schering, Fr.†; Schering, Ital.
Hydroxyprogesterone hexanoate (p.1448·1); oestradiol valerate (p.1455·2).
Habitual abortion; threatened abortion.

Gravibinon
Schering, Aust.; Schering, Ger.; Schering, Switz.†.
Hydroxyprogesterone hexanoate (p.1448·1); oestradiol valerate (p.1455·2).
Habitual or threatened abortion.

Gravidex Almirall, Spain.
Dinoprostone (p.1414·3).
Hydatidiform mole; labour induction; termination of pregnancy.

Gravigard SPA, Ital.
Copper-wound plastic (p.1337·3).
Intra-uterine contraceptive device.

Gravigen Byk Gulden, Ital.
Multivitamin and mineral preparation.

Gravindex Ortho Diagnostic, UK†.
Pregnancy test (p.1621·2).

Gravistat Jenapharm, Ger.
Ethinyloestradiol (p.1445·1); levonorgestrel (p.1454·1).
Combined oral contraceptive; menstrual disorders.

Gravitamon
Organon, Belg.†; Chefaro, Neth.†.
Multivitamin and mineral preparation.

Gravol Carter Horner, Canad.
Dimenhydrinate (p.408·2).
Nausea; vertigo; vomiting.

Green Antiseptic Mouthwash & Gargle Lee-Adams, Canad.
Alcohol (p.1099·1); cetylpyridinium chloride (p.1106·2).

Green Lipped Mussel Suisse, Austral.†.
Green-lipped mussel (p.1586·3); desert yucca; sea plants; bech de mer; devil's claw (p.27·2).
Adjuvant in arthritis.

Greenlife Formula Cantassium Co., UK†.
Multivitamin and mineral preparation.

Gregoderm Unigreg, UK.
Neomycin sulphate (p.229·2); polymyxin B sulphate (p.239·1); hydrocortisone (p.1043·3); nystatin (p.386·1).
Infected skin disorders.

Greosin Allen, Spain.
Griseofulvin (p.380·2).
Fungal skin and nail infections.

Gricin
Dresden, Ger.; LAW, Ger.
Griseofulvin (p.380·2).
Fungal skin infections.

Grietalgen Diviser Aquilea, Spain.
Peru balsam (p.1617·2); bismuth subnitrate (p.1180·2); ergocalciferol (p.1367·1); oestrone (p.1458·2); benzocaine (p.1286·2); retinol (p.1358·1).
Skin disorders.

Grietalgen Hidrocort Diviser Aquilea, Spain.
Bismuth subnitrate (p.1180·2); cholecalciferol (p.1366·3); oestrone (p.1458·2); benzocaine (p.1286·2); retinol (p.1358·1); hydrocortisone glycyrrhetinate (p.1044·2); neomycin sulphate (p.229·2).
Skin disorders.

Grifulvin V Ortho Dermatological, USA.
Griseofulvin (microsize) (p.380·2).
Fungal skin infections.

Grinal Hidrocortisona Zyma, Spain†.
Boric acid (p.1554·2); phenylmercuric borate; hydrocortisone acetate (p.1043·3); tuna-liver oil; talc; zinc oxide (p.1096·2).
Skin disorders.

Gripakin Fournier SA, Spain.
Chlorpheniramine maleate (p.405·1); paracetamol (p.72·2).
Cold symptoms; nasal congestion.

Gripalgine Pharmethic, Belg.
Aspirin (p.16·1); codeine phosphate (p.26·1); ascorbic acid (p.1365·2).
Fever; pain.

Gripavac *Pasteur Merieux, Spain.*
An influenza vaccine (p.1515·2).
Active immunisation.

Gripex *Lambda, USA.*
Guaiphenesin (p.1061·3); dextromethorphan hydrobromide (p.1057·3); phenylephrine hydrochloride (p.1066·2).
Coughs.

Grippal *Bayer, Spain.*
Aspirin (p.16·1); chlorpheniramine maleate (p.405·1); phenylpropanolamine (p.1067·2).
Influenza and cold symptoms; nasal congestion.

Grippalgine N *DP-Medica, Switz.*
Paracetamol (p.72·2); salicylamide (p.82·3); caffeine (p.749·3).
Cold and influenza symptoms.

Grippalin & C *Multi-Pro, Canad.*
Chlorpheniramine maleate (p.405·1); paracetamol (p.72·2); ascorbic acid (p.1365·2).

Grippefloran *Bioflora, Aust.*
Salix purpurea (p.82·3); tilia flower (p.1637·3); vitamin C (p.1365·2).
Cold symptoms.

Grippe-Gastreu R6 *Reckeweg, Ger.*
Homoeopathic preparation.

Grippetee Dr Zeidler *Apotheke Erzengel Michael, Aust.*
Tilia flower (p.1637·3); sambucus flower (p.1627·2); rose fruit (p.1365·2); thyme leaf (p.1636·3); drosera (p.1574·1).
Cold symptoms.

Grippetee EF-EM-ES *Smetana, Aust.*
Sambucus flower (p.1627·2); tilia flower (p.1637·3); plantago lanceolata.
Cold symptoms.

Grippe-Tee Stada *Stada, Ger.†.*
Paeonia officinalis; liquorice (p.1197·1); peppermint leaf (p.1208·1); verbascum flowers; chamomile (p.1561·2); meadowsweet (p.1599·1); tilia (p.1637·3); sambucus (p.1627·2); salix (p.82·3).
Cold symptoms; influenza.

Gripp-Heel *Heel, Ger.*
Homoeopathic preparation.

Grippin-Merz *Merz, Ger.*
Amantadine sulphate (p.1129·2).
Influenza A.

Grippinon *Nycomed, Aust.*
Aspirin (p.16·1); ascorbic acid (p.1365·2).
Cold symptoms.

Grippogran *Synpharma, Aust.*
Sambucus flower (p.1627·2); tilia flower (p.1637·3); centaury (p.1561·1).
Cold symptoms.

Grippon
Mer-National, S.Afr.
Capsules: Paracetamol (p.72·2); caffeine (p.749·3); ascorbic acid (p.1365·2); phenylephrine hydrochloride (p.1066·2); chlorpheniramine maleate (p.405·1).
Cold and influenza symptoms.

Mer-National, S.Afr.; Propan, S.Afr.
Syrup: Paracetamol (p.72·2); chlorpheniramine maleate (p.405·1); ephedrine (p.1059·3).
Cold and influenza symptoms.

Gripponyl *Pierre Fabre, Fr.†.*
Acetanilide (p.12·2); phenacetin (p.78·1); caffeine (p.749·3); theobromine (p.765·1); quinine sulphate (p.439·2); aconite (p.1542·2); belladonna (p.457·1); colchicine (p.393·1); Dover's powder; boldo (p.1554·1); kola (p.1645·1); cinchona (p.1564·1); calcium phosphate (p.1155·3).
Fever.

Grippostad
Stada, Ger.†.
DL-2-diethylaminoethyl-(2-cyclohexylbutyrate); diphenhydramine hydrochloride (p.409·1); caffeine (p.749·3); propyphenazone (p.81·3); salicylamide (p.82·3).
Cold symptoms.

Stada, Ger.
Paracetamol (p.72·2).
Cold symptoms; pain.

Grippostad C
Note. This name is used for preparations of different composition.
Stada, Ger.
Paracetamol (p.72·2); ascorbic acid (p.1365·2); caffeine (p.749·3); chlorpheniramine maleate (p.405·1).
Cold symptoms; influenza.

Stada, Switz.
Paracetamol (p.72·2); ascorbic acid (p.1365·2).
Cold symptoms.

Gripps *Pascoe, Ger.*
Homoeopathic preparation.

Grisactin *Wyeth-Ayerst, USA.*
Griseofulvin (microsize) (p.380·2).
Fungal skin infections.

Grisactin Ultra *Wyeth-Ayerst, USA.*
Griseofulvin (ultramicrosize) (p.380·2).
Fungal skin infections.

Grisefuline *Sanofi Winthrop, Fr.*
Griseofulvin (p.380·2).
Algodystrophies; fungal infections; Raynaud's syndrome.

Griseo *CT, Ger.*
Griseofulvin (p.380·2).
Fungal skin infections.

Griseoderm *Clonmel, Irl.†.*
Griseofulvin (p.380·2).
Fungal skin infections.

Griseomed *Waldheim, Aust.*
Griseofulvin (p.380·2).

Griseostatin *Schering-Plough, Austral.*
Griseofulvin (p.380·2).
Fungal infections of the skin and nails.

Grisetin *Lasa, Spain.*
Flutamide (p.537·1).
Prostatic cancer.

Grisol *Gebro, Switz.*
Griseofulvin (p.380·2).
Tinea pedis.

Grisovin
Glaxo Wellcome, Aust.; Sigma, Austral.; Roberts, Canad.; Glaxo Wellcome, S.Afr.†; Glaxo Wellcome, Swed.†; Glaxo Wellcome, Switz.†; Glaxo, UK.
Griseofulvin (p.380·2).
Fungal infections of the skin and nails.

Grisovina *Teofarma, Ital.*
Griseofulvin (p.380·2).
Fungal infections of the skin and nails.

Gris-PEG
Wander, Switz.†; Allergan Herbert, USA.
Griseofulvin (p.380·2).
Fungal infections.

Grocreme *Grossmann, Switz.†.*
Dequalinium chloride (p.1112·1).
Skin infections.

Grodurex *Grossmann, Switz.*
Hydrochlorothiazide (p.885·2); amiloride hydrochloride (p.819·2).
Hypertension; oedema.

Grofenac *Grossmann, Switz.*
Diclofenac sodium (p.31·2).
Gout; inflammation; musculoskeletal, joint, and periarticular disorders; pain.

Groliberin *Kabi, Swed.†.*
Sermorelin (p.1260·3).
Test for growth hormone secretion.

Gromazol *Grossmann, Switz.*
Clotrimazole (p.376·3).
Fungal foot infections.

Groprim *Grossmann, Switz.*
Co-trimoxazole (p.196·3).
Bacterial infections; blastomycosis; Pneumocystis carinii pneumonia.

Grorm
Serono, Ger.†; Serono, Ital.†.
Somatropin (p.1249·3).
Growth hormone deficiency.

Grotanat *Schulke & Mayr, Ger.*
Chlorocresol (p.1110·3); clorophene (p.1111·2); orthophenylphenol (p.1120·3).
Instrument disinfection.

Grovixim *Torlan, Spain.*
Carnitine chloride; cobamamide; cocarboxylase.
Tonic.

Gruncef *Grunenthal, Ger.*
Cefadroxil (p.163·3).
Bacterial infections.

Grune Nervensalbe *Doerr, Ger.†.*
Rosemary oil (p.1626·2); camphor baum oil; camphor (p.1557·2); chlorophyll (p.1000·1); pumilio pine oil (p.1623·3).
Nerve and joint pain.

Grune Salbe "Schmidt" N *Wider, Ger.*
Urea (p.1095·2); silver (p.1629·2); magnesium chloride (p.1157·2).
Ulcers; wounds.

Grunlicht Hingfong Essenz *Lichtenheldt, Ger.*
Peppermint oil (p.1208·1); anise oil (p.1550·1); cassia oil (p.1560·2); fennel oil (p.1579·2); rosemary oil (p.1626·2); thyme oil (p.1637·1); menthol (p.1600·2); camphor (p.1557·2); peppermint leaf (p.1208·1); bay leaf; arnica (p.1550·3); tilia (p.1637·3); chamomile (p.1561·2); aniseed (p.1549·3); fennel (p.1579·1); calamus (p.1556·1); valerian (p.1643·1).
Cold symptoms; nausea; nervous disorders; neuralgias; rheumatic disorders.

G.Test *Theranol-Deglaude, Fr.*
Pregnancy test (p.1621·2).

Guabeta N *OTW, Ger.†.*
Tolbutamide (p.333·2).
Diabetes mellitus.

Guafen *Agepha, Aust.*
Guaiphenesin (p.1061·3).
Catarrh; coughs.

guafrenon *Hefa, Ger.†.*
Guaiphenesin (p.1061·3).
Coughs.

Guaiacalcium Complex *Celsius, Ital.*
Dropropizine (p.1059·2); sodium benzoate (p.1102·3); calcium gluceptate (p.1155·1); potassium guaiacolsulfonate (p.1068·3); ephedrine hydrochloride (p.1059·3).
Respiratory-tract disorders.

Guaiadomus *Medici Domus, Ital.†.*
Guaiacol (p.1061·2); terpin hydrate (p.1070·2); ephedrine (p.1059·3); sodium benzoate (p.1102·3).
Respiratory disorders.

Guaiaspir *Lampugnani, Ital.*
Guacetisal (p.1061·2).
Respiratory disorders.

Guaifed *Muro, USA.*
Pseudoephedrine hydrochloride (p.1068·3); guaiphenesin (p.1061·3).
Coughs; nasal congestion.

Guaifed-PD *Muro, USA.*
Pseudoephedrine hydrochloride (p.1068·3); guaiphenesin (p.1061·3).
Coughs; nasal congestion.

Guaifenesin AC *Morton Grove, USA.*
Codeine phosphate (p.26·1); guaiphenesin (p.1061·3).

Guaifenesin DAC *Cypress, USA.*
Codeine phosphate (p.26·1); pseudoephedrine hydrochloride (p.1068·3); guaiphenesin (p.1061·3).
Coughs and associated respiratory-tract disorders.

Guaifenesin DM *Morton Grove, USA.*
Guaiphenesin (p.1061·3); dextromethorphan hydrobromide (p.1057·3).

Guaifenex *Ethex, USA.*
Guaiphenesin (p.1061·3); phenylpropanolamine hydrochloride (p.1067·2); phenylephrine hydrochloride (p.1066·2).
Coughs.

Guaifenex DM *Ethex, USA.*
Guaiphenesin (p.1061·3); dextromethorphan hydrobromide (p.1057·3).
Coughs.

Guaifenex LA *Ethex, USA.*
Guaiphenesin (p.1061·3).
Coughs.

Guaifenex PPA *Ethex, USA.*
Guaiphenesin (p.1061·3); phenylpropanolamine hydrochloride (p.1067·2).
Coughs.

Guaifenex PSE *Ethex, USA.*
Guaiphenesin (p.1061·3); pseudoephedrine hydrochloride (p.1068·3).
Coughs.

Guaifenex Rx *Ethex, USA.*
Blue tablets, guaiphenesin (p.1061·3); pseudoephedrine hydrochloride (p.1068·3); green tablets, guaiphenesin; dextromethorphan (p.1057·3).
Coughs.

Guaifenex Rx DM *Ethex, USA.*
Guaiphenesin (p.1061·3); pseudoephedrine hydrochloride (p.1068·3).
Coughs.

Guaimax-D *Schwarz, USA.*
Guaiphenesin (p.1061·3); pseudoephedrine hydrochloride (p.1068·3).
Coughs.

Guaipax *Eon, USA.*
Guaiphenesin (p.1061·3); phenylpropanolamine hydrochloride (p.1067·2).
Coughs.

Guaitab *Muro, USA.*
Guaiphenesin (p.1061·3); pseudoephedrine hydrochloride (p.1068·3).
Coughs; nasal congestion.

Guaivent *Ethex, USA.*
Guaiphenesin (p.1061·3); pseudoephedrine hydrochloride (p.1068·3).
Coughs.

Guai-Vent/PSE *Dura, USA.*
Guaiphenesin (p.1061·3); pseudoephedrine hydrochloride (p.1068·3).
Coughs.

Guajabronc *Molteni, Ital.*
Guacetisal (p.1061·2).
Respiratory disorders.

Guakalin *Stada, Ger.†.*
Oral drops: Ephedrine hydrochloride (p.1059·3); guaiphenesin (p.1061·3); camphor (p.1557·2); menthol (p.1600·2); anise oil (p.1550·1); primula root; fennel (p.1579·1); thyme (p.1636·3); wild thyme; castanea vulgaris; chamomile (p.1561·2).
Oral liquid: Guaiphenesin (p.1061·3); primula root; fennel (p.1579·1); thyme (p.1636·3); wild thyme; castanea vulgaris; chamomile (p.1561·2).
Respiratory-tract disorders.

Guanor *Rosemont, UK.*
Diphenhydramine hydrochloride (p.409·1); ammonium chloride (p.1055·2); sodium citrate (p.1153·2); menthol (p.1600·2).
Coughs.

Guar Verlan *Verla, Ger.*
Guar gum (p.321·3).
Diabetes mellitus; hyperlipidaemias.

Guarem
Stroschein, Ger.†; Rybar, Irl.; Orion, Switz.†; Shire, UK.
Guar gum (p.321·3).
Diabetes mellitus; hyperlipidaemias.

Guargel *Guidotti, Ital.†.*
Guar gum (p.321·3).
Constipation; diabetes mellitus; diverticulosis; hyperlipidaemias.

Guarina
Norgine, Austral.†; Norgine, UK†.
Guar gum (p.321·3).
Diabetes mellitus.

Guastil *Uriach, Spain.*
Sulpiride (p.692·3).
Psychoses; vertigo.

Guaxan *Boehringer Mannheim, Spain.*
Nimesulide (p.63·2).
Fever; inflammation; pain.

Guayaciclina *Novag, Spain†.*
Tetracycline guaiacolsulfonate.
Bacterial infections.

Gubamine *Gubler, Switz.*
Paracetamol (p.72·2); caffeine (p.749·3); propyphenazone (p.81·3).
Fever; pain.

Guethural *Elerte, Fr.*
Lozenges; oral granules: Guethol carbonate (p.1062·1).
Tablets: Guaietolin (p.1061·3).
Respiratory-tract congestion.

Gufen N *Steigerwald, Ger.*
Guaiphenesin (p.1061·3).
Respiratory-tract disorders.

GuiaCough CF *Schein, USA.*
Phenylpropanolamine hydrochloride (p.1067·2); dextromethorphan hydrobromide (p.1057·3); guaiphenesin (p.1061·3).
Coughs.

GuiaCough PE *Schein, USA.*
Pseudoephedrine hydrochloride (p.1068·3); guaiphenesin (p.1061·3).
Coughs.

Guiatex *Rugby, USA.*
Phenylephrine hydrochloride (p.1066·2); phenylpropanolamine hydrochloride (p.1067·2); guaiphenesin (p.1061·3).
Coughs.

Guiatex LA *Rugby, USA.*
Phenylpropanolamine hydrochloride (p.1067·2); guaiphenesin (p.1061·3).
Coughs.

Guiatex PSE *Rugby, USA.*
Pseudoephedrine hydrochloride (p.1068·3); guaiphenesin (p.1061·3).
Coughs.

Guiatuss CF *Barre-National, USA.*
Phenylpropanolamine hydrochloride (p.1067·2); dextromethorphan hydrobromide (p.1057·3); guaiphenesin (p.1061·3).
Coughs.

Guiatuss PE *Barre-National, USA.*
Pseudoephedrine hydrochloride (p.1068·3); guaiphenesin (p.1061·3).
Coughs.

Guiatussin with Codeine Expectorant *Rugby, USA.*
Codeine phosphate (p.26·1); guaiphenesin (p.1061·3).
Coughs.

Guiatussin DAC *Rugby, USA.*
Pseudoephedrine hydrochloride (p.1068·3); guaiphenesin (p.1061·3); codeine phosphate (p.26·1).
Coughs.

Guiatussin with Dextromethorphan *Rugby, USA.*
Dextromethorphan hydrobromide (p.1057·3); guaiphenesin (p.1061·3).
Coughs.

Gumbaral *Asta Medica, Ger.*
Ademetionine tosylate bis(sulphate) (p.1543·1).
Degenerative joint disorders.

Gumbix
Solvay, Aust.; Solvay, Ger.
Aminomethylbenzoic acid (p.711·2).
Haemorrhage.

Gum-Ese *McGloin, Austral.*
Lignocaine hydrochloride (p.1293·2); benzalkonium chloride (p.1101·3).
Mouth ulcers.

Gumilk *Diepal, Fr.*
Ceratonia (p.1472·2); maltodextrin (p.1350·2).
Regurgitation in infants.

Gunevax *Biocine, Ital.*
A rubella virus (Wistar RAA 27/3 strain) (p.1532·3).
Active immunisation.

Gurfix *Zyma, Aust.*
Hexetidine (p.1116·1).
Mouth and throat inflammation.

Gurgellosung-ratiopharm *Ratiopharm, Ger.*
Dequalinium chloride (p.1112·1).
Mouth and throat infections.

Guronamin *Chugai, Jpn.*
Glucuronamide.
Eclampsia; hyperbilirubinaemia; skin disorders; vomiting of pregnancy.

Guronsan
Note. This name is used for preparations of different composition.
Exel, Belg.; Lyocentre, Fr.
Glucuronamide; ascorbic acid (p.1365·2); caffeine (p.749·3).
Tonic.

Chugai, Jpn.
Glucurolactone or sodium glucuronate.
Eclampsia; hyperbilirubinaemia; skin disorders; vomiting of pregnancy.

Inibsa, Spain†.
Glucuronamide; ascorbic acid (p.1365·2).
Tonic.

Guronsan C *Lennon, S.Afr.†.*
Glucuronolactone; glucuronamide; ascorbic acid; caffeine.
Tonic.

Gustase *Geriatric Pharm. Corp., USA.*
Standardised amylolytic enzyme (Gerilase) (p.1549·1); standardised proteolytic enzyme (Geriprotase); standardised cellulolytic enzyme (Gericellulase) (p.1561·1).
Gastro-intestinal disorders.

Gustase Plus *Geriatric Pharm. Corp., USA.*
Phenobarbitone (p.350·2); homatropine methobromide (p.462·2); standardised amylolytic enzyme (Gerilase)

(p.1549·1); standardised proteolytic enzyme (Geriprotase); standardised cellulolytic enzyme (Gericellulase) (p.1561·1).
Gastro-intestinal disorders.

Gutalax *Fher, Spain.*
Sodium picosulphate (p.1213·2).
Constipation.

Gutnacht *Salushaus, Ger.*
Oral liquid: Valerian (p.1643·1); hypericum (p.1590·1); rosemary; melissa (p.1600·1); chamomile (p.1561·2); peppermint leaf (p.1208·1).
Tablets: Valerian (p.1643·1); passion flower (p.1615·3); lupulus (p.1597·2); hypericum (p.1590·1); melissa (p.1600·1); rhiz. jatamansi.
Nervousness; sleep disorders.

Gutron
Hafslund Nycomed, Aust.; Nycomed, Fr.; Nycomed, Ger.; Guidotti, Ital.; Nycomed, Switz.
Midodrine hydrochloride (p.910·1).
Ejaculation disorders; hypotension; urinary incontinence.

Guttacor *Galenika, Ger.*
Convallaria (p.1567·2); crataegus (p.1568·2); valerian (p.1643·1).
Cardiac disorders.

Guttacor-Balsam N *Galenika, Ger.*
Rosemary oil (p.1626·2); camphor (p.1557·2).
Guttacor-Balsam formerly contained crataegus, valerian, arnica, rosemary oil, mustard oil, menthol, bornyl valerate, and camphor.
Cardiovascular disorders.

Guttae 20 Hustentropfen N *Palmicol, Ger.*
Thyme (p.1636·3); wild thyme; primrose flower.
Catarrh; coughs.

Guttalax
Bender, Aust.; Wolfs, Belg.; Boehringer Ingelheim, Ital.; Byk, Switz.
Sodium picosulphate (p.1213·2).
Bowel evacuation; constipation; stool softener.

Guttaplast *Beiersdorf, Ger.*
Salicylic acid (p.1090·2).
Hyperkeratosis.

G-well *Goldline, USA.*
Lindane (p.1407·2).
Pediculosis; scabies.

GX *Pharmacia Upjohn, Ger.; Delta, Ger.; Serum-Werk Bernburg, Ger.*
Carbohydrate infusion.
Parenteral nutrition.

GX E *Pharmacia Upjohn, Ger.; Delta, Ger.*
Carbohydrate and electrolyte infusion.
Parenteral nutrition.

Gyan *Loves, Ger.†.*
Salicylic acid (p.1090·2).
Vaginitis.

Gynaedron *Cassella-med, Ger.†.*
Sulphanilamide (p.256·3); chlorphenesin (p.376·2).
Vaginitis.

Gynasan *Bastian, Ger.*
Oestriol (p.1457·2).
Oestrogenic.

Gynasol *Wild, Switz.*
Tartaric acid (p.1634·3); aluminium lactate (p.1548·1); aluminium sulphate (p.1548·1); anhydrous glucose (p.1343·3); sodium bicarbonate (p.1153·2).
Vaginal disorders.

Gynatren *Strathmann, Ger.*
A trichomonal vaccine (p.1536·3).

Gynecort *Combe, USA.*
Hydrocortisone acetate (p.1043·3).
Skin disorders.

Gynecrise *Bouteille, Fr.†.*
Ovary extract (p.1458·2).
Ovarian-hormone deficiency.

Gynecure *Pfizer, Canad.*
Tioconazole (p.388·3).
Vulvovaginal candidiasis.

Gynedron *Noristan, S.Afr.†.*
Sulphasomidine (p.257·1); borax (p.1554·2).
Vaginal infections.

Gynefix *Family Planning Sales, UK.*
Copper beads (p.1337·3).
Intra-uterine contraceptive device.

Gynegella *Guieu, Ital.†.*
Salicaria; whey.
Vaginal douche.

Gynegella P *Guieu, Ital.*
Salicaria; α-ketoglutaric acid.
Vaginal douche.

Gyne-Lotrimin
Schering-Plough, Austral.; Schering-Plough, USA.
Clotrimazole (p.376·3).
Vulvovaginal candidiasis.

Gyne-Moistrin
Schering-Plough, Canad.; Schering-Plough, USA†.
Polyglyceryl methacrylate; propylene glycol (p.1622·1).
Vaginal dryness.

Gynera *Schering, Switz.*
Gestodene (p.1447·2); ethinyloestradiol (p.1445·1).
Combined oral contraceptive.

Gynergen
Sandoz, Canad.†; Sandoz, Ger.†; Sandoz, Ital.†.
Ergotamine tartrate (p.445·3).
Migraine.

Gynergene Cafeine *Sandoz, Fr.*
Ergotamine tartrate (p.445·3); caffeine (p.749·3).
Migraine.

Gynergeno *Sandoz, Spain†.*
Ergotamine tartrate (p.445·3).
Glaucoma; migraine; neurocirculatory disorders; ocular herpes zoster; orthostatic hypotension; ozaena; tachycardia; uterine bleeding; uterine hypotonicity.

Gynescal *CCD, Fr.*
Paraformaldehyde (p.1121·1); salicylic acid (p.1090·2); benzoic acid (p.1102·3); borax (p.1554·2); sodium bicarbonate (p.1153·2).
Topical antiseptic.

Gynestrel *Recordati, Ital.*
Naproxen sodium (p.61·2).
Gynaecological disorders.

Gyne-Sulf *G & W, USA.*
Sulphathiazole (p.257·1); sulphacetamide (p.252·2); sulfabenzamide (p.251·1).
Vaginitis due to Gardnerella vaginalis.

Gyne-T
Janssen-Ortho, Canad.; Janssen-Cilag, Fr.; Janssen-Cilag, Ger.; Janssen-Cilag, Neth.
Copper-wound plastic (p.1337·3).
Intra-uterine contraceptive device.

Gynezol *Parke-Med, S.Afr.*
Clotrimazole (p.376·3).
Vaginal fungal infections.

Gyn-Hydralin *Nicholas, Fr.*
Glycine (p.1345·2).
Pruritus.

Gynintim Film *Piette, Belg.*
Nonoxinol 9 (p.1326·1).
Contraceptive.

Gynipral
Hafslund Nycomed, Aust.; Nycomed, Switz.
Hexoprenaline sulphate (p.754·1).
Premature labour.

Gyno Oceral *Asta Medica, Aust.*
Oxiconazole nitrate (p.386·3).
Fungal and Gram-positive vaginal infections.

Gyno-Canesten
Bayer, Ger.; Bayer, Ital.
Clotrimazole (p.376·3).
Balanitis; fungal vulvovaginal infections.

Gyno-Canestene *Bayer, Belg.*
Clotrimazole (p.376·3).
Vulvovaginal candidiasis.

Gynocastus *Zilly, Ger.*
Vitex agnus castus (p.1544·2).
Menstrual disorders.

Gyno-Daktar *Janssen-Cilag, Ger.*
Miconazole nitrate (p.384·3).
Balanitis; fungal vaginal infections.

Gyno-Daktarin
Janssen-Cilag, Aust.; Janssen-Cilag, Austral.; Janssen, Belg.; Janssen-Cilag, Fr.; Janssen-Cilag, Irl.; Janssen-Cilag, Neth.; Janssen-Cilag, S.Afr.; Janssen-Cilag, UK.
Miconazole nitrate (p.384·3).
Vaginal candidiasis and superinfection with Gram-positive bacteria.

Gynodian *Schering, Aust.*
Prasterone enanthate (p.1455·2); oestradiol valerate (p.1459·2).
Menopausal disorders.

Gynodian Depot
Schering, Ger.; Schering, Ital.; Schering, Spain; Schering, Switz.
Oestradiol valerate (p.1455·2); prasterone enanthate (p.1459·2).
Menopausal disorders.

Gynoflor
Pharmacia Upjohn, Aust.; Prospa, Belg.; Nourypharma, Ger.
Lactobacillus acidophilus (p.1594·1); oestriol (p.1457·2).
Vaginal disorders.

Gynoflor E *Medinova, Switz.*
Lactobacillus acidophilus (p.1594·1); oestriol (p.1457·2).
Restoration of vaginal flora; vaginal disorders.

Gynofug *Wolff, Ger.*
Ibuprofen (p.44·1).
Fever; inflammation; pain.

Gynogella *Searle, Switz.†.*
Lactic acid (p.1593·3); milk serum; sage (p.1627·1); α-ketoglutaric acid.
Vaginal disorders.

Gynogen *Forest Pharmaceuticals, USA†.*
Oestradiol valerate (p.1455·2).
Female castration; female hypogonadism; menopausal vasomotor symptoms; prevention of breast engorgement; primary ovarian failure; prostatic cancer; vulval and vaginal atrophy.

Gynokadin *Kade, Ger.*
Oestradiol valerate (p.1455·2).
Menopausal disorders.

Gynol *Ortho Pharmaceutical, USA.*
Nonoxinol 9 (p.1326·1).
Contraceptive.

Gynol II
Janssen-Cilag, Irl.; Cilag, UK.
Nonoxinol 9 (p.1326·1).
Contraceptive.

Gyno-Liderman *Jacoby, Aust.*
Oxiconazole nitrate (p.386·3).
Fungal and Gram-positive vaginal infections.

Gyno-Monistat *Janssen-Cilag, Ger.*
Miconazole nitrate (p.384·3).
Balanitis; fungal vaginal infections.

Gyno-Montril *Prospa, Belg.†.*
Mepartricin sodium lauryl sulphate (p.384·2).
Fungal vulvovaginal infections.

Gyno-Myfungar *Klinge, Switz.*
Oxiconazole nitrate (p.386·3).
Vaginal infections.

Gynomyk
Will-Pharma, Belg.; Cassenne, Fr.; Will-Pharma, Neth.
Butoconazole nitrate (p.376·1).
Fungal vulvovaginal infections.

Gyno-Mykotral *Rosen, Ger.*
Miconazole nitrate (p.384·3).
Fungal infections.

Gyno-Pevaryl
Janssen-Cilag, Aust.; Janssen-Cilag, Belg.; Janssen-Cilag, Fr.; Janssen-Cilag, Ger.; Janssen-Cilag, Irl.; Roche, S.Afr.; Pensa, Spain; Janssen-Cilag, Switz.; Cilag, UK.
Econazole nitrate (p.377·2).
Fungal balanitis; fungal vulvovaginal infections.

Gynophase *Schering, Fr.†.*
Norethisterone acetate (p.1453·1); ethinyloestradiol (p.1445·1).
Combined oral contraceptive; dysmenorrhoea.

Gynoplix *Doms-Adrian, Fr.†.*
Acetarsol (p.578·2); boric acid (p.1554·2).
Trichomoniasis.

Gynoplix Theraplix *Vaillant, Ital.*
Acetarsol (p.578·2).
Vaginal dryness.

Gynospasmine *Synthelabo, Fr.*
Paracetamol (p.72·2).
Fever; pain.

Gynospor *Garec, S.Afr.*
Miconazole nitrate (p.384·3).
Vaginal fungal infections.

Gynosyl *Homberger, Switz.*
Homoeopathic preparation.

Gyno-Tardyferon *Robapharm, Switz.*
Ferrous sulphate (p.1340·2); folic acid (p.1340·3); mucoproteose.
Iron and folic acid deficiency; iron-deficiency anaemia.

Gyno-Terazol
Janssen-Cilag, Belg.; Janssen-Cilag, Neth.; Janssen-Cilag, Switz.
Terconazole (p.388·2).
Fungal vulvovaginal infections.

Gynotherax *Bouchard, Fr.†.*
Chlorquinaldol (p.185·1).
Vaginal infections.

Gyno-Travogen
Schering, Aust.; Schering, Austral.†; Schering, Belg.; Schering, Irl.†; Schering, Neth.†; Schering, S.Afr.†; Schering, Switz.
Isoconazole nitrate (p.381·2).
Fungal and Gram-positive vaginal infections.

Gyno-Trosyd
Pfizer, Aust.; Pfizer, Canad.†; Pfizer, Fr.; Pfizer, S.Afr.; Pfizer, Switz.
Tioconazole (p.388·3).
Fungal vaginal infections; vaginal trichomoniasis.

Gynovin
Schering, Aust.; Schering, Spain.
Ethinyloestradiol (p.1445·1); gestodene (p.1447·2).
Combined oral contraceptive.

Gynovite Plus *Optimox, USA.*
Multivitamin and mineral preparation with iron and folic acid.

Gynovlane *Schering, Fr.†.*
Norethisterone acetate (p.1453·1); ethinyloestradiol (p.1445·1).
Combined oral contraceptive; dysmenorrhoea.

Gypsona *Smith & Nephew, Fr.†.*
Dried calcium sulphate (p.1557·2).
External splinting.

Gyramid
Parke, Davis, Aust.; Parke, Davis, Ger.†.
Enoxacin (p.203·3).
Bacterial infections.

H 1 *Esoform, Ital.*
Glutaraldehyde (p.1114·3).
Instrument disinfection.

H 2 Blocker *Ratiopharm, Ger.*
Cimetidine (p.1183·2) or cimetidine hydrochloride (p.1185·3).
Aspiration syndromes; gastro-intestinal haemorrhage; gastro-oesophageal reflux; hypersensitivity reactions; peptic ulcer; Zollinger-Ellison syndrome.

H_2 Oxyl *Stiefel, Ger.†.*
Benzoyl peroxide (p.1079·2).
Acne.

H Tussan *Inibsa, Spain.*
Anise oil (p.1550·1); hedera helix; thyme oil (p.1637·1).
Coughs.

Habekacin *Meiji, Jpn.*
Arbekacin sulphate (p.154·3).
Staphylococcal infections.

Habitrol
Ciba, Canad.; Basel, USA.
Nicotine (p.1607·2).
Aid to smoking withdrawal.

Habstal-Cor N *Steierl, Ger.*
Homoeopathic preparation.

Habstal-Nerv N *Steierl, Ger.*
Passion flower (p.1615·3); valerian root (p.1643·1).
Insomnia; nervous disorders.

Habstal-Pulm N *Steierl, Ger.*
Homoeopathic preparation.

HAC *Zeneca, Belg.*
Cetrimonium bromide (p.1106·1); chlorhexidine gluconate (p.1107·2).
Burns; disinfection of skin, instruments, textiles, and surfaces; wounds.

Hacdil-S *Zeneca, Belg.*
Cetrimonium bromide (p.1106·1); chlorhexidine gluconate (p.1107·2).
Disinfection of wounds and instruments.

Hachemina Fuerte *Medea, Spain.*
Aminobenzoic acid (p.1486·3).
Skin disorders.

Hacko-Kloster-Krautertee *Klever, Ger.†.*
Liquorice (p.1197·1); saponaria; senna (p.1212·2); parietaria officinalis; melissa (p.1600·1); peppermint leaf (p.1208·1); frangula bark (p.1193·2); fennel (p.1579·1); coriander (p.1567·3); viola tricolor; sassafras.
Herbal tea.

Hadensa
Kolassa, Aust.; Ferrer, Spain.
Chlorocarvacrol; ichthammol (p.1083·3); menthol (p.1600·2).
Anorectal disorders.

Kolassa, Aust.
Suppositories: Chlorocarvacrol; ichthammol (p.1083·3); chamomile oil; menthol (p.1600·2).
Anorectal disorders.

Hadiel *Piam, Ital.*
Bezafibrate (p.1268·2).
Hyperlipidaemias.

H-Adiftal *ISM, Ital.*
An adsorbed diphtheria vaccine (p.1507·3).
Active immunisation.

H-Adiftetal *ISM, Ital.*
An adsorbed diphtheria and tetanus vaccine (p.1508·1).
Active immunisation.

Haelan
Dista, Irl.; Dista, UK.
Flurandrenolone (p.1042·2).
Skin disorders.

Haelan-C *Dista, UK†.*
Flurandrenolone (p.1042·2); clioquinol (p.193·2).
Infected skin disorders.

Haemaccel
Hoechst, Aust.; Hoechst Marion Roussel, Austral.; Hoechst Marion Roussel, Belg.; Hoechst, Fr.; Asid Bonz, Ger.; Hoechst Marion Roussel, Irl.; Behring, Neth.; Behring, Norw.; Hoechst Marion Roussel, S.Afr.; Hoechst Marion Roussel, Swed.; Centeon, Switz.; Hoechst Marion Roussel, UK.
Polygeline (p.727·1) with electrolytes.
Extracorporeal circulation; organ perfusion; plasma exchange; plasma volume expansion.

Haemanal *Sigmapharm, Aust.*
Hydrastinine hydrochloride; chlorocarvacrol; zinc oxide (p.1096·2); tannic acid (p.1634·2); menthol (p.1600·2).
Anorectal disorders.

Haemate
Centeon, Ger.; Centeon, Ital.; Centeon, Neth.; Hoechst, Spain†; Centeon, Swed.; Centeon, Switz.; Centeon, UK.
A factor VIII preparation (p.720·3).
Haemorrhagic disorders.

Haematicum Glausch *Terramin, Aust.*
Iron; manganese.
Tonic.

Haemiton *Dresden, Ger.*
Clonidine hydrochloride (p.841·2).
Hypertension.

Haemiton compositum *Dresden, Ger.*
Clonidine hydrochloride (p.841·2); triamterene (p.957·2); hydrochlorothiazide (p.885·2).
Hypertension.

Haemiton-Augentropfen *ankerpharm, Ger.†.*
Clonidine hydrochloride (p.841·2).
Glaucoma.

Haemo Duoform *Mauermann, Ger.*
Hamamelis leaves (p.1587·1).
Haemorrhoids.

Haemocomplettan
Centeon, Aust.; Centeon, Ger.; Centeon, Switz.
Fibrinogen (p.722·3).
Haemorrhagic disorders; hypofibrinogenaemia.

Haemocomplettan P *Centeon, UK.*
Fibrinogen (p.722·3).
Fibrinogen disorders.

Haemocortin *Streuli, Switz.*
Ointment: Hydrocortisone acetate (p.1043·3); bismuth oxychloride (p.1181·1); lignocaine hydrochloride (p.1293·2); zinc oxide (p.1096·2).
Suppositories: Hydrocortisone acetate (p.1043·3); bismuth oxychloride (p.1181·1); lignocaine hydrochloride (p.1293·2); zinc oxide (p.1096·2); ethacridine lactate (p.1098·3); menthol (p.1600·2); adrenaline hydrochloride (p.813·3); hamamelis (p.1587·1); peru balsam (p.1617·2).
Anorectal disorders.

Haemoctin SDH *Biotest, Ger.*
A factor VIII preparation (p.720·3).
Haemorrhagic disorders.

Haemodyn *Klinge, Aust.*
Oxpentifylline (p.925·3).
Peripheral vascular disorders.

HAEMO-Exhirud *Sanofi Winthrop, Ger.*
Leech extract (p.897·2); allantoin (p.1078·2); laureth 9 (p.1325·2).
Anorectal disorders; urogenital venous disorders.

Haemofusin *Pharmacia Upjohn, Ger.*
Pentastarch (p.725·2) in sodium chloride.
Plasma volume expansion.

Haemoglukotest 20-800
Boehringer Mannheim, Ital.; Boehringer Mannheim, S.Afr.
Test for glucose in blood (p.1585·1).

Haemolan *Streuli, Switz.*
Ointment: Lignocaine hydrochloride (p.1293·2); bismuth oxychloride (p.1181·1); zinc oxide (p.1096·2); menthol (p.1600·2); peru balsam (p.1617·2).
Suppositories: Lignocaine hydrochloride (p.1293·2); bismuth oxychloride (p.1181·1); zinc oxide (p.1096·2); menthol (p.1600·2); peru balsam (p.1617·2); ethacridine lactate (p.1098·3); ephedrine hydrochloride (p.1059·3); hamamelis (p.1587·1).
Anorectal disorders.

Haemomac *CT, Ger.*
Bufexamac (p.22·2); lignocaine hydrochloride (p.1293·2); bismuth subgallate (p.1180·2); titanium dioxide (p.1093·3).
Haemorrhoids.

Haemonase P *SA Druggists Self Med, S.Afr.†.*
Bromelains (p.1555·1); *dl*-alpha tocopheryl acetate (p.1369·2).
Anorectal disorders; inflammation; oedema.

Haemoprotect *Brenner-Efeka, Ger.*
Ferrous sulphate (p.1340·2).
Iron deficiency; iron-deficiency anaemia.

Haemo-Red Formula *Eagle, Austral.*
Multivitamin and mineral preparation with yellow dock and nettle.

Haemorrhoid Cream *Nelson, UK.*
Homoeopathic preparation.

Haemosolvate *NBI, S.Afr.*
Factor VIII (p.720·3).
Factor VIII deficiency.

Haemosolvex *NBI, S.Afr.*
Factor IX (p.721·3).
Coagulation disorders.

Haemovex *Hospamed, Swed.*
Electrolytes; glucose (p.1151·1).
Haemofiltration.

Haemovital *Pharmadass, UK.*
Vitamin, mineral, and nutritional preparation.

Haenal *Strathmann, Ger.*
Dimethisoquin hydrochloride (p.1292·2).
Anorectal disorders; insect stings.

HAES *Leopold, Aust.*
Pentastarch (p.725·2).
Haemodilution; plasma volume expansion; shock.

HAES-steril
Fresenius, Belg.; Fresenius, Ger.; Fresenius, Norw.; Intramed, S.Afr.; Meda, Swed.; Fresenius, Switz.; Fresenius, UK.
Pentastarch (p.725·2) in sodium chloride.
Haemodilution; plasma volume expansion; shock.

Haimabig *ISI, Ital.*
A hepatitis B immunoglobulin (p.1512·3).
Passive immunisation.

Haima-D *ISI, Ital.*
An anti-D immunoglobulin (p.1503·2).
Prevention of rhesus sensitisation.

Haimaferone *ISI, Ital.*
Interferon alfa (p.615·3).
Malignant neoplasms; viral infections.

Haimagamma *Aima, Ital.†.*
A normal immunoglobulin (p.1522·1).
Agammaglobulinaemia; hypogammaglobulinaemia; passive immunisation.

Haima-Morbil *Aima, Ital.†.*
A measles immunoglobulin (p.1517·3).
Passive immunisation.

Haima-Parot *ISI, Ital.*
A mumps immunoglobulin (p.1521·2).
Passive immunisation.

Haimapertus *ISI, Ital.*
A pertussis immunoglobulin (p.1525·3).
Passive immunisation.

Haimaplex *Aima, Ital.†.*
Factor IX (p.721·3).
Blood-clotting factor deficiencies.

Haimarab *ISI, Ital.*
A rabies immunoglobulin (p.1530·2).
Passive immunisation.

Haimaros *Aima, Ital.†.*
A rubella immunoglobulin (p.1532·3).
Passive immunisation.

Haimaserum *ISI, Ital.*
Plasma protein fraction (p.726·3).
Hypoproteinaemia; hypovolaemia.

Haima-Tetanus *ISI, Ital.*
A tetanus immunoglobulin (p.1535·2).
Passive immunisation.

Haimaven *ISI, Ital.*
A normal immunoglobulin (p.1522·1).
Idiopathic thrombocytopenic purpura; immunodeficiency; passive immunisation.

4 Hair *Marlyn, USA.*
Multivitamin, mineral, and amino-acid preparation.

Hair Booster *Nature's Bounty, USA.*
Vitamin B substances with minerals, iron, and folic acid.

Hair and Nail Formula *Suisse, Austral.†.*
Equisetum (p.1575·1); silicon dioxide (p.1474·3); calcium salts (p.1155·1); magnesium (p.1157·2).
Tonic.

Hair Nutrition *Cantassium Co., UK.*
Multivitamin and mineral preparation.

Hair and Scalp *ICN, Canad.*
Pyrithione zinc (p.1089·3).
Medicated lotion.

Hair and Skin Formula *Vitaplex, Austral.*
Calcium pantothenate (p.1352·3); inositol (p.1591·1); aminobenzoic acid (p.1486·3); ascorbic acid (p.1365·2); *dl*-alpha tocopheryl acetate (p.1369·2).
Multivitamin preparation.

Hair-vit *Pharmadass, UK.*
Multivitamin, mineral, and trace element preparation.

HAL *Delta, Aust.†.*
Allergen extracts (p.1545·1).
Hyposensitisation.

Halamid
Note. This name is used for preparations of different composition.
Asta Medica, Ger.
Nedocromil sodium (p.756·2).
Obstructive airways disease.

Dox-Al, Ital.†.
Chloramine (p.1106·3).
Disinfection of skin, wounds, instruments, and surfaces.

Halbmond *Much, Ger.*
Diphenhydramine hydrochloride (p.409·1).
Sleep disorders.

Halcicomb *Westwood-Squibb, Canad.†.*
Halcinonide (p.1043·2); nystatin (p.386·1); neomycin sulphate (p.229·2).
Infected skin disorders.

Halciderm
Note. This name is used for preparations of different composition.
Bristol-Myers Squibb, Austral.; Bristol-Myers Squibb, Ital.; Squibb, Neth.†; Squibb, Switz.†; Squibb, UK.
Halcinonide (p.1043·2).
Skin disorders.

Bristol-Myers Squibb, Ital.; Squibb, Switz.†.
Tincture: Halcinonide (p.1043·2); benzoxonium chloride (p.1103·3); salicylic acid (p.1090·2).
Skin disorders.

Halciderm Combi *Bristol-Myers Squibb, Ital.*
Halcinonide (p.1043·2); neomycin sulphate (p.229·2); nystatin (p.386·1).
Infected skin disorders.

Halciderm comp *Squibb, Switz.†.*
Halcinonide (p.1043·2); nystatin (p.386·1); neomycin (p.229·2).
Infected skin disorders.

Halcimat *Bristol-Myers Squibb, Ger.†.*
Halcinonide (p.1043·2).
Skin disorders.

Halcion
Pharmacia Upjohn, Aust.; Pharmacia Upjohn, Austral.; Pharmacia Upjohn, Belg.; Pharmacia Upjohn, Canad.; Pharmacia Upjohn, Fr.; Pharmacia Upjohn, Ger.; Pharmacia Upjohn, Irl.; Pharmacia Upjohn, Ital.; Pharmacia Upjohn, Neth.; Pharmacia Upjohn, S.Afr.; Upjohn, Spain; Pharmacia Upjohn, Swed.; Pharmacia Upjohn, Switz.; Upjohn, USA.
Triazolam (p.696·3).
Insomnia.

Haldol
Janssen-Cilag, Aust.; Janssen-Cilag, Austral.; Janssen-Cilag, Belg.; Janssen-Ortho, Canad.; Janssen-Cilag, Fr.; Janssen-Cilag, Ger.; Janssen-Cilag, Irl.; Janssen-Cilag, Ital.; Janssen-Cilag, Neth.; Janssen-Cilag, Norw.; Janssen-Cilag, Swed.; Janssen-Cilag, Switz.; Janssen, UK; McNeil Pharmaceutical, USA.
Haloperidol (p.673·3), haloperidol decanoate (p.673·3), or haloperidol lactate (p.674·2).
Alcohol withdrawal syndrome; childhood behaviour disorders; extrapyramidal disorders; hyperkinesias; intractable hiccup; motor tics; nausea; pain; psychoses; psychosomatic symptoms; stuttering; Tourette syndrome; vomiting.

Haldrone *Lilly, USA†.*
Paramethasone acetate (p.1047·3).

Halenol *Halsey, USA.*
Paracetamol (p.72·2).
Fever; pain.

Haley's M-O *Sterling Health, USA.*
Magnesium hydroxide (p.1198·2); liquid paraffin (p.1382·1).
Constipation.

Half Betadur CR *Monmouth, UK.*
Propranolol hydrochloride (p.937·1).

Half Beta-Prograne *Tillomed, UK.*
Propranolol hydrochloride (p.937·1).
Angina pectoris; anxiety; essential tremor; hyperthyroidism; migraine; prophylaxis of gastro-intestinal bleeding.

Half Inderal
Zeneca, Irl.; Zeneca, UK.
Propranolol hydrochloride (p.937·1).
Angina pectoris; anxiety; essential tremor; hypertension; hyperthyroidism; migraine; myocardial infarction; upper gastro-intestinal haemorrhage.

Half Securon *Knoll, UK.*
Verapamil hydrochloride (p.960·3).
Angina pectoris; hypertension; myocardial infarction.

Half Sinemet
Du Pont, Irl.; Du Pont Pharmaceuticals, UK.
Levodopa (p.1137·1); carbidopa (p.1136·1).
These ingredients can be described by the British Approved Name Co-careldopa.
Parkinsonism.

Halfan
SmithKline Beecham, Aust.; SK-RIT, Belg.; SmithKline Beecham, Fr.; SmithKline Beecham, Ger.; SmithKline Beecham, Neth.; SmithKline Beecham, S.Afr.; Smith Kline & French, Spain; SmithKline Beecham, Switz.; SmithKline Beecham, UK; SmithKline Beecham, USA.
Halofantrine hydrochloride (p.430·3).
Malaria.

Halfprin *Kramer, USA.*
Aspirin (p.16·1).
Fever; inflammation; myocardial infarction; pain; transient ischaemic attacks.

Haliborange
Boots, Austral.†; Eurospital, Ital.; Glaxo Wellcome, S.Afr.†; Inibsa, Spain; Seven Seas, UK.
Vitamins A, C, and D.

Halibut
Note. This name is used for preparations of different composition.
Zyma, Spain.
Benzethonium chloride (p.1102·3); retinol (p.1358·1); zinc oxide (p.1096·2).
Skin disorders.

Adroka, Switz.
Halibut-liver oil (p.1345·3).
Tonic; vitamin A and D deficiency.

Halibut Hidrocortisona *Zyma, Spain.*
Hydrocortisone acetate (p.1043·3); retinol (p.1358·1); zinc oxide (p.1096·2); benzethonium chloride (p.1102·3).
Insect bites; skin disorders.

Halibut Multivit *Adroka, Switz.†.*
Halibut-liver oil with multivitamins.

Halicar *DHU, Ger.*
Homoeopathic preparation.

Halitol *Septa, Spain.*
Amoxycillin trihydrate (p.151·3).
Bacterial infections.

Halitran *Roche Nicholas, Neth.*
Retinol (p.1358·1); cholecalciferol (p.1366·3).
Vitamin A and D deficiency.

Halivite *Whitehall, Fr.*
Cod-liver oil (p.1337·3); vitamin A palmitate (p.1359·2); zinc oxide (p.1096·2).
Skin disorders.

Halivol *Warner-Lambert, Austral.*
Retinol; ergocalciferol (p.1367·1).
Vitamin A and D deficiency.

Halloo-Wach N *Roland, Ger.*
Caffeine (p.749·3); glucose monohydrate.
Fatigue.

Halls *Adams, Canad.*
Eucalyptus oil (p.1578·1); menthol (p.1600·2).
Coughs; nasal congestion.

Hall's Sugar Free Mentho-Lyptus *Warner-Lambert, USA.*
Menthol (p.1600·2); eucalyptus oil (p.1578·1).
Sore throats.

Halls Zinc Defense *Warner-Lambert, USA.*
Zinc acetate (p.1646·2).
Zinc supplement.

Halls-Plus Maximum Strength *Warner-Lambert, USA.*
Menthol (p.1600·2).

Halofed *Halsey, USA.*
Pseudoephedrine hydrochloride (p.1068·3).
Nasal congestion.

Halog
Bristol-Myers Squibb, Aust.; Westwood-Squibb, Canad.; Bristol-Myers Squibb, Fr.; Bristol-Myers Squibb, Ger.; Bristol-Myers Squibb, Norw.; Squibb, Spain; Westwood-Squibb, USA.
Halcinonide (p.1043·2).
Skin disorders.

Halog Neomycine *Bristol-Myers Squibb, Fr.*
Halcinonide (p.1043·2); neomycin sulphate (p.229·2).
Infected skin disorders.

Halog Tri *Bristol-Myers Squibb, Ger.*
Halcinonide (p.1043·2); neomycin sulphate (p.229·2); nystatin (p.386·1).
Infected skin disorders.

Halogedol *Fardi, Spain.*
Camphor (p.1557·2); methyl salicylate (p.55·2).
Muscle and joint pain.

Halomycetin *Kwizda, Aust.*
Chloramphenicol (p.182·1).
Bacterial eye infections.

Haloper *CT, Ger.*
Haloperidol (p.673·3).
Psychoses.

Haloral
Hal, Ger.; HAL, Neth.
Allergen extracts (p.1545·1).
Hyposensitisation.

Halospor *Ciba, Switz.†.*
Cefotiam hydrochloride (p.170·2).
Lignocaine hydrochloride (p.1293·2) is included in the intramuscular injection to alleviate the pain of injection.
Bacterial infections.

Halotestin
Upjohn, Austral.†; Pharmacia Upjohn, Canad.; Pharmacia Upjohn, Fr.; Pharmacia Upjohn, Ital.; Pharmacia Upjohn, Neth.; Pharmacia Upjohn, Norw.; Pharmacia Upjohn, S.Afr.; Upjohn, Swed.†; Upjohn, USA.
Fluoxymesterone (p.1447·1).
Breast cancer; delayed puberty; male hypogonadism; menstrual disorders; osteoporosis; postpartum breast engorgement.

Halotex *Westwood, USA.*
Haloprogin (p.381·2).
Fungal skin infections.

Halotussin *Halsey, USA.*
Guaiphenesin (p.1061·3).
Coughs.

Halotussin-DM *Halsey, USA.*
Dextromethorphan hydrobromide (p.1057·3); guaiphenesin (p.1061·3).
Coughs.

Halperon *Quantum, USA†.*
Haloperidol (p.673·3).

Halset
Zyma, Aust.; Stroschein, Ger.†.
Cetylpyridinium chloride (p.1106·2).
Mouth and throat infections.

Halstabletten-ratiopharm *Ratiopharm, Ger.†.*
Cetylpyridinium chloride (p.1106·2).
Inflammatory disorders and infections of the oropharynx.

Haltran *Roberts, USA.*
Ibuprofen (p.44·1).
Fever; osteoarthritis; pain; rheumatoid arthritis.

Halycitrol *Laboratories for Applied Biology, UK.*
Vitamin A and D substances.

Hamadin *Schwabe, Ger.; Spitzner, Ger.*
Saccharomyces boulardii (p.1594·1).
Acne; diarrhoea.

Hamamelide P *UPSA, Fr.†.*
Hamamelis (p.1587·1); leucocianidol (p.1580·2).
Peripheral vascular disorders.

Hamamelis Complex *Blackmores, Austral.*
Hamamelis (p.1587·1); collinsonia; plantain seed (p.1208·3); rhubarb (p.1212·1); ascorbic acid (p.1365·2); rutin (p.1580·2); hesperidin (p.1580·2).
Haemorrhoids.

Hamamilla *Pharmasette, Ital.*
Benzalkonium chloride (p.1101·3); hamamelis (p.1587·1); chamomile (p.1561·2); hypromellose (p.1473·1).
Eye disinfection; eye irritation.

Hamarin *Roche, UK†.*
Allopurinol (p.390·2).
Gout; hyperuricaemia.

Hamasana *Robugen, Ger.*
Hamamelis (p.1587·1).
Haemorrhoids; skin disorders.

Hamatopan
Wolff, Ger.
Ferrous sulphate (p.1340·2).
Iron deficiency; iron-deficiency anaemia.

Hamatopan F *Wolff, Ger.*
Dried ferrous sulphate (p.1340·2); folic acid (p.1340·3).
Iron-deficiency; iron-deficiency anaemia.

Hametum
Austroplant, Aust.; Spitzner, Ger.; Schwabe, Ger.; Schwabe, Switz.
Hamamelis (p.1587·1).
Bleeding gums; epistaxis; haemorrhoids; skin disorders.

Hametum-N
Note. This name is used for preparations of different composition.
Spitzner, Ger.; Schwabe, Ger.
Hamamelis (p.1587·1); aesculus (p.1543·3).
Anorectal disorders; haemorrhoids.

Schwabe, Switz.
Hamamelis (p.1587·1).
Haemorrhoids.

Hamevis *Truw, Ger.†.*
Hamamelis (p.1587·1).
Haemorrhoids; skin disorders.

HAMFL *Leopold, Aust.*
A range of electrolyte infusions with or without glucose (p.1151·1).
Haemofiltration.

Hamilton Bath Oil *Hamilton, Austral.*
Light liquid paraffin (p.1382·1).
Dry skin; eczema; psoriasis.

Hamilton Body Wash *Hamilton, Austral.*
Soap substitute.

Hamilton Lip Balm *Hamilton, Austral.*
Ethylhexyl *p*-methoxycinnamate (p.1487·1); avobenzone (p.1486·3).
Dry chapped lips; sunscreen.

Hamilton Sensitive Broad Spectrum Milk
Hamilton, Austral.
SPF 15: Ethylhexyl *p*-methoxycinnamate (p.1487·1); titanium dioxide (p.1093·3).
Sunscreen.

Hamilton Shower Oil *Hamilton, Austral.†.*
Light liquid paraffin (p.1382·1).
Dry skin; eczema; psoriasis.

Hamilton Skin Cream *Hamilton, Austral.*
Urea (p.1095·2).
Dry skin.

Hamilton Skin Lotion *Hamilton, Austral.*
Liquid paraffin (p.1382·1); glycerol (p.1585·2).
Dry skin.

Hamilton Skin Repair Cream *Hamilton, Austral.*
Dimethicone (p.1384·2); cetrimide (p.1105·2).
Dermatitis; dry skin.

Hamilton Solastick Broad Spectrum *Hamilton, Austral.*
SPF 15: Ethylhexyl *p*-methoxycinnamate (p.1487·1); avobenzone (p.1486·3).
SPF 30+: Ethylhexyl *p*-methoxycinnamate (p.1487·1); avobenzone (p.1486·3); oxybenzone (p.1487·3); titanium dioxide (p.1093·3).
Sunscreen.

Hamilton Sportblock Broad Spectrum Milk *Hamilton, Austral.*
SPF 30+: Ethylhexyl *p*-methoxycinnamate (p.1487·1); 3-(4-methylbenzylidene)bornan-2-one (p.1487·2); avobenzone (p.1486·3); titanium dioxide (p.1093·3).
Sunscreen.

Hamilton Sunscreen Clear Lotion Broad Spectrum *Hamilton, Austral.*
SPF 15: Ethylhexyl *p*-methoxycinnamate (p.1487·1); oxybenzone (p.1487·3); avobenzone (p.1486·3).
Sunscreen.

Hamilton Sunscreen Cream Broad Spectrum *Hamilton, Austral.*
SPF 15: Ethylhexyl *p*-methoxycinnamate (p.1487·1); octyl salicylate (p.1487·3); avobenzone (p.1486·3).
SPF 30+: Ethylhexyl *p*-methoxycinnamate (p.1487·1); 3-(4-methylbenzylidene)bornan-2-one (p.1487·2); avobenzone (p.1486·3); titanium dioxide (p.1093·3).
Sunscreen.

Hamilton Sunscreen 4 Hour *Hamilton, Austral.†.*
Ethylhexyl *p*-methoxycinnamate (p.1487·1); oxybenzone (p.1487·3); padimate O (p.1488·1); titanium dioxide (p.1093·3).
Sunscreen.

Hamilton Sunscreen Low Allergy *Hamilton, Austral.†.*
Ethylhexyl *p*-methoxycinnamate (p.1487·1); titanium dioxide (p.1093·3).
Sunscreen.

Hamilton Sunscreen Milk Broad Spectrum *Hamilton, Austral.*
SPF 15: Ethylhexyl *p*-methoxycinnamate (p.1487·1); avobenzone (p.1486·3); 3-(4-methylbenzylidene)bornan-2-one (p.1487·2).
SPF 30+: Ethylhexyl *p*-methoxycinnamate (p.1487·1); 3-(4-methylbenzylidene)bornan-2-one (p.1487·2); avobenzone (p.1486·3); titanium dioxide (p.1093·3).
Sunscreen.

Hamilton Sunscreen Milky Lotion *Hamilton, Austral.†.*
Sunscreen preparation.

Hamilton Superblock Broad Spectrum Milk SPF 30+ *Hamilton, Austral.*
Ethylhexyl *p*-methoxycinnamate (p.1487·1); 3-(4-methylbenzylidene)bornan-2-one (p.1487·2); avobenzone (p.1486·3); titanium dioxide (p.1093·3).
Sunscreen.

Hamilton Watersport Broad Spectrum Milk *Hamilton, Austral.*
SPF 30+: Ethylhexyl *p*-methoxycinnamate (p.1487·1); 3-(4-methylbenzylidene)bornan-2-one (p.1487·2); titanium dioxide (p.1093·3).
Sunscreen.

Hamoagil *Agil, Ger.†.*
Aesculus (p.1543·3); bismuth subnitrate (p.1180·2); zinc oxide (p.1096·2); dequalinium salicylate (p.1112·1); laureth 9 (p.1325·2); heparin (p.879·3).
Anorectal disorders.

Hamo-Europuran N *Scheurich, Ger.*
Laureth 9 (p.1325·2).
Hamo-Europuran formerly contained dequalinium salicylate, heparin, and laureth 9.
Anorectal disorders.

Hamofiltrasol *Alte Kreis, Aust.*
Anhydrous glucose; electrolytes (p.1151·1).
Haemofiltration solution.

Hamolind *Pharmakon, Switz.†.*
Plexus venosus haemorrhoidalis.
Haemorrhoids.

Hamo-ratiopharm *Ratiopharm, Ger.*
Ointment: Butoxycaine hydrochloride (p.1289·1); zinc oxide (p.1096·2); chamomile (p.1561·2).
Suppositories: Bismuth subgallate (p.1180·2); zinc oxide (p.1096·2); chamomile (p.1561·2).
Anal fissure; haemorrhoids.

Hamorrhoidal-Zapfchen *Weleda, Aust.*
Antimony.
Anorectal disorders.

Hamos N *Dr Janssen, Ger.*
Menthol (p.1600·2); aesculus (p.1543·3).
Haemorrhoids.

Hamos-Tropfen-S *Dr Janssen, Ger.*
Aesculus (p.1543·3).
Vascular disorders.

Hamovannad *Bastian, Ger.*
Inositol nicotinate (p.891·3).
Haemorrhoids; peripheral vascular disorders.

Hamo-Vibolex *Chephasaar, Ger.*
Cyanocobalamin (p.1363·3).
Hyperchromic anaemia.

Handexin *Ciba, Ital.*
Chlorhexidine gluconate (p.1107·2); aminoxide.
Hand disinfection.

Hands Dry *Chancellor, UK†.*
Aluminium chlorohydrate (p.1078·3); polyethylene glycol.
Sweaty palms.

Hanoartin *Hanosan, Ger.†.*
Allium sativum (p.1583·1); conium maculatum; kalium jodatum; chelidonium majus; sulfur.
Arteriosclerosis; hypertension.

Hanooxygen *Hanosan, Ger.†.*
Sodium citrate (p.1153·2); citric acid (p.1564·3); dibasic potassium phosphate (p.1159·2); iron and vitamin B substances.
Electrolyte disorders; metabolic alkalosis.

Hanotoxin N *Hanosan, Ger.*
Homoeopathic preparation.

Hansamed *Beiersdorf, Aust.†.*
Dexpanthenol (p.1570·3); chlorhexidine gluconate (p.1107·2).
Burns; wounds.

Hansamed Balsam *Beiersdorf, Ger.†.*
Dexpanthenol (p.1570·3); chlorhexidine gluconate (p.1107·2).
Burns; wounds.

Hansamed Spray *Beiersdorf, Ger.*
Chlorhexidine gluconate (p.1107·2).
Wound disinfection.

Hansaplast *Beiersdorf, Ger.*
Methacrylate copolymer (p.1603·2).
Wounds.

Hapeka 39 (Heparcholin) *Presselin, Ger.†.*
Herbal and homoeopathic preparation.

Harmogen
Abbott, Irl.; Upjohn, UK.
Estropipate (p.1444·3).
Menopausal disorders.

Harmomed *Kwizda, Aust.*
Dothiepin hydrochloride (p.283·1); diazepam (p.661·1).
Depression.

Harmonet
Wyeth Lederle, Belg.; Wyeth, Fr.; Wyeth, Ital.; Wyeth, Neth.
Gestodene (p.1447·2); ethinyloestradiol (p.1445·1).
Combined oral contraceptive.

Harnal *Yamanouchi, Jpn.*
Tamsulosin hydrochloride (p.951·2).
Benign prostatic hyperplasia.

Harnosal *TAD, Ger.*
Sulphaethidole; sulphamethizole (p.254·2).
Urinary-tract infections.

Harnsauretropfen N *Syxyl, Ger.*
Homoeopathic preparation.

Harntee *Steiner, Ger.*
Silver birch (p.1553·3); orthosiphon (p.1592·2); solidago virgaurea.
Urinary-tract disorders.

Harntee 400 *TAD, Ger.*
Birch leaf (p.1553·3); calendula officinalis; equisetum (p.1575·1); fennel (p.1579·1); couch-grass (p.1567·3); juniper (p.1592·2); liquorice (p.1197·1); ononis (p.1610·2); orthosiphon (p.1592·2); phaseolus vulgaris; solidago virgaurea; bearberry (p.1552·2).
Urinary-tract infections.

Harntreibender Tee *Salus, Aust.*
Urtica (p.1642·3); silver birch (p.1553·3); taraxacum (p.1634·2); prunus spinosa; ononis (p.1610·2).
Diuretic.

Harolan *Merz, Ger.†.*
Benzbromarone (p.392·3).
Gout; hyperuricaemia.

Harongan *Schwabe, Ger.*
Haronga.
Digestive system disorders.

Harpadol *Arkopharma, Fr.*
Harpagophytum procumbens (p.27·2).
Joint pain.

Harpagin *Merz, Ger.*
Benzbromarone (p.392·3); allopurinol (p.390·2).
Hyperuricaemia.

Harpagofito Orto *Normon, Spain.*
Harpagophytum procumbens (p.27·2).
Musculoskeletal and joint disorders.

Harpagoforte Asmedic *Dyckerhoff, Ger.*
Harpagophytum (p.27·2).
Gastro-intestinal disorders; musculoskeletal and joint disorders.

Harpagophytum Complex *Blackmores, Austral.*
Salix alba (p.82·3); cimicifuga racemosa (p.1563·3); harpagophytum procumbens (p.27·2); bryonia alba (p.1555·2); vitamins and minerals; hesperidin (p.1580·2); rutin (p.1580·2).
Musculoskeletal and joint disorders.

Hartiosen *Inkeysa, Spain.*
Harpagophytum procumbens (p.27·2).
Musculoskeletal and joint disorders.

Hartmannsche *Enzypharm, Aust.*
Electrolyte infusion (p.1147·1).
Fluid and electrolyte disorders.

Harzer Hustenelixier *Wernigerode, Ger.*
Ribwort.
Catarrh; mouth and throat inflammation.

Harzer Hustenloser *Wernigerode, Ger.*
Thyme (p.1636·3); primula root.
Cold symptoms.

Harzol *Hoyer, Ger.*
Sitosterol (p.1279·3).
Benign prostatic hyperplasia.

HA-Tabletten N *Thomae, Ger.*
Aspirin (p.16·1); paracetamol (p.72·2); caffeine (p.749·3).
Cold symptoms; fever; neuralgia; pain; rheumatism.

H-Atetal *ISM, Ital.*
An adsorbed tetanus vaccine (p.1535·3).
Active immunisation.

Hausmann-Amin *Braun, Switz.†.*
Amino-acid infusion with or without electrolytes.
Parenteral nutrition.

Hausmann-Amin Vacu-Mix *Hausmann, Switz.†.*
Amino-acid, carbohydrate, and electrolyte infusion.
Parenteral nutrition.

Hautplus N Dr Hagedorn *Naturarzneimittel, Ger.*
Homoeopathic preparation.

Haut-Vital *Twardy, Ger.*
Vitamins; calcium lactate (p.1155·2); Saccharomyces cerevisiae (p.1373·1); lecithin (p.1595·2).
Hair, skin, and nail disorders.

Haven *Dolorgiet, Ger.†.*
Aescin (p.1543·3); heparin sodium (p.879·3).
Skin trauma.

Havlane *Diamant, Fr.*
Loprazolam mesylate (p.675·3).
Insomnia.

Havrix
SmithKline Beecham, Aust.; SmithKline Beecham, Austral.; SK-RIT, Belg.; SmithKline Beecham, Canad.; SmithKline Beecham, Fr.; SmithKline Beecham, Ger.; SSW, Ger.; SmithKline Beecham, Irl.; SmithKline Beecham, Ital.; SmithKline Beecham, Neth.; SmithKline Beecham, Norw.; SmithKline Beecham, S.Afr.; Smith Kline & French, Spain; SmithKline Beecham, Swed.; SmithKline Beecham, Switz.; SmithKline Beecham, UK; SmithKline Beecham, USA.
An adsorbed inactivated hepatitis A vaccine (HM 175 strain) (p.1512·2).
Active immunisation.

Hawaiian Tropic
Note. This name is used for preparations of different composition.
Tanning Research, Canad.
SPF 10: Menthyl anthranilate (p.1487·2); ethylhexyl *p*-methoxycinnamate (p.1487·1); oxybenzone (p.1487·3).
SPF 30; SPF 45: Ethylhexyl *p*-methoxycinnamate (p.1487·1); octyl salicylate (p.1487·3); titanium dioxide (p.1093·3).
Sunscreen.

Tanning Research, USA.
SPF 8+; SPF 10+: Ethylhexyl *p*-methoxycinnamate (p.1487·1); oxybenzone (p.1487·3); menthyl anthranilate (p.1487·2).
Gel SPF 15+: Ethylhexyl *p*-methoxycinnamate (p.1487·1); octocrylene (p.1487·3); oxybenzone (p.1487·3); menthyl anthranilate (p.1487·2).
Lotion SPF 15+: Ethylhexyl *p*-methoxycinnamate (p.1487·1); oxybenzone (p.1487·3); menthyl anthranilate (p.1487·2).
SPF 30+: Ethylhexyl *p*-methoxycinnamate (p.1487·1); menthyl anthranilate (p.1487·2); oxybenzone (p.1487·3); octyl salicylate (p.1487·3); homosalate (p.1487·2).
SPF 45+: Ethylhexyl *p*-methoxycinnamate (p.1487·1); oxybenzone (p.1487·3); octyl salicylate (p.1487·3); titanium dioxide (p.1093·3); menthyl anthranilate (p.1487·2).
SPF 45+: Ethylhexyl *p*-methoxycinnamate (p.1487·1); octocrylene (p.1487·3); oxybenzone (p.1487·3); octyl salicylate (p.1487·3); titanium dioxide (p.1093·3).
Sunscreen.

Hawaiian Tropic Baby Faces
Note. This name is used for preparations of different composition.
Tanning Research, Canad.
SPF 35; SPF 50: Ethylhexyl *p*-methoxycinnamate (p.1487·1); octyl salicylate (p.1487·3); titanium dioxide (p.1093·3).
Sunscreen.

Tanning Research, USA.
SPF 20: Ethylhexyl *p*-methoxycinnamate (p.1487·1); octocrylene (p.1487·3); oxybenzone (p.1487·3); menthyl anthranilate (p.1487·2).
SPF 35; SPF 50: Ethylhexyl *p*-methoxycinnamate (p.1487·1); octocrylene (p.1487·3); oxybenzone (p.1487·3); octyl salicylate (p.1487·3); titanium dioxide (p.1093·3).
Sunscreen.

Hawaiian Tropic Bioshield *Tanning Research, Canad.*
SPF 15: Ethylhexyl *p*-methoxycinnamate (p.1487·1); octyl salicylate (p.1487·3); oxybenzone (p.1487·3).
SPF 30: Ethylhexyl *p*-methoxycinnamate (p.1487·1); octocrylene (p.1487·3); octyl salicylate (p.1487·3); titanium dioxide (p.1093·3).
Sunscreen.

Hawaiian Tropic Cool Aloe with I.C.E. *Tanning Research, USA.*
Lignocaine (p.1293·2); menthol (p.1600·2); aloe (p.1177·1).

Hawaiian Tropic Dark Tanning
Note. This name is used for preparations of different composition.
Tanning Research, Canad.
Lotion SPF 4: Ethylhexyl *p*-methoxycinnamate (p.1487·1); menthyl anthranilate (p.1487·2).
Oil SPF 4: Ethylhexyl *p*-methoxycinnamate (p.1487·1); padimate O (p.1488·1).
Sunscreen.

Tanning Research, USA.
Gel SPF 2; gel SPF 4: 2-Phenyl-1*H*-benzimidazole-5-sulphonic acid (p.1488·2).
Oil SPF 2; oil SPF 4: Ethylhexyl *p*-methoxycinnamate (p.1487·1); padimate O (p.1488·1).
Sunscreen.

Hawaiian Tropic Herbal *Tanning Research, Canad.*
SPF 4: Ethylhexyl *p*-methoxycinnamate (p.1487·1); oxybenzone (p.1487·3).
SPF 2; SPF 15: 2-Phenyl-1*H*-benzimidazole-5-sulphonic acid (p.1488·2); sulisobenzone (p.1488·3).
Sunscreen.

Hawaiian Tropic Just For Kids
Note. This name is used for preparations of different composition.
Tanning Research, Canad.
SPF 30: Ethylhexyl *p*-methoxycinnamate (p.1487·1); octyl salicylate (p.1487·3); titanium dioxide (p.1093·3).
Sunscreen.

Tanning Research, USA.
SPF 30: Ethylhexyl *p*-methoxycinnamate (p.1487·1); oxybenzone (p.1487·3); octyl salicylate (p.1487·3); homosalate (p.1487·2).
SPF 45: Ethylhexyl *p*-methoxycinnamate (p.1487·1); oxybenzone (p.1487·3); octyl salicylate (p.1487·3); octocrylene (p.1487·3); titanium dioxide (p.1093·3).
Sunscreen.

Hawaiian Tropic Lipbalm *Tanning Research, Canad.*
SPF 45: Ethylhexyl *p*-methoxycinnamate (p.1487·1); menthyl anthranilate (p.1487·2); octyl salicylate (p.1487·3); oxybenzone (p.1487·3); titanium dioxide (p.1093·3).
Sunscreen.

Hawaiian Tropic Protective Tanning *Tanning Research, USA.*
SPF 6: Titanium dioxide (p.1093·3).
Sunscreen.

Hawaiian Tropic Protective Tanning Dry *Tanning Research, USA.*
Gel SPF 6: 2-Phenyl-1*H*-benzimidazole-5-sulphonic acid (p.1488·2); sulisobenzone (p.1488·3).
Oil SPF 6: Ethylhexyl *p*-methoxycinnamate (p.1487·1); homosalate (p.1487·2); menthyl anthranilate (p.1487·2).
Sunscreen.

Hawaiian Tropic Self Tanning Sunblock *Tanning Research, USA.*
Ethylhexyl *p*-methoxycinnamate (p.1487·1); oxybenzone (p.1487·3).
Sunscreen.

Hawaiian Tropic Sport
Note. This name is used for preparations of different composition.
Tanning Research, Canad.
SPF 8: Ethylhexyl *p*-methoxycinnamate (p.1487·1); octocrylene (p.1487·3); oxybenzone (p.1487·3).
SPF 30: Ethylhexyl *p*-methoxycinnamate (p.1487·1); octocrylene (p.1487·3); octyl salicylate (p.1487·3); oxybenzone (p.1487·3); titanium dioxide (p.1093·3).
Sunscreen.

Tanning Research, USA.
SPF 15: Ethylhexyl *p*-methoxycinnamate (p.1487·1); octocrylene (p.1487·3); oxybenzone (p.1487·3).
SPF 30: Ethylhexyl *p*-methoxycinnamate (p.1487·1); octocrylene (p.1487·3); oxybenzone (p.1487·3); octyl salicylate (p.1487·3); titanium dioxide (p.1093·3).
Sunscreen.

Hay Fever
Homeocan, Canad.; Hylands, Canad.
Homoeopathic preparation.

Hay Fever Symptoms Relief *Brauer, Austral.*
Homoeopathic preparation.

Hay-Crom
Norton Waterford, Irl.; Norton, S.Afr.; Baker Norton, UK.
Sodium cromoglycate (p.762·1).
Formerly known as Eye-Crom in the *UK*.
Allergic conjunctivitis.

Hayfebrol *Scot-Tussin, USA.*
Pseudoephedrine hydrochloride (p.1068·3); chlorpheniramine maleate (p.405·1).
Upper respiratory-tract symptoms.

Haymine *Pharmax, UK.*
Chlorpheniramine maleate (p.405·1); ephedrine hydrochloride (p.1059·3).
Nasal congestion.

H-BIG *Abbott, USA.*
A hepatitis B immunoglobulin (p.1512·3).
Passive immunisation.

H-B-Vax
Merck Sharp & Dohme, Ital.†; Pasteur Merieux, Swed.
A hepatitis B vaccine (recombinant DNA) (p.1513·1).
Active immunisation.

H-B-Vax II
CSL, Austral.; Merck Sharp & Dohme, Belg.; Pasteur Merieux, Irl.; Merck Sharp & Dohme, S.Afr.; Pasteur Merieux, UK.
A hepatitis B vaccine (recombinant DNA) (p.1513·1).
Active immunisation.

HB-Vax-DNA *Pasteur Vaccins, Fr.*
A hepatitis B vaccine (recombinant DNA) (p.1513·1).
Active immunisation.

Hc45
Boots Healthcare, Irl.; Crookes Healthcare, UK.
Hydrocortisone acetate (p.1043·3).
Dermatitis; insect bites.

HC Derma-Pax *Recsei, USA.*
Hydrocortisone acetate (p.1043·3); mepyramine maleate (p.414·1); chlorpheniramine maleate (p.405·1).
Skin disorders.

HCG-Nostick *Organon Teknika, UK†; Organon Teknika, USA†.*
Pregnancy test (p.1621·2).

HD 85 *Lafayette, USA.*
Barium sulphate (p.1003·1).
Contrast medium for gastro-intestinal radiography.

HD 200 Plus *Lafayette, USA.*
Barium sulphate (p.1003·1).
Contrast medium for gastro-intestinal radiography.

Head Cold Relief *Brauer, Austral.*
Homoeopathic preparation.

Head & Shoulders
Procter & Gamble, Canad.; Procter & Gamble, USA.
Pyrithione zinc (p.1089·3).
Seborrhoeic dermatitis of the scalp.

Head & Shoulders Intensive Treatment *Procter & Gamble, USA.*
Selenium sulphide (p.1091·1).
Dandruff; pityriasis versicolor; seborrhoeic dermatitis.

Headache Complex *Brauer, Austral.*
Homoeopathic preparation.

Headache & Migraine *Homeocan, Canad.*
Homoeopathic preparation.

Headache Tablets
Note. This name is used for preparations of different composition.
Brauer, Austral.
Homoeopathic preparation.
Romilo, Canad.
Aspirin (p.16·1).

Headarest *Medinex, Canad.†.*
Paracetamol (p.72·2).
Fever; pain.

Headclear *Richardson-Vicks, Austral.†.*
Pseudoephedrine hydrochloride (p.1068·3); paracetamol (p.72·2); chlorpheniramine maleate (p.405·1).
Cold or influenza symptoms.

Headmaster *Seton, Irl.*
Phenothrin (p.1409·2).
Pediculosis.

Healfas NMF *Czarniak, Austral.†.*
Amino acids and vitamin B substances.
Skin disorders.

Healing Ointment *Nelson, UK.*
Homoeopathic preparation.

Healon
Pharmacia Upjohn, Austral.; Pharmacia Upjohn, Belg.; Pharmacia Upjohn, Canad.; Pharmacia Upjohn, Fr.; Pharmacia Upjohn, Ger.; Pharmacia Upjohn, Ital.; Pharmacia, Neth.†; Pharmacia Upjohn, Norw.; Pharmacia Upjohn, S.Afr.; Pharmacia Upjohn, Swed.; Kabi Pharmacia, USA.
Sodium hyaluronate (p.1630·3).
Adjunct in eye surgery.

Healon GV *Kabi Pharmacia, USA.*
Sodium hyaluronate (p.1630·3).

Healon Yellow
Pharmacia, Canad.†; Pharmacia Upjohn, Ital.; Pharmacia, Swed.†; Kabi Pharmacia, USA.
Sodium hyaluronate (p.1630·3); fluorescein sodium (p.1581·1).
Adjunct in eye surgery.

Healonid
Pharmacia Upjohn, Aust.; Pharmacia Upjohn, Fr.†; Pharmacia Upjohn, Irl.; Pharmacia, UK.
Sodium hyaluronate (p.1630·3).
Adjunct in eye surgery.

Healonid Yellow *Pharmacia Upjohn, Aust.*
Sodium hyaluronate (p.1630·3); fluorescein sodium (p.1581·1).
Adjunct in eye surgery.

HealthAid Boldo-Plus *Pharmadass, UK.*
Boldo (p.1554·1); taraxacum (p.1634·2); bladderwrack (p.1554·1); clivers (p.1565·2); bearberry (p.1552·2); juniper oil (p.1592·3); vitamin B_6 (p.1362·3).
Formerly known as HealthAid AquaFall.
Water retention.

HealthAid FemmeVit PMS Formula *Pharmadass, UK.*
Multivitamin and mineral preparation.

Healthy Feet *Pickles, UK.*
Undecenoic acid (p.389·2); dibromopropamidine isethionate (p.1112·2).
Fungal skin infections.

Heartburn Relief *Stanley, Canad.*
Aluminium hydroxide (p.1177·3); alginic acid (p.1470·3).

Heartline *BDI, USA.*
Aspirin (p.16·1).
Myocardial infarction.

Heb *Pilkington Barnes-Hind, USA†.*
Vehicle for topical preparations.

Hebagam IM *NBI, S.Afr.*
Hepatitis B immunoglobulin (p.1512·3).
Passive immunisation.

Hebucol *Logeais, Fr.*
Cyclobutyrol sodium (p.1569·2).
Dyspepsia.

HEC
Note. This name is used for preparations of different composition.
Chauvin, Fr.
Tannic acid (p.1634·2); hamamelis (p.1587·1); phenazone (p.78·2).
Haemorrhoids; nose bleeds; wounds.
Novopharma, Switz.
Tannin (p.1634·2); pectin (p.1474·1); peru balsam (p.1617·2); hamamelis (p.1587·1).
Mucous membrane disorders of the nose.

Hectonona *Milo, Spain.*
Algeldrate (p.1177·3); magnesium carbonate (p.1198·1); sodium bicarbonate (p.1153·2); tartaric acid (p.1634·3).
Formerly contained bismuth subnitrate, magnesium oxide, and sodium bicarbonate.
Gastro-intestinal hyperacidity.

Hedelix *Meuselbach, Ger.*
Hedera helix.
Respiratory-tract disorders.

Hederix
Note. This name is used for preparations of different composition.
Saba, Ital.
Codeine hydrobromide (p.27·1); hedera helix.
Coughs.
Plan, Switz.
Noscapine hydrochloride (p.1065·2); hedera; senega (p.1069·3); helenium (p.1059·2); iridis; marrubium (p.1063·3).
Coughs.

Hederka *Amino, Switz.†.*
Hedera helix; thyme oil (p.1637·1); mint oil; cinnamon oil (p.1564·2); fennel oil (p.1579·2).
Coughs.

Hedex
SmithKline Beecham, Irl.†; Sterling, Neth.†; Sterling Winthrop, Spain†; Sterling Health, UK.
Paracetamol (p.72·2).
Fever; pain.

Hedex Extra *Sterling Health, UK.*
Paracetamol (p.72·2); caffeine (p.749·3).
Fever; pain.

Hedex Headcold *Sterling Health, UK.*
Oral powder: Paracetamol (p.72·2); phenylephrine (p.1066·2); ascorbic acid (p.1365·2).
Tablets: Paracetamol (p.72·2); phenylephrine (p.1066·2); ascorbic acid (p.1365·2); caffeine (p.749·3).

Hedonin *Gerot, Aust.*
Phenylpropanol (p.1617·3); moxaverine hydrochloride (p.1604·3).
Biliary-tract disorders; gastro-intestinal disorders.

Heemex *Lane, UK.*
Hamamelis (p.1587·1); compound benzoin tincture; zinc oxide (p.1096·2).
Haemorrhoids.

Heer-More *Eagle, Austral.*
Homoeopathic preparation.

Heet
Whitehall-Robins, Canad.; Whitehall, USA.
Methyl salicylate (p.55·2); camphor (p.1557·2); capsaicin (p.24·2).
Muscle, joint, and soft-tissue pain; neuralgia.

hefasolon *Hefa, Ger.*
Prednisolone (p.1048·1) or prednisolone sodium phosphate (p.1048·1).
Corticosteroid.

Hegama *Alter, Spain†.*
Liver extract; cyanocobalamin (p.1363·3).
Anaemias; tonic.

Hegor
Note. This name is used for preparations of different composition.
Procter & Gamble, Aust.
Shampoo.
Scalp and hair disorders.
Procter & Gamble, Belg.†.
d-Phenothrin (p.1409·2).
Pediculosis.

Hegor Antipoux *Lachartre, Fr.†.*
d-Phenothrin (p.1409·2).
Pediculosis.

Hegrimarin *Strathmann, Ger.*
Silybum marianum (p.993·3).
Liver disorders.

Heilit *Heilit, Ger.*
Camphor (p.1557·2); methyl salicylate (p.55·2); benzyl nicotinate (p.22·1).
Musculoskeletal and joint disorders.

Heilit Rheuma-Bad N-Kombi *Pierre Fabre, Ger.†.*
Camphor (p.1557·2); menthol (p.1600·2); glycol salicylate (p.43·1).
Bath additive; musculoskeletal and joint disorders.

Heilit Rheuma-Olbad *Heilit, Ger.*
Camphor (p.1557·2); menthol (p.1600·2); methyl salicylate (p.55·2).
Bath additive; musculoskeletal and joint disorders.

Heitrin *Abbott, Ger.*
Terazosin hydrochloride (p.952·1).
Hypertension.

Hekbilin Kapseln *Strathmann, Ger.*
Cynara (p.1569·2).
Dyspepsia.

Hektulose *Stroschein, Ger.†.*
Lactulose (p.1195·3).
Constipation; gastro-enteritis; liver disorders.

Helago-oel N *Helago, Ger.*
Chamomile (p.1561·2); sage (p.1627·1).
Inflammatory disorders of the oropharynx.

Helastop *Hamilton, Austral.*
Propolis (p.1621·3).
Herpes labialis.

Heldis *Delagrange, Fr.†.*
Permethrin (p.1409·2); piperonyl butoxide (p.1409·3).
Pediculosis.

Helfergin *Promonta, Ger.*
Meclofenoxate hydrochloride (p.1599·1).
Cerebral insufficiency; cerebrovascular disorders.

Helianthus comp *Plantina, Ger.*
Homoeopathic preparation.

Helicidine *Sodip, Switz.†.*
Helix pomatia extract (p.1062·1).
Coughs and associated respiratory-tract disorders.

Helicocin *Biochemie, Aust.*
Oval tablet, amoxycillin trihydrate (p.151·3); round tablet, metronidazole (p.585·1).
Helicobacter pylori infection.

Helidac
Pharmacia Upjohn, Austral.; Procter & Gamble, USA.
Chewable tablets, bismuth citrate (p.1180·1) or bismuth salicylate (p.1180·1); tablets, metronidazole (p.585·1); capsules, tetracycline hydrochloride (p.259·1).
Peptic ulcer.

Heligoid *Allergopharma, Ger.†.*
Allergen extracts (p.1545·1).
Hyposensitisation.

Helimox *Essex, Ital.*
Amoxycillin (p.151·3).
Bacterial infections.

Helinol *Duphar, Spain†.*
Tripotassium dicitratobismuthate (p.1180·2).
Gastritis associated with Helicobacter pylori; peptic ulcer.

Heliomycort *Pfleger, Ger.†.*
Nystatin (p.386·1); neomycin sulphate (p.229·2); gramicidin (p.215·2); prednisolone acetate (p.1048·1).
Inflammatory skin disorders with fungal or bacterial infection.

Helios *Medici Domus, Ital.†.*
Cetylpyridinium chloride (p.1106·2).
Eye disorders.

Heliplant *Kanoldt, Ger.*
Silybum marianum (p.993·3).
Liver disorders.

Helipur
Braun, Belg.†; Braun, Ger.; Braun, Ital.
Chlorocresol (p.1110·3); clorophene (p.1111·2); orthophenylphenol (p.1120·3).
Surface and instrument disinfection.

Helipur H plus *Braun, Ger.*
Glyoxal (p.1115·1); glutaraldehyde (p.1114·3).
Instrument disinfection.

Helirad *Allen, Aust.*
Ranitidine bismutrex (p.1211·2).
Peptic ulcer.

Helis *Farmacologico Milanese, Ital.*
Benzalkonium chloride (p.1101·3).
Eye disinfection.

Helisal
Cortecs, Irl.; Cortecs, UK.
Diagnostic test for *Helicobacter pylori* in blood.

Helistat *Marion Merrell Dow, USA.*
Absorbable collagen sponge (p.1566·3).
Haemostatic.

Helix I *Braun, Ital.*
Sodium *o*-phenylphenol (p.1120·3).
Instrument disinfection.

Helixate
Centeon, Ger.; Bayer, Neth.; Centeon, Spain; Centeon, Swed.; Centeon, UK; Armour, USA.
A factor VIII preparation (p.720·3).
Haemophilia A.

Helixor
Germania, Aust.; Helixor, Ger.
Mistletoe (p.1604·1) from fir trees, pine trees, or apple trees.
Malignant neoplasms.

Helmex *Pfizer, Ger.*
Pyrantel embonate (p.109·3).
Worm infections.

Helmine *Inibsa, Spain.*
Ondansetron hydrochloride (p.1206·2).
Nausea and vomiting.

Helmintox *Innotech, Fr.*
Pyrantel embonate (p.109·3).
Intestinal nematode infections.

Helo-acid
Note. This name is used for preparations of different composition.
Rosch & Handel, Aust.
Citric acid (p.1564·3); tartaric acid (p.1634·3); lactic acid (p.1593·3); pepsin (p.1616·3).
Digestive disorders.
Helopharm, Ger.†.
Citric acid (p.1564·3); tartaric acid (p.1634·3).
Gastro-intestinal disorders.

Helo-acid compositum *Helopharm, Ger.†.*
White tablets, citric acid (p.1564·3); tartaric acid (p.1634·3); brown tablets, a porcine pancreatin (p.1612·1).
Gastro-intestinal disorders.

Helol *Italfarmaco, Spain.*
Tripotassium dicitratobismuthate (p.1180·2).
Gastritis; peptic ulcer.

Helonias Compound *Gerard House, UK.*
Helonias (p.1587·2); parsley (p.1615·3); black cohosh (p.1563·3); raspberry leaf (p.1624·2).
Fluid retention.

Helopanflat
Rosch & Handel, Aust.; Knoll, Switz.
Pancreatin (p.1612·1); simethicone (p.1213·1).
Adjunct in radiography; digestive disorders; flatulence; Roemheld syndrome.

Helopanflat N *Knoll, Ger.*
Porcine pancreatin (p.1612·1); simethicone (p.1213·1).
Digestive system disorders.

Helopanzym
Rosch & Handel, Aust.; Helopharm, Ger.†.
Pepsin (p.1616·3); pancreatin (p.1612·1); porcine bile (p.1553·2).
Digestive system disorders.

Helopyrin *Rosch & Handel, Aust.*
Etenzamide (p.35·3); ascorbic acid (p.1365·2); flavonoids (p.1580·1); rutin (p.1580·2); ephedrine hydrochloride (p.1059·3).
Cold symptoms.

Helpin *Berlin-Chemie, Ger.*
Brivudine (p.606·2).
Herpes and varicella infections.

Helvamox *Helvepharm, Switz.*
Amoxycillin trihydrate (p.151·3).
Bacterial infections.

Helvecin *Helvepharm, Switz.*
Indomethacin (p.45·2).
Gout; musculoskeletal, joint, and peri-articular disorders.

Helvedoclyn *Helvepharm, Switz.*
Doxycycline hydrochloride (p.202·3).
Bacterial infections.

Helvegeron *Helvepharm, Switz.*
Amino-acid, multivitamin and mineral preparation with ginseng and lecithin.
Tonic.

Helvemycin *Helvepharm, Switz.*
Erythromycin ethyl succinate (p.204·2) or erythromycin stearate (p.204·2).
Bacterial infections.

Helveprim *Helvepharm, Switz.*
Co-trimoxazole (p.196·3).
Bacterial infections; blastomycosis; malaria; Pneumocystis carinii pneumonia.

Helver Sal *Bauxili, Spain.*
Aspirin (p.16·1).
Fever; musculoskeletal, joint, and peri-articular disorders; pain; thrombo-embolism prophylaxis.

Hem Antih *Llorens, Spain.*
Chlorpheniramine maleate (p.405·1); dexamethasone sodium succinate (p.1037·3).
Eye disorders.

Hem Fe *Wakefield, USA†.*
Ferrous fumarate (p.1339·3); vitamin B_{12} (p.1363·3); desiccated gastric substance.
Ascorbic acid (p.1365·2) is included in this preparation to increase the absorption and availability of iron.
Docusate sodium (p.1189·3) is included in this preparation to reduce the constipating effects of iron.
Iron deficiency anaemias.

Hemabate
Upjohn, UK; Upjohn, USA.
Carboprost trometamol (p.1414·1).
Postpartum haemorrhage; termination of pregnancy.

Hema-Chek
Bayer Diagnostics, UK; Bayer, USA.
Test for occult blood in faeces.

Hema-Combistix
Bayer Diagnostics, Austral.; Ames, Irl.; Miles, Ital.†; Bayer Diagnostics, UK; Bayer, USA.
Test for pH, protein, glucose, and blood in urine.

Hemagene Tailleur *Elerte, Fr.*
Aspirin (p.16·1); phenacetin (p.78·1); menthol (p.1600·2); methyl nonyl ketone.
Gynaecological disorders.

Hemapep *SA Druggists Self Med, S.Afr.†.*
Potassium chloride; sodium chloride; calcium carbonate; glucose (p.1152·3).
Oral rehydration therapy.

Hemarexin *Technilab, Canad.†.*
Multivitamins; minerals; kola (p.1645·1); liver extract.
Tonic.

Hemaspan *Sanofi Winthrop, USA.*
Ferrous fumarate (p.1339·3).
Vitamin C (p.1365·2) is included in this preparation to increase the absorption and availability of iron.
Docusate sodium (p.1189·3) is included in this preparation to reduce the constipating effects of iron.
Iron-deficiency anaemias.

Hemastix
Bayer Diagnostics, Austral.; Miles, Canad.†; Bayer Diagnostics, Fr.; Ames, Irl.; Bayer Diagnostici, Ital.; Bayer Diagnostics, UK; Bayer, USA.
Test for blood in urine.

Hematest
Bayer Diagnostics, Austral.; Bayer, Canad.; Ames, S.Afr.; Ames, UK†; Bayer, USA.
Test for blood in faeces.

Hematinic *Solgar, UK.*
Liver (desiccated); vitamin B_{12} (p.1363·3); iron (p.1346·1); calcium ascorbate (p.1365·2); folic acid (p.1340·3).
Dietary supplement.

Hematon *Dexo, Fr.*
Arginine aspartate; cobalt gluconate; manganese gluconate.
Tonic.

Hematone *Thuna, Canad.*
Vitamin B substances, vitamin C, and iron.

Hemcort HC *Technilab, Canad.*
Hydrocortisone acetate (p.1043·3); zinc sulphate (p.1373·2).
Anorectal disorders.

Hemedonine *Creme d'Orient, Fr.*
Haematoporphyrin (p.1587·1).
Tonic.

Hemeran
Note. This name is used for preparations of different composition.
Ciba-Geigy, Aust.; Zyma, Belg.; Zyma, Switz.
A heparinoid (p.882·3).
Haematomas; thrombophlebitis; venous insufficiency.
Zyma, Ger.
Heparin sodium (p.879·3).
Skin trauma; soft-tissue injury.

Hemerven *Lucchini, Switz.*
Diosmin (p.1580·1).
Peripheral vascular disorders.

HemeSelect *SmithKline Diagnostics, USA.*
Test for occult blood in faeces.

Hemet *Halsey, USA†.*
Diperodon hydrochloride (p.1292·3); mepyramine maleate (p.414·1); phenylephrine hydrochloride (p.1066·2); bismuth subcarbonate (p.1180·1); zinc oxide (p.1096·2).
Anorectal disorders.

Hemicraneal *Knoll, Spain.*
Caffeine (p.749·3); ergotamine tartrate (p.445·3); paracetamol (p.72·2).
Headache; migraine.

Hemi-Daonil
Hoechst, Fr.; Hoechst Marion Roussel, Neth.
Glibenclamide (p.319·3).
Diabetes mellitus.

Hemineurin *Astra, Austral.*
Chlormethiazole (p.647·2) or chlormethiazole edisylate (p.647·2).
Agitation states; alcohol withdrawal syndrome; sedative; status epilepticus.

Hemineurine
Debat, Fr.†; Debat, Switz.†.
Chlormethiazole edisylate (p.647·2).
Drug withdrawal syndromes; premedication; psychiatric disorders; status epilepticus.

Heminevrin
Astra, Irl.; Astra, Norw.; Astra, S.Afr.; Astra, Swed.; Astra, UK.
Chlormethiazole (p.647·2) or chlormethiazole edisylate (p.647·2).
Alcohol withdrawal syndrome; behaviour disorders in the elderly; insomnia; pre-eclamptic toxaemia; psychomotor agitation; sedative; status epilepticus.

Hemipralon *URPAC, Fr.*
Propranolol hydrochloride (p.937·1).
Cardiovascular disorders; migraine.

Hemo 141 *Esteve, Spain.*
Ethamsylate (p.720·1).
Haemorrhage.

Hemoal *Combe, Spain.*
Ephedrine (p.1059·3); benzocaine (p.1286·2).
Anorectal disorders.

Hemocaine *Mallard, USA†.*
Diperodon hydrochloride (p.1292·3); mepyramine maleate (p.414·1); phenylephrine hydrochloride (p.1066·2); bismuth subcarbonate (p.1180·1); zinc oxide (p.1096·2).
Anorectal disorders.

Hemocane
Note. This name is used for preparations of different composition.
Key, Austral.
Ointment: Lignocaine (p.1293·2); allantoin (p.1078·2); hamamelis (p.1587·1); zinc oxide (p.1096·2); chlorhexidine acetate (p.1107·2).
Suppositories: Lignocaine (p.1293·2); allantoin (p.1078·2); hamamelis (p.1587·1); zinc oxide (p.1096·2).
Anal pruritus; haemorrhoids.
Eastern Pharmaceuticals, UK.
Lignocaine hydrochloride (p.1293·2); zinc oxide (p.1096·2); bismuth oxide (p.1180·1); benzoic acid (p.1102·3); cinnamic acid (p.1111·1).
Haemorrhoids.

Hemocaprol
Delagrange, Fr.†; Delagrange, Spain†.
Aminocaproic acid (p.711·1).
Haemorrhage.

Hemoccult
Prevention et Biologie, Fr.; Rohm, S.Afr.; SmithKline Diagnostics, USA.
Test for blood in faeces.

Hemoclar *Sanofi Winthrop, Fr.*
Pentosan polysulphate (p.928·1).
Soft-tissue disorders; superficial vascular disorders.

Hemocoavit *Bio-Therabel, Belg.†.*
Ascorbic acid (p.1365·2); hesperidin methyl chalcone (p.1580·2); rutin (p.1580·2); esculoside (p.1543·3); menadione sodium bisulphite (p.1370·3).
Haemorrhage.

Hemocromo *Francia, Ital.*
Ferric sodium gluconate (p.1340·1).
Iron-deficiency anaemia.

Hemocyte *US Pharmaceutical, USA.*
Injection: Ferrous gluconate (p.1340·1); vitamin B substances.
Procaine hydrochloride (p.1299·2) is included in this preparation to alleviate the pain of injection.
Tablets: Ferrous fumarate (p.1339·3).
Iron-deficiency anaemias.

Hemocyte Plus *US Pharmaceutical, USA.*
Vitamin B substances with iron and folic acid.
Iron deficiency anaemias.

Hemocyte-F *US Pharmaceutical, USA.*
Ferrous fumarate (p.1339·3); folic acid (p.1340·3).
Iron-deficiency anaemias.

Hemocyte-V *US Pharmaceutical, USA.*
Ferrous gluconate (p.1340·1); vitamin B substances.
Iron-deficiency anaemias.

Hemodex *Pharmacia Upjohn, Fr.*
Dextran 60 (p.716·3) with electrolytes.
Blood volume expansion.

Hemodren Compuesto *Llorens, Spain.*
Bismuth subgallate (p.1180·2); aesculus (p.1543·3); hamamelis (p.1587·1); hydrocortisone acetate (p.1043·3); ruscogenin (p.1627·1); tyrothricin (p.267·2); amylocaine hydrochloride (p.1286·1); benzocaine (p.1286·2).
Anorectal disorders.

Hemodren Simple *Llorens, Spain.*
Ruscogenin (p.1627·1).
Anorectal disorders.

Hemofactor HT *Grifols, Spain.*
Factor IX (p.721·3); factor X; prothrombin; factor VII (p.720·2).
Clotting-factor deficiencies; haemorrhage.

Hemofibrine Spugna *Ogna, Ital.*
Fibrin (p.722·2).
Absorbable haemostatic for dental use.

Hemofil
Baxter, Fr.; Baxter, Ger.; Baxter, Ital.; Baxter, Spain; Baxter, Swed.; Baxter, UK; Hyland, USA.
A factor VIII preparation (p.720·3).
Haemorrhagic disorders.

Hemofiltrasol *Gambro, Swed.*
Anhydrous glucose; electrolytes (p.1151·1).
Haemofiltration solution.

Hemofiltrationslosning 401 *Baxter, Swed.*
Anhydrous glucose; sodium chloride; sodium lactate; calcium chloride; magnesium chloride; potassium chloride (p.1151·1).
Haemofiltration solution.

Hemohes
Braun, Ger.; Braun, Swed.; Braun, Switz.
Pentastarch (p.725·2) with electrolytes.
Extracorporeal perfusion; haemodilution; plasma volume expansion.

Hemoluol *Warner-Lambert, Fr.*
Aesculus (p.1543·3); capsella bursa pastoris; cypress.
Peripheral vascular disorders.

Hemopad *Astra, USA†.*
Purified bovine collagen (p.1566·3).
Haemostatic.

Hemorid For Women *Thompson, USA.*
Cream: White soft paraffin (p.1382·3); liquid paraffin (p.1382·1); pramoxine hydrochloride (p.1298·2); phenylephrine hydrochloride (p.1066·2); aloe vera (p.1177·1).
Lotion: Liquid paraffin (p.1382·1); yellow soft paraffin (p.1382·3); glycerol (p.1585·2).
Suppositories: Zinc oxide (p.1096·2); phenylephrine hydrochloride (p.1066·2).
Anorectal disorders.

Hemorrane *Byk Elmu, Spain.*
Aesculus (p.1543·3); benzocaine (p.1286·2); hydrocortisone acetate (p.1043·3); prednisone (p.1049·2).
Anorectal disorders.

Hemorrogel *Arkopharma, Fr.*
Capsules: Aesculus (p.1543·3).
Haemorrhoids; peripheral vascular disorders.
Rectal gel: Ficaire; aesculus (p.1543·3); marigold.
Haemorrhoids.

Hemosedan *Centrapharm, Belg.*
Prednisolone (p.1048·1); hexachlorophane (p.1115·2); cinchocaine hydrochloride (p.1289·2); belladonna (p.457·1).
Haemorrhoids.

Hemo-Somaton *Desbergers, Canad.*
Combination preparation: Oral solution, bovine plasma; tablets, multivitamins and minerals.
Tonic.

Hemo-Somaton with Vitamin C *Desbergers, Canad.*
Combination preparation: Oral solution, bovine plasma; tablets multivitamins and minerals.
Tonic.

Hemostatico Antisep Asen *Asens, Spain.*
Benzalkonium chloride (p.1101·3); phenazone (p.78·2); hamamelis water (p.1587·1).
Epistaxis; wounds.

Hemostatique Erce *Synthelabo, Fr.†.*
Thromboplastin (p.728·1).
Haemorrhage.

Hemotene *Astra, USA.*
Absorbable collagen (p.1566·3).
Haemostatic.

Hemotripsin *Farmitalia, Spain†.*
Ascorbic acid (p.1365·2); promethazine hydrochloride (p.416·2); chymotrypsin (p.1563·2); trypsin (p.1640·1).
Haemorrhoids.

Hemovas *Robert, Spain.*
Oxpentifylline (p.925·3).
Vascular disorders.

Hemovasal *Manetti Roberts, Ital.*
Heparan sulphate (p.879·2).
Soft-tissue disorders; superficial vascular disorders; thrombosis prophylaxis.

Hemoxier *Duopharm, Ger.†.*
Ferrous gluconate (p.1340·1); ferrous fumarate (p.1339·3); ferrous sodium citrate.
Iron-deficiency anaemias.

Hem-Prep *G & W, USA.*
Shark-liver oil; phenylmercuric nitrate (p.1122·2); bismuth subgallate (p.1180·2); zinc oxide (p.1096·2); benzocaine (p.1286·2).
Anorectal disorders.

Hemril *Upsher-Smith, USA.*
Bismuth subgallate (p.1180·2); bismuth resorcinol compound (p.1181·1); benzyl benzoate (p.1402·2); peru balsam (p.1617·2); zinc oxide (p.1096·2).

Hemril-HC *Upsher-Smith, USA.*
Hydrocortisone acetate (p.1043·3).

Hepa *Kolassa, Aust.*
Ornithine aspartate (p.1352·3).
Hyperammonaemia associated with liver disorders.

Hepa B 5 *Pierre Fabre, Fr.†.*
Choline pantothenate.
Dyspepsia.

Hepa Factor *Sigma-Tau, Spain.*
Folic acid (p.1340·3); cobamamide (p.1364·2).
Folic acid deficiency; liver disorders.

Hepabene *Merckle, Aust.*
Fumitory (p.1581·3); silybum marianum (p.993·3).
Biliary-tract disorders.

Hepabionta
Note. This name is used for preparations of different composition.
Cascan, Ger.†; Merck, S.Afr.
Injection: Orotic acid (p.1611·2); vitamin B substances.
Liver disorders.
Cascan, Ger.†.
Tablets: Rutin (p.1580·2); orotic acid (p.1611·2); thioctic acid (p.1636·2); inositol (p.1591·1); vitamins.
Liver disorders.

Hepabionta comp *Cascan, Ger.†.*
Brown capsules, thioctic acid (p.1636·2); choline orotate (p.1611·2); vitamins; orange capsules, ox bile (p.1553·2); pancreatin (p.1612·1).
Liver disorders.

Hepabuzone *Spirig, Switz.*
Heparin sodium (p.879·3); phenylbutazone (p.79·2).
Musculoskeletal, joint, peri-articular, and soft-tissue disorders; peripheral vascular disorders; thrombophlebitis.

Hepaccine-B *Biovac, S.Afr.*
A hepatitis B vaccine (p.1513·1).
Active immunisation.

Hepacholine Sorbitol *Synthelabo, Fr.*
Choline citrate (p.1337·1); sorbitol (p.1354·2).
Constipation; dyspepsia.

Hepacitol *Andromaco, Spain.*
Arginine timonacicate (p.1334·2).
Liver disorders.

Hepaclem *Clement Thionville, Fr.*
Cynara (p.1569·2); boldo (p.1554·1); combretum (p.1593·2); curcuma zanthorrhiza.
Digestive-system disorders; renal disorders.

Hepacoban B12 *Bohm, Spain.*
Vitamin B substances; liver extract.
Tonic; vitamin B deficiency.

Hepacolina *IBIS, Ital.†.*
Cascara sagrada (p.1183·1); artichoke (p.1569·2); rhubarb (p.1212·1).
Constipation.

Hepacomplet B12 1000 *Reig Jofre, Spain.*
Vitamin B substances; liver; adenine hydrochloride (p.1543·2).
Anaemias; tonic.

Hepacomplet B12 Triple *Reig Jofre, Spain.*
Vitamin B substances; liver; amino acids.
Anaemias; tonic.

Hepadial *Biocodex, Fr.*
Dimecrotic acid, magnesium salt.
Dyspepsia.

Hepadif *Reig Jofre, Spain.*
Oral solution: Carnitine orotate (p.1611·2); carnitine (p.1336·2); vitamin B substances; liver extract.
Tablets: Carnitine orotate (p.1611·2); vitamin B substances; liver extract; sorbitol (p.1354·2); adenine hydrochloride (p.1543·2).
Acetonaemia; hepatitis.

Hepadigest *Uriach, Spain.*
Cyclobutyrol calcium (p.1569·2); metoclopramide hydrochloride (p.1200·3); procaine (p.1299·2); tiopronin (p.997·2).
Dyspepsia; hepatobiliary disorders.

Hepaduran *Zwintscher, Ger.†.*
Orthosiphon stamineus leaf (p.1592·2); curcuma zanthorrhiza; berberis; silybum marianum (p.993·3); rubia tinctorum; acetylmethionine.
Liver disorders.

Hepa-Factor *Max Farma, Ital.*
Folinic acid (p.1342·2); hydroxocobalamin (p.1363·3).
Hyperchromic anaemia; liver disorders.

Hepa-Factor Complex *Sigma-Tau, Ital.†.*
Cobamamide (p.1364·2); folinic acid (p.1342·2); factor VIII (p.720·3).
Hyperchromic anaemia; liver disorders.

Hepafungin *Schwabe, Ger.†.*
Silybum marianum (p.993·3); taraxacum (p.1634·2).
Liver disorders.

Hepagallin N *Pfluger, Ger.*
Cynara (p.1569·2).
Dyspepsia.

Hepa-Gastreu R7 *Reckeweg, Ger.*
Homoeopathic preparation.

Hepa-Gel
Lichtenstein, Ger.; Spirig, Switz.
Heparin sodium (p.879·3).
Peripheral vascular disorders; soft-tissue disorders.

Hepaglobin *Tropon-Cutter, Ger.†.*
A hepatitis B immunoglobulin (p.1512·3).
Passive immunisation.

Hepagrisevit Forte-N *Pharmacia Upjohn, Ger.*
Injection: Cyanocobalamin (p.1363·3); folic acid (p.1340·3); nicotinamide (p.1351·2).
Lignocaine hydrochloride (p.1293·2) is included in this preparation to alleviate the pain of injection.
Tablets: Cyanocobalamin (p.1363·3); folic acid (p.1340·3); pyridoxine hydrochloride (p.1362·3).
Liver disorders.

Hepagrisevit SP *Farmitalia Carlo Erba, Ger.†.*
Cyanocobalamin; folic acid; nicotinamide.
Liver disorders.

Hepagrisevit-Depot *Pharmacia Upjohn, Ger.†.*
Ampoule 1, hydroxocobalamin (p.1363·3); ampoule 2, nicotinamide (p.1351·2); folic acid (p.1340·3).
Liver disorders.

Hepagrume *Synthelabo, Fr.*
Arginine (p.1334·1); betaine (p.1553·2); choline dihydrogen citrate (p.1337·1); inositol (p.1591·1); sorbitol (p.1354·2).
Constipation; dyspepsia.

Hepa-L *Divapharma, Ger.†.*
Blackberry leaf; matricaria flowers (p.1561·2); caraway (p.1559·3); taraxacum (p.1634·2); peppermint leaves (p.1208·1); orange flowers.
Herbal tea.

hepa-L 90 N *Loges, Ger.*
Homoeopathic preparation.

Hepalean *Organon Teknika, Canad.*
Heparin sodium (p.879·3).
Thrombo-embolic disorders; thrombosis prophylaxis.

Hepalean-Lok *Organon Teknika, Canad.*
Heparin sodium (p.879·3).
To maintain patency of intravenous injection devices.

Hepalipon N *Rhenomed, Ger.*
Methionine (p.984·2); choline hydrogen tartrate (p.1337·1); inositol (p.1591·1).
Liver disorders.

Hepalixier *Gripp, Ger.†.*
Chelidonium; silybum marianum (p.993·3); taraxacum (p.1634·2); frangula bark (p.1193·2); peppermint leaf (p.1208·1); senna (p.1212·2); choline dihydrogen citrate (p.1337·1); cysteine hydrochloride (p.1338·3); thiamine hydrochloride (p.1361·1).
Liver disorders.

Hepa-loges N *Loges, Ger.*
Silybum marianum (p.993·3).
Liver disorders.

Hepa-Merz *Merz, Ger.*
Enteric-coated tablets†: Ornithine aspartate (p.1352·3); porcine pancreatin (p.1612·1).
Digestive system disorders.
Injection; oral granules: Ornithine aspartate (p.1352·3).
Liver disorders.

Hepa-Merz KT *Merz, Ger.*
Ornithine aspartate (p.1352·3).
Liver disorders.

Hepa-Merz Lact *Merz, Ger.*
Lactulose (p.1195·3).
Constipation; liver disorders; salmonella enteritis.

Hepa-Merz Sil *Merz, Ger.*
Silybum marianum (p.993·3).
Liver disorders.

Hepaminohek *Hek, Ger.†.*
Amino-acid infusion.
Parenteral nutrition in liver disease.

Hepanephrol *Roso-Phytopharma, Fr.*
Cynara (p.1569·2).
Formerly contained cynara and hesperidin.
Dyspepsia; fluid retention.

Hepanutrin *Geistlich, UK.*
Amino-acid infusion.
Parenteral nutrition.

Hepaplus *Hexal, Ger.*
Heparin sodium (p.879·3).
Soft-tissue injury; superficial vascular disorders.

Hepa-POS *Ursapharm, Ger.*
Cynara (p.1569·2).
Dyspepsia.

Hepar 10% *Pharmacia Upjohn, Ger.*
Amino-acid preparation.
Liver disorders.

Hepar H *Pfluger, Ger.*
Homoeopathic preparation.

Hepar 202 N *Staufen, Ger.*
Homoeopathic preparation.

Hepar Pasc Mono *Koch, Aust.*
Silybum marianum (p.993·3).
Liver disorders.

The symbol † denotes a preparation no longer actively marketed

Hepar SL Serturner, Ger.
Cynara (p.1569·2).
Dyspepsia.

Heparano N Pfluger, Ger.
Silybum marianum (p.993·3).
Liver disorders.

Heparaxal Roland, Ger.†.
Cynara (p.1569·2); boldo (p.1554·1); silybum marianum (p.993·3); cascara (p.1183·1); taraxacum (p.1634·2); turmeric (p.1001·3); senna (p.1212·2); belladonna; orotic acid (p.1611·2); ox bile (p.1553·2).
Biliary disorders.

Heparbil Montefarmaco, Ital.†.
Sodium dehydrocholate (p.1570·3); rhubarb (p.1212·1); cascara (p.1183·1); boldo (p.1554·1); combretum (p.1593·2); cynara (p.1569·2); equisetum (p.1575·1); belladonna (p.457·1); chamomile (p.1561·2).
Liver and biliary-tract disorders.

Heparchofid S Fides, Ger.†.
Urtica (p.1642·3); hamamelis (p.1587·1); absinthium (p.1541·1); arnica (p.1550·3); silybum marianum (p.993·3); taraxacum (p.1634·2); cynara (p.1569·2); spirit. aether.; peppermint leaf (p.1208·1); hypericum; graphites; chelidonium; colocynthis; fel tauri.
Digestive disorders; liver and gall disorders.

Heparegen Drossapharm, Switz.
Timonacic (p.1638·1).
Liver disorders.

Heparexine Murat, Fr.
Fosforylcholine magnesium (p.1581·3).
Constipation; dyspepsia.

Hepargitol Elerte, Fr.
Arginine hydrochloride (p.1334·1); sorbitol (p.1354·2); anhydrous sodium sulphate (p.1213·3); sodium phosphate (p.1159·3); citric acid (p.1564·3).
Constipation; dyspepsia.

Heparilene Clariana, Spain†.
A heparinoid (p.882·3).
Arteriosclerosis; hyperlipidaemias.

Heparin Comp
CT, Ger.; Ratiopharm, Ger.†.
Heparin sodium (p.879·3); arnica (p.1550·3); aesculus (p.1543·3).
Soft-tissue injury; superficial vascular disorders.

Heparin 30 000-ratiopharm/ Heparin 50 000-ratiopharm Ratiopharm, Ger.†.
Heparin sodium (p.879·3); dexpanthenol (p.1570·3).
Skin trauma.

Heparinol Streuli, Switz.†.
Heparin sodium (p.879·3); thymol.
Haematomas; thrombophlebitis; ulcers; varicose veins.

Heparos Desbergers, Canad.
Cyanocobalamin (p.1363·3); ferric ammonium citrate (p.1339·2).
Iron-deficiency anaemias.

Hepar-Pasc Pascoe, Ger.
Silybum marianum (p.993·3).
Liver disorders.

Hepar-Pasc N Pascoe, Ger.
Methionine (p.984·2); chelidonium majus; silybum marianum (p.993·3).
Liver disorders.

Hepar-POS Ursapharm, Ger.
Cynara (p.1569·2).
Dyspepsia.

Heparsyx N Syxyl, Ger.
Silybum marianum (p.993·3).
Liver disorders.

Hepa-Salbe Lichtenstein, Ger.
Heparin sodium (p.879·3).
Inflammation; swelling.

Hepaselect Dreluso, Ger.†.
Homoeopathic preparation.

Hepasil Edmond Pharma, Ital.†.
Fencibutirol (p.1578·3).
Biliary-tract disorders.

Hepasil Composto Edmond Pharma, Ital.
Fencibutirol sodium (p.1578·3); rhubarb (p.1212·1); frangula (p.1193·2); cascara (p.1183·1); boldo (p.1554·1).
Constipation.

Hepasol G.P. Laboratories, Austral.
Vitamin and mineral preparation with liver extract.
Tonic.

Hepasteril Fresenius, Ger.†.
Injection: Arginine (p.1334·1); malic acid (p.1598·3); magnesium hydrogen aspartate (p.1157·2); cyanocobalamin (p.1363·3); folic acid (p.1340·3).
Tablets: Choline chloride dihydrogen phosphate, calcium salt; pancreatin (p.1612·1); ox bile (p.1553·2); pepsin (p.1616·3); vitamins.
Gastro-intestinal disorders; liver disorders.

Hepasteril A Fresenius, Ger.†.
Arginine (p.1334·1); electrolytes; sorbitol; vitamins; ethoxazorutoside (p.1580·1).
Liver disease.

Hepatamine
Kendall McGaw, Canad.†; McGaw, USA.
Amino-acid infusion.
Parenteral nutrition in hepatic encephalopathy.

Hepatect
Biotest, Aust.; Biotest, Ger.; Intra Pharma, Irl.; Biotest, Ital.; Biotest, Switz.
A hepatitis B immunoglobulin (p.1512·3).
Passive immunisation.

Hepathromb LAW, Ger.; Brenner-Efeka, Ger.
Heparin sodium (p.879·3).
Inflammation; swelling.

Hepathrombin Godecke, Ger.
Heparin sodium (p.879·3).
Skin trauma.

Hepathrombine Warner-Lambert, Switz.
Heparin sodium (p.879·3); allantoin (p.1078·2); dexpanthenol (p.1570·3).
Scars; soft-tissue injury; venous insufficiency.

Hepathrombin-Procto Godecke, Ger.†.
Heparin sodium (p.879·3); prednisolone acetate (p.1048·1); laureth 9 (p.1325·2).
Anorectal disorders.

Hepatic-Aid Baxter, Ital.†.
Food for special diets.
Liver disorders.

Hepatic-Aid II
Kendall, UK†; McGaw, USA.
Food for special diets.
Liver disease; porto-hepatic encephalopathy.

Hepaticum "Mletzko" Mletzko, Ger.†.
Turmeric (p.1001·3); curcuma zanthorrhiza; cynara (p.1569·2); chelidonium; cinchona bark (p.1564·1); frangula bark (p.1193·2); gentian (p.1583·3); galanga; aloes (p.1177·1); cysteine (p.1338·3); anhydrous orotic acid (p.1611·2).
Liver disorders.

Hepaticum novo Pascoe, Ger.
Curcuma zanthorrhiza; peppermint leaf (p.1208·1); absinthium (p.1541·1).
Biliary disorders.

Hepaticum-Divinal Divinal, Ger.†.
Oral liquid: Agrimony; boldo (p.1554·1); cnicus benedictus (p.1565·3); centaury (p.1561·1); chelidonium; frangula bark (p.1193·2); hedera helix; hypericum (p.1590·1); peppermint leaf (p.1208·1); taraxacum (p.1634·2); caraway oil (p.1559·3); fennel oil (p.1579·2); peppermint oil (p.1208·1); guaiazulene (p.1586·3).
Tablets: Agrimony; boldo (p.1554·1); chelidonium; frangula bark (p.1193·2); gentian (p.1583·3); hedera helix; senna (p.1212·2); taraxacum (p.1634·2); caraway oil (p.1559·3); fennel oil (p.1579·2); peppermint oil (p.1208·1); ox bile (p.1553·2); cholic acid; guaiazulene (p.1586·3); yogurt; docusate sodium (p.1189·3); orotic acid (p.1611·2).
Liver disorders.

Hepaticum-Lac-Medice Medice, Ger.
Lactulose (p.1195·3).
Constipation; liver disorders; salmonella enteritis.

Hepaticum-Medice H Medice, Ger.
Cinchona bark (p.1564·1); silybum marianum (p.993·3); chelidonium; gentian (p.1583·3); turmeric (p.1001·3).
Adjunct in skin disorders; biliary disorders; gastro-intestinal disorders.

Hepatimed N Medice, Ger.
Chelidonium majus; hydrastis (p.1588·2); silybum marianum (p.993·3).
Acne; biliary disorders; constipation.

Hepato Fardi Fardi, Spain.
Choline orotate (p.1611·2); almond milk.
Liver disorders.

Hepatoclamar Clariana, Spain†.
Vitamin B substances; suprarenal cortex extract (p.1050·1); liver.
Lignocaine hydrochloride (p.1293·2) is included in this preparation to alleviate the pain of injection.
Anaemias; tonic.

Hepatodoron
Weleda, Aust.; Weleda, Ger.
Fragaria vesca; vitis vinifera.
Constipation; eczema; liver disorders.

Hepatofalk Falk, Ger.
Choline orotate (p.1611·2); adenosine (p.812·3); cyanocobalamin (p.1363·3); hydroxocobalamin acetate (p.1364·2).
Lignocaine hydrochloride (p.1293·2) is included in the intramuscular injection to alleviate the pain of injection.
Liver disorders.

Hepatofalk Neu Falk, Ger.
Choline orotate (p.1611·2); cysteine hydrochloride (p.1338·3); vitamins; ox bile (p.1553·2); ammi visnaga (p.1593·2); absinthium (p.1541·1); boldo (p.1554·1); chelidonium; curcuma zanthorrhiza; cynara (p.1569·2); taraxacum (p.1634·2).
Liver and biliary-tract disorders.

Hepatofalk Planta Falk, Ger.
Silybum marianum (p.993·3); javanese turmeric; chelidonium.
Liver disorders.

Hepaton Steigerwald, Ger.†.
Aloes (p.1177·1); cinchona bark (p.1564·1); peppermint leaf (p.1208·1); silybum marianum (p.993·3); chelidonium; gentian (p.1583·3); turmeric (p.1001·3).
Biliary disorders; liver disorders.

Hepatorell Sanorell, Ger.
Silybum marianum (p.993·3).
Liver disorders.

Hepatorex Cooperation Pharmaceutique, Fr.†.
Boldo (p.1554·1); cynara (p.1569·2); combretum (p.1593·2); sodium sulphate decahydrate (p.1213·3); sodium citrate (p.1153·2).
Gastro-intestinal disorders.

Hepatos
Note. This name is used for preparations of different composition.
Hevert, Ger.
Silybum marianum (p.993·3).
Liver disorders.

Teofarma, Ital.
Cascara (p.1183·1); boldo (p.1554·1).
Constipation.

Hepatos B12 Teofarma, Ital.
Cascara sagrada (p.1183·1); boldo (p.1554·1); inositol (p.1591·1); cyanocobalamin (p.1363·3).
Constipation.

Hepatoum Hepatoum, Fr.
Oral liquid: Pulsatilla (p.1623·3); turmeric (p.1001·3); chloroform (p.1220·3); amyl acetate (p.1375·2); peppermint oil (p.1208·1).
Digestive disorders.
Tablets: Pepsin (p.1616·3); pancreatin (p.1612·1); amylase (p.1549·1).
Dyspepsia.

Hepatoxane Esplanade, Fr.
Tocamphyl.
Dyspepsia.

Hepa-Uvocal Stroschein, Ger.†.
Injection: Liver extract; cyanocobalamin (p.1363·3).
Anaemias; liver disorders.
Tablets: Liver extract; potassium hydrogen aspartate (p.1161·3); magnesium hydrogen aspartate (p.1157·2).
Liver disorders.

Hepa-Vibolex Rosen, Ger.†.
Ornithine L-aspartate (p.1352·3).
Hepatic encephalopathy.

Hepavimil B12 Garcia Suarez, Spain†.
Vitamin B substances; liver extract.
Tonic; vitamin B_{12} deficiency.

Hepavis Minden, Ger.†.
Cyanocobalamin (p.1363·3); choline orotate (p.1611·2); magnesium orotate (p.1611·2); dehydrocholic acid (p.1570·2).
Liver disorders.

Hepavit Frika, Aust.
Hydroxocobalamin acetate (p.1364·2).
Anaemias; neurologic disorders.

Hepavite Covan, S.Afr.
Choline bitartrate (p.1337·1); inositol (p.1591·1); methionine (p.984·2); vitamin B substances; bioflavonoids; magnesium sulphate; zinc sulphate; potassium chloride.
Hepatic disorders.

Hepax
Note. This name is used for preparations of different composition.
Sabex, Canad.†.
Oral liquid: Cynara (p.1569·2); kinkeliba (p.1593·2); bearberry (p.1552·2); boldo (p.1554·1); crataegus (p.1568·2); adonis vernalis (p.1543·3); peptone; magnesium chloride (p.1157·2); rosemary.
Tablets: Boldo (p.1554·1); cynara (p.1569·2); kinkeliba (p.1593·2); bearberry (p.1552·2); crataegus (p.1568·2); peptone; magnesium chloride (p.1157·2).
Biliary insufficiency; gastro-intestinal disturbances.

UPSA, Fr.
Cynara (p.1569·2); kinkéliba (p.1593·2); boldo (p.1554·1); rosemary.
Digestive disorders.

Hep-B-Gammagee Merck Sharp & Dohme, USA†.
A hepatitis B immunoglobulin (p.1512·3).
Passive immunisation.

Hep-Flush Leo, UK.
Heparin sodium (p.879·3).
To maintain patency of in-dwelling intravenous lines.

Hep-Forte Marlyn, USA.
Multivitamin and mineral preparation.

Heplant Spitzner, Ger.
Silybum marianum (p.993·3).
Liver disorders.

HeplexAmine Fresenius, UK.
Amino-acid infusion.
Parenteral nutrition.

Hep-Lock Elkins-Sinn, USA.
Heparin sodium (p.879·3).
To maintain patency of in-dwelling intravenous lines.

Heplok
Leo, Irl.; Leo, UK.
Heparin sodium (p.879·3).
To maintain patency of in-dwelling intravenous lines.

Hep-Pak Winthrop, USA†.
Heparin (p.879·3).

Heprecomb Berna, Switz.
A hepatitis B vaccine (recombinant DNA) (p.1513·1).
Active immunisation.

Hep-Rinse Leo, Irl.
Heparin sodium (p.879·3).
To maintain patency of intravenous lines.

Hepro Casen Fleet, Spain.
Allantoin hydrochloride (p.1078·2); aminacrine (p.1098·3); hydrocortisone hemisuccinate (p.1044·1); lignocaine hydrochloride (p.1293·2).
Anorectal disorders.

Heprone Inibsa, Spain†.
Sucralfate (p.1214·2).
Peptic ulcer.

Hepsal
CP Pharmaceuticals, Irl.; CP Pharmaceuticals, UK.
Heparin sodium (p.879·3).
To maintain patency of in-dwelling intravenous lines.

Hepsan Knoll, Ger.†.
Methionine (p.984·2); choline bitartrate (p.1337·1); yeast extract (p.1373·1); soya-lecithin (p.1595·2); vitamins.
Liver disorders.

Heptadon Ebewe, Aust.
Methadone hydrochloride (p.53·2).
Pain.

Heptalac Copley, USA.
Lactulose (p.1195·3).

Hept-A-Myl
Synthelabo, Belg.; Synthelabo, Fr.
Heptaminol (p.1587·2) or heptaminol hydrochloride (p.1587·2).
Hypotension.

Heptan Aguettant, Fr.
Minerals and trace element preparation.
Parenteral nutrition.

Hepuman
Berna, Belg.; Berna, Spain; Berna, Switz.
A hepatitis B immunoglobulin (p.1512·3).
Passive immunisation.

Hepuman B Berna, Ital.
A hepatitis B immunoglobulin (p.1512·3).
Passive immunisation.

Heracillin Astra, Swed.
Flucloxacillin magnesium (p.209·1) or flucloxacillin sodium (p.209·2).
Bacterial infections.

Heracline Charton, Canad.
Adrenal cortex extract (p.1050·1); testis extract (p.1464·1); liver extract.
Tonic.

Heralvent Luhr-Lehrs, Ger.
Homoeopathic preparation.

Herb and Honey Cough Elixir Weleda, UK.
Honey (p.1345·3); althaea (p.1546·3); cetraria island.; marrubium vulgare (p.1063·3); pimpinella anisum fruit; sambucus nigra flowers (p.1627·2); thyme (p.1636·3).
Coughs.

Herbadon Herbapharm, Ger.
Aconite (p.1542·2).
Musculoskeletal and joint disorders.

Herbagola Gricar, Ital.
Cetylpyridinium chloride (p.1106·2).
Oral disinfection.

Herbal Anxiety Formula Faulding, Austral.
Passion flower (p.1615·3); chamomile (p.1561·2).
Anxiety; nervous tension.

Herbal Arthritis Formula Faulding, Austral.
Ginkgo biloba (p.1584·1); harpagophytum procumbens (p.27·2).
Arthritis; rheumatism.

Herbal Booster Pharmadass, UK.
Kola (p.1645·1); bissy nut (p.1645·1); echinacea (p.1574·2); spirulina (p.1632·2); yellow dock; ginger (p.1193·2); liquorice (p.1197·1).

Herbal Capillary Care Faulding, Austral.
Ginkgo biloba (p.1584·1); aesculus (p.1543·3).
Nocturnal leg cramps; tinnitus; tired legs and feet.

Herbal Cleanse Vitaplex, Austral.
Aloes (p.1177·1); taraxacum (p.1634·2); psyllium (p.1194·2); rumex crispus; sarsaparilla (p.1627·2); lappa (p.1594·2); clivers (p.1565·2); hydrastis (p.1588·2); slippery elm (p.1630·1); echinacea purpurea (p.1574·2); ginger (p.1193·2); silybum marianum (p.993·3).
Constipation; liver disorders.

Herbal Cold & Flu Relief Faulding, Austral.
Echinacea angustifolia (p.1574·2); liquorice (p.1197·1); garlic (p.1583·1).
Catarrh; cold and influenza symptoms.

Herbal Cold Relief Jamieson, Canad.
Ephedra (p.1059·3); eucalyptus oil (p.1578·1); grindelia.

Herbal Cough Expectorant Jamieson, Canad.
Elm bark (p.1630·1); eucalyptus oil (p.1578·1); honey (p.1345·3); anise oil (p.1550·1); camphor oil.

Herbal Digestive Formula Faulding, Austral.
Liquorice (p.1197·1); turmeric (p.1001·3); ginger (p.1193·2).
Dyspepsia; flatulence.

Herbal Diuretic Complex Suisse, Austral.†.
L-lysine; parsley herb (p.1615·3); juniper berries (p.1592·2); barberry; equisetum (p.1575·1); celery seed (p.1561·1); water cress; taraxacum (p.1634·2); buchu (p.1555·2); kelp (p.1593·1).
Herbal diuretic.

Herbal Diuretic Formula Faulding, Austral.
Taraxacum (p.1634·2); bearberry (p.1552·2).
Fluid retention.

Herbal Eye Care Formula Faulding, Austral.
Myrtillus (p.1606·1).
Eye disorders.

Herbal Headache Relief Faulding, Austral.
Feverfew (p.447·3).
Headache.

Herbal Indigestion Naturtabs Cantassium Co., UK.
Scutellaria; valerian (p.1643·1); fennel (p.1579·1); myrrh (p.1606·1); papain (p.1614·1); capsicum oleoresin.

Herbal Laxative
Note. This name is used for preparations of different composition.
Vitaplex, Austral.
Senna (p.1212·2); ispaghula husk (p.1194·2); liquorice (p.1197·1).
Constipation.

Quest, Canad.
Cascara (p.1183·1); rhubarb (p.1212·1).

Shaklee, Canad.
Senna (p.1212·2); buckthorn (p.1182·1); leptandra virginica.
Constipation.

Swiss Herbal, Canad.
Senna leaves (p.1212·2); cascara (p.1183·1); rhubarb root (p.1212·1); gentian root (p.1583·3); liquorice root (p.1197·1); juniper berries (p.1592·2); buchu leaves (p.1555·2); peppermint oil (p.1208·1).
Constipation.

Nature's Bounty, USA.
Senna (p.1212·2); cascara (p.1183·1).
Constipation.

Herbal Liver Formula *Faulding, Austral.*
Silybum marianum (p.993·3).
Digestive disorders; liver disorders.

Herbal Nerve *Swiss Herbal, Canad.*
Valerian root (p.1643·1); scutellaria; gentian root (p.1583·3); liquorice (p.1197·1).

Herbal Pain Relief *Cantassium Co., UK.*
Willow bark (p.82·3); passion flower (p.1615·3); valerian (p.1643·1).
Pain.

Herbal PMS Formula *Faulding, Austral.*
Myrtillus (p.1606·1); liquorice (p.1197·1); cimicifuga (p.1563·3).
Menstrual disorders.

Herbal Powder No.8 *Gerard House, UK†.*
Dandelion leaf (p.1634·2); uva ursi (p.1552·2); couch-grass (p.1567·3); buchu (p.1555·2).
Fluid retention.

Herbal Sleep Formula *Faulding, Austral.*
Valerian (p.1643·1).
Insomnia.

Herbal Sleep Well *Swiss Herbal, Canad.†.*
Valerian root (p.1643·1); passion flower (p.1615·3); lupulus (p.1597·2); melissa (p.1600·1); tilia (p.1637·3).
Insomnia due to fatigue.

Herbal Stress Relief *Faulding, Austral.*
Ginseng (p.1584·2).
Stress.

Herbalax *Sante Naturelle, Canad.*
Cascara (p.1183·1); frangula (p.1193·2); rhubarb (p.1212·1); senna (p.1212·2); bile salts (p.1553·2).

Herbalax Forte *Sante Naturelle, Canad.*
Cascara (p.1183·1); phenolphthalein (p.1208·2); bile salts (p.1553·2); capsicum oleoresin; papain (p.1614·1).

Herbalene *Lusty, UK.*
Senna leaf (p.1212·2); buckthorn (p.1182·1); elder leaf; fennel (p.1579·1).
Constipation.

Herbaneurin *Herbapharm, Ger.*
Hypericum (p.1590·1).
Anxiety; depression.

Herbatar *Erredici, Ital.*
Cream: Pine oil; birch oil (p.1092·2); castor oil (p.1560·2); chamomile (p.1561·2); allantoin (p.1078·2).
Skin disorders.
Scalp application: Pine oil; birch oil (p.1092·2); cedar oil.
Seborrhoeic dermatitis.

Herbatar Plus *Erredici, Ital.*
Ammonium lactate (p.1079·1); tar (p.1092·3); allantoin (p.1078·2).
Hyperkeratosis.

Herbatorment *Herbapharm, Ger.*
Tormentil (p.1638·3).
Diarrhoea.

Herbavit *Erredici, Ital.*
Biotin (p.1336·1); a heparinoid (p.882·3); arnica (p.1550·3); urtica (p.1642·3); polyglycopolyamine; dexpanthenol (p.1570·3); menthol (p.1600·2).
Prevention of hair loss.

Herbe *Recordati, Ital.*
Benzalkonium chloride (p.1101·3); hamamelis (p.1587·1).
Eye disinfection.

Herbelax *Waldheim, Aust.*
Calcium sennoside A (p.1212·3); calcium sennoside B (p.1212·3); bran (p.1181·2); fig (p.1193·2).
Bowel evacuation; constipation; stool softener.

Herbelix *Lane, UK.*
Lobelia (p.1481·3); tolu solution (p.1071·1); sodium bicarbonate (p.1153·2).
Nasal congestion.

Herbesan *Phygiene, Fr.*
Senna (p.1212·2); aniseed (p.1549·3); peppermint leaf (p.1208·1); couch-grass (p.1567·3).
Constipation.

Herbesan Instantane *Phygiene, Fr.*
Sennosides B (p.1212·3).
Constipation.

Herbesser *Tanabe, Jpn.*
Diltiazem hydrochloride (p.854·2).
Angina pectoris; arrhythmias; hypertension.

Herbheal Ointment *Potter's, UK.*
Colophony (p.1567·1); starch (p.1356·2); sublimed sulphur (p.1091·2); zinc oxide (p.1096·2); marshmallow root (p.1546·3); chickweed.
Skin irritation.

Herbin-Stodin *Lorenz, Ger.†.*
Aspirin (p.16·1); paracetamol (p.72·2); caffeine (p.749·3).
Cold symptoms; fever; migraine; neuralgia; pain; rheumatism.

Herbogesic *Seroyal, Canad.*
Magnesium salicylate (p.51·1).

Herbolax *Seroyal, Canad.*
Cascara (p.1183·1); rhubarb (p.1212·1); senna (p.1212·2); liquorice (p.1197·1).

Herbopyrine *Herbes Universelles, Canad.*
Aspirin (p.16·1); caffeine citrate (p.749·3).

Herborex *Rolmex, Canad.*
Cascara (p.1183·1); rumex crispus.

Herbulax *English Grains, UK.*
Frangula bark (p.1193·2); taraxacum (p.1634·2).
Constipation.

Herceptin *Genentech, USA.*
Trastuzumab (p.568·1).
Breast cancer.

Heridasone *Rovi, Spain†.*
Hydrocortisone acetate (p.1043·3); neomycin sulphate (p.229·2).
Infected skin disorders.

Herisan *Rougier, Canad.*
Zinc oxide (p.1096·2).
Superficial skin irritations.

Hermal *Merck-Clevenot, Fr.*
Pyrithione zinc (p.1089·3).
Seborrhoeic dermatitis.

Hermalind
Merck, Aust.†; Hermal, Ger.
Dexpanthenol (p.1570·3); chlorhexidine gluconate (p.1107·2).
Burns; wounds.

Hermasept *Merck, Aust.*
Dexpanthenol (p.1570·3); chlorhexidine gluconate (p.1107·2).
Burns; infected wounds.

Hermes ASS *Hermes, Ger.*
Aspirin (p.16·1).
Fever; pain.

Hermes ASS plus *Hermes, Ger.*
Aspirin (p.16·1); caffeine (p.749·3).
Pain.

Hermes Cevitt *Hermes, Ger.*
Ascorbic acid (p.1365·2).
Vitamin C deficiency.

Hermes Cevitt + Calcium *Hermes, Ger.*
Ascorbic acid (p.1365·2); calcium carbonate (p.1182·1).
Vitamin C and calcium deficiency.

Hermes Drix Abfuhr-Tee *Hermes, Ger.*
Senna (p.1212·2).
Constipation.

Hermolepsin *Orion, Swed.*
Carbamazepine (p.339·2).
Alcohol withdrawal syndrome; epilepsy; trigeminal neuralgia.

Hernia-Tee *Steierl, Ger.*
Bearberry (p.1552·2); herniaria (p.1587·2); equisetum (p.1575·1).
Urinary-tract disorders.

Hernidisc *Eagle, Austral.*
Homoeopathic preparation.

Herniol *Steierl, Ger.*
Bearberry (p.1552·2); herniaria (p.1587·2).
Urinary-tract disorders.

Herpecin-L *Chattem, USA.*
Allantoin (p.1078·2); padimate O (p.1488·1).
Oral lesions.

Herpen *Sumitomo, Jpn.*
Ampicillin sodium (p.153·1).
Bacterial infections.

Herpes-Gel *Master Pharma, Ital.*
Ibacitabine (p.613·2).
Herpesvirus infections.

Herpetad
TAD, Ger.; Windsor, UK.
Aciclovir (p.602·3).
Herpes simplex infections.

Herpetrol *Alva, USA.*
Multivitamin preparation with zinc and lysine.

Herpex *Germania, Aust.*
Bacillus subtilis.
Herpes zoster infection.

Herphonal *Dresden, Ger.*
Trimipramine maleate (p.310·1).
Depression; pain.

Herpid *Yamanouchi, UK.*
Idoxuridine (p.613·2) in dimethyl sulphoxide.
Cutaneous herpes simplex and zoster infections.

Herpidu *Ciba Vision, Switz.†.*
Idoxuridine (p.613·2).
Herpes simplex infections of the eye.

Herpidu Chloramphenicol *Dispersa, Switz.†.*
Idoxuridine (p.613·2); chloramphenicol (p.182·1).
Herpes simplex infections of the eye.

Herplex
Allergan, Austral.†; Allergan, Canad.; Allergan, USA†.
Idoxuridine (p.613·2).
Herpes simplex keratitis.

Herplex-D
Allergan, Austral.; Allergan, Irl.†; Allergan, S.Afr.†.
Idoxuridine (p.613·2).
Herpes simplex lesions of the skin.

Herpofug *Wolff, Ger.*
Aciclovir (p.602·3).
Herpesvirus infections.

Herposicc *Nycomed, Aust.*
Benzocaine (p.1286·2); sulphur (p.1091·2); zinc oxide (p.1096·2); talc (p.1092·1); phenol (p.1121·2).
Herpes labialis.

Herpotern *Rentschler, Ger.*
Aciclovir sodium (p.602·3).
Herpes and varicella virus infections.

Herpoviric *Azupharma, Ger.*
Aciclovir (p.602·3).
Herpesvirus infections.

Herten *Vir, Spain.*
Enalapril maleate (p.863·2).
Heart failure; hypertension.

Herviros
Merck, Aust.; Hermal, Ger.
Amethocaine hydrochloride (p.1285·2); aminoquinuride hydrochloride (p.1101·2).
Infected mouth disorders.

Herwicard 0,8 *Herbert, Ger.†.*
Glyceryl trinitrate (p.874·3).
Angina pectoris; myocardial infarction.

Herz- und Kreislauftonikum Bioflora *Bioflora, Aust.*
Crataegus (p.1568·2); mistletoe (p.1604·1); melissa (p.1600·1); rosemary; lavender flower (p.1594·3).
Cardiovascular disorders.

HerzASS *Ratiopharm, Ger.*
Aspirin (p.16·1).
Thrombosis prophylaxis.

Herzotial *Reinecke, Ger.†.*
Homoeopathic preparation.

Herz-plus *Herzpunkt, Ger.†.*
Valerian (p.1643·1); crataegus (p.1568·2); lupulus (p.1597·2); melissa (p.1600·1); mistletoe (p.1604·1); rutin (p.1580·2).
Heart and nerve tonic.

Herz-plus Forte N *Herzpunkt, Ger.†.*
Valerian (p.1643·1); lupulus (p.1597·2).
Insomnia; nervousness.

Herz-Plus Nerven *Herzpunkt, Ger.†.*
Valerian (p.1643·1); crataegus (p.1568·2); lupulus (p.1597·2); melissa (p.1600·1); mistletoe (p.1604·1).
Nervous disorders; sleep disorders.

Herz-Punkt forte *Herzpunkt, Ger.†.*
Crataegus; melissa; ginseng; ferrous gluconate.
Tonic.

Herz-Punkt Vitaltonikum N *Herzpunkt, Ger.†.*
Crataegus; melissa; ferrous gluconate.
Tonic.

Herz-Starkung N *Jukunda, Ger.*
Crataegus (p.1568·2); lycopus virg.; cactus; kalmia latifolia; camphora.
Cardiac disorders.

Herztropfen Truw Gold *Truw, Ger.*
Homoeopathic preparation.

Hespan
Du Pont, Canad.†; Don Baxter, Ital.†; Du Pont Pharmaceuticals, UK; Du Pont, USA.
Hetastarch (p.724·1) in sodium chloride.
Extracorporeal circulation; leucopheresis; plasma volume expansion.

Hespander *Kyorin, Jpn.*
Hetastarch (p.724·1) in glucose with electrolytes.
Haemodiluent; plasma volume expansion.

Hespercorbin *Fides, Spain.*
Glucosamine sulphate (p.1585·1).
Athrosis.

Hesteril *Fresenius, Fr.*
Pentastarch (p.725·2).
Haemodilution; plasma volume expansion.

Hetrazan
Lederle, Austral.; Wyeth-Ayerst, Canad.; Lederle, Ger.†; Lederle, UK.
Diethylcarbamazine citrate (p.99·2).
Worm infections.

Hetrolgalen *Galenika, Ger.*
Hedera helix.
Catarrh.

Heumann Abfurhtee Solubilax N *Heumann, Ger.*
Senna (p.1212·2); frangula bark (p.1193·2).
Bowel evacuation; constipation.

Heumann Beruhigungsdragees Tenerval N *Heumann, Ger.†.*
Valerian root (p.1643·1); melissa (p.1600·1).
Agitation; sleep disorders.

Heumann Beruhigungstee Tenerval N *Heumann, Ger.*
Valerian root (p.1643·1); melissa (p.1600·1); valerian oil.
Sleep disorders.

Heumann Blasen- und Nierentee Solubitrat N *Heumann, Ger.*
Orthosiphon leaf (p.1592·2); solidago virgaurea; birch leaf; fennel oil (p.1579·2).
Urinary-tract disorders.

Heumann Bronchialtee Solubifix *Heumann, Ger.*
Althaea (p.1546·3); liquorice (p.1197·1); primula root; anise oil (p.1550·1); thyme oil (p.1637·1).
Coughs and associated respiratory-tract disorders.

Heumann Hustenstiller *Salus, Aust.*
Drosera (p.1574·1); thyme (p.1636·3).
Coughs and cold symptoms.

Heumann Leber- und Gallentee Solu-Hepar NT *Heumann, Ger.*
Boldo (p.1554·1); chelidonium; silybum marianum (p.993·3); peppermint oil (p.1208·1).
Biliary-tract disorders; liver disorders.

Heumann Magentee Solu-Vetan *Heumann, Ger.*
Liquorice root (p.1197·1); peppermint leaf (p.1208·1); peppermint oil (p.1208·1).
Gastro-intestinal disorders.

Heumann's Bronchial *Salus, Aust.*
Thyme (p.1636·3).
Catarrh; coughs.

Heumann's Bronchialtee *Salus, Aust.*
Althea (p.1546·3); liquorice (p.1197·1); primula root; anise oil (p.1550·1); thyme oil (p.1637·1).
Bronchitis; catarrh; coughs.

Heuschnupfen Systral *Asta Medica, Ger.†.*
Terfenadine (p.418·1).
Allergy; neurodermatitis.

Heuschnupfenmittel *DHU, Ger.*
Homoeopathic preparation.

Hevac *Merieux, Belg.†.*
A hepatitis B vaccine (plasma-derived) (p.1513·1).
Active immunisation.

Hevac B
Pfizer, Aust.; Merieux, Ger.†; Sanofi Winthrop, Switz.†.
A hepatitis B vaccine (plasma-derived) (p.1513·1).
Active immunisation.

Hevert Enzym Novo *Hevert, Ger.*
Dimethicone (p.1213·1); pancreatin (p.1612·1); trypsin (p.1640·1).
Hevert Enzym formerly contained thiamine hydrochloride, cholesterol, dimethicone, fel tauri, folic acid, pancreatin, papain, riboflavine, and trypsin.
Digestive system disorders.

Hevert-Aktivon Mono *Hevert, Ger.*
Ginseng (p.1584·2).
Tonic.

Hevert-Blasen- und Nieren- Tee *Hevert, Ger.*
Orthosiphon (p.1592·2); bearberry (p.1552·2); phaseolus vulgaris; birch leaf (p.1553·3); equisetum (p.1575·1); ononis (p.1610·2); couch-grass (p.1567·3); tilia (p.1637·3); centaurea cyanus.
Urinary-tract disorders.

Hevert-Card forte *Hevert, Ger.*
Herbal and homoeopathic preparation.

Hevert-Dorm *Hevert, Ger.*
Diphenhydramine hydrochloride (p.409·1).
Sleep disorders.

Hevert-Entwasserungs-Tee *Hevert, Ger.*
Pterocarpus santalinus; rosemary; juniper (p.1592·2); cynara; levisticum officinale (p.1597·2); ononis (p.1610·2); taraxacum (p.1634·2); rose fruit (p.1365·2); calendula officinalis; squill (p.1070·1); birch leaf (p.1553·3); buchu (p.1555·2); centaurea cyanus.
Cystitis; oedema; renal calculi.

Hevert-Erkaltungs-Tee *Hevert, Ger.*
Elder flower (p.1627·2); thyme (p.1636·3); willow bark (p.82·3).
Cold symptoms.

Hevert-Gall S *Hevert, Ger.*
Chelidonium; cnicus benedictus (p.1565·3); chamomile (p.1561·2); taraxacum (p.1634·2); caraway oil (p.1559·3); peppermint oil (p.1208·1); boldo (p.1554·1); calamus (p.1556·1); silybum marianum (p.993·3); turmeric (p.1001·3).
Biliary disorders; duodenal disorders; liver disorders.

Hevert-Gicht-Rheuma-Tee comp *Hevert, Ger.*
Salix (p.82·3); sambucus (p.1627·2); birch leaf (p.1553·3); juniper (p.1592·2); achillea (p.1542·2); liquorice (p.1197·1); ononis (p.1610·2).
Rheumatic disorders.

Hevertigon *Hevert, Ger.*
Homoeopathic preparation.

Hevert-Mag *Hevert, Ger.*
Magaldrate (p.1198·1).
Gastric hyperacidity; heartburn; peptic ulcer.

Hevert-Magen-Galle-Leber-Tee *Hevert, Ger.*
Calendula officinalis; fennel (p.1579·1); absinthium (p.1541·1); centaurea (p.1561·1); chelidonium; mylabris cichorii; achillea (p.1542·2); thyme (p.1636·3); calamus (p.1556·1).
Digestive system disorders.

Hevert-Migrane *Hevert, Ger.*
Homoeopathic preparation.

Hevert-Nerv plus Eisen *Hevert, Ger.*
Minerals; cola; ginseng; iron phosphate; lecithin.
Tonic.

Hevertnier Complex *Hevert, Ger.*
Homoeopathic preparation.

Hevert-Nier II *Hevert, Ger.*
Homoeopathic preparation.

Hevertnier spasmo *Hevert, Ger.*
Homoeopathic preparation.

Hevertolax Phyto *Hevert, Ger.*
Senna fruit (p.1212·2).
Constipation.

Hevertopect *Hevert, Ger.*
Anise oil (p.1550·1); eucalyptus oil (p.1578·1); fennel oil (p.1579·2); peppermint leaf (p.1208·1); pumilio pine oil (p.1623·3); turpentine oil (p.1641·1); ammi visnaga (p.1593·2); ephedrine hydrochloride (p.1059·3); eucalyptus (p.1578·1); thyme (p.1636·3); verbascum.
Respiratory-tract disorders.

Hevertotox *Hevert, Ger.*
Homoeopathic preparation.
Formerly known as Hevert-Tox.

Hevertoval mono *Hevert, Ger.*
Homoeopathic preparation.

Hevertozym *Hevert, Ger.*
Pancreatin (p.1612·1).
Pancreatic insufficiency.

Hevert-Vitan N *Hevert, Ger.*
Multivitamin and mineral preparation.
Calcium and vitamin deficiency.

Hewallergia *Hevert, Ger.*
Homoeopathic preparation.

Heweberberol-Tee *Hevert, Ger.*
Birch leaf; solidago virgaurea; ononis (p.1610·2); orthosiphon leaf (p.1592·2); pterocarpus santalinus; liquorice root (p.1197·1).
Urinary-tract disorders.

Hewechol Artischockendragees *Hevert, Ger.*
Cynara (p.1569·2).
Dyspepsia.

Hewedolor *Hevert, Ger.*
Rhus toxicodendron (p.1624·3); capsicum (p.1559·2); methyl salicylate (p.55·2).
Neuromuscular disorders; scars.

Hewedolor A *Hevert, Ger.†.*
Vitamin B substances.
Vitamin B deficiency.

Hewedolor B *Hevert, Ger.†.*
Cyanocobalamin (p.1363·3); sodium salamidacetate (p.82·3).
Migraine; musculoskeletal and joint disorders; neuralgia; neuritis; pain.

Hewedolor forte *Hevert, Ger.*
Sodium salamidacetate (p.82·3).
Nerve pain.

Hewedolor neuro *Hevert, Ger.*
Thiamine hydrochloride (p.1361·1); pyridoxine hydrochloride (p.1362·3); lignocaine hydrochloride (p.1293·2).
Nerve pain.

Hewedolor plus Coffein *Hevert, Ger.*
Procaine hydrochloride (p.1299·2); caffeine (p.749·3).
Nerve pain.

Hewedolor Procain *Hevert, Ger.*
Procaine hydrochloride (p.1299·2).
Pain.

Hewedolor propy *Hevert, Ger.†.*
Propyphenazone (p.81·3).
Pain.

Hewedormir *Hevert, Ger.*
Valerian (p.1643·1).
Nervousness; sleep disorders.

Heweformica *Hevert, Ger.*
Homoeopathic preparation.

Hewegingko *Hevert, Ger.*
Homoeopathic preparation.

Hewekliman *Hevert, Ger.*
Homoeopathic preparation.

Hewekzem novo *Hevert, Ger.*
Panthenol (p.1571·1); retinol palmitate (p.1359·2); alpha tocopheryl acetate (p.1369·2); chamomile oil; echinacea; sarsaparilla.
Skin disorders.

Hewelymphon *Hevert, Ger.*
Homoeopathic preparation.

Hewenephron duo *Hevert, Ger.*
Solidago virgaurea; echinacea (p.1574·2).
Renal calculi.

Heweneural *Hevert, Ger.*
Lignocaine hydrochloride (p.1293·2).
Migraine; nervous system disorders.

Hewepsychon duo *Hevert, Ger.*
Kava (p.1592·3); hypericum (p.1590·1).
Depression; dystonias; hypertension; menopausal disorders; migraine; nocturnal enuresis; tonic.

Hewepsychon uno *Hevert, Ger.*
Hypericum (p.1590·1).
Anxiety; psychiatric disorders.

Hewerheum *Hevert, Ger.*
Homoeopathic preparation.

Hewesabal comp. *Hevert, Ger.*
Homoeopathic preparation.

Hewesabal mono *Hevert, Ger.*
Homoeopathic preparation.

Heweselen mono *Hevert, Ger.*
Homoeopathic preparation.

Hewethyreon *Hevert, Ger.*
Homoeopathic preparation.

Hewetraumen *Hevert, Ger.*
Homoeopathic preparation.

Heweurat *Hevert, Ger.*
Homoeopathic preparation.

Heweven P 3 *Hevert, Ger.*
Hamamelis (p.1587·1); aesculus (p.1543·3); aescin (p.1543·3).
Vascular disorders.

Heweven P 7 *Hevert, Ger.*
Oral drops: Hamamelis (p.1587·1); aesculus (p.1543·3); aescin; aesculin; echinacea.
Tablets†: Hamamelis (p.1587·1); aesculus (p.1543·3); aescin; aesculin; hesperidin methyl chalcone (p.1580·2); rutoside (p.1580·2); bamethan sulphate (p.827·1).
Vascular disorders.

Hewletts *Kestrel, UK.*
Zinc oxide (p.1096·2); hydrous wool fat (p.1385·3); arachis oil (p.1550·2); white soft paraffin (p.1382·3).
Dry skin.

Hexa-Betalin
Lilly, Canad.†; Lilly, USA†.
Pyridoxine hydrochloride (p.1362·3).
Vitamin supplement.

Hexa-Blok *Hexal, S.Afr.*
Atenolol (p.825·3).
Angina pectoris; hypertension.

Hexabrix
Salus, Aust.; Mallinckrodt, Austral.; Codali, Belg.; Mallinckrodt, Canad.; Guerbet, Fr.; Guerbet, Ger.; Guerbet, Ital.; Guerbet, Neth.; Guerbet, Norw.; Rovi, Spain; Gothia, Swed.; Guerbet, Switz.; May & Baker, UK; Mallinckrodt, USA.
Meglumine ioxaglate (p.1008·3); sodium ioxaglate (p.1008·3).
Radiographic contrast medium.

Hexacillin *Garec, S.Afr.*
Ampicillin trihydrate (p.153·2).
Bacterial infections.

Hexacortone *Spirig, Switz.*
Prednisolone acetate (p.1048·1).
Skin disorders.

Hexacycline *Diamant, Fr.†.*
Tetracycline hydrochloride (p.259·1).
Bacterial infections.

Hexadreps *Diepha, Fr.*
Biclotymol (p.1104·2).
Mouth and throat infections.

Hexadrol
Organon Teknika, Canad.; Organon, USA.
Dexamethasone (p.1037·1) or dexamethasone sodium phosphate (p.1037·2).
Corticosteroid.

Hexafene *Vifor, Switz.*
Inositol nicotinate (p.891·3); buclizine hydrochloride (p.404·1); hydroxyzine hydrochloride (p.412·1).
Vertigo.

Hexafluid *Diepha, Fr.*
Carbocisteine (p.1056·3).
Respiratory-tract congestion.

Hexalen
Faulding, Austral.; Lilly, Canad.; US Bioscience, Norw.; Swedish Orphan, Swed.; Speywood, UK; US Bioscience, USA.
Altretamine (p.502·2).
Ovarian cancer.

Hexalense *Leurquin, Fr.*
Aminocaproic acid (p.711·1).
Inflammatory eye disorders.

Hexalyse *Doms-Adrian, Fr.*
Biclotymol (p.1104·2); muramidase hydrochloride (p.1604·3); enoxolone (p.35·2).
Formerly contained biclotymol, dequalinium chloride, muramidase, papain, and enoxolone.
Mouth and throat disorders.

Hexamet *Hexal, S.Afr.*
Cimetidine (p.1183·2).
Gastro-oesophageal reflux; peptic ulcer; Zollinger-Ellison syndrome.

Hexamon N *Beiersdorf-Lilly, Ger.*
Hexylresorcinol (p.1116·1); laureth 9 (p.1325·2).
Anorectal disorders.

Hexanicit
Promed, Ger.; Yoshitomi, Jpn†; Astra, Swed.
Inositol nicotinate (p.891·3).
Hyperlipidaemias; peripheral and central circulatory disorders.

Hexanios G+R *Anios, Fr.*
Polyhexanide (p.1123·1); didecyldimethylammonium chloride (p.1112·2).
Instrument disinfection.

Hexanitrat *Hexal, Aust.*
Isosorbide dinitrate (p.893·1).
Angina pectoris; heart failure; myocardial infarction; pulmonary hypertension.

Hexanium *Fides, Spain.*
Emepronium bromide (p.461·1).
Urinary-tract disorders.

Hexaphane *Biorga, Fr.*
Gelatin (p.723·2); cystine (p.1339·1); zinc gluconate (p.1373·2); vitamin B substances.
Fragile hair and nails.

Hexaphenyl *Ingram & Bell, Canad.*
Hexachlorophane sodium (p.1115·3).
Disinfection.

Hexapindol
Tika, Norw.; Tika, Swed.
Pindolol (p.931·1).
Angina pectoris; arrhythmias; hypertension.

Hexapneumine *Doms-Adrian, Fr.*
Adult suppositories; paediatric suppositories: Biclotymol (p.1104·2); cineole (p.1564·1); paracetamol (p.72·2); pholcodine (p.1068·1).
Coughs; fever.
Adult syrup; paediatric syrup: Biclotymol (p.1104·2); chlorpheniramine maleate (p.405·1); guaiphenesin (p.1061·3); pholcodine (p.1068·1).
Coughs.
Infant suppositories: Biclotymol (p.1104·2); cineole (p.1564·1); paracetamol (p.72·2).
Fever; respiratory-tract disorders.
Infant syrup: Biclotymol (p.1104·2); chlorpheniramine maleate (p.405·1); guaiphenesin (p.1061·3); paracetamol (p.72·2); tolu balsam (p.1071·1).
Coughs; fever.
Tablets: Biclotymol (p.1104·2); chlorpheniramine maleate (p.405·1); phenylephrine hydrochloride (p.1066·2).
Nasal congestion.

Hexapock *Dynathera, Fr.†.*
Biclotymol (p.1104·2).
Mouth and throat disorders.

Hexaquart L
Braun, Ger.; Braun, Ital.†.
Didecyldimethylammonium chloride (p.1112·2); benzalkonium chloride (p.1101·3).
Surface disinfection.

Hexaquart S *Braun, Ger.*
Didecyldimethylammonium chloride (p.1112·2); benzalkonium chloride (p.1101·3).
Fungal skin infection prophylaxis; surface disinfection.

Hexaquine *Gomenol, Fr.*
Quinine benzoate (p.441·2); thiamine hydrochloride (p.1361·1); niaouli oil (p.1607·1).
Muscle cramps.

Hexaretic *Hexal, S.Afr.*
Amiloride (p.819·3); hydrochlorothiazide (p.885·2).
Cardiac oedema; hypertension.

Hexaspray *Doms-Adrian, Fr.*
Biclotymol (p.1104·2).
Mouth and throat disorders.

Hexastat
Bellon, Fr.; Rhone-Poulenc Rorer, Ital.; Rhone-Poulenc Rorer, Neth.†; Rhone-Poulenc Rorer, Norw.
Altretamine (p.502·2).
Malignant neoplasms.

Hexatin *Agepha, Aust.*
Hexetidine (p.1116·1).
Mouth and throat inflammation.

Hexatrione *Lederle, Fr.*
Triamcinolone hexacetonide (p.1050·2).
Musculoskeletal and joint disorders.

Hexavitamin
ACO, Swed.†; Upsher-Smith, USA.
Multivitamin preparation.

Hexavitamins *Novopharm, Canad.*
Multivitamin preparation.

Hexetidin comp. *Ratiopharm, Ger.†.*
Hexetidine (p.1116·1); cetylpyridinium chloride (p.1106·2).
Inflammatory disorders of the oropharynx.

Hexidin
Note. This name is used for preparations of different composition.
Genericon, Aust.; Nycomed, Norw.
Chlorhexidine gluconate (p.1107·2).
Mouth infections; oral hygiene.

Allergan, Austral.
Chlorhexidine gluconate (p.1107·2); thiomersal (p.1126·3).
Soft contact lens disinfectant solution.

Hexifoam *Rougier, Canad.†.*
Chlorhexidine gluconate (p.1107·2).
Skin disinfection.

Hexifrice *Substantia, Fr.†.*
Hexetidine (p.1116·1).
Oral hygiene.

Hexigel
Parke, Davis, Fr.†; Warner-Lambert Consumer, Switz.
Hexetidine (p.1116·1).
Mouth disorders.

Hexinawas *Wasserman, Spain.*
Altretamine (p.502·2).
Lung cancer; ovarian cancer.

Hexit *Odan, Canad.*
Lindane (p.1407·2).
Pediculosis; scabies.

Hexobion *Merck, Ger.*
Pyridoxine hydrochloride (p.1362·3).
Vitamin B deficiency.

Hexogen *Antigen, Irl.*
Inositol nicotinate (p.891·3).
Peripheral and cerebral vascular disorders.

Hexo-Imotryl *Cassenne, Fr.*
Benzydamine hydrochloride (p.21·3); hexamidine isethionate (p.1115·3).
Mouth and throat disorders.

Hexol *Sigma, Austral.*
Chlorhexidine (p.1107·2).
Skin disinfection.

Hexoll *Asta Medica, Neth.*
Acetic acid (p.1541·2); citric acid (p.1564·3).
Pediculosis.

Hexomedin *Rhone-Poulenc Rorer, Spain.*
Hexamidine isethionate (p.1115·3).
Burns; skin infections; wounds.

Hexomedin N *Rhone-Poulenc Rorer, Ger.*
Hexamidine isethionate (p.1115·3).
Acne; paronychia.

Hexomedin transkutan *Rhone-Poulenc, Ger.†.*
Hexamidine isethionate (p.1115·3); aluminium lactate (p.1548·1).
Bacterial skin infections; fungal skin infections.

Hexomedine
Note. This name is used for preparations of different composition.
Rhone-Poulenc Rorer, Belg.; Theraplix, Fr.; Rhone-Poulenc Rorer, Neth.; Rhone-Poulenc Rorer, Switz.
Hexamidine isethionate (p.1115·3).
Infected skin disorders; skin and mucous membrane disinfection.

Theraplix, Fr.
Throat spray: Hexamidine isethionate (p.1115·3); amethocaine hydrochloride (p.1285·2).
Infections of the mouth and throat.

Hexopal
Sanofi Winthrop, Irl.; Sanofi Winthrop, UK.
Inositol nicotinate (p.891·3).
Intermittent claudication; Raynaud's syndrome.

Hexoral
Parke, Davis, Aust.; Warner-Wellcome, Ger.
Hexetidine (p.1116·1).
Inflammation and infection of the mouth and throat.

Hexoraletten N *Warner-Lambert, Ger.*
Chlorhexidine hydrochloride (p.1107·2); benzocaine (p.1286·2).
Mouth and throat disorders.

Hextril
Warner-Lambert Consumer, Belg.; Warner-Lambert, Fr.; Warner-Lambert, Neth.; Warner-Lambert Consumer, Switz.
Hexetidine (p.1116·1).
Mouth and throat disorders.

HF *Fresenius, Switz.*
A range of electrolyte infusions with or without glucose (p.1151·1).
Haemofiltration.

H-F Antidote *Pharmascience, Canad.†.*
Calcium gluconate (p.1155·2).
Hydrofluoric acid burns.

HHR *Geneva, USA†.*
Hydralazine hydrochloride (p.883·2); hydrochlorothiazide (p.885·2); reserpine (p.942·1).

Hi Potency Cal *Swiss Herbal, Canad.*
Calcium carbonate (p.1182·1).

Hiberix
SmithKline Beecham, Austral.; SmithKline Beecham, Ital.
A haemophilus influenzae conjugate vaccine (tetanus toxoid conjugate) (p.1511·1).
Active immunisation.

Hibernal *Rhone-Poulenc Rorer, Swed.*
Chlorpromazine embonate (p.649·1) or chlorpromazine hydrochloride (p.649·1).
Adjunct to analgesia; psychoses.

Hibersulfan *Ecobi, Ital.†.*
Amidopyrine (p.15·2); caffeine (p.749·3); pyrithyldione (p.689·3).
Influenza; rheumatic disorders.

HIBest *Pasteur Vaccins, Fr.*
A haemophilus influenzae conjugate vaccine (tetanus protein conjugate) (p.1511·1).
Active immunisation.

Hibicet
ICI, Austral.; Zeneca, Irl.; Zeneca, Ital.; Zeneca, S.Afr.
Chlorhexidine gluconate (p.1107·2); cetrimide (p.1105·2).
Disinfection of skin, wounds, burns, surfaces, instruments, and external genitalia.

Hibicet concentraat *Zeneca, Neth.*
Chlorhexidine gluconate (p.1107·2); cetrimide (p.1105·2).
Formerly known as Savlon.
Disinfection.

Hibicet Hospital Concentrate *Zeneca, UK.*
Chlorhexidine gluconate (p.1107·2); cetrimide (p.1105·2).
Formerly known as Savlon Hospital Concentrate.
Disinfection.

Hibicet verdunning *Zeneca, Neth.*
Chlorhexidine gluconate (p.1107·2); cetrimide (p.1105·2).
Formerly known as Savlodil.
Disinfection.

Hibiclens
ICI, Austral.; ICI, Ger.†; Zeneca, USA.
Chlorhexidine gluconate (p.1107·2).
Skin disinfection.

Hibicol *ICI, Austral.*
Chlorhexidine gluconate (p.1107·2); isopropyl alcohol (p.1118·2).
Hand disinfection.

Hibident
SmithKline Beecham, Aust.; SmithKline Beecham Consumer, Belg.; SmithKline Beecham, Fr.†; SmithKline Beecham, Neth.†; Zeneca, S.Afr.†.
Chlorhexidine gluconate (p.1107·2).
Mouth infections; oral hygiene.

Hibidil
Zeneca, Belg.; Zeneca, Canad.; Zeneca, Fr.; Zeneca, Irl.†; Zeneca, Ital.†; Zeneca, S.Afr.†; Zeneca, Switz.
Chlorhexidine gluconate (p.1107·2).
Skin, mucous membrane, wound, and instrument disinfection.

Hibigel *SmithKline Beecham Consumer, Belg.†; SmithKline Beecham, Neth.†.*
Chlorhexidine gluconate (p.1107·2).
Mouth infections.

Hibiguard *Zeneca, Belg.*
Chlorhexidine gluconate (p.1107·2).
Disinfection of hands and skin.

Hibimax *Zeneca, Spain.*
Chlorhexidine gluconate (p.1107·2).
Instrument disinfection; skin and wound disinfection.

Hibiscrub *Zeneca, Belg.; Zeneca, Fr.; Zeneca, Irl.; Zeneca, Ital.; Zeneca, Neth.; Zeneca, Norw.; Zeneca, S.Afr.; Zeneca, Spain; Zeneca, Swed.; Zeneca, Switz.; Zeneca, UK.*
Chlorhexidine gluconate (p.1107·2).
Skin disinfection.

Hibisol *Zeneca, Irl.; Zeneca, Neth.; Zeneca, UK.*
Chlorhexidine gluconate (p.1107·2); isopropyl alcohol (p.1118·2).
Skin disinfection.

Hibisprint *Zeneca, Fr.*
Chlorhexidine gluconate (p.1107·2).
Skin disinfection.

Hibistat *Zeneca, USA.*
Chlorhexidine gluconate (p.1107·2).
Skin disinfection.

Hibital *Zeneca, Switz.*
Chlorhexidine gluconate (p.1107·2); isopropyl alcohol (p.1118·2).
Skin and hand disinfection.

Hibitane
Note. This name is used for preparations of different composition.
ICI, Austral.; Zeneca, Belg.; Zeneca, Canad.; Zeneca, Fr.; Zeneca, Irl.; ICI, Ital.†; Zeneca, Neth.; SmithKline Beecham, Norw.†; Zeneca, Norw.; Zeneca, S.Afr.; SmithKline Beecham, Spain†; Zeneca, Swed.; Zeneca, Switz.; Zeneca, UK.
Chlorhexidine gluconate (p.1107·2) or chlorhexidine hydrochloride (p.1107·2).
Mouth infections; skin, wound, instrument, and surface disinfection.

ICI, Austral.
Tincture: Chlorhexidine gluconate (p.1107·2); isopropyl alcohol (p.1118·2).
Instrument disinfection; skin disinfection.

SmithKline Beecham Consumer, Belg.; SmithKline Beecham, Spain.
Pastilles: Chlorhexidine hydrochloride (p.1107·2); benzocaine hydrochloride (p.1286·2).
Mouth and throat disorders.

Hibitane Hautdesinfiziens *ICI, Ger.†.*
Chlorhexidine gluconate (p.1107·2); isopropyl alcohol (p.1118·2).
Skin disinfection.

HibTITER *Wyeth Lederle, Aust.; Lederle, Austral.; Wyeth Lederle, Belg.; Wyeth-Ayerst, Canad.; Lederle, Ger.; Wyeth, Irl.; Cyanamid, Ital.†; Wyeth, S.Afr.; Cyanamid, Spain; Wyeth Lederle, Swed.; Lederle, Switz.; Lederle, UK; Lederle-Praxis, USA.*
A haemophilus influenzae conjugate vaccine (diphtheria CRM$_{197}$ protein conjugate) (p.1511·1).
Active immunisation.

HIB-Vaccinol *Procter & Gamble, Ger.*
A haemophilus influenza conjugate vaccine (diphtheria toxoid conjugate) (p.1511·1).
Active immunisation.

Hi-Cal VM *NCI, USA.*
Supplemental nutrition bar for immunocompromised individuals.

Hicin *Douglas, Austral.*
Indomethacin (p.45·2).
Gout; inflammation; musculoskeletal, joint, peri-articular, and soft-tissue disorders; oedema; pain.

Hiconcil *Bristol-Myers Squibb, Belg.; Bristol-Myers Squibb, Fr.; Bristol-Myers Squibb, Irl.†.*
Amoxycillin trihydrate (p.151·3).
Bacterial infections.

Hiconcil-NS *Bristol-Myers Squibb, S.Afr.*
Amoxycillin trihydrate (p.151·3); nystatin (p.386·1).
Bacterial infections; candidiasis.

Hi-Cor *C & M, USA.*
Hydrocortisone (p.1043·3).
Skin disorders.

Hicoseen *Piraud, Switz.*
Butamyrate citrate (p.1056·2); dextromethorphan (p.1057·3); guaiphenesin (p.1061·3).
Bronchitis; coughs.

Hicoton *Medika, Ger.*
Ferric saccharose complex (p.1353·2); calcium glycerophosphate (p.1155·2); rhus toxicodendron (p.1624·3); lupulus (p.1597·2); cinchona bark (p.1564·1); lecithin (p.1595·2); camphor monobromide.
Urinary-tract disorders.

Hiderm *Baypharm, Austral.*
Clotrimazole (p.376·3).
Fungal skin and vulvovaginal infections.

Hidonac *Zambon, Ital.*
Acetylcysteine (p.1052·3).
Paracetamol poisoning.

Hidra *Rydelle, Fr.*
Amino-acid, fatty-acid, vitamin, and mineral preparation.
Skin disorders.

Hidralma *Wasserman, Spain.*
Hydrotalcite (p.1194·1).
Hyperacidity.

Hidro Tar *Restiva, Ital.†.*
Cocoylamido probylbetaine; willow oleoresin.
Greasy skin; seborrhoeic dermatitis.

Hidro Tar 30 *Restiva, Ital.†.*
Urea (p.1095·2); willow oleoresin.
Seborrhoeic dermatitis.

Hidroaltesona *Alter, Spain.*
Hydrocortisone (p.1043·3).
Corticosteroid.

Hidroc Cloranf *Ciba Vision, Spain.*
Chloramphenicol (p.182·1); hydrocortisone acetate (p.1043·3).
Eye disorders.

Hidroc Neomic *Ciba Vision, Spain.*
Hydrocortisone acetate (p.1043·3); neomycin sulphate (p.229·2).
Eye disorders.

Hidroferol *Faes, Spain.*
Calcifediol (p.1366·3).
Hypoparathyroidism; hypophosphataemia; osteodystrophy; osteomalacia; rickets.

Hidropolivit *Menarini, Spain.*
Multivitamin preparation.

Hidropolivit Mineral *Menarini, Spain.*
Multivitamins and minerals; orotic acid; hesperidin.
Tonic.

Hidrosaluretil *Alcala, Spain.*
Hydrochlorothiazide (p.885·2).
Diabetes insipidus; hypertension; oedema; renal calculi.

Hidrosol *Galderma, Austral.†.*
Aluminium chloride (p.1078·3).
Hyperhidrosis.

Hidroxil B12 B6 B1 *Almirall, Spain.*
Hydroxocobalamin (p.1363·3); pyridoxine hydrochloride (p.1362·3); thiamine hydrochloride (p.1361·1).
Vitamin B deficiency.

Hierco *Ern, Spain.*
Ferritin (p.1580·1).
Iron-deficiency anaemia.

Hi-Fluor *Alphapharm, Austral.†.*
Sodium fluoride (p.742·1).
Bone pain in multiple myeloma; osteoporosis; Paget's disease of bone.

Higadin *Inibsa, Spain†.*
Liver extract.
Vitamin B_{12} deficiency.

Higado Potenciado Medic *Medical, Spain.*
Vitamin B substances; glutathione (p.983·1); liver extract; procaine ascorbate (p.1299·2).
Tonic; vitamin B deficiency.

Higdil Nr. 100 Cardiosan *Evers, Ger.†.*
Herbal and homoeopathic preparation.

Higdil Nr. 100 Cardiosan forte *Evers, Ger.†.*
Herbal and homoeopathic preparation.

High Potency N-Vites *Nion, USA.*
Vitamin B substances with vitamin C.

Higrotona *Ciba-Geigy, Spain.*
Chlorthalidone (p.839·3).
Diabetes insipidus; hypertension; oedema; renal calculi.

Higrotona Reserpina *Ciba-Geigy, Spain.*
Chlorthalidone (p.839·3); reserpine (p.942·1).
Hypertension.

Hildicon *Trommsdorff, Ger.†.*
Vitamin B substances.
Vitamin B deficiency.

Hill's Balsam Adult Expectorant *Windsor, UK.*
Guaiphenesin (p.1061·3); capsicum tincture (p.1559·2); compound benzoin tincture (p.1634·1); acetic acid (p.1541·2); anise oil (p.1550·1).
Coughs.

Hill's Balsam Adult Suppressant *Windsor, UK.*
Pholcodine (p.1068·1); treacle; capsicum (p.1559·2); compound benzoin tincture; anise oil (p.1550·1); acetic acid (p.1541·2); peppermint oil (p.1208·1).
Coughs.

Hill's Balsam Expectorant Pastilles *Windsor, UK.*
Compound benzoin tincture; capsicum oleoresin; peppermint oil (p.1208·1); ipecacuanha (p.1062·2); lobelia (p.1481·3); menthol (p.1600·2).
Cough and cold symptoms.

Hills Balsam Extra Strong *Windsor, UK.*
Menthol (p.1600·2); ipecacuanha (p.1062·2); benzoin tincture (p.1634·1); peppermint oil (p.1208·1).
Coughs and cold symptoms.

Hill's Balsam Junior Expectorant *Windsor, UK.*
Citric acid (p.1564·3); ipecacuanha (p.1062·2); treacle; capsicum (p.1559·2); compound benzoin tincture; orange oil (p.1610·3).
Coughs.

Hima *Wander, Switz.†.*
Phenol (p.1121·2); precipitated sulphur (p.1091·2); zinc oxide (p.1096·2).
Herpes labialis.

Hima-Pasta nouvelle formule *Mundipharma, Switz.*
Zinc sulphate (p.1373·2); zinc oxide (p.1096·2).
Herpes labialis.

Himega *Sigma, Austral.*
Eicosapentaenoic acid (p.1276·1); docosahexaenoic acid (p.1276·1).
Dietary supplement.

H-Insulin *Hoechst, Ger.*
Insulin injection (human, highly purified) (p.322·1).
Diabetes mellitus.

Hioxyl *Croma, Aust.; Quinoderm, Irl.; Quinoderm, UK.*
Hydrogen peroxide (p.1116·2).
Skin infections; skin ulcers; wounds.

Hiperlex *Bristol-Myers, Spain.*
Fosinopril sodium (p.870·3).
Heart failure; hypertension.

Hipoartel *Kendall, Spain.*
Enalapril maleate (p.863·2).
Heart failure; hypertension.

Hipoartel Plus *Kendall, Spain.*
Enalapril maleate (p.863·2); hydrochlorothiazide (p.885·2).
Hypertension.

Hipotest *Marlop, USA.*
Multivitamin and mineral preparation with iron.

Hi-Po-Vites *Hudson, USA.*
Multivitamin and mineral preparation with iron and folic acid.

Hippophan *Weleda, Fr.*
Sea buckthorn.
Tonic.

Hippramine *3M, S.Afr.*
Hexamine hippurate (p.216·1).
Urinary-tract infections.

Hippuran *Orion, Swed.†.*
Hexamine hippurate (p.216·1).
Urinary-tract infections.

Hipputope *Squibb Diagnostics, USA.*
Iodine-131 (p.1424·1) as sodium iodohippurate.

Hipranol *Zurich, S.Afr.†.*
Propranolol hydrochloride (p.937·1).
Angina pectoris; arrhythmias; hypertension.

Hiprex *Salus, Aust.; 3M, Austral.; 3M, Belg.; 3M, Canad.; 3M, Ger.†; 3M, Irl.; 3M, Norw.; 3M, Swed.; 3M, UK; Hoechst Marion Roussel, USA.*
Hexamine hippurate (p.216·1).
Urinary-tract infections.

Hirtonin *Takeda, Jpn.*
Protirelin tartrate (p.1259·3).
Prolonged disturbance of consciousness; spinocerebellar degeneration.

Hirucreme *Nicholas, Fr.*
Hirudin (p.883·1).
Peripheral vascular disorders.

Hirudex *Celafar, Ital.*
Leech extract (p.897·2); esculoside (p.1543·3).
Bruises; inflammation; oedema; phlebitis; varices.

Hirudoid *Kwizda, Aust.; Sankyo, Austral.; Luitpold, Belg.; Luitpold, Ger.; Luitpold, Ital.; Luitpold, Neth.; Luitpold, Norw.; Alfarma, Spain; Selena, Swed.; Luitpold, Switz.; Panpharma, UK.*
A heparinoid (p.882·3).
Soft-tissue injury; thrombophlebitis; venous insufficiency; wounds.

Hisfedin *Wolff, Ger.*
Terfenadine (p.418·1).
Hypersensitivity reactions.

Hismacap *Janssen-Cilag, Switz.†.*
Astemizole (p.402·1).
Hypersensitivity reactions.

Hismadrin *Janssen-Cilag, Aust.*
Astemizole (p.402·1); pseudoephedrine hydrochloride (p.1068·3).
Hypersensitivity reactions.

Hismanal *Janssen-Cilag, Aust.; Janssen-Cilag, Austral.; Janssen-Cilag, Belg.; McNeil Consumer, Canad.; Janssen-Cilag, Fr.; Janssen-Cilag, Ger.; Janssen-Cilag, Irl.; Janssen-Cilag, Ital.; Janssen-Cilag, Neth.; Janssen-Cilag, S.Afr.; Janssen-Cilag, Spain; Janssen-Cilag, Switz.; Johnson & Johnson MSD Consumer, UK; Janssen, USA.*
Astemizole (p.402·1).
Hypersensitivity reactions.

Hismanal-D *Janssen-Cilag, S.Afr.†.*
Pseudoephedrine hydrochloride (p.1068·3); astemizole (p.402·1).
Hypersensitivity reactions.

Hispamicina Retard *Inkeysa, Spain.*
Ampicillin sodium (p.153·1); ampicillin benzathine (p.154·1).
Bacterial infections.

Histabid *Russ, USA†.*
Chlorpheniramine maleate (p.405·1); phenylpropanolamine hydrochloride (p.1067·2).

Histacon *Noristan, S.Afr.†.*
Paracetamol (p.72·2); phenylephrine hydrochloride (p.1066·2); chlorpheniramine maleate (p.405·1); caffeine (p.749·3).
Allergic rhinitis; cold symptoms.

Histacyl Compositum *Streuli, Switz.*
Diphenhydramine hydrochloride (p.409·1); mepyramine maleate (p.414·1).
Hypersensitivity reactions.

Histacyl Cutane *Streuli, Switz.†.*
Diphenhydramine hydrochloride (p.409·1); chloral hydrate (p.645·3); camphor (p.1557·2); menthol (p.1600·2); hyoscyamus oil (p.464·3).
Hypersensitivity reactions.

Histacylettes *Streuli, Switz.*
Diphenhydramine hydrochloride (p.409·1); mepyramine hydrochloride (p.414·1); caffeine (p.749·3).
Hypersensitivity reactions.

Histadestal *Biolmmun, Ger.*
A normal immunoglobulin (p.1522·1); histamine dihydrochloride (p.1587·3).
Hypersensitivity reactions.

Histadyl and ASA *Lilly, USA†.*
Chlorpheniramine maleate (p.405·1); aspirin (p.16·1).

Histafen *Berk, UK.*
Terfenadine (p.418·1).
Allergic rhinitis; dermatologic hypersensitivity reactions; hayfever.

Histafilin *Estedi, Spain.*
Theophylline (p.765·1).
Heart failure; obstructive airways disease; paroxysmal dyspnoea.

Histagesic Modified *Jones, USA.*
Phenylephrine hydrochloride (p.1066·2); paracetamol (p.72·2); chlorpheniramine maleate (p.405·1).
Upper respiratory-tract symptoms.

Histaglobin *Germania, Aust.; Mirren, S.Afr.; Biobasal, Switz.†.*
A normal immunoglobulin (p.1522·1); histamine dihydrochloride (p.1587·3).
Hypersensitivity reactions.

Histaglobine *Promedica, Fr.†; Llorente, Spain†.*
A normal immunoglobulin (p.1522·1); histamine dihydrochloride (p.1587·3).
Hypersensitivity reactions.

Histaject *Mayrand, USA†.*
Brompheniramine maleate (p.403·2).
Hypersensitivity reactions.

Histajodol N *Kattwiga, Ger.*
Nonivamide (p.63·2); salicylic acid (p.1090·2); rosemary oil (p.1626·2).
Circulatory disorders; neuralgia; rheumatism; sciatica.

Histalert *3M, Austral.†.*
Diphenylpyraline hydrochloride (p.409·3).
Hypersensitivity reactions; motion sickness.

Histalet *Solvay, USA.*
Pseudoephedrine hydrochloride (p.1068·3); chlorpheniramine maleate (p.405·1).
Upper respiratory-tract symptoms.

Histalet Forte *Solvay, USA.*
Phenylpropanolamine hydrochloride (p.1067·2); phenylephrine hydrochloride (p.1066·2); chlorpheniramine maleate (p.405·1); mepyramine maleate (p.414·1).
Upper respiratory-tract symptoms.

Histalet X *Solvay, USA.*
Pseudoephedrine hydrochloride (p.1068·3); guaiphenesin (p.1061·3).
Coughs.

Histalgane *Spirig, Switz.*
Nonivamide (p.63·2); benzyl nicotinate (p.22·1); glycol salicylate (p.43·1); dimethyl sulphoxide (p.1377·2).
Musculoskeletal, joint, and peri-articular pain.

Histalgane mite *Spirig, Switz.*
Glycol salicylate (p.43·1); dimethyl sulphoxide (p.1377·2).
Musculoskeletal, joint, and peri-articular pain.

Histalix
Note. This name is used for preparations of different composition.
Roche, S.Afr.
Diphenhydramine hydrochloride (p.409·1); codeine phosphate (p.26·1).
Coughs; nasal congestion.

Wallace Mfg Chem., UK.
Diphenhydramine hydrochloride (p.409·1); ammonium chloride (p.1055·2); sodium citrate (p.1153·2); menthol (p.1600·2).
Coughs.

Histalix-C *Roche, S.Afr.*
Dextromethorphan hydrobromide (p.1057·3); paracetamol (p.72·2); pseudoephedrine hydrochloride (p.1068·3); ascorbic acid (p.1365·2).
Cold symptoms.

Histalon *ICN, Canad.*
Chlorpheniramine maleate (p.405·1).

Histamed *Propan, S.Afr.*
Elixir: Chlorpheniramine maleate (p.405·1).
Hypersensitivity reactions.
Cream†: Mepyramine maleate (p.414·1).
Skin disorders.
Lotion: Diphenhydramine hydrochloride (p.409·1); calamine (p.1080·1); camphor (p.1557·2); benzocaine (p.1286·2).
Skin disorders.

Histamed Co *Propan, S.Afr.*
Chlorpheniramine maleate (p.405·1); ascorbic acid (p.1365·2); salicylamide (p.82·3); paracetamol (p.72·2); caffeine (p.749·3); phenylephrine hydrochloride (p.1066·2).
Cold symptoms.

Histamen *Polifarma, Ital.*
Astemizole (p.402·1).
Allergic conjunctivitis; rhinitis; urticaria.

Histamen-D *Polifarma, Ital.†.*
Astemizole (p.402·1); pseudoephedrine hydrochloride (p.1068·3).
Nasal congestion; rhinitis; sneezing.

Histaminos *Lesvi, Spain.*
Astemizole (p.402·1).
Hypersensitivity reactions.

Histantil *Pharmascience, Canad.*
Promethazine hydrochloride (p.416·2).
Antihistamine.

Histaspan-D *Rorer, USA†.*
Chlorpheniramine maleate (p.405·1); phenylephrine hydrochloride (p.1066·2); hyoscine methonitrate (p.463·1).
Cold and hay-fever symptoms.

Histatab Plus *Century, USA.*
Phenylephrine hydrochloride (p.1066·2); chlorpheniramine maleate (p.405·1).
Upper respiratory-tract symptoms.

Histaterfen *Azupharma, Ger.*
Terfenadine (p.418·1).
Hypersensitivity reactions.

Hista-Vadrin *Scherer, USA.*
Phenylpropanolamine hydrochloride (p.1067·2); phenylephrine hydrochloride (p.1066·2); chlorpheniramine maleate (p.405·1).
Upper respiratory-tract symptoms.

Histaverin *Estedi, Spain.*
Codeine phosphate (p.26·1).
Formerly contained ammonium chloride, codeine phosphate, diphenhydramine hydrochloride, phenylephrine hydrochloride, papaverine hydrochloride, sodium citrate, and menthol.
Cough; diarrhoea; pain.

Histaxin *Asta Medica, Aust.*
Diphenhydramine hydrochloride (p.409·1).
Dermatologic hypersensitivity reactions.

Histenol Cold *Zee, Canad.*
Pseudoephedrine hydrochloride (p.1068·3); dextromethorphan hydrobromide (p.1057·3); paracetamol (p.72·2).

Histergan *Norma, UK.*
Diphenhydramine hydrochloride (p.409·1).

Histerone *Roberts, USA; Hauck, USA.*
Testosterone (p.1464·1).
Androgen replacement therapy; delayed puberty.

Histilos *UCB, Swed.*
Nicotinic acid (p.1351·2); meclozine hydrochloride (p.413·3); hydroxyzine hydrochloride (p.412·1).
Ménière's disease.

Histine DM *Ethex, USA.*
Phenylpropanolamine hydrochloride (p.1067·2); brompheniramine maleate (p.403·2); dextromethorphan hydrobromide (p.1057·3).
Coughs.

Histinex HC *Ethex, USA.*
Hydrocodone tartrate (p.43·1); phenylephrine hydrochloride (p.1066·2); chlorpheniramine maleate (p.405·1).
Coughs.

Histinex PV *Ethex, USA.*
Hydrocodone tartrate (p.43·1); pseudoephedrine hydrochloride (p.1068·3); chlorpheniramine maleate (p.405·1).
Cough and cold symptoms.

Histinorm *A.S., Ger.†.*
Histidine (p.1345·3).
Rheumatic disorders.

Histiotone *Morrith, Spain†.*
Liver extract; gastric mucosal extract; muscle extract; embryo extract; liver extract (antitoxin fraction); hydroxocobalamin acetate (p.1364·2); carnitine orotate (p.1611·2); lysine ascorbate.
Tonic; vitamin B_{12} deficiency.

Histiplus *Gry, Ger.†.*
Histidine hydrochloride (p.1345·3).
Histidine-deficiency disorders; renal disorders.

Histoacryl *Davis & Geck, UK.*
Enbucrilate (p.1569·1).
Tissue adhesive for closure of minor wounds.

Histodor *Lennon, S.Afr.*
Cream: Mepyramine maleate (p.414·1); diphenhydramine hydrochloride (p.409·1).
Tablets: Mepyramine maleate (p.414·1); promethazine hydrochloride (p.416·2); caffeine (p.749·3).
Hypersensitivity reactions.

Histodor Expectorant *Lennon, S.Afr.*
Diphenhydramine hydrochloride (p.409·1); ammonium chloride (p.1055·2); sodium citrate (p.1153·2).
Coughs.

Histo-Fluine P *Richard, Fr.*
Aesculus (p.1543·3); hamamelis (p.1587·1); shepherds purse; pulsatilla (p.1623·3); esculoside (p.1543·3).
Peripheral vascular disorders.

Histofreezer
Hamilton, Austral.; Braun Biotrol, Fr.
Dimethyl ether (p.1165·1); propane (p.1166·3).
Warts.

Histolyn-CYL *ALK, USA.*
Histoplasmin (p.1588·1).
Diagnostic test.

Histophtal *Metochem, Aust.*
Naphazoline hydrochloride (p.1064·2); antazoline hydrochloride (p.401·3).
Eye disorders.

Histor-D *Roberts, USA.*
Phenylephrine hydrochloride (p.1066·2); chlorpheniramine maleate (p.405·1).
Upper respiratory-tract symptoms.

Histor-D Timecelles *Roberts, USA.*
Chlorpheniramine maleate (p.405·1); phenylephrine hydrochloride (p.1066·2); hyoscine methonitrate (p.463·1).
Upper respiratory-tract symptoms.

Histosal *Ferndale, USA.*
Phenylpropanolamine hydrochloride (p.1067·2); paracetamol (p.72·2); caffeine (p.749·3); mepyramine maleate (p.414·1).
Upper respiratory-tract symptoms.

Histryl
Wellcome, Irl.†; SmithKline Beecham Consumer, UK†.
Diphenylpyraline hydrochloride (p.409·3).
Hypersensitivity reactions.

Histussin D *Bock, USA.*
Hydrocodone tartrate (p.43·1); pseudoephedrine hydrochloride (p.1068·3).
Coughs; respiratory-tract congestion.

Histussin HC *Sanofi Winthrop, USA.*
Chlorpheniramine maleate (p.405·1); phenylephrine hydrochloride (p.1066·2); hydrocodone tartrate (p.43·1).
Coughs and cold symptoms.

Hi-Vegi-Lip *Freeda, USA.*
Pancreatin (p.1612·1); pancrelipase (p.1613·3).
Deficiency of digestive enzymes.

Hives *Hylands, Canad.*
Homoeopathic preparation.

Hivid
Roche, Aust.; Roche, Austral.; Roche, Belg.; Roche, Canad.; Roche, Fr.; Roche, Ger.; Roche, Irl.; Roche, Ital.; Roche, Neth.; Roche, Norw.; Roche, S.Afr.; Roche, Spain; Roche, Swed.; Roche, Switz.; Roche, UK; Roche, USA.
Zalcitabine (p.629·2).
HIV infection.

Hivita *Mega Vitamin, Austral.*
A range of multivitamin and mineral preparations.

Hivita Childvita *Mega Vitamin, Austral.*
Multivitamin and mineral preparation with enzymes.

Hi-Z *Otsuka, Jpn.*
Oryzanol (p.1611·2).
Head and neck injury; hyperlipidaemia; irritable bowel syndrome; menopausal disorders.

Hizaar *Merck Sharp & Dohme, Ital.*
Losartan potassium (p.899·1); hydrochlorothiazide (p.885·2).
Hypertension.

HMG *Farma Lepori, Spain; Organon, Spain.*
Menotrophin (p.1252·1).
Female infertility; male infertility.

HMS
Allergan, S.Afr.; Allergan, Switz.; Allergan, USA.
Medrysone (p.1045·3).
Inflammatory eye disorders.

HMS Liquifilm
Allergan, Aust.†; Allergan, Austral.; Allergan, Canad.†; Allergan, Neth.†.
Medrysone (p.1045·3).
Inflammatory eye disorders.

HN 25
Milupa, Fr.; Milupa, Irl.; Milupa, Switz.
Preparation for enteral nutrition.
Gastro-intestinal disorders.

Hocura-Diureticum *Pascoe, Ger.†.*
Potassium acetate (p.1161·1); juniper (p.1592·2); adonis vernalis (p.1543·3); squill (p.1070·1).
Diuretic.

Hocura-Femin F *Pascoe, Ger.†.*
Homoeopathic preparation.

Hocura-Spondylose novo *Pascoe, Ger.*
Hypericum oil (p.1590·1); camphor (p.1557·2).
Nerve and muscle pain.

Hodernal *Rottapharm, Spain.*
Liquid paraffin (p.1382·1).
Constipation.

Hoecutin Olbad *Hoernecke, Ger.*
Soya oil (p.1355·1).
Bath additive; dry skin; pruritus.

Hoecutin Olbad F *Hoernecke, Ger.*
Arachis oil (p.1550·2); light liquid paraffin (p.1382·1).
Bath additive; dry skin; pruritus.

Hoemarin Derma *Hoernecke, Ger.*
Ichthammol (p.1083·3); sage oil.
Bath additive; eczema.

Hoemarin Rheuma *Hoernecke, Ger.*
Methyl salicylate (p.55·2); turpentine oil (p.1641·1); eucalyptus oil (p.1578·1).
Bath additive; circulatory disorders; musculoskeletal and joint disorders; neuralgia.

Hoepixin Bad N *Hoernecke, Ger.*
Coal tar (p.1092·3).
Bath additive; pruritic skin disorders.

Hoepixin N *Hoernecke, Ger.*
Coal tar (p.1092·3); thyme oil (p.1637·1).
Bath additive; eczema; psoriasis.

Hoestsiroop *SAN, Neth.†.*
Mallow root; liquorice root (p.1197·1); thyme (p.1636·3); anise (p.1549·3).
Coughs.

Hoevenol *Hoernecke, Ger.*
Capsules: Aesculus (p.1543·3).
Soft-tissue injury; venous insufficiency.
Topical emulsion: Methyl salicylate (p.55·2); aesculus (p.1543·3).
Haemorrhoids; peripheral vascular disorders; venous insufficiency.

Hoevenol A *Hoernecke, Ger.*
Topical application: Arnica (p.1550·3).
Topical gel: Arnica (p.1550·3); aesculus (p.1543·3).
Circulatory disorders; phlebitis; venous insufficiency.

Hofcomant *Hofmann, Aust.*
Amantadine sulphate (p.1129·2).
Drug-induced extrapyramidal disorders; herpes zoster; parkinsonism.

Hofels Cod Liver Oil and Garlic *Seven Seas, UK†.*
Vitamin A acetate (p.1359·2); vitamin D (p.1366·3); vitamin E (p.1369·1); garlic oil; cod-liver oil (p.1337·3).

Hoggar N *Stada, Ger.*
Doxylamine succinate (p.410·1).
Sleep disorders.

Hokunalin *Hokuriku, Jpn.*
Tulobuterol (p.774·2) or tulobuterol hydrochloride (p.774·2).
Respiratory-tract disorders.

Hold DM *Menley & James, USA.*
Dextromethorphan hydrobromide (p.1057·3).
Coughs.

Holfungin *Hollborn, Ger.*
Clotrimazole (p.376·3).
Fungal and bacterial skin infections.

Hollihesive *Sigma, Austral.†.*
Skin barrier dressing.

Hollister Karaya Paste *Sigma, Austral.†.*
Sterculia (p.1214·1).
Barrier paste.

Hollister Skin Gel *Sigma, Austral.†.*
Barrier gel.

Holopon *Byk Gulden, Ger.†.*
Hyoscine methobromide (p.463·1).
Smooth muscle spasms.

Holoxan
Asta Medica, Aust.; Asta Medica, Austral.; Asta Medica, Belg.; Asta Medica, Fr.; Asta Medica, Ger.; Asta Medica, Ital.; Asta Medica, Neth.; Asta, Norw.; Hoechst Marion Roussel, S.Afr.; Asta Medica, Swed.; Asta Medica, Switz.
Ifosfamide (p.540·2).
Malignant neoplasms.

Holsten aktiv *Holsten, Ger.*
Ethyl chloride (p.1292·3).
Local anaesthesia.

Homat *Allergan, Austral.†.*
Homatropine hydrobromide (p.462·2).
Production of mydriasis and cycloplegia.

Homatrop *Llorens, Spain.*
Homatropine hydrobromide (p.462·2).
Production of mydriasis and cycloplegia.

Homeocoksinum *Homeocan, Canad.*
Homoeopathic preparation.

Homeodose
Dolisos, Canad.; Dolisos, Fr.
A range of homoeopathic preparations.

Homeogene
Boiron, Canad.; Boiron, Fr.
Homoeopathic preparation.

Homeogrippe *Boiron, Fr.†.*
Homoeopathic preparation.

Homeoplasmine *Boiron, Fr.*
Homoeopathic preparation.

Homeovox *Boiron, Canad.*
Homoeopathic preparation.

Hominex *Ross, USA.*
A range of methionine-free preparations for enteral nutrition including an infant feed.
Vitamin B_6-nonresponsive homocystinuria or hypermethioninaemia.

Homoclomin *Eisai, Jpn.*
Homochlorcyclizine hydrochloride (p.411·3).
Allergic rhinitis; pruritus; urticaria.

Homocodeina Timol *Wasserman, Spain†.*
Cineole (p.1564·1); pholcodine (p.1068·1); niaouli oil (p.1607·1); guaiphenesin (p.1061·3); paracetamol (p.72·2); thymol (p.1127·1); camphor (p.1557·2).
Respiratory-tract disorders.

Homoderma *Brauer, Austral.*
Homoeopathic preparation.

Homosten *Lepetit, Ital.†.*
Chorionic gonadotrophin (p.1243·1); testosterone (p.1464·1).
Hormonal imbalance.

Homovowen-N *Weber & Weber, Ger.†.*
Homoeopathic preparation.

Honey Lemon Cough Lozenges *Sutton, Canad.*
Menthol (p.1600·2).

Honey & Molasses *Lane, UK.*
Ipecacuanha liquid extract (p.1062·2); white horehound (p.1063·3); squill vinegar (p.1070·1); capsicum (p.1559·2); peppermint oil (p.1208·1); tolu solution (p.1071·1); honey (p.1345·3); molasses; glycerol (p.1585·2); liquorice (p.1197·1); anise oil (p.1550·1).
Coughs.

Honeyflu *Home, Ital.*
Paracetamol (p.72·2); dextromethorphan hydrobromide (p.1057·3).
Cough; fever.

Hongosan *Medea, Spain.*
Acedoben (p.1541·1); aluminium chlorohydrate (p.1078·3); cetrimonium bromide (p.1106·1); dexamethasone (p.1037·1); salicylic acid (p.1090·2).
Skin infections.

Hongoseril *Isdin, Spain.*
Itraconazole (p.381·3).
Fungal infections.

Honvan
Asta Medica, Aust.; Asta Medica, Austral.; Asta Medica, Belg.; Asta Medica, Ger.; Asta Medica, Ital.†; Asta Medica, Neth.; Asta, Norw.; Noristan, S.Afr.†; Pras, Spain; Asta Medica, Swed.†; Asta Medica, Switz.; Asta Medica, UK.
Fosfestrol (p.1447·1) or fosfestrol sodium (p.1447·1).
Prostatic cancer.

Honvol *Carter Horner, Canad.*
Fosfestrol sodium (p.1447·1).
Prostatic cancer.

Hopacem *Hommel, Ger.*
Mianserin hydrochloride (p.297·1).
Depression.

Hordenol *Aerocid, Fr.*
Hordenine sulphate; caffeine (p.749·3).
Diarrhoea.

Horehound and Aniseed Cough Mixture *Potter's, UK.*
Pleurisy root; elecampane (p.1059·2); horehound (p.1063·3); skunk cabbage; lobelia (p.1481·3).
Coughs.

Hormodausse *Charton, Canad.*
Multivitamins and minerals; liver extract; beef serum proteins.

Hormodausse plus Calcium and Vitamin D
Charton, Canad.
Multivitamin and mineral preparation.

Hormomed *Merckle, Ger.†.*
Oestriol (p.1457·2).
Oestrogenic.

Hormonin *Shire, UK.*
Oestriol (p.1457·2); oestrone (p.1458·2); oestradiol (p.1455·1).
Menopausal disorders.

Horm-Valin *Schiwa, Ger.†; Hormonchemie, Ger.†.*
Valine (p.1358·1).
Liver disease.

Horphagen uno *Wolfer, Ger.†.*
Saw palmetto (p.1462·1).
Benign prostatic hyperplasia.

Horse Radish and Garlic Tablets *Vita Glow, Austral.*
Cochlearia armoracia; garlic (p.1583·1); ascorbic acid (p.1365·2); zinc sulphate (p.1373·2).
Catarrh; coughs; hayfever; sinusitis; upper respiratory-tract congestion.

Hortemox *Hortel, Spain†.*
Amoxycillin trihydrate (p.151·3); bromhexine hydrochloride (p.1055·3).
Respiratory-tract infections.

Horton *Warner-Lambert Consumer, Belg.*
Bisacodyl (p.1179·3).
Bowel evacuation; constipation.

Horvilan N *Schoning-Berlin, Ger.*
Turmeric (p.1001·3); peppermint oil (p.1208·1); chelidonium majus.
Biliary-tract disorders.

Hosbocin *Hosbon, Spain†.*
Ceftriaxone sodium (p.176·1).
Lignocaine hydrochloride (p.1293·2) is included in this preparation to alleviate the pain of injection.
Bacterial infections.

Hosbogen *Hosbon, Spain†.*
Gentamicin sulphate (p.212·1).
Bacterial infections.

Hosboral *Hosbon, Spain.*
Capsules; tablets; oral suspension: Amoxycillin trihydrate (p.151·3).
Bacterial infections.

Hosboral Bronquial *Hosbon, Spain.*
Amoxycillin trihydrate (p.151·3); bromhexine hydrochloride (p.1055·3).
Respiratory-tract infections.

Hospidermin *Lysoform, Ger.*
Alcohol (p.1099·1); potassium thiocyanate; 5-chloro-2-hydroxybenzoic acid.
Skin disinfection.

Hospisept *Lysoform, Ger.*
Propyl alcohol (p.1124·2); alcohol (p.1099·1).
Hand disinfection; skin disinfection.

Hostacain *Hoechst, Ger.†.*
Butanilicaine hydrochloride (p.1288·3) or butanilicaine phosphate (p.1288·3).
Local anaesthesia.

Hostacyclin
Hoechst, Aust.; Hoechst, Ger.
Tetracycline hydrochloride (p.259·1).
Amoebiasis; bacterial infections.

Hostacycline
Hoechst Marion Roussel, Belg.; Hoechst Marion Roussel, Irl.; Noristan, S.Afr.†.
Tetracycline hydrochloride (p.259·1).
Bacterial infections.

Hot Coldrex *Sterling, Neth.†.*
Paracetamol (p.72·2); ascorbic acid (p.1365·2); sodium citrate (p.1153·2).
Cold symptoms.

Hot Lemon Powders *Numark, UK†.*
Paracetamol (p.72·2); ascorbic acid (p.1365·2).
Cold symptoms.

Hot Lemon Relief *Apotex, Canad.*
Phenylephrine hydrochloride (p.1066·2); pheniramine maleate (p.415·3); paracetamol (p.72·2); ascorbic acid (p.1365·2).

Hot Thermo *Durachemie, Ger.*
Glycol salicylate (p.43·1); benzyl nicotinate (p.22·1).
Bruising; musculoskeletal and joint disorders; sprains; superficial vascular disorders.

12 Hour Antihistamine Nasal Decongestant *URL, USA.*
Pseudoephedrine sulphate (p.1068·3); dexbrompheniramine maleate (p.403·2).
Upper respiratory-tract symptoms.

8-Hour Bayer Timed-Release *Glenbrook, USA.*
Aspirin (p.16·1).
Fever; inflammation; myocardial infarction; pain; transient ischaemic attacks.

12 Hour Cold
Note. This name is used for preparations of different composition.
Goldline, USA.
Pseudoephedrine sulphate (p.1068·3); dexbrompheniramine maleate (p.403·2).
Upper respiratory-tract symptoms.

Hudson, USA.
Phenylpropanolamine hydrochloride (p.1067·2); chlorpheniramine maleate (p.405·1).
Upper respiratory-tract symptoms.

12 Hour Sinarest *Ciba Consumer, USA.*
Oxymetazoline hydrochloride (p.1065·3).
Nasal congestion.

Hova
Zyma, Aust.; Zyma, Ger.†.
Lupulus (p.1597·2); valerian (p.1643·1).
Nervous disorders; sleep disorders.

Hovaletten *Zyma, Aust.†.*
Valerian (p.1643·1); lupulus (p.1597·2).
Nervous disorders; sleep disorders.

Hovaletten N *Zyma, Ger.*
Lupulus (p.1597·2); valerian (p.1643·1).
Nervous disorders; sleep disorders.

Hovnizym *Pfluger, Ger.†.*
Echinacea (p.1574·2); alchemilla vulgaris; chamomile (p.1561·2); achillea (p.1542·2); arnica (p.1550·3); aconitum; apis; bryonia; calcium jod.; crocus; crotalus; ferrum phosph.; kalium chlor.; kalium phosph.; kalium sulf.; lachesis; pulsatilla; sepia.
Tonic.

H_2Oxyl
Stiefel, Canad.; Stiefel, Switz.†.
Benzoyl peroxide (p.1079·2).
Acne.

H-R Lubricating Jelly *Wallace, USA.*
Vaginal lubricant.

HRF
Wyeth, Austral.; Wyeth Lederle, Belg.; Monmouth, Irl.; Wyeth, Ital.†; Wyeth, Neth.; Akromed, S.Afr.; Monmouth, UK.
Gonadorelin hydrochloride (p.1248·1).
Anovulatory infertility; sterility or delayed puberty due to hypogonadotrophic hypogonadism; test of hypothalamic function.

H-Tronin *Hoechst, Ger.*
Insulin injection (human) (p.322·1).
Diabetes mellitus.

H-Tuss-D *Cypress, USA.*
Hydrocodone tartrate (p.43·1); pseudoephedrine hydrochloride (p.1068·3).
Coughs.

Huberdilat *ICN, Spain.*
Cetiedil (p.839·1).
Peripheral vascular disorders.

Huberdina *ICN, Spain†.*
Famotidine (p.1192·1).
Gastro-oesophageal reflux; peptic ulcer; Zollinger-Ellison syndrome.

Huberdor *ICN, Spain†.*
Metamizole magnesium (p.35·1).
Fever; pain.

Huberdoxina *ICN, Spain.*
Ciprofloxacin hydrochloride (p.185·3) or ciprofloxacin lactate (p.185·3).
Bacterial infections.

Hubergrip *ICN, Spain.*
Suppositories: Caffeine (p.749·3); calcium pantothenate (p.1352·3); citiolone (p.1564·3); chlorpheniramine maleate (p.405·1); paracetamol (p.72·2); vitamin A (p.1358·1).
Tablets: Caffeine (p.749·3); chlorpheniramine maleate (p.405·1); propyphenazone (p.81·3); salicylamide (p.82·3).
Influenza and cold symptoms.

Huberlitren *ICN, Spain.*
Calcium lactate; citric acid; magnesium sulphate; potassium chloride; sodium citrate; sodium chloride; tribasic sodium phosphate; glucose (p.1152·3).
Oral rehydration therapy.

Hubermizol *ICN, Spain.*
Astemizole (p.402·1).
Hypersensitivity reactions.

Huberplex *ICN, Spain.*
Chlordiazepoxide hydrochloride (p.646·3).
Alcohol withdrawal syndrome; anxiety; insomnia.

Huile analgesique "Polar-Bar" *Panax, Switz.*
Mint oil (p.1604·1); camphor (p.1557·2); menthol (p.1600·2); eucalyptus oil (p.1578·1); methyl salicylate (p.55·2); thymol (p.1127·1).
Headache.

Huile de Bain Therapeutique *Atlas, Canad.*
Wool fat (p.1385·3); liquid paraffin (p.1382·1).

Huile de Haarlem *Lefevre, Fr.*
Sulphur (p.1091·2); linseed oil (p.1596·2); turpentine oil (p.1641·1).
Arthritic disorders; respiratory-tract disorders.

Huile de millepertuis A. Vogel (huile de St. Jean) *Bioforce, Switz.*
Hypericum (p.1590·1); sunflower oil (p.1634·1).
Superficial wounds.

Huile Gomenolee *Gomenol, Fr.*
Niaouli oil (p.1607·1).
Nasal infections.

Huile Po-Ho A. Vogel *Bioforce, Switz.*
Peppermint oil (p.1208·1); eucalyptus oil (p.1578·1); juniper oil (p.1592·3); caraway oil (p.1559·3); fennel oil (p.1579·2).
Cold symptoms; headache; muscular tension.

Huile Solaire Bronzage *Clarins, Canad.*
SPF 3: Ethylhexyl *p*-methoxycinnamate (p.1487·1); oxybenzone (p.1487·3).
Sunscreen.

Humagel
Parke, Davis, Fr.†; Parke, Davis, Spain†.
Paromomycin sulphate (p.235·3).
Infective diarrhoea.

Humaject 10/90, 20/80, 30/70, 40/60, 50/50 *Lilly, Neth.*
Mixture of insulin injection (human) and isophane insulin injection (human) respectively in the proportions indicated (p.322·1).
Diabetes mellitus.

Humaject I *Lilly, UK.*
Injection device containing Humulin I (p.322·1).
Diabetes mellitus.

Humaject M1, M2, M3, M4, M5 *Lilly, UK.*
Injection device containing Humulin M1, M2, M3, M4, and M5 respectively (p.322·1).
Diabetes mellitus.

Humaject NPH *Lilly, Neth.*
Isophane insulin injection (human) (p.322·1).
Diabetes mellitus.

Humaject Regular *Lilly, Neth.*
Insulin injection (human) (p.322·1).
Diabetes mellitus.

Humaject S *Lilly, UK.*
Injection device containing Humulin S (p.322·1).
Diabetes mellitus.

Humal *Rosch & Handel, Aust.*
Humic acid; salicylic acid (p.1090·2).
Rheumatism.

Humalog
Lilly, Aust.; Lilly, Austral.; Lilly, Fr.; Lilly, Ger.; Lilly, Irl.; Lilly, Neth.; Lilly, Norw.; Lilly, S.Afr.; Lilly, Swed.; Lilly, Switz.; Lilly, UK; Lilly, USA.
Insulin lispro (p.322·1).
Diabetes mellitus.

Human Actraphane
Novo Nordisk, Irl.†; Novo Nordisk, UK†.
Mixture of neutral insulin injection (human, pyr) 30% and isophane insulin injection (human, pyr) 70% (p.322·1).
Diabetes mellitus.

Human Actrapid *Novo Nordisk, UK.*
Neutral insulin injection (human, pyr) (p.322·1).
Diabetes mellitus.

Human Initard 50/50
Novo Nordisk, Irl.†; Wellcome, Irl.†; Novo Nordisk, UK†; Wellcome, UK†.
Mixture of neutral insulin injection (human, emp, highly purified) 50% and isophane insulin injection (human, emp, highly purified) 50% (p.322·1).
Diabetes mellitus.

Human Insulatard *Novo Nordisk, UK.*
Isophane insulin injection (human, pyr, highly purified) (p.322·1).
Formerly known as Human Protaphane.
Diabetes mellitus.

Human Mixtard 10, 20, 30, 40, and 50 *Novo Nordisk, UK.*
Mixture of neutral insulin injection (human, pyr, highly purified) 10, 20, 30, 40, or 50% and isophane insulin injection (human, pyr, highly purified) 90, 80, 70, 60, or 50% respectively (p.322·1).
Diabetes mellitus.

Human Monotard *Novo Nordisk, UK.*
Insulin zinc suspension (amorphous 30%, crystalline 70%) (human, pyr) (p.322·1).
Diabetes mellitus.

Human Protaphane *Novo Nordisk, Irl.†.*
Isophane insulin injection (human, emp, highly purified) (p.322·1).
Diabetes mellitus.

Human Ultratard *Novo Nordisk, UK.*
Insulin zinc suspension (crystalline) (human, pyr) (p.322·1).
Diabetes mellitus.

Human Velosulin
Novo Nordisk, Irl.†; Wellcome, Irl.†; Novo Nordisk, UK; Glaxo Wellcome, UK.
Neutral insulin injection (human, emp, highly purified) (p.322·1).
Diabetes mellitus.

Humana Disanal *Humana, Ital.*
Food for special diets.
Gastro-intestinal disorders.

Humana HA *Humana, Ital.*
Infant feed.
Food intolerance.

Humana SL *Humana, Ital.*
Infant feed.
Milk intolerance.

Humanalbin *Centeon, Ger.*
Albumin (p.710·1).
Hypovolaemia.

Humaplus 10/90, 20/80, 30/70, 40/60, 50/50 *Lilly, Spain.*
Mixtures of insulin injection (human) and isophane insulin injection (human) respectively in the proportions indicated (p.322·1).
Diabetes mellitus.

Humaplus NPH *Lilly, Spain.*
Isophane insulin injection (human) (p.322·1).
Diabetes mellitus.

Humaplus Regular *Lilly, Spain.*
Insulin injection (human) (p.322·1).
Diabetes mellitus.

Humate-P *Armour, USA.*
Pasteurised antihemophilic factor (p.720·3).
Haemophilia A.

Humatin
Parke, Davis, Aust.; Parke, Davis, Canad.; Parke, Davis, Ger.; Parke, Davis, Ital.; Parke, Davis, Spain; Parke, Davis, Switz.; Parke, Davis, USA.
Paromomycin sulphate (p.235·3).
Hepatic encephalopathy and coma; intestinal amoebiasis; preoperative intestinal sterilisation; taeniasis.

Humatrope
Lilly, Aust.; Aza, Austral.; Lilly, Belg.; Lilly, Canad.; Lilly, Ger.; Lilly, Ital.; Lilly, Neth.; Lilly, Norw.; Lilly, S.Afr.; Lilly, Spain; Lilly, Swed.; Lilly, Switz.; Lilly, UK; Lilly, USA.
Somatropin (p.1249·3).
Growth hormone deficiency; Turner's syndrome.

Humatro-Pen *Aza, Austral.*
Somatropin (p.1249·3).
Growth hormone deficiency.

Humectante *Cusi, Spain.*
Methylcellulose (p.1473·3); sodium chloride (p.1162·2).
Dry eyes in contact lens wearers.

Humegon
Organon, Aust.; Organon, Austral.; Organon, Belg.; Organon, Canad.; Organon, Fr.; Organon, Ger.; Organon, Irl.; Organon, Neth.; Organon, Norw.; Donmed, S.Afr.; Organon, Swed.†; Organon, Switz.; Organon, UK; Organon, USA.
Menotrophin (p.1252·1).
Male and female infertility.

Humex
Note. This name is used for preparations of different composition.
Urgo, Fr.
Adult syrup: Ethylmorphine hydrochloride (p.36·1); squill (p.1070·1); ipecacuanha (p.1062·2); belladonna (p.457·1).
Coughs.
Capsules: Carbinoxamine maleate (p.404·2); phenylpropanolamine hydrochloride (p.1067·2); paracetamol (p.72·2).
Upper respiratory-tract disorders.
Lozenges: Ethylmorphine hydrochloride (p.36·1); ipecacuanha (p.1062·2); belladonna (p.457·1).
Coughs.
Mouthwash†: Benzododecinium bromide (p.1103·2); acetarsol sodium (p.578·2); amylocaine hydrochloride (p.1286·1); glycerol (p.1585·2); sodium cyclamate (p.1338·3).
Mouth disorders.
Nasal solution: Benzododecinium bromide (p.1103·2); bergamot oil (p.1553·1).
Nasal infections.
Paediatric syrup: Pholcodine (p.1068·1); sodium benzoate (p.1102·3); drosera (p.1574·1); belladonna (p.457·1); tolu balsam (p.1071·1).
Coughs.
Throat spray: Benzalkonium chloride (p.1101·3); lignocaine hydrochloride (p.1293·2).
Mouth and throat disorders.

Fournier SA, Spain.
Dextromethorphan hydrobromide (p.1057·3).
Coughs.

Humex Expectorant *Urgo, Fr.*
Lozenges: Acetylcysteine (p.1052·3).
Syrup: Carbocisteine (p.1056·3).
Respiratory-tract congestion.

Humex Kinaldine *Urgo, Fr.*
Dequalinium chloride (p.1112·1); ascorbic acid (p.1365·2).
Mouth and throat disorders.

Humibid *Adams, USA.*
Guaiphenesin (p.1061·3).
Coughs.

Humibid DM *Adams, USA.*
Dextromethorphan hydrobromide (p.1057·3); guaiphenesin (p.1061·3).
Coughs.

Humiderm *ConvaTec, UK.*
Sodium pidolate (p.1091·2).
Dry skin disorders.

Huminsulin *Lilly, Ger.*
Insulin injection (human, prb) (p.322·1).
Diabetes mellitus.

Huminsulin Basal
Lilly, Aust.; Lilly, Ger.; Lilly, Switz.
Isophane insulin injection (human, prb) (p.322·1).
Diabetes mellitus.

Huminsulin Long
Lilly, Aust.; Lilly, Ger.; Lilly, Switz.
Insulin zinc suspension (crystalline 70%, amorphous 30%) (human, prb) (p.322·1).
Diabetes mellitus.

Huminsulin Normal
Lilly, Aust.; Lilly, Ger.; Lilly, Switz.
Insulin injection (human, prb) (p.322·1).
Diabetes mellitus.

Huminsulin Profil I, II, III, IV and V
Lilly, Aust.; Lilly, Ger.; Lilly, Switz.
Mixtures of insulin injection (human, prb) 10%, 20%, 30%, 40% and 50% and isophane insulin injection (human, prb) 90%, 80%, 70%, 60% and 50% respectively (p.322·1).
Diabetes mellitus.

Huminsulin Ultralong
Lilly, Aust.; Lilly, Ger.; Lilly, Switz.
Insulin zinc suspension (crystalline) (human, prb) (p.322·1).
Diabetes mellitus.

HuMist Nasal Mist *Scherer, USA.*
Sodium chloride (p.1162·2).
Nasal irritation.

Humoferon *Sigma-Tau, Ital.*
Interferon alfa-n1 (p.615·3).
Chronic hepatitis; leukaemias.

Humopin N *Schoning-Berlin, Ger.*
Salicylic acid (p.1090·2).
Bath additive; musculoskeletal and joint disorders.

Humorsol *Merck Sharp & Dohme, USA.*
Demecarium bromide (p.1390·3).
Open-angle glaucoma; strabismus.

Humoryl *Synthelabo, Fr.*
Toloxatone (p.308·2).
Depression.

Humotet *Wellcome, Irl.†.*
A tetanus immunoglobulin (p.1535·2).
Passive immunisation.

Humoxal *Fournier SA, Spain.*
Oxymetazoline hydrochloride (p.1065·3).
Nasal congestion; sinus congestion.

Humulin 10/90, 20/80, 30/70, 40/60, and 50/50
Aza, Austral.; Lilly, Canad.; Lilly, Ital.; Lilly, S.Afr.; Lilly, USA.
Mixtures of insulin injection (human, prb) and isophane insulin injection (human, prb) (p.322·1) respectively in the proportions indicated.
Diabetes mellitus.

Humulin BR *Lilly, USA†.*
Buffered regular human insulin (crb) (p.322·1).
Diabetes mellitus.

Humulin I
Lilly, Irl.; Lilly, Ital.; Lilly, UK.
Isophane insulin injection (human, prb) (p.322·1).
Diabetes mellitus.

Humulin L
Aza, Austral.; Lilly, Canad.; Lilly, Ital.; Lilly, S.Afr.; Lilly, USA.
Insulin zinc suspension (human) (p.322·1).
Diabetes mellitus.

Humulin Lente
Lilly, Irl.; Lilly, UK.
Insulin zinc suspension (30% amorphous, 70% crystalline) (human, prb) (p.322·1).
Diabetes mellitus.

Humulin M1, M2, M3, M4, M5
Lilly, Irl.; Lilly, UK.
Mixtures of insulin injection (human, prb) 10%, 20%, 30%, 40%, and 50% and isophane insulin injection (human, prb) 90%, 80%, 70%, 60%, and 50% respectively (p.322·1).
Diabetes mellitus.

Humulin Mix 10/90, 20/80, 30/70, 40/60, 50/50
Lilly, Norw.; Lilly, Swed.
Mixtures of insulin injection (human) and isophane insulin injection (human) respectively in the proportions indicated (p.322·1).
Diabetes mellitus.

Humulin N
Lilly, Canad.; Lilly, S.Afr.; Lilly, USA.
Isophane insulin injection (human) (p.322·1).
Diabetes mellitus.

Humulin NPH
Aza, Austral.; Lilly, Norw.; Lilly, Swed.
Isophane insulin injection (human, prb) (p.322·1).
Diabetes mellitus.

Humulin R
Aza, Austral.; Lilly, Canad.; Lilly, Ital.; Lilly, S.Afr.; Lilly, USA†.
Insulin injection (human) (p.322·1).
Diabetes mellitus.

Humulin Regular
Lilly, Norw.; Lilly, Swed.
Insulin injection (human) (p.322·1).
Diabetes mellitus.

Humulin S
Lilly, Irl.; Lilly, UK.
Insulin injection (human, prb) (p.322·1).
Diabetes mellitus.

Humulin U
Lilly, Canad.; Lilly, Ital.; Lilly, S.Afr.
Insulin zinc suspension (crystalline) (human, prb) (p.322·1).
Diabetes mellitus.

Humulin U Ultralente *Lilly, USA.*
Insulin zinc suspension, extended (human, crb) (p.322·1).
Diabetes mellitus.

Humulin UL *Aza, Austral.*
Insulin zinc suspension (crystalline) (human, prb) (p.322·1).
Diabetes mellitus.

Humulin Zn
Lilly, Irl.; Lilly, UK.
Insulin zinc suspension (crystalline) (human, prb) (p.322·1).
Diabetes mellitus.

Humulina 10:90, 20:80, 30:70, 40:60, 50:50 *Lilly, Spain.*
Mixture of insulin injection (human, prb) and isophane insulin injection (human, prb) (p.322·1) respectively in the proportions indicated.
Diabetes mellitus.

Humulina Lenta *Lilly, Spain.*
Insulin zinc suspension (human) (p.322·1).
Diabetes mellitus.

Humulina NPH *Lilly, Spain.*
Isophane insulin injection (human, prb) (p.322·1).
Diabetes mellitus.

Humulina Regular *Lilly, Spain.*
Insulin injection (human, prb) (p.322·1).
Diabetes mellitus.

Humulina Ultralenta *Lilly, Spain.*
Insulin zinc suspension (crystalline 70%, amorphous 30%) (human) (p.322·1).
Diabetes mellitus.

Humuline 10/90, 20/80, 30/70, 40/60, 50/50
Lilly, Belg.; Lilly, Neth.
Mixtures of neutral insulin injection (human, biosynthetic) and insulin suspension (human, biosynthetic) respectively in the proportions indicated (p.322·1).
Diabetes mellitus.

Humuline Long *Lilly, Belg.*
Insulin suspension (human, biosynthetic) (p.322·1).
Diabetes mellitus.

Humuline NPH
Lilly, Belg.; Lilly, Neth.
Isophane insulin injection (human) (p.322·1).
Diabetes mellitus.

Humuline Regular
Lilly, Belg.; Lilly, Neth.
Neutral insulin injection (human) (p.322·1).
Diabetes mellitus.

Humuline Ultralong *Lilly, Belg.*
Insulin suspension (human, biosynthetic) (p.322·1).
Diabetes mellitus.

Humuline Zink *Lilly, Neth.†.*
Insulin zinc suspension (crystalline, human) (p.322·1).
Diabetes mellitus.

Humutard *Lilly, Swed.*
Insulin zinc suspension (human) (amorphous 30%, crystalline 70%) (p.322·1).
Diabetes mellitus.

Hurricaine
Clarben, Spain; Beutlich, USA.
Benzocaine (p.1286·2).
Local anaesthesia.

Hustagil Erkaltungsbalsam *Dentinox, Ger.*
Thyme oil (p.1637·1); oleum pini sylvestris; eucalyptus oil (p.1578·1); clove oil (p.1565·2).
Coughs and associated respiratory-tract disorders.

Hustagil Thymian-Hustensaft *Dentinox, Ger.*
Thyme (p.1636·3).
Coughs and associated respiratory-tract disorders.

Hustazol *Yoshitomi, Jpn.*
Cloperastine fendizoate (p.1057·2) or cloperastine hydrochloride (p.1057·2).
Coughs.

Husten- und Fieber-Saft/Tabletten *Ratiopharm, Ger.*
Paracetamol (p.72·2); dextromethorphan hydrobromide (p.1057·3).
Coughs; fever.

Hustensaft Weleda *Weleda, Aust.*
Herbal and homoeopathic preparation.

Hustensaft-Dr Schmidgall *Schmidgall, Aust.†.*
Plantago lanceolata; thyme (p.1636·3); primula.
Catarrh; coughs and cold symptoms.

Hustenstiller N *Palmicol, Ger.*
Menthol (p.1600·2); benzocaine (p.1286·2).
Catarrh; coughs.

Hustentabs-ratiopharm *Ratiopharm, Ger.*
Bromhexine hydrochloride (p.1055·3).
Respiratory-tract disorders associated with increased or viscous mucus.

Hustex *Synpharma, Switz.†.*
Dextromethorphan hydrobromide (p.1057·3); chlorpheniramine maleate (p.405·1); ammonium chloride (p.1055·2); ipecacuanha (p.1062·2).
Coughs.

Husties *Eu Rho, Ger.*
Thyme (p.1636·3).
Catarrh; coughs.

HVP Chelated Cal-Mag plus Vitamins *Swiss Herbal, Canad.†.*
Vitamin and mineral preparation.

HVP Chelated Multi-Mineral *Swiss Herbal, Canad.†.*
Multimineral preparation.

Hyalart
Bayer, Ger.; FAB, Ital.
Sodium hyaluronate (p.1630·3).
Musculoskeletal and joint disorders.

Hyalase
Rhone-Poulenc Rorer, Austral.; Xixia, S.Afr.; CP Pharmaceuticals, UK.
Hyaluronidase (p.1588·1).
Enhancement of absorption of intramuscular and subcutaneous injections; haematomas; hypodermoclysis; oedema.

Hyalgan
Kolassa, Aust.; Fournier, Fr.; Fidia, Ital.; Shire, UK; Sanofi Winthrop, USA.
Sodium hyaluronate (p.1630·3).
Osteoarthritis of the knee.

Hyalistil *SIFI, Ital.*
Sodium hyaluronate (p.1630·3).
Eye irritation.

Hyalurectal *Doms-Adrian, Fr.†.*
Tube 1, hyaluronidase (p.1588·1); tube 2, aesculus (p.1543·3); hamamelis (p.1587·1); cypress; peru balsam (p.1617·2); phenazone (p.78·2); amylocaine hydrochloride (p.1286·1).
Anorectal disorders.

Hyanit N *Strathmann, Ger.*
Urea (p.1095·2).
Skin disorders.

Hyason *Organon, Neth.*
Hyaluronidase (p.1588·1).
Adjunct to local anaesthesia of the eye.

Hyate:C
Speywood, Switz.; Speywood, UK; Speywood, USA.
A porcine factor VIII:C preparation (p.720·3).
Haemophilia in patients with antibodies to human factor VIII.

Hy-Bio *Solgar, UK.*
Vitamin C with bioflavonoids.

Hybolin *Hyrex, USA.*
Nandrolone phenylpropionate (p.1452·2) or nandrolone decanoate (p.1452·2).
Anaemia in renal disease; breast cancer.

Hybrin *Kabi, Swed.†.*
Ascorbic acid (p.1365·2); sodium ascorbate (p.1365·2).
Vitamin C deficiency.

HY-C *Solgar, USA†.*
Ascorbic acid (p.1365·2); citrus bioflavonoid complex (p.1580·1); rutin (p.1580·2); hesperidin complex (p.1580·2).
Dietary supplement.

Hycaden *Schering, Ital.†.*
Haloprogin (p.381·2).
Fungal skin infections.

Hycal
SmithKline Beecham, Irl.; SmithKline Beecham Drinks, UK.
Glucose syrup solids (p.1343·3).
Food for special diets.

Hycamtin
SmithKline Beecham, Austral.; SmithKline Beecham, Ger.; SmithKline Beecham, Neth.; SmithKline Beecham, Swed.; SmithKline Beecham, UK; SmithKline Beecham, USA.
Topotecan hydrochloride (p.567·2).
Ovarian cancer.

HycoClear Tuss *Ethex, USA.*
Hydrocodone tartrate (p.43·1); guaiphenesin (p.1061·3).
Coughs.

Hycodan
Note. This name is used for preparations of different composition.
Du Pont, Canad.
Hydrocodone tartrate (p.43·1).
Coughs.

Du Pont, USA.
Hydrocodone tartrate (p.43·1); homatropine methobromide (p.462·2).
Coughs.

Hycomine
Note. This name is used for preparations of different composition.
Boots, Austral.
Hydrocodone tartrate (p.43·1); homatropine methobromide (p.462·2); mepyramine maleate (p.414·1); phenylephrine hydrochloride (p.1066·2); ammonium chloride (p.1055·2).
Coughs.

Du Pont, Canad.
Hydrocodone tartrate (p.43·1); mepyramine maleate (p.414·1); phenylephrine hydrochloride (p.1066·2); ammonium chloride (p.1055·2).
Coughs; upper respiratory-tract congestion.

Du Pont, USA.
Hydrocodone tartrate (p.43·1); phenylpropanolamine hydrochloride (p.1067·2).
Coughs and cold symptoms.

Hycomine Compound *Du Pont, USA.*
Hydrocodone tartrate (p.43·1); chlorpheniramine maleate (p.405·1); phenylephrine hydrochloride (p.1066·2); paracetamol (p.72·2); caffeine (p.749·3).
Coughs and cold symptoms.

Hycomine Pediatric *Du Pont, USA.*
Phenylpropanolamine hydrochloride (p.1067·2); hydrocodone tartrate (p.43·1).
Coughs and cold symptoms.

Hyco-Pap *Lunsco, USA.*
Hydrocodone tartrate (p.43·1); paracetamol (p.72·2).

Hycor *Sigma, Austral.*
Hydrocortisone (p.1043·3) or hydrocortisone acetate (p.1043·3).
Inflammatory eye disorders.

Hycort
ICN, Canad.; Everett, USA.
Hydrocortisone (p.1043·3).
Inflammatory diseases of the gastro-intestinal tract; skin disorders.

Hycotuss Expectorant *Du Pont, USA.*
Hydrocodone tartrate (p.43·1); guaiphenesin (p.1061·3).
Coughs.

Hydac *Hoechst Marion Roussel, Swed.*
Felodipine (p.867·3).
Hypertension.

Hydeltrasol *Merck Sharp & Dohme, USA.*
Prednisolone sodium phosphate (p.1048·1).
Corticosteroid.

Hydeltra-TBA *Merck Sharp & Dohme, USA†.*
Prednisolone tebutate (p.1048·2).
Acute gouty arthritis; acute nonspecific tenosynovitis; bursitis; cystic tumours; epicondylitis; post-traumatic osteoarthritis; rheumatoid arthritis; synovitis of osteoarthritis.

Hydergin
Sandoz, Aust.; Sandoz, Ger.; Novartis, Swed.
Co-dergocrine mesylate (p.1566·1).
Cerebral and peripheral vascular disorders; cervical syndrome; hypertensive crises; mental function impairment; migraine and other vascular headaches; shock.

Hydergina
Sandoz, Ital.; Sandoz, Spain.
Co-dergocrine mesylate (p.1566·1).
Hypertension; impaired mental function in the elderly; vascular disorders.

Hydergine
Sandoz, Belg.; Sandoz, Canad.; Sandoz, Fr.; Sandoz, Irl.; Novartis, Neth.; Sandoz, S.Afr.†; Sandoz, Switz.; Sandoz, UK; Sandoz, USA.
Co-dergocrine mesylate (p.1566·1).
Cerebrovascular disorders; senile dementia.

Hyderm *Taro, Canad.*
Hydrocortisone acetate (p.1043·3).
Skin disorders.

Hydiphen *Dresden, Ger.*
Clomipramine hydrochloride (p.281·2).
Depression; nocturnal enuresis; pain; psychoses.

Hydoftal *Agepha, Aust.*
Hydrocortisone (p.1043·3); hydrocortisone acetate (p.1043·3); neomycin sulphate (p.229·2).
Inflammatory eye disorders.

Hydol *Napp, Irl.*
Dihydrocodeine tartrate (p.34·1).
Pain.

Hydonan *Hermal, Ger.†.*
Propantheline bromide (p.468·1); aluminium chlorohydrate (p.1078·3).
Hyperhidrosis.

Hydopa *Alphapharm, Austral.*
Methyldopa (p.904·2).
Hypertension.

Hydra Perfecte *L'Oreal, Canad.*
SPF 10: Ethylhexyl *p*-methoxycinnamate (p.1487·1).
Sunscreen.

Hydracillin *SmithKline Beecham, Ger.*
Procaine penicillin (p.240·2); benzylpenicillin sodium (p.159·3).
Lignocaine hydrochloride (p.1293·2) is included in this preparation to alleviate the pain of injection.
Bacterial infections.

Hydracort *Galderma, Fr.*
Hydrocortisone (p.1043·3).
Skin disorders.

Hydraderm *Sigma, Austral.*
Moisturiser.

Hydralarm *Chauvin, Fr.†.*
Sodium chloride (p.1162·2).
Dry eyes.

Hydralin *Nicholas, Fr.*
Powder for topical solution: Sodium perborate (p.1125·2); borax (p.1554·2); sodium bicarbonate (p.1153·2); sodium carbonate anhydrous (p.1630·2).
Soap: Borax (p.1554·2).
Skin cleansing.

Hydramyn *Lu Chem, USA†.*
Diphenhydramine hydrochloride (p.409·1).
Coughs.

Hydrap-ES
Note. A similar name is used for preparations of different composition.
Parmed, USA.
Hydrochlorothiazide (p.885·2); reserpine (p.942·1); hydralazine hydrochloride (p.883·2).
Hypertension.

Hydrapres
Note. A similar name is used for preparations of different composition.
Rubio, Spain.
Hydralazine hydrochloride (p.883·2).
Heart failure; hypertension.

Hydrasorb *Knoll, Canad.*
Polyurethane foam dressing.
Wounds.

Hydrastis Complex *Blackmores, Austral.*
Liquorice (p.1197·1); althaea (p.1546·3); matricaria recutita (p.1561·2); hydrastis (p.1588·2); vitamin A acetate (p.1359·2).
Gastro-intestinal disorders.

Hydrastis Salbe *Steigerwald, Ger.*
Homoeopathic preparation.

Hydrate *Hyrex, USA.*
Dimenhydrinate (p.408·2).
Motion sickness.

Hydra-zide *Par, USA.*
Hydralazine hydrochloride (p.883·2); hydrochlorothiazide (p.885·2).

Hydrea
Bristol-Myers Squibb, Austral.; Bristol-Myers Squibb, Belg.; Squibb, Canad.; Bristol-Myers Squibb, Fr.; Bristol-Myers Squibb, Irl.; Bristol-Myers Squibb, Neth.; Bristol-Myers Squibb, S.Afr.; Squibb, UK; Immunex, USA.
Hydroxyurea (p.539·1).
Malignant neoplasms.

Hydrene *Alphapharm, Austral.*
Triamterene (p.957·2); hydrochlorothiazide (p.885·2).
Hypertension; oedema.

Hydrenox *Knoll, UK†.*
Hydroflumethiazide (p.889·2).
Hypertension; oedema.

Hydrex
Note. This name is used for preparations of different composition.
Unitech, Irl.; Adams, UK.
Chlorhexidine gluconate (p.1107·2).
Skin disinfection.

Rolab, S.Afr.
Frusemide (p.871·1).
Oedema.

Hydrisalic *Pedinol, USA†.*
Salicylic acid (p.1090·2).
Hyperkeratotic skin.

Hydrisea *Pedinol, USA.*
Emollient and moisturiser.

Hydrisinol *Pedinol, USA.*
Emollient and moisturiser.

Hydro Cobex *Pasadena, USA.*
Hydroxocobalamin (p.1363·3).
Schilling test; vitamin B_{12} deficiency.

Hydro Cordes *Ichthyol, Ger.*
Allantoin (p.1078·2); dexpanthenol (p.1570·3); ethyl linoleate.
Skin disorders.

Hydro-Adreson *Organon, Neth.*
Injection: Hydrocortisone sodium succinate (p.1044·1).
Corticosteroid.

Hydrobexan *Keene, USA†.*
Hydroxocobalamin (p.1363·3).
Schilling test; vitamin B_{12} deficiency.

Hydrocal
Bioglan, Irl.; Bioglan, UK†.
Hydrocortisone acetate (p.1043·3); calamine (p.1080·1).
Skin disorders.

Hydrocare
Allergan, Austral.; Allergan, Ger.; Allergan, USA.
Range of solutions for soft contact lenses.

Hydrocare Enzymatic Protein Remover *Allergan, Austral.*
Papain (p.1614·1).
Cleanser for soft and gas permeable contact lenses.

Hydro-Cebral *Ratiopharm, Ger.*
Co-dergocrine mesylate (p.1566·1).
Cervical disc syndrome; mental function disorders.

Hydrocet *Carnrick, USA.*
Hydrocodone tartrate (p.43·1); paracetamol (p.72·2).
Analgesic.

Hydro-Chlor *Vortech, USA.*
Hydrochlorothiazide (p.885·2).
Hypertension; oedema.

Hydrocil Instant *Solvay, USA.*
Psyllium hydrophilic mucilloid (p.1194·2).
Constipation.

Hydroclonazone *Promedica, Fr.*
Chloramine (p.1106·3).
Water purification.

Hydrocobamine *Byk, Neth.*
Hydroxocobalamin (p.1363·3).
Megaloblastic anaemia; vitamin B_{12} deficiency.

Hydrocodeinon *Streuli, Switz.*
Dihydrocodeine hydrochloride (p.34·2).
Coughs.

Hydrocodone CP *Morton Grove, USA.*
Hydrocodone tartrate (p.43·1); phenylephrine hydrochloride (p.1066·2); chlorpheniramine maleate (p.405·1).
Upper respiratory-tract symptoms.

Hydrocodone GF *Morton Grove, USA.*
Hydrocodone tartrate (p.43·1); guaiphenesin (p.1061·3).
Upper respiratory-tract symptoms.

Hydrocodone HD *Morton Grove, USA.*
Hydrocodone tartrate (p.43·1); phenylephrine hydrochloride (p.1066·2); chlorpheniramine maleate (p.405·1).
Upper respiratory-tract symptoms.

Hydrocodone PA *Morton Grove, USA.*
Hydrocodone tartrate (p.43·1); phenylpropanolamine hydrochloride (p.1067·2).
Upper respiratory-tract symptoms.

Hydrocomp *Sanorania, Ger.*
Amiloride hydrochloride (p.819·2); hydrochlorothiazide (p.885·2).
Hypertension; oedema.

Hydrocort *CT, Ger.*
Hydrocortisone acetate (p.1043·3).
Skin disorders.

Hydrocort Mild *CT, Ger.*
Hydrocortisone (p.1043·3).
Skin disorders.

Hydrocortancyl *Roussel, Fr.*
Prednisolone (p.1048·1) or prednisolone acetate (p.1048·1).
Corticosteroid.

Hydrocortimycin *Kolassa, Aust.*
Hydrocortisone acetate (p.1043·3); neomycin sulphate (p.229·2).
Inflammatory eye disorders.

Hydrocortisone comp *Streuli, Switz.*
Hydrocortisone acetate (p.1043·3); zinc stearate (p.1469·3).
Skin disorders.

Hydrocortistab *Knoll, UK.*
Hydrocortisone acetate (p.1043·3).
Corticosteroid; inflammatory skin disorders.

Hydrocortisyl
Hoechst Marion Roussel, Irl.; Hoechst Marion Roussel, UK.
Hydrocortisone (p.1043·3).
Skin disorders.

Hydrocortone
Merck Sharp & Dohme, Aust.; Merck Sharp & Dohme, Irl.; Merck Sharp & Dohme, Switz.; Merck Sharp & Dohme, UK; Merck Sharp & Dohme, USA.
Hydrocortisone (p.1043·3), hydrocortisone acetate (p.1043·3), or hydrocortisone sodium phosphate (p.1044·1).
Corticosteroid.

Hydrocream *Paddock, USA.*
Vehicle for topical preparations.

Hydro-Crysti-12 *Roberts, USA; Hauck, USA.*
Hydroxocobalamin (p.1363·3).
Schilling test; vitamin B_{12} deficiency.

Hydroderm
Aesca, Aust.; Karrer, Ger.
Hydrocortisone (p.1043·3).
Skin disorders.

Hydrodexan
Procter & Gamble, Aust.; Hermal, Ger.
Hydrocortisone (p.1043·3); urea (p.1095·2).
Skin and scalp disorders.

HydroDiuril
Merck Sharp & Dohme, Canad.; Merck Sharp & Dohme, USA.
Hydrochlorothiazide (p.885·2).
Hypertension; oedema.

Hydroform *Dermacare, Austral.*
Hydrocortisone (p.1043·3); clioquinol (p.193·2).
Inflammatory skin disorders.

Hydrogesic *Edwards, USA.*
Hydrocodone tartrate (p.43·1); paracetamol (p.72·2).
Pain.

Hydrokon *Nycomed, Norw.†.*
Hydrocodone tartrate (p.43·1).
Coughs.

Hydrol *Janssen-Cilag, S.Afr.*
Potassium chloride; sodium chloride; sodium citrate; glucose (p.1152·3).
Oral rehydration therapy.

Hydro-Less *Lennon, S.Afr.*
Indapamide (p.890·2).
Hypertension.

Hydrolid *Helvepharm, Switz.*
Amiloride hydrochloride (p.819·2); hydrochlorothiazide (p.885·2).
Hypertension; oedema.

Hydro-long *Sanorania, Ger.*
Chlorthalidone (p.839·3).
Diabetes insipidus; hypertension; oedema.

Hydromal *Hauck, USA.*
Hydrochlorothiazide (p.885·2).
Hypertension; oedema.

Hydromedin *Merck Sharp & Dohme, Ger.*
Ethacrynic acid (p.866·3) or sodium ethacrynate (p.866·3).
Ascites; oedema.

Hydromet
Note. This name is used for preparations of different composition.
Merck Sharp & Dohme, Irl.; Merck Sharp & Dohme, Neth.†; Logos, S.Afr.†; Merck Sharp & Dohme, Spain†; Merck Sharp & Dohme, Swed.; Merck Sharp & Dohme, UK†.
Hydrochlorothiazide (p.885·2); methyldopa (p.904·2).
Hypertension.

Barre-National, USA.
Hydrocodone tartrate (p.43·1); homatropine methobromide (p.462·2).
Coughs.

Hydromine *Warner Chilcott, USA†.*
Hydrocodone tartrate (p.43·1); phenylpropanolamine hydrochloride (p.1067·2).

Hydromol *Quinoderm, Irl.*
Cream: Sodium pidolate (p.1091·2); arachis oil (p.1550·2); isopropyl myristate (p.1384·1); liquid paraffin (p.1382·1); sodium lactate (p.1153·2).
Topical solution: Light liquid paraffin (p.1382·1); isopropyl myristate (p.1384·1).
Dry skin.

Hydromol Cream *Quinoderm, UK.*
Arachis oil (p.1550·2); isopropyl myristate (p.1384·1); liquid paraffin (p.1382·1); sodium pidolate (p.1091·2); sodium lactate (p.1153·2).
Dry skin conditions.

Hydromol Emollient *Quinoderm, UK.*
Light liquid paraffin (p.1382·1); isopropyl myristate (p.1384·1).
Dry skin conditions.

Hydromorph *Purdue Frederick, Canad.*
Hydromorphone hydrochloride (p.43·2).
Pain.

Hydromox *Lederle, USA.*
Quinethazone (p.938·3).
Hypertension; oedema.

Hy-Drop *Fidia, Ital.*
Sodium hyaluronate (p.1630·3).
Dry eyes.

Hydropane *Halsey, USA.*
Hydrocodone tartrate (p.43·1); homatropine methobromide (p.462·2).
Coughs.

Hydropel *C & M, USA.*
Topical barrier preparation.

Hydrophed *Rugby, USA.*
Theophylline (p.765·1); ephedrine sulphate (p.1059·3); hydroxyzine hydrochloride (p.412·1).
Bronchospasm.

Hydrophene DH *Morton Grove, USA.*
Hydrocodone tartrate (p.43·1); phenylephrine hydrochloride (p.1066·2); mepyramine maleate (p.414·1).

Hydrophil *Omega, Canad.*
Urea (p.1095·2); white soft paraffin (p.1382·3).
Dry skin.

Hydrophilic *Rugby, USA.*
Vehicle for topical preparations.

Hydropres
Merck Sharp & Dohme, Canad.; Merck Sharp & Dohme, USA.
Hydrochlorothiazide (p.885·2); reserpine (p.942·1).
Hypertension.

Hydro-rapid
Sanorania, Ger.; Sanorania, Switz.†.
Frusemide (p.871·1).
Hypertension; oedema; oliguria; varices.

HydroSaluric
Merck Sharp & Dohme, Irl.; Merck Sharp & Dohme, UK.
Hydrochlorothiazide (p.885·2).
Hypertension; oedema.

Hydrosarpan *Servier, Canad.†.*
Raubasine (p.941·3).
Cerebral ischaemia; peripheral vascular disorders.

Hydro-Serp *Rugby, USA.*
Hydrochlorothiazide (p.885·2); reserpine (p.942·1).
Hypertension.

Hydroserpine *Rugby, USA.*
Hydrochlorothiazide (p.885·2); reserpine (p.942·1).
Hypertension.

Hydrosine *Major, USA†.*
Hydrochlorothiazide (p.885·2); reserpine (p.942·1).

Hydrosol Polyvitamine *Roche, Fr.*
Multivitamin preparation.

Hydrosol Polyvitamine BON *Doms-Adrian, Fr.*
Multivitamin preparation.

Hydrosone *Technilab, Canad.*
Hydrocortisone (p.1043·3).

HydroStat IR *Richwood, USA.*
Hydromorphone hydrochloride (p.43·2).
Pain.

HydroTex *Syosset, USA.*
Hydrocortisone (p.1043·3).
Skin disorders.

Hydrotricine
Rhone-Poulenc Rorer, Belg.†; Rhone-Poulenc Rorer, Ital.
Tyrothricin (p.267·2).
Bacterial stomatitis.

Hydrotrix
Kolassa, Aust.; Medice, Ger.; Trommsdorff, Ger.; Medice, Switz.
Frusemide (p.871·1); triamterene (p.957·2).
Heart failure; hypertension; oedema.

Hydroxium *Knoll, Neth.†.*
Co-dergocrine mesylate (p.1566·1).
Alzheimer's disease.

Hydroxo
Lipha, Belg.; Lipha Sante, Fr.†; Rolland, Switz.†.
Hydroxocobalamin (p.1363·3).
Musculoskeletal and nerve pain.

Hydroxy-Cal *Sisu, Canad.*
Vitamin C and minerals.

Hydro-Z *Mayrand, USA.*
Hydrochlorothiazide (p.885·2).
Hypertension; oedema.

Hydrozide
Note. This name is used for preparations of different composition.
Douglas, Austral.
Hydrochlorothiazide (p.885·2); amiloride hydrochloride (p.819·2).
Hepatic cirrhosis with ascites; hypertension; oedema.

Williams, USA.
Hydrochlorothiazide (p.885·2).
Hypertension; oedema.

Hydrozole *Dermacare, Austral.*
Hydrocortisone (p.1043·3); clotrimazole (p.376·3).
Skin disorders.

Hygeol *Wampole, Canad.*
Sodium hypochlorite (p.1124·3).
Disinfection; wound cleansing.

Hygienist *Bayer, Ital.*
Chlorocresol (preventol CMK) (p.1110·3); clorophene (preventol BP) (p.1111·2); orthophenylphenol (preventol extra) (p.1120·3).
Surface disinfection.

Hygienist Pavimenti e Piastrelle *Bayer, Ital.*
Benzalkonium chloride (p.1101·3).
Surface disinfection.

Hygine In *Geymonat, Ital.*
Lactobacillus acidophilus (p.1594·1).
Disturbances of vaginal flora.

Hygiodermil *Vifor, Switz.*
Bornyl salicylate (p.22·1); neroli oil (p.1606·3); lavender oil (p.1594·3); menthol (p.1600·2).
Skin disorders.

Hygroton
Ciba-Geigy, Aust.; Novartis, Austral.; Ciba-Geigy, Belg.; Geigy, Canad.; Ciba-Geigy, Fr.; Ciba, Ger.; Ciba-Geigy, Irl.†; Novartis, Neth.; Geigy, Norw.; Novartis, S.Afr.; Ciba-Geigy, Swed.†; Geigy, Switz.; Alliance, UK; Rorer, USA.
Chlorthalidone (p.839·3).
Diabetes insipidus; heart failure; hypertension; oedema.

Hygroton-K
Ciba-Geigy, Irl.†; Ciba-Geigy, Swed.†; Geigy, Switz.†; Geigy, UK†.
Chlorthalidone (p.839·3); potassium chloride (p.1161·1).
Heart failure; hypertension; oedema.

Hygroton-Quart *Ciba-Geigy, Fr.†.*
Chlorthalidone (p.839·3).
Hypertension; oedema.

Hygroton-Reserpine
Geigy, Canad.†; Novartis, S.Afr.; Geigy, Switz.
Chlorthalidone (p.839·3); reserpine (p.942·1).
Hypertension.

Hykaten *Zeneca, Neth.†.*
Atenolol (p.825·3); hydrochlorothiazide (p.885·2); amiloride hydrochloride (p.819·2).
Hypertension.

Hylak *Merckle, Aust.*
Metabolic products of lactic-acid producing organisms (p.1594·1); lactic acid (p.1593·3); amino acids.
Gastro-intestinal disorders; liver disorders; skin disorders.

Hylak forte *Merckle, Aust.*
Metabolic products of lactic-acid producing organisms (p.1594·1); metabolic products of Gram-positive and Gram-negative intestinal flora; lactic acid (p.1593·3); amino acids.
Gastro-intestinal disorders; liver disorders; skin disorders.

Hylak forte N *Merckle, Ger.*
Metabolic products of: *Lactobacillus helveticus* (p.1594·1); *Escherichia coli*; *Lactobacillus acidophilus* (p.1594·1).
Gastro-intestinal disorders.

Hylak N *Merckle, Ger.*
Metabolic products of *Lactobacillus helveticus* (p.1594·1).
Gastro-intestinal disorders.

Hylakombun *Merckle, Aust.*
Phthalylsulphathiazole (p.237·1); ethaverine hydrochloride (p.1577·1); ox bile (p.1553·2); metabolic products of *Escherichia coli*; *Enterococcus faecalis* (p.1594·1); *Lactobacillus acidophilus* (p.1594·1).
Bacterial infections of the gastro-intestinal tract.

Hylakombun N *Merckle, Ger.†.*
Pancreatin (p.1612·1); fel tauri (p.1553·2); chloroxine (p.215·3); ethaverine hydrochloride (p.1577·1).
Gastro-intestinal disorders.

Hylands *Hylands, Canad.*
A range of homoeopathic preparations.

Hylase *Dessau, Ger.*
Hyaluronidase (p.1588·1).
Adjunct in ocular surgery; adjuvant to increase absorption and dispersion of drugs; inflammation; prevention of episiotomy.

Hylashield *I-Med, Canad.*
Hylan A (p.1631·1).
Eye disorders.

Hylidone *Major, USA.*
Chlorthalidone (p.839·3).
Hypertension; oedema.

Hylorel *Fisons, USA.*
Guanadrel sulphate (p.877·3).
Hypertension.

Hylutin *Hyrex, USA.*
Hydroxyprogesterone hexanoate (p.1448·1).
Abnormal uterine bleeding; amenorrhoea; metrorrhagia.

Hymecel
Ciba Vision, Ger.; Ciba Vision, Switz.†.
Hypromellose (p.1473·1).
Adjunct in intra-ocular surgery; moistening of artificial lenses.

Hyoscal N *Steierl, Ger.*
Scopolia carniolica root.
Smooth muscle spasm.

Hyosophen *Rugby, USA.*
Atropine sulphate (p.455·1); hyoscine hydrobromide (p.462·3); hyoscyamine hydrobromide (p.464·2) or hyoscyamine sulphate (p.464·2); phenobarbitone (p.350·2).
Gastro-intestinal disorders.

Hyospasmol *Intramed, S.Afr.; Lennon, S.Afr.*
Hyoscine butylbromide (p.462·3).
Gastro-intestinal spasm.

Hypadil *Kowa, Jpn†.*
Nipradilol (p.922·3).

Hypaque
Sanofi Winthrop, Canad.; Sanofi Winthrop, Irl.; Sanofi Winthrop, UK; Nycomed, USA.
Meglumine diatrizoate (p.1003·2) or sodium diatrizoate (p.1003·2).
Radiographic contrast medium.

Hypaque-M 76% *Sanofi Winthrop, Canad.*
Meglumine diatrizoate (p.1003·2); sodium diatrizoate (p.1003·2).
Radiographic contrast medium.

Hypaque-M, Hypaque-76 *Nycomed, USA.*
Meglumine diatrizoate (p.1003·2); sodium diatrizoate (p.1003·2).
Radiographic contrast medium.

Hyperab
CSL, Austral.†; Bayer, Canad.; Tropon-Cutter, Ger.†; Cutter, USA.
A rabies immunoglobulin (p.1530·2).
Passive immunisation.

Hyperamine
Braun, Fr.; Braun, UK.
Amino-acid infusion.
Parenteral nutrition.

Hypercal
Note. This name is used for preparations of different composition.
Sodietal, Fr.
Nutritional supplement.

Nelson, UK.
Homoeopathic preparation.

Hypercal-B *Carlton Laboratories, UK†.*
Rauwolfia alkaloids (p.941·3); amylobarbitone (p.641·3).
Hypertension.

Hypercard *Hotz, Ger.*
Olive leaves; mistletoe (p.1604·1); ginseng (p.1584·2); convallaria (p.1567·2); rauwolfia; silicea; sumbulus moschatus; conium.
Cardiovascular disorders.

Hyperesa *Dolorgiet, Ger.*
Valerian (p.1643·1); hypericum (p.1590·1).
Insomnia; nervous disorders.

Hyperex *Propan, S.Afr.†.*
Hydralazine hydrochloride (p.883·2).
Hypertension.

Hyperforat *Klein, Ger.*
Hypericum (p.1590·1).
Depression; migraine; nocturnal enuresis; stuttering.

Hyperforat-forte *Klein, Ger.*
Hypericum (p.1590·1); rauwolfia vomitoria (p.941·3).
Depression; excitation; irritability.

HyperHep
Bayer, Canad.; Cutter, USA.
A hepatitis B immunoglobulin (p.1512·3).
Passive immunisation.

Hyperiagil *Agil, Ger.†.*
Benzyl nicotinate (p.22·1); glycol salicylate (p.43·1); rosemary oil (p.1626·2); camphor (p.1557·2); isopropyl alcohol.
Cervical syndrome; circulatory disorders; neuralgia; rheumatism; sciatica.

Hypericaps *Duopharm, Ger.*
Hypericum (p.1590·1).
Anxiety.

Hyperidyst-A *Weber & Weber, Ger.†.*
Homoeopathic preparation.

Hyperiforce *Bioforce, Switz.*
Hypericum (p.1590·1); melissa (p.1600·1); lupulus (p.1597·2).
Exhaustion; irritability; sleep disorders.

Hyperium *Biopharma, Fr.*
Rilmenidine phosphate (p.943·1).
Hypertension.

Hyperlipen
Sanofi Winthrop, Belg.; Sanofi Winthrop, Switz.
Ciprofibrate (p.1270·3).
Hyperlipidaemias.

Hyperlite *Pharmacia Upjohn, Spain.*
Electrolyte infusion (p.1147·1).
Fluid and electrolyte depletion.

Hyperlyte *McGaw, USA.*
A range of electrolyte preparations (p.1147·1).
Fluid and electrolyte disorders.

Hyperphen *Lennon, S.Afr.*
Hydralazine hydrochloride (p.883·2).
Hypertension.

Hyperstat
Schering-Plough, Austral.†; Schering-Plough, Belg.; Schering, Canad.; Schering-Plough, Fr.; Schering-Plough, Ital.; Schering-Plough, Neth.; Schering-Plough, S.Afr.; Schering-Plough, Spain; Schering-Plough, Swed.; Essex, Switz.; Schering, USA.
Diazoxide (p.847·2).
Hypertension; hypoglycaemia.

Hypertane *Schwarz, UK†.*
Hydrochlorothiazide (p.885·2); amiloride hydrochloride (p.819·2).
These ingredients can be described by the British Approved Name Co-amilozide.
Ascites; heart failure; hypertension.

Hypertensin *Ciba, Ger.†.*
Angiotensin amide (p.824·1).
Shock.

Hypertensine *Ciba, Switz.†.*
Angiotensin amide (p.824·1).
Shock.

Hyper-Tet *Bayer, Canad.; Tropon-Cutter, Ger.†; Cutter, USA.*
A tetanus immunoglobulin (p.1535·2).
Passive immunisation.

Hypertonalum *Essex, Ger.*
Diazoxide (p.847·2).
Hypertension.

Hypertorr *Henning, Ger.*
Triamterene (p.957·2); hydrochlorothiazide (p.885·2).
Heart failure; hypertension; oedema.

Hypertussin *Fink, Ger.†.*
Paracetamol (p.72·2); codeine phosphate (p.26·1).
Coughs with fever; pain.

Hy-Phen *Ascher, USA.*
Hydrocodone tartrate (p.43·1); paracetamol (p.72·2).

Hypnasmine *Elerte, Fr.*
Caffeine (p.749·3); butobarbitone (p.645·1); theophylline (p.765·1).
Asthma.

Hypnocalm *Farmabel, Belg.†.*
Flunitrazepam (p.670·1).
Insomnia.

Hypnodin *Takeda, Jpn†.*
Perlapine.

Hypnodorm *Alphapharm, Austral.*
Flunitrazepam (p.670·1).
Insomnia.

Hypnomidate
Janssen-Cilag, Aust.; Janssen-Cilag, Belg.; Janssen-Cilag, Fr.; Janssen-Cilag, Ger.; Janssen-Cilag, Neth.; Janssen-Cilag, S.Afr.; Janssen-Cilag, Spain; Janssen-Cilag, Switz.; Janssen-Cilag, UK.
Etomidate (p.1223·2) or etomidate hydrochloride (p.1223·3).
General anaesthesia.

Hypnor *Rolab, S.Afr.*
Flunitrazepam (p.670·1).
Insomnia.

Hypnorex
Synthelabo, Ger.; Synthelabo, Switz.†.
Lithium carbonate (p.290·3).
Depression; mania.

Hypnovel
Roche, Austral.; Roche, Fr.; Roche, Irl.; Roche, UK.
Midazolam hydrochloride (p.679·3).
Induction of anaesthesia; premedication; sedative.

Hypoca *Yamanouchi, Jpn.*
Barnidipine hydrochloride (p.827·1).
Hypertension.

Hypochylin *Recip, Swed.*
Glutamic acid hydrochloride (p.1344·3).
Hypochylia.

Hypodyn *Sandoz, Aust.*
Dihydroergotamine mesylate (p.444·2); etilefrine hydrochloride (p.867·2).
Hypotension.

Hypoguard *Priory, Irl.*
Test for glucose in blood (p.1585·1).

Hypoguard GA *Hypoguard, UK.*
Test for glucose in blood (p.1585·1).

Hypol *Felton, Austral.*
Capsules: Cod-liver oil (p.1337·3).
Arthritis; cardiovascular disorders; cold and influenza symptoms; dietary supplement; inflammatory disorders.
Oral emulsion: Cod-liver oil (p.1337·3); soya oil (p.1355·1); calcium hypophosphate; sodium hypophosphate.
Vitamin and mineral supplement.
Tablets: Vitamin A (p.1358·1); cholecalciferol (p.1366·3); vitamin C (p.1365·2); calcium dihydrogen phosphate (p.1556·2).
Vitamin and calcium supplement.

Hypolac *Neo Abello, Ital.*
Infant feed.
Food intolerance.

Hypolar Retard *Lagap, UK.*
Nifedipine (p.916·2).
Angina pectoris; hypertension.

Hypolind *Lindopharm, Ger.†.*
Norfenefrine hydrochloride (p.925·1).
Formerly contained norfenefrine hydrochloride and sparteine sulphate.
Hypotension.

hypo-loges *Loges, Ger.†.*
Oxedrine tartrate (p.925·3); scoparium; adonis vernalis; cacti grandiflorus; camphor.
Hypotension.

Hypomide *Lennon, S.Afr.*
Chlorpropamide (p.319·1).
Diabetes mellitus.

Hypon *Calmic, UK†.*
Aspirin (p.16·1); codeine phosphate (p.26·1); caffeine (p.749·3).
Fever; pain.

Hyposedon N *Harras-Curarina, Ger.*
Kava (p.1592·3); passion flower (p.1615·3).
Sleep disorders.

Hypostamin *Zyma, Aust.†.*
Tritoqualine (p.421·1).
Hypersensitivity reactions.

Hypostamine
Promedica, Fr.; Zyma, Ital.†.
Tritoqualine (p.421·1).
Hypersensitivity reactions.

Hyposulfene *ACT, Fr.†.*
Sodium thiosulphate (p.996·2).
Gastro-intestinal disorders; heavy-metal poisoning; respiratory-tract disorders; skin disorders.

Hypotears
Note. This name is used for preparations of different composition.
Ciba Vision, Canad.; Ciba Vision, Spain.
Eye drops: Polyvinyl alcohol (p.1474·2).
Dry eyes.

Ciba Vision, Canad.; Iolab, USA.
Eye ointment: White soft paraffin (p.1382·3); light liquid paraffin (p.1382·1).
Dry eyes.

CooperVision, Irl.†; Ciba Vision, Ital.; Ciba Vision, UK; Iolab, USA.
Eye drops: Polyvinyl alcohol (p.1474·2); macrogol (p.1597·3).
Dry eyes.

Hypoten *Covan, S.Afr.*
Sodium nitroprusside (p.943·2).
Hypertension.

Hy-Po-Tone *Lennon, S.Afr.*
Methyldopa (p.904·2).
Hypertension.

Hypotonex *Phonix, Ger.†.*
Homoeopathic preparation.

Hypotonin *Steigerwald, Ger.†.*
Crataegus (p.1568·2); convallaria (p.1567·2); sparteine sulphate (p.1632·1); ephedrine hydrochloride (p.1059·3); camphor (p.1557·2).
Hypotension.

Hypotonin forte *Steigerwald, Ger.†.*
Nikethamide (p.1483·3); ephedrine hydrochloride (p.1059·3); sparteine sulphate (p.1632·1).
Hypotension.

Hypotonodynat *Rhenomed, Ger.†.*
Oral drops: Ephedrine (p.1059·3); caffeine and sodium salicylate (p.751·1).
Tablets: Ephedrine hydrochloride (p.1059·3); caffeine and sodium salicylate (p.751·1); arnica; cocculus.
Hypotension.

Hypovase
Invicta, Irl.; Invicta, UK.
Prazosin hydrochloride (p.932·3).
Benign prostatic hyperplasia; heart failure; hypertension; Raynaud's syndrome.

Hypren *Astra, Aust.*
Ramipril (p.941·1).
Heart failure; hypertension; myocardial infarction.

Hypren plus *Astra, Aust.*
Ramipril (p.941·1); hydrochlorothiazide (p.885·2).
Hypertension.

Hyprenan
Astra, Norw.; Hassle, Swed.
Prenalterol hydrochloride (p.934·1).
Hypotension; reversal of beta blockade; shock.

HypRho-D
Bayer, Canad.; Tropon-Cutter, Ger.†; Cutter, USA.
An anti-D immunoglobulin (p.1503·2).
Prevention of rhesus sensitisation.

Hyprim *Italchimici, Ital.*
Brodimoprim (p.162·1).
Otorhinolaryngeal disorders; respiratory-tract infections.

Hyprogest *Keene, USA†.*
Hydroxyprogesterone hexanoate (p.1448·1).
Abnormal uterine bleeding; amenorrhoea; metrorrhagia.

Hypurin Biphasic 30/70 *CP Pharmaceuticals, UK.*
Mixture of neutral insulin injection (porcine, highly purified) 30% and isophane insulin injection (porcine, highly purified) 70% (p.322·1).
Diabetes mellitus.

Hypurin Isophane
Rhone-Poulenc Rorer, Austral.; CP Pharmaceuticals, UK.
Isophane insulin injection (bovine or porcine, highly purified) (p.322·1).
Diabetes mellitus.

Hypurin Lente *CP Pharmaceuticals, UK.*
Insulin zinc suspension (30% amorphous, 70% crystalline) (bovine, highly purified) (p.322·1).
Diabetes mellitus.

Hypurin Neutral
Rhone-Poulenc Rorer, Austral.; CP Pharmaceuticals, UK.
Neutral insulin injection (bovine or porcine, highly purified) (p.322·1).
Diabetes mellitus.

Hypurin Protamine Zinc *CP Pharmaceuticals, UK.*
Protamine zinc insulin injection (bovine, highly purified) (p.322·1).
Diabetes mellitus.

Hyrexin *Hyrex, USA.*
Diphenhydramine hydrochloride (p.409·1).
Motion sickness; parkinsonism.

Hyrin *Merckle, Ger.*
Metoclopramide (p.1202·1).
Gastro-intestinal disorders.

Hyrvalan *Monot, Fr.*
Paracetamol (p.72·2); ascorbic acid (p.1365·2); chlorpheniramine maleate (p.405·1).
Upper respiratory-tract disorders.

Hyskon
Dermatech, Austral.; Pharmacia Upjohn, Canad.; Reusch, Ger.; Kabi, Irl.†; Medisan, Swed.; Pharmacia, UK; Pharmacia, USA.
Dextran 70 (p.717·1) in glucose.
Aid to hysteroscopy.

Hysone
Note. This name is used for preparations of different composition.
Alphapharm, Austral.
Hydrocortisone (p.1043·3).
Corticosteroid.

Roberts, USA.
Clioquinol (p.193·2); hydrocortisone (p.1043·3).
Inflammatory skin disorders.

Hytakerol
Sanofi Winthrop, Canad.; Sanofi Winthrop, USA.
Dihydrotachysterol (p.1366·3).
Hypoparathyroidism; postoperative and idiopathic tetany.

Hytinic *Hyrex, USA.*
Capsules: Polysaccharide-iron complex (p.1353·2).
Injection: Ferrous gluconate (p.1340·1); vitamin B substances.
Procaine hydrochloride (p.1299·2) is included in this preparation to alleviate the pain of injection.
Iron-deficiency anaemias.

Hytone *Dermik, USA.*
Hydrocortisone (p.1043·3).
Skin disorders.

Hytrast
Codali, Belg.†; Therapex, Canad.†; Guerbet, Fr.; Byk Gulden, Ger.; Byk Gulden, Ital.†; Guerbet, Neth.†.
Iopydol (p.1008·1); iopydone (p.1008·1).
Contrast medium for upper respiratory-tract radiography.

Hytrin
Abbott, Austral.; Abbott, Belg.; Abbott, Canad.; Abbott, Irl.; Abbott, Neth.; Abbott, S.Afr.; Abbott, UK; Abbott, USA; Wellcome, USA.
Terazosin hydrochloride (p.952·1).
Benign prostatic hyperplasia; hypertension.

Hytrin BPH
Abbott, Switz.; Abbott, UK.
Terazosin hydrochloride (p.952·1).
Benign prostatic hyperplasia.

Hytrinex *Astra, Swed.*
Terazosin hydrochloride (p.952·1).
Benign prostatic hyperplasia; hypertension.

Hytuss *Hyrex, USA.*
Guaiphenesin (p.1061·3).
Coughs.

Hyzaar
Merck Sharp & Dohme-Chibret, Fr.; Merck Sharp & Dohme, Neth.; Merck, USA.
Losartan potassium (p.899·1); hydrochlorothiazide (p.885·2).
Hypertension.

Hyzine *Hyrex, USA†.*
Hydroxyzine hydrochloride (p.412·1).
Anxiety; hypersensitivity reactions.

Hyzum N *Merckle, Ger.*
Arnica (p.1550·3).
Inflammation; muscle and joint pain; soft-tissue injury.

Ial *Fidia, Ital.*
Sodium hyaluronate (p.1630·3).
Adjunct in ocular surgery.

Ialugen *IBSA, Switz.*
Sodium hyaluronate (p.1630·3).
Burns; wounds.

Ialugen Plus *IBSA, Switz.*
Sodium hyaluronate (p.1630·3); silver sulphadiazine (p.247·3).
Infected wounds and burns.

Ialurex *Fidia, Ital.*
Sodium hyaluronate (p.1630·3).
Dry eyes.

Iba-Cide *Ingram & Bell, Canad.*
Chloroxylenol (p.1111·1); terpineol (p.1635·1); isopropyl alcohol (p.1118·2).
Antiseptic.

Ibaril
Hoechst, Belg.†; Bipharma, Neth.; Hoechst Marion Roussel, Norw.; Hoechst Marion Roussel, Swed.
Desoxymethasone (p.1037·1).
Skin disorders.

Ibaril med salicylsyra *Hoechst Marion Roussel, Swed.*
Desoxymethasone (p.1037·1); salicylic acid (p.1090·2).
Skin disorders.

Ibaril med salicylsyre *Hoechst Marion Roussel, Norw.*
Desoxymethasone (p.1037·1); salicylic acid (p.1090·2).
Skin disorders.

Ibenon *Prodes, Spain.*
Ibuprofen (p.44·1).
Fever; inflammation; musculoskeletal, joint, and periarticular disorders; pain.

Ibercal *BOI, Spain.*
Calcium pidolate (p.1155·3).
Hypocalcaemia; osteoporosis.

Iberet
Abbott, Canad.; Abbott, S.Afr.; Abbott, Spain; Abbott, USA.
Ferrous sulphate (p.1340·2); vitamin B substances.
Vitamin C (p.1365·2) is included in this preparation to increase the absorption and availability of iron.
Iron-deficiency anaemias.

Iberet-Folic-500 *Abbott, USA.*
Ferrous sulphate (p.1340·2); folic acid (p.1340·3); vitamin B substances.
Vitamin C (p.1365·2) is included in this preparation to increase the absorption and availability of iron.
Iron-deficiency anaemias.

Iberogast
Steigerwald, Ger.; Steigerwald, Switz.
Iberis amara; angelica; silybum marianum (p.993·3); cuminum cyminum; chamomile (p.1561·2); chelidonium; liquorice (p.1197·1); melissa (p.1600·1); peppermint leaf (p.1208·1).
Gastro-intestinal disorders.

Ibexone *Sandipro, Belg.*
Co-dergocrine mesylate (p.1566·1).
Mental function impairment.

Ibiamox
Fisons, Austral.†; Ibi, Ital.; Xixia, S.Afr.†.
Amoxycillin sodium (p.151·3) or amoxycillin trihydrate (p.151·3).
Bacterial infections.

Ibicyn *Ibi, Ital.†.*
Tetracycline hydrochloride (p.259·1).
Bacterial infections.

Ibidroxil *Ibi, Ital.†.*
Cefadroxil (p.163·3).
Bacterial infections.

Ibifon *Ampharco, USA.*
Ibuprofen (p.44·1).

Ibikin *IBP, Ital.†.*
Trimethobenzamide hydrochloride (p.420·1).
Nausea and vomiting.

Ibilex
Alphapharm, Austral.; Ibi, Ital.†.
Cephalexin (p.178·2).
Bacterial infections.

Ibiman *Ibi, Ital.†.*
Cephamandole nafate (p.180·1).
Bacterial infections.

Ibimicyn *Ibi, Ital.*
Capsules†; syrup†: Ampicillin trihydrate (p.153·2).
Injection: Ampicillin sodium (p.153·1).
Bacterial infections.

Ibol *Cascan, Ger.†; Cascapharm, Ger.†.*
Ibuprofen (p.44·1).
Fever; inflammation; musculoskeletal and joint disorders; pain.

Ibopain *Docmed, S.Afr.*
Ibuprofen (p.44·1).
Musculoskeletal and joint disorders.

Ibosure *Pharmatec, Neth.†.*
Ibuprofen (p.44·1).
Musculoskeletal, joint, and peri-articular disorders.

Ibrufhalal *Halal, UK.*
Ibuprofen (p.44·1).
Inflammation; pain.

Ibsesal *Ern, Spain†.*
Boldine (p.1554·1); inosine (p.1591·1); metoclopramide (p.1202·1); sodium bicarbonate (p.1153·2); dibasic sodium phosphate (p.1159·3); sodium sulphate (p.1213·3); magnesium sulphate (p.1157·3).
Hepatobiliary disorders; nausea and vomiting.

Ibu
Kade, Ger.; Boots, USA; Knoll, USA; Truxton, USA.
Ibuprofen (p.44·1).
Fever; inflammation; musculoskeletal and joint disorders; pain.

ibu-Attritin *SmithKline Beecham, Ger.†.*
Ibuprofen (p.44·1).
Inflammation; pain; rheumatism.

Ibubest *CT, Ger.*
Ibuprofen (p.44·1).
Fever; pain.

Ibubeta *Betapharm, Ger.*
Ibuprofen (p.44·1).
Gout; inflammation; musculoskeletal and joint disorders.

Ibu-Cream *Rhone-Poulenc Rorer, Austral.†.*
Ibuprofen (p.44·1).
Painful or rheumatic disorders of the muscles and joints.

Ibudol *Donau, Aust.*
Ibuprofen (p.44·1).
Fever; inflammation; musculoskeletal and joint disorders; pain.

Ibudros
Manetti Roberts, Ital.; Ferrer, Switz.†.
Ibuproxam (p.45·2).
Gout; lymphangitis; musculoskeletal, joint, peri-articular, and soft-tissue disorders; phlebitis; superficial thrombophlebitis.

Ibufac *DDSA Pharmaceuticals, UK.*
Ibuprofen (p.44·1).

Ibufarm *Noristan, S.Afr.†.*
Ibuprofen (p.44·1).
Musculoskeletal and joint disorders.

Ibufen-L *Amino, Switz.*
Suppositories: Ibuprofen lysine (p.44·3); lignocaine hydrochloride (p.1293·2).
Tablets: Ibuprofen lysine (p.44·3).
Gout; musculoskeletal, joint, and peri-articular disorders.

Ibuflam *Lichtenstein, Ger.*
Ibuprofen (p.44·1) or ibuprofen sodium (p.44·3).
Fever; gout; inflammation; musculoskeletal and joint disorders; pain.

Ibufug *Wolff, Ger.*
Suppositories†: Ibuprofen sodium (p.44·3).
Tablets, sustained-release tablets: Ibuprofen (p.44·1).
Gout; inflammation; musculoskeletal and joint disorders; pain.

Ibugel Mayrhofer, Aust.; Dermal Laboratories, Irl.; Medinova, Switz.; Dermal Laboratories, UK.
Ibuprofen (p.44·1).
Musculoskeletal, joint, peri-articular, and soft-tissue disorders; neuralgia.

Ibuhexal Hexal, Ger.
Ibuprofen (p.44·1) or ibuprofen sodium (p.44·3).
Fever; inflammation; musculoskeletal and joint disorders; pain.

Ibular Lagap, UK.
Ibuprofen (p.44·1).
Inflammation; pain.

Ibuleve Searle, S.Afr.; Dendron, UK.
Ibuprofen (p.44·1).
Musculoskeletal and joint disorders.

Ibulgan Lagap, Switz.†.
Ibuprofen (p.44·1).
Gout; musculoskeletal, joint, and peri-articular disorders; pain.

Ibumed SmithKline Beecham, S.Afr.; Helvepharm, Switz.; Bradford Chemists Alliance, UK†.
Ibuprofen (p.44·1).
Fever; musculoskeletal and joint disorders; pain.

Ibumerck Merck, Ger.
Ibuprofen (p.44·1).
Fever; gout; inflammation; musculoskeletal and joint disorders; pain.

Ibumetin Nycomed, Neth.†; Nycomed, Norw.; Nycomed, Swed.
Ibuprofen (p.44·1).
Fever; inflammation; musculoskeletal and joint disorders; pain.

Ibumousse Dermal Laboratories, UK.
Ibuprofen (p.44·1).
Musculoskeletal and joint pain; neuralgia.

Ibuphlogont Azupharma, Ger.
Ibuprofen (p.44·1).
Gout; inflammation; musculoskeletal and joint disorders; pain.

Ibuprin Thompson, USA.
Ibuprofen (p.44·1).
Fever; osteoarthritis; pain; rheumatoid arthritis.

Ibuprof CT, Ger.
Ibuprofen (p.44·1) or ibuprofen lysine (p.44·3).
Fever; inflammation; musculoskeletal and joint disorders; pain.

Ibuprohm Ohm, USA.
Ibuprofen (p.44·1).
Fever; osteoarthritis; pain; rheumatoid arthritis.

Ibupron Merckle, Aust.
Ibuprofen (p.44·1).
Fever; inflammation; musculoskeletal and joint disorders; pain.

Iburem Donau, Aust.
Ibuprofen (p.44·1).
Pain.

Ibu-Slow Bio-Therabel, Belg.
Ibuprofen (p.44·1).
Musculoskeletal, joint, and peri-articular disorders.

Ibuspray Dermal Laboratories, UK.
Ibuprofen (p.44·1).
Musculoskeletal, joint, and soft-tissue disorders; neuralgia.

Ibustrin Pharmacia Upjohn, Aust.; Pharmacia Upjohn, Ital.
Indobufen (p.891·1) or indobufen sodium (p.891·1).
Thrombo-embolic disorders; thrombosis prophylaxis.

Ibu-Tab Alra, USA†.
Ibuprofen (p.44·1).
Fever; osteoarthritis; pain; rheumatoid arthritis.

Ibutad TAD, Ger.
Ibuprofen (p.44·1) or ibuprofen sodium (p.44·3).
Inflammation; musculoskeletal and joint disorders; pain.

Ibutop Schoeller, Aust.; Chefaro, Belg.; Chefaro Ardeval, Fr.; Chefaro, Ger.
Ibuprofen (p.44·1).
Musculoskeletal, joint, peri-articular, and soft-tissue disorders.

Ibutop Cuprofen Seton, UK.
Ibuprofen (p.44·1).
Musculoskeletal, joint, and soft-tissue disorders.

Ibutop Ralgex Seton, UK.
Ibuprofen (p.44·1).
Inflammation; musculoskeletal pain.

Ibu-Vivimed Mann, Ger.
Ibuprofen (p.44·1).
Fever; pain.

Ibux Weifa, Norw.
Ibuprofen (p.44·1).
Fever; musculoskeletal and joint disorders; pain.

Icacine Bristol-Myers Squibb, Fr.†.
Dibekacin sulphate (p.201·3).
Bacterial infections.

Icaps Ciba Vision, Canad.; Ciba Vision, USA.
Multivitamin and mineral preparation.

Icavex Asta Medica, Fr.
Thymoxamine hydrochloride (p.952·2).
Impotence.

Icaz Sandoz, Fr.
Isradipine (p.894·2).
Hypertension.

Ice Gel Mentholatum, Austral.; Hyde, Canad.
Menthol (p.1600·2).
Muscular aches and pains.

Ice Gel Therapy Sunfresh, Canad.
Menthol (p.1600·2).

Ice Lipbalm Mentholatum, Canad.
SPF 12: Padimate O (p.1488·1).
Sunscreen.

Ice Therapy Stella, Canad.
Menthol (p.1600·2).
Muscle pain.

Iceland Moss Compound Gerard House, UK†.
Iceland moss; liquorice (p.1197·1); lobelia (p.1481·3).
Upper respiratory-tract congestion.

Icespray Rhone-Poulenc Rorer, Spain.
Menthol (p.1600·2).
Insect bites; pruritus; sprains.

Ic-Gel Germiphene, Canad.
Chlorhexidine gluconate (p.1107·2); isopropyl alcohol (p.1118·2).

ICG-Pulsion Pulsion, Ger.
Indocyanine green (p.1590·3).
Diagnostic agent.

Ichthalgan Ichthyol, Ger.
Heparin sodium (p.879·3); ictasol (p.1083·3).
Muscle, joint, and peri-articular disorders; neuritis; thrombophlebitis.

Ichthalgan forte Ichthyol, Aust.
Heparin sodium (p.879·3); ictasol (p.1083·3).
Musculoskeletal, joint, and peri-articular disorders.

Ichtho-Bad
Note. This name is used for preparations of different composition.
Ichthyol, Aust.; Ichthyol, Switz.
Ichthammol (p.1083·3).
Rheumatic, neurological, gynaecological, urologic, and dermatologic disorders.

Ichthyol, Ger.
Light ammonium bituminosulphonate (p.1083·3).
Bath additive; musculoskeletal and joint disorders; neuralgia; pelvic inflammatory disorders; skin disorders.

Ichtho-Bellol Ichthyol, Aust.; Ichthyol, Ger.
Ictasol (p.1083·3); atropine sulphate (p.455·1).
Pelvic disorders.

Ichtho-Bellol compositum S Ichthyol, Ger.
Ictasol (p.1083·3); atropine sulphate (p.455·1); propyphenazone (p.81·3).
Pelvic disorders.

Ichtho-Cadmin Ichthyol, Aust.; Ichthyol, Ger.†; Ichthyol, Switz.†.
Ictasol (p.1083·3); cadmium sulphide (p.1555·3).
Scalp disorders.

Ichtho-Cortin Ichthyol, Aust.; Ichthyol, Ger.
Hydrocortisone (p.1043·3) or hydrocortisone acetate (p.1043·3); ictasol (p.1083·3).
Skin disorders.

Ichthoderm Ichthyol, Ger.
Ictasol (p.1083·3).
Skin disorders.

Ichth-Oestren Ichthyol, Aust.
Oestradiol benzoate (p.1455·1); light ammonium bituminosulphonate (p.1083·3); urea (p.1095·2); lactose (p.1349·3).
Vaginal disorders.

Ichtho-Himbin Ichthyol, Ger.†.
Ictasol (p.1083·3); yohimbine hydrochloride (p.1645·3); benzyl nicotinate (p.22·1); atropine sulphate (p.455·1).
Impotence.

Ichtholan Ichthyol, Aust.; Ichthyol, Ger.; Ichthyol, Switz.
Ichthammol (p.1083·3).
Inflammatory skin disorders; musculoskeletal and joint disorders; thrombophlebitis.

Ichtholan Spezial Ichthyol, Ger.
Ichthammol (p.1083·3).
Musculoskeletal and joint disorders.

Ichtholan T Ichthyol, Ger.; Ichthyol, Switz.†.
Ictasol (p.1083·3).
Skin disorders.

Ichthopaste Smith & Nephew, Ital.; Smith & Nephew, UK.
Ichthammol (p.1083·3); zinc oxide (p.1096·2).
Medicated bandage.

Ichthoseptal Ichthyol, Ger.
Chloramphenicol (p.182·1); ictasol (p.1083·3).
Infected skin disorders.

Ichthosin Ichthyol, Ger.
Ictasol (p.1083·3).
Skin disorders.

Ichthospasmin N Ichthyol, Ger.†.
Hyoscine methobromide (p.463·1); moxaverine hydrochloride (p.1604·3); propyphenazone (p.81·3); ictasol (p.1083·3).
Pelvic disorders.

Ichthraletten Ichthyol, Aust.; Ichthyol, Ger.; Ichthyol, Switz.
Sodium bituminosulphonate (p.1083·3).
Mastitis; skin disorders.

Ichthraletten Doxy Ichthyol, Ger.†.
Doxycycline hydrochloride (p.202·3).
Bacterial infections.

Ichthyol Ichthyol, Ger.
Ichthammol (p.1083·3).
Skin disorders.

Ichtopur Ichthyol, Aust.
Ichthammol (p.1083·3).
Urogenital disorders.

Icht-Oral Ichthyol, Ger.
Minocycline hydrochloride (p.226·2).
Bacterial infections.

Ichtyosoft LED, Fr.
Cream: Ictasol (p.1083·3); ammonium lactate (p.1079·1); gamolenic acid (p.1582·1).
Skin disorders.
Shampoo: Ictasol (p.1083·3); ammonium lactate (p.1079·1); salicylic acid (p.1090·2).
Scalp disorders.

Iclados Panthox & Burck, Ital.†.
Doxycycline hydrochloride (p.202·3).
Bacterial infections.

Icol Cusi, Spain.
Chloramphenicol (p.182·1) or chloramphenicol succinate (p.184·2); dexamethasone sodium phosphate (p.1037·2).
Infected eye disorders.

ICR salvia Boehringer Mannheim, Ger.†.
Electrolyte infusion (p.1147·1).
Electrolyte disorders.

Ictan Cusi, Spain.
Clotrimazole (p.376·3).
Fungal skin infections.

Icthaband Boots, Austral.; Seton, UK.
Ichthammol (p.1083·3); zinc oxide (p.1096·2).
Medicated bandage.

Ictholin Hilarys, Canad.
Ichthammol (p.1083·3); phenol (p.1121·2).

Ictiomen Casen Fleet, Spain.
Ichthammol (p.1083·3); talc (p.1092·1); menthol (p.1600·2).
Skin disorders.

Ictom 3 ICT, Ital.
Omega-3 triglycerides (p.1276·1); vitamin E (p.1369·1).
Dry skin; psoriasis.

Ictotest Bayer Diagnostics, Austral.; Miles, Canad.†; Ames, Irl.; Bayer Diagnostici, Ital.; Ames, S.Afr.; Bayer Diagnostics, UK; Bayer, USA.
Test for bilirubin in urine.

Icy Hot Chattem, USA.
Methyl salicylate (p.55·2); menthol (p.1600·2).
Muscle, joint, and soft-tissue pain; neuralgia.

Idalon Hoechst Marion Roussel, Neth.
Floctafenine (p.41·2).
Pain.

Idalprem Zyma, Spain.
Lorazepam (p.675·3).
Alcohol withdrawal syndrome; anxiety; epilepsy; insomnia; nausea and vomiting.

Idamycin Pharmacia Upjohn, Canad.; Pharmacia Upjohn, USA.
Idarubicin hydrochloride (p.540·1).
Malignant neoplasms.

Idaptan Danval, Spain.
Trimetazidine hydrochloride (p.959·2).
Angina pectoris; neurosensorial ischaemia.

Idarac Hoechst Marion Roussel, Belg.; Sanofi Winthrop, Canad.; Diamant, Fr.; Hoechst Marion Roussel, Irl.; Hoechst Marion Roussel, Ital.; Roussel, Spain.
Floctafenine (p.41·2).
Pain.

Idasal Wellcome, Spain†.
Methoxamine hydrochloride (p.903·3).
Nasal congestion.

Idasal Antibiotico Wellcome, Spain†.
Methoxamine hydrochloride (p.903·3); neomycin sulphate (p.229·2); polymyxin B sulphate (p.239·1).
Nasal congestion and infection.

Idasal Nebulizador Warner-Lambert, Spain.
Oxymetazoline hydrochloride (p.1065·3).
Nasal congestion; sinus congestion.

Ideolaxyl SmithKline Beecham, Fr.
Aloes (p.1177·1); frangula bark (p.1193·2); hyoscyamus (p.464·3); senna (p.1212·2).
Constipation.

Ideolider IPFI, Ital.
Acetylaspartic acid; citrulline (p.1337·2).
Memory impairment.

Ideos Innothera, Fr.; Helsinn Birex, Irl.; Vita, Spain; Ferring, Swed.
Calcium carbonate (p.1182·1); cholecalciferol (p.1366·3).
Calcium and vitamin D deficiency; hypocalcaemia; hypoparathyroidism; osteoporosis.

IDM Solution Rougier, Canad.
Guaiphenesin (p.1061·3); potassium iodide (p.1493·1); ephedrine hydrochloride (p.1059·3); mepyramine maleate (p.414·1).
Cold symptoms.

Ido A 50 Byk Elmu, Spain†.
Vitamin A (p.1358·1).
Vitamin A deficiency.

Ido-C Abigo, Swed.
Ascorbic acid (p.1365·2).
Some tablets also contain sodium ascorbate.
Vitamin C deficiency.

I-Doc Mentholatum, UK.
Hamamelis (p.1587·1).
Sore eyes.

Idocyklin Roerig, Swed.†.
Doxycycline (p.202·3) or doxycycline hydrochloride (p.202·3).
Bacterial infections.

Ido-E Pharmacia Upjohn, Norw.; Pharmacia Upjohn, Swed.
Alpha tocopheryl acetate (p.1369·2).
Vitamin E deficiency.

Idom Kanoldt, Ger.
Dothiepin hydrochloride (p.283·1).
Depression.

Idomed Rowex, Irl.
Indomethacin (p.45·2).
Gout; musculoskeletal, joint, and peri-articular disorders; pain.

Idonor Roger, Spain†.
Plafibride (p.1277·1).
Hyperlipidaemias; thrombotic disorders.

Idopamil Therabel Pharma, Belg.
Ibopamine hydrochloride (p.889·3).
Heart failure.

Idorubina Ital Suisse, Ital.†.
Vitamin B substances.
Nerve pain and inflammation.

Idotrim Abigo, Swed.
Trimethoprim (p.265·1).
Urinary-tract infections.

Idoxene Spodefell, UK†.
Idoxuridine (p.613·2).
Herpes simplex infections of the eye.

Idracemi Farmigea, Ital.
Eye drops: Hydrocortisone sodium phosphate (p.1044·1).
Eye ointment: Hydrocortisone hemisuccinate (p.1044·1); neomycin sulphate (p.229·2); chloramphenicol (p.182·1).
Eye disorders.

Idracemi Eparina Farmigea, Ital.
Hydrocortisone sodium phosphate (p.1044·1); heparin sodium (p.879·3).
Eye disorders.

Idratante Samil Sandoz, Ital.
Emollient.

Idril Winzer, Ger.
Actinoquinol sodium (p.1543·1); naphazoline nitrate (p.1064·2).
Eye disorders.

Idril N Hexal, Ger.†.
Xylometazoline hydrochloride (p.1071·2).
Rhinitis.

Idro P2 Sanofi Winthrop, Ital.
Sulmarin sodium; ascorbic acid (p.1365·2).
Capillary disorders; haemorrhage.

Idrobamina Eurofarmaco, Ital.†.
Hydroxocobalamin (p.1363·3).
Megaloblastic anaemia; vitamin B_{12} deficiency.

Idro-C Blue Cross, Ital.
Ascorbic acid (p.1365·2).

Idrocet Lusofarmaco, Ital.
Hydrocortisone acetate (p.1043·3); neomycin sulphate (p.229·2).
Inflammatory eye and ear disorders.

Idrocol Lafon, Fr.
Poloxamer 188 (p.1326·3).
Constipation.

Idrocortigamma IBP, Ital.†.
Hydrocortisone acetate (p.1043·3).
Skin disorders.

Idrodiuvis Vis, Ital.†.
Hydrochlorothiazide (p.885·2).
Diuretic.

Idrolattone Zoja, Ital.
Spironolactone (p.946·1).
Hyperaldosteronism; hypertension; oedema.

Idrolone Sanofi Winthrop, Ital.
Fenquizone potassium (p.868·2).
Hypertension; oedema.

Idroneomicil Poli, Ital.
Neomycin sulphate (p.229·2); hydrocortisone acetate (p.1043·3); naphazoline nitrate (p.1064·2).
Infection and inflammation of the eye, nose, and ear.

Idropan B Lisapharma, Ital.
Vitamin B substances; calcium folinate (p.1342·2).
Deficiency states; megaloblastic anaemia.

Idroplurivit Menarini, Ital.
Multivitamin preparation.

Idropulmina ISI, Ital.
Guaiphenesin (p.1061·3).
Coughs; respiratory-tract disorders.

Idroquark Polifarma, Ital.
Ramipril (p.941·1); hydrochlorothiazide (p.885·2).
Hypertension.

Idroskin Mavi, Ital.
Collagen (p.1566·3).
Dry skin.

Idrossamina Salus, Ital.†.
Hydroxocobalamin (p.1363·3).
Deficiency states; megaloblastic anaemia; neuritis.

Idrotal Bayropharm, Ital.†.
Hydrotalcite (p.1194·1).
Gastric hyperacidity.

Idrovel *Savoma, Ital.*
Emollient.

Idrovit *Benvegna, Ital.†.*
Vitamin B substances with ascorbic acid.

Idrum *FIRMA, Ital.*
Electrolytes (p.1147·1); carmellose sodium (p.1471·2).
Dry mouth.

Idrurto A *Ripari-Gero, Ital.†.*
Vitamin A (p.1358·1).
Vitamin A deficiency.

Iducher *Farmigea, Ital.*
Idoxuridine (p.613·2).
Viral infections of the eye.

Iducol *SIFI, Ital.*
Idoxuridine (p.613·2); colistin sulphomethate sodium (p.196·1); rolitetracycline (p.247·1) or tetracycline (p.259·1); xanthopterin.
Herpesvirus infections of the eye.

Iducutit *Pharmagalen, Ger.*
Idoxuridine (p.613·2) in dimethyl sulphoxide.
Herpes simplex and zoster infections.

Idulanex *Schering-Plough, Spain.*
Azatadine maleate (p.402·3); pseudoephedrine sulphate (p.1068·3).
Allergic rhinitis.

Idulian *Schering-Plough, Ital.†.*
Azatadine maleate (p.402·3).
Hypersensitivity reactions.

Idu-Phor *Superfos Biosector, Norw.*
Iodine (p.1493·1).
Formerly known as Jodosan.
Disinfection of skin, wounds, surfaces, and instruments.

Iduridin
Geymonat, Ital.; Ferring, Norw.; Ferring, UK†.
Idoxuridine (p.613·2) in dimethyl sulphoxide.
Herpesvirus infections.

Idustatin
Delalande, Ital.
Ointment (1.5%): Idoxuridine (p.613·2); neomycin sulphate (p.229·2); cod-liver oil (p.1337·3).
Herpes simplex infections of the skin and mucous membranes.

Synthelabo, Ital.
Ointment (3%); topical solution: Idoxuridine (p.613·2).
Herpesvirus infections.

Iduviran *Chauvin, Fr.*
Idoxuridine (p.613·2).
Viral eye infections.

Iecatec *Tedec Meiji, Spain.*
Enalapril maleate (p.863·2).
Heart failure; hypertension.

Ietepar *Rottapharm, Ital.*
Betaine glucuronate (p.1553·2); diethanolamine glucuronate; nicotinamide ascorbate.
Liver disorders; poisoning.

Ifenec *Italfarmaco, Ital.*
Econazole (p.377·2) or econazole nitrate (p.377·2).
Fungal infections; Gram-positive bacterial infections.

Ifex
Bristol, Canad.; Mead Johnson Oncology, USA.
Ifosfamide (p.540·2).
Malignant neoplasms.

IFO-cell *Cell Pharm, Ger.*
Ifosfamide (p.540·2).
Malignant neoplasms.

Ig Vena N *Sclavo, Ital.*
A normal immunoglobulin (p.1522·1).
Hypogammaglobulinaemia; idiopathic thrombocytopenic purpura; passive immunisation.

Igabulin *Immuno, Aust.*
Immunoglobulin A (p.1522·3).
Prevention of necrotising enterocolitis in babies.

Igitur-antirheumatische *Apomedica, Aust.*
Diethylamine salicylate (p.33·1); salicylic acid (p.1090·2); benzyl nicotinate (p.22·1); camphor (p.1557·2).
Musculoskeletal, joint, and peri-articular disorders.

Igitur-Rheumafluid *Apomedica, Aust.†.*
Diethylamine salicylate (p.33·1); salicylic acid (p.1090·2); glycol salicylate (p.43·1); benzyl nicotinate (p.22·1); camphor (p.1557·2).
Musculoskeletal and joint disorders; peripheral vascular disorders.

Igril *Wellcome, Spain.*
Caffeine hydrate (p.750·1); cyclizine hydrochloride (p.407·1); ergotamine tartrate (p.445·3).
Headache; migraine.

Igroseles *Schwarz, Ital.*
Atenolol (p.825·3); chlorthalidone (p.839·3).
Hypertension.

Igroton *Ciba, Ital.*
Chlorthalidone (p.839·3).
Diuretic; hypertension.

Igroton-Lopresor *Ciba, Ital.*
Chlorthalidone (p.839·3); metoprolol tartrate (p.907·3).
Hypertension.

Igroton-Reserpina *Ciba, Ital.*
Chlorthalidone (p.839·3); reserpine (p.942·1).
Hypertension.

Ikaran
Exel, Belg.; Pierre Fabre, Fr.; Formenti, Ital.; Robapharm, Switz.
Dihydroergotamine mesylate (p.444·2).
Hypotension; migraine and vascular headache; venous insufficiency; vertigo.

Ikecrin *Iketon, Ital.†.*
Carbaryl (p.1403·1).
Pediculosis.

Ikelax *Iketon, Ital.†.*
Cascara (p.1183·1); frangula (p.1193·2); senna (p.1212·2); docusate sodium (p.1189·3).
Constipation.

Ikestatina *Iketon, Ital.*
Somatostatin acetate (p.1261·1).
Diabetic ketoacidosis; gastro-intestinal haemorrhage; gastro-intestinal radiography; prevention of complications following pancreatic surgery.

Iketoncid *Iketon, Ital.*
Glutaraldehyde (p.1114·3); cetrimide (p.1105·2).
Instrument disinfection.

Ikorel
Bellon, Fr.; Rhone-Poulenc Rorer, Neth.; Rhone-Poulenc Rorer, UK.
Nicorandil (p.915·3).
Angina pectoris.

Iktorivil *Roche, Swed.*
Clonazepam (p.343·3).
Epilepsy.

Ilacen *Rorer, Spain†.*
Diflunisal (p.33·2).
Inflammation; pain.

Ilagane *Daker Farmasimes, Spain.*
Naproxen (p.61·2).
Musculoskeletal, joint, and peri-articular disorders.

Ildamen
Asta Medica, Aust.; Asta Medica, Ger.; Asta Medica, Ital.†; Asta Medica, Spain†; Asta Medica, Switz.†.
Oxyfedrine hydrochloride (p.927·1).
Angina pectoris; bradycardia; myocardial infarction.

Ildor *Esteve, Spain.*
Nedocromil sodium (p.756·2).
Obstructive airways disease.

Iletin II Pork Lente *Lilly, Canad.*
Insulin zinc suspension (porcine) (p.322·1).
Diabetes mellitus.

Iletin II Pork NPH *Lilly, Canad.*
Isophane insulin injection (porcine) (p.322·1).
Diabetes mellitus.

Iletin II Pork Regular *Lilly, Canad.*
Neutral insulin injection (porcine) (p.322·1).
Diabetes mellitus.

Iletin Lente *Lilly, Canad.*
Insulin zinc suspension (bovine and porcine) (p.322·1).
Diabetes mellitus.

Iletin NPH *Lilly, Canad.*
Isophane insulin injection (bovine and porcine) (p.322·1).
Diabetes mellitus.

Iletin Regular *Lilly, Canad.*
Neutral insulin injection (bovine and porcine) (p.322·1).
Diabetes mellitus.

Iletin Semilente *Lilly, Canad.†.*
Insulin zinc suspension (bovine and porcine) (p.322·1).
Diabetes mellitus.

Iletin Ultralente *Lilly, Canad.†.*
Insulin zinc suspension (crystalline) (bovine and porcine) (p.322·1).
Diabetes mellitus.

Iliadin
E. Merck, Norw.; Merck, S.Afr.; Meda, Swed.
Oxymetazoline hydrochloride (p.1065·3).
Conjunctivitis; eye irritation; nasal congestion; otitis media; sinus congestion.

Iliadine *Merck-Clevenot, Fr.†.*
Oxymetazoline hydrochloride (p.1065·3).
Nasal congestion.

Ilio-Funkton *Robugen, Ger.*
Dimethicone (p.1213·1).
Reduction of gastro-intestinal gas.

Ilioton *Robugen, Ger.†.*
Camphor monobromide; ethaverine hydrochloride (p.1577·1); rhubarb (p.1212·1); aloes (p.1177·1); sapo med. (p.1468·2); fennel (p.1579·1); caraway (p.1559·3); fennel oil (p.1579·2); caraway oil (p.1559·3).
Gastro-intestinal disorders.

Ilja Rogoff *Woelm, Ger.†.*
Garlic (p.1583·1).
Tonic.

Ilja Rogoff mit Rutin *Woelm, Ger.†.*
Garlic; mistletoe; crataegus; sophora japonica; lupulus.
Tonic.

Illings Bozner Maycur-Tee *Esplanade, Aust.*
Senna (p.1212·2); magnesium sulphate (p.1157·3); chamomile (p.1561·2); fennel (p.1579·1).

Iloban *Merck, Ger.†.*
Vitamin B preparation with liver extract.
Macrocytic anaemias; secondary anaemias and anaemias of unclear aetiology.

Ilomedin
Schering, Aust.; Schering, Ger.; Schering, Ital.; Schering, Norw.; Schering, Swed.; Schering, Switz.
Iloprost trometamol (p.1419·1).
Peripheral vascular disorders; thromboangitis obliterans; thrombo-embolic disorders.

Ilomedine
Schering, Fr.; Schering, Neth.
Iloprost trometamol (p.1419·1).
Peripheral ischaemia; thromboangitis obliterans.

Ilon Abszess
Herchemie, Aust.; Redel, Ger.
Turpentine; turpentine oil (p.1641·1).
Infected skin disorders.

Ilopan *Adria, USA.*
Dexpanthenol (p.1570·3).
Intestinal atony; paralytic ileus.

Ilopan-Choline *Savage, USA.*
Dexpanthenol (p.1570·3); choline bitartrate (p.1337·1).
Flatulence.

Ilosone
Lilly, Aust.; Lilly, Austral.; Lilly, Belg.†; Lilly, Canad.; Dista, Irl.; Lilly, Ital.; Lilly, S.Afr.; Dista, Switz.†; Lilly, UK; Dista, USA.
Erythromycin estolate (p.204·1).
Bacterial infections.

Iloticina *Derly, Spain†.*
Erythromycin (p.204·1).
Skin infections.

Iloticina Anti Acne *Dista, Spain†.*
Erythromycin (p.204·1).
Acne.

Ilotycin
Lilly, Canad.; Lilly, S.Afr.; Lilly, Switz.; Dista, USA.
Erythromycin (p.204·1) or erythromycin gluceptate (p.204·2).
Bacterial infections.

Ilozyme *Adria, USA.*
Pancrelipase (p.1613·3).
Pancreatic enzyme deficiency.

Ilube
Alcon, Irl.; Alcon, UK.
Acetylcysteine (p.1052·3); hypromellose (p.1473·1).
Dry eye syndromes.

Ilvicaps *Merck, S.Afr.†.*
Carbocisteine (p.1056·3).
Respiratory-tract disorders.

Ilvico
Note. This name is used for preparations of different composition.
Merck, Ger.†.
Effervescent tablets: Aspirin (p.16·1); ascorbic acid (p.1365·2).
Cold symptoms; fever; pain.
Oral liquid: Brompheniramine maleate (p.403·2); DL-methylephedrine hydrochloride (p.1064·1); sodium ascorbate (p.1365·2); phenazone (p.78·2); sodium salicylate (p.85·1).
Cold symptoms.

E. Merck, Irl.
Brompheniramine maleate (p.403·2); calcium ascorbate (p.1365·2); paracetamol (p.72·2); caffeine hydrate (p.750·1).
Cold and influenza symptoms.

Merck, S.Afr.
Syrup: Brompheniramine maleate (p.403·2); sodium ascorbate (p.1365·2); methylephedrine hydrochloride (p.1064·1); phenazone (p.78·2); sodium salicylate (p.85·1); codeine phosphate (p.26·1).
Tablets: Brompheniramine maleate (p.403·2); calcium ascorbate (p.1365·2); propyphenazone (p.81·3); salicylamide (p.82·3); quinine hydrochloride (p.439·2); caffeine (p.749·3).
Allergic rhinitis; cold symptoms.

Merck, Spain.
Brompheniramine maleate (p.403·2); caffeine (p.749·3); paracetamol (p.72·2).
Cold and flu symptoms.

Ilvico mit Vitamin C *Merck, Aust.*
Paracetamol (p.72·2); ascorbic acid (p.1365·2).
Fever; pain.

Ilvico N *Merck, Ger.*
Brompheniramine maleate (p.403·2); calcium ascorbate (p.1365·2); caffeine (p.749·3); paracetamol (p.72·2).
Cold symptoms.

Ilvispect *Merck, S.Afr.†.*
Carbocisteine (p.1056·3).
Respiratory-tract disorders.

I-L-X *Kenwood, USA.*
A range of preparations containing iron (p.1346·1), liver extracts, and vitamin B substances.
Vitamin C (p.1365·2) is included in some preparations to increase the absorption and availability of iron.
Iron-deficiency anaemias.

I-L-X B_{12} *Kenwood, USA.*
Iron preparation with multivitamins.

Imacillin
Astra, Norw.; Astra, Swed.
Amoxycillin (p.151·3) or amoxycillin trihydrate (p.151·3).
Bacterial infections.

Imacort *Spirig, Switz.*
Clotrimazole (p.376·3); hexamidine isethionate (p.1115·3); prednisolone acetate (p.1048·1).
Infected skin disorders.

Imagent GI *Alliance, USA†.*
Perflubron (p.1617·1).
Adjunct to magnetic resonance imaging of the gastro-intestinal tract.

Imagopaque
Nycomed, Aust.; Nycomed, Ger.; Nycomed, Ital.; Nycomed Imaging, Norw.; Nycomed, Spain; Nycomed, Switz.
Iopentol (p.1007·2).
Radiographic contrast medium.

Imap
Janssen-Cilag, Belg.; Janssen-Ortho, Canad.; Janssen-Cilag, Ger.; Janssen-Cilag, Neth.; Janssen-Cilag, Norw.; Janssen-Cilag, Switz.
Fluspirilene (p.672·3).
Anxiety; schizophrenia.

Imaplus *MVM, Fr.*
Vegetable oils.
Gastro-intestinal disorders; hypercholesterolaemia.

Imazol
Note. This name is used for preparations of different composition.
Karrer, Ger.; Spirig, Switz.
Cream: Clotrimazole (p.376·3); hexamidine isethionate (p.1115·3).
Fungal skin infections.

Karrer, Ger.; Spirig, Switz.
Paste: Clotrimazole (p.376·3).
Fungal skin infections.

Imazol comp *Karrer, Ger.*
Clotrimazole (p.376·3); hexamidine isethionate (p.1115·3); prednisolone acetate (p.1048·1).
Fungal skin infections.

Imbak *Mucos, Ger.*
Acidophilus-milk powder (p.1594·1); yeast (p.1373·1); juniper (p.1592·2); ginger (p.1193·2).
Gastro-intestinal disorders.

Imbretil *Hormonchemie, Ger.†.*
Carbolonium bromide (p.1312·2).
Skeletal muscle relaxant.

Imbrilon
Berk, Irl.; Berk, UK.
Indomethacin (p.45·2).
Gout; inflammation; pain; musculoskeletal, joint, and peri-articular disorders.

Imbun
Merckle, Aust.; Merckle, Ger.
Ibuprofen (p.44·1) or ibuprofen lysine (p.44·3).
Fever; inflammation; musculoskeletal, joint, and peri-articular disorders; pain.

Imdin S *Wernigerode, Ger.*
Xylometazoline hydrochloride (p.1071·2).
Rhinitis.

Imdur
Recipe, Aust.; Astra, Austral.; Astra, Canad.; Astra, Irl.; Astra, Norw.; Astra, S.Afr.; Schering-Plough, Spain†; Hassle, Swed.; Astra, Switz.; Astra, UK; Key, USA.
Isosorbide mononitrate (p.893·3).
Angina pectoris.

Imegul *Arkopharma, Fr.*
Cascara (p.1183·1); ispaghula husk (p.1194·2).
Constipation.

Imeron *Byk Gulden, Ger.*
Iomeprol (p.1006·3).
Radiographic contrast medium.

Imeson
Desitin, Ger.; Cimex, Switz.†.
Nitrazepam (p.682·2).
Epilepsy; sleep disorders.

Imet *FIRMA, Ital.*
Indomethacin (p.45·2).
Musculoskeletal and joint disorders.

Imex *Merz, Ger.*
Tetracycline hydrochloride (p.259·1).
Acne.

Imexim *Cimex, Switz.*
Co-trimoxazole (p.196·3).
Bacterial infections.

Imferdex *Fisons, Switz.†.*
Iron dextran (p.1348·1).
Iron-deficiency anaemia.

Imferon
Fisons, Austral.†; Fisons, Belg.†; Fisons, Neth.†; Roche, S.Afr.†; Llorente, Spain; Fisons, UK†.
Iron dextran (p.1348·1).
Iron-deficiency anaemia.

Imferon B12 *Llorente, Spain†.*
Iron dextran (p.1348·1); hydroxocobalamin (p.1363·3).
Hypochromic anaemias.

Imidazyl *Recordati, Ital.*
Naphazoline nitrate (p.1064·2).
Conjunctivitis.

Imidazyl Antistaminico *Recordati, Ital.*
Naphazoline nitrate (p.1064·2); thonzylamine hydrochloride (p.419·2).
Conjunctivitis.

Imidin N *Wernigerode, Ger.*
Xylometazoline hydrochloride (p.1071·2).
Nasal congestion; rhinitis.

Imigran
Glaxo Wellcome, Aust.; Glaxo Wellcome, Austral.; Glaxo Wellcome, Ger.; Glaxo Wellcome, Irl.; Glaxo Wellcome, Ital.; Glaxo Wellcome, Neth.; Glaxo Wellcome, Norw.; Glaxo Wellcome, S.Afr.; Glaxo Wellcome, Spain; Glaxo Wellcome, Swed.; Glaxo Wellcome, Switz.; Glaxo Wellcome, UK.
Sumatriptan or sumatriptan succinate (p.450·1).
Cluster headache; migraine.

Imigrane *Glaxo Wellcome, Fr.*
Sumatriptan succinate (p.450·1).
Migraine; vascular facial pain.

Imiject *Glaxo Wellcome, Fr.*
Sumatriptan succinate (p.450·1).
Vascular facial pain.

Iminase *SmithKline Beecham, Spain.*
Anistreplase (p.824·2).
Myocardial infarction.

Imipem *Neopharmed, Ital.*
Imipenem (p.216·3); cilastatin sodium (p.185·2).

Lignocaine (p.1293·2) is included in the intramuscular injection to alleviate the pain of injection.
Bacterial infections.

Imiprex Lasa, Spain†.
Imipramine oxide hydrochloride (p.289·3).
Depression; nocturnal enuresis.

Imiprin CP Protea, Austral.†.
Imipramine hydrochloride (p.289·2).

Imitrex
Glaxo Wellcome, Belg.; Glaxo Wellcome, Canad.; Glaxo Wellcome, USA.
Sumatriptan (p.451·2) or sumatriptan succinate (p.450·1).
Cluster headache; migraine.

Imizol Farmigea, Ital.
Naphazoline nitrate (p.1064·2).
Eye irritation.

Immignost
Richter, Aust.; GN, Ger.
Tetanus toxoid; diphtheria toxoid; Streptococcal group C antigen; tuberculin (p.1640·2); Candida albicans antigen; Trichophyton mentagrophytes antigen; proteus mirabilis antigen.
Assessment of cell-mediated immunity.

Immubron Bruschettini, Ital.
Lysates of: *Staphylococcus aureus*; *Streptococcus pyogenes*; *Streptococcus viridans*; *Klebsiella pneumoniae*; *Klebsiella ozaenae*; *Haemophilus influenzae*; *Branhamella catarrhalis*; strains of *Diplococcus pneumoniae*.
Respiratory-tract infections.

ImmuCyst
Serotherapeutisches, Aust.; Rhone-Poulenc Rorer, Austral.; Connaught, Canad.; CytoChemia, Ger.; Wassermann, Ital.; Inibsa, Spain; Sanofi Winthrop, Switz.
A BCG vaccine (p.1504·3).
Bladder cancer.

Immucytal Pierre Fabre, Ital.
Ribosomal fractions of *Klebsiella pneumoniae*; *Diplococcus pneumoniae*; *Streptococcus pyogenes*; *Haemophilus influenzae*; membrane fraction of *Klebsiella pneumoniae*.
Bronchial infections; otorhinolaryngeal infections.

Immudynal Ardeypharm, Ger.
Homoeopathic preparation.

Immugrip Pierre Fabre, Fr.
An inactivated influenza vaccine (p.1515·2).
Active immunisation.

Immukin
Boehringer Ingelheim, Irl.; Boehringer Ingelheim, UK.
Interferon gamma-1b (rbe) (p.616·1).
Infections in chronic granulomatous disease.

Immukine Boehringer Ingelheim, Neth.
Interferon gamma-1b (p.616·1).
Infections in chronic granulomatous disease.

IMMUNace Vitabiotics, UK.
Multivitamin, mineral, and amino-acid preparation.

Immun-Aid McGaw, USA.
Preparation for enteral nutrition.
Immunosuppression.

Immunaps T APS, Ger.†.
Homoeopathic preparation.

Immunate
Immuno, Ger.; Immuno, Ital.; Immuno, Swed.; Immuno, Switz.
A factor VIII preparation (p.720·3).
Haemorrhagic disorders.

Immunex CRP Wampole, USA.
Test for C-reactive protein in serum.

Immunine
Osterreichisches Institut, Aust.; Immuno, Canad.†; Immuno, Ger.; Immuno, Ital.; Baxter, Swed.; Immuno, Switz.
A factor IX preparation (p.721·3).
Haemorrhagic disorders.

Immunja OTW, Ger.
Homoeopathic preparation.

ImmunoHBs ISI, Ital.
A hepatitis B immunoglobulin (p.1512·3).
Passive immunisation.

Immunol Sarm, Ital.†.
Levamisole hydrochloride (p.102·3).
Adjuvant in treatment of malignant neoplasms; immune system disorders.

Immunomega Larkhall Laboratories, UK.
Multivitamin and mineral preparation.

Immunomorb ISI, Ital.
A measles immunoglobulin (p.1517·3).
Passive immunisation.

Immunoparot ISI, Ital.
A mumps immunoglobulin (p.1521·2).
Passive immunisation.

Immunopertox ISI, Ital.
A pertussis immunoglobulin (p.1525·3).
Passive immunisation.

Immunopret Bionorica, Ger.
Echinacea purpurea (p.1574·2).
Respiratory- and urinary-tract infections.

Immunoprin Ashbourne, UK.
Azathioprine (p.505·3).
Inflammatory disorders; organ transplants.

Immunorho ISI, Ital.
An anti-D immunoglobulin (p.1503·2).
Prevention of rhesus sensitisation.

Immunoros ISI, Ital.
A rubella immunoglobulin (p.1532·3).
Passive immunisation.

Immunotetan ISI, Ital.
A tetanus immunoglobulin (p.1535·2).
Passive immunisation.

Immunovac Artu, Neth.
Allergen extracts (p.1545·1).
Hyposensitisation.

Immunozig ISI, Ital.
A varicella-zoster immunoglobulin (p.1538·1).
Passive immunisation.

Immunozima Salus, Ital.
Muramidase hydrochloride (p.1604·3).
Viral infections.

Immutone Pharmadass, UK.
Shark-liver oil.

Imocur Fournier, Fr.
Bacterial fractions of *Haemophilus influenzae*; *Diplococcus pneumoniae*; *Klebsiella ozaenae*; *Klebsiella pneumoniae*; *Staphylococcus aureus*; *Streptococcus viridans*; *Streptococcus pyogenes*; *Branhamella (Neisseria) catarrhalis*.
Prevention of upper respiratory-tract infection.

Imodium
Janssen-Cilag, Aust.; Janssen-Cilag, Austral.; Janssen-Cilag, Belg.; McNeil Consumer, Canad.; Janssen-Cilag, Fr.; Janssen-Cilag, Ger.; Woelm, Ger.; Janssen-Cilag, Irl.; Janssen-Cilag, Ital.; Janssen-Cilag, Neth.; Janssen-Cilag, Norw.; Janssen-Cilag, S.Afr.; Abello, Spain; Janssen-Cilag, Swed.; Janssen-Cilag, Switz.; Johnson & Johnson MSD Consumer, UK; McNeil Consumer, USA; Janssen, USA.
Loperamide hydrochloride (p.1197·2).
Control of intestinal transit time; diarrhoea; management of ileostomies.

Imofolin Pharmacia Upjohn, Ger.†.
Calcium folinate (p.1342·2).
Antidote to folic acid antagonists; folic acid deficiency.

Imogam
CSL, Austral.; Connaught, Canad.
A rabies immunoglobulin (p.1530·2).
Passive immunisation.

Imogam 16 Pasteur Merieux, Ital.†.
A normal immunoglobulin (p.1535·2).
Agammaglobulinaemia; hypogammaglobulinaemia; passive immunisation.

Imogam Rabia Rhone-Poulenc Rorer, Spain.
A rabies immunoglobulin (p.1530·2).
Passive immunisation.

Imogam Rabies Connaught, USA.
A rabies immunoglobulin (p.1530·2).

Imogam Tetano Pasteur Merieux, Ital.
A tetanus immunoglobulin (p.1535·2).
Passive immunisation.

Imogam Tetanos Rhone-Poulenc Rorer, Spain†.
A tetanus immunoglobulin (p.1535·2).
Passive immunisation.

Imogenil N Roland, Ger.†.
Multivitamin and mineral preparation.
Bone disorders.

Imosec Abello, Spain.
Loperamide hydrochloride (p.1197·2).
Diarrhoea.

Imossel Martin, Fr.
Loperamide hydrochloride (p.1197·2).
Diarrhoea.

Imovane
Rhone-Poulenc Rorer, Aust.; Rhone-Poulenc Rorer, Austral.; Rhone-Poulenc Rorer, Belg.; Rhone-Poulenc Rorer, Canad.; Specia, Fr.; Rhone-Poulenc Rorer, Ital.; Rhone-Poulenc Rorer, Neth.; Rhone-Poulenc Rorer, Norw.; Rhone-Poulenc Rorer, S.Afr.; Rhone-Poulenc Rorer, Swed.; Rhone-Poulenc Rorer, Switz.
Zopiclone (p.699·2).
Sleep disorders.

Imovax Merieux, Fr.
A mumps vaccine (Urabe Am 9 strain) (p.1521·2).
Active immunisation.

Imovax Antiparotiditis Rhone-Poulenc Rorer, Spain†.
A mumps vaccine (p.1521·2).
Active immunisation.

Imovax BCG Pasteur Merieux, Ital.
A BCG vaccine (p.1504·3).
Active immunisation.

Imovax Colera Pasteur Merieux, Ital.†.
A cholera vaccine (p.1506·2).
Active immunisation.

Imovax DPT Rhone-Poulenc Rorer, Spain†.
A diphtheria, tetanus, and pertussis vaccine (p.1509·1).
Active immunisation of infants and young children.

Imovax DT Pasteur Merieux, Ital.
A diphtheria and tetanus vaccine (p.1508·1).
Active immunisation.

Imovax DTP Pasteur Merieux, Ital.
A diphtheria, tetanus, and pertussis vaccine (p.1509·1).
Active immunisation.

Imovax Meningo A & C Rhone-Poulenc Rorer, S.Afr.
Meningococcal vaccine (p.1520·3).
Active immunisation.

Imovax Polio
Pasteur Merieux, Belg.; Pasteur Merieux, Ital.; Pasteur Merieux, Norw.; Pasteur Merieux, Swed.
An inactivated poliomyelitis vaccine (p.1528·2).
Active immunisation.

Imovax Rabbia Pasteur Merieux, Ital.
A rabies vaccine (p.1530·3).
Active immunisation.

Imovax Rabies Connaught, USA.
A rabies vaccine (human diploid cell) (p.1530·3).
Active immunisation.

Imovax Tetano Pasteur Merieux, Ital.
A tetanus vaccine (p.1535·3).
Active immunisation.

Impact
Wander, Ital.; Sandoz Nutrition, USA.
Preparation for enteral nutrition.

Imperacin
Zeneca, Irl.†; ICI, UK†.
Oxytetracycline (p.235·1).
Bacterial infections.

Impetex Roche, Ital.
Diflucortolone valerate (p.1039·3); chlorquinaldol (p.185·1).
Infected skin disorders.

Impletol Bayer, Ger.
Procaine hydrochloride (p.1299·2); caffeine (p.749·3).
Nervous system disorders.

Importal
Zyma, Aust.; Zyma, Belg.; Zyma, Fr.; Zyma, Ger.; Novartis Consumer, Neth.; Zyma, Norw.; Novartis Consumer, S.Afr.; Novartis, Swed.; Zyma, Switz.; Zyma, UK†.
Lactitol (p.1195·2).
Constipation; hepatic encephalopathy.

Imposit N Madaus, Ger.
Cetylpyridinium chloride (p.1106·2); benzocaine (p.1286·2).
Mouth and throat disorders.

Impregon Fleming, USA.
Tetrachlorosalicylanilide.
Napkin disinfection.

Impresial Zambon, Ital.†.
Pipemidic acid (p.237·2).
Bacterial infections of the urinary tract.

Impresso Isis Puren, Ger.
Oxprenolol hydrochloride (p.926·2); hydralazine hydrochloride (p.883·2); chlorthalidone (p.839·3).
Hypertension.

Impril ICN, Canad.
Imipramine hydrochloride (p.289·2).
Depression.

Impromen
Janssen-Cilag, Belg.; Janssen-Cilag, Ger.; Formenti, Ital.; Janssen-Cilag, Neth.
Bromperidol (p.643·2), bromperidol decanoate (p.643·2), or bromperidol lactate (p.643·2).
Psychoses.

Impronta l Fides, Spain.
Piroxicam (p.80·2).
Gout; musculoskeletal, joint, peri-articular, and soft-tissue disorders; pain.

Improved Analgesic Rugby, USA.
Methyl salicylate (p.55·2); menthol (p.1600·2).
Muscle, joint, and soft-tissue pain; neuralgia.

Improved Once A Day Quest, UK.
Multivitamin and mineral preparation.

Improvera Upjohn, UK.
28 Tablets, estropipate (p.1444·3); 12 tablets, medroxyprogesterone acetate (p.1448·3).
Menopausal disorders; postmenopausal osteoporosis.

Improvil Monsanto, Austral.
21 Tablets, norethisterone (p.1453·1); ethinyloestradiol (p.1445·1); 7 tablets, inert.
Triphasic oral contraceptive.

Improvit Pharmador, S.Afr.†.
Multivitamin and mineral preparation.

Imp-Tab Alra, USA.
Imipramine hydrochloride (p.289·2).

Impugan
Dumex-Alpharma, Swed.; Dumex, Switz.
Frusemide (p.871·1).
Hypertension; nephrotic syndrome; oedema; renal insufficiency.

Imtack
Astra, Irl.; Astra, UK†.
Isosorbide dinitrate (p.893·1).
Angina pectoris.

Imtrate Douglas, Austral.
Isosorbide mononitrate (p.893·3).
Angina pectoris.

Imuderm Goldshield, UK.
Cream: White soft paraffin (p.1382·3); fractionated coconut oil (p.1599·2); glycerol (p.1585·2).
Skin disorders.
Oil: Light liquid paraffin (p.1382·1); almond oil (p.1546·2).
Dry skin disorders.

Imudon Solvay, Fr.
Lysates of *Lactobacillus acidophilus* (p.1594·1); *Lactobacillus helveticus* (p.1594·1); *Lactobacillus lactis* (p.1594·1); *Lactobacillus fermentum* (p.1594·1); *Streptococcus pyogenes*; *Streptococcus faecium* (p.1594·1); *Streptococcus faecalis* (p.1594·1); *Streptococcus sanguis*; *Staphylococcus aureus*; *Klebsiella pneumoniae*; *Corynebacterium pseudodiphtheriticum*; *Fusiformis fusiformis*; *Candida albicans*.
Mouth disorders.

Imufor Bender, Aust.
Interferon gamma-1b (p.616·1).
Infections in chronic granulomatous disease.

Imukin
Bender, Aust.; Boehringer Ingelheim, Austral.; Boehringer Ingelheim, Fr.; Thomae, Ger.; Boehringer Ingelheim, Ital.; Boehringer Ingelheim, Norw.; Boehringer Ingelheim, Spain; Boehringer Ingelheim, Swed.; Boehringer Ingelheim, Switz.
Interferon gamma-1b (rbe) (p.616·1).
Infections in chronic granulomatous disease.

Imunovir
Newport, Irl.; Nycomed, UK.
Inosine pranobex (p.615·2).
Viral infections.

Imuprel Adcock Ingram, S.Afr.
Isoprenaline hydrochloride (p.892·1).
Bronchospasm; heart block; shock.

Imuran
Glaxo Wellcome, Austral.; Glaxo Wellcome, Belg.; Glaxo Wellcome, Canad.; Wellcome, Irl.; Wellcome, Ital.†; Glaxo Wellcome, Neth.; Glaxo Wellcome, S.Afr.; Wellcome, UK; Glaxo Wellcome, USA.
Azathioprine (p.505·3) or azathioprine sodium (p.506·2).
Auto-immune disorders; transplant rejection.

Imurek
Glaxo Wellcome, Aust.; Glaxo Wellcome, Ger.; Wellcome, Switz.
Azathioprine (p.505·3) or azathioprine sodium (p.506·2).
Auto-immune disorders; transplant rejection.

Imurel
Glaxo Wellcome, Fr.; Glaxo Wellcome, Norw.; Evans, Spain; Glaxo Wellcome, Swed.
Azathioprine (p.505·3).
Auto-immune disorders; transplant rejection.

Imuvac Nezel, Spain†.
An influenza vaccine (p.1515·2).
Active immunisation.

Imuvit Natura Line, Switz.
Multivitamins and minerals; ginseng (p.1584·2).
Tonic.

In A Wink Ciba Vision, Austral.
Naphazoline nitrate (p.1064·2); zinc sulphate (p.1373·2).
Conjunctivitis; eye irritation.

In A Wink Allergy Ciba Vision, Austral.
Antazoline hydrochloride (p.401·3); tetrahydrozoline hydrochloride (p.1070·2).
Allergic conjunctivitis; hay fever.

In A Wink Moisturing Ciba Vision, Austral.
Povidone (p.1474·2).
Dry eyes.

Inabrin
Pharmacia Upjohn, Belg.; Pharmacia Upjohn, Ital.†.
Ibuprofen (p.44·1).
Fever; pain.

Inacid Merck Sharp & Dohme, Spain.
Indomethacin (p.45·2) or indomethacin sodium (p.45·2).
Gout; inflammation; musculoskeletal, joint, peri-articular, and soft-tissue disorders; pain; patent ductus arteriosus.

Inacilin Inibsa, Spain†.
Pivampicillin hydrochloride (p.238·2).
Bacterial infections.

Inadine
Johnson & Johnson, Ger.; Johnson & Johnson, Irl.; Ethicon, Ital.; Johnson & Johnson, Swed.†; Johnson & Johnson Medical, UK.
Povidone-iodine (p.1123·3).
Burns; wounds.

Inadrox Logeais, Fr.†.
Hydroxocobalamin acetate (p.1364·2); thiamine hydrochloride (p.1361·1).
Nerve pain.

Inagen Llorente, Spain†.
Ethambutol hydrochloride (p.207·2).
Tuberculosis.

Inalgon Neu Laevosan, Aust.
Dipyrone (p.35·1).
Fever; pain.

Inalintra Diviser Aquilea, Spain.
Oxymetazoline (p.1066·1).
Nasal or sinus congestion.

Inalpin Qualiphar, Belg.
Codeine phosphate (p.26·1); bromoform (p.1620·3); potassium guaiacolsulfonate (p.1068·3); sodium camsylate; guaiacol (p.1061·2); aconite (p.1542·2).
Coughs.

Inamide Gerard, Irl.
Indapamide (p.890·2).
Hypertension.

Inapsin Janssen-Cilag, S.Afr.
Droperidol (p.668·2).
Neuroleptanalgesia; premedication.

Inapsine
Janssen-Ortho, Canad.; Janssen, USA.
Droperidol (p.668·2).
Ménière's disease; nausea and vomiting in surgical and diagnostic procedures; neuroleptanalgesia; premedication.

Inarub Frega, Canad.
Methyl salicylate (p.55·2); menthol (p.1600·2); cineole (p.1564·1).

Inaspir Berenguer Infale, Spain.
Salmeterol xinafoate (p.761·2).
Obstructive airways disease.

Inca's Gold Larkhall Laboratories, UK.
Jojoba oil.

Incefal Andreu, Spain†.
Ibuprofen (p.44·1).
Fever; pain.

Incidal
Bayer, Ital.; Bayer, Neth.†.
Mebhydrolin napadisylate (p.413·2).
Hypersensitivity reactions.

The symbol † denotes a preparation no longer actively marketed

Incidin Henkel, Ger.
Isopropyl alcohol (p.1118·2); propyl alcohol (p.1124·2); amphotenside.
Equipment disinfection.

Incidin Extra Henkel, Ger.
Benzalkonium chloride (p.1101·3); oligo(di(iminoimidocarbonyl)iminohexamethylene); orthophenylphenol (p.1120·3).
Surface disinfection.

Incidin GG Henkel, Ger.†.
Tributyltin benzoate; formaldehyde (p.1113·2); glyoxal (p.1115·1).
Surface disinfection; topical fungal infections.

Incidin M Spray Extra Henkel, Ger.
Tributyltin benzoate; isopropyl alcohol (p.1118·2).
Skin disinfection.

Incidin perfekt Henkel, Ger.
Formaldehyde (p.1113·2); glyoxal (p.1115·1); glutaraldehyde (p.1114·3); benzalkonium chloride (p.1101·3); oligo(di(iminoimidocarbonyl)iminohexamethylene).
Surface disinfection.

Incidin Plus Henkel, Ger.
Glucoprotamine.
Surface disinfection.

Incidin Spezial
Note. This name is used for preparations of different composition.
Henkel, Ger.
Formaldehyde (p.1113·2); glyoxal (p.1115·1); glutaraldehyde (p.1114·3); alcohol (p.1099·1).
Surface disinfection.

Henkel, Ital.
Alcohol (p.1099·1); glyoxal (p.1115·1); glutaraldehyde (p.1114·3); benzalkonium chloride (p.1101·3).
Surface disinfection.

Incidine Paragerm, Fr.
Glutaraldehyde (p.1114·3); formaldehyde (p.1113·2); glyoxal (p.1115·1).
Surface and instrument disinfection.

Incidur Henkel, Ger.
Glutaraldehyde (p.1114·3); glyoxal (p.1115·1).
Surface disinfection.

Incidur Spray Henkel, Ger.
Glutaraldehyde (p.1114·3); benzalkonium chloride (p.1101·3); 5-bromo-5-nitro-1,3-dioxacyclohexane; alcohol (p.1099·1); propyl alcohol (p.1124·2).
Surface disinfection.

Incital Pierre Fabre, Fr.†.
Mefenorex hydrochloride (p.1482·1).
Obesity.

Includal Basotherm, Ger.†.
Dodecyltriphenylphosphonium bromide; benzoxonium chloride (p.1103·3).
Surface disinfection.

Inconturina OTW, Ger.
Solidago virgaurea; clove (p.1565·2).
Urinary-tract disorders.

Incremin
Note. This name is used for preparations of different composition.
Lederle, Austral.†.
Multivitamin and mineral preparation.

Cyanamid, Ital.
Lysine hydrochloride (p.1350·1); vitamin B substances.

Incremin Iron Whitehall, Austral.
Ferric pyrophosphate (p.1339·2); vitamin B substances; lysine hydrochloride (p.1350·1).
Dietary supplement.

Incremin with Iron
Lederle Consumer, Canad.†.
Ferric pyrophosphate (p.1339·2); vitamin B substances.
Iron-deficiency anaemia.

Lederle, USA.
Ferric pyrophosphate (p.1339·2); vitamin B substances; L-lysine.
Iron-deficiency anaemias.

Incremin with Vitamin C Whitehall, Austral.
Vitamin B substances; lysine hydrochloride; vitamin C.
Dietary supplement.

Incut Basotherm, Ger.†.
Dexamethasone isonicotinate (p.1037·1); oxytetracycline (p.235·1); natamycin (p.385·3); amethocaine (p.1285·2).
External ear disorders.

Incutin Andreabal, Switz.
Benzyl nicotinate (p.22·1); glycol salicylate (p.43·1); methyl salicylate (p.55·2); camphor (p.1557·2); capsicum (p.1559·2); pine oil; rosemary oil (p.1626·2).
Musculoskeletal, joint, peri-articular, and soft-tissue pain and inflammation.

Indaco Ciba Vision, Ital.
Naphazoline nitrate (p.1064·2); zinc sulphate (p.1373·2).
Eye irritation.

Indaflex Lampugnani, Ital.
Indapamide (p.890·2).
Hypertension.

Indamol Rhone-Poulenc Rorer, Ital.
Indapamide (p.890·2).
Hypertension.

Inderal
Zeneca, Aust.; ICI, Austral.; Zeneca, Belg.; Wyeth-Ayerst, Canad.; Zeneca, Irl.; Zeneca, Ital.; Zeneca, Neth.; Zeneca, Norw.; Zeneca, S.Afr.; Zeneca, Swed.; Zeneca, Switz.; Zeneca, UK; Wyeth-Ayerst, USA.
Propranolol hydrochloride (p.937·1).
Angina pectoris; anxiety; arrhythmias; essential tremor; hypertension; hyperthyroidism; migraine; myocardial infarction; obstructive cardiomyopathy; phaeochromocytoma; prevention of gastro-intestinal haemorrhage.

Inderal comp Zeneca, Aust.
Propranolol hydrochloride (p.937·1); triamterene (p.957·2); hydrochlorothiazide (p.885·2).
Hypertension.

Inderetic
Zeneca, Aust.; Zeneca, Belg.; Zeneca, Irl.; Zeneca, Neth.; Zeneca, S.Afr.; Zeneca, Switz.; Zeneca, UK.
Propranolol hydrochloride (p.937·1); bendrofluazide (p.827·3).
Hypertension.

Inderex Zeneca, UK.
Propranolol hydrochloride (p.937·1); bendrofluazide (p.827·3).
Hypertension.

Inderide
Wyeth-Ayerst, Canad.; Wyeth-Ayerst, USA.
Propranolol hydrochloride (p.937·1); hydrochlorothiazide (p.885·2).
Hypertension.

Inderm
Luitpold, Belg.; Luitpold, Ger.; Luitpold, Neth.; Luitpold, Switz.
Erythromycin (p.204·1).
Acne.

Indertal Urbion, Spain†.
Bacitracin (p.157·3); hydrocortisone acetate (p.1043·3); neomycin sulphate (p.229·2).
Infected skin disorders.

Indian Brandee Potter's, UK.
Capsicum (p.1559·2); compound cardamom tincture (p.1560·1).
Dyspepsia.

Indicatest Polidis, Fr.
Pregnancy test (p.1621·2).

Indigestion Complex Brauer, Austral.
Homoeopathic preparation.

Indigestion and Flatulence Cantassium Co., UK.
Capsicum oleoresin; valerian (p.1643·1); fennel (p.1579·1); myrrh (p.1606·1); papain (p.1614·1).

Indigestion and Flatulence Tablets Healthcrafts, UK.
Peppermint oil (p.1208·1); fennel oil (p.1579·2); capsicum oleoresin.
Dyspepsia; flatulence.

Indigestion Mixture Potter's, UK.
Meadowsweet (p.1599·1); gentian (p.1583·3); euonymus (p.1192·1).
Dyspepsia; flatulence; heartburn.

Indigestion Relief Liquid Boots, UK.
Simethicone (p.1213·1); aluminium hydroxide (p.1177·3); magnesium hydroxide (p.1198·2).
Formerly known as Double Action Indigestion Mixture.
Dyspepsia.

Indigestion Relief Tablets Boots, UK.
Simethicone (p.1213·1); dried aluminium hydroxide gel (p.1177·3); magnesium hydroxide (p.1198·2).
Formerly known as Double Action Indigestion Tablets.
Dyspepsia.

Indigestion Tablets and Oral Spray Brauer, Austral.
Homoeopathic preparation.

Indo CT, Ger.
Indomethacin (p.45·2).
Gout; inflammation; musculoskeletal, joint, and soft-tissue disorders; oedema; pain.

Indo Framan Inexfa, Spain.
Indomethacin (p.45·2).
Gout; musculoskeletal, joint, and peri-articular disorders; pain.

Indo Top Ratiopharm, Ger.
Indomethacin (p.45·2).
Musculoskeletal, joint, and soft-tissue disorders; pain.

Indobloc Dresden, Ger.
Propranolol hydrochloride (p.937·1).
Anxiety; arrhythmias; essential tremor; hypertension; hyperthyroidism; migraine; myocardial infarction.

Indoblok Parke-Med, S.Afr.†.
Propranolol hydrochloride (p.937·1).
Angina pectoris; anxiety; arrhythmias; hypertension; phaeochromocytoma.

Indocaf Reig Jofre, Spain.
Indomethacin (p.45·2).
Aluminium hydroxide (p.1177·3) is included in the capsules in an attempt to limit adverse effects on the gastro-intestinal mucosa.
Gout; inflammation; musculoskeletal, joint, and peri-articular disorders; pain.

Indochron Inwood, USA.
Indomethacin (p.45·2).
Acute gouty arthritis; ankylosing spondylitis; bursitis; osteoarthritis; rheumatoid arthritis; tendinitis.

Indocid
Merck Sharp & Dohme, Aust.; Merck Sharp & Dohme, Austral.; Merck Sharp & Dohme, Belg.; Merck Sharp & Dohme, Canad.; Merck Sharp & Dohme-Chibret, Fr.; Morson, Irl.; Merck Sharp & Dohme, Ital.; Merck Sharp & Dohme, Neth.; Merck Sharp & Dohme, Norw.; Merck Sharp & Dohme, S.Afr.; Merck Sharp & Dohme, Switz.; Morson, UK.
Indomethacin (p.45·2) or indomethacin sodium (p.45·2).
Gout; inflammation; maintenance of mydriasis in cataract surgery; musculoskeletal, joint, and peri-articular disorders; pain; prevention of postoperative ocular inflammation following cataract surgery.

Indocid PDA
Merck Sharp & Dohme, Austral.; Merck Sharp & Dohme, Canad.; Morson, Irl.; Frosst, Neth.; Morson, UK.
Indomethacin sodium (p.45·2).
Closure of patent ductus arteriosus.

Indocin Merck Sharp & Dohme, USA.
Capsules; oral suspension; suppositories; sustained-release capsules: Indomethacin (p.45·2).
Acute gouty arthritis; ankylosing spondylitis; bursitis; osteoarthritis; rheumatoid arthritis; tendinitis.
Injection: Indomethacin sodium (p.45·2).
Closure of patent ductus arteriosus.

Indocollirio SIFI, Ital.
Indomethacin (p.45·2).
Prevention of miosis and inflammation during cataract surgery.

Indocollyre
Germania, Aust.; Ophtapharma, Canad.; Chauvin, Fr.
Indomethacin (p.45·2).
Prevention of intra-operative miosis; prevention of ocular oedema following eye surgery.

Indocontin Mundipharma, Ger.
Indomethacin (p.45·2).
Inflammation; musculoskeletal and joint disorders; pain.

Indoflam Compu, S.Afr.†.
Indomethacin (p.45·2).
Inflammation; musculoskeletal and joint disorders; pain.

Indoflex Laser, S.Afr.†.
Indomethacin (p.45·2).
Gout; inflammation; musculoskeletal and joint disorders; pain.

Indoftol Merck Sharp & Dohme, Spain.
Indomethacin (p.45·2).
Ocular surgery.

Indohexal Hexal, Aust.
Indomethacin (p.45·2).
Gout; inflammation; musculoskeletal, joint, and peri-articular disorders; oedema; pain.

Indolar SR Lagap, UK.
Indomethacin (p.45·2).
Inflammation; joint disorders; pain.

Indolgina Uriach, Spain.
Indomethacin (p.45·2).
Gout; musculoskeletal, joint, and peri-articular disorders; pain.

Indolin Virginia, Ital.
Indapamide (p.890·2).
Hypertension.

Indom Collirio INTES, Ital.
Indomethacin (p.45·2).
Prevention of miosis and inflammation during cataract surgery.

Indomax Ashbourne, UK.
Indomethacin (p.45·2).
Gout; inflammation; musculoskeletal and joint disorders; pain.

Indomed
Amrad, Austral.; Noristan, S.Afr.†.
Indomethacin (p.45·2).
Gout; inflammation; musculoskeletal, joint, and peri-articular disorders; oedema; pain.

Indomee Merck Sharp & Dohme, Swed.
Indomethacin (p.45·2).
Gout; musculoskeletal and joint disorders; peri-articular disorders.

Indomelan Lannacher, Aust.
Indomethacin (p.45·2).
Gout; inflammation; musculoskeletal, joint, and peri-articular disorders; oedema; pain.

Indo-Mepha Mepha, Switz.
Indomethacin (p.45·2).
Musculoskeletal, joint, peri-articular, and soft-tissue pain and inflammation.

Indomet-ratiopharm Ratiopharm, Ger.
Indomethacin (p.45·2).
Gout; inflammation; musculoskeletal, joint, peri-articular, and soft-tissue disorders; pain.

Indomisal Brenner-Efeka, Ger.
Indomethacin (p.45·2).
Gout; inflammation; musculoskeletal and joint disorders; pain.

Indomod
Pharmacia Upjohn, Irl.; Pharmacia, UK.
Indomethacin (p.45·2).
Gout; musculoskeletal, joint, and peri-articular disorders.

Indonilo Sigma-Tau, Spain.
Indomethacin (p.45·2).
Gout; inflammation; musculoskeletal, joint, and peri-articular disorders; oedema; pain.

Indo-paed Hexal, Ger.
Indomethacin (p.45·2).
Gout; inflammation; musculoskeletal, joint, peri-articular, and soft-tissue disorders; pain.

Indo-Phlogont Azupharma, Ger.
Indomethacin (p.45·2).
Gout; inflammation; musculoskeletal and joint disorders.

Indophtal Novopharma, Switz.
Indomethacin (p.45·2).
Eye disorders.

Indoptic Merck Sharp & Dohme, Switz.
Indomethacin (p.45·2).
Prevention of oedema after cataract surgery.

Indoptol
Merck Sharp & Dohme, Aust.; Sigma, Austral.; Merck Sharp & Dohme, Belg.; Chibret, Neth.
Indomethacin (p.45·2).
Inhibition of intra-operative miosis; prevention of cystoid macula oedema after cataract surgery.

Indorektal Sanorania, Ger.
Indomethacin (p.45·2).
Gout; inflammation; musculoskeletal and joint disorders; pain.

Indorene Lusofarmaco, Ital.†.
Indoramin hydrochloride (p.891·1).
Hypertension.

Indosolona Nezel, Spain†.
Indomethacin (p.45·2); muramidase hydrochloride (p.1604·3); prednisolone (p.1048·1).
Inflammation; pain.

Indospray Rhone-Poulenc Rorer, Austral.
Indomethacin (p.45·2).
Musculoskeletal, joint, peri-articular, and soft-tissue disorders.

Indo-Tablinen Sanorania, Ger.
Indomethacin (p.45·2).
Gout; inflammation; musculoskeletal and joint disorders; pain.

Indotal Pharmagen, S.Afr.†.
Indomethacin (p.45·2).
Gout; inflammation; musculoskeletal and joint disorders; pain.

Indotard Bartholomew Rhodes, UK.
Indomethacin (p.45·2).
Inflammation; musculoskeletal, joint, and peri-articular disorders; pain.

Indotec Technilab, Canad.
Indomethacin (p.45·2).
Gout; musculoskeletal and joint disorders; ovarian hyperstimulation syndrome; pain; renal calculi; renal colic.

Indoxen Sigma-Tau, Ital.
Indomethacin (p.45·2).
Musculoskeletal disorders.

Inductor Pharmagyne, Fr.†.
Menotrophin (p.1252·1).
Female and male infertility.

Indulfan Henkel, Ital.
Glyoxal (p.1115·1); benzalkonium chloride (p.1101·3).
Surface disinfection.

Indulfan plus Henkel, Ger.
Formaldehyde (p.1113·2); glyoxal (p.1115·1); glutaraldehyde (p.1114·3); benzalkonium chloride (p.1101·3).
Surface disinfection.

Indunox Laser, S.Afr.†.
Etodroxizine (p.670·1).
Hypersensitivity reactions.

Indurgan Solvay, Spain.
Omeprazole (p.1204·2).
Gastro-oesophageal reflux; peptic ulcer; Zollinger-Ellison syndrome.

Indusil
Recordati, Ital.; Rorer, Spain†.
Cobamamide (p.1364·2).
Vitamin B_{12} deficiency.

Indusil T Diamant, Fr.
Cobamamide (p.1364·2).
Tonic.

Inerpan Synthelabo, Fr.†.
Copolymer of leucine and methyl glutamate.
Burns.

Inexbron Inexfa, Spain.
Amoxycillin trihydrate (p.151·3).
Bacterial infections.

Inexbron Mucolitico Inexfa, Spain.
Amoxycillin trihydrate (p.151·3); bromhexine hydrochloride (p.1055·3).
Respiratory-tract infections.

Inexfal Inexfa, Spain.
Cytidine; muramidase hydrochloride (p.1604·3); uridine (p.1641·3).
Liver disorders.

Infacet Propharm, S.Afr.†.
Promethazine hydrochloride (p.416·2); phenylpropanolamine hydrochloride (p.1067·2); paracetamol (p.72·2); codeine phosphate (p.26·1).
Congestion; fever; pain.

Infacol
Warner-Lambert, Austral.; Pharmax, Irl.; Pharmax, UK.
Simethicone (p.1213·1).
Colic; flatulence.

Infacol-C Parke, Davis, Austral.†.
Dicyclomine hydrochloride (p.460·1); simethicone (p.1213·1).
Colic; flatulence; smooth muscle spasm.

Infaderm Goldshield, UK.
Light liquid paraffin (p.1382·1); almond oil (p.1546·2).
Dry skin disorders.

Infadol VCA Bergamon, Ital.†.
Vitamins A and D.

Infadrops Goldshield, UK.
Paracetamol (p.72·2).
Fever; pain.

Infalina *Berenguer Infale, Spain†.*
Bacitracin zinc (p.157·3); neomycin sulphate (p.229·2); tyrothricin (p.267·2); undecenoic acid (p.389·2); zinc undecenoate (p.389·2); zinc oxide (p.1096·2).
Skin infections.

Infalyte *Mead Johnson Nutritionals, USA.*
Electrolytes and rice syrup solids (p.1152·3).
Formerly known as Ricelyte.
Oral rehydration therapy.

Infanrix
SmithKline Beecham, Aust.; SmithKline Beecham, Austral.; SK-RIT, Belg.; SmithKline Beecham, Irl.; SmithKline Beecham, Ital.; SBL, Swed.; SmithKline Beecham, USA.
A diphtheria, tetanus, and acellular pertussis vaccine (p.1509·1).
Active immunisation.

Infanrix DTPa
SmithKline Beecham, Ger.; SmithKline Beecham, Switz.
A diphtheria, tetanus, and pertussis vaccine (p.1509·1).
Active immunisation.

Infanrix DTPa + Hib *SmithKline Beecham, Ger.*
A diphtheria, tetanus, pertussis, and haemophilus influenzae vaccine (p.1509·3).
Active immunisation.

Infant Calm *Brauer, Austral.*
Passion flower (p.1615·3); aconitum nap; belladonna; chamomilla.
Insomnia; irritability or restlessness in children.

Infant Colic *Brauer, Austral.†.*
Homoeopathic preparation.

Infant Gaviscon *Reckitt & Colman, S.Afr.*
Alginic acid (p.1470·3); magnesium trisilicate (p.1199·1); dried aluminium hydroxide gel (p.1177·3); sodium bicarbonate (p.1153·2).
Gastro-oesophageal reflux.

Infant Teething *Brauer, Austral.†.*
Homoeopathic preparation.

Infant Tonic *Brauer, Austral.*
Angelica; ascorbic acid (p.1365·2); kola (p.1645·1); hypericum (p.1590·1); ginseng (p.1584·2); urtica (p.1642·3); aurum mur.; calc. phos.; ferrum met.; ferrum phos.; kali phos.; mag. phos.; phosphoric acid.
Tonic.

Infantol *Carter Horner, Canad.*
Multivitamin preparation.
Dietary supplement.

Infants Tylenol Cold Decongestant & Fever Reducer *McNeil Consumer, USA.*
Paracetamol (p.72·2); pseudoephedrine hydrochloride (p.1068·3).
Congestion; fever; pain.

Infantussin N *Palmicol, Ger.*
Anise oil (p.1550·1); fennel oil (p.1579·2); thyme (p.1636·3); althaea (p.1546·3).
Coughs and cold symptoms.

Infapain *Schwulst, S.Afr.*
Paracetamol (p.72·2); codeine phosphate (p.26·1).
Fever; pain.

Infapain Forte *Schwulst, S.Afr.*
Paracetamol (p.72·2); codeine phosphate (p.26·1); promethazine hydrochloride (p.416·2).
Fever; pain.

Infasoy
Wyeth Health, Austral.; Cow & Gate, Irl.; Akromed, S.Afr.†; Cow & Gate, UK.
Food for special diets.
Formerly known as Nutrilon Soya in the *UK*.
Galactosaemia; milk and lactose intolerance.

Infasurf *Forest Pharmaceuticals, USA.*
Calfactant (p.1623·1).
Neonatal respiratory distress syndrome.

Infa-Tardyferon
Germania, Aust.; Robapharm, Switz.†.
Ferrous sulphate (p.1340·2).
Iron deficiency; iron-deficiency anaemia.

Infazinc *Atlas, Canad.*
Zinc oxide (p.1096·2).

InfectoBicillin *Infectopharm, Ger.*
Benzathine phenoxymethylpenicillin (p.159·2).
Bacterial infections.

Infectocef *Infectopharm, Ger.*
Cefaclor (p.163·2).
Bacterial infections.

Infectocillin *Infectopharm, Ger.*
Phenoxymethylpenicillin potassium (p.236·2).
Bacterial infections.

Infectocin *Pharmador, S.Afr.†.*
Erythromycin stearate (p.204·2).
Bacterial infections.

Infectodyspept *Infectopharm, Ger.*
Carrot (p.1644·3).
Dyspepsia.

Infectoflam *Ciba Vision, Switz.*
Fluorometholone (p.1042·1); gentamicin sulphate (p.212·1).
Bacterial eye infections; inflammatory eye disorders.

Infectogripp *Infectopharm, Ger.†.*
Amantadine hydrochloride (p.1129·2).
Influenza A.

Infectomox *Infectopharm, Ger.*
Amoxycillin (p.151·3).
Bacterial infections.

Infectomycin *Infectopharm, Ger.*
Erythromycin estolate (p.204·1).
Bacterial infections.

Infectosoor *Infectopharm, Ger.*
Miconazole (p.384·3).
Mouth and throat candidiasis.

Infectotrimet *Infectopharm, Ger.*
Trimethoprim (p.265·1).
Urinary-tract infections.

Infectrin *Poli, Ital.*
Ampicillin (p.153·1); flucloxacillin (p.209·1).
Bacterial infections.

Infectrol *Bausch & Lomb, USA†.*
Dexamethasone (p.1037·1); neomycin sulphate (p.229·2); polymyxin B sulphate (p.239·1).
Infected eye disorders.

INFeD *Schein, USA.*
Iron dextran (p.1348·1).
Iron deficiency.

Infekt-Komplex Ho-Fu-Complex *Liebermann, Ger.*
Homoeopathic preparation.

Infergen *Amgen, USA.*
Interferon alfacon-1 (p.615·3).
Hepatitis C.

Inferil *Pharmarecord, Ital.*
Ferric sodium gluconate (p.1340·1).
Iron-deficiency anaemias.

Infesol *Berlin-Chemie, Ger.*
Amino-acid, electrolyte, and xylitol infusion.
Protein and fluid deficiency.

Infestat *Opus, UK.*
Nystatin (p.386·1).
Gastro-intestinal candidiasis.

Infibran *Expanpharm, Fr.*
Wheat bran (p.1181·2).
Constipation.

Infi-tract N *Infirmarius-Rovit, Ger.*
Scopolia carniolica; carlina acaulis; curcuma zanthorrhiza; chelidonium; gentian (p.1583·3); angelica; manna (p.1199·1); saffron (p.1001·1); zedoary; myrrh (p.1606·1); ascorbic acid (p.1365·2).
Biliary disorders; digestive disorders; gastro-intestinal spasm.

Infla-Ban *Triomed, S.Afr.*
Diclofenac sodium (p.31·2).
Gout; inflammation; musculoskeletal and joint disorders.

Inflaced *Biotherapie, Fr.*
Piroxicam (p.80·2).
Musculoskeletal joint, and peri-articular disorders.

Inflam *Lichtenstein, Ger.*
Capsules; slow-release capsules; suppositories; topical spray: Indomethacin (p.45·2).
Fever; gout; inflammation; musculoskeletal and joint disorders; pain.
Ointment: Indomethacin (p.45·2); laureth 9 (p.1325·2).
Inflammation; musculoskeletal and joint disorders; pain.

Inflamac *Spirig, Switz.*
Diclofenac sodium (p.31·2).
Fever; gout; inflammation; musculoskeletal, joint, and peri-articular disorders; pain.

Inflamase
Ciba Vision, Canad.; Iolab, USA.
Prednisolone sodium phosphate (p.1048·1).
Inflammatory eye disorders.

Inflammide *Boehringer Ingelheim, S.Afr.*
Budesonide (p.1034·3).
Asthma.

Inflanefran *Allergan, Ger.*
Prednisolone acetate (p.1048·1).
Eye disorders.

Inflanegent *Allergan, Ger.*
Prednisolone acetate (p.1048·1); gentamicin sulphate (p.212·1).
Infected eye disorders.

Inflazone *Lennon, S.Afr.*
Phenylbutazone (p.79·2).
Ankylosing spondylitis.

Inflexal
Kwizda, Aust.; Berna, Ital.; Swisspharm, S.Afr.; Berna, Spain; Berna, Switz.
An influenza vaccine (p.1515·2).
Active immunisation.

Infloran
Note. This name is used for preparations of different composition.
Kwizda, Aust.; Berna, Switz.
Bifidobacterium infantis; *Lactobacillus acidophilus* (p.1594·1).
Diarrhoea; dyspepsia; restoration of gastro-intestinal flora.
Berna, Ital.; Berna, Spain.
Bifidobacterium bifidum (p.1594·1); *Lactobacillus acidophilus* (p.1594·1).
Diarrhoea; restoration of gastro-intestinal flora.

Influaforce *Bioforce, Switz.*
Homoeopathic preparation.

Influbene
Note. This name is used for preparations of different composition.
Merckle, Aust.
Paracetamol (p.72·2); etilefrine hydrochloride (p.867·2); butethamate citrate (p.1056·2); chlorpheniramine maleate (p.405·1).
Respiratory-tract infections.
Mepha, Switz.†.
Dipyrone (p.35·1); etilefrine hydrochloride (p.867·2); butethamate citrate (p.1056·2); chlorpheniramine maleate (p.405·1).
Cold symptoms.

Influbene C *Mepha, Switz.*
Paracetamol (p.72·2); ascorbic acid (p.1365·2).
Fever; pain.

Influbene N *Mepha, Switz.*
Paracetamol (p.72·2).
Fever; pain.

Infludo
Weleda, Aust.; Weleda, Fr.; Weleda, Ger.; Weleda, UK.
Homoeopathic preparation.

Influex *Steigerwald, Ger.*
Homoeopathic preparation.

Influmix *Ismunit, Ital.†.*
An influenza vaccine (p.1515·2).
Active immunisation.

Influpozzi *IVP, Ital.*
An influenza vaccine (p.1515·2).
Active immunisation.

Influrem *Edmond Pharma, Ital.*
Propyphenazone (p.81·3); caffeine (p.749·3); paracetamol (p.72·2).
Cold symptoms; pain.

Influsanbalm *Weimer, Ger.†.*
Camphor (p.1557·2); cineole (p.1564·1); menthol (p.1600·2); thymol (p.1127·1); turpentine oil (p.1641·1).
Coughs, colds, and associated respiratory-tract disorders.

Influsplit SSW *Dresden, Ger.; SmithKline Beecham, Ger.*
An influenza vaccine (p.1515·2).
Active immunisation.

Influtruw *Truw, Ger.*
Homoeopathic preparation.

Influvac
Solvay, Aust.; Solvay, Belg.; Solvay, Fr.; Solvay, Ger.; Solvay, Irl.; Solvay, Neth.; Solvay, S.Afr.; Solvay Duphar, Swed.; Solvay, Switz.; Solvay, UK.
An inactivated influenza vaccine (surface antigen) (p.1515·2).
Active immunisation.

Influvac S *Solvay, Ital.*
An influenza vaccine (p.1515·2).
Active immunisation.

Influvidon *Waldheim, Aust.*
Salicylamide (p.82·3); caffeine (p.749·3); propyphenazone (p.81·3); hesperidin phosphate (p.1580·2); calcium ascorbate (p.1365·2); piprin hydrate (p.416·1).
Cold and influenza symptoms.

Influvirus *Nuovo ISM, Ital.*
An influenza vaccine (p.1515·2).
Active immunisation.

Influvit
Note. This name is used for preparations of different composition.
DHU, Ger.
Homoeopathic preparation.
Recordati, Ital.
Paracetamol (p.72·2); ascorbic acid (p.1365·2); propyphenazone (p.81·3).
Fever; pain.

Infosan *Nycomed Imaging, Norw.*
Albumin (p.710·1).
Contrast medium for echocardiography.

Infoson *Nycomed, Swed.†.*
Albumin (p.710·1).
Contrast medium for echocardiography.

Infraline *Rolmex, Canad.*
Methyl salicylate (p.55·2); menthol (p.1600·2); cineole (p.1564·1).

Inframin *SIFRA, Ital.*
Amino-acid infusion.
Parenteral nutrition in renal failure.

infraRUB *Whitehall, USA.*
Methyl salicylate (p.55·2); menthol (p.1600·2).
Muscle, joint, and soft-tissue pain; neuralgia.

Infree *Eisai, Jpn.*
Indomethacin farnesil (p.46·3).
Musculoskeletal, joint, and peri-articular disorders.

Infrotto *Cassella-med, Ger.†.*
Glycol salicylate (p.43·1); turpentine oil (p.1641·1); volatile mustard oil (p.1605·3); camphor (p.1557·2); rosemary oil (p.1626·2).
Gout; myalgia; neuralgia; rheumatism.

Infrotto Ultra *Cassella-med, Ger.*
Glycol salicylate (p.43·1); nonivamide (p.63·2).
Muscular and neuromuscular disorders; rheumatic disorders.

Infukoll HES *Serum-Werk Bernburg, Ger.*
Hetastarch (p.724·1) in sodium chloride.
Hypovolaemia.

Infukoll M 40 *Serum-Werk Bernburg, Ger.*
Dextran 40 (p.716·2) in sodium chloride.
Hypovolaemia; thrombosis prophylaxis.

Infumorph *Elkins-Sinn, USA.*
Morphine sulphate (p.56·2).

Infunutrin *Hormonchemie, Ger.†; Schiwa, Ger.†.*
Amino-acid, carbohydrate, and electrolyte infusion.
Parenteral nutrition.

Infunutrin 10% *Hormonchemie, Ger.†; Schiwa, Ger.†.*
Amino-acid infusion.
Parenteral nutrition.

Infunutrin E *Hormonchemie, Ger.†; Schiwa, Ger.†.*
Amino-acid and electrolyte infusion.
Parenteral nutrition.

Infunutrin KHE *Hormonchemie, Ger.†; Schiwa, Ger.†.*
Amino-acid, carbohydrate, and electrolyte infusion.
Parenteral nutrition.

Ingastri *Kendall, Spain.*
Famotidine (p.1192·1).
Gastro-oesophageal reflux; peptic ulcers; Zollinger-Ellison syndrome.

Ingelan
Note. This name is used for preparations of different composition.
Germania, Aust.; Boehringer Ingelheim, Ger.
Topical gel: Isoprenaline sulphate (p.892·1).
Skin disorders.
Boehringer Ingelheim, Ger.
Topical powder: Isoprenaline sulphate (p.892·1); salicylic acid (p.1090·2).
Skin disorders.

Inglobin *Galepharma, Spain†.*
A normal immunoglobulin (p.1522·1).
Hypogammaglobulinaemia; passive immunisation.

Ingro *Farmacologico Milanese, Ital.*
Potassium guaiacolsulfonate (p.1068·3); dextromethorphan hydrobromide (p.1057·3); eucalyptus (p.1578·1).
Coughs.

Ingrown Toe Nail Salve *Cress, Canad.*
Boric acid (p.1554·2); camphor (p.1557·2); salicylic acid (p.1090·2).

Inhacort *Boehringer Ingelheim, Ger.*
Flunisolide (p.1040·3).
Asthma.

Inhalador *Fournier SA, Spain.*
Camphor (p.1557·2); methyl salicylate (p.55·2); oleum pinus sylvestris; sassafras oil (p.1627·3); menthol (p.1600·2).
Nasal congestion.

Inhalene *Synthelabo, Belg.*
Menthol (p.1600·2); cineole (p.1564·1).
Cold symptoms; laryngitis; sinusitis.

Inhibace
Merck, Aust.; Roche, Aust.; Bayer, Austral.; Roche, Belg.; Roche, Canad.; Roche, S.Afr.; Andreu, Spain; Roche, Swed.; Roche, Switz.
Cilazapril (p.840·3).
Heart failure; hypertension.

Inhibace comp *Roche, Swed.*
Cilazapril (p.840·3); hydrochlorothiazide (p.885·2).
Hypertension.

Inhibace Plus
Merck, Aust.; Roche, Aust.; Roche, S.Afr.; Andreu, Spain; Roche, Switz.
Cilazapril (p.840·3); hydrochlorothiazide (p.885·2).
Hypertension.

Inhibin *Asta Medica, Neth.*
Hydroquinine hydrobromide (p.1589·2).
Muscle cramps.

Inhibostamin *Zyma, Ger.†.*
Tritoqualine (p.421·1).
Minor allergic disorders; pruritus.

Inhiston *Biomedica, Ital.*
Pheniramine maleate (p.415·3).
Hypersensitivity reactions.

Inibace *Roche, Ital.*
Cilazapril (p.840·3).
Hypertension.

Inibace Plus *Roche, Ital.*
Cilazapril (p.840·3); hydrochlorothiazide (p.885·2).
Hypertension.

Inibil *Sclavo, Ital.†.*
Aprotinin (p.711·3).
Haemorrhage; post-operative disorders; shock.

Inipomp *Synthelabo, Fr.*
Pantoprazole sodium (p.1207·3).
Gastro-oesophageal reflux; peptic ulcer.

Iniprol
Bournonville, Belg.; Choay, Fr.†; Italfarmaco, Ital.†.
Aprotinin (p.711·3).
Hyperfibrinolysis; pancreatitis; shock.

Iniston *Warner-Lambert, Spain.*
Pseudoephedrine hydrochloride (p.1068·3); triprolidine hydrochloride (p.420·3).
Nasal congestion.

Iniston Antitusivo *Warner-Lambert, Spain.*
Dextromethorphan hydrobromide (p.1057·3); pseudoephedrine hydrochloride (p.1068·3); triprolidine hydrochloride (p.420·3).
Formerly contained codeine phosphate, pseudoephedrine hydrochloride, and triprolidine hydrochloride.
Coughs; nasal congestion.

Iniston Expectorante *Warner-Lambert, Spain.*
Guaiphenesin (p.1061·3); pseudoephedrine hydrochloride (p.1068·3); triprolidine hydrochloride (p.420·3).
Formerly contained codeine phosphate, guaiphenesin, pseudoephedrine hydrochloride, and triprolidine hydrochloride.
Coughs; nasal congestion.

Initard *Novo Nordisk, Switz.†.*
Mixture of insulin injection (porcine, highly purified) 50% and isophane insulin injection (porcine, highly purified) 50% (p.322·1).
Diabetes mellitus.

Initard 50/50
Novo Nordisk, Canad.†; Novo Nordisk, UK†; Wellcome, UK†.
Mixture of neutral insulin injection (porcine, highly purified) 50% and isophane insulin injection (porcine, highly purified) 50% (p.322·1).
Diabetes mellitus.

Initard Humaine *Novo Nordisk, Switz.†.*
Mixture of insulin injection (human) 50% and isophane insulin injection (human) 50% (p.322·1).
Diabetes mellitus.

Initard Human Novo Nordisk, Austral.†.
Mixture of neutral insulin injection (human, emp, highly purified) 50% and isophane insulin injection (human, emp, highly purified) 50% (p.322·1).
Diabetes mellitus.

Initard Humanum Novo Nordisk, Belg.†.
A mixture of insulin injection (human, emp, highly purified) 50% and isophane insulin suspension (human, emp, highly purified) 50% (p.322·1).
Diabetes mellitus.

Initiss Pharmacia Upjohn, Ital.
Cilazapril (p.840·3).
Hypertension.

Initiss Plus Pharmacia Upjohn, Ital.
Cilazapril (p.840·3); hydrochlorothiazide (p.885·2).
Hypertension.

Inkamil Kendall, Spain.
Ciprofloxacin hydrochloride (p.185·3).
Bacterial infections.

Inmunivirus Doble Evans, Spain†.
A measles and mumps vaccine (Schwarz and Urabe Am 9 strains respectively) (p.1519·2).
Active immunisation.

Inmunoferon Cantabria, Spain.
Glicofosfopeptical (p.1584·3).
Immunotherapy.

Inmunogamma Leti, Spain†.
A normal immunoglobulin (p.1522·1).
Hypogammaglobulinaemia; passive immunisation.

Inmunogamma Anti D Leti, Spain†.
An anti-D immunoglobulin (p.1503·2).
Prevention of rhesus sensitisation.

Inmunogamma Antirrabica Leti, Spain†.
A rabies immunoglobulin (p.1530·2).
Passive immunisation.

Inmunogamma Antitet Leti, Spain†.
A tetanus immunoglobulin (p.1535·2).
Passive immunisation.

Inmunoglob Anti D Byk Elmu, Spain†.
An anti-D immunoglobulin (p.1503·2).
Prevention of rhesus sensitisation.

Inmunovirus Triple Evans, Spain†.
A measles, mumps, and rubella vaccine (Schwarz, Urabe Am 9, and Wistar RA 27/3 strains respectively) (p.1519·3).
Active immunisation.

Inmupen Llorente, Spain.
Amoxycillin trihydrate (p.151·3); potassium clavulanate (p.190·2).
Bacterial infections.

Inner Fresh Tablets Healthcrafts, UK.
Frangula bark (p.1193·2).
Constipation.

Innerfresh Pro Murdock, USA.
Chlorophyllin copper complex (p.1000·1).

Innersource Quest, Canad.
Multivitamin and mineral preparation.

Inno Rheuma Strallhofer, Aust.
Cream: Camphor (p.1557·2); menthol (p.1600·2); rosemary oil (p.1626·2).
Oil: Lavender oil (p.1594·3); menthol (p.1600·2); rosemary oil (p.1626·2).
Musculoskeletal and joint disorders; nerve pain.

Innobrand Lab Francais du Fractionnement, Fr.
A complex of factor VIII and von Willebrand's factor (p.720·3).
Von Willebrand's disease.

InnoGel Plus Hogil, USA.
Pyrethrins; piperonyl butoxide (p.1409·3).

Innohep
Leo, Belg.; Leo, Canad.; Leo, Fr.; Braun, Ger.; Leo, Irl.; Formenti, Ital.; Leo, Neth.; Lovens, Swed.; Leo, UK.
Tinzaparin sodium (p.954·2).
Thrombo-embolic disorders.

Innolyre Innotech, Fr.†.
Oxytetracycline hydrochloride (p.235·1).
Bacterial eye infections.

Innovace
Merck Sharp & Dohme, Irl.; Merck Sharp & Dohme, UK.
Enalapril maleate (p.863·2).
Heart failure; hypertension; ischaemic heart disease.

Innovar
Janssen, Canad.†; Janssen, USA.
Fentanyl citrate (p.38·1); droperidol (p.668·2).
Anaesthesia; neuroleptanalgesia; premedication.

Innozide
Merck Sharp & Dohme, Irl.; Merck Sharp & Dohme, UK.
Enalapril maleate (p.863·2); hydrochlorothiazide (p.885·2).
Hypertension.

Inocar Nezel, Spain.
Cilazapril (p.840·3).
Hypertension.

Inocar Plus Nezel, Spain.
Cilazapril (p.840·3); hydrochlorothiazide (p.885·2).
Hypertension.

Inocor
Sanofi Winthrop, Belg.; Sanofi Winthrop, Canad.; Sanofi Winthrop, Fr.; Sanofi Winthrop, Ital.; Sanofi, Swed.; Winthrop, Switz.†; Sanofi Winthrop, USA.
Amrinone (p.823·2) or amrinone lactate (p.823·1).
Heart failure.

Inofer AJC, Fr.
Ferrous succinate (p.1340·2).
Succinic acid is included in this preparation to increase the absorption and availability of iron.
Anaemia.

Inolaxine
Debat, Fr.; Debat, Switz.
Sterculia (p.1214·1).
Constipation.

Inolaxol Selena, Swed.
Sterculia (p.1214·1).
Adjunct in treatment of diarrhoea; constipation.

Inolin Tanabe, Jpn.
Tretoquinol hydrochloride (p.774·2).
Obstructive airways disease.

Inongan Fumouze, Fr.
Salicylic acid (p.1090·2); menthol (p.1600·2); methyl salicylate (p.55·2); camphor (p.1557·2); isobornyl acetate; eucalyptus oil (p.1578·1).
Muscle pain.

Inopamil
Astra, Ital.; Zambon, Neth.
Ibopamine hydrochloride (p.889·3).
Heart failure.

Inopectol Christiaens, Belg.†.
Camphor (p.1557·2); cineole (p.1564·1); guaiacol (p.1061·2); menthol (p.1600·2).
Rhinitis; sinusitis.

Inosin comp. A.S., Ger.†.
Inosine (p.1591·1); sodium pyruvate (p.1631·3); alpha tocopheryl acetate (p.1369·1); nicotinamide (p.1351·2).
Peripheral and cerebral vascular disorders.

Inotyol
Note. This name is used for preparations of different composition.
Brady, Aust.; Fournier, Belg.; Hoechst Marion Roussel, Ital.; Fournier SA, Spain†.
Ointment: Ichthammol (p.1083·3); hamamelis (p.1587·1); zinc oxide (p.1096·2); titanium dioxide (p.1093·3).
Burns; skin disorders; wounds.

Brady, Aust.; Hoechst Marion Roussel, Ital.
Topical powder: Ichthammol (p.1083·3); hamamelis (p.1587·1); zinc oxide (p.1096·2).
Skin disorders.

Centrapharm, Belg.†; Debat, Fr.†.
Topical powder: Ichthammol (p.1083·3); zinc oxide (p.1096·2).
Skin disorders.

Debat, Norw.; Selena, Swed.
Ointment: Ichthammol (p.1083·3); zinc oxide (p.1096·2); titanium dioxide (p.1093·3).
Skin disorders.

Debat, Fr.
Ointment: Ichthammol (p.1083·3); hamamelis (p.1587·1); zinc oxide (p.1096·2); titanium dioxide (p.1093·3); siam benzoin (p.1628·3).
Skin disorders.

Inovan Kyowa, Jpn.
Dopamine hydrochloride (p.861·1).
Anuria; oliguria; shock.

Inoven Johnson & Johnson MSD Consumer, UK.
Ibuprofen (p.44·1).
Fever; inflammation; pain.

Inpersol Abbott, USA†.
Glucose; electrolytes (p.1151·1).
Peritoneal dialysis solution.

Insadol
Laroche Navarron, Belg.†; Expanpharm, Fr.; Syntex, Switz.
Maize.
Dental disorders.

Insect Bite Ointment Seton, UK†.
Antazoline hydrochloride (p.401·3).
Insect bites.

Insidon
Ciba-Geigy, Aust.; Ciba-Geigy, Belg.; Ciba-Geigy, Fr.; Geigy, Ger.; Geigy, Irl.; Ciba, Ital.; Novartis, Neth.; Geigy, Norw.†; Geigy, Switz.
Opipramol hydrochloride (p.301·1).
Anxiety disorders; depression; non-psychotic mental disorders.

Insig Sigma, Austral.
Indapamide (p.890·2).
Hypertension.

Insom Lennon, S.Afr.
Flunitrazepam (p.670·1).
Insomnia.

Insomnal Rougier, Canad.
Diphenhydramine hydrochloride (p.409·1).
Insomnia.

Insomnia Homeocan, Canad.
Homoeopathic preparation.

Insomnia Passiflora Homeocan, Canad.
Homoeopathic preparation.

Insomnyl Bouchara, Fr.†.
Promethazine hydrochloride (p.416·2); crataegus (p.1568·2).
Insomnia.

Inspirol Halsschmerztabletten Hotz, Ger.
Tyrothricin (p.267·2); benzocaine (p.1286·2); dequalinium chloride (p.1112·1).
Mouth and throat infections.

Inspirol Heilpflanzenol Hotz, Ger.
Peppermint oil (p.1208·1).
Cold symptoms; gastro-intestinal disorders.

Inspirol Mundwasser konzentrat Hotz, Ger.
Menthol (p.1600·2); eucalyptus oil (p.1578·1); peppermint oil (p.1208·1); pumilio pine oil (p.1623·3).
Mouth and throat disorders.

Inspirol P Hotz, Ger.
Myrrh (p.1606·1).
Mouth and throat inflammation.

Inspiryl Draco, Swed.
Salbutamol sulphate (p.758·2).
Obstructive airways disease.

Instacare Ciba Vision, Austral.
Cleaning and disinfectant solutions for soft contact lenses.

Instacyl Streuli, Switz.
Aspirin (p.16·1); ascorbic acid (p.1365·2).
Cold symptoms.

Instant Rub Pharmalab, Canad.
Methyl salicylate (p.55·2); menthol (p.1600·2).

Instantine Bayer, Canad.
Aspirin (p.16·1); caffeine (p.749·3).
Fever; headache; pain.

Instat
Johnson & Johnson, Aust.; Ethicon, Ital.; Johnson & Johnson, Switz.; Johnson & Johnson Medical, UK; Johnson & Johnson Medical, USA.
Collagen (bovine) (p.1566·3).
Bleeding in surgical procedures.

Instenon
Hafslund Nycomed, Aust.; Byk Gulden, Ger.†.
Hexobendine hydrochloride (p.883·1); ethamivan (p.1480·3); etofylline (p.753·1).
Cerebrovascular disorders.

Instillagel
Chemieprodukte, Aust.; Melisana, Belg.†; Farco, Ger.; Farco, Irl.; Kronans, Swed.; Almed, Switz.; CliniMed, UK.
Lignocaine hydrochloride (p.1293·2); chlorhexidine gluconate (p.1107·2).
Catheterisation; endoscopy.

Instrunet liquid Smith & Nephew, Fr.†.
Formaldehyde (p.1113·2); glutaraldehyde (p.1114·3); glyoxal (p.1115·1); didecyldimethylammonium chloride (p.1112·2).
Instrument and surface disinfection.

Instrunet machine Smith & Nephew, Fr.†.
Dioctyl diethyltriamine; trioctyl diethyltriamine.
Instrument disinfection.

Instrunet mains Smith & Nephew, Fr.†.
Orthophenylphenol (p.1120·3).
Hand disinfection.

Instrunet powder Smith & Nephew, Fr.†.
Dioctyl diethyltriamine; trioctyl diethyltriamine.
Instrument disinfection.

Instru-Safe Eagle, Austral.
Silicone (p.1384·2).
Instrument lubrication.

Insulatard
Novo Nordisk, Aust.†; Novo Nordisk, Ger.; Novo Nordisk, UK; Glaxo Wellcome, UK.
Isophane insulin injection (porcine, highly purified) (p.322·1).
Diabetes mellitus.

Novo Nordisk, Irl.; Novo Nordisk, Neth.; Novo Nordisk, Norw.; Novo Nordisk, Spain; Novo Nordisk, Swed.
Isophane insulin injection (human, pyr, highly purified) (p.322·1).
Formerly known as Human Insulatard in *Irl.* and as Protaphan Human in *Swed.*
Diabetes mellitus.

Insulatard HM
Novo Nordisk, Aust.; Novo Nordisk, Belg.; Novo Nordisk, Fr.†; Novo Nordisk, Switz.
Isophane insulin injection (human, monocomponent) (p.322·1).
Formerly known as Protaphane HM in *Switz.*
Diabetes mellitus.

Insulatard Human Novo Nordisk, Ger.
Isophane insulin injection (human) (p.322·1).
Diabetes mellitus.

Insulatard Humana Novo Nordisk, Spain†.
Isophane insulin injection (human) (p.322·1).
Diabetes mellitus.

Insulatard MC Novo Nordisk, Switz.
Isophane insulin injection (porcine, highly purified) (p.322·1).
Diabetes mellitus.

Insulatard Nordisk Novo Nordisk, Fr.†.
Isophane insulin injection (crystalline) (porcine, highly purified) (p.322·1).
Diabetes mellitus.

Insulatard Novolet Novo Nordisk, Spain.
Isophane insulin injection (human) (p.322·1).
Diabetes mellitus.

Insulatard NPH
Novo Nordisk, Canad.†; Nordisk, USA†.
Isophane insulin injection (porcine, highly purified) (p.322·1).
Diabetes mellitus.

Insulatard NPH Human
Novo Nordisk, Canad.†; Nordisk, USA†.
Isophane insulin suspension (human, emp) (p.322·1).
Diabetes mellitus.

Insulatard-X Humanum Novo Nordisk, Belg.†.
Isophane insulin injection (human, emp) (p.322·1).
Diabetes mellitus.

Insulin 2 Novo Nordisk, Austral.
Acid insulin injection (bovine) (p.322·1).
Diabetes mellitus.

Insulin Basal Hoechst Marion Roussel, Norw.
Isophane insulin injection (human, emp) (p.322·1).
Diabetes mellitus.

Insulin Infusat Hoechst Marion Roussel, Norw.
Insulin injection (human, emp) (p.322·1).
Diabetes mellitus.

Insulin Komb 25/75 Hoechst Marion Roussel, Norw.
Mixture of insulin injection (human, emp) and isophane insulin injection (human, emp) (p.322·1).
Diabetes mellitus.

Insulin Rapid Hoechst Marion Roussel, Norw.
Insulin injection (human, emp) (p.322·1).
Diabetes mellitus.

Insulin Reaction Sherwood, USA.
Glucose (p.1343·3).
Hypoglycaemia.

Insuline NPH Organon, Fr.†.
Isophane insulin injection (crystalline) (porcine, highly purified) (p.322·1).
Diabetes mellitus.

Insuline Semi Tardum Organon, Fr.
Insulin zinc suspension (amorphous) (porcine, highly purified) (p.322·1).
Diabetes mellitus.

Insuline Tardum MX Organon, Fr.
Mixture of insulin zinc suspension (amorphous) (porcine, highly purified) 30% and insulin zinc suspension (crystalline) (bovine, highly purified) 70% (p.322·1).
Diabetes mellitus.

Insuline Ultra Tardum Organon, Fr.
Insulin zinc suspension (crystalline) (bovine, highly purified) (p.322·1).
Diabetes mellitus.

Insulin-Toronto (Regular) Novo Nordisk, Canad.†.
Neutral insulin injection (bovine and porcine) (p.322·1).
Diabetes mellitus.

Insuman 25/75 Hoechst Marion Roussel, Irl.
A mixture of insulin injection (human, emp) 25% and isophane insulin injection (human, emp) 75% (p.322·1).
Diabetes mellitus.

Insuman Basal
Hoechst, Aust.; Hoechst Marion Roussel, Irl.
Isophane insulin injection (human, emp) (p.322·1).
Diabetes mellitus.

Insuman Infusat Hoechst, Aust.
Soluble insulin injection (human) (p.322·1).
Diabetes mellitus.

Insuman Intermediaire 25/75 Hoechst, Fr.
Mixture of insulin injection (human, emp, highly purified) 25% and isophane insulin injection (human, emp, highly purified) 75% (p.322·1).
Diabetes mellitus.

Insuman Intermediaire 100% Hoechst, Fr.
Isophane insulin injection (human, emp, highly purified) (p.322·1).
Diabetes mellitus.

Insuman komb Typ 15, Typ 25, and Typ 50
Hoechst, Aust.
Mixtures of soluble insulin injection (human) 15%, 25%, and 50% and isophane insulin injection (human) 85%, 75%, and 50% respectively (p.322·1).
Diabetes mellitus.

Insuman Rapid
Hoechst, Aust.; Hoechst Marion Roussel, Irl.
Neutral insulin injection (human, emp) (p.322·1).
Diabetes mellitus.

Insuman Rapide Hoechst, Fr.
Insulin injection (human, emp, highly purified) (p.322·1).
Diabetes mellitus.

Insup Smaller, Spain.
Enalapril maleate (p.863·2).
Heart failure; hypertension.

Insuven Berenguer Infale, Spain.
Diosmin (p.1580·1).
Haemorrhoids; vascular disorders.

Intal
Schoeller, Aust.; Rhone-Poulenc Rorer, Austral.; Rhone-Poulenc Rorer, Canad.; Fisons, Ger.; Rhone-Poulenc Rorer, Ger.; Rhone-Poulenc Rorer, Irl.; Casen Fisons, Spain; Fisons, UK; Fisons, USA.
Sodium cromoglycate (p.762·1).
Allergic rhinitis; asthma; bronchitis.

Intal compositum Fisons, Ger.†.
Sodium cromoglycate (p.762·1); isoprenaline sulphate (p.892·1).
Asthma; bronchitis.

Intal Compound Fisons, UK†.
Sodium cromoglycate (p.762·1); isoprenaline sulphate (p.892·1).
Asthma.

Intal Nasal Fisons, Switz.†.
Sodium cromoglycate (p.762·1).
Allergic rhinitis.

Inteban Sumitomo, Jpn†.
Indomethacin (p.45·2).
Inflammation.

Inteflora Restan, S.Afr.
Saccharomyces boulardii (p.1594·1).
Gastro-intestinal disorders.

Integrilin Cor Therapeutics, USA.
Eptifibatide (p.865·3).
Myocardial infarction.

Integrin
Sanofi Winthrop, Irl.†; Sterling Winthrop, UK†.
Oxypertine (p.684·1).
Now known as Oxypertine.
Anxiety; psychoses.

Intensain
Therabel Pharma, Belg.†; Hoechst, Ger.; Normon, Spain†.
Chromonar hydrochloride (p.840·1).
Cardiac disorders.

Intensain-Lanicor *Cassella-Riedel, Ger.†; Boehringer Mannheim, Ger.†.*
Chromonar hydrochloride (p.840·1); digoxin (p.849·3).
Cardiovascular disorders.

Intensain-Lanitop *Boehringer Mannheim, Ger.†; Cassella-Riedel, Ger.†.*
Chromonar hydrochloride (p.840·1); medigoxin (p.902·1).
Heart failure.

Intensol *Roxane, USA.*
Metoclopramide hydrochloride (p.1200·3).
Gastro-intestinal disorders.

Interacton *Enzypharm, Neth.*
Amine oxidase; glutaminase; allyl sulphide.
Asthma; bronchitis; hypersensitivity reactions; pertussis; sinusitis; skin disorders.

Interberin *Wyeth Lederle, Aust.*
Sargramostim (p.727·3).
Neutropenia after bone marrow transplantation.

Interceed
Johnson & Johnson Medical, Fr.; Johnson & Johnson, Ger.; Johnson & Johnson Medical, UK.
Oxidised cellulose (p.714·2).
Postoperative adhesions.

Interceed (TC7) *Johnson & Johnson Medical, USA.*
Oxidised cellulose (p.714·2).
Gynaecological surgery.

Interceptor *Isnardi, Ital.†.*
Orgotein (p.87·3).
Inflammatory disorders.

Intercron *Laphal, Fr.*
Sodium cromoglycate (p.762·1).
Food hypersensitivity.

Intercyton
Evans, Fr.; Semar, Spain.
Flavodate sodium (p.1580·1).
Peripheral vascular disorders.

Interderm *Interpharma, Spain.*
Gentamicin (p.214·1); nystatin (p.386·1); triamcinolone acetonide (p.1050·2).
Infected skin disorders.

Intermigran *Sanol, Ger.†.*
Propranolol hydrochloride (p.937·1).
Angina pectoris; anxiety; hypertension; migraine; tachycardia; tremor.

Intesticarbine *Goupil, Fr.†.*
Belladonna leaves (p.457·1); magnesium oxide (p.1198·3); activated charcoal (p.972·2); hexamine (p.216·1); betanaphthol (p.98·3); calcium mandelate (p.223·3); sodium thiosulphate (p.996·2).
Gastro-intestinal disorders.

Intestin-Euvernil N *Bristol-Myers Squibb, Ger.†.*
Calcium sulphaloxate (p.162·1).
Intestinal bacterial infections.

Intestinol *Rosch & Handel, Aust.*
Pancreatin (p.1612·1); sodium cholate; duodenum extract; charcoal (p.972·2).
Gastro-intestinal disorders.

Intetrix
Ipsen, Belg.; Beaufour, Fr.
Tiliquinol (p.594·1); tiliquinol lauryl sulphate (p.594·1); tilbroquinol (p.594·1).
Infective diarrhoea; intestinal amoebiasis.

Intetrix P *Beaufour, Fr.*
Tilbroquinol (p.594·1).
Formerly contained tilbroquinol and furoylbromomethyloxine.
Infective diarrhoea.

Intradermi Fluid N *Eberth, Ger.*
Dihydroxymethylrutoside; aesculus (p.1543·3); benzyl nicotinate (p.22·1).
Bath additive; circulatory disorders; musculoskeletal and joint disorders; neuromuscular disorders and trauma.

Intradermi N *Eberth, Ger.*
Ointment: Bovine ovarian extract (p.1458·2); bovine testicular extract (p.1464·1); bovine adrenal extract.
Musculoskeletal disorders; peripheral circulatory disorders.
Oral drops: Troxerutin (p.1580·2); aesculus (p.1543·3); scoparium (p.1628·1).
Brachialgia paraesthetica; circulatory disorders.

Intradermo Cort Ant Fung *Cederroth, Spain.*
Fluocinolone acetonide (p.1041·1); gramicidin (p.215·2); neomycin sulphate (p.229·2); nystatin (p.386·1).
Infected skin disorders.

Intradermo Corticosteroi *Cederroth, Spain†.*
Fluocinolone acetonide (p.1041·1).
Skin disorders.

Intrafat *Nihon, Jpn.*
Soya oil (p.1355·1).
Contains egg lecithin.
Lipid infusion for parenteral nutrition.

Intrafer *Geymonat, Ital.*
Iron polymaltose (p.1349·1).
Iron deficiency; iron-deficiency anaemia.

Intrafusin
Pharmacia Upjohn, Aust.; Pharmacia Upjohn, Ger.; Kabi, Irl.†; Pharmacia Upjohn, Switz.; Pharmacia Upjohn, UK.
Amino-acid infusion with or without electrolytes.
Parenteral nutrition.

Intrafusin SX-E *Kabi Pharmacia, Ger.†.*
Amino-acid, carbohydrate, and electrolyte infusion.
Parenteral nutrition.

Intragam
Serotherapeutisches, Aust.; CSL, Austral.; NBI, S.Afr.
A normal immunoglobulin (p.1522·1).
Passive immunisation against hepatitis A; primary immune deficiency syndromes.

Intraglobin
Biotest, Aust.; Biotest, Ger.†; Biotest, Ital.
A normal immunoglobulin (p.1522·1).
Hypogammaglobulinaemia; idiopathic thrombocytopenic purpura; passive immunisation.

Intraglobin F
Biotest, Ger.; Mednostica, S.Afr.; Biotest, Switz.
A normal immunoglobulin (p.1522·1).
Hypogammaglobulinaemia; idiopathic thrombocytopenic purpura; Kawasaki syndrome; passive immunisation.

Intrait de Marron D'Inde P *Synthelabo, Fr.*
Aesculus (p.1543·3); metesculetol sodium (p.1602·3).
Haemorrhoids.

Intralgin
3M, Belg.†; 3M, S.Afr.†; 3M, UK.
Benzocaine (p.1286·2); salicylamide (p.82·3).
Soft-tissue injury and pain; muscle pain.

Intralipid
Pharmacia Upjohn, Aust.; Baxter, Austral.; Pharmacia Upjohn, Belg.; Pharmacia Upjohn, Canad.; Pharmacia Upjohn, Ger.; Pharmacia Upjohn, Irl.; Pharmacia Upjohn, Ital.; Pharmacia Upjohn, Neth.; Pharmacia Upjohn, Norw.; Pharmacia Upjohn, S.Afr.; Pharmacia Upjohn, Swed.; Pharmacia Upjohn, Switz.; Pharmacia Upjohn, UK; Clintec, USA.
Soya oil (p.1355·1).
Contains egg phospholipids.
Lipid infusion for parenteral nutrition.

Intralipide *Pharmacia Upjohn, Fr.*
Soya oil (p.1355·1).
Contains egg lecithin.
Lipid infusion for parenteral nutrition.

Intramin *Pharmacia Upjohn, Ger.*
Amino-acid, carbohydrate, and electrolyte infusion.
Parenteral nutrition.

Intramin G *Pharmacia Upjohn, Aust.*
Amino-acid, electrolyte, and glucose infusion.
Parenteral nutrition.

Intrasite
Note. This name is used for preparations of different composition.
Smith & Nephew, Austral.; Smith & Nephew, Fr.; Smith & Nephew, S.Afr.
Crilanomer (p.1080·3).
Formerly contained carmellose sodium and polyisobutylene in *Fr.*
Leg ulcers; wound dressing.

Smith & Nephew, Irl.
Hydrogel starch copolymer.
Wounds.

Smith & Nephew, UK.
Carmellose (p.1471·2).
Formerly known as Scherisorb. Formerly contained hydrogel starch copolymer.
Wound dressing.

Intrasol *Worndli, Switz.*
Thymol iodide (p.1127·1).
Oral hygiene.

Intrastigmina *Lusofarmaco, Ital.*
Neostigmine methylsulphate (p.1394·1).
Abdominal distension; post-operative intestinal atony; urinary retention.

Intraval Sodium
Rhone-Poulenc Rorer, Irl.; Rhone-Poulenc Rorer, S.Afr.; May & Baker, UK.
Thiopentone sodium (p.1233·1).
Convulsive states; general anaesthesia.

Intra-Vite B Group plus Ascorbic Acid *Roche, Austral.*
Vitamin B substances with vitamin C.

Intrazig *ISI, Ital.*
A varicella-zoster immunoglobulin (p.1538·1).
Passive immunisation.

Intrazolina *Torlan, Spain.*
Cephazolin sodium (p.181·1).
Lignocaine hydrochloride (p.1293·2) is included in this preparation to alleviate the pain of injection.
Bacterial infections.

Introlan *Elan, USA.*
Lactose-free, gluten-free preparation for enteral nutrition.

Introlite
Abbott, UK; Ross, USA.
Preparation for enteral nutrition.

Intron A
Aesca, Aust.; Schering-Plough, Austral.; Schering-Plough, Belg.; Schering, Canad.; Essex, Ger.; Schering-Plough, Irl.; Schering-Plough, Ital.; Schering-Plough, Neth.; Schering-Plough, S.Afr.; Schering-Plough, Spain; Essex, Switz.; Schering-Plough, UK; Schering, USA.
Interferon alfa-2b (rbe) (p.615·3).
Anogenital warts; chronic hepatitis; malignant neoplasms.

Introna
Schering-Plough, Fr.; Schering-Plough, Norw.; Schering-Plough, Swed.
Interferon alfa-2b (p.615·3).
Chronic active hepatitis; malignant neoplasms.

Intropin
Boots, Austral.†; Du Pont, Canad.; Du Pont, Irl.; Sanofi Labaz, Neth.†; Boots, S.Afr.; Du Pont, Swed.; Du Pont Pharmaceuticals, UK†; Du Pont, USA.
Dopamine hydrochloride (p.861·1).
Heart failure; renal failure; shock.

Inutest
Laevosan, Aust.; Kemiflor, Swed.; Laevosan, Switz.†.
Polyfructosan (p.1591·3).
Determination of glomerular filtration rate.

Invenol *Hoechst, Aust.*
Carbutamide (p.319·1).
Diabetes mellitus.

Inversine *Merck Sharp & Dohme, USA.*
Mecamylamine hydrochloride (p.901·3).
Hypertension.

Invertos *Pharmacia Upjohn, Norw.*
Anhydrous glucose (p.1343·3); fructose (p.1343·2).
Carbohydrate source.

Invigan *Fournier SA, Spain.*
Famotidine (p.1192·1).
Gastro-oesophageal reflux; peptic ulcer; Zollinger-Ellison syndrome.

Invirase
Roche, Austral.; Roche, Canad.; Roche, Ger.; Roche, Irl.; Roche, Ital.; Roche, Neth.; Roche, S.Afr.; Roche, Spain; Roche, Swed.; Roche, Switz.; Roche, UK; Roche, USA.
Saquinavir mesylate (p.625·2).
HIV infection.

In-Vite *Leo, Irl.†.*
Multivitamin preparation.

Invite B₁ *Nelson, Austral.†.*
Thiamine hydrochloride (p.1361·1).

Invite B₆ *Nelson, Austral.†.*
Pyridoxine hydrochloride (p.1362·3).
Vitamin B_6 deficiency.

Invite B Plus with Vitamin C *Nelson, Austral.†.*
Vitamin B substances with ascorbic acid.

Invite C *Nelson, Austral.†.*
Ascorbic acid (p.1365·2).
Vitamin C deficiency.

Invite E *Nelson, Austral.†.*
Alpha tocopheryl acetate (p.1369·1).
Abrasions; burns; dry skin; vitamin E deficiency.

Invite E Forte *Nelson, Austral.†.*
Capsules: Vitamin E (p.1369·1); wheat-germ oil.
Tablets: Alpha tocopheryl acid succinate (p.1369·1).
Vitamin E deficiency.

Invite E Hi-Forte *Nelson, Austral.†.*
Vitamin E (p.1369·1); wheat-germ oil.
Vitamin E deficiency.

Invite Multi-Vitamin & Mineral Capsules *Nelson, Austral.†.*
Multivitamin and mineral preparation.

Inyesprin *Andromaco, Spain.*
Lysine aspirin (p.50·3).
Fever; musculoskeletal, joint, and peri-articular disorders; pain; thrombo-embolism prophylaxis.

Inza
Note. This name is used for preparations of different composition.
Alphapharm, Austral.
Naproxen (p.61·2).
Inflammation; musculoskeletal and joint disorders; pain.

Lennon, S.Afr.
Ibuprofen (p.44·1).
Musculoskeletal and joint disorders.

Inzelloval *Kohler-Pharma, Ger.*
Mineral preparation.

Inzitan *Boehringer Mannheim, Spain.*
Cyanocobalamin (p.1363·3); dexamethasone (p.1037·1); thiamine hydrochloride (p.1361·1).
Lignocaine hydrochloride (p.1293·2) is included in this preparation to alleviate the pain of injection.
Musculoskeletal and joint disorders.

Inzolen *Kohler, Ger.*
A range of electrolyte and trace element infusions (p.1147·1).
Electrolyte disorders; metabolic disorders.

Ioban 2 *3M, Fr.†.*
Copolymer of isooctyl acrylate and *N*-vinyl-2-pyrrolidone.
Antiseptic.

Iobid DM *Iomed, USA.*
Guaiphenesin (p.1061·3); dextromethorphan hydrobromide (p.1057·3).
Coughs.

Iocare Balanced Salt Solution
Ciba Vision, UK; Iolab, USA.
Electrolytes (p.1147·1).
Eye irrigation.

Iocare BSS *Ciba Vision, Ger.*
Electrolytes (p.1147·1).
Eye irrigation.

Iocon *Galderma, USA.*
Coal tar (p.1092·3).
Scalp disorders.

Iodal *Iomed, USA.*
Hydrocodone tartrate (p.43·1); phenylephrine hydrochloride (p.1066·2); chlorpheniramine maleate (p.405·1).
Upper respiratory-tract symptoms.

Iodalfa *MC, Ital.†.*
Laurylamide iodate complex.
Surface disinfection.

Iodaminol *Desbergers, Canad.†.*
Iodised casein (p.1493·1).
Hyperthyroidism.

Iode *Valmo, Canad.*
Iodine (p.1493·1); potassium iodide (p.1493·1).

Ioden *Pan Quimica, Spain†.*
Povidone-iodine (p.1123·3).
Mouth infections; skin and instrument disinfection.

Iodex
Note. This name is used for preparations of different composition.
Qualiphar, Belg.
Iodine (p.1493·1).
Superficial wounds.

Lee, USA.
Povidone-iodine (p.1123·3).
Skin disinfection.

Iodex Buccal *Qualiphar, Belg.*
Povidone-iodine (p.1123·3).
Mouth and throat infections.

Iodex Dermique *Qualiphar, Belg.*
Povidone-iodine (p.1123·3).
Disinfection of skin and instruments; infected skin disorders.

Iodex with Methyl Salicylate *Medtech, USA.*
Iodine (p.1493·1); methyl salicylate (p.55·2).
Muscle, joint, and soft-tissue pain; neuralgia.

Iodex MS *Qualiphar, Belg.†.*
Iodine (p.1493·1); methyl salicylate (p.55·2).
Soft-tissue pain and inflammation.

Iodina *Men, Spain.*
Povidone-iodine (p.1123·3).
Skin, wound, burn, and instrument disinfection.

Iodine Tri-Test *Drug Houses Austral., Austral.†.*
Povidone-iodine (p.1123·3).
Topical antiseptic.

Iodocafedrina *Parisis, Spain†.*
Caffeine (p.749·3); ephedrine hydrochloride (p.1059·3); lobelia inflata (p.1481·3); sodium benzoate (p.1102·3); sodium iodide (p.1493·2); euphorbia lathyris; belladonna (p.457·1); crataegus (p.1568·2); grindelia; marrubium vulgare (p.1063·3); polygala (p.1069·3); conium maculatum; cimicifuga racemosa (p.1563·3).
Respiratory-tract disorders.

Iodocid *Bergamon, Ital.*
Povidone-iodine (p.1123·3).
Skin disinfection.

Iodo-Cortifair *Pharmafair, USA†.*
Clioquinol (p.193·2); hydrocortisone (p.1043·3).

Iodoflex *Smith & Nephew Healthcare, UK.*
Cadexomer-iodine (p.1105·1).
Leg ulcers; wounds.

Iodo-Niacin *Forest Pharmaceuticals, USA†.*
Potassium iodide (p.1493·1); nicotinamide hydroiodide.

Iodopen *Lyphomed, USA.*
Sodium iodide (p.1493·2).
Additive for intravenous total parenteral nutrition solutions.

Iodorganine T *Augot, Fr.†.*
Thyroid (p.1496·3).
Hypothyroidism.

Iodoril *MC, Ital.†.*
Povidone-iodine (p.1123·3).
Skin and mucous membrane disinfection.

Iodosan *SmithKline Beecham, Ital.†.*
Dextromethorphan hydrobromide (p.1057·3); guaiphenesin (p.1061·3).
Cough.

Iodosan Collutorio *SmithKline Beecham, Ital.*
Iodine (p.1493·1).
Oral hygiene.

Iodosan Nasale Contac *SmithKline Beecham, Ital.†.*
Xylometazoline hydrochloride (p.1071·2); domiphen bromide (p.1112·3).
Nasal congestion.

Iodosan Raffreddore Contac *SmithKline Beecham, Ital.†.*
Paracetamol (p.72·2); isopropamide iodide (p.464·3); dimetofrine; caffeine (p.749·3); chlorpheniramine maleate (p.405·1); ascorbic acid (p.1365·2).
Cold symptoms; influenza.

Iodoscrub *IMS, Ital.†.*
Povidone-iodine (p.1123·3).
Hand disinfection.

Iodosorb
Lannacher, Aust.; Choay, Fr.†; Strathmann, Ger.; Valeas, Ital.; Daker Farmasimes, Spain; Perstorp, Swed.; Perstorp, Switz.; Smith & Nephew Healthcare, UK; Oclassen, USA†.
Cadexomer-iodine (p.1105·1).
Skin ulcers; wounds.

Iodosteril *IMS, Ital.†.*
Povidone-iodine (p.1123·3).
Skin disinfection.

Iodoten *Bergamon, Ital.*
Povidone-iodine (p.1123·3).
Wound disinfection.

Iodotope *Squibb Diagnostics, USA.*
Iodine-131 (p.1424·1) as sodium iodide.
Hyperthyroidism; thyroid cancer.

Iodovit *Novopharma, Switz.†.*
Vitamin B substances.
Eye disorders.

Iolducyl *Ciba Vision, Fr.†.*
Potassium iodide (p.1493·1); sodium iodide (p.1493·2).
Eye disorders.

Iofed *Iomed, USA.*
Brompheniramine maleate (p.403·2); pseudoephedrine hydrochloride (p.1068·3).
Upper respiratory-tract symptoms.

Iohist D *Iomed, USA.*
Phenylpropanolamine hydrochloride (p.1067·2); phenyltoloxamine citrate (p.416·1); mepyramine maleate (p.414·1); pheniramine maleate (p.415·3).
Respiratory-tract disorders.

Iohist DM *Iomed, USA.*
Dextromethorphan hydrobromide (p.1057·3); phenylpropanolamine hydrochloride (p.1067·2); brompheniramine maleate (p.403·2).
Upper respiratory-tract symptoms.

Iomeron
Gerot, Aust.; Byk, Belg.; Byk, Fr.; Bracco, Ital.; Eisai, Jpn; Byk, Neth.; Rovi, Spain; Astra Tech, Swed.
Iomeprol (p.1006·3).
Radiographic contrast medium.

Ionamin
Rhone-Poulenc Rorer, Canad.; Rhone-Poulenc Rorer, Irl.; Torbet Laboratories, UK; Medeva, USA.
Phentermine (as an ion-exchange resin complex) (p.1484·3).
Obesity.

Ionamine *Fisons, Switz.*
Phentermine (as an ion-exchange resin complex) (p.1484·3).
Obesity.

Ionarthrol *Picot, Fr.*
Manganese sulphate (p.1350·3); magnesium sulphate (p.1157·3); calcium chloride (p.1155·1); nickel chloride; ferrous sulphate (p.1340·2); sodium sulphate (p.1213·3).
Joint disorders.

Ionax *Galderma, USA; Owen, USA.*
Skin cleanser.
Acne.

Ionax Astringent *Owen, USA.*
Salicylic acid (p.1090·2); allantoin (p.1078·2).
Acne.

Ionax Foam *Owen, USA.*
Skin cleanser.
Acne.

Ionax Scrub
Galderma, Austral.; Galderma, Fr.; Galderma, Irl.; Alcon, S.Afr.†; Galderma, UK.
Polyethylene granules (abrasive) (p.1077·2).
Acne.

Ionax T *Galderma, Fr.*
Coal tar (p.1092·3); salicylic acid (p.1090·2).
Seborrhoeic dermatitis.

Ionil
Galderma, Canad.; Alcon, S.Afr.†; Galderma, USA.
Salicylic acid (p.1090·2).
Seborrhoeic dermatitis.

Ionil Plus *Galderma, USA.*
Salicylic acid (p.1090·2).
Scalp psoriasis; seborrhoeic dermatitis.

Ionil Rinse *Galderma, Austral.*
Hydrolised collagen proteins (p.1566·3).
Dry brittle hair.

Ionil Scalp Cleanser *Galderma, Austral.*
Salicylic acid (p.1090·2).
Scalp disorders.

Ionil-T
Note. This name is used for preparations of different composition.
Galderma, Austral.; Galderma, Irl.; Galderma, Ital.; Alcon, S.Afr.†; Galderma, UK; Galderma, USA.
Coal tar (p.1092·3); salicylic acid (p.1090·2).
Scalp disorders.

Galderma, Canad.
Coal tar (p.1092·3).
Scalp disorders.

Ionil-T Plus
Galderma, Austral.; Galderma, Canad.; Galderma, USA.
Coal tar (p.1092·3).
Scalp disorders.

Ionimag *Byk, Fr.*
Magnesium lactate (p.1157·3).
Magnesium deficiency.

Ionitan *Aguettant, Fr.*
Electrolyte infusion (p.1147·1).
Parenteral nutrition.

Ionyl *Medinat, Fr.*
Phosphoric acid (p.1618·1); sodium glycerophosphate (p.1586·2); magnesium glycerophosphate (p.1157·2); manganese glycerophosphate (p.1586·2).
Tonic.

Iopamiro
Bristol-Myers Squibb, Ger.†; Bracco, Ital.; Dagra, Neth.†; Astra Tech, Norw.; Rovi, Spain; Astra Tech, Swed.; Bracco, Switz.
Iopamidol (p.1007·1).
Radiographic contrast medium.

Iopamiron *Schering, Fr.*
Iopamidol (p.1007·1).
Radiographic contrast medium.

Iophen *Rugby, USA.*
Iodinated glycerol (p.1062·2).
Coughs.

Iopidine
Alcon, Aust.; Alcon, Austral.; Alcon, Belg.; Alcon, Canad.; Alcon, Fr.; Alcon-Thilo, Ger.; Alcon, Irl.; Alcon, Ital.; Alcon, Norw.; Alcon, S.Afr.; Alcon, Swed.; Alcon, UK; Alcon, USA.
Apraclonidine hydrochloride (p.824·3).
Control of intra-ocular pressure following eye surgery; glaucoma.

Iopimax *Alcon, Spain.*
Apraclonidine hydrochloride (p.824·3).
Glaucoma.

Iosal II *Iomed, USA.*
Pseudoephedrine (p.1068·3); guaiphenesin (p.1061·3).
Coughs.

Iosalide *Yamanouchi, Ital.*
Josamycin (p.220·2) or josamycin propionate (p.220·2).
Bacterial infections.

Iosimitan *Wider, Ger.†.*
Camphor (p.1557·2); menthol (p.1600·2); khellin (p.1593·1); turpentine oil (p.1641·1); terebinthina laricina; eucalyptus oil (p.1578·1); lavander oil (p.1594·3).
Coughs and associated respiratory-tract disorders.

Iosopan *Goldline, USA.*
Magaldrate (p.1198·1).
Hyperacidity.

Iosopan Plus *Goldline, USA.*
Magaldrate (p.1198·1); simethicone (p.1213·1).
Hyperacidity.

Iotussin HC *Iomed, USA.*
Hydrocodone tartrate (p.43·1); phenylephrine hydrochloride (p.1066·2); chlorpheniramine maleate (p.405·1).
Upper respiratory-tract symptoms.

Ipacef *IPA, Ital.*
Cefuroxime sodium (p.177·1).
Bacterial infections.

Ipacid *IPA, Ital.*
Cefonicid sodium (p.167·2).
Lignocaine hydrochloride (p.1293·2) is included in this preparation to alleviate the pain of injection.
Bacterial infections.

Ipalat *Pfleger, Ger.*
Ointment: Pumilio pine oil (p.1623·3); eucalyptus oil (p.1578·1).
Pastilles†: Primula root.
Syrup: Primula root; thyme (p.1636·3).
Respiratory-tract disorders.

Ipamicina *IPA, Ital.*
Injection†: Fosfomycin sodium (p.210·2).
Tablets: Fosfomycin calcium (p.210·2).
Bacterial infections.

Ipamix *Gentili, Ital.*
Indapamide (p.890·2).
Hypertension.

Iparen *NCSN, Ital.*
Heparan sulphate (p.879·2).
Thrombosis prophylaxis.

Ipatox *IPA, Ital.*
Glutathione sodium (p.983·1).
Alcohol and drug poisoning; radiation trauma.

Ipatrizina *IPA, Ital.*
Propylene glycol cefatrizine (p.164·2).
Bacterial infections.

Ipavit *IPA, Ital.*
Vitamin B substances with calcium folinate(p.1342·2).

Ipazone *IPA, Ital.*
Cefoperazone sodium (p.167·3).
Bacterial infections.

Ipcamox *Nat Druggists, S.Afr.*
Amoxycillin trihydrate (p.151·3).
Bacterial infections.

Ipeca *Amino, Switz.*
Emetine hydrochloride (p.582·2); ethylmorphine hydrochloride (p.36·1); ephedrine hydrochloride (p.1059·3); codeine phosphate (p.26·1); cherry-laurel water; tolu balsam (p.1071·1).
Respiratory-tract disorders.

Iper D3 *Zambon, Ital.†.*
Cholecalciferol (p.1366·3).
Vitamin D deficiency.

Ipercortis *AGIPS, Ital.*
Triamcinolone (p.1050·2).
Corticosteroid.

Iperplasin *Angelini, Aust.*
Mepartricin (p.384·2).
Benign prostatic hyperplasia.

Ipersed *Salus, Ital.†.*
Nitrazepam (p.682·2).
Insomnia.

Ipersulfidin *Francia, Ital.†.*
Sulfaperin.
Bacterial infections.

Iperten *Master Pharma, Ital.*
Manidipine dihydrochloride (p.900·2).
Hypertension.

Ipertrofan *SPA, Ital.*
Mepartricin (p.384·2).
Benign prostatic hyperplasia.

Ipervital *IDI, Ital.*
Nutritional supplement.

Ipesil *Antigen, Irl.*
Ipecacuanha (p.1062·2); squill (p.1070·1).
Coughs.

Ipetitrin *Agepha, Aust.*
Ipecacuanha (p.1062·2).
Bronchitis; coughs.

Ipnovel *Roche, Ital.*
Midazolam (p.679·3).
General anaesthesia; premedication; sedative.

Ipoazotal *SIT, Ital.*
Arginine hydrochloride (p.1334·1); ornithine hydrochloride (p.1352·3); citrulline (p.1337·2).
Hyperammonaemia.

Ipoazotal Complex *SIT, Ital.*
Arginine hydrochloride (p.1334·1); ornithine hydrochloride (p.1352·3); citrulline (p.1337·2); acetyl aspartate; aceglumic acid; calcium oxoglurate.
Hyperammonaemia.

Ipobar *Miba, Ital.†.*
Penbutolol sulphate (p.927·2).
Cardiac disorders; hypertension.

Ipocalcin *Salus, Ital.*
Salcatonin (p.735·3).
Hypercalcaemia; osteoporosis; Paget's disease of bone; reflex sympathetic dystrophy.

Ipocol *Lagap, Switz.†.*
Divistyramine (p.1272·3).
Biliary-tract disorders; hypercholesterolaemia.

Ipocromo *Ripari-Gero, Ital.*
Ferric sodium gluconate (p.1340·1).
Iron-deficiency anaemias.

Ipogen *Gentili, Ital.*
Dihydralazine tartrate (p.854·1); chlorothiazide (p.839·1).
Hypertension.

Ipol
CSL, Austral.; Connaught, USA.
An inactivated poliomyelitis vaccine (p.1528·2).
Active immunisation.

Ipolab *Finmedical, Ital.*
Labetalol hydrochloride (p.896·1).
Hypertension.

Ipolina *Lafare, Ital.†.*
Hydralazine hydrochloride (p.883·2).
Hypertension.

Iposeb *Rydelle, Fr.*
Amino-acid, vitamin, and mineral preparation.
Seborrhoea.

Ipotensium *Pierrel, Ital.†.*
Clonidine hydrochloride (p.841·2).
Hypertension.

Ipotex *Cyanamid, Ital.†.*
Quinethazone (p.938·3); reserpine (p.942·1).
Hypertension.

Ippi Verde *Henkel, Ital.*
Triclosan (Irgasan DP 300) (p.1127·2).
Skin and hand disinfection.

Ipradol
Hafslund Nycomed, Aust.; Continental Ethicals, S.Afr.; Lacer, Spain; Hafslund Nycomed, Switz.†.
Hexoprenaline (p.754·1), hexoprenaline hydrochloride (p.754·1), or hexoprenaline sulphate (p.754·1).
Obstructive airways disease; prevention of uterine contractions.

Iprafen *Chiesi, Ital.*
Fenoterol hydrobromide (p.753·2); ipratropium bromide (p.754·2).
Obstructive airways disease.

Ipral
Bristol-Myers Squibb, Irl.; Squibb, UK†.
Trimethoprim (p.265·1).
Bacterial urinary- and respiratory-tract infections.

Ipratin *Alphapharm, Austral.*
Ipratropium bromide (p.754·2).
Obstructive airways disease.

Ipren *Pharmacia Upjohn, Swed.*
Ibuprofen (p.44·1).
Fever; inflammation; musculoskeletal and joint disorders; pain.

Iproben *Mepha, Switz.*
Ibuprofen (p.44·1).
Fever; pain.

Iprogel *Mepha, Switz.*
Ibuprofen (p.44·1).
Musculoskeletal, joint, peri-articular and soft-tissue pain and inflammation.

Iprosten *Takeda, Ital.*
Ipriflavone (p.740·1).
Osteoporosis.

Ipsatol Cough Formula Liquid for Children and Adults *Kenwood, USA.*
Guaiphenesin (p.1061·3); dextromethorphan hydrobromide (p.1057·3); phenylpropanolamine hydrochloride (p.1067·2).
Coughs.

Ipser Europe *Pasteur Vaccins, Fr.*
A snake venom antiserum (*Vipera ammodytes, V. aspis,* and *V. berus*) (p.1534·1).
Viper bites.

Ipstyl *Ipsen, Ital.*
Lanreotide (p.1252·3).
Acromegaly; carcinoid tumour.

Ipvent *Cipla-Medpro, S.Afr.*
Ipratropium bromide (p.754·2).
Obstructive airways disease.

Ircon *Kenwood, USA.*
Ferrous fumarate (p.1339·3).
Iron-deficiency anaemias.

Ircon-FA *Kenwood, USA.*
Ferrous fumarate (p.1339·3); folic acid (p.1340·3).
Iron-deficiency anaemias.

Irdal *Clonmel, Irl.†.*
Flurazepam dihydrochloride (p.672·2).
Insomnia.

Irenat
Kolassa, Aust.; Bayer, Ger.
Sodium perchlorate (p.1496·3).
Adjunct in radionuclide brain scanning; hyperthyroidism.

Irfen *Mepha, Switz.*
Ibuprofen (p.44·1).
Musculoskeletal and joint disorders; pain.

Irgaman *Hoechst Marion Roussel, Ital.*
Triclosan (Irgasan DP 300) (p.1127·2).
Skin disinfection.

Irgamid
Dispersa, Ger.†; Ciba Vision, Neth.; Ciba Vision, Switz.
Sulfadicramide (p.251·1).
Eye disorders.

Iridina Due *Montefarmaco, Ital.*
Naphazoline hydrochloride (p.1064·2).
Eye irritation.

Iridina Light *Montefarmaco, Ital.*
Benzalkonium chloride (p.1101·3).
Eye disinfection; eye irritation.

Iriflor *Tipomark, Ital.†.*
Benzalkonium chloride (p.1101·3).
Eye irritation.

Irigate *Optopics, USA.*
Sodium chloride (p.1162·2).
Eye irrigation.

Iris Med Complex *Dynamit, Aust.*
Homoeopathic preparation.

Irish Moss Cough Syrup *Bonnington, Austral.†.*
Carrageenan (p.1471·3); camphor (p.1557·2); menthol (p.1600·2).
Coughs.

Irocombivit *Schmidgall, Aust.*
Multivitamin preparation.

Irocopar *Iromedica, Switz.†.*
Carbaspirin calcium (p.25·1); paracetamol (p.72·2); caffeine (p.749·3).
Aluminium hydroxide (p.1177·3) is included in this preparation in an attempt to limit adverse effects on the gastro-intestinal mucosa.
Fever; inflammation; pain.

Irocopar cC *Schmidgall, Aust.*
Carbaspirin calcium (p.25·1); paracetamol (p.72·2); codeine phosphate sesquihydrate (p.26·1).
Pain.

Irocophan *Schmidgall, Aust.*
Carbaspirin calcium (p.25·1); paracetamol (p.72·2); caffeine (p.749·3).
Fever; pain.

Irocovit C *Schmidgall, Aust.*
Vitamin C (p.1365·2).
Vitamin C deficiency.

Iromin
Schmidgall, Aust.; Iromedica, Switz.†.
Carbaspirin calcium (p.25·1).
Fever; inflammation; pain.

Iromin Chinin C *Schmidgall, Aust.*
Carbaspirin calcium (p.25·1); quinine hydrochloride (p.439·2); ascorbic acid (p.1365·2).
Cold symptoms; fever; pain.

Iromin-G *Mission Pharmacal, USA.*
Ferrous gluconate (p.1340·1); folic acid (p.1340·3); multivitamins and minerals.
Iron-deficiency anaemias.

Iron Complex *Jamieson, Canad.*
Multivitamin and mineral preparation.

Iron Jelloids *Seton, UK.*
Ferrous fumarate (p.1339·3); vitamin B substances.
Iron deficiency.

Iron Plus
Cenovis, Austral.; Vitelle, Austral.; Swiss Herbal, Canad.
Multivitamin preparation with iron.
Tonic; vitamin and iron supplement.

Iron Tonic *Phillips Yeast, UK†.*
Yeast, iron, and vitamin preparation.

Ironax *Caber, Ital.*
Ferrous gluconate (p.1340·1).
Iron deficiency; iron-deficiency anaemia.

Ironorm *Wallace Mfg Chem., UK.*
Capsules: Dried ferrous sulphate (p.1340·2); folic acid (p.1340·3); concentrated intrinsic factor; vitamin B and C substances.
Elixir: Ferric ammonium citrate (p.1339·2); vitamins and minerals; proteolysed liver extract.
Oral drops: Ferrous sulphate (p.1340·2).
Iron deficiency.

Irontona *Brauer, Austral.*
Angelica; ascorbic acid (p.1365·2); kola (p.1645·1); ferrous sulphate (p.1340·2); hypericum (p.1590·1); ginseng (p.1584·2); urtica (p.1642·3); aurum muriaticum; calcarea phosphorica; ferrum metallicum; ferrum phosphoricum; kali phosphoricum; magnesia phosphorica; phosphoric acid.
Tonic.

Irospan *Fielding, USA.*
Ferrous sulphate (p.1340·2).
Ascorbic acid (p.1365·2) is included in this preparation to increase the absorption and availability of iron.
Iron-deficiency anaemias.

Iroviton 12 *Iromedica, Switz.†.*
Multivitamin and mineral preparation.

Irradol-A *Parke, Davis, Austral.†.*
Multivitamin and mineral preparation.

Irriclens *ConvaTec, UK.*
Sodium chloride (p.1162·2).
Wound cleansing and irrigation.

Irri-Cor *Germania, Aust.†.*
Imolamine hydrochloride (p.890·2).
Angina pectoris; cardiac stenosis; myocardial infarction; peripheral vascular disorders.

Irritos *Faes, Spain.*
Phenylpropanolamine hydrochloride (p.1067·2); dextromethorphan hydrobromide (p.1057·3).
Coughs; nasal congestion.

Irritren
Byk, Aust.; Byk, Belg.†; Tosse, Ger.; Byk, Switz.†.
Lonazolac calcium (p.50·3).
Inflammation; musculoskeletal and joint disorders; pain.

Irrodan *Biomedica, Ital.*
Buflomedil hydrochloride (p.834·2).
Cerebral and peripheral vascular disorders.

IRS 19
Note. This name is used for preparations of different composition.
Triosol, Belg.†; Solvay, Fr.; Solvay, Switz.†.
Nasal spray: Lysate of: *Diplococcus pneumoniae*; *Streptococcus*; *Micrococcus pyogenes* (Staphylococci); *Gaffkya tetragena*; *Neisseria*; *Klebsiella pneumoniae*; *Moraxella*; *Haemophilus influenzae*.
Respiratory-tract disorders.

Hefa, Ger.
Lysate of: *Diplococcus pneumoniae*; *Streptococcus pyogenes*; *Streptococcus faecalis* (*Enterococcus faecalis*) (p.1594·1); *Staphylococcus aureus*; *Branhamella catarrhalis*; *Neisseria flava*; *Neisseria perflava*; *Haemophilus influenzae*; *Klebsiella pneumoniae*; *Gaffkya tetragena*; *Moraxella*.
Respiratory-tract infections.

Solvay, Switz.†.
Sublingual tablets: Diplococcus pneumoniae; *Streptococcus* groups A, C, D, and G; *Klebsiella pneumoniae*; *Moraxella*; *Micrococcus pyogenes*; *Gaffkya tetragena*; *Branhamella catarrhalis*; *Neisseria perflava*; *Neisseria flava*; *Haemophilus influenzae*.
Respiratory-tract disorders.

Irtan *Fisons, Ger.; Rhone-Poulenc Rorer, Ger.*
Nedocromil sodium (p.756·2).
Allergic conjunctivitis; allergic rhinitis.

Irtonin *Takeda, Ital.*
Protirelin tartrate (p.1259·3).
Mental function disorders.

Irudil *Roche, Aust.*
Hirudin (p.883·1).
Peripheral vascular disorders.

Iruxol
Knoll, Ger.; Knoll, Irl.†; Knoll, Ital.
Collagenase (p.1566·3); chloramphenicol (p.182·1).
Burns; skin disorders; wounds.

Iruxol Mono
Knoll, Irl.; Knoll, S.Afr.; Knoll, Spain; Knoll, Switz.
Collagenase (p.1566·3); proteases.
Ulcers; wounds.

Iruxol Neo *Knoll, Spain.*
Collagenase (p.1566·3); neomycin sulphate (p.229·2).
Burns; ulcers; wounds.

Iruxolum mono *Ebewe, Aust.*
Enzymes from *Clostridium histolyticum*.
Necrotic ulcers; wounds.

IS 5 Mono *Ratiopharm, Ger.*
Isosorbide mononitrate (p.893·3).
Angina pectoris; heart failure; myocardial infarction; pulmonary hypertension.

Isairon *Bioindustria, Ital.*
Chondroitin sulphate–iron complex (p.1337·1).
Iron deficiency; iron-deficiency anaemias.

Iscador
Weleda, Aust.; Weleda, Ger.
Mistletoe (p.1604·1) from apple trees or oak trees.
Malignant neoplasms.

Ischelium *Polifarma, Ital.*
Co-dergocrine mesylate (p.1566·1).
Cerebral and peripheral vascular disorders; hypertension.

Ischelium Papaverina *Polifarma, Ital.*
Co-dergocrine mesylate (p.1566·1); papaverine hydrochloride (p.1614·2).
Cerebral and peripheral vascular disorders; hypertension.

Ischemol A *Farmila, Ital.*
Tetrahydrozoline hydrochloride (p.1070·2); chlorpheniramine maleate (p.405·1).
Eye disorders.

Isclofen *Isis, UK.*
Diclofenac sodium (p.31·2).
Musculoskeletal and joint disorders.

Isdin *Medice, Ger.†.*
Isosorbide dinitrate (p.893·1).
Cardiac disorders.

Isdinex *Isdin, Spain.*
Benzethonium chloride (p.1102·3); diphenhydramine hydrochloride (p.409·1).
Pruritus.

Isdinium *Isdin, Spain.*
Hydrocortisone butyrate (p.1044·1) or hydrocortisone propionate (p.1044·2).
Skin disorders.

Isdol *Isdin, Spain.*
Ibuprofen (p.44·1).
Fever; inflammation; musculoskeletal, joint, and periarticular disorders; pain.

Isepacin *Schering-Plough, Ital.*
Isepamicin sulphate (p.218·1).
Bacterial infections.

Isepalline *Schering-Plough, Fr.*
Isepamicin sulphate (p.218·1).
Bacterial infections.

Isephca S *Iso, Ger.*
Thyme (p.1636·3).
Coughs.

Isib *Ashbourne, UK.*
Isosorbide mononitrate (p.893·3).
Angina pectoris.

Isi-Calcin *ISI, Ital.*
Elcatonin (p.735·3).
Hypercalcaemia; osteoporosis; Paget's disease of bone; reflex sympathetic dystrophy.

Isicom *Desitin, Ger.*
Carbidopa (p.1136·1); levodopa (p.1137·1).
Parkinsonism.

Isiferone *ISI, Ital.*
Interferon alfa (p.615·3).
Malignant neoplasms; viral infections.

Isiflu Zonale *ISI, Ital.*
An influenza vaccine (p.1515·2).
Active immunisation.

ISI-F/2/ST *ISI, Ital.*
Amino acids.
Nutritional supplement in renal insufficiency.

Isilung *Exel, Belg.*
Eprazinone hydrochloride (p.1060·3).
Respiratory-tract disorders.

Isimoxin *ISI, Ital.*
Amoxycillin (p.151·3).
Bacterial infections.

Isisfen *Isis, UK.*
Ibuprofen (p.44·1).
Inflammation; pain.

Isitab *Agepha, Aust.*
Disinfection tablets for soft contact lenses.

Isiven *ISI, Ital.*
A normal immunoglobulin (p.1522·1).
Hypogammaglobulinaemia; idiopathic thrombocytopenic purpura; passive immunisation.

Iskedyl
Pierre Fabre, Fr.; Pierre Fabre, Spain.
Dihydroergocristine mesylate (p.1571·3); raubasine (p.941·3).
Cerebrovascular disorders; mental function disorders of the elderly.

Isla-Mint
Salus, Aust.; Engelhard, Ger.; Ceuta, UK.
Iceland moss.
Respiratory-tract disorders.

Isla-Moos *Engelhard, Ger.*
Iceland moss.
Coughs and associated respiratory-tract disorders.

Ismelin
Ciba-Geigy, Aust.; Novartis, Austral.; Ciba, Canad.†; Ciba-Geigy, Irl.†; Ciba, Neth.†; Ciba-Geigy, S.Afr.†; Ciba Vision, Switz.; Alliance, UK; Ciba, USA.
Guanethidine monosulphate (p.878·1).
Hypertension; lid retraction in exophthalmos; open-angle glaucoma.

Ismelin Esidrix *Ciba, Canad.†.*
Guanethidine monosulphate (p.878·1); hydrochlorothiazide (p.885·2).
Hypertension.

Ismeline
Ciba Vision, Fr.; Dispersa, Switz.†.
Guanethidine monosulphate (p.878·1).
Eye disorders; hypertension.

Ismipur *ISM, Ital.*
Mercaptopurine (p.546·1).
Acute leukaemia.

Ismo
Wyeth-Ayerst, Canad.; Boehringer Mannheim, Ger.; Boehringer Mannheim, Ital.; Boehringer Mannheim, Neth.; Boehringer Mannheim, Norw.; Boehringer Mannheim, S.Afr.; Europharma, Spain†; Boehringer Mannheim, Swed.; Boehringer Mannheim, Switz.; Boehringer Mannheim, UK; Wyeth-Ayerst, USA.
Isosorbide mononitrate (p.893·3).
Heart failure; ischaemic heart disease; pulmonary hypertension.

Ismotic *Alcon, USA.*
Isosorbide (p.892·3).
Raised intra-ocular pressure.

Isnaderm *Isnardi, Ital.†.*
Fluocinolone acetonide (p.1041·1).
Skin disorders.

Isnamide *Isnardi, Ital.†.*
Sulpiride (p.692·3).
Gastric ulcers; psychiatric disorders; vomiting.

Iso *Lacer, Spain.*
Isosorbide dinitrate (p.893·1).
Angina pectoris; heart failure; myocardial infarction; peripheral vascular disorders.

Iso Mack
Mack, Illert., Ger.; Boots, S.Afr.†; Mack, Switz.
Isosorbide dinitrate (p.893·1).
Angina pectoris; heart failure; myocardial infarction; pulmonary hypertension; pulmonary oedema.

Isoamitil Sedante *Hosbon, Spain†.*
Amylobarbitone (p.641·3).
Anxiety; insomnia; nervous disorders.

ISO-Augentropfen C *Iso, Ger.*
Homoeopathic preparation.

Iso-B *Tyson, USA.*
Multivitamin preparation.

Isobar *Logeais, Fr.*
Methyclothiazide (p.904·1); triamterene (p.957·2).
Hypertension.

Iso-Betadine *Asta Medica, Belg.*
Povidone-iodine (p.1123·3).
Burns; disinfection of the skin and mucous membranes; mouth and throat infections; skin infections; vulvovaginal infections; wounds.

Iso-Bid *Geriatric Pharm. Corp., USA†.*
Isosorbide dinitrate (p.893·1).
Angina pectoris.

Isobranch *Bieffe, Ital.*
L-Isoleucine (p.1349·2); L-leucine (p.1350·1); L-valine (p.1358·1).
Hepatic encephalopathy; post-trauma disorders.

Isocaine *Novocol, USA.*
Mepivacaine hydrochloride (p.1297·2).
Levonordefrin (p.1596·2) is included in some injections as a vasoconstrictor to diminish absorption and localise the effect of the local anaesthetic.
Local anaesthesia.

Isocal
Mead Johnson, Austral.; Mead Johnson, Canad.; Bristol-Myers Squibb, UK†; Mead Johnson Nutritionals, USA.
A range of preparations for enteral nutrition.

Isocard
Note. A similar name is used for preparations of different composition.
Sintesa, Belg.; Schwarz, Fr.; Eastern Pharmaceuticals, UK.
Isosorbide dinitrate (p.893·1).
Angina pectoris.

Iso-Card
Note. A similar name is used for preparations of different composition.
Triomed, S.Afr.
Verapamil hydrochloride (p.960·3).
Angina pectoris; arrhythmias; hypertension.

Isocef *Recordati, Ital.*
Ceftibuten (p.175·1).
Bacterial infections.

IsoCell *Antonetto, Ital.*
Multivitamin and mineral preparation with plant extracts.

Isocet *Rugby, USA.*
Paracetamol (p.72·2); caffeine (p.749·3); butalbital (p.644·3).

Isochinol
Schwarzhaupt, Ger.; Pharmacal, Switz.
Dimethisoquin hydrochloride (p.1292·2).
Burns; haemorrhoids; skin disorders; wounds.

Isocillin *Hoechst, Ger.*
Phenoxymethylpenicillin potassium (p.236·2).
Bacterial infections.

Isoclar *Boniscontro & Gazzone, Ital.*
Heparin sodium (p.879·3).
Thrombo-embolic disorders.

Isoclor *Ciba, USA.*
Chlorpheniramine maleate (p.405·1); pseudoephedrine hydrochloride (p.1068·3).
Cold symptoms.

Isoclor Expectorant *Fisons, USA.*
Codeine phosphate (p.26·1); pseudoephedrine hydrochloride (p.1068·3); guaiphenesin (p.1061·3).
Coughs.

Isocolan
Giuliani, Ital.; Giuliani, Switz.
Macrogol 4000 (p.1598·2); electrolytes (p.1147·1).
Bowel evacuation; constipation.

Isocom *Nutripharm, USA.*
Isometheptene mucate (p.447·3); dichloralphenazone (p.668·1); paracetamol (p.72·2).
Vascular and tension headache.

Isoday *Tillotts, Switz.*
Isosorbide dinitrate (p.893·1).
Heart failure; ischaemic heart disease; myocardial infarction.

Isodine
Faulding, Austral.; Meiji, Jpn.
Povidone-iodine (p.1123·3).
Mouth infections; skin, mucous membrane, wound, and burn disinfection.

Isodinit *Hexal, Ger.*
Isosorbide dinitrate (p.893·1).
Angina pectoris; heart failure; pulmonary hypertension.

Isodiur *Italfarmaco, Spain.*
Torasemide (p.956·3) or torasemide sodium (p.956·3).
Hypertension; oedema.

Isodril *Monot, Fr.*
Chlorhexidine gluconate (p.1107·2); phenylephrine hydrochloride (p.1066·2).
Eye disorders.

Isodrink *Volchem, Ital.*
Isotonic rehydration solution.

Iso-Eremfat *Fatol, Ger.*
Rifampicin (p.243·2); isoniazid (p.218·1).
Tuberculosis.

Isoess *Bieffe, Ital.*
Amino-acid infusion.
Parenteral nutrition in renal failure.

Isoetam *Ferrer, Spain.*
Ethambutol (p.208·2); isoniazid (p.218·1).
Pyridoxine hydrochloride (p.1362·3) is included in this preparation for the prophylaxis of peripheral neuropathy.
Tuberculosis.

Isoflurane *Abbott, UK.*
Isoflurane (p.1225·1).
Formerly available as Forane.
General anaesthesia.

Isofor *Rhone-Poulenc Rorer, S.Afr.*
Isoflurane (p.1225·1).
General anaesthesia.

isoforce *RAN, Ger.†.*
Isosorbide dinitrate (p.893·1).
Cardiac disorders.

Isofort *Bieffe, Ital.*
Amino-acid infusion.
Parenteral nutrition.

Isofra *Bouchara, Fr.*
Framycetin sulphate (p.210·3).
Bacterial infections.

Isoftal *Agepha, Aust.*
Naphazoline hydrochloride (p.1064·2).
Conjunctivitis.

Isogaine *Clarben, Spain.*
Mepivacaine hydrochloride (p.1297·2).
Local anaesthesia.

Isogel
Allen & Hanburys, Irl.†; Charwell Pharmaceuticals, UK.
Ispaghula husk (p.1194·2).
Colostomy control; constipation; diarrhoea; irritable bowel syndrome.

Isogen *Wyeth, Austral.†.*
Isosorbide dinitrate (p.893·1).
Heart failure; ischaemic heart disease.

Isoginkgo *Durachemie, Ger.*
Ginkgo biloba (p.1584·1).
Cerebral circulatory disorders.

Isoglaucon
Bender, Aust.; Basotherm, Ger.; Boehringer Ingelheim, Ital.; Boehringer Ingelheim, Spain.
Clonidine hydrochloride (p.841·2).
Glaucoma.

Isogrow *Bieffe, Ital.*
Amino-acid infusion.
Parenteral nutrition in neonates.

Isogutt *Winzer, Ger.*
Eye drops: Monobasic sodium phosphate (p.1159·3); dibasic sodium phosphate (p.1159·3).
Eye ointment†: Monobasic potassium phosphate (p.1159·3); dibasic potassium phosphate (p.1159·2).
Ocular burns.

Isogyn *Crosara, Ital.*
Isoconazole nitrate (p.381·2).
Fungal infections.

Isohes
Laevosan, Aust.; Laevosan, Switz.
Pentastarch (p.725·2).
Haemodilution; plasma volume expansion.

Iso-K *San Carlo, Ital.†.*
Ketoprofen (p.48·2).
Musculoskeletal and joint disorders.

Isoket
Gebro, Aust.; Schwarz, Ger.; Schwarz, Irl.; Sanofi Omnimed, S.Afr.; Schwarz, Switz.; Schwarz, UK.
Isosorbide dinitrate (p.893·1).
Angina pectoris; coronary spasm; heart failure; myocardial infarction; pulmonary hypertension.

Isolan *Elan, USA.*
Lactose-free, gluten-free preparation for enteral nutrition.

Isollyl Improved *Rugby, USA†.*
Aspirin (p.16·1); caffeine (p.749·3); butalbital (p.644·3).
Pain.

Isolyt *CT, Ger.*
Glucose monohydrate; sodium chloride; sodium citrate; potassium chloride (p.1152·3).
Diarrhoea; oral rehydration therapy.

Isolyte *McGaw, USA.*
A range of electrolyte infusions (p.1147·1).
Fluid and electrolyte disorders.

Isolyte with Dextrose *McGaw, USA.*
A range of electrolyte infusions with glucose (p.1147·1).
Carbohydrate source; fluid and electrolyte disorders.

Isomack *Pfizer, Aust.*
Isosorbide dinitrate (p.893·1).
Angina pectoris; heart failure; myocardial infarction; pulmonary hypertension.

Isomel *Clonmel, Irl.*
Isosorbide mononitrate (p.893·3).
Angina pectoris; heart failure.

Isomeride
Bender, Aust.†; Servier, Belg.†; Ardix, Fr.†; Servier, Ger.†; Servier, Ital.†; Servier, Neth.†; Servier, Switz.†.
Dexfenfluramine hydrochloride (p.1479·2).
Obesity.

Isomide *Monmouth, UK.*
Disopyramide (p.858·1) or disopyramide phosphate (p.858·1).
Arrhythmias.

Isomil
Abbott, Austral.; Abbott, Canad.; Abbott, Ital.; Abbott, S.Afr.†; Abbott, UK; Ross, USA.
Infant feed.
Galactosaemia; lactose intolerance; milk intolerance.

Isomil DF *Ross, USA.*
Lactose-free soy protein infant feed.
Diarrhoea.

Isomil SF *Ross, USA.*
Lactose-free, sucrose-free soy protein infant feed.
Milk intolerance; sucrose intolerance.

Isomonat *Boehringer Mannheim, Aust.*
Isosorbide mononitrate (p.893·3).
Heart failure; ischaemic heart disease; pulmonary hypertension.

Isomonit *Hexal, Ger.*
Isosorbide mononitrate (p.893·3).
Ischaemic heart disease.

Isomonoreal *Realpharma, Ger.*
Isosorbide mononitrate (p.893·3).
Angina pectoris; heart failure; myocardial infarction; pulmonary hypertension.

Isomyrtine *Schwarz, Fr.*
Pholcodine (p.1068·1); isomyrtol.
Formerly contained oxytetracycline, isomyrtol, terpineol, and pholcodine.
Coughs.

Isonefrine *Allergan, Ital.*
Phenylephrine hydrochloride (p.1066·2).
Production of mydriasis.

Isonitril *Rubio, Spain.*
Isosorbide mononitrate (p.893·3).
Angina pectoris; heart failure.

Isopap *Geneva, USA; Marsam, USA.*
Isometheptene mucate (p.447·3); dichloralphenazone (p.668·1); paracetamol (p.72·2).
Tension and vascular headaches.

Isopaque *Nycomed, Belg.*
Calcium metrizoate (p.1009·2); magnesium metrizoate (p.1009·2); meglumine metrizoate (p.1009·2); sodium metrizoate (p.1009·2).
Radiographic contrast medium.

Isopaque 350 *Nycomed, UK†.*
Calcium metrizoate (p.1009·2); magnesium metrizoate (p.1009·2); meglumine metrizoate (p.1009·2); sodium metrizoate (p.1009·2).
Radiographic contrast medium.

Isopaque Amin *Nycomed, Swed.†.*
Calcium metrizoate (p.1009·2); meglumine metrizoate (p.1009·2).
Radiographic contrast medium.

Isopaque Amin 200 *Nycomed, UK†.*
Calcium metrizoate (p.1009·2); meglumine metrizoate (p.1009·2).
Radiographic contrast medium.

Isopaque Cerebral 280 *Nycomed, UK†.*
Calcium metrizoate (p.1009·2); meglumine metrizoate (p.1009·2).
Radiographic contrast medium.

Isopaque Coronar 370 *Nycomed, UK†.*
Calcium metrizoate (p.1009·2); meglumine metrizoate (p.1009·2); sodium metrizoate (p.1009·2).
Radiographic contrast medium.

Isopaque Cysto
Nycomed Imaging, Norw.; Nycomed, Swed.; Nycomed, UK.
Calcium metrizoate (p.1009·2); magnesium metrizoate (p.1009·2); meglumine metrizoate (p.1009·2); sodium metrizoate (p.1009·2).
Radiographic contrast medium.

Isopas *Lennon, S.Afr.†.*
Pyrazinamide (p.241·1).
Tuberculosis.

Isophyl *Ego, Austral.†.*
Salicylic acid (p.1090·2).
Miliaria rubra; pruritus.

Isophyllen *Laevosan, Aust.*
Diprophylline (p.752·1).
Cardiovascular disorders; Cheyne Stokes respiration; oedema.

Isoplasmal G *Braun, Spain.*
Amino-acid, carbohydrate, and electrolyte infusion.
Parenteral nutrition.

Isopredon *Albert-Roussel, Aust.*
Fluprednisolone (p.1042·2).
Corticosteroid.

Isoprinosina *Synthelabo, Ital.*
Inosine pranobex (p.615·2).
Viral infections.

Isoprinosine
Synthelabo, Belg.; Synthelabo, Fr.; Fisons, Ger.†.
Inosine pranobex (p.615·2).
Viral infections.

Isoprochin P *Merckle, Ger.*
Propyphenazone (p.81·3).
Fever; pain.

Isoprodian
Fatol, Aust.; Fatol, Ger.; Mer-National, S.Afr.†.
Isoniazid (p.218·1); prothionamide (p.241·1); dapsone (p.199·2).
Buruli ulcer; leprosy; tuberculosis.

Isoptin
Ebewe, Aust.; Knoll, Austral.; Searle, Canad.; Knoll, Canad.; Knoll, Ger.; Knoll, Irl.; Knoll, Ital.; Knoll, Neth.; Knoll, Norw.; Knoll, S.Afr.; Meda, Swed.; Knoll, Switz.; Knoll, USA.
Verapamil hydrochloride (p.960·3).
Angina pectoris; arrhythmias; coronary spasm; heart failure; hypertension; hypertrophic cardiomyopathy; myocardial infarction.

Isoptine
Knoll, Belg.; Knoll, Fr.
Verapamil hydrochloride (p.960·3).
Angina pectoris; arrhythmias; hypertension; myocardial infarction.

Isopto Alkaline
Alcon, Irl.; Alcon, UK; Alcon, USA.
Hypromellose (p.1473·1).
Dry eyes.

Isopto B 12 *Alcon, Spain.*
Cyanocobalamin (p.1363·3).
Corneal damage.

Isopto Biotic *Alcon, Swed.*
Polymyxin B sulphate (p.239·1); neomycin sulphate (p.229·2); phenylephrine hydrochloride (p.1066·2).
Bacterial eye infections.

Isopto Carpina *Alcon, Spain.*
Pilocarpine hydrochloride (p.1396·3).
Glaucoma; reversal of mydriasis.

Isopto Carpine
Alcon, Austral.; Alcon, Belg.; Alcon, Canad.; Alcon, Irl.; Alcon, Neth.†; Alcon, Norw.; Alcon, S.Afr.; Alcon, Switz.; Alcon, UK; Alcon, USA.
Pilocarpine hydrochloride (p.1396·3).
Glaucoma; ocular hypertension; reversal of mydriasis.

Isopto Cetamide
Alcon, Belg.; Alcon, USA.
Sulphacetamide sodium (p.252·2).
Eye infections.

Isopto Cetapred
Alcon, Belg.; Alcon, Switz.†; Alcon, USA.
Prednisolone acetate (p.1048·1); sulphacetamide sodium (p.252·2).
Infected eye disorders.

Isopto Dex *Alcon-Thilo, Ger.*
Dexamethasone (p.1037·1).
Eye disorders.

Isopto Epinal
Alcon, Belg.†; Alcon, Spain†.
Adrenaline (p.813·2).
Glaucoma.

Isopto Fenicol
Alcon, Belg.†; Alcon, Spain; Alcon, Swed.
Chloramphenicol (p.182·1).
Bacterial eye infections.

Isopto Flucon
Alcon-Thilo, Ger.; Alcon, Spain.
Fluorometholone (p.1042·1).
Eye disorders.

Isopto Fluid *Alcon-Thilo, Ger.*
Hypromellose (p.1473·1).
Dry eyes.

Isopto Frin
Alcon, Austral.; Synthelabo, Belg.; Alcon, Irl.; Alcon, UK; Alcon, USA.
Phenylephrine hydrochloride (p.1066·2).
Eye fatigue; eye irritation; wetting agent for hard contact lenses.

Isopto Karbakolin *Alcon, Swed.*
Carbachol (p.1390·1).
Glaucoma.

Isopto Max *Alcon-Thilo, Ger.*
Dexamethasone (p.1037·1); neomycin sulphate (p.229·2); polymyxin B sulphate (p.239·1).
Infected eye disorders.

Isopto Maxidex
Alcon, Norw.; Alcon, Swed.
Dexamethasone (p.1037·1).
Inflammatory eye disorders.

Isopto Naturale *Alcon-Thilo, Ger.*
Dextran 70 (p.717·1); hypromellose (p.1473·1).
Dry eyes.

Isopto Pilomin *Alcon-Thilo, Ger.*
Pilocarpine hydrochloride (p.1396·3); physostigmine salicylate (p.1395·3).
Glaucoma.

Isopto Plain
Alcon, Irl.; Alcon, S.Afr.†; Alcon, Swed.; Alcon, UK; Alcon, USA.
Hypromellose (p.1473·1).
Dry eyes.

Isopto Tears
Alcon, Austral.; Alcon, Belg.; Alcon, Canad.; Alcon, Switz.; Alcon, USA.
Hypromellose (p.1473·1).
Dry eyes.

Isopulsan *Sanofi Winthrop, Spain†.*
Minaprine hydrochloride (p.298·1).
Mental function disorders.

Isopuramin *Bieffe, Ital.*
A range of amino-acid infusions.
Parenteral nutrition.

Iso-Puren *Isis Puren, Ger.*
Isosorbide dinitrate (p.893·1).
Heart failure; ischaemic heart disease.

Isoram *Bieffe, Ital.*
L-Arginine (p.1334·1); L-isoleucine (p.1349·2); L-leucine (p.1350·1); L-valine (p.1358·1).
Hepatic encephalopathy; post-trauma disorders.

Isordil
Wyeth, Austral.; Wyeth Lederle, Belg.; Wyeth-Ayerst, Canad.; Monmouth, Irl.; Wyeth, Neth.; Akromed, S.Afr.; Inibsa, Spain†; Monmouth, UK; Wyeth-Ayerst, USA.
Isosorbide dinitrate (p.893·1).
Angina pectoris; heart failure; myocardial infarction.

Isorel *Novipharm, Aust.*
Mistletoe (p.1604·1) from fir trees, apple trees or pine trees.
Malignant neoplasms.

Isoren *Bieffe, Ital.*
Amino-acid infusion.
Parenteral nutrition in renal failure.

Isorythm *Merck-Clevenot, Fr.*
Disopyramide (p.858·1) or disopyramide phosphate (p.858·1).
Arrhythmias.

Isosal *Waldheim, Aust.*
Cream: Salicylamide (p.82·3).
Topical fluid: Salicylamide (p.82·3); camphor (p.1557·2).
Musculoskeletal, joint, and peri-articular disorders; neuralgia; soft-tissue injury.

Isosarpan *Menarini, Ital.†.*
Pipratecol (p.931·3); raubasine (p.941·3).
Cerebrovascular disorders.

Isoselect *Bieffe, Ital.*
Amino-acid infusion.
Hepatic encephalopathy; parenteral nutrition.

Isosource
Sandoz Nutrition, Canad.; Sandoz Nutrition, USA.
A range of lactose-free preparations for enteral nutrition.

Isostenase *Azupharma, Ger.*
Isosorbide dinitrate (p.893·1).
Cardiac disorders.

Isotamine *ICN, Canad.*
Isoniazid (p.218·1).
Tuberculosis.

Isotard
Note. A similar name is used for preparations of different composition.
Numark, UK.
Isosorbide mononitrate (p.893·3).
Angina pectoris.

Isotard MC
Note. A similar name is used for preparations of different composition.
Novo Nordisk, Austral.
Isophane insulin injection (bovine, monocomponent) (p.322·1).
Diabetes mellitus.

Isotein HN *Sandoz Nutrition, USA.*
Lactose-free, gluten-free preparation for enteral nutrition.

Isoten *Wyeth Lederle, Belg.*
Bisoprolol fumarate (p.833·1).
Angina pectoris; cardiac hyperkinetic syndrome; hypertension.

Isotiran *Zilliken, Ital.†.*
Isobutiacilic acid.
Hyperthyroidism.

Isotol *Diaco, Ital.*
Mannitol (p.900·3).
Raised intra-ocular pressure; raised intracranial pressure.

Isotone Kochsalz *Braun, Ger.; Pharmacia Upjohn, Ger.*
Sodium chloride (p.1162·2).
Fluid and electrolyte disorders.

Isotrate
Note. This name is used for preparations of different composition.
Parke, Davis, Austral.†; Hauck, USA.
Isosorbide dinitrate (p.893·1).
Angina pectoris.

Helsinn Birex, Irl.; Bioglan, Irl.; Bioglan, UK†.
Isosorbide mononitrate (p.893·3).
Angina pectoris.

Isotrex
Stiefel, Austral.; Stiefel, Canad.; Stiefel, Fr.; Stiefel, Ger.; Stiefel, Irl.; Stiefel, Ital.; Stiefel, S.Afr.; Stiefel, UK.
Isotretinoin (p.1084·1).
Acne.

Isotrexin *Stiefel, UK.*
Isotretinoin (p.1084·1); erythromycin (p.204·1).
Acne.

Isotrim *Ghimas, Ital.*
Co-trimoxazole (p.196·3).
Bacterial infections.

Isovex *US Pharmaceutical, USA†.*
Ethaverine hydrochloride (p.1577·1).
Cerebral and peripheral ischaemia; smooth muscle spasm.

Isoviral *Lenza, Ital.†.*
Inosine pranobex (p.615·2).
Viral infections.

Isovist
Schering, Aust.; Schering, Ger.; Schering, Ital.; Schering, Neth.; Schering, Norw.; Schering, S.Afr.; Schering, Swed.; Schering, Switz.; Schering, UK.
Iotrolan (p.1008·2).
Radiographic contrast medium.

Isovit *Teofarma, Ital.†.*
Multivitamin preparation.

Isovorin
Wyeth Lederle, Aust.; Lederle, Neth.; Wyeth, S.Afr.; Cyanamid, Spain; Wyeth Lederle, Swed.; Lederle, Switz.; Wyeth, UK.
Calcium folinate (p.1342·2).
Adjunct to methotrexate and fluorouracil; folic acid deficiency; megaloblastic anaemia.

Isovue
Squibb Diagnostics, Canad.; Squibb Diagnostics, USA.
Iopamidol (p.1007·1).
Radiographic contrast medium.

Isoxapen *Imeco, Swed.†.*
Flucloxacillin sodium (p.209·2).
Bacterial infections.

Isoxyl *Inibsa, Spain†.*
Thiocarlide (p.263·1).
Pulmonary tuberculosis.

I-Soyalac *Nutricia-Loma Lindar, USA.*
Corn- and lactose-free soy protein infant feed.

Isozid *Fatol, Ger.*
Isoniazid (p.218·1).
Tuberculosis.

Isozid-compositum *Fatol, Ger.*
Isoniazid (p.218·1).
Pyridoxine hydrochloride (p.1362·3) is included in this preparation for the prophylaxis of peripheral neuropathy.
Tuberculosis.

Isozid-H *Gebro, Aust.*
Hexetidine (p.1116·1).
Skin disinfection.

Ispenoral *Rosen, Ger.*
Phenoxymethylpenicillin potassium (p.236·2).
Bacterial infections.

Isquebral *Iquinosa, Spain.*
Dihydroergocristine mesylate (p.1571·3); raubasine (p.941·3).
Cerebral trauma; vascular disorders.

Issium *Zilliken, Ital.*
Flunarizine hydrochloride (p.411·1).
Migraine; vertigo.

Istaglobina *Chinoin, Ital.†.*
A normal immunoglobulin (p.1522·1); histamine dihydrochloride (p.1587·3); sodium thiosulphate (p.996·2).
Hypersensitivity reactions.

Istamyl *Monot, Fr.*
Isothipendyl hydrochloride (p.412·2).
Hypersensitivity reactions.

Isteropac *Bracco, Switz.*
Iodamide (p.1005·2).
Contrast medium for hysterosalpingography.

Isteropac ER *Bracco, Ital.*
Meglumine iodamide (p.1005·3).
Contrast medium for hysterosalpingography.

Istin
Pfizer, Irl.; Pfizer, UK.
Amlodipine besylate (p.822·3).
Angina pectoris; hypertension.

Istopar *Disperga, Aust.*
Mineral preparation with liver extract and thiamine hydrochloride.
Iron-deficiency anaemia; tonic.

Isudrine *Boehringer Ingelheim, Fr.*
Aluminium phosphate (p.1178·3); magnesium oxide (p.1198·3).
Gastro-intestinal disorders.

Isugran *Synpharma, Aust.*
Mistletoe (p.1604·1).
Circulatory disorders.

Isuhuman Basal
Hoechst Marion Roussel, Neth.; Hoechst Marion Roussel, Swed.
Isophane insulin injection (human, emp) (p.322·1).
Diabetes mellitus.

Isuhuman Comb 25/75, 50/50 *Hoechst Marion Roussel, Swed.*
Mixtures of insulin injection (human, emp) and isophane insulin injection (human, emp) respectively in the proportions indicated (p.322·1).
Diabetes mellitus.

Isuhuman Comb 15, Comb 25, Comb 50
Hoechst Marion Roussel, Neth.
Mixtures of isophane insulin injection (human) 85%, 75% and 50% and neutral insulin injection (human) 15%, 25% and 50% respectively (p.322·1).
Diabetes mellitus.

Isuhuman Infusat
Hoechst Marion Roussel, Neth.; Hoechst Marion Roussel, Swed.
Insulin injection (human, emp) (p.322·1).
Diabetes mellitus.

Isuhuman Rapid
Hoechst Marion Roussel, Neth.; Hoechst Marion Roussel, Swed.
Insulin injection (human, emp) (p.322·1).
Diabetes mellitus.

Isuprel
Abbott, Austral.; Sanofi Winthrop, Belg.; Sanofi Winthrop, Canad.; Sanofi Winthrop, Fr.; Winthrop, Switz.†; Sanofi Winthrop, USA.
Isoprenaline hydrochloride (p.892·1).
Adams-Stokes attacks; bronchospasm; cardiac arrest; heart block; heart failure; hypovolaemic, septic, and cardiogenic shock.

Itacortone *Ghimas, Ital.†.*
Prednisolone palmitate (p.1049·1).
Ear disorders.

Itahepar *ITA, Ital.†.*
Choline orotate (p.1611·2); potassium orotate (p.1611·2); methionine (p.984·2); phosphorylcolamine; vitamins.
Liver protectant.

Italprid *Teofarma, Ital.*
Tiapride hydrochloride (p.696·1).
Alcohol withdrawal syndrome; behaviour disorders; gastro-intestinal motility disorders; headache; movement disorders.

Itax Antipoux *Pierre Fabre, Fr.*
Shampoo: Phenothrin (p.1409·2).
Topical spray: Phenothrin (p.1409·2); tetramethrin (p.1410·3); piperonyl butoxide (p.1409·3).
Pediculosis.

Itax Preventif *Pierre Fabre, Fr.*
Repellent 3535.
Head lice repellent.

ITC *Asta Medica, Belg.*
Sodium iodide (p.1493·2); potassium iodide (p.1493·1); calcium chloride (p.1155·1); sodium thiosulphate (p.996·2).
Cataracts.

Itch-X *Ascher, USA.*
Pramoxine hydrochloride (p.1298·2); benzyl alcohol (p.1103·3).
Local anaesthesia.

Item Antipoux *Gandhour, Fr.*
Lotion; shampoo: Phenothrin (p.1409·2).
Pediculosis.

Item Repulsif Antipoux *Gandhour, Fr.*
Topical spray: Diethyltoluamide (p.1405·1).
Head lice repellent.

Iteor *Pierre Fabre Sante, Fr.*
A range of vitamin and mineral preparations.

Itinerol B_6 *Vifor, Switz.*
Meclozine hydrochloride (p.413·3); pyridoxine hydrochloride (p.1362·3); caffeine (p.749·3).
Nausea; vomiting.

Itorex *Parekh, Ital.*
Cefuroxime sodium (p.177·1).
Bacterial infections.

Itridal *Asta Medica, Ger.†.*
Prothipendyl hydrochloride (p.689·2); cyclobarbitone calcium (p.660·2).
Agitation; sleeplessness.

Itrin *Abbott, Ital.*
Terazosin hydrochloride (p.952·1).
Hypertension.

Itrop
Bender, Aust.; Boehringer Ingelheim, Ger.; Boehringer Ingelheim, Switz.†.
Ipratropium bromide (p.754·2).
Arrhythmias; bradycardia.

ituran *Promonta, Ger.†.*
Nitrofurantoin (p.231·3).
Urinary-tract infections.

Iuvacor *Inverni della Beffa, Ital.*
Ubidecarenone (p.1641·2).
Cardiac disorders; co-enzyme Q_{10} deficiency.

Ivacin *Wyeth Lederle, Swed.*
Piperacillin sodium (p.237·2).
Bacterial infections.

Ivadal
Synthelabo, Aust.; Cipharm, Fr.; Vita, Ital.
Zolpidem tartrate (p.698·3).
Insomnia.

I-Valex *Ross, USA.*
A range of leucine-free preparations for enteral nutrition including an infant feed.
Leucine catabolism disorders.

Ivamix *Pharmacia Upjohn, Norw.*
Amino-acid and lipid (from soya oil (p.1355·1)) infusion.
Parenteral nutrition.

Ivarest
Note. This name is used for preparations of different composition.
Blistex, Canad.†.
Calamine (p.1080·1); benzocaine (p.1286·2).
Pruritus.
Blistex, USA.
Calamine (p.1080·1); diphenhydramine hydrochloride (p.409·1).
Formerly contained calamine and benzocaine.
Minor skin irritation.

Iveegam
Immuno, Canad.†; Immuno, USA†.
A normal immunoglobulin (p.1522·1).
Hypogammaglobulinaemia; passive immunisation.

Ivel Schlaf *Knoll, Ger.*
Valerian (p.1643·1); lupulus (p.1597·2).
Restlessness; sleep disorders.

Ivelip
Clintec, Fr.; Clintec, Ital.; Clintec, Spain; Baxter, UK.
Soya oil (p.1355·1).
Contains egg lecithin.
Lipid infusion for parenteral nutrition.

Ivemix *Clintec, Fr.*
Amino-acid, lipid (from soya oil (p.1355·1)), and glucose infusion.
Contains egg lecithin.
Parenteral nutrition.

Ivepaque *Nycomed, Fr.*
Iopentol (p.1007·2).
Radiographic contrast medium.

Iversal *Bayer, Ger.†.*
Ambazone (p.1101·2).
Inflammatory disorders of the oropharynx.

Iversal-A cum anaesthetico *Bayer, Ger.†.*
Ambazone (p.1101·2); propyl hydroxybenzoate (p.1117·2).
Painful inflammation of the oropharynx.

Ivisol *Winthrop, Belg.†.*
Chlorocresol (p.1110·3); clorophene (p.1111·2).
Disinfection of instruments.

Ivracain *Sintetica, Switz.*
Chloroprocaine hydrochloride (p.1289·1).
Local anaesthesia.

Ivy Block *Enviroderm, USA.*
Bentoquatam (p.1079·2).
Prophylaxis against poison ivy-, oak-, or sumac-induced contact dermatitis.

Ivy-Chex *JMI, USA.*
Polyvinylpyrrolidone vinylacetate copolymers; methyl salicylate (p.55·2).
Minor skin irritation.

Ivy-Rid *Roberts, USA.*
Polyvinylpyrrolidone vinylacetate copolymers.
Minor skin irritation.

Ixertol *Cimex, Switz.†.*
Cinnarizine (p.406·1).
Peripheral and cerebral vascular disorders.

Ixoten
Asta Medica, Aust.; Asta Medica, Ger.; Schering, Ital.†.
Trofosfamide (p.568·2).
Malignant neoplasms.

Izacef *Intramed, S.Afr.*
Cephazolin sodium (p.181·1).
Bacterial infections.

Jaa Pyral *Jaapharm, Canad.*
Pyrantel embonate (p.109·3).

Jaaps Health Salt *Roche Consumer, UK.*
Sodium bicarbonate (p.1153·2); tartaric acid (p.1634·3); sodium potassium tartrate (p.1213·3).
Constipation; dyspepsia.

Jabon Antiseptico Asens *Asens, Spain.*
Hexachlorophane (p.1115·2).
Skin disinfection.

Jabon Borico *Imba, Spain†.*
Boric acid (p.1554·2).
Skin disinfection.

Jabon de Ictiol *Perez Gimenez, Spain†.*
Ichthammol (p.1083·3).
Skin disorders.

Jabon Fenicado *Perez Gimenez, Spain†.*
Phenol (p.1121·2).
Skin disinfection.

Jabon Oxician Merc *Imba, Spain†.*
Mercuric oxycyanide (p.1602·2).
Skin disinfection.

Jack and Jill Children's Formula Cough Syrup *Buckley, Canad.*
Dextromethorphan hydrobromide (p.1057·3); chlorpheniramine maleate (p.405·1).
Formerly known as Jack and Jill Children's DM Formula Cough Liquid.
Cold symptoms; coughs.

Jack and Jill Cough Syrup *Buckley, Canad.*
Guaiphenesin (p.1061·3); mepyramine maleate (p.414·1).
Cold symptoms; coughs.

Jack & Jill Rub *Buckley, Canad.*
Camphor (p.1557·2); menthol (p.1600·2); cineole (p.1564·1).
Cold symptoms.

Jackson's All Fours *Waterhouse, UK.*
Guaiphenesin (p.1061·3).
Coughs.

Jackson's Children's Cough Pastilles *Ernest Jackson, UK.*
Ipecacuanha (p.1062·2); squill (p.1070·1); citric acid (p.1564·3); honey (p.1345·3).
Coughs.

Jackson's Febrifuge *Waterhouse, UK.*
Sodium salicylate (p.85·1).
Cold symptoms; musculoskeletal and joint disorders.

Jacosulfon *Giulini, Ger.†.*
Ointment: Sulphanilamide (p.256·3); sulphapyridine (p.256·3); sulphaguanidine (p.254·1); urea (p.1095·2); cod-liver oil (p.1337·3).
Topical powder: Sulphanilamide (p.256·3); sulphapyridine (p.256·3); sulphaguanidine (p.254·1); urea (p.1095·2).
Infected skin disorders; wounds.

Jacutin
Merck, Aust.; Hermal, Ger.; Hermal, Neth.†; Hermal, Switz.
Lindane (p.1407·2).
Pediculosis; scabies.

Jacutin N *Hermal, Ger.*
Bioallethrin (p.1402·3); piperonyl butoxide (p.1409·3).
Pediculosis.

Jaikal *S & K, Ger.*
Sodium thiosulphate (p.996·2); salicylic acid (p.1090·2); resorcinol (p.1090·1).
Acne.

Jaikin N *Basotherm, Ger.*
Dimethicone (p.1384·2).
Acne.

Jalapa comp *Pfluger, Ger.*
Homoeopathic preparation.

Jalovis *Coli, Ital.*
Injection†: Hyaluronidase (p.1588·1).
Extension of local anaesthesia; improve absorption of subcutaneous or intramuscular injections; re-absorption of physiological fluids.
Ointment: Hyaluronidase (p.1588·1); chlorhexidine hydrochloride (p.1107·2).
Bruising; chilblains; haemorrhoids; skin ulceration; wounds.

Jaluran *Bioindustria, Ital.*
Hyaluronidase (p.1588·1).
Facilitates subcutaneous absorption of drugs.

Jamaica Sarsaparilla *Potter's, UK.*
Sarsaparilla root (p.1627·2); capsicum (p.1559·2); liquorice (p.1197·1); peppermint oil (p.1208·1).
Skin disorders.

Jamylene *Theraplix, Fr.*
Docusate sodium (p.1189·3).
Constipation.

Janimine *Abbott, USA.*
Imipramine hydrochloride (p.289·2).
Depression; nocturnal enuresis.

Janopen *Martin, Spain†.*
Metampicillin sodium (p.224·3).
Bacterial infections.

Japan Freeze-Dried Tuberculin *Vaccina, S.Afr.*
Tuberculin purified protein derivative (p.1640·2).
Tuberculosis test.

Japanol *Liebermann, Ger.*
Mint oil (p.1604·1).
Cold symptoms; dyspepsia; myalgia.

Jarabe Manceau *Alcor, Spain.*
Senna (p.1212·2); coriander (p.1567·3); matricaria (p.1561·2).
Constipation.

Jarabe Manzanas Siken *Diafarm, Spain.*
Senna (p.1212·2); coriander (p.1567·3); prune (p.1209·2); frangula (p.1193·2); fennel (p.1579·1).
Constipation.

Jardin *Rolab, S.Afr.*
Dothiepin hydrochloride (p.283·1).
Depression.

Jarsin *Lichtwer, Ger.*
Hypericum (p.1590·1).
Depression.

Jasicholin N *Bolder, Ger.*
Butinoline phosphate (p.1555·3); dimethicone (p.1213·1).
Gastro-intestinal disorders.

Jasimenth CN *Bolder, Ger.*
Dequalinium chloride (p.1112·1); ascorbic acid (p.1365·2).
Inflammatory disorders and infections of the oropharynx.

Jasivita *Bolder, Ger.†.*
Di-isopropylammonium dichloroacetate (p.854·1); inositol nicotinate (p.891·3); pentetrazol (p.1484·2); vitamin A acetate (p.1359·2); octotiamine (p.1360·3); pyridoxine phosphate (p.1363·1); alpha tocopheryl acetate (p.1369·1).
Atherosclerosis; hyperlipidaemias; intermittent claudication; peripheral, coronary, and cerebral vascular disorders.

Jatamansin *Medice, Ger.†.*
Rhiz. nardostachys jat.; silybum marianum (p.993·3); aesculus (p.1543·3); hamamelis (p.1587·1); chelidonium; arnica (p.1550·3); melilotus officinalus; liquorice (p.1197·1); pholedrine sulphate (p.930·2); trimethylhesperidin chalcone (p.1580·2); hordenine sulphate; sparteine sulphate (p.1632·1); thiamine nitrate; cyanocobalamin; calcium gluconate; ferrous gluconate; magnesium gluconate dihydrate.
Vascular disorders.

Jatroneural
Procter & Gamble, Aust.; Procter & Gamble, Ger.
Trifluoperazine hydrochloride (p.697·3).
Anxiety disorders.

Jatropur *Procter & Gamble, Ger.*
Triamterene (p.957·2).
Oedema.

Jatrosom *Rohm, Aust.†.*
Tranylcypromine sulphate (p.308·2); trifluoperazine hydrochloride (p.697·3).
Depression.

Jatrosom N *Procter & Gamble, Ger.*
Tranylcypromine sulphate (p.308·2).
Formerly contained tranylcypromine sulphate and trifluoperazine hydrochloride.
Depression.

Jatrox *Procter & Gamble, Ger.*
Bismuth salicylate (p.1180·1).
Gastritis; peptic ulcer; traveller's diarrhoea.

Jecobiase *Pionneau, Fr.*
Sodium sulphate (p.1213·3); sodium citrate (p.1153·2); sodium bicarbonate (p.1153·2); magnesium chloride (p.1157·2).
Gastro-intestinal disorders.

Jecoderm *Nycomed, Norw.†.*
Zinc oxide (p.1096·2); cod-liver oil (p.1337·3).
Cracked skin; minor burns; minor wounds.

Jecopeptol *SmithKline Beecham, Fr.*
Aluminium hydroxide (p.1177·3); calcium carbonate (p.1182·1); magnesium hydroxide (p.1198·2); sodium bicarbonate (p.1153·2); boldo (p.1554·1); kinkeliba (p.1593·2); euonymus (p.1192·1).
Digestive disorders.

Jectofer
Astra, Aust.; Astra, Canad.; Astra, Ger.; Astra, Irl.; Astra, Neth.; Astra, Norw.; Astra, Swed.; Astra, UK.
Iron sorbitol (p.1349·1).
Iron deficiency; iron-deficiency anaemia.

Jedipin *Jenapharm, Ger.*
Nifedipine (p.916·2).
Hypertension; ischaemic heart disease; Raynaud's syndrome.

Jellin *Grunenthal, Ger.*
Fluocinolone acetonide (p.1041·1).
Skin disorders.

Jellin polyvalent *Grunenthal, Ger.*
Fluocinolone acetonide (p.1041·1); neomycin sulphate (p.229·2); nystatin (p.386·1).
Skin disorders with bacterial or fungal infection.

Jellin-Neomycin *Grunenthal, Ger.*
Fluocinolone acetonide (p.1041·1); neomycin sulphate (p.229·2).
Infected skin disorders.

Jellisoft *Grunenthal, Ger.*
Fluocinolone acetonide (p.1041·1).
Skin disorders.

Jellisoft-Neomycin *Grunenthal, Ger.*
Fluocinolone acetonide (p.1041·1); neomycin sulphate (p.229·2).
Infected skin disorders.

Jelonet
Smith & Nephew, Austral.; Smith & Nephew, Fr.; Smith & Nephew, Ital.; Smith & Nephew, S.Afr.; Smith & Nephew, UK.
Soft paraffin (p.1382·3).
Wound dressing.

Jemalt 13+13 *Wander Health Care, Switz.*
Multivitamin and mineral preparation.

Jenabroxol *Jenapharm, Ger.*
Ambroxol hydrochloride (p.1054·3).
Respiratory disorders associated with viscous or excessive mucus.

Jenabroxol comp *Jenapharm, Ger.*
Doxycycline hydrochloride (p.202·3); ambroxol hydrochloride (p.1054·3).
Respiratory-tract infections.

Jenacard *Jenapharm, Ger.*
Isosorbide dinitrate (p.893·1).
Angina pectoris; heart failure; pulmonary hypertension.

Jenacillin A *Jenapharm, Ger.*
Benzylpenicillin sodium (p.159·3); procaine penicillin (p.240·2).
Bacterial infections.

Jenacillin O *Jenapharm, Ger.*
Procaine penicillin (p.240·2).
Bacterial infections.

Jenacillin V *Jenapharm, Ger.*
Phenoxymethylpenicillin potassium (p.236·2).
Bacterial infections.

Jenacyclin *Jenapharm, Ger.*
Doxycycline (p.202·3).
Bacterial infections.

Jenacysteine *Jenapharm, Ger.*
Acetylcysteine (p.1052·3).
Respiratory disorders associated with viscous or excessive mucus.

Jenafenac *Jenapharm, Ger.*
Diclofenac sodium (p.31·2).
Inflammation; musculoskeletal and joint disorders.

Jenamazol *Jenapharm, Ger.*
Clotrimazole (p.376·3).
Corynebacterium infections; fungal infections.

Jenametidin *Jenapharm, Ger.*
Cimetidine (p.1183·2).
Aspiration syndrome; gastro-oesophageal reflux; peptic ulcer; Zollinger-Ellison syndrome.

Jenamicin *Hauck, USA†.*
Gentamicin sulphate (p.212·1).
Bacterial infections.

Jenamoxazol *Jenapharm, Ger.*
Co-trimoxazole (p.196·3).
Bacterial infections.

Jenampin *Jenapharm, Ger.*
Ampicillin trihydrate (p.153·2).
Bacterial infections.

Jenapamil *Jenapharm, Ger.*
Verapamil hydrochloride (p.960·3).
Angina pectoris; hypertension; tachycardia.

Jenapirox *Jenapharm, Ger.*
Piroxicam (p.80·2).
Musculoskeletal and joint disorders.

Jenaprofen *Jenapharm, Ger.*
Ibuprofen (p.44·1).
Fever; gout; inflammation; musculoskeletal and joint disorders; pain.

Jenapurinol *Jenapharm, Ger.*
Allopurinol (p.390·2).
Gout; hyperuricaemia; renal calculi.

Jenaspiron *Jenapharm, Ger.*
Spironolactone (p.946·1).
Ascites; hyperaldosteronism; hypertension; oedema.

Jenatacin *Jenapharm, Ger.*
Indomethacin (p.45·2).
Gout; musculoskeletal, joint, and soft-tissue disorders; pain.

Jenatenol *Jenapharm, Ger.*
Atenolol (p.825·3).
Arrhythmias; hypertension; ischaemic heart disease.

Jenateren comp *Jenapharm, Ger.*
Triamterene (p.957·2); hydrochlorothiazide (p.885·2).
Heart failure; hypertension; oedema.

Jenest *Organon, USA.*
21 Tablets, norethisterone (p.1453·1); ethinyloestradiol (p.1445·1); 7 tablets, inert.
Biphasic oral contraceptive.

Jenoxifen *Jenapharm, Ger.*
Tamoxifen citrate (p.563·3).
Breast cancer.

Jephagynon *Jenapharm, Ger.*
Oestradiol benzoate (p.1455·1); progesterone (p.1459·3).
Amenorrhoea.

Jephoxin *Jenapharm, Ger.*
Amoxycillin (p.151·3) or amoxycillin trihydrate (p.151·3).
Bacterial infections.

Jeprolol *Jenapharm, Ger.*
Metoprolol tartrate (p.907·3).
Cardiac disorders; hypertension; migraine.

Jeridin *Berk, UK.*
Isosorbide dinitrate (p.893·1).
Angina pectoris; heart failure.

Jestryl *ankerpharm, Ger.*
Carbachol (p.1390·1).
Glaucoma; production of miosis.

Jets *Freeda, USA.*
Multivitamin preparation with lysine.

JE-Vax
Connaught, Canad.; Connaught, USA.
A Japanese encephalitis vaccine (p.1510·1).
Active immunisation.

Jevity
Abbott, Austral.; Abbott, Canad.; Abbott, Irl.; Ross, UK; Ross, USA.
Preparation for enteral nutrition.

Jexin *Medeva, UK†.*
Tubocurarine chloride (p.1322·3).
Competitive neuromuscular blocker.

Jezil *Alphapharm, Austral.*
Gemfibrozil (p.1273·3).
Hyperlipidaemias.

JHP Rodler Japanisches Heilpflanzenol *Rodler, Ger.*
Mint oil (p.1604·1).
Herbal preparation.

Jiffy Corn Plasters *Brovar, S.Afr.†.*
Salicylic acid (p.1090·2).
Calluses; corns; warts.

Jiffy Toothache Drops *Block, Canad.*
Benzocaine (p.1286·2); eugenol (p.1578·2).
Toothache.

Jodetten *Henning, Ger.*
Potassium iodide (p.1493·1).
Iodine-deficiency disorders.

Jodid *Merck, Ger.*
Potassium iodide (p.1493·1).
Iodine-deficiency disorders.

Jodlauge, Tolzer *Jodquellen, Ger.*
Anions: chloride, bromide, iodide, bicarbonate; cations: sodium, magnesium, potassium, calcium.
Circulatory disorders.

jodminerase *GN, Ger.*
Potassium iodide (p.1493·1).
Iodine-deficiency disorders.

Jodobac *Bode, Ger.*
Povidone-iodine (p.1123·3).
Catheter care; disinfection of the skin, mucous membranes, and hands; wounds.

Jodo-Calcio-Vitaminico *Bruschettini, Ital.*
Sodium iodide (p.1493·2); potassium iodide (p.1493·1); rubidium iodide (p.1626·3); calcium gluconate (p.1155·2); ascorbic acid (p.1365·2).
Eye disorders.

Jodocur *Farmacologico Milanese, Ital.*
Povidone-iodine (p.1123·3).
Disinfection of skin, wounds, and burns; mouth and throat infections; vaginal hygiene.

Jodoform *Lohmann, Ger.*
Iodoform (p.1118·2).
Wounds.

Jodogard *Gedis, Ital.*
Povidone-iodine (p.1123·3).
Skin and hand disinfection.

Jodonorm *Sandoz, Aust.*
Sodium iodide (p.1493·2).
Iodine-deficiency goitre.

Jodoplex *Streuli, Switz.*
Povidone-iodine (p.1123·3).
Burns; infected skin disorders; skin, hand, and mucous-membrane disinfection; ulcers; wounds.

Jodquellsalz, Tolzer *Jodquellen, Ger.†.*
Cations: sodium, potassium, magnesium, calcium; anions: chloride, bromide, iodide, bicarbonate.
Circulatory disorders.

Jodthyrox
Merck, Aust.; Merck, Ger.
Thyroxine sodium (p.1497·1); potassium iodide (p.1493·1).
Endemic goitre; iodine-deficiency disorders.

Jofurol *Upjohn, Spain†.*
Celiprolol hydrochloride (p.838·3).
Angina pectoris; hypertension.

Joggers *Solgar, UK.*
Multivitamin and mineral preparation with bee pollen and ginseng.

Joghurt Milkitten
Note. This name is used for preparations of different composition.
Apotheke Roten Krebs, Aust.
Yogurt; lactose (p.1349·3); senna (p.1212·2); fruit paste (plums and figs); wheat germ oil.
Constipation.

Medopharm, Ger.†.
Fruit paste (plums and figs); yogurt concentrate; senna (p.1212·2).
Constipation.

Johanniskrautol mit Lecithin *Twardy, Ger.*
Hypericum oil (p.1590·1); soya lecithin (p.1595·2).
Nervous disorders.

John Plunkett's Forte Maxiblock Sunscreen *Sunspot, Austral.†.*
Benzophenone; padimate O (Escalol 507) (p.1488·1).
Sunscreen.

John Plunkett's Protective Day Cream *Sunspot, Austral.*
Elastin; collagen (p.1566·3); vitamin A (p.1358·1); Dermasome SOD; Dermasome E; Megasol Complex; oxybenzone (p.1487·3); ethylhexyl*p*methoxycinnamate (p.1487·1).
Formerly contained elastin, collagen, vitamin A, Dermasome SOD, Dermasome E, and Megasol Complex.
Emollient; sunscreen.

John Plunkett's Sunspot Cream *Sunspot, Austral.†.*
Salicylic acid (p.1090·2).
Hard dry skin; solar keratosis.

John Plunkett's Super Wrinkle Cream *Sunspot, Austral.*
Active soluble elastin; active soluble collagen (p.1566·3).
Dry skin; wrinkles.

John Plunkett's Vita-Pore *Sunspot, Austral.*
Soluble bio-sulphur CLR (p.1091·2); vitamin B; hamamelis (p.1587·1).
Oily skin.

Johnson's Antiseptic Powder *Pharmedica, S.Afr.*
Benzethonium chloride (p.1102·3).
Skin disorders.

Johnson's Baby Nappy Rash Ointment *Pharmedica, S.Afr.*
Zinc oxide (p.1096·2).
Napkin rash.

Johnson's Baby Sunblock
Johnson & Johnson, Canad.†; Johnson & Johnson, USA.
SPF 15: Zinc oxide (p.1096·2); titanium dioxide (p.1093·3).
Sunscreen.

Johnson & Johnson, Canad.†; Johnson & Johnson, USA.
SPF 30: Oxybenzone (p.1487·3); ethylhexyl *p*-methoxycinnamate (p.1487·1) octyl salicylate (p.1487·3); titanium dioxide (p.1093·3).
Sunscreen.

Johnson's Baby Sunblock Broad Spectrum
Johnson & Johnson, Austral.
SPF15+: Ethylhexyl *p*-methoxycinnamate (p.1487·1); oxybenzone (p.1487·3); octyl salicylate (p.1487·3); avobenzone (p.1486·3).
Sunscreen.

Johnson's Clean & Clear Daily Facial Moisturiser *Johnson & Johnson, Austral.*
SPF 15+: Salicylic acid (p.1090·2); ethylhexyl *p*-methoxycinnamate (p.1487·1); 3-(4-methylbenzylidene)bornan-2-one (p.1487·2); avobenzone (p.1486·3).
Moisturiser; sunscreen.

Johnson's Clean & Clear Foaming Facial Wash *Johnson & Johnson, Austral.*
Triclosan (p.1127·2).
Acne; soap substitute.

Johnson's Clean & Clear Invisible Blemish Treatment *Johnson & Johnson, Austral.*
Salicylic acid (p.1090·2); alcohol (p.1099·1).
Acne.

Johnson's Clean & Clear Medicated Cleansing Bar *Johnson & Johnson, Austral.*
Triclosan (p.1127·2).
Acne.

Johnson's Clean & Clear Oil Controlling Toner *Johnson & Johnson, Austral.*
Salicylic acid (p.1090·2); alcohol (p.1099·1).
Acne.

Johnson's Clean & Clear Skin Balancing Moisturiser *Johnson & Johnson, Austral.*
Salicylic acid (p.1090·2).
Acne.

Johnson's Penaten Crema Disinfettante *Johnson & Johnson, Ital.*
Cetylpyridinium chloride (p.1106·2).
Nappy rash.

Joint & Muscle Complex *Brauer, Austral.*
Homoeopathic preparation.

Joint & Muscle Oral Spray and Tablets *Brauer, Austral.*
Homoeopathic preparation.

Joint & Muscle Relief Cream *Brauer, Austral.*
Homoeopathic preparation.

Jomax *Hexal, Ger.*
Bufexamac (p.22·2).
Skin disorders.

Jomethid *Cox, UK.*
Ketoprofen (p.48·2).
Gout; musculoskeletal, joint, and peri-articular disorders; pain.

Jonctum *Marion Merrell, Fr.*
Oxaceprol (p.1611·3).
Burns; keloids; leg ulcers; rheumatic disorders.

Jonil T *Galderma, Switz.*
Coal tar (p.1092·3); salicylic acid (p.1090·2); benzalkonium chloride (p.1101·3).
Scalp disorders.

Jonosteril *Fresenius, Ger.*
A range of electrolyte infusions with or without carbohydrate (p.1147·1).
Fluid and electrolyte disorders.

Jonozell *Fresenius, Ger.†.*
Electrolyte and trace element infusion with sorbitol (p.1147·1).
Electrolyte disorders.

Jopamiro *Gerot, Aust.*
Iopamidol (p.1007·1).
Radiographic contrast medium.

Jopinol *Bernhauer, Aust.*
Iodine (p.1493·1); pumilio pine oil (p.1623·3).
Catarrh.

Jorkil *Bohm, Spain.*
Silicone (p.1213·1); metoclopramide hydrochloride (p.1200·3); levoglutamide (p.1344·3); aluminium glycinate (p.1177·2); mannitol (p.900·3).
Dyspepsia; meteorism.

Josacine
Bellon, Fr.; Mack, Switz.
Josamycin (p.220·2) or josamycin propionate (p.220·2).
Bacterial infections.

Josalid *Biochemie, Aust.*
Josamycin (p.220·2).
Bacterial infections; toxoplasmosis.

Josamina *Novag, Spain.*
Josamycin (p.220·2) or josamycin propionate (p.220·2).
Bacterial infections.

Josamy *Yamanouchi, Jpn.*
Josamycin propionate (p.220·2).
Bacterial infections.

Josaxin
UCB, Ital.; Yamanouchi, Spain.
Josamycin (p.220·2) or josamycin propionate (p.220·2).
Bacterial infections.

Jossalind *Hexal, Ger.*
Sodium hyaluronate (p.1630·3).
Ulcers; wounds.

Jossathromb *Jossa-Arznei, Ger.†.*
Mixture: Castan.; hamamelis (p.1587·1); ascorbic acid; calcium gluconate; pulsatilla; nux vomica; camphora; rutoside sodium sulphate (p.1580·2).
Tablets: Aesculus (p.1543·3); rutoside sodium sulphate (p.1580·2); thiamine hydrochloride.
Topical gel: Aescin (p.1543·3); camphor (p.1557·2); heparin sodium (p.879·3); hamamelis (p.1587·1).
Vascular disorders.

Jouvence *Carmaran, Canad.*
Hydroquinone (p.1083·1).

Jouvence de l'Abbe Soury *Chefaro Ardeval, Fr.*
Hamamelis (p.1587·1); calamus (p.1556·1); piscidia; viburnum.
Peripheral vascular disorders.

Jowidarmin *Hanosan, Ger.†.*
Homoeopathic preparation.

Joy-Rides *Stafford-Miller, UK.*
Hyoscine hydrobromide (p.462·3).
Motion sickness.

Jsoskleran *Iso, Ger.*
Homoeopathic preparation.

Jsostoma *Iso, Ger.*
Homoeopathic preparation.

JuBronchan C *Jukunda, Ger.*
Homoeopathic preparation.

JuCholan S *Jukunda, Ger.*
Silybum marianum (p.993·3); hypericum (p.1590·1); taraxacum (p.1634·2); peppermint leaf (p.1208·1); cheldionium.
Liver and biliary-tract disorders.

JuCor *Jukunda, Ger.*
Homoeopathic preparation.

Jucurba N *Strathmann, Ger.*
Harpagophytum procumbens (p.27·2).
Musculoskeletal and joint disorders.

JuCystan S *Jukunda, Ger.*
Homoeopathic preparation.

Judolor
Note. This name is used for preparations of different composition.
Nycomed, Aust.†; Woelm, Ger.†.
Tablets: Fursultiamine (p.1360·3).
Myalgia; neuralgia; neuritis; vitamin B deficiency.

Woelm, Ger.†.
Ointment: Bentiamine lauryl sulphate; benzyl nicotinate (p.22·1).
Myalgia; neuralgia; neuritis.

Judolor comp. N *Woelm, Ger.†.*
Paracetamol (p.72·2); fursultiamine (p.1360·3).
Musculoskeletal and joint disorders; neuralgia; neuritis; pain.

JuDorm *Jukunda, Ger.*
Lupulus (p.1597·2); melissa (p.1600·1); valerian (p.1643·1); hypericum (p.1590·1).
Insomnia; stress.

JuGrippan *Jukunda, Ger.*
Echinacea (p.1574·2); centaury (p.1561·1); chamomile (p.1561·2); calendula officinalus; hamamelis; achillea; ysop; arnica; bryonia; aconit; belladonna; ferrum phos.; kalium chloratum; silicea; ammonium carb.
Cold symptoms.

JuHepan *Jukunda, Ger.*
Homoeopathic preparation.

JuLax S *Jukunda, Ger.*
Senna (p.1212·2).
Constipation.

JuMenstran *Jukunda, Ger.*
Homoeopathic preparation.

Jumex
Sanofi Winthrop, Aust.; Chiesi, Ital.
Selegiline hydrochloride (p.1144·2).
Parkinsonism.

Jumexal *Sanofi Winthrop, Switz.*
Selegiline hydrochloride (p.1144·2).
Parkinsonism.

Junamac *Cantassium Co., UK.*
Multivitamin and mineral preparation.

Junce *Inibsa, Spain.*
Ascorbic acid (p.1365·2).
Adjunct in treatment of iron supplementation; vitamin C deficiency.

JuNeuron S *Jukunda, Ger.*
Scopolaminum hydrobromic.; avena sativa; valerian (p.1643·1); passion flower (p.1615·3); lupulus (p.1597·2); hypericum (p.1590·1); melissa (p.1600·1).
Insomnia; nervousness.

Jungle Formula Insect Repellent *Chefaro, UK.*
Diethyltoluamide (p.1405·1).

Jungle Formula Insect Repellent Plus U.V. Sunscreens *Chefaro, UK.*
Padimate O (p.1488·1); oxybenzone (p.1487·3); diethyltoluamide (p.1405·1).

Jungle Formula Sting Relief Cream *Chefaro, UK.*
Hydrocortisone (p.1043·3).
Insect bites and stings.

Junicol Junior *Nelson, Austral.†.*
Phenylephrine hydrochloride (p.1066·2); pholcodine (p.1068·1); paracetamol (p.72·2); chlorpheniramine maleate (p.405·1).
Coughs and cold symptoms.

Junicol V *Nelson, Austral.†.*
Phenylephrine hydrochloride (p.1066·2); pholcodine (p.1068·1); paracetamol (p.72·2).
Coughs and cold symptoms.

Junifen
Salus, Aust.†; Boots Healthcare, Belg.; Crookes Healthcare, UK.
Ibuprofen (p.44·1).
Fever; inflammation; pain.

Junior Disprol *Reckitt & Colman, Austral.†.*
Paracetamol (p.72·2).
Fever; pain.

Junior Ideal Quota *Cantassium Co., UK.*
Multivitamin and mineral preparation.

Junior Kao-C *Torbet Laboratories, UK.*
Calcium carbonate (p.1182·1); light kaolin (p.1195·1).
Diarrhoea.

Junior Strength Cold DM *WestCan, Canad.*
Pseudoephedrine hydrochloride (p.1068·3); chlorpheniramine maleate (p.405·1); dextromethorphan hydrobromide (p.1057·3); paracetamol (p.72·2).

Junior Time C *Vitaplex, Austral.*
Vitamin C substances (p.1365·2).

Juniormen *Retrain, Spain.*
Nicametate; ginseng; pyritinol; rutin; vitamins; deanol acid tartrate.
Tonic.

Juniorvit *Pharmadass, UK.*
Multivitamin and mineral preparation.

Juniperus-Komplex-Injektopas *Pascoe, Ger.*
Homoeopathic preparation.

Junisana *Hotz, Ger.*
Althaea (p.1546·3); thyme (p.1636·3); guajacum; liquorice (p.1197·1); iron(III)-sucrose-complex; juniper (p.1592·2); calcium lactate (p.1155·2).
Bronchitis; catarrh; coughs.

Juno Junipah *Torbet Laboratories, UK.*
Oral powders: Sodium sulphate (p.1213·3); sodium phosphate (p.1159·3); sodium bicarbonate (p.1153·2); juniper oil (p.1592·3).
Tablets: Sodium sulphate (p.1213·3); sodium chloride (p.1162·2); sodium phosphate (p.1159·3); phenolphthalein (p.1208·2); juniper oil (p.1592·3).
Constipation.

JuPhlebon S *Jukunda, Ger.*
Melilotus; scoparium (p.1628·1); aesculus (p.1543·3); hamamelis; cuprum aceticum.
Venous insufficiency.

Justar *Intersan, Ger.*
Cicletanine hydrochloride (p.840·2).
Hypertension.

Justebarin *Juste, Spain.*
Barium sulphate (p.1003·1).
Contrast medium for gastro-intestinal radiography.

Justegas *Juste, Spain.*
Citric acid (p.1564·3); sodium bicarbonate (p.1153·2).
Gastro-intestinal hyperacidity.

Justelax *Juste, Spain.*
Sennosides A and B (p.1212·3).
Bowel evacuation.

Justogen mono *Wernigerode, Ger.*
Taraxacum (p.1634·2).
Biliary-tract disorders; dyspepsia; reduced appetite.

Justor *Logeais, Fr.*
Cilazapril (p.840·3).
Heart failure; hypertension.

Jutussin N R8 *Reckeweg, Ger.*
Homoeopathic preparation.

Jutussin neo *Koch, Aust.*
Plantago lanceolata; thyme (p.1636·3); verbascum.
Coughs.

Juv 110 *Phonix, Ger.†.*
Homoeopathic preparation.

Juveacne *Tebib, Spain†.*
Alcohol; sulphur (p.1091·2); propylene glycol; resorcinol (p.1090·1); zinc oxide (p.1096·2); bentonite; acetone.
Acne.

Juvela
Note. This name is used for preparations of different composition.
Nutricia, Irl.; Scientific Hospital Supplies, UK.
Gluten-free or low-protein food for special diets.
Gluten-sensitive enteropathies.
Eisai, Jpn.
Tocopheryl nicotinate (p.1280·1).
Arteriosclerosis; hyperlipidaemia.

Juven Tos *Juventus, Spain†.*
Citiolone (p.1564·3); chlorpromazine (p.649·1); diprophylline (p.752·1); niaouli oil (p.1607·1).
Respiratory-tract disorders.

Juvencalcio *Juventus, Spain†.*
Calcium gluceptate (p.1155·1); cholecalciferol (p.1366·3).
Deficiency of calcium and vitamins A and D.

Juvental *Hennig, Ger.*
Atenolol (p.825·3).
Cardiovascular disorders.

Juvepirine *Asta Medica, Fr.*
Aspirin (p.16·1).
Glycine (p.1345·2) is included in this preparation in an attempt to limit adverse effects on the gastro-intestinal mucosa.
Fever; musculoskeletal and joint disorders; pain.

JuViton *Jukunda, Ger.*
Crataegus (p.1568·2); rosemary; hypericum (p.1590·1); primrose flower; ginger (p.1193·2); primula veris; kola; cactus; kalmia; lilium tigrinum; ambra; aurum colloidale; lycopus virg.
Cardiovascular disorders.

Juwoment Sport *Serum-Werk Bernburg, Ger.*
Heparin sodium (p.879·3).
Soft-tissue injury.

K-10 *SmithKline Beecham, Canad.*
Potassium chloride (p.1161·1).
Potassium depletion.

K 1000 *Hanosan, Ger.*
Homoeopathic preparation.

K + 10 *Alra, USA.*
Potassium chloride (p.1161·1).
Hypokalaemia; potassium depletion.

K + 8 *Alra, USA.*
Potassium chloride (p.1161·1).
Hypokalaemia; potassium depletion.

K + Care *Alra, USA.*
Potassium chloride (p.1161·1).
Hypokalaemia; potassium depletion.

K_5 "spezial" *Nordmark, Ger.†.*
Benzyl nicotinate (p.22·1); tyrosine (p.1357·3); dexpanthenol (p.1570·3); salicylic acid (p.1090·2).
Scalp disorders.

K Thrombin *Fawns & McAllan, Austral.*
Menadione sodium bisulphite (p.1370·3).
Haemorrhagic disorders.

Kaban *Asche, Ger.*
Clocortolone pivalate (p.1035·3); clocortolone hexanoate (p.1035·3).
Burns; skin disorders.

Kabanimat *Asche, Ger.*
Clocortolone pivalate (p.1035·3); clocortolone hexanoate (p.1035·3).
Burns; skin disorders.

Kabi Mix E *Pharmacia Upjohn, Aust.*
Amino-acid, carbohydrate, lipid (from soya oil (p.1355·1)), and electrolyte infusion.
Contains egg lecithin.
Parenteral nutrition.

Kabigamma *Pierrel, Ital.†.*
A normal immunoglobulin (p.1522·1).
Hypogammaglobulinaemia; passive immunisation.

Kabiglobin *Kabi Pharmacia, Ger.†.*
A normal immunoglobulin (p.1522·1).
Hypogammaglobulinaemia; passive immunisation.

Kabiglobulin *KabiVitrum, UK.*
A normal immunoglobulin (p.1522·1).
Agammaglobulinaemia; hypogammaglobulinaemia; passive immunisation.

Kabikinase
Pharmacia Upjohn, Aust.; Pharmacia Upjohn, Austral.; Pharmacia Upjohn, Belg.; Pharmacia Upjohn, Canad.; Pharmacia Upjohn, Fr.; Pharmacia Upjohn, Ger.; Pharmacia Upjohn, Irl.; Pierrel, Ital.†; Pharmacia Upjohn, Neth.; Pharmacia Upjohn, Norw.; Pharmacia Upjohn, S.Afr.; Pharmacia Upjohn, Spain; Pharmacia Upjohn, Swed.; Pharmacia Upjohn, Switz.; Pharmacia, UK; Kabi Pharmacia, USA.
Streptokinase (p.948·2).
Thrombo-embolic disorders.

KabiMix
Pharmacia Upjohn, Fr.; Pharmacia Upjohn, Ital.; Pharmacia Upjohn, Neth.; Pharmacia Upjohn, Norw.; Pharmacia Upjohn, Spain; Pharmacia Upjohn, Swed.; Pharmacia Upjohn, UK.
Amino-acid, carbohydrate, lipid (from soya oil (p.1355·1)), and electrolyte infusion.
Contains egg lecithin.
Parenteral nutrition.

Kabolin *Legere, USA†.*
Nandrolone decanoate (p.1452·2).

Kacinth *Intramed, S.Afr.*
Amikacin sulphate (p.150·2).
Bacterial infections.

Kadalex *Diaco, Ital.*
Potassium chloride (p.1161·1).
Hypokalaemia.

KadeFungin *Kade, Ger.*
Clotrimazole (p.376·3).
Fungal and bacterial infections of the vagina.

Kadian
Knoll, Canad.; Zeneca, USA.
Morphine sulphate (p.56·2).
Pain.

Kadiur *GiEnne, Ital.*
Canrenoate potassium (p.836·2); buthiazide (p.835·2).
Hyperaldosteronism.

Kadol *Teofarma, Ital.*
Phenylbutazone (p.79·2).
Musculoskeletal and soft-tissue disorders; skin irritation.

Kadyn-C *IBP, Ital.†.*
Magnesium aspartate (p.1157·2); potassium aspartate (p.1161·3); ascorbic acid (p.1365·2).
Asthenia.

Kaergona Hidrosoluble *Llorente, Spain.*
Menadione (p.1370·3).
Haemorrhage.

Kafa *Pharmacal, Switz.*
Propyphenazone (p.81·3); paracetamol (p.72·2); caffeine (p.749·3).
Pain.

Kai Fu *Serturner, Ger.†.*
Harpagophytum (p.27·2).
Musculoskeletal and joint disorders.

Kainair *Pharmafair, USA†.*
Proxymetacaine hydrochloride (p.1300·1).

Kajos
Astra, Norw.; Hassle, Swed.
Potassium citrate (p.1153·1).
Hypokalaemia.

Kala *Freeda, USA.*
Lactobacillus acidophilus (p.1594·1).
Dietary supplement.

Kalantol-A *Phonix, Ger.†.*
Aloes (p.1177·1); myrrh (p.1606·1); gummi arabicum (p.1470·2); arnica (p.1550·3); rosemary; calendula officinalis; hypericum (p.1590·1); peru balsam (p.1617·2); cajuput oil (p.1556·1); antimonium crudum.
Inflammation; pain.

Kalantol-B *Phonix, Ger.†.*
Aloes (p.1177·1); myrrh (p.1606·1); gummi arabicum (p.1470·2); arnica (p.1550·3); rosemary; calendula officinalis; hypericum (p.1590·1); peru balsam (p.1617·2); cajuput oil (p.1556·1); antimonium crudum; arnica; camphor (p.1557·2); sage oil.
Joint disorders.

Kalcipos *Recip, Swed.*
Calcium carbonate (p.1182·1).
Calcium deficiency; hyperphosphataemia; osteoporosis.

Kalcipos-D *Recip, Swed.*
Calcium carbonate (p.1182·1); cholecalciferol (p.1366·3).
Calcium and vitamin D deficiencies; osteoporosis.

Kalcitena *ACO, Swed.*
Calcium carbonate (p.1182·1).
Calcium deficiency; hyperphosphataemia; osteoporosis.

Kaleorid
Leo, Fr.; Leo, Norw.; Lovens, Swed.
Potassium chloride (p.1161·1).
Hypokalaemia; potassium supplement.

Kalgut *Tanabe, Jpn.*
Denopamine (p.847·1).
Heart failure.

Kali Mag *Vitaplex, Austral.*
Potassium amino acid chelate; magnesium amino acid chelate.
Potassium and magnesium supplement.

Kalicitrine *Promedica, Fr.*
Choline citrate (p.1337·1); potassium citrate (p.1153·1).
Dyspepsia.

Kaliglutol *Streuli, Switz.*
Potassium chloride (p.1161·1).
Hypokalaemia.

Kaliklora Jod med *Queisser, Ger.*
Potassium iodide (p.1493·1).
Iodine deficiency.

Kalilente
Ciba, Norw.†; Ciba-Geigy, Swed.†.
Potassium chloride (p.1161·1).
Hypokalaemia; potassium supplement.

Kalimate *Nikken, Jpn.*
Calcium polystyrene sulphonate (p.974·3).
Hyperkalaemia.

Kalinor *Knoll, Ger.*
Potassium citrate (p.1153·1); potassium bicarbonate (p.1153·1).
Potassium deficiency, particularly in association with metabolic acidosis.

Kalinorm *Nycomed, Norw.*
Potassium chloride (p.1161·1).
Hypokalaemia.

Kalinor-retard P *Knoll, Ger.*
Potassium chloride (p.1161·1).
Potassium deficiency.

Kalioral *Leopold, Aust.*
Anhydrous potassium citrate (p.1153·1); potassium bicarbonate (p.1153·1); citric acid (p.1564·3).

Kalipor *Kabi, Swed.†.*
Potassium chloride (p.1161·1).
Hypokalaemia; potassium supplement.

Kalisyl *Solvay, Aust.*
Diethylamine salicylate (p.33·1); myrtecaine (p.1297·3).
Inflammation; pain.

Kalitabs *Lovens, Swed.*
Potassium chloride (p.1161·1).
Potassium deficiency; potassium supplement.

Kalitrans *Fresenius, Ger.*
Potassium bicarbonate (p.1153·1).
Potassium deficiency.

Kalitrans retard *Fresenius, Ger.*
Potassium chloride (p.1161·1).
Potassium deficiency.

Kalium *Apogepha, Ger.*
Potassium adipate.
Potassium deficiency.

Kalium Duretter *Hassle, Swed.*
Potassium chloride (p.1161·1).
Potassium deficiency; potassium supplement.

Kalium Durettes
Astra, Belg.; Astra, Neth.
Potassium chloride (p.1161·1).
Hypokalaemia; potassium supplement.

Kalium Durules *Astra, Canad.*
Potassium chloride (p.1161·1).
Potassium depletion.

Kalium Retard *Nycomed, Swed.*
Potassium chloride (p.1161·1).
Hypokalaemia; potassium supplement.

Kalium-Can *Ratiopharm, Ger.*
Canrenoate potassium (p.836·2).
Ascites; hyperaldosteronism; oedema.

Kalium-Duriles *Astra, Ger.*
Potassium chloride (p.1161·1).
Potassium deficiency.

Kalium-Magnesium *Apogepha, Ger.*
Potassium adipate; magnesium adipate.
Potassium and magnesium deficiency.

Kalium-Magnesium-Asparaginat *Berlin-Chemie, Ger.*
Potassium hydroxide (p.1621·1); magnesium oxide (p.1198·3); DL-aspartic acid (p.1335·1); xylitol (p.1372·3).
Cardiac disorders.

Kalius *Fermenti, Ital.*
Trimebutine maleate (p.1639·3).
Gastro-intestinal disorders.

Kalkurenal
Polcopharma, Austral.†; Muller Goppingen, Ger.†.
Berberis; rubia tinctorum; saxifraga.
Urinary-tract disorders.

Kalkurenal Goldrute *Muller Goppingen, Ger.*
Solidago virgaurea.
Renal calculi.

Kalma
Note. This name is used for preparations of different composition.
Alphapharm, Austral.
Alprazolam (p.640·3).
Anxiety; panic disorders.
Fresenius, Ger.
Tryptophan (p.310·2).
Depression; sleep disorders.
Schering-Plough, Spain.
Ibuprofen (p.44·1).
Fever; inflammation; musculoskeletal, joint, and periarticular disorders; pain.

Kalm-B *Cantassium Co., UK.*
Multivitamin and mineral preparation.

Kalms *Lane, UK.*
Lupulus (p.1597·2); valerian (p.1643·1); gentian (p.1583·3).
Stresses and strains.

Kalodil *Fidia, Ital.†.*
Di-isopropylammonium dichloroacetate (p.854·1).
Cardiovascular disorders.

Kaloplasmal *Braun, Ger.*
Glucose monohydrate (p.1343·3); xylitol (p.1372·3).
Parenteral nutrition.

Kaloplasmal E *Braun, Ger.*
Electrolyte infusion with glucose and xylitol (p.1147·1).
Parenteral nutrition.

Kalovowen-N *Weber & Weber, Ger.*
Homoeopathic preparation.

Kalsimin *Byk Elmu, Spain.*
Salcatonin (p.735·3).
Hypercalcaemia; metastatic bone pain; osteoporosis; Paget's disease of bone.

Kalspare *Dominion, UK.*
Chlorthalidone (p.839·3); triamterene (p.957·2).
Ascites; hypertension; oedema.

Kalten
Zeneca, Belg.; Zeneca, Spain; Zeneca, Switz.; Zeneca, UK.
Atenolol (p.825·3); amiloride (p.819·3) or amiloride hydrochloride (p.819·2); hydrochlorothiazide (p.885·2).
Hypertension.

Kaltocarb
Faulding, Austral.; ConvaTec, UK.
Calcium alginate (p.714·1); activated charcoal (p.972·2).
Skin ulcers; wounds.

Kaltoclude *BritCair, UK†.*
Calcium alginate (p.714·1).
Wounds.

Kaltostat
Note. This name is used for preparations of different composition.
Faulding, Austral.; ConvaTec, UK; Calgon Vestal, USA.
Calcium alginate (p.714·1).
Haemostatic wound dressing.
Convatec, Irl.; Convatec, Ital.; Bristol-Myers Squibb, S.Afr.
Calcium alginate (p.714·1); sodium alginate (p.1470·3).
Haemostatic wound dressing.

Kaluril *Alphapharm, Austral.*
Amiloride hydrochloride (p.819·2).
Hypertension; oedema.

Kalymin *Dresden, Ger.*
Pyridostigmine bromide (p.1398·1).
Antimuscarinic toxicity; myasthenia gravis; reversal of competitive neuromuscular blockade; smooth muscle atony.

Kalzan *Fink, Ger.†.*
Calcium citrate (p.1155·1); calcium hydrogen phosphate (p.1155·3).
Calcium deficiency.

Kalzonorm *Merck, Aust.†.*
Calcium carbonate (p.1182·1).
Hypocalcaemia; increased calcium requirements; osteoporosis.

Kamfeine *Wolfs, Belg.*
Sodium camsylate; ephedrine hydrochloride (p.1059·3); lobelia (p.1481·3); sodium benzoate (p.1102·3).
Convalescence after influenza; dyspnoea.

Kamillan plus *Wernigerode, Ger.*
Chamomile (p.1561·2); achillea (p.1542·2).
Burns; gastro-intestinal disorders; inflammation of mucous membranes; wounds.

Kamillan supra *Wernigerode, Ger.*
Chamomile (p.1561·2).
Gastro-intestinal disorders; inflammation and infections of the skin and mucous membranes; respiratory-tract disorders.

Kamille N *Spitzner, Ger.*
Chamomile (p.1561·2).
Gastro-intestinal disorders; inflammation of skin and mucous membranes; upper respiratory-tract inflammation.

Kamillen Spuman *Luitpold, Ger.†.*
Chamomile (p.1561·2).
Vaginal disorders.

Kamillen-Bad *Medipharm, Switz.*
Chamomile flowers (p.1561·2).
Skin disorders.

Kamillen-Bad N Ritsert *Ritsert, Ger.*
Chamomile oil.
Anorectal disorders; bath additive; inflammation of skin and mucous membranes.

Kamillen-Bad-Robugen *Robugen, Ger.*
Chamomile (p.1561·2).
Anorectal disorders; bath additive; dermatitis; wounds.

Kamillex *Streuli, Switz.†.*
Chamomile (p.1561·2).
Gastro-intestinal disorders; mouth and throat disorders; skin disorders.

Kamillobad *Asta Medica, Ger.*
Chamomile (p.1561·2); chamomile oil.
Bath additive; inflammation of skin and mucous membranes.

Kamilloderm *Serum-Werk Bernburg, Ger.*
Chamomile (p.1561·2).
Burns; skin irritation; wounds.

Kamillofluid *Amino, Switz.*
Chamomile (p.1561·2).
Mouth and throat disorders; skin disorders.

Kamillomed *Kottas-Heldenberg, Aust.*
Chamomile (p.1561·2).
Gastro-intestinal disorders; skin and mucous membrane inflammation.

Kamillosan
Note. This name is used for preparations of different composition.
Asta Medica, Aust.; Asta Medica, Belg.; Asta Medica, Ger.; Norgine, Irl.; Dagra, Neth.†; Norgine, S.Afr.; Asta Medica, Switz.; Norgine, UK.
Chamomile (p.1561·2).
Anal disorders; gastro-intestinal disorders; mouth and throat disorders; respiratory-tract disorders; skin disorders; vulvovaginal disorders.
Asta Medica, Switz.
Buccal spray: Chamomile (p.1561·2); peppermint oil (p.1208·1); anise oil (p.1550·1).
Mouth and throat disorders.
Asta Medica, Switz.
Topical gel: Vitamin A (p.1358·1); chlorhexidine gluconate (p.1107·2); chamomile (p.1561·2).
Skin disorders.

Kamillosan Mundspray *Asta Medica, Ger.*
Chamomile (p.1561·2); peppermint oil (p.1208·1); anise oil (p.1550·1).
Inflammatory disorders of the oropharynx.

Kamistad *Stada, Ger.†.*
Lignocaine hydrochloride (p.1293·2); thymol (p.1127·1); chamomile (p.1561·2).
Inflammatory disorders of the mouth.

Kamol *Whitehall, Fr.*
Capsicum oleoresin; menthol (p.1600·2); eucalyptus oil (p.1578·1); camphor (p.1557·2); chloroform (p.1220·3); methyl salicylate (p.55·2).
Soft-tissue disorders.

Kamu Jay *Jamieson, Canad.*
Ascorbic acid (p.1365·2).
Vitamin supplement.

Kamu Jay Multi Complex *Jamieson, Canad.*
Vitamin and mineral preparation.

Kamycine *Bristol-Myers Squibb, Fr.*
Kanamycin sulphate (p.220·3).
Bacterial infections.

Kana *Arkopharma, Fr.†.*
Olive.
Promotes diuresis.

Kanacolirio *Medical, Spain.*
Kanamycin sulphate (p.220·3).
Bacterial eye infections.

Kanaderm *FIRMA, Ital.†.*
Kanamycin sulphate (p.220·3); dexamethasone sodium phosphate (p.1037·2).
Infected skin disorders.

Kanafosal *Medical, Spain.*
Ephedrine hydrochloride (p.1059·3); kanamycin sulphate (p.220·3); naphazoline hydrochloride (p.1064·2); procaine hydrochloride (p.1299·2); sulphanilamide sodium mesylate (p.256·3).
Nasal congestion and infection.

Kanafosal Predni *Medical, Spain.*
Ephedrine hydrochloride (p.1059·3); kanamycin sulphate (p.220·3); naphazoline hydrochloride (p.1064·2); prednisone (p.1049·2); procaine hydrochloride (p.1299·2); sulphanilamide sodium mesylate (p.256·3).
Nasal congestion and infection.

Kanamytrex
Bristol-Myers Squibb, Belg.†; Basotherm, Ger.
Kanamycin sulphate (p.220·3).
Bacterial infections.

Kanapomada *Medical, Spain.*
Kanamycin sulphate (p.220·3); plasma; prednisolone (p.1048·1); trypsin (p.1640·1); urea (p.1095·2).
Infected skin disorders.

Kana-Stulln *Stulln, Ger.*
Kanamycin sulphate (p.220·3).
Eye infections.

Kanatrombina *Baldacci, Ital.†.*
Bovine thrombin (p.728·1); kanamycin acid sulphate (p.220·2).
Haemorrhage.

Kanavit *Medphano, Ger.*
Phytomenadione (p.1371·1).
Vitamin K deficiency.

Kanazone *SIT, Ital.*
Dexamethasone phosphate (p.1037·2); kanamycin sulphate (p.220·3); phenylephrine hydrochloride (p.1066·2).
Eye, nose, and ear disorders.

Kanbine *Rovi, Spain.*
Amikacin sulphate (p.150·2).
Bacterial infections.

Kanendomycin *Meiji, Jpn.*
Bekanamycin sulphate (p.158·2).
Bacterial infections.

Kanendos *Fournier, Ital.*
Bekanamycin sulphate (p.158·2).
Adjuvant in hyperammonaemia; intestinal infections.

Kanescin *Torlan, Spain.*
Kanamycin sulphate (p.220·3).
Bacterial infections.

Kaneuron *L'Arguenon, Fr.*
Phenobarbitone (p.350·2); caffeine (p.749·3); crataegus (p.1568·2); passion flower (p.1615·3).
Anxiety; epilepsy.

Kank-A
Note. This name is used for preparations of different composition.
Blistex, Canad.
Benzocaine (p.1286·2); cetylpyridinium chloride (p.1106·2).
Canker sores; mouth irritation.
Blistex, USA.
Benzocaine (p.1286·2); compound benzoin tincture.
Mouth disorders.

Kannasyn
Sanofi Winthrop, Irl.; Sanofi Winthrop, UK.
Kanamycin acid sulphate (p.220·2).
Bacterial infections.

Kanopan *Nordmark, Ger.†.*
Maprotiline hydrochloride (p.296·2).
Depression.

Kan-Ophtal *Winzer, Ger.*
Kanamycin sulphate (p.220·3).
Bacterial eye infections.

Kanrenol *Nordmark, Ital.*
Canrenoate potassium (p.836·2).
Hyperaldosteronism; hypertension.

Kantrex
Bristol-Myers, Spain; Apothecon, USA.
Kanamycin sulphate (p.220·3).
Bacterial infections.

Kantrexil *Opus, S.Afr.*
Kanamycin sulphate (p.220·3); dimevamide (p.460·3); pectin (p.1474·1); bismuth subcarbonate (p.1180·1); activated attapulgite (p.1178·3).
Diarrhoea.

Kao *Covan, S.Afr.*
Kaolin (p.1195·1); pectin (p.1474·1).
Formerly contained kaolin, bismuth subcarbonate, and dicyclomine hydrochloride.
Diarrhoea.

Kao Lectrolyte *Pharmacia Upjohn, USA.*
Oral rehydration solution (p.1152·3).
Diarrhoea; vomiting.

Kaobrol *SmithKline Beecham, Fr.*
Magnesium carbonate (p.1198·1); calcium carbonate (p.1182·1); heavy kaolin (p.1195·1).
Gastro-intestinal disorders.

Kaochlor
Pharmacia Upjohn, Canad.; Adria, USA.
Potassium chloride (p.1161·1).
Hypokalaemia; potassium depletion.

Kaodene *Knoll, UK.*
Codeine phosphate (p.26·1); light kaolin (p.1195·1).
Diarrhoea.

Kaodene Non-Narcotic *Pfeiffer, USA.*
Kaolin (p.1195·1); pectin (p.1474·1); bismuth salicylate (p.1180·1).
Diarrhoea.

Kaodyne *Prosana, Austral.†.*
Codeine phosphate (p.26·1); kaolin (p.1195·1); calcium carbonate (p.1182·1); magnesium trisilicate (p.1199·1).
Gastro-intestinal disorders.

Kaofort *Boots, Austral.†.*
Codeine phosphate (p.26·1); light kaolin (p.1195·1).
Diarrhoea.

Kaologeais *Logeais, Fr.*
Magnesium oxide (p.1198·3); meprobamate (p.678·1); magnesium sulphate (p.1157·3); kaolin (p.1195·1); sterculia (p.1214·1).
Gastro-intestinal disorders.

Kaomagma
Note. This name is used for preparations of different composition.
Whitehall, Austral.
Kaolin (p.1195·1); aluminium hydroxide (p.1177·3).
Diarrhoea.
Akromed, S.Afr.†.
Kaolin (p.1195·1); pectin (p.1474·1); aluminium hydroxide (p.1177·3).
Diarrhoea.

Kaomagma with Pectin *Whitehall, Austral.*
Kaolin (p.1195·1); pectin (p.1474·1); aluminium hydroxide (p.1177·3).
Diarrhoea.

Kaomuth *Bailly, Fr.*
Kaolin (p.1195·1); magnesium hydroxide (p.1198·2).
Gastro-intestinal disorders.

Kaomycin
Pharmacia Upjohn, Canad.†; Pharmacia Upjohn, S.Afr.†.
Neomycin sulphate (p.229·2); kaolin (p.1195·1); pectin (p.1474·1).
Diarrhoea.

Kaomycine *Upjohn, Switz.†.*
Neomycin sulphate (p.229·2); kaolin (p.1195·1); pectin citrate.
Diarrhoea.

Kaon
Pharmacia Upjohn, Canad.; Savage, USA.
Potassium gluconate (p.1161·1).
Hypokalaemia; potassium depletion.

Kaon-Cl *Savage, USA.*
Potassium chloride (p.1161·1).
Hypokalaemia; potassium depletion.

Kaoneo *Covan, S.Afr.†.*
Kaolin (p.1195·1); pectin (p.1474·1); dicyclomine hydrochloride (p.460·1); neomycin sulphate (p.229·2).
Diarrhoea.

Kaopectate
Note. This name is used for preparations of different composition.
Pharmacia Upjohn, Austral.; Pharmacia Upjohn, Belg.; Pharmacia Upjohn, Irl.; Pharmacia Upjohn, Switz.; Pharmacia Upjohn, UK†.
Kaolin (p.1195·1); pectin (p.1474·1).
Diarrhoea.
McNeil Consumer, Canad.
Attapulgite (p.1178·3).
Cramps; diarrhoea.

Kaopectate Advanced Formula *Upjohn, USA.*
Attapulgite (p.1178·3).
Diarrhoea.

Kaopectate II *Upjohn, USA.*
Loperamide hydrochloride (p.1197·2).
Diarrhoea.

Kaopectate Maximum Strength *Upjohn, USA.*
Attapulgite (p.1178·3).
Diarrhoea.

Kaopectate N *Upjohn, Ger.†.*
Neomycin sulphate (p.229·2); kaolin (p.1195·1); pectin (p.1474·1).
Infective diarrhoea.

Kaopectin *Mer-National, S.Afr.*
Kaolin (p.1195·1); pectin (p.1474·1).
Diarrhoea.

Kaoprompt-H *Pharmacia Upjohn, Ger.*
Kaolin (p.1195·1); pectin (p.1474·1).
Diarrhoea.

Kao-Pront *Lachifarma, Ital.*
Kaolin (p.1195·1).
Diarrhoea.

Kao-Spen *Century, USA.*
Kaolin (p.1195·1); pectin (p.1474·1).
Diarrhoea.

Kaostatex *Garec, S.Afr.*
Light kaolin (p.1195·1); pectin (p.1474·1); sodium lactate; potassium chloride; sodium chloride (p.1152·3).
Diarrhoea.

Kapake
Galen, Irl.; Galen, UK.
Paracetamol (p.72·2); codeine phosphate (p.26·1).
These ingredients can be described by the British Approved Name Co-codamol.
Pain.

Kapanol
Glaxo Wellcome, Aust.; Glaxo Wellcome, Austral.; Glaxo Wellcome, Neth.; Glaxo Wellcome, Norw.
Morphine sulphate (p.56·2).
Pain.

Kapodin *Efarmes, Spain.*
Minoxidil (p.910·3).
Alopecia.

Kappabi *Logifarm, Ital.†.*
Dibekacin sulphate (p.201·3).
Bacterial infections.

Kaput *Maxfarma, Spain.*
Povidone-iodine (p.1123·3).
Skin and instrument disinfection; skin disorders.

Karacil *ICN, Canad.*
Ispaghula husk (p.1194·2).

Karayal *Roques, Fr.*
Magnesium oxide (p.1198·3); magnesium sulphate (p.1157·3); kaolin (p.1195·1); sterculia (p.1214·1).
Gastro-intestinal disorders.

Karbinone *Bio-Therabel, Belg.†.*
Naftazone (p.725·2).
Vascular disorders.

Karbolytt *Pharmacia Upjohn, Norw.*
Electrolyte infusion with glucose (p.1147·1).
Carbohydrate source; fluid and electrolyte disorders.

Karbons *Eagle, Austral.*
Activated charcoal (p.972·2).
Digestive system disorders.

Kardegic
Synthelabo, Fr.; Synthelabo, Switz.
Lysine aspirin (p.50·3).
Thrombosis prophylaxis.

Karden *Laevosan, Aust.*
Nicardipine hydrochloride (p.915·1).
Angina pectoris; hypertension.

Kardiamed *Medice, Ger.*
β-Acetyldigoxin (p.812·3).
Arrhythmias; heart failure.

Kardil *Orion, Norw.*
Diltiazem hydrochloride (p.854·2).
Angina pectoris.

Karelyne *Urgo, Fr.*
Sweet almond oil peroxide (p.1546·2).
Anorectal disorders.

Karicare Food Thickener *Nutricia, Austral.*
Pregelatinised maize starch (p.1356·2).
Dysphagia in children and adults; gastro-oesophageal reflux in infants.

Karicare Nutrilon *Nutricia, Austral.*
Infant feed.
Cow's milk, lactose, and disaccharide intolerance; galactosaemia.

Karidina *Kerifarm, Spain.*
Cephazolin sodium (p.181·1).
Bacterial infections.

Karidium
Lorvic, Canad.; Lorvic, USA.
Sodium fluoride (p.742·1).
Dental caries prophylaxis.

Karigel *Lorvic, USA.*
Sodium fluoride (p.742·1).
Dental caries prophylaxis.

Karigel-N *Lorvic, USA.*
Sodium fluoride (p.742·1).
Dental caries prophylaxis.

Karil *Sandoz, Ger.*
Salcatonin acetate (p.736·3).
Bone and calcium disorders.

Karilexina *Farmapros, Spain.*
Cephalexin (p.178·2).
Bacterial infections.

Kariopha *Kario, Fr.†.*
Multivitamin, amino-acid, and trace element preparation.
Nutritional supplement; tonic.

Karison *Dermapharm, Ger.*
Clobetasol propionate (p.1035·2).
Skin disorders.

Karotena ACO *Kabi, Swed.†.*
Betacarotene (p.1335·2).

Karrer *Lisapharma, Ital.*
Carnitine (p.1336·2).
Carnitine deficiency; myocardial ischaemia.

Karvisin *Synpharma, Aust.*
Fennel (p.1579·1); chamomile (p.1561·2); caraway (p.1559·3).
Gastro-intestinal disorders.

Karvol
Note. This name is used for preparations of different composition.
Boots, Austral.
Menthol (p.1600·2); oleum pini sylvestris; pumilio pine oil (p.1623·3); terpineol (p.1635·1).
Nasal congestion.
Boots Healthcare, Irl.; Crookes Laboratories, UK.
Chlorbutol (p.1106·3); menthol (p.1600·2); oleum pini sylvestris; pumilio pine oil (p.1623·3); terpineol (p.1635·1); thymol (p.1127·1).
Respiratory-tract congestion.
Boots, S.Afr.
Chlorbutol (p.1106·3); menthol (p.1600·2); cinnamon oil (p.1564·2); pine oil; terpineol (p.1635·1); thymol (p.1127·1).
Upper respiratory-tract congestion.

Kas-Bah *Potter's, UK.*
Buchu (p.1555·2); clivers (p.1565·2); couch-grass (p.1567·3); equisetum (p.1575·1); uva ursi (p.1552·2); senna (p.1212·2).
Urinary and bladder discomfort.

Kasof *J&J-Merck, USA.*
Docusate potassium (p.1189·3).
Anorectal disorders; severe constipation.

Katabios *SIT, Ital.*
Multivitamin preparation.

Katadolon *Asta Medica, Ger.*
Flupirtine maleate (p.42·1).
Pain.

Katar *Berna, Ital.*
Diplococcus pneumoniae; *Staphylococcus aureus*; *Staphylococcus albus*; *Streptococcus*; *Klebsiella pneumoniae*; *Branhamella catarrhalis*; *Haemophilus influenzae*; *Corynebacterium pseudodiphtheriae*.
Respiratory-tract congestion.

Katarakton *Ursapharm, Ger.†.*
Potassium iodide (p.1493·1).
Corneal or lens cloudiness.

Katasma *Bruschettini, Ital.*
Diprophylline (p.752·1).
Obstructive airways disease.

Katasma Balsamico *Bruschettini, Ital.†.*
Diprophylline (p.752·1); sodium guaiacolglycolate (p.1061·2); cafaminol.
Broncho-pulmonary disorders.

Kataval *Cyanamid, Ital.*
Triamcinolone acetonide (p.1050·2); neomycin sulphate (p.229·2).
Anorectal disorders; otitis externa; skin disorders.

Kation *Searle, Ital.*
Potassium citrate (p.1153·1).
Hypokalaemia.

Kationen *Leopold, Aust.*
A trace element preparation (p.1147·1).
Parenteral nutrition.

Kato *ICN, USA†.*
Potassium chloride (p.1161·1).
Hypokalaemia; potassium depletion.

Katoderm *Deverge, Ital.*
Collagen (p.1566·3); silver (p.1629·2).
Skin cleansing.

Katogel *Deverge, Ital.*
Emollient.
Dry skin; skin irritation.

Katosilver *Deverge, Ital.*
Silver sucralfate; allantoin-polymethylmethacrylate resin (p.1078·2); capriloylhydroxyproline olamine; enoxolone (p.35·2).
Prevention of decubitus ulcers; skin irritation.

Katovit
Thomae, Ger.†; Fher, Spain; Boehringer Ingelheim, Switz.†.
Prolintane hydrochloride (p.1485·1); vitamins.
Tonic.

Katovit N *Thomae, Ger.†.*
Prolintane hydrochloride (p.1485·1).
Tonic.

Katoxyn *Deverge, Ital.*
Silver (p.1629·2); benzoyl peroxide (p.1079·2); kaolin (p.1195·1); calcium gluconate (p.1155·2).
Disinfection of wounds and burns.

Katrum *Smaller, Spain.*
Capsaicin (p.24·2).
Diabetic neuropathy; musculoskeletal and joint disorders; neuralgia.

Kattwilact *Kattwiga, Ger.*
Lactulose (p.1195·3).
Constipation; hepatic encephalopathy; salmonella enteritis.

Kattwilon N *Kattwiga, Ger.*
Isoprenaline sulphate (p.892·1).
Allergic rashes; midge bites; pruritus; vaccination pocks; varicella.

Katulcin *Kattwiga, Ger.†.*
Lactose; kaolin (p.1195·1); liquorice (p.1197·1); bismuth salicylate (p.1180·1); faex medicinalis (p.1373·1); argent. colloid.; herba teucrii; light magnesium carbonate (p.1198·1); papain (p.1614·1).
Gastro-intestinal disorders.

Katulcin-Rupha *Kattwiga, Ger.*
Bismuth subnitrate (p.1180·2); bismuth salicylate (p.1180·1).
Gastritis; hyperchlorhydria; peptic ulcer.

Kaukafin *Medopharm, Ger.†.*
Eleutherococcus senticosus (p.1584·2).
Tonic.

Kausalpunkt N *Biotherax, Ger.†.*
Benzyl nicotinate (p.22·1).
Formerly contained noradrenaline acid tartrate and benzyl nicotinate.
Muscle and joint pain.

Kavacur *Biocur, Ger.*
Kava (p.1592·3).
Anxiety disorders.

Kavaform *Sanabo, Aust.*
Kawain (p.1592·3); magnesium orotate (p.1611·2); with or without vitis vinifera rubra.
Tonic.

Kavaform N *Klinge, Ger.*
Kawain (p.1592·3).
Mental function disorders; psychiatric disorders.

Kavain Harras Plus *Harras-Curarina, Ger.*
Kawain (p.1592·3); kava (p.1592·3).
Anxiety disorders.

Kavasedon *Harras-Curarina, Ger.*
Kava (p.1592·3).
Anxiety disorders.

Kavatino *Bionorica, Ger.*
Kava (p.1592·3).
Anxiety disorders.

Kavavit *Sanabo, Aust.*
Kawain (p.1592·3); vitamins.
Tonic.

Kavepenin *Astra, Swed.*
Phenoxymethylpenicillin potassium (p.236·2).
Bacterial infections.

Kaveri *Lichtwer, Ger.*
Ginkgo biloba leaf (p.1584·1).
Cerebral and peripheral circulatory disorders.

Kavigeba *Presselin, Ger.†.*
Multivitamin and mineral preparation.
Calcium deficiency.

Kavitol *Lannacher, Aust.†.*
Menadione sodium bisulphite (p.1370·3).
Haemorrhage; overdosage with coumarin anticoagulants.

Kavosan
Oral-B, Ital.†.
Sodium monohydrate; anhydrous sodium bitartrate.
Oral hygiene.

Oral-B, Ital.
Sodium perborate (p.1125·2).
Formerly known as Oral-B Kavosan.
Oral hygiene.

Kavosporal *Polcopharma, Austral.†.*
Valerian (p.1643·1); lupulus (p.1597·2).
Anxiety and tension states.

Kavosporal comp *Muller Goppingen, Ger.*
Kava (p.1592·3); valerian (p.1643·1).
Anxiety disorders.

Kavosporal forte *Muller Goppingen, Ger.*
Kava (p.1592·3).
Anxiety disorders.

Kawaform *Wander, Switz.*
Kawain (p.1592·3); magnesium orotate (p.1611·2); vitis vinifera.
Insomnia; tension; tonic.

Kay Ciel
Schering, Austral.†; Forest Pharmaceuticals, USA.
Potassium chloride (p.1161·1).
Hypokalaemia; potassium depletion.

Kayadol *Syntex, Spain†.*
Maize.
Mouth disorders.

Kay-Cee-L
Geistlich, Irl.; Geistlich, UK.
Potassium chloride (p.1161·1).
Hypokalaemia; potassium depletion.

Kayexalate
Sanofi Winthrop, Canad.; Sanofi Winthrop, Fr.; Sanofi Winthrop, Ital.; Sanofi Winthrop, USA.
Sodium polystyrene sulphonate (p.995·3).
Hyperkalaemia.

Kayexalate Calcium *Sanofi Winthrop, Belg.*
Calcium polystyrene sulphonate (p.974·3).
Hyperkalaemia.

Kayexalate Sodium *Sanofi Winthrop, Belg.*
Sodium polystyrene sulphonate (p.995·3).
Hyperkalaemia.

Kaylixir *Lannett, USA.*
Potassium gluconate (p.1161·1).
Hypokalaemia; potassium depletion.

Kaysine *Kay, USA†.*
Adenosine phosphate (p.1543·2).
Varicose veins.

Kaytwo *Eisai, Jpn.*
Menatetrenone (p.1371·3).
Vitamin K deficiency.

Kaywan *Eisai, Jpn†.*
Phytomenadione (p.1371·1).
Vitamin K deficiency.

Kaz *McGloin, Austral.*
Menthol (p.1600·2).
Inhalation.

K-C *Century, USA.*
Kaolin (p.1195·1); pectin (p.1474·1); bismuth subcarbonate (p.1180·1).
Diarrhoea.

KCl-retard *Zyma, Ger.*
Potassium chloride (p.1161·1).
Hypokalaemia.

KDS Comply *Wyeth-Ayerst, Canad.†.*
Preparation for enteral nutrition.

KDS Pre-Attain *Wyeth-Ayerst, Canad.†.*
Preparation for enteral nutrition.

KDS Pro-fibre *Wyeth-Ayerst, Canad.†.*
Preparation for enteral nutrition.

K-Dur
Key, Canad.; Key, USA.
Potassium chloride (p.1161·1).
Hypokalaemia.

Keal *Biogalenique, Fr.*
Sucralfate (p.1214·2).
Peptic ulcer.

Kedacillina *Bracco, Ital.*
Sulbenicillin sodium (p.250·3).
Lignocaine hydrochloride (p.1293·2) is included in this preparation to alleviate the pain of injection.
Bacterial infections.

Keep Clear Anti-Dandruff Shampoo *Avon, Canad.*
Pyrithione zinc (p.1089·3).

Kefadim
Lilly, Belg.; Lilly, UK.
Ceftazidime (p.173·3).
Bacterial infections.

Kefadol
Lilly, Irl.; Dista, UK.
Cephamandole nafate (p.180·1).
Bacterial infections.

Kefamin *Lilly, Spain.*
Ceftazidime (p.173·3).
Bacterial infections.

Kefandol *Lilly, Fr.*
Cephamandole nafate (p.180·1).
Bacterial infections.

Kefazim *Lilly, Aust.*
Ceftazidime (p.173·3).
Bacterial infections.

Kefazon *Esseti, Ital.*
Cefoperazone sodium (p.167·3).
Lignocaine hydrochloride (p.1293·2) is included in this preparation to alleviate the pain of injection.
Bacterial infections.

Kefenid *SIT, Ital.†.*
Ketoprofen (p.48·2).
Musculoskeletal and joint disorders.

Kefexin *Orion, Irl.*
Cephalexin (p.178·2).
Bacterial infections.

Keflet *Dista, USA†.*
Cephalexin (p.178·2).
Bacterial infections.

Keflex
Lilly, Aust.; Lilly, Austral.; Lilly, Canad.; Lilly, Irl.; Lilly, Norw.; Lilly, S.Afr.; Lilly, Swed.; Lilly, Switz.; Lilly, UK; Dista, USA.
Cephalexin (p.178·2).
Bacterial infections.

Keflin
Lilly, Aust.; Lilly, Belg.†; Lilly, Canad.; Lilly, Fr.; Lilly, Irl.†; Lilly, Ital.; Lilly, Neth.; Lilly, Norw.; Lilly, S.Afr.; Lilly, Spain; Lilly, Swed.; Lilly, USA†.
Cephalothin sodium (p.179·1).
Bacterial infections.

Keflin N *Lilly, Switz.†.*
Cephalothin sodium (p.179·1).
Bacterial infections.

Keflin Neutral *Lilly, Austral.*
Cephalothin sodium (p.179·1).
Bacterial infections.

Keflodin *Lilly, Ital.†.*
Cephaloridine (p.179·1).
Bacterial infections.

Keflor *Alphapharm, Austral.*
Cefaclor (p.163·2).
Bacterial infections.

Kefloridina *Lilly, Spain.*
Cephalexin (p.178·2).
Bacterial infections.

Kefloridina Mucolitico *Lilly, Spain.*
Bromhexine hydrochloride (p.1055·3); cephalexin (p.178·2).
Respiratory-tract infections.

Kefol *Lilly, Spain.*
Cephazolin sodium (p.181·1).
Bacterial infections.

Kefolor *Lilly, Swed.*
Cefaclor (p.163·2).
Bacterial infections.

Keforal
Lilly, Belg.; Lilly, Fr.; Lilly, Ital.; Lilly, Neth.
Cephalexin (p.178·2).
Bacterial infections.

Kefox *CT, Ital.*
Cefuroxime sodium (p.177·1).
Bacterial infections.

Kefoxina *CT, Ital.*
Propylene glycol cefatrizine (p.164·2).
Bacterial infections.

Kefroxil *Wharton, Ital.†.*
Cefadroxil (p.163·3).
Bacterial infections.

Keftab *Dista, USA.*
Cephalexin hydrochloride (p.178·2).
Bacterial infections.

Keftid *Galen, UK.*
Cefaclor (p.163·2).
Bacterial infections.

Kefurox
Lilly, Belg.; Lilly, Canad.; Lilly, USA.
Cefuroxime sodium (p.177·1).
Bacterial infections.

Kefzim *Lilly, S.Afr.*
Ceftazidime (p.173·3).
Bacterial infections.

Kefzol
Lilly, Aust.; Lilly, Austral.; Lilly, Belg.; Lilly, Canad.; Lilly, Fr.; Lilly, Irl.†; Lilly, Neth.; Lilly, S.Afr.; Lilly, Switz.; Lilly, UK; Lilly, USA.
Cephazolin sodium (p.181·1).
Lignocaine hydrochloride (p.1293·2) is included in some intramuscular injections to alleviate the pain of injection.
Bacterial infections.

Keimax *Essex, Ger.*
Ceftibuten (p.175·1).
Bacterial infections.

Keimicina *Boehringer Mannheim, Ital.*
Kanamycin sulphate (p.220·3).
Genito-urinary bacterial infections.

Kelatin
Yamanouchi, Belg.; Yamanouchi, Neth.
Penicillamine (p.988·3).
Cystinuria; heavy-metal poisoning; rheumatoid arthritis; Wilson's disease.

Keldrin *Thiemann, Ger.†.*
Capsules: Ethaverine hydrochloride (p.1577·1); diphenhydramine hydrochloride (p.409·1); ephedrine thiocyanate; etofylline (p.753·1); khellin (p.1593·1); camphor (p.1557·2); menthol (p.1600·2).
Suppositories: Ethaverine hydrochloride (p.1577·1); diphenhydramine hydrochloride (p.409·1); ephedrine thiocyanate; etofylline (p.753·1); khellin (p.1593·1).
Suppositories for infants: Ethaverine hydrochloride (p.1577·1); diphenhydramine hydrochloride (p.409·1); ephedrine thiocyanate; etofylline (p.753·1); khellin (p.1593·1); phenobarbitone (p.350·2).
Tablets: Ethaverine hydrochloride (p.1577·1); diphenhydramine hydrochloride (p.409·1); proxyphylline (p.757·3); khellin (p.1593·1); methylephedrine hydrochloride (p.1064·1).
Asthma; bronchitic disorders; silicosis.

Kelfiprim *Pharmacia Upjohn, Ital.*
Trimethoprim (p.265·1); sulfametopyrazine (p.251·3).
Bacterial infections.

Kelfizina
Pharmacia Upjohn, Belg.; Pharmacia Upjohn, Ital.
Sulfametopyrazine (p.251·3).
Bacterial infections; toxoplasmosis.

Kelfizine W
Pharmacia Upjohn, Irl.; Pharmacia Upjohn, UK.
Sulfametopyrazine (p.251·3).
Bacterial infections.

Keli-med *Permamed, Switz.*
Garlic (p.1583·1); hyoscyamus (p.464·3); allantoin (p.1078·2); heparin sodium (p.879·3); avobenzone (p.1486·3); 3-(4-methylbenzylidene)bornan-2-one (p.1487·2).
Scars.

Kelnac *Sankyo, Jpn.*
Purified plau-noi extract (plaunotol) (p.1208·3).
Gastric ulcer; gastritis.

Kelocyanor
3M, Austral.†; L'Arguenon, Fr.; Lipha, Irl.; Restan, S.Afr.†; Cambridge, UK.
Dicobalt edetate (p.978·3).
Cyanide poisoning.

Kelofibrase *Azupharma, Ger.*
Urea (p.1095·2); heparin sodium (p.879·3); camphor (p.1557·2).
Keloids; scars.

Kelosal *Kendall, Spain.*
Cisapride (p.1187·1).
Gastro-oesophageal reflux; gastroparesis.

Kelosoft
Chemomedica, Aust.; Geistlich, Switz.
Hyoscyamus oil (p.464·3).
Nasal disorders; scars.

Kelp Plus 3 *Larkhall Laboratories, UK.*
Kelp (p.1593·1); vitamin B_6 (p.1362·3); soya lecithin (p.1595·2); cider vinegar.

Kelsef *Jumer, Fr.*
Cephradine (p.181·3).
Bacterial infections.

Kelsopen *Faes, Spain.*
Amoxycillin trihydrate (p.151·3); potassium clavulanate (p.190·2).
Bacterial infections.

Keltican N *Trommsdorff, Ger.*
Trisodium uridine triphosphate; disodium uridine diphosphate; disodium uridine phosphate; disodium cytidine phosphate.
Lignocaine hydrochloride (p.1293·2) is included in the injection to alleviate the pain of injection.
Neuralgia; neuritis; neuropathy.

Keltrol *Kelco International, UK.*
Xanthan gum (p.1475·3).
Pharmaceutical suspending agent.

Kelual *Ducray, Fr.†.*
Lotion: Keluamid (p.1086·2); zinc sulphate (p.1373·2).
Topical emulsion: Keluamid (p.1086·2).
Seborrhoeic dermatitis.

Kemadren *Glaxo Wellcome, Spain.*
Procyclidine hydrochloride (p.467·3).
Drug-induced extrapyramidal disorders; parkinsonism.

Kemadrin
Glaxo Wellcome, Aust.; Glaxo Wellcome, Austral.; Glaxo Wellcome, Belg.; Glaxo Wellcome, Canad.; Wellcome, Irl.; Glaxo Wellcome, Ital.; Glaxo Wellcome, Neth.; Wellcome, Norw.†; Glaxo Wellcome, Swed.; Wellcome, Switz.; Wellcome, UK; Glaxo Wellcome, USA.
Procyclidine hydrochloride (p.467·3).
Drug-induced extrapyramidal disorders; parkinsonism.

Kemeol *Interdelta, Switz.*
Ephedrine (p.1059·3); neroli oil (p.1610·3); eucalyptus oil (p.1578·1).
Nasal congestion.

Kemerhine *Interdelta, Switz.*
Ephedrine hydrochloride (p.1059·3); neroli oil (p.1610·3); eucalyptus oil (p.1578·1).
Nasal congestion.

Kemerhinose *Interdelta, Switz.*
Sodium chloride (p.1162·2); benzododecinium bromide (p.1103·2).
Nasal congestion.

Kemicetin *Pharmacia Upjohn, Aust.*
Chloramphenicol (p.182·1) or chloramphenicol sodium succinate (p.182·2).
Bacterial infections.

Kemicetina *Pharmacia Upjohn, Belg.*
Chloramphenicol (p.182·1).
Bacterial infections.

Kemicetine *Farmitalia Carlo Erba, UK.*
Chloramphenicol sodium succinate (p.182·2).
Bacterial infections.

Kemodyn *Esseti, Ital.*
Citicoline sodium (p.1564·3).
Cerebrovascular disorders; parkinsonism.

Kempi *Upjohn, Spain.*
Spectinomycin hydrochloride (p.248·3).
Gonorrhoea.

Kemsol *Carter Horner, Canad.*
Dimethyl sulphoxide (p.1377·2).
Scleroderma.

Kenacomb
Bristol-Myers Squibb, Austral.; Westwood-Squibb, Canad.; Bristol-Myers Squibb, Irl.; Bristol-Myers Squibb, S.Afr.
Triamcinolone acetonide (p.1050·2); neomycin sulphate (p.229·2); gramicidin (p.215·2); nystatin (p.386·1).
Infected skin disorders.

Kenacombin *Bristol-Myers Squibb, Swed.†.*
Triamcinolone acetonide (p.1050·2); neomycin sulphate (p.229·2); gramicidin (p.215·2); nystatin (p.386·1).
Infected skin disorders.

Kenacombin Novum *Bristol-Myers Squibb, Swed.*
Triamcinolone acetonide (p.1050·2); nystatin (p.386·1).
Fungal skin infections.

Kenacort
Bristol-Myers Squibb, Austral.†; Bristol-Myers Squibb, Belg.; Bristol-Myers Squibb, Fr.; Bristol-Myers Squibb, Irl.†; Squibb, Ital.†; Squibb, Neth.†; Bristol-Myers Squibb, Swed.†; Bristol-Myers Squibb, Switz.; Apothecon, USA.
Triamcinolone (p.1050·2) or triamcinolone acetonide (p.1050·2).
Corticosteroid.

Kenacort Solubile *Bristol-Myers Squibb, Belg.*
Triamcinolone acetonide dipotassium phosphate (p.1050·3).
Corticosteroid.

Kenacort-A
Note. This name is used for preparations of different composition.
Bristol-Myers Squibb, Austral.; Bristol-Myers Squibb, Belg.; Bristol-Myers Squibb, Irl.†; Bristol-Myers Squibb, Ital.; Bristol-Myers Squibb, Neth.; Squibb, Switz.
Triamcinolone acetonide (p.1050·2).
Corticosteroid.

Squibb, Switz.
Tincture: Triamcinolone acetonide (p.1050·2); salicylic acid (p.1090·2).
Topical lotion†: Triamcinolone acetonide (p.1050·2); zinc oxide (p.1096·2).
Skin disorders.

Kenacort-A Solubile
Squibb, Neth.†; Squibb, Switz.
Triamcinolone acetonide dipotassium phosphate (p.1050·3).
Corticosteroid.

Kenacort-T
Bristol-Myers Squibb, Norw.; Bristol-Myers Squibb, Swed.
Triamcinolone acetonide (p.1050·2).
Corticosteroid.

Kenacort-T comp
Bristol-Myers Squibb, Norw.; Bristol-Myers Squibb, Swed.
Triamcinolone acetonide (p.1050·2); salicylic acid (p.1090·2).
Otitis externa; skin disorders.

Kenacort-T med Graneodin *Bristol-Myers Squibb, Swed.†.*
Triamcinolone acetonide (p.1050·2); neomycin sulphate (p.229·2); gramicidin (p.215·2).
Infected skin disorders.

Kenacutan
Bristol-Myers Squibb, Norw.; Bristol-Myers Squibb, Swed.
Triamcinolone acetonide (p.1050·2); halquinol (p.215·3).
Infected skin disorders.

Kenaject Mayrand, USA.
Triamcinolone acetonide (p.1050·2).
Corticosteroid.

Kenalcol Bristol-Myers Squibb, Fr.
Triamcinolone acetonide (p.1050·2); salicylic acid (p.1090·2); benzalkonium chloride (p.1101·3).
Skin disorders.

Kenalog
Note. This name is used for preparations of different composition.
Westwood-Squibb, Canad.; Berlin-Chemie, Ger.; Bristol-Myers Squibb, Irl.; Squibb, UK; Westwood-Squibb, USA.
Triamcinolone acetonide (p.1050·2).
Corticosteroid.

Bristol-Myers Squibb, Neth.
Triamcinolone acetonide (p.1050·2); salicylic acid (p.1090·2).
Keratosis; psoriasis.

Kenalog in Orabase
Bristol-Myers Squibb, Austral.; Westwood-Squibb, Canad.; Bristol-Myers Squibb, S.Afr.; Apothecon, USA.
Triamcinolone acetonide (p.1050·2).
Oral lesions.

Kenalone Bristol-Myers Squibb, Austral.
Triamcinolone acetonide (p.1050·2).
Skin disorders.

Kendural Abbott, Switz.
Ferrous sulphate (p.1340·2).
Sodium ascorbate (p.1365·2) is included in this preparation to increase the absorption and availability of iron.
Iron deficiency; iron-deficiency anaemia.

Kendural C Abbott, Ger.
Ferrous sulphate (p.1340·2).
Ascorbic acid (p.1365·2) is included in this preparation to increase the absorption and availability of iron.
Iron-deficiency; iron-deficiency anaemias.

Kendural-Fol-500 Abbott, Ger.
Ferrous sulphate (p.1340·2); folic acid (p.1340·3).
Ascorbic acid (p.1365·2) is included in this preparation to increase the absorption and availability of iron.
Iron and folic acid deficiency; iron-deficiency anaemias.

Kendural-Plus Abbott, Ger.
Ferrous sulphate (p.1340·2); vitamins.
Iron deficiency.

Kenergon Inorgan, Switz.
Lignocaine (p.1293·2).
Premature ejaculation.

Kenesil Kendall, Spain.
Nimodipine (p.922·2).
Cerebrovascular disorders.

Kenoidal Bristol-Myers Squibb, Belg.†.
Triamcinolone acetonide (p.1050·2); lignocaine (p.1293·2).
Anogenital pain; skin disorders.

Kenonel Marnel, USA.
Triamcinolone acetonide (p.1050·2).
Skin disorders.

Kenwood Therapeutic Liquid Kenwood, USA.
Multivitamin and mineral preparation.

Kephalodoron Weleda, Aust.
Ferrous sulphate (p.1340·2); silicon dioxide (p.1474·3).

Kephalosan Berlin-Chemie, Ger.†.
Propyphenazone (p.81·3); phenazone (p.78·2); caffeine (p.749·3).
Fever; pain.

Kepinol Pfleger, Ger.
Co-trimoxazole (p.196·3).
Bacterial infections; Pneumocystis carinii pneumonia.

Keppur Drossapharm, Switz.
Cream: Heparin sodium (p.879·3); comfrey (p.1567·1); hypericum oil (p.1590·1); calendula oil.
Topical gel: Heparin sodium (p.879·3); comfrey (p.1567·1).
Musculoskeletal, joint, peri-articular, and soft-tissue disorders; peripheral vascular disorders.

Keprodol Merckle, Aust.
Ketoprofen (p.48·2).
Inflammation; musculoskeletal and joint disorders; pain.

Keptan S Pfleger, Ger.†.
Glycol salicylate (p.43·1); benzyl nicotinate (p.22·1).
Formerly contained glycol salicylate, benzyl nicotinate, and heparin sodium.
Muscle and joint disorders; neuralgia.

Kerafilm Pierre Fabre, Fr.
Salicylic acid (p.1090·2); lactic acid (p.1593·3).
Formerly contained salicylic acid, lactic acid, iodine, and butyl aminobenzoate.
Calluses; corns; verrucae.

Keraform Asta Medica, Belg.†.
Bibrocathol (p.1553·2).
Eye infections.

Keralyt
Westwood-Squibb, Canad.; Westwood-Squibb, USA.
Salicylic acid (p.1090·2).
Hyperkeratosis.

Keras Caber, Ital.†.
Phosphatidylserine (p.1618·1).
Cognitive disorders.

Kerasal Spirig, Switz.
Salicylic acid (p.1090·2); urea (p.1095·2).
Skin disorders.

Keratisdin Isdin, Spain.
Lactic acid (p.1593·3).
Skin disorders.

Kerato Biciron N S & K, Ger.
Calcium pantothenate (p.1352·3).
Corneal injury.

Keratosane Biorga, Fr.
Urea (p.1095·2); pentosan polysulphate (p.928·1).
Skin disorders.

Keratosis Widmer, Aust.
Urea (p.1095·2); dexpanthenol (p.1570·3).
Hyperkeratotic skin disorders.

Keratosis forte Widmer, Aust.
Urea (p.1095·2); dexpanthenol (p.1570·3); tretinoin (p.1093·3).
Skin disorders.

Keratotal Collagen, Ital.
Ammonium lactate (p.1079·1).
Dry skin; scalp disorders.

Keratyl
Chauvin, Fr.; ankerpharm, Ger.; Novopharma, Switz.
Nandrolone sodium sulphate (p.1452·2).
Corneal damage.

Keri
Bristol-Myers Squibb, UK; Westwood, USA.
Emollient and moisturiser.
Dry skin.

Keri Facial Westwood, USA†.
Soap-free skin cleanser.

Keri Lotion Bristol-Myers Squibb, Canad.
SPF 15: Ethylhexyl *p*-methoxycinnamate (p.1487·1); octyl salicylate (p.1487·3); oxybenzone (p.1487·3).
Sunscreen.

Keri Soap Bristol-Myers Squibb, Canad.
Emollient.

Kerledex Searle, USA.
Betaxolol hydrochloride (p.832·1); chlorthalidone (p.839·3).
Hypertension.

Kerlon
Synthelabo, Ital.; Lorex Synthelabo, Neth.; Searle, Swed.; Synthelabo, Switz.
Betaxolol hydrochloride (p.832·1).
Angina pectoris; hypertension.

Kerlone
Synthelabo, Belg.; Synthelabo, Fr.; Synthelabo, Ger.; Boots, Spain†; Lorex, UK; Searle, USA.
Betaxolol hydrochloride (p.832·1).
Angina pectoris; hypertension.

Kernit CT, Ital.
Carnitine (p.1336·2).
Carnitine deficiency; myocardial ischaemia.

Kernosan Elixir Kern, Switz.
Aniseed (p.1549·3); cochlearia armoracia; calamus (p.1556·1); fennel (p.1579·1); hedera helix; imperatoria root; Iceland moss; pimpinella root plantain seed (p.1208·3); oak bark (p.1609·3); primula root; liquorice (p.1197·1).
Bronchitis; catarrh; coughs.

Kernosan Heidelberger Poudre Kern, Switz.
Absinthium (p.1541·1); aniseed (p.1549·3); caraway (p.1559·3); fennel (p.1579·1); juniper (p.1592·2); achillea (p.1542·2); pimpinella root.
Digestive system disorders.

Kernosan Huile de Massage Kern, Switz.
Plum oil; camphor (p.1557·2); methyl salicylate (p.55·2); eucalyptus oil (p.1578·1); lavender oil (p.1594·3); mint oil (p.1604·1); rosemary oil (p.1626·2); sage oil; thyme oil (p.1637·1); turpentine oil (p.1641·1); hyoscyamus oil (p.464·3).
Musculoskeletal, joint, and peri-articular pain.

Keroderm Turimed, Switz.
Linoleic acid ethyl ester; triclosan (p.1127·2); cholesterol (p.1383·3); cod-liver oil (p.1337·3); zinc oxide (p.1096·2); titanium dioxide (p.1093·3).
Eczema; inflammation; minor skin lesions.

Kerodex
Miba, Ital.; Whitehall, USA.
Barrier cream.

Keromask Innoxa, UK.
A covering cream.
Concealment of birth marks, scars, and disfiguring skin disease.

Kesint Mendelejeff, Ital.
Cefuroxime sodium (p.177·1).
Bacterial infections.

Kessar
Pharmacia Upjohn, Aust.; Pharmacia Upjohn, Austral.; Pharmacia Upjohn, Fr.; Pharmacia Upjohn, Ger.; Pharmacia Upjohn, Ital.; Pharmacia Upjohn, S.Afr.; Pharmacia Upjohn, Switz.
Tamoxifen citrate (p.563·3).
Breast cancer; endometrial cancer.

Kest Torbet Laboratories, UK.
Magnesium sulphate (p.1157·3); phenolphthalein (p.1208·2).
Constipation.

Kestine
Fisons, Neth.; Rhone-Poulenc Rorer, Norw.; Rhone-Poulenc Rorer, Swed.
Ebastine (p.410·2).
Allergic conjunctivitis; allergic rhinitis; pruritus; urticaria.

Kestomatine
Synthelabo, Belg.; Synthelabo, Switz.†.
Algeldrate (p.1177·3); simethicone (p.1213·1).
Gastro-intestinal disorders.

Kestomatine Baby Synthelabo, Belg.
Simethicone (p.1213·1); ceratonia (p.1472·2).
Abdominal distension; flatulence; vomiting.

Kestomatine Bebe Synthelabo, Switz.
Dimethicone (p.1213·1); carob fruit and seed (p.1472·2).
Gastro-intestinal disorders.

Kestrone Hyrex, USA.
Oestrone (p.1458·2).
Abnormal uterine bleeding; breast cancer; female castration; female hypogonadism; menopausal vulval and vaginal atrophy; primary ovarian failure; prostatic cancer.

Ket IRBI, Ital.†.
Ketanserin tartrate (p.894·3).
Hypertension.

Ketalar
Parke, Davis, Aust.; Parke, Davis, Austral.; Parke, Davis, Belg.; Parke, Davis, Canad.; Parke, Davis, Fr.; Parke, Davis, Irl.; Parke, Davis, Ital.; Parke, Davis, Neth.; Warner-Lambert, Norw.; Parke, Davis, S.Afr.†; Parke, Davis, Swed.; Parke, Davis, Switz.; Parke, Davis, UK; Parke, Davis, USA.
Ketamine hydrochloride (p.1226·2).
General anaesthesia.

Ketalgin IBP, Ital.†.
Ketoprofen (p.48·2).
Muscular and soft tissue disorders.

Ketalgine Amino, Switz.
Methadone hydrochloride (p.53·2).
Pain.

Ketanest Parke, Davis, Ger.
Ketamine hydrochloride (p.1226·2).
General anaesthesia; regional anaesthesia; status asthmaticus.

Ketartrium Esseti, Ital.
Ketoprofen (p.48·2) or ketoprofen sodium (p.48·3).
Musculoskeletal and joint disorders; phlebitis; superficial thrombophlebitis.

Ketas Kyorin, Jpn.
Ibudilast (p.754·2).
Asthma; cerebrovascular disorders.

Ketasma Lesvi, Spain.
Ketotifen fumarate (p.755·2).
Allergic rhinitis; asthma.

Ketazon
Gerot, Aust.; Medphano, Ger.
Kebuzone (p.48·1) or kebuzone sodium (p.48·1).
Trimecaine (p.1301·3) is included in the injection to alleviate the pain of injection.
Gout; inflammation; musculoskeletal and joint disorders; neuralgia; neuritis; pain; thrombophlebitis.

Ketensin Pharmacia Upjohn, Neth.
Ketanserin tartrate (p.894·3).
Hypertension.

Ketesse Tecefarma, Spain.
Dexketoprofen trometamol.
Inflammation; pain.

Ketil Tillomed, UK.
Ketoprofen (p.48·2).
Dysmenorrhoea; musculoskeletal, joint, and peri-articular disorders.

Keto Bayropharm, Ital.†.
Ketoprofen (p.48·2).
Musculoskeletal and joint disorders.

Ketocid Trinity, UK.
Ketoprofen (p.48·2).
Gout; musculoskeletal, joint, and peri-articular disorders; pain.

Ketoderm Janssen-Cilag, Fr.
Ketoconazole (p.383·1).
Fungal skin infections.

Keto-Diabur Test 5000
Boehringer Mannheim, Austral.; Boehringer Mannheim, Fr.; Boehringer Mannheim Diagnostics, Irl.; Boehringer Mannheim, Ital.; Boehringer Mannheim, S.Afr.; Boehringer Mannheim Diagnostics, UK.
Test for glucose and ketones in urine.

Keto-Diastix
Bayer Diagnostics, Austral.; Bayer, Canad.; Bayer Diagnostics, Fr.; Ames, Irl.; Bayer Diagnostici, Ital.; Ames, S.Afr.; Bayer Diagnostics, UK; Bayer, USA.
Test for glucose and ketones in urine.

Ketodol Schiapparelli, Ital.
Ketoprofen (p.48·2).
Sucralfate (p.1214·2) is included in this preparation in an attempt to limit adverse effects on the gastro-intestinal mucosa.
Pain.

Ketodur Searle, Swed.
Ketobemidone hydrochloride (p.48·2).
Pain.

Ketof Hexal, Ger.
Ketotifen fumarate (p.755·2).
Hypersensitivity reactions.

Ketofen Del Saz & Filippini, Ital.
Ketoprofen lysine (p.48·3).
Musculoskeletal and joint pain.

Ketoflam Parke-Med, S.Afr.
Ketoprofen (p.48·2).
Musculoskeletal, joint, and peri-articular disorders; pain.

Ketogan
Lundbeck, Norw.; Searle, Swed.
Ketobemidone hydrochloride (p.48·2); N,N-dimethyl-4,4-diphenyl-3-buten-2-amine hydrochloride.
Pain.

Ketogan Novum Searle, Swed.
Ketobemidone hydrochloride (p.48·2).
Adjunct in regional anaesthesia; pain.

Ketoisdin Isdin, Spain.
Ketoconazole (p.383·1).
Fungal infections.

Ketolar Parke, Davis, Spain.
Ketamine hydrochloride (p.1226·2).
General anaesthesia.

Keton Medi-Test Macherey Nagel Duren, S.Afr.
Test for ketones in urine.

Ketonex Ross, USA.
A range of isoleucine-, leucine-, and valine-free preparations for enteral nutrition including an infant feed.
Maple syrup urine disease.

Ketorax Lundbeck, Norw.
Ketobemidone hydrochloride (p.48·2).
Pain.

Ketosolan Spyfarma, Spain.
Ketoprofen (p.48·2).
Gout; musculoskeletal, joint, and peri-articular disorders; pain.

Ketosteril
Leopold, Aust.; Fresenius, Belg.†; Fresenius, Fr.; Fresenius-Praxis, Ger.; Fresenius, Switz.
Amino-acid preparation.
Nutritional supplement in renal failure.

Ketostix
Bayer Diagnostics, Austral.; Bayer, Canad.; Ames, Irl.; Bayer Diagnostici, Ital.; Ames, S.Afr.; Bayer Diagnostics, UK; Bayer, USA.
Test for ketones in urine, serum, plasma, and milk.

Ketostrip Lab Line, Ital.†.
Test for ketones in urine.

Ketovail Approved Prescription Services, UK†.
Ketoprofen (p.48·2).
Inflammation; musculoskeletal and joint disorders; pain.

Ketovite
Clements Stansen, Austral.†; Paines & Byrne, Irl.; Paines & Byrne, UK.
Multivitamin preparation.

Ketozip Ashbourne, UK.
Ketoprofen (p.48·2).
Dysmenorrhoea; gout; musculoskeletal, joint, and peri-articular disorders; sciatica.

Ketrax
Zeneca, Irl.; IDIS, UK.
Levamisole hydrochloride (p.102·3).
Worm infections.

Ketrizin Esseti, Ital.
Propylene glycol cefatrizine (p.164·2).
Bacterial infections.

Ketum Menarini, Fr.
Ketoprofen (p.48·2).
Musculoskeletal, joint, and soft-tissue disorders.

Ketur-Test
Boehringer Mannheim, Ital.; Boehringer Mannheim Diagnostics, UK.
Test for ketones in urine.

Kevatril Bristol-Myers Squibb, Ger.; SmithKline Beecham, Ger.
Granisetron hydrochloride (p.1193·3).
Nausea and vomiting associated with cytotoxic therapy.

Kevis Shampoo Antiforfora Restiva, Ital.
Pyrithione magnesium (p.1089·3); iceland moss.
Seborrhoeic dermatitis.

Kevopril Rhone-Poulenc Rorer, Aust.
Quinupramine (p.307·1).
Depression.

Kexelate Adcock Ingram, S.Afr.
Sodium polystyrene sulphonate (p.995·3).
Hyperkalaemia.

K-Exit Valtec, Canad.†.
Sodium polystyrene sulphonate (p.995·3).
Hyperkalaemia.

Key-Plex Hyrex, USA.
Vitamin B substances and vitamin C.
Parenteral nutrition.

Key-Pred Hyrex, USA.
Prednisolone acetate (p.1048·1).
Corticosteroid.

Key-Pred-SP Hyrex, USA.
Prednisolone sodium phosphate (p.1048·1).
Corticosteroid.

K-Flebo Sclavo, Ital.
Potassium aspartate (p.1161·3).
Hyperammonaemia; hypokalaemia.

K-G Elixir Geneva, USA.
Potassium gluconate (p.1161·1).
Hypokalaemia; potassium depletion.

KH3
Schwarzhaupt, Aust.; Schwarzhaupt, Ger.; Torbet Laboratories, UK.
Procaine hydrochloride (p.1299·2); haematoporphyrin (p.1587·1).
Tonic.

KH3 Powel Kenfarma, Spain.
Procaine hydrochloride (p.1299·2); haematoporphyrin (p.1587·1).
Tonic.

Khellangan N Ardeypharm, Ger.
Ammi visnaga fruit (p.1593·2).
Cardiac disorders.

Kiddi *Pharmaton, S.Afr.†.*
Lysine monohydrochloride; vitamins; calcium glycerophosphate.
Tonic.

Kiddi Nouvelle formule *Pharmaton, Switz.*
Multivitamin and mineral preparation.

Kiddi Pharmaton *Windsor, Irl.*
Multivitamin and mineral preparation with lysine.
Tonic.

Kiddicrom *Boehringer Ingelheim, S.Afr.*
Sodium cromoglycate (p.762·1).
Asthma.

Kiddie Vite *Covan, S.Afr.*
Ferrous gluconate (p.1340·1); vitamin B_1 (p.1361·2).
Iron-deficiency anaemia.

Kiddiekof *Covan, S.Afr.*
Codeine phosphate (p.26·1); mepyramine maleate (p.414·1); ephedrine hydrochloride (p.1059·3).
Coughs.

Kiddy Chews *Schein, USA.*
A range of vitamin preparations.

Kiddyflu *Caps, S.Afr.*
Paracetamol (p.72·2); dextromethorphan hydrobromide (p.1057·3); phenylephrine hydrochloride (p.1066·2); chlorpheniramine maleate (p.405·1).
Cold and influenza symptoms.

Kiditard
Dagra, Neth.†; Delandale, UK†.
Quinidine bisulphate (p.938·3).
Arrhythmias.

Kidrolase
Rhone-Poulenc Rorer, Canad.; Bellon, Fr.
Asparaginase (p.504·3).
Malignant neoplasms.

Kidscreen *Hamilton, Austral.*
Ethylhexyl *p*-methoxycinnamate (p.1487·1); titanium dioxide (p.1093·3).
Sunscreen.

KIE *Laser, USA.*
Ephedrine hydrochloride (p.1059·3); potassium iodide (p.1493·1).
Coughs.

Kiel Bone Graft *Davis & Geck, UK†.*
Surgibone (p.1634·2).
Bone disorders.

Kiflone *Berk, UK.*
Cephalexin (p.178·2).
Bacterial infections.

Kilios *Pharmacia Upjohn, Ital.*
Aspirin (p.16·1).
Fever; pain.

Killavon *Lysoform, Ger.†.*
Benzalkonium chloride (p.1101·3).
Fungal infections of the feet; surface disinfection.

Killpan *Labitec, Spain.*
Camphor (p.1557·2); arnica (p.1550·3); capsicum (p.1559·2); aesculus (p.1543·3); scrophularia aquatica; menthol (p.1600·2); rosemary; turpentine oil (p.1641·1).
Rheumatic and muscle pain.

Kilmicene *Pharmacia Upjohn, Switz.†.*
Tolciclate (p.388·3).
Fungal skin infections.

Kilozim *AGIPS, Ital.†.*
Metoclopramide (p.1202·1); pepsin (p.1616·3); sodium dehydrocholate (p.1570·3); bromelain (p.1555·1); casein; amylase (p.1549·1); cellulase (p.1561·1); lipase; trypsin (p.1640·1); chymotrypsin (p.1563·2).
Gastro-intestinal disorders.

Kiminto *Rhone-Poulenc Rorer, UK.*
Peppermint oil (p.1208·1).

Kimotab *Mochida, Jpn†.*
Bromelains (p.1555·1); trypsin (p.1640·1).
Inflammation.

Kincare *Moraz, UK.*
Parsley (p.1615·3); garlic (p.1583·1).
Pediculosis.

Kinciclina *Kin, Spain.*
Tetracycline megallate (p.261·1).
Bacterial infections.

Kinder Finimal *Roche Nicholas, Neth.*
Paracetamol (p.72·2).
Fever; pain.

Kinder Luuf *Apomedica, Aust.*
Camphor (p.1557·2); menthol (p.1600·2); eucalyptus oil (p.1578·1); turpentine oil (p.1641·1); thymol (p.1127·1).
Catarrh; cold symptoms.

Kindercal *Mead Johnson Nutritionals, USA.*
Preparation for enteral nutrition.

Kindergen *Scientific Hospital Supplies, UK.*
Preparation for enteral nutrition.

Kindergen PROD *Scientific Hospital Supplies, Irl.*
Preparation for enteral nutrition.
Peritoneal dialysis in renal failure.

Kindian *Corvi, Ital.†.*
Methyl salicylate (p.55·2); eucalyptus oil (p.1578·1); camphor (p.1557·2); hyoscyamus (p.464·3); cajuput oil (p.1556·1).
Pain.

Kindivite *Wyeth Health, Austral.†.*
Vitamins and minerals with fat, protein and carbohydrate.

Kine B6 *Granata, Ital.†.*
Dimenhydrinate (p.408·2); pyridoxine (p.1363·1) or pyridoxine hydrochloride (p.1362·3).
Nausea.

Kinedak *Ono, Jpn.*
Epalrestat (p.319·2).
Diabetic neuropathy.

Kinesed *Stuart, USA†.*
Phenobarbitone (p.350·2); hyoscyamine sulphate (p.464·2); atropine sulphate (p.455·1); hyoscine hydrobromide (p.462·3).
Adjunct in gastro-intestinal disorders.

Kinet *Solvay, Spain.*
Cisapride (p.1187·1).
Gastro-oesophageal reflux; gastroparesis.

Kinetin *Schering, Ger.†.*
Hyaluronidase (p.1588·1).
Aspiration of viscous effusions; extension of local anaesthesia; haematomas; oedema; to improve the absorption of intramuscular and subcutaneous injections.

Kinevac
Squibb Diagnostics, Canad.; Squibb Diagnostics, USA.
Sincalide (p.1630·1).
Adjunct in biliary, pancreatic, and gastro-intestinal investigations; ileus.

Kinidin
Astra, Austral.; Astra, Irl.; Astra, Norw.; Hassle, Swed.; Kabi, Swed.†; Astra, Switz.; Astra, UK.
Quinidine bisulphate (p.938·3).
Arrhythmias.

Kinidine *Astra, Neth.*
Quinidine bisulphate (p.938·3).
Arrhythmias.

Kinidine Durettes *Astra, Belg.*
Quinidine bisulphate (p.938·3).
Arrhythmias.

Kinin *NM, Swed.*
Quinine hydrochloride (p.439·2).
Malaria; myotonia.

Kinocystol *Pierre Fabre, Fr.†.*
Esterified oleic triglycerides.
Gastro-intestinal disorders.

Kinogen *Geymonat, Ital.*
Tyrothricin (p.267·2); hydrocortisone sodium succinate (p.1044·1).
Vulvovaginal infections.

Kinolymphat *PGM, Ger.*
Homoeopathic preparation.

Kinot *Farex, Canad.*
Camphor (p.1557·2); expressed mustard oil (p.1605·3).

Kinson *Alphapharm, Austral.*
Levodopa (p.1137·1); carbidopa (p.1136·1).
Parkinsonism.

Kintavit *Giuliani, Switz.*
Multivitamin and mineral preparation with ginseng.

Kinupril *Bellon, Fr.*
Quinupramine (p.307·1).
Depression.

Kinurea H *Fuca, Fr.*
Quinine and urea hydrochloride (p.1624·2).
Anorectal disorders.

Kir Richter *Lepetit, Ital.*
Aprotinin (p.711·3).
Antidote to thrombolytics; haemorrhage; shock.

Kira
Lichtwer, Ger.; Lichtwer, UK.
Hypericum (p.1590·1).
Depression.

kirim *Hormosan, Ger.*
Bromocriptine mesylate (p.1132·2).
Acromegaly; amenorrhoea; female infertility; galactorrhoea; hyperprolactinaemia; lactation suppression; ovulation disorders; parkinsonism; premenstrual syndrome.

Kiro Rub *Prodemdis, Canad.*
Methyl salicylate (p.55·2); camphor (p.1557·2); menthol (p.1600·2); eucalyptus oil (p.1578·1).

Kisitan *Lambda, USA.*
Oral liquid: Phenylephrine tannate (p.1067·1); chlorpheniramine tannate (p.405·2); mepyramine tannate (p.414·1).
Tablets: Phenylephrine tannate (p.1067·1); chlorpheniramine tannate (p.405·2).

Kisitex *Lambda, USA.*
Phenylephrine hydrochloride (p.1066·2); phenylpropanolamine (p.1067·2); guaiphenesin (p.1061·3).
Coughs.

Kisolv *Ecupharma, Ital.*
Urokinase (p.959·3).
Thrombo-embolic disorders.

Kiton *Pulitzer, Ital.*
Isosorbide mononitrate (p.893·3).
Cardiac stenosis; ischaemic heart disease.

Klacid
Abbott, Aust.; Abbott, Austral.; Abbott, Ger.; Abbott, Irl.; Abbott, Ital.; Abbott, Neth.; Abbott, Norw.; Abbott, S.Afr.; Abbott, Spain; Abbott, Swed.; Abbott, Switz.
Clarithromycin (p.189·1) or clarithromycin lactobionate (p.190·1).
Bacterial infections.

Klaciped *Abbott, Switz.*
Clarithromycin (p.189·1).
Bacterial infections.

Klar *Hermes, Ger.†.*
Aspirin (p.16·1); ascorbic acid.
Pain.

Klaricid *Abbott, UK.*
Clarithromycin (p.189·1).
Bacterial infections.

Klariderm *Clariana, Spain.*
Fluocinonide (p.1041·2).
Skin disorders.

Klarivitina *Clariana, Spain.*
Cyproheptadine hydrochloride (p.407·2).
Allergic rhinitis; reduced appetite; urticaria.

Klaron *Dermik, USA.*
Sulphacetamide sodium (p.252·2).
Acne.

KLB6 *Nature's Bounty, USA.*
Pyridoxine hydrochloride (p.1362·3); soya lecithin (p.1595·2); kelp (p.1593·1); cider vinegar.

Klean-Prep
UCB, Aust.; Norgine, Belg.; Rivex, Canad.; Norgine, Fr.; Norgine, Ger.; Helsinn Birex, Irl.; Norgine, S.Afr.; UCB, Swed.; Norgine, Switz.; Norgine, UK.
Macrogol 3350 (p.1598·2); electrolytes (p.1147·1).
Bowel evacuation.

K-Lease *Adria, USA.*
Potassium chloride (p.1161·1).
Potassium deficiency.

Kleen-Handz *American Medical, USA.*
Alcohol (p.1099·1).
Hand disinfection.

Kleenocid *Agepha, Aust.*
Chlorhexidine acetate (p.1107·2).
Skin disinfection.

Kleenosept *Agepha, Aust.*
Hexetidine (p.1116·1).
Skin disinfection.

Kleer *Modern Health Products, UK.*
Echinacea (p.1574·2); urtica (p.1642·3); burdock root (p.1594·2).
Skin disorders.

Kleer Cream *Lane, UK.*
Hamamelis (p.1587·1); eucalyptus oil (p.1578·1); methyl salicylate (p.55·2); camphor (p.1557·2); ti-tree oil (p.1599·2); zinc oxide (p.1096·2).
Formerly known as Soothene.
Minor skin disorders.

Klerist-D *Nutripharm, USA.*
Pseudoephedrine hydrochloride (p.1068·3); chlorpheniramine maleate (p.405·1).
Upper respiratory-tract symptoms.

Klexane
Rhone-Poulenc Rorer, Norw.; Rhone-Poulenc Rorer, Swed.
Enoxaparin sodium (p.864·2).
Anticoagulation during haemodialysis or haemofiltration; thrombo-embolic disorders; thrombosis prophylaxis.

Klifem *Pekana, Ger.*
Homoeopathic preparation.

Klimadoral *Kabi, Switz.†.*
Oestriol (p.1457·2).
Menopausal disorders.

Klimadynon *Bionorica, Ger.*
Cimicifuga (p.1563·3).
Menopausal disorders.

Klimaktoplant
DHU, Ger.; Omida, Switz.
Homoeopathic preparation.

Klimasyx *Syxyl, Ger.*
Homoeopathic preparation.

Klimax-E *Fink, Ger.†.*
Oestriol (p.1457·2).
Oestrogenic.

Klimofol *Ivamed, Ger.*
Propofol (p.1229·3).
General anaesthesia.

Klimonorm *Jenapharm, Ger.*
9 Tablets, oestradiol valerate (p.1455·2); 12 tablets, oestradiol valerate; levonorgestrel (p.1454·1).
Menopausal disorders.

Klinitamin *Eisai, Jpn†.*
Amino-acid and carbohydrate infusion.
Parenteral nutrition.

Klinoc *Wyeth Lederle, Aust.*
Minocycline hydrochloride (p.226·2).
Acne.

Klinomycin *Lederle, Ger.*
Minocycline hydrochloride (p.226·2).
Bacterial infections.

Klinoren S *Fides, Ger.†.*
Homoeopathic preparation.

Klinotab *Cyanamid, Belg.†.*
Minocycline hydrochloride (p.226·2).
Bacterial infections.

Klinoxid *Lederle, Ger.*
Benzoyl peroxide (p.1079·2).
Acne.

Kliofem *Novo Nordisk, UK.*
Oestradiol (p.1455·1); norethisterone acetate (p.1453·1).
Oestrogen deficiency; postmenopausal osteoporosis.

Kliogest
Novo Nordisk, Aust.; Novo Nordisk, Austral.; Novo Nordisk, Belg.; Novo Nordisk, Fr.; Novo Nordisk, Irl.; Novo Nordisk, Ital.; Novo Nordisk, Neth.; Novo Nordisk, Norw.; Novo Nordisk, S.Afr.; Novo Nordisk, Swed.; Novo Nordisk, Switz.
Oestradiol (p.1455·1); norethisterone acetate (p.1453·1).
Formerly contained oestradiol, oestriol, and norethisterone acetate.
Menopausal disorders; osteoporosis.

Kliogest N *Novo Nordisk, Ger.*
Oestradiol (p.1455·1); norethisterone acetate (p.1453·1).
Formerly contained oestradiol, oestriol, and norethisterone acetate.
Menopausal disorders.

Kliovance *Novo Nordisk, UK.*
Oestradiol (p.1455·1); norethisterone acetate (p.1453·1).
Menopausal disorders.

Klipal *Robapharm, Fr.*
Paracetamol (p.72·2); codeine phosphate (p.26·1).
Pain.

Klismacort *Bene, Ger.*
Prednisolone (p.1048·1).
Rectal corticosteroid.

Klistier *Fresenius, Ger.*
Dibasic sodium phosphate (p.1159·3); monobasic sodium phosphate (p.1159·3).
Bowel evacuation; constipation.

KLN *Roche Consumer, UK.*
Kaolin (p.1195·1); pectin (p.1474·1); sodium citrate (p.1153·2); peppermint oil (p.1208·1).
Diarrhoea.

Klobamicina *Almirall, Spain†.*
Dibekacin sulphate (p.201·3).
Bacterial infections.

Kloclor *Adcock Ingram, S.Afr.*
Cefaclor (p.163·2).
Bacterial infections.

Klodin *Savio, Ital.*
Ticlopidine hydrochloride (p.953·1).
Thrombosis prophylaxis.

K-Long *Pharmacia, Canad.†.*
Potassium chloride (p.1161·1).
Potassium depletion.

Klonopin *Roche, USA.*
Clonazepam (p.343·3).
Epilepsy.

K-Lor
Abbott, Canad.; Abbott, USA.
Potassium chloride (p.1161·1).
Hypokalaemia; potassium depletion.

Klor-Con *Upsher-Smith, USA.*
Potassium chloride (p.1161·1).
Hypokalaemia.

Klor-Con/EF *Upsher-Smith, USA.*
Potassium bicarbonate (p.1153·1); potassium citrate (p.1153·1).

Kloref
Note. This name is used for preparations of different composition.
Knoll, S.Afr.
Betaine hydrochloride (p.1553·2); potassium bicarbonate (p.1153·1).
Hypokalaemia.

Cox, UK.
Betaine hydrochloride (p.1553·2); potassium bicarbonate (p.1153·1); potassium chloride (p.1161·1); potassium benzoate (p.1161·1).
Hypokalaemia; potassium depletion.

Kloref-S *Cox, UK.*
Betaine hydrochloride (p.1553·2); potassium bicarbonate (p.1153·1); potassium chloride (p.1161·1).
Hypokalaemia; potassium depletion.

Klor-Kleen *Medentech, Irl.*
Sodium dichloroisocyanurate (p.1124·3); sodium dodecylbenzenesulphonate.
Surface disinfection.

Klorsept *Medentech, Irl.*
Sodium dichloroisocyanurate (p.1124·3).
Surface disinfection.

Klorvess *Sandoz, USA.*
Effervescent tablets: Potassium chloride (p.1161·1); potassium bicarbonate (p.1153·1); lysine hydrochloride (p.1350·1).
Oral effervescent granules: Potassium chloride (p.1161·1); potassium bicarbonate (p.1153·1); potassium citrate (p.1153·1); lysine hydrochloride (p.1350·1).
Oral liquid: Potassium chloride (p.1161·1).
Hypokalaemic-hypochloraemic alkalosis; potassium depletion.

Klosterfrau Aktiv *Klosterfrau, Ger.*
Garlic; hypericum; retinol; alpha tocopheryl acetate.
Tonic.

Klosterfrau Magentonikum *Klosterfrau, Ger.†.*
Cynara; liquorice; angelica; inula helenium; ginger; galanga; melissa; gentian; dried bitter-orange peel; clove; senna; cinnamon bark; black pepper; cardamom; nutmeg; star anise; poplar buds; fennel; citrus sinensis.
Tonic.

Klosterfrau Melissengeist *Klosterfrau, Ger.*
Melissa; inula helenium; angelica; ginger; clove; gentian; fruct. piperis nigri; galanga; nutmeg; dried bitter-orange peel; cinnamon bark; senna; cardamom; ethanol.
Herbal preparation.

Klosterfrau Vitaltonikum (Energeticum)
Klosterfrau, Ger.†.
Arnica; cynara; liquorice; melissa; inula helenium; gentian; angelica; fruct. piperis nigri; dried bitter-orange peel; ginger; galanga; clove; senna; cinnamon bark; cardamom; nutmeg; star anise; fennel; liquorice; gem. populi; vitamins; sweet orange peel.
Tonic.

Klotrix *Apothecon, USA.*
Potassium chloride (p.1161·1).
Hypokalaemia; potassium depletion.

Klysma Salinisch
Pharmacia Upjohn, Aust.; Pharmacia Upjohn, Ger.
Monobasic sodium phosphate (p.1159·3); dibasic sodium phosphate (p.1159·3).
Bowel evacuation.

Klysma Sorbit *Pharmacia Upjohn, Ger.*
Sorbitol (p.1354·2); potassium sorbate (p.1125·2).
Bowel evacuation; constipation.

K-Lyte
Note. This name is used for preparations of different composition.
Roberts, Canad.
Potassium citrate (p.1153·1).
Potassium depletion.

Apothecon, USA.
Potassium bicarbonate (p.1153·1).
Potassium deficiency.

K-Lyte DS *Apothecon, USA.*
Potassium bicarbonate (p.1153·1); potassium citrate (p.1153·1).
Potassium deficiency.

K-Lyte/Cl
Note. This name is used for preparations of different composition.
Roberts, Canad.; Apothecon, USA.
Effervescent powder: Potassium chloride (p.1161·1).
Potassium deficiency.

Apothecon, USA.
Effervescent tablets: Potassium chloride (p.1161·1); potassium bicarbonate (p.1153·1).
Potassium deficiency.

Klyx
Ferring, Norw.; Ferring, Swed.
Docusate sodium (p.1189·3); sorbitol (p.1354·2).
Bowel evacuation; constipation.

Klyx Magnum *Ferring, Switz.*
Docusate sodium (p.1189·3); dried magnesium sulphate (p.1158·2); urea (p.1095·2).
Bowel evacuation; constipation.

Klyxenema salinisch *Ferring, Ger.†; Braun, Ger.†.*
Monobasic sodium phosphate (p.1159·3); dibasic sodium phosphate (p.1159·3).
Bowel evacuation; constipation.

KMA *Berlin-Chemie, Ger.*
Potassium hydroxide (p.1621·1); magnesium oxide (p.1198·3).
Cardiac disorders.

K-Mag *Vita Glow, Austral.*
Potassium aspartate (p.1161·3); magnesium aspartate (p.1157·2).
Potassium and magnesium supplement.

K-Med *Riva, Canad.*
Potassium chloride (p.1161·1); magnesium gluconate (p.1157·2).
Potassium supplement.

K-Med 900 *Riva, Canad.†.*
Potassium chloride (p.1161·1).
Potassium supplement.

K-MIC *Hassle, Swed.†.*
Potassium chloride (p.1161·1).
Hypokalaemia; potassium supplement.

Kneipp Abfuhr Dragees N *Kneipp, Ger.†.*
Aloes (p.1177·1); gentian (p.1583·3); rhubarb (p.1212·1); frangula bark (p.1193·2).
Constipation.

Kneipp Abfuhr Herbagran *Kneipp, Ger.*
Ispaghula husk (p.1194·2).
Constipation.

Kneipp Abfuhr Tee N *Kneipp, Ger.*
Senna (p.1212·2).
Constipation.

Kneipp Baldrian *Kneipp, Ger.*
Valerian (p.1643·1).
Anxiety disorders; sleep disorders.

Kneipp Baldrian-Pflanzensaft Nerventrost
Kneipp, Ger.
Valerian (p.1643·1).
Nervousness; sleep disorders.

Kneipp Balsamo *Fher, Spain.*
Camphor (p.1557·2); peru balsam (p.1617·2); cineole (p.1564·1); oleum pini sylvestris; thymol (p.1127·1); menthol (p.1600·2).
Upper-respiratory-tract disorders.

Kneipp Beruhigungs-Bad A *Kneipp, Ger.*
Valerian oil; citronella oil (p.1565·1).
Bath additive; nervous disorders; sleep disorders.

Kneipp Birkenblatter-Pflanzensaft *Kneipp, Ger.*
Silver birch (p.1553·3).
Diuretic.

Kneipp Blasen- und Nieren-Tee *Kneipp, Ger.*
Equisetum (p.1575·1); solidago virgaurea; silver birch (p.1553·3); ononis (p.1610·2).
Bladder and kidney disorders.

Kneipp Blutreinigungs-Tee *Kneipp, Ger.†.*
Juniper (p.1592·2); peppermint leaf (p.1208·1); silver birch (p.1553·3).
Blood disorders.

Kneipp Brennessel-Pflanzensaft *Kneipp, Ger.*
Urtica (p.1642·3).
Diuretic.

Kneipp Brunnenkresse-Pflanzensaft *Kneipp, Ger.*
Nasturtium.
Diuretic.

Kneipp Brustkaramellen *Kneipp, Ger.†.*
Menthol (p.1600·2); anise oil (p.1550·1); sage oil; honey (p.1345·3).
Coughs and associated throat disorders.

Kneipp Calcium compositum N *Kneipp, Ger.*
Multivitamin and mineral preparation.
Calcium deficiency.

Kneipp Drei-Pflanzen-Dragees *Kneipp, Ger.*
Combination pack: Tablets, Crataegus (p.1568·2); tablets, garlic (p.1583·1); tablets, mistletoe (p.1604·1).
Arteriosclerosis.

Kneipp Entschlackungs-Tee *Kneipp, Ger.*
Juniper (p.1592·2); peppermint leaf (p.1208·1); birch leaf (p.1553·3).
Diuretic.

Kneipp Entwasserungstee *Nycomed, Aust.*
Juniper (p.1592·2); peppermint leaf (p.1208·1); silver birch leaf (p.1553·3).
Diuretic.

Kneipp Erkaltungs-Bad *Kneipp, Ger.*
Thyme oil (p.1637·1).
Bath additive; cold symptoms.

Kneipp Erkaltungsbad Spezial *Kneipp, Ger.*
Eucalyptus oil (p.1578·1); camphor (p.1557·2).
Bath additive; catarrh.

Kneipp Erkaltungs-Balsam N *Kneipp, Ger.*
Eucalyptus oil (p.1578·1); siberian fir oil; rosemary oil (p.1626·2); pumilio pine oil (p.1623·3); thyme oil (p.1637·1); turpentine oil (p.1641·1).
Coughs and associated respiratory-tract disorders.

Kneipp Fichtennadel Franzbranntwein *Kneipp, Ger.*
Menthol (p.1600·2); alcohol (p.1099·1).
Peripheral circulatory disorders; soft-tissue disorders.

Kneipp Flatuol *Kneipp, Ger.*
Fennel (p.1579·1); caraway (p.1559·3); peppermint leaf (p.1208·1); gentian (p.1583·3).
Gastro-intestinal disorders.

Kneipp Galle- und Leber-Tee *Nycomed, Aust.*
Peppermint leaf (p.1208·1); turmeric (p.1001·3); taraxacum (p.1634·2).
Gallbladder and liver disorders.

Kneipp Galle- und Leber-Tee N *Kneipp, Ger.*
Peppermint leaf (p.1208·1); turmeric (p.1001·3); taraxacum (p.1634·2).
Herbal tea.

Kneipp Gastropressan *Kneipp, Ger.†.*
Chamomile (p.1561·2); liquorice (p.1197·1); hamamelis (p.1587·1); guaiazulene (p.1586·3); absinthium (p.1541·1); polygalactomannan.
Gastro-intestinal disorders.

Kneipp Ginsenetten *Kneipp, Ger.*
Ginseng (p.1584·2).
Tonic.

Kneipp Grippe-Tee *Nycomed, Aust.*
Tilia (p.1637·3); salix purpurea (p.82·3); plantago lanceolata; thyme (p.1636·3); chamomile (p.1561·2).
Cold symptoms.

Kneipp Herz- und Kreislauf-Tee *Kneipp, Ger.*
Rosemary leaves; crataegus; motherwort; hypericum; Paraguay tea.
Herbal tea.

Kneipp Herz- und Kreislauf-Unterstutzungs-Tee *Nycomed, Aust.*
Rosemary leaf; crataegus (p.1568·2); maté leaf (p.1645·1).
Cardiovascular disorders.

Kneipp Herzsalbe Unguentum Cardiacum Kneipp *Kneipp, Ger.*
Rosemary oil (p.1626·2); camphor (p.1557·2); menthol (p.1600·2).
Cardiac disorders.

Kneipp Heupack Herbatherm N *Kneipp, Ger.*
Cut grasses and flowers.
Biliary-tract, kidney, and bladder disorders; rheumatic and arthritic disorders.

Kneipp Husten- und Bronchial-Tee
Nycomed, Aust.; Kneipp, Ger.
Fennel (p.1579·1); primula flowers and calyx; thyme (p.1636·3); plantago lanceolata.
Bronchitis; catarrh; coughs.

Kneipp Hustensaft Spitzwegerich *Kneipp, Ger.*
Plantago lanceolata.
Catarrh.

Kneipp Johanniskrasut-Pflanzensaft N *Kneipp, Ger.*
Hypericum oil (p.1590·1).
Psychiatric disorders.

Kneipp Johanniskraut-Ol N *Kneipp, Ger.*
Hypericum oil (p.1590·1).
Burns; wounds.

Kneipp Knoblauch Dragees N *Kneipp, Ger.*
Garlic (p.1583·1).
Arteriosclerosis.

Kneipp Knoblauch-Pflanzensaft *Kneipp, Ger.*
Garlic (p.1583·1).
Arteriosclerosis; digestive system disorders; hypertension.

Kneipp Krauter Hustensaft N *Kneipp, Ger.*
Norway spruce oil; pumilio pine oil (p.1623·3); primula flower; thyme (p.1636·3).
Coughs and associated respiratory-tract disorders.

Kneipp Krauter Taschenkur Nerven und Schlaf N *Kneipp, Ger.*
Combination pack: Tablets, valerian (p.1643·1); tablets, hypericum (p.1590·1); tablets, melissa leaves (p.1600·1); citronella oil (p.1565·1); lemon grass oil (p.1595·3).
Nervous disorders.

Kneipp Kreislauf-Bad Rosmarin-Aquasan
Kneipp, Ger.
Camphor (p.1557·2); rosemary oil (p.1626·2).
Bath additive; circulatory disorders.

Kneipp Latschernkiefer Franzbranntwein
Kneipp, Ger.
Camphor (p.1557·2); oleum pini sylvestris; alcohol (p.1099·1).
Musculoskeletal and joint disorders; peripheral vascular disorders; soft-tissue disorders.

Kneipp Lowenzahn-Pflanzensaft *Kneipp, Ger.*
Taraxacum (p.1634·2).
Gall bladder and liver disorders.

Kneipp Magentrost *Kneipp, Ger.†.*
Hypericum (p.1590·1); achillea (p.1542·2); centaury (p.1561·1); juniper (p.1592·2); peppermint leaf (p.1208·1); absinthium (p.1541·1); gentian (p.1583·3).
Digestive system disorders.

Kneipp Melissen-Pflanzensaft *Kneipp, Ger.*
Melissa (p.1600·1).
Nervous disorders.

Kneipp Milch-Molke-Bad *Kneipp, Ger.*
Skimmed milk; whey; lactic acid (p.1593·3).
Bath additive; burns; skin disorders.

Kneipp Minzol *Kneipp, Ger.*
Mint oil (p.1604·1).
Cold symptoms; gastro-intestinal disorders; myalgia; neuralgia.

Kneipp Mistel-Pflanzensaft *Kneipp, Ger.*
Mistletoe (p.1604·1).
Hypertension.

Kneipp Nerven- und Schlaf-Tee *Nycomed, Aust.*
Melissa (p.1600·1); valerian (p.1643·1); citrus sinensis.
Nervous disorders; sleep disorders.

Kneipp Nerven- und Schlaf-Tee N *Kneipp, Ger.*
Melissa leaves (p.1600·1); valerian root (p.1643·1); sweet orange peel.
Nervous disorders.

Kneipp Neurodermatitis-Bad *Kneipp, Ger.*
Soya oil (p.1355·1).
Bath additive; dry skin; pruritus.

Kneipp Nieren- und Blasen-Tee *Nycomed, Aust.*
Silver birch (p.1553·3); equisetum (p.1575·1); solidago virgaurea; ononis (p.1610·2); peppermint leaf (p.1208·1); calendula officinalis.
Urinary-tract disorders.

Kneipp Nieren- und Blasen-Tee N *Kneipp, Ger.†.*
Bearberry (p.1552·2); hibiscus; silver birch (p.1553·3); equisetum (p.1575·1).
Kidney and bladder disorders.

Kneipp Petersilie N *Kneipp, Ger.*
Parsley (p.1615·3).
Diuretic.

Kneipp Pflanzendragees Brennessel *Kneipp, Ger.*
Urtica (p.1642·3).
Diuretic.

Kneipp Pflanzendragees Johanniskraut *Kneipp, Ger.*
Hypericum (p.1590·1).
Nervous disorders.

Kneipp Pflanzendragees Mistel *Kneipp, Ger.*
Mistletoe (p.1604·1).
Circulatory disorders.

Kneipp Pflanzendragees Weissdorn *Kneipp, Ger.*
Crataegus leaves, flowers, and fruit (p.1568·2).
Cardiac disorders.

Kneipp Pildoras *Fher, Spain†.*
Juniper (p.1592·2); aloes (p.1177·1); bile (p.1553·2); calamus root (p.1556·1); rhubarb root (p.1212·1).
Constipation.

Kneipp Rettich-Pflanzensaft *Kneipp, Ger.*
Raphanus.
Gall bladder and liver disorders.

Kneipp Rheuma Bad *Kneipp, Ger.*
Juniper oil (p.1592·3); sweet birch oil (p.55·3).
Bath additive; rheumatism and spinal disorders.

Kneipp Rheuma Salbe Capsicum Forte *Kneipp, Ger.*
Cayenne pepper.
Musculoskeletal and joint disorders; neuralgia; sciatica.

Kneipp Rheuma Stoffwechsel-Bad Heublumen-Aquasan *Kneipp, Ger.*
Coumarin (p.1568·1); peppermint oil (p.1208·1); caraway oil (p.1559·3); sage oil; thyme oil (p.1637·1).
Bath additive; tonic bath.

Kneipp Rheuma Tee N *Kneipp, Ger.*
Bittersweet stalk (p.1574·2); willow bark (p.82·3); elder leaf (p.1627·2); juniper berry (p.1592·2); red sandalwood.
Rheumatic disorders.

Kneipp Rosmarin-Pflanzensaft *Kneipp, Ger.*
Rosemary leaf.
Circulatory disorders.

Kneipp Schafgarbe-Pflanzensaft Frauentost N *Kneipp, Ger.*
Achillea (p.1542·2).
Anorexia; digestive system disorders.

Kneipp Schlankheits-Unterstutzungstee
Kneipp, Ger.†.
Senna (p.1212·2); peppermint leaf (p.1208·1); black tea (p.1645·1); solidago virgaurea; levisticum officinale (p.1597·2); hibiscus.
Obesity.

Kneipp Sedativ-Bad *Kneipp, Ger.†.*
Valerian oil; citronella oil (p.1565·1).
Bath additive; sedative.

Kneipp Spitzwegerich-Pflanzensaft Hustentrost *Kneipp, Ger.*
Plantago lanceolata.
Cold symptoms; coughs.

Kneipp Stoffwechsel-Unterstutzungs-Tee *Nycomed, Aust.*
Prunus spinosa; taraxacum (p.1634·2); peppermint leaf (p.1208·1); levisticum officinale (p.1597·2); hibiscus.
Stimulation of metabolic activity.

Kneipp Tonikum-Bad Fichtennadel-Aquasan *Kneipp, Ger.*
Norway spruce oil; eucalyptus oil (p.1578·1); turpentine oil (p.1641·1).
Bath additive; tonic bath.

Kneipp Verdauungs-Tee *Nycomed, Aust.*
Prunus spinosa; chamomile (p.1561·2); fennel (p.1579·1); centaury (p.1561·1).
Gastro-intestinal disorders.

Kneipp Verdauungs-Tee N *Kneipp, Ger.*
Chamomile (p.1561·2); fennel (p.1579·1); centaury (p.1561·1).
Gastro-intestinal disorders.

Kneipp Wacholderbeer-Pflanzensaft *Kneipp, Ger.*
Juniper (p.1592·2).
Diuretic; gastro-intestinal disorders.

Kneipp Weissdorn-Pflanzensaft Sebastianeum *Kneipp, Ger.*
Crataegus (p.1568·2).
Cardiac disorders.

Kneipp Woerisettes *Roche, Switz.*
Aloes (p.1177·1); plant extracts.
Constipation.

Kneipp Worisetten *Kneipp, Ger.†.*
Aloes (p.1177·1); fennel (p.1579·1).
Gastro-intestinal disorders.

Kneipp Worisetten S *Kneipp, Ger.*
Senna (p.1212·2).
Constipation.

Kneipp Zinnkraut-Pflanzensaft *Kneipp, Ger.*
Equisetum (p.1575·1).
Bronchitis; coughs.

Kneipplax N *Kneipp, Ger.*
Ispaghula husk (p.1194·2); senna (p.1212·2).
Constipation.

Knochenzement *Synthes, Aust.*
Methylmethacrylate/polymethylmethacrylate (p.1603·2).
Bone cement in orthopaedic surgery.

K-Norm *Fisons, USA.*
Potassium chloride (p.1161·1).
Hypokalaemia; potassium depletion.

Knufinke Blasen- und Nieren-Tee Uro-K *Divapharma, Ger.†.*
Rose fruit (p.1365·2); ononis (p.1610·2); matricaria flowers (p.1561·2); orthosiphon leaf (p.1592·2); equisetum (p.1575·1); juniper (p.1592·2); willow bark (p.82·3).
Urinary calculi.

Knufinke Broncholind K *Divapharma, Ger.†.*
Anise (p.1549·3); pimpinella; althaea (p.1546·3); fennel (p.1579·1); liquorice (p.1197·1); thyme (p.1636·3).
Colds.

Knufinke Gastrobin Magen- und Darm-Tee
Divapharma, Ger.†.
Fennel (p.1579·1); matricaria flowers (p.1561·2); coriander (p.1567·3); caraway (p.1559·3); peppermint leaf (p.1208·1); achillea (p.1542·2); liquorice (p.1197·1).
Digestive system disorders.

Knufinke Herz- und Kreislauf-Tee Arterio-K
Divapharma, Ger.†.
Crataegus (p.1568·2).
Cardiovascular disorders.

Knufinke Nervenruh Beruhigungs-Tee *Divapharma, Ger.†.*
Valerian root (p.1643·1); motherwort (p.1604·2); lupulus (p.1597·2); melissa leaves (p.1600·1); peppermint leaves (p.1208·1).
Nervous disorders.

Knufinke Sanguis-L *Divapharma, Ger.†.*
Birch leaf; orthosiphon leaf (p.1592·2).
Digestive disorders; diuretic.

Koate
Kolassa, Aust.; Bayer, Canad.; Bayer, Ger.†; Sclavo, Ital.; Bayer, Swed.†; Bayer, USA.; Cutter, USA†.
A factor VIII preparation (p.720·3).
Haemorrhagic disorders.

Kodan Spray F *Schulke & Mayr, Ger.†.*
Alcohol (p.1099·1); isopropyl alcohol (p.1118·2); orthophenylphenol (p.1120·3).
Skin disinfection.

Kodan Tinktur Forte *Schulke & Mayr, Ger.*
Isopropyl alcohol (p.1118·2); propyl alcohol (p.1124·2); orthophenylphenol (p.1120·3).
Skin disinfection.

Kodapon *Pharmagen, S.Afr.†.*
Paracetamol (p.72·2); codeine phosphate (p.26·1).
Fever; pain.

Kof-Eze *Roberts, USA.*
Menthol (p.1600·2).
Coughs; sore throats.

Koffazon *Recip, Swed.*
Caffeine (p.749·3); phenazone (p.78·2).
Pain.

Koffex DM *Rougier, Canad.*
Dextromethorphan hydrobromide (p.1057·3).
Coughs.

Koffex DM-D *Rougier, Canad.*
Dextromethorphan hydrobromide (p.1057·3); pseudoephedrine hydrochloride (p.1068·3).

Koffex Expectorant *Rougier, Canad.*
Guaiphenesin (p.1061·3).

Kofron *Abbott, Spain.*
Clarithromycin (p.189·1).
Bacterial infections.

Kogenate
Bayer, Aust.; Bayer, Austral.; Bayer, Canad.; Bayer, Fr.; Bayer, Ger.; Bayer, Irl.; Bayer, Ital.; Bayer, Neth.; Bayer, Norw.; Bayer, Spain; Bayer, Swed.; Bayer, Switz.; Bayer, UK; Bayer, USA.
A factor VIII preparation (recombinant) (p.720·3).
Haemorrhagic disorders.

Kohle-Compretten *Merck, Ger.*
Activated charcoal (p.972·2).
Acute poisoning; diarrhoea.

Kohle-Hevert *Hevert, Ger.*
Activated charcoal (p.972·2).
Acute poisoning; diarrhoea.

Kohlensaurebad Bastian *Bastian, Ger.*
Sodium bicarbonate (p.1153·2).
Bath additive; cardiac and circulatory disorders.

Kohle-Pulvis *Kohler, Ger.*
Activated charcoal (p.972·2).
Acute poisoning; diarrhoea.

Kohle-Tabletten *Michallik, Ger.; Boxo, Ger.*
Activated charcoal (p.972·2).
Acute poisoning; diarrhoea.

Kohrsolin *Bode, Ger.*
Glutaraldehyde (p.1114·3); 1,6-dihydroxy-2,5-dioxahexan; polymethylolurea derivative.
Surface and instrument disinfection.

Kohrsolin FF *Bode, Ger.*
Glutaraldehyde (p.1114·3); benzalkonium chloride (p.1101·3); didecyldimethylammonium chloride (p.1112·2).
Surface disinfection.

Kohrsolin iD *Bode, Ger.*
Glutaraldehyde (p.1114·3); 1,6-dihydroxy-2,5-dioxahexan; polymethylolurea derivative.
Instrument disinfection.

Kola-Dallmann *Dallmann, Ger.*
Kola (p.1645·1); caffeine (p.749·3).
Fatigue.

Kola-Dallmann mit Lecithin *Dallmann, Ger.*
Kola (p.1645·1); caffeine (p.749·3); egg lecithin (p.1595·2).
Fatigue.

Koladex *Laboratories for Applied Biology, UK.*
Caffeine (p.749·3); kola nut (p.1645·1).
Tonic.

Kolanticon
Hoechst Marion Roussel, Irl.; Hoechst Marion Roussel, UK.
Aluminium hydroxide (p.1177·3); dicyclomine hydrochloride (p.460·1); light magnesium oxide (p.1198·3); simethicone (p.1213·1).
Gastro-intestinal disorders.

Kolantyl *Mer-National, S.Afr.*
Oral gel: Dicyclomine hydrochloride (p.460·1); aluminium hydroxide gel (p.1177·3); magnesium oxide (p.1198·3); methylcellulose (p.1473·3).
Wafers: Dicyclomine hydrochloride (p.460·1); aluminium hydroxide gel (p.1177·3); magnesium hydroxide (p.1198·2); methylcellulose (p.1473·3); magnesium trisilicate (p.1199·1).
Gastro-intestinal disorders.

Kola-Traubenzucker Dallmann's *Dallmann, Ger.†.*
Glucose monohydrate (p.1343·3); kola (p.1645·1).
Fatigue.

Kolemed *Rosch & Handel, Aust.*
Activated charcoal (p.972·2).
Diarrhoea; flatulence.

Kolephrin *Pfeiffer, USA.*
Pseudoephedrine hydrochloride (p.1068·3); paracetamol (p.72·2); chlorpheniramine maleate (p.405·1).
Upper respiratory-tract symptoms.

Kolephrin GG/DM *Pfeiffer, USA.*
Dextromethorphan hydrobromide (p.1057·3); guaiphenesin (p.1061·3).
Coughs.

Kolephrin/DM *Pfeiffer, USA.*
Chlorpheniramine maleate (p.405·1); dextromethorphan hydrobromide (p.1057·3); paracetamol (p.72·2); pseudoephedrine hydrochloride (p.1068·3).
Coughs and cold symptoms.

Kollateral *Ursapharm, Ger.*
Moxaverine hydrochloride (p.1604·3).
Coronary disorders; peripheral and cerebral circulatory disorders.

Kollateral A + E *Ursapharm, Ger.*
Moxaverine hydrochloride (p.1604·3); vitamin A acetate (p.1359·2); alpha tocopheryl acetate (p.1369·1).
Cerebral, coronary, and ocular vascular disorders.

Kolotanino *Perez Gimenez, Spain†.*
Albumin tannate (p.1176·3); belladonna powder (p.457·1); dihydrostreptomycin sulphate (p.202·2); phthalylsulphathiazole (p.237·1); opium powder (p.70·3); sulphaguanidine (p.254·1).
Gastro-intestinal infections.

Kolpicortin *Kade, Ger.†.*
Cell products of *Staphylococcus aureus*; *Enterococcus faecalis* (p.1594·1); *Pseudomonas aeruginosa*; *Escherichia coli*; hydrocortisone (p.1043·3).
Vaginitis.

Kolpon *Organon, Austral.†.*
Oestrone (p.1458·2).
Vulvovaginal disorders.

Kolsuspension *Abigo, Swed.*
Activated charcoal (p.972·2).
Diarrhoea; poisoning.

Kolton bronchiale Erkaltungssaft *Promonta, Ger.*
Thyme (p.1636·3).
Bronchitis; catarrh; coughs.

Kolton grippale N *Byk Gulden, Ger.*
Tablets: Piprinhydrinate (p.416·1); paracetamol (p.72·2); etenzamide (p.35·3).
Oral liquid†: Piprinhydrinate (p.416·1); sodium salicylate (p.85·1); thyme (p.1636·3).
Formerly contained piprinhydrinate, paracetamol, ascorbic acid, sodium salicylate, hedera helix, and thyme.
Coughs and cold symptoms.

Kolyum *Fisons, USA.*
Potassium gluconate (p.1161·1); potassium citrate (p.1153·1).
Hypokalaemia; potassium depletion.

Kombetin
Boehringer Mannheim, Ger.; Boehringer Mannheim, Ital.
Strophanthin-K (p.951·1).
Cardiac disorders.

Komb-H-Insulin *Hoechst, Ger.*
Mixture of insulin injection (human) 50% and isophane insulin (human) 50% (p.322·1).
Diabetes mellitus.

Kombi-Kalz *Asta Medica, Aust.†.*
Calcium carbonate (p.1182·1); cholecalciferol (p.1366·3); ascorbic acid (p.1365·2).
Calcium metabolic disorders with vitamin D deficiency.

Kombinax *Bracco, Ital.*
Co-trimazine (p.196·3).
Bacterial infections.

Komb-Insulin
Hoechst, Aust.
Insulin injection (porcine) (p.322·1).
Diabetes mellitus.

Hoechst, Ger.
Insulin injection (chromatographically purified, bovine) (p.322·1).
Diabetes mellitus.

Komb-Insulin S *Hoechst, Ger.*
Insulin (chromatographically purified, porcine), comprising a mixture of Insulin S and Depot-Insulin S *(Hoechst, Ger.)* (p.322·1).
Diabetes mellitus.

Kombistrat *UCB, Swed.†.*
Hydroxyzine hydrochloride (p.412·1); oxyphencyclimine hydrochloride (p.466·3).
Gastro-intestinal disorders.

Kombi-Stulln *Stulln, Ger.*
Polymyxin B sulphate (p.239·1); neomycin sulphate (p.229·2); gramicidin (p.215·2).
Eye infections.

Kompensan
Pfizer, Ger.; Pfizer, Switz.
Dihydroxyaluminum sodium carbonate (p.1188·3).
Gastro-intestinal disorders associated with hyperacidity.

Kompensan-S *Pfizer, Ger.*
Dihydroxyaluminum sodium carbonate (hydrated) (p.1188·3); dimethicone (p.1213·1).
Gastro-intestinal disorders.

Kompensan-S forte *Pfizer, Ger.†.*
Dihydroxyaluminum sodium carbonate (hydrated) (p.1188·3); dimethicone (p.1213·1); aluminium hydroxide gel (p.1177·3); magnesium hydroxide (p.1198·2).
Gastro-intestinal disorders.

Konakion
Roche, Aust.; Roche, Austral.; Roche, Belg.; Roche, Canad.†; Roche, Ger.; Roche, Irl.; Roche, Ital.; Roche, Neth.; Roche, Norw.; Roche, S.Afr.; Roche, Spain; Roche, Swed.; Roche, Switz.; Roche, UK; Roche, USA.
Phytomenadione (p.1371·1).
Anticoagulant antidote; haemorrhagic disorders; vitamin K deficiency.

Kondon's Nasal *Kondon, USA.*
Ephedrine (p.1059·3).
Nasal congestion.

Kondremul *Fisons, USA.*
Liquid paraffin (p.1382·1).
Constipation.

Kondremul with Cascara *Fisons, USA†.*
Liquid paraffin (p.1382·1); cascara (p.1183·1).
Constipation.

Kondremul with Phenolphthalein *Fisons, USA.*
Liquid paraffin (p.1382·1); phenolphthalein (p.1208·2).
Constipation.

Kongress-Tabletten-Pascoe *Pascoe, Ger.†.*
Homoeopathic preparation.

Konjax *Murat, Fr.*
Glucomannan (p.1584·3).
Obesity.

Konjunktival Thilo *Alcon-Thilo, Ger.*
Naphazoline hydrochloride (p.1064·2); pheniramine maleate (p.415·3).
Eye disorders.

Konor *Italzama, Ital.*
Tar (p.1092·3).
Seborrhoeic dermatitis.

Konorderm *Italzama, Ital.*
Inositol, vitamin PP, vitamin E, betacarotene, selenium, L-cystine.
Antoxidant nutritional supplement.

Konstitutin *CytoChemia, Ger.*
Eleutherococcus senticosus (p.1584·2).
Tonic.

Konsyl
Note. This name is used for preparations of different composition.
Mepha, Switz.; Eastern Pharmaceuticals, UK.
Ispaghula husk (p.1194·2).
Constipation; diarrhoea; diverticulosis; irritable bowel syndrome.

Konsyl, USA.
Psyllium (p.1194·2).

Konsyl Fiber *Konsyl, USA.*
Polycarbophil calcium (p.1209·1).

Konsyl-D *Konsyl, USA.*
Psyllium hydrophilic mucilloid (p.1194·2).
Constipation.

Kontabletten *Michallik, Ger.†.*
Activated charcoal (p.972·2); albumin tannate (p.1176·3); bismuth tannate (p.1181·1); kaolin (p.1195·1).
Diarrhoea.

Kontagripp *Azuchemie, Ger.†.*
Paracetamol (p.72·2); salicylamide (p.82·3); caffeine (p.749·3); oxeladin citrate (p.1065·3); diphenhydramine hydrochloride (p.409·1).
Coughs and cold symptoms.

Kontagripp Mono *Azupharma, Ger.*
Ibuprofen (p.44·1).
Fever; pain.

Kontagripp-RR *Azuchemie, Ger.†.*
Paracetamol (p.72·2); salicylamide (p.82·3); caffeine (p.749·3); oxeladin citrate (p.1065·3); diphenhydramine hydrochloride (p.409·1); pholedrine sulphate (p.930·2).
Cold symptoms.

Kontakto Derm Lotio *CCM, Ger.*
Benzocaine (p.1286·2); benzyl benzoate (p.1402·2).
Eczema; pruritus.

Kontexin
Pharmacia Upjohn, Aust.; Pharmacia Upjohn, Switz.
Phenylpropanolamine hydrochloride (p.1067·2).
Urinary incontinence.

Konyne 80 *Bayer, USA.*
Factor IX complex (p.721·3).
Haemorrhagic disorders.

Kophane Cough and Cold Formula *Pfeiffer, USA.*
Phenylpropanolamine hydrochloride (p.1067·2); chlorpheniramine maleate (p.405·1); dextromethorphan hydrobromide (p.1057·3).
Coughs and cold symptoms.

Koreberon *Dresden, Ger.*
Sodium fluoride (p.742·1).
Osteoporosis.

Korec *Sanofi Winthrop, Fr.*
Quinapril hydrochloride (p.938·1).
Heart failure; hypertension.

Koretic *Sanofi Winthrop, Fr.*
Quinapril hydrochloride (p.938·1); hydrochlorothiazide (p.885·2).
Hypertension.

Korodin
Note. This name is used for preparations of different composition.
Robugen, Ger.
Camphor (p.1557·2); crataegus (p.1568·2).
Cardiac disorders; circulatory disorders.

Medipharm, Switz.
Chamomile (p.1561·2); crataegus (p.1568·2).
Cardiac disorders.

Koromex *QHP, USA.*
Vaginal cream: Octoxinol (p.1326·2).
Vaginal jelly; vaginal gel; condom: Nonoxinol 9 (p.1326·1).
Contraceptive.

Korsolex FF *Bode, Ger.*
Glutaraldehyde (p.1114·3); succindialdehyde; polyoxyethylene cocosamine.
Instrument disinfection.

Korsolex-Endo-Disinfectant *Bode, Ger.*
Glutaraldehyde (p.1114·3).
Disinfection of endoscopes.

Korticoid c. Neomycin-ratiopharm *Ratiopharm, Ger.†.*
Triamcinolone acetonide (p.1050·2); neomycin sulphate (p.229·2).
Skin disorders.

Kortikoid-ratiopharm *Ratiopharm, Ger.*
Triamcinolone acetonide (p.1050·2).
Burns; skin disorders.

Koryn *Weimer, Ger.†.*
Camphor (p.1557·2); ephedrine (p.1059·3); menthol (p.1600·2); rosemary oil (p.1626·2).
Catarrh.

Koryn mild *Weimer, Ger.†.*
Camphor (p.1557·2); ephedrine (p.1059·3); rosemary oil (p.1626·2).
Catarrh.

Kos *Crinos, Ital.*
Ibuprofen pyridoxine (p.44·3).
Musculoskeletal and joint disorders; pain.

Kovilen *Mediolanum, Ital.*
Nedocromil sodium (p.756·2).
Ocular hypersensitivity reactions.

Kovinal *Mediolanum, Ital.*
Nedocromil sodium (p.756·2).
Allergic rhinitis.

Kovitonic *Freeda, USA.*
Ferric pyrophosphate (p.1339·2); folic acid (p.1340·3); vitamin B substances with L-lysine.
Iron-deficiency anaemias.

KP 24 *Nelson, Austral.†.*
Malathion (Maldison) (p.1407·3).
Pediculosis.

K-Pek *Rugby, USA.*
Attapulgite (p.1178·3).
Diarrhoea.

K-Phen *Kay, USA.*
Promethazine hydrochloride (p.416·2).
Hypersensitivity reactions; motion sickness; nausea; postoperative pain (adjunct); sedative; vomiting.

K-Phos MF *Beach, USA.*
Monobasic potassium phosphate (p.1159·3); anhydrous monobasic sodium phosphate (p.1159·3).
Urinary acidification.

K-Phos Neutral *Beach, USA.*
Anhydrous dibasic sodium phosphate (p.1159·3); monobasic potassium phosphate (p.1159·3); monobasic sodium phosphate (p.1159·3).
Phosphorus supplement.

K-Phos No.2 *Beach, USA.*
Monobasic potassium phosphate (p.1159·3); anhydrous monobasic sodium phosphate (p.1159·3).
Urinary acidification.

K-Phos Original *Beach, USA.*
Monobasic potassium phosphate (p.1159·3).
Urinary acidification.

KPN *Freeda, USA.*
Multivitamin and mineral preparation with iron and folic acid.

Krama *Miba, Ital.*
Barrier cream.

Kratalgin *Kwizda, Aust.*
Ibuprofen (p.44·1).
Pain.

Kratofin *Kwizda, Aust.*
Paracetamol (p.72·2); aluminium aspirin (p.15·1); caffeine (p.749·3).
Fever; pain.

Kratofin simplex *Kwizda, Aust.*
Paracetamol (p.72·2).
Fever; pain.

Krauter Hustensaft *Apomedica, Aust.†.*
Thyme (p.1636·3); ononis (p.1610·2); primula root; liquorice (p.1197·1); castaneae vulgaris; sambucus (p.1627·2).
Catarrh; coughs.

Krauterdoktor Beruhigungstropfen *Kollerics, Aust.*
Lupulus (p.1597·2); melissa (p.1600·1); orange flower.
Anxiety; nervous disorders.

Krauterdoktor Entschlackungs-Elixier *Kollerics, Aust.*
Taraxacum (p.1634·2); viola tricolor; manna (p.1199·1); bitter-orange peel (p.1610·3); rose fruit (p.1365·2).
Tonic.

Krauterdoktor Entspannungs- und Einschlaftropfen *Kollerics, Aust.*
Valerian (p.1643·1); lupulus (p.1597·2); melissa (p.1600·1).
Anxiety disorders; sleep disorders.

Krauterdoktor Entwasserungs-Elixier *Kollerics, Aust.*
Silver birch (p.1553·3); equisetum (p.1575·1); urtica (p.1642·3).
Urinary-tract disorders.

Krauterdoktor Erkaltungstropfen *Kollerics, Aust.*
Sambucus (p.1627·2); tilia (p.1637·3); centaury (p.1561·1).
Cold symptoms.

Krauterdoktor Gallentreibende Tropfen *Kollerics, Aust.*
Taraxacum (p.1634·2); achillea (p.1542·2); absinthium (p.1541·1).
Biliary-tract disorders.

Krauterdoktor Harnstein- und Nierengriesstropfen *Kollerics, Aust.*
Ononis (p.1610·2); taraxacum (p.1634·2); centaury (p.1561·1).
Urinary-tract disorders.

Krauterdoktor Hustentropfen *Kollerics, Aust.*
Fennel (p.1579·1); primula root; thyme (p.1636·3).
Catarrh; coughs.

Krauterdoktor Krampf- und Reizhustensirup *Kollerics, Aust.*
Aniseed (p.1549·3); drosera (p.1574·1); thyme (p.1636·3).
Coughs.

Krauterdoktor Magen-Darmtropfen *Kollerics, Aust.*
Valerian (p.1643·1); caraway (p.1559·3); melissa (p.1600·1).
Gastro-intestinal disorders.

Krauterdoktor Nerven-Tonikum *Kollerics, Aust.*
Valerian (p.1643·1); lupulus (p.1597·2); melissa (p.1600·1).
Anxiety; nervousness; sleep disorders.

Krauterdoktor Rosmarin-Wein *Kollerics, Aust.*
Rosemary; melissa (p.1600·1).
Circulatory disorders.

Krauterdoktor Verdauungsfordernde Tropfen *Kollerics, Aust.*
Angelica; centaury (p.1561·1); absinthium (p.1541·1).
Gastro-intestinal disorders.

Krautergeist S *Jukunda, Ger.*
Melissa; sloe; ginger; melissa oil; rosemary oil; lavender oil; capsicum oil; cinnamon oil; clove oil.
Tonic.

Krauterhaus Mag Kottas Babytee *Kottas-Heldenberg, Aust.*
Chamomile (p.1561·2); mallow leaf; melissa (p.1600·1); caraway (p.1559·3); fennel (p.1579·1).
Gastro-intestinal disorders.

Krauterhaus Mag Kottas Blasentee *Kottas-Heldenberg, Aust.*
Silver birch (p.1553·3); orthosiphon (p.1592·2); herniaria (p.1587·2); couch-grass (p.1567·3); ononis (p.1610·2); peppermint leaf (p.1208·1).
Urinary-tract disorders.

Krauterhaus Mag Kottas Blutreinigungstee *Kottas-Heldenberg, Aust.*
Peppermint leaf (p.1208·1); urtica (p.1642·3); viola tricolor; taraxacum (p.1634·2); achillea (p.1542·2); calendula officinalis.
Tonic.

Krauterhaus Mag Kottas Entschlackungstee *Kottas-Heldenberg, Aust.*
Silver birch (p.1553·3); peppermint leaf (p.1208·1); taraxacum (p.1634·2); urtica (p.1642·3); ononis (p.1610·2); chamomile (p.1561·2).
Diuretic.

Krauterhaus Mag Kottas Entwasserungstee *Kottas-Heldenberg, Aust.*
Equisetum (p.1575·1); parsley root (p.1615·3); couch-grass (p.1567·3); solidago virgaurea; urtica (p.1642·3); peppermint leaf (p.1208·1); calendula officinalis.
Urinary-tract disorders.

Krauterhaus Mag Kottas Fruhjahrs- und Herbstkurtee *Kottas-Heldenberg, Aust.*
Peppermint leaf (p.1208·1); equisetum (p.1575·1); achillea (p.1542·2); urtica (p.1642·3); viola tricolor; calendula officinalis; mallow flower.
Tonic.

Krauterhaus Mag Kottas Gallen- und Lebertee *Kottas-Heldenberg, Aust.*
Mallow leaf; peppermint leaf (p.1208·1); menyanthes (p.1601·2); agrimony; taraxacum (p.1634·2); calendula officinalis.
Biliary-tract disorders.

Krauterhaus Mag Kottas Grippetee *Kottas-Heldenberg, Aust.*
Sambucus (p.1627·2); tilia (p.1637·3); plantago lanceolata; rose fruit (p.1365·2).
Cold symptoms.

Krauterhaus Mag Kottas Husten- und Bronchialtee *Kottas-Heldenberg, Aust.*
Verbascum flower; althaea (p.1546·3); plantago lanceolata; thyme (p.1636·3); mallow flower.
Catarrh; coughs; sore throat.

Krauterhaus Mag Kottas Magen- und Darmtee *Kottas-Heldenberg, Aust.*
Chamomile (p.1561·2); mallow leaf; melissa (p.1600·1); peppermint leaf (p.1208·1); achillea (p.1542·2); calendula officinalis.
Gastro-intestinal disorders.

Krauterhaus Mag Kottas milder Abfuhrtee *Kottas-Heldenberg, Aust.*
Prunus spinosa; fennel (p.1579·1); mallow leaf; peppermint leaf (p.1208·1); rose fruit (p.1365·2).
Constipation.

Krauterhaus Mag Kottas Nerven- und Schlaftee *Kottas-Heldenberg, Aust.*
Citrus aurantium; melissa (p.1600·1); peppermint leaf (p.1208·1); valerian (p.1643·1); lupulus (p.1597·2); calendula officinalis.
Anxiety disorders; sleep disorders.

Krauterhaus Mag Kottas Nierentee *Kottas-Heldenberg, Aust.*
Orthosiphon (p.1592·2); equisetum (p.1575·1); herniaria (p.1587·2); ononis (p.1610·2); rose fruit (p.1365·2); peppermint leaf (p.1208·1).
Urinary-tract disorders.

Krauterhaus Mag Kottas Tee fur die Verdauung *Kottas-Heldenberg, Aust.*
Mallow leaf; peppermint leaf (p.1208·1); caraway (p.1559·3); absinthium (p.1541·1); bitter-orange peel (p.1610·3); calendula officinalis.
Gastro-intestinal disorders.

Krauterhaus Mag Kottas Tee gegen Blahungen *Kottas-Heldenberg, Aust.*
Mallow leaf; peppermint leaf (p.1208·1); caraway (p.1559·3); fennel (p.1579·1); achillea (p.1542·2); calendula officinalis.
Flatulence.

Krauterhaus Mag Kottas Tee gegen Durchfall *Kottas-Heldenberg, Aust.*
Erwachsene Tee: Tormentil (p.1638·3); chamomile (p.1561·2); mallow leaf; myrtillus (p.1606·1); bitter-orange peel (p.1610·3); mallow flower.
Kinder Tee: Chamomile (p.1561·2); mallow leaf; myrtillus (p.1606·1); rubus fruticosus; aniseed (p.1549·3).
Diarrhoea.

Krauterhaus Mag Kottas Wechseltee *Kottas-Heldenberg, Aust.*
Melissa (p.1600·1); peppermint leaf (p.1208·1); achillea (p.1542·2); sage (p.1627·1); valerian (p.1643·1); chamomile (p.1561·2); calendula officinalis.
Menopausal disorders.

Krauterlax *Henk, Ger.†.*
Aloes (p.1177·1); senna (p.1212·2); curcuma zanthorrhiza; mandragora officinarum.
Constipation.

Krauterlax A *Dolorgiet, Ger.*
Aloes (p.1177·1).
Constipation.

Krauterlax-S *Henk, Ger.*
Sennoside (p.1212·3).
Constipation.

Krautertee Nr 1 *Neuners, Aust.*
Valerian (p.1643·1); lupulus (p.1597·2); melissa (p.1600·1); lavender flower (p.1594·3); chamomile (p.1561·2).
Nervous disorders.

Krautertee Nr 2 *Neuners, Aust.*
Silver birch (p.1553·3); levisticum root (p.1597·2); solidago virgaurea; couch-grass (p.1567·3); prunus spinosa; sambucus (p.1627·2); calendula officinalis.
Urinary tract disorders.

Krautertee Nr 3 *Neuners, Aust.*
Bearberry (p.1552·2); parsley (p.1615·3); veronica; solidago virgaurea; equisetum (p.1575·1); rosemary.
Urinary tract disorders.

Krautertee Nr 4 *Neuners, Aust.*
Equisetum (p.1575·1); juniper (p.1592·2); solidago virgaurea; parsley (p.1615·3); rose fruit (p.1365·2); peppermint leaf (p.1208·1).
Urinary tract disorders.

Krautertee Nr 7 *Neuners, Aust.*
Althaea (p.1546·3); plantago lanceolata; thyme (p.1636·3); aniseed (p.1549·3); marrubium vulgare (p.1063·3).
Catarrh; coughs.

Krautertee Nr 8 *Neuners, Aust.*
Urtica (p.1642·3); sage (p.1627·1); fennel (p.1579·1); peppermint leaf (p.1208·1); chamomile (p.1561·2).
Gastro-intestinal disorders.

Krautertee Nr 9 *Neuners, Aust.*
Centaury (p.1561·1); menyanthes (p.1601·2); valerian (p.1643·1); melissa (p.1600·1); chamomile (p.1561·2); fennel (p.1579·1).
Gastro-intestinal disorders.

Krautertee Nr 10 *Neuners, Aust.*
Tilia (p.1637·3); thyme (p.1636·3); sage (p.1627·1); sambucus (p.1627·2); aniseed (p.1549·3); fennel (p.1579·1).
Cold and influenza symptoms.

Krautertee Nr 11 *Neuners, Aust.*
Althaea (p.1546·3); plantago lanceolata; aniseed (p.1549·3); fennel (p.1579·1); galeopsidis ochroleuca.
Upper respiratory-tract disorders.

Krautertee Nr 14 *Neuners, Aust.*
Prunus spinosa; linaria vulgaris; fennel (p.1579·1); caraway (p.1559·3); centaury (p.1561·1); peppermint leaf (p.1208·1).
Gastro-intestinal disorders.

Krautertee Nr 16 *Neuners, Aust.*
Sage (p.1627·1); orange flowers; achillea (p.1542·2); melissa (p.1600·1); lupulus (p.1597·2); flos calendulae.
Menopausal disorders.

Krautertee Nr 17 *Neuners, Aust.*
Taraxacum (p.1634·2); turmeric (p.1001·3); centaury (p.1561·1); absinthium (p.1541·1); chamomile (p.1561·2); caraway (p.1559·3).
Liver and biliary disorders.

Krautertee Nr 18 *Neuners, Aust.*
Juniper (p.1592·2); parsley (p.1615·3); ononis (p.1610·2).
Urinary tract disorders.

Krautertee Nr 19 *Neuners, Aust.*
Silver birch (p.1553·3); urtica (p.1642·3); juniper (p.1592·2); levisticum root (p.1597·2); viola tricoloris.
Diuresis.

Krautertee Nr 20 *Neuners, Aust.*
Crataegus (p.1568·2); taraxacum (p.1634·2); gentian (p.1583·3); centaury (p.1561·1); mistletoe (p.1604·1); rosemary.
Cardiovascular disorders.

Krautertee Nr 25 *Neuners, Aust.*
Parsley (p.1615·3); silver birch (p.1553·3); ononis (p.1610·2); taraxacum (p.1634·2); rubus fructicosus; rose fruit (p.1365·2).
Tonic.

Krautertee Nr 28 *Neuners, Aust.*
Marrubium vulgare (p.1063·3); agrimony herb; absinthium (p.1541·1); cichorium intybus; angelica; peppermint leaf (p.1208·1).
Biliary disorders.

Krautertee Nr 29 *Neuners, Aust.*
Silver birch (p.1553·3); taraxacum (p.1634·2); juniper (p.1592·2); rosemary; flos bellidis.
Diuresis.

Krautertee Nr 30 *Neuners, Aust.*
Juniper (p.1592·2); ononis (p.1610·2); silver birch (p.1553·3); rosemary; absinthium (p.1541·1); herba majoranae.
Diuresis.

Krautertee Nr 31 *Neuners, Aust.*
Bearberry (p.1552·2); orthosiphon (p.1592·2); levisticum root (p.1597·2).
Diuresis.

Krautertee Nr 32 *Neuners, Aust.*
Mistletoe (p.1604·1); crataegus (p.1568·2); equisetum (p.1575·1); prunus spinosa.
Circulatory and metabolic disorders.

Krautertee Nr 44 *Neuners, Aust.*
Crataegus (p.1568·2); folium juglandis; achillea (p.1542·2); linaria vulgaris; angelica; flos calendulae.
Circulatory disorders; gastro-intestinal disorders.

Krautertee Nr 107 *Neuners, Aust.*
Angelica; sage (p.1627·1); caraway (p.1559·3); peppermint leaf (p.1208·1); aniseed (p.1549·3); sweet basil.
Gastro-intestinal disorders.

Krautertee Nr 124 *Neuners, Aust.*
Valerian (p.1643·1); achillea (p.1542·2); chamomile (p.1561·2); plantago lanceolata; peppermint leaf (p.1208·1).
Labour.

Krautertee Nr 126 *Neuners, Aust.*
Caraway (p.1559·3); aniseed (p.1549·3); fennel (p.1579·1); parsley (p.1615·3); thyme (p.1636·3).
Breast feeding.

Krautertee Nr 141 *Neuners, Aust.*
Lupulus (p.1597·2); valerian (p.1643·1); melissa (p.1600·1); lavender flower (p.1594·3); peppermint leaf (p.1208·1).
Nervous disorders.

Krautertee Nr 201 *Neuners, Aust.*
Melissa (p.1600·1); lavender flower (p.1594·3); lupulus (p.1597·2); peppermint leaf (p.1208·1); orange flower.
Nervous disorders.

Krautertee Nr 204 *Neuners, Aust.*
Silver birch (p.1553·3); ononis (p.1610·2); solidago virgaurea; bearberry (p.1552·2); peppermint leaf (p.1208·1).
Urinary tract disorders.

Krautertee Nr 207 *Neuners, Aust.*
Galeopsis ochroleuca; wild thyme; rose fruit (p.1365·2); calendula officinalis.
Catarrh; coughs.

Krautertee Nr 209 *Neuners, Aust.*
Chamomile (p.1561·2); peppermint leaf (p.1208·1); melissa (p.1600·1); orange flower.
Gastro-intestinal disorders.

Krautertee Nr 210 *Neuners, Aust.*
Tilia (p.1637·3); sambucus (p.1627·2); peppermint leaf (p.1208·1); bitter-orange peel (p.1610·3).
Cold symptoms.

Krautertee Nr 211 *Neuners, Aust.*
Thyme (p.1636·3); drosera (p.1574·1); aniseed (p.1549·3); verbascum flowers.
Catarrh; coughs.

Krautertee Nr 217 *Neuners, Aust.*
Chamomile (p.1561·2); fennel (p.1579·1); caraway (p.1559·3); peppermint leaf (p.1208·1); bitter-orange peel (p.1610·3).
Gastro-intestinal disorders.

Krautertee Nr 311 *Neuners, Aust.*
Peppermint leaf (p.1208·1); thyme (p.1636·3); chamomile (p.1561·2); sage (p.1627·1).
Catarrh; coughs.

Krebsilasi *IRBI, Ital.*
Pancrelipase (p.1613·3).
Cystic fibrosis; malabsorption syndromes.

Kredex
SK-RIT, Belg.; SmithKline Beecham, Ital.; SmithKline Beecham, Norw.; Morrith, Spain; SmithKline Beecham, Swed.; Boehringer Mannheim, Swed.
Carvedilol (p.838·1).
Angina pectoris; heart failure; hypertension.

Kreislauf Katovit *Thomae, Ger.*
Etilefrine hydrochloride (p.867·2).
Hypotension.

Kreislaufja *OTW, Ger.*
Homoeopathic preparation.

Kremulsion *Atzinger, Ger.†.*
Cod-liver oil (p.1337·3); peru balsam (p.1617·2).
Skin disorders.

Krenosin
Sanofi Winthrop, Fr.; Sanofi Winthrop, Ital.
Adenosine (p.812·3).
Diagnosis of arrhythmias; paroxysmal supraventricular tachycardia.

Krenosine *Sanofi Winthrop, Switz.*
Adenosine (p.812·3).
Supraventricular tachycardia.

Kreon
Solvay, Aust.; Solvay, Ger.; Solvay, Spain.
Pancreatin (p.1612·1).
Pancreatic insufficiency.

Kresse *Upjohn, Spain.*
Minoxidil (p.910·3).
Alopecia.

Krestin *Kureha, Jpn†.*
Polysaccharide K (p.1619·3).
Malignant neoplasms.

Kretussot *Truw, Ger.†.*
Fennel oil (p.1579·2); thyme (p.1636·3); liquorice (p.1197·1).
Catarrh; coughs.

Kreuzlinger Klosterliniment *Luond, Switz.*
Salicylic acid (p.1090·2); camphor (p.1557·2); plant extracts.
Musculoskeletal, joint, and soft-tissue disorders.

Kreuz-Tabletten *RAN, Ger.†.*
Paracetamol (p.72·2); caffeine (p.749·3); aspirin (p.16·1).
Cold symptoms; migraine; pain; rheumatism.

Kripton *Alphapharm, Austral.*
Bromocriptine mesylate (p.1132·2).
Acromegaly; hyperprolactinaemia; lactation inhibition; parkinsonism.

Kronofed-A *Ferndale, USA.*
Pseudoephedrine hydrochloride (p.1068·3); chlorpheniramine maleate (p.405·1).
Cold symptoms.

Krophan *Repha, Ger.†.*
Homoeopathic preparation.

Krophan N *Repha, Ger.*
Bladderwrack (p.1554·1); potassium iodide (p.1493·1); thyreoidinum.
Iodine-deficiency disorders.

Kruschels *Pharmethic, Belg.*
Dried magnesium sulphate (p.1158·2); sodium chloride (p.1162·2); anhydrous sodium sulphate (p.1213·3); potassium sulphate (p.1161·2); potassium chloride (p.1161·1).
Constipation.

Kruses Fluid Magnesia *Felton, Austral.*
Magnesium bicarbonate.
Gastro-intestinal disorders.

Kryobulin
Immuno, Aust.; Immuno, Ital.; Immuno, Spain; Immuno, Swed.†; Immuno, Switz.; Immuno, UK†.
A factor VIII preparation (p.720·3).
Haemophilia A; von Willebrand's disease.

Kryptocur
Hoechst, Aust.; Hoechst Marion Roussel, Belg.; Hoechst, Ger.; Hoechst Marion Roussel, Ital.; Hoechst Marion Roussel, Switz.
Gonadorelin (p.1247·2).
Cryptorchidism.

K-San *Prosana, Austral.†.*
Potassium chloride (p.1161·1).

KSR *Alphapharm, Austral.*
Potassium chloride (p.1161·1).
Hypokalaemia.

K-Tab *Abbott, USA.*
Potassium chloride (p.1161·1).
Hypokalaemia; potassium depletion.

Kudrox Double Strength *Schwarz, USA.*
Aluminium hydroxide (p.1177·3); magnesium hydroxide (p.1198·2); simethicone (p.1213·1).
Hyperacidity.

Kufaprim *Zambon, Ital.†.*
Fosfomycin (p.210·1); cephalexin (p.178·2).
Bacterial infections.

Kuhlprednon *Gerot, Aust.*
Prednisolone (p.1048·1).
Skin disorders.

Kulan *Gerlach, Ger.†.*
Dimethyl phthalate (p.1405·3); ethohexadiol (p.1406·1).

Kurgan *Normon, Spain.*
Cephazolin sodium (p.181·1).
Lignocaine hydrochloride (p.1293·2) is included in the intramuscular injection to alleviate the pain of injection.
Bacterial infections.

Kuson *Labitec, Spain.*
Potassium hydroxide (p.1621·1).
Verrucas; warts.

Kutapressin *Schwarz, USA.*
Liver-derivative complex.
Skin disorders.

Kutrase *Schwarz, USA.*
Lipase; amylase (p.1549·1); protease; cellulase (p.1561·1); hyoscyamine sulphate (p.464·2); phenyltoloxamine citrate (p.416·1).
Functional dyspepsia devoid of organic pathology (nervous dyspepsia).

Ku-Zyme
Richmond, Canad.†; Schwarz, USA.
Lipase; amylase (p.1549·1); protease; cellulase (p.1561·1).
Functional dyspepsia due to enzyme deficiency or imbalance.

Ku-Zyme HP *Schwarz, USA.*
Pancrelipase (p.1613·3).
Pancreatic deficiency.

Kwai
Kwizda, Aust.; Lederle, Austral.†; Lichtwer, Fr.†; Solvay, Ital.; Lichtwer, Switz.; Lichtwer, UK.
Garlic (p.1583·1).
Arteriosclerosis; cold and influenza symptoms.

Kwai N *Lichtwer, Ger.*
Garlic (p.1583·1).
Atherosclerosis; lipid disorders.

Kwelcof *Ascher, USA.*
Hydrocodone tartrate (p.43·1); guaiphenesin (p.1061·3).
Coughs.

Kwell Reed & Carnrick, USA†.
Lindane (p.1407·2).
Pediculosis; scabies.

Kwellada Reed & Carnrick, Canad.
Lindane (p.1407·2).
Pediculosis; scabies.

Kwells
Roche Consumer, Austral.; Roche Consumer, Irl.; Roche Consumer, UK.
Hyoscine hydrobromide (p.462·3).
Motion sickness.

K-Y
Johnson & Johnson Medical, Fr.; Ethicon, Ital.; Johnson & Johnson, Switz.; Johnson & Johnson, UK; Johnson & Johnson, USA.
Lubricating gel.
Aid in ultrasound scanning; catheterisation; endoscopy; lubrication of mucous membranes and instruments.

K-Y Personal Lubricant Johnson & Johnson, Canad.
Nonoxinol 9 (p.1326·1).
Contraceptive; vaginal lubricant.

Kyaugutt Krewel, Ger.
Crataegus (p.1568·2).
Heart failure.

Kyaugutt N Meuselbach, Ger.†.
Crataegus (p.1568·2); valerian (p.1643·1); camphor (p.1557·2).
Cardiac disorders.

Kybernin
Centeon, Ger.; Centeon, Ital.; Hoechst, Spain; Centeon, Switz.; Centeon, UK.
Antithrombin III (p.711·2).
Antithrombin III deficiency; disseminated intravascular coagulation.

Kynosina IRBI, Ital.†.
Aspirin (p.16·1).
Fever; inflammation; pain.

Kyolic
Note. A similar name is used for preparations of different composition.
Quest, UK.
Garlic (p.1583·1).

Kyolic 103
Note. A similar name is used for preparations of different composition.
Quest, Canad.
Calcium ascorbate (p.1365·2).
Dietary supplement.

Kyolic Formula 105
Note. A similar name is used for preparations of different composition.
Quest, Canad.
Betacarotene, selenium, vitamin C, and vitamin E.

Kytril
SmithKline Beecham, Aust.; Beecham, Belg.; SmithKline Beecham, Canad.; SmithKline Beecham, Fr.; SmithKline Beecham, Irl.; SmithKline Beecham, Ital.; SmithKline Beecham, Neth.; SmithKline Beecham, Norw.; SmithKline Beecham, S.Afr.; Smith Kline & French, Spain; SmithKline Beecham, Swed.; SmithKline Beecham, Switz.; SmithKline Beecham, UK; SmithKline Beecham, USA.
Granisetron hydrochloride (p.1193·3).
Nausea and vomiting.

Kytta Kytta, Ger.
Glycol salicylate (p.43·1).
Inflammation; pain.

Kytta Baume Whitehall-Robins, Switz.
Comfrey (p.1567·1); methyl nicotinate (p.55·1).
Musculoskeletal pain.

Kytta Pommade Whitehall-Robins, Switz.
Comfrey (p.1567·1); pine-needle oil; lavender oil (p.1594·3).
Musculoskeletal pain; soft-tissue injury; wounds.

Kytta-Balsam f Kytta, Ger.
Comfrey (p.1567·1); methyl nicotinate (p.55·1).
Local circulatory disorders; musculoskeletal, joint, and soft-tissue disorders.

Kytta-Cor Kytta, Ger.
Crataegus (p.1568·2).
Cardiac disorders.

Kytta-Femin Kytta, Ger.
Agnus castus (p.1544·2).
Mastalgia; menstrual disorders.

Kytta-Nagelsalbe Kytta, Ger.†.
Undecenoic acid (p.389·2); benzoic acid (p.1102·3); salicylic acid (p.1090·2); stib. sulf. nigr.; comfrey (p.1567·1); vitamin A acetate (p.1359·2); cholecalciferol (p.1366·3).
Nail disorders.

Kytta-Plasma f Kytta, Ger.
Comfrey (p.1567·1).
Soft-tissue disorders.

Kytta-Rheumabad N Kytta, Ger.
Noble fir oil; norway spruce oil.
Bath additive; rheumatism.

Kytta-Salbe f Kytta, Ger.
Comfrey (p.1567·1).
Soft-tissue disorders.

Kytta-Sedativum f Kytta, Ger.
Valerian (p.1643·1); lupulus (p.1597·2); passion flower (p.1615·3).
Nervous excitability; sleep disorders.

Kytta-Thermopack Moor-Fangoparaffin Kytta, Ger.
Peat; medicinal mud.
Hemiplegia; musculoskeletal, joint, and soft-tissue disorders; myelitis.

L 25 Lehning, Fr.
Homoeopathic preparation.

L 28 Lehning, Fr.
Homoeopathic preparation.

L 52 Lehning, Fr.
Homoeopathic preparation.

L 72 Lehning, Fr.
Homoeopathic preparation.

L 114 Lehning, Fr.
Homoeopathic preparation.

LA-12 Hyrex, USA.
Hydroxocobalamin (p.1363·3).
Schilling test; vitamin B_{12} deficiency.

Lab/A Tosi, Ital.
Lactobacillus (p.1594·1).
Vulvovaginal candidiasis.

Labello Active Beiersdorf, Canad.
SPF 15: Ethylhexyl *p*-methoxycinnamate (p.1487·1); oxybenzone (p.1487·3).
Sunscreen.

Labileno Faes, Spain.
Lamotrigine (p.347·2).
Epilepsy.

Labiogenine Magistra, Switz.†.
Mineral preparation with extracts of cola, cinchona, and malt.
Tonic.

Labisan Schutz, Aust.
Phenol (p.1121·2); zinc oxide (p.1096·2); precipitated sulphur (p.1091·2).
Fever blisters.

Labiton Laboratories for Applied Biology, UK.
Thiamine (p.1361·2); caffeine (p.749·3); kola nuts (p.1645·1); alcohol.
Tonic.

Labmist Laboratories for Applied Biology, UK.
Sodium chloride (p.1162·2).
Nasal dryness.

Labocaina CCM, Ital.
Benzocaine (p.1286·2); resorcinol (p.1090·1); chlorothymol (p.1111·1).
Pruritus.

Labocane CCM, Ger.
Benzocaine (p.1286·2); benzyl cinnamate; benzyl benzoate (p.1402·2).
Eczema; pruritus.

Labopal Morrith, Spain.
Benazepril hydrochloride (p.827·1).
Hypertension.

Labophylline Laboratories for Applied Biology, UK†.
Theophylline (p.765·1); lysine (p.1350·1).
Asthma.

Laboprin Laboratories for Applied Biology, UK†.
Lysine aspirin (p.50·3).
Fever; inflammation; musculoskeletal disorders; pain.

Labosept
Laboratories for Applied Biology, Irl.; Laboratories for Applied Biology, UK.
Dequalinium chloride (p.1112·1).
Mouth and throat infections.

Labrocol Lagap, UK.
Labetalol hydrochloride (p.896·1).
Angina pectoris; hypertension.

Labstix
Bayer Diagnostics, Austral.; Bayer, Canad.; Ames, Irl.; Bayer Diagnostici, Ital.; Ames, S.Afr.; Bayer Diagnostics, UK; Bayer, USA.
Test for pH, protein, glucose, ketones, and blood in urine.

Labstix SG
Bayer, Canad.; Bayer Diagnostics, UK.
Test for specific gravity, glucose, blood, ketones, protein, and pH in urine.

Laburide Wolfs, Belg.
Pheneturide (p.350·1).
Epilepsy.

Lac 4 n Parke, Davis, Ger.
Almasilate (p.1177·1).
Gastro-intestinal disorders.

Lacalut Pietrasanta, Ital.
Aluminium lactate (p.1548·1); aluminium fluoride; aluminium hydroxide (p.1177·3); silicon dioxide (p.1474·3).
Gum disorders; oral hygiene; sensitive teeth.

Laccoderme a l'huile de cade Pharmascience, Fr.†.
Rectified cade oil (p.1092·2); hyoscyamus oil (p.464·3); salicylic acid (p.1090·2).
Psoriatic skin disorders.

Laccoderme acide salicylique Pharmascience, Fr.†.
Salicylic acid (p.1090·2); zinc oxide (p.1096·2); titanium dioxide (p.1093·3).
Skin disorders.

Laccoderme Dalibour Pharmascience, Fr.†.
Copper sulphate (p.1338·1); zinc sulphate (p.1373·2); zinc oxide (p.1096·2); camphor (p.1557·2); miristalkonium chloride (p.1119·3); saffron (p.1001·1).
Infected skin disorders.

Laccoderme goudron de houille Pharmascience, Fr.†.
Coal tar (p.1092·3); zinc oxide (p.1096·2); titanium dioxide (p.1093·3).
Skin disorders.

Laccoderme oxyde de zinc Pharmascience, Fr.†.
Zinc oxide (p.1096·2); titanium dioxide (p.1093·3).
Skin disorders.

Lac-Dol Douglas, Austral.
Lactulose (p.1195·3).
Constipation; hepatic encephalopathy.

Laceran Beiersdorf, Ger.
Urea (p.1095·2).
Dry skin disorders.

Lacerdermol Lacer, Spain.
Biotin (p.1336·1); calcium pantothenate (p.1352·3); vitamin A (p.1358·1).
Blepharitis; fragile nails; glossitis; skin disorders.

Lacerdermol Complex Lacer, Spain.
Vitamin B substances; vitamin A (p.1358·1).
Seborrhoeic blepharitis; skin disorders.

Lacermucin Lacer, Spain.
Tyloxapol (p.1329·2).
Respiratory-tract disorders.

Lacerol Lacer, Spain.
Diltiazem hydrochloride (p.854·2).
Angina pectoris; hypertension; myocardial infarction.

Lacertral Lacer, Spain†.
Tripotassium dictratobismuthate (p.1180·2).
Gastritis; peptic ulcer.

Lachemistol Wiedemann, Ger.
Homoeopathic preparation.

Lac-Hydrin
Westwood-Squibb, Canad.; Westwood-Squibb, USA.
Ammonium lactate (p.1079·1).
Formerly contained lactic acid in *Canad.*
Skin disorders.

Lacimen Menarini, Spain.
Lacidipine (p.897·1).
Hypertension.

Lacipil
Glaxo Wellcome, Ital.; Glaxo Wellcome, Spain.
Lacidipine (p.897·1).
Angina pectoris; hypertension.

Lacirex Guidotti, Ital.
Lacidipine (p.897·1).
Hypertension.

Lacoerdin-N Weber & Weber, Ger.
Convallaria (p.1567·2); potassium aspartate (p.1161·3); magnesium aspartate (p.1157·2); magnesium phosphate trihydrate (p.1157·3); magnesium sulphate (p.1157·3); crataegus (p.1568·2).
Cardiovascular disorders.

Lac-Ophtal Winzer, Ger.
Povidone (p.1474·2).
Dry eye disorders.

Lacovin Galderma, Spain.
Minoxidil (p.910·3).
Alopecia.

Lacribase Allergan, Ital.
Benzalkonium chloride (p.1101·3).
Eye disinfection.

Lacrigel
Note. This name is used for preparations of different composition.
Winzer, Ger.
Hydroxyethylcellulose (p.1472·3).
Dry eyes.

Farmigea, Ital.; Europhta, Mon.
Carbomer 940 (p.1471·2).
Dry eyes.

Lacril
Allergan, Austral.†; Allergan, Canad.; Allergan, USA.
Hypromellose (p.1473·1).
Formerly contained methylcellulose in *Canad.*
Dry eyes.

Lacri-Lube
Allergan, Austral.; Allergan, Canad.; Allergan, Irl.; Allergan, Ital.; Allergan, S.Afr.; Allergan, UK; Allergan, USA.
White soft paraffin (p.1382·3); liquid paraffin (p.1382·1); wool fat (p.1385·3).
Dry eyes.

Allergan, Spain.
Soft paraffin (p.1382·3).
Eye disorders.

Lacrilux Allergan, Ital.
Polyvinyl alcohol (p.1474·2).
Dry eyes.

Lacrimal Allergan, Ger.
Polyvinyl alcohol (p.1474·2).
Dry eyes.

Lacrimal OK Allergan, Ger.
Polyvinyl alcohol (p.1474·2); povidone (p.1474·2).
Dry eyes.

Lacrimalfa INTES, Ital.
Sodium chloride; sodium bicarbonate; sodium acid phosphate; magnesium sulphate.
Dry eyes.

Lacrimart Baif, Ital.
Methylcellulose (p.1473·3).
Dry eyes; eye disinfection.

Lacrime Ogna, Ital.
Elixir: Oleum pini sylvestris; storax (p.1632·3); cineole (p.1564·1).
Pastilles: Oleum pini sylvestris; storax (p.1632·3); cineole (p.1564·1); menthol (p.1600·2).
Bronchial catarrh; coughs; sore throat.

Lacrimill Ottolenghi, Ital.
Hypromellose (p.1473·1).
Dry eyes; eye disinfection; eye irritation.

Lacrinorm
Chauvin, Fr.; Farmigea, Ital.; Novopharma, Switz.
Carbomer 940 (p.1471·2).
Dry eyes.

Lacrisert
Sigma, Austral.; Merck Sharp & Dohme, Canad.; Merck Sharp & Dohme-Chibret, Fr.; Merck Sharp & Dohme, Ital.; Chibret, Neth.; Merck Sharp & Dohme, Norw.; Logos, S.Afr.; Merck Sharp & Dohme, Swed.; Merck Sharp & Dohme, USA.
Hydroxypropylcellulose (p.1473·1).
Dry eyes.

Lacrisic
Note. This name is used for preparations of different composition.
Agepha, Aust.
Carbomer (p.1471·2).
Dry eyes.

Basotherm, Ger.
Hypromellose (p.1473·1); povidone (p.1474·2); glycerol (p.1585·2).
Dry eyes.

Lacrisifi SIFI, Ital.
Hypromellose (p.1473·1).
Dry eyes; eye disinfection.

Lacrisol Bruschettini, Ital.
Hypromellose (p.1473·1).
Dry eyes; eye disinfection.

Lacri-Stulln Stulln, Ger.
Povidone (p.1474·2).
Dry eyes.

Lacrypos
Alcon, Belg.†; Alcon, Fr.; Alcon, Switz.†.
Sodium chondroitin sulphate A (p.1562·2).
Dry eyes.

Lacrystat Asta Medica, Belg.
Hypromellose (p.1473·1); dextran 70 (p.717·1).
Dry eyes.

Lacrytube Asta Medica, Belg.
Liquid paraffin (p.1382·1); white soft paraffin (p.1382·3); wool fat (p.1385·3).
Corneal protection in comatose or anaesthetised patients; keratoconjunctivitis sicca.

Lacryvisc Alcon, Fr.
Carbomer 934P (p.1471·2).
Dry eyes.

Lacson Lennon, S.Afr.
Lactulose (p.1195·3).
Constipation.

Lactacyd
SmithKline Beecham Sante, Fr.; Sanofi Winthrop, Ger.†; Sterling Health, Switz.†.
Milk serum; lactic acid (p.1593·3).
Skin disorders.

Lactacyd Antibatterico Maggioni, Ital.
Triclosan (p.1127·2).
Skin disinfection.

Lactacyd Derma Maggioni, Ital.
Milk serum; lactic acid (p.1593·3).
Acne; soap substitute.

Lactacyd Intimo Maggioni, Ital.
Milk serum; lactic acid (p.1593·3).
Genital hygiene.

Lactagel Creme d'Orient, Fr.
Ammonium lactate (p.1079·1).
Skin disorders.

Lacta-Gynecogel Medgenix, Belg.
Lactic acid (p.1593·3).
Vulvovaginal infections.

Lactaid
Pharmachem, Austral.; McNeil Consumer, Canad.; Clonmel, Irl.; Iketon, Ital.; Myplan, UK; McNeil Consumer, USA.
Tilactase (p.1637·3).
Lactase insufficiency; lactose intolerance.

Lactal Kabi, Swed.
Lactic acid (p.1593·3); glycogen.
Bacterial vaginosis.

Lactar Creme d'Orient, Fr.
Ammonium lactate (p.1079·1); cade oil (p.1092·2).
Seborrhoeic dermatitis.

Lact-Easy Pharmotech, Austral.
Tilactase (p.1637·3).
Lactose intolerance.

Lacteol
Menarini, Belg.; Lacteol du Dr Boucard, Fr.; Bruschettini, Ital.; Ramon Sala, Spain; Lacteol, Switz.
Lactobacillus acidophilus (p.1594·1).
Diarrhoea.

Lacticare
Note. This name is used for preparations of different composition.
Stiefel, Austral.†; Stiefel, Canad.; Stiefel, Fr.†; Stiefel, Irl.; Stiefel, S.Afr.†; Stiefel, UK.
Lactic acid (p.1593·3); sodium pidolate (p.1091·2).
Dry skin disorders.

Stiefel, USA.
Emollient and moisturiser.

Lacticare-HC Stiefel, USA.
Hydrocortisone (p.1043·3); lactic acid (p.1593·3).
Skin disorders.

Lactidorm Galactopharm, Ger.
Lupulus (p.1597·2).
Anxiety; insomnia.

Lactinex Becton Dickinson, USA.
Lactobacillus acidophilus (p.1594·1); *Lactobacillus bulgaricus* (p.1594·1).
Dietary supplement.

Lactinium Roland, Ger.†.
Orotic acid (p.1611·2).
Gout; liver disorders.

Lactinol Pedinol, USA.
Lactic acid (p.1593·3).

Lactinol-E Pedinol, USA.
Lactic acid (p.1593·3); vitamin E (p.1369·1).

Lactipan Ibi, Ital.
Streptococcus lactis; Lactobacillus acidophilus (p.1594·1); *Lactobacillus bulgaricus* (p.1594·1).
Gastro-intestinal disorders.

Lactisan Galactopharm, Ger.
Sour milk whey concentrate (p.1593·3).
Skin disinfection.

Lactismine Serono, Spain†.
Bromocriptine mesylate (p.1132·2).
Acromegaly; amenorrhoea; galactorrhoea; lactation inhibition; parkinsonism.

Lactisol
Note. This name is used for preparations of different composition.
Galactopharm, Ger.
Sour milk whey concentrate.
Burns; gastro-intestinal disorders; tonic; wounds.
C & M, USA†.
Salicylic acid (p.1090·2); lactic acid (p.1593·3).
Removal of benign epithelial growths.

Lactisona Stiefel, Spain.
Hydrocortisone (p.1043·3).
Skin disorders.

Lactisporin Virginia, Ital.
Lactic-acid-producing organisms (p.1594·1); dried yeast (p.1373·1).
Restoration of normal gastro-intestinal flora.

Lactivis Fitobucaneve, Ital.
Capsules: Vitamins; *Lactobacillus acidophilus* (p.1594·1); dried yeast (p.1373·1); dried yogurt.
Powder for oral liquid: Vitamins; lactic-acid-producing organisms (p.1594·1).
Nutritional supplement.

Lacto Calamine
Note. This name is used for preparations of different composition.
Boots, S.Afr.; Schering-Plough, UK.
Lotion: Calamine (p.1080·1); zinc oxide (p.1096·2); hamamelis (p.1587·1); phenol (p.1121·2).
Skin irritation; sunburn.
Schering-Plough, UK.
Cream: Calamine (p.1080·1); zinc oxide (p.1096·2); hamamelis (p.1587·1).
Dry skin; sunburn.

Lacto Pregomine Milupa, Fr.
Infant feed.
Cow's milk intolerance.

Lactobin Biotest, Ger.†.
A hyperimmune bovine colostrum (p.1506·2).
Diarrhoea in immunodeficiency; haemolytic uraemic syndrome.

Lactocal-F Laser, USA.
Multivitamin and mineral preparation with iron and folic acid.
Supplement for pregnant or lactating women.

Lactocol Ogna, Ital.
Guaiacol (p.1061·2); lactic acid (p.1593·3); calcium phosphate (p.1155·3); calcium lactate (p.1155·2); codeine hydrochloride (p.26·1); aconite (p.1542·2).
Coughs.

Lactocol Expectorante Alcala, Spain.
Guaiphenesin (p.1061·3).
Formerly contained guaiphenesin, anise oil, and pinus sylvestris oil.
Coughs.

Lactocur Biocur, Ger.
Lactulose (p.1195·3).
Constipation; hepatic encephalopathy; salmonella enteritis.

Lactofalk Falk, Ger.
Lactulose (p.1195·3).
Constipation; liver disorders; salmonella enteritis.

Lactoferment nouvelle formule Zyma, Switz.
Lactobacillus acidophilus (p.1594·1).
Gastro-intestinal disorders.

Lactoferrina Morrith, Spain.
Iron succinyl-protein complex (p.1349·2).
Iron deficiency anaemia.

Lactofilus Llorente, Spain.
Lactobacillus acidophilus (p.1594·1).
Restoration of the gastro-intestinal flora.

Lactofree Mead Johnson Nutritionals, USA.
Lactose-free infant feed.

Lactoger Schwarz, Ital.
Lactulose (p.1195·3).
Gastro-intestinal infections; hepatic encephalopathy.

Lactogermine Humana, Ital.
Lactic-acid-producing organisms (p.1594·1); vitamins.
Nutritional supplement.

Lactogest Thompson, USA†.
Tilactase (p.1637·3).
Lactose intolerance.

Lactolavol Rosch & Handel, Aust.
Calcium lactate (p.1155·2); tartaric acid (p.1634·3); atropine sulphate (p.455·1).
Vaginal disorders.

Lactolaxine Coll, Spain†.
Agar (p.1470·3); phenolphthalein (p.1208·2); lactic-acid-producing organisms (p.1594·1); sodium cholate.
Constipation.

Lactolife Fitolife, Ital.
Dried yeast (p.1373·1); lactic-acid-producing organisms (p.1594·1).
Gastro-intestinal disorders; nutritional supplement.

Lactoliofil Juventus, Spain.
Lactobacillus acidophilus (p.1594·1).
Restoration of the gastro-intestinal flora.

Lactomicina-R Medici, Ital.†.
Lactobacillus acidophilus (p.1594·1).
Gastro-intestinal disorders.

Lactonorm Geymonat, Ital.
Lactobacillus acidophilus (p.1594·1).
Disturbances in vaginal flora.

Lactored Fides, Spain.
Tilactase (p.1637·3); lipase; silicone (p.1213·1).
Milk intolerance.

Lactosec Continental Ethicals, S.Afr.
Pyridoxine hydrochloride (p.1362·3).
Lactation inhibition; post-partum breast engorgement; vitamin deficiency.

Lactostrict Fresenius, Ger.†.
Leucine (p.1350·1); valine (p.1358·1); isoleucine (p.1349·2).
Liver disorders.

Lactovagan Winthrop, Switz.†.
Lactic acid (p.1593·3).
Vaginal disorders.

Lactovit Herbaline, Ital.
Dried yeast (p.1373·1); myrtillus (p.1606·1); *Lactobacillus acidophilus* (p.1594·1).
Nutritional supplement.

Lactrase
Rivex, Canad.; Schwarz, USA.
Tilactase (p.1637·3).
Lactase insufficiency; lactose intolerance.

Lactuflor Chephasaar, Ger.
Lactulose (p.1195·3).
Constipation; liver disorders; salmonella enteritis.

Lactugal Galen, UK.
Lactulose (p.1195·3).
Constipation; hepatic encephalopathy.

Lactulax Rougier, Canad.
Lactulose (p.1195·3).
Constipation.

Lactuverlan Verla, Ger.
Lactulose (p.1195·3).
Constipation; liver disorders; salmonella enteritis.

Ladazol Adcock Ingram, S.Afr.
Danazol (p.1441·3).
Endometriosis; hereditary angioedema; mastalgia.

Ladropen
Berk, Irl.; Berk, UK†.
Flucloxacillin (p.209·1) or flucloxacillin sodium (p.209·2).
Bacterial infections.

Ladymega Cantassium Co., UK.
Multivitamin and mineral preparation.

Ladytone Vitabiotics, UK.
Multivitamin and mineral preparation.

Ladyvital Pharmadass, UK.
Multivitamin, mineral, and nutritional preparation.

Laevadosin
Note. This name is used for preparations of different composition.
Laevosan, Aust.
Buccal tablets: Adenosine (p.812·3); guanosine; adenosine phosphate, disodium salt; disodium cytidine phosphate; guanosine monophosphate, disodium salt; disodium uridine monophosphate.
Myopathies; peripheral, cerebral, and coronary vascular disorders.
Laevosan, Aust.; Boehringer Mannheim, Ger.†.
Injection: Adenosine triphosphate, disodium salt (p.1543·2); adenosine phosphate, disodium salt; guanosine monophosphate, disodium salt; adenosine (p.812·3); inosine (p.1591·1); guanosine; uridine (p.1641·3).
Myopathies; peripheral, cerebral, and coronary vascular disorders.

Laev-Amin Laevosan, Aust.
Amino-acid, carbohydrate, and electrolyte infusion.
Parenteral nutrition.

Laevilac S SmithKline Beecham, Ger.
Lactulose (p.1195·3).
Constipation; liver disorders; salmonella enteritis.

Laevodex Laevosan, Aust.
Dextran 40 (p.716·2) or dextran 60 (p.716·3) in sodium chloride infusion.
Plasma volume expansion; thrombosis prophylaxis.

Laevofusin-Basis and -Isoton Laevosan, Aust.
Electrolyte infusion (p.1147·1).
Fluid and electrolyte disorders.

Laevofusin-Starter Laevosan, Aust.
Sodium, chloride, lactate, and acetate infusion (p.1147·1).

Laevolac
Laevosan, Aust.; Boehringer Mannheim, Ital.; Byk Madaus, S.Afr.; Laevosan, Switz.
Lactulose (p.1195·3).
Constipation; gastro-intestinal bacterial infections; hepatic encephalopathy.

Laevoral
Laevosan, Aust.; Laevosan, Switz.†.
Fructose (p.1343·2).
Carbohydrate source; gastro-intestinal disorders; glucose substitute; liver disorders.

Laevosan
Laevosan, Aust.; Boehringer Mannheim, Ital.
Fructose (p.1343·2).
Alcohol poisoning; asthenia; cardiac disorders; diabetes; glucose substitute; liver disorders; poisoning.

Laevostrophan Laevosan, Aust.
Strophanthin-K (p.951·1).
Angina; arrhythmias; heart failure.

Laevostrophan compositum Laevosan, Aust.
Strophanthin-K (p.951·1); diprophylline (p.752·1).
Heart failure.

Laevovit D_3 Laevosan, Aust.
Cholecalciferol (p.1366·3).
Osteomalacia; rickets; vitamin D supplementation.

Lafarin Lafare, Ital.
Cephalexin (p.178·2).
Bacterial infections.

Lafol Brenner-Efeka, Ger.; LAW, Ger.
Folic acid (p.1340·3).
Folic acid deficiency.

Lafurex Lafare, Ital.
Cefuroxime sodium (p.177·1).
Bacterial infections.

Lagaflex Lagap, Switz.†.
Carisoprodol (p.1312·3); paracetamol (p.72·2).
Musculoskeletal pain and spasm.

Lagarmicin Bohm, Spain.
Erythromycin stearate (p.204·2).
Bacterial infections.

Laidor Esseti, Ital.
Nimesulide (p.63·2).
Fever; inflammation; pain.

Laifem Syxyl, Ger.†.
Homoeopathic preparation.

Lait Auto-Bronzant Clarins, Canad.
SPF 6: Ethylhexyl *p*-methoxycinnamate (p.1487·1); oxybenzone (p.1487·3); titanium dioxide (p.1093·3).
Sunscreen.

Lait Bronzage Clarins, Canad.
SPF 6; SPF 10: Ethylhexyl *p*-methoxycinnamate (p.1487·1); oxybenzone (p.1487·3); titanium dioxide (p.1093·3).
SPF 19: Ethylhexyl *p*-methoxycinnamate (p.1487·1); oxybenzone (p.1487·3); 2-phenyl-1*H*-benzimidazole-5-sulphonic acid (p.1488·2); titanium dioxide (p.1093·3).
Sunscreen.

Lait Hydratant Bronzage Vichy, Canad.
SPF 8: Avobenzone (p.1486·3); 3-(4-methylbenzylidene)bornan-2-one (p.1487·2); terephthalylidene dicamphor sulphonic acid; titanium dioxide (p.1093·3).
Sunscreen.

Lait Protecteur Lancome, Canad.; Vichy, Canad.
SPF 15: Avobenzone (p.1486·3); 3-(4-methylbenzylidene)bornan-2-one (p.1487·2); terephthalylidene dicamphor sulphonic acid; titanium dioxide (p.1093·3).
Sunscreen.

Laitan
Schwabe, Ger.; Spitzner, Ger.; Schwabe, Switz.
Kava (p.1592·3).
Anxiety disorders; sleep disorders.

Lakriment Neu Dolorgiet, Ger.
Liquorice (p.1197·1).
Catarrh.

Laktipex Ipex, Swed.
Lactulose (p.1195·3).
Constipation; hepatic encephalopathy.

Laktulax Kali, Aust.†.
Lactulose (p.1195·3).
Constipation.

Lamaline Solvay, Fr.
Paracetamol (p.72·2); belladonna (p.457·1); opium (p.70·3); caffeine (p.749·3).
Pain.

Lambanol Zilliken, Ital.†.
Docusate sodium (p.1189·3).
Constipation.

Lamicitin Glaxo Wellcome, S.Afr.
Lamotrigine (p.347·2).
Epilepsy.

Lamictal
Glaxo Wellcome, Aust.; Glaxo Wellcome, Austral.; Glaxo Wellcome, Belg.; Glaxo Wellcome, Canad.; Glaxo Wellcome, Fr.; Glaxo Wellcome, Ger.; Desitin, Ger.; Wellcome, Irl.; Glaxo Wellcome, Ital.; Glaxo Wellcome, Neth.; Glaxo Wellcome, Norw.; Wellcome, Spain; Glaxo Wellcome, Swed.; Wellcome, Switz.; Wellcome, UK; Wellcome, USA.
Lamotrigine (p.347·2).
Epilepsy.

L-Aminosauren-Losung Serag-Wiessner, Ger.†.
Amino-acid, carbohydrate, and electrolyte infusion.
Parenteral nutrition.

Lamisil
Sanabo, Aust.; Novartis, Austral.; Wander, Belg.; Sandoz, Canad.; Sandoz, Fr.; Sandoz, Ger.; Sandoz, Irl.; Sandoz, Ital.; Novartis, Neth.; Sandoz, Norw.; Novartis, S.Afr.; Sandoz, Spain; Novartis, Swed.; Sandoz, Switz.; Sandoz, UK; Sandoz, USA.
Terbinafine (p.388·1) or terbinafine hydrochloride (p.387·3).
Fungal skin and nail infections.

Lamnotyl Farmasur, Spain.
Boric acid (p.1554·2); hamamelis (p.1587·1); ichthammol (p.1083·3); zinc oxide (p.1096·2).
Skin disorders.

Lamoryl
Leo, Norw.; Lovens, Swed.†.
Griseofulvin (p.380·2).
Fungal infections.

Lampit Bayer, Ger.
Nifurtimox (p.589·1).
Trypanosomiasis.

Lampocef Lampugnani, Ital.†.
Cephazolin sodium (p.181·1).
Bacterial infections.

Lampocillina Salus, Ital.
Ampicillin sodium (p.153·1).
Bacterial infections.

Lampoflex Lampugnani, Ital.
Piroxicam (p.80·2).
Musculoskeletal and joint disorders.

Lampomandol AGIPS, Ital.
Cephamandole nafate (p.180·1).
Lignocaine hydrochloride (p.1293·2) is included in this preparation to alleviate the pain of injection.
Bacterial infections.

Lampomicol Lebens, Ital.†.
Miconazole (p.384·3) or miconazole nitrate (p.384·3).
Fungal infections; Gram-positive bacterial infections.

Lamposporin Lebens, Ital.†.
Cefuroxime sodium (p.177·1).
Bacterial infections.

Lampotrix Lebens, Ital.†.
Propylene glycol cefatrizine (p.164·2).
Bacterial infections.

Lampren
Novartis, Neth.; Padro, Spain.
Clofazimine (p.194·1).
Leprosy.

Lamprene
Novartis, Austral.; Geigy, Irl.; Novartis, S.Afr.; Geigy, Switz.; Alliance, UK; Geigy, USA.
Clofazimine (p.194·1).
Leprosy.

Lamra Merckle, Ger.
Diazepam (p.661·1).
Anxiety.

Lamuran
Boehringer Mannheim, Aust.; Boehringer Mannheim, Ger.†; SIT, Ital.
Raubasine (p.941·3).
Cerebral and peripheral circulatory disorders.

Lanabiotic
Note. This name is used for preparations of different composition.
Combe, Canad.
Bacitracin (p.157·3); polymyxin B sulphate (p.239·1).
Wounds.
Combe, USA.
Polymyxin B sulphate (p.239·1); neomycin sulphate (p.229·2); bacitracin (p.157·3); lignocaine (p.1293·2).
Bacterial skin infections.

Lanacane
Combe, Spain; Combe, UK; Combe, USA.
Benzocaine (p.1286·2).
Skin disorders.

Lanacane Medicated Cream Combe, Canad.
Benzocaine (p.1286·2); resorcinol (p.1090·1).
Skin disorders.

Lanacane Medicated Powder Combe, UK.
Menthol (p.1600·2); zinc oxide (p.1096·2).
Skin irritation.

Lanacard Madaus, Ger.†.
Digoxin (p.849·3).
Heart failure.

Lanacine Lannacher, Aust.
Clindamycin hydrochloride (p.191·1).
Bacterial infections.

Lanacordin Glaxo Wellcome, Spain.
Digoxin (p.849·3).
Arrhythmias; heart failure.

Lanacort
Combe, Canad.; CCM, Ital.; Combe, UK; Combe, USA.
Hydrocortisone acetate (p.1043·3).
Skin disorders.

Lanacrist Tika, Swed.
Digoxin (p.849·3).
Arrhythmias; heart failure.

Lanadigin-EL Promonta, Ger.†.
Acetyldigoxin (p.812·3); potassium aspartate (p.1161·3); magnesium aspartate (p.1157·2).
Cardiac disorders.

Lanaphilic
Note. This name is used for preparations of different composition.
Medco, USA.
Urea (p.1095·2).
Dry skin; hyperkeratosis.
Medco, USA.
Vehicle for topical preparations.

Lanasting Combe, UK†.
Cream: Benzyl alcohol (p.1103·3); lignocaine (p.1293·2).
Topical spray: Benzocaine (p.1286·2); benzethonium chloride (p.1102·3).
Insect bites; skin irritation; stings.

Lanatilin Nycomed, Aust.
α-Acetyldigoxin (p.812·3).
Arrhythmias; heart failure.

Lancetina Uno, Ital.†.
Fosfomycin calcium (p.210·2).
Bacterial infections.

Lander Dandruff Control Lander, Canad.
Pyrithione zinc (p.1089·3).
Dandruff.

Lanexat Roche, Swed.
Flumazenil (p.981·1).
Benzodiazepine overdosage; reversal of benzodiazepine-induced sedation.

Langoran Marion Merrell, Fr.
Isosorbide dinitrate (p.893·1).
Angina pectoris; heart failure.

Laniazid *Lannett, USA.*
Isoniazid (p.218·1).
Tuberculosis.

Lanicor
Boehringer Mannheim, Aust.; Boehringer Mannheim, Ger.; Boehringer Mannheim, Ital.†.
Digoxin (p.849·3).
Arrhythmias; heart failure.

Lanirapid
Boehringer Mannheim, Jpn; Boehringer Mannheim, Spain.
Medigoxin (p.902·1).
Arrhythmias; heart failure.

Lanitop
Boehringer Mannheim, Aust.; Boehringer Mannheim, Belg.; Boehringer Mannheim, Ger.; Boehringer Mannheim, Ital.; Boehringer Mannheim, Switz.
Medigoxin (p.902·1).
Arrhythmias; heart failure.

Lanoc *Lannacher, Aust.*
Metoprolol tartrate (p.907·3).
Angina pectoris; arrhythmias; hypertension; migraine; myocardial infarction.

Lanofene *Augot, Fr.*
Zinc oxide (p.1096·2).
Eczema; nappy rash.

Lanohex *Rougier, Canad.*
Phenoxyethanol (p.1122·2).
Scalp disorders; skin cleansing.

Lanolelle *Warner-Lambert, Canad.*
Hydrous wool fat (p.1385·3).
Dry skin.

Lanolor *Squibb, USA.*
Emollient and moisturiser.

Lanophyllin *Lannett, USA.*
Theophylline (p.765·1).
Asthma; bronchospasm.

Lanorinal *Lannett, USA.*
Aspirin (p.16·1); caffeine (p.749·3); butalbital (p.644·3).
Pain.

Lanoxicaps *Wellcome, USA.*
Digoxin (p.849·3).
Atrial fibrillation and flutter; heart failure; paroxysmal supraventricular tachycardia.

Lanoxin
Glaxo Wellcome, Austral.; Glaxo Wellcome, Belg.; Glaxo Wellcome, Canad.; Wellcome, Irl.; Glaxo Wellcome, Ital.; Glaxo Wellcome, Neth.; Glaxo Wellcome, Norw.; Glaxo Wellcome, S.Afr.; Glaxo Wellcome, Swed.; Wellcome, Switz.; Wellcome, UK; Glaxo Wellcome, USA.
Digoxin (p.849·3).
Atrial fibrillation and flutter; heart failure; paroxysmal supraventricular tachycardia.

Lansox *Takeda, Ital.*
Lansoprazole (p.1196·2).
Gastro-oesophageal reflux disease; peptic ulcer; Zollinger-Ellison syndrome.

Lansoyl
Fournier, Belg.; Therabel Pharma, Belg.; Jouveinal, Canad.; Jouveinal, Fr.; Central, Irl.†; Jouveinal, Switz.
Liquid paraffin (p.1382·1).
Constipation.

Lantanon
Organon, Ital.; Donmed, S.Afr.; Organon, Spain; Intervet, Switz.†.
Mianserin hydrochloride (p.297·1).
Depression.

Lantarel *Lederle, Ger.*
Methotrexate sodium (p.547·1).
Psoriasis vulgaris; psoriatic arthritis; rheumatoid arthritis.

Lantigen B
Note. This name is used for preparations of different composition.
Overta, Aust.†; Cassenne, Fr.†; Bruschettini, Switz.
Antigens from: pneumococci; streptococci; *Branhamella catarrhalis*; staphylococci; *Klebsiella pneumoniae*; *Haemophilus influenzae*.
Respiratory-tract disorders.

COB, Belg.
Antigens from autolysate of: *Diplococcus pneumoniae*; *Streptococcus pyogenes*; *Branhamella catarrhalis*; *Staphylococcus aureus*; *Klebsiella pneumoniae*; *Haemophilus influenzae*.
Cold symptoms.

Bruschettini, Ital.
Antigen extracts of: *Streptococcus pneumoniae*; *Streptococcus pyogenes*; *Branhamella catarrhalis*; *Staphylococcus aureus*; *Klebsiella pneumoniae*; *Haemophilus influenzae* type b.
Upper respiratory-tract infections.

Lantogent *Plevifarma, Spain.*
Gentamicin sulphate (p.212·1).
Bacterial infections.

Lanuretic *Lannacher, Aust.*
Hydrochlorothiazide (p.885·2); amiloride hydrochloride (p.819·2).
Hypertension; oedema.

Lanvis
Glaxo Wellcome, Austral.; Glaxo Wellcome, Belg.; Glaxo Wellcome, Canad.; Wellcome, Irl.; Glaxo Wellcome, Neth.; Glaxo Wellcome, S.Afr.; Glaxo Wellcome, Swed.; Wellcome, Switz.; Wellcome, UK.
Thioguanine (p.566·2).
Bone-marrow transplantation; leukaemias; lymphoma; polycythaemia vera.

Lanzo
Wyeth, Norw.; Wyeth Lederle, Swed.; Orion, Swed.
Lansoprazole (p.1196·2).
Gastro-oesophageal reflux; peptic ulcer; Zollinger-Ellison syndrome.

Lanzor
Houde, Fr.; Albert-Roussel, Ger.; Hoechst, Ger.; Hoechst Marion Roussel, S.Afr.
Lansoprazole (p.1196·2).
Formerly known as Lanazor in *S.Afr.*
Gastro-oesophageal reflux; peptic ulcer; Zollinger-Ellison syndrome.

Lao-Dal *Synthelabo, Fr.*
Camphor (p.1557·2); menthol (p.1600·2); lignocaine hydrochloride (p.1293·2); chloroform (p.1220·3); methyl salicylate (p.55·2); turpentine oil (p.1641·1); glycol salicylate (p.43·1).
Soft-tissue disorders.

Lapices Epiderm Metadier *Prats, Spain.*
Dithranol (p.1082·1); salicylic acid (p.1090·2).
Skin disorders.

Lapidar *Swiss Herbal, Canad.*
Cascara (p.1183·1); frangula (p.1193·2); senna (p.1212·2).

Lapidar 10 *Kunzle, Switz.*
Capsules: Frangula bark (p.1193·2); cascara (p.1183·1); senna (p.1212·2).
Tablets: Frangula bark (p.1193·2); senna (p.1212·2); liquorice (p.1197·1).
Constipation.

Lapidar 14 *Kunzle, Switz.*
Frangula bark (p.1193·2); senna (p.1212·2); marian thistle (p.993·3).
Constipation.

Lapidar 10 plus *Kunzle, Switz.*
Frangula bark (p.1193·2); senna (p.1212·2); mint oil (p.1604·1); fennel oil (p.1579·2).
Constipation.

Lapiz Termo Compositum *Domenech Garcia, Spain†.*
Camphor (p.1557·2); capsicum oleoresin; methyl salicylate (p.55·2); salicylic acid (p.1090·2); suxibuzone (p.88·2); menthol (p.1600·2); turpentine oil (p.1641·1); lavender oil (p.1594·3); thyme oil (p.1637·1); eucalyptus oil (p.1578·1).
Rheumatic and muscle pain.

Laractone *Lagap, UK.*
Spironolactone (p.946·1).
Ascites; heart failure; hyperaldosteronism; oedema.

Larafen *Lagap, UK.*
Ketoprofen (p.48·2).
Musculoskeletal and joint disorders; pain.

Laraflex *Lagap, UK.*
Naproxen (p.61·2).
Gout; inflammation; musculoskeletal disorders; pain.

Larapam *Lagap, UK.*
Piroxicam (p.80·2).
Gout; inflammation; musculoskeletal disorders; pain.

Laratrim *Lagap, UK.*
Co-trimoxazole (p.196·3).
Bacterial infections.

Larch Resin comp. *Weleda, UK.*
Ananassa fruit; lavender oil (p.1594·3); larch resin.
Sore eyes.

Larex *Inibsa, Spain†.*
Polynoxylin (p.1123·1).
Mouth infections.

Largactil
Rhone-Poulenc Rorer, Aust.; Rhone-Poulenc Rorer, Austral.; Rhone-Poulenc Rorer, Belg.; Rhone-Poulenc Rorer, Canad.; Specia, Fr.; Rhone-Poulenc Rorer, Irl.; Rhone-Poulenc Rorer, Ital.; Rhone-Poulenc Rorer, Neth.; Rhone-Poulenc Rorer, Norw.; Rhone-Poulenc Rorer, S.Afr.; Rhone-Poulenc Rorer, Spain; Rhone-Poulenc Rorer, Switz.; May & Baker, UK.
Chlorpromazine (p.649·1), chlorpromazine embonate (p.649·1), or chlorpromazine hydrochloride (p.649·1).
Agitation; alcohol or opioid withdrawal syndrome; anxiety; behaviour disorders; eclampsia; induction of hypothermia; infantile neurotoxicosis; intractable hiccup; nausea and vomiting; porphyria; premedication; pruritus; psychoses; shock; sleep disorders.

Largal ultra *Septodont, Switz.*
Edetate sodium; cetrimonium bromide (p.1106·1).
Adjunct in dental surgery.

Largatrex *Rhone-Poulenc Rorer, Spain.*
Chlorpromazine (p.649·1); heptaminol (p.1587·2); benzhexol (p.458·1).
Aggression; anxiety; psychoses.

Largitor *Italfarmaco, Spain.*
Myrtillus (p.1606·1).
Vascular disorders.

Largon
Note. This name is used for preparations of different composition.
Klinge, Aust.
Kawain (p.1592·3).
Nervous disorders.

Wyeth-Ayerst, USA.
Propiomazine hydrochloride (p.417·3).
Sedative.

Lariam
Roche, Aust.; Roche, Austral.; Roche, Belg.; Roche, Canad.; Roche, Fr.; Roche, Ger.; Roche, Irl.; Roche, Ital.; Roche, Neth.; Roche, Norw.; Roche, S.Afr.; Roche, Swed.; Roche, Switz.; Roche, UK; Roche, USA.
Mefloquine hydrochloride (p.432·2).
Malaria.

Laridal *Elfar, Spain.*
Astemizole (p.402·1).
Hypersensitivity reactions.

Larifikehl *Sanum-Kehlbeck, Ger.*
Homoeopathic preparation.

Larilon *Bioprogress, Ital.*
Chlorhexidine gluconate (p.1107·2); benzododecinium chloride (p.1103·2).
Disinfection of wounds and burns.

Larmes Artificielles *Ciba Vision, Fr.*
Sodium chloride (p.1162·2).
Dry eyes.

Larobec *Roche, USA†.*
Vitamin B substances with vitamin C and folic acid.
Vitamin supplementation during levodopa therapy.

Larocal *Roche, Switz.†.*
Muramidase (p.1604·3); tyrothricin (p.267·2); lignocaine (p.1293·2); cetylpyridinium chloride (p.1106·2).
Mouth and throat disorders.

Larodopa
Roche, Canad.†; Roche, Fr.†; Roche, Irl.†; Roche, Ital.†; Roche, S.Afr.†; Cambridge, UK; Roche, USA.
Levodopa (p.1137·1).
Now known as Levodopa Tablets in the *UK.*
Parkinsonism.

Laroferon *Roche, Fr.*
Interferon alfa-2a (p.615·3).
Hepatitis C.

Laroscorbine *Roche, Fr.*
Ascorbic acid (p.1365·2).
Vitamin C deficiency.

Laroxyl
Roche, Fr.; Roche, Ger.†; Roche, Irl.†; Roche, Ital.
Amitriptyline hydrochloride (p.273·3).
Depression; nocturnal enuresis; pain.

Larydol *Dolisos, Canad.*
Homoeopathic preparation.

Larylin *Bayer, Ger.†.*
Lozenges: Guaiphenesin (p.1061·3).
Coughs and associated respiratory-tract disorders.

Larylin Heissgetrank gegen Schmerzen und Fieber *Bayer, Ger.*
Paracetamol (p.72·2).
Fever; pain.

Larylin Husten-Heissgetrank *Bayer, Ger.*
Ambroxol hydrochloride (p.1054·3).
Respiratory disorders associated with viscid or excessive mucus.

Larylin Hustenloser *Bayer, Ger.†.*
Dropropizine (p.1059·2); benzocaine (p.1286·2); cetylpyridinium chloride (p.1106·2); guaiphenesin (p.1061·3).
Coughs and associated respiratory-tract disorders.

Larylin Hustenpastillen-losend *Bayer, Ger.*
Ambroxol hydrochloride (p.1054·3).
Respiratory disorders associated with viscid or excessive mucus.

Larylin Hustensaft-losend *Bayer, Ger.*
Ambroxol hydrochloride (p.1054·3).
Respiratory disorders associated with viscid or excessive mucus.

Larylin Hustensirup N *Bayer, Ger.*
Dropropizine (p.1059·2).
Catarrh; coughs.

Larylin Husten-Stiller Pastillen *Bayer, Ger.*
Dropropizine (p.1059·2).
Coughs.

Larylin Nasenspray N *Bayer, Ger.*
Oxymetazoline hydrochloride (p.1065·3).
A similar preparation formerly contained naphazoline nitrate and pheniramine maleate.
Colds; middle ear inflammation; nasal congestion.

Laryngarsol
Couvreur, Belg.†.
Mouth and throat spray: Acetarsol (p.578·2).
Mouth and throat disorders.

Synthelabo, Belg.
Tablets: Ascorbic acid (p.1365·2); sodium ascorbate (p.1365·2); dequalinium chloride (p.1112·1).
Mouth and throat disorders.

Laryng-O-Jet *IMS, UK.*
Lignocaine hydrochloride (p.1293·2).
Local anaesthesia.

Laryngomedin N *Rhone-Poulenc Rorer, Ger.*
Hexamidine isethionate (p.1115·3).
A similar preparation formerly contained hexamidine isethionate and amethocaine hydrochloride.
Painful or inflammatory disorders of the oropharynx.

Laryngsan N *Opfermann, Ger.*
Camphor (p.1557·2); caffeine and sodium benzoate; ammonia solution (p.1548·3); peppermint oil (p.1208·1).
Coughs and cold symptoms; inflammatory disorders of the oropharynx.

Lasa Antiasmatico *Lasa, Spain.*
Aminophylline (p.748·1); potassium iodide (p.1493·1).
Obstructive airways disease.

Lasa Con Codeina *Lasa, Spain.*
Chlorpheniramine maleate (p.405·1); codeine phosphate (p.26·1); pseudoephedrine hydrochloride (p.1068·3).
Upper-respiratory-tract disorders.

Lasafort *Lifepharma, Ital.†.*
Aspirin (p.16·1); paracetamol (p.72·2); caffeine (p.749·3).
Cold symptoms; fever; pain.

Lasain *Inibsa, Spain.*
Metamizole magnesium (p.35·1).
Fever; pain.

Lasar *Biocur, Ger.*
dl-Alpha tocopheryl acetate (p.1369·2); magnesium oxide (p.1198·3).
Vitamin E or magnesium deficiency.

Lasar mono *Jossa-Arznei, Ger.†.*
Magnesium sulphate (p.1157·3).
Magnesium deficiency.

Laser *Tosi, Ital.*
Naproxen (p.61·2).
Gout; musculoskeletal and joint disorders; neuralgia.

Laser Slim 'n Trim *Laser, S.Afr.†.*
Cathine hydrochloride (p.1478·1).
Obesity.

Lasikal
Hoechst Marion Roussel, Irl.; Borg, UK.
Frusemide (p.871·1); potassium chloride (p.1161·1).
Oedema.

Lasilacton *Hoechst, Aust.*
Frusemide (p.871·1); spironolactone (p.946·1).
Oedema.

Lasilactone
Hoechst Marion Roussel, Switz.; Borg, UK.
Frusemide (p.871·1); spironolactone (p.946·1).
Hypertension; oedema.

Lasiletten *Hoechst Marion Roussel, Neth.*
Frusemide (p.871·1).
Hypertension; oedema.

Lasilix *Hoechst, Fr.*
Frusemide (p.871·1).
Hypertension; oedema.

Lasipressin *Hoechst, UK†.*
Frusemide (p.871·1); penbutolol sulphate (p.927·2).
Hypertension.

Lasitace *Hoechst, Aust.*
Ramipril (p.941·1); frusemide (p.871·1).
Heart failure; hypertension.

Lasitone *Hoechst Marion Roussel, Ital.*
Frusemide (p.871·1); spironolactone (p.946·1).
Oedema.

Lasix
Hoechst, Aust.; Hoechst Marion Roussel, Austral.; Hoechst Marion Roussel, Belg.; Hoechst Marion Roussel, Canad.; Hoechst, Ger.; Hoechst Marion Roussel, Irl.; Hoechst Marion Roussel, Ital.; Hoechst Marion Roussel, Neth.; Hoechst Marion Roussel, Norw.; Hoechst Marion Roussel, S.Afr.; Hoechst Marion Roussel, Swed.; Hoechst Marion Roussel, Switz.; Borg, UK; Hoechst Marion Roussel, USA.
Frusemide (p.871·1) or frusemide sodium (p.872·3).
Forced diuresis; heart failure; hypertension; oedema; renal failure.

Lasix + K
Hoechst Marion Roussel, Irl.†; Borg, UK†.
White tablets, frusemide (p.871·1); yellow tablets, potassium chloride (p.1161·1).
Oedema.

Lasix-Reserpin *Hoechst Marion Roussel, Ital.†.*
Frusemide (p.871·1); reserpine (p.942·1).
Hypertension.

Lasma
Pharmax, Irl.; Pharmax, UK.
Theophylline (p.765·1).
Obstructive airways disease.

Lasonil
Bayer, Aust.; Bayer, Austral.; Bayer, Belg.; Bayer, Fr.; Bayer, Ger.; Bayer, Ital.; Bayer, Neth.; Bayer, Spain; Bayer, Switz.†; Bayer, UK.
A heparinoid (p.882·3); hyaluronidase (p.1588·1).
Superficial tissue injuries.

Lasonil H *Bayer, Ital.*
A heparinoid (p.882·3); hyaluronidase (p.1588·1); vitamin A palmitate (p.1359·2); calcium pantothenate (p.1352·3); menthol (p.1600·2).
Anorectal disorders.

Lasoproct *Bayer, Ital.*
A heparinoid (p.882·3); hyaluronidase (p.1588·1); vitamin A palmitate (p.1359·2); calcium pantothenate (p.1352·3); dexamethasone (p.1037·1); amethocaine hydrochloride (p.1285·2); menthol (p.1600·2).
Anorectal disorders.

Lasoreuma *Bayer, Ital.*
A heparinoid (p.882·3); glycol salicylate (p.43·1); benzyl nicotinate (p.22·1).
Inflammation; pain.

Lasoride
Hoechst Marion Roussel, Irl.; Borg, UK.
Frusemide (p.871·1); amiloride hydrochloride (p.819·2).
These ingredients can be described by the British Approved Name Co-amilofruse.
Oedema.

Lasoven *Bayer, Ital.*
A heparinoid (p.882·3).
Peripheral vascular disorders; soft-tissue disorders.

Laspar *Intramed, S.Afr.*
Asparaginase (p.504·3).
Lymphoblastic leukaemias.

Lassatina *ISI, Ital.*
Senna (p.1212·2); cascara (p.1183·1); rhubarb (p.1212·1); liquorice (p.1197·1); belladonna (p.457·1); nux vomica (p.1609·3); aniseed (p.1549·3).
Constipation.

Lassifar *Lafare, Ital.*
Lactulose (p.1195·3).
Hepatic encephalopathy.

Lass-Med *Cassella-med, Ital.†.*
Cascara sagrada (p.1183·1); rhubarb (p.1212·1); aloes (p.1177·1).
Constipation.

Lastet *Pharmacia Upjohn, Ital.; Kayaku, Jpn; Pras, Spain.*
Etoposide (p.532·3).
Malignant neoplasms.

Lasticom *Asta Medica, Aust.*
Azelastine hydrochloride (p.403·1).
Asthma; bronchitis.

Late Orphon *Repha, Ger.†.*
Orthosiphon leaves (p.1592·2).
Urinary-tract disorders.

Latensin *Sanum-Kehlbeck, Ger.*
Bacillus cereus.
Immunotherapy.

Latepyrine *Solvay, Belg.†.*
Paracetamol (p.72·2); ethyl carbosalicylate; quinine camphosulfonate (p.441·2).
Fever; headache.

Latesyl *Solvay, Aust.*
Diethylamine salicylate (p.33·1); myrtecaine (p.1297·3).
Musculoskeletal and joint disorders; neuralgia.

Laticort *Medphano, Ger.*
Hydrocortisone butyrate (p.1044·1).
Skin disorders.

Latimit *Medphano, Ger.*
Hydrocortisone acetate (p.1043·3).
Skin disorders.

Latocef *Del Saz & Filippini, Ital.*
Propylene glycol cefatrizine (p.164·2).
Bacterial infections.

Latoral *Dukron, Ital.†.*
Cephalexin (p.178·2).
Bacterial infections.

Latorex *Dukron, Ital.†.*
Cephaloridine (p.179·1).
Bacterial infections.

Latoxacef *Magis, Ital.†.*
Latamoxef disodium (p.221·2).
Bacterial infections.

Latschenkiefer Franzbranntwein *Klosterfrau, Ger.*
Camphor (p.1557·2); pumilio pine oil (p.1623·3).
Muscle and joint pain; soft-tissue disorders.

Latycin
Biochemie, Aust.; Boucher & Muir, Austral.
Tetracycline hydrochloride (p.259·1).
Bacterial infections.

Laubeel *Desitin, Ger.*
Lorazepam (p.675·3).
Anxiety disorders; sleep disorders.

Laucalon *Europharma, Spain†.*
Butopiprine hydrobromide (p.1056·2).
Coughs.

Laudamonium *Henkel, Ger.*
Benzalkonium chloride (p.1101·3).
Skin and surface disinfection.

Lauracalm *Farmabel, Belg.†.*
Lorazepam (p.675·3).
Anxiety; insomnia.

Lauridin *Locatelli, Ital.†.*
Cephaloridine (p.179·1).
Bacterial infections.

Lauromicina *Lafare, Ital.*
Ointment: Fluocinolone acetonide (p.1041·1); erythromycin stearate (p.204·2).
Infected skin disorders.
Tablets: Lauryl sulphate salt of erythromycin stearate (p.204·2).
Bacterial infections.

Lauvir *Pierre Fabre, Fr.†.*
Chlorhexidine gluconate (p.1107·2).
Wound cleansing.

Lavaflac *Pharmacia Upjohn, Spain.*
Sodium chloride (p.1162·2).
Fluid and electrolyte disorders.

Lavagin *Mayrhofer, Aust.*
Lactic acid (p.1593·3); sodium lactate (p.1153·2).
Vaginal disorders.

Lavanda Sofar *Sofar, Ital.*
Anhydrous citric acid (p.1564·3); sodium citrate (p.1153·2); alum (p.1547·1); phenol (p.1121·2).
Vaginal disinfection.

Lavasept *Fresenius, Switz.*
Polyhexanide (p.1123·1).
Bone and soft-tissue infections; wounds.

Lavement au Phosphate *Norgine, Belg.*
Monobasic sodium phosphate (p.1159·3); dibasic sodium phosphate (p.1159·3).
Bowel evacuation.

Lavichthol *Ichthyol, Aust.*
Ictasol (p.1083·3).
Skin disorders.

Lavisa *Lesvi, Spain.*
Fluconazole (p.378·1).
Fungal infections.

Lavolax *Lavomat, Swed.†.*
Potassium chloride; sodium chloride; sodium bicarbonate; anhydrous sodium sulphate (p.1147·1).
Bowel evacuation.

Lavolen *Lacer, Spain.*
Trisodium polysaccharide sulphate; a nonoxinol (p.1326·1).
Contraceptive.

Lax Pills *G & W, USA.*
Yellow phenolphthalein (p.1208·2).
Constipation.

Laxa *Nobel, Canad.*
Aloin (p.1177·2); cascara (p.1183·1); phenolphthalein (p.1208·2); bile salts (p.1553·2).

Laxabon
Tika, Norw.; Tika, Swed.
Macrogol 3350 (p.1598·2); electrolytes (p.1147·1).
Bowel evacuation.

Laxadoron *Weleda, UK.*
Caraway (p.1559·3); clove (p.1565·2); centaury (p.1561·1); peppermint leaf (p.1208·1); yarrow (p.1542·2); senna leaf (p.1212·2); aniseed (p.1549·3); nectar hoyae carnosae.
Constipation.

Laxagel *Everest, Canad.*
Capsules: Docusate sodium (p.1189·3).
Oral powder: Ispaghula husk (p.1194·2).
Constipation.

Laxagetten *CT, Ger.*
Bisacodyl (p.1179·3).
Constipation.

Laxalind *Melisana, Switz.†.*
Frangula bark (p.1193·2); aloes (p.1177·1); cascara (p.1183·1); senna (p.1212·2).
Constipation.

Laxalpin *Kwizda, Aust.*
Senna (p.1212·2); frangula bark (p.1193·2); fennel (p.1579·1); chamomile (p.1561·2); guaiacum wood; liquorice (p.1197·1); sambucus (p.1627·2); adiantum capillus veneris; sodium potassium tartrate (p.1213·3).
Constipation; flatulence.

Laxamalt
Bouchara, Fr.; Bouchara, Switz.
Liquid paraffin (p.1382·1).
Constipation.

Laxanin N *Schwarzhaupt, Ger.*
Bisacodyl (p.1179·3).
Constipation.

Laxans *Schulke & Mayr, Aust.*
Ispaghula husk (p.1194·2).
Constipation.

Laxans-ratiopharm *Ratiopharm, Ger.*
Bisacodyl (p.1179·3).
Bowel evacuation; constipation.

Laxante Bescansa *Bescansa, Spain.*
Calcium carbonate (p.1182·1); carrageenan mucilage (p.1471·3); phenolphthalein (p.1208·2).
Constipation.

Laxante Bescansa Aloico *Bescansa, Spain.*
Aloin (p.1177·2); belladonna (p.457·1); phenolphthalein (p.1208·2); rhubarb (p.1212·1).
Constipation.

Laxante Derly *Derly, Spain.*
Cascara (p.1183·1); senna (p.1212·2).
Constipation.

Laxante Geve *Bama, Spain†.*
Aloin (p.1177·2); phenolphthalein (p.1208·2).
Constipation.

Laxante Olan *Puerto Galiano, Spain.*
Ipomoea (p.1194·2); phenolphthalein (p.1208·2); sodium bicarbonate; tartaric acid.
Constipation.

Laxante Richelet *Vitafarma, Spain†.*
Belladonna (p.457·1); bile (p.1553·2); boldo (p.1554·1); phenolphthalein (p.1208·2); frangula (p.1193·2); magnesium oxide (p.1198·3); sodium bicarbonate; methionine (p.984·2).
Constipation.

Laxante Salud *Boots, Spain.*
Aloes (p.1177·1); phenolphthalein (p.1208·2).
Constipation.

Laxante Sanatorium *Santiveri, Spain.*
Aloes (p.1177·1); aniseed (p.1549·3); sulphur (p.1091·2); senna (p.1212·2); matricaria (p.1561·2).
Constipation.

Laxarol *Therapex, Canad.*
Phenolphthalein (p.1208·2); liquid paraffin (p.1382·1).

Laxasan
Note. This name is used for preparations of different composition.
Dolisos, Canad.
Homoeopathic preparation.

Dolisos, Fr.
Senna (p.1212·2); tamarind (p.1217·3).
Constipation.

Gebro, Switz.
Sodium picosulphate (p.1213·2); fennel oil (p.1579·2); peppermint oil (p.1208·1).
Constipation.

Laxatan *Cassella-med, Ger.†.*
Aloes (p.1177·1).
Constipation.

Laxative Pills
Stanley, Canad.; Rugby, USA.
Yellow phenolphthalein (p.1208·2).
Constipation.

Laxativum *Giuliani, Switz.†.*
Rhubarb (p.1212·1); cascara (p.1183·1); boldo (p.1554·1); phenolphthalein (p.1208·2).
Constipation.

Laxativum Nouvelle Formule *Giuliani, Switz.*
Cascara (p.1183·1); boldo (p.1554·1); senna (p.1212·2).
Constipation.

Laxativum Truw *Truw, Ger.†.*
Senna (p.1212·2).
Constipation.

Laxatone *Richelin, S.Afr.†.*
Phenolphthalein (p.1208·2).
Constipation.

Laxavit *Wolfs, Belg.*
Docusate sodium (p.1189·3); glycerol (p.1585·2).
Constipation.

Laxbene
Note. This name is used for preparations of different composition.
Merckle, Aust.; Merckle, Ger.; Mepha, Switz.†.
Suppositories: Bisacodyl (p.1179·3).
Bowel evacuation; constipation.

Merckle, Aust.
Tablets: Bisacodyl (p.1179·3); dimethicone (p.1213·1).
Bowel evacuation; constipation.

Laxbene N *Merckle, Ger.*
Bisacodyl (p.1179·3).
Constipation.

Laxeersiroop *SAN, Neth.†.*
Lactulose (p.1195·3).
Constipation.

Laxen Busto *Fermentaciones y Sintesis, Spain.*
Phenolphthalein (p.1208·2).
Constipation.

Laxette *Medpro, S.Afr.*
Lactulose (p.1195·3).
Constipation; hepatic encephalopathy.

Laxettes *Mentholatum, Austral.*
Chocolate: Phenolphthalein (p.1208·2).
Tablets: Calcium sennoside A (p.1212·3); calcium sennoside B (p.1212·3).
Constipation.

Laxherba N *Kattwiga, Ger.†.*
Frangula (p.1193·2); aloes (p.1177·1); senna (p.1212·2).
Constipation.

Laxicaps *Propan-Vernleigh, S.Afr.†.*
Phenolphthalein (p.1208·2); ferrous sulphate (p.1340·2).
Constipation.

Laxil *Vis, Ital.†.*
Liquid paraffin (p.1382·1).
Constipation.

Laxilose *Technilab, Canad.*
Lactulose (p.1195·3).
Constipation.

Laxiplant cum Senna *Wander OTC, Switz.*
Ispaghula husk (p.1194·2); senna (p.1212·2).
Constipation.

Laxiplant Soft
Schwabe, Ger.; Wander OTC, Switz.
Ispaghula husk (p.1194·2).
Constipation; diarrhoea.

Laxiplant-N *Schwabe, Ger.†.*
Ispaghula husk (p.1194·2); senna (p.1212·2).
Constipation.

Laxisoft *Semar, Spain.*
Ispaghula husk (p.1194·2).
Constipation.

Laxitex *Andreu, Spain†.*
Sulisatin sodium (p.1215·1).
Constipation.

Lax-Lorenz *Lorenz, Ger.†.*
Aloes (p.1177·1); cascara sagrada (p.1183·1); phenolphthalein (p.1208·2); raphany root; gentian; galanga; myrrh; angelica; valerian; cinnamon; cardamom.
Constipation.

Laxo Vian *Alcala, Spain.*
Atropine sulphate (p.455·1); hyoscyamus (p.464·3); cascara (p.1183·1); phenolphthalein (p.1208·2); podophyllum (p.1089·1); sodium bicarbonate.
Constipation.

Laxoberal
Boehringer Ingelheim, Ger.; Windsor, Irl.; Ferring, Swed.; Windsor, UK.
Sodium picosulphate (p.1213·2).
Bowel evacuation; constipation.

Laxoberal Bisa *Boehringer Ingelheim, Ger.*
Bisacodyl (p.1179·3).
Constipation.

Laxoberon
Boehringer Ingelheim, Belg.; Boehringer Ingelheim, Neth.†; Boehringer Ingelheim, Switz.
Sodium picosulphate (p.1213·2).
Constipation.

Laxolind *Metochem, Aust.*
Senna (p.1212·2); frangula (p.1193·2); chamomile (p.1561·2).
Bowel regulation.

Laxomild *Renopharm, Switz.*
Calcium sennoside A (p.1212·3); calcium sennoside B (p.1212·3).
Constipation.

Laxomundin *Mundipharma, Ger.*
Lactulose (p.1195·3).
Constipation.

Laxonol *PQS, Spain†.*
Sodium picosulphate (p.1213·2).
Constipation.

Laxopol *Pohl, Ger.*
Castor oil (p.1560·2).
Constipation.

Laxose
Pinewood, Irl.; Berk, UK.
Lactulose (p.1195·3).
Constipation; hepatic encephalopathy.

Laxucil *Novopharm, Canad.*
Ispaghula husk (p.1194·2).

Laxulac *IRBI, Ital.†.*
Lactulose (p.1195·3).
Hepatic encephalopathy and coma.

Laxvital *Maxfarma, Spain.*
Carmellose (p.1471·2); docusate sodium (p.1189·3); casanthranol (p.1182·3).
Constipation.

Laxygocce *Ragionieri, Ital.†.*
Cascara (p.1183·1); cynara (p.1569·2).
Constipation.

Laxysat mono *Ysatfabrik, Ger.*
Buckthorn (p.1182·1).
Constipation.

Lazer *Pedinol, USA.*
Vitamin E (p.1369·1); vitamin A (p.1358·1).
Minor skin irritation.

Lazerformaldehyde *Pedinol, USA.*
Formaldehyde (p.1113·2).
Bromhidrosis (feet); hyperhidrosis; warts.

LazerSporin-C *Pedinol, USA.*
Neomycin sulphate (p.229·2); polymyxin B sulphate (p.239·1); hydrocortisone (p.1043·3).
Bacterial ear infections.

LBC-LAX *Murdock, USA.*
Cascara (p.1183·1).

LC-65
Allergan, Austral.; Allergan, USA.
Range of solutions for contact lenses.

L-Caine *Century, USA†.*
Lignocaine hydrochloride (p.1293·2).
Local anaesthesia.

L-Carn *Sigma-Tau, Ger.*
Carnitine (p.1336·2).
Carnitine deficiency.

L-Cimexyl *Cimex, Switz.*
Acetylcysteine (p.1052·3).
Respiratory-tract disorders.

L-Combur-5-Test *Boehringer Mannheim, Austral.*
Test for pH, protein, glucose, ketones, and blood in urine.

Le 100 B *Pharmalab, Canad.*
Cascara (p.1183·1); phenolphthalein (p.1208·2).

Le 500 D *Pharmalab, Canad.*
Cascara (p.1183·1).

Le Face Protection *Creative Brands, Austral.*
Ethylhexyl *p*-methoxycinnamate (p.1487·1); avobenzone (p.1486·3).
Sunscreen.

Le Stick a Levres *Duchesnay, Canad.*
Ethylhexyl *p*-methoxycinnamate (p.1487·1); allantoin (p.1078·2); vitamin A palmitate (p.1359·2).
Sunscreen.

Le Sucrine *Eurospital, Ital.†.*
Aspartame (p.1335·1).
Sugar substitute.

Le Tan Baby Sunblock *Australis, Austral.†.*
SPF15+: Ethylhexyl *p*-methoxycinnamate (p.1487·1); avobenzone (p.1486·3).
Sunscreen.

Le Tan Broad Spectrum *Creative Brands, Austral.*
SPF15+: Ethylhexyl *p*-methoxycinnamate (p.1487·1); avobenzone (p.1486·3).
Sunscreen.

Le Tan Burn Relief *Australis, Austral.†.*
Lignocaine hydrochloride (p.1293·2); panthenol (p.1571·1).
Skin irritation; sunburn.

Le Tan Fast *Creative Brands, Austral.*
Dihydroxyacetone (p.1081·2).
Artificial suntan.

Le Tan Fast Plus *Creative Brands, Austral.*
SPF15+: Ethylhexyl *p*-methoxycinnamate (p.1487·1); avobenzone (p.1486·3); dihydroxyacetone (p.1081·2).
Artificial suntan; sunscreen.

Le Tan Natural *Creative Brands, Austral.*
SPF 15+: Titanium dioxide (p.1093·3); zinc oxide (p.1096·2).
Sunscreen.

Le Tan Self Tan *Creative Brands, Austral.*
Dihydroxyacetone (p.1081·2).
Artificial suntan.

Le Tan Sport *Creative Brands, Austral.*
SPF 15+: Ethylhexyl *p*-methoxycinnamate (p.1487·1); oxybenzone (p.1487·3); avobenzone (p.1486·3).
Sunscreen.

Le Tan Sunblock Stick *Creative Brands, Austral.*
Ethylhexyl *p*-methoxycinnamate (p.1487·1); avobenzone (p.1486·3).
Sunscreen.

Le Tan Sunscreen Lotion *Creative Brands, Austral.*
SPF4; SPF8: Ethylhexyl *p*-methoxycinnamate (p.1487·1).
SPF15+: Ethylhexyl *p*-methoxycinnamate (p.1487·1); avobenzone (p.1486·3).
Sunscreen.

Le Tan Ultimate *Creative Brands, Austral.*
SPF8: Ethylhexyl *p*-methoxycinnamate (p.1487·1); benzophenone (p.1487·1).
SPF15+: Ethylhexyl *p*-methoxycinnamate (p.1487·1); avobenzone (p.1486·3); benzophenone (p.1487·1).
Sunscreen.

Le Trim-BM *Or-Dov, Austral.*
Benzocaine (p.1286·2); methylcellulose (p.1473·3); ferrous gluconate; vitamins.
Obesity.

Lealgin *Janssen-Cilag, Swed.*
Phenoperidine hydrochloride (p.79·1).
Adjunct in neuroleptanalgesia; pain in surgical procedures; respiratory depressant in intensive care.

Leaton fur Erwachsene *Pharmacia Upjohn, Aust.*
Multivitamins with caffeine (p.749·3).
Tonic.

Leaton fur Kinder *Pharmacia Upjohn, Aust.*
Multivitamins.
Tonic.

Leber- und Galletee *Salus, Aust.*
Absinthium (p.1541·1); calamus (p.1556·1); angelica; peppermint leaf (p.1208·1); bitter-orange leaf.
Liver and biliary disorders.

Leberam *Chephasaar, Ger.†.*
Arginine oxoglurate (p.1334·2).
Liver disorders.

Leberetic *Ern, Spain.*
Potassium sulphate (p.1161·2); sodium bicarbonate (p.1153·2); sodium sulphate (p.1213·3).
Liver disorders.

Leberinfusion *Leopold, Aust.*
Arginine (p.1334·1); malic acid (p.1598·3); sodium hydroxide (p.1631·1); potassium hydroxide (p.1621·1).
Liver disorders.

Lebersal *Ern, Spain.*
Magnesium sulphate (p.1157·3); sodium bicarbonate (p.1153·2); dibasic sodium phosphate (p.1159·3); sodium sulphate (p.1213·3).
Gastro-intestinal disorders; hepatic insufficiency.

Lebersana *Benvegna, Ital.†.*
Metochalcone (p.1603·2); glutathione (p.983·1); glucurolactone.
Liver and biliary-tract disorders.

Lebic *Isis Puren, Ger.*
Baclofen (p.1308·2).
Skeletal muscle spasm or spasticity.

Leblon *De Angeli, Ital.†.*
Pirenzepine hydrochloride (p.467·1).
Gastroduodenitis; peptic ulcer.

Lebopride *Spyfarma, Spain.*
Sulpiride (p.692·3).
Behaviour disorders; psychoses; vertigo.

Lebriton N *Zeppenfeldt, Ger.*
Homoeopathic preparation.

Lecibral *Nezel, Spain.*
Nicardipine hydrochloride (p.915·1).
Angina pectoris; cerebrovascular disorders; hypertension.

Lecicarbon
Note. This name is used for preparations of different composition.
Brady, Aust.
Potassium acid tartrate (p.1209·1); sodium bicarbonate (p.1153·2).
Constipation.

Athenstaedt, Ger.; Athenstaedt, Switz.
Sodium bicarbonate (p.1153·2); anhydrous monobasic sodium phosphate (p.1159·3).
Bowel evacuation; constipation.

Lecithin comp *Agepha, Aust.†.*
Lecithin (p.1595·2); caffeine (p.749·3).

Lecitone *Yves Ponroy, Fr.*
Nutritional supplement containing phospholipids and vitamins.
Tonic.

Lecitone Magnesium *Yves Ponroy, Fr.*
Nutritional supplement containing phospholipids and magnesium oxide.
Tonic.

Lecitone Vitalite *Yves Ponroy, Fr.*
Nutritional supplement containing phospholipids and vitamins.
Tonic.

Lecivital *Agepha, Aust.*
Oral solution: Lecithin (p.1595·2); caffeine (p.749·3).
Tablets: Lecithin (p.1595·2); vitamin E acetate (p.1369·1).
Tonic.

Lecrolyn *Leiras, Norw.; Santen, Swed.*
Sodium cromoglycate (p.762·1).
Allergic conjunctivitis.

Lectil *Bouchara, Fr.*
Betahistine hydrochloride (p.1553·1).
Vertigo.

Lectopam *Roche, Canad.*
Bromazepam (p.643·1).
Anxiety.

Ledclair
Sinclair, Irl.; Sinclair, UK.
Sodium calciumedetate (p.994·1).
Heavy metal poisoning.

Ledercillin VK
Wyeth-Ayerst, Canad.; Lederle, USA†.
Phenoxymethylpenicillin potassium (p.236·2).
Bacterial infections.

Ledercort
Note. This name is used for preparations of different composition.
Cyanamid, Belg.†.
Eye ointment: Triamcinolone acetonide (p.1050·2); neomycin sulphate (p.229·2).
Eye disorders.

Cyanamid, Belg.; Cyanamid, Ital.; Lederle, Neth.; Lederle, Norw.†; Wyeth, S.Afr.; Cyanamid, Spain; Wyeth Lederle, Swed.†; Lederle, Switz.; Lederle, UK.
Triamcinolone (p.1050·2), triamcinolone acetate (p.1050·2), or triamcinolone acetonide (p.1050·2).
Corticosteroid.

Lederderm *Lederle, Ger.*
Minocycline hydrochloride (p.226·2).
Bacterial infections.

Lederfen
Cyanamid, Aust.; Lederle, Ger.†; Wyeth, Irl.; Lederle, UK.
Fenbufen (p.37·1).
Musculoskeletal and joint disorders.

Lederfolat *Lederle, Ger.*
Calcium folinate (p.1342·2).
Folate deficiency.

Lederfolin
Cyanamid, Ital.; Cyanamid, Spain; Lederle, UK.
Calcium folinate (p.1342·2).
Drug-induced folic acid deficiency; megaloblastic anaemia; methotrexate overdose; potentiation of fluorouracil activity.

Lederfoline *Lederle, Fr.*
Calcium folinate (p.1342·2).
Adjunct to fluorouracil therapy for colorectal cancer; drug-induced megaloblastic anaemia; folic acid deficiency; prevention of methotrexate toxicity.

Lederlind *Lederle, Ger.*
Nystatin (p.386·1).
Fungal infections of the skin and mucous membranes.

Lederlon *Lederle, Ger.*
Triamcinolone hexacetonide (p.1050·2).
Parenteral corticosteroid.

Ledermicina *Cyanamid, Ital.*
Demeclocycline hydrochloride (p.201·2).
Bacterial infections.

Ledermix
Cyanamid, Aust.; Wyeth, Irl.; Wyeth, S.Afr.; Lederle, Switz.; Lederle, UK.
Paste, triamcinolone acetonide (p.1050·2); demeclocycline calcium (p.201·2); cement, triamcinolone acetonide; demeclocycline hydrochloride (p.201·2); solution, eugenol (p.1578·2).
Bacterial infection and inflammatory disorders in dentistry.

Ledermycin
Cyanamid, Aust.; Lederle, Austral.; Wyeth Lederle, Belg.; Wyeth, Irl.; Lederle, Neth.; Lederle, S.Afr.†; Lederle, UK.
Demeclocycline hydrochloride (p.201·2).
Bacterial infections; hyponatraemia; intestinal amoebiasis.

Lederpaediat *Lederle, Ger.*
Erythromycin ethyl succinate (p.204·2).
Bacterial infections.

Lederpax *Cyanamid, Spain.*
Erythromycin (p.204·1).
Acne.

Lederplatin *Wyeth Lederle, Swed.*
Cisplatin (p.513·3).
Malignant neoplasms.

Lederplex
Lederle, S.Afr.†.
Multivitamins; minerals; liver extracts.
Tonic.

Lederle, USA†.
Vitamin B substances.

Lederspan
Cyanamid, Aust.; Wyeth Lederle, Belg.; Wyeth, Irl.; Lederle, Neth.; Wyeth, Norw.; Wyeth, S.Afr.; Wyeth Lederle, Swed.; Lederle, UK.
Triamcinolone hexacetonide (p.1050·2).
Corticosteroid.

Ledertam
Cyanamid, Ital.; Wyeth Lederle, Swed.
Tamoxifen citrate (p.563·3).
Breast cancer.

Ledertepa
Wyeth Lederle, Belg.; Lederle, Neth.
Thiotepa (p.566·3).
Malignant neoplasms.

Ledertrexate
Lederle, Austral.; Wyeth Lederle, Belg.; Lederle, Fr.; Lederle, Neth.
Methotrexate (p.547·1) or methotrexate sodium (p.547·1).
Malignant neoplasms; mycosis fungoides; psoriasis; rheumatoid arthritis.

Ledervorin
Wyeth Lederle, Belg.; Lederle, Neth.
Calcium folinate (p.1342·2).
Adjunct to high-dose methotrexate therapy; folic acid deficiency; overdosage with folic acid antagonists.

Ledoren *Boniscontro & Gazzone, Ital.*
Nimesulide (p.63·2).
Fever; inflammation; pain.

Ledovit A *Bama, Spain†.*
Vitamin A (p.1358·1).
Vitamin A deficiency.

Ledovit C *Bama, Spain.*
Ascorbic acid (p.1365·2).
Adjunct in treatment of iron supplementation; vitamin C deficiency.

Ledovit C B12 *Bama, Spain†.*
Ascorbic acid (p.1365·2); cyanocobalamin (p.1363·3).
Deficiency of vitamins B_{12} and C.

Ledox *Weifa, Norw.*
Naproxen (p.61·2).
Gout; musculoskeletal and joint disorders; pain.

Ledoxid Acne *Lederle, Switz.*
Benzoyl peroxide (p.1079·2).
Acne.

Ledum Med Complex *Dynamit, Aust.*
Homoeopathic preparation.

Lefax
Asche, Ger.; Pharmacia Upjohn, Switz.
Simethicone (p.1213·1).
Anti-foaming agent in radiography of the gastro-intestinal tract; detergent intoxication; gastro-intestinal disorders associated with excess gas.

Lefaxin *Lannacher, Aust.*
Simethicone (p.1213·1).
Flatulence.

Lefcar *Glaxo Wellcome, Ital.*
Carnitine (p.1336·2) or carnitine hydrochloride (p.1336·2).
Carnitine deficiency; myocardial ischaemia.

Leferdivin *Hotz, Ger.*
Vitamin B substances; lecithin; ferrous citrate; glutamic acid.
Tonic.

Legalon
Note. This name is used for preparations of different composition.
Madaus, Aust.; Madaus, Fr.; Madaus, Ger.
Silybum marianum (p.993·3).
Liver disorders.

Ibi, Ital.; Byk Madaus, S.Afr.; Madaus, Spain; Madaus, Switz.
Silymarin (p.993·3).
Liver disorders.

Legalon SIL
Madaus, Belg.; Madaus, Ger.; Madaus, Switz.
Disodium silibinin dihemisuccinate (p.993·3).
Mushroom poisoning.

Legapas *Ebi, Switz.*
Cascara (p.1183·1).
Constipation.

Legapas comp *Pascoe, Ger.*
Cascara (p.1183·1); silybum marianum (p.993·3); chelidonium majus; taraxacum (p.1634·2).
Formerly known as Legapas N.
Liver disorders.

Legapas mono *Pascoe, Ger.*
Cascara (p.1183·1).
Constipation.

Legatrin *Columbia, USA†.*
Quinine sulphate (p.439·2).
Nocturnal leg cramps.

Legatrin PM *Columbia, USA.*
Paracetamol (p.72·2); diphenhydramine hydrochloride (p.409·1).
Insomnia.

Legatrin Rub *Columbia, USA.*
Menthol (p.1600·2); benzocaine (p.1286·2).

Legederm
Schering-Plough, Ital.; Schering-Plough, Swed.
Alclometasone dipropionate (p.1031·3).
Skin disorders.

Legendal
Zambon, Neth.; Inpharzam, Switz.
Lactulose (p.1195·3).
Constipation; hepatic encephalopathy.

Legofer *Asta Medica, Ital.*
Iron succinyl-protein complex (p.1349·2).
Anaemia; iron deficiency.

Legofer Folinico *Farmades, Ital.†.*
Iron succinyl-protein complex (p.1349·2); calcium folinate (p.1342·2).
Iron and folate deficiency.

Lehydan *Abigo, Swed.*
Phenytoin (p.352·3).
Epilepsy.

Leicester Retard *Polifarma, Ital.*
Isosorbide mononitrate (p.893·3).
Angina pectoris.

Leiguar
Roche, Ital.†; Labatec, Switz.
Guar (p.321·3).
Diabetes mellitus; hyperlipidaemias; obesity.

Leioderm *LAW, Ger.*
Hydroxyquinoline sulphate (p.1589·3).
Impetigo.

Leioderm P *LAW, Ger.*
Hydroxyquinoline sulphate (p.1589·3); prednisolone (p.1048·1).
Infected skin disorders.

Leios *Wyeth, Ger.*
Levonorgestrel (p.1454·1); ethinyloestradiol (p.1445·1).
Combined oral contraceptive.

Lejguar *Meta Fackler, Ger.*
Guar gum (p.321·3).
Diabetes mellitus; hyperlipidaemias.

Lektinol *Madaus, Ger.*
Mistletoe (p.1604·1).
Malignant neoplasms.

Lelong Contusions
Note. This name is used for preparations of different composition.
SmithKline Beecham Sante, Fr.
Ointment: Arnica (p.1550·3); tamus communis.
Soft-tissue disorders.

Sterling Midy, Fr.†.
Mousse for topical use: Pentosan polysulphate sodium (p.928·1).
Bruising; circulatory disorders.

Lelong Irritations *SmithKline Beecham Sante, Fr.*
Enoxolone (p.35·2); propanocaine hydrochloride (p.1299·3).
Inflammatory and pruritic skin disorders.

Lema C *Ern, Spain.*
Ascorbic acid (p.1365·2); borax (p.1554·2).
Halitosis; mouth and throat inflammation; pyorrhoea.

Lemazol
Petrasch, Aust.; Stark, Ger.†.
Ascorbic acid (p.1365·2); potassium orotate (p.1611·2); inositol (p.1591·1); sorbitol (p.1354·2).
Liver disorders.

Lemgrip *Reckitt & Colman, Belg.*
Paracetamol (p.72·2).
Fever; pain.

Lemivit *Kemiprogress, Ital.*
Vitamins; lecithin (p.1595·2).
Fatigue.

Lemocin
Note. This name is used for preparations of different composition.
Sanabo, Aust.; Sandoz, Ger.; Sandoz OTC, Switz.
Tyrothricin (p.267·2); cetrimonium bromide (p.1106·1); lignocaine (p.1293·2) or lignocaine hydrochloride (p.1293·2).
Mouth and throat disorders.

Wander, Belg.
Tyrothricin (p.267·2); cetrimide (p.1105·2); lignocaine (p.1293·2).
Mouth and throat disorders.

Lemocin CX *Sandoz, Ger.*
Chlorhexidine gluconate (p.1107·2).
Mouth infections.

Lemon Time *Buckley, Canad.*
Paracetamol (p.72·2); phenylephrine hydrochloride (p.1066·2); mepyramine maleate (p.414·1); ascorbic acid (p.1365·2).
Cold symptoms.

Lemonvit *Molteni, Ital.*
Ascorbic acid (p.1365·2).
Vitamin C deficiency.

Lem-Plus
Note. This name is used for preparations of different composition.
Brovar, S.Afr.†.
Paracetamol (p.72·2); ascorbic acid (p.1365·2).
Cold symptoms.

Adcock Ingram, UK.
Capsules: Paracetamol (p.72·2); caffeine (p.749·3); phenylephrine (p.1066·2).
Oral powder: Paracetamol (p.72·2); ascorbic acid (p.1365·2).
Cold symptoms.

Lemsip
Note. This name is used for preparations of different composition.
Reckitt & Colman, Austral.; Meda, Swed.
Paracetamol (p.72·2).
Cold and influenza symptoms.

Reckitts, Irl.
Paracetamol (p.72·2); sodium citrate (p.1153·2); ascorbic acid (p.1365·2).
Cold and influenza symptoms.

Reckitt & Colman, S.Afr.
Paracetamol (p.72·2); phenylephrine hydrochloride (p.1066·2); sodium citrate (p.1153·2).
Cold and influenza symptoms.

Reckitt & Colman, UK.
Paracetamol (p.72·2); ascorbic acid (p.1365·2) phenylephrine hydrochloride (p.1066·2).
Cold symptoms.

Lemsip Chesty Cough *Reckitt & Colman, UK.*
Guaiphenesin (p.1061·3); glycerol (p.1585·2); terpeneless lemon oil (p.1596·1).
Coughs.

Lemsip Cold Relief *Reckitt & Colman, UK†.*
Paracetamol (p.72·2); phenylephrine (p.1066·2); sodium citrate (p.1153·2); ascorbic acid (p.1365·2).
Cold symptoms.

Lemsip Dry Tickly Cough *Reckitt & Colman, UK.*
Honey (p.1345·3); terpeneless lemon oil (p.1596·1); glycerol (p.1585·2).
Coughs.

Lemsip Expectorant *Reckitt & Colman, UK†.*
Diphenhydramine hydrochloride (p.409·1); ammonium chloride (p.1055·2); sodium citrate (p.1153·2).
Catarrh; coughs.

Lemsip Flu *Reckitt & Colman, Austral.*
Paracetamol (p.72·2); pseudoephedrine hydrochloride (p.1068·3); dextromethorphan hydrobromide (p.1057·3); chlorpheniramine maleate (p.405·1).
Cold and influenza symptoms; coughs.

Lemsip Flu Strength *Reckitt & Colman, UK.*
Paracetamol (p.72·2); phenylephrine (p.1066·2); ascorbic acid (p.1365·2).
Cold and influenza symptoms.

Lemsip Junior Blackcurrant *Reckitt & Colman, UK†.*
Paracetamol (p.72·2); phenylephrine (p.1066·2); sodium citrate (p.1153·2); ascorbic acid (p.1365·2).
Cold symptoms.

Lemsip Linctus *Reckitt & Colman, UK†.*
Ipecacuanha (p.1062·2); honey (p.1345·3); terpeneless lemon oil (p.1596·1); glycerol (p.1585·2); citric acid monohydrate (p.1564·3).
Coughs; sore throat.

Lemsip Lozenges *Reckitt & Colman, Austral.*
Cetylpyridinium chloride (p.1106·2).
Sore throat.

Lemsip Menthol Extra Reckitt & Colman, UK.
Paracetamol (p.72·2); phenylephrine hydrochloride (p.1066·2); ascorbic acid (p.1365·2).
Cold and influenza symptoms.

Lemsip Night Time Reckitt & Colman, UK.
Dextromethorphan hydrobromide (p.1057·3); chlorpheniramine maleate (p.405·1); phenylpropanolamine hydrochloride (p.1067·2); paracetamol (p.72·2).
Influenza symptoms.

Lemsip with Phenylephrine Reckitts, Irl.
Paracetamol (p.72·2); phenylephrine hydrochloride (p.1066·2); ascorbic acid (p.1365·2).
Cold and influenza symptoms.

Lemsip Power + Reckitt & Colman, UK.
Ibuprofen (p.44·1); pseudoephedrine hydrochloride (p.1068·3).
Cold and flu symptoms.

Lemuval Bayer, Aust.
A heparinoid (p.882·3); hyaluronidase (p.1588·1); vitamin A palmitate (p.1359·2); calcium pantothenate (p.1352·3); menthol (p.1600·2).
Anorectal disorders.

Len V.K. Lennon, S.Afr.
Phenoxymethylpenicillin potassium (p.236·2).
Bacterial infections.

Lenadol Lennon, S.Afr.†.
Paracetamol (p.72·2); codeine phosphate (p.26·1); diphenhydramine hydrochloride (p.409·1); caffeine (p.749·3).
Fever; pain and associated tension.

Lenamet SA Druggists, S.Afr.
Cimetidine (p.1183·2).
Gastric hypersecretion; peptic ulcer.

Lenasone Intramed, S.Afr.
Betamethasone sodium phosphate (p.1033·3).
Corticosteroid.

Lenazine Lennon, S.Afr.
Promethazine hydrochloride (p.416·2).
Hypersensitivity reactions.

Lenazine Forte Lennon, S.Afr.
Promethazine hydrochloride (p.416·2); codeine phosphate (p.26·1); ephedrine hydrochloride (p.1059·3).
Coughs.

Len-B Co SA Druggists Self Med, S.Afr.†.
Vitamin B substances.

Lencid Christiaens, Belg.†.
Lindane (p.1407·2).
Pediculosis.

Lendorm Bender, Aust.
Brotizolam (p.643·2).
Sleep disorders.

Lendormin
Boehringer Ingelheim, Belg.; Boehringer Ingelheim, Ger.; Boehringer Ingelheim, Ital.; Boehringer Ingelheim, Jpn; Boehringer Ingelheim, Neth.; Boehringer Ingelheim, S.Afr.
Brotizolam (p.643·2).
Insomnia; premedication.

Lendormine Boehringer Ingelheim, Switz.
Brotizolam (p.643·2).
Sleep disorders.

Lenen
Note. This name is used for preparations of different composition.
Schering, Ger.; Scherax, Ger.
Fluocortin butyl (p.1041·3).
Rhinitis.

Schering, Ital.†.
Clocortolone pivalate (p.1035·3).
Skin disorders.

Leniartril San Carlo, Ital.
Naproxen (p.61·2).
Musculoskeletal and joint disorders; pain.

Lenicalm
Dolisos, Fr.; Dolisos, Ital.
Asperula odorata; crataegus (p.1568·2); tilia (p.1637·3).
Insomnia; nervous disorders.

Lenicet Athenstaedt, Ger.
Aluminium diacetate hydroxide; aluminium hydroxide (p.1177·3).
Skin disorders.

Lenident Zeta, Ital.
Procaine hydrochloride (p.1299·2).
Dental pain.

Leniderm
Note. This name is used for preparations of different composition.
Salus, Ital.†.
Fluocinolone acetonide (p.1041·1).
Skin disorders.

Inpharzam, Switz.†.
Vitamin A palmitate (p.1359·2); alpha tocopheryl acetate (p.1369·2); dexpanthenol (p.1570·3); allantoin (p.1078·2); titanium dioxide (p.1093·3).
Skin disorders.

Lenidermyl Oberlin, Fr.
Palmitoyl collagen acid (p.1566·3).
Skin disorders.

Lenidolor Menarini, Ital.
Meclofenamic acid (p.51·2) or meclofenamate sodium (p.51·1).
Musculoskeletal and joint disorders; pain.

Lenil Zeta, Ital.
Chlorhexidine hydrochloride (p.1107·2).
Disinfection of wounds and burns.

Leniline Erredici, Ital.
Vitamin E; vitamin C; ginkgo biloba; melilotus; bioflavonoids.
Nutritional supplement.

Lenipasta Novogaleno, Ital.
Zinc oxide (p.1096·2); rice starch (p.1356·2); enoxolone (p.35·2).
Skin irritation; wounds.

Lenirit Bonomelli, Ital.
Hydrocortisone acetate (p.1043·3).
Skin disorders.

Lenirose Novogaleno, Ital.
Sulphur (p.1091·2); titanium dioxide (p.1093·3); panthenol (p.1570·3); rusco; calendula; oryzanol (p.1611·2); enoxolone (p.35·2).
Rosacea; seborrhoeic dermatitis; skin irritation.

Lenisolone Lennon, S.Afr.
Prednisolone (p.1048·1).
Corticosteroid.

Lenisun Zeta, Ital.†.
Benzocaine (p.1286·2); triclosan (p.1127·2).
Local anaesthesia and disinfection.

Lenitral Besins-Iscovesco, Fr.
Glyceryl trinitrate (p.874·3).
Angina pectoris; heart failure; hypotension.

Lenium
SmithKline Beecham, Irl.; Johnson & Johnson MSD Consumer, UK.
Selenium sulphide (p.1091·1).
Dandruff; scalp seborrhoea.

Lenixil Eurospital, Ital.
Chlorhexidine gluconate (p.1107·2).
Disinfection of minor wounds and burns.

Lennacol Lennon, S.Afr.†.
Chloramphenicol (p.182·1).
Bacterial infections.

Lennamine Lennon, S.Afr.†.
Diphenhydramine hydrochloride (p.409·1); ammonium chloride (p.1055·2); sodium citrate (p.1153·2); menthol (p.1600·2).
Coughs; nasal congestion.

Lenocef SA Druggists, S.Afr.
Cephalexin (p.178·2).
Bacterial infections.

Lenolax Lennon, S.Afr.
Dibasic sodium phosphate (p.1159·3); monobasic sodium phosphate (p.1159·3).
Bowel evacuation; constipation.

Lenoltec with Codeine No 1, No 2, or No 3
Technilab, Canad.
Paracetamol (p.72·2); caffeine (p.749·3); codeine phosphate (p.26·1).
Cold symptoms; pain.

Lenoltec with Codeine No 4 Technilab, Canad.
Paracetamol (p.72·2); codeine phosphate (p.26·1).
Pain.

Lenoprel Intramed, S.Afr.†.
Isoprenaline hydrochloride (p.892·1).
Bronchospasm; shock.

Lenovate Lennon, S.Afr.
Betamethasone valerate (p.1033·3).
Corticosteroid.

Lenoxin Glaxo Wellcome, Ger.
Digoxin (p.849·3).
Heart failure; tachycardia.

Lens Fresh
Allergan, Aust.; Allergan, Ger.; Allergan, USA.
Range of solutions for contact lenses.

Lens Lubricant Bausch & Lomb, USA.
Wetting solution for hard contact lenses.

Lens Plus Allergan, USA.
Range of solutions for soft contact lenses.

Lens Plus Buffered Saline Solution Allergan, Canad.
Buffered sodium chloride (p.1162·2).
Rinsing solution for contact lenses.

Lens Plus Rewetting Drops Allergan, Canad.
Wetting solution for soft contact lenses.

Lens Tears Agepha, Aust.
Wetting solution for contact lenses.

Lens Wet Agepha, Aust.
Wetting solution for contact lenses.

Lensan A Ciba Vision, Aust.
Hydrogen peroxide (p.1116·2).
Disinfecting solution for contact lenses.

Lensan B Ciba Vision, Aust.
Catalase (p.1560·3).
Neutralising solution for contact lenses.

Lensch Ravensberg, Ger.†.
Bisdequalinium diacetate (p.1104·2); naphazoline acetate (p.1064·3).
Rhinitis.

Lensept
Ciba Vision, Aust.; Alcon, Austral.†; Ciba Vision, USA.
Hydrogen peroxide (p.1116·2).
Disinfecting solution for soft contact lenses.

Lensrins NT
Ciba Vision, Aust.; Alcon, Austral.†.
Rinsing and storage solution for soft contact lenses.

Lenstrip 2 Lennon, S.Afr.
Test for glucose and ketones in urine.

Lenstrip 3 Lennon, S.Afr.
Test for glucose, protein, and blood in urine.

Lenstrip 5 Lennon, S.Afr.
Test for glucose, ketones, protein, pH, and blood in urine.

Lenstrip 8 Lennon, S.Afr.
Test for glucose, ketones, protein, pH, blood, nitrite, bilirubin, and urobilinogen in urine.

Lenstrip B.G.2 Lennon, S.Afr.
Test for glucose in blood (p.1585·1).

Lenstrip Glucose Lennon, S.Afr.
Test for glucose in urine (p.1585·1).

Lenstrip Glyco Lennon, S.Afr.
Test for glucose in blood (p.1585·1).

Lenta MC Novo Nordisk, Ital.†.
Insulin zinc suspension (amorphous 30%, crystalline 70%) (bovine with porcine, monocomponent) (p.322·1).
Diabetes mellitus.

Lentard MC Novo Nordisk, UK.
Insulin zinc suspension (amorphous porcine 30%, crystalline bovine 70%, monocomponent) (p.322·1).
Diabetes mellitus.

Lentare Novartis, S.Afr.
Formestane (p.537·3).
Breast cancer.

Lentaron
Ciba-Geigy, Aust.; Ciba-Geigy, Belg.; Ciba, Canad.; Ciba-Geigy, Fr.; Ciba Cancer Care, Ger.; Ciba-Geigy, Irl.; Ciba, Ital.; Novartis, Neth.; Ciba-Geigy, Spain; Ciba, Switz.; Ciba, UK.
Formestane (p.537·3).
Breast cancer.

Lente
Novo Nordisk, Canad.†; Novo Nordisk, Ger.†; Novo Nordisk, USA.
Insulin zinc suspension (porcine, amorphous, 30%) (bovine, crystalline, 70%) (p.322·1).
Diabetes mellitus.

Lente Iletin I Lilly, USA.
Insulin zinc suspension (bovine and porcine) (p.322·1).
Diabetes mellitus.

Lente Iletin II Lilly, USA.
Insulin zinc suspension (porcine) (p.322·1).
Diabetes mellitus.

Lente L Novo Nordisk, USA.
Insulin zinc suspension (porcine) (p.322·1).
Diabetes mellitus.

Lente MC
Novo Nordisk, Aust.; Novo Nordisk, Austral.; Novo Nordisk, Belg.; Novo Nordisk, Fr.; Novo Nordisk, Spain; Novo Nordisk, Switz.
Insulin zinc suspension (porcine, amorphous, 30%) (bovine, crystalline, 70%) (p.322·1).
Diabetes mellitus.

Lenticor Kwizda, Aust.†.
Pentaerythritol tetranitrate (p.927·3); drotaverine hydrochloride (p.1574·2); ergotamine tartrate (p.445·3); meprobamate (p.678·1).
Coronary vascular disorders.

Lentinorm Neu Kanoldt, Ger.†.
Calcium lactate (p.1155·2); vitamins.
Eye disorders.

Lentizol
Parke, Davis, Irl.; Parke, Davis, UK.
Amitriptyline hydrochloride (p.273·3).
Depression.

Lentogesic Mer-National, S.Afr.
Capsules: Dextropropoxyphene hydrochloride (p.27·3); paracetamol (p.72·2); pemoline (p.1484·1); levoglutamide (p.1344·3).
Syrup: Paracetamol (p.72·2); codeine phosphate (p.26·1); promethazine hydrochloride (p.416·2).
Fever; pain.

Lentogest Amsa, Ital.
Hydroxyprogesterone hexanoate (p.1448·1).
Infertility; menstrual and menopausal disorders; threatened or habitual abortion.

Lento-Kalium Boehringer Mannheim, Ital.
Potassium chloride (p.1161·1).
Hypokalaemia.

Lentolith Mer-National, S.Afr.
Lithium carbonate (p.290·3).
Bipolar disorder; depression.

Lentoquine Berenguer Infale, Spain.
Hydroquinidine hydrochloride (p.889·3).
Arrhythmias.

Lentorsil Italfarmaco, Ital.
Ursodeoxycholic acid (p.1642·1).
Biliary disorders; cholesterol gallstones.

Lentostamin SIT, Ital.†.
Chlorpheniramine maleate (p.405·1).
Hypersensitivity reactions.

Lenurex-K Lennon, S.Afr.†.
Cyclopenthiazide (p.845·2); potassium chloride (p.1161·1).
Hypertension; oedema.

Lenzacef Lenza, Ital.†.
Cephradine (p.181·3).
Bacterial infections.

Leo K
Leo, Irl.†; Leo, UK†.
Potassium chloride (p.1161·1).
Hypokalaemia; potassium depletion.

Leodin Byk Elmu, Spain†.
Caffeine (p.749·3); propyphenazone (p.81·3).
Fever; pain.

Leokol Kabi, Swed.†.
Activated charcoal (p.972·2).
Diarrhoea; poisoning.

Leonal Byk Leo, Spain.
Ibuprofen (p.44·1).
Fever; musculoskeletal, joint, and peri-articular disorders; pain.

Leo-Pillen Cassella-med, Ger.†.
Aloes (p.1177·1).
Constipation.

Leopin Quest, Canad.
Vitamin B substances.
Dietary supplement.

Leotone Leo, Irl.†.
Vitamin B substances with caffeine(p.749·3).
Tonic.

Leotuss Leo, Irl.†.
Diphenhydramine hydrochloride (p.409·1); diprophylline (p.752·1); sodium citrate (p.1153·2); menthol (p.1600·2).
Coughs and congestion.

Leparan Italfarmaco, Ital.
Heparan sulphate.
Thrombosis prophylaxis.

Lepheton Pharmacia Upjohn, Swed.
Ethylmorphine hydrochloride (p.36·1); ephedrine hydrochloride (p.1059·3).
Bronchitis; coughs.

Lepinal Dresden, Ger.
Phenobarbitone (p.350·2).
Epilepsy.

Lepinaletten Dresden, Ger.
Phenobarbitone (p.350·2).
Epilepsy.

Leponex
Sandoz, Aust.; Sandoz, Belg.; Sandoz, Fr.; Wander, Ger.; Sandoz, Ital.; Novartis, Neth.; Sandoz, Norw.; Novartis, S.Afr.; Sandoz, Spain; Novartis, Swed.; Sandoz, Switz.
Clozapine (p.657·3).
Schizophrenia.

Leptanal
Janssen-Cilag, Norw.; Janssen-Cilag, Swed.
Fentanyl citrate (p.38·1).
Adjunct in neuroleptanalgesia; pain.

Leptanal comp Janssen, Swed.†.
Fentanyl citrate (p.38·1); droperidol (p.668·2).
Adjunct in neuroleptanalgesia; premedication.

Lepticur Diamant, Fr.
Tropatepine hydrochloride (p.469·2).
Extrapyramidal disorders; parkinsonism.

Leptilan Geigy, Ger.
Sodium valproate (p.361·2).
Epilepsy.

Leptilanil Ciba-Geigy, Aust.
Sodium valproate (p.361·2).
Epilepsy; febrile convulsions.

Leptilen Ciba-Geigy, Swed.†.
Sodium valproate (p.361·2).
Epilepsy.

Leptofen Pharmacia Upjohn, Ital.
Fentanyl (p.38·1); droperidol (p.668·2).
Neuroleptanalgesia; premedication.

Lerdip Byk, Neth.
Lercanidipine hydrochloride (p.897·3).
Hypertension.

Lergigan Recip, Swed.
Promethazine hydrochloride (p.416·2).
Alcoholism; anxiety; croup; hypersensitivity reactions; nausea; premedication; sedative; sleep disorders; tension; vertigo.

Lergigan comp Recip, Swed.
Promethazine hydrochloride (p.416·2); caffeine (p.749·3); ephedrine sulphate (p.1059·3).
Alcoholism; anxiety; croup; hypersensitivity reactions; nausea; premedication; sedative; sleep disorders; tension; vertigo.

Lergoban Riker, UK†.
Diphenylpyraline hydrochloride (p.409·3).
Hypersensitivity reactions.

Lergocil Juste, Spain.
Azatadine maleate (p.402·3).
Hypersensitivity reactions.

Lerisum Poli, Ital.†.
Medazepam (p.677·3).
Psychoses.

Leritine Frosst, Canad.
Anileridine hydrochloride (p.15·3) or anileridine phosphate (p.15·3).
Adjunct in general anaesthesia; anxiety; pain.

Lerivon
Organon, Austral.; Organon, Belg.
Mianserin hydrochloride (p.297·1).
Depression.

Lervipan Lersa, Spain.
Pivampicillin (p.238·2).
Bacterial infections.

Les Yeux 1 Bilosa, Aust.
Hydrogen peroxide (p.1116·2).
Disinfecting solution for gas-permeable contact lenses.

Les Yeux 2 Bilosa, Aust.
Catalase (p.1560·3).
Neutralising solution for gas-permeable contact lenses.

Lescol
Sandoz, Aust.; Novartis, Austral.; Sandoz, Belg.; Sandoz, Canad.; Sandoz, Fr.; Sandoz, Irl.; Sandoz, Ital.; Novartis, Neth.; Sandoz,

Norw.; Novartis, S.Afr.; Sandoz, Spain; Novartis, Swed.; Sandoz, Switz.; Sandoz, UK; Sandoz, USA.
Fluvastatin sodium (p.1273·2).
Atherosclerosis; hypercholesterolaemia.

Lespenefril *Nattermann, Spain.*
Lespecapitosides.
Uraemia.

Lespenephryl
UCB, Aust.†; Darcy, Fr.; UCB, Ger.†.
Lespedeza capitata.
Diuresis.

Lesporene *Creapharm, Fr.†.*
Tamoxifen citrate (p.563·3).
Breast cancer.

Lessmusec *Brunel, S.Afr.*
Carbocisteine (p.1056·3).
Respiratory-tract disorders.

Lesspain *Be-Tabs, S.Afr.*
Paracetamol (p.72·2); codeine phosphate (p.26·1); promethazine hydrochloride (p.416·2).
Fever; pain.

Lesten *Serono, Ital.†.*
Suprarenal cortex (p.1050·1); vitamin B substances and nicotinamide; lignocaine hydrochloride (p.1293·2).
Asthenia.

Lestid
Pharmacia Upjohn, Norw.; Pharmacia Upjohn, Swed.
Colestipol hydrochloride (p.1272·1).
Hyperlipidaemias.

Lethidrone *Wellcome, Austral.†.*
Nalorphine hydrobromide (p.986·2).
Opioid analgesic overdosage.

Lethyl *Lennon, S.Afr.*
Phenobarbitone (p.350·2).
Anxiety; insomnia; migraine.

Letoclar *Zyma, Ital.†.*
Letosteine (p.1063·2).
Bronchial hypersecretion.

Letofort *Salus, Ital.*
Letosteine (p.1063·2).
Respiratory-tract disorders associated with increased or viscous mucus.

Leuco-4 *Pharmascience, Fr.†.*
Injection: Ampoule 1, adenine hydrochloride (p.1543·2); ampoule 2. dibasic sodium phosphate (p.1159·3); anhydrous monobasic sodium phosphate (p.1159·3).
Tablets: Adenine (p.1543·2).
Leucopenia.

Leuco Dibios *Inibsa, Spain†.*
Dequalinium chloride (p.1112·1).
Vulvovaginal candidiasis; vulvovaginal trichomoniasis.

Leuco Hubber *ICN, Spain.*
Hydrocortisone acetate (p.1043·3); neomycin sulphate (p.229·2).
Vulvovaginal inflammatory disorders.

Leucobasal
Germania, Aust.; Biobasal, Switz.
Mequinol (p.1086·2).
Hyperpigmentation.

Leucodinine *Wolfs, Belg.†.*
Monobenzone (p.1088·3).
Hyperpigmentation.

Leucodinine B *Promedica, Fr.*
Mequinol (p.1086·2).
Hyperpigmentation.

Leucomax
Aesca, Aust.; Sandoz, Aust.; Sandoz, Belg.; Sandoz, Fr.; Sandoz, Ger.; Essex, Ger.; Sandoz, Irl.; Sandoz, Ital.; Novartis, Neth.; Schering-Plough, Norw.; Novartis, S.Afr.; Sandoz, Spain; Schering-Plough, Swed.; Novartis, Swed.; Essex, Switz.; Sandoz, Switz.; Sandoz, UK.
Molgramostim (p.725·1).
Neutropenia induced by antineoplastic agents, bone marrow transplantation, or ganciclovir.

Leucorsan *Zilliken, Ital.*
Vaginal capsules: Benzydamine hydrochloride (p.21·3); hydroxyquinoline sulphate (p.1589·3); hydroxyquinoline benzoate (p.1589·3).
Vaginal douche: Benzydamine hydrochloride (p.21·3); hydroxyquinoline sulphate (p.1589·3); hydroxyquinoline benzoate (p.1589·3); cetrimonium tosylate (p.1106·1).
Vaginal and cervical inflammation.

Leucotrofina
Note. This name is used for preparations of different composition.
Pharmacia Upjohn, Aust.
Bovine thymus extract.
Leucopenia.

Pierre Fabre, Ital.†.
Thymomodulin.
Hypersensitivity reactions; infections; leucopenia.

Leukase
Note. This name is used for preparations of different composition.
SmithKline Beecham, Aust.; SmithKline Beecham, Ger.†.
Ointment; topical powder; topical spray; instillation; topical application: Framycetin sulphate (p.210·3); trypsin (p.1640·1).
Burns; infected skin disorders; infected wounds.

SmithKline Beecham, Ger.†.
Topical dosage form: Framycetin sulphate (p.210·3); trypsin (p.1640·1); lignocaine hydrochloride (p.1293·2).
Infected skin disorders; infected wounds.

Leukase N *SmithKline Beecham, Ger.*
Topical gel: Framycetin sulphate (p.210·3); lignocaine hydrochloride (p.1293·2).
Topical powder; ointment: Framycetin sulphate (p.210·3).
Infected skin disorders; infected wounds.

Leukase-Kegel *SmithKline Beecham, Aust.*
Framycetin sulphate (p.210·3); trypsin (p.1640·1); lignocaine hydrochloride (p.1293·2).
Infective skin and mouth disorders.

Leukeran
Glaxo Wellcome, Aust.; Glaxo Wellcome, Austral.; Glaxo Wellcome, Belg.; Glaxo Wellcome, Canad.; Glaxo Wellcome, Ger.; Wellcome, Irl.; Glaxo Wellcome, Ital.; Glaxo Wellcome, Neth.; Glaxo Wellcome, Norw.; Glaxo Wellcome, S.Afr.; Glaxo Wellcome, Spain; Glaxo Wellcome, Swed.; Wellcome, Switz.; Wellcome, UK; Glaxo Wellcome, USA.
Chlorambucil (p.512·3).
Malignant neoplasms.

Leukichtan *Ichthyol, Aust.*
Ictasol (p.1083·3); cod-liver oil (p.1337·3).
Burns; skin disorders; wounds.

Leukichtan N *Ichthyol, Ger.*
Ictasol (p.1083·3).
Ulcers; wounds.

Leukine *Immunex, USA.*
Sargramostim (p.727·3).
Myeloid reconstitution after autologous bone marrow transplant.

leukominerase *GN, Ger.*
Lithium carbonate (p.290·3).
Bipolar disorder; depression; mania.

Leukona-Eukalpin-Bad *Atzinger, Ger.*
Norway spruce oil; eucalyptus oil (p.1578·1).
Bath additive; respiratory tract disorders.

Leukona-Jod-Bad
Richter, Aust.; Atzinger, Ger.
Iodine (p.1493·1).
Arteriosclerosis; bath additive; iodine-deficiency goitre; neuralgia; spinal disorders.

Leukona-Kreislauf-Bad *Atzinger, Ger.*
Rosemary oil (p.1626·2); camphor (p.1557·2); eucalyptus oil (p.1578·1).
Bath additive; circulatory disorders.

Leukona-Mintol *Atzinger, Ger.*
Peppermint oil (p.1208·1).
Gastro-intestinal disorders; respiratory-tract disorders.

Leukona-Rheuma-Bad *Richter, Aust.*
Pumilio pine oil (p.1623·3); camphor (p.1557·2); thyme oil (p.1637·1); turpentine oil (p.1641·1); methyl salicylate (p.55·2).
Musculoskeletal and joint disorders; prostatitis; skin disorders.

Leukona-Rheuma-Bad N *Atzinger, Ger.*
Methyl salicylate (p.55·2); turpentine oil (p.1641·1); Norway spruce oil.
Bath additive; rheumatic disorders.

Leukona-Rheumasalbe *Atzinger, Ger.*
Camphor (p.1557·2); turpentine oil (p.1641·1); rosemary oil (p.1626·2).
Cold symptoms; frostbite; rheumatism; soft-tissue injury.

Leukona-Sauna-Konzentrat *Atzinger, Ger.†.*
Thyme oil (p.1637·1); menthol (p.1600·2); camphor (p.1557·2); spruce oil; eucalyptus oil (p.1578·1).
Arthritis and rheumatism; circulatory disorders; respiratory-tract disorders.

Leukona-Sedativ-Bad *Atzinger, Ger.*
Chloral hydrate (p.645·3); lupulus (p.1597·2); valerian (p.1643·1).
Bath additive; nervous disorders; sleep disorders; spasmophilia.

Leukona-Sedativ-Bad sine Chloralhydrat *Atzinger, Ger.*
Valerian (p.1643·1); lupulus (p.1597·2).
Bath additive; nervous disorders; sleep disorders.

Leukona-Stoffwechsel-Bad *Atzinger, Ger.*
Juniper oil (p.1592·3).
Allergic skin disorders; bath additive; metabolic disorders.

Leukona-Sulfomoor-Bad *Richter, Aust.*
Sulphurated potash (p.1091·3); colloidal sulphur (p.1091·2); sodium humate; peat.
Musculoskeletal and joint disorders; skin disorders.

Leukona-Sulfomoor-Bad N *Atzinger, Ger.*
Sulphurated potash (p.1091·3); peat; sodium humate.
Bath additive; musculoskeletal and joint disorders; skin disorders.

Leukona-Tonikum-Bad *Atzinger, Ger.†.*
Eucalyptus oil (p.1578·1); camphor (p.1557·2); rosemary oil (p.1626·2).
Bath additive; neuromuscular disorders; peripheral circulatory disorders.

Leukona-Wundsalbe *Atzinger, Ger.*
Cod-liver oil (p.1337·3); hamamelis water (p.1587·1); allantoin (p.1078·2).
Skin ulcers; wounds.

LeukoNorm *CytoChemia, Ger.*
Leucocytes (p.724·3).
Immunotherapy.

Leunase
Rhone-Poulenc Rorer, Austral.; Kyowa, Jpn.
Asparaginase (p.504·3).
Malignant neoplasms.

Leuplin *Takeda, Jpn.*
Leuprorelin acetate (p.1253·1).
Endometriosis; precocious puberty; prostatic cancer.

Leustat *Janssen-Cilag, UK.*
Cladribine (p.515·3).
Hairy-cell leukaemia.

Leustatin
Janssen-Cilag, Austral.; Janssen-Ortho, Canad.; Janssen-Cilag, Neth.; Janssen-Cilag, Swed.; Ortho Biotech, USA.
Cladribine (p.515·3).
Hairy-cell leukaemia.

Leustatine *Janssen-Cilag, Fr.*
Cladribine (p.515·3).
Hairy-cell leukaemia.

Levaknel *Crinos, Ital.*
Zinc oxide (p.1096·2); chlorhexidine (p.1107·2); triclosan (Irgasan DP 300) (p.1127·2).
Seborrhoea.

Levaliver *Elmu, Spain.*
Aceglutamide (p.1541·2); amino acids; betaine hydrochloride (p.1553·2); cyclobutyrol sodium (p.1569·2); pyridoxal phosphate (p.1363·1); sorbitol (p.1354·2).
Liver disorders.

Levanxol
Strallhofer, Aust.; Pharmacia Upjohn, Belg.; Pharmacia, S.Afr.†.
Temazepam (p.693·3).
Anxiety disorders; sleep disorders.

Levaquin *McNeil Pharmaceutical, USA.*
Levofloxacin (p.221·2).
Bacterial infections.

Levate *ICN, Canad.*
Amitriptyline hydrochloride (p.273·3).
Depression.

Levatol *Schwarz, USA.*
Penbutolol sulphate (p.927·2).
Hypertension.

Levaxin *Nycomed, Swed.*
Thyroxine sodium (p.1497·1).
Hypothyroidism; thyroid cancer.

Levbid *Schwarz, USA.*
Hyoscyamine sulphate (p.464·2).
Biliary and renal colic; gastro-intestinal disorders; parkinsonism; rhinitis.

Levicor *Bioindustria, Ital.*
Metaraminol tartrate (p.903·1).
Hypotension.

Levisticum *Hanosan, Ger.†.*
Homoeopathic preparation.

Levlen
Schering, Aust.; Schering, Austral.; Berlex, USA.
Levonorgestrel (p.1454·1); ethinyloestradiol (p.1445·1).
28-Day packs also contain 7 inert tablets.
Combined oral contraceptive.

Levobren *GiEnne, Ital.*
Levosulpiride (p.693·1).
Gastro-intestinal disorders; headache; migraine; vertigo.

Levocarnil *Sigma-Tau, Fr.*
Carnitine (p.1336·2).
Carnitine deficiency.

Levocarvit *Mitim, Ital.*
Carnitine (p.1336·2).
Carnitine deficiency; myocardial ischaemia.

Levo-Dromoran
Roche, Canad.†; Roche, USA.
Levorphanol tartrate (p.50·2).
Pain; premedication.

Levofolene *Farmades, Ital.*
Calcium levofolinate (p.1342·3).
Antidote to folic acid antagonists; folate deficiency anaemia.

Levoglusalino Vitulia *Ern, Spain.*
Electrolyte infusion with fructose (p.1147·1).
Carbohydrate source; fluid and electrolyte depletion.

Levolac *Pharmacia Upjohn, Norw.*
Lactulose (p.1195·3).
Constipation; hepatic encephalopathy.

Levonova
Leiras, Norw.; Leiras, Swed.
Levonorgestrel (p.1454·1).
Menorrhagia; progestogen-only contraceptive.

Levophed
Abbott, Austral.; Sanofi Winthrop, Belg.; Sanofi Winthrop, Canad.; Sanofi Winthrop, Irl.; Abbott, UK; Sanofi Winthrop, USA.
Noradrenaline acid tartrate (p.924·1).
Cardiac arrest; hypotensive states.

Levophta
Chauvin, Fr.; Ciba Vision, Ger.; Winzer, Ger.
Levocabastine hydrochloride (p.412·3).
Allergic conjunctivitis.

Levopraid *Ravizza, Ital.*
Levosulpiride (p.693·1).
Gastro-intestinal disorders; headache; psychiatric disorders; vertigo.

Levoprome *Lederle, USA.*
Methotrimeprazine hydrochloride (p.679·1).
Pain; premedication.

Levora *SCS, USA.*
Ethinyloestradiol (p.1445·1); levonorgestrel (p.1454·1).
28-Day packs also contain 7 inert tablets.
Combined oral contraceptive.

Levorin *Wyeth Lederle, Aust.*
Calcium levofolinate (p.1342·3).
Enhancement of fluorouracil activity; methotrexate toxicity.

Levostab *Formenti, Ital.*
Levocabastine hydrochloride (p.412·3).
Allergic conjunctivitis; allergic rhinitis.

Levo-T
Pharmascience, Canad.; Lederle, USA.
Thyroxine sodium (p.1497·1).
Hypothyroidism; TSH suppression.

Levotensin *Simes, Ital.†.*
Levomoprolol hydrochloride (p.898·1).
Heart failure; hypertension.

Levothroid
Rhone-Poulenc Rorer, Spain; Rhone-Poulenc Rorer, USA; Forest Laboratories, USA.
Thyroxine sodium (p.1497·1).
Hypothyroidism; TSH suppression.

Levothym *Promonta Lundbeck, Ger.*
Oxitriptan (p.301·2).
Depression; neurological disorders; sleep disorders.

Levothyrox *Merck-Clevenot, Fr.*
Thyroxine sodium (p.1497·1).
Hypothyroidism.

Levotirox *IRBI, Ital.†.*
Thyroxine sodium (p.1497·1).
Hypothyroidism.

Levotonine *Panpharma, Fr.*
Oxitriptan (p.301·2).
Myoclonus.

Levotuss *Dompe, Ital.*
Levodropropizine (p.1059·2).
Coughs.

Levovist
Schering, Ger.; Schering, Ital.; Schering, Neth.; Schering, Swed.; Schering, Switz.; Schering, UK.
Galactose (p.1005·2).
Ultrasound contrast medium.

Levoxyl *Daniels, USA.*
Thyroxine sodium (p.1497·1).
Formerly known as Levoxine.
Hypothyroidism; TSH suppression.

Levsin
Rivex, Canad.; Schwarz, USA.
Hyoscyamine sulphate (p.464·2).
Adjunct to hypotonic duodenography; anticholinesterase poisoning; biliary and renal colic; gastro-intestinal disorders; improvement of radiological visibility of the kidneys; neuroegenic bladder; pancreatitis; parkinsonism; partial heart block associated with vagal activity; premedication; rhinitis.

Levsin with Phenobarbitone *Schwarz, USA.*
Phenobarbitone (p.350·2); hyoscyamine sulphate (p.464·2).
Gastro-intestinal disorders.

Levsinex *Schwarz, USA.*
Hyoscyamine sulphate (p.464·2).
Biliary and renal colic; gastro-intestinal disorders; parkinsonism; rhinitis.

Levudin *GD, Ital.*
Yeast (p.1373·1); betacarotene (p.1335·2).

Levugen *Travenol, UK.*
Fructose (p.1343·2).

Levulosalino Isot *Braun, Spain.*
Sodium chloride (p.1162·2); fructose (p.1343·2).
Carbohydrate source; fluid and electrolyte disorders.

Levupotasico *Ern, Spain.*
Fructose (p.1343·2); potassium chloride (p.1161·1).
Hypokalaemia.

Levurinetten *Zyma, Aust.*
Dried yeast (p.1373·1); vitamin B substances.
Skin disorders.

Levurinetten N *Zyma, Ger.*
Dried yeast (p.1373·1).
Appetite loss; skin disorders.

Levurinettes *Zyma, Switz.†.*
Vitamin B preparation with yeast.
Tonic.

Levusalino *Braun, Spain; Ern, Spain.*
Fructose (p.1343·2); sodium chloride (p.1162·2).
Fluid and electrolyte disorders.

Lexat *Eagle, Austral.*
Bile salts (p.1553·2); pancreatin (p.1612·1); boldo (p.1554·1); chelidonium; aloes (p.1177·1); agar (p.1470·3); sanguinaria (p.1627·2).
Digestive system disorders.

Lexatin *Andreu, Spain.*
Bromazepam (p.643·1).
Anxiety; insomnia.

Lexibiotico *Llano, Spain.*
Cephalexin (p.178·2).
Bacterial infections.

Lexil *Roche, Ital.*
Bromazepam (p.643·1); propantheline bromide (p.468·1).
Gastro-intestinal disorders.

Lexincef *Serra Pamies, Spain.*
Cephalexin (p.178·2).
Bacterial infections.

Lexinor *Astra, Swed.*
Norfloxacin (p.233·1).
Bacterial infections.

Lexobene *Merckle, Ger.*
Diclofenac sodium (p.31·2).
Lignocaine hydrochloride (p.1293·2) is included in this preparation to alleviate the pain of injection.
Inflammation; rheumatism.

Lexomil Roche, Fr.
Bromazepam (p.643·1).
Alcohol withdrawal syndrome; anxiety.

Lexostad Stada, Ger.
Bromazepam (p.643·1).
Anxiety disorders; insomnia.

Lexotan
Roche, Austral.; Roche, Belg.; Roche, Irl.; Roche, Ital.; Roche, S.Afr.; Roche, UK.
Bromazepam (p.643·1).
Anxiety.

Lexotanil
Roche, Aust.; Roche, Ger.; Roche, Neth.; Roche, Switz.
Bromazepam (p.643·1).
Anxiety disorders.

Lexpec Rosemont, UK.
Folic acid (p.1340·3).
Anaemias.

Lexpec with Iron Rosemont, UK.
Ferric ammonium citrate (p.1339·2); folic acid (p.1340·3).
Iron and folic acid deficiency.

Lexpec with Iron-M Rosemont, UK.
Ferric ammonium citrate (p.1339·2); folic acid (p.1340·3).
Iron and folic acid deficiency.

Lextron Lilly, USA†.
Iron with vitamin B complex.

Lexxel Astra Merck, USA.
Enalapril maleate (p.863·2); felodipine (p.867·3).
Hypertension.

LH-Color Organon, Switz.†.
Fertility test (p.1621·2).

Li 450 Ziethen, Ger.
Lithium carbonate (p.290·3).
Bipolar disorders; depression; mania.

Liaptene E. Merck, Switz.†.
Clofibrate (p.1271·1); nicotinyl alcohol tartrate (p.915·3).
Hyperlipidaemias.

Libanil Approved Prescription Services, UK†.
Glibenclamide (p.319·3).
Diabetes mellitus.

Libenar
SmithKline Beecham, Ital.; Sterling Health, Spain.
Sodium chloride (p.1162·2).
Nasal dryness; nasal hygiene.

Liberalgium Diviser Aquilea, Spain.
Diclofenac sodium (p.31·2).
Gout; inflammation; musculoskeletal, joint, and periarticular disorders; pain; renal colic.

Liberanas OTC, Spain.
Sodium chloride (p.1162·2).
Nasal congestion.

Liberbil Ferrer, Spain.
Cyclobutyrol sodium (p.1569·2); theophylline dehydrocholinate; metoclopramide hydrochloride (p.1200·3).
Hepatobiliary disorders.

Liberen Lisapharma, Ital.
Dextropropoxyphene hydrochloride (p.27·3).
Pain; renal and hepatic colic.

Liberol Galactina, Switz.
Camphor (p.1557·2); methyl salicylate (p.55·2); guaiacol (p.1061·2); mustard spirit (p.1605·3); pumilio pine oil (p.1623·3); thyme oil (p.1637·1); eucalyptus oil (p.1578·1); turpentine oil (p.1641·1); hyoscyamus oil (p.464·3).
Chilblains; cold symptoms; muscle and joint pain.

Libetist Opus, UK.
Salbutamol sulphate (p.758·2).
Asthma; bronchitis; emphysema.

Libetusin Dimportex, Spain†.
Bromhexine (p.1055·3); co-trimoxazole (p.196·3); potassium guaiacolsulfonate (p.1068·3).
Respiratory-tract infections.

Libexin Master Pharma, Ital.†.
Prenoxdiazine hybenzate (p.1068·3) or prenoxdiazine hydrochloride (p.1068·3).
Coughs.

Libexin Mucolitico Master Pharma, Ital.
Prenoxdiazine hybenzate (p.1068·3) or prenoxdiazine hydrochloride (p.1068·3); carbocisteine (p.1056·3).
Coughs.

Libexine Labatec, Switz.
Prenoxdiazine hybenzate (p.1068·3) or prenoxdiazine hydrochloride (p.1068·3).
Coughs.

Libexine Compositum Labatec, Switz.
Prenoxdiazine hydrochloride (p.1068·3); guaiphenesin (p.1061·3); terpin hydrate (p.1070·2).
Coughs.

Libidomega Cantassium Co., UK.
Amino-acid, vitamin, and mineral preparation.

Libratar UCB, Ital.†.
Chlorbenzoxamine hydrochloride (p.1183·2); bismuth subnitrate (p.1180·2); aluminium hydroxide (p.1177·3); magnesium carbonate (p.1198·1); calcium carbonate (p.1182·1).
Peptic ulcer.

Libratar Complex UCB, Ger.†.
Aluminium hydroxide (p.1177·3); magnesium carbonate (p.1198·1); calcium carbonate (p.1182·1); bismuth subnitrate (p.1180·2).
Formerly contained chlorbenzoxamine hydrochloride, aluminium hydroxide, magnesium carbonate, calcium carbonate and bismuth subnitrate.
Gastro-intestinal disorders.

Librax
Roche, Aust.; Roche, Austral.†; Roche, Belg.; Roche, Canad.; Roche, Fr.; Roche, Ger.†; Roche, Ital.; Roche, S.Afr.; Roche, Spain†; Roche, Swed.†; Roche, Switz.; Roche, USA.
Chlordiazepoxide (p.646·3) or chlordiazepoxide hydrochloride (p.646·3); clidinium bromide (p.459·2).
Dysmenorrhoea; irritable bowel syndrome; nocturnal enuresis; peptic ulcer (adjunct); smooth muscle spasm.

Libraxin Roche, Irl.†.
Chlordiazepoxide (p.646·3); clidinium bromide (p.459·2).
Colonic spasm; nervous dyspepsia; peptic ulcers.

Libritabs Roche Products, USA.
Chlordiazepoxide (p.646·3).
Anxiety.

Librium
Roche, Austral.†; Roche, Belg.†; Roche, Canad.†; Roche, Fr.†; Roche, Ger.†; Roche, Irl.; Roche, Ital.; Roche, Neth.†; Roche, S.Afr.; Roche, Swed.†; Roche, Switz.†; ICN, UK; Roche Products, USA.
Chlordiazepoxide (p.646·3) or chlordiazepoxide hydrochloride (p.646·3).
Alcohol withdrawal syndrome; anxiety; skeletal muscle spasm.

Librofem
Zyma, Spain†; Zyma, UK.
Ibuprofen (p.44·1).
Fever; pain.

Licain Curasan, Ger.
Lignocaine hydrochloride (p.1293·2).
Local anaesthesia.

Licarpin Allergan, Swed.
Pilocarpine nitrate (p.1396·3).
Glaucoma.

Lice Enz
Richmond, Canad.†; Copley, USA†.
Pyrethrins; piperonyl butoxide (p.1409·3).
Pediculosis.

Lice Rid Florafaun, Austral.
Malathion (Maldison) (p.1407·3).
Pediculosis.

Licoplex DS Keene, USA.
Ferrous gluconate (p.1340·1); vitamin B substances.
Procaine hydrochloride (p.1299·2) is included in this preparation to alleviate the pain of injection.
Iron-deficiency anaemias.

Licor Amoniacal Asens, Spain.
Alcohol (p.1099·1); ammonia (p.1548·3); ammonium carbonate (p.1055·1).
Exhaustion; nausea; shock.

Lidaltrin Lacer, Spain.
Quinapril hydrochloride (p.938·1).
Heart failure; hypertension.

Lidaltrin Diu Lacer, Spain.
Quinapril hydrochloride (p.938·1); hydrochlorothiazide (p.885·2).
Hypertension.

Lida-Mantle-HC Miles, USA.
Hydrocortisone acetate (p.1043·3); lignocaine (p.1293·2).
Skin disorders.

Lidaprim
Hafslund Nycomed, Aust.; Nycomed, Ger.†; Lisapharma, Ital.
Sulfametrole (p.252·1); trimethoprim (p.265·1).
Bacterial infections.

Lidazon Demopharm, Switz.
Lozenges: Cetylpyridinium chloride (p.1106·2); dichlorobenzyl alcohol (p.1112·2); chlorquinaldol (p.185·1); lignocaine (p.1293·2).
Oral liquid; oral spray: Cetylpyridinium chloride (p.1106·2); dichlorobenzyl alcohol (p.1112·2); lignocaine (p.1293·2) or lignocaine hydrochloride (p.1293·2).
Mouth and throat disorders.

Lid-Care Ciba Vision, Austral.
Eyelid cleanser.

Lidecomb Syntex, Canad.†.
Fluocinonide (p.1041·2); neomycin sulphate (p.229·2); gramicidin (p.215·2); nystatin (p.386·1).
Infected skin disorders.

Lidemol Syntex, Canad.†.
Fluocinonide (p.1041·2).
Skin disorders.

Lident Adrenalina Warner-Lambert, Ital.
Lignocaine hydrochloride (p.1293·2).
Adrenaline acid tartrate (p.813·3) is included in this preparation as a vasoconstrictor to diminish absorption and localise the effect of the local anaesthetic.
Local anaesthesia in dentistry.

Lident Andrenor Warner-Lambert, Ital.
Lignocaine hydrochloride (p.1293·2).
Adrenaline acid tartrate (p.813·3) and noradrenaline acid tartrate (p.924·1) are included in this preparation as vasoconstrictors to diminish absorption and localise the effect of the local anaesthetic.
Local anaesthesia in dentistry.

Liderfeme Farmalider, Spain†.
Ibuprofen (p.44·1).
Fever; pain.

Liderflex Farmalider, Spain.
Camphor (p.1557·2); methyl salicylate (p.55·2); menthol (p.1600·2).
Muscular and joint pain.

Liderman Jacoby, Aust.
Oxiconazole nitrate (p.386·3).
Fungal skin infections.

Lidesthesin Ritsert, Ger.
Lignocaine hydrochloride (p.1293·2).
Local anaesthesia.

Lidex
Yamanouchi, Belg.; Roche, Canad.; Syntex, USA.
Fluocinonide (p.1041·2).
Skin disorders.

Lidifen Berk, UK.
Ibuprofen (p.44·1).
Fever; inflammation; musculoskeletal and joint disorders; pain.

Lidobama Complex Bama, Spain.
Cellulase (p.1561·1); cyclobutyrol (p.1569·2); dimethicone (p.1213·1); lignocaine hydrochloride (p.1293·2); pancreatin (p.1612·1).
Digestive-system disorders.

Lidobama Plus Bama, Spain†.
Cellulase (p.1561·1); cyclobutyrol (p.1569·2); chlorquinaldol (p.185·1); dimethicone (p.1213·1); lignocaine hydrochloride (p.1293·2); pancreatin (p.1612·1).
Digestive-system disorders.

Lidocaton
Weimer, Ger.; Swisspharm, S.Afr.†; Weimer, Switz.
Lignocaine hydrochloride (p.1293·2).
Adrenaline (p.813·2) is included in this preparation as a vasoconstrictor to diminish absorption and localise the effect of the local anaesthetic.
Local anaesthesia.

Lidocorit Gebro, Aust.
Lignocaine hydrochloride (p.1293·2).
Arrhythmias.

Lidodan Odan, Canad.
Lignocaine (p.1293·2) or lignocaine hydrochloride (p.1293·2).
Local anaesthesia.

Lidohex Bichsel, Switz.
Lignocaine hydrochloride (p.1293·2); chlorhexidine gluconate (p.1107·2).
Catheterisation; endoscopy.

Lido-Hyal
Ogna, Ital.; Wild, Switz.
Hyaluronidase (p.1588·1); lignocaine hydrochloride (p.1293·2).
Local anaesthesia; prophylaxis of soft-tissue disorders.

Lidoject
Hexal, Ger.; Mayrand, USA.
Lignocaine hydrochloride (p.1293·2).
Local anaesthesia.

Lidomyxin Sabex, Canad.
Polymyxin B sulphate (p.239·1); lignocaine hydrochloride (p.1293·2).
Ear infections, pain, and pruritus.

LidoPen Survival Technology, USA.
Lignocaine hydrochloride (p.1293·2).
Arrhythmias.

LidoPosterine Kade, Ger.
Lignocaine (p.1293·2).
Anorectal disorders.

Lidosporin Glaxo Wellcome, Canad.; Warner-Lambert, Canad.
Cream: Polymyxin B sulphate (p.239·1); gramicidin (p.215·2); lignocaine hydrochloride (p.1293·2).
Skin disorders.
Ear drops: Polymyxin B sulphate (p.239·1); lignocaine hydrochloride (p.1293·2).
Ear infections.

Lidox Major, USA.
Chlordiazepoxide hydrochloride (p.646·3); clidinium bromide (p.459·2).
Irritable bowel syndrome; peptic ulcer (adjunct).

Lidrian Bieffe, Ital.
Lignocaine hydrochloride (p.1293·2).
Local anaesthesia.

Lidrone Serra Pamies, Spain.
Phenylephrine hydrochloride (p.1066·2); naphazoline nitrate (p.1064·2); prednisolone (p.1048·1); cetrimide (p.1105·2).
Nasal congestion and infection.

Liedasi Radiumfarma, Ital.†.
Di-isopropylammonium dichloroacetate (p.854·1); cocarboxylase (p.1361·2); cyanocobalamin (p.1363·3).
Neuralgia; neuritis.

Lievigran Bifarma, Ital.†.
Dried yeast (p.1373·1); wheat germ.

Lievistar Lampugnani, Ital.
Dried yeast (p.1373·1); cynara (p.1569·2).
Nutritional supplement.

Lievital Lampugnani, Ital.†.
Dried yeast (p.1373·1); cynara (p.1569·2); vitamin B substances.

Lievitosohn Antonetto, Ital.
Saccharomyces cerevisiae (p.1373·1); vitamin B substances.
Restoration of normal gastro-intestinal flora.

Lievitovit Gazzoni, Ital.
Dried yeast (p.1373·1); vitamin B substances.
Restoration of normal gastro-intestinal flora.

Lievitovit 300 Gazzoni, Ital.
Dried yeast (p.1373·1).

Lifaton B12 Sobater, Spain.
Cyanocobalamin (p.1363·3).
Vitamin B12 deficiency.

Life Brand Cough Lozenges Sutton, Canad.
Menthol (p.1600·2).

Life Brand Natural Source Tanning Research, Canad.
SPF 25: Titanium dioxide (p.1093·3).
Sunscreen.

Life Brand Sunblock Tanning Research, Canad.
SPF 30: Ethylhexyl *p*-methoxycinnamate (p.1487·1); avobenzone (p.1486·3); homosalate (p.1487·2).
Sunscreen.

Life Drops
Note. A similar name is used for preparations of different composition.
Potter's, UK.
Capsicum (p.1559·2); sambucus (p.1627·2); peppermint oil (p.1208·1).
Cold symptoms; sore throat.

Lifedrops
Note. A similar name is used for preparations of different composition.
Lifeplan, UK.
Sambucus (p.1627·2); peppermint (p.1208·1).
Coughs and cold symptoms; flatulence.

Liferitin IBYS, Spain†.
Erythromycin estolate (p.204·1).
Bacterial infections.

Lifestyles Ansell, Canad.
Nonoxinol 9 (p.1326·1).
Contraceptive.

Lifesystem Herbal Formula 1 Arthritic Aid
Cenovis, Austral.
Celery (p.1561·1); juniper (p.1592·2); harpagophytum procumbens (p.27·2); salix (p.82·3).
Arthritic and rheumatic pain.

Lifesystem Herbal Formula 7 Liver Tonic Cenovis, Austral.
Silybum marianum (p.993·3); taraxacum (p.1634·2); cynara (p.1569·2); garlic (p.1583·1).
Digestive disorders; liver tonic.

Lifesystem Herbal Formula 6 For Peripheral Circulation Cenovis, Austral.
Ginkgo biloba (p.1584·1); crataegus (p.1568·2); zanthoxylum (p.1645·3); capsicum (p.1559·2); rutin (p.1580·2); hesperidin (p.1580·2).
Peripheral vascular disorders.

Lifesystem Herbal Formula 12 Willowbark
Cenovis, Austral.
Scutellaria; harpagophytum procumbens (p.27·2); salix (p.82·3).
Headache.

Lifesystem Herbal Formula 4 Women's Formula Cenovis, Austral.
Angelica; cimicifuga (p.1563·3); caulophyllum; pulsatilla (p.1623·3); agnus castus (p.1544·2).
Menstrual disorders.

Lifesystem Herbal Plus Formula 8 Echinacea Cenovis, Austral.
Echinacea (p.1574·2); *d*-alpha tocopheryl acid succinate (p.1369·2); betacarotene (p.1335·2); ascorbic acid (p.1365·2); sodium ascorbate (p.1365·2); zinc amino acid chelate (p.1373·3).
Minor upper respiratory-tract disorders; skin disorders; wounds.

Lifesystem Herbal Plus Formula 5 Eye Relief
Cenovis, Austral.
Euphrasia officinalis; ginkgo biloba (p.1584·1); betacarotene (p.1335·2); *d*-alpha tocopheryl acid succinate (p.1369·2); ascorbic acid (p.1365·2); rutin (p.1580·2); hesperidin (p.1580·2).
Eye strain; tired eyes.

Lifesystem Herbal Plus Formula 9 Fatty Acids And Vitamin E Cenovis, Austral.
d-Alpha tocopherol (p.1369·1); evening primrose oil (p.1582·1); omega-3 marine triglycerides (p.1276·1).
Dietary supplement.

Lifesystem Herbal Plus Formula 11 Ginkgo
Cenovis, Austral.
Ginkgo biloba (p.1584·1); ginger (p.1193·2); dibasic potassium phosphate (p.1159·2); magnesium oxide (p.1198·3).
Peripheral vascular disorders; tonic.

Lifesystem Herbal Plus Formula 3 Male Formula Cenovis, Austral.
Eleutherococcus senticosus; equisetum; sarsaparilla; liquorice; damiana; zinc amino acid chelate; betacarotene; pyridoxine hydrochloride; *d*-alpha tocopheryl acid succinate; magnesium oxide.
Tonic.

Lifesystem Herbal Plus Formula 2 Valerian
Cenovis, Austral.
Valerian (p.1643·1); scutellaria; passion flower (p.1615·3); dibasic potassium phosphate (p.1159·2); magnesium oxide (p.1198·3).
Nervous tension; sleep disorders.

Lifesystem Mineral Plus Formula 10 Osteoporosis Cenovis, Austral.
Calcium carbonate (p.1182·1); cholecalciferol (p.1366·3).
Calcium deficiency; osteoporosis.

Lifril Casen Fleet, Spain.
Pirlindole (p.306·3).
Depression.

Lifurox
Lilly, Norw.; Lilly, Swed.
Cefuroxime sodium (p.177·1).
Bacterial infections.

Liga Jacobs, UK.
Gluten-free food for special diets.

Lightning Cough Remedy Potter's, UK.
Liquorice (p.1197·1); anise oil (p.1550·1).
Coughs.

Lignospan Septodont, Switz.
Lignocaine hydrochloride (p.1293·2).

Adrenaline acid tartrate (p.813·3) is included in this preparation as a vasoconstrictor to diminish absorption and localise the effect of the local anaesthetic.
Local anaesthesia.

Lignostab-A *Astra, UK.*
Lignocaine hydrochloride (p.1293·2).
Adrenaline (p.813·2) is included in this preparation as a vasoconstrictor to diminish absorption and localise the effect of the local anaesthetic.
Local anaesthesia.

Lignostab-N *Astra, UK†.*
Lignocaine hydrochloride (p.1293·2).
Noradrenaline (p.924·1) is included in this preparation as a vasoconstrictor to diminish absorption and localise the effect of the local anaesthetic.
Local anaesthesia.

Ligvites *Gerard House, UK.*
Guaiacum (p.1586·3); black cohosh (p.1563·3); white willow bark (p.82·3); sarsaparilla (p.1627·2); poplar bark (p.1620·1).
Inflammation; pain.

Li-iL Rheuma-Bad *Li-il, Ger.*
Glycol salicylate (p.43·1); methyl salicylate (p.55·2).
Bath additive; musculoskeletal, joint, and soft-tissue disorders.

Likacin *Lisapharma, Ital.*
Amikacin sulphate (p.150·2).
Bacterial infections.

Likuden M *Hoechst, Ger.*
Griseofulvin (microfine) (p.380·2).
Fungal infections.

Lilacillin *Takeda, Jpn.*
Sulbenicillin sodium (p.250·3).
Mepivacaine hydrochloride (p.1297·2) is included in the intramuscular injection to alleviate the pain of injection.
Bacterial infections.

Li-Liquid *Rosemont, UK.*
Lithium citrate (p.290·3).
Depression; mania; psychoses.

Lilium Med Complex *Dynamit, Aust.*
Homoeopathic preparation.

Lillypen Profil 10, 20, 30, and 40 *Lilly, Fr.*
Mixtures of insulin injection (human, prb) 10%, 20%, 30%, and 40% and isophane insulin injection (human, prb) 90%, 80%, 70%, and 60% respectively (p.322·1).
Diabetes mellitus.

Lillypen Protamine Isophane *Lilly, Fr.*
Isophane insulin injection (human, prb) (p.322·1).
Diabetes mellitus.

Lillypen Rapide *Lilly, Fr.*
Insulin injection (human, prb) (p.322·1).
Diabetes mellitus.

Liman
Solvay, Aust.; Solvay, Ger.
Tenoxicam (p.88·2).
Gout; musculoskeletal and joint disorders.

Limbao *Kanoldt, Ger.*
Kava (p.1592·3).
Anxiety disorders.

Limbatril *Roche, Ger.*
Amitriptyline hydrochloride (p.273·3); chlordiazepoxide (p.646·3).
Dystonias; non-psychotic mental disorders.

Limbial *Chiesi, Ital.*
Oxazepam (p.683·2).
Anxiety; insomnia; nervous disorders.

Limbitrol
Roche, Aust.; Roche, Belg.; Roche, Irl.†; Roche, Neth.†; Roche, S.Afr.; Roche, Switz.; Roche, UK†; Roche, USA.
Amitriptyline hydrochloride (p.273·3); chlordiazepoxide (p.646·3).
Mixed anxiety depressive states.

Limbitryl *Roche, Ital.*
Amitriptyline hydrochloride (p.273·3); chlordiazepoxide (p.646·3).
Mixed anxiety depressive states.

Limclair
Sinclair, Irl.; Sinclair, UK.
Trisodium edetate (p.980·2).
Calcareous corneal opacities; digitalis-induced arrhythmias; hypercalcaemia; parathyroidism.

Limethason *Green Cross, Jpn.*
Dexamethasone palmitate (p.1037·3).
Rheumatoid arthritis.

Limican *Synthelabo, Ital.*
Alizapride hydrochloride (p.1176·3).
Nausea and vomiting.

Limifen *Janssen-Cilag, Spain.*
Alfentanil hydrochloride (p.12·3).
General anaesthesia.

Liminate *Modern Health Products, UK.*
Turkey rhubarb (p.1212·1); senna leaf (p.1212·2); chondrus (p.1471·3).
Constipation.

Limit-X *UB Interpharm, Switz.*
Cathine hydrochloride (p.1478·1).
Obesity.

Limonal *Falqui, Ital.*
Light magnesium carbonate (p.1198·1); anhydrous citric acid (p.1564·3).
Constipation.

Limone *CliniMed, UK.*
A deodorant spray for stoma care.

Limovan *Rhone-Poulenc Rorer, Spain.*
Zopiclone (p.699·2).
Insomnia.

Limpidex *Sigma-Tau, Ital.*
Lansoprazole (p.1196·2).
Gastro-oesophageal reflux; peptic ulcer; Zollinger-Ellison syndrome.

Limptar
Hoechst, Aust.; Cassella-med, Ger.; Hoechst Marion Roussel, Switz.
Quinine sulphate (p.439·2); aminophylline (p.748·1).
Leg cramp.

Limptar N *Cassella-med, Ger.*
Quinine sulphate (p.439·2).
Night cramp.

Linaris *RAN, Ger.*
Co-trimoxazole (p.196·3).
Bacterial infections.

Lincil *Funk, Spain.*
Nicardipine hydrochloride (p.915·1).
Angina pectoris; cerebrovascular disorders; hypertension.

Lincocin
Pharmacia Upjohn, Austral.; Pharmacia Upjohn, Belg.; Pharmacia Upjohn, Canad.; Upjohn, Irl.†; Pharmacia Upjohn, Ital.; Pharmacia Upjohn, Neth.; Pharmacia Upjohn, Norw.†; Pharmacia Upjohn, S.Afr.; Upjohn, Spain; Pharmacia Upjohn, Swed.; Pharmacia Upjohn, Switz.; Upjohn, USA.
Lincomycin hydrochloride (p.222·1).
Bacterial infections.

Lincocine *Pharmacia Upjohn, Fr.*
Lincomycin hydrochloride (p.222·1).
Bacterial infections.

Lincorex *Hyrex, USA.*
Lincomycin hydrochloride (p.222·1).
Bacterial infections.

Linctifed
Wellcopharm, Ger.†; Wellcome, Irl.†; Glaxo Wellcome, S.Afr.
Triprolidine hydrochloride (p.420·3); pseudoephedrine hydrochloride (p.1068·3); codeine phosphate (p.26·1); guaiphenesin (p.1061·3).
Coughs.

Linctodyl *Pharmaceutical Enterprises, S.Afr.*
Dextromethorphan hydrobromide (p.1057·3); ephedrine hydrochloride (p.1059·3); ammonium chloride (p.1055·2).
Coughs.

Linctosan *Garec, S.Afr.*
Diphenhydramine hydrochloride (p.409·1); ammonium chloride (p.1055·2); sodium citrate (p.1153·2); menthol (p.1600·2).
Coughs; nasal congestion.

Linctus Tussi Infans *Propan, S.Afr.*
Ipecacuanha (p.1062·2); squill (p.1070·1); tolu (p.1071·1).
Coughs.

Lindemil *Knoll, Spain.*
Alum (p.1547·1); benzalkonium chloride (p.1101·3).
Vaginal antiseptic; vulvovaginal trichomoniasis (adjuvant).

Lindigoa S *Brenner-Efeka, Ger.; LAW, Ger.*
Aesculus (p.1543·3); troxerutin (p.1580·2).
Vascular disorders.

Lindilane *Cipharm, Fr.*
Paracetamol (p.72·2); codeine phosphate (p.26·1).
Pain.

Lindocetyl *Lindopharm, Ger.†.*
Acetylcysteine (p.1052·3).
Respiratory-tract disorders associated with increased or viscous mucus.

Lindofluid N *Lindopharm, Ger.*
Bornyl acetate (p.1555·1) α-pinene; arnica (p.1550·3); melissa (p.1600·1).
Muscle, joint, and nerve pain.

Lindotab *Lindopharm, Ger.*
Tiaprofenic acid (p.89·1).
Inflammation; musculoskeletal, joint, and soft-tissue disorders.

Lindoxyl *Lindopharm, Ger.*
Ambroxol hydrochloride (p.1054·3).
Respiratory-tract disorders associated with increased or viscous mucus.

Linea *Valeas, Ital.*
Diethylpropion hydrochloride (p.1479·3).
Obesity.

Linea F *Angelini, Ital.*
Benzalkonium chloride (p.1101·3); benzydamine hydrochloride (p.21·3).
Disinfection of wounds and burns.

Lineafarm *Wyeth, Spain.*
Nonoxinol 9 (p.1326·1).
Contraceptive.

Linervidol *Interdelta, Switz.*
Paracetamol (p.72·2); pyridoxine hydrochloride (p.1362·3); promethazine hydrochloride (p.416·2).
Agitation; fever; pain.

Linfoglobulina *Rhone-Poulenc Rorer, Spain.*
Antilymphocyte immunoglobulin (horse) (p.504·2).
Organ transplant rejection.

Linfolysin *Nuovo ISM, Ital.*
Chlorambucil (p.512·3).
Chronic lymphoid leukaemia; Hodgkin's disease; lymphoma.

Lingraine
Sanofi Winthrop, Irl.; Sanofi Winthrop, UK.
Ergotamine tartrate (p.445·3).
Migraine and other vascular headaches.

Lini-Bombe *Thepenier, Fr.*
Veratrol; menthol (p.1600·2); chloral hydrate (p.645·3); salicylic acid (p.1090·2).
Formerly contained veratrol, menthol, chloral hydrate, and phenazone gentisate.
Musculoskeletal and joint disorders.

Linimento Bertelli *Kelemata, Ital.†.*
Camphor (p.1557·2); cineole (p.1564·1); methyl salicylate (p.55·2); ethyl nicotinate (p.36·1).
Soft-tissue disorders.

Linimento Klari *Clariana, Spain.*
Camphor (p.1557·2); capsicum (p.1559·2); amyl salicylate (p.15·3); rosemary oil (p.1626·2); sassafras oil (p.1627·3); turpentine oil (p.1641·1).
Rheumatic and muscle pain.

Linimento Naion *Puerto Galiano, Spain.*
Camphor (p.1557·2); alcohol (p.1099·1); salicylic acid (p.1090·2); turpentine; menthol (p.1600·2); soft soap (p.1468·1); capsicum (p.1559·2); methyl salicylate (p.55·2); rosemary; lavender (p.1594·3).
Rheumatic and muscle pain.

Linimento Sloan *Warner-Lambert, Spain.*
Ammonia (p.1548·3); capsicum (p.1559·2); methyl salicylate (p.55·2); oleum pini sylvestris; sassafras; turpentine oil (p.1641·1); camphor (p.1557·2).
Rheumatic and muscle pain.

Liniplant *Spitzner, Ger.*
Eucalyptus oil (p.1578·1); cajuput oil (p.1556·1).
Upper respiratory-tract disorders.

Linitul *Bama, Spain.*
Medicated dressing: Peru balsam (p.1617·2); beeswax; paraffin; castor oil; soft paraffin.
Ointment: Peru balsam (p.1617·2); beeswax; castor oil.
Skin disorders.

Linitul Antibiotico *Bama, Spain.*
Acexamic acid (p.1542·1); bacitracin (p.157·3); neomycin sulphate (p.229·2); polymyxin B sulphate (p.239·1).
Skin disorders.

Link
Alpharma, Norw.; Dumex-Alpharma, Swed.
Aluminium hydroxide-magnesium carbonate co-dried gel (p.1178·2).
Dyspepsia; gastric hyperacidity; gastritis; heartburn; peptic ulcer.

Links-Glaukosan *Woelm, Ger.†.*
Adrenaline acid tartrate (p.813·3); adrenalone hydrochloride (p.1543·3).
Glaucoma; inflammatory eye disorders.

Linoforce
Bioforce, Canad.†; Bioforce, Switz.
Linseed (p.1596·2); senna (p.1212·2); frangula bark (p.1193·2).
Constipation.

Linola
Note. This name is used for preparations of different composition.
Montavit, Aust.
Fatty acids, betacarotene, cholecalciferol-cholesterin, vitamin E.
Skin disorders.

Wolff, Ger.; Cimex, Switz.
Linoleic acid (p.1582·1); 9,11-octadecadienoic acid.
Skin disorders.

Linola gras *Cimex, Switz.*
Linoleic acid (p.1582·1); betacarotene (p.1335·2); cholecalciferol (p.1366·3); tocopheryl acetate (p.1369·2).
Skin disorders.

Linola mi-gras *Cimex, Switz.*
Linoleic acid (p.1582·1); 9,11-octadecadienoic acid.
Skin disorders.

Linoladiol
Note. This name is used for preparations of different composition.
Montavit, Aust.
Oestradiol (p.1455·1).
Vaginal disorders.

Cimex, Switz.
Oestradiol (p.1455·1); linoleic acid (p.1582·1); 9,11-octadecadienoic acid.
Vulvovaginal disorders.

Linoladiol N *Wolff, Ger.*
Oestradiol (p.1455·1).
Skin disorders; vaginal disorders.

Linoladiol-H N *Wolff, Ger.*
Oestradiol (p.1455·1); prednisolone (p.1048·1).
Acne; ulcus cruris; vaginal disorders.

Linola-Fett 2000 *Wolff, Ger.*
Linoleic acid (p.1582·1).
Skin disorders.

Linola-Fett N *Wolff, Ger.*
Linoleic acid (p.1582·1); 9,11-octadecadienoic acid.
Skin disorders.

Linola-Fett-N Olbad *Wolff, Ger.*
Bath additive; emollient.

Linola-H N *Wolff, Ger.*
Prednisolone (p.1048·1).
Skin disorders.

Linola-H-compositum N *Wolff, Ger.*
Prednisolone (p.1048·1); neomycin sulphate (p.229·2).
Burns; infected skin disorders.

Linola-H-Fett N *Wolff, Ger.*
Prednisolone (p.1048·1).
Skin disorders.

Linola-sept *Wolff, Ger.*
Clioquinol (p.193·2).
Infected skin disorders.

Linotar
Linotar, Austral.; MZ, S.Afr.
Coal tar (p.1092·3).
Skin disorders.

Linsal *Sigma, Austral.*
Methyl salicylate (p.55·2).
Rubefacient and topical analgesic.

L-Insulin *Berlin-Chemie, Ger.*
Neutral insulin suspension (porcine) (p.322·1).
Diabetes mellitus.

Linusit *Dietavigor, Ital.†.*
Linseed (p.1596·2).
Nutritional supplement.

Linusit Creola *Fink, Ger.*
Linseed (p.1596·2).
Gastro-intestinal disorders.

Linusit Darmaktiv Leinsamen *Fink, Ger.*
Linseed (p.1596·2).
Gastro-intestinal disorders.

Linusit Gold *Drogenhansa, Aust.*
Linseed (p.1596·2).
Gastro-intestinal disorders.

Linvite *Linton, S.Afr.*
Multivitamin and mineral preparation.

Liobifar *Lifepharma, Ital.†.*
Antibiotic-resistant *Bacillus subtilis* spores.
Disturbances in gastric flora.

Liocarpina *SIFI, Ital.*
Pilocarpine hydrochloride (p.1396·3).
Glaucoma; ocular hypertension.

Lio-Crio *ISM, Ital.†.*
A factor VIII preparation (p.720·3).
Haemorrhagic disorders.

Lioftal s. T. *Hennig, Ger.†.*
Inositol nicotinate (p.891·3); etofylline (p.753·1); etaverine (p.1577·1).
Hyperlipidaemias; peripheral vascular disorders.

Liogynon *Schering, Aust.*
Levonorgestrel (p.1454·1); ethinyloestradiol (p.1445·1).
Triphasic oral contraceptive.

Liometacen
Gerot, Aust.; Chiesi, Ital.
Meglumine indomethacin (p.46·3).
Gout; musculoskeletal and joint disorders; pain; renal and biliary colic; thrombophlebitis.

Lio-Morbillo *Nuovo ISM, Ital.*
A measles vaccine (Schwarz strain) (p.1517·3).
Active immunisation.

Lioresal
Ciba-Geigy, Aust.; Novartis, Austral.; Ciba-Geigy, Belg.; Ciba, Canad.; Ciba-Geigy, Fr.; Geigy, Ger.; Ciba-Geigy, Irl.; Ciba, Ital.; Novartis, Neth.; Ciba, Norw.; Novartis, S.Afr.; Ciba-Geigy, Spain; Novartis, Swed.; Geigy, Switz.; Novartis, UK; Geigy, USA.
Baclofen (p.1308·2).
Skeletal muscle spasm or spasticity.

Liosiero *Nuovo ISM, Ital.*
A botulism antitoxin (types A, B, and E) (p.1506·1).
Botulism.

Lioton *Sanofi Winthrop, Ital.*
Heparin sodium (p.879·3).
Peripheral vascular disorders; soft-tissue disorders.

Liotoxid *Recordati, Ital.†.*
Cogalactoisomerase sodium (p.1566·2).
Liver disorders.

Liotropina *SIFI, Ital.*
Atropine sulphate (p.455·1).
Eye disorders.

Liozim *Farmanova, Ital.*
Fructose (p.1343·2); acacia honey (p.1345·3); lactic-acid-producing organisms (p.1594·1).
Nutritional supplement.

Lip Block Sunscreen *Norwood, Canad.*
SPF 15: Ethylhexyl *p*-methoxycinnamate (p.1487·1); oxybenzone (p.1487·3); titanium dioxide (p.1093·3).
Sunscreen.

Lip Medex
Blistex, Canad.; Blistex, USA.
Camphor (p.1557·2); phenol (p.1121·2).
Dry, cracked lips; herpes labialis.

Lip Tone *Blistex, USA.*
SPF 15: Ethylhexyl *p*-methoxycinnamate (p.1487·1); menthyl anthranilate (p.1487·2).
Sunscreen.

Lipactin
Novartis Consumer, Canad.; Zyma, Ger.; Widmer, Switz.
Heparin sodium (p.879·3); zinc sulphate (p.1373·2).
Herpes labialis.

Lipanor *Sanofi Winthrop, Fr.*
Ciprofibrate (p.1270·3).
Hyperlipidaemias.

Lipanthyl
Fournier, Belg.; Fournier, Fr.; Fournier, Ger.; Puropharma, Ital.; Fournier, Switz.
Fenofibrate (p.1273·1).
Hyperlipidaemias.

Lipantil *Fournier, UK.*
Fenofibrate (p.1273·1).
Hyperlipidaemias.

Liparison *Zyma, Spain.*
Fenofibrate (p.1273·1).
Hyperlipidaemias.

Liparmonyl *Yves Ponroy, Fr.†.*
Omega-3 marine triglycerides (p.1276·1); wheat-germ oil.
Nutritional supplement.

Liparoid *Guidotti, Ital.†.*
A heparinoid (p.882·3).
Vascular disorders.

Lipase-Se Enzyme Cantassium Co., UK†.
Lipase; selenium yeast (p.1353·3).

Lipaten Merck, S.Afr.
Clofibrate (p.1271·1); nicotinyl alcohol tartrate (p.915·3).
Hyperlipidaemias.

Lipavil Farmades, Ital.†.
Clofibrate (p.1271·1).
Hyperlipidaemias.

Lipavlon Zeneca, Fr.
Clofibrate (p.1271·1).
Hyperlipidaemias.

Lipaxan Italfarmaco, Ital.
Fluvastatin sodium (p.1273·2).
Hypercholesterolaemia.

Lipazil Douglas, Austral.
Gemfibrozil (p.1273·3).
Hyperlipdaemias.

Lipbalm with Sunscreen Hyde, Canad.
Padimate O (p.1488·1).
Sunscreen.

Lipcor Nycomed, Aust.†.
Fenofibrate (p.1273·1).
Hyperlipidaemias.

Lipemol Squibb, Spain.
Pravastatin sodium (p.1277·1).
Hyperlipidaemias.

Lipenan Bouchara, Fr.†.
Clofibride (p.1272·1).
Hyperlipidaemias.

Lipex Amrad, Austral.
Simvastatin (p.1278·2).
Hyperlipidaemias.

Lip-Eze
Note. This name is used for preparations of different composition.
Nyal, Austral.†.
Roxadimate (p.1488·2).
Cracked or chapped lips.

SmithKline Beecham Consumer, Austral.
SPF15+: Ethylhexyl *p*-methoxycinnamate (p.1487·1); avobenzone (p.1486·3).
Dry, cracked, and chapped lips; sunscreen.

Lipguard Nelson, Austral.†.
Dimethicone; chlorhexidine acetate (p.1107·2); padimate O (p.1488·1); allantoin (p.1078·2).
Dry, cracked, or chapped lips; sunscreen.

Lipidax UCB, Ital.†.
Fenofibrate (p.1273·1).
Hyperlipidaemias.

Lipidem Braun, Switz.
Soya oil (p.1355·1).
Contains egg lecithin.
Lipid infusion for parenteral nutrition.

Lipidil
Fournier, Canad.; Fournier, Ger.
Fenofibrate (p.1273·1).
Hyperlipidaemias.

Lipil Ibirn, Ital.†.
Fenofibrate (p.1273·1).
Hyperlipidaemias.

Lipiodol
Salus, Aust.; Mallinckrodt, Austral.; Codali, Belg.; Guerbet, Fr.; Byk Gulden, Ger.; Guerbet, Ital.; Guerbet, Neth.; Guerbet, Norw.; May & Baker, UK.
Iodised oil (p.1006·1).
Radiographic contrast medium.

Lipiscor Sanum-Kehlbeck, Ger.
Marine fish oil (p.1276·1).
Hyperlipidaemias.

Lipisorb
Mead Johnson, Austral.; Mead Johnson, Canad.; Mead Johnson Nutritionals, USA.
Preparation for enteral nutrition.
Malabsorption syndromes.

Lipitor
Parke, Davis, Austral.; Warner-Lambert, Ital.; Parke, Davis, Neth.; Parke, Davis, S.Afr.; Parke, Davis, Swed.; Pfizer, Swed.; Parke, Davis, UK; Parke, Davis, USA.
Atorvastatin calcium (p.1268·1).
Hypercholesterolaemia.

Liplat Esteve, Spain.
Pravastatin sodium (p.1277·1).
Hyperlipidaemias.

Liple Green Cross, Jpn.
Alprostadil (p.1412·2).
Maintenance of patent ductus arteriosus; peripheral vascular disorders; skin ulcers.

Lipo Cordes Ichthyol, Ger.
Allantoin (p.1078·2); dexpanthenol (p.1570·3); ethyl linoleate.
Skin disorders.

Lipo Sol Widmer, Switz.
Triclosan (p.1127·2).
Acne; seborrhoea.

Lipobalsamo Teofarma, Ital.
Cineole (p.1564·1); guaiacol (p.1061·2).
Respiratory-tract disorders.

Lipobase
Yamanouchi, Irl.; Yamanouchi, UK.
Cetostearyl alcohol (p.1383·2); cetomacrogol (p.1325·1); liquid paraffin (p.1382·1); white soft paraffin (p.1382·3).
Diluent for Locoid Lipocream.

Lipobay
Bayer, Neth.; Bayer, Swed.; Bayer, UK.
Cerivastatin sodium (p.1269·3).
Hypercholesterolaemia.

Lipoclar Crinos, Ital.
Fenofibrate (p.1273·1).
Hyperlipidaemias.

Lipoclin
Kwizda, Aust.; Sumitomo, Jpn.
Clinofibrate (p.1271·1).
Hyperlipidaemias.

Lipocol Merz, Ger.
Cholestyramine (p.1269·3).
Hypercholesterolaemia.

Lipodel Synthelabo, Ital.
Pantethine (p.1276·3).
Lipid disorders.

Lipofacton Nourypharma, Ger.†.
Clofibrate (p.1271·1); nicotinyl alcohol tartrate (p.915·3).
Lipid disorders.

Lipofene Teofarma, Ital.
Fenofibrate (p.1273·1).
Hyperlipidaemias.

Lipoflavonoid
Lipomed, UK†; Numark, USA.
Multivitamin preparation with lemon bioflavonoids (p.1580·1).

Lipofren Abello, Spain.
Lovastatin (p.1275·1).
Hyperlipidaemias.

Lipofundin
Braun, Aust.; Braun, Ger.; Braun, UK.
Soya oil (p.1355·1).
Lipid infusion for parenteral nutrition.

Lipofundin MCT
Braun, Aust.; Braun, Ital.; Braun, Switz.
Soya oil (p.1355·1); medium-chain triglycerides.
Contains egg phospholipids.
Lipid infusion for parenteral nutrition.

Lipofundin MCT/LCT
Omnimed, S.Afr.; Braun, UK.
Soya oil (p.1355·1); medium-chain triglycerides.
Contains egg lecithin.
Lipid infusion for parenteral nutrition.

Lipofundin S
Braun, Irl.; Braun, Ital.
Soya oil (p.1355·1).
Lipid infusion for parenteral nutrition.

Lipofundina MCT/LCT Braun, Spain.
Soya oil (p.1355·1).
Lipid infusion for parenteral nutrition.

Lipogen Goldline, USA.
Vitamin B substances.
It may also contain vitamin C.

Lipoglutaren Recordati, Ital.†.
Meglutol (p.1275·3).
Lipid disorders.

Lipograsil Uriach, Spain.
Cynara (p.1569·2); cascara (p.1183·1); phenolphthalein (p.1208·2); fucus (p.1554·1).
Formerly contained cynara, cascara, phenolphthalein, fucus, caffeine citrate, thyroid extract, magnesium chloride and sodium bicarbonate.
Obesity.

Lipo-Merz
Kolassa, Aust.; Merz, Ger.; Merz, Switz.
Etofibrate (p.1272·3).
Hyperlipidaemias.

Lipomul Roberts, USA.
High calorie preparation containing maize oil for enteral nutrition(p.1598·3).

Liponet UCB, Spain.
Pantethine (p.1276·3).
Hyperlipidaemias.

Lipo-Nicin ICN, USA†.
Nicotinic acid (p.1351·2); vitamins B and C.
Nicotinic acid deficiency.

Liponol Rugby, USA.
Vitamin B substances with methionine.

Liponorm Gentili, Ital.
Simvastatin (p.1278·2).
Coronary arteriosclerosis; hypercholesterolaemia; ischaemic heart disease.

Lipopill Roussel, Ital.†.
Phentermine resinate (p.1484·3).
Obesity.

Liporex Synthelabo, Fr.†.
Choline citrate (p.1337·1); betaine (p.1553·2); inositol (p.1591·1); sorbitol (p.1354·2); arginine (p.1334·1); vitamin B substances.
Constipation; dyspepsia.

Liposit
Note. This name is used for preparations of different composition.
Merz, Ger.
Sitosterol (p.1279·3).
Hyperlipidaemias.

SIT, Ital.†.
Fenofibrate (p.1273·1).
Hyperlipidaemias.

Liposom Fidia, Ital.
Hypothalamic phospholipid liposomes (p.1599·1).
Neuroendocrine disorders.

Lipostabil
Note. This name is used for preparations of different composition.
Nattermann, Ger.
Essential phospholipids.
Lipid disorders.

Rhone-Poulenc Rorer, Ital.
Phosphatidyl choline (p.1618·1).
Fat emboli; hyperlipidaemias.

Rhone-Poulenc Rorer, S.Afr.
Capsules: Essential phospholipids; multivitamins; theophylline (p.765·1).
Atherosclerosis; diabetic angiopathies; hyperlipidaemias.
Injection: Essential phospholipids; multivitamins; adenosine phosphate (p.1543·2).
Atherosclerosis; hyperlipidaemias; thrombo-embolic disorders.

Lipostabil Forte Nattermann, Spain†.
Etofylline (p.753·1); phospholipids.
Arteriosclerosis; hyperlipidaemias; post-myocardial infarction circulatory disorders.

Lipostat
Note. This name is used for preparations of different composition.
Bristol-Myers Squibb, Irl.; Bristol-Myers Squibb, UK.
Pravastatin sodium (p.1277·1).
Atherosclerosis; hypercholesterolaemia; myocardial infarction.

Del Saz & Filippini, Ital.
A heparinoid (p.882·3).
Thrombosis prophylaxis.

Lipostop Francia, Ital.
A heparinoid (p.882·3).
Thrombosis prophylaxis.

Liposyn
Abbott, Canad.†; Abbott, Ital.; Abbott, Swed.
Fractionated safflower oil (p.1353·3); fractionated soya oil (p.1355·1).
Contains fractionated egg lecithin.
Lipid infusion for parenteral nutrition.

Liposyn II Abbott, USA.
Safflower oil (p.1353·3); soya oil (p.1355·1).
Contains egg phospholipids.
Lipid infusion for parenteral nutrition.

Liposyn III Abbott, USA.
Soya oil (p.1355·1).
Contains egg phospholipids.
Lipid infusion for parenteral nutrition.

Lipotalon Merckle, Ger.
Dexamethasone palmitate (p.1037·3).
Rheumatic disorders.

Lipotrend Cholesterol Boehringer Mannheim, Ital.
Test for cholesterol in blood.

Lipotriad
Lipomed, UK†.
Multivitamin preparation.

Numark, USA.
Multivitamin and mineral preparation.

Lipotropic Factors Solgar, UK.
Choline bitartrate (p.1337·1); inositol (p.1591·1); methionine (p.984·2).
Dietary supplement.

Lipovas Daker Farmasimes, Spain†.
Fenofibrate (p.1273·1).
Hyperlipidaemias.

Lipoven Fresenius, Fr.
Soya oil (p.1355·1).
Contains egg lecithin.
Lipid infusion for parenteral nutrition.

Lipovenoes Fresenius, Belg.
Soya oil (p.1355·1).
Contains egg lecithin.
Lipid infusion for parenteral nutrition.

Lipovenos
Leopold, Aust.; Fresenius, Ger.; SIFRA, Ital.; Fresenius, Norw.; Mein, Spain; Meda, Swed.; Fresenius, Switz.; Fresenius, UK.
Soya oil (p.1355·1).
Contains egg lecithin.
Lipid infusion for parenteral nutrition.

Lipovenous Intramed, S.Afr.
Soya oil (p.1355·1).
Contains egg lecithin.
Lipid infusion for parenteral nutrition.

Lipovit Brunel, S.Afr.
Multivitamin preparation.

Lipovite Rugby, USA†.
Vitamin B substances and choline.

Lipox TAD, Ger.
Bezafibrate (p.1268·2).
Hyperlipidaemias.

Lipozet Zwintscher, Ger.†.
Aloes (p.1177·1); senna (p.1212·2); orthosiphon (p.1592·2); bladderwrack (p.1554·1); crataegus (p.1568·2); khellin; camphor; sapo med.
Constipation.

Lipozid Poli, Ital.
Gemfibrozil (p.1273·3).
Hyperlipidaemias.

Liprevil Schwarz, Ger.
Pravastatin sodium (p.1277·1).
Hyperlipidaemias.

Liprocil
Note. This name is used for preparations of different composition.
Clintec, Fr.
Medium-chain triglycerides; vitamins.
Nutritional supplement.

Roussel, S.Afr.†.
Medium chain triglyceride oil.
Fat intolerance; nutritional supplement.

Lip-Sed
Note. This name is used for preparations of different composition.
Parke, Davis, Austral.†.
Lotion: Lignocaine (p.1293·2); chlorhexidine acetate (p.1107·2); salol (p.83·1).
Cracked lips; herpes labialis.

Parke, Davis, Austral.
Medicated stick: Ethylhexyl *p*-methoxycinnamate (p.1487·1); oxybenzone (p.1487·3); avobenzone (p.1486·3).
Chapped, cracked, or blistered lips; sunscreen.

Warner-Lambert, Austral.†.
Topical gel: Padimate O (p.1488·1).
Dry, cracked, or chapped lips; sunscreen.

Lipshield Lipbalm Mentholatum, Canad.
SPF 21: Padimate O (p.1488·1); ethylhexyl *p*-methoxycinnamate (p.1487·1); oxybenzone (p.1487·3).
Sunscreen.

Lipsin
Nycomed, Aust.; Hoechst Marion Roussel, S.Afr.
Fenofibrate (p.1273·1).
Hyperlipidaemias.

Lipur Parke, Davis, Fr.
Gemfibrozil (p.1273·3).
Hyperlipidaemias.

Liquemin
Roche, Aust.; Roche, Ital.; Roche, Neth.†.
Heparin (p.879·3) or heparin sodium (p.879·3).
Thrombo-embolic disorders.

Liquemin N Roche, Ger.
Heparin sodium (p.879·3).
Thrombo-embolic disorders.

Liquemine
Roche, Belg.; Roche, Fr.†; Roche, Switz.
Heparin sodium (p.879·3).
Hyperlipidaemias; thrombo-embolic disorders.

Liqufruta Cough Medicine LRC Products, UK.
Ipecacuanha (p.1062·2); menthol (p.1600·2); glucose (p.1343·3).
Coughs.

Liqufruta Garlic Cough Medicine LRC Products, UK.
Garlic oil; guaiphenesin (p.1061·3).
Coughs.

Liquibid Ion, USA.
Guaiphenesin (p.1061·3).

Liquibid-D Ion, USA.
Guaiphenesin (p.1061·3); phenylephrine hydrochloride (p.1066·2).
Upper respiratory-tract symptoms.

Liquicard Duopharm, Ger.
Crataegus (p.1568·2).
Circulatory disorders; heart failure.

Liqui-Char
Oxford Pharmaceuticals, UK; Jones, USA.
Activated charcoal (p.972·2).
Emergency treatment of poisoning.

Liquid B Complex Jamieson, Canad.
Vitamin B substances.

Liquid Pred Muro, USA.
Prednisone (p.1049·2).
Corticosteroid.

Liquid Soap Pre-Op Delta, Austral.
Triclosan (p.1127·2).
Skin cleansing.

Liquidepur Woelm, Ger.
Senna (p.1212·2).
Constipation.

Liqui-Doss Ferndale, USA.
Liquid paraffin (p.1382·1).
Constipation.

Liquifer
Abbott, Aust.; Abbott, Ger.†; Abbott, Ital.; Abbott, Neth.; Abbott, S.Afr.†; Abbott, Switz.
Ferrous polystyrene sulphonate or ferrous sulphate (p.1340·2).
Ascorbic acid (p.1365·2) may be included in this preparation to increase the absorption and availability of iron.
Anaemia.

Liquifilm
Allergan, Aust.; Allergan, Austral.; Allergan, Belg.; Allergan, Canad.; Allergan, Fr.; Allergan, Ger.; Allergan, Irl.; Allergan, Neth.†; Allergan, S.Afr.; Allergan, Switz.; Allergan, USA.
Polyvinyl alcohol (p.1474·2).
Dry eyes; wetting and lubricating solution for contact lenses.

Liquifilm Lagrimas Allergan, Spain.
Polyvinyl alcohol (p.1474·2).
Dry eyes.

Liquifilm Tears Allergan, UK.
Polyvinyl alcohol (p.1474·2).
Dry eyes.

Liquifilm Wetting Allergan, USA.
Wetting solution for hard contact lenses.

Liquifresh Allergan, Spain.
Polyvinyl alcohol (p.1474·2); povidone (p.1474·2).
Contact lens discomfort; dry eyes.

Liquigen
Scientific Hospital Supplies, Austral.; Scientific Hospital Supplies, Irl.; Scientific Hospital Supplies, UK.
Medium chain triglycerides.
Enteral nutrition.

Liquigesic Co *Paedpharm, Austral.*
Paracetamol (p.72·2); codeine phosphate (p.26·1).
Pain.

Liqui-Histine DM *Liquipharm, USA.*
Dextromethorphan hydrobromide (p.1057·3); phenylpropanolamine hydrochloride (p.1067·2); brompheniramine maleate (p.403·2).
Upper respiratory-tract symptoms.

Liquimat *Owen, USA.*
Sulphur (p.1091·2).
Acne; oily skin.

Liquipake *Lafayette, USA.*
Barium sulphate (p.1003·1).
Contrast medium for gastro-intestinal radiography.

Liquipom Dexa Antib *Iquinosa, Spain.*
Dexamethasone sodium phosphate (p.1037·2); neomycin sulphate (p.229·2); polymyxin B sulphate (p.239·1).
Infected eye and ear disorders.

Liquipom Dexa Const *Iquinosa, Spain.*
Dexamethasone sodium phosphate (p.1037·2); phenylephrine hydrochloride (p.1066·2).
Eye disorders.

Liquipom Dexamida *Iquinosa, Spain.*
Dexamethasone sodium phosphate (p.1037·2); phenylephrine hydrochloride (p.1066·2); sulphacetamide sodium (p.252·2).
Infected eye disorders.

Liquipom Medrisone *Iquinosa, Spain.*
Medrysone (p.1045·3).
Eye disorders.

Liquiprin *Menley & James, USA.*
Paracetamol (p.72·2).
Fever; pain.

Liquirit N *Loges, Ger.*
Algeldrate (p.1177·3); magnesium carbonate (p.1198·1); liquorice (p.1197·1).
Gastro-intestinal disorders.

Liquisorb *E. Merck, UK†.*
Gluten-free, low-lactose preparation for enteral nutrition.

Liquisorb B vit *Kabi Pharmacia, Ger.†.*
Multivitamin and mineral preparation.

Liquisorb K *Kabi Pharmacia, Ger.†.*
Potassium chloride (p.1161·1); potassium bicarbonate (p.1153·1); monobasic potassium phosphate (p.1159·3).
Potassium deficiency.

Liquisorbon MCT
Nutricia, Irl.; Nutricia, UK.
Gluten- and fructose-free, low-lactose preparation for enteral nutrition.
Fat malabsorption.

Liruptin *Fides, Ger.†.*
Solidago virgaurea; equisetum (p.1575·1); scoparium (p.1628·1); urtica (p.1642·3); birch leaf (p.1553·3); ononis (p.1610·2); rubia tinctorum; echinacea (p.1574·2); bearberry (p.1552·2); tilia (p.1637·3); acid benz.; calculi ren.; acid. oxalic.
Urinary-tract disorders.

Lis *Lisapharma, Ital.*
Lactulose (p.1195·3).
Constipation; disturbances of the gastro-intestinal flora; hepatic cirrhosis; hepatic encephalopathy.

Lisa *Lisapharma, Ital.*
Cefonicid sodium (p.167·2).
Lignocaine hydrochloride (p.1293·2) is included in the intramuscular injection to alleviate the pain of injection.
Bacterial infections.

Lisabutina *Lisapharma, Ital.†.*
Phenylbutazone (p.79·2); tripelennamine hydrochloride (p.420·2).
Musculoskeletal and joint disorders; neuralgia; neuritis.

Lisacef *Lisapharma, Ital.*
Cephradine (p.181·3).
Lignocaine hydrochloride (p.1293·2) is included in the intramuscular injection to alleviate the pain of injection.
Bacterial infections.

Lisal *Pharmacia, Swed.†.*
Sodium chloride (p.1162·2).
Contact lens care; eye wash.

Lisanirc *Lisapharma, Ital.*
Nicardipine hydrochloride (p.915·1).
Angina pectoris; cerebrovascular disorders; heart failure; hypertension; Ménière's disease.

Lisenteral *Lisapharma, Ital.*
Lysates of various *E. coli* strains and other coliform bacteria.
Colibacilliary gastro-intestinal and genito-urinary infections.

Liserdol
Wyeth, Ger.; Pharmacia Upjohn, Ital.; Pharmacia Upjohn, S.Afr.; Wyeth, Switz.
Metergoline (p.1142·3).
Galactorrhoea; gastric motility disorders; hyperprolactinaemia; lactation inhibition; menstrual disorders; migraine.

Lisi-Budol *Merck Sharp & Dohme, Spain†.*
Ibuprofen lysine (p.44·3).
Fever; inflammation; pain.

Lisiflen *Pulitzer, Ital.†.*
A heparinoid (p.882·3); aminopropylone (p.15·2).
Inflammation; pain.

Lisil *KBR, Ital.*
Carbocisteine (p.1056·3).
Respiratory-tract disorders associated with increased or viscous mucus.

Lisino *Essex, Ger.*
Loratadine (p.413·1).
Hypersensitivity reactions.

Lisiofer *Cortissone, Ital.*
Ferric sodium gluconate (p.1340·1).
Anaemia.

Lisi-Vigor *Ripari-Gero, Ital.†.*
Vitamin B substances.

Liskantin *Desitin, Ger.*
Primidone (p.358·3).
Epilepsy.

Liskonum *SmithKline Beecham, UK.*
Lithium carbonate (p.290·3).
Bipolar disorder; mania.

Lismol *Lesvi, Spain.*
Cholestyramine (p.1269·3).
Hyperlipidaemias.

Lisolipin *Bracco, Ital.†.*
Dextrothyroxine sodium (p.1272·2).
Hypercholesterolaemia.

Lisomucil *Synthelabo, Ital.*
Carbocisteine (p.1056·3).
Respiratory-tract disorders.

Lisomucil Teofillina *Lirca, Ital.†.*
Carbocisteine (p.1056·3); theophylline (p.765·1).
Respiratory-tract disorders.

Lisopulm *Esseti, Ital.*
Ambroxol hydrochloride (p.1054·3).
Respiratory-tract disorders.

Listerex *Warner-Lambert, USA†.*
Salicylic acid (p.1090·2).
Acne.

Listerfluor *Parke, Davis, S.Afr.*
Sodium fluoride (p.742·1).
Dental caries prophylaxis.

Listerine
Note. This name is used for preparations of different composition.
Warner-Lambert, Canad.
Lozenges†: Hexylresorcinol (p.1116·1); menthol (p.1600·2); cineole (p.1564·1).
Sore throat.
Mouthwash: Cineole (p.1564·1); thymol (p.1127·1); menthol (p.1600·2).
Dental plaque prophylaxis; oral hygiene.
Warner-Lambert, Irl.; Warner-Lambert, UK; Warner-Wellcome, USA.
Cineole (p.1564·1); menthol (p.1600·2); methyl salicylate (p.55·2); thymol (p.1127·1).
Dental plaque prophylaxis; oral hygiene.

Listermint *Warner-Lambert, UK.*
Cetylpyridinium chloride (p.1106·2); zinc chloride (p.1373·1).
Oral hygiene.

Listermint Arctic Mint Mouthwash *Warner-Wellcome, USA.*
Glycerol (p.1585·2).

Listermint with Fluoride
Note. This name is used for preparations of different composition.
Warner-Lambert, Irl.; Warner-Lambert, UK.
Sodium fluoride (p.742·1); cetylpyridinium chloride (p.1106·2).
Oral hygiene.
Warner-Lambert, USA†.
Sodium fluoride (p.742·1).
Dental caries prophylaxis.

Listomin *Lion, Jpn†.*
Butoctamide hemisuccinate.

Listran *Uriach, Spain.*
Nabumetone (p.60·1).
Musculoskeletal and joint disorders.

Litalir
Bristol-Myers Squibb, Ger.; Bristol-Myers Squibb, Switz.
Hydroxyurea (p.539·1).
Malignant neoplasms.

Litarek *Kendall, Spain.*
Gemfibrozil (p.1273·3).
Hyperlipidaemias.

Litarex
Dumex, Neth.†; Astra, Norw.; Astra, Swed.†; Dumex, Switz.; Dumex, UK.
Lithium citrate (p.290·3).
Bipolar disorder; mania.

Lithane *Pfizer, Canad.*
Lithium carbonate (p.290·3).
Bipolar disorder.

Lithiabyl *Plantes et Medecines, Fr.*
Berberis vulgaris; urtica (p.1642·3); taraxacum (p.1634·2).
Formerly contained berberis and hexamine.
Digestive disorders.

Lithiagel *Cochon, Fr.*
Basic aluminium carbonate (p.1177·2).
Diagnosis of hyperparathyroidism; hyperphosphataemia due to chronic renal failure.

Lithias-cyl Ho-Len-Complex *Liebermann, Ger.*
Homoeopathic preparation.

Lithicarb *Rhone-Poulenc Rorer, Austral.*
Lithium carbonate (p.290·3).
Bipolar disorder.

Lithines *Rovi, Spain†.*
Lithium carbonate (p.290·3); sodium bicarbonate (p.1153·2); tartaric acid (p.1634·3).
Gastro-intestinal hyperacidity.

Lithines Magnesies *Sorin-Maxim, Fr.†.*
Lithium carbonate (p.290·3); magnesium chloride (p.1157·2); tartaric acid (p.1634·3); sodium bicarbonate (p.1153·2).
Adjunct in lithium therapy.

Lithiofor *Vifor, Switz.*
Lithium sulphate (p.295·1).
Bipolar disorders; depression.

Lithionit
Astra, Norw.; Astra, Swed.
Lithium sulphate (p.295·1).
Bipolar disorder; mania.

Lithizine *Technilab, Canad.*
Lithium carbonate (p.290·3).
Bipolar disorder.

Lithobid *Solvay, USA.*
Lithium carbonate (p.290·3).
Bipolar disorder.

Lithofalk
Merck, Aust.†; Falk, Ger.; Falk, Switz.; Thames, UK†.
Chenodeoxycholic acid (p.1562·1); ursodeoxycholic acid (p.1642·1).
Cholesterol gallstones.

Lithonate
Approved Prescription Services, UK; Solvay, USA.
Lithium carbonate (p.290·3).
Bipolar disorder; depression; mania.

Lithostat *Mission Pharmacal, USA.*
Acetohydroxamic acid (p.1541·3).
Urinary-tract infection with urea-splitting organisms.

Lithotabs *Solvay, USA.*
Lithium carbonate (p.290·3).
Bipolar disorder.

Lithurex *Phonix, Ger.*
Pyridoxine hydrochloride; magnesium citrate pentahydrate (p.1198·2); citric acid monohydrate (p.1564·3); sodium citrate (p.1153·2); potassium citrate (p.1153·1).
Urinary-tract disorders.

Litiax *Novag, Spain.*
Quercus infectoria (p.1582·1).
Renal calculi.

Litican
Synthelabo, Belg.; Lorex Synthelabo, Neth.
Alizapride hydrochloride (p.1176·3).
Nausea; vomiting.

Liticon *Lagap, Ital.†.*
Pentazocine lactate (p.75·1).
Pain.

Liticum *Delagrange, Spain†.*
Alizapride hydrochloride (p.1176·3).
Gastro-oesophageal reflux; gastroparesis; nausea and vomiting.

Litinoides *Serra Pamies, Spain†.*
Lithium carbonate (p.290·3); sodium bicarbonate (p.1153·2); tartaric acid (p.1634·3).
Gastro-intestinal hyperacidity.

Litobile *Poli, Ital.*
Magnesium trihydrate salt of chenodeoxycholic (p.1562·1) and ursodeoxycholic acids (p.1642·1).
Biliary dyspepsia; gallstones.

Litoff *Caber, Ital.*
Ursodeoxycholic acid (p.1642·1).
Biliary-tract disorders.

Litosmil *Evans, Fr.*
Diosmin (p.1580·1).
Peripheral vascular disorders.

Litoxol *SmithKline Beecham Sante, Fr.*
Sulphaguanidine (p.254·1); aluminium salicylate.
Infective diarrhoea.

Litrison *Roche, Ital.*
Choline bitartrate (p.1337·1); DL-methionine (p.984·2); vitamin B substances.
Liver disorders.

Little Trimmers Herbal Formula SL28 *Suisse, Austral.†.*
Mandrake; gotu cola; gentian; fennel; boldo; walnut; hawthorn; bearberry; kola nut; buchu; bladderwrack; dandelion; alfalfa; golden seal; sarsaparilla root; emukra; chickweed; liquorice root; echinacea; safflower; lecithin; apple cider vinegar; papaya; chlorophyll; spirulina; great northern white bean; soy bean protein.
Herbal supplement for dieting.

Litursol *Crinos, Ital.*
Ursodeoxycholic acid (p.1642·1).
Biliary-tract disorders.

Liv 52 *Ebi, Switz.*
Capparis spinosa; cichorium intybus; solanum nigrum; cassia occidentalis; terminalia arjuna; achillea millefolium; tamarix gallica; ferrum bhasma.
Gastro-intestinal disorders; tonic.

Livadex *Restan, S.Afr.*
Vitamin B substances; liver extracts; caffeine.
Tonic.

Livaid *Lagamed, S.Afr.†.*
Vitamin B substances; liver extracts.
Tonic.

Livamine *Bioceuticals, UK.*
Multivitamin and mineral preparation.

Livartil *Sodip, Switz.†.*
Cynara (p.1569·2); kinkéliba (p.1593·2); boldo (p.1554·1); orthosiphon (p.1592·2).
Gastro-intestinal disorders.

Liv-Detox *Blackmores, Austral.*
DL-Methionine (p.984·2); choline bitartrate (p.1337·1); inositol (p.1591·1); levoglutamide (p.1344·3); pyridoxine hydrochloride (p.1362·3); riboflavine (p.1362·1); sodium sulphate (p.1213·3).
Liver disorders.

Liver Tonic Capsules *Vita Glow, Austral.*
Silybum marianum (p.993·3).
Antioxidant supplement; dyspepsia; liver tonic.

Liver Tonic Herbal Formula 6 *Vitelle, Austral.*
Silybum marianum (p.993·3); taraxacum (p.1634·2); cynara (p.1569·2); garlic (p.1583·1).
Digestive disorders; liver tonic.

Liverasi *Francia, Ital.*
Cogalactoisomerase sodium (p.1566·2).
Liver disorders.

Liverasten *UCB, Ital.†.*
Suprarenal cortex (p.1050·1); cyanocobalamin (p.1363·3); calcium folinate (p.1342·2); cytidine; uridine (p.1641·3).
Lignocaine hydrochloride (p.1293·2) is included in this preparation to alleviate the pain of injection.
Deficiency states.

Liver-Atox Dus *Ist. Chim. Inter., Ital.†.*
Multivitamin preparation with inosine (p.1591·1).

Liverchin *Salus, Ital.†.*
Cynarine (p.1569·3); solanum melongena; sorbitol (p.1354·2).
Digestive disorders; liver and biliary-tract disorders.

Livercrom *Byk Elmu, Spain.*
Arginine timonacicate (p.1334·2).
Liver disorders.

Liverest *Farmacologico Milanese, Ital.†.*
Inosine (p.1591·1); folic acid (p.1340·3); cyanocobalamin (p.1363·3).
Anaemia; deficiency states.

Liverguard *Pharmadass, UK.*
Capparis spinosa; achorium intybus; solanum nigrum; cassia occidentalis; terminalia arjuna; achillea millifolium (p.1542·2); tamarix gallica; mandur bhasma.

Livial
Organon, Belg.; Organon, Irl.; Organon, Ital.; Organon, Neth.; Organon, UK.
Tibolone (p.1466·3).
Menopausal disorders; osteoporosis.

Liviane Compuesto *Knoll, Spain.*
Aescin (p.1543·3); thiocolchicoside (p.1322·1).
Musculoskeletal lesions; peripheral vascular disorders.

Liviel *Organon, Aust.*
Tibolone (p.1466·3).
Menopausal disorders.

Livifem *Donmed, S.Afr.*
Tibolone (p.1466·3).
Menopausal disorders.

Livitamin *SmithKline Beecham Consumer, USA†.*
Capsules; liquid: Iron (p.1346·1); liver (desiccated or fraction); vitamin B substances; copper.
Vitamin C (p.1365·2) is included in the capsules to increase the absorption and availability of iron.
Chewable tablets: Ferrous fumarate (p.1339·3); vitamin B substances.
Vitamin C (p.1365·2) is included in this preparation to increase the absorption and availability of iron.
Iron-deficiency anaemias.

Livitamin with Intrinsic Factor *SmithKline Beecham Consumer, USA†.*
Ferrous fumarate (p.1339·3); intrinsic factor; liver (desiccated); vitamin B substances; copper.
Vitamin C (p.1365·2) is included in this preparation to increase the absorption and availability of iron.
Anaemias.

Liviton *Restan, S.Afr.*
Vitamins; minerals; caffeine; liver extracts.
Tonic.

Livitrinsic-f *Goldline, USA.*
Ferrous fumarate (p.1339·3); folic acid (p.1340·3); intrinsic factor; vitamin B_{12} substances (p.1363·3).
Vitamin C (p.1365·2) is included in this preparation to increase the absorption and availability of iron.
Anaemias.

Livocab
Janssen-Cilag, Ger.; Taxandria, Neth.; Janssen-Cilag, Spain.
Levocabastine hydrochloride (p.412·3).
Allergic conjunctivitis; allergic rhinitis.

Livolex *Legere, USA†.*
Vitamins and iron preparation.

Livostin
Janssen-Cilag, Aust.; Janssen-Cilag, Austral.; Janssen-Cilag, Belg.; Janssen-Ortho, Canad.; Janssen-Cilag, Ital.; Janssen-Cilag, Norw.; Janssen-Cilag, S.Afr.; Janssen-Cilag, Swed.; Janssen-Cilag, Switz.; Ciba Vision, UK; Iolab, USA.
Levocabastine hydrochloride (p.412·3).
Allergic conjunctivitis; allergic rhinitis.

Lixacol *Schering-Plough, Spain.*
Mesalazine (p.1199·2).
Ulcerative colitis.

Lixidol *Roche, Ital.*
Ketorolac trometamol (p.49·1).
Pain.

Lixir *Abigo, Swed.*
Multivitamins; caffeine.

Lizipaina *Upsamedica, Spain.*
Bacitracin (p.157·3); muramidase (p.1604·3); papain (p.1614·1).
Mouth and throat inflammation.

LKV-Drops *Freeda, USA.*
Multivitamin preparation.

Llorentecaina Noradrenal *Llorente, Spain.*
Lignocaine hydrochloride (p.1293·2).
Noradrenaline acid tartrate (p.924·1) is included in this preparation as a vasoconstrictor to diminish absorption and localise the effect of the local anaesthetic.
Local anaesthesia.

Lloyd's Cream *Seton, UK.*
Diethylamine salicylate (p.33·1).
Muscular pain.

Lobac
Note. This name is used for preparations of different composition.
Sanofi Winthrop, Norw.†; Sterling Winthrop, Swed.†.
Chlormezanone (p.648·3); paracetamol (p.72·2).
Pain; skeletal muscle spasm.

Seatrace, USA.
Salicylamide (p.82·3); phenyltoloxamine (p.416·1); paracetamol (p.72·2).
Musculoskeletal pain.

Lobak
Sanofi Winthrop, Irl.†; Zurich, S.Afr.; Sanofi Winthrop, UK†.
Chlormezanone (p.648·3); paracetamol (p.72·2).
Pain; skeletal muscle spasm.

Lobamine-Cysteine
Pierre Fabre, Fr.; Actipharm, Switz.
Methionine (p.984·2); cysteine hydrochloride (p.1338·3).
Hair and nail disorders.

Lobana *Ulmer, USA.*
Soap-free skin cleanser.

Lobana Body *Ulmer, USA.*
Emollient and moisturiser.

Lobana Derm-Ade *Ulmer, USA.*
Vitamin A (p.1358·1); vitamin D (p.1366·3); vitamin E (p.1369·1).
Skin disorders.

Lobana Peri-Garde *Ulmer, USA.*
Vitamin A (p.1358·1); vitamin D (p.1366·3); vitamin E (p.1358·1); chloroxylenol (p.1111·1).
Skin disorders.

Lobelia Compound *Gerard House, UK.*
Lobelia (p.1481·3); gum ammoniacum; squill (p.1070·1).
Cough and cold symptoms.

Lobelia Med Complex *Dynamit, Aust.*
Homoeopathic preparation.

Lobione *Rhone-Poulenc Rorer, Belg.*
Betahistine mesylate (p.1553·1).
Vertigo.

Locabiosol
Bender, Aust.; Servier, Ger.
Fusafungine (p.210·3).
Upper respiratory-tract infection and inflammation.

Locabiotal
Eutherapie, Belg.; Therval, Fr.; Servier, Irl.; Stroder, Ital.; Servier, S.Afr.; Servier, Switz.; Servier, UK.
Fusafungine (p.210·3).
Upper respiratory-tract infection and inflammation.

Locacid *Pierre Fabre, Fr.*
Tretinoin (p.1093·3).
Acne.

Locacorten
Ciba, Canad.; Zyma, Ger.; Novartis, Neth.; Ciba, Norw.†; Ciba-Geigy, Swed.†; Max Ritter, Switz.
Flumethasone pivalate (p.1040·3).
Skin disorders.

Locacorten c. Neomycin *Zyma, Switz.†.*
Flumethasone pivalate (p.1040·3); neomycin sulphate (p.229·2).
Infected skin disorders.

Locacorten mit Neomycin *Ciba-Geigy, Aust.*
Flumethasone pivalate (p.1040·3); neomycin sulphate (p.229·2).
Infected skin disorders.

Locacorten Tar
Ciba-Geigy, Aust.; Ciba-Geigy, S.Afr.†; Ciba-Geigy, Swed.†; Max Ritter, Switz.
Flumethasone pivalate (p.1040·3); coal tar (p.1092·3); salicylic acid (p.1090·2).
Skin disorders.

Locacorten Triclosan *Max Ritter, Switz.*
Flumethasone pivalate (p.1040·3); triclosan (p.1127·2).
Infected skin disorders.

Locacorten Vioform
Ciba-Geigy, Aust.; Novartis, Austral.; Ciba, Canad.; Zyma, Ger.; Novartis, Neth.; Ciba, Norw.; Novartis, S.Afr.; Ciba-Geigy, Swed.; Zyma, Switz.†.
Flumethasone pivalate (p.1040·3); clioquinol (p.193·2).
External ear disorders; infected skin disorders.

Locacortene
Note. This name is used for preparations of different composition.
Zyma, Belg.
Flumethasone pivalate (p.1040·3).
Skin disorders.

Ciba-Geigy, Fr.†.
Flumethasone pivalate (p.1040·3); neomycin sulphate (p.229·2).
Infected skin disorders.

Locacortene Tar *Zyma, Belg.*
Flumethasone pivalate (p.1040·3); coal tar (p.1092·3); salicylic acid (p.1090·2).
Skin disorders.

Locacortene Vioforme
Zyma, Belg.; Ciba-Geigy, Fr.†.
Flumethasone pivalate (p.1040·3); clioquinol (p.193·2).
External ear disorders; infected skin disorders.

Localone *Pierre Fabre, Fr.*
Triamcinolone acetonide (p.1050·2); salicylic acid (p.1090·2).
Skin disorders.

Localyn *Recordati, Ital.*
Ear drops: Fluocinolone acetonide (p.1041·1); neomycin sulphate (p.229·2).
Formerly contained fluocinolone acetonide, neomycin sulphate, polymyxin B sulphate, and ketocaine hydrochloride.
Ear disorders.
Lotion; ointment; topical solution: Fluocinolone acetonide (p.1041·1).
Skin disorders.
Nasal spray: Fluocinolone acetonide (p.1041·1); clonazoline hydrochloride (p.1057·1).
Nasal inflammation and hypersensitivity.

Localyn SV *Recordati, Ital.*
Fluocinolone acetonide (p.1041·1).
Nasal inflammation and hypersensitivity.

Localyn-Neomicina *Recordati, Ital.*
Fluocinolone acetonide (p.1041·1); neomycin sulphate (p.229·2).
Infected skin disorders.

Locapred
Pierre Fabre, Fr.; Pierre Fabre, Switz.
Desonide (p.1036·3).
Skin disorders.

Locasalen
Ciba-Geigy, Aust.; Zyma, Belg.; Ciba, Canad.; Zyma, Ger.; Novartis, Neth.; Ciba, Norw.; Ciba-Geigy, Swed.†; Max Ritter, Switz.
Flumethasone pivalate (p.1040·3); salicylic acid (p.1090·2).
Skin disorders.

Locasalene *Ciba-Geigy, Fr.†.*
Flumethasone pivalate (p.1040·3); salicylic acid (p.1090·2).
Skin disorders.

Locaseptil *Syntex, Switz.†.*
Phenylmercuric benzoate; prednisolone acetate (p.1048·1); cinchocaine benzoate (p.1289·3).
Nasal or buccal lesions.

Locaseptil-Neo *Drossapharm, Switz.*
Prednisolone acetate (p.1048·1) cinchocaine (p.1289·2).
Nasal and buccal lesions.

Locasil *Locatelli, Ital.*
Silymarin (p.993·3).
Liver disorders.

Locasol
Nutricia, Austral.; Cow & Gate, UK.
Low-calcium infant feed.
Formerly known as Locasol New Formula in *Austral.*
Hypercalcaemia.

Locasol New Formula *Cow & Gate, Irl.*
Low-calcium food for special diets.

Locatop *Pierre Fabre, Fr.*
Desonide (p.1036·3).
Skin disorders.

Loceptin *Nycomed, Swed.*
Morphine sulphate (p.56·2).
Pain.

Loceryl
Roche, Aust.; Roche, Austral.; Roche, Belg.; Roche, Fr.; Roche, Ger.; Roche, Irl.; Roche, Norw.; Roche, S.Afr.; Roche, Swed.; Roche, Switz.; Roche, UK.
Amorolfine hydrochloride (p.372·1).
Fungal infections of the skin and nails.

Locetar *Andreu, Spain.*
Amorolfine hydrochloride (p.372·1).
Fungal nail infections.

Locid N *Rohm, Ger.†.*
Calcium carbonate (p.1182·1); magnesium hydroxide (p.1198·2); aluminium hydroxide gel (p.1177·3).
Gastro-intestinal disorders.

Locilan *Monsanto, Austral.*
Norethisterone (p.1453·1).
Progestogen-only contraceptive.

Lockolys *Dicamed, Swed.*
Anhydrous glucose; sodium chloride; sodium lactate; calcium chloride; magnesium chloride (p.1151·1).
Peritoneal dialysis solution.

Locobase
Yamanouchi, Ital.; Yamanouchi, Switz.; Brocades, UK†.
Emollient.
Diluents for Locoid preparations.

Locoid
Yamanouchi, Belg.; Yamanouchi, Fr.; Yamanouchi, Irl.; Yamanouchi, Neth.; Yamanouchi, Norw.; Pharmaplan, S.Afr.; Yamanouchi, Swed.; Yamanouchi, Switz.; Yamanouchi, UK; Ferndale, USA.
Hydrocortisone butyrate (p.1044·1).
Skin disorders.

Locoid C
Yamanouchi, Irl.; 3M, S.Afr.†; Yamanouchi, UK.
Hydrocortisone butyrate (p.1044·1); chlorquinaldol (p.185·1).
Skin disorders with bacterial or fungal infection.

Locoid Crelo *Yamanouchi, Swed.*
Hydrocortisone butyrate (p.1044·1).
Skin disorders.

Locoidol *Yamanouchi, Norw.*
Hydrocortisone butyrate (p.1044·1); chlorquinaldol (p.185·1).
Infected skin disorders.

Locoidon
Angelini, Aust.; Yamanouchi, Ital.
Hydrocortisone butyrate (p.1044·1).
Skin disorders.

LOCOL *Sandoz, Ger.*
Fluvastatin sodium (p.1273·2).
Hyperlipidaemias.

Locorten
Novartis Consumer, Ital.
Ear drops; oral drops: Flumethasone pivalate (p.1040·3); clioquinol (p.193·2).
Gingivitis; oral inflammatory lesions; otitis.
Lotion: Flumethasone pivalate (p.1040·3).
Otitis externa; skin disorders.

Zyma, Ital.
Cream; ointment: Flumethasone pivalate (p.1040·3); neomycin sulphate (p.229·2).
Otitis externa; skin disorders.

Locorten Neomicina *Zyma, Ital.†.*
Flumethasone pivalate (p.1040·3); neomycin sulphate (p.229·2).
Skin disorders.

Locorten Tar *Zyma, Ital.*
Flumethasone pivalate (p.1040·3); salicylic acid (p.1090·2); coal tar (p.1092·3).
Skin disorders.

Locorten Vioform *Zyma, UK.*
Flumethasone pivalate (p.1040·3); clioquinol (p.193·2).
Inflammatory disorders of the ear with bacterial or fungal infection; otorrhoea.

Locorten Vioformio *Novartis Consumer, Ital.*
Flumethasone pivalate (p.1040·3); clioquinol (p.193·2).
Skin disorders.

Locortene *Zyma, Spain.*
Flumethasone pivalate (p.1040·3).
Skin disorders.

Locortene Vioformo *Zyma, Spain.*
Clioquinol (p.193·2); flumethasone pivalate (p.1040·3).
Infected skin disorders.

Lodales *Sanofi Winthrop, Fr.*
Simvastatin (p.1278·2).
Hypercholesterolaemia.

Lodema *Hamilton, Austral.*
Coumarin (p.1568·1).
Lymphoedema and elephantitis associated with filariasis; oedema.

Loderix *EGIS, Hung.*
Setastine hydrochloride (p.417·3).
Hypersensitivity reactions.

Loderm *Vinas, Spain.*
Erythromycin (p.204·1) or erythromycin lauryl sulphate.
Acne.

Loderm Retinoico *Vinas, Spain.*
Erythromycin lauryl sulphate; tretinoin (p.1093·3).
Acne.

Lodiar *Ashbourne, UK.*
Loperamide hydrochloride (p.1197·2).
Diarrhoea.

Lodine
Kwizda, Aust.†; Wyeth, Fr.; Wyeth, Ital.; Wyeth, Switz.; Monmouth, UK; Wyeth-Ayerst, USA.
Etodolac (p.36·2).
Musculoskeletal, joint, and peri-articular disorders; pain.

Lodis *Eugal, Ital.*
Loperamide hydrochloride (p.1197·2).
Diarrhoea.

Lodixal *Knoll, Belg.*
Verapamil hydrochloride (p.960·3).
Hypertension.

Lodopin *Fujisawa, Jpn.*
Zotepine (p.700·1).
Schizophrenia.

Lodosyn *Merck, USA.*
Carbidopa (p.1136·1).
Parkinsonism.

Lodrane *ECR, USA.*
Pseudoephedrine hydrochloride (p.1068·3); brompheniramine maleate (p.403·2).
Allergic rhinitis; nasal congestion.

Lodronat *Boehringer Mannheim, Aust.*
Disodium clodronate (p.737·3).
Hypercalcaemia of malignancy; osteolysis of malignancy.

Loesfer *Searle, Switz.*
Ferrous gluconate dihydrate (p.1340·1).
Ascorbic acid (p.1365·2) is included in this preparation to increase the absorption and availability of iron.
Iron deficiency; iron-deficiency anaemia.

Loesfer + acide folique *Searle, Switz.*
Ferrous gluconate dihydrate (p.1340·1); folic acid (p.1340·3).
Ascorbic acid (p.1365·2) is included in this preparation to increase the absorption and availability of iron.
Folic acid deficiency; iron deficiency; iron-deficiency anaemia.

Loestrin
Parke, Davis, UK; Parke, Davis, USA.
Norethisterone acetate (p.1453·1); ethinyloestradiol (p.1445·1).
Combined oral contraceptive.

Loestrin 1.5/30 *Parke, Davis, Canad.*
Norethisterone acetate (p.1453·1); ethinyloestradiol (p.1445·1).
Combined oral contraceptive.

Loestrin Fe *Parke, Davis, USA.*
21 Tablets, norethisterone acetate (p.1453·1); ethinyloestradiol (p.1445·1); 7 tablets, ferrous fumarate (p.1339·3).
Combined oral contraceptive.

Lofenalac
Mead Johnson, Austral.; Bristol-Myers Squibb, Belg.; Mead Johnson, Canad.; Bristol-Myers Squibb, Fr.; Bristol-Myers Squibb, Irl.; Mead Johnson, Ital.; Mead Johnson Nutritionals, UK; Mead Johnson Nutritionals, USA.
Food for special diets.
Phenylketonuria.

Lofenoxal *Monsanto, Austral.*
Diphenoxylate hydrochloride (p.1189·1).
Atropine sulphate (p.455·1) is included in this preparation to discourage abuse.
Diarrhoea.

Lofensaid *Opus, UK.*
Diclofenac sodium (p.31·2).
Inflammation; musculoskeletal, joint, and peri-articular disorders; pain.

Lofoxin *Locatelli, Ital.*
Fosfomycin calcium (p.210·2).
Bacterial infections.

Loftan *Cascan, Ger.; Cascapharm, Ger.*
Salbutamol sulphate (p.758·2).
Obstructive airways disease.

Lofton *Abbott, Spain.*
Buflomedil hydrochloride (p.834·2).
Peripheral vascular disorders.

Loftran *SmithKline Beecham, Canad.†.*
Ketazolam (p.675·2).
Anxiety.

Loftyl
Abbott, Aust.; Abbott, Belg.; Abbott, Fr.; Abbott, Ital.; Abbott, Neth.; Abbott, S.Afr.; Abbott, Switz.
Buflomedil hydrochloride (p.834·2).
Peripheral vascular disorders.

Logacron *Inexfa, Spain.*
Mercurochrome (p.1119·2).
Wound disinfection.

Logamel
Ciba, Norw.†; Zyma, Spain†; Zyma, Switz.†.
Flumethasone pivalate (p.1040·3); triclosan (p.1127·2).
Infected skin disorders.

Logamicyl *CPB, Belg.†.*
Doxycycline hydrochloride (p.202·3).
Bacterial infections.

Logan *Ist. Chim. Inter., Ital.*
Citicoline sodium (p.1564·3).
Arteriosclerosis; cerebral vascular disorders; parkinsonism.

Logastric *Bio-Therabel, Belg.*
Omeprazole (p.1204·2).
Gastro-oesophageal reflux; peptic ulcer; Zollinger-Ellison syndrome.

Logecine *Logeais, Fr.*
Erythromycin (p.204·1).
Bacterial infections.

Logen *Goldline, USA.*
Diphenoxylate hydrochloride (p.1189·1).
Atropine sulphate (p.455·1) is included in this preparation to discourage abuse.
Diarrhoea.

Logicin Chest Rub *Sigma, Austral.*
Menthol (p.1600·2); camphor (p.1557·2); eucalyptus oil (p.1578·1); thymol (p.1127·1); clove oil (p.1565·2); cedar wood oil; turpentine oil (p.1641·1).
Nasal congestion.

Logicin Cough & Cold *Sigma, Austral.*
Codeine phosphate (p.26·1); paracetamol (p.72·2); pseudoephedrine hydrochloride (p.1068·3).
Cold and influenza symptoms.

Logicin Cough Mixture for Congested Chesty Coughs *Sigma, Austral.*
Guaiphenesin (p.1061·3); pseudoephedrine hydrochloride (p.1068·3).
Coughs; nasal congestion.

Logicin Cough Mixture for Dry Coughs *Sigma, Austral.*
Dextromethorphan hydrobromide (p.1057·3); pseudoephedrine hydrochloride (p.1068·3).
Coughs; nasal congestion.

Logicin Flu Strength *Sigma, Austral.*
Dextromethorphan hydrobromide (p.1057·3); pseudoephedrine hydrochloride (p.1068·3); paracetamol (p.72·2).
Cold and influenza symptoms.

Logicin Flu Strength Day & Night *Sigma, Austral.*
Daytime tablets, paracetamol (p.72·2); pseudoephedrine hydrochloride (p.1068·3); dextromethorphan hydrobromide (p.1057·3); night-time tablets, paracetamol; pseudoephedrine hydrochloride; chlorpheniramine maleate (p.405·1).
Cold and influenza symptoms.

Logicin Hay Fever *Sigma, Austral.*
Paracetamol (p.72·2); pseudoephedrine hydrochloride (p.1068·3); chlorpheniramine maleate (p.405·1).
Hay fever.

Logicin Junior Childrens Cough Mixture *Sigma, Austral.*
Dextromethorphan hydrobromide (p.1057·3); pseudoephedrine hydrochloride (p.1068·3).
Coughs; nasal congestion.

Logicin Sinus *Sigma, Austral.*
Pseudoephedrine hydrochloride (p.1068·3).
Upper respiratory-tract congestion.

Logiflox *Monsanto, Fr.*
Lomefloxacin hydrochloride (p.222·2).
Cystitis in women.

Logimat *Astra, Belg.*
Felodipine (p.867·3); metoprolol succinate (p.908·2).
Hypertension.

Logimax
Astra, Aust.; Astra, Fr.; Astra, Norw.; Astra, Spain; Hassle, Swed.; Astra, Switz.
Felodipine (p.867·3); metoprolol succinate (p.908·2).
Hypertension.

Logiparin
Novo Nordisk, Aust.; CSL, Austral.†; Novo Nordisk, Ital.†; Novo Nordisk, S.Afr.†; Novo Nordisk, Swed.†; Novo Nordisk, UK†.
Tinzaparin sodium (p.954·2).
Thrombo-embolic disorders.

Logirene *Pharmacia Upjohn, Fr.*
Frusemide (p.871·1); amiloride hydrochloride (p.819·2).
Heart failure.

Logoderm *Schering-Plough, Austral.*
Alclometasone dipropionate (p.1031·3).
Skin disorders.

Logomed Abfuhr-Dragees *Logomed, Ger.†.*
Bisacodyl (p.1179·3).
Constipation.

Logomed Akne-Gel *Logomed, Ger.†.*
Benzoyl peroxide (p.1079·2).
Acne.

Logomed Allergie-Gel *Logomed, Ger.†.*
Diphenhydramine hydrochloride (p.409·1).
Allergic skin disorders; insect stings; pruritus; sunburn.

Logomed Allergie-Tabletten *Logomed, Ger.*
Terfenadine (p.418·1).
Hypersensitivity reactions.

Logomed Beruhigungs-Tabletten *Logomed, Ger.*
Diphenhydramine hydrochloride (p.409·1).
Sleep disorders.

Logomed Desinfektions-Salbe *Logomed, Ger.*
Povidone-iodine (p.1123·3).
Infected skin disorders; skin ulceration; wounds.

Logomed Durchfall-Kapseln *Logomed, Ger.*
Loperamide hydrochloride (p.1197·2).
Diarrhoea.

Logomed Ekzem-Salbe *Logomed, Ger.*
Bufexamac (p.22·2).
Eczema; neurodermatitis.

Logomed Erkaltungs-Balsam *Logomed, Ger.*
Camphor (p.1557·2); eucalyptus oil (p.1578·1); oleum pini sylvestris; turpentine oil (p.1641·1).
Upper respiratory-tract disorders.

Logomed Galle-Dragees *Logomed, Ger.*
Hymecromone (p.1589·3).
Biliary disorders.

Logomed Hamorrhoiden *Logomed, Ger.*
Bufexamac (p.22·2); lignocaine hydrochloride (p.1293·2); bismuth subgallate (p.1180·2); titanium dioxide (p.1093·3).
Haemorrhoids.

Logomed Hautpilz-Salbe *Logomed, Ger.*
Clotrimazole (p.376·3).
Fungal skin infections.

Logomed Herz *Logomed, Ger.*
Crataegus (p.1568·2).
Cardiac disorders.

Logomed Heuschnupfen-Spray *Logomed, Ger.*
Sodium cromoglycate (p.762·1).
Allergic rhinitis.

Logomed Husten *Logomed, Ger.*
Ambroxol hydrochloride (p.1054·3).
Respiratory disorders associated with viscid or excessive mucus.

Logomed Juckreiz *Logomed, Ger.*
Gel: Diphenhydramine hydrochloride (p.409·1).
Allergic skin disorders; insect stings; pruritus; sunburn.
Tablets†: Terfenadine (p.418·1).
Hypersensitivity reactions.

Logomed Kreislauf-Tabletten *Logomed, Ger.*
Etilefrine hydrochloride (p.867·2).
Hypotension.

Logomed Leber-Kapseln *Logomed, Ger.*
Silybum marianum (p.993·3).
Liver disorders.

Logomed Magen *Logomed, Ger.*
Magaldrate (p.1198·1).
Gastric hyperacidity; peptic ulcer.

Logomed Nasen-Tropfen *Logomed, Ger.*
Xylometazoline hydrochloride (p.1071·2).
Nasal congestion.

Logomed Neuro-Aktiv-Tabletten *Logomed, Ger.*
Pyritinol hydrochloride (p.1624·1).
Cerebrovascular disorders; mental function disorders.

Logomed Prostata-Kapseln *Logomed, Ger.*
Urtica (p.1642·3).
Micturition disorders associated with prostatic cancer.

Logomed Reise-Tabletten *Logomed, Ger.*
Dimenhydrinate (p.408·2).
Motion sickness; nausea and vomiting; vertigo.

Logomed Schmerz *Logomed, Ger.*
Ibuprofen (p.44·1).
Fever; pain.

Logomed Schmerz- /Fieber *Logomed, Ger.*
Paracetamol (p.72·2).
Fever; pain.

Logomed Sport-Gel *Logomed, Ger.*
Heparin sodium (p.879·3).
Soft-tissue injury.

Logomed Venen-Salbe *Logomed, Ger.*
Heparin sodium (p.879·3).
Soft-tissue injury.

Logomed Verdauungs-Kapseln *Logomed, Ger.†.*
Turmeric (p.1001·3).
Biliary disorders.

Logomed Wund-Heilbalsam *Logomed, Ger.†.*
Dexpanthenol (p.1570·3).
Skin lesions.

Logopharm Immun *Logomed, Ger.*
Echinacea purpura (p.1574·2).
Respiratory- and urinary-tract infections.

Logradin *Juste, Spain.*
Loratadine (p.413·1); pseudoephedrine sulphate (p.1068·3).
Allergic rhinitis.

Logroton
Recipe, Aust.; Ciba-Geigy, Belg.; Ciba-Geigy, Fr.; Novartis, Neth.; Ciba-Geigy, S.Afr.†; Ciba, Switz.
Metoprolol tartrate (p.907·3); chlorthalidone (p.839·3).
Hypertension.

Logryx *SCAT, Fr.†.*
Minocycline hydrochloride (p.226·2).
Bacterial infections.

Logynon
Schering, Austral.; Schering, Irl.; Schering, S.Afr.; Schering, UK.
Levonorgestrel (p.1454·1); ethinyloestradiol (p.1445·1).
28-Day packs also contain 7 inert tablets.
Triphasic oral contraceptive.

Loitin *Vita, Spain.*
Fluconazole (p.378·1).
Fungal infections.

Lokalicid *Dermapharm, Ger.*
Clotrimazole (p.376·3).
Fungal skin infections.

Lokalison-antimikrobiell Creme N *Dermapharm, Ger.*
Dexamethasone (p.1037·1); neomycin sulphate (p.229·2); nystatin (p.386·1).
Infected skin disorders.

Lokilan *Roche, Norw.*
Flunisolide (p.1040·3).
Rhinitis.

Lokilan Nasal *Roche, Swed.*
Flunisolide (p.1040·3).
Allergic rhinitis.

Lolum *Lifepharma, Ital.†.*
Labetalol hydrochloride (p.896·1).
Hypertension.

Lomabronchin N *Lomapharm, Ger.*
Homoeopathic preparation.

Lomaherpan
Madaus, Aust.; Lomapharm, Ger.
Melissa (p.1600·1).
Herpesvirus infections.

Lomahypericum *Lomapharm, Ger.*
Hypericum (p.1590·1).
Formerly known as Lophakomp-Hypericum.
Psychiatric disorders.

Lomapect *TAD, Ger.†.*
Yellow tablets, prenoxdiazine hydrochloride (p.1068·3); blue tablets, diphenhydramine hydrochloride (p.409·1); prenoxdiazine hydrochloride.
Coughs.

Lomarheumin N *Lomapharm, Ger.*
Homoeopathic preparation.

Lomarin *Geymonat, Ital.*
Dimenhydrinate (p.408·2).
Nausea; vertigo; vomiting.

Lomasatin M *Lomapharm, Ger.*
Myrrh (p.1606·1).
Mouth and throat inflammation.

Lomatol *Lomapharm, Ger.*
Oral drops: Peppermint leaf (p.1208·1); fennel (p.1579·1); caraway (p.1559·3); absinthium (p.1541·1).
Formerly known as Anethol 36 Lohmann.
Tablets: Absinthium (p.1541·1); caraway (p.1559·3); peppermint leaf (p.1208·1); caraway oil (p.1559·3); peppermint oil (p.1208·1).
Formerly known as Anethol 36 Lohmann.
Gastro-intestinal disorders.

Lomatuell H *Lohmann, Ital.*
White soft paraffin (p.1382·3).
Wound dressing.

Lomazell forte N *Lomapharm, Ger.*
Benzyl nicotinate (p.22·1); nonivamide (p.63·2); bovine placental extract.
Circulatory disorders of the skin.

Lombriareu *Areu, Spain.*
Pyrantel embonate (p.109·3).
Worm infections.

Lomeblastin *Pharmacia Upjohn, Ger.†.*
Lomustine (p.544·1).
Malignant neoplasms.

Lomeflon *Senju, Jpn.*
Lomefloxacin hydrochloride (p.222·2).
Bacterial eye and ear infections.

Lomexin
Angelini, Aust.; Effik, Fr.; S & K, Ger.; Recordati, Ital.; Dominion, UK.
Fenticonazole nitrate (p.377·3).
Fungal infections.

Lomide *Alcon, Austral.*
Lodoxamide trometamol (p.756·1).
Allergic conjunctivitis; vernal keratoconjunctivitis.

Lomir
Sandoz, Aust.; Sandoz, Belg.; Wander, Ger.; Sandoz, Ital.; Novartis, Neth.; Sandoz, Norw.; Sandoz, Spain; Novartis, Swed.; Sandoz, Switz.
Isradipine (p.894·2).
Hypertension.

Lomisat *Fher, Spain†.*
Clobutinol hydrochloride (p.1057·1).
Coughs.

Lomisat Compositum *Fher, Spain†.*
Ammonium chloride (p.1055·2); clobutinol hydrochloride (p.1057·1); orciprenaline sulphate (p.756·3); sodium benzoate (p.1102·3).
Respiratory-tract disorders.

Lomodex 40 *CP Pharmaceuticals, UK†.*
Dextran 40 (p.716·2) in glucose.
Intravascular sludging; plasma volume expansion.

Lomodex 70 *CP Pharmaceuticals, UK†.*
Dextran 70 (p.717·1) in glucose or sodium chloride.
Plasma volume expansion; thrombosis prophylaxis.

Lomol *Du Pont, Fr.†.*
Pentastarch (p.725·2) in sodium chloride.
Hypovolaemia.

Lomont *Rosemont, UK.*
Lofepramine hydrochloride (p.296·1).
Depression.

Lomotil
Searle, Austral.; Searle, Canad.; Searle, Irl.; Searle, S.Afr.; Searle, UK; Searle, USA.
Diphenoxylate hydrochloride (p.1189·1).
Atropine sulphate (p.455·1) is included in this preparation to discourage abuse.
These ingredients can be described by the British Approved Name Co-phenotrope.
Diarrhoea.

Lomper *Esteve, Spain.*
Mebendazole (p.104·1).
Worm infections.

Lomudal
Fisons, Belg.; Specia, Fr.; Italchimici, Ital.; Fisons, Neth.; Rhone-Poulenc Rorer, Norw.; Rhone-Poulenc Rorer, S.Afr.; Rhone-Poulenc Rorer, Swed.; Fisons, Switz.
Sodium cromoglycate (p.762·1).
Allergic conjunctivitis; allergic rhinitis; asthma; bronchial hypersensitivity; food hypersensitivity; inflammatory bowel disease.

Lomudal Comp *Rhone-Poulenc Rorer, S.Afr.†.*
Sodium cromoglycate (p.762·1); isoprenaline sulphate (p.892·1).
Bronchospasm.

Lomudal Compositum *Fisons, Neth.†.*
Sodium cromoglycate (p.762·1); isoprenaline sulphate (p.892·1).
Asthma.

Lomupren *Fisons, Ger.*
Sodium cromoglycate (p.762·1).
Allergic rhinitis.

Lomupren compositum *Fisons, Ger.*
Sodium cromoglycate (p.762·1); xylometazoline hydrochloride (p.1071·2).
Allergic rhinitis.

Lomusol
Sigmapharm, Aust.; Fisons, Belg.; Specia, Fr.; Fisons, Neth.; Fisons, Switz.
Sodium cromoglycate (p.762·1).
Allergic conjunctivitis; allergic rhinitis.

Lomusol comp *Sigmapharm, Aust.*
Sodium cromoglycate (p.762·1); xylometazoline hydrochloride (p.1071·2).
Allergic rhinitis.

Lomusol plus Xylometazoline *Fisons, Belg.*
Sodium cromoglycate (p.762·1); xylometazoline hydrochloride (p.1071·2).
Allergic rhinitis.

Lomusol-X *Fisons, Switz.*
Sodium cromoglycate (p.762·1); xylometazoline hydrochloride (p.1071·2).
Allergic rhinitis; nasal congestion.

Lomuspray *Italchimici, Ital.*
Sodium cromoglycate (p.762·1).
Asthma.

Lonalac *Mead Johnson Nutritionals, USA.*
Preparation for enteral nutrition.

Lonarid
Boehringer Ingelheim, Ger.; Boehringer Ingelheim, Ital.
Paracetamol (p.72·2); codeine phosphate (p.26·1).
Pain.

Lonarid Mono
Boehringer Ingelheim, Belg.; Boehringer Ingelheim, Ger.†.
Paracetamol (p.72·2).
Fever; pain.

Lonarid N
Boehringer Ingelheim, Belg.; Boehringer Ingelheim, Ger.†.
Paracetamol (p.72·2); codeine phosphate (p.26·1); caffeine (p.749·3).
Pain.

Lonavar *CSL, Austral.*
Oxandrolone (p.1458·3).
Anabolic.

London Drugs Baby Sunblock *Tanning Research, Canad.*
SPF 30: Ethylhexyl *p*-methoxycinnamate (p.1487·1); homosalate (p.1487·2); octyl salicylate (p.1487·3); oxybenzone (p.1487·3).
Sunscreen.

London Drugs Dark Tanning *Tanning Research, Canad.*
SPF 4: Menthyl anthranilate (p.1487·2); ethylhexyl *p*-methoxycinnamate (p.1487·1).
Sunscreen.

London Drugs Sport *Tanning Research, Canad.*
SPF 15: Ethylhexyl *p*-methoxycinnamate (p.1487·1); oxybenzone (p.1487·3).
SPF 30: Ethylhexyl *p*-methoxycinnamate (p.1487·1); octyl salicylate (p.1487·3); oxybenzone (p.1487·3).
Sunscreen.

London Drugs Sunblock *Tanning Research, Canad.*
SPF 15: Ethylhexyl *p*-methoxycinnamate (p.1487·1); oxybenzone (p.1487·3).
SPF 30: Ethylhexyl *p*-methoxycinnamate (p.1487·1); homosalate (p.1487·2); octyl salicylate (p.1487·3); oxybenzone (p.1487·3).
Sunscreen.

London Drugs Sunscreen *Tanning Research, Canad.*
SPF 8: Ethylhexyl *p*-methoxycinnamate (p.1487·1); oxybenzone (p.1487·3).
Sunscreen.

Longachin *Teofarma, Ital.*
Quinidine arabogalactane sulphate (p.940·2).
Arrhythmias.

Longacor
Procter & Gamble, Belg.†; Procter & Gamble, Fr.; Rovi, Spain; Nativelle, Switz.
Quinidine arabogalactane sulphate (p.940·2).
Arrhythmias.

Longalgic *Evans, Fr.*
Benorylate (p.21·2).
Pain.

Longastatina *Italfarmaco, Ital.*
Octreotide (p.1255·2).
Acromegaly; diarrhoea associated with immunodeficiency; malignant neoplasms; pancreatic disorders.

Longasteril 40 *Fresenius-Klinik, Ger.*
Dextran 40 (p.716·2) in glucose or sodium chloride.
Plasma volume expansion; thrombosis prophylaxis; vascular disorders.

Longasteril 70 *Fresenius-Klinik, Ger.*
Dextran 70 (p.717·1) with electrolytes.
Plasma volume expansion; thrombosis prophylaxis.

Longatren
Bayer, Aust.; Bayropharm, Ital.†.
Azidocillin sodium (p.155·2).
Bacterial infections.

Longazem *Ripari-Gero, Ital.*
Diltiazem hydrochloride (p.854·2).
Hypertension; ischaemic heart disease.

Longdigox *Trommsdorff, Ger.†.*
β-Acetyldigoxin (p.812·3).
Cardiac disorders.

Longevital *Sanitalia, Ital.*
Pollen; royal jelly (p.1626·3).
Nutritional supplement.

Longifene
Bios, Belg.; Covan, S.Afr.; UCB, Switz.
Buclizine hydrochloride (p.404·1).
Hypersensitivity reactions; motion sickness; nausea; vomiting.

Longivol *Medical, Spain.*
Embryo extract; methyltestosterone; vitamins; caffeine; calcium magnesium phytate; ethinyloestradiol.
Tonic.

Longopax *Essex, Ger.†.*
Perphenazine (p.685·2); amitriptyline hydrochloride (p.273·3).
Psychiatric disorders.

Longtussin *Klinge, Aust.*
Day capsules, etamiphylline hydrochloride (p.753·1); guaiphenesin (p.1061·3); night capsules, codeine (p.26·1); chlorphenoxamine hydrochloride (p.405·3).
Bronchitis; cough.

Longum
Pharmacia Upjohn, Belg.; Pharmacia Upjohn, Ger.; Farmitalia, Spain†.
Sulfametopyrazine (p.251·3).
Bacterial infections; malaria; toxoplasmosis.

Loniten
Pharmacia Upjohn, Aust.; Pharmacia Upjohn, Austral.; Pharmacia Upjohn, Canad.; Pharmacia Upjohn, Irl.; Pharmacia Upjohn, Ital.; Pharmacia Upjohn, S.Afr.; Upjohn, Spain; Pharmacia Upjohn, Switz.; Upjohn, UK; Upjohn, USA.
Minoxidil (p.910·3).
Alopecia androgenetica; hypertension.

Lonnoten
Pharmacia Upjohn, Belg.; Pharmacia Upjohn, Neth.
Minoxidil (p.910·3).
Hypertension.

Lonol *Garec, S.Afr.*
Allopurinol (p.390·2).
Gout; hyperuricaemia.

Lonolox *Pharmacia Upjohn, Ger.*
Minoxidil (p.910·3).
Hypertension.

Lonoten *Pharmacia Upjohn, Fr.*
Minoxidil (p.910·3).
Hypertension.

Lonox *Geneva, USA.*
Diphenoxylate hydrochloride (p.1189·1).
Atropine sulphate (p.455·1) is included in this preparation to discourage abuse.
Diarrhoea.

Lonseren *Rhone-Poulenc Rorer, Spain.*
Pipothiazine palmitate (p.687·1).
Psychoses.

Lo/Ovral *Wyeth-Ayerst, USA.*
Norgestrel (p.1454·1); ethinyloestradiol (p.1445·1).
28-Day packs also contain 7 inert tablets.
Combined oral contraceptive.

Lopalind *Lindopharm, Ger.*
Loperamide hydrochloride (p.1197·2).
Diarrhoea.

Lop-Dia *Gastropharm, Ger.; Philopharm, Ger.*
Loperamide hydrochloride (p.1197·2).
Diarrhoea.

Lopedium
Hexal, Ger.; Hexal, S.Afr.
Loperamide hydrochloride (p.1197·2).
Diarrhoea.

Lopelin *Fumouze, Fr.*
Loperamide hydrochloride (p.1197·2).
Diarrhoea.

Lopemid *Gentili, Ital.*
Loperamide hydrochloride (p.1197·2).
Diarrhoea; ileostomy management.

Loperacap *ICN, Canad.*
Loperamide hydrochloride (p.1197·2).

LoperaGen *Norgine, UK.*
Loperamide hydrochloride (p.1197·2).
Diarrhoea.

Loperam *Septa, Spain†.*
Loperamide (p.1197·3).
Diarrhoea.

Loperamerck *Merck, Ger.*
Loperamide hydrochloride (p.1197·2).
Diarrhoea.

Loperastat *Be-Tabs, S.Afr.*
Loperamide hydrochloride (p.1197·2).
Diarrhoea.

Loperhoe *Betapharm, Ger.*
Loperamide hydrochloride (p.1197·2).
Diarrhoea.

Loperol *Rolab, S.Afr.*
Loperamide hydrochloride (p.1197·2).
Diarrhoea.

Loperyl *SmithKline Beecham, Ital.*
Loperamide hydrochloride (p.1197·2).
Diarrhoea.

Lopetrans *Fresenius-Praxis, Ger.*
Loperamide hydrochloride (p.1197·2).
Diarrhoea.

Lophakomp-B1 *Lomapharm, Ger.*
Thiamine hydrochloride (p.1361·1).
Vitamin B_1 deficiency.

Lophakomp-B6 *Lomapharm, Ger.*
Pyridoxine hydrochloride (p.1362·3).
Vitamin B_6 deficiency.

Lophakomp-B 12 *Lomapharm, Ger.*
Cyanocobalamin (p.1363·3).
Vitamin B_{12} deficiency.

Lophakomp-B 12 Depot *Lomapharm, Ger.*
Hydroxocobalamin acetate (p.1364·2).
Vitamin B_{12} deficiency.

Lophakomp-Echinacea H *Lomapharm, Ger.*
Homoeopathic preparation.

Lophakomp-Hamamelis H *Lomapharm, Ger.*
Homoeopathic preparation.

Lophakomp-Procain N *Lomapharm, Ger.*
Procaine hydrochloride (p.1299·2).
Nervous system disorders.

Lopid
Parke, Davis, Austral.; Parke, Davis, Belg.; Parke, Davis, Canad.; Parke, Davis, Irl.; Parke, Davis, Ital.; Parke, Davis, Neth.; Parke, Davis, S.Afr.; Parke, Davis, Spain; Parke, Davis, Swed.; Parke, Davis, UK; Parke, Davis, USA†.
Gemfibrozil (p.1273·3).
Hyperlipidaemias.

Lopimed *Ecosol, Switz.*
Loperamide hydrochloride (p.1197·2).
Diarrhoea.

Lopirin
Bristol-Myers Squibb, Aust.; Bristol-Myers Squibb, Switz.
Captopril (p.836·3).
Diabetic nephropathy; heart failure; hypertension; myocardial infarction.

Lopirin Cor *Bristol-Myers Squibb, Ger.*
Captopril (p.836·3).
Diabetic nephropathy; heart failure; hypertension.

Lopranol LA *Opus, UK.*
Propranolol hydrochloride (p.937·1).
Angina pectoris; hypertension.

Lopresor
Recipe, Aust.; Novartis, Austral.; Ciba-Geigy, Belg.; Geigy, Canad.; Ciba, Ger.; Geigy, Irl.; Ciba, Ital.; Novartis, Neth.; Novartis, S.Afr.; Padro, Spain; Ciba, Switz.; Geigy, UK.
Metoprolol fumarate (p.908·2) or metoprolol tartrate (p.907·3).
Angina pectoris; arrhythmias; hypertension; hyperthyroidism; migraine; myocardial infarction.

Lopresor Oros *Ciba-Geigy, S.Afr.†.*
Metoprolol fumarate (p.908·2).
Angina pectoris; arrhythmias; hypertension; myocardial infarction.

Lopresoretic
Ciba-Geigy, Irl.†; Geigy, UK†.
Metoprolol tartrate (p.907·3); chlorthalidone (p.839·3).
Hypertension.

Lopressor
Ciba-Geigy, Fr.; Geigy, USA.
Metoprolol tartrate (p.907·3).
Angina pectoris; arrhythmias; hypertension; migraine; myocardial infarction.

Lopressor HCT *Geigy, USA.*
Metoprolol tartrate (p.907·3); hydrochlorothiazide (p.885·2).
Hypertension.

Lopril *Bristol-Myers Squibb, Fr.*
Captopril (p.836·3).
Diabetic nephropathy; heart failure; hypertension; myocardial infarction.

Loprofin
Nutricia, Fr.†; Cow & Gate, Irl.
A range of lactose-free, gluten-free, low-phenylalanine, low-protein foods.
Amino-acid abnormalities including phenylketonuria; liver disorders; renal failure.

Loprox
Hoechst Marion Roussel, Canad.; Bipharma, Neth.; Hoechst Marion Roussel, USA.
Ciclopirox olamine (p.376·2).
Fungal skin infections.

Loptomit *Bournonville, Neth.*
Timolol maleate (p.953·3).
Glaucoma; raised intra-ocular pressure.

Lopurin *Boots, USA†.*
Allopurinol (p.390·2).
Calcium oxalate calculi; gout; hyperuricaemia.

Lorabid
Lilly, Aust.; Lilly, S.Afr.; Lilly, Swed.; Lilly, USA.
Loracarbef (p.222·3).
Bacterial infections.

Loradur *Merckle, Aust.*
Amiloride hydrochloride dihydrate (p.819·2); hydrochlorothiazide (p.885·2).
Hypertension; oedema.

Lorafem *Lilly, Ger.*
Loracarbef (p.222·3).
Bacterial infections.

Loraga *Parke, Davis, Swed.*
Lactulose (p.1195·3).
Constipation; hepatic encephalopathy.

Loramet
Wyeth Lederle, Belg.; Wyeth, Irl.; Wyeth, Neth.; Akromed, S.Afr.; Wyeth, Spain; Wyeth, Switz.
Lormetazepam (p.677·1).
Sedative; sleep disorders.

Lorans *Searle, Ital.*
Lorazepam (p.675·3).
Anxiety; insomnia.

Lorasifar *Siphar, Switz.*
Lorazepam (p.675·3).
Anxiety; sedative; sleep disorders.

Lorastyne *Schering-Plough, Austral.*
Loratadine (p.413·1).
Allergic rhinitis; dermatological hypersensitivity reactions; urticaria.

Lorax
Lilly, Aust.; Lilly, Neth.
Loracarbef (p.222·3).
Bacterial infections.

Loraz *Quantum, USA†.*
Lorazepam (p.675·3).

Lorcet *UAD, USA.*
Hydrocodone tartrate (p.43·1); paracetamol (p.72·2).
Pain.

Lorelco
Nordic, Canad.†; Merrell Dow, USA†.
Probucol (p.1277·3).
Hypercholesterolaemia.

Lorenzo's Oil *Scientific Hospital Supplies, UK.*
Glycerol trioleate; glycerol trierucate (p.1597·1).
Adrenoleucodystrophy.

Lorestat *Recordati, Ital.†.*
Tolrestat (p.333·3).
Diabetic neuropathy.

Loretam *Wyeth, Ger.*
Lormetazepam (p.677·1).
Insomnia; premedication.

Loretic *Xixia, S.Afr.*
Triamterene (p.957·2); hydrochlorothiazide (p.885·2).
Hypertension; oedema.

Lorexane *Zeneca, Irl.†.*
Lindane (p.1407·2).
Pediculosis; scabies.

Lorexina *Crosara, Ital.†.*
Cephalexin (p.178·2).
Bacterial infections.

Loricin *Sigma-Tau, Ital.*
Sulbactam sodium (p.250·3); ampicillin sodium (p.153·1).
Lignocaine hydrochloride (p.1293·2) is included in the intramuscular injection to alleviate the pain of injection.
Bacterial infections.

Loridem *Sandipro, Belg.*
Lorazepam (p.675·3).
Anxiety; insomnia; premedication.

Lorien *Lennon, S.Afr.*
Fluoxetine hydrochloride (p.284·1).
Bulimia nervosa; depression.

Lorinden *Medphano, Ger.†.*
Flumethasone pivalate (p.1040·3).
Skin disorders.

Lorinden T *Medphano, Ger.*
Flumethasone pivalate (p.1040·3); coal tar (p.1092·3); salicylic acid (p.1090·2).
Skin disorders.

Loron
Boehringer Mannheim, Irl.; Boehringer Mannheim, UK.
Disodium clodronate (p.737·3).
Hypercalcaemia of malignancy; tumour-induced osteolysis and bone pain.

Loroxide
Dermik, Canad.; Dermik, USA.
Benzoyl peroxide (p.1079·2).
Acne.

Lortaan *Merck Sharp & Dohme, Ital.*
Losartan potassium (p.899·1).
Hypertension.

Lortab *UCB, USA.*
Hydrocodone tartrate (p.43·1); paracetamol (p.72·2).
Pain.

Lortab ASA *UCB, USA.*
Hydrocodone tartrate (p.43·1); aspirin (p.16·1).
Pain.

Lorzaar *MSD Chibropharm, Ger.*
Losartan potassium (p.899·1).
Hypertension.

Losalen
Novartis Consumer, Ital.; Zyma, Spain.
Flumethasone pivalate (p.1040·3); salicylic acid (p.1090·2).
Skin disorders.

Losan Fe *Hexal, Ger.*
Ferrous gluconate (p.1340·1).
Iron deficiency.

Losapan *Divinal, Ger.†.*
Chelidonium; frangula bark (p.1193·2); boldo (p.1554·1); hedera helix; peppermint leaf (p.1208·1); agrimony; cnicus benedictus (p.1565·3); centaury (p.1561·1); hypericum (p.1590·1).
Biliary disorders; gallstones; gastro-intestinal disorders.

Losaprex *Sigma-Tau, Ital.*
Losartan potassium (p.899·1).
Hypertension.

Losazid *Sigma-Tau, Ital.*
Losartan potassium (p.899·1); hydrochlorothiazide (p.885·2).
Hypertension.

Loscalcon *Beiersdorf-Lilly, Ger.*
Calcium carbonate (p.1182·1).
Calcium deficiency.

Loscon *Basotherm, Ger.*
Medicated shampoo†: Colloidal sulphur (p.1091·2).
Tincture: Thioxolone (p.1093·3); benzoxonium chloride (p.1103·3).
Scalp disorders.

Losec
Astra, Aust.; Astra, Austral.; Astra, Belg.; Astra, Canad.; Astra, Irl.; Schering-Plough, Ital.; Astra, Neth.; Astra, Norw.; Astra, S.Afr.; Schering-Plough, Spain; Hassle, Swed.; Astra, UK.
Omeprazole (p.1204·2), omeprazole magnesium (p.1205·3), or omeprazole sodium (p.1204·2).
Aspiration syndrome; gastro-oesophageal reflux; peptic ulcer; Zollinger-Ellison syndrome.

Losec Helicopak *Astra, Austral.*
Capsules, omeprazole (Losec) (p.1204·2); capsules, amoxycillin trihydrate (Alphamox) (p.151·3); tablets, metronidazole (Metrogyl) (p.585·1).
Peptic ulcer associated with Helicobacter pylori infection.

Losferon *Besins-Iscovesco, Fr.*
Ferrous gluconate (p.1340·1).
Iron deficiency anaemia.

Losferron
Asta Medica, Aust.; Prospa, Belg.; Beiersdorf-Lilly, Ger.; SPA, Ital.; Will-Pharma, Neth.
Ferrous gluconate (p.1340·1).
Ascorbic acid (p.1365·2) may be included in this preparation to increase the absorption and availability of iron.
Iron-deficiency anaemia.

Losferron-Fol *Asta Medica, Aust.*
Ferrous gluconate (p.1340·1); folic acid (p.1340·3).
Ascorbic acid (p.1365·2) is included in this preparation to increase the absorption and availability of iron.
Iron and folic acid deficiency anaemias.

Losnesium *Beiersdorf-Lilly, Ger.*
Magnesium carbonate (p.1198·1); magnesium oxide (p.1198·3).
Magnesium deficiency.

Lotagen *Byk, Belg.*
Metacresolsulphonic acid-formaldehyde (p.725·1).
Gynaecological disorders.

Lotanal *Fher, Spain†.*
Bamethan sulphate (p.827·1); propyphenazone (p.81·3); hyoscine butylbromide (p.462·3).
Dysmenorrhoea.

Lotem *Adcock Ingram, S.Afr.*
Ibuprofen (p.44·1); paracetamol (p.72·2).
Fever; pain.

Lotemax *Bausch & Lomb, USA.*
Loteprednol etabonate (p.1045·3).
Eye disorders.

Lotensin
Ciba, Canad.; Ciba, USA.
Benazepril hydrochloride (p.827·1).
Hypertension.

Lotensin HCT *Ciba-Geigy, USA.*
Benazepril hydrochloride (p.827·1); hydrochlorothiazide (p.885·2).
Hypertension.

Lotharin *Berk, UK.*
Diphenoxylate hydrochloride (p.1189·1).
Atropine sulphate (p.455·1) is included in this preparation to discourage abuse.
The ingredients in this preparation can be described by the British Approved Name Co-phenotrope.
Diarrhoea.

Loticort *Cassella-med, Ital.†.*
Fluorometholone (p.1042·1); aminoquinuride hydrochloride (p.1101·2); resorcinol (p.1090·1); precipitated sulphur (p.1091·2).
Acne; seborrhoeic eczema.

Lotil *Original Additions, UK.*
Emollient.
Dry skin.

Lotio Artesan *Cassella-med, Ger.†.*
Zinc oxide (p.1096·2).
Skin disorders.

Lotio decapans *Widmer, Switz.*
Resorcinol (p.1090·1); salicylic acid (p.1090·2).
Scalp disorders.

Lotio Hermal *Hermal, Ger.†.*
Zinc oxide (p.1096·2); lecithin (p.1595·2); glycerol (p.1585·2).
Skin disorders.

Lotion pour Feux Sauvages
Note. This name is used for preparations of different composition.
Atlas, Canad.
Camphor (p.1557·2); zinc salicylate.

Sabex, Canad.
Benzoin (p.1634·1); camphor (p.1557·2); menthol (p.1600·2); myrrh (p.1606·1).

Valmo, Canad.
Benzoin (p.1634·1); camphor (p.1557·2); menthol (p.1600·2).

Lotocreme *Abbott, S.Afr.†.*
Hexachlorophane (p.1115·2).
Skin disorders.

Lo-Tone *Rolab, S.Afr.†.*
Oxprenolol hydrochloride (p.926·2).
Cardiovascular disorders.

Lotrel *Ciba-Geigy, USA.*
Amlodipine besylate (p.822·3); benazepril hydrochloride (p.827·1).
Hypertension.

Lotremin *Schering-Plough, Austral.†.*
Clotrimazole (p.376·3).
Fungal skin infections.

Lotricomb *Essex, Ger.*
Betamethasone dipropionate (p.1033·3); clotrimazole (p.376·3).
Skin disorders with fungal infections.

Lotriderm
Schering-Plough, Belg.; Schering, Canad.; Schering-Plough, Irl.; Schering-Plough, S.Afr.; Dominion, UK.
Betamethasone dipropionate (p.1033·3); clotrimazole (p.376·3).
Fungal skin infections.

Lotrimin *Schering, USA.*
Clotrimazole (p.376·3).
Fungal skin infections.

Lotrimin AF *Schering-Plough, USA.*
Cream; lotion; topical solution: Clotrimazole (p.376·3).
Powder; spray: Miconazole nitrate (p.384·3).
Fungal skin infections.

Lotrisone *Schering, USA.*
Betamethasone dipropionate (p.1033·3); clotrimazole (p.376·3).
Fungal skin infections.

Lotusix *Torlan, Spain.*
Phenylephrine hydrochloride (p.1066·2); guaiphenesin (p.1061·3); co-trimoxazole (p.196·3).
Respiratory-tract infections.

Lotussin
Note. This name is used for preparations of different composition.
Searle, Irl.†.
Diphenhydramine hydrochloride (p.409·1); dextromethorphan hydrobromide (p.1057·3).
Coughs.

Searle, S.Afr.
Diphenhydramine hydrochloride (p.409·1); dextromethorphan hydrobromide (p.1057·3); ephedrine hydrochloride (p.1059·3); guaiphenesin (p.1061·3).
Coughs.

Lotussin Expectorant *Searle, S.Afr.*
Diphenhydramine (p.409·1); aminophylline (p.748·1); ammonium chloride (p.1055·2).
Coughs.

Lo-Uric *Rolab, S.Afr.*
Allopurinol (p.390·2).
Gout; hyperuricaemia.

Lovan *Amrad, Austral.*
Fluoxetine hydrochloride (p.284·1).
Depression; obsessive-compulsive disorder.

Lovelle
Organon, Ger.; Intervet, Switz.†.
Desogestrel (p.1443·3); ethinyloestradiol (p.1445·1).
Combined oral contraceptive.

Lovenox
Gerot, Aust.; Rhone-Poulenc Rorer, Canad.; Bellon, Fr.; Rhone-Poulenc Rorer, USA.
Enoxaparin sodium (p.864·2).
Thrombosis prophylaxis.

Lovitran *Tendem-Haco, Neth.†.*
Vitamin A (p.1358·1); vitamin D (p.1366·3).

Low Liquemine *Roche, Switz.*
Dalteparin sodium (p.845·3).
Anticoagulant during haemodialysis or haemofiltration; thrombo-embolic disorders.

Lowasa *Central, Irl.*
Aspirin (p.16·1).
Cardiovascular disorders; myocardial infarction.

Lowgan *Yamanouchi, Jpn.*
Amosulalol hydrochloride (p.823·1).
Hypertension.

Lowila Cake *Westwood-Squibb, USA.*
Skin cleanser.

Lowsium Plus *Rugby, USA.*
Magaldrate (p.1198·1); simethicone (p.1213·1).
Hyperacidity.

Loxapac
Wyeth Lederle, Belg.; Wyeth-Ayerst, Canad.; Lederle, Fr.; Wyeth, Irl.; Cyanamid, Ital.†; Lederle, Neth.†; Cyanamid, Spain†; Wyeth, UK.
Loxapine (p.677·1), loxapine hydrochloride (p.677·1), or loxapine succinate (p.677·1).
Psychoses.

Loxazol
Glaxo Wellcome, Neth.; Wellcome, Switz.
Permethrin (p.1409·2).
Pediculosis; scabies.

Loxen *Sandoz, Fr.*
Nicardipine hydrochloride (p.915·1).
Hypertension.

Loxitane *Lederle, USA.*
Loxapine succinate (p.677·1).
Psychoses.

Loxonin *Sankyo, Jpn.*
Loxoprofen sodium (p.50·3).
Inflammation; pain.

Lozide *Servier, Canad.*
Indapamide (p.890·2).
Hypertension.

Lozione Cruz Verde con Erogatore *Fastfarm, Ital.†.*
Pyrethrum (p.1410·1); piperonyl butoxide (p.1409·3); diethyltoluamide (p.1405·1).
Insect repellent; insecticide.

Lozione Cruz Verde Zanzara *Fastfarm, Ital.†.*
Diethyltoluamide (p.1405·1).
Insect repellent.

Lozione Same AS *Savoma, Ital.*
Methionine (p.984·2); zinc sulphate (p.1373·2); pyridoxine (p.1363·1).
Seborrhoea.

Lozione Vittoria *Ottolenghi, Ital.*
Benzalkonium chloride (p.1101·3).
Skin cleansing.

Lozol *Rhone-Poulenc Rorer, USA.*
Indapamide (p.890·2).
Heart failure; hypertension.

LP Mix *Braun, Fr.*
Amino-acid and lipid infusion.
Parenteral nutrition.

L.P.C. Shampoo *Schwulst, S.Afr.†.*
Coal tar (p.1092·3).
Scalp disorders.

L-Polamidon *Hoechst, Ger.*
Levomethadone hydrochloride (p.50·1).
Pain.

LP-Truw *Truw, Ger.†.*
Safflower oil (p.1353·3); vitamins; silybum marianum (p.993·3); chelidonium; choline hydrogen tartrate; nicotinyl alcohol (p.915·3).
Lipid disorders.

LP-Truw mono *Truw, Ger.*
Sitosterol (p.1279·3).
Hyperlipidaemias.

LPV *CSL, Austral.*
Phenoxymethylpenicillin potassium (p.236·2).
Bacterial infections.

LSP *Seroyal, Canad.*
Calcium aspartate; magnesium aspartate (p.1157·2).

Luan *Molteni, Ital.*
Lignocaine hydrochloride (p.1293·2).
Local anaesthesia.

Luase *Alfarma, Spain.*
Diclofenac sodium (p.31·2).
Gout; inflammation; musculoskeletal, joint, and peri-articular disorders; pain; renal colic.

Lubafax *Douglas, Austral.*
Lubricant for skin or for medical instruments.

Lubalix *Drossapharm, Switz.*
Cloxazolam (p.657·3).
Anxiety disorders; insomnia.

Lubarol *Biovital, Austral.*
Nonoxinol 9 (p.1326·1).
Contraceptive.

Lubentyl
Note. This name is used for preparations of different composition.
Synthelabo, Fr.
Liquid paraffin (p.1382·1); hard paraffin (p.1382·1).
Constipation.

Kramer, Switz.†.
Liquid paraffin (p.1382·1).
Constipation.

Lubentyl a la Magnesie
Note. This name is used for preparations of different composition.
Synthelabo, Fr.
Liquid paraffin (p.1382·1); hard paraffin (p.1382·1); magnesium hydroxide (p.1198·2).
Constipation.

Kramer, Switz.†.
Liquid paraffin (p.1382·1); magnesium hydroxide (p.1198·2).
Constipation.

Lubex *Permamed, Switz.*
Sodium sulphosuccinated undecenoic acid monoethanolamide (p.389·2).
Skin disorders.

Lubexyl *Permamed, Switz.*
Benzoyl peroxide (p.1079·2).
Acne.

Lubo *Synthelabo, Switz.†.*
Guar mucilage (p.321·3).
Lubricant.

Lubogliss *Streuli, Switz.*
Lignocaine hydrochloride (p.1293·2).
Catheterisation; endoscopy.

Luborant
Antigen, Irl.; Antigen, UK.
Electrolytes (p.1147·1); carmellose sodium (p.1471·2); sorbitol (p.1354·2).
Saliva substitute.

Lubraseptic Jelly *Guardian, USA†.*
Phenylphenol (p.1120·3); amylphenol.
Lubricant; sterile dressing.

LubraSol *Pharmaceutical Specialties, USA.*
Emollient.

Lubricante Urol *Organon, Spain†.*
Amethocaine hydrochloride (p.1285·2).
Local anaesthesia.

Lubricating Gel *Lake, USA†.*
Vaginal lubricant.

Lubricating Jelly *Lake, USA.*
Vaginal lubricant.

Lubriderm
Note. This name is used for preparations of different composition.
Warner-Lambert, Canad.
Wool fat (p.1385·3); liquid paraffin (p.1382·1).
Skin disorders.

Warner-Lambert, USA.
Emollient and moisturiser.

Lubriderm AHA *Warner-Lambert, Canad.*
Lactic acid (p.1593·3).

Lubriderm Daily UV Defense *Warner-Lambert, Canad.*
SPF 15: Wool fat (p.1385·3); liquid paraffin (p.1382·1); avobenzone (p.1486·3); ethylhexyl *p*-methoxycinnamate (p.1487·1); phenylbenzimidazole sulphonic acid (p.1488·2).
Sunscreen.

Lubrifilm
Cusi, Spain; Cusi, UK†.
Yellow soft paraffin (p.1382·3); liquid paraffin (p.1382·1); wool fat (p.1385·3).
Eye disorders.

Lubrilax *Normon, Spain.*
Sodium picosulphate (p.1213·2).
Constipation.

Lubrilent *SIFI, Ital.*
Wetting solution for hard contact lenses.

Lubrin *Kenwood, USA.*
Tricaprylin (p.1639·1); glycerol (p.1585·2); laureth 23 (p.1325·2).
Vaginal lubricant.

Lubrirhin *Basotherm, Ger.*
Bromhexine (p.1055·3).
Rhinitis.

Lubri-Tears
Alcon, UK; Bausch & Lomb, USA.
Eye ointment: White soft paraffin (p.1382·3); liquid paraffin (p.1382·1); wool fat (p.1385·3).
Dry eyes.

Bausch & Lomb, USA.
Eye drops: Hypromellose (p.1473·1); dextran 70 (p.717·1).
Dry eyes.

Lucenfal *Farma Lepori, Spain.*
Nicardipine hydrochloride (p.915·1).
Angina pectoris; cerebrovascular disorders; hypertension.

Lucibran *Bracco, Ital.*
Alfoscerate olamine.
Anxiety; confusion.

Lucidril
Kolassa, Aust.; Lipha Sante, Fr.; Dainippon, Jpn†.
Meclofenoxate hydrochloride (p.1599·1).
Cerebral function disorders.

Lucil *Efarmes, Spain†.*
Calcium pantothenate (p.1352·3); mercuric chloride (p.1601·2); pilocarpine hydrochloride (p.1396·3); resorcinol acetate (p.1090·1); salicylic acid (p.1090·2).
Hair and scalp disorders.

Lucisan *Ircafarm, Ital.*
Naphazoline nitrate (p.1064·2); hamamelis (p.1587·1); boric acid (p.1554·2); borax (p.1554·2).
Eye irritation.

Lucosil
Lundbeck, Aust.; Lundbeck, Belg.†; Lundbeck, Norw.†.
Sulphamethizole (p.254·2) or sulphamethizole monoethanolamine (p.254·2).
Ear infections; eye disorders; urinary-tract infections.

Lucostin *Lundbeck, Aust.†.*
Lomustine (p.544·1).
Malignant neoplasms.

Lucostine
Lundbeck, Norw.†; Lundbeck, Swed.†.
Lomustine (p.544·1).
Malignant neoplasms.

Lucrin
Abbott, Austral.; Abbott, Belg.; Abbott, Fr.; Abbott, Neth.; Abbott, S.Afr.; Abbott, Switz.
Leuprorelin (p.1253·1) or leuprorelin acetate (p.1253·1).
Adjunct in anovulatory infertility; endometriosis; prostatic cancer; uterine fibromas.

Lucrusanum *Molitor, Ger.†.*
Bibrocathol (p.1553·2); benzocaine (p.1286·2).
Burns; ulcers; wounds.

Luctor *Sanofi Winthrop, Ger.*
Naftidrofuryl oxalate (p.914·2).
Peripheral vascular disorders.

Ludilat *Organon, Aust.*
Bencyclane fumarate (p.827·3).
Peripheral and cerebral vascular disorders.

Ludiomil
Ciba-Geigy, Aust.; Ciba-Geigy, Belg.; Ciba, Canad.; Ciba-Geigy, Fr.; Geigy, Ger.; Ciba-Geigy, Irl.†; Ciba, Ital.; Novartis, Neth.; Novartis, S.Afr.; Ciba-Geigy, Spain; Novartis, Swed.; Geigy, Switz.; Ciba, UK; Ciba, USA.
Maprotiline hydrochloride (p.296·2) or maprotiline mesylate (p.296·3).
Depression.

Ludoxin *Woelm, Ger.†.*
Celandine; boldo leaves (p.1554·1); Javanese turmeric; wahoo root-bark (p.1192·1); cynara leaves (p.1569·2); ox bile (p.1553·2); scopolia root; cape aloe (p.1177·1); peppermint oil (p.1208·1).
Liver disorders.

Luffa comp-Heel Nasentropfen *Heel, Ger.*
Homoeopathic preparation.

Luffa compositum *Heel, Ger.*
Homoeopathic preparation.

Luffa comp.-Tropfen-Pascoe N *Pascoe, Ger.*
Homoeopathic preparation.

Luffa Med Complex *Dynamit, Aust.*
Homoeopathic preparation.

luffa-loges *Loges, Ger.*
Homoeopathic preparation.

Luforan *Serono, Spain.*
Gonadorelin (p.1247·2).
Hypothalamic-pituitary dysfunction.

Lufyllin *Wallace, USA.*
Diprophylline (p.752·1).
Bronchial asthma; reversible bronchospasm.

Lufyllin-EPG *Wallace, USA.*
Diprophylline (p.752·1); ephedrine hydrochloride (p.1059·3); guaiphenesin (p.1061·3); phenobarbitone (p.350·2).
Bronchospasm.

Lufyllin-GG *Wallace, USA.*
Diprophylline (p.752·1); guaiphenesin (p.1061·3).
Bronchial asthma; reversible bronchospasm.

Lugro *Molitor, Ger.†.*
Ichthammol (p.1083·3); resorcinol (p.1090·1); zinc oxide (p.1096·2).
Skin disorders.

Luiflex
Kwizda, Aust.; Luitpold, Belg.
Indomethacin (p.45·2).
Musculoskeletal, joint, peri-articular, and soft-tissue disorders.

Luitase *Sankyo, Ital.*
Pancrelipase (p.1613·3).
Cystic fibrosis; malabsorption.

Luivac *Luitpold, Ger.*
Lysate of *Staphylococcus aureus*; *Streptococcus mitis*; *Streptococcus pyogenes*; *Streptococcus pneumoniae*; *Klebsiella pneumoniae*; *Branhamella catarrhalis*; *Haemophilus influenzae*.
Respiratory-tract infections.

Luizym
Note. This name is used for preparations of different composition.
Luitpold, Ger.
Enzyme extract from *Aspergillus oryzae*.
Digestive system disorders.

Luitpold, Ital.
Protease; cellulase (p.1561·1); amylase (p.1549·1).
Digestive disorders.

Lukadin *San Carlo, Ital.*
Amikacin sulphate (p.150·2).
Gram-negative bacterial infections.

Lumbago-Gastreu R11 *Reckeweg, Ger.*
Homoeopathic preparation.

Lumbalgine *Cooperation Pharmaceutique, Fr.*
Glycol salicylate (p.43·1); menthol (p.1600·2); camphor (p.1557·2); turpentine oil (p.1641·1); benzyl nicotinate (p.22·1).
Muscular disorders.

Lumbaxol Para *Aldo, Spain.*
Chlormezanone (p.648·3); paracetamol (p.72·2).
Dysmenorrhoea; neuralgias; peri-articular disorders; premenstrual syndrome.

Lumbinon *Lichtenstein, Ger.*
Glycol salicylate (p.43·1).
Formerly contained methyl nicotinate, glycol salicylate, colloidal sulphur, sodium chondroitin sulphate, and heparin.
Migraine; musculoskeletal, joint, and soft-tissue disorders; neuralgia.

Lumexon *Merckle, Ger.†.*
Methotrexate (p.547·1).
Malignant neoplasms; psoriasis vulgaris; psoriatic arthritis.

Lumifurex *Irex, Fr.*
Nifuroxazide (p.231·3).
Diarrhoea.

Lumin *Alphapharm, Austral.*
Mianserin hydrochloride (p.297·1).
Depression.

Luminal
Desitin, Ger.; Bayer, Spain; E. Merck, Switz.; Sanofi Winthrop, USA.
Phenobarbitone (p.350·2) or phenobarbitone sodium (p.350·2).
Adjunct in the treatment of poisoning; epilepsy; insomnia; premedication.

Luminale *Bracco, Ital.*
Phenobarbitone (p.350·2) or phenobarbitone sodium (p.350·2).
Barbiturate withdrawal; epilepsy; sedative.

Luminaletas *Bayer, Spain.*
Phenobarbitone (p.350·2).
Epilepsy.

Luminalette *Bracco, Ital.*
Phenobarbitone (p.350·2).
Barbiturate withdrawal; epilepsy; sedative.

Luminaletten *Desitin, Ger.*
Phenobarbitone (p.350·2).
Epilepsy.

Lumirelax
Gallier, Fr.†.
Ointment: Methocarbamol (p.1316·1); methyl nicotinate (p.55·1).

Jumer, Fr.
Tablets: Methocarbamol (p.1316·1).
Musculoskeletal and joint disorders.

Lumirem
Salus, Aust.; Guerbet, Fr.; Guerbet, Ger.; Guerbet, Ital.; Guerbet, Neth.; Gothia, Swed.; Guerbet, Switz.
Ferumoxsil (p.1004·2).
Contrast medium for magnetic resonance imaging of the gastro-intestinal tract.

Lumitens *Solvay, Fr.*
Xipamide (p.971·2).
Hypertension; oedema.

Lumota *Thomae, Ger.†.*
Apalcillin sodium.
Bacterial infections.

Lunadon *Singer, Switz.*
Tolazoline hydrochloride (p.956·1); drofenine hydrochloride (p.460·3); diphenhydramine hydrochloride (p.409·1).
Nervous disorders; sleep disorders.

Lundiran *Vir, Spain.*
Naproxen (p.61·2).
Gout; musculoskeletal, joint, and peri-articular disorders; pain.

Lunelax
Tika, Norw.; Tika, Swed.
Ispaghula husk (p.1194·2).
Adjunct in treatment of diarrhoea; bowel evacuation; constipation; irritable bowel syndrome.

Lunelax comp. *Tika, Swed.*
Ispaghula husk (p.1194·2); sennosides (p.1212·3).
Constipation.

Lunerin
Astra, Norw.†; Tika, Swed.
Brompheniramine maleate (p.403·2); phenylpropanolamine hydrochloride (p.1067·2).
Rhinitis.

Lunibron-A *Valeas, Ital.*
Flunisolide (p.1040·3).
Hypersensitivity disorders of the respiratory tract.

Lunis *Valeas, Ital.*
Flunisolide (p.1040·3).
Rhinitis.

Luostyl *UPSA, Fr.†.*
Difemerine hydrochloride (p.460·3).
Smooth-muscle spasms.

Lupidon *Seid, Spain.*
Calcium pantothenate (p.1352·3); dimethicone (p.1213·1); magnesium polygalacturonate.
Flatulence.

Lupidon G *Bruschettini, Ital.*
A herpes simplex type 2 vaccine (p.1515·2).
Active immunisation.

Lupidon H *Bruschettini, Ital.*
A herpes simplex type 1 vaccine (p.1515·2).
Active immunisation.

Lupidon H+G *Hermal, Switz.*
Lupidon H, a herpes simplex vaccine (type I); Lupidon G, a herpes simplex vaccine (type II) (p.1515·2).
Herpes simplex infections.

Lupovalin *Selz, Ger.*
Diphenhydramine hydrochloride (p.409·1).
Insomnia.

Lupron
Abbott, Canad.; TAP, USA.
Leuprorelin acetate (p.1253·1).
Endometriosis; precocious puberty; prostatic cancer.

Luret *Sanofi Winthrop, Ger.*
Azosemide (p.826·3).
Oedema.

Lurgyl *Boehringer Ingelheim, Switz.†.*
Tramazoline hydrochloride (p.1071·1); chlorhexidine gluconate (p.1107·2); aluminium lactate (p.1548·1).
Mouth and throat disorders.

Luride *Colgate-Hoyt, USA.*
Sodium fluoride (p.742·1).
Dental caries prophylaxis.

Lurline PMS *Fielding, USA.*
Paracetamol (p.72·2); pamabrom (p.927·1); pyridoxine (p.1363·1).
Premenstrual syndrome.

Luroscrub *Dial, USA†.*
Chlorhexidine gluconate (p.1107·2).
Antimicrobial skin cleanser.

Lurselle
Chepharin, Aust.†; Hoechst Marion Roussel, Austral.; Marion Merrell, Fr.†; Hoechst, Ger.; Lepetit, Ital.†; Mer-National, S.Afr.; Marion Merrell Dow, Switz.†; Hoechst Marion Roussel, UK†.
Probucol (p.1277·3).
Hypercholesterolaemia.

Lusadol *Lundbeck, S.Afr.†.*
Doxylamine succinate (p.410·1); paracetamol (p.72·2); codeine phosphate (p.26·1); caffeine (p.749·3).
Pain and associated tension.

Lusap *Interdelta, Switz.*
Malathion (p.1407·3).
Pediculosis.

Lustral
Invicta, Irl.; Invicta, UK.
Sertraline hydrochloride (p.307·2).
Anxiety; depression; obsessive-compulsive disorder.

Lutenyl
Schering, Ital.; Theramex, Mon.
Nomegestrol acetate (p.1452·3).
Endometriosis; fibromas; menopausal disorders; menstrual disorders.

Luteolas *Serono, Ital.†.*
Ethynodiol (p.1445·3); mestranol (p.1450·2).
Oestrogenic; progestogenic.

Luteonorm *Serono, Ital.†.*
Ethynodiol diacetate (p.1445·3).
Progestogenic.

Luteran *Solymes, Fr.*
Chlormadinone acetate (p.1439·1).
Endometriosis; fibromas; menstrual disorders.

Lutestral *Cassenne, Fr.*
Chlormadinone acetate (p.1439·1); ethinyloestradiol (p.1445·1).
Menstrual disorders.

Lutex-E *Farmigea, Ital.†.*
Progesterone (p.1459·3); *dl*-alpha tocopheryl acetate (p.1369·2).
Progestogenic.

Lutionex *Roussel, Fr.*
Demegestone (p.1443·3).
Endometriosis; fibromas; menstrual disorders.

Lutometrodiol *Monsanto, Fr.*
Ethynodiol diacetate (p.1445·3).
Endometriosis; fibromas; mastopathy; menstrual disorders; progestogen-only oral contraceptive.

Lutoral *Sanofi Winthrop, Ital.*
Medroxyprogesterone acetate (p.1448·3).
Menstrual disorders; premature labour; prostatic hyperplasia; threatened abortion.

Lutrefact *Hoechst Marion Roussel, Norw.†.*
Gonadorelin (p.1247·2).
Amenorrhoea; diagnosis of fertility disorders; hypogonadism.

Lutrelef
Sigmapharm, Aust.; Ferring, Belg.†; Ferring, Fr.; Ferring, Ger.; Ferring, Ital.; Ferring, Neth.; Ferring, Norw.†; Ferring, Swed.; Ferring, Switz.
Gonadorelin acetate (p.1248·1).
Delayed puberty; hypogonadal hypogonadism; investigation of hypothalamic-pituitary function; male and female infertility; polycystic ovary syndrome.

Lutrepulse
Ferring, Canad.; Ferring, USA.
Gonadorelin acetate (p.1248·1).
Hypothalamic amenorrhoea.

Luuf Balsam *Apomedica, Aust.*
Camphor (p.1557·2); menthol (p.1600·2); eucalyptus oil (p.1578·1); turpentine oil (p.1641·1); pumilio pine oil (p.1623·3); oleum pini sylvestris; thymol (p.1127·1).
Respiratory-tract disorders.

Luuf-Erkaltungsol *Apomedica, Aust.*
Oleum pini sylvestris; eucalyptus oil (p.1578·1); pumilio pine oil (p.1623·3).
Respiratory-tract disorders.

Luuf-Heilpflanzenol *Apomedica, Aust.*
Eucalyptus oil (p.1578·1); peppermint oil (p.1208·1); cajuput oil (p.1556·1).
Digestive disorders; flatulence; pain; respiratory tract disorders; soft-tissue injury.

Luuf-Nasenspray *Apomedica, Aust.*
Naphazoline hydrochloride (p.1064·2); diphenhydramine hydrochloride (p.409·1).
Colds; hay fever; sinusitis.

Luvased
Wyeth Lederle, Aust.; Brenner-Efeka, Ger.; LAW, Ger.
Valerian (p.1643·1); lupulus (p.1597·2).
Anxiety disorders; sleep disorders.

Luvased-Tropfen N *Brenner-Efeka, Ger.; LAW, Ger.*
Valerian (p.1643·1); lupulus (p.1597·2); melissa (p.1600·1); passion flower (p.1615·3).
Nervous disorders; sleep disorders.

Luvatren
Cilag, Swed.†; Janssen-Cilag, Switz.†.
Moperone hydrochloride (p.682·1).
Alcohol withdrawal syndrome; epilepsy; psychoses.

Luvenil *Ellem, Ital.†.*
Vinburnine phosphate (p.1644·1).
Cerebrovascular disorders.

Luvion *GiEnne, Ital.*
Canrenone (p.836·2) or canrenoate potassium (p.836·2).
Hyperaldosteronism; hypertension.

Luvos Heilerde *Luvos, Ger.*
Natural loess.
Gastro-intestinal disorders; skin disorders.

Luvox
Solvay, Austral.; Solvay, Canad.; Solvay, S.Afr.; Solvay, USA.
Fluvoxamine maleate (p.288·3).
Depression; obsessive-compulsive disorder.

Luxazone *Allergan, Ital.*
Dexamethasone (p.1037·1).
Eye disorders.

Luxazone Eparina *Allergan, Ital.*
Dexamethasone (p.1037·1); heparin sodium (p.879·3).
Eye disorders.

Luxoben *Asta Medica, Ital.*
Tiapride hydrochloride (p.696·1).
Anxiety; dyskinesia.

Luzone *Sigma-Tau, Spain.*
Sulodexide sulphate (p.951·1).
Atherosclerosis; hyperlipidaemias; thrombo-embolic disorders.

Lyasin *MC, Ital.*
Chlorhexidine gluconate (p.1107·2).
Hand disinfection.

Lyban *Rhone-Poulenc Rorer, Austral.*
Pyrethrins; piperonyl butoxide (p.1409·3).
Pediculosis.

Lycamed *UCB, Ital.*
Lysine calcium citrate hydrochloride.
Calcium supplement.

Lycaon *Boehringer Ingelheim, Fr.†.*
Colloidal aluminium phosphate (p.1178·3); mannitol (p.900·3).
Gastro-intestinal disorders.

Lycia Luminique *Esoform, Ital.*
Benzalkonium chloride (p.1101·3); hamamelis (p.1587·1); chamomile (p.1561·2).
Eye disinfection; eye irritation.

Lycimin Tonic for Children with Iron *Nelson, Austral.†.*
Lysine hydrochloride; vitamin B substances; iron.

Lycimin Tonic for Children with Vitamin C *Nelson, Austral.†.*
Lysine hydrochloride; vitamin B substances; ascorbic acid.

Lyclear
Warner-Lambert, Austral.; Warner-Lambert, Irl.; Wellcome, Irl.; Glaxo Wellcome, S.Afr.; Warner-Lambert, UK.
Permethrin (p.1409·2).
Pediculosis; scabies.

Lycoaktin *Steigerwald, Ger.*
Injection: Homoeopathic preparation.
Tablets†; oral liquid†: Lycopi virgin.; leonuri card.; crataegi oxyac.; rosmarini; monobasic potassium phosphate.
Hyperthyroidism.

Lycoaktin M *Steigerwald, Ger.*
Lycopus virginicus.
Hyperthyroidism with nervous disorders.

Lycovowen-N *Weber & Weber, Ger.*
Homoeopathic preparation.

Lyderm *Taro, Canad.*
Fluocinonide (p.1041·2).
Skin disorders.

Lyeton *Lebens, Ital.†.*
Ursodeoxycholic acid (p.1642·1).
Biliary-tract disorders.

Lygal *Desitin, Ger.*
Prednisolone (p.1048·1); salicylic acid (p.1090·2); dexpanthenol (p.1570·3).
Scalp disorders; skin disorders.

Lygal N *Desitin, Ger.*
Salicylic acid (p.1090·2).
Lygal scalp ointment formerly contained sulphur and salicylic acid.
Scalp disorders.

Lyman *Drossapharm, Switz.*
Tablets†: Aloxiprin (p.15·1).
Thrombo-embolism prophylaxis.
Topical gel; cream: Heparin sodium (p.879·3); allantoin (p.1078·2); dexpanthenol (p.1570·3); lavender oil (p.1594·3).
Soft-tissue disorders.

Lymetel *Daker Farmasimes, Spain.*
Fluvastatin sodium (p.1273·2).
Hypercholesterolaemia.

Lymphaden *Hevert, Ger.*
Homoeopathic preparation.

Lymphadenomtropfen N *Syxyl, Ger.†.*
Homoeopathic preparation.

Lymphazurin *Hirsch, USA.*
Sulphan blue (p.1633·3).
Adjunct to lymphography.

Lymphdiaral *Pascoe, Ger.*
Homoeopathic preparation.

Lymphex *Drossapharm, Switz.*
Coumarin (p.1568·1).
Lymphoedema.

Lymphoglobulin *Merieux, Ger.*
Antilymphocyte immunoglobulin (horse) (p.504·2).
Aplastic anaemia; organ transplantation.

Lymphoglobuline
Pasteur Merieux, Belg.; Imtix, Fr.; Imtix, Ital.; Imtix, Neth.; Rhone-Poulenc Rorer, S.Afr.; Pasteur Merieux, Switz.
An antilymphocyte immunoglobulin (horse) (p.504·2).
Formerly known as Lymfoglobuline in *Neth.*
Aplastic anaemia; organ transplantation.

Lympholact *Pfluger, Ger.†.*
Homoeopathic preparation.

Lymphomyosot *Heel, Ger.*
Homoeopathic preparation.

Lymphoser
Berna, Ital.†; Berna, Spain†; Berna, Switz.†.
An antilymphocyte immunoglobulin (horse) (p.504·2).
Aplastic anaemia; organ transplantation.

Lymphozil *Redel, Ger.*
Echinaceae pallida (p.1574·2); calc. carbonic. hahn.; lachesis.
Tonic.

Lynandron *Nourypharma, Ger.†.*
Oestradiol benzoate (p.1455·1); oestradiol phenylpropionate (p.1455·2); testosterone propionate (p.1464·2); testosterone phenylpropionate (p.1464·2); testosterone isocaproate (p.1464·2).
Menopausal disorders.

Lyndac *Eurofarmaco, Ital.*
Sulindac (p.86·3).
Gout; musculoskeletal and joint disorders; neuritis; soft-tissue injury.

Lyndiol
Organon, Aust.; Organon, Belg.; Organon, Ger.; Organon, Neth.†; Organon, Norw.†; Donmed, S.Afr.†; Organon, Swed.†.
Lynoestrenol (p.1448·2); ethinyloestradiol (p.1445·1).
Combined oral contraceptive; menstrual disorders.

Lyndiol 2.5 *Organon, Spain†.*
Lynoestrenol (p.1448·2); mestranol (p.1450·2).
Combined oral contraceptive; menstrual disorders.

Lyndiol E *Ravasini, Ital.†.*
Lynoestrenol (p.1448·2); ethinyloestradiol (p.1445·1).
Combined oral contraceptive.

Lyndiolett *Organon, Swed.*
Lynoestrenol (p.1448·2); ethinyloestradiol (p.1445·1).
Combined oral contraceptive.

Lynoral *Organon, Neth.*
Ethinyloestradiol (p.1445·1).
Breast cancer; menstrual disorders; oestrogen deficiency; postcoital contraceptive; prostatic cancer.

Lyn-ratiopharm *Ratiopharm, Ger.*
Lynoestrenol (p.1448·2); ethinyloestradiol (p.1445·1).
Combined oral contraceptive; menstrual disorders.

Lyn-ratiopharm-Sequenz *Ratiopharm, Ger.*
7 Capsules, ethinyloestradiol (p.1445·1); 15 capsules, lynoestrenol (p.1448·2); ethinyloestradiol.
Sequential-type oral contraceptive.

Lyobalsam *Truw, Ger.*
Camphor (p.1557·2); eucalyptus oil (p.1623·3).
Respiratory-tract disorders.

Lyobalsam N *Neos-Donner, Ger.†.*
Camphor (p.1557·2); thymol (p.1127·1); menthol (p.1600·2); eucalyptus oil (p.1578·1); pine needle oil (p.1623·3).
Respiratory-tract disorders.

Lyobalsam N ohne Menthol *Neos-Donner, Ger.†.*
Camphor (p.1557·2); thymol (p.1127·1); eucalyptus oil (p.1578·1); pine needle oil (p.1623·3).
Colds; respiratory-tract disorders.

Lyobex retard *Bristol, Ger.†.*
Noscapine (p.1065·2).
Coughs and associated respiratory-tract disorders.

Lyo-Bifidus *GNR, Fr.*
Bifidobacterium bifidus (Bacillus bifidus) (p.1594·1).
Diarrhoea.

Lyodura *Davis & Geck, UK†.*
Collagenous fibres developed from homologous human dura mater cerebri (p.1566·3).
Repair of lesions and reinforcement of body tissue.

Lyofoam *Seton, UK.*
Polyurethane foam dressing.
Ulcers; wounds.

Lyofoam C *Seton, UK.*
Activated charcoal (p.972·2).
Malodorous wounds.

Lyogen
Promonta Lundbeck, Ger.; Byk, Switz.†.
Fluphenazine decanoate (p.671·2) or fluphenazine hydrochloride (p.671·3).
Psychoses.

Lyoginseng *Chefaro Ardeval, Fr.†.*
Ginseng (p.1584·2).
Tonic.

Lyophytum *Chefaro Ardeval, Fr.†.*
Harpagophytum procumbens root (p.27·2).
Joint pain; sprains; tendinitis.

Lyorodin *Rodleben, Ger.; UCB, Ger.*
Fluphenazine decanoate (p.671·2) or fluphenazine hydrochloride (p.671·3).
Psychoses.

Lyostypt
Braun Surgical, Switz.; Davis & Geck, UK.
Collagen (p.1566·3).
Haemorrhage.

Lyovac Cosmegen
Merck Sharp & Dohme, Belg.; Merck Sharp & Dohme, Ger.; Merck Sharp & Dohme, Neth.
Dactinomycin (p.527·2).
Malignant neoplasms.

Lyphocin *Lyphomed, USA.*
Vancomycin hydrochloride (p.267·2).
Bacterial infections.

Lypholyte *Lyphomed, USA.*
A range of electrolyte preparations (p.1147·1).
Fluid and electrolyte disorders.

Lyprinol *Nutraceuticals, UK.*
Green-lipped mussel (p.1586·3).

Lypsyl Cold Sore Gel *Zyma, UK.*
Lignocaine hydrochloride (p.1293·2); zinc sulphate (p.1373·2); cetrimide (p.1105·2).

Lyptocodine *Monot, Fr.*
Adult and paediatric syrup: Pholcodine (p.1068·1); codeine camsylate (p.27·1); cineole (p.1564·1); potassium guaiacolsulfonate (p.1068·3); magnesium sulphate (p.1157·3).
Infant syrup: Calcium bromide (p.1620·3); guaiphenesin (p.1061·3); mannitol (p.900·3); syrup diacode.
Suppositories†: Pholcodine (p.1068·1); codeine camsylate (p.27·1); cineole (p.1564·1).
Coughs.

Lysalgo *SIT, Ital.*
Mefenamic acid (p.51·2).
Inflammation; pain.

Lysanxia
Parke, Davis, Belg.; Parke, Davis, Fr.
Prazepam (p.687·2).
Alcohol withdrawal syndrome; anxiety.

Lysatec rt-PA *Boehringer Ingelheim, Canad.†.*
Alteplase (p.818·1).
Thrombo-embolic disorders.

Lysbex *Provita, Aust.*
Bibenzonium bromide (p.1055·3).
Coughs.

Lysedem *Knoll, Fr.*
Coumarin (p.1568·1).
Post-mastectomy lymphoedema.

Lysedil *Vifor, Switz.*
Promethazine hydrochloride (p.416·2); belladonna (p.457·1).
Coughs; gastro-intestinal disorders; hypersensitivity reactions; sedative.

Lysedil compositum *Vifor, Switz.*
Promethazine hydrochloride (p.416·2); belladonna (p.457·1); paracetamol (p.72·2).
Coughs; fever; gastro-intestinal disorders; hypersensitivity reactions; pain; sedative.

Lyseen
Hommel, Ger.; Zyma, Ital.
Pridinol mesylate (p.1318·2).
Skeletal muscle spasm.

Lyseen New *Therabel Pharma, Belg.†.*
Chlormezanone (p.648·3).
Formerly contained pridinol mesylate.
Skeletal muscle spasm.

Lysetol FF *Schulke & Mayr, Ger.*
Glutaraldehyde (p.1114·3); ethylhexanal.
Disinfection of instruments.

Lysetol V *Schulke & Mayr, Ger.*
Formaldehyde (p.1113·2); glutaraldehyde (p.1114·3); ethylhexanal.
Disinfection of instruments.

Lysinotol *Asta Medica, Spain.*
Lysine aspirin (p.50·3).
Fever; musculoskeletal, joint, and peri-articular disorders; pain; thrombo-embolism prophylaxis.

Lysivit B_{12} a l'inositol *Sarget, Fr.*
Lysine hydrochloride; inositol; cyanocobalamin.
Tonic.

Lyso-6
Darcy, Fr.; UCB, Switz.
Muramidase hydrochloride (p.1604·3); pyridoxine hydrochloride (p.1362·3).
Mouth and throat disorders.

Lysobex Bracco, Ital.†.
Bibenzonium bromide (p.1055·3).
Coughs.

Lysocalm Darcy, Fr.
Muramidase hydrochloride (p.1604·3); menthol (p.1600·2).
Mouth and throat infections.

Lysocline
Note. This name is used for preparations of different composition.
Parke, Davis, Fr.
Methacycline hydrochloride (p.225·1).
Formerly contained methacycline hydrochloride and muramidase hydrochloride.
Bacterial infections.

Wild, Switz.†.
Methacycline hydrochloride (p.225·1); muramidase hydrochloride (p.1604·3).
Bacterial infections.

Lysodren Bristol, Canad.; Bristol-Myers Oncology, USA.
Mitotane (p.553·2).
Adrenal cortical cancer.

Lysofon Lafon, Fr.
Lozenges: Tricarbaurinium (p.1639·1); amethocaine hydrochloride (p.1285·2).
Throat spray: Tricarbaurinium (p.1639·1).
Mouth and throat disorders.

Lysoform Lysoform, Ger.; Rovi, Spain†.
Formaldehyde (p.1113·2).
Hyperhidrosis; skin infections; surface and linen disinfection.

Lysoform Killavon Lysoform, Ger.
Benzalkonium chloride (p.1101·3).
Disinfection of skin, mucous membranes, and surfaces; skin disorders.

Lysoformin Lysoform, Ger.
Formaldehyde (p.1113·2); glutaraldehyde (p.1114·3).
Surface disinfection.

Lysoformin 3000 Lysoform, Ger.
Glyoxal (p.1115·1); glutaraldehyde (p.1114·3); didecyldimethylammonium chloride (p.1112·2).
Disinfection of instruments and surfaces.

Lysoformin spezial Lysoform, Ger.
Guanidine derivative; didecyldimethylammonium chloride (p.1112·2).
Disinfection of surfaces.

Lysokana Zambon, Spain.
Kanamycin sulphate (p.220·3); muramidase hydrochloride (p.1604·3); papain (p.1614·1).
Mouth and throat inflammation.

Lysolac Simes, Ital.†.
Tilactase (p.1637·3).
Lactose intolerance.

Lysolin Schulke & Mayr, Ger.†.
Orthophenylphenol (p.1120·3); chlorocresol (p.1110·3).
Skin disinfection; surface disinfection.

Lysomucil Zambon, Belg.
Acetylcysteine (p.1052·3).
Paracetamol overdose; respiratory-tract disorders associated with viscous mucus.

Lysopaine
Boehringer Ingelheim, Fr.; Wild, Switz.
Muramidase hydrochloride (p.1604·3); papain (p.1614·1); bacitracin (p.157·3).
Mouth and throat disorders.

Lysotan Maggioni, Ital.†.
Dimethylalkyl coconut oil; cinnamaldehyde.
Water purification.

Lysox Menarini, Belg.
Acetylcysteine (p.1052·3).
Respiratory-tract disorders associated with viscous secretions.

Lyspafen
Roche, S.Afr.†; Janssen-Cilag, Switz.
Difenoxin hydrochloride (p.1188·3).
Atropine sulphate (p.455·1) is included in this preparation to discourage abuse.
Diarrhoea.

Lyspamin Bracco, Ital.†.
Nicofetamide (p.1607·2).
Gastro-intestinal disorders; smooth muscle spasm.

Lyssagam Serotherapeutisches, Aust.†.
A rabies immunoglobulin (p.1530·2).
Passive immunisation.

Lyssavac N
Berna, Ital.; Berna, Switz.
A rabies vaccine (p.1530·3).
Active immunisation.

Lyssipoll Lyssia, Ger.†.
Diphenylpyraline hydrochloride (p.409·3).
Rhinitis.

Lyssuman Berna, Spain.
A rabies immunoglobulin (p.1530·2).
Passive immunisation.

Lysthenon
Hafslund Nycomed, Aust.; Nycomed, Ger.; Nycomed, Switz.
Suxamethonium chloride (p.1319·1).
Depolarising neuromuscular blocker.

Lysuron Boehringer Mannheim, Switz.
Allopurinol (p.390·2).
Gout; hyperuricaemia; renal calculi.

Lyteca Zurich, S.Afr.†.
Paracetamol (p.72·2).
Pain.

Lyteprep Therapex, Canad.
Electrolyte solution (p.1147·1).
Gastro-intestinal lavage.

Lytos
Boehringer Mannheim, Aust.; Boehringer Mannheim, Fr.
Disodium clodronate (p.737·3).
Malignant hypercalcaemia; malignant osteolysis; Paget's disease of bone.

Lytren
Mead Johnson, Canad.
Glucose; potassium citrate; sodium chloride; sodium citrate; citric acid (p.1152·3).
Diarrhoea; oral rehydration therapy.

Mead Johnson, Fr.
Maltodextrin; glucose; potassium citrate; sodium chloride; citric acid; sodium citrate; calcium gluconate; magnesium phosphate (p.1152·3).
Diarrhoea; oral rehydration therapy.

Lytren RHS Mead Johnson, Canad.
Citric acid; potassium citrate; sodium chloride; sodium citrate (p.1152·3).

M C Therapex, Canad.†.
Hypromellose (p.1473·1).
Adjunct in small bowel radiography.

M & M Malam, UK.
Dressing: Cod-liver oil (p.1337·3); purified honey (p.1345·3).

M 40 N Madaus, Ger.†.
Aloes (p.1177·1); frangula bark (p.1193·2).
Constipation.

M2 Woelm Rorer, Ger.†.
Honey (p.1345·3).
Tonic.

Maagersan Cermak, Aust.
Vitamin A (p.1358·1); cholecalciferol (p.1366·3).
Vitamin A and D deficiency.

Maalox
Gerot, Aust.; Rhone-Poulenc Rorer, Belg.; Novartis Consumer, Canad.; Theraplix, Fr.; Rhone-Poulenc Rorer, Ger.; Nattermann, Ger.; Rhone-Poulenc Rorer, Irl.; Rhone-Poulenc Rorer, Ital.; Nattermann, Neth.; Rhone-Poulenc Rorer, S.Afr.; Rhone-Poulenc Rorer, Spain; Rhone-Poulenc Rorer, UK; Rhone-Poulenc Rorer, USA.
Aluminium hydroxide (p.1177·3); magnesium hydroxide (p.1198·2).
These ingredients can be described by the British Approved Name Co-magaldrox.
Gastro-intestinal hyperacidity.

Maalox Antacid Rhone-Poulenc Rorer, USA.
Calcium carbonate (p.1182·1).
Hyperacidity.

Maalox Anti-Diarrheal Rhone-Poulenc Rorer, USA.
Loperamide hydrochloride (p.1197·2).
Diarrhoea.

Maalox Anti-Gas Rhone-Poulenc Rorer, USA.
Simethicone (p.1213·1).
Flatulence.

Maalox Daily Fiber Rhone-Poulenc Rorer, USA.
Psyllium hydrophilic mucilloid (p.1194·2).

Maalox GRF Novartis Consumer, Canad.
Simethicone (p.1213·1).
Dyspepsia; flatulence.

Maalox Heartburn Relief Rhone-Poulenc Rorer, USA.
Aluminium hydroxide-magnesium carbonate co-dried gel (p.1178·2); magnesium carbonate (p.1198·1).
Hyperacidity.

Maalox HRF Novartis Consumer, Canad.
Aluminium hydroxide-magnesium carbonate co-dried gel (p.1178·2); magnesium alginate (p.1470·3); magnesium carbonate (p.1198·1).
Dyspepsia; gastro-oesophageal reflux; heartburn.

Maalox Plus
Novartis Consumer, Canad.; Rorer, Irl.; Rhone-Poulenc Rorer, Ital.; Nattermann, Neth.; Rhone-Poulenc Rorer, S.Afr.; Rhone-Poulenc Rorer, UK; Rhone-Poulenc Rorer, USA.
Aluminium hydroxide (p.1177·3); magnesium hydroxide (p.1198·2); simethicone (p.1213·1).
Flatulence; gastro-intestinal hyperacidity; gastro-oesophageal reflux.

Maalox TC
Novartis Consumer, Canad.; Rhone-Poulenc Rorer, Ital.; Rhone-Poulenc Rorer, UK.
Aluminium hydroxide (p.1177·3); magnesium hydroxide (p.1198·2).
Formerly known as Maalox Concentrate in the *UK*.
These ingredients can be described by the British Approved Name Co-magaldrox.
Gastro-intestinal hyperacidity.

Maaloxan
Rhone-Poulenc Rorer, Ger.; Nattermann, Ger.; Piraud, Switz.
Aluminium hydroxide (p.1177·3); magnesium hydroxide (p.1198·2).
Gastro-intestinal disorders associated with gastric hyperacidity.

Maaloxan Ca Piraud, Switz.
Aluminium hydroxide (p.1177·3); magnesium hydroxide (p.1198·2); calcium carbonate (p.1182·1).
Formerly known as Camalox.
Gastric hyperacidity.

Mab Whitehall, Fr.
Magnesium carbonate (p.1198·1); calcium carbonate (p.1182·1); sodium bicarbonate (p.1153·2).
Gastro-intestinal disorders.

Mabogastrol Tedec Meiji, Spain.
Anethole (p.1549·3); aluminium hydroxide (p.1177·3); magnesium carbonate (p.1198·1); sodium bicarbonate (p.1153·2).
Formerly contained anethole, bismuth subnitrate, magnesium carbonate, and sodium bicarbonate.
Gastro-intestinal hyperacidity; meteorism; peptic ulcer.

Mabosil Mabo, Spain.
Magnesium trisilicate (p.1199·1).
Gastro-intestinal hyperacidity.

Maboterpen
Note. This name is used for preparations of different composition.
Mabo, Spain.
Suppositories: Camphor (p.1557·2); cineole (p.1564·1); dextromethorphan (p.1057·3); niaouli oil (p.1607·1); guaiacol (p.1061·2).
Respiratory-tract disorders.

Tedec Meiji, Spain.
Syrup: Tolu balsam (p.1071·1); diphenhydramine hydrochloride (p.409·1); ephedrine hydrochloride (p.1059·3); niaouli oil (p.1607·1); pinus sylvestris; sodium benzoate (p.1102·3); bitter orange; potassium guaiacolsulfonate (p.1068·3).
Upper-respiratory-tract disorders.

Mabthera Roche, UK.
Rituximab (p.560·3).
Follicular lymphoma.

Mac
Note. This name is used for preparations of different composition.
Hamilton, Austral.†.
Aminacrine (p.1098·3); cod-liver oil (p.1337·3).
Burns; paronychia; ulcers; whitlows; wounds.

Manetti Roberts, Ital.†.
Amylmetacresol (p.1101·3).
Coughs; sore throat.

Ernest Jackson, UK.
Amylmetacresol (p.1101·3); menthol (p.1600·2).
Sore throat.

Mac Extra Ernest Jackson, UK.
Hexylresorcinol (p.1116·1).
Sore throat.

Macaine Adcock Ingram, S.Afr.
Bupivacaine hydrochloride (p.1286·3).
Adrenaline (p.813·2) is included in some injections as a vasoconstrictor to diminish absorption and localise the effect of the local anaesthetic.
Local anaesthesia.

Macalvit
Note. This name is used for preparations of different composition.
Sandoz, Aust.; Sandoz, Ital.†; Novartis, Swed.
Ascorbic acid (p.1365·2); calcium lactate gluconate (p.1155·2); calcium carbonate (p.1182·1).
Calcium and vitamin C deficiency.

Sandoz, Ger.
Effervescent tablets: Ascorbic acid (p.1365·2); calcium lactate gluconate (p.1155·2); calcium phosphinate.
Cold and influenza symptoms; tonic.

Sandoz, Spain.
Multivitamin and mineral preparation.

Machlor Eagle, Austral.
Magnesium chloride (p.1157·2); magnesium oxide (p.1198·3); magnesium amino acid chelate.
Magnesium supplement.

Mack Pen Pfizer, Aust.
Phenoxymethylpenicillin potassium (p.236·2).
Bacterial infections.

Mackenzies Cox, UK.
Ammonia (p.1548·3); eucalyptus oil (p.1578·1).
Catarrh; colds.

Mackenzies Menthoids BML, Austral.
Phenolphthalein (p.1208·2); potassium nitrate (p.1123·1); methylene blue (p.984·3).
Backache; rheumatic pain.

Macladin Guidotti, Ital.
Clarithromycin (p.189·1).
Bacterial infections.

Maclar Abbott, Aust.
Clarithromycin (p.189·1).
Opportunistic mycobacterial infections.

Maclean Indigestion Tablets SmithKline Beecham Consumer, UK.
Calcium carbonate (p.1182·1); light magnesium carbonate (p.1198·1); aluminium hydroxide (p.1177·3).
Gastro-intestinal disorders.

Macleans Mouthguard SmithKline Beecham Consumer, UK.
Cetylpyridinium chloride (p.1106·2); sodium fluoride (p.742·1).
Oral hygiene.

Macleans Sensitive SmithKline Beecham Consumer, Austral.
Sodium fluoride (p.742·1); strontium acetate.
Dental caries prophylaxis; pain associated with sensitive teeth.

Macmiror
Salus, Aust.; Poli, Ital.; Farma Lepori, Spain; Poli, Switz.
Nifuratel (p.589·1).
Genito-urinary-tract infections; trichomoniasis.

Macmiror Complex Poli, Ital.
Nifuratel (p.589·1); nystatin (p.386·1).
Vulvovaginal infections.

Macocyn Mack, Illert., Ger.†.
Oxytetracycline hydrochloride (p.235·1).
Bacterial infections.

Macosil Vifor, Switz.
Aluminium hydroxide (p.1177·3); magnesium hydroxide (p.1198·2); simethicone (p.1213·1).
Gastro-intestinal disorders.

Macro Antioxidant Whitehall, Austral.
Vitamin and mineral preparation.
Dietary supplement.

Macro Anti-Stress Whitehall, Austral.
Vitamin B substances, ascorbic acid, and valerian (p.1643·1).
Dietary supplement; stress.

Macro B Whitehall, Austral.
Vitamin B substances.
Dietary supplement.

Macro C Whitehall, Austral.
Ascorbic acid (p.1365·2); calcium ascorbate (p.1365·2); bioflavonoids (p.1580·1); rutin (p.1580·2); hesperidin (p.1580·2).

Macro C + Garlic with Zinc Whitehall, Austral.
Ascorbic acid (p.1365·2); calcium ascorbate (p.1365·2); zinc (p.1373·1); garlic (p.1583·1).
Cold and influenza symptoms; zinc and vitamin C deficiencies.

Macro E Whitehall, Austral.
d-Alpha tocopherol (p.1369·1).
Vitamin E deficiency; vitamin E supplement.

Macro Garlic Whitehall, Austral.
Odourless Arizona garlic (p.1583·1).
Cold and influenza symptoms.

Macro Go Whitehall, Austral.
Vitamin B substances with ascorbic acid.
Dietary supplement.

Macro Liquical Lederle, Austral.†.
Calcium carbonate (p.1182·1).
Calcium supplement.

Macro M Whitehall, Austral.
Multivitamin and mineral preparation.
Dietary supplement.

Macro Maxepa Whitehall, Austral.
Eicosapentaenoic acid (p.1276·1); docosahexaenoic acid (p.1276·1); *d*-alpha tocopheryl acetate.
Omega-3 fatty acid supplement.

Macro Natural Vitamin E Cream Whitehall, Austral.
d-Alpha tocopheryl acetate (p.1369·2); vitamin A palmitate (p.1359·2); panthenol (p.1571·1); allantoin (p.1078·2).
Dry skin; minor skin disorders.

Macro Paks Suisse, Austral.†.
Multivitamin, mineral, and amino acid preparation.

Macro PMT Whitehall, Austral.
Vitamins B and C and mineral preparation.
Dietary supplement.

Macro Sports Supplement Whitehall, Austral.†.
Multivitamin, mineral, electrolyte and nutritional supplement preparation.

Macrobid
Procter & Gamble, Canad.; Procter & Gamble, Irl.; Procter & Gamble, UK; Procter & Gamble, USA.
Nitrofurantoin (p.231·3).
Urinary-tract infections.

Macrocide Macarthys, UK†.
Antiseptic skin cleanser.

Macrodantin
Pharmacia Upjohn, Austral.; Procter & Gamble, Canad.; Procter & Gamble, Irl.; Formenti, Ital.; SmithKline Beecham, S.Afr.; Procter & Gamble, UK; Procter & Gamble, USA.
Nitrofurantoin (p.231·3).
Urinary-tract infections.

Macrodex
Kabi Pharmacia, Aust.; Pharmacia Upjohn, Austral.; Pharmacia Upjohn, Canad.; Reusch, Ger.; Kabi, Irl.†; Don Baxter, Ital.†; Pharmacia Upjohn, Norw.; Pharmacia Upjohn, S.Afr.; Antibioticos, Spain; Medisan, Swed.; Braun, Switz.; Pharmacia, UK; Pharmacia, USA.
Dextran 60 (p.716·3) or dextran 70 (p.717·1) in glucose or sodium chloride.
Plasma volume expansion; thrombosis prophylaxis.

Macrodoxine Lagamed, S.Afr.†.
Vitamin B substances with vitamin C.

Macrolate Pharmagen, S.Afr.†.
Erythromycin estolate (p.204·1).
Bacterial infections.

Macrolax Carlo Erba OTC, Ital.
Docusate sodium (p.1189·3); sorbitol (p.1354·2).
Constipation.

Macromycine Farmabel, Belg.†.
Erythromycin ethyl succinate (p.204·2).
Bacterial infections.

Macropen Xixia, S.Afr.
Amoxycillin (p.151·3); flucloxacillin (p.209·1).
Bacterial infections.

Macroral Malesci, Ital.
Midecamycin acetate (p.226·2).
Bacterial infections.

Macrosil Faes, Spain.
Roxithromycin (p.247·1).
Bacterial infections; toxoplasmosis.

Macrotec Squibb Diagnostics, USA.
Technetium-99m (p.1425·1) labelled albumin.

Mactam Coli, Ital.
Latamoxef disodium (p.221·2).
Gram-negative bacterial infections.

Madar Ravizza, Ital.
Nordazepam (p.682·3).
Sleep disorders.

Madecassol
Kolassa, Aust.; Laroche Navarron, Belg.; Syntex, Canad.†; Nicholas, Fr.; Laroche Navarron, Neth.†; Syntex, Switz.
Centella (p.1080·3).
Burns; keloids; scars; wounds.

Madecassol Neomycine Hydrocortisone Nicholas, Fr.
Centella (p.1080·3); neomycin sulphate (p.229·2); hydrocortisone acetate (p.1043·3).
Skin disorders; wounds.

Madecassol Tulgras Nicholas, Fr.
Centella (p.1080·3).
Ulcers; wounds.

Maderan Nycomed, Switz.
Sulfametrole (p.252·1); trimethoprim (p.265·1).
Bacterial infections.

Madicure Taxandria, Neth.
Mebendazole (p.104·1).
Enterobiasis.

Madopar
Roche, Aust.; Roche, Austral.; Roche, Ger.; Roche, Irl.; Roche, Ital.; Roche, Neth.; Roche, Norw.; Roche, S.Afr.; Syntex, Spain; Roche, Switz.; Roche, UK.
Levodopa (p.1137·1); benserazide hydrochloride (p.1132·1).
These ingredients can be described by the British Approved Name Co-beneldopa.
Parkinsonism.

Madopark Roche, Swed.
Levodopa (p.1137·1); benserazide hydrochloride (p.1132·1).
Parkinsonism.

Madurase Tecnobio, Spain.
Clebopride malate (p.1188·2).
Adjunct in gastro-intestinal radiography and intubation; gastro-oesophageal reflux; gastroparesis; nausea and vomiting.

Maffee N Togal, Switz.†.
Aloes (p.1177·1); frangula bark (p.1193·2); taraxacum (p.1634·2).
Constipation.

Mafu Bayer, Ital.
Tetramethrin (p.1410·3); piperonyl butoxide (p.1409·3).
Insecticide.

Mag-200 Optimox, USA.
Magnesium oxide (p.1198·3).
Magnesium deficiency.

Mag 2
Charton, Canad.; Theraplix, Fr.; Synthelabo, Ital.; Casen Fisons, Spain; Roche, Switz.
Magnesium pidolate (p.1157·3).
Eclampsia; magnesium deficiency; muscular cramp; nervous disorders.

Mag 50 Vitaplex, Austral.
Magnesium amino acid chelate.
Magnesium supplement.

Mag Doskar's Leber-Galletonikum Doskar, Aust.
Cynara (p.1569·2); taraxacum (p.1634·2); peppermint leaf (p.1208·1).
Liver and biliary-tract disorders.

Mag Doskar's Magentonikum Doskar, Aust.
Chamomile (p.1561·2); peppermint leaf (p.1208·1); melissa (p.1600·1).
Gastro-intestinal disorders.

Mag Doskar's Nerventonikum Doskar, Aust.
Valerian (p.1643·1); lupulus (p.1597·2); melissa (p.1600·1); chamomile (p.1561·2).
Nervous disorders.

Mag Doskar's Nieren- und Blasentonikum Doskar, Aust.
Urtica (p.1642·3); equisetum (p.1575·1); silver birch (p.1553·3).
Renal and bladder disorders.

Mag Kottas Baby-Tee Kottas-Heidenberg, Aust.
Chamomile (p.1561·2); mallow leaves; spearmint (p.1632·1); caraway (p.1559·3); fennel (p.1579·1).
Gastro-intestinal disorders.

Mag Kottas Beruhigungstee Kottas-Heidenberg, Aust.
Tea: Melissa (p.1600·1); spearmint (p.1632·1); valerian (p.1643·1); flos aurantii; mallow leaves; rose fruit (p.1365·2); mallow flowers.
Tea bags: Melissa (p.1600·1); spearmint (p.1632·1); valerian (p.1643·1); flos aurantii; mallow leaves; rose fruit (p.1365·2).
Nervous disorders.

Mag Kottas Blahungs-Verdauungstee Kottas-Heidenberg, Aust.
Tea: Mallow leaves; peppermint leaf (p.1208·1); caraway (p.1559·3); fennel (p.1579·1); centaury (p.1561·1); calendula officinalis.
Tea bags: Mallow leaves; peppermint leaf (p.1208·1); caraway (p.1559·3); fennel (p.1579·1); centaury (p.1561·1).
Gastro-intestinal disorders.

Mag Kottas Entschlackungstee Kottas-Heidenberg, Aust.
Tea: Silver birch (p.1553·3); peppermint leaf (p.1208·1); urtica (p.1642·3); violae tricoloris; taraxacum (p.1634·2); calendula officinalis.
Tea bags: Silver birch (p.1553·3); peppermint leaf (p.1208·1); urtica (p.1642·3); violae tricoloris; taraxacum (p.1634·2).
Tonic.

Mag Kottas Entwasserungstee Kottas-Heidenberg, Aust.
Tea: Orthosiphon (p.1592·2); equisetum (p.1575·1); herniaria (p.1587·2); taraxacum (p.1634·2); peppermint leaf (p.1208·1); calendula officinalis.
Tea bags: Orthosiphon (p.1592·2); equisetum (p.1575·1); herniaria (p.1587·2); taraxacum (p.1634·2); peppermint leaf (p.1208·1).
Renal and bladder disorders.

Mag Kottas Grippe-Tee Kottas-Heidenberg, Aust.
Tea: Sambucus (p.1627·2); tilia (p.1637·3); plantago lanceolata; rose fruit (p.1365·2).
Tea bags: Sambucus (p.1627·2); tilia (p.1637·3); plantago lanceolata; orris; rose fruit (p.1365·2).
Cold symptoms.

Mag Kottas Herz- und Kreislauftee Kottas-Heidenberg, Aust.
Flos aurantii; crataegus (p.1568·2); maté leaves (p.1645·1); peppermint leaf (p.1208·1); rosemary.
Cardiovascular disorders.

Mag Kottas Husten-Bronchialtee Kottas-Heidenberg, Aust.
Tea: Althaea leaves and root (p.1546·3); plantago lanceolata; thyme (p.1636·3); aniseed (p.1549·3); verbascum flowers.
Respiratory-tract disorders.
Tea bags: Plantago lanceolata; thyme (p.1636·3); aniseed (p.1549·3); althaea root (p.1546·3); iceland moss.
Catarrh; cough.

Mag Kottas Krauterexpress-Nerven-Schlaf-Tee Kottas-Heidenberg, Aust.
Lupulus (p.1597·2); flos aurantii; melissa (p.1600·1); peppermint leaf (p.1208·1); valerian (p.1643·1).
Nervous disorders.

Mag Kottas Leber-Gallentee Kottas-Heidenberg, Aust.
Tea: Mallow leaves; peppermint leaf (p.1208·1); menyanthes (p.1601·2); cnicus benedictus (p.1565·3); taraxacum (p.1634·2); calendula officinalis.
Biliary disorders; gastro-intestinal disorders.
Tea bags: Chamomile (p.1561·2); peppermint leaf (p.1208·1); menyanthes (p.1601·2); herba teucrii; taraxacum (p.1634·2).
Biliary disorders.

Mag Kottas Magen-Darmtee Kottas-Heidenberg, Aust.
Tea: Mallow leaves; melissa (p.1600·1); peppermint leaf (p.1208·1); chamomile (p.1561·2); calamus (p.1556·1); calendula officinalis.
Tea bags: Chamomile (p.1561·2); mallow leaves; peppermint leaf (p.1208·1); centaury (p.1561·1); calamus (p.1556·1); fennel (p.1579·1).
Gastro-intestinal disorders.

Mag Kottas Nerven-Beruhigungstee Kottas-Heidenberg, Aust.
Melissa (p.1600·1); peppermint leaf (p.1208·1); valerian (p.1643·1); flos aurantii; mistletoe (p.1604·1); calendula officinalis.
Nervous disorders.

Mag Kottas Nieren-Blasentee Kottas-Heidenberg, Aust.
Tea: Peppermint leaf (p.1208·1); orthosiphon (p.1592·2); equisetum (p.1575·1); herniaria (p.1587·2); bearberry (p.1552·2); calendula officinalis.
Tea bags: Peppermint leaf (p.1208·1); orthosiphon (p.1592·2); equisetum (p.1575·1); herniaria (p.1587·2); ononis (p.1610·2).
Renal and bladder disorders.

Mag Kottas Schlaftee Kottas-Heidenberg, Aust.
Lupulus (p.1597·2); flos aurantii; melissa (p.1600·1); peppermint leaf (p.1208·1); valerian (p.1643·1).
Nervous disorders.

Mag Kottas Tee fur stillende Mutter Kottas-Heidenberg, Aust.
Tea: Melissa (p.1600·1); mallow leaves; peppermint leaf (p.1208·1); caraway (p.1559·3); fennel (p.1579·1); calendula officinalis.
Tea bags: Melissa (p.1600·1); mallow leaves; peppermint leaf (p.1208·1); caraway (p.1559·3); fennel (p.1579·1).
Gastro-intestinal disorders during lactation.

Mag Kottas Wechseltee Kottas-Heidenberg, Aust.
Tea: Melissa (p.1600·1); peppermint leaf (p.1208·1); chamomile (p.1561·2); potentilla anserina; valerian (p.1643·1).
Tea bags: Melissa (p.1600·1); peppermint leaf (p.1208·1); chamomile (p.1561·2); achillea (p.1542·2); valerian (p.1643·1).
Menopausal disorders.

Magagel Genpharm, S.Afr.
Aluminium oxide (p.1077·2); magnesium trisilicate (p.1199·1).
Gastro-oesophageal reflux; peptic ulcer.

Magalan Invamed, USA.
Aluminium hydroxide (p.1177·3); magnesium hydroxide (p.1198·2); simethicone (p.1213·1).

Magalba Salters, S.Afr.
Magnesium sulphate (p.1157·3); magnesium carbonate (p.1198·1).
Constipation.

Magalox Plus Invamed, USA.
Aluminium hydroxide (p.1177·3); magnesium hydroxide (p.1198·2); simethicone (p.1213·1).

Magalphil Philopharm, Ger.
Magaldrate (p.1198·1).
Gastro-intestinal disorders associated with hyperacidity.

Magan Savage, USA.
Magnesium salicylate (p.51·1).
Fever; osteoarthritis; pain; rheumatoid arthritis.

Magasan Gastropharm, Ger.
Magaldrate (p.1198·1).
Gastric hyperacidity.

Magastron Hexal, Ger.
Magaldrate (p.1198·1).
Gastric hyperacidity; peptic ulcer.

Mag-Cal Mega Freeda, USA.
Magnesium (p.1157·2); calcium (p.1155·1).
Dietary supplement.

Magcal Plus Blackmores, Austral.†.
Magnesium phosphate (p.1157·3); calcium phosphate (p.1155·3); dibasic potassium phosphate (p.1159·2); iron phosphate; dibasic sodium phosphate (p.1159·3).

Magenal Synpharma, Switz.†.
Aluminium hydroxide (p.1177·3); magnesium hydroxide (p.1198·2).
Gastro-intestinal disorders associated with hyperacidity.

Magen-Darm Rowopan (Rowo-837) Pharmakon, Ger.†.
Homoeopathic preparation.

Magenpulver Hafter Streuli, Switz.
Bismuth subnitrate (p.1180·2); calcium carbonate (p.1182·1); magnesium peroxide (p.1119·1).
Gastric hyperacidity.

Magentabletten Hafter Streuli, Switz.
Bismuth subnitrate (p.1180·2); calcium carbonate (p.1182·1); magnesium carbonate (p.1198·1).
Gastric hyperacidity.

Magentee
Note. This name is used for preparations of different composition.
Salus, Aust.
Chamomile (p.1561·2); peppermint leaf (p.1208·1); caraway (p.1559·3); valerian (p.1643·1).
Gastro-intestinal disorders.
Weleda, Aust.
Angelica; gentian (p.1583·3); menyanthes (p.1601·2); caraway (p.1559·3); parsley (p.1615·3); achillea (p.1542·2).
Gastro-intestinal disorders.

Magentee EF-EM-ES Smetana, Aust.
Absinthium (p.1541·1); centaury (p.1561·1); taraxacum (p.1634·2); skin powder; cort. aurantii dulc; hypericum (p.1590·1).
Gastro-intestinal disorders.

Magen-Tee Stada N Stada, Ger.
Chamomile (p.1561·2); peppermint leaf (p.1208·1); achillea (p.1542·2).
Gastro-intestinal disorders.

Mag-G Cypress, USA.
Magnesium gluconate (p.1157·2).
Dietary supplement.

Maghen Savio, Ital.†.
Pirenzepine hydrochloride (p.467·1).
Gastritis; peptic ulcer.

Magic Mix Taranis, Fr.
Maize starch (p.1356·2).
Dietary aid; gastro-oesophageal reflux in infants.

Magicul Alphapharm, Austral.
Cimetidine (p.1183·2).
Gastro-oesophageal reflux; peptic ulcer; Zollinger-Ellison syndrome.

Magion Ern, Spain.
Magaldrate (p.1198·1).
Hyperacidity.

Magisbile Magis, Ital.
Fencibutirol (p.1578·3); boldo (p.1554·1); rhubarb (p.1212·1); cascara (p.1183·1); sorbitol (p.1354·2).
Constipation; dyspepsia; haemorrhoids.

Magisgel Morado, Ital.†.
Royal jelly (p.1626·3).
Nutritional supplement.

Magium Hexal, Ger.
Magnesium aspartate (p.1157·2).
Magnesium deficiency.

Magium E Hexal, Ger.
dl-Alpha tocopheryl acetate (p.1369·2); magnesium oxide (p.1198·3).
Vitamin E and magnesium deficiency.

Magium K Hexal, Ger.
Potassium aspartate (p.1161·3); magnesium aspartate (p.1157·2).
Potassium and magnesium deficiency.

Maglid CPB, Belg.
Aluminium hydroxide (p.1177·3); magnesium hydroxide (p.1198·2).
Gastro-intestinal disorders associated with hyperacidity.

Maglucate Pharmascience, Canad.
Magnesium gluconate (p.1157·2).
Hypomagnesaemia.

Magluphen Nycomed, Aust.†.
Diclofenac sodium (p.31·2).
Gout; inflammation; musculoskeletal and joint disorders; pain; renal and biliary colic.

Maglut Magis, Ital.
Glutathione (p.983·1).
Alcohol and drug poisoning; radiation trauma.

Magmed Lichtenstein, Ger.
Magaldrate (p.1198·1).
Gastric hyperacidity; peptic ulcer.

Magmin
Vita Glow, Austral.; Selmag, Switz.
Magnesium aspartate (p.1157·2).
Magnesium deficiency; magnesium supplement.

Magnacal
Wyeth-Ayerst, Canad.†; Sherwood, USA.
Preparation for enteral nutrition.

Magnalox Schein, USA.
Aluminium hydroxide (p.1177·3); magnesium hydroxide (p.1198·2).
Hyperacidity.

Magnapen Beecham Research, UK.
Capsules: Ampicillin trihydrate (p.153·2); flucloxacillin sodium (p.209·2).
These ingredients can be described by the British Approved Name Co-fluampicil.
Injection: Ampicillin sodium (p.153·1); flucloxacillin sodium (p.209·2).
These ingredients can be described by the British Approved Name Co-fluampicil.
Syrup: Ampicillin trihydrate (p.153·2); flucloxacillin magnesium (p.209·1).
These ingredients can be described by the British Approved Name Co-fluampicil.
Bacterial infections.

Magnaprin Rugby, USA.
Aspirin (p.16·1).
Aluminium hydroxide (p.1177·3), calcium carbonate (p.1182·1), and magnesium hydroxide (p.1198·2) are included in this preparation in an attempt to limit adverse effects on the gastro-intestinal mucosa.
Fever; inflammation; myocardial infarction; pain; transient ischaemic attacks.

Magnaspart Rosen, Ger.
Magnesium aspartate (p.1157·2).
Magnesium deficiency.

Magnatex Propan, S.Afr.
Ibuprofen (p.44·1).
Musculoskeletal and joint disorders.

Magnatol Sterling Health, UK.
Potassium bicarbonate (p.1153·1); alexitol sodium (p.1176·3); magnesium carbonate (p.1198·1).
Gastro-oesophageal reflux.

Magne-B$_6$ Sanofi Winthrop, Fr.
Oral solution: Magnesium lactate (p.1157·3); magnesium pidolate (p.1157·3); pyridoxine hydrochloride (p.1362·3).
Tablets: Magnesium lactate (p.1157·3); pyridoxine hydrochloride (p.1362·3).
Anxiety attacks; magnesium deficiency.

Magnecyl Pharmacia Upjohn, Swed.
Aspirin (p.16·1).
Fever; inflammation; pain.

Magnecyl-koffein Pharmacia Upjohn, Swed.
Aspirin (p.16·1); caffeine (p.749·3).
Fever; inflammation; pain.

Magnerot A Worwag, Ger.
Magnesium aspartate (p.1157·2).
Magnesium deficiency.

Magnerot Ampullen Worwag, Ger.†.
Magnesium gluconate (p.1157·2).
Magnesium deficiency.

Magnerot Classic Worwag, Ger.
Magnesium orotate (p.1611·2).
Magnesium deficiency.

Magnerot N Worwag, Ger.
Magnesium phosphate (p.1157·3); magnesium citrate (p.1198·2).
Magnesium deficiency.

Magnesan Montefarmaco, Ital.†.
Magnesium oxide (p.1198·3); magnesium carbonate (p.1198·1); aluminium hydroxide (p.1177·3).
Gastro-intestinal disorders associated with hyperacidity.

Magnesia Bisurata Wyeth, Ital.
Magnesium carbonate (p.1198·1); sodium bicarbonate (p.1153·2); kaolin (p.1195·1).
Gastro-intestinal disorders associated with hyperacidity.

Magnesia Bisurata Aromatic Wyeth, Ital.
Magnesium carbonate (p.1198·1); sodium bicarbonate (p.1153·2); calcium carbonate (p.1182·1).
Gastro-intestinal hyperacidity.

Magnesia Effervescente Sanitas Sanitas, Ital.†.
Magnesium hydroxide (p.1198·2); sodium bicarbonate (p.1153·2); tartaric acid (p.1634·3).
Constipation; gastro-intestinal hyperacidity.

Magnesia Effervescente Sella Sella, Ital.
Magnesium hydroxide (p.1198·2); tartaric acid (p.1634·3); sodium bicarbonate (p.1153·2).
Constipation; gastro-intestinal hyperacidity.

Magnesia komp ACO, Swed.†.
Calcium carbonate (p.1182·1); heavy magnesium carbonate (p.1198·1).
Heartburn.

Magnesia S Pellegrino
Synthelabo, Ital.; Saprochi, Switz.
Magnesium hydroxide (p.1198·2).
Constipation; gastro-intestinal hyperacidity.

Magnesia san Pellegrino Seid, Spain.
Magnesium hydroxide (p.1198·2); sodium bicarbonate (p.1153·2).
Constipation; gastro-intestinal hyperacidity.

Magnesia Validada Domenech Garcia, Spain†.
Anise oil (p.1550·1); magnesium carbonate (p.1198·1); sodium bicarbonate (p.1153·2); tartaric acid (p.1634·3); menthol valerate; menthol (p.1600·2).
Nausea; vomiting.

Magnesia Volta *Edmond Pharma, Ital.*
Magnesium hydroxide (p.1198·2).
Constipation; gastro-intestinal hyperacidity.

Magnesie Abismuree *Whitehall, Fr.†.*
Magnesium carbonate (p.1198·1); calcium carbonate (p.1182·1); sodium bicarbonate (p.1153·2).
Gastro-intestinal disorders.

Magnesie Plus *Whitehall, Belg.*
Magnesium carbonate (p.1198·1); sodium bicarbonate (p.1153·2); calcium carbonate (p.1182·1).
Gastro-intestinal disorders associated with hyperacidity.

Magnesioboi *BOI, Spain.*
Magnesium lactate (p.1157·3).
Magnesium depletion.

Magnesiocard
Verla, Ger.; Verla, Switz.
Magnesium aspartate hydrochloride (p.1158·2).
Magnesium deficiency; magnesium supplement.

Magnesit *Byk Madaus, S.Afr.*
Magnesium l-aspartate hydrochloride (p.1158·2).
Hypomagnesaemia.

Magnesium Biomed *Verla, Switz.*
Coated tablets: Magnesium glutamate; magnesium citrate (p.1198·2).
Granules for oral liquid: Magnesium aspartate (p.1157·2).
Magnesium deficiency; magnesium supplement.

Magnesium Complexe *Golaz, Switz.*
Magnesium chloride (p.1157·2); magnesium glutamate; magnesium glycerophosphate (p.1157·2); magnesium orotate (p.1611·2); magnesium aspartate (p.1157·2).
Magnesium deficiency; magnesium supplement.

Magnesium compositum *OPW, Ger.*
Magnesium adipate; magnesium nicotinate.
Circulatory disorders.

Magnesium Diasporal
Nycomed, Aust.; Protina, Ger.; Protina, Switz.
Magnesium carbonate (p.1198·1), magnesium citrate (p.1198·2), magnesium laevulinate (p.1158·2), magnesium oxide (p.1198·3), or magnesium sulphate (p.1158·2).
Magnesium deficiency.

Magnesium Glycocolle Lafarge *Labomed, Fr.*
Magnesium chloride (p.1157·2); glycine (p.1345·2).
Anxiety; magnesium deficiency.

Magnesium Plus *Cenovis, Austral.; Vitelle, Austral.*
Magnesium orotate (p.1611·2); magnesium oxide (p.1198·3); magnesium amino acid chelate; monobasic potassium phosphate (p.1159·3); calcium hydrogen phosphate (p.1155·3).
Mineral supplement.

Magnesium Pyre *Salvat, Spain.*
Magnesium bromide; magnesium chloride (p.1157·2); magnesium fluoride; magnesium iodide.
Magnesium depletion.

Magnesium Tonil *APS, Ger.*
Capsules: Heavy magnesium oxide (p.1198·3); *dl*-alpha tocopheryl acetate (p.1369·2).
Magnesium or vitamin E deficiency.
Injection: Magnesium sulphate (p.1157·3).
Magnesium deficiency.

Magnesium Tonil N *APS, Ger.*
Magnesium citrate (p.1198·2).
Magnesium deficiency.

Magnesium Tonil Vitamin E *Richter, Aust.*
Magnesium oxide (p.1198·3); *dl*-alpha tocopheryl acetate (p.1369·2).
Vitamin E and magnesium deficiency.

Magnesium-Eufidol *Medopharm, Ger.*
Potassium aspartate (p.1161·3); magnesium aspartate (p.1157·2).
Cardiac disorders; magnesium or potassium deficiency.

Magnesium-OK *Wassen, UK.*
Magnesium oxide (p.1198·3); minerals; multivitamins.

Magnesium-OK Donna *Wassen, Ital.*
Magnesium; vitamins; minerals.
Nutritional supplement.

Magnesium-Plus-Hevert *Hevert, Ger.*
Magnesium oxide (p.1198·3); *d*-alpha tocopherol (p.1369·1).
Magnesium or vitamin E deficiency.

Magnespasmyl
Meuse, Belg.; Fisons, Fr.; Sanofi Winthrop, Switz.
Magnesium lactate (p.1157·3).
Magnesium deficiency; magnesium supplement.

Magneston *Berenguer Infale, Spain†.*
Magnesium gluceptate (p.1157·2).
Magnesium depletion.

Magnetrans *Fresenius, Ger.†.*
Magnesium aspartate (p.1157·2).
Magnesium deficiency.

Magnetrans forte *Fresenius-Praxis, Ger.*
Magnesium oxide (p.1198·3).
Magnesium deficiency.

Magnevist
Schering, Aust.; Berlex, Canad.; Schering, Fr.; Schering, Ger.; Schering, Ital.; Schering, Neth.; Schering, Norw.; Schering, Spain; Schering, Swed.; Schering, Switz.; Schering, UK; Berlex, USA.
Meglumine gadopentetate (p.1004·3).
Contrast medium for magnetic resonance imaging.

Magnezie *Lifeplan, UK.*
Vitamin and mineral preparation.

Magnezyme *Reckitt & Colman, Belg.†.*
Magnesium carbonate (p.1198·1).
Fatigue.

Magnofit *Asta Medica, Aust.*
Chewable tablets: Magnesium citrate (p.1198·2); magnesium carbonate (p.1198·1).
Effervescent tablets: Magnesium oxide (p.1198·3),.
Magnesium deficiency.

Magnogene
Note. This name is used for preparations of different composition.
Monal, Fr.; Interdelta, Switz.
Magnesium chloride (p.1157·2).
Magnesium deficiency; magnesium supplement.

Berenguer Infale, Spain.
Magnesium bromide; magnesium chloride (p.1157·2); magnesium fluoride; magnesium iodide.
Magnesium depletion.

Magnograf *Juste, Spain.*
Gadopentetic acid (p.1004·3).
Radiographic contrast medium.

Magnolax *Wampole, Canad.*
Magnesium hydroxide (p.1198·2); liquid paraffin (p.1382·1).
Constipation.

Magnolex *Sante Naturelle, Canad.*
Magnesium gluceptate (p.1157·2).

Magnoplasm *Faulding, Austral.*
Glycerol (p.1585·2); magnesium sulphate (p.1157·3).
Poultice for abscesses, boils, and carbuncles.

Magnorbin *Merck, Ger.*
Magnesium ascorbate (p.1157·2).
Magnesium deficiency.

Magnorol *Rolmex, Canad.*
Magnesium gluceptate (p.1157·2).

Magnoscorbol *Roche Nicholas, Fr.*
Magnesium chloride (p.1157·2); ascorbic acid (p.1365·2).
Anxiety attacks; magnesium deficiency.

Magnosolv *Asta Medica, Aust.*
Precipitated magnesium carbonate (p.1198·1); magnesium oxide (p.1198·3).
Magnesium deficiency.

Magnox *Lennod, USA.*
Aluminium hydroxide (p.1177·3); magnesium hydroxide (p.1198·2).
Hyperacidity.

Magnurol *Esteve, Spain.*
Terazosin hydrochloride (p.952·1).
Benign prostatic hyperplasia; hypertension.

Magocrus *Mago, Ger.†.*
Allantoin (p.1078·2); methylbenzethonium chloride (p.1119·3); wheat-germ; *Aspergillus oryzae*.
Ulcers.

Magonate *Fleming, USA.*
Magnesium gluconate (p.1157·2).
Dietary supplement.

Magopsor *Strathmann, Ger.*
Ointment: Dexamethasone (p.1037·1); allantoin (p.1078·2); retinol palmitate (p.1359·2); alpha tocopheryl acetate (p.1369·1).
Skin disorders.

Mag-Ox *Blaine, USA.*
Magnesium oxide (p.1198·3).
Hyperacidity; magnesium deficiency.

Magsal *US Pharmaceutical, USA.*
Magnesium salicylate (p.51·1); phenyltoloxamine citrate (p.416·1).
Pain.

Mag-Tab SR *Niche, USA.*
Magnesium lactate (p.1157·3).
Magnesium deficiency.

Magtrate *Mission Pharmacal, USA.*
Magnesium gluconate (p.1157·2).
Dietary supplement.

Magtrom *Trommsdorff, Ger.*
Magnesium aspartate (p.1157·2).
Magnesium deficiency.

Magvital
Panderma, Aust.; Vifor, Switz.
Magnesium aspartate (p.1157·2), magnesium hydrogen aspartate (p.1157·2), or magnesium sulphate (p.1157·3).
Eclampsia; magnesium deficiency; premature labour.

Mahiou *Vectem, Spain.*
Phenolphthalein (p.1208·2); vitamin F.
Skin disorders.

Maind *Also, Ital.†.*
Pyritinol hydrochloride (p.1624·1).
Cerebrovascular disorders; mental function disorders.

Maiorad *Rotta, Ital.*
Tiropramide hydrochloride (p.1638·2).
Smooth muscle spasm.

Majeptil
Rhone-Poulenc Rorer, Belg.; Rhone-Poulenc Rorer, Canad.; Specia, Fr.; Rhone-Poulenc Rorer, Spain.
Thioproperazine mesylate (p.695·1).
Psychoses.

Majocarmin *Hevert, Ger.†.*
Caraway oil (p.1559·3); fennel oil (p.1579·2); melissa oil (p.1600·1); peppermint oil (p.1208·1); absinthium (p.1541·1); cinnamon (p.1564·2); gentian (p.1583·3); myrrh (p.1606·1); pimpinella; rhubarb (p.1212·1); ginger (p.1193·2); citrus sinensis; calamus (p.1556·1); cinchona bark (p.1564·1); condurango (p.1567·2).
Gastro-intestinal disorders.

Majocarmin mite *Hevert, Ger.†.*
Absinthium (p.1541·1); calamus (p.1556·1); cinchona bark (p.1564·1); gentian (p.1583·3); valerian (p.1643·1); peppermint leaf (p.1208·1).
Dyspepsia; hypochlorhydria; loss of appetite.

Majocarmin-Tee *Hevert, Ger.*
Anise (p.1549·3); fennel (p.1579·1); caraway (p.1559·3); chamomile (p.1561·2); peppermint leaf (p.1208·1).
Gastro-intestinal disorders.

Majolat *Klinge, Aust.*
Nifedipine (p.916·2).
Angina pectoris; hypertension.

Major-Con *Major, USA.*
Simethicone (p.1213·1).
Flatulence.

Major-gesic *Major, USA.*
Phenyltoloxamine citrate (p.416·1); paracetamol (p.72·2).
Upper respiratory-tract symptoms.

Majorpen *Cyanamid, Ital.†.*
Amoxycillin sodium (p.151·3) or amoxycillin trihydrate (p.151·3).
Bacterial infections.

Makatussin
Note. This name is used for preparations of different composition.
Gebro, Aust.
Ointment: Camphor (p.1557·2); menthol (p.1600·2); cypress oil; eucalyptus oil (p.1578·1); pumilio pine oil (p.1623·3); oleum pini sylvestris; turpentine oil (p.1641·1); thyme oil (p.1637·1); peppermint oil (p.1208·1).
Respiratory-tract disorders.

Makara, Ger.†.
Guaiphenesin (p.1061·3); sodium dibunate (p.1070·1).
Bronchitis.

Gebro, Switz.
Ointment: Camphor (p.1557·2); menthol (p.1600·2); cypress oil; eucalyptus oil (p.1578·1); pumilio pine oil (p.1623·3); oleum pini sylvestris; turpentine oil (p.1641·1); thyme oil (p.1637·1).
Oral drops: Drosera (p.1574·1); liquorice (p.1197·1); pimpinella; senega root (p.1069·3); thyme (p.1636·3); anise oil (p.1550·1); eucalyptus oil (p.1578·1); camphor (p.1557·2); menthol (p.1600·2).
Syrup: Drosera (p.1574·1); liquorice (p.1197·1); senega root (p.1069·3); thyme (p.1636·3).
Respiratory-tract disorders.

Makatussin Balsam Mild *Roland, Ger.†.*
Eucalyptus oil (p.1578·1); thyme oil (p.1637·1).
Bronchitis; catarrh.

Makatussin Balsam mit Menthol *Roland, Ger.*
Eucalyptus oil (p.1578·1); menthol (p.1600·2); thyme oil (p.1637·1).
Bronchitis; catarrh.

Makatussin forte
Note. This name is used for preparations of different composition.
Makara, Ger.†.
Dihydrocodeine hydrochloride (p.34·2); diphenhydramine hydrochloride (p.409·1); guaiphenesin (p.1061·3).
Bronchitis; coughs.

Gebro, Switz.
Dihydrocodeine hydrochloride (p.34·2); drosera (p.1574·1); liquorice (p.1197·1); pimpinella; senega root (p.1069·3); thyme (p.1636·3); anise oil (p.1550·1); eucalyptus oil (p.1578·1); camphor (p.1557·2); menthol (p.1600·2).
Bronchitis; coughs.

Makatussin Inhalat Menthol *Roland, Ger.†.*
Eucalyptus oil (p.1578·1); peppermint oil (p.1208·1); thyme oil (p.1637·1).
Bronchitis; catarrh.

Makatussin Inhalat Mild *Roland, Ger.†.*
Eucalyptus oil (p.1578·1); thyme oil (p.1637·1).
Bronchitis; catarrh.

Makatussin Saft *Roland, Ger.*
Thyme (p.1636·3).
Bronchitis; catarrh.

Makatussin Saft Drosera *Roland, Ger.*
Drosera (p.1574·1).
Coughs.

Makatussin Saft forte *Roland, Ger.†.*
Drosera (p.1574·1); codeine phosphate (p.26·1).
Bronchitis.

Makatussin Tetra *Makara, Ger.†.*
Tetracycline hydrochloride (p.259·1); guaiphenesin (p.1061·3); papaverine hydrochloride (p.1614·2).
Bacterial infections of the respiratory tract.

Makatussin Tropfen *Roland, Ger.*
Thyme (p.1636·3); star anise oil.
Bronchitis; catarrh.

Makatussin Tropfen Drosera *Roland, Ger.*
Drosera (p.1574·1).
Coughs.

Makatussin Tropfen forte *Roland, Ger.*
Dihydrocodeine hydrochloride (p.34·2); drosera (p.1574·1).
Coughs.

Makinil *Mickan, Ger.†.*
Glycol salicylate (p.43·1); menthol (p.1600·2); rosemary oil (p.1626·2).
Musculoskeletal and joint pain; soft-tissue disorders; sports injuries.

Malafene *Knoll, Belg.*
Ibuprofen (p.44·1).
Fever; inflammation; pain.

Malandil *Bohm, Spain.*
Carnitine hydrochloride (p.1336·2); cobamamide (p.1364·2); lysine hydrochloride (p.1350·1).
Anaemias; tonic.

Malarone
Glaxo Wellcome, Austral.; Glaxo Wellcome, Swed.; Glaxo Wellcome, UK.
Atovaquone (p.579·3); proguanil hydrochloride (p.435·3).
Malaria.

Malatal *Hauck, USA†.*
Atropine sulphate (p.455·1); hyoscine hydrobromide (p.462·3); hyoscyamine hydrobromide (p.464·2) or hyoscyamine sulphate (p.464·2); phenobarbitone (p.350·2).
Gastro-intestinal disorders.

Malatex *Norton, UK†.*
Benzoic acid (p.1102·3); malic acid (p.1598·3); salicylic acid (p.1090·2); propylene glycol (p.1622·1).
Skin ulcers.

Malaviron *Wallace Mfg Chem., UK.*
Chloroquine phosphate (p.426·3).
Malaria.

Male Formula Herbal Plus Formula 2 *Vitelle, Austral.*
Eleutherococcus senticosus; equisetum; sarsaparilla; liquorice; damiana; zinc amino acid chelate; betacarotene; pyridoxine hydrochloride; *d*-alpha tocopheryl acid succinate; magnesium oxide.
Tonic.

Malex *Schieffer, Switz.†.*
Paracetamol (p.72·2); aspirin (p.16·1); calcium hydrogen phosphate (p.1155·3); caffeine and sodium salicylate (p.751·1); colloidal aluminium hydroxide (p.1177·3).
Fever; musculoskeletal and joint disorders; pain.

Malex N *Schieffer, Switz.†.*
Paracetamol (p.72·2).
Fever; pain.

Malexin *BASF, Ger.*
Naproxen (p.61·2).
Gout; inflammation; musculoskeletal and joint disorders; pain.

Malfesto *Boileau & Boyd, Irl.†.*
Malathion (p.1407·3).
Pediculosis; scabies.

Malgis *SmithKline Beecham, Fr.†.*
Paracetamol (p.72·2).
Fever; pain.

Maliasin
Ebewe, Aust.; Knoll, Ger.; Ravizza, Ital.; Knoll, Switz.
Barbexaclone (p.339·1).
Epilepsy.

Malimed *Ecosol, Switz.*
Cimetidine (p.1183·2).
Gastric hyperacidity; gastro-intestinal haemorrhage; gastro-oesophageal reflux; peptic ulcer; Zollinger-Ellison syndrome.

Malinert *Strathmann, Ger.*
Aspirin (p.16·1); paracetamol (p.72·2).
Formerly known as Malinert N Tablets.
Inflammation; pain.

Malipuran *Heumann, Ger.*
Bufexamac (p.22·2).
Skin disorders.

Malivan *Recordati, Ital.†.*
Amidopyrine (p.15·2).
Fever; pain.

Malix *Lagap, UK.*
Glibenclamide (p.319·3).
Diabetes mellitus.

Mallamint *Roberts, USA.*
Calcium carbonate (p.1182·1).
Hyperacidity.

Mallazine *Roberts, USA; Hauck, USA.*
Tetrahydrozoline hydrochloride (p.1070·2).
Minor eye irritation.

Mallebrin
Note. This name is used for preparations of different composition.
Krewel, Ger.
Hexaurea aluminium chloride.
Formerly known as Mallebrinetten.
Mouth and throat disorders.

Krewel, Switz.†.
Aluminium chloride (p.1078·3).
Mouth and throat disorders.

Mallebrin Fertiglosung *Krewel, Ger.†.*
Hexetidine (p.1116·1).
Mouth and throat infections.

Mallebrin Konzentrat *Krewel, Ger.*
Aluminium chloride (p.1078·3).
Inflammatory disorders and infections of the oropharynx.

Mallebrinettes *Krewel, Switz.†.*
Hexaurea aluminium chloride.
Mouth and throat disorders.

Mallisol *Hauck, USA.*
Povidone-iodine (p.1123·3).
Skin disinfection.

Mallorol *Novartis, Swed.*
Thioridazine (p.695·1) or thioridazine hydrochloride (p.695·1).
Alcohol withdrawal syndrome; pain; psychoses.

Malocide *Specia, Fr.*
Pyrimethamine (p.436·3).
Toxoplasmosis.

Malogen Aqueous *Germiphene, Canad.*
Testosterone (p.1464·1).
Androgenic.

Malogen in Oil *Germiphene, Canad.*
Testosterone propionate (p.1464·2).
Androgenic.

Malogex *Germiphene, Canad.*
Testosterone enanthate (p.1464·1).
Androgenic.

Maloprim
Glaxo Wellcome, Austral.; Wellcome, Belg.†; Wellcome, Irl.; Glaxo Wellcome, S.Afr.; Wellcome, UK.
Pyrimethamine (p.436·3); dapsone (p.199·2).
Malaria.

Maltlevol *Carter Horner, Canad.*
Multivitamin preparation with ferric ammonium citrate (p.1339·2).
Food supplement; iron-deficiency anaemia.

Maltlevol-M *Carter Horner, Canad.*
Multivitamin and mineral preparation.

Malto Mannite Magnesiaca *Molteni, Ital.†.*
Magnesium hydroxide (p.1198·2); maltose (p.1350·2); mannitol (p.900·3); sodium citrate (p.1153·2); sorbitol (p.1354·2).
Gastro-intestinal disorders.

Maltofer
Lucien, Fr.; Therabel, Fr.; Vifor International, Switz.
Iron polymaltose (p.1349·1).
Formerly known as Fer Lucien in *Fr.*
Iron deficiency; iron-deficiency anaemias.

Maltofer Fol *Vifor International, Switz.*
Iron polymaltose (p.1349·1); folic acid (p.1340·3).
Iron and folic acid deficiency.

Maltogen *Nestle, Austral.†.*
Infant feed supplement.
Anorexia; constipation.

Maltovis *Volchem, Ital.*
Maltodextrin (p.1350·2).
Carbohydrate source.

Maltsupex *Wallace, USA.*
Malt extract (p.1350·1).
Constipation.

Maltyl *Merckle, Ger.*
Dequalinium chloride (p.1112·1).
Inflammatory disorders and infections of the oropharynx.

Malun *Temmler, Ger.†.*
Monalazone disodium (p.1120·1); oestradiol benzoate (p.1455·1).
Vaginal infections; vaginitis.

Malun N *Temmler, Ger.†.*
Monalazone disodium (p.1120·1).
Vaginal infections.

Malvedrin *Adroka, Switz.*
Ointment: Mallow leaves; vitamin A (p.1358·1); vitamin D (p.1366·3); chamomile oil; hypericum oil (p.1590·1); linseed oil (p.1596·2).
Skin irritation; superficial wounds.
Topical liquid: Mallow leaves.
Mouth and throat disorders; superficial wounds.

Malveol *Magistra, Switz.*
Althaea leaves (p.1546·3); mallow leaves; salicylic acid (p.1090·2); mint oil (p.1604·1).
Mouth and throat disorders.

Malvitona *Lovens, Swed.*
Vitamin B substances; caffeine.

Mamellin *Frika, Aust.*
Vitamin F; peru balsam (p.1617·2); alpha-tocopheryl acetate (p.1369·1).
Skin damage.

Mammol *Abbott, USA.*
Bismuth subnitrate (p.1180·2); castor oil (p.1560·2); peru balsam (p.1617·2).
Nipple care.

Man Formula *Avon, Canad.*
Multivitamin and mineral preparation.

Manceau *SmithKline Beecham Consumer, Belg.*
Senna (p.1212·2); mali comm. syrup.
Constipation.

Mancef *Lafare, Ital.*
Cephamandole nafate (p.180·1).
Lignocaine hydrochloride (p.1293·2) is included in this preparation to alleviate the pain of injection.
Bacterial infections.

Mandarine *Boiron, Canad.*
Homoeopathic preparation.

Mandelamine
Warner-Lambert, Austral.†; Parke, Davis, Canad.; Parke, Davis, Ger.; Warner-Lambert, Switz.; Parke, Davis, USA†.
Hexamine mandelate (p.216·1).
Urinary-tract infections.

Mandocarbine *Monal, Fr.†.*
Activated charcoal (p.972·2).
Formerly contained vegetable charcoal, magnesium hydroxide, and calcium mandelate.
Gastro-intestinal disorders.

Mandokef
Lilly, Aust.; Lilly, Ger.; Lilly, Ital.; Lilly, S.Afr.; Lilly, Spain; Lilly, Switz.
Cephamandole nafate (p.180·1).
Lignocaine hydrochloride (p.1293·2) may be included in the intramuscular injection to alleviate the pain of injection.
Bacterial infections.

Mandol
Lilly, Austral.; Lilly, Belg.; Lilly, Canad.; Lilly, Neth.; Lilly, USA†.
Cephamandole nafate (p.180·1).
Bacterial infections.

Mandolsan *San Carlo, Ital.*
Cephamandole nafate (p.180·1).
Lignocaine hydrochloride (p.1293·2) is included in the intramuscular injection to alleviate the pain of injection.
Bacterial infections.

Mandragora Med Complex *Dynamit, Aust.*
Homoeopathic preparation.

Mandro-Angin *Henk, Ger.†.*
Tyrothricin (p.267·2); cetylpyridinium chloride (p.1106·2); benzocaine (p.1286·2).
Mouth and throat disorders.

Mandrogallan *Henk, Ger.†.*
Mandragora officinarum root; atropine sulphate (p.455·1); ox bile (p.1553·2); papaverine hydrochloride (p.1614·2); cholic acid; curcuma zanthorrhiza rhizome; aloes (p.1177·1); jalap (p.1195·1).
Biliary disorders; dyspepsia.

Mandrogripp
Note. A similar name is used for preparations of different composition.
Dolorgiet, Ger.
Paracetamol (p.72·2).
Fever; pain.

Mandro-Gripp
Note. A similar name is used for preparations of different composition.
Henk, Ger.†.
Paracetamol (p.72·2); ephedrine hydrochloride (p.1059·3); dextromethorphan hydrobromide (p.1057·3).
Cold and influenza symptoms.

Mandrolax *Dolorgiet, Ger.*
Bisacodyl (p.1179·3).
Constipation.

Mandrolax Lactu *Dolorgiet, Ger.*
Lactulose (p.1195·3).
Constipation; hepatic encephalopathy; salmonella enteritis.

Mandrolax Pico *Dolorgiet, Ger.*
Sodium picosulphate (p.1213·2).
Constipation.

Mandrorhinon *Henk, Ger.†.*
Calcium lactate (p.1155·2); calcium hydrogen phosphate (p.1155·3); propyphenazone (p.81·3); ephedrine hydrochloride (p.1059·3); potassium iodide (p.1493·1); mandragora officinarum root; scopolia carniolica root; nicotinamide (p.1351·2).
Upper respiratory tract infections.

Mandros *Henk, Ger.†.*
Aspirin (p.16·1); caffeine (p.749·3); thiamine nitrate.
Cold symptoms; fever; pain.

Mandros Diarstop *Dolorgiet, Ger.*
Loperamide hydrochloride (p.1197·2).
Diarrhoea.

Mandros Reise *Dolorgiet, Ger.*
Dimenhydrinate (p.408·2).
Motion sickness; nausea; vertigo; vomiting.

Mandros-forte *Henk, Ger.†.*
Paracetamol (p.72·2); caffeine (p.749·3); codeine phosphate (p.26·1); papaverine hydrochloride (p.1614·2).
Migraine; pain.

Mandro-Zep *Henk, Ger.†.*
Diazepam (p.661·1).
Psychiatric disorders.

Maneon *Poli, Ital.*
Amineptine hydrochloride (p.273·2).
Depression.

Manerix
Roche, Canad.; Roche, Irl.; Andreu, Spain; Roche, UK.
Moclobemide (p.298·3).
Depression.

Manevac *Galen, UK.*
Ispaghula (p.1194·2); senna fruit (p.1212·2).
A similar product was formerly marketed in the *UK* under the name Agiolax.
Bowel evacuation; constipation.

Mangamac *Cantassium Co., UK†.*
Manganese aspartate; vitamins and minerals.

Mangaplexe *Lehning, Fr.*
Manganese gluconate (p.1351·1).
Hypersensitivity.

Mangatrace *Rorer, Austral.†.*
Manganese chloride (p.1350·3).
Parenteral nutrition.

Manialit *ISF, Ital.†.*
Lithium carbonate (p.290·3).
Bipolar disorder.

Manicol *Martin, Fr.*
Mannitol (p.900·3).
Bowel evacuation; constipation; dyspepsia.

Manidon *Knoll, Spain.*
Verapamil hydrochloride (p.960·3).
Angina pectoris; arrhythmias; hypertension.

Manimon *Dresden, Ger.*
Propranolol hydrochloride (p.937·1); triamterene (p.957·2); hydrochlorothiazide (p.885·2).
Hypertension.

Maninil *Berlin-Chemie, Ger.*
Glibenclamide (p.319·3).
Diabetes mellitus.

Maniprex *Wolfs, Belg.*
Lithium carbonate (p.290·3).
Bipolar disorder; depression.

Manir *Byk, Fr.†.*
Oxyphencyclimine hydrochloride (p.466·3).
Gastro-intestinal disorders; peptic ulcer.

Mannest *Manne, USA†.*
Conjugated oestrogens (p.1457·3).

Mannex *Bioceuticals, UK.*
Multivitamin and mineral preparation.

Mannistol *Bieffe, Ital.*
Mannitol (p.900·3).
Cranial and ocular hypertension.

Mannite *Saprochi, Switz.*
Mannitol (p.900·3).
Constipation.

Mannit-Losung *Serag-Wiessner, Ger.*
Mannitol (p.900·3).
Forced diuresis; oedema; renal failure.

Manns Knoblauch Pillen Plus *Mann, Ger.†.*
Garlic (p.1583·1); mistletoe (p.1604·1); crataegus (p.1568·2); lupulus (p.1597·2); chlorophyllin copper complex sodium.
Circulatory disorders; gastro-intestinal disorders.

Manoderm *Propan-Vernleigh, S.Afr.†.*
Clioquinol (p.193·2); hydrocortisone (p.1043·3).
Skin disorders.

Manoplax
Boots, UK†; Boots, USA†.
Flosequinan (p.870·2).
Heart failure.

Mansal *Vita, Spain.*
Cimetidine (p.1183·2).
Acid aspiration; gastro-intestinal haemorrhage; gastro-oesophageal reflux; peptic ulcer; Zollinger-Ellison syndrome.

Mantadan *Boehringer Ingelheim, Ital.*
Amantadine hydrochloride (p.1129·2).
Influenza A; mental function impairment; parkinsonism.

Mantadil *Wellcome, USA†.*
Chlorcyclizine hydrochloride (p.404·3); hydrocortisone acetate (p.1043·3).

Mantadix
Du Pont, Belg.; Du Pont, Fr.
Amantadine hydrochloride (p.1129·2).
Influenza A; parkinsonism.

Manusept
Note. This name is used for preparations of different composition.
Bode, Ger.
Orthophenylphenol (p.1120·3).
Hand disinfection.

Houghs Healthcare, UK.
Triclosan (p.1127·2); isopropyl alcohol (p.1118·2).
Skin disinfection.

Manusept HD *Bode, Ger.*
Alcohol (p.1099·1).
Hand disinfection.

Maolate *Upjohn, USA.*
Chlorphenesin carbamate (p.1313·1).
Musculoskeletal pain.

Maox *Manne, USA.*
Magnesium oxide (p.1198·3).
Hyperacidity.

Mapap *Major, USA.*
Paracetamol (p.72·2).
Fever; pain.

Mapap Cold Formula *Major, USA.*
Paracetamol (p.72·2); chlorpheniramine maleate (p.405·1); pseudoephedrine hydrochloride (p.1068·3); dextromethorphan hydrobromide (p.1057·3).

Mapox *Fresenius-Praxis, Ger.*
Aciclovir (p.602·3) or aciclovir sodium (p.602·3).
Herpesvirus infections.

Mapro-GRY *Gry, Ger.*
Maprotiline hydrochloride (p.296·2).
Depression.

Maprolit *Magis, Ital.†.*
Maprotiline hydrochloride (p.296·2) or maprotiline mesylate (p.296·3).
Anxiety; depression; insomnia.

Maprolu *Hexal, Ger.*
Maprotiline hydrochloride (p.296·2).
Depression.

Mapro-Tablinen *Sanorania, Ger.†.*
Maprotiline hydrochloride (p.296·2).
Depression.

Mapurit *Sanum-Kehlbeck, Ger.*
dl-Alpha tocopheryl acetate (p.1369·2); magnesium oxide (p.1198·3).
Magnesium or vitamin E deficiency.

Maquil *Pharmaton, Ger.*
Cynara (p.1569·2).
Dyspepsia.

Marament Balsam W *Wider, Ger.*
Camphor (p.1557·2); methyl salicylate (p.55·2); benzyl nicotinate (p.22·1).
Neuralgia; rheumatism; sciatica; sprains.

Marament-N *Amino, Switz.*
Camphor (p.1557·2); methyl salicylate (p.55·2); benzyl nicotinate (p.22·1); oleum pini sylvestris.
Musculoskeletal, joint, and soft-tissue disorders.

Maranon H *Henkel, Ger.*
Sodium hypochlorite (p.1124·3).
Instrument disinfection.

Maranox *Dent, USA.*
Paracetamol (p.72·2).
Fever; pain.

Marax
Note. This name is used for preparations of different composition.
Asche, Ger.
Magaldrate (p.1198·1).
Gastro-intestinal disorders associated with hyperacidity.

Roerig, USA.
Ephedrine sulphate (p.1059·3); theophylline (p.765·1); hydroxyzine hydrochloride (p.412·1).
Bronchospastic disorders.

Marbagelan *Behringwerke, Ger.†.*
Gelatin (p.723·2).
Haemorrhagic disorders.

Marbec *Marlyn, USA†.*
Vitamin B substances with vitamin C.

Marblen *Fleming, USA.*
Calcium carbonate (p.1182·1); magnesium carbonate (p.1198·1).
Hyperacidity.

Marcain
Astra, Austral.; Astra, Irl.; Astra, Norw.; Astra, Swed.; Astra, UK.
Bupivacaine hydrochloride (p.1286·3).
Adrenaline (p.813·2) or adrenaline acid tartrate (p.813·3) is included in some injections as a vasoconstrictor to diminish absorption and localise the effect of the local anaesthetic.
Local anaesthesia.

Marcain plus Fentanyl *Astra, Austral.*
Bupivacaine hydrochloride (p.1286·3); fentanyl citrate (p.38·1).
Epidural analgesia.

Marcain plus Pethidine *Astra, Austral.*
Bupivacaine hydrochloride (p.1286·3); pethidine hydrochloride (p.76·1).
Epidural analgesia.

Marcain Spinal Heavy *Astra, Austral.*
Bupivacaine hydrochloride (p.1286·3) in hyperbaric glucose solution.
Local anaesthesia.

Marcaina *Astra, Ital.*
Bupivacaine hydrochloride (p.1286·3).
Adrenaline acid tartrate (p.813·3) is included in some injections as a vasoconstrictor to diminish absorption and localise the effect of the local anaesthetic.
Local anaesthesia.

Marcaine
Astra, Belg.; Sanofi Winthrop, Canad.; Astra, Fr.; Astra, Neth.; Sanofi Winthrop, USA.
Bupivacaine hydrochloride (p.1286·3).
Adrenaline (p.813·2) or adrenaline acid tartrate (p.813·3) is included in some injections as a vasoconstrictor to diminish absorption and localise the effect of the local anaesthetic.
Analgesia; local anaesthesia.

Marcaine glucose *Astra, Neth.*
Bupivacaine hydrochloride (p.1286·3) in glucose.
Spinal anaesthesia.

Marcelle Multi-Defense *Professional Health, Canad.*
SPF 15: Menthyl anthranilate (p.1487·2); ethylhexyl *p*-methoxycinnamate (p.1487·1); 2-phenyl-1*H*-benzimidazole-5-sulphonic acid (p.1488·2).
Sunscreen.

Marcelle Protective Block *Professional Health, Canad.*
SPF 15: Titanium dioxide (p.1093·3).
SPF 25: Titanium dioxide (p.1093·3); zinc oxide (p.1096·2).
Sunscreen.

Marcelle Sunblock *Professional Health, Canad.*
SPF 8: Ethylhexyl *p*-methoxycinnamate (p.1487·1); oxybenzone (p.1487·3).
SPF 15; SPF 20: Ethylhexyl *p*-methoxycinnamate (p.1487·1); octyl salicylate (p.1487·3); oxybenzone (p.1487·3).
Sunscreen.

Marcen *Pharmacia Upjohn, Spain.*
Ketazolam (p.675·2).
Anxiety; insomnia.

Marciderm *Sanofi Winthrop, Switz.†.*
Benzoic acid (p.1102·3); salicylic acid (p.1090·2); tartaric acid (p.1634·3).
Skin disorders.

Marcillin *Marnel, USA.*
Ampicillin trihydrate (p.153·2).

Marco Rub Camphorated *Marc-O, Canad.*
Camphor (p.1557·2); menthol (p.1600·2); cineole (p.1564·1).

Marcocid *Willvonseder, Aust.*
Propyl alcohol (p.1124·2); isopropyl alcohol (p.1118·2).
Skin disinfection.

Marcof *Marnel, USA.*
Hydrocodone tartrate (p.43·1); potassium guaiacolsulfonate (p.1068·3).
Coughs.

Marcoumar
Roche, Aust.; Roche, Belg.; Roche, Neth.; Roche, Switz.
Phenprocoumon (p.929·3).
Thrombo-embolic disorders.

Marcumar
Roche, Ger.; Roche, Spain†.
Phenprocoumon (p.929·3).
Thrombo-embolic disorders; thrombosis prophylaxis.

Marduk *S & K, Ger.*
Benzoyl peroxide (p.1079·2).
Acne.

Mareen *Krewel, Ger.*
Doxepin hydrochloride (p.283·2).
Anxiety disorders; depression; sleep disorders; withdrawal syndromes.

Marespin *Abiogen, Ital.*
Sulfenazone sodium (p.252·1).
Respiratory-tract infections.

Marevan
Boots, Austral.; Bio-Therabel, Belg.; Nycomed, Norw.; Goldshield, UK.
Warfarin sodium (p.964·2).
Thrombo-embolic disorders.

Marezine *Himmel, USA.*
Cyclizine hydrochloride (p.407·1).
Motion sickness.

Margesic *Marnel, USA.*
Butalbital (p.644·3); paracetamol (p.72·2); caffeine (p.749·3).

Margesic H *Marnel, USA.*
Hydrocodone tartrate (p.43·1); paracetamol (p.72·2).
Pain.

Margesic No. 3 *Marnel, USA†.*
Paracetamol (p.72·2); codeine phosphate (p.26·1).
Pain.

Marianon *Klein, Ger.*
Silybum marianum (p.993·3); chelidonium majus; achillea (p.1542·2); absinthium (p.1541·1); hypericum (p.1590·1).
Biliary disorders.

Mariazeller *Apotheke Gnadenmutter, Aust.*
Cinnamon (p.1564·2); frangula bark (p.1193·2); cinchona bark (p.1564·1); dried bitter-orange peel (p.1610·3); clove (p.1565·2); flos aurantii; chamomile (p.1561·2); melissa (p.1600·1); menyanthes (p.1601·2); cardamom fruit (p.1560·1); fructus aurantii immat; coriander (p.1567·3); absinthium (p.1541·1); cnicus benedictus (p.1565·3); centaury (p.1561·1); achillea moschata; achillea (p.1542·2); guaiacum wood; juniper (p.1592·2); galanga; gentian (p.1583·3); ginger (p.1193·2); nutmeg (p.1609·2); rhubarb (p.1212·1).
Gastro-intestinal disorders.

Marie Rose *Sterling Midy, Fr.†.*
Lotion: Pyrethrins; acetic acid (p.1541·2).
Shampoo: Pyrethrum (p.1410·1); piperonyl butoxide (p.1409·3).
Topical spray: Pyrethrins; piperonyl butoxide (p.1409·3).
Pediculosis.

Marienbader Pillen N *Palmicol, Ger.*
Bisacodyl (p.1179·3).
Constipation.

Mariendistel Curarina *Harras-Curarina, Ger.*
Silybum marianum (p.993·3).
Liver disorders.

Marine Lipid Concentrate *Vitaline, USA.*
Omega-3 marine triglycerides with vitamin E (p.1276·1).
Dietary supplement.

Marinepa *Lifeplan, UK.*
Omega-3 marine triglycerides (p.1276·1).
Nutritional supplement.

Marinol
Note. This name is used for preparations of different composition.
Sanofi Winthrop, Canad.; Roxane, USA.
Dronabinol (p.1191·2).
Appetite stimulant; nausea and vomiting associated with cancer chemotherapy.
Pharmadeveloppement, Fr.
Iodine (p.1493·1); marine algae; calcium dihydrogen phosphate (p.1556·2); tannic acid (p.1634·2); phosphoric acid (p.1618·1); sea water.
Tonic.

Markalakt
Koch, Aust.; Pascoe, Ger.
Chamomile (p.1561·2).
Allergic disorders; gastro-intestinal disorders; skin disorders.

Marlidan *Vinas, Spain.*
Liver extract.
Tonic.

Marlin Salt System *Marlin, USA.*
Sodium chloride (p.1162·2).
Rinsing and storage solution for soft contact lenses.

Marlyn Formula 50 *Marlyn, USA.*
Amino acids; pyridoxine hydrochloride (p.1362·3).
Fungal nail infections; postnatal hair-loss; splitting nails.

Marly-Skin *Sandoz, Ital.*
Barrier preparation.

Marmine *Vortech, USA.*
Dimenhydrinate (p.408·2).
Motion sickness.

Marnal *Vortech, USA.*
Aspirin (p.16·1); caffeine (p.749·3); butalbital (p.644·3).
Pain.

Marnatal-F *Marnel, USA.*
Multivitamin and mineral preparation with iron and folic acid.

Marocid *Lifepharma, Ital.†.*
Erythromycin estolate (p.204·1).
Bacterial infections.

Marolderm *Dermapharm, Ger.*
Dexpanthenol (p.1570·3).
Burns; skin ulceration; sunburn; wounds.

Marplan
Roche, Irl.†; Roche, Ital.†; Cambridge, UK; Roche, USA.
Isocarboxazid (p.290·3).
Now known as Isocarboxazid Tablets in the *UK*.
Depression.

Marpres *Marnel, USA.*
Hydrochlorothiazide (p.885·2); reserpine (p.942·1); hydralazine hydrochloride (p.883·2).
Hypertension.

Marrubene Codethyline *Lemoine, Fr.*
Elecampane (p.1059·2); marrubium (p.1063·3); terpin (p.1070·2); sodium benzoate (p.1102·3); ethylmorphine hydrochloride (p.36·1).
Respiratory-tract congestion.

Marsil *Crosara, Ital.*
Silybum marianum (p.993·3).
Liver disorders.

Marsilid *Roche, Fr.*
Iproniazid phosphate (p.290·2).
Depression.

Marthritic *Marnel, USA.*
Salsalate (p.83·1).

Marticassol *Ciba Vision, Fr.†.*
Centella (Madecassol) (p.1080·3).
Ocular scarring.

Marti-Contact *Ciba Vision, Fr.†.*
Cleansing and disinfecting solution for soft and hard contact lenses.

Martigene *Ciba Vision, Fr.*
Phenylephrine hydrochloride (p.1066·2); brompheniramine maleate (p.403·2).
Allergic conjunctivitis.

Martigenta *Ciba Vision, Fr.†.*
Gentamicin sulphate (p.212·1).
Bacterial eye infections.

Martimil *Alonga, Spain.*
Nortriptyline hydrochloride (p.300·2).
Depression.

Martindale Methadone Mixture DTF *Martindale Pharmaceuticals, UK.*
Methadone hydrochloride (p.53·2).
It contains hydroxybenzoate esters as preservatives.
NOTE. There is no connection between Martindale, The Complete Drug Reference and Martindale Pharmaceuticals.
Opioid withdrawal.

Martisol *Ciba Vision, Fr.†.*
Neomycin sulphate (p.229·2); prednisolone metasulphobenzoate (p.1049·1).
Allergic eye conditions; bacterial eye infections.

Martos-10 *Otsuka, Jpn.*
Maltose (p.1350·2).
Carbohydrate source; diabetes mellitus.

Marvelon
Organon, Aust.; Organon, Austral.; Organon, Belg.; Organon, Canad.; Organon, Ger.; Organon, Neth.; Organon, Norw.; Donmed, S.Afr.; Organon, Switz.; Organon, UK.
Desogestrel (p.1443·3); ethinyloestradiol (p.1445·1).
28-Day packs also contain 7 inert tablets.
Combined oral contraceptive.

Marvina *Muller Goppingen, Ger.†.*
Arnica; cinchona bark; condurango; dried bitter-orange peel; fresh lemon peel; gentian; calamus; calcium phosphinate.
Tonic.

Marviol *Organon, Irl.*
Desogestrel (p.1443·3); ethinyloestradiol (p.1445·1).
Combined oral contraceptive.

Marzine
Glaxo Wellcome, Aust.; Glaxo Wellcome, Canad.; Wellcome, Fr.†; Wellcome, Ital.†; Glaxo Wellcome, Neth.†; Warner-Lambert, Norw.; Glaxo Wellcome, Swed.; Wellcome, Switz.
Cyclizine hydrochloride (p.407·1) or cyclizine lactate (p.407·1).
Ménière's disease; motion sickness; nausea; vertigo; vomiting.

Marzine RF *Wellcome, UK†.*
Cinnarizine (p.406·1).
Marzine formerly contained cyclizine hydrochloride.
Vestibular disorders.

Masacin *Boehringer Mannheim, Ital.†.*
Procaterol hydrochloride (p.757·3).
Obstructive airways disease.

Masagil *Calmante Vitaminado, Spain.*
Liniment: Camphor (p.1557·2); ammonia (p.1548·3); methyl salicylate (p.55·2); rosemary oil (p.1626·2); turpentine oil (p.1641·1).
Topical spray: Camphor (p.1557·2); methyl salicylate (p.55·2); turpentine oil (p.1641·1); menthol (p.1600·2).
Rheumatic and muscle pain.

Masdil *Esteve, Spain.*
Diltiazem hydrochloride (p.854·2).
Angina pectoris; arrhythmias; hypertension; myocardial infarction.

Masern-Impfstoff Merieux *Pasteur Merieux, Ger.*
A live measles vaccine (attenuated Schwarz strain) (p.1517·3).
Active immunisation.

Masern-Lebend-Impfstoff *Chiron Behring, Ger.*
A live measles vaccine (more attenuated Enders strain) (p.1517·3).
Active immunisation.

Masern-Vaccinol *Procter & Gamble, Ger.*
A live measles vaccine (attenuated Schwarz strain) (p.1517·3).
Active immunisation.

Masern-Virus-Impfstoff *Chiron Behring, Ger.*
A live measles vaccine (more attenuated Enders strain) (p.1517·3).
Active immunisation.

Masigel K *Boehringer Ingelheim, Ger.*
Dimagnesium aluminium trisilicate.
Gastro-intestinal disorders.

Maskam Krauter-Tee *Duopharm, Ger.*
Senna (p.1212·2).
Constipation; exogenous obesity.

Masmoran *Pfizer, Ger.†.*
Hydroxyzine embonate (p.411·3).
Psychiatric disorders.

Masnoderm *Dominion, UK.*
Clotrimazole (p.376·3).
Fungal infections.

Masor *Formenti, Ital.*
Stepronin lysine (p.1070·1).
Respiratory-tract disorders.

Massage Balm Arnica *Weleda, UK.*
Arnica flower oil; birch leaf oil (p.55·3); lavender oil (p.1594·3); rosemary oil (p.1626·2).
Rheumatic and muscular pain.

Massage Balm Calendula *Weleda, UK.*
Calendula officinalis; betula alba (p.1553·3); lavender oil (p.1594·3).
Muscle tension.

Masse
Janssen-Cilag, Austral.†; Ortho, Canad.†; Janssen-Cilag, Irl.; Janssen-Cilag, S.Afr.†; Janssen-Cilag, UK†; Advanced Care, USA.
Emollient and moisturiser.
Sore or cracked nipples.

Massengill *SmithKline Beecham Consumer, USA.*
Concentrated solution: Lactic acid (p.1593·3); sodium lactate (p.1153·2); sodium bicarbonate (p.1153·2); alcohol (p.1099·1); octoxinol 9 (p.1326·2).
Powder: Ammonium alum; phenol (p.1121·2); methyl salicylate (p.55·2); eucalyptus oil (p.1578·1); menthol (p.1600·2); thymol (p.1127·1); sodium chloride (p.1162·2).
Vaginal disorders.

Massengill Disposable
SmithKline Beecham Consumer, USA.
Alcohol (p.1099·1); lactic acid (p.1593·3); sodium lactate (p.1153·2); octoxinol 9 (p.1326·2); propylene glycol (p.1622·1); cetylpyridinium chloride (p.1106·2); diazolidinyl urea.
Vaginal disorders.
SmithKline Beecham Consumer, USA.
Vinegar (p.1541·2).
Vaginal disorders.

Massengill Feminine Cleansing Wash *SmithKline Beecham Consumer, USA.*
Vaginal cleanser.

Massengill Medicated
Note. This name is used for preparations of different composition.
SmithKline Beecham Consumer, Canad.; SmithKline Beecham Consumer, USA.
Vaginal douche: Povidone-iodine (p.1123·3).
Vaginal disorders.
SmithKline Beecham Consumer, USA.
Soft cloth towelette: Hydrocortisone (p.1043·3).
Corticosteroid.

Massorax *RTA, Switz.*
Methyl salicylate (p.55·2); isopropyl nicotinate; capsicum (p.1559·2); camphor (p.1557·2); turpentine oil (p.1641·1); eucalyptus oil (p.1578·1); lavender oil (p.1594·3).
Musculoskeletal, joint, and soft-tissue disorders.

Master Cortex 200 *Coli, Ital.†.*
Suprarenal cortex (p.1050·1).
Anaemia; asthenia.

Masteron *Syntex, Belg.†.*
Drostanolone propionate (p.1444·2).
Breast cancer.

Mastia *Inexfa, Spain.*
Aspirin (p.16·1); caffeine (p.749·3).
Contains thiamine.
Fever; pain.

Mastical *Nycomed, Spain.*
Calcium carbonate (p.1182·1).
Hypocalcaemia; osteoporosis.

Mastiol *Bama, Spain.*
Chlorhexidine acetate (p.1107·2); benzocaine (p.1286·2); retinol (p.1358·1).
Mastitis.

Mastodanatrol *Sterling Winthrop, Fr.†.*
Danazol (p.1441·3).
Benign breast disorders.

Mastodynon *Bionorica, Ger.*
Homoeopathic preparation.

Mastu NH *Stada, Ger.†.*
Aesculus (p.1543·3); suprarenal cortex (p.1050·1); butoxycaine hydrochloride (p.1289·1); bismuth subnitrate (p.1180·2); zinc oxide (p.1096·2).
Anal fissures; haemorrhoids.

Mastu S *Stada, Ger.*
Bufexamac (p.22·2); bismuth subgallate (p.1180·2); titanium dioxide (p.1093·3); lignocaine hydrochloride (p.1293·2).
Anorectal disorders.

Materna
Wyeth-Ayerst, Canad.; Lederle, USA†.
Multivitamin and mineral preparation.
Dietary supplement during pregnancy and lactation.

Materna Nova *Lederle, Switz.*
Multivitamin and mineral preparation.

Maternity One *Swiss Herbal, Canad.*
Multivitamin and mineral preparation.

Mathieu Cough Syrup *Mathieu, Canad.*
Ammonium chloride (p.1055·2); potassium iodide (p.1493·1).

Mathoine *Wolfs, Belg.*
Phenytoin (p.352·3); methylphenobarbitone (p.349·2).
Epilepsy.

Matiga *Pierre Fabre, Fr.*
Arachis oil (p.1550·2); menthol (p.1600·2).
Musculoskeletal, joint, peri-articular, and soft-tissue disorders.

Matmille *Ritsert, Ger.*
Bath additive: Chamomile (p.1561·2); chamomile oil.
Ointment; oral liquid: Chamomile (p.1561·2).
Gastro-intestinal disorders; skin and mucous membrane disorders.

Mato *Hevert, Ger.*
Homoeopathic preparation.

Matrabec *Warner-Lambert, Spain†.*
Multivitamin and mineral preparation.

Matrix *IRBI, Ital.*
A heparinoid (p.882·3).
Osteoarthritis.

Matulane *Roche, USA.*
Procarbazine hydrochloride (p.559·2).
Malignant neoplasms.

Mature Balance *Pharmavite, Canad.*
Multivitamin and mineral preparation.

Maudor *Searle, Ger.†.*
Ruscus aculeatus; esculoside (p.1543·3).
Vascular disorders.

Mauran *Coli, Ital.†.*
Ranitidine hydrochloride (p.1209·3).
Gastro-intestinal disorders associated with hyperacidity.

Maveral *Farmades, Ital.*
Fluvoxamine maleate (p.288·3).
Depression; obsessive-compulsive disorder.

Mavid *Abbott, Ger.*
Clarithromycin (p.189·1).
Mycobacterial infections.

Mavigen Sebo *Mavi, Ital.*
Cystine (p.1339·1).
Seborrhoea.

Mavik *Knoll, USA.*
Trandolapril (p.957·1).
Heart failure following myocardial infarction; hypertension.

Mavipiu *Mavi, Ital.*
Colamin; zinc oxide (p.1096·2); oryzanol (p.1611·2).
Skin irritation.

Maxadol *Restan, S.Afr.*
Capsules: Paracetamol (p.72·2); codeine phosphate (p.26·1).
Syrup: Paracetamol (p.72·2); codeine phosphate (p.26·1); promethazine hydrochloride (p.416·2).
Fever; pain.

Maxadol Forte *Restan, S.Afr.*
Paracetamol (p.72·2); codeine phosphate (p.26·1); caffeine (p.749·3); meprobamate (p.678·1).
Pain.

Maxadol-P *Restan, S.Afr.*
Paracetamol (p.72·2).
Fever; pain.

Maxair
3M, Canad.; Jouveinal, Canad.; 3M, Fr.†; 3M, Switz.; 3M, USA.
Pirbuterol acetate (p.757·2).
Obstructive airways disease.

Maxalt
Merck Sharp & Dohme, UK; Merck, USA.
Rizatriptan benzoate (p.449·3).
Migraine.

Maxamaid MSUD
Scientific Hospital Supplies, Irl.; Scientific Hospital Supplies, UK; Ross, USA†.
Food for special diets.
Homocystinuria; hypermethioninaemia; maple syrup urine disease.

Maxamaid RVHB
Scientific Hospital Supplies, Irl.; Scientific Hospital Supplies, UK.
Methionine-free food.
Homocystinuria; hypermethioninaemia.

Maxamaid XLYS, TRY *Scientific Hospital Supplies, UK.*
Lysine- and tryptophan-free food.
Glutaric aciduria.

Maxamaid XMET *Ross, USA†.*
Food for special diets.
Homocystinuria.

Maxamaid XMET, THRE, VAL, ISOLEU
Scientific Hospital Supplies, UK; Ross, USA†.
Food for special diets.
Methylmalonic acidaemia; propionic acidaemia.

Maxamaid XP
Taranis, Fr.†; Scientific Hospital Supplies, Irl.; Medifood-Trufood, Ital.; Scientific Hospital Supplies, UK; Ross, USA†.
Food for special diets.
Phenylketonuria.

Maxamaid XPHEN, TYR Scientific Hospital Supplies, UK; Ross, USA†.
Food for special diets.
Tyrosinaemia.

Maxamum MSUD Ross, USA†.
Food for special diets.
Maple syrup urine disease.

Maxamum XP
Taranis, Fr.†; Scientific Hospital Supplies, Irl.; Medifood-Trufood, Ital.; Scientific Hospital Supplies, UK; Ross, USA†.
Food for special diets.
Phenylketonuria.

Maxamum XPhen, Tyr Scientific Hospital Supplies, Austral.
Food for special diets.
Tyrosinaemia.

Maxaquin
Searle, Ital.; Searle, S.Afr.; Searle, Switz.; Searle, USA.
Lomefloxacin hydrochloride (p.222·2).
Bacterial infections.

Max-Caro Marlyn, USA†.
Betacarotene (p.1335·2).
Erythropoietic protoporphyria.

Maxcil Triomed, S.Afr.
Amoxycillin trihydrate (p.151·3).
Bacterial infections.

Maxenal McNeil Consumer, Canad.†.
Pseudoephedrine hydrochloride (p.1068·3).
Nasal congestion.

Maxepa
Cenovis, Austral.; Vitelle, Austral.; Pierre Fabre, Fr.; Zyma, Ital.; Seven Seas, UK; Solgar, USA.
Omega-3 marine triglycerides (p.1276·1).
Dietary supplement; lipid disorders.

Maxepa & EPO Vitaplex, Austral.
Marine fish oil (p.1276·1); evening primrose oil (p.1582·1).
Dietary supplement.

Maxepa Plus Vita Glow, Austral.
Marine fish oil (p.1276·1); magnesium phosphate (p.1157·3).
Psoriasis; rheumatoid arthritis.

Maxeran Hoechst Marion Roussel, Canad.
Metoclopramide hydrochloride (p.1200·3).
Adjunct in gastro-intestinal radiography; delayed gastric emptying; facilitation of small bowel intubation; postoperative vomiting.

Maxi-6 Desbergers, Canad.
Multivitamin preparation.

Maxi-10 Desbergers, Canad.
Multivitamin preparation.

Maxi-B
Sanofi Winthrop, Belg.; Sanofi Winthrop, Neth.
Vitamin B substances.
Neurological or rheumatic pain.

Maxicaine Synthelabo, Fr.
Parethoxycaine hydrochloride (p.1298·2).
Throat disorders.

Maxi-calc Searle, Switz.
Calcium carbonate (p.1182·1).
Calcium deficiency; calcium supplement.

Maxicilina Pharmacia Upjohn, Spain.
Injection: Ampicillin sodium (p.153·1); ampicillin benzathine (p.154·1).
Bacterial infections.

Maxicortex 2000 Manetti Roberts, Ital.†.
Natural corticosteroids.
Adrenal insufficiency; endotoxic shock.

Maxidex
Alcon, Austral.; Alcon, Belg.; Alcon, Canad.; Alcon, Fr.; Alcon, Irl.; Alcon, Neth.†; Alcon, S.Afr.; Alcon, Spain; Alcon, Switz.; Alcon, UK; Alcon, USA.
Dexamethasone (p.1037·1) or dexamethasone sodium phosphate (p.1037·2).
Inflammatory eye and external ear disorders.

Maxidon Astra, Swed.
Morphine sulphate (p.56·2).
Pain.

Maxidrol Alcon, Fr.
Dexamethasone (p.1037·1); neomycin sulphate (p.229·2); polymyxin B sulphate (p.239·1).
Infected eye disorders.

Maxiflor Allergan Herbert, USA.
Diflorasone diacetate (p.1039·3).
Skin disorders.

Maxijul
Note. This name is used for preparations of different composition.
Scientific Hospital Supplies, Austral.
Maltodextrin (p.1350·2).
Carbohydrate food supplement.

Scientific Hospital Supplies, Irl.; Scientific Hospital Supplies, UK.
Gluten-, lactose-, and fructose-free preparation for enteral nutrition.

Maxi-Kalz Asta Medica, Aust.
Calcium monocitrate (p.1155·1); calcium dicitrate (p.1155·1).
Calcium supplementation.

Maxilase
Sanofi Winthrop, Fr.; Sanofi Winthrop, Spain.
Amylase (p.1549·1).
Oedema; upper respiratory-tract congestion.

Maxilase Antibiotica Lesvi, Spain†.
Alpha amylase (p.1549·1); benzydamine (p.21·3); metampicillin (p.224·3).
Bacterial infections.

Maxilase-Bacitracine Sanofi Winthrop, Fr.
Alpha-amylase (p.1549·1); bacitracin (p.157·3).
Bacterial infections of the mouth and throat.

Maxilube Mission Pharmacal, USA.
Dimethicone (p.1384·2); glycerol (p.1585·2); carbomer 934 (p.1471·2); triethanolamine (p.1639·1); sodium lauryl sulphate (p.1468·3).
Vaginal lubricant.

Maximal Ecobi, Ital.†.
Cobamamide (p.1364·2).
Vitamin B12 deficiency states.

Maximet SR Opus, UK.
Indomethacin (p.45·2).
Inflammation; musculoskeletal, joint, and peri-articular disorders; pain.

Maximum Blue Label Vitaline, USA.
Multivitamin and mineral preparation.

Maximum Green Label Vitaline, USA.
Multivitamin and mineral preparation.

Maximum Red Label Vitaline, USA.
Multivitamin and mineral preparation with iron and folic acid.

Maximum Strength Allergy Drops Bausch & Lomb, USA.
Naphazoline hydrochloride (p.1064·2); hypromellose (p.1473·1).
Minor eye irritation.

Maximum Strength Anbesol Whitehall, USA.
Benzocaine (p.1286·2); alcohol (p.1099·1).
Local anaesthesia.

Maximum Strength Aqua-Ban Thompson, USA.
Pamabrom (p.927·1).
Premenstrual water retention.

Maximum Strength Arthriten Alva, USA.
Paracetamol (p.72·2); magnesium salicylate (p.51·1); caffeine (p.749·3).

Maximum Strength Dermarest Dricort Del, USA.
Hydrocortisone acetate (p.1043·3).

Maximum Strength Desenex Antifungal Ciba, USA.
Miconazole nitrate (p.384·3).

Maximum Strength Dristan Cold Whitehall, USA.
Paracetamol (p.72·2); pseudoephedrine hydrochloride (p.1068·3); brompheniramine maleate (p.403·2).
Cold symptoms; nasal congestion.

Maximum Strength Dynafed BDI, USA.
Paracetamol (p.72·2); pseudoephedrine hydrochloride (p.1068·3).
Upper respiratory-tract symptoms.

Maximum Strength Flexall 454 Chattem, USA.
Menthol (p.1600·2); aloe vera (p.1177·1); eucalyptus oil (p.1578·1); methyl salicylate (p.55·2); thyme oil (p.1578·1).
Musculoskeletal disorders; pain.

Maximum Strength KeriCort-10 Bristol-Myers Squibb, USA.
Hydrocortisone (p.1043·3).

Maximum Strength Midol Multi-Symptom Formula Glenbrook, USA†.
Paracetamol (p.72·2); mepyramine maleate (p.414·1).
Menstrual symptoms.

Maximum Strength Midol PMS Glenbrook, USA†.
Paracetamol (p.72·2); pamabrom (p.927·1); mepyramine maleate (p.414·1).
Premenstrual syndrome.

Maximum Strength Nasal Decongestant Taro, USA.
Oxymetazoline hydrochloride (p.1065·3).
Nasal congestion.

Maximum Strength Ornex Menley & James, USA.
Pseudoephedrine hydrochloride (p.1068·3); paracetamol (p.72·2).
Upper respiratory-tract symptoms.

Maximum Strength Sine-Aid McNeil Consumer, USA.
Pseudoephedrine hydrochloride (p.1068·3); paracetamol (p.72·2).
Upper respiratory-tract symptoms.

Maximum Strength Sinutab Without Drowsiness Warner-Lambert, USA.
Pseudoephedrine hydrochloride (p.1068·3); paracetamol (p.72·2).
Upper respiratory-tract symptoms.

Maximum Strength Sleepinal Thompson, USA.
Diphenhydramine hydrochloride (p.409·1).
Insomnia.

Maximum Strength TheraFlu Non-Drowsy Sandoz, USA.
Paracetamol (p.72·2); dextromethorphan hydrobromide (p.1057·3); pseudoephedrine hydrochloride (p.1068·3).
Coughs and cold symptoms.

Maximum Strength Tylenol Allergy Sinus McNeil Consumer, USA.
Pseudoephedrine hydrochloride (p.1068·3); chlorpheniramine maleate (p.405·1); paracetamol (p.72·2).
Upper respiratory-tract symptoms.

Maximum Strength Tylenol Allergy Sinus NightTime McNeil Consumer, USA.
Pseudoephedrine hydrochloride (p.1068·3); diphenhydramine hydrochloride (p.409·1); paracetamol (p.72·2).

Maximum Strength Tylenol Sinus McNeil Consumer, USA.
Pseudoephedrine hydrochloride (p.1068·3); paracetamol (p.72·2).
Upper respiratory-tract symptoms.

Maximum Strength Unisom SleepGels Pfizer, USA.
Diphenhydramine hydrochloride (p.409·1).
Insomnia.

Maxipime
Bristol-Myers Squibb, Aust.; Aesca, Aust.; Bristol-Myers Squibb, Austral.; Bristol-Myers Squibb, Belg.; Bristol-Myers Squibb, Canad.; Bristol-Myers Squibb, Ger.; SmithKline Beecham, Ger.; Bristol-Myers Squibb, Ital.; Bristol-Myers Squibb, Neth.; Bristol-Myers Squibb, S.Afr.; Bristol-Myers, Spain; Bristol-Myers Squibb, Swed.; Bristol-Myers Squibb, Switz.; Bristol-Myers Squibb, USA.
Cefepime hydrochloride (p.165·1).
Bacterial infections.

Maxipro HBV
Scientific Hospital Supplies, Irl.; Scientific Hospital Supplies, UK.
Food for special diets.
Hypoproteinaemia.

Maxisorb
Scientific Hospital Supplies, Irl.; Scientific Hospital Supplies, UK.
Food for special diets.

Maxisporin Yamanouchi, Neth.
Cephradine (p.181·3).
Bacterial infections.

Maxitone Brunel, S.Afr.
Haematoporphyrin; cyanocobalamin; caffeine; rose hip; yeast.
Tonic.

Maxitrol
Alcon, Belg.; Alcon, Canad.; Alcon, Irl.; Alcon, Neth.†; Alcon, Norw.; Alcon, S.Afr.; Alcon, Spain; Alcon, Switz.; Alcon, UK; Alcon, USA.
Dexamethasone (p.1037·1); neomycin sulphate (p.229·2); polymyxin B sulphate (p.239·1).
Inflammatory eye infections.

Maxi-Tyro Goupil, Fr.†.
Parethoxycaine hydrochloride (p.1298·2); tyrothricin (p.267·2).
Mouth and throat disorders.

Maxivate Westwood-Squibb, USA.
Betamethasone dipropionate (p.1033·3).
Skin disorders.

Maxivent Ashbourne, UK.
Salbutamol (p.758·2).
Asthma; bronchospasm.

Maxivit Pfizer, Switz.
Multivitamin and mineral preparation.

Maxi-Vite Goldline, USA.
Multivitamin, mineral, and amino-acid preparation.

Maxolon
SmithKline Beecham, Austral.; Monmouth, Irl.; SmithKline Beecham, S.Afr.; Monmouth, UK; SmithKline Beecham, USA.
Metoclopramide hydrochloride (p.1200·3).
Adjunct to gastro-intestinal x-ray or intubation; gastro-intestinal motility disorders; gastro-oesophageal reflux; nausea and vomiting.

Maxomat Sanofi Winthrop, Fr.
Somatropin (p.1249·3).
Growth-hormone deficiency; Turner's syndrome.

Maxovite Tyson, USA.
Multivitamin and mineral preparation.
Premenstrual syndrome.

Maxsoten Wyeth Lederle, Belg.
Bisoprolol fumarate (p.833·1); hydrochlorothiazide (p.885·2).
Hypertension.

Maxtrex Farmitalia Carlo Erba, UK.
Tablets: Methotrexate (p.547·1).
Malignant neoplasms.

Maxzide
Wyeth Lederle, Belg.; Lederle, USA.
Triamterene (p.957·2); hydrochlorothiazide (p.885·2).
Hypertension; oedema.

Maycor
Note. This name is used for preparations of different composition.
Parke, Davis, Ger.†; Godecke, Ger.†.
Oral spray: Glyceryl trinitrate (p.874·3).
Cardiac disorders.

Parke, Davis, Ger.; Godecke, Ger.; Parke, Davis, Spain.
Tablets; sustained-release capsules: Isosorbide dinitrate (p.893·1).
Angina pectoris; heart failure; myocardial infarction; peripheral vascular disorders.

May-Cur-Tee Gersthofer, Aust.
Frangula bark (p.1193·2); senna (p.1212·2); fennel (p.1579·1); chamomile (p.1561·2); magnesium sulphate (p.1157·3).
Bowel evacuation; constipation.

Maydil Parke, Davis, Aust.
Isosorbide dinitrate (p.893·1).
Angina pectoris; heart failure; myocardial infarction.

Mayfit akut Mayrhofer, Aust.
Methyl salicylate (p.55·2); camphor (p.1557·2); menthol (p.1600·2).
Musculoskeletal and joint disorders.

Mayfit chronisch Mayrhofer, Aust.
Methyl salicylate (p.55·2); capsicum (p.1559·2); turpentine oil (p.1641·1).
Musculoskeletal and joint disorders.

Mayfung Mayrhofer, Aust.
Bath additive: Disodium sulphosuccinated undecenoic acid monoethanolamide (p.389·2).
Ointment†: Undecenoic acid diethanolamide (p.389·2).
Topical solution: Undecenoic acid monoethanolamide (p.389·2).
Fungal infections.

Maygace Bristol-Myers, Spain.
Megestrol acetate (p.1449·3).
Breast cancer; endometrial cancer.

Maylaktin Mayrhofer, Aust.†.
Bromocriptine mesylate (p.1132·2).
Hyperprolactinaemia.

Maynar Novag, Spain.
Aciclovir (p.602·3) or aciclovir sodium (p.602·3).
Herpesvirus infections.

Mayogel Propan, S.Afr.
Aluminium hydroxide (p.1177·3); magnesium oxide (p.1198·3).
Gastro-intestinal disorders.

May-Vita Mayrand, USA.
Vitamin B substances with minerals.

Mazanor Wyeth-Ayerst, USA.
Mazindol (p.1482·1).
Obesity.

Mazon Medicated Cream Nasmark, Canad.
Coal tar (p.1092·3); resorcinol (p.1090·1); salicylic acid (p.1090·2).
Skin disorders.

Mazon Medicated Shampoo Nasmark, Canad.
Coal tar (p.1092·3); salicylic acid (p.1090·2); sulphur (p.1091·2).
Scalp disorders.

Mazon Medicated Soap Nasmark, Canad.
Coal tar (p.1092·3).
Skin disorders.

MB-Combi Ciba-Geigy, S.Afr.†.
30 capsules, clofazimine (p.194·1); 2 capsules, rifampicin (p.243·2); 28 tablets, dapsone (p.199·2).
Leprosy.

MB-Tab Alra, USA.
Meprobamate (p.678·1).

M-Caps Pal-Pak, USA.
Methionine (p.984·2).
Odour, dermatitis, and ulceration in incontinent adults.

MCP Hexal, Ger.; Isis Puren, Ger.; CT, Ger.
Metoclopramide (p.1202·1) or metoclopramide hydrochloride (p.1200·3).
Gastro-intestinal disorders.

MCP-ratiopharm Ratiopharm, Ger.
Metoclopramide (p.1202·1) or metoclopramide hydrochloride (p.1200·3).
Gastro-intestinal disorders.

MCR-50 Tillotts, UK.
Isosorbide mononitrate (p.893·3).
Angina pectoris.

MCT
Medifood-Trufood, Ital.; Mead Johnson Nutritionals, USA.
Medium-chain triglycerides.
Adjunct in the management of disorders of fat absorption and transport.

MCT Duocal
Scientific Hospital Supplies, Austral.†; Scientific Hospital Supplies, UK.
Medium-chain triglycerides.
Fat malabsorption.

MCT Oil
Mead Johnson, Austral.; Nutricia, Austral.; Mead Johnson, Canad.; Mead Johnson Nutritionals, UK; Cow & Gate, UK.
Medium chain triglycerides.
Ketogenic diets; malabsorption syndromes; type I hyperlipoproteinaemia.

MCT Pepdite
Scientific Hospital Supplies, Irl.; Scientific Hospital Supplies, UK.
Medium-chain triglyceride and protein preparation.
Disorders of fat absorption; protein intolerance.

mct Psycho Dragees N Eurim, Ger.
Hypericum (p.1590·1).
Anxiety disorders; depression.

MD-60, MD-76
Mallinckrodt, Austral.; Mallinckrodt, Canad.; Mallinckrodt, USA.
Meglumine diatrizoate (p.1003·2); sodium diatrizoate (p.1003·2).
Radiographic contrast medium.

MD-Gastroview
Mallinckrodt, Austral.; Mallinckrodt, USA.
Meglumine diatrizoate (p.1003·2); sodium diatrizoate (p.1003·2).
Contrast medium for gastro-intestinal radiography.

MDP-Squibb Squibb Diagnostics, USA.
Technetium-99m medronate (p.1425·1).

MDR AM MDR, USA†.
Multivitamin and mineral preparation.

MDR PM MDR, USA†.
Multivitamin and mineral preparation.

Measavax Merieux, UK†.
A measles vaccine (Schwarz strain) (p.1517·3).
Active immunisation.

Measlegam NBI, S.Afr.
Measles immunoglobulin (p.1517·3).
Passive immunisation.

Meaverin Rhone-Poulenc Rorer, Ger.
Injection: Mepivacaine hydrochloride (p.1297·2). Adrenaline acid tartrate (p.813·3) is included in some injections as a vasoconstrictor to diminish absorption and localise the effect of the local anaesthetic.
Local anaesthesia.

Topical gel: Mepivacaine hydrochloride (p.1297·2); laureth 9 (p.1325·2).
Catheterisation; intubation; local anaesthesia.

Meaverin "A" mit Adrenalin *Rhone-Poulenc Rorer, Ger.*
Mepivacaine hydrochloride (p.1297·2).
Adrenaline acid tartrate (p.813·3) is included in this preparation as a vasoconstrictor to diminish absorption and localise the effect of the local anaesthetic.
Local anaesthesia.

Meaverin hyperbar *Rhone-Poulenc Rorer, Ger.*
Mepivacaine hydrochloride (p.1297·2).
Local anaesthesia.

Meaverin "N" mit Noradrenaline *Rhone-Poulenc Rorer, Ger.*
Mepivacaine hydrochloride (p.1297·2).
Noradrenaline acid tartrate (p.924·1) is included in this preparation as a vasoconstrictor to diminish absorption and localise the effect of the local anaesthetic.
Local anaesthesia.

Mebaral *Sanofi Winthrop, USA.*
Methylphenobarbitone (p.349·2).
Anxiety; epilepsy.

Mebendan *Tedec Meiji, Spain.*
Mebendazole (p.104·1).
Worm infections.

Mebonat *Boehringer Mannheim, Spain.*
Disodium clodronate (p.737·3).
Hypercalcaemia of malignancy.

Mebron *Daiichi, Jpn.*
Epirizole (p.35·3).
Inflammation; pain.

Mebucaine *Wander OTC, Switz.*
Cetylpyridinium chloride (p.1106·2); oxybuprocaine hydrochloride (p.1298·1); tyrothricin (p.267·2).
Mouth and throat disorders.

Mebutan *SmithKline Beecham, Neth.*
Nabumetone (p.60·1).
Osteoarthritis; rheumatoid arthritis.

Mebutina *Formenti, Ital.†.*
Mebutamate (p.901·3).
Hypertension.

Mecain *Curasan, Ger.*
Mepivacaine hydrochloride (p.1297·2).
Local anaesthesia.

Mecca *Mentholatum, Canad.*
Camphor (p.1557·2); phenol (p.1121·2); zinc oxide (p.1096·2).

Mechol *Manne, USA†.*
Vitamin B substances with vitamin C and soy protein.

Mechovit *Streuli, Switz.*
DL-methionine (p.984·2); vitamins.
Liver disorders.

Meclan *Ortho Dermatological, USA.*
Meclocycline sulfosalicylate (p.224·1).
Acne.

Meclocil *Esseti, Ital.†.*
Meclocycline sulfosalicylate (p.224·1); vitamins.
Skin infections.

Meclocil Desa *Esseti, Ital.†.*
Dexamethasone valerate (p.1037·3); meclocycline sulfosalicylate (p.224·1); vitamins.
Skin disorders.

Meclocil Ovuli *Esseti, Ital.†.*
Meclocycline sulfosalicylate (p.224·1).
Vulvovaginal infections.

Mecloderm *Istoria, Ital.*
Meclocycline sulfosalicylate (p.224·1).
Skin infections.

Mecloderm Antiacne *Istoria, Ital.*
Meclocycline sulfosalicylate (p.224·1).
Acne; seborrhoeic dermatitis.

Mecloderm F *Istoria, Ital.*
Meclocycline sulfosalicylate (p.224·1); fluocinolone acetonide (p.1041·1).
Infected skin disorders.

Mecloderm Ovuli *Istoria, Ital.*
Meclocycline sulfosalicylate (p.224·1).
Vulvovaginal and cervical infections.

Mecloderm Polvere Aspersoria *Schwarz, Ital.*
Meclocycline sulfosalicylate (p.224·1).
Skin infections.

Meclodium *Quantum, USA†.*
Meclofenamate sodium (p.51·1).

Meclodol *Parke, Davis, Ital.*
Meclofenamate sodium (p.51·1).
Musculoskeletal and joint disorders; pain.

Meclomen
Parke, Davis, Aust.; Parke, Davis, Ital.†; Parke-Med, S.Afr.; Parke, Davis, Spain; Parke, Davis, Switz.†; Parke, Davis, USA†.
Meclofenamate sodium (p.51·1).
Menorrhagia; musculoskeletal, joint, and peri-articular disorders; pain.

Meclon *Farmigea, Ital.*
Clotrimazole (p.376·3); metronidazole (p.585·1).
Vulvovaginal and cervical infections.

Meclosorb *S & K, Ger.*
Meclocycline sulfosalicylate (p.224·1).
Bacterial skin infections.

Meclutin *ABC, Ital.*
Meclocycline sulfosalicylate (p.224·1); fluocinolone acetonide (p.1041·1).
Infected skin disorders.

Meclutin Semplice *ABC, Ital.*
Meclocycline sulfosalicylate (p.224·1).
Bacterial skin infections.

Mectizan
Merck Sharp & Dohme-Chibret, Fr.; Merck Sharp & Dohme, USA.
Ivermectin (p.101·1).
Veterinary names include: Eqvalan; Ivomec; Oramec.
Onchocerciasis.

Meda *Circle, USA.*
Paracetamol (p.72·2).
Fever; pain.

Meda Syrup Forte *Dal-Med, USA†.*
Dextromethorphan hydrobromide (p.1057·3); guaiphenesin (p.1061·3); phenylephrine hydrochloride (p.1066·2); chlorpheniramine maleate (p.405·1).

Medacaps N *Palmicol, Ger.*
Deanol hydrogen tartrate (p.1478·2).
Medacaps formerly contained inositol nicotinate, deanol hydrogen tartrate, crataegus, procaine hydrochloride, haematoporphyrin, hesperidin, and alpha tocopheryl acetate.
Tonic.

Medacote *Dal-Med, USA.*
Mepyramine maleate (p.414·1); dimethicone (p.1384·2); zinc oxide (p.1096·2); menthol (p.1600·2); camphor (p.1557·2).
Pruritus.

Medactin (PPSB) *Medac, Ger.†.*
Factor IX (p.721·3).
Haemorrhagic disorders.

Medadyne *Dal-Med, USA†.*
Oral liquid: Methylbenzethonium chloride (p.1119·3); benzocaine (p.1286·2); tannic acid (p.1634·2); camphor (p.1557·2); chlorothymol (p.1111·1); menthol (p.1600·2); benzyl alcohol (p.1103·3).
Oral disorders.
Throat spray: Lignocaine (p.1293·2); cetyldimethylammonium chloride.

Medamet *Caps, S.Afr.*
Metronidazole (p.585·1).
Anaerobic bacterial infections; protozoal infections.

Medamint *Dal-Med, USA†.*
Benzocaine (p.1286·2).

Medasond *Fresenius, Norw.†.*
Preparation for enteral nutrition.

Medaspor *Medpro, S.Afr.*
Clotrimazole (p.376·3).
Fungal infections.

Medatussin *Dal-Med, USA†.*
Dextromethorphan (p.1057·3); guaiphenesin (p.1061·3).

Medatussin Plus *Dal-Med, USA†.*
Dextromethorphan (p.1057·3); chlorpheniramine maleate (p.405·1); phenylpropanolamine hydrochloride (p.1067·2); phenyltoloxamine citrate (p.416·1); guaiphenesin (p.1061·3); L-menthol (p.1600·2).

Medazine *Medpro, S.Afr.*
Cyclizine hydrochloride (p.407·1).
Nausea and vomiting.

Medazyme *Dal-Med, USA†.*
Cellulase (p.1561·1); amylase (p.1549·1); protease; lipase; simethicone (p.1213·1).

Medebar *Medefield, Austral.*
Barium sulphate (p.1003·1).
Radiographic contrast medium.

Medebiotin *Medea, Spain.*
Biotin sodium.
Biotin deficiency.

Medecitral *Medea, Spain.*
Belladonna alkaloids (p.457·1); sodium bromide (p.1620·3); sodium citrate (p.1153·2).
Vomiting.

Medefizz *Medefield, Austral.*
Potassium bicarbonate; citric acid.
Effervescent system for double-contrast radiography.

Medefoam-2 *Medefield, Austral.*
Simethicone (p.1213·1).
Antifoaming agent for barium radiography.

Medemycin *Meiji, Jpn.*
Midecamycin (p.226·2).
Bacterial infections.

Medenorex *Medea, Spain.*
Cyproheptadine hydrochloride (p.407·2); amino acids and vitamins.
Tonic.

Mede-Prep *Medefield, Austral.*
Mannitol (p.900·3).
Bowel preparation before radiography or surgery.

Mederebro *Medea, Spain†.*
Cyanocobalamin (p.1363·3); cerebral medullary neuropeptides; thiamine nitrate (p.1361·1).
Neurological disorders.

Mederebro Compuesto *Medea, Spain.*
Cyanocobalamin (p.1363·3); cerebral medullary neuropeptides; pyridoxine hydrochloride (p.1362·3); phosphoserine; thiamine nitrate (p.1361·1); levoglutamide (p.1344·3).
Neurological disorders.

Mederma *Merz, Ger.†.*
Tablets: Citiolone (p.1564·3); echinacea (p.1574·2); pancreatin (p.1612·1); vitamin A (p.1358·1); vitamin E succinate; dried yeast (p.1373·1).
Topical application: Dequalinium undecenoate (p.1112·1); allantoin hydroxyaluminium lactate (p.1078·2); colloidal sulphur (p.1091·2).
Skin disorders.

Mederreumol *Medea, Spain.*
Indomethacin (p.45·2).
Gout; inflammation; musculoskeletal, joint, and peri-articular disorders; pain; renal colic.

Medescan *Medefield, Austral.*
Barium sulphate (p.1003·1).
Radiographic contrast medium.

Medesup *Medea, Spain.*
Bisacodyl (p.1179·3).
Bowel evacuation; constipation.

Medevac *Medefield, Austral.*
Arachis oil (p.1550·2); sorbitol (p.1354·2).
Gallbladder evacuant for oral cholecystography.

Medi Creme *Warner-Lambert, Austral.*
Chlorhexidine acetate (p.1107·2); cetrimide (p.1105·2); hexamidine isethionate (p.1115·3); allantoin (p.1078·2); lignocaine (p.1293·2).
Abrasions; cuts; insect bites and stings; minor burns; skin irritation.

Medi Pulv *Warner-Lambert, Austral.*
Hexamidine isethionate (p.1115·3); chlorhexidine hydrochloride (p.1107·2); allantoin (p.1078·2).
Cuts; minor burns and scalds.

Mediabet *Medice, Ger.*
Metformin hydrochloride (p.330·1).
Diabetes mellitus.

Medialipide
Braun, Belg.; Braun, Fr.
Soya oil (p.1355·1); medium-chain triglycerides.
Contains egg lecithin.
Lipid infusion for parenteral nutrition.

Mediamox *Biohorm, Spain†.*
Amoxycillin trihydrate (p.151·3).
Bacterial infections.

Medianox *Grossmann, Switz.*
Chloral hydrate (p.645·3).
Nervousness; sleep disorders.

Medianut *Braun, Fr.*
Amino-acid and lipid infusion.
Parenteral nutrition.

Mediatensyl *Inergie, Fr.*
Urapidil (p.959·2).
Hypertension.

Mediator *Biopharma, Fr.*
Benfluorex hydrochloride (p.1268·2).
Adjunct in asymptomatic diabetes; hyperlipidaemias.

Mediaven
Will-Pharma, Belg.; Drossapharm, Switz.
Naftazone (p.725·2).
Diabetic retinopathy; venous insufficiency.

Mediaxal
Servier, Ital.; Servier, Switz.
Benfluorex hydrochloride (p.1268·2).
Hyperlipidaemias.

Medibronc *Monot, Fr.*
Carbocisteine (p.1056·3).
Respiratory-tract congestion.

Medica *Qualiphar, Belg.*
Chlorhexidine gluconate (p.1107·2); lignocaine hydrochloride (p.1293·2).
Throat disorders.

Medical Pic *Artsana, Ital.*
Chlorhexidine gluconate (p.1107·2); parahydroxybenzoate phenoxyethanol.
Wound and burn disinfection.

Medicament Sinus *Prodemdis, Canad.*
Pseudoephedrine hydrochloride (p.1068·3); paracetamol (p.72·2).

Medicanol *Medica, Neth.†.*
Chlorhexidine gluconate (p.1107·2); alcohol (p.1099·1).
Hand disinfection.

Medicated Analgesic Cream *Prodemdis, Canad.*
Methyl salicylate (p.55·2); camphor (p.1557·2); menthol (p.1600·2); eucalyptus oil (p.1578·1).

Medicated Chest Rub *Hyde, Canad.; Sunfresh, Canad.*
Camphor (p.1557·2); eucalyptus oil (p.1578·1); menthol (p.1600·2).

Medichol *Medice, Ger.†.*
Anethole (p.1549·3); carvone; (+)-fenchone; DL-limonene; menthol (p.1600·2); menthone; phenylpropanol (p.1617·3); *dl*-alpha tocopherol (p.1369·2); chelidonium; silybum marianum (p.993·3); turmeric (p.1001·3).
Biliary disorders; digestive disorders; gallstones.

Medichrom *Qualiphar, Belg.*
Mercurochrome (p.1119·2).
Disinfection of minor wounds.

Medicinal Gargle *Weleda, UK.*
Rhatany (p.1624·3); myrrh (p.1606·1); clove oil (p.1565·2); eucalyptus oil (p.1578·1); geranium oil (p.1584·1); lavender oil (p.1594·3); peppermint oil (p.1208·1); sage oil; aesculus; argentum nitricum; calcium fluoricum; magnesium sulphuricum.
Mouth and throat disorders.

Mediclear *Boots, UK.*
Benzoyl peroxide (p.1079·2).
Acne.

Medicoal *Concord, UK.*
Activated charcoal (p.972·2).
Acute poisoning; drug overdosage.

Medicod *Propan-Vernleigh, S.Afr.†.*
Paracetamol (p.72·2); codeine phosphate (p.26·1); caffeine (p.749·3).
Pain.

Medicone *Dickinson, USA.*
Yeast extract (p.1373·1); shark-liver oil.

Medicone Derma *Medicone, USA.*
Benzocaine (p.1286·2); zinc oxide (p.1096·2); hydroxyquinoline sulphate (p.1589·3); ichthammol (p.1083·3); menthol (p.1600·2).
Skin disorders.

Medicone Dressing *Medicone, USA.*
Benzocaine (p.1286·2); zinc oxide (p.1096·2); hydroxyquinoline sulphate (p.1589·3); cod-liver oil (p.1337·3); menthol (p.1600·2).
Skin disorders.

Medicone Rectal *Medicone, USA.*
Ointment: Benzocaine (p.1286·2); hydroxyquinoline sulphate (p.1589·3); zinc oxide (p.1096·2); menthol (p.1600·2); castor oil (p.1560·2); peru balsam (p.1617·2).
Suppositories: Benzocaine (p.1286·2); hydroxyquinoline sulphate (p.1589·3); zinc oxide (p.1096·2); menthol (p.1600·2); peru balsam (p.1617·2).
Anorectal disorders.

Mediconet *Medicone, USA.*
Hamamelis (p.1587·1).
Perianal cleansing.

Medicreme *Medice, Ger.†.*
Cetylpyridinium chloride (p.1106·2); neomycin hydrochloride (p.230·1).
Infected skin disorders.

Medicrucin-blau *Medice, Ger.†.*
Neomycin hydrochloride (p.230·1); bacitracin (p.157·3); methylene blue (p.984·3).
Wounds.

Medicrucin-gelb N *Medice, Ger.†.*
Neomycin hydrochloride (p.230·1); bacitracin (p.157·3).
Infected skin disorders; wounds.

Medicrucin-rose *Medice, Ger.†.*
Tribromophenol bismuth (p.1180·2); bismuth oxyiodide (p.1181·1); neomycin hydrochloride (p.230·1); zinc oxide (p.1096·2).
Infected skin disorders; wounds.

Medicyclomine *Brunel, S.Afr.*
Dicyclomine hydrochloride (p.460·1).
Gastro-intestinal spasm; urinary-tract spasm.

Medi-Dan *Mahdeen, Canad.*
Coal tar (p.1092·3); benzalkonium chloride (p.1101·3); salicylic acid (p.1090·2).

Mediderm *Ego, Austral.†.*
Lignocaine hydrochloride (p.1293·2); phenoxypropanol (p.1122·2); cetrimide (p.1105·2); chlorhexidine gluconate (p.1107·2); allantoin (p.1078·2).
Cuts; minor burns; pruritus due to haemorrhoids.

Medidral *Medifood-Trufood, Ital.†.*
Oral rehydration solution (p.1152·3).

Medifed *Medpro, S.Afr.*
Triprolidine hydrochloride (p.420·3); pseudoephedrine hydrochloride (p.1068·3); dextromethorphan hydrobromide (p.1057·3).
Coughs.

Medifeed *Roussel, S.Afr.†.*
Preparation for enteral nutrition.

Mediflex *Crown, S.Afr.*
Indomethacin (p.45·2).
Musculoskeletal and joint disorders.

Mediflor Tisane Antirhumatismale No 2
Monot, Fr.
Birch; ash; meadowsweet (p.1599·1); strawberry plant; parietaria; couch-grass (p.1567·3); asparagus; juniper (p.1592·2); bearberry (p.1552·2); black currant (p.1365·2); tilia (p.1637·3); frangula bark (p.1193·2).
Muscular pain; rheumatic pain.

Mediflor Tisane Calmante Troubles du Sommeil No 14 *Monot, Fr.*
Passion flower (p.1615·3); bitter orange (p.1610·3); crataegus (p.1568·2); melissa (p.1600·1); tilia (p.1637·3); valerian (p.1643·1).
Insomnia; nervous disorders.

Mediflor Tisane Circulation du Sang No 12
Monot, Fr.
Aesculus (p.1543·3); red vine; hyssop; valerian (p.1643·1); hamamelis (p.1587·1); cypress nut; mistletoe (p.1604·1); willow leaf (p.82·3); melissa (p.1600·1); crataegus (p.1568·2); frangula bark (p.1193·2).
Peripheral vascular disorders.

Mediflor Tisane Contre la Constipation Passagere No 7 *Monot, Fr.*
Senna (p.1212·2); ash; fennel (p.1579·1); liquorice (p.1197·1); rosemary.
Formerly known as Mediflor Tisane Laxative.
Constipation.

Mediflor Tisane Dietetique *Monot, Fr.†.*
Fucus vesiculosus (p.1554·1); senna (p.1212·2); frangula (p.1193·2); rosemary; ash; hyssop; red vine.
Obesity.

Mediflor Tisane Digestive No 3 *Monot, Fr.*
Aniseed (p.1549·3); mint (p.1208·1); angelica; lavender (p.1594·3); orange leaf; rosemary; elecampane (p.1059·2); fennel (p.1579·1); coriander (p.1567·3); hyssop.
Digestive disorders.

Mediflor Tisane Diuretique *Monot, Fr.†.*
Asparagus; fennel (p.1579·1); couch-grass (p.1567·3); bearberry (p.1552·2); ash; ulmaria (p.1599·1); strawberry root; althaea leaf (p.1546·3); liquorice (p.1197·1).
Diuresis; renal calculi.

Mediflor Tisane Hepatique No 5 *Monot, Fr.*
Boldo (p.1554·1); combretum (p.1593·2); elecampane root (p.1059·2); rosemary; liquorice (p.1197·1); berberis; mercury herb; mallow leaves; senna leaves (p.1212·2).
Digestive disorders; liver disorders.

Mediflor Tisane Hypotensive *Monot, Fr.†.*
Olive; mistletoe (p.1604·1); crataegus (p.1568·2); red vine; hamamelis (p.1587·1); marrubium vulgare (p.1063·3); orange; fumitory (p.1581·3); ash; senna (p.1212·2).
Hypertension.

Mediflor Tisane Pectorale d'Alsace *Monot, Fr.†.*
Mallow; althaea flowers (p.1546·3); poppy (p.1068·2); coltsfoot flowers and leaves (p.1057·2); verbascum flowers and leaves; catsfoot; althaea herb and root (p.1546·3); calendula officinalis; wild thyme; ground ivy; liquorice (p.1197·1); melissa (p.1600·1); ulmaria (p.1599·1); couch-grass (p.1567·3).
Respiratory-tract disorders.

Medi-Flu *Parke, Davis, USA.*
Chlorpheniramine maleate (p.405·1); dextromethorphan hydrobromide (p.1057·3); paracetamol (p.72·2); pseudoephedrine hydrochloride (p.1068·3).
Coughs and cold symptoms.

Medigel
Note. This name is used for preparations of different composition.
Medice, Ger.
Bamethan sulphate (p.827·1); ephedrine sulphate (p.1059·3); laureth 9 (p.1325·2).
Soft-tissue injury; venous insufficiency.

Medifood-Trufood, Ital.
Nutritional supplement.
Vomiting.

Propan, S.Afr.; Mer-National, S.Afr.
Dicyclomine hydrochloride (p.460·1); aluminium hydroxide gel (p.1177·3); magnesium oxide (p.1198·3); simethicone (p.1213·1); sodium lauryl sulphate (p.1468·3); methylcellulose (p.1473·3).
Formerly contained dicyclomine hydrochloride, aluminium hydroxide gel, magnesium oxide, and simethicone.
Gastro-intestinal disorders.

Medigesic *US Pharmaceutical, USA.*
Butalbital (p.644·3); paracetamol (p.72·2); caffeine (p.749·3).
Pain.

Medihaler-duo *3M, UK†.*
Isoprenaline hydrochloride (p.892·1); phenylephrine bitartrate (p.1066·2).
Bronchospasm.

Medihaler-Epi
3M, Austral.; 3M, Canad.†; 3M, S.Afr.†; 3M, Switz.; 3M, UK†; 3M, USA†.
Adrenaline acid tartrate (p.813·3).
Anaphylaxis; asthma.

Medihaler-Ergotamine
3M, Canad.†; 3M, UK.
Ergotamine tartrate (p.445·3).
Migraine and other vascular headaches; occipital neuralgia.

Medihaler-Iso
Salus, Aust.; 3M, Austral.†; 3M, Belg.; 3M, Neth.; 3M, S.Afr.†; 3M, UK†; 3M, USA.
Isoprenaline sulphate (p.892·1).
Bronchospasm.

Medijel
Key, Austral.; DDD, UK.
Lignocaine hydrochloride (p.1293·2); aminacrine hydrochloride (p.1098·3).
Mouth ulcers; sore gums.

Medikasma *Propan, S.Afr.*
Amylobarbitone (p.641·3); ephedrine hydrochloride (p.1059·3); aminophylline (p.748·1).
Asthma.

Medi-Keel A *Restan, S.Afr.*
Lozenges: Cetylpyridinium chloride (p.1106·2); benzocaine (p.1286·2).
Sore throat.
Mouthwash†: Cetylpyridinium chloride (p.1106·2).
Mouth and throat infections.
Throat spray: Phenol (p.1121·2).
Mouth and throat infections.

Medikol *Selena, Swed.*
Activated charcoal (p.972·2).
Diarrhoea; poisoning.

Medi-Kord *Medirel, Switz.*
Adrenaline hydrochloride (p.813·3); zinc phenolsulphonate octahydrate (p.1096·3).
Adjunct in dental procedures.

Medil *Crosara, Ital.*
Buflomedil hydrochloride (p.834·2).
Cerebral and peripheral vascular disorders.

Medilan *Westbrook, UK.*
Wool fat (p.1385·3).

Medilave *Martindale Pharmaceuticals, UK†.*
Benzocaine (p.1286·2); cetylpyridinium chloride (p.1106·2).
NOTE. There is no connection between Martindale, The Complete Drug Reference and Martindale Pharmaceuticals.
Mouth pain.

Medilax *Mission Pharmacal, USA.*
Phenolphthalein (p.1208·2).
Constipation.

Medilet *Medice, Ger.*
Lactulose (p.1349·3).
Constipation.

Medilyn *Medpro, S.Afr.*
Diphenhydramine hydrochloride (p.409·1); ammonium chloride (p.1055·2); sodium citrate (p.1153·2).
Coughs.

Mediment *Krewel, Ger.†.*
Camphor (p.1557·2); benzyl nicotinate (p.22·1); glycol salicylate (p.43·1).
Muscle, nerve, and joint pain.

Medimonth *Marpa, Austral.†.*
Paracetamol (p.72·2); codeine phosphate (p.26·1); phenolphthalein (p.1208·2); belladonna (p.457·1).
Cramps; dysmenorrhoea; griping pain; headache.

Medinait *Procter & Gamble, Spain.*
Dextromethorphan hydrobromide (p.1057·3); doxylamine succinate (p.410·1); ephedrine sulphate (p.1059·3); paracetamol (p.72·2).
Cold and influenza symptoms.

Medinat Esten *Bioglan, Austral.*
Vitamins; minerals; equisetum (p.1575·1); eleutherococcus senticosus (p.1584·2); damiana (p.1570·2); cimicifuga (p.1563·3); angelica.
Menopausal disorders.

Medinat PMT-Eze *Bioglan, Austral.*
Pyridoxine hydrochloride (p.1362·3); cyanocobalamin (p.1363·3); ferrous fumarate (p.1339·3); buchu (p.1555·2); bearberry (p.1552·2); parsley (p.1615·3); juniper oil (p.1592·3); evening primrose oil (p.1582·1).
Premenstrual syndrome.

Medinex *Whitehall, UK.*
Diphenhydramine hydrochloride (p.409·1).
Insomnia.

Medinol *Seton, UK.*
Paracetamol (p.72·2).
Formerly known as Cupanol.
Fever; pain.

Medinox Mono *Pfleger, Ger.†.*
Pentobarbitone sodium (p.685·1).
Sleep disorders.

Mediocard *Medice, Ger.†.*
Homoeopathic preparation.

Mediolax *Medice, Ger.*
Bisacodyl (p.1179·3).
Mediolax N formerly contained senna, aloes, and bisacodyl.
Constipation.

Mediosept *Medice, Ger.†.*
Benzethonium chloride (p.1102·3); sage oil.
Pre-operative skin disinfection.

Mediovit N *Medice, Ger.†.*
Multivitamin and mineral preparation.

Medipain *Medi-Plex, USA†.*
Hydrocodone tartrate (p.43·1); paracetamol (p.72·2).

Medipax *Pharmatec, S.Afr.†.*
Diphenhydramine hydrochloride (p.409·1); ammonium chloride (p.1055·2).
Coughs.

Medipect *Vernleigh, S.Afr.†.*
Kaolin (p.1195·1); pectin (p.1474·1); electrolytes (p.1152·3); dextrose.
Diarrhoea.

Mediper *Medici, Ital.†.*
Cefoperazone sodium (p.167·3).
Lignocaine hydrochloride (p.1293·2) is included in this preparation to alleviate the pain of injection.
Gram-negative bacterial infections.

Mediphon *Medice, Ger.†.*
Hexachlorophane (p.1115·2); laureth 9 (p.1325·2); zinc undecenoate (p.389·2).
Skin disorders.

Mediplant *Roche, Aust.*
Ointment: Menthol (p.1600·2); camphor (p.1557·2); eucalyptus oil (p.1578·1).
Pastilles: Menthol (p.1600·2); eucalyptus oil (p.1578·1).
Respiratory-tract disorders.

Mediplant Inhalations *Roche, Aust.*
Menthol (p.1600·2); camphor (p.1557·2); eucalyptus oil (p.1578·1).
Respiratory-tract disorders.

Mediplant Krauter *Roche, Aust.*
Althaea (p.1546·3); thyme (p.1636·3); ammonium chloride (p.1055·2).
Respiratory-tract disorders.

Mediplast *Beiersdorf, USA.*
Salicylic acid (p.1090·2).
Hyperkeratosis.

Mediplex *US Pharmaceutical, USA.*
Multivitamin and mineral preparation.

Medipo *Mediolanum, Ital.*
Simvastatin (p.1278·2).
Coronary arteriosclerosis; hypercholesterolaemia; ischaemic heart disease.

Medipramine *Propan-Vernleigh, S.Afr.†.*
Imipramine hydrochloride (p.289·2).
Depression; nocturnal enuresis.

Medipren
McNeil Consumer, Canad.†; Johnson & Johnson, Spain†; McNeil Consumer, USA†.
Ibuprofen (p.44·1).
Fever; osteoarthritis; pain; rheumatoid arthritis.

Medi-Prep *Seton, UK.*
Cetrimide (p.1105·2).
Skin disinfection.

Medi-Quik
Note. This name is used for preparations of different composition.
Mentholatum, Canad.
Aerosol: Benzalkonium chloride (p.1101·3); camphor (p.1557·2); lignocaine (p.1293·2).
Topical spray: Benzalkonium chloride (p.1101·3); lignocaine (p.1293·2).

Mentholatum, USA.
Aerosol†: Lignocaine hydrochloride (p.1293·2); benzalkonium chloride (p.1101·3).
Skin disorders.
Ointment†: Polymyxin B sulphate (p.239·1); neomycin sulphate (p.229·2); bacitracin (p.157·3).
Bacterial skin infections.
Topical spray: Lignocaine (p.1293·2); benzalkonium chloride (p.1101·3).
Skin disorders.

Medised *Seton, UK.*
Paracetamol (p.72·2); promethazine hydrochloride (p.416·2).
Fever; pain.

Medisense G2 *Medisense, UK.*
Test for glucose in blood (p.1585·1).

Medismon *Medice, Ger.*
Erythromycin stinoprate (p.206·2).
Bacterial infections.

Medi-Sol *Mykal, UK.*
Adhesive remover.

Medi-Swab *Seton, UK.*
Isopropyl alcohol (p.1118·2).
Pre-injection swab.

Medi-Swab H *Seton, UK.*
Isopropyl alcohol (p.1118·2); chlorhexidine acetate (p.1107·2).
Pre-injection swab.

Medi-Tab *Marpa, Austral.†.*
Dexchlorpheniramine maleate (p.405·1); pseudoephedrine hydrochloride (p.1068·3); ephedrine hydrochloride (p.1059·3).
Allergic asthma; hay fever; sinusitis.

Meditar *Yamanouchi, Ital.*
Coal tar (Stantar) (p.1092·3).
Seborrhoeic dermatitis of the scalp.

Medi-Test Combi 2 *BHR, UK.*
Test for glucose and protein in urine.

Medi-Test Combi 5 *Ascot, Austral.*
Test for glucose, blood, ascorbic acid, protein, and pH in urine.

Medi-Test Combi 7 *Ascot, Austral.*
Test for glucose, blood, ketones, ascorbic acid, nitrite, protein, and pH in urine.

Medi-Test Combi 9
Ascot, Austral.; BHR, UK.
Test for glucose, ascorbic acid, ketones, blood, protein, nitrite, pH, bilirubin, and urobilinogen in urine.

Medi-Test Combi 3A *Ascot, Austral.*
Test for glucose, protein, pH, and ascorbic acid in urine.

Medi-Test Combi 4A *Ascot, Austral.*
Test for nitrite, blood, protein, pH, and ascorbic acid in urine.

Medi-Test Combi 5N *Ascot, Austral.*
Test for pH, glucose, blood, ascorbic acid, protein, and nitrite in urine.

Medi-Test Combi 6A *Ascot, Austral.*
Test for blood, bilirubin, protein, ketones, ascorbic acid, glucose, and pH in urine.

Medi-Test Glucose
Ascot, Austral.; BHR, UK.
Test for glucose in urine (p.1585·1).

Medi-Test Glucose 2 *Ascot, Austral.*
Test for glucose and ascorbic acid in urine.

Medi-Test Glucose 3 *Ascot, Austral.*
Test for glucose, ketones, and ascorbic acid in urine.

Medi-Test Glycaemie C *BHR, UK.*
Test for glucose in blood (p.1585·1).

Medi-Test Keton *Ascot, Austral.*
Test for ketones in urine.

Medi-Test Nitrit *Ascot, Austral.*
Test for nitrite in urine.

Medi-Test Protein 2 *Ascot, Austral.*
Test for protein and pH in urine.

Medi-Test Urbi *Ascot, Austral.*
Test for urobilinogen and bilirubin in urine.

Medi-Tissue *Seton, UK.*
Alcohol (p.1099·1); benzalkonium chloride (p.1101·3).
Skin and instrument disinfection.

Meditonsin H *Medice, Ger.*
Homoeopathic preparation.

Meditox *Marpa, Austral.†.*
Pyrethrin; piperonyl butoxide (p.1409·3).
Pediculosis.

Medituss
Note. A similar name is used for preparations of different composition.
Crown, S.Afr.
Mepyramine maleate (p.414·1); ammonium chloride (p.1055·2); sodium citrate (p.1153·2); cetrimide (p.1105·2); menthol (p.1600·2); ephedrine hydrochloride (p.1059·3).
Respiratory-tract congestion.

Medi-Tuss
Note. A similar name is used for preparations of different composition.
Warner Chilcott, USA†.
Guaiphenesin (p.1061·3).
Coughs.

Medi-Tuss AC *Warner Chilcott, USA†.*
Codeine phosphate (p.26·1); guaiphenesin (p.1061·3).
Coughs.

Medi-Tuss DAC *Warner Chilcott, USA†.*
Guaiphenesin (p.1061·3); pseudoephedrine hydrochloride (p.1068·3); codeine phosphate (p.26·1).
Coughs.

Medi-Tuss DM *Warner Chilcott, USA†.*
Guaiphenesin (p.1061·3); dextromethorphan hydrobromide (p.1057·3).
Coughs.

Medium *Kwizda, Aust.†.*
Meprobamate (p.678·1); belladonna (p.457·1); ergotamine tartrate (p.445·3).
Migraine; nervous disorders.

Medivarsin *Medice, Ger.†.*
Aesculus (p.1543·3); melilotus.
Formerly contained mofebutazone, liquorice, magnesium gluconate, trimethylhesperidin chalcone, chamomile, aesculus, and melilotus.
Post-thrombotic syndrome; vascular disorders.

Mediveine *Elerte, Fr.*
Diosmin (p.1580·1).
Haemorrhoids; peripheral vascular disorders.

Medivitan N *Medice, Ger.*
Hydroxocobalamin (p.1363·3); sodium folate (p.1341·2); pyridoxine hydrochloride (p.1362·3).
Lignocaine hydrochloride (p.1293·2) is included in this preparation to alleviate the pain of injection.
Alcoholism; anaemias; cachexia; peripheral neuropathies; vitamin deficiency.

Medivitan N Neuro *Medice, Ger.*
Thiamine hydrochloride (p.1361·1); pyridoxine hydrochloride (p.1362·3).
Neuralgia; neuritis; polyneuropathies.

Medi-Wipe *Seton, UK.*
Chlorhexidine gluconate (p.1107·2); alcohol (p.1099·1).

Medixin *Pierrel, Ital.*
Co-trimoxazole (p.196·3).
Bacterial infections.

Medizinalbad *Synpharma, Aust.†.*
Camphor (p.1557·2); anise oil (p.1550·1); eucalyptus oil (p.1578·1); methyl salicylate (p.55·2); niaouli oil (p.1607·1); citronella oil (p.1565·1); peppermint oil (p.1208·1); rosemary oil (p.1626·2); thyme oil (p.1637·1).
Musculoskeletal and joint disorders.

Medobiotin
Apotheke Roten Krebs, Aust.; Medopharm, Ger.
Biotin (p.1336·1).
Hair and nail disorders.

Medocarnitin *Medosan, Ital.*
Carnitine (p.1336·2).
Carnitine deficiency; myocardial ischaemia.

Medocodene *Medo, UK†.*
Paracetamol (p.72·2); codeine phosphate (p.26·1).
These ingredients can be described by the British Approved Name Co-codamol.
Fever; pain.

Medomet *DDSA Pharmaceuticals, UK.*
Methyldopa (p.904·2).

Medomycin *Medosan, Ital.†.*
Methacycline hydrochloride (p.225·1).
Bacterial infections.

Medopal *A.L., Norw.†.*
Methyldopa (p.904·2).
Hypertension.

Medopam *Schwulst, S.Afr.*
Oxazepam (p.683·2).
Alcohol withdrawal syndrome; anxiety.

Medophyll *Li-il, Ger.*
Thymol (p.1127·1).
Skin ulceration; superficial skin disorders; wounds.

Medopren *Malesci, Ital.*
Methyldopa (p.904·2).
Hypertension.

Medosalgon *Loges, Ger.†.*
Apple pectin; chamomile (p.1561·2); methiosulfonium chloride (p.1603·1).
Gastro-intestinal disorders.

Medotar *Medco, USA.*
Coal tar (p.1092·3); zinc oxide (p.1096·2).
Skin disorders.

Medoxim *Medici, Ital.*
Cefuroxime sodium (p.177·1).
Bacterial infections.

Medozide *Malesci, Ital.*
Methyldopa (p.904·2); hydrochlorothiazide (p.885·2).
Hypertension.

Medphlem *Medpro, S.Afr.*
Carbocisteine (p.1056·3).
Respiratory-tract disorders.

Medpramol *Schwulst, S.Afr.*
Paracetamol (p.72·2).
Fever; pain.

Medralone *Keene, USA.*
Methylprednisolone acetate (p.1046·1).
Corticosteroid.

Medramil *Farmigea, Ital.*
Medrysone (p.1045·3); tetrahydrozoline hydrochloride (p.1070·2); pheniramine maleate (p.415·3).
Eye disorders.

Medramine retard *Mepha, Switz.*
Dimenhydrinate (p.408·2); pyridoxine hydrochloride (p.1362·3).
Nausea; vomiting.

Medramine-B_6 Rectocaps *Mepha, Switz.*
Dimenhydrinate (p.408·2); pyridoxine hydrochloride (p.1362·3); caffeine (p.749·3).
Nausea; vomiting.

Medrate *Pharmacia Upjohn, Ger.*
Methylprednisolone (p.1046·1) or methylprednisolone sodium succinate (p.1046·1).
Corticosteroid.

Medrate Akne-Lotio *Upjohn, Ger.†.*
Methylprednisolone acetate (p.1046·1); sulphur (p.1091·2); aluminium chlorohydrate (p.1078·3).
Acne; eczema.

Medricol *Cusi, Spain.*
Chloramphenicol (p.182·1); medroxyprogesterone acetate (p.1448·3).
Eye disorders.

Medriusar *Difa, Ital.†.*
Medrysone (p.1045·3).
Eye disorders.

Medrivas *Cusi, Spain.*
Medroxyprogesterone acetate (p.1448·3); tetrahydrozoline hydrochloride (p.1070·2).
Eye disorders.

Medrivas Antib *Cusi, Spain.*
Chloramphenicol succinate (p.184·2); medroxyprogesterone acetate (p.1448·3); tetrahydrozoline hydrochloride (p.1070·2).
Infected eye disorders.

Medrol
Upjohn, Austral.†; Pharmacia Upjohn, Belg.; Pharmacia Upjohn, Canad.; Pharmacia Upjohn, Fr.; Pharmacia Upjohn, Ital.; Upjohn, Neth.†; Pharmacia Upjohn, Norw.; Pharmacia Upjohn, S.Afr.; Pharmacia Upjohn, Swed.; Pharmacia Upjohn, Switz.; Upjohn, USA.
Methylprednisolone (p.1046·1) or methylprednisolone acetate (p.1046·1).
Corticosteroid.

Medrol Acetate *Upjohn, USA†.*
Methylprednisolone acetate (p.1046·1).
Corticosteroid.

Medrol Acne Lotion
Upjohn, Austral.†; Pharmacia Upjohn, Canad.
Methylprednisolone acetate (p.1046·1); aluminium chlorohydrate complex (p.1078·3); sulphur (p.1091·2).
Acne; seborrhoeic dermatitis.

Medrol Lozione Antiacne *Pharmacia Upjohn, Ital.*
Methylprednisolone acetate (p.1046·1); aluminium chlorohydrate (p.1078·3); colloidal sulphur (p.1091·2).
Acne.

Medrol Veriderm
Pharmacia Upjohn, Canad.; Pharmacia Upjohn, Ital.†.
Methylprednisolone acetate (p.1046·1).
Formerly called Medrol Topical in *Canad.*
Skin disorders.

Medrone
Pharmacia Upjohn, Irl.; Upjohn, Swed.†; Upjohn, UK.
Methylprednisolone (p.1046·1) or methylprednisolone acetate (p.1046·1).
Corticosteroid.

MED-Rx *Iomed, USA.*
Blue tablets, pseudoephedrine hydrochloride (p.1068·3); guaiphenesin (p.1061·3); white tablets, guaiphenesin.
Upper respiratory-tract symptoms.

MED-Rx DM *Iomed, USA.*
Blue tablets, pseudoephedrine hydrochloride (p.1068·3); guaiphenesin (p.1061·3); green tablets, guaiphenesin; dextromethorphan hydrobromide (p.1057·3).
Upper respiratory-tract symptoms.

Medyn *Medice, Ger.*
Pyridoxine hydrochloride (p.1362·3); folic acid (p.1340·3); cyanocobalamin (p.1363·3).
Prevention of elevated homocysteine concentration.

Mefac *Rowex, Irl.*
Mefenamic acid (p.51·2).
Musculoskeletal and joint disorders; pain.

Mefalgic *Rolab, S.Afr.*
Mefenamic acid (p.51·2).
Dysmenorrhoea; fever; pain.

Mefenacide *Streuli, Switz.*
Mefenamic acid (p.51·2).
Influenza symptoms; pain.

Mefic *Parke, Davis, Austral.*
Mefenamic acid (p.51·2).
Menorrhagia; pain; primary dysmenorrhoea.

Meflam *Trinity, UK.*
Mefenamic acid (p.51·2).
Fever; inflammation; pain.

Mefoxin
Merck Sharp & Dohme, Austral.; Merck Sharp & Dohme, Belg.; Merck Sharp & Dohme, Canad.; Merck Sharp & Dohme-Chibret, Fr.; Merck Sharp & Dohme, Irl.; Merck Sharp & Dohme, Ital.; Merck Sharp & Dohme, Neth.; Merck Sharp & Dohme, S.Afr.; Merck Sharp & Dohme, UK; Merck Sharp & Dohme, USA.
Cefoxitin sodium (p.170·3).
Lignocaine hydrochloride (p.1293·2) may be included in the intramuscular injection to alleviate the pain of injection.
Bacterial infections.

Mefoxitin
Merck Sharp & Dohme, Aust.; Merck Sharp & Dohme, Ger.; Merck Sharp & Dohme, Norw.; Merck Sharp & Dohme, Spain; Merck Sharp & Dohme, Swed.; Merck Sharp & Dohme, Switz.
Cefoxitin sodium (p.170·3).
Lignocaine hydrochloride (p.1293·2) may be included in the intramuscular injection to alleviate the pain of injection.
Bacterial infections.

Mefren Incolore *Zyma, Belg.*
Chlorhexidine gluconate (p.1107·2).
Disinfection of minor wounds; disinfection of the skin.

Mefren Pastilles *Zyma, Belg.*
Chlorhexidine hydrochloride (p.1107·2).
Mouth and throat infections.

Mega-13 *Vita Health, Canad.†.*
Multivitamin preparation.

Mega 65 *Arkopharma, Fr.*
Fish oil (p.1276·1).
Nutritional supplement.

Mega B
Sisu, Canad.; Quest, Canad.; Quest, UK; Arco, USA.
Vitamin B substances.

Mega B Extra Strength *Cenovis, Austral.*
Vitamin B substances; ascorbic acid.
Vitamin B deficiency.

Mega B Slow Release *Vita Glow, Austral.*
Vitamin B substances; ascorbic acid.
Dietary supplement.

Mega Balance *Pharmavite, Canad.*
Multivitamin and mineral preparation.

Mega C *Vita Glow, Austral.†.*
Calcium ascorbate (p.1365·2); ascorbic acid (p.1365·2).
Vitamin C deficiency.

Mega Capsule *Quest, Canad.*
Multivitamin and mineral preparation.

Mega E *Cenovis, Austral.*
dl-Alpha tocopheryl acetate (p.1369·2).
Vitamin E supplement.

Mega Multi *Cenovis, Austral.*
Vitamin and mineral preparation.

Mega Stress Vitamins *Vita Pharm, Canad.*
Multivitamin and mineral preparation.

Mega Swiss One *Swiss Herbal, Canad.†.*
Multivitamin and mineral preparation.

Mega Vim *Jamieson, Canad.*
Multivitamin and mineral preparation.

Mega VM *Nature's Bounty, USA.*
Multivitamin and mineral preparation.

Mega-Ade *Vita Health, Canad.†.*
Multivitamin preparation with lecithin.

Megabyl *Martin, Fr.*
Di-isopromine hydrochloride (p.1189·1); sorbitol (p.1354·2).
Constipation; dyspepsia.

Mega-Cal *Jamieson, Canad.†.*
Calcium carbonate (p.1182·1).
Mineral supplement.

Mega-Calcium *Sandoz, Aust.*
Calcium lactate gluconate (p.1155·2); calcium carbonate (p.1182·1).
Calcium deficiency.

Megace
Bristol-Myers Squibb, Aust.; Bristol, Canad.; Bristol-Myers Squibb, Fr.; Bristol-Myers Squibb, Irl.; Bristol-Myers Squibb, Ital.; Bristol-Myers Squibb, Neth.; Bristol-Myers Squibb, Norw.; Bristol-Myers Squibb, Swed.; Bristol-Myers Squibb, UK; Bristol-Myers Oncology, USA.
Megestrol acetate (p.1449·3).
Anorexia, cachexia, or unexplained significant weight loss in AIDS patients; breast cancer; endometrial cancer.

Megacillin
Note. This name is used for preparations of different composition.
Grunenthal, Aust.
Phenoxymethylpenicillin potassium (p.236·2).
Bacterial infections.

Frosst, Canad.
Benzathine penicillin (p.158·3) or benzylpenicillin potassium (p.159·2).
Bacterial infections.

Megacillin forte *Grunenthal, Ger.†.*
Benzylpenicillin sodium (p.159·3); clemizole penicillin (p.191·1).
Lignocaine hydrochloride (p.1293·2) is included in this preparation to alleviate the pain of injection.
Bacterial infections.

Megacillin for Injection *Grunenthal, Ger.†.*
Clemizole penicillin (p.191·1).
Bacterial infections.

Megacillin oral *Grunenthal, Ger.*
Phenoxymethylpenicillin potassium (p.236·2).
Bacterial infections.

Megacilline *Grunenthal, Switz.*
Injection: Clemizole penicillin (p.191·1).
Syrup; tablets: Phenoxymethylpenicillin potassium (p.236·2).
Bacterial infections.

Megacort *Uno, Ital.*
Dexamethasone sodium phosphate (p.1037·2).
Musculoskeletal and joint disorders.

Mega-Dolor *Lorenz, Ger.†.*
Aspirin (p.16·1); codeine phosphate (p.26·1); caffeine (p.749·3).
Cold symptoms; fever; pain.

Megadose *Arco, USA†.*
Multivitamin and mineral preparation.

Megadoxa *Restan, S.Afr.*
Vitamin B substances.

Megafol *Alphapharm, Austral.*
Folic acid (p.1340·3).
Folic acid deficiency; megaloblastic anaemia.

Megagrisevit mono *Pharmacia Upjohn, Ger.*
Clostebol acetate (p.1440·2).
Anabolic; fractures; osteoporosis.

Megal *IFI, Ital.†.*
Propyphenazone (p.81·3); barbitone (p.642·3); caffeine (p.749·3).
Pain.

Megalac *Meuselbach, Ger.*
Almasilate (p.1177·1).
Gastro-intestinal disorders.

Megalax *Propan, S.Afr.*
Bisacodyl (p.1179·3).
Bowel evacuation; constipation.

Megalip *Biotrading, Ital.†.*
Metochalcone (p.1603·2).
Biliary disorders.

Megalocin *Kyorin, Jpn.*
Fleroxacin (p.209·1).
Bacterial infections.

Megalotect
Intra Pharma, Irl.; Mednostica, S.Afr.; Lovens, Swed.
A cytomegalovirus immunoglobulin (p.1507·1).
Passive immunisation.

Megamag *Mayoly-Spindler, Fr.*
Magnesium aspartate (p.1157·2).
Magnesium deficiency.

Mega-MaxEPA *Solgar, USA†.*
Omega-3 marine triglycerides (p.1276·1).
Dietary supplement.

Megamilbedoce *Andromaco, Spain.*
Hydroxocobalamin (p.1363·3).
Vitamin B12 deficiency.

Mega-Min *Vita Health, Canad.†.*
Multimineral preparation.

Megamino MM *Cantassium Co., UK†.*
Amino-acid and mineral preparation.

Megamox *Garec, S.Afr.*
Ampicillin (p.153·1); cloxacillin (p.195·2).
Bacterial infections.

Meganest *Clarben, Spain.*
Carticaine.
Adrenaline (p.813·2) is included in this preparation as a vasoconstrictor to diminish absorption and localise the effect of the local anaesthetic.
Local anaesthesia in dentistry.

Megapen *Garec, S.Afr.*
Amoxycillin (p.151·3); flucloxacillin (p.209·1).
Bacterial infections.

Megapyn *Compu, S.Afr.*
Syrup: Paracetamol (p.72·2); codeine phosphate (p.26·1); promethazine hydrochloride (p.416·2).
Fever; pain.
Tablets: Paracetamol (p.72·2); codeine phosphate (p.26·1); caffeine (p.749·3); meprobamate (p.678·1).
Pain and associated tension.

Megareal *Sodietal, Fr.*
Preparation for enteral nutrition.

Megast *Schiapparelli Searle, Ital.†.*
Carbenoxolone sodium (p.1182·2); metoclopramide hydrochloride (p.1200·3).
Gastro-intestinal disorders associated with hyperacidity.

Mega-Star *Lenza, Ital.†.*
Methylprednisolone (p.1046·1) or methylprednisolone sodium hemisuccinate (p.1046·1).
Cardiovascular disorders; hypersensitivity reactions; joint disorders.

Megasthenyl *Byk, Fr.*
Ribonucleic acid (p.1624·3); manganese gluconate (p.1351·1).
Tonic.

Megaton *Hyrex, USA.*
Vitamin B substances with minerals.

Megavac *Omega, Canad.†.*
Vaccine containing *Staphylococcus aureus*; *Staphylococcus albus*; *Streptococcus*; *Diplococcus pneumoniae*; *Moraxella (Branhamella) catarrhalis*; *Klebsiella pneumoniae*; *Haemophilus influenzae*.
Bacterial infections of the respiratory tract.

Megavit B Complex *Vitaplex, Austral.†.*
Vitamin B substances.

Megavit C 1000 *Vitaplex, Austral.†.*
Ascorbic acid and mixed ascorbates (p.1365·2).

Megavit Natural E *Vitaplex, Austral.†.*
d-Alpha tocopherol (p.1369·1).

Megavit Supa-Boost *Vitaplex, Austral.†.*
Multivitamin preparation with minerals and herbs.

Megavites *ICN, Canad.*
Vitamin B substances and vitamin C.

Megefren *Pras, Spain.*
Megestrol acetate (p.1449·3).
Breast cancer; endometrial cancer.

Megel *SAN, Ital.†.*
Royal jelly (p.1626·3).

Megental Pediatrico *Menarini, Ital.†.*
Gentamicin sulphate (p.212·1).
Bacterial infections.

Megestat
Bristol-Myers Squibb, Ger.; Bristol-Myers Squibb, Switz.
Megestrol acetate (p.1449·3).
Breast cancer; endometrial cancer.

Megestil *Boehringer Mannheim, Ital.*
Megestrol acetate (p.1449·3).
Breast cancer; endometrial cancer.

Meggezones
Schering-Plough, Canad.; Schering-Plough, UK.
Menthol (p.1600·2).
Catarrh; coughs; sore throats.

Megimide *Inibsa, Spain†.*
Bemegride (p.1478·1).
Barbiturate intoxication.

Meglucon *Hexal, Ger.*
Metformin hydrochloride (p.330·1).
Diabetes mellitus.

Megostat
Bristol-Myers Squibb, Austral.; Squibb, Spain.
Megestrol acetate (p.1449·3).
Anorexia; breast cancer.

Megral
Note. This name is used for preparations of different composition.
Glaxo Wellcome, Canad.
Ergotamine tartrate (p.445·3); cyclizine hydrochloride (p.407·1); caffeine hydrate (p.750·1).
Migraine and other vascular headaches.

Wasserman, Spain†.
Caffeine (p.749·3); propyphenazone (p.81·3).
Fever; pain.

Megrin *Yoshitomi, Jpn†.*
Nicotinyl hepronicate (p.883·1).
Peripheral vascular disease.

Meiact *Meiji, Jpn.*
Cefditoren pivoxil (p.164·3).
Bacterial infections.

Meicelin *Meiji, Jpn.*
Cefminox sodium (p.167·1).
Bacterial infections.

Meilax *Meiji, Jpn.*
Ethyl loflazepate (p.669·3).

Meinfusona *Mein, Spain.*
Electrolyte infusion with vitamin B substances (p.1147·1).
Electrolyte depletion; vitamin B deficiency.

Meinfusona Trofica *Mein, Spain†.*
Amino-acid, electrolyte, sorbitol, vitamin and rutin infusion.
Hypoproteinaemia.

Meinvenil Fisiologico *Mein, Spain.*
Sodium chloride (p.1162·2).
Fluid and electrolyte disorders.

Meinvenil Glucosalina *Mein, Spain.*
Glucose (p.1343·3); sodium chloride (p.1162·2).
Carbohydrate source; fluid and electrolyte disorders.

Mejoral *Sterling Health, Spain.*
Aspirin (p.16·1); caffeine (p.749·3).
Fever; pain.

Mejoral Infantil *Sterling Health, Spain.*
Aspirin (p.16·1).
Fever; musculoskeletal and joint disorders; pain; periarticular disorders; thrombo-embolism prophylaxis.

Melabon
Note. This name is used for preparations of different composition.
Provita, Aust.; Lacer, Spain.
Paracetamol (p.72·2); propyphenazone (p.81·3); caffeine (p.749·3) or caffeine citrate (p.749·3).
Fever; pain.

Oramon, Ger.†.
Aspirin (p.16·1).
Arthritis; cold symptoms; fever; pain; rheumatism.

Agpharm, Switz.†.
Etenzamide (p.35·3); propyphenazone (p.81·3); benzyl mandelate; caffeine (p.749·3).
Cold symptoms; pain.

Melabon Infantil *Lacer, Spain.*
Paracetamol (p.72·2).
Fever; pain.

Melabon N
Note. This name is used for preparations of different composition.
Oramon, Ger.†.
Paracetamol (p.72·2); salicylamide (p.82·3); caffeine (p.749·3).
Cold symptoms; migraine; pain.

Agpharm, Switz.
Aspirin (p.16·1); paracetamol (p.72·2); caffeine (p.749·3).
Cold symptoms; pain.

Melabon plus C *Oramon, Ger.†.*
Aspirin (p.16·1); ascorbic acid.
Cold symptoms; fever; pain.

Melactone *Clonmel, Irl.*
Spironolactone (p.946·1).
Heart failure; hepatic cirrhosis; hypertension; idiopathic oedema; nephrotic syndrome.

Meladinine
Promedica, Fr.; Basotherm, Ger.; Boehringer Ingelheim, Neth.†; Basotherm, Switz.
Methoxsalen (p.1086·3).
Mycosis fungoides; psoriasis; vitiligo.

Melaforte *Agpharm, Switz.†.*
Etenzamide (p.35·3); propyphenazone (p.81·3); benzyl mandelate; caffeine (p.749·3).
Cold symptoms; pain.

Melanex
Note. This name is used for preparations of different composition.
Boehringer Mannheim, S.Afr.
Raubasine (p.941·3).
Vascular disorders.

Neutrogena, USA.
Hydroquinone (p.1083·1).
Hyperpigmentation.

Melanex Duo *Paraphar, Fr.*
Hydroquinone (p.1083·1); alpha hydroxy acids.
Skin hyperpigmentation.

Melbetese *Clonmel, Irl.*
Glibenclamide (p.319·3).
Diabetes mellitus.

Mel-C *Leopold, Aust.*
Sodium ascorbate (p.1365·2).
Vitamin C deficiency.

Melcain *Rorer, Ger.†.*
Procaine hydrochloride (p.1299·2); natural honey.
Nervous system disorders.

Meldopa *Clonmel, Irl.*
Methyldopa (p.904·2).
Hypertension.

Meleril *Sandoz, Spain.*
Thioridazine (p.695·1) or thioridazine hydrochloride (p.695·1).
Anxiety; psychoses.

Melex *Sankyo, Jpn.*
Mexazolam (p.679·3).
Anxiety disorders; psychosomatic disorders; sleep disorders.

Melfen *Clonmel, Irl.*
Ibuprofen (p.44·1).
Musculoskeletal, joint, and peri-articular disorders.

Melfiat *Solvay, USA†.*
Phendimetrazine tartrate (p.1484·2).
Obesity.

Mel-H *Leopold, Aust.*
Multivitamin and amino-acid preparation.

Meli Rephastasan *Repha, Ger.*
Melilotus officinalis.
Haemorrhoids; thrombophlebitis; venous insufficiency.

Meliane
Schering, Belg.; Schering, Fr.; Schering, Neth.
Gestodene (p.1447·2); ethinyloestradiol (p.1445·1).
Combined oral contraceptive.

Melicedin *Wolfer, Ger.†.*
Crataegus (p.1568·2).
Cardiac disorders.

Melior *Giuliani, Switz.†.*
Ephedrine hydrochloride (p.1059·3); potassium guaiacolsulfonate (p.1068·3); sodium benzoate (p.1102·3); belladonna tincture (p.457·1); althaea (p.1546·3); helenium (p.1059·2); polygala amara (p.1069·3); viola.
Coughs.

Melipramine *Boucher & Muir, Austral.*
Imipramine hydrochloride (p.289·2).
Depression.

Melisana
Note. This name is used for preparations of different composition.
Melisana, Belg.†.
Melissa oil; lemon oil (p.1595·3); bitter-orange oil; cinnamon oil (p.1564·2); cardamom oil (p.1560·1); nutmeg oil (p.1609·3); angelica oil; coriander oil (p.1567·3).
Digestive disorders; nervous disorders.

Pan Quimica, Spain†.
Calamus (p.1556·1); lemon tincture; melissa (p.1600·1); orange tincture; nutmeg (p.1609·2); cinnamon (p.1564·2).
Anxiety; insomnia; nervous disorders; pain.

Meliseptol
Braun, Belg.†; Braun, Ger.
Propyl alcohol (p.1124·2); glyoxal (p.1115·1).
Surface disinfection.

Melisol *Max Ritter, Switz.*
Soya oil (p.1355·1); liquid paraffin (p.1382·1).
Dry skin.

Melissa comp. *Weleda, UK.*
Archangelica root; cinnamon (p.1564·2); melissa leaf (p.1600·1); nutmeg (p.1609·2).
Nausea.

Melissa Tonic *Geistlich, Switz.*
Melissa (p.1600·1); monarda; rosemary; red-poppy petal (p.1001·1); hibiscus; valerian (p.1643·1); passion flower (p.1615·3).
Agitation; nervousness; sleep disorders.

Melissin *Surf Ski International, UK.*
Guaiphenesin (p.1061·3); menthol (p.1600·2); glycerol (p.1585·2); melissa (p.1600·1); benzoic acid (p.1102·3); citric acid (p.1564·3).
Colds; coughs.

Melix
Pharmador, S.Afr.†; Lagap, Switz.†.
Glibenclamide (p.319·3).
Diabetes mellitus.

Melixeran *Lusofarmaco, Ital.†.*
Melitracen hydrochloride (p.296·3).
Depression.

Melizide *Alphapharm, Austral.*
Glipizide (p.320·3).
Diabetes mellitus.

Mellaril
Sandoz, Canad.; Sandoz, USA.
Thioridazine (p.695·1) or thioridazine hydrochloride (p.695·1).
Depression with anxiety; hyperactivity in children; psychoses; severe behavioural problems in children.

Mellerette *Sandoz, Ital.*
Thioridazine (p.695·1) or thioridazine hydrochloride (p.695·1).
Anxiety; behaviour disorders.

Melleretten
Sandoz, Aust.; Sandoz, Ger.; Novartis, Neth.
Thioridazine (p.695·1) or thioridazine hydrochloride (p.695·1).
Anxiety disorders; behaviour disorders; depression; sleep disorders.

Mellerettes *Sandoz, Switz.*
Thioridazine hydrochloride (p.695·1).
Agitation; anxiety disorders; depression; psychoses; sleep disorders.

Melleril
Sandoz, Aust.; Novartis, Austral.; Wander, Belg.; Sandoz, Fr.; Sandoz, Ger.; Sandoz, Irl.; Sandoz, Ital.; Novartis, Neth.; Sandoz, Norw.; Novartis, S.Afr.; Sandoz, Switz.; Novartis, UK.
Thioridazine (p.695·1) or thioridazine hydrochloride (p.695·1).
Agitation; alcohol withdrawal syndrome; anxiety disorders; behaviour disorders in children; bipolar disorders; depression; psychoses; sleep disorders.

Mellin HA *Mellin, Ital.*
Infant feed.
Food intolerance.

Melocin *Curasan, Ger.*
Mezlocillin sodium (p.225·3).
Bacterial infections.

Meloka *Lacer, Spain.*
Benfotiamine (p.1360·3); caffeine (p.749·3); codeine phosphate (p.26·1); paracetamol (p.72·2); propyphenazone (p.81·3).
Fever; pain.

Melopat *Medopharm, Ger.*
Betahistine mesylate (p.1553·1).
Ménière's syndrome; vestibular disorders.

Melostrophan *Rorer, Ger.†.*
Ouabain (p.925·2).
Cardiac disorders.

Melpaque HP *Stratus, USA.*
Hydroquinone (p.1083·1).

Melquin HP *Stratus, USA.*
Hydroquinone (p.1083·1).

Melrose *Roberts & Sheppey, UK.*
Hydrous wool fat (p.1385·3); yellow soft paraffin (p.1382·3); hard paraffin (p.1382·1).
Emollient.

Melrosum *Nattermann, Neth.*
Honey (p.1345·3).
Coughs.

Melrosum Codein Hustensirup *Nattermann, Ger.*
Codeine phosphate (p.26·1); honey (p.1345·3).
Coughs and catarrh.

Melrosum Extra Sterk *Nattermann, Neth.*
Codeine phosphate (p.26·1); vegetable extracts.
Coughs.

Melrosum Hustensirup Forte *Nattermann, Ger.*
Thyme (p.1636·3).
Bronchitis; catarrh; cough.

Melrosum Hustensirup N *Nattermann, Ger.*
Grindelia; pimpinella; primula root; rose petals (p.1001·1); thyme (p.1636·3).
Catarrh.

Melrosum Inhalationstropfen *Nattermann, Ger.†.*
Eucalyptus oil (p.1578·1); oleum pini sylvestris.
Cold symptoms.

Melrosum Medizinalbad *Nattermann, Ger.*
Thyme oil (p.1637·1); oleum pini sylvestris.
Bath additive; respiratory-tract disorders.

Melsept
Braun, Ger.; Braun, Ital.
Formaldehyde (p.1113·2); glutaraldehyde (p.1114·3); glyoxal (p.1115·1).
Surface disinfection.

Melsept SF
Braun, Ger.; Braun, Ital.
Glutaraldehyde (p.1114·3); glyoxal (p.1115·1); didecyldimethylammonium chloride (p.1112·2).
Surface disinfection.

Melsept Spray *Braun, Ital.*
Alcohol (p.1099·1); glyoxal (p.1115·1).
Disinfection of minor wounds and surfaces.

Melsitt
Braun, Belg.†; Braun, Ger.
Formaldehyde (p.1113·2); glutaraldehyde (p.1114·3); didecyldimethylammonium chloride (p.1112·2).
Surface disinfection.

Meltus Baby *Seton, UK.*
Dilute acetic acid (p.1541·2).
Coughs.

Meltus Cough Control *Seton, UK.*
Dextromethorphan (p.1057·3).
Dry coughs.

Meltus Dry Cough *Seton, UK.*
Dextromethorphan hydrobromide (p.1057·3); pseudoephedrine hydrochloride (p.1068·3).
Coughs.

Meltus Expectorant *Seton, UK.*
Guaiphenesin (p.1061·3); cetylpyridinium chloride (p.1106·2).
Coughs.

Meltus Expectorant with Decongestant *Seton, UK.*
Guaiphenesin (p.1061·3); pseudoephedrine hydrochloride (p.1068·3); menthol (p.1600·2).

Meltus Honey & Lemon *Seton, UK.*
Guaiphenesin (p.1061·3); honey (p.1345·3); glycerol (p.1585·2); terpeneless lemon oil (p.1596·1).
Coughs.

Melvit *Beta, Ital.*
Multivitamin and mineral preparation.

Melzine *Clonmel, Irl.*
Thioridazine hydrochloride (p.695·1).
Agitation; anxiety disorders; childhood behaviour disorders; psychoses; senile confusion; tension.

Memac *Bracco, Ital.*
Donepezil hydrochloride (p.1391·2).
Alzheimer's disease.

membranoSome *Vitorgan, Ger.†.*
Chorion fet.; hepar fet.; mucosa intestinalis crassi fet.; mucosa intestinalis tenuis fet.; electrolytes; thymus juv.; glandula lymphonodi; lien; procaine hydrochloride.
Supportive tumour therapy; tonic.

Memo-Puren *Isis Puren, Ger.*
Piracetam (p.1619·1).
Mental function disorders.

Memoq *Godecke, Ger.; Parke, Davis, Ger.*
Nicergoline (p.1607·1).
Mental function disorders.

Memoril *Recordati, Ital.*
Levoglutamide (p.1344·3).
Mental function impairment.

Memorino *Vita, Spain.*
Piracetam (p.1619·1); pyritinol hydrochloride (p.1624·1).
Cerebrovascular disorders; mental function impairment.

Memory Plus *Life Essence, UK.*
Becopa.
Memory impairment.

Memoserina S *Rhone-Poulenc Rorer, Ital.*
DL-Phosphoserine; levoglutamide (p.1344·3); cyanocobalamin (p.1363·3); protein hydrolysate.
Tonic.

Memosprint *Poli, Ital.*
Pyridoxine phosphoserinate (p.1363·1).
Mental function impairment; tonic.

Memovisus *Carlo Erba OTC, Ital.*
Myrtillus (p.1606·1); cobamamide (p.1364·2); DL-phosphoserine; aceglutamide (p.1541·2).
Tonic.

Memovit B12 *Magis, Ital.*
Levoglutamide (p.1344·3); DL-phosphoserine; cyanocobalamin (p.1363·3).
Tonic.

Menabil Complex
Note. This name is used for preparations of different composition.
Menarini, Ital.†.
Syrup: Meburamide sodium; fenipentol sodium hemisuccinate (p.1579·1); cyclobutyrol nicotinamide (p.1569·2); ox bile extract (p.1553·2); rhubarb (p.1212·1); boldo (p.1554·1); cascara (p.1183·1); belladonna (p.457·1); star anise; cynara (p.1569·2).
Tablets: Meburamide; fenipentol hemisuccinate (p.1579·1); cyclobutyrol nicotinamide (p.1569·2); ox bile extract (p.1553·2); rhubarb (p.1212·1); cynara (p.1569·2); belladonna (p.457·1); boldo (p.1554·1); cascara (p.1183·1).
Biliary and hepatic disorders; constipation.

Menarini, Spain.
Cynara scolymus (p.1569·2); boldine (p.1554·1); cyclobutyrol (p.1569·2); methionine phenylbutyrate; rhubarb (p.1212·1); bile salts (p.1553·2); fenipentol sodium hemisuccinate (p.1579·1); belladonna (p.457·1); cascara (p.1183·1).
Constipation; hepatobiliary disorders.

Menacor *Menarini, Ital.†.*
Cloridarol (p.845·1).
Hyperlipidaemias; ischaemic heart disease.

Menaderm
Menarini, Ital.; Menarini, Spain.
Beclomethasone dipropionate (p.1032·1); neomycin sulphate (p.229·2).
Infected skin disorders.

Menaderm Clio *Menarini, Spain.*
Beclomethasone dipropionate (p.1032·1); clioquinol (p.193·2).
Infected skin disorders.

Menaderm Otologico *Menarini, Spain.*
Beclomethasone dipropionate (p.1032·1); clioquinol (p.193·2).
External ear disorders.

Menaderm Simple *Menarini, Spain.*
Beclomethasone dipropionate (p.1032·1).
Skin disorders.

Menaderm Simplex *Menarini, Ital.*
Beclomethasone dipropionate (p.1032·1).
Skin disorders.

Menadol *Rugby, USA.*
Ibuprofen (p.44·1).

Menalation *McGloin, Austral.*
Menthol (p.1600·2); pumilio pine oil (p.1623·3).
Cold symptoms.

Menalcol *Men, Spain.*
Alcohol (p.1099·1); chlorhexidine gluconate (p.1107·2).
Skin and wound disinfection.

Menalgil B6 *Menarini, Spain.*
Cyanocobalamin (p.1363·3); di-isopropylammonium dichloroacetate (p.854·1); thiamine monophosphate (p.1361·2); pyridoxine hydrochloride (p.1362·3).
Lignocaine (p.1293·2) is included in the injection to alleviate the pain of injection.
Vitamin B deficiency.

Menalgon *Menarini, Ital.*
Thiamine monophosphate (p.1361·2); cyanocobalamin (p.1363·3).
Neuritis.

Menalgon B6 *Menarini, Ital.*
Thiamine monophosphate (p.1361·2); pyridoxine hydrochloride (p.1362·3); cyanocobalamin (p.1363·3).
Nerve and muscle pain and inflammation.

Menalmina *Men, Spain.*
Chlorhexidine gluconate (p.1107·2).
Skin and wound disinfection.

Menaval *Legere, USA†.*
Oestradiol valerate (p.1455·2).

Menaven *Menarini, Spain.*
Heparin sodium (p.879·3).
Peripheral vascular disorders.

Mencalisvit *Menarini, Spain.*
Calcium lactate (p.1155·2); cholecalciferol (p.1366·3).
Vitamin D and calcium deficiency.

Mencevax ACWY
SmithKline Beecham, Aust.; SmithKline Beecham, Austral.; SK-RIT, Belg.; SmithKline Beecham, Ger.; SSW, Ger.; SmithKline Beecham, Ital.
A meningococcal vaccine (groups A, C, W, and Y) (p.1520·3).
Active immunisation.

Mencortex *Menarini, Ital.†.*
Suprarenal cortex (p.1050·1).
Adrenal insufficiency; hypotension; toxicosis.

Mencortex B6 *Menarini, Ital.†.*
Suprarenal cortex (p.1050·1); pyridoxine hydrochloride (p.1362·3).
Toxicosis; vomiting.

Mendrome *Bristol-Myers Squibb, S.Afr.†.*
Fluphenazine hydrochloride (p.671·3); bendrofluazide (p.827·3).
Premenstrual syndrome.

Meneparol *Menarini, Spain.*
Amino acids; cyanocobalamin (p.1363·3); liver extract.
Liver disorders.

Meneparol Sol *Menarini, Spain†.*
Amino acids; cyanocobalamin (p.1363·3); sorbitol (p.1354·2); liver extract.
Liver disorders.

Menest *SmithKline Beecham, USA.*
Esterified oestrogens (p.1458·1).
Breast cancer; female castration; female hypogonadism; menopausal vasomotor symptoms; primary ovarian failure; prostatic cancer; vulval and vaginal atrophy.

Mengivac (A+C)
Pasteur Merieux, Irl.; Pasteur Merieux, UK.
A meningococcal vaccine (groups A and C) (p.1520·3).
Active immunisation.

Meni-D *Seatrace, USA.*
Meclozine hydrochloride (p.413·3).
Motion sickness; vertigo.

Meningokokken-Impfstoff A + C *Merieux, Ger.*
A meningococcal vaccine (groups A and C) (p.1520·3).
Active immunisation.

Meningovax A+C
Pasteur Merieux, Neth.; Pasteur Merieux, Norw.; Pasteur Merieux, Swed.
A meningococcal vaccine (groups A and C) (p.1520·3).
Active immunisation.

Meniodina *Men, Spain†.*
Povidone-iodine (p.1123·3).
Skin and mucous membrane disinfection; skin infections.

Menobiol *Yves Ponroy, Fr.*
Multivitamin and mineral preparation with fatty acids.
Menopausal disorders.

Menodoron
Weleda, Aust.; Weleda, UK.
Capsella bursa pastoris; majorana; achillea (p.1542·2); oak (p.1609·3); urtica (p.1642·3).
Menstrual disorders.

Menoflush *Pharmaceutical Enterprises, S.Afr.*
Ethinyloestradiol (p.1445·1); multivitamins.
Menopausal disorders.

Menoflush + ¼ *Pharmaceutical Enterprises, S.Afr.*
Ethinyloestradiol (p.1445·1); multivitamins; phenobarbitone (p.350·2).
Formerly known as Menoflush-Menogloed + ¼.
Menopausal disorders.

Menogen *Breckenridge, USA.*
Esterified oestrogens (p.1458·1); methyltestosterone (p.1450·3).
Menopausal disorders.

Menogon Ferring, Ger.; Ferring, UK.
Menotrophin (p.1252·1).
Male and female infertility.

Meno-implant Organon, Neth.
Oestradiol (p.1455·1).
Oestrogen deficiency.

Menomune CSL, Austral.; Pasteur Merieux, Ital.; Connaught, USA.
A meningococcal vaccine (groups A, C, Y and W-135) (p.1520·3).
Active immunisation.

Menopace Vitabiotics, UK.
Multivitamin and mineral preparation.

Menopause Homeocan, Canad.
Homoeopathic preparation.

Menophase Searle, Irl.; Searle, UK.
15 Tablets, mestranol (p.1450·2); 13 tablets, mestranol; norethisterone (p.1453·1).
Menopausal disorders; osteoporosis.

Menoplex Fiske, USA.
Paracetamol (p.72·2); phenyltoloxamine citrate (p.416·1).
Pain.

Menoprem Wyeth, Austral.
Maroon tablets, conjugated oestrogens (p.1457·3); blue tablets, medroxyprogesterone acetate (p.1448·3).
Menopausal disorders; osteoporosis.

Menorest Rhone-Poulenc Rorer, Austral.; Specia, Fr.; Rhone-Poulenc Rorer, Ger.; Rhone-Poulenc Rorer, Irl.; Rhone-Poulenc Rorer, Ital.; Rhone-Poulenc Rorer, Neth.; Rhone-Poulenc Rorer, Norw.; Rhone-Poulenc Rorer, S.Afr.; Rhone-Poulenc Rorer, Spain; Rhone-Poulenc Rorer, Swed.; Rhone-Poulenc Rorer, Switz.; Rhone-Poulenc Rorer, UK.
Oestradiol (p.1455·1).
Menopausal disorders; osteoporosis.

Menosan Bioforce, Switz.
Homoeopathic preparation.

Menoselect Dreluso, Ger.
Homoeopathic preparation.

Menova Merck, Ger.†.
Chlormadinone acetate (p.1439·1); ethinyloestradiol (p.1445·1).
Dysfunctional uterine bleeding; menstrual disorders.

Menovis Teofarma, Ital.
Oestradiol benzoate (p.1455·1); progesterone (p.1459·3).
Menstrual disorders.

Menoxicor Tecefarma, Spain.
Cloridarol (p.845·1).
Ischaemic heart disease.

Menpovax 4 Chiron, Ital.†.
A meningococcal vaccine (groups A, C, W, and Y) (p.1520·3).
Active immunisation.

Menpovax A+C Sclavo, Ital.†.
A meningococcal vaccine (groups A and C) (p.1520·3).
Active immunisation.

Menpros Continental, Spain.
Misoprostol (p.1419·3).
Peptic ulcer.

Menrium Roche Products, USA†.
Chlordiazepoxide (p.646·3); esterified oestrogens (p.1458·1).
Menopausal symptoms.

Mensiso Menarini, Ital.
Sissomicin sulphate (p.248·1).
Bacterial infections.

Mensoton Berlin-Chemie, Ger.
Ibuprofen (p.44·1).
Pain.

Menstrualin Diabetylin, Ger.†.
Yeast (p.1373·1); capsella bursa pastoris; alchemilla; hypericum (p.1590·1); sulphur (p.1091·2).
Dysmenorrhoea.

Menstruasan Bioforce, Switz.
Homoeopathic preparation.

Mensuosedyl Plantes et Medecines, Fr.†.
Paracetamol (p.72·2); anemone (p.1623·3); crataegus (p.1568·2).
Migraine; pain.

Mentacur Asche, Ger.
Peppermint oil (p.1208·1).
Irritable bowel syndrome.

Mental Alertness Homeocan, Canad.
Homoeopathic preparation.

Mentalgina Ragionieri, Ital.†.
Phenazone (p.78·2); caffeine (p.749·3).
Pain.

Mentamida Kin, Spain.
Benzydamine hydrochloride (p.21·3); hexetidine (p.1116·1).
Mouth and throat inflammation.

Mentax Kaken, Jpn; Penederm, USA.
Butenafine hydrochloride (p.376·1).
Fungal skin infections.

Menthacin Mentholatum, USA.
Capsaicin (p.24·2); menthol (p.1600·2).
Arthritis.

Menthamel (Rowo-211) Pharmakon, Ger.†.
Homoeopathic preparation.

Menthol and Wintergreen Heat Product Seton, UK†.
Methyl salicylate (p.55·2); camphor (p.1557·2); menthol (p.1600·2); eucalyptus oil (p.1578·1); volatile mustard oil (p.1605·3).
Rheumatic pain.

Mentholatum Balm Mentholatum, UK†.
Menthol (p.1600·2); camphor (p.1557·2); eucalyptus oil (p.1578·1); pumilio pine oil (p.1623·3); methyl salicylate (p.55·2).
Cold symptoms.

Mentholatum Cherry Chest Rub Mentholatum, USA.
Camphor (p.1557·2); menthol (p.1600·2); eucalyptus oil (p.1578·1).
Coughs and cold symptoms.

Mentholatum Cherry Ice Mentholatum, USA.
SPF 11: Padimate O (p.1488·1); dimethicone (p.1384·2).
Dry lips; sunscreen.

Mentholatum Cough Drops Mentholatum, Canad.
Eucalyptus oil (p.1578·1); menthol (p.1600·2).

Mentholatum Extra Strength Ointment Mentholatum, Canad.
Camphor (p.1557·2); eucalyptus oil (p.1578·1); menthol (p.1600·2).

Mentholatum Nasal Inhaler Mentholatum, UK.
Menthol (p.1600·2); camphor (p.1557·2); methyl salicylate (p.55·2).
Nasal congestion.

Mentholatum Natural Ice Mentholatum, USA.
SPF 14: Padimate O (p.1488·1); dimethicone (p.1384·2).
Dry lips; sunscreen.

Mentholatum Natural Ice Lip Protectant Mentholatum, USA.
Menthol (p.1600·2); camphor (p.1557·2).
Dry lips.

Mentholatum Ointment
Note. This name is used for preparations of different composition.
Mentholatum, Canad.
Camphor (p.1557·2); menthol (p.1600·2).

Mentholatum, USA.
Camphor (p.1557·2); menthol (p.1600·2); eucalyptus oil (p.1578·1).
Coughs and cold symptoms.

Mentholatum Softlips Mentholatum, USA.
Dimethicone (p.1384·2).
Dry lips.

Mentholatum Softlips Lipbalm Mentholatum, USA.
Dimethicone (p.1384·2); padimate O (p.1488·1).
Dry lips.

Mentholatum Softlips Lipbalm (UV) Mentholatum, USA.
Ethylhexyl *p*-methoxycinnamate (p.1487·1); padimate O (p.1488·1); oxybenzone (p.1487·3); dimethicone (p.1384·2).
Dry lips; sunscreen.

Menthol-Balsam Doerr, Ger.†.
Peppermint oil (p.1208·1); clove oil (p.1565·2); camphor oil.
Bronchitis; cold symptoms; insect stings; migraine; rheumatic disorders.

Mentholease Warner-Lambert, UK.
Menthol (p.1600·2); eucalyptus oil (p.1578·1).
Hay fever.

Mentholon Original N Schoning-Berlin, Ger.
Menthol (p.1600·2); camphor (p.1557·2); eucalyptus oil (p.1578·1).
Catarrh.

Mentho-lyptus Warner-Lambert Confectionery, UK.
Menthol (p.1600·2); eucalyptus oil (p.1578·1).
Cold symptoms; sore throat.

Mentholyptus Vaporiser Fluid Nelson, Austral.†.
Menthol (p.1600·2); eucalyptus oil (p.1578·1); camphor salicylate.
Cold symptoms.

Menthoneurin
Byk, Aust.; Byk, Neth.
Liniment: Glycol salicylate (p.43·1); benzyl nicotinate (p.22·1).
Formerly contained glycol salicylate, benzyl nicotinate, and methyl nicotinate in *Neth.*
Musculoskeletal and joint disorders; neuralgia.

Byk, Aust.; Byk, Neth.
Ointment: Glycol salicylate (p.43·1); menthol (p.1600·2).
Headache; musculoskeletal and joint disorders; neuralgia.

Menthoneurin-Salbe Tosse, Ger.
Glycol salicylate (p.43·1); menthol (p.1600·2).
Muscular and neuromuscular disorders; rheumatic disorders; soft-tissue disorders.

Menthoneurin-Vollbad N Tosse, Ger.
Glycol salicylate (p.43·1); benzyl nicotinate (p.22·1); methyl nicotinate (p.55·1).
Bath additive; musculoskeletal and joint disorders.

MenthoRub Schein, USA.
Menthol (p.1600·2); camphor (p.1557·2).
Muscle, joint, and soft-tissue pain; neuralgia.

Menthymin Mono ankerpharm, Ger.
Thyme (p.1636·3).
Upper respiratory-tract disorders.

Mentis Menarini, Spain.
Pyrisuccideanol dimaleate (p.1619·2).
Cerebrovascular impairment; senility.

Mentium Guidotti, Ital.
Pirisudanol maleate (p.1619·2).
Mental function disorders.

Mentobox
Alcala, Spain.
Tablets: Camphor (p.1557·2); tolu balsam (p.1071·1); cineole (p.1564·1); drosera (p.1574·1); thyme (p.1636·3); menthol (p.1600·2); sodium benzoate (p.1102·3).
Upper respiratory-tract disorders.

Ale, Spain†.
Ointment: Camphor (p.1557·2); Cedrus deodora oil; cineole (p.1564·1); methyl salicylate (p.55·2); thymol (p.1127·1); turpentine.
Upper respiratory-tract disorders.

Mentobox Antitusivo Alcala, Spain.
Dextromethorphan hydrobromide (p.1057·3); benzocaine (p.1286·2); guaiphenesin (p.1061·3); menthol (p.1600·2).
Respiratory-tract disorders.

Mentol Sedans Sulfamidad Orravan, Spain†.
Camphor (p.1557·2); bismuth subnitrate (p.1180·2); boric acid (p.1554·2); sulphanilamide (p.256·3); thymol (p.1127·1); zinc oxide (p.1096·2); menthol (p.1600·2); phenol (p.1121·2); alcohol; lavender essence; talc.
Skin infections.

Mentopin
Note. This name is used for preparations of different composition.
Brady, Aust.
Lavender flower (p.1594·3); sage (p.1627·1); peppermint leaf (p.1208·1); paprika (p.1559·2); urtica (p.1642·3); pine; camphor (p.1557·2); menthol (p.1600·2); pumilio pine oil (p.1623·3); peppermint oil (p.1208·1).
Musculoskeletal and joint disorders; neuralgia.

Hermes, Ger.
Acetylcysteine (p.1052·3).
Coughs; respiratory disorders associated with viscid or excessive mucus.

Mentopin Echinacea Hermes, Ger.
Echinacea purpura (p.1574·2).
Respiratory- and urinary-tract infections.

Mentopin Erkaltungsbalsam Hermes, Ger.
Eucalyptus oil (p.1578·1); pine needle oil.
Cold symptoms.

Mentopin Gurgellosung Hermes, Ger.
Chlorhexidine gluconate (p.1107·2).
Inflammation and infection of the mouth and throat.

Mentopin Hustenstiller Hermes, Ger.
Clobutinol hydrochloride (p.1057·1).
Catarrh; coughs.

Mentopin Nasenspray Hermes, Ger.
Xylometazoline hydrochloride (p.1071·2).
Nasal congestion; sinusitis.

Mentopin Vitamin C + ASS Hermes, Ger.
Aspirin (p.16·1); ascorbic acid (p.1365·2).
Fever; pain.

Mentor Lifeplan, UK.
Ginkgo biloba (p.1584·1).

Menutil Hoechst Marion Roussel, Belg.
Diethylpropion hydrochloride (p.1479·3).
Obesity.

Menzol Schwarz, UK†.
Norethisterone (p.1453·1).
Menstrual disorders.

282 Mep Frosst, Canad.
Aspirin (p.16·1); caffeine citrate (p.749·3); codeine phosphate (p.26·1); meprobamate (p.678·1).
Anxiety; inflammation; pain; skeletal muscle spasm.

Mepalax ABC, Ital.
Boldo (p.1554·1); rhubarb (p.1212·1); cascara (p.1183·1).
Constipation.

Mepentil Recordati, Ital.†.
Thymopentin (p.1637·2).
Immunodeficiency disorders.

Mepergan Wyeth-Ayerst, USA.
Pethidine hydrochloride (p.76·1); promethazine hydrochloride (p.416·2).
Preanaesthetic medication.

Mephamesone Mepha, Switz.
Dexamethasone sodium phosphate (p.1037·2).
Corticosteroid.

Mephanol Mepha, Switz.
Allopurinol (p.390·2).
Gout; hyperuricaemia; renal calculi.

Mephaquine Mepha, Switz.
Mefloquine hydrochloride (p.432·2).
Malaria.

Mephathiol Mepha, Switz.
Carbocisteine (p.1056·3).
Respiratory-tract disorders associated with increased mucus.

Mephaxine Mepha, Switz.
Prenoxdiazine hydrochloride (p.1068·3) or prenoxdiazine hybenzate (p.1068·3).
Coughs.

Mephaxine Compositum Mepha, Switz.
Prenoxdiazine hydrochloride (p.1068·3); guaiphenesin (p.1061·3); terpin hydrate (p.1070·2).
Coughs.

Mephyton Merck Sharp & Dohme, USA.
Phytomenadione (p.1371·1).
Coagulation disorders due to faulty formation of factors II, VII, IX, and X.

Mepicain Monico, Ital.
Mepivacaine hydrochloride (p.1297·2).
Adrenaline acid tartrate (p.813·3) is included in some injections as a vasoconstrictor to diminish absorption and localise the effect of the local anaesthetic.
Local anaesthesia.

Mepicaton Weimer, Ger.; Weimer, Switz.
Mepivacaine hydrochloride (p.1297·2).
Local anaesthesia.

Mepicor Corvi, Ital.†.
Mepindolol sulphate (p.902·3).
Cardiovascular disorders.

Mepident Warner-Lambert, Ital.
Mepivacaine hydrochloride (p.1297·2).
Adrenaline acid tartrate (p.813·3) is included in some injections as a vasoconstrictor to diminish absorption and localise the effect of the local anaesthetic.
Local anaesthesia in dentistry.

Mepidium Recordati, Ital.†.
Timepidium bromide (p.469·1).
Smooth muscle spasm.

Mepiforan Bieffe, Ital.
Mepivacaine hydrochloride (p.1297·2).
Adrenaline acid tartrate (p.813·3) is included in some injections as a vasoconstrictor to diminish absorption and localise the effect of the local anaesthetic.
Local anaesthesia.

Mepihexal Hexal, Ger.
Mepivacaine hydrochloride (p.1297·2).
Local anaesthesia.

Mepi-Mynol Molteni, Ital.
Mepivacaine hydrochloride (p.1297·2).
Adrenaline acid tartrate (p.813·3) is included in some injections as a vasoconstrictor to diminish absorption and localise the effect of the local anaesthetic.
Local anaesthesia.

Mepivastesin Espe, Ger.
Mepivacaine hydrochloride (p.1297·2).
Local anaesthesia.

Mepivastesin forte Espe, Ger.†.
Mepivacaine hydrochloride (p.1297·2).
Adrenaline hydrochloride (p.813·3) is included in this preparation as a vasoconstrictor to diminish absorption and localise the effect of the local anaesthetic.
Local anaesthesia.

Mepral Bracco, Ital.
Omeprazole (p.1204·2).
Gastro-oesophageal reflux disease; peptic ulcer; Zollinger-Ellison syndrome.

Mepranix Ashbourne, UK.
Metoprolol tartrate (p.907·3).
Angina pectoris; arrhythmias; hypertension; myocardial infarction.

Meprate DDSA Pharmaceuticals, UK.
Meprobamate (p.678·1).

Meprepose Pharmalab, S.Afr.†.
Meprobamate (p.678·1).
Anxiety; muscle relaxant.

Mepril Kwizda, Aust.
Enalapril maleate (p.863·2).
Hypertension.

Meprodil Streuli, Switz.
Meprobamate (p.678·1).
Anxiety; muscle relaxant; sedative.

Meprofen AGIPS, Ital.
Ketoprofen (p.48·2).
Musculoskeletal, joint, peri-articular, and soft-tissue disorders.

Meprogesic Propan, S.Afr.
Paracetamol (p.72·2); codeine phosphate (p.26·1); meprobamate (p.678·1).
Pain; tension-type headache.

Meprolol TAD, Ger.
Metoprolol tartrate (p.907·3).
Arrhythmias; hypertension; ischaemic heart disease; migraine; myocardial infarction.

Mepromol Propan, S.Afr.
Paracetamol (p.72·2); codeine phosphate (p.26·1); caffeine (p.749·3); meprobamate (p.678·1).
Pain.

Mepron Glaxo Wellcome, Canad.; Glaxo Wellcome, USA.
Atovaquone (p.579·3).
Pneumocystis carinii pneumonia.

Mepronizine Sanofi Winthrop, Fr.
Meprobamate (p.678·1); aceprometazine maleate (p.640·2).
Insomnia.

Meprospan Inibsa, Spain†; Wallace, USA†.
Meprobamate (p.678·1).
Anxiety; insomnia; skeletal muscle spasm.

Meptid Wyeth, Ger.; Monmouth, Irl.; Monmouth, UK.
Meptazinol (p.53·1) or meptazinol hydrochloride (p.52·2).
Pain.

Meptidol Wyeth Lederle, Aust.
Meptazinol hydrochloride (p.52·2).
Pain.

Meptin Otsuka, Jpn.
Procaterol hydrochloride (p.757·3).
Obstructive airways disease.

Mepyrimal Propan, S.Afr.
Mepyramine maleate (p.414·1).
Skin disorders.

Meracote *Sigma, Austral.*
Alginic acid (p.1470·3); aluminium hydroxide (p.1177·3); magnesium trisilicate (p.1199·1); sodium bicarbonate (p.1153·2).
Gastric reflux; heartburn.

Meral *Darci, Belg.†.*
Magnesium trisilicate (p.1199·1); sodium bicarbonate (p.1153·2); calcium carbonate (p.1182·1); calcium hydrogen phosphate (p.1155·3); sodium tartrate (p.1214·1).
Gastro-intestinal disorders.

Meralop
Merck Sharp & Dohme, Ital.; Thea, Spain.
Keracyanin (p.1593·1).
Disorders of vision.

Meralops *Thea, Fr.*
Keracyanin (p.1593·1).
Visual impairment.

Merankol Gel *Lepetit, Ital.†.*
Dicyclomine hydrochloride (p.460·1); methylcellulose; sodium lauryl sulphate; magnesium hydroxide (p.1198·2); dried aluminium hydroxide (p.1177·3).
Gastro-intestinal disorders.

Merankol Pastiglie *Bruno, Ital.*
Dicyclomine hydrochloride (p.460·1); methylcellulose; sodium lauryl sulphate; magnesium hydroxide (p.1198·2); dried aluminium hydroxide (p.1177·3); magnesium trisilicate (p.1199·1).
Gastro-intestinal disorders.

Merasyn *Mer-National, S.Afr.*
Aluminium hydroxide gel (p.1177·3); magnesium hydroxide (p.1198·2); simethicone (p.1213·1); methylcellulose (p.1473·3).
Formerly contained aluminium hydroxide gel, magnesium hydroxide, and simethicone.
Flatulence; hyperchlorhydria.

Merbentul *Marion Merrell Dow, Ger.†.*
Chlorotrianisene (p.1439·2).
Prostatic cancer.

Merbentyl
Hoechst Marion Roussel, Austral.; Hoechst Marion Roussel, Irl.; Mer-National, S.Afr.; Florizel, UK.
Dicyclomine hydrochloride (p.460·1).
Gastro-intestinal spasm.

Mercalm *Phygiene, Fr.*
Caffeine (p.749·3); dimenhydrinate (p.408·2).
Motion sickness.

Mercap *Medac, Ger.*
Mercaptopurine (p.546·1).
Acute lymphatic leukaemia; non-Hodgkin's lymphoma.

Mercaptyl *Knoll, Switz.*
Penicillamine (p.988·3).
Biliary cirrhosis; cystinuria; heavy-metal poisoning; hepatitis; pulmonary fibrosis; rheumatoid arthritis; scleroderma.

Mercilon
Organon, Aust.; Organon, Belg.; Organon, Fr.; Organon, Irl.; Organon, Ital.; Organon, Neth.; Donmed, S.Afr.; Organon, Swed.; Organon, Switz.; Organon, UK.
Desogestrel (p.1443·3); ethinyloestradiol (p.1445·1).
28-Day packs also contain 7 inert tablets.
Combined oral contraceptive.

Merck Skin Testing Solutions *E. Merck, UK†.*
Allergen extracts (single and mixed) (p.1545·1).
Hyposensitisation.

Mercodol with Decapryn *Hoechst Marion Roussel, Canad.*
Hydrocodone tartrate (p.43·1); etafedrine hydrochloride (p.1061·1); sodium citrate (p.1153·2); doxylamine succinate (p.410·1).
Coughs.

Mercromina *Lainco, Spain.*
Mercurochrome (p.1119·2).
Wound disinfection.

Mercrotona *Orravan, Spain.*
Mercurochrome sodium (p.1119·2); alcohol (p.1099·1).
Wound disinfection.

Mercroverk *Verkos, Spain†.*
Mercurochrome sodium (p.1119·2).
Wound disinfection.

Mercryl Lauryle
Menarini, Fr.; Sanofi Winthrop, Spain.
Mercurobutol (p.1119·1).
Skin and mucous membrane disinfection.

Mercuchrom *Krewel, Ger.*
Mercurochrome (p.1119·2).
Burns; skin disinfection; wounds.

Mercufila Coaltar *Seid, Spain†.*
Coal tar (p.1092·3); quillaia (p.1328·2).
Skin disorders; vaginitis.

Mercurin *Monik, Spain.*
Mercurochrome sodium (p.1119·2).
Wound disinfection.

Mercurio Rojo *Perez Gimenez, Spain†.*
Mercurochrome (p.1119·2).
Wound disinfection.

Mercurobromo *Spyfarma, Spain.*
Mercurochrome (p.1119·2).
Wound disinfection.

Mercutina Brota *Escaned, Spain.*
Mercurochrome (p.1119·2).
Wound disinfection.

Mercuval *GN, Ger.*
Unithiol (p.998·2).
Lead poisoning; mercury poisoning.

Meregon *Malesci, Ital.†.*
Bunaftine citrate (p.835·1) or bunaftine hydrochloride (p.835·1).
Arrhythmias.

Mereprine
Hoechst Marion Roussel, Belg.; Marion Merrell, Fr.; Cassella-med, Ger.; Hoechst Marion Roussel, Switz.
Doxylamine succinate (p.410·1).
Hypersensitivity reactions; restlessness and excitement in children; sleep disorders.

Meresa
Schoeller, Aust.; Dolorgiet, Ger.
Sulpiride (p.692·3).
Depression; Ménière's disease; psychoses.

Merfen N *Zyma, Ger.†.*
Phenylmercuric acetate (p.1122·2); isopropyl alcohol (p.1118·2); propyl alcohol (p.1124·2).
Hand disinfection.

Merfen nouveau *Max Ritter, Switz.*
Chlorhexidine gluconate (p.1107·2) or chlorhexidine hydrochloride (p.1107·2); benzoxonium chloride (p.1103·3).
Skin and wound disinfection.

Merfene *Zyma, Fr.*
Chlorhexidine gluconate (p.1107·2).
Formerly contained phenylmercuric borate.
Wound disinfection.

Merfen-Orange N *Zyma, Ger.†.*
Phenylmercuric acetate (p.1122·2).
Antiseptic.

Merfluan Sali Dentali *Colgate-Palmolive, Ital.*
Sodium fluoride (p.742·1); minerals.
Dental caries prophylaxis.

Meridia *Knoll, USA.*
Sibutramine (p.1485·2).
Obesity.

Meridol *Marion Merrell, Spain.*
Aluminium aspirin (p.15·1); caffeine (p.749·3); chlorpheniramine maleate (p.405·1); paracetamol (p.72·2).
Influenza and cold symptoms; nasal congestion.

Meridol-D *Pharmaceutical Enterprises, S.Afr.*
Paracetamol (p.72·2); codeine phosphate (p.26·1); diphenhydramine (p.409·1).
Fever; pain.

Merieux Inactivated Rabies Vaccine *Pasteur Merieux, UK.*
An inactivated rabies vaccine (Wistar PM/WI 38 1503-3M strain) (p.1530·3).
Active immunisation.

Merinax *Sanofi Winthrop, Belg.†.*
Hexapropymate (p.675·1).
Insomnia.

Merislon *Eisai, Jpn.*
Betahistine mesylate (p.1553·1).
Ménière's disease; vertigo.

Meritene
Sandoz Nutrition, Canad.; Wander, Ital.; Novartis, Norw.; Wander, S.Afr.†; Novartis Nutrition, Swed.; Wander Health Care, Switz.; Sandoz Nutrition, USA.
Preparation for enteral nutrition.

Merlit *Ebewe, Aust.*
Lorazepam (p.675·3).
Anxiety disorders; sleep disorders.

Merluzzina *Scherer, Ital.†.*
Cod-liver oil (p.1337·3).
Vitamin A and D supplement.

Merocaine
Seton, Irl.; Hoechst Marion Roussel, UK.
Benzocaine (p.1286·2); cetylpyridinium chloride (p.1106·2).
Mouth and throat disorders.

Merocet *Hoechst Marion Roussel, UK.*
Cetylpyridinium chloride (p.1106·2); alcohol (p.1099·1).
Oral cleansing.

Merocets
Seton, Irl.; Hoechst Marion Roussel, UK.
Cetylpyridinium chloride (p.1106·2).
Sore throat.

Merol *Medecine Vegetale, Fr.*
Eucalyptus (p.1578·1); bitter-orange (p.1610·3); potassium guaiacolsulfonate (p.1068·3); codeine (p.26·1).
Coughs.

Meromycin *Merckle, Aust.*
Erythromycin ethyl succinate (p.204·2) or erythromycin stearate (p.204·2).
Bacterial infections.

Meronem
Zeneca, Belg.; Zeneca, Ger.; Grunenthal, Ger.; Zeneca, Irl.; Zeneca, Neth.; Zeneca, S.Afr.; Zeneca, Spain; Zeneca, Swed.; Zeneca, Switz.; Zeneca, UK.
Meropenem (p.224·2).
Bacterial infections.

Meropen *Sumitomo, Jpn.*
Meropenem (p.224·2).
Bacterial infections.

Merothol *Hoechst Marion Roussel, UK.*
Cetylpyridinium chloride (p.1106·2); menthol (p.1600·2); eucalyptus oil (p.1578·1).
Mouth and throat infections; nasal congestion.

Merovit *Marion Merrell Dow, UK†.*
Cetylpyridinium chloride (p.1106·2); ascorbic acid (p.1365·2).
Sore throat.

Merrem
ICI, Austral.; Zeneca, Canad.; Zeneca, Ital.; Zeneca, USA.
Meropenem (p.224·2).
Bacterial infections.

Mersol
Note. This name is used for preparations of different composition.
Ratiopharm, Ger.
Nicotinamide (p.1351·2); folic acid (p.1340·3).
Photosensitivity.

Century, USA.
Thiomersal (p.1126·3).
Skin disinfection.

Mersyndol *Hoechst Marion Roussel, Austral.*
Paracetamol (p.72·2); codeine phosphate (p.26·1); doxylamine succinate (p.410·1).
Fever; pain.

Mersyndol with Codeine *Hoechst Marion Roussel, Canad.*
Paracetamol (p.72·2); codeine phosphate (p.26·1); doxylamine succinate (p.410·1).
Cold symptoms; pain.

Mersyndol Daystrength *Hoechst Marion Roussel, Austral.*
Paracetamol (p.72·2); codeine phosphate (p.26·1).
Fever; pain.

Merthiolate
Lilly, Ital.†; Lilly, S.Afr.; Lilly, Spain†.
Thiomersal (p.1126·3).
Skin and wound disinfection.

Meruvax II
CSL, Austral.; Merck Sharp & Dohme, Belg.†; Pasteur Merieux, Ital.†; Pasteur Merieux, Swed.; Pro Vaccine, Switz.; Morson, UK†; Merck Sharp & Dohme, USA.
A rubella vaccine (Wistar RA 27/3 strain) (p.1532·3).
Active immunisation.

Mervan
Continental Pharma, Belg.†; Continental Pharma, Switz.†.
Alclofenac (p.12·3) or alclofenac aminoethanol (p.12·3).
Lignocaine hydrochloride (p.1293·2) is included in the intramuscular injection to alleviate the pain of injection.
Inflammation; musculoskeletal, joint, and peri-articular disorders; pain.

Merz Spezial *Medra, Aust.*
Multivitamin and mineral preparation.

Merz Spezial Dragees SN *Merz, Ger.*
Multivitamin preparation with iron and acetylmethionine.

Mes-Acton *Sudmedica, Ger.†.*
Thymus extract; liver extract; spleen extract.
Immunotherapy.

Mesantoin
Sandoz, Canad.†; Sandoz, USA.
Methoin (p.349·1).
Epilepsy.

Mesasal
SmithKline Beecham, Austral.; SmithKline Beecham, Canad.; SmithKline Beecham, Norw.; SmithKline Beecham, Swed.
Mesalazine (p.1199·2).
Inflammatory bowel disease.

Mescolor *Horizon, USA.*
Chlorpheniramine maleate (p.405·1); pseudoephedrine hydrochloride (p.1068·3); hyoscine methonitrate (p.463·1).
Upper respiratory-tract symptoms.

Mescorit *Boehringer Mannheim, Ger.*
Metformin hydrochloride (p.330·1).
Diabetes mellitus.

Mesid *Janssen-Cilag, Ital.*
Nimesulide (p.63·2).
Fever; inflammation; pain.

M-Eslon *Rhone-Poulenc Rorer, Canad.*
Morphine sulphate (p.56·2).
Pain.

Mesnex *Mead Johnson Oncology, USA.*
Mesna (p.983·3).
Prevention of ifosfamide-induced haemorrhagic cystitis.

Mesocaine *GNR, Fr.*
Lignocaine hydrochloride (p.1293·2).
Local anaesthesia.

Mespafin *Merckle, Ger.*
Doxycycline hydrochloride (p.202·3).
Bacterial infections.

Mestacine *Novalis, Fr.*
Minocycline hydrochloride (p.226·2).
Bacterial infections.

Mestinon
Roche, Aust.; Roche, Austral.†; Roche, Belg.; ICN, Canad.; Roche, Fr.; Roche, Ger.; Roche, Irl.; Roche, Ital.; Roche, Neth.; Roche, Norw.; Roche, S.Afr.; Roche, Spain; Roche, Swed.; Roche, Switz.; ICN, UK; ICN, USA.
Pyridostigmine bromide (p.1398·1).
Myasthenia gravis; paralytic ileus; postoperative urinary retention; reversal of competitive neuromuscular blockade.

Mestoranum
Schering, Norw.; Schering, Swed.
Mesterolone (p.1450·1).
Hypogonadism.

Mesulid
Therabel Pharma, Belg.; LPB, Ital.
Nimesulide (p.63·2) or nimesulide betadex (p.63·2).
Fever; inflammation; joint disorders; pain.

Meta Framan *Oftalmiso, Spain.*
Metampicillin sodium (p.224·3).
Bacterial infections.

metabiarex *Meta Fackler, Ger.*
Homoeopathic preparation.

Metabola B *Eagle, Austral.†.*
Vitamin and mineral preparation.
Vitamin B supplementation.

Metabolic Mineral Mixture
Scientific Hospital Supplies, Austral.; Scientific Hospital Supplies, UK.
Essential mineral salts.
Mineral supplementation for enteral diets.

Metabolic Mineral Mixture-Calcium Citrate
Scientific Hospital Supplies, Austral.†.
Mineral and trace element preparation.

Metabolicum *Novag, Spain.*
Sodium cytidine monophosphate; cobamamide (p.1364·2); hydroxocobalamin (p.1363·3).
Megaloblastic anaemias; neuritis; tonic.

Metaboline *Desbergers, Canad.†.*
Methandienone (p.1450·2); multivitamins and nutrients.
Anabolic; osteoporosis.

Metacaf *Chong Kun Dang, Ital.*
Cefmetazole sodium (p.166·2).
Lignocaine hydrochloride (p.1293·2) is included in the intramuscular injection to alleviate the pain of injection.
Bacterial infections.

Metacen *Chiesi, Ital.*
Indomethacin (p.45·2).
Musculoskeletal and joint disorders.

Metaclarben *Clarben, Spain†.*
Metampicillin sodium (p.224·3).
Bacterial infections.

Metacuprol *Lemoine, Fr.*
Copper sulphate (p.1338·1).
Skin and mucous membrane infections.

Metadomus *Medici Domus, Ital.†.*
Methacycline hydrochloride (p.225·1).
Bacterial infections.

Metadoxil *Baldacci, Ital.*
Metadoxine (p.1363·1).
Alcoholism; hepatic failure.

Metadyne *Pharmavite, Canad.*
Povidone-iodine (p.1123·3).

Metafar *Lafare, Ital.*
Cefmetazole sodium (p.166·2).
Lignocaine hydrochloride (p.1293·2) is included in the intramuscular injection to alleviate the pain of injection.
Bacterial infections.

metaginkgo *Meta Fackler, Ger.*
Homoeopathic preparation.

Metagliz *Prodes, Spain.*
Metoclopramide glycyrrhizinate (p.1202·1).
Gastro-oesophageal reflux disease; gastroparesis; nausea and vomiting.

Metagliz Bismutico *Prodes, Spain.*
Bismuth subnitrate (p.1180·2); metoclopramide glycyrrhizinate (p.1202·1).
Gastritis; peptic ulcer; vomiting.

Metahydrin *Hoechst Marion Roussel, USA.*
Trichlormethiazide (p.958·2).
Hypertension; oedema.

metakaveron *Meta Fackler, Ger.*
Homoeopathic preparation.

Metakelfin *Pharmacia Upjohn, Ital.*
Sulfametopyrazine (p.251·3); pyrimethamine (p.436·3).
Malaria.

Metakes *Inexfa, Spain.*
Metampicillin sodium (p.224·3).
Bacterial infections.

Metalcaptase
Heyl, Ger.; Knoll, S.Afr.
Penicillamine (p.988·3).
Cystine calculi; cystinuria; heavy-metal poisoning; hepatitis; rheumatoid arthritis; scleroderma; Wilson's disease.

Metalcor *Alcor, Spain†.*
Metampicillin (p.224·3).
Bacterial infections.

Metalon *Caps, S.Afr.*
Metoclopramide hydrochloride (p.1200·3).
Gastro-intestinal motility disorders; vomiting.

Metalpha *Ashbourne, UK.*
Methyldopa (p.904·2).

metamagnesol *Meta Fackler, Ger.*
Magnesium aspartate (p.1157·2).
Magnesium deficiency.

Metamas *Tafir, Spain†.*
Metampicillin sodium (p.224·3).
Bacterial infections.

Metamicina *Rottapharm, Ital.†.*
Methacycline hydrochloride (p.225·1).
Bacterial infections.

Metamucil
Procter & Gamble, Aust.; Procter & Gamble, Austral.; Procter & Gamble, Belg.; Procter & Gamble, Canad.; Wick, Ger.; Searle, Irl.†; Searle, Neth.; Searle, S.Afr.; Procter & Gamble, Spain; Procter & Gamble,

Swed.†; Procter & Gamble, Switz.; Procter & Gamble (H&B Care), UK†; Procter & Gamble, USA.
Ispaghula husk (p.1194·2).
Constipation; dietary fibre supplement; diverticular disease; haemorrhoids; stool softener.

Metandren *Ciba, Canad.*
Methyltestosterone (p.1450·3).
Androgen replacement therapy; breast cancer.

Metanium
Bengue, Irl.; Roche Consumer, UK.
Titanium dioxide (p.1093·3); titanium peroxide (p.1093·3); titanium salicylate (p.1093·3).
Napkin rash and related disorders.

metaossylen *Meta Fackler, Ger.*
Homoeopathic preparation.

Metaphen *Abbott, Austral.†.*
Nitromersol (p.1120·1).
Antiseptic in pre-operative skin preparation.

Metaplexan
Rhone-Poulenc Rorer, Aust.; Rhone-Poulenc Rorer, Ger.
Mequitazine (p.414·2).
Hypersensitivity disorders.

Metaprel *Sandoz, USA.*
Orciprenaline sulphate (p.756·3).
Bronchial asthma; reversible bronchospasm.

Metasal *Salus, Ital.*
Cefmetazole sodium (p.166·2).
Lignocaine hydrochloride (p.1293·2) is included in the intramuscular injection to alleviate the pain of injection.
Bacterial infections.

Metasedin *Esteve, Spain.*
Methadone hydrochloride (p.53·2).
Opiate withdrawal; pain.

metasolidago *Meta Fackler, Ger.*
Homoeopathic preparation.

Metasolvens *Hogapharm, Switz.*
Bromhexine hydrochloride (p.1055·3).
Respiratory-tract disorders associated with increased mucus.

Metaspirine *SmithKline Beecham Sante, Fr.*
Aspirin (p.16·1); caffeine (p.749·3).
Fever; pain.

Metastron
Amersham, Canad.; Amersham, Fr.; Amersham, Ital.; Amersham, Spain; Amersham International, UK; Medi-Physics, USA; Amersham, USA.
Strontium-89 (p.1425·1) in the form of strontium chloride.
Metastatic bone pain.

Metatensin *Hoechst Marion Roussel, USA.*
Trichlormethiazide (p.958·2); reserpine (p.942·1).
Hypertension.

Metatone
Warner-Lambert, Irl.; Parke, Davis, Switz.†; Warner-Lambert, UK.
Calcium glycerophosphate; manganese glycerophosphate; potassium glycerophosphate; sodium glycerophosphate; thiamine hydrochloride.
Tonic.

metavirulent *Meta Fackler, Ger.*
Homoeopathic preparation.

Metaxol *Propan, S.Afr.; Mer-National, S.Afr.*
Theophylline (p.765·1); codeine phosphate (p.26·1); mepyramine maleate (p.414·1).
Coughs.

Metazem *Bioglan, Irl.; Clonmel, Irl.*
Diltiazem hydrochloride (p.854·2).
Angina pectoris.

Metazol
Note. This name is used for preparations of different composition.
CT, Ital.
Cefmetazole sodium (p.166·2).
Lignocaine hydrochloride (p.1293·2) is included in the intramuscular injection to alleviate the pain of injection.
Bacterial infections.

Schwulst, S.Afr.
Metronidazole (p.585·1).
Anaerobic bacterial infections; protozoal infections.

Metcon *Docmed, S.Afr.*
Metoclopramide hydrochloride (p.1200·3).
Gastro-intestinal disorders; nausea and vomiting.

Meted
GenDerm, Canad.; Helsinn Birex, Irl.; Euroderma, UK; GenDerm, USA.
Salicylic acid (p.1090·2); sulphur (p.1091·2).
Scalp disorders.

Metenix 5 *Borg, UK.*
Metolazone (p.907·2).
Ascites; hypertension; oedema.

Meteophyt *OTW, Ger.†.*
Capsules: Ox bile (p.1553·2); turmeric (p.1001·3); aloes (p.1177·1); papain (p.1614·1); porcine pancreatin (p.1612·1); caraway oil (p.1559·3); fennel oil (p.1579·2); orange oil (p.1610·3); peppermint oil (p.1208·1); chamomile oil.
Oral drops: Ox bile (p.1553·2); turmeric (p.1001·3); fennel (p.1579·1); caraway (p.1559·3); chamomile (p.1561·2); peppermint leaf (p.1208·1); dried bitter-orange peel (p.1610·3); aloes (p.1177·1).
Digestive system disorders.

Meteophyt forte *OTW, Ger.*
Pancreatin (p.1612·1).
Pancreatic disorders.

Meteophyt N *OTW, Ger.*
Turmeric (p.1001·3).
Dyspepsia.

Meteophyt S *OTW, Ger.*
Chamomile (p.1561·2); peppermint leaf (p.1208·1); dried bitter-orange peel (p.1610·3); caraway (p.1559·3).
Dyspepsia; loss of appetite.

Meteophyt-V *OTW, Ger.†.*
Bromelains (p.1555·1); porcine pancreatin (p.1612·1); papain (p.1614·1); ox bile (p.1553·2); aloes (p.1177·1); curcuma zanthorrhiza; caraway oil (p.1559·3); fennel oil(p.1579·2); orange oil (p.1610·3); peppermint oil (p.1208·1); chamomile oil; dimethicone (p.1213·1).
Digestive system disorders.

Meteoril *Salvat, Spain.*
Simethicone (p.1213·1); magnesium trisilicate (p.1199·1); aluminium glycinate (p.1177·2).
Formerly contained simethicone, magnesium trisilicate, aluminium glycinate, and metoclopramide hydrochloride.
Flatulence; gastro-intestinal hyperacidity.

Meteosan *Zyma, Ger.*
Dimethicone (p.1213·1).
Gastro-intestinal disorders.

Meteospasmyl *Mayoly-Spindler, Fr.*
Alverine citrate (p.1548·1); simethicone (p.1213·1).
Formerly contained alverine citrate and methionine.
Gastro-intestinal disorders.

Meteoxane *Solvay, Fr.*
Simethicone (p.1213·1); phloroglucinol (p.1618·1).
Formerly contained atropine, hyoscyamine, amylobarbitone, and dimethicone.
Gastro-intestinal disorders.

Meteozym *Zyma, Ger.*
Pancreatin (p.1612·1); simethicone (p.1213·1).
Digestive system disorders.

Meterfolic *Sinclair, UK†.*
Ferrous fumarate (p.1339·3); folic acid (p.1340·3).
Iron and folic acid deficiency in pregnancy; neural tube defect prophylaxis.

Metex *Medac, Ger.*
Methotrexate sodium (p.547·1).
Arthritis; psoriasis.

Metforal *Guidotti, Ital.*
Metformin hydrochloride (p.330·1).
Diabetes mellitus.

Methabid *Pharmador, S.Afr.†.*
Indomethacin (p.45·2).
Fever; musculoskeletal and joint disorders.

Methacin *Mentholatum, Canad.*
Menthol (p.1600·2); capsaicin (p.24·2).

Methaderm *Taiho, Jpn†.*
Dexamethasone propionate (p.1037·3).
Skin disorders.

Methadose
Rosemont, UK; Mallinckrodt, USA.
Methadone hydrochloride (p.53·2).
Opioid withdrawal; pain.

Methagual *Gordon, USA.*
Methyl salicylate (p.55·2); guaiacol (p.1061·2).
Muscle, joint, and soft-tissue pain; neuralgia.

Methalgen *Alra, USA.*
Methyl salicylate (p.55·2); menthol (p.1600·2); camphor (p.1557·2); mustard oil (p.1605·3).
Musculoskeletal and joint pain.

Methamax *Garec, S.Afr.*
Indomethacin (p.45·2).
Gout; musculoskeletal and joint disorders.

Methatropic *Goldline, USA.*
Vitamin B substances with methionine.

Methergin
Sandoz, Aust.; Sandoz, Belg.; Sandoz, Fr.; Sandoz, Ger.; Sandoz, Ital.; Novartis, Neth.; Sandoz, Norw.; Sandoz, Spain; Novartis, Swed.; Sandoz, Switz.
Methylergometrine maleate (p.1603·1).
Postpartum haemorrhage; uterine atony; uterine haemorrhage.

Methergine *Sandoz, USA.*
Methylergometrine maleate (p.1603·1).
Postpartum atony; postpartum haemorrhage.

Methex *Generics, UK.*
Methadone hydrochloride (p.53·2).
Formerly known as Methodex.
Opioid withdrawal.

Methitoral *Fuji, Jpn.*
Neticonazole hydrochloride (p.386·1).
Fungal infections.

Methnine *Medical Research, Austral.*
Methionine (p.984·2).
Liver disorders; paracetamol overdosage.

Methoblastin
Pharmacia Upjohn, Austral.; Pharmacia Upjohn, S.Afr.
Methotrexate (p.547·1).
Malignant neoplasms; psoriasis; rheumatoid arthritis.

Methocaps *Caps, S.Afr.*
Indomethacin (p.45·2).
Gout; musculoskeletal and joint disorders.

Methocel
Ciba Vision, Ger.; Ciba Vision, Ital.; Restan, S.Afr.
Hypromellose (p.1473·1).
Lubricating and disinfecting drops for use with contact lenses; ophthalmic diagnostic procedures.

Methocel Dispersa *Ciba Vision, Ger.*
Hypromellose (p.1473·1).
Comfort solution for hard contact lenses.

Methopt *Sigma, Austral.*
Hypromellose (p.1473·1).
Dry eyes.

Methycobal *Eisai, Jpn.*
Mecobalamin (p.1364·2).
Megaloblastic anaemia; peripheral neuropathies.

Methyl Salicylate Compound Liniment *McGloin, Austral.*
Methyl salicylate (p.55·2); menthol (p.1600·2); eucalyptus oil (p.1578·1).
Muscle pain.

Methyl Salicylate Ointment Compound *McGloin, Austral.*
Methyl salicylate (p.55·2); menthol (p.1600·2); cineole (p.1564·1); cajuput oil (p.1556·1).
Muscle pain.

Methylan *Vifor, Switz.†.*
Histamine dihydrochloride (p.1587·3); methyl nicotinate (p.55·1); glycol salicylate (p.43·1); camphor (p.1557·2); juniper oil (p.1592·3); rosemary oil (p.1626·2).
Musculoskeletal and joint disorders.

Methylergobrevin *Dresden, Ger.; Wernigerode, Ger.*
Methylergometrine maleate (p.1603·1).
Postpartum haemorrhage; third-stage labour; uterine atony.

Methyl-Gag *Riom, Fr.†.*
Mitoguazone dihydrochloride (p.552·1).
Leukaemias.

Methyment *Pharmonta, Aust.*
Aluminium acetotartrate (p.1547·3); aluminium formate.
Inflammation and infection of the mouth and throat.

Meticortelone
Schering-Plough, Ital.; Schering-Plough, S.Afr.
Prednisolone (p.1048·1).
Corticosteroid.

Meticorten
Schering-Plough, S.Afr.; Schering, USA.
Prednisone (p.1049·2).
Corticosteroid.

Metifarma *Merck, Spain.*
Amoxycillin trihydrate (p.151·3).
Bacterial infections.

Metifarma Mucolit *Merck, Spain.*
Capsules: Amoxycillin trihydrate (p.151·3); bromhexine hydrochloride (p.1055·3); guaiphenesin (p.1061·3).
Oral suspension†: Amoxycillin trihydrate (p.151·3); bromhexine (p.1055·3).
Respiratory-tract infections.

Metifex *Cassella-med, Ger.*
Ethacridine lactate (p.1098·3).
Diarrhoea; gastro-enteritis; spastic constipation.

Metifex-L *Cassella-med, Ger.*
Loperamide hydrochloride (p.1197·2).
Diarrhoea.

Metiguanide *Pharmacia Upjohn, Ital.*
Metformin hydrochloride (p.330·1).
Diabetes mellitus.

Metilbetasone Solubile *Coli, Ital.*
Methylprednisolone acetate (p.1046·1).
Injectable corticosteroid.

Metimyd
Note. This name is used for preparations of different composition.
Schering, Canad.; Schering-Plough, Swed.; Schering, USA.
Eye drops; ear drops: Prednisolone acetate (p.1048·1); sulphacetamide sodium (p.252·2).
Ear infections; eye infections.

Schering, Canad.†.
Eye ointment: Prednisolone acetate (p.1048·1); sulphacetamide sodium (p.252·2); neomycin sulphate (p.229·2).
Eye disorders.

Metina *Fournier, Ital.*
Carnitine hydrochloride (p.1336·2).
Carnitine deficiency; myocardial ischaemia.

Metinal-Idantoina *Bayer, Ital.*
Phenytoin (p.352·3); methylphenobarbitone (p.349·2).
Epilepsy.

Metinal-Idantoina L *Bayer, Ital.*
Phenytoin (p.352·3); methylphenobarbitone (p.349·2); phenobarbitone (p.350·2).
Epilepsy.

Metinox *Lennon, S.Afr.†.*
Tin (p.1638·1); tin oxide (p.1638·1).
Acne; boils.

Metivirol *Ripari-Gero, Ital.*
Inosine pranobex (p.615·2).
Viral infections.

Metixen *Berlin-Chemie, Ger.*
Methixene hydrochloride (p.465·1).
Drug-induced extrapyramidal disorders.

Metizol *Glenwood, USA†.*
Metronidazole (p.585·1).

Meto *BASF, Ger.; Isis Puren, Ger.*
Metoprolol tartrate (p.907·3).
Arrhythmias; hypertension; ischaemic heart disease; migraine; myocardial infarction.

Metobeta *Betapharm, Ger.*
Metoprolol tartrate (p.907·3).
Arrhythmias; hypertension; ischaemic heart disease; migraine; myocardial infarction.

Metoclamid *Hexal, Ger.†.*
Metoclopramide hydrochloride (p.1200·3).
Gastro-intestinal disorders.

Metocobil *Vita, Ital.†.*
Metoclopramide hydrochloride (p.1200·3).
Gastro-intestinal disorders.

Meto-comp *Ratiopharm, Ger.*
Metoprolol tartrate (p.907·3); hydrochlorothiazide (p.885·2).
Hypertension.

Metocor *Rowa, Irl.*
Metoprolol tartrate (p.907·3).
Angina pectoris; arrhythmias; hypertension; hyperthyroidism; migraine; myocardial infarction.

Metocyl *Rowa, Irl.*
Metoclopramide hydrochloride (p.1200·3).
Gastro-intestinal disorders.

Metodura *Durachemie, Ger.*
Metoprolol tartrate (p.907·3).
Arrhythmias; hypertension; ischaemic heart disease; migraine; myocardial infarction.

Metodura comp *Durachemie, Ger.*
Metoprolol tartrate (p.907·3); hydrochlorothiazide (p.885·2).
Hypertension.

Metogastron *Hexal, Aust.*
Metoclopramide hydrochloride (p.1200·3).
Nausea and vomiting; upper gastro-intestinal motility disorders.

Metohexal
Hexal, Aust.; Hexal, Austral.; Hexal, Ger.
Metoprolol tartrate (p.907·3).
Angina pectoris; arrhythmias; hypertension; hyperthyroidism; migraine; myocardial infarction.

Metohexal Comp *Hexal, Ger.*
Metoprolol tartrate (p.907·3); hydrochlorothiazide (p.885·2).
Hypertension.

Metolol *Merckle, Aust.*
Metoprolol tartrate (p.907·3).
Angina pectoris; arrhythmias; hypertension; hyperthyroidism; migraine; myocardial infarction.

Metolol compositum *Merckle, Aust.*
Metoprolol tartrate (p.907·3); hydrochlorothiazide (p.885·2).
Hypertension.

Metomerck *Merck, Ger.*
Metoprolol tartrate (p.907·3).
Arrhythmias; hypertension; ischaemic heart disease; migraine; myocardial infarction.

Metop *Gerard, Irl.*
Metoprolol tartrate (p.907·3).
Angina pectoris; arrhythmias; hypertension; hyperthyroidism; migraine; myocardial infarction.

Metopiron
Ciba, Ger.†; Novartis, Neth.; Ciba, Norw.; Novartis, Swed.
Metyrapone (p.1603·3).
Cushing's syndrome; diagnosis of ACTH deficiencies or adrenocortical hyperfunction; hyperaldosteronism; oedema.

Metopirone
Novartis, Austral.; Ciba, Canad.†; Ciba-Geigy, Fr.; Ciba-Geigy, Irl.; Ciba, Switz.; Alliance, UK; Ciba, USA.
Metyrapone (p.1603·3).
Cushing's syndrome; diagnosis of ACTH deficiencies or adrenocortical hyperfunction; hyperaldosteronism; oedema.

Metoproferm *Fermenta, Swed.†.*
Metoprolol tartrate (p.907·3).
Cardiovascular disorders; migraine.

Metorene *Sanofi Winthrop, Spain.*
Naftazone (p.725·2).
Peripheral vascular disorders.

Metorfan *Coli, Ital.*
Dextromethorphan hydrobromide (p.1057·3).
Coughs.

Metoros *Ciba-Geigy, Aust.*
Metoprolol fumarate (p.908·2).
Angina pectoris; hypertension.

Metostad Comp *Stada, Ger.*
Metoprolol tartrate (p.907·3); hydrochlorothiazide (p.885·2).
Hypertension.

Metosyn
Zeneca, Irl.; Zeneca, Norw.; Bioglan, UK.
Fluocinonide (p.1041·2).
Skin and scalp disorders.

Meto-Tablinen *Sanorania, Ger.*
Metoprolol tartrate (p.907·3).
Angina pectoris; arrhythmias; hypertension; migraine; myocardial infarction.

Meto-thiazid *CT, Ger.*
Metoprolol tartrate (p.907·3); hydrochlorothiazide (p.885·2).
Hypertension.

Metra *Forest Laboratories, USA†.*
Phendimetrazine tartrate (p.1484·2).
Obesity.

Metramid *Nicholas, UK†.*
Metoclopramide hydrochloride (p.1200·3).
Gastro-intestinal motility disorders; nausea and vomiting.

Metrazole *Docmed, S.Afr.*
Metronidazole (p.585·1).
Anaerobic bacterial infections; protozoal infections.

Metreton *Schering, Canad.*
Prednisone acetate (p.1049·3); chlorpheniramine maleate (p.405·1); ascorbic acid (p.1365·2).
Hypersensitivity disorders.

Metric *Fielding, USA†.*
Metronidazole (p.585·1).
Trichomoniasis.

Metrizol Lederle, Switz.†.
Metronidazole (p.585·1).
Rosacea.

Metro McGaw, USA.
Metronidazole (p.585·1).
Amoebiasis; anaerobic bacterial infections; trichomoniasis.

Metrocream Galderma, Canad.
Metronidazole (p.585·1).
Rosacea.

Metrodin
Serono, Austral.; Serono, Belg.†; Serono, Canad.; Serono, Irl.; Serono, Ital.; Serono, Neth.; Research Labs, S.Afr.; Serono, Switz.; Serono, UK; Serono, USA.
Urofollitrophin (p.1263·1).
Female infertility; ovarian stimulation for fertilisation in vitro; stimulation of spermatogenesis.

Metrodine Serono, Fr.
Urofollitrophin (p.1263·1).
Female infertility; ovarian stimulation for fertilisation in vitro.

Metrogel
Galderma, Canad.; Bioglan, Irl.; Boots Healthcare, Neth.; Sandoz, UK; 3M, USA.
Metronidazole (p.585·1).
Bacterial vaginosis; rosacea.

Metrogyl Alphapharm, Austral.
Metronidazole (p.585·1).
Anaerobic bacterial infections; protozoal infections.

Metrolag Lagap, Switz.†.
Metronidazole (p.585·1) or metronidazole benzoate (p.585·1).
Anaerobic bacterial infections; protozoal infections.

Metrolyl Lagap, UK.
Metronidazole (p.585·1).
Anaerobic bacterial infections.

Metronide Clonmel, Irl.
Metronidazole (p.585·1).
Anaerobic bacterial infections; protozoal infections.

Metronom Merckle, Aust.
Propafenone hydrochloride (p.935·3).
Arrhythmias.

Metrostat Propan, S.Afr.
Metronidazole (p.585·1).
Anaerobic bacterial infections; protozoal infections.

Metrotonin Temmler, Ger.†.
Amylobarbitone (p.641·3); dimetamfetamine.
Nervous disorders.

Metrotop
Pharmacia Upjohn, Irl.; Seton, UK.
Metronidazole (p.585·1).
Acne; fungating tumours.

Metrozine Searle, Austral.
Metronidazole (p.585·1).
Anaerobic bacterial infections; protozoal infections.

Metrozol Parkfields, UK.
Metronidazole (p.585·1).

Met-Rx Met-Rx, USA.
Preparations for enteral nutrition.

Metryl Lagamed, S.Afr.†.
Metronidazole (p.585·1).
Anaerobic bacterial infections.

Metsal 3M, Austral.
Menthol (p.1600·2); eucalyptus oil (p.1578·1); methyl salicylate (p.55·2).
Pain of rheumatism, arthritis, sprains, and strains.

Metsal Analgesic 3M, Austral.
Triethanolamine salicylate (p.1639·2); menthol (p.1600·2).
Muscle pain.

Metsal AR Analgesic 3M, Austral.
Triethanolamine salicylate (p.1639·2).
Musculoskeletal and joint pain.

Metsal AR Heat Rub 3M, Austral.
Methyl salicylate (p.55·2); eucalyptus oil (p.1578·1); menthol (p.1600·2).
Musculoskeletal and joint pain.

Metsal Heat Rub 3M, Austral.
Methyl salicylate (p.55·2); eucalyptus oil (p.1578·1); menthol (p.1600·2).
Musculoskeletal and joint pain.

Metubine
Lilly, Canad.; Dista, USA.
Metocurine iodide (p.1316·2).
Competitive neuromuscular blocker.

Metypred Orion, Ger.
Methylprednisolone (p.1046·1), methylprednisolone acetate (p.1046·1), or methylprednisolone sodium succinate (p.1046·1).
Corticosteroid.

Metypresol Intramed, S.Afr.
Methylprednisolone sodium succinate (p.1046·1).
Corticosteroid.

Metysolon Dermapharm, Ger.
Methylprednisolone (p.1046·1).
Corticosteroid.

Mevacor
Merck Sharp & Dohme, Aust.; Merck Sharp & Dohme, Canad.; Merck Sharp & Dohme, Norw.; Merck Sharp & Dohme, Spain; Merck Sharp & Dohme, USA.
Lovastatin (p.1275·1).
Hypercholesterolaemia.

Mevalon Guidotti, Ital.
Meglutol (p.1275·3).
Hyperlipidaemia.

Mevalotin
Luitpold, Ger.; Sankyo, Jpn; Luitpold, Switz.
Pravastatin sodium (p.1277·1).
Hypercholesterolaemia.

Mevaso Llorens, Spain†.
Medrysone (p.1045·3); tetrahydrozoline hydrochloride (p.1070·2).
Eye disorders.

Mevilin-L Medeva, UK.
A measles vaccine (Schwarz strain) (p.1517·3).
Active immunisation.

Mevinacor Merck Sharp & Dohme, Ger.
Lovastatin (p.1275·1).
Hypercholesterolaemia.

Mexalen Merckle, Aust.
Paracetamol (p.72·2).
Fever; pain.

Mexavit Merckle, Aust.
Paracetamol (p.72·2); ascorbic acid (p.1365·2).
Cold symptoms.

Mexe N Merckle, Ger.
Codeine phosphate (p.26·1); paracetamol (p.72·2).
Pain.

Mexitil
Bender, Aust.; Boehringer Ingelheim, Austral.; Boehringer Ingelheim, Belg.; Boehringer Ingelheim, Canad.; Boehringer Ingelheim, Fr.; Boehringer Ingelheim, Ger.; Boehringer Ingelheim, Irl.; Boehringer Ingelheim, Ital.; Boehringer Ingelheim, Neth.; Boehringer Ingelheim, Norw.; Boehringer Ingelheim, S.Afr.; Boehringer Ingelheim, Spain; Boehringer Ingelheim, Swed.; Boehringer Ingelheim, Switz.; Boehringer Ingelheim, UK; Boehringer Ingelheim, USA.
Mexiletine hydrochloride (p.908·3).
Ventricular arrhythmias.

Mexsana Schering-Plough, USA.
Kaolin (p.1195·1); eucalyptus oil (p.1578·1); camphor (p.1557·2); corn starch (p.1356·2); lemon oil (p.1595·3); zinc oxide (p.1096·2).
Nappy rash.

Mezen Errekappa, Ital.
Promelase (p.1621·3).
Inflammation; oedema.

Mezenol Pharmador, S.Afr.†.
Co-trimoxazole (p.196·3).
Bacterial infections.

Mezinc
Abigo, Swed.
Plaster: Zinc oxide (p.1096·2); zinc resin (p.1373·1).
Wound dressing.

Molnlycke, Swed.†.
Compress: Zinc oxide (p.1096·2).
Wound dressing.

Meziv Euroderm, Ital.
Methionine (p.984·2); vitamin B substances; zinc sulphate (p.1373·2).
Hair loss.

Mezlin Miles, USA.
Mezlocillin sodium (p.225·3).
Bacterial infections.

Meztardia Humana 50/50 Novo Nordisk, Spain†.
Mixture of insulin injection (human) 50% and isophane insulin injection (human) 50% (p.322·1).
Diabetes mellitus.

Mezym F Berlin-Chemie, Ger.
Pancreatin (p.1612·1).
Pancreatic disorders.

MF 110 Max Farma, Ital.
Nimesulide (p.63·2).
Fever; inflammation; pain.

MFV-Ject Pasteur Merieux, UK.
An inactivated influenza vaccine (split virion) (p.1515·2).
Active immunisation.

MG400 Triton, USA.
Salicylic acid (p.1090·2); sulphur (p.1091·2).
Seborrhoea.

MG 50 Terapeutico, Ital.
Magnesium proteinate.
Magnesium deficiency; magnesium supplement.

MG Cold Sore Formula Outdoor Recreations, USA.
Menthol (p.1600·2); lignocaine (p.1293·2).

MG217 Dual Triton, USA.
Coal tar (p.1092·3).
Skin disorders.

Mg 5-Granoral Vifor International, Switz.
Magnesium aspartate (p.1157·2).
Magnesium deficiency; magnesium supplement.

Mg 5-Granulat Artesan, Ger.; Cassella-med, Ger.
Magnesium aspartate (p.1157·2).
Magnesium deficiency.

Mg 5-Longoral
Kolassa, Aust.; Artesan, Ger.; Cassella-med, Ger.; Vifor International, Switz.
Magnesium aspartate (p.1157·2).
Magnesium deficiency; magnesium supplement.

MG217 Medicated Triton, USA.
Conditioner: Coal tar (p.1092·3).
Shampoo; ointment: Coal tar (p.1092·3); salicylic acid (p.1090·2); colloidal sulphur (p.1091·2).
Skin disorders.

Mg 5-Oraleff Vifor International, Switz.
Magnesium aspartate (p.1157·2).
Magnesium deficiency; magnesium supplement.

Mg 5-Sulfat
Artesan, Ger.; Cassella-med, Ger.; Vifor International, Switz.
Magnesium sulphate (p.1157·3).
Arrhythmias; eclampsia; fetal hypotrophy; magnesium deficiency; pre-eclampsia; premature labour.

Mg-nor Knoll, Ger.
Magnesium aspartate (p.1157·2).
Magnesium deficiency.

Miacalcic
Novartis, Austral.; Sandoz, Belg.; Sandoz, Fr.; LPB, Ital.; Sandoz, Norw.; Novartis, S.Afr.; Sandoz, Spain; Novartis, Swed.; Sandoz, Switz.; Sandoz, UK.
Salcatonin (p.735·3).
Familial hyperphosphatasia; hypercalcaemia; hyperparathyroidism; metastatic bone pain; osteolysis of malignancy; osteoporosis; Paget's disease of bone; reflex sympathetic dystrophy; vitamin D intoxication.

Miacalcin Sandoz, USA.
Salcatonin (p.735·3).
Osteoporosis.

Mi-Acid Major, USA.
Aluminium hydroxide (p.1177·3); magnesium hydroxide (p.1198·2); simethicone (p.1213·1).
Hyperacidity.

Mi-Acid Gelcaps Major, USA.
Calcium carbonate (p.1182·1); magnesium carbonate (p.1198·1).
Hyperacidity.

Miadenil Francia, Ital.
Salcatonin (p.735·3).
Hypercalcaemia; osteoporosis; Paget's disease of bone; reflex sympathetic dystrophy.

Mialin Biomedica, Ital.
Alprazolam (p.640·3).
Anxiety disorders.

Miambutol Cyanamid, Ital.
Ethambutol hydrochloride (p.207·2).
Tuberculosis.

Mianeurin Hexal, Ger.
Mianserin hydrochloride (p.297·1).
Depression.

Miazide Cyanamid, Ital.
Ethambutol hydrochloride (p.207·2); isoniazid (p.218·1).
Tuberculosis.

Miazide B6 Cyanamid, Ital.
Ethambutol hydrochloride (p.207·2); isoniazid (p.218·1); pyridoxine hydrochloride (p.1362·3).
Tuberculosis.

Mibrox Nycomed, Ger.†.
Ambroxol hydrochloride (p.1054·3).
Respiratory disorders associated with viscid or excessive mucus.

Mibrox comp Nycomed, Ger.†.
Doxycycline hydrochloride (p.202·3); ambroxol hydrochloride (p.1054·3).
Respiratory disorders associated with viscid or excessive mucus.

Micanol
Evans Medical, Irl.; Bioglan, Norw.; Bioglan, Swed.; Medeva, UK; Bioglan, USA.
Dithranol (p.1082·1).
Psoriasis.

Micatin
McNeil Consumer, Canad.; Ortho Pharmaceutical, USA.
Miconazole nitrate (p.384·3).
Fungal skin infections.

Micaveen Rydelle, Ital.
Avena (p.1551·3).
Soap substitute.

Micebrina Derly, Spain.
Multivitamin and mineral preparation.

Micebrina Ginseng Derly, Spain.
Multivitamins and minerals; rutin; ginseng root (p.1584·2).
Tonic.

Micelle A Bioglan, Austral.†.
Vitamin A (p.1358·1).

Micetal Uriach, Spain.
Flutrimazole (p.380·2).
Fungal skin infections.

Micexin Miba, Ital.†.
Cefmolexin lysine.
Bacterial infections.

Michalon N Rorer, Ger.†.
Homoeopathic preparation.

Micifrona Iquinosa, Spain.
Lespedeza capitata.
Uraemia.

Miclast Pierre Fabre, Ital.
Ciclopirox olamine (p.376·2).
Fungal skin and vaginal infections.

Micoclorina Zambon, Ital.†.
Chloramphenicol (p.182·1) or chloramphenicol glycinate (p.184·2).
Bacterial infections.

Micoderm Kemyos, Ital.
Miconazole nitrate (p.384·3).
Fungal and bacterial infections.

Micodry Zambon, Ital.†.
Chloramphenicol palmitoylglycolate (p.184·2).
Bacterial infections.

Micoespec Centrum, Spain.
Econazole nitrate (p.377·2).
Fungal skin and nail infections.

Micogin Crosara, Ital.
Econazole nitrate (p.377·2).
Fungal and bacterial infections.

Micolette
Dominion, Irl.; Dexcel, UK.
Sodium citrate (p.1153·2); sodium lauryl sulphoacetate (p.1468·3); glycerol (p.1585·2).
Bowel evacuation; constipation.

Micomax Max Farma, Ital.
Miconazole pivoxil chloride (p.385·2).
Fungal infections; Gram-positive bacterial superinfections.

Micomicen Synthelabo, Ital.
Ciclopirox olamine (p.376·2).
Vulvovaginal candidiasis.

Micomisan
Propan, S.Afr.; Hosbon, Spain†.
Clotrimazole (p.376·3).
Fungal skin infections; vaginal candidiasis.

Micomplex Schiapparelli Searle, Ital.†.
Pyrrolnitrin (p.387·1); betamethasone valerate (p.1033·3); bekanamycin sulphate (p.158·2).
Skin infections.

Miconal
Note. This name is used for preparations of different composition.
Ecobi, Ital.
Miconazole (p.384·3) or miconazole nitrate (p.384·3).
Fungal infections; secondary Gram-positive bacterial infections.

Bioglan, USA.
Dithranol (p.1082·1).
Psoriasis.

Micoren Zyma, Ital.
Prethcamide (p.1485·1).
Respiratory insufficiency.

Micos AGIPS, Ital.
Econazole (p.377·2) or econazole nitrate (p.377·2).
Fungal infections; Gram-positive bacterial infections.

Micoseptil Reig Jofre, Spain.
Econazole nitrate (p.377·2).
Fungal skin and nail infections.

Micosona Schering, Spain.
Naftifine hydrochloride (p.385·3).
Fungal skin infections.

Micosten Bergamon, Ital.†.
Econazole nitrate (p.377·2).
Fungal infections; Gram-positive bacterial infections.

Micotar Dermapharm, Ger.
Miconazole (p.384·3) or miconazole nitrate (p.384·3).
Fungal infections.

Micotef LPB, Ital.
Miconazole (p.384·3) or miconazole nitrate (p.384·3).
Fungal infections; Gram-positive bacterial infections.

Micoter Cusi, Spain†.
Clotrimazole (p.376·3).
Fungal skin infections.

Micoticum Vita, Spain.
Ketoconazole (p.383·1).
Fungal infections.

Micoxolamina Mastelli, Ital.
Ciclopirox olamine (p.376·2).
Fungal infections.

Micrainin Wallace, USA.
Aspirin (p.16·1); meprobamate (p.678·1).
Pain.

Micral Test Boehringer Mannheim, S.Afr.
Test for microalbuminuria.

Micral Test II
Boehringer Mannheim, Austral.; Boehringer Mannheim Diagnostics, UK.
Test for microalbuminuria in diagnosis of diabetic nephropathy.
Formerly known as Micral Test.

Micralax
Pharmacia Upjohn, Spain; Medeva, UK.
Sodium citrate (p.1153·2); sodium lauryl sulphoacetate (p.1468·3).
Bowel evacuation; constipation; painful defaecation.

Micranet Ogna, Ital.
Propyphenazone (p.81·3); paracetamol (p.72·2); caffeine (p.749·3).
Migraine; toothache.

MICRhoGAM Ortho Pharmaceutical, USA.
An anti-D immunoglobulin (p.1503·2).
Prevention of rhesus sensitisation.

Micristin OPW, Ger.
Aspirin (p.16·1).
Myocardial infarction; thrombosis prophylaxis; vascular disorders.

Micro + Sabex, Canad.
A range of trace element preparations.

Micro Cr Sabex, Canad.
Chromium trichloride (p.1337·1).
Trace element additive.

Micro Cu Sabex, Canad.
Copper sulphate (p.1338·1).
Trace element additive.

Micro I Sabex, Canad.
Sodium iodide (p.1493·2).
Trace element additive.

Micro Mn Sabex, Canad.
Manganese sulphate (p.1350·3).
Trace element additive.

Micro Se *Sabex, Canad.*
Selenious acid (p.1353·3).
Trace element additive.

Micro Zn *Sabex, Canad.*
Zinc sulphate (p.1373·2).
Trace element additive.

Microbac *Propan-Vernleigh, S.Afr.†.*
Co-trimoxazole (p.196·3).
Bacterial infections.

Microbamat *Waldheim, Aust.*
Meprobamate (p.678·1).
Anxiety disorders; sleep disorders.

Microbar *Rooster, Neth.†.*
Barium sulphate (p.1003·1).
Contrast medium for gastro-intestinal radiography.

Microbar-Colon *Bracco, Switz.*
Barium sulphate (p.1003·1).
Contrast medium for gastro-intestinal radiography.

Microbar-HD (E-Z-HD) *Bracco, Switz.*
Barium sulphate (p.1003·1).
Contrast medium for gastro-intestinal double-contrast radiography.

Microbumintest *Bayer Diagnostici, Ital.*
Test for albumin in urine.

Microcal *Eurospital, Ital.†.*
Aspartame (p.1335·1).
Sugar substitute.

Microcid *Bioglan, Swed.*
Hydrogen peroxide (p.1116·2).
Impetigo.

Microcidal *Lennon, S.Afr.*
Griseofulvin (p.380·2).
Fungal infections of the skin and nails.

Microclisma Evacuante AD-BB *Sofar, Ital.*
Glycerol (p.1585·2).

Microclismi Marco Viti *Boots, Ital.*
Glycerol (p.1585·2).
Bowel evacuation; constipation.

Microclismi Sella *Sella, Ital.*
Glycerol (p.1585·2).
Bowel evacuation; constipation.

Microdiol *Organon, Spain.*
Ethinyloestradiol (p.1445·1); desogestrel (p.1443·3).
Combined oral contraceptive; menstrual disorders.

Microdoine *Gomenol, Fr.*
Nitrofurantoin (p.231·3).
Bacterial infections of the urinary tract.

Microgel *Restan, S.Afr.*
Oral suspension: Dicyclomine hydrochloride (p.460·1); aluminium hydroxide (p.1177·3); magnesium oxide (p.1198·3); simethicone (p.1213·1).
Tablets: Calcium carbonate (p.1182·1); magnesium carbonate (p.1198·1); magnesium trisilicate (p.1199·1); simethicone (p.1213·1); sodium hexametaphosphate.
Gastro-intestinal disorders.

Micro-Guard *Sween, USA†.*
Chloroxylenol (p.1111·1).
Fungal skin infections.

Microgynon
Schering, Aust.; Schering, Austral.; Schering, Belg.; Schering, Ger.; Schering, Irl.; Schering, Ital.; Schering, Neth.; Schering, Norw.; Schering, Spain; Schering, Switz.; Schering, UK.
Levonorgestrel (p.1454·1); ethinyloestradiol (p.1445·1).
28-Day packs also contain 7 inert tablets.
Combined oral contraceptive.

Micro-K
Wyeth-Ayerst, Canad.; Continental Ethicals, S.Afr.†; Robins, USA.
Potassium chloride (p.1161·1).
Hypokalaemia; potassium depletion.

Microkaleorid *Leo, Fr.†.*
Potassium chloride (p.1161·1).
Hypokalaemia.

Micro-Kalium *Lannacher, Aust.*
Potassium chloride (p.1161·1).
Potassium deficiency.

Microklist
Pharmacia Upjohn, Aust.; Pharmacia Upjohn, Ger.; Pharmacia Upjohn, Switz.
Sodium citrate (p.1153·2); sodium lauryl sulphoacetate (p.1468·3); sorbitol (p.1354·2).
Bowel evacuation; constipation.

Microlax
Pharmacia Upjohn, Austral.; SmithKline Beecham Consumer, Belg.; Pharmacia Upjohn, Canad.; Sanofi Winthrop, Fr.; Pharmacia Upjohn, Irl.; Pharmacia Upjohn, Neth.; Pharmacia Upjohn, Norw.; Pharmacia Upjohn, S.Afr.; Pharmacia Upjohn, Swed.
Sodium citrate (p.1153·2); sodium lauryl sulphoacetate (p.1468·3); sorbitol (p.1354·2).
Bowel evacuation; constipation.

Microlev *Ido, Fr.*
Dried yeast (p.1373·1).
Vitamin B deficiency.

Microlipid *Sherwood, USA.*
High calorie preparation containing safflower oil (p.1353·3) for enteral nutrition.

Microlut
Schering, Austral.; Schering, Belg.; Schering, Ger.; Schering, Irl.†; Schering, Ital.; Schering, Switz.
Levonorgestrel (p.1454·1).
Progestogen-only oral contraceptive.

Microluton *Schering, Norw.*
Levonorgestrel (p.1454·1).
Progestogen-only oral contraceptive.

Micronase *Upjohn, USA.*
Glibenclamide (p.319·3).
Diabetes mellitus.

microNefrin *Bird, USA.*
Racepinephrine hydrochloride (p.815·2).
Bronchospasm.

Micronor
Janssen-Cilag, Austral.; Janssen-Ortho, Canad.; Janssen-Cilag, Irl.; Cilag, UK; Ortho Pharmaceutical, USA.
Norethisterone (p.1453·1).
Progestogen-only oral contraceptive.

Micronor.HRT *Ortho-Cilag, UK.*
Norethisterone (p.1453·1).
Menopausal disorders.

Micronovum
Janssen-Cilag, Aust.; Janssen-Cilag, Ger.; Janssen-Cilag, S.Afr.; Janssen-Cilag, Switz.
Norethisterone (p.1453·1).
Progestogen-only oral contraceptive.

Micropaque
Salus, Aust.; Codali, Belg.; Guerbet, Fr.; Guerbet, Ger.; Guerbet, Neth.; Pan Quimica, Spain; Guerbet, Switz.; Bioglan, UK.
Barium sulphate (p.1003·1).
Contrast medium for gastro-intestinal radiography.

Microphta *Europhta, Mon.*
Micronomicin sulphate (p.226·2).
Bacterial eye infections.

Microphyllin *Rhone-Poulenc Rorer, S.Afr.*
Theophylline (p.765·1).
Asthma; bronchospasm.

Microplex *Pharmatec, S.Afr.†.*
Multivitamin and mineral preparation.

Micropur
Sirmeta, Austral.; Katadyn, Fr.
Silver chloride complex (p.1629·2).
Water disinfection.

Microsan N *GN, Ger.*
Multivitamin and magnesium preparation.

Microser *Formenti, Ital.*
Betahistine hydrochloride (p.1553·1).
Ménière's disease; vertigo; vestibular disorders.

Microshield Antiseptic *Johnson & Johnson, Austral.*
Cetrimide (p.1105·2); chlorhexidine gluconate (p.1107·2).
Skin, wound, burn, and instrument disinfection.

Microshield Handrub *Johnson & Johnson, Austral.*
Chlorhexidine gluconate (p.1107·2); alcohol (p.1099·1).
Skin disinfection.

Microshield PVP *Johnson & Johnson, Austral.*
Povidone-iodine (p.1123·3).
Skin disinfection.

Microshield PVP Plus *Johnson & Johnson, Austral.*
Povidone-iodine (p.1123·3); triclosan (p.1127·2).
Skin disinfection.

Microshield PVP-S *Johnson & Johnson, Austral.*
Povidone-iodine (p.1123·3).
Bacterial or fungal skin and mucous membrane infections; skin, wound, and burn disinfection.

Microshield T *Johnson & Johnson, Austral.*
Triclosan (p.1127·2).
Skin disinfection.

Microshield Tincture *Johnson & Johnson, Austral.*
Chlorhexidine gluconate (p.1107·2); alcohol (p.1099·1).
Skin, surface, and instrument disinfection.

Microsol *Herbaxt, Fr.*
A range of trace element and mineral preparations.

Microstix-3 *Bayer, USA.*
Test for nitrite in urine and for bacterial growth.

Microtrast
Salus, Aust.; Guerbet, Fr.; Guerbet, Ger.; Nicholas, UK†.
Barium sulphate (p.1003·1).
Contrast medium for gastro-intestinal radiography.

Microtrim *Rosen, Ger.*
Co-trimoxazole (p.196·3).
Bacterial infections.

Microval
Wyeth, Austral.; Wyeth Lederle, Belg.; Wyeth, Fr.; John Wyeth, Irl.†; Akromed, S.Afr.; Wyeth, UK.
Levonorgestrel (p.1454·1).
Progestogen-only oral contraceptive.

Microzide *Watson, USA.*
Hydrochlorothiazide (p.885·2).
Hypertension; oedema.

Mictasol
Note. This name is used for preparations of different composition.
Medgenix, Belg.
Camphor monobromide; hexamine (p.216·1); malva purpurea fruit; esculoside (p.1543·3); rutin (p.1580·2).
Anorectal disorders; urinary-tract disorders.

Martin, Fr.
Malva purpurea; camphor monobromide; hexamine (p.216·1).
Urinary-tract infections.

Zoja, Ital.†.
Malva purpurea; hexamine (p.216·1).
Genito-urinary tract infections; haemorrhoids.

Mictasol Bleu
Note. This name is used for preparations of different composition.
Martin, Fr.
Malva purpurea; camphor monobromide; methylene blue (p.984·3).
Urinary-tract infections.

Zoja, Ital.
Malva purpurea; methylene blue (p.984·3).
Genito-urinary tract disorders; haemorrhoids.

Mictasone *Zoja, Ital.*
Hydrocortisone acetate (p.1043·3); tetracycline hydrochloride (p.259·1); mallow flowers; mallow leaves.
Genito-urinary tract infections; haemorrhoids.

Mictonetten *Apogepha, Ger.*
Propiverine hydrochloride (p.468·2).
Bladder disorders; urinary incontinence.

Mictonorm *Apogepha, Ger.*
Propiverine hydrochloride (p.468·2).
Bladder disorders; urinary incontinence.

Mictral
Sanofi Winthrop, Irl.; Sanofi Winthrop, UK.
Nalidixic acid (p.228·2); sodium citrate (p.1153·2); citric acid (p.1564·3); sodium bicarbonate (p.1153·2).
Urinary-tract infections.

Mictrin *Econo Med, USA.*
Hydrochlorothiazide (p.885·2).
Hypertension; oedema.

Mictrol
Kabi, Swed.†; Kabi, Switz.†.
Terodiline hydrochloride (p.468·3).
Bladder disorders.

Micturin *Kabivitrum, Irl.†.*
Terodiline hydrochloride (p.468·3).
Formerly known as Terolin.
Neurogenic bladder; urinary incontinence.

Micturol Sedante *Knoll, Spain.*
Phenazopyridine hydrochloride (p.78·3); sulphamethizole (p.254·2).
Urinary-tract infections.

Micur BT *Boehringer Mannheim Diagnostics, UK†.*
Test for antibacterials in urine.

Micutrin *Searle, Ital.*
Pyrrolnitrin (p.387·1).
Fungal skin infections.

Micutrin Beta *Searle, Ital.*
Pyrrolnitrin (p.387·1); betamethasone valerate (p.1033·3).
Inflammatory fungal skin infections; onychomycosis.

Midacina *Lensa, Spain.*
Fluocinolone acetonide (p.1041·1); gramicidin (p.215·2); neomycin (p.229·2).
Infected skin disorders.

Midalgan
Welcker-Lyster, Canad.; SmithKline Beecham Consumer, Switz.
Histamine dihydrochloride (p.1587·3); capsicum (p.1559·2); glycol salicylate (p.43·1); methyl nicotinate (p.55·1).
Musculoskeletal and joint disorders.

Midamor
Merck Sharp & Dohme, Aust.; Merck Sharp & Dohme, Austral.; Merck Sharp & Dohme, Canad.; Merck Sharp & Dohme, Neth.; Merck Sharp & Dohme, Norw.; Merck Sharp & Dohme, Swed.; Merck Sharp & Dohme, Switz.; Merck Sharp & Dohme, UK†; Merck Sharp & Dohme, USA.
Amiloride hydrochloride (p.819·2).
Ascites; heart failure; hypertension; oedema.

Midarine
Glaxo Wellcome, Ital.; Wellcome, Switz.
Suxamethonium chloride (p.1319·1).
Depolarising neuromuscular blocker.

Midaten *Farmacusi, Spain.*
Piretanide (p.931·3).
Hypertension; oedema.

Midchlor *Schein, USA.*
Isometheptene mucate (p.447·3); dichloralphenazone (p.668·1); paracetamol (p.72·2).
Tension and vascular headaches.

Midecin *Farmaka, Ital.*
Midecamycin (p.226·2).
Bacterial infections.

Miderm *Mendelejeff, Ital.*
Miconazole (p.384·3) or miconazole nitrate (p.384·3).
Fungal and bacterial infections.

Midium *Teofarma, Ital.*
Vitamin A palmitate (p.1359·2); tocopheryl acetate (p.1369·1); pyridoxine hydrochloride (p.1362·3).
Metabolic disorders.

Midol *Glenbrook, USA†.*
Aspirin (p.16·1); caffeine (p.749·3); cinnamedrine hydrochloride.
Pain.

Midol Douche *Bayer, Canad.*
Acetic acid (p.1541·2).
Vaginal cleansing.

Midol Extra Strength *Bayer, Canad.†.*
Paracetamol (p.72·2); pamabrom (p.927·1); mepyramine maleate (p.414·1).
Dysmenorrhoea.

Midol IB *Glenbrook, USA.*
Ibuprofen (p.44·1).
Formerly known as Midol 200.
Fever; osteoarthritis; pain; rheumatoid arthritis.

Midol Maximum Strength Multi-Symptom Menstrual *Sterling Health, USA.*
Paracetamol (p.72·2); mepyramine maleate (p.414·1).
Pain.

Midol Multi-Symptom *Bayer, Canad.*
Paracetamol (p.72·2); caffeine (p.749·3); mepyramine maleate (p.414·1).
Backache; bloating; dysmenorrhoea; headache.

Midol Original *Bayer, Canad.*
Aspirin (p.16·1); cinnamedrine; caffeine (p.749·3).
Pain.

Midol PM *Sterling, USA.*
Paracetamol (p.72·2); diphenhydramine (p.409·1).

Midol PMS *Glenbrook, USA.*
Paracetamol (p.72·2); pamabrom (p.927·1); mepyramine maleate (p.414·1).
Pain.

Midol PMS Extra Strength *Bayer, Canad.*
Paracetamol (p.72·2); pamabrom (p.927·1); mepyramine maleate (p.414·1).
Premenstrual syndrome.

Midol Regular *Bayer, Canad.*
Aspirin (p.16·1); caffeine (p.749·3).
Pain.

Midon *Monmouth, Irl.*
Midodrine hydrochloride (p.910·1).
Orthostatic hypotension.

Midoride *Amrad, Austral.*
Amiloride hydrochloride (p.819·2).
Ascites; hypertension; oedema.

Midorm AR *Piam, Ital.†.*
Flurazepam dihydrochloride (p.672·2).
Insomnia.

Midotens *Boehringer Ingelheim, Swed.*
Lacidipine (p.897·1).
Hypertension.

Midran
Manetti Roberts, Ital.†; Novo Nordisk, S.Afr.†.
Aprotinin (p.711·3).
Antidote to fibrinolytics; haemorrhage; pancreatitis.

Midriatic *Llorens, Spain.*
Atropine sulphate (p.455·1); hyoscine hydrobromide (p.462·3); phenylephrine hydrochloride (p.1066·2).
Eye disorders; production of mydriasis.

Midrid *Shire, UK.*
Isometheptene mucate (p.447·3); paracetamol (p.72·2).
Formerly contained dichloralphenazone, isometheptene mucate, and paracetamol.
Migraine.

Midrin *Carnrick, USA.*
Isometheptene mucate (p.447·3); dichloralphenazone (p.668·1); paracetamol (p.72·2).
Tension and vascular headaches.

Midro
Note. This name is used for preparations of different composition.
Wolfs, Belg.
Senna (p.1212·2).
Constipation.

Vaillant, Ital.
Senna (p.1212·2); liquorice (p.1197·1); peppermint leaves (p.1208·1); caraway (p.1559·3).
Constipation.

Midro Abfuhr *Midro, Ger.*
Senna (p.1212·2).
Constipation.

Midro N *Midro, Ger.*
Senna (p.1212·2).
Constipation.

Midro-Tee *Salus, Aust.*
Senna (p.1212·2); peppermint leaf (p.1208·1); caraway (p.1559·3); liquorice (p.1197·1); delphinium consolida; mallow flowers.
Bowel evacuation; constipation.

Midy Vitamine C *SmithKline Beecham Sante, Fr.*
Ascorbic acid (p.1365·2).
Tonic; vitamin C deficiency.

Midysalb *Sanofi Winthrop, Ger.*
Glycol salicylate (p.43·1); methyl nicotinate (p.55·1); histamine dihydrochloride (p.1587·3).
Formerly contained mephenesin, glycol salicylate, methyl nicotinate, and histamine hydrochloride.
Musculoskeletal and joint disorders; neuralgia.

Miegel *SAN, Ital.*
Honey (p.1345·3); royal jelly (p.1626·3).

Mielocol *Herbes Universelles, Canad.*
Guaiphenesin (p.1061·3); aralia racemosa; cineole (p.1564·1); honey (p.1345·3); poplar buds (p.1620·1); sanguinaria (p.1627·2); white pine; wild cherry (p.1644·3).

Mielogen *Schering-Plough, Ital.*
Molgramostim (p.725·1).
Neutropenia induced by antineoplastics, bone marrow transplant, or ganciclovir.

Mifegyne
Roussel, Fr.; Hoechst Marion Roussel, Swed.; Roussel, UK.
Mifepristone (p.1451·1).
Termination of pregnancy.

Migergot *G & W, USA.*
Ergotamine tartrate (p.445·3); caffeine (p.749·3).

Miglucan *Boehringer Mannheim, Fr.*
Glibenclamide (p.319·3).
Diabetes mellitus.

Migpriv
Synthelabo, Belg.; Synthelabo, Fr.
Lysine aspirin (p.50·3); metoclopramide hydrochloride (p.1200·3).
Migraine.

Migracin *SmithKline Beecham, Ital.*
Amikacin sulphate (p.150·2).
Bacterial infections.

Migradon *Schmidgall, Aust.*
Propyphenazone (p.81·3); paracetamol (p.72·2); caffeine (p.749·3).
Fever; pain.

Migraeflux Sodip, Switz.†.
Dimenhydrinate (p.408·2); paracetamol (p.72·2); codeine phosphate (p.26·1).
Migraine and other vascular headaches.

Migraeflux N Hennig, Ger.
Orange tablets, dimenhydrinate (p.408·2); paracetamol (p.72·2); green tablets, paracetamol; codeine phosphate (p.26·1).
Migraine and other vascular headaches.

Migraeflux orange N Hennig, Ger.
Dimenhydrinate (p.408·2); paracetamol (p.72·2).
Migraine and other vascular headaches.

Migrafen Chatfield Laboratories, UK.
Ibuprofen (p.44·1).

Migrafin Lorex Synthelabo, Neth.
Lysine aspirin (p.50·3); metoclopramide (p.1202·1).
Migraine.

Migraine-Kranit
Note. This name is used for preparations of different composition.
Codali, Belg.†.
Ethaverine hydrochloride (p.1577·1); caffeine (p.749·3); propyphenazone (p.81·3); paracetamol (p.72·2); phenobarbitone (p.350·2).
Migraine.

Krewel, Switz.
Paracetamol (p.72·2); caffeine (p.749·3); chlorpheniramine maleate (p.405·1).
Migraine and other vascular headaches.

Migraine-Kranit Nova Codali, Belg.
Caffeine (p.749·3); paracetamol (p.72·2); propyphenazone (p.81·3).
Migraine.

Migral Glaxo Wellcome, Austral.
Ergotamine tartrate (p.445·3); cyclizine hydrochloride (p.407·1); caffeine (p.749·3).
Migraine.

Migralam Lambda, USA.
Isometheptene mucate (p.447·3); caffeine (p.749·3); paracetamol (p.72·2).
Vascular and tension headaches.

Migralave N Temmler, Ger.
Buclizine hydrochloride (p.404·1); paracetamol (p.72·2).
Migraine and other vascular headaches.

Migraleve
Note. This name is used for preparations of different composition.
Charwell Pharmaceuticals, Irl.; Charwell Pharmaceuticals, UK.
Pink tablets, buclizine hydrochloride (p.404·1); paracetamol (p.72·2); codeine phosphate (p.26·1); yellow tablets, paracetamol; codeine phosphate.
Migraine.

Llorens, Spain.
Buclizine hydrochloride (p.404·1); codeine phosphate (p.26·1); docusate sodium (p.1189·3); paracetamol (p.72·2).
Migraine and other vascular headaches.

Unipharma, Switz.
Paracetamol (p.72·2); codeine phosphate (p.26·1); buclizine hydrochloride (p.404·1).
Migraine and other vascular headaches.

Migralgine Martin, Fr.
Phenazone (p.78·2); amylocaine hydrochloride (p.1286·1); codeine (p.26·1); caffeine (p.749·3).
Pain.

Migralift Charwell Pharmaceuticals, UK.
Pink tablets, buclizine hydrochloride (p.404·1); paracetamol (p.72·2); codeine phosphate (p.26·1); yellow tablets, paracetamol; codeine phosphate.
Migraine.

Migranal
Novartis, Ital.; Novartis, UK; Novartis, USA.
Dihydroergotamine mesylate (p.444·2).
Migraine.

Migranat Rowa, Irl.
Caffeine (p.749·3); ergotamine tartrate (p.445·3); pipoxolan hydrochloride (p.1618·3).
Migraine and other vascular headaches.

Migrane-Gastreu R16 Reckeweg, Ger.
Homoeopathic preparation.

Migrane-Kranit mono Krewel, Ger.
Phenazone (p.78·2).
Pain.

Migrane-Kranit N Krewel, Ger.
Suppositories: Ethaverine hydrochloride (p.1577·1); paracetamol (p.72·2); propyphenazone (p.81·3).
Tablets: Paracetamol (p.72·2); propyphenazone (p.81·3); codeine phosphate (p.26·1).
Headache including migraine.

Migrane-Kranit spezial N Krewel, Ger.†.
Ergotamine tartrate (p.445·3); cyclizine hydrochloride (p.407·1).
Migraine.

Migrane-Neuridal Krewel, Ger.
Paracetamol (p.72·2); metoclopramide hydrochloride (p.1200·3).
Migraine and other vascular headaches.

Migranerton Dolorgiet, Ger.
Paracetamol (p.72·2); metoclopramide hydrochloride (p.1200·3).
Migraine and other vascular headaches.

Migranex Jossa-Arznei, Ger.†.
Gelsemium (p.1583·2); hypericum (p.1590·1); magnesium citrate tetradecahydrate (p.1198·2); dehydrocholic acid (p.1570·2); phenazone and caffeine citrate (p.78·2).
Headache including migraine.

Migranex spezial N Jossa-Arznei, Ger.†.
Ergotamine tartrate (p.445·3); gelsemium (p.1583·2); papaverine hydrochloride (p.1614·2); inositol nicotinate (p.891·3); propyphenazone (p.81·3).
Headache including migraine.

Migran-eze Medinat, Austral.†.
Aloxiprin (p.15·1); gelsemium (p.1583·2); humulus (p.1597·2); thiamine hydrochloride (p.1361·1); pyridoxine hydrochloride (p.1362·3); iris versicolor; viola odorata; sanguinaria.
Migraine.

Migranin Cassella-med, Ger.
Phenazone (p.78·2); caffeine (p.749·3).
Migraine; pain.

Migratan S Berlin-Chemie, Ger.
Ergotamine tartrate (p.445·3); propyphenazone (p.81·3).
Migraine and other vascular headaches.

Migratine Major, USA.
Isometheptene mucate (p.447·3); dichloralphenazone (p.668·1); paracetamol (p.72·2).
Tension and vascular headaches.

Migravess Bayer, UK.
Aspirin (p.16·1); metoclopramide hydrochloride (p.1200·3).
Migraine.

Migrex Pink Woods, Austral.†.
Paracetamol (p.72·2); codeine phosphate (p.26·1); buclizine hydrochloride (p.404·1); docusate sodium (p.1189·3).
Migraine; tension headaches.

Migrex Yellow Woods, Austral.†.
Paracetamol (p.72·2); codeine phosphate (p.26·1); docusate sodium (p.1189·3).
Migraine; tension headache.

Migrexa
Note. This name is used for preparations of different composition.
Sanorania, Ger.
Ergotamine tartrate (p.445·3).
Cluster headache; migraine.

Sanorania, Switz.
Ergotamine tartrate (p.445·3); caffeine (p.749·3).
Dysmenorrhoea; migraine and other vascular headaches.

Migril
Glaxo Wellcome, Aust.; Wellcome, Belg.†; Wellcome, Irl.; Glaxo Wellcome, Neth.†; Glaxo Wellcome, S.Afr.; Wellcome, Switz.; Glaxo Wellcome, UK.
Ergotamine tartrate (p.445·3); cyclizine hydrochloride (p.407·1); caffeine hydrate (p.750·1).
Migraine.

Migristene Rhone-Poulenc Rorer, Spain.
Dimethothiazine mesylate (p.408·3).
Migraine.

Migwell Glaxo Wellcome, Fr.
Ergotamine tartrate (p.445·3); caffeine (p.749·3); cyclizine hydrochloride (p.407·1).
Migraine.

Mijal Juste, Spain.
Butibufen (p.24·1).
Musculoskeletal, joint, and peri-articular disorders; pain.

Mijex Pickles, UK.
Gel: Diethyltoluamide (p.1405·1).
Topical stick; topical spray; topical liquid: Diethyltoluamide (p.1405·1); calcium oxide (p.1557·1).
Insect repellent.

Mijex Extra Pickles, UK.
Butylacetylamino propionate.
Insect repellent.

Mikan Boniscontro & Gazzone, Ital.
Amikacin sulphate (p.150·2).
Bacterial infections.

mikanil N Mickan, Ger.
Glycol salicylate (p.43·1); benzyl nicotinate (p.22·1); Norway spruce oil.
Muscle and joint pain; soft-tissue disorders.

Mikavir Salus, Ital.
Amikacin sulphate (p.150·2).
Gram-negative bacterial infections.

Mikelan
Lipha Sante, Fr.; Otsuka, Jpn; Hoechst Marion Roussel, S.Afr.; Miquel Otsuka, Spain.
Carteolol hydrochloride (p.837·3).
Angina pectoris; arrhythmias; glaucoma; hypertension; ocular hypertension.

Mikium Vinas, Spain†.
Ciclopirox olamine (p.376·2).
Fungal infections of the skin and mucous membranes.

Mikro-30 Wyeth, Ger.
Levonorgestrel (p.1454·1).
Progestogen-only oral contraceptive.

Mikrobac Bode, Ger.
Benzalkonium chloride (p.1101·3); dodecylbispropylenetriamine.
Surface disinfection.

Mikroplex Jod Galmeda, Ger.†.
Iodine (p.1493·1).
Hyperthyroidism; hypothyroidism.

Mikrozid Schulke & Mayr, Ger.
Alcohol (p.1099·1); propyl alcohol (p.1124·2).
Formerly contained alcohol, propyl alcohol, glutaraldehyde, and 2-ethylhexanal.
Surface disinfection.

Mikutan N Streuli, Switz.
Aluminium acetate (p.1547·3); zinc oxide (p.1096·2).
Skin disorders.

Milavir Zyma, Spain.
Aciclovir (p.602·3).
Herpes simplex infections.

Milax Berlin-Chemie, Ger.
Glycerol (p.1585·2).
Constipation.

Milbedoce Anabolico Andromaco, Spain.
Cobamamide (p.1364·2); hydroxocobalamin acetate (p.1364·2).
Tonic.

Mildison
Yamanouchi, Irl.; Yamanouchi, Neth.; Yamanouchi, Norw.; Yamanouchi, Swed.; Yamanouchi, UK.
Hydrocortisone (p.1043·3).
Skin disorders.

Miles Nervine Miles, USA.
Diphenhydramine hydrochloride (p.409·1).
Insomnia.

milgamma Worwag, Ger.
Benfotiamine (p.1360·3); pyridoxine hydrochloride (p.1362·3).
Neurological symptoms associated with vitamin B deficiency.

milgamma N Worwag, Ger.
Thiamine hydrochloride (p.1361·1); pyridoxine hydrochloride (p.1362·3); cyanocobalamin (p.1363·3).
Myalgia; neuralgia; neuritis; polyneuropathy.

milgamma-NA Worwag, Ger.
Benfotiamine (p.1360·3); pyridoxine hydrochloride (p.1362·3).
Neurological symptoms associated with vitamin B deficiency.

Milid
Waldheim, Aust.; Opfermann, Ger.; Rottapharm, Ital.; Ethimed, S.Afr.†.
Proglumide (p.1209·2).
Gastro-intestinal disorders.

Miliken Mucol Med Retard Knoll, Spain.
Ampicillin sodium (p.153·1); ampicillin benzathine (p.154·1); bromhexine hydrochloride (p.1055·3).
Lignocaine hydrochloride (p.1293·2) is included in this preparation to alleviate the pain of injection.
Respiratory-tract infections.

Miliken Mucol Retard Knoll, Spain.
Ampicillin sodium (p.153·1); ampicillin benzathine (p.154·1); bromhexine hydrochloride (p.1055·3); guaiphenesin hydrochloride (p.1061·3).
Lignocaine hydrochloride (p.1293·2) is included in this preparation to alleviate the pain of injection.
Respiratory-tract infections.

Miliken Mucolitico Knoll, Spain.
Ampicillin sodium (p.153·1); bromhexine hydrochloride (p.1055·3); guaiphenesin (p.1061·3).
Lignocaine hydrochloride (p.1293·2) is included in this preparation to alleviate the pain of injection.
Respiratory-tract infections.

Milk of Magnesia
SmithKline Beecham, Irl.; Winthrop, Switz.†; Sterling Health, UK.
Magnesium hydroxide (p.1198·2).
Constipation; dyspepsia.

Milkinol Schwarz, USA.
Liquid paraffin (p.1382·1).
Constipation.

Milkitten Abfuhrdragees Medopharm, Ger.†.
Bisacodyl (p.1179·3); chelidonium.
Constipation.

Milkitten S Medopharm, Ger.†.
Senna (p.1212·2); bisacodyl (p.1179·3); chelidonium.
Constipation.

Milkitten-Fruchtewurfel Medopharm, Ger.†.
Senna (p.1212·2).
Constipation.

Milla Ilex, Ital.
Chamomile (p.1561·2).

Millaterol Andreu, Spain†.
Tiadenol (p.1279·3).
Hyperlipidaemias.

Millerspas Lennon, S.Afr.
Hyoscyamine sulphate (p.464·2); atropine sulphate (p.455·1); hyoscine hydrobromide (p.462·3); phenobarbitone (p.350·2).
Peptic ulcer; reduction of respiratory and gastro-intestinal secretions; renal and biliary colic.

Millevit Nordmark, Ger.†.
Cyanocobalamin (p.1363·3).
Vitamin B deficiency.

Milli Anovlar Schering, Fr.
Norethisterone acetate (p.1453·1); ethinyloestradiol (p.1445·1).
Combined oral contraceptive; dysmenorrhoea.

Millibar Lisapharma, Ital.
Indapamide (p.890·2).
Hypertension.

Millicortene Ciba, Switz.
Dexamethasone (p.1037·1).
Corticosteroid.

Millicorten-Vioform Zyma, Ger.
Dexamethasone pivalate (p.1037·3); clioquinol (p.193·2).
Infected skin disorders.

Milligynon Schering, Fr.
Norethisterone acetate (p.1453·1).
Progestogen-only oral contraceptive.

Millisrol Kayaku, Jpn.
Glyceryl trinitrate (p.874·3).
Angina pectoris; heart failure; hypertension during surgery; maintenance of hypotension during surgery.

Millypar Adcock Ingram Self Medication, S.Afr.
Magnesium hydroxide (p.1198·2); liquid paraffin (p.1382·1).
Constipation.

Milontin
Parke, Davis, Austral.†; Parke, Davis, USA.
Phensuximide (p.352·2).
Absence seizures.

Milophene Milex, USA†.
Clomiphene citrate (p.1439·2).
Anovulatory infertility.

Mil-Par
SmithKline Beecham, Irl.; Sterling Health, UK.
Magnesium hydroxide (p.1198·2); liquid paraffin (p.1382·1).
Constipation.

Milrosina Biogalenica, Spain.
Resorcinol (p.1090·1); borax (p.1554·2).
Formerly contained resorcinol, borax, and calcium ascorbate.
Mouth ulcers.

Milrosina Hidrocort Biogalenica, Spain†.
Hydrocortisone hemisuccinate (p.1044·1); resorcinol (p.1090·1); borax (p.1554·2).
Formerly contained hydrocortisone hemisuccinate, resorcinol, borax, and calcium ascorbate.
Mouth ulcers.

Milrosina Nistatina Biogalenica, Spain.
Hydrocortisone hemisuccinate (p.1044·1); nystatin (p.386·1).
Oral candidiasis.

Miltaun Byk, Aust.
Meprobamate (p.678·1).
Anxiety disorders; premedication; skeletal muscle spasticity; sleep disorders.

Miltex
Asta Medica, Ger.; Asta Medica, Swed.
Miltefosine (p.551·3).
Skin metastases of breast cancer.

Milton
Lachartre, Fr.; Procter & Gamble, Irl.; Procter & Gamble (H&B Care), UK.
Sterilising tablets: Sodium dichloroisocyanurate (p.1124·3).
Disinfection.

Lachartre, Fr.; Procter & Gamble, Irl.; Procter & Gamble, Ital.; Procter & Gamble (H&B Care), UK.
Sterilising fluid: Sodium hypochlorite (p.1124·3).
Decontamination of fruit and vegetables; sterilisation of feeding bottles; water purification.

Milton Anti-Bacterial Procter & Gamble, Austral.
Sodium dichloroisocyanurate (p.1124·3) or sodium hypochlorite (p.1124·3).
Disinfection of infant feeding equipment; disinfection of surfaces, equipment, and drinking water.

Milton Infa-Care Procter & Gamble, Austral.†.
Soap substitute.

Milton Milgard Procter & Gamble, Austral.†.
Emollient cleanser.
Nappy rash.

Miltown
Inibsa, Spain†; Wallace, USA.
Meprobamate (p.678·1).
Anxiety; insomnia; skeletal muscle spasm.

Milumil Milupa, Ital.
Infant feed.
Gastro-oesophageal disorders.

Milupa Wyeth-Ayerst, Canad.
A range of foods for special diets.

Milupa Biber-C Milupa, Ital.
Carbohydrate, amino-acid, lipid, and mineral preparation with vitamin C.
Nutritional supplement.

Milupa Biberfrutta Milupa, Ital.
Carbohydrate, amino-acid, and lipid preparation with vitamin C and iron.
Nutritional supplement.

Milupa GES
Milupa, Aust.; Milupa, Ital.
Potassium chloride; sodium chloride; sodium bicarbonate; anhydrous glucose (p.1152·3).
Diarrhoea; oral rehydration therapy.

Milupa HIST
Milupa, Fr.†; Milupa, Ital.
Food for special diets.
Histidinaemia.

Milupa Hn 25 Milupa, Ital.
Nutritional supplement.
Diarrhoea.

Milupa HOM
Milupa, Fr.†; Milupa, Ital.
Food for special diets.
Homocystinuria.

Milupa lpd
Milupa, Irl.; Milupa, UK.
Low-protein food.
Disorders of amino-acid metabolism in childhood.

Milupa Lpf Milupa, Ital.
Food for special diets.
Protein metabolism disorders; renal impairment.

Milupa LYS
Milupa, Fr.†; Milupa, Ital.
Food for special diets.
Hyperlysinaemia.

Milupa MSUD *Milupa, Fr.†; Milupa, Ital.*
Food for special diets.
Maple syrup urine disease.

Milupa Neo *Milupa, Ital.†.*
Benzethonium chloride (p.1102·3); hamamelis (p.1587·1).
Nipple care during breast feeding.

Milupa OS
Milupa, Fr.†; Milupa, Ital.
Food for special diets.
Methylmalonic aciduria; propionic acidaemia.

Milupa PKU
Milupa, Fr.†; Milupa, Irl.; Milupa, Ital.
Food for special diets.
Hyperphenylalaninaemia; phenylketonuria.

Milupa Pregomin *Milupa, Ital.*
Preparation for enteral nutrition.
Diarrhoea; disorders of fructose and galactose metabolism; food hypersensitivity; gastro-intestinal resection; milk and soya intolerance.

Milupa Som *Milupa, Ital.*
Food for special diets.
Disaccharide deficiency; fructosaemia; galactosaemia; milk intolerance.

Milupa TYR
Milupa, Fr.†; Milupa, Ital.
Food for special diets.
Hypertyrosinaemia.

Milupa UCD
Milupa, Fr.†; Milupa, Ital.
Food for special diets.
Argininosuccinic aciduria; citrullinaemia; hyperammonaemia; hyperargininaemia; ornithinaemia.

Milurit *Thiemann, Ger.*
Allopurinol (p.390·2).
Gout; hyperuricaemia.

Milvane
Schering, Ital.; Schering, Switz.
Gestodene (p.1447·2); ethinyloestradiol (p.1445·1).
Triphasic oral contraceptive.

Mimedran *Esteve, Spain.*
Piperazine sultamate (p.108·1).
Hyperlipidaemias.

Minachlor *Esoform, Ital.*
Chloramine (p.1106·3).
Disinfection of wounds, burns, and external genitalia.

Minadex *Seven Seas, UK.*
Multivitamin and mineral preparation.

Minadex Mix *Grifols, Spain.*
Multivitamin and mineral preparation.

Minadex Mix Ginseng *Grifols, Spain.*
Multivitamins and minerals; ginseng (p.1584·2).

Minafen
Medifood-Trufood, Ital.†; Cow & Gate, UK†.
Food for special diets.
Phenylketonuria.

Minakne *Hexal, Ger.*
Minocycline hydrochloride (p.226·2).
Skin disorders.

Minalfene *Bouchara, Fr.*
Alminoprofen (p.15·1).
Inflammation; pain.

Minalgin *Streuli, Switz.*
Dipyrone (p.35·1).
Colic; fever; pain.

Minalka *Cedar Health, UK.*
Mineral preparation.
Musculoskeletal and joint disorders.

Minamino
MPS, Austral.; Lagamed, S.Afr.; Chancellor, UK.
Vitamins, minerals, and amino acids with liver, spleen, and gastric mucosa.
Dietary supplement.

Minard's Liniment *SmithKline Beecham Consumer, Canad.*
Camphor (p.1557·2); ammonium hydroxide; turpentine.

Minax *Alphapharm, Austral.*
Metoprolol tartrate (p.907·3).
Angina pectoris; hypertension; migraine; myocardial infarction.

Mincifit *Arkopharma, Fr.*
Black currant leaves (p.1365·2) green tea (p.1645·1).
Obesity.

Mindaril
Dispersa, Ger.†; Dispersa, Switz.†.
Oxyphenbutazone (p.72·1); chloramphenicol (p.182·1).
Infected eye disorders.

Min-Detox-C *Eagle, Austral.†.*
Ascorbic acid (p.1365·2); calcium ascorbate (p.1365·2); sodium ascorbate (p.1365·2); hesperidin (p.1580·2); zinc sulphate (p.1373·2).
Vitamin C deficiency.

Mindiab
Pharmacia Upjohn, Norw.; Pharmacia Upjohn, Swed.
Glipizide (p.320·3).
Diabetes mellitus.

Mindol-Merck *Bracco, Ital.*
Propyphenazone (p.81·3); caffeine (p.749·3); ethylmorphine hydrochloride (dionina) (p.36·1).
Pain.

Minedil *Formenti, Ital.†.*
Homonicotinic acid (p.1274·3).
Hypercholesterolaemia.

Minestril *Parke, Davis, Belg.*
Norethisterone acetate (p.1453·1); ethinyloestradiol (p.1445·1).
Combined oral contraceptive; gynaecological disorders.

Minestrin *Parke, Davis, Canad.*
Norethisterone acetate (p.1453·1); ethinyloestradiol (p.1445·1).
28-Day packs also contain 7 inert tablets.
Combined oral contraceptive.

Minha *Vifor, Switz.*
Naphazoline nitrate (p.1064·2).
Eye disorders.

28 Mini *Jenapharm, Ger.*
Levonorgestrel (p.1454·1).
Progestogen-only oral contraceptive.

Mini New Gen *Roche, Ital.*
Vitamin, mineral, and carbohydrate preparation.
Nutritional supplement.

Mini Ovulo Lanzas *Lanzas, Spain.*
Benzalkonium chloride (p.1101·3).
Contraceptive.

Mini Pregnon *Nourypharma, Neth.*
22 Tablets, lynoestrenol (p.1448·2); ethinyloestradiol (p.1445·1); 6 tablets, inert.
Combined oral contraceptive.

Mini Thin Asthma Relief *BDI, USA.*
Ephedrine hydrochloride (p.1059·3); guaiphenesin (p.1061·3).

Mini Thin Pseudo *BDI, USA.*
Pseudoephedrine hydrochloride (p.1068·3).
Nasal congestion.

Minias *Farmades, Ital.*
Lormetazepam (p.677·1).
Insomnia.

Miniasal *OPW, Ger.*
Aspirin (p.16·1).
Thrombo-embolism prophylaxis.

Minidalton *Hoechst Marion Roussel, Ital.*
Parnaparin sodium (p.927·1).
Thrombosis prophylaxis.

Minidiab
Pharmacia Upjohn, Aust.; Pharmacia Upjohn, Austral.; Pharmacia Upjohn, Belg.; Pharmacia Upjohn, Fr.; Pharmacia Upjohn, Ital.; Pharmacia Upjohn, S.Afr.
Glipizide (p.320·3).
Diabetes mellitus.

Minidine *Sigma, Austral.*
Povidone-iodine (p.1123·3).
Herpes labialis; pre-operative antisepsis; sore throat; wounds.

Minidox *CT, Ital.†.*
Doxycycline hydrochloride (p.202·3).
Bacterial infections.

Minidril *Wyeth, Fr.*
Levonorgestrel (p.1454·1); ethinyloestradiol (p.1445·1).
Combined oral contraceptive; dysmenorrhoea.

Minidyne *Pedinol, USA.*
Povidone-iodine (p.1123·3).
Skin disinfection.

Miniflu *Alfa Biotech, Ital.†.*
An influenza vaccine (p.1515·2).
Active immunisation.

Minifom
Tika, Norw.; Draco, Swed.
Dimethicone 1000 (p.1213·1).
Adjunct to gastro-intestinal radiography and endoscopy; colic; flatulence.

Mini-Gamulin Rh *Armour, USA.*
An anti-D immunoglobulin (p.1503·2).
Prevention of rhesus sensitisation.

Mini-Gravigard *SPA, Ital.*
Copper (p.1337·3).
Intra-uterine contraceptive device.

Minihep
Leo, Irl.; Leo, Neth.; Leo, UK.
Heparin sodium (p.879·3) or heparin calcium (p.879·3).
Thrombo-embolic disorders.

Miniluteolas *Serono, Ital.†.*
Ethynodiol (p.1445·3); ethinyloestradiol (p.1445·1).
Combined oral contraceptive; menstrual disorders.

Minims Artificial Tears
Smith & Nephew, Austral.; Chauvin, Irl.; Chauvin, UK.
Hydroxyethylcellulose (p.1472·3); sodium chloride (p.1162·2).
Dry eyes.

Mini-Pe *Searle, Swed.*
Norethisterone (p.1453·1).
Progestogen-only oral contraceptive.

Miniphase *Schering, Fr.*
Norethisterone acetate (p.1453·1); ethinyloestradiol (p.1445·1).
Biphasic oral contraceptive; dysmenorrhoea.

Minipres *Pfizer, Spain.*
Prazosin hydrochloride (p.932·3).
Benign prostatic hyperplasia; heart failure; hypertension; Raynaud's syndrome.

Minipress
Pfizer, Aust.; Pfizer, Austral.; Roerig, Belg.; Pfizer, Canad.; Pfizer, Fr.; Pfizer, Ger.; Pfizer, Ital.†; Pfizer, Neth.; Pfizer, S.Afr.; Pfizer, Switz.; Pfizer, USA.
Prazosin hydrochloride (p.932·3).
Benign prostatic hyperplasia; heart failure; hypertension; Raynaud's syndrome.

Minirin
Sigmapharm, Aust.; Rhone-Poulenc Rorer, Austral.; Ferring, Belg.; Ferring, Fr.; Ferring, Ger.; Ferring, Norw.; Ferring, Swed.; Ferring, Switz.
Desmopressin acetate (p.1245·2).
Diabetes insipidus; nocturnal enuresis; polydipsia; polyuria; prolonged haemorrhage; stimulation of factor VIII activity; test of renal concentrating capacity.

Minirin/DDAVP *Ferring, Ital.*
Desmopressin acetate (p.1245·2).
Diabetes insipidus; polydipsia; polyuria; renal function tests.

Miniscap *Vifor, Switz.*
Cathine hydrochloride (p.1478·1).
Obesity.

Mini-sintrom *Ciba-Geigy, Fr.*
Nicoumalone (p.916·1).
Thrombo-embolic disorders.

Minisiston *Jenapharm, Ger.*
Ethinyloestradiol (p.1445·1); levonorgestrel (p.1454·1).
Combined oral contraceptive; menstrual disorders.

Minisone *IDI, Ital.†.*
Betamethasone (p.1033·2).
Corticosteroid.

Ministat
Organon, Belg.; Organon, Neth.
Lynoestrenol (p.1448·2); ethinyloestradiol (p.1445·1).
Combined oral contraceptive; menstrual disorders.

Minitran
Byk, Aust.; 3M, Austral.; 3M, Belg.; 3M, Canad.; Synthelabo, Ital.; 3M, Neth.; 3M, Norw.; 3M, Spain; 3M, Swed.; 3M, Switz.; 3M, UK; Riker, USA.
Glyceryl trinitrate (p.874·3).
Angina pectoris; maintenance of venous patency at peripheral infusion sites.

MinitranS *3M, Ger.*
Glyceryl trinitrate (p.874·3).
Ischaemic heart disease.

Minit-Rub *Bristol-Myers Products, USA.*
Methyl salicylate (p.55·2); menthol (p.1600·2); camphor (p.1557·2).
Muscle, joint, and soft-tissue pain; neuralgia.

Minizide *Pfizer, USA.*
Prazosin hydrochloride (p.932·3); polythiazide (p.932·1).
Hypertension.

Mino-50 *Wyeth Lederle, Belg.*
Minocycline hydrochloride (p.226·2).
Acne.

Mino T *Wyeth, S.Afr.*
Minocycline hydrochloride (p.226·2).
Acne; bacterial infections.

Minobese *Restan, S.Afr.*
Phentermine hydrochloride (p.1484·3).
Obesity.

Minocin
Cyanamid, Aust.; Wyeth Lederle, Belg.; Wyeth-Ayerst, Canad.; Wyeth, Irl.; Cyanamid, Ital.; Lederle, Neth.; Cyanamid, Spain; Lederle, Switz.; Wyeth, UK; Lederle, USA.
Minocycline hydrochloride (p.226·2).
Bacterial infections.

Minoclir *Jenapharm, Ger.*
Minocycline hydrochloride (p.226·2).
Bacterial infections.

Minodiab
Kenfarma, Spain; Farmitalia Carlo Erba, UK.
Glipizide (p.320·3).
Diabetes mellitus.

Minodyl *Quantum, USA†.*
Minoxidil (p.910·3).

Minogal *Galen, UK.*
Minocycline (p.227·1).

Minogalen *Pharmagalen, Ger.*
Minocycline hydrochloride (p.226·2).
Acne.

Minolip *Master Pharma, Ital.†.*
Benfluorex hydrochloride (p.1268·2).
Glucose metabolic disorders; hyperlipidaemias; obesity.

Minolis *Pharmascience, Fr.*
Minocycline hydrochloride (p.226·2).
Bacterial infections.

Minomycin
Lederle, Austral.; Wyeth, S.Afr.
Minocycline hydrochloride (p.226·2).
Bacterial infections.

Minoplus *Rosen, Ger.*
Minocycline hydrochloride (p.226·2).
Bacterial infections.

Minoremed *Lichtenstein, Ger.†.*
Amiloride hydrochloride (p.819·2); hydrochlorothiazide (p.885·2).
Ascites; hypertension; oedema.

Minorplex *Abigo, Swed.*
Multivitamin preparation.

Minotab
Wyeth Lederle, Belg.; Lederle, Neth.
Minocycline hydrochloride (p.226·2).
Bacterial infections.

Minotabs *Hexal, S.Afr.*
Minocycline hydrochloride (p.226·2).
Acne; bacterial infections.

Minoton *Madaus, Spain.*
Magaldrate (p.1198·1).
Gastro-intestinal hyperacidity.

Minotricon *Ragionieri, Ital.†.*
Minoxidil (p.910·3).
Androgenic alopecia.

Minovital *Terapeutico, Ital.*
Minoxidil (p.910·3).
Alopecia.

Minovlar ED *Schering, S.Afr.†.*
21 Tablets, norethisterone acetate (p.1453·1); ethinyloestradiol (p.1445·1); 7 tablets, inert.
Combined oral contraceptive.

Min-Ovral *Wyeth-Ayerst, Canad.*
Levonorgestrel (p.1454·1); ethinyloestradiol (p.1445·1).
28-Day packs also contain 7 inert tablets.
Combined oral contraceptive.

Mino-Wolff *Wolff, Ger.*
Minocycline hydrochloride (p.226·2).
Acne.

Minox *Rowex, Irl.*
Minocycline (p.227·1).
Bacterial infections.

Minoxigaine *Kenral, Canad.*
Minoxidil (p.910·3).
Alopecia androgenetica.

Minoximen *Menarini, Ital.*
Minoxidil (p.910·3).
Alopecia.

Minozinan *Rhone-Poulenc Rorer, Switz.*
Methotrimeprazine maleate (p.679·1).
Anxiety; asthma; excitement; hypersensitivity reactions; insomnia; psychoses.

Minprog
Pharmacia Upjohn, Aust.; Pharmacia Upjohn, Ger.
Alprostadil (p.1412·2).
Maintenance of ductus arteriosus patency.

Minprostin
Pharmacia Upjohn, Norw.; Pharmacia Upjohn, Swed.
Dinoprostone (p.1414·3).
Labour induction.

Minprostin E_2 *Pharmacia Upjohn, Ger.*
Dinoprostone (p.1414·3).
Labour induction.

Minprostin $F_2\alpha$ *Pharmacia Upjohn, Ger.*
Dinoprost trometamol (p.1414·2).
Uterine bleeding.

Minrin *Ferring, Neth.*
Desmopressin acetate (p.1245·2).
Diabetes insipidus; haemorrhagic disorders; nocturnal enuresis; polyuria; test of renal concentrating capacity; uraemia.

Mint Sensodyne *Block, USA.*
Potassium nitrate (p.1123·1).
Hypersensitive teeth.

Mintec
SmithKline Beecham Consumer, Austral.; Monmouth, UK.
Peppermint oil (p.1208·1).
Irritable bowel syndrome; spastic colon.

Mintetten S *Truw, Ger.†.*
Thyme (p.1636·3); liquorice (p.1197·1); menthol (p.1600·2); eucalyptus oil (p.1578·1); peppermint oil (p.1208·1).
Coughs and associated respiratory-tract disorders.

Mintetten Truw *Truw, Ger.*
Primula rhizome; drosera (p.1574·1); thyme (p.1636·3).
Catarrh; cough.

Mintezol
Merck Sharp & Dohme, Austral.; Merck Sharp & Dohme, Canad.; Merck Sharp & Dohme, Irl.; Logos, S.Afr.†; Merck Sharp & Dohme, UK; Merck Sharp & Dohme, USA.
Thiabendazole (p.110·1).
Worm infections.

Mintox *Major, USA.*
Aluminium hydroxide (p.1177·3); magnesium hydroxide (p.1198·2).
Hyperacidity.

Mintox Plus *Major, USA.*
Aluminium hydroxide (p.1177·3); magnesium hydroxide (p.1198·2); simethicone (p.1213·1).
Hyperacidity.

Minulet
Wyeth Lederle, Aust.; Wyeth, Austral.; Wyeth Lederle, Belg.; Wyeth, Fr.; Wyeth, Ger.; Wyeth, Irl.; Wyeth, Ital.; Wyeth, Neth.; Wyeth, Spain; Wyeth, Switz.; Wyeth, UK.
Gestodene (p.1447·2); ethinyloestradiol (p.1445·1).
28-Day packs also contain 7 inert tablets.
Combined oral contraceptive.

Minulette *Akromed, S.Afr.*
21 Tablets, gestodene (p.1447·2); ethinyloestradiol (p.1445·1); 7 tablets, inert.
Combined oral contraceptive.

Minuric *Sanofi Omnimed, S.Afr.*
Benzbromarone (p.392·3).
Gout; hyperuricaemia.

Minurin *Ferring, Spain.*
Desmopressin (p.1245·1).
Diabetes insipidus; nocturnal enuresis.

Minusten *Zambon, Ital.†.*
Levomoprolol hydrochloride (p.898·1); mebutizide (p.901·3).
Hypertension.

Minute-Gel *Oral-B, USA.*
Acidulated phosphate fluoride (p.742·1).
Dental caries prophylaxis.

Minutil Henkel, Ger.
Formaldehyde (p.1113·2); glyoxal (p.1115·1); glutaraldehyde (p.1114·3).
Surface disinfection.

MinVitin Wander Health Care, Switz.
Food for special diets.
Obesity.

Minx-med Pino, Ger.†.
Mint oil (p.1604·1).
Cold symptoms; gastro-intestinal disorders; myalgia; neuralgia.

Miocamen Menarini, Ital.
Midecamycin acetate (p.226·2).
Bacterial infections.

Miocardin Magis, Ital.
Carnitine (p.1336·2).
Carnitine deficiency; myocardial ischaemia.

Miocarpine Ciba Vision, Canad.
Pilocarpine hydrochloride (p.1396·3).
Open-angle glaucoma.

Miochol
Ciba Vision, Austral.; Bournonville, Belg.; Ciba Vision, Canad.; Ciba Vision, Ger.; Ciba Vision, Ital.; Bournonville, Neth.†; MCM, S.Afr.; Ciba Vision, Swed.; Ciba Vision, UK; Iolab, USA.
Acetylcholine chloride (p.1389·1).
Production of miosis in eye surgery.

Miocor Ecobi, Ital.
Carnitine (p.1336·2).
Carnitine deficiency; myocardial ischaemia.

Miocrin Rubio, Spain.
Sodium aurothiomalate (p.83·2).
Lupus erythematosus; rheumatoid arthritis.

Miocuril Terapeutico, Ital.
Sodium uridine triphosphate.
Heart failure; muscular disorders.

Miodene Bioprogress, Ital.
Ubidecarenone (p.1641·2).
Cardiac disorders.

Mioflex Braun, Spain.
Suxamethonium chloride (p.1319·1).
Depolarising neuromuscular blocker.

Miokacin FIRMA, Ital.
Midecamycin acetate (p.226·2).
Bacterial infections.

Miokalium Bama, Spain.
Injection: Magnesium chloride (p.1157·2); potassium aspartate (p.1161·3); potassium chloride (p.1161·1).
Tablets†: Aspartic acid; magnesium chloride; potassium aspartate (p.1161·3); potassium bicarbonate (p.1153·1); potassium chloride (p.1161·1).
Potassium depletion.

Miol Robert, Spain.
Omeprazole (p.1204·2) or omeprazole sodium (p.1204·2).
Gastro-oesophageal reflux; peptic ulcer; Zollinger-Ellison syndrome.

Miolene Lusofarmaco, Ital.
Ritodrine hydrochloride (p.1625·3).
Premature labour; threatened abortion.

Mionevrasi Boehringer Mannheim, Ital.
Cyanocobalamin (p.1363·3); pyridoxine hydrochloride (p.1362·3); cocarboxylase (p.1361·2).
Lignocaine hydrochloride (p.1293·2) is included in this preparation to alleviate the pain of injection.
Neuralgia; neuritis; vitamin B deficiencies.

Mionevrasi Forte Boehringer Mannheim, Ital.†.
Sodium uridine triphosphate; cyanocobalamin (p.1363·3); cocarboxylase (p.1361·2); pyridoxine hydrochloride (p.1362·3).
Neuralgia; neuritis; neuropathy.

Miopat Poliformo, Ital.
Medigoxin (p.902·1).
Heart failure.

Miophen Robugen, Ger.†.
Codeine phosphate (p.26·1); caffeine (p.749·3); aspirin (p.16·1).
Pain.

Miopos-POS stark Ursapharm, Ger.†.
Pilocarpine nitrate (p.1396·3); physostigmine salicylate (p.1395·3).
Postoperative increase in intra-ocular pressure.

Miopotasio Bama, Spain†.
Potassium chloride (p.1161·1).
Potassium depletion.

Miorel Lederle, Fr.
Thiocolchicoside (p.1322·1).
Skeletal muscle spasm.

Mios INTES, Ital.
Pilocarpine hydrochloride (p.1396·3); carbachol (p.1390·1); paraoxon (p.1395·3); procaine hydrochloride (p.1299·2).
Raised intra-ocular pressure.

Miosal Charton, Canad.
Triethanolamine salicylate (p.1639·2).
Pain.

Miosen Belmac, Spain.
Dipyridamole (p.857·1).
Thrombo-embolism prophylaxis.

Miostat
Alcon, Austral.; Alcon, Belg.; Alcon, Canad.; Alcon, Neth.†; Alcon, Switz.; Alcon, USA.
Carbachol (p.1390·1).
Production of miosis.

Miotic Double Asta Medica, Belg.
Physostigmine salicylate (p.1395·3); pilocarpine hydrochloride (p.1396·3).
Glaucoma; herniated iris.

Miotonal Caber, Ital.
Carnitine (p.1336·2).
Carnitine deficiency; myocardial ischaemia.

Miotyn Ibirn, Ital.
Ubidecarenone (p.1641·2).
Cardiac disorders.

Miovisin Farmigea, Ital.
Acetylcholine chloride (p.1389·1).
Production of miosis in eye surgery.

Miowas
IFI, Ital.†; Wasserman, Spain†.
Methocarbamol (p.1316·1).
Skeletal muscle spasm.

Miowas G Wasserman, Spain.
Gallamine triethiodide (p.1315·2).
Competitive neuromuscular blocker.

Miozets Semar, Spain.
Benzocaine (p.1286·2); tyrothricin (p.267·2).
Mouth and throat disorders.

Mipralin Lennon, S.Afr.†.
Imipramine hydrochloride (p.289·2).
Depression.

Mirabol Volchem, Ital.
Preparation for enteral nutrition.

Miracef Tosi, Ital.
Propylene glycol cefatrizine (p.164·2).
Bacterial infections.

Miraclar Iquinosa, Spain.
Naphazoline hydrochloride (p.1064·2).
Eye disorders.

Miraclid Mochida, Jpn†.
Ulinastatin (p.1641·3).
Circulatory failure; pancreatitis.

Miraclin Farmacologico Milanese, Ital.
Doxycycline hydrochloride (p.202·3).
Bacterial infections.

Miracorten
Zyma, Aust.; Max Ritter, Switz.
Halobetasol propionate (p.1043·2).
Skin disorders.

Miradol Durbin, UK.
Paracetamol (p.72·2).

Miradon Schering, USA.
Anisindione (p.824·2).
Thrombo-embolic disorders.

Miraflow
Ciba Vision, Austral.; Ciba Vision, USA.
Range of solutions for contact lenses.

Miranax
Grunenthal, Aust.; Syntex, Swed.
Naproxen sodium (p.61·2).
Gout; inflammation; musculoskeletal, joint, and peri-articular disorders; pain.

Miranova Schering, Ger.
Ethinyloestradiol (p.1445·1); levonorgestrel (p.1454·1).
Combined oral contraceptive.

Mirantal Ciba Vision, Spain.
Phenylephrine hydrochloride (p.1066·2); medrysone (p.1045·3); neomycin sulphate (p.229·2); zinc sulphate (p.1373·2).
Infected eye disorders.

Mirapex Pharmacia Upjohn, USA.
Pramipexole (p.1143·2).
Parkinsonism.

Mirapront Pfizer, Aust.
Phentermine resinate (p.1484·3).
Obesity.

Mirapront N Mack, Illert., Ger.
Cathine polystyroldivinylbenzol-sulphonic acid (p.1478·1).
Obesity.

MiraSept Alcon, USA.
Hydrogen peroxide (p.1116·2).
Disinfecting solution for soft contact lenses.

Miraxid
Merck, Aust.†; Rorer, Ger.†; Lovens, Swed.†; Leo, Switz.†; Fisons, UK†.
Pivmecillinam (p.238·3) or pivmecillinam hydrochloride (p.239·1); pivampicillin (p.238·2).
Bacterial infections.

Mirazul Fardi, Spain.
Phenylephrine hydrochloride (p.1066·2).
Eye disorders.

Mirbanil Boehringer Ingelheim, Spain†.
Sulpiride (p.692·3).
Behaviour disorders; psychoses; vertigo.

Mircol
Rhone-Poulenc Rorer, Belg.; Rhone-Poulenc Rorer, Neth.†; Italfarmaco, Spain.
Mequitazine (p.414·2).
Hypersensitivity reactions.

Mirena
Schering, Belg.; Schering, Neth.; Pharmacia Upjohn, Switz.; Schering, UK.
Levonorgestrel (p.1454·1).
Progestogen-releasing intra-uterine contraceptive device.

Mirfat Merckle, Ger.
Clonidine hydrochloride (p.841·2).
Hypertension.

Mirfudorm Merckle, Ger.
Oxazepam (p.683·2).
Formerly contained carbromal.
Anxiety; sleep disorders.

Mirfulan
Merckle, Aust.
Cod-liver oil (p.1337·3); zinc oxide (p.1096·2); hamamelis (p.1587·1); urea (p.1095·2).
Skin disorders.

Merckle, Ger.
Cod-liver oil (p.1337·3); zinc oxide (p.1096·2); hamamelis (p.1587·1); urea (p.1095·2).
Wounds.

Mirfulan Spray N Merckle, Ger.
Cod-liver oil (p.1337·3); zinc oxide (p.1096·2); levomenol (p.1596·1).
Skin disorders; wounds.

Mirfusot Merckle, Ger.
Thyme (p.1636·3).
Coughs and associated respiratory-tract disorders.

Mirfusot N mit Kodein Merckle, Ger.†.
Codeine phosphate (p.26·1); thyme (p.1636·3).
Coughs and associated respiratory-tract disorders.

Mirocor Medipharm, Switz.†.
Crataegus (p.1568·2); menthol (p.1600·2); camphor (p.1557·2); valerian (p.1643·1).
Cardiovascular disorders.

Miroton Knoll, Ger.
Squill (p.1070·1); convallaria (p.1567·2); nerium oleander (p.1610·1); adonis vernalis (p.1543·3).
Cardiovascular disorders.

Miroton N Knoll, Ger.
Adonis vernalis (p.1543·3); convallaria (p.1567·2); squill (p.1070·1).
Cardiac disorders.

Mirpan Dolorgiet, Ger.
Maprotiline hydrochloride (p.296·2).
Depression.

Mirsol Permamed, Switz.
Zipeprol hydrochloride (p.1071·3).
Adjunct in bronchial examination; coughs.

Mirtex P DMG, Ital.
Vitamin, mineral, and lipid preparation with myrtillus.
Nutritional supplement.

Mirtilene SIFI, Ital.
Myrtillus (p.1606·1); betacarotene (p.1335·2); *dl*-alpha tocopheryl acetate (p.1369·2).
Capillary disorders; eye disorders.

Mirtilene Forte SIFI, Ital.
Myrtillus (p.1606·1).
Eye disorders.

Mirtilus Llorens, Spain.
Betacarotene (p.1335·2); myrtillus (p.1606·1).
Eye disorders.

Mirtilvedo C Fitobucaneve, Ital.
Vitamin preparation with betacarotene, myrtillus, carrot, and rose fruit.
Nutritional supplement.

Miscidon Torlan, Spain.
Spironolactone (p.946·1); hydrochlorothiazide (p.885·2).
Hypertension; oedema.

Misfans Lennon, S.Afr.†.
Ipecacuanha tincture (p.1062·2); aniseed (p.1549·3); prune (p.1209·2); squill tincture (p.1070·1); tolu syrup (p.1071·1).
Coughs.

Misodex Sepharma, Ital.
Misoprostol (p.1419·3).
NSAID-induced peptic ulcer.

Misofenac Sepharma, Ital.
Diclofenac sodium (p.31·2).
Misoprostol (p.1419·3) is included in this preparation in an attempt to limit adverse effects on the gastro-intestinal mucosa.
Musculoskeletal and joint disorders.

Mission Prenatal Mission Pharmacal, USA.
A range of multivitamin and mineral preparations with iron and folic acid.
Iron-deficiency anaemias; prenatal and postpartum supplement.

Mission Surgical Supplement Mission Pharmacal, USA.
Ferrous gluconate (p.1340·1); multivitamins and minerals.
Dietary supplement for pre- and postsurgical patients; iron-deficiency anaemias.

Mistabron
UCB, Aust.; Bios, Belg.; UCB, Neth.; UCB, S.Afr.; UCB, Switz.
Mesna (p.983·3).
Respiratory-tract disorders.

Mistabronco UCB, Ger.
Mesna (p.983·3).
Respiratory-tract disorders.

Mistamine Galderma, UK.
Mizolastine (p.414·3).
Allergic rhinoconjunctivitis; urticaria.

Mistel Curarina Harras-Curarina, Ger.
Mistletoe (p.1604·1).
Cardiovascular disorders.

Mistelan Reinecke, Ger.
Mistletoe (p.1604·1); rose fruit (p.1365·2); equisetum (p.1575·1); eriodictyon (p.1060·3); rauwolfia serpentina (p.941·3); avena (p.1551·3); crataegus (p.1568·2); angust.; angelica; damiana; ginseng.
Arteriosclerosis; hypertension.

Mistel-Krautertabletten Salushaus, Ger.
Mistletoe (p.1604·1).
Cardiovascular disorders.

Mistelol-Kapseln Twardy, Ger.
Mistletoe oil (p.1604·1).
Cardiovascular disorders.

Mistosil McGloin, Austral.
Magnesium trisilicate (p.1199·1); calcium carbonate (p.1182·1); magnesium carbonate (p.1198·1).
Hyperacidity.

Misulban
Nuovo ISM, Ital.; Techni-Pharma, Mon.†.
Busulphan (p.509·3).
Malignant neoplasms.

Mitalolo Ellem, Ital.†.
Labetalol hydrochloride (p.896·1).
Hypertension; hypertensive crisis.

Mitchell Expel Anti Lice Spray Mitchell, UK.
Carbaryl (p.1403·1).
Pediculosis.

Mithracin
Pfizer, Neth.†; Pfizer, Norw.; Pfizer, UK†; Miles, USA.
Plicamycin (p.558·2).
Hypercalcaemia of malignancy; hypercalciuria of malignancy; Paget's disease of bone; testicular cancer.

Mithracine
Pfizer, Fr.; Pfizer, Switz.†.
Plicamycin (p.558·2).
Hypercalcaemia of malignancy; malignant neoplasms.

Mitidin Savoma, Ital.†.
Nitrazepam (p.682·2).
Anxiety; insomnia.

Mitil Lennon, S.Afr.
Prochlorperazine maleate (p.687·3).
Migraine; nausea and vomiting; nonpsychotic mental disorders; vestibular disorders.

Mitocor Zambon, Ital.
Ubidecarenone (p.1641·2).
Cardiac disorders.

Mito-medac Medac, Ger.
Mitomycin (p.552·2).
Malignant neoplasms.

Mitosyl
Note. This name is used for preparations of different composition.
Delagrange, Belg.
Cod-liver oil (p.1337·3); zinc oxide (p.1096·2); methyl salicylate (p.55·2).
Burns; skin disorders; wounds.

Synthelabo, Fr.; Synthelabo, Ger.; Delagrange, Spain; Delagrange, Switz.†.
Cod-liver oil (p.1337·3); zinc oxide (p.1096·2).
Anorectal disorders; skin disorders; wounds.

Mitoxana Asta Medica, UK.
Ifosfamide (p.540·2).
Malignant neoplasms.

Mitran Hauck, USA.
Chlordiazepoxide hydrochloride (p.646·3).
Alcohol withdrawal syndrome; anxiety.

Mitrolan
Whitehall-Robins, Canad.†; Robins, USA.
Polycarbophil calcium (p.1209·1).
Constipation; diarrhoea.

Mittoval Schering, Ital.
Alfuzosin hydrochloride (p.817·2).
Benign prostatic hyperplasia.

Mivacron
Glaxo Wellcome, Aust.; Glaxo Wellcome, Austral.; Glaxo Wellcome, Belg.; Glaxo Wellcome, Canad.; Glaxo Wellcome, Fr.; Glaxo Wellcome, Ger.; Zeneca, Ger.; Wellcome, Irl.; Glaxo Wellcome, Ital.; Glaxo Wellcome, Neth.; Glaxo Wellcome, Norw.; Glaxo Wellcome, S.Afr.; Wellcome, Spain; Glaxo Wellcome, Swed.; Wellcome, Switz.; Wellcome, UK; Wellcome, USA.
Mivacurium chloride (p.1316·3).
Competitive neuromuscular blocker.

mivitase 2000 GN, Ger.
Multivitamin and mineral preparation.

Mixer Biomedica, Ital.
Atenolol (p.825·3); nifedipine (p.916·2).
Angina pectoris; hypertension.

Mixobar
Byk Gulden, Ital.; Astra Tech, Norw.; Astra Tech, Swed.
Barium sulphate (p.1003·1).
Contrast medium for gastro-intestinal radiography.

Mixogen Donmed, S.Afr.
Injection: Oestradiol benzoate (p.1455·1); oestradiol phenylpropionate (p.1455·2); testosterone propionate (p.1464·2); testosterone phenylpropionate (p.1464·2); testosterone isocaproate (p.1464·2).
Oestrogen deficiency.
Tablets†: Ethinyloestradiol (p.1445·1); methyltestosterone (p.1450·3).
Androgenic; oestrogenic.

Mixotone Teofarma, Ital.
Polymyxin B sulphate (p.239·1); neomycin sulphate (p.229·2); hydrocortisone sodium succinate (p.1044·1); lignocaine hydrochloride (p.1293·2).
Formerly contained tetracycline hydrochloride, polymyxin B sulphate, neomycin sulphate, hydrocortisone sodium succinate, tetrahydrozoline hydrochloride, and lignocaine hydrochloride.
Bacterial infections of the ear.

Mix-O-Vit Asta Medica, Belg.†.
Multivitamin preparation.

Mixtard
Novo Nordisk, Aust.†; Novo Nordisk, Canad.†; Nordisk, Fr.†; Novo Nordisk, Ger.; Novo Nordisk, Switz.; Nordisk, USA†.
Mixture of insulin injection (porcine, highly-purified) 30% and isophane insulin (porcine, highly-purified) 70% (p.322·1).
Diabetes mellitus.

Mixtard 10/90, 15/85, 20/80, 30/70, 40/60, 50/50
Novo Nordisk, Aust.; Novo Nordisk, Austral.; Novo Nordisk, Canad.†; Novo Nordisk, Ger.; Novo Nordisk, Neth.; Novo Nordisk, Norw.; Novo Nordisk, S.Afr.; Novo Nordisk, Spain; Novo Nordisk, Swed.; Nordisk, USA†.
Mixtures of insulin injection (human, monocomponent) and isophane insulin injection (human, monocomponent) respectively in the proportions indicated (p.322·1).
Diabetes mellitus.

Mixtard 10, 20, 30, 40, and 50
Novo Nordisk, Belg.; Novo Nordisk, Fr.; Novo Nordisk, Irl.; Novo Nordisk, Spain; Novo Nordisk, Switz.
Mixtures of insulin injection (human) 10%, 20%, 30% 40%, and 50% and isophane insulin injection (human) 90%, 80%, 70%, 60%, and 50% respectively (p.322·1).
Diabetes mellitus.

Mixtard-X Humanum *Novo Nordisk, Belg.†.*
A mixture of isophane insulin suspension (human, emp) 70% and neutral insulin injection (human, emp) 30% (p.322·1).
Diabetes mellitus.

Mizollen
Lorex Synthelabo, Neth.; Lorex, UK.
Mizolastine (p.414·3).
Allergic rhinoconjunctivitis; urticaria.

M-KYA *Nature's Bounty, USA†.*
Quinine sulphate (p.439·2).
Nocturnal leg cramps.

ML 20 *Blackmores, Austral.*
Magnesium phosphate (p.1157·3); dibasic potassium phosphate (p.1159·2); dried yeast (p.1373·1); lecithin (p.1595·2); *d*-alpha tocopheryl acid succinate (p.1369·2).
Magnesium deficiency.

ML Cu 250
CCD, Fr.; Parke, Davis, Ital.†.
Copper-wound plastic (p.1337·3).
Intra-uterine contraceptive device.

ML Cu 375 *CCD, Fr.*
Copper-wound plastic (p.1337·3).
Intra-uterine contraceptive device.

"Mletzko" Tropfen *Mletzko, Ger.†.*
Turmeric (p.1001·3); curcuma zanthorrhiza; cinchona bark (p.1564·1); gentian (p.1583·3); galanga; frangula bark (p.1193·2); calamus (p.1556·1); aloes (p.1177·1).
Gastro-intestinal disorders.

M-long *Grunenthal, Ger.; Hexal, Ger.*
Morphine sulphate (p.56·2).
Pain.

M-M Vax
Merck Sharp & Dohme, Aust.; CSL, Austral.†; Chiron Behring, Ger.; Pro Vaccine, Switz.
A measles and mumps vaccine (Enders' attenuated Edmonston and Jeryl Lynn (level B) strains respectively) (p.1519·2).
Active immunisation.

MMR II
CSL, Austral.; Merck Sharp & Dohme, Canad.; Pasteur Merieux, Irl.; Pasteur Merieux, Ital.; Merck Sharp & Dohme, S.Afr.; Pasteur Merieux, Swed.; Pro Vaccine, Switz.; Pasteur Merieux, UK; Merck Sharp & Dohme, USA.
A measles, mumps, and rubella vaccine (Enders' attenuated Edmonston, Jeryl Lynn (B level), and Wistar RA 27/3 strains respectively) (p.1519·3).
Active immunisation.

MMR Triplovax *Pasteur Merieux, Ger.*
A measles, mumps, and rubella vaccine (More attenuated Enders', Jeryl Lynn, and Wistar RA 27/3 strains respectively) (p.1519·3).
Active immunisation.

MMR Vax
Merck Sharp & Dohme, Aust.; Merck Sharp & Dohme, Belg.; Chiron Behring, Ger.
A measles, mumps, and rubella vaccine (Enders' attenuated Edmonston or Moraten, Jeryl Lynn, and Wistar RA 27/3 strains respectively) (p.1519·3).
Active immunisation.

Mnemina Fosforo *Lagap, Ital.†.*
Levoglutamide (p.1344·3); cyanocobalamin (p.1363·3); pyridoxal phosphate (p.1363·1); DL-phosphoserine.
Tonic.

Mnemo Organico *Blue Cross, Ital.*
Royal jelly (p.1626·3); liver.
Nutritional supplement.

Mnemo Organico Plus *Blue Cross, Ital.†.*
Royal jelly (p.1626·3); soya lecithin (p.1595·2).
Nutritional supplement.

Mnesis *Takeda, Ital.*
Idebenone (p.1590·2).
Cerebrovascular disorders.

Moban *Gate, USA; Du Pont, USA.*
Molindone hydrochloride (p.681·3).
Psychoses.

Mobec *Thomae, Ger.*
Meloxicam (p.52·1).
Musculoskeletal and joint disorders.

Mobenol *Horner, Canad.†.*
Tolbutamide (p.333·2).
Diabetes mellitus.

Mobic
Boehringer Ingelheim, Aust.; Boehringer Ingelheim, Belg.; Boehringer Ingelheim, Fr.; Boehringer Ingelheim, Irl.; Boehringer Ingelheim, Ital.; Boehringer Ingelheim, S.Afr.; Boehringer Ingelheim, Swed.; Boehringer Ingelheim, UK.
Meloxicam (p.52·1).
Ankylosing spondylitis; osteoarthritis; rheumatoid arthritis.

Mobicox *Boehringer Ingelheim, Switz.*
Meloxicam (p.52·1).
Arthroses; rheumatoid arthritis.

Mobidin *Ascher, USA.*
Magnesium salicylate (p.51·1).
Fever; inflammation; pain.

Mobiflex
Roche, Canad.; Roche, Irl.; Roche, UK.
Tenoxicam (p.88·2).
Musculoskeletal, joint, peri-articular, and soft-tissue disorders.

Mobiforton *Sanofi Winthrop, Ger.*
Tetrazepam (p.694·3).
Skeletal muscle spasm; spasticity.

Mobigesic *Ascher, USA.*
Magnesium salicylate (p.51·1); phenyltoloxamine citrate (p.416·1).
Pain.

Mobilan *Galen, UK†.*
Indomethacin (p.45·2).
Gout; inflammation; musculoskeletal disorders; pain.

Mobilat
Note. This name is used for preparations of different composition.
Kwizda, Aust.; Luitpold, Belg.; Luitpold, Ger.; Byk Madaus, S.Afr.; Luitpold, Switz.
Suprarenal extract (p.1050·1); a heparinoid (p.882·3); salicylic acid (p.1090·2).
Joint and soft-tissue disorders.

Luitpold, Ger.
Tablets: Ibuprofen (p.44·1).
Fever; pain.
Topical spray: Indomethacin (p.45·2).
Musculoskeletal, joint, and soft-tissue disorders.

Luitpold, Ital.
Hydrocortisone (p.1043·3); a heparinoid (p.882·3); salicylic acid (p.1090·2).
Musculoskeletal and joint trauma; peri-articular and soft-tissue disorders.

Luitpold, Neth.
A heparinoid (p.882·3); salicylic acid (p.1090·2).
Soft-tissue injuries; sports injuries.

Mobilis *Alphapharm, Austral.*
Piroxicam (p.80·2).
Ankylosing spondylitis; osteoarthritis; rheumatoid arthritis.

Mobilisin
Kwizda, Aust.; Luitpold, Belg.; Luitpold, Ger.; Luitpold, Ital.; Luitpold, Switz.
Flufenamic acid (p.41·3); glycol salicylate (p.43·1) or salicylic acid (p.1090·2); a heparinoid (p.882·3).
Musculoskeletal, joint, peri-articular, and soft-tissue disorders; neuralgias.

Mobilisin plus *Kwizda, Aust.*
Flufenamic acid (p.41·3); glycol salicylate (p.43·1); a heparinoid (p.882·3); benzyl nicotinate (p.22·1).
Musculoskeletal and joint disorders.

Mobisyl *Ascher, USA.*
Triethanolamine salicylate (p.1639·2).
Muscle, joint, and soft-tissue pain; neuralgia.

Moclamine *Roche, Fr.*
Moclobemide (p.298·3).
Depression.

Moctanin *Ethitek, USA.*
Monoctanoin (p.1604·2).
Gallstones.

Mod *IRBI, Ital.*
Domperidone (p.1190·3).
Gastro-intestinal disorders.

Modalim
Sanofi Winthrop, Neth.; Sanofi Winthrop, UK.
Ciprofibrate (p.1270·3).
Hyperlipidaemias.

Modalina *Sanofi Winthrop, Ital.*
Trifluoperazine hydrochloride (p.697·3).
Psychiatric disorders.

Modamide *Merck Sharp & Dohme-Chibret, Fr.*
Amiloride hydrochloride (p.819·2).
Ascites; hypertension; oedema.

Modane
Note. This name is used for preparations of different composition.
Cooperation Pharmaceutique, Fr.
Calcium pantothenate (p.1352·3); senna (p.1212·2).
Formerly contained calcium pantothenate and danthron.
Constipation.

Reig Jofre, Spain.
Calcium pantothenate (p.1352·3); calcium sennoside A (p.1212·3); calcium sennoside B (p.1212·3).
Constipation.

Savage, USA.
Phenolphthalein (p.1208·2).
Constipation.

Modane Bulk *Adria, USA.*
Psyllium hydrophilic mucilloid (p.1194·2).
Constipation.

Modane Plus *Adria, USA.*
Phenolphthalein (p.1208·2); docusate sodium (p.1189·3).
Constipation.

Modane Soft *Adria, USA.*
Docusate sodium (p.1189·3).
Constipation.

Modantis *Surf Ski International, UK.*
Antazoline hydrochloride (p.401·3); titanium dioxide (p.1093·3); allantoin (p.1078·2); cetrimide (p.1105·2).
Minor burns and scalds; sunburn.

Modaplate *Berk, UK.*
Dipyridamole (p.857·1).
Thrombo-embolism prophylaxis.

Modecate
Bristol-Myers Squibb, Austral.; Squibb, Canad.; Sanofi Winthrop, Fr.; Bristol-Myers Squibb, Irl.; Bristol-Myers Squibb, S.Afr.; Squibb, Spain; Sanofi Winthrop, UK.
Fluphenazine decanoate (p.671·2).
Psychoses.

Modecate Acutum *Bristol-Myers Squibb, S.Afr.*
Fluphenazine hydrochloride (p.671·3).
Psychoses.

Modenol
Note. This name is used for preparations of different composition.
Boehringer Mannheim, Aust.; Boehringer Mannheim, Switz.†.
Buthiazide (p.835·2); reserpine (p.942·1); rescinnamine (p.942·1); raubasine (p.941·3); potassium chloride (p.1161·1).
Hypertension.

Boehringer Mannheim, Ger.
Buthiazide (p.835·2); reserpine (p.942·1).
Hypertension.

Moderatan *Theranol-Deglaude, Fr.*
Diethylpropion hydrochloride (p.1479·3).
Obesity.

Moderator *Faes, Spain.*
Celiprolol hydrochloride (p.838·3).
Angina pectoris; hypertension.

Moderil *Pfizer, USA†.*
Rescinnamine (p.942·1).
Hypertension.

Moderin Acne *Upjohn, Spain.*
Aluminium chlorohydrate (p.1078·3); sulphur (p.1091·2); methylprednisolone acetate (p.1046·1).
Acne.

Modicon
Janssen-Cilag, Neth.; Ortho Pharmaceutical, USA.
Norethisterone (p.1453·1); ethinyloestradiol (p.1445·1).
28-Day packs also contain 7 inert tablets.
Combined oral contraceptive.

Modiem *Piam, Ital.*
Cefonicid sodium (p.167·2).
Lignocaine hydrochloride (p.1293·2) is included in this preparation to alleviate the pain of injection.
Bacterial infections.

Modifast
Novartis, Austral.; Wander Health Care, Switz.; Kent, UK†.
Food for special diets.
Obesity.

Modified Seravit *Scientific Hospital Supplies, Austral.†.*
Multivitamin and mineral preparation.

Modilac AR *Sodilac, Fr.*
Infant feed.
Regurgitation in infants.

ModimMunal *OM, Ger.*
Escherichia coli antigens.
Arthritis.

Modiodal *Lafon, Fr.*
Modafinil (p.1483·3).
Narcoleptic syndrome.

Modip *Promed, Ger.; Astra, Ger.*
Felodipine (p.867·3).
Hypertension.

Modisal
Note. This name is used for preparations of different composition.
Lagap, Switz.†.
Amiloride hydrochloride (p.819·2); hydrochlorothiazide (p.885·2).
Hypertension; oedema.

Lagap, UK.
Isosorbide mononitrate (p.893·3).
Angina pectoris.

Modiscop *Brady, Aust.*
Morphine hydrochloride (p.56·1); ethylmorphine hydrochloride (p.36·1); hyoscine hydrobromide (p.462·3).
Pain.

Moditen
Sanofi Winthrop, Belg.†; Squibb, Canad.; Sanofi Winthrop, Fr.; Bristol-Myers Squibb, Irl.; Sanofi Labaz, Neth.†; Sanofi Winthrop, Switz.†; Sanofi Winthrop, UK.
Fluphenazine enanthate (p.671·3) or fluphenazine hydrochloride (p.671·3).
Anxiety; behaviour disorders; psychoses.

Moditen Depot *Bristol-Myers Squibb, Ital.*
Fluphenazine decanoate (p.671·2).
Psychoses.

Modivid
Medac, Ger.†; Hoechst Marion Roussel, Irl.; Hoechst Marion Roussel, Ital.
Cefodizime sodium (p.167·1).
Lignocaine hydrochloride (p.1293·2) may be included in the intramuscular injection to alleviate the pain of injection.
Bacterial infections.

Modizide *Amrad, Austral.*
Amiloride hydrochloride (p.819·2); hydrochlorothiazide (p.885·2).
Ascites; hypertension; oedema.

Modopar *Roche, Fr.*
Levodopa (p.1137·1); benserazide hydrochloride (p.1132·1).
Parkinsonism.

Modraderm *Schering-Plough, Belg.†.*
Alclometasone dipropionate (p.1031·3).
Skin disorders.

Modrasone
Schering-Plough, Irl.; Dominion, UK.
Alclometasone dipropionate (p.1031·3).
Skin disorders.

Modrastane *Winthrop, USA†.*
Trilostane (p.1639·2).
Cushing's syndrome.

Modrenal *Wanskerne, UK.*
Trilostane (p.1639·2).
Breast cancer; Cushing's syndrome; hyperaldosteronism.

Moducal
Mead Johnson, Canad.†; Mead Johnson Nutritionals, USA.
Glucose polymers.
Carbohydrate source.

Moducren
Merck Sharp & Dohme-Chibret, Fr.; Morson, Irl.; Merck Sharp & Dohme, Neth.; Merck Sharp & Dohme, S.Afr.; Merck Sharp & Dohme, Switz.; Morson, UK.
Amiloride hydrochloride (p.819·2); hydrochlorothiazide (p.885·2); timolol maleate (p.953·3).
Hypertension.

Moducrin
Merck Sharp & Dohme, Aust.; Merck Sharp & Dohme, Ger.
Amiloride hydrochloride (p.819·2); hydrochlorothiazide (p.885·2); timolol maleate (p.953·3).
Hypertension.

Modula *Antonetto, Ital.*
Polycarbophil calcium (p.1209·1).
Constipation; diarrhoea.

Modulamin *Braun, Switz.*
Amino-acid infusion with or without electrolytes.
Parenteral nutrition.

Modulase *IRBI, Ital.†.*
Trimebutine (p.1639·3) or trimebutine maleate (p.1639·3).
Gastro-intestinal disorders.

Modulator *Servier, Spain.*
Benfluorex hydrochloride (p.1268·2).
Diabetes; hypercholesterolaemia; hypertriglyceridaemia; hyperuricaemia of obesity.

Modulite *Eurorga, Fr.*
Trimebutine (p.1639·3); sorbitol (p.1354·2).
Constipation.

Modulon
Jouveinal, Canad.; Eurorga, Fr.
Trimebutine maleate (p.1639·3).
Irritable bowel syndrome; postoperative paralytic ileus.

Modu-Puren *Isis Puren, Ger.*
Amiloride hydrochloride (p.819·2); hydrochlorothiazide (p.885·2).
Hypertension; oedema.

Moduret
Merck Sharp & Dohme, Canad.; Du Pont, Irl.; Du Pont Pharmaceuticals, UK.
Amiloride hydrochloride (p.819·2); hydrochlorothiazide (p.885·2).
These ingredients can be described by the British Approved Name Co-amilozide.
Ascites; heart failure; hypertension; oedema.

Moduretic
Merck Sharp & Dohme, Aust.; Merck Sharp & Dohme, Austral.; Merck Sharp & Dohme, Belg.; Du Pont, Fr.; Du Pont, Irl.; Merck Sharp & Dohme, Ital.; Merck Sharp & Dohme, Neth.; Merck Sharp & Dohme, S.Afr.; Merck Sharp & Dohme, Swed.; Merck Sharp & Dohme, Switz.; Du Pont Pharmaceuticals, UK; Merck Sharp & Dohme, USA.
Amiloride hydrochloride (p.819·2); hydrochlorothiazide (p.885·2).
These ingredients can be described by the British Approved Name Co-amilozide.
Ascites; heart failure; hypertension; oedema.

Moduretic Mite *Merck Sharp & Dohme, Norw.*
Amiloride hydrochloride (p.819·2); hydrochlorothiazide (p.885·2).
Hypertension; oedema.

Moduretik *Du Pont, Ger.*
Amiloride hydrochloride (p.819·2); hydrochlorothiazide (p.885·2).
Ascites; hypertension; oedema.

Modus
Note. This name is used for preparations of different composition.
Scharper, Ital.†.
Papaveroline (p.927·1).
Cardiovascular disorders; cerebrovascular disorders, musculoskeletal disorders; circulatory disorders.

Berenguer Infale, Spain.
Nimodipine (p.922·2).
Cerebrovascular disorders.

Modustatina *Sanofi Winthrop, Ital.*
Somatostatin acetate (p.1261·1).
Adjunct in gastro-intestinal radiography; diabetic ketoacidosis; gastro-intestinal haemorrhage; pancreatic disorders.

Modustatine
Sanofi Winthrop, Belg.; Sanofi Winthrop, Fr.
Somatostatin acetate (p.1261·1).
Aid to gastro-intestinal examinations; gastro-intestinal haemorrhage; postoperative gastro-intestinal fistulae.

Mofesal Medice, Ger.
Mofebutazone (p.56·1).
Rheumatism; superficial thrombophlebitis.

Mofesal N Medice, Ger.
Mofebutazone sodium (p.56·1).
Lignocaine hydrochloride (p.1293·2) is included in this preparation to alleviate the pain of injection.
Rheumatism; superficial thrombophlebitis.

Mogadan Roche, Ger.†.
Nitrazepam (p.682·2).
Sleep disorders.

Mogadon
Roche, Aust.; Roche, Austral.; Roche, Belg.; Roche, Canad.; Roche, Fr.; Roche, Irl.; Roche, Ital.; Roche, Neth.; Roche, Norw.; Roche, S.Afr.; Roche, Spain†; Roche, Swed.; Roche, Switz.; Roche, UK.
Nitrazepam (p.682·2).
Epilepsy; sleep disorders.

Mogil OTW, Ger.†.
Paracetamol (p.72·2).
Fever; pain.

Moi-Stir
Solvay, Canad.; Kingswood, USA.
Carmellose sodium (p.1471·2); electrolytes (p.1147·1); sorbitol (p.1354·2).
Dry mouth.

Moisture Drops
Note. This name is used for preparations of different composition.
Bausch & Lomb, Canad.
Hypromellose (p.1473·1); glycerol (p.1585·2); povidone (p.1474·2).
Dry eye; eye irritation.
Bausch & Lomb, USA.
Hypromellose (p.1473·1); dextran 70 (p.717·1); glycerol (p.1585·2).
Dry eyes.

Moisture Eyes Co-Pharma, UK.
Hypromellose (p.1473·1).
Keratoconjunctivitis sicca; lubrication of artificial eyes and hard contact lenses.

Moisturel
Westwood-Squibb, Canad.; Westwood-Squibb, USA†.
White soft paraffin (p.1382·3); dimethicone (p.1384·2).
Dry skin disorders.

Molagar Substantia, Fr.†.
Light liquid paraffin (p.1382·1); agar (p.1470·3).
Constipation.

Molcer Wallace Mfg Chem., UK.
Docusate sodium (p.1189·3).
Ear wax.

Moldina Juventus, Spain.
Bifonazole (p.375·3).
Fungal skin and nail infections.

Molevac
Parke, Davis, Aust.; Parke, Davis, Ger.; Parke, Davis, Switz.
Viprynium embonate (p.111·2).
Enterobiasis.

Molidex Clintec, Ital.†.
Anhydrous glucose (p.1343·3); hydrocortisone (p.1043·3).
Parenteral nutrition.

Molipaxin
Hoechst Marion Roussel, Irl.; Roussel, S.Afr.; Hoechst Marion Roussel, UK.
Trazodone hydrochloride (p.308·3).
Depression.

Mol-Iron Schering-Plough, USA.
Ferrous sulphate (p.1340·2).
Iron-deficiency anaemias.

Mollifene Pfeiffer, USA.
Urea hydrogen peroxide (p.1127·3).
Ear wax removal.

Mollipect Tika, Swed.
Bromhexine hydrochloride (p.1055·3); ephedrine hydrochloride (p.1059·3).
Coughs.

Moloco Manzoni, Ital.†.
Placenta extract.
Lactation insufficiency.

Moloco T Manzoni, Ital.†.
Placenta extract; thyroid extract (p.1496·3).
Lactation insufficiency.

Molsicor Betapharm, Ger.
Molsidomine (p.912·2).
Angina pectoris.

Molsidain Hoechst, Spain.
Molsidomine (p.912·2).
Angina pectoris.

Molsidolat
Albert-Roussel, Aust.†; Hoechst Marion Roussel, Ital.†.
Molsidomine (p.912·2).
Angina pectoris.

Molsihexal Hexal, Ger.
Molsidomine (p.912·2).
Angina pectoris.

Molsiton Edmond Pharma, Ital.†.
Molsidomine (p.912·2).
Angina pectoris.

Molybdene Injectable Aguettant, Fr.
Ammonium molybdate (p.1351·1).
Parenteral nutrition.

Molypen Lyphomed, USA.
Ammonium molybdate (p.1351·1).
Parenteral nutrition.

Mom Lozione Preventiva Candioli, Ital.
Benzyl benzoate (p.1402·2).
Insect repellent.

Mom Piretro Emulsione Candioli, Ital.
Tetramethrin (p.1410·3); piperonyl butoxide (p.1409·3).
Pediculosis.

Mom Shampoo Antiparassitario Candioli, Ital.
Tetramethrin (p.1410·3); phenothrin (p.1409·2).
Pediculosis.

Mom Shampoo Schiuma Candioli, Ital.
Phenothrin (p.1409·2).
Pediculosis.

Mom Zanzara Candioli, Ital.
Benzyl benzoate (p.1402·2); ethyl hexanediol.
Insect repellent.

Moment Angelini, Ital.
Ibuprofen (p.44·1).
Fever; pain.

Momentol Squibb, Spain.
Co-trimoxazole (p.196·3).
Bacterial infections; Pneumocystis carinii pneumonia.

Momentum
Note. This name is used for preparations of different composition.
Salus, Aust.; Whitehall, Neth.
Paracetamol (p.72·2).
Fever; pain.
Whitehall, USA.
Aspirin (p.16·1); phenyltoloxamine citrate (p.416·1).
Backache.

Momentum Analgetikum Much, Ger.
Paracetamol (p.72·2).
Fever; pain.

Momentum Muscular Backache Formula
Whitehall, USA.
Magnesium salicylate (p.51·1).
Pain.

Momicine Morrith, Spain.
Midecamycin acetate (p.226·2).
Bacterial infections.

Momorsyx Forte Syxyl, Ger.†.
Homoeopathic preparation.

Monacant Rorer, Ger.†.
Dihydrocodeine hydrochloride (p.34·2); paracetamol (p.72·2); sodium salicylate (p.85·1).
Fever; pain.

Monafed Monarch, USA.
Guaiphenesin (p.1061·3).
Coughs.

Monafed DM Monarch, USA.
Guaiphenesin (p.1061·3); dextromethorphan hydrobromide (p.1057·3).
Coughs.

Monapax Nattermann, Ger.
Homoeopathic preparation.

Monapax mit Dihydrocodein Rorer, Ger.†.
Dihydrocodeine hydrochloride (p.34·2); ipecacuanha tincture (p.1062·2); hedera helix; drosera; hyoscyamus.
Coughs.

Monapax N Rorer, Ger.†.
Eucalyptus oil (p.1578·1); pumilio pine oil (p.1623·3); camphor (p.1557·2).
Coughs and associated respiratory-tract disorders.

Monasin Medinova, Switz.†.
Metronidazole (p.585·1).
Anaerobic bacterial infections; protozoal infections.

Monaspor
Grunenthal, Aust.; Ciba, Neth.†; Ciba, UK†.
Cefsulodin sodium (p.173·2).
Bacterial infections.

Moneva Schering, Fr.
Gestodene (p.1447·2); ethinyloestradiol (p.1445·1).
Combined oral contraceptive.

Moni BASF, Ger.; Sanorania, Ger.
Isosorbide mononitrate (p.893·3).
Angina pectoris; heart failure; pulmonary hypertension.

Monicor Pierre Fabre, Fr.
Isosorbide mononitrate (p.893·3).
Angina pectoris; heart failure.

Moni-Gynedron Noristan, S.Afr.†.
Sulphasomidine (p.257·1); borax (p.1554·2).
Vaginal candidiasis.

Monilac Chugai, Jpn.
Lactulose (p.1195·3).
Constipation; hyperammonaemia.

Monistat
Janssen-Cilag, Austral.; McNeil Consumer, Canad.; Janssen-Cilag, Switz.; Ortho Pharmaceutical, USA.
Miconazole nitrate (p.384·3).
Fungal infections.

Monit Lorex, UK.
Isosorbide mononitrate (p.893·3).
Angina pectoris.

Monitan Wyeth-Ayerst, Canad.
Acebutolol hydrochloride (p.809·3).
Angina pectoris; hypertension.

Monit-Puren Isis Puren, Ger.
Isosorbide mononitrate (p.893·3).
Heart failure; ischaemic heart disease; myocardial infarction; pulmonary hypertension.

Mono Baycuten Bayropharm, Ger.†.
Clotrimazole (p.376·3).
Fungal infections.

Mono Demetrin Godecke, Ger.; Parke, Davis, Ger.
Prazepam (p.687·2).
Anxiety disorders; sleep disorders.

Mono & Disaccharide Free Diet Powder (Product 3232A) Mead Johnson, Austral.
Preparation for enteral nutrition.
Impaired glucose transport; intractable diarrhoea; lactase, sucrase, or maltase deficiency; test for fructose utilisation.

Mono Mack
Pfizer, Aust.; Mack, Illert., Ger.; Mack, Neth.†; Boots, S.Afr.†.
Isosorbide mononitrate (p.893·3).
Angina pectoris; heart failure; myocardial infarction; pulmonary hypertension.

Mono Maycor Parke, Davis, Ger.; Godecke, Ger.
Isosorbide mononitrate (p.893·3).
Cardiac disorders.

Mono Praecimed Molimin, Ger.
Paracetamol (p.72·2).
Fever; pain.

monobeltin Schwarz, Ger.†.
Aspirin (p.16·1).
Thrombo-embolic disorders.

Monobeta Betapharm, Ger.
Isosorbide mononitrate (p.893·3).
Angina pectoris; heart failure.

Monobios CT, Ital.
Cefonicid sodium (p.167·2).
Lignocaine hydrochloride (p.1293·2) is included in this preparation to alleviate the pain of injection.
Bacterial infections.

Monocaps Freeda, USA.
Multivitamin and mineral preparation with iron and folic acid.

Mono-Cedocard
Byk, Neth.; Tillotts, UK.
Isosorbide mononitrate (p.893·3).
Angina pectoris.

Monocete Pedinol, USA†.
Monochloroacetic acid.
Verrucae.

Mono-Chlor Gordon, USA†.
Monochloroacetic acid.
Verrucae.

Monocid
Beecham, Belg.; Procter & Gamble, Ital.; Smith Kline & French, Spain; SmithKline Beecham, USA.
Cefonicid sodium (p.167·2).
Lignocaine hydrochloride (p.1293·2) may be included in the intramuscular injection to alleviate the pain of injection.
Bacterial infections.

Monocilline Andreabal, Switz.
Phenoxymethylpenicillin potassium (p.236·2).
Bacterial infections.

Monocinque Lusofarmaco, Ital.
Isosorbide mononitrate (p.893·3).
Cardiac disorders.

Monoclair Hennig, Ger.
Isosorbide mononitrate (p.893·3).
Cardiac disorders.

Monoclate-P
Centeon, Aust.; Centeon, Ger.; Centeon, Irl.; Rhone-Poulenc Rorer, Spain; Centeon, Swed.; Centeon, UK; Armour, USA.
A factor VIII preparation (p.720·3).
Haemorrhagic disorders.

Monocline Doms-Adrian, Fr.
Doxycycline hydrochloride (p.202·3).
Bacterial infections.

Monocor Lederle, UK.
Bisoprolol fumarate (p.833·1).
Angina pectoris; hypertension.

Monocortin
Grunenthal, Ger.†; Grunenthal, Switz.†.
Paramethasone acetate (p.1047·3).
Corticosteroid.

Monodox Oclassen, USA.
Doxycycline (p.202·3).
Acne.

Monodoxin Crosara, Ital.
Doxycycline hydrochloride (p.202·3).
Bacterial infections.

Monodral Sanofi Winthrop, Austral.†.
Penthienate bromide (p.466·3).
Gastro-intestinal disorders.

Monodur Astra, Austral.
Isosorbide mononitrate (p.893·3).
Angina pectoris.

Mono-Embolex NM Sandoz, Ger.
Certoparin sodium (p.839·1).
Postoperative thrombosis prophylaxis.

Monofed Garec, S.Afr.
Pseudoephedrine hydrochloride (p.1068·3).
Upper respiratory-tract congestion.

Monofeme Wyeth, Austral.
21 Tablets, ethinyloestradiol (p.1445·1); levonorgestrel (p.1454·1); 7 tablets, inert.
Combined oral contraceptive.

Monoflam Lichtenstein, Ger.
Diclofenac sodium (p.31·2).
Gout; inflammation; musculoskeletal and joint disorders; neuralgia; neuritis; pain.

Monofoscin CEPA, Spain.
Fosfomycin trometamol (p.210·2).
Enterocolitis; staphylococcal infections; urinary-tract infections.

Monogen Scientific Hospital Supplies, UK.
Preparation for enteral nutrition.
Lipid and lymphatic disorders.

Mono-Gesic Schwarz, USA.
Salsalate (p.83·1).
Fever; osteoarthritis; pain; rheumatoid arthritis.

Monogestin Wyeth Lederle, Aust.
Gestodene (p.1447·2); ethinyloestradiol (p.1445·1).
Combined oral contraceptive.

mono-glycocard RAN, Ger.†.
Digitoxin (p.848·3).
Cardiac disorders.

Monohaem Bayer Diagnostics, Austral.†.
Test for occult blood in faeces.

mono-Hepagrisevit Farmitalia Carlo Erba, Ger.†.
Cyanocobalamin (p.1363·3); folic acid (p.1340·3); nicotinamide (p.1351·2); lignocaine hydrochloride (p.1293·2).
Liver disorders.

Monoket
Gebro, Aust.; Chiesi, Ital.; Pharmacia Upjohn, Norw.; Pharmacia Upjohn, Swed.; Schwarz, USA.
Isosorbide mononitrate (p.893·3).
Angina pectoris; heart failure; myocardial infarction; pulmonary hypertension.

Mono-Latex Wampole, USA.
Test for infectious mononucleosis.

Monolong Isis, Ger.
Isosorbide mononitrate (p.893·3).
Coronary heart disease; heart failure.

Monomax Trinity, UK.
Isosorbide mononitrate (p.893·3).
Angina pectoris.

Monomycin
Grunenthal, Aust.; Grunenthal, Ger.
Erythromycin (p.204·1) or erythromycin ethyl succinate (p.204·2).
Bacterial infections.

Monomycine Grunenthal, Switz.
Erythromycin ethyl succinate (p.204·2).
Bacterial infections.

Mononine
Centeon, Ger.; Centeon, Irl.; Centeon, Ital.; Centeon, Spain; Urgentum, Swed.; Centeon, UK; Armour, USA.
A factor IX preparation (p.721·3).
Haemophilia B.

Monoparin
CP Pharmaceuticals, Irl.; CP Pharmaceuticals, UK.
Heparin calcium (p.879·3) or heparin sodium (p.879·3).
Thrombo-embolic disorders.

Monopina Bioindustria, Ital.
Amlodipine besylate (p.822·3).
Angina pectoris; hypertension.

Monopress Bayer, Spain.
Nitrendipine (p.923·1).
Angina pectoris; hypertension; Raynaud's syndrome.

Monopril
Bristol-Myers Squibb, Austral.; Bristol-Myers Squibb, Canad.; Bristol-Myers Squibb, S.Afr.; Bristol-Myers Squibb, Swed.; Bristol-Myers Squibb, USA.
Fosinopril sodium (p.870·3).
Heart failure; hypertension.

Monopril comp Bristol-Myers Squibb, Swed.
Fosinopril sodium (p.870·3); hydrochlorothiazide (p.885·2).
Hypertension.

Monoprim Hafslund Nycomed, Aust.
Trimethoprim (p.265·1).
Urinary and respiratory-tract bacterial infections.

Monopur Pohl, Ger.
Isosorbide mononitrate (p.893·3).
Cardiac disorders.

Monores Valeas, Ital.
Clenbuterol hydrochloride (p.752·1).
Obstructive airways disease.

Monos Selvi, Ital.
Rufloxacin hydrochloride.
Bacterial infections.

Monosorb Dexcel, UK.
Isosorbide mononitrate (p.893·3).
Angina pectoris.

Monostenase Azupharma, Ger.
Isosorbide mononitrate (p.893·3).
Cardiac disorders.

MonoStep Asche, Ger.
Ethinyloestradiol (p.1445·1); levonorgestrel (p.1454·1).
Combined oral contraceptive.

Monostop Delagrange, Spain.
Bifonazole (p.375·3).
Fungal skin and nail infections.

Monotard
Novo Nordisk, Irl.; Novo Nordisk, Neth.; Novo Nordisk, Norw.; Novo Nordisk, Spain; Novo Nordisk, Swed.
Insulin zinc suspension (amorphous 30%, crystalline 70%) (human, monocomponent) (p.322·1).
Formerly known as Human Monotard in *Irl.* and as Monotard HM in *Spain*.
Diabetes mellitus.

Monotard HM
Novo Nordisk, Aust.; Novo Nordisk, Austral.; Novo Nordisk, Belg.;

Novo Nordisk, Fr.; Novo Nordisk, Ger.; Novo Nordisk, Ital.; Novo Nordisk, S.Afr.; Novo Nordisk, Switz.
Insulin zinc suspension (amorphous 30%, crystalline 70%) (human, monocomponent) (p.322·1).
Diabetes mellitus.

Monotest Serotherapeutisches, Aust.; Merieux, Fr.; Pasteur Merieux, Ital.; Rhone-Poulenc Rorer, S.Afr.; Pasteur Merieux, Swed.; Merieux, Switz.†.
Tuberculin PPD (p.1640·2).
Sensitivity test.

Mono-Tildiem Synthelabo, Fr.
Diltiazem hydrochloride (p.854·2).
Angina pectoris; hypertension.

Monotrean
Note. This name is used for preparations of different composition.
Luitpold, Ger.
Dimenhydrinate (p.408·2).
Formerly contained quinine hydrochloride and papaverine.
Dizziness; nausea; vomiting.

Luitpold, Ital.; Luitpold, Switz.†.
Papaverine (p.1614·2); quinine hydrochloride (p.439·2).
Cerebrovascular disorders; Ménière's disease; nocturnal cramps; vertigo.

Mono-Tridin Opfermann, Ger.
Sodium monofluorophosphate (p.743·3).
Osteoporosis.

Monotrim Solvay, Irl.; Gea, Neth.†; Mono, S.Afr.†; Gea, Switz.; Solvay, UK.
Trimethoprim (p.265·1) or trimethoprim lactate (p.266·2).
Bacterial infections.

Mono-Trimedil Zyma, Ger.†.
Paracetamol (p.72·2).
Fever; pain.

Monotussin Beige, S.Afr.
Codeine phosphate (p.26·1); mepyramine maleate (p.414·1); ephedrine hydrochloride (p.1059·3).
Coughs.

Monovacc-Test Pasteur Merieux, Belg.; Connaught, USA.
Old tuberculin (p.1640·2).
Test for tuberculin sensitivity.

Monovax Merieux, Fr.
A BCG vaccine (p.1504·3).
Active immunisation.

Monovent Lagap, UK.
Terbutaline sulphate (p.764·1).
Premature labour; reversible airways obstruction.

Mono-Wolff Wolff, Ger.
Isosorbide mononitrate (p.893·3).
Cardiac disorders.

Monozide Lederle, UK.
Bisoprolol fumarate (p.833·1); hydrochlorothiazide (p.885·2).
Hypertension.

Monphytol Laboratories for Applied Biology, Irl.; Laboratories for Applied Biology, UK.
Methyl undecenoate (p.389·2); propyl undecenoate (p.389·2); salicylic acid (p.1090·2); methyl salicylate (p.55·2); propyl salicylate; chlorbutol (p.1106·3).
Fungal skin and nail infections.

Montalen Pharmonta, Aust.
Magnesium trisilicate (p.1199·1); aluminium hydroxide (p.1177·3); peppermint oil (p.1208·1).
Gastro-intestinal disorders associated with hyperacidity.

Montamed Montavit, Aust.
Salverine hydrochloride (p.1627·2); propyphenazone (p.81·3); caffeine (p.749·3).
Pain.

Montana
Note. This name is used for preparations of different composition.
Pharmonta, Aust.
Lupulus (p.1597·2); gentian (p.1583·3); cinnamon (p.1564·2); bitter-orange peel (p.1610·3); caraway (p.1559·3); taraxacum (p.1634·2); peppermint oil (p.1208·1); pterocarpus santalinus.
Gastro-intestinal disorders.

EGS, Ger.
Juniper (p.1592·2); caraway (p.1559·3); cardamom (p.1560·1); bitter-orange peel; cinnamon (p.1564·2); peppermint oil (p.1208·1); senna (p.1212·2); menyanthes (p.1601·2); pterocarpus santalinus; sassafras; centaury (p.1561·1); absinthium (p.1541·1); calamus (p.1556·1); gentian (p.1583·3); valerian (p.1643·1); rhubarb (p.1212·1); sarsaparilla (p.1627·2); aloes (p.1177·1).
Gastro-intestinal disorders.

Montavon Aerocid, Fr.
Pilocarpine nitrate (p.1396·3); antimony potassium tartrate (p.98·1).
Alcohol withdrawal syndrome.

Montricin Prospa, Belg.; SPA, Ital.
Mepartricin sodium lauryl sulphate (p.384·2).
Fungal infections.

Monuril Strallhofer, Aust.; Madaus, Belg.; Zambon, Fr.; Madaus, Ger.; Pharmax, Irl.; Zambon, Ital.; Zambon, Neth.; Inpharzam, Switz.; Pharmax, UK†.
Fosfomycin trometamol (p.210·2).
Urinary-tract infections.

Monurol Pharmazam, Spain; Forest Pharmaceuticals, USA.
Fosfomycin trometamol (p.210·2).
Enterocolitis; staphylococcal infections; urinary-tract infections.

Monydrin Tika, Norw.; Tika, Swed.
Phenylpropanolamine hydrochloride (p.1067·2).
Rhinitis.

Monzal Thomae, Ger.†.
Vetrabutine hydrochloride (p.1644·1).
Facilitates parturition.

Moorbad-Saar N CPF, Ger.
Salicylic acid (p.1090·2); sodium humate.
Bath additive; gynaecological disorders; musculoskeletal and joint disorders; neuralgia.

Moorhumin Torfwerk Einfeld, Ger.†.
Peat.
Bath additive; eczema; gynaecological disorders; rheumatism.

Moorland Torbet Laboratories, UK.
Bismuth aluminate (p.1180·1); magnesium trisilicate (p.1199·1); dried aluminium hydroxide gel (p.1177·3); heavy magnesium carbonate (p.1198·1); light kaolin (p.1195·1); calcium carbonate (p.1182·1).
Dyspepsia.

Moorlauge Bastian Bastian, Ger.
Medicinal mud.
Bath additive; rheumatic disorders.

Moorocoll Sagitta, Ger.†; Schonenberger, Switz.†.
Peat.
Bath additive; circulatory disorders; gynaecological disorders; musculoskeletal and joint disorders.

Moorparaffin Bastian Bastian, Ger.†.
Peat.
Neuritis; rheumatism.

Mopen FIRMA, Ital.
Amoxycillin trihydrate (p.151·3).
Bacterial infections.

Mopral Astra, Fr.; Astra, Spain.
Omeprazole (p.1204·2) or omeprazole sodium (p.1204·2).
Gastro-oesophageal reflux; peptic ulcer; Zollinger-Ellison syndrome.

Mopsoralen Wolfs, Belg.
Methoxsalen (p.1086·3).
Mycosis fungoides; psoriasis; vitiligo.

Moradorm Bouhon, Ger.
Valerian (p.1643·1); passion flower (p.1615·3); diphenhydramine hydrochloride (p.409·1).
Nervousness; sleep disorders.

Moradorm S Bouhon, Ger.
Valerian (p.1643·1); passion flower (p.1615·3); lupulus (p.1597·2).
Nervous disorders; sleep disorders.

Moradorm-A Bouhon, Ger.†.
Diphenhydramine hydrochloride (p.409·1).
Sleep disorders.

Morapid Mundipharma, Aust.
Morphine sulphate (p.56·2).
Pain.

Moraten Berna, Ital.; Swisspharm, S.Afr.; Berna, Spain†; Berna, Switz.
A measles vaccine (attenuated Edmonston-Zagreb strain) (p.1517·3).
Active immunisation.

Morbil Biagini, Ital.
A measles immunoglobulin (p.1517·3).
Passive immunisation.

Morbilvax Biocine, Ital.; Biovac, S.Afr.
A measles vaccine (attenuated Schwarz strain) (p.1517·3).
Active immunisation.

Morbulin Immuno, Ital.†.
A measles immunoglobulin (p.1517·3).
Passive immunisation.

Morcap Faulding, UK.
Morphine sulphate (p.56·2).
Pain.

Morde X Vitafarma, Spain.
Alcohol (p.1099·1); sucrose octa-acetate (p.1633·2).
Nail biting.

MoreDophilus Freeda, USA.
Acidophilus-carrot derivative (p.1594·1).
Dietary supplement.

Morfina Miro Palex, Spain†.
Morphine hydrochloride (p.56·1).
Dyspnoea; pain; premedication.

Morfina Serra Serra Pamies, Spain.
Morphine hydrochloride (p.56·1).
Dyspnoea; pain; premedication.

Morgenxil Llorente, Spain.
Amoxycillin trihydrate (p.151·3).
Bacterial infections.

Morhulin Seton, Irl.; Seton, UK.
Cod-liver oil (p.1337·3); zinc oxide (p.1096·2).
Skin disorders.

Morniflu Master Pharma, Ital.
Morniflumate (p.56·1).
Fever; inflammation; pain.

Moronal Bristol-Myers Squibb, Ger.
Nystatin (p.386·1).
Fungal infections.
Combination pack†: 1 Tablet, nystatin (p.386·1); 1 pessary, nystatin; ointment, nystatin; triamcinolone acetonide (p.1050·2).
Vaginal candidiasis.

Moronal V Bristol-Myers Squibb, Ger.
Nystatin (p.386·1); triamcinolone acetonide (p.1050·2).
Skin disorders with fungal infection.

Moronal V N Bristol-Myers Squibb, Ger.†.
Nystatin (p.386·1); triamcinolone acetonide (p.1050·2).
Skin disorders with fungal infection.

Morphalgin Fawns & McAllan, Austral.
Morphine hydrochloride (p.56·1); aspirin (p.16·1).
Pain.

Morphitec Technilab, Canad.
Morphine hydrochloride (p.56·1).
Pain.

Morrhulan Streuli, Switz.
Cod-liver oil (p.1337·3).
Minor skin lesions.

Morsep Napp, Irl.†; Napp, UK†.
Cetrimide (p.1105·2); vitamin A palmitate (p.1359·2); ergocalciferol (p.1367·1).
Sore skin conditions.

Morstel Clonmel, Irl.
Morphine sulphate (p.56·2).
Pain.

Mortha Woods, Austral.†.
Morphine sulphate (p.56·2); tacrine hydrochloride (p.1399·1).
Pain.

Morton Salt Substitute Morton Salt, USA.
Low sodium dietary salt substitute.

Morubel Biocine, Ital.†.
A measles and rubella vaccine (Schwarz and Wistar RA 27/3 strains respectively) (p.1519·2).
Active immunisation.

Moruman Berna, Ital.; Berna, Switz.
A measles immunoglobulin (p.1517·3).
Passive immunisation.

Morupar Biocine, Ital.
A measles, mumps, and rubella vaccine (Schwarz, Wistar RA 27/3, and Urabe AM9 strains, respectively) (p.1519·3).
Active immunisation.

MoRu-Viraten Berna, Canad.
A measles and rubella vaccine (p.1519·2).
Active immunisation.

MOS ICN, Canad.
Morphine hydrochloride (p.56·1) or morphine sulphate (p.56·2).
Pain.

Mosaro Klinge, Aust.†.
Kawain (p.1592·3).
Nervous disorders.

Mosco Medtech, Canad.; Medtech, USA.
Salicylic acid (p.1090·2).
Hyperkeratosis.

Moscontin Asta Medica, Fr.
Morphine sulphate (p.56·2).
Pain.

Mosegor Wander, Belg.†; Wander, Ger.; Sandoz, Spain; Sandoz, Switz.
Pizotifen malate (p.449·1).
Anorexia; migraine; tonic.

Mosil
Note. This name is used for preparations of different composition.
Menarini, Fr.
Midecamycin acetate (p.226·2).
Bacterial infections.

Fournier SA, Spain†.
Almasilate (p.1177·1).
Gastro-intestinal hyperacidity.

Moskill SCT, Ital.†.
Pyrethrum (p.1410·1).
Insecticide.

Mostarina Pharmacia, Spain†.
Prednimustine (p.559·2).
Malignant neoplasms.

Mostazola Byly, Spain†.
Camphor (p.1557·2); capsicum oleoresin; lavender oil (p.1594·3); methyl salicylate (p.55·2); mustard oil (p.1605·3); turpentine oil (p.1641·1).
Soft-tissue and muscular disorders; upper-respiratory-tract disorders.

Motens Boehringer Ingelheim, Belg.; Boehringer Ingelheim, Neth.; Boehringer Ingelheim, Spain; Boehringer Ingelheim, Switz.; Boehringer Ingelheim, UK.
Lacidipine (p.897·1).
Hypertension.

Mother's and Children's Vitamin Drops Houghs Healthcare, UK.
Vitamins A, C, and D.

Motherwort Compound Gerard House, UK.
Passion flower (p.1615·3); motherwort (p.1604·2); lime flowers (p.1637·3).
Stresses and strains.

Motiax Neopharmed, Ital.
Famotidine (p.1192·1).
Gastro-oesophageal reflux; peptic ulcer; Zollinger-Ellison syndrome.

Motifene Panpharma, UK.
Diclofenac sodium (p.31·2).
Inflammation; musculoskeletal and joint disorders; pain.

Motilex Guidotti, Ital.
Clebopride malate (p.1188·2).
Gastro-intestinal disorders.

Motilium Janssen-Cilag, Aust.; Janssen-Cilag, Austral.; Janssen-Cilag, Belg.; Janssen-Ortho, Canad.; Janssen-Cilag, Fr.; Byk Gulden, Ger.; Janssen-Cilag, Irl.; Janssen-Cilag, Ital.; Janssen-Cilag, Neth.; Janssen-Cilag, S.Afr.; Esteve, Spain; Janssen-Cilag, Switz.; Sanofi Winthrop, UK.
Domperidone (p.1190·3) or domperidone maleate (p.1191·1).
Gastro-intestinal disorders.

Motipress Bristol-Myers Squibb, Irl.; Sanofi Winthrop, UK.
Fluphenazine hydrochloride (p.671·3); nortriptyline hydrochloride (p.300·2).
Mixed anxiety depressive states.

Motival Sanofi Winthrop, Fr.; Bristol-Myers Squibb, Irl.; Bristol-Myers Squibb, S.Afr.; Sanofi Winthrop, UK.
Fluphenazine hydrochloride (p.671·3); nortriptyline hydrochloride (p.300·2).
Mixed anxiety depressive states.

Motivan Faes, Spain.
Paroxetine hydrochloride (p.301·2).
Depression.

Motofen Carnrick, USA.
Difenoxin hydrochloride (p.1188·3).
Atropine sulphate (p.455·1) is included in this preparation to discourage abuse.
Diarrhoea.

Motolon Labatec, Switz.†.
Methaqualone (p.678·3); diphenhydramine hydrochloride (p.409·1).
Sedative; sleep disorders.

Motosol Europharma, Spain.
Ambroxol hydrochloride (p.1054·3).
Respiratory-tract disorders.

Motozina Biomedica, Ital.
Dimenhydrinate (p.408·2).
Formerly contained cyclizine hydrochloride.
Motion sickness.

Motrim Lannacher, Aust.
Trimethoprim (p.265·1).
Bacterial infections.

Motrin Pharmacia Upjohn, Belg.; McNeil Consumer, Canad.; Pharmacia Upjohn, Canad.; Pharmacia Upjohn, Switz.; Pharmacia Upjohn, UK; McNeil Consumer, USA; Upjohn, USA.
Ibuprofen (p.44·1).
Formerly known as Pediaprofen in the *USA*.
Fever; gout; inflammation; musculoskeletal, joint, and peri-articular disorders; oedema; pain.

Motrin IB Sinus Upjohn, USA.
Pseudoephedrine hydrochloride (p.1068·3); ibuprofen (p.44·1).

Mousticreme Sterling Midy, Fr.†.
Parethoxycaine hydrochloride (p.1298·2); dimethyl phthalate (p.1405·3).
Mosquito bites.

Mouth Gel Numark, UK†.
Lignocaine hydrochloride (p.1293·2).

MouthKote Parnell, USA.
Artificial saliva.

MouthKote F/R Parnell, USA.
Sodium fluoride (p.742·1).

MouthKote O/R Unimed, USA.
Oral rinse: Benzyl alcohol (p.1103·3); menthol (p.1600·2).
Topical solution: Cetylpyridinium chloride (p.1106·2); diphenhydramine (p.409·1).
Sore throat.

MouthKote P/R Unimed, USA.
Ointment: Diphenhydramine hydrochloride (p.409·1).
Oral lesions.
Topical solution: Diphenhydramine (p.409·1); cetylpyridinium chloride (p.1106·2).
Minor mouth or throat irritation.

Mouthrinse Arjo, Canad.
Cetylpyridinium chloride (p.1106·2); sodium benzoate (p.1102·3).
Mouth and throat disorders; oral hygiene.

Mouthwash National Care, Canad.
Cetylpyridinium chloride (p.1106·2).

Mouthwash Antiseptic & Gargle Lander, Canad.
Alcohol (p.1099·1); eucalyptus oil (p.1578·1); menthol (p.1600·2); thymol (p.1127·1).
Oral hygiene.

Mouthwash & Gargle Scott, Canad.
Cetylpyridinium chloride (p.1106·2); domiphen bromide (p.1112·3).

Mouthwash Mint/Peppermint Lander, Canad.
Cetylpyridinium chloride (p.1106·2); domiphen bromide (p.1112·3).

Mova Nitrat Lindopharm, Ger.
Silver nitrate (p.1629·2).
Eye disorders.

Movalis
Bender, Aust.; Boehringer Ingelheim, Spain.
Meloxicam (p.52·1).
Musculoskeletal and joint disorders.

Movecil Carlo Erba, Ital.†.
Pyricarbate (p.1624·1).
Vascular disorders.

Movelat
Sankyo, Austral.; Panpharma, UK.
A heparinoid (p.882·3); salicylic acid (p.1090·2).
Formerly contained a heparinoid, adrenocortical extract, and salicylic acid in the *UK*.
Musculoskeletal and joint pain; sprains; strains.

Movens Inverni della Beffa, Ital.
Meclofenamate sodium (p.51·1) or meclofenamic acid (p.51·2).
Musculoskeletal and joint disorders; pain.

Mover Mitsubishi, Jpn.
Actarit (p.12·2).
Rheumatoid arthritis.

Movergan Orion, Ger.
Selegiline hydrochloride (p.1144·2).
Parkinsonism.

Movicard Ravensberg, Ger.
Oral drops: Magnesium aspartate (p.1157·2); potassium aspartate (p.1161·3); troxerutin (p.1580·2).
Tablets†: Magnesium aspartate (p.1157·2); potassium aspartate (p.1161·3); adenosine triphosphate disodium salt (p.1543·2); troxerutin (p.1580·2); mistletoe (p.1604·1); crataegus (p.1568·2).
Cardiovascular disorders.

Movicol
Norgine, Fr.; Norgine, Ger.; Norgine, Ital.; Norgine, S.Afr.; Norgine, UK.
Macrogol 3350 (p.1598·2); electrolytes (p.1147·1).
Constipation; faecal impaction.

Movicox Boehringer Ingelheim, Neth.
Meloxicam (p.52·1).
Osteoarthritis; rheumatoid arthritis.

Moviflex
Kwizda, Aust.; Luitpold, Switz.
Phenylephrine hydrochloride (p.1066·2); a heparinoid (p.882·3); glycol salicylate (p.43·1).
Musculoskeletal, joint, peri-articular, and soft-tissue disorders.

Movilat Alfarma, Spain.
A heparinoid (p.882·3); salicylic acid (p.1090·2); suprarenal extract (p.1050·1).
Rheumatic and muscular pain.

Movilisin Alfarma, Spain.
Flufenamic acid (p.41·3); a heparinoid (p.882·3); glycol salicylate (p.43·1) or salicylic acid (p.1090·2).
Myalgia; peri-articular disorders; soft-tissue disorders.

Moxacef
Note. This name is used for preparations of different composition.
Bristol-Myers Squibb, Belg.; Bristol-Myers Squibb, Neth.†.
Cefadroxil (p.163·3).
Bacterial infections.

Pulitzer, Ital.†.
Latamoxef disodium (p.221·2).
Gram-negative bacterial infections.

Moxacin
Note. This name is used for preparations of different composition.
CSL, Austral.
Amoxycillin sodium (p.151·3) or amoxycillin trihydrate (p.151·3).
Bacterial infections.

Ibirn, Ital.†.
Amoxycillin trihydrate (p.151·3); fosfomycin calcium (p.210·2).
Bacterial infections.

Moxalactam
Lilly, Fr.†; Lilly, Ger.†.
Latamoxef disodium (p.221·2).
Bacterial infections.

Moxaline Bristol-Myers Squibb, Belg.†.
Amoxycillin trihydrate (p.151·3).
Bacterial infections.

Moxan Garec, S.Afr.
Amoxycillin (p.151·3).
Bacterial infections.

Moxatres Radiumfarma, Ital.†.
Latamoxef disodium (p.221·2).
Gram-negative bacterial infections.

Moxipin Rottapharm, Spain†.
Amoxycillin trihydrate (p.151·3).
Bacterial infections.

Moxipin Mucolitico Rottapharm, Spain†.
Amoxycillin trihydrate (p.151·3); bromhexine hydrochloride (p.1055·3).
Respiratory-tract infections.

Moxiprim Zambon, Ital.†.
Fosfomycin (p.210·1); amoxycillin (p.151·3).
Bacterial infections.

Moxiral Pharmacia Upjohn, Aust.
Minoxidil (p.910·3).
Alopecia androgenetica.

Moxydar Serozym, Fr.
Aluminium hydroxide (p.1177·3); magnesium hydroxide (p.1198·2); aluminium phosphate (p.1178·3); guar gum (p.321·3).
Gastro-intestinal disorders.

Moxymax Parke-Med, S.Afr.
Amoxycillin (p.151·3).
Bacterial infections.

Moxypen Lennon, S.Afr.
Amoxycillin trihydrate (p.151·3).
Bacterial infections.

MPA Hexal, Ger.
Medroxyprogesterone acetate (p.1448·3).
Malignant neoplasms.

M-P-Cil Brovar, S.Afr.†.
Ampicillin trihydrate (p.153·2).
Bacterial infections.

M-Prednisol Pasadena, USA.
Methylprednisolone acetate (p.1046·1).
Corticosteroid.

Mr. Multy Vitalia, UK.
Multivitamin and mineral preparation.

Mrs Cullen's Powders Cullen & Davison, UK.
Aspirin (p.16·1); caffeine (p.749·3).
Fever; pain.

MRV Stallergenes, Switz.†.
Staphylococcus aureus; *Staphylococcus albus*; streptococci; *Diplococcus pneumoniae*; *Moraxella (Branhamella) catarrhalis*; *Klebsiella pneumoniae*; *Haemophilus influenzae*.
Respiratory-tract infections.

M-R-Vax II Merck Sharp & Dohme, USA.
A measles and rubella vaccine (more attenuated Enders' attenuated Edmonston, and Wistar RA 27/3 strains respectively) (p.1519·2).
Active immunisation.

MRX Mahdeen, Canad.
Benzethonium chloride (p.1102·3); camphor (p.1557·2); alcohol (p.1099·1); benzoic acid (p.1102·3).

MS Contin
Pharmacia Upjohn, Austral.; Asta Medica, Belg.; Purdue Frederick, Canad.; Asta Medica, Ital.; Asta Medica, Neth.; Purdue Frederick, USA.
Morphine sulphate (p.56·2).
Pain.

MSI Mundipharma, Ger.
Morphine sulphate (p.56·2).
Pain.

MSIR
Purdue Frederick, Canad.; Purdue Frederick, USA.
Morphine sulphate (p.56·2).
Pain.

MS/L Richwood, USA.
Morphine sulphate (p.56·2).
Pain.

MSR Mundipharma, Ger.
Morphine sulphate (p.56·2).
Pain.

MS/S Richwood, USA.
Morphine sulphate (p.56·2).
Pain.

MST Continus
Mundipharma, Ger.; Napp, Irl.; Adcock Ingram, S.Afr.; Asta Medica, Spain; Mundipharma, Switz.; Napp, UK.
Morphine sulphate (p.56·2).
Pain.

MSTA Connaught, USA.
Mumps skin test (p.1604·3).
Assessment of cell-mediated immunity; detection of delayed hypersensitivity to mumps.

MSUD Aid
Scientific Hospital Supplies, Austral.; Scientific Hospital Supplies, UK.
Food for special diets.
Errors of branched-chain amino acid metabolism; maple syrup urine disease.

MSUD Maxamaid Scientific Hospital Supplies, Austral.
Food for special diets.
Maple syrup urine disease.

MTE Lyphomed, USA.
A range of trace element preparations.
Additive for intravenous total parenteral nutrition solutions.

MTX Hexal, Ger.
Methotrexate sodium (p.547·1).
Arthritis; malignant neoplasms; psoriasis.

Mucabrox Streuli, Switz.
Ambroxol hydrochloride (p.1054·3).
Respiratory-tract disorders associated with increased or viscous mucus.

Mucaderma Merz, Ger.
Zinc oxide (p.1096·2); titanium dioxide (p.1093·3).
Ulcers; wounds.

Mucaine
Whitehall, Austral.; Axcan, Canad.; Wyeth, Irl.; Akromed, S.Afr.; Wyeth, UK.
Aluminium hydroxide (p.1177·3); magnesium hydroxide (p.1198·2); oxethazaine (p.1298·1).
Gastritis; gastro-oesophageal reflux; heartburn; peptic ulcer.

Mucaine 2 in 1 Whitehall, Austral.
Aluminium hydroxide (p.1177·3); magnesium hydroxide (p.1198·2); simethicone (p.1213·1).
Dyspepsia; flatulence.

Mucal
Note. This name is used for preparations of different composition.
Bournonville, Belg.
Aluminium silicate (p.1178·3); magnesium silicate (p.1473·3); calcium silicate (p.1182·2).
Peptic ulcer.

Irex, Fr.
Aluminium sodium silicate (p.1178·3); aluminium magnesium silicate (p.1471·1); aluminium calcium silicate (p.1178·3).
Gastro-intestinal disorders.

OM, Ger.
Aluminium magnesium silicate (p.1471·1); aluminium calcium silicate (p.1178·3).
Gastro-intestinal disorders.

Mucantil Serpero, Ital.
Aerosol; elixir; oral drops: Iodinated glycerol (p.1062·2); phenylpropanolamine hydrochloride (p.1067·2).
Capsules: Iodinated glycerol (p.1062·2); phenylpropanolamine hydrochloride (p.1067·2); peppermint oil (p.1208·1).
Respiratory-tract disorders.

Mucasept-A Merz, Ger.
Isopropyl alcohol (p.1118·2); alcohol (p.1099·1).
Hand disinfection.

Mucedokehl Sanum-Kehlbeck, Ger.
Homoeopathic preparation.

Mucibron Hosbon, Spain.
Ambroxol hydrochloride (p.1054·3).
Respiratory-tract disorders.

Muciclar
Note. This name is used for preparations of different composition.
Parke, Davis, Fr.
Carbocisteine (p.1056·3).
Respiratory-tract congestion.

Piam, Ital.
Ambroxol hydrochloride (p.1054·3).
Respiratory-tract disorders.

Mucidan
Note. This name is used for preparations of different composition.
Solvay, Aust.; Kali-Chemie, Ger.†; Meda, Swed.†.
Tablets: Hexamine calcium thiocyanate (p.216·2); ammonium chloride (p.1055·2); liquorice (p.1197·1).
Coughs; dry mouth or throat.

Kali-Chemie, Ger.†.
Nasal ointment: Hexamine calcium thiocyanate (p.216·2); camphor (p.1557·2); menthol (p.1600·2).
Catarrh; rhinitis.

Mucilar Spirig, Switz.
Ispaghula husk (p.1194·2).
Gastro-intestinal disorders; obesity.

Mucilar Avena Spirig, Switz.
Ispaghula husk (p.1194·2); avena (p.1551·3).
Constipation; obesity.

Mucilax Douglas, Austral.
Ispaghula husk (p.1194·2).
Constipation.

Mucilloid Lalco, Canad.
Ispaghula husk (p.1194·2).

Mucinol Sanofi Winthrop, Ger.
Anethole trithione (p.1549·3).
Dry mouth.

Mucinum
Note. This name is used for preparations of different composition.
Pharmethic, Belg.
Bisacodyl (p.1179·3).
Formerly contained phenolphthalein, senna, cascara, boldo, aniseed, pancreas extract, erepsin, enterokinase, ox bile extract, belladonna, ipomoea resin, and dried magnesium sulphate.
Constipation.

Sabex, Canad.
Phenolphthalein (p.1208·2); senna (p.1212·2).
Constipation.

Innothera, Fr.
Phenolphthalein (p.1208·2); whole bile (p.1553·2); belladonna leaf (p.457·1); senna leaf (p.1212·2); frangula bark (p.1193·2); boldo (p.1554·1); ipomoea (p.1194·2); aniseed (p.1549·3).
Constipation.

Mucinum a l'Extrait de Cascara Innothera, Fr.
Cascara (p.1183·1); senna leaf (p.1212·2); boldo (p.1554·1); aniseed (p.1549·3).
Constipation.

Mucinum Herbal Sabex, Canad.†.
Senna (p.1212·2).
Constipation.

Muciplasma Alcala, Spain.
Methylcellulose (p.1473·3).
Constipation.

Mucipulgite
Ipsen, Belg.; Beaufour, Fr.; Beaufour, Switz.
Activated attapulgite (p.1178·3); guar gum (p.321·3).
Gastro-intestinal disorders.

Mucisol Deca, Ital.
Acetylcysteine (p.1052·3).
Respiratory-tract disorders.

Muciteran Farmasan, Ger.
Acetylcysteine (p.1052·3).
Ear and respiratory-tract disorders associated with increased or viscous mucus.

Mucitux
Riom, Fr.; Recordati, Ital.†.
Eprazinone hydrochloride (p.1060·3).
Respiratory-tract congestion.

Mucivital
Arkopharma, Fr.; Arkofarm, Ital.
Ispaghula husk (p.1194·2).
Constipation; diarrhoea; stool softener.

Muclox Sigma-Tau, Spain.
Famotidine (p.1192·1).
Gastro-oesophageal reflux; peptic ulcer; Zollinger-Ellison syndrome.

Muco4 Sanofi Winthrop, Ital.
Neltenexine (p.1065·1).
Respiratory-tract disorders.

Muco Panoral Lilly, Ger.
Bromhexine hydrochloride (p.1055·3); cefaclor (p.163·2).
Bacterial infections of the respiratory tract.

Muco Sanigen Thiemann, Ger.
Acetylcysteine (p.1052·3).
Respiratory-tract disorders associated with increased or viscous mucus.

Muco Teolixir Biogalenica, Spain†.
Citiolone (p.1564·3); theophylline (p.765·1).
Obstructive airways disease.

Muco-Aspecton Krewel, Ger.
Ambroxol hydrochloride (p.1054·3).
Respiratory-tract disorders associated with increased or viscous mucus.

Mucobene Merckle, Aust.
Acetylcysteine (p.1052·3).
Respiratory-tract disorders associated with viscous mucus.

Mucobron OFF, Ital.
Ambroxol hydrochloride (p.1054·3).
Respiratory-tract disorders.

Mucobronchyl Pharmacal, Switz.
Isoprenaline sulphate (p.892·1); phenylephrine hydrochloride (p.1066·2).
Bronchitis.

Mucobroxol Mundipharma, Ger.
Ambroxol hydrochloride (p.1054·3).
Respiratory-tract disorders associated with increased or viscous mucus.

Mucocaps Roche, S.Afr.
Carbocisteine (p.1056·3).
Respiratory-tract disorders.

Mucocedyl 3M, Ger.
Acetylcysteine (p.1052·3).
Respiratory-tract disorders associated with increased or viscous mucus.

Mucocil Novartis, Neth.
Acetylcysteine (p.1052·3).
Respiratory-tract disorders.

Mucocis Crosara, Ital.
Carbocisteine (p.1056·3).
Respiratory-tract disorders.

Mucocit A Merz, Ger.†.
Propyl alcohol (p.1124·2); glyoxal (p.1115·1); glutaraldehyde (p.1114·3).
Surface disinfection.

Mucoclear Mundipharma, Ger.†.
Ambroxol hydrochloride (p.1054·3).
Respiratory-tract disorders associated with increased or viscous mucus.

Muco-Dest Klus, Switz.
Peppermint oil (p.1208·1); camphor oil.
Nasal disorders.

Mucodil Valeas, Ital.
Stepronin lysine (p.1070·1).
Respiratory-tract disorders.

Mucodyne
Rhone-Poulenc Rorer, Irl.; Nattermann, Neth.; Rorer, UK.
Carbocisteine (p.1056·3).
Respiratory-tract congestion.

Mucofalk Falk, Ger.
Psyllium (p.1194·2).
Gastro-intestinal disorders.

Muco-Fen Wakefield, USA.
Guaiphenesin (p.1061·3).
Coughs.

Muco-Fen-DM Wakefield, USA.
Guaiphenesin (p.1061·3); dextromethorphan hydrobromide (p.1057·3).
Coughs.

Muco-Fen-LA Wakefield, USA.
Guaiphenesin (p.1061·3).
Coughs.

Mucofim Vitalpharma, Belg.†.
Acetylcysteine (p.1052·3).
Respiratory-tract disorders associated with viscous mucus.

Muco-Fips Lichtenstein, Ger.
Ambroxol hydrochloride (p.1054·3).
Respiratory-tract disorders associated with increased or viscous mucus.

Mucoflem Xixia, S.Afr.
Carbocisteine (p.1056·3).
Respiratory-tract disorders.

Mucofluid
Note. This name is used for preparations of different composition.
Bios, Belg.†; UCB, Fr.; UCB, Ger.†; UCB, Ital.; UCB, Spain.
Mesna (p.983·3).
Respiratory-tract disorders.

Spirig, Switz.
Acetylcysteine (p.1052·3).
Respiratory-tract disorders.

Mucofor Vifor, Switz.
Erdosteine (p.1060·3).
Respiratory-tract disorders associated with excess mucus.

Mucogel Pharmax, UK.
Aluminium hydroxide (p.1177·3); magnesium hydroxide (p.1198·2).
These ingredients can be described by the British Approved Name Co-magaldrox.
Gastro-intestinal hyperacidity.

Mucogen *Antigen, Irl.*
Carbocisteine (p.1056·3).
Lower respiratory-tract disorders with excessive or viscous mucus.

Mucojet *Lilly, Ital.*
Carbocisteine (p.1056·3).
Respiratory-tract disorders.

Mucokehl *Sanum-Kehlbeck, Ger.*
Homoeopathic preparation.

Mucolair *3M, Belg.*
Acetylcysteine (p.1052·3).
Adjuvant in respiratory-tract infections.

Mucolase *Lampugnani, Ital.*
Carbocisteine (p.1056·3).
Respiratory-tract disorders.

Mucolator
Labima, Belg.; Abbott, Fr.
Acetylcysteine (p.1052·3).
Paracetamol overdose; respiratory-tract disorders associated with excess or viscous mucus.

Mucolene *Formenti, Ital.*
Mesna (p.983·3).
Respiratory-tract disorders associated with excess or viscous mucus.

Mucoless *Parke-Med, S.Afr.*
Carbocisteine (p.1056·3).
Respiratory-tract disorders.

Mucolex *Parke, Davis, Irl.*
Carbocisteine (p.1056·3).
Respiratory-tract disorders with excessive or viscous mucus.

Mucolinct *Propan, S.Afr.*
Carbocisteine (p.1056·3).
Respiratory-tract disorders.

Mucolitico Maggioni *Sanofi Winthrop, Ital.*
Domiodol (p.1058·3).
Respiratory-tract congestion.

Mucolysin
Farmila, Ital.; Interdelta, Switz.
Tiopronin (p.997·2).
Respiratory-tract disorders.

Mucolysin Antibiotico *Proter, Ital.†.*
Erythromycin (p.204·1); tiopronin sodium (p.997·3).
Respiratory-tract infections.

Mucolyticum "Lappe" *Bristol, Ger.†.*
Acetylcysteine (p.1052·3).
Respiratory-tract disorders associated with increased or viscous mucus.

Mucolytisches Expectorans *SmithKline Beecham, Ger.†.*
Iodinated glycerol (p.1062·2); phenylpropanolamine hydrochloride (p.1067·2).
Respiratory-tract disorders.

Muco-Mepha *Mepha, Switz.*
Acetylcysteine (p.1052·3).
Respiratory-tract disorders associated with increased or viscous mucus.

Mucomist *Bristol, Ital.†.*
Acetylcysteine (p.1052·3).
Respiratory-tract disorders.

Mucomyst
Bristol-Myers Squibb, Aust.; Bristol-Myers Squibb, Austral.; Bristol-Myers Squibb, Belg.; Roberts, Canad.; Bristol-Myers Squibb, Fr.; Bristol-Myers Squibb, Neth.; Astra, Norw.; Draco, Swed.; Apothecon, USA.
Acetylcysteine (p.1052·3) or acetylcysteine sodium (p.1053·1).
Dry eyes; paracetamol poisoning; respiratory-tract disorders.

Muconorm *Prospa, Ital.*
Telmesteine (p.1070·2).
Respiratory-tract disorders.

Mucopan *Propan, S.Afr.*
Carbocisteine (p.1056·3).
Respiratory-tract disorders.

Muco-Perasthman N *Polypharm, Ger.*
Acetylcysteine (p.1052·3).
Respiratory-tract disorders associated with increased or viscous mucus.

Mucophlogat *Azupharma, Ger.*
Ambroxol hydrochloride (p.1054·3).
Respiratory-tract disorders associated with increased or viscous mucus.

Mucoplex *ICN, USA†.*
Vitamin B substances.

Mucoplexil *Theraplix, Fr.*
Carbocisteine (p.1056·3).
Respiratory-tract congestion.

Mucopront
Mack, Illert., Ger.; Madaus, S.Afr.†.
Carbocisteine (p.1056·3) or carbocisteine sodium (p.1056·3).
Respiratory-tract disorders associated with increased or viscous mucus.

Mucorama *Boehringer Mannheim, Spain.*
Phenylpropanolamine hydrochloride (p.1067·2); iodinated glycerol (p.1062·2).
Obstructive airways disease.

Mucorama TS *Pharmalab, Spain.*
Iodinated glycerol (p.1062·2); co-trimoxazole (p.196·3).
Respiratory-tract infections.

Mucorex *Berenguer Infale, Spain.*
Citiolone (p.1564·3).
Respiratory-tract disorders.

Mucorex Ampicilina *Berenguer Infale, Spain.*
Capsules; tablets: Ampicillin (p.153·1); citiolone (p.1564·3).
Injection: Ampicillin sodium (p.153·1); ampicillin benzathine (p.154·1); citiolone (p.1564·3).
Lignocaine hydrochloride (p.1293·2) is included in this preparation to alleviate the pain of injection.
Respiratory-tract infections.

Mucorex Ciclin *Berenguer Infale, Spain.*
Citiolone (p.1564·3); tartaric acid (p.1634·3); tetracycline hydrochloride (p.259·1).
Respiratory-tract infections.

Mucorhinyl *Synthelabo, Belg.*
Phenylephrine hydrochloride (p.1066·2); chlorpheniramine maleate (p.405·1); sulphanilamide (p.256·3).
Rhinitis; rhinopharyngitis; sinusitis.

Mucosan
Note. This name is used for preparations of different composition.
Fher, Spain.
Ambroxol hydrochloride (p.1054·3).
Respiratory-tract disorders.

Resinag, Switz.†.
Aluminium formate; aluminium hydroxide (p.1177·3); cineole (p.1564·1); chamomile (p.1561·2); sage (p.1627·1); arnica (p.1550·3); amethocaine hydrochloride (p.1285·2).
Mouth disorders.

Muco-Sana *Klus, Switz.*
Peppermint oil (p.1208·1); camphor oil; lavender oil (p.1594·3).
Nasal disorders.

Mucoseptal *Actipharm, Switz.*
Carbocisteine (p.1056·3).
Respiratory-tract disorders.

Mucosil *Dey, USA.*
Acetylcysteine sodium (p.1053·1).
Mucolytic in bronchopulmonary disorders.

Mucosirop *Roche, S.Afr.*
Carbocisteine (p.1056·3).
Respiratory-tract disorders.

Mucosodine *Soekami, Fr.†.*
Sodium perborate (p.1125·2); sodium bicarbonate (p.1153·2); sodium chloride (p.1162·2); borax (p.1554·2).
Mouth infections.

Mucosol
Tosi, Ital.†; Be-Tabs, S.Afr.†.
Carbocisteine (p.1056·3).
Respiratory-tract disorders.

Mucosolvan
Bender, Aust.; Thomae, Ger.; Boehringer Ingelheim, Ital.
Ambroxol hydrochloride (p.1054·3).
Respiratory-tract disorders.

Mucosolvon *Boehringer Ingelheim, Switz.*
Ambroxol hydrochloride (p.1054·3).
Respiratory-tract disorders.

Mucospas *Bender, Aust.*
Ambroxol hydrochloride (p.1054·3); clenbuterol hydrochloride (p.752·1).
Respiratory-tract disorders.

Mucospect *Triomed, S.Afr.*
Carbocisteine (p.1056·3).
Respiratory-tract disorders.

Mucosta *Otsuka, Jpn.*
Rebamipide (p.1211·3).
Gastric ulcer; gastritis.

Mucosteine *Medgenix, Belg.*
Carbocisteine (p.1056·3).
Respiratory-tract disorders associated with viscous mucus.

Mucosyt *Bioprogress, Ital.*
Tiopronin (p.997·2).
Respiratory-tract disorders associated with increased or viscous mucus.

Mucotablin *Sanorania, Ger.*
Ambroxol hydrochloride (p.1054·3).
Respiratory-tract disorders associated with increased or viscous mucus.

Muco-Tablinen *Sanorania, Ger.*
Ambroxol hydrochloride (p.1054·3).
Respiratory-tract disorders associated with increased or viscous mucus.

Mucotectan
Bender, Aust.; Thomae, Ger.
Ambroxol hydrochloride (p.1054·3); doxycycline hydrochloride (p.202·3).
Bacterial infections of the respiratory tract.

Mucotherm *Lannacher, Aust.*
Ethyl nicotinate (p.36·1).
Anorectal disorders; prostatitis.

Mucothiol
SCAT, Fr.; Geymonat, Ital.
Methyl diacetylcysteinate (p.1064·1).
Respiratory-tract congestion.

Mucotreis *Ecobi, Ital.*
Carbocisteine (p.1056·3).
Respiratory-tract disorders.

Muco-Trin *Klus, Switz.*
Xylometazoline hydrochloride (p.1071·2); peppermint oil (p.1208·1); camphor oil.
Nasal congestion.

Mucovent *Byk Gulden, Ger.†.*
Ambroxol hydrochloride (p.1054·3).
Respiratory-tract disorders associated with increased or viscous mucus.

Mucovital *Berenguer Infale, Spain.*
Carbocisteine lysine (p.1056·3).
Respiratory-tract congestion.

Mucoxin *Wyeth, Ital.*
Oral suspension: Oxethazaine (p.1298·1); aluminium hydroxide (p.1177·3); magnesium oxide (p.1198·3).
Tablets: Oxethazaine (p.1298·1); algeldrate (p.1177·3); magnesium carbonate (p.1198·1).
Gastro-intestinal disorders associated with hyperacidity.

Mucret
Astra, Aust.; Stern, Ger.
Acetylcysteine (p.1052·3).
Respiratory-tract disorders associated with increased or viscous mucus.

Mu-Cron
Zyma, Irl.; Zyma, UK.
Paracetamol (p.72·2); phenylpropanolamine hydrochloride (p.1067·2).
Catarrh; fever; nasal congestion; sinus pain.

Mu-Cron Junior *Zyma, UK.*
Phenylpropanolamine hydrochloride (p.1067·2); ipecacuanha (p.1062·2).
Nasal congestion.

Mudd Acne *Chattem, Canad.*
Salicylic acid (p.1090·2).
Acne.

Mudrane *ECR, USA.*
Potassium iodide (p.1493·1); aminophylline (p.748·1); phenobarbitone (p.350·2); ephedrine hydrochloride (p.1059·3).
Bronchospasm.

Mudrane-2 *ECR, USA†.*
Potassium iodide (p.1493·1); aminophylline (p.748·1).
Bronchospasm.

Mudrane GG *ECR, USA.*
Elixir†: Guaiphenesin (p.1061·3); theophylline (p.765·1); phenobarbitone (p.350·2); ephedrine hydrochloride (p.1059·3).
Tablets: Guaiphenesin (p.1061·3); aminophylline (p.748·1); phenobarbitone (p.350·2); ephedrine hydrochloride (p.1059·3).
Bronchospasm.

Mudrane GG-2 *ECR, USA.*
Guaiphenesin (p.1061·3); aminophylline (p.748·1).
Bronchospasm.

Mulgatol
Woelm, Ger.
Multivitamin preparation.

Rhone-Poulenc Rorer, S.Afr.†.
Multivitamin and mineral preparation.

Mulgatol Gelee N *Woelm, Ger.*
Multivitamin and mineral preparation.

Mulimen *Fides, Ger.*
Homoeopathic preparation.

Mulkine *Beaufour, Fr.*
Montmorillonite; guar gum (p.321·3).
Constipation.

Mullersche Tabletten *Staufen, Ger.†.*
Homoeopathic preparation.

Mulmicor *Lappe, Ger.*
Camphor (p.1557·2).
Hypotension.

Mulsal A Megadosis *Vitafarma, Spain.*
Vitamin A (p.1358·1).
Skin disorders.

Mulsal N *Mucos, Ger.*
Trypsin (p.1640·1); papain (p.1614·1); bromelain (p.1555·1).
Inflammation; musculoskeletal and joint disorders; oedema.

Multaben *Priorin, Switz.†.*
d-Alpha tocopherol (p.1369·1); wheat-germ oil.
Vitamin E deficiency.

Multene *Clintec, Fr.*
Amino acid preparation.
Parenteral nutrition.

Multe-Pak *SoloPak, USA.*
A range of trace element preparations.
Parenteral nutrition.

Multi-12 *Sabex, Canad.*
A multivitamin preparation.
Parenteral nutrition.

Multi 75 *Fibertone, USA.*
Multivitamin and mineral preparation.

Multi 1000 *Sabex, Canad.*
Multivitamin preparation.
Parenteral nutrition.

Multi B *Seroyal, Canad.*
Vitamin B substances.

Multi B Complex *Quest, UK.*
Vitamin B and C preparation.

Multi Cal-Mag *Seroyal, Canad.*
Vitamin and mineral preparation.

Multi Formula for Men 50+ *Jamieson, Canad.*
Multivitamin and mineral preparation.

Multi Forte 29 *Stanley, Canad.*
Multivitamin and mineral preparation.

Multi II *Solgar, UK.*
Amino-acid, multivitamin, and mineral preparation.

Multi II IV VI *Sisu, Canad.*
Multivitamin and mineral preparation.

Multi Vit Drops with Iron *Barre-National, USA.*
Multivitamin preparation with iron.

Multi for Women *Jamieson, Canad.*
Multivitamin and mineral preparation.

Multi-B Forte *G.P. Laboratories, Austral.*
Vitamin B substances and vitamin C.

Multibionta
Merck, Aust.; Merck, Ger.; E. Merck, Irl.; Merck, S.Afr.†; Merck, Spain; E. Merck, Switz.; E. Merck, UK.
Multivitamin preparation.
Parenteral nutrition.

Multibionta Junior *Merck, Aust.*
Multivitamin preparation with calcium.

Multibionta Mineral *Merck, Spain.*
Multivitamin and mineral preparation.

Multibionta plus Mineral *Merck, Ger.*
Multivitamin and mineral preparation.

Multibionta plus Mineralien *Merck, Aust.*
Multivitamin and mineral preparation.

Multibionta-Eisen *Merck, Ger.†.*
Red-brown capsules, multivitamin preparation with rutoside; green capsules, ferrous succinate (p.1340·2).
Iron and vitamin deficiency; iron-deficiency anaemia.

Multibret Hematinic *Copley, USA†.*
Ferrous sulphate (p.1340·2); vitamin B substances with vitamin C.
Iron-deficiency anaemias.

Multibret-Folic *Copley, USA†.*
Ferrous sulphate (p.1340·2); folic acid (p.1340·3); vitamin B substances with vitamin C.
Iron-deficiency anaemias.

Multicentrum *Whitehall, Ital.*
Vitamin, mineral, and trace-element preparation.
Nutritional supplement.

Multi-Day *Nature's Bounty, USA.*
A range of vitamin preparations.

Multifluorid *DMG, Ger.*
Sodium fluoride (p.742·1); olaflur (p.1610·1); dectaflur (p.1570·2).
Dental caries prophylaxis; hypersensitive teeth.

Multifungin
Note. This name is used for preparations of different composition.
Ebewe, Aust.
Topical powder: Bromochlorosalicylanilide (p.375·3).
Fungal skin and nail infections.

Ebewe, Aust.; Nordmark, Ger.†; Knoll, Irl.†; Knoll, S.Afr.†; Knoll, Spain†.
Bromochlorosalicylanilide (p.375·3); bamipine lactate (p.403·2) or bamipine salicylate (p.403·2).
Fungal skin and nail infections.

Multifungin H *Knoll, Irl.†.*
Bromochlorosalicylanilide (p.375·3); bamipine lactate (p.403·2); hydrocortisone acetate (p.1043·3).
Inflamed fungal skin disorders.

Multiglyco *Seroyal, Canad.*
Vitamin B substances, vitamin C, and minerals.

Multilac *Dieterba, Ital.†.*
Food for special diets.
Milk intolerance.

Multilase *Sigma-Tau, Ital.*
Anistreplase (p.824·2).
Myocardial infarction.

Multilens Solution *Agepha, Aust.*
Disinfection and storage solution for hard contact lenses.

Multilex *Rugby, USA.*
A range of vitamin preparations.

Multilind
Bristol-Myers Squibb, Ger.; Bristol-Myers Squibb, Switz.
Nystatin (p.386·1); zinc oxide (p.1096·2).
Fungal skin infections.

Multiload
Organon, Austral.; Nourypharma, Ger.; Organon, Irl.; Organon, Neth.; Donmed, S.Afr.; Organon, Switz.; Organon, UK.
Copper-wound plastic (p.1337·3).
Intra-uterine contraceptive device.

Multilyte *Lyphomed, USA.*
A range of electrolyte preparations (p.1147·1).
Fluid and electrolyte disorders.

Multi-min *Neo-Life, Austral.*
Mineral and trace element preparation.

Multi-Mins *Seroyal, Canad.*
Mineral preparation.

Multi-Mulsin N *Mucos, Ger.*
Multivitamin preparation.

Multiparin
CP Pharmaceuticals, Irl.; CP Pharmaceuticals, UK.
Heparin sodium (p.879·3).
Thrombo-embolic disorders.

Multipax *Rhone-Poulenc Rorer, Canad.*
Hydroxyzine hydrochloride (p.412·1).
Anxiety.

Multi-Phyto *Pharmavite, Canad.*
Multivitamin and mineral preparation.

Multiplex 1 *Plantina, Ger.†.*
Homoeopathic preparation.

Multiron *Vitabiotics, UK.*
Multivitamin and mineral preparation.

Multi-Sanasol *Vifor, Switz.*
Multivitamin and mineral preparation.

Multi-Sanostol *Roland, Ger.*
Multivitamin and mineral preparation.

Multi-Sanosvit mit Eisen Roland, Ger.
Multivitamin preparation with minerals including iron.

Multisoy Dieterba, Ital.
Infant feed.
Milk intolerance.

Multistix
Bayer Diagnostics, Austral.; Bayer, Canad.; Bayer Diagnostici, Ital.; Bayer, USA.
Test for glucose, protein, blood, ketones, bilirubin, urobilinogen, and pH in urine.

Multistix 2
Bayer, Canad.; Miles, Ital.†; Bayer, USA.
Test for nitrites and leucocytes in urine.

Multistix 5
Bayer Diagnostics, Austral.; Bayer, Canad.
Test for glucose, blood, protein, nitrites, and leucocytes in urine.

Multistix 7
Bayer Diagnostics, Austral.; Bayer, USA.
Test for glucose, protein, blood, ketones, nitrites, leucocytes, and pH in urine.

Multistix 9
Bayer Diagnostics, Austral.; Ames, S.Afr.; Bayer, USA.
Test for pH, protein, glucose, ketones, bilirubin, blood, urobilinogen, nitrites, and leucocytes in urine.

Multistix GP Bayer Diagnostics, UK.
Test for specific gravity, pH, protein, glucose, ketones, blood, nitrites, and leucocytes in urine.

Multistix SG
Bayer Diagnostics, Austral.; Bayer, Canad.; Ames, Irl.; Ames, S.Afr.; Bayer Diagnostics, UK; Bayer, USA.
Test for pH, protein, glucose, ketones, bilirubin, blood, urobilinogen, and specific gravity in urine.

Multistix 8 SG
Bayer, Canad.; Bayer Diagnostics, Fr.; Bayer Diagnostics, UK; Bayer, USA.
Test for glucose, protein, blood, ketones, nitrites, leucocytes, pH, and specific gravity in urine.

Multistix 9 SG Bayer, USA.
Test for glucose, protein, blood, ketones, bilirubin, nitrites, leucocytes, pH, and specific gravity in urine.

Multistix 10 SG
Bayer Diagnostics, Austral.; Bayer, Canad.; Bayer Diagnostics, Fr.; Ames, Irl.; Bayer Diagnostici, Ital.; Ames, S.Afr.; Bayer Diagnostics, UK; Bayer, USA.
Test for pH, protein, glucose, ketones, bilirubin, blood, urobilinogen, nitrites, leucocytes, and specific gravity in urine.

Multi-Symptom Tylenol Cold McNeil Consumer, USA.
Chlorpheniramine maleate (p.405·1); dextromethorphan hydrobromide (p.1057·3); paracetamol (p.72·2); pseudoephedrine hydrochloride (p.1068·3).
Coughs and cold symptoms.

Multi-Symptom Tylenol Cough McNeil Consumer, USA.
Dextromethorphan hydrobromide (p.1057·3); paracetamol (p.72·2).
Formerly known as Maximum Strength Tylenol Cough.
Coughs.

Multi-Symptom Tylenol Cough with Decongestant McNeil Consumer, USA.
Pseudoephedrine hydrochloride (p.1068·3); dextromethorphan hydrobromide (p.1057·3); paracetamol (p.72·2).
Formerly known as Maximum Strength Tylenol Cough with Decongestant.
Coughs and cold symptoms.

Multi-Tar Plus ICN, Canad.
Cade oil (p.1092·2); tar (p.1092·3); coal tar (p.1092·3); pyrithione zinc (p.1089·3).
Seborrhoeic dermatitis.

Multitest
Serotherapeutisches, Aust.; Pasteur Merieux, Belg.; Pasteur Merieux, Ger.
Tetanus antigen; diphtheria antigen; streptococcus antigen; tuberculin antigen (p.1640·2); candida albicans antigen; trichophyton antigen; proteus mirabilis antigen.
Assessment of cell-mediated immunity.

Multitest CMI
CSL, Austral.; Connaught, Canad.; Imtix, Neth.; Rhone-Poulenc Rorer, S.Afr.; Connaught, USA.
Tetanus antigen; diphtheria antigen; streptococcus antigen; tuberculin antigen (p.1640·2); candida albicans antigen; trichophyton antigen; proteus mirabilis antigen.
Assessment of cell-mediated immunity.

Multitest IMC
Imtix, Fr.; Imtix, Ital.; Rhone-Poulenc Rorer, Spain; Merieux, Switz.†.
Tetanus antigen; diphtheria antigen; streptococcus antigen; tuberculin antigen (p.1640·2); candida albicans antigen; trichophyton antigen; proteus mirabilis antigen.
Assessment of cell-mediated immunity.

Multiton Biochimici, Ital.
Multivitamin and mineral preparation.

Multitrace-5 Concentrate American Regent, USA.
Trace element preparation.

Multi-Vi-Min Sisu, Canad.
Multivitamin and mineral preparation.

Multivit Biovital Schieffer, Switz.
Multivitamin and mineral preparation with plant extracts.

Multivitamin Phytopharma V OTW, Ger.
Multivitamin preparation.

Multivitamin-Dragees-Pascoe Pascoe, Ger.
Multivitamin preparation.

Multivitamines Gisand, Switz.
Multivitamin and mineral preparation.

Multivit-B Lannacher, Aust.
Vitamin B substances.

Multi-Vite Seroyal, Canad.
Multivitamin and mineral preparation.

Multivite Plus Duncan, Flockhart, Irl.†.
Ferrous fumarate (p.1339·3); folic acid (p.1340·3); vitamins and calcium.
Prophylaxis of deficiencies during pregnancy.

Multivitol Hermes, Ger.
Multivitamin and mineral preparation.

Multodrin Montavit, Aust.
Dexamethasone (p.1037·1); diphenhydramine hydrochloride (p.409·1).
Skin disorders.

Multojod-Gastreu N R12 Reckeweg, Ger.
Homoeopathic preparation.

Multosin Takeda, Ger.
Estramustine meglumine phosphate or estramustine sodium phosphate (p.532·2).
Prostatic cancer.

Multum
Note. This name is used for preparations of different composition.
Rosen, Ger.
Chlordiazepoxide (p.646·3).
Anxiety disorders; sleep disorders.

Lampugnani, Ital.
Benzydamine hydrochloride (p.21·3).
Gynaecological disorders; mouth and throat disorders; musculoskeletal, joint, peri-articular, and soft-tissue disorders.

Mulvidren-F Softab Stuart, USA.
Sodium fluoride (p.742·1) with multivitamins.
Dental caries prophylaxis in children.

Mumaten
Berna, Ital.; Swisspharm, S.Afr.; Berna, Switz.
A mumps vaccine (attenuated Rubini strain) (p.1521·2).
Active immunisation.

Mumpsvax
Merck Sharp & Dohme, Aust.; CSL, Austral.†; Merck Sharp & Dohme, Belg.†; Merck Sharp & Dohme, Canad.; Chiron Behring, Ger.; Pasteur Merieux, Irl.; Pasteur Merieux, Ital.; Pro Vaccine, Switz.; Pasteur Merieux, UK; Merck Sharp & Dohme, USA.
A mumps vaccine (Jeryl Lynn (B level) strain) (p.1521·2).
Active immunisation.

Munari Chepharin, Aust.†.
Allyl isothiocyanate (p.1605·3); capsicum (p.1559·2); wheat-germ oil; alpha tocopheryl acetate (p.1369·1); kaolin (p.1195·1).
Inflammation; pain.

Mundicycline Mundipharma, Aust.
Doxycycline fosfatex (p.202·3).
Bacterial infections.

Mundidol Mundipharma, Aust.
Morphine sulphate pentahydrate (p.56·2).
Pain.

Mundil Mundipharma, Ger.
Captopril (p.836·3).
Heart failure; hypertension.

Mundiphyllin Mundipharma, Aust.
Aminophylline (p.748·1).
Respiratory-tract disorders.

Mundisal
Mundipharma, Aust.; Mundipharma, Ger.; Mundipharma, Switz.
Choline salicylate (p.25·2); cetalkonium chloride (p.1105·2).
Mouth and throat disorders.

Municaps Schwarzhaupt, Ger.
Multivitamin preparation.
Tonic.

Munitren H Robugen, Ger.
Hydrocortisone (p.1043·3).
Anogenital pruritus; skin disorders.

Munleit Hommel, Ger.
Doxylamine succinate (p.410·1).
Insomnia.

Munobal
Hoechst, Aust.; Hoechst, Ger.; Hoechst Marion Roussel, Switz.
Felodipine (p.867·3).
Angina pectoris; hypertension.

Munvatten Kabi, Swed.†.
Salol (p.83·1); terpineol (p.1635·1); menthol (p.1600·2).
Mouthwash.

Muphoran
Servier, Aust.; Servier, Fr.
Fotemustine (p.538·1).
Cerebral cancer; disseminated malignant melanoma.

Murazyme Prospa, Belg.
Muramidase (p.1604·3).
Herpesvirus infections.

Murelax Wyeth, Austral.
Oxazepam (p.683·2).
Alcohol withdrawal syndrome; anxiety.

Murine
Note. This name is used for preparations of different composition.
Abbott, Austral.
Berberine chloride (p.1553·1).
Sore eyes.

Abbott, Canad.; Ross, USA.
Ear drops: Urea hydrogen peroxide (p.1127·3).
Ear wax removal.

Abbott, Canad.; Ross, USA.
Eye drops: Povidone (p.1474·2); polyvinyl alcohol (p.1474·2).
Dry eyes.

Abbott, UK.
Naphazoline hydrochloride (p.1064·2).
Eye irritation.

Murine Clear Eyes Abbott, S.Afr.
Naphazoline hydrochloride (p.1064·2).
Eye irritation.

Murine Plus Ross, USA.
Polyvinyl alcohol (p.1474·2); povidone (p.1474·2); tetrahydrozoline hydrochloride (p.1070·2).
Minor eye irritation.

Murine Sore Eyes Abbott, Austral.
Tetrahydrozoline hydrochloride (p.1070·2); hypromellose (p.1473·1).
Formerly known as Sore Eyes.
Eye irritation.

Murine Supplemental Tears Abbott, Canad.
Benzalkonium chloride (p.1101·3); disodium edetate (p.980·1).

Muripsin
Norgine, Austral.†; Norgine, UK†.
Glutamic acid hydrochloride (p.1344·3).
Formerly contained pepsin and glutamic acid hydrochloride in the *UK*.
Gastric acid deficiency.

Muro 128
Bausch & Lomb, Canad.; Bausch & Lomb, USA.
Sodium chloride (p.1162·2).
Corneal oedema.

Murocel
Bausch & Lomb, Canad.; Bausch & Lomb, USA.
Methylcellulose (p.1473·3).
Dry eyes.

Murocoll-2 Bausch & Lomb, USA.
Hyoscine hydrobromide (p.462·3); phenylephrine hydrochloride (p.1066·2).
Induction of mydriasis and cycloplegia; uveitis.

Murode ICN, Spain.
Diflorasone diacetate (p.1039·3).
Skin disorders.

Muroptic Optopics, USA.
Sodium chloride (p.1162·2).
Corneal oedema.

Muro's Opcon Bausch & Lomb, USA.
Naphazoline hydrochloride (p.1064·2); hypromellose (p.1473·1).
Minor eye irritation.

Murri Antidolorifico Bracco, Ital.
Aspirin (p.16·1); paracetamol (p.72·2); caffeine (p.749·3).
Fever; pain.

Musapam Krewel, Ger.
Tetrazepam (p.694·3).
Skeletal muscle tension and spasm.

Musaril Sanofi Winthrop, Ger.
Tetrazepam (p.694·3).
Skeletal muscle spasm.

Muscalm Kayaku, Jpn†.
Tolperisone hydrochloride (p.1322·2).
Muscle relaxant; muscle tension; spastic paralysis.

Muscaran Christiaens, Belg.
Bethanechol chloride (p.1389·3).
Urinary bladder atony; urinary retention.

Muscarsan Sanum-Kehlbeck, Ger.
Homoeopathic preparation.

Muscle Rub Schein, USA.
Methyl salicylate (p.55·2); menthol (p.1600·2).
Muscle, joint, and soft-tissue pain; neuralgia.

Muscoril Inverni della Beffa, Ital.
Thiocolchicoside (p.1322·1).
Muscle spasticity; neuromuscular pain; parkinsonism.

Muse
Astra, UK; Vivus, USA.
Alprostadil (p.1412·2).
Impotence.

Muskel Trancopal Sanofi Winthrop, Ger.†.
Chlormezanone (p.648·3).
Skeletal muscle spasm.

Muskel Trancopal compositum Sanofi Winthrop, Ger.†.
Chlormezanone (p.648·3); paracetamol (p.72·2).
Skeletal muscle spasm.

Muskel Trancopal cum codeino Sanofi Winthrop, Ger.†.
Chlormezanone (p.648·3); paracetamol (p.72·2); codeine phosphate (p.26·1).
Skeletal muscle spasm.

Muskelat Azupharma, Ger.
Tetrazepam (p.694·3).
Skeletal muscle tension and spasm.

Muskol Schering-Plough, Canad.
SPF 6: Diethyltoluamide (p.1405·1); padimate O (p.1488·1).
Insect repellent; sunscreen.

Mus-Lax Jones, USA†.
Chlorzoxazone (p.1313·1); paracetamol (p.72·2).
Musculoskeletal pain.

Mussera Stark, Ger.†.
Sodium salamidacetate (p.82·3); paracetamol (p.72·2); benzyl nicotinate (p.22·1).
Chilblains; muscle, nerve, and joint pain; peripheral vascular disorders.

Mustargen
Merck Sharp & Dohme, Aust.; Merck Sharp & Dohme, Canad.; Merck Sharp & Dohme, Switz.; Merck Sharp & Dohme, USA.
Mustine hydrochloride (p.555·1).
Malignant neoplasms; mycosis fungoides; polycythaemia vera.

Musterole Schering-Plough, USA.
Methyl salicylate (p.55·2); menthol (p.1600·2); methyl nicotinate (p.55·1).
Muscle, joint, and soft-tissue pain; neuralgia.

Musterole Extra Schering-Plough, USA.
Methyl salicylate (p.55·2); camphor (p.1557·2); menthol (p.1600·2); mustard oil (p.1605·3).
Muscle, joint, and soft-tissue pain; neuralgia.

Mutabase Schering-Plough, Spain.
Perphenazine (p.685·2); amitriptyline hydrochloride (p.273·3).
Depression.

Mutabon Schering-Plough, Ital.
Perphenazine (p.685·2); amitriptyline hydrochloride (p.273·3).
Psychiatric disorders.

Mutabon A/D/F Schering-Plough, Neth.†.
Perphenazine (p.685·2); amitriptyline (p.273·2).
Anxiety; depression; psychoses.

Mutabon D Schering-Plough, Austral.
Perphenazine (p.685·2); amitriptyline hydrochloride (p.273·3).
Mixed anxiety depressive states.

Mutaflor
Emonta, Aust.; Ardeypharm, Ger.; Ardeypharm, Switz.†.
Escherichia coli.
Gastro-intestinal disorders.

Mutagrip
Sanofi Winthrop, Belg.; Pasteur Vaccins, Fr.; Pasteur Merieux, Ger.; Pasteur Merieux, Ital.; Sanofi Winthrop, Neth.†; Rhone-Poulenc Rorer, Spain.
An influenza vaccine (p.1515·2).
Active immunisation.

Mutamycin
Bristol, Canad.; Bristol-Myers Squibb, Neth.†; Bristol-Myers Squibb, Norw.; Bristol-Myers Squibb, Swed.; Bristol-Myers Oncology, USA.
Mitomycin (p.552·2).
Malignant neoplasms.

Mutamycine Bristol-Myers Squibb, Switz.
Mitomycin (p.552·2).
Malignant neoplasms.

Mutan Lannacher, Aust.
Fluoxetine hydrochloride (p.284·1).
Anxiety disorders; bulimia nervosa; depression.

Mutellon Klein, Ger.
Lycopus europaeus; motherwort (p.1604·2); valerian (p.1643·1).
Hyperthyroidism.

Mutesa Wyeth, Fr.
Aluminium hydroxide (p.1177·3); magnesium oxide (p.1198·3); oxethazaine (p.1298·1).
Gastro-oesophageal pain.

Muthesa
Whitehall, Belg.; Wyeth, Switz.
Aluminium hydroxide (p.1177·3); magnesium hydroxide (p.1198·2), magnesium carbonate (p.1198·1), or magnesium oxide (p.1198·3); oxethazaine (p.1298·1).
Gastro-intestinal disorders.

Muthesa N Whitehall, Neth.
Aluminium hydroxide (p.1177·3); magnesium hydroxide (p.1198·2).
Eructation; heartburn.

Muvial AGIPS, Ital.
Timonacic methyl hydrochloride (p.1638·1).
Otorhinolaryngeal disorders; respiratory-tract disorders.

Muxol
Note. This name is used for preparations of different composition.
Leurquin, Fr.
Ambroxol hydrochloride (p.1054·3).
Respiratory-tract congestion.

Vifor, Switz.
Bisacodyl (p.1179·3).
Constipation.

MVC Lyphomed, USA†.
Multivitamin infusion.
Parenteral nutrition.

MVI
Rhone-Poulenc Rorer, Canad.; Astra, USA.
Multivitamin infusion.
Parenteral nutrition.

MVI-12
Rhone-Poulenc Rorer, Austral.; Astra, USA.
Multivitamin preparation.
Parenteral nutrition.

MVI Paediatric Rhone-Poulenc Rorer, Austral.
Multivitamin preparation.
Parenteral nutrition.

MVI Pediatric Astra, USA.
Multivitamin preparation.
Parenteral nutrition.

MVM Tyson, USA.
Multivitamin and mineral preparation.

MXL
Napp, Irl.; Napp, UK.
Morphine sulphate (p.56·2).
Pain.

Myacyne Schur, Ger.
Topical powder; ointment: Neomycin sulphate (p.229·2).
Topical powder spray: Neomycin sulphate (p.229·2); tyrothricin (p.267·2).
Infected skin disorders.

Myadec
Warner-Lambert, Austral.; Parke, Davis, USA.
Multivitamin and mineral preparation.

Myalgesic Wolfs, Belg.
Salicylamide (p.82·3); benzocaine (p.1286·2).
Local anaesthesia.

Myalgol N Robugen, Ger.
Glycol salicylate (p.43·1); benzyl nicotinate (p.22·1).
Formerly contained salicylic acid, camphor, glycol salicylate, benzyl nicotinate, and capsicum.
Circulatory disorders of the skin; muscle and joint pain; soft-tissue disorders.

Myambutol
Cyanamid, Aust.; Lederle, Austral.; Wyeth Lederle, Belg.; Wyeth-Ayerst, Canad.; Lederle, Fr.; Lederle, Ger.; Wyeth, Irl.; Lederle, Neth.; Wyeth, S.Afr.; Cyanamid, Spain; Wyeth Lederle, Swed.; Lederle, Switz.; Wyeth, UK†; Lederle, USA.
Ethambutol hydrochloride (p.207·2).
Opportunistic mycobacterial infections; tuberculosis.

Myambutol-INH
Cyanamid, Aust.; Lederle, Ger.; Lederle, Switz.
Ethambutol hydrochloride (p.207·2); isoniazid (p.218·1).
Tuberculosis.

Myapap Gen-King, USA.
Paracetamol (p.72·2).
Fever; pain.

Mycanden Schering, S.Afr.†.
Haloprogin (p.381·2).
Fungal skin infections.

Mycardol
Sanofi Winthrop, Irl.; Sanofi Winthrop, UK.
Pentaerythritol tetranitrate (p.927·3).
Angina pectoris.

Mycatox Brenner-Efeka, Ger.
Dequalinium chloride (p.1112·1); hexylresorcinol (p.1116·1); sage (p.1627·1).
Bath additive; fungal infections.

Mycatox N Brenner-Efeka, Ger.†.
Ointment: Hexylresorcinol (p.1116·1); thymol (p.1127·1); zinc oxide (p.1096·2).
Topical liquid: Hexylresorcinol (p.1116·1); thymol (p.1127·1); 4-hydroxybenzoic acid.
Fungal infections.

Mycelex Bayer, USA.
Clotrimazole (p.376·3).
Fungal infections.

Mycelex-7 Combination Pack Bayer, USA.
Cream and vaginal tablet: Clotrimazole (p.376·3).
Vulvovaginal candidiasis.

Mycetin Farmigea, Ital.
Chloramphenicol (p.182·1).
Bacterial eye infections.

Mycifradin
Pharmacia Upjohn, Canad.; Pharmacia Upjohn, Irl.; Pharmacia Upjohn, S.Afr.; Upjohn, UK; Upjohn, USA.
Neomycin sulphate (p.229·2).
Hepatic coma; pre-operative bowel preparation.

Myciguent
Pharmacia Upjohn, Canad.; Upjohn, Irl.†; Upjohn, USA.
Neomycin sulphate (p.229·2).
Bacterial skin infections.

Mycil
Note. This name is used for preparations of different composition.
Boots, Austral.; Roberts, Canad.; Salusa, S.Afr.†.
Chlorphenesin (p.376·2).
Fungal skin infections.

Boots Healthcare, Irl.; Crookes Healthcare, UK.
Ointment: Tolnaftate (p.389·1); benzalkonium chloride (p.1101·3).
Fungal skin infections.

Boots Healthcare, Irl.; Crookes Healthcare, UK.
Topical powder: Tolnaftate (p.389·1); chlorhexidine hydrochloride (p.1107·2).
Fungal skin infections.

Boots Healthcare, Irl.; Crookes Healthcare, UK.
Topical spray: Tolnaftate (p.389·1).
Fungal skin infections.

Mycil Gold Crookes Healthcare, UK.
Clotrimazole (p.376·3).
Fungal skin infections.

Mycinette Pfeiffer, USA.
Phenol (p.1121·2); alum (p.1547·1).
Sore throat.

Mycinettes Pfeiffer, USA.
Benzocaine (p.1286·2).
Sore throat.

Mycinopred
Allergan, Ger.†; Allergan, Switz.
Prednisolone acetate (p.1048·1); polymyxin B sulphate (p.239·1); neomycin sulphate (p.229·2).
Infected eye disorders.

Myci-Spray Misemer, USA.
Phenylephrine hydrochloride (p.1066·2); mepyramine maleate (p.414·1).
Nasal congestion.

Mycitracin
Upjohn, Austral.†; Upjohn, USA.
Bacitracin (p.157·3); neomycin sulphate (p.229·2); polymyxin B sulphate (p.239·1).
Bacterial eye infections; bacterial skin infections.

Mycitracin Plus Upjohn, USA.
Bacitracin (p.157·3); neomycin sulphate (p.229·2); polymyxin B sulphate (p.239·1); lignocaine (p.1293·2).
Bacterial skin infections.

Myclo-Derm Boehringer Ingelheim, Canad.
Clotrimazole (p.376·3).
Fungal skin infections.

Myclo-Gyne Boehringer Ingelheim, Canad.
Clotrimazole (p.376·3).
Vaginal candidiasis.

Mycoban Vesta, S.Afr.
Clotrimazole (p.376·3).
Fungal skin infections; vulvovaginal candidiasis.

Myco-Biotic II Moore, USA.
Triamcinolone acetonide (p.1050·2); nystatin (p.386·1).
Skin disorders.

Mycobutin
Pharmacia Upjohn, Aust.; Pharmacia Upjohn, Austral.; Pharmacia Upjohn, Canad.; Pharmacia Upjohn, Ger.; Pharmacia Upjohn, Ital.; Pharmacia Upjohn, Neth.; Pharmacia Upjohn, S.Afr.; Pharmacia Upjohn, UK; Adria, USA.
Rifabutin (p.242·2).
Opportunistic mycobacterial infections; tuberculosis.

Mycobutine Pharmacia Upjohn, Switz.
Rifabutin (p.242·2).
Mycobacterial infections.

Mycocide NS Woodward, USA.
Benzalkonium chloride (p.1101·3).
Skin disinfection.

Mycocort Merck, Aust.†.
Fluprednidene acetate (p.1042·2); miconazole nitrate (p.384·3).
Infected skin disorders.

Mycocur Schering, Ital.†.
Fluocortolone (p.1041·3); fluocortolone hexanoate (p.1041·3); nystatin (p.386·1); neomycin sulphate (p.229·2).
Skin disorders.

Mycodecyl Diepha, Fr.
Cream: Undecenoic acid (p.389·2); zinc undecenoate (p.389·2).
Topical powder: Undecenoic acid (p.389·2); zinc undecenoate (p.389·2); calcium undecenoate (p.389·2).
Topical solution: Undecenoic acid (p.389·2).
Fungal skin infections.

Mycoderm
Note. This name is used for preparations of different composition.
Merck, Aust.†.
Miconazole nitrate (p.384·3).
Skin infections.

Ego, Austral.
Cream: Salicylic acid (p.1090·2); undecylenic alkanolamide (p.389·2); sodium propionate (p.387·1); butyl hydroxybenzoate (p.1117·2).
Fungal and bacterial skin infections.
Powder: Salicylic acid (p.1090·2); sodium propionate (p.387·1); butyl hydroxybenzoate (p.1117·2).
Fungal skin infections.

Mycodermil Vifor, Switz.
Fenticonazole nitrate (p.377·3).
Fungal skin infections.

Mycofug
Merck, Aust.†; Hermal, Ger.
Clotrimazole (p.376·3).
Fungal infections.

Mycogel Biorga, Fr.†.
Copper pidolate; zinc pidolate; melaleuca oil (p.1599·2).
Skin cleanser.

Mycogen II Goldline, USA.
Triamcinolone acetonide (p.1050·2); nystatin (p.386·1).
Skin disorders.

Mycohaug C Betapharm, Ger.
Clotrimazole (p.376·3).
Fungal skin infections.

Myco-Intradermi Eberth, Ger.†.
Nystatin (p.386·1); zinc oxide (p.1096·2).
Fungal infections.

Myco-Jellin Grunenthal, Ger.†.
Cream: Fluocinolone acetonide (p.1041·1); chlormidazole hydrochloride (p.376·2).
Topical solution: Fluocinolone acetonide (p.1041·1); chlormidazole hydrochloride (p.376·2); salicylic acid (p.1090·2).
Fungal infections with inflammatory symptoms.

Mycolog
Note. This name is used for preparations of different composition.
Sanofi Winthrop, Belg.; Sanofi Winthrop, Neth.; Sanofi Winthrop, Switz.
Triamcinolone acetonide (p.1050·2); gramicidin (p.215·2); neomycin sulphate (p.229·2); nystatin (p.386·1).
Infected skin disorders.

Bristol-Myers Squibb, Fr.
Triamcinolone acetonide (p.1050·2); neomycin sulphate (p.229·2); nystatin (p.386·1).
Infected skin disorders.

Mycolog-II Westwood-Squibb, USA.
Triamcinolone acetonide (p.1050·2); nystatin (p.386·1).
Cutaneous candidiasis.

Mycomnes Fumouze, Fr.
Nifuratel (p.589·1); nystatin (p.386·1).
Vaginal infections.

Myconel Marnel, USA.
Triamcinolone acetonide (p.1050·2); nystatin (p.386·1).
Skin disorders.

Mycopol Nycomed, Aust.
Undecenoic acid (p.389·2); benzoic acid (p.1102·3); isopropyl alcohol (p.1118·2).
Fungal infections.

Mycopril Anatomia, UK†.
Calcium magnesium caprylate complex.
Formerly known as Capricin.
Dietary supplement.

Mycospor
Bayer, Austral.; Bayer, Belg.; Bayer, Ger.; Bayer, Neth.; Bayer, Norw.; Bayer, S.Afr.; Bayer, Spain.
Bifonazole (p.375·3).
Fungal skin infections.

Mycospor Carbamid Bayer, Norw.
Bifonazole (p.375·3); urea (p.1095·2).
Fungal nail infections.

Mycospor Nagelset Bayer, Ger.
Bifonazole (p.375·3); urea (p.1095·2).
Fungal nail infections.

Mycospor Onicoset Bayer, Spain.
Bifonazole (p.375·3); urea (p.1095·2).
Fungal nail infections.

Mycosporan Bayer, Swed.
Bifonazole (p.375·3).
Fungal skin infections.

Mycosporan-Karbamid Bayer, Swed.
Bifonazole (p.375·3); urea (p.1095·2).
Fungal nail infections.

Mycosporin Bayer, Aust.
Bifonazole (p.375·3).
Fungal skin and nail infections.

Mycostatin
Bristol-Myers Squibb, Aust.; Bristol-Myers Squibb, Austral.; Squibb, Canad.; Bristol-Myers Squibb, Irl.; Bristol-Myers Squibb, Ital.; Bristol-Myers Squibb, Norw.; Bristol-Myers Squibb, S.Afr.; Squibb, Spain; Bristol-Myers Squibb, Swed.; Apothecon, USA; Bristol-Myers Oncology, USA; Mead Johnson Laboratories, USA; Westwood-Squibb, USA.
Nystatin (p.386·1).
Candidiasis.

Mycostatin V Bristol-Myers Squibb, Aust.
Triamcinolone acetonide (p.1050·2); neomycin sulphate (p.229·2); gramicidin (p.215·2); nystatin (p.386·1).
Infected skin disorders.

Mycostatine
Bristol-Myers Squibb, Fr.; Sanofi Winthrop, Switz.
Nystatin (p.386·1).
Candidiasis.

Mycostatin-Zinkoxid Bristol-Myers Squibb, Aust.
Nystatin (p.386·1); zinc oxide (p.1096·2).
Candidiasis.

Mycoster Pierre Fabre, Fr.
Ciclopirox (p.376·2) or ciclopirox olamine (p.376·2).
Fungal infections of the skin and nails.

Myco-Synalar
Note. This name is used for preparations of different composition.
Grunenthal, Aust.; Grunenthal, Switz.
Cream: Fluocinolone acetonide (p.1041·1); chlormidazole hydrochloride (p.376·2).
Fungal skin infections.

Grunenthal, Aust.; Yamanouchi, Spain; Grunenthal, Switz.
Topical solution: Fluocinolone acetonide (p.1041·1); chlormidazole hydrochloride (p.376·2); salicylic acid (p.1090·2).
Fungal skin infections.

Mycota
Note. This name is used for preparations of different composition.
Boots, S.Afr.; Seton, UK.
Cream; topical powder: Undecenoic acid (p.389·2); zinc undecenoate (p.389·2).
Fungal skin infections.

Boots, S.Afr.; Seton, UK.
Topical spray: Undecenoic acid (p.389·2); dichlorophen (p.99·2).
Fungal skin infections.

Myco-Triacet II Lemmon, USA.
Triamcinolone acetonide (p.1050·2); nystatin (p.386·1).
Skin disorders.

Myco-Ultralan Schering, Fr.
Fluocortolone (p.1041·3); fluocortolone hexanoate (p.1041·3); nystatin (p.386·1); neomycin sulphate (p.229·2).
Infected skin disorders.

Mycozol Warner-Lambert, Austral.
Salicylic acid (p.1090·2); benzoic acid (p.1102·3).
Fungal skin infections.

Mycrol Rolab, S.Afr.†.
Ethambutol hydrochloride (p.207·2).
Tuberculosis.

Mydalgan Asche, Ger.†.
Methyl nicotinate (p.55·1); benzyl nicotinate (p.22·1); histamine dihydrochloride (p.1587·3); capsicum (p.1559·2); nonivamide (p.63·2); glycol salicylate (p.43·1).
Bruising; muscle and joint disorders.

Mydfrin
Alcon, Canad.; Alcon, USA.
Phenylephrine hydrochloride (p.1066·2).
Funduscopy; open-angle glaucoma; ophthalmic examination; pupil dilatation during surgery; refraction without cycloplegia; uveitis.

Mydocalm
Gebro, Aust.; Strathmann, Ger.; Labatec, Switz.
Tolperisone hydrochloride (p.1322·2).
Lignocaine hydrochloride (p.1293·2) is included in the injection to alleviate the pain of injection.
Peripheral vascular disease; skeletal muscle spasticity and spasm.

Mydral Ocusoft, USA.
Tropicamide (p.469·2).

Mydriacil Alcon, Irl.
Tropicamide (p.469·2).
Production of mydriasis and cycloplegia.

Mydriacyl
Alcon, Austral.; Alcon, Belg.†; Alcon, Canad.; Alcon, S.Afr.; Alcon, Swed.; Alcon, UK; Alcon, USA.
Tropicamide (p.469·2).
Production of mydriasis and cycloplegia.

Mydrial Winzer, Ger.
Phenylephrine hydrochloride (p.1066·2).
Production of mydriasis.

Mydrial-Atropin Winzer, Ger.†.
Tyramine hydrochloride (p.1641·2); atropine borate (p.456·1); adrenaline acid tartrate (p.813·3).
Eye disorders.

Mydrian Ciba Vision, Norw.
Tropicamide (p.469·2).
Production of mydriasis.

Mydriaticum
Agepha, Aust.; Bournonville, Belg.; Merck Sharp & Dohme-Chibret, Fr.; Stulln, Ger.; Restan, S.Afr.; Ciba Vision, Switz.
Tropicamide (p.469·2).
Production of mydriasis and cycloplegia.

Mydrilate
Boehringer Ingelheim, Irl.; Boehringer Ingelheim, UK.
Cyclopentolate hydrochloride (p.459·3).
Iritis; production of mydriasis and cycloplegia; uveitis.

Mydrum ankerpharm, Ger.
Tropicamide (p.469·2).
Aid in eye examination; production of mydriasis.

Myelobromol
Enzypharm, Aust.; Sinclair, UK.
Mitobronitol (p.551·3).
Available on a named-patient basis only in the *UK*.
Chronic myeloid leukaemia.

Myelografin Schering, Ital.†.
Meglumine ioserate.
Contrast medium.

Myelostim Italfarmaco, Ital.
Lenograstim (p.724·3).
Mobilisation of autologous peripheral blood progenitor cells; neutropenia induced by bone-marrow transplantation or cytotoxic chemotherapy.

Myfedrine Morton Grove, USA.
Paediatric liquid: Pseudoephedrine hydrochloride (p.1068·3).
Syrup: Pseudoephedrine hydrochloride (p.1068·3); guaiphenesin (p.1061·3); dextromethorphan hydrobromide (p.1057·3).

Myfedrine Plus Morton Grove, USA.
Pseudoephedrine hydrochloride (p.1068·3); chlorpheniramine maleate (p.405·1).

Myfungar
Wyeth, Ger.; Brenner-Efeka, Ger.; Klinge, Switz.
Oxiconazole nitrate (p.386·3).
Fungal skin infections.

Mygale compositum Weleda, Aust.
Homoeopathic preparation.

Mygdalon DDSA Pharmaceuticals, UK.
Metoclopramide hydrochloride (p.1200·3).

Mygel Geneva, USA.
Aluminium hydroxide (p.1177·3); magnesium hydroxide (p.1198·2); simethicone (p.1213·1).
Hyperacidity.

Myidyl Pharmaceutical Basics, USA†.
Triprolidine hydrochloride (p.420·3).
Hypersensitivity reactions.

Myk Cassenne, Fr.
Sulconazole nitrate (p.387·2).
Fungal skin infections.

Myk-1
Will-Pharma, Belg.; Will-Pharma, Neth.
Sulconazole nitrate (p.387·2).
Fungal skin infections.

Myko Cordes
Note. This name is used for preparations of different composition.
Ichthyol, Aust.; Ichthyol, Ger.
Cream; topical solution: Clotrimazole (p.376·3).
Fungal skin infections.

Ichthyol, Aust.
Paste: Clotrimazole (p.376·3); zinc oxide (p.1096·2).
Fungal skin infections.

Myko Cordes Plus Ichthyol, Ger.
Clotrimazole (p.376·3); zinc oxide (p.1096·2).
Fungal skin infections.

Mykoderm Engelhard, Ger.
Nystatin (p.386·1).
Fungal skin infections.

Mykofungin Wyeth, Ger.
Clotrimazole (p.376·3).
Fungal infections of skin and genito-urinary tract.

Mykohaug *Betapharm, Ger.*
Clotrimazole (p.376·3).
Fungal and bacterial vaginal infections; vaginal trichomoniasis.

Mykontral *LAW, Ger.*
Tioconazole (p.388·3).
Fungal skin infections.

MykoPosterine N *Kade, Ger.*
Nystatin (p.386·1).
Fungal infections.

mykoproct *Squibb-Heyden, Ger.†.*
Nystatin (p.386·1); triamcinolone acetonide (p.1050·2); lignocaine hydrochloride (p.1293·2).
Anorectal fungal infections.

mykoproct sine *Bristol-Myers Squibb, Ger.*
Nystatin (p.386·1); triamcinolone acetonide (p.1050·2).
Infected eczema.

Mykotin mono *Ardeypharm, Ger.*
Miconazole nitrate (p.384·3).
Fungal skin infections.

Mykozem *Schoeller, Aust.*
Undecenoic acid (p.389·2); urea (p.1095·2); zinc stearate (p.1469·3).
Fungal skin infections.

Mykrox *Fisons, USA.*
Metolazone (p.907·2).
Formerly known as Microx.
Hypertension.

Mykundex *Biocur, Ger.*
Nystatin (p.386·1).
Fungal infections.

Mykundex Heilsalbe *Biocur, Ger.*
Nystatin (p.386·1); zinc oxide (p.1096·2).
Fungal infections.

Mykundex Ovula *Jossa-Arznei, Ger.†.*
Nystatin (p.386·1).
Fungal vaginal infections.

Mylagen *Goldline, USA.*
Capsules: Calcium carbonate (p.1182·1); magnesium carbonate (p.1198·1).
Oral liquid: Aluminium hydroxide (p.1177·3); magnesium hydroxide (p.1198·2); simethicone (p.1213·1).
Hyperacidity.

Mylanta
Note. This name is used for preparations of different composition.
Warner-Lambert, Austral.; Janssen-Cilag, Belg.; Warner-Lambert, Canad.; Parke, Davis, Ital.†; J&J-Merck, USA.
Tablets: Aluminium hydroxide (p.1177·3); magnesium hydroxide (p.1198·2); simethicone (p.1213·1).
Flatulence; hyperacidity.

J&J-Merck, USA.
Lozenges: Calcium carbonate (p.1182·1).
Hyperacidity.

Mylanta Gas *J&J-Merck, USA.*
Simethicone (p.1213·1).
Flatulence.

Mylanta Gelcaps *J&J-Merck, USA.*
Calcium carbonate (p.1182·1); magnesium carbonate (p.1198·1).
Hyperacidity.

Mylanta Natural Fiber *J&J-Merck, USA.*
Psyllium hydrophilic mucilloid (p.1194·2).

Mylanta Plain *Warner-Lambert, Canad.*
Aluminium hydroxide (p.1177·3); magnesium hydroxide (p.1198·2).
Gastro-intestinal disorders associated with hyperacidity.

Mylanta Plus *Warner-Lambert, Austral.*
Oral liquid: Aluminium hydroxide (p.1177·3); magnesium hydroxide (p.1198·2); calcium carbonate (p.1182·1); sodium bicarbonate (p.1153·2); alginic acid (p.1470·3).
Tablets: Magaldrate (p.1198·1); alginic acid (p.1470·3); sodium bicarbonate (p.1153·2).
Dyspepsia; gastro-oesophageal reflux.

Mylanta-II *ICI, Neth.†.*
Algeldrate (p.1177·3); magnesium hydroxide (p.1198·2); simethicone (p.1213·1).
Gastro-intestinal disorders.

Mylepsinum *Zeneca, Ger.*
Primidone (p.358·3).
Epilepsy.

Myleran
Glaxo Wellcome, Aust.; Glaxo Wellcome, Austral.; Glaxo Wellcome, Belg.; Glaxo Wellcome, Canad.; Glaxo Wellcome, Ger.; Wellcome, Irl.; Glaxo Wellcome, Ital.; Glaxo Wellcome, Neth.; Glaxo Wellcome, Norw.; Glaxo Wellcome, S.Afr.; Glaxo Wellcome, Swed.; Wellcome, Switz.; Wellcome, UK; Glaxo Wellcome, USA.
Busulphan (p.509·3).
Chronic myeloid leukaemia; myelofibrosis; polycythaemia vera; primary thrombocythaemia.

Mylicon
Parke, Davis, Austral.†; Warner-Lambert, Ital.; J&J-Merck, USA.
Simethicone (p.1213·1).
Flatulence.

Mylocort *Triomed, S.Afr.*
Hydrocortisone acetate (p.1043·3).
Skin disorders.

Mylol *Boots, S.Afr.*
Topical liquid: Diethyltoluamide (p.1405·1); dimethyl phthalate (p.1405·3); dibutyl phthalate (p.1404·2).
Topical spray: Diethyltoluamide (p.1405·1).
Insect repellent.

Mylproin *Desitin, Ger.*
Valproic acid (p.361·2).
Epilepsy.

Myminic Expectorant *Morton Grove, USA.*
Phenylpropanolamine hydrochloride (p.1067·2); guaiphenesin (p.1061·3).
Coughs.

Myminic Syrup *Morton Grove, USA.*
Phenylpropanolamine hydrochloride (p.1067·2); chlorpheniramine maleate (p.405·1).

Myminicol *Morton Grove, USA.*
Phenylpropanolamine hydrochloride (p.1067·2); chlorpheniramine maleate (p.405·1); dextromethorphan hydrobromide (p.1057·3).
Coughs and cold symptoms.

Mynah
Wyeth, S.Afr.; Lederle, UK†.
Ethambutol hydrochloride (p.207·2); isoniazid (p.218·1).
Tuberculosis.

Mynatal *ME Pharmaceuticals, USA.*
Multivitamin and mineral preparation with iron and folic acid.

Mynate 90 Plus *ME Pharmaceuticals, USA.*
Multivitamin and mineral preparation.

Mynocine *Lederle, Fr.*
Minocycline hydrochloride (p.226·2).
Bacterial infections.

Myo Hermes *Organon, Spain.*
Bethanechol chloride (p.1389·3).
Gastro-intestinal motility disorders; urinary retention.

Myocardetten *Byk Gulden, Ger.†.*
Aminophylline hydrate (p.748·1); phenobarbitone (p.350·2); papaverine hydrochloride (p.1614·2); atropine methonitrate (p.455·1); glyceryl trinitrate (p.874·3).
Cardiac disorders.

Myocardon *Byk, Aust.*
Aminophylline hydrochloride (p.748·2); papaverine hydrochloride (p.1614·2); atropine methonitrate (p.455·1); glyceryl trinitrate (p.874·3).
Angina pectoris; heart failure; myocardial infarction.

Myocardon mono *Byk, Aust.*
Isosorbide mononitrate (p.893·3).
Angina pectoris; heart failure; myocardial infarction.

Myocardon N *Byk Gulden, Ger.*
Theophylline (p.765·1).
Formerly contained aminophylline hydrate, phenobarbitone, papaverine hydrochloride, atropine methonitrate, and glyceryl trinitrate.
Cardiac disorders.

Myocholine
Croma, Aust.; Glenwood, Ger.; Glenwood, Switz.
Bethanechol chloride (p.1389·3).
Antimuscarinic effects of tricyclic antidepressants; dysphagia; gastro-oesophageal reflux; urinary retention.

Myochrysine
Rhone-Poulenc Rorer, Canad.; Merck Sharp & Dohme, USA†.
Sodium aurothiomalate (p.83·2).
Rheumatoid arthritis.

Myocrisin
Rhone-Poulenc Rorer, Austral.; Rhone-Poulenc Rorer, Irl.; Rhone-Poulenc Rorer, Norw.; Rhone-Poulenc Rorer, S.Afr.; Rhone-Poulenc Rorer, Swed.; JHC Healthcare, UK.
Sodium aurothiomalate (p.83·2).
Juvenile chronic arthritis; lupus erythematosus; rheumatoid arthritis.

Myo-Echinacin *Madaus, Aust.*
Echinaceae purpureae (p.1574·2).
Urinary and respiratory-tract infections.

Myofedrin *Apogepha, Ger.*
Oxyfedrine hydrochloride (p.927·1).
Cardiac disorders.

Myoflex
Note. This name is used for preparations of different composition.
Bayer, Canad.; Fisons, USA.
Triethanolamine salicylate (p.1639·2).
Muscle, joint, and soft-tissue pain; neuralgia.

Pharmacare Consumer, S.Afr.
Paracetamol (p.72·2); chlormezanone (p.648·3).
Pain and associated tension.

Sodip, Switz.†.
Chlormezanone (p.648·3).
Skeletal muscle spasm.

Myoflex Ice *Bayer, Canad.*
Menthol (p.1600·2).
Pain.

Myoflex Ice Plus *Bayer, Canad.*
Triethanolamine salicylate (p.1639·2); menthol (p.1600·2).
Muscle pain.

Myogeloticum N *Hanosan, Ger.*
Homoeopathic preparation.

Myogesic *Lambda, USA.*
Magnesium salicylate (p.51·1); phenyltoloxamine citrate (p.416·1).

Myogit *Pfleger, Ger.*
Diclofenac sodium (p.31·2).
Inflammation; rheumatism.

Myolastan
Sanofi Winthrop, Aust.; Sanofi Winthrop, Belg.; Sanofi Winthrop, Fr.; Sanofi Winthrop, Spain.
Tetrazepam (p.694·3).
Skeletal muscle spasm.

Myolin *Roberts, USA; Hauck, USA.*
Orphenadrine citrate (p.465·2).
Musculoskeletal pain.

Myolosyx *Syxyl, Ger.*
Homoeopathic preparation.

Myo-Melcain *Rorer, Ger.†.*
Procaine hydrochloride (p.1299·2); honey.
Muscular and neuromuscular disorders; sympathetic nerve blockade.

Myonal *Eisai, Jpn.*
Eperisone hydrochloride (p.1315·2).
Skeletal muscle spasm; spasticity.

Myonasan *Hanosan, Ger.†.*
Crataegus (p.1568·2); spigelia; camphora (p.1557·2); aurum chloratum; kalmia; veratrum; arnica (p.1550·3); melissa (p.1600·1); cactus; strophanthus (p.951·1); ignatia; calf-heart extract.
Cardiovascular disorders.

Myophen *Teral, USA.*
Orphenadrine citrate (p.465·2).

Myoplegine *Christiaens, Belg.*
Suxamethonium chloride (p.1319·1).
Depolarising neuromuscular blocker.

Myo-Prolixan *Jacoby, Aust.†.*
Azapropazone (p.20·3); phenprobamate (p.686·1).

Myoquin *Fawns & McAllan, Austral.*
Quinine bisulphate (p.439·1).
Malaria; nocturnal cramps.

Myoscain *Waldheim, Aust.*
Guaiphenesin (p.1061·3).
Coughs.

Myoscint *Byk Gulden, Ital.*
Indium (^{111}In) imciromab pentetate (p.1423·3).
Diagnosis of myocardial infarction.

Myospasmal *TAD, Ger.*
Tetrazepam (p.694·3).
Skeletal muscle tension and spasm.

Myotenlis *Pharmacia Upjohn, Ital.*
Suxamethonium chloride (p.1319·1).
Depolarising neuromuscular blocker.

Myotonachol
Glenwood, Canad.; Glenwood, USA.
Bethanechol chloride (p.1389·3).
Gastro-oesophageal reflux; neurogenic bladder; urinary retention.

Myotonine *Glenwood, UK.*
Bethanechol chloride (p.1389·3).
Gastro-intestinal motility disorders; gastro-oesophageal reflux; urinary retention.

Myotrol *Legere, USA†.*
Orphenadrine citrate (p.465·2).

Myoview
Amersham, Fr.; Sorin, Ital.; Amersham, Spain; Amersham International, UK.
Technetium-99m tetrofosmin (p.1425·1).
Myocardial perfusion imaging.

Myoviton *Therabel, Fr.*
Pyridoxine hydrochloride (p.1362·3); adenosine triphosphate, disodium salt (p.1543·2).
Tonic.

Myoxam *Menarini, Spain.*
Midecamycin acetate (p.226·2).
Bacterial infections.

Mypaid *Restan, S.Afr.*
Ibuprofen (p.44·1); paracetamol (p.72·2).
Fever; pain.

Myphetane DC *Morton Grove, USA.*
Phenylpropanolamine hydrochloride (p.1067·2); codeine phosphate (p.26·1); brompheniramine maleate (p.403·2).
Coughs and cold symptoms.

Myphetane DX *Morton Grove, USA.*
Pseudoephedrine hydrochloride (p.1068·3); brompheniramine maleate (p.403·2); dextromethorphan hydrobromide (p.1057·3).
Coughs and cold symptoms.

Myphetapp *Morton Grove, USA.*
Phenylpropanolamine hydrochloride (p.1067·2); brompheniramine maleate (p.403·2).

Myprodol *Adcock Ingram, S.Afr.*
Ibuprofen (p.44·1); paracetamol (p.72·2); codeine phosphate (p.26·1).
Inflammation; pain.

Myproflam *Adcock Ingram, S.Afr.*
Ketoprofen (p.48·2).
Musculoskeletal, joint, and peri-articular disorders.

Myrin *Wyeth, S.Afr.*
Ethambutol hydrochloride (p.207·2); isoniazid (p.218·1); rifampicin (p.243·2).
Tuberculosis.

Myrol *Dorom, Ital.*
Dihydroergocryptine mesylate (p.1571·3).
Dementia; hyperprolactinaemia; lactation inhibition; parkinsonism; vascular headache.

Myrrhinil-Intest *Repha, Ger.*
Myrrh (p.1606·1); carbo coffeae (p.1645·1); chamomile (p.1561·2).
Gastro-intestinal disorders.

Myrtaven *IBSA, Switz.*
Vaccinium myrtillus (p.1606·1).
Peripheral vascular disorders.

Myrtilen *Synpharma, Aust.*
Myritillus (p.1606·1); caraway (p.1559·3); rice starch (p.1356·2).
Diarrhoea.

Mysca *Martin, Fr.†.*
Menthol (p.1600·2); cade oil (p.1092·2); zinc oxide (p.1096·2); thyme oil (p.1637·1); camphor (p.1557·2); resorcinol (p.1090·1).
Skin irritation.

Myser *Mitsubishi, Jpn.*
Difluprednate (p.1039·3).
Skin disorders.

Mysoline
Zeneca, Aust.; ICI, Austral.; Zeneca, Belg.; Wyeth-Ayerst, Canad.; Zeneca, Fr.; Zeneca, Irl.; SIT, Ital.; Zeneca, Neth.; Zeneca, Norw.; Zeneca, S.Afr.; Zeneca, Spain; Zeneca, Swed.; Zeneca, Switz.; Zeneca, UK; Wyeth-Ayerst, USA.
Primidone (p.358·3).
Formerly known as Mylepsin in *Swed.*
Epilepsy; essential tremor.

Mysteclin
Note. This name is used for preparations of different composition.
Bristol-Myers Squibb, Aust.; Bristol-Myers Squibb, Ger.; Squibb-Heyden, Ger.†.
Tetracycline (p.259·1) or tetracycline hydrochloride (p.259·1); amphotericin (p.372·2).
Vaginal infections.

Bristol-Myers Squibb, Austral.
Tetracycline hydrochloride (p.259·1).
Bacterial infections.

Squibb, UK†.
Tetracycline hydrochloride (p.259·1); nystatin (p.386·1).
Bacterial infections.

Mysteclin-F *Bristol-Myers Squibb, Irl.†.*
Tetracycline (p.259·1); amphotericin (p.372·2).
Mixed bacterial/candidal infections.

Mysteclin-V
Note. This name is used for preparations of different composition.
Bristol-Myers Squibb, Austral.
Tetracycline (p.259·1); nystatin (p.386·1).
Bacterial infections.

Bristol-Myers Squibb, S.Afr.†.
Tetracycline (p.259·1); amphotericin (p.372·2).
Bacterial infections.

Mytelase
Sanofi Winthrop, Fr.; Sanofi, Swed.; Sanofi Winthrop, USA.
Ambenonium chloride (p.1389·2).
Myasthenia gravis.

Mytex *Morton Grove, USA.*
Phenylephrine hydrochloride (p.1066·2); phenylpropanolamine hydrochloride (p.1067·2); guaiphenesin (p.1061·3).

Mytobrin *Intramed, S.Afr.*
Tobramycin sulphate (p.264·1).
Bacterial infections.

Mytolac *Procter & Gamble, Swed.†.*
Benzoyl peroxide (p.1079·2).
Acne.

Mytrex *Savage, USA.*
Triamcinolone acetonide (p.1050·2); nystatin (p.386·1).
Skin disorders.

Mytussin *Morton Grove, USA.*
Guaiphenesin (p.1061·3).
Coughs.

Mytussin AC *Morton Grove, USA.*
Codeine phosphate (p.26·1); guaiphenesin (p.1061·3).
Coughs.

Mytussin CF *Morton Grove, USA.*
Guaiphenesin (p.1061·3); phenylpropanolamine hydrochloride (p.1067·2); dextromethorphan hydrobromide (p.1057·3).

Mytussin DAC *Morton Grove, USA.*
Pseudoephedrine hydrochloride (p.1068·3); guaiphenesin (p.1061·3); codeine phosphate (p.26·1).
Coughs.

Mytussin DM *Morton Grove, USA.*
Dextromethorphan hydrobromide (p.1057·3); guaiphenesin (p.1061·3).
Coughs.

Mytussin PE *Morton Grove, USA.*
Guaiphenesin (p.1061·3); pseudoephedrine hydrochloride (p.1068·3).

My-Vitalife *ME Pharmaceuticals, USA.*
Multivitamin and mineral preparation.

Myvlar *Schering, Aust.*
Gestodene (p.1447·2); ethinyloestradiol (p.1445·1).
Combined oral contraceptive.

Myxal *Basotherm, Ger.†.*
Topical liquid: Dodecyltriphenylphosphonium bromide; benzoxonium chloride (p.1103·3).
Topical powder: Dodecyltriphenylphosphonium bromide; benzoxonium chloride (p.1103·3); aluminium chlorohydrate (p.1078·3).
Fungal infections.

Myxal S *Basotherm, Ger.†.*
Dodecyltriphenylphosphonium bromide.
Disinfection.

Myxofat *Fatol, Ger.*
Acetylcysteine (p.1052·3).
Respiratory-tract disorders associated with increased or viscous mucus.

M-Zole 7 Dual Pack *Alpharma, USA.*
Miconazole nitrate (p.384·3).
Vulvovaginal candidiasis.

N32 Collutorio *Esoform, Ital.*
Chlorhexidine gluconate (p.1107·2).
Oral disinfection.

N D Clear *Seatrace, USA.*
Pseudoephedrine hydrochloride (p.1068·3); chlorpheniramine maleate (p.405·1).
Upper respiratory-tract symptoms.

Naabak *Thea, Fr.*
Sodium isospaglumate (p.1591·3).
Allergic conjunctivitis.

Naaprep
SmithKline Beecham Consumer, Belg.; SmithKline Beecham Consumer, Switz.
Sodium chloride (p.1162·2).
Cleansing of eyelids; nasal irrigation; rinsing solution for contact lenses.

Naaxia
Ciba Vision, Belg.†; Thea, Fr.; Ciba Vision, Ger.; Ciba Vision, Ital.; Ciba Vision, Spain.
Magnesium spaglumate (p.1591·3) or sodium spaglumate.
Allergic conjunctivitis.

Naaxia Nouvelle formule *Ciba Vision, Switz.*
Sodium isospaglumate (p.1591·3); spaglumate decahydrate.
Allergic keratoconjunctivitis.

Nabact *Pharmador, S.Afr.†.*
Metronidazole (p.585·1).
Anaerobic bacterial infections.

Nabuser *Procter & Gamble, Ital.*
Nabumetone (p.60·1).
Musculoskeletal, joint, and peri-articular disorders.

NAC *Zambon, Ger.; CT, Ger.; Ratiopharm, Ger.*
Acetylcysteine (p.1052·3).
Respiratory-tract disorders associated with increased or viscous mucus.

Nacha *Lineafarm, Spain.*
A nonoxinol (p.1326·1).
Contraceptive.

Naclof
Gebro, Aust.†; Ciba Vision, Neth.; Ciba Vision, Norw.†; Restan, S.Afr.; Ciba Vision, Swed.†.
Diclofenac sodium (p.31·2).
Eye inflammation following cataract surgery.

Naclon *Teofarma, Ital.*
Sodium hypochlorite (p.1124·3).
Disinfection of skin, wounds, external genitalia, and drinking water.

Nacom *Du Pont, Ger.*
Carbidopa (p.1136·1); levodopa (p.1137·1).
Parkinsonism.

Nacor *Nezel, Spain.*
Enalapril maleate (p.863·2).
Heart failure; hypertension.

Nacton *Pharmark, UK†.*
Poldine methylsulphate (p.467·2).
Gastric hyperacidity; peptic ulcer.

Nad *Medical, Spain.*
Nadide (p.1606·1).
Vertigo.

Nadex
Zyma, Belg.; Zyma, Switz.
Pirisudanol maleate (p.1619·2).
Asthenia; depression; mental function impairment.

Nadinola *Nadinola, Canad.*
Hydroquinone (p.1083·1).

Nadir *Recordati, Ital.†.*
Metoclopramide hydrochloride (p.1200·3).
Gastro-intestinal disorders.

Nadisan *Boehringer Mannheim, Ger.†.*
Carbutamide (p.319·1).
Diabetes mellitus.

Nadopen-V *Nadeau, Canad.*
Phenoxymethylpenicillin potassium (p.236·2).
Bacterial infections.

Nadostine *Nadeau, Canad.*
Nystatin (p.386·1).
Candidiasis.

Nafasol *Lennon, S.Afr.*
Naproxen (p.61·2).
Dysmenorrhoea; gout; musculoskeletal and joint disorders.

Nafazair *Bausch & Lomb, USA.*
Naphazoline hydrochloride (p.1064·2).
Minor eye irritation.

Nafazair A *Bausch & Lomb, USA.*
Naphazoline hydrochloride (p.1064·2); pheniramine maleate (p.415·3).
Eye irritation.

Nafcil *Apothecon, USA.*
Nafcillin sodium (p.228·1).
Bacterial infections.

Naferon *Sclavo, Ital.*
Interferon beta (p.616·1).
Malignant neoplasms; viral infections.

Nafrine *Schering, Canad.*
Oxymetazoline hydrochloride (p.1065·3).

Naftazolina *Bruschettini, Ital.*
Naphazoline hydrochloride (p.1064·2).
Eye congestion; eye irritation.

Nafti *CT, Ger.; Isis Puren, Ger.*
Naftidrofuryl oxalate (p.914·2).
Peripheral vascular disorders.

Naftifin Zinkpaste *Biochemie, Aust.*
Naftifine hydrochloride (p.385·3); zinc oxide (p.1096·2).
Fungal skin infections.

Naftilong *Hexal, Ger.*
Naftidrofuryl oxalate (p.914·2).
Peripheral vascular disorders.

Naftilux *Therabel, Fr.*
Naftidrofuryl oxalate (p.914·2).
Mental function impairment in the elderly; peripheral vascular and cerebrovascular disorders.

Naftin
Allergan, Canad.; Allergan Herbert, USA.
Naftifine hydrochloride (p.385·3).
Fungal skin infections.

Nafti-ratiopharm *Ratiopharm, Ger.*
Naftidrofuryl oxalate (p.914·2).
Peripheral vascular disorders.

Naftocol *Panthox & Burck, Ital.†.*
Oxybromonaftoic acid (p.1612·1).
Liver and biliary-tract disorders.

Naftodril *Arcana, Aust.*
Naftidrofuryl oxalate (p.914·2).
Peripheral and cerebral vascular disorders.

Nagar *Mibo, Ital.†.*
Argitiopronin.
Liver disorders.

Nagel Batrafen *Hoechst, Ger.*
Ciclopirox (p.376·2).
Fungal nail infections.

Nail Nutrition *Cantassium Co., UK.*
Multivitamins; minerals; amino acids.

4 Nails *Marlyn, USA.*
Multivitamin, mineral, and amino-acid preparation.

Nail-vit *Pharmadass, UK.*
Multivitamin, mineral, and trace element preparation.

Nalador
Schering, Aust.; Schering, Fr.; Schering, Ger.; Schering, Ital.; Schering, Neth.; Schering, Switz.
Sulprostone (p.1420·3).
Cervical dilatation; postpartum haemorrhage; termination of pregnancy.

Nalcrom
Rhone-Poulenc Rorer, Canad.; Rhone-Poulenc Rorer, Irl.; Italchimici, Ital.; Fisons, Neth.; Rhone-Poulenc Rorer, S.Afr.; Casen Fisons, Spain; Fisons, Switz.; Pantheon, UK.
Sodium cromoglycate (p.762·1).
Food hypersensitivity; proctitis; ulcerative colitis.

Nalcron *Specia, Fr.*
Sodium cromoglycate (p.762·1).
Food hypersensitivity.

Naldec Pediatric *Bioline, USA†.*
Phenylpropanolamine hydrochloride (p.1067·2); phenylephrine hydrochloride (p.1066·2); phenyltoloxamine citrate (p.416·1); chlorpheniramine maleate (p.405·1).

Naldecol *Bristol, Ger.†.*
Phenylpropanolamine hydrochloride (p.1067·2); phenylephrine hydrochloride (p.1066·2); phenyltoloxamine citrate (p.416·1); carbinoxamine maleate (p.404·2).
Rhinitis; sinusitis; sore throat; tracheitis.

Naldecon *Apothecon, USA.*
Phenylpropanolamine hydrochloride (p.1067·2); phenylephrine hydrochloride (p.1066·2); phenyltoloxamine citrate (p.416·1); chlorpheniramine maleate (p.405·1).
Nasal congestion.

Naldecon CX *Apothecon, USA.*
Phenylpropanolamine hydrochloride (p.1067·2); guaiphenesin (p.1061·3); codeine phosphate (p.26·1).
Coughs and cold symptoms.

Naldecon DX *Apothecon, USA.*
Phenylpropanolamine hydrochloride (p.1067·2); guaiphenesin (p.1061·3); dextromethorphan hydrobromide (p.1057·3).
Coughs.

Naldecon EX *Apothecon, USA.*
Phenylpropanolamine hydrochloride (p.1067·2); guaiphenesin (p.1061·3).
Coughs and cold symptoms.

Naldecon Senior DX *Apothecon, USA.*
Guaiphenesin (p.1061·3); dextromethorphan hydrobromide (p.1057·3).
Coughs.

Naldecon Senior EX *Apothecon, USA.*
Guaiphenesin (p.1061·3).
Coughs and cold symptoms.

Naldelate DX Adult *Barre-National, USA.*
Phenylpropanolamine hydrochloride (p.1067·2); dextromethorphan hydrobromide (p.1057·3); guaiphenesin (p.1061·3).
Coughs.

Nalfon
Lilly, Aust.; Lilly, Canad.; Dista, USA.
Fenoprofen calcium (p.37·2).
Fever; gout; musculoskeletal and joint disorders; pain.

Nalgesic *Lilly, Fr.*
Fenoprofen calcium (p.37·2).
Pain.

Nalgest *Major, USA.*
Phenylpropanolamine hydrochloride (p.1067·2); phenylephrine hydrochloride (p.1066·2); chlorpheniramine maleate (p.405·1); phenyltoloxamine citrate (p.416·1).
Upper respiratory-tract symptoms.

Nalgisa *ISF, Ital.†.*
Diflunisal (p.33·2).
Pain.

Nalicidin *Rhone-Poulenc, Ital.†.*
Nalidixic acid (p.228·2).
Gram-negative urinary-tract infections.

Nalidixin *NCSN, Ital.*
Nalidixic acid (p.228·2).
Gram-negative genito-urinary tract infections.

Naligram *Geymonat, Ital.*
Nalidixic acid (p.228·2).
Gram-negative genito-urinary tract infections.

Nalion *Lesvi, Spain.*
Norfloxacin (p.233·1).
Bacterial infections.

Nalissina *Rhone-Poulenc Rorer, Ital.*
Nalidixic acid (p.228·2).
Gram-negative urinary-tract infections.

Nallpen *SmithKline Beecham, USA.*
Nafcillin sodium (p.228·1).
Bacterial infections.

Nalone *SERB, Fr.*
Naloxone hydrochloride (p.986·2).
Diagnosis of opioid dependence; diagnosis of toxic coma; opioid overdosage; opioid-induced respiratory depression.

Nalorex
Du Pont, Fr.; Du Pont, Irl.; Du Pont, Ital.; Du Pont Pharmaceuticals, UK.
Naltrexone hydrochloride (p.988·1).
Opioid withdrawal.

Nalspan DX *Morton Grove, USA.*
Phenylpropanolamine hydrochloride (p.1067·2); guaiphenesin (p.1061·3); dextromethorphan hydrobromide (p.1057·3).

Nalspan Pediatric *Morton Grove, USA.*
Phenylpropanolamine hydrochloride (p.1067·2); phenylephrine hydrochloride (p.1066·2); phenyltoloxamine citrate (p.416·1); chlorpheniramine maleate (p.405·1).

Nalspan Senior DX *Morton Grove, USA.*
Dextromethorphan hydrobromide (p.1057·3); guaiphenesin (p.1061·3).

Nanbacine *Bellon, Fr.*
Xibornol (p.270·3).
Mouth and throat infections; respiratory-tract disorders.

Nani Pre Dental *Alter, Spain.*
Saffron (p.1001·1); guaiazulene (p.1586·3); lignocaine hydrochloride (p.1293·2); myrrh (p.1606·1); menthol (p.1600·2).
Toothache.

Nanotiv
Pharmacia Upjohn, Ger.†; Pharmacia Upjohn, Norw.; Pharmacia Upjohn, Swed.
A factor IX preparation (p.721·3).
Haemorrhagic disorders.

Nansius *Berenguer Infale, Spain.*
Potassium clorazepate (p.657·1).
Anxiety; insomnia.

Napacod *Propan, S.Afr.*
Paracetamol (p.72·2); codeine phosphate (p.26·1).
Fever; pain.

Napageln *Lederle, Jpn.*
Felbinac (p.37·1).
Inflammation; musculoskeletal, joint, and peri-articular disorders; pain.

Napamide *Douglas, Austral.*
Indapamide (p.890·2).
Hypertension.

Napamol *Propan, S.Afr.*
Paracetamol (p.72·2).
Fever; pain.

Na-PAS *Kabi, Swed.†.*
Sodium aminosalicylate (p.151·1).
Tuberculosis.

Napflam *Noristan, S.Afr.†.*
Naproxen (p.61·2).
Dysmenorrhoea; musculoskeletal and joint disorders.

Napharzol *Pharmacal, Switz.†.*
Naphazoline nitrate (p.1064·2); mild silver protein.
Cold symptoms; sinusitis.

Naphazole-A *Major, USA.*
Naphazoline hydrochloride (p.1064·2); pheniramine maleate (p.415·3).
Eye irritation.

Naphazoline Plus *Parmed, USA.*
Naphazoline hydrochloride (p.1064·2); pheniramine maleate (p.415·3).
Minor eye irritation.

Naphcon
Alcon, Austral.; Alcon, Belg.†; Alcon, Canad.; Alcon, USA.
Naphazoline hydrochloride (p.1064·2).
Eye irritation.

Naphcon-A
Alcon, Austral.; Alcon, Belg.†; Alcon, Canad.; Alcon, USA.
Naphazoline hydrochloride (p.1064·2); pheniramine maleate (p.415·3).
Eye irritation.

Naphensyl *Propan, S.Afr.*
Phenylephrine hydrochloride (p.1066·2).
Respiratory-tract disorders.

Naphoptic-A *Optopics, USA.*
Naphazoline hydrochloride (p.1064·2); pheniramine maleate (p.415·3).
Eye irritation.

Napmel *Clonmel, Irl.*
Naproxen (p.61·2).
Dysmenorrhoea; gout; musculoskeletal and joint disorders.

Nappy Rash Powder *Sigma, Austral.*
Chlorphenesin (p.376·2).
Chafing; nappy rash; prickly heat.

Nappy Rash Relief Cream *Brauer, Austral.*
Calendula officinalis; clematis recta; daphne mezereum; hypericum (p.1590·1); chamomile (p.1561·2).
Nappy rash.

Nappy-Mate *Ethicare, Austral.*
Aluminium chlorohydrate (p.1078·3); zinc oxide (p.1096·2); benzoin tincture (p.1634·1); silicone (p.1384·2).
Nappy rash.

Napratec *Searle, UK.*
Naproxen (p.61·2).
Misoprostol (p.1419·3) is included in this preparation in an attempt to limit adverse effects on the gastro-intestinal mucosa.
Ankylosing spondylitis; osteoarthritis; rheumatoid arthritis.

Naprel *Brunel, S.Afr.*
Naproxen (p.61·2).
Dysmenorrhoea; gout; musculoskeletal and joint disorders.

Naprelan
Meda, Swed.†; Wyeth-Ayerst, USA.
Naproxen sodium (p.61·2).
Gout; musculoskeletal, joint, and peri-articular disorders; pain.

Napren *Nycomed, Norw.; AFI, Norw.*
Naproxen (p.61·2).
Gout; musculoskeletal and joint disorders; pain.

Naprex *Pinewood, Irl.*
Naproxen (p.61·2).
Dysmenorrhoea; gout; musculoskeletal and joint disorders.

Napril *Randob, USA†.*
Pseudoephedrine hydrochloride (p.1068·3); chlorpheniramine maleate (p.405·1).
Upper respiratory-tract symptoms.

Naprilene
Sigma-Tau, Ital.; Sigma-Tau, Spain.
Enalapril maleate (p.863·2).
Angina pectoris; heart failure; hypertension.

Naprium *Radiumfarma, Ital.†.*
Naproxen (p.61·2).
Musculoskeletal and joint disorders; neuralgias.

Naprius *Aesculapius, Ital.*
Naproxen (p.61·2).
Fever; inflammation; musculoskeletal, joint, peri-articular, and soft-tissue disorders; pain.

Naprobene *Merckle, Aust.*
Naproxen (p.61·2).
Gout; inflammation; musculoskeletal and joint disorders; pain.

Naprocoat *Roche, Neth.*
Naproxen (p.61·2).
Musculoskeletal and joint disorders.

Naprodol *Upsamedica, Ital.*
Naproxen sodium (p.61·2).
Pain.

Napro-Dorsch *Nycomed, Ger.†.*
Naproxen (p.61·2).
Inflammation; pain.

Naprogesic *Roche Consumer, Austral.*
Naproxen sodium (p.61·2).
Dysmenorrhoea.

Naprokes *Inexfa, Spain.*
Naproxen (p.61·2).
Gout; musculoskeletal, joint, and peri-articular disorders; pain.

Naprolag *Lagap, Switz.†.*
Naproxen (p.61·2).
Musculoskeletal, joint, and peri-articular disorders.

Naprorex *Lampugnani, Ital.*
Naproxen sodium (p.61·2).
Inflammation; musculoskeletal and joint disorders; pain.

Naproscript *Searle, S.Afr.†.*
Naproxen (p.61·2).
Dysmenorrhoea; musculoskeletal and joint disorders.

Naprosyn
Syntex, Austral.; Roche, Canad.; Roche, Irl.; Recordati, Ital.; Roche, Norw.; Roche, S.Afr.; Syntex, Spain; Syntex, Swed.; Roche, Switz.; Roche, UK; Syntex, USA.
Naproxen (p.61·2) or naproxen sodium (p.61·2).
Gout; musculoskeletal, joint, peri-articular, and soft-tissue disorders; pain.

Naprosyne
Roche, Belg.; Cipharm, Fr.; Roche, Neth.
Naproxen (p.61·2).
Fever; gout; inflammation; musculoskeletal and joint disorders; pain.

Naproval *Septa, Spain.*
Naproxen (p.61·2).
Gout; musculoskeletal, joint, and peri-articular disorders; pain.

Naprovite *Roche, Neth.*
Naproxen sodium (p.61·2).
Fever; inflammation; musculoskeletal and joint disorders; pain.

Naqua *Schering, USA.*
Trichlormethiazide (p.958·2).
Hypertension; oedema.

Naramig
Glaxo Wellcome, Swed.; Glaxo Wellcome, UK.
Naratriptan hydrochloride (p.448·3).
Migraine.

Naranocor Pfluger, Ger.
Crataegus (p.1568·2).
Arrhythmias; heart failure.

Naranocut H Pfluger, Ger.
Homoeopathic preparation.

Naranofem Pfluger, Ger.
Homoeopathic preparation.

Naranopect P Pfluger, Ger.
Hedera helix.
Respiratory-tract disorders.

Naranotox Pfluger, Ger.
Homoeopathic preparation.

Narbalek Soekami, Fr.†.
Vitamin B substances, iron, and mineral preparation.
Tonic.

Narbel Chugai, Jpn†.
Tetrahydrozoline nitrate (p.1070·3).
Eye congestion; nasal congestion.

Narcan
Boots, Austral.; Du Pont, Belg.; Du Pont, Canad.; Du Pont, Fr.; Du Pont, Irl.; Crinos, Ital.; Boots, S.Afr.; Du Pont, Switz.; Du Pont Pharmaceuticals, UK; Du Pont, USA.
Naloxone hydrochloride (p.986·2).
Opioid overdosage; reversal of opioid depression.

Narcanti
Torrex, Aust.; Du Pont, Ger.; Du Pont, Norw.; Meda, Swed.
Naloxone hydrochloride (p.986·2).
Opioid overdosage; reversal of opioid depression.

Narcaricin Heumann, Ger.
Benzbromarone (p.392·3).
Gout; hyperuricaemia.

Narcolo Lusofarmaco, Ital.†.
Dextromoramide tartrate (p.27·2).
Pain.

Narcoral Crinos, Ital.
Naltrexone hydrochloride (p.988·1).
Opioid overdosage; opioid withdrawal.

Narcozep Roche, Fr.†.
Flunitrazepam (p.670·1).
General anaesthesia; premedication.

Nardelzine
Parke, Davis, Belg.; Parke, Davis, Spain†.
Phenelzine sulphate (p.302·1).
Anxiety; bulimia; depression.

Nardil
Parke, Davis, Austral.; Parke, Davis, Canad.; Parke, Davis, Irl.; Hansam, UK; Parke, Davis, USA.
Phenelzine sulphate (p.302·1).
Depression; phobic states.

Nardyl Vifor, Switz.
Promethazine hydrochloride (p.416·2); hyoscyamine sulphate (p.464·2); atropine sulphate (p.455·1); hyoscine hydrobromide (p.462·3).
Anxiety; neuroses; sleep disorders; tension.

Narfen Alter, Spain.
Ibuprofen (p.44·1).
Fever; musculoskeletal, joint, and peri-articular disorders; pain.

Naride Amrad, Austral.
Indapamide (p.890·2).
Hypertension.

Narifresh Rappai, Switz.
Sea salt (p.1162·2); chamomile (p.1561·2).
Nasal disorders.

Narilet Fher, Spain.
Ipratropium bromide (p.754·2).
Rhinorrhoea.

Narine Schering-Plough, Spain.
Pseudoephedrine sulphate (p.1068·3); loratadine (p.413·1).
Allergic rhinitis.

Narium Hamilton, Austral.
Sodium chloride (p.1162·2).
Nasal irritation and inflammation.

Narixan Schiapparelli, Ital.
Pseudoephedrine hydrochloride (p.1068·3).
Rhinitis; upper respiratory-tract congestion.

Narlisim Baldacci, Ital.
Muramidase hydrochloride (p.1604·3); phenolpropamine iodide; thonzylamine hydrochloride (p.419·2).
Nasal congestion.

Narobic Schwulst, S.Afr.
Metronidazole (p.585·1).
Anaerobic bacterial infections; protozoal infections.

Narol Almirall, Spain.
Buspirone hydrochloride (p.643·3).
Anxiety.

Narop Astra, Swed.
Ropivacaine hydrochloride (p.1300·2).
Local anaesthesia.

Naropin
Astra, Aust.; Astra, Austral.; Astra, Ger.; Astra, Irl.; Astra, Neth.; Astra, UK; Astra, USA.
Ropivacaine hydrochloride (p.1300·2).
Local anaesthesia.

Naropina Astra, Ital.
Ropivacaine hydrochloride (p.1300·2).
Epidural anaesthesia; local anaesthesia; pain.

Narphen Napp, UK.
Phenazocine hydrobromide (p.78·1).
Pain.

Nasa-12 Glaxo Wellcome, Belg.
Pseudoephedrine hydrochloride (p.1068·3).
Rhinitis.

Nasabid Abana, USA.
Pseudoephedrine hydrochloride (p.1068·3); guaiphenesin (p.1061·3).
Cough; nasal congestion.

Nasacor Rhone-Poulenc Rorer, S.Afr.
Triamcinolone acetonide (p.1050·2).
Hypersensitivity reactions.

Nasacort
Rhone-Poulenc Rorer, Canad.; Rhone-Poulenc Rorer, UK; Rhone-Poulenc Rorer, USA.
Triamcinolone acetonide (p.1050·2).
Allergic rhinitis.

Nasahist B Keene, USA†.
Brompheniramine maleate (p.403·2).
Hypersensitivity reactions.

NaSal Sterling Health, USA.
Sodium chloride (p.1162·2).
Nasal congestion.

Nasal Inhaler Pickles, UK.
Eucalyptus (p.1578·1); menthol (p.1600·2); methyl salicylate (p.55·2); pumilio pine oil (p.1623·3).
Nasal congestion.

Nasal Jelly
Note. This name is used for preparations of different composition.
Thuna, Canad.
Ephedrine hydrochloride (p.1059·3); methyl salicylate (p.55·2); thymol (p.1127·1).

Kondon, USA.
Phenol (p.1121·2); camphor (p.1557·2); menthol (p.1600·2); eucalyptus oil (p.1578·1); lavender oil (p.1594·3).
Nasal congestion.

Nasal Moist Blairex, USA.
Sodium chloride (p.1162·2).
Inflammation and dryness of nasal membranes.

Nasal Relief Rugby, USA.
Oxymetazoline hydrochloride (p.1065·3).
Nasal congestion.

Nasal Rovi Rovi, Spain†.
Diphenhydramine hydrochloride (p.409·1); hydrocortisone (p.1043·3); lignocaine hydrochloride (p.1293·2); naphazoline nitrate (p.1064·2).
Nasal congestion.

Nasal & Sinus Relief Stanley, Canad.
Pseudoephedrine hydrochloride (p.1068·3).

Nasal Spray for Hayfever Unichem, UK.
Beclomethasone dipropionate (p.1032·1).
Hayfever.

Nasalate Paedpharm, Austral.
Chlorhexidine (p.1107·2); phenylephrine hydrochloride (p.1066·2).
Epistaxis; nasal surgery; vestibulitis.

Nasal-Bec Norton, UK.
Beclomethasone dipropionate (p.1032·1).
Rhinitis.

Nasalcrom McNeil Consumer, USA.
Sodium cromoglycate (p.762·1).
Allergic rhinitis.

Nasalemed SmithKline Beecham, Ital.
Xylometazoline hydrochloride (p.1071·2); domiphen bromide (p.1112·3).
Nasal congestion.

Nasaleze Healtheze, UK.
Cellulose (p.1472·2).
Allergic rhinitis.

Nasalgon Labopharma, Ger.†.
Ephedrine hydrochloride (p.1059·3); hydroxyquinoline (p.1589·3); echinaceae angustifolia (p.1574·2); terpin hydrate (p.1070·2).
Rhinitis.

Nasalide
Cassenne, Fr.; Syntex, USA.
Flunisolide (p.1040·3).
Allergic rhinitis.

Nasaltex Bristol-Myers, Spain†.
Oxymetazoline hydrochloride (p.1065·3).
Nasal congestion.

Nasan Hexal, Ger.
Xylometazoline hydrochloride (p.1071·2).
Formerly contained tetrahydrozoline hydrochloride.
Rhinitis.

Nasanal Brady, Aust.
Aluminium acetotartrate (p.1547·3); pumilio pine oil (p.1623·3).
Nasal disorders.

Nasapert
Searle, Belg.; Astra, Neth.†.
Brompheniramine maleate (p.403·2); phenylpropanolamine hydrochloride (p.1067·2).
Allergic rhinitis.

Nasarel Roche, USA.
Flunisolide (p.1040·3).
Rhinitis.

Nasatab LA ECR, USA.
Guaiphenesin (p.1061·3); pseudoephedrine hydrochloride (p.1068·3).
Coughs.

Nasatuss Abana, USA.
Hydrocodone tartrate (p.43·1); phenylephrine hydrochloride (p.1066·2); chlorpheniramine maleate (p.405·1).
Coughs and congestion.

Nasben Demopharm, Switz.
Xylometazoline hydrochloride (p.1071·2).
Nasal congestion.

Nasben soft Demopharm, Switz.
Sodium chloride (p.1162·2).
Nasal disorders.

Nascobal Schwarz, USA.
Cyanocobalamin (p.1363·3).
Vitamin B_{12} deficiency.

Nasdro Mer-National, S.Afr.
Phenylephrine hydrochloride (p.1066·2); naphazoline nitrate (p.1064·2).
Nasal congestion.

Nasello Synpharma, Switz.
Calcium laevulinate (p.1155·2); camphor (p.1557·2); ephedrine hydrochloride (p.1059·3); menthol (p.1600·2); pheniramine maleate (p.415·3); procaine hydrochloride (p.1299·2); hydroxyquinoline (p.1589·3).
Rhinitis.

Nasengel Ratiopharm, Ger.
Xylometazoline hydrochloride (p.1071·2).
Catarrh; colds; sinusitis.

Nasengel AL Aliud, Ger.
Xylometazoline hydrochloride (p.1071·2).
Rhinitis.

Nasenol-ratiopharm Ratiopharm, Ger.†.
Anhydrous ephedrine (p.1059·3); eucalyptus oil (p.1578·1); menthol (p.1600·2); camphor (p.1557·2).
Cold symptoms.

Nasenspray AL Aliud, Ger.
Xylometazoline hydrochloride (p.1071·2).
Rhinitis.

Nasenspray E Ratiopharm, Ger.
Xylometazoline hydrochloride (p.1071·2).
Catarrh; rhinitis; sinusitis.

Nasenspray K Ratiopharm, Ger.
Xylometazoline hydrochloride (p.1071·2).
Catarrh; rhinitis; sinusitis.

Nasentropfen AL Aliud, Ger.
Xylometazoline hydrochloride (p.1071·2).
Rhinitis.

Nasentropfen E Ratiopharm, Ger.
Xylometazoline hydrochloride (p.1071·2).
Catarrh; rhinitis; sinusitis.

Nasentropfen K Ratiopharm, Ger.
Xylometazoline hydrochloride (p.1071·2).
Catarrh; rhinitis; sinusitis.

Naseptin
Zeneca, Irl.; Zeneca, S.Afr.; Bioglan, UK.
Chlorhexidine hydrochloride (p.1107·2); neomycin sulphate (p.229·2).
Nasal carriage of staphylococci; staphylococcal infections.

Nasex DP-Medica, Switz.
Phenylephrine hydrochloride (p.1066·2); cetylpyridinium chloride (p.1106·2).
Nasal disorders.

Nasicortin
Merck, Ger.†; Bracco, Ital.
Dexamethasone tebutate (p.1037·3); oxymetazoline hydrochloride (p.1065·3).
Conjunctivitis; nasal polyps; rhinitis; rhinopharyngitis; sinusitis.

Nasimild Merck, Aust.†.
Benzalkonium chloride (p.1101·3); polysorbate 80 (p.1327·3).
Nasal disorders.

Nasin Tika, Swed.
Oxymetazoline hydrochloride (p.1065·3).
Rhinitis; sinusitis.

Nasivin
Merck, Aust.; Bracco, Ital.; E. Merck, Neth.
Oxymetazoline hydrochloride (p.1065·3).
Nasal congestion; rhinitis; sinus disorders.

Nasivin gegen Heuschnupfen Merck, Ger.†.
Sodium cromoglycate (p.762·1).
Allergic disorders; conjunctivitis.

Nasivin gegen Schnupfen Merck, Ger.
Oxymetazoline hydrochloride (p.1065·3).
Catarrh; otitis media; rhinitis.

Nasivin Intensiv-Bad N Merck, Ger.
Eucalyptus oil (p.1578·1); thyme oil (p.1637·1); camphor (p.1557·2).
Respiratory-tract congestion.

Nasivin Intensiv-Balsam Merck, Ger.†.
Eucalyptus oil (p.1578·1); camphor (p.1557·2); menthol (p.1600·2); pumilio pine oil (p.1623·3).
Coughs and colds.

Nasivin Kinderbad Merck, Ger.
Eucalyptus oil (p.1578·1).
Respiratory-tract congestion.

Nasivine Asta Medica, Switz.
Oxymetazoline hydrochloride (p.1065·3).
Catarrh; rhinitis; sinusitis.

Nasivinetten Asta Medica, Switz.
Oxymetazoline hydrochloride (p.1065·3).
Catarrh; rhinitis; sinusitis.

Nasivinetten gegen Schnupfen Merck, Ger.
Oxymetazoline hydrochloride (p.1065·3).
Catarrh; otitis media; rhinitis.

Naska Lifepharma, Ital.†.
Propenidazole (p.592·2).
Protozoal and fungal infections of the genito-urinary tract.

Naso Pekamin Medical, Spain.
Phenylephrine hydrochloride (p.1066·2); kanamycin sulphate (p.220·3); trypsin (p.1640·1).
Nasal congestion and infection.

Nasobec Baker Norton, UK.
Beclomethasone dipropionate (p.1032·1).
Rhinitis.

Nasobol Sodip, Switz.
Benzoic acid (p.1102·3); peru balsam (p.1617·2); verbena oil; eucalyptus oil (p.1578·1); lavender oil (p.1594·3); wild thyme oil.
Respiratory-tract disorders.

Nasoferm Nordic, Swed.
Xylometazoline hydrochloride (p.1071·2).
Rhinitis; sinusitis.

Nasokey Inkeysa, Spain†.
Phenylephrine hydrochloride (p.1066·2); hydrocortisone acetate (p.1043·3); neomycin sulphate (p.229·2).
Congestion and infection of the nose and ear.

Nasomixin
Note. This name is used for preparations of different composition.
Fournier, Ital.
Phenylephrine hydrochloride (p.1066·2); phenylpropanolamine hydrochloride (p.1067·2); hydrocortisone (p.1043·3); neomycin sulphate (p.229·2).
Cold symptoms; rhinitis; sinusitis.

Hoechst Marion Roussel, S.Afr.
Phenylephrine hydrochloride (p.1066·2); phenylpropanolamine hydrochloride (p.1067·2); hydrocortisone (p.1043·3); neomycin sulphate (p.229·2); menthol (p.1600·2).
Rhinitis; sinusitis.

Nasonex
Schering-Plough, Swed.; Schering-Plough, UK; Schering, USA.
Mometasone furoate (p.1047·2).
Rhinitis.

Nasopomada Medical, Spain.
Bismuth subgallate (p.1180·2); prednisolone (p.1048·1); rutin (p.1580·2); sulphanilamide (p.256·3); tetracycline hydrochloride (p.259·1); urea; benzocaine (p.1286·2).
Nasal furunculosis; sinusitis.

Nasotic Oto Juventus, Spain.
Betamethasone valerate (p.1033·3); neomycin sulphate (p.229·2); papain (p.1614·1); polymyxin B sulphate (p.239·1).
Ear disorders; rhinitis.

Nasovalda Sterling Health, Spain.
Oxymetazoline hydrochloride (p.1065·3).
Nasal congestion; sinus congestion.

Nastoren Lepetit, Ital.
Somatostatin acetate (p.1261·1).
Gastro-intestinal haemorrhage; prevention of postoperative complications following pancreatic surgery.

Nasulind Steierl, Ger.
Peppermint oil (p.1208·1); thyme oil (p.1637·1).
Nasal congestion.

Natabec
Parke, Davis, Aust.; Warner-Lambert, Ger.; Warner-Lambert Consumer, Switz.
Multivitamin and mineral preparation.

Natabec F Warner-Lambert, Ger.
Multivitamin and mineral preparation with sodium fluoride (p.742·1).

Natabec Rx Parke, Davis, USA†.
Multivitamin and mineral preparation with iron and folic acid.

Natabec-F.A. with Fluoride Parke, Davis, S.Afr.†.
Multivitamin and mineral preparation.

Natacyn
Alcon, S.Afr.; Alcon, USA.
Natamycin (p.385·3).
Fungal eye infections.

Natafucin Yamanouchi, Ital.
Natamycin (p.385·3).
Fungal skin infections.

NatalCare Plus Ethex, USA.
Multivitamin and mineral preparation.

Natalins Mead Johnson Nutritionals, USA.
Multivitamin and mineral preparation with iron and folic acid.
Dietary supplement during pregnancy and lactation.

Natarex Prenatal Major, USA.
Multivitamin and mineral preparation with iron and folic acid.

Natecal 600 Italfarmaco, Spain.
Calcium carbonate (p.1182·1).
Hypocalcaemia; osteoporosis.

Naticardina Asta Medica, Ital.
Quinidine polygalacturonate (p.938·3).
Arrhythmias.

Nati-K Centrapharm, Fr.
Potassium tartrate (p.1161·2).
Hypokalaemia.

Natil 3M, Ger.
Cyclandelate (p.845·2).
Cerebral metabolic and vascular disorders; migraine; retinopathy; vestibular disorders.

Natirose Procter & Gamble, Fr.†.
Glyceryl trinitrate (p.874·3).
Angina pectoris; pulmonary oedema.

Natisedina Teofarma, Ital.; Berenguer Infale, Spain†.
Quinidine phenylethylbarbiturate (p.940·2).
Arrhythmias.

Natisedine
Note. This name is used for preparations of different composition.
Sabex, Canad.; Giulini, Ger.†; Sanofi Labaz, Neth.†.
Quinidine phenylethylbarbiturate (p.940·2).
Nervous disorders with arrhythmia.

Procter & Gamble, Fr.
Phenobarbitone (p.350·2); passion flower (p.1615·3). Formerly contained quinidine phenylethylbarbiturate.
Anxiety; insomnia; palpitations.

Natispray
Procter & Gamble, Fr.; Teofarma, Ital.; Nativelle, Switz.
Glyceryl trinitrate (p.874·3).
Angina pectoris; pulmonary oedema.

Nativa HA Guigoz, Ital.
Infant feed.
Milk intolerance.

Na-To-Caps SIT, Ital.
Mixed tocopherols (p.1369·1).
Vitamin E deficiency.

Natracalm English Grains, UK.
Passiflora incarnata (p.1615·3).
Tension.

Natraleze English Grains, UK.
Slippery elm bark (p.1630·1); meadowsweet (p.1599·1); liquorice (p.1197·1).
Dyspepsia; flatulence; heartburn.

Natramid Trinity, UK.
Indapamide (p.890·2).
Hypertension.

Natrasleep English Grains, UK.
Lupulus (p.1597·2); valerian (p.1643·1).
Insomnia.

Natrilix
Servier, Austral.; Servier, Ger.; Servier, Irl.; Servier, Ital.; Servier, S.Afr.; Servier, UK.
Indapamide (p.890·2).
Hypertension.

Natrioxen Benedetti, Ital.
Naproxen sodium (p.61·2).
Lignocaine hydrochloride (p.1293·2) is included in the intramuscular injection to alleviate the pain of injection.
Inflammation; musculoskeletal and joint disorders; pain.

Natrocitral Chemdorf, Spain.
Oxethazaine (p.1298·1); sodium citrate (p.1153·2); aluminium glycinate (p.1177·2).
Gastro-intestinal disorders.

Natron Berlin-Chemie, Ger.†.
Sodium carbonate (p.1153·2).
Urinary-tract disorders.

Natuderm Leo, UK†.
Emollient.

Natudolor Duopharm, Ger.
Potentilla anserina.
Dysmenorrhoea.

Natudophilus Cantassium Co., UK.
Lactobacillus acidophilus (p.1594·1); *Bifidobacterium bifidum* (p.1594·1).

Natudor Plantes et Medecines, Fr.
Crataegus (p.1568·2); passion flower (p.1615·3).
Anxiety; insomnia; palpitations.

Natulan
Roche, Aust.; Roche, Austral.; Roche, Belg.; Roche, Canad.; Roche, Fr.; Roche, Ger.; Roche, Ital.; Roche, Neth.; Roche, Norw.; Roche, S.Afr.; Roche, Spain; Roche, Switz.; Cambridge, UK.
Procarbazine hydrochloride (p.559·2).
Now known as Procarbazine Capsules in the *UK*.
Malignant neoplasms.

Natulanar Roche, Swed.†.
Procarbazine hydrochloride (p.559·2).
Malignant neoplasms.

Natulax Lichtenstein, Ger.
Lactulose (p.1195·3).
Constipation; hepatic encephalopathy; salmonella enteritis.

Natur B12 Panthox & Burck, Ital.†.
Hydroxocobalamin (p.1363·3).
Lignocaine hydrochloride (p.1293·2) is included in this preparation to alleviate the pain of injection.
Megaloblastic anaemia; neuralgias; neuritis.

Natura Medica Dolisos, Fr.
A range of herbal extracts.

Natural Fibre Cenovis, Austral.; Vitelle, Austral.
Psyllium (p.1194·2).
Constipation; dietary supplement.

Natural Source Laxative Adams, Canad.
Ispaghula husk (p.1194·2).
Constipation; fibre supplementation.

Natural Vegetable Alkaliniser Vitaplex, Austral.†.
Celery (p.1561·1); peppermint leaf (p.1208·1); cochlearia armoracia; rorippa nasturtium aquaticum; parsley (p.1615·3); silver birch (p.1553·3).
Herbal diuretic.

Natural Zanzy Montefarmaco, Ital.
Geranium oil (p.1584·1); lavender oil (p.1594·3); citronella oil (p.1565·1).
Insect repellent.

Naturalyte UBI, USA.
Glucose; electrolytes (p.1152·3).
Diarrhoea; oral rehydration therapy.

Naturcil London Drugs, Canad.
Ispaghula husk (p.1194·2).

Nature Ferm Thermalife, Austral.†.
Chamomile/protein/trace metal complex.
Musculoskeletal and joint pain; soft-tissue injury.

Nature's Bounty 1 Nature's Bounty, USA†.
Multivitamin and mineral preparation with iron and folic acid.

Natures Remedy
Block, Canad.; SmithKline Beecham Consumer, USA.
Cascara (p.1183·1); aloes (p.1177·1).
Constipation.

Nature's Tears Rugby, USA.
Hypromellose (p.1473·1); dextran 70 (p.717·1).
Dry eyes.

Naturest
Note. This name is used for preparations of different composition.
Vita Glow, Austral.
Valerian (p.1643·1); passion flower (p.1615·3); scutellaria; verbena officinalis; magnesium oxide (p.1198·3); calcium phosphate (p.1155·3).
Insomnia.

Lane, UK.
Passion flower (p.1615·3).
Insomnia.

Naturetin
Squibb, Canad.; Apothecon, USA.
Bendrofluazide (p.827·3).
Hypertension; oedema.

Naturgen terre silice Marbot, Switz.
Medicinal mud.
Bronchitis; coughs; musculoskeletal and joint disorders; phlebitis.

Naturgen terre volcanique Marbot, Switz.
Medicinal volcanic mud.
Digestive-system disorders.

Naturine Leo, Fr.
Bendrofluazide (p.827·3).
Hypertension; oedema.

Naturlix Fides, Spain†.
Ispaghula husk (p.1194·2).
Constipation.

Naturvite Solgar, UK.
Multivitamin and mineral preparation.

Natusan
Organon, Spain.
Glyceroborate complex; boric acid (p.1554·2); borax (p.1554·2).
Formerly contained glyceroborate complex, lanolin, paraffin, and titanium dioxide.
Skin disorders.

Innovex, UK†.
Boric acid (p.1554·2); borax (p.1554·2).
Napkin rash.

Natuscap retard Vifor, Switz.
Chlorpheniramine maleate (p.405·1); codeine phosphate (p.26·1); phenylephrine hydrochloride (p.1066·2).
Coughs and associated respiratory-tract disorders.

Natuvit
Roche Nicholas, Fr.; Asta Medica, Neth.
Nutritional supplement.

Natyl Interdelta, Switz.
Dipyridamole (p.857·1).
Thrombo-embolism prophylaxis.

Naudicelle
Key, Austral.; Swiss Herbal, Canad.; Bio-Oil Research, Irl.; Bio-Oil Research, UK.
Evening primrose oil (p.1582·1).
Dietary supplement.

Naudicelle Forte Bio-Oil Research, UK.
Borage oil (p.1582·1); marine fish oil (p.1276·1).

Naudicelle Marine Key, Austral.
Evening primrose oil (p.1582·1); marine fish oil (p.1276·1).
Dietary supplement.

Naudicelle Plus
Key, Austral.†; Bio-Oil Research, UK.
Evening primrose oil (p.1582·1); marine fish oil (p.1276·1).
Dietary supplement.

Naudicelle plus Epanoil Key, Austral.†.
Evening primrose oil (p.1582·1); marine fish oil (p.1276·1).
Dietary supplement.

Naudicelle SL Bio-Oil Research, UK.
Salmon oil (p.1276·1); lecithin (p.1595·2).

Naudicelle Super Key, Austral.†.
Borage oil (p.1582·1); evening primrose oil (p.1582·1).
Nutritional fatty acid supplement.

Naudivite Bio-Oil Research, UK.
A range of vitamin, mineral, and nutritional supplements.

Naupathon Staufen, Ger.
Homoeopathic preparation.

Naus-A-Way Roberts, USA†.
Glucose (p.1343·3); fructose (p.1343·2); phosphoric acid (p.1618·1).
Nausea and vomiting.

Nausea Complex Brauer, Austral.
Homoeopathic preparation.

Nauseatol Sabex, Canad.
Dimenhydrinate (p.408·2).
Nausea and vomiting.

Nausex
Asta Medica, Aust.; Nobel, Canad.
Dimenhydrinate (p.408·2).
Ménière's disease; motion sickness; nausea and vomiting; vestibular disorders.

Nausicalm Brothier, Fr.
Dimenhydrinate (p.408·2).
Motion sickness; nausea and vomiting.

Nausigon Mundipharma, Aust.
Metoclopramide hydrochloride (p.1200·3).
Gastro-intestinal ulcers; intractable hiccups; nausea and vomiting; upper gastro-intestinal motility disorders.

Nausilen Baldacci, Ital.
Alizapride hydrochloride (p.1176·3).
Nausea and vomiting.

Nausyn
Weleda, Aust.; Weleda, UK.
Homoeopathic preparation.

Nautamine Synthelabo, Fr.
Diphenhydramine di(acefyllinate) (p.409·1).
Motion sickness; nausea and vomiting.

Nautisan Salus, Aust.
Chlorbutol (p.1106·3); caffeine (p.749·3).
Nausea and vomiting.

Nauzelin Janssen-Cilag, Spain.
Domperidone (p.1190·3).
Gastroparesis; nausea and vomiting.

Nauzine Be-Tabs, S.Afr.
Cyclizine hydrochloride (p.407·1).
Nausea and vomiting; vertigo.

Navane
Pfizer, Austral.; Pfizer, Canad.; Pfizer, Neth.; Roerig, Swed.†; Roerig, USA.
Thiothixene (p.695·3).
Psychoses.

Navarrofilina Navarro, Spain†.
Aminophylline (p.748·1); phenobarbitone sodium (p.350·2).
Obstructive airways disease.

Navelbine
Bender, Aust.; Asta Medica, Austral.; Glaxo Wellcome, Canad.; Pierre Fabre, Fr.; Pierre Fabre, Ger.; Pierre Fabre, Ital.; Pierre Fabre, Spain; Pierre Fabre, Swed.; Robapharm, Switz.; Pierre Fabre, UK; Glaxo Wellcome, USA.
Vinorelbine tartrate (p.571·2).
Breast cancer; non-small cell lung cancer.

Navicalm
Note. This name is used for preparations of different composition.
UCB, Neth.
Hydroxyzine hydrochloride (p.412·1).
Nervous tension; pruritus; urticaria.

UCB, Spain.
Meclozine hydrochloride (p.413·3).
Motion sickness.

Navidrex
Ciba-Geigy, Austral.†; Ciba-Geigy, Irl.†; Ciba, Neth.†; Ciba, Switz.†; Alliance, UK.
Cyclopenthiazide (p.845·2).
Heart failure; hypertension; oedema.

Navidrex-K
Ciba-Geigy, Irl.†; Ciba-Geigy, S.Afr.†.
Cyclopenthiazide (p.845·2); potassium chloride (p.1161·1).
Heart failure; hypertension; oedema.

Navispare
Ciba-Geigy, Irl.; Ciba, UK.
Cyclopenthiazide (p.845·2); amiloride hydrochloride (p.819·2).
Hypertension.

Navoban
Sanabo, Aust.; Novartis, Austral.; Sandoz, Fr.; Sandoz, Ger.; Asta Medica, Ger.; Sandoz, Irl.; Sandoz, Ital.; Sandoz, Norw.; Novartis, S.Afr.; Sandoz, Spain; Novartis, Swed.; Sandoz, Switz.; Sandoz, UK.
Tropisetron hydrochloride (p.1217·3).
Nausea and vomiting induced by cytotoxic therapy; postoperative nausea and vomiting.

Naxen
Alphapharm, Austral.†; Syncare, Canad.; Rolab, S.Afr.
Naproxen (p.61·2).
Dysmenorrhoea; gout; musculoskeletal and joint disorders.

Naxidine Lilly, Neth.
Nizatidine (p.1203·2).
Gastro-oesophageal reflux; peptic ulcer.

Naxogin
Farmitalia Carlo Erba, Aust.; Pharmacia Upjohn, Belg.; Carlo Erba, Ital.†; Pharmacia, S.Afr.†.
Nimorazole (p.589·3).
Acute ulcerative gingivitis; amoebiasis; giardiasis; vaginal trichomoniasis.

Naxogyn Pharmacia Upjohn, Fr.
Nimorazole (p.589·3).
Trichomoniasis.

Naxpa Novag, Spain.
Ambroxol hydrochloride (p.1054·3).
Respiratory-tract disorders.

Naxy Sanofi Winthrop, Fr.
Clarithromycin (p.189·1).
Bacterial infections.

Nazene-Z Restan, S.Afr.
Oxymetazoline hydrochloride (p.1065·3); zinc sulphate (p.1373·2).
Allergic rhinitis; nasal congestion; sinusitis.

Nazophyl Medecine Vegetale, Fr.
Eucalyptus oil (p.1578·1); pine oil.
Nose and throat infections.

NB-Tee N Eu Rho, Ger.
Birch leaf (p.1553·3); orthosiphon leaf (p.1592·2).
Urinary-tract disorders.

NB-tee Siegfried Siegfried, Ger.†.
Bearberry (p.1552·2); birch leaf (p.1553·3); juniper (p.1592·2); solidago virgaurea; couch-grass (p.1567·3); equisetum (p.1575·1); ononis (p.1610·2); orthosiphon (p.1592·2).
Urinary-tract disorders.

N-Combur Test Boehringer Mannheim, Austral.
Test for nitrite, protein, glucose, and pH in urine.

ND Stat Hyrex, USA†.
Brompheniramine maleate (p.403·2).
Hypersensitivity reactions.

ND-Gesic Hyrex, USA.
Phenylephrine hydrochloride (p.1066·2); paracetamol (p.72·2); chlorpheniramine maleate (p.405·1); mepyramine maleate (p.414·1).
Upper respiratory-tract symptoms.

NE 300 Miba, Ital.†.
Uridine (p.1641·3); cytidine; guanosine; inosine (p.1591·1); cobamamide (p.1364·2); suprarenal cortex (p.1050·1); nicotinamide (p.1351·2); calcium folinate (p.1342·2); lignocaine hydrochloride (p.1293·2).
Adjunct in antibiotic therapy; anaemias; anorexia; liver disorders; tonic.

Nealgon Laevosan, Aust.†.
Dipyrone (p.35·1); tropine benzilate hydrochloride (p.469·3).
Smooth muscle spasm.

Nealorin Pras, Spain.
Carboplatin (p.510·3).
Malignant neoplasms.

Neatenol Fides, Spain.
Atenolol (p.825·3).
Angina pectoris; arrhythmias; hypertension; myocardial infarction.

Neatenol Diu Fides, Spain.
Bendrofluazide (p.827·3); atenolol (p.825·3).
Hypertension.

Neatenol Diuvas Fides, Spain.
Bendrofluazide (p.827·3); hydralazine hydrochloride (p.883·2); atenolol (p.825·3).
Hypertension.

Nebacetin
Tyrol, Aust.; Yamanouchi, Ger.; Lundbeck, Neth.†; Byk Gulden, S.Afr.†; Lundbeck, Swed.†; Eumedica, Switz.†.
Neomycin (p.229·2) or neomycin sulphate (p.229·2); bacitracin (p.157·3) or bacitracin zinc (p.157·3).
Bacterial infections.

Nebacetin N Yamanouchi, Ger.
Neomycin sulphate (p.229·2).
Wounds.

Nebacetine Eumedica, Belg.†.
Neomycin sulphate (p.229·2); bacitracin (p.157·3).
Cystitis; eye disorders; otitis externa; rhinitis; skin disorders; surgical wound irrigation.

Nebcin
Lilly, Austral.; Lilly, Canad.; Lilly, Irl.; Lilly, S.Afr.; Lilly, UK; Lilly, USA.
Tobramycin (p.264·1) or tobramycin sulphate (p.264·1).
Bacterial infections.

Nebcina
Lilly, Norw.; Lilly, Swed.
Tobramycin sulphate (p.264·1).
Bacterial infections.

Nebcine Lilly, Fr.
Tobramycin sulphate (p.264·1).
Bacterial infections.

Nebicina Lilly, Ital.
Tobramycin sulphate (p.264·1).
Bacterial infections.

Nebilet
Janssen-Cilag, Aust.; Berlin-Chemie, Ger.; Menarini, Neth.
Nebivolol hydrochloride (p.914·3).
Hypertension.

Neblik Knoll, Spain.
Eformoterol fumarate (p.752·3).
Obstructive airways disease.

Nebris Celafar, Ital.
Olax dissitiflora; chamomile (p.1561·2).
Dry skin.

Nebris Junior Inverni della Beffa, Ital.†.
Calendula officinalis.
Acne; greasy skin.

Nebulasma Urbion, Spain.
Sodium cromoglycate (p.762·1).
Allergic rhinitis; asthma.

Nebulcrom Casen Fisons, Spain.
Sodium cromoglycate (p.762·1).
Allergic rhinitis; asthma.

Nebulicina Fher, Spain.
Oxymetazoline hydrochloride (p.1065·3).
Formerly contained fenoxazoline hydrochloride.
Nasal congestion.

NebuPent Lyphomed, USA.
Pentamidine isethionate (p.590·2).
Pneumocystis carinii pneumonia.

Necon Watson, USA.
Norethisterone (p.1453·1); ethinyloestradiol (p.1445·1).
28-Day packs also contain 7 inert tablets.
Combined oral contraceptive.

Necopen Esteve, Spain.
Cefixime (p.165·3).
Bacterial infections.

Necthar Cal *Level, Spain†.*
Calcium phosphate (p.1155·3); calcium glycerophosphate (p.1155·2); calcium lactate (p.1155·2); calcium pantothenate; magnesium phosphate; sodium fluoride (p.742·1); ergocalciferol (p.1367·1); vitamin A (p.1358·1).
Bone and dental disorders; calcium deficiency; osteomalacia; rickets.

Necyrane *Evans, Fr.*
Ritiometan magnesium (p.1124·2).
Nose and throat infections.

Neda Fruchtewurfel
Note. This name is used for preparations of different composition.
Zyma, Aust.
Senna (p.1212·2); fig (p.1193·2); tamarind (p.1217·3).
Constipation.
Zyma, Ger.
Senna (p.1212·2).
Constipation.

Neda Krautertabletten *Zyma, Aust.†.*
Senna (p.1212·2).
Constipation.

Neda Lactiv Importal *Zyma, Ger.*
Lactitol (p.1195·2).
Constipation.

Nedeltran *Rhone-Poulenc Rorer, Neth.*
Trimeprazine tartrate (p.419·3).
Hypersensitivity reactions; psychoses.

Nedios *Byk, Neth.*
Acipimox (p.1267·3).
Hyperlipidaemias.

Nedolon A *Merck, Ger.†.*
Aspirin (p.16·1); codeine phosphate (p.26·1).
Pain.

Nedolon P *Merck, Ger.*
Paracetamol (p.72·2); codeine phosphate (p.26·1).
Pain.

NEE 1/35 *Lexis, USA.*
Ethinyloestradiol (p.1445·1); norethisterone (p.1453·1).
28-Day packs also contain 7 inert tablets.
Combined oral contraceptive.

Nefadar
Bristol-Myers Squibb, Norw.; Bristol-Myers Squibb, Swed.
Nefazodone hydrochloride (p.299·3).
Depression.

Nefadol *Zilliken, Ital.*
Nefopam hydrochloride (p.62·3).
Pain.

Nefam *Biagini, Ital.*
Nefopam hydrochloride (p.62·3).
Pain.

Nefluan *Molteni, Ital.*
Lignocaine hydrochloride (p.1293·2); neomycin sulphate (p.229·2); fluocinolone acetonide (p.1041·1).
Endoscopy.

Nefrocarnit *Medice, Ger.*
Carnitine (p.1336·2).
Carnitine deficiency.

Nefrolan *May & Baker, S.Afr.†.*
Clorexolone.
Hypertension; oedema; premenstrual syndrome.

Nefrolit *Vitafarma, Spain†.*
Convallaria (p.1567·2); glucurolactone; khellin (p.1593·1); rubia tinctorum; salicylamide (p.82·3); solidago virgaurea; carzenide (p.1560·2); potassium hyaluronate.
Renal calculi.

Negaban *Beecham, Belg.*
Temocillin sodium (p.258·3).
Gram-negative bacterial infections.

Negaderm *Byk Gulden, Ital.†.*
Metacresolsulphonic acid-formaldehyde (p.725·1).
Skin disorders.

Negatol
Byk, Fr.; Byk Gulden, Ital.; Juventus, Spain; Byk, Switz.
Metacresolsulphonic acid-formaldehyde (p.725·1).
Formerly contained cresol in *Spain.*
Burns; minor haemorrhage; ulcers; vaginal disorders; wounds.

Negatol Dental *Wild, Switz.*
Metacresolsulphonic acid-formaldehyde (p.725·1).
Aphthous stomatitis; gingival haemorrhage.

NegGram
Sanofi Winthrop, Canad.; Sanofi Winthrop, Ital.; Sanofi Winthrop, USA.
Nalidixic acid (p.228·2).
Gram-negative urinary-tract infections.

Negram
Sanofi Winthrop, Austral.; Sanofi Winthrop, Fr.; Sanofi Winthrop, Irl.; Winthrop, Neth.†; Sanofi Winthrop, Norw.; Sanofi, Swed.†; Winthrop, Switz.†; Sanofi Winthrop, UK.
Nalidixic acid (p.228·2).
Gram-negative urinary- and gastro-intestinal-tract infections.

Nehydrin
Woldheim, Aust.; TAD, Ger.†.
Dihydroergocristine mesylate (p.1571·3).
Cerebral, metabolic, and circulatory disorders.

Nehydrin N *TAD, Ger.*
Co-dergocrine mesylate (p.1566·1).
Mental function disorders.

Nelex
Byk Gulden, Norw.†; Byk Madaus, S.Afr.; Pharmacia Upjohn, Swed.
Metacresolsulphonic acid-formaldehyde (p.725·1).
Anogenital warts; cervical erosion; external urethral erosion; vaginitis; wounds.

Nelova 10/11 *Warner Chilcott, USA.*
Norethisterone (p.1453·1); ethinyloestradiol (p.1445·1).
28-Day packs also contain 7 inert tablets.
Biphasic oral contraceptive.

Nelova 0.5/35E and 1/35E *Warner Chilcott, USA.*
Norethisterone (p.1453·1); ethinyloestradiol (p.1445·1).
28-Day packs also contain 7 inert tablets.
Combined oral contraceptive.

Nelova 1/50M *Warner Chilcott, USA.*
Norethisterone (p.1453·1); mestranol (p.1450·2).
28-Day packs also contain 7 inert tablets.
Combined oral contraceptive.

Nelulen *Watson, USA†.*
Ethynodiol diacetate (p.1445·3); ethinyloestradiol (p.1445·1).
28-Day packs also contain 7 inert tablets.
Combined oral contraceptive.

Nemactil *Rhone-Poulenc Rorer, Spain.*
Pericyazine (p.685·2).
Anxiety; behaviour disorders; psychoses.

Nemasol *ICN, Canad.*
Sodium aminosalicylate (p.151·1).
Tuberculosis.

Nematorazine *Millot-Solac, Fr.†.*
Piperazine sebacate (p.108·1).
Ascariasis; enterobiasis.

Nembutal
Abbott, Canad.; Abbott, USA.
Pentobarbitone sodium (p.685·1).
Epilepsy; insomnia; premedication; sedative.

Nemdyn *Hamilton, Austral.*
Neomycin undecenoate (p.229·2); bacitracin zinc (p.157·3).
Fungal or bacterial ear infections.

Nemestran
Hoechst Marion Roussel, Neth.; Roussel, Spain; Hoechst Marion Roussel, Switz.
Gestrinone (p.1447·3).
Endometriosis.

Nemexin
Willvonseder, Aust.; Du Pont, Ger.; Du Pont, Switz.
Naltrexone hydrochloride (p.988·1).
Opioid withdrawal.

Neo *Neo Laboratories, UK.*
Cream: Cetrimide (p.1105·2); benzalkonium chloride (p.1101·3).
Napkin rash; skin irritation.
Oral mixture: Dill oil (p.1572·1); ginger (p.1193·2); sodium bicarbonate (p.1153·2).

Neo Amphocort *Squibb, Switz.†.*
Amphotericin (p.372·2); triamcinolone acetonide (p.1050·2).
Infected skin disorders.

Neo Analsona *Casen Fisons, Spain.*
Benzocaine (p.1286·2); fluocinolone acetonide (p.1041·1); neomycin sulphate (p.229·2); ruscogenin (p.1627·1).
Anorectal disorders.

Neo Aritmina *Solvay, Ital.*
Prajmalium bitartrate (p.932·2).
Arrhythmias.

Neo Artrol *Recordati Elmu, Spain.*
Flurbiprofen (p.42·1).
Musculoskeletal, joint, and peri-articular disorders; pain.

Neo Atromid *Zeneca, Spain.*
Clofibrate (p.1271·1).
Hyperlipidaemias.

Neo Baby Mixture *Neo Laboratories, UK.*
Dill oil (p.1572·1); ginger essence (p.1193·2); sodium bicarbonate (p.1153·2).
Colic; teething.

Neo Bace *Pharmavite, Canad.*
Bacitracin (p.157·3); polymyxin B sulphate (p.239·1).

Neo Bacitrin *Fides, Spain.*
Ointment: Bacitracin (p.157·3); neomycin sulphate (p.229·2); zinc oxide (p.1096·2).
Topical powder: Bacitracin (p.157·3); neomycin sulphate (p.229·2).
Skin infections.

Neo Bacitrin Hidrocortis *Fides, Spain.*
Bacitracin (p.157·3); hydrocortisone acetate (p.1043·3); neomycin sulphate (p.229·2); zinc oxide (p.1096·2).
Infected skin disorders.

Neo Borocillina *Schiapparelli, Ital.*
Dichlorobenzyl alcohol (p.1112·2); sodium benzoate (p.1102·3).
Mouth and throat disinfection.

Neo Borocillina Balsamica *Schiapparelli, Ital.*
Dichlorobenzyl alcohol (p.1112·2); terpin hydrate (p.1070·2); menglytate (p.1063·3).
Mouth and throat disinfection; respiratory-tract infections.

Neo Borocillina C *Schiapparelli, Ital.*
Dichlorobenzyl alcohol (p.1112·2); ascorbic acid (p.1365·2).
Mouth and throat disinfection.

Neo Borocillina Collutorio *Schiapparelli, Ital.*
Dichlorobenzyl alcohol (p.1112·2).
Mouth and throat disinfection.

Neo Borocillina Spray *Schiapparelli, Ital.*
Dichlorobenzyl alcohol (p.1112·2).
Mouth and throat disinfection.

Neo Borocillina Tosse Compresse *Schiapparelli, Ital.*
Dextromethorphan hydrobromide (p.1057·3); guaiphenesin (p.1061·3); menglytate (p.1063·3); dichlorobenzyl alcohol (p.1112·2).
Coughs; mouth and throat disinfection.

Neo Borocillina Tosse Gocce *Schiapparelli, Ital.†.*
Dextromethorphan hydrobromide (p.1057·3); guaiphenesin (p.1061·3); menglytate (p.1063·3).
Coughs.

Neo Borocillina Tosse Sciroppo *Schiapparelli, Ital.*
Dextromethorphan hydrobromide (p.1057·3); guaiphenesin (p.1061·3); menglytate (p.1063·3).
Coughs.

Neo Cal *Neolab, Canad.*
Calcium carbonate (p.1182·1).

Neo Cal D *Neolab, Canad.*
Calcium carbonate (p.1182·1); vitamin D (p.1366·3).

Neo Carbone Belloc *Vaillant, Ital.*
Activated charcoal (p.972·2).
Diarrhoea; flatulence.

Neo Cardiol *Francia, Ital.*
Carnitine (p.1336·2).
Carnitine deficiency; myocardial ischaemia.

Neo Cepacol Collutorio *Lepetit, Ital.*
Cetylpyridinium chloride (p.1106·2); sodium phosphate; sodium diphosphate; disodium edetate; methyl salicylate; cineole; cinnamon oil; mint oil; menthol.
Dental plaque prevention; mouth and throat disinfection.

Neo Cepacol Pastiglie *Hoechst Marion Roussel, Ital.*
Cetylpyridinium chloride (p.1106·2).
Mouth and throat disinfection.

Neo Citran
Sanabo, Aust.; Sandoz, Canad.; Wander OTC, Switz.
Paracetamol (p.72·2); pheniramine maleate (p.415·3); phenylephrine hydrochloride (p.1066·2); ascorbic acid (p.1365·2).
Cold symptoms.

Neo Citran A *Sandoz, Canad.*
Phenylephrine hydrochloride (p.1066·2); pheniramine maleate (p.415·3); ascorbic acid (p.1365·2).

Neo Citran Daycaps *Sandoz, Canad.*
Pseudoephedrine hydrochloride (p.1068·3); dextromethorphan hydrobromide (p.1057·3); paracetamol (p.72·2).

Neo Citran DM *Sandoz, Canad.*
Phenylephrine hydrochloride (p.1066·2); pheniramine maleate (p.415·3); dextromethorphan hydrobromide (p.1057·3).

Neo Citran Nutrasweet *Sandoz, Canad.*
Phenylephrine hydrochloride (p.1066·2); pheniramine maleate (p.415·3); paracetamol (p.72·2).

Neo Citran Sinus *Sandoz, Canad.*
Phenylephrine hydrochloride (p.1066·2); paracetamol (p.72·2).

Neo Colecisto Test *IMS, Ital.†.*
Radiographic examination of gallbladder function.

Neo Confetto Falqui *Falqui, Ital.†.*
Senna (p.1212·2).
Constipation.

Neo Coricidin *Schering-Plough, Ital.*
Chlorpheniramine maleate (p.405·1); aspirin (p.16·1); caffeine (p.749·3).
Cold symptoms.

Neo Coricidin Gola *Schering-Plough, Ital.*
Cetylpyridinium chloride (p.1106·2).
Mouth and throat disinfection.

Neo Decabutin *Inkeysa, Spain.*
Indomethacin (p.45·2).
Gout; inflammation; musculoskeletal, joint, and peri-articular disorders; oedema; pain.

Neo Diftepertus *Evans, Spain†.*
A diphtheria, tetanus, and pertussis vaccine (p.1509·1).
Active immunisation in infants and young children.

Neo Dohyfral *Solvay, Neth.*
Cholecalciferol (p.1366·3).
Vitamin D deficiency.

Neo Eblimon *Guidotti, Ital.*
Naproxen (p.61·2).
Inflammation; musculoskeletal and joint disorders; pain.

Neo Elixifilin *Morrith, Spain.*
Theophylline (p.765·1).
Heart failure; obstructive airways disease.

Neo Endofren *Bama, Spain†.*
Diiodotyrosine (p.1493·1); reserpine (p.942·1); methimazole (p.1495·3).
Hyperthyroidism.

Neo Esoformolo *Esoform, Ital.*
Sodium *o*-phenylphenol (p.1120·3).
Disinfection of waste materials.

Neo Eubalsamina *Milanfarma, Ital.†.*
Methyl salicylate (p.55·2); eucalyptus oil (p.1578·1); camphor (p.1557·2); turpentine oil (p.1641·1).
Rheumatism.

Neo Expectan *Wander OTC, Switz.*
Acetylcysteine (p.1052·3).
Respiratory-tract disorders associated with increased or viscous mucus.

Neo Fertinorm *Serono, Spain.*
Urofollitrophin (p.1263·1).
Female infertility.

Neo Foille Pomata Disinfettante *Isnardi, Ital.†.*
Hydroxyquinoline sulphate (p.1589·3); colloidal sulphur (p.1091·2); menthol (p.1600·2).
Skin irritation; wound disinfection.

Neo Formitrol *Novartis, Ital.*
Cetylpyridinium chloride (p.1106·2).
Oral disinfection.

Neo Gastrausil *Searle, Ital.*
Cimetidine (p.1183·2).
Gastro-intestinal disorders associated with hyperacidity.

Neo Genyl *Meuse, Belg.*
Injection: Liver extract.
Vitamin B_{12} deficiency.
Oral liquid†: Cyanocobalamin (p.1363·3); folic acid (p.1340·3); ferric glycerophosphate (p.1586·2); sodium methylarsinate (p.1631·2).
Anaemias; tonic.

Neo Gilurytmal *Lacer, Spain.*
Prajmalium bitartrate (p.932·2).
Arrhythmias.

Neo Ginsana *IBP, Ital.†.*
Panax ginseng (p.1584·2).
Tonic.

Neo Gola Sel *Sella, Ital.†.*
Cetylpyridinium chloride (p.1106·2).
Disinfection.

Neo Gratusminal *Simes, Ital.†.*
Proscillaridin (p.938·1); quinalbarbitone (p.690·2).
Cardiac disorders; insomnia.

Neo H2 *Boehringer Ingelheim, Ital.*
Roxatidine acetate hydrochloride (p.1212·1).
Gastro-intestinal disorders associated with hyperacidity.

Neo Hubber *ICN, Spain.*
Hydrocortisone acetate (p.1043·3); neomycin sulphate (p.229·2).
External ear disorders; rhinitis.

Neo Iloticina *Dista, Spain.*
Erythromycin estolate (p.204·1).
Bacterial infections.

Neo Intol Plus *Carlo Erba, Ital.†.*
Orthophenylphenol (p.1120·3); didecyldimethylammonium chloride (p.1112·2).
Vaginal douche.

Neo Kodan *Schulke & Mayr, Ger.*
Octenidine hydrochloride (p.1120·2); propyl alcohol (p.1124·2); isopropyl alcohol (p.1118·2).
Skin disinfection.

Neo Lacrim *Alcon, Spain.*
Phenylephrine hydrochloride (p.1066·2).
Eye irritation.

Neo Lactoflorene *Montefarmaco, Ital.*
Lactic-acid-producing organisms (p.1594·1); vitamins.
Nutritional supplement.

Neo Lyndiol *Organon, Spain.*
Ethinyloestradiol (p.1445·1); lynoestrenol (p.1448·2).
Combined oral contraceptive; menstrual disorders.

Neo Makatussin N *Gebro, Switz.*
Dihydrocodeine hydrochloride (p.34·2); diphenhydramine hydrochloride (p.409·1).
Bronchitis; coughs.

Neo Melubrina *Hoechst, Spain.*
Dipyrone (p.35·1).
Fever; pain.

Neo Moderin *Upjohn, Spain.*
Methylprednisolone acetate (p.1046·1); neomycin sulphate (p.229·2).
Infected skin disorders.

Neo Mom *Candioli, Ital.*
Tetramethrin (p.1410·3); phenothrin (p.1409·2).
Pediculosis.

Neo Nisidina C-Fher *Boehringer Ingelheim, Ital.*
Aspirin (p.16·1); paracetamol (p.72·2); ascorbic acid (p.1365·2).
Cold symptoms; pain.

Neo Nisidina-FHER *Boehringer Ingelheim, Ital.*
Aspirin (p.16·1); paracetamol (p.72·2); caffeine (p.749·3).
Cold symptoms; fever; pain.

neo OPT *Optimed, Ger.*
Bromazepam (p.643·1).
Anxiety; sleep disorders.

Neo Penprobal *Knoll, Spain†.*
Ampicillin sodium (p.153·1); ampicillin benzathine (p.154·1); guaiphenesin (p.1061·3).
Lignocaine hydrochloride (p.1293·2) is included in this preparation to alleviate the pain of injection.
Respiratory-tract infections.

Neo Rinactive *Farmacusi, Spain.*
Budesonide (p.1034·3).
Nasal polyps; rhinitis.

Neo Silvikrin *Doetsch, Grether, Switz.*
Wheat-germ oil; millet extract; keratin; L-cysteine; vitamins.
Hair disorders.

Neo Soluzione Sulfo Balsamica *Deca, Ital.*
Sodium sulphide; sodium bromide (p.1620·3); cineole (p.1564·1).
Catarrhal sore throat; rhinitis.

Neo Synalar *Yamanouchi, Spain.*
Fluocinolone acetonide (p.1041·1); neomycin sulphate (p.229·2).
Infected skin disorders.

Neo Togram *Llorente, Spain*†.
Metampicillin sodium (p.224·3).
Bacterial infections.

Neo Tomizol *Robert, Spain.*
Carbimazole (p.1491·2).
Hyperthyroidism.

Neo Topico Giusto *Milupa, Ital.*
Benzethonium chloride (p.1102·3); hamamelis (p.1587·1).
Nipple care during breast feeding; wound disinfection.

Neo Trefogel *Panthox & Burck, Ital.*†.
Wheat germ; ginseng (p.1584·2); royal jelly (p.1626·3); honey (p.1345·3).
Nutritional supplement.

Neo Uniplus *Angelini, Ital.*
Aspirin (p.16·1); paracetamol (p.72·2).
Cold symptoms; pain.

Neo Uniplus C *Angelini, Ital.*
Aspirin (p.16·1); paracetamol (p.72·2); ascorbic acid (p.1365·2).
Cold symptoms; pain.

Neo Urgenin *Madaus, Spain.*
Echinacea angustifolia (p.1574·2); prunus africana; saw palmetto (p.1462·1).
Prostatic disorders.

Neo Visage *Miquel Otsuka, Spain.*
Sulphur (p.1091·2); dexpanthenol (p.1570·3); hexachlorophane (p.1115·2); hydrocortisone acetate (p.1043·3); placenta extract; basic zinc carbonate (p.1096·1).
Acne.

Neo Zeta-Foot *Zeta, Ital.*
Cream: Usnic acid (p.1643·1); salicylic acid (p.1090·2); undecenoic acid (p.389·2); aluminium acetate (p.1547·3).
Topical powder: Usnic acid (p.1643·1); undecenoic acid (p.389·2); aluminium oxide (p.1077·2); zinc stearate (p.1469·3); zinc oxide (p.1096·2); kaolin (p.1195·1); magnesium carbonate (p.1198·1); thyme oil (p.1637·1).
Foot infections.

Neo-Alcos-Anal *Will-Pharma, Belg.*
Sodium oleate (p.1469·1); laureth 9 (p.1325·2).
Haemorrhoids.

Neo-Aminomel *Geistlich, Switz.*†.
Amino-acid and electrolyte infusion.
Parenteral nutrition.

Neo-Ampiplus *Menarini, Ital.*
Amoxycillin trihydrate (p.151·3).
Bacterial infections.

Neo-Angin
Note. This name is used for preparations of different composition.
Klosterfrau, Aust.
Dichlorobenzyl alcohol (p.1112·2); amylmetacresol (p.1101·3); anise oil (p.1550·1); peppermint oil (p.1208·1); menthol (p.1600·2).
Mouth and throat disorders.

Divapharma, Ger.
Hexetidine (p.1116·1); benzalkonium chloride (p.1101·3).
Mouth and throat infection and inflammation.

Neo-Angin au miel et citron *Doetsch, Grether, Switz.*
Dichlorobenzyl alcohol (p.1112·2); amylmetacresol (p.1101·3); honey (p.1345·3); lemon oil (p.1595·3); mint oil (p.1604·1).
Sore throat.

Neo-Angin avec vitamin C exempt de sucre *Doetsch, Grether, Switz.*
Dichlorobenzyl alcohol (p.1112·2); amylmetacresol (p.1101·3); menthol (p.1600·2); ascorbic acid (p.1365·2).
Sore throat.

Neo-Angin exempt de sucre *Doetsch, Grether, Switz.*
Dichlorobenzyl alcohol (p.1112·2); amylmetacresol (p.1101·3); menthol (p.1600·2); anethole (p.1549·3); mint oil (p.1604·1); rectified camphor oil.
Sore throat.

Neo-Angin Lido *Doetsch, Grether, Switz.*
Cetylpyridinium chloride (p.1106·2); lignocaine hydrochloride (p.1293·2).
Mouth and throat disorders.

Neo-Angin N *Divapharma, Ger.*
Dichlorobenzyl alcohol (p.1112·2); menthol (p.1600·2); amylmetacresol (p.1101·3).
Mouth and throat infections; sore throat.

Neo-Audiocort *Cyanamid, Ital.*
Triamcinolone acetonide hemisuccinate (p.1050·3); neomycin sulphate (p.229·2).
Ear disorders.

Neobac *Dermapharm, Ger.*
Neomycin sulphate (p.229·2); bacitracin (p.157·3).
Fungal skin and nose infections.

Neobacitracine *Bencard, Belg.*
Bacitracin (p.157·3); neomycin sulphate (p.229·2).
Bacterial infections.

Neo-Ballistol *Klever, Ger.*
Capsules: Potassium oleate; peppermint oil (p.1208·1); anise oil (p.1550·1); caraway oil (p.1559·3).
Oral liquid: Potassium oleate; ammonium oleate; peppermint oil (p.1208·1); anise oil (p.1550·1).
Gastro-intestinal disorders.

Neo-Bex *Neolab, Canad.*
Vitamin B substances.

Neo-Bex Forte *Neolab, Canad.*
Vitamin B substances with ascorbic acid and zinc.

Neobiphyllin
Jacoby, Aust.†; *Trommsdorff, Ger.; Zyma, Switz.*
Diprophylline (p.752·1); proxyphylline (p.757·3); theophylline (p.765·1).
Cor pulmonale; obstructive airways disease.

Neo-Biphyllin Special *Zyma, Switz.*†.
Etamiphylline camsylate (p.753·1); diprophylline (p.752·1); proxyphylline (p.757·3).
Obstructive airways disease.

Neobiphyllin-Clys *Trommsdorff, Ger.*
Diprophylline (p.752·1); proxyphylline (p.757·3); theophylline (p.765·1).
Obstructive airways disease.

Neo-Boldolaxine *Bouchara, Fr.*†.
Bisacodyl (p.1179·3); docusate sodium (p.1189·3); boldo (p.1554·1); aloin (p.1177·2); belladonna (p.457·1).
Constipation.

Neobonsen *Duopharm, Ger.*
Evening primrose oil (p.1582·1).
Eczema.

Neo-Bradoral *Ciba-Geigy, Switz.*†.
Domiphen bromide (p.1112·3).
Mouth and throat infections.

Neobron *Pfizer, Switz.*
Multivitamin and mineral preparation.

neo-bronchol *Divapharma, Ger.*
Ambroxol hydrochloride (p.1054·3).
Respiratory-tract disorders.

Neobrufen *Knoll, Spain.*
Ibuprofen (p.44·1).
Fever; musculoskeletal, joint, and peri-articular disorders; pain.

Neo-Bucosin *Synpharma, Switz.*
Dequalinium chloride (p.1112·1); lignocaine hydrochloride (p.1293·2).
Mouth and throat disorders.

Neo-C *Neo-Life, Austral.*
Ascorbic acid (p.1365·2); Neo-Plex Concentrate; dried whole citrus juice; flavedo; mesocarp; endocarp; citrus protopectin; flavonoid complex; rutin; hesperidin; lemon bioflavonoid complex.
Vitamin C deficiency.

Neocalcigenol *Darci, Belg.*†.
Calcium phosphate (p.1155·3); ergocalciferol (p.1367·1); sodium fluoride (p.742·1); sodium ascorbate (p.1365·2).
Bone fractures; calcium supplement; dental caries prophylaxis.

Neocalcigenol Forte *Darci, Belg.*†.
Calcium phosphate (p.1155·3); sodium methylarsinate (p.1631·2); sodium fluoride (p.742·1).
Bone fractures; calcium supplement; dental caries prophylaxis.

Neocalcit comp *Pfleger, Ger.*†.
Multivitamin and mineral preparation.
Calcium deficiency.

Neo-Calglucon *Sandoz, USA.*
Calcium glubionate (p.1155·1).
Calcium deficiency; inadequate dietary calcium intake.

Neocapil *Spirig, Switz.*
Minoxidil (p.910·3).
Androgenic alopecia.

Neo-Castaderm *Lannett, USA*†.
Resorcinol (p.1090·1); boric acid (p.1554·2); phenol (p.1121·2).

Neocate
Scientific Hospital Supplies, Austral.; Scientific Hospital Supplies, Irl.; Scientific Hospital Supplies, UK.
Infant feed.
Gastro-intestinal disorders; malabsorption; protein intolerance.

Neocate One + *SHS, USA.*
Preparation for enteral nutrition.

Neocefal *Metapharma, Ital.*
Cephamandole nafate sodium (p.180·1).
Lignocaine (p.1293·2) is included in this preparation to alleviate the pain of injection.
Bacterial infections.

Neocepacilina *CEPA, Spain.*
Benzylpenicillin sodium (p.159·3); procaine penicillin (p.240·2); benzathine penicillin (p.158·3).
Bacterial infections; rheumatic fever.

Neochinidin *Brocchieri, Ital.*†.
Quinidine polygalacturonate (p.938·3).
Arrhythmias.

Neochinosol *Chinosolfabrik, Ger.*
Ethacridine lactate (p.1098·3).
Mouth and throat disorders.

Neo-Cholex *Horner, Canad.*†.
Cottonseed oil (p.1567·3).
Adjuvant in cholecystography.

Neocibalena *Zyma, Spain.*
Aspirin (p.16·1); caffeine (p.749·3); paracetamol (p.72·2).
Fever; pain.

Neo-Cibalgin *Zyma, Switz.*
Aspirin (p.16·1); paracetamol (p.72·2); caffeine (p.749·3).
Fever; pain.

Neo-Cibalgina *Zyma, Ital.; Novartis Consumer, Ital.*
Aspirin (p.16·1); paracetamol (p.72·2); caffeine (p.749·3).
Fever; pain.

Neo-Cimexon *Cimex, Switz.*
Multivitamin and mineral preparation.

Neo-Cimexon G *Cimex, Switz.*
Multivitamin and mineral preparation with ginseng.

Neocin *Ocusoft, USA.*
Polymyxin B (p.239·3); neomycin (p.229·2); bacitracin (p.157·3).
Bacterial eye infections.

Neocitran
Note. A similar name is used for preparations of different composition.
Sandoz, Fr.
Paracetamol (p.72·2); pseudoephedrine hydrochloride (p.1068·3).
Rhinitis.

NeoCitran
Note. A similar name is used for preparations of different composition.
Sandoz, Ger.
Paracetamol (p.72·2).
Fever; pain.

Neo-Cleanse *Neo-Life, Austral.*
Senna leaves (p.1212·2); buckthorn bark (p.1182·1); liquorice root (p.1197·1); prune (p.1209·2); alfalfa leaf (p.1544·2); rhubarb root (p.1212·1); culvers root; blue malva flowers; asparagus; aniseed (p.1549·3).
Constipation.

Neoclym *Poli, Ital.*
Cyclofenil (p.1440·2).
Infertility; menopausal disorders; menstrual disorders.

Neo-Codion
Note. This name is used for preparations of different composition.
Therabel Pharma, Belg.
Codeine camsylate (p.27·1); ethylmorphine camsylate (p.36·1); potassium guaiacolsulfonate (p.1068·3).
Coughs.

Bouchara, Fr.
Infant syrup: Sodium benzoate (p.1102·3); grindelia; senega (p.1069·3).
Respiratory-tract congestion.
Paediatric syrup: Codeine camsylate (p.27·1); sodium benzoate (p.1102·3).
Suppositories; paediatric suppositories: Codeine camsylate (p.27·1); cineole (p.1564·1).
Syrup: Codeine camsylate (p.27·1).
Tablets: Codeine camsylate (p.27·1); potassium guaiacolsulfonate (p.1068·3); grindelia.
Coughs.

Fatol, Ger.†.
Codeine camsylate (p.27·1); ethylmorphine camsylate (p.36·1); verbascum; grindelia; marrubium album (p.1063·3).
Coughs.

Bouchara, Switz.†.
Suppositories: Codeine camsylate (p.27·1); ethylmorphine camsylate (p.36·1); cineole (p.1564·1).
Tablets: Codeine camsylate (p.27·1); ethylmorphine camsylate (p.36·1); potassium guaiacolsulfonate (p.1068·3); grindelia; erysimum officinale; marrubium vulgare (p.1063·3).
Coughs.

Neo-Codion Adultes *Bouchara, Switz.*†.
Ascorbic acid (p.1365·2); codeine camsylate (p.27·1); ethylmorphine camsylate (p.36·1); aconite root (p.1542·2); bromoform (p.1620·3); cherry-laurel; magnesium sulphate (p.1157·3); tolu balsam (p.1071·1); ipecacuanha (p.1062·2).
Coughs.

Neo-Codion Enfants *Bouchara, Switz.*†.
Ascorbic acid (p.1365·2); codeine camsylate (p.27·1); ethylmorphine camsylate (p.36·1); sodium bromide (p.1620·3); sodium benzoate (p.1102·3); drosera (p.1574·1); belladonna (p.457·1); magnesium sulphate (p.1157·3); tolu balsam (p.1071·1); ipecacuanha (p.1062·2).
Coughs.

Neo-Codion N
Note. This name is used for preparations of different composition.
Fatol, Ger.†.
Codeine camsylate (p.27·1); ethylmorphine camsylate (p.36·1).
Coughs.

Bouchara, Switz.
Infant syrup†*:* Sodium benzoate (p.1102·3); ascorbic acid (p.1365·2); grindelia; red-poppy; wild thyme; polygala amara (p.1069·3).
Syrup: Codeine camsylate (p.27·1); ascorbic acid (p.1365·2); ipecacuanha (p.1062·2); tolu balsam (p.1071·1).
Tablets: Codeine camsylate (p.27·1); potassium guaiacolsulfonate (p.1068·3); grindelia.
Coughs.

Neo-Codion NN *Fatol, Ger.*
Codeine camsylate (p.27·1).
Coughs.

Neo-Codion Nourrisons *Bouchara, Switz.*†.
Ascorbic acid (p.1365·2); sodium bromide (p.1620·3); sodium benzoate (p.1102·3); drosera (p.1574·1); grindelia; wild thyme; red-poppy; polygala (p.1069·3); maidenhair fern.
Coughs.

Neocolan *Seid, Spain.*
Dicyclomine hydrochloride (p.460·1); metochalcone (p.1603·2); procaine hydrochloride (p.1299·2).
Hepatobiliary disorders.

Neocon *Janssen-Cilag, Neth.*
Norethisterone (p.1453·1); ethinyloestradiol (p.1445·1).
Combined oral contraceptive.

Neocon 1/35 *Cilag, UK*†.
Norethisterone (p.1453·1); ethinyloestradiol (p.1445·1).
Combined oral contraceptive.

Neocones
Austrodent, Aust.; Prats, Spain; Septodont, Switz.
Amethocaine hydrochloride (p.1285·2); neomycin sulphate (p.229·2); polymyxin B sulphate (p.239·1); tyrothricin (p.267·2).
Dental disorders.

Neocontrast *Bama, Spain.*
Iopanoic acid (p.1007·1).
Contrast medium for biliary-tract radiography.

Neo-Cortef
Pharmacia Upjohn, Canad.; Pharmacia Upjohn, Irl.; Dominion, UK; Upjohn, USA†.
Hydrocortisone (p.1043·3) or hydrocortisone acetate (p.1043·3); neomycin sulphate (p.229·2).
Infected eye, ear, or skin disorders.

Neocortigamma *IBP, Ital.*†.
Hydrocortisone (p.1043·3); neomycin (p.229·2).
Skin disorders and infections.

Neo-Cortofen *Ripari-Gero, Ital.*
Dexamethasone (p.1037·1); neomycin sulphate (p.229·2).
Eczema; nasal mucosal inflammation; rhinitis.

Neo-Cortofen "Antrax" *Ripari-Gero, Ital.*†.
Dexamethasone (p.1037·1); neomycin sulphate (p.229·2); coal tar (p.1092·3).
Eczema.

Neocortovol *IBP, Ital.*†.
Hydrocortisone (p.1043·3); neomycin sulphate (p.229·2).
Vaginal bacterial infections.

Neo-Cranimal *Dagra, Neth.*†.
Ergotamine tartrate (p.445·3); caffeine monohydrate (p.750·1); meclozine hydrochloride (p.413·3).
Migraine and other vascular headaches.

Neo-Cratylen
Madaus, Aust.; Madaus, Ger.
Crataegus (p.1568·2).
Cardiac disorders.

Neo-Cromaton Bicomplesso *Menarini, Ital.*
Vitamin B substances.
Deficiency states; macrocytic anaemias.

Neo-Cromaton Bicomplesso Ferro *Menarini, Ital.*†.
Vitamin B substances; ferric ammonium citrate (p.1339·2).
Deficiency states; macrocytic anaemias; microcytic anaemias.

Neo-Cromaton Cortex *Menarini, Ital.*†.
Suprarenal cortex (p.1050·1); cyanocobalamin (p.1363·3); calcium folinate (p.1342·2).
Anaemia; tonic.

Neo-Cultol *Fisons, USA.*
Liquid paraffin (p.1382·1).
Constipation.

Neo-Cutigenol *Centrapharm, Belg.*
Chlorhexidine acetate (p.1107·2); vitamin A palmitate (p.1359·2).
Formerly contained hydroxyquinoline sulphate, vitamin A palmitate, titanium dioxide, zinc oxide, and cod-liver oil.
Burns; skin disorders; wounds.

Neocutis *Pentaderm, Ital.*
Azelaic acid (p.1079·1); jaluramina.
Acne; seborrhoea.

Neo-Cytamen
DBL, Austral.; Evans Medical, Irl.; Teofarma, Ital.; Medeva, UK.
Hydroxocobalamin (p.1363·3).
Leber's optic atrophy; macrocytic anaemias; tobacco amblyopia.

Neo-Dagracycline *Asta Medica, Neth.*
Doxycycline fosfatex (p.202·3).
Bacterial infections.

Neo-Debiol AD3 *Meuse, Belg.*
Vitamin A acetate (p.1359·2); cholecalciferol (p.1366·3).
Vitamin A and D deficiency.

NeoDecadron
Merck Sharp & Dohme, Canad.; Merck Sharp & Dohme, USA.
Dexamethasone sodium phosphate (p.1037·2); neomycin sulphate (p.229·2).
Eye or ear inflammation with bacterial infection; inflammatory skin disorders with secondary infection.

Neo-Decongestine *Roche, Switz.*†.
Kaolin (p.1195·1); glycerol (p.1585·2); guaiacol salicylate; methyl salicylate (p.55·2).
Soft-tissue disorders.

Neo-Delphicort *Cyanamid, Aust.*
Triamcinolone acetonide (p.1050·2); neomycin sulphate (p.229·2).
Ear or eye infection and inflammation.

Neodemusin *Bama, Spain*†.
Albumin tannate (p.1176·3); ethylmorphine hydrochloride (p.36·1); neomycin sulphate (p.229·2).
Gastro-intestinal infections.

Neoderm
Note. This name is used for preparations of different composition.
Desbergers, Canad.
Zinc oxide (p.1096·2); zinc peroxide (p.1127·3).
Minor abrasions, wounds, and burns.

Propan, S.Afr.
Hydrocortisone acetate (p.1043·3); neomycin sulphate (p.229·2).
Skin disorders.

Neoderm Ginecologico *Crosara, Ital.*
Fluocinolone acetonide (p.1041·1).
Vulvovaginitis.

Neodes *Benvegna, Ital.†.*
Dexamethasone sodium phosphate (p.1037·2); neomycin sulphate (p.229·2).
Eye disorders.

Neodesfila *Kin, Spain.*
Cresol (p.1111·2); eugenol (p.1578·2); hydroxyquinoline sulphate (p.1589·3); lignocaine hydrochloride (p.1293·2).
Toothache.

Neo-Desogen *Hoechst Marion Roussel, Ital.*
Benzalkonium chloride (p.1101·3).
Instrument disinfection; skin, burn, and wound disinfection.

Neo-Destomygen *Stomygen, Ital.*
Chlorhexidine gluconate (p.1107·2).
Oral hygiene.

Neodexa *Llorens, Spain.*
Dexamethasone phosphate (p.1037·2); neomycin sulphate (p.229·2).
Infected eye disorders.

Neo-Dexair *Bausch & Lomb, USA.*
Dexamethasone sodium phosphate (p.1037·2); neomycin sulphate (p.229·2).
Eye inflammation with bacterial infection.

Neo-Dexameth *Major, USA.*
Dexamethasone sodium phosphate (p.1037·2); neomycin sulphate (p.229·2).
Eye inflammation with bacterial infection.

Neodexaplast *Llorens, Spain†.*
Dexamethasone (p.1037·1); neomycin sulphate (p.229·2).
Infected skin disorders.

Neodexon *Bournonville, Belg.*
Dexamethasone sodium phosphate (p.1037·2); neomycin sulphate (p.229·2).
Infected inflammatory eye disorders.

Neo-Diaral *Roberts, USA.*
Loperamide (p.1197·3).
Diarrhoea.

Neo-Diophen *Hamilton, Austral.*
Mepyramine maleate (p.414·1); phenylpropanolamine hydrochloride (p.1067·2); dextromethorphan hydrobromide (p.1057·3); atropine sulphate (p.455·1).
Asthma; bronchitis; coughs and cold symptoms; hay fever.

Neodolpasse *Leopold, Aust.*
Diclofenac sodium (p.31·2); orphenadrine citrate (p.465·2).
Inflammation; musculoskeletal and joint disorders; pain.

Neodone *IFCI, Ital.*
Paracetamol (p.72·2); aspirin (p.16·1); caffeine (p.749·3).
Fever; pain.

Neodorm *Nordmark, Ger.†.*
Pentobarbitone (p.684·3).
Nervous disorders; sleeplessness.

Neodorm SP *Knoll, Ger.*
Temazepam (p.693·3).
Sleep disorders.

Neodox *Rosen, Ger.*
Doxycycline hydrochloride (p.202·3).
Bacterial infections.

Neodualestrepto *Antibioticos, Spain†.*
Streptomycin pantothenate (p.250·1); streptomycin sulphate (p.249·3).
Bacterial infections.

Neoduplamox *Procter & Gamble, Ital.*
Amoxycillin trihydrate (p.151·3); potassium clavulanate (p.190·2).
Bacterial infections.

Neo-Durabolic *Hauck, USA.*
Nandrolone decanoate (p.1452·2).
Anaemia in renal disease.

Neodyn *Sepharma, Ital.*
Sachets: Vitamin, mineral, and carbohydrate preparation with creatine.
Tablets: Carbohydrate, amino-acid, and fatty-acid preparation with creatine.
Nutritional supplement.

Neo-Emedyl *Montavit, Aust.*
Dimenhydrinate (p.408·2); caffeine (p.749·3).
Motion sickness; nausea and vomiting; vestibular disorders.

Neo-Emocicatrol *Bouty, Ital.*
Tannic acid (p.1634·2); benzalkonium chloride (p.1101·3).

Neo-Emoform *Byk Gulden, Ital.*
Sodium monofluorophosphate (p.743·3).
Gingivitis; oral hygiene.

Neo-Epa *Vis, Ital.†.*
Adenosine (p.812·3); cytidine; guanosine; uridine (p.1641·3); cyanocobalamin (p.1363·3); cynarine (p.1569·3); inositol (p.1591·1).
Liver disorders.

Neo-Eparbiol *Ecobi, Ital.*
Inosine (p.1591·1); cyanocobalamin (p.1363·3).
Anaemias; tonic.

Neoeserin *ankerpharm, Ger.†.*
Neostigmine bromide (p.1393·3).
Glaucoma; miosis.

Neo-Estrone *Neolab, Canad.†.*
Esterified oestrogens (p.1458·1).
Oestrogenic.

Neo-Eunomin *Grunenthal, Ger.*
Ethinyloestradiol (p.1445·1); chlormadinone acetate (p.1439·1).
Acne; alopecia; biphasic oral contraceptive; hirsutism; seborrhoea.

Neo-Eunomine *Janssen-Cilag, Switz.*
Ethinyloestradiol (p.1445·1); chlormadinone acetate (p.1439·1).
Biphasic oral contraceptive.

Neofazol *Rubio, Spain.*
Cephazolin sodium (p.181·1).
Lignocaine hydrochloride (p.1293·2) is included in this preparation to alleviate the pain of injection.
Bacterial infections.

Neofed *Propan, S.Afr.*
Triprolidine hydrochloride (p.420·3); pseudoephedrine hydrochloride (p.1068·3); guaiphenesin (p.1061·3); codeine phosphate (p.26·1).
Coughs.

Neofen *MC, Ital.†.*
Benzalkonium chloride (p.1101·3); cetrimonium chloride (p.1106·1); didecyldimethylammonium chloride (p.1112·2); alcohol (p.1099·1).
Skin disinfection.

Neofenox *Boots Healthcare, Belg.*
Phenylephrine hydrochloride (p.1066·2); dichlorobenzyl alcohol (p.1112·2); naphazoline nitrate (p.1064·2).
Adjuvant in sinusitis; nasal congestion.

Neo-Fepramol *Istoria, Ital.*
Paracetamol (p.72·2).
Fever; pain.

Neo-Fer
Neolab, Canad.; Nycomed, Norw.
Ferrous fumarate (p.1339·3).
Iron deficiency; iron-deficiency anaemia.

Neo-Fluimucil *Zambon, Ger.†.*
Acetylcysteine (p.1052·3).
Respiratory-tract disorders associated with increased or viscous mucus.

Neofocin *Medici, Ital.†.*
Fosfomycin calcium (p.210·2).
Bacterial infections.

Neo-fradin *Pharma Tek, USA.*
Neomycin sulphate (p.229·2).

Neofrin *Ocusoft, USA.*
Phenylephrine hydrochloride (p.1066·2).

Neo-Furadantin *Formenti, Ital.*
Nitrofurantoin (p.231·3).
Bacterial infections of the genito-urinary tract.

Neo-Gallonorm *Mauermann, Ger.†.*
Agrimony; silybum marianum (p.993·3); chelidonium; curcuma zanthorrhiza; taraxacum (p.1634·2); frangula bark (p.1193·2); peppermint leaf (p.1208·1); turmeric (p.1001·3); wheat germ; belladonna; vitamins; ox bile (p.1553·2); hepar.; heparin sodium (p.879·3); pancreatin (p.1612·1).
Digestive disorders; liver and biliary-tract disorders.

Neogama *Hormosan, Ger.*
Sulpiride (p.692·3).
Psychiatric disorders; vestibular disorders.

Neo-Gepan *Pohl, Ger.†.*
Paracetamol (p.72·2); aspirin (p.16·1); caffeine (p.749·3).
Influenza; migraine; neuralgia; pain; rheumatism.

Neo-Gepan C *Pohl, Ger.†.*
Paracetamol (p.72·2); aspirin (p.16·1); caffeine (p.749·3); ascorbic acid (p.1365·2).
Fever; pain.

Neogest *Schering, UK.*
Norgestrel (p.1454·1).
Progestogen-only oral contraceptive.

Neo-Geynevral *Geymonat, Ital.*
Thiamine diphosphate hydrochloride; pyridoxine hydrochloride (p.1362·3); cyanocobalamin (p.1363·3).
Neuritis.

Neo-Gilurytmal
Solvay, Aust.; Solvay, Ger.; Solvay, Switz.†.
Prajmalium bitartrate (p.932·2).
Arrhythmias.

Neogluconin *Waldheim, Aust.*
Glibenclamide (p.319·3).
Diabetes mellitus.

Neo-Golaseptine *SMB, Belg.†.*
Sulphacetamide sodium (p.252·2); benzethonium chloride (p.1102·3).
Mouth and throat disorders.

Neogonadil *Bruco, Ital.†.*
Chorionic gonadotrophin (p.1243·1).
Amenorrhoea; cryptorchidism; infertility.

Neogram *SIFI, Ital.*
Neomycin sulphate (p.229·2); gramicidin (p.215·2).
Eye infections.

Neo-Gravidtest *Lab Line, Ital.†.*
Pregnancy test (p.1621·2).

Neogynon
Schering, Aust.; Schering, Ger.; Schering, Neth.; Schering, Switz.
Levonorgestrel (p.1454·1); ethinyloestradiol (p.1445·1).
Combined oral contraceptive; endometriosis; menstrual disorders.

Neogynona *Schering, Spain.*
Ethinyloestradiol (p.1445·1); levonorgestrel (p.1454·1).
Combined oral contraceptive; menstrual disorders.

Neo-Helvagit *Helvepharm, Switz.†.*
Ibuprofen (p.44·1).
Fever; pain.

Neo-Heparbil *Montefarmaco, Ital.*
Fencibutirol (p.1578·3); frangula (p.1193·2); rhubarb (p.1212·1); cascara sagrada (p.1183·1); belladonna (p.457·1).
Constipation.

Neo-Hydro *Streuli, Switz.*
Hydrocortisone acetate (p.1043·3); neomycin sulphate (p.229·2).
Inflammation and infection of the eye, nose, or ear.

Neo-Intol *Carlo Erba OTC, Ital.*
Cetrimonium tosylate (p.1106·1).
External genital disinfection.

Neoiodarsolo *Baldacci, Ital.*
Amino-acid preparation with vitamin B substances.
Tonic.

Neo-Istafene *UCB, Ital.†.*
Meclozine hydrochloride (p.413·3).
Antihistamine.

Neokratin *Laevosan, Aust.*
Paracetamol (p.72·2); propyphenazone (p.81·3); caffeine (p.749·3).
Fever; pain.

Neo-Lapitrypsin *Truw, Ger.*
Oleum pini sylvestris; pumilio pine oil (p.1623·3); melissa oil; spike lavender oil (p.1632·2); juniper oil (p.1592·3); fennel oil (p.1579·2); peppermint oil (p.1208·1).
Biliary disorders; gallstones; renal calculi.

Neo-Laryngobis *Bio-Chemical, Canad.†.*
Bismuth dipropylacetate (p.1181·1).
Throat infections.

Neo-Levulase Fortius *Zambeletti, Ital.†.*
Vitamin B substances.
Dyspepsia; vitamin deficiency.

Neo-Lidocaton
Weimer, Ger.; Dentalica, Ital.†; Pharmaton, Switz.†.
Lignocaine hydrochloride (p.1293·2).
Lypressin (p.1263·2) or vasopressin (p.1263·2) and noradrenaline (p.924·1) are included in this preparation as vasoconstrictors to diminish absorption and localise the effect of the local anaesthetic.
Local anaesthesia.

Neo-Liniment *Neomed, Switz.†.*
Methyl salicylate (p.55·2); camphor (p.1557·2); benzyl nicotinate (p.22·1); dimethyl sulphoxide (p.1377·2); thyme oil (p.1637·1); eucalyptus oil (p.1578·1); oleum pini sylvestris.
Musculoskeletal and joint disorders.

Neolog *Zyma, Ital.†.*
Flumethasone pivalate (p.1040·3); triclosan (p.1127·2).
Infected skin disorders.

Neoloid
Bradley, Canad.; Kenwood, USA.
Castor oil (p.1560·2).
Bowel evacuation; constipation; diarrhoea.

Neo-Lotan *Neopharmed, Ital.*
Losartan potassium (p.899·1).
Hypertension.

Neo-Lotan Plus *Neopharmed, Ital.*
Losartan potassium (p.899·1); hydrochlorothiazide (p.885·2).
Hypertension.

Neolutin Depositum *Medici, Ital.†.*
Algestone acetophenide (p.1439·1).
Acne.

Neo-Medrate Akne-Lotio *Upjohn, Ger.†.*
Methylprednisolone acetate (p.1046·1); neomycin sulphate (p.229·2); aluminium chlorohydrate (p.1078·3); sulphur (p.1091·2).
Acne; eczema.

Neo-Medrol
Pharmacia Upjohn, Austral.; Pharmacia Upjohn, S.Afr.; Upjohn, Switz.†.
Methylprednisolone acetate (p.1046·1); neomycin sulphate (p.229·2); aluminium chlorohydrate (p.1078·3); colloidal sulphur (p.1091·2).
Acne.

Neo-Medrol Acne *Pharmacia Upjohn, Canad.*
Methylprednisolone acetate (p.1046·1); neomycin sulphate (p.229·2); aluminium chlorohydrate (p.1078·3); colloidal sulphur (p.1091·2).
Acne; seborrhoeic dermatitis.

Neo-Medrol Lozione Antiacne *Pharmacia Upjohn, Ital.†.*
Methylprednisolone acetate (p.1046·1); neomycin sulphate (p.229·2); aluminium chlorohydrate (p.1078·3); colloidal sulphur (p.1091·2).
Acne.

Neo-Medrol Veriderm
Pharmacia Upjohn, Canad.; Pharmacia Upjohn, Ital.
Methylprednisolone acetate (p.1046·1); neomycin sulphate (p.229·2).
Infected skin disorders.

Neo-Medrone
Note. This name is used for preparations of different composition.
Pharmacia Upjohn, Irl.; Upjohn, UK†.
Cream: Methylprednisolone acetate (p.1046·1); neomycin sulphate (p.229·2).
Inflamed skin infections.

Pharmacia Upjohn, Irl.
Topical lotion: Methylprednisolone acetate (p.1046·1); neomycin sulphate (p.229·2); aluminium chlorohydrate (p.1078·3); sulphur (p.1091·2).
Acne; rosacea; seborrhoeic dermatitis.

Neo-Mercazole
Roche, Austral.; Nicholas, Fr.; Roche, Irl.; Roche, Norw.; Lagamed, S.Afr.; Nicholas, Swed.†; Roche, Switz.; Roche, UK.
Carbimazole (p.1491·2).
Hyperthyroidism.

Neomercurochromo *SIT, Ital.*
Ointment; topical powder: Chlorhexidine gluconate (p.1107·2).
Wound disinfection.
Topical solution: Chloroxylenol (p.1111·1).
Skin disinfection.

Neomeritine *Janssen-Cilag, Belg.*
Ambucetamide hydrochloride (p.1548·2); aspirin (p.16·1); paracetamol (p.72·2); codeine phosphate (p.26·1); caffeine (p.749·3).
Gynaecological pain.

Neo-Mindol *Bracco, Ital.*
Ibuprofen (p.44·1).
Pain.

Neo-Minophagen C *Minophagen, Jpn.*
Ammonium glycyrrhizinate (p.1055·2).
Liver disorders; skin disorders; stomatitis.

Neomixin *Hauck, USA.*
Polymyxin B sulphate (p.239·1); neomycin sulphate (p.229·2); bacitracin (p.157·3).
Bacterial skin infections.

neo-morphazole *Nicholas, Ger.†.*
Carbimazole (p.1491·2).
Hyperthyroidism.

Neomyrt Plus *Baif, Ital.*
Myrtillus (p.1606·1); fish-liver oil; centella (p.1080·3); selenium (p.1353·3).
Nutritional supplement.

Neo-NaClex *Goldshield, UK.*
Bendrofluazide (p.827·3).
Hypertension; oedema.

Neo-NaClex-K *Goldshield, UK.*
Bendrofluazide (p.827·3); potassium chloride (p.1161·1).
Hypertension; oedema.

Neo-Nevral *Hoechst Marion Roussel, Ital.*
Paracetamol (p.72·2); aspirin (p.16·1); caffeine (p.749·3).
Fever; pain.

Neoniagar *Sintesa, Belg.*
Mebutizide (p.901·3).
Hypertension; oedema.

neo-Novutox *Braun, Ger.†.*
Lignocaine hydrochloride (p.1293·2).
Adrenaline acid tartrate (p.813·3) is included in some injections as a vasoconstrictor to diminish absorption and localise the effect of the local anaesthetic.
Local anaesthesia.

Neo-Optalidon *Novartis, Ital.*
Paracetamol (p.72·2); propyphenazone (p.81·3); caffeine (p.749·3).
Fever; pain.

NeoOstrogynal *Asche, Ger.*
Oestradiol valerate (p.1455·2); oestriol (p.1457·2).
Menopausal disorders; oestrogenic.

Neopan *Propan, S.Afr.*
Neomycin sulphate (p.229·2); sodium propionate (p.387·1).
Ear infections.

Neopap *PolyMedica, USA.*
Paracetamol (p.72·2).
Fever; pain.

Neoparyl *Ciba Vision, Fr.†.*
Phenylephrine and meglumine heparinate.
Eye irritation.

Neoparyl Framycetine *Ciba Vision, Fr.*
Phenylephrine and meglumine heparinate; framycetin sulphate (p.210·3).
Eye infections and burns.

Neoparyl-B_{12} *Ciba Vision, Fr.†.*
Phenylephrine and meglumine heparinate; heparin sodium (p.879·3); hydroxocobalamin acetate (p.1364·2).
Eye irritation.

Neo-Pause *Neolab, Canad.†.*
Testosterone enanthate (p.1464·1); oestradiol valerate (p.1455·2).
Androgenic; oestrogenic.

Neopax *Janssen-Cilag, Ital.†.*
Sodium picosulphate (p.1213·2).
Constipation.

Neopec *Propan-Vernleigh, S.Afr.†.*
Kaolin (p.1195·1); pectin (p.1474·1); neomycin sulphate (p.229·2).
Diarrhoea.

Neopelle *Also, Ital.*
Collagen (p.1566·3).
Wound dressing.

Neopenyl *Andromaco, Spain.*
Benzylpenicillin sodium (p.159·3); clemizole penicillin (p.191·1).
Lignocaine hydrochloride (p.1293·2) is included in this preparation to alleviate the pain of injection.
Bacterial infections.

Neoperborina Gola *Pagni, Ital.†.*
Cetylpyridinium chloride (p.1106·2); dequalinium chloride (p.1112·1); thymol (p.1127·1); cineole; menthol; mint oil.
Oral disinfection.

Neo-Pergonal *Serono, Fr.*
Menotrophin (p.1252·1).
Male and female infertility.

Neopermease *Sanabo, Aust.*
Hyaluronidase (p.1588·1).
Adjunct with chemotherapy for malignant neoplasms.

Neophedan *Intramed, S.Afr.*
Tamoxifen citrate (p.563·3).
Breast cancer.

Neo-Phlogicid *Waldheim, Aust.*
Aluminium acetotartrate (p.1547·3); camphor (p.1557·2); methyl salicylate (p.55·2); salicylic acid (p.1090·2); menthol (p.1600·2); eucalyptus oil (p.1578·1).
Frostbite; inflammation; musculoskeletal and joint disorders; sciatica.

Neopiran *Panthox & Burck, Ital.†.*
Nifenazone (p.63·1).
Joint disorders; migraine; musculoskeletal and joint disorders; myalgia; neuritis.

Neo-Planotest
Organon Teknika, Austral.; Organon Teknika, UK.
Pregnancy test (p.1621·2).

Neoplatin *Bristol-Myers, Spain.*
Cisplatin (p.513·3).
Malignant neoplasms.

Neoplex
Medicopharm, Aust.; Madaus, Ger.†.
Albumin tannate (p.1176·3); liquorice (p.1197·1); magnesium trisilicate (p.1199·1).
Gastro-intestinal disorders.

Neoplus *Terapeutico, Ital.*
Royal jelly (p.1626·3); pollen; ginseng (p.1584·2).
Nutritional supplement.

Neopons *Baxenden, UK.*
A range of alkyl sulphates.

Neo-Pregnosticon *Organon Teknika, Austral.*
Pregnancy test (p.1621·2).

Neo-Prunex *Neolab, Canad.*
Phenolphthalein (p.1208·2).
Constipation.

Neopurghes *Janssen-Cilag, Ital.†.*
Phenolphthalein (p.1208·2).
Constipation.

Neo-Pyodron *Cassella-med, Ger.*
Zinc oxide (p.1096·2); almasilate (p.1177·1); dequalinium chloride (p.1112·1).
Infected skin disorders; pyoderma.

Neopyrin *Knoll, Ger.*
Paracetamol (p.72·2); caffeine (p.749·3).
Pain.

Neopyrin-N *Nordmark, Ger.†.*
Etenzamide (p.35·3); paracetamol (p.72·2); isometheptene mucate (p.447·3); octamylamine mucate.
Cold symptoms; fever; pain.

Neoral
Novartis, Austral.; Sandoz, Fr.; Sandoz, Irl.; Novartis, Neth.; Sandoz, UK; Sandoz, USA.
Cyclosporin (p.519·1).
Atopic dermatitis; nephrotic syndrome; prevention of graft-versus-host disease; psoriasis; rheumatoid arthritis; transplant rejection.

Neoral-Sandimmun *Sandoz, Belg.*
Cyclosporin (p.519·1).
Auto-immune disorders; transplant rejection.

NeoRecormon
Boehringer Mannheim, Swed.; Boehringer Mannheim, UK.
Epoetin beta (p.718·3).
Formerly known as Recormon in *Swed.*
Anaemias; autologous blood transfusion.

Neoreserpan *Panthox & Burck, Ital.†.*
Syrosingopine (p.951·2).
Hypertension.

NeoRespin *Murdock, USA.*
Ephedrine hydrochloride (p.1059·3); guaiphenesin (p.1061·3).

Neorgine *Cantabria, Spain.*
Cinnarizine (p.406·1); co-dergocrine mesylate (p.1566·1).
Cerebrovascular disorders.

Neoride *Hosbon, Spain†.*
Sulpiride adamantanecarboxylate.
Behaviour disorders; psychoses; vertigo.

Neo-Rinoleina *Synthelabo, Ital.*
Xylometazoline hydrochloride (p.1071·2).
Nasal congestion.

Neorlest
Parke, Davis, Aust.; Parke, Davis, Ger.
Ethinyloestradiol (p.1445·1); norethisterone acetate (p.1453·1).
Combined oral contraceptive.

Neorutin *Stada, Switz.*
Rutin (p.1580·2).
Venous insufficiency.

neos nitro OPT *Optimed, Ger.*
Glyceryl trinitrate (p.874·3).
Cardiac disorders.

Neo-Sabenyl *SmithKline Beecham Consumer, Belg.*
Clorophene (p.1111·2); triethanolamine lauryl sulphate (p.1468·3).
Disinfection of skin, hands, mucous membranes, instruments, and materials; irrigation in ear, nose, and throat procedures; skin disorders; wound irrigation.

Neosalid *Bruco, Ital.†.*
Sodium salamidacetate (p.82·3).
Fever; inflammation; pain.

Neosar *Adria, USA.*
Cyclophosphamide (p.516·2).
Malignant neoplasms.

Neosidantoina *Squibb, Spain.*
Phenytoin sodium (p.352·3).
Epilepsy.

Neo-Sinedol *Wild, Switz.*
Lignocaine hydrochloride (p.1293·2); dehydrated alcohol.
Local anaesthesia.

Neo-Soyal *Nutricia, Ital.*
Infant feed.
Galactosaemia; milk intolerance.

Neosporin
Note. This name is used for preparations of different composition.
Glaxo Wellcome, Austral.; Glaxo Wellcome, Canad.; Wellcome, Irl.; Glaxo Wellcome, Neth.†; Wellcome, Switz.; Dominion, UK; Glaxo Wellcome, USA.
Cream; eye and ear drops: Neomycin sulphate (p.229·2); polymyxin B sulphate (p.239·1); gramicidin (p.215·2).
Bacterial eye and ear infections; bacterial skin infections.

Glaxo Wellcome, Austral.; Glaxo Wellcome, Canad.; Glaxo Wellcome, S.Afr.; Glaxo Wellcome, USA.
Topical aerosol; topical ointment; eye ointment: Neomycin sulphate (p.229·2); polymyxin B sulphate (p.239·1); bacitracin (p.157·3) or bacitracin zinc (p.157·3).
Superficial bacterial eye or skin infections.

Glaxo Wellcome, Canad.; Glaxo Wellcome, USA.
Bladder irrigation; cream: Neomycin sulphate (p.229·2); polymyxin B sulphate (p.239·1).
Bacterial urinary-tract infections; skin infections.

Neosporin GU *Glaxo Wellcome, USA.*
Neomycin sulphate (p.229·2); polymyxin B sulphate (p.239·1).
Prevention of catheter-associated urinary-tract infections.

Neosporin Plus *Glaxo Wellcome, USA.*
Cream: Neomycin (p.229·2); polymyxin B sulphate (p.239·1); lignocaine (p.1293·2).
Ointment: Neomycin (p.229·2); polymyxin B sulphate (p.239·1); lignocaine (p.1293·2); bacitracin zinc (p.157·3).

Neosporin-B *Wellcome, Switz.†.*
Neomycin sulphate (p.229·2); polymyxin B sulphate (p.239·1); bacitracin zinc (p.157·3).
Bacterial eye infections.

Neospray *Salud, Spain†.*
Benzalkonium chloride (p.1101·3); lignocaine hydrochloride (p.1293·2).
Skin infections.

Neo-Stediril
Wyeth Lederle, Aust.; Wyeth Lederle, Belg.; Wyeth, Ger.; Wyeth, Neth.; Wyeth, Switz.
Ethinyloestradiol (p.1445·1); levonorgestrel (p.1454·1).
Combined oral contraceptive.

Neostigmine Min-I-Mix *IMS, USA.*
Neostigmine methylsulphate (p.1394·1).
Atropine sulphate (p.455·1) is included in this preparation to protect against muscarinic actions.
Reversal of competitive neuromuscular blockade.

Neostix-3 *Bayer Diagnostics, Austral.†.*
Test for protein, glucose, and blood in urine.

Neostix-N *Bayer Diagnostics, Austral.*
Test for protein, glucose, blood, and nitrite in urine.

Neo-Stomygen *Stomygen, Ital.*
Mouthwash: Sodium monofluorophosphate (p.743·3); cetylpyridinium chloride (p.1106·2); enoxolone (p.35·2); xylitol (p.1372·3).
Formerly contained chlorhexidine gluconate, cetylpyridinium chloride, and sodium monofluorophosphate.
Toothpaste: Sodium monofluorophosphate (p.743·3); propolis (p.1621·3); enoxolone (p.35·2); cetylpyridinium chloride (p.1106·2).
Formerly contained chlorhexidine gluconate and cetylpyridinium chloride.
Oral disinfection; oral hygiene.

Neostrata *Canderm, Canad.*
A range of preparations containing glycolic acid (p.1083·1) or gluconolactone.
Skin disorders.

Neostrata AHA *NeoStrata, USA.*
Hydroquinone (p.1083·1).
Skin hyperpigmentation.

Neostrata HQ *Canderm, Canad.*
Hydroquinone (p.1083·1).
Skin hyperpigmentation.

Neosulf *Alphapharm, Austral.*
Neomycin sulphate (p.229·2).
Bowel sterilisation before surgery.

Neosultrin *Cilag, Ger.†.*
Sulfabenzamide (p.251·1); sulphathiazole (p.257·1); sulphacetamide (p.252·2); urea.
Vaginitis.

Neo-Synalar
Syntex, Belg.†; Syntex, USA†.
Fluocinolone acetonide (p.1041·1); neomycin sulphate (p.229·2).
Infected skin disorders.

Neosyncarpine *Ciba Vision, Fr.†.*
Pilocarpine nitrate (p.1396·3); phenylephrine hydrochloride (p.1066·2).
Production of miosis; raised intra-ocular pressure.

Neo-Synephrine
Sanofi Winthrop, Austral.; Abbott, Austral.; Sanofi Winthrop, Belg.; Sanofi Winthrop, Canad.; Sanofi Winthrop, Ger.†; Teofarma, Ital.; Sanofi, Swed.; Winthrop, Switz.†; Sanofi Winthrop, USA.
Phenylephrine hydrochloride (p.1066·2).
Eye disorders; nasal congestion; paroxysmal supraventricular tachycardia; production of mydriasis; to maintain blood pressure during anaesthesia; vascular failure.

Neo-Synephrine 12 Hour *Sterling Health, USA.*
Oxymetazoline hydrochloride (p.1065·3).
Nasal congestion.

Neosynephrin-POS *Ursapharm, Ger.*
Phenylephrine hydrochloride (p.1066·2).
Eye disorders.

Neo-Synodorm *Synpharma, Switz.*
Diphenhydramine (p.409·1).
Agitation; nervousness; sleep disorders.

Neo-Tabs *Pharma Tek, USA.*
Neomycin sulphate (p.229·2).

Neotal *Hauck, USA.*
Polymyxin B sulphate (p.239·1); neomycin sulphate (p.229·2); bacitracin zinc (p.157·3).
Eye infections.

Neotensin *CEPA, Spain.*
Enalapril maleate (p.863·2).
Heart failure; hypertension.

Neotensin Diu *CEPA, Spain.*
Hydrochlorothiazide (p.885·2); enalapril maleate (p.863·2).
Hypertension.

Neotest
Merieux, Fr.; Merieux, Switz.†.
Tuberculin PPD (p.1640·2).
Sensitivity testing.

Neotetranase *Rottapharm, Ital.*
Amoxycillin trihydrate (p.151·3).
Bacterial infections.

Neothyllin *Metochem, Aust.*
Diprophylline (p.752·1).
Heart failure; hypertension; obstructive airways disease.

Neothylline *Lemmon, USA†.*
Diprophylline (p.752·1).
Asthma; bronchospasm.

Neothylline-GG *Lemmon, USA†.*
Diprophylline (p.752·1); guaiphenesin (p.1061·3).
Bronchospasm.

Neo-Thyreostat *Herbrand, Ger.; Berlin-Chemie, Ger.*
Carbimazole (p.1491·2).
Hyperthyroidism.

Neotigason
Roche, Aust.; Roche, Austral.; Roche, Belg.; Roche, Ger.; Roche, Irl.; Roche, Neth.; Roche, Norw.; Roche, S.Afr.; Andreu, Spain; Roche, Swed.; Roche, Switz.; Roche, UK.
Acitretin (p.1077·3).
Keratinisation disorders; psoriasis.

Neo-Tinic *Neolab, Canad.*
Multivitamins and iron.

Neo-Tizide
Pharmacia Upjohn, Aust.; Carlo Erba, Ital.†.
Methaniazide calcium (p.225·1).
Tuberculosis.

Neoton *Searle, Ital.*
Fosfocreatine sodium.
Cardiac disorders.

Neotopic *Technilab, Canad.*
Polymyxin B sulphate (p.239·1); bacitracin zinc (p.157·3); neomycin sulphate (p.229·2).
Bacterial skin infections.

Neotrace *Lyphomed, USA.*
Trace element preparation.
Additive for intravenous total parenteral nutrition solutions.

Neotracin
Ciba Vision, Ger.; Ciba Vision, Switz.
Neomycin sulphate (p.229·2); bacitracin (p.157·3).
Bacterial eye infections.

Neo-Treupine *Asta Medica, Switz.†.*
Paracetamol (p.72·2).
Tocopheryl acetate (p.1369·1) is included in this preparation to reduce the hepatotoxicity of paracetamol.
Fever; pain.

Neotri *Beiersdorf-Lilly, Ger.*
Xipamide (p.971·2); triamterene (p.957·2).
Hypertension; oedema.

Neotricin *Bausch & Lomb, USA†.*
Neomycin sulphate (p.229·2); bacitracin zinc (p.157·3); polymyxin B sulphate (p.239·1).
Eye infections.

Neotricin HC *Bausch & Lomb, USA.*
Neomycin sulphate (p.229·2); bacitracin zinc (p.157·3); polymyxin B sulphate (p.239·1); hydrocortisone acetate (p.1043·3).
Eye inflammation with bacterial infection.

Neo-Trim *Neo-Life, Austral.*
Blend of plant fibre.
Obesity.

Neotrizine *Lilly, USA†.*
Sulphadiazine (p.252·3); sulfamerazine (p.251·3); sulphadimidine (p.253·2).

Neotroparin *Chinoin, Hung.*
Drotaverine hydrochloride (p.1574·2); homatropine methobromide (p.462·2).
Smooth muscle spasm.

Neotul *Fides, Spain†.*
Famotidine (p.1192·1).
Peptic ulcer; Zollinger-Ellison syndrome.

Neo-Tuss *Neolab, Canad.*
Dextromethorphan hydrobromide (p.1057·3); chlorpheniramine maleate (p.405·1); phenylephrine hydrochloride (p.1066·2); sodium citrate (p.1153·2); guaiphenesin (p.1061·3).
Coughs; respiratory tract congestion.

NeoTussan *Sandoz, Ger.*
Dextromethorphan polistirex (p.1058·2).
Coughs.

Neotyf *Biocine, Ital.*
A typhoid vaccine (p.1536·3).
Active immunisation.

Neo-Urtisan *Synpharma, Switz.*
Pheniramine maleate (p.415·3); lignocaine hydrochloride (p.1293·2); calcium gluconate (p.1155·2); chlorhexidine gluconate (p.1107·2).
Hypersensitivity reactions of the skin.

Neo-Ustiol *INTES, Ital.*
Sodium citrate (p.1153·2); aminobenzoic acid (p.1486·3); procaine (p.1299·2); cod-liver oil (p.1337·3).
Ophthalmic burns.

Neovis *Searle, Ital.*
Vitamin, carbohydrate, and mineral preparation with creatine.
Nutritional supplement.

Neo-Vites *Neolab, Canad.*
Multivitamins or multivitamins and minerals.

Neo-Vivactil *Sanofi Winthrop, Switz.*
Amino-acid, mineral, and vitamin C preparation.

Neovletta *Schering, Swed.*
Levonorgestrel (p.1454·1); ethinyloestradiol (p.1445·1).
Combined oral contraceptive.

Neoxene *Ecobi, Ital.*
Chlorhexidine gluconate (p.1107·2).
Disinfection of skin, hands, wounds, burns, and vagina.

Neoxidil
Galderma, Belg.; Galderma, Fr.
Minoxidil (p.910·3).
Androgenic alopecia.

Neoxinal *Farmec, Ital.*
Chlorhexidine gluconate (p.1107·2).
Disinfection of skin, wounds, and burns.

Neo-Xylestesin *Espe, Aust.*
Lignocaine hydrochloride (p.1293·2).
Adrenaline hydrochloride (p.813·3) is included in this preparation as a vasoconstrictor to diminish absorption and localise the effect of the local anaesthetic.
Local anaesthesia in dentistry.

Neo-Xylestesin forte and Neo-Xylestesin special *Espe, Aust.*
Lignocaine hydrochloride (p.1293·2).
Adrenaline hydrochloride (p.813·3) and noradrenaline hydrochloride (p.924·2) are included in this preparation as vasoconstrictors to diminish absorption and localise the effect of the local anaesthetic.
Local anaesthesia in dentistry.

Neo-Zol *Neolab, Canad.*
Clotrimazole (p.376·3).

Nepatim *San Carlo, Ital.†.*
Sodium fructose-1,6-diphosphate; calcium folinate (p.1342·2); cyanocobalamin (p.1363·3).
Anaemias; tonic.

Nepenthe *Medeva, UK†.*
Morphine (p.56·1); opium (p.70·3).
Pain.

Nephlex Rx *Nephro-Tech, USA.*
Vitamin B substances and vitamin C.

Nephral *Pfleger, Ger.*
Triamterene (p.957·2); hydrochlorothiazide (p.885·2).
Hypertension; oedema.

Nephramine
Fresenius, Fr.; Pharmacia Upjohn, Spain; Fresenius, UK; McGaw, USA.
Amino-acid infusion.
Parenteral nutrition in renal impairment.

Nephrex *Rhone-Poulenc Rorer, Austral.*
Calcium acetate (p.1155·1).
Hyperphosphataemia.

Nephril
Pfizer, Irl.; Pfizer, UK.
Polythiazide (p.932·1).
Hypertension; oedema.

Nephrisan P *Ziethen, Ger.*
Squill (p.1070·1).
Cardiac disorders.

Nephrisol *Redel, Ger.†.*
Herniaria (p.1587·2); bearberry (p.1552·2); boldo (p.1554·1).
Urinary-tract disorders.

Nephrisol mono *Redel, Ger.*
Solidago virgaurea.
Urinary-tract disorders.

Nephro-Calci *R&D, USA.*
Calcium carbonate (p.1182·1).
Calcium deficiency; dietary supplement.

Nephrocaps *Fleming, USA.*
Vitamin B substances with vitamin C.
Vitamin deficiency in renal dialysis.

Nephro-Derm *R&D, USA†.*
Emollient and moisturiser.

Nephro-Fer *R&D, USA.*
Ferrous fumarate (p.1339·3).
Iron-deficiency anaemias.

Nephro-Fer Rx *R&D, USA.*
Folic acid (p.1340·3); iron (p.1346·1).

Nephrolith mono *Biomo, Ger.*
Solidago virgaurea.
Renal calculi.

Nephrolithol N *Pfluger, Ger.*
Homoeopathic preparation.

nephro-loges *Loges, Ger.*
Equisetum (p.1575·1); solidago virgaurea; ononis (p.1610·2); parsley root (p.1615·3).
Urinary-tract disorders.

Nephron *Nephron, USA.*
Racepinephrine hydrochloride (p.815·2).
Bronchospasm.

Nephron FA *Nephro-Tech, USA.*
Multivitamin preparation with iron and folic acid.
Docusate sodium (p.1189·3) is included in this preparation to reduce the constipating effects of iron.

Nephronorm Med *APS, Ger.*
Tablets: Orthosiphon leaf (p.1592·2).
Tea: Silver birch (p.1553·3); solidago virgaurea; orthosiphon (p.1592·2); ononis (p.1610·2); rose fruit (p.1365·2); cornflower; calendula officinalis.
Urinary-tract disorders.

Nephro-Pasc *Pascoe, Ger.*
Solidago virgaurea; birch leaf (p.1553·3); orthosiphon (p.1592·2).
Urinary-tract disorders.

Nephroplasmal N *Braun, Ger.*
Amino-acid and glycerol infusion.
Parenteral nutrition in renal disease.

Nephropur tri *Repha, Ger.*
Solidago virgaurea; betula (p.1553·3); orthosiphon (p.1592·2).
Urinary-tract disorders.

Nephroselect M *Dreluso, Ger.*
Solidago virgaurea; equisetum (p.1575·1); birch leaf (p.1553·3); ononis (p.1610·2); levisticum officinale (p.1597·2); tropaeolum majus; saw palmetto (p.1462·1).
Urinary-tract disorders.

Nephrosolid N *Bioforce, Switz.*
Solidago virgaurea; silver birch (p.1553·3); ononis (p.1610·2); equisetum (p.1575·1).
Urinary-tract disorders.

Nephros-Strath *Strath-Labor, Ger.†.*
Belladonna (p.457·1); gratiola officinalis; maize.
Bladder disorders.

Nephrosteril
Fresenius, Belg.; Fresenius-Klinik, Ger.†; Fresenius, Switz.
Amino-acid infusion.
Parenteral nutrition in renal disease.

Nephrotect *Fresenius-Klinik, Ger.*
Amino-acid infusion.
Parenteral nutrition in renal failure.

Nephrotrans
Medice, Ger.; Salmon, Switz.
Sodium bicarbonate (p.1153·2).
Metabolic acidosis.

Nephro-Vite *R&D, USA.*
A range of vitamin preparations.

Nephro-Vite Rx +Fe *R&D, USA.*
Multivitamin preparation with iron and folic acid.

Nephrox *Fleming, USA.*
Aluminium hydroxide (p.1177·3).
Hyperacidity.

Nephrubin *Weber & Weber, Ger.*
Herbal tea: Salix (p.82·3); aesculus (p.1543·3); sambucus (p.1627·2); tilia (p.1637·3); birch leaf (p.1553·3); parsley (p.1615·3); centaury (p.1561·1); herniaria (p.1587·2); guaiacum wood; celery (p.1561·1); orthosiphon staminei leaf (p.1592·2).
Tablets: Birch leaf (p.1553·3); orthosiphon (p.1592·2). Formerly contained benzoic acid, khellin, and rubia tinctorum.
Urinary-tract disorders.

Nephulon E *Redel, Ger.†.*
Sodium lauryl sulphate (p.1468·3); guaiphenesin (p.1061·3); ammonium thiocyanate; ammonium glycyrrhizinate (p.1055·2); chamomile (p.1561·2); menthol (p.1600·2); bergamot oil (p.1553·1).
Bronchitis; laryngitis; tracheitis.

Nephulon G *Redel, Ger.*
Guaiphenesin (p.1061·3).
Cough and cold symptoms.

Nephur-Test + Leucocytes
Boehringer Mannheim, Austral.; Boehringer Mannheim Diagnostics, UK.
Test for leucocytes, nitrites, pH, protein, glucose, and blood in urine.

Nepituss *Pfizer, Ital.*
Nepinalone hydrochloride (p.1065·1).
Coughs.

Nepresol
Ciba-Geigy, Aust.; Ciba-Geigy, Belg.; Ciba, Ger.; Ciba, Ital.†; Ciba, Neth.†; Novartis, Neth.; Ciba, Norw.; Novartis, S.Afr.; Novartis, Swed.; Ciba, Switz.
Dihydralazine mesylate (p.854·1) or dihydralazine sulphate (p.854·1).
Heart failure; hypertension.

Nepressol *Ciba-Geigy, Fr.*
Dihydralazine sulphate (p.854·1).
Heart failure; hypertension.

Nepro
Abbott, Austral.; Abbott, Canad.; Abbott, UK; Ross, USA.
Preparation for enteral nutrition in renal dialysis patients.

Neptal *Procter & Gamble, Ger.*
Acebutolol hydrochloride (p.809·3).
Cardiac disorders; hypertension.

Neptazane
Storz, Austral.; Storz, Canad.; Lederle, USA.
Methazolamide (p.903·2).
Glaucoma.

Nerdipina *Ferrer, Spain.*
Nicardipine hydrochloride (p.915·1).
Angina pectoris; cerebrovascular disorders; hypertension.

Nerex *Farmanova, Ital.*
Royal jelly (p.1626·3); honey (p.1345·3); myrtillus (p.1606·1); fructose.
Nutritional supplement.

Nergadan *Uriach, Spain.*
Lovastatin (p.1275·1).
Hyperlipidaemias.

Nerial *Simes, Ital.†.*
Peruvoside (p.928·3).
Cardiac disorders.

Neribas
Schering, Ger.; Schering, Switz.
Emollient.
Skin disorders.

Nericur *Schering, UK.*
Benzoyl peroxide (p.1079·2).
Acne.

Neriforte
Schering, Aust.; Schering, Switz.†.
Diflucortolone valerate (p.1039·3).
Skin disorders.

Neriquinol *Schering, Aust.*
Diflucortolone valerate (p.1039·3); chlorquinaldol (p.185·1).
Infected skin disorders.

Nerisalic
Stiefel, Canad.; Schering, Fr.
Diflucortolone valerate (p.1039·3); salicylic acid (p.1090·2).
Skin disorders.

Nerisona
Schering, Aust.; Schering, Belg.; Schering, Ger.; Schering, Ital.; Schering, Neth.; Schering, Switz.
Diflucortolone valerate (p.1039·3).
Skin disorders.

Nerisona C
Schering, Ger.; Schering, Ital.
Diflucortolone valerate (p.1039·3); chlorquinaldol (p.185·1).
Infected skin disorders.

Nerisone
Stiefel, Canad.; Schering, Fr.; Schering, Irl.†; Schering, S.Afr.; Schering, UK.
Diflucortolone valerate (p.1039·3).
Skin disorders.

Nerisone C *Schering, Fr.*
Diflucortolone valerate (p.1039·3); chlorquinaldol (p.185·1).
Infected skin disorders.

Nerofen *Boots Healthcare, Neth.†.*
Ibuprofen (p.44·1).
Fever; pain.

Nerpemide *Morrith, Spain.*
Proteolytic enzymes.
Herpesvirus infections; neuritis.

Nervade *Vesta, S.Afr.*
Caffeine (p.749·3); sodium glycerophosphate (p.1586·2); magnesium glycerophosphate (p.1157·2); potassium glycerophosphate (p.1586·2); glycerophosphoric acid (p.1586·2); potassium citrate (p.1153·1); yeast extract.
Tonic.

Nervan *Rosch & Handel, Aust.*
Paracetamol (p.72·2); propyphenazone (p.81·3); caffeine citrate (p.749·3).
Fever; pain.

Nerva-Phos *Stotzer, Switz.†.*
Calcium magnesium phytate trihydrate; thiamine hydrochloride (p.1361·1); ascorbic acid (p.1365·2).
Tonic.

Nervatona *Brauer, Austral.*
Homoeopathic preparation.

Nervatona Plus *Brauer, Austral.*
Homoeopathic preparation.

Nervauxan *Pfluger, Ger.†.*
Testicular extract (p.1464·1).
Impotence.

Nervencreme S *Fides, Ger.*
Peppermint oil (p.1208·1); eucalyptus oil (p.1578·1).
Pain.

Nervendragees
Note. This name is used for preparations of different composition.
Rosch & Handel, Aust.
Valerian (p.1643·1); lupulus (p.1597·2); melissa (p.1600·1); orange flowers; rosemary.
Nervous disorders; sleep disorders.

Ratiopharm, Ger.
Valerian root (p.1643·1); passion flower (p.1615·3); lupulus (p.1597·2).
Anxiety disorders; insomnia.

Nervenja *OTW, Ger.*
Homoeopathic preparation.

Nervenruh
Note. This name is used for preparations of different composition.
Klosterfrau, Aust.
Valerian (p.1643·1); passion flower (p.1615·3); lupulus (p.1597·2).
Anxiety disorders; sleep disorders.

Divapharma, Ger.†.
Valerian root (p.1643·1); lupulus (p.1597·2).
Nervous disorders.

Nerventee *Smetana, Aust.*
Valerian (p.1643·1); lupulus (p.1597·2); hypericum (p.1590·1); peppermint leaf (p.1208·1); calluna vulgaris; delphinium consolida.
Anxiety disorders; sleep disorders.

Nerven-Tee Stada N *Stada, Ger.*
Passion flower (p.1615·3); peppermint leaf (p.1208·1); melissa (p.1600·1); valerian (p.1643·1).
Sedative; sleep disorders.

Nervfluid S *Fides, Ger.*
Camphor (p.1557·2); eucalyptus oil (p.1578·1); pumilio pine oil (p.1623·3).
Nerve, muscle, and joint pain.

Nervidox *Teral, USA.*
Vitamin B_{12} (p.1363·3); vitamin B_1 (p.1361·2).

Nervidox 6 *Teral, USA.*
Vitamin B_{12} (p.1363·3); vitamin B_1 (p.1361·2); vitamin B_6 (p.1362·3).

Nervifene *Interdelta, Switz.*
Chloral hydrate (p.645·3).
Agitation; insomnia.

Nervifloran *Bioflora, Aust.*
Valerian (p.1643·1); lupulus (p.1597·2); melissa (p.1600·1); orange flowers; rosemary.
Nervous disorders; sleep disorders.

Nerviguttum *Molitor, Ger.†.*
Rauwolfia serpentina (p.941·3); menyanthes (p.1601·2); melissa (p.1600·1); veronica; rose fruit (p.1365·2); valerian (p.1643·1); folia aurantii; lupulus (p.1597·2).
Psychiatric disorders.

Nervine *Mathieu, Canad.*
Aspirin (p.16·1); caffeine (p.749·3).

Nervinetten *Eurim, Ger.*
Valerian (p.1643·1); lupulus (p.1597·2).
Agitation; sleep disorders.

Nervinfant *Jossa-Arznei, Ger.†.*
Oral liquid: Thiamine hydrochloride (p.1361·1); lupulus (p.1597·2); passion flower (p.1615·3); piscidia erythrina; mistletoe (p.1604·1); sodium phytate (p.995·3); guaiphenesin (p.1061·3); sodium glycerophosphate (p.1586·2).
Nervous disorders.
Suppositories: Valerian (p.1643·1); guaiphenesin (p.1061·3).
Agitation; excitability; sleep disorders.

Nervinfant comp *Jossa-Arznei, Ger.†.*
Paracetamol (p.72·2); guaiphenesin (p.1061·3); valerian (p.1643·1).
Fever; influenza; pain.

Nervinfant N *Biocur, Ger.*
Lupulus (p.1597·2); passion flower (p.1615·3).
Agitation; sleep disorders.

Nervinum Felke *Truw, Ger.†.*
Homoeopathic preparation.

Nervinum Stada *Stada, Ger.†.*
Aprobarbital (p.642·2); valerian tincture (p.1643·1).
Sedative; sleep disorders.

Nervipan
Note. This name is used for preparations of different composition.
Medopharm, Ger.
Valerian (p.1643·1).
Anxiety.

Gazzoni, Ital.†.
Valepotriates (p.1643·1).
Insomnia.

Nervipane *Apotheke Roten Krebs, Aust.*
Valepotriates (p.1643·1).
Nervous disorders.

Nervisal *Bristol, Ger.†.*
Aprobarbital (p.642·2); valerian (p.1643·1); lupulus (p.1597·2); quebracho; thiamine hydrochloride; pyridoxine; cyanocobalamin.
Nervous disorders; sleep disorders.

Nervita *Boiron, Canad.*
Homoeopathic preparation.

nervo OPT mono *Optimed, Ger.†.*
Barbitone sodium (p.642·3).
Chronic fatigue syndrome; insomnia; nervous disorders.

nervo OPT N *Optimed, Ger.*
Diphenhydramine hydrochloride (p.409·1).
Sleep disorders.

Nervobaldon V *Zwintscher, Ger.†.*
Homoeopathic preparation.

Nervobion *Merck, Spain.*
Cyanocobalamin (p.1363·3); pyridoxine (p.1363·1) or pyridoxine hydrochloride (p.1362·3); thiamine (p.1361·2).
Vitamin B deficiency.

Nervocaine *Keene, USA.*
Lignocaine hydrochloride (p.1293·2).
Local anaesthesia.

Nervogastrol *Heumann, Ger.*
Bismuth subnitrate (p.1180·2); bismuth subgallate (p.1180·2); heavy magnesium carbonate (p.1198·1); calcium carbonate (p.1182·1); sodium bicarbonate (p.1153·2); chelidonium; condurango (p.1567·2); scopolia carniolica.
Gastro-intestinal disorders.

Nervoid *Hanosan, Ger.†.*
Homoeopathic preparation.

Nervolitan *3M, Ger.†.*
Aprobarbital sodium (p.642·2); secbutobarbitone sodium (p.692·1).
Nervous disorders; sleep disorders.

Nervolitan S *3M, Ger.†.*
Phenobarbitone sodium (p.350·2).
Nervous disorders; sleep disorders.

Nervonocton N *Pfluger, Ger.†.*
Kava (p.1592·3).
Nervous disorders.

Nervo.opt *Truw, Ger.†.*
Barbitone sodium (p.642·3); phenobarbitone (p.350·2); calcium gluconate; valerian (p.1643·1); lupulus (p.1597·2).
Nervous disorders; sleep disorders.

Nervopax au Silicea *Lehning, Fr.*
Homoeopathic preparation.

Nervoregin *Pfluger, Ger.*
Arnica montana; avena (p.1551·3); crataegus (p.1568·2); passion flower (p.1615·3); hypericum perforatum; anamirta cocculus; acidum phosphoricum; viscum album.
Psychiatric disorders.

Nervoregin forte *Pfluger, Ger.*
Valerian (p.1643·1); lupulus (p.1597·2); passion flower (p.1615·3).
Nervous disorders.

Nervoregin H *Pfluger, Ger.*
Homoeopathic preparation.

Nervosana *Hotz, Ger.*
Achillea (p.1542·2); liquorice (p.1197·1); melissa (p.1600·1); peppermint leaf (p.1208·1); rubus fruticosus; chamomille (p.1561·2); tilia (p.1637·3); valerian (p.1643·1); absinthium (p.1541·1).
Nervous disorders; sleeplessness.

Nervospur *Syxyl, Ger.†.*
Cactus grand.; flores arnicae; radix arnicae; cortex chinae; nuces moschat; cortex hamamelidis; folia hamamelidis; herba rutae; flores chamomillae; herba visci albi; fructus cynosbati; herba passiflorae; stramentum avenae; nuces colae; abrotanum; acid. phosphoric.; mangan. acetic.; arsenic. jodat.; yohimbinum; calcium carbonic.; calcium fluorat.; ferrum metallic.; magnesium phosph.; platinum; selenium; silicea; testis; damiana; ginseng; lecithinum; cobalt; molybdenum.
Nerve tonic.

Nervpin N *Schoning-Berlin, Ger.*
Menthol (p.1600·2); noble fir oil.
Nerve and joint pain; skin trauma; sprains.

Nervuton N *Redel, Ger.*
Homoeopathic preparation.

Nesacain *Astra, Switz.*
Chloroprocaine hydrochloride (p.1289·1).
Local anaesthesia.

Nesacaine
Astra, Canad.; Astra, USA.
Chloroprocaine hydrochloride (p.1289·1).
Local anaesthesia.

Nesdonal
Rhone-Poulenc Rorer, Belg.; Specia, Fr.†; Rhone-Poulenc Rorer, Neth.
Thiopentone sodium (p.1233·1).
General anaesthesia.

Nesfare Antibiotico *Madaus, Spain.*
Human placenta; framycetin sulphate (p.210·3); triamcinolone acetonide (p.1050·2); chamomile oil; calendula oil.
Infected skin disorders.

Nesivine *Merck-Belgolabo, Belg.*
Oxymetazoline hydrochloride (p.1065·3).
Eustachian-tube inflammation; nasal disorders; pharyngolaryngitis.

Nesporac *Cusi, Spain†.*
Fluconazole (p.378·1).
Fungal infections.

Nestabs *Fielding, USA.*
Multivitamin and mineral preparation with iron and folic acid.
Multivitamin and mineral supplement for pregnancy and lactation.

Nestabs FA *Fielding, USA.*
Ferrous fumarate (p.1339·3); folic acid (p.1340·3); multivitamins and minerals.
Iron-deficiency anaemias.

Nestargel
Nestle, S.Afr.†; Nestle, Switz.; Nestle, UK.
Ceratonia (p.1472·2).
Infant feed thickener.

Nesthakchen *Schulke & Mayr, Aust.*
Fennel (p.1579·1); aniseed (p.1549·3); caraway (p.1559·3); chamomile (p.1561·2); liquorice (p.1197·1); fennel oil (p.1579·2); anise oil (p.1550·1); caraway oil (p.1559·3); chamomile oil.
Gastro-intestinal disorders.

Nestosyl
Note. This name is used for preparations of different composition.
Pharmethic, Belg.
Benzocaine (p.1286·2); butyl aminobenzoate (p.1289·1); resorcinol (p.1090·1); zinc oxide (p.1096·2).
Minor wounds; skin disorders.

Jumer, Fr.
Benzocaine (p.1286·2); butyl aminobenzoate (p.1289·1); resorcinol (p.1090·1); hydroxyquinoline (p.1589·3); zinc oxide (p.1096·2).
Local anaesthesia; sunburn; superficial burns.

Sanofi Midy, Neth.†.
Pramoxine hydrochloride (p.1298·2); zinc oxide (p.1096·2).
Skin disorders.

Nestrex *Fielding, USA.*
Pyridoxine hydrochloride (p.1362·3).
Pyridoxine deficiency.

Nestrovit *Roche, Switz.†.*
Multivitamin and mineral preparation.

Nethaprin Dospan *Mer-National, S.Afr.*
Bufylline (p.749·3); doxylamine succinate (p.410·1); etafedrine hydrochloride (p.1061·1); phenylephrine hydrochloride (p.1066·2).
Coughs; obstructive airways disease.

Nethaprin Expectorant *Mer-National, S.Afr.*
Bufylline (p.749·3); doxylamine succinate (p.410·1); etafedrine hydrochloride (p.1061·1); guaiphenesin (p.1061·3).
Obstructive airways disease.

Netillin
Schering-Plough, Irl.; Schering-Plough, UK.
Netilmicin sulphate (p.231·1).
Bacterial infections.

Netilyn
Schering-Plough, Norw.; Schering-Plough, Swed.
Netilmicin sulphate (p.231·1).
Bacterial infections.

Netox *Vita, Ital.†.*
Cogalactoisomerase sodium (p.1566·2).
Liver disorders.

Netrocin *Schering-Plough, Spain.*
Netilmicin sulphate (p.231·1).
Bacterial infections.

Netromicine *Schering-Plough, Fr.*
Netilmicin sulphate (p.231·1).
Bacterial infections.

Netromycin
Schering-Plough, Austral.; Schering, Canad.; Schering-Plough, S.Afr.; Schering, USA.
Netilmicin sulphate (p.231·1).
Bacterial infections.

Netromycine
Schering-Plough, Belg.; Schering-Plough, Neth.; Essex, Switz.
Netilmicin sulphate (p.231·1).
Bacterial infections.

Nettacin *Schering-Plough, Ital.*
Netilmicin sulphate (p.231·1).
Bacterial infections.

Nettinerv *Iso, Ger.*
Homoeopathic preparation.

Netux *Nicholas, Fr.*
Codeine (p.26·1); phenyltoloxamine (p.416·1).
Coughs.

Neucalm 50 *Legere, USA†.*
Hydroxyzine hydrochloride (p.412·1).

Neucor *CT, Ital.*
Nicardipine hydrochloride (p.915·1).
Angina pectoris; heart failure; hypertension.

Neuer *Daiichi, Jpn.*
Cetraxate hydrochloride (p.1183·1).
Gastric ulcer; gastritis.

Neugen *Bioprogress, Ital.*
Nicergoline (p.1607·1).
Cerebrovascular disorders.

Neugra N *Hermes, Ger.*
Multivitamin and mineral preparation.

Neulactil
Rhone-Poulenc Rorer, Austral.; Rhone-Poulenc Rorer, Irl.; Rhone-Poulenc Rorer, Norw.; Rhone-Poulenc Rorer, S.Afr.; Rhone-Poulenc Rorer, Swed.†; JHC Healthcare, UK.
Pericyazine (p.685·2).
Anxiety disorders; behaviour disorders in children; pain; psychoses.

Neulente *Wellcome, Irl.†.*
Insulin zinc suspension (bovine, purified) (p.322·1).
Diabetes mellitus.

Neuleptil
Rhone-Poulenc Rorer, Aust.; Rhone-Poulenc Rorer, Belg.; Rhone-Poulenc Rorer, Canad.; Specia, Fr.; Rhone-Poulenc Rorer, Ital.; Rhone-Poulenc Rorer, Neth.; Rhone-Poulenc Rorer, Switz.
Pericyazine (p.685·2), pericyazine mesylate (p.685·2), or pericyazine tartrate (p.685·2).
Psychoses.

Neumega *Genetics Institute, USA.*
Oprelvekin (p.725·2).
Thrombocytopenia.

Neumobiot *Reig Jofre, Spain.*
Benzylpenicillin sodium (p.159·3); niaouli oil (p.1607·1); guaiphenesin (p.1061·3).
Lignocaine hydrochloride (p.1293·2) is included in this preparation to alleviate the pain of injection.
Respiratory-tract infections.

Neumobronquial *Bama, Spain†.*
Amoxycillin trihydrate (p.151·3); bromhexine (p.1055·3).
Respiratory-tract infections.

Neumopectolina *Inkeysa, Spain.*
Guaiphenesin (p.1061·3); sodium benzoate (p.1102·3); co-trimoxazole (p.196·3).
Respiratory-tract infections.

Neupan *Smith Kline & French, Ital.†.*
Oxiracetam (p.1611·3).
Mental function impairment.

Neuphane *Wellcome, Irl.†.*
Isophane insulin injection (bovine, purified) (p.322·1).
Diabetes mellitus.

Neupogen
Roche, Aust.; Amgen, Austral.; Roche, Belg.; Amgen, Canad.; Roche, Fr.; Amgen, Ger.; Roche, Ger.; Roche, Irl.; Dompe Biotec, Ital.; Roche, Neth.; Roche, Norw.; Roche, S.Afr.; Roche, Spain; Amgen, Swed.; Roche, Switz.; Roche, UK; Amgen, USA.
Filgrastim (p.723·1).
Mobilisation of blood progenitor cells; neutropenia.

Neupramir *Lusofarmaco, Ital.*
Pramiracetam sulphate (p.1621·2).
Mental function impairment.

Neuquinon *Eisai, Jpn.*
Ubidecarenone (p.1641·2).
Heart failure.

Neuraben *Bioindustria, Ital.*
BT-851; pyridoxine hydrochloride (p.1362·3); cyanocobalamin (p.1363·3).
Joint disorders; neuritis.

Neuracen *Promonta, Ger.†.*
Beclamide (p.339·2).
Behavioural disorders; epilepsy.

Neuractiv *Ciba, Ital.*
Oxiracetam (p.1611·3).
Mental function impairment.

Neuralgin *Pfleger, Ger.*
Aspirin (p.16·1); paracetamol (p.72·2); caffeine (p.749·3).
Pain.

Neuralysan S *Steigerwald, Ger.*
Thiamine hydrochloride (p.1361·1); pyridoxine hydrochloride (p.1362·3).
Neuralgia; neuritis.

Neuramag P *CT, Ger.*
Paracetamol (p.72·2); caffeine (p.749·3).
Pain.

Neuramate *Halsey, USA.*
Meprobamate (p.678·1).
Anxiety.

Neuramide Sherman *Difa, Ital.*
Neuramide.
Herpesvirus infections.

Neur-Amyl *Fawns & McAllan, Austral.*
Amylobarbitone (p.641·3).
Hypnotic; sedative.

Neuranidal *LAW, Ger.*
Aspirin (p.16·1); paracetamol (p.72·2); caffeine (p.749·3).
Pain.

Neuranidal Duo *LAW, Ger.*
Aspirin (p.16·1); caffeine (p.749·3).
Fever; pain.

Neurapas *Pascoe, Ger.*
Hypericum (p.1590·1); valerian (p.1643·1); passion flower (p.1615·3); larkspur; eschscholtzia californ..
Psychiatric disorders.

Neurarmonil *Rhone-Poulenc, Ital.†.*
Amitriptylinoxide (p.278·1).
Depression.

Neuraston *Pfluger, Ger.†.*
Ginseng (p.1584·2); passion flower (p.1615·3); lupulus (p.1597·2); aconitum nap.; asa foetida; aurum chloratum; belladonna; ferrum phosphoricum; ignatia; kalium phosphoricum; manganum met.; selenium met.; zincum met.; arnica; avena sativa; cuprum aceticum; damiana.
Psychiatric disorders.

NeuRecover *NeuroGenesis, USA.*
A range of multivitamin, mineral, and amino-acid preparations.

Neurex *Salus, Ital.*
Citicoline sodium (p.1564·3).
Cerebrovascular disorders; parkinsonism.

Neuri-cyl N Ho-Len-Complex *Liebermann, Ger.*
Homoeopathic preparation.

Neuridon *Synthelabo, Belg.*
Paracetamol (p.72·2).
Fever; pain.

Neuridon Forte *Synthelabo, Belg.*
Paracetamol (p.72·2); propyphenazone (p.81·3); codeine phosphate (p.26·1).
Fever; pain.

Neuriherpes *Iquinosa, Spain†.*
Proteolytic enzymes.
Herpes; neuritis.

Neuril *Schoeller, Aust.†.*
Melperone hydrochloride (p.677·3).
Anxiety disorders; drug and alcohol withdrawal syndrome; psychoses; senile dementia; sleep disorders.

Neuriplege *Genevrier, Fr.*
Ointment: Chlorproethazine hydrochloride (p.649·1); cymene (p.27·2).
Tablets†; injection†: Chlorproethazine hydrochloride (p.649·1).
Painful skeletal muscle spasm.

Neurium *Hexal, Ger.*
Thioctic acid (p.1636·2) or ethylenediamine thioctate (p.1636·2).
Diabetic polyneuropathy.

Neuro *Rotexmedica, Ger.†.*
Vitamin B substances.
Vitamin B deficiency.

Neuro B-12 *Lambda, USA.*
Vitamin B_{12} (p.1363·3); vitamin B_1 (p.1361·2).

Neuro B-12 Forte *Lambda, USA.*
Vitamin B substances and ascorbic acid.

Neuro Calme *Geistlich, Switz.*
Vitamin B substances and mineral preparation.
Tonic.

Neuro Nutrients *Solgar, UK.*
Amino-acid preparation with vitamin B substances, vitamin C, and ginkgo biloba.

Neuro-AS *A.S., Ger.†.*
Vitamin B substances.
Lignocaine hydrochloride (p.1293·2) is included in this preparation to alleviate the pain of injection.
Vitamin B deficiency.

Neuro-AS N *A.S., Ger.*
Thiamine hydrochloride (p.1361·1); pyridoxine hydrochloride (p.1362·3).
Vitamin B deficiency.

Neuro-B forte *Biomo, Ger.*
Thiamine hydrochloride (p.1361·1); pyridoxine hydrochloride (p.1362·3).
Neurological system disorders.

Neurobiol *Teofarma, Ital.*
Sodium bromide (p.1620·3); phenobarbitone (p.350·2); passion flower (p.1615·3); crataegus (p.1568·2).
Insomnia; nervous disorders.

Neurobion
Merck, Aust.; Merck-Belgolabo, Belg.; Merck, Ger.; E. Merck, Irl.; E. Merck, Neth.; Merck, S.Afr.; Meda, Swed.; E. Merck, Switz.†; Alba, USA.
Vitamin B substances.
Neuralgias; neuritis; neuropathy; vitamin B deficiency.

Neurobionta *Bracco, Ital.*
Thiamine hydrochloride (p.1361·1); pyridoxine hydrochloride (p.1362·3); cyanocobalamin (p.1363·3).
Herpes zoster; neuralgias; neuritis.

Neurobore Pur *Bouteille, Fr.†.*
Potassium borotartrate (p.1620·2).
Bromide deficiency.

Neuro-Brachont N *Azuchemie, Ger.†.*
Dipyrone (p.35·1).
Lignocaine hydrochloride (p.1293·2) is included in the injection to alleviate the pain of injection.
Pain.

Neurocalcium *Biologiques de l'Ile-de-France, Fr.*
Syrup: Calcium bromide (p.1620·3); calcium chloride (p.1155·1); calcium gluconogluceptate.
Tablets: Calcium gluconate (p.1155·2); calcium bromide (p.1620·3); phenobarbitone (p.350·2).
Anxiety; insomnia; palpitations.

Neurocatavin Dexa *Llorente, Spain.*
Vitamin B substances; dexamethasone disodium phosphate (p.1037·2); suprarenal cortex (p.1050·1).
Lignocaine (p.1293·2) is included in this preparation to alleviate the pain of injection.
Myalgia; neuralgia; neuritis; rheumatism.

Neurochol C *Kytta, Ger.*
Chelidonium majus; taraxacum (p.1634·2); absinthium (p.1541·1).
Gastro-intestinal disorders.

Neurocil *Bayer, Ger.*
Methotrimeprazine hydrochloride (p.679·1) or methotrimeprazine maleate (p.679·1).
Psychiatric disorders.

Neurocordin *Nezel, Spain†.*
Aceglutamide (p.1541·2); gamma-aminobutyric acid (p.1582·1); magnesium pemoline (p.1484·2); pyritinol.
Hyperactivity; mental function impairment.

Neurocynesine *Boiron, Fr.†.*
Homoeopathic preparation.

Neurodavur *Belmac, Spain.*
Vitamin B substances.
Lignocaine hydrochloride (p.1293·2) is included in the intramuscular injection to alleviate the pain of injection.
Vitamin B deficiency.

Neurodavur Plus *Belmac, Spain.*
Vitamin B substances; dexamethasone sodium phosphate (p.1037·2).
Lignocaine hydrochloride (p.1293·2) is included in this preparation to alleviate the pain of injection.
Myalgia; neuralgia; neuritis.

Neuro-Demoplas
Adenylchemie, Ger.†.
Tablets: Propyphenazone (p.81·3); phenylbutazone (p.79·2); vitamin B substances; aesculus (p.1543·3).
Acute ankylosing spondylitis; rheumatism.

Godecke, Ger.†.
Injection: Ampoule 1, phenylbutazone sodium (p.79·3) ampoule 2, cyanocobalamin (p.1363·3).
Lignocaine hydrochloride (p.1293·2) is included in this preparation to alleviate the pain of injection.
Acute ankylosing spondylitis; rheumatism.

Neurodep *Med. Prod. Panam., USA.*
Capsules: Vitamin B substances.
Injection: Vitamin B substances and vitamin C.

Neurodif *Vinas, Spain.*
Lysine aspirin (p.50·3); vitamin B substances.
Lignocaine hydrochloride (p.1293·2) is included in the intramuscular injection to alleviate the pain of injection.
Musculoskeletal and joint disorders; neuritis.

Neuro-Do *Grasler, Ger.*
Homoeopathic preparation.

Neurodynamicum *Faes, Spain.*
Citicoline sodium (p.1564·3).
Cerebrovascular disorders.

Neuro-Effekton *Brenner-Efeka, Ger.†.*
Diclofenac sodium (p.31·2); vitamin B substances.
Inflammation; pain; rheumatism.

Neuro-Europan *Kwizda, Aust.*
Etenzamide (p.35·3); propyphenazone (p.81·3); vitamin B substances.
Musculoskeletal and joint disorders; neuralgia; neuritis.

Neuro-F *Leppin, S.Afr.†.*
Vitamin B substances and folic acid.

Neurofenac
Merck, Aust.; Cascan, Ger.†; Cascapharm, Ger.†.
Diclofenac sodium (p.31·2); vitamin B substances.
Gout; musculoskeletal and joint disorders; neuralgia; neuritis; pain.

Neuro-Fibraflex N *Nycomed, Ger.†.*
Vitamin B substances.
Vitamin B deficiency.

Neuroflorine *Fuca, Fr.*
Passion flower (p.1615·3); crataegus (p.1568·2); valerian (p.1643·1).
Anxiety; insomnia; palpitations.

Neuro-Fortamin *Asche, Ger.†.*
Dipyrone (p.35·1); lignocaine hydrochloride (p.1293·2).
Pain.

Neuro-Fortamin S *Asche, Ger.†.*
Dipyrone (p.35·1).
Pain.

Neuroftal *INTES, Ital.*
Injection: Thiamine hydrochloride (p.1361·1); nicotinamide (p.1351·2); strychnine glycerophosphate.
Procaine hydrochloride (p.1299·2) is included in this preparation to alleviate the pain of injection.
Tablets: Thiamine hydrochloride (p.1361·1); riboflavine (p.1362·1); nicotinamide (p.1351·2); strychnine nitrate (p.1633·1); sodium glycerophosphate (p.1586·2).
Optic nerve atrophy.

Neuroglutamin *Pharmonta, Aust.*
Glutamic acid (p.1344·3).
Memory and concentration disorders.

Neurogobens *Normon, Spain.*
Lysine aspirin (p.50·3); vitamin B substances.
Lignocaine hydrochloride (p.1293·2) is included in this preparation to alleviate the pain of injection.
Pain.

Neurogrisevit N *Pharmacia Upjohn, Ger.*
Thiamine nitrate (p.1361·1); pyridoxine hydrochloride (p.1362·3).
Vitamin B deficiency.

Neurol
Note. This name is used for preparations of different composition.
SIT, Ital.
Sodium valerate; sodium glycerophosphate (p.1586·2).
Tonic.

Abigo, Swed.
Valerian (p.1643·1).
Insomnia; nervous disorders.

Neurolepsin *Kwizda, Aust.*
Lithium carbonate (p.290·3).
Depression; mania.

Neuro-Lichtenstein *Lichtenstein, Ger.*
Vitamin B substances.
Vitamin B deficiency.

Neurolid *Recipe, Aust.*
Lignocaine hydrochloride (p.1293·2).
Local anaesthesia.

Neurolite
Du Pont, Fr.; Du Pont, Spain.
Technetium-99m bicisate (p.1425·1).
Cerebral perfusion imaging.

Neurolithium
Therabel Pharma, Belg.†; Labcatal, Fr.; Labcatal, Switz.
Lithium gluconate (p.295·1).
Bipolar disorder; hypomania; mania.

Neurolytril *Dorsch, Ger.†.*
Diazepam (p.661·1).
Muscular disorders; psychiatric disorders; sleep disorders.

Neuromade *Knoll, Spain.*
Cyanocobalamin (p.1363·3); thiamine hydrochloride (p.1361·1); pyridoxine hydrochloride (p.1362·3).
Lignocaine hydrochloride (p.1293·2) is included in the intramuscular injection to alleviate the pain of injection.
Vitamin B deficiency.

Neuromet *SmithKline Beecham, Ital.*
Oxiracetam (p.1611·3).
Mental function impairment.

Neuromultivit *Lannacher, Aust.*
Vitamin B substances.
Neuropathy.

Neuronika *Klinge, Ger.*
Kawain (p.1592·3).
Alcohol withdrawal syndrome; psychiatric disorders.

Neurontin
Parke, Davis, Aust.; Parke, Davis, Austral.; Parke, Davis, Canad.; Parke, Davis, Fr.; Parke, Davis, Ger.; Parke, Davis, Irl.; Parke, Davis, Ital.; Warner-Lambert, Norw.; Parke, Davis, S.Afr.; Parke, Davis, Spain; Parke, Davis, Swed.; Parke, Davis, Switz.; Parke, Davis, UK; Parke, Davis, USA.
Gabapentin (p.346·3).
Epilepsy.

Neuropax *Sterling Midy, Fr.†.*
Passion flower (p.1615·3); crataegus (p.1568·2); phenobarbitone (p.350·2).
Anxiety; insomnia.

Neuroplant *Spitzner, Ger.*
Hypericum (p.1590·1).
Psychiatric disorders.

Neuro-Presselin *Presselin, Ger.†.*
Passion flower (p.1615·3); hypericum (p.1590·1); ether; acid. phosph.; ignatia; guaiphenesin (p.1061·3); chlorophyllin (p.1000·1).
Nervous disorders; sleep disorders.

Neuro-ratiopharm *Ratiopharm, Ger.*
Vitamin B substances.
Vitamin B deficiency.

Neuro-Rotexmedica N *Rotexmedica, Ger.†.*
Thiamine hydrochloride (p.1361·1); pyridoxine hydrochloride (p.1362·3).
Vitamin B deficiency.

Neurorubine Nouvelle formule *Mepha, Switz.*
Vitamin B substances.
Neuralgias; neuritis; neuropathy.

Neurosido *Knoll, Spain†.*
Disodium cytidine triphosphate; dexamethasone (p.1037·1); thiocolchicoside (p.1322·1); disodium uridine triphosphate.
Inflammation; pain.

NeuroSlim *NeuroGenesis, USA; Matrix, USA.*
Multivitamin, mineral, and amino-acid preparation.

Neurospas *Rolab, S.Afr.†.*
Baclofen (p.1308·2).
Skeletal muscle spasm or spasticity.

Neuro-Spondyril S *Dorsch, Ger.†.*
Propyphenazone (p.81·3); vitamin B substances.
Musculoskeletal and joint disorders; neuralgia; neuritis; rheumatism.

Neurosthenol *Richard, Fr.*
Cerebral cortex extract (pork); glutamic acid; phosphoric acid; electrolytes.
Tonic.

Neurostop *Lacer, Spain.*
Benfotiamine (p.1360·3).
Vitamin B1 deficiency.

Neurostop Complex *Lacer, Spain.*
Benfotiamine (p.1360·3); hydroxocobalamin acetate (p.1364·2); pyridoxine hydrochloride (p.1362·3).
Vitamin B deficiency.

Neurotensyl *Sciencex, Fr.*
Crataegus (p.1568·2); passion flower (p.1615·3); valerian (p.1643·1).
Anxiety; insomnia; palpitations.

Neurothioct *Knoll, Ger.*
Thioctic acid (p.1636·2).
Diabetic polyneuropathy.

Neurotisan *Hanosan, Ger.*
Hypericum (p.1590·1).
Psychiatric disorders.

Neuroton *NCSN, Ital.*
Citicoline sodium (p.1564·3).
Cerebrovascular disorders; parkinsonism.

Neurotop *Gerot, Aust.*
Carbamazepine (p.339·2).
Alcohol withdrawal syndrome; bipolar disorder; diabetes insipidus; diabetic neuropathy; epilepsy; trigeminal neuralgia.

Neurotrat
Knoll, Ger.; Knoll, Switz.
Vitamin B substances.
Neuralgias; neuritis; neuropathies; vitamin B deficiency.

Neurotropan *Phonix, Ger.*
Choline citrate (p.1337·1).
Liver disorders.

Neurotropan-Hy *Phonix, Ger.†.*
Ampoule 1, choline citrate (p.1337·1); procaine hydrochloride (p.1299·2); ampoule 2, hyaluronidase (p.1588·1).
Musculoskeletal and joint disorders.

Neurotropan-M *Phonix, Ger.†.*
Choline citrate (p.1337·1); procaine hydrochloride (p.1299·2).
Liver disorders.

Neurovegetalin *Verla, Ger.*
Hypericum (p.1590·1).
Formerly contained ergotamine tartrate, ergotoxine phosphate, hyoscyamine, hyoscine hydrobromide, and phenobarbitone.
Psychiatric disorders.

Neuro-Vibolex *Chephasaar, Ger.*
Injection: Thiamine hydrochloride (p.1361·1); pyridoxine hydrochloride (p.1362·3); cyanocobalamin (p.1363·3).
Tablets: Thiamine hydrochloride (p.1361·1); pyridoxine hydrochloride (p.1362·3).
Neuralgia; neuritis; neuropathy.

Neurovitan *Fujisawa, Jpn.*
Octotiamine (p.1360·3); riboflavine (p.1362·1); pyridoxine hydrochloride (p.1362·3); cyanocobalamin (p.1363·3).
Vitamin B deficiency.

Neusinol *Labima, Belg.*
Naphazoline (p.1064·2).
Nasal congestion.

Neut *Abbott, USA.*
Sodium bicarbonate (p.1153·2).
Neutralising additive solution for acidic intravenous infusions.

Neutrafillina *Roussel, Ital.†.*
Diprophylline (p.752·1).
Respiratory-tract disorders.

Neutragel *Propan, S.Afr.*
Dicyclomine hydrochloride (p.460·1); dried aluminium hydroxide (p.1177·3); light magnesium oxide (p.1198·3).
Gastro-intestinal hyperacidity.

Neutralca-S *Desbergers, Canad.*
Aluminium hydroxide (p.1177·3); magnesium hydroxide (p.1198·2).
Gastric hyperacidity; peptic ulcer.

Neutralon *Schering, Ital.†.*
Aluminium sodium silicate (p.1178·3).
Gastro-intestinal disorders.

Neutralon Con Belladonna *Schering, Ital.†.*
Aluminium sodium silicate (p.1178·3); belladonna herb (p.457·1).
Gastro-intestinal disorders.

Neutra-Phos *Baker Norton, USA.*
Monobasic and dibasic sodium and potassium phosphates (p.1159·2).
Phosphorus supplement.

Neutra-Phos-K *Baker Norton, USA.*
Monobasic and dibasic potassium phosphates (p.1159·2).
Phosphorus supplement.

Neutrasid *Chinosolfabrik, Ger.†.*
Aluminium hydroxide (p.1177·3); magnesium oxide (p.1198·3); calcium hydrogen phosphate (p.1155·3).
Gastro-intestinal disorders.

Neutrexin
Lilly, Canad.; IPSEN Biotech, Fr.; Ipsen, Irl.; Ipsen, Ital.; Swedish Orphan, Swed.; Speywood, UK; US Bioscience, USA.
Trimetrexate glucuronate (p.568·1).
Pneumocystis carinii pneumonia.

Neutrogena
Note. This name is used for preparations of different composition.
Faulding, Austral.
Soap substitute.

Neutrogena, USA.
SPF 8: Ethylhexyl *p*-methoxycinnamate (p.1487·1); methyl anthranilate; titanium dioxide (p.1093·3).
SPF 15: Ethylhexyl *p*-methoxycinnamate (p.1487·1); octyl salicylate (p.1487·3); methyl anthranilate; titanium dioxide (p.1093·3).
SPF 25: Ethylhexyl *p*-methoxycinnamate (p.1487·1); oxybenzone (p.1487·3); octyl salicylate (p.1487·3).
SPF 30: Ethylhexyl *p*-methoxycinnamate (p.1487·1); octocrylene (p.1487·3); methyl anthranilate; zinc oxide (p.1096·2).
Sunscreen.

Neutrogena Dermatologics, USA.
Skin cleanser; emollient and moisturiser.

Neutrogena Acne Mask
Faulding, Austral.; Professional Health, Canad.; Neutrogena Dermatologics, USA.
Benzoyl peroxide (p.1079·2).
Acne.

Neutrogena Acne Skin Cleanser *Faulding, Austral.*
Triclosan (p.1127·2).
Acne; oily skin.

Neutrogena Antiseptic *Neutrogena, USA.*
Skin cleanser.

Neutrogena Chemical-Free *Neutrogena, USA.*
SPF 17: Titanium dioxide (p.1093·3).
Sunscreen.

Neutrogena Dermatological Cream *Neutrogena, UK.*
Glycerol (p.1585·2); cetostearyl alcohol (p.1383·2).
Dry skin.

Neutrogena Drying *Neutrogena Dermatologics, USA.*
Hamamelis (p.1587·1).

Neutrogena Glow *Neutrogena, USA.*
SPF 8: Ethylhexyl *p*-methoxycinnamate (p.1487·1).
Sunscreen.

Neutrogena Healthy Scalp Anti-Dandruff *Professional Health, Canad.*
Salicylic acid (p.1090·2).

Neutrogena Intensified *Neutrogena, USA.*
SPF 15: Ethylhexyl *p*-methoxycinnamate (p.1487·1); 2-phenyl-1*H*-benzimidazole-5-sulphonic acid (p.1488·2); titanium dioxide (p.1093·3).
Sunscreen.

Neutrogena Lip *Neutrogena, USA.*
SPF 15: Ethylhexyl *p*-methoxycinnamate (p.1487·1); oxybenzone (p.1487·3).
Sunscreen.

Neutrogena Long Lasting Dandruff Control
Johnson & Johnson, UK.
Ketoconazole (p.383·1).
Dandruff.

Neutrogena Moisture *Neutrogena, USA.*
SPF 5: Ethylhexyl *p*-methoxycinnamate (p.1487·1).
SPF 15: Ethylhexyl *p*-methoxycinnamate (p.1487·1); oxybenzone (p.1487·3).
Sunscreen.

Neutrogena No-Stick *Neutrogena, USA.*
Ethylhexyl *p*-methoxycinnamate (p.1487·1); homosalate (p.1487·2); oxybenzone (p.1487·3); octyl salicylate (p.1487·3).
Sunscreen.

Neutrogena No-Stick Sunblock *Professional Health, Canad.*
SPF 30: Ethylhexyl *p*-methoxycinnamate (p.1487·1); homosalate (p.1487·2); octyl salicylate (p.1487·3); oxybenzone (p.1487·3).
Sunscreen.

Neutrogena On-The-Spot Acne Lotion *Professional Health, Canad.*
Benzoyl peroxide (p.1079·2).
Acne.

Neutrogena Sunblocker *Professional Health, Canad.*
SPF 17: Titanium dioxide (p.1093·3).
Sunscreen.

Neutrogena T/Derm *Neutrogena, USA.*
Coal tar (p.1092·3).
Skin disorders.

Neutrogena T/Gel
Faulding, Austral.; Professional Health, Canad.; Neutrogena, USA.
Coal tar (p.1092·3).
Scalp disorders.

Neutrogena T/Sal
Faulding, Austral.; Neutrogena Dermatologics, USA.
Salicylic acid (p.1090·2); coal tar (p.1092·3).
Scalp disorders; seborrhoeic dermatitis.

Neutrogena T/Scalp *Neutrogena Dermatologics, USA.*
Hydrocortisone (p.1043·3).
Pruritus of the scalp.

Neutrogin *Chugai, Jpn.*
Lenograstim (p.724·3).
Neutropenia.

Neutrolac *Bayer, Ital.*
Powdered milk; aluminium hydroxide (p.1177·3); calcium carbonate (p.1182·1); magnesium trisilicate (p.1199·1).
Gastro-intestinal disorders associated with hyperacidity.

Neutromed *Kwizda, Aust.*
Cimetidine (p.1183·2) or cimetidine hydrochloride (p.1185·3).
Acid aspiration syndrome; gastro-intestinal erosions; gastro-intestinal haemorrhage; gastro-oesophageal reflux; peptic ulcer; Zollinger-Ellison syndrome.

Neutromil *Farmitalia Carlo Erba, Ger.†.*
Buzepide metiodide (p.459·2); cyamemazine (p.660·2); papaverine hydrochloride (p.1614·2); activated attapulgite (p.1178·3); light magnesium oxide (p.1198·3); dried aluminium hydroxide gel (p.1177·3).
Gastro-intestinal disorders.

Neutronorm *Ebewe, Aust.*
Cimetidine (p.1183·2).
Gastro-intestinal erosions; gastro-intestinal haemorrhage; gastro-oesophageal reflux; peptic ulcer; Zollinger-Ellison syndrome.

Neutrose S Pellegrino *Synthelabo, Ital.*
Calcium carbonate (p.1182·1); magnesium carbonate (p.1198·1); kaolin (p.1195·1); magnesium trisilicate (p.1199·1).
Gastro-intestinal disorders associated with hyperacidity.

Neutroses
Pharmethic, Belg.; DB, Fr.; DB, Switz.
Calcium carbonate (p.1182·1); magnesium carbonate (p.1198·1); kaolin (p.1195·1); magnesium trisilicate (p.1199·1).
Bloating; flatulence; gastric hyperacidity.

Neu-Up *Kyowa, Jpn.*
Nartograstim (p.725·2).
Neutropenia.

Neuvita *Fujisawa, Jpn.*
Octotiamine (p.1360·3).
Vitamin B_1 deficiency.

Neuzym *Eisai, Jpn.*
Muramidase hydrochloride (p.1604·3).
Chronic sinusitis; haemorrhage; respiratory-tract congestion.

Nevadral Retard *Kabi, Swed.†.*
Norfenefrine hydrochloride (p.925·1).
Hypotension.

Nevanil *Dermalife, Ital.†.*
Quercetin (p.1580·2); troxerutin (p.1580·2); hesperidin methyl chalcone (p.1580·2); calcium ascorbate (p.1365·2).
Capillary impairment.

Nevasona *Cantabria, Spain†.*
Dimethicone (p.1384·2); lanolin; talc; vitamin F; zinc oxide (p.1096·2).
Skin disorders.

Neverill *Schuck, Ger.†.*
Homoeopathic preparation.

Neviran *Coli, Ital.*
Aciclovir (p.602·3).
Herpesvirus infections.

Nevrazon *Panthox & Burck, Ital.†.*
Amidopyrine ascorbate (p.15·2); thiamine monophosphate; cyanocobalamin; adenosine phosphate.
Musculoskeletal and joint disorders; neuritis; pain.

Nevril *Tosi, Ital.*
Thiamine phosphate monochloride (p.1361·2); hydroxocobalamin (p.1363·3).
Megaloblastic anaemia; neuralgias; neuritis.

Nevrine Codeine *Pharmacobel, Belg.*
Paracetamol (p.72·2); caffeine hydrate (p.750·1); codeine phosphate (p.26·1).
Fever; pain.

Nevrostenina B12 *Zoja, Ital.†.*
Sodium glycerophosphate (p.1586·2); potassium glycerophosphate (p.1586·2); magnesium glycerophosphate (p.1157·2); glycine (p.1345·2); cyanocobalamin (p.1363·3).
Tonic.

Nevrosthenine *3M, Switz.†.*
Sodium glycerophosphate; potassium glycerophosphate; magnesium glycerophosphate; glycine.
Tonic.

Nevrosthenine Glycocolle Freyssinge
3M, Belg.; 3M, Fr.
Glycine; sodium glycerophosphate; potassium glycerophosphate; magnesium glycerophosphate.
Tonic.

Nevrotal *Vinas, Spain†.*
Bovine cerebral cortical gangliosides (p.1582·3).
Peripheral neuropathy.

Nevrum *Vis, Ital.†.*
Thiamine hydrochloride (p.1361·1); pyridoxine hydrochloride (p.1362·3); cyanocobalamin (p.1363·3).
Neuritis.

New Acute Cold Formula *Invamed, USA.*
Chlorpheniramine maleate (p.405·1); phenylpropanolamine hydrochloride (p.1067·2); dextromethorphan hydrobromide (p.1057·3); paracetamol (p.72·2).

New De Witt's Pills *Fleet, Austral.*
Bearberry (p.1552·2); buchu (p.1555·2).
Fluid retention.

New Decongestant Pediatric *Goldline, USA.*
Phenylpropanolamine hydrochloride (p.1067·2); phenylephrine hydrochloride (p.1066·2); chlorpheniramine maleate (p.405·1); phenyltoloxamine citrate (p.416·1).
Upper respiratory-tract symptoms.

New Era Biochemic Tissue Salts *Seven Seas, UK.*
A range of mineral preparations.

New Era Calm & Clear *Seven Seas, UK.*
Dibasic potassium phosphate (p.1159·2).

New Era Combination Tissue Salts *Seven Seas, UK.*
A range of multimineral preparations.

New Era Elasto *Seven Seas, UK.*
Calcium fluoride (p.1556·3); calcium phosphate (p.1155·3); iron phosphate; magnesium phosphate (p.1157·3).

New Era Hymosa *Seven Seas, UK.*
Ferrous phosphate; potassium chloride (p.1161·1); potassium sulphate (p.1161·2); calcium sulphate (p.1557·1); silica (p.1474·3).

New Era Nervone *Seven Seas, UK.*
Calcium phosphate (p.1155·3); magnesium phosphate (p.1157·3); potassium chloride (p.1161·1); sodium phosphate; potassium phosphate.

New Era Zief *Seven Seas, UK.*
Iron phosphate; silica (p.1474·3); sodium phosphate; sodium sulphate (p.1213·3).

New Freshness *Fleet, USA†.*
Vinegar (p.1541·2); octoxinol 9 (p.1326·2); sorbic acid (p.1125·2).
Vaginal disorders.

New Gen Mix *Roche, Ital.*
Multivitamin and mineral preparation.
Nutritional supplement.

NewAce *Bristol-Myers Squibb, Neth.*
Fosinopril sodium (p.870·3).
Heart failure; hypertension.

Newderm *Wolfs, Belg.*
Zinc oxide (p.1096·2); vitamin A (p.1358·1); vitamin D (p.1366·3); cod-liver oil (p.1337·3).
Skin irritation.

New-Gonavislide *Mochida, Jpn†.*
Pregnancy test (p.1621·2).

Newral *Dojin Iyaku, Jpn.*
Neticonazole hydrochloride (p.386·1).
Fungal skin infections.

Newrelax *Potter's, UK.*
Lupulus (p.1597·2); scullcap; valerian (p.1643·1); vervain.
Tension.

New-Skin *Medtech, USA.*
Topical barrier preparation.

NeyArthros *Vitorgan, Ger.*
Articuli fet.; cartilago; synovia.
Inflammatory and degenerative joint disorders.

NeyArthros-Liposome *Vitorgan, Ger.*
Cartilago articuli; synovia; articuli fet.; thymus fet.; funicul. umbilical.; methenolone acetate; prednisolone acetate; lipid extract of cartilago articuli/synovia/articuli fet.; zinc sulphate manganese sulphate; magnesium chloride; potassium chloride; calcium chloride; columna vertebralis fet.; capsula articuli fet.; musculi fet.; gland. suprarenal.
Inflammatory and degenerative joint disorders.

NeyCalm *Vitorgan, Ger.*
Animal tissue extract: cortex cerebri; diencephalon; epiphyse; placenta mat.
Psychiatric disorders.

NeyChondrin *Vitorgan, Ger.*
Thymus fet.; hypophyse; diencephalon; medulla spinal.; gland. suprarenal.; testes juvenil; hepar; pancreas; musculi; columna vertebral fet.; articuli fet.; ren; placenta; nucleus pulp.
Muscular, neuromuscular, and joint disorders.

NeyChondrin "N" (Revitorgan-Dilutionen "N" Nr. 68) *Vitorgan, Ger.*
Animal tissue extracts (NeyChondrin) (p.1599·1); methenolone acetate (p.1450·3); prednisolone acetate

(p.1048·1); alpha tocopheryl acetate (p.1369·1); procaine hydrochloride (p.1299·2).
Muscular, neuromuscular, and joint disorders.

NeyChondrin-Tropfen (Revitorgan-Lingual Nr. 68) Vitorgan, Ger.
Animal tissue extracts (NeyChondrin); methenolone acetate; prednisolone acetate; alpha tocopheryl acetate; procaine hydrochloride.
Muscular, neuromuscular, and joint disorders.

NeyCorenar Vitorgan, Ger.
Protein extracts from animal heart.
Cardiovascular disorders.

NeyDesib Vitorgan, Ger.
Lysates of thymus fet.; lien fet.; lymphonodi; gland. suprarenal.
Allergies; auto-immune disorders.

NeyDigest Vitorgan, Ger.†.
Preparations of intestinal mucosa.
Gastro-intestinal disorders.

Neydin-F Vitorgan, Ger.
Lysates of chorion; cutis fet.; ovary; amnion; hepar; gland. supraren.; liquor amnii; yeast.
Circulatory disorders of skin and soft tissue.

Neydin-M Vitorgan, Ger.
Placenta mat.; testes juvenil; cutis fet.; amnion; hepar; gland. supraren.; liquor amnii; faex.
Hypersensitivity; inflammation.

NeyDop Vitorgan, Ger.
Cortex cerebri; diencephalon; cerebellum; placenat fet.
Central nervous system disorders.

NeyDop "N" (Revitorgan-Dilutionen "N" Nr. 97) Vitorgan, Ger.
Cortex cerebri; diencephalon; cerebellum; placenta fet.; ascorbic acid (p.1365·2); lithium chloride (p.295·1); levodopa (p.1137·1).
Central nervous system disorders.

NeyDop-Tropfen (Revitorgan-Lingual Nr. 97) Vitorgan, Ger.
Animal tissue extracts (NeyDop); ascorbic acid; lithium chloride; levodopa.
Central nervous system disorders.

NeyFaexan Vitorgan, Ger.
Mucosa intestinal.; muc. vesicae urinal.; mucosa vesicae felleae; muc. nasopharyngeal.
Gastro-intestinal disorders.

NeyFegan Vitorgan, Ger.
Liver extract.
Liver disorders.

NeyGeront "N" (Revitorgan-Dilutionen "N" Nr. 64) Vitorgan, Ger.
Animal tissue extracts (NeyGeront); heparin (p.879·3); methenolone acetate (p.1450·3); liothyronine hydrochloride; vitamins; procaine hydrochloride.
Tonic.

NeyGeront (Revitorgan Dilution Nr. 64) Vitorgan, Ger.
Embryo total.; placenta; amnion; funiculus umbilical.; cor; ren; pancreas; mucosa intestinal; lien; thymus juvenil.; gland. suprarenal.; gland. parathyreoid.; testes juvenil.; hypophyse tot.; diencephalon; cort. cerebri.
Tonic.

NeyGeront-Tropfen (Revitorgan-Lingual Nr. 64) Vitorgan, Ger.
Animal tissue extracts (NeyGeront); heparin; methenolone acetate; liothyronine hydrochloride; vitamins; procaine hydrochloride.
Tonic.

NeyGeront-Vitalkapseln Vitorgan, Ger.
Animal tissue extracts; heparin; methenolone acetate; liothyronine hydrochloride; procaine hydrochloride; lecithin; trace elements and vitamins.
Tonic.

NeyImmun Vitorgan, Ger.
Standardised animal protein extract (placenta; umbilical cord; thymus).
Tonic.

NeyMan Vitorgan, Ger.†.
Mammalian tissue extract (ren, medulla spinalis, testes, prostata, corpus cavernosum, vesicula seminalis, mucosa vesic. urinar., cor, aorta, vasae fet., placenta, hepar, lien, pancreas, thyreoidea, diencephalon, cortex cerebri).
Prostatic disorders.

NeyMan "N" (Revitorgan-Dilutionen "N" Nr. 35) Vitorgan, Ger.†.
Mammalian tissue extract; multivitamins.
Prostatic disorders.

Neyman-Tropfen (Revitorgan-Lingual Nr. 35) Vitorgan, Ger.†.
Animal tissue extracts (NeyMan); multivitamins.
Prostatic disorders.

NeyNormin Vitorgan, Ger.
Thymus fet.; gland. suprarenal.; lymphonodi gland.; parathyreoidea; hepar; ren; pancreas; lien; vasae fet.; funiculus umbilical.; hypophyse; diencephalon; mucosae miscae; cutis; medulla ossium.
Allergic diathesis; insufficiency of the diencephalon-pituitary-adrenal system; intestinal disorders; rheumatism; vegetative dystonias; virus infection.

NeyNormin "N" (Revitorgan-Dilutionen "N" Nr. 65) Vitorgan, Ger.
Animal tissue extracts (NeyNormin); prednisolone acetate (p.1048·1); liothyronine hydrochloride (p.1495·2); oestradiol benzoate (p.1455·1); chorionic gonadotrophin (p.1243·1); alpha tocopheryl acetate (p.1369·1); cyanocobalamin (p.1363·3).
Allergic diathesis; insufficiency of the diencephalon-pituitary-adrenal system; intestinal disorders; rheumatism; vegetative dystonias; virus infection.

NeyNormin-Tropfen (Revitorgan-Lingual Nr. 65) Vitorgan, Ger.
Animal tissue extracts (NeyNormin); prednisolone acetate; liothyronine hydrochloride; oestradiol benzoate; chorionic gonadotrophin; alpha tocopheryl acetate; cyanocobalamin.
Allergic diathesis; insufficiency of the diencephalon-pituitary-adrenal system; intestinal disorders; rheumatism; vegetative dystonias; viral infections.

NeyParadent-Liposome Vitorgan, Ger.
Protein extracts from crista dentalis; placenta; diencephalon; methenolone acetate; alpha tocopheryl acetate; procaine hydrochloride; lipid extract from crista dentalis; sodium salicylate; ascorbic acid; chamomile; arnica; myrrh; sea salt.
Mouth disorders.

NeyPsorin Vitorgan, Ger.
Animal skin extract.
Skin disorders.

NeyPulpin Vitorgan, Ger.
Crista dental. fet.; placenta; diencephalon.
Dental disorders.

NeyPulpin "N" (Revitorgan-Dilutionen "N" Nr. 10) Vitorgan, Ger.
Crista dentalis; placenta; diencephalon; methenolone acetate (p.1450·3); alpha tocopheryl acetate (p.1369·2); ascorbic acid (p.1365·2); procaine hydrochloride (p.1299·2).
Dental disorders.

Neythymun Vitorgan, Ger.
Thymus extract.
Allergic disorders; immunosuppressant in rheumatic disorders; immunotherapy.

NeyTroph Vitorgan, Ger.
Musculi juv.; musculi fet.; cor fet.; thymus; medulla spinal.; cortex cerebri; epiphyse; diencephalon.
Muscular and nervous disorders.

NeyTumorin Vitorgan, Ger.
Diencephalon; placenta matern.; funiculus umbilical.; thymus juvenil.; epiphysis; testes juvenil.; gland. suprarenal.; thyreoidea; medulla oss. pulmo; hepar; pancreas; ren; lien; mucosa intestinal.
Neoplasms.

NeyTumorin "N" (Revitorgan-Dilutionen Nr. 66) Vitorgan, Ger.
Animal tissue extracts (NeyTumorin) (p.1599·1); methenolone acetate (p.1450·3); prednisolone acetate (p.1048·1); liothyronine hydrochloride (p.1495·1); alpha tocopheryl acetate (p.1369·1); cyanocobalamin (p.1363·3).
Neoplasms.

NeyTumorin-Tropfen (Revitorgan-Lingual Nr. 66) Vitorgan, Ger.
Animal tissue extracts (NeyTumorin) (p.1599·1); methenolone acetate; prednisolone acetate; liothyronine hydrochloride; alpha tocopheryl acetate; cyanocobalamin.
Neoplasms.

Nezeril
Astra, Neth.†; Draco, Swed.
Oxymetazoline hydrochloride (p.1065·3).
Nasal congestion; rhinitis; sinusitis.

NF Cough Syrup with Codeine Stanley, Canad.
Pseudoephedrine hydrochloride (p.1068·3); codeine phosphate (p.26·1); guaiphenesin (p.1061·3).

NGT Geneva, USA.
Triamcinolone acetonide (p.1050·2); nystatin (p.386·1).
Skin disorders.

Nia Novo Nordisk, Aust.
Megestrol acetate (p.1449·3).
Breast cancer; endometrial cancer.

Nia-Bid Roberts, USA; Hauck, USA.
Nicotinic acid (p.1351·2).
Hyperlipidaemia (adjunct); nicotinic acid deficiency; pellagra.

Niacels Roberts, USA†.
Nicotinic acid (p.1351·2).
Hyperlipidaemia (adjunct); nicotinic acid deficiency; pellagra.

Niacor Upsher-Smith, USA.
Nicotinic acid (p.1351·2).
Hyperlipidaemia (adjunct); nicotinic acid deficiency; pellagra.

Niagestin
Novo Nordisk, Ger.†; Novo Nordisk, Swed.†.
Megestrol acetate (p.1449·3).
Malignant neoplasms.

Niagestine
Novo Nordisk, Belg.†; Novo Nordisk, Switz.†.
Megestrol acetate (p.1449·3).
Malignant neoplasms.

Nialen Novag, Spain.
Ibuproxam (p.45·2).
Musculoskeletal, joint, peri-articular, and soft-tissue disorders; pain.

Niamid Roerig, Belg.
Nialamide (p.300·2).
Depression.

Niamide Pfizer, Fr.†.
Nialamide (p.300·2).
Depression.

Niaplus Tyson, USA†.
Nicotinic acid (p.1351·2).

Niaspan KOS, USA.
Nicotinic acid (p.1351·2).
Hyperlipidaemias.

Nibiol
Debat, Fr.; Fournier SA, Spain†.
Nitroxoline (p.233·1).
Bacterial infections of the urinary tract.

Nicabate
Hoechst Marion Roussel, Austral.; Hoechst Marion Roussel, UK†.
Nicotine (p.1607·2).
Aid to smoking withdrawal.

Nicagel Vifor, Switz.†.
Methyl nicotinate (p.55·1); glycol salicylate (p.43·1).
Joint pain; peri-articular and soft-tissue disorders.

Nican
Note. This name is used for preparations of different composition.
Marion Merrell, Fr.†.
Codeine (p.26·1); sodium benzoate (p.1102·3); aconite (p.1542·2); belladonna herb (p.457·1); grindelia; bromoform (p.1620·3).
Respiratory disorders.
Uhlmann-Eyraud, Switz.
Codeine (p.26·1); belladonna (p.457·1); drosera (p.1574·1); grindelia; plantaginis; thyme (p.1636·3); sodium benzoate (p.1102·3).
Coughs.

Nicangin Astra, Swed.
Nicotinic acid (p.1351·2).
Hyperlipidaemias.

Nicant Piam, Ital.
Nicardipine hydrochloride (p.915·1).
Angina pectoris; heart failure; hypertension.

Nicaphlogyl Vifor, Switz.
Propyphenazone (p.81·3); etenzamide (p.35·3).
Inflammation; pain.

Nicapress Boehringer Ingelheim, Ital.
Nicardipine hydrochloride (p.915·1).
Angina pectoris; heart failure; hypertension.

Nicardal Italfarmaco, Ital.
Nicardipine hydrochloride (p.915·1).
Angina pectoris; heart failure; hypertension.

Nicardium Drug Research, Ital.
Nicardipine hydrochloride (p.915·1).
Angina pectoris; cerebrovascular disorders; heart failure; hypertension; Ménière's disease.

Nicarpin San Carlo, Ital.
Nicardipine hydrochloride (p.915·1).
Hypertension; ischaemic heart disease.

Nicazide IFI, Ital.†.
Isoniazid (p.218·1).
Tuberculosis.

N'ice SmithKline Beecham Consumer, USA.
Lozenges: Menthol (p.1600·2).
Throat spray: Menthol (p.1600·2); glycerol (p.1585·2).
Sore throat.

N'ice 'n Clear SmithKline Beecham Consumer, USA.
Menthol (p.1600·2).

N'ice Vitamin C SmithKline Beecham Consumer, USA.
Ascorbic acid (p.1365·2).
Scurvy; vitamin C deficiency.

Nicef Galen, UK.
Cephradine (p.181·3).
Bacterial infections.

Nicene Adcock Ingram, S.Afr.
Nitroxoline (p.233·1); sulphamethizole (p.254·2); pyridoxine hydrochloride (p.1362·3).
Urinary-tract infections.

Nicene forte Chephasaar, Ger.†.
Nitroxoline (p.233·1).
Urinary-tract infections.

Nicene N Chephasaar, Ger.†.
Nitroxoline (p.233·1); sulphamethizole (p.254·2).
Urinary-tract infections.

Nicer Ist. Chim. Inter., Ital.
Nicergoline (p.1607·1).
Cerebrovascular disorders.

Nicergolyn ICT-Lodi, Ital.†.
Nicergoline (p.1607·1).
Vascular disorders.

Nicerium Hexal, Ger.
Nicergoline (p.1607·1).
Cerebrovascular disorders.

Nicetile Sigma-Tau, Ital.
Acetylcarnitine hydrochloride (p.1542·1).
Cerebrovascular disorders; nerve disorders.

Nicholin
Cyanamid, Ital.; Takeda, Jpn.
Citicoline (p.1564·3).
Cerebral disorders; pancreatitis; parkinsonism.

Nicicalcium Lipha, Fr.†.
Vitamin and mineral preparation.
Tonic.

Nicizina Pharmacia Upjohn, Ital.
Isoniazid (p.218·1).
Tuberculosis.

Niclocide Miles, USA†.
Niclosamide (p.105·3).
Taeniasis.

Nico-400 Jones, USA.
Nicotinic acid (p.1351·2).
Hyperlipidaemia (adjunct); nicotinic acid deficiency; pellagra.

Nico Hepatocyn Uriach, Spain.
Cynara (p.1569·2); aloes (p.1177·1); boldo (p.1554·1); cascara (p.1183·1).
Formerly contained cynara, bile extract, boldo, cascara, nicotinamide, podophyllum resin, and euonymus.
Constipation.

Nicobid Tempules Rorer, USA.
Nicotinic acid (p.1351·2).
Hyperlipidaemia (adjunct); nicotinic acid deficiency; pellagra.

Nicobion
Astra, Fr.; Merck, Ger.
Nicotinamide (p.1351·2).
Burns; pellagra; vitamin B deficiency.

Nicobrevin Robinson, UK.
Menthyl valerate; anhydrous quinine (p.439·1); camphor (p.1557·2); eucalyptus oil (p.1578·1).
Aid to smoking withdrawal.

Nicodan Wernigerode, Ger.
Propyl nicotinate (p.81·3).
Pain; peripheral circulatory disorders.

Nicodan N LAW, Ger.†.
Propyl nicotinate (p.81·3).
Pain.

Nicodent Nicodent, Austral.†.
Sodium monofluorophosphate (p.743·3).
Dentifrice.

Nicoderm
Hoechst Marion Roussel, Canad.; SmithKline Beecham Consumer, USA.
Nicotine (p.1607·2).
Aid to smoking withdrawal.

Nicodisc Lacer, Spain.
Nicotine (p.1607·2).
Aid to smoking withdrawal.

Nicodrasi Bruco, Ital.†.
Nadide (p.1606·1).
Disturbance of cellular respiration; heart disease; hepatitis.

Nicolan
Solvay, Aust.; Meda, Swed.
Nicotine (p.1607·2).
Aid to smoking withdrawal.

Nicolar Rhone-Poulenc Rorer, USA.
Nicotinic acid (p.1351·2).
Hyperlipidaemia (adjunct); nicotinic acid deficiency; pellagra.

Nicolip Hennig, Ger.
Inositol nicotinate (p.891·3).
Hyperlipidaemias.

Nicolsint Epifarma, Ital.
Citicoline (p.1564·3).
Cerebrovascular disorders; parkinsonism.

Nicomax Pensa, Spain.
Nicotine polacrilex (p.1608·1).
Aid to smoking withdrawal.

Niconacid Wander, Ger.†.
Nicotinic acid (p.1351·2).
Hyperlipidaemias; nicotinic acid deficiency.

Niconil
Elan, Irl.; Elan, UK.
Nicotine (p.1607·2).
Aid to smoking withdrawal.

Nico-Padutin Bayropharm, Ger.†.
Kallidinogenase (Kallikrein) (p.1592·3); inositol nicotinate (p.891·3).
Peripheral and cerebral vascular disorders.

Nicopatch Pierre Fabre, Fr.
Nicotine (p.1607·2).
Aid to smoking withdrawal.

Nicoplectal Schwab, Ger.†.
Nicotinic acid (p.1351·2); aesculus (p.1543·3).
Peripheral and cerebral vascular disorders.

Nicoprive
Theranol-Deglaude, Fr.; IFI, Ital.
Quinine ascorbate (p.1624·2); vitamins; crataegus (p.1568·2).
Aid to smoking withdrawal.

Nicopyron Trommsdorff, Ger.†.
Nifenazone (p.63·1).
Pain.

Nicorette
Pharmacia Upjohn, Aust.; Pharmacia Upjohn, Austral.; Pharmacia Upjohn, Belg.; Hoechst Marion Roussel, Canad.; Pharmacia Upjohn, Fr.; Pharmacia Upjohn, Ger.; Pharmacia Upjohn, Irl.; Carlo Erba OTC, Ital.; Pharmacia Upjohn, Neth.; Pharmacia Upjohn, Norw.; Restan, S.Afr.; Pharmacia Upjohn, Spain; Pharmacia Upjohn, Swed.; Pharmacia Upjohn, Switz.; Pharmacia Upjohn, UK; SmithKline Beecham Consumer, USA.
Nicotine (p.1607·2), nicotine betadex, or nicotine resin complex (p.1608·1).
Aid to smoking withdrawal.

Nicosterolo Guidotti, Ital.†.
Sorbinicate (p.1279·3).
Hyperlipidaemias.

Nicostop TTS Drossapharm, Switz.
Nicotine (p.1607·2).
Aid to smoking withdrawal.

Nicotibine Hoechst Marion Roussel, Belg.
Isoniazid (p.218·1).
Tuberculosis.

Nicotinell
Zyma, Aust.; Novartis, Austral.; Ciba-Geigy, Belg.; Ciba-Geigy, Fr.; Zyma, Ger.; Zyma, Irl.; Zyma, Ital.; Novartis Consumer, Neth.; Novartis, Norw.; Novartis Consumer, S.Afr.; Zyma, Spain; Novartis, Swed.; Geigy, Switz.; Zyma, UK.
Nicotine (p.1607·2) or nicotine resin (p.1608·1).
Aid to smoking withdrawal.

Nicotinex Fleming, USA.
Nicotinic acid (p.1351·2).
Hyperlipidaemia (adjunct); nicotinic acid deficiency; pellagra.

Nicotrans Recordati, Ital.; Pharmacia Upjohn, Spain.
Nicotine (p.1607·2).
Aid to smoking withdrawal.

Nicotrol Pharmacia Upjohn, Aust.; McNeil Consumer, Canad.; Pharmacia Upjohn, Spain; McNeil Consumer, USA.
Nicotine (p.1607·2).
Aid to smoking withdrawal.

Nico-Vert Edwards, USA.
Meclozine (p.413·3).
Formerly contained dimenhydrinate.
Motion sickness.

Nicovitol Lannacher, Aust.
Nicotinamide (p.1351·2).
Nicotinamide deficiency.

Nicozid Piam, Ital.
Isoniazid (p.218·1).
Tuberculosis.

NidaGel Ferring, Canad.
Metronidazole (p.585·1).
Bacterial vaginosis.

Nidal HA Nestle, Fr.
Infant feed.
Potential hypersensitivity to cows milk.

Nidatron Propan, S.Afr.
Metronidazole (p.585·1).
Amoebiasis; anaerobic bacterial infections; giardiasis; trichomoniasis.

Nide Ibirn, Ital.
Nimesulide (p.63·2).
Fever; inflammation; pain.

Nidina H.A. Nestle, Ital.
Infant feed.
Food hypersensitivity.

Nidol Damor, Ital.
Nimesulide (p.63·2).
Fever; inflammation; pain.

Nidran Sankyo, Jpn.
Nimustine hydrochloride (p.556·2).
Malignant neoplasms.

Nidrel Specia, Fr.
Nitrendipine (p.923·1).
Hypertension.

Nidryl Geneva, USA†.
Diphenhydramine hydrochloride (p.409·1).
Insomnia; motion sickness; parkinsonism.

Nieral Schuck, Ger.
Solidago virgaurea.
Urinary-tract infections.

Nierano HM Pfluger, Ger.
Homoeopathic preparation.

Nierentee Smetana, Aust.
Ononis (p.1610·2); equisetum (p.1575·1); herb. polygonii.
Urinary-tract disorders.

Nieren-Tee Syxyl, Ger.†.
Phaseolus vulgaris; delphinium consolida; calendula; centaurea cyanus; mallow flowers; herniaria (p.1587·2); stoechados; birch leaf; orthosiphon (p.1592·2); rosemary; bearberry (p.1552·2); rose fruit (p.1365·2); juniper (p.1592·2); equisetum (p.1575·1); ononis (p.1610·2).
Herbal tea.

Nierentee 2000 Heumann, Ger.
Birch leaves (p.1553·3); orthosiphon (p.1592·2); juniper berry oil (p.1592·3); fennel oil (p.1579·2).
Urinary-tract disorders.

Nierofu Hoyer, Ger.†.
Nitrofurantoin (p.231·3).
Urinary-tract infections.

Nieron Blasen- und Nieren-Tee VI Hoyer, Ger.
Birch leaf; orthosiphon leaf (p.1592·2); solidago virgaurea; peppermint leaf (p.1208·1); liquorice root (p.1197·1); ononis (p.1610·2).
Urinary-tract disorders.

Nieron S Hoyer, Ger.
Solidago virgaurea; taraxacum (p.1634·2).
Urinary-tract disorders.

Nieron-Tee N Hoyer, Ger.
Birch leaf; equisetum (p.1575·1); taraxacum (p.1634·2); ononis (p.1610·2).
Urinary-tract disorders.

Nieroxin N Osterholz, Ger.
Mate leaf (p.1645·1); solidago virgaurea; juniper oil (p.1592·3).
Urinary-tract disorders.

Nif-Atenil Ecosol, Switz.
Atenolol (p.825·3); nifedipine (p.916·2).
Hypertension.

Nife CT, Ger.; BASF, Ger.; Isis Puren, Ger.
Nifedipine (p.916·2).
Hypertension; ischaemic heart disease; Raynaud's syndrome.

nife-basan Schonenberger, Switz.
Nifedipine (p.916·2).
Hypertension; ischaemic heart disease.

Nifebene Merckle, Aust.
Nifedipine (p.916·2).
Angina pectoris; hypertension; Raynaud's syndrome.

Nifecard Asta Medica, Aust.; Sigma, Austral.
Nifedipine (p.916·2).
Angina pectoris; hypertension.

Nifeclair Hennig, Ger.
Nifedipine (p.916·2).
Angina pectoris; hypertension; Raynaud's syndrome.

Nifecor Betapharm, Ger.
Nifedipine (p.916·2).
Angina pectoris; hypertension; Raynaud's syndrome.

Nifed Rowex, Irl.
Nifedipine (p.916·2).
Angina pectoris; hypertension; peripheral vascular disorders.

Nifedalat Hexal, S.Afr.
Nifedipine (p.916·2).
Angina pectoris; hypertension; Raynaud's syndrome.

Nifedicor Searle, Ital.; Streuli, Switz.
Nifedipine (p.916·2).
Hypertension; ischaemic heart disease; Raynaud's syndrome.

Nifedin Benedetti, Ital.
Nifedipine (p.916·2).
Hypertension; ischaemic heart disease; Raynaud's syndrome.

Nifedipat Azupharma, Ger.
Nifedipine (p.916·2).
Angina pectoris; hypertension.

Nifedipress Dexcel, UK.
Nifedipine (p.916·2).
Angina pectoris; hypertension.

Nifedotard Bartholomew Rhodes, UK.
Nifedipine (p.916·2).
Angina pectoris; hypertension.

Nifehexal Hexal, Ger.
Nifedipine (p.916·2).
Hypertension; ischaemic heart disease; Raynaud's syndrome.

Nifehexal Sali Hexal, Ger.
Nifedipine (p.916·2); mefruside (p.902·2).
Hypertension.

Nifelat TAD, Ger.
Nifedipine (p.916·2).
Angina pectoris; hypertension; Raynaud's syndrome.

Nifelate Biogalenique, Fr.†.
Nifedipine (p.916·2).
Angina pectoris; hypertension; Raynaud's syndrome.

Nifelease Lennon, UK.
Nifedipine (p.916·2).
Angina pectoris; hypertension.

Nifensar Rhone-Poulenc Rorer, Irl.
Nifedipine (p.916·2).
Angina pectoris; hypertension.

Nifensar XL Rhone-Poulenc Rorer, UK†.
Nifedipine (p.916·2).
Hypertension.

Nife-Puren Isis Puren, Ger.
Nifedipine (p.916·2).
Angina pectoris; hypertension.

Niferex Landmark, Canad.; Central, Irl.†; Warner-Wellcome, Spain†; Tillotts, UK; Schwarz, USA.
Polysaccharide-iron complex (p.1353·2).
Iron-deficiency anaemias.

Niferex Daily Schwarz, USA.
Multivitamin and mineral preparation.

Niferex Forte Central Pharmaceuticals, USA†.
Polysaccharide-iron complex (p.1353·2); folic acid (p.1340·3); cyanocobalamin (p.1363·3).
Iron-deficiency anaemias.

Niferex with Vitamin C Schwarz, USA†.
Polysaccharide-iron complex (p.1353·2).
Vitamin C (p.1365·2) is included in this preparation to increase the absorption and availability of iron.
Iron-deficiency anaemias.

Niferex-PN Schwarz, USA.
Multivitamin and mineral preparation with iron and folic acid.
Iron-deficiency anaemias.

Nife-Wolff Wolff, Ger.
Nifedipine (p.916·2).
Hypertension; ischaemic heart disease; Raynaud's syndrome.

Nifical Sanorania, Ger.
Nifedipine (p.916·2).
Cardiac disorders; hypertension; Raynaud's syndrome.

Nifidine Rolab, S.Afr.
Nifedipine (p.916·2).
Angina pectoris.

Nifint Merckle, Aust.; Merckle, Ger.
Menthol (p.1600·2).
Upper respiratory-tract catarrh.

Niflactol Upsamedica, Spain.
Morniflumate (p.56·1).
Musculoskeletal, joint, and peri-articular disorders; pain.

Niflactol Topico Upsamedica, Spain.
Niflumic acid (p.63·1).
Peri-articular and soft-tissue disorders.

Niflam Upsamedica, Ital.
Capsules; cream; topical gel: Niflumic acid (p.63·1).
Suppositories: Morniflumate (p.56·1).
Inflammation; pain.

Niflan Yoshitomi, Jpn; Senju, Jpn.
Pranoprofen (p.81·2).
Fever; inflammation; pain.

Niflugel Upsamedica, Belg.; UPSA, Fr.; Upsamedica, Switz.
Niflumic acid (p.63·1).
Musculoskeletal, joint, peri-articular and soft-tissue disorders.

Nifluril
Note. This name is used for preparations of different composition.
Upsamedica, Belg.; UPSA, Fr.; Upsamedica, Switz.
Capsules; ointment: Niflumic acid (p.63·1).
Inflammation; musculoskeletal, joint, and peri-articular disorders; pain.

UPSA, Fr.
Dental gel: Niflumic acid glycinamide (p.63·1); hexetidine (p.1116·1).
Gingivitis; inflammatory mouth disorders.

UPSA, Fr.; Upsamedica, Switz.
Suppositories: Morniflumate (p.56·1).
Inflammation; musculoskeletal, joint, and peri-articular disorders; pain.

Nifreal Realpharma, Ger.
Nifedipine (p.916·2).
Hypertension; ischaemic heart disease; Raynaud's syndrome.

Nif-Ten Zeneca, Aust.; Zeneca, Ger.; Zeneca, Irl.; Zeneca, Ital.; Zeneca, Neth.; Zeneca, Switz.
Atenolol (p.825·3); nifedipine (p.916·2).
Angina pectoris; hypertension.

Nifucin Apogepha, Ger.
Topical gel: Nitrofurazone (p.232·3).
Burns; wounds.
Topical liquid: Nitrofurazone (p.232·3); propipocaine hydrochloride (p.1300·1).
Bacterial skin infections; burns.

Nifur Lafon-Ratiopharm, Fr.
Nifuroxazide (p.231·3).
Diarrhoea.

Nifuran Jenapharm, Ger.
Furazolidone (p.583·1).
Vaginal infections.

Nifurantin Apogepha, Ger.
Nitrofurantoin (p.231·3).
Urinary-tract infections.

Nifurantin B 6 Apogepha, Ger.
Nitrofurantoin (p.231·3); pyridoxine hydrochloride (p.1362·3).
Urinary-tract infections.

Nifuretten Apogepha, Ger.
Nitrofurantoin (p.231·3).
Urinary-tract infections.

Nigersan Sanum-Kehlbeck, Ger.
Homoeopathic preparation.

Night Cast Regular Formula Seres, USA†.
Sulphur (p.1091·2); salicylic acid (p.1090·2).
Acne.

Night Cast S Dormer, Canad.†.
Sulphur (p.1091·2); resorcinol (p.1090·1).
Acne.

Night Cast Special Formula Seres, USA†.
Sulphur (p.1091·2); resorcinol (p.1090·1).
Acne.

Night Cold Comfort Boots, UK.
Paracetamol (p.72·2); pseudoephedrine hydrochloride (p.1068·3); diphenhydramine hydrochloride (p.409·1); pholcodine (p.1068·1).
Cold symptoms.

Night Cough Pastilles Ernest Jackson, UK.
Codeine phosphate (p.26·1); wild cherry bark (p.1644·3).
Coughs.

Night Leg Cramp Relief Invamed, USA.
Quinine sulphate (p.439·2).

Night Nurse SmithKline Beecham Consumer, Irl.; SmithKline Beecham Consumer, UK.
Paracetamol (p.72·2); promethazine hydrochloride (p.416·2); dextromethorphan hydrobromide (p.1057·3).
Cold and influenza symptoms.

Night Time Healthcrafts, UK.
Valerian (p.1643·1); lupulus (p.1597·2); passion flower (p.1615·3).
Sleep disturbances.

Night-Care CT, Ger.
Pumilio pine oil (p.1623·3); thyme oil (p.1637·1); eucalyptus oil (p.1578·1); menthol (p.1600·2).
Catarrh.

Nighttime Cold & Flu Stanley, Canad.
Pseudoephedrine hydrochloride (p.1068·3); doxylamine succinate (p.410·1); dextromethorphan hydrobromide (p.1057·3); paracetamol (p.72·2).

Night-Time Effervescent Cold Goldline, USA.
Phenylpropanolamine hydrochloride (p.1067·2); diphenhydramine citrate (p.409·1); aspirin (p.16·1).
Upper respiratory-tract symptoms.

Nighttime Pamprin Chattem, USA.
Diphenhydramine hydrochloride (p.409·1); paracetamol (p.72·2).
Insomnia.

NightTime Theraflu Sandoz, USA.
Paracetamol (p.72·2); dextromethorphan hydrobromide (p.1057·3); pseudoephedrine hydrochloride (p.1068·3); chlorpheniramine maleate (p.405·1).
Coughs and cold symptoms.

Nigrantyl Lacteol du Dr Boucard, Fr.
Black currant (p.1365·2); sodium citrate (p.1153·2).
Capillary fragility.

Nigroids Ernest Jackson, UK.
Liquorice (p.1197·1); menthol (p.1600·2).

Nikacid Rhone-Poulenc Rorer, Austral.†.
Nicotinic acid (p.1351·2).

Nikesanol Rowa, Irl.†.
Multivitamin preparation.

nikofrenon Hefa, Ger.
Nicotine (p.1607·2).
Aid to smoking withdrawal.

Nikotugg ACO, Swed.
Nicotine resin (p.1608·1).
Aid to smoking withdrawal.

Nilandron Hoechst Marion Roussel, USA.
Nilutamide (p.556·2).
Prostatic cancer.

Nilevar Laphal, Fr.
Norethandrolone (p.1452·3).
Medullary aplasia.

NilnOcen Zeppenfeldt, Ger.
Paracetamol (p.72·2).
Fever; pain.

Nilodor Cussons, UK.
A deodorant liquid for use with colostomies and ileostomies.

Nilstat Wyeth, Austral.; Wyeth Lederle, Belg.; Stiefel, Canad.; Lederle, USA.
Nystatin (p.386·1).
Candidiasis.

Nilstim De Witt, UK†.
Methylcellulose 2500 (p.1473·3); microcrystalline cellulose (p.1472·1).
Obesity.

Nimbex Glaxo Wellcome, Aust.; Glaxo Wellcome, Austral.; Glaxo Wellcome, Fr.; Glaxo Wellcome, Ger.; Zeneca, Ger.; Wellcome, Irl.; Glaxo Wellcome, Ital.; Glaxo Wellcome, Neth.; Glaxo Wellcome, Norw.; Glaxo Wellcome, S.Afr.; Wellcome, Spain; Glaxo Wellcome, Swed.; Wellcome, UK; Glaxo Wellcome, USA.
Cisatracurium besylate (p.1304·3).
Competitive neuromuscular blocker.

Nimbisan Solvay, Ital.
Brotizolam (p.643·2).
Insomnia.

Nimbus Biomerica, USA.
Pregnancy test (p.1621·2).

Nimedex Italfarmaco, Ital.
Nimesulide betadex (p.63·2).
Fever; inflammation; pain.

Nimesulene Guidotti, Ital.
Nimesulide (p.63·2).
Fever; inflammation; pain.

Nimicor Formenti, Ital.
Nicardipine hydrochloride (p.915·1).
Angina pectoris; heart failure; hypertension.

Nimodrel Opus, UK.
Nifedipine (p.916·2).
Angina pectoris; hypertension.

Nimopect Hevert, Ger.
Thyme (p.1636·3).
Coughs.

Nimotop Bayer, Aust.; Bayer, Austral.; Bayer, Belg.; Bayer, Canad.; Bayer, Fr.; Bayer, Ger.; Bayer, Irl.; Bayer, Ital.; Bayer, Neth.; Bayer, Norw.; Bayer, S.Afr.; Bayer, Spain; Bayer, Swed.; Bayer, Switz.; Bayer, UK; Bayer, USA.
Nimodipine (p.922·2).
Cerebral disorders in the elderly; neurological deficit following cerebral vasospasm or subarachnoid haemorrhage.

Nims Caber, Ital.
Nimesulide (p.63·2).
Fever; inflammation; pain.

Nina Medichemie, Switz.
Paracetamol (p.72·2).
Fever; pain.

Nina cum Diphenhydramino Medichemie, Switz.
Paracetamol (p.72·2); diphenhydramine hydrochloride (p.409·1).
Fever; pain.

Ni-No-Fluid N Hotz, Ger.
Peppermint oil (p.1208·1).
Cold symptoms; gastro-intestinal disorders.

Niocitran Sandoz, Belg.
Paracetamol (p.72·2); pseudoephedrine hydrochloride (p.1068·3).
Cold symptoms.

Niong retard Rhone-Poulenc Rorer, Switz.
Glyceryl trinitrate (p.874·3).
Angina pectoris; heart failure.

Niopam E. Merck, Irl.; E. Merck, UK.
Iopamidol (p.1007·1).
Radiographic contrast medium.

Niotal Synthelabo, Ital.
Zolpidem tartrate (p.698·3).
Insomnia.

Nipaxon Pharmacia Upjohn, Swed.
Noscapine (p.1065·2).
Coughs.

Nipent Cyanamid, Belg.†; Parke, Davis, Canad.†; Lederle, Fr.; Lederle, Ger.; Parke, Davis, Ital.; Cyanamid, Spain; Lederle, UK; Supergen, USA.
Pentostatin (p.557·3).
Hairy-cell leukaemia.

Nipiozim Malesci, Ital.†.
Pepsinogen.
Digestive insufficiency.

Nipolept
Ebewe, Aust.; Rhone-Poulenc Rorer, Ger.
Zotepine (p.700·1).
Schizophrenia.

Nipride
Roche, Belg.†; Roche, Canad.; Roche, Fr.†; Roche, Irl.; Roche, Neth.†; Roche, Swed.†; Roche, Switz.†; Roche, UK†.
Sodium nitroprusside (p.943·2).
Controlled hypotension; ergotamine intoxication; heart failure; hypertensive crisis.

Niprina Pensa, Spain.
Nitrendipine (p.923·1).
Angina pectoris; hypertension; Raynaud's syndrome.

nipruss Schwarz, Ger.
Sodium nitroprusside (p.943·2).
Controlled hypotension; hypertension.

NiQuitin CQ SmithKline Beecham, UK.
Nicotine (p.1607·2).
Aid to smoking withdrawal.

Nirason N Ravensberg, Ger.
Pentaerythritol tetranitrate (p.927·3).
Formerly contained pentaerythritol tetranitrate, phenobarbitone, theophylline, and procaine hydrochloride.
Cardiovascular disorders.

Nirolex for Chesty Coughs Boots, UK.
Guaiphenesin (p.1061·3); ephedrine hydrochloride (p.1059·3); menthol (p.1600·2).
Coughs.

Nirolex for Dry Coughs Boots, UK.
Dextromethorphan hydrobromide (p.1057·3).
Coughs.

Nirox Medici, Ital.
Piroxicam (p.80·2).
Musculoskeletal and joint disorders.

Nirvanil
Recordati, Ital.; Sodip, Switz.†.
Valnoctamide (p.698·1).
Nervous disorders.

Nisaid-25 Schwulst, S.Afr.
Indomethacin (p.45·2).
Gout; inflammation; musculoskeletal and joint disorders; pain.

Nisal Epifarma, Ital.
Nimesulide (p.63·2).
Fever; inflammation; pain.

Nisapulvol Mayoly-Spindler, Fr.
Methyl hydroxybenzoate (p.1117·2); ethyl hydroxybenzoate (p.1117·2); propyl hydroxybenzoate (p.1117·2); benzyl hydroxybenzoate (p.1117·2); zinc oxide (p.1096·2).
Intertrigo; pruritus.

Nisaseptol Mayoly-Spindler, Fr.
Propyl hydroxybenzoate (p.1117·2); benzyl hydroxybenzoate (p.1117·2).
Intertrigo; pruritus.

Nisasol Mayoly-Spindler, Fr.
Methyl hydroxybenzoate (p.1117·2); ethyl hydroxybenzoate (p.1117·2); propyl hydroxybenzoate (p.1117·2).
Infected skin disorders.

Niscodil Janssen-Cilag, Ital.†.
Pentaerythritol tetranitrate (p.927·3).
Angina pectoris.

Nisicur Apomedica, Aust.
Etenzamide (p.35·3); diphenhydramine hydrochloride (p.409·1); caffeine (p.749·3); ascorbic acid (p.1365·2).
Cold and influenza symptoms.

Nisita
Engelhard, Ger.
Sodium chloride (p.1162·2); sodium bicarbonate (p.1153·2).
Nasal disorders.

Engelhard, Switz.
Sal ems.
Nasal disorders.

Nisolid Master Pharma, Ital.
Flunisolide (p.1040·3).
Obstructive airways disease; rhinitis.

Nisulid Wyeth, Switz.
Nimesulide (p.63·2).
Fever; inflammation; pain.

Nisylen DHU, Ger.
Homoeopathic preparation.

Nite Time Cold Formula Barre-National, USA.
Pseudoephedrine hydrochloride (p.1068·3); dextromethorphan hydrobromide (p.1057·3); doxylamine succinate (p.410·1); paracetamol (p.72·2).
Coughs and cold symptoms.

Nitecall Restan, S.Afr.
Paracetamol (p.72·2); dextromethorphan hydrobromide (p.1057·3); chlorpheniramine maleate (p.405·1); phenylpropanolamine hydrochloride (p.1067·2).
Cold and influenza symptoms.

Nitens Pulitzer, Ital.
Naproxen cetrimonium (p.62·1).
Gynaecological disorders.

Nitepax Lagamed, S.Afr.
Noscapine (as resin complex) (p.1065·2).
Coughs.

Nitesco S Celafar, Ital.
Ruscus aculeatus; hedera helix; aesculus hippocastanum triterpene saponin (p.1543·3); aescin (p.1543·3).
Stretch marks.

Nitoman
Virgo Healthcare, Austral.; Roche, Irl.†; Roche, Norw.†; Roche, UK†.
Tetrabenazine (p.694·2).
Movement disorders.

Nitorol Eisai, Jpn.
Isosorbide dinitrate (p.893·1).
Angina pectoris; ischaemic heart disease; myocardial infarction.

Nitossil Zyma, Ital.
Cloperastine fendizoate (p.1057·2) or cloperastine hydrochloride (p.1057·2).
Coughs.

Nitradisc
Searle, Austral.; Heumann, Ger.; Searle, Norw.; Searle, S.Afr.; Searle, Spain.
Glyceryl trinitrate (p.874·3).
Angina pectoris.

Nitrados Berk, Irl.†.
Nitrazepam (p.682·2).
Insomnia.

Nitrangin Isis, Ger.
Glyceryl trinitrate (p.874·3).
Angina pectoris; coronary spasm; myocardial infarction.

Nitrangin compositum Isis, Ger.
Glyceryl trinitrate (p.874·3); valerian (p.1643·1).
Angina pectoris.

Nitrangin forte Wernigerode, Ger.
Glyceryl trinitrate (p.874·3).
Angina pectoris; coronary spasm; myocardial infarction.

Nitrazep CT, Ger.
Nitrazepam (p.682·2).
Insomnia.

Nitrazepan Prodes, Spain.
Nitrazepam (p.682·2).
Insomnia.

Nitrazine Paper Apothecon, USA.
Test for pH in urine.

Nitrek Bertek, USA.
Glyceryl trinitrate (p.874·3).
Angina pectoris.

Nitrendepat Azupharma, Ger.
Nitrendipine (p.923·1).
Hypertension.

Nitrepress Hexal, Ger.
Nitrendipine (p.923·1).
Hypertension.

Nitrex Essex, Ital.
Isosorbide mononitrate (p.893·3).
Angina pectoris.

Nitriate L'Arguenon, Fr.
Sodium nitroprusside (p.943·2).
Controlled hypotension; heart failure; hypertensive crisis.

Nitriderm TTS Novartis, Fr.
Glyceryl trinitrate (p.874·3).
Angina pectoris.

Nitrisken Wander, Ger.†.
Isosorbide dinitrate (p.893·1); pindolol (p.931·1).
Angina pectoris.

Nitrit Medi-Test Macherey Nagel Duren, S.Afr.
Test for nitrite in urine.

Nitro Dur Schering-Plough, Spain.
Glyceryl trinitrate (p.874·3).
Angina pectoris.

Nitro Mack
Pfizer, Aust.; Mack, Illert., Ger.; Mack, Switz.
Glyceryl trinitrate (p.874·3).
Adjuvant in biliary-tract endoscopy; cardiovascular disorders.

Nitro Pohl
Pohl, Ger.†; Pohl, Neth.
Glyceryl trinitrate (p.874·3).
Heart failure.

Nitro Rorer Rorer, Ger.†.
Glyceryl trinitrate (p.874·3).
Cardiac disorders.

Nitrobaat
Organon, Belg.†; Nourypharma, Neth.
Glyceryl trinitrate (p.874·3).
Angina pectoris.

Nitro-Bid
Hoechst Marion Roussel, Austral.; Hoechst Marion Roussel, Canad.†; Marion Merrell Dow, USA.
Glyceryl trinitrate (p.874·3).
Angina pectoris; controlled hypotension; heart failure; perioperative hypertension.

Nitrocine
Schwarz, Irl.; Sanofi Omnimed, S.Afr.; Schwarz, UK.
Glyceryl trinitrate (p.874·3).
Angina pectoris; controlled hypotension; heart failure; hypertension during cardiac surgery; myocardial ischaemia during cardiovascular surgery.

Nitrocit Genpharm, S.Afr.
Potassium citrate (p.1153·1).
Urinary alkalinisation.

Nitrocod Be-Tabs, S.Afr.
Paracetamol (p.72·2); codeine phosphate (p.26·1).
Fever; pain.

Nitrocontin Continus
Napp, Irl.†; Asta Medica, UK†.
Glyceryl trinitrate (p.874·3).
Angina pectoris.

Nitrocor Recordati, Ital.†.
Glyceryl trinitrate (p.874·3).
Angina pectoris.

Nitro-Crataegutt Schwabe, Ger.
Pentaerythritol tetranitrate (p.927·3); crataegus (p.1568·2).
Heart failure.

Nitroderm
Ciba-Geigy, Aust.; Ciba-Geigy, Belg.; Ciba, Ger.; Ciba, Ital.; Novartis, S.Afr.; Ciba-Geigy, Spain; Ciba, Switz.; Reuabuen, USA.
Glyceryl trinitrate (p.874·3).
Angina pectoris; prevention of phlebitis and extravasation during intravenous infusion.

Nitrodex
Dexo, Fr.; Dexo, Switz.
Pentaerythritol tetranitrate (p.927·3).
Angina pectoris; heart failure.

Nitrodisc Roberts, USA.
Glyceryl trinitrate (p.874·3).
Angina pectoris.

Nitro-Dur
Ebewe, Aust.; Schering-Plough, Austral.; Key, Canad.; Schering-Plough, Irl.; Sigma-Tau, Ital.; Schering-Plough, Neth.; Schering-Plough, Norw.; Essex, Switz.; Schering-Plough, UK; Key, USA.
Glyceryl trinitrate (p.874·3).
Angina pectoris; heart failure.

Nitrodurat Pohl, Ger.†.
Glyceryl trinitrate (p.874·3); isosorbide dinitrate (p.893·1).
Cardiac disorders.

Nitro-Dyl Bio-Therabel, Belg.
Glyceryl trinitrate (p.874·3).
Angina pectoris.

Nitroflu Beige, S.Afr.
Aspirin (p.16·1); caffeine (p.749·3); ascorbic acid (p.1365·2); chlorpheniramine maleate (p.405·1).
Cold and influenza symptoms.

Nitrofurantoin comp. Ratiopharm, Ger.†.
Nitrofurantoin (p.231·3); sulphadiazine (p.252·3).
Urinary-tract infections.

Nitrofurin G.W. Panthox & Burck, Ital.†.
Nitrofurantoin (p.231·3).
Bacterial infections of the urinary tract.

Nitrogard
Astra, Canad.†; Forest Pharmaceuticals, USA.
Glyceryl trinitrate (p.874·3).
Angina pectoris.

Nitro-Gesanit Rorer, Ger.†.
Glyceryl trinitrate (p.874·3).
Cardiac disorders.

Nitroglin Stadapharm, Ger.†.
Glyceryl trinitrate (p.874·3).
Cardiac disorders.

Nitroglyn
Pharmacia, Swed.†; Kenwood, USA.
Glyceryl trinitrate (p.874·3).
Angina pectoris.

Nitroina Parisis, Spain.
Acetic acid (p.1541·2); chelidonium; salicylic acid (p.1090·2); iodine tincture (p.1493·1); thuya occidentalis (p.1636·3).
Warts.

Nitroject Omega, Canad.†.
Glyceryl trinitrate (p.874·3).
Cardiac disorders; perioperative hypertension; surgical hypotension.

Nitrokapseln-ratiopharm Ratiopharm, Ger.
Glyceryl trinitrate (p.874·3).
Angina pectoris.

Nitrol
Note. This name is used for preparations of different composition.
Rhone-Poulenc Rorer, Canad.; Savage, USA.
Glyceryl trinitrate (p.874·3).
Angina pectoris.

SmithKline Beecham Sante, Fr.
Celandine; thuja (p.1636·3); iodine (p.1493·1); salicylic acid (p.1090·2); glacial acetic acid (p.1541·2).
Warts.

Nitrolan Elan, USA.
Lactose-free, gluten-free preparation for enteral nutrition.

Nitrolate Roche, Austral.†.
Glyceryl trinitrate (p.874·3).
Angina pectoris.

Nitrolingual
Salus, Aust.; Rhone-Poulenc Rorer, Austral.; Codali, Belg.; Rhone-Poulenc Rorer, Canad.; Pohl, Ger.; Lipha, Irl.; Pohl, Neth.; Pohl, Norw.; Mer-National, S.Afr.; Meda, Swed.; Pohl, Switz.; Lipha, UK; Rhone-Poulenc Rorer, USA.
Glyceryl trinitrate (p.874·3).
Angina pectoris; biliary colic; hypertensive crisis; pulmonary oedema; smooth muscle spasm.

Nitromaxitate Ris, Ital.†.
Mannityl hexanitrate (p.901·3); glyceryl trinitrate (p.874·3).
Cardiovascular disorders.

Nitromex
Dumex, Norw.; Dumex-Alpharma, Swed.
Glyceryl trinitrate (p.874·3).
Cardiovascular disorders; control of blood pressure during surgery.

Nitromin Servier, UK.
Glyceryl trinitrate (p.874·3).
Angina pectoris.

Nitromint Rhone-Poulenc Rorer, Switz.
Glyceryl trinitrate (p.874·3).
Angina pectoris; coronary artery spasm.

Nitronal
Salus, Aust.; Pohl, Ger.; Lipha, Irl.; Mer-National, S.Afr.†; Pohl, Switz.; Lipha, UK.
Glyceryl trinitrate (p.874·3).
Angina pectoris; control of blood pressure during surgery; heart failure; myocardial infarction; pulmonary oedema.

Nitrong
Chemomedica, Aust.; Rhone-Poulenc Rorer, Belg.; Rhone-Poulenc Rorer, Canad.; Rhone-Poulenc, Ital.†; Rhone-Poulenc Rorer, Norw.†; May & Baker, S.Afr.†; Orion, Swed.; Rhone-Poulenc Rorer, USA.
Glyceryl trinitrate (p.874·3).
Angina pectoris; heart failure.

Nitro-Novodigal Beiersdorf-Lilly, Ger.†.
β-Acetyldigoxin (p.812·3); pentaerythritol tetranitrate (p.927·3).
Heart failure.

Nitro-Obsidan Isis, Ger.
Pentaerythritol tetranitrate (p.927·3); propranolol hydrochloride (p.937·1).
Angina pectoris; hypertension.

Nitropacin Juste, Spain.
Glyceryl trinitrate (p.874·3).
Angina pectoris; heart failure; myocardial infarction.

nitroperlinit RAN, Ger.†.
Glyceryl trinitrate (p.874·3).
Cardiovascular disorders.

Nitro-Pflaster-ratiopharm Ratiopharm, Ger.
Glyceryl trinitrate (p.874·3).
Angina pectoris.

Nitroplast Lacer, Spain.
Glyceryl trinitrate (p.874·3).
Angina pectoris.

Nitro-Praecordin N Roland, Ger.
Glyceryl trinitrate (p.874·3); benzyl nicotinate (p.22·1).
Angina pectoris; coronary vascular disorders.

Nitropress Abbott, USA.
Sodium nitroprusside (p.943·2).
Controlled hypotension; hypertensive crisis.

Nitroprussiat Fides, Spain.
Sodium nitroprusside (p.943·2).
Controlled hypotension; heart failure; hypertension.

Nitrorectal Pohl, Ger.†.
Glyceryl trinitrate (p.874·3).
Cardiac disorders.

Nitroretard
Byk Gulden, Ital.†; Dumex, Norw.†; Dumex-Alpharma, Swed.†.
Glyceryl trinitrate (p.874·3).
Angina pectoris.

Nitrosorbide Lusofarmaco, Ital.
Isosorbide dinitrate (p.893·1).
Cardiac disorders.

Nitrosorbon Pohl, Ger.
Isosorbide dinitrate (p.893·1).
Cardiac disorders.

Nitrospan Rorer, USA†.
Glyceryl trinitrate (p.874·3).
Angina pectoris.

Nitro-Spray Drug Houses Austral., Austral.†.
Isosorbide dinitrate (p.893·1).
Angina pectoris.

Nitrostat
Parke, Davis, Canad.; Parke, Davis, Neth.; Parke, Davis, USA.
Glyceryl trinitrate (p.874·3).
Angina pectoris.

Nitrosylon Knoll, Ital.
Glyceryl trinitrate (p.874·3).
Angina pectoris.

Nitro-Tablinen Sanorania, Ger.
Isosorbide dinitrate (p.893·1).
Cardiac disorders.

Nitrotard Berenguer Infale, Spain.
Glyceryl trinitrate (p.874·3).
Angina pectoris; heart failure; myocardial infarction.

Nitro-Time Time-Cap, USA.
Glyceryl trinitrate (p.874·3).
Angina pectoris.

Nitrourean Pras, Spain.
Carmustine (p.511·3).
Malignant neoplasms.

Nitroven Pohl, Norw.
Glyceryl trinitrate (p.874·3).
Angina pectoris; blood pressure control during cardiac surgery; heart failure.

Nitrozell
Byk, Aust.; Byk Gulden, Ger.†; Byk, Neth.†.
Glyceryl trinitrate (p.874·3).
Angina pectoris; myocardial infarction.

Nitrumon
Sintesa, Belg.; Simes, Ital.†.
Carmustine (p.511·3).
Malignant neoplasms.

Nitur Test Boehringer Mannheim, Austral.†.
Test for nitrites in urine.

Nitux Inpharzam, Switz.
Morclofone (p.1064·2).
Coughs.

Nivabetol Jumer, Fr.
Betaine (p.1553·2); acetylmethionine; sorbitol (p.1354·2).
Constipation; dyspepsia.

Nivadil
Klinge, Ger.; Klinge, Irl.; Fujisawa, Jpn.
Nilvadipine (p.922·1).
Hypertension; stroke.

Nivador Menarini, Spain.
Cefuroxime axetil (p.177·1).
Bacterial infections.

Nivalin Waldheim, Aust.
Galantamine hydrobromide (p.1393·1).
Alzheimer's disease; cerebrovascular disorders; glaucoma; myasthenia gravis; myelitis; neuritis; poliomyelitis; reversal of competitive neuromuscular blockade; smooth muscle atony.

Nivalina UCB, Ital.†.
Galantamine hydrobromide (p.1393·1).
Reversal of competitive neuromuscular blockade.

Nivaquine
Rhone-Poulenc Rorer, Austral.†; Rhone-Poulenc Rorer, Belg.; Specia, Fr.; Rhone-Poulenc Rorer, Irl.; Rhone-Poulenc Rorer, Neth.; Rhone-Poulenc Rorer, S.Afr.; Rhone-Poulenc Rorer, Switz.; May & Baker, UK.
Chloroquine sulphate (p.426·3).
Giardiasis; hepatic amoebiasis; light-sensitive skin conditions; lupus erythematosus; malaria; rheumatoid arthritis.

Nivaten Cox, UK.
Nifedipine (p.916·2).

Nivea Beiersdorf, USA.
A range of emollient, cleansing, and moisturising preparations.

Nivea Sun Beiersdorf, USA.
SPF 15: Ethylhexyl *p*-methoxycinnamate (p.1487·1); octyl salicylate (p.1487·3); oxybenzone (p.1487·3); 2-phenyl-1*H*-benzimidazole-5-sulphonic acid (p.1488·2).
Sunscreen.

Nivemycin Knoll, UK.
Neomycin sulphate (p.229·2).
Bowel preparation; hepatic coma.

Niven Pulitzer, Ital.
Nicardipine hydrochloride (p.915·1).
Angina pectoris; heart failure; hypertension.

Nix
Warner-Lambert, Austral.; Warner-Lambert Consumer, Belg.; Warner-Wellcome, Canad.; Glaxo Wellcome, Canad.; Warner-Lambert, Fr.; Warner-Lambert, Ital.; Warner-Lambert, Norw.; Glaxo Wellcome, Swed.; Warner-Lambert, Swed.; Wellcome, USA.
Permethrin (p.1409·2).
Pediculosis; scabies.

Nixyn Organon, Spain.
Capsules; suppositories: Isonixin (p.48·1).
Gout; musculoskeletal, joint, and peri-articular disorders; pain.
Cream: Isonixin (p.48·1); methyl salicylate (p.55·2).
Peri-articular and soft-tissue disorders.

Nizacol Benedetti, Ital.
Miconazole (p.384·3) or miconazole nitrate (p.384·3).
Fungal infections; Gram-positive bacterial infections.

Nizax
Lilly, Ger.; Lilly, Ital.; Lilly, Swed.
Nizatidine (p.1203·2).
Gastro-oesophageal reflux; peptic ulcer.

Nizaxid Norgine, Fr.
Nizatidine (p.1203·2).
Gastro-oesophageal reflux; peptic ulcer.

Nizcreme Janssen-Cilag, S.Afr.
Ketoconazole (p.383·1).
Fungal skin infections.

Nizoral
Janssen-Cilag, Aust.; Janssen-Cilag, Austral.; Janssen-Cilag, Belg.; Janssen-Ortho, Canad.; Janssen-Cilag, Fr.; Janssen-Cilag, Ger.; Janssen-Cilag, Irl.; Janssen-Cilag, Ital.; Janssen-Cilag, Neth.; Janssen-Cilag, S.Afr.; Janssen-Cilag, Switz.; Janssen-Cilag, UK; Johnson & Johnson MSD Consumer, UK; Janssen, USA.
Ketoconazole (p.383·1).
Dandruff; fungal infections; seborrhoeic dermatitis.

Nizovules Janssen-Cilag, S.Afr.
Ketoconazole (p.383·1).
Vaginal candidiasis.

Nizshampoo Janssen-Cilag, S.Afr.
Ketoconazole (p.383·1).
Fungal scalp infections.

N-Labstix
Ames, Irl.; Bayer Diagnostics, UK.
Test for glucose, protein, pH, ketones, blood, and nitrites in urine.

N-Multistix
Bayer Diagnostics, Austral.; Bayer, USA.
Test for glucose, protein, blood, ketones, bilirubin, urobilinogen, nitrites, and pH in urine.

N-Multistix SG
Bayer Diagnostics, Austral.; Bayer, Canad.; Ames, Irl.; Bayer Diagnostici, Ital.; Bayer Diagnostics, UK; Bayer, USA.
Test for pH, specific gravity, proteins, glucose, ketones, blood, nitrites, bilirubin, and urobilinogen in urine.

No 440 Herbes Universelles, Canad.
Vitamins A, C, and D.

No Doz Key, Austral.
Caffeine (p.749·3).
Fatigue.

No Doz Plus Key, Austral.
Caffeine (p.749·3); vitamin B substances; glucose (p.1343·3).
Fatigue.

No Drowsiness Sinarest Ciba, USA.
Pseudoephedrine hydrochloride (p.1068·3); paracetamol (p.72·2).
Upper respiratory-tract symptoms.

No Gas Key, Austral.
Activated charcoal (p.972·2); simethicone (p.1213·1).
Diarrhoea; drug poisoning; excess gastro-intestinal gas.

No Grip Vifor, Switz.
Salicylamide (p.82·3); noscapine hydrochloride (p.1065·2); mepyramine maleate (p.414·1); ascorbic acid (p.1365·2); hesperidin methyl chalcone (p.1580·2).
Cold symptoms.

no more burn Johnson & Johnson Medical, USA†.
Lignocaine hydrochloride (p.1293·2).

no more germies Johnson & Johnson Medical, USA†.
Soap: Triclosan (p.1127·2).
Towelettes: Benzalkonium chloride (p.1101·3).

no more itchies Johnson & Johnson Medical, USA†.
Hydrocortisone (p.1043·3).

no more ouchies Johnson & Johnson Medical, USA†.
Lignocaine hydrochloride (p.1293·2).

No Name Cough Lozenge Sutton, Canad.
Menthol (p.1600·2).

No Odor Suisse, Austral.†.
Chlorophyll (p.1000·1).
Nutritional supplement.

No Pain-HP Young Again Products, USA.
Capsaicin (p.24·2).
Pain.

NO-AD Babies Solar, Canad.
SPF 30; SPF 45: Ethylhexyl *p*-methoxycinnamate (p.1487·1); octyl salicylate (p.1487·3); oxybenzone (p.1487·3).
Sunscreen.

NO-AD Kids Solar, Canad.
SPF 30: Ethylhexyl *p*-methoxycinnamate (p.1487·1); octyl salicylate (p.1487·3); oxybenzone (p.1487·3).
Sunscreen.

NO-AD Sport Solar, Canad.
SPF 15; SPF 30: Ethylhexyl *p*-methoxycinnamate (p.1487·1); octyl salicylate (p.1487·3); oxybenzone (p.1487·3).
Sunscreen.

NO-AD Sunblock Solar, Canad.
SPF 15; SPF 30; SPF 45: Ethylhexyl *p*-methoxycinnamate (p.1487·1); octyl salicylate (p.1487·3); oxybenzone (p.1487·3).
Sunscreen.

NO-AD Sunscreen Solar, Canad.
SPF 8: Ethylhexyl *p*-methoxycinnamate (p.1487·1); oxybenzone (p.1487·3).
Sunscreen.

No-Alcool Sella Sella, Ital.†.
Cetylpyridinium chloride (p.1106·2).
Disinfection.

Noaldol Lampugnani, Ital.†.
Diflunisal (p.33·2).
Musculoskeletal disorders; pain.

Noalgil Pharmacia Upjohn, Spain.
Ibuprofen (p.44·1).
Fever; inflammation; musculoskeletal, joint, and peri-articular disorders; pain.

Noan Ravizza, Ital.
Diazepam (p.661·1).
Anxiety; epilepsy; insomnia.

Nobacter Boots Healthcare, Fr.
Triclocarban (p.1127·2).
Skin cleansing and disinfection.

Nobecutan
Astra, Ger.; Astra, Neth.†; Astra Tech, Norw.†; Astra, Switz.†.
Thiram (p.1636·2).
Antiseptic aerosol dressing.

Nobecutane
Astra, Austral.†; Astra, Belg.; Simes, Ital.†; Astra Tech, UK†.
Thiram (p.1636·2).
Antiseptic aerosol dressing.

Nobese No. 1 Restan, S.Afr.
Cathine hydrochloride (p.1478·1).
Obesity.

Nobligan
Boehringer Mannheim, Aust.; Searle, Swed.
Tramadol hydrochloride (p.90·1).
Pain.

Nobliten Lacer, Spain.
A nonoxinol (p.1326·1).
Contraceptive.

Nobritol Andreu, Spain.
Amitriptyline hydrochloride (p.273·3); medazepam (p.677·3).
Depression.

Nobrium
Roche, Irl.†; Roche, Ital.†; Roche, Neth.†; Roche, Switz.†; Roche, UK†.
Medazepam (p.677·3).
Anxiety disorders.

Noceptin Christiaens, Neth.
Morphine sulphate (p.56·2).
Pain.

Nocertone
Sanofi Winthrop, Belg.; Sanofi Winthrop, Fr.; Sanofi Winthrop, Spain†.
Oxetorone fumarate (p.449·1).
Cluster headache; migraine.

Noctal UCB, Ger.†.
Ibomal (p.675·2).
Sleep disorders.

Noctamid
Schering, Aust.; Schering, Belg.; Schering, Ger.; Asche, Ger.; Schering, Irl.; Schering, Ital.†; Schering, Neth.; Schering, S.Afr.; Schering, Spain; Schering, Switz.
Lormetazepam (p.677·1).
Premedication; sleep disorders.

Noctamide Schering, Fr.
Lormetazepam (p.677·1).
Insomnia.

Noctazepam Brenner-Efeka, Ger.
Oxazepam (p.683·2).
Anxiety; sleep disorders.

Noctec
Bristol-Myers Squibb, Austral.†; Bristol-Myers Squibb, UK†.
Chloral hydrate (p.645·3).
Insomnia; premedication.

Noctis Bouty, Ital.
Valerian (p.1643·1); passion flower (p.1615·3); crataegus (p.1568·2).
Sleep disorders.

Noctisan Dolisos, Fr.
Crataegus (p.1568·2); tilia (p.1637·3); valerian (p.1643·1).
Insomnia.

Noctran Menarini, Fr.
Potassium clorazepate (p.657·1); acepromazine (p.640·1); aceprometazine (p.640·2).
Insomnia.

Noctura Nelson, UK.
Homoeopathic preparation.

Nocvalene Arkopharma, Fr.
Crataegus (p.1568·2); red-poppy petal (p.1001·1); passion flower (p.1615·3).
Insomnia.

Node Tar Piam, Ital.
Coal tar (p.1092·3); cade oil (p.1092·2); selenium sulphide (p.1091·1); salicylic acid (p.1090·2).
Scalp disorders.

Nodex Brothier, Fr.
Dextromethorphan hydrobromide (p.1057·3).
Coughs.

Nodol Del Saz & Filippini, Ital.†.
Ranitidine hydrochloride (p.1209·3).
Gastro-intestinal disorders associated with hyperacidity.

NoDoz Bristol-Myers Products, USA.
Caffeine (p.749·3).
Fatigue.

No-Drowsiness Allerest Ciba, USA.
Pseudoephedrine hydrochloride (p.1068·3); paracetamol (p.72·2).
Upper respiratory-tract symptoms.

Noemin N Trommsdorff, Ger.
Bismuth aluminate (p.1180·1).
Gastro-intestinal disorders.

Nofedol Rhone-Poulenc Rorer, Spain.
Paracetamol (p.72·2).
Fever; pain.

No-Flu Klinge, Switz.
Paracetamol (p.72·2); dextromethorphan hydrobromide (p.1057·3); phenylephrine hydrochloride (p.1066·2).
Cold symptoms.

Noflu F Siegfried, Ger.†.
Paracetamol (p.72·2); dextromethorphan hydrobromide (p.1057·3); phenylephrine hydrochloride (p.1066·2).
Cold symptoms.

Nofum Faes, Spain.
Lobeline sulphate (p.1481·3).
Aid to smoking withdrawal.

No-Gas Giuliani, Ital.
Dimethicone (p.1213·1); activated charcoal (p.972·2).
Gastro-intestinal disorders associated with excess gas.

Nogram Sanofi Winthrop, Ger.†.
Nalidixic acid (p.228·2).
Bacterial infections of the urinary tract.

No-Gravid Irmed, Ital.
Copper (p.1337·3).
Intra-uterine contraceptive device.

No-Hist Dunhall, USA.
Phenylephrine hydrochloride (p.1066·2); phenylpropanolamine hydrochloride (p.1067·2); pseudoephedrine hydrochloride (p.1068·3).
Nasal congestion.

Noiafren Hoechst, Spain.
Clobazam (p.656·3).
Anxiety; insomnia.

Noivy Hilarys, Canad.
Calamine (p.1080·1); camphor (p.1557·2); menthol (p.1600·2); benzocaine (p.1286·2).

Nokhel Promesa, Spain†.
Amikhelline hydrochloride (p.1548·2).
Renal and hepatic colic.

Noktone Gea, Norw.
Ranitidine hydrochloride (p.1209·3).
Aspiration syndrome; gastro-oesophageal reflux; peptic ulcer; Zollinger-Ellison syndrome.

Nolahist Carnrick, USA.
Phenindamine tartrate (p.415·2).
Allergic rhinitis.

Nolamine Carnrick, USA.
Phenindamine tartrate (p.415·2); chlorpheniramine maleate (p.405·1); phenylpropanolamine hydrochloride (p.1067·2).
Nasal decongestant.

Noleptan Thomae, Ger.†.
Fominoben hydrochloride (p.1061·2).
Respiratory disorders.

Nolex LA Carnrick, USA†.
Phenylpropanolamine hydrochloride (p.1067·2); guaiphenesin (p.1061·3).
Symptoms associated with nasal congestion and viscous mucous.

Nolgen Antigen, Irl.
Tamoxifen citrate (p.563·3).
Breast cancer.

Nolipax Salus, Ital.
Fenofibrate (p.1273·1).
Diabetic retinopathy; hyperlipidaemias; xanthomatosis.

Nolipid Samil, Ital.
Colextran hydrochloride (p.1272·2).
Hyperlipidaemia.

Nolol Docmed, S.Afr.
Propranolol hydrochloride (p.937·1).
Angina pectoris; anxiety; arrhythmias; hypertension; hyperthyroidism; phaeochromocytoma.

Nolotil Europharma, Spain.
Metamizole magnesium (p.35·1).
Fever; pain.

Nolotil Compositum Europharma, Spain.
Metamizole magnesium (p.35·1); hyoscine butylbromide (p.462·3).
Gastro-intestinal spasm; pain.

Noltam Lederle, UK†.
Tamoxifen citrate (p.563·3).
Anovulatory infertility; breast cancer.

Nolvadex
Zeneca, Aust.; ICI, Austral.; Zeneca, Belg.; Zeneca, Canad.; Zeneca, Fr.; Zeneca, Ger.; Zeneca, Irl.; Zeneca, Ital.; Zeneca, Neth.; Zeneca, Norw.; Zeneca, S.Afr.; Zeneca, Spain; Zeneca, Swed.; Zeneca, Switz.; Zeneca, UK; Zeneca, USA.
Tamoxifen citrate (p.563·3).
Anovulatory infertility; breast cancer; endometrial cancer.

Nomapam Amrad, Austral.
Temazepam (p.693·3).
Insomnia.

Nomon Mono Hoyer, Ger.
Cucurbita (p.1569·1).
Urinary-tract disorders.

Non Acid FIRMA, Ital.
Oral granules: Sodium citrate (p.1153·2); potassium citrate (p.1153·1); tribasic sodium phosphate (p.1160·1); tartaric acid (p.1634·3); sodium bicarbonate (p.1153·2).
Tablets: Sodium citrate (p.1153·2); potassium citrate (p.1153·1); tribasic sodium phosphate (p.1160·1).
Gastro-intestinal disorders.

No-Name Dandruff Treatment Sutton, Canad.
Pyrithione zinc (p.1089·3).

Nonan Aguettant, Fr.
Mineral preparation.
Parenteral nutrition.

Nonflamin Yoshitomi, Jpn.
Tinoridine hydrochloride (p.89·2).
Inflammation; pain.

Non-Ovlon Jenapharm, Ger.
Ethinyloestradiol (p.1445·1); norethisterone acetate (p.1453·1).
Combined oral contraceptive; menstrual disorders.

Noodis UCB, Belg.
Piracetam (p.1619·1).
Childhood learning difficulties.

Nootrop UCB, Ger.
Piracetam (p.1619·1).
Mental function disorders.

Nootropil
UCB, Aust.; UCB, Belg.; UCB, Ital.; UCB, Neth.; UCB, S.Afr.; UCB, Spain; UCB, Switz.; UCB, UK.
Piracetam (p.1619·1).
Alcoholism; cerebrovascular disorders; dyslexia; mental function impairment; myoclonus; vertigo.

Nootropyl UCB, Fr.
Piracetam (p.1619·1).
Dyslexia in children; mental function impairment in the elderly; stroke; vertigo.

Nooxine Exel, Belg.†.
Vincamine (p.1644·1).
Mental function disorders.

Nopar Lilly, Ital.
Pergolide mesylate (p.1142·3).
Parkinsonism.

Noparin Novo Nordisk, Swed.†.
Heparin sodium (p.879·3).
Thrombo-embolic disorders.

Nopika Vinas, Spain.
Menthol (p.1600·2).
Insect stings; muscle sprains and strains; pruritus.

Nopil Mepha, Switz.
Co-trimoxazole (p.196·3).
Bacterial infections; Pneumocystis carinii pneumonia.

Nopron
Synthelabo, Fr.; Sanofi Winthrop, Ital.
Niaprazine (p.415·1).
Insomnia.

Nopyn Rolab, S.Afr.
Paracetamol (p.72·2); codeine phosphate (p.26·1); caffeine (p.749·3); meprobamate (p.678·1).
Pain associated with tension.

Noquema Faes, Spain.
Cetylpyridinium chloride (p.1106·2); cholecalciferol (p.1366·3); benzocaine (p.1286·2); retinol (p.1358·1).
Burns.

Norabromol N Michallik, Ger.
Sodium 3,5-dibromo-4-hydroxybenzenesulphonate.
Wounds.

Noradran Norma, UK.
Diphenhydramine hydrochloride (p.409·1); diprophylline (p.752·1); ephedrine hydrochloride (p.1059·3); guaiphenesin (p.1061·3).
Coughs.

Noradrec Recordati, Ital.†.
Noradrenaline acid tartrate (p.924·1).
Hypotension.

Norakin N Hexal, Ger.
Biperiden hydrochloride (p.458·3).
Blepharospasm; dystonias; parkinsonism; torticollis.

Nor-Anaesthol Merz, Ger.
Lignocaine hydrochloride (p.1293·2).
Noradrenaline (p.924·1) is included in this preparation as a vasoconstrictor to diminish absorption and localise the effect of the local anaesthetic.
Local anaesthesia.

Noravid Hoechst Marion Roussel, Ital.
Defibrotide (p.847·1).
Thrombo-embolic disorders.

Norbiline
Bellon, Fr.; Rhone-Poulenc Rorer, Ital.; Semar, Spain†.
Prozapine hydrochloride (p.1622·3); sorbitol (p.1354·2).
Biliary-tract disorders; gastro-intestinal disorders.

Norcept-E Gynopharma, USA†.
Norethisterone (p.1453·1); ethinyloestradiol (p.1445·1).
Combined oral contraceptive.

Norcet Abana, USA†.
Hydrocodone tartrate (p.43·1); paracetamol (p.72·2).
Pain.

Norco Watson, USA.
Hydrocodone tartrate (p.43·1); paracetamol (p.72·2).
Pain.

Norcristine Noristan, S.Afr.†.
Vincristine sulphate (p.570·1).
Malignant neoplasms.

Norcuron
Organon, Aust.; Organon Teknika, Austral.; Organon Teknika, Belg.; Organon, Canad.; Organon Teknika, Ger.; Organon Teknika, Irl.; Organon Teknika, Ital.; Organon Teknika, Neth.; Organon Teknika, Norw.; Sanofi Omnimed, S.Afr.; Organon Teknika, Spain; Organon Teknika, Swed.; Organon Teknika, Switz.; Organon Teknika, UK; Organon, USA.
Vecuronium bromide (p.1323·1).
Competitive neuromuscular blocker.

Nordapanin N Michallik, Ger.
Benzocaine (p.1286·2); acriflavine (p.1098·3).
Mouth and throat disorders.

Nordathricin N Michallik, Ger.
Tyrothricin (p.267·2); cetylpyridinium chloride (p.1106·2); benzocaine (p.1286·2).
Mouth and throat disorders.

Nordaz Bouchara, Fr.
Nordazepam (p.682·3).
Alcohol withdrawal syndrome; anxiety.

Norden Byk Gulden, Ital.†.
Octopamine hydrochloride (p.925·1).
Hypotension.

Nordette
Wyeth, Austral.; Akromed, S.Afr.; Wyeth Lederle, Swed.†; Wyeth-Ayerst, USA.
Levonorgestrel (p.1454·1); ethinyloestradiol (p.1445·1).
28-Day packs also contain 7 inert tablets.
Combined oral contraceptive; menstrual disorders.

Nordicort Ascot, Austral.
Hydrocortisone sodium succinate (p.1044·1).
Corticosteroid.

Nordimmun Novo Nordisk, Swed.†.
A normal immunoglobulin (p.1522·1).
Hypogammaglobulinaemia; idiopathic thrombocytopenic purpura.

Nordiol
Wyeth, Austral.; Akromed, S.Afr.
Levonorgestrel (p.1454·1); ethinyloestradiol (p.1445·1).
28-Day packs also contain 7 inert tablets.
Combined oral contraceptive; menstrual disorders.

Norditropin
Novo Nordisk, Aust.; Novo Nordisk, Austral.; Novo Nordisk, Belg.; Novo Nordisk, Ger.; Novo Nordisk, Irl.; Novo Nordisk, Ital.; Novo Nordisk, Neth.; Novo Nordisk, Norw.; Novo Nordisk, S.Afr.; Novo Nordisk, Spain; Novo Nordisk, Swed.; Novo Nordisk, UK; Novo Nordisk, USA.
Somatropin (p.1249·3).
Growth hormone deficiency; growth retardation due to chronic renal disease; Turner's syndrome.

Norditropine
Novo Nordisk, Fr.; Novo Nordisk, Switz.
Somatropin (p.1249·3).
Growth hormone deficiency; growth retardation in renal failure; Turner's syndrome.

Nordolce Vegetal, Ital.
Acero canadese.
Nutritional supplement.

Nordox Panpharma, UK†.
Doxycycline hydrochloride (p.202·3).
Bacterial infections.

Nordryl Vortech, USA.
Diphenhydramine hydrochloride (p.409·1).
Insomnia; motion sickness; parkinsonism.

Norel US Pharmaceutical, USA.
Phenylephrine hydrochloride (p.1066·2); phenylpropanolamine hydrochloride (p.1067·2); guaiphenesin (p.1061·3).
Upper respiratory-tract symptoms.

Norel Plus US Pharmaceutical, USA.
Phenylpropanolamine hydrochloride (p.1067·2); paracetamol (p.72·2); chlorpheniramine maleate (p.405·1); phenyltoloxamine citrate (p.416·1).
Upper respiratory-tract symptoms.

Norethin 1/35E Schiapparelli Searle, USA.
Norethisterone (p.1453·1); ethinyloestradiol (p.1445·1).
28-Day packs also contain 7 inert tablets.
Combined oral contraceptive.

Norethin 1/50M Schiapparelli Searle, USA.
Norethisterone (p.1453·1); mestranol (p.1450·2).
28-Day packs also contain 7 inert tablets.
Combined oral contraceptive.

Norfemac Hoechst Marion Roussel, Canad.
Bufexamac (p.22·2).
Anorectal disorders; inflammatory skin disorders; phlebitis; vulval disorders.

Norfenazin Reig Jofre, Spain.
Nortriptyline hydrochloride (p.300·2); perphenazine (p.685·2).
Depression.

Norflex
Salus, Aust.; 3M, Austral.; 3M, Belg.; 3M, Canad.; 3M, Ger.; 3M, S.Afr.; 3M, Swed.; 3M, Switz.; 3M, UK†; 3M, USA.
Orphenadrine citrate (p.465·2).
Drug-induced extrapyramidal disorders; hiccups; musculoskeletal and joint disorders; parkinsonism; skeletal muscle spasm; tension headache.

Norflex Co 3M, S.Afr.
Orphenadrine citrate (p.465·2); paracetamol (p.72·2).
Fever; pain; skeletal muscle spasm.

Norfor SmithKline Beecham, Fr.†.
Norethisterone (p.1453·1).
Breast cancer; endometrial cancer.

Norforms Fleet, USA.
Pessaries: Vaginal deodorant.
Topical powder: Corn starch (p.1356·2); zinc oxide (p.1096·2).
Vaginal irritation.

Norgagil Norgine, Fr.
Sterculia (p.1214·1); attapulgite (p.1178·3); meprobamate (p.678·1).
Gastro-intestinal disorders.

Norgalax
Norgine, Belg.; Norgine, Fr.; Norgine, Ger.; Norgine, Irl.; Norgine, Switz.; Norgine, UK.
Docusate sodium (p.1189·3).
Bowel evacuation; constipation.

Norgesic
Note. This name is used for preparations of different composition.
Salus, Aust.; 3M, Austral.; 3M, Irl.; 3M, Norw.†; 3M, Swed.; 3M, Switz.
Orphenadrine citrate (p.465·2); paracetamol (p.72·2).
Skeletal muscle pain and spasm.

3M, Canad.; 3M, USA.
Orphenadrine citrate (p.465·2); aspirin (p.16·1); caffeine (p.749·3).
Skeletal muscle pain.

3M, Ger.†.
Glycol salicylate (p.43·1).
Muscular and neuromuscular pain; rheumatism.

Norgesic N 3M, Ger.
Injection†: Dipyrone (p.35·1).
Pain.
Tablets: Orphenadrine citrate (p.465·2); propyphenazone (p.81·3).
Dysmenorrhoea; headache; musculoskeletal pain.

Norgeston Schering, UK.
Levonorgestrel (p.1454·1).
Progestogen-only oral contraceptive.

Norglicem Rottapharm, Spain.
Glibenclamide (p.319·3).
Diabetes mellitus.

Norglycin Upjohn, Ger.†.
Tolazamide (p.333·2).
Diabetes mellitus.

Norgotin Helsinn Birex, Irl.†.
Ephedrine hydrochloride (p.1059·3); amethocaine hydrochloride (p.1285·2); chlorhexidine acetate (p.1107·2).
Otitis.

Norica Ottolenghi, Ital.
Benzalkonium chloride (p.1101·3).
Room disinfection and deodorization.

Noricaven Bionorica, Ger.†.
Asperula odorata; silybum marianum (p.993·3); crataegus (p.1568·2); rue; echinacea (p.1574·2).
Vascular disorders.

Noricaven novo Bionorica, Ger.
Aesculus (p.1543·3).
Venous insufficiency.

Noriclan Lilly, Spain.
Dirithromycin (p.202·2).
Bacterial infections.

Noriday
Searle, Austral.; Searle, Irl.; Searle, UK.
Norethisterone (p.1453·1).
Progestogen-only oral contraceptive.

Noriel Biogalenique, Fr.†.
Flunitrazepam (p.670·1).
Insomnia.

Norifortan Hoechst Marion Roussel, S.Afr.
Avapyrazone; dipyrone (p.35·1).
Painful smooth muscle spasm.

Norilax Ethimed, S.Afr.†.
Docusate sodium (p.1189·3); danthron (p.1188·2).
Constipation.

Noriline Noristan, S.Afr.†.
Amitriptyline hydrochloride (p.273·3).
Depression; nocturnal enuresis.

Norimin
Monsanto, Austral.; Searle, UK.
Norethisterone (p.1453·1); ethinyloestradiol (p.1445·1).
28-Day packs also contain 7 inert tablets.
Combined oral contraceptive.

Norimode
Noristan, S.Afr.†; Tillomed, UK.
Loperamide hydrochloride (p.1197·2).
Diarrhoea; ostomy management.

Norimox Noristan, S.Afr.†.
Amoxycillin (p.151·3).
Bacterial infections.

Norincol Volchem, Ital.
Carbohydrate, lipid, amino-acid, and dietary fibre preparation.
Nutritional supplement.

Norinyl-1
Searle, Austral.; Searle, Irl.; Syntex, S.Afr.; Searle, UK.
Norethisterone (p.1453·1); mestranol (p.1450·2).
28-Day packs also contain 7 inert tablets.
Combined oral contraceptive; menstrual disorders.

Norinyl 1/50 Searle, Canad.
Norethisterone (p.1453·1); mestranol (p.1450·2).
28-Day packs also contain 7 inert tablets.
Combined oral contraceptive.

Norinyl 1 + 50 Syntex, USA.
Norethisterone (p.1453·1); mestranol (p.1450·2).
28-Day packs also contain 7 inert tablets.
Combined oral contraceptive.

Norinyl 1 + 35 Syntex, USA.
Norethisterone (p.1453·1); ethinyloestradiol (p.1445·1).
28-Day packs also contain 7 inert tablets.
Combined oral contraceptive.

Norinyl 2 mg Syntex, USA†.
Norethisterone (p.1453·1); mestranol (p.1450·2).
Combined oral contraceptive.

Noripam Noristan, S.Afr.†.
Oxazepam (p.683·2).
Alcohol withdrawal syndrome; anxiety disorders.

Norisep Noristan, S.Afr.†.
Co-trimoxazole (p.196·3).
Bacterial infections.

Norisodrine Aerotrol Abbott, USA†.
Isoprenaline hydrochloride (p.892·1).
Asthma; bronchiectasis; bronchitis; bronchospasm; emphysema.

Norisodrine with Calcium Iodide Abbott, USA.
Isoprenaline sulphate (p.892·1); calcium iodide (p.1056·2).
Coughs.

Noristerat
Schering, Fr.; Schering, Ger.; Schering, Ital.†; Schering, UK.
Norethisterone enanthate (p.1453·1).
Progestogen-only injectable contraceptive.

Norit
Wolfs, Belg.; Norit, Neth.
Activated charcoal (p.972·2).
Diarrhoea; treatment of poisoning.

Noritate
Dermik, Canad.; Kestrel, UK; Dermik, USA.
Metronidazole (p.585·1).
Acne; rosacea.

Norit-Carbomix Wolfs, Belg.
Activated charcoal (p.972·2).
Diarrhoea; treatment of poisoning.

Noritren
Lundbeck, Ital.; Lundbeck, Norw.; Lundbeck, Swed.†.
Nortriptyline hydrochloride (p.300·2).
Depression.

Norivite Hoechst Marion Roussel, S.Afr.
Vitamin B substances.

Norivite-12 Ethimed, S.Afr.
Cyanocobalamin (p.1363·3).
Anaemias; tonic.

Norizine Noristan, S.Afr.†.
Cyclizine hydrochloride (p.407·1).
Nausea and vomiting; vestibular disorders.

Norkotral N Desitin, Ger.†.
Oxazepam (p.683·2).
Formerly contained pentobarbitone calcium and promazine phosphate.
Sleep disorders.

Norkotral Tema Desitin, Ger.
Temazepam (p.693·3).
Sleep disorders.

Norlac Rx Solvay, USA†.
Multivitamin and mineral preparation with iron and folic acid.

Norlestrin Parke, Davis, Canad.†.
Norethisterone acetate (p.1453·1); ethinyloestradiol (p.1445·1).
Combined oral contraceptive.

Norlipol Ifesa, Spain†.
Tiadenol (p.1279·3).
Hyperlipidaemias.

Norlutate
Parke, Davis, Canad.; Parke, Davis, USA†.
Norethisterone acetate (p.1453·1).
Abnormal uterine bleeding; amenorrhoea; endometriosis.

Norluten SmithKline Beecham, Fr.
Norethisterone (p.1453·1).
Endometriosis; fibromas; menstrual disorders.

Normabrain Hoechst, Ger.
Piracetam (p.1619·1).
Mental function disorders.

Normacidine Synthelabo, Belg.
Calcium carbonate (p.1182·1); aluminium glycinate (p.1177·2).
Gastro-intestinal disorders associated with hyperacidity.

Normacol
Note. This name is used for preparations of different composition.
Norgine, Belg.; Rivex, Canad.; Norgine, Fr.; Norgine, Irl.; Norgine, S.Afr.; Norgine, Switz.; Norgine, UK.
Sterculia (p.1214·1).
Formerly known as Normacol Special in the *UK*.
Constipation; diverticular disease; ingestion of foreign bodies; ostomy management.

Asche, Ger.†.
Bassorin; frangula bark (p.1193·2).
Constipation.

Schering, Ital.†.
Tragacanth (p.1475·2); frangula bark (p.1193·2).
Constipation.

Normacol a la Bourdaine Norgine, Fr.
Sterculia (p.1214·1); frangula bark (p.1193·2).
Constipation.

Normacol a la Dipropyline Norgine, Fr.†.
Sterculia (p.1214·1); alverine citrate (p.1548·1).
Gastro-intestinal disorders.

Normacol Antispasmodique Norgine, Belg.
Sterculia (p.1214·1); alverine citrate (p.1548·1).
Constipation.

Normacol (avec bourdaine) Norgine, Switz.
Sterculia (p.1214·1); frangula (p.1193·2).
Constipation.

Normacol Forte Stafford-Miller, Spain.
Sterculia (p.1214·1); frangula bark (p.1193·2).
Constipation.

Normacol Granulat Berlin-Chemie, Ger.†.
Sterculia (p.1214·1); frangula bark (p.1193·2).
Constipation.

Normacol Lavement Norgine, Fr.
Monobasic sodium phosphate (p.1159·3); dibasic sodium phosphate (p.1159·3).
Bowel evacuation.

Normacol Plus
Norgine, Austral.; Norgine, Belg.; Norgine, Irl.; Norgine, S.Afr.; Norgine, UK.
Sterculia (p.1214·1); frangula (p.1193·2).
Formerly known as Normacol Standard in *Irl.* and *UK*.
Constipation; diverticulitis.

Normaform Sodip, Switz.
Phentermine resin (as an ion-exchange resin complex) (p.1484·3).
Obesity.

Normalax Herbaline, Ital.
Rhamnus alpinus; globularia vulgaris; chamomile (p.1561·2); red-poppy petal (p.1001·1); liquorice (p.1197·1); fennel (p.1579·1).
Constipation.

Normalene Montefarmaco, Ital.
Bisacodyl (p.1179·3).
Constipation.

Normalin Noristan, S.Afr.†.
Procaterol hydrochloride (p.757·3).
Bronchospasm.

NormaLine Antonetto, Ital.
Glucomannan (p.1584·3).
Dietary supplement in diabetes mellitus and hyperlipidaemias; obesity.

Normalip Knoll, Ger.
Fenofibrate (p.1273·1).
Hyperlipidaemias.

Normaloe Tillomed, UK.
Loperamide hydrochloride (p.1197·2).
Diarrhoea.

Normase Molteni, Ital.
Lactulose (p.1195·3).
Constipation; gastro-intestinal disorders; hepatic encephalopathy.

Normasol Seton, UK.
Sodium chloride (p.1162·2).
Irrigation solution.

Normastigmin Sigmapharm, Aust.
Neostigmine bromide (p.1393·3) or neostigmine methylsulphate (p.1394·1).
Gastro-intestinal atony; glaucoma; myasthenia gravis; pre- and post-operative lowering of intra-ocular pressure; reversal of competitive neuromuscular blockade; reversal of mydriasis and cycloplegia; urinary retention.

The symbol † denotes a preparation no longer actively marketed

Normastigmine mit Pilocarpin Sigmapharm, Aust.
Neostigmine bromide (p.1393·3); pilocarpine hydrochloride (p.1396·3).
Glaucoma; pre- and post-operative lowering of intra-ocular pressure; reversal of mydriasis and cycloplegia.

Normatens Solvay, Neth.
Moxonidine (p.913·1).
Hypertension.

Normax Medeva, UK.
Danthron (p.1188·2); docusate sodium (p.1189·3).
These ingredients can be described by the British Approved Name Co-danthrusate.
Constipation.

Normegon Organon, UK.
Human menopausal gonadotrophins (p.1252·1).
Infertility.

Normensan Dispergo, Aust.
Papaverine hydrochloride (p.1614·2); hyoscyamine (p.464·2); propyphenazone (p.81·3).
Dysmenorrhoea; migraine; smooth muscle spasm.

Normhydral Asta Medica, Aust.†.
Anhydrous glucose; sodium chloride; sodium bicarbonate; potassium chloride (p.1152·3).
Diarrhoea; oral rehydration therapy.

Normicina Tedec Meiji, Spain.
Midecamycin acetate (p.226·2).
Bacterial infections.

Normide Inibsa, Spain†.
Chlordiazepoxide (p.646·3).
Alcohol withdrawal syndrome; anxiety; insomnia.

Normiflo Wyeth-Ayerst, USA.
Ardeparin sodium (p.825·2).
Thrombosis prophylaxis.

Normin Searle, Irl.
Norethisterone (p.1453·1); ethinyloestradiol (p.1445·1).
Combined oral contraceptive.

Normi-Nox Herbrand, Ger.†.
Methaqualone (p.678·3).
Sleep disorders.

Normison
Wyeth, Austral.; Wyeth Lederle, Belg.; Wyeth, Fr.; Wyeth, Irl.; Wyeth, Ital.; Wyeth, Neth.; Akromed, S.Afr.; Wyeth, Switz.; Wyeth, UK.
Temazepam (p.693·3).
Insomnia; premedication.

Normix Wassermann, Ital.
Rifaximin (p.246·3).
Gastro-intestinal bacterial infections; hyperammonaemia.

Normo Gastryl Sabex, Canad.
Sodium bicarbonate (p.1153·2); sodium sulphate (p.1213·3); sodium phosphate (p.1159·3).
Gastric hyperacidity.

Normo Nar Zambon, Spain.
Muramidase hydrochloride (p.1604·3); thonzylamine hydrochloride (p.419·2); methylethylaminophenol hydriodide.
Nasal congestion.

Normobren Medosan, Ital.
Acetylcarnitine hydrochloride (p.1542·1).
Cerebrovascular disorders.

Normoc Merckle, Ger.
Bromazepam (p.643·1).
Anxiety; sleep disorders.

Normo-Calcium Maggioni, Ital.†.
Carnitine hydrochloride (p.1336·2); calcium lactobionate (p.1155·2); multivitamins.
Disorders associated with calcium and vitamin deficiency.

Normodyne Schering, USA.
Labetalol hydrochloride (p.896·1).
Hypertension.

Normofenicol Normon, Spain.
Chloramphenicol (p.182·1) or chloramphenicol sodium succinate (p.182·2).
Lignocaine hydrochloride (p.1293·2) is included in the injection to alleviate the pain of injection.
Bacterial infections.

Normofundin G-5 Braun, Ger.
Electrolyte infusion with glucose (p.1147·1).
Carbohydrate source; fluid and electrolyte disorders.

Normofundin OP Braun, Ger.
Electrolyte infusion (p.1147·1).
Fluid and electrolyte disorders.

Normofundin sKG Braun, Ger.
Potassium-free electrolyte infusion with glucose (p.1147·1).
Carbohydrate source; fluid and electrolyte disorders.

Normofundin X Braun, Ger.
Electrolyte infusion with xylitol (p.1147·1).
Carbohydrate source; fluid and electrolyte disorders.

Normogam ICT, Ital.
Gamolenic acid (p.1582·1).
Gamolenic acid deficiency; nutritional supplement.

Normogamma Nuovo ISM, Ital.
A normal immunoglobulin (p.1522·1).
Passive immunisation.

Normogastryl
Upsamedica, Belg.; UPSA, Fr.; Upsamedica, Spain; Upsamedica, Switz.
Sodium bicarbonate (p.1153·2); anhydrous sodium sulphate (p.1213·3); monobasic sodium phosphate (p.1159·3).
Gastro-intestinal disorders.

Normogin Baldacci, Ital.
Bacilli vaginalis culture.
Vaginal bacterial infections.

Normoglaucon
Tramedico, Belg.; Mann, Ger.; Mann, Neth.
Metipranolol hydrochloride (p.906·3); pilocarpine hydrochloride (p.1396·3).
Glaucoma; ocular hypertension.

Normoglic Salfa, Ital.†.
Chlorpropamide (p.319·1).
Diabetes mellitus.

Normoglucon Klinge, Aust.
Glibenclamide (p.319·3).
Diabetes mellitus.

Normolyt Gebro, Aust.
Anhydrous glucose; sodium chloride; sodium citrate; potassium chloride (p.1152·3).
Diarrhoea; oral rehydration therapy.

Normolytoral Gebro, Switz.
Anhydrous glucose; sodium chloride; sodium citrate; potassium chloride (p.1152·3).
Diarrhoea; oral rehydration therapy.

Normonal Eisai, Jpn.
Tripamide (p.959·2).
Hypertension.

Normonsona Normon, Spain.
Prednisolone (p.1048·1).
Corticosteroid.

Normoparin Caber, Ital.
Heparin sodium (p.879·3).
Thrombo-embolic disorders.

Normophasic Nourypharma, Switz.
7 Tablets, ethinyloestradiol (p.1445·1); 15 tablets, ethinyloestradiol; lynoestrenol (p.1448·2).
Sequential-type oral contraceptive.

Normopresil Semar, Spain.
Chlorthalidone (p.839·3); atenolol (p.825·3).
Hypertension.

Normopress
Note. This name is used for preparations of different composition.
Caber, Ital.
Atenolol (p.825·3); indapamide (p.890·2).
Hypertension.

Schwulst, S.Afr.
Methyldopa (p.904·2).
Hypertension.

Normo-real Sodietal, Fr.
A range of preparations for enteral nutrition.

Normorix
AFI, Norw.; Nycomed, Swed.
Hydrochlorothiazide (p.885·2); amiloride hydrochloride (p.819·2).
Hypertension; liver cirrhosis with ascites; oedema.

Normosang Orphan, Fr.
Haem arginate (p.983·1).
Acute porphyria.

Normosedin Inexfa, Spain†.
Diiodotyrosine (p.1493·1); sodium fluoride (p.742·1).
Hyperthyroidism.

Normosol Abbott, USA.
A range of electrolyte infusions (p.1147·1).
Fluid and electrolyte disorders.

Normosol and Dextrose Abbott, USA.
A range of electrolyte infusions with glucose (p.1147·1).
Carbohydrate source; fluid and electrolyte disorders.

Normosol M 900 Cal Abbott, Ital.
Electrolyte infusion with glucose and fructose (p.1147·1).
Carbohydrate source; fluid and electrolyte disorders.

Normosol M Con Glucosio 5% Abbott, Ital.
Electrolyte infusion with glucose (p.1147·1).
Fluid and electrolyte disorders.

Normosol R Abbott, Ital.
Electrolyte infusion (p.1147·1).
Fluid and electrolyte disorders.

Normosol R Con Glucosio 5% Abbott, Ital.
Electrolyte infusion with glucose (p.1147·1).
Carbohydrate source; fluid and electrolyte disorders.

Normosol R/K Con Glucosio 5% Abbott, Ital.
Electrolyte infusion with glucose (p.1147·1).
Carbohydrate source; fluid and electrolyte disorders.

Normospor Propan, S.Afr.
Clotrimazole (p.376·3).
Fungal infections of the skin; vulvovaginal fungal infections.

Normotensin Hoechst, Aust.
Penbutolol sulphate (p.927·2); frusemide (p.871·1).
Hypertension.

Normothen Bioindustria, Ital.
Doxazosin mesylate (p.862·3).
Hypertension.

Normotin OTW, Ger.†.
Scoparium; convallaria; crataegus; adonis vernalis; cereus grandiflorus; sparteine sulphate (p.1632·1); camphor; ephedrine hydrochloride (p.1059·3).
Hypotension.

Normotin VI OTW, Ger.
Crataegus (p.1568·2).
Cardiac disorders.

Normotin-P OTW, Ger.†.
Ethamivan (p.1480·3); norfenefrine hydrochloride (p.925·1); heptaminol hydrochloride (p.1587·2).
Hypotension.

Normotin-R OTW, Ger.
Ethamivan (p.1480·3); norfenefrine hydrochloride (p.925·1); heptaminol hydrochloride (p.1587·2).
Hypotension.

Normovite Antianem Iny Normon, Spain.
Folic acid (p.1340·3); ferrous gluceptate (p.1339·3).
Lignocaine hydrochloride (p.1293·2) is included in this preparation to alleviate the pain of injection.
Anaemias; tonic.

Normovite Antianemico Normon, Spain.
Folic acid (p.1340·3); ferrous gluceptate (p.1339·3).
Iron and folic acid deficiency.

Normovlar ED Schering, S.Afr.
21 Tablets, levonorgestrel (p.1454·1); ethinyloestradiol (p.1445·1); 7 tablets, inert.
Biphasic oral contraceptive; menstrual disorders.

Normoxidil Medosan, Ital.
Minoxidil (p.910·3).
Alopecia.

Normoxin Asta Medica, Aust.
Moxonidine (p.913·1).
Hypertension.

Normozide Schering, USA†.
Labetalol hydrochloride (p.896·1); hydrochlorothiazide (p.885·2).
Hypertension.

Normum Serpero, Ital.
Sulpiride (p.692·3).
Dysthymia; psychoses.

No-Roma Salt, UK.
A deodorant liquid for use with colostomies and ileostomies.
Formerly known as Saltair No-Roma.

Noroxin
Merck Sharp & Dohme, Austral.; Merck Sharp & Dohme, Canad.; Merck Sharp & Dohme, Ital.; Merck Sharp & Dohme, Neth.; Merck Sharp & Dohme, S.Afr.; Merck Sharp & Dohme, Spain; Merck Sharp & Dohme, Switz.; Merck Sharp & Dohme, UK†; Merck Sharp & Dohme, USA.
Norfloxacin (p.233·1).
Bacterial infections.

Noroxine Merck Sharp & Dohme-Chibret, Fr.
Norfloxacin (p.233·1).
Bacterial infections of the urinary tract; gonococcal cervicitis; gonococcal urethritis.

Nor-Pa Salus, Ital.
Atenolol (p.825·3); indapamide (p.890·2).
Hypertension.

Norpace
Searle, Austral.; Roberts, Canad.; Heumann, Ger.; Searle, S.Afr.; Searle, Switz.; Searle, USA.
Disopyramide phosphate (p.858·1).
Arrhythmias.

Norphen
Byk, Aust.†; Byk Gulden, Ger.†.
Octopamine hydrochloride (p.925·1) or octopamine tartrate (p.925·1).
Cardiac disease; hypotension.

Norphenovit N Byk Gulden, Ger.†.
Octopamine tartrate (p.925·1); thiamine nitrate; riboflavine; cyanocobalamin; nicotinamide; ascorbic acid.
Hypotension.

Norphyllin SR Norton, UK.
Aminophylline (p.748·1).
Bronchospasm.

Norplant
Wyeth-Ayerst, Canad.; Leiras, Swed.; Hoechst Marion Roussel, UK; Wyeth-Ayerst, USA.
Levonorgestrel (p.1454·1).
Progestogen-only implantable contraceptive.

Norplatin Noristan, S.Afr.†.
Cisplatin (p.513·3).
Malignant neoplasms.

Norpramin
Note. This name is used for preparations of different composition.
Hoechst Marion Roussel, Canad.; Hoechst Marion Roussel, USA.
Desipramine hydrochloride (p.282·2).
Depression.

CEPA, Spain.
Omeprazole (p.1204·2).
Gastro-oesophageal reflux; peptic ulcer; Zollinger-Ellison syndrome.

Norpro Noristan, S.Afr.†.
Propranolol hydrochloride (p.937·1).
Anxiety disorders; cardiovascular disorders.

Norprolac
Sandoz, Aust.; Sandoz, Fr.; Sandoz, Ger.; Novartis, Neth.; Sandoz, Norw.; Novartis, S.Afr.; Sandoz, Spain; Novartis, Swed.; Sandoz, Switz.; Sandoz, UK.
Quinagolide hydrochloride (p.1143·3).
Hyperprolactinaemia.

Nor-QD Syntex, USA.
Norethisterone (p.1453·1).
Progestogen-only oral contraceptive.

Norquentiel SmithKline Beecham, Fr.†.
15 Tablets, ethinyloestradiol (p.1445·1); 6 tablets, ethinyloestradiol; norethisterone (p.1453·1).
Sequential-type oral contraceptive.

Nortab Bristol-Myers Squibb, Austral.†.
Nortriptyline hydrochloride (p.300·2).
Depression.

Nortase Asche, Ger.
Rizolipase; protease and amylase from *Aspergillus oryzae*.
Digestive system disorders.

Nortem Norton Waterford, Irl.
Temazepam (p.693·3).
Insomnia.

Nortensin Hoechst, Ger.†.
Reserpine (p.942·1); frusemide (p.871·1).
Hypertension.

Nor-Tet Vortech, USA.
Tetracycline hydrochloride (p.259·1).
Bacterial infections.

Nortimil Chiesi, Ital.
Desipramine hydrochloride (p.282·2).
Depression; psychoses.

Nortrilen
Lundbeck, Aust.; Lundbeck, Belg.; Promonta Lundbeck, Ger.; Lundbeck, Neth.; Lundbeck, Switz.
Nortriptyline hydrochloride (p.300·2).
Depression.

Nortron Dista, Spain.
Dirithromycin (p.202·2).
Bacterial infections.

Nortussine
Note. This name is used for preparations of different composition.
Norgine, Belg.; Norgine, Fr.
Syrup: Dextromethorphan hydrobromide (p.1057·3); mepyramine maleate (p.414·1); phenylephrine hydrochloride (p.1066·2); guaiphenesin (p.1061·3).
Coughs.

Norgine, Fr.
Paediatric syrup: Dextromethorphan hydrobromide (p.1057·3); mepyramine maleate (p.414·1); guaiphenesin (p.1061·3).
Coughs.

Noruxol Knoll, Ital.
Collagenase (p.1566·3).
Necrotic wounds and ulcers.

Norval Bencard, UK†.
Mianserin hydrochloride (p.297·1).
Depression.

Norvas Pfizer, Spain.
Amlodipine besylate (p.822·3).
Angina pectoris; hypertension.

Norvasc
Pfizer, Aust.; Pfizer, Austral.; Pfizer, Canad.; Pfizer, Ger.; Mack, Illert., Ger.; Pfizer, Ital.; Pfizer, Neth.; Pfizer, Norw.; Pfizer, S.Afr.; Pfizer, Swed.; Pfizer, Switz.; Pfizer, USA.
Amlodipine besylate (p.822·3).
Angina pectoris; hypertension.

Norvedan
Boehringer Mannheim, Aust.; LPB, Ital.†.
Fentiazac (p.41·1) or fentiazac calcium (p.41·1).
Inflammation; musculoskeletal and joint disorders; pain.

Norvir
Abbott, Austral.; Abbott, Ital.; Abbott, Neth.; Abbott, Spain; Abbott, Swed.; Abbott, Switz.; Abbott, UK; Abbott, USA.
Ritonavir (p.625·1).
HIV infection.

Norvital Zyma, Ital.†.
Nutritional supplement.

Norwich Extra Strength Procter & Gamble, USA.
Aspirin (p.16·1).
Fever; inflammation; myocardial infarction; pain; transient ischaemic attacks.

Norzetam Chemil, Ital.
Piracetam (p.1619·1).
Mental function impairment.

Norzine Purdue Frederick, USA.
Thiethylperazine maleate (p.419·2).
Nausea and vomiting.

Norzol Rosemont, UK.
Metronidazole benzoate (p.585·1).
Bacterial infections.

NoSalt Norcliff Thayer, USA†.
Low sodium dietary salt substitute.

Noscaflex Wolfs, Belg.
Paediatric syrup: Noscapine camsylate (p.1065·2).
Syrup: Noscapine hydrochloride (p.1065·2); guaiphenesin (p.1061·3).
Tablets: Noscapine hydrochloride (p.1065·2).
Coughs.

Noscal Sankyo, Jpn.
Troglitazone (p.334·1).
Diabetes mellitus.

Noscalin Sauter, Switz.†.
Noscapine (p.1065·2); menthol (p.1600·2).
Coughs.

Noscorex Interdelta, Switz.
Noscapine hydrochloride (p.1065·2); guaiphenesin (p.1061·3).
Coughs; upper-respiratory-tract inflammation.

Nose Fresh Rappai, Switz.
Sea salt (p.1162·2).
Nasal disorders.

Nosebo Ottolenghi, Ital.
Sulphur (p.1091·2).
Acne; skin cleansing.

Nosenil Farbo, Ital.
Ginkgo biloba (p.1584·1); eleutherococcus (p.1584·2); kola (p.1645·1); equisetum (p.1575·1); urtica (p.1642·3).

Nose-X Pharmco, S.Afr.†.
Oxymetazoline hydrochloride (p.1065·3).
Nasal congestion.

Nosor Nose Balm Pickles, UK.
Dibromopropamidine isethionate (p.1112·2); wheatgerm oil; camphor (p.1557·2); menthol (p.1600·2); eucalyptus (p.1578·1).

No-spa *Chinoin, Hung.*
Drotaverine hydrochloride (p.1574·2).
Peptic ulcer; smooth muscle spasm.

Nospilin *Ciba Vision, Switz.†.*
Antazoline sulphate (p.402·1); xylometazoline hydrochloride (p.1071·2).
Eye irritation.

Nossacin *Benedetti, Ital.*
Cinoxacin (p.185·2).
Bacterial infections of the urinary tract.

Nostril
Note. This name is used for preparations of different composition.
Boehringer Ingelheim, Fr.†.
Chlorhexidine gluconate (p.1107·2); cetrimonium bromide (p.1106·1).
Nose and throat infections.

Ciba, USA.
Phenylephrine hydrochloride (p.1066·2).
Nasal congestion.

Nostrilla *Ciba Consumer, USA.*
Oxymetazoline hydrochloride (p.1065·3).
Nasal congestion.

Nostroline *Bioglan, UK†.*
Menthol (p.1600·2).
Nasal congestion.

Notakehl *Sanum-Kehlbeck, Ger.*
Homoeopathic preparation.

Noten *Alphapharm, Austral.*
Atenolol (p.825·3).
Angina pectoris; arrhythmias; hypertension; myocardial infarction.

Notens *Farge, Ital.†.*
Bendrofluazide (p.827·3); syrosingopine (p.951·2).
Kidney disorders.

Notezine *Pharmacie Centrale des Hopitaux, Fr.†.*
Diethylcarbamazine citrate (p.99·2).
Filariasis.

Notul *Mendelejeff, Ital.*
Cimetidine hydrochloride (p.1185·3).
Gastro-intestinal disorders associated with hyperacidity.

Nourilax *Chefaro, Neth.†.*
Bisacodyl (p.1179·3).
Constipation.

Nourishake *Neo-Life, Austral.*
Nutritional supplement.

Noury Hoofdlotion *Chefaro, Neth.†.*
Malathion (p.1407·3).
Pediculosis.

Nourymag *Nourypharma, Ger.*
Racemic magnesium aspartate (p.1157·2).
Magnesium deficiency.

Nourytam *Nourypharma, Ger.*
Tamoxifen citrate (p.563·3).
Breast cancer.

Nova Perfecting Lotion *Avon, Canad.*
Salicylic acid (p.1090·2).
Acne.

Nova Rectal *Sabex, Canad.*
Pentobarbitone sodium (p.685·1).
Insomnia; sedative.

Novaban
Sandoz, Belg.; Novartis, Neth.
Tropisetron hydrochloride (p.1217·3).
Nausea and vomiting.

Novabritine *Bencard, Belg.*
Amoxycillin sodium (p.151·3) or amoxycillin trihydrate (p.151·3).
Bacterial infections.

Novacef *IFI, Ital.*
Propylene glycol cefatrizine (p.164·2).
Bacterial infections.

Novacet *GenDerm, USA.*
Sulphacetamide sodium (p.252·2); sulphur (p.1091·2).
Acne; seborrhoeic dermatitis.

Novacetol *Pharmastra, Fr.*
Aspirin (p.16·1); paracetamol (p.72·2); codeine hydrochloride (p.26·1).
Fever; pain.

Novaclens *Johnson & Johnson, Austral.†.*
Chlorhexidine gluconate (p.1107·2).
Skin disinfection; wounds.

Novacnyl *Esseti, Ital.*
Meclocycline sulfosalicylate (p.224·1).
Skin infections.

Novacol *Johnson & Johnson, Austral.†.*
Chlorhexidine gluconate (p.1107·2).
Skin, surface and instrument disinfection.

Novacort
Note. This name is used for preparations of different composition.
Pulitzer, Ital.†.
Suprarenal cortex (p.1050·1).
Adrenal insufficiency; endotoxic shock; tonic.

Syntex, Switz.†.
Cloprednol (p.1035·3).
Corticosteroid.

Novacrom *Novopharma, Switz.†.*
Sodium cromoglycate (p.762·1).
Allergic eye disorders.

Nova-Dec *Rugby, USA.*
Multivitamin and mineral preparation with iron and folic acid.

Novaderm *Johnson & Johnson, Austral.†.*
Triclosan (Irgasan DP300) (p.1127·2).
Skin disinfection.

Novadine *Johnson & Johnson, Austral.†.*
Povidone-iodine (p.1123·3).
Abrasions; burns; skin disinfection; skin infections.

Novadral
Parke, Davis, Aust.; Godecke, Ger.; Warner-Lambert, Switz.
Norfenefrine hydrochloride (p.925·1).
Hypotension.

Novafed *Marion Merrell Dow, USA†.*
Pseudoephedrine hydrochloride (p.1068·3).
Nasal congestion.

Novafed A *Hoechst Marion Roussel, USA.*
Pseudoephedrine hydrochloride (p.1068·3); chlorpheniramine maleate (p.405·1).
Upper respiratory-tract symptoms.

Novagard *Pharmacia Upjohn, UK†.*
Copper-wound plastic (p.1337·3).
Intra-uterine contraceptive device.

Novagcilina *Novag, Spain.*
Amoxycillin sodium (p.151·3) or amoxycillin trihydrate (p.151·3).
Bacterial infections.

Novagest Expectorant with Codeine *Major, USA.*
Guaiphenesin (p.1061·3); pseudoephedrine hydrochloride (p.1068·3); codeine phosphate (p.26·1).
Coughs.

Novahaler *3M, Spain.*
Beclomethasone dipropionate (p.1032·1).
Asthma.

Novahistex *Merrell Dow, Canad.†.*
Nasal spray: Xylometazoline hydrochloride (p.1071·2).
Capsules: Pseudoephedrine hydrochloride (p.1068·3); chlorpheniramine maleate (p.405·1).
Respiratory-tract congestion.

Novahistex C *Hoechst Marion Roussel, Canad.*
Codeine phosphate (p.26·1); phenylephrine hydrochloride (p.1066·2).
Coughs.

Novahistex DH *Hoechst Marion Roussel, Canad.*
Hydrocodone tartrate (p.43·1); phenylephrine hydrochloride (p.1066·2).
Coughs.

Novahistex DH Expectorant *Hoechst Marion Roussel, Canad.*
Phenylephrine hydrochloride (p.1066·2); hydrocodone tartrate (p.43·1); guaiphenesin (p.1061·3).
Coughs.

Novahistex DM *Hoechst Marion Roussel, Canad.*
Dextromethorphan hydrobromide (p.1057·3); pseudoephedrine hydrochloride (p.1068·3).
Formerly contained dextromethorphan hydrobromide and phenylephrine hydrochloride.
Coughs; nasal/sinus congestion.

Novahistex DM Expectorant *Hoechst Marion Roussel, Canad.*
Dextromethorphan hydrobromide (p.1057·3); guaiphenesin (p.1061·3); pseudoephedrine hydrochloride (p.1068·3).
Formerly contained dextromethorphan hydrobromide, phenylephrine hydrochloride, and guaiphenesin.
Coughs; nasal/sinus congestion.

Novahistex Expectorant *Hoechst Marion Roussel, Canad.*
Guaiphenesin (p.1061·3); pseudoephedrine hydrochloride (p.1068·3).
Formerly contained phenylephrine hydrochloride and guaiphenesin.
Respiratory-tract congestion.

Novahistex Sinus *Merrell Dow, Canad.†.*
Paracetamol (p.72·2); pseudoephedrine hydrochloride (p.1068·3).
Sinus headache and congestion.

Novahistine
Note. This name is used for preparations of different composition.
Hoechst Marion Roussel, Canad.
Phenylephrine hydrochloride (p.1066·2).
Nasal/sinus congestion.

SmithKline Beecham, USA†.
Phenylephrine hydrochloride (p.1066·2); chlorpheniramine maleate (p.405·1).
Upper respiratory-tract symptoms.

Novahistine DH
Note. This name is used for preparations of different composition.
Hoechst Marion Roussel, Canad.
Hydrocodone tartrate (p.43·1); phenylephrine hydrochloride (p.1066·2).
Coughs.

SmithKline Beecham, USA†.
Codeine phosphate (p.26·1); pseudoephedrine hydrochloride (p.1068·3); chlorpheniramine maleate (p.405·1).
Coughs; nasal congestion.

Novahistine DM *Hoechst Marion Roussel, Canad.*
Dextromethorphan hydrobromide (p.1057·3); pseudoephedrine hydrochloride (p.1068·3).
Formerly contained dextromethorphan hydrobromide and phenylephrine hydrochloride.
Coughs; nasal/sinus congestion.

Novahistine DM Expectorant *Hoechst Marion Roussel, Canad.*
Dextromethorphan hydrobromide (p.1057·3); guaiphenesin (p.1061·3); pseudoephedrine hydrochloride (p.1068·3).
Formerly contained dextromethorphan hydrobromide, phenylephrine hydrochloride, and guaiphenesin.
Coughs; nasal/sinus congestion.

Novahistine DMX *SmithKline Beecham, USA†.*
Pseudoephedrine hydrochloride (p.1068·3); dextromethorphan hydrobromide (p.1057·3); guaiphenesin (p.1061·3).
Coughs.

Novahistine Expectorant *SmithKline Beecham, USA†.*
Codeine phosphate (p.26·1); pseudoephedrine hydrochloride (p.1068·3); guaiphenesin (p.1061·3).
Coughs; respiratory congestion.

Novain *Agepha, Aust.*
Oxybuprocaine hydrochloride (p.1298·1).
Local anaesthesia.

Novalac Diarelac *Novalac, Fr.*
Infant feed.
Diarrhoea.

Novalgin
Hoechst, Aust.; Hoechst, Ger.; Hoechst Marion Roussel, Neth.; Hoechst Marion Roussel, Swed.
Dipyrone (p.35·1).
Fever; pain.

Novalgina *Hoechst Marion Roussel, Ital.*
Dipyrone (p.35·1).
Fever; pain.

Novalgine
Hoechst Marion Roussel, Belg.; Hoechst, Fr.†; Hoechst Marion Roussel, Switz.
Dipyrone (p.35·1).
Fever; pain.

Novalm *LDM, Fr.*
Meprobamate (p.678·1).
Anxiety.

Novalucol *Hassle, Swed.*
Chewable tablets†: Aluminium hydroxide (p.1177·3); magnesium carbonate (p.1198·1).
Mixture: Aluminium hydroxide (p.1177·3); magnesium hydroxide (p.1198·2).
Heartburn; peptic ulcer.

Novalucol Novum *Hassle, Swed.*
Calcium carbonate (p.1182·1); magnesium hydroxide (p.1198·2).
Heartburn.

Novalucol S *Hassle, Swed.†.*
Aluminium hydroxide (p.1177·3); magnesium carbonate (p.1198·1); magnesium subcarbonate.
Antacid.

Novaluzid
Hassle, Norw.; Hassle, Swed.
Magnesium hydroxide (p.1198·2); magnesium carbonate (p.1198·1); aluminium hydroxide (p.1177·3).
Dyspepsia; gastritis; heartburn; hyperacidity; peptic ulcer.

Novamilor *Novopharm, Canad.*
Amiloride hydrochloride (p.819·2); hydrochlorothiazide (p.885·2).
Hypertension; oedema.

Novamina *PQS, Spain.*
Benzalkonium chloride (p.1101·3).
Instrument disinfection; skin and wound disinfection.

Novamine *Clintec, USA.*
Amino-acid infusion.
Parenteral nutrition.

Novamoxin *Novopharm, Canad.*
Amoxycillin trihydrate (p.151·3).
Bacterial infections.

Novanaest *Gebro, Aust.*
Procaine hydrochloride (p.1299·2).
Local anaesthesia.

Novaneurina B12 *ISI, Ital.*
Thiamine monophosphate monochloride (p.1361·2); cyanocobalamin (p.1363·3).
Neuritis; vitamin supplement.

Novanox *Pfleger, Ger.*
Nitrazepam (p.682·2).
Sleep disorders.

Novantron
Wyeth Lederle, Aust.; Lederle, Ger.; Lederle, Switz.
Mitozantrone hydrochloride (p.553·3).
Malignant neoplasms.

Novantrone
Lederle, Austral.; Wyeth Lederle, Belg.; Wyeth-Ayerst, Canad.; Lederle, Fr.; Wyeth, Irl.; Cyanamid, Ital.; Lederle, Neth.; Wyeth, Norw.; Wyeth, S.Afr.; Cyanamid, Spain; Wyeth Lederle, Swed.; Lederle, UK; Immunex, USA.
Mitozantrone hydrochloride (p.553·3).
Malignant neoplasms.

Novapamyl *Novalis, Fr.*
Verapamil hydrochloride (p.960·3).
Hypertension.

Novapen
Note. This name is used for preparations of different composition.
Pinewood, Irl.
Ampicillin (p.153·1).
Bacterial infections.

IBP, Ital.†.
Dicloxacillin sodium (p.202·1).
Gram-positive bacterial infections.

Novapirina *Zyma, Ital.*
Diclofenac sodium (p.31·2).
Fever; pain.

Novaprin *Pharmexco, UK.*
Ibuprofen (p.44·1).

Novarok *Schering, Jpn.*
Imidapril hydrochloride (p.890·2).
Hypertension.

Novaruca *Bioglan, UK†.*
Glutaraldehyde (p.1114·3).
Viral warts.

Novasen *Novopharm, Canad.*
Aspirin (p.16·1).
Inflammation; pain.

Novasil Plus *Seton, UK†.*
Aluminium hydroxide (p.1177·3); magnesium hydroxide (p.1198·2); simethicone (p.1213·1).
Gastro-intestinal disorders.

Novasone *Schering-Plough, Austral.*
Mometasone furoate (p.1047·2).
Skin disorders.

Novasrub *Johnson & Johnson, Austral.†.*
Povidone-iodine (p.1123·3); triclosan (p.1127·2).
Skin disinfection.

Novastan *Mitsubishi, Jpn.*
Argatroban (p.825·3).
Thrombo-embolic disorders.

Nova-T
Berlex, Canad.; Schering, Fr.; Schering, Ger.; Schering, Ital.; Schering, Neth.; Schering, S.Afr.; Schering, Switz.; Schering, UK.
Copper-wound plastic (p.1337·3) with a silver core (p.1629·2).
Intra-uterine contraceptive device.

Novatane *Johnson & Johnson, Austral.†.*
Chlorhexidine gluconate (p.1107·2).
Instrument disinfection; skin disinfection; wounds.

Novatec
Merck Sharp & Dohme, Belg.; Merck Sharp & Dohme, Neth.
Lisinopril (p.898·2).
Heart failure; hypertension; myocardial infarction.

Novatox *Pulitzer, Ital.*
Glutathione (p.983·1).
Alcohol and drug poisoning; radiation trauma.

Novatropina *Asta Medica, Ital.†.*
Homatropine methobromide (p.462·2).
Smooth muscle spasm.

Novazam *Genevrier, Fr.*
Diazepam (p.661·1).
Alcohol withdrawal syndrome; anxiety.

Novazyd
Merck Sharp & Dohme, Belg.; Merck Sharp & Dohme, Neth.
Lisinopril (p.898·2); hydrochlorothiazide (p.885·2).
Hypertension.

Novelciclina *Sabater, Spain.*
Doxycycline hydrochloride (p.202·3).
Bacterial infections.

Novelian *Prodes, Spain.*
Sumatriptan succinate (p.450·1).
Cluster headache; migraine.

Noventerol *Laves, Ger.†; Chefaro, Ger.†.*
Activated charcoal (p.972·2); kaolin (p.1195·1); pectin (p.1474·1); fresh milk powder; lactose.
Diarrhoea.

Noveril
Sandoz, Aust.; Wander, Belg.†; Wander, Ger.; Sandoz, Ital.†; Wander, Neth.†; Sandoz, S.Afr.†; Sandoz, Switz.
Dibenzepin hydrochloride (p.282·3).
Depression; nocturnal enuresis.

Novesin
Restan, S.Afr.; Ciba Vision, Switz.
Oxybuprocaine hydrochloride (p.1298·1).
Local anaesthesia.

Novesina *Sandoz, Ital.*
Oxybuprocaine hydrochloride (p.1298·1).
Local anaesthesia.

Novesine
Bournonville, Belg.; Merck Sharp & Dohme-Chibret, Fr.; Ciba Vision, Ger.; Wander, Switz.†.
Oxybuprocaine hydrochloride (p.1298·1).
Local anaesthesia.

Novesine 1% *Wander, Ger.*
Oxybuprocaine hydrochloride (p.1298·1).
Local anaesthesia.

Novesine 1% KNO *Bournonville, Neth.†.*
Oxybuprocaine hydrochloride (p.1298·1).
Local anaesthesia.

Novid *Nycomed, Norw.*
Aspirin (p.16·1).
Fever; pain.

Novidol *Synpharma, Switz.*
Salicylamide (p.82·3); propyphenazone (p.81·3); caffeine (p.749·3).
Fever; pain.

Novidroxin *Fatol, Ger.*
Hydroxocobalamin acetate (p.1364·2).
Vitamin B deficiency.

Noviform
Ciba Vision, Ger.; Meda, Swed.; Ciba Vision, Switz.
Bibrocathol (p.1553·2).
Eye disorders.

Noviform-Aethylmorphin *Dispersa, Ger.†.*
Bibrocathol (p.1553·2); ethylmorphine hydrochloride (p.36·1).
Eye disorders.

Noviforme *Novopharma, Switz.*
Bibrocathol (p.1553·2).
Eye disorders.

Novifort *Ciba Vision, Ger.*
Bibrocathol (p.1553·2); hydrocortisone acetate (p.1043·3).
Allergic and inflammatory disorders of the eye.

Novilax *Eurospital, Ital.*
Sodium lauryl sulphate (p.1468·3); sodium citrate (p.1153·2); glycerol (p.1585·2); sorbitol (p.1354·2).
Formerly known as Microlax.
Constipation.

Novim *Lalco, Canad.*
Multivitamin and mineral preparation.

Novipec *Montavit, Aust.*
Salverine (p.1627·2); ephedrine (p.1059·3); spike lavender oil (p.1632·2).
Respiratory-tract disorders.

Novirell B *Sanorell, Ger.*
Thiamine hydrochloride (p.1361·1); pyridoxine hydrochloride (p.1362·3); cyanocobalamin (p.1363·3).
Lignocaine hydrochloride (p.1293·2) is included in this preparation to alleviate the pain of injection.
Dermatoses; neuralgia; neuritis; rheumatic disorders; spinal disorders.

Noviserum Antitet *IBYS, Spain†.*
A tetanus immunoglobulin (p.1535·2).
Passive immunisation.

Novitan *Theranol-Deglaude, Fr.*
Procaine hydrochloride (p.1299·2); haematoporphyrin (p.1587·1).
Tonic.

Novo AC and C *Novopharm, Canad.*
Aspirin (p.16·1); caffeine (p.749·3); codeine phosphate (p.26·1).
Pain.

Novo Aerofil Sedante *Panto, Spain.*
Dimethicone (p.1213·1); metoclopramide hydrochloride (p.1200·3); oxazepam (p.683·2).
Gastro-intestinal disorders.

Novo B *Novopharm, Canad.*
Vitamin B substances and vitamin C.

Novo Dermoquinona *Llorente, Spain.*
Mequinol (p.1086·2).
Hyperpigmentation.

Novo E *Novopharm, Canad.*
d-Alpha tocopheryl acetate (p.1369·2) or *dl*-alpha tocopheryl acetate (p.1369·2).

Novo Mandrogallan N *Dolorgiet, Ger.*
Chelidonium; taraxacum (p.1634·2); absinthium (p.1541·1).
Biliary-tract disorders; dyspepsia.

Novo Melanidina *Llorente, Spain.*
Psoralen.
Suntanning; vitiligo.

Novo Petrin *OTW, Ger.*
Paracetamol (p.72·2); propyphenazone (p.81·3); caffeine (p.749·3).
Fever; pain.

Novo V-K *Novo Nordisk, S.Afr.*
Phenoxymethylpenicillin potassium (p.236·2).
Bacterial infections.

Novo-Alprazol *Novopharm, Canad.*
Alprazolam (p.640·3).
Anxiety; sedative.

Novo-Atenol *Novopharm, Canad.*
Atenolol (p.825·3).
Angina pectoris; hypertension.

Novo-AZT *Novopharm, Canad.*
Zidovudine (p.630·2).
HIV infection.

Novobedouze
Therabel Pharma, Belg.; Bouchara, Fr.†; Bouchara, Switz.†.
Hydroxocobalamin acetate (p.1364·2).
Neuralgia; vitamin B_{12} deficiency.

Novobiocyl *Francia, Ital.*
Cefoperazone sodium (p.167·3).
Lignocaine hydrochloride (p.1293·2) is included in this preparation to alleviate the pain of injection.
Bacterial infections.

Novo-Butamide *Novopharm, Canad.*
Tolbutamide (p.333·2).
Diabetes mellitus.

Novo-Butazone *Novopharm, Canad.*
Phenylbutazone (p.79·2).
Arthritis; inflammation.

Novocain
Sanofi Winthrop, Canad.; Hoechst, Ger.; Sanofi Winthrop, USA.
Procaine hydrochloride (p.1299·2).
Local anaesthesia.

Novo-Carbamaz *Novopharm, Canad.*
Carbamazepine (p.339·2).
Epilepsy.

Novo-Card-Fludilat *Thiemann, Ger.†.*
Bencyclane fumarate (p.827·3); β-acetyldigoxin (p.812·3).
Cardiovascular disorders.

Novo-Cerusol *Novopharma, Switz.*
Xylene (p.1381·3).
Ear wax removal.

Novocetam *Beiersdorf-Lilly, Ger.*
Piracetam (p.1619·1).
Mental function disorders.

Novo-Chlorocap *Novopharm, Canad.*
Chloramphenicol (p.182·1).
Bacterial infections.

Novo-Cholamine *Novopharm, Canad.*
Cholestyramine (p.1269·3).
Bile-acid induced diarrhoea; hypercholesterolaemia; pruritus associated with partial biliary obstruction.

Novocholin *Adler, Aust.*
Herba teucrii; agrimony herb; rhubarb (p.1212·1); peppermint oil (p.1208·1).
Biliary disorders.

Novocillin *Novo Nordisk, S.Afr.*
Procaine penicillin (p.240·2).
Bacterial infections.

Novo-Cimetine *Novopharm, Canad.*
Cimetidine (p.1183·2).
Histamine H_2 receptor antagonist.

Novo-Clopamine *Novopharm, Canad.*
Clomipramine hydrochloride (p.281·2).
Depression.

Novo-Clopate *Novopharm, Canad.*
Potassium clorazepate (p.657·1).
Anxiety; sedative.

Novo-Cloxin *Novopharm, Canad.*
Cloxacillin sodium (p.195·2).
Bacterial infections.

Novo-Cycloprine *Novopharm, Canad.*
Cyclobenzaprine hydrochloride (p.1313·2).
Skeletal muscle spasm.

Novo-Difenac *Novopharm, Canad.*
Diclofenac sodium (p.31·2).
Osteoarthritis; rheumatoid arthritis.

Novodigal
Asta Medica, Aust.; Asta Medica, Belg.; Beiersdorf-Lilly, Ger.
β-Acetyldigoxin (p.812·3) or digoxin (p.849·3).
Arrhythmias; heart failure.

Novodil
Note. This name is used for preparations of different composition.
Augot, Fr.
Cyclandelate (p.845·2).
Mental function impairment in the elderly.
OFF, Ital.
Dipyridamole (p.857·1).
Thrombo-embolic disorders.

Novo-Diltazem *Novopharm, Canad.*
Diltiazem hydrochloride (p.854·2).
Angina pectoris.

Novo-Dimenate *Novopharm, Canad.*
Dimenhydrinate (p.408·2).
Nausea and vomiting; vertigo.

Novo-Dipam *Novopharm, Canad.*
Diazepam (p.661·1).

Novo-Dipiradol *Novopharm, Canad.*
Dipyridamole (p.857·1).
Cardiac disorders.

Novodone *AGIPS, Ital.†.*
Amidopyrine guaiacolglycolate (p.15·2); calcium monoethylcamphorate; vitamin A; ergocalciferol.
Fever; pain.

Novo-Doparil *Novopharm, Canad.*
Methyldopa (p.904·2); hydrochlorothiazide (p.885·2).
Hypertension.

Novodorm *Rubio, Spain†.*
Triazolam (p.696·3).
Insomnia.

Novo-Doxylin *Novopharm, Canad.*
Doxycycline hydrochloride (p.202·3).
Bacterial infections.

Novo-Ferrogluc *Novopharm, Canad.*
Ferrous gluconate (p.1340·1).
Iron-deficiency anaemia.

Novo-Ferrosulfate *Novopharm, Canad.*
Ferrous sulphate (p.1340·2).
Iron-deficiency anaemia.

Novo-Fibrate *Novopharm, Canad.*
Clofibrate (p.1271·1).
Hyperlipidaemias.

Novo-Fibre *Novopharm, Canad.*
Grain and citrus fibre.
Bowel disorders; constipation; fibre supplement.

Novofilin *Ferrer, Spain.*
Diprophylline (p.752·1); proxyphylline (p.757·3); theophylline (p.765·1).
Obstructive airways disease.

Novofluen *Engelhard, Ger.†.*
Co-dergocrine mesylate (p.1566·1).
Adjuvant for mental function disorders; cervical disc syndrome; hypertension.

Novo-Flupam *Novopharm, Canad.*
Flurazepam hydrochloride (p.672·2).
Insomnia.

Novo-Flurazine *Novopharm, Canad.*
Trifluoperazine hydrochloride (p.697·3).

Novo-Flurprofen *Novopharm, Canad.*
Flurbiprofen (p.42·1).
Inflammation; pain.

Novo-Folacid *Novopharm, Canad.*
Folic acid (p.1340·3).
Anaemias.

Novo-Fumar *Novopharm, Canad.*
Ferrous fumarate (p.1339·3).
Iron deficiency anaemias.

Novo-Furan *Novopharm, Canad.*
Nitrofurantoin (p.231·3).
Bacterial infections of the urinary tract.

Novogel *Morado, Ital.*
Royal jelly (p.1626·3); liver extract.
Nutritional supplement.

Novogent *Temmler, Ger.*
Ibuprofen (p.44·1).
Musculoskeletal and joint disorders.

Novo-Gesic *Novopharm, Canad.*
Paracetamol (p.72·2).
Fever; pain.

Novo-Gesic C *Novopharm, Canad.*
Paracetamol (p.72·2); caffeine (p.749·3); codeine phosphate (p.26·1).
Fever; pain.

Novogyn *Schering, Ital.*
Levonorgestrel (p.1454·1); ethinyloestradiol (p.1445·1).
Combined oral contraceptive.

Novo-Helisen
Chemomedica, Aust.†; Allergopharma, Ger.; Allergopharma, Switz.
Allergen extracts (p.1545·1).
Hyposensitisation.

Novo-Hexidyl *Novopharm, Canad.*
Benzhexol hydrochloride (p.457·3).

Novo-Hydrazide *Novopharm, Canad.*
Hydrochlorothiazide (p.885·2).
Hypertension; oedema.

Novo-Hydrocort *Novopharm, Canad.*
Hydrocortisone (p.1043·3) or hydrocortisone acetate (p.1043·3).
Topical corticosteroid.

Novo-Hylazin *Novopharm, Canad.*
Hydralazine hydrochloride (p.883·2).
Hypertension.

Novo-Ipramide *Novopharm, Canad.*
Ipratropium bromide (p.754·2).
Bronchodilator.

Novo-Keto *Novopharm, Canad.*
Ketoprofen (p.48·2).
Fever; pain.

Novo-Lexin *Novopharm, Canad.*
Cephalexin (p.178·2).
Bacterial infections.

Novolin 10/90, 20/80, 30/70, 40/60, 50/50
Novo Nordisk, Canad.; Novo Nordisk, USA.
Mixtures of insulin injection (human) and isophane insulin injection (human) in the proportions indicated (p.322·1).
Diabetes mellitus.

Novolin L *Novo Nordisk, USA.*
Insulin zinc suspension (human, crb) (p.322·1).
Diabetes mellitus.

Novolin Lente *Novo Nordisk, Canad.*
Insulin zinc suspension (crystalline 70%) (human, pyr) (p.322·1).
Diabetes mellitus.

Novolin N *Novo Nordisk, USA.*
Isophane insulin suspension (human, crb) (p.322·1).
Diabetes mellitus.

Novolin NPH *Novo Nordisk, Canad.*
Isophane insulin injection (human, pyr) (p.322·1).
Diabetes mellitus.

Novolin R *Novo Nordisk, USA.*
Insulin injection (human, crb) (p.322·1).
Diabetes mellitus.

Novolin Toronto *Novo Nordisk, Canad.*
Neutral insulin injection (human, pyr) (p.322·1).
Diabetes mellitus.

Novolin Ultralente *Novo Nordisk, Canad.*
Insulin zinc suspension (crystalline) (human, pyr) (p.322·1).
Diabetes mellitus.

Novo-Lorazem *Novopharm, Canad.*
Lorazepam (p.675·3).
Anxiety; sedative.

Novo-Medopa *Novopharm, Canad.*
Methyldopa (p.904·2).
Hypertension.

Novo-Meprazine *Novopharm, Canad.*
Methotrimeprazine maleate (p.679·1).
Insomnia; nausea; pain; psychoses; vomiting.

Novo-Mepro *Novopharm, Canad.*
Meprobamate (p.678·1).
Anxiety.

Novo-Methacin *Novopharm, Canad.*
Indomethacin (p.45·2).
Inflammation; pain.

Novo-Metoprol *Novopharm, Canad.*
Metoprolol tartrate (p.907·3).
Angina pectoris; hypertension.

Novomina *Spitzner, Ger.†.*
Dimenhydrinate (p.408·2).
Hypersensitivity reactions; migraine; motion sickness; nausea; vertigo; vomiting.

Novomina infant *Spitzner, Ger.†.*
Dimenhydrinate (p.408·2); pyridoxine hydrochloride (p.1362·3).
Motion sickness; vomiting.

Novomint N *Demopharm, Switz.*
Cetylpyridinium chloride (p.1106·2); lignocaine hydrochloride (p.1293·2); menthol (p.1600·2).
Mouth and throat disorders.

Novo-Mucilax *Novopharm, Canad.*
Ispaghula husk (p.1194·2).
Constipation.

Novo-Naprox *Novopharm, Canad.*
Naproxen (p.61·2) or naproxen sodium (p.61·2).
Inflammation; pain.

Novonausin *Camps, Spain.*
Sodium citrate (p.1153·2); cerium oxalate (p.1183·1).
Nausea and vomiting.

Novo-Nidazol *Novopharm, Canad.*
Metronidazole (p.585·1).
Trichomoniasis.

Novo-Nifedin *Novopharm, Canad.*
Nifedipine (p.916·2).
Angina pectoris.

Novonorm *Novo Nordisk, UK.*
Repaglinide (p.331·1).
Diabetes mellitus.

Novopen *Novo Nordisk, S.Afr.*
Benzylpenicillin sodium (p.159·3).
Bacterial infections.

Novo-Pen-G *Novopharm, Canad.*
Benzylpenicillin potassium (p.159·2).
Bacterial infections.

Novo-Pen-VK *Novopharm, Canad.*
Phenoxymethylpenicillin potassium (p.236·2).
Bacterial infections.

Novo-Peridol *Novopharm, Canad.*
Haloperidol (p.673·3).
Psychoses.

Novophen *Amino, Switz.†.*
Lignocaine hydrochloride (p.1293·2); phenosalyl. cod. gall.; fumariae; salviae.
Mouth and throat disorders.

Novo-Pheniram *Novopharm, Canad.*
Chlorpheniramine maleate (p.405·1).

Novopin MIG *Schoning-Berlin, Ger.*
Menthol (p.1600·2).
Headache including migraine.

Novo-Pindol *Novopharm, Canad.*
Pindolol (p.931·1).
Angina pectoris; hypertension.

Novo-Pirocam *Novopharm, Canad.*
Piroxicam (p.80·2).
Inflammation; pain.

Novo-Plus *Novopharm, Canad.*
Lactose (p.1349·3).
Placebo.

Novo-Poxide *Novopharm, Canad.*
Chlordiazepoxide hydrochloride (p.646·3).

Novo-Pramine *Novopharm, Canad.*
Imipramine hydrochloride (p.289·2).
Depression.

Novo-Pranol *Novopharm, Canad.*
Propranolol hydrochloride (p.937·1).
Cardiac disorders; hypertension; migraine headache; phaeochromocytoma.

Novo-Prazin *Novopharm, Canad.*
Prazosin hydrochloride (p.932·3).
Hypertension.

Novo-Profen *Novopharm, Canad.*
Ibuprofen (p.44·1).
Inflammation; pain.

Novo-Propamide *Novopharm, Canad.*
Chlorpropamide (p.319·1).
Diabetes mellitus.

Novo-Propoxyn *Novopharm, Canad.*
Dextropropoxyphene hydrochloride (p.27·3).
Pain.

Novoprotect *Wyeth, Ger.*
Amitriptyline hydrochloride (p.273·3).
Depression.

Novoptine
Allergan, Fr.†; Allergan, Switz.†.
Cetylpyridinium chloride (p.1106·2).
Eye infections.

Novo-Purol *Novopharm, Canad.*
Allopurinol (p.390·2).

Novo-Pyrazone *Novopharm, Canad.*
Sulphinpyrazone (p.395·2).

Novo-Ranidine *Novopharm, Canad.*
Ranitidine hydrochloride (p.1209·3).
Gastro-intestinal disorders.

Novo-Renal *Novopharm, Canad.*
Multivitamin and mineral preparation for dialysis patients.

Novo-Ridazine *Novopharm, Canad.*
Thioridazine hydrochloride (p.695·1).
Psychiatric disorders.

Novo-Rythro *Novopharm, Canad.*
Erythromycin (p.204·1), erythromycin estolate (p.204·1), erythromycin ethyl succinate (p.204·2), or erythromycin stearate (p.204·2).
Bacterial infections.

Novosal *Zyma, Ital.*
Low sodium dietary salt substitute.

Novo-Salmol *Novopharm, Canad.*
Salbutamol (p.758·2) or salbutamol sulphate (p.758·2).
Obstructive airways disease.

Novo-Semide *Novopharm, Canad.*
Frusemide (p.871·1).
Oedema.

NovoSeven
Novo Nordisk, Fr.; Novo Nordisk, Ger.; Novo Nordisk, Irl.; Novo Nordisk, Ital.; Novo Nordisk, Neth.; Novo Nordisk, Norw.; Novo Nordisk,

Spain; Novo Nordisk, Swed.; Novo Nordisk, Switz.; Novo Nordisk, UK.
Activated eptacog alfa (p.720·2).
Haemorrhagic disorders.

Novo-Sorbide Novopharm, Canad.
Isosorbide dinitrate (p.893·1).
Angina pectoris.

Novo-Soxazole Novopharm, Canad.
Sulphafurazole (p.253·3).

Novo-Spiroton Novopharm, Canad.
Spironolactone (p.946·1).
Hyperaldosteronism.

Novo-Spirozine Novopharm, Canad.
Hydrochlorothiazide (p.885·2); spironolactone (p.946·1).
Hypertension; oedema.

Novospray Peters, Fr.
Mixed amphoteric and quaternary ammonium salts; polyhexanide (p.1123·1); alcohol (p.1099·1); isopropyl alcohol (p.1118·2).
Disinfection.

Novostrep Novo Nordisk, S.Afr.
Streptomycin sulphate (p.249·3).
Bacterial infections.

Novo-Sucralate Novopharm, Canad.
Sucralfate (p.1214·2).
Peptic ulcer.

Novo-Sundac Novopharm, Canad.
Sulindac (p.86·3).
Inflammation; pain.

Novoter Farmacusi, Spain.
Fluocinonide (p.1041·2).
Skin disorders.

Novoter Gentamicina Cusi, Spain.
Fluocinonide (p.1041·2); gentamicin sulphate (p.212·1).
Infected skin disorders.

Novo-Tetra Novopharm, Canad.
Tetracycline hydrochloride (p.259·1).
Bacterial infections.

Novo-Thalidone Novopharm, Canad.
Chlorthalidone (p.839·3).
Hypertension; oedema.

Novothyral
Merck, Aust.; Merck-Belgolabo, Belg.; Merck, Ger.; E. Merck, Switz.
Liothyronine sodium (p.1495·1); thyroxine sodium (p.1497·1).
Adjunct to antithyroid therapy; euthyroid goitre; hypothyroidism; thyroiditis.

Novo-Timol Novopharm, Canad.
Timolol maleate (p.953·3).
Angina pectoris; glaucoma; hypertension.

Novotossil Zambon, Belg.
Cloperastine fendizoate (p.1057·2) or cloperastine hydrochloride (p.1057·2).
Coughs.

Novo-Triamzide Novopharm, Canad.
Triamterene (p.957·2); hydrochlorothiazide (p.885·2).
Hypertension; oedema.

Novo-Trimel Novopharm, Canad.
Co-trimoxazole (p.196·3).
Bacterial infections.

Novo-Triolam Novopharm, Canad.
Triazolam (p.696·3).
Insomnia; sedative.

Novo-Triphyl Novopharm, Canad.
Choline theophyllinate (p.751·3).

Novo-Tripramine Novopharm, Canad.
Trimipramine maleate (p.310·1).
Depression.

Novo-Triptyn Novopharm, Canad.
Amitriptyline hydrochloride (p.273·3).
Depression.

Novo-Veramil Novopharm, Canad.
Verapamil hydrochloride (p.960·3).
Angina pectoris; arrhythmias; hypertension.

Novo-Vites Novopharm, Canad.
Multivitamin preparation with or without iron.

Novoxapam Novopharm, Canad.
Oxazepam (p.683·2).

Novo-Zolamide Novopharm, Canad.
Acetazolamide (p.810·3).

Novuxol
Note. This name is used for preparations of different composition.
Knoll, Ger.
Clostridium histolyticum.
Cleansing of skin ulcers.

Nordmark, Neth.
Collagenase (p.1566·3).
Wounds.

Noxacorn
Note. This name is used for preparations of different composition.
Roche Nicholas, Neth.
Lignocaine (p.1293·2); salicylic acid (p.1090·2).
Calluses; corns; warts.

Cox, UK†.
Salicylic acid (p.1090·2).
Corns.

Noxenur Disperga, Aust.
Atropine sulphate (p.455·1); ephedrine hydrochloride (p.1059·3); thiamine hydrochloride (p.1361·1).
Nocturnal enuresis.

Noxenur N Galenika, Ger.†.
Atropine sulphate (p.455·1); ephedrine hydrochloride (p.1059·3); thiamine hydrochloride.
Urinary-tract disorders.

Noxenur S Galenika, Ger.
Atropine sulphate (p.455·1).
Nocturnal enuresis.

Noxigram FIRMA, Ital.
Cinoxacin (p.185·2).
Bacterial infections of the urinary tract.

Noxitem Amrad, Austral.
Tamoxifen citrate (p.563·3).
Breast cancer.

Noxom S Fides, Ger.
Homoeopathic preparation.

Noxotab Fides, Ger.
Homoeopathic preparation.

Noxyflex Innothera, Fr.
Noxythiolin (p.1120·2).
Intraperitoneal infections.

Noxyflex S
Geistlich, Irl.; Geistlich, UK.
Noxythiolin (p.1120·2).
Fungal and bacterial infections.

Noxylin Inibsa, Spain†.
Polynoxylin (p.1123·1).
Skin infections.

Nozid Vitalpharma, Belg.
Aluminium hydroxide-magnesium carbonate co-dried gel (p.1178·2); magnesium hydroxide (p.1198·2) or magnesium oxide (p.1198·3).
Digestive disorders associated with hyperacidity.

Nozinan
Gerot, Aust.; Rhone-Poulenc Rorer, Belg.; Rhone-Poulenc Rorer, Canad.; Specia, Fr.; Rhone-Poulenc Rorer, Irl.; Rhone-Poulenc Rorer, Ital.; Rhone-Poulenc Rorer, Neth.; Pharmacia Upjohn, Norw.; Rhone-Poulenc Rorer, Swed.; Rhone-Poulenc Rorer, Switz.; Link, UK.
Methotrimeprazine (p.679·1), methotrimeprazine embonate (p.679·2), methotrimeprazine hydrochloride (p.679·1), or methotrimeprazine maleate (p.679·1).
Tablets were formerly known as Veractil in the *UK*.
Alcohol withdrawal syndrome; anxiety; depression; general anaesthesia; insomnia; nausea and vomiting; pain; premedication; pruritus; psychoses.

NP-27 Thompson, USA†.
Tolnaftate (p.389·1).
Fungal skin infections.

NPH Iletin I Lilly, USA.
Isophane insulin suspension (bovine and porcine) (p.322·1).
Diabetes mellitus.

NPH Iletin II Lilly, USA.
Isophane insulin suspension (porcine) (p.322·1).
Diabetes mellitus.

NSA CSL, Austral.
Human albumin (p.710·1).
Burns; cardiopulmonary bypass; haemodialysis; hypoproteinaemia; hypovolaemia; plasma exchange; respiratory distress syndrome; shock.

NTR Teofarma, Ital.
Phenylephrine hydrochloride (p.1066·2); thenyldiamine hydrochloride (p.419·1).
Cold symptoms.

n-Tricidine Warner-Lambert, Belg.†.
Tyrothricin (p.267·2); lignocaine hydrochloride (p.1293·2).
Mouth and throat disorders.

NTS Hercon, USA.
Glyceryl trinitrate (p.874·3).

NTZ Long Acting Nasal Sterling Health, USA.
Oxymetazoline hydrochloride (p.1065·3).
Nasal congestion.

Nu-Alpraz Nu-Pharm, Canad.
Alprazolam (p.640·3).
Anxiety; sedative.

Nu-Amilzide Nu-Pharm, Canad.
Hydrochlorothiazide (p.885·2); amiloride hydrochloride (p.819·2).
Hypertension; oedema.

Nu-Amoxi Nu-Pharm, Canad.
Amoxycillin trihydrate (p.151·3).
Bacterial infections.

Nu-Ampi Nu-Pharm, Canad.
Ampicillin trihydrate (p.153·2).
Bacterial infections.

Nuardin Bencard, Belg.
Cimetidine (p.1183·2).
Gastro-intestinal disorders associated with hyperacidity.

Nu-Atenol Nu-Pharm, Canad.
Atenolol (p.825·3).
Angina pectoris; hypertension.

Nu-Baclo Nu-Pharm, Canad.
Baclofen (p.1308·2).
Muscle relaxation; skeletal muscle spasticity.

Nubain
Torrex, Aust.; Du Pont, Canad.; Du Pont, Fr.; Du Pont, Ger.; Boots, S.Afr.; Du Pont, Switz.; Du Pont Pharmaceuticals, UK; Du Pont, USA.
Nalbuphine hydrochloride (p.60·2).
Adjunct to anaesthesia; pain; premedication.

Nubee 12 Propan, S.Afr.†.
Cyanocobalamin (p.1363·3).
Macrocytic anaemias.

Nubee Co Propan-Vernleigh, S.Afr.†.
Vitamin B substances.

Nubral
AB-Consult, Aust.; Galderma, Ger.
Urea (p.1095·2).
Dry skin.

Nubral 4 HC Galderma, Ger.
Hydrocortisone (p.1043·3); urea (p.1095·2); sodium chloride (p.1162·2).
Skin disorders.

Nu-Cal Odan, Canad.
Calcium (p.1155·1).
Calcium deficiency.

Nu-Capto Nu-Pharm, Canad.
Captopril (p.836·3).
ACE inhibitor.

Nu-Cephalex Nu-Pharm, Canad.
Cephalexin (p.178·2).
Bacterial infections.

Nu-Cimet Nu-Pharm, Canad.
Cimetidine (p.1183·2).
Histamine H_2-receptor inhibitor.

Nucleo CMP Ferrer, Spain.
Sodium cytidine monophosphate; disodium uridine diphosphate; disodium uridilic acid; sodium uridine triphosphate.
Formerly contained sodium cytidine monophosphate, hydroxocobalamin or hydroxocobalamin acetate, and sodium uridine triphosphate.
Neuralgias; neuritis.

Nucleo-Cortex Rhone-Poulenc Rorer, Ital.†.
Suprarenal cortex (p.1050·1); vitamins and nucleosides; lignocaine hydrochloride (p.1293·2).
Tonic.

Nucleodoxina Baldacci, Ital.†.
Adenosine monophosphate potassium (p.1543·2); uridine monophosphate potassium; taurine (p.1635·1); pyridoxine hydrochloride (p.1362·3); cyanocobalamin (p.1363·3).
Taurine (p.1635·1); inosine (p.1591·1); uridine (p.1641·3); pyridoxine hydrochloride (p.1362·3); cyanocobalamin (p.1363·3).
Metabolic disorders.

Nucleonevrina Ist. Chim. Inter., Ital.†.
Hydroxocobalamin (p.1363·3); thiamine monophosphate (p.1361·2); nucleosides; lignocaine hydrochloride (p.1293·2).
Neuritis, neuralgias.

Nucleserina Medea, Spain.
Pyridoxine hydrochloride (p.1362·3); ribonucleic acid (p.1624·3); phosphoserine; levoglutamide (p.1344·3).
Mental function impairment; tonic.

Nuclevit
Synthelabo, Belg.†; Synthelabo, Switz.†.
Mineral and nucleotide preparation.
Tonic.

Nuclevit B_{12} Synthelabo, Fr.
Nucleotide preparation with cyanocobalamin (p.1363·3).
Tonic.

Nuclosina ICN, Spain.
Omeprazole (p.1204·2).
Gastro-oesophageal reflux; peptic ulcer; Zollinger-Ellison syndrome.

Nu-Cloxi Nu-Pharm, Canad.
Cloxacillin sodium (p.195·2).
Bacterial infections.

Nucoa Llorente, Spain.
Isopropyl myristate (p.1384·1).
Skin disorders.

Nucofed Roberts, USA.
Codeine phosphate (p.26·1); pseudoephedrine hydrochloride (p.1068·3).
Coughs and cold symptoms.

Nucofed Expectorant Roberts, USA.
Codeine phosphate (p.26·1); pseudoephedrine hydrochloride (p.1068·3); guaiphenesin (p.1061·3).
Coughs and cold symptoms.

Nucosef Sugar Free SmithKline Beecham Consumer, Austral.
Codeine phosphate (p.26·1); pseudoephedrine hydrochloride (p.1068·3).
Congestion; coughs.

Nu-Cotrimox Nu-Pharm, Canad.
Co-trimoxazole (p.196·3).
Bacterial infections.

Nucotuss Expectorant Barre-National, USA.
Pseudoephedrine hydrochloride (p.1068·3); guaiphenesin (p.1061·3); codeine phosphate (p.26·1).
Coughs.

Nuctalon Takeda, Fr.
Estazolam (p.669·2).
Insomnia.

Nu-Diclo Nu-Pharm, Canad.
Diclofenac sodium (p.31·2).
Inflammation; pain.

Nu-Diltiaz Nu-Pharm, Canad.
Diltiazem hydrochloride (p.854·2).
Angina pectoris.

Nudopa Douglas, Austral.
Methyldopa (p.904·2).
Hypertension.

Nuelin
3M, Austral.; 3M, Irl.; 3M, Norw.; 3M, S.Afr.; 3M, UK.
Theophylline (p.765·1) or theophylline sodium glycinate (p.772·2).
Obstructive airways disease.

Nu-Gel
Note. This name is used for preparations of different composition.
Johnson & Johnson Medical, Fr.
Povidone (p.1474·2).
Burns; wounds.

Johnson & Johnson, Ger.
Sodium alginate (p.1470·3); carmellose (p.1471·2); hydroxyethylcellulose (p.1472·3).
Burns; skin ulcers; wounds.

Nu-Hydral Nu-Pharm, Canad.
Hydralazine hydrochloride (p.883·2).
Hypertension.

Nuicalm Stafford-Miller Continental, Belg.
Diphenhydramine hydrochloride (p.409·1).
Insomnia.

Nuidor Sterling Midy, Fr.†.
Phenobarbitone (p.350·2); passion flower (p.1615·3); crataegus (p.1568·2).
Anxiety; insomnia.

Nu-Indo Nu-Pharm, Canad.
Indomethacin (p.45·2).
Inflammation; pain.

Nu-Iron Mayrand, USA.
Polysaccharide-iron complex (p.1353·2).
Iron-deficiency anaemias.

Nu-Iron Plus Mayrand, USA.
Polysaccharide-iron complex (p.1353·2); cyanocobalamin (p.1363·3); folic acid (p.1340·3).
Iron-deficiency anaemias.

Nu-Iron V Mayrand, USA.
Polysaccharide-iron complex (p.1353·2); folic acid (p.1340·3); multivitamins and minerals.
Iron-deficiency anaemias.

Nujol
Schering-Plough, Canad.; Fumouze, Fr.
Liquid paraffin (p.1382·1).
Constipation.

Nu-K Consolidated Chemicals, UK†.
Potassium chloride (p.1161·1).
Hypokalaemia; potassium depletion.

Nulacin Goldshield, UK.
Magnesium trisilicate (p.1199·1); heavy magnesium oxide (p.1198·3); calcium carbonate (p.1182·1); heavy magnesium carbonate (p.1198·1); peppermint oil (p.1208·1).
Gastro-intestinal hyperacidity.

Nulacin Fermentos Seid, Spain.
Amylolytic enzymes; proteolytic enzymes; lipolytic enzymes (p.1612·1); dehydrocholic acid (p.1570·2); procaine (p.1299·2).
Digestive enzyme deficiency.

Nulcerin Andromaco, Spain.
Famotidine (p.1192·1).
Gastro-oesophageal reflux; peptic ulcer; Zollinger-Ellison syndrome.

Nuleron Teofarma, Ital.
Magnesium polygalacturonate; calcium pantothenate (p.1352·3); promethazine hydrochloride (p.416·2); dimethicone (p.1213·1).
Gastro-intestinal disorders associated with excess gas.

Nulicaine Kay, USA.
Lignocaine hydrochloride (p.1293·2).
Local anaesthesia.

Nullatuss Wernigerode, Ger.
Clobutinol hydrochloride (p.1057·1).
Coughs.

Nullo Chattem, USA†.
Chlorophyllin copper complex (p.1000·1).
Control of body odour.

Nu-Loraz Nu-Pharm, Canad.
Lorazepam (p.675·3).
Anxiety; sedative.

NuLytely Braintree, USA.
Macrogol 3350 (p.1598·2); electrolytes (p.1147·1).
Bowel evacuation.

Numatol Spyfarma, Spain.
Citicoline sodium (p.1564·3).
Cerebrovascular disorders; tonic.

Nu-Medopa Nu-Pharm, Canad.
Methyldopa (p.904·2).
Hypertension.

Nu-Metop Nu-Pharm, Canad.
Metoprolol tartrate (p.907·3).
Angina pectoris; hypertension.

Numidan Therabel, Ital.
Naproxen piperazine (p.62·1).
Musculoskeletal, joint, peri-articular, and soft-tissue disorders.

Numobid Teral, USA.
Guaiphenesin (p.1061·3).

Numobid DM Teral, USA.
Guaiphenesin (p.1061·3); dextromethorphan hydrobromide (p.1057·3).

Numonyl Teral, USA.
Guaiphenesin (p.1061·3); phenylephrine hydrochloride (p.1066·2).

Numorphan
Du Pont, Canad.; Du Pont, USA.
Oxymorphone hydrochloride (p.72·1).
Adjunct to general anaesthesia; pain; premedication.

Numotac 3M, UK†.
Isoetharine hydrochloride (p.755·1).
Bronchospasm.

Numzident Goodys, USA.
Benzocaine (p.1286·2).
Oral lesions.

Numzit
Note. This name is used for preparations of different composition.
Beige, S.Afr.
Benzocaine (p.1286·2); menthol (p.1600·2).
Teething pain.

Goodys, USA.
Lotion: Benzocaine (p.1286·2); glycerol (p.1585·2).
Topical gel: Benzocaine (p.1286·2); clove oil (p.1565·2).
Oral lesions.

Nu-Naprox Nu-Pharm, Canad.
Naproxen (p.61·2).
Inflammation; pain.

Nu-Nifed Nu-Pharm, Canad.
Nifedipine (p.916·2).
Angina pectoris.

Nuovo Andrews Maggioni, Ital.†.
Sodium bicarbonate (p.1153·2); dried magnesium sulphate (p.1158·2); anhydrous citric acid (p.1564·3); tartaric acid (p.1634·3).
Gastro-intestinal disorders.

Nuovo Snelling Silk Farmades, Ital.†.
Dietary fibre supplement.
Disorders of lipid and glucose metabolism.

Nu-Pen-VK Nu-Pharm, Canad.
Phenoxymethylpenicillin potassium (p.236·2).
Bacterial infections.

Nupercainal
Note. This name is used for preparations of different composition.
Ciba-Geigy, Aust.†; Novartis Consumer, Canad.; Zyma, Switz.; Zyma, UK; Ciba, USA.
Cream; ointment: Cinchocaine (p.1289·2) or cinchocaine hydrochloride (p.1289·2).
Anal fissures; haemorrhoids; insect bites; pain; premature ejaculation; pruritus.

Ciba Self Medication, Canad.†.
Suppositories: Cinchocaine (p.1289·2); zinc oxide (p.1096·2); bismuth subgallate (p.1180·2).
Pain; pruritus.

Novartis Consumer, Canad.
Cream: Cinchocaine (p.1289·2); domiphen bromide (p.1112·3).
Pain; pruritus.

Ciba, USA.
Suppositories: Zinc oxide (p.1096·2).
Anorectal disorders.

Nupercaine Heavy Astra, Austral.
Cinchocaine hydrochloride (p.1289·2).
Spinal anaesthesia.

Nu-Pindol Nu-Pharm, Canad.
Pindolol (p.931·1).
Angina pectoris; hypertension.

Nu-Pirox Nu-Pharm, Canad.
Piroxicam (p.80·2).
Inflammation; pain.

Nu-Prazo Nu-Pharm, Canad.
Prazosin hydrochloride (p.932·3).
Hypertension.

Nuprin Bristol-Myers Products, USA.
Ibuprofen (p.44·1).
Fever; osteoarthritis; pain; rheumatoid arthritis.

Nuprin Backache Bristol-Myers Products, USA.
Magnesium salicylate (p.51·1).
Pain.

Nu-Prochlor Nu-Pharm, Canad.
Prochlorperazine maleate (p.687·3).
Psychoses; vomiting.

Nuquin HP Stratus, USA.
Cream: Hydroquinone (p.1083·1); dioxybenzone (p.1487·1); oxybenzone (p.1487·3).
Gel: Hydroquinone (p.1083·1); dioxybenzone (p.1487·1).

Nuran Frosst, Ger.†.
Cyproheptadine hydrochloride (p.407·2).
Reduced appetite.

Nuran BC forte Frosst, Ger.†.
Cyproheptadine hydrochloride (p.407·2); vitamin B substances; ascorbic acid.
Reduced appetite.

Nu-Ranit Nu-Pharm, Canad.
Ranitidine hydrochloride (p.1209·3).
Histamine H_2-receptor antagonist.

Nurdelin Zambon, Ger.†.
Cyproheptadine hydrochloride (p.407·2); cobamamide (p.1364·2).
Reduced appetite.

Nureflex Boots Healthcare, Fr.
Ibuprofen (p.44·1).
Fever; juvenile chronic arthritis; pain.

Nuril Prodes, Spain.
Pipemidic acid (p.237·2).
Urinary-tract infections.

Nuriphasic Nourypharma, Ger.
Blue tablets, ethinyloestradiol (p.1445·1); white tablets, lynoestrenol (p.1448·2); ethinyloestradiol.
Menorrhagia; menstrual disorders.

Nur-Isterate Schering, S.Afr.
Norethisterone enanthate (p.1453·1).
Injectable contraceptive.

Nurocain Astra, Austral.
Lignocaine hydrochloride (p.1293·2).
Adrenaline (p.813·2) is included in this preparation as a vasoconstrictor to diminish absorption and localise the effect of the local anaesthetic.
Local anaesthesia.

Nurocain with Sympathin Astra, Austral.†.
Lignocaine hydrochloride (p.1293·2).
Adrenaline (p.813·2) and noradrenaline (p.924·1) are included in this preparation as vasoconstrictors to diminish absorption and localise the effect of the local anaesthetic.
Local anaesthesia.

Nurofen
Salus, Aust.; Boots, Austral.; Boots Healthcare, Belg.; Boots Healthcare, Fr.; Boots Healthcare, Irl.; Boots Healthcare, Ital.; Boots Healthcare, Neth.; Boots, S.Afr.; Boots, Spain; Astra, Swed.; Boots, Switz.; Crookes Healthcare, UK.
Ibuprofen (p.44·1).
Formerly called Nerofen in *Belg.*
Fever; musculoskeletal, joint, and peri-articular disorders; pain.

Nurofen Advance Crookes Healthcare, UK.
Ibuprofen lysine (p.44·3).

Nurofen Cold & Flu
Boots, S.Afr.; Crookes Healthcare, UK.
Ibuprofen (p.44·1); pseudoephedrine hydrochloride (p.1068·3).
Cold and influenza symptoms.

Nurofen Plus Crookes Healthcare, UK.
Ibuprofen (p.44·1); codeine phosphate (p.26·1).
Pain.

Nurogrip Boots Healthcare, Spain.
Ibuprofen (p.44·1); pseudoephedrine hydrochloride (p.1068·3).
Cold and influenza symptoms.

Nuromax
Glaxo Wellcome, Canad.; Wellcome, USA.
Doxacurium chloride (p.1315·1).
Competitive neuromuscular blocker.

Nurse Harvey's Gripe Mixture Harvey-Scruton, UK.
Dill oil (p.1572·1); caraway oil (p.1559·3); sodium bicarbonate (p.1153·2).
Colic.

Nurse Sykes Balsam Waterhouse, UK.
Guaiphenesin (p.1061·3).
Coughs.

Nurse Sykes Powders Waterhouse, UK.
Aspirin (p.16·1); paracetamol (p.72·2); caffeine (p.749·3).
Fever; pain.

Nursoy
Wyeth-Ayerst, Canad.; Wyeth-Ayerst, USA†.
Soy protein infant formula.
Lactose intolerance; sensitivity to cow's milk.

Nu-Salt Cumberland, USA.
Low sodium dietary salt substitute.

Nu-Seals
Lilly, Irl.; Lilly, UK.
Aspirin (p.16·1).
Fever; inflammation; pain; thrombo-embolic disorders.

Nu-Tears Optopics, USA.
Polyvinyl alcohol (p.1474·2).
Dry eyes.

Nu-Tears II Optopics, USA.
Polyvinyl alcohol (p.1474·2); macrogol 400 (p.1598·2).
Dry eyes.

Nu-Tetra Nu-Pharm, Canad.
Tetracycline hydrochloride (p.259·1).
Bacterial infections.

Nutra Nutrabain Galderma, Fr.
Soap substitute.
Dry skin.

Nutra Nutraderme Galderma, Fr.
Liquid paraffin (p.1382·1).
Dry skin.

Nutra Nutraplus Galderma, Fr.
Urea (p.1095·2).
Dry skin.

Nutra Tear Dakryon, USA†.
Vitamin B_{12} (p.1363·3); polyvinyl alcohol (p.1474·2).
Dry eyes.

Nutracel
Note. This name is used for preparations of different composition.
Isdin, Spain.
Guanosine; inosine (p.1591·1); miconazole nitrate (p.384·3); vitamin F.
Skin disorders.

Baxter, UK.
Glucose and electrolyte infusion.
Parenteral nutrition.

Nutracort Galderma, USA.
Hydrocortisone (p.1043·3).
Skin disorders.

Nutra-D Galderma, Austral.
Emollient.

Nutraderm
Galderma, Canad.; Alcon, S.Afr.†; Galderma, USA.
Emollient.
Dry skin.

Nutradex Pharmacia Upjohn, Swed.
Carbohydrate and electrolyte infusion.
Parenteral nutrition.

Nutraflow Alcon, Fr.
Rinsing, neutralising, and storage solution for soft contact lenses.

Nutraloric Nutraloric, USA.
Preparation for enteral nutrition.

Nutramigen
Mead Johnson, Austral.; Mead Johnson, Fr.; Bristol-Myers Squibb, Irl.; Mead Johnson, Ital.; Bristol-Myers Squibb, Norw.†; Bristol-Myers Squibb, S.Afr.†; Mead Johnson Nutritionals, UK; Mead Johnson Nutritionals, USA.
Protein hydrolysate preparation.
Cow's milk, soya, or lactose intolerance; galactokinase deficiency; galactosaemia; lactose or sucrose intolerance; protein sensitivity.

Nutra-Plex Medi-Plex, USA†.
Vitamin B preparation with minerals.

Nutraplus
Galderma, Austral.; Galderma, Canad.†; Galderma, Irl.; Alcon, S.Afr.†; Galderma, Switz.; Galderma, UK; Galderma, USA.
Urea (p.1095·2).
Dry skin; hyperkeratosis.

Nutra-Soothe Pertussin, USA.
Emollient.

Nutrasorb Galderma, Austral.
Acrylate copolymer; glycerol (p.1585·2); menthol (p.1600·2).
Acne; oily skin.

Nutrated Propan, S.Afr.†.
Ethylenediamine hydrate; aminophylline (p.748·1).
Respiratory-tract disorders.

Nutrauxil Kabivitrum, Irl.†.
Preparation for enteral nutrition.

Nutrazest Pharmatec, S.Afr.†.
Multivitamin preparation.

Nutren Clintec, USA.
Lactose-free, gluten-free preparation for enteral nutrition.

Nutrex Beta, Ital.
Royal jelly (p.1626·3); pollen; ginkgo biloba (p.1584·1); eleutherococcus (p.1584·2).
Nutritional supplement.

Nutri 2000 (Nutrinaut) Nutricia, Ital.
Preparation for enteral nutrition.

Nutri Twin Pharmacia Upjohn, Ger.
Amino acid, electrolyte, and carbohydrate solution.
Parenteral nutrition.

Nu-Triazide Nu-Pharm, Canad.
Triamterene (p.957·2); hydrochlorothiazide (p.885·2).
Hypertension; oedema.

Nu-Triazo Nu-Pharm, Canad.†.
Triazolam (p.696·3).
Insomnia; sedative.

Nutrical Nutricia, Ital.
Preparation for enteral nutrition.

Nutricap Yves Ponroy, Fr.
Amino-acid, fatty-acid, vitamin, and mineral preparation.
Hair and nail disorders.

Nutricomp
Braun, Irl.; Braun, Ital.
A range of preparations for enteral nutrition.

Nutricon Pasadena, USA.
Multivitamin and mineral preparation with iron and folic acid.

Nutricremal Sodietal, Fr.
High-protein nutritional supplement.

Nutrideen Bioceuticals, UK.
Marine protein extract with vitamin C and zinc.

Nutridoral Sodietal, Fr.
High-protein nutritional supplement.

Nutridrink
Nutricia, Fr.; Nutricia, Ital.
Preparation for enteral nutrition.

Nutrifer Plus Whitehall-Robins, Canad.†.
Multivitamins and minerals.

Nutriflex
Germania, Aust.; Braun, Belg.; Braun, Ger.; Braun, Swed.; Vifor Medical, Switz.; Braun, UK.
Amino-acid, carbohydrate, and electrolyte infusion.
Parenteral nutrition.

Nutrifundin Braun, Ger.†.
Amino-acid, carbohydrate, and lipid (from soya oil (p.1355·1)) infusion.
Parenteral nutrition.

Nutrigel Farbo, Ital.
Fructose; soya lecithin (p.1595·2); honey (p.1345·3); royal jelly (p.1626·3).

Nutrigene GNR, Fr.
Yellow tablets, deoxyribonucleic acid (p.1570·3); vitamin B substances; alpha tocopherol acetate; blue tablets, ribonucleic acid (p.1624·3).
The yellow tablets were formerly brown, and the blue tablets formerly contained adenosine triphosphate, ribonucleic acid, magnesium iodide, and horse muscle extract.
Painful arthritic disorders.

Nutrigil Diepal, Fr.
A range of preparations for enteral nutrition.

Nutri-Junior Nutricia, Ital.
Infant feed.
Hypersensitivity disorders.

Nutrilamine Braun, Fr.
Amino-acid infusion.
Parenteral nutrition.

Nutrilan Elan, USA.
Lactose-free preparation for enteral nutrition.

Nutrilon AR Nutricia, Ital.
A range of infant feeds.
Gastro-oesophageal reflux.

Nutrilon Pepti Cow & Gate, Irl.
Infant feed.
Cow's milk intolerance.

Nutrilyte American Regent, USA.
A range of electrolyte preparations (p.1147·1).
Fluid and electrolyte disorders.

Nutrimed Nutrimed, Fr.
Preparation for enteral nutrition.

Nutri-Min Chlorella, UK.
Mineral and trace element preparation.

Nutrineal PD4
Baxter, Spain; Baxter, Swed.; Baxter, Switz.; Baxter, UK.
Sodium chloride; calcium chloride; magnesium chloride; sodium lactate; amino acids (p.1151·1).
Peritoneal dialysis.

Nutrineal PD2 and PD4 Baxter, Ital.
Calcium chloride; magnesium chloride; sodium lactate; sodium chloride; amino acids (p.1151·1).
Peritoneal dialysis solution.

Nutrison
Nutricia, Fr.; Nutricia, Irl.; Nutricia, Ital.; Nutricia, UK.
A range of preparations for enteral nutrition.
Formerly known as Fortison in the *UK.*

Nutrisond Nutricia, Ital.†.
Preparation for enteral nutrition.

Nutrisource Sandoz Nutrition, Canad.
Preparation for enteral nutrition.

NutriTwin G Pharmacia Upjohn, Aust.
Amino-acid; carbohydrate and electrolyte infusion.
Parenteral nutrition.

Nutrivimin med jarn Hassle, Swed.†.
Multivitamin and iron preparation.
Iron-deficiency anaemia.

Nutrizym
Note. This name is used for preparations of different composition.
Merck, Aust.†; Merck, S.Afr.†; E. Merck, Switz.†.
Pancreatin (p.1612·1); bromelains (p.1555·1); ox bile (p.1553·2).
Pancreatic insufficiency.

E. Merck, Irl.; E. Merck, UK.
Pancreatin (p.1612·1).
Pancreatic insufficiency.

Nutrizym N Cascan, Ger.; Cascapharm, Ger.
Pancreatin (p.1612·1).
Pancreatic insufficiency.

Nutrodrip
Wander, Ital.; Wander Health Care, Switz.†.
Range of preparations for enteral nutrition.

Nutrol A D Rolmex, Canad.
Vitamin A (p.1358·1); vitamin D (p.1366·3).

Nutrol E plus Zinc & Selenium Rolmex, Canad.
Vitamin E, zinc, and selenium.

Nutrol No I Rolmex, Canad.
Multivitamin and mineral preparation.

Nutrol V Rolmex, Canad.
Betacarotene, selenium, vitamin C, and vitamin E.

Nutropin Genentech, USA.
Somatropin (p.1249·3).
Growth hormone deficiency.

Nutrox Tyson, USA.
Multivitamin, mineral, and amino-acid preparation.

Nuvacthen Depot Padro, Spain.
Tetracosactrin hexa-acetate (p.1261·3).
Hypersensitivity disorders; inflammation; suprarenal cortex stimulation.

Nuvapen CEPA, Spain.
Ampicillin sodium (p.153·1) or ampicillin trihydrate (p.153·2).
Bacterial infections.

Nuvapen Mucolitico Retard CEPA, Spain†.
Acetylcysteine (p.1052·3); ampicillin sodium (p.153·1); ampicillin benzathine (p.154·1).
Respiratory-tract infections.

Nuvapen Retard CEPA, Spain†.
Ampicillin sodium (p.153·1); ampicillin benzathine (p.154·1).
Bacterial infections.

Nuvelle
Schering, Irl.; Schering, Ital.; Schering, UK.
16 Tablets, oestradiol valerate (p.1455·2); 12 tablets, oestradiol valerate; levonorgestrel (p.1454·1).
Menopausal disorders; osteoporosis.

Nuvelle TS Schering, UK.
Phase I patches, oestradiol (p.1455·1); phase II patches, oestradiol; levonorgestrel (p.1454·1).
Menopausal disorders.

Nu-Verap Nu-Pharm, Canad.
Verapamil hydrochloride (p.960·3).
Angina pectoris; arrhythmias; hypertension.

Nux ISO Iso, Ger.
Homoeopathic preparation.

Nux Med Complex Dynamit, Aust.
Homoeopathic preparation.

Nuxil Dolisos, Canad.
Homoeopathic preparation.

Nyaderm Taro, Canad.
Nystatin (p.386·1).
Fungal and bacterial infections.

Nyal Bronchitis *SmithKline Beecham Consumer, Austral.*
Ammonium chloride (p.1055·2); squill (p.1070·1); liquorice (p.1197·1); senega (p.1069·3).
Cough; upper respiratory-tract congestion.

Nyal Cold Sore
SmithKline Beecham Consumer, Austral.
Cream: Menthol (p.1600·2); camphor (p.1557·2).
Cracked lips; herpes labialis.
Topical lotion: Benzoin (p.1634·1); menthol (p.1600·2); camphor (p.1557·2).
Herpes labialis.
Sterling Health, Austral.†.
Topical liquid: Povidone-iodine (p.1123·3).
Herpes labialis.

Nyal Decongestant *SmithKline Beecham Consumer, Austral.*
Phenylephrine hydrochloride (p.1066·2).
Nasal congestion.

Nyal Dry Cough *SmithKline Beecham Consumer, Austral.*
Pentoxyverine citrate (p.1066·1).
Coughs.

Nyal Medithroat Anaesthetic Lozenges *SmithKline Beecham Consumer, Austral.*
Hexylresorcinol (p.1116·1).
Sore mouth and throat.

Nyal Medithroat Gargle *SmithKline Beecham Consumer, Austral.*
Povidone-iodine (p.1123·3).
Sore throat.

Nyal Toothache Drops *SmithKline Beecham Consumer, Austral.*
Benzocaine (p.1286·2); phenol (p.1121·2).
Toothache.

Nycopren
Nycomed, Aust.; Farmabel, Belg.†; Sanofi Winthrop, Neth.; Nycomed, Switz.; Ardern, UK.
Naproxen (p.61·2).
Gout; inflammation; musculoskeletal, joint, and peri-articular disorders; pain.

Nycto *Pierre Fabre, Fr.†.*
Phenylephrine hydrochloride (p.1066·2).
Ocular congestion.

Nydrazid *Apothecon, USA.*
Isoniazid (p.218·1).
Tuberculosis.

Nyefax *Douglas, Austral.*
Nifedipine (p.916·2).
Hypertension.

Nylax *Crookes Healthcare, UK.*
Phenolphthalein (p.1208·2); senna leaf (p.1212·2); bisacodyl (p.1179·3).
Constipation.

Nylax with Senna *Crookes Healthcare, UK.*
Senna (p.1212·2).
Constipation.

Nymix Mucolytikum *Dolorgiet, Ger.*
Ambroxol hydrochloride (p.1054·3).
Respiratory-tract disorders associated with increased or viscous mucus.

Nymix-amid N *Dolorgiet, Ger.†.*
Co-trimoxazole (p.196·3).
Formerly contained sulphadiazine and guaiphenesin.
Bacterial infections of the respiratory tract.

Nymix-cyclin N *Dolorgiet, Ger.†.*
Doxycycline hydrochloride (p.202·3).
Bacterial infections.

Nyolol
Ciba Vision, Fr.; Ciba Vision, Spain.
Timolol maleate (p.953·3).
Glaucoma; ocular hypertension.

Nyquil *Procter & Gamble, Canad.*
Dextromethorphan hydrobromide (p.1057·3); doxylamine succinate (p.410·1); pseudoephedrine hydrochloride (p.1068·3); paracetamol (p.72·2).
Coughs and cold symptoms.

NyQuil Hot Therapy *Richardson-Vicks, USA.*
Paracetamol (p.72·2); pseudoephedrine hydrochloride (p.1068·3); dextromethorphan hydrobromide (p.1057·3); doxylamine succinate (p.410·1).
Coughs and cold symptoms.

NyQuil Nighttime Cold/Flu *Richardson-Vicks, USA.*
Pseudoephedrine hydrochloride (p.1068·3); doxylamine succinate (p.410·1); dextromethorphan hydrobromide (p.1057·3); paracetamol (p.72·2).
Coughs and cold symptoms.

Nyrene *Planta, Canad.*
Melissa (p.1600·1); valerian (p.1643·1).
Insomnia.

Nysconitrine *Bio-Therabel, Belg.*
Glyceryl trinitrate (p.874·3).
Angina pectoris; heart failure.

Nyspes *DDSA Pharmaceuticals, UK.*
Nystatin (p.386·1).
Vaginal candidiasis.

Nystacid *Lennon, S.Afr.*
Nystatin (p.386·1).
Candidiasis.

Nystacortone *Spirig, Switz.*
Prednisolone acetate (p.1048·1); nystatin (p.386·1); chlorhexidine hydrochloride (p.1107·2).
Infected skin disorders.

Nystaderm *Dermapharm, Ger.*
Nystatin (p.386·1).
Fungal infections.

Nystaderm Comp *Dermapharm, Ger.*
Nystatin (p.386·1); hydrocortisone acetate (p.1043·3).
Infected skin disorders.

Nystadermal *Squibb, UK.*
Nystatin (p.386·1); triamcinolone acetonide (p.1050·2).
Inflammatory candidiasis.

Nystaform
Bayer, Irl.; Bayer, UK.
Nystatin (p.386·1); chlorhexidine hydrochloride (p.1107·2).
Fungal and bacterial skin infections.

Nystaform-HC
Bayer, Irl.; Bayer, UK.
Nystatin (p.386·1); chlorhexidine acetate (p.1107·2) or chlorhexidine hydrochloride (p.1107·2); hydrocortisone (p.1043·3).
Infected skin disorders.

Nystalocal
Nourypharma, Ger.; Medinova, Switz.
Dexamethasone (p.1037·1); chlorhexidine hydrochloride (p.1107·2); nystatin (p.386·1).
Infected skin disorders.

Nystamont *Rosemont, UK.*
Nystatin (p.386·1).
Formerly known as Arpistatin.
Candidiasis.

Nystan *Squibb, UK.*
Nystatin (p.386·1).
Fungal infections.

Nystatin-Dome *Lagap, UK.*
Nystatin (p.386·1).
Candidiasis.

Nystex *Savage, USA.*
Nystatin (p.386·1).
Candidiasis.

Nystop *Paddock, USA.*
Nystatin (p.386·1).
Candidiasis.

Nytcold Medicine *Rugby, USA.*
Pseudoephedrine hydrochloride (p.1068·3); dextromethorphan hydrobromide (p.1057·3); doxylamine succinate (p.410·1); paracetamol (p.72·2).
Coughs and cold symptoms.

Nytol
Stafford-Miller, Austral.†; Block, Canad.; Block, Ger.; Stafford-Miller, UK; Block, USA.
Diphenhydramine hydrochloride (p.409·1).
Insomnia.

Nytol Herbal *Stafford-Miller, UK.*
Lupulus (p.1597·2); piscidia erythrina; passion flower (p.1615·3); pulsatilla (p.1623·3); wild lettuce (p.1645·1).
Insomnia.

Nytol Natural Source *Block, Canad.*
Valerian (p.1643·1).
Insomnia.

O A R *Colgate Oral Care, Austral.*
Sodium nitrite (p.995·2).
Rust prevention in disinfecting solutions. Not for use on human skin.

O-4 Cycline *Garec, S.Afr.*
Oxytetracycline hydrochloride (p.235·1).
Bacterial infections.

Oasil Relax *Daker Farmasimes, Spain†.*
Phenobarbitone (p.350·2); meprobamate (p.678·1).
Anxiety; bronchial asthma; hypersensitivity reactions of the skin; insomnia; skeletal muscle spasm.

Oasil Simes *Daker Farmasimes, Spain.*
Meprobamate (p.678·1).
Anxiety; insomnia; skeletal muscle spasm.

OB Thera *Legere, USA†.*
Multivitamin preparation.

Obalan *Lannett, USA.*
Phendimetrazine tartrate (p.1484·2).
Obesity.

Obaron *Mepha, Switz.*
Benzbromarone (p.392·3).
Gout; hyperuricaemia.

Obducti laxativi vegetabiles S *Hanseler, Switz.*
Aloes (p.1177·1); belladonna (p.457·1); frangula bark (p.1193·2); senna (p.1212·2).
Constipation.

Obe-Nix *Holloway, USA.*
Phentermine hydrochloride (p.1484·3).
Obesity.

Obephen *Hauck, USA†.*
Phentermine hydrochloride (p.1484·3).
Obesity.

Oberdol *Diafarm, Spain†.*
Chlorpheniramine maleate (p.405·1); phenylephrine hydrochloride (p.1066·2); paracetamol (p.72·2).
Cold symptoms; nasal congestion.

Obesaic *Manetti Roberts, Ital.†.*
Thyroid (p.1496·3); lipocaic.
Obesity.

Obesan-X *Technicon, S.Afr.*
Phendimetrazine bitartrate (p.1484·2).
Obesity.

Obetine *Tecnobio, Spain.*
Almagate (p.1177·1).
Hyperacidity.

Obeval *Vale, USA†.*
Phendimetrazine tartrate (p.1484·2).
Obesity.

Obex-LA *Adcock Ingram, S.Afr.*
Phendimetrazine bitartrate (p.1484·2).
Obesity.

Obifax *PQS, Spain†.*
Glycerol (p.1585·2).
Constipation.

Obiron *Pfizer, Austral.*
Multivitamin and iron preparation.

Oblioser
Serono, Ital.†; Serono, Spain.
Morphine sulphate (p.56·2).
Pain.

Obliterol *Faes, Spain.*
Pantethine (p.1276·3).
Hyperlipidaemias.

Oblivon *Doetsch, Grether, Switz.*
Methylpentynol (p.679·3).
Nervous disorders.

Obracin
Lilly, Belg.; Lilly, Neth.; Lilly, Switz.
Tobramycin sulphate (p.264·1).
Bacterial infections.

Obron-F *Pfizer, Switz.†.*
Multivitamin and mineral preparation.

Obron-N *Pfizer, Ger.†.*
Multivitamin and mineral preparation.

Obsidan *Isis, Ger.*
Propranolol hydrochloride (p.937·1).
Angina pectoris; anxiety; arrhythmias; hypertension; hyperthyroidism; migraine; myocardial infarction; tremor.

Obsilazin N *Isis, Ger.*
Propranolol hydrochloride (p.937·1); dihydralazine sulphate (p.854·1).
Hypertension.

Obstilax *Sanico, Belg.*
Sodium picosulphate (p.1213·2).
Constipation.

Obstinol *Thiemann, Ger.*
Liquid paraffin (p.1382·1); phenolphthalein (p.1208·2).
Bowel evacuation; constipation.

Obstinol mild *Thiemann, Ger.*
Liquid paraffin (p.1382·1).
Bowel regulation.

Obstinoletten *Thiemann, Ger.†; Chefaro, Ger.†.*
Aloes (p.1177·1); frangula bark (p.1193·2); cascara (p.1183·1); bovine gallbladder; caraway oil (p.1559·3); fennel oil (p.1579·2).
Constipation.

Oby-Cap *Richwood, USA.*
Phentermine hydrochloride (p.1484·3).
Obesity.

Oby-Trim 30 *Rexar, USA.*
Phentermine hydrochloride (p.1484·3).

Ocal *Sopar, Belg.†.*
Mercuric oxycyanide (p.1602·2); boric acid (p.1554·2); sodium chloride (p.1162·2).
Conjunctival inflammation and irritation.

O-Cal FA *Pharmics, USA.*
Multivitamin and mineral preparation with iron and folic acid.

Occlucort *GenDerm, Canad.*
Betamethasone dipropionate (p.1033·3).
Skin disorders.

Occlusal
GenDerm, Canad.; Helsinn Birex, Irl.; Euroderma, UK; GenDerm, USA.
Salicylic acid (p.1090·2).
Warts.

Ocean *Fleming, USA.*
Sodium chloride (p.1162·2).
Nasal irritation.

Ocean-A/S *Fleming, USA†.*
Atropine sulphate (p.455·1).
Coughs; post nasal drip; snoring due to mucus formation.

Oceantone *Cantassium Co., UK.*
Green-lipped mussel (p.1586·3).

Oceral
Asta Medica, Aust.; Siegfried, Switz.
Oxiconazole nitrate (p.386·3).
Fungal infections; mixed fungal and Gram-positive bacterial infections.

Oceral GB *Yamanouchi, Ger.*
Oxiconazole nitrate (p.386·3).
Fungal infections.

Ociter *Bracco, Ital.†.*
Ornicarbase (p.1611·1).
Liver disorders.

OCL *Abbott, USA.*
Macrogol 3350 (p.1598·2); electrolytes (p.1147·1).
Bowel evacuation.

Octacosanol *Cantassium Co., UK.*
Vitamin E (p.1369·1); octacosanol.

Octadon *Thiemann, Ger.†.*
Salacetamide (p.82·3); paracetamol (p.72·2); ethenzamide (p.35·3); caffeine (p.749·3).
Cold symptoms; fever; neuralgia; neuritis; pain; rheumatism.

Octadon N *Thiemann, Ger.†.*
Paracetamol (p.72·2).
Fever; pain.

Octadon P *Thiemann, Ger.*
Paracetamol (p.72·2); caffeine (p.749·3).
Pain.

Octagam
Octapharma, Aust.; Octapharma, Ger.; Octapharma, Norw.; Octapharma, Swed.; Octapharma, Switz.; Octapharma, UK.
A normal immunoglobulin (p.1522·1).
Bone-marrow transplantation; hypogammaglobulinaemia; idiopathic thrombocytopenic purpura; immunodeficiency; Kawasaki disease; passive immunisation.

Octamide *Adria, USA.*
Metoclopramide hydrochloride (p.1200·3).
Nausea and vomiting.

Octanyne
Octapharma, Ger.; Octapharma, Norw.
A factor IX preparation (p.721·3).
Haemorrhagic disorders.

Octaplas
Octapharma, Aust.; Octapharma, Ger.; Octapharma, UK.
Plasma (p.725·3).
Haemorrhagic disorders.

Octavi
Octapharma, Ger.; Octapharma, Norw.; Octapharma, Swed.†.
A factor VIII preparation (p.720·3).
Haemorrhagic disorders.

Octavit *Serturner, Ger.†.*
Nicametate citrate.
Peripheral and cerebrovascular disorders.

Octeniderm *Schulke & Mayr, Switz.†.*
Octenidine hydrochloride (p.1120·2); propyl alcohol (p.1124·2); isopropyl alcohol (p.1118·2).
Skin disinfection.

Octenisept
Schulke & Mayr, Aust.; Schulke & Mayr, Ger.; Schulke & Mayr, Switz.
Octenidine hydrochloride (p.1120·2); phenoxyethanol (p.1122·2).
Skin and mucous membrane disinfection.

Octicair *Bausch & Lomb, USA.*
Hydrocortisone (p.1043·3); neomycin sulphate (p.229·2); polymyxin B (p.239·3).
Bacterial ear infections.

Octilia *SIFI, Ital.*
Tetrahydrozoline hydrochloride (p.1070·2).
Eye irritation and congestion.

Octilia Bagnio Oculare *SIFI, Ital.†.*
Matricaria; lime; monobasic potassium phosphate; sodium phosphate; disodium edetate; polysorbate 80; chlorhexidine gluconate.
Eye irritation.

Octinum
Knoll, Ital.†; Knoll, Switz.
Isometheptene mucate (p.447·3) or isometheptene hydrochloride (p.447·3).
Migraine; smooth muscle spasm; vegetative dystonia.

Octocaine *Novocol, USA.*
Lignocaine hydrochloride (p.1293·2).
Adrenaline (p.813·2) is included in this preparation as a vasoconstrictor to diminish absorption and localise the effect of the local anaesthetic.
Local anaesthesia.

Octofene
Debat, Fr.; Hoechst Marion Roussel, Ital.
Clofoctol (p.195·1).
Otorhinolaryngeal infections; respiratory-tract infections.

Octonativ-M
Pharmacia Upjohn, Norw.; Pharmacia Upjohn, Swed.
A factor VIII preparation (p.720·3).
Haemorrhagic disorders.

Octonox *Pharmethic, Belg.*
Phenobarbitone sodium (p.350·2); quinalbarbitone sodium (p.690·2); amylobarbitone sodium (p.641·3).
Insomnia.

Octostim
Rhone-Poulenc Rorer, Austral.; Ferring, Canad.; Ferring, Neth.; Ferring, Norw.; Ferring, Swed.; Ferring, Switz.
Desmopressin acetate (p.1245·2).
Diabetes insipidus; haemorrhagic disorders; test of renal concentrating capacity.

Octovit *Goldshield, UK.*
Multivitamin and mineral preparation.

Octreoscan *Byk Gulden, Ital.*
Indium-111 pentetreotide (p.1423·3).
Detection and location of neuroendocrine tumours.

Octron *Lambda, USA.*
Vitamin B substances and iron.

Octron Plus *Lambda, USA.*
Ferric cacodylate.

Octron$_s$ *Lambda, USA.*
Vitamin B substances and iron.

Ocu-caine *Ocumed, USA.*
Proxymetacaine hydrochloride (p.1300·1).

OcuCaps *Akorn, USA.*
Antioxidant, vitamin, and mineral supplement.

Ocu-Carpine *Ocumed, USA.*
Pilocarpine hydrochloride (p.1396·3).
Glaucoma; raised intra-ocular pressure; reversal of mydriasis.

Ocuclear
Schering, Canad.; Schering-Plough, USA.
Oxymetazoline hydrochloride (p.1065·3).
Minor eye irritation.

Ocucoat
Note. This name is used for preparations of different composition.
Storz, Belg.; Storz, Fr.†; Storz, Norw.†; Storz, Swed.†; Storz, UK; Storz, USA.
Hypromellose (p.1473·1).
Adjunct in ocular surgery.

Storz, USA.
Eye drops: Dextran 70 (p.717·1); hypromellose (p.1473·1).
Dry eyes.

Ocudex *Charton, Canad.†.*
Dexamethasone sodium phosphate (p.1037·2).
Corticosteroid.

Ocufen
Allergan, Austral.; Allergan, Canad.; Allergan, Fr.; Allergan, Irl.; Allergan, Ital.; Allergan, S.Afr.; Allergan, UK; Allergan, USA.
Flurbiprofen sodium (p.42·1).
Intra-operative miosis inhibition; postoperative anterior eye inflammation; prevention of cystoid macular oedema.

Ocuflox
Allergan, Austral.; Allergan, Canad.; Allergan, USA.
Ofloxacin (p.233·3).
Bacterial conjunctivitis.

Ocuflur
Allergan, Aust.; Allergan, Belg.; Allergan, Ger.; Allergan, Spain; Allergan, Switz.
Flurbiprofen sodium (p.42·1).
Intra-operative miosis inhibition; postoperative eye inflammation; prevention of macular oedema after cataract surgery.

Ocufri *Allergan, Norw.*
Polyvinyl alcohol (p.1474·2).
Dry eyes.

Ocugram *Charton, Canad.*
Gentamicin sulphate (p.212·1).
Bacterial infections.

Oculinum *Allergan, USA†.*
Botulinum A toxin (p.1310·1).
Strabismus and blepharospasm associated with dystonia.

Oculoforte *Restan, S.Afr.*
Zinc sulphate (p.1373·2); phenylephrine hydrochloride (p.1066·2); tetrahydrozoline hydrochloride (p.1070·2).
Eye irritation.

Oculosan
Note. This name is used for preparations of different composition.
Restan, S.Afr.
Zinc sulphate (p.1373·2); naphazoline nitrate (p.1064·2).
Eye irritation.

Ciba Vision, Switz.
Zinc sulphate (p.1373·2); naphazoline nitrate (p.1064·2); hamamelis (p.1587·1); euphrasia; neroli oil (p.1606·3); lavender oil (p.1594·3).
Eye irritation.

Oculosan forte *Ciba Vision, Switz.*
Zinc sulphate (p.1373·2); phenylephrine hydrochloride (p.1066·2); tetrahydrozoline hydrochloride (p.1070·2); hamamelis (p.1587·1).
Eye irritation.

Oculosan N *Ciba Vision, Ger.*
Zinc sulphate (p.1373·2); naphazoline nitrate (p.1064·2).
Inflammatory and allergic disorders of the eye.

Oculotect
Note. This name is used for preparations of different composition.
Ciba Vision, Aust.; Ciba Vision, Neth.
Povidone (p.1474·2).
Dry eyes.

Ciba Vision, Ger.; Ciba Vision, Switz.
Vitamin A palmitate (p.1359·2).
Corneal damage; dry eyes.

Oculotect Fluid *Ciba Vision, Ger.*
Povidone (p.1474·2).
Dry eyes.

Oculube *Charton, Canad.*
White soft paraffin (p.1382·3); liquid paraffin (p.1382·1).
Dry eyes.

Ocupress *Otsuka, USA.*
Carteolol hydrochloride (p.837·3).
Glaucoma; ocular hypertension.

Ocusert
Allergan, Austral.; Dominion, UK; Alza, USA.
Pilocarpine (p.1396·3).
Glaucoma; raised intra-ocular pressure.

Ocusoft VMS *Ocusoft, USA.*
Multivitamin and mineral preparation.

Ocustil *SIFI, Ital.*
Sodium hyaluronate (p.1630·3).
Eye protection.

Ocusulf-10 *Optopics, USA.*
Sulphacetamide sodium (p.252·2).
Eye infections.

Ocutears *Charton, Canad.*
Hypromellose (p.1473·1); dextran 40 (p.716·2).
Dry eyes.

Ocutricin *Bausch & Lomb, USA.*
Eye drops: Polymyxin B sulphate (p.239·1); neomycin sulphate (p.229·2); gramicidin (p.215·2).
Eye ointment: Polymyxin B sulphate (p.239·1); neomycin sulphate (p.229·2); bacitracin zinc (p.157·3).
Eye infections.

Ocutrien *Cantassium Co., UK.*
Multivitamin and mineral preparation.

Ocutrulan *Truw, Ger.*
Homoeopathic preparation.

Ocu-Vinc *Alcon-Thilo, Ger.†.*
Vincamine (p.1644·1).
Circulatory disorders of the retina; Ménière's disease.

Ocuvite
Wyeth-Ayerst, Canad.; Storz, UK; Storz, USA.
Multivitamin and mineral preparation.

Odaban
Petrus, Austral.; Bracey, UK.
Aluminium chloride (p.1078·3).
Hyperhidrosis.

Odala wern *Wernigerode, Ger.*
Chamomile (p.1561·2); sage (p.1627·1); benzocaine (p.1286·2).
Inflammatory mouth disorders.

Odamida *Pelayo, Spain.*
Benzalkonium chloride (p.1101·3); zinc chloride (p.1373·1).
Formerly contained alum, sulphanilamide, and zinc chloride.
Gingivitis; oral hygiene; pyorrhoea.

Oddibil
Gerot, Aust.; Theraplix, Fr.; Nattermann, Ger.
Fumitory (p.1581·3).
Biliary disorders; digestive and renal disorders.

Oddispasmol *Merckle, Aust.*
Fumitory (p.1581·3).
Biliary disorders.

Odemase *Azupharma, Ger.*
Frusemide (p.871·1).
Hypertension; oedema.

Odemo-Genat *Azuchemie, Ger.†.*
Chlorthalidone (p.839·3).
Hypertension; oedema.

Odenil Unas *Isdin, Spain.*
Amorolfine hydrochloride (p.372·1).
Fungal nail infections.

Odol Med Dental *SmithKline Beecham, Spain.*
Chlorhexidine gluconate (p.1107·2).
Bacterial mouth infections.

Odontalg *Giovanardi, Ital.*
Lignocaine hydrochloride (p.1293·2).
Local anaesthesia.

Odontalgico Dr. Knapp con Vit. B1 *Montefarmaco, Ital.*
Paracetamol (p.72·2); propyphenazone (p.81·3); thiamine hydrochloride (p.1361·1); caffeine (p.749·3).
Pain.

Odontocromil c Sulfamida *Kin, Spain.*
Ascorbic acid (p.1365·2); chlorophyllin copper complex sodium; phenol (p.1121·2); sulphanilamide sodium (p.256·3); zinc chloride (p.1373·1); methyl salicylate (p.55·2); peppermint oil (p.1208·1); anise oil (p.1550·1).
Mouth inflammation; mouth wounds.

Odonton-Echtroplex *Weber & Weber, Ger.*
Homoeopathic preparation.

Odontoxina *Molteni, Ital.*
Chlorhexidine gluconate (p.1107·2); melissa oil; geranium oil; carnation oil; peppermint oil; spearmint oil.
Oral disinfection.

Odourless Garlic *Vitaplex, Austral.*
Garlic (p.1583·1); echinacea purpurea (p.1574·2); zinc gluconate (p.1373·2); betacarotene (p.1335·2).
Upper respiratory-tract congestion.

Odrik
Hoechst Marion Roussel, Austral.; Roussel, Fr.; Hoechst Marion Roussel, Irl.; Alter, Spain; Roussel, UK.
Trandolapril (p.957·1).
Hypertension; left ventricular dysfunction following myocardial infarction.

O-Due *Teofarma, Ital.*
Taurine (p.1635·1).
Vascular disorders.

Oecotrim *Laevosan, Aust.*
Co-trimoxazole (p.196·3).
Bacterial infections; Pneumocystis carinii pneumonia.

Oecozol *Laevosan, Aust.*
Metronidazole (p.585·1).
Anaerobic bacterial infections.

Oedemex *Mepha, Switz.*
Frusemide (p.871·1).
Forced diuresis; hypertension; oedema.

OeKolp *Kade, Ger.*
Oestriol (p.1457·2).
Menopausal disorders; vaginal disorders.

Oenobiol *Oenobiol, Fr.*
A range of nutritional supplements.

Oesclim *Fournier, Fr.*
Oestradiol (p.1455·1).
Menopausal disorders.

Oesto-Mins *Tyson, USA.*
Multivitamin and mineral preparation.

Oestraclin *Seid, Spain.*
Oestradiol (p.1455·1).
Amenorrhoea; female hypogonadism; menopausal disorders; osteoporosis; prostatic cancer; uterine hypoplasia.

Oestradiol Implants *Organon, UK.*
Oestradiol (p.1455·1).
Menopausal disorders.

Oestrifen *Ashbourne, UK.*
Tamoxifen citrate (p.563·3).
Anovulatory infertility; breast cancer.

Oestrilin *Desbergers, Canad.*
Oestrone (p.1458·2).
Kraurosis vulvae; pruritus vulvae; vaginitis.

Oestrilir N *Ardeypharm, Ger.†.*
Oestriol (p.1457·2).
Oestrogenic.

Oestring *Pharmacia Upjohn, Swed.*
Oestradiol (p.1455·1).
Vaginal disorders due to oestrogen deficiency.

Oestrodose *Besins-Iscovesco, Fr.*
Oestradiol (p.1455·1).
Menopausal disorders.

Oestro-Feminal
Pfizer, Aust.; Mack, Illert., Ger.
Conjugated oestrogens (p.1457·3).
Menopausal disorders.

Mack, Switz.
Esterified oestrogens (p.1458·1).
Menopausal disorders.

Oestrogel
Piette, Belg.; Besins-Iscovesco, Fr.; Hoechst Marion Roussel, Irl.; Golaz, Switz.; Hoechst Marion Roussel, UK.
Oestradiol (p.1455·1).
Menopausal disorders; osteoporosis.

Oestro-Gynaedron
Cassella-med, Ger.†; Artesan, Switz.†.
Sulphanilamide (p.256·3); chlorphenesin (p.376·2); ethinyloestradiol (p.1445·1).
Vaginal disorders.

Oestro-Gynaedron M *Artesan, Ger.; Cassella-med, Ger.*
Oestriol (p.1457·2).
Vaginal disorders.

Oestro-Gynaedron Nouveau *Artesan, Switz.*
Oestriol (p.1457·2).
Adjunct in vaginal surgery; oestrogen deficiency.

Oestro-Gynedron *Noriston, S.Afr.†.*
Stilboestrol dipropionate (p.1462·3); sulphasomidine (p.257·1); borax (p.1554·2).
Vaginal discharge; vaginitis.

OestroTricho N *Kade, Ger.†.*
Chlorphenesin (p.376·2); oestriol (p.1457·2).
Vaginal infections.

Oestrugol N *Atzinger, Ger.*
Oestriol (p.1457·2); urea (p.1095·2); thymol (p.1127·1).
Vaginitis.

Off-Ezy
Del, Canad.; Del, USA.
Salicylic acid (p.1090·2).
Calluses; corns; warts.

Ofil *Pharmazam, Spain.*
Pollen fractions.
Prostatitis.

O-Flam *MDM, Ital.*
Fentiazac (p.41·1).
Inflammation; oedema.

Oflocet
Hoechst Marion Roussel, Austral.; Diamant, Fr.
Ofloxacin (p.233·3).
Bacterial infections.

Oflocin *Glaxo Wellcome, Ital.*
Ofloxacin (p.233·3).
Respiratory-tract infections; urinary-tract infections.

Oflovir *Vir, Spain.*
Ofloxacin (p.233·3).
Bacterial infections.

Oftaciclox *Alcon, Spain.*
Ciprofloxacin hydrochloride (p.185·3).
Bacterial eye infections.

Oftalar *Cusi, Spain.*
Pranoprofen (p.81·2).
Eye disorders.

Oftalmil *Bruschettini, Ital.*
Naphazoline hydrochloride (p.1064·2); zinc phenolsulphonate (p.1096·3).
Eye irritation.

Oftalmo
Note. This name is used for preparations of different composition.
Funk, Spain†.
Eye drops: Gramicidin (p.215·2); hydrocortisone (p.1043·3); neomycin sulphate (p.229·2); polymyxin B sulphate (p.239·1); pseudoephedrine hydrochloride (p.1068·3); tetrahydrozoline hydrochloride (p.1070·2); phenazone (p.78·2).
Eye disorders.

Medical, Spain.
Eye ointment: Hydrocortisone acetate (p.1043·3); neomycin sulphate (p.229·2).
Infected eye disorders.

Oftalmol Dexa *Reig Jofre, Spain.*
Boric acid (p.1554·2); dexamethasone sodium metasulphobenzoate (p.1037·2); mercuric cyanide (p.1602·2); naphazoline nitrate (p.1064·2); trinitrophenol (p.1639·3); procaine hydrochloride (p.1299·2).
Eye disorders.

Oftalmol Ocular *Reig Jofre, Spain.*
Boric acid (p.1554·2); mercuric cyanide (p.1602·2); naphazoline nitrate (p.1064·2); trinitrophenol (p.1639·3); procaine hydrochloride (p.1299·2).
Eye congestion; infected eye disorders.

Oftalmosporin *Wellcome, Ital.†.*
Polymyxin B sulphate (p.239·1); neomycin sulphate (p.229·2); hydrocortisone (p.1043·3).
Eye infections.

Oftalmotrim *Cusi, Spain.*
Polymyxin B sulphate (p.239·1); trimethoprim (p.265·1).
Eye infections.

Oftalmotrim Dexa *Cusi, Spain.*
Dexamethasone sodium (p.1037·3); polymyxin B sulphate (p.239·1); trimethoprim (p.265·1).
Bacterial eye infections.

Oftalmowell *Evans, Spain.*
Gramicidin (p.215·2); neomycin sulphate (p.229·2); polymyxin B sulphate (p.239·1).
Eye infections.

Oftalzina *SIT, Ital.*
Procaine hydrochloride (p.1299·2); naphazoline nitrate (p.1064·2).
Conjunctival congestion.

Oftan
Leiras, Norw.; Ciba Vision, Switz.
Timolol maleate (p.953·3).
Glaucoma; ocular hypertension.

Oftapinex *Santen, Swed.*
Dipivefrine hydrochloride (p.1572·3).
Open-angle glaucoma.

Oftargol *Pons, Spain†.*
Mild silver protein.
Eye infections.

Oftimolo *Farmila, Ital.*
Timolol maleate (p.953·3).
Glaucoma; ocular hypertension.

Oftinal *Schering-Plough, Spain.*
Oxymetazoline hydrochloride (p.1065·3).
Eye irritation.

Oftisone *Locatelli, Ital.†.*
Medrysone (p.1045·3); neomycin sulphate (p.229·2).
Eye infections.

Oftyll Desoxydrop *Omisan, Ital.*
Disinfecting solution for contact lens.

OG (Odontalgico Gazzoni) *Gazzoni, Ital.†.*
Anaesthetic ether (p.1223·1).
Toothache.

Ogast *Takeda, Fr.*
Lansoprazole (p.1196·2).
Gastro-oesophageal reflux; peptic ulcer; Zollinger-Ellison syndrome.

Ogen
Pharmacia Upjohn, Austral.; Pharmacia Upjohn, Canad.; Abbott, USA.
Estropipate (p.1444·3).
Female hypogonadism; menopausal disorders; osteoporosis.

Ogestane *Besins-Iscovesco, Fr.*
A vitamin, mineral, and fish oil preparation.

Ogostal *Lilly, Ger.†.*
Capreomycin sulphate (p.162·1).
Tuberculosis.

Ogyline *Roussel, Fr.*
Norgestrienone (p.1455·1).
Progestogen-only oral contraceptive.

OH B12 *Poli, Ital.*
Hydroxocobalamin (p.1363·3).
Anaemias; liver disorders; neuralgia; neuritis.

OH B12 B1 *Poli, Ital.*
Hydroxocobalamin (p.1363·3); thiamine monophosphate chloride (p.1361·2).
Anaemias; neuralgia; neuritis.

OIF *Otsuka, Jpn.*
Interferon alfa (p.615·3).
Hepatitis; renal cancer.

Oil Bleo *Kayaku, Jpn†.*
Bleomycin sulphate (p.507·3).
Malignant neoplasms.

Oil of Olay *Procter & Gamble, USA.*
SPF 15: Ethylhexyl *p*-methoxycinnamate (p.1487·1); titanium dioxide (p.1093·3); 2-phenyl-1*H*-benzimidazole-5-sulphonic acid (p.1488·2).
Sunscreen.

Oilatum
Stiefel, Canad.; Stiefel, Spain.
Emollient.

Oilatum Bar *Stiefel, Austral.*
Soap substitute.

Oilatum Cream
Stiefel, Irl.; Stiefel, S.Afr.†; Stiefel, UK.
Arachis oil (p.1550·2).
Dry skin disorders.

Oilatum Emollient
Stiefel, Austral.; Stiefel, Irl.; Stiefel, S.Afr.†; Stiefel, UK.
Liquid paraffin (p.1382·1); acetylated wool alcohols (p.1385·2).
Dry skin conditions.

Oilatum Fragrance Free *Stiefel, UK.*
Light liquid paraffin (p.1382·1).
Dry skin disorders.

Oilatum Gel
Stiefel, Irl.; Stiefel, UK.
Light liquid paraffin (p.1382·1).
Dry skin disorders.

Oilatum Plus
Stiefel, Austral.; Stiefel, UK.
Light liquid paraffin (p.1382·1); triclosan (p.1127·2); benzalkonium chloride (p.1101·3).
Eczema.

Oilatum Skin Therapy *Stiefel, UK.*
Light liquid paraffin (p.1382·1).
Dry skin.

Oilatum Soap
Note. This name is used for preparations of different composition.
Stiefel, S.Afr.†.
Arachis oil (p.1550·2).
Soap substitute.

Stiefel, UK.
Liquid paraffin (p.1382·1).
Dry skin disorders.

Stiefel, USA.
Skin cleanser.

Oil-Free Acne Wash *Professional Health, Canad.*
Salicylic acid (p.1090·2).
Acne.

Oil-Free Sunblock *Clinique, Canad.*
SPF 15: Ethylhexyl *p*-methoxycinnamate (p.1487·1); octocrylene (p.1487·3); octyl salicylate (p.1487·3); oxybenzone (p.1487·3).
Sunscreen.

Oil-Free Sunscreen *Avon, Canad.*
SPF 15: Ethylhexyl *p*-methoxycinnamate (p.1487·1); octocrylene (p.1487·3); octyl salicylate (p.1487·3).
Sunscreen.

Oil-Free Sunspray *Estee Lauder, Canad.*
SPF 10; SPF 15: Ethylhexyl *p*-methoxycinnamate (p.1487·1); homosalate (p.1487·2); octyl salicylate (p.1487·3); oxybenzone (p.1487·3).
Sunscreen.

Ojosbel *Collado, Spain.*
Hamamelis water (p.1587·1); naphazoline hydrochloride (p.1064·2).
Eye irritation.

Ojosbel Azul *Collado, Spain.*
Hamamelis water (p.1587·1); methylene blue (p.984·3); naphazoline hydrochloride (p.1064·2).
Eye irritation.

Okacin *Ciba Vision, Switz.*
Lomefloxacin hydrochloride (p.222·2).
Bacterial eye infections.

Okal *Puerto Galiano, Spain.*
Aspirin (p.16·1); caffeine (p.749·3).
Glycine (p.1345·2) is included in this preparation in an attempt to limit adverse effects on the gastro-intestinal mucosa.
Fever; inflammation; pain.

Okal Infantil *Puerto Galiano, Spain.*
Aspirin (p.16·1).
Fever; musculoskeletal and joint disorders; pain; thrombosis prophylaxis.

Okavena *Rovi, Spain†.*
Leucocianidol (p.1580·2).
Vascular disorders.

Oki *Dompe, Ital.*
Ketoprofen lysine (p.48·3).
Inflammation; pain.

Okokit II *Hughes & Hughes, UK.*
Test for faecal occult blood.

Okoubarell *Sanorell, Ger.*
Homoeopathic preparation.

Okoubasan *Sanum-Kehlbeck, Ger.*
Homoeopathic preparation.

Okuzell *Hafslund Nycomed, Aust.*
Hypromellose (p.1473·1).
Eye irritation.

O-Lac
Mead Johnson, Austral.; Mead Johnson, Ital.
Infant feed.
Galactosaemia; lactose intolerance; sucrose intolerance.

Oladerm *Sodip, Switz.†.*
Bath additive.
Skin disorders.

Olamin P *Delta BKB, Ital.*
Piroctone olamine (p.1089·1).
Seborrhoeic dermatitis.

Ol-Amine *Meuse, Belg.*
Multivitamin and mineral preparation.

Olbad Cordes
Ichthyol, Aust.; Ichthyol, Ger.; Ichthyol, Switz.†.
Soya oil (p.1355·1).
Bath additive; skin disorders.

Olbad Cordes comp *Ichthyol, Aust.*
Soya oil (p.1355·1); shale oil.
Bath additive; skin disorders.

Olbad Cordes F *Ichthyol, Ger.*
Arachis oil (p.1550·2).
Bath additive; skin disorders.

Olbas
Note. This name is used for preparations of different composition.
Synpharma, Switz.
Inhaler: Peppermint oil (p.1208·1); eucalyptus oil (p.1578·1); menthol (p.1600·2); cineole (p.1564·1).
Oil: Peppermint oil (p.1208·1); eucalyptus oil (p.1578·1); cajuput oil (p.1556·1); sweet birch oil (p.55·3); juniper oil (p.1592·3); clove oil (p.1565·2).
Ointment: Peppermint oil (p.1208·1); eucalyptus oil (p.1578·1); cajuput oil (p.1556·1); sweet birch oil (p.55·3); turpentine oil (p.1641·1); clove oil (p.1565·2).
Cold symptoms; nasal congestion.

Lane, UK.
Inhaler: Cajuput oil (p.1556·1); menthol (p.1600·2); peppermint oil (p.1208·1); eucalyptus oil (p.1578·1).
Oil: Cajuput oil (p.1556·1); eucalyptus oil (p.1578·1); sweet birch oil (p.55·3); clove oil (p.1565·2); juniper oil (p.1592·3); menthol (p.1600·2); dementholised mint oil (p.1604·1).
Pastilles: Eucalyptus oil (p.1578·1); peppermint oil (p.1208·1); menthol (p.1600·2); juniper oil (p.1592·3); sweet birch oil (p.55·3); clove oil (p.1565·2).
Cold symptoms; coughs.

Olbemox *Pharmacia Upjohn, Ger.*
Acipimox (p.1267·3).
Lipid disorders.

Olbetam
Pharmacia Upjohn, Aust.; Pharmacia Upjohn, Belg.; Pharmacia Upjohn, Irl.; Pharmacia Upjohn, Ital.; Pharmacia Upjohn, S.Afr.; Pharmacia Upjohn, Switz.; Pharmacia Upjohn, UK.
Acipimox (p.1267·3).
Hyperlipidaemias.

Olbiacor *Salus, Ital.*
Fendiline hydrochloride (p.868·1).
Ischaemic heart disease; myocardial infarction.

Olcadil *Sanabo, Aust.*
Cloxazolam (p.657·3).
Alcohol withdrawal syndrome; anxiety disorders; premedication; sleep disorders.

Olcam *Irex, Fr.*
Piroxicam (p.80·2).
Musculoskeletal and joint disorders.

Olcenon *Lederle, Jpn.*
Tretinoin tocopheryl.
Skin ulcers.

Oldamin *Fuji, Jpn.*
Ethanolamine oleate (p.1576·2).
Oesophageal varices.

Oldan *Europharma, Spain.*
Acemetacin (p.12·2).
Musculoskeletal, joint, and peri-articular disorders.

Older *Sagitta, Ger.†.*
Diprophylline (p.752·1); isoprenaline sulphate (p.892·1); diphenhydramine hydrochloride (p.409·1); guaiphenesin (p.1061·3); primula root; thyme; plantago lanceolata; pulmonaria.
Asthma; bronchitis; coughs; emphysema.

Oleatum *Stiefel, Ger.*
Light liquid paraffin (p.1382·1).
Skin disorders.

Oleatum fett *Stiefel, Switz.†.*
Liquid paraffin (p.1382·1).
Skin disorders.

Oleobal *Pierre Fabre Medikosma, Ger.*
Soya oil (p.1355·1); light liquid paraffin (p.1382·1).
Bath additive; skin disorders.

Oleocalcium AD *Lisapharma, Ital.†.*
Calcium oleate; vitamin A (p.1358·1); ergocalciferol (p.1367·1).
Bone disorders.

Oleomycetin
Agepha, Aust.; Winzer, Ger.
Chloramphenicol (p.182·1).
Bacterial eye infections.

Oleomycetin-Prednison
Agepha, Aust.; Winzer, Ger.
Chloramphenicol (p.182·1); prednisone (p.1049·2).
Infected eye disorders.

Oleosint *Apomedica, Aust.*
Diethanolamine oleate; soya oil (p.1355·1).
Skin disorders.

Oleosorbate
Bournonville, Belg.; Merck Sharp & Dohme-Chibret, Fr.†.
Polysorbate 80 (p.1327·3).
Nasal and aural suppuration; removal of ear wax; rhinitis.

Oleovit *Laevosan, Aust.*
Vitamin A palmitate (p.1359·2); dexpanthenol (p.1570·3).
Eye disorders.

Oleovit A *Laevosan, Aust.*
Capsules: Vitamin A palmitate (p.1359·2).
Ear disorders; gastro-intestinal disorders; hyperthyroidism; respiratory-tract disorders; skin disorders; urogenital disorders.
Oral drops: Vitamin A (p.1358·1); betacarotene (p.1335·2).
Vitamin A deficiency.

Oleovit A + D *Laevosan, Aust.*
Capsules: Vitamin A palmitate (p.1359·2); cholecalciferol (p.1366·3).
Oral drops: Vitamin A (p.1358·1); betacarotene (p.1335·2); cholecalciferol (p.1366·3).
Rickets; vitamin A and D supplementation.

Oleovit D_3 *Laevosan, Aust.*
Cholecalciferol (p.1366·3).
Hypoparathyroidism; rickets.

Oleum Rhinale *Weleda, UK.*
Calendula; merc. sulph.; peppermint oil (p.1208·1); eucalyptus oil (p.1578·1).
Catarrh; sinus congestion.

Olfen *Mepha, Switz.*
Diclofenac sodium (p.31·2).
Lignocaine hydrochloride (p.1293·2) is included in the intramuscular injection to alleviate the pain of injection.
Inflammation; musculoskeletal, joint, peri-articular, and soft-tissue disorders; pain.

Olfex *Ifidesa Aristegui, Spain.*
Budesonide (p.1034·3).
Asthma; insect bites; nasal polyps; rhinitis; skin disorders.

Olicard
Solvay, Ger.; Nezel, Spain; Solvay, Switz.†.
Isosorbide mononitrate (p.893·3).
Heart failure; ischaemic heart disease.

Olicardin *Solvay, Aust.*
Isosorbide mononitrate (p.893·3).
Angina pectoris; heart failure; myocardial infarction; pulmonary hypertension.

Oligobs *CCD, Fr.*
A range of multivitamin and mineral preparations.

Oligocean *Ido, Fr.*
Trace element and mineral preparation derived from shellfish.
Tonic.

Oligocure *Labcatal, Fr.*
Manganese gluconate; copper gluconate; colloidal gold.
Tonic.

Oligoderm *Labcatal, Fr.*
Manganese gluconate (p.1351·1); copper gluconate (p.1338·1).
Cracked nipples.

Oligo-elements Aguettant *Aguettant, Fr.*
Trace element preparation.
Parenteral nutrition.

Oligofer *Sabex, Canad.*
Mineral preparation with vitamin B_{12}.

Oligoforme *Ido, Fr.*
A range of nutritional supplements.

Oligogranul *Boiron, Fr.*
A range of trace element and mineral preparations.

Oligomarine *Sessa, Ital.†.*
Marine protein and trace element preparation.

Oligophytum *Holistica, Fr.*
A range of mineral-rich plant extracts.

Oligosol
Labcatal, Fr.; Labcatal, Switz.
A range of trace element and mineral preparations.

Oligostim *Dolisos, Fr.*
A range of trace element and mineral preparations.

Oliviase *UPSA, Fr.*
Olive leaves.
Diuresis.

Olivysat *Ysatfabrik, Ger.*
Olive leaves.
Prevention of atherosclerosis.

Olmifon *Lafon, Fr.*
Adrafinil (p.1477·2).
Mental function impairment in the elderly.

Ologyn *Labatec, Switz.*
Norgestrel (p.1454·1); ethinyloestradiol (p.1445·1).
Combined oral contraceptive; menstrual disorders.

Olren *Heumann, Ger.†.*
Scopolia carniolica; ethaverine hydrochloride (p.1577·1).
Urinary-tract disorders.

Olren N *Heumann, Ger.*
Scopolia carniolica.
Urinary-tract disorders.

Olynth
Parke, Davis, Aust.; Warner-Lambert, Ger.; Warner-Lambert Consumer, Switz.
Xylometazoline hydrochloride (p.1071·2).
Nasal congestion.

Omacor *Pharmacia Upjohn, Norw.*
Omega-3 marine triglycerides (p.1276·1).
Hyperlipidaemia.

Omadine *Erredici, Ital.*
Pyrithione disulphide (p.1089·3); urtica (p.1642·3).
Seborrhoeic dermatitis.

Omapren *Vita, Spain.*
Omeprazole (p.1204·2) or omeprazole sodium (p.1204·2).
Gastro-oesophageal reflux; peptic ulcers; Zollinger-Ellison syndrome.

Ombolan *Esteve, Spain†.*
Droxicam (p.35·2).
Ankylosing spondylitis; arthritis; inflammation.

Ombrelle *Dermtek, Canad.*
SPF 30: Avobenzone (p.1486·3); ethylhexyl *p*-methoxycinnamate (p.1487·1); oxybenzone (p.1487·3).
Sunscreen.

Ombrelle Extreme *Dermtek, Canad.*
SPF 30: Avobenzone (p.1486·3); ethylhexyl *p*-methoxycinnamate (p.1487·1); oxybenzone (p.1487·3); titanium dioxide (p.1093·3).
Sunscreen.

Ombrelle for Kids *Dermtek, Canad.*
SPF 30: Avobenzone (p.1486·3); ethylhexyl *p*-methoxycinnamate (p.1487·1); 2-phenyl-1*H*-benzimidazole-5-sulphonic acid (p.1488·2); 3-(4-methylbenzylidene)bornan-2-one (p.1487·2).
Sunscreen.

Ombrelle, Ombrelle Sport Spray *Dermtek, Canad.*
SPF 15: Avobenzone (p.1486·3); ethylhexyl *p*-methoxycinnamate (p.1487·1); oxybenzone (p.1487·3).
Sunscreen.

Omca *Bristol-Myers Squibb, Ger.*
Fluphenazine hydrochloride (p.671·3).
Psychiatric disorders.

Omca Nacht *Squibb-Heyden, Ger.†.*
Fluphenazine hydrochloride (p.671·3); pentobarbitone sodium (p.685·1).
Angina pectoris; gastro-intestinal disorders; psychiatric disorders; sleep disorders.

Omega *Schmidgall, Aust.*
Proxyphylline (p.757·3); crataegus (p.1568·2); convallaria (p.1567·2).
Cardiac disorders.

Omega-3 *Gisand, Switz.*
Omega-3 marine triglycerides (p.1276·1).
Dietary supplement; hyperlipidaemia.

Omegacoeur *Holistica, Fr.*
Omega-3 triglycerides (p.1276·1); herbs.
Circulatory disorders.

Omega-H3
Vitabiotics, Irl.; Vitabiotics, UK.
Multivitamin and mineral preparation.

Omegaline *Holistica, Fr.*
Borage oil (p.1582·1).
Nutritional supplement.

Omeprazen *Malesci, Ital.*
Omeprazole (p.1204·2) or omeprazole sodium (p.1204·2).
Gastro-oesophageal reflux; peptic ulcer; Zollinger-Ellison syndrome.

Omeril *Bayer, Ger.*
Mebhydrolin napadisylate (p.413·2).
Hypersensitivity reactions.

Omida Gel Antirhumatismal *Omida, Switz.*
Homoeopathic preparation.

Omida Granules Relaxants *Omida, Switz.*
Homoeopathic preparation.

Omida Spray Nasal *Omida, Switz.*
Homoeopathic preparation.

Omiderm *Dormer, Canad.†.*
Polyurethane foam dressing.
Wounds.

Omifin *Marion Merrell, Spain.*
Clomiphene citrate (p.1439·2).
Anovulatory infertility; male infertility.

Omix *Yamanouchi, Fr.*
Tamsulosin hydrochloride (p.951·2).
Benign prostatic hyperplasia.

Omnadin *Hermal, Ger.†.*
Proteins (metabolic products of *Bacillus mycoides* and *Sarcina flava*); bovine bile extract (p.1553·2); lipids.
Immunotherapy.

Omnalio *Estedi, Spain.*
Chlordiazepoxide hydrochloride (p.646·3).
Alcohol withdrawal syndrome; anxiety; insomnia.

Omniadol *Montefarmaco, Ital.*
Propyphenazone (p.81·3); paracetamol (p.72·2); caffeine (p.749·3).
Cold symptoms; pain.

Omniapharm *Merckle, Ger.*
Bromhexine hydrochloride (p.1055·3).
Respiratory-tract disorders associated with increased or viscous mucus.

Omnibionta
Merck, Aust.
Multivitamin preparation.

Merck-Belgolabo, Belg.; Meda, Swed.
Brown/red capsules, multivitamins; yellow/ochre capsules, minerals.

Omnic
Yamanouchi, Ger.; Yamanouchi, Irl.; Yamanouchi, Ital.; Yamanouchi, Neth.
Tamsulosin hydrochloride (p.951·2).
Benign prostatic hyperplasia.

Omnicare
Allergan, Aust.; Allergan, Austral.; Allergan, Ger.†.
Solution, hydrogen peroxide (p.1116·2); tablets, neutraliser.
Disinfecting and neutralising system for soft contact lenses.

Omnicef *Parke, Davis, USA.*
Cefdinir (p.164·3).
Bacterial infections.

Omniderm *Face, Ital.*
Fluocinolone acetonide (p.1041·1).
Inflammatory skin disorders.

Omniflora
Zyma, Aust.; Med Fabrik, Ger.†.
Lactobacillus acidophilus (p.1594·1); *Lactobacterium bifidum* (p.1594·1); *Escherichia coli.*
Gastro-intestinal disorders.

Omniflora N *Zyma, Ger.*
Lactobacillus gasseri; Bifidobacterium longum.
Gastro-intestinal disorders.

Omnigel *CTS Dental, UK†.*
Stannous fluoride (p.1632·2).
Dental caries prophylaxis.

Omnigraf *Juste, Spain.*
Iohexol (p.1006·3).
Radiographic contrast medium.

OmniHIB *SmithKline Beecham, USA.*
A haemophilus influenzae conjugate vaccine (tetanus toxoid conjugate) (p.1511·1).
Active immunisation.

OMNIhist LA *WE, USA.*
Phenylephrine hydrochloride (p.1066·2); chlorpheniramine maleate (p.405·1); hyoscine methonitrate (p.463·1).
Upper respiratory-tract symptoms.

Omnilan *Schering, Aust.*
Fluocortolone pivalate (p.1041·3).
Skin disorders.

Omnipaque
Schering, Aust.; Nycomed, Austral.; Nycomed, Belg.; Sanofi Winthrop, Canad.; Nycomed, Fr.; Schering, Ger.; Nycomed, Ital.; Nycomed, Neth.†; Nycomed Imaging, Norw.; Nycomed, Swed.; Schering, Switz.; Nycomed, UK; Nycomed, USA.
Iohexol (p.1006·3).
Radiographic contrast medium.

Omnipen *Wyeth-Ayerst, USA.*
Ampicillin (p.153·1).
Bacterial infections.

Omnipen-N *Wyeth-Ayerst, USA.*
Ampicillin sodium (p.153·1).
Bacterial infections.

Omniplex *Vitaplex, Austral.*
Multivitamin and mineral supplement with herbs.
Dietary supplement.

Omniscan
Nycomed, Aust.; Nycomed, Austral.; Nycomed, Belg.; Sanofi Winthrop, Canad.; Nycomed, Ger.; Nycomed, Ital.; Nycomed, Neth.†; Nycomed Imaging, Norw.; Nycomed, Spain; Nycomed, Swed.; Nycomed, Switz.; Nycomed, UK; Sanofi Winthrop, USA.
Gadodiamide (p.1004·3).
Contrast medium for magnetic resonance imaging.

Omnisept *Synthelabo, Ger.*
Lactobacillus acidophilus (p.1594·1).
Diarrhoea.

Omnitrace *Lifeplan, UK.*
Trace element preparation.

Omnitrast *Schering, Spain.*
Iohexol (p.1006·3).
Radiographic contrast medium.

Omni-Tuss *Rhone-Poulenc Rorer, Canad.*
Codeine resin (p.26·1); phenyltoloxamine resin (p.416·1); chlorpheniramine resin (p.405·2); ephedrine resin (p.1059·3); guaiacol carbonate (p.1061·2).
Coughs.

Omnival *Nordmark, Ger.†.*
Multivitamin and mineral preparation.

Omnopon
Intramed, S.Afr.; Roche, UK†.
Papaveretum (p.71·1) (containing morphine hydrochloride, codeine hydrochloride, and papaverine hydrochloride).
NOTE. This preparation was reformulated to exclude the noscapine component.
Pain; premedication.

Ompranyt *Boehringer Mannheim, Spain.*
Omeprazole (p.1204·2).
Gastro-oesophageal reflux; peptic ulcer; Zollinger-Ellison syndrome.

OMS Concentrate *Upsher-Smith, USA.*
Morphine sulphate (p.56·2).

Omsat *Boehringer Mannheim, Ger.†.*
Co-trimoxazole (p.196·3).
Bacterial infections.

Onagre *Sante Naturelle, Canad.*
Evening primrose oil (p.1582·1).

Onaka *Max Farma, Ital.*
Poditimod (p.1618·3).
Immunostimulant.

Oncaspar *Enzon, USA.*
Pegaspargase (p.505·1).
Acute lymphoblastic leukaemia.

Once-a-Day
Quest, Canad.; Quest, UK.
Multivitamin and mineral preparation.

Oncet *Wakefield, USA.*
Hydrocodone tartrate (p.43·1); paracetamol (p.72·2).
Cough and cold symptoms.

Onco Tiotepa *Pras, Spain.*
Thiotepa (p.566·3).
Malignant neoplasms.

Onco-Carbide *Teofarma, Ital.*
Hydroxyurea (p.539·1).
Chronic myeloid leukaemia.

Oncosal *Inibsa, Spain.*
Flutamide (p.537·1).
Prostatic cancer.

OncoScint CR 103
CIS, Ital.; Chiron, Spain; Eurocetus, UK†.
Indium (^{111}In) satumomab pendetide (p.1423·3).
Diagnosis of colorectal cancer.

OncoScint CR/OV *Cytogen, USA.*
Indium (^{111}In) satumomab pendetide (p.1423·3).
Detection of colorectal and ovarian metastases.

Oncotam *Mayoly-Spindler, Fr.*
Tamoxifen citrate (p.563·3).
Breast cancer.

OncoTICE
Organon, Aust.; Organon Teknika, Austral.; Organon Teknika, Canad.; Apogepha, Ger.; Organon Teknika, Ital.; Organon Teknika, Neth.; Organon Teknika, Norw.; Organon Teknika, Swed.; Organon Teknika, Switz.
A BCG vaccine (p.1504·3).
Bladder cancer.

Oncovin
Lilly, Aust.; Lilly, Austral.; Lilly, Belg.; Lilly, Canad.; Lilly, Fr.; Lilly, Irl.; Lilly, Neth.; Lilly, Norw.; Lilly, S.Afr.; Lilly, Swed.; Lilly, Switz.; Lilly, UK; Lilly, USA.
Vincristine sulphate (p.570·1).
Idiopathic thrombocytopenic purpura; malignant neoplasms.

Oncovite *Mission Pharmacal, USA.*
Multivitamin preparation with zinc.

Onctose *Monot, Fr.*
Diphenhydramine methylsulphate (p.409·2); lignocaine hydrochloride (p.1293·2).
Pruritus.

Onctose a l'Hydrocortisone *Denolin, Belg.*
Hydrocortisone acetate (p.1043·3); diphenhydramine methylsulphate (p.409·2); lignocaine hydrochloride (p.1293·2).
Cutaneous hypersensitivity reactions; insect stings; pruritus.

Onctose Hydrocortisone *Monot, Fr.*
Diphenhydramine methylsulphate (p.409·2); lignocaine hydrochloride (p.1293·2); hydrocortisone acetate (p.1043·3).
Pruritus.

Ondroly-A *Boffi, Ital.*
Peppermint oil (p.1208·1); clove oil (p.1565·2); menthol (p.1600·2); benzoin tincture (p.1628·3); phenol (p.1121·2).
Dentistry.

Ondrox *Unimed, USA.*
Multivitamin, mineral, and amino acid preparation.

One A Day
Bayer, Canad.; Bayer, Ital.; Miles Consumer Healthcare, USA.
Vitamin, multivitamin, or multivitamin and mineral preparations.

One Touch
Lifescan, Fr.; LifeScan, USA.
Test for glucose in blood (p.1585·1).

One-Alpha
Leo, Canad.; Leo, Irl.; Adcock Ingram, S.Afr.; Leo, UK.
Alfacalcidol (p.1366·3).
Hyperparathyroidism; hypoparathyroidism; hypophosphataemia; neonatal hypocalcaemia; osteomalacia; osteoporosis; renal osteodystrophy; rickets.

One-Step hCG *Wampole, USA†.*
Pregnancy test (p.1621·2).

One-Tablet-Daily *Goldline, USA.*
A range of vitamin preparations with or without minerals.

Onguent nasal Ruedi *Spirig, Switz.*
Mint oil (p.1604·1); camphor oil.
Nasal dryness.

Onico Fitex *Belmac, Spain.*
Borogallic acid; salicylic acid (p.1090·2).
Fungal nail infections.

Oniria *Lifepharma, Ital.†.*
Quazepam (p.689·3).
Insomnia.

Onkohas *Braun, Ger.†.*
A hydroxyethyl ether starch (p.724·2) in sodium chloride.
Plasma volume expansion.

Onkovertin
Braun, Aust.; Braun, Ger.
Dextran 60 (p.716·3) in sodium chloride.
Plasma volume expansion; pre-operative haemodilution; thrombo-embolism prophylaxis.

Onkovertin N
Braun, Aust.; Braun, Ger.
Dextran 40 (p.716·2) in sodium chloride.
Thrombo-embolism prophylaxis; vascular disorders.

Only One *Sisu, Canad.*
Multivitamin and mineral preparation.

Onopordon Comp B *Weleda, UK.*
Onopordon; primula officinalis; hyoscyamus (p.464·3).
Cardiac disorders.

Onoprose *Ono, Jpn.*
Promelase (p.1621·3).
Inflammation; respiratory-tract congestion.

Onoton *Maggioni, Ital.†.*
Pancreatin (p.1612·1); hemicellulase (p.1561·1); ox bile extract (p.1553·2); dimethicone (p.1213·1).
Digestive-system disorders.

Onrectal *Herbes Universelles, Canad.*
Benzocaine (p.1286·2); bismuth subcarbonate (p.1180·1); bismuth subgallate (p.1180·2); hamamelis (p.1587·1); naphazoline hydrochloride (p.1064·2); zinc oxide (p.1096·2).
Haemorrhoids.

Onsukil
Syntex, Ger.†; Miquel Otsuka, Spain.
Procaterol or procaterol hydrochloride (p.757·3).
Obstructive airways disease.

Ontosein *Tedec Meiji, Spain.*
Orgotein (p.87·3).
Arthropathies; cystitis; secondary effects of radiotherapy.

Onycho Phytex
Note. This name is used for preparations of different composition.
Rupertus, Aust.
Sorbic acid (p.1125·2); tannic acid (p.1634·2); methyl salicylate (p.55·2); salicylic acid (p.1090·2); acetic acid (p.1541·2).
Fungal nail infections.

UCB, Switz.†.
Borogallic acid; glacial acetic acid (p.1541·2); salicylic acid (p.1090·2).
Fungal skin infections.

Onychomal *Hermal, Ger.*
Urea (p.1095·2).
Nail disorders.

Ony-Clear *Pedinol, USA.*
Miconazole nitrate (p.384·3).
Formerly called Ony-Clear Nail and contained triacetin, cetylpyridinium chloride, and chloroxylenol.
Fungal nail infections.

Onymyken *Schuck, Ger.†.*
Clotrimazole (p.376·3).
Fungal infections.

Onymyken S *Schuck, Ger.†.*
Propionic acid (p.387·1); salicylic acid (p.1090·2); undecenoic acid (p.389·2); 5-chlorocarvacrol; chlorothymol (p.1111·1); 5,5′-dibrom-2,2′-dihydroxybenzil; hexylresorcinol (p.1116·1); methyl salicylate (p.55·2).
Fungal infections.

Onysin *Lambda, USA.*
Vitamin B substances and lysine.

Onyvul *Stiefel, Canad.†.*
Urea (p.1095·2).
Nail avulsion.

Opacinan *Alcon, Fr.†.*
Vitamin B substances.
Alcoholism; pain; vitamin B deficiency.

Opacist ER
Bracco, Ital.; Bracco, Switz.
Meglumine iodamide (p.1005·3).
Contrast medium for urinary-tract radiography.

Opalgyne *Innothera, Fr.*
Benzydamine hydrochloride (p.21·3).
Vaginitis.

Opalia *Ecobi, Ital.*
Royal jelly (p.1626·3).
Nutritional supplement.

Opalmon *Ono, Jpn.*
Limaprost alfadex (p.1419·2).
Thromboangiitis obliterans.

Opas
Note. This name is used for preparations of different composition.
Leo, Irl.†.
Sodium bicarbonate (p.1153·2); calcium carbonate (p.1182·1); magnesium carbonate (p.1198·1).
Dyspepsia; flatulence; heartburn.

Shire, UK.
Sodium bicarbonate (p.1153·2); calcium carbonate (p.1182·1); magnesium carbonate (p.1198·1); magnesium trisilicate (p.1199·1).
Gastro-intestinal disorders.

Opazimes *Shire, UK.*
Aluminium hydroxide (p.1177·3); light kaolin (p.1195·1); belladonna (p.457·1); morphine hydrochloride (p.56·1).
Gastro-intestinal disorders.

Opcon *Bausch & Lomb, Canad.†.*
Naphazoline hydrochloride (p.1064·2).
Eye congestion.

Opcon-A
Bausch & Lomb, Canad.; Bausch & Lomb, USA.
Naphazoline hydrochloride (p.1064·2); pheniramine maleate (p.415·3).
Eye irritation.

Opdensit *Stroschein, Ger.†.*
Papaverine hydrochloride (p.1614·2).
Impotence; Peyronie's disease.

Operand *Redi-Products, USA.*
Povidone-iodine (p.1123·3).
Skin disinfection; vaginal disorders.

Operidine
Janssen-Cilag, Austral.; Janssen-Cilag, UK†.
Phenoperidine hydrochloride (p.79·1).
Adjunct in neuroleptanalgesia; pain; respiratory depressant in intensive care.

Ophcillin N *Medicopharm, Aust.*
Benzylpenicillin sodium (p.159·3); sulphadiazine (p.252·3).

Ophdilvas N *Mann, Ger.*
Vincamine (p.1644·1).
Formerly contained vincamine and papaverine hydrochloride.
Cerebral and peripheral vascular disorders; circulatory disorders of the eye.

Ophtacortine *Cusi, Spain†.*
Hydrocortisone acetate (p.1043·3); neomycin sulphate (p.229·2).
Infected eye disorders.

Ophtadil *Chauvin, Fr.*
Buphenine hydrochloride (p.1555·3); ethoxazorutoside (p.1580·1); sodium ascorbate (p.1365·2); tocophersolan (p.1370·1).
Ocular vascular disorders.

Ophtagram
Chauvin, Fr.; ankerpharm, Ger.; Novopharma, Switz.
Gentamicin sulphate (p.212·1).
Bacterial eye infections.

Ophtaguttal *Agepha, Aust.*
Naphazoline hydrochloride (p.1064·2); zinc sulphate (p.1373·2); boric acid (p.1554·2).
Conjunctival irritation.

Ophtal *Winzer, Ger.*
Idoxuridine (p.613·2).
Herpes infections of the eye.

Ophtalmin *Winzer, Ger.*
Oxedrine tartrate (p.925·3); naphazoline hydrochloride (p.1064·2); antazoline hydrochloride (p.401·3).
Eye disorders.

Ophtalmine *Specia, Fr.*
Boric acid (p.1554·2); borax (p.1554·2); red vine; rose water (p.1001·1); peppermint water (p.1208·1); hamamelis water (p.1587·1); thymol (p.1127·1).
Eye irritation.

Ophtalmotrim *Asta Medica, Belg.*
Trimethoprim (p.265·1); polymyxin B sulphate (p.239·1).
Bacterial eye infections.

Ophtamedine *Bournonville, Belg.*
Hexamidine isethionate (p.1115·3).
Eye disorders; otitis; rhinitis.

Ophtasiloxane *Alcon, Fr.*
Dimethicone (p.1384·2).
Corneal burns; prevention of corneal adhesions.

Ophtasone *Novopharma, Switz.*
Betamethasone disodium phosphate (p.1033·3); gentamicin sulphate (p.212·1).
Infected eye disorders.

Ophtergine *Allergan, Fr.†.*
Yellow mercuric oxide (p.1601·3).
Parasitic eye infections.

Ophthaine
Bristol-Myers Squibb, Austral.†; Bristol-Myers Squibb, Irl.; Squibb, UK; Apothecon, USA†; Squibb, USA†.
Proxymetacaine hydrochloride (p.1300·1).
Local anaesthesia.

Ophthalgan *Wyeth-Ayerst, USA.*
Glycerol (p.1585·2).
Corneal oedema.

Ophthalin
Ciba Vision, Austral.; Ciba Vision, UK.
Sodium hyaluronate (p.1630·3).
Adjunct in ocular surgery.

Ophthetic
Allergan, Austral.; Allergan, Canad.; Allergan, Ger.†; Allergan, S.Afr.; Allergan, USA.
Proxymetacaine hydrochloride (p.1300·1).
Local anaesthesia.

Ophthifluor *Deklerht, USA.*
Fluorescein sodium (p.1581·1).
Ophthalmic diagnostic agent.

Ophtho-Bunolol *Kenral, Canad.*
Levobunolol hydrochloride (p.897·3).
Glaucoma.

Ophtho-Chloram *Kenral, Canad.*
Chloramphenicol (p.182·1).
Eye infections.

Ophthocort
Parke, Davis, Canad.; Parke, Davis, USA†.
Chloramphenicol (p.182·1); hydrocortisone acetate (p.1043·3); polymyxin B sulphate (p.239·1).
Infected eye disorders.

Ophtho-Sulf *Kenral, Canad.*
Sulphacetamide sodium (p.252·2).
Eye infections.

Ophtho-Tate *Kenral, Canad.*
Prednisolone acetate (p.1048·1).
Eye disorders.

Ophtim *Thea, Fr.*
Timolol maleate (p.953·3).
Glaucoma; ocular hypertension.

Ophtocain *Winzer, Ger.*
Amethocaine hydrochloride (p.1285·2); naphazoline hydrochloride (p.1064·2).
Ophthalmic procedures.

Ophtocortin *Winzer, Ger.*
Medrysone (p.1045·3).
Inflammatory disorders of the eye.

Ophtol-A *Winzer, Ger.*
Vitamin A palmitate (p.1359·2).
Eye disorders.

Ophtomydrol *Winzer, Ger.†.*
Cyclopentolate hydrochloride (p.459·3); naphazoline hydrochloride (p.1064·2).
Eye disorders.

Ophtopur-N *Winzer, Ger.*
Zinc borate (p.1554·3); naphazoline hydrochloride (p.1064·2).
Eye disorders.

Ophtorenin *Winzer, Ger.†.*
Bupranolol (p.835·2).
Glaucoma.

Ophtosan *Winzer, Ger.*
Vitamin A palmitate (p.1359·2).
Eye disorders.

Ophtosol *Winzer, Ger.†.*
Bromhexine hydrochloride (p.1055·3).
Dry eye disorders.

Ophtovitol *Winzer, Ger.†.*
Stanolone (p.1462·2); adenosine (p.812·3); multivitamins.
Corneal disorders.

Ophtrivin-A *Ciba Vision, Canad.*
Xylometazoline hydrochloride (p.1071·2); antazoline sulphate (p.402·1).
Eye disorders.

Opilon
Parke, Davis, Irl.; Hansam, UK.
Thymoxamine hydrochloride (p.952·2).
Peripheral vascular disorders; Raynaud's syndrome.

Opino
Note. This name is used for preparations of different composition.
Kolassa, Aust.
Tablets: Buphenine hydrochloride (p.1555·3); aescin (p.1543·3).
Topical gel: Buphenine hydrochloride (p.1555·3); aescin (p.1543·3); rosemary oil (p.1626·2); pumilio pine oil (p.1623·3); melissa oil.
Vascular disorders.
Bayropharm, Ital.†.
Buphenine hydrochloride (p.1555·3); aescin (p.1543·3); rosemary oil (p.1626·2); pumilio pine oil (p.1623·3); melissa oil.
Contusions; ecchymoses; haematomas; peripheral vascular disorders.

opino heparinoid *Tropon, Ger.†.*
A heparinoid (p.882·3); aescin (p.1543·3); buphenine hydrochloride (p.1555·3); rosemary oil (p.1626·2); pumilio pine oil (p.1623·3); melissa oil.
Skin trauma.

opino N *Gepepharm, Ger.*
Aescin (p.1543·3).
Bruises; haematoma; peripheral vascular disorders.

opino N spezial *Gepepharm, Ger.*
Buphenine hydrochloride (p.1555·3); aescin (p.1543·3).
Bruises; haematoma; peripheral vascular disorders.

Opiren *Almirall, Spain.*
Lansoprazole (p.1196·2).
Gastro-oesophageal reflux; peptic ulcer.

Opobyl
Note. This name is used for preparations of different composition.
Bailly, Fr.
Boldo (p.1554·1); aloes (p.1177·1).
Formerly contained bile and liver extracts, boldo, combretum, euonymine, aloes, belladonna, and hyoscyamus.
Constipation.
Medipharma, Ger.†; Sanofi Labaz, Neth.†.
Bile acids and salts (p.1553·2); boldo (p.1554·1); aloes (p.1177·1); belladonna leaf (p.457·1); hyoscyamus leaf (p.464·3).
Constipation.
Uriach, Spain.
Aloes (p.1177·1); boldo (p.1554·1).
Formerly contained bile extract, boldo, combretum micranthum, euonymus, and podophyllum.
Constipation.
Interdelta, Switz.
Aloes (p.1177·1); boldo (p.1554·1); ox bile (p.1553·2).
Constipation.

Opobyl-phyto *Medipharma, Ger.*
Chelidonium majus; turmeric (p.1001·3).
Biliary-tract disorders.

Opogastrina Fortius *Zambeletti, Ital.†.*
Gastric mucosal extract.
Gastro-intestinal disorders.

Oponaf *Juste, Spain.*
Lactitol (p.1195·2).
Constipation; hepatic encephalopathy.

Opo-Veinogene *Gallier, Fr.†.*
Red vine; aesculus (p.1543·3); esculoside (p.1543·3).
Haemorrhoids; peripheral vascular disorders.

Opragen *Lohmann, Ger.*
Collagen (p.1566·3).
Haemorrhage; skin ulcers; wounds.

Opram *Pinewood, Irl.†.*
Metoclopramide hydrochloride (p.1200·3).
Gastro-intestinal disorders.

Opridan *Locatelli, Ital.*
Bromopride hydrochloride (p.1181·3).
Gastro-intestinal disorders.

O'Prin *Dolisos, Canad.*
Homoeopathic preparation.

Oprisine *Opus, UK.*
Azathioprine (p.505·3).
Chronic active hepatitis; dermatomyositis; haemolytic anaemia; idiopathic thrombocytopenic purpura; immunosuppressant in organ and tissue transplantation; pemphigus; polyarteritis nodosa; pyoderma gangrenosa; rheumatoid arthritis; systemic lupus erythematosus.

Opsite
Smith & Nephew, Austral.; Smith & Nephew, Fr.; Smith & Nephew, S.Afr.; Smith & Nephew, UK.
Polyurethane dressing.
Burns; wounds.

Opsonat *Pekana, Ger.*
Homoeopathic preparation.

Optalgin *Inibsa, Spain.*
Dipyrone (p.35·1).
Fever; pain.

Optalia *Boiron, Canad.*
Homoeopathic preparation.

Optalidon
Note. This name is used for preparations of different composition.
Wander, Belg.; Sandoz, Spain.
Propyphenazone (p.81·3); caffeine (p.749·3).
Fever; pain.
Sandoz, Ger.
Ibuprofen (p.44·1) or ibuprofen lysine (p.44·3).
Fever; pain.
Novartis, Ital.
Propyphenazone (p.81·3); caffeine (p.749·3); butalbital (p.644·3).
Neuralgia; pain.

Optalidon a la Noramidopyrine *Sandoz, Fr.*
Caffeine (p.749·3); dipyrone (p.35·1).
Formerly contained caffeine, butalbital, and dipyrone.
Pain.

Optalidon N *Sandoz, Ger.*
Propyphenazone (p.81·3); caffeine (p.749·3).
Pain.

Optalidon special Noc *Sandoz, Ger.*
Dihydroergotamine mesylate (p.444·2); propyphenazone (p.81·3).
Vascular headache.

Optamide *McGloin, Austral.*
Sulphacetamide sodium (p.252·2).
Bacterial eye infections.

Optamine *Theraplix, Fr.*
Co-dergocrine mesylate (p.1566·1).
Cerebral vascular disorders; mental function impairment in the elderly.

Optanox *Byk, Fr.†.*
Vinylbitone (p.698·2).
Insomnia.

Optavite *Dioptic, Canad.; Akorn, Canad.*
Vitamin and mineral preparation.

Optazine
Note. This name is used for preparations of different composition.
Whitehall, Austral.
Naphazoline hydrochloride (p.1064·2).
Eye irritation.
Uhlmann-Eyraud, Switz.
Naphazoline nitrate (p.1064·2); digitoxin (p.848·3); rutin (p.1580·2); aesculus (p.1543·3); hamamelis (p.1587·1).
Eye irritation.

Optazine A *Whitehall, Austral.†.*
Naphazoline hydrochloride (p.1064·2); antazoline sulphate (p.402·1); zinc sulphate (p.1373·2).
Eye irritation.

Optenyl *Stroschein, Ger.†.*
Papaverine hydrochloride (p.1614·2).
Smooth muscle spasms.

Opteron *Therabel, Ital.*
Ticlopidine hydrochloride (p.953·1).
Thrombosis prophylaxis.

Optibiol *Yves Ponroy, Fr.*
Nutritional supplement with fatty acids.
Visual disorders.

Optical *Strallhofer, Aust.*
Multivitamin preparation with calcium carbonate.

Optical mit Eisen *Strallhofer, Aust.*
Multivitamin preparation with calcium carbonate and ferrous gluconate.

Opticare PMS *Standard Drug, USA.*
Multivitamin and mineral preparation with iron and folic acid.

Opticet *Propan, S.Afr.†.*
Sulphacetamide sodium (p.252·2).
Eye infections.

Opti-Clean *Alcon, USA.*
Range of solutions for contact lenses.

Opti-Clean II *Alcon, Canad.*
Cleaning solution for hard and soft contact lenses.

Opticrom
Fisons, Aust.; Rhone-Poulenc Rorer, Austral.; Fisons, Belg.; Rhone-Poulenc Rorer, Canad.; Fisons, Ger.; Rhone-Poulenc Rorer, Irl.; Fisons, Neth.; Rhone-Poulenc Rorer, S.Afr.; Fisons, Switz.; Fisons, UK; Fisons, USA.
Sodium cromoglycate (p.762·1).
Allergic conjunctivitis; keratoconjunctivitis.

Opticron *Specia, Fr.*
Sodium cromoglycate (p.762·1).
Allergic eye disorders.

Opticyl *Optopics, USA.*
Tropicamide (p.469·2).
Production of mydriasis and cycloplegia.

Optiderm
Hermal, Ger.; Bruschettini, Ital.; Hermal, Switz.
Urea (p.1095·2); laureth 9 (p.1325·2).
Dry and pruritic skin disorders.

Optidex *Fisons, Fr.†.*
Neomycin sulphate (p.229·2); polymyxin B sulphate (p.239·1); dexamethasone sodium metasulphobenzoate (p.1037·2).
Inflammation and infections of the eye.

Optifen *Spirig, Switz.*
Ibuprofen (p.44·1).
Fever; inflammation; musculoskeletal, joint, and periarticular disorders; pain.

Opti-Free
Alcon, Aust.; Alcon, Canad.; Alcon, Fr.; Alcon, USA.
Cleaning, rinsing, disinfecting, and storage solution, cleaning tablets, and rewetting drops for soft contact lenses.

Opti-Free Comfort *Alcon, Austral.*
Cleansing and lubricating solution for contact lenses.

Opti-Free Daily *Alcon, Austral.*
Cleansing solution for soft contact lenses.

Opti-Free Enzymatic *Alcon, Austral.*
Pancreatin (p.1612·1).
Cleanser for soft contact lenses.

Opti-Free Express *Alcon, UK.*
Cleansing, rinsing, disinfecting, and storage solution for soft contact lenses.

Opti-Free Multi-Action *Alcon, Austral.*
Rinsing, disinfecting and storing solution for soft and disposable contact lenses.
Formerly known as Opti-Free Rinsing, Disinfecting and Storing.

Optigene *Pfeiffer, USA.*
Electrolytes (p.1147·1).
Eye irrigation.

Optigene 3 *Pfeiffer, USA.*
Tetrahydrozoline hydrochloride (p.1070·2).
Minor eye irritation.

Optilast *Asta Medica, UK.*
Azelastine hydrochloride (p.403·1).
Allergic conjunctivitis.

Optilax *Phytomed, Switz.*
Linseed (p.1596·2); senna (p.1212·2); frangula bark (p.1193·2); rhubarb (p.1212·1); malt extract (p.1350·1); chamomile (p.1561·2).
Constipation.

Optilets *Abbott, USA.*
Multivitamin preparation.

Optilets-M *Abbott, USA.*
Multivitamin and mineral preparation with iron.

Optilube *Dioptic, Canad.*
Wool fat (p.1385·3); liquid paraffin (p.1382·1); soft paraffin (p.1382·3).

Optilube PVA *Dioptic, Canad.*
Polyvinyl alcohol (p.1474·2).

Optima *Stanley, Canad.*
Multivitamin and mineral preparations.

Optima 50 Plus *Unichem, UK.*
Multivitamin preparation with ginkgo and ginseng.

Optimax
Note. This name is used for preparations of different composition.
E. Merck, Irl.
Tryptophan (p.310·2); pyridoxine hydrochloride (p.1362·3); ascorbic acid (p.1365·2).
Depression.
E. Merck, UK.
Tryptophan (p.310·2).
Formerly contained tryptophan, pyridoxine hydrochloride, and ascorbic acid.
Depression.

Optimin *Juste, Spain.*
Loratadine (p.413·1).
Hypersensitivity reactions.

Optimine
Schering-Plough, Belg.; Schering, Canad.; Essex, Ger.†; Schering-Plough, Irl.; Schering-Plough, S.Afr.; Schering-Plough, UK; Schering, USA.
Azatadine maleate (p.402·3).
Hypersensitivity reactions.

Optimoist *Colgate-Palmolive, USA.*
Hydroxyethylcellulose (p.1472·3); electrolytes (p.1147·1); sodium monofluorophosphate (p.743·3); xylitol (p.1372·3).
Dry mouth.

Optimol
Alphapharm, Austral.; Santen, Swed.
Timolol maleate (p.953·3).
Glaucoma; raised intra-ocular pressure.

Optimox Prenatal *Optimox, USA†.*
Multivitamin and mineral preparation with iron and folic acid.

Optimycin *Biochemie, Aust.*
Methacycline hydrochloride (p.225·1).
Bacterial infections.

Optimycin S *Biochemie, Aust.*
Methacycline hydrochloride (p.225·1); guaiphenesin (p.1061·3).
Lower respiratory-tract bacterial infections.

Optimyd *Schering, USA.*
Prednisolone sodium phosphate (p.1048·1); sulphacetamide sodium (p.252·2).
Eye inflammation with bacterial infection.

Optimyxin *Sabex, Canad.*
Eye ointment: Polymyxin B sulphate (p.239·1); bacitracin zinc (p.157·3).
Eye/ear drops: Polymyxin B sulphate (p.239·1); gramicidin (p.215·2).
Eye or ear infections.

Optimyxin Plus *Sabex, Canad.*
Polymyxin B sulphate (p.239·1); gramicidin (p.215·2); neomycin sulphate (p.229·2).
Eye or ear infections.

Optinem *Zeneca, Aust.*
Meropenem (p.224·2).
Bacterial infections.

Optipect
Thiemann, Ger.
Acetylcysteine (p.1052·3).
Respiratory-tract disorders with excess mucus.
Thiemann, Ger.†.
Balsam: Camphor (p.1557·2); eucalyptus oil (p.1578·1); juniper oil (p.1592·3); pumilio pine oil (p.1623·3); oleum pini sylvestris; turpentine oil (p.1641·1); thymol (p.1127·1).
Oral drops: Ammonium chloride (p.1055·2); camphor (p.1557·2); ephedrine hydrochloride (p.1059·3); liquorice (p.1197·1); ammonia solution (p.1548·3); menthol (p.1600·2); eucalyptus oil (p.1578·1); peppermint oil (p.1208·1); saponin; eucalyptus (p.1578·1); sage (p.1627·1).
Syrup: Ammonium chloride (p.1055·2); camphor (p.1557·2); ephedrine hydrochloride (p.1059·3); thyme (p.1636·3); liquorice (p.1197·1); ammonia solution (p.1548·3); menthol (p.1600·2); eucalyptus oil (p.1578·1); peppermint oil (p.1208·1); sage oil; saponin.
Tablets: Ammonium chloride (p.1055·2); camphor (p.1557·2); ephedrine hydrochloride (p.1059·3); liquorice (p.1197·1); menthol (p.1600·2); anise oil (p.1550·1); eucalyptus oil (p.1578·1); peppermint oil (p.1208·1); saponin; sage oil.
Coughs and associated respiratory-tract disorders.

Optipect Kodein *Thiemann, Ger.*
Codeine (p.26·1).
Coughs.

Optipect mit Kodein *Thiemann, Ger.†.*
Oral drops: Ammonium chloride (p.1055·2); camphor (p.1557·2); ephedrine hydrochloride (p.1059·3); liquorice (p.1197·1); ammonia solution (p.1548·3); menthol (p.1600·2); eucalyptus oil (p.1578·1); peppermint oil (p.1208·1); saponin; eucalyptus (p.1578·1); sage (p.1627·1); codeine (p.26·1).
Syrup: Ammonium chloride (p.1055·2); camphor (p.1557·2); ephedrine hydrochloride (p.1059·3); thyme (p.1636·3); liquorice (p.1197·1); ammonia solution (p.1548·3); menthol (p.1600·2); eucalyptus oil (p.1578·1); peppermint oil(p.1208·1); sage oil; saponin; codeine phosphate (p.26·1).
Coughs and associated respiratory-tract disorders.

Optipect N *Thiemann, Ger.*
Camphor (p.1557·2); menthol (p.1600·2); peppermint oil (p.1208·1).
Respiratory-tract disorders.

Optipect Neo *Thiemann, Ger.*
Camphor (p.1557·2); menthol (p.1600·2); peppermint oil (p.1208·1).
Respiratory-tract disorders.

Opti-Plus
Alcon, Austral.; Alcon, Fr.
Pancreatin (p.1612·1).
Soft contact lens cleaner.

OptiPranolol *Bausch & Lomb, USA.*
Metipranolol hydrochloride (p.906·3).
Glaucoma; ocular hypertension.

Optipyrin Neu *Pfleger, Ger.*
Paracetamol (p.72·2); codeine phosphate (p.26·1).
Pain.

Optipyrin S *Pfleger, Ger.†.*
Etenzamide (p.35·3); codeine phosphate (p.26·1); trospium chloride (p.1640·1).
Smooth muscle spasms.

Optiray
Mallinckrodt, Aust.; Mallinckrodt, Austral.; Codali, Belg.; Mallinckrodt, Canad.; Guerbet, Fr.; Byk Gulden, Ital.; Mallinckrodt, Spain; Gothia, Swed.†; Guerbet, Switz.; Mallinckrodt, USA.
Ioversol (p.1008·3).
Radiographic contrast medium.

Optisen *Allergan, Ital.*
Carbohydrate, vitamin, and mineral preparation.
Antoxidant nutritional supplement.

Opti-Soak
Alcon, Aust.; Alcon, Austral.; Alcon, Canad.
Wetting, disinfection and storage of hard and gas permeable contact lenses.

Opti-Soft *Alcon, USA.*
Rinsing and storage solution for soft contact lenses.

Optistin *Allergan, Ital.†.*
Phenylephrine hydrochloride (p.1066·2).
Allergic conjunctivitis; ocular irritation.

Opti-Tears
Alcon, Aust.; Alcon, Canad.; Alcon, USA.
Range of solutions for contact lenses.

Optivite PMT *Optimox, USA.*
Multivitamin and mineral preparation.
Premenstrual syndrome.

Optizor *Inergie, Fr.*
Glyceryl trinitrate (p.874·3).
Angina pectoris.

Opti-Zyme
Alcon, Canad.; Alcon, USA.
Pancreatin (p.1612·1).
Contact lens cleaner.

Opto Vit-E *Pharmacal, Switz.*
Alpha tocopheryl acetate (p.1369·1).
Vitamin E deficiency.

Optocain *Molteni, Ital.*
Mepivacaine hydrochloride (p.1297·2).
Adrenaline acid tartrate (p.813·3) is included in some preparations as a vasoconstrictor to diminish absorption and localise the effect of the local anaesthetic.
Local anaesthesia.

Optochinidin retard *Boehringer Mannheim, Ger.*
Quinidine sulphate (p.939·1).
Arrhythmias.

Optocillin
Bayer, Aust.; Bayer, Ger.
Mezlocillin sodium (p.225·3); oxacillin sodium (p.234·2).
Bacterial infections.

Optocor *Kanoldt, Ger.*
Crataegus (p.1568·2).
Heart failure.

Optovit *Hermes, Ger.*
d-Alpha tocopherol (p.1369·1).
Vitamin E deficiency.

Optovit-E *Hermes, Ger.†.*
Alpha tocopheryl acetate (p.1369·1).
Vitamin E deficiency.

Optovite B12 *Normon, Spain.*
Cyanocobalamin (p.1363·3).
Vitamin B_{12} deficiency.

Optovite B C *Normon, Spain†.*
Vitamin B substances and ascorbic acid.

Optrex
Boots, Austral.; Etris, Fr.; Boots Healthcare, Irl.; Boots, Ital.; Boots, Spain; Cassella-med, Switz.; Crookes Healthcare, UK.
Hamamelis (p.1587·1).
Eye irritation.

Optrex Clear Eyes *Crookes Healthcare, UK.*
Hamamelis (p.1587·1); naphazoline hydrochloride (p.1064·2).
Formerly known as Optrex Clearine.
Eye irritation.

Optrex Eye Dew *Crookes Healthcare, UK.*
Hamamelis (p.1587·1); naphazoline hydrochloride (p.1064·2).

Optrex Hayfever Allergy Eye Drops *Crookes Healthcare, UK.*
Sodium cromoglycate (p.762·1).
Ocular symptoms of allergic rhinitis.

Optrex Medicated *Boots, Austral.*
Hamamelis (p.1587·1); naphazoline hydrochloride (p.1064·2).
Eye irritation; sore, tired eyes.

Opturem *Kade, Ger.*
Ibuprofen (p.44·1) or ibuprofen sodium (p.44·3).
Inflammation; musculoskeletal and joint disorders.

Opumide *Opus, UK.*
Indapamide (p.890·2).
Hypertension.

Opustan *Opus, UK.*
Mefenamic acid (p.51·2).
Menorrhagia; pain.

OPV-Merieux *Rhone-Poulenc Rorer, S.Afr.*
An oral poliomyelitis vaccine (p.1528·2).
Active immunisation.

ORA5 *McHenry, USA.*
Copper sulphate (p.1338·1); potassium iodide (p.1493·1); iodine (p.1493·1).
Minor mouth or throat irritation.

Orabase
Convatec, Austral.; Squibb, Canad.; Bristol-Myers Squibb, Irl.; ConvaTec, UK.
Carmellose sodium (p.1471·2); pectin (p.1474·1); gelatin (p.723·2).
Oral and perioral lesions; stoma care.

Orabase Baby *Colgate-Hoyt, USA.*
Benzocaine (p.1286·2).
Mouth disorders.

Orabase Gel *Colgate-Oral, USA.*
Benzocaine (p.1286·2).

Orabase HCA *Colgate-Hoyt, USA.*
Hydrocortisone acetate (p.1043·3).
Oral inflammatory and ulcerative lesions.

Orabase Lip *Colgate-Hoyt, USA.*
Benzocaine (p.1286·2); allantoin (p.1078·2); menthol (p.1600·2); camphor (p.1557·2); phenol (p.1121·2).
Minor irritation.

Orabase-B *Colgate-Palmolive, USA.*
Benzocaine (p.1286·2).
Oral lesions.

Orabet
Note. This name is used for preparations of different composition.
Laevosan, Aust.; Lagap, UK.
Metformin hydrochloride (p.330·1).
Diabetes mellitus.

Berlin-Chemie, Ger.
Tolbutamide (p.333·2).
Diabetes mellitus.

Orabetic *Dorsch, Ger.†.*
Glibenclamide (p.319·3).
Diabetes mellitus.

Orabolin
Organon, Austral.†; Organon, Belg.†; Donmed, S.Afr.†.
Ethyloestrenol (p.1445·3).
Anabolic.

Oracef *Lilly, Ger.*
Cephalexin (p.178·2).
Bacterial infections.

Oracefal *Bristol-Myers Squibb, Fr.*
Cefadroxil (p.163·3).
Bacterial infections.

Oracillin VK *Pharmalab, S.Afr.†.*
Phenoxymethylpenicillin potassium (p.236·2).
Bacterial infections.

Oracilline
Rhone-Poulenc Rorer, Belg.; Schwarz, Fr.
Phenoxymethylpenicillin (p.236·2) or benzathine phenoxymethylpenicillin (p.159·2).
Bacterial infections.

Oracit *Carolina, USA.*
Sodium citrate (p.1153·2); citric acid (p.1564·3).
Chronic metabolic acidosis; urine alkalinising agent.

Oracort *Taro, Canad.*
Triamcinolone acetonide (p.1050·2).
Oral lesions.

Oracyclin *Wyeth Lederle, Aust.*
Minocycline hydrochloride dihydrate (p.226·2).
Acne.

Oradex-C *Del, USA†.*
Dyclocaine hydrochloride (p.1292·3).
Sore throat.

Oradexon
Organon, Belg.†; Nourypharma, Neth.; Donmed, S.Afr.; Organon, Switz.
Dexamethasone (p.1037·1) or dexamethasone sodium phosphate (p.1037·2).
Corticosteroid.

Oradroxil *Lampugnani, Ital.*
Cefadroxil (p.163·3).
Bacterial infections.

Oradyne-Z *Stafford-Miller, Ital.*
Benzalkonium saccharinate (p.1102·1); dodequinium bromide.
Oral disinfection.

Orafen *Technilab, Canad.*
Ketoprofen (p.48·2).
Musculoskeletal and joint disorders; pain.

Oragalin *Lacer, Spain†.*
Azintamide (p.1551·3); cellulase (p.1561·1); pancreatin (p.1612·1).
Hepatobiliary disorders.

Oragalin Espasmolitico *Lacer, Spain.*
Azintamide (p.1551·3); hyoscine methobromide (p.463·1).
Hepatobiliary disorders.

Ora-Gallin
Hafslund Nycomed, Aust.; Truw, Ger.†.
Azintamide (p.1551·3); pancreatin (p.1612·1); cellulase (p.1561·1).
Liver and biliary disorders.

Ora-Gallin compositum *Hafslund Nycomed, Aust.*
Azintamide (p.1551·3); papaverine hydrochloride (p.1614·2).
Gastro-intestinal disorders; liver and biliary disorders.

Ora-Gallin purum *Hafslund Nycomed, Aust.*
Azintamide (p.1551·3).
Liver and biliary disorders.

Oragallin S *Truw, Ger.*
Azintamide (p.1551·3); hyoscine methobromide (p.463·1).
Biliary disorders; diarrhoea; spastic constipation.

Oragard *Colgate-Palmolive, UK.*
Lignocaine hydrochloride (p.1293·2); cetylpyridinium chloride (p.1106·2).
Mouth disorders.

Oragrafin
Squibb Diagnostics, Canad.†; Squibb Diagnostics, USA.
Calcium iopodate (p.1007·3) or sodium iopodate (p.1007·3).
Radiographic contrast medium for cholecystography.

Orahesive
Convatec, Austral.; Squibb, Canad.; ConvaTec, UK.
Carmellose sodium (p.1471·2); pectin (p.1474·1); gelatin (p.723·2).
Oral and perioral lesions; stoma care.

Orajel
Del, Canad.; Del, Switz.; Del, USA.
Benzocaine (p.1286·2).
Minor mouth or throat irritation; toothache.

Orajel Mouth Aid
Del, Canad.; Del, USA.
Topical gel: Benzocaine (p.1286·2); benzalkonium chloride (p.1101·3); zinc chloride (p.1373·1).
Mouth and lip sores.

Del, USA.
Topical liquid: Benzocaine (p.1286·2); cetylpyridinium chloride (p.1106·2).
Mouth and throat disorders.

Orajel Perioseptic *Del, USA.*
Urea hydrogen peroxide (p.1127·3).
Oral hygiene; oral inflammation.

Oral Rehidr Sal Farmasur *Farmasur, Spain.*
Glucose; potassium iodide; sodium bicarbonate; sodium chloride (p.1152·3).
Oral rehydration therapy.

Oralamid *CaDiGroup, Ital.*
Food for special diets.
Diarrhoea.

Oralav *Braun, Ger.*
Macrogol 4000 (p.1598·2); electrolytes (p.1147·1).
Bowel evacuation.

Oral-B Anti-Bacterial with Fluoride *Oral-B, Canad.*
Cetylpyridinium chloride (p.1106·2); sodium fluoride (p.742·1).

Oral-B Anti-Cavity Dental Rinse *Oral-B, Canad.*
Sodium fluoride (p.742·1).

Oral-B Collutorio per la Protezione di Denti e Gengive *Oral-B, Ital.*
Cetylpyridinium chloride (p.1106·2); sodium fluoride (p.742·1).
Prevention of dental disorders.

Oral-B Collutorio Protezione Anti-Carie Fluorinse *Oral-B, Ital.*
Sodium fluoride (p.742·1).
Dental caries prophylaxis.

Oral-B Fluoride *Oral-B, UK†.*
Sodium fluoride (p.742·1).
Dental caries prophylaxis.

Oral-B Sensitive *Oral-B, Austral.*
Potassium nitrate (p.1123·1); sodium fluoride (p.742·1).
Dental caries prophylaxis; sensitive teeth.

Oralbalance *Ethical Research, Irl.*
Xylitol (p.1372·3).
Saliva substitute.

Oralcer
Vitabiotics, Irl.; Vitabiotics, UK.
Clioquinol (p.193·2); ascorbic acid.
Mouth ulcers.

Oralcon *Alcon, Swed.*
Dichlorphenamide (p.848·2).
Glaucoma; preoperative control of intra-ocular pressure.

Oralcrom *Searle, Spain.*
Sodium cromoglycate (p.762·1).
Food hypersensitivity; gastro-intestinal hypersensitivity reactions; inflammatory bowel disease.

Oraldene
Warner-Lambert, Irl.; Warner-Lambert, UK.
Hexetidine (p.1116·1).
Oral hygiene.

Oraldettes *Parke, Davis, S.Afr.†.*
Benzalkonium chloride (p.1101·3).
Mouth and throat infections.

Oraldex *ISM, Ital.†.*
Plant allergen extracts (p.1545·1).
Hyposensitisation.

Oraldine
Parke, Davis, S.Afr.; Warner-Lambert, Spain.
Hexetidine (p.1116·1).
Mouth infections.

Oralesper *Pharmacia Upjohn, Spain.*
Magnesium chloride hexahydrate; potassium chloride; monobasic potassium phosphate; sodium chloride; sodium phosphate dodecahydrate; sodium lactate; glucose (p.1152·3).
Oral rehydration therapy.

Oralfene *Pierre Fabre, Fr.*
Ibuprofen (p.44·1).
Fever; pain.

Oralgan *Pierre Fabre, Fr.*
Paracetamol (p.72·2).
Fever; pain.

Oralgan Codeine *Pierre Fabre, Fr.*
Paracetamol (p.72·2); codeine phosphate (p.26·1).
Fever; pain.

Oralgar *Marc-O, Canad.*
Benzocaine (p.1286·2); camphor (p.1557·2); chlorbutol (p.1106·3).

Oralgen *Artu, Neth.*
Allergen extracts (p.1545·1).
Hyposensitisation.

Oralgen β *Artu, Neth.†.*
Bacterial allergen extracts (p.1545·1).
Hyposensitisation.

Oralife Peppermint *Delta, Austral.*
Peppermint oil (p.1208·1); chlorhexidine gluconate (p.1107·2).
Dry lips and mouth.

Oral-K *Sclavo, Ital.*
dl-Potassium aspartate (p.1161·3); *dl*-magnesium aspartate (p.1157·2).

Oralone Dental *Thames, USA.*
Triamcinolone acetonide (p.1050·2).
Oral lesions.

Oralovite *Meda, Swed.*
Vitamin B substances with vitamin C.
Alcoholism; polyneuropathy; vitamin deficiency.

Oralpadon
Leopold, Aust.
Glucose monohydrate; sodium chloride; potassium bicarbonate (p.1152·3).
Gastro-intestinal disorders; oral rehydration therapy.

Fresenius-Praxis, Ger.; Fresenius, Switz.
Glucose monohydrate; sodium chloride; potassium chloride; sodium acid citrate (p.1152·3).
Diarrhoea; oral rehydration therapy.

Oralsan *Bioprogress, Ital.*
Chlorhexidine hydrochloride (p.1107·2); sodium fluoride (p.742·1); sodium monofluorophosphate (p.743·3).
Oral disinfection.

Oralsone *Vinas, Spain.*
Hydrocortisone hemisuccinate (p.1044·1).
Mouth ulcers.

Oralsone B C *Vinas, Spain.*
Ascorbic acid (p.1365·2); hydrocortisone hemisuccinate (p.1044·1); pyridoxine (p.1363·1); riboflavine (p.1362·1).
Mouth ulcers.

Oralspray *Warner-Lambert, Spain.*
Hexetidine (p.1116·1).
Mouth and throat infections.

Oralvac *SmithKline Beecham, Ger.*
Allergen extracts (p.1545·1).
Hyposensitisation.

Oral-Virelon *Chiron Behring, Ger.*
An oral poliomyelitis vaccine (p.1528·2).
Active immunisation.

Oralvite *Bencard, Neth.†.*
Vitamin B substances with vitamin C.

Oramil *Ganassini, Ital.*
Rose honey (p.1345·3).
Oral disinfection.

Oraminic II *Vortech, USA.*
Brompheniramine maleate (p.403·2).
Hypersensitivity reactions.

Oramond *Lennon, S.Afr.†.*
Thymol (p.1127·1); menthol (p.1600·2).
Mouth and throat disorders.

Oramorph
Bender, Aust.; Boehringer Ingelheim, Canad.; Boehringer Ingelheim, Irl.; Boehringer Ingelheim, Swed.; Boehringer Ingelheim, UK; Roxane, USA.
Morphine sulphate (p.56·2).
Pain.

Oramox *Antigen, Irl.*
Amoxycillin trihydrate (p.151·3).
Bacterial infections.

Orangel *Paraphar, Fr.*
Gelatin (p.723·2).
Hair and nail tonic.

Oranol *Piraud, Switz.*
Multivitamin and mineral preparation.

Orap
Janssen-Cilag, Aust.; Janssen-Cilag, Austral.; Janssen-Cilag, Belg.; Janssen-Ortho, Canad.; Janssen-Cilag, Fr.; Janssen-Cilag, Ger.; Janssen-Cilag, Irl.; Janssen-Cilag, Ital.; Janssen-Cilag, Neth.; Janssen-Cilag, Norw.; Janssen-Cilag, S.Afr.; Janssen-Cilag, Spain; Janssen-Cilag, Swed.; Janssen-Cilag, Switz.; Janssen-Cilag, UK; Gate, USA.
Pimozide (p.686·2).
Mania; personality disorders; psychoses; Tourette syndrome.

Orapen *Be-Tabs, S.Afr.†.*
Phenoxymethylpenicillin potassium (p.236·2).
Bacterial infections.

Oraphen-PD *Great Southern, USA.*
Paracetamol (p.72·2).
Fever; pain.

Orascan *Germiphene, Canad.*
Tolonium chloride (p.1638·2).
Diagnosis of oral cancer.

Ora-Sed Jel *Parke, Davis, Austral.†.*
Choline salicylate (p.25·2).
Mouth lesions.

Ora-Sed Lotion *Parke, Davis, Austral.†.*
Lignocaine (p.1293·2).
Mouth lesions.

Orasedon *Oramon, Ger.†.*
Valerian (p.1643·1).
Anxiety; sleep disorders.

Orasept *Pharmakon, USA.*
Oral liquid: Tannic acid (p.1634·2); methylbenzethonium chloride (p.1119·3).
Throat spray: Benzocaine (p.1286·2); methylbenzethonium chloride (p.1119·3); menthol (p.1600·2).
Sore throat.

Oraseptic
Note. This name is used for preparations of different composition.
Prodemdis, Canad.
Domiphen bromide (p.1112·3).

Warner-Lambert, Ital.
Hexetidine (p.1116·1).
Mouth and throat disorders.

Oraseptic Gola *Warner-Lambert, Ital.*
Cetylpyridinium chloride (p.1106·2); dichlorobenzyl alcohol (p.1112·2).
Mouth and throat disorders.

Orasol *Goldline, USA.*
Benzocaine (p.1286·2); phenol (p.1121·2); alcohol (p.1099·1); povidone-iodine (p.1123·3).

Orasone *Solvay, USA.*
Prednisone (p.1049·2).
Corticosteroid.

Orasorbil
Rottapharm, Ger.; Rottapharm, Ital.
Isosorbide mononitrate (p.893·3).
Angina pectoris.

Oraspor *Ciba, Ital.†.*
Cefroxadine (p.173·2).
Bacterial infections.

Orastel *Clintec, Fr.*
Preparations for enteral nutrition.

Orasthin *Hoechst, Ger.*
Oxytocin (p.1257·2).
Induction and maintenance of labour; postpartum haemorrhage.

Oratect *MGI, USA†.*
Benzocaine (p.1286·2).
Stomatitis.

Oratrol
Alcon, Belg.; Alcon, Spain; Alcon, Switz.
Dichlorphenamide (p.848·2).
Glaucoma; raised intra-ocular pressure.

Oravil *Streuli, Switz.*
Vitamin A acetate (p.1359·2); *d*-alpha tocopheryl acetate (p.1369·2).
Dietary supplement.

Oraxim *Malesci, Ital.*
Cefuroxime axetil (p.177·1).
Bacterial infections.

Orazinc *Mericon, USA.*
Zinc sulphate (p.1373·2).
Dietary supplement.

Orbenin
SmithKline Beecham, Austral.†; Beecham, Belg.; Wyeth-Ayerst, Canad.†; SmithKline Beecham, Irl.; SmithKline Beecham, Neth.; SmithKline Beecham, S.Afr.; SmithKline Beecham, Spain; Forley, UK†.
Cloxacillin sodium (p.195·2).
Bacterial infections.

Orbenine SmithKline Beecham, Fr.
Cloxacillin sodium (p.195·2).
Bacterial infections.

Orbinamon Pfizer, Ger.†.
Thiothixene (p.695·3).
Psychiatric disorders.

Orbis Blasen- und Nierentee Mack, Illert., Ger.†.
Orthosiphon (p.1592·2); mate (p.1645·1); solidago virgaurea; melissa (p.1600·1); liquorice (p.1197·1).
Diuretic.

Orbis Husten- und Bronchial-tee Mack, Illert., Ger.†.
Fennel oil (p.1579·2); anise oil (p.1550·1); peppermint oil (p.1208·1); coltsfoot leaf (p.1057·2); liquorice (p.1197·1); fennel (p.1579·1); aniseed (p.1549·3); rose fruit (p.1365·2); peppermint leaf (p.1208·1).
Coughs.

Orbis Nerven- und Beruhigungstee Mack, Illert., Ger.†.
Melissa oil; peppermint oil (p.1208·1); angelica oil; lupulus (p.1597·2); melissa (p.1600·1); peppermint leaf (p.1208·1); angelica; crataegus (p.1568·2); calluna vulgaris.
Sedative.

Ordinal Forte Asche, Ger.
Octodrine camsylate (p.925·1); norfenefrine hydrochloride (p.925·1).
Hypotension.

Ordinal retard Asche, Ger.†.
Octodrine camsylate (p.925·1); norfenefrine hydrochloride (p.925·1); adenosine (p.812·3).
Hypotension.

Ordinator Synthelabo, Fr.
Fenozolone (p.1481·3).
Intellectual and physical impairment.

Ordine Pharmacia Upjohn, Austral.
Morphine hydrochloride (p.56·1).
Insomnia associated with pain; pain.

Ordov Chesty Cough Or-Dov, Austral.
Guaiphenesin (p.1061·3); bromhexine hydrochloride (p.1055·3).
Coughs.

Ordov Congested Cough Or-Dov, Austral.
Guaiphenesin (p.1061·3); pseudoephedrine hydrochloride (p.1068·3).
Respiratory-tract congestion.

Ordov Dry Tickly Cough Or-Dov, Austral.
Pholcodine (p.1068·1).
Coughs.

Ordov Extra Day & Night Cold and Flu Or-Dov, Austral.
16 Daytime tablets, codeine phosphate (p.26·1); paracetamol (p.72·2); pseudoephedrine hydrochloride (p.1068·3); 8 night-time tablets, paracetamol; chlorpheniramine maleate (p.405·1).
Cold and influenza symptoms.

Ordov Febrideine Or-Dov, Austral.
Paracetamol (p.72·2); codeine phosphate (p.26·1).
Fever; pain.

Ordov Febrigesic Or-Dov, Austral.
Paracetamol (p.72·2).
Pain.

Ordov Migradol Or-Dov, Austral.
Paracetamol (p.72·2); codeine phosphate (p.26·1); doxylamine succinate (p.410·1).
Pain.

Ordov Sinudec Or-Dov, Austral.
Oxymetazoline hydrochloride (p.1065·3).
Nasal congestion.

Ordov Sinus & Hayfever Or-Dov, Austral.
Paracetamol (p.72·2); pseudoephedrine hydrochloride (p.1068·3); chlorpheniramine maleate (p.405·1).
Upper respiratory-tract disorders.

Ordrine AT Extended-Release Eon, USA.
Phenylpropanolamine hydrochloride (p.1067·2); caramiphen edisylate (p.1056·2).
Coughs.

Orelox
Hoechst Marion Roussel, Austral.; Diamant, Fr.; Albert-Roussel, Ger.; Hoechst, Ger.; Corvi, Ital.; Hoechst Marion Roussel, Neth.; Hoechst Marion Roussel, S.Afr.; Hosbon, Spain; Hoechst Marion Roussel, Swed.; Hoechst Marion Roussel, Switz.; Hoechst Marion Roussel, UK.
Cefpodoxime proxetil (p.172·1).
Bacterial infections.

Oretic Abbott, USA.
Hydrochlorothiazide (p.885·2).
Hypertension; oedema.

Oreticyl Abbott, USA†.
Hydrochlorothiazide (p.885·2); deserpidine (p.847·2).
Hypertension.

Oreton Methyl Schering, USA.
Methyltestosterone (p.1450·3).
Androgen replacement therapy; breast cancer; male hypogonadism; postpartum breast engorgement; postpubertal cryptorchidism.

Orexin Roberts, USA.
Vitamin B preparation.

Orfen Wyeth, Spain.
Aluminium hydroxide (p.1177·3); magnesium oxide (p.1198·3).
Hyperacidity.

Orfenace Kinsmor, Canad.
Orphenadrine citrate (p.465·2).
Skeletal muscle spasm.

Orfidal Wyeth, Spain.
Lorazepam (p.675·3).
Alcohol withdrawal syndrome; anxiety; epilepsy; insomnia; nausea; vomiting.

Orfidora Wyeth, Spain.
Indoramin (p.891·2).
Benign prostatic hyperplasia; hypertension.

Orfiril
Desitin, Ger.; Desitin, Norw.; Desitin, Swed.; Desitin, Switz.
Sodium valproate (p.361·2).
Formerly known as Orfilept in *Swed.*
Bipolar disorder; epilepsy.

Orgafol Organon, UK.
Urofollitrophin (p.1263·1).
Fertility disorders.

Orgametril
Organon, Aust.; Organon, Belg.; Organon, Fr.; Organon, Ger.; Organon, Neth.; Organon, Spain; Organon, Swed.; Organon, Switz.
Lynoestrenol (p.1448·2).
Benign mammary dysplasia; endometrial cancer; endometriosis; menstrual disorders; progestogen-only oral contraceptive.

Organex Sante Naturelle, Canad.
d-Alpha tocopheryl acetate (p.1369·2).

Organic Zinc Amino Acid Chelate Complex Suisse, Austral.†.
Multivitamin and mineral preparation.

Organidin
Note. This name is used for preparations of different composition.
Horner, Canad.†.
Iodinated glycerol (p.1062·2).
Bronchitis.

Wallace, USA.
Guaiphenesin (p.1061·3).
Formerly contained iodinated glycerol.
Coughs.

Organoderm Mundipharma, Ger.†.
Malathion (p.1407·3).
Pediculosis.

Organon LH Color Organon, UK†.
Fertility test (p.1621·2).

Orgaplasma Ardeypharm, Ger.
Ginseng (p.1584·2).
Tonic.

Orgaran
Organon, Austral.; Organon, Canad.; Nourypharma, Neth.; Organon, Swed.; Durbin, UK; Organon, USA.
Danaparoid sodium (p.846·1).
Thrombosis prophylaxis.

Orgastyptin Organon, Ger.†.
Oestriol sodium succinate (p.1457·2).
Oestrogenic.

Orgasuline 30/70 Organon, Fr.
Mixture of insulin injection (human, emp, highly purified) 30% and isophane insulin injection (human, emp, highly purified) 70% (p.322·1).
Diabetes mellitus.

Orgasuline N.P.H. Organon, Fr.
Isophane insulin injection (human, emp, highly purified) (p.322·1).
Diabetes mellitus.

Orgasuline Rapide Organon, Fr.
Insulin injection (human, emp, highly purified) (p.322·1).
Diabetes mellitus.

Orgo-M Max Farma, Ital.†.
Orgotein (p.87·3).
Cystitis; musculoskeletal and joint disorders.

Oribiox Bohm, Spain.
Oxolinic acid (p.235·1).
Urinary-tract infections.

Oricant Luhr-Lehrs, Ger.
Homoeopathic preparation.

Oricillin Grunenthal, Ger.†.
Propicillin potassium (p.240·3).
Bacterial infections.

Oriens Proter, Ital.†.
Acetoxolone aluminium (p.1176·2).
Gastro-intestinal disorders.

Orifer F Hoechst Marion Roussel, Canad.
Multivitamin and mineral preparation.
Prenatal supplement.

Original Wassen, Ital.
Multivitamin and mineral preparation.
Nutritional supplement.

Original Alka-Seltzer Effervescent Tablets Bayer, USA.
Sodium bicarbonate (p.1153·2); citric acid (p.1564·3); aspirin (p.16·1).
Hyperacidity.

Original Eclipse Triangle, USA†.
SPF 10: Padimate O (p.1488·1); lisadimate (p.1487·2).
Sunscreen.

Original Midol Multi-Symptom Formula Glenbrook, USA†.
Paracetamol (p.72·2); mepyramine maleate (p.414·1).
Menstrual disorders.

Original Sensodyne Block, USA.
Strontium chloride (p.1633·1).
Hypersensitive teeth.

Original-Hico-Gallenheil Reinecke, Ger.†.
Capsella bursa pastoris; equisetum (p.1575·1); rorippa nasturtium aquaticum; frangula bark (p.1193·2); birch leaf (p.1553·3); peppermint leaf (p.1208·1); senna (p.1212·2); chelidonium; taraxacum (p.1634·2); angust.; curcuma; card. mar.; millefol.: abrotan.; absinth.; anhydrous sodium sulphate (p.1213·3); sodium potassium tartrate (p.1213·3); sodium bicarbonate (p.1153·2).
Biliary disorders; liver disorders.

Original-Tinktur "Truw" Truw, Ger.
Homoeopathic preparation.

Orimeten
Ciba-Geigy, Aust.; Ciba-Geigy, Belg.; Ciba Cancer Care, Ger.; Ciba-Geigy, Irl.; Ciba, Ital.; Novartis, Neth.; Ciba, Norw.; Novartis, S.Afr.; Ciba-Geigy, Spain; Novartis, Swed.; Ciba, UK.
Aminoglutethimide (p.502·3).
Breast cancer; Cushing's syndrome; ectopic ACTH production; prostatic cancer.

Orimetene
Ciba-Geigy, Fr.; Ciba, Switz.
Aminoglutethimide (p.502·3).
Breast cancer; Cushing's syndrome; hyperaldosteronism; prostatic cancer.

Orimune Lederle-Praxis, USA.
An oral poliomyelitis vaccine (p.1528·2).
Active immunisation.

Orinase
Hoechst Marion Roussel, Canad.; Upjohn, USA.
Tolbutamide (p.333·2).
Diabetes mellitus.

Orinase Diagnostic Upjohn, USA.
Tolbutamide sodium (p.333·3).
Diagnosis of pancreatic adenoma.

ORLAAM BioDevelopment, USA.
Levomethadyl acetate hydrochloride (p.50·2).
Opioid withdrawal.

Orlept CP Pharmaceuticals, UK.
Sodium valproate (p.361·2).
Epilepsy.

Orlest
Parke, Davis, Aust.; Parke, Davis, Ger.†.
Ethinyloestradiol (p.1445·1); norethisterone acetate (p.1453·1).
Combined oral contraceptive.

Ormazine Hauck, USA†.
Chlorpromazine hydrochloride (p.649·1).
Acute intermittent porphyria; adjunct in tetanus; hiccups; nausea and vomiting; premedication; psychoses; severe behavioural disorders in children.

Ormobyl Novartis Consumer, Ital.†.
Phenolphthalein (p.1208·2); rhubarb (p.1212·1); boldo (p.1554·1).
Constipation.

Ormodon Pharmaceutical Enterprises, S.Afr.
Nitrazepam (p.682·2).
Insomnia.

Ornade
Note. This name is used for preparations of different composition.
SmithKline Beecham Consumer, Belg.; SmithKline Beecham Consumer, Canad.; SmithKline Beecham Consumer, USA†.
Chlorpheniramine maleate (p.405·1); phenylpropanolamine hydrochloride (p.1067·2).
Cold symptoms; rhinitis.

Syntex, Spain.
Cinnarizine (p.406·1); phenylpropanolamine hydrochloride (p.1067·2); isopropamide iodide (p.464·3).
Nasal congestion.

Ornade Expectorant SmithKline Beecham Consumer, Canad.
Chlorpheniramine maleate (p.405·1); phenylpropanolamine hydrochloride (p.1067·2); guaiphenesin (p.1061·3).
Coughs and cold symptoms.

Ornade-DM SmithKline Beecham Consumer, Canad.
Chlorpheniramine maleate (p.405·1); phenylpropanolamine hydrochloride (p.1067·2); dextromethorphan hydrobromide (p.1057·3).
Coughs and cold symptoms.

Ornasec Smith Kline & French, Spain†.
Diphenylpyraline hydrochloride (p.409·3); phenylpropanolamine hydrochloride (p.1067·2); isopropamide iodide (p.464·3).
Nasal congestion.

Ornatos
Note. This name is used for preparations of different composition.
Procter & Gamble, Aust.
Chlorpheniramine maleate (p.405·1); phenylpropanolamine hydrochloride (p.1067·2).
Cold symptoms; hay fever.

Rohm, Ger.†.
Chlorpheniramine maleate (p.405·1); phenylpropanolamine hydrochloride (p.1067·2); isopropamide iodide (p.464·3).
Colds; hay fever; vasomotor rhinitis.

Ornatos N Procter & Gamble, Ger.†.
Chlorpheniramine maleate (p.405·1); phenylpropanolamine hydrochloride (p.1067·2).
Cold symptoms; hay fever; vasomotor rhinitis.

Ornel Lennon, S.Afr.†.
Oxprenolol hydrochloride (p.926·2).
Angina pectoris; hypertension.

Ornex Menley & James, USA.
Pseudoephedrine hydrochloride (p.1068·3); paracetamol (p.72·2).
Upper respiratory-tract symptoms.

Ornex Severe Cold No Drowsiness Menley & James, USA†.
Pseudoephedrine hydrochloride (p.1068·3); dextromethorphan hydrobromide (p.1057·3); paracetamol (p.72·2).
Coughs and cold symptoms.

Ornicetil
Ebewe, Aust.; Logeais, Fr.; Intersan, Ger.†; Geymonat, Ital.; Semar, Spain; Interdelta, Switz.
Ornithine oxoglurate (p.1352·3).
Hyperammonaemia; liver disorders; nausea induced by cancer chemotherapy.

Ornicetil S Geymonat, Ital.
Ornithine oxoglurate (p.1352·3).
Mental function impairment.

Ornidyl Marion Merrell Dow, USA.
Eflornithine hydrochloride (p.581·3).
African trypanosomiasis.

Ornil Volchem, Ital.
L-Ornithine (p.1352·3).
Adjunct in dietary management of hypercholesterolaemia.

Ornil KG Volchem, Ital.
L-Ornithine oxoglurate (p.1352·3).
Stress.

Ornitaine Schwarz, Fr.
Ornithine hydrochloride (p.1352·3); betaine (p.1553·2); sorbitol (p.1354·2); citric acid monohydrate (p.1564·3) magnesium oxide (p.1198·3).
Dyspepsia.

Oro B12 Ripari-Gero, Ital.
Orotic acid (p.1611·2); cyanocobalamin (p.1363·3); folic acid (p.1340·3).
Nutritional supplement.

Oroacid Rosch & Handel, Aust.
Betaine hydrochloride (p.1553·2); pepsin (p.1616·3).
Hypochlorhydria; loss of appetite.

Orobicin Fulton, Ital.
Bacitracin (p.157·3); neomycin sulphate (p.229·2).
Gastro-intestinal infections; pre-operative bowel preparation.

Orocaine Beige, S.Afr.
Cetrimide (p.1105·2); benzocaine (p.1286·2).
Mouth and throat infections.

Orocal Theramex, Mon.
Calcium carbonate (p.1182·1).
Calcium deficiency; osteoporosis.

Orocal Vitamine D_3 Theramex, Mon.
Calcium carbonate (p.1182·1); cholecalciferol (p.1366·3).
Calcium and vitamin D deficiency; osteoporosis.

Orochlor Triomed, S.Afr.
Benzocaine (p.1286·2); chlorhexidine gluconate (p.1107·2).
Mouth and throat disorders.

Orochol Berna, Switz.
An oral cholera vaccine (p.1506·2).
Active immunisation.

Orocholin Rosch & Handel, Aust.
Choline dihydrogen citrate (p.1337·1); calcium citrate (p.1155·1).
Liver protection.

Oro-Clense Germiphene, Canad.
Chlorhexidine gluconate (p.1107·2).
Gingivitis.

Or-O-Derm Giuliani, Ital.
Vitamin and mineral preparation.
Antioxidant nutritional supplement.

Orodine Colgate Oral Care, Austral.†.
Povidone-iodine (p.1123·3).
Disinfection of suction systems.

Orofar
Note. This name is used for preparations of different composition.
Zyma, Belg.
Benzoxonium chloride (p.1103·3).
Mouth and throat disorders.

Zyma, Switz.
Benzoxonium chloride (p.1103·3); lignocaine hydrochloride (p.1293·2).
Mouth and throat disorders.

Orofar Lidocaine Zyma, Belg.
Benzoxonium chloride (p.1103·3); lignocaine hydrochloride (p.1293·2).
Mouth and throat disorders.

Orofluor Colgate Oral Care, Austral.
Acidulated phosphate fluoride or sodium fluoride (p.742·1).
Dental caries prophylaxis; sensitive teeth.

Oroken Bellon, Fr.
Cefixime (p.165·3).
Otitis media; pyelonephritis; respiratory-tract infections; urinary-tract infections.

Oromag B12 Pulitzer, Ital.†.
Potassium orotate (p.1611·2); cyanocobalamin (p.1363·3); folic acid (p.1340·3).
Nutritional supplement.

Oromedine Sanofi Winthrop, Fr.
Hexamidine isethionate (p.1115·3); amethocaine hydrochloride (p.1285·2).
Mouth and throat disorders.

Oro-Min Germiphene, Canad.†.
Minerals.
Dental caries prophylaxis.

Oromone Solvay, Fr.
Oestradiol (p.1455·1).
Menopausal disorders; osteoporosis.

Oro-NaF Germiphene, Canad.
Sodium fluoride (p.742·1).
Dental caries prophylaxis.

Oro-Pivalone Uhlmann-Eyraud, Switz.
Tixocortol pivalate (p.1050·1); bacitracin zinc (p.157·3).
Mouth and throat disorders.

Oropivalone Bacitracine Jouveinal, Fr.
Tixocortol pivalate (p.1050·1); bacitracin zinc (p.157·3).
Mouth and throat disorders.

Orosept
Note. This name is used for preparations of different composition.
Triomed, S.Afr.
Chlorhexidine gluconate (p.1107·2).
Mouth disorders.
OroClean, Switz.
Isopropyl alcohol (p.1118·2); propyl alcohol (p.1124·2); didecyldiammonium chloride.
Hand disinfection.

Oroseptol SmithKline Beecham Sante, Fr.
Tablets: Dequalinium chloride (p.1112·1); amethocaine hydrochloride (p.1285·2).
Throat spray: Hexamidine isethionate (p.1115·3); amethocaine hydrochloride (p.1285·2).
Mouth and throat disorders.

Oroseptol Lysozyme SmithKline Beecham Sante, Fr.
Dequalinium chloride (p.1112·1); amethocaine hydrochloride (p.1285·2); muramidase hydrochloride (p.1604·3).
Mouth and throat disorders.

Orostat Gingi-Pak, Switz.
Adrenaline hydrochloride (p.813·3).
Dental haemorrhage and leakage of fluid from tissues.

Oroticon Lisina Also, Ital.†.
Vitamin B substances; lysine hydrochloride (p.1350·1); orotic acid (p.1611·2).
Nutritional supplement.

Orotofalk Falk, Ger.†.
Choline orotate (p.1611·2); vitamins; curcuma zanthorrhiza; cynara (p.1569·2).
Liver disorders.

Orotric Vita, Spain.
Succinimide (p.1633·2).
Hyperoxaluria; renal calculi.

Orotrix San Carlo, Ital.
Propylene glycol cefatrizine (p.164·2).
Bacterial infections.

Orovite
SmithKline Beecham, Austral.†; Seton, Irl.; Seton, UK.
Vitamin B substances with ascorbic acid.

Orovite '7' Seton, UK.
Multivitamin preparation.

Orovite Complement B_6 Seton, UK.
Pyridoxine hydrochloride (p.1362·3).
Isoniazid-induced peripheral neuritis; sideroblastic anaemia; vitamin B_6 deficiency.

Oroxine Glaxo Wellcome, Austral.
Thyroxine sodium (p.1497·1).
Hypothyroidism; suppression of thyrotrophin.

Orpec Orion, Switz.
Ipecacuanha (p.1062·2).
Poisoning.

Orphengesic Martec, USA.
Orphenadrine citrate (p.465·2); aspirin (p.16·1); caffeine (p.749·3).
Musculoskeletal pain.

Orphol Opfermann, Ger.
Co-dergocrine mesylate (p.1566·1).
Cognitive impairment in the elderly.

Orpidan-150 Heumann, Ger.†.
Chlorazanil hydrochloride.
Oedema.

Orravina Prodes, Spain.
Aspirin (p.16·1).
Fever; musculoskeletal, joint, and peri-articular disorders; pain; thrombo-embolism prophylaxis.

Orstanorm Novartis, Swed.
Dihydroergotamine mesylate (p.444·2).
Migraine; orthostatic hypotension.

Orstanorm med heparin Sandoz, Swed.†.
Dihydroergotamine mesylate (p.444·2); heparin sodium (p.879·3); lignocaine hydrochloride (p.1293·2).
Postoperative thrombo-embolic disorders.

Ortacrone Sanofi Winthrop, Spain†.
Amiodarone hydrochloride (p.820·1).
Cardiac disorders.

Ortenal Specia, Fr.
Phenobarbitone (p.350·2); amphetamine sulphate (p.1477·3).
Epilepsy.

Ortensan Cimex, Switz.
Paracetamol (p.72·2).
Fever; pain.

Orthangin N Promonta Lundbeck, Ger.
Crataegus (p.1568·2).
Cardiovascular disorders.

Orthangin Novo Promonta Lundbeck, Ger.
Crataegus (p.1568·2).
Cardiac disorders.

Ortho Janssen-Cilag, Irl.
Dienoestrol (p.1444·1).
Atrophic vaginitis; kraurosis vulvae.

Ortho 0.5/35 Janssen-Ortho, Canad.
Norethisterone (p.1453·1); ethinyloestradiol (p.1445·1).
28-Day packs also contain 7 inert tablets.
Combined oral contraceptive.

Ortho 1/35 Janssen-Ortho, Canad.
Norethisterone (p.1453·1); ethinyloestradiol (p.1445·1).
28-Day packs also contain 7 inert tablets.
Combined oral contraceptive.

Ortho 7/7/7 Janssen-Ortho, Canad.
Norethisterone (p.1453·1); ethinyloestradiol (p.1445·1).
28-Day packs also contain 7 inert tablets.
Triphasic oral contraceptive.

Ortho 10/11 Janssen-Ortho, Canad.
Norethisterone (p.1453·1); ethinyloestradiol (p.1445·1).
28-Day packs also contain 7 inert tablets.
Biphasic oral contraceptive.

Ortho Cyclen Ortho Pharmaceutical, USA.
Norgestimate (p.1453·3); ethinyloestradiol (p.1445·1).
28-Day packs also contain 7 inert tablets.
Combined oral contraceptive.

Ortho Gynest Depot Janssen-Cilag, Ital.
Oestriol (p.1457·2).
Menopausal disorders.

Ortho Gyne-T
Janssen-Cilag, Irl.; Ortho, UK.
Copper-wound plastic (p.1337·3).
Intra-uterine contraceptive device.

Ortho Tri-Cyclen Ortho Pharmaceutical, USA.
Norgestimate (p.1453·3); ethinyloestradiol (p.1445·1).
28-Day packs also contain 7 inert tablets.
Triphasic oral contraceptive.

Orthocardon-N Tosse, Ger.
Crataegus (p.1568·2).
Cardiovascular disorders.

Ortho-Cept
Janssen-Ortho, Canad.; Ortho Pharmaceutical, USA.
Desogestrel (p.1443·3); ethinyloestradiol (p.1445·1).
28-Day packs also contain 7 inert tablets.
Combined oral contraceptive.

Orthoclone OKT3
Janssen-Cilag, Austral.; Janssen-Cilag, Belg.; Janssen-Ortho, Canad.; Janssen-Cilag, Fr.; Janssen-Cilag, Ger.; Janssen-Cilag, Ital.; Janssen-Cilag, Neth.; Janssen-Cilag, Norw.; Janssen-Cilag, Swed.; Janssen-Cilag, Switz.; Ortho Biotech, USA.
Muromonab-CD3 (p.554·2).
Acute renal, cardiac, or hepatic allograft rejection.

Ortho-Creme
Janssen-Cilag, Austral.; Janssen-Cilag, Irl.; Cilag, UK; Ortho Pharmaceutical, USA†.
Nonoxinol 9 (p.1326·1).
Contraceptive.

Ortho-Dienoestrol Janssen-Cilag, Belg.
Dienoestrol (p.1444·1).
Vulvovaginal disorders.

Ortho-Est
Janssen-Cilag, S.Afr.; Ortho Pharmaceutical, USA.
Estropipate (p.1444·3).
Female hypogonadism; menopausal disorders; osteoporosis.

Orthoforms
Janssen-Cilag, Irl.; Cilag, UK.
Nonoxinol 9 (p.1326·1).
Contraceptive.

Ortho-Gastrine Brunet, Fr.†.
Anhydrous sodium sulphate (p.1213·3); anhydrous dibasic sodium phosphate (p.1159·3); sodium bicarbonate (p.1153·2); sodium citrate (p.1153·2).
Constipation; dyspepsia.

Ortho-Gel Janssen-Cilag, Ger.
Nonoxinol 9 (p.1326·1).
Contraceptive.

Ortho-Gynest
Janssen-Cilag, Aust.; Janssen-Cilag, Belg.; Janssen-Cilag, Ger.; Janssen-Cilag, Irl.; Cilag, Neth.†; Janssen-Cilag, Switz.; Cilag, UK.
Oestriol (p.1457·2).
Atrophic vaginitis; kraurosis vulvae; pruritus vulvae.

Ortho-Gynol
Janssen-Cilag, Austral.; Janssen-Cilag, Switz.†; Ortho Pharmaceutical, USA.
Octoxinol 9 (p.1326·2).
Contraceptive.
McNeil Consumer, Canad.; Cilag, Ger.†; Cilag, Neth.†; Cilag, UK†.
p-Di-isobutyl-phenoxypolyethoxyethanol (p.1324·3).
Contraceptive.

Ortho-Gynol II Johnson & Johnson, Canad.
Nonoxinol 9 (p.1326·1).
Contraceptive.

Orthoheptamin Giulini, Ger.†.
Etifelmine hydrochloride; heptaminol hydrochloride (p.1587·2).
Hypotension.

Ortholan Pharmasal, Ger.†.
Nicoboxil (p.63·1); nonivamide (p.63·2); pine needle oil (p.1623·3); salicylamide (p.82·3); cayenne pepper.
Muscle, joint, and nerve disorders.

Ortholan mit Salicylester Medopharm, Ger.
Glycol salicylate (p.43·1); benzyl nicotinate (p.22·1).
Musculoskeletal, joint, and soft-tissue disorders; peripheral vascular disorders.

Ortho-Maren retard Lubapharm, Switz.
Pholedrine sulphate (p.930·2); norfenefrine hydrochloride (p.925·1).
Hypotension.

Ortho-Neo-T Janssen-Cilag, Ital.†.
Copper (p.1337·3).
Intra-uterine contraceptive device.

Orthonett Novum Janssen-Cilag, Swed.
Norethisterone (p.1453·1); ethinyloestradiol (p.1445·1).
Combined oral contraceptive.

Ortho-Novin Janssen-Cilag, Irl.
Norethisterone (p.1453·1); mestranol (p.1450·2).
Combined oral contraceptive.

Ortho-Novin 1/50 Janssen-Cilag, UK†.
Norethisterone (p.1453·1); mestranol (p.1450·2).
Combined oral contraceptive; menstrual disorders.

Ortho-Novum Janssen-Cilag, Aust.
Norethisterone (p.1453·1); mestranol (p.1450·2).
Combined oral contraceptive.

Ortho-Novum 1/35
Janssen-Cilag, Fr.; Ortho Pharmaceutical, USA.
Norethisterone (p.1453·1); ethinyloestradiol (p.1445·1).
28-Day packs also contain 7 inert tablets.
Combined oral contraceptive.

Ortho-Novum 1/50
Janssen-Cilag, Austral.†; Janssen-Cilag, Belg.; Janssen-Ortho, Canad.; Janssen-Cilag, Ger.; Cilag, Neth.†; Janssen-Cilag, Switz.; Ortho Pharmaceutical, USA.
Norethisterone (p.1453·1); mestranol (p.1450·2).
28-Day packs also contain 7 inert tablets.
Combined oral contraceptive; endometriosis; menstrual disorders.

Ortho-Novum 1/80 Ortho, Canad.†.
Norethisterone (p.1453·1); mestranol (p.1450·2).
Endometriosis; menstrual disorders.

Ortho-Novum 7/7/7 Ortho Pharmaceutical, USA.
Norethisterone (p.1453·1); ethinyloestradiol (p.1445·1).
28-Day packs also contain 7 inert tablets.
Triphasic oral contraceptive.

Ortho-Novum 10/11 Ortho Pharmaceutical, USA.
Norethisterone (p.1453·1); ethinyloestradiol (p.1445·1).
28-Day packs also contain 7 inert tablets.
Biphasic oral contraceptive.

Ortho-Novum 0.5 mg Ortho, Canad.†.
Norethisterone (p.1453·1); mestranol (p.1450·2).
Endometriosis; menstrual disorders.

Ortho-Novum 2 mg Ortho, Canad.†.
Norethisterone (p.1453·1); mestranol (p.1450·2).
Endometriosis; menstrual disorders.

Ortho-Novum SQ Cilag, Belg.†.
14 Tablets, mestranol (p.1450·2); 7 tablets, mestranol; norethisterone (p.1453·1).
Sequential-type oral contraceptive.

Orthoxicol
Note. This name is used for preparations of different composition.
Upjohn, Austral.†.
Aspirin (p.16·1); codeine phosphate (p.26·1); methoxyphenamine hydrochloride (p.1063·3); pseudoephedrine (p.1068·3).
Cold symptoms.
Pharmacia Upjohn, Belg.
Dextromethorphan hydrobromide (p.1057·3); methoxyphenamine hydrochloride (p.1063·3).
Coughs.
Upjohn, Irl.†; Pharmacia Upjohn, S.Afr.
Codeine phosphate (p.26·1); methoxyphenamine hydrochloride (p.1063·3).
Coughs.

Orthoxicol 1 Johnson & Johnson, Austral.†.
Paracetamol (p.72·2); pseudoephedrine hydrochloride (p.1068·3); dextromethorphan hydrobromide (p.1057·3).
Cold and influenza symptoms.

Orthoxicol 2 Johnson & Johnson, Austral.†.
Paracetamol (p.72·2); pseudoephedrine hydrochloride (p.1068·3).
Cold symptoms.

Orthoxicol 3 Johnson & Johnson, Austral.†.
Paracetamol (p.72·2); pseudoephedrine hydrochloride (p.1068·3); chlorpheniramine maleate (p.405·1).
Sinus disorders.

Orthoxicol 8 and 9 Johnson & Johnson, Austral.†.
Paracetamol (p.72·2); dextromethorphan hydrobromide (p.1057·3).
Cold symptoms; cough.

Orthoxicol 4 and 6 Johnson & Johnson, Austral.†.
Paracetamol (p.72·2); guaiphenesin (p.1061·3); pseudoephedrine hydrochloride (p.1068·3).
Cold symptoms.

Orthoxicol 5 and 7 Johnson & Johnson, Austral.†.
Guaiphenesin (p.1061·3); pseudoephedrine hydrochloride (p.1068·3).
Chest congestion; nasal congestion.

Orthoxicol for Children Nightrest Johnson & Johnson, Austral.
Chlorpheniramine maleate (p.405·1); dextromethorphan hydrobromide (p.1057·3).
Cold symptoms; coughs.

Orthoxicol Cold & Flu Johnson & Johnson, Austral.
Paracetamol (p.72·2); pseudoephedrine hydrochloride (p.1068·3); dextromethorphan hydrobromide (p.1057·3).
Cold and influenza symptoms.

Orthoxicol Congested Cough Johnson & Johnson, Austral.
Guaiphenesin (p.1061·3); pseudoephedrine hydrochloride (p.1068·3).
Cold symptoms.

Orthoxicol Cough Roberts, USA.
Phenylpropanolamine hydrochloride (p.1067·2); chlorpheniramine maleate (p.405·1); dextromethorphan hydrobromide (p.1057·3).
Coughs and cold symptoms.

Orthoxicol Cough Suppressant Upjohn, Austral.†.
Codeine phosphate (p.26·1); methoxyphenamine hydrochloride (p.1063·3); sodium citrate (p.1153·2).
Coughs.

Orthoxicol Cough Suppressant For Children Upjohn, Austral.†.
Dextromethorphan hydrobromide (p.1057·3); methoxyphenamine hydrochloride (p.1063·3); sodium citrate (p.1153·2).
Coughs.

Orthoxicol Day & Night Cold & Flu Johnson & Johnson, Austral.
Daytime caplets, paracetamol (p.72·2); pseudoephedrine hydrochloride (p.1068·3); dextromethorphan hydrobromide (p.1057·3); night-time caplets, paracetamol; dextromethorphan hydrobromide; chlorpheniramine maleate (p.405·1).
Cold and influenza symptoms.

Orthoxicol Dry Cough Johnson & Johnson, Austral.
Paracetamol (p.72·2); dextromethorphan hydrobromide (p.1057·3).
Cold symptoms.

Orthoxicol Expectorant Upjohn, Austral.†.
Dextromethorphan hydrobromide (p.1057·3); guaiphenesin (p.1061·3); methoxyphenamine hydrochloride (p.1063·3).
Coughs; respiratory congestion.

Orthoxicol Expectorant (with antihistamine) Upjohn, Austral.†.
Chlorpheniramine maleate (p.405·1); dextromethorphan hydrobromide (p.1057·3); guaiphenesin (p.1061·3); methoxyphenamine hydrochloride (p.1063·3).
Coughs; nasal congestion; respiratory congestion.

Orthoxicol Headcold Johnson & Johnson, Austral.
Paracetamol (p.72·2); pseudoephedrine hydrochloride (p.1068·3).
Cold and influenza symptoms.

Orthoxicol Infant Johnson & Johnson, Austral.
Pseudoephedrine hydrochloride (p.1068·3).
Cold symptoms; nasal congestion.

Orthoxicol Nasal Relief Upjohn, Austral.†.
Pseudoephedrine hydrochloride (p.1068·3); methoxyphenamine hydrochloride (p.1063·3).
Sinus and nasal congestion.

Orthoxicol Nasal Relief with Antihistamine
Upjohn, Austral.†.
Pseudoephedrine hydrochloride (p.1068·3); methoxyphenamine hydrochloride (p.1063·3); chlorpheniramine maleate (p.405·1).
Sinus and nasal congestion.

Orti B Seroyal, Canad.
Vitamin B substances.

Ortic C Seroyal, Canad.
Ascorbic acid (p.1365·2).

Ortisan
Note. This name is used for preparations of different composition.
Ortis, Ital.
Senna (p.1212·2); tamarind (p.1217·3).
Constipation.
Cedar Health, UK.
Fruit and fibre preparation.
Constipation.

Ortitruw Truw, Ger.
Homoeopathic preparation.

Orto Dermo P Normon, Spain.
Povidone-iodine (p.1123·3).
Instrument disinfection; skin, mucous membrane, and wound disinfection.

Orto Nasal Normon, Spain.
Cineole (p.1564·1); oxymetazoline hydrochloride (p.1065·3); menthol (p.1600·2).
Nasal congestion.

Ortodermina Salus, Ital.
Lignocaine hydrochloride (p.1293·2).
Surface anaesthesia of skin and mucous membranes.

Ortoton Bastian, Ger.
Methocarbamol (p.1316·1).
Skeletal muscle spasm and tension.

Ortoton Plus Bastian, Ger.
Methocarbamol (p.1316·1); aspirin (p.16·1).
Skeletal muscle spasm and tension.

Or-Tyl Ortega, USA.
Dicyclomine hydrochloride (p.460·1).
Functional bowel/irritable bowel syndrome.

Orucote Rhone-Poulenc Rorer, S.Afr.
Ketoprofen (p.48·2).
Orucote Gel was formerly known as Orugel.
Dysmenorrhoea; gout; musculoskeletal, joint, and peri-articular disorders.

Orudis
Rhone-Poulenc Rorer, Austral.; Rhone-Poulenc Rorer, Canad.; Rhone-Poulenc Rorer, Ger.; Rhone-Poulenc Rorer, Irl.; Rhone-Poulenc Rorer, Ital.; Rhone-Poulenc Rorer, Neth.; Rhone-Poulenc Rorer, Norw.; May & Baker, S.Afr.†; Rhone-Poulenc Rorer, Spain; Rhone-Poulenc Rorer, Swed.; Rhone-Poulenc Rorer, Switz.; May & Baker, UK; Wyeth-Ayerst, USA.
Ketoprofen (p.48·2) or ketoprofen sodium (p.48·3).
Gout; inflammation; musculoskeletal, joint, peri-articular, and soft-tissue disorders; pain.

Orugesic *Rhone-Poulenc Rorer, Irl.*
Ketoprofen (p.48·2).
Musculoskeletal, joint, peri-articular, and soft-tissue disorders.

Oruject *Rhone-Poulenc Rorer, S.Afr.*
Ketoprofen (p.48·2).
Gout; musculoskeletal, joint, and peri-articular disorders.

Orulop *Llorente, Spain.*
Loperamide hydrochloride (p.1197·2).
Diarrhoea.

Oruvail
Rhone-Poulenc Rorer, Austral.; May & Baker, Canad.; Rhone-Poulenc Rorer, Irl.; Rhone-Poulenc Rorer, S.Afr.; May & Baker, UK; Wyeth-Ayerst, USA.
Ketoprofen (p.48·2).
Gout; musculoskeletal, joint, peri-articular, and soft-tissue disorders; pain.

Osa *Piraud, Switz.*
Salicylamide (p.82·3); lignocaine hydrochloride (p.1293·2); calcium pantothenate (p.1352·3); calcium phosphate (p.1155·3).
Gum pain.

Osa Gel de dentition aux plantes *Piraud, Switz.*
Mint oil (p.1604·1); chamomile oil; sage oil; clove oil (p.1565·2); propolis (p.1621·3).
Inflammatory dental disorders.

Osangin *Antonetto, Ital.*
Dequalinium chloride (p.1112·1).
Mouth and throat disinfection.

Osanit
Zeppenfeldt, Ger.; Piraud, Switz.†.
Homoeopathic preparation.

Os-Cal
Wyeth-Ayerst, Canad.; SmithKline Beecham Consumer, USA.
Calcium carbonate (p.1182·1).
Calcium supplement.

Os-Cal D *Wyeth-Ayerst, Canad.*
Calcium carbonate (p.1182·1); cholecalciferol (p.1366·3).
Calcium and vitamin D supplement.

Os-Cal + D *SmithKline Beecham Consumer, USA.*
Calcium carbonate (p.1182·1); vitamin D (p.1366·3).
Calcium supplement.

Os-Cal Forte *SmithKline Beecham Consumer, USA.*
Multivitamin and mineral preparation with iron.

Os-Cal Fortified *SmithKline Beecham Consumer, USA.*
Multivitamin and mineral preparation with calcium and iron.

Os-Cal Plus *SmithKline Beecham, USA.*
Multivitamin and mineral preparation with iron.

Oscevitin-A *Grasler, Ger.*
Calcium phosphate (p.1155·3); vitamin A acetate; cholecalciferol; ascorbic aid.
Calcium deficiency.

Oscillococcinum
Boiron, Canad.; Boiron, Fr.; Boiron, Switz.
Homoeopathic preparation.

Oscorel *Rhone-Poulenc Rorer, Neth.*
Ketoprofen (p.48·2).
Musculoskeletal and joint disorders.

Oseototal *Faes, Spain.*
Salcatonin (p.735·3).
Hypercalcaemia; metastatic bone pain; Paget's disease of bone; postmenopausal osteoporosis.

Osfolate
Asta Medica, Fr.; Mayoly-Spindler, Switz.
Calcium folinate (p.1342·2).
Drug-induced megaloblastic anaemias; folate deficiency; prevention of folic-acid antagonist toxicity.

Osfolato *Lusofarmaco, Ital.*
Calcium folinate (p.1342·2).
Folate deficiency; reversal of methotrexate toxicity.

Osiren
Hoechst, Aust.
Injection: Canrenoate potassium (p.836·2).
Hyperaldosteronism.

Hoechst, Aust.; Hoechst Marion Roussel, Switz.†.
Tablets: Spironolactone (p.946·1).
Cardiac oedema; hyperaldosteronism; hypertension; liver cirrhosis with ascites; nephrotic syndrome.

Osmasept *Chinosolfabrik, Ger.†.*
Osmaron-amidosulphonate (a high molecular weight aliphatic amine).
Skin disinfection.

Osmil *Sandoz, Ger.*
16 Tablets, oestradiol (p.1455·1); 12 tablets, oestradiol; medroxyprogesterone acetate (p.1448·3).
Menopausal disorders; osteoporosis.

Osmitrol
Baxter, Austral.; Baxter, Canad.; Baxter, USA.
Mannitol (p.900·3).
Cerebral oedema; early renal failure; raised intra-ocular pressure.

Osmofundin 10%
Braun, Aust.; Braun, Ger.
Mannitol (p.900·3); sodium acetate (p.1153·1); sodium chloride (p.1162·2).
Cataract surgery; cerebral oedema; forced diuresis; oliguria; renal failure.

Osmofundin 15% *Braun, Ger.*
Mannitol (p.900·3).
Fluid retention; renal failure.

Osmofundin 20%
Note. This name is used for preparations of different composition.
Braun, Aust.
Mannitol (p.900·3).
Cataract surgery; cerebral oedema; forced diuresis; oliguria; renal failure.

Braun, Ger.†.
Mannitol (p.900·3); sorbitol (p.1354·2).
Fluid retention; renal failure.

Osmogel
Merck-Clevenot, Fr.; Merck-Clevenot, Switz.†.
Magnesium sulphate (p.1157·3); lignocaine hydrochloride (p.1293·2).
Soft-tissue disorders.

Osmoglyn *Alcon, USA.*
Glycerol (p.1585·2).
Glaucoma; raised intra-ocular pressure before ophthalmic surgery.

Osmohes *Laevosan, Aust.*
Pentastarch (p.725·2).
Hypovolaemic shock.

Osmolac *Sanofi Winthrop, Ital.*
Lactulose (p.1195·3).
Adjunct in gastro-intestinal bacterial infections; hepatic encephalopathy.

Osmoleine *Pharmethic, Belg.*
Precipitated sulphur (p.1091·2); boric acid (p.1554·2).
Rhinitis; sinusitis.

Osmolite
Abbott, Austral.; Abbott, Fr.; Abbott, Irl.; Abbott, Ital.; Abbott, Switz.; Abbott, UK; Ross, USA.
A range of preparations for enteral nutrition.

Osmolite HN *Abbott, Canad.*
Preparation for enteral nutrition.

Osmopak-Plus *Charton, Canad.*
Hydrated magnesium sulphate (p.1157·3); benzocaine (p.1286·2).
Superficial inflammatory conditions.

Osmorich *Abbott, Ital.*
Preparation for enteral nutrition.

Osmosteril 10% *Fresenius, Ger.*
Mannitol (p.900·3); sodium lactate (p.1153·2).
Fluid retention; renal failure.

Osmosteril 20% *Fresenius, Ger.*
Mannitol (p.900·3).
Forced diuresis; renal failure.

Osmotan G *Aguettant, Fr.*
Electrolyte infusion with glucose (p.1147·1).
Carbohydrate source; fluid and electrolyte disorders.

Osmotol *Chauvin, Fr.*
Resorcinol (p.1090·1); ephedrine hydrochloride (p.1059·3).
Otitis externa.

Osmovist
Berlex, Canad.; Berlex, USA†.
Iotrolan (p.1008·2).
Radiographic contrast medium.

Osnervan *Glaxo Wellcome, Ger.*
Procyclidine hydrochloride (p.467·3).
Drug-induced extrapyramidal disorders; parkinsonism.

Ospamox *Biochemie, Aust.*
Amoxycillin trihydrate (p.151·3).
Bacterial infections.

Ospen
Biochemie, Aust.; Sandoz, Fr.; Sandoz, Ger.†; Sandoz, Switz.
Benzathine phenoxymethylpenicillin (p.159·2), phenoxymethylpenicillin (p.236·2), or phenoxymethylpenicillin potassium (p.236·2).
Bacterial infections.

Ospexin *Biochemie, Aust.*
Cephalexin (p.178·2).
Bacterial infections.

Ospocard *Unipack, Aust.*
Nifedipine (p.916·2).
Angina pectoris; hypertension; Raynaud's syndrome.

Ospolot
Bayer, Austral.; Desitin, Ger.; Bayropharm, Ital.†.
Sulthiame (p.359·3).
Behavioural disorders; epilepsy.

Ospronim *Intramed, S.Afr.*
Pentazocine lactate (p.75·1).
Pain.

Ospur *Henning, Ger.*
Calcium carbonate (p.1182·1).
Calcium deficiency; osteoporosis.

Ospur D$_3$ *Henning, Ger.*
Cholecalciferol (p.1366·3).
Vitamin D deficiency.

Ospur F *Henning, Ger.*
Sodium fluoride (p.742·1).
Bone metastases; osteoporosis.

Ossian *Bioindustria, Ital.†.*
Oxolinic acid (p.235·1).
Gram-negative urinary-tract infections.

Ossidal N *Bilgast, Ger.*
Homoeopathic preparation.

Ossin
Grunenthal, Ger.; Grunenthal, Switz.
Sodium fluoride (p.742·1).
Bone metastases; osteoporosis.

Ossiplex
Gebro, Aust.; Synthelabo, Ger.; Segix, Ital.
Sodium fluoride (p.742·1); ascorbic acid (p.1365·2).
Osteoporosis.

Ossiten *Boehringer Mannheim, Ital.*
Disodium clodronate (p.737·3).
Multiple myeloma; osteolytic tumours; postmenopausal osteoporosis; primary hyperparathyroidism.

Ossofluor *Streuli, Switz.*
Sodium fluoride (p.742·1).
Osteoporosis.

Ossofortin *Strathmann, Ger.*
Calcium phosphate (p.1155·3); calcium gluconate (p.1155·2); cholecalciferol (p.1366·3).
Calcium and vitamin D deficiency.

Ossopan
Germania, Aust.; Eumedica, Belg.†; Robapharm, Fr.; Pierre Fabre, Ger.; Sanofi Winthrop, Irl.; Berna, Spain; Robapharm, Switz.; Sanofi Winthrop, UK.
Microcrystalline hydroxyapatite (p.1589·2).
Calcium and phosphorus deficiency; dental caries prophylaxis; fractures; growth disorders; osteomalacia; osteoporosis; rickets.

Osspulvit S *Madaus, Ger.*
Calcium phosphate (p.1155·3); cholecalciferol (p.1366·3).
Calcium deficiency.

Osspulvit S forte *Madaus, Ger.*
Calcium preparation with vitamins.

Osspulvit Vitaminado *Madaus, Spain†.*
Hydroxyapatite (p.1589·2); yeast (p.1373·1); vitamins.
Bone and dental disorders; calcium deficiency; osteomalacia; rickets; tonic.

Oss-regen *Pekana, Ger.*
Homoeopathic preparation.

Ossyl *Mayrhofer, Aust.†.*
Hydroxyapatite (p.1589·2).
Calcium deficiency; fractures; osteoporosis.

Ostac
Boehringer Mannheim, Belg.; Boehringer Mannheim, Canad.; Boehringer Mannheim, Ger.; Boehringer Mannheim, Neth.; Boehringer Mannheim, Norw.; Boehringer Mannheim, S.Afr.; Boehringer Mannheim, Swed.; Boehringer Mannheim, Switz.
Disodium clodronate (p.737·3).
Hypercalcaemia of malignancy; osteolysis of malignancy.

Osteine C *Zambon, Fr.†.*
Ascorbic acid and mineral preparation.
Tonic.

Ostelin
Boots, Austral.; Teofarma, Ital.
Ergocalciferol (p.1367·1).
Hypoparathyroidism; osteomalacia; rickets; vitamin D deficiency.

Osten *Takeda, Jpn.*
Ipriflavone (p.740·1).
Osteoporosis.

Osteo *Quest, Canad.*
Calcium, magnesium, vitamin C, vitamin D, and silicon.

Osteobion *Merck, Spain.*
Salcatonin (p.735·3).
Hypercalcaemia; metastatic bone pain; osteoporosis; Paget's disease of bone.

Osteocalcil *Dolisos, Canad.*
Homoeopathic preparation.

Osteocalcin
Tosi, Ital.; Arcola, USA.
Salcatonin (p.735·3).
Hypercalcaemia; osteoporosis; Paget's disease of bone; reflex sympathetic dystrophy.

Osteocare *Vitabiotics, UK.*
Calcium carbonate (p.1182·1); calcium lactate (p.1155·2); calcium citrate (p.1155·1); magnesium hydroxide (p.1198·2); zinc sulphate (p.1373·2); vitamin D (p.1366·3).

Osteochondrin S *Dyckerhoff, Ger.*
Ribonucleic acids from cattle and yeast (p.1624·3).
Bone disorders.

Osteocynesine
Boiron, Canad.; Boiron, Fr.; Boiron, Switz.†.
Homoeopathic preparation.

Osteodidronel *Procter & Gamble, Belg.*
Disodium etidronate (p.738·3).
Postmenopausal osteoporosis.

Osteofix *Chiesi, Ital.*
Ipriflavone (p.740·1).
Postmenopausal osteoporosis.

Osteofluor
Merck, Aust.†; Merck-Clevenot, Fr.
Sodium fluoride (p.742·1).
Osteoporosis.

Osteogen *Richard, Fr.*
Pyridoxine phosphate (p.1363·1); calcium ascorbate (p.1365·2); magnesium deoxyribonucleinate (p.1570·3); deoxyribonucleic acid (p.1570·3).
Osteopathies; senile debility.

Osteogenon *Germania, Aust.*
Hydroxyapatite (p.1589·2).
Calcium deficiency; fractures; osteoporosis.

Osteomineral *Yves Ponroy, Fr.†.*
Mineral preparation.

Osteoplex *Vitaplex, Austral.*
Mineral, vitamin, enzyme, and herb preparation.
Calcium deficiency.

Osteopor *Pierre Fabre, Spain.*
Hydroxyapatite (p.1589·2).
Calcium deficiency; osteoporosis.

Osteopor-F *Hausmann, Switz.†.*
Sodium fluoride (p.742·1).
Osteoporosis.

Osteoporosis Mineral Plus Formula 9 *Vitelle, Austral.*
Calcium carbonate (p.1182·1); cholecalciferol (p.1366·3).
Calcium deficiency; osteoporosis.

Osteos *TAD, Ger.*
Salcatonin acetate (p.736·3).
Hypercalcaemia; malignant osteolysis; osteoporosis; Paget's disease of bone; reflex sympathetic dystrophy.

OsteoScan *Mallinckrodt, USA.*
Technetium-99m disodium oxidronate (p.1425·1).
Bone scanning agent.

Osteosil *Ghimas, Ital.*
Equisetum (p.1575·1).
Nutritional supplement.

Osteoton *Herbaline, Ital.*
Food for special diets.
Bone disorders.

Osteotonina *Menarini, Ital.*
Salcatonin (p.735·3).
Hypercalcaemia; osteoporosis; Paget's disease of bone; reflex sympathetic dystrophy.

Osteovis *NCSN, Ital.*
Salcatonin (p.735·3).
Hypercalcaemia; osteoporosis; Paget's disease of bone; reflex sympathetic dystrophy.

Osteovit *Pharmadass, UK.*
Multivitamin, mineral, and trace element preparation.

Ostersoy
Crookes, Irl.†; Farley, UK†.
Gluten-, sucrose-, and lactose-free food for special diets.
Cow's milk protein sensitivity; galactokinase deficiency; galactosaemia; lactose and sucrose intolerance.

Osteum *Vinas, Spain.*
Disodium etidronate (p.738·3).
Ectopic ossification; osteoporosis; Paget's disease of bone.

Ostiderm *Pedinol, USA.*
Lotion: Aluminium sulphate (p.1548·1); zinc oxide (p.1096·2).
Formerly contained aluminium sulphate and phenol.
Roll-on: Aluminium chlorohydrate (p.1078·3); camphor (p.1557·2).
Foot odour; hyperhidrosis.

Ostobon *Coloplast, UK.*
A deodorant powder for use with ostomies.

Ostochont *Godecke, Ger.*
Liniment: Glycol salicylate (p.43·1); benzyl nicotinate (p.22·1); nonivamide (p.63·2).
Ointment; topical gel: Heparin (p.879·3); glycol salicylate (p.43·1); benzyl nicotinate (p.22·1).
Bruising; musculoskeletal and joint disorders; neuralgia.

Ostoforte *Frosst, Canad.*
Ergocalciferol (p.1367·1).
Hypoparathyroidism; phosphataemia; rickets.

Ostostabil *Jenapharm, Ger.*
Salcatonin (p.735·3).
Hypercalcaemia; osteolysis of malignancy; osteoporosis; Paget's disease of bone; reflex sympathetic dystrophy.

Ostram
Merck-Clevenot, Fr.; Faes, Spain; E. Merck, UK.
Calcium phosphate (p.1155·3).
Calcium deficiency; osteoporosis.

Ostrolut *Schering, Aust.*
Hydroxyprogesterone hexanoate (p.1448·1); oestradiol benzoate (p.1455·1).
Secondary amenorrhoea.

Ostronara *Asche, Ger.*
16 Tablets, oestradiol valerate (p.1455·2); 12 tablets, oestradiol valerate; levonorgestrel (p.1454·1).
Menopausal disorders.

Ostro-Primolut
Schering, Aust.†; Schering, Ger.
Norethisterone acetate (p.1453·1); ethinyloestradiol (p.1445·1).
Menstrual disorders.

Osvical *Alter, Spain.*
Ascorbic acid (p.1365·2); calcium hypophosphite; calcium laevulinate (p.1155·2); cholecalciferol (p.1366·3).
Bone and dental disorders; calcium deficiency; osteomalacia; rickets.

Osvical Lisina *Alter, Spain†.*
Calcium ascorbate (p.1365·2); vitamin B substances and amino acids; ergocalciferol (p.1367·1); calcium adipate; calcium hypophosphite; calcium carbonate (p.1182·1); calcium citrate hydrochloride.
Bone and dental disorders; calcium deficiency; osteomalacia; rickets.

Osyrol *Hoechst, Ger.*
Canrenoate potassium (p.836·2) or spironolactone (p.946·1).
Hyperaldosteronism; hypertension; liver cirrhosis and ascites; oedema.

Osyrol Lasix *Hoechst, Ger.*
Spironolactone (p.946·1); frusemide (p.871·1).
Ascites; hyperaldosteronism; liver cirrhosis; oedema.

Otalgan
Note. This name is used for preparations of different composition.
Willvonseder, Aust.; Wolfs, Belg.
Lignocaine hydrochloride (p.1293·2); phenazone (p.78·2).
Formerly contained procaine hydrochloride and phenazone in *Belg*.
Earache; otitis.
Sudmedica, Ger.; Berna, Ital.; Berna, Spain; Medichemie, Switz.
Procaine hydrochloride (p.1299·2); phenazone (p.78·2).
Earache; otitis media.
Medichemie, Neth.
Lignocaine hydrochloride (p.1293·2).
Earache.

Otalgicin Sudmedica, Ger.
Xylometazoline hydrochloride (p.1071·2).
Nasal congestion.

Otazul Ottolenghi, Ital.
Benzalkonium chloride (p.1101·3); azulene (p.1552·1); hamamelis (p.1587·1).
Eye disinfection; eye irritation.

O-Tet Docmed, S.Afr.
Oxytetracycline hydrochloride (p.235·1).
Bacterial infections.

Otex Dendron, UK.
Urea hydrogen peroxide (p.1127·3).
Ear wax removal.

Otic Domeboro Miles, USA.
Acetic acid (p.1541·2); aluminium acetate (p.1547·3).
Superficial infections of the external auditory canal.

Oticane Parke, Davis, Austral.†.
Benzocaine (p.1286·2); sodium propionate (p.387·1); salicylic acid (p.1090·2); chlorhexidine acetate.
Bacterial or fungal otitis externa.

Otic-Care Parmed, USA.
Hydrocortisone (p.1043·3); neomycin sulphate (p.229·2); polymyxin B sulphate (p.239·1).
Bacterial ear infections.

Oticin HC Teral, USA.
Polymyxin B sulphate (p.239·1); neomycin sulphate (p.229·2); hydrocortisone (p.1043·3).

Oti-Med Hyrex, USA.
Pramoxine hydrochloride (p.1298·2); hydrocortisone (p.1043·3).
Ear disorders.

Otipax
Biocodex, Fr.; Inpharzam, Switz.
Lignocaine hydrochloride (p.1293·2); phenazone (p.78·2).
Earache.

Otised Propan, S.Afr.
Phenazone (p.78·2); benzocaine (p.1286·2).
Ear infections.

Otitex Sudmedica, Ger.
Docusate sodium (p.1189·3).
Removal of ear wax.

OtiTricin Bausch & Lomb, USA.
Hydrocortisone (p.1043·3); neomycin sulphate (p.229·2); polymyxin B (p.239·3).
Bacterial ear infections.

Otix Farmacusi, Spain.
Dexamethasone phosphate (p.1037·2); polymyxin B sulphate (p.239·1); trimethoprim (p.265·1).
Otitis externa.

Oto -cyl Ho-Len-Complex Liebermann, Ger.
Homoeopathic preparation.

Oto Difusor Medical, Spain.
Benzocaine (p.1286·2); hyaluronidase (p.1588·1); hydrocortisone acetate (p.1043·3); neomycin sulphate (p.229·2); sulphanilamide sodium mesylate (p.256·3).
Ear disorders.

Oto Neomicin Calm Ale, Spain.
Benzocaine (p.1286·2); hydrocortisone acetate (p.1043·3); neomycin sulphate (p.229·2); sulphacetamide sodium (p.252·2).
Ear disorders.

Oto Vitna Quimifar, Spain†.
Dexamethasone (p.1037·1); benzocaine (p.1286·2); hydrocortisone acetate (p.1043·3); neomycin sulphate (p.229·2).
External ear disorders.

Otobacid N Asche, Ger.
Dexamethasone (p.1037·1); cinchocaine hydrochloride (p.1289·2).
Ear disorders.

Otobiotic
Note. This name is used for preparations of different composition.
UCB, Ital.†.
Colistin sulphate (p.195·3); neomycin sulphate (p.229·2); hydrocortisone acetate (p.1043·3); lignocaine (p.1293·2).
Ear disorders.
Schering, USA.
Polymyxin B sulphate (p.239·1); hydrocortisone (p.1043·3).
Bacterial ear infections.

Otocain Abana, USA.
Benzocaine (p.1286·2).
Earache.

Otocaina Mendelejeff, Ital.†.
Chlorbutol (p.1106·3); guaiacol (p.1061·2); boric acid (p.1554·2); sulphanilamide (p.256·3); urea (p.1095·2).
Ear disorders.

Otocalm Parmed, USA.
Benzocaine (p.1286·2); phenazone (p.78·2).
Earache.

Otocalmine Pharmacobel, Belg.
Phenazone (p.78·2); procaine hydrochloride (p.1299·2).
Ear disorders.

Otocerum Reig Jofre, Spain.
Phenol (p.1121·2); chlorbutol (p.1106·3); benzocaine (p.1286·2); turpentine oil (p.1641·1); castor oil (p.1560·2).
Removal of ear wax.

Otocomb Otic Bristol-Myers Squibb, Austral.
Triamcinolone acetonide (p.1050·2); neomycin sulphate (p.229·2); nystatin (p.386·1); gramicidin (p.215·2).
Otitis externa.

Otocort Lemmon, USA.
Hydrocortisone (p.1043·3); neomycin sulphate (p.229·2); polymyxin B (p.239·3).
Bacterial ear infections.

Otocusi Enzimatico Cusi, Spain†.
Betamethasone sodium phosphate (p.1033·3); hyaluronidase (p.1588·1); polymyxin B sulphate (p.239·1); amethocaine hydrochloride (p.1285·2); tetracycline hydrochloride (p.259·1); trypsin (p.1640·1).
External ear disorders.

Otodex Qualimed, Austral.
Framycetin sulphate (p.210·3); gramicidin (p.215·2); dexamethasone (p.1037·1).
Ear disorders.

Otodolor Ursapharm, Ger.
Phenazone (p.78·2); procaine hydrochloride (p.1299·2).
Inflammatory ear disorders.

Otofa
Bouchara, Fr.; Bouchara, Switz.
Rifamycin sodium (p.246·2).
Otitis.

Oto-Flexiole N Mann, Ger.
Amethocaine hydrochloride (p.1285·2).
Oto-Flexiole formerly contained amethocaine hydrochloride and phenazone.
Earache; otitis.

Otofluor SIT, Ital.
Sodium fluoride (p.742·1); calcium gluconate (p.1155·2).
Otosclerosis.

Otogen Belmac, Spain†.
Lithium carbonate (p.290·3); potassium bromide (p.1620·3); potassium iodide (p.1493·1); thiamine (p.1361·2).
Ear disorders; nervous disorders.

Otogen Calmante Belmac, Spain.
Benzalkonium chloride (p.1101·3); clove oil (p.1565·2); phenol (p.1121·2); amethocaine hydrochloride (p.1285·2); menthol (p.1600·2).
Ear disorders.

Otogen Hydrocortisona Belmac, Spain†.
Hydrocortisone (p.1043·3); neomycin sulphate (p.229·2); tyrothricin (p.267·2).
Ear disorders.

Otogen Prednisolona Belmac, Spain†.
Neomycin sulphate (p.229·2); prednisolone (p.1048·1); tyrothricin (p.267·2).
Ear disorders.

Otoial Fidia, Ital.
Sodium hyaluronate (p.1630·3).
Tympanic membrane lesions.

Otolitan N farblos 3M, Ger.
Dequalinium chloride (p.1112·1); lignocaine hydrochloride (p.1293·2).
Earache; otitis.

Otolitan N mit Rivanol 3M, Ger.
Ethacridine lactate (p.1098·3); lignocaine hydrochloride (p.1293·2).
Earache; otitis.

Otolysine Chauvin, Fr.
Triethanolamine caprylate.
Removal of ear wax.

Otomar-HC Marnel, USA.
Chloroxylenol (p.1111·1); hydrocortisone (p.1043·3); pramoxine hydrochloride (p.1298·2).
Ear disorders.

Otomicetina Deca, Ital.
Chloramphenicol (p.182·1); neomycin sulphate (p.229·2); tuaminoheptane sulphate (p.1071·1).
Ear infections.

Otomide L'Arguenon, Fr.
Hexamidine isethionate (p.1115·3); lignocaine hydrochloride (p.1293·2).
Formerly contained sulfasuccinamide sodium and amylocaine hydrochloride.
Otitis.

Otomidone SIT, Ital.
Phenazone (p.78·2); procaine hydrochloride (p.1299·2).
Formerly contained amidopyrine, procaine hydrochloride, and chlorbutol.
Earache.

Otomidrin Fardi, Spain.
Fluocinolone acetonide (p.1041·1); framycetin sulphate (p.210·3); lignocaine hydrochloride (p.1293·2).
Ear disorders.

Otomize
Stafford-Miller, Irl.; Stafford-Miller, UK.
Dexamethasone (p.1037·1); neomycin sulphate (p.229·2).
Otitis externa.

Otomycin-HPN Misemer, USA.
Hydrocortisone (p.1043·3); neomycin sulphate (p.229·2); polymyxin B (p.239·3).
Bacterial ear infections.

Otonasal Diftersa, Spain.
Ephedrine hydrochloride (p.1059·3); procaine (p.1299·2); sulphanilamide (p.256·3).
Congestion and infection of the nose and ear.

Otone Lennon, S.Afr.†.
Oxyphenbutazone (p.72·1).
Ankylosing spondylitis.

Otonina Berna, Spain.
Benzocaine (p.1286·2); neomycin sulphate (p.229·2); prednisolone (p.1048·1).
Ear disorders.

Otopax Vaillant, Ital.
Procaine hydrochloride (p.1299·2); phenazone (p.78·2).
Earache.

Oto-Phen Mer-National, S.Afr.
Phenazone (p.78·2).
Earache; otitis.

Oto-Phen Forte Mer-National, S.Afr.
Benzocaine (p.1286·2); ephedrine hydrochloride (p.1059·3); phenazone (p.78·2); potassium hydroxyquinoline sulphate (p.1621·1).
Earache; otitis.

Otoralgyl
Note. This name is used for preparations of different composition.
Rhone-Poulenc Rorer, Belg.; Martin, Fr.
Lignocaine hydrochloride (p.1293·2).
Earache.
Martin, Switz.
Sulfasuccinamide sodium (p.252·1); lignocaine hydrochloride (p.1293·2).
Earache; otitis.

Otoralgyl sulfamide Martin, Fr.
Sulfasuccinamide sodium (p.252·1); lignocaine hydrochloride (p.1293·2).
Earache; otitis externa.

Otormon F (Femminile) Farmades, Ital.†.
Methandriol; xenyethanol; vitamin A palmitate (p.1359·2); vitamin E (p.1369·1); guaiacol (p.1061·2); pumilio pine oil (p.1623·3); niaouli oil (p.1607·1); cineole (p.1564·1).
Ear disorders.

Otosan Streuli, Switz.
Procaine hydrochloride (p.1299·2); phenazone (p.78·2).
Ear disorders; earache.

Otosan Gocce Auricolari Otosan, Ital.
Almond oil (p.1546·2); alcohol (p.1099·1); cajuput oil (p.1556·1); geranium oil (p.1584·1); juniper oil (p.1592·3); chamomile (p.1561·2).
Ear wax removal.

Otosedol Pensa, Spain.
Phenazone (p.78·2); procaine hydrochloride (p.1299·2).
Earache.

Otosedol Biotico Pensa, Spain.
Chloramphenicol (p.182·1); benzocaine (p.1286·2); tyrothricin (p.267·2).
Ear disorders.

Otoseptil Ethimed, S.Afr.†.
Neomycin undecenoate (p.229·2); tyrothricin (p.267·2); hydrocortisone (p.1043·3).
Ear disorders.

Otosmo Aristegui, Spain†.
Phenazone (p.78·2); procaine hydrochloride (p.1299·2).
Earache.

Otosporin
Note. This name is used for preparations of different composition.
Glaxo Wellcome, Aust.; Warner-Lambert Consumer, Belg.; Glaxo Wellcome, Ger.; Wellcome, Irl.; Glaxo Wellcome, Neth.; Glaxo Wellcome, S.Afr.; Glaxo Wellcome, Spain; Wellcome, Switz.; Wellcome, UK; Calmic, USA.
Polymyxin B sulphate (p.239·1); neomycin sulphate (p.229·2); hydrocortisone (p.1043·3).
Bacterial infections of the outer ear.
Warner-Lambert, Ital.
Neomycin sulphate (p.229·2); polymyxin B sulphate (p.239·1).
Formerly contained hydrocortisone, neomycin sulphate, and polymyxin B sulphate.
Bacterial infections of the external ear.

Otospray Stafford-Miller, Switz.
Neomycin sulphate (p.229·2); dexamethasone (p.1037·1).
Ear disorders.

Otothricinol Plan, Switz.
Tyrothricin (p.267·2); phenazone (p.78·2); cetylpyridinium chloride (p.1106·2).
Ear disorders.

Otovowen Weber & Weber, Ger.
Homoeopathic preparation.

Otowaxol Norgine, Ger.
Docusate sodium (p.1189·3).
Removal of ear wax.

Otreon
Luitpold, Aust.; Luitpold, Ital.; Alfarma, Spain.
Cefpodoxime proxetil (p.172·1).
Bacterial infections.

Otrinol Zyma, Switz.
Pseudoephedrine hydrochloride (p.1068·3).
Nasal congestion.

Otrisal Zyma, Aust.
Sodium chloride (p.1162·2).
Nasal and pharyngeal dryness; nasal congestion.

Otriven Ciba Vision, Ger.
Xylometazoline hydrochloride (p.1071·2).
Conjunctival disorders.

Otriven gegen Schnupfen Zyma, Ger.
Xylometazoline hydrochloride (p.1071·2).
Catarrh; nasal congestion; rhinitis.

Otriven H Zyma, Ger.
Sodium cromoglycate (p.762·1).
Allergic disorders of the conjunctiva; allergic rhinitis.

Otriven-Millicorten Ciba, Ger.†.
Xylometazoline hydrochloride (p.1071·2); dexamethasone pivalate (p.1037·3).
Allergic rhinitis.

Otrivin
Zyma, Aust.; Novartis, Austral.; Novartis Consumer, Canad.; Zyma, Ital.; Novartis Consumer, Neth.; Novartis, Norw.; Ciba-Geigy, S.Afr.; Zyma, Spain; Novartis, Swed.; Zyma, Switz.; Ciba Consumer, USA.
Xylometazoline hydrochloride (p.1071·2).
Nasal congestion; otitis; rhinitis; sinusitis.

Otrivin Menthol Novartis, Swed.
Xylometazoline hydrochloride (p.1071·2); menthol (p.1600·2); cineole (p.1564·1).
Rhinitis.

Otrivine
Zyma, Belg.; Zyma, Irl.; Zyma, UK.
Xylometazoline hydrochloride (p.1071·2).
Nasal congestion; rhinitis; sinusitis.

Otrivine-Antistin
Ciba Vision, Irl.; Ciba Vision, UK.
Xylometazoline hydrochloride (p.1071·2); antazoline sulphate (p.402·1).
Allergic conjunctivitis.

Otsuka MV Otsuka, Jpn.
Multivitamin preparation.

Ottimal ICT-Lodi, Ital.†.
Tiemonium methylsulphate (p.468·3).
Smooth muscle spasm.

Ottoclor Ottolenghi, Ital.
Chloramine (p.1106·3).
Wound disinfection.

Ottovis Fitolife, Ital.
Royal jelly (p.1626·3); ginseng (p.1584·2); wheatgerm oil; soya lecithin (p.1595·2); pollen.
Tonic.

Ottovit Valeas, Ital.†.
Multivitamin preparation.

Otylol Bridoux, Fr.
Procaine hydrochloride (p.1299·2); amethocaine hydrochloride (p.1285·2); phenol (p.1121·2); ephedrine hydrochloride (p.1059·3); thyme oil (p.1637·1).
Ear disorders.

Ouate Hemostatique Qualiphar, Belg.
Ferric chloride (p.1579·3); phenazone (p.78·2).
Haemorrhage.

Ouate Hemostatique U.S. Pharmastra, Fr.†.
Calcium alginate (p.714·1).
Haemorrhage.

Out of Africa Sunfresh, Canad.
Pyrithione zinc (p.1089·3).

Outgro
Whitehall-Robins, Canad.; Whitehall, USA.
Tannic acid (p.1634·2); chlorbutol (p.1106·3).
Ingrown toenails.

Out-of-Sorts Potter's, UK.
Tinnevelly senna (p.1212·2); cape aloe (p.1177·1); cascara bark (p.1183·1); taraxacum (p.1634·2); fennel seed (p.1579·1).
Constipation.

Ovanon
Organon, Aust.; Aaciphar, Belg.; Organon, Fr.; Nourypharma, Ger.; Nourypharma, Neth.; Donmed, S.Afr.†; Ercopharm, Switz.
7 Tablets, ethinyloestradiol (p.1445·1); 15 tablets, ethinyloestradiol; lynoestrenol (p.1448·2).
28-Day packs also contain 6 inert tablets.
Dysmenorrhoea; sequential-type oral contraceptive.

Ovaras Serono, Ital.†.
Mestranol (p.1450·2); ethynodiol diacetate (p.1445·3).
Menopausal disorders; menstrual disorders.

Ovastat Medac, Ger.
Treosulfan (p.568·1).
Ovarian cancer.

Ovatest OTW, Ger.†.
Oestradiol benzoate (p.1455·1); bovine ovaries; bovine testes.
Menopausal disorders; prostatic adenoma.

Ovcon 35 Mead Johnson Laboratories, USA.
Norethisterone (p.1453·1); ethinyloestradiol (p.1445·1).
28-Day packs also contain 7 inert tablets.
Combined oral contraceptive.

Overal Lusofarmaco, Ital.
Roxithromycin (p.247·1).
Bacterial infections.

Ovesterin
Organon, Norw.; Organon, Swed.
Oestriol (p.1457·2).
Vulvovaginal disorders due to oestrogen deficiency.

Ovestin
Organon, Aust.; Organon, Austral.; Organon, Fr.†; Organon, Ger.; Organon, Irl.; Organon, Ital.; Organon, Neth.†; Organon, Switz.; Organon, UK.
Oestriol (p.1457·2).
Vulvovaginal disorders due to oestrogen deficiency.

Ovestinon Organon, Spain.
Oestriol (p.1457·2).
Oestrogen deficiency.

Ovex Johnson & Johnson MSD Consumer, UK.
Mebendazole (p.104·1).
Enterobiasis.

Ovibion
Klinge, Aust.; Schwab, Ger.†.
Porcine ovarian extract (p.1458·2).
Menopausal disorders; menstrual disorders.

Ovide GenDerm, USA.
Malathion (p.1407·3).
Pediculosis.

Ovidol
Aaciphar, Belg.; Nourypharma, Neth.; Nourypharma, Switz.
7 Tablets, ethinyloestradiol (p.1445·1); 15 tablets, ethinyloestradiol; desogestrel (p.1443·3).
Sequential-type oral contraceptive.

Oviol Nourypharma, Ger.
7 Tablets, ethinyloestradiol (p.1445·1); 15 tablets, ethinyloestradiol; desogestrel (p.1443·3).
28-Day packs also contain 6 inert tablets.
Sequential-type oral contraceptive.

Ovis Parke, Davis, Ger.†.
Dichlorophen (p.99·2); zinc oxide (p.1096·2).
Fungal infections.

Ovis Neu Warner-Lambert, Ger.
Clotrimazole (p.376·3).
Fungal infections.

Ovol Carter Horner, Canad.
Simethicone (p.1213·1).
Flatulence; infant colic.

Ovoplex Wyeth, Spain.
Ethinyloestradiol (p.1445·1); levonorgestrel (p.1454·1).
Combined oral contraceptive; menstrual disorders.

Ovoquinol Nadeau, Canad.†.
Di-iodohydroxyquinoline (p.581·1); sulphadiazine (p.252·3); undecenoic acid (p.389·2).
Cervicitis; vaginitis.

Ovoresta Organon, Ger.
Lynoestrenol (p.1448·2); ethinyloestradiol (p.1445·1).
Combined oral contraceptive; menstrual disorders.

Ovoresta M Organon, Ger.
Lynoestrenol (p.1448·2); ethinyloestradiol (p.1445·1).
Combined oral contraceptive; menstrual disorders.

Ovoresta Micro Organon, Spain†.
Lynoestrenol (p.1448·2); ethinyloestradiol (p.1445·1).
Combined oral contraceptive; menstrual disorders.

Ovosiston Jenapharm, Ger.
Mestranol (p.1450·2); chlormadinone acetate (p.1439·1).
Combined oral contraceptive; menstrual disorders.

Ovostat
Organon, Belg.; Organon, Neth.; Donmed, S.Afr.; Organon, Switz.
Lynoestrenol (p.1448·2); ethinyloestradiol (p.1445·1).
28-Day packs also contain 7 inert tablets.
Combined oral contraceptive; menstrual disorders.

Ovo-Vinces Wolff, Ger.
Oestriol (p.1457·2).
Menopausal disorders.

Ovowop Hor-Fer-Vit, Ger.†.
Ethinyloestradiol (p.1445·1); oestrone (p.1458·2).
Menopausal disorders.

Ovral
Wyeth-Ayerst, Canad.; Akromed, S.Afr.; Wyeth-Ayerst, USA.
Norgestrel (p.1454·1); ethinyloestradiol (p.1445·1).
28-Day packs also contain 7 inert tablets.
Combined oral contraceptive; menstrual disorders.

Ovran
Wyeth, Irl.; Wyeth, UK.
Ethinyloestradiol (p.1445·1); levonorgestrel (p.1454·1).
Combined oral contraceptive; endometriosis; menstrual disorders.

Ovran 30
Wyeth, Irl.; Wyeth, UK.
Ethinyloestradiol (p.1445·1); levonorgestrel (p.1454·1).
Combined oral contraceptive; gynaecological disorders.

Ovranet Wyeth, Ital.
Ethinyloestradiol (p.1445·1); levonorgestrel (p.1454·1).
Combined oral contraceptive.

Ovranette
Kwizda, Aust.†; Wyeth, Irl.; Wyeth, UK.
Ethinyloestradiol (p.1445·1); levonorgestrel (p.1454·1).
Combined oral contraceptive; endometriosis; menstrual disorders.

Ovrette Wyeth-Ayerst, USA.
Norgestrel (p.1454·1).
Progestogen-only oral contraceptive.

OvuGen BioGenex, USA.
Fertility test (p.1621·2).

Ovukit
MediMar, UK.; Monoclonal Antibodies, USA.
Fertility test (p.1621·2).

Ovulen
Searle, Austral.; Searle, Belg.; Searle, Neth.†; Searle, Switz.
Ethynodiol diacetate (p.1445·3); ethinyloestradiol (p.1445·1).
28-Day packs also contain 7 inert tablets.
Combined oral contraceptive; menstrual disorders.

Ovules Sedo-Hemostatiques du Docteur Jouve Gerda, Fr.
Phenazone (p.78·2); calcium chloride (p.1155·1).
Dysmenorrhoea; gynaecological examination; minor gynaecological surgery.

Ovuquick
MediMar, UK; Monoclonal Antibodies, USA.
Fertility test (p.1621·2).

Ovuthricinol Plan, Switz.†.
Tyrothricin (p.267·2); sulphanilamide (p.256·3).
Genito-urinary tract disorders.

Ovysmen
Janssen-Cilag, Aust.; Janssen-Cilag, Belg.; Janssen-Cilag, Ger.; Janssen-Cilag, Irl.; Janssen-Cilag, Switz.; Cilag, UK.
Norethisterone (p.1453·1); ethinyloestradiol (p.1445·1).
Combined oral contraceptive.

Owbridges for Chesty Coughs Chefaro, UK.
Guaiphenesin (p.1061·3).
Coughs.

Owbridges for Children Chefaro, UK†.
Sodium citrate (p.1153·2); menthol (p.1600·2); diphenhydramine hydrochloride (p.409·1).
Congestion; coughs.

Owbridges for Dry Tickly Coughs Chefaro, UK†.
Dextromethorphan hydrobromide (p.1057·3).
Coughs.

oxa CT, Ger.
Oxazepam (p.683·2).
Anxiety disorders; sleep disorders.

Oxacant mono Klein, Ger.
Crataegus (p.1568·2).
Heart failure.

Oxacant N Klein, Ger.
Crataegus (p.1568·2); hypericum (p.1590·1); convallaria (p.1567·2); adonis vernalis (p.1543·3); cereus grandiflorus; scoparium (p.1628·1); mellisa (p.1600·1); valerian (p.1643·1); motherwort (p.1604·2).
Cardiac disorders.

Oxacant-forte N Klein, Ger.
Crataegus (p.1568·2); convallaria (p.1567·2); adonis vernalis (p.1543·3); cereus grandiflorus.
Cardiac disorders.

Oxacant-Khella N Klein, Ger.
Crataegus (p.1568·2); convallaria (p.1567·2); adonis vernalis (p.1543·3); cereus grandiflorus; ammi visnaga (p.1593·2).
Cardiac disorders.

Oxacant-sedativ Klein, Ger.
Crataegus (p.1568·2); motherwort (p.1604·2); melissa (p.1600·1); valerian (p.1643·1).
Nervous disorders.

Oxacef Gibipharma, Ital.†.
Latamoxef disodium (p.221·2).
Bacterial infections.

Oxadilene Evans, Fr.
Butalamine hydrochloride (p.835·2); papaverine hydrochloride (p.1614·2).
Cerebrovascular disorders.

Oxadol ISI, Ital.
Nefopam hydrochloride (p.62·3).
Pain.

Oxahexal Hexal, Aust.
Oxazepam (p.683·2).
Anxiety disorders; sleep disorders.

Oxaline Rolab, S.Afr.
Oxazepam (p.683·2).
Alcohol withdrawal syndrome; anxiety disorders.

Oxalyt Madaus, Aust.
Potassium sodium hydrogen citrate.
Renal calculi.

Oxalyt-C
Madaus, Ger.†; Madaus, Switz.†.
Potassium sodium hydrogen citrate.
Urinary-tract disorders.

Oxandrin BTG, USA.
Oxandrolone (p.1458·3).
Bone pain associated with osteoporosis; protein catabolism; weight loss.

Oxapam Lilly, Ital.
Oxazepam (p.683·2).
Anxiety disorders.

Oxaprim Otifarma, Ital.†.
Co-trimoxazole (p.196·3).
Bacterial infections; Pneumocystis carinii pneumonia.

Oxa-Puren Klinge-Nattermann, Ger.†.
Oxazepam (p.683·2).
Anxiety; sleep disorders.

Oxascand Enapharm, Swed.
Oxazepam (p.683·2).
Alcohol withdrawal syndrome; anxiety; sleep disorders.

Oxatokey Inkeysa, Spain.
Oxatomide (p.415·1).
Hypersensitivity reactions.

Oxbarukain ankerpharm, Ger.
Oxybuprocaine hydrochloride (p.1298·1).
Local anaesthesia.

OxBipp Oxford Pharmaceuticals, UK.
Bismuth subnitrate (p.1180·2); iodoform (p.1118·2).

Oxeprax Wyeth, Spain.
Tamoxifen (p.564·3).
Breast cancer.

Oxicebral Pfizer, Spain†.
Vincamine (p.1644·1).
Cerebral trauma; cerebrovascular disorders.

Oxiderma Galderma, Spain.
Benzoyl peroxide (p.1079·2).
Acne.

Oxidermiol Antihist Farmasur, Spain.
Benzocaine (p.1286·2); tyrothricin (p.267·2); tripelennamine hydrochloride (p.420·2).
Cutaneous hypersensitivity reactions.

Oxidermiol Enzima Farmasur, Spain.
Bacitracin (p.157·3); neomycin sulphate (p.229·2); trypsin (p.1640·1).
Skin infections.

Oxidermiol Fuerte Farmasur, Spain.
Fluocinolone acetonide (p.1041·1).
Skin disorders.

Oxidermiol Lassar Farmasur, Spain.
Starch; salicylic acid (p.1090·2); soft paraffin; zinc oxide (p.1096·2).
Skin disorders.

Oxido Amari Cusi, Spain.
Mercuric chloride (p.1601·2); mercuric oxide (p.1601·3).
Eye disorders.

Oxi-Freeda Freeda, USA.
Multivitamin, mineral, and amino-acid preparation.

Oxilin Allergan, Ital.
Oxymetazoline hydrochloride (p.1065·3).
Conjunctivitis; eye congestion.

Oxilium
Labor, Aust.; Oxo, Switz.
Tetrachlorodecaoxide (p.1635·1).
Burns; skin disinfection; wounds.

Oximen Men, Spain.
Hydrogen peroxide (p.1116·2).
Haemostasis; skin and mucous membrane disinfection.

Oxinorm Zambeletti, Ital.†.
Orgotein (p.87·3).
Cystitis; musculoskeletal and joint disorders; Peyronie's disease.

Oxipor
Whitehall-Robins, Canad.; Whitehall, Irl.†.
Coal tar (p.1092·3); salicylic acid (p.1090·2); benzocaine (p.1286·2).
Skin disorders.

Oxipor VHC Whitehall, USA.
Coal tar (p.1092·3).
Formerly contained coal tar, salicylic acid, and benzocaine.
Psoriasis.

Oxis
Astra, Irl.; Astra, Neth.; Draco, Swed.; Astra, UK.
Eformoterol fumarate (p.752·3).
Asthma.

Oxistat Glaxo Wellcome, USA.
Oxiconazole nitrate (p.386·3).
Fungal skin infections.

Oxitimol Arzo, Spain†.
Alcohol; glycerol; thymol (p.1127·1); hydrogen peroxide (p.1116·2).
Aural hygiene; oral hygiene; wound disinfection.

Oxitover Llorente, Spain.
Mebendazole (p.104·1).
Worm infections.

Oxivel Zeller, Switz.
Ginkgo biloba (p.1584·1).
Tonic.

Oxivent
Bender, Aust.; Boehringer Ingelheim, Belg.; Boehringer Ingelheim, Irl.; Boehringer Ingelheim, Ital.; Boehringer Ingelheim, UK.
Oxitropium bromide (p.757·1).
Obstructive airways disease.

Oxleti Leti, Spain.
Oxatomide (p.415·1).
Hypersensitivity reactions.

Oxodal Synthelabo Delagrange, Spain.
Betaxolol hydrochloride (p.832·1).
Hypertension.

Oxoferin Yamanouchi, Ger.
Reaction product of sodium chlorite, sodium hypochlorite, sulphuric acid, potassium chlorate, sodium carbonate-hydrogen peroxide, and sodium peroxide.
Wounds.

Oxoinex Inexfa, Spain.
Oxolinic acid (p.235·1).
Urinary-tract infections.

Oxosint Medivis, Ital.
Co-tetroxazine (p.196·3).
Bacterial infections; Pneumocystis carinii pneumonia.

Oxovinca Schering, Fr.†.
Vincamine oxoglurate (p.1644·1).
Mental function impairment in the elderly.

Oxsoralen
Gerot, Aust.; Dermatech, Austral.; ICN, Canad.; Italfarmaco, Ital.; Elder, Neth.†; Restan, S.Afr.; Galderma, Spain; ICN, USA.
Methoxsalen (p.1086·3).
Psoriasis; vitiligo.

Oxsoralon Wolfs, Belg.
Methoxsalen (p.1086·3).
Psoriasis.

Oxy
Note. This name is used for preparations of different composition.
Reckitt & Colman, Austral.; SmithKline Beecham Consumer, Canad.; SmithKline Beecham Consumer, UK; SmithKline Beecham Consumer, USA.
Benzoyl peroxide (p.1079·2).
Acne.

Triomed, S.Afr.
Oxytetracycline hydrochloride (p.235·1).
Bacterial infections.

Oxy Biciron S & K, Ger.
Oxytetracycline hydrochloride (p.235·1); tramazoline hydrochloride (p.1071·1).
Bacterial eye infections.

Oxy Clean Facial Scrub SmithKline Beecham Consumer, UK.
Borax (p.1554·2); triclosan (p.1127·2).
Acne.

Oxy Clean Lathering Norcliff Thayer, USA†.
Abrasive skin cleanser.

Oxy Clean Medicated SmithKline Beecham, USA†.
Salicylic acid (p.1090·2); alcohol (p.1099·1).
Acne.

Oxy Clean Soap Norcliff Thayer, USA†.
Salicylic acid (p.1090·2); borax (p.1554·2).
Acne.

Oxy Cleanser SmithKline Beecham Consumer, UK.
Regular: Triclosan (p.1127·2); salicylic acid (p.1090·2); alcohol (p.1099·1).
Formerly called Oxy Clean Medicated Cleanser.
Sensitive: Salicylic acid (p.1090·2); alcohol (p.1099·1).
Acne.

Oxy Control SmithKline Beecham Consumer, Canad.
Salicylic acid (p.1090·2).
Acne.

Oxy Deep Pore SmithKline Beecham Consumer, Canad.
Salicylic acid (p.1090·2).
Acne.

Oxy Duo Pads SmithKline Beecham Consumer, UK.
Regular: Triclosan (p.1127·2); salicylic acid (p.1090·2); alcohol (p.1099·1).
Sensitive: Salicylic acid (p.1090·2); alcohol (p.1099·1).
Acne.

Oxy Facial Wash SmithKline Beecham Consumer, UK.
Triclosan (p.1127·2).
Formerly called Oxy Clean Facial Wash.
Skin disorders.

Oxy Fissan Fink, Ger.; Zyma, Ger.
Benzoyl peroxide (p.1079·2).
Acne.

Oxy Gentle SmithKline Beecham Consumer, Canad.
Triclosan (p.1127·2).
Acne.

Oxy Medicated Soap
SmithKline Beecham Consumer, Canad.; SmithKline Beecham, USA.
Triclosan (p.1127·2).
Acne.

Oxy Night Watch
SmithKline Beecham Consumer, Canad.; SmithKline Beecham Consumer, USA.
Salicylic acid (p.1090·2).
Acne.

Oxy Power Pads SmithKline Beecham Consumer, Canad.
Salicylic acid (p.1090·2).
Acne.

Oxy ResiDon't SmithKline Beecham, USA†.
Triclosan (p.1127·2); diazolidinyl urea.

Oxy Skin Wash Reckitt & Colman, Austral.
Triclosan (p.1127·2).
Acne; skin cleanser.

Oxyboldine Cooperation Pharmaceutique, Fr.
Boldine (p.1554·1); anhydrous sodium sulphate (p.1213·3); monobasic sodium phosphate (p.1159·3).
Dyspepsia.

Oxybutyn ICN, Canad.
Oxybutynin hydrochloride (p.466·1).

Oxycardin
Note. This name is used for preparations of different composition.
Schwarz, Fr.†.
Isosorbide mononitrate (p.893·3).
Angina pectoris; heart failure.

Schwarz, Ger.†.
Bupranolol hydrochloride (p.835·2); isosorbide dinitrate (p.893·1).
Cardiac disorders.

Oxy-Care Agepha, Aust.
Hydrogen peroxide (p.1116·2); sodium chloride (p.1162·2).
Disinfecting, cleaning, and storage solution for hard and soft contact lenses.

Oxycel
Associated Hospital Supply, UK; Becton Dickinson, USA.
Oxidised cellulose (p.714·2).
Bleeding in surgical procedures.

Oxyclean Allergan, Austral.†.
Cleansing solution for contact lenses.

Oxycocet Technilab, Canad.
Oxycodone hydrochloride (p.71·2); paracetamol (p.72·2).
Fever; pain.

Oxycodan Technilab, Canad.
Oxycodone hydrochloride (p.71·2); aspirin (p.16·1).
Fever; inflammation; pain.

Oxycontin
Purdue Frederick, Canad.; Purdue Frederick, USA.
Oxycodone hydrochloride (p.71·2).
Pain.

Oxyderm ICN, Canad.
Benzoyl peroxide (p.1079·2).
Hyperkeratosis.

Oxydermine Wild, Switz.
Zinc oxide (p.1096·2); laureth 9 (p.1325·2).
Burns; skin disorders; wounds.

Oxydess II Vortech, USA.
Dexamphetamine sulphate (p.1478·2).
Attention deficit disorder with hyperactivity; narcoleptic syndrome; obesity.

Oxy-Dumocyclin
Dumex, Norw.†; Dumex-Alpharma, Swed.†.
Oxytetracycline hydrochloride (p.235·1).
Bacterial infections.

Oxyfan Coli, Ital.
Oxitriptan (p.301·2).
Depression; nervous system disorders.

Oxygenabund Herbert, Ger.†.
Thiamine hydrochloride (p.1361·1); dipyridamole (p.857·1); magnesium orotate (p.1611·2).
Tonic.

Oxygeron
Boehringer Mannheim, Aust.; Drossapharm, Switz.
Vincamine (p.1644·1).
Cerebrovascular disorders; circulatory eye disorders; vertigo.

OxyIR Purdue Frederick, USA.
Oxycodone hydrochloride (p.71·2).
Pain.

Oxylin
Allergan, Neth.†; Allergan, S.Afr.
Oxymetazoline hydrochloride (p.1065·3).
Conjunctivitis; eye irritation.

Oxymycin
Lennon, S.Afr.†; DDSA Pharmaceuticals, UK.
Oxytetracycline (p.235·1) or oxytetracycline hydrochloride (p.235·1).
Bacterial infections.

Oxynol SIT, Ital.†.
Hydroxyquinoline sulphate (p.1589·3).
Formerly known as Neo Mercurochromo Intimo.
Feminine hygiene.

Oxypan Propan, S.Afr.
Oxytetracycline hydrochloride (p.235·1).
Bacterial infections.

Oxypangam Sanorania, Ger.
Di-isopropylammonium dichloroacetate (p.854·1).
Hypoxia due to circulatory disorders.

Oxyperol Lemoine, Fr.
Peru balsam (p.1617·2); zinc oxide (p.1096·2).
Eczema.

Oxyplastine
Note. This name is used for preparations of different composition.
Bournonville, Belg.
Zinc oxide (p.1096·2); peru balsam (p.1617·2); calcium hydroxide (p.1556·3).
Barrier cream; skin disorders.

Parke, Davis, Fr.; Wild, Switz.
Zinc oxide (p.1096·2).
Skin disorders.

Oxyprenix Ashbourne, UK.
Oxprenolol hydrochloride (p.926·2).
Angina pectoris; anxiety; hypertension.

Oxysept
Note. This name is used for preparations of different composition.
Allergan, Aust.
Oxysept 1 solution, hydrogen peroxide (p.1116·2); Oxysept 2 solution, catalase (p.1560·3).
Disinfecting, neutralising, and storage system for soft contact lenses.

Allergan, Austral.
Part I, hydrogen peroxide (p.1116·2); part II, rinsing and storage solution.
Disinfecting, rinsing, and storage solution for soft contact lenses.

Allergan, Canad.
Cleaning and disinfecting solution for soft contact lenses.

Allergan, Ger.
Oxysept 1, hydrogen peroxide 3% (p.1116·2); Oxysept 2, disodium edetate (p.980·1).
Disinfecting and neutralising system for soft contact lenses.

Allergan, USA.
Hydrogen peroxide (p.1116·2).
Disinfecting solution for soft contact lenses.

Oxysept Comfort
Allergan, Aust.; Allergan, Ger.
Solution, hydrogen peroxide 3% (p.1116·2); tablets, catalase (p.1560·3).
Disinfection and neutralisation of soft contact lenses.

Oxysept Light Allergan, Ger.†.
Solution, hydrogen peroxide 3% (p.1116·2); tablets, catalase (p.1560·3).
Disinfection and neutralisation of soft contact lenses.

Oxysept Quick
Allergan, Aust.; Allergan, Ger.†.
Catalase (p.1560·3).
Neutralisation of hydrogen peroxide contact lens disinfecting solution.

Oxytetral
Alpharma, Norw.; Dumex-Alpharma, Swed.
Oxytetracycline hydrochloride (p.235·1).
Bacterial infections.

Oxytetramix Ashbourne, UK.
Oxytetracycline (p.235·1).
Bacterial infections.

Oxy-thymoline Meyer, Fr.†.
Borax (p.1554·2); thymol (p.1127·1); phenol (p.1121·2); chloral hydrate (p.645·3); rhatany (p.1624·3).
Infections of the mouth and throat.

Oxythyol Richard, Fr.
Starch (p.1356·2); zinc oxide (p.1096·2); ichthammol (p.1083·3); white soft paraffin (p.1382·3); wool fat (p.1385·3).
Burns; eczema.

Oxytoko Vitafarma, Spain†.
Benzoyl peroxide (p.1079·2).
Acne.

Oxyzal Gordon, USA.
Hydroxyquinoline sulphate (p.1589·3); benzalkonium chloride (p.1101·3).
Minor skin infections.

Oyo Polypharm, Ger.
Sodium pangamate (p.1614·1).
Cerebral and peripheral vascular disorders; ischaemic heart disease; migraine.

Oysco Rugby, USA.
Calcium carbonate (p.1182·1).
Calcium deficiency; dietary supplement.

Oysco D Rugby, USA.
Calcium with vitamin D.
Calcium deficiency; dietary supplement.

Oyst-Cal Goldline, USA.
Calcium carbonate (p.1182·1).
Calcium deficiency; dietary supplement.

Oyst-Cal-D Goldline, USA.
Calcium with vitamin D.
Calcium deficiency; dietary supplement.

Oyster Calcium Nature's Bounty, USA.
Calcium with vitamins A and D.
Calcium deficiency; dietary supplement.

Oyster Calcium with Vitamin D Nion, USA.
Calcium with vitamin D.
Calcium deficiency; dietary supplement.

Oyster Shell Stanley, Canad.†.
Calcium with vitamin D.
Calcium deficiency; dietary supplement.

Oyster Shell Calcium Vangard, USA.
Calcium carbonate (p.1182·1).
Calcium deficiency; dietary supplement.

Oyster Shell Calcium with Vitamin D Major, USA.
Calcium with vitamin D.
Calcium deficiency; dietary supplement.

Oystercal Nature's Bounty, USA.
Calcium carbonate (p.1182·1).
Calcium deficiency; dietary supplement.

Oystercal-D Nature's Bounty, USA.
Calcium with vitamin D.
Calcium deficiency; dietary supplement.

Oz Aleph, Ital.
Zinc oxide (p.1096·2).
Skin disorders.

Ozabran N Redel, Ger.†.
Paracetamol (p.72·2); propyphenazone (p.81·3); caffeine (p.749·3).
Formerly contained salicylamide, paracetamol, propyphenazone, caffeine, ascorbic acid, diphenylpyraline hydrochloride, and phenylephrine hydrochloride.
Cold symptoms; pain.

Ozidia Pfizer, Fr.
Glipizide (p.320·3).
Diabetes mellitus.

Ozonol Bayer, Canad.
Phenol (p.1121·2); zinc oxide (p.1096·2).
Bites and stings; burns; cuts; skin irritation.

Ozonol Antibiotic Plus Bayer, Canad.
Polymyxin B (p.239·1); bacitracin (p.157·3); lignocaine hydrochloride (p.1293·2).
Minor cuts and burns; skin irritation.

Ozopulmin Geymonat, Ital.
Injection: Verbenone.
Suppositories: Verbenone; pine oil.
Respiratory-system disorders.

Ozopulmin Antiasmatico Wasserman, Spain†.
Dexamethasone phosphate (p.1037·2); diprophylline (p.752·1); pinus sylvestris oil; turpentine oil (p.1641·1).
Obstructive airways disease.

Ozopulmin Antipiretico ICT-Lodi, Ital.†.
Verbenone; *trans*-verbenol; myrtenol; myrtenal; *trans*-pinocarveol; *cis*-pinenol; pine oil; propyphenazone (p.81·3).
Respiratory-system disorders.

Ozopulmin Diprofillina ICT-Lodi, Ital.†.
Suppositories: Verbenone; *trans*-verbenol; myrtenol; myrtenal; *trans*-pinocarveol; *cis*-pinenol; pine oil; diprophylline (p.752·1).
Tablets; injection: Verbenone; *trans*-verbenol; myrtenol; myrtenal; *trans*-pinocarveol; *cis*-pinenol; diprophylline (p.752·1).
Respiratory-system disorders.

Ozopulmin G Geymonat, Ital.
Suppositories: Verbenone; pine oil.
Syrup: Verbenone; dextromethorphan hydrobromide (p.1057·3).
Topical gel: Verbenone.
Respiratory system disorders.

Ozothin SmithKline Beecham, Ger.
Injection; inhalation: Oxidation product of turpentine oil "Landes" (p.1641·1); terpin hydrate (p.1070·2).
Suppositories: Paracetamol (p.72·2); oxidation product of turpentine oil "Landes" (p.1641·1); oleum pini sylvestris.
Tablets: Diprophylline (p.752·1); oxidation products of turpentine oil "Landes" (p.1641·1).
Respiratory-tract disorders.

Ozothine SCAT, Fr.
Suppositories: Oxidation products of turpentine oil (p.1641·1).
Syrup: Oxidation products of turpentine oil (p.1641·1); ethylmorphine hydrochloride (p.36·1); sodium benzoate (p.1102·3).
Respiratory-tract disorders.

Ozothine a la Diprophylline SCAT, Fr.
Oxidation products of turpentine oil (p.1641·1); diprophylline (p.752·1).
Asthma; bronchospastic disorders.

Ozovit
Koch, Aust.; Pascoe, Ger.
Magnesium peroxide (p.1119·1).
Gastro-intestinal disorders.

Ozym
Note. This name is used for preparations of different composition.
Procter & Gamble, Aust.
Amylase from *Aspergillus oryzae* (p.1549·1); papain (p.1614·1); fel suis (p.1553·2); pancreatin (p.1612·1).
Gastro-intestinal disorders.

Trommsdorff, Ger.
Pancreatin (p.1612·1).
Formerly contained amylase from aspergillus, papain, fel suis, and pancreatin.
Pancreatic insufficiency.

P 10 Pulitzer, Ital.†.
Betamethasone valero-acetate (p.1034·1).
Skin disorders.

P & S
Baker Cummins, Canad.; Baker Cummins, USA.
Scalp application: Liquid phenol (p.1121·2).
Psoriasis; seborrhoeic dermatitis.

Baker Cummins, Canad.; Baker Cummins, USA.
Shampoo: Salicylic acid (p.1090·2).
Psoriasis; seborrhoea.

P & S Plus
Baker Cummins, Canad.; Baker Cummins, USA.
Coal tar (p.1092·3); salicylic acid (p.1090·2).
Psoriasis; seborrhoeic dermatitis.

P. Veinos Augot, Fr.
Aesculus (p.1543·3); cypress; hamamelis (p.1587·1).
Peripheral vascular disorders.

Pabalate Robins, USA.
Sodium salicylate (p.85·1); sodium aminobenzoate.
Pain.

Pabalate-SF Robins, USA†.
Potassium salicylate; potassium aminobenzoate (p.1620·1).
Pain.

Pabanol ICN, Canad.†.
Aminobenzoic acid (p.1486·3).
Sunscreen.

Pabasun Jumer, Fr.
Aminobenzoic acid (p.1486·3).
Sunscreen.

Pabenol Gentili, Ital.†.
Deanol acetamidobenzoate (p.1478·2).
Mental function disorders.

Pabina Pharmalab, S.Afr.†.
Aminobenzoic acid (p.1486·3).
Sunscreen.

Pablum Sobee Mead Johnson, Canad.†.
Soya-based infant feed.
Hypersensitivity to cow's milk or wheat flour.

Pabrinex
Link, Irl.; Link, UK.
Vitamin B and C substances.
Vitamin deficiency.

P-A-C Upjohn, USA.
Aspirin (p.16·1); caffeine (p.749·3).
Pain.

Pac Merieux Pasteur Merieux, Ger.
An acellular pertussis vaccine (p.1526·1).
Active immunisation.

Pacaps Lunsco, USA.
Butalbital (p.644·3); caffeine (p.749·3); paracetamol (p.72·2).

Pacerone Upsher-Smith, USA.
Amiodarone hydrochloride (p.820·1).
Arrhythmias.

Paceum Orion, Switz.
Diazepam (p.661·1).
Convulsions; non-psychotic mental disorders; premedication; skeletal muscle spasm; sleep disorders.

Pacifene Sussex, UK.
Ibuprofen (p.44·1).
Fever; pain.

Pacifenity Vitaplex, Austral.
Passion flower (p.1615·3); mistletoe (p.1604·1); avena (p.1551·3); valerian (p.1643·1); gentian (p.1583·3); lupulus (p.1597·2); scutellaria; leonurus cardiaca (p.1604·2).
Herbal relaxant.

Pacimol Nat Druggists, S.Afr.
Paracetamol (p.72·2).
Fever; pain.

Pacinol
Schering-Plough, Norw.†; Schering-Plough, Swed.
Fluphenazine hydrochloride (p.671·3).
Alcohol or opioid withdrawal syndromes; psychoses.

Pacinone
Byk, Belg.†; Delagrange, Neth.†.
Halazepam (p.673·2).
Anxiety.

Pacis Faulding, Canad.
A BCG vaccine (p.1504·3).
Bladder cancer.

Pacium Uriach, Spain.
Diazepam (p.661·1).
Contains pyridoxine hydrochloride.
Alcohol withdrawal syndrome; anxiety; febrile convulsions; insomnia; skeletal muscle spasm.

Padamin Leopold, Aust.
Amino-acid infusion.
Parenteral nutrition.

Paderyl Gerda, Fr.
Syrup: Codeine phosphate (p.26·1).
Formerly contained papaverine hydrobromide, codeine hydrobromide, cinnamaverine hydrochloride, belladonna, hyoscyamus, and mistletoe.
Tablets: Codeine phosphate (p.26·1).
Formerly contained papaverine hydrobromide, codeine hydrobromide, cinnamaverine hydrochloride, belladonna, hyoscyamus, hyssop, and valerian.
Coughs.

Padiafusin
Pharmacia Upjohn, Aust.; Pharmacia Upjohn, Ger.
Electrolyte infusion with glucose (p.1147·1).
Carbohydrate source; fluid and electrolyte disorders.

Padiafusin OP Pharmacia Upjohn, Ger.
Potassium-free electrolyte infusion with glucose (p.1147·1).
Carbohydrate source; fluid and electrolyte disorders.

Padiamox Plantorgan, Ger.†.
Amoxycillin trihydrate (p.151·3).
Bacterial infections.

Padilclorina Blue Cross, Ital.†.
Paratoluenechlorosulphonamide sodium.
Skin and wound disinfection; surface disinfection.

Padma 28
Padma, Switz.; Padma, UK.
Aegle sepiar fructus; amomi fructus; aquilegiae herba; calendula flos; cardamomi fructus; caryophylli flos; costi amari radix; hedychii rhizoma; lactucae sativae herba; lichen islandicus; liquiritiae radix; meliae tousand fructus; myrobalani fructus; plantaginis herba; polygoni herba; potentillae aureae herba; santali rubri lignum; sidae cordifoliae herba; aconiti tuber; valerianae radix; calcium sulphate; camphor.
Circulatory disorders.

Padma-Lax Padma, Switz.
Aloes (p.1177·1); kaolin (p.1195·1); calumba radix (p.1557·2); condurango (p.1567·2); enulae radix; gentian (p.1583·3); myrobalan; sodium bicarbonate (p.1153·2); anhydrous sodium sulphate (p.1213·3); piper longum; frangula bark (p.1193·2); cascara (p.1183·1); rhubarb (p.1212·1); nux vomica (p.1609·3); ginger (p.1193·2).
Constipation.

Padrin Fujisawa, Jpn.
Prifinium bromide (p.467·2).
Gastro-intestinal spasm.

Padutin
Bayer, Aust.; Bayer, Ger.
Kallidinogenase (Kallikrein) (p.1592·3).
Male infertility.

Paedamin Paedpharm, Austral.
Diphenhydramine hydrochloride (p.409·1); phenylephrine hydrochloride (p.1068·3).
Upper respiratory-tract disorders.

Paedavit Antigen, Irl.†.
Multivitamin preparation.

Paedialgon Chephasaar, Ger.
Paracetamol (p.72·2).
Fever; pain.

Paediasure
Abbott, Irl.; Abbott, UK.
Preparation for enteral nutrition.

Paediathrocin Abbott, Ger.
Erythromycin (p.204·1) or erythromycin ethyl succinate (p.204·2).
Bacterial infections.

Paediatric Seravit
Scientific Hospital Supplies, Austral.; Scientific Hospital Supplies, UK.
Multivitamin, mineral, and trace element preparation.
Dietary supplement; metabolic disorders.

Paedisup Chephasaar, Ger.
Paracetamol (p.72·2); doxylamine succinate (p.410·1).
Fever; pain.

Paf Lofarma, Ital.
Bucarbetene; chlorbutol (p.1106·3).
Scabies.

Paidenur Juventus, Spain†.
Atropine sulphate (p.455·1); aminohydroxybutyric acid (p.339·1); imipramine hydrochloride (p.289·2).
Nocturnal enuresis.

Paididont Metochem, Aust.
Chamomile (p.1561·2); cetylpyridinium chloride (p.1106·2); laureth 9 (p.1325·2).
Teething pain.

Paidocin Master Pharma, Ital.
Rokitamycin (p.246·3).
Bacterial infections.

Paidocol *IBIS, Ital.†.*
Vitamin B substances.

Paidoflor *Ardeypharm, Ger.*
Lactobacillus acidophilus (p.1594·1).
Gastro-intestinal disorders.

Paidomal *Malesci, Ital.*
Lysine theophyllinate.
Obstructive airways disease.

Paidorinovit *SIT, Ital.*
Ephedrine (p.1059·3); cineole (p.1564·1); niaouli oil (p.1607·1).
Nasal congestion.

Paidoterin Descongestivo *Aldo, Spain†.*
Chlorpheniramine maleate (p.405·1); diphenhydramine hydrochloride (p.409·1); phenylephrine hydrochloride (p.1066·2); guaiphenesin (p.1061·3); choline salicylate (p.25·2); sodium citrate (p.1153·2).
Upper-respiratory-tract disorders.

Paidozim *Juventus, Spain.*
Amylase (p.1549·1); cellulase (p.1561·1); lipase; metoclopramide (p.1202·1); protease.
Digestive enzyme insufficiency; dyspepsia.

Paigastrol *Orravan, Spain.*
Pancreatin (p.1612·1); pepsin (p.1616·3).
Digestive enzyme insufficiency.

Pain Aid *Zee, Canad.*
Aspirin (p.16·1); caffeine (p.749·3).

Pain Aid Free *Zee, Canad.*
Paracetamol (p.72·2).

Pain Buster *Prodemdis, Canad.*
Methyl salicylate (p.55·2); camphor (p.1557·2); menthol (p.1600·2); eucalyptus oil (p.1578·1).

Pain Bust-R II *Continental, USA.*
Methyl salicylate (p.55·2); menthol (p.1600·2).
Musculoskeletal and joint disorders.

Pain Doctor *Fougera, USA.*
Capsaicin (p.24·2); methyl salicylate (p.55·2); menthol (p.1600·2).
Pain.

Pain And Fever Relief *Brauer, Austral.*
Homoeopathic preparation.

Pain Gel Plus *Mentholatum, USA.*
Menthol (p.1600·2).
Pain.

Pain Patch *Mentholatum, USA.*
Menthol (p.1600·2).
Musculoskeletal and joint pain.

Pain Relief Syrup for Children *Unichem, UK.*
Paracetamol (p.72·2).
Fever; pain.

Pain Reliever *Rugby, USA.*
Paracetamol (p.72·2); aspirin (p.16·1); caffeine (p.749·3).
Pain.

Pain X *Ascher, USA.*
Capsaicin (p.24·2); menthol (p.1600·2); camphor (p.1557·2).
Pain.

Painagon *Be-Tabs, S.Afr.*
Syrup: Paracetamol (p.72·2); codeine phosphate (p.26·1); promethazine hydrochloride (p.416·2).
Tablets: Paracetamol (p.72·2); codeine phosphate (p.26·1); meprobamate (p.678·1); caffeine (p.749·3).
Fever; pain; pain associated with tension.

Painamol *Be-Tabs, S.Afr.*
Paracetamol (p.72·2).
Fever; pain.

Painamol Plus *Be-Tabs, S.Afr.*
Paracetamol (p.72·2); codeine phosphate (p.26·1).
Fever; pain.

Paincod *Crown, S.Afr.*
Aspirin (p.16·1); paracetamol (p.72·2); codeine phosphate (p.26·1).
Fever; pain.

Paineze *Nelson, Austral.†.*
Paracetamol (p.72·2); codeine phosphate (p.26·1).
Pain.

Painguard *Nelson, Austral.†.*
Methyl salicylate (p.55·2); menthol (p.1600·2); camphor (p.1557·2); capsicum oleoresin; eucalyptus oil (p.1578·1).
Sprains.

Painrite *Columbia, S.Afr.*
Paracetamol (p.72·2); codeine phosphate (p.26·1); caffeine (p.749·3); meprobamate (p.678·1).
Pain and associated tension.

Painrite SA *Columbia, S.Afr.*
Paracetamol (p.72·2); codeine phosphate (p.26·1).
Fever; pain.

Pains-of *Eagle, Austral.*
Multivitamin and amino acid preparation.
Pain.

Painstop *Paedpharm, Austral.*
Paracetamol (p.72·2); promethazine hydrochloride (p.416·2); codeine phosphate (p.26·1).
Pain.

Palacos *Essex, Switz.*
Methylmethacrylate co-polymer (p.1603·2).
Bone cement for orthopaedic surgery.

Palacos avec Garamycin *Essex, Switz.*
Methylmethacrylate co-polymer (p.1603·2); gentamicin sulphate (p.212·1).
Bone cement for orthopaedic surgery.

Palacos avec Gentamicine *Schering-Plough, Fr.*
Methylmethacrylate/methacrylate copolymer (p.1603·2); gentamicin sulphate (p.212·1).
Bone cement for orthopaedic surgery.

Palacos cum gentamicin
Schering-Plough, Norw.; Schering-Plough, Swed.
Polymethylmethacrylate (p.1603·2); gentamicin sulphate (p.212·1).
Bone cement for orthopaedic surgery.

Palacos E with Garamycin *Schering-Plough, Austral.*
Methylmethacrylate methyl acrylate copolymer (p.1603·2); gentamicin sulphate (p.212·1).
Bone cement for orthopaedic surgery.

Palacos LV with Gentamicin *Schering-Plough, UK.*
Methylmethacrylate/methylacrylate copolymer (p.1603·2); gentamicin sulphate (p.212·1).
Bone cement for orthopaedic surgery.

Palacos R
Merck, Ger.; Schering-Plough, UK.
Methylmethacrylate/methylacrylate copolymer (p.1603·2).
Bone cement for orthopaedic surgery.

Palacos R with Garamycin
Schering-Plough, Austral.; Schering-Plough, S.Afr.
Methylmethacrylate/methylacrylate copolymer (p.1603·2); gentamicin sulphate (p.212·1).
Bone cement for orthopaedic surgery.

Palacos R with Gentamicin
Schering-Plough, Irl.; Schering-Plough, UK.
Methylmethacrylate/methylacrylate copolymer (p.1603·2); gentamicin sulphate (p.212·1).
Bone cement for orthopaedic surgery.

Palacos R Gentamicine *Schering-Plough, Fr.*
Methylmethacrylate/methylacrylate copolymer (p.1603·2); gentamicin sulphate (p.212·1).
Bone cement for orthopaedic surgery.

Palacos R met gentamicine *Schering-Plough, Neth.*
Methylmethacrylate/methylacrylate copolymer (p.1603·2); gentamicin sulphate (p.212·1).
Bone cement for orthopaedic surgery.

Palacril Lotio *Warner-Lambert, Ger.*
Diphenhydramine hydrochloride (p.409·1); zinc oxide (p.1096·2).
Skin disorders.

Paladac with Minerals *Parke, Davis, Austral.†.*
Multivitamin and mineral preparation.

Paladac Solu *Parke, Davis, Spain†.*
Multivitamin preparation.

Palafer *SmithKline Beecham, Canad.*
Ferrous fumarate (p.1339·3).
Iron deficiency; iron supplement; iron-deficiency anaemias.

Palafer CF *SmithKline Beecham, Canad.*
Ferrous fumarate (p.1339·3); folic acid (p.1340·3).
Ascorbic acid (p.1365·2) is included in this preparation to increase the absorption and availability of iron.
Prenatal supplement.

Palaprin
Roche, Aust.; Nicholas, Irl.†.
Aloxiprin (p.15·1).
Pain.

Palatol *Pascoe, Ger.*
Distillate: Peppermint oil (p.1208·1); niaouli oil (p.1607·1); cajuput oil (p.1556·1); eucalyptus oil (p.1578·1).
Catarrh.
Ointment†: Echinacea angustifolia (p.1574·2); arnica (p.1550·3); hamamelis (p.1587·1); peppermint oil (p.1208·1); niaouli oil (p.1607·1); cajuput oil (p.1556·1); eucalyptus oil (p.1578·1).
Respiratory-tract disorders.

Palatol N *Pascoe, Ger.*
Eucalyptus oil (p.1578·1); peppermint oil (p.1208·1); niaouli oil (p.1607·1); cajuput oil (p.1556·1); hamamelis (p.1587·1).
Catarrh.

Paldesic *Rosemont, UK.*
Paracetamol (p.72·2).
Fever; pain.

Palfium
Faulding, Austral.; Janssen-Cilag, Belg.; Synthelabo, Fr.; Antigen, Irl.; Asta Medica, Neth.; Boehringer Mannheim, UK.
Dextromoramide tartrate (p.27·2).
Pain.

Paliuryl *Richelet, Fr.*
Rhamnus paliurus.
Azotaemia; stimulation of renal water excretion.

Palladone
Napp, Irl.; Napp, UK.
Hydromorphone hydrochloride (p.43·2).
Pain.

Palliacol N *Wander, Ger.†.*
Dried aluminium hydroxide gel (p.1177·3); magnesium hydroxide (p.1198·2).
Gastro-intestinal disorders.

Pallidan *Berna, Spain.*
Methaqualone (p.678·3).
Insomnia.

Palmi *Medecine Vegetale, Fr.*
Boldo (p.1554·1); combretum (p.1593·2); gentian (p.1583·3).
Digestive disorders.

Palmicol *Palmicol, Ger.*
Heavy magnesium carbonate (p.1198·1).
Gastro-intestinal disorders.

Palmil *Cantabria, Spain.*
Castor oil (p.1560·2).
Bowel evacuation.

Palmisan *Palmicol, Ger.*
Homoeopathic preparation.

Palmitate-A 5000 *Akorn, USA.*
Vitamin A (p.1358·1).

Palmofen *Zambon, Ital.†.*
Fosfomycin calcium (p.210·2).
Bacterial infections.

Palmolive UV *Palmolive Skincare, Austral.†.*
Ethylhexyl *p*-methoxycinnamate (p.1487·1); octyl salicylate (p.1487·3); octocrylene (p.1487·3); avobenzone (p.1486·3).
Sunscreen.

Palohex *Winthrop, Neth.†.*
Inositol nicotinate (p.891·3).
Peripheral vascular disorders.

Palpipax *Bouchard, Fr.*
Meprobamate (p.678·1); valerian (p.1643·1).
Formerly contained sparteine sulphate and meprobamate.
Nervous disorders.

Pals
Glenwood, Canad.†; Glenwood, USA.
Chlorophyllin copper complex (p.1000·1).
Odour control in ostomy and incontinent patients.

Paludrine
Zeneca, Aust.; ICI, Austral.; Zeneca, Belg.; Wyeth-Ayerst, Canad.; Zeneca, Fr.; Zeneca, Ger.; Zeneca, Irl.; Zeneca, Ital.; Zeneca, Neth.; Zeneca, Norw.; Zeneca, S.Afr.; Zeneca, Swed.; Zeneca, Switz.; Zeneca, UK.
Proguanil hydrochloride (p.435·3).
Malaria.

Paluther *Rhone-Poulenc Rorer, Fr.*
Artemether (p.425·2).
Malaria.

Pamba *OPW, Ger.*
Aminomethylbenzoic acid (p.711·2).
Haemorrhage.

Pamed-C *Permamed, Switz.†.*
Paracetamol (p.72·2); ascorbic acid (p.1365·2).
Fever; pain.

Pameion *Astra, Ital.†.*
Papaverine hydrochloride (p.1614·2).
Vascular disorders.

Pamelor *Sandoz, USA.*
Nortriptyline hydrochloride (p.300·2).
Depression.

Pamergan *Rhone-Poulenc Rorer, Canad.†.*
Pethidine hydrochloride (p.76·1); promethazine hydrochloride (p.416·2).
Pain; premedication.

Pamergan P100 *Martindale Pharmaceuticals, UK.*
Pethidine hydrochloride (p.76·1); promethazine hydrochloride (p.416·2).
NOTE. There is no connection between Martindale, The Complete Drug Reference and Martindale Pharmaceuticals.
Pain; premedication.

Pameton *SmithKline Beecham, UK.*
Paracetamol (p.72·2); DL-methionine (p.984·2).
Fever; pain.

Pamica *Eagle, Austral.†.*
Di-isopropylammonium dichloroacetate (p.854·1); calcium gluconate (p.1155·2).

Pamine *Kenwood, USA.*
Hyoscine methobromide (p.463·1).
Peptic ulcer (adjunct).

Pamocil *Uno, Ital.*
Amoxycillin trihydrate (p.151·3).
Bacterial infections.

Pamol *Docmed, S.Afr.*
Paracetamol (p.72·2).
Fever; pain.

Pamoxan *Uriach, Spain.*
Viprynium embonate (p.111·2).
Worm infections.

Pamprin
Chattem, Canad.; Chattem, USA.
Paracetamol (p.72·2); pamabrom (p.927·1); mepyramine maleate (p.414·1).
Pain; premenstrual syndrome.

Pan *Merckle, Ger.†.*
Heparin sodium (p.879·3); dexpanthenol (p.1570·3).
Skin trauma.

Pan C *Freeda, USA.*
Hesperidin (p.1580·2); citrus bioflavonoids complex (p.1580·1); vitamin C (p.1365·2).
Capillary bleeding.

Panacef *Lilly, Ital.*
Cefaclor (p.163·2).
Bacterial infections.

Panacet *ECR, USA.*
Hydrocodone tartrate (p.43·1); paracetamol (p.72·2).

Panacete *Prosana, Austral.†.*
Paracetamol (p.72·2).
Fever; pain.

Panadeine
Note. This name is used for preparations of different composition.
Sanofi Winthrop, Austral.; SmithKline Beecham Consumer, Austral.; SmithKline Beecham Consumer, Irl.; Sterling Health, UK.
Paracetamol (p.72·2); codeine phosphate (p.26·1).
Formerly known as Panadeine Co in the *UK*.
These ingredients can be described by the British Approved Name Co-codamol.
Fever; pain.

SmithKline Beecham Consumer, Belg.
Paracetamol (p.72·2); caffeine (p.749·3); codeine phosphate (p.26·1).
Fever; pain.

Panadeine Plus *SmithKline Beecham Consumer, Austral.*
Paracetamol (p.72·2); codeine phosphate (p.26·1); doxylamine succinate (p.410·1).
Fever; pain.

Panado *Restan, S.Afr.*
Paracetamol (p.72·2).
Fever; pain.

Panadoc *Saphar, S.Afr.†.*
Polysorbate 20 (p.1327·3); ammonium chloride (p.1055·2).
Coughs.

Pando-Co *Restan, S.Afr.*
Paracetamol (p.72·2); codeine phosphate (p.26·1).
Fever; pain.

Panadol
SmithKline Beecham Consumer, Austral.; SmithKline Beecham Consumer, Belg.; SmithKline Beecham Consumer, Canad.; SmithKline Beecham Sante, Fr.; SmithKline Beecham Consumer, Irl.; Maggioni, Ital.; SmithKline Beecham Consumer, Neth.; Sterling Health, Spain; SmithKline Beecham Consumer, Switz.; Sterling Health, UK; Glenbrook, USA; Sterling Health, USA.
Paracetamol (p.72·2).
Fever; pain.

Panadol Allergy Sinus *SmithKline Beecham Consumer, Austral.*
Paracetamol (p.72·2); pseudoephedrine hydrochloride (p.1068·3); chlorpheniramine maleate (p.405·1).
Formerly known as Panadol Sinus Relief with Antihistamine.
Allergic symptoms; pain; sinus congestion.

Panadol Children's Cold *SmithKline Beecham Consumer, Austral.*
Paracetamol (p.72·2); pseudoephedrine hydrochloride (p.1068·3); chlorpheniramine maleate (p.405·1).
Cold symptoms; fever; pain.

Panadol Codeine
SmithKline Beecham Consumer, Belg.; SmithKline Beecham Sante, Fr.
Paracetamol (p.72·2); codeine phosphate (p.26·1).
Fever; pain.

Panadol Cold and Flu *SmithKline Beecham Consumer, Austral.*
Paracetamol (p.72·2); pseudoephedrine hydrochloride (p.1068·3); dextromethorphan hydrobromide (p.1057·3).
Cold and influenza symptoms.

Panadol Elixir with Promethazine *SmithKline Beecham Consumer, Austral.†.*
Paracetamol (p.72·2); promethazine hydrochloride (p.416·2).
Fever; pain.

Panadol Extra *Sterling Health, UK.*
Paracetamol (p.72·2); caffeine (p.749·3).
Fever; pain.

Panadol Night
SmithKline Beecham Consumer, Austral.; SmithKline Beecham Consumer, UK.
Paracetamol (p.72·2); diphenhydramine hydrochloride (p.409·1).
Insomnia; pain.

Panadol Plus *SmithKline Beecham Consumer, Neth.*
Paracetamol (p.72·2); caffeine (p.749·3).
Fever; pain.

Panadol Sinus *SmithKline Beecham Consumer, Austral.*
Paracetamol (p.72·2); pseudoephedrine hydrochloride (p.1068·3).
Pain; sinus congestion.

Panadol Sinus Day/Night *SmithKline Beecham Consumer, Austral.*
Day caplets, paracetamol (p.72·2); pseudoephedrine hydrochloride (p.1068·3); night caplets, paracetamol; pseudoephedrine hydrochloride; chlorpheniramine maleate (p.405·1).
Cold symptoms; fever.

Panadol Ultra *Sterling Health, UK.*
Paracetamol (p.72·2); codeine phosphate (p.26·1).
These ingredients can be described by the British Approved Name Co-codamol.
Pain.

Panadol-C *Sterling Health, Switz.†.*
Paracetamol (p.72·2); ascorbic acid (p.1365·2).
Fever; pain.

Panafcort
Rhone-Poulenc Rorer, Austral.; Propan, S.Afr.
Prednisone (p.1049·2).
Corticosteroid.

Panafcortelone *Rhone-Poulenc Rorer, Austral.*
Prednisolone (p.1048·1).
Corticosteroid.

Panafil *Rystan, USA.*
Papain (p.1614·1); urea (p.1095·2); chlorophyllin copper complex (p.1000·1).
Treatment of wounds, ulcers, and traumatic lesions.

Panafil-White *Rystan, USA.*
Papain (p.1614·1); urea (p.1095·2).
Treatment of wounds, ulcers, and traumatic lesions.

Panaleve *Pinewood, UK.*
Paracetamol (p.72·2).
Fever; pain.

Panalgesic
Note. This name is used for preparations of different composition.
Sanofi Winthrop, Austral.
Paracetamol (p.72·2); codeine phosphate (p.26·1); doxylamine succinate (p.410·1).
Pain with agitation.

Robins, USA; Poythress, USA.
Methyl salicylate (p.55·2); menthol (p.1600·2).
Muscle, joint, and soft-tissue pain; neuralgia.

Panalgesic Gold *ECR, USA.*
Methyl salicylate (p.55·2); menthol (p.1600·2); camphor (p.1557·2).
Muscle, joint, and soft-tissue pain; neuralgia.

Panamax *Sanofi Winthrop, Austral.*
Paracetamol (p.72·2).
Fever; pain.

Panamax Co *Sanofi Winthrop, Austral.*
Paracetamol (p.72·2); codeine phosphate (p.26·1).
Fever; pain.

Panamor *Lagamed, S.Afr.*
Diclofenac sodium (p.31·2).
Gout; inflammation; musculoskeletal and joint disorders; pain.

Panasal *ECR, USA.*
Hydrocodone tartrate (p.43·1); aspirin (p.16·1).

Panasma *Propan, S.Afr.*
Aminophylline (p.748·1); ephedrine hydrochloride (p.1059·3); amylobarbitone (p.641·3).
Asthma.

Panasol-S *Seatrace, USA.*
Prednisone (p.1049·2).
Corticosteroid.

Panax
Note. This name is used for preparations of different composition.
Willvonseder, Aust.
Paracetamol (p.72·2); butethamate citrate (p.1056·2); caffeine (p.749·3).
Fever; pain.

Medichemie, Switz.†.
Dipyrone (p.35·1); butethamate citrate (p.1056·2); caffeine (p.749·3).
Pain.

Panax Complex *Blackmores, Austral.*
Avena (p.1551·3); fenugreek (p.1579·3); alfalfa (p.1544·2); ginseng (p.1584·2); multivitamins.
Tonic.

Panax N *Medichemie, Switz.*
Ibuprofen (p.44·1).
Fever; pain.

Panaxid *Lilly, Belg.*
Nizatidine (p.1203·2).
Gastro-intestinal disorders associated with hyperacidity.

Panbesy *Bio-Therabel, Belg.*
Phentermine hydrochloride (p.1484·3).
Obesity.

Panbetal *Biotekfarma, Ital.†.*
Vitamin B substances.

Pancardiol *Almirall, Spain.*
Isosorbide mononitrate (p.893·3).
Angina pectoris; heart failure.

Pancebrin
Lilly, Aust.; Lilly, S.Afr.
Multivitamin preparation.

Panchelidon N *Kanoldt, Ger.*
Chelidonium.
Smooth muscle spasms.

Pancholtruw N *Truw, Ger.*
Pancreatin (p.1612·1).
Pancholtruw formerly contained pancreatin, bromelains, dehydrocholic acid, chelidonium, and silybum marianum.
Digestive system disorders.

Pancof-HC *Pan America, USA.*
Hydrocodone tartrate (p.43·1); chlorpheniramine (p.405·2); pseudoephedrine (p.1068·3).
Coughs.

Pancreal Kirchner *Iderne, Fr.*
Pancreatin (porcine) (p.1612·1).
Dyspepsia.

Pancrease
Note. This name is used for preparations of different composition.
Janssen-Cilag, Austral.; Janssen-Cilag, Belg.; Janssen-Ortho, Canad.; Janssen-Cilag, Ital.; Janssen-Cilag, Neth.; Janssen-Cilag, Norw.; Janssen-Cilag, Spain; Janssen-Cilag, Swed.; McNeil Pharmaceutical, USA.
Pancrelipase (p.1613·3).
Pancreatic insufficiency.

Janssen-Cilag, Irl.; Cilag, UK.
Pancreatin (p.1613·3).
Pancreatic insufficiency.

Pancrease HL
Janssen-Cilag, Neth.; Cilag, UK.
Pancreatin (p.1612·1).
Pancreatic insufficiency.

Pancreasmit *Sigma-Tau, Ital.†.*
Dried pancreas.
Cystic fibrosis; malabsorption syndromes; pancreatic insufficiency.

Pancrelase *Byk, Fr.*
Pancreas (porcine); pancreatin (porcine) (p.1612·1); fungal cellulase (p.1561·1); tannic acid (p.1634·2).
Dyspepsia; pancreatic insufficiency.

Pancreoflat *Solvay, Ital.*
Pancreatin (p.1612·1); dimethicone (p.1213·1).
Digestive system disorders.

Pancreolauryl-Test
Salus, Aust.; Geymonat, Ital.; Inibsa, Spain†; Charwell Pharmaceuticals, UK.
Combination pack: 1 Blue capsule, fluorescein dilaurate (p.1581·1); 1 red capsule, fluorescein sodium (p.1581·1).
Evaluation of pancreatic function.

Pancreolauryl-Test N *Temmler, Ger.*
Combination pack: Blue capsules, fluorescein dilaurate (p.1581·1); red capsules, fluorescein sodium (p.1581·1).
Evaluation of pancreatic function.

Pancreon *Solvay, Ital.*
Pancreatin (p.1612·1).
Cystic fibrosis; malabsorption syndromes.

Pancreon Compositum *Solvay, Ital.*
Pancreatin (p.1612·1); ox bile extract (p.1553·2).
Digestive system disorders.

Pancresil *Edmond Pharma, Ital.*
Dimethicone (p.1213·1); pancreatin (p.1612·1).
Digestive system disorders.

Pancrex
Paines & Byrne, Irl.; Samil, Ital.; Paines & Byrne, UK.
Pancreatin (p.1612·1).
Pancreatic insufficiency.

Pancrex V *Clements Stansen, Austral.†.*
Pancreatin (p.1612·1).
Pancreatic insufficiency.

Pancrezyme 4X *Vitaline, USA.*
Pancreatin (p.1612·1); pancrelipase (p.1613·3).
Pancreatic insufficiency.

Pancrin *Solvay, Aust.*
Pancreatin (p.1612·1).
Pancreatic insufficiency.

Pancrophil *Inibsa, Spain†.*
Pancreas.
Digestive enzyme deficiency; malabsorption; pancreatitis.

Pancrotanon *Geymonat, Ital.*
Pancreatin (p.1612·1).
Digestive system disorders.

Panda Baby Cream *Thornton & Ross, UK.*
Zinc oxide (p.1096·2); castor oil (p.1560·2).
Dry skin; nappy rash.

Pandel
Basotherm, Ger.; Savage, USA.
Hydrocortisone buteprate (p.1044·2).
Skin disorders.

Pandermin Cicatrizante *Vinas, Spain†.*
Sodium hyaluronate (p.1630·3).
Wound healing.

Pandigal *Beiersdorf, Ger.†.*
Lanatoside A (p.897·2); lanatoside B (p.897·2); lanatoside C (p.897·2).
Cardiac disorders.

Panectyl *Rhone-Poulenc Rorer, Canad.*
Trimeprazine tartrate (p.419·3).
Coughs; dyspnoea; pruritus.

Paneraj *Biomedica, Ital.†.*
Pastilles: Peru balsam (p.1617·2); tolu balsam (p.1071·1); tridace; narceine (p.62·2).
Syrup: Peru balsam (p.1617·2); tolu balsam (p.1071·1); liquorice (p.1197·1); tridace; narceine phosphate (p.62·2); ephedrine hydrochloride (p.1059·3); sodium benzoate.
Coughs.

Panerel *Cox, UK.*
Paracetamol (p.72·2); codeine phosphate (p.26·1).
Fever; pain.

Panergon *Mack, Illert., Ger.†.*
Papaverine hydrochloride (p.1614·2).
Cerebral vascular disorders; coronary vascular disorders; diabetic angiopathy; Ménière's disease; migraine; peripheral vascular disease; retinopathy.

Panesclerina *Berenguer Infale, Spain†.*
Probucol (p.1277·3).
Hyperlipidaemias.

Panex *Roberts, USA.*
Paracetamol (p.72·2).
Fever; pain.

Panflavin *Chinosolfabrik, Ger.*
Acriflavine (p.1098·3).
Infections of the oropharynx.

Panfungol *Esteve, Spain.*
Ketoconazole (p.383·1).
Fungal infections.

Panfurex *Bouchara, Fr.*
Nifuroxazide (p.231·3).
Diarrhoea.

Pangamma *IBP, Ital.†.*
Zinc oxide (p.1096·2).
Skin disorders.

Pangamox *Alonga, Spain.*
Amoxycillin trihydrate (p.151·3); potassium clavulanate (p.190·2).
Bacterial infections.

Pangel *Pannoc, Belg.*
Benzoyl peroxide (p.1079·2).
Acne.

Pangen *Fournier, Ger.*
Collagen (p.1566·3).
Haemorrhagic disorders.

Pangramin *Epipharm, Aust.†.*
Allergen extracts (p.1545·1).
Hypersensitivity reactions.

Pangrol *Berlin-Chemie, Ger.*
Pancreatin (p.1612·1).
Pancreatic insufficiency.

Panhematin
Abbott, Austral.; Abbott, USA.
Haematin (p.983·1).
Porphyria.

Panimycin *Meiji, Jpn.*
Dibekacin sulphate (p.201·3).
Bacterial infections.

Paniodal *Adivar, Ital.*
Povidone-iodine (p.1123·3).
Skin and wound disinfection.

Paniodine *Angelini, Ital.*
Povidone-iodine (p.1123·3).
Skin and wound disinfection.

Panix *Research Labs, S.Afr.*
Alprazolam (p.640·3).
Anxiety.

Pankreaden *Knoll, Ital.*
Pancrelipase (p.1613·3).
Pancreatic insufficiency.

Pankreaplex N *Schaper & Brummer, Ger.†.*
Silybum marianum (p.993·3); syzygium jambolanum; condurango (p.1567·2); sarsaparilla (p.1627·2); pancreatin hydrolysate (p.1612·1).
Digestive system disorders.

Pankreaplex Neu *Schaper & Brummer, Ger.*
Silybum marianum (p.993·3); syzygium jambolana; condurango (p.1567·2); sarsaparilla (p.1627·2).
Gastro-intestinal disorders.

Pankreas M *Hanosan, Ger.†.*
Homoeopathic preparation.

Pankreas S *Hanosan, Ger.†.*
Pancreatin (p.1612·1); fruct. phaseoli; herb. galegae; iris; abrotanum; sulfur; syzyg. jamb.; armoracia; capsicum.
Digestive system disorders.

Pankrease *Janssen-Cilag, S.Afr.*
Pancrelipase (p.1613·3).
Pancreatic disorders.

Pankreatan *Zyma, Ger.*
Pancreatin (p.1612·1).
Digestive system disorders.

Pankreaticum *Hevert, Ger.*
Injection: Homoeopathic preparation.
Oral drops: Boldo (p.1554·1); curcuma (p.1001·3); eichhornia; myrtillus; okoubaka; quassia; syzygium; sanguinaria; tanacetum; taraxacum.
Biliary disorders; digestive disorders; pancreatitis.

Pankreatin comp. N *Brunnengraber, Ger.†.*
Pancreatin (p.1612·1); bile acids (p.1553·2).
Digestive system disorders.

Pankreoflat
Solvay, Aust.; Solvay, Ger.; Solvay, S.Afr.; Solvay, Spain; Solvay, Switz.†.
Pancreatin (p.1612·1); dimethicone (p.1213·1).
Aerophagia; flatulence; preparation for gastro-intestinal ultrasound or radiography.

Pankreoflat Sedante *Kalifarma, Spain†.*
Dimethicone (p.1213·1); oxazepam (p.683·2); pancreatin (p.1612·1).
Aerophagia; delayed digestion; flatulence.

Pankreon
Solvay, Ger.; Solvay, Norw.; Solvay, Spain; Solvay Duphar, Swed.
Pancreatin (p.1612·1).
Cystic fibrosis; pancreatic insufficiency.

Pankreon comp. forte *Kali-Chemie, Swed.†.*
Pancreatin (p.1612·1); ox bile extract (p.1553·2).
Bile insufficiency; pancreatic insufficiency.

Pankreon compositum
Solvay, Aust.; Solvay, Belg.†; Kali-Chemie, Ger.†.
Pancreatin (p.1612·1); ox bile (p.1553·2).
Digestive system disorders; pancreatic insufficiency.

Pankreon forte
Solvay, Aust.; Kali-Chemie, Ger.
Pancreatin (p.1612·1).
Digestive system disorders; pancreatic insufficiency.

Pankreon Fuerte *Kalifarma, Spain†.*
Pancreatin (p.1612·1); ox bile (p.1553·2).
Dyspepsia; pancreatic insufficiency.

Pankreon fur Kinder *Kali-Chemie, Ger.†.*
Pancreatin (p.1612·1); retinol; cyanocobalamin; folic acid.
Digestive system disorders.

Pankre-Uvocal *Stroschein, Ger.†.*
Pancreatic extract.
Pancreatic hypofunction; subacute pancreatitis.

Pankrevowen *Weber & Weber, Ger.*
Homoeopathic preparation.

Pankrotanon *Vifor, Switz.†.*
Pancreatin (p.1612·1).
Gastro-intestinal disorders.

Panmist JR *Pan America, USA.*
Pseudoephedrine (p.1068·3); guaiphenesin (p.1061·3).
Coughs.

Panmycin *Upjohn, USA.*
Tetracycline hydrochloride (p.259·1).
Bacterial infections.

Panmycin P *Upjohn, Austral.†.*
Tetracycline hydrochloride (p.259·1).
Bacterial infections.

Pannaz *Pan America, USA.*
Phenylpropanolamine (p.1067·2); chlorpheniramine (p.405·2); hyoscine (p.462·3).
Upper respiratory-tract disorders.

Pan-Nerventonikum *Merckle, Ger.†.*
Rhizoma gelsemii (p.1583·2); lupulus (p.1597·2); hypericum (p.1590·1); lavender (p.1594·3); melissa (p.1600·1); pulsatilla anserina; valerian (p.1643·1); rosemary.
Depression; nervousness.

Pannocort *Pannoc, Belg.*
Hydrocortisone acetate (p.1043·3).
Skin disorders.

Pannogel *CS, Fr.*
Benzoyl peroxide (p.1079·2).
Acne.

Panocaine *Hoechst Marion Roussel, Canad.*
Benzocaine (p.1286·2); amethocaine hydrochloride (p.1285·2).
Local anaesthesia in dentistry.

Panocod *Sanofi, Swed.*
Paracetamol (p.72·2); codeine phosphate (p.26·1).
Pain.

Panodil
SmithKline Beecham, Norw.; Sterling Health, Swed.
Paracetamol (p.72·2).
Fever; pain.

Pan-Ophtal *Winzer, Ger.*
Dexpanthenol (p.1570·3).
Eye disorders.

Panoral *Lilly, Ger.*
Cefaclor (p.163·2).
Bacterial infections.

Panorex *Glaxo Wellcome, Ger.*
Edrecolomab (p.531·3).
Colorectal cancer.

Panotile
Note. This name is used for preparations of different composition.
Zambon, Belg.; Zambon, Fr.; Zambon, Neth.; Inpharzam, Switz.
Polymyxin B sulphate (p.239·1); neomycin sulphate (p.229·2); fludrocortisone acetate (p.1040·1); lignocaine hydrochloride (p.1293·2).
Ear disorders.

Zambon, Spain.
Polymyxin B sulphate (p.239·1); neomycin sulphate (p.229·2); fludrocortisone acetate (p.1040·1); furaltadone hydrochloride (p.210·3); lignocaine hydrochloride (p.1293·2).
Ear disorders.

Panotile N *Zambon, Ger.*
Polymyxin B sulphate (p.239·1); fludrocortisone acetate (p.1040·1); lignocaine hydrochloride (p.1293·2).
Ear disorders.

PanOxyl
Salus, Aust.; Stiefel, Austral.; Stiefel, Canad.; Stiefel, Fr.; Stiefel, Ger.; Stiefel, Irl.; Stiefel, Ital.; Stiefel, Norw.; Stiefel, S.Afr.; Stiefel, Spain; Stiefel, Switz.; Stiefel, UK; Stiefel, USA.
Benzoyl peroxide (p.1079·2).
Acne.

Panpeptal N *Gastropharm, Ger.*
Pancreatin (p.1612·1).
Pancreatic insufficiency.

Panpur *Knoll, Ger.*
Porcine pancreatin (p.1612·1).
Digestive system disorders.

Panpurol *Shinyaku, Jpn.*
Pipethanate ethobromide (p.467·1).
The injection contains benzyl alcohol (p.1103·3) to alleviate the pain of injection.
Smooth muscle spasm.

Panquil *Warner-Lambert, Austral.*
Promethazine hydrochloride (p.416·2); paracetamol (p.72·2).
Fever; insomnia; pain.

Panrectal *Quimifar, Spain†.*
Paracetamol (p.72·2).
Fever; pain.

Pansan
Note. This name is used for preparations of different composition.
Solvay, Aust.
Stomach enzymes (p.1616·3); glutamic acid hydrochloride (p.1344·3).
Gastro-intestinal disorders.

Kali-Chemie, Ger.†.
Oral liquid: Pepsin (p.1616·3); glycine (p.1345·2).
Tablets: Pepsin (p.1616·3); glutamic acid hydrochloride (p.1344·3).
Gastro-intestinal disorders.

Panscol *Baker Cummins, USA.*
Salicylic acid (p.1090·2).
Hyperkeratosis.

Pansecoff *Asta Medica, Aust.*
Ergotamine tartrate (p.445·3); caffeine (p.749·3).
Migraine and other vascular headaches.

Panseptil *Gedis, Ital.*
Chlorhexidine gluconate (p.1107·2); cetrimide (p.1105·2); alcohol (p.1099·1); isopropyl alcohol (p.1118·2).
Surface disinfection.

Pansoral
Inava, Fr.; Pierre Fabre, Switz.
Choline salicylate (p.25·2); cetalkonium chloride (p.1105·2).
Mouth disorders.

Pansporin *Takeda, Jpn.*
Cefotiam hydrochloride (p.170·2) or cefotiam hexetil hydrochloride (p.170·2).

Mepivacaine hydrochloride (p.1297·2) is included in the intramuscular injection to alleviate the pain of injection.
Bacterial infections.

Pansporine Therabel Pharma, Belg.†.
Cefotiam hydrochloride (p.170·2).
Bacterial infections.

Pansteryl Sanofi Winthrop, Belg.
Benzalkonium chloride (p.1101·3).
Disinfection of instruments, materials, and hands; storage of sterile materials.

Pantecta
Ravizza, Ital.; Pharmacia Upjohn, Spain.
Pantoprazole sodium (p.1207·3).
Gastro-oesophageal reflux; peptic ulcer.

Pantederm Hexal, Ger.
Zinc oxide (p.1096·2); dexpanthenol (p.1570·3).
Burns; wounds.

Pantelmin Janssen-Cilag, Aust.
Mebendazole (p.104·1).
Worm infections.

Pantenil Quimica Medica, Spain.
Tablets†: Calcium pantothenate (p.1352·3).
Topical application: Calcium pantothenate (p.1352·3); mercuric chloride (p.1601·2); aminobenzoic acid (p.1486·3).
Hair, scalp, and skin disorders.

Pantestone Organon, Fr.
Testosterone undecanoate (p.1464·2).
Male hypogonadism.

Pantetina Sanofi Winthrop, Ital.
Pantethine (p.1276·3).
Hypertriglyceridaemia.

Pantheline CP Protea, Austral.†.
Propantheline bromide (p.468·1).

Panthenol Jenapharm, Ger.; Braun, Ger.; Lichtenstein, Ger.; LAW, Ger.; ankerpharm, Ger.
Dexpanthenol (p.1570·3).
Eye disorders; inflammatory disorders of the gastro-intestinal tract; pantothenic acid deficiency; paraesthesias; paralytic ileus; postoperative gastro-intestinal atony; respiratory-tract disorders; wounds.

Panthoderm Jones, USA.
Dexpanthenol (p.1570·3).
Skin disorders.

Panthogenat Azupharma, Ger.
Dexpanthenol (p.1570·3).
Wounds.

Pantinol Gerot, Aust.
Aprotinin (p.711·3).
Hyperfibrinolysis; prevention of postoperative complications; shock.

Pantobamin Medix, Spain.
Cyproheptadine (p.407·3); amino acids and vitamins.
Anorexia; tonic.

Panto-Bi Zambon, Ital.†.
Vitamin B substances.

Pantobionta Merck, Spain.
Multivitamin and mineral preparation.

Pantocrinale Simons, Ger.
Hydrocortisone sodium phosphate (p.1044·1); salicylic acid (p.1090·2).
Scalp disorders.

Pantodrin Abbott, Spain.
Erythromycin (p.204·1).
Acne.

Pantogar
Note. This name is used for preparations of different composition.
Salus, Aust.
Calcium pantothenate (p.1352·3); cystine (p.1339·1).
Hair and nail disorders.
Agpharm, Switz.
Thiamine nitrate (p.1361·1); calcium pantothenate (p.1352·3); medicinal yeast (p.1373·1); cystine (p.1339·1); keratin; aminobenzoic acid (p.1486·3).
Hair and nail disorders.

Pantok Lacer, Spain.
Simvastatin (p.1278·2).
Hyperlipidaemias.

Pantolax Schwabe-Curamed, Ger.
Suxamethonium chloride (p.1319·1).
Depolarising neuromuscular blocker.

Pantoloc
Byk, Aust.; Byk Madaus, S.Afr.; Nycomed, Swed.
Pantoprazole sodium (p.1207·3).
Gastro-oesophageal reflux; peptic ulcer.

Pantomicina Abbott, Spain.
Erythromycin ethyl succinate (p.204·2), erythromycin lactobionate (p.204·2), or erythromycin stearate (p.204·2).
Bacterial infections.

Pantona Beiersdorf, Ger.†.
Multivitamin and mineral preparation with iron, folic acid, and liver extract; orotic acid (p.1611·2); caffeine (p.749·3).
Iron or vitamin deficiency; tonic.

Pantonate Eagle, Austral.
Calcium pantothenate (p.1352·3).
Vitamin B_5 supplement.

Pantopan Pharmacia Upjohn, Ital.
Pantoprazole sodium (p.1207·3).
Gastro-oesophageal reflux; peptic ulcer.

Pantopon
Roche, Canad.†; Roche, USA.
Hydrochlorides of mixed opium alkaloids (p.71·1).
Hypnotic; pain; sedative.

Pantorc Byk Gulden, Ital.
Pantoprazole sodium.
Gastro-oesophageal reflux; peptic ulcer.

Pantosin Daiichi, Jpn.
Pantethine (p.1276·3).
Blood disorders; constipation; eczema; hyperlipidaemia; pantothenic acid deficiency; pantothenic acid supplement; streptomycin and kanamycin toxicity.

Pantosse Vis, Ital.†.
Ephedrine hydrochloride (p.1059·3); calcium guaiacolsulfonate (p.1068·3); ammonium camphorate (p.1055·2); caffeine and sodium benzoate; ethylmorphine hydrochloride (p.36·1); tolu balsam (p.1071·1); pumilio pine oil (p.1623·3).
Respiratory-tract disorders.

Pantothen
Hafslund Nycomed, Aust.; Streuli, Switz.
Panthenol (p.1571·1) or calcium pantothenate (p.1352·3).
Alcoholism; gastro-intestinal tract disorders; liver disorders; muscle cramps; neuropathies; respiratory-tract disorders; skin disorders; sweating.

Pantovigar Simons, Ger.
Thiamine nitrate (p.1361·1); calcium pantothenate (p.1352·3); medicinal yeast (p.1373·1); cystine (p.1339·1); keratin; aminobenzoic acid (p.1486·3).
Disorders of the hair and nails.

Pantovit
Salus, Aust.; Logifarm, Ital.†.
Multivitamin preparation.

Pantovit Vital Salus, Aust.
Multivitamin, iron, and mineral preparation.

Pantozol
Byk, Belg.; Byk Gulden, Ger.; Byk, Neth.
Pantoprazole sodium (p.1207·3).
Gastro-oesophageal reflux; peptic ulcer.

Pantozyme Wander, Switz.†.
Pancreatin (p.1612·1); cellulase (p.1561·1); pepsin (p.1616·3).
Digestive system disorders.

Pantrop
Lundbeck, Aust.; Tropon, Ger.†.
Amitriptyline hydrochloride (p.273·3); chlordiazepoxide (p.646·3).
Depression; sleep disorders.

Panwarfin Abbott, USA†.
Warfarin sodium (p.964·2).
Pulmonary embolism; venous thrombosis.

Panxeol IPRAD, Fr.
Eschscholtzia californica; passion flower (p.1615·3).
Insomnia; nervous disorders.

Panzid Duncan, Ital.†.
Ceftazidime (p.173·3).
Bacterial infections.

Panzynorm
Note. This name is used for preparations of different composition.
Ebewe, Aust.
Pancreatin (p.1612·1).
Nordmark, Ger.†.
Porcine pancreatin (p.1612·1); porcine stomach extract; ox bile (p.1553·2); porcine pylorus extract.
Digestive system disorders.

Panzynorm forte Nordmark, Ger.†.
Porcine pancreatin (p.1612·1); porcine stomach extract; ox bile (p.1553·2); glycine hydrochloride (p.1345·2).
Digestive system disorders.

Panzynorm forte-N Knoll, Ger.
Pancreatin (p.1612·1).
Pancreatic insufficiency.

Panzytrat
Knoll, Ger.; Knoll, Irl.; Nordmark, Neth.; Knoll, Switz.; Knoll, UK†.
Pancreatin (p.1612·1).
Pancreatic insufficiency.

Papaine DB, Fr.
Carica papaya.
Dyspepsia.

Papaverine Hydrochloride Boots, UK; Penn, UK; Martindale Pharmaceuticals, UK.
Papaverine hydrochloride (p.1614·2).
Impotence.

Papaya Enzyme Nature's Bounty, USA.
Papain (p.1614·1); amylase (p.1549·1).
Gastro-intestinal disorders.

Papaya Plus Gerard House, UK.
Charcoal (p.972·3); papain (p.1614·1); slippery elm (p.1630·1); hydrastis (p.1588·2).
Digestive disorders.

Papayasanit-N Weber & Weber, Ger.
Homoeopathic preparation.

Paplex Medicis, USA†.
Salicylic acid (p.1090·2); lactic acid (p.1593·3).

Paplex Ultra Medicis, USA†.
Salicylic acid (p.1090·2).

Paps Richard, Fr.
Sulphur (p.1091·2); zinc undecenoate (p.389·2); bismuth subgallate (p.1180·2); menthol (p.1600·2); camphor (p.1557·2); salicylic acid (p.1090·2); zinc oxide (p.1096·2); boric acid (p.1554·2); labiatae oil.
Bacterial and fungal skin infections.

Papulex
Knoll, Austral.; GenDerm, Canad.; Helsinn Birex, Irl.; Euroderma, UK.
Nicotinamide (p.1351·2).
Acne.

Par Decon Par, USA†.
Phenylpropanolamine hydrochloride (p.1067·2); phenylephrine hydrochloride (p.1066·2); phenyltoloxamine citrate (p.416·1); chlorpheniramine maleate (p.405·1).

Par Glycerol Par, USA.
Iodinated glycerol (p.1062·2).
Coughs.

Para
Qualiphar, Belg.; Charton, Canad.
Bioallethrin (p.1402·3); piperonyl butoxide (p.1409·3).
Pediculosis.

Para Lentes SCAT, Fr.
Acetic acid (p.1541·2).
Pediculosis.

Para Muc Merz, Ger.†.
Hexylresorcinol (p.1116·1); chlorocarvacrol; amethocaine hydrochloride (p.1285·2); myrrh (p.1606·1).
Inflammatory disorders of the mouth.

Para Plus SCAT, Fr.
Permethrin (p.1409·2); malathion (p.1407·3); piperonyl butoxide (p.1409·3).
Pediculosis.

Para Repulsif SCAT, Fr.
Piperonal (p.1409·3).
Head lice repellent.

para sanol Sanol, Ger.†.
Aluminium glycinate (p.1177·2); xenytropium bromide (p.469·3); meprobamate (p.678·1).
Gastro-intestinal disorders.

Para Special Poux SCAT, Fr.
Bioallethrin (p.1402·3); piperonyl butoxide (p.1409·3).
Pediculosis.

Parabolan Negma, Fr.
Trenbolone hexahydrobenzylcarbonate (p.1467·2).
Anabolic; osteoporosis.

Paracefan
Boehringer Ingelheim, Belg.†; Boehringer Ingelheim, Ger.
Clonidine (p.842·2) or clonidine hydrochloride (p.841·2).
Alcohol withdrawal syndrome; Gilles de la Tourette syndrome; opiate withdrawal syndrome.

Paracet Weifa, Norw.
Paracetamol (p.72·2).
Fever; pain.

Paracet Comp CT, Ger.
Paracetamol (p.72·2); codeine phosphate (p.26·1).
Pain.

Paracetacod
Note. This name is used for preparations of different composition.
Ratiopharm, Ger.
Paracetamol (p.72·2); codeine phosphate (p.26·1).
Pain.
Mer-National, S.Afr.
Paracetamol (p.72·2); codeine phosphate (p.26·1); ascorbic acid (p.1365·2).
Pain.

Paracetamol Comp Stada, Ger.
Paracetamol (p.72·2); codeine phosphate (p.26·1).
Pain.

Paracetamolplus Ratiopharm, Ger.
Paracetamol (p.72·2); caffeine (p.749·3).
Pain.

Paracets Sussex, UK.
Paracetamol (p.72·2).
Fever; pain.

Parachoc Paedpharm, Austral.
Methylcellulose (p.1473·3); liquid paraffin (p.1382·1).
Constipation.

Paraclear Roche Consumer, UK.
Paracetamol (p.72·2).

Paracodin
Note. This name is used for preparations of different composition.
Ebewe, Aust.
Oral drops: Dihydrocodeine thiocyanate (p.34·2); thyme (p.1636·3); castanea vulgaris.
Syrup: Dihydrocodeine tartrate (p.34·1); althaea (p.1546·3); grindelia.
Coughs.
Ebewe, Aust.; Knoll, Austral.; Knoll, Ger.; Knoll, Irl.; Knoll, S.Afr.; Knoll, Switz.
Dihydrocodeine tartrate (p.34·1) or dihydrocodeine thiocyanate (p.34·2).
Formerly contained dihydrocodeine tartrate, althaea, and grindelia in *S.Afr.*
Coughs; diarrhoea.

Paracodin N Knoll, Ger.
Dihydrocodeine tartrate (p.34·1) or dihydrocodeine thiocyanate (p.34·2).
Coughs.

Paracodin retard
Knoll, Ger.; Knoll, Ger.†; Knoll, Switz.
Dihydrocodeine tartrate (p.34·1); dihydrocodeine resin (p.34·2).
Coughs; diarrhoea.

Paracodina
Knoll, Ital.; Knoll, Spain.
Dihydrocodeine tartrate (p.34·1) or dihydrocodeine thiocyanate (p.34·2).
Coughs; pain.

Paracodine Knoll, Belg.
Oral drops†: Dihydrocodeine thiocyanate (p.34·2); thyme (p.1636·3); aesculus (p.1543·3).
Syrup: Dihydrocodeine tartrate (p.34·1); grindelia; althaea (p.1546·3).
Tablets: Dihydrocodeine tartrate (p.34·1).
Coughs.

Paracodol
Roche Consumer, Irl.; Roche, S.Afr.†; Roche Consumer, UK.
Paracetamol (p.72·2); codeine phosphate (p.26·1).
These ingredients can be described by the British Approved Name Co-codamol.
Fever; pain.

Paractol Asta Medica, Ger.
Chewable tablets: Simethicone (p.1213·1); aluminium hydroxide gel (p.1177·3).
Oral suspension: Simethicone (p.1213·1); aluminium hydroxide gel (p.1177·3); magnesium hydroxide (p.1198·2).
Gastro-intestinal disorders.

Paradenton Medicopharm, Aust.
Myrrh (p.1606·1); sage leaf (p.1627·1); chamomile flowers (p.1561·2); tannic acid (p.1634·2).
Aphthous ulcers; bleeding gums; bruised gums; gingivitis; periodontitis.

Paraderm Whitehall, Austral.
Bufexamac (p.22·2).
Skin disorders.

Paraderm Plus Whitehall, Austral.
Chlorhexidine gluconate (p.1107·2); lignocaine hydrochloride (p.1293·2); bufexamac (p.22·2).
Minor skin lesions.

Paradex Rhone-Poulenc Rorer, Austral.
Dextropropoxyphene hydrochloride (p.27·3); paracetamol (p.72·2).
Pain.

Paradiol Pfleger, Ger.†.
Olive oil (p.1610·1); arachis oil (p.1550·2); cetaceum; cera alba (p.1383·1).
Skin disorders.

Paradione Abbott, USA†.
Paramethadione (p.350·1).
Absence seizures.

Paradote Penn, UK.
Paracetamol (p.72·2); methionine (p.984·2).
Fever; pain.

Paraflex
Janssen-Cilag, S.Afr.†; Astra, Swed.; McNeil Pharmaceutical, USA.
Chlorzoxazone (p.1313·1).
Headache; premedication; skeletal muscle spasm.

Paraflex comp. Astra, Swed.
Chlorzoxazone (p.1313·1); aspirin (p.16·1); dextropropoxyphene napsylate (p.27·3).
Headache; skeletal muscle spasm.

Paraflex spezial Cilag, Ger.†.
Chlorzoxazone (p.1313·1); paracetamol (p.72·2).
Skeletal muscle pain.

Parafon
Janssen-Cilag, Aust.; J&J, S.Afr.†; Janssen-Cilag, Switz.
Chlorzoxazone (p.1313·1); paracetamol (p.72·2).
Pain; skeletal muscle spasm.

Parafon Forte Johnson & Johnson, Canad.
Chlorzoxazone (p.1313·1); paracetamol (p.72·2).
Pain; skeletal muscle spasm.

Parafon Forte C8 Johnson & Johnson, Canad.
Chlorzoxazone (p.1313·1); paracetamol (p.72·2); codeine phosphate (p.26·1).
Pain; skeletal muscle spasm.

Parafon Forte DSC McNeil Pharmaceutical, USA.
Chlorzoxazone (p.1313·1).
Musculoskeletal pain.

Paragar Spirig, Switz.
Liquid paraffin (p.1382·1); agar (p.1470·3); phenolphthalein (p.1208·2).
Constipation.

Paragard T380A Gynopharma, USA.
Copper-wound plastic (p.1337·3).
Intra-uterine contraceptive device.

Paragerm AK Promedica, Fr.†.
A mixture of natural balsams and antiseptics.
House dust mite allergies (adjuvant); surface disinfection.

Paragip Boiron, Canad.
Homoeopathic preparation.

Paragol Streuli, Switz.
Liquid paraffin (p.1382·1); phenolphthalein (p.1208·2).
Bowel evacuation; constipation.

Paragrippe Boiron, Fr.
Homoeopathic preparation.

Para-Hist AT Pharmics, USA†.
Phenylephrine hydrochloride (p.1066·2); promethazine hydrochloride (p.416·2); codeine phosphate (p.26·1).
Coughs.

Para-Hist HD Pharmics, USA.
Phenylephrine hydrochloride (p.1066·2); chlorpheniramine maleate (p.405·1); hydrocodone tartrate (p.43·1).
Coughs and cold symptoms.

Parahypon Calmic, Irl.
Paracetamol (p.72·2); caffeine (p.749·3); codeine phosphate (p.26·1).
Pain.

Parakapton Rosch & Handel, Aust.
Paracetamol (p.72·2).
Pain, fever.

Parake Galen, UK.
Paracetamol (p.72·2); codeine phosphate (p.26·1).

These ingredients can be described by the British Approved Name Co-codamol.
Pain.

Paral Forest Pharmaceuticals, USA.
Paraldehyde (p.684·1).
Sedative.

Paralergin Vita, Spain.
Astemizole (p.402·1).
Hypersensitivity reactions.

Paralgesic Poythress, USA.
Methyl salicylate (p.55·2); menthol (p.1600·2); camphor (p.1557·2).

Paralgin
Note. This name is used for preparations of different composition.
Fawns & McAllan, Austral.
Paracetamol (p.72·2).
Fever; pain.

Weifa, Norw.
Codeine phosphate (p.26·1); paracetamol (p.72·2).
Pain.

Paralice Fleet, Austral.
Bioallethrin (p.1402·3); piperonyl butoxide (p.1409·3).
Pediculosis.

Paralief Clonmel, Irl.
Paracetamol (p.72·2).
Fever; pain.

Paralink Rice Steele, Irl.
Paracetamol (p.72·2).
Fever; pain.

Paralyoc Farmalyoc, Fr.
Paracetamol (p.72·2).
Fever; pain.

Paramax
Lorex Synthelabo, Irl.; Lorex, UK.
Paracetamol (p.72·2); metoclopramide hydrochloride (p.1200·3).
Migraine.

Paramettes Whitehall-Robins, Canad.
Multivitamin and mineral preparation.

Paramettes Children Whitehall-Robins, Canad.†.
Multivitamin preparation.

Paramettes Childrens Plus Iron Whitehall-Robins, Canad.†.
Multivitamin preparation with iron.

Paramettes Teens Whitehall-Robins, Canad.†.
Multivitamin preparation with iron.

Paramin Wallis, UK.
Paracetamol (p.72·2).
Fever; pain.

Paraminan Jumer, Fr.
Aminobenzoic acid (p.1486·3).
Skin disorders.

Paramol
Galen, Irl.; Seton, UK.
Paracetamol (p.72·2); dihydrocodeine tartrate (p.34·1).
Fever; pain.

Paran Noriston, S.Afr.†.
Paracetamol (p.72·2); codeine phosphate (p.26·1).
Pain.

Paranico Elerte, Fr.
Nicotinamide (p.1351·2); quinine ascorbate (p.1624·2); thiamine hydrochloride (p.1361·1).
Aid to smoking withdrawal.

Paranorm Wallace Mfg Chem., UK.
Dextromethorphan hydrobromide (p.1057·3); ephedrine hydrochloride (p.1059·3); guaiphenesin (p.1061·3).
Coughs.

Paranthil Xixia, S.Afr.
Albendazole (p.96·2).
Worm infections.

Paraplatin
Bristol-Myers Squibb, Aust.; Bristol-Myers Squibb, Austral.†; Bristol-Myers Squibb, Belg.; Bristol, Canad.; Bristol-Myers Squibb, Irl.; Bristol-Myers Squibb, Ital.; Bristol-Myers Squibb, Neth.; Bristol-Myers Squibb, Norw.; Bristol-Myers Squibb, S.Afr.; Bristol-Myers, Spain; Bristol-Myers Squibb, Swed.; Bristol-Myers Squibb, UK; Bristol-Myers Oncology, USA.
Carboplatin (p.510·3).
Malignant neoplasms.

Paraplatine
Bristol-Myers Squibb, Fr.; Bristol-Myers Squibb, Switz.
Carboplatin (p.510·3).
Malignant neoplasms.

Parapsyllium Pharmygiene, Fr.
Ispaghula husk (p.1194·2); light liquid paraffin (p.1382·1).
Constipation.

Paraseptine Qualiphar, Belg.†.
Sulphanilamide (p.256·3).
Bacterial infections of skin, wounds, and mucous membranes.

Parasidose Gilbert, Fr.†.
Lotion†: Bioallethrin (p.1402·3); piperonyl butoxide (p.1409·3).
Shampoo: Phenothrin (p.1409·2).
Pediculosis.

Parasin Nelson, Austral.†.
Paracetamol (p.72·2).
Fever; pain.

Parasol Rice Steele, Irl.†.
Paracetamol (p.72·2).
Fever; pain.

Para-Speciaal SCAT, Neth.
Bioallethrin (p.1402·3); piperonyl butoxide (p.1409·3).
Pediculosis.

Paraspen Parke, Davis, Austral.†.
Paracetamol (p.72·2).
Fever; pain.

Parasthman Polypharm, Ger.†.
Theophylline (p.765·1).
Obstructive airways disease.

Parathar Rorer, USA.
Teriparatide acetate (p.744·1).
Diagnosis of hypoparathyroidism.

Paratulle Seton, UK.
Yellow soft paraffin (p.1382·3).
Wounds.

Paraxin Boehringer Mannheim, Ger.
Capsules†; *instillation*†; *ear drops*†; *ointment*†: Chloramphenicol (p.182·1).
Injection: Chloramphenicol sodium succinate (p.182·2).
Oral liquid†: Chloramphenicol steaglate (p.184·2).
Bacterial infections.

Parcaine Ocusoft, USA.
Proxymetacaine hydrochloride (p.1300·1).

Pardale Martindale Pharmaceuticals, UK†.
Paracetamol (p.72·2); codeine phosphate (p.26·1); caffeine (p.749·3).
NOTE. There is no connection between Martindale, The Complete Drug Reference and Martindale Pharmaceuticals.
Fever; pain.

Pardec Warner-Lambert, Canad.†.
Multivitamin preparation.

Pardelprin Cox, UK.
Indomethacin (p.45·2).
Dysmenorrhoea; musculoskeletal, joint, and peri-articular disorders.

Par-Drix Parmed, USA†.
Pseudoephedrine sulphate (p.1068·3); dexbrompheniramine maleate (p.403·2).
Upper respiratory-tract symptoms.

Pa-Real Lampugnani, Ital.
Royal jelly (p.1626·3).
Nutritional supplement.

Parecid Proge, Ital.
Cefonicid sodium (p.167·2).
Lignocaine hydrochloride (p.1293·2) is included in this preparation to alleviate the pain of injection.
Bacterial infections.

Paredrine Pharmics, USA.
Hydroxyamphetamine hydrobromide (p.1589·2).
Production of mydriasis.

Paregorique Lafran, Fr.
Prepared opium (p.70·3); benzoic acid (p.1102·3); anise oil (p.1550·1); camphor (p.1557·2).
Diarrhoea.

Paremyd Allergan, USA.
Hydroxyamphetamine hydrobromide (p.1589·2); tropicamide (p.469·2).
Induction of mydriasis with partial cycloplegia.

Parentamin
Serag-Wiessner, Ger.; Pharmacia Upjohn, Ital.
Amino-acid infusion.
Parenteral nutrition.

Parentamin E Serag-Wiessner, Ger.
Amino-acid and electrolyte infusion.
Parenteral nutrition.

Parentamin EAS Serag-Wiessner, Ger.†.
Amino-acid infusion.
Parenteral nutrition in renal impairment.

Parentamin G E Serag-Wiessner, Ger.
Amino-acid, electrolyte, and glucose infusion.
Parenteral nutrition.

Parentamin GX E Serag-Wiessner, Ger.
Amino-acid, electrolyte, glucose, and xylitol infusion.
Parenteral nutrition.

Parentamin L Serag-Wiessner, Ger.†.
Amino-acid, carbohydrate, electrolyte, and vitamin infusion.
Parenteral nutrition.

Parentamin X-E Serag-Wiessner, Ger.
Amino-acid, electrolyte, and xylitol infusion.
Parenteral nutrition.

Parenteral Serag-Wiessner, Ger.
Electrolyte infusion (p.1147·1).
Fluid and electrolyte disorders.

Parenteral BG 5 Serag-Wiessner, Ger.
Electrolyte infusion with glucose (p.1147·1).
Carbohydrate source; fluid and electrolyte disorders.

Parenteral B-S Serag-Wiessner, Ger.†.
Electrolyte infusion with sorbitol (p.1147·1).
Carbohydrate source; fluid and electrolyte disorders.

Parenteral BX Serag-Wiessner, Ger.
Electrolyte and xylitol infusion (p.1147·1).
Carbohydrate source; fluid and electrolyte disorders.

Parenteral D 40 Serag-Wiessner, Ger.†.
Dextran 40 (p.716·2) in sorbitol or with electrolytes.
Plasma volume expansion; vascular disorders.

Parenteral EK Cal GX Serag-Wiessner, Ger.†.
Electrolyte infusion with glucose and xylitol (p.1147·1).
Carbohydrate source; fluid and electrolyte disorders.

Parenteral EK G5 Serag-Wiessner, Ger.
Electrolyte infusion with glucose (p.1147·1).
Carbohydrate source; fluid and electrolyte disorders.

Parenteral EK X Serag-Wiessner, Ger.
Electrolyte and xylitol infusion (p.1147·1).
Carbohydrate source; fluid and electrolyte disorders.

Parenteral G5 Serag-Wiessner, Ger.
Electrolyte infusion with glucose (p.1147·1).
Carbohydrate source; fluid and electrolyte disorders.

Parenteral HG5 Serag-Wiessner, Ger.
Electrolyte infusion with glucose (p.1147·1).
Carbohydrate source; fluid and electrolyte disorders.

Parenteral HL 5 Serag-Wiessner, Ger.†.
Electrolyte infusion with fructose (p.1147·1).
Carbohydrate source; fluid and electrolyte disorders.

Parenteral HX5 Serag-Wiessner, Ger.
Electrolyte infusion with xylitol (p.1147·1).
Carbohydrate source; fluid and electrolyte disorders.

Parenteral L 5 Serag-Wiessner, Ger.†.
Electrolyte infusion with fructose (p.1147·1).
Carbohydrate source; fluid and electrolyte disorders.

Parenteral OP Serag-Wiessner, Ger.
Electrolyte infusion (p.1147·1).
Fluid and electrolyte disorders.

Parenteral X5 Serag-Wiessner, Ger.
Electrolyte infusion with xylitol (p.1147·1).
Carbohydrate source; fluid and electrolyte disorders.

Parentrovite
SmithKline Beecham, Austral.†; Bencard, Belg.†; Bencard, Irl.†; Bencard, Neth.†; Bencard, S.Afr.†; SmithKline Beecham, Swed.†; Bencard, UK†.
Vitamin B substances with vitamin C.
Alcoholism; polyneuropathy; vitamin deficiency.

Parepectolin Rorer, USA.
Paregoric USP (p.70·3); pectin (p.1474·1); kaolin (p.1195·1).
Diarrhoea.

Par-F Pharmics, USA.
Multivitamin and mineral preparation with iron and folic acid.

Parfenac
Wyeth Lederle, Aust.; Whitehall, Fr.; Lederle, Ger.; Lederle, Neth.; Whitehall, S.Afr.; Whitehall-Robins, Switz.; Lederle, UK†.
Bufexamac (p.22·2).
Skin disorders.

Parfenac Basisbad Lederle, Ger.
Arachis oil (p.1550·2); light liquid paraffin (p.1382·1).
Dry, pruritic skin disorders.

Parfenal Cyanamid, Ital.
Bufexamac (p.22·2).
Skin disorders.

Par-Gamma Biagini, Ital.
A mumps immunoglobulin (p.1521·2).
Passive immunisation.

Pargin Metapharma, Ital.
Econazole nitrate (p.377·2).
Fungal infections.

Pargitan Abigo, Swed.
Benzhexol hydrochloride (p.457·3).
Drug-induced extrapyramidal disorders; parkinsonism; spasms in children.

Parhist SR Parmed, USA.
Phenylpropanolamine hydrochloride (p.1067·2); chlorpheniramine maleate (p.405·1).
Upper respiratory-tract symptoms.

Pariet Eisai, UK.
Rabeprazole (p.1209·2).
Gastro-oesophageal reflux; peptic ulcer.

Pariorix
SmithKline Beecham, Aust.†; SmithKline Beecham, Austral.†; SmithKline Beecham, Switz.†.
A mumps vaccine (Urabe Am 9 strain) (p.1521·2).
Active immunisation.

Par-Isalon Godecke, Ger.†.
2-(*N*-(2-Diethylaminoethyl)methylamino)-1-phenyl-1-propanol-bis(dihydrogen phosphate); ephedrine hydrochloride (p.1059·3); theophylline (p.765·1); theobromine (p.765·1); caffeine (p.749·3); phenazone (p.78·2).
Asthma; bronchitis; respiratory tract disorders.

Parizac Lacer, Spain.
Omeprazole (p.1204·2) or omeprazole sodium (p.1204·2).
Gastro-oesophageal reflux; peptic ulcers; Zollinger-Ellison syndrome.

Parke Davis Laxative Parke, Davis, Austral.†.
Senna (p.1212·2); fibre.
Constipation.

Parkelanta Warner-Wellcome, Spain†.
Aluminium hydroxide (p.1177·3); magnesium hydroxide (p.1198·2); simethicone (p.1213·1).
Gastro-intestinal hyperacidity and flatulence.

Parkelase Parke, Davis, Spain.
Deoxyribonuclease (p.1059·1); plasmin (p.932·1).
Wound healing.

Parkelase Chloromycetin Parke, Davis, Spain.
Chloramphenicol (p.182·1); deoxyribonuclease (p.1059·1); plasmin (p.932·1).
Abscesses; burns; cervicitis; ulcers; vaginitis.

Parkemed
Parke, Davis, Aust.; Parke, Davis, Ger.; Parke, Davis, Ital.†.
Mefenamic acid (p.51·2).
Fever; inflammation; musculoskeletal and joint disorders; pain.

Parkevit-Fe Parke, Davis, Ger.†.
Multivitamin preparation with iron and folic acid.
Anaemias; iron and folic acid deficiencies.

Parkinane Lederle, Fr.
Benzhexol hydrochloride (p.457·3).
Parkinsonism.

Parkipan L'Arguenon, Fr.
Ointment: Trypan blue; amylocaine hydrochloride (p.1286·1); titanium dioxide (p.1093·3).
Topical solution: Trypan blue.
Viral infections of the skin and mucous membranes.

Parkopan Hexal, Ger.
Benzhexol hydrochloride (p.457·3).
Parkinsonism.

Parkotil
Lilly, Aust.†; Lilly, Ger.
Pergolide mesylate (p.1142·3).
Parkinsonism.

Parks Hommel, Ger.
Pridinol hydrochloride (p.1318·2).
Extrapyramidal disorders; parkinsonism.

Parks-Plus Hommel, Ger.†.
Pridinol hydrochloride (p.1318·2); amitriptyline hydrochloride (p.273·3).
Movement disorders; parkinsonism.

Parlax Soekami, Fr.†.
Liquid paraffin (p.1382·1).
Constipation.

Parlax Compose Soekami, Fr.†.
Liquid paraffin (p.1382·1); olive oil (p.1610·1); passion flower (p.1615·3).
Formerly contained liquid paraffin, olive oil, passion flower, and combretum altum.
Constipation.

Parlodel
Sandoz, Aust.; Novartis, Austral.; Sandoz, Belg.; Sandoz, Canad.; Sandoz, Fr.; Sandoz, Irl.; Sandoz, Ital.; Sandoz, Jpn; Novartis, Neth.; Sandoz, Norw.; Novartis, S.Afr.; Sandoz, Spain; Sandoz, Switz.; Sandoz, UK; Sandoz, USA.
Bromocriptine mesylate (p.1132·2).
Acromegaly; benign breast disorders; female infertility; hyperprolactinaemia; lactation inhibition; male hypogonadism; parkinsonism; polycystic ovary syndrome; premenstrual disorders; prolactinoma.

Parmecal
Geymonat, Ital.; Geymonat, Switz.
Food for special diets.
Colic; diarrhoea.

Parmentier Therabel Pharma, Belg.
Caffeine (p.749·3); phenazone (p.78·2).
Headache; migraine; pain.

Parmid Lagap, UK.
Metoclopramide hydrochloride (p.1200·3).
Gastro-intestinal disorders; migraine.

Parmodalin Sanofi Winthrop, Ital.
Tranylcypromine sulphate (p.308·2); trifluoperazine hydrochloride (p.697·3).
Depression.

Par-Natal Plus 1 Improved Parmed, USA.
Multivitamin and mineral preparation with iron and folic acid.

Parnate
SmithKline Beecham, Austral.; SmithKline Beecham, Canad.; Procter & Gamble, Ger.; SmithKline Beecham, Irl.; SmithKline Beecham, S.Afr.; Smith Kline & French, Spain; SmithKline Beecham, UK; SmithKline Beecham, USA.
Tranylcypromine sulphate (p.308·2).
Depression.

Paro Hoechst Marion Roussel, Ital.
Hydrocortisone acetate (p.1043·3).
Skin disorders.

Parocin Almirall, Spain.
Meloxicam (p.52·1).
Osteoarthritis; rheumatoid arthritis.

Parodium Pierre Fabre Sante, Fr.
Chlorhexidine gluconate (p.1107·2); rhubarb (p.1212·1); formaldehyde (p.1113·2).
Gum disorders.

Parodontal Serum-Werk Bernburg, Ger.
Chamomile (p.1561·2); sage (p.1627·1); lignocaine (p.1293·2).
Mouth inflammation.

Parodontal F5 med Wernigerode, Ger.
Salol (p.83·1); thymol (p.1127·1); mint oil; cineole (p.1564·1); clove oil (p.1565·2); sage oil.
Mouth inflammation.

Parodontax Madaus, Aust.
Mouthwash: Echinacea purpurea (p.1574·2); chamomile (p.1561·2); myrrh (p.1606·1); menthol (p.1600·2); clove oil (p.1565·2); caraway oil (p.1559·3); sage oil; peppermint oil (p.1208·1); mint oil (p.1604·1).
Bleeding gums; inflammation of the mouth and gums; oral hygiene.
Toothpaste: Echinacea purpurea (p.1574·2); sodium bicarbonate (p.1153·2); chamomile (p.1561·2); myrrh (p.1606·1); rhatany root (p.1624·3); sage oil; peppermint oil (p.1208·1).
Dental caries prophylaxis; oral hygiene.

Paronal Christiaens, Belg.
Asparaginase (p.504·3).
Acute leukaemia.

Paroven
Novartis, Austral.; Zyma, Irl.; Novartis Consumer, S.Afr.; Zyma, UK.
Oxerutins (p.1580·2).
Chronic venous insufficiency; haemorrhoids.

Parsal Brenner-Efeka, Ger.
Ibuprofen (p.44·1).
Fever; gout; inflammation; musculoskeletal and joint disorders; pain.

Parsilid *Crinos, Ital.*
Ticlopidine hydrochloride (p.953·1).
Thrombosis prophylaxis.

Parsitan *Rhone-Poulenc Rorer, Canad.*
Ethopropazine hydrochloride (p.461·1).
Drug-induced extrapyramidal disorders; parkinsonism.

Parstelin
SmithKline Beecham, Austral.†; SmithKline Beecham, Irl.; SmithKline Beecham, UK.
Tranylcypromine sulphate (p.308·2); trifluoperazine hydrochloride (p.697·3).
Mixed anxiety depressive states.

Partapp TD *Parmed, USA.*
Phenylpropanolamine hydrochloride (p.1067·2); phenylephrine hydrochloride (p.1066·2); brompheniramine maleate (p.403·2).
Upper respiratory-tract symptoms.

Partenelle *Arkopharma, Switz.†.*
Feverfew (p.447·3).
Migraine.

Partobulin
Immuno, Aust.; Immuno, Ger.; Immuno, Ital.; Immuno, UK.
An anti-D immunoglobulin (p.1503·2).
Prevention of rhesus sensitisation.

Partobuline *Immuno, Switz.†.*
An anti-D immunoglobulin (p.1503·2).
Prevention of rhesus sensitisation.

Partocon *Ferring, Swed.*
Oxytocin (p.1257·2).
Abortion induction; labour induction; promotion of lactation.

Parto-Gamma *Biagini, Ital.*
An anti-D immunoglobulin (p.1503·2).
Prevention of rhesus sensitisation.

Partogloman *Octapharma, Aust.†.*
An anti-D immunoglobulin (p.1503·2).
Prevention of rhesus sensitisation.

Partrim *Parke-Med, S.Afr.†.*
Co-trimoxazole (p.196·3).
Bacterial infections.

Partusisten
Boehringer Ingelheim, Ger.; Boehringer Ingelheim, Neth.; Vifor, Switz.
Fenoterol hydrobromide (p.753·2).
Fetal distress; premature labour.

Partuss LA *Parmed, USA.*
Phenylpropanolamine hydrochloride (p.1067·2); guaiphenesin (p.1061·3).
Coughs.

Paruman
Berna, Ital.; Berna, Switz.
A mumps immunoglobulin (p.1521·2).
Passive immunisation.

Parvisedil *SIT, Ital.*
Aminohydroxybutyric acid (p.339·1); valerian (p.1643·1); passion flower (p.1615·3); chamomile (p.1561·2); crataegus (p.1568·2).
Restlessness and insomnia in infants.

Parvlex *Freeda, USA.*
Ferrous fumarate (p.1339·3); folic acid (p.1340·3); vitamin B substances with vitamin C.
Iron-deficiency anaemias.

Parvolex
DBL, Austral.; Bioniche, Canad.; Evans Medical, Irl.; Glaxo Wellcome, S.Afr.; Medeva, UK.
Acetylcysteine (p.1052·3).
Paracetamol overdosage.

Pasaden
Note. This name is used for preparations of different composition.
Asta Medica, Belg.†.
Homofenazine (p.675·2).
Anxiety; neurovegetative states; sedative.

Farmades, Ital.
Etizolam (p.669·3).
Anxiety; insomnia.

Pascallerg *Pascoe, Ger.*
Homoeopathic preparation.

Pascobilin novo *Pascoe, Ger.*
Peppermint leaf (p.1208·1); taraxacum (p.1634·2); cynara (p.1569·2).
Biliary-tract disorders.

Pascodolor Tropfen *Pascoe, Ger.*
Homoeopathic preparation.

Pascofemin *Pascoe, Ger.*
Homoeopathic preparation.

Pascohepan novo *Pascoe, Ger.*
Chelidonium; silybum marianum (p.993·3); taraxacum (p.1634·2).
Pascohepan formerly contained chelidonium, quassia, silybum marianum, and taraxacum.
Liver disorders.

Pascoletten N *Pascoe, Ger.*
Aloes (p.1177·1); chamomile (p.1561·2).
Pascoletten formerly contained cascara bark, frangula bark, rhubarb, aloes, and chamomile.
Constipation.

Pascoleucyn *Pascoe, Ger.*
Homoeopathic preparation.

Pascolibrin *Pascoe, Ger.*
Homoeopathic preparation.

Pascomag *Pascoe, Ger.*
Bismuth subnitrate (p.1180·2); German chamomile flowers (p.1561·2); linseed (p.1596·2).
Gastro-intestinal disorders.

Pascomucil
Koch, Aust.; Pascoe, Ger.
Ispaghula husk (p.1194·2).
Constipation; diarrhoea.

Pasconal forte *Pascoe, Ger.*
Homoeopathic preparation.

Pasconal Nerventropfen N *Pascoe, Ger.*
Homoeopathic preparation.

Pasconeural-Injektopas *Pascoe, Ger.*
Procaine hydrochloride (p.1299·2); caffeine (p.749·3).
Local anaesthesia.

Pasconeural-Injektopas 1% *Pascoe, Ger.*
Procaine hydrochloride (p.1299·2).
Local anaesthesia.

Pascopankreat
Note. This name is used for preparations of different composition.
Koch, Aust.
Condurango (p.1567·2); silybum marianum (p.993·3); fennel fruit (p.1579·1); caraway oil (p.1559·3); chamomile oil.
Dyspepsia.

Pascoe, Ger.†.
Yellow tablets, papain (p.1614·1); absinthium (p.1541·1); fennel (p.1579·1); cinchona bark (p.1564·1); condurango (p.1567·2); vegetable charcoal (p.972·3); red tablets, pancreatin (p.1612·1); cascara (p.1183·1); ox bile (p.1553·2); silybum marianum (p.993·3); aniseed (p.1549·3); sarsaparilla (p.1627·2); syzygium jamb.; chamomile oil.
Digestive system disorders.

Pascopankreat S *Pascoe, Ger.*
Pancreatin; caraway oil (p.1559·3); chamomile oil; condurango; sarsaparilla; cholesterin.; menthol; ol. anisi; card. mar.; foenic.; syzyg. jamb.
Digestive system disorders.

Pascopnakreat novo *Pascoe, Ger.*
Combination pack: Yellow tablets, absinthium (p.1541·1); condurango (p.1567·2); red tablets, pancreatin (p.1612·1).
Oral drops: Caraway oil (p.1559·3); chamomile oil; condurango (p.1567·2); silybum marianum (p.993·3); fennel (p.1579·1).
Gastro-intestinal disorders.

Pascorenal *Pascoe, Ger.*
Homoeopathic preparation.

Pascosabal N *Pascoe, Ger.*
Homoeopathic preparation.

Pascosedon S *Pascoe, Ger.*
Valerian (p.1643·1); lupulus (p.1597·2); melissa (p.1600·1).
Anxiety; sleep disorders.

Pascossan *Pascoe, Ger.†.*
Homoeopathic preparation.

Pascotox *Pascoe, Ger.*
Oral drops: Echinacea angustifolia (p.1574·2); baptisia; bryonia; eupatorium perfoliatum; arnica; ferr. phosphoric.; thuja; china; lachesis; cupr; sulfuric.
Tablets: Echinacea angustifolia (p.1574·2); baptisia; bryonia; eupatorium perfoliatum; thuja; lachesis.
Tonic.

Pascotox forte-Injektopas *Pascoe, Ger.*
Echinacea angustifolia (p.1574·2).
Tonic.

Pascotox mono *Pascoe, Ger.*
Echinacea angustifolia (p.1574·2).
Tonic.

Pascotox-Injektopas *Pascoe, Ger.†.*
Echinacea angustifolia (p.1574·2); apis; viscum alb.; ferr. met.; cupr. met.; formica rufa; achat.
Tonic.

Pascovenol novo *Pascoe, Ger.*
Aesculus (p.1543·3); mellilotus; hamamelis (p.1587·1).
Vascular disorders.

Pascovenol S *Pascoe, Ger.†.*
Oral drops: Aesculus (p.1543·3); silybum marianum fruit (p.993·3); melilot; rutoside sodium sulphate (p.1580·2); hamamelis (p.1587·1).
Tablets: Hamamelis leaves (p.1587·1); aesculus (p.1543·3); silybum marianum fruit (p.993·3); melilot; rutin (p.1580·2).
Vascular disorders.

Paser *Jacobus, USA.*
Aminosalicylic acid (p.151·1).
Tuberculosis.

Pas-Fatol N *Fatol, Ger.*
Sodium aminosalicylate (p.151·1).
Tuberculosis.

Pasgensin *Pascoe, Ger.*
Vitamins; oxedrine tartrate (p.925·3).
Hypotension; tonic.

Pasisana *Hotz, Ger.*
Herbal and homoeopathic preparation.

Pasivital h *Hotz, Ger.*
Homoeopathic preparation.

Pasmol *Ram, USA†.*
Ethaverine hydrochloride (p.1577·1).

Paspat
Note. This name is used for preparations of different composition.
Luitpold, Ger.
Autolysate of: *Staphylococcus aureus*; *Staphylococcus albus*; *Streptococcus viridans*; *Streptococcus haemolyt.*; *Diplococcus pneumoniae*; *Moraxella (Branhamella) catarrhalis*; *Haemophilus influenzae*; *Candida albicans.*
Immunotherapy in respiratory-tract infections.

Luitpold, Ital.
Lysate of *Staphylococcus aureus*, *Streptococcus mitis*, *Streptococcus pyogenes*, *Streptococcus pneumoniae*, *Klebsiella pneumoniae*, *Branhamella catarrhalis*, and *Haemophilus influenzae*.
Respiratory-tract infections.

Paspertase
Solvay, Aust.; Solvay, Ger.
Metoclopramide hydrochloride (p.1200·3); pancreatin (p.1612·1).
Gastro-intestinal disorders.

Paspertin
Solvay, Aust.; Solvay, Ger.; Solvay, Switz.
Metoclopramide (p.1202·1) or metoclopramide hydrochloride (p.1200·3).
Adjunct in gastro-intestinal radiography; gastro-intestinal disorders.

Pasrin *Lennon, S.Afr.*
Buspirone hydrochloride (p.643·3).
Anxiety.

Passedan *Austroplant, Aust.*
Passion flower (p.1615·3); melissa leaf (p.1600·1).
Dystonias; menopausal disorders; sleep disorders.

Passedyl *Urgo, Fr.*
Drosera (p.1574·1); grindelia; sodium benzoate (p.1102·3); potassium bromide (p.1620·3); potassium guaiacolsulfonate (p.1068·3); orange-flower water; terpin (p.1070·2); tolu balsam (p.1071·1); senega (p.1069·3).
Respiratory-tract congestion.

Passelyt *Smetana, Aust.*
Passion flower (p.1615·3); melissa leaf (p.1600·1).
Anxiety disorders; sleep disorders.

Passiflora Complex
Note. This name is used for preparations of different composition.
Blackmores, Austral.
Passion flower (p.1615·3); lupulus (p.1597·2); scutellaria; valerian (p.1643·1); multivitamins.
Anxiety; insomnia; stress symptoms.

Dolisos, Canad.
Homoeopathic preparation.

Passiflora GHL *Lehning, Fr.*
Homoeopathic preparation.

Passiflorine
Note. This name is used for preparations of different composition.
Parke, Davis, Fr.
Passion flower (p.1615·3); crataegus (p.1568·2).
Insomnia; nervous disorders.

Teofarma, Ital.; Wasserman, Spain.
Passion flower (p.1615·3); crataegus (p.1568·2); salix alba (p.82·3).
Anxiety; insomnia; menopausal disorders.

Passinevryl *Thera, Fr.†.*
Passion flower (p.1615·3); willow (p.82·3); crataegus (p.1568·2); valerian (p.1643·1).
Insomnia.

Passionflower Plus *Eagle, Austral.*
Passion flower (p.1615·3); valerian (p.1643·1); scutellaria; lupulus (p.1597·2).
Anxiety; insomnia.

Passiorin
Note. This name is used for preparations of different composition.
Simons, Ger.†.
Crataegus (p.1568·2); passion flower (p.1615·3); willow (p.82·3); thiamine hydrochloride (p.1361·1).
Nervous disorders.

Agpharm, Switz.†.
Crataegus (p.1568·2); passion flower (p.1615·3).
Agitation; nervous disorders; sleep disorders; tension.

Passiorin N *Simons, Ger.*
Crataegus (p.1568·2); passion flower (p.1615·3).
Nervous disorders; sleep disorders.

Past Ail *Medecine Vegetale, Fr.*
Garlic (p.1583·1).
Capillary fragility; circulatory disorders.

Pasta boli *Spirig, Switz.*
Salicylic acid (p.1090·2); eucalyptus oil (p.1578·1); peppermint oil (p.1208·1); methyl salicylate (p.55·2).
Musculoskeletal, joint, peri-articular, and soft-tissue disorders.

Pasta Cool *Apomedica, Aust.*
Heparin sodium (p.879·3); salicylic acid (p.1090·2).
Musculoskeletal and joint disorders; peri-articular disorders; soft-tissue injury.

Pasta Dicofarm *Dicofarm, Ital.*
Zinc oxide (p.1096·2); titanium dioxide (p.1093·3); vitamin E (p.1369·1); vitamin F.
Skin irritation.

Pasta Lactisol *Galactopharm, Ger.*
Sour milk whey concentrate.
Skin disorders.

Pasta Lassar Imba *Imba, Spain.*
Almond oil (p.1546·2); lanolin; zinc oxide (p.1096·2).
Skin disorders.

Pasta Lassar Orravan *Orravan, Spain.*
Salicylic acid (p.1090·2); soft paraffin; zinc oxide (p.1096·2).
Skin disorders.

Pasta Plumbi *Salus, Aust.*
Lead (p.1595·1).
Insect bites and stings.

Pasta Prura *Propan-Vernleigh, S.Afr.†.*
Coal tar (p.1092·3); zinc oxide (p.1096·2); calamine (p.1080·1).
Skin disorders.

Pasta rubra salicylata *Apomedica, Aust.*
Diethylamine salicylate (p.33·1); salicylic acid (p.1090·2); methyl salicylate (p.55·2).
Gout; rheumatism; sciatica; soft-tissue injury; tendinitis.

Pastaba *Pastaba, Fr.†.*
Magnesium hydroxide (p.1198·2); sodium benzoate (p.1102·3); potassium chlorate (p.1620·3); silver protein (p.1629·3); lupulin.
Aid to smoking withdrawal.

Pastariso *General Dietary, UK†.*
Gluten-free pasta.
Gluten-sensitive enteropathies.

Pastiglie al Pumilene *Montefarmaco, Ital.†.*
Dequalinium chloride (p.1112·1).
Sore throat.

Pastiglie Valda *Valda, Ital.*
Cicliomenol; enoxolone (p.35·2); menthol (p.1600·2); cineole (p.1564·1).
Catarrh; mouth and throat irritation.

Pastillas Dr Andreu *Roche Nicholas, Spain.*
Dextromethorphan hydrobromide (p.1057·3); sodium benzoate.
Cough.

Pastillas Juanola *Juanola, Spain.*
Cineole (p.1564·1); liquorice (p.1197·1); terpin (p.1070·2); menthol (p.1600·2).
Coughs; throat irritation.

Pastillas Koki Ment Tivo *Perez Gimenez, Spain.*
Benzocaine (p.1286·2); tyrothricin (p.267·2); menthol (p.1600·2).
Sore throat.

Pastillas Pectoral Kely *Boots, Spain.*
Cineole (p.1564·1); niaouli oil (p.1607·1); senega (p.1069·3); liquorice (p.1197·1); sodium benzoate (p.1102·3); potassium guaiacolsulfonate (p.1068·3); terpin monohydrate (p.1070·2).
Respiratory-tract disorders.

Pastillas Vicks Limon *Procter & Gamble, Spain†.*
Ascorbic acid; cetylpyridinium chloride (p.1106·2); citric acid; menthol (p.1600·2).
Throat irritation.

Pastillas Vicks Mentol *Procter & Gamble, Spain†.*
Camphor (p.1557·2); benzyl alcohol; tolu balsam (p.1071·1); thymol (p.1127·1); menthol (p.1600·2); eucalyptus (p.1578·1); cetylpyridinium chloride (p.1106·2).
Throat irritation.

Pastilles d'Ems *Siemens, Switz.*
Sal ems.
Cold symptoms; upper-respiratory-tract inflammation.

Pastilles Jessel *Jessel, Fr.†.*
Vitamin A (p.1358·1); ergocalciferol (p.1367·1); iron (p.1346·1); berberine sulphate (p.1553·1); zinc phosphate (p.1373·3); strychnine sulphate (p.1633·1).
Nutritional supplement.

Pastilles M.B.C *Monal, Fr.†.*
Menthol (p.1600·2); amylocaine hydrochloride (p.1286·1); procaine hydrochloride (p.1299·2); mint oil (p.1604·1); borax (p.1554·2); potassium chlorate (p.1620·3).
Mouth and throat disorders.

Pastilles Monleon *Toulade, Fr.*
Methylene blue (p.984·3); tolu balsam (p.1071·1); drosera (p.1574·1); aconite (p.1542·2); hamamelis (p.1587·1); ipecacuanha (p.1062·2).
Coughs; mouth and throat disorders.

Pastilles pour la gorge no 535 *Renapharm, Switz.*
Dequalinium disalicylate (p.1112·1).
Mouth and throat disorders.

Pastilles Valda *Valda, Canad.*
Guaiacol (p.1061·2); cineole (p.1564·1); menthol (p.1600·2); terpin hydrate (p.1070·2); thymol (p.1127·1).

Pastimmun *Pasteur Merieux, Belg.*
A BCG vaccine (p.1504·3).
Bladder cancer.

Pasuma *Merck, S.Afr.†.*
Injection: Testosterone propionate (p.1464·2); vitamin E (p.1369·1); yohimbine glycerophosphate (p.1645·3); strychnine glycerophosphate.
Tablets: Methyltestosterone (p.1450·3); vitamin E (p.1369·1); yohimbine hydrochloride (p.1645·3); strychnine glycerophosphate; caffeine (p.749·3); ephedrine hydrochloride (p.1059·3).
Male loss of libido.

Pasuma-Dragees *Herchemie, Aust.*
Methyltestosterone (p.1450·3); alpha tocopheryl acetate (p.1369·1); yohimbine hydrochloride (p.1645·3); strychnine glycerophosphate; caffeine (p.749·3); oxedrine tartrate (p.925·3).

Patanol *Alcon, USA.*
Olopatadine hydrochloride (p.415·1).
Allergic conjunctivitis.

Pate a l'Eau Roche-Posay *Roche-Posay, Fr.*
Zinc oxide (p.1096·2); titanium dioxide (p.1093·3); borax (p.1554·2).
Eczema.

Pate d'Unna *Rougier, Canad.*
Zinc oxide (p.1096·2).

Pate Iodoforme du Prof Dr Walkhoff *Haupt, Switz.*
Iodoform (p.1118·2); parachlorophenol (p.1120·3); camphor (p.1557·2); menthol (p.1600·2).
Dental inflammation.

Patentex
Medra, Aust.; Frere, Belg.; CCD, Fr.; Patentex, Ger.†; Brovar, S.Afr.†.
Nonoxinol 9 (p.1326·1).
Contraceptive.

Patentex Oval N
Patentex, Ger.; Patentex, Switz.
Nonoxinol 9 (p.1326·1).
Contraceptive.

Patentex Ovuli Milanfarma, Ital.†.
Nonoxinol (p.1326·1).
Contraception.

Pates Pectorales Oberlin, Fr.
Codeine (p.26·1); tolu balsam (p.1071·1); cherry-laurel.
Coughs.

Pathilon Lederle, USA.
Tridihexethyl chloride (p.469·2).
Peptic ulcer (adjunct).

Pathocil Wyeth-Ayerst, USA.
Dicloxacillin sodium (p.202·1).
Bacterial infections.

Patriot Agropharm, UK.
Pyrethrins; piperonyl butoxide (p.1409·3).
Insecticide and repellent.

Patussol Andreabal, Switz.
Oral drops: Dextromethorphan hydrobromide (p.1057·3); chlorpheniramine maleate (p.405·1); ipecacuanha (p.1062·2); senega (p.1069·3).
Syrup: Dextromethorphan hydrobromide (p.1057·3); chlorpheniramine maleate (p.405·1); ammonium chloride (p.1055·2); ipecacuanha (p.1062·2).
Coughs.

Paucisone ITA, Ital.†.
Betamethasone sodium phosphate (p.1033·3).
Corticosteroid.

Pavabid Hoechst Marion Roussel, USA.
Papaverine hydrochloride (p.1614·2).
Cerebral and peripheral ischaemia; smooth muscle spasm.

Pa-Vaccinol Procter & Gamble, Ger.
A pertussis vaccine (p.1526·1).
Active immunisation.

Pavacol-D Boehringer Ingelheim, UK.
Pholcodine (p.1068·1).
Coughs.

Pavarine Vortech, USA.
Papaverine hydrochloride (p.1614·2).
Cerebral and peripheral ischaemia; smooth muscle spasm.

Pavased Hauck, USA†.
Papaverine hydrochloride (p.1614·2).
Cerebral and peripheral ischaemia; smooth muscle spasm.

Pavatine Major, USA†.
Papaverine hydrochloride (p.1614·2).
Cerebral and peripheral ischaemia; smooth muscle spasm.

Pavecef IBP, Ital.†.
Cephamandole nafate sodium (p.180·1).
Bacterial infections.

Paveciclina IBP, Ital.†.
Methacycline hydrochloride (p.225·1).
Bacterial infections.

Pavephos IBP, Ital.†.
Levoglutamide; DL-phosphoserine; cyanocobalamin.
Tonic.

Paveriwern Wernigerode, Ger.
Papaver somniferum.
Gastro-intestinal spasm.

Paverolan Lannett, USA.
Papaverine hydrochloride (p.1614·2).
Cerebral and peripheral ischaemia; smooth muscle spasm.

Paveron Karlspharma, Ger.†.
Injection: Papaverine hydrochloride (p.1614·2).
Sustained-release tablets: Papaverine hydrochloride (p.1614·2); ethoxazorutoside (p.1580·1); ascorbic acid (p.1365·2).
Cerebral, ocular, coronary, and peripheral vascular disorders.

Paverysat Burger Ysatfabrik, Ger.†.
Capita papaveris immaturi.
Smooth muscle spasms.

Paverysat forte Ysatfabrik, Ger.
Chelidonium; turmeric (p.1001·3).
Biliary-tract spasm.

Pavulon
Organon, Aust.; Organon Teknika, Austral.; Organon, Canad.; Organon Teknika, Irl.; Organon Teknika, Ital.; Organon Teknika, Neth.; Organon Teknika, Norw.; Sanofi Omnimed, S.Afr.; Organon, Spain; Organon Teknika, Swed.; Organon Teknika, Switz.; Organon Teknika, UK; Organon, USA.
Pancuronium bromide (p.1317·2).
Competitive neuromuscular blocker.

Pawa-Rutan Hanosan, Ger.
Homoeopathic preparation.

Pax Intramed, S.Afr.
Diazepam (p.661·1).
Alcohol withdrawal syndrome; anxiety; premedication.

Paxadorm Schwulst, S.Afr.
Nitrazepam (p.682·2).
Insomnia.

Paxam Alphapharm, Austral.
Clonazepam (p.343·3).
Epilepsy.

Paxarel Circle, USA.
Acetylcarbromal.
Anxiety; insomnia; sedative; spastic colitis.

Paxeladine
Ipsen, Belg.†; Beaufour, Fr.
Oxeladin citrate (p.1065·3).
Coughs.

Paxeladine Noctee Beaufour, Fr.
Oxeladin citrate (p.1065·3); promethazine hydrochloride (p.416·2).
Coughs.

Paxical Intramed, S.Afr.
Droperidol (p.668·2).
Nausea and vomiting; neuroleptanalgesia; premedication.

Paxidal
Note. This name is used for preparations of different composition.
Propan, S.Afr.
Paracetamol (p.72·2); doxylamine succinate (p.410·1); caffeine (p.749·3); codeine phosphate (p.26·1).
Pain and associated tension.

Wallace Mfg Chem., UK.
Caffeine (p.749·3); meprobamate (p.678·1); paracetamol (p.72·2).

Paxil
SmithKline Beecham, Canad.; SmithKline Beecham, USA.
Paroxetine hydrochloride (p.301·2).
Depression; panic disorders.

Paxipam
Schering-Plough, Ital.; Schering, USA†.
Halazepam (p.673·2).
Anxiety.

Paxom Synlab, Fr.†.
Cobamamide (p.1364·2).
Neuralgia; neuropathy.

Paxtibi Dista, Spain.
Nortriptyline hydrochloride (p.300·2).
Depression.

Paxyl Faulding, Austral.
Lignocaine (p.1293·2) or lignocaine hydrochloride (p.1293·2); benzalkonium chloride (p.1101·3); allantoin (p.1078·2).
Burns; chapped skin; insect bites; skin abrasions; sunburn; windburn.

Payagastron Weber & Weber, Ger.†.
Homoeopathic preparation.

Pazbronquial Cinfa, Spain.
Codeine phosphate (p.26·1); ephedrine hydrochloride (p.1059·3); sodium benzoate (p.1102·3); sodium citrate (p.1153·2); potassium guaiacolsulfonate (p.1068·3); thiamine hydrochloride (p.1361·1); pyridoxine hydrochloride (p.1362·3); menthol (p.1600·2); drosera (p.1574·1); lobelia inflata (p.1481·3); thyme (p.1636·3); origanum vulgare.
Coughs.

Pazo Bristol-Myers Products, USA.
Benzocaine (p.1286·2); ephedrine sulphate (p.1059·3); zinc oxide (p.1096·2); camphor (p.1557·2).
Haemorrhoids.

PBZ Geigy, USA.
Tripelennamine citrate (p.420·2) or tripelennamine hydrochloride (p.420·2).
Hypersensitivity reactions.

PC Arthri-Spray Procare, Austral.
Copper salicylate; methyl salicylate (p.55·2).
Musculoskeletal, joint, and peri-articular disorders.

PC 30 N Terra-Bio, Ger.
Chamomile (p.1561·2).
Skin disorders.

PC Regulax Procare, Austral.
Peppermint leaf (p.1208·1); ispaghula husk (p.1194·2); slippery elm (p.1630·1); ginger (p.1193·2); pectin (p.1474·1).
Gastro-intestinal disorders; hyperlipidaemias; varicose veins.

PC Rei-shi Procare, Austral.
Rei-shi; shi-taki.
Nutritional supplement.

PC 30 V Terra-Bio, Ger.
Aesculus (p.1543·3); dexpanthenol (p.1570·3); chamomile (p.1561·2).
Skin disorders; ulcers; wounds.

PC-Cap Alra, USA.
Dextropropoxyphene hydrochloride (p.27·3); aspirin (p.16·1); caffeine (p.749·3).

PCE
Abbott, Canad.; Abbott, USA.
Erythromycin (p.204·1).
Bacterial infections.

PCF Ritsert, Ger.
Homoeopathic preparation.

P-Cortin Farge, Ital.†.
Suprarenal cortex (p.1050·1); sodium pantothenate (p.1353·1); ascorbic acid (p.1365·2).
Adrenocortical insufficiency.

PDF Pharmascience, Canad.†.
Sodium fluoride (p.742·1).
Dental caries prophylaxis.

PDP Liquid Protein Wesley, USA.
Tryptophan (p.310·2); hydrolysed animal collagen (p.1566·3).
Dietary supplement.

PE Alcon, USA.
Pilocarpine hydrochloride (p.1396·3); adrenaline acid tartrate (p.813·3).
Glaucoma; raised intra-ocular pressure.

PE pfrimmer Pfrimmer, Ger.†.
Amino-acid, carbohydrate, electrolyte, and vitamin infusion.
Parenteral nutrition.

Peacetime Lifeplan, UK.
Nutritional supplement.

Peauline Bipharma, Neth.†.
Benzoyl peroxide (p.1079·2).
Acne.

Pe-Ce Gebro, Aust.
Turpentine oil (p.1641·1); eucalyptus oil (p.1578·1); nutmeg oil (p.1609·3); cedar leaf oil; camphor (p.1557·2); thymol (p.1127·1).
Coughs and cold symptoms.

Pe-Ce Ven N Terra-Bio, Ger.
Aescin (p.1543·3); heparin sodium (p.879·3).
Vascular disorders.

Pecram Zyma, UK.
Aminophylline hydrate (p.748·1).
Bronchospasm; cardiac asthma and failure.

Pect Hustenloser Rentschler, Ger.
Ambroxol hydrochloride (p.1054·3).
Respiratory-tract disorders associated with increased or viscous mucus.

Pectamol
Malesci, Ital.†; Alpharma, Norw.
Oxeladin citrate (p.1065·3).
Coughs.

Pectapas novo Pascoe, Ger.
Homoeopathic preparation.

Pectibran Yves Ponroy, Fr.†.
Dietary fibre supplement.

Pectikon Be-Tabs, S.Afr.
Light kaolin (p.1195·1); apple pectin (p.1474·1).
Diarrhoea.

Pectinfant N Pharminfant, Ger.†.
Codeine phosphate (p.26·1); diphenylpyraline hydrochloride (p.409·3).
Coughs and associated respiratory-tract disorders.

Pectin-K PD Pharm, S.Afr.
Kaolin (p.1195·1); apple pectin (p.1474·1).
Diarrhoea.

Pectipar Cooperation Pharmaceutique, Fr.†.
Opium (p.70·3); heavy kaolin (p.1195·1).
Diarrhoea.

Pecto 6 Pierre Fabre, Fr.†.
Adult syrup: Codeine (p.26·1); ethylmorphine hydrochloride (p.36·1); potassium guaiacolsulfonate (p.1068·3); sodium benzoate (p.1102·3); drosera (p.1574·1); aconite (p.1542·2); eucalyptus (p.1578·1).
Paediatric syrup: Codeine (p.26·1); potassium guaiacolsulfonate (p.1068·3); aconite (p.1542·2); belladonna (p.457·1); sodium benzoate (p.1102·3).
Coughs; upper respiratory-tract disorders.

Pecto-Baby Pharmacal, Switz.
Guaiphenesin (p.1061·3); pholcodine (p.1068·1); chlorpheniramine maleate (p.405·1).
Coughs.

Pectobal Dextro Clariana, Spain.
Dextromethorphan hydrobromide (p.1057·3); mepyramine maleate (p.414·1).
Respiratory-tract disorders.

Pectobloc Siegfried, Ger.†.
Pindolol (p.931·1).
Cardiac disorders; hypertension.

Pectocalmine Pharmacal, Switz.
Codeine phosphate (p.26·1); guaiphenesin (p.1061·3); ephedrine hydrochloride (p.1059·3); opium (p.70·3); senega (p.1069·3).
Coughs and associated respiratory-tract disorders.

Pectocalmine Baby Couvreur, Belg.†.
Sodium bromide (p.1620·3); potassium guaiacolsulfonate (p.1068·3); pholcodine (p.1068·1); chlorpheniramine maleate (p.405·1).
Coughs.

Pectocalmine Gommes Couvreur, Belg.†.
Codeine phosphate (p.26·1).
Coughs.

Pectocalmine Junior
Note. This name is used for preparations of different composition.
Couvreur, Belg.†.
Codeine phosphate (p.26·1); aconite (p.1542·2); cherry-laurel water; tolu balsam (p.1071·1); rhubarb (p.1212·1).
Coughs.

Pharmacal, Switz.
Codeine phosphate (p.26·1); cherry-laurel; tolu balsam (p.1071·1); red-poppy; anethole (p.1549·3).
Coughs and associated respiratory-tract disorders.

Pectocalmine Sirop Couvreur, Belg.†.
Ephedrine hydrochloride (p.1059·3); codeine phosphate (p.26·1); potassium guaiacolsulfonate (p.1068·3); red-poppy petal.
Coughs.

Pectocor N LAW, Ger.
Camphor (p.1557·2).
Cardiac disorders.

Pectoderme Plantes et Medecines, Fr.
α-Pinene; β-pinene; myrtol; lavender oil (p.1594·3); terpineol (p.1635·1); eugenol (p.1578·2); camphor (p.1557·2); cineole (p.1564·1).
Respiratory-tract congestion.

Pectofree Couvreur, Belg.†.
Dextromethorphan hydrobromide (p.1057·3).
Coughs.

Pectolin Noristan, S.Afr.†.
Kaolin (p.1195·1); apple pectin (p.1474·1); electrolytes (p.1152·3).
Diarrhoea.

Pectolitan mit Codein Kettelhack Riker, Ger.†.
Pimpinella; ipecacuanha (p.1062·2); camphor (p.1557·2); codeine (p.26·1); liq. ammon. anis.
Coughs and associated respiratory-tract disorders.

Pectomucil Qualiphar, Belg.
Acetylcysteine (p.1052·3).
Paracetamol poisoning; respiratory-tract disorders associated with viscous secretions.

Pectoral Wenig, Aust.
Ephedrine hydrochloride (p.1059·3); α-phenylethylaceticacid-β-diethylaminoethanolester dihydrogen citrate.
Coughs.

Pectoral Brum Brum, Spain.
Aconite (p.1542·2); tolu balsam (p.1071·1); ipecacuanha (p.1062·2); orange; sodium benzoate (p.1102·3); potassium guaiacolsulfonate (p.1068·3).
Respiratory-tract disorders.

Pectoral Edulcor Pierre Fabre, Fr.
Codeine phosphate (p.26·1).
Formerly contained belladonna, aconite, codeine phosphate, cherry-laurel, bromoform, and glycerol.
Coughs.

Pectoral Funk Antitus Funk, Spain.
Carbocisteine (p.1056·3); chlorpheniramine maleate (p.405·1); phenylephrine hydrochloride (p.1066·2); oxolamine citrate (p.1065·3).
Respiratory-tract disorders.

Pectoral N Mepha, Switz.
Ipecacuanha, plantain, primula; senega root (p.1069·3); thyme (p.1636·3).
Pectoral formerly contained ipecacuanha, plantain, primula, polygala, and thyme.
Cold symptoms; coughs.

Pectoris Llorens, Spain†.
Capobenic acid (p.836·3).
Ischaemic heart disease.

Pectosan Cooperation Pharmaceutique, Fr.
Potassium guaiacolsulfonate (p.1068·3); codeine (p.26·1); bromoform (p.1620·3); sodium camsylate.
Formerly contained potassium guaiacolsulfonate, pholcodine, ethylmorphine hydrochloride, belladonna, senega, and sodium benzoate.
Coughs.

Pectosan Ampicilina Pharmalab, Spain.
Ampicillin trihydrate (p.153·2); ephedrine hydrochloride (p.1059·3).
Respiratory-tract infections.

Pectosorin Richter, Aust.
Potassium guaiacolsulfonate (p.1068·3).
Bronchitis; catarrh; coughs.

Pectospir Soekami, Fr.†.
Codeine (p.26·1); bromoform (p.1620·3); aconite (p.1542·2); belladonna (p.457·1); opium (p.70·3); grindelia; tolu balsam (p.1071·1); iris florentina.
Colds; coughs; hoarseness.

Pectothymin Planta, Canad.
Aniseed (p.1549·3); thyme (p.1636·3); primula.
Coughs.

Pectovox Soekami, Fr.†.
Codeine (p.26·1); bromoform (p.1620·3); aconite (p.1542·2); belladonna (p.457·1); opium (p.70·3); grindelia; tolu balsam (p.1071·1); iris florentina.
Coughs and cold symptoms.

Pectox
Woelm, Ger.; Italfarmaco, Spain; Piraud, Switz.
Carbocisteine (p.1056·3) or carbocisteine lysine (p.1056·3).
Respiratory-tract congestion.

Pectox Ampicilina Italfarmaco, Spain.
Ampicillin (p.153·1); carbocisteine (p.1056·3).
Respiratory-tract infections.

Pectramin Streuli, Switz.
Diphenhydramine hydrochloride (p.409·1); ammonium chloride (p.1055·2); menthol (p.1600·2).
Coughs.

Pectrolyte Restan, S.Afr.
Kaolin (p.1195·1); pectin (p.1474·1); chloroform and morphine tincture (p.56·1); sodium lactate; potassium chloride; sodium chloride (p.1152·3).
Colic; diarrhoea.

Pedamed Rice Steele, Irl.†.
Zinc undecenoate (p.389·2); zinc oxide (p.1096·2); alum (p.1547·1); allantoin (p.1078·2); chlorhexidine hydrochloride (p.1107·2).
Fungal infections.

Pedameth Forest Pharmaceuticals, USA.
Methionine (p.984·2).
Control of odour, dermatitis, and ulceration in incontinent adults; nappy rash.

Ped-El
Kabi Pharmacia, Ger.†; Kabivitrum, Irl.†; Pharmacia, Neth.†; Pharmacia, S.Afr.†; Pharmacia, Swed.†; Kabi, Switz.†; KabiVitrum, UK.
Electrolyte and trace element preparation (p.1147·1).
Parenteral nutrition.

PediaCare Allergy Formula McNeil Consumer, USA.
Chlorpheniramine maleate (p.405·1).

PediaCare Cold-Allergy McNeil Consumer, USA†.
Pseudoephedrine hydrochloride (p.1068·3); chlorpheniramine maleate (p.405·1).
Allergic rhinitis; cold symptoms.

PediaCare Cough-Cold *McNeil Consumer, USA.*
Pseudoephedrine hydrochloride (p.1068·3); chlorpheniramine maleate (p.405·1); dextromethorphan hydrobromide (p.1057·3).
Coughs and cold symptoms.

PediaCare Infant's Decongestant *McNeil Consumer, USA.*
Pseudoephedrine hydrochloride (p.1068·3).
Nasal congestion.

PediaCare NightRest Cough-Cold Formula *McNeil Consumer, USA.*
Pseudoephedrine hydrochloride (p.1068·3); chlorpheniramine maleate (p.405·1); dextromethorphan hydrobromide (p.1057·3).
Coughs and cold symptoms.

Pediacof *Sanofi Winthrop, USA.*
Codeine phosphate (p.26·1); phenylephrine hydrochloride (p.1066·2); chlorpheniramine maleate (p.405·1); potassium iodide (p.1493·1).
Coughs.

Pediacon DX *Goldline, USA.*
Phenylpropanolamine hydrochloride (p.1067·2); guaiphenesin (p.1061·3); dextromethorphan hydrobromide (p.1057·3).
Coughs.

Pediacon EX *Goldline, USA.*
Phenylpropanolamine (p.1067·2); guaiphenesin (p.1061·3).
Coughs.

Pediaflor *Ross, USA.*
Sodium fluoride (p.742·1).
Dental caries prophylaxis in children.

Pedialyte
Abbott, Canad.
Glucose; potassium citrate; sodium chloride; sodium citrate (p.1152·3).
Diarrhoea; oral rehydration therapy.

Abbott, Ital.
Sodium lactate; sodium citrate dihydrate; sodium chloride; potassium chloride; magnesium chloride hexahydrate; calcium chloride dihydrate; anhydrous glucose (p.1152·3).
Oral rehydration therapy.

Ross, USA.
Electrolytes; glucose (p.1152·3).
Diarrhoea; oral rehydration therapy.

Pediaphyllin PL *Galephar, Neth.†.*
Theophylline (p.765·1).
Bronchospasm.

Pediapirin *Sandoz, Spain.*
Paracetamol (p.72·2).
Fever; pain.

Pediapred
Rhone-Poulenc Rorer, Canad.; Fisons, USA.
Prednisolone sodium phosphate (p.1048·1).
Corticosteroid.

PediaProfen *McNeil Consumer, USA.*
Ibuprofen (p.44·1).
Fever; osteoarthritis; pain; rheumatoid arthritis.

PediaSure
Abbott, Austral.; Abbott, Canad.; Abbott, Ital.; Ross, USA.
Preparation for enteral nutrition.

Pediatric Cough Syrup *Technilab, Canad.*
Pseudoephedrine hydrochloride (p.1068·3); dextromethorphan hydrobromide (p.1057·3).

Pediatrivite *Seroyal, Canad.*
Multivitamin and mineral preparation.

Pediatrix *Technilab, Canad.*
Paracetamol (p.72·2).
Fever; pain.

Pediavax *Merck Sharp & Dohme, Belg.†.*
A haemophilus influenzae conjugate vaccine (meningococcal protein conjugate) (p.1511·1).
Active immunisation.

Pedia-Vit *Roerig, Belg.†.*
Multivitamin preparation.

Pediazole
Abbott, Canad.; Abbott, Fr.; Abbott, S.Afr.; Abbott, Switz.; Ross, USA.
Erythromycin ethyl succinate (p.204·2); acetyl sulphafurazole (p.253·3).
Otitis media.

Pedi-Bath *Pedinol, USA.*
Emollient.

Pedi-Boro Soak Paks *Pedinol, USA.*
Aluminium sulphate (p.1548·1); calcium acetate (p.1155·1).
Inflammatory skin disorders.

Pedi-Cort V *Pedinol, USA.*
Hydrocortisone (p.1043·3); clioquinol (p.193·2).
Skin disorders.

Pedi-Dent *Stanley, Canad.*
Sodium fluoride (p.742·1).
Dental caries prophylaxis.

Pediderm *Nelson, Austral.†.*
Tolnaftate (p.389·1).
Fungal skin infections.

Pedi-Dri *Pedinol, USA.*
Nystatin (p.386·1); menthol (p.1600·2).
Hyperhidrosis and bromhidrosis of the feet; tinea pedis.

Pedigesic *Parke-Med, S.Afr.*
Paracetamol (p.72·2); codeine phosphate (p.26·1); promethazine hydrochloride (p.416·2).
Fever; pain.

Pedikurol *Merckle, Aust.*
Clotrimazole (p.376·3).
Fungal skin and nail infections.

Pedil *Salters, S.Afr.*
Zinc undecenoate (p.389·2); undecenoic acid (p.389·2).
Fungal skin infections.

Pedimed *Restan, S.Afr.*
Aluminium oxide (p.1077·2); magnesium oxide (p.1198·3); methylpolysiloxane (p.1213·1).
Flatulence associated with hyperacidity.

Pedimycose *Scholl, Fr.†.*
Tolnaftate (p.389·1).
Fungal skin infections.

Pediotic *Glaxo Wellcome, USA.*
Hydrocortisone (p.1043·3); neomycin sulphate (p.229·2); polymyxin B sulphate (p.239·1).
Bacterial ear infections.

Pedi-Pro *Pedinol, USA.*
Aluminium chlorohydrate (p.1078·3); chloroxylenol (p.1111·1); menthol (p.1600·2); zinc undecenoate (p.389·2).
Fungal skin infections; minor skin disorders.

Pedisafe *BASF, Ger.*
Clotrimazole (p.376·3).
Fungal infections.

Peditrace
Pharmacia Upjohn, Aust.; Pharmacia Upjohn, Ger.; Pharmacia Upjohn, Irl.; Pharmacia Upjohn, Ital.; Pharmacia Upjohn, Neth.; Pharmacia Upjohn, Norw.; Pharmacia Upjohn, Swed.; Pharmacia Upjohn, Switz.; Pharmacia Upjohn, UK.
Trace-element preparation (p.1147·1).
Parenteral nutrition.

Pedituss Cough *Major, USA.*
Phenylephrine hydrochloride (p.1066·2); chlorpheniramine maleate (p.405·1); codeine phosphate (p.26·1); potassium iodide (p.1493·1).
Coughs.

Pedi-Vit-A *Pedinol, USA.*
Vitamin A (p.1358·1).
Irritated or dry skin.

Pedopur *Jacoby, Aust.*
Vitis vinifera.
Peripheral vascular disorders.

Pedoz *Hamilton, Austral.*
Tetrabromocresol (p.1126·3); undecenoic acid (p.389·2); zinc undecenoate (p.389·2); zinc oxide (p.1096·2).
Hyperhidrosis; skin irritation; tinea pedis.

Pedpain *Columbia, S.Afr.*
Paracetamol (p.72·2); codeine phosphate (p.26·1); promethazine hydrochloride (p.416·2).
Fever; pain.

Pedriachol *Propan, S.Afr.*
Phenobarbitone (p.350·2); pipenzolate bromide (p.467·1).
Gastro-intestinal disorders.

PedTE-PAK *SoloPak, USA.*
Trace element preparation.
Parenteral nutrition.

Pedtrace *Lyphomed, USA.*
Trace element preparation.
Parenteral nutrition.

PedvaxHIB
CSL, Austral.; Merck Sharp & Dohme, Canad.; Chiron Behring, Ger.; Merck Sharp & Dohme, Neth.†; Pasteur Merieux, Swed.; Merck Sharp & Dohme, Switz.†; Merck Sharp & Dohme, USA.
A haemophilus influenzae conjugate vaccine (meningococcal protein conjugate) (p.1511·1).
Active immunisation.

Peerless Composition Essence *Potter's, UK.*
Oak bark (p.1609·3); pinus canadensis; poplar bark (p.1620·1); prickly ash bark (p.1645·3); bayberry bark.
Colds.

Peflacin
Rhone-Poulenc Rorer, Ger.; Rhone-Poulenc Rorer, Ital.; Rhone-Poulenc Rorer, Neth.†.
Pefloxacin mesylate (p.236·1).
Bacterial infections.

Peflacine
Rhone-Poulenc Rorer, Aust.†; Rhone-Poulenc Rorer, Belg.;; Bellon, Fr.; Rhone-Poulenc Rorer, Spain.
Pefloxacin mesylate (p.236·1).
Bacterial infections.

Peflox *Formenti, Ital.*
Pefloxacin mesylate (p.236·1).
Bacterial infections.

Pefrakehl *Sanum-Kehlbeck, Ger.*
Homoeopathic preparation.

Peganone
Abbott, Norw.†; Abbott, USA.
Ethotoin (p.345·3).
Epilepsy.

Peglyte *Pharmascience, Canad.*
Macrogol 3350 (p.1598·2); electrolytes (p.1147·1).
Gastro-intestinal lavage.

Peinfort *Ebewe, Aust.†.*
Paracetamol (p.72·2).
Fever; pain.

Peitel *Novag, Spain.*
Prednicarbate (p.1047·3).
Skin disorders.

Pekamin *Medical, Spain.*
Benzylpenicillin sodium (p.159·3).
Bacterial infections.

Pekolin *Antigen, Irl.†.*
Light kaolin (p.1195·1); pectin (p.1474·1).
Diarrhoea.

Pektan N *Steigerwald, Ger.†.*
Cortex quercus (p.1609·3); fructus mali; kaolin (p.1195·1); semen cacao (p.1636·2).
Diarrhoea.

Pela Moorlauge *Pino, Ger.†.*
Peat.
Bath additive; peripheral circulatory disorders; rheumatism.

Pelamine *Major, USA†.*
Tripelennamine hydrochloride (p.420·2).
Hypersensitivity reactions.

Pelargon *Nestle, Fr.*
Infant feed.
Constipation; digestive disorders; regurgitation.

Pelarol *Qualiphar, Belg.†.*
Lotion: Resorcinol (p.1090·1); thymol (p.1127·1); menthol (p.1600·2); methyl salicylate (p.55·2); benzoic acid (p.1102·3); linoleyl linoleate.
Ointment: Resorcinol (p.1090·1); cade oil (p.1092·2); menthol (p.1600·2); camphor (p.1557·2); salicylic acid (p.1090·2); zinc oxide (p.1096·2); vitamin A substances (p.1358·1); ergocalciferol (p.1367·1); linoleyl linoleate.
Skin disorders.

Pelina *Rosen, Ger.*
Dexpanthenol (p.1570·3).
Skin and mucous membrane lesions.

Pellisal-Gel *Woelm, Ger.*
Diphenhydramine hydrochloride (p.409·1).
Allergic skin reactions; insect stings; minor burns; skin rashes; sunburn.

Pellit *Engelhard, Switz.†.*
Diphenhydramine hydrochloride (p.409·1); diethyltoluamide (p.1405·1); dimethyl phthalate (p.1405·3).
Insect bites; insect repellent; skin disorders.

Pellit Insektenstich, Pellit Sonnenallergie *Engelhard, Ger.*
Diphenhydramine hydrochloride (p.409·1).
Formerly contained diphenhydramine hydrochloride, diethyltoluamide, and dimethyl phthalate.
Allergic skin reactions; insect stings; minor burns.

Pellit Sonnenbrand *Engelhard, Ger.*
Hamamelis (p.1587·1).
Skin lesions and inflammation; sunburn.

Pellit Wund- und Heilsalbe *Engelhard, Ger.*
Tyrothricin (p.267·2); fomocaine hydrochloride; diphenhydramine hydrochloride (p.409·1).
Infected skin disorders.

Pelsano
Note. This name is used for preparations of different composition.
Schmidgall, Aust.; Iromedica, Switz.
Bath oil: Sunflower oil (p.1634·1); undecenoic acid (p.389·2).
Skin disorders.

Schmidgall, Aust.; Iromedica, Switz.
Ointment: Sunflower oil (p.1634·1); dexpanthenol (p.1570·3).
Skin disorders.

Schmidgall, Aust.
Topical powder: Zinc undecenoate (p.389·2).
Skin disorders.

Wolfs, Belg.
Undecenoic acid (p.389·2); zinc stearate (p.1469·3).
Skin disorders.

Pelson *Berenguer Infale, Spain.*
Nitrazepam (p.682·2).
Insomnia.

Pelsonfilina *Berenguer Infale, Spain†.*
Nitrazepam (p.682·2); theophylline glycinate (p.772·2).
Dyspnoea; insomnia.

Pelvichthol *Ichthyol, Aust.*
Ictasol (p.1083·3); benzyl nicotinate (p.22·1); homofenazine hydrochloride (p.675·2).
Urogenital disorders.

Pelvichthol N *Ichthyol, Ger.*
Ictasol (p.1083·3); benzyl nicotinate (p.22·1).
Pelvichthol formerly contained ictasol, benzyl nicotinate, and homofenazine hydrochloride.
General pelvic symptoms.

Pelvis *Coli, Ital.†.*
Oxolinic acid (p.235·1).
Bacterial infections of the urinary tract.

Pelvo Magnesium
3M, Belg.; 3M, Fr.†.
Onion (p.1610·2); magnesium carbonate (p.1198·1) or magnesium chloride (p.1157·2).
Painful pelvic congestion in females; prostate and micturition disorders in men.

Pemine *Lilly, Ital.*
Penicillamine hydrochloride (p.991·1).
Cystinuria; lead poisoning; rheumatoid arthritis; Wilson's disease.

PE-Mix *Leopold, Aust.*
Amino-acid, carbohydrate, electrolyte, and lipid (as soya oil (p.1355·1)).
Contains egg lecithin.
Parenteral nutrition.

Pemix *Prodes, Spain.*
Pirozadil (p.1277·1).
Hyperlipidaemias.

Pen 2 *MediSense, Canad.†.*
Test for glucose in blood (p.1585·1).

Penadur
SK-RIT, Belg.; Wyeth, Switz.†.
Benzathine penicillin (p.158·3).
Prevention of acute flares of rheumatoid arthritis; streptococcal infections of the throat; syphilis.

Penadur 6-3-3 *Wyeth, Switz.†.*
Benzathine penicillin (p.158·3); procaine penicillin (p.240·2); benzylpenicillin potassium (p.159·2).
Bacterial infections.

Penadur VK Mega *Wyeth, Switz.†.*
Phenoxymethylpenicillin potassium (p.236·2).
Bacterial infections.

Penampil *Nuovo, Ital.†.*
Ampicillin (p.153·1).
Bacterial infections.

Penaten
Note. This name is used for preparations of different composition.
Hilarys, Canad.
Hamamelis (p.1587·1); zinc oxide (p.1096·2).

Johnson & Johnson, Ital.
Cetylpyridinium chloride (p.1106·2).
Skin disinfection.

Pen-BASF *BASF, Ger.*
Phenoxymethylpenicillin potassium (p.236·2).
Bacterial infections.

Penbene *Merckle, Aust.*
Phenoxymethylpenicillin potassium (p.236·2).
Bacterial infections.

Penbeta *Betapharm, Ger.*
Phenoxymethylpenicillin potassium (p.236·2).
Bacterial infections.

Pen-Bristol *Grunenthal, Ger.†.*
Ampicillin sodium (p.153·1) or ampicillin trihydrate (p.153·2).
Bacterial infections.

Penbritin
SmithKline Beecham, Austral.†; Bencard, Belg.; Wyeth-Ayerst, Canad.; SmithKline Beecham, Irl.; SmithKline Beecham, S.Afr.; Beecham Research, UK.
Ampicillin sodium (p.153·1) or ampicillin trihydrate (p.153·2).
Bacterial infections.

Pencloxin *Lagap, Switz.†.*
Ampicillin trihydrate (p.153·2); cloxacillin sodium (p.195·2).
Bacterial infections.

Pendramine *Asta Medica, UK.*
Penicillamine (p.988·3).
Cystinuria; heavy-metal poisoning; hepatitis; rheumatoid arthritis; Wilson's disease.

Pendysin *Jenapharm, Ger.*
Benzathine penicillin (p.158·3).
Lignocaine hydrochloride (p.1293·2) is included in this preparation to alleviate the pain of injection.
Chronic streptococcal infections; syphilis.

Penecare
Penederm, Canad.; Reed & Carnrick, USA.
Emollient.

Penecort *Allergan Herbert, USA.*
Hydrocortisone (p.1043·3).
Skin disorders.

Penederm *Pharmascience, Canad.*
Cream: Lactic acid (p.1593·3); light liquid paraffin (p.1382·1).
Lotion: Lactic acid (p.1593·3).
Dry skin.

Penetradol *Fournier, Fr.†.*
Papain (p.1614·1); phenylbutazone (p.79·2).
Inflammation; pain.

Penetrating Rub *Golden Pride, Canad.; Rawleigh, Canad.*
Methyl salicylate (p.55·2); menthol (p.1600·2); eucalyptus oil (p.1578·1); cajuput oil (p.1556·1) expressed mustard oil (p.1605·3).

Penetrex *Warner-Lambert, USA.*
Enoxacin (p.203·3).
Gonorrhoea; urinary-tract infections.

Penetrol *Seton, UK.*
Inhalation: Menthol (p.1600·2); cajuput oil (p.1556·1); lavender oil (p.1594·3); otto lavend; eucalyptus oil (p.1578·1); peppermint oil (p.1208·1).
Lozenges: Ammonium chloride (p.1055·2); phenylephrine hydrochloride (p.1066·2); creosote (p.1057·3); menthol (p.1600·2).
Nasal congestion.

Peneytol *Wolfs, Belg.†.*
Zinc oxide (p.1096·2); bismuth subnitrate (p.1180·2); boric acid (p.1554·2); salicylic acid (p.1090·2); cod-liver oil (p.1337·3).
Skin irritation.

Penferm *Fermenta, Swed.†.*
Phenoxymethylpenicillin potassium (p.236·2).
Bacterial infections.

Penglobe
Astra, Aust.; Astra, Belg.; Astra, Canad.; Astra, Fr.; Astra, Ger.; Astra, Ital.; Astra, Neth.†; Astra, Spain; Astra, Swed.
Bacampicillin hydrochloride (p.157·2).
Bacterial infections.

Penhexal *Hexal, Ger.*
Phenoxymethylpenicillin potassium (p.236·2).
Bacterial infections.

Peniazol *Winzer, Ger.†.*
Tyrothricin (p.267·2); sulphathiazole (p.257·1).
Bacterial infections of the eye.

Penibiot *Normon, Spain.*
Benzylpenicillin sodium (p.159·3).
Bacterial infections.

Penibiot Lidocaina *Normon, Spain.*
Benzylpenicillin sodium (p.159·3).
Lignocaine hydrochloride (p.1293·2) is included in this preparation to alleviate the pain of injection.
Bacterial infections.

Penibiot Retard *Reig Jofre, Spain†.*
Benzylpenicillin sodium (p.159·3); procaine penicillin (p.240·2).
Bacterial infections; rheumatic fever.

Penicillat *Azupharma, Ger.*
Phenoxymethylpenicillin potassium (p.236·2).
Bacterial infections.

Penicilloral *Terapeutico, Ital.†.*
Phenethicillin sodium (p.236·2).
Bacterial infections.

Penicline *Delagrange, Fr.†.*
Ampicillin (p.153·1) or ampicillin sodium (p.153·1).
Bacterial infections.

Penidural
John Wyeth, Irl.†; Yamanouchi, Neth.; Wyeth, UK†.
Benzathine penicillin (p.158·3).
Bacterial infections.

Penidural D/F *Yamanouchi, Neth.*
Benzathine penicillin (p.158·3); procaine penicillin (p.240·2); benzylpenicillin potassium (p.159·2).
Bacterial infections.

Penilente Forte *Novo Nordisk, S.Afr.*
Benzathine penicillin (p.158·3); procaine penicillin (p.240·2); benzylpenicillin sodium (p.159·3).
Bacterial infections.

Penilente LA *Novo Nordisk, S.Afr.*
Benzathine penicillin (p.158·3).
Bacterial infections.

Penilevel *Ern, Spain.*
Capsules; oral sachets: Phenoxymethylpenicillin potassium (p.236·2).
Injection: Benzylpenicillin sodium (p.159·3).
Bacterial infections.

Penilevel Retard *Ern, Spain.*
Benzylpenicillin sodium (p.159·3); benzathine penicillin (p.158·3); phenoxymethylpenicillin calcium (p.236·2).
Bacterial infections; glomerulonephritis; rheumatic fever.

Penimox *IBSA, Switz.*
Amoxycillin (p.151·3) or amoxycillin trihydrate (p.151·3).
Bacterial infections.

Penimycin *Winzer, Ger.†.*
Tyrothricin (p.267·2); dihydrostreptomycin sulphate (p.202·2).
Eye infections.

Peni-Oral *Wyeth, Belg.†.*
Phenoxymethylpenicillin potassium (p.236·2).
Bacterial infections.

Peniroger *UCB, Spain.*
Benzylpenicillin sodium (p.159·3).
Bacterial infections.

Peniroger Procain *Roger, Spain†.*
Benzylpenicillin sodium (p.159·3); procaine penicillin (p.240·2).
Bacterial infections; rheumatic fever.

Peniroger Retard *Roger, Spain†.*
Benzathine penicillin (p.158·3).
Bacterial infections; rheumatic fever.

Penisintex Bronquial *Jorba, Spain.*
Ampicillin sodium (p.153·1); ampicillin benzathine (p.154·1); bromhexine (p.1055·3).
Lignocaine hydrochloride (p.1293·2) is included in this preparation to alleviate the pain of injection.
Respiratory-tract infections.

Penisol *Ecosol, Switz.*
Phenoxymethylpenicillin potassium (p.236·2).
Bacterial infections.

Penitardon *Rorer, Ger.†.*
Buphenine hydrochloride (p.1555·3).
Central and peripheral vascular disorders.

Pen-Kera *Ascher, USA.*
Emollient and moisturiser.

Penles *Lederle, Jpn.*
Lignocaine (p.1293·2).
Pain of inserting intravenous needles.

PenMix 10/90, 20/80, 30/70, 40/60, 50/50 *Novo Nordisk, UK†.*
Mixtures of insulin injection (human, pyr) and isophane insulin suspension (human, pyr) respectively in the proportions indicated (p.322·1).
Diabetes mellitus.

Penmox *Compu, S.Afr.*
Amoxycillin (p.151·3).
Bacterial infections.

Pennine *Thornton & Ross, UK†.*
Zinc sulphate (p.1373·2); hamamelis (p.1587·1); benzalkonium chloride (p.1101·3).
Eye irritation.

Penntuss *Rhone-Poulenc Rorer, Canad.*
Codeine polistirex (p.27·1); chlorpheniramine polistirex (p.405·2).
Allergic rhinitis; coughs and cold symptoms.

Pen-Os *Biochemie, Aust.*
Benzathine phenoxymethylpenicillin (p.159·2).
Bacterial infections.

Penrite *Columbia, S.Afr.*
Ampicillin trihydrate (p.153·2).
Bacterial infections.

Pensacaine with Adrenaline *Astra, UK†.*
Lignocaine hydrochloride (p.1293·2).
Adrenaline (p.813·2) is included in this preparation as a vasoconstrictor to diminish absorption and localise the effect of the local anaesthetic.
Local anaesthesia.

Pensatron *Pensa, Spain†.*
Droxicam (p.35·2).
Ankylosing spondylitis; arthritis; inflammation.

Pensig *Sigma, Austral.†.*
Phenethicillin potassium (p.236·2).
Bacterial infections.

Penstabil *Medphano, Ger.†.*
Ampicillin trihydrate (p.153·2).
Bacterial infections.

Penstapho
Bristol-Myers Squibb, Belg.; Bristol-Myers Squibb, Ital.
Oxacillin sodium (p.234·2).
Gram-positive bacterial infections.

Penstapho N *Bristol-Myers Squibb, Belg.*
Cloxacillin sodium (p.195·2).
Staphylococcal infections.

Pensulvit *SIFI, Ital.*
Tetracycline (p.259·1); sulfamethylthiazole (p.251·3).
Bacterial eye infections.

Penta-3B *Sabex, Canad.*
Thiamine hydrochloride (p.1361·1); pyridoxine hydrochloride (p.1362·3); cyanocobalamin (p.1363·3).
Alcoholism; neuritis; vitamin B supplement.

Penta-3B + C *Sabex, Canad.*
Thiamine hydrochloride (p.1361·1); pyridoxine hydrochloride (p.1362·3); cyanocobalamin (p.1363·3); ascorbic acid (p.1365·2).
Alcoholism; neuritis; vitamin supplement.

Penta-3B Plus *Sabex, Canad.*
Multivitamin preparation.

Pentabil *OFF, Ital.*
Fenipentol (p.1579·1).
Hepatic and biliary-tract disorders.

Pentacard *Byk, Belg.*
Isosorbide mononitrate (p.893·3).
Angina pectoris.

Pentacarinat
Gerot, Aust.; Rhone-Poulenc Rorer, Austral.†; Rhone-Poulenc Rorer, Belg.; Rhone-Poulenc Rorer, Canad.; Bellon, Fr.; Rhone-Poulenc Rorer, Ger.; Glaxo Wellcome, Ger.; Rhone-Poulenc Rorer, Irl.; Rhone-Poulenc Rorer, Ital.; Rhone-Poulenc Rorer, Neth.; Rhone-Poulenc Rorer, Norw.; Rhone-Poulenc Rorer, S.Afr.; Rhone-Poulenc Rorer, Spain; Rhone-Poulenc Rorer, Swed.; Rhone-Poulenc Rorer, Switz.; Rhone-Poulenc Rorer, UK; Armour, USA.
Pentamidine isethionate (p.590·2).
African trypanosomiasis; leishmaniasis; Pneumocystis carinii pneumonia.

Pentacin *Farmaka, Ital.†.*
Pentamycin (p.386·3).
Vulvovaginal infections.

Pentacine *Vifor, Switz.*
Pentamycin (p.386·3).
Vaginitis.

Pentacol *Sofar, Ital.*
Mesalazine (p.1199·2).
Inflammatory bowel disease.

Pentacoq *Merieux, Fr.*
Vial, a haemophilus influenzae conjugate vaccine (tetanus toxoid conjugate) (Act-HIB) (p.1511·1); syringe, a diphtheria, tetanus, pertussis, and poliomyelitis vaccine (Tetracoq) (p.1509·3).
Active immunisation.

Pentafen *Zoja, Ital.*
Pentazocine lactate (p.75·1).
Pain.

Pentagamma *IBP, Ital.†.*
Dithranol (p.1082·1); cade oil (p.1092·2); precipitated sulphur (p.1091·2).
Skin disorders.

Pentaglobin
Biotest, Aust.; Biotest, Ger.; Biotest, Ital.; Biotest, Switz.
A normal immunoglobulin (p.1522·1).
Immunoglobulin deficiency; passive immunisation.

Pental Col *Cederroth, Spain†.*
Alcohol (p.1099·1); benzethonium chloride (p.1102·3).
Skin disinfection.

Pental Forte *Cederroth, Spain.*
Benzalkonium chloride (p.1101·3); mafenide (p.223·2); sulphanilamide (p.256·3); zinc oxide (p.1096·2).
Skin infections.

Pentalgina *Pierrel, Ital.*
Pentazocine lactate (p.75·1).
Pain.

Pentalmicina *Cederroth, Spain.*
Enoxolone (p.35·2); mafenide (p.223·2); neomycin sulphate (p.229·2); sulphanilamide (p.256·3).
Skin infections.

Pentalong *Isis, Ger.*
Pentaerythritol tetranitrate (p.927·3).
Angina pectoris; heart failure.

Pentam 300 *Lyphomed, USA.*
Pentamidine isethionate (p.590·2).
Pneumocystis carinii pneumonia.

Pentamycetin *Sabex, Canad.*
Chloramphenicol (p.182·1).
Eye infections.

Pentamycetin-HC *Sabex, Canad.*
Chloramphenicol (p.182·1); hydrocortisone acetate (p.1043·3).
Eye and ear infections.

Pentaneural *Wyeth, Ger.†.*
Meprobamate (p.678·1); pentaerythritol tetranitrate (p.927·3).
Angina pectoris.

Pentasa
Sigmapharm, Aust.; Yamanouchi, Belg.; Hoechst Marion Roussel, Canad.; Ferring, Fr.; Ferring, Ger.; Yamanouchi, Irl.; Yamanouchi, Ital.; Yamanouchi, Neth.; Ferring, Norw.; Ferring, Swed.; Ferring, Switz.; Ferring, UK; Marion Merrell Dow, USA.
Mesalazine (p.1199·2).
Inflammatory bowel disease.

Pentaspan
Du Pont, Canad.; Du Pont Pharmaceuticals, UK; Du Pont, USA.
Pentastarch (p.725·2).
Leucopheresis; plasma volume expansion.

Penta-Thion *Sabex, Canad.*
Ascorbic acid (p.1365·2); thiamine (p.1361·2).
Vitamin supplement.

Pentatop *Life, Ger.*
Sodium cromoglycate (p.762·1).
Hypersensitivity reactions.

Pentavac *Pasteur Merieux, Swed.*
A diphtheria, tetanus, pertussis, poliomyelitis, and haemophilus influenzae vaccine.
Active immunisation.

Pentavenon *Godecke, Ger.†.*
Ointment: Aesculus (p.1543·3); troxerutin (p.1580·2); heparin (p.879·3).
Oral drops: Aesculus (p.1543·3); adenosine (p.812·3); troxerutin (p.1580·2).
Tablets: Aesculus (p.1543·3); inositol nicotinate (p.891·3); adenosine (p.812·3); rutoside (p.1580·2); pholedrine sulphate (p.930·2).
Skin trauma; vascular disorders.

Penta-Vite *Roche Consumer, Austral.*
Multivitamin preparation.

Penta-Vite Chewable Multi Vitamins with Minerals *Roche Consumer, Austral.*
Multivitamin and mineral preparation.

Pentavitol *Hafslund Nycomed, Aust.*
Multivitamin preparation.

Pentazine *Century, USA†.*
Promethazine hydrochloride (p.416·2).
Hypersensitivity reactions; motion sickness; nausea; postoperative pain (adjunct); sedative; vomiting.

Pentazine VC with Codeine *Century, USA.*
Promethazine hydrochloride (p.416·2); codeine phosphate (p.26·1).
Coughs and cold symptoms.

Pent-HIBest *Pasteur Vaccins, Fr.*
Vial, a haemophilus influenzae conjugate vaccine (tetanus toxoid conjugate) (HIBest) (p.1511·1); syringe, a diphtheria, tetanus, pertussis, and poliomyelitis vaccine (DTCP) (p.1509·3).
Active immunisation.

Penthrane
Abbott, Austral.†; Abbott, Ger.†; Abbott, USA†.
Methoxyflurane (p.1228·2).
General anaesthesia.

Penticort
Lederle, Fr.; Cyanamid, Ital.†.
Amcinonide (p.1032·1).
Skin disorders.

Penticort Neomycine *Lederle, Fr.*
Amcinonide (p.1032·1); neomycin sulphate (p.229·2).
Infected skin disorders.

Pentids *Apothecon, USA†.*
Benzylpenicillin potassium (p.159·2).
Bacterial infections.

Pentoderm *Biosarto, Spain†.*
Arnica (p.1550·3); boric acid (p.1554·2); dexpanthenol (p.1570·3); sodium polygalacturonate sulphonate; undecenoic acid (p.389·2); phenoxyethanol (p.1122·2); ovolecithin.
Fungal skin infections.

Pentoflux *Bouchara, Fr.*
Oxpentifylline (p.925·3).
Intermittent claudication; mental function impairment in the elderly.

Pentohexal *Hexal, Ger.*
Oxpentifylline (p.925·3).
Peripheral vascular disorders.

Pentolair *Bausch & Lomb, USA.*
Cyclopentolate hydrochloride (p.459·3).

Pentomer *Merckle, Aust.*
Oxpentifylline (p.925·3).
Cerebral, ocular and peripheral vascular disorders; ear disorders.

Pento-Puren *Isis Puren, Ger.*
Oxpentifylline (p.925·3).
Peripheral vascular disorders.

Pentostam *Wellcome, UK.*
Sodium stibogluconate (p.578·3).
Leishmaniasis.

Pentothal
Abbott, Austral.; Abbott, Belg.; Abbott, Canad.; Abbott, Ital.; Abbott, Norw.; Abbott, Spain; Abbott, Swed.; Abbott, Switz.; Abbott, USA.
Thiopentone sodium (p.1233·1).
Convulsions; general anaesthesia; sedative.

Pentovena *Boehringer Mannheim, Spain.*
Diosmin (p.1580·1).
Peripheral vascular disorders.

Pentox *CT, Ger.*
Oxpentifylline (p.925·3).
Peripheral vascular disorders.

Pentoxi
Genericon, Aust.; Mepha, Switz.
Oxpentifylline (p.925·3).
Vascular disorders.

Pentran *Berk, UK.*
Phenytoin sodium (p.352·3).
Epilepsy; trigeminal neuralgia.

Pentrax
Note. This name is used for preparations of different composition.
GenDerm, Canad.; Helsinn Birex, Irl.; Euroderma, UK; GenDerm, USA.
Coal tar (Fractar) (p.1092·3).
Scalp disorders.
Rydelle, Ital.
Coal tar (Fractar) (p.1092·3); salicylic acid (p.1090·2).
Seborrhoeic dermatitis.

Pentrax Gold *GenDerm, USA.*
Coal tar (p.1092·3).
Scalp disorders.

Pentrex *Bristol-Myers Squibb, S.Afr.†.*
Ampicillin trihydrate (p.153·2).
Bacterial infections.

Pentrex-F *Bristol-Myers Squibb, S.Afr.†.*
Ampicillin (p.153·1); nystatin (p.386·1).
Bacterial infections; candidiasis.

Pentrexyl
Bristol-Myers Squibb, Belg.; Bristol-Myers Squibb, Irl.†; Bristol-Myers Squibb, Ital.; Bristol-Myers Squibb, Neth.; Bristol-Myers Squibb, Norw.; Bristol-Myers Squibb, Swed.
Ampicillin (p.153·1), ampicillin sodium (p.153·1), or ampicillin trihydrate (p.153·2).
Bacterial infections.

Pentrones *Rhone Poulenc Chemicals, UK.*
A range of non-ionic and anionic surfactants.

Pentylan *Lannett, USA.*
Pentaerythritol tetranitrate (p.927·3).
Angina pectoris.

Pen-V *Goldline, USA†.*
Phenoxymethylpenicillin potassium (p.236·2).
Bacterial infections.

pen-V-basan *Sagitta, Ger.†.*
Phenoxymethylpenicillin potassium (p.236·2).
Bacterial infections.

Pen-Vee *Lioh, Canad.*
Benzathine phenoxymethylpenicillin (p.159·2) or phenoxymethylpenicillin (p.236·2).
Bacterial infections.

Pen-Vee K *Wyeth-Ayerst, USA.*
Phenoxymethylpenicillin potassium (p.236·2).
Bacterial infections.

Peobe *Sanofi Winthrop, Spain†.*
Piracetam (p.1619·1); pyridoxine hydrochloride (p.1362·3).
Alcoholism; mental function impairment; vertigo.

PEP *Galpharm, UK.*
Glucose (p.1343·3); caffeine (p.749·3).
Fatigue.

Pepcid
Amrad, Austral.; Merck Sharp & Dohme, Canad.; Johnson & Johnson, Canad.; Morson, Irl.; Pharmacia Upjohn, Neth.; Pharmacia Upjohn, Norw.; Merck Sharp & Dohme, S.Afr.; Pharmacia Upjohn, Swed.; Johnson & Johnson MSD Consumer, UK; Merck Sharp & Dohme, USA.
Famotidine (p.1192·1).
Dyspepsia; gastro-oesophageal reflux; heartburn; peptic ulcer; Zollinger-Ellison syndrome.

Pepcidac *Martin, Fr.*
Famotidine (p.1192·1).
Gastro-oesophageal reflux.

Pepcidin
Merck Sharp & Dohme, Neth.; Merck Sharp & Dohme, Norw.; Merck Sharp & Dohme, Swed.
Famotidine (p.1192·1).
Gastro-oesophageal reflux; peptic ulcer; Zollinger-Ellison syndrome.

Pepcidine
Merck Sharp & Dohme, Aust.; Merck Sharp & Dohme, Austral.; Merck Sharp & Dohme, Belg.; Merck Sharp & Dohme, Switz.
Famotidine (p.1192·1).
Gastro-oesophageal reflux; peptic ulcer; Zollinger-Ellison syndrome.

Pepdine *Merck Sharp & Dohme-Chibret, Fr.*
Famotidine (p.1192·1).
Gastro-oesophageal reflux; peptic ulcer; Zollinger-Ellison syndrome.

Pepdite
Scientific Hospital Supplies, Irl.; Scientific Hospital Supplies, UK.
Infant feed.
Bowel disorders; malabsorption syndromes; protein or lactose intolerance.

Pepdul *MSD Chibropharm, Ger.*
Famotidine (p.1192·1).
Peptic ulcer; upper gastro-intestinal haemorrhage; Zollinger-Ellison syndrome.

Pepleo *Kayaku, Jpn.*
Peplomycin sulphate (p.558·1).
Malignant neoplasms.

Pepp *Theranol-Deglaude, Fr.*
Dimethicone (p.1213·1); aluminium hydroxide (p.1177·3); magnesium hydroxide (p.1198·2).
Gastro-intestinal disorders.

Pepsaldra Engelhard, Ger.†.
Pepsin (p.1616·3); glutamic acid hydrochloride (p.1344·3).
Gastro-intestinal disorders.

Pepsaldra compositum N Engelhard, Ger.†.
Pepsin (p.1616·3); pancreas powder (p.1612·1).
Gastro-intestinal disorders.

Pepsaletten N Palmicol, Ger.
Glutamic acid hydrochloride (p.1344·3).
Gastro-intestinal disorders.

Pepsamar Sanofi Winthrop, Spain.
Aluminium hydroxide (p.1177·3).
Gastro-intestinal hyperacidity; hyperphosphataemia.

Pepsane
Rosa-Phytopharma, Fr.; Rosa-Phytopharma, Switz.†.
Guaiazulene (p.1586·3); dimethicone (p.1213·1).
Gastro-intestinal disorders.

Pepsillide Cambridge Laboratories, Austral.†.
Bismuth subnitrate (p.1180·2); magnesium carbonate (p.1198·1); sodium bicarbonate (p.1153·2); frangula bark (p.1193·2); liquorice (p.1197·1).
Gastro-intestinal disorders.

Pepsiton Unipack, Aust.
Pepsin (p.1616·3); absinthium (p.1541·1).
Gastro-intestinal disorders.

Peptac Norton, UK.
Sodium alginate (p.1470·3); sodium bicarbonate (p.1153·2); calcium carbonate (p.1182·1).
Gastro-oesophageal reflux; heartburn; hiatus hernia.

Peptamen
Clintec, Irl.; Clintec, Ital.; Nestle, UK; Carnation, USA.
Preparation for enteral nutrition.
Gastro-intestinal disorders.

Peptard Riker, UK†.
Hyoscyamine sulphate (p.464·2).
Gastro-intestinal hypersecretion; gastro-intestinal spasm.

Peptarom Fresenius, Ger.†.
Ursodeoxycholic acid (p.1642·1).
Dyspepsia; gallstones.

Peptavlon
Zeneca, Aust.; Wyeth-Ayerst, Canad.; Zeneca, Fr.; Zeneca, Irl.†; Zeneca, Norw.†; Zeneca, Swed.†; Zeneca, Switz.; Cambridge, UK; Ayerst, USA.
Pentagastrin (p.1616·3).
Now known as Pentagastrin Injection in the *UK*.
Test of gastric secretory function.

Peptazol Boehringer Mannheim, Ital.
Pantoprazole sodium (p.1207·3).
Gastro-oesophageal reflux; peptic ulcer.

Pepti-2000 LF
Nutricia, Irl.; Nutricia, UK.
Gluten-free preparation for enteral nutrition.
Formerly known as Nutranel in the *UK*.

Peptichemio Nuovo ISM, Ital.
Multialchilpeptide (p.554·2).
Myeloproliferative disorders.

Pepticum Andromaco, Spain.
Omeprazole (p.1204·2).
Gastro-oesophageal reflux; peptic ulcer; Zollinger-Ellison syndrome.

Pepti-Junior
Nutricia, Fr.; Cow & Gate, Irl.; Nutricia, Ital.; Cow & Gate, UK.
Food for special diets.
Diarrhoea; food intolerance; malabsorption.

Peptimax Ashbourne, UK.
Cimetidine (p.1183·2).
Gastro-intestinal disorders.

Peptinaut
Nutricia, Fr.†; Nutricia, Ital.
Preparation for enteral nutrition.

Peptireal Sodietal, Fr.
A range of preparations for enteral nutrition.

Peptison
Nutricia, Fr.†; Nutricia, Ital.
Preparation for enteral nutrition.

Peptisorb
Pfrimmer Nutricia, Switz.; E. Merck, UK†.
Range of preparations for enteral nutrition.

Peptisorbon E. Merck, UK†.
Fructose- and gluten-free, low-lactose preparation for enteral nutrition.

Pepto Diarrhea Control Procter & Gamble, USA.
Loperamide hydrochloride (p.1197·2).
Diarrhoea.

Pepto Pancreasi Composta Serono, Ital.†.
Pepsin (p.1616·3); pancreatin (p.1612·1); amylase (p.1549·1).
Digestive system disorders.

Pepto-Bismol
Note. This name is used for preparations of different composition.
Procter & Gamble, Canad.; Procter & Gamble (H&B Care), UK; Procter & Gamble, USA.
Caplets; chewable tablets; oral liquid: Bismuth salicylate (p.1180·1).
Diarrhoea; dyspepsia; nausea; upset stomach.

Procter & Gamble, Canad.
Tablets: Calcium carbonate (p.1182·1); bismuth salicylate (p.1180·1).
Diarrhoea; dyspepsia; nausea; upset stomach.

Peptol Carter Horner, Canad.
Cimetidine (p.1183·2).
Gastric acid hypersecretion.

Pepto-Pancreasi Whitehall, Ital.
Pepsin (p.1616·3); pancreatin (p.1612·1).
Digestive system disorders.

Pep-uls-ade Cambridge Laboratories, Austral.†.
Bismuth subnitrate (p.1180·2); magnesium carbonate (p.1198·1); sodium bicarbonate (p.1153·2); frangula bark (p.1193·2).
Gastro-intestinal disorders.

Pepzitrat Berlin-Chemie, Ger.
Pepsin (p.1616·3); citric acid (p.1564·3).
Gastro-intestinal disorders.

Peracan Solvay, Belg.†.
Isoaminile (p.1063·2).
Coughs.

Peracel Monot, Fr.
Loperamide hydrochloride (p.1197·2).
Diarrhoea.

Peracil Boniscontro & Gazzone, Ital.
Piperacillin sodium (p.237·2).
Lignocaine hydrochloride (p.1293·2) is included in this preparation to alleviate the pain of injection.
Bacterial infections.

Peracon
Kali, Aust.; Solvay, Ger.; Hoechst Marion Roussel, S.Afr.
Isoaminile citrate (p.1063·2) or isoaminile cyclamate (p.1063·2).
Coughs.

Peracon Expectorant Hoechst Marion Roussel, S.Afr.
Isoaminile cyclamate (p.1063·2); ammonium chloride (p.1055·2).
Coughs.

Peragit AFI, Norw.†.
Benzhexol hydrochloride (p.457·3).
Parkinsonism.

Peralgon Sarm, Ital.†.
Indomethacin (p.45·2).
Musculoskeletal and joint disorders.

Peran BASF, Ger.
Acemetacin (p.12·2).
Gout; inflammation; musculoskeletal, joint, and periarticular disorders.

Perasthman N Polypharm, Ger.
Theophylline (p.765·1).
Obstructive airways disease.

Perative Abbott, UK.
Preparation for enteral nutrition.

Perazolin Zenyaku, Jpn.
Sobuzoxane (p.561·3).
Leukaemia; lymphoma.

Perbilen Hoechst, Spain.
Piretanide (p.931·3).
Hypertension; oedema.

Perborina Pagni, Ital.†.
Anhydrous sodium percarbonate.
Oral and genital disinfection.

Percase Millot-Solac, Fr.†.
Heparin (p.879·3).
Haemorrhoids and other rectal disorders; superficial phlebitis.

Perchloracap Mallinckrodt, USA.
Potassium perchlorate (p.1496·1).
To reduce accumulation of pertechnetate by the choroid plexus, salivary glands, and thyroid.

Perclar Parke, Davis, Ital.
Mesoglycan sodium (p.1602·3).
Thrombosis prophylaxis.

Perclodin Pinewood, Irl.†.
Dipyridamole (p.857·1).
Platelet disorders.

Perclusone SERB, Fr.
Clofezone (p.25·3); clofexamide hydrochloride (p.25·3).
Musculoskeletal, joint, peri-articular, and soft-tissue disorders; superficial phlebitis.

Percocet
Du Pont, Canad.; Du Pont, USA.
Oxycodone hydrochloride (p.71·2); paracetamol (p.72·2).
Fever; pain.

Percodan
Note. This name is used for preparations of different composition.
Boots, Austral.†.
Oxycodone hydrochloride (p.71·2); aspirin (p.16·1); paracetamol (p.72·2).
Pain.

Du Pont, Canad.
Oxycodone hydrochloride (p.71·2); aspirin (p.16·1).
Fever; inflammation; pain.

Du Pont, USA.
Oxycodone hydrochloride (p.71·2); oxycodone terephthalate (p.71·3); aspirin (p.16·1).
Pain.

Percoffedrinol N Passauer, Ger.
Caffeine (p.749·3).
Fatigue.

Percogesic Richardson-Vicks, USA.
Paracetamol (p.72·2); phenyltoloxamine citrate (p.416·1).
Fever; pain.

Percorina Boehringer Ingelheim, Spain.
Isosorbide mononitrate (p.893·3).
Angina pectoris; heart failure.

Percorten Ciba-Geigy, Aust.†.
Deoxycortone acetate (p.1036·2).
Corticosteroid.

Percutacrine Thyroxinique Besins-Iscovesco, Fr.†.
Thyroxine (p.1498·3).
Local treatment of excess adipose tissue.

Percutafeine Pierre Fabre, Fr.
Caffeine (p.749·3).
Obesity.

Percutalgine
Piette, Belg.; Besins-Iscovesco, Fr.
Dexamethasone (p.1037·1) or dexamethasone acetate (p.1037·1); salicylamide (p.82·3); glycol salicylate (p.43·1).
Musculoskeletal, joint, peri-articular, and soft-tissue disorders.

Percutalin Berenguer Infale, Spain.
Dexamethasone (p.1037·1) or dexamethasone acetate (p.1037·1) salicylamide (p.82·3); glycol salicylate (p.43·1); methyl nicotinate (p.55·1).
Musculoskeletal, joint, peri-articular, and soft-tissue disorders.

Percutase N Godecke, Ger.
Glycol salicylate (p.43·1); benzyl nicotinate (p.22·1).
Formerly contained glycol salicylate, heparin, benzyl nicotinate, and nonivamide.
Musculoskeletal and joint disorders.

Percutol
Rorer, Irl.†; Dominion, UK.
Glyceryl trinitrate (p.874·3).
Angina pectoris.

Percyl Bergamon, Ital.†.
Chlorhexidine gluconate (p.1107·2).
Disinfection.

Perdiem Rhone-Poulenc Rorer, USA.
Psyllium (p.1194·2); senna (p.1212·2).
Constipation.

Perdiem Fiber Rhone-Poulenc Rorer, USA.
Psyllium (p.1194·2).
Constipation.

Perdiphen Spitzner, Ger.; Schwabe, Ger.
Ephedrine hydrochloride (p.1059·3); paracetamol (p.72·2); diphenylpyraline hydrochloride (p.409·3).
Influenza symptoms.

Perdiphen phyto Spitzner, Ger.; Schwabe, Ger.
Primula rhizome; thyme (p.1636·3).
Cold symptoms.

Perdiphen-N Spitzner, Ger.†; Schwabe, Ger.†.
Paracetamol (p.72·2); thyme (p.1636·3); primula.
Coughs with feverish colds.

Perdipina Sandoz, Ital.
Nicardipine hydrochloride (p.915·1).
Angina pectoris; heart failure; hypertension.

Perdipine Yamanouchi, Jpn.
Nicardipine hydrochloride (p.915·1).
Cerebrovascular disorders; hypertension.

Perdix Schwarz, UK.
Moexipril hydrochloride (p.912·1).
Hypertension.

Perdolan Janssen-Cilag, Belg.
Suppositories (baby and infant): Aspirin (p.16·1); paracetamol (p.72·2); codeine phosphate (p.26·1).
Tablets; suppositories (adult): Aspirin (p.16·1); paracetamol (p.72·2); caffeine (p.749·3); codeine phosphate (p.26·1).
Fever; pain.

Perdolan Duo Janssen-Cilag, Belg.
Paracetamol (p.72·2); codeine phosphate (p.26·1).
Pain.

Perdolan Mono Janssen-Cilag, Belg.
Paracetamol (p.72·2).
Fever; pain.

Perdolan Mono C Janssen-Cilag, Belg.
Paracetamol (p.72·2); ascorbic acid (p.1365·2).
Fever; pain.

Perduretas Codeina Medea, Spain.
Codeine phosphate (p.26·1).
Cough; diarrhoea; pain.

Perebron
Angelini, Ital.; Farma Lepori, Spain.
Oxolamine citrate (p.1065·3) or oxolamine phosphate (p.1065·3).
Adjunct in obstructive airways disease; coughs.

Pereflat Solvay, Fr.
Dimethicone (p.1213·1); pancreas extract (porcine).
Dyspepsia.

Peremesin
Note. This name is used for preparations of different composition.
Bristol-Myers Squibb, Ger.
Meclozine hydrochloride (p.413·3).
Nausea; vertigo; vomiting.

Bristol-Myers Squibb, Norw.
Meclozine hydrochloride (p.413·3); caffeine (p.749·3).
Nausea; vertigo; vomiting.

Peremesin N Bristol-Myers Squibb, Ger.
Meclozine hydrochloride (p.413·3).
Formerly contained meclozine hydrochloride and caffeine.
Nausea; vertigo; vomiting.

Peremesine Squibb, Switz.†.
Suppositories: Meclozine hydrochloride (p.413·3).
Tablets: Meclozine hydrochloride (p.413·3); caffeine (p.749·3).
Nausea; vertigo; vomiting.

Peremin Sandoz, Aust.
Paracetamol (p.72·2); pheniramine maleate (p.415·3); phenylephrine hydrochloride (p.1066·2); ascorbic acid (p.1365·2).
Cold and influenza symptoms.

Perenan Sanofi Winthrop, Fr.
Co-dergocrine mesylate (p.1566·1).
Mental function impairment in the elderly.

Perennia Wyeth Lederle, Aust.
Red-brown tablets, conjugated oestrogens (p.1457·3); white tablets, medroxyprogesterone acetate (p.1448·3).
Menopausal disorders.

Perenterol
Thiemann, Ger.; Biocodex, Switz.
Saccharomyces boulardii (p.1594·1).
Acne; diarrhoea.

Peresal
Henkel, Ger.; Henkel, Ital.
Peracetic acid (p.1121·1); hydrogen peroxide (p.1116·2).
Instrument disinfection.

Perfadex Medisan, Swed.
Dextran 40 (p.716·2) in electrolytes.
Organ perfusion before transplantation.

Perfan
Hoechst Marion Roussel, Belg.; Hoechst, Ger.; Hoechst Marion Roussel, Irl.; Lepetit, Ital.; Hoechst Marion Roussel, Neth.; Hoechst Marion Roussel, UK.
Enoximone (p.865·1).
Heart failure.

Perfane Marion Merrell, Fr.
Enoximone (p.865·1).
Heart failure.

Perfectil Vitabiotics, UK.
Multivitamin, amino-acid, and mineral preparation.

Perflamint Pfleger, Ger.†.
Peppermint oil (p.1208·1); menthol (p.1600·2); acriflavine (p.1098·3).
Coughs and cold symptoms; infections of the oropharynx.

Perflux Leopold, Aust.
Electrolyte infusion (p.1147·1).
Forced diuresis.

Perfolate Asta Medica, Fr.
Calcium folinate (p.1342·2).
Drug-induced megaloblastic anaemia; folate deficiency; prevention of methotrexate toxicity.

Perfolin Gambar, Ital.
Calcium folinate (p.1342·2).
Anaemias; antidote to folic acid antagonists; folate deficiency.

Perform Schulke & Mayr, Ger.
Potassium peroxymonosulphate.
Surface disinfection.

Perfudal Schering-Plough, Spain.
Felodipine (p.867·3).
Angina pectoris; hypertension.

Perfudan Piam, Ital.
Buflomedil hydrochloride (p.834·2).
Cerebral and peripheral vascular disorders.

Perfus Multivitaminico Rius, Spain.
Carbazochrome (p.714·1); vitamins; electrolytes.
Haemorrhage; skeletal muscle disorders.

Perfusion de PAS Bichsel, Switz.
Sodium aminosalicylate (p.151·1).
Tuberculosis.

Perfusion mixte Streuli, Switz.
Sodium chloride (p.1162·2) infusion with glucose.
Dehydration.

Pergagel Albert-Roussel, Ger.†.
Sodium apolate (p.943·2).
Skin trauma.

Pergalen
Hoechst, Austral.†; Hoechst, Fr.†; Albert-Roussel, Ger.†.
Sodium apolate (p.943·2); benzyl nicotinate (p.22·1).
Peripheral vascular disorders; soft tissue disorders.

Perganit Astra, Ital.
Glyceryl trinitrate (p.874·3).
Angina pectoris; hypertension; pulmonary oedema.

Pergastric Prodes, Spain.
Dimethicone (p.1213·1).
Flatulence.

Perginol Gambar, Ital.
Sodium tetrachloroiodite.
Gynaecological infections.

Pergogreen
Serono, Ital.; Serono, Swed.†; Serono, Switz.
Menotrophin (p.1252·1).
Male and female infertility.

Pergonal
Serono, Aust.; Serono, Austral.†; Serono, Belg.†; Serono, Canad.; Serono, Ger.; Serono, Irl.; Serono, Ital.†; Serono, Neth.; Serono, Norw.†; Research Labs, S.Afr.; Serono, Spain; Serono, Swed.†; Serono, Switz.; Serono, UK; Serono, USA.
Menotrophin (p.1252·1).
Male and female infertility.

Pergotime
Serono, Belg.†; Serono, Fr.; Serono, Ger.; Serono, Norw.; Serono, Swed.
Clomiphene citrate (p.1439·2).
Anovulatory infertility.

Perhepar Lepetit, Ital.†.
Vitamin B substances.

Periactin
Merck Sharp & Dohme, Aust.; Merck Sharp & Dohme, Austral.; Merck Sharp & Dohme, Belg.; Johnson & Johnson, Canad.; Merck Sharp & Dohme, Irl.; Neopharmed, Ital.; Merck Sharp & Dohme, Neth.; Merck Sharp & Dohme, Norw.†; Merck Sharp & Dohme, S.Afr.; Sigma-Tau, Spain; Merck Sharp & Dohme, Swed.; Merck Sharp & Do-

hme, Switz.; Merck Sharp & Dohme, UK; Merck Sharp & Dohme, USA.
Cyproheptadine hydrochloride (p.407·2).
Hypersensitivity reactions; migraine; pruritus; reduced appetite; vascular headache.

Periactin B-C Logos, S.Afr.†.
Cyproheptadine hydrochloride (p.407·2); vitamin B substances with vitamin C.
Reduced appetite.

Periactin Vita Logos, S.Afr.†.
Cyproheptadine hydrochloride (p.407·2); multivitamins.
Reduced appetite.

Periactine Merck Sharp & Dohme-Chibret, Fr.
Cyproheptadine hydrochloride (p.407·2).
Hypersensitivity reactions; pruritus.

Periactinol Frosst, Ger.†.
Cyproheptadine hydrochloride (p.407·2).
Hypersensitivity reactions; vascular headache including migraine.

Periamin G
Pharmacia Upjohn, Aust.; Pharmacia Upjohn, Ger.
Amino-acid, carbohydrate, and electrolyte infusion.
Parenteral nutrition.

Periamin X Pharmacia Upjohn, Ger.
Amino-acid, xylitol, and electrolyte infusion.
Parenteral nutrition.

Peribilan Lannacher, Aust.†.
Oral powder: Ox bile (p.1553·2); pig bile (p.1553·2); atropine sulphate (p.455·1); peppermint oil (p.1208·1).
Suppositories: Ox bile (p.1553·2); pig bile (p.1553·2); atropine sulphate (p.455·1).
Constipation; gastro-intestinal motility disorders.

Periblastine Intramed, S.Afr.
Vinblastine sulphate (p.569·1).
Malignant neoplasms.

Pericam Clonmel, Irl.
Piroxicam (p.80·2).
Dysmenorrhoea; gout; musculoskeletal, joint, and peri-articular disorders.

Pericel Celafar, Ital.
Flavodate sodium (p.1580·1).
Vascular disorders.

Pericephal Hofmann, Aust.
Cinnarizine (p.406·1).
Cerebral and peripheral vascular disorders.

Peri-Colace
Roberts, Canad.; Apothecon, USA.
Casanthranol (p.1182·3); docusate sodium (p.1189·3).
Constipation.

Pericristine Intramed, S.Afr.
Vincristine sulphate (p.570·1).
Malignant neoplasms.

Peridex
Procter & Gamble, Canad.; Procter & Gamble, USA.
Chlorhexidine gluconate (p.1107·2).
Gingivitis.

Peridil-Heparine Pharmy, Fr.†.
Monoethanolamine nicotinate; heparin sodium (p.879·3); procaine (p.1299·2).
Peripheral vascular disorders; rheumatic pain.

Peridin-C Beutlich, USA.
Hesperidin methyl chalcone (p.1580·2); hesperidin complex (p.1580·2); ascorbic acid (p.1365·2).
Capillary bleeding.

Peridol Technilab, Canad.
Haloperidol (p.673·3).
Behaviour disorders; psychoses; Tourette syndrome.

Peridon Italchimici, Ital.
Domperidone (p.1190·3).
Gastro-intestinal disorders.

Peri-Dos Softgels Goldline, USA.
Docusate sodium (p.1189·3); casanthranol (p.1182·3).
Constipation.

Peridys Robapharm, Fr.
Domperidone (p.1190·3).
Dyspepsia; nausea and vomiting.

Perifazo Pharmacia Upjohn, Fr.
Amino-acid infusion.
Parenteral nutrition.

Periflex Scientific Hospital Supplies, UK.
Preparation for enteral nutrition.

Perifusin
Kabi, Irl.†; KabiVitrum, UK†.
Amino acid and electrolyte infusion.
Parenteral nutrition.

Perihemin Lederle, USA†.
Cyanocobalamin (p.1363·3); intrinsic factor concentrate; ferrous fumarate (p.1339·3); folic acid (p.1340·3); ascorbic acid (p.1365·2).
Anaemias.

Perikursal
Wyeth Lederle, Aust.; Wyeth, Ger.
Levonorgestrel (p.1454·1); ethinyloestradiol (p.1445·1).
Biphasic oral contraceptive.

Perilax Lennon, S.Afr.†.
Bisacodyl (p.1179·3).
Bowel evacuation; constipation.

Perilox Drossapharm, Switz.
Metronidazole (p.585·1).
Rosacea.

Perinal
Dermal Laboratories, Irl.; Dermal Laboratories, UK.
Hydrocortisone (p.1043·3); lignocaine hydrochloride (p.1293·2).
Anal and perianal pain and pruritus.

Perinorm Nat Druggists, S.Afr.
Metoclopramide hydrochloride (p.1200·3).
Gastro-intestinal disorders.

Periochip
Procter & Gamble, UK; Astra, USA.
Chlorhexidine (p.1107·2) or chlorhexidine gluconate (p.1107·2).
Periodontal disease.

Periogard
Note. This name is used for preparations of different composition.
Colgate-Palmolive, Ital.
Oral drops: Sanguinaria (p.1627·2).
Toothpaste: Sanguinaria (p.1627·2); sodium monofluorophosphate (p.743·3).
Gum disorders; halitosis; oral hygiene.

Colgate-Oral, USA.
Chlorhexidine gluconate (p.1107·2); alcohol (p.1099·1).
Mouth disorders.

Peripherin
Asta Medica, Aust.; Asta Medica, Ger.†.
Ephedrine (p.1059·3); etofylline (p.753·1); theophylline hydrate (p.765·1).
Cerebral vascular disorders; orthostatic circulatory disorders.

Periphramine Pharmacia Upjohn, Spain.
Amino-acid infusion.
Parenteral nutrition.

Periplasmal Braun, Ger.
Amino-acid, carbohydrate, and electrolyte infusion.
Parenteral nutrition.

Periplasmal G Braun, Spain.
Amino-acid, carbohydrate and electrolyte infusion.
Parenteral nutrition.

Periplum Italfarmaco, Ital.
Nimodipine (p.922·2).
Cerebrovascular disorders.

Peripress
Pfizer, Norw.†; Pfizer, Swed.†.
Prazosin hydrochloride (p.932·3).
Benign prostatic hyperplasia; heart failure; hypertension; Raynaud's syndrome.

Peristaltine Zyma, Fr.
Cascara (p.1183·1).
Constipation.

Peritinic Lederle, USA†.
Multivitamin preparation with iron; docusate sodium (p.1189·3).

Peritofundin Braun, Aust.
Electrolytes; glucose (p.1151·1).
Peritoneal dialysis solution.

Peritol Medphano, Ger.
Cyproheptadine hydrochloride (p.407·2).
Hypersensitivity reactions; pruritus; reduced appetite.

Peritolys med glukos Baxter, Swed.†.
Anhydrous glucose; electrolytes (p.1151·1).
Peritoneal dialysis solution.

Peritrast Kohler, Ger.
Lysine diatrizoate (p.1004·1).
Radiographic contrast medium.

Peritrast comp Kohler, Ger.
Sodium diatrizoate (p.1003·2); lysine diatrizoate (p.1004·1).
Radiographic contrast medium.

Peritrast-Infusio Kohler, Ger.
Sodium diatrizoate (p.1003·2); lysine diatrizoate (p.1004·1).
Radiographic contrast medium.

Peritrast-Oral CT Kohler, Ger.
Lysine diatrizoate (p.1004·1); sodium diatrizoate (p.1003·2).
Contrast medium for computer tomography of the abdominal cavity.

Peritrast-Oral-G I Kohler, Ger.
Lysine diatrizoate (p.1004·1).
Contrast medium for gastro-intestinal radiography.

Peritrast-RE Kohler, Ger.
Lysine diatrizoate (p.1004·1).
Radiographic contrast medium.

Peritrate
Parke, Davis, Canad.; Substantia, Fr.†; Teofarma, Ital.; Parke, Davis, S.Afr.†; Parke, Davis, Spain†; Parke, Davis, USA†.
Pentaerythritol tetranitrate (p.927·3).
Angina pectoris; heart failure; myocardial infarction.

Perivar Intersan, Ger.
Ointment: Heparin sodium (p.879·3).
Formerly contained sparteine sulphate and adrenaline.
Sustained-release tablets: Aesculus (p.1543·3).
Formerly contained sparteine sulphate and calcium glycerophosphate.
Soft-tissue injury; vascular disorders.

Perivar N Intersan, Ger.
Troxerutin (p.1580·2); heptaminol hydrochloride (p.1587·2); ginkgo biloba (p.1584·1).
Vascular disorders.

Perkamillon
Robugen, Ger.†; Medipharm, Switz.
Ointment: Chamomile (p.1561·2); hamamelis (p.1587·1).
Minor wounds.

Robugen, Ger.; Medipharm, Switz.
Liquid: Chamomile (p.1561·2).
Inflammatory disorders of the skin or mucous membranes.

Perketan Inverni della Beffa, Ital.
Ketanserin tartrate (p.894·3).
Hypertension.

Perkod Biogalenique, Fr.†.
Dipyridamole (p.857·1).
Coronary disorders.

Perles d'huile de foie de morue du Dr Geistlich Geistlich, Switz.
Cod-liver oil (p.1337·3); halibut-liver oil (p.1345·3).
Vitamin A and D deficiency.

Perlinganit
Nycomed, Aust.; Schwarz, Ger.; Orion, Swed.; Schwarz, Switz.
Glyceryl trinitrate (p.874·3).
Cardiovascular disorders; controlled hypotension.

Perlinsol Cutaneo Medea, Spain.
Acedoben sodium (p.1541·1); vitamin F.
Skin disorders.

Perliver Sanico, Belg.†.
Liver extract.
Anaemias; weak states.

Perlutex Leo, Norw.
Medroxyprogesterone acetate (p.1448·3).
Endometrial cancer; endometriosis; menopausal disorders; test of ovarian function.

Permapen Roerig, USA.
Benzathine penicillin (p.158·3).
Bacterial infections.

Permax
Lilly, Aust.; Lilly, Austral.; Lilly, Belg.; Draxis, Canad.; Lilly, Neth.; Lilly, S.Afr.; Athena Neurosciences, USA.
Pergolide mesylate (p.1142·3).
Parkinsonism.

Permease Sanabo, Aust.
Hyaluronidase (p.1588·1).
Haematomas; increase absorption and reduce discomfort of injections; reduce viscosity of secretions and discharge.

Permitabs Bioglan, UK.
Potassium permanganate (p.1123·2).
Wound cleansing.

Permitil Schering, USA.
Fluphenazine hydrochloride (p.671·3).
Psychoses.

Permixon
Germania, Aust.; Pierre Fabre, Fr.; Pierre Fabre, Ital.; Pierre Fabre, Spain.
Saw palmetto (p.1462·1).
Prostatic adenoma; prostatic hyperplasia.

Permixon Novum Robapharm, Switz.
Saw palmetto (p.1462·1).
Prostatic hyperplasia.

Pernaemon Organon, Belg.†.
Liver extract.
Anaemias due to vitamin B_{12} deficiency.

Pernaemyl Biosyn, Ger.
Bovine liver extract; cyanocobalamin (p.1363·3).
Liver disorders; megaloblastic anaemia; vitamin B_{12} deficiency.

Pernazene Synthelabo, Fr.
Tymazoline hydrochloride (p.1071·2).
Nasal congestion.

Pernexin Schering, Ital.
Iron succinyl-protein complex (p.1349·2).
Anaemias; iron deficiency.

Pernicream Salusa, S.Afr.†.
Amethocaine (p.1285·2); menthol (p.1600·2).
Chilblains.

Pernionin Krewel, Ger.
Methyl salicylate (p.55·2); benzyl nicotinate (p.22·1); methyl nicotinate (p.55·1).
Musculoskeletal and joint disorders; peripheral vascular disorders.

Pernionin N Krewel, Ger.
Methyl salicylate (p.55·2); sage oil.
Circulatory disorders.

Pernionin Teil-Bad N Krewel, Ger.
Methyl salicylate (p.55·2); benzyl nicotinate (p.22·1); methyl nicotinate (p.55·1).
Bath additive; musculoskeletal and joint disorders; peripheral circulatory disorders.

Pernionin Voll-Bad N Krewel, Ger.
Norway spruce oil; benzyl nicotinate (p.22·1); methyl nicotinate (p.55·1).
Bath additive; musculoskeletal and joint disorders; peripheral circulatory disorders.

Pernivit Salusa, S.Afr.†.
Acetomenaphthone (p.1370·3); nicotinic acid (p.1351·2).
Chilblains.

Pernox
Westwood-Squibb, Canad.; Westwood, USA.
Polyethylene granules (abrasive) (p.1077·2); sulphur (p.1091·2); salicylic acid (p.1090·2).
Acne; oily skin.

Pernutrin Grifols, Spain.
Amino-acid, carbohydrate, electrolyte, and vitamin infusion.
Parenteral nutrition.

Pernyzol Recordati, Ital.
Metronidazole benzoate (p.585·1).
Bacterial mouth infections.

Pero Opfermann, Ger.
Glycerol (p.1585·2); bleached wax.
Skin disorders.

Perocef Pulitzer, Ital.
Cefoperazone sodium (p.167·3).
Lignocaine hydrochloride (p.1293·2) is included in this preparation to alleviate the pain of injection.
Bacterial infections.

Perocur Biocur, Ger.
Saccharomyces boulardii (p.1594·1).
Diarrhoea.

Peroxacne Isdin, Spain.
Benzoyl peroxide (p.1079·2).
Acne.

Peroxiben Isdin, Spain.
Benzoyl peroxide (p.1079·2).
Acne.

Peroxin Dermol, USA.
Benzoyl peroxide (p.1079·2).
Acne.

Peroxinorm
Grunenthal, Aust.†; Grunenthal, Ger.†; Andromaco, Spain†.
Orgotein (p.87·3).
Treatment of inflammatory symptoms.

Peroxyl
Colgate-Palmolive, UK; Colgate-Palmolive, USA.
Hydrogen peroxide (p.1116·2).
Mouth and gum irritation.

Perozon Erkaltungsbad Schoeller, Aust.
Eucalyptus oil (p.1578·1); camphor (p.1557·2); menthol (p.1600·2).
Bath additive; cold symptoms; rheumatic disorders.

Perozon Heublumen Schoeller, Aust.
Thyme oil (p.1637·1); hay flowers.
Bath additive.

Perozon Rosmarin-Olbad mono Spitzner, Ger.
Rosemary oil (p.1626·2).
Bath additive; peripheral vascular disorders.

Perpain Medinat, Austral.†.
Aloxiprin (p.15·1); codeine phosphate (p.26·1); viburnum opulus; chamomile (p.1561·2); cimicifuga (p.1563·3).
Dysmenorrhoea; premenstrual uterine congestion.

Perpector Grossmann, Switz.
Codeine phosphate (p.26·1); ephedrine hydrochloride (p.1059·3); potassium iodide (p.1493·1); primula root; valerian (p.1643·1).
Coughs.

Perphyllon Asta Medica, Aust.
Etofylline (p.753·1); theophylline hydrate (p.765·1); papaverine hydrochloride (p.1614·2); atropine methonitrate (p.455·1).
Asthma; bronchitis; emphysema.

Perphyllone Asta Medica, Belg.†.
Etofylline (p.753·1); theophylline hydrate (p.765·1); papaverine hydrochloride (p.1614·2); atropine methonitrate (p.455·1); phenobarbitone (p.350·2).
Angina pectoris; coronary and cerebral perfusion disorders; pulmonary disorders.

Persa-Gel Ortho Dermatological, USA.
Benzoyl peroxide (p.1079·2).
Acne.

Persantin
Bender, Aust.; Boehringer Ingelheim, Austral.; Thomae, Ger.; Boehringer Ingelheim, Irl.; Boehringer Ingelheim, Ital.; Boehringer Ingelheim, Neth.; Boehringer Ingelheim, Norw.; Boehringer Ingelheim, S.Afr.; Boehringer Ingelheim, Spain; Boehringer Ingelheim, Swed.; Boehringer Ingelheim, UK.
Dipyridamole (p.857·1) or dipyridamole hydrochloride (p.857·3).
Angina pectoris; diagnostic aid; heart failure; myocardial infarction; thrombosis prophylaxis.

Persantine
Boehringer Ingelheim, Belg.; Boehringer Ingelheim, Canad.; Boehringer Ingelheim, Fr.; Boehringer Ingelheim, Switz.; Boehringer Ingelheim, USA.
Dipyridamole (p.857·1).
Adjunct in thallium myocardial perfusion imaging; angina pectoris; thrombo-embolism prophylaxis.

Persivate Lagamed, S.Afr.
Betamethasone valerate (p.1033·3).
Skin disorders.

Perskindol Singer, Switz.
Menthol (p.1600·2).
Muscle and joint pain.

Persol
Note. This name is used for preparations of different composition.
Dreveny, Aust.
Hydrogen peroxide (p.1116·2).
Cleaning and disinfecting solution for hard and soft contact lenses.

Horner, Canad.
Benzoyl peroxide (p.1079·2); colloidal sulphur (p.1091·2).
Acne; rosacea.

Persolv Richter Lepetit, Ital.
Urokinase (p.959·3).
Thrombo-embolic disorders.

Personnelle Contre le Rhume Therapex, Canad.
Pseudoephedrine hydrochloride (p.1068·3); dextromethorphan hydrobromide (p.1057·3); paracetamol (p.72·2).

Personnelle DM Therapex, Canad.
Pseudoephedrine hydrochloride (p.1068·3); dextromethorphan hydrobromide (p.1057·3).

Perspiran N Godecke, Ger.†.
Theophylline (p.765·1) or theophylline hydrate (p.765·1); ephedrine hydrochloride (p.1059·3).
Bronchospastic disorders.

Persumbran
Bender, Aust.†; Thomae, Ger.†.
Dipyridamole (p.857·1); oxazepam (p.683·2).
Angina; heart failure.

Persumbrax Boehringer Ingelheim, Ital.
Dipyridamole (p.857·1); oxazepam (p.683·2).
Cardiovascular disorders.

Pert Plus Procter & Gamble, Canad.
Pyrithione zinc (p.1089·3).
Seborrhoeic dermatitis.

Pertensal Vinas, Spain.
Nifedipine (p.916·2).
Angina pectoris; hypertension.

pertenso Schwarz, Ger.†.
Bemetizide (p.827·1); triamterene (p.957·2); bupranolol hydrochloride (p.835·2); dihydralazine sulphate (p.854·1).
Hypertension.

Pertenso N Fournier, Ger.
Propranolol hydrochloride (p.937·1); hydralazine hydrochloride (p.883·2); bendrofluazide (p.827·3).
Hypertension.

Pertil Astra, Spain.
Isosorbide mononitrate (p.893·3).
Angina pectoris; heart failure.

Pertin Solvay, Aust.
Metoclopramide hydrochloride (p.1200·3).
Gastro-intestinal motility disorders; nausea and vomiting.

Pertiroid Piam, Ital.
Potassium perchlorate (p.1496·1).
Hyperthyroidism.

Pertix
Note. This name is used for preparations of different composition.
Hommel, Ger.
Pentoxyverine (p.1066·1) or pentoxyverine citrate (p.1066·1).
Oral liquid†: Butethamate citrate (p.1056·2).
Suppositories†: Butethamate citrate (p.1056·2); guaiacol phenylbutyrate (p.1061·2).
Coughs and associated respiratory-tract disorders.

Glaxo Allen, Ital.†.
Menadiol calcium diphosphate; butethamate citrate (p.1056·2).
Coughs; laryngospasm.

Pertix-S Hommel, Ger.†.
Menadiol calcium diphosphate; butethamate citrate (p.1056·2).
Coughs.

Pertix-Solo Hommel, Ger.
Menadiol calcium diphosphate.
Coughs.

Pertofran
Ciba-Geigy, Aust.; Novartis, Austral.; Ciba-Geigy, Belg.; Ciba-Geigy, Fr.; Geigy, Ger.; Ciba-Geigy, Irl.†; Novartis, Neth.; Ciba-Geigy, S.Afr.†; Geigy, Switz.†; Novartis, UK†.
Desipramine hydrochloride (p.282·2).
Depression.

Pertofrane
Geigy, Canad.; Rorer, USA†.
Desipramine hydrochloride (p.282·2).
Depression.

Pertoglobulin Nuovo ISM, Ital.
A pertussis immunoglobulin (p.1525·3).
Passive immunisation.

Pertranquil
Note. This name is used for preparations of different composition.
Hoechst, Aust.; Hoechst Marion Roussel, Belg.
Meprobamate (p.678·1).
Anxiety disorders; neurodermatitis; sedative; skeletal muscle spasm; sleep disorders.

Llorente, Spain.
Diazepam (p.661·1); aminohydroxybutyric acid (p.339·1).
Anxiety; insomnia.

Pertrombon Gerot, Aust.
Sodium nicotinate; heparin (p.879·3).
Decubitus ulcer; promote resorption of excess fluid; soft-tissue injury; thrombophlebitis; ulcus cruris; varices.

Pertropin Lannett, USA.
Linolenic acid, vitamin E substances, and essential fatty acids.
Dietary supplement.

Pertudoron
Weleda, Aust.; Weleda, Fr.
Homoeopathic preparation.

Pertus-Gamma Biagini, Ital.
A human pertussis immunoglobulin (p.1525·3).
Passive immunisation.

Pertussetten Schmidgall, Aust.†.
Thyme (p.1636·3); primula; ephedrine hydrochloride (p.1059·3).

Pertussex Compositum Uhlmann-Eyraud, Switz.
Codeine phosphate (p.26·1); ephedrine hydrochloride (p.1059·3); drosera; galeopsis; thyme; lichen islandicus; primula.
Coughs and associated respiratory-tract disorders.

Pertussin
Note. This name is used for preparations of different composition.
Schmidgall, Aust.†.
Balsam: Amber oil; eucalyptus oil (p.1578·1); turpentine oil; thyme oil (p.1637·1).
Oral drops: Thyme (p.1636·3); galeopsis ochroleuca; iceland moss; primula rhizome; ephedrine hydrochloride (p.1059·3).
Syrup: Thyme (p.1636·3).
Coughs.

Polcopharma, Austral.†; Fink, Ger.†.
Thyme (p.1636·3); drosera (p.1574·1).
Asthma; bronchial congestion; cough.

Pertussin, USA.
Dextromethorphan hydrobromide (p.1057·3).
Coughs.

Pertussin All-Night PM Pertussin, USA†.
Paracetamol (p.72·2); doxylamine succinate (p.410·1); pseudoephedrine hydrochloride (p.1068·3); dextromethorphan hydrobromide (p.1057·3).

Pertussin AM Pertussin, USA†.
Pseudoephedrine hydrochloride (p.1068·3); dextromethorphan hydrobromide (p.1057·3); guaiphenesin (p.1061·3).

Pertussin N Fink, Ger.†.
Thyme (p.1636·3).
Catarrh; coughs.

Pertuvac Chiron Behring, Ger.
A pertussis vaccine (p.1526·1).
Active immunisation.

Perubare Mayoly-Spindler, Switz.
Peru balsam (p.1617·2); thymol (p.1127·1); thyme oil (p.1637·1); rosemary oil (p.1626·2); lavender oil (p.1594·3).
Upper-respiratory-tract disorders.

Perubore
Note. This name is used for preparations of different composition.
ACP, Belg.
Peru balsam (p.1617·2); thyme oil (p.1637·1); rosemary oil (p.1626·2); thymol (p.1127·1).
Rhinitis; sinusitis.

Mayoly-Spindler, Fr.
Thyme oil (p.1637·1); rosemary oil (p.1626·2); lavender oil (p.1594·3); thymol (p.1127·1); peru balsam (p.1617·2).
Respiratory-tract congestion.

Perudent Dreveny, Aust.
Peru balsam (p.1617·2).
Dental preparation.

Peru-Lenicet Athenstaedt, Ger.
Aluminium diacetate hydroxide; aluminium hydroxide gel (p.1177·3); peru balsam (p.1617·2).
Skin disorders.

Perultid Procter & Gamble, Ital.†.
Niperotidine hydrochloride (p.1203·2).
Gastro-intestinal disorders associated with hyperacidity.

Pervasum Lesvi, Spain.
Cinnarizine (p.406·1).
Migraine; motion sickness; vascular disease; vestibular disorders.

Perventil Malesci, Ital.†.
Theophylline (p.765·1); salbutamol (p.758·2).
Obstructive airways disease.

Pervin Piam, Ital.†.
Vincamine (p.1644·1) or vincamine hydrochloride (p.1644·1).
Mental function disorders.

Pervincamine
Synthelabo, Belg.†; Synthelabo, Fr.; Synthelabo, Switz.†.
Vincamine (p.1644·1).
Cerebrovascular disorders; mental function disorders; vertigo.

Perviolona Hortel, Spain†.
Adenine; vitamin B substances; amino acids.
Tonic.

Pervita Lifeplan, UK.
Betacarotene (p.1335·2).
Nutritional supplement.

Perycit
Inibsa, Spain†; Astra, Swed.
Niceritrol (p.915·2).
Angina pectoris; hyperlipidaemias; peripheral vascular disorders.

Pesalin Prodes, Spain†.
Alizapride hydrochloride (p.1176·3).
Gastro-oesophageal reflux; gastroparesis; nausea and vomiting.

Pesendorfer Iso, Ger.
Homoeopathic preparation.

Pesos Valeas, Ital.†.
Fenfluramine hydrochloride (p.1480·3).
Obesity.

Petadolex Weber & Weber, Ger.
Petasites officinalis.
Smooth muscle spasms.

Petaforce V Bioforce, Ger.
Petasites officinalis.
Migraine; urinary-tract pain.

Pe-Tam Qualiphar, Belg.
Paracetamol (p.72·2).
Fever; pain.

Peteha Fatol, Ger.
Injection: Prothionamide (p.241·1); nicotinamide (p.1351·2).
Tablets: Prothionamide (p.241·1).
Tuberculosis.

Peter Pote's Restan, S.Afr.†.
Bismuth citrate (p.1180·1); potassium hydroxide (p.1621·1); pepsin (p.1616·3); belladonna (p.457·1); nux vomica (p.1609·3); ammonia solution (p.1548·3).
Gastro-intestinal disorders.

Petercillin Intramed, S.Afr.; Lennon, S.Afr.
Ampicillin sodium (p.153·1) or ampicillin trihydrate (p.153·2).
Bacterial infections.

Peterkaien Intramed, S.Afr.
Lignocaine hydrochloride (p.1293·2).
Arrhythmias; local anaesthesia.

Peterpect Lennon, S.Afr.†.
Kaolin (p.1195·1); citrus pectin (p.1474·1); bismuth subcarbonate (p.1180·1).
Diarrhoea; gastro-enteritis.

Peterphyllin
Intramed, S.Afr.; Lennon, S.Afr.†.
Aminophylline (p.748·1).
Heart failure; obstructive airways disease; oedema; paroxysmal nocturnal dyspnoea.

Peterphyllin Co. Lennon, S.Afr.†.
Aminophylline (p.748·1); ephedrine hydrochloride (p.1059·3); phenobarbitone (p.350·2).
Allergic rhinitis; bronchospasm.

Peter's Sirop Monot, Fr.
Ammoniated anise (p.1549·3); ethylmorphine hydrochloride (p.36·1); aconite (p.1542·2); belladonna (p.457·1); cherry laurel.
Respiratory-tract disorders.

Pethic Berna, Ital.†.
Diplococcus pneumoniae; *Streptococcus*; *Staphylococcus*; *Haemophilus influenzae*.
Respiratory-tract disorders.

Petidion
Gerot, Aust.; Gerot, Switz.
Ethadione (p.344·3).
Absence seizures; myoclonic seizures.

Petigan Miro Braun, Spain†.
Pethidine hydrochloride (p.76·1); promethazine hydrochloride (p.416·2).
Nausea; pain; premedication; shock (prophylaxis).

Petinimid
Gerot, Aust.; Gerot, Switz.
Ethosuximide (p.344·3).
Absence seizures.

Petinutin
Parke, Davis, Aust.; Parke, Davis, Ger.; Parke, Davis, Switz.
Methsuximide (p.349·1).
Epilepsy.

Petites Pilules Carters pour le Foie Fumouze, Fr.
Boldine (p.1554·1); aloes (p.1177·1).
Constipation.

Petnidan Desitin, Ger.
Ethosuximide (p.344·3).
Absence seizures.

Petogen Intramed, S.Afr.
Medroxyprogesterone acetate (p.1448·3).
Injectable contraceptive.

Petrolagar Whitehall, UK†.
Liquid paraffin (p.1382·1); light liquid paraffin (p.1382·1).
Constipation.

Petrolagar No. 1 Whitehall, Irl.†.
Liquid paraffin (p.1382·1); light liquid paraffin (p.1382·1).
Constipation.

Petrolagar No. 2 Whitehall, Irl.
Liquid paraffin (p.1382·1); light liquid paraffin (p.1382·1); phenolphthalein (p.1208·2).
Constipation.

Petrolagar with Phenolphthalein Whitehall, Irl.
Light liquid paraffin (p.1382·1); liquid paraffin (p.1382·1); phenolphthalein (p.1208·2).
Constipation.

Petroleum Med Complex Dynamit, Aust.
Homoeopathic preparation.

Petylyl Dresden, Ger.
Desipramine hydrochloride (p.282·2).
Depression.

Pevalip Janssen-Cilag, Aust.
Econazole (p.377·2).
Fungal skin and nail infections.

Pevaryl
Note. This name is used for preparations of different composition.
Janssen-Cilag, Aust.; SmithKline Beecham Consumer, Austral.; Janssen-Cilag, Belg.; Janssen-Cilag, Fr.; Janssen-Cilag, Irl.; Janssen-Cilag, Ital.; Janssen-Cilag, Neth.; Janssen-Cilag, Norw.; Roche, S.Afr.; Pensa, Spain; Janssen-Cilag, Swed.; Janssen-Cilag, Switz.; Cilag, UK.
Econazole (p.377·2) or econazole nitrate (p.377·2).
Fungal and Gram-positive bacterial infections.

Janssen-Cilag, Aust.
Paste; topical powder; topical powder spray: Econazole nitrate (p.377·2); zinc oxide (p.1096·2).
Fungal skin and nail infections; Gram-positive infections.

Pevaryl TC Cilag, UK.
Econazole nitrate (p.377·2); triamcinolone acetonide (p.1050·2).
Skin disorders with bacterial or fungal infection.

Pevisone
Janssen-Cilag, Aust.; Janssen-Cilag, Belg.; Janssen-Cilag, Fr.; Janssen-Cilag, Ital.; Janssen-Cilag, Norw.; Roche, S.Afr.; Janssen-Cilag, Swed.; Janssen-Cilag, Switz.
Econazole nitrate (p.377·2); triamcinolone acetonide (p.1050·2).
Infected skin disorders.

Pexan E Worwag, Ger.
d-Alpha tocopherol (p.1369·1) or alpha-tocopherol acetate (p.1369·1).
Vitamin E deficiency.

Pexid
Sigma, Austral.; Hoechst Marion Roussel, Belg.; Marion Merrell, Fr.†; Marion Merrell Dow, Ger.†.
Perhexiline maleate (p.928·1).
Angina pectoris.

pezetamid Hefa, Ger.†.
Pyrazinamide (p.241·1).
Tuberculosis.

Pfefferminz-Lysoform Lysoform, Ger.
Formaldehyde (p.1113·2); peppermint oil (p.1208·1); menthol (p.1600·2).
Infections of the oropharynx.

Pfeiffer's Allergy Pfeiffer, USA.
Chlorpheniramine maleate (p.405·1).
Hypersensitivity reactions.

Pfeiffer's Cold Sore Pfeiffer, USA.
Sumatra benzoin (p.1634·1); camphor (p.1557·2); menthol (p.1600·2); cineole (p.1564·1).
Oral lesions.

Pfeil Stada, Ger.
Ibuprofen (p.44·1).
Formerly contained etenzamide and propyphenazone.
Pain.

Pfizerpen Roerig, USA.
Benzylpenicillin potassium (p.159·2).
Bacterial infections.

Pfizerpen-AS Roerig, USA†.
Procaine penicillin (p.240·2).
Bacterial infections.

PG 53 Bouty, Ital.
Fertility test (p.1621·2).

pH 550 Restan, S.Afr.
Suspension: Dicyclomine hydrochloride (p.460·1); aluminium hydroxide gel (p.1177·3); magnesium oxide (p.1198·3); calcium carbonate (p.1182·1); dimethicone (p.1213·1).
Tablets: Calcium carbonate (p.1182·1); magnesium carbonate (p.1198·1); magnesium trisilicate (p.1199·1).
Flatulence; gastric hyperacidity; hiatus hernia; peptic ulcer.

PH 3 Compuesto Salvat, Spain†.
Magnesium polygalacturonate; liquorice (p.1197·1); aluminium glycinate (p.1177·2); hyoscine methobromide (p.463·1).
Gastro-intestinal spasms; hyperacidity; peptic ulcer.

Phaeva Schering, Fr.
Gestodene (p.1447·2); ethinyloestradiol (p.1445·1).
Triphasic oral contraceptive.

Phakan Chauvin, Fr.
Combination pack: Oral solution, glycine (p.1345·2); glutamic acid (p.1344·3); pyridoxine hydrochloride (p.1362·3); capsules, cysteine hydrochloride (p.1338·3); ascorbic acid (p.1365·2).
Cataracts.

Phakolen Novopharma, Switz.
Combination pack: White capsules, glycine (p.1345·2); L-glutamic acid (p.1344·3); pyridoxine hydrochloride (p.1362·3); blue capsules, L-cysteine (p.1338·3); ascorbic acid (p.1365·2).
Prevention of cataract formation.

Phanacol Pharmakon, USA.
Phenylpropanolamine hydrochloride (p.1067·2); dextromethorphan hydrobromide (p.1057·3); guaiphenesin (p.1061·3); paracetamol (p.72·2).

Phanadex Cough Pharmakon, USA.
Phenylpropanolamine hydrochloride (p.1067·2); dextromethorphan hydrobromide (p.1057·3); mepyramine maleate (p.414·1); guaiphenesin (p.1061·3).
Coughs.

Phanatuss Cough Pharmakon, USA.
Dextromethorphan hydrobromide (p.1057·3); guaiphenesin (p.1061·3).
Coughs.

Phapax Lehning, Fr.
Homoeopathic preparation.

Phardol 10 Kreussler, Ger.†.
Glycol salicylate (p.43·1); benzyl nicotinate (p.22·1).
Musculoskeletal, joint, and nerve disorders.

Phardol Mono Kreussler, Ger.
Glycol salicylate (p.43·1).
Musculoskeletal, joint, soft-tissue, and nerve disorders.

Phardol N Balsam Kreussler, Ger.†.
Camphor (p.1557·2); glycol salicylate (p.43·1); pumilio pine oil (p.1623·3); benzyl nicotinate (p.22·1); eucalyptus oil (p.1578·1); rosemary oil (p.1626·2); turpentine oil (p.1641·1).
Muscle and joint disorders.

Phardol Rheuma Kreussler, Ger.
Glycol salicylate (p.43·1); oleum pini sylvestris; benzyl nicotinate (p.22·1).
Musculoskeletal, joint, soft-tissue, and nervous disorders.

Pharken Lilly, Spain.
Pergolide mesylate (p.1142·3).
Parkinsonism.

Pharmacaine Brovar, S.Afr.†.
Lignocaine hydrochloride (p.1293·2).

Adrenaline (p.813·2) is included in some injections as a vasoconstrictor to diminish absorption and localise the effect of the local anaesthetic.
Local anaesthesia.

Pharmacal *Pharmadex, Canad.†.*
Calcium carbonate (p.1182·1).
Calcium supplement.

Pharmacilline *Monot, Fr.*
Gramicidin (p.215·2).
Infections of the mouth, nose, and throat.

Pharmacol DM *Therapex, Canad.*
Phenylpropanolamine hydrochloride (p.1067·2); pheniramine maleate (p.415·3); mepyramine maleate (p.414·1); dextromethorphan hydrobromide (p.1057·3).

Pharma-Col Junior *Warner-Lambert, Austral.*
Dextromethorphan hydrobromide (p.1057·3); pseudoephedrine hydrochloride (p.1068·3); paracetamol (p.72·2).
Coughs and cold symptoms.

Pharmacreme *Young, USA†.*
Vehicle and diluent.

Pharmadose alcool *Gilbert, Fr.*
Alcohol (p.1099·1).
Skin and wound disinfection.

Pharmadose mercuresceine *Gilbert, Fr.*
Mercurochrome (p.1119·2).
Wound and burn disinfection.

Pharmadose teinture d'arnica *Gilbert, Fr.*
Arnica (p.1550·3).
Ecchymoses.

Pharmaethyl *Austrodent, Aust.*
Dichlorotetrafluoroethane (p.1164·3).
Local anaesthesia in dentistry.

Pharmaflam *Pharmador, S.Afr.†.*
Diclofenac sodium (p.31·2).
Inflammation; musculoskeletal and joint disorders; pain.

Pharmaflex *Braun, Belg.*
Metronidazole (p.585·1).
Anaerobic bacterial infections; protozoal infections.

Pharmaflur *Pharmics, USA.*
Sodium fluoride (p.742·1).
Dental caries prophylaxis.

Pharmalax *Pharmascience, Canad.†.*
Docusate calcium (p.1189·3).
Constipation.

Pharmalgen
Epipharm, Aust.†; ALK, Swed.; Trimedal, Switz.; Pharmacia, UK; ALK, USA.
Venoms of bee, wasp, hornet, yellow jacket, and mixed vespids (p.1545·1).
Hyposensitisation.

Pharmalose *Pharmascience, Canad.†.*
Lactulose (p.1195·3).
Constipation; hepatic encephalopathy.

Pharmalyn *Pharma Plus, Switz.†.*
Diphenhydramine hydrochloride (p.409·1); dextromethorphan hydrobromide (p.1057·3); sodium citrate (p.1153·2); menthol (p.1600·2).
Coughs.

Pharmamox *Rivopharm, Switz.†.*
Amoxycillin (p.151·3).
Bacterial infections.

Pharmaprim *Pharma Plus, Switz.†.*
Co-trimoxazole (p.196·3).
Bacterial infections; Pneumocystis carinii pneumonia.

Pharmaquine *Pharma Plus, Switz.†.*
Chloroquine phosphate (p.426·3).
Malaria.

Pharmatex *Innothera, Fr.*
Pessaries; soap; tampons; vaginal cream: Benzalkonium chloride (p.1101·3).
Contraceptive; skin hygiene.
Topical gel: Hydroxyethylmethylcellulose (p.1472·3); benzalkonium chloride (p.1101·3); glycerol (p.1585·2).
Vaginal lubricant.

Pharmaton
Boehringer Ingelheim, Austral.; Boehringer Ingelheim, Fr.; Windsor, Irl.; Windsor, UK.
Multivitamins and minerals; ginseng; lecithin; deanol bitartrate.
Tonic.

Pharmaton Complex *Fher, Spain.*
Multivitamins and minerals; ginseng; lecithin; deanol bitartrate.
Tonic.

Pharmaton SA *Boehringer Ingelheim, S.Afr.*
Multivitamins and minerals; ginseng; lecithin; rutin.
Tonic.

Pharmatovit
Bender, Aust.; Pharmaton, Switz.
Multivitamin and mineral preparation.

Pharmatrocin *Pharma Plus, Switz.†.*
Erythromycin ethyl succinate (p.204·2).
Bacterial infections.

Pharmet *Pharmador, S.Afr.†.*
Methyldopa (p.904·2).
Hypertension.

Pharmetapp *Therapex, Canad.*
Phenylephrine hydrochloride (p.1066·2); phenylpropanolamine hydrochloride (p.1067·2); brompheniramine maleate (p.403·2).

Pharmilin-DM *Therapex, Canad.*
Dextromethorphan hydrobromide (p.1057·3).

Pharminicol DM *Therapex, Canad.*
Phenylpropanolamine hydrochloride (p.1067·2); pheniramine maleate (p.415·3); mepyramine maleate (p.414·1); dextromethorphan hydrobromide (p.1057·3).

Pharminil DM *Therapex, Canad.*
Dextromethorphan hydrobromide (p.1057·3).

Pharmitussin DM *Therapex, Canad.*
Dextromethorphan hydrobromide (p.1057·3); guaiphenesin (p.1061·3).

Pharmorubicin
Pharmacia Upjohn, Austral.; Pharmacia Upjohn, Canad.; Pharmacia Upjohn, Irl.; Pharmacia Upjohn, UK.
Epirubicin hydrochloride (p.532·1).
Malignant neoplasms.

Pharmoxin *Pharmador, S.Afr.†.*
Amoxycillin trihydrate (p.151·3).
Bacterial infections.

Pharyngine a la Vitamine C *Salver, Fr.†.*
Tyrothricin (p.267·2); amethocaine hydrochloride (p.1285·2); ascorbic acid (p.1365·2).
Infections of the mouth and throat.

Pharyngocin *Upjohn, Ger.†.*
Erythromycin (p.204·1).
Bacterial infections.

Pharyngor *Rappai, Switz.*
Potassium chloride; sodium chloride; magnesium chloride; calcium chloride; potassium acid phosphate (p.1147·1); chamomile.
Dry mouth and throat.

Pharysyx *Syxyl, Ger.*
Homoeopathic preparation.

Phasal *Lagap, UK†.*
Lithium carbonate (p.290·3).
Bipolar disorder; depression; mania.

Phazyme
Stafford-Miller, Austral.; Reed & Carnrick, Canad.; Reed & Carnrick, USA.
Simethicone (p.1213·1).
Some preparations in *Austral.* formerly contained pancreatin.
Gastro-intestinal disorders.

Phena-Chlor *Warner Chilcott, USA†.*
Phenylpropanolamine hydrochloride (p.1067·2); phenylephrine hydrochloride (p.1066·2); phenyltoloxamine citrate (p.416·1); chlorpheniramine maleate (p.405·1).

Phenacon *Teral, USA.*
Phenylephrine hydrochloride (p.1066·2); chlorpheniramine maleate (p.405·1); hyoscine methonitrate (p.463·1).
Coughs.

Phenadex Cough/Cold *Barre-National, USA.*
Phenylpropanolamine hydrochloride (p.1067·2); dextromethorphan hydrobromide (p.1057·3); guaiphenesin (p.1061·3).
Cough and cold symptoms.

Phenadex Senior *Barre-National, USA.*
Dextromethorphan hydrobromide (p.1057·3); guaiphenesin (p.1061·3).
Coughs.

Phenaemal *Desitin, Ger.*
Phenobarbitone (p.350·2).
Epilepsy.

Phenaemaletten *Desitin, Ger.*
Phenobarbitone (p.350·2).
Epilepsy.

Phenahist-TR *Williams, USA.*
Phenylpropanolamine hydrochloride (p.1067·2); phenylephrine hydrochloride (p.1066·2); chlorpheniramine maleate (p.405·1); hyoscyamine sulphate (p.464·2); hyoscine hydrobromide (p.462·3); atropine sulphate (p.455·1).
Upper respiratory-tract symptoms.

Phenameth *Major, USA†.*
Promethazine hydrochloride (p.416·2).
Hypersensitivity reactions; motion sickness; nausea; postoperative pain (adjunct); sedative; vomiting.

Phenameth DM *Major, USA.*
Promethazine hydrochloride (p.416·2); dextromethorphan hydrobromide (p.1057·3).
Coughs and cold symptoms.

Phenamin *Nycomed, Norw.*
Dexchlorpheniramine maleate (p.405·1).
Hypersensitivity reactions; pruritus.

Phenapap Sinus Headache & Congestion *Rugby, USA.*
Pseudoephedrine hydrochloride (p.1068·3); paracetamol (p.72·2); chlorpheniramine maleate (p.405·1).
Upper respiratory-tract symptoms.

Phenaphen *Robins, USA†.*
Paracetamol (p.72·2).

Phenaphen with Codeine
Note. This name is used for preparations of different composition.
Wyeth-Ayerst, Canad.
Aspirin (p.16·1); phenobarbitone (p.350·2); codeine phosphate (p.26·1).
Pain.

Robins, USA.
Paracetamol (p.72·2); codeine phosphate (p.26·1).
Pain.

Phenaseptic *Rugby, USA†.*
Phenol (p.1121·2); borax (p.1554·2); glycerol (p.1585·2); menthol (p.1600·2); thymol (p.1127·1).
Minor mouth or throat irritation.

Phenate *Roberts, USA; Hauck, USA.*
Phenylpropanolamine hydrochloride (p.1067·2); chlorpheniramine maleate (p.405·1); paracetamol (p.72·2).
Upper respiratory-tract symptoms.

Phenazine
Note. This name is used for preparations of different composition.
Keene, USA.
Promethazine hydrochloride (p.416·2).
Hypersensitivity reactions; motion sickness; nausea; postoperative pain (adjunct); sedative; vomiting.

Legere, USA†.
Phendimetrazine tartrate (p.1484·2).

Phenazo *ICN, Canad.*
Phenazopyridine hydrochloride (p.78·3).
Urinary-tract pain.

Phenazodine *Lannett, USA†.*
Phenazopyridine hydrochloride (p.78·3).
Irritation of the lower urinary tract.

Phenchlor SHA *Rugby, USA.*
Phenylpropanolamine hydrochloride (p.1067·2); phenylephrine hydrochloride (p.1066·2); chlorpheniramine maleate (p.405·1); hyoscyamine sulphate (p.464·2); hyoscine hydrobromide (p.462·3); atropine sulphate (p.455·1).
Upper respiratory-tract symptoms.

Phendex *Garec, S.Afr.*
Triprolidine hydrochloride (p.420·3); pseudoephedrine hydrochloride (p.1068·3); guaiphenesin (p.1061·3); codeine phosphate (p.26·1).
Coughs.

Phendry *Lu Chem, USA.*
Diphenhydramine hydrochloride (p.409·1).
Insomnia; motion sickness; parkinsonism.

Phenephrin *Nelson, Austral.†.*
Codeine phosphate (p.26·1); phenylephrine hydrochloride (p.1066·2); menthol (p.1600·2); guaiphenesin (p.1061·3).
Congestion; coughs.

Phenerbel-S *Rugby, USA.*
Phenobarbitone (p.350·2); ergotamine tartrate (p.445·3); belladonna (p.457·1).

Phenergan
Note. This name is used for preparations of different composition.
Rhone-Poulenc Rorer, Aust.†; Rhone-Poulenc Rorer, Austral.; Rhone-Poulenc Rorer, Belg.; Rhone-Poulenc Rorer, Canad.; Evans, Fr.; Rhone-Poulenc Rorer, Irl.; Rhone-Poulenc Rorer, Neth.; Rhone-Poulenc Rorer, Norw.; Rhone-Poulenc Rorer, S.Afr.; Rhone-Poulenc Rorer, Switz.; Rhone-Poulenc Rorer, UK; Wyeth-Ayerst, USA.
Promethazine (p.416·2) or promethazine hydrochloride (p.416·2).
Hypersensitivity reactions; insomnia; motion sickness; nausea; parkinsonism; premedication; skin disorders; vomiting.

Rhone-Poulenc Rorer, Austral.†; Rhone-Poulenc Rorer, S.Afr.†.
Cream: Promethazine (p.416·2); dibromopropamidine isethionate (p.1112·2).
Burns; insect bites; scalds; stings.

Phenergan with Codeine *Wyeth-Ayerst, USA.*
Promethazine hydrochloride (p.416·2); codeine phosphate (p.26·1).
Coughs and cold symptoms.

Phenergan with Dextromethorphan *Wyeth-Ayerst, USA.*
Promethazine hydrochloride (p.416·2); dextromethorphan hydrobromide (p.1057·3).
Coughs and cold symptoms.

Phenergan Expectorant
Note. This name is used for preparations of different composition.
Rhone-Poulenc Rorer, Belg.; Rhone-Poulenc Rorer, Neth.†.
Promethazine hydrochloride (p.416·2); potassium guaiacolsulfonate (p.1068·3); ipecacuanha (p.1062·2).
Coughs.

Ciba Self Medication, Canad.
Promethazine hydrochloride (p.416·2); potassium guaiacolsulfonate (p.1068·3).
Coughs.

Rhone-Poulenc Rorer, Switz.
Promethazine hydrochloride (p.416·2); guaiphenesin (p.1061·3); ipecacuanha (p.1062·2).
Coughs.

Phenergan Expectorant with Codeine *Ciba Self Medication, Canad.*
Promethazine hydrochloride (p.416·2); potassium guaiacolsulfonate (p.1068·3); codeine phosphate (p.26·1).
Coughs.

Phenergan VC *Wyeth-Ayerst, USA.*
Promethazine hydrochloride (p.416·2); phenylephrine hydrochloride (p.1066·2).
Nasal congestion and cold symptoms.

Phenergan VC with Codeine *Wyeth-Ayerst, USA.*
Promethazine hydrochloride (p.416·2); phenylephrine hydrochloride (p.1066·2); codeine phosphate (p.26·1).
Coughs, nasal congestion and cold symptoms.

Phenergan VC Expectorant *Ciba Self Medication, Canad.*
Promethazine hydrochloride (p.416·2); phenylephrine hydrochloride (p.1066·2); potassium guaiacolsulfonate (p.1068·3).
Coughs.

Phenergan VC Expectorant with Codeine
Ciba Self Medication, Canad.
Promethazine hydrochloride (p.416·2); phenylephrine hydrochloride (p.1066·2); potassium guaiacolsulfonate (p.1068·3); codeine phosphate (p.26·1).
Coughs.

Phenergan-D *Wyeth-Ayerst, USA†.*
Promethazine hydrochloride (p.416·2); pseudoephedrine hydrochloride (p.1068·3).
Nasal congestion and cold symptoms.

Phenetron *Lannett, USA†.*
Chlorpheniramine maleate (p.405·1).
Hypersensitivity reactions.

Phenex *Ross, USA.*
A range of phenylalanine-free preparations for enteral nutrition including an infant feed.
Phenylketonuria.

Phenhalal *Halal, UK.*
Promethazine hydrochloride (p.416·2).

Phenhist DH with Codeine *Rugby, USA.*
Pseudoephedrine hydrochloride (p.1068·3); chlorpheniramine maleate (p.405·1); codeine phosphate (p.26·1).
Coughs and cold symptoms.

Phenhist Expectorant *Rugby, USA.*
Pseudoephedrine hydrochloride (p.1068·3); guaiphenesin (p.1061·3); codeine phosphate (p.26·1).
Coughs.

Phenhydan
Gerot, Aust.; Desitin, Ger.; Desitin, Switz.
Phenytoin (p.352·3) or phenytoin sodium (p.352·3).
Arrhythmias; epilepsy; trigeminal neuralgia.

Phenistix
Bayer Diagnostics, Austral.†; Miles, Ital.†; Ames, S.Afr.; Ames, USA†.
Test for phenylketonuria and urinary salicylates.

Phenobarb Vitalet *Adcock Ingram, S.Afr.†.*
Phenobarbitone (p.350·2); vitamin B substances.
Epilepsy; insomnia.

Phenocillin *Streuli, Switz.*
Benzathine phenoxymethylpenicillin (p.159·2) or phenoxymethylpenicillin (p.236·2).
Bacterial infections.

Phenoject *Mayrand, USA†.*
Promethazine hydrochloride (p.416·2).
Hypersensitivity reactions; motion sickness; nausea; postoperative pain (adjunct); sedative; vomiting.

Phenolax *Upjohn, USA.*
Phenolphthalein (p.1208·2).
Constipation.

Phenoptic *Optopics, USA.*
Phenylephrine hydrochloride (p.1066·2).
Funduscopy; open-angle glaucoma; ophthalmic examination; pupil dilatation during surgery; refraction without cycloplegia; uveitis.

Phenoris *Stickley, Canad.*
Clioquinol (p.193·2); allantoin (p.1078·2); phenol (p.1121·2).
Topical antiseptic.

Phenoro
Roche, Fr.; Sauter, Switz.†.
Betacarotene (p.1335·2); canthaxanthin (p.999·3).
Lupus erythematosus; photosensitivity; porphyrias.

Phenoxine *Lannett, USA.*
Phenylpropanolamine hydrochloride (p.1067·2).
Obesity.

Phenpro *Ratiopharm, Ger.*
Phenprocoumon (p.929·3).
Thrombo-embolic disorders.

Phensedyl
Note. This name is used for preparations of different composition.
Rhone-Poulenc Rorer, Austral.
Promethazine hydrochloride (p.416·2); pholcodine (p.1068·1); pseudoephedrine hydrochloride (p.1068·3).
Coughs.

Rhone-Poulenc Rorer, S.Afr.
Promethazine hydrochloride (p.416·2); codeine phosphate (p.26·1); ephedrine hydrochloride (p.1059·3).
Coughs.

Rhone-Poulenc Rorer, UK†.
Promethazine hydrochloride (p.416·2); codeine phosphate (p.26·1).
Coughs.

Phensedyl Plus *Rhone-Poulenc Rorer, UK.*
Pholcodine (p.1068·1); pseudoephedrine hydrochloride (p.1068·3); promethazine hydrochloride (p.416·2).
Congestion; coughs; sore throats.

Phensic *SmithKline Beecham Consumer, UK.*
Aspirin (p.16·1); caffeine (p.749·3).
Fever; pain.

Phensic Soluble *SmithKline Beecham Consumer, UK†.*
Aspirin (p.16·1).
Calcium carbonate (p.1182·1) is included in this preparation in an attempt to limit adverse effects on the gastro-intestinal mucosa.
Fever; pain.

Phentrol *Vortech, USA†.*
Phentermine hydrochloride (p.1484·3).
Obesity.

Phenurin *Merckle, Ger.†.*
Nitrofurantoin (p.231·3).
Urinary-tract infections.

Phenurone *Abbott, USA†.*
Phenacemide (p.350·1).
Epilepsy.

Phenyldrine *Rugby, USA.*
Phenylpropanolamine hydrochloride (p.1067·2).
Obesity.

Phenylfenesin LA *Goldline, USA.*
Phenylpropanolamine hydrochloride (p.1067·2); guaiphenesin (p.1061·3).
Coughs.

Phenyl-Free *Mead Johnson, Ital.*
Food for special diets.
Disorders of phenylalanine metabolism; phenylketonuria.

Phenylgesic *Goldline, USA.*
Phenyltoloxamine citrate (p.416·1); paracetamol (p.72·2).
Upper respiratory-tract symptoms.

Phenzine *Hauck, USA†.*
Phendimetrazine tartrate (p.1484·2).
Obesity.

Pherajod *Boots, Ger.†.*
Potassium iodide (p.1493·1); sodium thiosulphate (p.996·2).
Eye disorders.

Pheramin N *Kanoldt, Ger.*
Diphenhydramine hydrochloride (p.409·1).
Allergic disorders of the conjunctiva.

Pherarutin *Kanoldt, Ger.*
Troxerutin (p.1580·2).
Retinal disorders.

Pherazine with Codeine *Halsey, USA.*
Promethazine hydrochloride (p.416·2); codeine phosphate (p.26·1).
Coughs and cold symptoms.

Pherazine DM *Halsey, USA.*
Promethazine hydrochloride (p.416·2); dextromethorphan hydrobromide (p.1057·3).
Coughs and cold symptoms.

Pherazine VC *Halsey, USA.*
Promethazine hydrochloride (p.416·2); phenylephrine hydrochloride (p.1066·2).
Upper respiratory-tract symptoms.

Pherazine VC with Codeine *Halsey, USA.*
Promethazine hydrochloride (p.416·2); phenylephrine hydrochloride (p.1066·2); codeine phosphate (p.26·1).
Coughs and cold symptoms.

pH5-Eucerin *Beiersdorf, Ger.*
Emollient.
Skin disorders.

Phicon *Williams, USA.*
Pramoxine hydrochloride (p.1298·2); vitamin A (p.1358·1); vitamin E (p.1369·1).
Local anaesthesia.

Phicon-F *Williams, USA.*
Pramoxine hydrochloride (p.1298·2); undecenoic acid (p.389·2).
Fungal skin infections.

Philcociclina *Biotrading, Ital.†.*
Doxycycline hydrochloride (p.202·3).
Bacterial infections.

Phillips' Chewable *Sterling, USA.*
Magnesium hydroxide (p.1198·2).
Hyperacidity.

Phillips Gelcaps *Bayer, Canad.*
Docusate sodium (p.1189·3); phenolphthalein (p.1208·2).
Constipation.

Phillips' Laxative Gelcaps *Sterling, USA.*
Docusate sodium (p.1189·3); phenolphthalein (p.1208·2).

Phillips' Laxcaps *Glenbrook, USA.*
Docusate sodium (p.1189·3); phenolphthalein (p.1208·2).
Constipation.

Phillips' Milk of Magnesia
Bayer, Canad.; Sterling Health, USA.
Magnesium hydroxide (p.1198·2).
Constipation; hyperchlorhydria; peptic ulcer.

Phillips P.T.Y. Yeast Tablets *Phillips Yeast, UK.*
Yeast (p.1373·1); vitamin B substances.
Formerly known as Tonic Yeast.

Phimetin *BHR, UK.*
Cimetidine (p.1183·2).
Gastro-intestinal disorders associated with hyperacidity.

pHisoDerm
Sterling, Canad.†; Cilag, UK; Chattem, USA.
Skin cleanser.

pHisoHex
Sanofi Winthrop, Canad.; Maggioni, Ital.†; Sanofi Winthrop, USA.
Entsufon sodium (p.1574·3); hexachlorophane (p.1115·2).
Skin disinfection.

Phisohex Face Wash *SmithKline Beecham Consumer, Austral.*
Triclosan (p.1127·2).
Formerly known as Phisohex Reformulated.
Acne; skin infections.

pHiso-MED *Sanofi Winthrop, UK.*
Chlorhexidine gluconate (p.1107·2).
Formerly contained hexachlorophane.
Skin disinfection.

Phlebex *Thomae, Ger.†.*
Cream; topical gel: Pentosan polysulphate sodium (p.928·1); aescin (p.1543·3); camphor (p.1557·2).
Topical liquid: Pentosan polysulphate sodium (p.928·1); aescin (p.1543·3).
Vascular disorders.

Phlebodril
Note. This name is used for preparations of different composition.
Pierre Fabre, Ger.
Ruscus aculeatus; trimethylhesperidin chalcone (p.1580·2).
Vascular disorders.

Robapharm, Switz.
Capsules: Ruscus aculeatus; hesperidin methyl chalcone (p.1580·2); ascorbic acid (p.1365·2).
Cream†: Ruscus aculeatus; melilotus officinalis.
Vascular disorders.

Phlebodril N *Pierre Fabre, Ger.*
Ruscus aculeatus rhizome; melilotus officinalis; dextran sulphate (p.1571·1).
Vascular disorders.

Phlebogel *Lipha Sante, Fr.*
Aescin (p.1543·3); buphenine hydrochloride (p.1555·3).
Peripheral vascular disorders.

Phlebostasin *Klinge, Switz.*
Aesculus (p.1543·3).
Peripheral vascular disorders.

Phlexy *Scientific Hospital Supplies, Austral.*
Food for special diets.
Phenylketonuria.

Phlogantine *Streuli, Switz.†.*
Camphor (p.1557·2); methyl salicylate (p.55·2); eucalyptus oil (p.1578·1); mint oil; kaolin (p.1195·1).
Bronchitis; musculoskeletal inflammation; skin disorders.

Phlogase *Godecke, Ger.†.*
Oxyphenbutazone (p.72·1); heparin sodium (p.879·3).
Musculoskeletal and joint disorders; superficial phlebitis.

Phlogenzym *Mucos, Ger.*
Bromelains (p.1555·1); trypsin (p.1640·1); rutin (p.1580·2).
Inflammation; oedema.

Phlogidermil *Vifor, Switz.*
Ichthammol (p.1083·3); hamamelis (p.1587·1); guaiazulene (p.1586·3); cod-liver oil (p.1337·3); lavender oil (p.1594·3); zinc oxide (p.1096·2).
Inflammation; muscular pain.

Phlogont *Azupharma, Ger.*
Tablets†: Oxyphenbutazone (p.72·1).
Acute ankylosing spondylitis; gout.
Topical liquid: Glycol salicylate (p.43·1).
Musculoskeletal, joint, and soft-tissue disorders.

Phlogont Rheuma *Azupharma, Ger.*
Glycol salicylate (p.43·1) or methyl salicylate (p.55·2).
Musculoskeletal, joint, and soft-tissue disorders.

Phlogont-Thermal *Azupharma, Ger.*
Glycol salicylate (p.43·1); benzyl nicotinate (p.22·1).
Muscle and joint disorders; sports injuries.

Phocytan *Aguettant, Fr.*
Glucose-1-phosphate disodium, tetrahydrate.
Hypophosphataemia; parenteral nutrition.

Pholcolin
Rhone-Poulenc Rorer, Austral.†; Antigen, Irl.
Pholcodine (p.1068·1).
Coughs.

Pholcolinct *Propan, S.Afr.*
Pholcodine (p.1068·1).
Cough.

Pholcomed *Medo, UK.*
Pholcodine (p.1068·1).
Formerly contained pholcodine and papaverine hydrochloride.
Coughs.

Pholco-Mereprine *Hoechst Marion Roussel, Belg.*
Doxylamine succinate (p.410·1); pholcodine (p.1068·1); potassium guaiacolsulfonate (p.1068·3); sodium benzoate (p.1102·3).
Respiratory-tract disorders.

Pholcones *Cooperation Pharmaceutique, Fr.*
Quinine sulphate (p.439·2); camphor (p.1557·2); cineole (p.1564·1); pholcodine (p.1068·1); amylocaine hydrochloride (p.1286·1).
Coughs; respiratory disorders.

Pholcones Bismuth *Cooperation Pharmaceutique, Fr.*
Guaiphenesin (p.1061·3); bismuth succinate (p.1181·1); cineole (p.1564·1).
Respiratory-tract congestion.

Pholcones Bismuth-Quinine *Cooperation Pharmaceutique, Fr.†.*
Pholcodine (p.1068·1); bismuth succinate (p.1181·1); cineole (p.1564·1); guaiphenesin (p.1061·3); camphor (p.1557·2); quinine sulphate (p.439·2).
Coughs; throat disorders.

Pholcones Guaiphenesine-Quinine *Cooperation Pharmaceutique, Fr.†.*
Pholcodine (p.1068·1); cineole (p.1564·1); camphor (p.1557·2); guaiphenesin (p.1061·3); quinine sulphate (p.439·2).
Throat disorders.

Pholprin *Marion Merrell Dow, Switz.†.*
Pholcodine (p.1068·1); doxylamine succinate (p.410·1); guaiphenesin (p.1061·3).
Coughs.

Pholtex *Riker, S.Afr.*
Pholcodine resin complex (p.1068·1); phenyltoloxamine resin complex (p.416·1).
Coughs.

Pholtrate *McGloin, Austral.*
Pholcodine (p.1068·1).
Coughs.

Phol-Tussil *Interdelta, Switz.*
Pholcodine (p.1068·1); sodium benzoate (p.1102·3); tolu balsam (p.1071·1).
Coughs.

Phol-Tux *Interdelta, Switz.*
Pholcodine (p.1068·1); ethylmorphine hydrochloride (p.36·1); potassium guaiacolsulfonate (p.1068·3); belladonna (p.457·1); senega root (p.1069·3); sodium benzoate (p.1102·3).
Coughs.

Phonal *Knoll, Spain.*
Lozenges: Bacitracin (p.157·3); benzocaine (p.1286·2); neomycin sulphate (p.229·2); polymyxin B sulphate (p.239·1).
Mouth and throat disorders.
Throat spray: Benzalkonium chloride (p.1101·3); dexamethasone disodium phosphate (p.1037·2).
Mouth and throat inflammation.

Phonix Antitox *Phonix, Ger.*
Homoeopathic preparation.

Phonix Arthrophon *Phonix, Ger.*
Homoeopathic preparation.

Phonix Aurum III/012B *Phonix, Ger.*
Herbal and homoeopathic preparation.

Phonix Bronchophon *Phonix, Ger.*
Homoeopathic preparation.

Phonix Cuprum I/0178A *Phonix, Ger.†.*
Homoeopathic preparation.

Phonix Ferrum 032 A *Phonix, Ger.*
Homoeopathic preparation.

Phonix Gastriphon *Phonix, Ger.*
Artemisia abrotanum; absinthium (p.1541·1); centaury (p.1561·1); gentian (p.1583·3).
Gastro-intestinal disorders.

Phonix Hydrargyrum II/027A *Phonix, Ger.*
Homoeopathic preparation.

Phonix Kalium nitricum 05 *Phonix, Ger.†.*
Homoeopathic preparation.

Phonix Kalophon *Phonix, Ger.†.*
Aloes (p.1177·1); myrrh; gummi arabicum; arnica (p.1550·3); rosemary; calendula officinalis; hypericum (p.1590·1); peru balsam; cajuput oil; antimonium crudum.
Skin disorders.

Phonix Lymphophon *Phonix, Ger.*
Homoeopathic preparation.

Phonix Phonohepan *Phonix, Ger.*
Homoeopathic preparation.

Phonix Phonomigral *Phonix, Ger.†.*
Homoeopathic preparation.

Phonix Plumbum 024 A *Phonix, Ger.*
Homoeopathic preparation.

Phonix Solidago II/035 B *Phonix, Ger.*
Homoeopathic preparation.

Phonix Spongia 013 B *Phonix, Ger.†.*
Homoeopathic preparation.

Phonix Tartarus III/020 *Phonix, Ger.*
Homoeopathic preparation.

Phor Pain *Goldshield, UK.*
Ibuprofen (p.44·1).
Cold symptoms; pain.

PhosChol *American Lecithin, USA.*
Phosphatidyl choline (p.1618·1).
Nutritional supplement.

Phoscortil *Kolassa, Aust.*
Prednisolone sodium metasulphobenzoate (p.1048·1); aluminium phosphate (p.1178·3).

Phosetamin *Kohler-Pharma, Ger.*
Calcium, magnesium, and potassium salts of phosphorylcolamine.
Electrolyte disorders.

Phos-Ex
Vitaline, Norw.; Spectra Nova, Swed.; Vitaline, UK; Vitaline, USA†.
Calcium acetate (p.1155·1).
Calcium deficiency; hyperphosphataemia.

Phos-Flur
Colgate Oral Care, Austral.; Colgate-Hoyt, USA.
Acidulated phosphate fluoride or sodium fluoride (p.742·1).
Dental caries prophylaxis.

PhosLo *Braintree, USA.*
Calcium acetate (p.1155·1).
Hyperphosphataemia.

Phosoforme
Monin, Fr.; Pharmacie de France, Switz.†.
Ethylphosphoric acid; phosphoric acid (p.1618·1).
Urinary-tract disorders.

Phosoveol Vitamine C *Fournier, Fr.†.*
Concentrated phosphoric acid (p.1618·1); ascorbic acid (p.1365·2); calcium gluceptate (p.1155·1).
Tonic.

pHos-pHaid *Guardian, USA†.*
Ammonium biphosphate (p.1549·1); monobasic sodium phosphate (p.1159·3); sodium acid pyrophosphate.
Urine acidifier for prevention of renal calculi.

Phosphalugel
Kolassa, Aust.; Yamanouchi, Belg.; Yamanouchi, Fr.; Yamanouchi, Ger.; Wild, Switz.
Aluminium phosphate (p.1178·3).
Gastro-intestinal disorders associated with hyperacidity.

Phospharome *Plantes et Medecines, Fr.*
Kola (p.1645·1); gentian (p.1583·3); cinchona (p.1564·1); minerals.
Tonic.

Phosphate-Sandoz
Novartis, Austral.; Sandoz, Canad.; Sandoz, Irl.; Novartis, S.Afr.; Sandoz, UK.
Monobasic sodium phosphate (p.1159·3); sodium bicarbonate (p.1153·2); potassium bicarbonate (p.1153·1).
Hypercalcaemia; hypophosphataemia.

Phosphocholine *Soekami, Fr.†.*
Dibasic sodium phosphate (p.1159·3); choline citrate (p.1337·1); trisodium citrate (p.1153·2).
Dyspepsia.

Phosphocol *Mallinckrodt, USA.*
Phosphorus-32 (p.1424·3) in the form of chromic phosphate.
Malignant neoplasms.

Phospho-Lax *Sofar, Ital.*
Monobasic sodium phosphate (p.1159·3); dibasic sodium phosphate (p.1159·3).
Constipation.

Phospholine *Biobasal, Switz.†.*
Ecothiopate iodide (p.1392·1).
Convergent strabismus; glaucoma.

Phospholine Iodide
Storz, Austral.; Storz, Belg.; Storz, Canad.; Promedica, Fr.; Chinoin, Ital.†; Wyeth, Neth.; Dominion, UK; Wyeth-Ayerst, USA.
Ecothiopate iodide (p.1392·1).
Available on a named-patient basis only in the *UK*.
Convergent strabismus; glaucoma.

Phospholinjodid *Winzer, Ger.†.*
Ecothiopate iodide (p.1392·1).
Glaucoma.

Phosphoneuros *Doms-Adrian, Fr.*
Phosphoric acid (p.1618·1); calcium dihydrogen phosphate (p.1556·2); dibasic sodium phosphate (p.1159·3); magnesium glycerophosphate (p.1157·2).
Hypercalciuria; hypophosphataemic rickets; osteoporosis.

Phosphonorm
Medice, Ger.; Salmon, Switz.
Aluminium chlorohydrate (p.1078·3).
Hyperphosphataemia.

Phosphore-Sandoz *Sandoz, Fr.*
Monoammonium phosphate (p.1549·1); monobasic potassium phosphate (p.1159·3); manganese glycerophosphate (p.1586·2).
Bone loss during immobilisation; hypercalciuria; osteoporosis; rickets.

Phosphorus Med Complex *Dynamit, Aust.*
Homoeopathic preparation.

Phospho-Soda Fleet *Sofar, Ital.†.*
Monobasic sodium phosphate (p.1159·3); dibasic sodium phosphate (p.1159·3).
Constipation.

Phosphotec *Squibb Diagnostics, USA.*
Technetium-99m pyrophosphate (p.1425·1).

Photoderm Latte *Piam, Ital.*
Ethylhexyl *p*-methoxycinnamate (p.1487·1); avobenzone (p.1486·3).
Sunscreen.

Photofrin
Ligand, Canad.; Sanofi Winthrop, USA.
Porfimer sodium (p.559·1).
Oesophageal cancer; papillary bladder cancer.

Photoplex
Note. This name is used for preparations of different composition.
Allergan, Canad.
SPF 15: Avobenzone (p.1486·3); octyl salicylate (p.1487·3); octocrylene (p.1487·3); oxybenzone (p.1487·3).
Sunscreen.

Allergan Herbert, USA.
Avobenzone (p.1486·3); padimate O (p.1488·1).
Sunscreen.

Phrenilin *Carnrick, USA.*
Butalbital (p.644·3); paracetamol (p.72·2).
Tension headache.

Phthazol *Rhone-Poulenc Rorer, Austral.†.*
Phthalylsulphathiazole (p.237·1).
Gastro-intestinal bacterial infections.

pHygiene *Galderma, Canad.†.*
Lactic acid (p.1593·3).
Skin cleanser; skin disorders.

Phylarm *LCA, Fr.*
Sodium chloride (p.1162·2); borax (p.1554·2); boric acid (p.1554·2).
Eye wash.

Phylletten *Rorer, Ger.†.*
Dequalinium chloride (p.1112·1).
Inflammatory disorders and infections of the oropharynx.

Phyllocontin
Purdue Frederick, Canad.; Napp, Irl.; Lagamed, S.Afr.; Napp, UK; Purdue Frederick, USA.
Aminophylline (p.748·1) or aminophylline hydrate (p.748·1).
Asthma; chronic bronchitis; emphysema; heart failure.

Phyllosan *Seton, UK.*
Multivitamin and mineral preparation.

Phyllotemp
Mundipharma, Ger.; Mundipharma, Switz.
Aminophylline (p.748·1) or aminophylline hydrate (p.748·1).
Obstructive airways disease.

Phylorinol *Schaffer, USA.*
Mouthwash: Phenol (p.1121·2); methyl salicylate (p.55·2).
Minor mouth or throat irritation.

Topical solution: Phenol (p.1121·2); boric acid (p.1554·2); strong iodine solution (p.1493·1).
Oral wounds and infections.

Physeptone *Glaxo Wellcome, Austral.; Wellcome, Irl.; Glaxo Wellcome, S.Afr.; Wellcome, UK.*
Methadone hydrochloride (p.53·2).
Cough; pain.

Physex *Leo, Norw.†; Byk Elmu, Spain.*
Chorionic gonadotrophin (p.1243·1).
Cryptorchidism; delayed puberty; impotence; male and female infertility; metrorrhagia; threatened and habitual abortion.

Physiogel *Braun, Switz.*
Modified gelatin (p.723·2) with electrolytes.
Hypovolaemia.

Physiogesic *Herbert, Canad.*
Diethylamine salicylate (p.33·1).

Physiogine *Organon, Fr.*
Oestriol (p.1457·2).
Oestrogen deficiency.

Physiolax *Medipharm, Switz.*
Aloes (p.1177·1); belladonna (p.457·1).
Constipation; stool softener.

Physiologica *Qualiphar, Belg.; Gifrer Barbezat, Fr.; Pharmacal, Switz.*
Sodium chloride (p.1162·2).
Eye wash; nasal irrigation.

Physiolyte *McGaw, USA.*
Electrolytes (p.1147·1).
Irrigation solution.

Physiomenthol *Herbert, Canad.*
Menthol (p.1600·2).

Physiomer *Sanofi Winthrop, Fr.*
Sea water (p.1162·2).
Nasal irrigation.

Physiomint *Koch, Aust.*
Mint oil (p.1604·1).
Gastro-intestinal disorders; headache; migraine; respiratory-tract disorders; rheumatic disorders; soft-tissue and muscle injury.

Physiomycine *Lophal, Fr.*
Methacycline hydrochloride (p.225·1).
Bacterial infections.

Physiorhine *Rhone-Poulenc Rorer, Belg.*
Sodium chloride (p.1162·2).
Cleansing of nasal passages and eyelids.

Physio-Rub *Herbert, Canad.*
Methyl salicylate (p.55·2); menthol (p.1600·2); cineole (p.1564·1).

Physiosoin *Chauvin, Fr.*
Sodium chloride (p.1162·2).
Eye wash; nasal irrigation.

PhysioSol *Abbott, USA.*
Electrolytes (p.1147·1).
Irrigation solution.

Physiospir *Soekami, Fr.†.*
Sodium chloride (p.1162·2).
Nose and eye irrigation.

Physiostat *Organon, Fr.*
7 Tablets, ethinyloestradiol (p.1445·1); 15 tablets, ethinyloestradiol; lynoestrenol (p.1448·2).
Dysmenorrhoea; sequential-type oral contraceptive.

Physiotens *Solvay, Fr.; Solvay, Ger.; Solvay, Switz.; Solvay, UK.*
Moxonidine (p.913·1).
Hypertension.

Physium *Boiron, Canad.*
Sodium chloride (p.1162·2).
Nasal congestion; nasal hygiene.

Phytat *Cochon, Fr.*
Sodium phytate (p.995·3).
Hypercalciuria.

Phytemag *Lesourd, Fr.*
Magnesium silicate (p.1473·3); magnesium glycerophosphate (p.1157·2); chlorophyll (p.1000·1); parsley, thyme and buchu powder; equisetum, wild celery, and ginger powder; oxides of zinc, copper, and nickel.
Tonic.

Phytex
Note. This name is used for preparations of different composition.
Rupertus, Aust.
Sorbic acid (p.1125·2); tannic acid (p.1634·2); methyl salicylate (p.55·2); salicylic acid (p.1090·2); acetic acid (p.1541·2).
Fungal infections of the feet.
Rhone-Poulenc Rorer, Austral.†; Pharmax, Irl.; Pharmax, UK.
Borotannic complex (p.1634·2 and p.1554·2); salicylic acid (p.1090·2); methyl salicylate (p.55·2); acetic acid (p.1541·2).
Fungal skin and nail infections.

Phytoberidin *Synpharma, Switz.*
Valerian (p.1643·1); hypericum (p.1590·1); passion flower (p.1615·3); guaiazulene (p.1586·3); lupulus (p.1597·2); melissa (p.1600·1).
Insomnia; nervous disorders.

Phytobronchin *Steigerwald, Ger.*
Syrup†: Althaea (p.1546·3).
Coughs.
Tablets; liquid; tincture; lozenges: Primula rhizome; thyme (p.1636·3).
Cold symptoms.

Phytocalm *UPSA, Fr.*
Valerian (p.1643·1); ballota; crataegus (p.1568·2); passion flower (p.1615·3).
Insomnia; nervous disorders.

Phytocean *Ido, Fr.*
Nutritional supplement.

Phytocil *Fisons, UK†.*
Cream: Phenoxypropanol (p.1122·2); chlorophenoxyethanol (p.1122·2); salicylic acid (p.1090·2); menthol (p.1600·2).
Topical powder: Zinc undecenoate (p.389·2); chlorophenoxyethanol (p.1122·2); phenoxypropanol (p.1122·2).
Fungal skin infections.

Phytocoltar *Phytosolba, Fr.†.*
Coal tar (p.1092·3); chelidonium; groundsel; sage (p.1627·1); cypress oil; cajuput oil (p.1556·1); rosemary oil (p.1626·2).
Seborrhoeic dermatitis.

Phytocortal *Steierl, Ger.*
Homoeopathic preparation.

Phytodolor *Madaus, Aust.; Steigerwald, Ger.*
Populus tremula leaf and bark (p.1620·1); fraxinus excelsior bark; solidago virgaurea.
Neuralgia; rheumatism.

Phytoestrol N *Muller Goppingen, Ger.*
Rhubarb (p.1212·1).
Endometritis; juvenile oligomenorrhoea and dysmenorrhoea; menopausal disorders; primary and secondary amenorrhoea.

Phytofibre *Plantes et Medecines, Fr.*
Ispaghula (p.1194·2).
Constipation.

Phytogran
Note. This name is used for preparations of different composition.
Synpharma, Aust.
Valerian root (p.1643·1); lupulus (p.1597·2); melissa leaf (p.1600·1).
Anxiety; sleep disorders.
Grandel-Synpharma, Ger.; Biorex, Switz.†.
Lupulin; hypericum (p.1590·1).
Agitation; insomnia.

Phytohepar *Steigerwald, Ger.*
Silybum marianum (p.993·3).
Liver disorders.

Phyto-Hypophyson C *Steierl, Ger.*
Homoeopathic preparation.

Phyto-Hypophyson L *Steierl, Ger.*
Homoeopathic preparation.

Phytolax
Note. This name is used for preparations of different composition.
Sante Naturelle, Canad.
Cascara (p.1183·1); phenolphthalein (p.1208·2); bile salts (p.1553·2); capsicum oleoresin; papain (p.1614·1).
Synpharma, Switz.
Aloes (p.1177·1); frangula (p.1193·2); belladonna (p.457·1).
Constipation.

Phytolife Plus *Blackmores, UK.*
Calcium (p.1155·1); soya (p.1355·1).
Menopausal disorders.

Phytomed Cardio *Phytomed, Switz.*
Crataegus (p.1568·2); cereus grandiflorus; passion flower (p.1615·3); rosemary.
Cardiac disorders.

Phytomed Gastro *Phytomed, Switz.*
Angelica; centaury (p.1561·1); chamomile (p.1561·2); peppermint leaf (p.1208·1); caraway (p.1559·3); potato.
Digestive disorders.

Phytomed Hepato *Phytomed, Switz.*
Absinthium (p.1541·1); cynara (p.1569·2); peppermint leaf (p.1208·1); raphanus sativus var. nigra; silybum marianum (p.993·3); taraxacum (p.1634·2).
Digestive disorders.

Phytomed Nephro *Phytomed, Switz.*
Silver birch (p.1553·3); solidago virgaurea; orthosiphon stamineus (p.1592·2); juniper (p.1592·2); ononis (p.1610·2); taraxacum (p.1634·2).
Urinary-tract disorders.

Phytomed Prosta *Phytomed, Switz.*
Echinacea purpurea (p.1574·2); poplar buds (p.1620·1); saw palmetto (p.1462·1); solidago virgaurea.
Prostatic pain; urinary disorders.

Phytomed Rhino *Phytomed, Switz.*
Cinchona bark (p.1564·1); echinacea purpurea (p.1574·2); salix (p.82·3); solidago virgaurea.
Cold symptoms; sinusitis.

Phytomed Somni *Phytomed, Switz.*
Valerian (p.1643·1); passion flower (p.1615·3); lupulus (p.1597·2); lavandula angustifolia.
Sleep disorders.

Phytomelis *Lehning, Fr.*
Hamamelis (p.1587·1); aesculus (p.1543·3).
Haemorrhoids; peripheral vascular disorders.

Phytonoctu *Steigerwald, Ger.*
Melissa (p.1600·1); passion flower (p.1615·3); valerian (p.1643·1).
Nervous disorders; sleep disorders.

Phytonoxon N *Steigerwald, Ger.*
Corydalis cava; eschscholtzia californica.
Sleep disorders.

Phytophanere *Phytosolba, Fr.*
Wheat-germ oil; carrot oil; borage oil (p.1582·1); rice-bran oil; salmon oil; yeast (p.1373·1); antilles cherries; fish roe.
Fragile hair and nails.

Phytopure *Nobel, Canad.*
Multivitamin and mineral preparation.

Phytorin *Phytopharma, Ger.†.*
Homoeopathic preparation.

Phytotherapie Boribel no 8 *Dietetique et Sante, Fr.*
Tilia (p.1637·3); passion flower (p.1615·3); valerian (p.1643·1).
Insomnia; nervous disorders.

Phytotherpie Boribel no 9 *Dietetique et Sante, Fr.*
Fraxinus excelsior; bladderwrack (p.1554·1).
Obesity.

Phytotux *Lehning, Fr.*
Tolu balsam (p.1071·1); Desessartz syrup.
Coughs.

Phytotux H *Homeocan, Canad.*
Homoeopathic preparation.

Phytpulmon *Bionorica, Ger.†.*
Aniseed (p.1549·3); inula helenium rhizome (p.1059·2); hyssop; orris; lichen islandicus; liquorice (p.1197·1); achillea (p.1542·2); pulmonaria; sage (p.1627·1); verbena; viola odorata.
Respiratory-tract disorders.

Piantanol *Milanfarma, Ital.†.*
Ceratonia (p.1472·2).
Gastro-intestinal disorders.

Piascledine *Pharmascience, Fr.; ABC, Ital.*
Avocado oil; soya oil (p.1355·1).
Gum disorders; musculoskeletal and joint disorders; phlebitis; skin disorders; skin ulceration.

Piazofolina *Bracco, Ital.*
Morinamide hydrochloride (p.227·2).
Tuberculosis.

Picariz *Picot, Fr.*
Food for special diets.
Diarrhoea.

Picibanil *Chugai, Jpn.*
Lyophilised powder of *Streptococcus pyogenes.*
Malignant neoplasms.

Picillin *CT, Ital.*
Piperacillin sodium (p.237·2).
Lignocaine hydrochloride (p.1293·2) is included in this preparation to alleviate the pain of injection.
Bacterial infections.

Pickles Antiseptic Cream *Pickles, UK.*
Dibromopropamide isethionate (p.1112·2).
Skin disinfection.

Pickles Corn Caps *Pickles, UK.*
Salicylic acid (p.1090·2); colophony (p.1567·1).

Pickles Foot Ointment *Pickles, UK.*
Salicylic acid (p.1090·2).
Calluses; corns.

Pickles Toothache Tincture *Pickles, UK.*
Clove oil (p.1565·2); lignocaine (p.1293·2).

Picolax
Note. This name is used for preparations of different composition.
Ferring, Irl.; Nordic, UK.
Sodium picosulphate (p.1213·2); magnesium citrate (p.1198·2).
Bowel evacuation; constipation.
Falqui, Ital.†.
Sodium picosulphate (p.1213·2).
Constipation.

Picolaxine *Pharmethic, Belg.*
Sodium picosulphate (p.1213·2).
Constipation.

Pico-Salax *Ferring, Norw.; Ferring, Swed.; Ferring, Switz.*
Sodium picosulphate (p.1213·2); magnesium oxide (p.1198·3); citric acid (p.1564·3).
Bowel evacuation.

Picot *Picot, Fr.*
Dextrin (p.1339·1); maltose (p.1350·2).
Sugar substitute.

Picten *Miquel Otsuka, Spain†.*
Hydrochlorothiazide (p.885·2); methyldopa (p.904·2); reserpine (p.942·1); triamterene (p.957·2).
Hypertension.

Pidilat *Solvay, Ger.*
Nifedipine (p.916·2).
Angina pectoris; hypertension; Raynaud's syndrome.

Pidocal *Sanofi Winthrop, Switz.*
Calcium pidolate (p.1155·3); calcium carbonate (p.1182·1).
Calcium deficiency; osteoporosis.

Pielograf *Juste, Spain.*
Meglumine diatrizoate (p.1003·2); sodium diatrizoate (p.1003·2).
Radiographic contrast medium.

Pielografin *Schering, Ital.†.*
Sodium diatrizoate (p.1003·2); meglumine diatrizoate (p.1003·2).
Radiographic contrast medium.

Pierami *Fournier, Ital.*
Amikacin sulphate (p.150·2).
Bacterial infections.

Pierminox *Pierrel, Ital.†.*
Minoxidil (p.910·3).
Alopecia androgenetica.

Pigenil *Inverni della Beffa, Ital.*
Pygeum africanum (p.1461·3).
Prostatic hyperplasia.

Pigitil *Dorom, Ital.*
Pidotimod (p.1618·3).
Immunostimulant.

Pigmanorm
Note. This name is used for preparations of different composition.
Widmer, Ger.
Hydroquinone (p.1083·1); tretinoin (p.1093·3); hydrocortisone (p.1043·3).
Skin hyperpigmentation.
Widmer, Switz.
Hydroquinone (p.1083·1); tretinoin (p.1093·3); dexamethasone (p.1037·1); dexpanthenol (p.1570·3); ethylhexyl *p*-methoxycinnamate (p.1487·1); avobenzone (p.1486·3).
Skin hyperpigmentation.

Piladren *Alcon-Thilo, Ger.†.*
Pilocarpine (p.1396·3); adrenaline (p.813·2).
Glaucoma.

Pilagan *Allergan, USA.*
Pilocarpine nitrate (p.1396·3).
Glaucoma; reversal of mydriasis.

Pilder *Quimifar, Spain.*
Gemfibrozil (p.1273·3).
Hyperlipidaemias.

Pildoras Ferrug Sanatori *Santiveri, Spain.*
Sulphur (p.1091·2); ferrous sulphate (p.1340·2); cinchona (p.1564·1); rhubarb (p.1212·1).
Anaemias.

Pildoras Zeninas *Puerto Galiano, Spain.*
Aloes (p.1177·1); belladonna (p.457·1); cascara (p.1183·1); jalap (p.1195·1); podophyllum (p.1089·1); phenolphthalein (p.1208·2); liquorice (p.1197·1).
Constipation.

Pileabs *Lane, UK.*
Slippery elm bark (p.1630·1); cascara sagrada (p.1183·1).
Haemorrhoids.

Piletabs *Potter's, UK.*
Pilewort; agrimony; cascara (p.1183·1); collinsonia.
Haemorrhoids.

Pilewort Compound *Gerard House, UK.*
Pilewort; senna leaf (p.1212·2); geum maculatum; cascara (p.1183·1).
Constipation.

Pil-Food *Serra Pamies, Spain.*
Multivitamins and amino acids; lactoalbumin; panicum miliaceum.

Pil-Food Nouvelle formule *Golaz, Switz.*
Multivitamins and amino acids; protein hydrolysate; millet.
Hair and nail disorders.

Pilfor P *BASF, Ger.*
Paracetamol (p.72·2); codeine phosphate (p.26·1).
Pain.

Pilison *Schering, Aust.*
Fluocortolone pivalate (p.1041·3); salicylic acid (p.1090·2).
Skin disorders.

Pilka *Zyma, Aust.; Ferrer, Spain; Zyma, Switz.*
Drosera (p.1574·1); thyme (p.1636·3).
Pilka suppositories formerly contained camphor, cineole, drosera, niaouli oil, paracetamol, thyme, and cholesterol in *Spain.*
Coughs.

Pilka Forte *Zyma, Aust.*
Thyme (p.1636·3); drosera (p.1574·1); ephedrine hydrochloride (p.1059·3).
Coughs.

Pillole Fattori *Ogna, Ital.*
Cape aloes (p.1177·1); rhubarb (p.1212·1); cascara (p.1183·1).
Constipation.

Pillole Frerichs Maldifassi *Procemsa, Ital.†.*
Rhubarb (p.1212·1); socotrine aloes (p.1177·1); calamus (p.1556·1); gentian (p.1583·3).
Constipation.

Pillole Lassative Aicardi *Schiapparelli, Ital.†.*
Aloes (p.1177·1); cascara (p.1183·1); phenolphthalein (p.1208·2).
Constipation.

Pillole Schias *AFOM, Ital.†.*
Rhubarb (p.1212·1); gentian (p.1583·3); boldo (p.1554·1); nux vomica (p.1609·3); cascara (p.1183·1); inositol (p.1591·1); phenolphthalein (p.1208·2).
Constipation.

Pilo *Asta Medica, Belg.; Chauvin, Fr.; Ciba Vision, Norw.; Novopharma, Switz.*
Pilocarpine hydrochloride (p.1396·3) or pilocarpine nitrate (p.1396·3).
Glaucoma; ocular hypertension; reversal of mydriasis.

Pilocar *Iolab, USA.*
Pilocarpine hydrochloride (p.1396·3).
Glaucoma; raised intra-ocular pressure; reversal of mydriasis.

Pilocarpol *Mayrhofer, Aust.†; Winzer, Ger.*
Pilocarpine (p.1396·3).
Glaucoma; production of miosis.

Pilodren *Farmila, Ital.*
Pilocarpine hydrochloride (p.1396·3); adrenaline acid tartrate (p.813·3).
Open-angle glaucoma.

Pilo-Eserin *Ciba Vision, Ger.*
Pilocarpine hydrochloride (p.1396·3); physostigmine salicylate (p.1395·3).
Glaucoma.

Pilofrine *Novopharma, Switz.†.*
Pilocarpine nitrate (p.1396·3); phenylephrine hydrochloride (p.1066·2).
Glaucoma; ocular hypertension.

Piloftal *Agepha, Aust.*
Pilocarpine (p.1396·3).
Glaucoma; ophthalmic surgery.

Pilogel
Alcon, Aust.; Alcon-Thilo, Ger.; Alcon, Irl.; Alcon, Ital.; Alcon, Neth.†; Alcon, S.Afr.; Alcon, UK.
Pilocarpine hydrochloride (p.1396·3).
Glaucoma; ocular hypertension.

Pilogel HS *Alcon, Switz.*
Pilocarpine hydrochloride (p.1396·3).
Glaucoma.

Pilomann *Mann, Ger.*
Pilocarpine hydrochloride (p.1396·3).
Glaucoma.

Pilomann-Ol *Mann, Ger.*
Pilocarpine (p.1396·3).
Glaucoma.

Pilopine HS
Alcon, Canad.; Alcon, USA.
Pilocarpine hydrochloride (p.1396·3).
Glaucoma; raised intra-ocular pressure; reversal of mydriasis.

Pilopos *Ursapharm, Ger.*
Pilocarpine nitrate (p.1396·3).
Glaucoma; production of miosis.

Pilopt *Sigma, Austral.*
Pilocarpine hydrochloride (p.1396·3).
Glaucoma.

Piloptic *Optopics, USA.*
Pilocarpine hydrochloride (p.1396·3).
Glaucoma; reversal of mydriasis.

Pilopto-Carpine *Lebeh, USA.*
Pilocarpine hydrochloride (p.1396·3).
Glaucoma; raised intra-ocular pressure; reversal of mydriasis.

Pilostat *Bausch & Lomb, USA.*
Pilocarpine hydrochloride (p.1396·3).
Glaucoma; raised intra-ocular pressure; reversal of mydriasis.

Pilostigmin Puroptal *Metochem, Aust.*
Neostigmine bromide (p.1393·3); pilocarpine hydrochloride (p.1396·3).
Glaucoma; production of miosis.

Pilo-Stulln *Stulln, Ger.*
Pilocarpine hydrochloride (p.1396·3).
Glaucoma.

Pilosuryl *Pierre Fabre, Fr.*
Pilosella; phyllanthus.
Water retention.

Pilotonina *Farmila, Ital.*
Pilocarpine hydrochloride (p.1396·3).
Ocular hypertension; production of miosis.

Pilovital *Lesvi, Spain.*
Minoxidil (p.910·3).
Alopecia androgenetica.

Pilowal *Apotheke Heiligen Brigitta, Aust.†.*
Benzyl nicotinate (p.22·1); dexpanthenol (p.1570·3).

Pilule Dupuis *Synthelabo, Fr.*
Bisacodyl (p.1179·3); aloes (p.1177·1); frangula bark (p.1193·2).
Constipation.

Pilules de Vichy *Spiphar, Belg.*
Sodium picosulphate (p.1213·2); electrolytes (p.1147·1).
Formerly contained danthron and electrolytes.
Constipation.

Piluno *Roche, Switz.†.*
Multivitamins; millet; wheat-germ oil; yeast; cystine; dexpanthenol.
Hair disorders; peripheral vascular disorders.

Pilzcin
Kolassa, Aust.; Merz, Ger.; Shionogi, Jpn.
Croconazole hydrochloride (p.377·1).
Fungal skin infections.

Pima *Fleming, USA.*
Potassium iodide (p.1493·1).
Chronic pulmonary diseases.

Pima Biciron *Basotherm, Ger.†.*
Chloramphenicol (p.182·1); natamycin (p.385·3).
Bacterial and fungal eye infections.

Pima Biciron N *Basotherm, Ger.*
Natamycin (p.385·3).
Fungal eye infections.

Pimafucin
Yamanouchi, Belg.; Basotherm, Ger.; Brocades, UK†.
Natamycin (p.385·3).
Fungal infections; trichomoniasis.

Pimafucort
Note. This name is used for preparations of different composition.
Yamanouchi, Belg.; Yamanouchi, Ger.; Brocades, Ital.†; Yamanouchi, Neth.
Hydrocortisone (p.1043·3); natamycin (p.385·3); neomycin sulphate (p.229·2).
Infected skin disorders.

Yamanouchi, Fr.†.
Dexamethasone (p.1037·1); natamycin (p.385·3); neomycin sulphate (p.229·2); bacitracin (p.157·3).
Infected skin disorders.

Pimarektal *Basotherm, Ger.†.*
Natamycin (p.385·3); hydrocortisone (p.1043·3); 3-benzhydryloxy-8-isopropyl-$1\alpha H,5\alpha H$-nortropan methanesulphonate; benzalkonium chloride (p.1101·3).
Anorectal disorders.

Pimexone *Formenti, Ital.*
Mepixanox (p.1482·2).
Respiratory disorders.

Pinal N *Atzinger, Ger.*
Zinc oxide (p.1096·2); N-(2-hydroxyethyl)-10-undecenamide; salicylic acid (p.1090·2).
Skin disorders.

Pin-Alcol *Schoning-Berlin, Ger.*
Menthol (p.1600·2); pine oil (p.1623·3).
Neuromuscular and joint disorders; pruritus; soft-tissue injury.

Pinalgesic *Pinewood, Irl.*
Mefenamic acid (p.51·2).
Menorrhagia; pain.

Pinamet *Pinewood, Irl.*
Cimetidine (p.1183·2).
Gastric hyperacidity; peptic ulcer; Zollinger-Ellison syndrome.

Pinamox *Pinewood, Irl.*
Amoxycillin (p.151·3).
Bacterial infections.

Pinbetol *Dolorgiet, Ger.†.*
Pindolol (p.931·1).
Cardiac disorders; hypertension.

Pindac *Leo, Irl.*
Pinacidil (p.930·3).
Hypertension.

Pindione *Lipha Sante, Fr.*
Phenindione (p.928·3).
Thrombo-embolic disorders.

Pindoptan *Kanoldt, Ger.*
Pindolol (p.931·1).
Glaucoma.

Pindoreal *Realpharma, Ger.*
Pindolol (p.931·1).
Arrhythmias; hypertension; ischaemic heart disease.

Pinedrin *Lisapharma, Ital.*
Pumilio pine oil (p.1623·3); thyme (p.1636·3).
Respiratory system disorders.

Pinefedrina *Lisapharma, Ital.†.*
Ephedrine hydrochloride (p.1059·3); vitamin A palmitate (p.1359·2); pumilio pine (p.1623·3); thyme (p.1636·3).
Coughs.

Pinetarsol *Ego, Austral.*
Tar (p.1092·3).
Skin disorders.

Pinex *Alpharma, Norw.*
Paracetamol (p.72·2).
Fever; pain.

Pinex Forte *Alpharma, Norw.*
Codeine phosphate (p.26·1); paracetamol (p.72·2).
Pain.

Pinifed *Pinewood, Irl.*
Nifedipine (p.916·2).
Hypertension; ischaemic heart disease.

Pinikehl *Sanum-Kehlbeck, Ger.*
Homoeopathic preparation.

Piniment *Austroplant, Aust.*
Balsam: Camphor (p.1557·2); eucalyptus oil (p.1578·1); oleum pini sylvestris; pumilio pine oil (p.1623·3); turpentine oil (p.1641·1); guaiazulene (p.1586·3).
Coughs; gastro-intestinal spasm; respiratory-tract disorders.
Nasal ointment: Ephedrine hydrochloride (p.1059·3); camphor (p.1557·2); eucalyptus oil (p.1578·1); oleum pini sylvestris; pumilio pine oil (p.1623·3); turpentine oil (p.1641·1); sage oil; sunflower oil (p.1634·1).
Nasal congestion.
Ointment: Camphor (p.1557·2); menthol (p.1600·2); eucalyptus oil (p.1578·1); Norway spruce oil; pumilio pine oil (p.1623·3); turpentine oil (p.1641·1).
Catarrh,; cold and influenza symptoms; cough.

Pinimenthol
Note. This name is used for preparations of different composition.
Schoeller, Aust.†.
Ointment: Camphor (p.1557·2); menthol (p.1600·2); eucalyptus oil (p.1578·1); norway spruce oil; pumilio pine oil (p.1623·3); turpentine oil (p.1641·1).
Topical solution: Camphor (p.1557·2); menthol (p.1600·2); eucalyptus oil (p.1578·1); pumilio pine oil (p.1623·3); turpentine oil (p.1641·1); pine oil.
Coughs and cold symptoms; musculoskeletal and joint disorders.

Rovi, Spain†.
Camphor (p.1557·2); cineole (p.1564·1); pinus sylvestris oil; turpentine oil (p.1641·1); menthol (p.1600·2); pinus pinaster oil.
Upper-respiratory-tract disorders.

Piniol, Switz.
Camphor (p.1557·2); menthol (p.1600·2); orange oil (p.1610·3); pine cone oil; eucalyptus oil (p.1578·1); pumilio pine oil (p.1623·3); turpentine oil (p.1641·1); pine-needle oil.
Influenza; muscle and joint pain; neuralgia.

Pinimenthol Bad N *Spitzner, Ger.*
Camphor (p.1557·2); eucalyptus oil (p.1578·1); menthol (p.1600·2).
Bath additive.

Pinimenthol N *Spitzner, Ger.*
Eucalyptus oil (p.1578·1); pine needle oil; menthol (p.1600·2).
Respiratory-tract disorders.

Pinimenthol-Oral N *Spitzner, Ger.*
Anethole (p.1549·3); cineole (p.1564·1); pumilio pine oil (p.1623·3).
Asthma; bronchitis.

Pinimenthol-S *Spitzner, Ger.*
Eucalyptus oil (p.1578·1); oleum pini sylvestris.
Respiratory-tract disorders.

Piniol
Note. This name is used for preparations of different composition.
Schoeller, Aust.†.
Balsam: Camphor (p.1557·2); eucalyptus oil (p.1578·1); pine oil; pumilio pine oil (p.1623·3); turpentine oil (p.1641·1); guaiazulene (p.1586·3).
Coughs and cold symptoms; pain; urinary frequency.
Nasal ointment: Ephedrine hydrochloride (p.1059·3); sunflower oil (p.1634·1); camphor (p.1557·2); eucalyptus oil (p.1578·1); pine oil; pumilio pine oil (p.1623·3); turpentine oil (p.1641·1); sage oil.
Cold symptoms; nasal congestion.

Spitzner, Ger.
Naphazoline hydrochloride (p.1064·2).
Rhinitis.

Piniol N *Spitzner, Ger.*
Camphor (p.1557·2); eucalyptus oil (p.1578·1); oleum pini sylvestris.
Respiratory-tract disorders.

Pink Biscoat *Invamed, USA.*
Bismuth salicylate (p.1180·1).

Pinofit *Pino, Ger.†.*
Glycol salicylate (p.43·1); menthol (p.1600·2); mint oil (p.1604·1).
Inflammatory disorders; soft tissue injuries.

Pinoidal-Bad *Pino, Ger.†.*
Norway spruce oil; camphor (p.1557·2); menthol (p.1600·2).
Bath additive.

Pino-Pak Fangoparaffin *Pino, Ger.†.*
Hard paraffin; medicinal mud.
Rheumatic disorders; trauma.

Pinorhinol *Bouchara Sante, Fr.*
Menthol (p.1600·2); camphor (p.1557·2); cineole (p.1564·1).
Nose and throat infections.

Pin-Rid *Apothecary, USA.*
Pyrantel embonate (p.109·3).

Pinselina Dr. Knapp *Montefarmaco, Ital.*
Benzocaine (p.1286·2); phenol (p.1121·2); thymol (p.1127·1); menthol (p.1600·2).
Mouth disorders.

Pintacrom *Diafarm, Spain.*
Mercurochrome (p.1119·2).
Wound disinfection.

Pinthym *Centrapharm, Belg.†.*
Camphor (p.1557·2); creosote (p.1057·3); cineole (p.1564·1); mint oil (p.1604·1); menthol (p.1600·2); pine oil; rosemary oil (p.1626·2); wild thyme oil; thyme oil (p.1637·1).
Rhinitis; sinusitis.

Pinus-Strath *Strath-Labor, Ger.†.*
Turiones pini; plantago lanceolata; thyme (p.1636·3).
Respiratory-tract disorders.

Pin-X *Effcon, USA.*
Pyrantel embonate (p.109·3).

Pioral Pasta *Teofarma, Ital.*
Chlorothymol (p.1111·1).
Oral disinfection.

Piorlis *Aristegui, Spain.*
Cineole (p.1564·1); eugenol (p.1578·2); peppermint oil; methyl salicylate (p.55·2); thymol (p.1127·1); tyrothricin (p.267·2).
Gingivitis; mouth ulcers; pyorrhoea.

Piorreol *Boots, Spain†.*
Chlorhexidine acetate (p.1107·2); tyrothricin (p.267·2).
Mouth infections.

Pip-A-Ray *Vernleigh, S.Afr.†.*
Piperazine hydrate (p.107·2) or piperazine phosphate (p.107·2).
Ascariasis; enterobiasis.

Pipcil
Wyeth Lederle, Belg.; Lederle, Neth.
Piperacillin sodium (p.237·2).
Bacterial infections.

Pipeacid *Del Saz & Filippini, Ital.*
Pipemidic acid (p.237·2).
Urinary-tract infections.

Pipedac *Teofarma, Ital.*
Pipemidic acid (p.237·2).
Urinary-tract infections.

Pipedase *Logifarm, Ital.†.*
Pipemidic acid (p.237·2).
Urinary-tract infections.

Pipefort *Lampugnani, Ital.*
Pipemidic acid (p.237·2).
Urinary-tract infections.

Pipemid *Gentili, Ital.*
Pipemidic acid (p.237·2).
Urinary-tract infections.

Piper *Panthox & Burck, Ital.†.*
Pipenzolate bromide (p.467·1).
Peptic ulcers.

Piperilline *Lederle, Fr.*
Piperacillin sodium (p.237·2).
Bacterial infections.

Piperital *Ibi, Ital.*
Piperacillin sodium (p.237·2).
Lignocaine hydrochloride (p.1293·2) is included in this preparation to alleviate the pain of injection.
Bacterial infections.

Piperonil *Lusofarmaco, Ital.*
Pipamperone hydrochloride (p.687·1).
Psychiatric disorders.

Piperzam *Zambon, Spain.*
Piperacillin sodium (p.237·2).
Bacterial infections.

Piportil
Rhone-Poulenc Rorer, Belg.; Specia, Fr.; Rhone-Poulenc Rorer, Irl.; Rhone-Poulenc Rorer, Neth.; Rhone-Poulenc Rorer, S.Afr.; Rhone-Poulenc Rorer, Switz.; JHC Healthcare, UK.
Pipothiazine (p.687·1) or pipothiazine palmitate (p.687·1).
Psychoses.

Piportil L4 *Rhone-Poulenc Rorer, Canad.*
Pipothiazine palmitate (p.687·1).
Schizophrenia.

Piportyl *Rhone-Poulenc Rorer, Norw.†.*
Pipothiazine palmitate (p.687·1).
Psychoses.

Pipracil
Wyeth-Ayerst, Canad.; Lederle, USA.
Piperacillin sodium (p.237·2).
Bacterial infections.

Pipracin *IRBI, Ital.*
Piperacillin sodium (p.237·2).
Lignocaine hydrochloride (p.1293·2) is included in the intramuscular injection to alleviate the pain of injection.
Bacterial infections.

Pipralen *Lennon, S.Afr.*
Piperazine hydrate (p.107·2).
Ascariasis; enterobiasis.

Pipram
Rhone-Poulenc Rorer, Belg.; Bellon, Fr.; Rhone-Poulenc Rorer, Ital.; Rhone-Poulenc Rorer, Neth.
Pipemidic acid (p.237·2).
Urinary-tract infections.

Pipril
Cyanamid, Aust.; Lederle, Austral.; Lederle, Ger.; Wyeth, Irl.; Wyeth, S.Afr.; Cyanamid, Spain; Lederle, Switz.; Lederle, UK.
Piperacillin sodium (p.237·2).
Lignocaine (p.1293·2) may be included in the intramuscular injection to alleviate the pain of injection.
Bacterial infections.

Piprine *Be-Tabs, S.Afr.*
Piperazine citrate (p.107·2).
Ascariasis; enterobiasis.

Piprol *Elfar, Spain.*
Ciprofloxacin hydrochloride (p.185·3).
Bacterial infections.

Piproxen *Nuovo ISM, Ital.*
Naproxen piperazine (p.62·1).
Gout; musculoskeletal, joint, and peri-articular disorders; neuralgia.

Piptal
Sigma, Austral.†; Rhone-Poulenc, Ital.†; Boehringer Mannheim, UK†.
Pipenzolate bromide (p.467·1).
Gastro-intestinal spasm.

Piptalin *Boehringer Mannheim, UK†.*
Pipenzolate bromide (p.467·1); simethicone (p.1213·1).
Gastro-intestinal disorders.

Pipurin *NCSN, Ital.*
Pipemidic acid (p.237·2).
Urinary-tract infections.

Pirabene *Merckle, Aust.*
Piracetam (p.1619·1).
Alcohol withdrawal syndrome; organic brain disorders.

Piracebral *Hexal, Ger.*
Piracetam (p.1619·1).
Mental function disorders.

Piracetam Complex *Berenguer Infale, Spain.*
Co-dergocrine mesylate (p.1566·1); piracetam (p.1619·1).
Cerebrovascular disorders.

Piracetrop *Holsten, Ger.*
Piracetam (p.1619·1).
Mental-function impairment.

Piraldina *Bracco, Ital.*
Pyrazinamide (p.241·1).
Tuberculosis.

Piralone *Ferrer, Spain.*
Lorazepam pivalate (p.676·3).
Alcohol withdrawal syndrome; anxiety; epilepsy; insomnia; nausea and vomiting.

Piramox *Radiumfarma, Ital.†.*
Amoxycillin (p.151·3) or amoxycillin sodium (p.151·3).
Bacterial infections.

Pirehexal *Hexal, Ger.*
Pirenzepine hydrochloride (p.467·1).
Gastro-intestinal disorders.

Pirem *Godecke, Ger.†.*
Carbuterol hydrochloride (p.751·3).
Asthma; bronchospastic disorders.

piren-basan *Schonenberger, Switz.*
Pirenzepine hydrochloride (p.467·1).
Gastro-intestinal disorders associated with hyperacidity.

Pirenex *Hoechst Marion Roussel, Switz.*
Piretanide (p.931·3) or piretanide sodium (p.931·3).
Hypertension; oedema; poisoning; renal disorders.

Pirenil Rectal *Prodes, Spain†.*
Dipyrone (p.35·1).
Fever; pain.

Pireuma *Terapeutico, Ital.*
Propyphenazone (p.81·3).
Fever; pain.

Pirfalin *Farmigea, Ital.*
Pirenoxine sodium (p.1619·1).
Cataracts.

Piricef *CT, Ital.†.*
Cefapirin sodium (p.164·1).
Bacterial infections.

Piridasmin *Ifesa, Spain†.*
Theophylline (p.765·1).
Heart failure; obstructive airways disease; paroxysmal dyspnoea.

Piridolan *Janssen, Swed.†.*
Piritramide (p.80·2).
Pain.

Pirifedrina *Funk, Spain.*
Codeine phosphate (p.26·1); ephedrine hydrochloride (p.1059·3); paracetamol (p.72·2).
Influenza and cold symptoms.

Pirilene *Marion Merrell, Fr.*
Pyrazinamide (p.241·1).
Tuberculosis.

Pirinasol *Bayer, Spain.*
Paracetamol (p.72·2).
Fever; pain.

Piriton
Boots, Austral.†; Allen & Hanburys, Irl.; Stafford-Miller, UK.
Chlorpheniramine maleate (p.405·1).
Hypersensitivity reactions.

Pirobeta *Betapharm, Ger.*
Piroxicam (p.80·2).
Gout; musculoskeletal, joint, and peri-articular disorders.

Pirobiotic *Clariana, Spain†.*
Metampicillin sodium (p.224·3).
Lignocaine hydrochloride (p.1293·2) is included in this preparation to alleviate the pain of injection.
Bacterial infections.

Pirocam
Merckle, Aust.; Spirig, Switz.
Piroxicam (p.80·2).
Gout; inflammation; musculoskeletal, joint, and peri-articular disorders; pain.

Pirodal *SIT, Ital.†.*
Piromidic acid (p.238·2).
Bacterial infections.

Piroflam
Lichtenstein, Ger.; Opus, UK.
Piroxicam (p.80·2).
Gout; musculoskeletal and joint disorders.

Pirofosfasi *Benvegna, Ital.†.*
Cocarboxylase (p.1361·2).

Piroftal *Bruschettini, Ital.*
Piroxicam (p.80·2).
Eye inflammation; ocular oedema.

Pirom *Solmer, Switz.*
Balm: Camphor (p.1557·2); menthol (p.1600·2); methyl salicylate (p.55·2); eucalyptus oil (p.1578·1); cinnamon oil (p.1564·2).
Embrocation: Camphor (p.1557·2); menthol (p.1600·2); methyl salicylate (p.55·2); eucalyptus oil (p.1578·1); sweet birch oil (p.55·3); citrus oil.
Cold symptoms; headache; insect bites and stings; muscle and joint pain; sports injuries.

Piro-Phlogont *Azupharma, Ger.*
Piroxicam (p.80·2).
Musculoskeletal and joint disorders.

Piro-Puren *Isis Puren, Ger.*
Piroxicam (p.80·2).
Musculoskeletal and joint disorders.

Piroreumal *Medosan, Ital.†.*
Amidopyrine hydroxyisophthalate (p.15·2).
Musculoskeletal and joint disorders.

Pirorheum *Hexal, Ger.*
Piroxicam (p.80·2).
Gout; musculoskeletal, joint, and peri-articular disorders.

Pirorheuma *Hexal, Ger.*
Piroxicam (p.80·2).
Musculoskeletal, joint, peri-articular, and soft-tissue disorders.

Pirosal *Teral, USA.*
Sodium thiosalicylate (p.85·2).

Pirosol *Ecosol, Switz.*
Piroxicam (p.80·2).
Inflammation; musculoskeletal, joint, and peri-articular disorders; pain.

Pirox
G.P. Laboratories, Austral.; CT, Ger.; Alpharma, Norw.
Piroxicam (p.80·2).
Dysmenorrhoea; gout; musculoskeletal and joint disorders.

Piroximerck *Merck, Ger.*
Piroxicam (p.80·2).
Gout; musculoskeletal and joint disorders.

Pirox-Spondyril *Nycomed, Ger.†.*
Piroxicam (p.80·2).
Gout; musculoskeletal and joint disorders.

Pirozip *Ashbourne, UK.*
Piroxicam (p.80·2).
Gout; musculoskeletal and joint disorders.

Piruvasi *Isnardi, Ital.†.*
Cocarboxylase (p.1361·2); nadide (p.1606·1); coenzyme A (p.1566·2); sodium glycerophosphate (p.1586·2); thioctic acid (p.1636·2).
Vitamin B1 deficiency.

Pirxane *Lisapharma, Ital.*
Buflomedil pyridoxal phosphate compound (p.834·2).
Vascular disorders.

Piscin *Muller Goppingen, Ger.†.*
Homoeopathic preparation.

Pisol *Roussel, Ital.†.*
Cloracetadol (p.26·1); promethazine trimethoxybenzoate.
Fever; pain.

Pitocin
Parke, Davis, Aust.; Parke, Davis, Ger.†; Warner-Lambert, Norw.; Parke, Davis, USA.
Oxytocin (p.1257·2) or oxytocin citrate (p.1258·1).
Incomplete or inevitable abortion; induction and maintenance of labour; postpartum haemorrhage.

Piton-S *Organon, Neth.†.*
Oxytocin (p.1257·2).
Labour induction; postpartum haemorrhage; promotion of lactation.

Pitressin
Note. This name is used for preparations of different composition.
Parke, Davis, Austral.; Parke, Davis, Ger.; Parke, Davis, Irl.; Goldshield, UK; Parke, Davis, USA.
Argipressin (p.1263·2).
Aid in abdominal radiography; diabetes insipidus; postoperative abdominal distension; variceal haemorrhage.

Parke, Davis, Canad.†.
Vasopressin (p.1263·2).
Adjunct in abdominal radiography; diabetes insipidus; postoperative abdominal distension.

Pitrex *Taro, Canad.*
Tolnaftate (p.389·1).
Fungal skin infections.

Pivacef *FIRMA, Ital.†.*
Cephalexin pivalate hydrochloride (p.238·3).
Bacterial infections.

Pivalone
Jouveinal, Fr.; Dagra, Neth.†; Uhlmann-Eyraud, Switz.
Tixocortol pivalate (p.1050·1).
Nasal polyps; rhinitis.

Pivalone compositum *Uhlmann-Eyraud, Switz.*
Tixocortol pivalate (p.1050·1); neomycin sulphate (p.229·2).
Infected nasal disorders.

Pivalone Neomycine *Jouveinal, Fr.*
Tixocortol pivalate (p.1050·1); neomycin sulphate (p.229·2).
Rhinitis; sinusitis.

Pivaloxicam *Chiesi, Ital.*
Piroxicam pivalate (p.81·1).
Musculoskeletal and joint disorders.

Pivamiser *Serra Pamies, Spain.*
Pivampicillin hydrochloride (p.238·2).
Bacterial infections.

Pivanozolo *Ripari-Gero, Ital.*
Miconazole pivoxil chloride (p.385·2).
Fungal infections; Gram-positive bacterial superinfections.

Pixfix *Hoernecke, Ger.*
Coal tar (p.1092·3).
Skin disorders.

Pixicam *Hexal, S.Afr.*
Piroxicam (p.80·2).
Gout; musculoskeletal and joint disorders.

Pixidin *Sanico, Belg.*
Chlorhexidine hydrochloride (p.1107·2).
Formerly contained tar, benzocaine, menthol, cineole, senna, and red-poppy petal.
Mouth and throat disorders.

Pixol *Cortecs, UK†.*
Tar (p.1092·3); coal tar (p.1092·3); cade oil (p.1092·2).
Skin disorders.

Pixor Stick Anti-acne N *Doetsch, Grether, Switz.*
Salicylic acid (p.1090·2); triclosan (p.1127·2).
Acne.

Piz Buin
Note. This name is used for preparations of different composition.
Johnson & Johnson, Austral.†.
SPF8; cream SPF 15+; topical milk SPF 15+: Ethylhexyl *p*-methoxycinnamate (p.1487·1); avobenzone (p.1486·3); titanium dioxide (p.1093·3).
Stick SPF 15+: Ethylhexyl *p*-methoxycinnamate (p.1487·1); avobenzone (p.1486·3).
Sunscreen.

Zyma, UK.
Oxybenzone (p.1487·3); ethylhexyl *p*-methoxycinnamate (p.1487·1); avobenzone (p.1486·3); titanium dioxide (p.1093·3).
Sunscreen.

PK Aid
Scientific Hospital Supplies, Austral.; Scientific Hospital Supplies, Irl.; Scientific Hospital Supplies, UK.
Amino-acid preparation without phenylalanine.
Phenylketonuria.

PK-Merz
Kolassa, Aust.; Merz, Ger.; Merz, Switz.
Amantadine sulphate (p.1129·2).
Coma; parkinsonism; postherpetic neuralgia.

PKU *Milupa, UK.*
Food for special diets.
Phenylketonuria.

PKU 2 and 3 *Milupa, UK.*
Food for special diets.
Phenylketonuria.

PKU 1 Mix *Milupa, Ital.*
Food for special diets.
Hyperphenylalaninaemia; phenylketonuria.

Placacid *Recordati, Ital.†.*
Clormecaine hydrochloride (p.1289·3); sodium lauryl sulphate; aluminium glycinate (p.1177·2); magnesium oxide (p.1198·3); magnesium trisilicate (p.1199·1); carmellose sodium (p.1471·2).
Gastric hyperacidity; peptic ulcers.

Placatus *Zilliken, Ital.*
Nepinalone hydrochloride (p.1065·1).
Coughs.

placentapur *Feldhoff, Ger.†.*
Placental extract.
Skin disorders.

Placentex *Mastelli, Ital.*
Polydeoxyribonucleotide (p.1570·3).
Inflammatory and degenerative disorders.

Placentina *INTES, Ital.*
Placenta extract.
Inflammation; rheumatic disorders.

Placentormon *Labopharma, Ger.†.*
Bovine placenta extract (p.1599·1).
Skin disorders.

Placidex *De Witt, UK.*
Paracetamol (p.72·2).
Pain.

Placidyl
Abbott, Canad.†; Abbott, USA.
Ethchlorvynol (p.669·2).
Insomnia.

Placil *Alphapharm, Austral.*
Clomipramine hydrochloride (p.281·2).
Depression; narcoleptic syndrome; obsessive-compulsive disorder; phobias.

Placinoral *Robert, Spain.*
Lorazepam pivalate (p.676·3).
Alcohol withdrawal syndrome; anxiety; epilepsy; insomnia; nausea and vomiting.

Placis *Wasserman, Spain.*
Cisplatin (p.513·3).
Malignant neoplasms.

Plactidil *Samil, Ital.*
Picotamide (p.930·2).
Thrombo-embolic disorders.

Plak Out
Byk, Aust.; Byk Gulden, Ital.
Chlorhexidine gluconate (p.1107·2).
Oral disinfection.

Plander *Pharmacia Upjohn, Ital.*
Dextran 70 (p.717·1) in sodium chloride.
Plasma volume expansion.

Plander R *Pharmacia Upjohn, Ital.*
Dextran 40 (p.716·2) in sodium chloride.
Extracorporeal perfusion; plasma volume expansion; thrombosis prophylaxis.

Planor *Roussel, Fr.*
Norgestrienone (p.1455·1); ethinyloestradiol (p.1445·1).
Combined oral contraceptive; endometriosis; mastalgia; menstrual disorders; polycystic ovary syndrome.

Planosec
Organon, Austral.†; Donmed, S.Afr.†.
Pregnancy test (p.1621·2).

Planphylline *Asta Medica, Fr.*
Aminophylline (p.748·1).
Asthma; obstructive airways disease.

Plant Spray *Dolisos, Canad.*
Homoeopathic preparation.

Planta Lax *Hoveler, Aust.*
Senna leaf and pod (p.1212·2); frangula bark (p.1193·2); blackberry leaf; chamomile flowers (p.1561·2); coriander (p.1567·3); fennel (p.1579·1).
Bowel evacuation; constipation; stool softener.

Plantaben *Madaus, Spain.*
Ispaghula (p.1194·2).
Constipation.

Plantacard *Madaus, Ger.*
Homoeopathic preparation.

Plantago Complex *Blackmores, Austral.†.*
Psyllium (p.1194·2); rhubarb (p.1212·1); whey; gentian (p.1583·3); cascara (p.1183·1).
Constipation.

Planten *Whitehall, Ital.*
Ispaghula husk (p.1194·2).
Constipation.

Plantiodine Plus *Blackmores, Austral.*
Kelp (p.1593·1); alfalfa (p.1544·2); protibel yeast (p.1373·1); rose hip (p.1365·2); lecithin (p.1595·2).
Tonic.

Plantival *Schwabe, Switz.*
Valerian (p.1643·1); passion flower (p.1615·3).
Anxiety disorders.

Plantival N and forte *Schwabe, Ger.†.*
Valerian (p.1643·1); passion flower (p.1615·3).
Nervous disorders; sleep disorders.

Plantival Novo *Schwabe, Ger.*
Valerian (p.1643·1); melissa (p.1600·1).
Agitation; sleep disorders.

Plantival plus *Schwabe, Ger.†.*
Carbromal (p.645·2); diphenhydramine hydrochloride (p.409·1); valerian (p.1643·1); passion flower (p.1615·3).
Sleep disorders.

Plantmobil *Plantina, Ger.*
Camphor (p.1557·2); eucalyptus oil (p.1578·1); turpentine oil (p.1641·1).
Cold symptoms; musculoskeletal and joint disorders.

Plantocur *Biocur, Ger.*
Ispaghula husk (p.1194·2).
Constipation.

Plantoletten *Robugen, Ger.*
Rhubarb (p.1212·1); aloes (p.1177·1).
Constipation.

Planum
Note. This name is used for preparations of different composition.
Pharmacia Upjohn, Ger.; Pharmacia Upjohn, Switz.
Temazepam (p.693·3).
Sleep disorders.

Menarini, Ital.
Desogestrel (p.1443·3); ethinyloestradiol (p.1445·1).
Combined oral contraceptive.

Plaqacide *Oral-B, Austral.*
Chlorhexidine gluconate (p.1107·2).
Oral disorders; prevention of dental plaque.

Plaquefarbetabletten *Blend-a-med, Ger.†.*
Erythrosine (p.1000·2).
Disclosing agent for dental plaque.

Plaquenil
Kwizda, Aust.†; Sanofi Winthrop, Austral.; Sanofi Winthrop, Belg.; Sanofi Winthrop, Canad.; Sanofi Winthrop, Fr.; Sanofi Winthrop, Irl.; Sanofi Winthrop, Ital.; Sanofi Winthrop, Neth.; Sanofi Winthrop, Norw.; Sanofi, Swed.; Sanofi Winthrop, Switz.; Sanofi Winthrop, UK; Sanofi Winthrop, USA.
Hydroxychloroquine sulphate (p.431·2).
Lupus erythematosus; malaria; photodermatoses; rheumatoid arthritis; Sjögren's syndrome.

Plas-Amino *Otsuka, Jpn.*
Amino-acid and carbohydrate infusion.
Parenteral nutrition.

Plasbumin
Bayer, Canad.; Cutter, USA.
Albumin (p.710·1).
Hypoalbuminaemia; hypovolaemia; neonatal hyperbilirubinaemia.

Plasil *Lepetit, Ital.*
Metoclopramide hydrochloride (p.1200·3).
Gastro-intestinal disorders.

Plasil Enzimatico *Lepetit, Ital.†.*
Metoclopramide hydrochloride (p.1200·3); sodium dehydrocholate (p.1570·3); bromelains (p.1555·1); pancreatin (p.1612·1); dimethicone (p.1213·1).
Gastro-intestinal disorders.

Plasimine *Isdin, Spain.*
Mupirocin (p.227·2).
Bacterial skin infections.

Plaskine Neomicina *Lasa, Spain.*
Lysine acexamate (p.1542·1); neomycin undecenoate (p.229·2).
Burns; ulcers; wounds.

Plasma Marin Hypertonique *Aqualab, Fr.*
Mineral preparation.

Plasmacair *Clintec, Fr.*
Dextran 40 (p.716·2) with electrolytes.
Haemodilution; hypotension; shock.

Plasmaclar *Lacer, Spain.*
Xanthinol nicotinate (p.971·1); pentosan polysulphate sodium (p.928·1).
Hyperlipidaemias.

Plasmafusin HES *Pharmacia Upjohn, Ger.*
Hetastarch (p.724·1) in sodium chloride.
Plasma volume expansion.

Plasmagel *Bellon, Fr.*
Gelatin (p.723·2) with electrolytes or glucose.
Hypotension; shock.

Plasmagelan *Braun, Switz.†.*
Modified gelatin (p.723·2).
Extracorporeal circulation; hypovolaemia; shock.

Plasma-Lyte
Baxter, Austral.; Baxter, UK; Baxter, USA.
A range of electrolyte infusions with or without glucose (p.1147·1).
Fluid and electrolyte disorders.

Plasma-Lyte 148 *Baxter, Spain.*
Electrolyte infusion (p.1147·1).
Fluid and electrolyte disorders.

Plasmanate
Bayer, Canad.; Cutter, USA.
Plasma protein fraction (p.726·3).
Hypoproteinaemia; hypovolaemia.

Plasma-Plex *Armour, USA.*
Plasma protein fraction (p.726·3).
Hypoproteinaemia; hypovolaemia.

Plasmarine *Pharmadeveloppement, Fr.*
Mineral preparation.
Tonic.

Plasmasteril *Leopold, Aust.; Fresenius, Belg.; Fresenius, Ger.; Fresenius, Switz.*
Hetastarch (p.724·1) in sodium chloride.
Plasma volume expansion.

Plasmatein *Alpha Therapeutic, UK†; Alpha Therapeutic, USA.*
Plasma protein fraction (p.726·3).
Hypoproteinaemia; hypovolaemia.

Plasmaviral *ISI, Ital.*
Plasma protein fraction (p.726·3).
Hypoproteinaemia; shock.

Plasmion *Bellon, Fr.*
Gelatin (p.723·2) with electrolytes.
Hypotension; shock.

Plasmodex *Pharmacia Upjohn, Norw.; Medisan, Swed.*
Dextran 60 (p.716·3) with electrolytes.
Plasma volume expansion.

Plasmoid *Grifols, Spain†.*
Electrolyte infusion with povidone (p.1474·2 and p.1147·1).
Hypovolaemia.

Plasmonsoy *Plasmon, Ital.*
Infant feed.
Cow's milk intolerance.

Plasmoquine *Medchem, S.Afr.*
Chloroquine sulphate (p.426·3).
Malaria.

Plasmutan *Wasserman, Spain†.*
Calcium acexamate (p.1542·1); aluminium phosphate (p.1178·3).
Gastritis; hiatus hernia; peptic ulcer.

Plast Apyr Fisio Irrigac *Mein, Spain.*
Sodium chloride (p.1162·2).
Urological irrigation.

Plast Apyr Fisiologico *Mein, Spain.*
Sodium chloride (p.1162·2).
Fluid and electrolyte disorders.

Plastenan *Bournonville, Belg.; Isopharm, Fr.; Wasserman, Spain†.*
Calcium acexamate (p.1542·1) or sodium acexamate (p.1542·1).
Bone disorders; wounds.

Plastenan Neomicina *Wasserman, Spain†.*
Sodium acexamate (p.1542·1); neomycin sulphate (p.229·2).
Ulcers; wounds.

Plastenan Neomycine *Bournonville, Belg.†; Isopharm, Fr.*
Sodium acexamate (p.1542·1); neomycin sulphate (p.229·2).
Infected wounds and burns.

Plastodermo *Sanofi Winthrop, Spain†.*
Chloramphenicol (p.182·1).
Skin infections.

Plastolin Poultice *Lennon, S.Afr.†.*
Glycerol (p.1585·2); kaolin (p.1195·1).
Counter irritation.

Plastufer *Wyeth, Ger.*
Ferrous sulphate (p.1340·2).
Iron deficiency; iron-deficiency anaemia.

Plastulen N *Wyeth, Ger.*
Ferrous sulphate (p.1340·2); folic acid (p.1340·3).
Iron and folic acid deficiency.

Platamine *Pharmacia Upjohn, Ital.; Pharmacia Upjohn, S.Afr.*
Cisplatin (p.513·3).
Malignant neoplasms.

Platelet *IBIS, Ital.†.*
Dipyridamole (p.857·1).
Platelet function disorders.

Platet *Nicholas, UK†.*
Aspirin (p.16·1).
Cardiovascular disorders.

Platiblastin *Pharmacia Upjohn, Aust.; Pharmacia Upjohn, Ger.*
Cisplatin (p.513·3).
Malignant neoplasms.

Platiblastine-S *Pharmacia Upjohn, Switz.*
Cisplatin (p.513·3).
Malignant neoplasms.

Platinex *Bristol-Myers Squibb, Ger.; Bristol-Myers Squibb, Ital.*
Cisplatin (p.513·3).
Malignant neoplasms.

Platinol *Bristol-Myers Squibb, Aust.; Bristol-Myers Squibb, Belg.; Bristol, Canad.; Bristol-Myers Squibb, Neth.; Bristol-Myers Squibb, Norw.; Bristol-Myers Squibb, Swed.; Bristol-Myers Squibb, Switz.; Bristol-Myers Oncology, USA.*
Cisplatin (p.513·3).
Malignant neoplasms.

Platinwas *Wasserman, Spain.*
Carboplatin (p.510·3).
Malignant neoplasms.

Platistil *Kenfarma, Spain.*
Cisplatin (p.513·3).
Malignant neoplasms.

Platistin *Pharmacia Upjohn, Norw.; Pharmacia Upjohn, Swed.†.*
Cisplatin (p.513·3).
Malignant neoplasms.

Plato *Lennon, S.Afr.*
Dipyridamole (p.857·1).
Platelet function inhibition.

Platocillina *Crosara, Ital.*
Ampicillin (p.153·1).
Bacterial infections.

Platosin *Pharmachemie, S.Afr.*
Cisplatin (p.513·3).
Malignant neoplasms.

Platrix *Smith & Nephew, Fr.†.*
Calcium sulphate (p.1557·2).
External splinting.

Plaucina *Tecnobio, Spain†.*
Enoxaparin sodium (p.864·2).
Thrombo-embolic disorders.

Plausitin *Carlo Erba OTC, Ital.*
Morclofone (p.1064·2).
Coughs.

Plavix *Sanofi Winthrop, UK; Bristol-Myers Squibb, UK; Sanofi Winthrop, USA.*
Clopidogrel bisulphate (p.844·3).
Atherosclerosis.

Plax
Note. This name is used for preparations of different composition.
Pfizer, Canad.
Sodium benzoate (p.1102·3); sodium lauryl sulphate (p.1468·3); sodium salicylate (p.85·1).
Colgate-Palmolive, Ital.
Triclosan (p.1127·2); sodium fluoride (p.742·1).
Dental plaque prevention.

Plazenta-Uvocal *Mulli, Ger.†.*
Protein-free placenta extract.
Tonic.

Plebe *Pharmadeveloppement, Fr.*
Vitamin and mineral preparation.
Tonic.

Plecton *Guidotti, Ital.†.*
Cicloxilic acid (p.1563·3).
Liver disorders.

Pleegzuster *Tendem-Haco, Neth.†.*
Ferric ammonium citrate (p.1339·2); calcium glycerophosphate (p.1155·2).
Tonic.

Plegicil *Clin Midy, Fr.†.*
Acepromazine (p.640·1).
Anxiety; vomiting.

Plegine *Wyeth, Ital.; Wyeth-Ayerst, USA†.*
Phendimetrazine tartrate (p.1484·2).
Obesity.

Plegisol *Abbott, USA.*
Electrolytes (p.1147·1).
Cardioplegic solution.

Plegivex *Ivex, UK.*
Electrolyte solution for coronary instillation (p.1147·1).
Induction of arrest during cardiothoracic surgery.

Pleiabil *Guidotti, Ital.†.*
Cicloxilic acid (p.1563·3); cascara (p.1183·1).
Digestive system disorders.

Pleiamide *Guidotti, Ital.*
Chlorpropamide (p.319·1); metformin hydrochloride (p.330·1).
Diabetes mellitus.

Plendil *Astra, Aust.; Astra, Austral.; Astra, Belg.; Astra, Canad.; Astra, Irl.; Astra, Ital.; Astra, Neth.; Astra, Norw.; Astra, S.Afr.; Astra, Spain; Hassle, Swed.; Astra, Switz.; Astra, UK; Astra Merck, USA.*
Felodipine (p.867·3).
Angina pectoris; hypertension.

Plenigraf *Juste, Spain.*
Calcium diatrizoate (p.1004·1); meglumine diatrizoate (p.1003·2); sodium diatrizoate (p.1003·2).
Radiographic contrast medium.

Plenish-K *Lennon, S.Afr.*
Potassium chloride (p.1161·1).
Potassium deficiencies.

Plenolyt *Madaus, Spain.*
Ciprofloxacin hydrochloride (p.185·3).
Bacterial infections.

Plenosol N *Madaus, Ger.*
Mistletoe (p.1604·1).
Joint disorders.

Plenumil *Merck, Spain†.*
Aminohydroxybutyric acid (p.339·1); pyritinol hydrochloride (p.1624·1).
Cerebrovascular disorders; mental function impairment.

Plenur *Lasa, Spain.*
Lithium carbonate (p.290·3).
Bipolar disorder; depression; neutropenia.

Plenyl *Oberlin, Fr.*
Vitamin and mineral preparation.

Pleo Vitamin *Inibsa, Spain.*
Multivitamins and minerals; orotic acid, diethylaminoethanol salt; adenosine.
Formerly known as Pleo Vitamin Geriat.
Tonic.

Pleocortex *Retrain, Spain.*
Suprarenal cortex (p.1050·1).
Adrenal insufficiency; tonic.

Pleocortex B6 *Retrain, Spain.*
Suprarenal cortex (p.1050·1); pyridoxine hydrochloride (p.1362·3).
Vomiting.

Pleomix-Alpha *Illa, Ger.*
Thioctic acid (p.1636·2) or trometamol thioctate (p.1640·1).
Diabetic polyneuropathy.

Pleomix-B *Trommsdorff, Ger.*
Vitamin B substances.
Vitamin B deficiency.

Pleon *Lacer, Spain.*
Adenine; vitamin B substances; carnitine orotate; fructose diphosphate magnesium; potassium orotate; xanthine.
Tonic.

Pleon RA *Henning, Ger.*
Sulphasalazine (p.1215·2).
Polyarthritis.

Plesial *Ichthyol, Ger.†.*
Dithranol (p.1082·1); salicylic acid (p.1090·2).
Psoriasis.

Plesmet *Nelson, Austral.†; Link, Irl.; Link, UK.*
Ferrous glycine sulphate (p.1340·1).
Iron-deficiency anaemia.

Pletaal *Otsuka, Jpn.*
Cilostazol (p.841·1).
Ischaemic symptoms in arterial occlusion.

Plexium *Lehning, Fr.*
Selenium (p.1353·3).
Muscular disorders; skin disorders.

Plexocardio *Benvegna, Ital.†.*
Benziodarone (p.393·1).
Coronary vascular disorders.

Plexoton B12 *Coli, Ital.*
Vitamin B substances.
Anaemias; liver disorders; tonic.

Pliagel *Alcon, Austral.*
Poloxamer 407 (p.1326·3).
Soft contact lens cleaner.

Plissamur forte *Ardeypharm, Ger.*
Aesculus (p.1543·3).
Venous insufficiency.

Plitican *Synthelabo, Fr.; Synthelabo, Switz.*
Alizapride hydrochloride (p.1176·3).
Nausea; vomiting.

Pluralane *Ardeypharm, Ger.†.*
Silver nitrate (p.1629·2).
Vaginitis.

Pluravit Multi *Sterling Health, Austral.†.*
Multivitamin and mineral preparation.

Pluravit Super *Sterling Health, Austral.†.*
Multivitamin and mineral preparation.

Pluravit Super B *Sterling Health, Austral.†.*
Vitamin B substances with ascorbic acid.
Vitamin B supplement.

Plurexid *Evans, Fr.*
Chlorhexidine gluconate (p.1107·2).
Disinfection of skin and mucous membranes.

Pluribios *Madariaga, Spain.*
Multivitamin preparation with cocarboxylase.
Eye disorders.

Pluriderm *Guieu, Ital.*
Thyme (p.1636·3); carrot (p.1644·3); sage oil; whey; lactic acid (p.1593·3).
Skin disinfection.

Plurifactor *Gomenol, Fr.*
Vitamin B substances; deoxyribonucleic acid; glycine.
Tonic.

Plurimen *Asta Medica, Spain.*
Selegiline hydrochloride (p.1144·2).
Parkinsonism.

Plurisalina *Grifols, Spain.*
Electrolyte injection (p.1147·1) with sodium lactate (p.1153·2).
Fluid and electrolyte disorders.

Pluriviron *Asche, Ger.†.*
Mesterolone (p.1450·1); yohimbine hydrochloride (p.1645·3).
Androgenic.

Pluryl *Leo, Neth.†.*
Bendrofluazide (p.827·3).
Hypertension; oedema.

Plus Kalium retard *Amino, Switz.*
Potassium chloride (p.1161·1).
Hypokalaemia.

Plusdermona *Bama, Spain†.*
Silver sulphadiazine (p.247·3).
Wound infections.

Pluserix *SmithKline Beecham, Austral.†; SmithKline Beecham, Ger.†; Smith Kline & French, Irl.†; Smith Kline & French, Ital.†; SmithKline Beecham, Switz.†.*
A measles, mumps, and rubella vaccine (Schwarz, Urabe Am 9, and RA 27/3 strains respectively) (p.1519·3).
Active immunisation.

pM *Promedica, Fr.*
Aluminium chlorohydrate (p.1078·3).
Hyperhidrosis.

PMB *Akromed, S.Afr.†; Wyeth-Ayerst, USA.*
Conjugated oestrogens (p.1457·3); meprobamate (p.678·1).
Menopausal disorders.

P-Mega-Tablinen *Sanorania, Ger.*
Phenoxymethylpenicillin potassium (p.236·2).
Bacterial infections.

PMS *Homeocan, Canad.*
Homoeopathic preparation.

PMS L21 *Homeocan, Canad.*
Homoeopathic preparation.

PMS Support *Vitaplex, Austral.*
Vitamins; minerals; viburnum; buchu (p.1555·2); ginger (p.1193·2); evening primrose oil (p.1582·1).
Muscular cramps; oedema.

PMS-Artificial Tears *Pharmascience, Canad.*
Polyvinyl alcohol (p.1474·2).
Dry eyes.

PMS-Artificial Tears Plus *Pharmascience, Canad.*
Polyvinyl alcohol (p.1474·2); povidone (p.1474·2).
Dry eyes.

PMS-Dicitrate *Pharmascience, Canad.*
Sodium citrate dihydrate (p.1153·2); citric acid monohydrate (p.1564·3).
Neutralising buffer; systemic alkaliniser.

PMS-Egozinc *Pharmascience, Canad.*
Zinc sulphate (p.1373·2).
Zinc supplement.

PMS-Levazine *Pharmascience, Canad.*
Perphenazine (p.685·2); amitriptyline hydrochloride (p.273·3).
Depression; psychoses.

PMS-Phosphates *Pharmascience, Canad.*
Monobasic sodium phosphate (p.1159·3); dibasic sodium phosphate (p.1159·3).
Constipation.

PMS-Prolactase *Pharmascience, Canad.†.*
Tilactase from *Aspergillus oryzae* or *Kluyveromyces lactis* (p.1637·3).
Lactase insufficiency.

PMT Complex
Note. This name is used for preparations of different composition.
Brauer, Austral.
Homoeopathic preparation.
Cenovis, Austral.; Vitelle, Austral.
Vitamins; minerals; ginger (p.1193·2); viburnum; agnus castus (p.1544·2); cimicifuga (p.1563·3); kelp (p.1593·1).
Premenstrual syndrome.

PMT Formula *Vitalia, UK.*
Evening primrose oil (p.1582·1); vitamins; minerals; valerian (p.1643·1); passion flower (p.1615·3).
Premenstrual syndrome.

PMT Tablets and Oral Spray *Brauer, Austral.*
Homoeopathic preparation.

PMT-EZE *Rhone-Poulenc Rorer, Austral.†.*
Vitamins, minerals; bearberry (p.1552·2); parsley (p.1615·3); juniper (p.1592·2); viburnum opulus.
Premenstrual syndrome.

Pneucid *Divpharm, S.Afr.*
Sodium citrate (p.1153·2); citric acid monohydrate (p.1564·3).
Buffering agent for increasing gastric pH before anaesthesia.

Pneumaseptic *Cochon, Fr.*
Potassium guaiacolsulfonate (p.1068·3); sodium benzoate (p.1102·3).
Respiratory-tract congestion.

Pneumo 23 *Pasteur Vaccins, Fr.; Pasteur Merieux, Ital.*
A pneumococcal vaccine (23-valent) (p.1527·3).
Active immunisation.

Pneumodoron *Weleda, Aust.*
Homoeopathic preparation.

Pneumogeine *Labomed, Fr.*
Theophylline (p.765·1); caffeine (p.749·3); potassium iodide (p.1493·1); sodium benzoate (p.1102·3).
Asthma; obstructive airways disease.

Pneumogenol *Pharmethic, Belg.†.*
Caffeine hydrate (p.750·1); theophylline hydrate (p.765·1); sodium iodide (p.1493·2).
Obstructive airways disease.

Pneumomist *ECR, USA.*
Guaiphenesin (p.1061·3).

Pneumonium LA *Wala, Ger.†.*
Petasites officinalis root.
Asthma; bronchitis.

Pneumopan
Note. This name is used for preparations of different composition.
Gebro, Aust.
Thyme (p.1636·3); equisetum (p.1575·1); plantago lanceolata; potassium guaiacolsulfonate (p.1068·3).
Coughs.
SmithKline Beecham Sante, Fr.
Codeine (p.26·1); chlorpheniramine maleate (p.405·1); bromoform (p.1620·3); sodium benzoate (p.1102·3).
Coughs.

Pneumopect *Gebro, Aust.†.*
Noscapine (p.1065·2); thyme (p.1636·3); viola.
Coughs.

Pneumopent *Fisons, Canad.†; Italchimici, Ital.*
Pentamidine isethionate (p.590·2).
Pneumocystis carinii pneumonia.

Pneumoplasme *Augot, Fr.*
Black-mustard-flour paper (p.1605·3).
Respiratory-tract congestion.

Pneumoplasme a l'Histamine *Augot, Fr.*
Black-mustard-flour paper (p.1605·3); histamine dihydrochloride (p.1587·3).
Respiratory-tract congestion.

Pneumorel
Eutherapie, Belg.; Biopharma, Fr.; Stroder, Ital.
Fenspiride hydrochloride (p.1579·3).
Respiratory-tract disorders.

Pneumotussin HC *ECR, USA.*
Hydrocodone tartrate (p.43·1); guaiphenesin (p.1061·3).
Coughs.

Pneumovax
Merck Sharp & Dohme, Aust.; CSL, Austral.; Pasteur Merieux, Belg.; Merck Sharp & Dohme, Canad.; Chiron Behring, Ger.; Pasteur Merieux, Irl.; Pasteur Merieux, Norw.; Merck Sharp & Dohme, S.Afr.; Pasteur Merieux, Swed.; Pro Vaccine, Switz.; Pasteur Merieux, UK; Merck Sharp & Dohme, USA.
A pneumococcal vaccine (23-valent) (p.1527·3).
Active immunisation.

Pneumune
Wyeth Lederle, Belg.; Lederle, Neth.
A pneumococcal vaccine (23-valent) (p.1527·3).
Active immunisation.

Pnu-Imune
Wyeth Lederle, Swed.; Wyeth, UK; Lederle-Praxis, USA.
A pneumococcal vaccine (23-valent) (p.1527·3).
Active immunisation.

P.O. 12 *Boehringer Ingelheim, Fr.*
Enoxolone (p.35·2).
Inflammatory skin disorders.

Pockinal *Mauermann, Ger.*
Hedera helix.
Bronchitis.

Poconeol *Plantes et Medecines, Fr.*
A range of homoeopathic preparations.

Pocyl *Lacer, Spain.*
Ibuprofen (p.44·1).
Fever; musculoskeletal, joint, and peri-articular disorders; pain.

Pod-Ben-25 *C & M, USA†.*
Podophyllum resin (p.1089·1).
Warts.

Podertonic *Inkeysa, Spain.*
Ferrocholinate (p.1339·2).
Iron-deficiency anaemia.

Podine *Pharmacare Consumer, S.Afr.*
Povidone-iodine (p.1123·3).
Oral hygiene; skin disorders; wounds.

Podium *Torlan, Spain.*
Diazepam (p.661·1).
Contains pyridoxine hydrochloride.
Alcohol withdrawal syndrome; anxiety; febrile convulsions; insomnia; skeletal muscle spasm.

Podocon *Paddock, USA.*
Podophyllum resin (p.1089·1).
Epitheliomatosis; genital warts and other papillomas; keratosis.

Podofilm *Pharmascience, Canad.*
Podophyllum resin (p.1089·1).
Warts.

Podofin *Syosset, USA.*
Podophyllum resin (p.1089·1).
Epitheliomatosis; genital warts; keratoses.

Podomexef
Luitpold, Ger.; Luitpold, Switz.
Cefpodoxime proxetil (p.172·1).
Bacterial infections.

Poikicholan *Lomapharm, Ger.*
Silybum marianum (p.993·3).
Liver disorders.

Poikicin *Lomapharm, Ger.†.*
Diphenylpyraline hydrochloride (p.409·3); caffeine (p.749·3); quinine dihydrochloride (p.439·1); ascorbic acid (p.1365·2); salicylamide (p.82·3).
Fever; influenza.

Poikigastran N *Lomapharm, Ger.*
Algeldrate (p.1177·3); magnesium hydroxide (p.1198·2).
Gastro-intestinal disorders.

Poikigeron *Lomapharm, Ger.*
Procaine hydrochloride; adenosine phosphate; haematoporphyrin; minerals; ginkgo biloba.
Tonic.

Poikilocard N *Lomapharm, Ger.*
Crataegus (p.1568·2).
Cardiac disorders.

Poikiloton *Lomapharm, Ger.†.*
Oral drops: Ephedrine hydrochloride (p.1059·3); etofylline (p.753·1); proxyphylline (p.757·3); pentetrazol (p.1484·2).
Tablets: Nikethamide calcium thiocyanate (p.1483·3); pentetrazol (p.1484·2); etilefrine hydrochloride (p.867·2); kola (p.1645·1); vitamins.
Hypotension.

Poikiven T *Lomapharm, Ger.*
Homoeopathic preparation.

Point-Two *Colgate-Hoyt, USA.*
Sodium fluoride (p.742·1).
Dental caries prophylaxis.

Poison Antidote Kit *Bowman, USA.*
Combination pack: Syrup, ipecacuanha (p.1062·2); suspension, charcoal (p.972·2).
Emergency treatment of poisoning.

Poladex *Major, USA†.*
Dexchlorpheniramine maleate (p.405·1).
Hypersensitivity reactions.

Polamin *Schering-Plough, Ital.*
Dexchlorpheniramine maleate (p.405·1).
Hypersensitivity reactions.

Polar Ice *Scott, Canad.*
Menthol (p.1600·2).
Musculoskeletal and joint pain.

Polaramin
Aesca, Aust.; Schering-Plough, Ital.; Schering-Plough, Norw.; Schering Plough, Swed.
Dexchlorpheniramine maleate (p.405·1).
Hypersensitivity reactions; pruritus.

Polaramin Espettorante *Schering-Plough, Ital.*
Dexchlorpheniramine maleate (p.405·1); guaiphenesin (p.1061·3); pseudoephedrine sulphate (p.1068·3).
Colds; coughs.

Polaramine
Schering-Plough, Austral.; Schering-Plough, Belg.; Schering, Canad.; Schering-Plough, Fr.; Schering-Plough, Neth.; Schering-Plough, S.Afr.; Schering-Plough, Spain; Essex, Switz.; Schering, USA.
Dexchlorpheniramine maleate (p.405·1).
Hypersensitivity reactions; migraine; pruritus.

Polaramine Expectorant
Schering-Plough, Belg.; Schering, USA.
Dexchlorpheniramine maleate (p.405·1); guaiphenesin (p.1061·3); pseudoephedrine sulphate (p.1068·3).
Coughs and cold symptoms.

Polaramine Expectorante *Schering-Plough, Spain.*
Dexchlorpheniramine maleate (p.405·1); guaiphenesin (p.1061·3); pseudoephedrine sulphate (p.1068·3).
Upper-respiratory-tract disorders.

Polaramine Infant Compound *Schering-Plough, Austral.†.*
Chlorpheniramine maleate (p.405·1); paracetamol (p.72·2).
Formerly contained dexchlorpheniramine maleate and sodium salicylate.
Cold symptoms; pruritus; teething.

Polaramine Pectoral *Schering-Plough, Fr.*
Dexchlorpheniramine maleate (p.405·1); pseudoephedrine sulphate (p.1068·3); guaiphenesin (p.1061·3); sodium benzoate (p.1102·3).
Coughs and cold symptoms; respiratory-tract disorders.

Polaramine Topico *Schering-Plough, Spain.*
Allantoin (p.1078·2); dexchlorpheniramine maleate (p.405·1).
Cutaneous hypersensitivity reactions.

Polaratyne *Schering-Plough, S.Afr.*
Loratadine (p.413·1).
Allergic rhinitis; urticaria.

Polaratyne D *Schering-Plough, S.Afr.*
Loratadine (p.413·1); pseudoephedrine sulphate (p.1068·3).
Upper respiratory-tract congestion.

Polaronil
Note. This name is used for preparations of different composition.
Aesca, Aust.; Essex, Ger.
Dexchlorpheniramine maleate (p.405·1).
Hypersensitivity reactions.

Schering-Plough, Belg.
Dexamethasone (p.1037·1); dexchlorpheniramine maleate (p.405·1); ascorbic acid (p.1365·2).
Hypersensitivity reactions.

Polase *Wyeth, Ital.*
Potassium aspartate hemihydrate (p.1161·3); magnesium aspartate tetrahydrate (p.1157·2).
Potassium and magnesium deficiency.

Polcortolon TC *Medphano, Ger.*
Triamcinolone acetonide (p.1050·2); tetracycline hydrochloride (p.259·1).
Infected skin disorders.

Poledin *Ciba Vision, Spain.*
Sodium cromoglycate (p.762·1).
Eye disorders.

Polery *Veyron-Froment, Fr.*
Paediatric syrup: Ethylmorphine hydrochloride (p.36·1); sodium bromide (p.1620·3); sodium benzoate (p.1102·3); codeine (p.26·1); belladonna (p.457·1); erysimin; senega (p.1069·3).
Syrup: Ethylmorphine hydrochloride (p.36·1); sodium bromide (p.1620·3); sodium benzoate (p.1102·3); codeine (p.26·1); aconite (p.1542·2); belladonna (p.457·1); erysimin; senega (p.1069·3); cherry-laurel.
Coughs.

Poli ABE *Vita, Spain.*
Pyridoxine hydrochloride (p.1362·3); placenta extract; vitamin A palmitate (p.1359·2); tocopheryl acetate (p.1369·1).
Deficiency of vitamins A and E.

Poli Biocatines *Garcia Suarez, Spain†.*
Multivitamins; isoniazid (p.218·1).
Vitamin deficiency.

Polial
Plasmon, Ital.; Ultrapharm, UK.
Food for special diets.
Egg intolerance; gluten intolerance; milk intolerance.

Poliantib *Cusi, Spain.*
Chlortetracycline hydrochloride (p.185·1); polymyxin B sulphate (p.239·1).
Bacterial eye infections.

Polibar
Codali, Belg.†; E-Z-EM, Neth.†; E-Z-EM, UK.
Barium sulphate (p.1003·1).
Formerly known as Polibar ACB in the *UK*.
Contrast medium for gastro-intestinal radiography.

Polibar Liquid *Therapex, Canad.†.*
Barium sulphate (p.1003·1).
Simethicone (p.1213·1) is included in this preparation to eliminate gas from the gastro-intestinal tract before radiography.
Radiographic contrast medium.

Polibar Plus *Therapex, Canad.†.*
Barium sulphate (p.1003·1).
Simethicone (p.1213·1) is included in this preparation to eliminate gas from the gastro-intestinal tract before radiography.
Radiographic contrast medium.

Polibar Rapid
Therapex, Canad.†; E-Z-EM, UK.
Barium sulphate (p.1003·1).
Contrast medium for gastro-intestinal radiography.

Polibar Viscous *E-Z-EM, UK.*
Barium sulphate (p.1003·1).
Contrast medium for gastro-intestinal radiography.

Polibar-ACB *Bracco, Switz.*
Barium sulphate (p.1003·1).
Contrast medium for gastro-intestinal radiography.

Polibeta B12 *Ceccarelli, Ital.*
Vitamin B substances with gastric mucosa.
Nutritional supplement.

Polibutin *Juste, Spain.*
Trimebutine (p.1639·3) or trimebutine maleate (p.1639·3).
Gastro-intestinal spasm; nausea and vomiting.

Policolinosil *Medea, Spain.*
Amino acids; liver extract; pangamic acid (p.1614·1); ribonucleic acid (p.1624·3); thioctic acid (p.1636·2); inositol (p.1591·1); vitamin B substances.
Liver disorders; tonic.

Polidasa *Almirall, Spain.*
Amylase (p.1549·1); cellulase (p.1561·1); dimethicone (p.1213·1); tilactase (p.1637·3); lipase.
Formerly contained amylase, bromelains, cellulase, dimethicone, tilactase, lipase, and metoclopramide.
Digestive-system disorders.

Polides *Farmigea, Ital.*
Polydeoxyribonucleotide (p.1570·3).
Gynaecological disorders.

Poliglicol Anti Acne *Kin, Spain.*
Sulphur (p.1091·2); calamine (p.1080·1); resorcinol acetate (p.1090·1); triclosan (p.1127·2); zinc oxide (p.1096·2).
Acne.

Poliglobin N *Bayer, Spain.*
A normal immunoglobulin (p.1522·1).
Idiopathic thrombocytopenia; immunodeficiency disorders.

Polijodurato *Farmigea, Ital.*
Sodium iodide (p.1493·2); potassium iodide (p.1493·1); rubidium iodide (p.1626·3); calcium chloride (p.1155·1).
Cataracts.

Polilevo *Poli, Ital.*
Arginine hydrochloride (p.1334·1); ornithine hydrochloride (p.1352·3); citrulline (p.1337·2); vitamin B substances.
Liver disorders.

Polimod *Poli, Ital.*
Pidotimod (p.1618·3).
Immunostimulant.

Polimoxal *Herdel, Ital.†.*
Latamoxef disodium (p.221·2).
Bacterial infections.

Polimucil *Poli, Ital.*
Carbocisteine (p.1056·3); sobrerol (p.1069·3).
Respiratory-tract disorders.

Polinazolo *Guieu, Ital.*
Econazole nitrate (p.377·2).
Vulvovaginal candidiasis.

Polineural *Biotekfarma, Ital.*
Citicoline sodium (p.1564·3).
Mental function impairment; parkinsonism.

Polinorm *Zeneca, Aust.*
Atenolol (p.825·3); chlorthalidone (p.839·3); hydralazine hydrochloride (p.883·2).
Hypertension.

Polio Sabin (Orale) *SmithKline Beecham, Ital.*
An oral poliomyelitis vaccine (p.1528·2).
Active immunisation.

Poliodine *Gifrer Barbezat, Fr.*
Povidone-iodine (p.1123·3).
Wound and skin disinfection.

poliomyelan *Feldhoff, Ger.*
Bovine testicular extract (p.1464·1); bovine placental extract.
Musculoskeletal disorders; peripheral circulatory disorders.

Polioral
Biocine, Ital.; Biovac, S.Afr.
An oral poliomyelitis vaccine (p.1528·2).
Active immunisation.

Polio-Vaccinol *Procter & Gamble, Ger.*
An oral poliomyelitis vaccine (p.1528·2).
Active immunisation.

Polipirox *Biologici Italia, Ital.*
Piroxicam (p.80·2).
Rheumatic disorders.

Poliplacen *Farmigea, Ital.†.*
Polydeoxyribonucleotide (p.1570·3).
Gynaecological disorders.

Polirino *Wasserman, Spain†.*
Phenylephrine hydrochloride (p.1066·2); hydrocortisone hemisuccinate (p.1044·1); lignocaine hydrochloride (p.1293·2); muramidase hydrochloride (p.1604·3); naphazoline nitrate (p.1064·2); neomycin sulphate (p.229·2); tripelennamine hydrochloride (p.420·2).
Nasal congestion and infection.

Polisan *Milana, Ital.*
Benzalkonium chloride (p.1101·3).
Surface disinfection.

Polisilan Gel *Upsamedica, Spain.*
Aluminium hydroxide (p.1177·3); dimethicone (p.1213·1); sorbitol (p.1354·2).
Gastro-intestinal hyperacidity and flatulence.

Polisilon *Upsamedica, Ital.*
Dimethicone (p.1213·1).
Aerophagia; gastro-intestinal disorders associated with hyperacidity.

Polistin Pad *Trommsdorff, Ger.*
Carbinoxamine maleate (p.404·2).
Hypersensitivity reactions.

Polistin T-Caps *Trommsdorff, Ger.*
Carbinoxamine maleate (p.404·2).
Hypersensitivity reactions; pruritus.

Politintura Schias *AFOM, Ital.†.*
Rhubarb (p.1212·1); boldo (p.1554·1); cascara (p.1183·1); inositol (p.1591·1).
Constipation; digestive system disorders.

Politosse *Poli, Ital.*
Cloperastine fendizoate (p.1057·2).
Coughs.

Polividona Yodada *Calmante Vitaminado, Spain; Neusc, Spain.*
Povidone-iodine (p.1123·3).
Skin and body cavity disinfection; skin infections.

Polivitaendil Mineral *Wasserman, Spain†.*
Multivitamins and minerals; adenosine triphosphate; glycine.

Poliwit *Radiumfarma, Ital.*
Multivitamin and mineral preparation.

Polixima *Sifarma, Ital.*
Cefuroxime sodium (p.177·1).
Bacterial infections.

Pollalin *HAL, Neth.*
Grass pollen allergen extracts(p.1545·1).
Hyposensitisation.

Pollcapsan M *Alsitan, Ger.*
Pollen.
Tonic.

Pollen Pearls *Suisse, Austral.†.*
Bee collected pollen; royal jelly; propolis; honeycomb capping; ginseng; foti; gotu cola.
Nutritional supplement.

Pollen Royal *Ido, Fr.*
Pollen; propolis (p.1621·3); royal jelly (p.1626·3).
Nutritional supplement.

Pollen-B *Wassen, UK.*
Pollen; dolomite.

Pollenna *Nelson, UK.*
Homoeopathic preparation.

Pollinex
Stallergenes, Belg.; Bencard, Canad.; Kallergen, Ital.†; Kalopharma, Ital.†; Artu, Neth.
Plant allergen extracts (p.1545·1).
Hyposensitisation.

Pollingel *Bracco, Ital.*
Heart; pollen; royal jelly (p.1626·3).
Nutritional supplement.

Pollinil *Dolisos, Canad.*
Homoeopathic preparation.

Pollinosan
Bioforce, Ger.; Bioforce, Switz.
Homoeopathic preparation.

Pollinose S *Alsitan, Ger.*
Pollen.
Pollen hypersensitivity.

Pollon-eze *Johnson & Johnson MSD Consumer, UK.*
Astemizole (p.402·1).
Hay fever; urticaria.

Pollonis *Janssen-Cilag, Aust.*
Astemizole (p.402·1).
Hay fever.

Pollstimol *Strathmann, Ger.*
Grass pollen extracts.
Benign prostatic hyperplasia.

Pollyferm *Nordic, Swed.*
Sodium cromoglycate (p.762·1).
Allergic rhinitis and conjunctivitis.

Polocaine
Astra, Canad.; Astra, USA.
Mepivacaine hydrochloride (p.1297·2).
Levonordefrin hydrochloride is included in some injections as a vasoconstrictor to diminish absorption and localise the effect of the local anaesthetic.
Local anaesthesia.

Poloral *Berna, Switz.*
An oral poliomyelitis vaccine (p.1528·2).
Active immunisation.

Poloris *Block, Ger.*
Coal tar (p.1092·3); allantoin (p.1078·2).
Skin disorders.

Poloris HC *Block, Ger.*
Coal tar (p.1092·3); allantoin (p.1078·2); hydrocortisone (p.1043·3).
Psoriasis.

Polvac *Teomed, Switz.*
Pollen allergen extracts (p.1545·1).
Hyposensitisation.

Polvere Cruz Verde *Fastfarm, Ital.†.*
Dicophane (p.1404·3).
Pediculosis.

Polvere Disinfettante *Isnardi, Ital.†.*
Hydroxyquinoline (p.1589·3); colloidal sulphur (p.1091·2).
Skin disinfection; skin irritation.

Polvos Wilfe *Calmante Vitaminado, Spain.*
Sulphanilamide (p.256·3); sulphathiazole (p.257·1).
Skin infections.

Poly Pred *Allergan, Spain.*
Neomycin sulphate (p.229·2); polymyxin B sulphate (p.239·1); prednisolone acetate (p.1048·1).
Infected eye disorders.

Polyanion *Sigmapharm, Aust.*
Pentosan polysulphate sodium (p.928·1).
Hyperlipidaemias; thrombo-embolic disorders.

Polybactrin
Glaxo Wellcome, Aust.; Wellcopharm, Ger.†; Wellcome, Irl.; Fresenius, Switz.†; Calmic, UK†.
Neomycin sulphate (p.229·2); polymyxin B sulphate (p.239·1); bacitracin (p.157·3) or bacitracin zinc (p.157·3).
Bacterial skin infections.

Polybactrin Solubile *Fresenius, Switz.†.*
Neomycin sulphate (p.229·2); polymyxin B sulphate (p.239·1); bacitracin (p.157·3).
Irrigating solution for bacterial infections; wounds.

Polybactrin Soluble *Wellcome, Irl.†.*
Neomycin sulphate (p.229·2); polymyxin B sulphate (p.239·1); bacitracin zinc (p.157·3).
Urinary-tract infections.

Polybion
Merck, Ger.; Bracco, Ital.; Meda, Swed.†.
Vitamin B substances.
Alcoholism; polyneuropathy; vitamin B deficiency.

Polybion Forte *Merck, Ger.*
Vitamin B substances.
Vitamin B deficiency.

Polycal
Nutricia, Irl.; Nutricia, UK.
Food for special diets.
Formerly known as Fortical in the *UK*.

Polycare *Alcon, Fr.*
Sodium dichloroisocyanurate (p.1124·3).
Soft contact-lens cleanser.

Polycid N *Grunenthal, Ger.†.*
Chlormidazole hydrochloride (p.376·2); tyrothricin (p.267·2); tetracycline hydrochloride (p.259·1); hydrocortisone (p.1043·3).
Skin disorders.

Polycidin *Ciba Vision, Canad.*
Eye ointment: Bacitracin zinc (p.157·3); polymyxin B sulphate (p.239·1).
Eye/ear drops: Gramicidin (p.215·2); polymyxin B sulphate (p.239·1).
Eye and ear infections.

Polycillin *Apothecon, USA†.*
Ampicillin trihydrate (p.153·2).
Bacterial infections.

Polycillin-N *Apothecon, USA†.*
Ampicillin sodium (p.153·1).
Bacterial infections.

Polycillin-PRB *Apothecon, USA†.*
Ampicillin trihydrate (p.153·2).
Probenecid (p.394·3) is included in this preparation to reduce renal tubular excretion of ampicillin.
Bacterial infections.

Polycin-B *Ocusoft, USA.*
Bacitracin zinc (p.157·3); polymyxin B sulphate (p.239·1).
Bacterial eye infections.

Polycitra *Willen, USA.*
Potassium citrate (p.1153·1); sodium citrate (p.1153·2); citric acid monohydrate (p.1564·3).
Chronic metabolic acidosis; urine alkalinising agent.

Polycitra-K
Note. This name is used for preparations of different composition.
Baker Cummins, Canad.
Potassium citrate (p.1153·1).
Hypokalaemia.

Willen, USA.
Potassium citrate (p.1153·1); citric acid monohydrate (p.1564·3).
Chronic metabolic acidosis; urine alkalinising agent.

Polycitra-LC *Willen, USA.*
Potassium citrate (p.1153·1); sodium citrate (p.1153·2); citric acid monohydrate (p.1564·3).
Chronic metabolic acidosis; urine alkalinising agent.

Polyclean *Alcon, Fr.*
Cleansing solution for contact lenses.

Polyclens *Alcon, Austral.*
Cleaning liquid for contact lenses.

Polycose
Abbott, Austral.; Abbott, Canad.; Abbott, Ital.; Abbott, UK; Ross, USA.
Glucose polymers.
Nutritional carbohydrate supplement.

Polycrol
Note. This name is used for preparations of different composition.
Nicholas, Irl.†.
Oral gel: Simethicone (p.1213·1); magnesium hydroxide (p.1198·2); aluminium hydroxide gel (p.1177·3).
Tablets: Simethicone (p.1213·1); magnesium hydroxide (p.1198·2); aluminium hydroxide-magnesium carbonate co-dried gel (p.1178·2).
Dyspepsia; flatulence; heartburn; hiatus hernia; hyperchlorhydria.

Zurich, S.Afr.†.
Aluminium hydroxide (p.1177·3); light magnesium oxide (p.1198·2); simethicone (p.1213·1).
Gastro-intestinal hyperacidity.

Polyderm *Taro, Canad.*
Bacitracin zinc (p.157·3); polymyxin B sulphate (p.239·1).
Burns; minor wounds.

Poly-Dex *Ocusoft, USA.*
Dexamethasone (p.1037·1); neomycin sulphate (p.229·2); polymyxin B sulphate (p.239·1).
Infected eye disorders.

Polydexa
Note. This name is used for preparations of different composition.
Therabel Pharma, Belg.; Bouchara, Fr.; Bouchara, Switz.
Ear drops: Neomycin sulphate (p.229·2); polymyxin B sulphate (p.239·1); dexamethasone sodium metasulphobenzoate (p.1037·2).
Otitis.

Bouchara, Switz.†.
Nasal solution: Neomycin sulphate (p.229·2); polymyxin B sulphate (p.239·1); dexamethasone sodium metasulphobenzoate (p.1037·2); phenylephrine hydrochloride (p.1066·2).
Rhinitis; sinusitis.

Polydexa a la Phenylephrine *Bouchara, Fr.*
Neomycin sulphate (p.229·2); polymyxin B sulphate (p.239·1); dexamethasone sodium metasulphobenzoate (p.1037·2); phenylephrine hydrochloride (p.1066·2).
Nose and throat disorders.

Polydiet HC *DHN, Fr.*
Preparation for enteral nutrition.

Polydine *Century, USA.*
Povidone-iodine (p.1123·3).
Skin disinfection.

Polydona *Hexal, Ger.*
Povidone-iodine (p.1123·3).
Burns; skin ulcers; wounds.

Polydurat N *Pohl, Ger.†.*
Multivitamin preparation.

Polyerga *Merz, Ger.*
Polypeptides derived from spleen.
Adjuvant tumour therapy.

Polyfax
Wellcome, Irl.; Dominion, UK.
Polymyxin B sulphate (p.239·1); bacitracin zinc (p.157·3).
Bacterial infections of the skin and eye.

Polyfen *Chinosolfabrik, Ger.†.*
Neomycin hydrochloride (p.230·1); aminoquinuride hydrochloride (p.1101·2).
Bacterial infections of the oropharynx.

Polyferon *Rentschler, Ger.†.*
Interferon gamma (rbe) (p.616·1).
Arthritis.

Polyflam *Farmabel, Belg.†.*
Diclofenac sodium (p.31·2).
Inflammation; musculoskeletal, joint, and peri-articular disorders; pain.

Polyfra *Alcon, Fr.*
Eye drops: Framycetin sulphate (p.210·3); polymyxin B sulphate (p.239·1); oxedrine hydrochloride (p.925·3).
Eye ointment: Framycetin sulphate (p.210·3); polymyxin B sulphate (p.239·1).
Formerly contained muramidase hydrochloride, framycetin sulphate, and polymyxin B sulphate.
Bacterial eye infections.

Polygam
NBI, S.Afr.; American Red Cross, USA†.
A normal immunoglobulin (p.1522·1).
Hypogammaglobulinaemia.

Polygamma *Association Nationale, Fr.†.*
A normal immunoglobulin (p.1522·1).
Passive immunisation.

Polyglobin *Bayer, Swed.†.*
A normal immunoglobulin (p.1522·1).
Hypogammaglobulinaemia; idiopathic thrombocytopenic purpura; Kawasaki syndrome.

Polyglobin N *Bayer, Ger.*
A normal immunoglobulin (p.1522·1).
Hypogammaglobulinaemia; idiopathic thrombocytopenic purpura; passive immunisation.

Polygris *Essex, Ger.†.*
Griseofulvin (ultramicronised) (p.380·2).
Fungal infections.

Poly-Gynaedron *Artesan, Ger.†.*
Chlorindanol (p.1562·2); chlorphenesin (p.376·2); ethinyloestradiol (p.1445·1).
Infective vaginitis.

Polygynax
Darci, Belg.; Innothera, Fr.; UCB, Ger.
Neomycin sulphate (p.229·2); nystatin (p.386·1); polymyxin B sulphate (p.239·1).
Vulvovaginal infections.

Polygynax Virgo *Innothera, Fr.*
Neomycin sulphate (p.229·2); nystatin (p.386·1); polymyxin B sulphate (p.239·1).
Vulvovaginitis.

Poly-Gynedron *Noristan, S.Afr.†.*
Sulphasomidine (p.257·1); acetarsol sodium (p.578·2); borax (p.1554·2); stilboestrol dipropionate (p.1462·3).
Vaginal infections.

Poly-Histine *Sanofi Winthrop, USA.*
Phenyltoloxamine citrate (p.416·1); mepyramine maleate (p.414·1); pheniramine maleate (p.415·3).
Allergic rhinitis.

Poly-Histine CS CV *Sanofi Winthrop, USA.*
Codeine phosphate (p.26·1); phenylpropanolamine hydrochloride (p.1067·2); brompheniramine maleate (p.403·2).
Coughs and cold symptoms.

Poly-Histine D *Sanofi Winthrop, USA.*
Phenylpropanolamine hydrochloride (p.1067·2); phenyltoloxamine citrate (p.416·1); mepyramine maleate (p.414·1); pheniramine maleate (p.415·3).
Allergic rhinitis; nasal congestion.

Poly-Histine DM *Sanofi Winthrop, USA.*
Dextromethorphan hydrobromide (p.1057·3); phenylpropanolamine hydrochloride (p.1067·2); brompheniramine maleate (p.403·2).
Coughs and cold symptoms.

Poly-Joule *Sharpe, Austral.*
Dextrin (p.1339·1).
Nutritional supplement.

Poly-Karaya
Synthelabo, Fr.; Kramer, Switz.
Sterculia (p.1214·1); povidone (p.1474·2).
Constipation; diarrhoea; meteorism.

Polymox
Bristol-Myers Squibb, S.Afr.†; Apothecon, USA†.
Amoxycillin trihydrate (p.151·3).
Bacterial infections.

Poly-Mulsin *Mucos, Ger.†.*
Multivitamin preparation.

Polyneural *Stroschein, Ger.†.*
Vitamin B substances.
Vitamin B deficiency.

Polypharm-Zahnungsgel N *Polypharm, Ger.*
Sage (p.1627·1); lignocaine hydrochloride (p.1293·2).
Toothache.

Polypirine *Lehning, Fr.*
Propyphenazone (p.81·3); phenicarbazide (p.79·1); phenacetin (p.78·1); caffeine citrate (p.749·3); cinnamon (p.1564·2); ipecacuanha (p.1062·2); squill (p.1070·1).
Fever; pain.

Poly-Pred *Allergan, USA.*
Prednisolone acetate (p.1048·1); neomycin sulphate (p.229·2); polymyxin B sulphate (p.239·1).
Eye inflammation with bacterial infection.

Polypress *Pfizer, Ger.*
Prazosin hydrochloride (p.932·3); polythiazide (p.932·1).
Hypertension.

Polyrinse *Alcon, Fr.*
Sodium chloride (p.1162·2).
Rinsing and soaking solution for contact lenses.

Polyrinse Desinfektionssystem *Alcon, Aust.*
Sodium dichloroisocyanurate (p.1124·3).
Disinfection and rinsing of soft contact lenses.

Polyrinse-Aufnahmelosung *Alcon, Aust.*
Sodium chloride (p.1162·2).
Storage solution for soft contact lenses.

Polyrinse-Augenelement *Alcon, Aust.*
Sodium chloride (p.1162·2); boric acid (p.1554·2).
Comfort drops for contact lenses.

Poly-Rivitin *Clinced, Aust.*
Multivitamin preparation.

Polyseptol *Qualiphar, Belg.*
Filtrate from culture of: *Staphylococcus aureus, Streptococcus pyogenes, Pseudomonas aeruginosa*, and *Escherichia coli*; sulphanilamide (p.256·3); cod-liver oil (p.1337·3).
Infected skin disorders.

Polysilane
Clin Midy, Fr.†; Sanofi Labaz, Neth.†; Upsamedica, Switz.
Dimethicone (p.1213·1).
Gastro-intestinal disorders.

Polysilane Comp *Sanofi Labaz, Neth.†.*
Liquorice (p.1197·1); aluminium glycinate (p.1177·2); algeldrate (p.1177·3); magnesium trisilicate (p.1199·1); calcium carbonate (p.1182·1); simethicone (p.1213·1).
Gastro-intestinal disorders.

Polysilane Joullie *Synthelabo, Fr.*
Chewable tablets/lozenges: Simethicone (p.1213·1); aluminium hydroxide (p.1177·3).
Gastro-intestinal disorders.
Paediatric oral granules: Simethicone (p.1213·1); ceratonia (p.1472·2).
Gastro-oesophageal reflux.

Polysilane Midy *Sanofi Winthrop, Switz.†.*
Dimethicone (p.1213·1); galactomannan.
Gastro-intestinal disorders.

Polysilane Reglisse *Clin Midy, Fr.†.*
Dimethicone (p.1213·1); liquorice (p.1197·1); aluminium glycinate (p.1177·2); aluminium hydroxide (p.1177·3); magnesium trisilicate (p.1199·1); calcium carbonate (p.1182·1).
Gastric hyperacidity.

Polysilon *Upsamedica, Belg.*
Dimethicone (p.1213·1).
Gastro-intestinal disorders associated with hyperacidity.

Polysorb *Fougera, USA.*
Emollient and moisturiser.

Polyspectran *Alcon-Thilo, Ger.*
Eye and ear drops: Polymyxin B sulphate (p.239·1); neomycin sulphate (p.229·2); gramicidin (p.215·2).
Ointment: Polymyxin B sulphate (p.239·1); bacitracin (p.157·3); neomycin sulphate (p.229·2).
Bacterial infections of the eye, ear, and nose.

Polyspectran B *Thilo, Neth.†.*
Neomycin sulphate (p.229·2); polymyxin B sulphate (p.239·1); bacitracin (p.157·3).
Bacterial eye infections.

Polyspectran G *Thilo, Neth.†.*
Neomycin sulphate (p.229·2); gramicidin (p.215·2); polymyxin B sulphate (p.239·1).
Bacterial eye infections.

Polyspectran HC *Alcon-Thilo, Ger.*
Polymyxin B sulphate (p.239·1); bacitracin (p.157·3); hydrocortisone acetate (p.1043·3).
Bacterial and inflammatory eye disorders; otitis media; skin disorders.

Polyspectran OS *Alcon-Thilo, Ger.†.*
Polymyxin B sulphate (p.239·1); bacitracin (p.157·3); neomycin sulphate (p.229·2); hydrocortisone acetate (p.1043·3).
Ear disorders.

Polysporin
Note. This name is used for preparations of different composition.
Warner-Lambert, Canad.
Cream; eye/ear drops: Polymyxin B sulphate (p.239·1); gramicidin (p.215·2).
Bacterial contamination prophylaxis; eye and ear infections; infected skin disorders.

Warner-Lambert, Canad.; Glaxo Wellcome, S.Afr.; Glaxo Wellcome, USA.
Eye ointment; ointment; topical powder: Polymyxin B sulphate (p.239·1); bacitracin (p.157·3) or bacitracin zinc (p.157·3).
Eye and ear infections; infected lesions.

Wellcome, Norw.†.
Polymyxin B sulphate (p.239·1); neomycin sulphate (p.229·2); gramicidin (p.215·2).
Eye infections.

Polysporin Burn Formula *Warner-Lambert, Canad.*
Polymyxin B sulphate (p.239·1); gramicidin (p.215·2); lignocaine hydrochloride (p.1293·2).
Infected burns; skin pain.

Polysporin Triple Antibiotic *Warner-Wellcome, Canad.*
Polymyxin B sulphate (p.239·1); bacitracin (p.157·3); gramicidin (p.215·2).
Burns; minor wounds.

Polytabs-F *Major, USA.*
Multivitamin preparation with fluoride(p.742·1).
Dental caries prophylaxis; dietary supplement.

Polytar
Stiefel, Austral.; Stiefel, Canad.; Stiefel, Fr.†; Stiefel, Ger.; Stiefel, Irl.; Stiefel, Ital.; Stiefel, S.Afr.; Stiefel, Spain; Stiefel, Switz.†; Stiefel, USA.
Tar (p.1092·3); cade oil (p.1092·2); coal tar (p.1092·3).
Skin and scalp disorders.

Polytar AF
Note. This name is used for preparations of different composition.
Stiefel, Canad.
Coal tar (p.1092·3); pyrithione disulphide (p.1089·3); salicylic acid (p.1090·2); menthol (p.1600·2).
Scalp disorders.

Stiefel, UK.
Tar (p.1092·3); cade oil (p.1092·2); coal tar (p.1092·3); pyrithione zinc (p.1089·3).
Scalp disorders.

Polytar Emollient
Stiefel, Irl.; Stiefel, UK.
Tar (p.1092·3); cade oil (p.1092·2); coal tar (p.1092·3); liquid paraffin (p.1382·1).
Aid to ointment and paste removal in psoriasis; skin disorders.

Polytar Liquid *Stiefel, UK.*
Tar (p.1092·3); cade oil (p.1092·2); coal tar (p.1092·3).
Aid to ointment and paste removal in psoriasis; scalp disorders.

Polytar Plus
Stiefel, Irl.; Stiefel, UK.
Tar (p.1092·3); cade oil (p.1092·2); coal tar (p.1092·3).
Aid to ointment removal in psoriasis; scalp disorders.

Poly-Tears *Alcon, Austral.*
Hypromellose (p.1473·1); dextran 70 (p.717·1).
Dry eyes.

Polytinic *Pharmics, USA.*
Ferrous fumarate (p.1339·3); folic acid (p.1340·3).
Ascorbic acid (p.1365·2) is included in this preparation to improve the absorption and availability of iron.

Polytonyl
Upsamedica, Belg.; UPSA, Fr.; Upsamedica, Switz.
Vitamin, mineral, and amino-acid preparation.
Tonic.

Polytopic *Technilab, Canad.*
Polymyxin B sulphate (p.239·1); bacitracin (p.157·3).
Infected lesions.

Polytracin *Metapharma, Canad.*
Polymyxin B sulphate (p.239·1); bacitracin zinc (p.157·3).
Bacterial infections.

Polytrim
Glaxo Wellcome, Aust.; Glaxo Wellcome, Belg.; Allergan, Canad.;

Wellcome, Ital.†; Glaxo Wellcome, Neth.; Allergan, S.Afr.; Dominion, UK; Allergan, USA.
Trimethoprim (p.265·1) or trimethoprim sulphate (p.266·2); polymyxin B sulphate (p.239·1).
Bacterial eye and skin infections.

Polyvalent Snake Antivenom *CSL, Austral.*
A snake antiserum of king brown snake, tiger snake, brown snake, death adder, and taipan (p.1534·1).
Passive immunisation.

Poly-Vi-Flor
Mead Johnson, Canad.; Mead Johnson Nutritionals, USA.
A range of vitamin preparations with fluoride(p.742·1).
Dental caries prophylaxis; dietary supplement.

Poly-Vi-Sol
Bristol-Myers Squibb, Belg.†; Mead Johnson, Canad.; Mead Johnson Nutritionals, USA.
A range of vitamin preparations.

Polyvit *Propan, S.Afr.*
Multivitamin preparation.

Polyvita *Piette, Belg.*
Multivitamin, mineral, and amino-acid preparation.

Poly-Vitamin Plus *Chephasaar, Ger.*
Multivitamin and mineral preparation.

Polyxan-Blau *Ritsert, Ger.*
Homoeopathic preparation.

Polyxan-Blau comp. *Ritsert, Ger.*
Homoeopathic preparation.

Polyxan-Gelb *Ritsert, Ger.*
Homoeopathic preparation.

Polyxan-Grun *Ritsert, Ger.*
Homoeopathic preparation.

Polyzym
Alcon, Aust.; Alcon, Austral.; Alcon, Fr.
Pancreatin (p.1612·1).
Hard and soft contact lens cleanser.

Pomada Antibiotica *Knoll, Spain.*
Bacitracin (p.157·3); neomycin sulphate (p.229·2); polymyxin B sulphate (p.239·1).
Skin infections.

Pomada Balsamica *Alcala, Spain.*
Camphor (p.1557·2); cedrus deodora oil; cineole (p.1564·1); methyl salicylate (p.55·2); thymol (p.1127·1); turpentine.
Cold symptoms.

Pomada Heridas *Asens, Spain.*
Benzalkonium chloride (p.1101·3); phenazone (p.78·2); sulphanilamide (p.256·3); zinc oxide (p.1096·2).
Skin infections.

Pomada Infantil Vera *Labitec, Spain.*
Bismuth subnitrate (p.1180·2); boric acid (p.1554·2); talc (p.1092·1); zinc oxide (p.1096·2).
Skin irritation.

Pomada Llorens Sulfaclor *Llorens, Spain†.*
Chloramphenicol (p.182·1); sulphacetamide sodium (p.252·2).
Skin infections.

Pomada Mercurial *Orravan, Spain†.*
Mercuric oxide (p.1601·3).
Skin disinfection.

Pomada Oftalm Antisep *Asens, Spain†.*
Boric acid (p.1554·2); methylene blue (p.984·3); procaine hydrochloride (p.1299·2).
Bacterial eye infections.

Pomada Orravan Prec Amar *Orravan, Spain†.*
Mercuric oxide (p.1601·3); soft paraffin.
Skin disorders.

Pomada Pptado Blanc Brum *Byly, Spain†.*
Mercuric chloride (p.1601·2); soft paraffin.
Skin disorders.

Pomada Pptado Blanc Orra *Orravan, Spain†.*
Mercuric chloride (p.1601·2); soft paraffin.
Skin disorders.

Pomada Revulsiva *Orravan, Spain.*
Camphor (p.1557·2); capsicum oleoresin; eugenol (p.1578·2); methyl salicylate (p.55·2); turpentine oil (p.1641·1).
Musculoskeletal, joint, peri-articular, and soft-tissue disorders.

Pomada Sulfamida Orravan *Orravan, Spain†.*
Sulphanilamide (p.256·3).
Skin infections.

Pomada Wilfe *Calmante Vitaminado, Spain.*
Sulphanilamide (p.256·3); sulphathiazole (p.257·1).
Skin infections.

Pomata Midy *Midy, Ital.†.*
Benzocaine (p.1286·2); hamamelis (p.1587·1); aesculus (p.1543·3).
Anorectal disorders.

Pomata Midy HC *Maggioni, Ital.*
Benzocaine (p.1286·2); hamamelis (p.1587·1); aesculus (p.1543·3); hydrocortisone acetate (p.1043·3).
Anorectal disorders.

Pommade au The des Bois *Valmo, Canad.*
Methyl salicylate (p.55·2); camphor (p.1557·2); menthol (p.1600·2); cineole (p.1564·1).

Pommade Kytta *Whitehall-Robins, Switz.†.*
Comfrey (p.1567·1); pumilio pine oil (p.1623·3); lavender oil (p.1594·3).
Muscle and joint pain; wounds.

Pommade Lelong *SmithKline Beecham Sante, Fr.*
Peru balsam (p.1617·2); sulphapyridine (p.256·3); vitamin A (p.1358·1).
Skin disorders.

Pommade Midy
Welcker-Lyster, Canad.; Clin Midy, Fr.†.
Amylocaine hydrochloride (p.1286·1); benzocaine (p.1286·2); hamamelis (p.1587·1); aesculus (p.1543·3).
Haemorrhoids and other anal disorders.

Pommade Mo Cochon *Cochon, Fr.*
Salicylic acid (p.1090·2).
Callus; corns; verrucae.

Pommade nasale Ruedi *Stotzer, Switz.*
Camphorated oil (p.1557·2); mint oil (p.1604·1).
Nasal dryness.

Pommade Po-Ho N A Vogel *Bioforce, Switz.*
Hypericum (p.1590·1); peppermint oil (p.1208·1); hamamelis (p.1587·1); peppermint leaf (p.1208·1); calendula officinalis; lemon oil (p.1595·3).
Catarrh; cold and influenza symptoms; sinus disorders.

Ponac *Pharmacare Consumer, S.Afr.*
Mefenamic acid (p.51·2).
Musculoskeletal, joint, and soft-tissue disorders; pain.

Ponalar *Godecke, Ger.*
Mefenamic acid (p.51·2).
Inflammation; musculoskeletal and joint disorders; pain.

Ponalgic *Antigen, Irl.*
Mefenamic acid (p.51·2).
Menorrhagia; musculoskeletal and joint disorders; pain.

Ponaris *Jamol, USA†.*
Cajuput oil (p.1556·1); eucalyptus oil (p.1578·1); peppermint oil (p.1208·1).
Nasal congestion.

Ponderal
Eutherapie, Belg.†; Servier, Canad.†; Biopharma, Fr.†; Servier, Ital.†; Servier, Neth.†; Danval, Spain†.
Fenfluramine hydrochloride (p.1480·3).
Obesity.

Ponderax
Servier, Aust.†; Servier, Austral.†; Servier, Ger.†; Servier, Irl.†; Servier, S.Afr.†; Servier, UK†.
Fenfluramine hydrochloride (p.1480·3).
Obesity.

Pondimin
Wyeth-Ayerst, Canad.†; Robins, USA†.
Fenfluramine hydrochloride (p.1480·3).
Obesity.

Pondinil *Sauter, Switz.†.*
Mefenorex hydrochloride (p.1482·1).
Obesity.

Pondocillin
Merck, Aust.; Leo, Canad.; Leo, Irl.; Leo, Norw.; Adcock Ingram, S.Afr.; Lovens, Swed.; Leo, UK†.
Pivampicillin (p.238·2).
Bacterial infections.

Pondocillin Plus *Leo, UK†.*
Pivmecillinam hydrochloride (p.239·1); pivampicillin (p.238·2).
Bacterial infections.

Ponds Prevent *Lever Pond's, Canad.*
Ethylhexyl *p*-methoxycinnamate (p.1487·1); oxybenzone (p.1487·3).
Sunscreen.

Ponflural *Servier, Switz.†.*
Fenfluramine hydrochloride (p.1480·3).
Obesity.

Ponmel *Clonmel, Irl.*
Mefenamic acid (p.51·2).
Pain.

Ponoxylan
Rhone-Poulenc Rorer, Austral.†; Roche, S.Afr.†.
Polynoxylin (p.1123·1).
Bacterial and fungal skin infections.

Ponstan
Parke, Davis, Austral.; Parke, Davis, Canad.; Elan, Irl.; Parke, Davis, S.Afr.; Parke, Davis, Switz.; Elan, UK.
Mefenamic acid (p.51·2).
Fever; inflammation; menorrhagia; pain.

Ponstel
Parke-Med, S.Afr.; Parke, Davis, USA.
Mefenamic acid (p.51·2).
Fever; menorrhagia; pain.

Ponstyl *Parke, Davis, Fr.*
Mefenamic acid (p.51·2).
Fever; pain.

Pontocaine
Sanofi Winthrop, Canad.; Sanofi Winthrop, USA.
Amethocaine (p.1285·2) or amethocaine hydrochloride (p.1285·2).
Local anaesthesia.

Pontuc
Sanabo, Aust.; Sandoz, Aust.; Sandoz, Ger.
Co-dergocrine mesylate (p.1566·1); nifedipine (p.916·2).
Hypertension.

Pool 8 *Fiori, Ital.*
Amino-acid preparation.
Nutritional supplement.

Po-Pon-S *Shionogi, USA.*
Multivitamin and mineral preparation.

POR 8
Sandoz, Aust.; Novartis, Austral.; Sandoz, Ger.; Sandoz, S.Afr.†; Sandoz, Switz.
Ornipressin (p.1257·1).
Reduction of bleeding during surgery; variceal haemorrhage.

Porcelana
Lavoris-Dep, Canad.; DEP, USA.
Hydroquinone (p.1083·1).
Hyperpigmentation.

Porcelana with Sunscreen
Note. This name is used for preparations of different composition.
Lavoris-Dep, Canad.
Hydroquinone (p.1083·1); ethylhexyl *p*-methoxycinnamate (p.1487·1).
DEP, USA.
Hydroquinone (p.1083·1); padimate O (p.1488·1).
Hyperpigmentation.

Porfanil *Prodes, Spain†.*
Tiapride hydrochloride (p.696·1).
Behaviour disorders; headache.

Porfirin 12 *Zilliken, Ital.*
Injection†: Haematoporphyrin dihydrochloride (p.1587·1); cyanocobalamin (p.1363·3).
Oral liquid: Haematoporphyrin dihydrochloride (p.1587·1); cyanocobalamin (p.1363·3); inositol (p.1591·1).
Tonic.

Pork Mixtard 30 *Novo Nordisk, UK.*
Mixture of neutral insulin injection (porcine, highly purified) 30% and isophane insulin injection (porcine, highly purified) 70% (p.322·1).
Formerly known as Mixtard 30/70.
Diabetes mellitus.

Porosan *Reig Jofre, Spain†.*
Camphor (p.1557·2); lavender oil (p.1594·3); methyl salicylate (p.55·2); rosemary oil (p.1626·2); turpentine oil (p.1641·1); eucalyptus oil (p.1578·1).
Soft-tissue and muscular disorders; upper-respiratory-tract disorders.

Porosis D *Cedar Health, UK.*
Calcium citrate (p.1155·1); magnesium citrate (p.1198·2); boron; vitamin D (p.1366·3).

Porostenina *Savio, Ital.*
Salcatonin (p.735·3).
Hypercalcaemia; osteoporosis; Paget's disease of bone; reflex sympathetic dystrophy.

Porphyrin *Zilliken, Ital.†.*
Haematoporphyrin (p.1587·1).
Tonic.

Porriver *Ogna, Ital.*
Trichloroacetic acid (p.1639·1).
Verrucae; warts.

Portagen
Mead Johnson, Austral.; Mead Johnson, Canad.; Bristol-Myers Squibb, Irl.; Bristol-Myers Squibb, S.Afr.; Mead Johnson Nutritionals, UK†; Mead Johnson Nutritionals, USA.
Preparation for enteral nutrition.
Impaired fat absorption; lactose intolerance.

Portolac
Zyma, Aust.†; Zyma, Belg.; Zyma, Ital.
Lactitol (p.1195·2).
Liver disorders.

Posalfilin
Norgine, Austral.; Norgine, Irl.; Norgine, S.Afr.; Norgine, UK.
Podophyllum resin (p.1089·1); salicylic acid (p.1090·2).
Warts.

Posebor *Galderma, Fr.†.*
Alcloxa (p.1078·2); hexamidine isethionate (p.1115·3); DL-lysine monohydrochloride.
Acne.

Posedrine *Laso, Spain.*
Beclamide (p.339·2).
Epilepsy.

Posicor
Roche, Austral.†; Roche, Irl.†; Roche, Neth.†; Roche, UK†; Roche, USA†.
Mibefradil dihydrochloride (p.910·1).
Angina pectoris; hypertension.

Posicycline *Alcon, Fr.*
Oxytetracycline hydrochloride (p.235·1).
Bacterial eye infections.

Posifenicol *Ursapharm, Ger.*
Azidamfenicol (p.155·2).
Bacterial eye infections.

Posifenicol C *Ursapharm, Ger.*
Chloramphenicol (p.182·1).
Bacterial eye infections.

Posiformin *Ursapharm, Ger.*
Bibrocathol (p.1553·2).
Inflammatory eye disorders.

Posiject
Boehringer Ingelheim, Irl.; Boehringer Ingelheim, UK.
Dobutamine hydrochloride (p.860·1).
Agent for cardiac stress testing; heart failure.

Posilent *Ursapharm, Ger.*
Cytidine.
Eye disorders.

Posine *Alcon, Fr.*
Oxedrine hydrochloride (p.925·3); boric acid (p.1554·2); rose water; hamamelis (p.1587·1).
Conjunctival irritation.

Positex *Ursapharm, Ger.†.*
Prednisolone sodium metasulphobenzoate (p.1048·1); chloramphenicol (p.182·1).
Allergic and inflammatory eye disorders.

Positon *Iquinosa, Spain.*
Neomycin sulphate (p.229·2); nystatin (p.386·1); triamcinolone (p.1050·2) or triamcinolone acetonide (p.1050·2).
Formerly contained gramicidin, neomycin sulphate, nystatin, and triamcinolone acetonide.
Infected skin disorders.

Posorutin *Ursapharm, Ger.*
Troxerutin (p.1580·2).
Haemorrhoids; ophthalmic disorders; venous insufficiency.

Postacne *Dermik, Canad.*
Colloidal sulphur (p.1091·2).
Acne; oily skin.

Postacton *Ferring, Swed.†.*
Lypressin (p.1263·2).
Diabetes insipidus; haemorrhage; test of pituitary function.

Postadoxin *UCB, Ger.†.*
Meclozine (p.413·3); pyridoxine.
Motion sickness; nausea; vomiting.

Postadoxin N *Rodleben, Ger.*
Meclozine hydrochloride (p.413·3).
Motion sickness; nausea; vomiting.

Postadoxine *UCB, Belg.*
Meclozine (p.413·3); vitamin B_6 (p.1362·3).
Nausea and vomiting.

Postafen
UCB, Ger.; UCB, Norw.; UCB, Swed.
Meclozine (p.413·3) or meclozine hydrochloride (p.413·3).
Hypersensitivity reactions; nausea; vertigo; vomiting.

Postafene *Darci, Belg.*
Meclozine hydrochloride (p.413·3).
Hypersensitivity reactions; motion sickness; nausea and vomiting; pruritus.

Posterine *Kade, Ger.*
Hamamelis (p.1587·1).
Anorectal disorders.

Posterine Corte *Kade, Ger.*
Hydrocortisone acetate (p.1043·3).
Anorectal disorders.

Posterisan
Mayrhofer, Aust.; Kade, Ger.; Rhone-Poulenc Rorer, S.Afr.†.
Cell contents and metabolic products of *Escherichia coli*.
Anorectal disorders.

Posterisan forte *Kade, Ger.*
Cell contents and metabolic products of *Escherichia coli*; hydrocortisone (p.1043·3).
Anorectal disorders.

Posti N *Kade, Ger.*
Rutoside (p.1580·2); esculoside (p.1543·3).
Vascular disorders.

Postinor-2 *Medimpex, UK.*
Levonorgestrel (p.1454·1).
Available on a named-patient basis only.
Postcoital oral contraception.

PostMI *Ashbourne, UK.*
Aspirin (p.16·1).
Angina; ischaemic heart disease; myocardial infarction.

Postoval *Akromed, S.Afr.*
11 Tablets, oestradiol valerate (p.1455·2); 10 tablets, oestradiol valerate; norgestrel (p.1454·1); 7 tablets, inert.
Menopausal disorders; menstrual disorders.

Posture *Whitehall, USA.*
Calcium phosphate (p.1155·3).
Calcium supplement.

Posture-D *Whitehall, USA.*
Calcium phosphate (p.1155·3); vitamin D (p.1366·3).
Calcium supplement.

Potaba
Croma, Aust.; Glenwood, Canad.; Glenwood, Ger.; Glenwood, Switz.; Glenwood, UK; Glenwood, USA.
Potassium aminobenzoate (p.1620·1).
Dermatomyositis; linear scleroderma; morphoea; pemphigus; Peyronie's disease; scleroderma.

Potable Aqua *Wisconsin Pharmacal, USA.*
Tetraglycine hydroperiodide (p.1126·3).
Disinfection of drinking water.

Potacol-R *Otsuka, Jpn.*
Carbohydrate and electrolyte infusion.
Carbohydrate source; compensation of metabolic acidosis; fluid and electrolyte disorders.

Potasalan *Lannett, USA.*
Potassium chloride (p.1161·1).
Hypokalaemia; potassium depletion.

Potasion *Delagrange, Spain.*
Potassium chloride (p.1161·1) or potassium gluceptate (p.1161·3).
Potassium depletion.

Potassion
Note. This name is used for preparations of different composition.
Delagrange, Fr.†.
Potassium gluceptate (p.1161·3).
Hypokalaemia.
Miba, Ital.
Potassium succinate; potassium malate; potassium citrate (p.1153·1); potassium acid tartrate (p.1209·1); potassium bicarbonate (p.1153·1).
Acidosis; potassium deficiency.

Potassium Iodide and Stramonium Compound *McGloin, Austral.*
Potassium iodide (p.1493·1); stramonium (p.468·2); lobelia (p.1481·3); liquorice (p.1197·1).
Coughs; respiratory-tract congestion.

Potassium-Sandoz *Sandoz, Canad.*
Potassium chloride (p.1161·1); potassium bicarbonate (p.1153·1).
Potassium depletion; potassium load tests.

Potenciator *Iquinosa, Spain.*
Arginine aspartate (p.1334·2).
Tonic.

Potendal *Zambon, Spain.*
Ceftazidime (p.173·3).
Bacterial infections.

Potent C *Vita Glow, Austral.†.*
Ascorbic acid (p.1365·2).
Vitamin C deficiency.

Potsilo *Stark, Ger.*
Bisacodyl (p.1179·3); docusate sodium (p.1189·3); calcium pantothenate (p.1352·3); benzyl mandelate.
Constipation.

Potter's Pastilles *Ernest Jackson, UK.*
Sylvestris pine oil; pumilio pine oil (p.1623·3); eucalyptus oil (p.1578·1); creosote (p.1057·3); menthol (p.1600·2); thymol (p.1127·1); marshmallow (p.1546·3).
Cough and cold symptoms.

Poudre de proteines *Fresenius, Switz.†.*
Protein, fat, carbohydrate and mineral preparation.

Povanyl *Warner-Lambert, Fr.*
Viprynium embonate (p.111·2).
Enterobiasis.

Poviderm *Farmec, Ital.*
Povidone-iodine (p.1123·3).
Skin and wound disinfection.

Povidex *Morton Grove, USA.*
Povidone-iodine (p.1123·3).

Powdered C *Neo-Life, Austral.*
Ascorbic acid and other vitamin C substances.
Vitamin C deficiency.

Powergel *Searle, UK.*
Ketoprofen (p.48·2).
Inflammation; pain.

Powerin *Whitehall, UK.*
Aspirin (p.16·1); caffeine (p.749·3); paracetamol (p.72·2).
Fever; pain.

PowerLean *SwissHealth, UK.*
Conjugate linoleic acid (p.1582·1).
Nutritional supplement.

PowerMate *Green Turtle Bay Vitamin Co., USA.*
Vitamins; minerals; green tea extract; ginkgo biloba extract; glutathione; acetylcysteine; echinacea; golden seal root; pine bark extract.
Tonic.

PowerVites *Green Turtle Bay Vitamin Co., USA.*
Vitamins; minerals; aminobenzoic acid; inositol; bioflavonoids; bee pollen; folic acid.
Tonic.

Poxider *Martin, Spain.*
Fluocinolone acetonide (p.1041·1); gramicidin (p.215·2); neomycin sulphate (p.229·2).
Infected skin disorders.

Poysept *Dermapharm, Ger.*
Povidone-iodine (p.1123·3).
Burns; skin and mucous membrane disinfection; skin ulcers; wounds.

PP-Cap *Alra, USA.*
Dextropropoxyphene hydrochloride (p.27·3).

PPD Tine Test *Wyeth, S.Afr.*
Tuberculin (p.1640·2).
Diagnosis of tuberculosis.

PPS *Immuno, Ital.*
Plasma protein fraction (p.726·3).
Burns; hypovolaemia; shock.

PPSB *Bio-Transfusion, Fr.†.*
A factor IX preparation (p.721·3).
Haemorrhagic disorders.

PPSB Konzentrat hepatitissicher *Biotest, Aust.†.*
A factor IX preparation (p.721·3).
Haemorrhagic disorders.

PPSB-Komplex *Alpha Therapeutic, Ger.†.*
A factor IX preparation (p.721·3).
Haemorrhagic disorders.

PPSB-Tropon *Tropon-Cutter, Ger.†.*
A factor IX preparation (p.721·3).
Haemorrhagic disorders.

PR 100 *Farmacologico Milanese, Ital.*
Desonide pivalate (p.1036·3).
Skin disorders.

PR 100-Cloressidina *Farmacologico Milanese, Ital.*
Desonide pivalate (p.1036·3); chlorhexidine (p.1107·2).
Skin disorders.

PR Freeze Spray *Crookes Healthcare, UK.*
Dimethyl ether (p.1165·1); dimethoxymethane (p.1572·1).
Formerly contained trichlorofluoromethane and dichlorodifluoromethane.
Muscular pain and stiffness.

PR Heat Spray *Crookes Healthcare, UK.*
Methyl salicylate (p.55·2); ethyl nicotinate (p.36·1); camphor (p.1557·2).
Bruises; muscular and rheumatic pain; sprains.

Pra-Brexidol *Pharmacia Upjohn, Ger.*
Piroxicam (p.80·2).
Gout; musculoskeletal and joint disorders.

Practazin *Cardel, Fr.*
Spironolactone (p.946·1); althiazide (p.819·1).
Hypertension; oedema.

Practil *Organon, Ital.*
Desogestrel (p.1443·3); ethinyloestradiol (p.1445·1).
Combined oral contraceptive.

Practo-Clyss
Braun, Belg.; Fresenius-Praxis, Ger.; Fresenius-Klinik, Ger.; Vifor Medical, Switz.
Monobasic sodium phosphate (p.1159·3); dibasic sodium phosphate (p.1159·3).
Bowel evacuation; constipation.

Practomil *Vifor Medical, Switz.*
Glycerol (p.1585·2).
Bowel evacuation; constipation.

Practon *Cardel, Fr.*
Spironolactone (p.946·1).
Hyperaldosteronism; hypertension; myasthenia; oedema.

Pradif *Boehringer Ingelheim, Ital.*
Tamsulosin hydrochloride (p.951·2).
Benign prostatic hyperplasia.

Praecicor *Molimin, Ger.*
Verapamil hydrochloride (p.960·3).
Angina pectoris; arrhythmias; hypertension.

Praeciglucon *Pfleger, Ger.*
Glibenclamide (p.319·3).
Diabetes mellitus.

Praecimal *Pfleger, Ger.†.*
Ergotamine tartrate (p.445·3); caffeine (p.749·3); nicotinamide (p.1351·2); mepyramine maleate (p.414·1).
Headache including migraine.

Praecimed N *Molimin, Ger.†.*
Aspirin (p.16·1); paracetamol (p.72·2); codeine phosphate (p.26·1).
Coughs and cold symptoms; neuralgia; pain.

Praecimycin *Molimin, Ger.†.*
Erythromycin ethyl succinate (p.204·2) or erythromycin stearate (p.204·2).
Bacterial infections.

Praecineural *Pfleger, Ger.*
Aspirin (p.16·1); codeine phosphate (p.26·1).
Pain; rheumatism.

Praecipect *Molimin, Ger.*
Thyme (p.1636·3); primula rhizome.
Formerly contained thyme, primula rhizome, and ephedrine hydrochloride.
Respiratory-tract disorders.

Praecivenin *Pfleger, Ger.†.*
Tablets; capsules: Aesculus (p.1543·3); troxerutin (p.1580·2).
Vascular disorders.
Topical gel; ointment: Heparin sodium (p.879·3).
Skin trauma.

Praecordin S *Roland, Ger.*
Strong camphor oil; menthol (p.1600·2); benzyl nicotinate (p.22·1).
Cardiac disorders.

Praedex *Leopold, Aust.*
Dextran 1 (p.716·1).
Prevention of anaphylactic reactions to infusions of dextrans.

Praefeminon plus *Redel, Ger.*
Ferric ammonium citrate (p.1339·2); pulsatilla; valeriana.
Gynaecological disorders.

Praesidin *Medopharm, Ger.*
Lignocaine hydrochloride (p.1293·2); diphenhydramine methylsulphate (p.409·2); titanium dioxide (p.1093·3).
Skin disorders.

Praesidium *Bonomelli, Ital.†.*
Phospholipids, essential fatty acids, vitamin E, and selenium.

Pragman
Klosterfrau, Aust.; Albert-Roussel, Ger.†; Cassella-med, Ital.†.
Tolpropamine hydrochloride (p.419·3).
Skin irritation.

Pragmarel *UPSA, Fr.†.*
Trazodone hydrochloride (p.308·3).
Depression.

Pragmatar
Bioglan, Irl.; Bioglan, UK.
Coal tar (p.1092·3); sulphur (p.1091·2); salicylic acid (p.1090·2).
Skin disorders.

Prairie Gold *Larkhall Laboratories, UK.*
Vitamin E (p.1369·1).

Pralifan *Inibsa, Spain.*
Mitozantrone hydrochloride (p.553·3).
Malignant neoplasms.

Pramace
Astra, Irl.†; Hassle, Swed.
Ramipril (p.941·1).
Heart failure; hypertension.

PrameGel
GenDerm, Canad.; GenDerm, USA.
Pramoxine hydrochloride (p.1298·2); menthol (p.1600·2).
Pruritus.

Pramet FA *Ross, USA†.*
Multivitamin and mineral preparation with iron and folic acid.

Pramilet FA *Ross, USA.*
Multivitamin and mineral preparation with iron and folic acid.

Pramin *Alphapharm, Austral.*
Metoclopramide hydrochloride (p.1200·3).

Pramino *Janssen-Cilag, Ger.*
Norgestimate (p.1453·3); ethinyloestradiol (p.1445·1).
Triphasic oral contraceptive.

Pramistar *FIRMA, Ital.*
Pramiracetam sulphate (p.1621·2).
Anxiety disorders; mental function impairment.

Pramosone *Ferndale, USA.*
Hydrocortisone acetate (p.1043·3); pramoxine (p.1298·2).

Pramox HC *Dermtek, Canad.*
Hydrocortisone acetate (p.1043·3); pramoxine hydrochloride (p.1298·2).
Skin disorders.

Prandase *Bayer, Canad.*
Acarbose (p.317·2).
Diabetes mellitus.

Prandin *Novo Nordisk, USA.*
Repaglinide (p.331·1).
Diabetes mellitus.

Prandin E_2 *Pharmacia Upjohn, S.Afr.*
Dinoprostone (p.1414·3).
Labour induction.

Prandiol *Theraplix, Fr.†.*
Dipyridamole (p.857·1).
Coronary disorders.

Prandium *Schiapparelli Searle, Ital.†.*
Bromelains (p.1555·1); prozapine hydrochloride (p.1622·3); dimethicone (p.1213·1); pancreatin (p.1612·1); dehydrocholic acid (p.1570·2).
Digestive system disorders.

Pranolol *Alpharma, Norw.*
Propranolol hydrochloride (p.937·1).
Angina pectoris; arrhythmias; hypertension; hyperthyroidism; migraine; myocardial infarction; tremor.

Pranox *Asta Medica, Belg.*
Pranoprofen (p.81·2).
Eye inflammation.

Pranoxen *Propan, S.Afr.*
Naproxen (p.61·2).
Dysmenorrhoea; gout; musculoskeletal and joint disorders.

Pranoxen Continus *Napp, UK†.*
Naproxen (p.61·2).
Inflammation; pain.

Prantal
Schering-Plough, Austral.; Schering-Plough, Ital.
Diphemanil methylsulphate (p.460·3).
Hyperhidrosis.

Pranzo *Vinas, Spain.*
Cyproheptadine hydrochloride (p.407·2); amino acids.
Tonic.

Prareduct *Alfarma, Spain.*
Pravastatin sodium (p.1277·1).
Hypercholesterolaemia; myocardial infarction.

Prasig *Sigma, Austral.*
Prazosin hydrochloride (p.932·3).
Benign prostatic hyperplasia; heart failure; hypertension; Raynaud's syndrome.

Prasterol *Malesci, Ital.*
Pravastatin sodium (p.1277·1).
Arteriosclerosis; cardiovascular disorders; hypercholesterolaemia.

Praticef *Caber, Ital.*
Cefonicid sodium (p.167·2).
Lignocaine hydrochloride (p.1293·2) is included in this preparation to alleviate the pain of injection.
Bacterial infections.

Pratsiol *Lagamed, S.Afr.*
Prazosin hydrochloride (p.932·3).
Hypertension.

Prava
Note. This name is used for preparations of different composition.
Bristol-Myers Squibb, S.Afr.
Pravastatin sodium (p.1277·1).
Hypercholesterolaemia.

Bristol-Myers Squibb, Switz.
Lomustine (p.544·1).
Malignant neoplasms.

Pravachol
Bristol-Myers Squibb, Aust.; Bristol-Myers Squibb, Austral.; Squibb, Canad.; Bristol-Myers Squibb, Norw.; Bristol-Myers Squibb, Swed.; Bristol-Myers Squibb, USA.
Pravastatin sodium (p.1277·1).
Hypercholesterolaemia.

Pravaselect *Menarini, Ital.*
Pravastatin sodium (p.1277·1).
Arteriosclerosis; cardiovascular disorders; hypercholesterolaemia.

Pravasin *Bristol-Myers Squibb, Ger.*
Pravastatin sodium (p.1277·1).
Hypercholesterolaemia.

Pravasine *Bristol-Myers Squibb, Belg.*
Pravastatin sodium (p.1277·1).
Hypercholesterolaemia.

Pravidel
Sandoz, Ger.; Novartis, Swed.
Bromocriptine mesylate (p.1132·2).
Acromegaly; amenorrhoea; breast disorders; galactorrhoea; hyperprolactinaemia; infertility; lactation inhibition; ovulation disorders; parkinsonism; premenstrual syndrome.

Prax *Ferndale, USA.*
Pramoxine hydrochloride (p.1298·2).
Local anaesthesia.

Praxadium *Theraplix, Fr.†.*
Nordazepam (p.682·3).
Alcohol withdrawal syndrome; anxiety.

Praxenol *Biotekfarma, Ital.†.*
Naproxen aminobutanol (p.62·1).
Musculoskeletal and joint disorders.

Praxilene
Lipha, Belg.; Lipha Sante, Fr.; Lipha, Irl.; Formenti, Ital.; Faes, Spain; Lipha, Switz.; Lipha, UK.
Naftidrofuryl oxalate (p.914·2).
Cerebral and peripheral vascular disorders.

Praxinor *Lipha Sante, Fr.*
Theodrenaline hydrochloride (p.1636·2); cafedrine hydrochloride (p.835·3).
Hypotension.

Praxiten
Wyeth Lederle, Aust.; Wyeth, Ger.
Oxazepam (p.683·2).
Anxiety disorders; sleep disorders.

Prazene *Parke, Davis, Ital.*
Prazepam (p.687·2).
Anxiety disorders; psychoneurotic disorders.

Prazine
Wyeth Lederle, Belg.; Wyeth, Switz.
Promazine embonate (p.689·1) or promazine hydrochloride (p.689·1).
Behaviour disorders in children; hiccups; nausea; psychoses; sedative; tetany; vomiting.

Prazinil *Pierre Fabre, Fr.*
Carpipramine hydrochloride (p.645·2).
Anxiety; psychoses.

Pre Nutrison *Nutricia, Ital.*
Preparation for enteral nutrition.

Pre-Attain *Sherwood, USA.*
Lactose-free preparation for enteral nutrition.

Prebon *Alba, USA.*
Multivitamin and mineral preparation.

Precef *Bristol-Myers Squibb, Belg.*
Ceforanide (p.168·2).
Bacterial infections.

Precision
Wander, Ital.; Wander, S.Afr.†; Sandoz Nutrition, USA.
A range of preparations for enteral nutrition.

Precitene MCT 50 *Wander Health Care, Switz.*
Preparation for enteral nutrition.

Preconativ
Kabi Pharmacia, Ger.†; Pierrel, Ital.†; Kabi, Swed.†.
A factor IX preparation (p.721·3).
Haemorrhagic disorders.

Preconceive *Lane, UK.*
Folic acid (p.1340·3).
Prevention of neural tube defects in pregnancy.

Precopen *Fides, Spain.*
Amoxycillin trihydrate (p.151·3).
Bacterial infections.

Precopen Mucolitico *Fides, Spain.*
Amoxycillin trihydrate (p.151·3); bromhexine hydrochloride (p.1055·3).
Respiratory-tract infections.

Precortalon aquosum *Organon, Swed.*
Prednisolone sodium succinate (p.1048·2).
Corticosteroid.

Precortisyl
Roussel, Irl.†; Hoechst Marion Roussel, UK.
Prednisolone (p.1048·1).
Corticosteroid.

Precosa *Astra, Swed.*
Saccharomyces boulardii (p.1594·1).
Antibiotic-associated colitis.

Precosol *Wolfs, Belg.*
Macrogol 4000 (p.1598·2); electrolytes (p.1147·1).
Bowel evacuation.

Prectal *Artesan, Ger.; Cassella-med, Ger.*
Prednisolone acetate (p.1048·1).
Bronchitis; hypersensitivity reactions; laryngotracheal stenosis.

Precurgen *Knoll, Spain.*
Cytosine inosinate.
Liver disorders.

Precurson *SPA, Ital.†.*
Sodium phosphogluconate.
Hypercholesterolaemias.

Precyclan *Leo, Fr.*
Meprobamate (p.678·1); bendrofluazide (p.827·3); medroxyprogesterone acetate (p.1448·3).
Formerly contained meprobamate, bendrofluazide, and flumedroxone acetate.
Premenstrual syndrome.

Pred *Alcon, USA.*
Prednisolone acetate (p.1048·1).
Inflammatory eye disorders.

Pred Forte
Allergan, Belg.; Allergan, Canad.; Allergan, Irl.; Allergan, Neth.†; Allergan, S.Afr.†; Allergan, Switz.; Allergan, UK.
Prednisolone acetate (p.1048·1).
Inflammatory eye disorders.

Pred G
Allergan, S.Afr.; Allergan, Switz.; Allergan, USA.
Prednisolone acetate (p.1048·1); gentamicin sulphate (p.212·1).
Infected eye disorders.

Pred Mild
Allergan, Canad.; Allergan, Irl.; Allergan, S.Afr.; Allergan, Switz.
Prednisolone acetate (p.1048·1).
Corneal burns; inflammatory or allergic eye disorders.

Predaject *Mayrand, USA†.*
Prednisolone acetate (p.1048·1).
Corticosteroid.

Predalon *Organon, Ger.*
Chorionic gonadotrophin (p.1243·1).
Cryptorchidism; delayed puberty; stimulation of gonadal function.

Predalone *Forest Laboratories, USA.*
Prednisolone acetate (p.1048·1).
Corticosteroid.

Predate *Legere, USA†.*
Prednisolone acetate (p.1048·1), prednisolone sodium phosphate (p.1048·1), or prednisolone tebutate (p.1048·2).
Corticosteroid.

Pred-Clysma
Leiras, Norw.; Leiras, Swed.
Prednisolone sodium phosphate (p.1048·1).
Proctitis; ulcerative colitis.

Predcor *Hauck, USA.*
Prednisolone acetate (p.1048·1).
Corticosteroid.

Predeltilone *Noristan, S.Afr.†.*
Prednisolone (p.1048·1).
Corticosteroid.

Predeltin *Noristan, S.Afr.†.*
Prednisone (p.1049·2).
Corticosteroid.

Predenema
Pharmax, Irl.; Pharmax, UK.
Prednisolone sodium metasulphobenzoate (p.1048·1).
Ulcerative colitis.

Predfoam
Pharmax, Irl.; Pharmax, UK.
Prednisolone sodium metasulphobenzoate (p.1048·1).
Proctitis; ulcerative colitis.

Predictor
British Pharmaceuticals, Austral.; Organon, Austral.; Chefaro Ardeval, Fr.; Angelini, Ital.; Chefaro, UK.
Pregnancy test (p.1621·2).

Predmix *Royal Childrens Hospital, Austral.*
Prednisolone sodium phosphate (p.1048·1).
Corticosteroid.

Predmycin *Allergan, Belg.*
Prednisolone acetate (p.1048·1); polymyxin B sulphate (p.239·1); neomycin sulphate (p.229·2).
Eye disorders.

Predmycin-P Liquifilm *Allergan, Neth.†.*
Prednisolone acetate (p.1048·1); polymyxin B sulphate (p.239·1); neomycin sulphate (p.229·2).
Eye infections.

Prednabene *Merckle, Ger.*
Prednisolone sodium phosphate (p.1048·1).
Parenteral corticosteroid.

Prednefrin *Allergan, Austral.*
Prednisolone acetate (p.1048·1); phenylephrine hydrochloride (p.1066·2).
Eye inflammation.

Prednesol
Glaxo Wellcome, Irl.; Glaxo, UK.
Prednisolone sodium phosphate (p.1048·1).
Corticosteroid.

Predni *Lichtenstein, Ger.*
Prednisolone acetate (p.1048·1).
Corticosteroid.

Predni aquos. in der Ophtiole *Mann, Ger.†.*
Prednisolone sodium phosphate (p.1048·1); neomycin sulphate (p.229·2).
Inflammatory disorders and bacterial infections of the eye.

Predni Azuleno *Lacer, Spain.*
Chloramphenicol (p.182·1); guaiazulene (p.1586·3); prednisolone (p.1048·1).
Infected skin disorders.

Prednicen-M *Schwarz, USA†.*
Prednisone (p.1049·2).
Corticosteroid.

Predni-Coelin *Pfleger, Ger.†.*
Tablets: Prednisolone (p.1048·1).
Oral corticosteroid.

Prednicort
Note. This name is used for preparations of different composition.
Continental Pharma, Belg.
Prednisone (p.1049·2).
Corticosteroid.

Cortec, Swed.†.
Prednisolone (p.1048·1).
Corticosteroid.

Prednicortelone *Continental Pharma, Belg.*
Prednisolone (p.1048·1).
Corticosteroid.

Predni-F-Tablinen *Sanorania, Ger.*
Dexamethasone (p.1037·1).
Oral corticosteroid.

Prednigamma *IBP, Ital.†.*
Bacitracin (p.157·3); neomycin (p.229·2); prednisolone (p.1048·1).
Dermatitis; eczema.

Predni-H *Sanorania, Ger.*
Prednisolone (p.1048·1) or prednisolone acetate (p.1048·1).
Corticosteroid.

Predni-Helvacort *Helvepharm, Switz.*
Prednisolone (p.1048·1).
Corticosteroid.

Prednihexal
Hexal, Aust.; Hexal, Ger.
Prednisolone (p.1048·1) or prednisolone acetate (p.1048·1).
Corticosteroid.

Prednilen *Lenza, Ital.†.*
Methylprednisolone (p.1046·1).
Corticosteroid.

Predniment *Ferring, Ger.†.*
Prednisone (p.1049·2).
Proctitis; ulcerative colitis.

Predni-M-Tablinen *Sanorania, Ger.*
Methylprednisolone (p.1046·1).
Oral corticosteroid.

Predni-POS *Ursapharm, Ger.*
Prednisolone acetate (p.1048·1).
Eye disorders.

Prednis Neomic *Cusi, Spain.*
Neomycin sulphate (p.229·2); prednisone (p.1049·2).
Infected eye disorders.

Prednisol *Pasadena, USA.*
Prednisolone tebutate (p.1048·2).
Corticosteroid.

Prednisolut *Jenapharm, Ger.*
Prednisolone hemisuccinate (p.1048·1).
Corticosteroid.

Predni-Tablinen *Sanorania, Ger.*
Prednisone (p.1049·2).
Oral corticosteroid.

Prednitop
Albert-Roussel, Aust.; Knoll, Switz.
Prednicarbate (p.1047·3).
Inflammatory skin disorders.

Prednitracin
Ciba Vision, Ger.; Ciba Vision, Switz.
Prednisolone acetate (p.1048·1); neomycin sulphate (p.229·2); bacitracin (p.157·3).
Infected eye disorders.

Predopa *Kyowa, Jpn.*
Dopamine hydrochloride (p.861·1).
Shock.

Predsol
Sigma, Austral.; Evans Medical, Irl.; Glaxo Wellcome, S.Afr.; Medeva, UK.
Prednisolone sodium phosphate (p.1048·1).
Crohn's disease; inflammatory disorders of the ear or eye; proctitis; ulcerative colitis.

Predsol-N *Medeva, UK.*
Prednisolone sodium phosphate (p.1048·1); neomycin sulphate (p.229·2).
Inflammatory disorders of the ear or eye with bacterial infection.

Prefagyl *Oberlin, Fr.*
Magnesium chloride (p.1157·2); sodium bicarbonate (p.1153·2); anhydrous sodium sulphate (p.1213·3); dibasic sodium phosphate (p.1159·3).
Formerly contained magnesium chloride, sodium bicarbonate, sodium sulphate, dibasic sodium phosphate, and sodium bromide.
Gastro-intestinal disorders.

Prefakehl *Sanum-Kehlbeck, Ger.†.*
Homoeopathic preparation.

Prefamone
Asta Medica, Belg.; Dexo, Fr.; Dexo, Switz.
Diethylpropion hydrochloride (p.1479·3).
Obesity.

Preferid
Yamanouchi, Belg.; Yamanouchi, Irl.; Yamanouchi, Ital.; Yamanouchi, Neth.; Yamanouchi, Norw.; Yamanouchi, Swed.†; Yamanouchi, Switz.; Brocades, UK†.
Budesonide (p.1034·3).
Skin disorders.

Prefil *Norgine, UK.*
Sterculia (p.1214·1).
Obesity.

Prefin *Miquel Otsuka, Spain.*
Buprenorphine hydrochloride (p.22·2).
Pain.

Prefine *Pierre Fabre, Fr.*
Sterculia (p.1214·1).
Obesity.

Preflex *Alcon, Austral.†.*
Cleaning solution for soft contact lenses.

Preflex Daily Cleaner *Alcon, USA.*
Cleansing solution for soft contact lenses.

Prefolic *Knoll, Ital.*
Calcium mefolinate (p.1342·3).
Antidote to folic acid antagonists; folate deficiency; reduction of aminopterin and methotrexate toxicity.

Prefrin
Allergan, Austral.; Allergan, Irl.†; Allergan, S.Afr.
Phenylephrine hydrochloride (p.1066·2).
Eye irritation.

Prefrin A
Allergan, Aust.; Allergan, Canad.; Allergan, Irl.†; Allergan, S.Afr.†.
Mepyramine maleate (p.414·1); phenylephrine hydrochloride (p.1066·2).
Eye inflammation; eye irritation.

Prefrin Liquifilm
Allergan, Aust.; Allergan, Canad.; Allergan, USA.
Phenylephrine hydrochloride (p.1066·2).
Eye irritation.

Prefrin Z *Allergan, Austral.*
Zinc sulphate (p.1373·2); phenylephrine hydrochloride (p.1066·2).
Eye irritation.

Prefrinal med mepyramin *Allergan, Swed.†.*
Mepyramine maleate (p.414·1); phenylephrine hydrochloride (p.1066·2).
Allergic conjunctivitis.

Pregaday *Medeva, UK.*
Ferrous fumarate (p.1339·3); folic acid (p.1340·3).
Prophylaxis of iron and folic acid deficiency in pregnancy.

Pregamal *Glaxo Wellcome, S.Afr.*
Folic acid (p.1340·3); ferrous fumarate (p.1339·3).
Anaemias.

Pregcolor
Organon, Austral.†; Donmed, S.Afr.
Pregnancy test (p.1621·2).

Pregestimil
Mead Johnson, Austral.; Mead Johnson, Fr.; Bristol-Myers Squibb, Irl.; Mead Johnson, Ital.; Bristol-Myers Squibb, Norw.†; Mead Johnson Nutritionals, UK; Mead Johnson Nutritionals, USA.
Food for special diets.
Cow's milk intolerance; galactokinase deficiency; galactosaemia; impaired fat absorption; lactose or sucrose and protein intolerance; soya intolerance.

Preglandin *Ono, Jpn.*
Gemeprost (p.1418·3).
Termination of pregnancy.

Pregnacare *Vitabiotics, UK.*
Multivitamin and mineral preparation.

Pregna-Cert *Merlin, UK.*
Pregnancy test (p.1621·2).

Pregna-Sure HCG *Merlin, UK.*
Pregnancy test (p.1621·2).

Pregnavit *Merckle, Aust.*
Multivitamin and iron preparation.

Pregnavit F *Merckle, Ger.*
Multivitamin preparation.

Pregnavite Forte F
Bencard, Irl.†; Goldshield, UK.
Dried ferrous sulphate (p.1340·2); folic acid (p.1340·3); vitamins; calcium phosphate.
Prophylaxis of neural tube defects in pregnancy.

Pregnazon *Pharmadass, UK.*
Multivitamin, mineral, and trace element preparation.

Pregnesin *Serono, Ger.*
Chorionic gonadotrophin (p.1243·1).
Cryptorchidism; delayed puberty in males; infertility in females and males.

Pregnifer *Weifa, Norw.*
Ferrous sulphate (p.1340·2); folic acid (p.1340·3).
Iron and folic acid supplement during pregnancy and lactation.

Pregnon *Nourypharma, Neth.†.*
22 Tablets, lynoestrenol (p.1448·2); ethinyloestradiol (p.1445·1); 6 tablets, inert.
Combined oral contraceptive.

Pregnon L *Nourypharma, Ger.*
Lynoestrenol (p.1448·2); ethinyloestradiol (p.1445·1).
Combined oral contraceptive.

Pregnosis
Key, Austral.; Roche, Canad.†; Roche, USA.
Pregnancy test (p.1621·2).

Pregnospia Duoclon *Organon Teknika, UK.*
Pregnancy test (p.1621·2).

Pregnosticon 'All In' *Organon Teknika, UK†.*
Pregnancy test (p.1621·2).

Pregnosticon Planotest *Organon Teknika, UK†.*
Pregnancy test (p.1621·2).

Pregnyl
Organon, Aust.; Organon, Austral.; Organon, Belg.; Organon, Canad.; Organon, Irl.; Ravasini, Ital.†; Organon, Neth.; Organon, Norw.; Donmed, S.Afr.; Organon, Spain; Organon, Swed.; Organon, Switz.; Organon, UK; Organon, USA.
Chorionic gonadotrophin (p.1243·1).
Cryptorchidism; delayed puberty; hypogonadotrophic hypogonadism; male and female infertility; uterine haemorrhage.

Pregomin *Milupa, Switz.*
Infant feed.
Carbohydrate malabsorption syndromes; cow's-milk-protein intolerance; digestive system disorders; soya-milk-protein intolerance.

Pregomine *Milupa, Fr.*
Nutritional supplement.
Gastro-intestinal disorders.

Pregstik
Donmed, S.Afr.; Organon, UK†.
Pregnancy test (p.1621·2).

Pre-H-Cal *Williams, USA†.*
Multivitamin and mineral preparation with iron and folic acid.

Prehist *Marnel, USA.*
Phenylephrine hydrochloride (p.1066·2); chlorpheniramine maleate (p.405·1).
Upper respiratory-tract symptoms.

Prehist D *Marnel, USA.*
Phenylephrine hydrochloride (p.1066·2); chlorpheniramine maleate (p.405·1); hyoscine methonitrate (p.463·1).
Upper respiratory-tract symptoms.

Prejomin
Milupa, Irl.; Milupa, UK.
Gluten-free preparation for enteral nutrition.
Galactokinase deficiency; galactosaemia; protein intolerance; sucrose, fructose, or lactose intolerance.

Prelafel *Akromed, S.Afr.*
Multivitamin and mineral preparation.

Prelief *AkPharma, USA.*
Calcium glycerophosphate (p.1155·2).
Dyspepsia.

Prelis *Ciba, Ger.*
Metoprolol tartrate (p.907·3).
Cardiac disorders; hypertension; migraine.

Prelis comp *Ciba, Ger.*
Metoprolol tartrate (p.907·3); chlorthalidone (p.839·3).
Hypertension.

Prelloran *Zyma, Switz.*
A heparinoid (p.882·3); glycol salicylate (p.43·1).
Haematomas; musculoskeletal pain and inflammation; peripheral vascular disorders; phlebitis.

Prelone
Vesta, S.Afr.; Muro, USA.
Prednisolone (p.1048·1).
Corticosteroid.

Prelu-2 *Roxane, USA.*
Phendimetrazine tartrate (p.1484·2).
Obesity.

Preludin Endurets *Boehringer Ingelheim, USA†.*
Phenmetrazine hydrochloride (p.1484·3).
Obesity.

Premandol *Spirig, Switz.*
Prednisolone acetate (p.1048·1); almond oil (p.1546·2); zinc oxide (p.1096·2).
Skin disorders.

Premarin
Wyeth Lederle, Aust.; Wyeth, Austral.; Wyeth Lederle, Belg.; Wyeth-Ayerst, Canad.; Wyeth, Fr.; Wyeth, Irl.; Wyeth, Ital.; Wyeth, Neth.; Wyeth, S.Afr.; Wyeth, Spain; Wyeth, Switz.; Wyeth, UK; Wyeth-Ayerst, USA.
Conjugated oestrogens (p.1457·3).
Acne; amenorrhoea; breast cancer; dysfunctional uterine haemorrhage; female infertility; menopausal disorders; oestrogen deficiency; osteoporosis; prostatic cancer.

Premarin compositum *Wyeth Lederle, Aust.*
16 Tablets, conjugated oestrogens (p.1457·3); 12 tablets, conjugated oestrogens; medrogestone (p.1448·2).
Oestrogen deficiency.

Premarin with Methyltestosterone *Wyeth-Ayerst, USA.*
Conjugated oestrogens (p.1457·3); methyltestosterone (p.1450·3).
Menopausal disorders; postpartum breast engorgement.

Premarin Plus
Kwizda, Aust.†; Wyeth, Neth.; Wyeth, Switz.
28 Tablets, conjugated oestrogens (p.1457·3); 12 tablets, medrogestone (p.1448·2).
Menopausal disorders; oestrogen deficiency; osteoporosis.

Premarina *Wyeth Lederle, Swed.*
Conjugated oestrogens (p.1457·3).
Hypogenitalism; menopausal disorders; osteoporosis.

Premarin-MPA *Wyeth Lederle, Aust.*
Conjugated oestrogens (p.1457·3); medroxyprogesterone acetate (p.1448·3).
Oestrogen deficiency.

Premella
Wyeth Lederle, Aust.; Wyeth, Switz.
Conjugated oestrogens (p.1457·3); medroxyprogesterone acetate (p.1448·3).
Menopausal disorders; osteoporosis.

Premelle
Wyeth, Neth.; Wyeth Lederle, Swed.
Conjugated oestrogens (p.1457·3); medroxyprogesterone acetate (p.1448·3).
Atrophic urethritis; atrophic vaginitis; menopausal disorders; osteoporosis.

Premelle Cycle *Wyeth, Neth.*
14 Tablets, conjugated oestrogens (p.1457·3); 14 tablets, conjugated oestrogens; medroxyprogesterone acetate (p.1448·3).
Atrophic urethritis; atrophic vaginitis; menopausal disorders; osteoporosis.

Premelle S *Wyeth, Ital.*
14 Tablets, conjugated oestrogens (p.1457·3); 14 tablets, conjugated oestrogens; medroxyprogesterone acetate (p.1448·3).
Menopausal disorders; osteoporosis.

Premence *Vitabiotics, UK.*
Multivitamin and mineral preparation.

Prementaid *Potter's, UK.*
Vervain; motherwort (p.1604·2); pulsatilla (p.1623·3); bearberry (p.1552·2); valerian (p.1643·1).
Premenstrual fluid retention.

Premidan Adult *Monot, Fr.†.*
Pholcodine (p.1068·1); belladonna (p.457·1); aconite (p.1542·2); cherry laurel; opium (p.70·3); senega (p.1069·3); ipecacuanha (p.1062·2).
Upper respiratory-tract disorders.

Premidan Infant *Monot, Fr.†.*
Pholcodine (p.1068·1); aconite (p.1542·2); drosera (p.1574·1); ipecacuanha (p.1062·2).
Respiratory-tract disorders.

Premique Cycle
Wyeth, Irl.; Wyeth, UK.
Conjugated oestrogens (p.1457·3); medroxyprogesterone acetate (p.1448·3).
Menopausal disorders.

Premium *SIT, Ital.†.*
Hesperidin methyl chalcone (p.1580·2); troxerutin (p.1580·2); myrtillus (p.1606·1); aescin (p.1543·3); calcium ascorbate (p.1365·2).
Altered capillary permeability; capillary fragility.

Premium Prenatal Quest, Canad.
Multivitamin and mineral preparation.

Premiums Newton, UK†.
Magnesium trisilicate (p.1199·1); aluminium hydroxide (p.1177·3); magnesium carbonate (p.1198·1); creta (p.1182·1); peppermint oil (p.1208·1).
Dyspepsia.

Premofil M ZLB, Switz.
A factor VIII preparation (p.720·3).
Haemorrhagic disorders.

Prempac Sekvens Wyeth Lederle, Swed.
28 tablets, conjugated oestrogens (p.1457·3); 14 tablets, medroxyprogesterone acetate (p.1448·3).
Oestrogen deficiency; osteoporosis.

Prempak Wyeth, Ital.
Conjugated oestrogens (p.1457·3).
Atrophic urethritis; menopausal disorders; oestrogen deficiency; osteoporosis; vaginitis.

Prempak N Wyeth, S.Afr.
21 Tablets, conjugated oestrogens (p.1457·3); 10 tablets, medrogestone (p.1448·2).
Menopausal disorders; osteoporosis.

Prempak-C
Wyeth, Irl.; Wyeth, Neth.; Wyeth, UK.
28 Tablets, conjugated oestrogens (p.1457·3); 12 tablets, norgestrel (p.1454·1).
Menopausal disorders; osteoporosis.

Premphase Wyeth-Ayerst, USA.
Maroon tablets, conjugated oestrogens (p.1457·3); purple tablets, medroxyprogesterone acetate (p.1448·3).
Menopausal disorders.

Premplus Wyeth Lederle, Belg.
White tablets, medrogestone (p.1448·2); red tablets, conjugated oestrogens (p.1457·3).
Oestrogen deficiency.

Prempro Wyeth-Ayerst, USA.
Conjugated oestrogens (p.1457·3); medroxyprogesterone acetate (p.1448·3).
Menopausal disorders.

Premsyn PMS Chattem, USA.
Paracetamol (p.72·2); pamabrom (p.927·1); mepyramine maleate (p.414·1).
Pain.

Premus Ciba Vision, Aust.
Storage and disinfecting solution for contact lenses.

Prenacid SIFI, Ital.
Desonide sodium phosphate (p.1036·3).
Inflammatory eye disorders.

Prenalex Servier, Ger.
Tertatolol hydrochloride (p.952·2).
Hypertension.

Pre-Nan Nestle, Austral.
Feed for low birth-weight infants.

Prenatal
Bio-Sante, Canad.; Jamieson, Canad.; Quest, Canad.; Stanley, Canad.; Lederle, Ger.†; Cyanamid, Ital.†.
Multivitamin and mineral preparation.

Prenatal with Folic Acid Geneva, USA.
Multivitamin and mineral preparation with iron and folic acid.

Prenatal Maternal Ethex, USA.
Multivitamin and mineral preparation with calcium and iron.

Prenatal MR 90 Ethex, USA.
Multivitamin and mineral preparation.

Prenatal Nutrients Solgar, UK.
Multivitamin and mineral preparation.

Prenatal One Eon, USA†.
Multivitamin and mineral preparation with iron and folic acid.

Prenatal Plus Rugby, USA; Goldline, USA.
Multivitamin and mineral preparation with calcium and iron.

Prenatal Plus-Improved Rugby, USA.
Multivitamin and mineral preparation with iron and folic acid.

Prenatal Z Ethex, USA.
Multivitamin and mineral preparation with calcium and iron.

Prenatal-S Goldline, USA.
Multivitamin and mineral preparation with iron and folic acid.

Prenate Sanofi Winthrop, USA.
Multivitamin and mineral preparation with iron and folic acid.

Prenavite
Roberts, Canad.; Rugby, USA.
Multivitamin and mineral preparation.
Dietary supplement during pregnancy and lactation.

Prenoxan au phenobarbital Schering-Plough, Fr.
Phenobarbitone (p.350·2); aspirin (p.16·1).
Fever; pain.

Prent
Gepepharm, Ger.; Bayer, Ital.; Bayer, Neth.†; Bayer, Switz.†.
Acebutolol hydrochloride (p.809·3).
Angina pectoris; arrhythmias; hypertension.

Prepacol
Salus, Aust.; Codali, Belg.; Guerbet, Fr.; Guerbet, Ger.
Combination pack: Tablets, bisacodyl (p.1179·3); oral solution, dibasic sodium phosphate (p.1159·3); monobasic sodium phosphate (p.1159·3).
Bowel evacuation.

Prepadine Berk, UK.
Dothiepin hydrochloride (p.283·1).
Depression.

Pre-Par
Kali, Aust.†; Solvay, Belg.; Solvay, Fr.; Solvay, Ger.; Solvay, Ital.; Solvay, Neth.; Duphar, Spain.
Ritodrine hydrochloride (p.1625·3).
Premature labour; prevention of fetal distress; relaxation of the uterus.

Preparacion H Wyeth, Spain.
Yeast extract (p.1373·1); shark-liver oil.
Haemorrhoids.

Preparation H
Note. This name is used for preparations of different composition.
Whitehall, Austral.; Whitehall-Robins, Canad.; Whitehall, Irl.; Whitehall, UK; Whitehall, USA.
Live yeast cell derivative (p.1373·1); shark-liver oil.
Haemorrhoids.

Whitehall, Fr.
Rectal cream: Yeast (p.1373·1); halibut-liver oil (p.1345·3).
Suppositories: Butyl aminobenzoate (p.1289·1); yeast (p.1373·1); esculoside (p.1543·3); halibut-liver oil (p.1345·3).
Haemorrhoids.

Preparation H Cleansing Pads Whitehall-Robins, Canad.
Hamamelis (p.1587·1).
Anal and vaginal hygiene; anal irritation; haemorrhoids.

Preparation H Hydrocortisone Whitehall, USA.
Hydrocortisone (p.1043·3).
Anal pruritus.

Preparation H Sperti Whitehall, Belg.
Dried yeast (p.1373·1).
Haemorrhoids.

Preparation H Veinotonic Whitehall, Fr.
Diosmin (p.1580·1).
Haemorrhoids.

Preparazione Antiemorroidaria Giuliani, Ital.
Hydrocortisone acetate (p.1043·3); benzocaine (p.1286·2).
Haemorrhoids.

Preparazione H Whitehall, Ital.
Live yeast cell extract (p.1373·1).
Haemorrhoids.

Prepcat Lafayette, USA.
Barium sulphate (p.1003·1).
Contrast medium for gastro-intestinal radiography.

Pre-Pen
Rivex, Canad.; Biolac, Swed.; Bayer, USA.
Penicilloyl-polylysine (p.1616·2).
Diagnosis of penicillin hypersensitivity.

Prepidil
Pharmacia Upjohn, Aust.; Pharmacia Upjohn, Belg.; Pharmacia Upjohn, Canad.; Pharmacia Upjohn, Fr.; Pharmacia Upjohn, Ger.; Pharmacia Upjohn, Irl.; Pharmacia Upjohn, Ital.; Pharmacia Upjohn, Neth.; Pharmacia Upjohn, S.Afr.; Upjohn, Spain; Pharmacia Upjohn, Switz.; Upjohn, UK; Upjohn, USA.
Dinoprostone (p.1414·3).
Labour induction.

Prepulsid
Janssen-Cilag, Aust.; Janssen-Cilag, Austral.; Janssen-Cilag, Belg.; Janssen-Ortho, Canad.; Janssen-Cilag, Fr.; Janssen-Cilag, Irl.; Janssen-Cilag, Ital.; Janssen-Cilag, Neth.; Janssen-Cilag, Norw.; Janssen-Cilag, S.Afr.; Janssen-Cilag, Spain; Janssen-Cilag, Swed.; Janssen-Cilag, Switz.; Janssen-Cilag, UK.
Cisapride (p.1187·1).
Dyspepsia; gastro-oesophageal reflux; impaired gastric motility.

Prepurex
Wellcome, Irl.†; Glaxo Wellcome, S.Afr.†; Wellcome Diagnostics, UK.
Pregnancy test (p.1621·2).

Pres Boehringer Ingelheim, Ger.
Enalapril maleate (p.863·2).
Heart failure; hypertension.

Pres iv Boehringer Ingelheim, Ger.
Enalaprilat (p.863·2).
Heart failure; hypertension.

Pres plus Boehringer Ingelheim, Ger.
Enalapril maleate (p.863·2); hydrochlorothiazide (p.885·2).
Hypertension.

Presalin Hauck, USA.
Aspirin (p.16·1); paracetamol (p.72·2); salicylamide (p.82·3); aluminium hydroxide (p.1177·3).
Pain.

Prescaina Llorens, Spain.
Oxybuprocaine hydrochloride (p.1298·1).
Local anaesthesia.

Prescal
Ciba-Geigy, Irl.; Ciba, UK.
Isradipine (p.894·2).
Angina pectoris; hypertension.

Prescription Strength Desenex Ciba, USA.
Cream: Clotrimazole (p.376·3).
Topical spray: Miconazole nitrate (p.384·3).
Fungal infections.

Presept
Ethicon, Ital.; Johnson & Johnson Medical, UK.
Sodium dichloroisocyanurate (p.1124·3).
Instrument and surface disinfection.

Preservex UCB, UK.
Aceclofenac (p.12·1).
Musculoskeletal and joint disorders.

Presinol
Bayer, Aust.; Bayer, Belg.†; Bayer, Ger.; Bayropharm, Ital.†.
Methyldopa (p.904·2).
Hypertension.

Preslow Astra, Spain.
Felodipine (p.867·3).
Angina pectoris; hypertension.

Presolol Alphapharm, Austral.
Labetalol hydrochloride (p.896·1).
Hypertension.

Presomen
Note. This name is used for preparations of different composition.
Kali-Chemie, Ger.†.
Conjugated oestrogens (p.1457·3).
Uterine bleeding.

Solvay, Ger.
Extract from pregnant mare's urine.
Menopausal disorders.

Presomen compositum Kali-Chemie, Ger.
Combination pack: 10 Tablets, extract from pregnant mare's urine; 11 tablets, medrogestone (p.1448·2); extract from pregnant mare's urine.
Menopausal disorders; menstrual disorders.

Presomen spezial Kali-Chemie, Ger.†.
Conjugated oestrogens (p.1457·3).
Menopausal disorders.

Pressalolo Locatelli, Ital.
Labetalol hydrochloride (p.896·1).
Hypertension.

Pressalolo Diuretico Locatelli, Ital.
Labetalol hydrochloride (p.896·1); chlorthalidone (p.839·3).
Hypertension.

Pressamina Teofarma, Ital.
Dimetofrine hydrochloride (p.857·1).
Hypotension.

Pressanol Propan-Vernleigh, S.Afr.†.
Propranolol hydrochloride (p.937·1).
Cardiovascular disorders.

Presselin 214 Presselin, Ger.†.
Cinnamon (p.1564·2); frangula bark (p.1193·2); clove (p.1565·2); chamomile (p.1561·2); lavender (p.1594·3); mace; sage (p.1627·1); star anise; cardamom (p.1560·1); caraway (p.1559·3); coriander (p.1567·3); fennel (p.1579·1); juniper (p.1592·2); absinthium (p.1541·1); achillea (p.1542·2); angelica; gentian (p.1583·3); liquorice (p.1197·1); ginger (p.1193·2); calamus (p.1556·1); glechoma hederaceum.
Gastro-intestinal disorders.

Presselin BN Nieren-Blasen Presselin, Ger.
Homoeopathic preparation.

Presselin Chol Presselin, Ger.†.
Homoeopathic preparation.

Presselin Cpl 87 N Presselin, Ger.
Homoeopathic preparation.

Presselin 20 F Presselin, Ger.
Homoeopathic preparation.

Presselin Gold N Presselin, Ger.
Homoeopathic preparation.

Presselin Heilozon Presselin, Ger.†.
Magnesium preparation with vitamins.

Presselin Hepaticum P Presselin, Ger.
Taraxacum (p.1634·2); chelidonium; silybum marianum (p.993·3).
Liver and biliary-tract disorders.

Presselin HK Herz-Kreislauf Presselin, Ger.
Homoeopathic preparation.

Presselin K 1 N Presselin, Ger.
Hypericum (p.1590·1); valerian (p.1643·1); lupulus (p.1597·2); passion flower (p.1615·3).
Depression; nervous disorders; sleep disorders.

Presselin K12 NE Presselin, Ger.
Homoeopathic preparation.

Presselin 20 M Presselin, Ger.
Homoeopathic preparation.

Presselin 52 N Presselin, Ger.
Chamomile (p.1561·2) lavender (p.1594·3); sage (p.1627·1); caraway (p.1559·3); cardamom (p.1560·1); coriander (p.1567·3); fennel (p.1579·1); absinthium (p.1541·1); ginger (p.1193·2).
Liver disorders.

Presselin 218 N Presselin, Ger.
Homoeopathic preparation.

Presselin Nervennahrung N Presselin, Ger.
Homoeopathic preparation.

Presselin Olin 1 Presselin, Ger.†.
Echinacea angustifolia; aconitum; belladonna; eupatorium perf.; baptisia; bryonia; fucus vesiculosus; peppermint oil; mercurius solubilis; lachesis; silicon dioxide; ascorbic acid; rutin.
Tonic.

Presselin Olin 2 Presselin, Ger.†.
Iron preparation with minerals and herbs.
Anaemias; iron deficiency.

Presselin Olin 5 Presselin, Ger.
Homoeopathic preparation.

Presselin Osmo Presselin, Ger.†.
Citric acid (p.1564·3); dried magnesium sulphate (p.1158·2); tartaric acid (p.1634·3); sodium bicarbonate (p.1153·2); ascorbic acid (p.1365·2).
Gastro-intestinal disorders; metabolic disorders.

Presselin Stoffwechseltee Presselin, Ger.†.
Calendula officinalis; senna (p.1212·2); fennel (p.1579·1); phaseolus vulgaris; pirus aucuparia; juniper (p.1592·2); rose fruit (p.1365·2); stoechados; bellis perennis; red-poppy petal (p.1001·1); chamomile (p.1561·2); prunus spinosa; feverfew (p.447·3); equisetum (p.1575·1); buckthorn (p.1182·1); berberis; couchgrass (p.1567·3).
Constipation.

Presselin Telagut Presselin, Ger.†.
Multivitamin and mineral preparation.
Bone disorders.

Presselin Thyre Presselin, Ger.†.
Homoeopathic preparation.

Presselin VE Presselin, Ger.
Melilotus officinalis.
Venous disorders.

Pressimed Wild, Switz.
Dihydroergocristine mesylate (p.1571·3); bendrofluazide (p.827·3); reserpine (p.942·1).
Hypertension.

Pressimedin Kwizda, Aust.
Dihydroergocristine mesylate (p.1571·3); bendrofluazide (p.827·3); reserpine (p.942·1).
Hypertension.

Pressimmun
Behringwerke, Ger.†; Behring, Ital.†.
Antilymphocyte immunoglobulin (horse) (p.504·2).
Organ transplant rejection.

Pressimmune Hoechst, UK†.
Antilymphocyte immunoglobulin (horse) (p.504·2).
Organ transplant rejection.

Pressin Alphapharm, Austral.
Prazosin hydrochloride (p.932·3).
Benign prostatic hyperplasia; heart failure; hypertension; Raynaud's syndrome.

Pressionorm Marion Merrell Dow, Ger.†.
Gepefrine tartrate (p.874·3).
Orthostatic hypotension.

Pressitan Iquinosa, Spain.
Enalapril maleate (p.863·2).
Heart failure; hypertension.

Pressitan Plus Iquinosa, Spain.
Enalapril maleate (p.863·2); hydrochlorothiazide (p.885·2).
Hypertension.

Pressural Polifarma, Ital.
Indapamide (p.890·2).
Hypertension.

Pressyn Ferring, Canad.
Vasopressin (p.1263·2).
Adjunct in abdominal radiography; diabetes insipidus; postoperative abdominal distension.

Prestim
Leo, Irl.; Leo, Neth.; Leo, UK.
Timolol maleate (p.953·3); bendrofluazide (p.827·3).
Hypertension.

Prestole SmithKline Beecham, Fr.
Triamterene (p.957·2); hydrochlorothiazide (p.885·2).
Hypertension.

Presun
Note. This name is used for preparations of different composition.
Westwood-Squibb, Canad.; Westwood, USA.
SPF 8; SPF 39: Padimate O (p.1488·1); oxybenzone (p.1487·3).
Sunscreen.

Westwood-Squibb, Canad.; Westwood, USA.
Cream SPF 15: Padimate O (p.1488·1); oxybenzone (p.1487·3).
Sunscreen.

Westwood-Squibb, Canad.; Westwood, USA.
Lotion SPF 15: Aminobenzoic acid (p.1486·3); padimate O (p.1488·1); oxybenzone (p.1487·3).
Sunscreen.

Westwood-Squibb, Canad.
SPF 21: Titanium dioxide (p.1093·3).
SPF 29: Ethylhexyl *p*-methoxycinnamate (p.1487·1); octyl salicylate (p.1487·3); oxybenzone (p.1487·3).
SPF 30: Ethylhexyl *p*-methoxycinnamate (p.1487·1); octyl salicylate (p.1487·3); oxybenzone (p.1487·3); avobenzone (p.1486·3).
Sunscreen.

Presun Active Bristol-Myers Products, USA.
SPF 15; SPF 30: Ethylhexyl *p*-methoxycinnamate (p.1487·1); oxybenzone (p.1487·3); octyl salicylate (p.1487·3).
Sunscreen.

Presun Facial Westwood, USA.
SPF 15: Padimate O (p.1488·1); oxybenzone (p.1487·3).
Sunscreen.

Presun for Kids Westwood, USA; Bristol-Myers Products, USA.
Ethylhexyl *p*-methoxycinnamate (p.1487·1); oxybenzone (p.1487·3); octyl salicylate (p.1487·3).
Sunscreen.

Presun Lip Stick Westwood, USA.
SPF 15: Padimate O (p.1488·1); oxybenzone (p.1487·3).
Sunscreen.

Presun Moisturizing Bristol-Myers Products, USA.
SPF 46: Padimate O (p.1488·1); oxybenzone (p.1487·3).
Sunscreen.

Presun Moisturizing with Keri Bristol-Myers Products, USA.
SPF 15: Padimate O (p.1488·1); oxybenzone (p.1487·3).

SPF 25: Ethylhexyl *p*-methoxycinnamate (p.1487·1); oxybenzone (p.1487·3); octyl salicylate (p.1487·3).
Sunscreen.

Presun Sensitive Skin *Westwood, USA; Bristol-Myers Products, USA.*
SPF 15; SPF 29: Ethylhexyl *p*-methoxycinnamate (p.1487·1); oxybenzone (p.1487·3); octyl salicylate (p.1487·3).
Sunscreen.

Presun Spray Mist *Bristol-Myers Products, USA.*
SPF 23: Ethylhexyl *p*-methoxycinnamate (p.1487·1); padimate O (p.1488·1); oxybenzone (p.1487·3); octyl salicylate (p.1487·3).
Sunscreen.

PreSun Ultra *Westwood-Squibb, USA.*
Avobenzone (p.1486·3); ethylhexyl *p*-methoxycinnamate (p.1487·1); octyl salicylate (p.1487·3); oxybenzone (p.1487·3).
Sunscreen.

Pretts Diet Aid *Milance, USA.*
Alginic acid (p.1470·3); carmellose sodium (p.1471·2); sodium bicarbonate (p.1153·2).

Pretuval *Roche, Switz.*
Dextromethorphan hydrobromide (p.1057·3); pseudoephedrine hydrochloride (p.1068·3); paracetamol (p.72·2).
Cold symptoms.

Pretuval C *Roche, Switz.*
Dextromethorphan hydrobromide (p.1057·3); pseudoephedrine hydrochloride (p.1068·3); paracetamol (p.72·2); ascorbic acid (p.1365·2).
Cold symptoms.

Pre-Tycin *Dista, S.Afr.†.*
Soap substitute.

Pretz *Parnell, USA.*
Sodium chloride (p.1162·2).
Inflammation and dryness of nasal membranes.

Pretz-D *Parnell, USA.*
Ephedrine sulphate (p.1059·3).
Nasal congestion.

Prevacid
Abbott, Canad.; TAP, USA.
Lansoprazole (p.1196·2).
Gastro-oesophageal reflux; peptic ulcer; Zollinger-Ellison syndrome.

Prevalite *Upsher-Smith, USA.*
Cholestyramine (p.1269·3).

Prevalon *Abello, Spain.*
Multivitamin and amino-acid preparation.
Tonic.

Preven *Gynetics, USA.*
Levonorgestrel (p.1454·1); ethinyloestradiol (p.1445·1).
Postcoital oral contraceptive.

Prevencal *Lalco, Canad.*
Calcium carbonate (p.1182·1).

Prevencal & D *Lalco, Canad.*
Calcium carbonate (p.1182·1); vitamin D (p.1366·3).

Prevencal & D & Fer *Lalco, Canad.*
Calcium carbonate (p.1182·1); vitamin D (p.1366·3); ferrous fumarate (p.1339·3).

Prevencal & D & Magnesium *Lalco, Canad.*
Calcium carbonate (p.1182·1); vitamin D (p.1366·3); magnesium oxide (p.1198·3).

Prevent *Agropharm, UK.*
Pyrethrins; piperonyl butoxide (p.1409·3); d'lemonin.
Insecticide.

Prevenzyme *Legere, USA†.*
Pancreatin (p.1612·1); pepsin (p.1616·3); amylase (p.1549·1); papain (p.1614·1); glutamic acid hydrochloride (p.1344·3); betaine hydrochloride (p.1553·2).

Prevex
Note. This name is used for preparations of different composition.
Trans Canaderm, Canad.
Cream: Cyclomethicone; yellow soft paraffin (p.1382·3).
Barrier cream for hands.
Lotion; body oil: Moisturiser.

Schering-Plough, Ital.
Felodipine (p.867·3).
Angina pectoris; hypertension.

Prevex B *Trans Canaderm, Canad.*
Betamethasone valerate (p.1033·3).
Skin disorders.

Prevex Diaper Rash Cream *Trans Canaderm, Canad.*
Zinc oxide (p.1096·2).
Barrier cream.

Prevex HC *Trans Canaderm, Canad.*
Hydrocortisone (p.1043·3).
Skin disorders.

Prevident *Colgate-Hoyt, USA.*
Sodium fluoride (p.742·1).
Dental caries prophylaxis.

Preview Urine *Carter-Wallace, Austral.†.*
Pregnancy test (p.1621·2).

Previgrip *Cassenne, Fr.*
Inactivated influenza vaccine (p.1515·2).
Active immunisation.

Previscan *Procter & Gamble, Fr.*
Fluindione (p.870·2).
Thrombo-embolic disorders.

Prevision *Midy, Ital.†.*
Pregnancy test (p.1621·2).

Prevpac *TAP, USA.*
Capsules, lansoprazole (Prevacid) (p.1196·2); capsules, amoxycillin trihydrate (Trimox) (p.151·3); tablets, clarithromycin (Biaxin) (p.189·1).
Duodenal ulcer associated with Helicobacter pylori infection.

Prexan *Lafare, Ital.*
Naproxen (p.61·2).
Musculoskeletal, joint, peri-articular, and soft-tissue disorders; neuralgias.

Prexene *Herbaline, Ital.*
Garlic (p.1583·1); crataegus (p.1568·2); olive oil (p.1610·1); silver birch (p.1553·3).
Hypertension; tachycardia.

Prexidil *Bioindustria, Ital.†.*
Minoxidil (p.910·3).
Hypertension.

Prexidine *Pred, Fr.*
Chlorhexidine gluconate (p.1107·2).
Mouth infections.

Prezal *Hoechst Marion Roussel, Neth.*
Lansoprazole (p.1196·2).
Gastro-oesophageal reflux; peptic ulcer.

Priadel
Fisons, Austral.†; Synthelabo, Belg.; Delandale, Irl.; Lorex Synthelabo, Neth.; Riker, S.Afr.†; Synthelabo, Switz.; Delandale, UK.
Lithium carbonate (p.290·3) or lithium citrate (p.290·3).
Affective disorders; aggression; bipolar disorder; depression; mania.

Priamide *Janssen-Cilag, Belg.*
Isopropamide iodide (p.464·3).
Diarrhoea; gastro-intestinal spasm.

Priatan *Minden, Ger.†.*
Oral drops: (−)-3,4-Dimethyl-5-phenyl-2-thiazolidinimine hydrochloride; ephedrine hydrochloride (p.1059·3); dihydrocodeine hydrochloride (p.34·2); thyme (p.1636·3); althaea (p.1546·3).
Oral liquid: Dimethylphenyliminothiazolidine hydrorhodanide; ephedrine thiocyanate; ammonium bromide (p.1620·3); potassium bromide (p.1620·3); sodium bromide (p.1620·3); thyme (p.1636·3); althaea (p.1546·3).
Coughs and associated respiratory-tract disorders.

Priatan-N *Minden, Ger.†.*
Dimethylphenyliminothiazolidine hydrorhodanide; ephedrine thiocyanate; theophylline (p.765·1).
Asthma.

Priaxim *Ravizza, Ital.*
Flunoxaprofen (p.41·3).
Gynaecological inflammation; musculoskeletal, joint, peri-articular, and soft-tissue disorders; venous disorders.

Priciasol *Labima, Belg.*
Naphazoline (p.1064·2).
Nasal congestion.

Prickly Heat Powder *Carter-Wallace, Austral.*
Zinc oxide (p.1096·2).
Chafed skin; eczema; heat rash; prickly heat.

Prid *Corvi, Ital.†.*
Cinchona calisaya (p.1564·1); rhubarb (p.1212·1); kola (p.1645·1).
Digestive system disorders.

Prid con Boldo *Corvi, Ital.†.*
Boldo (p.1554·1); cinchona calisaya (p.1564·1); rhubarb (p.1212·1); kola (p.1645·1).
Digestive system disorders.

Pridio *Quimifar, Spain.*
Caffeine (p.749·3); chlorpheniramine maleate (p.405·1); paracetamol (p.72·2); salicylamide (p.82·3).
Influenza and cold symptoms.

Priftin *Hoechst Marion Roussel, USA.*
Rifapentine (p.246·3).
Tuberculosis.

Prilagin *Gambar, Ital.*
Miconazole (p.384·3) or miconazole nitrate (p.384·3).
Candidiasis; Gram-positive bacterial infections.

Prilosec *Astra Merck, USA.*
Omeprazole (p.1204·2).
Gastro-oesophageal reflux; peptic ulcer; Zollinger-Ellison syndrome.

Priltam *Vinas, Spain.*
Capsaicin (p.24·2).
Diabetic neuropathy; musculoskeletal and joint disorders; postherpetic neuralgia.

Primacine *Pinewood, Irl.*
Erythromycin ethyl succinate (p.204·2) or erythromycin stearate (p.204·2).
Bacterial infections.

Primacor
Sanofi Winthrop, Austral.; Sanofi Winthrop, Canad.; Sanofi Winthrop, UK; Sanofi Winthrop, USA.
Milrinone lactate (p.910·2).
Heart failure.

Primaderm-B *Arrow, USA.*
Benzocaine (p.1286·2); zinc oxide (p.1096·2); cod-liver oil (p.1337·3).
Anorectal disorders.

Primafen *Hoechst, Spain.*
Cefotaxime sodium (p.168·2).
Lignocaine (p.1293·2) is included in the intramuscular injection to alleviate the pain of injection.
Bacterial infections.

Primahex *ConvaTec, UK.*
Chlorhexidine (p.1107·2); alcohol (p.1099·1).
Skin disinfection.

Primalan
Inava, Fr.; Rhone-Poulenc Rorer, Irl.; Rhone-Poulenc Rorer, Ital.; May & Baker, UK.
Mequitazine (p.414·2).
Hypersensitivity reactions.

Primamed *Sanofi Winthrop, Ger.*
Aluminium chlorohydrate (p.1078·3).
Skin disorders; wounds.

Primanol *Jamieson, Canad.*
Evening primrose oil (p.1582·1).

Primanol-Borage *Jamieson, Canad.*
A range of borage oil (p.1582·1) preparations.

Primasept M *Maggioni, Ital.†.*
Propyl alcohol (p.1124·2); isopropyl alcohol (p.1118·2); orthophenylphenol (p.1120·3).
Skin disinfection.

Primasept Med *Schulke & Mayr, Ger.*
Propyl alcohol (p.1124·2); isopropyl alcohol (p.1118·2); orthophenylphenol (p.1120·3).
Hand disinfection.

Primatene *Whitehall, USA.*
Theophylline (p.765·1); ephedrine hydrochloride (p.1059·3).
Bronchial asthma.

Primatene Dual Action *Whitehall, USA.*
Theophylline (p.765·1); ephedrine hydrochloride (p.1059·3); guaiphenesin (p.1061·3).
Asthma.

Primatene Mist *Whitehall, USA.*
Adrenaline (p.813·2).
Bronchial asthma.

Primatene Mist Suspension *Whitehall, USA.*
Adrenaline acid tartrate (p.813·3).
Bronchial asthma.

Primatour
Bio-Therabel, Belg.†; Asta Medica, Neth.
Chlorcyclizine hydrochloride (p.404·3); cinnarizine (p.406·1).
Motion sickness.

Primatuss Cough Mixture 4 *Rugby, USA.*
Chlorpheniramine maleate (p.405·1); dextromethorphan hydrobromide (p.1057·3).
Coughs and cold symptoms.

Primatuss Cough Mixture 4D *Rugby, USA.*
Pseudoephedrine hydrochloride (p.1068·3); dextromethorphan hydrobromide (p.1057·3); guaiphenesin (p.1061·3).
Coughs.

Primavit *IBP, Ital.†.*
Vitamin A acetate (p.1359·2).

Primaxin
Merck Sharp & Dohme, Austral.; Merck Sharp & Dohme, Canad.; Merck Sharp & Dohme, UK; Merck Sharp & Dohme, USA.
Imipenem (p.216·3); cilastatin sodium (p.185·2).
Bacterial infections.

Primbactam *Menarini, Ital.*
Aztreonam (p.156·3).
Bacterial infections.

Prime Time *Quest, Canad.*
Multivitamin and mineral preparation.

Primene
Clintec, Canad.; Clintec, Fr.; Baxter, Ger.; Baxter, Irl.; Clintec, Spain; Baxter, UK.
Amino-acid infusion.
Parenteral nutrition in infants.

Primer Unna Boot *Glenwood, USA.*
Zinc oxide (p.1096·2); acacia; glycerol; castor oil; white soft paraffin.
Venous insufficiency.

Primeral *Master Pharma, Ital.*
Naproxen sodium (p.61·2).
Musculoskeletal and joint disorders; pain.

Primesin *Knoll, Ital.*
Fluvastatin sodium (p.1273·2).
Hypercholesterolaemia.

Primobolan
Schering, Aust.; Schering, Austral.; Schering, Belg.†; Schering, Ger.; Schering, Ital.; Schering, Neth.; Schering, Norw.; Schering, S.Afr.; Schering, Spain; Schering, Switz.†.
Methenolone acetate (p.1450·3) or methenolone enanthate (p.1450·3).
Anabolic; anaemias; breast cancer; female genital cancer; liver disorders; osteoporosis.

Primodian Depot
Schering, Aust.; Schering, Austral.†; Schering, Ger.†; Schering, Ital.†; Schering, S.Afr.; Schering, Switz.†.
Oestradiol valerate (p.1455·2); testosterone enanthate (p.1464·1).
Menopausal disorders.

Primodium *Janssen-Cilag, Swed.*
Loperamide oxide (p.1197·3).
Diarrhoea.

Primofenac *Streuli, Switz.*
Diclofenac sodium (p.31·2).
Gout; inflammation; musculoskeletal, joint, and periarticular disorders; pain.

Primogonyl
Schering, Ger.; Schering, Switz.†.
Chorionic gonadotrophin (p.1243·1).
Cryptorchidism, hypogonadism, delayed puberty, and impotence in males; infertility in females.

Primogyn C *Schering, Austral.†.*
Ethinyloestradiol (p.1445·1).
Amenorrhoea; oestrogen deficiency.

Primogyn Depot
Schering, Austral.; Schering, S.Afr.
Oestradiol valerate (p.1455·2).
Amenorrhoea; menorrhagia; oestrogen deficiency; uterine hypoplasia.

Primolut Depot
Schering, Irl.†; Schering, Norw.†; Schering, S.Afr.
Hydroxyprogesterone hexanoate (p.1448·1).
Amenorrhoea; female infertility; habitual and threatened abortion; uterine hypoplasia.

Primolut N
Schering, Austral.; Schering, Irl.; Schering, Neth.; Schering, Norw.; Schering, S.Afr.; Schering, Switz.; Schering, UK.
Norethisterone (p.1453·1).
Endometriosis; menopausal disorders; menorrhagia; menstrual disorders; uterine hypoplasia.

Primolut-Nor
Schering, Aust.; Schering, Belg.; Schering, Fr.; Schering, Ger.; Schering, Ital.; Schering, Spain; Schering, Swed.; Schering, Switz.
Norethisterone acetate (p.1453·1).
Breast cancer; endometriosis; female infertility; mastopathy; menorrhagia; menstrual disorders; progestogen-only oral contraceptive; uterine hypoplasia.

Primosept *Andreabal, Switz.*
Trimethoprim (p.265·1).
Urinary-tract infections.

Primosiston
Note. This name is used for preparations of different composition.
Schering, Aust.; Schering, Ger.; Schering, Ital.†; Schering, Neth.†; Schering, Spain; Schering, Switz.
Tablets: Norethisterone acetate (p.1453·1); ethinyloestradiol (p.1445·1).
Menstrual disorders.

Schering, Ger.†; Schering, Switz.
Injection: Hydroxyprogesterone hexanoate (p.1448·1); oestradiol benzoate (p.1455·1).
Metrorrhagia.

Primoteston Depot
Schering, Austral.; Schering, Norw.; Schering, S.Afr.†; Schering, UK.
Testosterone enanthate (p.1464·1).
Some injections also contain testosterone propionate.
Androgenic; breast cancer; genital cancer in females; male androgen deficiency.

Primotussan *Galenika, Ger.*
Primula rhizome; thyme (p.1636·3).
Cold symptoms.

Primotussin N mit Codein *Galenika, Ger.†.*
Codeine phosphate (p.26·1); primula root; thyme (p.1636·3); drosera (p.1574·1).
Bronchitis; bronchopneumonia; pertussis.

Primoxan *Delagrange, Switz.†.*
Metoclopramide (p.1202·1); simethicone (p.1213·1).
Gastro-intestinal disorders.

Primoxil *Bayer, Ital.*
Moexipril hydrochloride (p.912·1).
Hypertension.

Primperan
Synthelabo, Belg.; Synthelabo, Fr.; Berk, Irl.; Lorex Synthelabo, Neth.; Synthelabo, Norw.; Roche, S.Afr.†; Delagrange, Spain; Tika, Swed.; Synthelabo, Switz.; Berk, UK.
Metoclopramide (p.1202·1) or metoclopramide hydrochloride (p.1200·3).
Gastro-intestinal disorders.

Primperan Complex *Delagrange, Spain.*
Dimethicone (p.1213·1); metoclopramide (p.1202·1); sorbitol (p.1354·2).
Aerophagia; dyspepsia; hiatus hernia; meteorism; vomiting.

Primperoxane *Synthelabo, Fr.*
Metoclopramide (p.1202·1); dimethicone (p.1213·1).
Dyspepsia.

Primyxine *Thera, Fr.*
Oxytetracycline hydrochloride (p.235·1); polymyxin B sulphate (p.239·1).
Acne; skin and wound infections.

Prinactizide *Dakota, Fr.*
Althiazide (p.819·1); spironolactone (p.946·1).
Hypertension; oedema.

Princi B1 + B6 *Sanofi Winthrop, Neth.*
Thiamine hydrochloride (p.1361·1); pyridoxine hydrochloride (p.1362·3).
Vitamin B deficiency associated with alcoholism.

Princi-B
Bournonville, Belg.; Sanofi Winthrop, Switz.†.
Vitamin B substances.
Alcoholism; cardiovascular disorders; drug intoxication; neurogenic pain; rheumatic pain.

Princi-B Fort *Labomed, Fr.*
Vitamin B substances.
Neuromuscular pain; vitamin B deficiency.

Principen
Squibb, Ital.†; Apothecon, USA.
Ampicillin sodium (p.153·1) or ampicillin trihydrate (p.153·2).
Bacterial infections.

Principen with Probenecid *Squibb, USA†.*
Ampicillin trihydrate (p.153·2).
Probenecid (p.394·3) is included in this preparation to reduce renal tubular excretion of ampicillin.
Gonorrhoea.

Prindex Mucolitico *Hosbon, Spain†.*
Bromhexine hydrochloride (p.1055·3); cephalexin (p.178·2).
Respiratory-tract infections.

Prinil *Merck Sharp & Dohme, Switz.*
Lisinopril (p.898·2).
Heart failure; hypertension.

Prinivil
Merck Sharp & Dohme, Aust.; Amrad, Austral.; Merck Sharp & Dohme, Canad.; Du Pont, Fr.; Du Pont, Ital.; Merck Sharp & Dohme, S.Afr.; Du Pont, Spain; Merck Sharp & Dohme, USA.
Lisinopril (p.898·2).
Heart failure; hypertension; myocardial infarction.

Prinivil Plus Du Pont, Spain.
Lisinopril (p.898·2); hydrochlorothiazide (p.885·2).
Hypertension.

Prinsyl Coventry, UK.
Chloroxylenol (p.1111·1).

Printania Clintec, Fr.
High protein nutritional supplement.

Printol Coventry, UK.
Tar acids (p.1126·2).

Prinzide
Merck Sharp & Dohme, Aust.; Merck Sharp & Dohme, Canad.; Du Pont, Fr.; Du Pont, Ital.; Merck Sharp & Dohme, Switz.; Merck Sharp & Dohme, USA.
Lisinopril (p.898·2); hydrochlorothiazide (p.885·2).
Hypertension.

Prioderm
Asta Medica, Belg.; Sarget, Fr.; Seton, Irl.; Dagra, Neth.; Norpharma, Norw.; Abigo, Swed.; Mundipharma, Switz.; Seton, UK.
Malathion (p.1407·3).
Pediculosis; scabies.

Priolatt San Carlo, Ital.†.
Latamoxef disodium (p.221·2).
Bacterial infections.

Priomicina San Carlo, Ital.†.
Fosfomycin calcium (p.210·2).
Bacterial infections.

Priorin
Roche Nicholas, Ger.; Roche, Ital.
Wheat-germ oil; millet; calcium pantothenate; cystine.
Hair and nail disorders; skin disorders.

Priorin Biotin Roche Nicholas, Ger.
Biotin (p.1336·1).
Biotin deficiency.

Priorin N Roche, Switz.
Millet; wheat-germ oil; cystine; calcium pantothenate.
Hair and nail disorders.

Priorix SmithKline Beecham, UK.
A measles, mumps, and rubella vaccine (attenuated Schwarz, Jeryl Lynn, and Wistar RA 27/3 strains respectively) (p.1519·3).
Active immunisation.

Priory Cleansing Herbs Gerard House, UK†.
Senna leaf (p.1212·2); frangula (p.1193·2); fennel (p.1579·1); psyllium seeds (p.1194·2).
Constipation.

Priovit 12 SIT, Ital.
Multivitamin preparation.

Pripsen
Note. This name is used for preparations of different composition.
Seton, Irl.; Seton, UK.
Oral powder: Piperazine phosphate (p.107·2); senna (p.1212·2).
Ascariasis; enterobiasis.

Seton, UK.
Elixir: Piperazine citrate (p.107·2).
Ascariasis; enterobiasis.

Seton, UK.
Tablets: Mebendazole (p.104·1).
Enterobiasis.

Priscol
Ciba Vision, Ger.; Ciba Vision, Switz.†.
Tolazoline hydrochloride (p.956·1).
Vascular eye disorders.

Priscoline
Novartis, Austral.; Ciba, Canad.†; Ciba, USA.
Tolazoline hydrochloride (p.956·1).
Peripheral vascular disorders; persistent pulmonary hypertension of the newborn.

Prisdal Prodes, Spain.
Citalopram hydrobromide (p.281·1).
Depression.

Prisma
Note. This name is used for preparations of different composition.
Thiemann, Ger.
Mianserin hydrochloride (p.297·1).
Depression.

Mediolanum, Ital.
Mesoglycan sodium (p.1602·3).
Thrombosis prophylaxis.

Privin
Ciba-Geigy, Aust.; Ciba, Ger.
Naphazoline nitrate (p.1064·2).
Aid to cystoscopy and rhinoscopy; nasal congestion.

Privina Ciba-Geigy, Spain.
Naphazoline nitrate (p.1064·2).
Nasal congestion.

Privine
Ciba Self Medication, Canad.†; Ciba, USA.
Naphazoline hydrochloride (p.1064·2).
Nasal congestion.

Pro Dunhall, USA.
Promethazine hydrochloride (p.416·2).
Hypersensitivity reactions; motion sickness; nausea; postoperative pain (adjunct); sedative; vomiting.

Pro Dorm Synthelabo, Ger.
Lorazepam (p.675·3).
Anxiety; sleep disorders.

Pro Skin Marlyn, USA.
Multivitamin and mineral preparation.

Proacid Procare, Austral.
Glycine (p.1345·2); calcium carbonate (p.1182·1); aloes (p.1177·1).
Gastric hyperacidity.

Pro-Actidil
Glaxo Wellcome, Aust.; Wellcopharm, Ger.†; Wellcome, Irl.†; Glaxo Wellcome, S.Afr.†; Wellcome, Spain; Wellcome, Switz.†; Wellcome, UK†.
Triprolidine hydrochloride (p.420·3).
Hypersensitivity reactions.

Pro-Air Parke, Davis, Canad.†.
Procaterol hydrochloride (p.757·3).
Bronchospasm.

Proaller Pekana, Ger.
Homoeopathic preparation.

ProAmatine Roberts, USA.
Midodrine hydrochloride (p.910·1).
Orthostatic hypotension.

Proampi Leo, Fr.
Pivampicillin (p.238·2).
Bacterial infections.

Probalan Lannett, USA†.
Probenecid (p.394·3).
Adjunct to beta-lactam antibacterials; gout.

Probamide Mallard, USA†.
Propantheline bromide (p.468·1).
Adjunct in peptic ulcer.

Pro-Banthine
Searle, Austral.; Searle, Belg.; Roberts, Canad.; Monsanto, Fr.; Baker Norton, Irl.; Searle, Neth.; Searle, S.Afr.†; Searle, Swed.; Searle, Switz.; Hansam, UK; Schiapparelli Searle, USA.
Propantheline bromide (p.468·1).
Gastro-intestinal spasm; hyperhidrosis; neurogenic bladder; nocturnal enuresis; peptic ulcer; renal colic.

Probaphen Bene, Ger.†.
Pentosan polysulphate sodium (p.928·1); glycol salicylate (p.43·1); menthol (p.1600·2).
Rheumatic disorders; superficial phlebitis.

Probase 3 Schering-Plough, UK.
Emollient.
Dry skin.

Probax Fischer, USA.
Propolis (p.1621·3).
Skin disorders.

Probecid
Astra, Norw.; Astra, Swed.
Probenecid (p.394·3).
Adjunct to beta-lactam antibacterials; gout.

Probec-T J&J-Merck, USA.
Vitamin B substances with vitamin C.

Proben Noristan, S.Afr.†.
Probenecid (p.394·3).
Gout.

Proben-C Rugby, USA†.
Probenecid (p.394·3); colchicine (p.393·1).
Gout.

Probeta
Note. A similar name is used for preparations of different composition.
Allergan, Canad.
Levobunolol hydrochloride (p.897·3); dipivefrine hydrochloride (p.1572·3).
Glaucoma; ocular hypertension.

Probeta LA
Note. A similar name is used for preparations of different composition.
Trinity, UK.
Propranolol hydrochloride (p.937·1).
Angina pectoris; hypertension.

Probigol Biohorma, Ital.
Propolis (p.1621·3); echinacea (p.1574·2).
Oral hygiene.

Probilin
Godecke, Ger.†; Parke, Davis, Ger.†; Parke, Davis, Ital.†.
Piprozolin (p.1619·1).
Biliary-tract disorders; dyspepsia.

Pro-Bionate Natren, USA.
Lactobacillus acidophilus (p.1594·1).
Dietary supplement.

Probiophyt V OTW, Ger.
Silybum marianum (p.993·3).
Liver disorders.

Probucard Astra, Neth.†.
Glyceryl trinitrate (p.874·3).
Angina pectoris.

Pro-C Procare, Austral.
Ascorbic acid (p.1365·2).
Vitamin C supplement.

Procadil Recordati, Ital.
Procaterol hydrochloride (p.757·3).
Obstructive airways disease.

Procal Christiaens, Belg.
Sodium fluoride (p.742·1).
Osteoporosis.

ProcalAmine McGaw, USA.
Amino-acid and electrolyte infusion.
Parenteral nutrition.

Procalmadiol Hoechst Marion Roussel, Belg.
Meprobamate (p.678·1).
Anxiety; insomnia; premedication; tension.

Pro-Cal-Sof Vangard, USA.
Docusate calcium (p.1189·3).
Constipation.

Procamide Zambon, Ital.
Procainamide hydrochloride (p.934·1).
Arrhythmias.

Procan Parke, Davis, Canad.
Procainamide hydrochloride (p.934·1).
Arrhythmias.

Procanbid Parke, Davis, USA.
Procainamide hydrochloride (p.934·1).
Formerly called Procan SR.
Arrhythmias.

Procaneural RAN, Ger.
Procaine hydrochloride (p.1299·2).
Nervous system disorders.

Procaptan Stroder, Ital.
Perindopril erbumine (p.928·2).
Hypertension.

Procardia Pfizer, USA.
Nifedipine (p.916·2).
Angina pectoris; hypertension.

Prociclide Crinos, Ital.
Defibrotide (p.847·1).
Thrombosis prophylaxis.

Procillin Caps, S.Afr.
Procaine penicillin (p.240·2).
Bacterial infections.

Procof Columbia, S.Afr.
Diphenhydramine hydrochloride (p.409·1); pholcodine (p.1068·1); guaiphenesin (p.1061·3).
Coughs.

Procol
SmithKline Beecham Consumer, Irl.; SmithKline Beecham, UK.
Phenylpropanolamine hydrochloride (p.1067·2).
Nasal congestion.

Procold Procare, Austral.
Ascorbic acid (p.1365·2); cochlearia armoracia; verbascum thapsus; euphorbia hirta; garlic (p.1583·1).
Respiratory-tract disorders.

Procomfrin Planta, Canad.
Comfrey (p.1567·1).
Bruises; sprains; wounds.

Procordal Gold Staufen, Ger.
Homoeopathic preparation.

Procordal Weiss Staufen, Ger.
Homoeopathic preparation.

Procort Roberts, USA.
Hydrocortisone (p.1043·3).
Corticosteroid.

Procorum
Ebewe, Aust.; Knoll, Ger.; Knoll, Ital.
Gallopamil hydrochloride (p.874·2).
Arrhythmias; hypertension; ischaemic heart disease; myocardial infarction.

Procoutol Spirig, Switz.
Triclosan (p.1127·2).
Skin disorders.

Procren
Abbott, Norw.; Abbott, Swed.
Leuprorelin acetate (p.1253·1).
Formerly known as Lupron in *Swed.*
Prostatic cancer.

Procrin Abbott, Spain.
Leuprorelin acetate (p.1253·1).
Endometriosis; prostatic cancer; uterine fibroma.

Procrit Ortho Biotech, USA.
Epoetin alfa (p.718·3).
Anaemia in cancer patients on chemotherapy; anaemia in zidovudine-treated HIV-infected patients; anaemia of chronic renal failure; pre-operative anaemias.

Proctalgen BC Lutz, Switz.
Hamamelis (p.1587·1); diethylamine salicylate (p.33·1).
Anorectal disorders.

Proctidol Zyma, Ital.
Hydrocortisone acetate (p.1043·3); benzocaine (p.1286·2).
Haemorrhoids.

Proctium Esteve, Spain.
Calcium dobesilate (p.1556·3); lignocaine hydrochloride (p.1293·2); prednisolone (p.1048·1).
Anorectal disorders.

Proctocort
Note. This name is used for preparations of different composition.
Cassenne, Austral.†.
Cinchocaine hydrochloride (p.1289·2); hydrocortisone (p.1043·3).
Anorectal disorders.

Boehringer Ingelheim, Fr.; Monarch, USA.
Hydrocortisone (p.1043·3) or hydrocortisone acetate (p.1043·3).
Anorectal disorders.

Schering, Ital.†.
Fluocortolone pivalate (p.1041·3); fluocortolone hexanoate (p.1041·3); pramoxine hydrochloride (p.1298·2); chlorquinaldol (p.185·1); troxerutin (p.1580·2).
Anorectal disorders.

Proctocream HC
Stafford-Miller, UK; Schwarz, USA.
Hydrocortisone acetate (p.1043·3); pramoxine hydrochloride (p.1298·2).
Anorectal disorders.

Proctofibe Roussel, UK†.
Fibrous grain and citrus extract (p.1181·2).
Constipation.

Proctofoam
Note. This name is used for preparations of different composition.
Searle, S.Afr.
Hydrocortisone acetate (p.1043·3); pramoxine hydrochloride (p.1298·2).
Anorectal disorders.

Schwarz, USA.
Pramoxine hydrochloride (p.1298·2).
Anorectal disorders.

Proctofoam-HC
Reed & Carnrick, Canad.; Trommsdorff, Ger.†; Stafford-Miller, Irl.; Reed & Carnrick, Neth.†; Stafford-Miller, UK; Schwarz, USA.
Hydrocortisone acetate (p.1043·3); pramoxine hydrochloride (p.1298·2).
Anorectal disorders.

Procto-Glyvenol
Ciba-Geigy, Aust.; Zyma, Switz.
Tribenoside (p.1638·3); lignocaine (p.1293·2) or lignocaine hydrochloride (p.1293·2).
Haemorrhoids.

Procto-Jellin Grunenthal, Ger.
Fluocinolone acetonide (p.1041·1); lignocaine hydrochloride (p.1293·2).
Anorectal disorders.

Procto-Kaban Asche, Ger.
Clocortolone pivalate (p.1035·3); clocortolone hexanoate (p.1035·3); cinchocaine hydrochloride (p.1289·2).
Anorectal disorders.

Proctolog
Jouveinal, Fr.; Juste, Spain.
Ruscogenin (p.1627·1); trimebutine (p.1639·3).
Anorectal disorders.

Proctolyn Recordati, Ital.
Fluocinolone acetonide (p.1041·1); ketocaine hydrochloride (p.1293·2).
Anorectal disorders.

Proctonide Recordati, Ital.†.
Fluocinonide (p.1041·2); ketocaine hydrochloride (p.1293·2).
Anorectal disorders.

Proctoparf Much, Ger.
Bufexamac (p.22·2); bismuth subgallate (p.1180·2); lignocaine hydrochloride (p.1293·2); titanium dioxide (p.1093·3).
Anorectal disorders.

Proctor's Pinelyptus Ernest Jackson, UK.
Eucalyptus oil (p.1578·1); menthol (p.1600·2); sylvestris pine oil; abietis oil.
Coughs; throat irritation.

Proctosedyl
Note. This name is used for preparations of different composition.
Hoechst Marion Roussel, Austral.; Hoechst Marion Roussel, UK.
Cinchocaine hydrochloride (p.1289·2); hydrocortisone (p.1043·3).
Anorectal disorders.

Hoechst Marion Roussel, Canad.; Hoechst Marion Roussel, Irl.; Hoechst Marion Roussel, Norw.; Roussel, S.Afr.; Hoechst Marion Roussel, Swed.; Roussel, Switz.†.
Cinchocaine hydrochloride (p.1289·2); hydrocortisone (p.1043·3); framycetin sulphate (p.210·3); esculoside (p.1543·3).
Anorectal disorders.

Roche, Ital.
Ointment: Amylocaine (p.1286·1); benzocaine (p.1286·2); hydrocortisone acetate (p.1043·3); esculoside (p.1543·3).
Suppositories: Benzocaine (p.1286·2); hydrocortisone acetate (p.1043·3); esculoside (p.1543·3).
Anal pruritus; haemorrhoids.

Hoechst Marion Roussel, Neth.
Cinchocaine hydrochloride (p.1289·2); hydrocortisone (p.1043·3); framycetin sulphate (p.210·3).
Haemorrhoids.

Proctosoll Schiapparelli, Ital.
Benzocaine (p.1286·2); hydrocortisone acetate (p.1043·3); heparin sodium (p.879·3).
Haemorrhoids.

Proctosone Technilab, Canad.
Cinchocaine hydrochloride (p.1289·2); hydrocortisone acetate (p.1043·3); neomycin sulphate (p.229·2); esculoside (p.1543·3).
Anorectal disorders.

Proctospre
Hennig, Ger.; Sodip, Switz.
Cinchocaine (p.1289·2); chlorquinaldol (p.185·1); diphenylpyraline (p.410·1).
Anogenital disorders.

Proctosteroid Aldo, Spain.
Triamcinolone diacetate (p.1050·2).
Proctitis; proctosigmoiditis; ulcerative colitis.

Procto-Synalar
Note. This name is used for preparations of different composition.
Grunenthal, Aust.
Fluocinolone acetonide (p.1041·1); lignocaine hydrochloride (p.1293·2).
Anorectal disorders.

Yamanouchi, Belg.
Fluocinolone acetonide (p.1041·1); lignocaine hydrochloride (p.1293·2); bismuth subgallate (p.1180·2); menthol (p.1600·2).
Anorectal disorders.

Procto-Synalar N Grunenthal, Switz.
Fluocinolone acetonide (p.1041·1); lignocaine hydrochloride (p.1293·2).
Procto-Synalar formerly contained fluocinolone acetonide, lignocaine hydrochloride, menthol, and bismuth subgallate.
Anorectal disorders.

Proculens N Mann, Ger.†.
Panthenol (p.1571·1); naphazoline nitrate (p.1064·2).
Contact lens care.

Proculin ankerpharm, Ger.
Naphazoline hydrochloride (p.1064·2).
Conjunctivitis.

Procutan Schering-Plough, S.Afr.
Hydrocortisone (p.1043·3).
Skin disorders.

Pro-Cute Ferndale, USA.
Emollient and moisturiser.

Procutene Bouty, Ital.†.
Triclocarban (p.1127·2).
Infected skin disorders.

ProCycle Gold Cyclin, USA.
Multivitamin, mineral and nutritional preparation.

Procyclid ICN, Canad.
Procyclidine hydrochloride (p.467·3).
Parkinsonism.

Procyclo Organon, Ger.
11 Tablets, oestradiol valerate (p.1455·2); 10 tablets, oestradiol valerate; medroxyprogesterone acetate (p.1448·3).
Menopausal disorders.

Procytox Carter Horner, Canad.
Cyclophosphamide (p.516·2).
Malignant neoplasms.

Pro-Dafalgan
Upsamedica, Belg.; UPSA, Fr.; Upsamedica, Switz.
Propacetamol hydrochloride (p.81·2).
Fever; pain.

Prodafem
Pharmacia Upjohn, Aust.; Pharmacia Upjohn, Switz.
Medroxyprogesterone acetate (p.1448·3).
Amenorrhoea; endometriosis; menopausal disorders; menorrhagia.

Prodalix Forte Cough Linctus Nelson, Austral.†.
Promethazine hydrochloride (p.416·2); pseudoephedrine hydrochloride (p.1068·3); codeine phosphate (p.26·1); guaiphenesin (p.1061·3); ipecacuanha (p.1062·2).
Coughs and congestion.

Prodalix Forte Cough Linctus-New Formula
Nelson, Austral.†.
Promethazine hydrochloride (p.416·2); pseudoephedrine hydrochloride (p.1068·3); dextromethorphan hydrobromide (p.1057·3); guaiphenesin (p.1061·3).
Coughs and congestion.

Prodamox Rubio, Spain.
Proglumetacin maleate (p.81·2).
Gout; musculoskeletal, joint, and peri-articular disorders; pain.

Prodasone Pharmacia Upjohn, Fr.
Medroxyprogesterone acetate (p.1448·3).
Breast and endometrial cancers.

Prodeine Sanofi Winthrop, Austral.
Paracetamol (p.72·2); codeine phosphate (p.26·1).
Fever; pain.

Proderm Dow, USA.
Castor oil (p.1560·2); peru balsam (p.1617·2).
Decubitus ulcers.

Prodessal Prodes, Spain.
Cyanocobalamin (p.1363·3); cyclobutyrol (p.1569·2); cytidine; electrolytes (p.1147·1); uridine (p.1641·3).
Liver disorders; oral hygiene.

Pro-Diaban
Bayer, Aust.; Bayer, Ger.
Glisoxepide (p.321·2).
Diabetes mellitus.

Prodiarrhoea Procare, Austral.
Activated charcoal (p.972·2).
Diarrhoea; flatulence.

Prodicard Astra, Neth.
Isosorbide dinitrate (p.893·1).
Angina pectoris.

Prodiem Plain Novartis Consumer, Canad.
Psyllium hydrophilic mucilloid (p.1194·2).
Constipation; fibre supplement.

Prodiem Plus Novartis Consumer, Canad.
Psyllium hydrophilic mucilloid (p.1194·2); senna pod (p.1212·2).
Constipation.

Prodis Procare, Austral.
Multivitamins, amino acids, ginseng, and minerals.
Dietary supplement.

Prodium
Note. This name is used for preparations of different composition.
Propan, S.Afr.
Loperamide hydrochloride (p.1197·2).
Diarrhoea; ostomy management.

Breckenridge, USA.
Phenazopyridine hydrochloride (p.78·3).
Irritation of the lower urinary tract.

Prodon Tika, Swed.
Ketoprofen (p.48·2).
Musculoskeletal and joint disorders.

Prodorol Be-Tabs, S.Afr.
Propranolol hydrochloride (p.937·1).
Angina pectoris; anxiety; arrhythmias; hypertension; hyperthyroidism; phaeochromocytoma.

Prodrox 250 Legere, USA†.
Hydroxyprogesterone hexanoate (p.1448·1).

Product Code 889 Scientific Hospital Supplies, Austral.
Preparation for enteral nutrition.
Methylmalonic acidaemia; propionic acidaemia.

Proechina Procare, Austral.
Echinacea angustifolia (p.1574·2).

Pro-Efferalgan Upsamedica, Ital.
Propacetamol hydrochloride (p.81·2).
Pain.

Proendotel Fidia, Ital.
Cloricromen hydrochloride (p.845·1).
Formerly called Cromocap.
Thrombotic disorders.

Proesten Procare, Austral.
Vitamins; minerals; garlic (p.1583·1); cimicifuga (p.1563·3); viburnum opulus; passion flower (p.1615·3); sarsaparilla (p.1627·2).
Dietary supplement; menopausal disorders.

Profact Hoechst, Ger.
Buserelin (p.1242·1) or buserelin acetate (p.1241·3).
Prostatic cancer.

Profasi
Serono, Aust.; Serono, Austral.; Serono, Belg.†; Serono, Irl.; Serono, Neth.; Serono, Norw.; Research Labs, S.Afr.; Serono, Swed.; Serono, Switz.; Serono, UK; Serono, USA.
Chorionic gonadotrophin (p.1243·1).
Cryptorchidism; delayed puberty; hypogonadotrophic hypogonadism; male and female infertility.

Profasi HP
Serono, Canad.; Serono, Ital.; Serono, Spain.
Chorionic gonadotrophin (p.1243·1).
Cryptorchidism; hypogonadotrophic hypogonadism; male and female infertility; metrorrhagia; threatened and recurrent abortion.

Profen Wakefield, USA.
Phenylpropanolamine hydrochloride (p.1067·2); guaiphenesin (p.1061·3).
Upper respiratory-tract symptoms.

Profen II Wakefield, USA.
Phenylpropanolamine hydrochloride (p.1067·2); guaiphenesin (p.1061·3).
Coughs.

Profen II DM Wakefield, USA.
Phenylpropanolamine hydrochloride (p.1067·2); guaiphenesin (p.1061·3); dextromethorphan hydrobromide (p.1057·3).
Coughs.

Profenal Alcon, USA.
Suprofen (p.88·1).
Inhibition of intra-operative miosis.

Profenda Jamieson, Canad.
Betacarotene, vitamin C, and vitamin E.

Profenid
Gerot, Aust.; Specia, Fr.; Rhone-Poulenc Rorer, Switz.†.
Ketoprofen (p.48·2).
Musculoskeletal, joint, peri-articular, and soft-tissue disorders; pain.

Profenil Drug Research, Ital.†.
Ketoprofen (p.48·2).
Musculoskeletal, joint, and soft-tissue disorders.

Profer Tedec Meiji, Spain.
Ferritin (p.1580·1).
Iron-deficiency anaemia.

Profiber Sherwood, USA.
Lactose-free preparation for enteral nutrition.

Pro-fibre Wyeth-Ayerst, Canad.†.
Preparation for enteral nutrition.

Profilate
Alpha Therapeutic, Ger.; Alfa Farmaceutici, Ital.†; Alpha Therapeutic, Swed.†; Alpha Therapeutic, USA†.
A factor VIII preparation (p.720·3).
Haemorrhagic disorders.

Profilnine
Alpha Therapeutic, Ger.†; Alpha Therapeutic, USA.
A factor IX preparation (p.721·3).
Haemorrhagic disorders.

Proflex
Zyma, Irl.; Zyma, UK.
Ibuprofen (p.44·1).
Inflammation; musculoskeletal, joint, and peri-articular disorders; pain.

Proflo Procare, Austral.
Vitamins; minerals; bioflavonoids (p.1580·1); ruscus aculeatus; aesculus (p.1543·3); hamamelis (p.1587·1); pulsatilla (p.1623·3).
Dietary supplement; peripheral vascular disorders.

Profluid Procare, Austral.
Taraxacum (p.1634·2); parsley piert; bearberry (p.1552·2); juniper (p.1592·2).
Bladder disorders; cystitis; fluid retention.

ProFree Allergan, USA.
Papain (p.1614·1).
Cleansing solution for contact lenses.

Progan Nelson, Austral.†.
Promethazine hydrochloride (p.416·2).
Hypersensitivity reactions; sedative.

Progandol Almirall, Spain.
Doxazosin mesylate (p.862·3).
Benign prostatic hyperplasia; heart failure; hypertension.

Progastrit Hexal, Ger.
Aluminium hydroxide (p.1177·3); magnesium hydroxide (p.1198·2).
Gastro-intestinal disorders.

Progeffik Effik, Spain.
Progesterone (p.1459·3).
Dysfunctional uterine bleeding; menopausal disorders; menstrual disorders.

Progeril
Midy, Ital.†; Sanofi Winthrop, Switz.
Co-dergocrine mesylate (p.1566·1).
Hypertension; migraine; vascular disorders.

Progeril Papaverina Midy, Ital.†.
Co-dergocrine mesylate (p.1566·1); papaverine (p.1614·2) or papaverine hydrochloride (p.1614·2).
Hypertension; vascular disorders.

Progesic
Note. A similar name is used for preparations of different composition.
Lilly, Irl.†; Lilly, UK†.
Fenoprofen calcium (p.37·2).
Fever; musculoskeletal and joint disorders; pain.

Pro-gesic
Note. A similar name is used for preparations of different composition.
Nastech, USA.
Triethanolamine salicylate (p.1639·2).
Musculoskeletal and joint disorders.

Progestan Nourypharma, Neth.
Progesterone (p.1459·3).
Endometrial cancer; endometrial hyperplasia; menopausal disorders.

Progestasert
Theraplix, Fr.; Alza, USA.
Progesterone (p.1459·3).
Progestogen-only intra-uterine contraceptive device.

Progesterone-retard Pharlon Schering, Fr.
Hydroxyprogesterone hexanoate (p.1448·1).
Female infertility; premature labour; progestogen; threatened and habitual abortion.

Progestogel
Piette, Belg.; Besins-Iscovesco, Fr.; Kade, Ger.; Lusofarmaco, Ital.; Seid, Spain; Golaz, Switz.
Progesterone (p.1459·3).
Benign breast disorders.

Progestol Synthelabo, Ital.
Progesterone (p.1459·3).
Acne; seborrhoea; seborrhoeic alopecia.

Progestosol
Besins-Iscovesco, Fr.; Besins-Iscovesco, Switz.†.
Progesterone (p.1459·3).
Seborrhoea.

Progevera Upjohn, Spain.
Medroxyprogesterone acetate (p.1448·3).
Endometriosis; female infertility; menometrorrhagia; menopausal disorders; menstrual disorders.

Progevera 250 Upjohn, Spain.
Medroxyprogesterone acetate (p.1448·3).
Malignant neoplasms.

Proginkgo Procare, Austral.
Ginkgo biloba (p.1584·1).
Cerebral and peripheral vascular disorders; tonic.

Proglan Procare, Austral.
Black currant seed oil.
Dietary supplement; source of polyunsaturated fatty acids.

Proglicem
Schering-Plough, Fr.; Essex, Ger.; Schering-Plough, Ital.; Schering-Plough, Neth.; Essex, Switz.
Diazoxide (p.847·2).
Hypertension; hypoglycaemia.

Proglycem
Schering, Canad.; Baker Norton, USA.
Diazoxide (p.847·2).
Hypoglycaemia.

Pro-Gola Ghimas, Ital.
Propolis (p.1621·3).

Progout Alphapharm, Austral.
Allopurinol (p.390·2).
Gout; hyperuricaemia; renal calculi.

Prograf
Janssen-Cilag, Austral.; Fujisawa, Canad.; Fujisawa, Fr.; Fujisawa, Ger.; Fujisawa, Irl.; Fujisawa, Jpn; Fujisawa, Spain; Fujisawa, Swed.; Fujisawa, UK; Fujisawa, USA.
Tacrolimus (p.562·2).
Graft-versus-host disease; organ transplant rejection.

Progress Procare, Austral.
Ginseng; garlic; multivitamins; minerals; kelp; cramp bark.
Dietary supplement.

Proguval Eberth, Ger.
Plantago lanceolata.
Catarrh; mouth and throat inflammation.

Progylut Schering, Ger.†.
11 Tablets, ethinyloestradiol (p.1445·1); 10 tablets, ethinyloestradiol; norethisterone acetate (p.1453·1).
Menstrual disorders.

Progyluton Schering, Spain.
11 Tablets, oestradiol valerate (p.1455·2); 10 tablets, oestradiol valerate; norgestrel (p.1454·1).
Female infertility; menopausal disorders; menstrual disorders.

Progynon
Schering, Aust.; Schering, Swed.
Oestradiol valerate (p.1455·2).
Amenorrhoea; menopausal disorders; menorrhagia; osteoporosis.

Progynon C
Schering, Aust.; Schering, Ger.; Schering, Switz.†.
Ethinyloestradiol (p.1445·1).
Menstrual disorders; oestrogen deficiency.

Progynon Depot
Schering, Ital.; Schering, Spain.
Oestradiol valerate (p.1455·2).
Menstrual disorders; oestrogen deficiency.

Progynon Depot 10
Schering, Ger.; Schering, Neth.; Schering, Switz.
Oestradiol valerate (p.1455·2).
Menstrual disorders; oestrogen deficiency; uterine hypoplasia.

Progynon Depot 40 Schering, Ger.†.
Oestradiol valerate (p.1455·2).
Postmenopausal breast cancer.

Progynon Depot 100
Schering, Ger.†; Schering, Neth.†; Schering, Switz.†.
Oestradiol undecanoate (p.1455·2).
Prostatic cancer.

Progynova
Schering, Aust.; Schering, Austral.; Schering, Belg.; Schering, Fr.; Schering, Ger.; Schering, Irl.†; Schering, Ital.; Schering, Neth.; Schering, Norw.; Schering, S.Afr.; Schering, Spain; Schering, Switz.; Schering, UK.
Oestradiol (p.1455·1) or oestradiol valerate (p.1455·2).
Menopausal disorders; oestrogen deficiency; osteoporosis.

Prohance
Squibb Diagnostics, Canad.; Byk Gulden, Ger.; Bracco, Ital.; Byk, Neth.; Bristol-Myers Squibb, Swed.†; Bracco, Switz.; Bracco, UK; Bracco, USA.
Gadoteridol (p.1005·1).
Contrast medium for magnetic resonance imaging.

Prohepar Nordmark, Ger.†.
Bovine liver extract; choline hydrogen tartrate; cysteine (p.1338·3); inositol (p.1591·1); cyanocobalamin (p.1363·3).
Liver disorders.

ProHIBiT
Serotherapeutisches, Aust.; Pasteur Merieux, Austral.†; Pasteur Merieux, Swed.†; Berna, Switz.; Connaught, USA.
A haemophilus influenzae conjugate vaccine (diphtheria toxoid conjugate) (p.1511·1).
Active immunisation.

ProHIBiT-DPT Berna, Switz.
A diphtheria, tetanus, pertussis, and Haemophilus influenzae vaccine (p.1509·3).
Active immunisation.

Prohist Be-Tabs, S.Afr.
Promethazine hydrochloride (p.416·2).
Nausea and vomiting; premedication; sedative.

Prokids Procare, Austral.
Multivitamin and mineral preparation.

Prokine Hoechst, USA†.
Sargramostim (p.727·3).
Myeloid reconstitution after autologous bone marrow transplant.

Prokinyl Techni-Pharma, Mon.
Metoclopramide hydrochloride (p.1200·3).
Aid to gastro-intestinal examination; dyspepsia; nausea and vomiting.

Prol Procare, Austral.
Silybum marianum (p.993·3).
Liver disorders.

Prolac International Research, Austral.†.
Multivitamin, carbohydrate and protein preparation.

Prolacam Schering, Aust.
Lysuride maleate (p.1142·1).
Acromegaly; amenorrhoea; female infertility; galactorrhoea; lactation inhibition; mastitis.

Prolactase Pharmascience, Canad.†.
Tilactase (p.1637·3).
Lactose intolerance.

Proladone Knoll, Austral.
Oxycodone pectinate (p.71·3).
Pain.

Prolair 3M, Fr.
Beclomethasone dipropionate (p.1032·1).
Asthma.

Prolan Procare, Austral.
Multivitamin and mineral preparation.
Anxiety; dietary supplement.

Prolastin
Bayer, Canad.; Bayer, Ger.; Bayer, USA.
Alpha$_1$ antitrypsin (p.1546·2).
Congenital alpha$_1$ antitrypsin deficiency.

Prolastina Bayer, Spain.
Alpha$_1$ antitrypsin (p.1546·2).
Congenital alpha$_1$ antitrypsin deficiency.

Prolax
Note. A similar name is used for preparations of different composition.
Procare, Austral.
Senna (p.1212·2); prune (p.1209·2).
Constipation.

Pro-Lax
Note. A similar name is used for preparations of different composition.
Rivex, Canad.
Polyethylene glycol (p.1597·3); electrolytes (p.1147·1).
Constipation.

Prolert Pensa, Spain.
Caffeine (p.749·3).
Fatigue.

Proleukin
Laevosan, Aust.; Ligand, Canad.; Chiron, Fr.; Chiron Behring, Ger.; Chiron, Ital.; Chiron, Neth.; Chiron, Spain; Roche, Switz.; Chiron, UK; Chiron, USA.
Aldesleukin (p.541·3).
Metastatic renal-cell carcinoma.

Prolief Propan, S.Afr.
Paracetamol (p.72·2).
Fever; pain.

Prolifen *Chiesi, Ital.*
Clomiphene citrate (p.1439·2).
Anovulatory infertility.

Prolipase
Janssen-Cilag, Aust.; Janssen-Cilag, Switz.
Pancrelipase (p.1613·3).
Dyspepsia; pancreatic insufficiency.

Prolixan
Jacoby, Aust.; Siegfried, Ger.†; Asta Medica, Neth.; Siegfried, Switz.
Azapropazone (p.20·3).
Inflammation; musculoskeletal, joint, and peri-articular disorders; pain.

Prolixana *Siegfried, Swed.*
Azapropazone (p.20·3).
Musculoskeletal and joint disorders.

Prolixin *Apothecon, USA; Princeton, USA.*
Fluphenazine decanoate (p.671·2), fluphenazine enanthate (p.671·3), or fluphenazine hydrochloride (p.671·3).
Psychoses.

Proloid *Parke, Davis, S.Afr.†.*
Thyroglobulin (p.1496·3).
Hypothyroidism.

Proloide *Parke, Davis, Spain†.*
Thyroglobulin (p.1496·3).
Hypothyroidism.

Prolopa
Roche, Belg.; Roche, Canad.
Levodopa (p.1137·1); benserazide hydrochloride (p.1132·1).
Parkinsonism.

Proloprim
Glaxo Wellcome, Canad.; Glaxo Wellcome, S.Afr.†; Glaxo Wellcome, USA.
Trimethoprim (p.265·1).
Bacterial infections of the urinary tract.

Prolugol-liquid N *Atzinger, Ger.†.*
Thymol (p.1127·1); iodine (p.1493·1); urea (p.1095·2).
Vaginal infections; vaginitis.

Proluton
Schering, Aust.; Schering, Austral.; Schering, Belg.†; Schering, Ger.; Schering, Ital.; Schering, Neth.; Schering, Spain; Schering, Switz.; Schering, UK.
Progesterone (p.1459·3) or hydroxyprogesterone hexanoate (p.1448·1).
Formerly known as Primolut Depot in the *UK*.
Amenorrhoea; female infertility; habitual and threatened abortion; metrorrhagia; progestogen deficiency; uterine hypoplasia.

Promahist *Propan-Vernleigh, S.Afr.†.*
Promethazine hydrochloride (p.416·2).
Coughs; nausea; vomiting.

Promal *Propan-Vernleigh, S.Afr.†.*
Chloroquine phosphate (p.426·3).
Malaria.

Promani *SmithKline Beecham, Canad.*
Triclosan (p.1127·2).
Dry or irritated skin.

Promanum N *Braun, Ger.*
Alcohol (p.1099·1); isopropyl alcohol (p.1118·2).
Hand disinfection.

Promaquid *Rhone-Poulenc Rorer Consumer, Canad.†.*
Dimethothiazine mesylate (p.408·3).
Asthma; headaches; hypersensitivity reactions.

Promatussin DM *Lioh, Canad.*
Promethazine hydrochloride (p.416·2); dextromethorphan hydrobromide (p.1057·3); pseudoephedrine (p.1068·3).
Coughs.

Promaxol *Esteve, Spain.*
Procaterol hydrochloride (p.757·3).
Obstructive airways disease.

Promeal *Volchem, Ital.*
Preparation for enteral nutrition.

Promedrol
Pharmacia Upjohn, Aust.; Pharmacia Upjohn, Switz.
Methylprednisolone suleptanate (p.1046·2).
Corticosteroid.

Promega *Parke, Davis, USA.*
Omega-3 marine triglycerides with vitamin E (p.1276·1).
Dietary supplement.

Promelatonin *Pharma-Natura, Ital.*
Tryptophan; niacin; calcium; magnesium.
Nutritional supplement; sleep disorders.

Promet 50 *Legere, USA†.*
Promethazine hydrochloride (p.416·2).

Prometa *Muro, USA.*
Orciprenaline sulphate (p.756·3).

Prometh *Seatrace, USA†.*
Promethazine hydrochloride (p.416·2).
Hypersensitivity reactions; motion sickness; nausea; postoperative pain (adjunct); sedative; vomiting.

Prometh with Dextromethorphan *Barre-National, USA.*
Promethazine hydrochloride (p.416·2); dextromethorphan hydrobromide (p.1057·3).
Coughs and cold symptoms.

Prometh VC Plain *Warner Chilcott, USA; Goldline, USA; Barre-National, USA.*
Promethazine hydrochloride (p.416·2); phenylephrine hydrochloride (p.1066·2).
Allergic rhinitis; nasal congestion.

Promethazine VC with Codeine *Warner Chilcott, USA.*
Promethazine hydrochloride (p.416·2); phenylephrine hydrochloride (p.1066·2); codeine phosphate (p.26·1).

Promethegan *G & W, USA.*
Promethazine (p.416·2).

Promethist with Codeine *Rahslog, USA.*
Phenylephrine hydrochloride (p.1066·2); codeine phosphate (p.26·1); promethazine hydrochloride (p.416·2).
Coughs and cold symptoms.

Prometrium
Schering, Canad.; Solvay, USA.
Progesterone (p.1459·3).
Adjunct to oestrogen replacement therapy.

Prominal
Sanofi Winthrop, Austral.; Merck, Spain; Sanofi Winthrop, UK.
Methylphenobarbitone (p.349·2).
Epilepsy.

Promincil *Chefaro Ardeval, Fr.*
Fucus (p.1554·1); meadowsweet (p.1599·1); equisetum (p.1575·1).
Herbal slimming preparation.

Prominol *MCR, USA.*
Butalbital (p.644·3); paracetamol (p.72·2).
Pain.

Promise *Block, USA†.*
Potassium nitrate (p.1123·1); sodium monofluorophosphate (p.743·3).
Sensitive teeth.

Promit
Torrex, Aust.; Pharmacia Upjohn, Austral.; Kabi Pharmacia, Canad.†; Pharmacia Upjohn, Fr.; Reusch, Ger.; Braun, Switz.; Pharmacia, USA.
Dextran 1 (p.716·1).
Prevention of anaphylactic reactions to infusions of dextrans.

Promiten
Pharmacia Upjohn, Norw.; Medisan, Swed.
Dextran 1 (p.716·1).
Prevention of anaphylactic reactions to infusions of dextrans.

Promkiddi *Weimer, Ger.†.*
Promethazine hydrochloride (p.416·2).
Hypersensitivity reactions; sedative.

Promocard
Astra, Belg.; Astra, Neth.
Isosorbide mononitrate (p.893·3).
Angina pectoris.

ProMod
Abbott, Austral.; Abbott, Canad.; Abbott, UK; Ross, USA.
Dietary protein supplement.

Promonta Nervennahrung *Promonta, Ger.†.*
Lecithin; vitamins; iron; rutin; minerals.
Tonic.

Promoxil *Medpro, S.Afr.*
Amoxycillin (p.151·3).
Bacterial infections.

Promune *Procare, Austral.*
Multivitamins, amino acids, and minerals with thymus extract.
Dietary supplement.

Pro-Nat *Pro-Nat, Fr.*
A range of organ extracts (bovine) (p.1599·1).

Pronaxen *Orion, Swed.*
Naproxen (p.61·2).
Musculoskeletal and joint disorders; pain.

Prondol
John Wyeth, Irl.†; Wyeth, UK†.
Iprindole hydrochloride (p.290·2).
Depression.

Pronemia Hematinic *Lederle, USA.*
Ferrous fumarate (p.1339·3); intrinsic factor concentrate; vitamin B_{12} substances (p.1363·3); folic acid (p.1340·3).
Vitamin C (p.1365·2) is included in this preparation to increase the absorption and availability of iron.
Anaemias.

Pronerv *Gerot, Aust.*
Thiamine hydrochloride (p.1361·1) or thiamine mononitrate (p.1361·1); pyridoxine hydrochloride (p.1362·3); cyanocobalamin (p.1363·3).
Neuralgia; neuritis; neuropathies.

Pronervon N *Lappe, Ger.†.*
Melissa leaves (p.1600·1); valerian root (p.1643·1); angelica root; passion flowers (p.1615·3); calluna vulgaris; sodium phosphate; barbitone (p.642·3) or barbitone and barbitone sodium (p.642·3).
Nervous disorders.

Pronervon Phyto *Lappe, Ger.*
Valerian (p.1643·1); passion flower (p.1615·3); melissa (p.1600·1).
Agitation; sleep disorders.

Pronervon T *Lappe, Ger.*
Temazepam (p.693·3).
Sleep disorders.

Pronestyl
Bristol-Myers Squibb, Austral.; Bristol-Myers Squibb, Belg.†; Squibb, Canad.; Bristol-Myers Squibb, Irl.; Bristol-Myers Squibb, Neth.; Bristol-Myers Squibb, S.Afr.; Bristol-Myers Squibb, Switz.; Squibb, UK; Apothecon, USA.
Procainamide hydrochloride (p.934·1).
Arrhythmias.

Pronitol *Fournier SA, Spain.*
Prunus africana.
Prostatic adenoma.

Pronovan *AFI, Norw.*
Propranolol hydrochloride (p.937·1).
Angina pectoris; arrhythmias; hypertension; hyperthyroidism; migraine; myocardial infarction; tremor.

Prontal *Robapharm, Spain†.*
Codeine (p.26·1); ephedrine (p.1059·3); salicylamide (p.82·3); terpin (p.1070·2).
Respiratory-tract disorders.

Prontalgin *SPA, Ital.†.*
Ibuprofen (p.44·1).
Fever; pain.

Prontalgine *Boehringer Ingelheim, Fr.*
Paracetamol (p.72·2); dimethyl-*N*-octyl-(β-benzoyl-ethyl) ammonium bromide; codeine phosphate (p.26·1); caffeine (p.749·3).
Formerly contained paracetamol, amylobarbitone, dimethyl-*N*-octyl-(β-benzoyl-ethyl) ammonium bromide, codeine phosphate, and caffeine.
Pain.

Prontamid *SIT, Ital.*
Sulphacetamide sodium (p.252·2).
Eye infections.

Prontina *Abello, Spain†.*
Paracetamol (p.72·2).
Fever; pain.

Pronto
Note. This name is used for preparations of different composition.
Del, Canad.; Del, USA.
Shampoo: Pyrethrins; piperonyl butoxide (p.1409·3).
Pediculosis.

Del, USA.
Surface spray: Phenothrin (p.1409·2).
Lice infestation.

Pronto Emoform *Byk Gulden, Ital.*
Sodium monofluorophosphate (p.743·3); sodium fluoride (p.742·1).
Oral hygiene.

Pronto G *Edmond Pharma, Ital.†.*
Cetylpyridinium chloride (p.1106·2).
Mouth and throat infections.

Pronto Platamine *Pharmacia Upjohn, Ital.*
Cisplatin (p.513·3).
Malignant neoplasms.

Pronto Red *3M, Ital.†.*
Mercurochrome (p.1119·2).
Wound disinfection.

Prontobario
Gerot, Aust.; Bracco, Ital.
Barium sulphate (p.1003·1).
Simethicone (p.1213·1) is included in some preparations to eliminate gas from the gastro-intestinal tract before radiography.
Contrast medium for gastro-intestinal radiography.

Prontocalcin *Dompe, Ital.†.*
Salcatonin (p.735·3).
Osteoporosis; Paget's disease of bone.

Prontoclisma *Ecobi, Ital.†.*
Sorbitol (p.1354·2); docusate sodium (p.1189·3).
Constipation.

Prontogest *Amsa, Ital.*
Progesterone (p.1459·3).
Formerly known as Gestone.
Adjunct in gynaecological surgery; habitual abortion; menstrual disorders; postnatal depression; threatened abortion.

Prontokef *Master Pharma, Ital.*
Cefoperazone sodium (p.167·3).
Lignocaine hydrochloride (p.1293·2) is included in this preparation to alleviate the pain of injection.
Bacterial infections.

Prontolax *Streuli, Switz.*
Bisacodyl (p.1179·3).
Bowel evacuation; constipation.

Prontomucil *Francia, Ital.*
Guacetisal (p.1061·2).
Cold and flu symptoms; respiratory-tract congestion.

Prontopyrin plus *Mack, Illert., Ger.*
Paracetamol (p.72·2); caffeine (p.749·3).
Cold symptoms; pain.

Prontovent *Salus, Ital.*
Clenbuterol hydrochloride (p.752·1).
Obstructive airways disease.

Propa PH
Del, Canad.; Del, USA.
Salicylic acid (p.1090·2).
Acne.

Propabloc *Azupharma, Ger.*
Propranolol hydrochloride (p.937·1).
Angina pectoris; anxiety; arrhythmias; essential tremor; hypertension; hyperthyroidism; migraine.

Propac *Sherwood, USA.*
Dietary protein supplement.

Propacet *Lemmon, USA.*
Dextropropoxyphene napsylate (p.27·3); paracetamol (p.72·2).
Pain.

Propaderm
Roberts, Canad.; Glaxo Allen, Ital.†; Allen & Hanburys, S.Afr.†; Glaxo, UK.
Beclomethasone dipropionate (p.1032·1).
Skin disorders.

Propaderm-C
Glaxo Wellcome, Canad.†; Allen & Hanburys, S.Afr.†.
Beclomethasone dipropionate (p.1032·1); clioquinol (p.193·2).
Infected skin disorders.

Propafen *BASF, Ger.*
Propafenone hydrochloride (p.935·3).
Arrhythmias.

Propagest *Reed & Carnrick, USA.*
Phenylpropanolamine hydrochloride (p.1067·2).
Nasal congestion.

Propain
Note. This name is used for preparations of different composition.
Restan, S.Afr.
Syrup: Promethazine hydrochloride (p.416·2); paracetamol (p.72·2).
Pain and associated tension.

Restan, S.Afr.; Panpharma, UK.
Tablets: Paracetamol (p.72·2); codeine phosphate (p.26·1); diphenhydramine hydrochloride (p.409·1); caffeine (p.749·3).
Fever; pain and associated tension.

Propain Forte *Restan, S.Afr.*
Paracetamol (p.72·2); codeine phosphate (p.26·1); diphenhydramine (p.409·1); caffeine (p.749·3); phenobarbitone (p.350·2).
Pain and associated tension.

Propalgina Plus *Roche Nicholas, Spain.*
Ascorbic acid (p.1365·2); chlorpheniramine maleate (p.405·1); dextromethorphan hydrobromide (p.1057·3); phenylephrine hydrochloride (p.1066·2); paracetamol (p.72·2).
Formerly known as Propalgina.
Upper respiratory-tract disorders.

Propalgina PS Hot Lemon *Roche Nicholas, Spain.*
Dextromethorphan hydrobromide (p.1057·3); paracetamol (p.72·2); pseudoephedrine hydrochloride (p.1068·3).
Upper-respiratory-tract disorders.

Propamerck *Merck, Ger.*
Propafenone hydrochloride (p.935·3).
Arrhythmias.

Propan Gel-S *Propan, S.Afr.*
Aluminium hydroxide (p.1177·3); magnesium oxide (p.1198·3); dicyclomine hydrochloride (p.460·1); dimethicone (p.1213·1).
Gastro-intestinal disorders associated with hyperacidity.

Propanix *Ashbourne, UK.*
Propranolol hydrochloride (p.937·1).
Anxiety; cardiovascular disorders; essential tremor; migraine.

Propanthel *ICN, Canad.*
Propantheline bromide (p.468·1).
Anticholinergic.

Propa-Oramon *Oramon, Ger.†.*
Propafenone hydrochloride (p.935·3).
Arrhythmias.

PROPApH *Del, USA.*
Salicylic acid (p.1090·2).

Propaphenin *Rodleben, Ger.*
Chlorpromazine hydrochloride (p.649·1).
Anxiety; hiccups; nausea; pain; premedication; pruritus; psychoses; sleep disorders; vomiting.

Proparakain-POS *Ursapharm, Ger.*
Proxymetacaine hydrochloride (p.1300·1).
Local anaesthesia.

Propargile *Holistica, Fr.*
Propolis (p.1621·3); pollen; clay.
Digestive disorders.

Propastad *Stada, Ger.*
Propafenone hydrochloride (p.935·3).
Arrhythmias.

Propavan *Sanofi, Swed.*
Propiomazine maleate (p.417·3).
Sleep disorders.

Propecia *Merck, USA.*
Finasteride (p.1446·1).
Alopecia androgenetica.

Pro-Pecton Balsam *Lappe, Ger.†.*
Pulmonaria; galeopsis; plantago lanceolata; wild thyme; coltsfoot leaf (p.1057·2); guaiphenesin (p.1061·3); pumilio pine oil (p.1623·3); turpentine oil (p.1641·1); eucalyptus oil (p.1578·1); camphor (p.1557·2); menthol (p.1600·2).
Respiratory-tract disorders.

Pro-Pecton Codein Hustentropfen *Lappe, Ger.†.*
Pulmonaria; galeopsis; plantago lanceolata; wild thyme; coltsfoot leaf(p.1057·2); guaiphenesin (p.1061·3); ascorbic acid (p.1365·2); ephedrine hydrochloride (p.1059·3); codeine phosphate (p.26·1).
Coughs and associated respiratory-tract disorders.

Pro-Pecton Forte Hustensaft *Lappe, Ger.†.*
Pulmonaria; galeopsis; plantago lanceolata; wild thyme; coltsfoot leaf (p.1057·2); guaiphenesin (p.1061·3); ascorbic acid (p.1365·2); ephedrine hydrochloride (p.1059·3).
Coughs and associated respiratory-tract disorders.

Pro-Pecton Hustensaft *Lappe, Ger.†.*
Pulmonaria; galeopsis; plantago lanceolata; wild thyme; coltsfoot leaf (p.1057·2); guaiphenesin (p.1061·3); ascorbic acid (p.1365·2).
Coughs and colds.

Pro-Pecton Hustentropfen *Lappe, Ger.†.*
Pulmonaria; galeopsis; plantago lanceolata; wild thyme; coltsfoot leaf (p.1057·2); guaiphenesin (p.1061·3); ascorbic acid; ephedrine hydrochloride (p.1059·3).
Coughs and associated respiratory-tract disorders.

Propess
Ferring, Swed.; Ferring, UK.
Dinoprostone (p.1414·3).

Formerly known as Propess-RS in the *UK*.
Labour induction.

Pro-Phree Ross, USA.
Protein-free infant feed supplement.

Prophthal Procare, Austral.
Myrtillus (p.1606·1); ginkgo biloba (p.1584·1).

Prophyllen Streuli, Switz.†.
Diprophylline (p.752·1).
Obstructive airways disease.

Prophyllin Rystan, USA.
Sodium propionate (p.387·1); chlorophyllin copper complex (p.1000·1).
Contact dermatoses; dermatophytosis; eczemas; minor burns.

Prophylux Hennig, Ger.
Propranolol hydrochloride (p.937·1).
Angina pectoris; anxiety; arrhythmias; essential tremor; migraine; myocardial infarction.

Propiazol IBIS, Ital.†.
Sodium propionate (p.387·1); sulphathiazole sodium (p.257·1).
Eye infections.

Propimex Ross, USA.
A range of methionine- and valine-free preparations for enteral nutrition including an infant feed.
Methylmalonic acidaemia; propionic acidaemia.

Propine
Allergan, Austral.; Allergan, Belg.; Allergan, Canad.; Allergan, Fr.; Allergan, Irl.; Allergan, Ital.; Allergan, Norw.; Allergan, S.Afr.; Allergan, Swed.; Allergan, UK; Allergan, USA.
Dipivefrine hydrochloride (p.1572·3).
Ocular hypertension; open-angle glaucoma.

Propiocine
Roussel, Fr.; Roussel, Switz.†.
Erythromycin propionate (p.204·2).
Bacterial infections.

Propionat Farmigea, Ital.
Sodium propionate (p.387·1).
Eye disorders.

Proplex Baxter, UK.
A factor IX preparation (p.721·3).
Haemophilia B.

Proplex T
Baxter, Spain; Hyland, USA.
A factor IX preparation (p.721·3).
Haemorrhagic disorders.

Pro-Plus Roche Consumer, UK.
Caffeine (p.749·3).

Propofan Marion Merrell, Fr.
Dextropropoxyphene (p.27·3); paracetamol (p.72·2); caffeine (p.749·3).
Formerly contained dextropropoxyphene, carbaspirin calcium, paracetamol, chlorpheniramine maleate, and caffeine.
Pain.

Propolcream Bucaneve, Ital.
Propolis (p.1621·3).

Propolgel SAN, Ital.†.
Propolis (p.1621·3).

Proporal Biomedical, Ital.†.
Propolis (p.1621·3).
Oral hygiene.

Propra CT, Ger.
Propranolol hydrochloride (p.937·1).
Angina pectoris; arrhythmias; hypertension; hyperthyroidism; tremor.

Propra comp Ratiopharm, Ger.
Propranolol hydrochloride (p.937·1); triamterene (p.957·2); hydrochlorothiazide (p.885·2).
Hypertension.

Proprahexal Hexal, Aust.
Propranolol hydrochloride (p.937·1).
Angina pectoris; anxiety disorders; arrhythmias; hypertension; hyperthyroidism; migraine; phaeochromocytoma; tremor.

Propranur Henning, Ger.
Propranolol hydrochloride (p.937·1).
Angina pectoris; arrhythmias; hypertension; hyperthyroidism.

Propra-ratiopharm Ratiopharm, Ger.
Propranolol (p.937·2) or propranolol hydrochloride (p.937·1).
Angina pectoris; arrhythmias; hypertension; hyperthyroidism; tremor.

Pro-PS Procare, Austral.
Cream: Disodium fumarate (p.1083·1); cetrimide (p.1105·2); chlorhexidine gluconate (p.1107·2).
Tablets: Disodium fumarate (p.1083·1); fumaric acid (p.1083·1); vitamins; minerals.
Psoriasis.

Propulm Istoria, Ital.
Procaterol hydrochloride (p.757·3).
Obstructive airways disease.

Propulsid Janssen, USA.
Cisapride (p.1187·1).
Gastro-oesophageal reflux.

Propulsin Janssen-Cilag, Ger.
Cisapride (p.1187·1).
Gastro-intestinal disorders.

Propycil Solvay, Ger.
Propylthiouracil (p.1496·2).
Hyperthyroidism.

Propyl-Thyracil Frosst, Canad.
Propylthiouracil (p.1496·2).
Hyperthyroidism.

Propyre T Salvat, Spain.
Aspirin (p.16·1); caffeine (p.749·3); theobromine (p.765·1).
Fever; inflammation; pain.

Prorex Hyrex, USA†.
Promethazine hydrochloride (p.416·2).
Hypersensitivity reactions; motion sickness; nausea; postoperative pain (adjunct); sedative; vomiting.

Prorhinel
Monal, Fr.; Stiefel, Ger.; Monal, Neth.†; Interdelta, Switz.
Benzododecinium bromide (p.1103·2); polysorbate 80 (p.1327·3).
Nose and throat disorders.

Prorynorm Hexal, Ger.
Propafenone hydrochloride (p.935·3).
Arrhythmias.

Prosaid BHR, UK.
Naproxen (p.61·2).
Musculoskeletal and joint disorders.

Prosanon Cidan, Spain†.
Hydrochlorothiazide (p.885·2); papain (p.1614·1); quercetin (p.1580·2); retinol acetate (p.1359·2).
Vascular disorders.

Prosbis Llorente, Spain†.
Amoxycillin trihydrate (p.151·3); bromhexine hydrochloride (p.1055·3).
Respiratory-tract infections.

Proscar
Merck Sharp & Dohme, Aust.; Merck Sharp & Dohme, Austral.; Merck Sharp & Dohme, Belg.; Merck Sharp & Dohme, Canad.; MSD Chibropharm, Ger.; Merck Sharp & Dohme, Irl.; Merck Sharp & Dohme, Ital.; Merck Sharp & Dohme, Neth.; Merck Sharp & Dohme, Norw.; Merck Sharp & Dohme, S.Afr.; Merck Sharp & Dohme, Spain; Merck Sharp & Dohme, Swed.; Merck Sharp & Dohme, Switz.; Merck Sharp & Dohme, UK; Merck Sharp & Dohme, USA.
Finasteride (p.1446·1).
Benign prostatic hyperplasia.

Prosed/DS Star, USA.
Hexamine (p.216·1); salol (p.83·1); methylene blue (p.984·3); benzoic acid (p.1102·3); atropine sulphate (p.455·1); hyoscyamine sulphate (p.464·2).
Pain and discomfort of the urinary tract.

Prosed-X Procare, Austral.
Valerian (p.1643·1); lupulus (p.1597·2); passion flower (p.1615·3).
Anxiety; insomnia.

Proser Ibirn, Ital.
Saw palmetto (p.1462·1).
Prostatic hyperplasia.

Prosiston Schering, Ger.
Norethisterone acetate (p.1453·1); ethinyloestradiol (p.1445·1).
Menstrual disorders.

Proskin
Note. This name is used for preparations of different composition.
Procare, Austral.
Multivitamin and mineral preparation.
Dietary supplement; skin disorders.

Upsamedica, Spain.
Dimethicone (p.1384·2); thiomersal (p.1126·3); zinc oxide (p.1096·2).
Skin disorders.

Proslender Procare, Austral.
Glymnema sylvestre.
Obesity.

Proslim-Lipid Procare, Austral.
Purified bile extract (p.1553·2).
Obesity.

Prosobee
Mead Johnson, Austral.; Mead Johnson, Canad.; Mead Johnson, Fr.; Bristol-Myers Squibb, Irl.; Mead Johnson, Ital.; Bristol-Myers Squibb, Norw.†; Mead Johnson Nutritionals, UK; Mead Johnson Nutritionals, USA.
Infant feed.
Cow's milk intolerance; galactokinase deficiency; galactosaemia; lactose or sucrose intolerance.

Pro-Sof Plus Vangard, USA.
Docusate sodium (p.1189·3); casanthranol (p.1182·3).
Constipation.

ProSol Baxter, USA.
Amino-acid infusion.
Parenteral nutrition.

Prosom
Abbott, Canad.†; Abbott, USA.
Estazolam (p.669·2).
Insomnia.

Prospan
Salus, Aust.; Engelhard, Ger.; Engelhard, Switz.
Hedera helix.
Respiratory-tract disorders associated with excess viscous mucus.

Prospervital Provita, Aust.
Deanol bitartrate (p.1478·2); orotic acid (p.1611·2); pentetrazol (p.1484·2); inositol nicotinate (p.891·3).

Prosplen Stroschein, Ger.†.
Extract of cow spleen.
Hypersensitivity reactions; immunostimulant; radiation injury.

Prost-1 Procare, Austral.
Vitamins; amino acids; minerals; harpagophytum procumbens (p.27·2); yucca; salix (p.82·3); green-lipped mussel (p.1586·3); bromelains (p.1555·1); papain (p.1614·1).
Dietary supplement; musculoskeletal and joint disorders.

Prost-2 Procare, Austral.
Vitamins; minerals; green-lipped mussel (p.1586·3); bromelains (p.1555·1); papain (p.1614·1).
Dietary supplement.

Prosta Procare, Austral.
Saw palmetto (p.1462·1).
Benign prostatic hyperplasia.

Prosta Fink forte Fink, Ger.; Kade, Ger.
Cucurbita (p.1569·1).
Prostatic disorders.

Prosta Fink N Fink, Ger.; Kade, Ger.
Saw palmetto (p.1462·1); cucurbita (p.1569·1).
Prostatic disorders.

Prosta-Caps Chassot N Ebi, Switz.
Cucurbita (p.1569·1); cucurbita oil; saw palmetto (p.1462·1); echinacea angustifolia (p.1574·2); rubia tinctorum; orthosiphon (p.1592·2); ononis (p.1610·2).
Benign prostatic hyperplasia.

Prosta-Caps Fink SmithKline Beecham Consumer, Switz.
Cucurbita (p.1569·1); cucurbita oil; saw palmetto (p.1462·1).
Benign prostatic hyperplasia.

Prostacur Pras, Spain.
Flutamide (p.537·1).
Prostatic cancer.

Prostadilat Pfizer, Aust.
Doxazosin mesylate (p.862·3).
Benign prostatic hyperplasia; hypertension.

Prostaflor
Schoeller, Aust.; Schieffer, Switz.
Pollen extracts.
Benign prostatic hyperplasia.

Prostaforton Plantorgan, Ger.
Urtica root (p.1642·3).
Prostatic disorders.

Prostagalen Galenika, Ger.
Urtica root (p.1642·3).
Prostagalen N formerly contained serenoa serrulata, hamamelis, urtica root, and ononis.
Prostatic disorders.

Prostagutt Austroplant, Aust.
Saw palmetto (p.1462·1); populi trem. (p.1620·1); urtica dioica (p.1642·3).
Benign prostatic hyperplasia; bladder disorders.

Prostagutt forte Schwabe, Ger.
Sago palm; urtica (p.1642·3).
Prostatic disorders.

Prostagutt mono Schwabe, Ger.
Sago palm.
Prostatic disorders.

Prostagutt Tropfen Schwabe, Ger.†.
Saw palmetto (p.1462·1); urtica (p.1642·3); poplar buds (p.1620·1).
Prostatic disorders.

Prostagutt uno Schwabe, Ger.
Sago palm.
Prostatic disorders.

Prostagutt-F Schwabe, Switz.
Saw palmetto (p.1462·1); urtica (p.1642·3).
Benign prostatic hyperplasia.

Prostaherb Cucurbitae Redel, Ger.
Cucurbita (p.1569·1).
Prostatic disorders.

Prostaherb N Redel, Ger.
Urtica root (p.1642·3).
Prostatic disorders.

Prostal
Note. This name is used for preparations of different composition.
Teikoku, Jpn.
Chlormadinone acetate (p.1439·1).
Prostatic cancer; prostatic hyperplasia.

Rolab, S.Afr.
Metoclopramide hydrochloride (p.1200·3).
Gastro-intestinal disorders.

Prostalog Tosse, Ger.
Cucurbita (p.1569·1).
Prostatic disorders.

Prostamal Prodes, Spain.
Prunus africana.
Prostatic adenoma.

Prostamed Klein, Ger.
Cucurbita (p.1569·1); solidago virgaurea; poplar buds (p.1620·1).
Urinary-tract disorders.

Prostamol uno Berlin-Chemie, Ger.†.
Saw palmetto (p.1462·1).
Prostatic hyperplasia.

Prostandin Ono, Jpn.
Alprostadil alfadex (p.1413·1).
Peripheral vascular disorders.

Prostaneurin Heumann, Ger.
Urtica (p.1642·3).
Prostatic hyperplasia.

Prostap
Wyeth, Irl.; Lederle, UK.
Leuprorelin acetate (p.1253·1).
Endometriosis; prostatic cancer; uterine fibroids.

Prostaphlin Apothecon, USA†.
Oxacillin sodium (p.234·2).
Bacterial infections.

Prostarmon.E Ono, Jpn†.
Dinoprostone β-cyclodextrin clathrate (p.1416·2).
Induction and augmentation of labour.

Prostarmon.F Ono, Jpn†.
Dinoprost (p.1414·2).
Ileus; induction and augmentation of labour; intestinal paralysis following surgery; termination of pregnancy.

Prostasal TAD, Ger.
Sitosterol (p.1279·3).
Prostatic disorders.

Prostasan N Bioforce, Switz.
Saw palmetto (p.1462·1).
Benign prostatic hyperplasia.

Prostaselect Dreluso, Ger.
Homoeopathic preparation.

Prostaserene Therabel Pharma, Belg.
Saw palmetto (p.1462·1).
Micturition disorders due to benign prostatic hyperplasia.

Prostasyx Syxyl, Ger.
Homoeopathic preparation.

Prostata-Echtroplex Weber & Weber, Ger.†.
Homoeopathic preparation.

Prostata-Entoxin N Klein & Steube, Ger.†.
Homoeopathic preparation.

Prostata-Gastreu N R25 Reckeweg, Ger.
Homoeopathic preparation.

Prostata-Komplex N Ho-Fu-Complex Liebermann, Ger.
Homoeopathic preparation.

Prostata-Kurbis S Twardy, Ger.
Cucurbita (p.1569·1); cucurbita oil; sago palm.
Urinary-tract disorders.

Prostatin F Kanoldt, Ger.
Bearberry (p.1552·2); urtica root (p.1642·3).
Prostatitis.

Prostatin N Kanoldt, Ger.†.
Etenzamide (p.35·3); bearberry (p.1552·2); urtica root (p.1642·3).
Urinary-tract disorders.

Prostatin N Liquidum Kanoldt, Ger.†.
Urtica root (p.1642·3); saw palmetto (p.1462·1); bearberry (p.1552·2).
Urinary-tract disorders.

Prostatonin
Bender, Aust.; Pharmaton, Switz.
Pygeum africanum (p.1461·3); urtica (p.1642·3).
Benign prostatic hyperplasia.

Prostaturol Homberger, Switz.†.
Homoeopathic preparation.

Prosta-Urgenin
Madaus, Belg.; Madaus, Ger.
Saw palmetto (p.1462·1).
Prostatic hyperplasia.

Prosta-Urgenine Madaus, Switz.
Saw palmetto (p.1462·1).
Benign prostatic hyperplasia.

Prostavasin
Gebro, Aust.; Schwarz, Ger.; Schwarz, Ital.
Alprostadil alfadex (p.1413·1).
Peripheral vascular disorders.

Prostawern Wernigerode, Ger.
Urtica (p.1642·3).
Prostatic disorders.

Prosteo Procare, Austral.
Calcium gluconate (p.1155·2); calcium carbonate (p.1182·1); cholecalciferol (p.1366·3); dolomite.
Calcium supplement.

Prostep
Glaxo Wellcome, Austral.; Boehringer Ingelheim, Canad.; Lederle, USA.
Nicotine (p.1607·2).
Aid to smoking withdrawal.

Prostess TAD, Ger.
Saw palmetto (p.1462·1).
Benign prostatic hyperplasia.

Prostetin Takeda, Jpn.
Oxendolone.
Prostatic hyperplasia.

Prostide Sigma-Tau, Ital.
Finasteride (p.1446·1).
Benign prostatic hyperplasia.

Prostigmin
Roche, Aust.; Roche, Austral.†; ICN, Canad.; Roche, Ger.†; Roche, Irl.; Roche, Neth.; Roche, Norw.; Roche, S.Afr.†; Roche, UK†; ICN, USA.
Neostigmine bromide (p.1393·3) or neostigmine methylsulphate (p.1394·1).
Myasthenia gravis; paralytic ileus; postoperative distension and urinary retention; reversal of competitive neuromuscular blockade.

Prostigmina Roche, Ital.
Neostigmine methylsulphate (p.1394·1).
Anticholinesterase; parasympathomimetic.

Prostigmine
Roche, Belg.; Roche, Fr.; Roche, Spain; Roche, Switz.
Neostigmine methylsulphate (p.1394·1).
Ileus; meteorism; myasthenia gravis; postoperative intestinal atony; postoperative urinary retention; reversal of competitive neuromuscular blockade.

Prostin Upjohn, Swed.†.
Dinoprost trometamol (p.1414·2).
Termination of pregnancy.

Prostin E2
Pharmacia Upjohn, Aust.; Pharmacia Upjohn, Austral.; Pharmacia Upjohn, Belg.; Pharmacia Upjohn, Canad.; Pharmacia Upjohn, Irl.;

Pharmacia Upjohn, Ital.; Pharmacia Upjohn, Neth.; Pharmacia Upjohn, S.Afr.; Pharmacia Upjohn, Switz.; Upjohn, UK; Upjohn, USA.
Dinoprostone (p.1414·3).
Hydatidiform mole; intra-uterine death; labour induction; termination of pregnancy.

Prostin F2 Alpha
Pharmacia Upjohn, Austral.; Pharmacia Upjohn, Irl.; Pharmacia Upjohn, Ital.†; Pharmacia Upjohn, S.Afr.; Upjohn, UK.
Dinoprost trometamol (p.1414·2).
Labour induction; termination of pregnancy.

Prostin VR
Pharmacia Upjohn, Austral.; Pharmacia Upjohn, Belg.; Pharmacia Upjohn, Canad.; Pharmacia Upjohn, Ital.; Pharmacia Upjohn, Neth.; Pharmacia Upjohn, S.Afr.; Pharmacia Upjohn, Switz.; Upjohn, UK; Upjohn, USA.
Alprostadil (p.1412·2).
Maintenance of patent ductus arteriosus.

Prostine E_2 *Pharmacia Upjohn, Fr.*
Dinoprostone (p.1414·3).
Hydatidiform mole; labour induction; termination of pregnancy.

Prostine F_2 Alpha *Pharmacia Upjohn, Fr.*
Dinoprost trometamol (p.1414·2).
Labour induction.

Prostine VR *Pharmacia Upjohn, Fr.*
Alprostadil (p.1412·2).
Maintenance of patent ductus arteriosus.

Prostinfenem *Pharmacia Upjohn, Swed.*
Carboprost trometamol (p.1414·1).
Postpartum haemorrhage; termination of pregnancy.

Prostin/15M *Pharmacia Upjohn, Neth.*
Carboprost trometamol (p.1414·1).
Intra-uterine death; termination of pregnancy.

Prostivas
Pharmacia Upjohn, Norw.; Pharmacia Upjohn, Swed.
Alprostadil (p.1412·2).
Maintenance of patent ductus arteriosus.

Prostogenat *Azupharma, Ger.*
Flutamide (p.537·1).
Prostatic cancer.

Prosturol *Knoll, Spain.*
Benzydamine hydrochloride (p.21·3); prunus africana.
Prostatic adenoma.

Prost-X *Homeocan, Canad.*
Homoeopathic preparation.

Prosulf *CP Pharmaceuticals, UK.*
Protamine sulphate (p.993·1).
Neutralisation of heparin activity.

Pro-Symbioflor
Peithner, Aust.; Symbiopharm, Ger.
Autolysates of: *Escherichia coli*; *Enterococcus faecalis* (p.1594·1).
Gastro-intestinal disorders.

Protactyl *Wyeth, Ger.*
Promazine hydrochloride (p.689·1).
Psychiatric disorders.

Protagens *Thilo, Neth.†.*
Povidone (p.1474·2).
Dry eyes.

Protagent
Agepha, Aust.; Bournonville, Belg.; Alcon-Thilo, Ger.; Alcon, Switz.
Povidone (p.1474·2).
Dry eyes; eye irritation.

Protalgia *Reig Jofre, Spain.*
Fosfosal (p.42·3).
Pain.

Protamide *Therabel Pharma, Belg.*
Stomach extract.
Postherpetic neuralgia.

Protamine Zinc Insulin MC *Novo Nordisk, Austral.†.*
Protamine zinc insulin suspension (bovine, monocomponent) (p.322·1).
Diabetes mellitus.

Protangix *Soekami, Fr.†.*
Dipyridamole (p.857·1).
Coronary disorders; thrombo-embolic disorders.

Protaphan HM *Novo Nordisk, Ger.*
Neutral isophane insulin injection (human) (p.322·1).
Diabetes mellitus.

Protaphane HM
Novo Nordisk, Austral.; Novo Nordisk, Ital.; Novo Nordisk, S.Afr.
Isophane insulin injection (human, monocomponent) (p.322·1).
Diabetes mellitus.

Protar Protein *Dermol, USA.*
Coal tar (p.1092·3).

Protasol *Agepha, Aust.*
Comfort drops for hard contact lenses.

Protat *Potter's, UK.*
Corn silk; kava (p.1592·3).
Bladder discomfort.

Protaxil *Rottapharm, Spain.*
Proglumetacin maleate (p.81·2).
Gout; musculoskeletal, joint, and peri-articular disorders; pain.

Protaxon
Mayrhofer, Aust.; Opfermann, Ger.
Proglumetacin maleate (p.81·2).
Gout; musculoskeletal, joint, peri-articular, and soft-tissue disorders.

Proteamin *Tanabe, Jpn.*
Amino-acid and carbohydrate infusion.
Parenteral nutrition.

Protec *Protec, UK.*
Dioctyl adipate (p.1405·3).
Formerly known as Gurkha.
Insect repellent.

Pro-Tec Sport *Allergan, Canad.*
SPF 20: Ethylhexyl *p*-methoxycinnamate (p.1487·1); octyl salicylate (p.1487·3); oxybenzone (p.1487·3).
Sunscreen.

ProTech *Triton, USA.*
Povidone-iodine (p.1123·3); lignocaine hydrochloride (p.1293·2).
Burns; cuts.

Protecor *Duopharm, Ger.*
Crataegus (p.1568·2); magnesium complex with acid hydrolysate of corn starch; alpha tocopheryl acetate (p.1369·2).
Cardiovascular disorders.

Protectaid *Axcan, Canad.*
Nonoxinol 9 (p.1326·1); sodium cholate; benzalkonium chloride (p.1101·3).
Contraceptive.

Protecteur Levres *Lancome, Canad.*
SPF 15: Ethylhexyl *p*-methoxycinnamate (p.1487·1); titanium dioxide (p.1093·3).
Sunscreen.

Protectin-OPT *Truw, Ger.†.*
Aspirin (p.16·1).
Thrombo-embolic disorders.

Protective Healing Cream *Numark, UK†.*
Zinc oxide (p.1096·2).

Protecto *National Care, Canad.*
Benzethonium chloride (p.1102·3); zinc oxide (p.1096·2).
Barrier cream.

Protecto-Derm *Ingram & Bell, Canad.*
Silicone (p.1384·2).
Barrier cream.

Protectol *Daniels, USA.*
Calcium undecenoate (p.389·2).
Bromhidrosis; fungal skin infections; hyperhidrosis; minor skin irritation; nappy rash.

Protecton *Fink, Ger.†.*
Selenium with vitamin E.

Protector *Syntex, Spain.*
Diphenoxylate hydrochloride (p.1189·1).
Atropine sulphate (p.455·1) is included in this preparation to discourage abuse.
Diarrhoea.

Protegra *Lederle, USA.*
Multivitamin and mineral preparation.

Protein Free Diet (Product 80056) *Mead Johnson, Austral.*
Preparation for infant enteral nutrition.
Disorders of amino acid metabolism.

Protein 2 Medi-Test *Macherey Nagel Duren, S.Afr.*
Test for protein and pH in urine.

Protein Plus *Nutricia, Austral.*
High protein enteral feed.

Protein-Free *Mead Johnson, Ital.*
Food for low-protein diets.

Proteinsteril *Fresenius, Switz.†.*
Amino-acid infusion with or without electrolytes.
Parenteral nutrition.

Proteinsteril Hepa *Fresenius, Belg.*
Amino-acid infusion.
Parenteral nutrition in liver failure.

Proteinsteril KE *Fresenius, Belg.*
Amino-acid infusion with electrolytes.
Parenteral nutrition.

Proteinsteril KE Nephro *Fresenius, Belg.†.*
Amino-acid infusion.
Parenteral nutrition in kidney failure.

Protemp *Procare, Austral.*
Vitamins; minerals; bearberry (p.1552·2); parsley (p.1615·3); juniper (p.1592·2); viburnum opulus.
Dietary supplement; premenstrual syndrome.

Proten plus *Fresenius, Switz.†.*
Preparation for enteral nutrition.

Protenate *Hyland, USA.*
Plasma protein fraction (p.726·3).
Hypoproteinaemia; hypovolaemia.

Protensin-M *Bristol-Myers Squibb, S.Afr.*
Hydroflumethiazide (p.889·2); reserpine (p.942·1).
Hypertension.

Proteoferrina *Bayer, Ital.*
Iron succinyl-protein complex (p.1349·2).
Iron deficiency; iron-deficiency anaemia.

Proteolis *Benvegna, Ital.†.*
Bromelains (p.1555·1).
Inflammation and oedema.

Proteoseryl *Splenodex, Fr.†.*
Horse blood extract.
Wounds.

Proteosulfan *Gallier, Fr.†.*
Sulphur proteolysate (p.1091·2); aspirin (p.16·1).
Musculoskeletal and joint disorders.

Proteozym *Wiedemann, Ger.*
Bromelains (p.1555·1).
Inflammation; oedema.

Protergan Geriat *Andreu, Spain†.*
Vitamin B substances; magnesium oxoglurate; timonacic sodium; timonacic; amino acids; suprarenal cortex.
Tonic.

Protergan Pediat *Andreu, Spain†.*
Vitamin B substances; magnesium oxoglurate; timonacic; amino acids; thioctic acid.
Tonic.

Proteroxyna *Proter, Ital.†.*
Oxytetracycline (p.235·1); lignocaine (p.1293·2).
Bacterial infections.

Proterytrin *Proter, Ital.†.*
Erythromycin estolate (p.204·1) or erythromycin ethyl succinate (p.204·2).
Bacterial infections.

Prothanon
ankerpharm, Ger.†.
Eye drops; nose drops: Dioxopromethazine hydrochloride (p.417·1); naphazoline hydrochloride (p.1064·2).
Conjunctivitis; rhinitis.

LAW, Ger.
Topical gel: Dioxopromethazine hydrochloride (p.417·1).
Skin disorders.

Prothanon Cromo *ankerpharm, Ger.*
Sodium cromoglycate (p.762·1).
Allergic conjunctivitis; allergic rhinitis.

Prothazin *Rodleben, Ger.; UCB, Ger.; Wernigerode, Ger.*
Promethazine hydrochloride (p.416·2).
Allergic disorders; anxiety; biliary spasm; insomnia; premedication; psychoses; vomiting.

Prothazine
Rhone-Poulenc Rorer, Austral.†; Vortech, USA.
Promethazine hydrochloride (p.416·2).
Hypersensitivity reactions; motion sickness; nausea; postoperative pain (adjunct); sedative; vomiting.

Prothera *ICN, USA†.*
Skin cleanser.

Prothiaden
Knoll, Austral.; Knoll, Belg.; Knoll, Fr.; Knoll, Irl.; Knoll, Neth.; Knoll, S.Afr.; Alter, Spain; Knoll, UK.
Dothiepin hydrochloride (p.283·1).
Depression; mixed anxiety depressive states.

Prothil *Solvay, Ger.*
Medrogestone (p.1448·2).
Menopausal disorders; menstrual disorders; threatened and habitual abortion.

Prothiucil *Donau, Aust.*
Propylthiouracil (p.1496·2).
Hyperthyroidism; ulcerative colitis.

Prothromplex
Immuno, Aust.; Immuno, Ger.; Omnimed, S.Afr.; Immuno, Swed.†; Immuno, Switz.; Immuno, UK.
A factor IX preparation (p.721·3).
Haemorrhagic disorders.

Prothyrid
Mayrhofer, Aust.†; Henning, Ger.
Thyroxine sodium (p.1497·1); liothyronine hydrochloride (p.1495·2).
Hypothyroidism; thyroiditis.

Prothyrysat *Ysatfabrik, Ger.*
Lycopus europaeus.
Hyperthyroidism.

Protiaden
Nordmark, Ital.; Knoll, Switz.
Dothiepin hydrochloride (p.283·1).
Depression; mixed anxiety depressive states.

Protid *Lunsco, USA.*
Paracetamol (p.72·2); chlorpheniramine maleate (p.405·1); phenylephrine hydrochloride (p.1066·2).

Protidepar *Zilliken, Ital.†.*
Cyanocobalamin (p.1363·3); folic acid (p.1340·3); nicotinamide (p.1351·2); ascorbic acid (p.1365·2); inositol (p.1591·1).
Anaemias; liver disorders; neuralgias; neuritis; tonic.

Protidepar 100 *Zilliken, Ital.†.*
Cyanocobalamin (p.1363·3); folic acid (p.1340·3); nicotinamide (p.1351·2); ascorbic acid (p.1365·2); inositol (p.1591·1); suprarenal cortex (p.1050·1).
Anaemias; liver disorders; neuralgias; neuritis; tonic.

Protifar
Nutricia, Irl.; Nutricia, Ital.; Nutricia, UK.
Food for special diets.
Hypoproteinaemia.

Protifortf *Pharmygiene, Fr.*
Preparation for enteral nutrition.

Protil *Diepal, Fr.*
High protein nutritional supplement.

Protilase *Rugby, USA.*
Pancrelipase (p.1613·3).
Pancreatic enzyme deficiency.

Protina G *Torre, Ital.*
Preparation for enteral nutrition.

Protina Torre MP *Torre, Ital.*
Preparation for enteral nutrition.

Protinutril *Pharmacia Upjohn, Fr.*
Amino-acid, vitamin, and mineral infusion.
Parenteral nutrition.

Protipharm *DHN, Fr.*
A range of nutritional supplements.

Protireal *Sodietal, Fr.*
Preparation for enteral nutrition.

Protitis *Molitor, Ger.†.*
Suppositories: Saw palmetto (p.1462·1); echinacea (p.1574·2); belladonna (p.457·1); chelidonium majus; ichthammol (p.1083·3); guaiazulene (p.1586·3).
Tablets: Scopolia carniolica root; echinacea (p.1574·2); chelidonium majus; ononis (p.1610·2); equisetum (p.1575·1); aesculus (p.1543·3); benzyl mandelate; docusate sodium (p.1189·3); vitamins.
Urinary-tract disorders.

Protium
Knoll, Irl.; Knoll, UK.
Pantoprazole sodium (p.1207·3).
Gastro-oesophageal reflux; peptic ulcer.

Protoferron *UCB, Spain†.*
Ferritin (p.1580·1).
Iron-deficiency anaemia.

Protol *Procare, Austral.*
Vitamins; minerals; garlic (p.1583·1).
Dietary supplement; viral infections.

Protopam
Wyeth-Ayerst, Canad.; Ayerst, USA.
Pralidoxime chloride (p.992·2).
Anticholinesterase antagonist; organophosphorus insecticide poisoning.

Protopanyl *Romigal, Ger.†.*
Lecithin; vitamins; minerals; hop flower.
Tonic.

Protostat *Ortho Pharmaceutical, USA.*
Metronidazole (p.585·1).
Amoebiasis; anaerobic bacterial infections; trichomoniasis.

Prototapen *Bristol-Myers Squibb, Fr.†.*
Ampicillin trihydrate (p.153·2).
Probenecid (p.394·3) is included in this preparation to reduce renal tubular excretion of ampicillin.
Gonorrhoea.

Protovit
Roche, Aust.†; Roche, Belg.; Roche, Ital.; Roche Nicholas, Spain.
Multivitamin preparation.

Protovit N *Roche, Switz.†.*
Multivitamin preparation.

Protraz *Propan-Vernleigh, S.Afr.†.*
Nitrazepam (p.682·2).
Insomnia.

Protromplex TIM 3 *Immuno, Ital.*
Factor IX (p.721·3).
Deficiency of factors II, IX, and X.

Protropin
Roche, Canad.; Genentech, USA.
Somatrem (p.1249·3).
Growth hormone deficiency.

Protuss *Horizon, USA.*
Hydrocodone tartrate (p.43·1); potassium guaiacolsulfonate (p.1068·3).

Protuss DM *Horizon, USA.*
Guaiphenesin (p.1061·3); pseudoephedrine hydrochloride (p.1068·3); dextromethorphan hydrobromide (p.1057·3).
Coughs.

Protuss-D *Horizon, USA.*
Hydrocodone tartrate (p.43·1); pseudoephedrine hydrochloride (p.1068·3); potassium guaiacolsulfonate (p.1068·3).
Coughs.

Pro-Uro *Ghimas, Ital.*
Pipemidic acid (p.237·2).
Urinary-tract infections.

Provames *Cassenne, Fr.*
Oestradiol (p.1455·1).
Menopausal disorders; osteoporosis.

Provascul *Gerot, Aust.*
Bamethan succinate (p.827·1).
Peripheral vascular disorders.

Provatene *Solgar, USA†.*
Betacarotene (p.1335·2).
Erythropoietic protoporphyria.

Provelle *Pharmacia Upjohn, Austral.*
28 Tablets, conjugated oestrogens (p.1457·3); 14 or 28 tablets, medroxyprogesterone acetate (p.1448·3).
Menopausal disorders; osteoporosis.

Provenal *Pulitzer, Ital.*
A heparinoid (p.882·3).
Vascular disorders with a risk of thrombosis.

Proveno N *Madaus, Ger.*
Aescin (p.1543·3).
Vascular disorders.

Pro-Vent *Wellcome, Irl.*
Theophylline (p.765·1).
Bronchospasm.

Proventil *Schering, USA; Key, USA.*
Salbutamol (p.758·2) or salbutamol sulphate (p.758·2).
Bronchospasm.

Provera
Pharmacia Upjohn, Aust.; Pharmacia Upjohn, Austral.; Pharmacia Upjohn, Belg.; Pharmacia Upjohn, Canad.; Pharmacia Upjohn, Irl.; Pharmacia Upjohn, Ital.; Pharmacia Upjohn, Neth.; Pharmacia Upjohn, Norw.; Pharmacia Upjohn, S.Afr.; Pharmacia Upjohn, Swed.; Pharmacia Upjohn, Switz.; Pharmacia Upjohn, UK; Upjohn, USA.
Medroxyprogesterone acetate (p.1448·3).
Endometriosis; malignant neoplasms; menopausal disorders; menorrhagia; secondary amenorrhoea.

Provertin-UM TIM 3 *Immuno, Ital.*
Factor VII (p.720·2).
Factor VII deficiency.

Provide *Rowa, Irl.*
Gluten-, lactose-, and milk-free food for special diets.
Bowel disorders; nutritional supplement.

Provigil *Cephalon, UK.*
Modafinil (p.1483·3).
Narcoleptic syndrome.

Provimicina Sabater, Spain†.
Demeclocycline (p.201·2).
Bacterial infections.

Proviodine Rougier, Canad.
Povidone-iodine (p.1123·3).
Burns; skin and mucous membrane disinfection; vaginal infections; wounds.

Provipen Sabater, Spain†.
Benzylpenicillin (p.159·2); procaine penicillin (p.240·2); benzathine penicillin (p.158·3).
Bacterial infections; rheumatic fever.

Provipen Benzatina Sabater, Spain†.
Benzathine penicillin (p.158·3).
Bacterial infections; rheumatic fever.

Provipen Procaina Sabater, Spain†.
Procaine penicillin (p.240·2).
Bacterial infections.

Proviron
Schering, Aust.; Schering, Austral.; Schering, Belg.; Schering, Fr.; Schering, Ger.; Schering, Ital.; Schering, Neth.; Schering, S.Afr.; Schering, Spain; Schering, Switz.; Schering, UK.
Mesterolone (p.1450·1).
Anaemia; androgenic; hypogonadism; impotence; male infertility.

Provisc
Alcon, Aust.; Alcon, Austral.; Alcon, Belg.; Alcon, Fr.; Alcon-Thilo, Ger.; Alcon, Ital.; Alcon, Norw.†; Alcon, S.Afr.; Alcon, Swed.; Alcon, UK.
Sodium hyaluronate (p.1630·3).
Adjunct in eye surgery.

Provitamin A-E Cielle, Ital.
Vitamin A (p.1358·1); vitamin E (p.1369·1); royal jelly (p.1626·3).
Nutritional supplement.

Provocholine Roche, USA.
Methacholine chloride (p.1393·2).
Diagnosis of bronchial hyperreactivity.

Provotest Hoechst, Ger.
Dichlorodifluoromethane (p.1164·3).
Diagnostic agent.

Prowess Harley Street Supplies, UK.
Yohimbine hydrochloride (p.1645·3); pemoline (p.1484·1); methyltestosterone (p.1450·3).
Sexual disorders.

Prowess Plain Harley Street Supplies, UK.
Yohimbine hydrochloride (p.1645·3).
Impotence.

ProWohl Eurim, Ger.
Magaldrate (p.1198·1).
Gastro-intestinal disorders.

Proxen
Grunenthal, Aust.; Macarthur, Austral.; Syntex, Ger.; Roche, Ger.; Garec, S.Afr.; Berenguer Infale, Spain; Grunenthal, Switz.
Naproxen (p.61·2) or naproxen lysine (p.62·1).
Fever; gout; musculoskeletal, joint, peri-articular, and soft-tissue disorders; pain.

Proxidin Procare, Austral.
Vitamins; minerals; garlic; eleutherococcus senticosus.
Dietary supplement.

Proxigel Reed & Carnrick, USA.
Urea hydrogen peroxide (p.1127·3).
Oral inflammation.

Proxil Rottapharm, Ital.
Proglumetacin dimaleate (p.81·2).
Inflammation; pain.

Proxine Del Saz & Filippini, Ital.
Naproxen (p.61·2).
Musculoskeletal and joint disorders; pain.

Proxy Parmed, USA†.
Dextropropoxyphene hydrochloride (p.27·3); paracetamol (p.72·2).

Proxy-Retardoral Artesan, Ger.†.
Proxyphylline (p.757·3).
Asthmatic disorders; bronchospastic disorders; emphysema.

Proyeast Procare, Austral.
Garlic (p.1583·1); echinacea (p.1574·2); ascorbic acid (p.1365·2); chapparal (p.1562·1); zinc gluconate (p.1373·2); vitamin A (p.1358·1); pau d'arco.
Candidiasis.

Prozac
Lilly, Austral.; Lilly, Belg.; Lilly, Canad.; Lilly, Fr.; Dista, Irl.; Lilly, Irl.; Lilly, Ital.; Lilly, Neth.; Lilly, S.Afr.; Dista, Spain; Dista, UK; Dista, USA.
Fluoxetine hydrochloride (p.284·1).
Bulimia nervosa; depression; obsessive-compulsive disorder.

Prozef Bristol-Myers Squibb, S.Afr.
Cefprozil (p.172·3).
Bacterial infections.

Proziere Ashbourne, UK.
Prochlorperazine maleate (p.687·3).

Prozin Lusofarmaco, Ital.
Chlorpromazine hydrochloride (p.649·1).
Hiccups; pain; premedication; psychiatric disorders; vomiting.

Prozine
Note. This name is used for preparations of different composition.
Propan-Vernleigh, S.Afr.
Carbamazepine (p.339·2).
Epilepsy; trigeminal neuralgia.

Hauck, USA.
Promazine hydrochloride (p.689·1).
Psychoses.

Prozyme Procare, Austral.
Outer layer, pepsin (p.1616·3); bromelains (p.1555·1); glutamic acid hydrochloride (p.1344·3); inner layer, pancreatin (p.1612·1); papain (p.1614·1); bromelains.
Dyspepsia.

Prozyn Adcock Ingram, S.Afr.
Fluoxetine hydrochloride (p.284·1).
Bulimia nervosa; mixed anxiety depressive states; obsessive-compulsive disorder.

Pruina Faes, Spain.
Senna (p.1212·2); cassia fistula (p.1183·1); coriander (p.1567·3); tamarind (p.1217·3).
Constipation.

Prulet Mission Pharmacal, USA.
Phenolphthalein (p.1208·2).
Constipation.

Prunasine Christiaens, Belg.
Senna fruit (p.1212·2).
Constipation.

Prunetta Byk Gulden, Ital.†.
Phenolphthalein (p.1208·2).
Constipation.

Prunogil Diepal, Fr.
Dietary fibre supplement.
Constipation.

Prunus-Bad Weleda, Aust.
Prunus spinosa.
Tonic.

Prurex Agepha, Aust.
Diphenhydramine hydrochloride (p.409·1).
Burns; hypersensitivity reactions; insect bites; pruritus; sunburn.

Pruriderm ultra Declimed, Ger.†.
Prednisolone acetate (p.1048·1); promethazine hydrochloride (p.416·2); laureth 9 (p.1325·2).
Anogenital inflammatory skin disorders.

Pruri-med Permamed, Switz.
Sodium sulphosuccinated undecenoic acid monoethanolamide (p.389·2); laureth 9 (p.1325·2).
Skin disorders.

Prurimix Metochem, Aust.
Talc (p.1092·1); zinc oxide (p.1096·2); laureth 9 (p.1325·2); menthol (p.1600·2); diphenylpyraline hydrochloride (p.409·3).
Skin disorders.

Prurivax Qualiphar, Belg.†.
Diphenhydramine hydrochloride (p.409·1); calcium pantothenate (p.1352·3).
Skin irritation.

Pryleugan Dresden, Ger.
Imipramine hydrochloride (p.289·2).
Depression; nocturnal enuresis; pain.

Prysma UCB, Spain.
Omeprazole (p.1204·2).
Gastro-oesophageal reflux; peptic ulcer; Zollinger-Ellison syndrome.

Pselac Laevosan, Aust.
Lactitol (p.1195·2).
Constipation; hepatic encephalopathy.

Pserhofer's Agepha, Aust.
Aloes (p.1177·1); frangula (p.1193·2).

Pseudo Major, USA.
Pseudoephedrine hydrochloride (p.1068·3).
Nasal congestion.

Pseudo-Car DM Geneva, USA.
Pseudoephedrine hydrochloride (p.1068·3); carbinoxamine maleate (p.404·2); dextromethorphan hydrobromide (p.1057·3).
Coughs and cold symptoms.

Pseudocef
Grunenthal, Aust.; Takeda, Ger.
Cefsulodin sodium (p.173·2).
Lignocaine hydrochloride (p.1293·2) is included in the intramuscular injection to alleviate the pain of injection.
Bacterial infections.

Pseudo-Chlor Geneva, USA; Major, USA.
Pseudoephedrine hydrochloride (p.1068·3); chlorpheniramine maleate (p.405·1).
Upper respiratory-tract symptoms.

Pseudofrin Trianon, Canad.
Pseudoephedrine hydrochloride (p.1068·3).
Congestion.

Pseudo-Gest Major, USA.
Pseudoephedrine hydrochloride (p.1068·3).
Nasal congestion.

Pseudo-Gest Plus Major, USA.
Pseudoephedrine hydrochloride (p.1068·3); chlorpheniramine maleate (p.405·1).
Upper respiratory-tract symptoms.

Pseudophage Servier, Fr.
Sodium alginate (p.1470·3); gelidium corneum (p.1470·3).
Obesity.

Psico Blocan Estedi, Spain.
Chlordiazepoxide hydrochloride (p.646·3); hyoscine methobromide (p.463·1).
Smooth muscle spasm.

Psicoben Ravizza, Ital.†.
Benperidol (p.642·3).
Psychiatric disorders.

Psicocen Centrum, Spain.
Sulpiride (p.692·3).
Behaviour disorders; psychoses; vertigo.

Psicofar Sifarma, Ital.
Chlordiazepoxide hydrochloride (p.646·3).
Anxiety disorders; behaviour disorders in children.

Psicoperidol Lusofarmaco, Ital.†.
Trifluperidol hydrochloride (p.698·1).
Schizophrenia.

Psicosoma
Trommsdorff, Ger.†; Ferrer, Spain†.
Magnesium glutamate hydrobromide (p.1598·3).
Anxiety; behaviour disorders; insomnia; nervous disorders associated with magnesium deficiency; vascular headache.

Psicoterina Francia, Ital.†.
Chlordiazepoxide hydrochloride (p.646·3).
Psychoses.

Psilo-Balsam N Stada, Ger.
Diphenhydramine hydrochloride (p.409·1); cetylpyridinium chloride (p.1106·2).
Formerly contained diphenhydramine hydrochloride, cetylpyridinium chloride, and butoxycaine hydrochloride.
First-degree burns; insect stings; nettle rash; skin irritation; sunburn; wind burns.

Psiquiwas Wasserman, Spain†.
Oxazepam (p.683·2).
Alcohol withdrawal syndrome; anxiety; insomnia.

Psocortene Ciba-Geigy, Fr.†.
Flumethasone pivalate (p.1040·3); salicylic acid (p.1090·2); coal tar (p.1092·3).
Skin disorders.

Psoil Basotherm, Ger.†.
Thioxolone (p.1093·3); hydrocortisone (p.1043·3).
Psoriasis of the scalp.

Psomaglobin N Bayer, Ger.†.
A pseudomonas immunoglobulin (*Pseudomonas aeruginosa*) (p.1530·1).
Passive immunisation.

Psoraderm 5
Sun Life, Fr.; Pharmacal, Switz.
5-Methoxypsoralen (p.1088·3).
Psoriasis.

Psoradexan
Procter & Gamble, Aust.; Hermal, Ger.; Procter & Gamble, Switz.
Dithranol (p.1082·1); urea (p.1095·2).
Psoriasis.

Psoradrate
Procter & Gamble, Irl.; Procter & Gamble, UK†.
Dithranol (p.1082·1); urea (p.1095·2).
Psoriasis.

Psoralon MT
Hermal, Ger.; Hermal, Switz.†.
Dithranol (p.1082·1); salicylic acid (p.1090·2).
Psoriasis.

Psorantral Isdin, Spain.
Dithranol (p.1082·1); salicylic acid (p.1090·2).
Psoriasis.

Psor-a-set Hogil, USA.
Salicylic acid (p.1090·2).

Psor-asist Sunspot, Austral.
Cream: Sulphur (p.1091·2); salicylic acid (p.1090·2); coal tar (p.1092·3).
Lotion: Sulphur (p.1091·2); salicylic acid (p.1090·2); aloes (p.1177·1); urea (p.1095·2).
Psoriasis.

Psorasolv Potter's, UK.
Starch (p.1356·2); sublimed sulphur (p.1091·2); zinc oxide (p.1096·2); poke root; clivers (p.1565·2).
Psoriasis.

Psorcon Dermik, USA.
Diflorasone diacetate (p.1039·3).
Skin disorders.

Psorcutan
Schering, Aust.; Schering, Ger.; Schering, Ital.
Calcipotriol (p.1080·2).
Psoriasis.

Psoriacen Centrum, Spain†.
Polypodium leucotomos.
Skin disorders.

Psoriasdin Isdin, Spain.
Coal tar (p.1092·3).
Skin disorders.

Psoriasis-Bad Balneopharm, Ger.
Fumaric acid (p.1083·1); disodium fumarate (p.1083·1).
Bath additive; psoriasis.

Psoriasis-Salbe M Balneopharm, Ger.
Fumaric acid (p.1083·1); coal tar (p.1092·3); allantoin (p.1078·2); methyl salicylate (p.55·2); salicylic acid (p.1090·2).
Psoriasis.

Psoriasis-Solution Balneopharm, Ger.
Disodium fumarate (p.1083·1).
Psoriasis.

Psoriasis-Tabletten Balneopharm, Ger.
Sodium fumarate (p.1083·1).
Psoriasis.

Psoriasol Lalco, Canad.
Tar (p.1092·3).
Psoriasis.

Psoricreme Schering-Plough, Neth.
Dithranol (p.1082·1).
Psoriasis.

Psoriderm
Note. This name is used for preparations of different composition.
Dermal Laboratories, Irl.; Dermal Laboratories, UK.
Coal tar (p.1092·3).
Psoriasis.

Istoria, Ital.
Dithranol (p.1082·1).
Psoriasis.

Psorigel
Galderma, Austral.; Galderma, Canad.; Galderma, Irl.; Galderma, S.Afr.; Galderma, UK; Galderma, USA.
Coal tar (p.1092·3).
Eczema; psoriasis.

Psorigerb N Redel, Ger.
Salicylic acid (p.1090·2); coal tar (p.1092·3); urea (p.1095·2).
Eczema; psoriasis.

Psorimed Wolff, Ger.
Salicylic acid (p.1090·2).
Scalp disorders.

Psorin
Note. This name is used for preparations of different composition.
MPS, Austral.†; Thames, UK.
Ointment: Dithranol (p.1082·1); salicylic acid (p.1090·2); coal tar (p.1092·3).
Psoriasis.

Thames, UK.
Scalp gel: Dithranol (p.1082·1); salicylic acid (p.1090·2); methyl salicylate (p.55·2).
Psoriasis.

PsoriNail Summers, USA.
Coal tar (p.1092·3).
Psoriasis.

Psorion ICN, USA.
Betamethasone dipropionate (p.1033·3).

Psorispray Medice, Ger.†.
Coal tar (p.1092·3); undecenoic acid (p.389·2); salicylic acid (p.1090·2); dithranol (p.1082·1).
Skin disorders.

Psychatrin Jossa-Arznei, Ger.†.
Hypericum (p.1590·1).
Psychiatric disorders.

Psychobald Sigmapharm, Aust.
Valerian (p.1643·1).
Anxiety disorders; sleep disorders.

Psychoneuroticum (Rowo-578) Pharmakon, Ger.
Homoeopathic preparation.
Lignocaine hydrochloride (p.1293·2) is included in this preparation to alleviate the pain of injection.

Psychopax
Sigmapharm, Aust.; Sigmapharm, Switz.
Diazepam (p.661·1).
Anxiety; skeletal muscle spasm; sleep disorders.

Psychotonin Madaus, Aust.
Hypericum (p.1590·1).
Depression.

Psychotonin forte Steigerwald, Ger.
Hypericum (p.1590·1).
Psychiatric disorders.

Psychotonin M Steigerwald, Ger.
Hypericum (p.1590·1).
Psychiatric disorders.

Psychotonin-sed. Steigerwald, Ger.
Hypericum (p.1590·1); valerian (p.1643·1).
Psychiatric disorders.

Psychoverlan Verla, Ger.†.
Magnesium glutamate hydrobromide (p.1598·3).
Nervous system disorders.

Psycoton Esseti, Ital.
Piracetam (p.1619·1).
Mental function impairment.

Psylia Techni-Pharma, Mon.
Psyllium (p.1194·2).
Constipation.

Psymion Desitin, Ger.
Maprotiline hydrochloride (p.296·2).
Depression.

Psyquil
Bristol-Myers Squibb, Aust.; Sanofi Winthrop, Ger.; Squibb, Switz.†.
Fluopromazine (p.670·3) or fluopromazine hydrochloride (p.670·3).
Agitation; nausea and vomiting; neuroleptanalgesia; premedication; schizophrenia.

Psyquil compositum Squibb-Heyden, Ger.†.
Fluopromazine hydrochloride (p.670·3); pethidine hydrochloride (p.76·1).
Pain; premedication; sedative.

PSY-stabil Pekana, Ger.
Homoeopathic preparation.

PT 105 Legere, USA†.
Phendimetrazine (p.1484·2); phendimetrazine tartrate (p.1484·2).

PTE Lyphomed, USA.
A range of trace element preparations.
Parenteral nutrition.

Puamin Schwarzhaupt, Ger.
Lign. muira puama; yohimbe; nicametate citrate monohydrate; alpha tocopheryl acetate.
Male impotence; tonic.

Pudan-Lebertran-Zinksalbe Bano, Aust.
Zinc oxide (p.1096·2); peru balsam (p.1617·2); codliver oil (p.1337·3).
Burns; decubitus ulcer; nappy rash; wounds.

Puernol *Formenti, Ital.*
Paracetamol (p.72·2).
Fever; pain.

Puerzym *FIRMA, Ital.*
Pepsinogen.
Digestive system disorders.

Pufolic *Mavi, Ital.*
Folic acid; omega 6 and omega 3 triglycerides.
Nutritional supplement.

Puhlmann-Tee *Strunz & Korber, Aust.†.*
Coltsfoot leaf (p.1057·2); galeopsis ochroleuca; pulmonaria.

Pularin *Allen & Hanburys, S.Afr.†.*
Heparin (p.879·3).
Thrombo-embolic disorders.

Pulbil *Klinge, Ger.*
Sodium cromoglycate (p.762·1).
Asthma.

Pulmadil
3M, Belg.; 3M, Neth.; 3M, S.Afr.†; 3M, UK†.
Rimiterol hydrobromide (p.758·1).
Bronchospasm.

Pulmarin *NCSN, Ital.*
Potassium guaiacolsulfonate (p.1068·3); cineole (p.1564·1); pine oil; menthol (p.1600·2).
Catarrh.

Pulmax *Zyma, Fr.*
Peru balsam (p.1617·2); camphor (p.1557·2); eucalyptus oil (p.1578·1); rosemary oil (p.1626·2).
Respiratory-tract congestion.

Pulmaxan *Astra, Ital.*
Budesonide (p.1034·3).
Asthma.

Pulmeno *Sandoz, Spain.*
Theophylline (p.765·1).
Heart failure; obstructive airways disease; paroxysmal dyspnoea.

Pulmex
Note. This name is used for preparations of different composition.
Zyma, Aust.†.
Eucalyptus oil (p.1578·1); rosemary oil (p.1626·2); camphor (p.1557·2); peru balsam (p.1617·2).
Coughs.

Zyma, Belg.
Benzyl benzoate (p.1402·2); benzyl cinnamate; peru balsam (p.1617·2); camphor (p.1557·2); rosemary oil (p.1626·2); eucalyptus oil (p.1578·1).
Cold symptoms.

Zyma, Switz.
Ointment; capsules for inhalation: Peru balsam (p.1617·2); camphor (p.1557·2); eucalyptus oil (p.1578·1); rosemary oil (p.1626·2).
Cold symptoms; coughs.
Stick†: Peru balsam (p.1617·2); camphor (p.1557·2); eucalyptus oil (p.1578·1); rosemary oil (p.1626·2); menthol (p.1600·2).
Respiratory-tract disorders.

Pulmex Baby
Note. This name is used for preparations of different composition.
Zyma, Belg.
Benzyl benzoate (p.1402·2); benzyl cinnamate; peru balsam (p.1617·2); rosemary oil (p.1626·2); eucalyptus oil (p.1578·1).
Cold symptoms.

Zyma, Switz.
Peru balsam (p.1617·2); eucalyptus oil (p.1578·1); rosemary oil (p.1626·2).
Cold symptoms; coughs.

Pulmicort
Astra, Aust.; Astra, Austral.; Astra, Belg.; Astra, Canad.; Astra, Fr.; Astra, Ger.; Stern, Ger.; Astra, Irl.; Astra, Neth.; Astra, Norw.; Astra, S.Afr.; Astra, Spain; Draco, Swed.; Astra, Switz.; Astra, UK; Astra, USA.
Budesonide (p.1034·3).
Allergic rhinitis; asthma; croup; nasal polyps; obstructive airways disease.

Pulmicret *Stern, Ger.*
Acetylcysteine (p.1052·3).
Respiratory-tract disorders associated with increased or viscous mucus.

Pulmictan *Faes, Spain.*
Budesonide (p.1034·3).
Asthma.

Pulmidur
Astra, Aust.; Stern, Ger.
Theophylline (p.765·1).
Obstructive airways disease.

Pulmilide *Bender, Aust.*
Flunisolide hemihydrate (p.1040·3).
Asthma.

Pulminflamatoria *Faes, Spain.*
Ampicillin sodium (p.153·1); ampicillin benzathine (p.154·1); bromhexine hydrochloride (p.1055·3).
Respiratory-tract infections.

Pulmo Bailly
Bengue, Irl.; Roche Consumer, UK.
Codeine (p.26·1) or codeine phosphate (p.26·1); guaiacol (p.1061·2).
Coughs.

Pulmo Borbalan *Spyfarma, Spain.*
Amoxycillin trihydrate (p.151·3); bromhexine hydrochloride (p.1055·3).
Respiratory-tract infections.

Pulmo -cyl Ho-Len-Complex *Liebermann, Ger.*
Homoeopathic preparation.

Pulmo Grey Balsam *Orravan, Spain.*
Camphor (p.1557·2); allyl sulphide; cineole (p.1564·1); niaouli oil (p.1607·1); guaiacol (p.1061·2).
Respiratory-tract disorders.

Pulmo Menal *Alacan, Spain.*
Bromhexine hydrochloride (p.1055·3); guaiphenesin (p.1061·3); sodium benzoate (p.1102·3); co-trimoxazole (p.196·3).
Respiratory-tract infections.

Pulmocare
Abbott, Austral.; Abbott, Canad.; Abbott, Irl.; Abbott, Ital.; Abbott, UK; Ross, USA.
Preparation for enteral nutrition.
Respiratory system disorders.

Pulmoclase
Bios, Belg.; UCB, Ger.†; UCB, Irl.; UCB, Neth.
Carbocisteine (p.1056·3).
Respiratory-tract disorders associated with production of viscous mucus.

Pulmocordio forte *Hevert, Ger.*
Ammi visnaga; belladonna; ipecacuanha; kalium jodat.; thyme (p.1636·3); castanae; ephedrine hydrochloride (p.1059·3); potassium guaiacolsulfonate (p.1068·3).
Coughs and associated respiratory-tract disorders.

Pulmocordio mite SL *Hevert, Ger.*
Anise oil (p.1550·1); fennel oil (p.1579·2); liquorice (p.1197·1); thyme (p.1636·3).
Respiratory-tract disorders.

Pulmocure *Medinova, Switz.†.*
Dihydrocodeine tartrate (p.34·1); ephedrine hydrochloride (p.1059·3); guaiphenesin (p.1061·3).
Respiratory-tract disorders.

Pulmofasa *Sabater, Spain.*
Ammonium camphocarbonate diaminopyridine carboxylate (p.1477·3); calcium pantothenate (p.1352·3); cineole (p.1564·1); senega (p.1069·3); sodium benzoate (p.1102·3); potassium guaiacolsulfonate (p.1068·3); tolu balsam (p.1071·1); pinus sylvestris; anethole (p.1549·3).
Respiratory-tract disorders.

Pulmofasa Antihist *Sabater, Spain.*
Ammonium camphocarbonate (p.1477·3); calcium pantothenate (p.1352·3); cineole (p.1564·1); diphenhydramine hydrochloride (p.409·1); sodium benzoate (p.1102·3); potassium guaiacolsulfonate (p.1068·3); senega (p.1069·3); tolu balsam (p.1071·1); pinus sylvestris; anethole (p.1549·3).
Upper respiratory-tract disorders.

Pulmofluide Enfants *Phygiene, Fr.†.*
Terpin (p.1070·2); sodium benzoate (p.1102·3); guaiphenesin (p.1061·3); pholcodine (p.1068·1); Dessessartz syrup; tolu balsam (p.1071·1).
Coughs.

Pulmofluide Ephedrine *Phygiene, Fr.†.*
Ephedrine hydrochloride (p.1059·3); terpin (p.1070·2); cineole (p.1564·1); sodium benzoate (p.1102·3); guaiphenesin (p.1061·3); codeine (p.26·1); ipecacuanha (p.1062·2).
Asthma; chronic bronchitis.

Pulmofluide Simple *Phygiene, Fr.*
Terpin (p.1070·2); cineole (p.1564·1); sodium benzoate (p.1102·3); guaiphenesin (p.1061·3).
Formerly contained terpin, cineole, sodium benzoate, guaiphenesin, codeine, and ipecacuanha.
Respiratory-tract congestion.

Pulmofor *Vifor, Switz.*
Dextromethorphan hydrobromide (p.1057·3).
Coughs.

Pulmoll *SmithKline Beecham Sante, Fr.*
Terpin (p.1070·2); menthol (p.1600·2); amylocaine hydrochloride (p.1286·1).
Throat disorders.

Pulmoll au menthol et a l'eucalyptus *SmithKline Beecham Sante, Fr.*
Menthol (p.1600·2); peppermint oil (p.1208·1); eucalyptus oil (p.1578·1).
Throat disorders.

Pulmonal S *Schaper & Brummer, Ger.*
Ambroxol hydrochloride (p.1054·3).
Respiratory-tract disorders associated with increased or viscous mucus.

Pulmonase *Monin, Fr.*
Codeine (p.26·1); sodium benzoate (p.1102·3); cherry-laurel; aconite root (p.1542·2); drosera (p.1574·1); tolu balsam (p.1071·1).
Coughs.

Pulmonilo Synergium *Aristegui, Spain.*
Oxytetracycline (p.235·1); calcium guaiacolate; niaouli oil (p.1607·1); cineole (p.1564·1).
Respiratory-tract infections.

Pulmonium N *Wala, Ger.*
Plantago lanceolata; Norway spruce; petasites officinalis.
Respiratory-tract disorders.

Pulmophyllin *Propan, S.Afr.*
Theophylline (p.765·1).
Obstructive airways disease.

Pulmophylline *Riva, Canad.*
Theophylline (p.765·1).
Bronchoconstriction.

Pulmorex DM *Prodemdis, Canad.*
Diphenhydramine hydrochloride (p.409·1); dextromethorphan hydrobromide (p.1057·3); ammonium chloride (p.1055·2).

Pulmorphan *Riva, Canad.*
Dextromethorphan hydrobromide (p.1057·3); guaiphenesin (p.1061·3); pheniramine maleate (p.415·3); phenylephrine hydrochloride (p.1066·2).
Coughs.

Pulmorphan Pediatrique *Riva, Canad.*
Dextromethorphan hydrobromide (p.1057·3); pheniramine maleate (p.415·3); phenylephrine hydrochloride (p.1066·2).
Coughs.

Pulmosepta *Septa, Spain†.*
Aconite (p.1542·2); codeine phosphate (p.26·1); ipecacuanha (p.1062·2); pyridoxine hydrochloride (p.1362·3); potassium guaiacolsulfonate (p.1068·3).
Respiratory-tract disorders.

Pulmoserum *Bailly, Fr.*
Codeine (p.26·1); guaiacol (p.1061·2); phosphoric acid (p.1618·1).
Coughs.

Pulmosodyl *Bridoux, Fr.*
Ethylmorphine hydrochloride (p.36·1); bromoform (p.1620·3); potassium guaiacolsulfonate (p.1068·3); sodium benzoate (p.1102·3); cherry-laurel; tolu balsam (p.1071·1).
Coughs.

Pulmospin *Spyfarma, Spain.*
Guaiphenesin (p.1061·3); ampicillin trihydrate (p.153·2).
Respiratory-tract infections.

Pulmospir *Soekami, Fr.†.*
Codeine (p.26·1); ethylmorphine (p.36·1); belladonna (p.457·1); aconite (p.1542·2); sodium benzoate (p.1102·3); potassium sulphoguaiacolate; tolu balsam (p.1071·1).
Coughs.

Pulmosterin Duo *Normon, Spain.*
Bromhexine (p.1055·3); guaiphenesin (p.1061·3); co-trimoxazole (p.196·3).
Respiratory-tract infections.

Pulmosterin Meta *Normon, Spain.*
Bromhexine (p.1055·3); guaiphenesin (p.1061·3); metampicillin sodium (p.224·3).
Lignocaine hydrochloride (p.1293·2) is included in this preparation to alleviate the pain of injection.
Respiratory-tract infections.

Pulmosterin Retard *Normon, Spain.*
Ampicillin sodium (p.153·1); ampicillin benzathine (p.154·1); guaiphenesin (p.1061·3).
Respiratory-tract infections.

Pulmothiol *Soekami, Fr.†.*
Aconite (p.1542·2); crataegus (p.1568·2); eucalyptus (p.1578·1); senega (p.1069·3); lobelia (p.1481·3); belladonna (p.457·1); terpin (p.1070·2); potassium guaiacolsulfonate (p.1068·3); sodium bromide (p.1620·3); sodium benzoate (p.1102·3); tolu balsam (p.1071·1); Desessartz; bromoform (p.1620·3); codeine (p.26·1); white poppy; cherry-laurel.
Coughs.

Pulmo-Timelets *Temmler, Ger.*
Theophylline (p.765·1).
Obstructive airways disease.

Pulmotin *Serum-Werk Bernburg, Ger.*
Thyme (p.1636·3); guaiphenesin (p.1061·3).
Bronchitis; catarrh; coughs.

Pulmotin-N *Serum-Werk Bernburg, Ger.*
Anise oil (p.1550·1); camphor (p.1557·2); eucalyptus oil (p.1578·1); thyme oil (p.1637·1); conifer oil; thymol (p.1127·1).
Respiratory-tract disorders.

Pulmotrim *Farge, Ital.†.*
Co-trimoxazole (p.196·3); oxolamine citrate (p.1065·3).
Respiratory-tract infections.

Pulmotropic *Robert, Spain.*
Doxycycline guaiacolsulfonate (p.203·2); muramidase hydrochloride (p.1604·3).
Respiratory-tract infections.

Pulmovent *Bender, Aust.*
Acetylcysteine (p.1052·3).
Respiratory-tract disorders.

Pulmovirolo *Blue Cross, Ital.*
Potassium guaiacolsulfonate (p.1068·3).
Respiratory-tract disorders.

Pulmozyme
Roche, Aust.; Roche, Austral.; Roche, Belg.; Roche, Canad.; Roche, Fr.; Roche, Ger.; Roche, Irl.; Roche, Ital.; Roche, Neth.; Roche, Norw.; Roche, S.Afr.; Roche, Spain; Roche, Swed.; Roche, Switz.; Roche, UK; Genentech, USA.
Dornase alfa (p.1059·1).
Cystic fibrosis.

Pulpomixine *Septodont, Switz.*
Dexamethasone acetate (p.1037·1); framycetin sulphate (p.210·3); polymyxin B sulphate (p.239·1).
Dental disorders.

Pulsan *Yamanouchi, Jpn.*
Indenolol hydrochloride (p.891·1).
Angina pectoris; arrhythmias; hypertension.

Pulsar *Medosan, Ital.*
Colextran hydrochloride (p.1272·2).
Glucose metabolic disorders; hyperlipidaemia; obesity.

Pulsatilla Med Complex *Dynamit, Aust.*
Homoeopathic preparation.

Pulsitil *Janssen-Cilag, Aust.*
Cisapride (p.1187·1).
Constipation; dyspepsia; gastro-oesophageal reflux; intestinal pseudo-obstruction.

Pulsnorma *Giulini, Ger.†.*
Ajmaline (p.817·1); sparteine sulphate (p.1632·1); antazoline hydrochloride (p.401·3); phenobarbitone (p.350·2).
Arrhythmias.

Pulsti *Cassenne, Fr.†.*
Gonadorelin (p.1247·2).
Female infertility.

Pulveol *Laleuf, Fr.†.*
Menthol (p.1600·2); cineole (p.1564·1); terpin (p.1070·2); boric acid (p.1554·2).
Respiratory-tract congestion.

Pulverizador Nasal *Collado, Spain.*
Phenylephrine hydrochloride (p.1066·2).
Nasal congestion.

Pulverodil *Sanofi Winthrop, Spain†.*
Neomycin sulphate (p.229·2); nystatin (p.386·1); tyrothricin (p.267·2); triamcinolone acetonide (p.1050·2).
Skin infections with inflammation.

Pulvhydrops D *Lomapharm, Ger.*
Equisetum (p.1575·1).
Oedema; urinary-tract disorders.

Pulvicrus *Mago, Ger.†.*
Hexachlorophane (p.1115·2); guaiazulene (p.1586·3); alpha tocopheryl acetate (p.1369·1); wheatgerm; *Aspergillus oryzae* fermented with wheat bran.
Ulcers.

Pulvis-3 *Bayer, Ital.*
Propoxur (p.1410·1).
Pediculosis.

Pulvispray *Peters, Fr.*
Mixed aldehydes; alcohol (p.1099·1); isopropyl alcohol (p.1118·2).
Disinfection.

Pulvo *Fournier, Ger.*
Catalase (p.1560·3); hexamidine isethionate (p.1115·3).
Ulcers; wounds.

Pulvo 47
Note. This name is used for preparations of different composition.
Fournier, Belg.
Catalase (p.1560·3); hexachlorophane (p.1115·2).
Burns; skin irritation; ulcers; wounds.

Fournier, Fr.
Catalase (p.1560·3); hexamidine isethionate (p.1115·3).
Burns; wounds.

Pulvo Neomycin *Fournier, Ger.*
Catalase (p.1560·3); neomycin sulphate (p.229·2).
Burns; infected skin disorders; ulcers; wounds.

Pulvo Neomycine *Fournier, Belg.*
Catalase (p.1560·3); neomycin sulphate (p.229·2).
Burns; skin irritation; wounds.

Pulvo 47 Neomycine *Fournier, Fr.*
Catalase (p.1560·3); neomycin sulphate (p.229·2).
Infected wounds and burns.

Pumilen-Balsam *Tosse, Ger.†.*
Eucalyptus oil (p.1578·1); pumilio pine oil (p.1623·3); oleum pini sylvestris; turpentine oil (p.1641·1); thymol (p.1127·1); menthol (p.1600·2); glycol salicylate (p.43·1).
Coughs and associated respiratory-tract disorders.

Pumilene *Montefarmaco, Ital.†.*
Pumilio pine oil (p.1623·3); guaiphenesin (p.1061·3).
Respiratory-tract congestion.

Pumilen-N *Tosse, Ger.*
Eucalyptus oil (p.1578·1); pumilio pine oil (p.1623·3); oleum pini sylvestris; peppermint oil (p.1208·1); thymol (p.1127·1).
Colds; nasal congestion.

Pumilsan *Montefarmaco, Ital.*
Dequalinium chloride (p.1112·1).
Mouth and throat disinfection.

Pump-Hep
Leo, Irl.†; Leo, UK.
Heparin sodium (p.879·3).
Thrombo-embolic disorders.

Puncto E *Asta Medica, Ger.*
d-Alpha tocopherol (p.1369·1).
Vitamin E deficiency.

Pungino *Whitehall, Ital.*
Vitamin B_1 (p.1361·2) citronella oil (p.1565·1).
Insect repellent.

Punktyl
Mayrhofer, Aust.†; Krewel, Ger.
Lorazepam (p.675·3).
Anxiety; sleep disorders.

Puntual *Lainco, Spain.*
Calcium sennoside A (p.1212·3); calcium sennoside B (p.1212·3).
Constipation.

Puntualex *Lainco, Spain.*
Calcium sennoside A (p.1212·3); calcium sennoside B (p.1212·3).
Bowel evacuation.

Puodermina Hidrocor *Promesa, Spain†.*
Bacitracin (p.157·3); hydrocortisone acetate (p.1043·3); neomycin sulphate (p.229·2).
Infected skin disorders.

Pupilla *Schiapparelli, Ital.*
Naphazoline nitrate (p.1064·2).
Inflammatory and allergic eye disorders.

Pupilla Antistaminico *Schiapparelli, Ital.*
Naphazoline nitrate (p.1064·2); thonzylamine hydrochloride (p.419·2).
Inflammatory and allergic eye disorders.

Pupilla Light *Schiapparelli, Ital.*
Benzalkonium chloride (p.1101·3); hypromellose; chamomile water; hyssop water; rose water; plantaginis water; mallow water; myrtillus water.
Eye disinfection; eye irritation.

Puralube *Fougera, USA.*
Eye drops: Polyvinyl alcohol (p.1474·2).
Eye ointment: White soft paraffin (p.1382·3); light liquid paraffin (p.1382·1).
Dry eyes.

Purata *Lennon, S.Afr.*
Oxazepam (p.683·2).
Alcohol withdrawal syndrome; anxiety.

Puraya *Delalande, Ger.†.*
Sterculia (p.1214·1).
Constipation.

Purazine *SA Druggists Self Med, S.Afr.†.*
Cinnarizine (p.406·1).
Nausea; vertigo; vomiting.

Purbac *Intramed, S.Afr.*
Co-trimoxazole (p.196·3).
Bacterial infections.

Pur-Bloka *Lennon, S.Afr.*
Propranolol hydrochloride (p.937·1).
Angina pectoris; arrhythmias; hypertension; hyperthyroidism; migraine; phaeochromocytoma.

Pure Omega *BritHealth, UK.*
Fish oil concentrate (p.1276·1).

Pureduct *Rosen, Ger.*
Allopurinol (p.390·2).
Hyperuricaemia.

Puregon
Organon, Austral.; Organon, Ger.; Organon, Irl.; Organon, Ital.; Organon, Neth.; Organon, Norw.; Organon, Swed.; Organon, UK.
Follitropin beta (p.1247·1).
Female infertility.

Pureness Blemish Control *Shiseido, Canad.*
Sulphur (p.1091·2).
Acne.

Puresis *Lennon, S.Afr.*
Frusemide (p.871·1).
Hypertension; oedema.

Purethal
Hal, Ger.; HAL, Neth.
Grass or tree pollen allergen extracts(p.1545·1).
Hyposensitisation.

Purganol *Saunier-Daguin, Fr.*
Phenolphthalein (p.1208·2).
Constipation.

Purgante *Orravan, Spain.*
Phenolphthalein (p.1208·2).
Constipation.

Purgazen *Wenig, Aust.*
Bisacodyl (p.1179·3); dimethicone (p.1213·1).
Bowel evacuation; constipation.

Purge *Fleming, USA.*
Castor oil (p.1560·2).
Constipation.

Purgestol *Blue Cross, Ital.†.*
Phenolphthalein (p.1208·2).
Constipation.

Purgo-Pil *Qualiphar, Belg.*
Bisacodyl (p.1179·3).
Bowel evacuation; constipation.

Purgoxin *Lennon, S.Afr.*
Digoxin (p.849·3).
Cardiac disorders.

Purianta *Apomedica, Aust.*
Thyme (p.1636·3); guaiphenesin (p.1061·3).
Coughs and cold symptoms.

Puri-Clens *Sween, USA.*
Methylbenzethonium chloride (p.1119·3).
Wound cleanser.

Puricos *SA Druggists, S.Afr.*
Allopurinol (p.390·2).
Gout; hyperuricaemia.

Purigoa *Salus, Aust.*
Bisacodyl (p.1179·3); docusate sodium (p.1189·3).
Constipation.

Purimmun *Armour, Ger.†.*
A normal immunoglobulin (p.1522·1).
Hypogammaglobulinaemia; passive immunisation.

Pur-in Isophane *CP Pharmaceuticals, UK†.*
Isophane insulin suspension (human, emp) (p.322·1).
Diabetes mellitus.

Pur-in Mix 15/85, 25/75, 50/50 *CP Pharmaceuticals, UK†.*
Mixtures of neutral insulin injection (human, emp) and isophane insulin injection (human, emp) respectively in the proportions indicated (p.322·1).
Diabetes mellitus.

Pur-in Neutral *CP Pharmaceuticals, UK†.*
Neutral insulin (human, emp) (p.322·1).
Diabetes mellitus.

Puri-Nethol
Glaxo Wellcome, Aust.; Glaxo Wellcome, Austral.; Glaxo Wellcome, Belg.; Glaxo Wellcome, Canad.; Glaxo Wellcome, Fr.; Glaxo Wellcome, Ger.; Wellcome, Irl.; Glaxo Wellcome, Ital.; Glaxo Wellcome, Neth.; Glaxo Wellcome, Norw.; Glaxo Wellcome, S.Afr.; Glaxo Wellcome, Swed.; Wellcome, Switz.; Wellcome, UK; Wellcome, USA.
Mercaptopurine (p.546·1).
Leukaemias.

Purinol
Merckle, Aust.; Horner, Canad.†; Pinewood, Irl.
Allopurinol (p.390·2).
Gout; hyperuricaemia; prophylaxis of uric acid and calcium oxalate stones.

Purisole *Fresenius, Switz.*
Sorbitol (p.1354·2); mannitol (p.900·3).
Bladder irrigation.

Puritabs *Dermatech, Austral.*
Sodium dichloroisocyanurate (p.1124·3).
Water disinfection.

Purmycin *Lennon, S.Afr.*
Erythromycin estolate (p.204·1).
Bacterial infections.

Purochin *Sclavo, Ital.*
Urokinase (p.959·3).
Thrombo-embolic disorders.

Puromylon *Lennon, S.Afr.*
Nalidixic acid (p.228·2).
Urinary-tract infections.

Puroptal *Metochem, Aust.*
Hypromellose (p.1473·1).
Eye irritation.

Purostrophan *Kali-Chemie, Ger.†.*
Ouabain (p.925·2).
Heart failure.

Purostrophyll *Kali-Chemie, Ger.†.*
Ouabain (p.925·2); diprophylline (p.752·1).
Cardiac disorders.

Purporent *Rowa, Irl.†.*
Nicotinaldehyde; liquid ammonii anisatus; eucalyptus oil (p.1578·1); camphor (p.1557·2); pine oil; rosemary oil (p.1626·2); aroma oils.
Bronchitis; coughs; laryngitis; respiratory-tract congestion.

Purpose *Johnson & Johnson, USA; Merck, USA.*
A range of emollient, cleansing, and moisturising preparations.

Pur-Rutin *Andreabal, Switz.*
Troxerutin (p.1580·2).
Peripheral vascular disorders.

Pursenid *Sandoz, Spain.*
Calcium sennoside A (p.1212·3); calcium sennoside B (p.1212·3).
Constipation.

Pursennid
Note. This name is used for preparations of different composition.
Sandoz, Aust.; Novartis, Ital.; Novartis, Norw.
Calcium sennoside A (p.1212·3); calcium sennoside B (p.1212·3).
Bowel evacuation; constipation.

Sandoz, Ger.†; Novartis, Swed.
Senna leaf (p.1212·2).
Bowel evacuation; constipation.

Pursennid Complex *Novartis, Ital.*
Senna (p.1212·2); polycarbophil calcium (p.1209·1).
Constipation.

Pursennid Fibra *Novartis, Ital.*
Polycarbophil calcium (p.1209·1).
Constipation; diarrhoea.

Pursennide
Wander, Belg.†; Sandoz, Fr.; Wander, Neth.†; Sandoz OTC, Switz.
Calcium sennoside A (p.1212·3); calcium sennoside B (p.1212·3).
Bowel evacuation; constipation.

Pursept A *Merz, Ger.*
Alcohol (p.1099·1); glyoxal (p.1115·1); quaternary ammonium compounds.
Surface and instrument disinfection.

Pursept N *Merz, Ger.†.*
Glutaraldehyde (p.1114·3); glyoxal (p.1115·1); quaternary ammonium compounds.
Surface disinfection.

Purtego *Goldschmidt, Ger.†.*
Mixture of alkyloligoamines and alkyloligoamine carbonic acids.
Surface disinfection.

Puvasoralen *Crawford, UK.*
Methoxsalen (p.1086·3).
Available on a named-patient basis only.
Mycosis fungoides; psoriasis; vitiligo.

PV Carpine
Allergan, Austral.; Allergan, Irl.†; Allergan, S.Afr.; Allergan, Switz.†.
Pilocarpine hydrochloride (p.1396·3) or pilocarpine nitrate (p.1396·3).
Glaucoma; reversal of mydriasis.

PVF *Frosst, Canad.*
Benzathine phenoxymethylpenicillin (p.159·2).
Bacterial infections.

PVFK *Frosst, Canad.*
Phenoxymethylpenicillin potassium (p.236·2).
Bacterial infections.

PVK *Lilly, Austral.*
Phenoxymethylpenicillin potassium (p.236·2).
Bacterial infections.

P-V-Tussin *Solvay, USA.*
Syrup: Hydrocodone tartrate (p.43·1); pseudoephedrine hydrochloride (p.1068·3); chlorpheniramine maleate (p.405·1).
Coughs and cold symptoms.
Tablets: Hydrocodone tartrate (p.43·1); phenindamine tartrate (p.415·2); guaiphenesin (p.1061·3).
Coughs.

Pyal *Sanico, Belg.*
Sulphanilamide (p.256·3); sulphathiazole (p.257·1); cod-liver oil (p.1337·3); cholecalciferol (p.1366·3).
Burns; wounds.

Pygmal *Astier, Fr.*
2,4,5-Trichlorophenol complex with tri-isobutyl phosphate; zinc oxide (p.1096·2); zinc carbonate (p.1096·1).
Acne.

Pygnoforton *Plantorgan, Ger.†.*
Strandkiefernrinden.
Vascular disorders.

Pykaryl T *Rodleben, Ger.*
Benzyl nicotinate (p.22·1).
Peripheral vascular disorders; rheumatic disorders; soft-tissue injuries.

Pykno *Procare, Austral.*
Vitis vinifera; myrtillus (p.1606·1).
Peripheral vascular disorders; tonic.

Pyknolepsinum *Desitin, Ger.*
Ethosuximide (p.344·3).
Absence seizures.

Pylorid
Glaxo Wellcome, Irl.; Glaxo Wellcome, Ital.; Glaxo Wellcome, Neth.; Glaxo, UK.
Ranitidine bismutrex (p.1211·2).
Peptic ulcer.

Pyloriset *Orion, USA.*
Test for gastro-intestinal disorders.

Pylorisin *Glaxo Wellcome, Aust.*
Ranitidine bismutrex (p.1211·2).
Peptic ulcer.

Pynmed *Medpro, S.Afr.*
Syrup: Paracetamol (p.72·2); codeine phosphate (p.26·1); promethazine hydrochloride (p.416·2).
Tablets: Paracetamol (p.72·2); codeine phosphate (p.26·1); caffeine (p.749·3); meprobamate (p.678·1).
Pain and associated tension.

Pynstop *Adcock Ingram Self Medication, S.Afr.*
Paracetamol (p.72·2); codeine phosphate (p.26·1); caffeine (p.749·3); doxylamine succinate (p.410·1).
Fever; pain and associated tension.

Pyocefal *Takeda, Fr.*
Cefsulodin sodium (p.173·2).
Lignocaine (p.1293·2) is included in the intramuscular injection to alleviate the pain of injection.
Bacterial infections.

Pyocidin-Otic *Forest Pharmaceuticals, USA†.*
Polymyxin B sulphate (p.239·1); hydrocortisone (p.1043·3).
Superficial bacterial infections of the external auditory canal.

Pyodron *Cassella-med, Ger.†.*
Sulphanilamide (p.256·3); zinc oxide (p.1096·2).
Pyogenic skin disorders.

Pyogenium N *Hanosan, Ger.†.*
Homoeopathic preparation.

Pyolysin *Serum-Werk Bernburg, Ger.*
Extract of staphylococci, streptococci, escherichia coli, pseudomonas aeruginosa, micrococcus-ovis-Buillon; zinc oxide (p.1096·2); salicylic acid (p.1090·2).
Infected skin disorders; wounds.

Pyopen
Wyeth-Ayerst, Canad.†; Link, UK†.
Carbenicillin sodium (p.162·3).
Bacterial infections.

Pyoredol *Roussel, Fr.*
Phenytoin sodium (p.352·3).
Gum disorders.

Pyorex *Bailly, Fr.*
Ethacridine lactate (p.1098·3); sodium ricinoleate.
Formerly contained ethacridine lactate, acetarsol lithium, and sodium ricinoleate.
Oral hygiene.

Pyostacine
Rhone-Poulenc Rorer, Belg.; Specia, Fr.
Pristinamycin (p.240·2).
Bacterial infections.

Pyr *Zeta, Ital.†.*
Pyrethrum (p.1410·1); piperonyl butoxide (p.1409·3); dicophane (p.1404·3).
Pediculosis.

Pyracod *Propan-Vernleigh, S.Afr.†.*
Potassium guaiacolsulfonate (p.1068·3); mepyramine maleate (p.414·1); codeine phosphate (p.26·1); sodium citrate (p.1153·2).
Coughs.

Pyradol
Note. This name is used for preparations of different composition.
Gallier, Fr.†.
Morpholine salicylate (p.60·1).
Formerly contained pranosal salicylate.
Pain.

Xixia, S.Afr.
Paracetamol (p.72·2).
Fever; pain.

Pyrafat
Kolassa, Aust.; Fatol, Ger.
Pyrazinamide (p.241·1).
Tuberculosis.

Pyragamma *Worwag, Ger.†.*
Pyridoxine hydrochloride (p.1362·3).
Vitamin B_6 deficiency.

Pyragesic *Noristan, S.Afr.†.*
Paracetamol (p.72·2).
Fever; pain.

Pyralin *Kenral, Austral.*
Sulphasalazine (p.1215·2).
Crohn's disease; rheumatoid arthritis; ulcerative colitis.

Pyralvex
Kwizda, Aust.; Norgine, Austral.; Norgine, Belg.; Norgine, Fr.; Norgine, Ger.; Norgine, Irl.; Norgine, Ital.; Norgine, S.Afr.; Berna, Spain; Norgine, Switz.; Norgine, UK.
Rhubarb (p.1212·1); salicylic acid (p.1090·2).
Formerly known as Peralvex in the *UK*.
Mouth and throat disorders.

Pyramine *Propan-Vernleigh, S.Afr.†.*
Mepyramine maleate (p.414·1).
Hypersensitivity reactions.

Pyrazide *Hoechst Marion Roussel, S.Afr.*
Pyrazinamide (p.241·1).
Tuberculosis.

Pyrazol *Compu, S.Afr.†.*
Allopurinol (p.390·2).
Gout; hyperuricaemia.

Pyrcon *Meuselbach, Ger.*
Viprynium embonate (p.111·2).
Oxyuriasis.

Pyreazid *Salvat, Spain.*
Isoniazid (p.218·1).
Tuberculosis.

Pyreflor *Clement, Fr.*
Lotion: Permethrin (p.1409·2); piperonyl butoxide (p.1409·3); enoxolone (p.35·2).
Shampoo: Permethrin (p.1409·2); piperonyl butoxide (p.1409·3).
Pediculosis.

Pyreses *Berenguer Infale, Spain.*
Aloglutamol (p.1177·2).
Gastro-intestinal hyperacidity; peptic ulcer.

Pyrethane *Gerda, Fr.*
Dipyrone (p.35·1).
Pain.

Pyrethrum Spray *Nelson, UK.*
Homoeopathic preparation.

Pyribenzamine *Novartis Consumer, Canad.*
Tripelennamine hydrochloride (p.420·2).
Hypersensitivity reactions.

Pyridamel *Clonmel, Irl.†.*
Dipyridamole (p.857·1).
Platelet disorders.

Pyriderm *Schering-Plough, Belg.*
Pyrethrum (p.1410·1); piperonyl butoxide (p.1409·3).
Pediculosis.

Pyridiate *Rugby, USA.*
Phenazopyridine hydrochloride (p.78·3).
Irritation of the lower urinary tract.

Pyridium
Parke, Davis, Canad.; Servier, Fr.†; Parke, Davis, Ger.†; Parke, Davis, S.Afr.; Parke, Davis, USA.
Phenazopyridine hydrochloride (p.78·3).
Pain and irritation of the urinary tract.

Pyridium Plus *Parke, Davis, USA†.*
Phenazopyridine hydrochloride (p.78·3); hyoscyamine hydrobromide (p.464·2); butalbital (p.644·3).
Urinary-tract pain and spasm, with apprehension.

Pyridoscorbine *Synthelabo, Fr.†.*
Ascorbic acid (p.1365·2); pyridoxine (p.1363·1).
Cold symptoms; tonic.

Pyrifin *Hoechst Marion Roussel, S.Afr.*
Rifampicin (p.243·2); isoniazid (p.218·1); pyrazinamide (p.241·1).
Tuberculosis.

Pyrifoam *Dermatech, Austral.*
Permethrin (p.1409·2).
Formerly contained pyrethrins I and II and piperonyl butoxide.
Pediculosis.

Pyrilax *Berlin-Chemie, Ger.*
Bisacodyl (p.1179·3).
Bowel evacuation; constipation.

Pyrinex *Ambix, USA.*
Pyrethrins; piperonyl butoxide (p.1409·3).
Pediculosis.

Pyrinyl II *Barre-National, USA.*
Pyrethrins; piperonyl butoxide technical (p.1409·3).
Pediculosis.

Pyrinyl Plus *Rugby, USA.*
Pyrethrins; piperonyl butoxide (p.1409·3).
Pediculosis.

Pyriped *Propan-Vernleigh, S.Afr.†.*
Mepyramine maleate (p.414·1).
Antihistaminic.

Pyrisept *Weifa, Norw.*
Cetylpyridinium chloride (p.1106·2).
Disinfection of hands and skin; minor skin infections.

Pyrocaps *Be-Tabs, S.Afr.*
Piroxicam (p.80·2).
Gout; musculoskeletal and joint disorders.

Pyrogastrone
Note. This name is used for preparations of different composition.
Sanofi Winthrop, Irl.; Sanofi Winthrop, UK.
Tablets: Carbenoxolone sodium (p.1182·2); alginic acid (p.1470·3); aluminium hydroxide (p.1177·3); magnesium trisilicate (p.1199·1); sodium bicarbonate (p.1153·2).
Flatulence; gastro-oesophageal reflux; heartburn; hiatus hernia; peptic ulcer.

Sanofi Winthrop, UK.
Oral suspension: Carbenoxolone sodium (p.1182·2); aluminium hydroxide (p.1177·3); sodium alginate (p.1470·3); potassium bicarbonate (p.1153·1).
Gastro-oesophageal reflux.

Pyrogenium N *Hanosan, Ger.*
Homoeopathic preparation.

Pyromed S *Sanofi Winthrop, Ger.*
Paracetamol (p.72·2).
Fever; pain.

Pyroxin *Rhone-Poulenc Rorer, Austral.*
Pyridoxine hydrochloride (p.1362·3).
Alcoholism; anaemias; homocystinuria; nausea and vomiting in pregnancy; premenstrual syndrome; radiation sickness.

PZI Iletin *Lilly, Canad.*†.
Protamine zinc insulin suspension (bovine and porcine) (p.322·1).
Diabetes mellitus.

Qari *Mediolanum, Ital.*
Rufloxacin hydrochloride (p.247·3).
Bacterial infections.

QM Integratore *Mavi, Ital.*
Trace-element preparation with vitamin B substances and vitamin C.
Nutritional supplement.

Q-Mazine *Seton, UK.*
Promethazine hydrochloride (p.416·2).
Motion sickness; urticaria.

QT *Schering-Plough, USA.*
SPF 2: Ethylhexyl *p*-methoxycinnamate (p.1487·1); dihydroxyacetone (p.1081·2).
Sunscreen.

QTest *Quidel, USA.*
Pregnancy test (p.1621·2).

QTest Ovulation *Quidel, USA.*
Fertility test (p.1621·2).

Quack *Esoform, Ital.*†.
Benzalkonium chloride (p.1101·3).
Surface disinfection.

Quadblock *Hamilton, Austral.*
Cream; topical milk: Ethylhexyl *p*-methoxycinnamate (p.1487·1); titanium dioxide (p.1093·3); 3-(4-methylbenzylidene)bornan-2-one (p.1487·2).
Formerly contained oxybenzone, ethylhexyl*p*-methoxycinnamate, padimate O, and titanium dioxide.
Stick: Oxybenzone (p.1487·3); ethylhexyl *p*-methoxycinnamate (p.1487·1); avobenzone (p.1486·3); titanium dioxide (p.1093·3).
Sunscreen.

Quadra Hist *Schein, USA.*
Phenylpropanolamine hydrochloride (p.1067·2); phenylephrine hydrochloride (p.1066·2); chlorpheniramine maleate (p.405·1); phenyltoloxamine citrate (p.416·1).
Upper respiratory-tract symptoms.

Quadramet *Du Pont, USA.*
Samarium-153 (p.1424·3) in the form of samarium lexidronam.
Metastatic bone pain.

Quadriderm
Schering-Plough, S.Afr.; Essex, Switz.
Betamethasone valerate (p.1033·3); gentamicin sulphate (p.212·1); tolnaftate (p.389·1); clioquinol (p.193·2).
Infected skin disorders.

Quadrinal *Knoll, USA.*
Ephedrine hydrochloride (p.1059·3); phenobarbitone (p.350·2); theophylline calcium salicylate (p.772·2); potassium iodide (p.1493·1).
Chronic respiratory disease.

Quadronal *Asta Medica, Switz.*†.
Paracetamol (p.72·2); propyphenazone (p.81·3); caffeine (p.749·3).
Fever; pain.

Quadronal ASS Comp *Asta Medica, Ger.*
Aspirin (p.16·1); caffeine (p.749·3).
Quadronal AS formerly contained aspirin, etenzamide, and caffeine.
Pain.

Quadronal Comp *Asta Medica, Ger.*
Paracetamol (p.72·2); caffeine (p.749·3).
Formerly contained propyphenazone, paracetamol, and caffeine.
Pain.

Quait *SIT, Ital.*
Lorazepam (p.675·3).
Anxiety disorders; premedication.

Quaname *Wyeth, Belg.*†.
Meprobamate (p.678·1).
Lumbago; mood disorders; muscular contractures; torticollis.

Quanil *Wyeth, Ital.*
Meprobamate (p.678·1).
Anxiety disorders.

Quantaffirm *Organon Teknika, USA.*
Test for infectious mononucleosis.

Quantalan
Bristol-Myers Squibb, Aust.; Bristol-Myers Squibb, Ger.; Bristol-Myers Squibb, Switz.
Cholestyramine (p.1269·3).
Diarrhoea; hypercholesterolaemia; poisoning with phenprocoumon; pruritus associated with biliary obstruction.

Quanto *Mediolanum, Ital.*†.
Pepsin (p.1616·3); metoclopramide hydrochloride (p.1200·3); fenipentol hemisuccinate (p.1579·1); dimethicone (p.1213·1); trypsin (p.1640·1); chymotrypsin (p.1563·2); amylase (p.1549·1); lipase.
Gastro-intestinal disorders.

Quantor *Almirall, Spain.*
Ranitidine hydrochloride (p.1209·3).
Acid aspiration; gastro-intestinal haemorrhage; gastro-oesophageal reflux; peptic ulcer; Zollinger-Ellison syndrome.

Quarelin *Chinoin, Hung.*
Dipyrone (p.35·1); caffeine (p.749·3); drotaverine hydrochloride (p.1574·2).
Migraine.

Quark *Polifarma, Ital.*
Ramipril (p.941·1).
Heart failure; hypertension.

Quartamon *Schulke & Mayr, Ger.*†.
Benzalkonium chloride (p.1101·3).
Skin disinfection.

Quartan *Schulke & Mayr, Ger.*†.
N-(2-hydroxyethyl)-N-(2-lauroyloxy-ethyl)-*N*-methylbenzylammonium chloride; guaiazulene (p.1586·3).
Mastitis.

Quartasept Konz *Maggioni, Ital.*†.
N,N-Dimethyl-*N*-lauryl-*N*-benzylammonium chloride.
Surface disinfection.

Quartasept Konz R *Maggioni, Ital.*†.
Methyloxyethyldodecyloxyethylbenzylammonium chloride.
Surface disinfection.

Quarzan *Roche, USA.*
Clidinium bromide (p.459·2).
Peptic ulcer (adjunct).

Quasar *Ravizza, Ital.*
Verapamil hydrochloride (p.960·3).
Hypertension.

Quatohex *Braun, Ger.*
Didecyldimethylammonium chloride (p.1112·2); benzalkonium chloride (p.1101·3); biguanidinium acetate; polymeric biguanides.
Surface disinfection.

Quazium *Schering-Plough, Ital.*
Quazepam (p.689·3).
Insomnia.

Quelfas A *Czarniak, Austral.*†.
Methyl salicylate (p.55·2); menthol (p.1600·2); camphor (p.1557·2); eucalyptus oil (p.1578·1).
Arthritic pain; muscular pain.

Quelicin
Abbott, Canad.; Abbott, USA.
Suxamethonium chloride (p.1319·1).
Depolarising neuromuscular blocker.

Quelidrine *Abbott, USA.*
Dextromethorphan hydrobromide (p.1057·3); chlorpheniramine maleate (p.405·1); ephedrine hydrochloride (p.1059·3); phenylephrine hydrochloride (p.1066·2); ammonium chloride (p.1055·2); ipecac fluidextract (p.1062·2).
Coughs.

Quell P *Searle, S.Afr.*†.
Pyrethrins; piperonyl butoxide (p.1409·3).
Pediculosis.

Quellada
Note. This name is used for preparations of different composition.
Stafford-Miller, Austral.
Permethrin (p.1409·2).
Quellada lotion formerly contained lindane.
Pediculosis; scabies.

Stafford-Miller Continental, Belg.; Stafford-Miller, Irl.; Searle, S.Afr.; Stafford-Miller, UK†.
Lindane (p.1407·2).
Pediculosis; scabies.

Quellada H *Block, Ger.*
Lindane (p.1407·2).
Pediculosis.

Quellada P *Block, Ger.*
Pyrethrum flower (p.1410·1); piperonyl butoxide (p.1409·3).
Pediculosis.

Quellada-M *Stafford-Miller, UK.*
Malathion (p.1407·3).
Pediculosis.

Quenobilan *Estedi, Spain.*
Chenodeoxycholic acid (p.1562·1).
Gallstones.

Quenocol *Zambon, Spain.*
Chenodeoxycholic acid (p.1562·1).
Gallstones.

Quensyl *Sanofi Winthrop, Ger.*
Hydroxychloroquine sulphate (p.431·2).
Chronic polyarthritis; lupus erythematosus; malaria.

Quentakehl *Sanum-Kehlbeck, Ger.*
Homoeopathic preparation.

Queratil *Septa, Spain.*
Cineole (p.1564·1); ichthammol (p.1083·3); trinitrophenol (p.1639·3); ergocalciferol (p.1367·1); tannic acid (p.1634·2); zinc oxide (p.1096·2); retinol (p.1358·1).
Burns.

Quercetol Hemostatico *Ferrer, Spain.*
Carbazochrome (p.714·1); quercetin (p.1580·2); creatinine sulphate.
Haemorrhage.

Quercetol K *Ferrer, Spain.*
Ascorbic acid (p.1365·2); calcium gluconate (p.1155·2); carbazochrome (p.714·1); menadione sodium bisulphite (p.1370·3); quercetin (p.1580·2).
Capillary fragility; haemorrhage.

Querto *Byk Gulden, Ger.*
Carvedilol (p.838·1).
Hypertension.

Questran
Bristol-Myers Squibb, Austral.; Bristol-Myers Squibb, Belg.; Bristol, Canad.; Bristol-Myers Squibb, Fr.; Bristol-Myers Squibb, Irl.; Bristol-Myers Squibb, Ital.; Bristol-Myers Squibb, Neth.; Bristol-Myers Squibb, Norw.; Bristol-Myers Squibb, S.Afr.; Bristol-Myers, Spain; Bristol-Myers Squibb, Swed.; Bristol-Myers Squibb, UK; Bristol, USA.
Cholestyramine (p.1269·3).
Adjunct in organophosphorus pesticide poisoning; diarrhoea; hypercholesterolaemia; pruritus associated with biliary obstruction.

Quibron *Apothecon, USA.*
Theophylline (p.765·1); guaiphenesin (p.1061·3).
Bronchospasm.

Quibron-T
Bristol, Canad.; Roberts, USA.
Theophylline (p.765·1).
Obstructive airways disease.

Quick Pep *Thompson, USA.*
Caffeine (p.749·3).
Fatigue.

Quick-Cillin *Genpharm, S.Afr.*†.
Procaine penicillin (p.240·2).
Bacterial infections.

Quickmicina *Panthox & Burck, Ital.*†.
Methacycline hydrochloride (p.225·1).
Bacterial infections.

QuickVue *Quidel, USA.*
Pregnancy test (p.1621·2).

Quiedorm *Menarini, Spain.*
Quazepam (p.689·3).
Insomnia.

Quiess *Forest Laboratories, USA*†.
Hydroxyzine hydrochloride (p.412·1).
Anxiety; hypersensitivity reactions.

Quiet Days *Cantassium Co., UK.*
Scutellaria; lupulus (p.1597·2); valerian (p.1643·1).

Quiet Life *Lane, UK.*
Motherwort (p.1604·2); wild lettuce (p.1645·1); lupulus (p.1597·2); passion flower (p.1615·3); valerian (p.1643·1); thiamine hydrochloride (p.1361·1); riboflavine (p.1362·1); nicotinamide (p.1351·2).
Stresses and strains.

Quiet Night *Healthcrafts, UK.*
Valerian (p.1643·1); lupulus (p.1597·2); passion flower (p.1615·3).
Sleep disturbances.

Quiet Nite *Cantassium Co., UK.*
Valerian (p.1643·1); lupulus (p.1597·2); lettuce (p.1645·1); passion flower (p.1615·3).
Insomnia.

Quiet Tyme *Cantassium Co., UK.*
Scutellaria; lupulus (p.1597·2); passion flower (p.1615·3); valerian (p.1643·1); gentian (p.1583·3); vitamin B substances.

Quietan *Roche, Ital.*
Valerian (p.1643·1); passion flower (p.1615·3); crataegus (p.1568·2).
Insomnia.

Quietival *Chefaro Ardeval, Fr.*†.
Passion flower (p.1615·3); valerian (p.1643·1); melissa (p.1600·1).
Sleep disorders.

Quilibrex *Delalande, Ital.*†.
Oxazepam (p.683·2).
Anxiety disorders; insomnia.

Quilla simplex *Pharmacia Upjohn, Swed.*
Ammonium chloride (p.1055·2); quillaia (p.1328·2).
Respiratory-tract disorders.

Quilonorm
SmithKline Beecham, Aust.; SmithKline Beecham, Switz.
Lithium acetate (p.295·1) or lithium carbonate (p.290·3).
Bipolar disorder; depression; mania.

Quilonum
SmithKline Beecham, Ger.; SmithKline Beecham, S.Afr.
Lithium acetate (p.295·1) or lithium carbonate (p.290·3).
Cluster headache; depression; mania.

Quimocyclin N *Rhone-Poulenc, Ger.*†.
Tetracycline hydrochloride (p.259·1).
Bacterial infections.

Quimodril *Italfarmaco, Spain.*
Trypsin (p.1640·1); chymotrypsin (p.1563·2); teclothiazide potassium (p.951·3).
Oedema.

Quimotrase *Cusi, Spain.*
Chymotrypsin (p.1563·2).
Ocular surgery.

Quimpe Amida *Quimpe, Spain.*
Sulphanilamide (p.256·3); zinc oxide (p.1096·2).
Skin infections.

Quimpe Antibiotico *Quimpe, Spain.*
Tetracycline hydrochloride (p.259·1).
Bacterial infections.

Quimpe Vitamin *Quimpe, Spain.*
Vitamin B substances and amino-acid preparation.

Quimpedor *Quimpe, Spain.*
Caffeine (p.749·3); phenazone (p.78·2); pyridoxine hydrochloride (p.1362·3); propyphenazone (p.81·3); thiamine hydrochloride (p.1361·1).
Fever; pain.

Quinaband
Boots, Austral.; Seton, UK.
Calamine (p.1080·1); clioquinol (p.193·2); zinc oxide (p.1096·2).
Leg ulcers; medicated bandage.

Quinaglute
Berlex, Canad.†*; Schering, Ital.*†*; Schering, S.Afr.; Berlex, USA.*
Quinidine gluconate (p.938·3).
Arrhythmias.

Quinalan *Lannett, USA.*
Quinidine gluconate (p.938·3).
Arrhythmias.

Quinamm *Marion Merrell Dow, USA*†.
Quinine sulphate (p.439·2).
Nocturnal leg cramps.

Quinate
Note. This name is used for preparations of different composition.
Rhone-Poulenc Rorer, Austral.
Quinine sulphate (p.439·2).
Diagnosis of myasthenia gravis; malaria; muscle cramps; myotonia congenita.

Rougier, Canad.
Quinidine gluconate (p.938·3).
Arrhythmias.

Quinazide *Malesci, Ital.*
Quinapril hydrochloride (p.938·1); hydrochlorothiazide (p.885·2).
Hypertension.

Quinazil *Malesci, Ital.*
Quinapril hydrochloride (p.938·1).
Heart failure; hypertension.

Quinbisul *Alphapharm, Austral.*
Quinine bisulphate (p.439·1).
Malaria; nocturnal leg cramps.

Quindan *Danbury, USA*†.
Quinine sulphate (p.439·2).

Quinicardina *Berenguer Infale, Spain.*
Quinidine sulphate (p.939·1).
Arrhythmias.

Quinidex
Whitehall, Austral.†*; Wyeth-Ayerst, Canad.; Robins, USA.*
Quinidine sulphate (p.939·1).
Arrhythmias.

Quinidurule *Astra, Fr.*
Quinidine bisulphate (p.938·3).
Arrhythmias.

Quinimax *Sanofi Winthrop, Fr.*
Quinine hydrochloride (p.439·2); quinidine hydrochloride; cinchonine hydrochloride; cinchonidine hydrochloride.
Formerly contained quinine-resorcinol dihydrochloride, quinidine-resorcinol dihydrochloride, cinchonine-resorcinol dihydrochloride, and cinchonidine-resorcinol dihydrochloride.
Malaria.

Quinisedine *Le Marchand, Fr.*
Quinine benzoate (p.441·2); crataegus (p.1568·2).
Formerly contained quinine valerianate, marrubium, crataegus, and phenobarbitone.
Cramps.

Quinobarb *Rougier, Canad.*
Quinidine phenylethylbarbiturate (p.940·2).
Arrhythmias; sedative.

Quinocarbine *Bouchara, Fr.*
Aluminium orthoxyquinoleate; activated charcoal (p.972·2).
Diarrhoea; meteorism.

Quinocort
Quinoderm, Irl.; Quinoderm, UK.
Hydrocortisone (p.1043·3); potassium hydroxyquinoline sulphate (p.1621·1).
Infected skin disorders.

Quinoctal *Fawns & McAllan, Austral.*
Quinine sulphate (p.439·2).
Malaria; nocturnal leg cramps.

Quinoderm
Quinoderm, Irl.; Ethimed, S.Afr.†*; Quinoderm, Switz.; Quinoderm, UK.*
Benzoyl peroxide (p.1079·2); potassium hydroxyquinoline sulphate (p.1621·1).
Acne; folliculitis; rosacea.

Quinoderm Antibacterial Face Wash *Quinoderm, UK.*
Chlorhexidine gluconate (p.1107·2); cetrimide (p.1105·2); detergents.
Skin cleanser; soap substitute.

Quinoderm Hydrocortisone
Quinoderm, Switz.†*; Quinoderm, UK*†.
Benzoyl peroxide (p.1079·2); potassium hydroxyquinoline sulphate (p.1621·1); hydrocortisone (p.1043·3).
Acne; folliculitis; rosacea.

Quinoderm-H *Hoechst Marion Roussel, S.Afr.*
Benzoyl peroxide (p.1079·2); potassium hydroxyquinoline sulphate (p.1621·1); hydrocortisone (p.1043·3).
Skin disorders.

Quinodis
Grunenthal, Aust.; Roche, Belg.; Roche, Ger.; Grunenthal, Ger.; Grunenthal, Switz.
Fleroxacin (p.209·1).
Bacterial infections.

Quinoforme *Synthelabo, Fr.*
Basic quinine formate (p.441·2).
Malaria.

Quinoped *Quinoderm, UK.*
Benzoyl peroxide (p.1079·2); potassium hydroxyquinoline sulphate (p.1621·1).
Fungal skin infections.

Quinora *Key, USA.*
Quinidine sulphate (p.939·1).
Arrhythmias.

Quinortar *Iquinosa, Spain.*
Coal tar (p.1092·3); chlorquinaldol (p.185·1); titanium dioxide (p.1093·3).
Skin disorders.

Quinsana Plus *Mennen, USA.*
Tolnaftate (p.389·1).
Fungal skin infections.

Quinsul *Alphapharm, Austral.*
Quinine sulphate (p.439·2).
Malaria; nocturnal leg cramps.

Quintabs *Freeda, USA.*
A range of vitamin preparations.

Quintasa
Ferring, Canad.; Ferring, Spain.
Mesalazine (p.1199·2).
Inflammatory bowel disease.

Quintex *Bio-Therabel, Belg.*
Dioxethedrin hydrochloride (p.1572·2); promethazine hydrochloride (p.416·2); codeine phosphate (p.26·1).
Coughs; respiratory-tract disorders.

Quintex Pediatrique *Bio-Therabel, Belg.*
Dioxethedrin hydrochloride (p.1572·2); promethazine hydrochloride (p.416·2); pholcodine (p.1068·1); potassium guaiacolsulfonate (p.1068·3).
Coughs.

Quinton *Neopharmed, Ital.†.*
Lysine aspirin (p.50·3).
Inflammation; pain.

Quintonine *SmithKline Beecham Sante, Fr.*
Cinnamon (p.1564·2); kola (p.1645·1); dried bitter-orange peel (p.1610·3); cinchona bark (p.1564·1); quassia (p.1624·1); gentian (p.1583·3); calcium glycerophosphate (p.1155·2); nux vomica (p.1609·3).
Asthenia.

Quintopan Adult *SmithKline Beecham Sante, Fr.*
Codeine (p.26·1); ethylmorphine (p.36·1); bromoform (p.1620·3); sodium benzoate (p.1102·3); grindelia; polygala (p.1069·3); bryonia (p.1555·2); aconite (p.1542·2).
Coughs.

Quintopan Enfant *SmithKline Beecham Sante, Fr.*
Promethazine hydrochloride (p.416·2); pholcodine (p.1068·1); potassium guaiacolsulfonate (p.1068·3); dioxethedrin hydrochloride (p.1572·2).
Coughs.

Quiphile *Geneva, USA†.*
Quinine sulphate (p.439·2).
Nocturnal leg cramps.

Quipro *Andromaco, Spain.*
Ciprofloxacin hydrochloride (p.185·3).
Bacterial infections.

Quiralam *Lilly, Spain.*
Dexketoprofen trometamol.
Inflammation; pain.

Quiridil *Zoja, Ital.*
Sulpiride (p.692·3).
Dysthymia; psychoses.

Quit *Lemstam, Austral.†.*
Silver nitrate (p.1629·2).
Aid to smoking withdrawal.

Quitaxon
Boehringer Mannheim, Belg.; Boehringer Mannheim, Fr.
Doxepin hydrochloride (p.283·2).
Depression.

Quitt *Meda, Swed.†.*
Nicotine resin (p.1608·1).
Aid to smoking withdrawal.

Quocin *Isdin, Spain.*
Acetic acid (p.1541·2); salicylic acid (p.1090·2).
Callosities.

Quoderm *Isdin, Spain.*
Meclocycline sulfosalicylate (p.224·1).
Acne.

Quosten *Ibi, Ital.*
Salcatonin (p.735·3).
Hypercalcaemia; osteoporosis; Paget's disease of bone; reflex sympathetic dystrophy.

Quotane
Bellon, Belg.†; Evans, Fr.
Dimethisoquin hydrochloride (p.1292·2).
Pruritus.

Quotivit O.E. *Theraplix, Fr.*
Multivitamin and mineral preparation.

QV *Ego, Austral.*
Soap substitute; bath additive; emollient.
Skin disorders.

QV Lip Balm *Ego, Austral.*
Ethylhexyl*p*-methoxycinnamate (p.1487·1); avobenzone (p.1486·3).
Dry, cracked, or chapped lips.

QV Tar *Ego, Austral.†.*
Liquid paraffin (p.1382·1); tar (p.1092·3).
Emollient.

Qvar *3M, UK.*
Beclomethasone dipropionate (p.1032·1).
Asthma.

Q-Vax *CSL, Austral.*
An inactivated Q fever vaccine (p.1530·1).
Active immunisation.

Q-Vel *Ciba Consumer, USA†.*
Quinine sulphate (p.439·2).
Nocturnal leg cramps.

R 1406 *Janssen-Cilag, Fr.*
Phenoperidine hydrochloride (p.79·1).
Analgesia in anaesthesia.

R & C
Reed & Carnrick, Canad.; Reed & Carnrick, USA.
Pyrethrins; piperonyl butoxide (p.1409·3).
Pediculosis; surface and textile insecticide.

R Calm *Labima, Belg.*
Diphenhydramine hydrochloride (p.409·1).
Bites and stings; skin disorders.

R Calm + B6 *Labima, Belg.*
Dimenhydrinate (p.408·2); pyridoxine (p.1363·1).
Motion sickness; urticaria.

RA Lotion *Medco, USA.*
Resorcinol (p.1090·1); calamine (p.1080·1); borax (p.1554·2).
Acne.

Rabarbaroni *Max Farma, Ital.*
Rhubarb (p.1212·1); cinchona (p.1564·1); bitter orange (p.1610·3); liquorice (p.1197·1).
Constipation.

RabAvert *Chiron, USA.*
A rabies vaccine (p.1530·3).
Active immunisation.

Rabies-Imovax *Pasteur Merieux, Swed.*
A rabies vaccine (Wistar PM/WI 38-1503-3M) (p.1530·3).
Active immunisation.

Rabigam *NBI, S.Afr.*
A rabies immunoglobulin (p.1530·2).
Passive immunisation.

Rabipur
Hoechst, Aust.; Chiron Behring, Ger.
A rabies vaccine (Flury strain grown on chicken fibroblast cultures) (p.1530·3).
Active immunisation.

Rabivac *Chiron Behring, Ger.*
A rabies vaccine (Pitman-Moore strain grown on human diploid cell cultures) (p.1530·3).
Active immunisation.

Raboldo *Vaillant, Ital.*
Cascara (p.1183·1); boldo (p.1554·1); rhubarb (p.1212·1).
Constipation.

Rabro
Note. This name is used for preparations of different composition.
Schoeller, Aust.†.
Calcium carbonate (p.1182·1); liquorice (p.1197·1); magnesium oxide (p.1198·3); frangula bark (p.1193·2).
Gastritis; hyperacidity.

Granelli, Ital.†.
Calcium carbonate (p.1182·1); liquorice (p.1197·1); magnesium oxide (p.1198·3); frangula bark (p.1193·2).
Dyspepsia.

Vitafarma, Spain.
Calcium carbonate (p.1182·1); dimethicone (p.1213·1); frangula bark (p.1193·2); magnesium oxide (p.1198·3); liquorice (p.1197·1).
Flatulence; gastritis; hyperchlorhydria; peptic ulcer.

Rabro N *Fink, Ger.*
Calcium carbonate (p.1182·1); magnesium oxide (p.1198·3); liquorice (p.1197·1).
Gastritis; hyperchlorhydria.

Rabuman
Kwizda, Aust.; Berna, Ital.; Berna, Switz.
A rabies immunoglobulin (p.1530·2).
Passive immunisation.

Racestyptin *Austrodent, Aust.*
Aluminium chloride (p.1078·3); hydroxyquinoline sulphate (p.1589·3).
Adjunct in dental procedures.

Racestyptine *Septodont, Switz.*
Solution: Aluminium chloride (p.1078·3).
Thread: Aluminium chloride (p.1078·3); lignocaine (p.1293·2); hydroxyquinoline (p.1589·3).
Dental and gum disorders.

Ra-Cliss *SIFRA, Ital.*
Monobasic sodium phosphate (p.1159·3); dibasic sodium phosphate (p.1159·3).
Bowel evacuation; constipation.

Radacor *Hanseler, Switz.†.*
Cereus grandiflorus; flos monardae; melissa (p.1600·1); mint leaf; crataegus (p.1568·2).
Cardiac disorders.

Radalgin *Streuli, Switz.*
Nonivamide (p.63·2); methyl nicotinate (p.55·1); glycol salicylate (p.43·1); histamine dihydrochloride (p.1587·3).
Musculoskeletal pain; sports injuries.

Radanil *Roche, Arg.*
Benznidazole (p.580·2).
Protozoal infections.

Radecol *Dresden, Ger.*
Nicotinyl alcohol tartrate (p.915·3).
Hyperlipidaemias; vascular disorders.

Radedorm *Dresden, Ger.*
Nitrazepam (p.682·2).
Sleep disorders.

Radenarcon *Dresden, Ger.*
Etomidate (p.1223·2).
General anaesthesia.

Radepur *Dresden, Ger.*
Chlordiazepoxide (p.646·3).
Anxiety disorders; insomnia.

Radialar 280 *Juste, Spain.*
Meglumine diatrizoate (p.1003·2).
Radiographic contrast medium.

Radian *Roche, S.Afr.*
Cream: Menthol (p.1600·2); camphor (p.1557·2); methyl salicylate (p.55·2); capsicum oleoresin; camphor oil.
Liniment: Menthol (p.1600·2); aspirin (p.16·1); camphor (p.1557·2); methyl salicylate (p.55·2).
Pain.

Radian-B
Note. This name is used for preparations of different composition.
Roche Consumer, Austral.
Liniment: Menthol (p.1600·2); camphor (p.1557·2); ammonium salicylate (p.15·2); methyl salicylate (p.55·2); ethyl salicylate (p.36·1).
Musculoskeletal and joint disorders; soft-tissue disorders.

Roche Consumer, Austral.; Roche Consumer, Irl.; Roche Consumer, UK.
Topical rub: Menthol (p.1600·2); camphor (p.1557·2); methyl salicylate (p.55·2); capsicum oleoresin.
Musculoskeletal, joint, and soft-tissue disorders; pain.

Roche Consumer, Irl.; Roche Consumer, UK.
Liniment; topical spray: Menthol (p.1600·2); camphor (p.1557·2); ammonium salicylate (p.15·2); salicylic acid (p.1090·2).
Musculoskeletal and joint disorders; pain.

Radikal
Note. This name is used for preparations of different composition.
Sandipro, Belg.
Malathion (p.1407·3).
Pediculosis.

Maurer, Ger.
Clotrimazole (p.376·3).
Fungal infections.

Radikal-Salicylcollodicum *Herzpunkt, Ger.†.*
Salicylic acid (p.1090·2).
Skin disorders.

Radio Salil *Vinas, Spain.*
Ointment: Camphor (p.1557·2); methyl nicotinate (p.55·1); methyl salicylate (p.55·2); salicylic acid (p.1090·2); menthol (p.1600·2).
Spray: Camphor (p.1557·2); diethylamine salicylate (p.33·1); menthol (p.1600·2).
Musculoskeletal, joint, peri-articular, and soft-tissue disorders.

Radioced *Interfarma, Ital.*
Dimethicone (p.1384·2).
Barrier preparation.

Radiocillina *Radiumfarma, Ital.†.*
Ampicillin (p.153·1).
Bacterial infections.

Radiocin *Radiumfarma, Ital.†.*
Fluocinolone acetonide (p.1041·1).
Skin disorders.

Radiogardase-Cs *Heyl, Ger.*
Prussian blue (p.993·3).
Reduction in body-half-life of radiocaesium.

Radiopaque *Schering, Fr.†.*
Barium sulphate (p.1003·1).
Contrast medium for radiography.

Radioselectan *Schering, Fr.*
Sodium diatrizoate (p.1003·2); meglumine diatrizoate (p.1003·2).
Contrast medium for radiography.

Radiostol *Glaxo Wellcome, Canad.†.*
Ergocalciferol (p.1367·1).

Radix *Streuli, Switz.†.*
Peppermint leaf (p.1208·1); hedera helix; aniseed (p.1549·3); cardamom fruit (p.1560·1); juniper (p.1592·2); fennel (p.1579·1); thyme (p.1636·3); pulmonaria; polygala amara (p.1069·3); angelica; liquorice (p.1197·1); saponaria; pini summitates; pini turiones; diphenhydramine hydrochloride (p.409·1).
Coughs.

Radolor *Hanseler, Switz.†.*
Phenazone (p.78·2); propyphenazone (p.81·3).
Fever; pain.

Rado-Salil *Will-Pharma, Belg.*
Ethyl salicylate (p.36·1); methyl salicylate (p.55·2); glycol salicylate (p.43·1); salicylic acid (p.1090·2); camphor (p.1557·2); menthol (p.1600·2); capsicum oleoresin.
Lumbago; muscle and joint pain.

Radox *Radiumfarma, Ital.†.*
Doxycycline hydrochloride (p.202·3).
Bacterial infections.

Rafen *Alphapharm, Austral.*
Ibuprofen (p.44·1).
Dysmenorrhoea; musculoskeletal and joint disorders; pain with inflammation; soft-tissue injuries.

Raffreddoremed *Iodosan, Ital.*
Paracetamol (p.72·2); isopropamide iodide (p.464·3); dimetofrine; caffeine (p.749·3); chlorpheniramine maleate (p.405·1); ascorbic acid (p.1365·2).
Cold and influenza symptoms.

Rafton *Ferring, Canad.*
Alginic acid (p.1470·3) or sodium alginate (p.1470·3); aluminium hydroxide (p.1177·3).
Heartburn.

Ragaden *Ganassini, Ital.*
Cetylpyridinium chloride (p.1106·2).
Nipple disinfection.

Ragonil *Roche, Ecuad.*
Benznidazole (p.580·2).
Protozoal infections.

Ralena *Zyma, Ger.†.*
Yellow-white capsules, betamethasone (p.1033·2); dimethindene maleate (p.408·3); white capsules, dimethindene maleate.
Allergic disorders.

Ralgex *Seton, UK.*
Cream: Methyl nicotinate (p.55·1); capsicum oleoresin.
Topical spray: Glycol monosalicylate (p.43·1); ethyl salicylate (p.36·1); methyl salicylate (p.55·2); methyl nicotinate (p.55·1).
Topical stick: Glycol salicylate (p.43·1); ethyl salicylate (p.36·1); methyl salicylate (p.55·2); capsicum oleoresin; menthol (p.1600·2).
Musculoskeletal and joint disorders; pain.

Ralgex Freeze Spray *Seton, UK.*
Isopentane; dimethyl ether (p.1165·1); glycol monosalicylate (p.43·1).
Musculoskeletal and joint disorders; pain.

Ralgex (low-odour) *Seton, UK.*
Glycol monosalicylate (p.43·1); methyl nicotinate (p.55·1).
Musculoskeletal and joint disorders; pain.

Ralicid *Waldheim, Aust.*
Indomethacin (p.45·2).
Gout; inflammation; musculoskeletal, joint, and peri-articular disorders; oedema; pain.

Ralofekt *Dresden, Ger.*
Oxpentifylline (p.925·3).
Peripheral vascular disorders; vascular disorders of the eye or ear.

Ralogaine *Kenral, Austral.*
Minoxidil (p.910·3).
Alopecia androgenetica.

Ralone *Llorens, Spain†.*
Zeranol (p.1467·3).
Lactation inhibition; menopausal disorders; menstrual disorders.

Ralovera *Kenral, Austral.*
Medroxyprogesterone acetate (p.1448·3).
Abnormal uterine bleeding; adjunct to oestrogen therapy; amenorrhoea; breast cancer; endometrial cancer; endometriosis; renal cancer.

Ralozam *Pharmacia Upjohn, Austral.*
Alprazolam (p.640·3).
Anxiety; panic disorders.

Ralur *Drossapharm, Switz.*
Heparin sodium (p.879·3); indomethacin (p.45·2); laureth 9 (p.1325·2).
Musculoskeletal, joint, peri-articular, and soft-tissue disorders.

Ramace
Astra, Austral.; Astra, Belg.; Astra, S.Afr.
Ramipril (p.941·1).
Heart failure; hypertension.

Ramatocina *Prats, Spain†.*
Betamethasone (p.1033·2); indomethacin (p.45·2); paracetamol (p.72·2); thiamine (p.1361·2).
Inflammation; pain.

Ramend *Schieffer, Ger.*
Senna (p.1212·2).
Constipation.

Ramend Krauter *Schieffer, Ger.*
Senna (p.1212·2); maté (p.1645·1); coriander (p.1567·3); fennel (p.1579·1); aniseed (p.1549·3).
Constipation.

Ramet Cade *CS, Fr.*
Cade oil (p.1092·2).
Skin disorders.

Ramet Dalibour *CS, Fr.*
Copper sulphate (p.1338·1); zinc sulphate (p.1373·2).
Skin cleaning and disinfection.

Ramet Pain *CS, Fr.*
Copper sulphate (p.1338·1); zinc sulphate (p.1373·2).
Skin cleansing and disinfection.

Rami Hoeststroop *Warner-Lambert, Neth.†.*
Codeine (p.26·1); antimony potassium tartrate (p.98·1).
Coughs.

Rami Hoeststroop voor Kinderen *Warner-Lambert, Neth.†.*
Codeine (p.26·1).
Coughs.

Rami Slijmoplossende *Warner-Lambert, Neth.*
Carbocisteine (p.1056·3).
Coughs.

Ramno-Flor *Medifood-Trufood, Ital.*
Lactic-acid-producing organisms (p.1594·1).
Nutritional supplement.

Ramp *MediMar, UK.*
Pregnancy test (p.1621·2).

Ramses
Schmid, Canad.; Schmid, USA.
Nonoxinol 9 (p.1326·1).
Contraceptive.

Ramysis *Isis, UK.*
Doxycycline hydrochloride (p.202·3).
Bacterial infections.

Ran *Corvi, Ital.†.*
Naphazoline hydrochloride (p.1064·2).
Conjunctival congestion; nasal congestion.

Ran H2 *Seid, Spain.*
Ranitidine hydrochloride (p.1209·3).
Acid aspiration; gastro-intestinal haemorrhage; gastro-oesophageal reflux disease; peptic ulcer; Zollinger-Ellison syndrome.

Ranacid *Nycomed, Norw.*
Ranitidine hydrochloride (p.1209·3).
Acid aspiration syndrome; gastro-oesophageal reflux; peptic ulcer; Zollinger-Ellison syndrome.

Ranamp *Ranbaxy, S.Afr.*
Ampicillin trihydrate (p.153·2).
Bacterial infections.

Ranaps *Approved Prescription Services, UK.*
Ranitidine hydrochloride (p.1209·3).
Acid aspiration; dyspepsia; gastro-intestinal haemorrhage; gastro-oesophageal reflux; peptic ulcer; Zollinger-Ellison syndrome.

Ranceph *Ranbaxy, S.Afr.*
Cephalexin (p.178·2).
Bacterial infections.

Randa *Kayaku, Jpn.*
Cisplatin (p.513·3).
Malignant neoplasms.

Randum *Hoechst Marion Roussel, Ital.*
Metoclopramide hydrochloride (p.1200·3).
Gastro-intestinal disorders.

Ranestol *Parke, Davis, Neth.†.*
Bevantolol hydrochloride (p.832·3).
Angina pectoris; hypertension.

Ranezide *Parke, Davis, Neth.†.*
Bevantolol hydrochloride (p.832·3); hydrochlorothiazide (p.885·2).
Hypertension.

Ranfen *Ranbaxy, S.Afr.*
Ibuprofen (p.44·1).
Fever; inflammation; musculoskeletal, joint, and soft-tissue disorders; pain.

Rangozona *Farmasur, Spain†.*
Feprazone (p.41·2).
Fever; inflammation; pain.

Rani *BASF, Ger.; Isis Puren, Ger.; Sanorania, Ger.*
Ranitidine hydrochloride (p.1209·3).
Aspiration syndrome; gastro-intestinal haemorrhage; gastro-oesophageal reflux; peptic ulcer; Zollinger-Ellison syndrome.

Rani 2 *Alphapharm, Austral.*
Ranitidine hydrochloride (p.1209·3).
Gastro-oesophageal reflux; peptic ulcer; Zollinger-Ellison syndrome.

Raniben *FIRMA, Ital.*
Ranitidine hydrochloride (p.1209·3).
Gastro-intestinal disorders associated with hyperacidity.

Raniberl *Berlin-Chemie, Ger.*
Ranitidine hydrochloride (p.1209·3).
Aspiration syndrome; gastro-oesophageal reflux; peptic ulcer; Zollinger-Ellison syndrome.

Ranibeta *Betapharm, Ger.*
Ranitidine hydrochloride (p.1209·3).
Aspiration syndrome; gastro-intestinal haemorrhage; gastro-oesophageal reflux; peptic ulcer; Zollinger-Ellison syndrome.

Ranibloc
Wolff, Ger.; Glaxo Allen, Ital.
Ranitidine hydrochloride (p.1209·3).
Aspiration syndrome; gastro-intestinal haemorrhage; gastro-oesophageal reflux; peptic ulcer; Zollinger-Ellison syndrome.

Ranic *Glaxo Wellcome, Belg.*
Ranitidine hydrochloride (p.1209·3).
Gastro-oesophageal reflux.

Ranicux *TAD, Ger.*
Ranitidine hydrochloride (p.1209·3).
Aspiration syndrome; gastro-intestinal haemorrhage; gastro-oesophageal reflux; peptic ulcer; Zollinger-Ellison syndrome.

Ranidil *Menarini, Ital.*
Ranitidine hydrochloride (p.1209·3).
Gastro-intestinal disorders associated with hyperacidity.

Ranidin *Faes, Spain.*
Ranitidine hydrochloride (p.1209·3).
Acid aspiration; gastro-intestinal haemorrhage; gastro-oesophageal reflux disease; peptic ulcer; Zollinger-Ellison syndrome.

Ranidura *Durachemie, Ger.*
Ranitidine hydrochloride (p.1209·3).
Aspiration syndrome; gastro-intestinal haemorrhage; gastro-oesophageal reflux; peptic ulcer; Zollinger-Ellison syndrome.

Ranilonga *Alonga, Spain.*
Ranitidine hydrochloride (p.1209·3).
Acid aspiration; gastro-intestinal haemorrhage; gastro-oesophageal reflux disease; peptic ulcer; Zollinger-Ellison syndrome.

Ranimerck *Merck, Ger.*
Ranitidine hydrochloride (p.1209·3).
Aspiration syndrome; gastro-oesophageal reflux; peptic ulcer; Zollinger-Ellison syndrome.

Rani-nerton *Dolorgiet, Ger.*
Ranitidine hydrochloride (p.1209·3).
Aspiration syndrome; gastro-intestinal haemorrhage; gastro-oesophageal reflux; peptic ulcer; Zollinger-Ellison syndrome.

Raniplex *Fournier, Fr.*
Ranitidine hydrochloride (p.1209·3).
Gastro-oesophageal reflux; peptic ulcer; Zollinger-Ellison syndrome.

Raniprotect *Brenner-Efeka, Ger.; LAW, Ger.*
Ranitidine hydrochloride (p.1209·3).
Aspiration syndrome; gastro-intestinal haemorrhage; gastro-oesophageal reflux; peptic ulcer; Zollinger-Ellison syndrome.

Rani-Q *Scand Pharm, Swed.*
Ranitidine hydrochloride (p.1209·3).
Gastro-intestinal disorders associated with hyperacidity.

Ranitic *Hexal, Ger.*
Ranitidine hydrochloride (p.1209·3).
Aspiration syndrome; gastro-intestinal haemorrhage; gastro-oesophageal reflux; peptic ulcer; Zollinger-Ellison syndrome.

Ranix *Knoll, Spain.*
Ranitidine hydrochloride (p.1209·3).
Acid aspiration; gastro-intestinal haemorrhage; gastro-oesophageal reflux disease; peptic ulcer; Zollinger-Ellison syndrome.

Ranmoxy *Ranbaxy, S.Afr.*
Amoxycillin trihydrate (p.151·3).
Bacterial infections.

Rantec *Berk, UK.*
Ranitidine hydrochloride (p.1209·3).
Acid aspiration; dyspepsia; gastro-intestinal haemorrhage; gastro-oesophageal reflux; peptic ulcer; Zollinger-Ellison syndrome.

Rantudil *Bayer, Ger.*
Acemetacin (p.12·2).
Gout; inflammation; musculoskeletal, joint, and peri-articular disorders; thrombophlebitis.

Ranuber *ICN, Spain.*
Ranitidine hydrochloride (p.1209·3).
Acid aspiration; gastro-intestinal haemorrhage; gastro-oesophageal reflux disease; peptic ulcer; Zollinger-Ellison syndrome.

Ranvil *Gentili, Ital.*
Nicardipine hydrochloride (p.915·1).
Angina pectoris; heart failure; hypertension.

Ranzol *Ranbaxy, S.Afr.*
Cephazolin sodium (p.181·1).
Bacterial infections.

Rapako S *Truw, Ger.*
Homoeopathic preparation.

Rapako xylo *Truw, Ger.*
Xylometazoline hydrochloride (p.1071·2).
Rhinitis.

Rap-eze *Roche Consumer, UK.*
Calcium carbonate (p.1182·1).
Dyspepsia.

Raphanus S Potier *Pharmethic, Belg.*
Raphanus sativus niger.
Dyspepsia associated with biliary dyskinesia.

Rapicort *Malesci, Ital.*
Hydrocortisone sodium succinate (p.1044·1).
Shock.

Rapidal *Aristegui, Spain.*
Terfenadine (p.418·1).
Hypersensitivity reactions.

Rapidocaine *Sintetica, Switz.*
Lignocaine hydrochloride (p.1293·2).
Adrenaline hydrochloride (p.813·3) is included in some injections as a vasoconstrictor to diminish absorption and localise the effect of the local anaesthetic.
Arrhythmias; local anaesthesia.

Rapidol *Pharmonta, Aust.*
Paracetamol (p.72·2); propyphenazone (p.81·3); caffeine (p.749·3).
Fever; pain.

Rapidosept *Bayer, Ger.†.*
Dichlorobenzyl alcohol (p.1112·2); isopropyl alcohol (p.1118·2); butyl glycol.
Hand disinfection.

RapidVue *Quidel, USA.*
Pregnancy test (p.1621·2).

Rapifen
Janssen-Cilag, Aust.; ICI, Austral.; Janssen-Cilag, Belg.; Janssen-Cilag, Fr.; Janssen-Cilag, Ger.; Janssen-Cilag, Irl.; Janssen-Cilag, Neth.; Janssen-Cilag, Norw.; Janssen-Cilag, S.Afr.; Janssen-Cilag, Swed.; Janssen-Cilag, Switz.; Janssen, UK.
Alfentanil hydrochloride (p.12·3).
Induction of general anaesthesia; pain during surgical procedures.

Rapignost Amylase *Hoechst Marion Roussel, Irl.†.*
Test for amylase in urine.

Rapignost Basic Screen Plus *Hoechst Marion Roussel, Irl.*
Test for ascorbic acid, glucose, protein, blood, pH, and nitrites in urine.

Rapignost Diabetes Profile *Hoechst Marion Roussel, Irl.*
Test for ketones, ascorbic acid, and glucose in urine.

Rapignost Total Screen L *Hoechst Marion Roussel, Irl.*
Test for bilirubin, urobilinogen, pH, glucose, protein, ketones, blood, nitrite, ascorbic acid, and leucocytes in urine.

Rapilysin
Boehringer Mannheim, Fr.; Boehringer Mannheim, Ger.; Boehringer Mannheim, Swed.; Boehringer Mannheim, UK.
Reteplase (p.942·3).
Myocardial infarction.

Rapi-snooze *Medinaturals, UK.*
Melatonin (p.1599·3); pyridoxine (p.1363·1); valerian (p.1643·1).

Rapitard *Novo Nordisk, Ger.*
Biphasic insulin injection (bovine with porcine, monocomponent) (p.322·1).
Diabetes mellitus.

Rapitard MC
Novo Nordisk, Aust.†; CSL-Novo, Austral.†; Novo Nordisk, Fr.; Novo Nordisk, Ital.†; Novo Nordisk, Switz.; Novo Nordisk, UK†.
Biphasic insulin injection (bovine with porcine, monocomponent) (p.322·1).
Diabetes mellitus.

Rapitil *Fisons, UK.*
Nedocromil sodium (p.756·2).
Allergic conjunctivitis.

Rapitux *Boehringer Ingelheim, Ital.*
Levodropropizine (p.1059·2).
Coughs.

Rapolyte
Helsinn Birex, Irl.; Janssen, UK†.
Sodium chloride; potassium chloride; sodium citrate; glucose (p.1152·3).
Diarrhoea; oral rehydration therapy.

Rappell *Charwell Pharmaceuticals, UK.*
Piperonal (p.1409·3).
Pediculosis.

Rapura *Globopharm, Switz.*
Peru balsam (p.1617·2); camphor (p.1557·2); thymol (p.1127·1); zinc oxide (p.1096·2).
Minor skin lesions.

RAS *Wiedemann, Ger.*
Antireticular serum (rabbit).
Tonic.

Rasal *Kendall, Spain.*
Olsalazine sodium (p.1204·1).
Ulcerative colitis.

Rasayana *Bioforce, Switz.†.*
Cnicus benedictus (p.1565·3); cichorium; fumitory (p.1581·3); aloes (p.1177·1); frangula bark (p.1193·2).
Constipation; stool softener.

Rashaway *Czarniak, Austral.†.*
Zinc oxide (p.1096·2); Germall 115; cod-liver oil (p.1337·3).
Skin disorders.

Rasilvax *Biocine, Ital.*
A rabies vaccine (human diploid cell) (p.1530·3).
Active immunisation.

Rastinon
Hoechst, Aust.; Hoechst Marion Roussel, Austral.; Hoechst Marion Roussel, Belg.; Hoechst, Ger.; Hoechst Marion Roussel, Irl.; Hoechst Marion Roussel, Ital.; Hoechst Marion Roussel, Neth.; Hoechst Marion Roussel, S.Afr.; Hoechst, Spain; Hoechst, Swed.†; Hoechst Marion Roussel, Switz.; Hoechst Marion Roussel, UK†.
Tolbutamide (p.333·2).
Diabetes mellitus.

Hoechst, Ger.†.
Injection: Tolbutamide sodium (p.333·3).
Diagnostic agent.

Rathimed *Pfleger, Ger.†.*
Metronidazole (p.585·1).
Bacterial infections.

Rathimed N *Pfleger, Ger.†.*
Metronidazole (p.585·1).
Trichomoniasis.

Rationale *Manetti Roberts, Ital.*
Colextran hydrochloride (p.1272·2).
Hyperlipidaemias.

Rationasal *Ratiopharm, Spain.*
Xylometazoline hydrochloride (p.1071·2).
Nasal congestion; sinusitis.

Raudopen *Alter, Spain.*
Amoxycillin trihydrate (p.151·3).
Bacterial infections.

Raudosal *Pharmethic, Belg.†.*
Rauwolfia vomitoria (p.941·3).
Hypertension.

Rau-D-Tablinen *Sanorania, Ger.†.*
Reserpine (p.942·1); benzylhydrochlorothiazide.
Hypertension.

Raufluin *Crosara, Ital.†.*
Hydrochlorothiazide (p.885·2); reserpine (p.942·1).
Hypertension.

Raufuncton N *Knoll, Ger.*
Rauwolfiae vomitoria (p.941·3); squill (p.1070·1); convallaria (p.1567·2); adonis vernalis (p.1543·3).
Arrhythmias; hypertension.

Raunova Plus *SmithKline Beecham, Ital.†.*
Syrosingopine (p.951·2); hydrochlorothiazide (p.885·2).
Hypertension.

Rautrax
Bristol-Myers Squibb, Irl.†; Bristol-Myers Squibb, S.Afr.†.
Hydroflumethiazide (p.889·2); rauwolfia serpentina (p.941·3); potassium chloride (p.1161·1).
Hypertension.

Rauverid *Forest Pharmaceuticals, USA†.*
Rauwolfia serpentina (p.941·3).
Hypertension; psychosis.

RauwolfiaViscomp *Schuck, Ger.*
Homoeopathic preparation.

Rauwolsan H *Pfluger, Ger.*
Homoeopathic preparation.

Rauwoplant *Schwabe, Ger.*
Rauwolfia (p.941·3); crataegus (p.1568·2).
Hypertension.

Rauzide *Apothecon, USA.*
Rauwolfia serpentina (p.941·3); bendrofluazide (p.827·3).
Hypertension.

Ravalgen *Fink, Ger.*
Garlic oil.
Arteriosclerosis.

Ravamil *Merck, S.Afr.*
Verapamil hydrochloride (p.960·3).
Angina pectoris; arrhythmias; hypertension.

Ravenol *Caber, Ital.*
A heparinoid (p.882·3).
Vascular disorders with a risk of thrombosis.

Raveron
Germania, Aust.; Robapharm, Ger.†; Berna, Spain†.
Prostatic extract.
Prostatic disorders.

Ravigona *Roche Nicholas, Spain.*
Vitamin A palmitate (p.1359·2); tocopheryl acetate (p.1369·1).
Eye disorders; male infertility.

Ravocaine and Novocain *Cook-Waite, USA.*
Propoxycaine hydrochloride (p.1300·1); procaine (p.1299·2).
Noradrenaline (p.924·1) is included as a vasoconstrictor to diminish absorption and localise the effect of the local anaesthetic.
Local anaesthesia.

Raxar
Glaxo Wellcome, UK; Glaxo Wellcome, USA.
Grepafloxacin hydrochloride (p.215·3).
Bacterial infections.

Ray Block *Del-Ray, USA.*
SPF 15: Padimate O (p.1488·1); oxybenzone (p.1487·3).
Sunscreen.

Raygard *Australis, Austral.†.*
Ethylhexyl *p*-methoxycinnamate (p.1487·1); avobenzone (p.1486·3).
Sunscreen.

Raygard Quadgard *Australis, Austral.†.*
Ethylhexyl *p*-methoxycinnamate (p.1487·1); avobenzone (p.1486·3); titanium dioxide (p.1093·3).
Sunscreen.

Raykit *Boots, Austral.†.*
Combination pack: 3 Tablets, bisacodyl (p.1179·3); 1 suppository, bisacodyl; 1 sachet of powder, magnesium citrate (p.1198·2).
Bowel evacuation.

Rayvist
Schering, Aust.; Schering, Ger.†; Schering, Ital.†; Schering, Switz.
Meglumine ioglicate (p.1006·2) or meglumine ioglicate and sodium ioglicate (p.1006·2).
Radiographic contrast medium.

Razoxin *Cambridge, UK.*
Razoxane (p.560·2).
Now known as Razoxane Tablets.
Malignant neoplasms.

RBC
Rybar, Irl.; Shire, UK.
Antazoline hydrochloride (p.401·3); calamine (p.1080·1); cetrimide (p.1105·2).
Insect stings; pruritus; skin irritation.

RCF
Abbott, Austral.†; Ross, USA.
Carbohydrate-free soy protein infant feed.

Reabilan
Clintec, Fr.; Clintec, Irl.; Nestle, UK; Elan, USA.
A range of preparations for enteral nutrition.

Reach *Johnson & Johnson, UK†.*
Cetylpyridinium chloride (p.1106·2); sodium fluoride (p.742·1).
Oral hygiene.

Reach Junior Fluoride *Johnson & Johnson, Irl.*
Sodium fluoride (p.742·1).
Dental care.

Reactenol *Lafare, Ital.†.*
Methylprednisolone (p.1046·1).
Corticosteroid.

Reactine *Pfizer, Canad.*
Cetirizine hydrochloride (p.404·2).
Allergic rhinitis; urticaria.

Reactivan
Cascan, Ger.†; Merck, S.Afr.
Fencamfamin hydrochloride (p.1480·3); vitamins.
Tonic.

Reactovalone *Jouveinal, Canad.†.*
Tixocortol pivalate (p.1050·1).
Ulcerative colitis; ulcerative proctitis.

Readi-Cat *Therapex, Canad.†.*
Barium sulphate (p.1003·1).
Radiographic contrast medium.

Realderm *Reall, Switz.*
Zinc oxide (p.1096·2); glycerol (p.1585·2); aluminium acetotartrate (p.1547·3).
Nappy rash; skin irritation.

Realmentyl *Clintec-Sopharga, Fr.†.*
Preparation for enteral nutrition.

Reapam *Parke, Davis, Neth.*
Prazepam (p.687·2).
Anxiety.

Reasec
Janssen-Cilag, Belg.; Janssen-Cilag, Ger.; Janssen-Cilag, Ital.; Janssen-Cilag, Switz.
Diphenoxylate hydrochloride (p.1189·1).
Atropine sulphate (p.455·1) is included in this preparation to discourage abuse.
Diarrhoea.

Rebetron *Schering, USA.*
Injection, interferon alfa-2b (Intron A) (p.615·3); capsules, tribavirin (Rebetol) (p.626·2).
Chronic hepatitis C.

Rebif *Serono, UK.*
Interferon beta-1a (p.616·1).
Multiple sclerosis.

Reca *Cantabria, Spain.*
Enalapril maleate (p.863·2).
Heart failure; hypertension.

Recaps-Depot *Sanol, Ger.†.*
Red tablets, procaine; adenosine phosphate; haematoporphyrin; yellow tablets, vitamins; hesperidin complex.
Tonic.

Recaps-Depot H 3 forte *Sanol, Ger.†.*
Procaine hydrochloride; procaine; adenosine phosphate; haematoporphyrin; vitamins; hesperidin complex.
Tonic.

Recarcin *Sanum-Kehlbeck, Ger.*
Bacillus firmus.
Immunotherapy.

Recatol *Woelm, Ger.†.*
Cathine hydrochloride (p.1478·1); thiamine hydrochloride (p.1361·1); pyridoxine hydrochloride (p.1362·3); ascorbic acid (p.1365·2).
Obesity.

Recatol N *Woelm, Ger.*
Phenylpropanolamine hydrochloride (p.1067·2); thiamine hydrochloride (p.1361·1); pyridoxine hydrochloride (p.1362·3); ascorbic acid (p.1365·2).
Obesity.

Recef *Uno, Ital.*
Cephazolin sodium (p.181·1).
Bacterial infections.

Recefril *Lacer, Spain†.*
Amoxycillin trihydrate (p.151·3).
Bacterial infections.

Receptozine *Be-Tabs, S.Afr.*
Promethazine hydrochloride (p.416·2).
Hypersensitivity.

Recessan
Note. This name is used for preparations of different composition.
Provita, Aust.
Tyrothricin (p.267·2); thymol (p.1127·1); pancreatin (p.1612·1); laureth 9 (p.1325·2).
Infections and pain of the mouth and lips.

Kreussler, Ger.
Laureth 9 (p.1325·2).
Inflammatory disorders of the oropharynx.

Reclomide *Major, USA.*
Metoclopramide hydrochloride (p.1200·3).
Nausea and vomiting.

Recofol
Leiras, Norw.; Leiras, Swed.
Propofol (p.1229·3).
General anaesthesia.

Recombinate
CSL, Austral.; Baxter, Belg.; Baxter, Fr.; Baxter, Ger.; Baxter, Ital.; Baxter, Spain; Baxter, Swed.; ZLB, Switz.; Baxter, UK; Hyland, USA.
A factor VIII preparation (recombinant) (p.720·3).
Haemorrhagic disorders.

Recombivax HB
Merck Sharp & Dohme, Canad.; Pasteur Merieux, Ital.; Pasteur Merieux, Spain; Merck Sharp & Dohme, USA.
A hepatitis B vaccine (recombinant DNA) (p.1513·1).
Active immunisation.

Recordil
Meram, Fr.†; Recordati, Ital.†.
Efloxate (p.863·1).
Cardiovascular disorders.

Recormon
Boehringer Mannheim, Aust.; Boehringer Mannheim, Belg.; Boehringer Mannheim, Fr.; Boehringer Mannheim, Ger.; Boehringer Mannheim, Irl.; Boehringer Mannheim, Neth.†; Boehringer Mannheim, Norw.; Boehringer Mannheim, S.Afr.; Boehringer Mannheim, Switz.; Boehringer Mannheim, UK.
Epoetin beta (p.718·3).
Anaemias; autologous blood transfusions.

Recosenin *Robapharm, Ger.†.*
Whole heart extract.
Cardiovascular disorders.

Recovery Food *Milupa, Irl.*
Food for special diet.

Rectagene II *Pfeiffer, USA†.*
Bismuth subgallate (p.1180·2); bismuth resorcinol compound (p.1181·1); benzyl benzoate (p.1402·2); zinc oxide (p.1096·2); bismuth oxyiodide (p.1181·1); calcium phosphate (p.1155·3); peru balsam (p.1617·2).
Haemorrhoids.

Rectagene Medicated Balm *Pfeiffer, USA.*
Yeast (p.1373·1); shark-liver oil.
Haemorrhoids.

Rectagene Medicated Rectal Balm *Pfeiffer, USA.*
Benzocaine (p.1286·2); phenylephrine hydrochloride (p.1066·2); bismuth subgallate (p.1180·2); zinc oxide (p.1096·2); mepyramine maleate (p.414·1).
Anorectal disorders.

Rectalad *Carter-Wallace, Austral.*
Docusate sodium (p.1189·3).
Bowel evacuation; constipation.

Rectamigdol *Diviser Aquilea, Spain†.*
Bismuth camphocarbonate (p.1181·1).
Sore throat.

Rectinol *G.P. Laboratories, Austral.*
Adrenaline (p.813·2); benzocaine (p.1286·2); zinc oxide (p.1096·2).
Anorectal disorders.

Recto Menaderm
Note. This name is used for preparations of different composition.
Menarini, Ital.†.
Beclomethasone dipropionate (p.1032·1); clioquinol (p.193·2); heparin sodium (p.879·3); lignocaine hydrochloride (p.1293·2).
Anorectal disorders.

Menarini, Spain.
Beclomethasone dipropionate (p.1032·1); clioquinol (p.193·2); heparin (p.879·3); cod-liver oil (p.1337·3); lignocaine hydrochloride (p.1293·2).
Anorectal disorders.

Recto Mugolio *Warner-Lambert, Ital.*
Pumilio pine oil (p.1623·3).
Respiratory-tract disorders.

Rectocoricidin *Schering-Plough, Ital.†.*
Chlorpheniramine maleate (p.405·1); paracetamol (p.72·2); fenalamide (p.1578·3).
Cold symptoms.

Rectocort *Welcker-Lyster, Canad.*
Hydrocortisone acetate (p.1043·3).
Skin disorders.

Rectodelt *Trommsdorff, Ger.*
Prednisone (p.1049·2).
Rectal corticosteroid.

Rectolax *Martin, Fr.†.*
Mannitol (p.900·3); carrageenan (p.1471·3).
Bowel evacuation; constipation.

Rectolmin Antiterm *Zyma, Spain†.*
Paracetamol (p.72·2); propyphenazone (p.81·3).
Fever; pain.

Rectopanbiline *Sarget, Fr.*
Bile extract (p.1553·2); gelatin (p.723·2); glycerol (p.1585·2).
Formerly contained bile extract, hepatica, and boldo.
Bowel evacuation; constipation.

Rectoparin *Dorsch, Ger.†.*
Suppositories: Bismuth subnitrate (p.1180·2); procaine hydrochloride (p.1299·2); panthenol (p.1571·1).
Topical gel: Procaine hydrochloride (p.1299·2); panthenol (p.1571·1).
Anorectal disorders; skin disorders.

Rectoparin N *Dorsch, Ger.†.*
Lignocaine hydrochloride (p.1293·2); dexpanthenol (p.1570·3).
Anorectal disorders.

Rectophedrol *Martin, Fr.*
Cineole (p.1564·1); guaiacol carbonate (p.1061·2); wild thyme oil; camphor (p.1557·2); ephedrine (p.1059·3); procaine hydrochloride (p.1299·2).
Respiratory-tract disorders.

Rectoplexil
Rhone-Poulenc Rorer, Belg.; Theraplix, Fr.
Oxomemazine (p.415·2); guaiphenesin (p.1061·3); sodium benzoate (p.1102·3); paracetamol (p.72·2).
Coughs.

Rectopyrine *Synpharma, Switz.†.*
Codeine phosphate (p.26·1); emetine hydrochloride (p.582·2); dipyrone (p.35·1); drosera (p.1574·1); echinacea (p.1574·2).
Cold symptoms.

Rectoquintyl *Sodip, Switz.*
Ethyl orthoformate (p.1061·1); wild thyme oil; cineole (p.1564·1).
Coughs.

Rectoquintyl-Promethazine *Sodip, Switz.*
Ethyl orthoformate (p.1061·1); promethazine (p.416·2); wild thyme oil; cineole (p.1564·1).
Coughs.

Rectoquotane *Evans, Fr.*
Dimethisoquin hydrochloride (p.1292·2); cetrimide (p.1105·2).
Formerly contained dimethisoquin hydrochloride, esculoside, ephedrine hydrochloride, and cetrimonium bromide.
Anorectal disorders.

Recto-Reparil *Naturwaren, Ital.*
Aescin (p.1543·3); amethocaine hydrochloride (p.1285·2).
Formerly contained aescin, belladonna, and amethocaine hydrochloride.
Anorectal disorders.

Rectosalyl *Bouty, Ital.†.*
Aspirin (p.16·1).
Fever; pain.

Rectosan *Terramin, Aust.*
Naphazoline hydrochloride (p.1064·2); menthol (p.1600·2); benzocaine (p.1286·2).
Anorectal disorders.

Rectosan 'A' *Lennon, S.Afr.†.*
Zinc oxide (p.1096·2); resorcinol (p.1090·1); bismuth subgallate (p.1180·2); peru balsam (p.1617·2); belladonna (p.457·1); benzocaine (p.1286·2).
Haemorrhoids.

Rectosellan *Mann, Ger.*
Aesculus (p.1543·3); melilotus officinalis.
Haemorrhoids.

Rectosellan H *Mann, Ger.*
Ointment: Laureth 9 (p.1325·2); zinc oxide (p.1096·2).
Suppositories: Zinc oxide (p.1096·2); benzocaine (p.1286·2).
Anorectal disorders.

Rectosellan N *Mann, Ger.†.*
Guaiazulene (p.1586·3); menthol (p.1600·2); allantoin (p.1078·2); aluminium hydroxide salicylate; camphor (p.1557·2); laureth 9 (p.1325·2); cod-liver oil (p.1337·3); zinc oxide (p.1096·2).
Anorectal disorders.

Rectoseptal-Neo bismuthe *Actipharm, Switz.*
Bismuth succinate (p.1181·1); cineole (p.1564·1); terpin hydrate (p.1070·2); potassium hydroxyquinoline sulphate hydrate (p.1621·1).
Pharyngeal disorders.

Rectoseptal-Neo Pholcodine *Actipharm, Switz.*
Guaiacol (p.1061·2); cineole (p.1564·1); terpin hydrate (p.1070·2); pholcodine (p.1068·1).
Respiratory-tract disorders.

Rectoseptal-Neo simple *Actipharm, Switz.*
Guaiacol (p.1061·2); cineole (p.1564·1); terpin hydrate (p.1070·2); potassium hydroxyquinoline sulphate hydrate (p.1621·1).
Respiratory-tract disorders.

Rectovalone
Jouveinal, Canad.; Jouveinal, Fr.; Byk, Neth.; Juste, Spain.
Tixocortol pivalate (p.1050·1).
Crohn's disease; haemorrhagic rectocolitis; ulcerative colitis.

Rectovasol *Qualiphar, Belg.*
Bismuth subgallate (p.1180·2); bismuth oxyiodogallate (p.1181·1); zinc oxide (p.1096·2); aesculus (p.1543·3); hamamelis (p.1587·1); amylocaine (p.1286·1); peru balsam (p.1617·2).
Haemorrhoids.

Recvalysat *Ysatfabrik, Ger.*
Valerian (p.1643·1).
Nervous disorders.

Red Away *Rivex, Canad.*
Naphazoline hydrochloride (p.1064·2).

Red Cross Canker Sore Medication *Mentholatum, USA.*
Benzocaine (p.1286·2).
Canker sores.

Red Cross Toothache *Mentholatum, USA.*
Eugenol (p.1578·2).
Toothache.

Red Kooga *English Grains, UK.*
Ginseng (p.1584·2).
Tonic.

Red Kooga Betalife *English Grains, UK.*
Multivitamin preparation with ginseng, selenium, and fish oil.

Red Kooga Sport *English Grains, UK.*
Multivitamin preparation with ginseng, iron, and glucose.
Tonic.

Red Oil *Nello, UK.*
Methyl nicotinate (p.55·1); volatile mustard oil (p.1605·3); clove oil (p.1565·2); arachis oil (p.1550·2).
Muscle pain.

Red Point *Synpharma, Aust.†.*
Camphor (p.1557·2); citral; anise oil (p.1550·1); eucalyptus oil (p.1578·1); methyl salicylate (p.55·2); citronella oil (p.1565·1); niaouli oil (p.1607·1); rosemary oil (p.1626·2); thyme oil (p.1637·1); peppermint oil (p.1208·1); cayenne pepper; mustard oil (p.1605·3); arnica (p.1550·3).
Musculoskeletal and joint disorders.

Redactiv *Schiapparelli, Ital.*
Rifaximin (p.246·3).
Bacterial skin infections.

Redaxa Fit *Palmicol, Ger.*
Equisetum (p.1575·1).
Water retention.

Redaxa Lax *Palmicol, Ger.*
Rhubarb (p.1212·1); aloes (p.1177·1).
Constipation.

Redeptin
SmithKline Beecham, Irl.; Janssen-Cilag, UK†.
Fluspirilene (p.672·3).
Schizophrenia.

Redinon Cortex *Bracco, Ital.†.*
Suprarenal cortex (p.1050·1); cyanocobalamin (p.1363·3); inosine (p.1591·1); ferrocholinate (p.1339·2).
Anaemias; tonic.

Redomex *Lundbeck, Belg.*
Amitriptyline hydrochloride (p.273·3).
Depression; pain.

Redox-Injektopas *Pascoe, Ger.*
Multivitamin preparation.
Procaine hydrochloride (p.1299·2) is included in this preparation to alleviate the pain of injection.

Redoxon
Roche, Aust.; Roche Consumer, Austral.; Roche, Belg.; Roche, Canad.; Roche Consumer, Irl.; Roche, Ital.; Roche Nicholas, Neth.; Roche, S.Afr.; Roche Nicholas, Spain; Roche, Switz.; Roche Consumer, UK.
Ascorbic acid (p.1365·2), calcium ascorbate (p.1365·2), or sodium ascorbate (p.1365·2).
Malabsorption syndromes; methaemoglobinaemia; vitamin C deficiency; vitamin C supplement.

Redoxon Calciovit *Roche Nicholas, Spain.*
Ascorbic acid (p.1365·2); calcium carbonate (p.1182·1); ergocalciferol (p.1367·1); pyridoxine hydrochloride.
Bone and dental disorders; calcium deficiency; osteomalacia; rickets.

Redoxon Complex *Roche Nicholas, Spain.*
Multivitamin and mineral preparation.

Redoxon Double Action *Roche Consumer, UK.*
Vitamin C (p.1365·2); zinc (p.1373·1).

Redoxon Protector *Roche Consumer, UK.*
Betacarotene; ascorbic acid; dl-alpha tocopheryl acetate.

Redoxon-B *Roche, Canad.*
Ascorbic acid; vitamin B substances; magnesium salts.
Nutritional supplement.

Redoxon-Cal *Roche, Canad.*
Ascorbic acid; ergocalciferol; pyridoxine hydrochloride; calcium carbonate.
Bone and dental disorders; delayed wound and fracture healing; nutritional supplement; osteomalacia; osteoporosis.

Reducdyn *Nordmark, Ger.†.*
Citiolone (p.1564·3); cysteine (p.1338·3); fructose (p.1343·2).
Liver disorders.

Reducealin *Propan, S.Afr.*
Propylhexedrine (p.1485·1); vitamin B substances.
Obesity.

Reducelle *Alsitan, Ger.*
Aloes (p.1177·1); birch leaf (p.1553·3); cascara (p.1183·1); ononis (p.1610·2); phaseolus vulgaris.
Bowel evacuation; constipation.

Reducterol *Elfar, Spain.*
Bezafibrate (p.1268·2).
Hyperlipidaemias.

Reducto *Salus, Aust.*
Monobasic potassium phosphate (p.1159·3); dibasic sodium phosphate dihydrate (p.1159·3).
Calcium oxalate stones; hypercalcaemia.

Reducto-special *Asta Medica, Switz.*
Monobasic potassium phosphate (p.1159·3); dibasic sodium phosphate dihydrate (p.1159·3).
Calcium oxalate stones; hypercalcaemia; phosphate supplement.

Reducto-spezial *Temmler, Ger.*
Monobasic potassium phosphate (p.1159·3); dibasic sodium phosphate dihydrate (p.1159·3).
Calcium oxalate stones; hypercalcaemia; phosphate supplement.

Redufen *Zollweiden, Switz.*
Ibuprofen (p.44·1).
Fever; pain.

Redul *Schering, Ger.†.*
Glymidine (p.321·2).
Diabetes mellitus.

Reduligne *Chefaro Ardeval, Fr.†.*
Fucus (p.1554·1); taraxacum (p.1634·2); equisetum (p.1575·1).
Herbal slimming preparation.

Redupres *Leti, Spain.*
Verapamil hydrochloride (p.960·3).
Angina pectoris; arrhythmias; hypertension.

Redurate *Schwulst, S.Afr.*
Allopurinol (p.390·2).
Gout; hyperuricaemia.

Redutemp *International Ethical, USA.*
Paracetamol (p.72·2).

Redutona *Faes, Spain.*
Phenytoin (p.352·3); phenobarbitone (p.350·2); aminohydroxybutyric acid (p.339·1); pyridoxine hydrochloride (p.1362·3).
Epilepsy.

Reduvit *Technicon, S.Afr.*
Multivitamin and mineral preparation.

Reef Tanning Lotion *Boots, Austral.*
SPF6: Ethylhexyl *p*-methoxycinnamate (p.1487·1).
SPF15+: Ethylhexyl *p*-methoxycinnamate (p.1487·1); oxybenzone (p.1487·3).
Sunscreen.

Reef Tanning Oil *Boots, Austral.*
SPF6: Ethylhexyl *p*-methoxycinnamate (p.1487·1); oxybenzone (p.1487·3).
SPF15+: Ethylhexyl *p*-methoxycinnamate (p.1487·1); octocrylene (p.1487·3).
Sunscreen.

Reemplazante Gastric *Mein, Spain.*
Ammonium chloride; potassium chloride; sodium chloride (p.1147·1).
Formerly known as Sol Reemplazante Gastric.
Fluid and electrolyte depletion.

Reemplazante Intesti *Mein, Spain.*
Glucose; potassium chloride; sodium chloride; sodium lactate (p.1152·3).
Formerly known as Sol Reemplazante Intesti.
Fluid depletion.

Reese's Pinworm *Reese, USA.*
Pyrantel embonate (p.109·3).
Worm infections.

Refagan *Bayer, Ital.†.*
Salicylamide (p.82·3); aspirin (p.16·1); caffeine (p.749·3); mebhydrolin (p.413·2).
Cold symptoms.

Refagan N *Bayropharm, Ger.†.*
Salicylamide (p.82·3); aspirin (p.16·1); caffeine (p.749·3).
Cold symptoms.

Refesan T *Hanosan, Ger.*
Homoeopathic preparation.

Reflex
Note. This name is used for preparations of different composition.
Boots Healthcare, Fr.
Picolamine salicylate (p.80·1).
Musculoskeletal and joint pain.

Boots Healthcare, Spain.
Camphor (p.1557·2); methyl salicylate (p.55·2); turpentine oil (p.1641·1); menthol (p.1600·2).
Rheumatic and muscle pain.

Reflexspray Boots Healthcare, Belg.
Methyl salicylate (p.55·2); turpentine oil (p.1641·1); camphor (p.1557·2); menthol (p.1600·2).
Muscle, joint, and peri-articular disorders.

Reflex-Zonen-Salbe (RZS) (Rowo-333) Pharmakon, Ger.†.
Poppy-seed oil (p.1620·1); mace oil (p.1597·3); hyoscyamus oil (p.464·3); melissa oil.
Tonic.

Reflocheck
Boehringer Mannheim, Ital.; Boehringer Mannheim Diagnostics, UK†.
Test for glucose in blood (p.1585·1).

Reflotron Boehringer Mannheim, Irl.
Test for a range of cardiac risk factors in blood, serum, or plasma.

Refludan
Hoechst Marion Roussel, Neth.; Hoechst Marion Roussel, Swed.; Hoechst Marion Roussel, UK; Hoechst Marion Roussel, USA.
Lepirudin (p.883·1).
Thrombo-embolic disorders.

Reflux IPS, Neth.
Hexamine mandelate (p.216·1).
Urinary-tract infections.

Refluxine Spirig, Switz.
Alginic acid (p.1470·3); sodium bicarbonate (p.1153·2); aluminium hydroxide-magnesium carbonate co-dried gel (p.1178·2).
Gastro-oesophageal reflux.

Refobacin
Merck, Aust.; Merck, Ger.
Gentamicin sulphate (p.212·1).
Bacterial infections.

Refobacin-Palacos R
Merck, Aust.; Merck, Ger.
Gentamicin sulphate (p.212·1); methylacrylate copolymer/methylmethacrylate (p.1603·2).
Bone cement for orthopaedic surgery.

Refolinon
Pharmacia Upjohn, S.Afr.; Farmitalia Carlo Erba, UK.
Folinic acid (p.1342·2) or calcium folinate (p.1342·2).
Antidote to folic acid antagonists; megaloblastic anaemia.

Refosporin Merck, Ger.†.
Cefazedone sodium (p.164·2).
Bacterial infections.

Refresh
Allergan, Austral.; Allergan, Canad.; Allergan, S.Afr.; Allergan, UK; Allergan, USA.
Polyvinyl alcohol (p.1474·2); povidone (p.1474·2).
Dry eyes.

Refresh Night Time Allergan, UK.
White soft paraffin (p.1382·3); liquid paraffin (p.1382·1); wool alcohols (p.1385·2).
Dry eyes.

Refresh Plus Allergan, USA.
Carmellose sodium (p.1471·2).

Refresh PM Allergan, USA.
White soft paraffin (p.1382·3); liquid paraffin (p.1382·1); wool alcohols (p.1385·2).
Dry eyes.

Refulgin Spyfarma, Spain.
Adenosine triphosphate (p.1543·2); hydroxocobalamin acetate (p.1364·2); pyritinol hydrochloride (p.1624·1); prosultiamine (p.1360·3).
Mental function impairment.

Refusal Artu, Neth.
Disulfiram (p.1573·1).
Alcoholism.

Regadrin B Berlin-Chemie, Ger.
Bezafibrate (p.1268·2).
Hyperlipidaemias.

Regain NCI, USA.
Lactose-free preparation for enteral nutrition.
Impaired renal function.

Regaine
Pharmacia Upjohn, Aust.; Pharmacia Upjohn, Austral.; Pharmacia Upjohn, Belg.; Pharmacia Upjohn, Fr.; Pharmacia Upjohn, Irl.; Pharmacia Upjohn, Ital.; Pharmacia Upjohn, Neth.; Pharmacia Upjohn, Norw.; Pharmacia Upjohn, S.Afr.; Upjohn, Spain; Pharmacia Upjohn, Swed.; Pharmacia Upjohn, Switz.; Pharmacia Upjohn, UK.
Minoxidil (p.910·3).
Alopecia androgenetica.

Regal Cantabria, Spain.
Styrax tonkinensis tincture; myrrh tincture (p.1606·1); rhatany tincture (p.1624·3); resorcinol (p.1090·1); zinc chloride (p.1373·1); zinc phenolsulphonate (p.1096·3); methyl salicylate (p.55·2); menthol (p.1600·2).
Halitosis; mouth inflammation.

Regalen Eisai, Jpn.
Chenodeoxycholic acid (p.1562·1).
Cholesterol gallstones.

Regard Smith & Nephew, S.Afr.
Glycerol (p.1585·2).
Lubrication.

Regasinum Rowa, Ger.
A range of homoeopathic preparations.

Regastrol Sarm, Ital.†.
Metoclopramide hydrochloride (p.1200·3).
Gastro-intestinal disorders.

Regavasal N Rowa, Ger.
Homoeopathic preparation.

Regelan
Zeneca, Aust.; Zeneca, Switz.
Clofibrate (p.1271·1).
Hyperlipidaemias.

Regelan N Zeneca, Ger.
Clofibrate (p.1271·1).
Hyperlipidaemias.

Regenaplex Regenaplex, Ger.
A range of homoeopathic preparations.

Regender Alacan, Spain.
Polypodium leucotomos.
Skin disorders.

Regenerin Schoeller, Aust.
Procaine hydrochloride (p.1299·2); vitamin A (p.1358·1); vitamin E (p.1369·1).
Reduced mental and physical capacity in the elderly.

Regeneron Rovi, Spain†.
Vitamin and amino-acid preparation.
Tonic.

Regenon
Salus, Aust.; Trenker, Belg.; Temmler, Ger.; Asta Medica, Switz.
Diethylpropion hydrochloride (p.1479·3).
Obesity.

Regenon A Temmler, Ger.†.
Diethylpropion hydrochloride (p.1479·3); docusate sodium (p.1189·3).
Obesity.

Regenprostat Iquinosa, Spain†.
Prunus africana.
Prostatic adenoma.

Regepar Enzypharm, Aust.
Selegiline hydrochloride (p.1144·2).
Parkinsonism.

Regepithel Alcon-Thilo, Ger.
Multivitamin preparation.
Eye disorders.

Regibloc Intramed, S.Afr.
Bupivacaine hydrochloride (p.1286·3).
Local anaesthesia.

Regina Royal Concorde Regina, UK.
Royal jelly (p.1626·3); ginseng (p.1584·2); damiana aphrodisiaca (p.1570·2); saw palmetto (p.1462·1).

Regina Royal Five Regina, UK.
Royal jelly (p.1626·3); bee pollen; pure honey (p.1345·3).

Regina Royal One Hundred Regina, UK.
Royal jelly (p.1626·3).

Reginerton Dolorgiet, Ger.†.
Metoclopramide hydrochloride (p.1200·3).
Nausea and vomiting.

Regison Dietetique et Sante, Fr.†.
Bran (p.1181·2).
Dietary fibre supplement.

Regitin Ciba, Ger.†.
Phentolamine mesylate (p.930·1).
Phaeochromocytoma.

Regitine
Novartis, Austral.; Ciba-Geigy, Belg.; Novartis, Neth.; Ciba-Geigy, S.Afr.†; Ciba, Switz.; Ciba, USA.
Phentolamine mesylate (p.930·1).
Dermal necrosis and sloughing following intravenous administration of noradrenaline; phaeochromocytoma.

Regium Hormosan, Ger.†.
Meprobamate (p.678·1); belladonna (p.457·1); ergotamine tartrate (p.445·3).
Dysmenorrhoea; menopausal disorders; psychiatric disorders; respiratory disorders; sleep disorders.

Regivital Togal, Switz.†.
Valerian (p.1643·1).
Agitation; sleep disorders.

Regla pH
Note. This name is used for preparations of different composition.
Darci, Belg.
Algeldrate (p.1177·3); light magnesium oxide (p.1198·3).
Gastro-intestinal disorders associated with hyperacidity.

UCB, Neth.
Algeldrate (p.1177·3); magnesium carbonate (p.1198·1) or magnesium hydroxide (p.1198·2).
Gastro-intestinal disorders.

UCB, Switz.
Suspension: Aluminium hydroxide (p.1177·3); light magnesium oxide (p.1198·3); aluminium hydroxide-magnesium carbonate co-dried gel (p.1178·2).
Tablets: Aluminium hydroxide-magnesium carbonate co-dried gel (p.1178·2); glycine (p.1345·2).
Gastric hyperacidity; peptic ulcer.

Reglan
Wyeth-Ayerst, Canad.; Robins, USA.
Metoclopramide hydrochloride (p.1200·3).
Gastric motility disorders; nausea and vomiting.

Regomed Interpharm, Aust.
Enalapril maleate (p.863·2).
Heart failure; hypertension.

Regonol
Organon, Canad.; Organon, USA.
Pyridostigmine bromide (p.1398·1).
Myasthenia gravis; reversal of competitive neuromuscular blockade.

Regranex Ortho McNeil, USA.
Becaplermin (p.1079·2).
Diabetic neuropathic ulcers.

Regroton Rhone-Poulenc Rorer, USA.
Chlorthalidone (p.839·3); reserpine (p.942·1).
Hypertension.

Regubil Riva, Canad.
Biliary salts (p.1553·2); dehydrocholic acid (p.1570·2); deoxycholic acid.
Biliary-tract disorders.

Regulace Republic, USA.
Docusate sodium (p.1189·3); casanthranol (p.1182·3).
Constipation.

Regulacor Ursapharm, Ger.
Crataegus (p.1568·2).
Cardiac disorders.

Regulan
Procter & Gamble, Irl.; Procter & Gamble (H&B Care), UK.
Ispaghula husk (p.1194·2).
Constipation; diverticular disease; irritable bowel syndrome.

Regular Pharkos, Ital.†.
Cascara sagrada (p.1183·1); rhubarb (p.1212·1); boldo (p.1554·1); bitter orange (p.1610·3).
Constipation; liver disorders.

Regular Iletin I Lilly, USA.
Insulin injection (bovine and porcine) (p.322·1).
Diabetes mellitus.

Regular Iletin II Lilly, USA.
Insulin injection (porcine) (p.322·1).
Diabetes mellitus.

Regular Strength Anbesol Whitehall, USA.
Benzocaine (p.1286·2); phenol (p.1121·2); alcohol (p.1099·1).
Dental pain.

Regular Strength Bayer Sterling Health, USA.
Aspirin (p.16·1).
Formerly known as Therapy Bayer.
Fever; inflammation; myocardial infarction; pain; transient ischaemic attacks.

Regulax N Meuselbach, Ger.
Senna (p.1212·2).
Constipation.

Regulax Picosulfat Meuselbach, Ger.
Sodium picosulphate (p.1213·2).
Constipation.

Regulax SS Republic, USA.
Docusate sodium (p.1189·3).
Constipation.

Reguletts
Husler, Switz.; Seton, UK.
Phenolphthalein (p.1208·2).
Constipation.

Regulex Whitehall-Robins, Canad.
Docusate sodium (p.1189·3).
Constipation.

Regulex-D Whitehall-Robins, Canad.
Danthron (p.1188·2); docusate sodium (p.1189·3).
Constipation.

Reguloid Rugby, USA.
Psyllium hydrophilic mucilloid (p.1194·2).
Constipation.

Regulose Sandoz, UK.
Lactulose (p.1195·3).
Constipation.

Regulton
Knoll, Belg.; Knoll, Ger.
Amezinium methylsulphate (p.819·1).
Hypotension.

Regunon Schering, Swed.
Levonorgestrel (p.1454·1); ethinyloestradiol (p.1445·1).
Combined oral contraceptive.

Regutol Schering-Plough, USA†.
Docusate sodium (p.1189·3).
Constipation.

Rehibin Serono, UK†.
Cyclofenil (p.1440·2).
Anovulatory infertility.

Rehidrat
Searle, Irl.; Searle, UK.
Sodium chloride; potassium chloride; sodium bicarbonate; citric acid; glucose; sucrose; fructose (p.1152·3).
Diarrhoea; oral rehydration therapy.

Searle, S.Afr.
Sodium chloride; potassium chloride; sodium bicarbonate; glucose; sucrose (p.1152·3).
Diarrhoea; oral rehydration therapy.

Rehydralyte
Ross, Canad.; Ross, USA.
Glucose; potassium citrate; sodium chloride; sodium citrate (p.1152·3).
Diarrhoea; oral rehydration therapy.

Rehydrex med glucos Pharmacia Upjohn, Swed.
Electrolyte infusion with anhydrous glucose (p.1147·1).
Fluid and electrolyte disorders.

Reidrax Bonomelli, Ital.
Electrolytes; vitamins; glucose (p.1152·3).
Oral rehydration therapy.

Reise Superpep-K Pharmacal, Switz.
Dimenhydrinate (p.408·2).
Motion sickness; nausea; vertigo; vomiting.

Reisedragee Eu Rho Eu Rho, Ger.
Diphenhydramine hydrochloride (p.409·1); 8-chlorotheophylline.
Nausea; vomiting.

Reisegold Much, Ger.
Sugar-coated tablets: Diphenhydramine hydrochloride (p.409·1); caffeine (p.749·3); 8-chlorotheophylline; pyridoxine hydrochloride (p.1362·3).
Tablets: Dimenhydrinate (p.408·2).
Motion sickness.

Reisetabletten-ratiopharm Ratiopharm, Ger.
Dimenhydrinate (p.408·2).
Motion sickness; nausea; vertigo; vomiting.

Rekawan
Solvay, Aust.; Solvay, Ger.
Potassium chloride (p.1161·1).
Potassium deficiency.

Rekomill Pino, Ger.†.
Chamomile flowers (p.1561·2).
Inflammatory disorders.

Rekont Madaus, Aust.
Trospium chloride (p.1640·1).
Bladder function disorders.

Rekord B12 Sigma-Tau, Ital.
Amino-acid and vitamin B substances.
Tonic.

Rekord B12 Ferro Sigma-Tau, Ital.†.
Amino-acid, vitamin, and ferritin preparation (p.1580·1).
Anaemias.

Rekord Ferro Sigma-Tau, Ital.
Iron succinyl-protein complex (p.1349·2).
Anaemias; iron-deficiency.

Rela Schering, USA†.
Carisoprodol (p.1312·3).

Relafen
SmithKline Beecham, Canad.; SmithKline Beecham, USA.
Nabumetone (p.60·1).
Osteoarthritis; rheumatoid arthritis.

Relastef Italfarmaco, Ital.†.
Tretinoin (p.1093·3).
Acne; photo-ageing.

Relaten Herbaline, Ital.
Chamomile (p.1561·2); crataegus (p.1568·2); eschscholtzia californica; red-poppy (p.1001·1).
Agitation; anxiety; insomnia.

Relax B^+ Vitalia, UK.
Valerian (p.1643·1); lupulus (p.1597·2); passion flower (p.1615·3); vitamin B substances.

Relaxadon Geneva, USA†.
Atropine sulphate (p.455·1); hyoscine hydrobromide (p.462·3); hyoscyamine hydrobromide (p.464·2) or hyoscyamine sulphate (p.464·2); phenobarbitone (p.350·2).
Gastro-intestinal disorders.

Relaxaplex Vitaplex, Austral.
Valerian (p.1643·1); scutellaria; passion flower (p.1615·3); lupulus (p.1597·2); gentian (p.1583·3).
Herbal sedative.

Relaxar Bouty, Ital.
Liniment: Mephenesin (p.1315·3); methyl nicotinate (p.55·1).
Neuromuscular pain; soft-tissue disorders.
Tablets†: Mephenesin (p.1315·3).
Skeletal muscle spasm.

Relaxa-Tabs Woods, Austral.
Mepyramine maleate (p.414·1).
Insomnia; nervous tension.

Relaxedans Salvat, Spain.
Chlordiazepoxide (p.646·3); pyridoxine (p.1363·1).
Anxiety.

Relaxibys Antibioticos, Spain.
Carisoprodol (p.1312·3); paracetamol (p.72·2).
Musculoskeletal spasticity.

Relaxine
Trenker, Belg.; Phygiene, Fr.
Valerian (p.1643·1).
Insomnia; nervous disorders.

Relaxit
Note. This name is used for preparations of different composition.
Abigo, Swed.
Sodium bicarbonate (p.1153·2); potassium acid tartrate (p.1209·1); calcium silicate (p.1182·2).
Constipation.

Crawford, UK.
Sodium citrate (p.1153·2); sodium lauryl sulphate (p.1468·3); sorbic acid (p.1125·2); glycerol (p.1585·2); sorbitol (p.1354·2).
Constipation.

Relaxoddi Leurquin, Fr.
Butacaine (p.1288·3); oleic acid (p.1384·2).
Dyspepsia.

Relaxyl
Note. This name is used for preparations of different composition.
Hafslund Nycomed, Aust.
Dibasic sodium phosphate dodecahydrate (p.1159·3); monobasic sodium phosphate dihydrate (p.1159·3).
Bowel evacuation; constipation.

Seton, UK.
Alverine citrate (p.1548·1).
Irritable bowel syndrome.

Relcofen Cox, UK.
Ibuprofen (p.44·1).

Releaf Lake, USA.
A range of vitamin and mineral preparations.

Relefact LH-RH
Hoechst, Aust.; Hoechst, Austral.†; Hoechst, Ger.; Hoechst Marion Roussel, Irl.; Hoechst Marion Roussel, Neth.; Hoechst Marion Roussel, UK.
Gonadorelin (p.1247·2).
Diagnosis of hypothalamic-pituitary-gonadal dysfunction.

Relefact LH-RH/TRH Hoechst, UK†.
Gonadorelin (p.1247·2); protirelin (p.1259·1).
Diagnosis of pituitary-gonadal dysfunction.

Relefact TRH
Hoechst, Aust.; Hoechst Marion Roussel, Canad.; Hoechst, Ger.; Hoechst Marion Roussel, Neth.; Hoechst Marion Roussel, Switz.
Protirelin (p.1259·1).
Diagnosis of thyroid and pituitary dysfunction.

Reless
Epipharm, Aust.†; Scherax, Ger.
Bee venom extract or wasp venom extract.
Hyposensitisation.

Reless-Wespengiftprotein Epipharm, Aust.†.
Wasp venom.
Diagnosis of wasp sting hypersensitivity; hyposensitisation.

Reliaseal Barrere, Austral.†.
Polyisobutylene compound.
Ostomy adhesive.

Reliberan Geymonat, Ital.
Chlordiazepoxide hydrochloride (p.646·3).
Anxiety disorders.

Relief Allergan, USA.
Phenylephrine hydrochloride (p.1066·2).
Minor eye irritation.

Relief-Coff PD Pharm, S.Afr.
Diphenhydramine hydrochloride (p.409·1); ammonium chloride (p.1055·2); sodium citrate (p.1153·2).
Coughs.

Relif Smith Kline & French, Spain.
Nabumetone (p.60·1).
Osteoarthritis; rheumatoid arthritis.

Relifen SmithKline Beecham, S.Afr.
Nabumetone (p.60·1).
Musculoskeletal, joint, and soft-tissue disorders.

Relifex
Bencard, Belg.†; SmithKline Beecham, Irl.; SmithKline Beecham, Ital.†; SmithKline Beecham, Norw.; SmithKline Beecham, Swed.; SmithKline Beecham, UK.
Nabumetone (p.60·1).
Gout; musculoskeletal and joint disorders.

Relipain Pharmacia Upjohn, Ital.†.
Morphine sulphate (p.56·2).
Pain.

Relisan Xixia, S.Afr.
Nabumetone (p.60·1).
Musculoskeletal and joint disorders.

Relisorm Serono, Canad.
Gonadorelin acetate (p.1248·1).
Diagnosis of hypothalamic-pituitary-gonadal dysfunction.

Relisorm L
Serono, Ital.†; Serono, Switz.
Gonadorelin acetate (p.1248·1).
Test of hypothalamic-pituitary-gonadal function.

Relitone Garec, S.Afr.
Nabumetone (p.60·1).
Musculoskeletal and joint disorders.

Reliv Recip, Swed.
Paracetamol (p.72·2).
Fever; pain.

Relivora Komplex Sanum-Kehlbeck, Ger.
Homoeopathic preparation.

Reloxyl
Note. This name is used for preparations of different composition.
RDC, Ital.
Benzoyl peroxide (p.1079·2).
Acne; skin disinfection.

Cheminova, Spain.
Amoxycillin trihydrate (p.151·3).
Bacterial infections.

Reloxyl Mucolitico Cheminova, Spain.
Amoxycillin trihydrate (p.151·3); guaiphenesin (p.1061·3).
Respiratory-tract infections.

Relsyne Sanofi Winthrop, Ital.†.
Somatorelin acetate (p.1260·3).
Diagnosis of growth hormone deficiency.

Relvene Pharmascience, Fr.
Oxerutins (p.1580·2).
Chronic venous insufficiency.

Remcol Cold Shionogi, USA.
Phenylpropanolamine hydrochloride (p.1067·2); chlorpheniramine maleate (p.405·1); paracetamol (p.72·2).
Upper respiratory-tract symptoms.

Remcol-C Shionogi, USA.
Chlorpheniramine maleate (p.405·1); dextromethorphan hydrobromide (p.1057·3); paracetamol (p.72·2).
Coughs and cold symptoms.

Remdue Biomedica, Ital.
Flurazepam dihydrochloride (p.672·2).
Insomnia.

Remedacen Rhone-Poulenc Rorer, Ger.
Dihydrocodeine polistirex (p.34·2).
Coughs.

Remedeine Napp, UK.
Paracetamol (p.72·2); dihydrocodeine tartrate (p.34·1).
Pain.

Remederm Widmer, Ger.
Urea (p.1095·2); vitamin A palmitate (p.1359·2); α-tocopheryl acetate (p.1369·1); dexpanthenol (p.1570·3); hard paraffin (p.1382·1); white soft paraffin (p.1382·3); light liquid paraffin (p.1382·1).
Skin disorders.

Remederm HC Widmer, Ger.
Hydrocortisone (p.1043·3).
Skin disorders.

Remedial Kwizda, Aust.†.
Vinpocetine (p.1644·2).
Mental function disorders in the elderly.

Remeflin
Recordati, Ital.; Zambon, Spain†.
Dimefline hydrochloride (p.1480·1).
Respiratory and circulatory disorders.

Remegel
Warner-Lambert, Irl.; Warner-Lambert, Ital.; Warner-Lambert, UK.
Calcium carbonate (p.1182·1).
Gastric hyperacidity.

Remen Parke, Davis, Ital.
Pramiracetam sulphate (p.1621·2).
Mental function impairment.

Remergil Organon, Ger.; Thiemann, Ger.
Mirtazapine (p.298·2).
Depression.

Remeron
Organon, Aust.; Organon, Ital.; Nourypharma, Neth.; Organon, Swed.; Organon, USA.
Mirtazapine (p.298·2).
Depression.

Remestan
Wyeth Lederle, Aust.; Wyeth, Ger.
Temazepam (p.693·3).
Sleep disorders.

Remicade Centocor, USA.
Infliximab (p.1194·2).
Crohn's disease.

Remicaine Adcock Ingram Generics, S.Afr.
Lignocaine hydrochloride (p.1293·2).
Arrhythmias; local anaesthesia.

Remicard Adcock Ingram Generics, S.Afr.
Lignocaine hydrochloride (p.1293·2).
Arrhythmias.

Remicyclin D Schaper & Brummer, Ger.†.
Doxycycline hydrochloride (p.202·3).
Bacterial infections.

Remid TAD, Ger.
Allopurinol (p.390·2).
Gout; hyperuricaemia.

Remifemin
Schaper & Brummer, Ger.; Asta Medica, Switz.
Cimicifuga (p.1563·3).
Menopausal and menstrual disorders.

Remifemin plus Schaper & Brummer, Ger.
Hypericum (p.1590·1); cimicifuga (p.1563·3).
Menstrual and menopausal disorders.

Remigeron Schaper & Brummer, Ger.†.
Saw palmetto (p.1462·1).
Benign prostatic hyperplasia.

Remiprostan Uno Schaper & Brummer, Ger.
Saw palmetto (p.1462·1).
Benign prostatic hyperplasia.

Remisan Vir, Spain.
Amoxycillin trihydrate (p.151·3).
Bacterial infections.

Remisan Mucolitico Vir, Spain.
Amoxycillin trihydrate (p.151·3); bromhexine hydrochloride (p.1055·3).
Respiratory-tract infections.

Remivox Janssen, Ger.†.
Lorcainide hydrochloride (p.899·1).
Arrhythmias.

Remnos DDSA Pharmaceuticals, UK.
Nitrazepam (p.682·2).
Insomnia.

Remontal Vita, Spain.
Nimodipine (p.922·2).
Cognitive impairment in the elderly; neurological deficit following subarachnoid haemorrhage.

Remoplexe Lehning, Fr.
Copper gluconate (p.1338·1).
Musculoskeletal and joint disorders; viral infections.

Remotiv
Bayer, Ger.; Zeller, Switz.
Hypericum (p.1590·1).
Anxiety disorders; depression; sleep disorders.

Remotrox Pharmaceutical Enterprises, S.Afr.
Dicyclomine hydrochloride (p.460·1); dried aluminium hydroxide gel (p.1177·3); light magnesium oxide (p.1198·3).
Gastro-intestinal disorders.

Remov Piam, Ital.
Nimesulide (p.63·2).
Fever; inflammation; pain.

Remove Smith & Nephew, Austral.
Dipropylene glycol methyl ether.
Adhesive remover.

Remular-S International Ethical, USA.
Chlorzoxazone (p.1313·1).
Musculoskeletal pain.

Remy Sella, Ital.
Camphor (p.1557·2); ethyl salicylate (p.36·1); menthol (p.1600·2); capsicum oleoresin.
Rheumatism.

Remydrial Winzer, Ger.
Dapiprazole hydrochloride (p.1570·2).
Production of mydriasis.

Remysal N DCG, Swed.†.
Diethylamine salicylate (p.33·1); benzyl nicotinate (p.22·1).
Topical pain relief.

Renacidin
Note. This name is used for preparations of different composition.
Guardian, Canad.†.
Anhydrous citric acid (p.1564·3); gluconic acid (primarily as gluconolactone); calcium carbonate (p.1182·1); dibasic magnesium citrate; magnesium hydroxycarbonate (p.1198·1).
Urinary-tract disorders.

Guardian, USA.
Anhydrous citric acid (p.1564·3); gluconic acid.
Renal calculi.

Renacor Dieckmann, Ger.
Enalapril maleate (p.863·2); hydrochlorothiazide (p.885·2).
Hypertension.

Renal Care Abbott, Ital.
Preparation for enteral nutrition in renal failure.

Renal (Rowo-121) Pharmakon, Ger.†.
Homoeopathic preparation.

Renalin Dialyzer Reprocessing Concentrate
Renal Systems, USA.
Hydrogen peroxide (p.1116·2); acetic acid (p.1541·2); peracetic acid (p.1121·1).

RenAmin Clintec, USA.
Amino-acid infusion.
Parenteral nutrition in renal impairment.

Renapur Schering-Plough, Swed.
Anhydrous potassium citrate (p.1153·1); anhydrous sodium citrate (p.1153·2); anhydrous citric acid (p.1564·3).
Renal calculi.

Renascin
Mack, Illert., Ger.†; IFI, Ital.†.
Tocopheryl nicotinate (p.1280·1).
Hyperlipidaemias; mental function impairment; vascular disorders.

Renedil
Hoechst Marion Roussel, Belg.; Hoechst Marion Roussel, Canad.; Hoechst Marion Roussel, Neth.
Felodipine (p.867·3).
Angina pectoris; hypertension.

Renese
Pfizer, Belg.; Pfizer, Norw.†; Pfizer, Swed.†; Pfizer, USA.
Polythiazide (p.932·1).
Hypertension; oedema.

Renese R Pfizer, USA.
Polythiazide (p.932·1); reserpine (p.942·1).
Hypertension.

Reneuron Juste, Spain.
Fluoxetine hydrochloride (p.284·1).
Bulimia; depression; obsessive-compulsive disorder.

Renezide Lennon, S.Afr.
Triamterene (p.957·2); hydrochlorothiazide (p.885·2).
Hypertension; oedema.

Renidone Rolab, S.Afr.†.
Chlorthalidone (p.839·3).
Hypertension; oedema.

Renilan Mochida, Jpn†.
Cefpimizole sodium (p.171·2).
Bacterial infections.

Renitec
Merck Sharp & Dohme, Aust.; Merck Sharp & Dohme, Austral.; Merck Sharp & Dohme, Belg.; Merck Sharp & Dohme-Chibret, Fr.; Merck Sharp & Dohme, Neth.; Merck Sharp & Dohme, Norw.; Merck Sharp & Dohme, S.Afr.; Merck Sharp & Dohme, Spain; Merck Sharp & Dohme, Swed.
Enalapril maleate (p.863·2) or enalaprilat (p.863·2).
Heart failure; hypertension.

Renitec Comp Merck Sharp & Dohme, Norw.
Enalapril maleate (p.863·2); hydrochlorothiazide (p.885·2).
Hypertension.

Renitec Plus Merck Sharp & Dohme, Neth.
Enalapril maleate (p.863·2); hydrochlorothiazide (p.885·2).
Hypertension.

Reniten Merck Sharp & Dohme, Switz.
Enalapril maleate (p.863·2) or enalaprilat (p.863·2).
Heart failure; hypertension.

Rennie
Roche, Belg.; Roche Nicholas, Fr.; Roche Nicholas, Ger.; Roche, Ital.; dRoche Nicholas, Neth.; Roche, Swed.; Roche, Switz.; Roche Consumer, UK.
Calcium carbonate (p.1182·1); magnesium carbonate (p.1198·1).
Dyspepsia; flatulence.

Rennie Defarin Roche Nicholas, Ger.
Calcium carbonate (p.1182·1); magnesium carbonate (p.1198·1); simethicone (p.1213·1).
Gastro-intestinal disorders with meteorism.

Rennie Deflatine
Roche Nicholas, Fr.; Roche Nicholas, Neth.; Roche, Switz.; Roche Consumer, UK.
Simethicone (p.1213·1); calcium carbonate (p.1182·1); magnesium carbonate (p.1198·1).
Bloating; dyspepsia; flatulence; trapped gas.

Rennie Gold Roche Consumer, UK.
Calcium carbonate (p.1182·1).
Dyspepsia; flatulence.

Rennie Rap-Eze Roche Consumer, Irl.
Calcium carbonate (p.1182·1).
Gastric hyperacidity; heartburn.

Renob Blasen- und Nierentee Pfleger, Ger.
Birch leaves (p.1553·3); couch-grass rhizome (p.1567·3); solidago virgaurea; ononis (p.1610·2); liquorice root (p.1197·1).
Urinary-tract disorders.

Renografin
Squibb Diagnostics, Canad.; Squibb Diagnostics, USA.
Meglumine diatrizoate (p.1003·2); sodium diatrizoate (p.1003·2).
Radiographic contrast medium.

Reno-M
Squibb Diagnostics, Canad.; Squibb Diagnostics, USA.
Meglumine diatrizoate (p.1003·2).
Radiographic contrast medium.

Renoquid Glenwood, USA.
Sulfacytine (p.251·1).
Bacterial infections.

Renormax Sandoz, USA.
Spirapril (p.946·1).
Hypertension.

Renova
Janssen-Ortho, Canad.; Ortho Dermatological, USA.
Tretinoin (p.1093·3).
Acne; photoageing of the skin.

Renovist Squibb Diagnostics, USA.
Meglumine diatrizoate (p.1003·2); sodium diatrizoate (p.1003·2).
Radiographic contrast medium.

Renovue Squibb Diagnostics, USA.
Meglumine iodamide (p.1005·3).
Radiographic contrast medium.

Rentamine Pediatric Major, USA.
Phenylephrine tannate (p.1067·1); ephedrine tannate (p.1060·1); chlorpheniramine tannate (p.405·2); pentoxyverine tannate (p.1066·2).
Coughs and cold symptoms.

Rentibloc Rentschler, Ger.
Sotalol hydrochloride (p.945·1).
Arrhythmias.

Rentylin Rentschler, Ger.
Oxpentifylline (p.925·3).
Peripheral and ocular vascular disorders.

Renu
Bausch & Lomb, Fr.; Bausch & Lomb, USA.
Range of solutions for soft contact lenses.

Renu Enzymatic Cleaner Bausch & Lomb, USA.
Subtilisin-A.
Cleansing solution for soft contact lenses.

Renu Multiplus Bausch & Lomb, UK.
Solution for cleansing, disinfecting, and removal of protein from contact lenses.

Renutryl Germania, Aust.
Preparation for enteral nutrition.

Renutryl 500 Clintec, Fr.
Nutritional supplement.

Renzepin Bergamon, Ital.†.
Pirenzepine hydrochloride (p.467·1).
Peptic ulcer.

Reocol Also, Ital.
Tartaric acid; sodium bicarbonate (p.1153·2); anhydrous citric acid; magnesium sulphate (p.1157·3).
Constipation; dyspepsia.

Reoflus Pulitzer, Ital.
Heparin calcium (p.879·3).
Thrombo-embolic disorders.

Reolase Pulitzer, Ital.
Telmesteine (p.1070·2).
Respiratory-tract disorders.

Reolina IFI, Ital.†.
Bile extract (p.1553·2); phenolphthalein (p.1208·2); cascara (p.1183·1); rhubarb (p.1212·1).
Constipation.

Reomax Bioindustria, Ital.
Ethacrynic acid (p.866·3) or sodium ethacrynate (p.866·3).
Oedema.

Reomucil Astra, Ital.
Carbocisteine (p.1056·3) or carbocisteine sodium (p.1056·3).
Respiratory-tract congestion.

ReoPro
Lilly, Austral.; Lilly, Fr.; Beiersdorf-Lilly, Ger.; Lilly, Irl.; Lilly, Ital.; Lilly, Neth.; Centocor, Norw.; Lilly, S.Afr.; Lilly, Spain; Lilly, Swed.; Lilly, Switz.; Lilly, UK; Centocor, USA; Lilly, USA.
Abciximab (p.804·3).
Prevention of ischaemic cardiac complications during angioplasty.

Reoxyl Tosse, Ger.†.
Mephenesin (p.1315·3).
Muscular disorders.

Repalyte Rhone-Poulenc Rorer, Austral.
Sodium chloride; potassium chloride; sodium acid citrate; glucose (p.1152·3).
Diarrhoea; oral rehydration therapy.

Repan Everett, USA.
Butalbital (p.644·3); caffeine (p.749·3); paracetamol (p.72·2).
Pain.

Repan CF Everett, USA.
Paracetamol (p.72·2); butalbital (p.644·3).
Pain.

Reparil
Note. This name is used for preparations of different composition.

Madaus, Aust.; Madaus, Belg.; Madaus, Fr.†; Madaus, Ger.; Naturwaren, Ital.; Madaus, S.Afr.†; Madaus, Switz.†.
Injection: Sodium aescinate (p.1543·3).
Back pain; inflammation; oedema; vascular disorders.

Madaus, Aust.; Madaus, Belg.; Madaus, Fr.†; Madaus, Ger.; Naturwaren, Ital.; Madaus, Switz.
Tablets: Aescin (p.1543·3).
Inflammation; oedema; pain; vascular disorders.

Madaus, Aust.; Byk Madaus, S.Afr.
Topical gel: Aescin (p.1543·3); diethylamine salicylate (p.33·1).
Muscle and joint pain; soft-tissue injury.

Madaus, Belg.; Madaus, Fr.; Madaus, Switz.
Topical gel: Aescin (p.1543·3); sodium aescin polysulphate (p.1543·3); diethylamine salicylate (p.33·1).
Venous, oedematous, and inflammatory disorders.

Naturwaren, Ital.
Topical gel: Aescin (p.1543·3); heparin sodium (p.879·3); diethylamine salicylate (p.33·1).
Soft-tissue disorders.

Reparil N Madaus, Switz.
Aescin (p.1543·3); diethylamine salicylate (p.33·1).
Soft-tissue injury.

Reparil-Gel N, Reparil-Sportgel Madaus, Ger.
Aescin (p.1543·3); diethylamine salicylate (p.33·1).
Inflammation.

Repasma Pharmador, S.Afr.
Amylobarbitone (p.641·3); aminophylline (p.748·1); ephedrine hydrochloride (p.1059·3).
Asthma.

Repeltin Pierre Fabre, Ger.
Trimeprazine (p.419·3).
Bronchial asthma or asthma-like complaints; pruritus.

Repervit IDI, Ital.
Vitamin A palmitate (p.1359·2).
Vitamin A deficiency.

Repha Orphon Repha, Ger.
Orthosiphon (p.1592·2).
Gout; rheumatism; urinary-tract disorders.

Rephacimin Repha, Ger.
Homoeopathic preparation.

Rephacratin Repha, Ger.
Crataegus (p.1568·2).
Cardiac disorders.

Rephahyval Repha, Ger.
Hypericum (p.1590·1).
Anxiety disorders; depression.

Rephalgin Repha, Ger.
Homoeopathic preparation.

Rephalysin C Repha, Ger.
Escherichia coli.
Gastro-intestinal disorders.

Rephamen N Repha, Ger.†.
Homoeopathic preparation.

Repha-Os Repha, Ger.
Tormentil root (p.1638·3); rhatany root (p.1624·3); myrrh (p.1606·1); anise oil (p.1550·1); eucalyptus oil (p.1578·1); peppermint oil (p.1208·1); clove oil (p.1565·2); menthol (p.1600·2).
Inflammatory disorders of the oropharynx.

Rephaprossan Repha, Ger.
Homoeopathic preparation.

Rephastasan Repha, Ger.
Ointment: Homoeopathic preparation.
Topical liquid†: Aesculus (p.1543·3); arnica (p.1550·3); hamamelis (p.1587·1); chelidonium majus; card. mar.; calc. fluorat.; symphytum; lachesis.
Vascular disorders.

Replace Sabax, S.Afr.†.
Preparation for enteral nutrition.

Replenate BPL, UK.
A factor VIII preparation (p.720·3).
Formerly known as 8SM.
Haemophilia A.

Replenine BPL, UK.
A factor IX preparation (p.721·3).
Haemophilia B.

Replens
Sanofi Winthrop, Austral.; Roberts, Canad.; Solymes, Fr.; Ethical Research, Irl.; Janssen-Cilag, Ital.; Logos, S.Afr.; Lanzas, Spain; Unipath, UK; Warner-Lambert, USA.
Polycarbophil (p.1209·1).
Vaginal dryness.

Replete Clintec, USA.
Lactose-free, gluten-free preparation for enteral nutrition.

Repocal Desitin, Ger.†.
Lormetazepam (p.677·1).
Formerly contained pentobarbitone calcium.
Sleep disorders.

Reposans Wesley, USA.
Chlordiazepoxide hydrochloride (p.646·3).
Alcohol withdrawal syndrome; anxiety.

Reposo-Mono Medgenix, Belg.
Meprobamate (p.678·1).
Insomnia.

Repowine Truw, Ger.
Scoparium (p.1628·1).
Cardiac disorders.

Repowinon Truw, Ger.
Homoeopathic preparation.

Represil Llorens, Spain†.
Feprazone (p.41·2).
Fever; inflammation; pain.

Reprol Lirca, Ital.†.
Reproterol hydrochloride (p.758·1).
Asthma; bronchitis.

Repronex Ferring, USA.
Menotrophin (p.1252·1).
Infertility.

Reproven Hanosan, Ger.
Homoeopathic preparation.

Reptilase
Dispergo, Aust.; Pharmadeveloppement, Fr.; Knoll, Ger.†; Difa, Ital.; Llorente, Spain.
Haemocoagulase (p.712·3).
Haemorrhage.

Repursan M Boots, Ger.
Cort. yohimbe.; nuces colae; lign. muir. puam.; testes; vitamins; minerals.
Tonic.

Repursan ST Biokanol, Ger.
Pausinystalia yohimbe; kola (p.1645·1); ephedra (p.1059·3); vitamins; minerals.
Sexual fatigue.

Requiesan Klein, Ger.
Eschscholtzia californica; avena (p.1551·3).
Sleep disorders.

Requip
SmithKline Beecham, Fr.; SmithKline Beecham, Irl.; SmithKline Beecham, Ital.; SmithKline Beecham, Neth.; SmithKline Beecham, Swed.; SmithKline Beecham, UK; SmithKline Beecham, USA.
Ropinirole hydrochloride (p.1144·1).
Parkinsonism.

Resaid Geneva, USA.
Phenylpropanolamine hydrochloride (p.1067·2); chlorpheniramine maleate (p.405·1).
Upper respiratory-tract symptoms.

Resalt Compu, S.Afr.
Sodium chloride; potassium chloride; glucose; sodium bicarbonate (p.1152·3).
Diarrhoea; oral rehydration therapy.

Resaltex
Procter & Gamble, Aust.; Procter & Gamble, Ger.
Reserpine (p.942·1); hydrochlorothiazide (p.885·2); triamterene (p.957·2).
Hypertension.

Resan Mucolitico Alacan, Spain.
Ampicillin sodium (p.153·1); bromhexine (p.1055·3).
Lignocaine (p.1293·2) is included in this preparation to alleviate the pain of injection.
Respiratory-tract infections.

Resan Retard Alacan, Spain.
Ampicillin sodium (p.153·1); ampicillin benzathine (p.154·1); bromhexine hydrochloride (p.1055·3).
Lignocaine hydrochloride (p.1293·2) is included in this preparation to alleviate the pain of injection.
Respiratory-tract infections.

Rescaps-D SR Geneva, USA.
Phenylpropanolamine hydrochloride (p.1067·2); caramiphen edisylate (p.1056·2).
Coughs.

Rescon Ion, USA.
Capsules: Pseudoephedrine hydrochloride (p.1068·3); chlorpheniramine maleate (p.405·1).
Liquid: Phenylpropanolamine hydrochloride (p.1067·2); chlorpheniramine maleate (p.405·1).
Upper respiratory-tract symptoms.

Rescon-DM Ion, USA.
Dextromethorphan hydrobromide (p.1057·3); pseudoephedrine hydrochloride (p.1068·3); chlorpheniramine maleate (p.405·1).
Coughs and cold symptoms.

Rescon-ED Ion, USA.
Pseudoephedrine hydrochloride (p.1068·3); chlorpheniramine maleate (p.405·1).
Upper respiratory-tract symptoms.

Rescon-GG Ion, USA.
Phenylephrine hydrochloride (p.1066·2); guaiphenesin (p.1061·3).
Coughs.

Rescriptor
Pharmacia Upjohn, Austral.; Pharmacia Upjohn, USA.
Delavirdine mesylate (p.607·2).
HIV infection.

Rescula Ueno, Jpn.
Unoprostone isopropyl (p.1421·3).
Glaucoma; ocular hypertension.

Rescuvolin
Medac, Ger.; Nycomed, Norw.; Pharmachemie, S.Afr.; Nycomed, Swed.
Folinic acid (p.1342·2) or calcium folinate (p.1342·2).
Adjunct to fluorouracil in colorectal cancer; antidote to folic acid antagonists.

Resdan Whitehall-Robins, Canad.
Cetrimide (p.1105·2).
Dandruff.

Resdan Rx Whitehall, Neth.†.
Coal tar (p.1092·3); menthol (p.1600·2).
Scalp disorders.

Resectal Leopold, Aust.
Sorbitol (p.1354·2); mannitol (p.900·3).
Bladder and prostate surgery.

Resectisol Kendall McGaw, USA.
Mannitol (p.900·3).
Urological irrigation solution.

Resedorm Bristol, Ger.†.
Oral liquid: Secbutobarbitone (p.692·1); aprobarbital (p.642·2).
Tablets: Secbutobarbitone (p.692·1); aprobarbital (p.642·2); butethamate citrate (p.1056·2).
Sleep disorders.

Reseril Mead Johnson, Ital.
Nefazodone hydrochloride (p.299·3).
Depression.

Reset Biomedica, Ital.
Aniracetam (p.1549·3).
Mental function impairment.

Resfolin Piam, Ital.
Calcium folinate (p.1342·2).
Anaemias; antidote to folic acid antagonists; folate deficiency; reduction of aminopterin and methotrexate toxicity.

Residex P55 Agropharm, UK.
Permethrin (p.1409·2).
Mosquito repellent for nets and clothing.

Resimatil Sanofi Winthrop, Ger.
Primidone (p.358·3).
Epilepsy.

Resina Carbolica Dentilin Ghimas, Ital.
Guaiacol (p.1061·2); lignocaine hydrochloride (p.1293·2); alcohol (p.1099·1); camphor (p.1557·2); thymol (p.1127·1).
Dental disinfection; dental pain.

Resinaluminio Rubio, Spain†.
Aluminium polystyrene sulphonate.
Hyperkalaemia.

Resincalcio Rubio, Spain.
Calcium polystyrene sulphonate (p.974·3).
Hyperkalaemia.

Resincolestiramina Rubio, Spain.
Cholestyramine (p.1269·3).
Hyperlipidaemias.

Resinol Mentholatum, USA.
Calamine (p.1080·1); zinc oxide (p.1096·2); resorcinol (p.1090·1).
Minor skin irritation.

Resinsodio Rubio, Spain.
Sodium polystyrene sulphonate (p.995·3).
Hyperkalaemia.

Resistan Lichtwer, Ger.
Homoeopathic preparation.

Resisten Retard Smaller, Spain.
Ampicillin sodium (p.153·1); ampicillin benzathine (p.154·1); bromhexine hydrochloride (p.1055·3).
Lignocaine hydrochloride (p.1293·2) is included in this preparation to alleviate the pain of injection.
Respiratory-tract infections.

Resiston One Fisons, UK.
Sodium cromoglycate (p.762·1); xylometazoline hydrochloride (p.1071·2).
Allergic rhinitis.

Resistone QD Rhone Poulenc Chemicals, UK.
Alkylaryltrialkylammonium chloride (p.1101·2).
Disinfection.

Resivit
Note. This name is used for preparations of different composition.
UPSA, Fr.†.
Leucocianidol (p.1580·2).
Haemorrhoids; vascular disorders.

Rhone-Poulenc Rorer, Spain.
Multivitamin preparation.

Resnedal Byk Elmu, Spain.
Chlorthalidone (p.839·3); spironolactone (p.946·1); reserpine (p.942·1).
Hypertension.

Resochin
Bayer, Aust.; Bayer, Ger.; Bayer, Spain.
Chloroquine phosphate (p.426·3).
Amoebiasis; malaria; rheumatoid arthritis; systemic lupus erythematosus.

Resochine Bayer, Switz.
Chloroquine phosphate (p.426·3).
Amoebiasis; lupus erythematosus; malaria; rheumatoid arthritis.

Resoferix Brunnengraber, Ger.†.
Ferrous sulphate (p.1340·2).
Iron-deficiency; iron-deficiency anaemias.

Resoferon
Ciba-Geigy, Belg.; Geigy, Switz.
Ferrous sulphate (p.1340·2).
Succinic acid is included to increase the absorption and availability of iron.
Iron deficiency; iron-deficiency anaemia.

Resoferon fol B Geigy, Switz.†.
Ferrous sulphate (p.1340·2); folic acid (p.1340·3); cyanocobalamin (p.1363·3).
Succinic acid is included in this preparation to increase the absorption and availability of ferrous sulphate.
Iron and folic acid deficiency.

Resol
Note. This name is used for preparations of different composition.
Terramin, Aust.
Camphor (p.1557·2); terpineol (p.1635·1); eucalyptus oil (p.1578·1); pumilio pine oil (p.1623·3); menthol (p.1600·2); thymol (p.1127·1).
Catarrh; rheumatism.

Wyeth-Ayerst, USA.
Glucose; sodium chloride; potassium citrate; citric acid; sodium phosphate; magnesium chloride; calcium chloride; sodium citrate (p.1152·3).
Diarrhoea; oral rehydration therapy.

Resolution Phoenix Health, UK.
Nicotine (p.1607·2); vitamins.
Aid to smoking withdrawal.

Resolutivo Regium Miquel Garriga, Spain.
Boldo (p.1554·1); chumbera; equisetum (p.1575·1); xanthium; sideritide; rosemary; cynodon; hepatica; saxifraga; arenaria; lithospermum; melissa (p.1600·1).
Formerly contained anethole, borneol, camphene, rubia tinctorum, oxidised terpenes, pinenes, fenchone, cineole, atropine sulphate and papaverine hydrochloride.
Hyperuricaemia; renal calculi.

Resolve Seton, UK.
Paracetamol (p.72·2); sodium bicarbonate (p.1153·2); potassium bicarbonate (p.1153·1).

Resolve/GP Allergan, USA.
Cleansing solution for hard and gas permeable contact lenses.

Resonium Sanofi, Swed.
Sodium polystyrene sulphonate (p.995·3).
Hyperkalaemia.

Resonium A
Sanofi Winthrop, Aust.; Sanofi Winthrop, Austral.; Sanofi Winthrop, Ger.; Sanofi Winthrop, Irl.; Sanofi Winthrop, Neth.; Sanofi Winthrop, Switz.; Sanofi Winthrop, UK.
Sodium polystyrene sulphonate (p.995·3).
Hyperkalaemia.

Resonium Calcium
Sanofi Winthrop, Canad.; Sanofi Winthrop, Norw.; Sanofi, Swed.; Winthrop, Switz.†.
Calcium polystyrene sulphonate (p.974·3).
Hyperkalaemia.

Resorbane Spirig, Switz.
Cineole (p.1564·1); camphor (p.1557·2); niaouli oil (p.1607·1).
Respiratory-tract disorders.

Resorborina Belmac, Spain.
Mouthwash: Benzalkonium chloride (p.1101·3); dexamethasone (p.1037·1); resorcinol (p.1090·1); amethocaine hydrochloride (p.1285·2).
Throat spray: Benzalkonium chloride (p.1101·3); betamethasone (p.1033·2); amethocaine hydrochloride (p.1285·2).
Mouth and throat inflammation.

Resorpil Reig Jofre, Spain†.
Calcium pantothenate (p.1352·3); mercuric chloride (p.1601·2); pilocarpine chloride (p.1396·3); resorcinol acetate (p.1090·1).
Hair, scalp, and skin disorders.

Resource
Sandoz Nutrition, Canad.; Sandoz, USA.
Preparation for enteral nutrition.

Resp Murdock, USA.
Ephedrine hydrochloride (p.1059·3).

Respacal
Bios, Belg.; UCB, UK.
Tulobuterol hydrochloride (p.774·2).
Bronchospasm.

Respa-DM Respa, USA.
Dextromethorphan hydrobromide (p.1057·3); guaiphenesin (p.1061·3).

Respa-GF Respa, USA.
Guaiphenesin (p.1061·3).

Respahist Respa, USA.
Pseudoephedrine hydrochloride (p.1068·3); brompheniramine maleate (p.403·2).

Respaire Laser, USA.
Pseudoephedrine hydrochloride (p.1068·3); guaiphenesin (p.1061·3).
Coughs and cold symptoms; nasal congestion.

Respalis Nestle, Fr.
Preparation for enteral nutrition.
Respiratory insufficiency.

Respalor Mead Johnson Nutritionals, USA.
Lactose-free preparation for enteral nutrition.
Respiratory system disorders.

Respa-1st Respa, USA.
Pseudoephedrine hydrochloride (p.1068·3); guaiphenesin (p.1061·3).

Respatona Brauer, Austral.
Ammonia (p.1548·3); anise oil (p.1550·1); althaea (p.1546·3); bryonia (p.1555·2); lichen islandicus; chamomile (p.1561·2); thyme (p.1636·3); urtica (p.1642·3); aconitum napellus; coccus cacti; corallium rubrum; drosera rotundifolia; ipecacuanha; kali bich.; kreosotum; spongia tosta; sticta pulmonaria.
Coughs.

Respatona Plus with Echinacea Brauer, Austral.
Anise oil (p.1550·1); althaea (p.1546·3); bryonia (p.1555·2); iceland moss; echinacea angustifolia (p.1574·2); chamomile (p.1561·2); thyme (p.1636·3); urtica (p.1642·3); aconitum napellus; coccus cacti; corallium rubrum; drosera rotundifolia; ipecacuanha; kali bich.; kreosotum; spongia tosta; sticta pulmonaria.
Coughs.

Respax Pharmacia Upjohn, Austral.
Salbutamol sulphate (p.758·2).
Obstructive airways disease.

Respbid Boehringer Ingelheim, USA.
Theophylline (p.765·1).
Reversible bronchospasm.

Respibien Cinfa, Spain.
Oxymetazoline hydrochloride (p.1065·3).
Nasal congestion.

Respicort Mundipharma, Switz.†.
Triamcinolone acetonide (p.1050·2).
Asthma.

Respicur
Byk, Aust.; Byk Gulden, Ital.
Theophylline (p.765·1).
Obstructive airways disease.

RespiGam *Medimmune, USA.*
Respiratory syncytial virus immunoglobulins (p.1532·1).
Passive immunisation.

Respilene *Sanofi Winthrop, Fr.*
Pholcodine (p.1068·1).
Formerly contained zipeprol hydrochloride.
Respiratory-tract disorders.

Respinol *Pharmaceutical Enterprises, S.Afr.*
Phenylephrine hydrochloride (p.1066·2); chlorpheniramine maleate (p.405·1); hyoscine methonitrate (p.463·1).
Cold symptoms; sinusitis; vasomotor rhinitis.

Respinol Compound *Pharmaceutical Enterprises, S.Afr.*
Pholcodine (p.1068·1); pseudoephedrine hydrochloride (p.1068·3); chlorpheniramine maleate (p.405·1); hyoscine methonitrate (p.463·1).
Cold symptoms; coughs; rhinitis; sinusitis.

Respir *Schering-Plough, Spain.*
Oxymetazoline hydrochloride (p.1065·3).
Nasal congestion.

Respir Balsamico *Schering-Plough, Spain.*
Camphor (p.1557·2); cineole (p.1564·1); oxymetazoline hydrochloride (p.1065·3) menthol (p.1600·2).
Nasal congestion.

Respirase *Gibipharma, Ital.†.*
Zipeprol (p.1071·3) or zipeprol hydrochloride (p.1071·3).
Coughs.

Respirex *Sanofi Winthrop, Spain†.*
Zipeprol hydrochloride (p.1071·3).
Coughs.

Respiride *Schiapparelli Searle, Ital.†.*
Fenspiride hydrochloride (p.1579·3).
Bronchopneumopathy; inflammation of the respiratory tract.

Respiro *Byk Gulden, Ital.*
Xylometazoline hydrochloride (p.1071·2); cineole (p.1564·1); menthol (p.1600·2); chlorbutol (p.1106·3).
Nasal congestion.

Respirol *Tika, Swed.†.*
Terbutaline sulphate (p.764·1).
Bronchodilator.

Respiroma *Fournier SA, Spain.*
Iodinated glycerol (p.1062·2); salbutamol sulphate (p.758·2).
Respiratory-tract disorders.

Respisniffers *Pharmacare Consumer, S.Afr.*
Cineole (p.1564·1); pine oil; chloroxylenol (p.1111·1); turpentine oil (p.1641·1); menthol (p.1600·2).
Bronchitis; cold symptoms; nasal congestion.

Respitol *Cinfa, Spain.*
Sodium chloride (p.1162·2).
Nasal congestion.

Resplant *Spitzner, Ger.*
Echinacea purpurea (p.1574·2).
Respiratory- and urinary-tract infections.

Resplen *Chugai, Jpn†.*
Eprazinone hydrochloride (p.1060·3).
Coughs.

Respocort *3M, Austral.*
Beclomethasone dipropionate (p.1032·1).
Obstructive airways disease.

Respolin *3M, Austral.*
Salbutamol sulphate (p.758·2).
Bronchospasm.

Respontin *Glaxo Wellcome, UK.*
Ipratropium bromide (p.754·2).
Obstructive airways disease.

Resprim *Alphapharm, Austral.*
Co-trimoxazole (p.196·3).
Bacterial infections; Pneumocystis carinii pneumonia.

Resprin *Rice Steele, Irl.*
Aspirin (p.16·1).
Fever; inflammation; pain.

Res-Q *Boyle, USA†.*
Activated charcoal (p.972·2); magnesium hydroxide (p.1198·2); tannic acid (p.1634·2).
Emergency treatment of poisoning.

Restaid *Nelson, Austral.†.*
Doxylamine succinate (p.410·1).
Insomnia.

Restameth-SR *Restan, S.Afr.*
Indomethacin (p.45·2).
Gout; musculoskeletal and joint disorders.

Restandol
Organon, Irl.; Organon, UK.
Testosterone undecanoate (p.1464·2).
Male hypogonadism; osteoporosis.

Restas *Sumitomo, Jpn†; Kanebo, Jpn†.*
Flutoprazepam (p.673·1).

Restaslim *Restan, S.Afr.*
Phenylpropanolamine hydrochloride (p.1067·2).
Obesity.

Restavit *Woods, Austral.*
Doxylamine succinate (p.410·1).
Insomnia.

Restenil *Recip, Swed.*
Meprobamate (p.678·1).
Anxiety; headache; skeletal muscle spasm; sleep disorders.

Restid
UCB, Ital.†; UCB, Spain†.
Oxametacin (p.71·1).
Musculoskeletal, joint, and peri-articular disorders.

Restin *Laser, S.Afr.*
Valerian (p.1643·1); vitamin B substances; ascorbic acid.
Nonpsychotic mental disorders.

Restore *InAgra, USA.*
Psyllium hydrophilic mucilloid (p.1194·2).

Restoril
Sandoz, Canad.; Sandoz, USA.
Temazepam (p.693·3).
Insomnia.

Restovar
Organon, Aust.; Donmed, S.Afr.†; Organon, Swed.
Lynoestrenol (p.1448·2); ethinyloestradiol (p.1445·1).
Combined oral contraceptive.

Restrical *Cooperation Pharmaceutique, Fr.*
Liquid paraffin (p.1382·1).
Constipation.

Restructa forte 5 *Fides, Ger.†.*
Homoeopathic preparation.

Restwell *Mer-National, S.Afr.*
Doxylamine succinate (p.410·1).
Insomnia.

Resulax *Tika, Swed.*
Sorbitol (p.1354·2).
Bowel evacuation; constipation.

Resulin *Ist. Chim. Inter., Ital.*
Nimesulide (p.63·2).
Fever; inflammation; pain.

Resurmide *Ibi, Ital.*
Somatostatin acetate (p.1261·1).
Gastro-intestinal haemorrhage.

Resyl
Zyma, Aust.; Ciba Self Medication, Canad.†; Zyma, Ital.; Novartis, Swed.; Zyma, Switz.
Guaiphenesin (p.1061·3).
Coughs.

Resyl DM *Zyma, Ital.*
Guaiphenesin (p.1061·3); dextromethorphan hydrobromide (p.1057·3).
Coughs.

Resyl mit Codein *Zyma, Aust.*
Guaiphenesin (p.1061·3); codeine phosphate (p.26·1).
Coughs.

Resyl Plus *Zyma, Switz.*
Guaiphenesin (p.1061·3); codeine phosphate (p.26·1).
Coughs.

Retabolin forte *Cimex, Switz.*
Vitamin B substances.
Neuralgia; neuritis.

Retacillin *Jenapharm, Ger.*
Benzylpenicillin sodium (p.159·3); procaine penicillin (p.240·2); benzathine penicillin (p.158·3).
Bacterial infections.

Retacnyl *Galderma, Fr.*
Tretinoin (p.1093·3).
Acne; keratinisation disorders.

Retarcyl *Delagrange, Fr.†.*
Morpholine salicylate (p.60·1).
Pain.

Retarpen
Note. This name is used for preparations of different composition.
Biochemie, Aust.
Benzathine penicillin (p.158·3).
Bacterial infections.

Septa, Spain.
Ampicillin sodium (p.153·1); ampicillin benzathine (p.154·1).
Lignocaine (p.1293·2) is included in this preparation to alleviate the pain of injection.
Bacterial infections.

Retarpen Balsamico *Septa, Spain.*
Ampicillin sodium (p.153·1); ampicillin benzathine (p.154·1); cineole (p.1564·1); guaiphenesin (p.1061·3).
Lignocaine hydrochloride (p.1293·2) is included in this preparation to alleviate the pain of injection.
Respiratory-tract infections.

Retarpen compositum *Biochemie, Aust.*
Benzylpenicillin sodium (p.159·3); procaine penicillin (p.240·2); benzathine penicillin (p.158·3).
Bacterial infections.

Retarpen Mucolitico *Septa, Spain.*
Ampicillin sodium (p.153·1); ampicillin benzathine (p.154·1); bromhexine hydrochloride (p.1055·3).
Lignocaine hydrochloride (p.1293·2) is included in this preparation to alleviate the pain of injection.
Respiratory-tract infections.

Retavase *Boehringer Mannheim, USA.*
Reteplase (p.942·3).
Myocardial infarction.

Retcin *DDSA Pharmaceuticals, UK.*
Erythromycin (p.204·1).

Retef *Galderma, Ger.*
Hydrocortisone aceponate (p.1044·2).
Skin disorders.

Retencal *UCB, Spain.*
Imidazole ketoglutarate (p.740·1).
Bone formation disorders; calcium metabolism disorders; osteoporosis; Paget's disease of bone; thrombo-embolic disorders.

Retens *Wasserman, Spain.*
Doxycycline hydrochloride (p.202·3).
Bacterial infections.

Reticulex *Lilly, USA†.*
Liver-stomach concentrate; vitamin B_{12}; ferrous sulphate (p.1340·2); ascorbic acid (p.1365·2); folic acid (p.1340·3).

Reticulogen *Lilly, Ital.*
Cyanocobalamin (p.1363·3).
Megaloblastic anaemia; vitamin B_{12} deficiency.

Reticulogen Fortific *Lilly, Spain.*
Cyanocobalamin (p.1363·3).
Formerly contained cyanocobalamin, liver extract, and thiamine hydrochloride.
Vitamin B_{12} deficiency.

Reticus *Farmila, Ital.*
Desonide (p.1036·3).
Skin disorders.

Reticus Antimicotico *Farmila, Ital.†.*
Desonide (p.1036·3); clioquinol (p.193·2).
Skin disorders with fungal infection.

Retimax *Cusi, Spain.*
Oxpentifylline (p.925·3).
Cerebral and peripheral vascular disorders.

Retin-A
Janssen-Cilag, Aust.; Janssen-Cilag, Austral.; Janssen-Ortho, Canad.; Janssen-Cilag, Fr.; Janssen-Cilag, Irl.; Janssen-Cilag, Ital.; Janssen-Cilag, S.Afr.; Janssen-Cilag, Switz.; Janssen-Cilag, UK; Ortho Dermatological, USA.
Tretinoin (p.1093·3).
Acne; photo-ageing of the skin.

Retinol *INTES, Ital.*
Vaccinium myrtillus (p.1606·1).
Eye disorders.

Retinol-A *Young Again Products, USA.*
Vitamin A palmitate (p.1359·2).
Minor skin disorders.

Retinosio Vitaminico *Difa, Ital.†.*
Fructose (p.1343·2); alpha tocopherol (p.1369·2).
Diabetic retinopathy.

Retinova
RoC, Fr.; Johnson & Johnson, Swed.; Ortho-Cilag, UK.
Tretinoin (p.1093·3).
UV-induced skin damage.

Retinovix *Difa, Ital.†.*
Melanocyte-stimulating hormone (p.1254·1); thiamine (p.1361·2); strychnine nitrate (p.1633·1).
Loss of retinal sensitivity.

Retirides *OTC, Spain.*
Tretinoin (p.1093·3).
Acne.

Retisol-A *Stiefel, Canad.*
Tretinoin (p.1093·3).
Acne.

Retitop *Roche-Posay, Fr.*
Tretinoin (p.1093·3).
Acne; keratinisation disorders.

Retolen *Byk Elmu, Spain.*
Astemizole (p.402·1).
Hypersensitivity reactions.

ReTrieve *Dermatech, Austral.*
Tretinoin (p.1093·3).
Dry skin.

Retrovir
Glaxo Wellcome, Aust.; Glaxo Wellcome, Austral.; Glaxo Wellcome, Belg.; Glaxo Wellcome, Canad.; Glaxo Wellcome, Fr.; Glaxo Wellcome, Ger.; Wellcome, Irl.; Glaxo Wellcome, Ital.; Glaxo Wellcome, Neth.; Glaxo Wellcome, Norw.; Glaxo Wellcome, S.Afr.; Glaxo Wellcome, Spain; Glaxo Wellcome, Swed.; Wellcome, Switz.; Glaxo Wellcome, UK; Glaxo Wellcome, USA.
Zidovudine (p.630·2).
HIV infection.

Retterspitz Aerosol *Retterspitz, Ger.*
Ephedrine hydrochloride (p.1059·3); pumilio pine oil (p.1623·3); siberian fir oil; thyme oil (p.1637·1); eucalyptus oil (p.1578·1); menthol (p.1600·2).
Respiratory-tract infections.

Retterspitz Ausserlich *Retterspitz, Ger.*
Rosemary oil (p.1626·2); citric acid (p.1564·3); tartaric acid (p.1634·3); alum (p.1547·1); thymol (p.1127·1).
Inflammatory disorders.

Retterspitz Gelee *Retterspitz, Ger.*
Thymol (p.1127·1); allantoin (p.1078·2); rosemary oil (p.1626·2); tartaric acid (p.1634·3); alum (p.1547·1); citric acid (p.1564·3).
Skin disorders.

Retterspitz Heilsalbe *Retterspitz, Ger.*
Pumilio pine oil (p.1623·3); siberian fir oil; thymol (p.1127·1); allantoin (p.1078·2).
Haemorrhoids; skin disorders.

Retterspitz Innerlich *Retterspitz, Ger.*
Citric acid (p.1564·3); tartaric acid (p.1634·3); alum (p.1547·1); thyme oil (p.1637·1).
Gastro-intestinal disorders.

Retterspitz Quick *Retterspitz, Ger.*
Rosemary oil (p.1626·2); camphor (p.1557·2); menthol (p.1600·2); thymol (p.1127·1).
Chest disorders; joint disorders; myalgia.

Reucam *CT, Ital.*
Piroxicam (p.80·2).
Musculoskeletal and joint disorders.

Reudene *ABC, Ital.*
Piroxicam (p.80·2).
Musculoskeletal and joint disorders.

Reuflodol *Nattermann, Spain.*
Pinazone (p.41·2).
Musculoskeletal, joint, and peri-articular disorders; pain.

Reuflos *Roussel, Ital.†.*
Diflunisal (p.33·2).
Pain.

Reumacort *Teofarma, Ital.*
Hydrocortisone acetate (p.1043·3); methyl gentisate (p.55·1).
Musculoskeletal and joint pain.

Reumagil *KBR, Ital.*
Piroxicam (p.80·2).
Musculoskeletal and joint disorders.

Reumaless *Pharmaton, Ger.*
Balsam: Methyl salicylate (p.55·2); benzyl nicotinate (p.22·1).
Musculoskeletal, joint, and soft-tissue disorders; neuralgia.
Capsules: Urtica (p.1642·3).
Rheumatism.

Reumatosil *Saba, Ital.*
Nifenazone (p.63·1).
Neuralgias; neuritis; rheumatic disorders.

Reumo *UCB, Spain.*
Indomethacin (p.45·2).
Gout; musculoskeletal, joint, and peri-articular disorders; pain.

Reumoquin *Nattermann, Spain.*
Ketoprofen (p.48·2).
Gout; musculoskeletal, joint, and peri-articular disorders; pain.

Reumyl
Note. This name is used for preparations of different composition.
Lenza, Ital.†.
Sulindac (p.86·3).
Musculoskeletal and joint disorders.

Hassle, Swed.†.
Aspirin (p.16·1).
Fever; inflammation; pain.

Reuprofen *Terapeutico, Ital.*
Ketoprofen (p.48·2).
Musculoskeletal, joint, peri-articular, and soft-tissue disorders.

Reused *Corvi, Ital.†.*
Amidopyrine (p.15·2); sodium salicylate (p.85·1); caffeine (p.749·3).
Rheumatic disorders.

Reusin *Alfarma, Spain.*
Indomethacin (p.45·2).
Gout; musculoskeletal, joint, peri-articular, and soft-tissue disorders; pain.

Reutenox *Kalifarma, Spain.*
Tenoxicam (p.88·2).
Calcium stones; musculoskeletal, joint, and peri-articular disorders.

Reutol *Errekappa, Ital.†.*
Tolmetin sodium (p.89·3).
Inflammation.

Revalid
Geymonat, Ital.; Vifor, Switz.
Amino acids; millet; wheat-germ; dried yeast; soya protein; minerals; vitamins.
Skin, hair, and nail disorders.

Revanil *Cambridge, UK.*
Lysuride maleate (p.1142·1).
Parkinsonism.

Revasc *Rhone-Poulenc Rorer, UK.*
Desirudin (p.883·1).
Venous thrombosis prophylaxis.

Revaton *Pharmco, S.Afr.*
Haematoporphyrin (p.1587·1); vitamin B_{12} (p.1363·3); ascorbic acid (p.1365·2); yeast extract (p.1373·1).
Tonic.

Reve *Vaillant, Ital.*
Valerian (p.1643·1); passion flower (p.1615·3).
Insomnia.

Reveal *BR Pharmaceuticals, UK.*
Pregnancy test (p.1621·2).

Revelatest *Pierre Fabre, Fr.*
Pregnancy test (p.1621·2).

Reverin
Hoechst, Aust.; Hoechst, Austral.†; Hoechst, Belg.†; Hoechst Marion Roussel, Canad.; Hoechst, Ger.†; Hoechst Marion Roussel, Irl.†; Hoechst Marion Roussel, Ital.†; Hoechst Marion Roussel, S.Afr.†.
Rolitetracycline (p.247·1).
Lignocaine hydrochloride (p.1293·2) may be included in the intramuscular injection to alleviate the pain of injection.
Bacterial infections.

Reversol *Organon, USA.*
Edrophonium chloride (p.1392·2).
Diagnosis of myasthenia gravis; evaluation of emergency treatment of myasthenic crises; reversal of competitive neuromuscular blockade.

Revex *Ohmeda, USA.*
Nalmefene hydrochloride (p.985·3).
Opioid poisoning.

Rev-Eyes
Storz, Canad.†; Lederle, USA; Storz, USA.
Dapiprazole hydrochloride (p.1570·2).
Reversal of mydriasis and cycloplegia.

Revia
Torrex, Aust.; Du Pont, Canad.; Du Pont, Fr.
Naltrexone hydrochloride (p.988·1).
Alcohol withdrawal syndromes; opioid withdrawal syndromes.

Revic *Cusi, Spain.*
Carbomer (p.1471·2).
Dry eyes.

Revicain *Wiedemann, Ger.*
Procaine hydrochloride (p.1299·2); vitamins.
Tonic.

Revicain Comp *Wiedemann, Ger.*
Procaine hydrochloride (p.1299·2); aescin (p.1543·3); minerals.
Tonic.

Revicain Comp Plus *Wiedemann, Ger.*
Procaine hydrochloride (p.1299·2); aescin (p.1543·3); haematoporphyrin (p.1587·1); vitamins; minerals.
Tonic.

Revimine *Rhone-Poulenc Rorer, Canad.†.*
Dopamine hydrochloride (p.861·1).
Shock.

Revit *ICN, Canad.*
Multivitamin preparation.

Revitaleyes *Allergan, Canad.*
Polyvinyl alcohol (p.1474·2).
Dry eyes.

Revitalose *Darcy, Fr.*
Ampoule A, magnesium aspartate (p.1157·2); L-leucine (p.1350·1); L-lysine hydrochloride (p.1350·1); L-phenylalanine (p.1353·1); L-valine (p.1358·1); ampoule B, sodium ascorbate (p.1365·2).
Asthenia.

Revitalose C
Note. This name is used for preparations of different composition.
Rivex, Canad.
Ascorbic acid (p.1365·2).
Vitamin C supplement.
UCB, Switz.
Amino acids; vitamin C.
Tonic.

Revitalose C 1000 *Darci, Belg.*
Amino acids and sodium ascorbate.
Tonic.

Revitex *Gerbex, Canad.*
Multivitamin preparation preparation with calcium and iron.

Revitonil *Lichtwer, UK.*
Echinacea (p.1574·2); peppermint (p.1208·1); clove (p.1565·2); aniseed (p.1549·3); liquorice (p.1197·1); fennel (p.1579·1); eucalyptus (p.1578·1).
Cold symptoms.

Revitonus C *Sabex, Canad.*
Ascorbic acid (p.1365·2); suprarenal cortex extract (p.1050·1); testicular extract (p.1464·1); brain extract (p.1599·1).
Vitamin C supplement.

Revivan *Astra, Ital.*
Dopamine hydrochloride (p.861·1).
Shock.

Revive *Allergan, UK.*
Carmellose (p.1471·2).
Comfort drops for use with soft contact lenses.

Revivona *Hafslund Nycomed, Aust.*
Multivitamin preparation.

Revocyl *Sanico, Belg.†.*
Amyl salicylate (p.15·3); camphor (p.1557·2); capsicum (p.1559·2); menthol (p.1600·2); chloroform (p.1220·3); belladonna (p.457·1).
Muscular and rheumatic pain.

Rewodina *Dresden, Ger.*
Diclofenac sodium (p.31·2).
Inflammation; musculoskeletal and joint disorders; pain.

Rex *LPB, Ital.*
Calcium lactate gluconate (p.1155·2); calcium carbonate (p.1182·1).
Bone disorders; hypocalcaemia.

Rexachlor *Be-Tabs, S.Afr.*
Paracetamol (p.72·2); chlormezanone (p.648·3).
Pain and associated tension.

Rexalgan *Dompe, Ital.*
Tenoxicam (p.88·2).
Musculoskeletal and joint disorders.

Rexan *Ist. Chim. Inter., Ital.*
Aciclovir (p.602·3).
Herpesvirus infections.

Rexgenta *Areu, Spain.*
Gentamicin sulphate (p.212·1).
Bacterial infections.

Rexidina Otoiatrica *Bouty, Ital.†.*
Prednisolone metasulphobenzoate (p.1049·1); chlorhexidine gluconate (p.1107·2).
Otitis; otorrhoea.

Rexigen *Pharmador, S.Afr.†.*
Propranolol hydrochloride (p.937·1).
Anxiety; cardiovascular disorders.

Rexigen Forte *Ion, USA.*
Phendimetrazine tartrate (p.1484·2).

Rexiluven S *Sandoz, Ger.*
Aesculus (p.1543·3).
Venous insufficiency.

Rexitene
Boehringer Mannheim, Aust.; LPB, Ital.†.
Guanabenz acetate (p.877·3).
Hypertension.

Rexitene Plus *LPB, Ital.†.*
Guanabenz acetate (p.877·3); mefruside (p.902·2).
Hypertension.

Rexolate *Hyrex, USA.*
Sodium thiosalicylate (p.85·2).
Gout; pain; rheumatic fever.

Rexophtal *Novopharma, Switz.*
Chlorhexidine gluconate (p.1107·2); phenylephrine hydrochloride (p.1066·2).
Eye disorders.

Rexort *Takeda, Fr.*
Citicoline (p.1564·3).
Cerebrovascular disorders.

Rexorubia
Homeocan, Canad.; Lehning, Fr.
Homoeopathic preparation.

Rezamid
Rhone-Poulenc Rorer Consumer, Canad.†; Summers, USA.
Resorcinol (p.1090·1); sulphur (p.1091·2).
Acne.

Rezine *Marnel, USA.*
Hydroxyzine hydrochloride (p.412·1).

Rezulin *Parke, Davis, USA.*
Troglitazone (p.334·1).
Diabetes mellitus.

R-Flex *Rolab, S.Afr.*
Sulindac (p.86·3).
Musculoskeletal and joint disorders.

R-Gel *Healthline, USA.*
Capsaicin (p.24·2).

R-Gen *Goldline, USA.*
Iodinated glycerol (p.1062·2).
Coughs.

R-Gene *Kabivitrum, USA.*
Arginine hydrochloride (p.1334·1).
Test to assess pituitary reserve for growth hormone.

RH 50 Antirheumatikum *Hormosan, Ger.†.*
Red ant extract; echinacea (p.1574·2).
Neuromuscular and joint disorders.

RH 50 percutan *Hormosan, Ger.†.*
Red ant extract; echinacea (p.1574·2); methyl nicotinate (p.55·1).
Arthroses; inflammatory disorders; neuralgia; rheumatic joint disorders.

Rhabarex B *Palmicol, Ger.*
Bisacodyl (p.1179·3).
Constipation; stool softener.

Rheaban Maximum Strength *Pfizer, USA.*
Activated attapulgite (p.1178·3).
Diarrhoea.

Rhefluin
Kytta, Ger.; Siegfried, Switz.
Amiloride hydrochloride (p.819·2); hydrochlorothiazide (p.885·2).
Ascites; hypertension; oedema.

Rheila Hustenstiller *Diedenhofen, Ger.†.*
Dextromethorphan hydrobromide (p.1057·3).
Coughs.

Rheila Medicated Cough Drops *Hilarys, Canad.*
Liquorice (p.1197·1); menthol (p.1600·2).

Rheila Stringiet N *Diedenhofen, Ger.*
Benzalkonium chloride (p.1101·3).
Mouth and throat infections.

Rhenus *APS, Ger.*
Aesculus (p.1543·3).
Haemorrhoids; venous insufficiency.

Rheobral *Niverpharm, Fr.*
Troxerutin (p.1580·2); vincamine (p.1644·1).
Mental function impairment in the elderly.

Rheoflux *Niverpharm, Fr.*
Troxerutin (p.1580·2).
Haemorrhoids; venous insufficiency.

Rheofusin
Pharmacia Upjohn, Aust.; Kabi Pharmacia, Ger.†.
Dextran 40 (p.716·2) in sorbitol, sodium chloride, or with electrolytes.
Thrombosis prophylaxis; vascular disorders.

Rheogen N *Robugen, Ger.*
Rhubarb (p.1212·1); aloes (p.1177·1).
Constipation.

Rheohes *Braun, Ger.*
Pentastarch (p.725·2).
Circulatory disorders; plasma volume expansion.

Rheolind *Rhenomed, Ger.†.*
Bisacodyl (p.1179·3); docusate sodium (p.1189·3).
Constipation.

Rheomacrodex
Torrex, Aust.; Pharmacia Upjohn, Austral.; Medisan, Canad.; Pharmacia Upjohn, Fr.; Reusch, Ger.; Kabi, Irl.†; Baxter, Ital.†; Pharmacia Upjohn, Norw.; Pharmacia Upjohn, S.Afr.; Pharmacia Upjohn, Spain; Medisan, Swed.; Braun, Switz.; Cambridge, UK; Pharmacia, USA.
Dextran 40 (p.716·2) in glucose, sorbitol, or sodium chloride.
Cerebral oedema; extracorporeal circulation; plasma volume expansion; thrombosis prophylaxis; vascular disorders.

rheotromb *Curasan, Ger.*
Urokinase (p.959·3).
Thrombo-embolic disorders.

Rhesogam *Chiron Behring, Ger.; Centeon, Ger.*
An anti-D immunoglobulin (p.1503·2).
Prevention of rhesus sensitisation.

Rhesogamma
Behring, Ital.†; Centeon, Norw.; Centeon, Swed.
Anti-D immunoglobulin (p.1503·2).
Prevention of rhesus sensitisation.

Rhesonativ
Pharmacia Upjohn, Ger.†; Pierrel, Ital.†; Pharmacia Upjohn, Norw.; Pharmacia Upjohn, Swed.; Kabivitrum, USA†.
An anti-D immunoglobulin (p.1503·2).
Prevention of rhesus sensitisation.

Rhesugam *NBI, S.Afr.*
An anti-D immunoglobulin (p.1503·2).
Prevention of rhesus sensitisation.

Rhesuman
Berna, Belg.; Berna, Ital.; Berna, Spain; Berna, Switz.
An anti-D immunoglobulin (p.1503·2).
Prevention of rhesus sensitisation.

Rheu *Salvator, Aust.*
Homoeopathic preparation.

Rheubalmin *Hoernecke, Ger.*
Diethylamine salicylate (p.33·1); benzyl nicotinate (p.22·1).
Musculoskeletal and joint disorders; neuralgia.

Rheubalmin Bad *Hoernecke, Ger.*
Methyl salicylate (p.55·2); isobornyl acetate; camphor (p.1557·2).
Bath additive; circulatory disorders; musculoskeletal, joint, and soft-tissue disorders; neuralgia; respiratory-tract disorders.

Rheubalmin Bad Nico *Hoernecke, Ger.*
Benzyl nicotinate (p.22·1).
Bath additive; circulatory disorders; musculoskeletal and joint disorders; neuralgia.

Rheubalmin Indo *Hoernecke, Ger.*
Indomethacin (p.45·2).
Musculoskeletal, joint, and soft-tissue disorders.

Rheubalmin N *Hoernecke, Ger.*
Glycol salicylate (p.43·1).
Musculoskeletal and joint disorders; neuralgia.

Rheubalmin Thermo *Hoernecke, Ger.*
Ointment: Glycol salicylate (p.43·1); benzyl nicotinate (p.22·1).
Musculoskeletal, joint, and soft-tissue disorders; peripheral vascular disorders.
Topical solution: Glycol salicylate (p.43·1); benzyl nicotinate (p.22·1); camphor (p.1557·2).
Musculoskeletal and joint disorders; neuralgia; peripheral vascular disorders.

Rheucostan M *Hanosan, Ger.*
Homoeopathic preparation.

Rheu-Do *Neos-Donner, Ger.†.*
Glycol salicylate (p.43·1); benzyl nicotinate (p.22·1).
Frostbite; musculoskeletal and joint disorders; sports injuries.

Rheu-Do mite *Neos-Donner, Ger.†.*
Glycol salicylate (p.43·1).
Musculoskeletal and joint disorders.

Rheufenac *Helvepharm, Switz.*
Diclofenac sodium (p.31·2).
Gout; inflammation; musculoskeletal, joint, and periarticular disorders; oedema; pain; renal and biliary colic.

Rheuflex *Goldcrest, UK†.*
Naproxen (p.61·2).
Gout; musculoskeletal and joint disorders.

Rheugesal *Solvay, Aust.*
Diethylamine salicylate (p.33·1); flufenamic acid (p.41·3); myrtecaine (p.1297·3).
Musculoskeletal, joint, peri-articular, and soft-tissue disorders.

Rheugesic *Medpro, S.Afr.*
Piroxicam (p.80·2).
Gout; musculoskeletal and joint disorders; pain.

Rheuma *Weleda, Aust.*
Aconitum napellus (p.1542·2); arnica (p.1550·3); betula folium (p.1553·3); mandragora radix; formica; rosemary oil (p.1626·2).
Musculoskeletal and joint disorders.

Rheuma Bad *Eu Rho, Ger.*
Glycol salicylate (p.43·1); benzyl nicotinate (p.22·1); camphor (p.1557·2); diethylamine salicylate (p.33·1).
Cold symptoms; musculoskeletal and joint disorders; neuralgia; peripheral vascular disorders.

Rheuma Lindofluid *Lindopharm, Ger.*
Flufenamic acid (p.41·3).
Musculoskeletal, joint, peri-articular, and soft-tissue disorders.

Rheuma Liquidum *Eu Rho, Ger.*
Glycol salicylate (p.43·1); benzyl nicotinate (p.22·1); nonivamide (p.63·2).
Musculoskeletal, joint, peri-articular, and soft-tissue disorders; neuralgia; peripheral vascular disorders.

Rheumabad N *Lichtenstein, Ger.†.*
Methyl salicylate (p.55·2).
Rheumatic disorders.

Rheumabene *Merckle, Ger.*
Dimethyl sulphoxide (p.1377·2).
Musculoskeletal and joint disorders.

Rheumacin *CP Pharmaceuticals, UK.*
Indomethacin (p.45·2).
Inflammation; pain.

Rheumadoron
Note. This name is used for preparations of different composition.
Weleda, Fr.
Homoeopathic preparation.
Weleda, UK.
Ointment: Aconitum napellus; arnica montana (p.1550·3); betula alba (p.1553·3); mandragora root; rosemary oil (p.1626·2).
Oral drops: Aconitum napellus; arnica montana (p.1550·3); betula alba (p.1553·3); mandragora root.
Rheumatic and muscular pain.

Rheumadrag *Schuck, Ger.†.*
Sodium gentisate (p.85·1); betula; urtica; thiamine hydrochloride; salicylamide (p.82·3).
Joint and muscle pain; neuralgia; neuritis; sciatica.

Rheumagel *Schmidgall, Aust.†.*
Diethylamine salicylate (p.33·1).
Musculoskeletal, joint, peri-articular, and soft-tissue disorders.

Rheuma-Gel *Ratiopharm, Ger.*
Etofenamate (p.36·3).
Musculoskeletal, joint, and soft-tissue disorders.

Rheumagutt-Bad N *Pino, Ger.†.*
Salicylic acid (p.1090·2).
Bath additive; musculoskeletal and joint disorders.

Rheuma-Hek *Strathmann, Ger.*
Urtica (p.1642·3).
Musculoskeletal and joint disorders.

Rheuma-Hevert *Hevert, Ger.*
Homoeopathic preparation.

Rheumajecta *Enzypharm, Neth.†.*
Sulfurylase sulfokinase; choline acetyltransferase; catalase (p.1560·3).
Rheumatic disorders.

Rheumakaps *Steigerwald, Ger.*
Salix (p.82·3).
Fever; headache; musculoskeletal and joint disorders.

Rheumalan *Hilarys, Canad.*
Methyl salicylate (p.55·2); camphor (p.1557·2); menthol (p.1600·2); belladonna (p.457·1); capsicum oleoresin croton oil (p.1188·2); eucalyptus oil (p.1578·1); expressed mustard oil (p.1605·3); salicylic acid (p.1090·2).

Rheumaliment *Galenika, Ger.†.*
Methyl salicylate (p.55·2); salicylic acid (p.1090·2); capsaicin (p.24·2); rosemary oil (p.1626·2); volatile mustard oil (p.1605·3); camphor (p.1557·2).
Circulatory disorders; nerve, muscle, and joint disorders.

Rheumaliment N *Galenika, Ger.*
Camphor (p.1557·2); eucalyptus oil (p.1578·1); turpentine oil (p.1641·1).
Musculoskeletal and joint pain.

rheuma-loges *Loges, Ger.*
Homoeopathic preparation.

rheuma-loges N Balsam *Loges, Ger.†.*
Benzyl nicotinate (p.22·1); oleum pini sylvestris; rosemary oil.
Circulatory disorders; neuromuscular disorders; rheumatic disorders; sports injuries.

rheumamed *Feldhoff, Ger.†.*
Bovine extract of testes and placenta (p.1464·1) (p.1599·1); benzyl nicotinate (p.22·1).
Arthroses; rheumatism; sciatica; spondyloses.

Rheuma-Pasc *Pascoe, Ger.*
Homoeopathic preparation.

Rheuma-Pasc N *Pascoe, Ger.*
Rosemary oil (p.1626·2); methyl salicylate (p.55·2); hamamelis (p.1587·1).
Neuralgia; neuritis.

Rheuma-Plantina *Plantina, Ger.*
Homoeopathic preparation.

Rheumaplast N *Beiersdorf, Ger.*
Cayenne pepper.
Musculoskeletal and joint disorders.

Rheumasalbe *CT, Ger.*
Nonivamide (p.63·2); benzyl nicotinate (p.22·1); eucalyptus oil (p.1578·1).
Musculoskeletal, joint, and soft-tissue disorders; neuralgia.

Rheuma-Salbe *Stada, Ger.*
Glycol salicylate (p.43·1); benzyl nicotinate (p.22·1).
Musculoskeletal, joint, and soft-tissue disorders; peripheral vascular disorders.

Rheumasalbe Capsicum *Kneipp, Ger.†.*
Capsicum (p.1559·2); meadowsweet oil.
Muscular, neuromuscular, and joint disorders.

Rheuma-Salbe Lichtenstein *Lichtenstein, Ger.*
Glycol salicylate (p.43·1); benzyl nicotinate (p.22·1); camphor (p.1557·2).
Neuralgia; rheumatic pain; sports injuries; tenosynovitis.

Rheumasan
Note. This name is used for preparations of different composition.
Kwizda, Aust.†.
Salicylic acid (p.1090·2); sodium humate; norway spruce oil; camphor (p.1557·2); eucalyptus oil (p.1578·1); menthol (p.1600·2).
Cold symptoms; musculoskeletal and joint disorders.
Plantorgan, Ger.†.
Ethanolamine salicylate; benzyl nicotinate (p.22·1); nonivamide (p.63·2); camphor (p.1557·2); pine needle oil (p.1623·3); spike lavender oil (p.1632·2).
Bruising; frostbite; joint, nerve, and muscle disorders; peripheral vascular disorders.

Rheumasan Bad *Sanofi Winthrop, Ger.*
Diethylamine salicylate (p.33·1); sodium humate.
Formerly contained ethanolamine salicylate, ethanolamine humate, menthol, camphor, eucalyptus oil, and siberian fir oil.
Bath additive; musculoskeletal and joint disorders.

Rheumasan D *Sanofi Winthrop, Ger.†.*
Diclofenac sodium (p.31·2).
Inflammation; musculoskeletal and joint disorders; pain.

Rheumasan N *Sanofi Winthrop, Ger.*
Ointment: Salicylic acid (p.1090·2); methyl nicotinate (p.55·1).
Rheumasan contained ethanolamine salicylate, camphor, and methyl nicotinate.
Topical rub: Salicylic acid (p.1090·2); benzyl nicotinate (p.22·1).
Bruising; musculoskeletal, joint, and nerve disorders.

Rheumaselect *Dreluso, Ger.*
Homoeopathic preparation.

Rheuma-Sern *Serturner, Ger.*
Harpagophytum procumbens (p.27·2).
Musculoskeletal and joint disorders.

Rheumasit *Medice, Ger.*
Dexamethasone (p.1037·1); benzyl nicotinate (p.22·1).
Muscle, joint, and soft-tissue disorders.

Rheumasol *English Grains, UK.*
Guaiacum resin (p.1586·3); prickly ash bark (p.1645·3).
Rheumatic and muscular pain and stiffness.

Rheumatab Salicis *Schuck, Ger.*
Salix (p.82·3).
Headache; rheumatic disorders.

Rheuma-Tee *Romigal, Ger.†.*
Radix harpagophyti (p.27·2).
Herbal preparation.

Rheuma-Teufelskralle HarpagoMega *Twardy, Ger.*
Harpagophytum procumbens (p.27·2).
Appetite loss; dyspepsia; musculoskeletal and joint disorders.

Rheumatex *Wampole, USA.*
Test for rheumatoid factor in serum.

Rheumat-Eze *Medinat, Austral.†.*
Aloxiprin (p.15·1); codeine (p.26·1); silica; manganese chelate; rhus tox; arnica; hypericum.
Arthritic conditions; rheumatic conditions.

Rheumatic Pain *Cantassium Co., UK.*
Guaiacum resin (p.1586·3); taraxacum (p.1634·2); celery (p.1561·1); buckbean (p.1601·2).
Muscle and joint pain.

Rheumatic Pain Remedy *Potter's, UK.*
Bogbean (p.1601·2); burdock root (p.1594·2); yarrow (p.1542·2); guaiacum resin (p.1586·3).
Rheumatic pain.

Rheumatic Pain Tablets *Healthcrafts, UK.*
Guaiacum resin (p.1586·3); bogbean (p.1601·2); celery seed (p.1561·1).
Rheumatic pain.

Rheumatica *Nelson, UK.*
Homoeopathic preparation.

Rheumatism Rhus Tox *Homeocan, Canad.*
Homoeopathic preparation.

Rheumatisme *Gerbex, Canad.*
Methyl salicylate (p.55·2); camphor (p.1557·2); capsicum oleoresin; trimethylcyclohexanol.

Rheumatol *Tosse, Ger.†.*
Bumadizone calcium (p.22·2).
Acute ankylosing spondylitis; rheumatism.

Rheumaton
Carter-Wallace, Switz.; Wampole, USA.
Test for rheumatoid factor in serum or synovial fluid.

Rheumatrex
Wyeth-Ayerst, Canad.; Lederle, USA.
Methotrexate (p.547·1) or methotrexate sodium (p.547·1).
Psoriasis; rheumatoid arthritis.

Rheumavincin *Schur, Ger.†.*
Choline salicylate (p.25·2).
Musculoskeletal and joint disorders; pleuritis.

Rheumax *Hoernecke, Ger.*
Methyl salicylate (p.55·2).
Musculoskeletal and joint disorders.

Rheumed *Phytomed, Switz.*
Homoeopathic preparation.

Rheumeda *Madaus, Ger.*
Homoeopathic preparation.

Rheumesser *Gerot, Aust.*
Kebuzone (p.48·1); salamidacetic acid (p.82·3); dexamethasone (p.1037·1); cyanocobalamin (p.1363·3) or hydroxocobalamin acetate (p.1364·2).
Also contains lignocaine (p.1293·2).
Musculoskeletal and joint disorders.

Rheumex
Note. This name is used for preparations of different composition.
Gebro, Aust.
Glycol salicylate (p.43·1); benzyl nicotinate (p.22·1); allantoin (p.1078·2).
Musculoskeletal and joint disorders; sports injuries.

Labopharma, Ger.†.
Bath additive: Diethylamine salicylate (p.33·1); rosemary oil (p.1626·2); arnica (p.1550·3); aesculus (p.1543·3).
Cream: Diethylamine salicylate (p.33·1); rosemary oil (p.1626·2); benzyl nicotinate (p.22·1).
Tea: Phaseolis vulgaris; salix (p.82·3); gnaphalium alba; birch leaf (p.1553·3); peppermint oil (p.1208·1); senna (p.1212·2); aniseed (p.1549·3); caraway (p.1559·3); coriander (p.1567·3); rose fruit (p.1365·2); fennel (p.1579·1); juniper (p.1592·2); equisetum (p.1575·1); meadowsweet (p.1599·1); taraxacum (p.1634·2); urtica (p.1642·3); levisticum root (p.1597·2); ononis (p.1610·2); stipites dulcamara (p.1574·2).
Musculoskeletal and joint disorders; peripheral circulatory disorders; sports injuries.

Rheumichthol Bad *Ichthyol, Ger.*
Light ammonium bituminosulphonate (p.1083·3); glycol salicylate (p.43·1); diethylamine salicylate (p.33·1).
Bath additive; musculoskeletal and joint disorders.

Rheumitin *Krewel, Ger.*
Piroxicam (p.80·2).
Gout; musculoskeletal, joint, and soft-tissue disorders.

Rheumon
Kolassa, Aust.; Bayer, Ger.; Bayer, Switz.
Etofenamate (p.36·3).
Musculoskeletal, joint, peri-articular, and soft-tissue disorders.

Rheumox
Wyeth, Irl.; Continental Ethicals, S.Afr.†; Lagamed, S.Afr.†; Goldshield, UK.
Azapropazone (p.20·3).
Acute gout; musculoskeletal and joint disorders.

Rheumyl *3M, Ger.†.*
Diethylamine salicylate (p.33·1); benzyl nicotinate (p.22·1).
Muscle, joint, and nerve disorders.

Rheumyl N *3M, Ger.†.*
Diethylamine salicylate (p.33·1); benzyl nicotinate (p.22·1).
Muscle, joint, and nerve disorders.

Rheunerton *Dolorgiet, Ger.†.*
Glycol salicylate (p.43·1).
Musculoskeletal and joint disorders.

Rheunervol N *LAW, Ger.*
Camphor (p.1557·2).
Rheunervol formerly contained camphor, bornyl acetate, and propyl nicotinate.
Musculoskeletal and joint disorders.

Rheutrop *Kolassa, Aust.*
Acemetacin (p.12·2).
Gout; inflammation; musculoskeletal and joint disorders; thrombophlebitis; vasculitis.

Rhinaaxia
Zyma, Aust.; Zyma, Belg.†; Zyma, Fr.; Zambon, Ital.; Inpharzam, Switz.
Magnesium isospaglumate (p.1591·3) or sodium spaglumate.
Rhinitis.

Rhinadvil *Whitehall, Fr.*
Ibuprofen (p.44·1); pseudoephedrine hydrochloride (p.1068·3).
Fever; headache; rhinitis with nasal congestion.

Rhinalair *Inava, Fr.*
Pseudoephedrine hydrochloride (p.1068·3).
Nasal congestion.

Rhinalar
Syntex, Austral.†; Roche, Canad.
Flunisolide (p.1040·3).
Allergic rhinitis.

Rhinalene a la framycetine *SmithKline Beecham Sante, Fr.*
Framycetin sulphate (p.210·3).
Nasal infections.

Rhinall *Scherer, USA.*
Phenylephrine hydrochloride (p.1066·2).
Nasal congestion.

Rhinamide
Note. This name is used for preparations of different composition.
Sopar, Belg.†.
Diphenylpyraline hydrochloride (p.409·3); sulphanilamide (p.256·3); ephedrine hydrochloride (p.1059·3).
Nasal congestion.

Bailly, Fr.
Sulphanilamide (p.256·3); ephedrine hydrochloride (p.1059·3); butacaine sulphate (p.1288·3); benzoic acid (p.1102·3).
Congestion of the nose and throat.

Rhinaris *Pharmascience, Canad.*
Macrogol (p.1597·3); propylene glycol (p.1622·1).
Rhinitis.

Rhinaris-F *Pharmascience, Canad.†.*
Flunisolide (p.1040·3).
Allergic rhinitis.

Rhinaspray *Boehringer Ingelheim, Austral.†.*
Tramazoline hydrochloride (p.1071·1).
Eustachian-tube congestion; nasal congestion.

Rhinatate *Major, USA.*
Phenylephrine tannate (p.1067·1); chlorpheniramine tannate (p.405·2); mepyramine tannate (p.414·1).
Upper respiratory-tract symptoms.

Rhinathiol
Synthelabo, Fr.; Lorex Synthelabo, Neth.; Synthelabo, Switz.
Carbocisteine (p.1056·3).
Respiratory-tract disorders associated with viscous mucus.

Rhinathiol Antitussivum *Synthelabo, Belg.*
Dextromethorphan hydrobromide (p.1057·3).
Coughs.

Rhinathiol Mucolyticum *Synthelabo, Belg.*
Carbocisteine (p.1056·3).
Respiratory-tract disorders associated with abnormal mucus production.

Rhinathiol Promethazine
Synthelabo, Fr.; Synthelabo, Switz.
Carbocisteine (p.1056·3); promethazine hydrochloride (p.416·2).
Respiratory-tract disorders.

RhinATP *Synthelabo, Fr.*
Adenosine triphosphate, disodium salt (p.1543·2); sulfasuccinamide (p.252·1).
Infections of the nose and throat.

Rhinergal
Wander, S.Afr.†; Wander, Switz.†.
Clemastine (p.406·2) or clemastine hydrogen fumarate (p.406·2); phenylpropanolamine hydrochloride (p.1067·2).
Cold symptoms; nasal congestion; rhinitis.

Rhinex *Wernigerode, Ger.*
Naphazoline hydrochloride (p.1064·2).
Nasal congestion; rhinitis; sinusitis.

rhinicept *Sanol, Ger.†.*
Phenylpropanolamine hydrochloride (p.1067·2); chlorpheniramine maleate (p.405·1).
Colds.

Rhinidine *Warner-Lambert Consumer, Belg.*
Xylometazoline hydrochloride (p.1071·2).
Nasal congestion and irritation.

Rhinipan *Pharmacal, Switz.*
Phenylephrine hydrochloride (p.1066·2); dequalinium diacetate (p.1112·1); chlorhexidine gluconate (p.1107·2).
Catarrh; rhinitis; sinusitis.

Rhinitin *Piraud, Switz.†.*
Diphenhydramine hydrochloride (p.409·1); caffeine (p.749·3).
Allergic rhinitis; cold symptoms.

Rhino-Blache *Gallier, Fr.†.*
Chlorhexidine gluconate (p.1107·2).
Infections of the nose and throat.

Rhinocap
Note. This name is used for preparations of different composition.
Inibsa, Spain†.
Phenylephrine hydrochloride (p.1066·2); carbinoxamine maleate (p.404·2).
Nasal congestion.

Grossmann, Switz.
Phenylephrine hydrochloride (p.1066·2); dimenhydrinate (p.408·2); caffeine (p.749·3).
Allergic rhinitis; cold symptoms; nasal congestion; sinus congestion.

Rhinocaps
Note. This name is used for preparations of different composition.
Vemedia, Neth.
Camphor (p.1557·2); chlorothymol (p.1111·1); cineole (p.1564·1); menthol (p.1600·2); terpineol (p.1635·1).
Cold symptoms.

Ferndale, USA.
Phenylpropanolamine hydrochloride (p.1067·2); aspirin (p.16·1); paracetamol (p.72·2).
Upper respiratory-tract symptoms.

Rhinocillin B *Medicopharm, Aust.*
Bacitracin (p.157·3).
No indications given.

Rhinocort
Astra, Austral.; Astra, Belg.; Astra, Canad.; Astra, Irl.; Astra, Neth.; Astra, Norw.; Astra, S.Afr.; Astra, Spain; Tika, Swed.; Astra, Switz.; Astra, UK; Astra, USA.
Budesonide (p.1034·3).
Nasal polyps; rhinitis.

Rhinocortol *Astra, Aust.*
Budesonide (p.1034·3).
Nasal polyps; rhinitis.

Rhinocure *Medibel, Switz.*
Polysorbate 80 (p.1327·3); sodium chloride (p.1162·2); matricaria (p.1561·2); benzethonium chloride (p.1102·3).
Rhinopharyngeal disorders.

Rhinocure Simplex *Medibel, Switz.*
Polysorbate 80 (p.1327·3); sodium chloride (p.1162·2); benzethonium chloride (p.1102·3).
Rhinopharyngeal disorders.

Rhinodrin *Montavit, Aust.*
Diphenhydramine hydrochloride (p.409·1); naphazoline hydrochloride (p.1064·2).
Rhinitis.

Rhinofebral
Martin, Fr.; Martin, Switz.
Paracetamol (p.72·2); chlorpheniramine maleate (p.405·1); ascorbic acid (p.1365·2).
Cold symptoms; rhinopharyngeal disorders.

Rhinofebryl *Rhone-Poulenc Rorer, Belg.*
Chlorpheniramine maleate (p.405·1); paracetamol (p.72·2).
Rhinitis with fever and/or headache.

Rhinofed *Noriston, S.Afr.†.*
Triprolidine hydrochloride (p.420·3); pseudoephedrine hydrochloride (p.1068·3).
Nasal congestion.

Rhinofluimucil *Zambon, Fr.*
Acetylcysteine (p.1052·3); tuaminoheptane sulphate (p.1071·1); benzalkonium chloride (p.1101·3).
Rhinopharyngeal congestion.

Rhinofluine *Pharmethic, Belg.†.*
Pilocarpine hydrochloride (p.1396·3); procaine (p.1299·2).
Nasal congestion; rhinitis.

Rhino-Gastreu R49 *Reckeweg, Ger.*
Homoeopathic preparation.

Rhinogesic *Pal-Pak, USA.*
Phenylephrine hydrochloride (p.1066·2); paracetamol (p.72·2); chlorpheniramine maleate (p.405·1); salicylamide (p.82·3).
Upper respiratory-tract symptoms.

Rhinoguttae pro Infantibus *Leyh, Ger.*
Ephedrine hydrochloride (p.1059·3); silver protein acetyl tannate.
Bacterial nose infections.

Rhinoinfant *Pharminfant, Ger.†.*
Buphenine hydrochloride (p.1555·3); diphenylpyraline hydrochloride (p.409·3); sodium salamidacetate (p.82·3).
Colds.

Rhino-Lacteol *Lacteol du Dr Boucard, Fr.*
Lactobacillus acidophilus (p.1594·1).
Infections of the nose and throat.

Rhinolar *McGregor, USA†.*
Phenylpropanolamine hydrochloride (p.1067·2); chlorpheniramine maleate (p.405·1); hyoscine methonitrate (p.463·1).
Upper respiratory-tract symptoms.

Rhinolar-EX *McGregor, USA.*
Phenylpropanolamine hydrochloride (p.1067·2); chlorpheniramine maleate (p.405·1).
Upper respiratory-tract symptoms.

Rhinolast
Astra, Ger.; Stern, Ger.; Orion, Irl.; Vesta, S.Afr.; Asta Medica, UK.
Azelastine hydrochloride (p.403·1).
Allergic rhinitis.

rhino-loges N *Loges, Ger.†.*
Guaiazulene (p.1586·3); eucalyptus oil (p.1578·1); sage oil; pumilio pine oil (p.1623·3).
Colds; nasal congestion.

Rhinomer
Zyma, Ger.; Zyma, Switz.; Novartis Consumer, UK.
Sodium chloride (p.1162·2).
Nasal congestion; rhinitis.

Rhino-Mex *Charton, Canad.*
Naphazoline hydrochloride (p.1064·2); amylocaine hydrochloride (p.1286·1).
Nasal congestion.

Rhino-Mex-N *Charton, Canad.*
Naphazoline hydrochloride (p.1064·2).
Nasal congestion.

Rhinon *Petrasch, Aust.*
Nasal ointment: Naphazoline hydrochloride (p.1064·2); sulphadiazine (p.252·3).
Nose drops: Naphazoline hydrochloride (p.1064·2).
Rhinitis; sinusitis.

Rhinoperd *Agepha, Aust.*
Naphazoline hydrochloride (p.1064·2).
Rhinitis; sinusitis.

Rhinoperd comp *Agepha, Aust.*
Naphazoline hydrochloride (p.1064·2); diphenhydramine hydrochloride (p.409·1).
Cold symptoms; rhinitis.

Rhinopront
Note. This name is used for preparations of different composition.
Pfizer, Aust.; Mack, Belg.; Mack, Illert., Ger.; Mack, Switz.
Capsules: Carbinoxamine maleate (p.404·2); phenylephrine hydrochloride (p.1066·2).
Colds; nasal catarrh; rhinitis.

Pfizer, Aust.; Mack, Illert., Ger.; Mack, Switz.
Oral liquid: Carbinoxamine polistirex (p.404·2); phenylpropanolamine polistirex (p.1067·3).
Colds; nasal catarrh; rhinitis.

Mack, Illert., Ger.
Nasal spray: Tetrahydrozoline hydrochloride (p.1070·2).
Catarrh; colds; hay fever.

Rhinopront Top *Mack, Switz.*
Tetrahydrozoline hydrochloride (p.1070·2).
Rhinopharyngeal disorders.

Rhinopten *Debat, Fr.*
Antigens of: *Staphylococcus aureus* 634, 636, 659; *Streptococcus* 147; *Streptococcus pyogenes* 155, 1178; *Diplococcus pneumoniae* 209, 210; *Moraxella (Branhamella) catarrhalis* 987.
Disorders of the ear, nose, and throat.

Rhinoptil *Promonta, Ger.†.*
Cafaminol.
Colds; nasal congestion.

Rhinosovil *Eu Rho, Ger.*
Naphazoline nitrate (p.1064·2); pheniramine maleate (p.415·3).
Nasal congestion; rhinitis.

Rhinospray
Boehringer Ingelheim, Belg.; Thomae, Ger.; Boehringer Ingelheim, Neth.†; Fher, Spain.
Tramazoline hydrochloride (p.1071·1).
Nasal congestion; rhinitis.

Rhinospray Plus *Bender, Aust.*
Tramazoline hydrochloride (p.1071·1); cineole (p.1564·1); menthol (p.1600·2); camphor (p.1557·2).
Nasal congestion.

Rhino-stas *Stada, Ger.*
Xylometazoline hydrochloride (p.1071·2).
Rhinitis; sinusitis.

Rhino-Sulforgan *Jolly-Jatel, Fr.†.*
Sulphurated oil; butyl aminobenzoate (p.1289·1); Labrafil; cineole (p.1564·1).
Infections of the nose and throat.

Rhino-Sulfuryl *Aerocid, Fr.*
Sodium thiosulphate (p.996·2); ephedrine hydrochloride (p.1059·3).
Rhinopharyngeal congestion.

Rhinosyn *Great Southern, USA.*
Pseudoephedrine hydrochloride (p.1068·3); chlorpheniramine maleate (p.405·1).
Upper respiratory-tract symptoms.

Rhinosyn-DM *Great Southern, USA.*
Pseudoephedrine hydrochloride (p.1068·3); chlorpheniramine maleate (p.405·1); dextromethorphan hydrobromide (p.1057·3).
Coughs and cold symptoms.

Rhinosyn-DMX *Great Southern, USA.*
Dextromethorphan hydrobromide (p.1057·3); guaiphenesin (p.1061·3).
Coughs.

Rhinosyn-X *Great Southern, USA.*
Pseudoephedrine hydrochloride (p.1068·3); dextromethorphan hydrobromide (p.1057·3); guaiphenesin (p.1061·3).
Coughs.

Rhino-Tantum *Roche, Switz.†.*
Benzydamine hydrochloride (p.21·3).
Nasal congestion.

Rhinothricinol *Plan, Switz.*
Tyrothricin (p.267·2); eucalyptus oil (p.1578·1).
Rhinopharyngeal infections.

Rhinotrophyl *Jolly-Jatel, Fr.*
Thenoate ethanolamine (p.262·2); framycetin sulphate (p.210·3).
Infections of the nose and throat.

Rhinotussal
Note. This name is used for preparations of different composition.
Mack, Illert., Ger.; Madaus, S.Afr.†; Mack, Switz.
Capsules: Dextromethorphan hydrobromide (p.1057·3); phenylephrine hydrochloride (p.1066·2); carbinoxamine maleate (p.404·2).
Coughs and associated respiratory-tract disorders.
Mack, Illert., Ger.; Mack, Switz.
Oral liquid: Dextromethorphan polistirex (p.1058·2); phenylpropanolamine polistirex (p.1067·3); carbinoxamine polistirex (p.404·2).
Coughs and associated respiratory-tract disorders.
Ethimed, S.Afr.†.
Syrup: Dextromethorphan hydrobromide (p.1057·3); phenylpropanolamine hydrochloride (p.1067·2); carbinoxamine maleate (p.404·2).
Coughs.

Rhinotussal E Balsam *Mack, Illert., Ger.†.*
Camphor (p.1557·2); oleum pini sylvestris; pumilio pine oil (p.1623·3); peppermint oil (p.1208·1); eucalyptus oil (p.1578·1); rosemary oil (p.1626·2).
Coughs and associated respiratory-tract disorders.

Rhinotussal S Balsam *Mack, Illert., Ger.†.*
Camphor (p.1557·2); oleum pini sylvestris; eucalyptus oil (p.1578·1); turpentine oil (p.1641·1); guaiazulene (p.1586·3).
Coughs and associated respiratory-tract disorders.

Rhinovalon *Sintesa, Belg.*
Tixocortol pivalate (p.1050·1).
Rhinitis.

Rhinovalon Neomycine *Sintesa, Belg.*
Tixocortol pivalate (p.1050·1); neomycin sulphate (p.229·2).
Infective rhinitis.

Rhinovent *Boehringer Ingelheim, Switz.*
Ipratropium bromide (p.754·2).
Rhinitis.

Rhinox *Nycomed, Norw.*
Oxymetazoline hydrochloride (p.1065·3).
Nasal congestion.

Rhinureflex *Boots Healthcare, Fr.*
Ibuprofen (p.44·1); pseudoephedrine hydrochloride (p.1068·3).
Rhinitis.

Rhinyl *Pierre Fabre Sante, Fr.*
Framycetin sulphate (p.210·3); sodium propionate (p.387·1).
Colds.

Rhodacine *Rhodiapharm, Canad.*
Indomethacin (p.45·2).
Gout; musculoskeletal and joint disorders.

Rhodalbumin *Merieux, Ger.†.*
Albumin (p.710·1).
Hypoproteinaemia; hypovolaemia.

Rhodialax *Rhodiapharm, Canad.†.*
Lactulose (p.1195·3).
Constipation.

Rhodialose *Rhodiapharm, Canad.†.*
Lactulose (p.1195·3).
Hepatic encephalopathy.

Rhodiglobin *Pasteur Merieux, Swed.†.*
A normal immunoglobulin (p.1522·1).
Hypogammaglobulinaemia; passive immunisation.

Rhodine *Rhone-Poulenc Rorer, Belg.*
Aspirin (p.16·1).
Dental pain; fever; headache; rheumatic pain.

Rhodis *Rhodiapharm, Canad.*
Ketoprofen (p.48·2).
Musculoskeletal and joint disorders.

Rhoditest-Tuberkulin *Pasteur Merieux, Swed.†.*
Tuberculin (PPD) (p.1640·2).
Sensitivity testing.

Rhodogil *Rhone-Poulenc Rorer, Spain.*
Spiramycin (p.249·2); metronidazole (p.585·1).
Bacterial infections.

Rhodurea *Rhodiapharm, Canad.†.*
Urea (p.1095·2).
Dry skin disorders; hyperkeratosis.

RhoGAM *Ortho Pharmaceutical, USA.*
An anti-D immunoglobulin (p.1503·2).
Prevention of rhesus sensitisation.

Rhoival *Tosse, Ger.*
Agrimony; solidago virgaurea; hypericum (p.1590·1); capsella bursa pastoris; arnica (p.1550·3); valerian (p.1643·1).
Urinary-tract disorders.

Rholosone *Rhodiapharm, Canad.†.*
Betamethasone valerate (p.1033·3).
Scalp disorders; skin disorders.

Rhonal
Rhone-Poulenc Rorer, Belg.; Theraplix, Fr.; Nattermann, Neth.†; Rhone-Poulenc Rorer, Spain; Rhone-Poulenc Rorer, Switz.†.
Aspirin (p.16·1).
Fever; musculoskeletal, joint and peri-articular disorders; pain; thrombo-embolism prophylaxis.

Rhophylac *ZLB, Switz.*
An anti-D immunoglobulin (p.1503·2).
Prevention of rhesus sensitisation.

Rhoprolene *Rhodiapharm, Canad.†.*
Betamethasone dipropionate (p.1033·3).
Skin disorders.

Rhoprosone *Rhodiapharm, Canad.†.*
Betamethasone dipropionate (p.1033·3).
Skin disorders.

Rhotral *Rhodiapharm, Canad.*
Acebutolol hydrochloride (p.809·3).
Angina pectoris; hypertension.

Rhotrimine *Rhodiapharm, Canad.*
Trimipramine maleate (p.310·1).
Depression.

Rhovail *Rho-Pharm, Canad.*
Ketoprofen (p.48·2).
Musculoskeletal and joint disorders.

Rhovane *Rhodiapharm, Canad.*
Zopiclone (p.699·2).
Insomnia.

Rhuaka *Waterhouse, UK.*
Cascara (p.1183·1); rhubarb (p.1212·1); senna (p.1212·2).
Constipation.

Rhuli Gel *Rydelle, USA.*
Benzyl alcohol (p.1103·3); menthol (p.1600·2); camphor (p.1557·2).
Minor skin irritation.

Rhuli Spray *Rydelle, USA.*
Calamine (p.1080·1); camphor (p.1557·2); benzocaine (p.1286·2).
Minor skin irritation.

Rhumalgan
Lagap, Switz.†; Lagap, UK.
Diclofenac sodium (p.31·2).
Gout; inflammation; musculoskeletal disorders; pain.

Rhus Med Complex *Dynamit, Aust.*
Homoeopathic preparation.

Rhus Toxicodendron Oligoplex *Madaus, Ger.*
Homoeopathic preparation.

Rhus-Rheuma-Gel N *DHU, Ger.*
Rhus toxicodendron (p.1624·3); ledum; symphytum (p.1567·1).
Muscle and joint disorders.

Rhythmochin I *Promonta, Ger.†.*
Quinidine (p.938·3); procainamide hydrochloride (p.934·1); crataegus (p.1568·2).
Arrhythmias.

Rhythmochin II (cum sedativo) *Promonta, Ger.†.*
Quinidine (p.938·3); procainamide hydrochloride (p.934·1); crataegus (p.1568·2); phenobarbitone (p.350·2).
Arrhythmias.

Rhythmocor *Solvay, Aust.*
Propafenone hydrochloride (p.935·3).
Arrhythmias.

Riabal
Logeais, Fr.; Ibi, Ital.
Prifinium bromide (p.467·2).
Smooth muscle spasm.

Riacen *Chiesi, Ital.*
Piroxicam (p.80·2).
Musculoskeletal and joint disorders.

Ribalgilasi *Italfarmaco, Ital.†.*
Ribonuclease (p.1624·3).
Musculoskeletal and joint pain and inflammation.

Ribatran *Leurquin, Fr.*
Trypsin (p.1640·1); ribonuclease (p.1624·3); chymotrypsinogen.
Oedema following trauma or surgery; respiratory-tract inflammation.

Ribbeck *Ziethen, Ger.†.*
Codeine phosphate (p.26·1); diphenhydramine hydrochloride (p.409·1); papaverine hydrochloride (p.1614·2).
Coughs and associated respiratory-tract disorders.

Ribelfan *Pharmacia Upjohn, Ital.*
Propyphenazone (p.81·3); noscapine (p.1065·2).
Cold and influenza symptoms.

Ribex Flu *Ircafarm, Ital.*
Diclofenac sodium (p.31·2).
Fever; influenza symptoms; pain.

Ribex Gola *Ircafarm, Ital.*
Benzethonium chloride (p.1102·3).
Mouth disinfection.

Ribex Tosse *Ircafarm, Ital.*
Dropropizine (p.1059·2).
Coughs.

Ribexen con Espettorante *Ircafarm, Ital.*
Dropropizine (p.1059·2); guaiphenesin (p.1061·3).
Coughs.

Ribocarbo *Ribosepharm, Ger.*
Carboplatin (p.510·3).
Malignant neoplasms.

Ribociclina *Formenti, Ital.*
Doxycycline hydrochloride (p.202·3); trypsin (p.1640·1); chymotrypsin (p.1563·2); ribonuclease (p.1624·3).
Bacterial infections.

Ribocort B12 *Lagap, Ital.†.*
Suprarenal cortex (p.1050·1); cyanocobalamin (p.1363·3); inosine (p.1591·1).
Adrenal insufficiency; anaemias; hepatic insufficiency; tonic.

Ribofluor *Ribosepharm, Ger.*
Fluorouracil (p.534·3).
Malignant neoplasms.

Ribofolin
Schoeller, Aust.; Ribosepharm, Ger.
Calcium folinate (p.1342·2).
Antidote to folic acid antagonists.

Ribolac
Zyma, Ger.†; Gebro, Switz.
Lactobacillus acidophilus (p.1594·1); vitamins.
Diarrhoea.

Ribomed *Maggioni, Ital.†.*
Ribostamycin sulphate (p.242·2).
Gastro-intestinal infections.

Ribomicin *Farmigea, Ital.*
Gentamicin sulphate (p.212·1).
Bacterial eye infections.

Ribomunyl
Germania, Aust.; Inava, Fr.; Pierre Fabre, Ger.; Pierre Fabre, Spain; Robapharm, Switz.
Ribosomes of *Klebsiella pneumoniae*; *Streptococcus pneumoniae*; *Streptococcus pyogenes*; *Haemophilus influenzae*; membrane fraction of *Klebsiella pneumoniae*.
Respiratory-tract infections.

Ribomustin *Ribosepharm, Ger.*
Bendamustine hydrochloride.
Malignant neoplasms.

Ribon *Therabel Pharma, Belg.*
Riboflavine (p.1362·1).
Muscle cramps; vitamin B_2 deficiency.

Ribostamin *Delalande, Ital.†.*
Ribostamycin sulphate (p.242·2).
Bacterial infections.

Ribostat *Valeas, Ital.*
Ribostamycin sulphate (p.242·2).
Gastro-intestinal infections.

Ribosten *IBP, Ital.†.*
Vitamin B substances.

Ribotrex *Pierre Fabre, Ital.*
Azithromycin (p.155·2).
Bacterial infections.

Ribovir *Plants, Ital.*
Royal jelly (p.1626·3); echinacea (p.1574·2); black currant (p.1365·2).
Nutritional supplement.

Ribo-Wied *Wiedemann, Ger.*
Spleen; liver; heart; placenta (p.1599·1).
Tonic.

Ribrain *Yamanouchi, Ger.*
Betahistine mesylate (p.1553·1).
Ménière's disease.

Ribusol *Wasserman, Spain.*
Budesonide (p.1034·3).
Asthma; nasal polyps; rhinitis; skin disorders.

Riccomycine *Kropf, Switz.*
Neomycin sulphate (p.229·2); ichthammol (p.1083·3); matricaria (p.1561·2); vitamin A palmitate (p.1359·2); ergocalciferol (p.1367·1); hamamelis (p.1587·1).
Burns; superficial infected wounds.

Riccovitan *Kropf, Switz.*
Vitamin A palmitate (p.1359·2); ergocalciferol (p.1367·1); ichthammol (p.1083·3); hamamelis (p.1587·1); chamomile (p.1561·2); zinc oxide (p.1096·2).
Burns; skin inflammation; superficial wounds.

Ricerca System Anagen *Rydelle, Ital.*
Multivitamin, mineral, and amino-acid preparation.
Skin, hair, and nail disorders.

Ricerca System Elios *Rydelle, Ital.*
Multivitamin, mineral, and amino-acid preparation.
Sunlight-induced skin damage.

Ricerca System Hidra *Rydelle, Ital.*
Antoxidants; polyunsaturated fatty acids.
Dry skin.

Ricerca System Iposeb *Rydelle, Ital.*
Multivitamin, mineral, and amino-acid preparation.
Seborrhoea.

Richelet *Therabel Pharma, Belg.†.*
Jugland. reg.; nasturtii officinal.; cochlear. armorac.; cochlear. officin.; menyanth. (p.1601·2); cinnamon. (p.1564·2); citr. vulgar.; colombo tincture (p.1557·2); kal. iod. (p.1493·1); iod. (p.1493·1); magnes. chlorid. (p.1157·2); magnes. bromid.; nicotinamid. (p.1351·2).
Haemorrhoids; phlebitis; varices.

Ricino Koki *Calmante Vitaminado, Spain.*
Castor oil (p.1560·2).
Bowel evacuation.

Ricobid *Rico, USA.*
Chlorpheniramine tannate (p.405·2); phenylephrine tannate (p.1067·1).

Ricobid D *Rico, USA.*
Phenylephrine tannate (p.1067·1).

Ricobid H *Rico, USA.*
Chlorpheniramine tannate (p.405·2).

Ricolind *3M, Ger.†.*
Diphenylpyraline (p.410·1); panthenol (p.1571·1).
Burns; skin disorders.

Ricoliver *Mendelejeff, Ital.†.*
Inosine (p.1591·1); cyanocobalamin (p.1363·3).
Anaemia; liver impairment.

Ricortex *Proter, Ital.†.*
Inosine (p.1591·1); cyanocobalamin (p.1363·3); suprarenal cortex (p.1050·1).
Hepatic insufficiency; megaloblastic anaemia; tonic.

Ricridene *Lipha Sante, Fr.*
Nifurzide (p.231·3).
Diarrhoea.

Ricura *Pekana, Ger.*
Homoeopathic preparation.

RID *Leeming, USA; Pfizer, USA.*
Pyrethrins; piperonyl butoxide (p.1409·3).
Pediculosis.

Rid-a-Pain *Pfeiffer, USA†.*
Benzocaine (p.1286·2); menthol (p.1600·2); cineole (p.1564·1).
Oral lesions.

Rid-a-Pain with Codeine *Pfeiffer, USA.*
Codeine phosphate (p.26·1); paracetamol (p.72·2); caffeine (p.749·3); aspirin (p.16·1); salicylamide (p.82·3).
Pain.

Ridaura
SmithKline Beecham, Aust.; SmithKline Beecham, Austral.; SK-RIT, Belg.; SmithKline Beecham, Canad.; Yamanouchi, Ger.; SmithKline Beecham, Irl.; SmithKline Beecham, Ital.; Yamanouchi, Neth.; SmithKline Beecham, Norw.; SmithKline Beecham, S.Afr.; Recordati Elmu, Spain; SmithKline Beecham, Swed.; SmithKline Beecham, Switz.; Yamanouchi, UK; SmithKline Beecham, USA.
Auranofin (p.19·3).
Juvenile chronic arthritis; psoriatic arthritis; rheumatoid arthritis.

Ridauran *Robapharm, Fr.*
Auranofin (p.19·3).
Rheumatoid arthritis.

Ridazine *Rolab, S.Afr.*
Thioridazine hydrochloride (p.695·1).
Alcohol withdrawal syndrome; depression; psychoses.

Ridenol *R.I.D., USA.*
Paracetamol (p.72·2).

Rideril *DDSA Pharmaceuticals, UK.*
Thioridazine (p.695·1).

Ridutox *SoSe, Ital.*
Glutathione (p.983·1).
Alcohol and drug poisoning; radiation sickness.

Riesal *Distriborg, Fr.†.*
A range of gluten-free foods.

Rifa *Grunenthal, Ger.*
Rifampicin (p.243·2) or rifampicin sodium (p.245·3).
Tuberculosis.

Rifacol *Formenti, Ital.*
Rifaximin (p.246·3).
Adjuvant in hyperammonaemia; gastro-intestinal infections.

Rifadin
Hoechst Marion Roussel, Austral.; Hoechst Marion Roussel, Canad.; Hoechst Marion Roussel, Irl.; Lepetit, Ital.; Hoechst Marion Roussel, Neth.; Pharmacia Upjohn, Norw.; Hoechst Marion Roussel, S.Afr.; Hoechst Marion Roussel, Swed.; Hoechst Marion Roussel, UK; Hoechst Marion Roussel, USA.
Rifampicin (p.243·2) or rifampicin sodium (p.245·3).
Leprosy; prophylaxis of Haemophilus influenzae type B infection; prophylaxis of meningococcal infection; tuberculosis.

Rifadine
Hoechst Marion Roussel, Belg.; Marion Merrell, Fr.
Rifampicin (p.243·2) or rifampicin sodium (p.245·3).
Brucellosis; meningococcal meningitis; tuberculosis and other mycobacterial infections.

Rifagen *Llorente, Spain.*
Rifampicin (p.243·2).
Meningitis; mycobacterial infections; tuberculosis.

Rifa/INH *Grunenthal, Ger.†.*
Combination pack: Tablets, rifampicin (p.243·2); tablets, isoniazid (p.218·1).
Tuberculosis.

Rifaldin *Marion Merrell, Spain.*
Rifampicin (p.243·2) or rifampicin sodium (p.245·3).
Meningitis; mycobacterial infections; tuberculosis.

Rifamate *Hoechst Marion Roussel, USA.*
Rifampicin (p.243·2); isoniazid (p.218·1).
Pulmonary tuberculosis.

Rifanicozid *Piam, Ital.*
Rifampicin (p.243·2); isoniazid (p.218·1).
Tuberculosis.

Rifapiam *Piam, Ital.*
Rifampicin (p.243·2).
Bacterial infections including tuberculosis.

Rifater
Albert-Roussel, Aust.; Hoechst Marion Roussel, Canad.; Marion Merrell, Fr.; Grunenthal, Ger.; Hoechst Marion Roussel, Irl.; Lepetit, Ital.; Hoechst Marion Roussel, S.Afr.; Merrell Dow, Spain; Hoechst Marion Roussel, Switz.; Hoechst Marion Roussel, UK; Hoechst Marion Roussel, USA.
Rifampicin (p.243·2); isoniazid (p.218·1); pyrazinamide (p.241·1).
Tuberculosis.

Rifazida *Pharmacia Upjohn, Spain†.*
Isoniazid (p.218·1); rifampicin (p.243·2).
Tuberculosis.

Rifcin *Rolab, S.Afr.*
Rifampicin (p.243·2).
Tuberculosis.

Rifedot *Alacan, Spain.*
Astemizole (p.402·1).
Hypersensitivity reactions.

Rifinah
Marion Merrell, Fr.; Grunenthal, Ger.; Hoechst Marion Roussel, Irl.; Lepetit, Ital.; Hoechst Marion Roussel, Neth.; Hoechst Marion Roussel, S.Afr.; Merrell Dow, Spain; Hoechst Marion Roussel, Switz.; Hoechst Marion Roussel, UK.
Rifampicin (p.243·2); isoniazid (p.218·1).
Tuberculosis.

Rifloc *Marion Merrell Dow, Ger.†.*
Isosorbide dinitrate (p.893·1).
Cardiac disorders.

Rifocin
Albert-Roussel, Aust.; Lepetit, Ital.
Rifamycin sodium (p.246·2).
Gram-positive bacterial infections; tuberculosis.

Rifocina *Merrell Dow, Spain.*
Rifampicin sodium (p.245·3).
Asymptomatic carriers of Neisseria meningitidis; bacterial infections; tuberculosis.

Rifocine
Hoechst Marion Roussel, Belg.; Marion Merrell, Fr.; Marion Merrell Dow, Switz.†.
Rifamycin (p.246·3) or rifamycin sodium (p.246·2).
Lignocaine hydrochloride (p.1293·2) is included in the intramuscular injection to alleviate the pain of injection.
Bacterial infections.

Rifoldin *Albert-Roussel, Aust.*
Rifampicin (p.243·2).
Asymptomatic Haemophilus influenzae carriers; asymptomatic meningococcal carriers; brucellosis; leprosy; staphylococcal infections; tuberculosis.

Rifoldin INH *Albert-Roussel, Aust.*
Rifampicin (p.243·2); isoniazid (p.218·1).
Tuberculosis.

Rifoldine *Hoechst Marion Roussel, Switz.*
Tablets; syrup: Rifampicin (p.243·2).
Injection†: Rifampicin sodium (p.245·3).
Bacterial infections including tuberculosis and leprosy.

Rifoldine-INH *Marion Merrell Dow, Switz.†.*
Rifampicin (p.243·2); isoniazid (p.218·1).
Tuberculosis.

Rifun *Schwarz, Ger.; Isis, Ger.*
Pantoprazole sodium (p.1207·3).
Gastro-oesophageal reflux; peptic ulcer.

Rigoletten *Tendem, Neth.*
Aluminium hydroxide-magnesium carbonate co-dried gel (p.1178·2); magnesium hydroxide (p.1198·2).
Gastro-intestinal disorders associated with hyperacidity.

Rigoran *Vita, Spain.*
Ciprofloxacin hydrochloride (p.185·3) or ciprofloxacin lactate (p.185·3).
Bacterial infections.

Riker Antibiotic-Spray *Salus, Aust.*
Bacitracin zinc (p.157·3); neomycin sulphate (p.229·2); polymyxin B sulphate (p.239·1).
Bacterial infections.

Riker Silicone-Spray *Salus, Aust.*
Aluminium hydroxide (p.1177·3); allantoin (p.1078·2); silicone (p.1384·2); cetylpyridinium chloride (p.1106·2).
Colostomy hygiene; decubitus ulcers; nappy rash.

Riker Sport *3M, Ger.†.*
Glycol salicylate (p.43·1); benzyl nicotinate (p.22·1).
Musculoskeletal and joint disorders.

Rikerspray *Riker, S.Afr.†.*
Aldioxa (p.1078·2); cetylpyridinium chloride (p.1106·2); terpineol (p.1635·1); dimethicone (p.1384·2).
Skin disorders.

Rikodeine *3M, Austral.*
Dihydrocodeine tartrate (p.34·1).
Coughs.

Rikoderm *3M, Austral.*
Light liquid paraffin (p.1382·1); dewaxed wool fat (p.1385·3).
Dry skin disorders.

Rikosilver *3M, Ital.†.*
Silver protein (p.1629·3); chlorhexidine acetate (p.1107·2).
Wound disinfection.

Rikosol *3M, Belg.†.*
Neomycin sulphate (p.229·2); bacitracin zinc (p.157·3); polymyxin B sulphate (p.239·1).
Prophylaxis of bacterial infections in surgery.

Rikosol Silicone *3M, Belg.†.*
Aldioxa (p.1078·2); dimethicone (p.1384·2).
Barrier preparation; colostomy hygiene; decubitus ulcer.

Rikospray *3M, Ital.*
Aldioxa (p.1078·2); cetylpyridinium chloride (p.1106·2); terpineol (p.1635·1); dimethicone (p.1384·2).
Barrier preparation; skin disinfection.

Rilance *Schwarz, Ital.†.*
Vitamin B substances.

Rilaprost *Guidotti, Ital.*
Saw palmetto (p.1462·1).
Prostatic hyperplasia.

Rilaten *Guidotti, Ital.*
Rociverine (p.1626·1).
Smooth muscle spasm.

Rilatine *Ciba-Geigy, Belg.*
Methylphenidate hydrochloride (p.1483·1).
Attention deficit hyperactivity disorder; narcoleptic syndrome.

Rilex *Lindopharm, Ger.*
Tetrazepam (p.694·3).
Skeletal muscle spasticity; skeletal muscle tension.

Rilfit *Apomedica, Aust.†.*
Aspirin (p.16·1); paracetamol (p.72·2); salicylamide (p.82·3); caffeine (p.749·3).
Fever; pain.

Rilutek
Rhone-Poulenc Rorer, Aust.; Specia, Fr.; Rhone-Poulenc Rorer, Ger.; Rhone-Poulenc Rorer, Irl.; Rhone-Poulenc Rorer, Ital.; Rhone-Poulenc Rorer, Neth.; Rhone-Poulenc Rorer, Swed.; Rhone-Poulenc Rorer, UK.
Riluzole (p.1625·1).
Amyotrophic lateral sclerosis.

Rim *Bracco, Ital.†.*
Phenolphthalein (p.1208·2); sodium citrate (p.1153·2).
Constipation.

Rimacid *Rima, UK.*
Indomethacin (p.45·2).

Rimacillin *Rima, UK.*
Ampicillin (p.153·1).
Bacterial infections.

Rimactan
Ciba-Geigy, Aust.; Ciba-Geigy, Belg.; Ciba-Geigy, Fr.; Ciba, Ger.; Ciba, Ital.†; Novartis, Neth.; Ciba, Norw.; Ciba-Geigy, Spain; Swedish Orphan, Swed.; Ciba, Switz.
Rifampicin (p.243·2) or rifampicin sodium (p.245·3).
Bacterial infections including tuberculosis; brucellosis.

Rimactan + INH *Ciba-Geigy, Aust.*
Rifampicin (p.243·2); isoniazid (p.218·1).
Tuberculosis.

Rimactane
Ciba, Canad.; Ciba-Geigy, Irl.; Novartis, S.Afr.; Ciba, UK; Ciba, USA.
Rifampicin (p.243·2) or rifampicin sodium (p.245·3).
Meningococcal meningitis; mycobacterial infections; staphylococcal infections.

Rimactane/INH Dual Pack *Ciba, USA†.*
Combination pack: 60 capsules, Rimactane (p.243·2); 30 tablets, isoniazid (p.218·1).
Tuberculosis.

Rimactazid
Ciba-Geigy, Irl.; Ciba-Geigy, Spain; Ciba, UK.
Rifampicin (p.243·2); isoniazid (p.218·1).
Tuberculosis.

Rimactazide *Ciba, Switz.*
Rifampicin (p.243·2); isoniazid (p.218·1).
Tuberculosis.

Rimactazide + Z *Ciba, Switz.*
Blisters containing tablets, rifampicin (p.243·2); isoniazid (p.218·1); tablets, pyrazinamide (p.241·1).
Tuberculosis.

Rimafen *Rima, UK.*
Ibuprofen (p.44·1).

Rimafungol *Belmac, Spain.*
Ciclopirox olamine (p.376·2).
Fungal infections.

Rimapam *Rima, UK.*
Diazepam (p.661·1).

Rimapen *Rima, UK.*
Phenoxymethylpenicillin potassium (p.236·2).

Rimapurinol *Rima, UK.*
Allopurinol (p.390·2).

Rimargen *SIT, Ital.†.*
Chlorhexidine gluconate (p.1107·2).
Wound disinfection.

Rimarin *Rima, UK.*
Chlorpheniramine (p.405·2).

Rimasal *Rima, UK.*
Salbutamol (p.758·2).

Rimatil *Santen, Jpn†.*
Bucillamine (p.1555·2).
Rheumatoid arthritis.

Rimbol *Esteve, Spain.*
Astemizole (p.402·1).
Hypersensitivity reactions.

Rimevax
SmithKline Beecham, Aust.; SmithKline Beecham, Austral.†; SK-RIT, Belg.; SmithKline Beecham, Ital.; SmithKline Beecham, S.Afr.; Smith Kline & French, Spain; SmithKline Beecham, Switz.
A measles vaccine (Schwarz strain) (p.1517·3).
Active immunisation.

Rimidol *UCB, Swed.*
Naphazoline hydrochloride (p.1064·2).
Conjunctivitis.

Rimifon
Roche, Belg.†; Roche, Fr.; Roche, Spain; Roche, Switz.; Cambridge, UK.
Isoniazid (p.218·1).
Tuberculosis and other mycobacterial infections.

Rimoxallin *Rima, UK.*
Amoxycillin trihydrate (p.151·3).
Bacterial infections.

Rimoxyn *Rima, UK.*
Naproxen (p.61·2).

Rimparix
SmithKline Beecham, Ger.†; SmithKline Beecham, Switz.†.
A measles and mumps vaccine (Schwarz and Urabe Am 9 strains respectively) (p.1519·2).
Active immunisation.

Rimso
Roberts, Canad.; Britannia Pharmaceuticals, UK; Research Industries Corp., USA.
Dimethyl sulphoxide (p.1377·2).
Interstitial cystitis.

Rimycin *Alphapharm, Austral.*
Rifampicin (p.243·2).
Leprosy; prophylaxis of Haemophilus influenzae type B infection; prophylaxis of meningococcal infection; tuberculosis.

Rin Up *Astra, Spain†.*
Phenylephrine hydrochloride (p.1066·2).
Upper respiratory-tract congestion.

Rinactive *Farmacusi, Spain.*
Budesonide (p.1034·3).
Nasal polyps; rhinitis.

Rinade BID *Econo Med, USA.*
Pseudoephedrine hydrochloride (p.1068·3); chlorpheniramine maleate (p.405·1).
Upper respiratory-tract symptoms.

Rinafort *Schering-Plough, Belg.*
Dexbrompheniramine maleate (p.403·2); pseudoephedrine sulphate (p.1068·3).
Mucous membrane congestion; otorhinolaryngological disorders; respiratory-tract disorders.

Rinantipiol *Antipiol, Ital.*
Silver protein (p.1629·3); resorcinol (p.1090·1); niaouli oil (p.1607·1); adrenaline hydrochloride (p.813·3); procaine hydrochloride (p.1299·2).
Respiratory-tract disorders.

Rinatec
Boehringer Ingelheim, Irl.; Boehringer Ingelheim, UK.
Ipratropium bromide (p.754·2).
Rhinitis.

Rinaze *Boehringer Ingelheim, S.Afr.*
Beclomethasone dipropionate (p.1032·1).
Allergic rhinitis.

Rinazina *Maggioni, Ital.*
Naphazoline nitrate (p.1064·2).
Nasal congestion.

Rince Bouche Antiseptique *Atlas, Canad.*
Cetylpyridinium chloride (p.1106·2).

Rinedrone *Deca, Ital.*
Dexamethasone (p.1037·1); thonzonium bromide (p.1636·3).
Rhinitis; rhinosinusitis.

Rinex *Triomed, S.Afr.*
Chlorpheniramine maleate (p.405·1); phenylpropanolamine hydrochloride (p.1067·2); phenylephrine hydrochloride (p.1066·2).
Allergic rhinitis; cold and influenza symptoms.

Rinexin
Pharmacia Upjohn, Norw.; Recip, Swed.
Phenylpropanolamine hydrochloride (p.1067·2).
Rhinitis; sinusitis; urinary incontinence.

Ring N *Mack, Illert., Ger.*
Aspirin (p.16·1); caffeine (p.749·3); ascorbic acid.
Cold symptoms; fever; pain.

Ringworm Ointment *Douglas, Austral.*
Tolnaftate (p.389·1).
Fungal skin infections.

Rinil *Recip, Swed.*
Sodium cromoglycate (p.762·1).
Allergic conjunctivitis; allergic rhinitis.

Rino Calyptol *Rhone-Poulenc Rorer, Ital.*
Oxymetazoline hydrochloride (p.1065·3).
Nasal congestion.

Rino Clenil
Chiesi, Ital.; Chiesi, Neth.†.
Beclomethasone dipropionate (p.1032·1).
Rhinitis.

Rino Dexa *Cusi, Spain.*
Chlorpheniramine maleate (p.405·1); dexamethasone sodium phosphate (p.1037·2); muramidase hydrochloride (p.1604·3); neomycin sulphate (p.229·2).
Formerly known as Rinocusi Dexa.
Rhinitis; rhinopharyngeal infection; sinusitis.

Rino Ebastel *Almirall, Spain.*
Pseudoephedrine hydrochloride (p.1068·3); ebastine (p.410·2).
Allergic rhinitis.

Rino Naftazolina *Bruschettini, Ital.*
Naphazoline hydrochloride (p.1064·2).
Nasal congestion.

Rino Pumilene *Montefarmaco, Ital.†.*
Ephedrine hydrochloride (p.1059·3).
Nasal congestion; rhinitis.

Rino Vitna *Quimifar, Spain†.*
Dexamethasone (p.1037·1); diphenhydramine hydrochloride (p.409·1); hydrocortisone acetate (p.1043·3); neomycin sulphate (p.229·2).
Rhinitis and nasal infection.

Rinobalsamiche *Farmatre, Ital.; Iema, Ital.; Morigi, Ital.; Nova Argentia, Ital.; Ramini, Ital.; Sella, Ital.; Eugal, Ital.*
Menthol (p.1600·2); niaouli oil (p.1607·1).
Nasal congestion.

Rinobanedif *Roche Nicholas, Spain.*
Antazoline (p.402·1); bacitracin zinc (p.157·3); phenylephrine hydrochloride (p.1066·2); neomycin sulphate (p.229·2); prednisolone (p.1048·1); cineole (p.1564·1); niaouli oil (p.1607·1).
Upper respiratory tract disorders.

Rinoberen *Berenguer Infale, Spain†.*
Ipratropium bromide (p.754·2).
Rhinorrhoea.

Rinobios *Pharkos, Ital.†.*
Tetrahydrozoline hydrochloride (p.1070·2).
Cold symptoms; nasal congestion; rhinitis.

Rinoblanco Dexa Antibio *Alcon, Spain.*
Dexamethasone sodium phosphate (p.1037·2); neomycin sulphate (p.229·2); xylometazoline hydrochloride (p.1071·2).
Rhinitis and nasal infection.

Rinocidina *Valeas, Ital.*
Tyrothricin (p.267·2); naphazoline nitrate (p.1064·2).
Rhinitis; sinusitis.

Rinocorin *Cusi, Spain.*
Oxymetazoline hydrochloride (p.1065·3).
Nasal congestion; sinusitis.

Rinocusi Descong *Cusi, Spain†.*
Diphenhydramine hydrochloride (p.409·1); phenylephrine hydrochloride (p.1066·2); hydrocortisone acetate (p.1043·3); neomycin sulphate (p.229·2).
Rhinitis and nasal infection.

Rinocusi Vitaminico *Cusi, Spain.*
Vitamin A (p.1358·1).
Formerly contained choline hydrochloride, vitamin A and vitamin E.
Nasal congestion.

Rinodif *Roche Nicholas, Spain.*
Oxymetazoline hydrochloride (p.1065·3).
Nasal congestion; sinusitis.

Rinofan *Akromed, S.Afr.†.*
Carbocisteine (p.1056·3).
Respiratory-tract disorders.

Rinofil *Vis, Ital.†.*
Menthol (p.1600·2); niaouli oil (p.1607·1).
Inflammation of the upper-respiratory tract.

Rinofluimucil
Zambon, Ital.; Zambon, Spain; Inpharzam, Switz.
Acetylcysteine (p.1052·3); tuaminoheptane sulphate (p.1071·1).
Formerly contained acetylcysteine, tuaminoheptane sulphate, and betamethasone in *Ital.*
Rhinitis; sinusitis.

Rinofluimucil-S *Zambon, Ger.*
Acetylcysteine (p.1052·3); tuaminoheptane sulphate (p.1071·1).
Rhinitis; sinusitis.

Rinofol *Hosbon, Spain†.*
Oxymetazoline hydrochloride (p.1065·3).
Nasal congestion.

Rinofrenal
Note. This name is used for preparations of different composition.
Searle, Ital.
Sodium cromoglycate (p.762·1); chlorpheniramine maleate (p.405·1).
Rhinitis.

Sigma-Tau, Spain.
Sodium cromoglycate (p.762·1).
Rhinitis.

Rinofrenal Plus *Sigma-Tau, Spain.*
Chlorpheniramine maleate (p.405·1); sodium cromoglycate (p.762·1).
Hay fever; rhinitis.

Rinoftal *Wassermann, Ital.†.*
Naphazoline nitrate (p.1064·2).
Nasal and conjunctival congestion.

Rinogutt Antiallergico Spray *Boehringer Ingelheim, Ital.*
Tramazoline hydrochloride (p.1071·1); chlorpheniramine maleate (p.405·1).
Allergic rhinitis.

Rinogutt Eucalipto-Fher *Boehringer Ingelheim, Ital.*
Tramazoline hydrochloride (p.1071·1); cineole (p.1564·1); menthol (p.1600·2); camphor (p.1557·2).
Nasal congestion.

Rinogutt Spray-Fher *Boehringer Ingelheim, Ital.*
Tramazoline hydrochloride (p.1071·1).
Nasal congestion.

Rinojet *Valeas, Ital.*
Betamethasone (p.1033·2); phenylephrine hydrochloride (p.1066·2).
Formerly contained betamethasone, neomycin sulphate, polymyxin B sulphate, and phenylephrine hydrochloride.
Rhinitis; rhinopharyngitis; sinusitis.

Rinojet SF *Valeas, Ital.*
Neomycin sulphate (p.229·2); polymyxin B sulphate (p.239·1).
Rinojet SF senza Fenilefrina formerly contained betamethasone, neomycin sulphate, and polymyxin B sulphate.
Infections of the upper-respiratory tract.

Rinoleina Adulti *Granelli, Ital.†.*
Ephedrine camphocarbonate; amylocaine hydrochloride (p.1286·1); thymol (p.1127·1); sozoiodol zinc (p.1125·3).
Cold symptoms.

Rinoleina Bambini *Granelli, Ital.†.*
Thymol (p.1127·1); sozoiodol zinc (p.1125·3).
Cold symptoms.

Rinomar
Note. This name is used for preparations of different composition.
Janssen-Cilag, Belg.
Cinnarizine (p.406·1); phenylpropanolamine hydrochloride (p.1067·2); isopropamide iodide (p.464·3).
Rhinitis.

Pharmacia Upjohn, Norw.; Recip, Swed.
Cinnarizine (p.406·1); phenylpropanolamine hydrochloride (p.1067·2).
Nasal congestion; vasomotor rhinitis.

Rinomicine Fardi, Spain.
Oral sachets: Ascorbic acid (p.1365·2); caffeine (p.749·3); chlorpheniramine maleate (p.405·1); phenylephrine hydrochloride (p.1066·2); paracetamol (p.72·2); salicylamide (p.82·3).
Tablets: Caffeine (p.749·3); chlorpheniramine maleate (p.405·1); phenylephrine hydrochloride (p.1066·2); paracetamol (p.72·2); salicylamide (p.82·3).
Influenza and cold symptoms; nasal congestion.

Rinomicine Activada Fardi, Spain.
Caffeine (p.749·3); chlorpheniramine maleate (p.405·1); phenylephrine hydrochloride (p.1066·2); paracetamol (p.72·2); salicylamide (p.82·3).
Influenza and cold symptoms; nasal congestion.

Rinopaidolo Deca, Ital.
Niaouli oil (p.1607·1); eucalyptus oil (p.1578·1).
Nasal congestion.

Rinopanteina DMG, Ital.
Dexpanthenol (p.1570·3); vitamin A (p.1358·1).
Nasal hygiene.

Rinoretard Pfizer, Spain.
Carbinoxamine (p.404·2); phenylpropanolamine (p.1067·2).
Nasal congestion.

Rinos Molteni, Ital.
Xylometazoline hydrochloride (p.1071·2); thymol (p.1127·1); cineole (p.1564·1).
Nasal congestion.

Rinosedin Streuli, Switz.
Xylometazoline hydrochloride (p.1071·2).
Adjunct in rhinoscopy; cold symptoms; otitis; sinus disorders.

Rinosil Zeta, Ital.
Cetylpyridinium chloride (p.1106·2); chlorbutol; menthol; cineole; camphor.
Nasal disinfection.

Rinospray Recordati, Ital.
Dequalinium chloride (p.1112·1); naphazoline hydrochloride (p.1064·2).
Disinfection and decongestion of the upper-respiratory tract.

Rinostil Deca, Ital.
Eucalyptus oil (p.1578·1); camphor (p.1557·2); thymol (p.1127·1); menthol (p.1600·2).
Rhinopharyngeal congestion.

Rinosular Morrith, Spain†.
Diphenhydramine (p.409·1); naphazoline hydrochloride (p.1064·2); prednisolone phosphate (p.1049·1); sulphanilamide sodium mesylate (p.256·3).
Rhinitis and nasal infection.

Rinotiazol Fenilefri Andreu, Spain†.
Atropine sulphate (p.455·1); cineole (p.1564·1); phenylephrine hydrochloride (p.1066·2); niaouli oil (p.1607·1); sulphathiazole (p.257·1); cholesterol (p.1383·3).
Nasal congestion and infection.

Rinotricina SIT, Ital.
Tyrothricin (p.267·2).
Rhinitis; sinusitis.

Rinovagos Valeas, Ital.
Ipratropium bromide (p.754·2).
Rhinitis.

Rinovel Ern, Spain.
Naphazoline nitrate (p.1064·2); neomycin sulphate (p.229·2); prednisolone (p.1048·1).
Congestion and infection of the nose and ear.

Rinovit SIT, Ital.
Ephedrine (p.1059·3); cineole (p.1564·1); niaouli oil (p.1607·1).
Nasal congestion.

Rinovit Nube SIT, Ital.
Silver protein (p.1629·3); naphazoline nitrate (p.1064·2); niaouli oil (p.1607·1).
Congestion of the upper-respiratory tract.

Rinsoderm Nycomed, Norw.
Pyrethrum extract (p.1410·1); piperonyl butoxide (p.1409·3).
Pediculosis.

Rinstead Schering-Plough, UK.
Contact pastille: Lignocaine hydrochloride (p.1293·2).
Mouth irritation; mouth ulcers.
Pastilles: Menthol (p.1600·2); chloroxylenol (p.1111·1).
Mouth ulcers.
Topical gel: Benzocaine (p.1286·2); chloroxylenol (p.1111·1).
Mouth ulcers; teething pain.

Rinstead Teething Gel Schering-Plough, UK.
Lignocaine (p.1293·2); cetylpyridinium chloride (p.1106·2).

Rinurel Warner-Lambert, Fr.
Phenylpropanolamine hydrochloride (p.1067·2); phenyltoloxamine citrate (p.416·1); paracetamol (p.72·2).
Disorders of the ear, nose, and throat.

Rinutan Warner-Lambert, Fr.
Paracetamol (p.72·2); phenylpropanolamine hydrochloride (p.1067·2); phenyltoloxamine citrate (p.416·1).
Disorders of the ear, nose, and throat.

Rio-Josipyrin N CPF, Ger.
Aspirin (p.16·1); paracetamol (p.72·2); caffeine (p.749·3).
Headache; influenza; neuralgia.

Riopan
Byk, Aust.; Byk, Belg.; Whitehall-Robins, Canad.; Byk Gulden, Ger.; Roland, Ger.; Byk Gulden, Ital.; Byk, Neth.; Byk, Switz.; Whitehall, USA.
Magaldrate (p.1198·1).
Gastritis; gastro-oesophageal reflux; hyperacidity; peptic ulcer.

Riopan Plus
Whitehall-Robins, Canad.; Whitehall, USA.
Magaldrate (p.1198·1); simethicone (p.1213·1).
Gastro-intestinal disorders.

Riopone Akromed, S.Afr.
Magaldrate (p.1198·1).
Gastro-intestinal hyperacidity.

Riosol F Funk, Spain†.
Cresol (p.1111·2); phenol (p.1121·2); mercuric stearate (p.1602·2); salicylic acid (p.1090·2).
Skin disorders.

Riostatin Adcock Ingram, S.Afr.
Tetracycline hydrochloride (p.259·1); nystatin (p.386·1); vitamin B substances; ascorbic acid.
Bacterial infections.

Riotapen Fermentaciones y Sintesis, Spain.
Amoxycillin sodium (p.151·3) or amoxycillin trihydrate (p.151·3).
Bacterial infections.

Ripason Robapharm, Ger.†.
Liver extract.
Liver disorders.

Ripix
Ciba Vision, Ital.; Ciba Vision, Switz.
Pilocarpine hydrochloride (p.1396·3); metipranolol (p.906·2).
Glaucoma; ocular hypertension.

Risatarun Ravensberg, Ger.
Deanol aceglumate (p.1478·2).
Nervous system disorders.

Riscalon Boehringer Mannheim, Spain.
Fentiazac (p.41·1).
Musculoskeletal, joint, peri-articular, and soft-tissue disorders.

Rischiaril Piam, Ital.
Deanol hemisuccinate (p.1478·2).
Mental function impairment.

Risicordin Heumann, Ger.
Spironolactone (p.946·1); hydrochlorothiazide (p.885·2).
Ascites; hyperaldosteronism; hypertension; liver cirrhosis; oedema.

Risocon ankerpharm, Ger.†.
Ephedrine (p.1059·3); thymol (p.1127·1); camphor (p.1557·2).
Rhinitis.

Risoltuss Magis, Ital.
Cloperastine fendizoate (p.1057·2).
Coughs.

Risordan Specia, Fr.
Isosorbide dinitrate (p.893·1).
Angina pectoris; heart failure; pulmonary oedema.

Risperdal
Janssen-Cilag, Aust.; Janssen-Cilag, Austral.; Janssen-Cilag, Belg.; Janssen-Ortho, Canad.; Janssen-Cilag, Fr.; Janssen-Cilag, Ger.; Organon, Ger.; Janssen-Cilag, Irl.; Janssen-Cilag, Ital.; Janssen-Cilag, Neth.; Janssen-Cilag, Norw.; Janssen-Cilag, S.Afr.; Janssen-Cilag, Spain; Janssen-Cilag, Swed.; Organon, Swed.; Janssen-Cilag, Switz.; Janssen-Cilag, UK; Janssen, USA.
Risperidone (p.690·3).
Psychoses.

Rispolin Janssen-Cilag, Aust.
Risperidone (p.690·3).
Psychoses.

Rispran Smith Kline & French, Spain†.
Carbuterol hydrochloride (p.751·3).
Obstructive airways disease.

Ristalen Juventus, Spain.
Enalapril maleate (p.863·2).
Heart failure; hypertension.

Ristofact Behringwerke, Ger.†.
Factor VIII (p.720·3); fibrinogen (p.722·3).
Haemorrhagic disorders.

Risulpir Lisapharma, Ital.†.
Sulphadimethoxine (p.253·2).
Bacterial infections.

Risumic Dainippon, Jpn.
Amezinium methylsulphate (p.819·1).
Hypotension.

Risunal A Inibsa, Spain†.
Carbachol (p.1390·1); ergocalciferol (p.1367·1); neostigmine bromide (p.1393·3); thiamine (p.1361·2).
Musculoskeletal and joint disorders.

Risunal B Inibsa, Spain†.
Carbachol (p.1390·1); ergocalciferol (p.1367·1); oestrone (p.1458·2); neostigmine bromide (p.1393·3); progesterone (p.1459·3).
Musculoskeletal and joint disorders.

Ritalin
Novartis, Austral.; Ciba, Canad.; Geigy, Ger.; Ciba-Geigy, Irl.†; Novartis, Neth.; Ciba, Norw.; Novartis, S.Afr.; Novartis, UK; Ciba, USA.
Methylphenidate hydrochloride (p.1483·1).
Attention deficit disorders; narcoleptic syndrome.

Ritaline
Ciba-Geigy, Fr.; Ciba, Switz.
Methylphenidate hydrochloride (p.1483·1).
Attention deficit disorders; narcoleptic syndrome.

Ritarsulfa Benvegna, Ital.†.
Sulphadimethoxine (p.253·2).
Bacterial infections.

Riteban Centrum, Spain.
Minoxidil (p.910·3).
Alopecia androgenetica.

Rite-Diet
Nutricia, Fr.†; Nutricia, Irl.; Nutricia, UK.
A range of gluten-free and low-protein foods.
Gluten sensitivity; liver disorders; phenylketonuria; renal failure.

Rition Piam, Ital.
Glutathione sodium (p.983·1).
Alcohol and drug poisoning; radiation trauma.

Ritmocor Malesci, Ital.
Quinidine polygalacturonate (p.938·3).
Arrhythmias.

Ritmodan Hoechst Marion Roussel, Ital.
Disopyramide (p.858·1) or disopyramide phosphate (p.858·1).
Arrhythmias.

Ritmoforine Hoechst Marion Roussel, Neth.
Disopyramide phosphate (p.858·1).
Arrhythmias.

Ritmogel Terapeutico, Ital.
Royal jelly (p.1626·3).
Nutritional supplement.

Ritmos Inverni della Beffa, Ital.†.
Ajmaline (p.817·1).
Arrhythmias.

Ritmos Elle Inverni della Beffa, Ital.†.
Lorajmine hydrochloride (p.898·3).
Arrhythmias.

Ritmosedina Inverni della Beffa, Ital.†.
Ajmaline phenobarbitone (p.351·3).
Arrhythmias.

Ritmusin Gebro, Aust.†.
Aprindine hydrochloride (p.825·1).
Arrhythmias.

Ritro Fournier, Ital.
Flurithromycin ethyl succinate (p.210·1).
Bacterial infections.

Rituxan IDEC, USA.
Rituximab (p.560·3).
Non-Hodgkin's lymphoma.

Rivacide Rivadis, Fr.†.
Hydroxyquinoline sulphate (p.1589·3).
Skin disinfection.

Rivadescin Schaper & Brummer, Ger.†.
Rauwolfia serpentina (p.941·3).
Hypertension.

Rivagerme Rivadis, Fr.†.
A range of disinfectant preparations.

Rivanol Chinosolfabrik, Ger.
Ethacridine lactate (p.1098·3).
Antiseptic.

Rivasone Riva, Canad.
Betamethasone valerate (p.1033·3).
Skin disorders.

Rivela Beiersdorf, Ital.
Pregnancy test (p.1621·2).

Rivescal Tar Pergam, Ital.
Coal tar (p.1092·3); salicylic acid (p.1090·2).
Seborrhoeic dermatitis.

Rivescal ZPT Pergam, Ital.
Pyrithione zinc (p.1089·3).
Seborrhoeic dermatitis.

Rivistel Delagrange, Port.†.
Alpiropride (p.444·2).
Migraine.

Rivitin BC Lannacher, Aust.
Vitamin B substances and vitamin C.

Rivoclox Rivopharm, Switz.†.
Cloxacillin sodium (p.195·2).
Gram-positive bacterial infections.

Rivogel Rivopharm, Switz.†.
Aluminium hydroxide (p.1177·3); magnesium hydroxide (p.1198·2).
Gastric hyperacidity.

Rivogel + Dimethicone Rivopharm, Switz.†.
Aluminium hydroxide (p.1177·3); magnesium hydroxide (p.1198·2); dimethicone (p.1213·1).
Flatulence; gastric hyperacidity.

Rivolyn Rivopharm, Switz.†.
Diphenhydramine hydrochloride (p.409·1); dextromethorphan hydrobromide (p.1057·3); sodium citrate (p.1153·2); menthol (p.1600·2).
Coughs.

Rivomag Rivopharm, Switz.†.
Magnesium hydroxide (p.1198·2).
Constipation; gastric hyperacidity.

Rivopen-V Rivopharm, Switz.
Phenoxymethylpenicillin potassium (p.236·2).
Bacterial infections.

Rivosil Benvegna, Ital.†.
Hydroflumethiazide (p.889·2).
Production of diuresis.

Rivostatin Rivopharm, Switz.
Nystatin (p.386·1).
Fungal infections.

Rivotril
Roche, Aust.; Roche, Austral.; Roche, Belg.; Roche, Canad.; Roche, Fr.; Roche, Ger.; Roche, Irl.; Roche, Ital.; Roche, Neth.; Roche, Norw.; Roche, S.Afr.; Syntex, Spain; Roche, Switz.; Roche, UK.
Clonazepam (p.343·3).
Epilepsy.

Rivovit Rivopharm, Switz.†.
Multivitamin preparation.

Rivoxicillin Rivopharm, Switz.
Amoxycillin (p.151·3).
Bacterial infections.

Rivozol Rivopharm, Switz.
Metronidazole (p.585·1) or metronidazole benzoate (p.585·1).
Anaerobic bacterial infections; protozoal infections.

Riwa Franzbranntwein Gerlach, Ger.
Camphor (p.1557·2); alcohol (p.1099·1).
Musculoskeletal, joint, and soft-tissue disorders; poor circulation.

α-Rix SK-RIT, Belg.
An influenza vaccine (p.1515·2).
Active immunisation.

Rixapen Menarini, Belg.
Clometocillin potassium (p.195·1).
Bacterial infections; prevention of flares of rheumatoid arthritis.

Rizaben Kissei, Jpn.
Tranilast (p.774·1).
Allergic rhinitis; asthma; atopic dermatitis; keloids.

Rize Yoshitomi, Jpn.
Clotiazepam (p.657·2).
Anxiety states; autonomic disorders; premedication; sleep disorders.

Rizen Formenti, Ital.
Clotiazepam (p.657·2).
Anxiety disorders; sleep disorders.

RMS
Note. This name is used for preparations of different composition.
Reith & Petrasch, Ger.
Lactic acid (p.1593·3) or calcium lactate (p.1155·2).
Skin disorders.
Upsher-Smith, USA.
Morphine sulphate (p.56·2).
Pain.

RN13 Regeneresen Dyckerhoff, Ger.
Ribonucleic acid (p.1624·3).
Tonic.

Roaccutan
Roche, Aust.; Roche, Ger.; Roche, Ital.
Isotretinoin (p.1084·1).
Acne.

Roaccutane
Roche, Austral.; Roche, Belg.; Roche, Fr.; Roche, Irl.; Roche, Neth.; Roche, S.Afr.; Roche, Switz.; Roche, UK.
Isotretinoin (p.1084·1).
Acne.

Roacutan Andreu, Spain.
Isotretinoin (p.1084·1).
Acne.

Ro-A-Vit Cambridge, UK.
Vitamin A palmitate (p.1359·2).
Now known as Vitamin A Palmitate Ampoules.
Vitamin A deficiency.

Robadin Robapharm, Ger.†.
Extracts from stomach and duodenal mucous membranes.
Gastro-intestinal disorders.

Robafen AC Cough Major, USA.
Guaiphenesin (p.1061·3); codeine phosphate (p.26·1).
Coughs.

Robafen CF Major, USA.
Phenylpropanolamine hydrochloride (p.1067·2); dextromethorphan hydrobromide (p.1057·3); guaiphenesin (p.1061·3).
Coughs.

Robafen DAC Major, USA.
Pseudoephedrine hydrochloride (p.1068·3); codeine phosphate (p.26·1); guaiphenesin (p.1061·3).
Coughs.

Robafen DM Major, USA.
Dextromethorphan hydrobromide (p.1057·3); guaiphenesin (p.1061·3).
Coughs.

Robal No.2 Aqueous Chugai, Jpn†.
Sodium hexestrol diphosphate.
Menopausal disorders; menstrual disorders; prostatic hyperplasia.

Robalate Wyeth-Ayerst, Canad.†.
Aluminium glycinate (p.1177·2).
Gastro-intestinal disorders.

Robatar Rougier, Canad.
Tar (p.1092·3).
Skin disorders of the scalp.

RoBathol Pharmaceutical Specialties, USA.
Emollient.

Robaxacet Whitehall-Robins, Canad.
Methocarbamol (p.1316·1); paracetamol (p.72·2).
Musculoskeletal, peri-articular, and soft-tissue pain.

Robaxacet-8 Whitehall-Robins, Canad.
Methocarbamol (p.1316·1); paracetamol (p.72·2); codeine phosphate (p.26·1).
Musculoskeletal pain.

Robaxin
Whitehall, Austral.†; Whitehall-Robins, Canad.; Continental Ethicals, S.Afr.; Lasa, Spain; Wyeth Lederle, Swed.; Shire, UK; Robins, USA.
Methocarbamol (p.1316·1).
Musculoskeletal pain.

Robaxisal
Whitehall-Robins, Canad.; Shire, Irl.; Continental Ethicals, S.Afr.; Lasa, Spain; Robins, USA.
Methocarbamol (p.1316·1); aspirin (p.16·1).
Musculoskeletal pain.

Robaxisal Compuesto Laso, Spain.
Methocarbamol (p.1316·1); paracetamol (p.72·2).
Musculoskeletal pain.

Robaxisal Forte
Wyeth Lederle, Swed.; Shire, UK†.
Methocarbamol (p.1316·1); aspirin (p.16·1).
Musculoskeletal pain and spasm.

Robaxisal-C Whitehall-Robins, Canad.
Methocarbamol (p.1316·1); aspirin (p.16·1); codeine phosphate (p.26·1).
Musculoskeletal pain.

Roberfarin Robert, Spain.
Dequalinium chloride (p.1112·1); enoxolone (p.35·2); hydrocortisone acetate (p.1043·3); oxethazaine (p.1298·1); tyrothricin (p.267·2).
Mouth and throat inflammation.

Robervital Robert, Spain.
Oxaceprol (p.1611·3); tocopheryl sodium succinate.
Dermatomyositis; musculoskeletal and joint disorders.

Robicillin VK Robins, USA†.
Phenoxymethylpenicillin potassium (p.236·2).
Bacterial infections.

Robidex Whitehall-Robins, Canad.†.
Dextromethorphan hydrobromide (p.1057·3).
Coughs.

Robidone Wyeth-Ayerst, Canad.
Hydrocodone tartrate (p.43·1).
Coughs.

Robidrine Whitehall-Robins, Canad.
Pseudoephedrine hydrochloride (p.1068·3).
Nasal congestion.

Robigesic Whitehall-Robins, Canad.
Paracetamol (p.72·2).
Fever; pain.

Robimycin Robitabs Robins, USA.
Erythromycin (p.204·1).
Bacterial infections.

Robinia Med Complex Dynamit, Aust.
Homoeopathic preparation.

Robinia Ro-Plex (Rowo-99) Pharmakon, Ger.
Homoeopathic preparation.

Robinul
Salus, Aust.; Wyeth, Austral.; Wyeth Lederle, Belg.; Wyeth-Ayerst, Canad.; Brenner-Efeka, Ger.; Wyeth, Neth.; Wyeth, Norw.; Intramed, S.Afr.; Wyeth Lederle, Swed.; Wyeth, Switz.; Wyeth, UK; Robins, USA.
Glycopyrronium bromide (p.461·3).
Adjunct in peptic ulcer; hyperhidrosis; intra-operative management of cardiac vagal reflexes; premedication; protection against muscarinic effects of anticholinesterases used to reverse neuromuscular blockade.

Robinul-Neostigmin
Wyeth, Norw.; Wyeth Lederle, Swed.
Neostigmine methylsulphate (p.1394·1).
Glycopyrronium bromide (p.461·3) is included in this preparation to protect against the muscarinic actions.
Reversal of competitive neuromuscular blockade.

Robinul-Neostigmine
Wyeth Lederle, Belg.; Wyeth, Switz.; Wyeth, UK.
Neostigmine methylsulphate (p.1394·1).
Glycopyrronium bromide (p.461·3) is included in this preparation to protect against the muscarinic actions.
Reversal of competitive neuromuscular blockade.

Robitet Robicaps Robins, USA†.
Tetracycline hydrochloride (p.259·1).
Bacterial infections.

Robitussin
Whitehall, Austral.†; Whitehall-Robins, Canad.; Whitehall, Ital.†; Wyeth, Spain; Whitehall, Swed.†; Robins, USA.
Guaiphenesin (p.1061·3).
Coughs.

Robitussin AC
Note. This name is used for preparations of different composition.
Whitehall-Robins, Canad.
Guaiphenesin (p.1061·3); pheniramine maleate (p.415·3); codeine phosphate (p.26·1).
Coughs.

Robins, USA.
Guaiphenesin (p.1061·3); codeine phosphate (p.26·1).
Coughs.

Robitussin CF
Whitehall-Robins, Canad.†; Robins, USA.
Guaiphenesin (p.1061·3); phenylpropanolamine hydrochloride (p.1067·2); dextromethorphan hydrobromide (p.1057·3).
Coughs; nasal congestion.

Robitussin for Chesty Coughs Whitehall, UK.
Guaiphenesin (p.1061·3).
Coughs.

Robitussin for Chesty Coughs with Congestion Whitehall, UK.
Guaiphenesin (p.1061·3); pseudoephedrine hydrochloride (p.1068·3).
Formerly known as Robitussin Plus.
Coughs.

Robitussin with Codeine Whitehall-Robins, Canad.
Guaiphenesin (p.1061·3); pheniramine maleate (p.415·3); codeine phosphate (p.26·1).
Coughs.

Robitussin Cold & Cough Robins, USA.
Guaiphenesin (p.1061·3); pseudoephedrine hydrochloride (p.1068·3); dextromethorphan hydrobromide (p.1057·3).

Robitussin Cough Calmers Robins, USA.
Dextromethorphan hydrobromide (p.1057·3).
Coughs.

Robitussin Cough & Cold Whitehall-Robins, Canad.
Guaiphenesin (p.1061·3); dextromethorphan hydrobromide (p.1057·3); pseudoephedrine hydrochloride (p.1068·3).
Coughs and cold symptoms.

Robitussin Cough Cold & Flu Whitehall-Robins, Canad.
Guaiphenesin (p.1061·3); dextromethorphan hydrobromide (p.1057·3); pseudoephedrine hydrochloride (p.1068·3); paracetamol (p.72·2).
Cold and flu symptoms; coughs.

Robitussin Cough Drops Robins, USA.
Menthol (p.1600·2); eucalyptus oil (p.1578·1).

Robitussin Cough Soother Whitehall, Irl.
Dextromethorphan hydrobromide (p.1057·3).
Coughs.

Robitussin DAC Robins, USA.
Guaiphenesin (p.1061·3); pseudoephedrine hydrochloride (p.1068·3); codeine phosphate (p.26·1).
Coughs.

Robitussin DM
Whitehall, Austral.; Whitehall-Robins, Canad.; Robins, USA.
Guaiphenesin (p.1061·3); dextromethorphan hydrobromide (p.1057·3).
Coughs.

Robitussin DM Antitusivo Wyeth, Spain.
Dextromethorphan hydrobromide (p.1057·3).
Coughs.

Robitussin DM-P Whitehall, Austral.
Dextromethorphan hydrobromide (p.1057·3); pseudoephedrine hydrochloride (p.1068·3).
Coughs; nasal and sinus congestion.

Robitussin for Dry Coughs Whitehall, UK.
Dextromethorphan hydrobromide (p.1057·3).
Formerly known as Robitussin Cough Soother.
Coughs.

Robitussin EX Whitehall, Austral.
Guaiphenesin (p.1061·3).
Coughs.

Robitussin Expectorant
Note. This name is used for preparations of different composition.
Whitehall, Irl.
Guaiphenesin (p.1061·3).
Coughs.

Whitehall-Robins, Switz.
Acetylcysteine (p.1052·3).
Coughs with viscous mucus.

Robitussin Expectorant Plus Whitehall, Irl.
Guaiphenesin (p.1061·3); pseudoephedrine hydrochloride (p.1068·3).
Coughs; nasal congestion.

Robitussin Junior Whitehall, UK.
Dextromethorphan hydrobromide (p.1057·3).
Coughs.

Robitussin Maximum Strength Cough & Cold Robins, USA.
Dextromethorphan hydrobromide (p.1057·3); pseudoephedrine hydrochloride (p.1068·3).
Coughs and cold symptoms.

Robitussin Night Relief Robins, USA.
Pseudoephedrine hydrochloride (p.1068·3); dextromethorphan hydrobromide (p.1057·3); mepyramine maleate (p.414·1); paracetamol (p.72·2).
Coughs and cold symptoms.

Robitussin Night-Time Whitehall, UK.
Brompheniramine; codeine phosphate (p.26·1); pseudoephedrine (p.1068·3).
Coughs; nasal congestion.

Robitussin PE
Whitehall-Robins, Canad.†; Robins, USA.
Pseudoephedrine hydrochloride (p.1068·3); guaiphenesin (p.1061·3).
Coughs; nasal congestion.

Robitussin Pediatric
Whitehall-Robins, Canad.; Robins, USA.
Dextromethorphan hydrobromide (p.1057·3).
Coughs.

Robitussin Pediatric Cough & Cold
Whitehall-Robins, Canad.; Robins, USA.
Dextromethorphan hydrobromide (p.1057·3); pseudoephedrine hydrochloride (p.1068·3).
Coughs and cold symptoms.

Robitussin PS Whitehall, Austral.
Guaiphenesin (p.1061·3); pseudoephedrine hydrochloride (p.1068·3).
Coughs; nasal congestion.

Robitussin Severe Congestion Robins, USA.
Guaiphenesin (p.1061·3); pseudoephedrine hydrochloride (p.1068·3).

Robuden Ascot, Austral.†.
Protein-free stomach and intestine extracts.
Gastro-intestinal disorders.

Robugen-Kamillensalbe Schmidgall, Aust.†.
Chamomile (p.1561·2); hamamelis (p.1587·1).

Roburis Ripari-Gero, Ital.
Ubidecarenone (p.1641·2).
Cardiac disorders; coenzyme Q10 deficiency.

Roburvit Echo, Ital.
Royal jelly (p.1626·3).

Robusanon Robugen, Ger.†.
Paste: Hexachlorophane (p.1115·2); heparin sodium (p.879·3); ichthammol (p.1083·3); vitamin E.
Powder: Crystal violet (p.1111·2); digitalis (p.848·3); glycine (p.1345·2).
Abscesses; ulcers; wounds.

Robuvalen Robugen, Ger.
Zinc oxide (p.1096·2).
Eczema; skin lesions.

RoC Sunscreen Stick Roc, UK.
Dibenzoylmethane (p.1487·1); a cinnamic ester.
Sunscreen.

RoC Total Sunblock Roc, UK.
Ethylhexyl *p*-methoxycinnamate (p.1487·1); oxybenzone (p.1487·3); dibenzoylmethane (p.1487·1); titanium dioxide (p.1093·3).
Sunscreen.

Rocaltrol
Roche, Aust.; Roche, Austral.; Roche, Belg.; Roche, Canad.; Roche, Fr.; Roche, Ger.; Roche, Irl.; Roche, Ital.; Roche, Neth.; Roche, Norw.; Roche, S.Afr.; Syntex, Spain; Roche, Swed.; Roche, Switz.; Roche, UK; Roche, USA.
Calcitriol (p.1366·3).
Hypocalcaemia; hypoparathyroidism; osteomalacia; osteoporosis; renal osteodystrophy; rickets; secondary hyperparathyroidism; vitamin D deficiency.

Rocanal Imediat Medirel, Switz.
Povidone-iodine (p.1123·3).
Dental disinfection.

Rocanal Permanent Gangrene Medirel, Switz.
Powder, hydrocortisone acetate (p.1043·3); paraformaldehyde (p.1121·1); zinc oxide (p.1096·2); zinc stearate (p.1469·3); zinc acetate (p.1646·2); liquid, eugenol (p.1578·2).
Dental infections.

Rocanal Permanent Vital Medirel, Switz.
Powder, paraformaldehyde (p.1121·1); zinc oxide (p.1096·2); zinc stearate (p.1469·3); zinc acetate (p.1646·2); liquid, eugenol (p.1578·2).
Dental disorders.

Rocap Rolab, S.Afr.
Oxytetracycline hydrochloride (p.235·1).
Bacterial infections.

RO-Carpine Richmond Ophthalmics, Canad.†.
Pilocarpine hydrochloride (p.1396·3).
Cholinergic; production of miosis.

Roccal
Sanofi Winthrop, Irl.; Schein, UK.
Benzalkonium chloride (p.1101·3).
Skin disinfection.

Rocefalin Roche, Spain.
Ceftriaxone sodium (p.176·1).
Lignocaine (p.1293·2) is included in the intramuscular injection to alleviate the pain of injection.
Bacterial infections.

Rocefin Roche, Ital.
Ceftriaxone sodium (p.176·1).
Lignocaine hydrochloride (p.1293·2) is included in the intramuscular injection to alleviate the pain of injection.
Bacterial infections.

Rocephalin
Roche, Norw.; Roche, Swed.
Ceftriaxone sodium (p.176·1).
Lignocaine hydrochloride (p.1293·2) is included in some injections to alleviate the pain of injection.
Bacterial infections.

Rocephin
Biochemie, Aust.; Roche, Aust.; Roche, Austral.; Roche, Canad.; Roche, Ger.; Roche, Irl.; Roche, Neth.; Roche, S.Afr.; Roche, UK; Roche, USA.
Ceftriaxone sodium (p.176·1).
Lignocaine hydrochloride (p.1293·2) may be included in the intramuscular injection to alleviate the pain of injection.
Bacterial infections.

Rocephine
Roche, Belg.; Roche, Fr.; Roche, Switz.
Ceftriaxone sodium (p.176·1).
Lignocaine hydrochloride (p.1293·2) may be included in the intramuscular injection to alleviate the pain of injection.
Bacterial infections.

Roceron Roche, Norw.
Interferon alfa-2a (p.615·3).
Chronic active hepatitis B; chronic hepatitis C; malignant neoplasms.

Rocgel Roques, Fr.
Boehmite.
Gastro-intestinal disorders.

Rochagan Roche, Braz.
Benznidazole (p.580·2).
Protozoal infections.

Roche Syntex, Canad.
Naproxen sodium (p.61·2).
Inflammation; pain.

Roche Super B Roche, Austral.†.
Vitamin B substances with calcium ascorbate.

Roche Super B Stress Tablets Roche, Austral.†.
Vitamin B substances with ascorbic acid and minerals.

Rochevit Roche Nicholas, Spain.
Multivitamin and mineral preparation.

Rociclyn Zambon, Neth.
Tolfenamic acid (p.89·3).
Osteoarthritis; rheumatoid arthritis.

Rocilin Rosco, Norw.
Phenoxymethylpenicillin potassium (p.236·2).
Bacterial infections.

Rocillin Rolab, S.Afr.
Amoxycillin trihydrate (p.151·3).
Bacterial infections.

Rocmalat Stroschein, Ger.†.
Arginine (p.1334·1) or arginine hydrochloride (p.1334·1); malic acid (p.1598·3).
Liver disorders.

Rocmaline
Frika, Aust.; Roques, Fr.
Arginine (p.1334·1); malic acid (p.1598·3).
Liver disorders.

Rocodin Brunel, S.Afr.
Paracetamol (p.72·2); codeine phosphate (p.26·1).
Fever; pain.

Rocornal
Rentschler, Ger.; UCB, Ger.; Mochida, Jpn†.
Trapidil (p.957·2).
Angina pectoris; cerebral haemorrhage; stroke.

Rodavan
Laevosan, Aust.; Asta Medica, Ger.
Chlorphenoxamine hydrochloride (p.405·3); caffeine (p.749·3); 8-chlorotheophylline.
Motion sickness; nausea; vertigo; vomiting.

Rodazol Rodleben, Ger.†.
Aminoglutethimide (p.502·3).
Breast cancer; Cushing's syndrome.

Rodex Legere, USA†.
Pyridoxine hydrochloride (p.1362·3).

Rodex TD Legere, USA†.
Pyridoxine (p.1363·1).

RO-Dexsone Richmond Ophthalmics, Canad.†.
Dexamethasone sodium phosphate (p.1037·2).
Corticosteroid.

Rodogyl Specia, Fr.
Spiramycin (p.249·2); metronidazole (p.585·1).
Bacterial mouth infections.

RO-Dry Eyes Richmond Ophthalmics, Canad.
Polyvinyl alcohol (p.1474·2).
Dry eyes.

RO-Eye Drops Richmond Ophthalmics, Canad.
Tetrahydrozoline hydrochloride (p.1070·2).

RO-Eyewash Richmond Ophthalmics, Canad.
Boric acid (p.1554·2).

Rofact ICN, Canad.
Rifampicin (p.243·2).
Tuberculosis.

Rofanten Belmac, Spain†.
Naproxen (p.61·2).
Gout; musculoskeletal, joint and peri-articular disorders; pain.

Rofatuss Rosen, Ger.
Clobutinol hydrochloride (p.1057·1).
Coughs.

Rofen Rolab, S.Afr.
Ibuprofen (p.44·1).
Fever; pain.

Rofenid Rhone-Poulenc Rorer, Belg.
Ketoprofen (p.48·2).
Inflammation; musculoskeletal, joint, and peri-articular disorders; oedema; pain.

Roferon-A
Roche, Aust.; Roche, Austral.; Roche, Belg.; Roche, Canad.; Roche, Fr.; Roche, Ger.; Roche, Irl.; Roche, Ital.; Roche, Neth.; Roche, S.Afr.; Roche, Spain; Roche, Swed.; Roche, Switz.; Roche, UK; Roche, USA.
Interferon alfa-2a (p.615·3).
Formerly known as Receron-A in *Swed.*
AIDS-related Kaposi's sarcoma; chronic myeloid leukaemia; hairy-cell leukaemia; hepatitis B; hepatitis C; malignant melanoma; non-Hodgkin's lymphoma; renal-cell cancer; T-cell lymphoma; thrombocytosis.

Roflatol Phyto (Rowo-146) Pharmakon, Ger.
Chamomile (p.1561·2); caraway oil (p.1559·3); fennel oil (p.1579·2); peppermint oil (p.1208·1).
Gastro-intestinal disorders.

Roflual Roche, Fr.†.
Rimantadine hydrochloride (p.624·2).
Influenza prophylaxis.

Rogaine
Pharmacia Upjohn, Canad.; Pharmacia Upjohn, USA.
Minoxidil (p.910·3).
Alopecia androgenetica.

Roge Pastor Farina, Ital.
Anhydrous citric acid (p.1564·3); magnesium carbonate (p.1198·1).
Constipation.

RO-Gentycin Richmond Ophthalmics, Canad.†.
Gentamicin sulphate (p.212·1).
Eye infections.

Rogitine
Ciba, Canad.; Ciba-Geigy, Irl.†; Alliance, UK.
Phentolamine mesylate (p.930·1).
Dermal necrosis and sloughing following intravenous administration of noradrenaline; phaeochromocytoma.

Rogorin Saba, Ital.†.
Bromelains (p.1555·1).
Oedema and inflammation.

rohasal Roha, Ger.
Absinthium (p.1541·1); aniseed (p.1549·3); kaolin (p.1195·1); calcium phosphate (p.1155·3); dried magnesium sulphate (p.1158·2); calcium carbonate (p.1182·1); heavy magnesium carbonate (p.1198·1); sodium bicarbonate (p.1153·2).
Gastro-intestinal disorders.

Rohipnol Andreu, Spain.
Flunitrazepam (p.670·1).
Anxiety; general anaesthesia; insomnia.

Rohypnol
Roche, Aust.; Roche, Austral.; Roche, Belg.; Roche, Fr.; Roche, Ger.;

Roche, Irl.; Roche, Neth.; Roche, Norw.; Roche, S.Afr.; Roche, Swed.; Roche, Switz.; Roche, UK.
Flunitrazepam (p.670·1).
General anaesthesia; insomnia; premedication.

Roidhemo *Cusi, Spain.*
Benzyl phenol; benzyl salicylate; aesculus (p.1543·3); ephedrine hydrochloride (p.1059·3); hamamelis (p.1587·1); lactic acid (p.1593·3).
Anorectal disorders.

Roipnol *Roche, Ital.*
Flunitrazepam (p.670·1).
Insomnia.

Roiten *Schering, Ital.†.*
Vincamine oxoglurate (p.1644·1).
Disorders of cerebral circulation.

Rokan *Intersan, Ger.*
Ginkgo biloba leaf (p.1584·1).
Mental function disorders; peripheral circulatory disorders.

Rokital *Formenti, Ital.*
Rokitamicin (p.246·3).
Bacterial infections.

Rolaids *Adams, Canad.*
Calcium carbonate (p.1182·1); magnesium hydroxide (p.1198·2).
Dyspepsia.

Rolatuss Expectorant *Huckaby, USA.*
Phenylephrine hydrochloride (p.1066·2); codeine phosphate (p.26·1); chlorpheniramine maleate (p.405·1); ammonium chloride (p.1055·2).
Coughs.

Rolatuss with Hydrocodone *Major, USA.*
Phenylpropanolamine hydrochloride (p.1067·2); phenylephrine hydrochloride (p.1066·2); mepyramine maleate (p.414·1); pheniramine maleate (p.415·3); hydrocodone tartrate (p.43·1).
Coughs and cold symptoms.

Rolatuss Plain *Major, USA.*
Phenylephrine hydrochloride (p.1066·2); chlorpheniramine maleate (p.405·1).
Upper respiratory-tract symptoms.

Rolazine *Rolab, S.Afr.*
Hydralazine hydrochloride (p.883·2).
Hypertension.

Roleca Wacholder *Serturner, Ger.*
Juniper oil (p.1592·3).
Diuretic.

Rolene *Riva, Canad.*
Betamethasone dipropionate (p.1033·3).
Skin disorders.

Roliwol *Stada, Switz.*
Methyl salicylate (p.55·2); camphor (p.1557·2); methyl nicotinate (p.55·1); menthol (p.1600·2); turpentine oil (p.1641·1); eucalyptus oil (p.1578·1); mint oil (p.1604·1); thymol (p.1127·1); nutmeg oil (p.1609·3).
Musculoskeletal and joint pain; sports injuries.

Roliwol B *Stada, Switz.*
Glycol salicylate (p.43·1); camphor (p.1557·2); diethylamine salicylate (p.33·1); pine oil.
Musculoskeletal, joint, and peri-articular pain.

Roliwol S *Stada, Switz.*
Glycol salicylate (p.43·1); benzyl nicotinate (p.22·1); nonivamide (p.63·2).
Musculoskeletal, joint, and peri-articular disorders.

Roll-bene *Mepha, Switz.*
Heparin sodium (p.879·3); dimethyl sulphoxide (p.1377·2); dexpanthenol (p.1570·3).
Inflammation; musculoskeletal, joint, peri-articular, and soft-tissue disorders; pain; peripheral vascular disorders.

Rollkur Godecke *Godecke, Ger.†; Parke, Davis, Ger.†.*
Silver-white acetyltannate.
Gastro-intestinal disorders.

Roll-On *Shaklee, Canad.*
Aluminium chlorohydrate (p.1078·3).
Hyperhidrosis.

Romadin *Medinsa, Spain.*
Astemizole (p.402·1).
Hypersensitivity reactions.

Roma-nol *Jamol, USA†.*
Iodine solution (p.1493·1).
Skin and mucous membrane infections.

Romarene *Beaufour, Fr.*
Rosemary; taraxacum (p.1634·2); combretum (p.1593·2); sodium potassium tartrate (p.1213·3); sodium citrate (p.1153·2).
Gastro-intestinal disorders.

Romarinex-Choline *Aerocid, Fr.*
Rosemary; cynara (p.1569·2); boldo (p.1554·1); taraxacum (p.1634·2); combretum (p.1593·2); choline citrate (p.1337·1).
Gastro-intestinal disorders.

Romazicon *Roche, USA.*
Flumazenil (p.981·1).
Formerly known as Mazicon.
Benzodiazepine overdosage; reversal of benzodiazepine-induced sedation.

Rombay *Apotheke Heiligen Dreifaltigkeit, Aust.*
Talc (p.1092·1); zinc oxide (p.1096·2); peru balsam (p.1617·2).
Skin irritation.

Rombellin *Simons, Ger.*
Biotin (p.1336·1).
Biotin deficiency.

Romet *Mitsubishi, Jpn†.*
Repirinast (p.758·1).
Asthma.

Romigal N *Romigal, Ger.†.*
Salicylamide (p.82·3); aspirin (p.16·1); caffeine with citric acid (p.749·3).
Influenza; neuritis; pain.

Romilar
Note. This name is used for preparations of different composition.
Roche Consumer, Belg.†.
Dextromethorphan hydrobromide (p.1057·3); ammonium chloride (p.1055·2); dexpanthenol (p.1570·3).
Coughs.

Roche, Ital.
Dextromethorphan hydrobromide (p.1057·3); ammonium chloride (p.1055·2).
Coughs.

Roche Nicholas, Spain.
Dextromethorphan hydrobromide (p.1057·3).
Coughs.

Romilar Antitussivum *Roche, Belg.*
Dextromethorphan hydrobromide (p.1057·3).
Coughs.

Romilar Expectorante *Roche, Spain†.*
Dextromethorphan hydrobromide (p.1057·3); ammonium chloride (p.1055·2); dexpanthenol (p.1570·3).
Respiratory-tract disorders.

Romilar Mucolyticum *Roche, Belg.*
Carbocisteine (p.1056·3).
Respiratory-tract disorders associated with accumulation of mucus.

Romin *Rolab, S.Afr.*
Minocycline hydrochloride (p.226·2).
Acne; bacterial infections.

Rommix *Ashbourne, UK.*
Erythromycin (p.204·1).

Romozin *Glaxo Wellcome, UK†.*
Troglitazone (p.334·1).
Diabetes mellitus.

Romycin *Ocusoft, USA†.*
Erythromycin (p.204·1).
Eye infections.

RO-Naphz *Richmond Ophthalmics, Canad.*
Naphazoline hydrochloride (p.1064·2).
Eye congestion.

Rondamine-DM *Major, USA.*
Pseudoephedrine hydrochloride (p.1068·3); dextromethorphan hydrobromide (p.1057·3); carbinoxamine maleate (p.404·2).
Coughs and cold symptoms.

Rondec
Abbott, Ital.; Abbott, S.Afr.†; Abbott, Spain; Dura, USA.
Carbinoxamine maleate (p.404·2); pseudoephedrine hydrochloride (p.1068·3).
Allergic and vasomotor rhinitis; nasal congestion.

Rondec Chewable *Dura, USA.*
Brompheniramine maleate (p.403·2); pseudoephedrine hydrochloride (p.1068·3).
Upper respiratory-tract disorders.

Rondec-DM *Dura, USA.*
Carbinoxamine maleate (p.404·2); pseudoephedrine hydrochloride (p.1068·3); dextromethorphan hydrobromide (p.1057·3).
Coughs and cold symptoms; respiratory symptoms of allergy.

Rondimen *Asta Medica, Ger.*
Mefenorex hydrochloride (p.1482·1).
Obesity.

Rondomycin
Parke, Davis, Austral.; Roerig, Swed.†.
Methacycline hydrochloride (p.225·1).
Bacterial infections.

Rondomycine *Roerig, Belg.†.*
Methacycline hydrochloride (p.225·1).
Bacterial infections.

Roniacol Supraspan *Roche, Canad.†.*
Nicotinyl alcohol tartrate (p.915·3).
Angina pectoris; circulatory disorders.

Ronicol
Roche, Ger.†; Roche, Irl.†; Roche, Ital.†; Roche, Neth.†; Roche, Swed.†; Roche, Switz.†; Tillomed, UK.
Nicotinyl alcohol tartrate (p.915·3).
Hyperlipidaemias; vascular disorders.

Ronmix *Ashbourne, UK.*
Erythromycin (p.204·1).

Ronpirin APCQ *Mitchell, UK.*
Paracetamol (p.72·2); aspirin (p.16·1); caffeine (p.749·3); quinine hydrochloride (p.439·2).

Ronpirin Cold Remedy *Mitchell, UK.*
Promethazine hydrochloride (p.416·2); dextromethorphan hydrochloride; paracetamol (p.72·2).
Cold symptoms.

RO-Parcaine *Richmond Ophthalmics, Canad.†.*
Proxymetacaine hydrochloride (p.1300·1).
Local anaesthesia.

Rophelin *Rolmex, Canad.*
Ammonium chloride (p.1055·2); tolu balsam (p.1071·1); white pine compound; wild cherry bark (p.1644·3).

RO-Predphate *Richmond Ophthalmics, Canad.†.*
Prednisolone sodium phosphate (p.1048·1).
Inflammatory disorders of the eye.

R.O.R. *Merieux, Fr.*
A measles, mumps, and rubella vaccine (Edmonston 749D, Jeryl Lynn, and Wistar RA 27/3 strains respectively) (p.1519·3).
Active immunisation.

Rosaced *Pierre Fabre, Fr.*
Metronidazole (p.585·1).
Rosacea.

Rosacin *Master Pharma, Ital.†.*
Acrosoxacin (p.150·1).
Gonococcal urethritis.

Rosal *Ibi, Ital.†.*
Rosaprostol (p.1420·3).
Gastro-duodenal inflammation; peptic ulcer.

Rosalgin *Farma Lepori, Spain.*
Benzydamine hydrochloride (p.21·3).
Vaginitis.

Rosalox *Drossapharm, Switz.*
Metronidazole (p.585·1).
Rosacea.

Rosarthron *Steierl, Ger.*
Rosemary oil (p.1626·2); pumilio pine oil (p.1623·3).
Circulatory disorders; gout; musculoskeletal and joint disorders; neuritis; respiratory-tract disorders.

Rosarthron forte *Steierl, Ger.*
Rosemary oil (p.1626·2); methyl salicylate (p.55·2); benzyl nicotinate (p.22·1).
Circulatory disorders; gout; musculoskeletal and joint disorders; neuritis; respiratory-tract disorders.

Roscopenin *Hydro, Swed.†.*
Phenoxymethylpenicillin potassium (p.236·2).
Bacterial infections.

Rose Hips C *Swiss Herbal, Canad.†.*
Vitamin C (p.1365·2); lemon bioflavonoids (p.1580·1); hesperidin (p.1580·2); rutin (p.1580·2).
Dietary supplement.

Roseomix *Farmigea, Ital.†.*
Kanamycin sulphate (p.220·3); polymyxin B sulphate (p.239·1).
Bacterial eye infections.

Rosetin *Benvegna, Ital.†.*
Amidopyrine ethiodide (p.15·2).
Neuritis; rheumatism; sciatica.

Rosets *Akorn, USA.*
Rose bengal sodium (p.1626·1).
Ophthalmic diagnostic agent.

Rosig *Sigma, Austral.*
Piroxicam (p.80·2).
Ankylosing spondylitis; osteoarthritis; rheumatoid arthritis.

Rosils *Boots Healthcare, Belg.*
Noscapine (p.1065·2); phenylephrine hydrochloride (p.1066·2).
Coughs; upper respiratory-tract congestion.

Rosimon-Neu *Ravensberg, Ger.†.*
Morazone hydrochloride (p.56·1); salicylamide (p.82·3); dextropropoxyphene hydrochloride (p.27·3).
Influenza; pain; spasm.

Rosken Silk *Warner-Lambert, Austral.†.*
Ethylhexyl *p*-methoxycinnamate (p.1487·1); oxybenzone (p.1487·3); avobenzone (p.1486·3).
Emollient; sunscreen.

Rosken Skin Repair *Warner-Lambert, Austral.*
Dimethicone (p.1384·2).
Dermatitis; dry skin.

Rosken Solar Block *Mentholatum, Austral.*
Lotion: Ethylhexyl *p*-methoxycinnamate (p.1487·1); avobenzone (p.1486·3); octyl triazone; titanium dioxide (p.1093·3).
Sportstick: Ethylhexyl *p*-methoxycinnamate (p.1487·1); 3-(4-methylbenzylidene)bornan-2-one (p.1487·2); avobenzone (p.1486·3).
Sunstick: Padimate O (p.1488·1); oxybenzone (p.1487·3); avobenzone (p.1486·3).
Sunscreen.

Rosken Solar Block Concentrated *Mentholatum, Austral.*
Padimate O (p.1488·1); 3-(4-methylbenzylidene)bornan-2-one (p.1487·2); avobenzone (p.1486·3).
Sunscreen.

Rosken Solar Block Toddler *Mentholatum, Austral.*
Ethylhexyl *p*-methoxycinnamate (p.1487·1); avobenzone (p.1486·3); octyl triazone; titanium dioxide (p.1093·3).
Sunscreen.

Rosmarinsalbe *Doerr, Ger.†.*
Rosemary oil (p.1626·2); camphor oil; chlorophyll (p.1000·1).
Joint pain; rheumatic disorders.

Rosol-Gamma *Biagini, Ital.*
A rubella immunoglobulin (p.1532·3).
Passive immunisation.

Rosone *Riva, Canad.*
Betamethasone dipropionate (p.1033·3).
Skin disorders.

Rosovax *Nuovo ISM, Ital.*
A rubella vaccine (Wistar RA 27/3 strain) (p.1532·3).
Active immunisation.

Ross SLD *Ross, USA†.*
Low-fat low-residue food.

Rossepar *KBR, Ital.*
Ferric sodium gluconate (p.1340·1).
Iron deficiency; iron-deficiency anaemias.

Rossitrol *Corvi, Ital.*
Roxithromycin (p.247·1).
Bacterial infections.

Rossocorten *Caber, Ital.†.*
Inosine (p.1591·1); suprarenal cortex (p.1050·1); cyanocobalamin (p.1363·3).
Anaemias; tonic.

Rossomicina *Pierrel, Ital.†.*
Erythromycin ethyl succinate (p.204·2) or erythromycin stearate (p.204·2).
Amoebiasis; bacterial infections.

Ro-Strumal NEU (Rowo-221) *Pharmakon, Ger.*
Spongia tosta; putamen ovi tosta; magnesium hydrogen phosphate; anhydrous sodium phosphate; terra silicea purificata.
Hyperthyroidism.

RotaShield *Wyeth-Ayerst, USA.*
A rotavirus vaccine (p.1532·2).
Active immunisation.

Roter
Note. This name is used for preparations of different composition.
Four Macs, Austral.†; Maurer, Ger.†; Boots Healthcare, Neth.†; Roterpharma, UK.
Bismuth subnitrate (p.1180·2); magnesium carbonate (p.1198·1); sodium bicarbonate (p.1153·2); frangula bark (p.1193·2).
Gastro-intestinal disorders.

Bournonville, Belg.†; Farma Lepori, Spain†.
Bismuth subnitrate (p.1180·2); magnesium carbonate (p.1198·1); sodium bicarbonate (p.1153·2); frangula bark (p.1193·2); calamus root (p.1556·1).
Gastro-intestinal disorders.

Boots, S.Afr.†.
Bismuth subcarbonate (p.1180·1); magnesium carbonate (p.1198·1); sodium bicarbonate (p.1153·2); frangula bark (p.1193·2).
Dyspepsia; peptic ulcer.

Roter APC *Boots Healthcare, Neth.†.*
Aspirin (p.16·1); paracetamol (p.72·2); caffeine (p.749·3).
Fever; pain.

Roter Complex *Farma Lepori, Spain.*
Bismuth subnitrate (p.1180·2); magnesium carbonate (p.1198·1); sodium bicarbonate (p.1153·2); frangula bark (p.1193·2); calamus root (p.1556·1); sulpiride (p.692·3).
Duodenitis; gastritis; hyperchlorhydria; peptic ulcer.

Roter Keel *Boots Healthcare, Neth.†.*
Chlorhexidine hydrochloride (p.1107·2).
Sore throats.

Roter Noscapect *Boots Healthcare, Neth.†.*
Noscapine hydrochloride (p.1065·2).
Coughs.

Roter Paracof *Boots Healthcare, Neth.†.*
Paracetamol (p.72·2); caffeine (p.749·3).
Fever; pain.

Rotersept
Note. This name is used for preparations of different composition.
Bournonville, Belg.†.
Chlorhexidine hydrochloride (p.1107·2).
Mouth and throat infections.

Maurer, Ger.†; Roterpharma, Irl.; Roterpharma, UK†.
Chlorhexidine gluconate (p.1107·2).
Cracked nipples; mastitis; skin disinfection.

Rotesan *Knoll, Spain.*
Roxithromycin (p.247·1).
Bacterial infections.

Rotet *Rolab, S.Afr.*
Tetracycline hydrochloride (p.259·1).
Bacterial infections.

Roth's RKT Tropfen *Infirmarius-Rovit, Ger.*
Homoeopathic preparation.

Roth's Ropulmin N *Infirmarius-Rovit, Ger.*
Homoeopathic preparation.

Roth's Rotacard *Infirmarius-Rovit, Ger.*
Homoeopathic preparation.

Rotil *Bioprogress, Ital.*
Niperotidine hydrochloride (p.1203·2).
Peptic ulcer.

Rotilen *Terapeutico, Ital.*
Methacycline hydrochloride (p.225·1).
Bacterial infections.

Rotol *Jukunda, Ger.*
Hypericum (p.1590·1).
Joint pain; nervous disorders; wounds.

Rotramin *Evans, Spain.*
Roxithromycin (p.247·1).
Bacterial infections.

RO-Tropamide *Richmond Ophthalmics, Canad.†.*
Tropicamide (p.469·2).
Production of mydriasis and cycloplegia.

Rot-Wellcovax *Wellcopharm, Ger.†.*
A rubella vaccine (Wistar RA 27/3 strain) (p.1532·3).
Active immunisation.

Roubac *Rougier, Canad.*
Co-trimoxazole (p.196·3).
Bacterial infections.

Rouhex-G *Rougier, Canad.*
Chlorhexidine gluconate (p.1107·2).
Acne; skin disinfection; surface and instrument disinfection.

Rounox *Rougier, Canad.*
Paracetamol (p.72·2).
Fever; pain.

Rouvax
Merieux, Fr.; Pasteur Merieux, Ital.; Rhone-Poulenc Rorer, S.Afr.; Rhone-Poulenc Rorer, Spain†.
A measles vaccine (Schwarz strain) (p.1517·3).
Active immunisation.

Rovaktivit *Rowa, Irl.†.*
Melissa (p.1600·1); eugenol (p.1578·2); soya lecithin (p.1595·2); alcohol.
Tonic.

Rovamicina *Rhone-Poulenc Rorer, Ital.*
Spiramycin (p.249·2).
Bacterial infections.

Rovamycin
Gerot, Aust.; Rhone-Poulenc Rorer, Norw.; Rhone-Poulenc Rorer, Swed.†.
Spiramycin (p.249·2).
Bacterial infections; toxoplasmosis.

Rovamycine
Rhone-Poulenc Rorer, Belg.; Rhone-Poulenc Rorer, Canad.; Specia, Fr.; Rhone-Poulenc Rorer, Ger.; Rhone-Poulenc Rorer, Neth.; Rhone-Poulenc Rorer, Spain; Rhone-Poulenc Rorer, Switz.
Spiramycin (p.249·2) or spiramycin adipate (p.249·2).
Bacterial infections; prevention of flares of rheumatoid arthritis; toxoplasmosis.

Rovigon
Roche, Aust.; Roche, Belg.; Roche Nicholas, Fr.; Roche, Ital.; Roche, Switz.
Vitamin A palmitate (p.1359·2); *dl*-alpha tocopheryl acetate (p.1369·2).
Vitamin A and E deficiency.

Rovigon G *Roche Nicholas, Ger.*
Vitamin A palmitate (p.1359·2); alpha tocopheryl acetate (p.1369·1).
Vitamin A and E deficiency.

Rovilax *Rovi, Spain†.*
Docusate sodium (p.1189·3).

Rowachol
Note. This name is used for preparations of different composition.
Rosch & Handel, Aust.; Rowa, UK.
Capsules: Menthol (p.1600·2); menthone; α-pinene; β-pinene; camphene; borneol; cineol (p.1564·1).
Biliary-tract disorders; dyspepsia.
Rosch & Handel, Aust.; Ist. Chim. Inter., Ital.†.
Oral drops: Menthol (p.1600·2); menthone; α-pinene; β-pinene; camphene; borneol; cineol (p.1564·1); rheochrysin.
Biliary-tract disorders; dyspepsia.
Rowa, Ger.; Rowa, Irl.
Capsules; oral drops: Menthol (p.1600·2); menthone; α-pinene; β-pinene; borneol; camphene; cineole (p.1564·1).
Biliary-tract disorders.
Diviser Aquilea, Spain.
Menthol (p.1600·2); pinenes; borneol; camphene; cineole (p.1564·1); emodin; oxidised terpenes.
Anorexia; hepatobiliary disorders.

Rowachol comp. *Rowa, Ger.*
Menthol (p.1600·2); menthone; α-pinene; β-pinene; borneol; camphene; cineole (p.1564·1); deanol benzilate hydrochloride (p.1478·2).
Biliary-tract disorders.

Rowachol-Digestiv *Rowa, Ger.*
Menthol (p.1600·2); menthone; α-pinene; β-pinene; borneol; camphene; cineole (p.1564·1).
Digestive system disorders; hepatobiliary disorders.

Rowacylat *Rowa, Irl.†.*
Paracetamol (p.72·2); codeine phosphate (p.26·1); chlormezanone (p.648·3); pipoxolan hydrochloride (p.1618·3).
Pain and associated stress; premenstrual syndrome; rheumatism.

Rowadermat *Rosch & Handel, Aust.*
Carbenoxolone disodium (p.1182·2).
Aphthous ulcers; herpes labialis.

Rowalind
Rosch & Handel, Aust.; Rowa, Ger.; Rowa, Irl.
Nicotinaldehyde; ammonia solution (p.1548·3); ammonium chloride (p.1055·2); camphor (p.1557·2); menthol (p.1600·2); rosemary oil (p.1626·2); lavender oil (p.1594·3).
Musculoskeletal and joint disorders; neuralgia; neuritis.

Rowanefrin *Funk, Spain.*
Anethole (p.1549·3); borneol; camphene; rubia tinctorum; oxidised terpenes; pinenes; fenchone; cineole (p.1564·1).
Renal calculi; urinary-tract disorders.

Rowapraxin
Rowa, Ger.; Rowa, Irl.
Pipoxolan (p.1618·3) or pipoxolan hydrochloride (p.1618·3).
Smooth muscle spasm.

Rowarolan
Note. This name is used for preparations of different composition.
Rowa, Ger.
Calcium carbonate (p.1182·1); colloidal silicon dioxide (p.1475·1).
Ulcers.
Rowa, Irl.
Calcium carbonate (p.1182·1).
Adsorbent in ulcers and sores.

Rowasa
Solvay, Fr.; Solvay, USA.
Mesalazine (p.1199·2).
Inflammatory bowel disease.

Rowatanal *Rowa, Irl.*
Bismuth subgallate (p.1180·2); zinc oxide (p.1096·2); menthol (p.1600·2).
Anal irritation; haemorrhoids.

Rowatin *Ist. Chim. Inter., Ital.†.*
α-Pinene; β-pinene; camphene; borneol; anethole (p.1549·3); fenchone; cineole (p.1564·1).
Renal calculi; renal colic.

Rowatinex
Rosch & Handel, Aust.; Rowa, Ger.; Rowa, Irl.; Monmouth, UK.
α-Pinene; β-pinene; camphene; borneol; anethole (p.1549·3); fenchone; cineole (p.1564·1).
Renal calculi; renal disorders; urolithiasis.

Rowo-52 *Pharmakon, Ger.*
Homoeopathic preparation.
Lignocaine hydrochloride (p.1293·2) is included in this preparation to alleviate the pain of injection.

Rowo-215 *Pharmakon, Ger.†.*
Homoeopathic preparation.

Rowo-216 *Pharmakon, Ger.*
Homoeopathic preparation.
Lignocaine hydrochloride (p.1293·2) is included in this preparation to alleviate the pain of injection.

Rowo-298 *Pharmakon, Ger.*
Homoeopathic preparation.
Lignocaine hydrochloride (p.1293·2) is included in this preparation to alleviate the pain of injection.

Rowo-Galphimia Komplex (Rowo-2) *Pharmakon, Ger.†.*
Homoeopathic preparation.

Rowok *Ono, Jpn†.*
Ornoprostil (p.1420·3).

Rowo-Rytesthin (Rowo-576) *Pharmakon, Ger.*
Homoeopathic preparation.

Rowo-Sedaphin (Rowo-138) *Pharmakon, Ger.*
Homoeopathic preparation.

Rowo-Spasmol (Rowo-140) *Pharmakon, Ger.†.*
Homoeopathic preparation.

Roxalia *Boiron, Canad.*
Homoeopathic preparation.

Roxane *Albert-Roussel, Aust.†.*
Roxatidine acetate hydrochloride (p.1212·1).
Gastro-oesophageal reflux; peptic ulcer.

Roxanol *Roxane, USA.*
Morphine sulphate (p.56·2).
Pain.

Roxene *Benedetti, Ital.*
Piroxicam (p.80·2).
Musculoskeletal, joint, peri-articular, and soft-tissue disorders.

Roxenil *Caber, Ital.*
Piroxicam (p.80·2).
Musculoskeletal and joint disorders.

Roxiam
Astra, Aust.; Astra, Neth.†; Astra, Swed.†; Astra, UK†.
Remoxipride hydrochloride (p.690·3).
Psychoses.

Roxicam *Rolab, S.Afr.*
Piroxicam (p.80·2).
Inflammation; musculoskeletal and joint disorders; pain.

Roxicet
Boehringer Ingelheim, Canad.; Roxane, USA.
Oxycodone hydrochloride (p.71·2); paracetamol (p.72·2).
Pain.

Roxicodone *Roxane, USA.*
Oxycodone hydrochloride (p.71·2).
Pain.

Roxiden *Pulitzer, Ital.*
Piroxicam (p.80·2).
Musculoskeletal and joint disorders.

Roxillin *Rowex, Irl.*
Amoxycillin trihydrate (p.151·3).
Bacterial infections.

Roxilox *Roxane, USA.*
Oxycodone hydrochloride (p.71·2); paracetamol (p.72·2).
Pain.

Roxim *Bergamon, Ital.†.*
Piroxicam (p.80·2).
Rheumatic disorders.

Roxiprin *Roxane, USA.*
Oxycodone hydrochloride (p.71·2); oxycodone terephthalate (p.71·3); aspirin (p.16·1).
Pain.

Roxit
Albert-Roussel, Ger.; Hoechst, Ger.; Hoechst Marion Roussel, Ital.; Knoll, Neth.; Hoechst Marion Roussel, S.Afr.
Roxatidine acetate hydrochloride (p.1212·1).
Gastro-oesophageal reflux; peptic ulcer.

Roxiwas *Wasserman, Spain.*
Roxatidine acetate (p.1212·2).
Gastro-oesophageal reflux; peptic ulcer.

Roxochemil *Chemil, Ital.†.*
Erythromycin estolate (p.204·1).
Bacterial infections.

Roxy *Adcock Ingram, S.Afr.*
Oxytetracycline hydrochloride (p.235·1).
Bacterial infections.

Roxyne *Roerig, Belg.†.*
Doxycycline hydrochloride (p.202·3).
Bacterial infections.

Royal E *Cielle, Ital.*
Royal jelly (p.1626·3); vitamin E (p.1369·1).
Nutritional supplement.

Royal Galanol *Lifeplan, UK.*
Evening primrose oil (p.1582·1); royal jelly (p.1626·3).
Nutritional supplement.

Royal Life *Bioceuticals, UK.*
Multivitamin, mineral, and amino-acid preparation.

Royal Mille *Blue Cross, Ital.†.*
Royal jelly (p.1626·3); panax ginseng (p.1584·2).
Nutritional supplement.

Royal Zolfo *Irmed, Ital.†.*
Colloidal sulphur (p.1091·2).
Cleansing of greasy skin.

Roychlor *Waymar, Canad.*
Potassium chloride (p.1161·1).
Potassium deficiency.

Royen *Rubio, Spain.*
Calcium acetate (p.1155·1).
Hyperphosphataemia in patients with renal insufficiency.

Royflex *Waymar, Canad.*
Triethanolamine salicylate (p.1639·2).
Musculoskeletal and joint disorders.

Royl 6 *Vesta, S.Afr.*
Vitamin B substances with vitamin C.

Royl-Fibre *Vesta, S.Afr.†.*
Mineral and fibre preparation.

Royvac Kit *Waymar, Canad.*
Oral solution, magnesium citrate (p.1198·2); 3 tablets, bisacodyl (p.1179·3); 1 suppository, bisacodyl.
Bowel evacuation.

Rozagel *Biorga, Fr.*
Metronidazole (p.585·1).
Rosacea.

Rozex
Galderma, Austral.; Galderma, Belg.; Galderma, Fr.; Galderma, Irl.; Galderma, Ital.; Galderma, Neth.; Galderma, S.Afr.; Galderma, Spain; Galderma, Switz.; Stafford-Miller, UK.
Metronidazole (p.585·1).
Rosacea.

Rozide *Rolab, S.Afr.*
Pyrazinamide (p.241·1).
Tuberculosis.

RR-plus *Godecke, Ger.†.*
Sparteine sulphate (p.1632·1); ephedrine hydrochloride (p.1059·3); convallaria (p.1567·2); crataegus (p.1568·2); caffeine (p.749·3); aesculus (p.1543·3).
Hypotension; tonic.

R/S Lotion *Summers, USA.*
Sulphur (p.1091·2); resorcinol (p.1090·1).
Acne.

R-Tannamine *Qualitest, USA.*
Phenylephrine tannate (p.1067·1); chlorpheniramine tannate (p.405·2); mepyramine tannate (p.414·1).
Upper respiratory-tract symptoms.

R-Tannate *Warner Chilcott, USA; Copley, USA; Schein, USA.*
Phenylephrine tannate (p.1067·1); chlorpheniramine tannate (p.405·2); mepyramine tannate (p.414·1).
Allergic rhinitis; nasal congestion.

Rubacina *Rubio, Spain.*
Famotidine (p.1192·1).
Gastro-oesophageal reflux; peptic ulcer; Zollinger-Ellison syndrome.

Rubavax *Merieux, UK†.*
A rubella vaccine (Wistar RA 27/3 strain) (p.1532·3).
Active immunisation.

9 Rubbing Oils *Potter's, UK.*
Amber oil; clove oil (p.1565·2); eucalyptus oil (p.1578·1); linseed oil (p.1596·2); methyl salicylate (p.55·2); volatile mustard oil (p.1605·3); turpentine oil (p.1641·1); thyme oil (p.1637·1); peppermint oil (p.1208·1).
Rheumatic and muscular pain.

Rubeaten
Kwizda, Aust.; Berna, Ital.; Swisspharm, S.Afr.; Berna, Spain; Berna, Switz.
A rubella vaccine (Wistar RA 27/3 strain) (p.1532·3).
Active immunisation.

Rubegam *NBI, S.Afr.†.*
A rubella immunoglobulin (p.1532·3).
Passive immunisation.

Rubellabulin *Immuno, Ital.†.*
A rubella immunoglobulin (p.1532·3).
Passive immunisation.

Rubellovac *Chiron Behring, Ger.*
A rubella vaccine (Wistar RA 27/3 strain) (p.1532·3).
Active immunisation.

Rubesal *Hamilton, Austral.*
Diethylamine salicylate (p.33·1); camphor (p.1557·2); menthol (p.1600·2).
Muscular pain.

Rubesol-1000 *Central Pharmaceuticals, USA†.*
Cyanocobalamin (p.1363·3).
Schilling test; vitamin B_{12} deficiency.

Rubeuman
Berna, Ital.; Berna, Spain†; Berna, Switz.
A rubella immunoglobulin (p.1532·3).
Passive immunisation.

Rubex
Note. This name is used for preparations of different composition.
Rice Steele, Irl.
Ascorbic acid (p.1365·2).
Anaemias; infections; rheumatic disorders; scurvy; wounds and fractures.
Bristol-Myers Oncology, USA.
Doxorubicin hydrochloride (p.529·2).
Malignant neoplasms.

Rubia Paver *Medical, Spain.*
Atropine sulphate (p.455·1); papaverine hydrochloride (p.1614·2); rubia tinctorum.
Renal calculi.

Rubicin *Steigerwald, Ger.†.*
Homoeopathic preparation.

Rubicolan S *Syxyl, Ger.*
Homoeopathic preparation.

Rubidazone *Bellon, Fr.†.*
Zorubicin hydrochloride (p.572·3).
Leukaemias.

Rubidiosin Composto *SIT, Ital.*
Rubidium iodide (p.1626·3); potassium iodide (p.1493·1); testosterone hemisuccinate (p.1465·3); lignocaine (p.1293·2); heparin sodium (p.879·3).
Cataracts.

Rubifen *Rubio, Spain.*
Methylphenidate hydrochloride (p.1483·1).
Behaviour disorders; depression; hyperactivity; narcoleptic syndrome.

Rubimycin *Pharmador, S.Afr.†.*
Erythromycin stearate (p.204·2).
Bacterial infections.

Rubinorm *IFI, Ital.†.*
Rubidium chloride (p.307·2).
Depression.

Rubisan
DHU, Ger.; Omida, Switz.
Homoeopathic preparation.

Rubistenol *Fermenti, Ital.*
Rubidium iodide (p.1626·3); sodium iodide (p.1493·2); potassium iodide (p.1493·1); sodium formate (p.1581·3); strychnine glycerophosphate.
Eye disorders.

Rubiulcer *Rubio, Spain.*
Ranitidine hydrochloride (p.1209·3).
Acid aspiration; gastro-intestinal haemorrhage; peptic ulcer; Zollinger-Ellison syndrome gastro-oesophageal reflux.

Rubizon-Rheumagel *Makara, Aust.*
Glycol salicylate (p.43·1); camphor (p.1557·2); benzyl nicotinate (p.22·1); capsaicin (p.24·2).
Frostbite; musculoskeletal and joint disorders; neuralgia; sport massage.

Rubjovit *SIFI, Ital.*
Rubidium iodide (p.1626·3); sodium iodide (p.1493·2); calcium formate (p.1581·3); sodium ascorbate (p.1365·2); thiamine hydrochloride (p.1361·1).
Cataracts.

Rubozinc *Labcatal, Fr.*
Zinc gluconate (p.1373·2).
Acne; acrodermatitis enteropathica.

Rubragel *Adcock Ingram, S.Afr.†.*
Dried aluminium hydroxide gel (p.1177·3); magnesium oxide (p.1198·3); simethicone (p.1213·1).
Gastro-intestinal hyperacidity with flatulence.

Rubragel-D *Keatings, S.Afr.†.*
Dicyclomine hydrochloride (p.460·1); dried aluminium hydroxide gel (p.1177·3); magnesium oxide (p.1198·3); simethicone (p.1213·1); sodium lauryl sulphate; hypromellose.
Gastro-intestinal disorders.

Rubramin *Squibb, Canad.*
Vitamin B_{12} (p.1363·3).
Schilling test; vitamin B_{12} deficiency.

Rubramin PC *Apothecon, USA.*
Cyanocobalamin (p.1363·3).
Vitamin B_{12} deficiency.

Rubraton *Bristol-Myers Squibb, Belg.†.*
Cyanocobalamin (p.1363·3); folic acid (p.1340·3); ferric ammonium citrate (p.1339·2).
Folate deficiency; iron-deficiency anaemias; vitamin B_{12} deficiency.

Rubratope *Squibb Diagnostics, USA.*
Cobalt-58 (p.1423·2) as cyanocobalamin.

Rubriment
Note. This name is used for preparations of different composition.
Ebewe, Aust.
Benzyl nicotinate (p.22·1); nonivamide (p.63·2); glycol salicylate (p.43·1); salicylamide (p.82·3); camphor (p.1557·2); turpentine oil (p.1641·1).
Frostbite; joint, muscle, and nerve disorders; peripheral vascular disorders; sport massage.
Knoll, Ger.
Bath additive: Benzyl nicotinate (p.22·1).
Ointment: Benzyl nicotinate (p.22·1); nonivamide (p.63·2).
Inflammation; peripheral vascular disorders; rheumatism.

Rubriment-N *Knoll, Ger.*
Benzyl nicotinate (p.22·1); glycol salicylate (p.43·1); camphor (p.1557·2).
Frostbite; peripheral vascular disorders; rheumatism.

Rubrocalcium *Caber, Ital.*
Calcium laevulinate (p.1155·2).
Calcium deficiency.

Rubrociclina *DMG, Ital.*
Demeclocycline hydrochloride (p.201·2); erythromycin (p.204·1) or erythromycin estolate (p.204·1).
Bacterial infections.

Rubrocortex *Chemil, Ital.†.*
Suprarenal cortex (p.1050·1); cyanocobalamin (p.1363·3); meglumine (p.1599·2); electrolytes; inosine (p.1591·1).
Anaemias.

Rubrocortin *Farma Lepori, Spain.*
Cyanocobalamin (p.1363·3); suprarenal cortex extract (p.1050·1); liver extract; inosine (p.1591·1).
Anaemias; tonic.

Rubroferrina *NCSN, Ital.*
Ferric sodium gluconate (p.1340·1).
Anaemias.

Rubus Complex *Blackmores, Austral.*
Raspberry leaf (p.1624·2); spirulina (p.1632·2); ascorbic acid; mitchella repens; hesperidin (p.1580·2); rutin

(p.1580·2); *d*-alpha tocopheryl acid succinate; vitamin B substances; choline bitartrate; inositol.
Obstetric and gynaecological disorders.

Rudi-Rouvax *Merieux, Fr.*
A measles and rubella vaccine (Schwarz and Wistar RA 27/3 strains respectively) (p.1519·2).
Active immunisation.

Rudistrol *Boiron, Canad.*
Homoeopathic preparation.

Rudivax
Merieux, Fr.; Pasteur Merieux, Ital.; Rhone-Poulenc Rorer, S.Afr.
A rubella vaccine (Wistar RA 27/3 strain) (p.1532·3).
Active immunisation.

Rudocaine *Streuli, Switz.*
Carticaine hydrochloride (p.1289·1).
Adrenaline hydrochloride (p.813·3) is included in this preparation as a vasoconstrictor to diminish absorption and localise the effect of the local anaesthetic.
Local anaesthesia.

Rudocycline *Streuli, Switz.*
Doxycycline hydrochloride (p.202·3).
Bacterial infections.

Rudolac *Streuli, Switz.*
Lactulose (p.1195·3).
Constipation; hepatic encephalopathy.

Rudotel *OPW, Ger.*
Medazepam (p.677·3).
Anxiety disorders.

Rufen *Boots, USA†.*
Ibuprofen (p.44·1).
Fever; osteoarthritis; pain; rheumatoid arthritis.

Rufol
Debat, Fr.; Roussel, Ital.†.
Sulphamethizole (p.254·2).
Bacterial infections of the urinary tract.

Ru-lets *Rugby, USA†.*
A range of vitamin preparations.

Rulicalcin *Hoechst Marion Roussel, Ital.*
Salcatonin (p.735·3).
Hypercalcaemia; osteoporosis; Paget's disease of bone; reflex sympathetic dystrophy.

Rulid
Hoechst Marion Roussel, Belg.; Roussel, Fr.; Hoechst, Ger.; Hoechst Marion Roussel, Ital.; Hoechst Marion Roussel, Switz.
Roxithromycin (p.247·1).
Bacterial infections.

Rulide
Albert-Roussel, Aust.; Hoechst Marion Roussel, Austral.; Hoechst Marion Roussel, Neth.; Hoechst Marion Roussel, S.Afr.; Roussel, Spain.
Roxithromycin (p.247·1).
Bacterial infections.

Rulofer *Lomapharm, Ger.†.*
Iron(III)-saccharose complex (p.1353·2); folic acid (p.1340·3); cyanocobalamin (p.1363·3).
Iron deficiency.

Rulofer G *Lomapharm, Ger.*
Ferrous gluconate (p.1340·1).
Iron deficiency.

Rulofer N *Lomapharm, Ger.*
Ferrous fumarate (p.1339·3).
Iron deficiency.

RuLox *Rugby, USA.*
Aluminium hydroxide (p.1177·3); magnesium hydroxide (p.1198·2).
Hyperacidity.

RuLox Plus *Rugby, USA.*
Aluminium hydroxide (p.1177·3); magnesium hydroxide (p.1198·2); simethicone (p.1213·1).
Hyperacidity.

Rulun *Lacer, Spain.*
Hydrochlorothiazide (p.885·2); rauwolfia (p.941·3); trichlormethiazide (p.958·2); xanthinol nicotinate (p.971·1); pentosan polysulphate (p.928·1).
Hypertension.

Rumafluor *Zyma, Fr.†.*
Sodium fluoride (p.742·1).
Vertebral osteoporosis.

Rumalon
Germania, Aust.; Ascot, Austral.†; Eumedica, Belg.†; Robapharm, Fr.†; Robapharm, Switz.†.
Cartilage; bone marrow.
Joint disorders.

Rumatral *Wander, Switz.†.*
Aloxiprin (p.15·1).
Musculoskeletal and joint disorders.

Rumicine *Schering-Plough, Fr.*
Aspirin (p.16·1); chlorpheniramine maleate (p.405·1); caffeine (p.749·3).
Fever; pain.

Rumitard *Zurich, S.Afr.†.*
Indomethacin (p.45·2).
Musculoskeletal and joint disorders.

Rumitex *Beckerath, Ger.*
Homoeopathic preparation.

Rum-K *Fleming, USA.*
Potassium chloride (p.1161·1).
Hypokalaemia.

Rupton Chronules
Dexo, Fr.; Dexo, Switz.
Brompheniramine maleate (p.403·2); phenylpropanolamine hydrochloride (p.1067·2).
Upper-respiratory-tract disorders.

Ruscorectal
Heumann, Ger.; Juste, Spain.
Ruscogenin (p.1627·1).
Anorectal disorders.

Ruscoroid *Inverni della Beffa, Ital.*
Ruscogenin (p.1627·1); amethocaine hydrochloride (p.1285·2).
Anorectal disorders.

Ruscovarin *Alpinamed, Switz.*
Heparin (p.879·3).
Peripheral vascular disorders.

Ruscus *Llorens, Spain.*
Cinchocaine hydrochloride (p.1289·2); prednisolone (p.1048·1); ruscogenin (p.1627·1); zinc oxide (p.1096·2); menthol (p.1600·2).
Anorectal disorders.

Russian Athletic Formula *Suisse, Austral.†.*
Multivitamin and mineral preparation.

Rusyde *CP Pharmaceuticals, UK.*
Frusemide (p.871·1).
Oedema.

Rutibal *Pfluger, Ger.†.*
Cyanocobalamin (p.1363·3); procaine hydrochloride (p.1299·2); nicotinamide (p.1351·2); 3′,4′,7′-tris(O-hydroxymethyl)rutoside; caffeine (p.749·3).
Liver disorders; peripheral circulatory disorders; tonic.

Ruticalzon *Brady, Aust.*
Cholecalciferol (p.1366·3); rutin (p.1580·2); vitamin C (p.1365·2); calcium citrate (p.1155·1).
Haemorrhage; infections.

Ruticalzon N *SmithKline Beecham, Ger.†.*
Rutin (p.1580·2); ascorbic acid (p.1365·2); calcium citrate (p.1155·1).
Haemorrhagic disorders.

Rutice Fuerte *Faes, Spain.*
Ascorbic acid (p.1365·2); rutin (p.1580·2).
Vascular disorders.

Rutinion *Biomo, Ger.*
Rutin (p.1580·2).
Capillary impairment; venous insufficiency.

Rutisan CE *Carlo Erba OTC, Ital.*
Rutin (p.1580·2); vitamin C (p.1365·2); vitamin E (p.1369·1).
Vascular disorders.

Rutiscorbin *Frika, Aust.*
Rutin (p.1580·2); ascorbic acid (p.1365·2).
Haemorrhage; infections.

Rutisept Extra *Henkel, Ger.*
Isopropyl alcohol (p.1118·2); triclosan (p.1127·2).
Hand disinfection.

Rutovincine *Synthelabo, Fr.†.*
Vinca alkaloids; troxerutin (p.1580·2); ascorbic acid (p.1365·2).
Cerebrovascular disorders; mental function impairment.

Ru-Tuss *Boots, USA.*
Oral liquid: Phenylephrine hydrochloride (p.1066·2); chlorpheniramine maleate (p.405·1).
Tablets: Phenylephrine hydrochloride (p.1066·2); phenylpropanolamine hydrochloride (p.1067·2); chlorpheniramine maleate (p.405·1); hyoscyamine sulphate (p.464·2); atropine sulphate (p.455·1); hyoscine hydrobromide (p.462·3).
Upper respiratory-tract symptoms.

Ru-Tuss DE *Boots, USA.*
Pseudoephedrine hydrochloride (p.1068·3); guaiphenesin (p.1061·3).
Coughs.

Ru-Tuss Expectorant *Boots, USA.*
Pseudoephedrine hydrochloride (p.1068·3); dextromethorphan hydrobromide (p.1057·3); guaiphenesin (p.1061·3).
Coughs.

Ru-Tuss with Hydrocodone *Boots, USA.*
Hydrocodone tartrate (p.43·1); phenylephrine hydrochloride (p.1066·2); phenylpropanolamine hydrochloride (p.1067·2); pheniramine maleate (p.415·3); mepyramine maleate (p.414·1).
Cough, cold, and hay fever symptoms.

Ru-Tuss II *Boots, USA.*
Chlorpheniramine maleate (p.405·1); phenylpropanolamine hydrochloride (p.1067·2).
Cold symptoms.

Ruvenas *Mepha, Switz.†.*
Troxerutin (p.1580·2); esculoside (p.1543·3); hesperidin sodium phosphate (p.1580·2).
Vascular disorders.

Ru-Vert-M *Solvay, USA.*
Meclozine (p.413·3) or meclozine hydrochloride (p.413·3).
Motion sickness; vertigo.

RV PABA Stick *ICN, Canad.†.*
Aminobenzoic acid (p.1486·3).
Sunscreen.

RV Paque
ICN, Canad.; ICN, USA.
Zinc oxide (p.1096·2); cinoxate (p.1487·1).
Sunscreen.

R.V.C. *Lennon, S.Afr.†.*
Acetarsol (p.578·2).
Vaginal trichomoniasis.

RVHB Maxamaid *Scientific Hospital Supplies, Austral.*
Food for special diets.
Homocystinuria; hypermethioninaemia.

Ryccard *Propan, S.Afr.*
Cyclizine hydrochloride (p.407·1).
Nausea; vestibular disorders; vomiting.

Rydene *Roche, Belg.*
Nicardipine hydrochloride (p.915·1).
Angina pectoris; hypertension.

Rymed *Edwards, USA.*
Pseudoephedrine hydrochloride (p.1068·3); guaiphenesin (p.1061·3).
Coughs.

Rymed-TR *Edwards, USA.*
Phenylpropanolamine hydrochloride (p.1067·2); guaiphenesin (p.1061·3).
Coughs.

Ryna *Wallace, USA.*
Pseudoephedrine hydrochloride (p.1068·3); chlorpheniramine maleate (p.405·1).
Upper respiratory-tract symptoms.

Ryna-C *Wallace, USA.*
Pseudoephedrine hydrochloride (p.1068·3); chlorpheniramine maleate (p.405·1); codeine phosphate (p.26·1).
Coughs and cold symptoms.

Rynacrom
Rhone-Poulenc Rorer, Austral.; Rhone-Poulenc Rorer, Canad.; Rhone-Poulenc Rorer, Irl.; Rhone-Poulenc Rorer, S.Afr.; Pantheon, UK.
Sodium cromoglycate (p.762·1).
Allergic rhinitis.

Rynacrom Compound
Rhone-Poulenc Rorer, Irl.; Pantheon, UK.
Sodium cromoglycate (p.762·1); xylometazoline hydrochloride (p.1071·2).
Allergic rhinitis; nasal congestion.

Ryna-CX *Wallace, USA.*
Pseudoephedrine hydrochloride (p.1068·3); guaiphenesin (p.1061·3); codeine phosphate (p.26·1).
Coughs.

Rynatan *Wallace, USA.*
Phenylephrine tannate (p.1067·1); chlorpheniramine tannate (p.405·2); mepyramine tannate (p.414·1).
Cold symptoms.

Rynatuss *Wallace, USA.*
Pentoxyverine tannate (p.1066·2); chlorpheniramine tannate (p.405·2); ephedrine tannate (p.1060·1); phenylephrine tannate (p.1067·1).
Coughs.

Ryped *Propan, S.Afr.*
Erythromycin estolate (p.204·1).
Bacterial infections.

Rythmodan
Albert-Roussel, Aust.; Hoechst Marion Roussel, Austral.; Hoechst Marion Roussel, Belg.; Hoechst Marion Roussel, Canad.; Roussel, Fr.; Hoechst Marion Roussel, Irl.; Hoechst Marion Roussel, Neth.; Hoechst Marion Roussel, S.Afr.; Borg, UK.
Disopyramide (p.858·1) or disopyramide phosphate (p.858·1).
Arrhythmias.

Rythmodul *Albert-Roussel, Ger.; Hoechst, Ger.*
Disopyramide phosphate (p.858·1).
Arrhythmias.

Rythmol
Knoll, Canad.; Knoll, Fr.; Knoll, S.Afr.; Knoll, USA.
Propafenone hydrochloride (p.935·3).
Arrhythmias.

Rytmogenat *Azupharma, Ger.*
Propafenone hydrochloride (p.935·3).
Arrhythmias.

Rytmonorm
Knoll, Belg.; Knoll, Ger.; Knoll, Ital.; Knoll, Neth.; Knoll, Spain; Meda, Swed.; Knoll, Switz.
Propafenone hydrochloride (p.935·3).
Arrhythmias.

Rytmonorma *Ebewe, Aust.*
Propafenone hydrochloride (p.935·3).
Arrhythmias.

S-2 *Nephron, USA.*
Racepinephrine hydrochloride (p.815·2).
Bronchospasm.

S.8 *Chefaro, Ger.*
Diphenhydramine hydrochloride (p.409·1).
Sleep disorders.

S 13 *Salvat, Spain†.*
Silicone (p.1384·2); hexachlorophane (p.1115·2); isopropyl myristate; acedoben (p.1541·1); cinnamic acid.
Skin disorders.

S Amet *Europharma, Spain.*
Ademetionine (p.1543·1).
Depression; liver disorders.

Saave *Matrix, USA†.*
Amino acids; pyridoxal phosphate (p.1363·1).
Nutritional deficiencies.

SAB *Parke, Davis, Aust.*
Simethicone (p.1213·1); magnesium hydroxide (p.1198·2); aluminium hydroxide (p.1177·3).
Flatulence, dyspepsia; peptic ulcer.

SAB Simplex
Parke, Davis, Aust.; Parke, Davis, Ger.; Warner-Lambert, Switz.
Simethicone (p.1213·1).
Detergent intoxication; meteorism; reduction of intestinal gas before or after gastro-intestinal procedures.

Saba *Lampugnani, Ital.*
Saw palmetto (p.1462·1).
Prostatic hyperplasia.

Sabadilla Med Complex *Dynamit, Aust.*
Homoeopathic preparation.

Sabal *Ducray, Fr.*
Keluamid (p.1086·2); saw palmetto (p.1462·1); piroctone olamine (p.1089·1).
Seborrhoea.

Sabalia *Boiron, Canad.*
Homoeopathic preparation.

Sabalin *Lichtwer, UK.*
Saw palmetto (p.1462·1).
Male urinary discomfort.

Sabanotropico *Calmante Vitaminado, Spain.*
Bismuth subgallate (p.1180·2); dexamethasone disodium phosphate (p.1037·2); phenol (p.1121·2); sulphathiazole (p.257·1); tannic acid (p.1634·2); menthol (p.1600·2).
Skin disorders.

Sabatif *Apomedica, Aust.†.*
Simethicone (p.1213·1); activated charcoal (p.972·2); sulphur (p.1091·2); rhubarb (p.1212·1); senna leaf (p.1212·2); caraway oil (p.1559·3); fennel oil (p.1579·2).
Dyspepsia; flatulence; laxative.

Sabax Calcium *Sabax, S.Afr.†.*
Calcium gluconate (p.1155·2); calcium laevulinate (p.1155·2); calcium D-saccharate (p.1557·1).
Calcium deficiency; hypocalcaemia; lead colic; tetany.

Sabax Fosenema *Adcock Ingram, S.Afr.*
Monobasic sodium phosphate (p.1159·3); dibasic sodium phosphate (p.1159·3).
Bowel evacuation.

Sabax Gentamix *Adcock Ingram, S.Afr.*
Gentamicin sulphate (p.212·1).
Bacterial infections.

Sabidal *Zyma, Belg.†.*
Choline theophyllinate (p.751·3).
Bronchospasm.

Sabidal Rectiol *Zyma, Ital.†.*
Theophylline (p.765·1).
Asthma; bronchospastic disorders.

Sabidal SR
Zyma, Ital.†; Zyma, UK†.
Choline theophyllinate (p.751·3).
Asthma; chronic bronchitis; emphysema.

Sabin *SK-RIT, Belg.*
An oral poliomyelitis vaccine (p.1528·2).
Active immunisation.

Sabortonic *Lasa, Spain†.*
Hydroxybenzylhypophosphorous acid; ascorbic acid; calcium gluceptate; glucose.
Tonic.

Sabril
Hoechst, Aust.; Hoechst Marion Roussel, Austral.; Hoechst Marion Roussel, Belg.; Hoechst Marion Roussel, Canad.; Marion Merrell, Fr.; Hoechst, Ger.; Hoechst Marion Roussel, Irl.; Corvi, Ital.; Yamanouchi, Neth.; Hoechst Marion Roussel, S.Afr.; Hoechst Marion Roussel, Switz.; Hoechst Marion Roussel, UK.
Vigabatrin (p.364·3).
Epilepsy.

Sabrilex
Astra, Norw.; Marion Merrell, Spain; Astra, Swed.
Vigabatrin (p.364·3).
Epilepsy.

Saburgen-N *Weber & Weber, Ger.*
Homoeopathic preparation.

Saburlan *Weber & Weber, Ger.†.*
Cucurbita (p.1569·1); saw palmetto (p.1462·1).
Benign prostatic hyperplasia.

S-A-C *Lannett, USA.*
Paracetamol (p.72·2); salicylamide (p.82·3); caffeine (p.749·3).
Pain.

S-Acide *Pharmascience, Fr.†.*
(Methoxy-3′-hydroxy-4′) benzal bis(thio-2-ethanol).
Skin disinfection.

Sacnel
Note. This name is used for preparations of different composition.
URPAC, Fr.†.
Cream: Sublimed sulphur (p.1091·2); dithiosalicylic acid (p.1081·3); hamamelis (p.1587·1); ethyl linoleate; menthol (p.1600·2); cholesterol (p.1383·3).
Acne.

URPAC, Fr.†; Teofarma, Ital.
Lotion: Sublimed sulphur (p.1091·2); dithiosalicylic acid (p.1081·3); zinc oxide (p.1096·2); titanium dioxide (p.1093·3); hamamelis (p.1587·1).
Acne; seborrhoeic dermatitis.

Sacolene *Monsanto, Fr.*
Methylenated milk proteins.
Diarrhoea.

Sacsol *Eagle, Austral.*
Hexane (p.1379·1); camphor (p.1557·2).
Surgical cement solvent for stoma patients.

Sacsol NF *Eagle, Austral.*
Trichloroethane (p.1381·2); camphor (p.1557·2).
Non-flammable surgical cement solvent for stoma patients.

Sadefen *Roche Nicholas, Spain.*
Ibuprofen (p.44·1).
Fever; inflammation; musculoskeletal, joint, and peri-articular disorders; pain.

Saf-Clens *Calgon Vestal, USA.*
Wound cleanser.

Safe Tussin 30 *Kramer, USA.*
Guaiphenesin (p.1061·3); dextromethorphan hydrobromide (p.1057·3).
Coughs.

Safeway Cough Lozenges Sutton, Canad.
Menthol (p.1600·2).

Sagamicin Kyowa, Jpn.
Micronomicin sulphate (p.226·2).
Bacterial infections.

Sagamicina Allergan, Ital.
Micronomicin sulphate (p.226·2).
Bacterial eye infections.

Sagittacin N BASF, Ger.
Tetracycline hydrochloride (p.259·1).
Respiratory-tract infections.

Sagittacortin BASF, Ger.
Hydrocortisone (p.1043·3) or hydrocortisone acetate (p.1043·3).
Skin disorders.

Sagittamuc BASF, Ger.
Ambroxol hydrochloride (p.1054·3); doxycycline hydrochloride (p.202·3).
Respiratory-tract infections.

Sagittaproct BASF, Ger.
Injection: Quinine dihydrochloride (p.439·1).
Haemorrhoids.
Suppositories; ointment: Hamamelis (p.1587·1); bismuth subgallate (p.1180·2).
Haemorrhoids.
Topical gel: Lignocaine hydrochloride (p.1293·2).
Local anaesthesia.

Sagittaproct S BASF, Ger.
Laureth 9 (p.1325·2); zinc oxide (p.1096·2); bismuth subnitrate (p.1180·2).
Haemorrhoids.

Sagrada-Lax Folqui, Ital.
Cascara sagrada (p.1183·1).
Constipation.

Sagrosept Schulke & Mayr, Ger.
Lotion: Isopropyl alcohol (p.1118·2); propyl alcohol (p.1124·2); lactic acid (p.1593·3).
Medicated wipes: Isopropyl alcohol (p.1118·2); propyl alcohol (p.1124·2); benzoic acid (p.1102·3); lactic acid (p.1593·3).
Skin disinfection; surface disinfection.

Sagrotan Med Schulke & Mayr, Ger.
Benzalkonium chloride (p.1101·3).
Skin and wound disinfection.

Saintbois nouvelle formule Vifor, Switz.
Ethylmorphine hydrochloride (p.36·1); potassium guaiacolsulfonate (p.1068·3); sodium benzoate (p.1102·3); belladonna (p.457·1); hyssopus officinalis; tolu balsam (p.1071·1).
Coughs; respiratory-tract disorders.

Saizen
Serono, Aust.; Serono, Austral.; Serono, Belg.†; Serono, Canad.; Serono, Fr.; Serono, Ger.; Serono, Irl.; Serono, Ital.; Serono, Norw.; Research Labs, S.Afr.; Serono, Spain; Serono, Swed.; Serono, Switz.; Serono, UK.
Somatropin (p.1249·3).
Growth failure due to renal failure; growth hormone deficiency; Turner's syndrome.

Sal de Frutas Eno SmithKline Beecham, Spain.
Citric acid (p.1564·3); sodium bicarbonate (p.1153·2); sodium carbonate (p.1630·2).
Gastro-intestinal disorders.

Salac
GenDerm, Canad.; GenDerm, USA.
Salicylic acid (p.1090·2).
Acne.

Sal-Acid Pedinol, USA.
Salicylic acid (p.1090·2).
Hyperkeratosis.

Salact Knoll, Austral.
Salicylic acid (p.1090·2).
Acne.

Salactic Film Pedinol, USA.
Salicylic acid (p.1090·2).
Verrucas.

Salactol
Dermal Laboratories, Irl.; Dermal Laboratories, UK.
Salicylic acid (p.1090·2); lactic acid (p.1593·3); flexible collodion.
Calluses; corns; verrucas; warts.

Salagen
Chiron, Irl.; Chiron, Neth.; Chiron, UK; MGI, USA.
Pilocarpine hydrochloride (p.1396·3).
Dry mouth.

Salagesic Blackmores, Austral.
Salix (p.82·3); wood betony; cimicifuga (p.1563·3); amino acids and minerals.
Pain.

Salamol Norton, UK.
Salbutamol (p.758·2) or salbutamol sulphate (p.758·2).
Asthma; bronchospasm.

Salatac
Dermal Laboratories, Irl.; Dermal Laboratories, UK.
Salicylic acid (p.1090·2); lactic acid (p.1593·3).
Calluses; corns; verrucas; warts.

Salazopyrin
Pharmacia Upjohn, Aust.; Pharmacia Upjohn, Austral.; Pharmacia Upjohn, Canad.; Pharmacia Upjohn, Irl.; Pharmacia Upjohn, Ital.; Pharmacia Upjohn, Norw.; Pharmacia Upjohn, S.Afr.; Pharmacia Upjohn, Swed.; Pharmacia Upjohn, Switz.; Pharmacia Upjohn, UK.
Sulphasalazine (p.1215·2).
Inflammatory bowel disease; pyoderma gangrenosum; rheumatoid arthritis.

Salazopyrina Pharmacia Upjohn, Spain.
Sulphasalazine (p.1215·2).
Proctitis; ulcerative colitis.

Salazopyrine
Pharmacia Upjohn, Belg.; Pharmacia Upjohn, Fr.; Pharmacia Upjohn, Neth.
Sulphasalazine (p.1215·2).
Inflammatory bowel disease; rheumatoid arthritis.

Salbei-Halspastillen Globopharm, Aust.
Sage oil; calcium pantothenate (p.1352·3); chlorhexidine hydrochloride (p.1107·2).
Mouth and throat disorders.

Salbu BASF, Ger.; Orion, Ger.
Salbutamol (p.758·2) or salbutamol sulphate (p.758·2).
Obstructive airways disease.

Salbufax Master Pharma, Ital.
Salbutamol sulphate (p.758·2).
Asthma; bronchospastic disorders.

Salbuhexal Hexal, Ger.
Salbutamol (p.758·2) or salbutamol sulphate (p.758·2).
Obstructive airways disease.

Salbulair 3M, Ger.; Asta Medica, Ger.
Salbutamol sulphate (p.758·2).
Obstructive airways disease.

Salbulin
3M, S.Afr.; 3M, UK.
Salbutamol (p.758·2).
Obstructive airways disease.

Salbumol Glaxo Wellcome, Fr.
Salbutamol sulphate (p.758·2).
Asthma; premature labour.

Salbutard Lusofarmaco, Ital.
Salbutamol sulphate (p.758·2).
Asthma; bronchospastic disorders.

Salbuvent
Nycomed, Norw.; Tillotts, UK†.
Salbutamol (p.758·2) or salbutamol sulphate (p.758·2).
Obstructive airways disease.

Salcacam Salvat, Spain.
Piroxicam (p.80·2).
Gout; musculoskeletal, joint, and peri-articular disorders; pain.

Salcatyn Ibirn, Ital.†.
Salcatonin (p.735·3).
Paget's disease of bone; postmenopausal osteoporosis.

Salcedogen Fardi, Spain.
Citric acid (p.1564·3); magnesium chloride (p.1157·2); sodium bicarbonate (p.1153·2); sodium citrate (p.1153·2); mannitol (p.900·3).
Constipation; hepatobiliary disorders; hypomagnesaemia; lithiasis; uric acidaemia.

Salcedol Fardi, Spain.
Potassium sulphate (p.1161·2); sodium bicarbonate (p.1153·2); sodium sulphate (p.1213·3); tartaric acid (p.1634·3).
Gastro-intestinal disorders; hepatobiliary disorders.

Salcemetic Fardi, Spain.
Cyclobutyrol (p.1569·2); metoclopramide hydrochloride (p.1200·3); mannitol (p.900·3).
Gastro-intestinal disorders.

Sal-Clens C & M, USA.
Salicylic acid (p.1090·2).
Acne.

Saldac Douglas, Austral.
Sulindac (p.86·3).
Musculoskeletal and joint disorders; pain with inflammation.

Saldeva Roche Nicholas, Spain.
Caffeine (p.749·3); dimenhydrinate (p.408·2); paracetamol (p.72·2).
Dysmenorrhoea.

Sale Misura Plasmon, Ital.†.
Low sodium dietary salt substitute.

Sale Sohn Antonetto, Ital.†.
Low sodium dietary salt substitute.

Sales de Frutas P G Perez Gimenez, Spain.
Citric acid (p.1564·3); sodium bicarbonate (p.1153·2); tartaric acid (p.1634·3).
Gastro-intestinal disorders.

Sales de Frutas Verkos Verkos, Spain†.
Potassium acetotartrate; sodium bicarbonate (p.1153·2); sodium citrate (p.1153·2); sodium tartrate (p.1214·1); tartaric acid (p.1634·3).
Gastro-intestinal disorders.

Sales Fruta Mag Viviar Viviar, Spain.
Magnesium carbonate (p.1198·1); sodium bicarbonate (p.1153·2); tartaric acid (p.1634·3).
Gastro-intestinal disorders.

Sales Gras Quimifar, Spain†.
Silicic acid (p.1474·3); aluminium sulphate (p.1548·1); ferric sulphate.
Skin disorders.

Sales Orto Normon, Spain.
Citric acid (p.1564·3); sodium bicarbonate (p.1153·2); tartaric acid (p.1634·3).
Gastro-intestinal disorders.

Saleto Roberts, USA.
Paracetamol (p.72·2); aspirin (p.16·1); salicylamide (p.82·3); caffeine (p.749·3).
The name Saleto is also used for a preparation containing ibuprofen.
Pain.

Saleto-200, -400, -600, -800 Roberts, USA.
Ibuprofen (p.44·1).
The name Saleto is also used for a preparation containing paracetamol, aspirin, salicylamide, and caffeine.
Fever; osteoarthritis; pain; rheumatoid arthritis.

Saleto-D Roberts, USA.
Phenylpropanolamine hydrochloride (p.1067·2); paracetamol (p.72·2); caffeine (p.749·3); salicylamide (p.82·3).
Upper respiratory-tract symptoms.

Saleton Syntex, Spain†.
Diphenoxylate hydrochloride (p.1189·1); furazolidone (p.583·1); neomycin sulphate (p.229·2).
Atropine sulphate (p.455·1) is included in this preparation to discourage abuse.
Diarrhoea.

Salflex Carnrick, USA.
Salsalate (p.83·1).
Fever; osteoarthritis; pain; rheumatoid arthritis.

Salf-Pas Salf, Ital.
Sodium aminosalicylate (p.151·1).
Tuberculosis.

Salgydal a la noramidopyrine Doms-Adrian, Fr.
Dipyrone (p.35·1); paracetamol (p.72·2); codeine phosphate (p.26·1).
Pain.

Salhumin
Note. This name is used for preparations of different composition.
Schoeller, Aust.; Bastian, Switz.†.
Bath additive: Sodium humate; salicylic acid (p.1090·2).
Rheumatic disorders.

Schoeller, Aust.
Liniment: Sodium humate; capsicum (p.1559·2); salicylic acid (p.1090·2); eucalyptus oil (p.1578·1); rosemary oil (p.1626·2); turpentine oil (p.1641·1); camphor (p.1557·2).
Circulatory disorders; muscle, joint, and nerve pain.

Salhumin Gel N Bastian, Ger.
Glycol salicylate (p.43·1); benzyl nicotinate (p.22·1); camphor (p.1557·2).
Neuralgia; peripheral vascular disorders; rheumatism; sports injuries.

Salhumin Rheuma-Bad Bastian, Ger.
Salicylic acid (p.1090·2); sodium humate.
Bath additive; musculoskeletal and joint disorders.

Salhumin Sitzbad Bastian, Ger.
Salicylic acid (p.1090·2); sodium humate.
Bath additive; gynaecological disorders.

Salhumin Teilbad N Bastian, Ger.
Salicylic acid (p.1090·2); sodium humate; esculoside (p.1543·3).
Bath additive; circulatory disorders.

Sali Catapresan Boehringer Ingelheim, Spain†.
Cyclothiazide (p.845·3); clonidine hydrochloride (p.841·2).
Hypertension.

Sali Chianciano Epatobiliari Terme di Chianciano, Ital.†.
Sodium sulphate (p.1213·3); sodium bicarbonate (p.1153·2); magnesium sulphate (p.1157·3).
Liver disorders.

Sali Ciccarelli Ciccarelli, Ital.†.
Mineral salt preparation.
Astringent footbath.

Sali D'Achille Terme di Salsomaggiore, Ital.
Mineral salt preparation.
Sore feet.

Sali di Salsomaggiore Terme di Salsomaggiore, Ital.
Mineral salt preparation.
Gynaecological disorders; mouth and throat disorders.

Sali Iodati di Montecatini Terme di Montecatini, Ital.
Mineral salt preparation.
Constipation.

Sali Lassativi di Chianciano Terme di Chianciano, Ital.
Mineral salt preparation.
Constipation; digestive-system disorders.

Sali Tamerici di Montecatini Terme di Montecatini, Ital.
Mineral salt preparation.
Constipation.

Sali-Adalat Bayer, Ger.
Nifedipine (p.916·2); mefruside (p.902·2).
Hypertension.

Sali-Aldopur
Kwizda, Aust.; Hormosan, Ger.
Spironolactone (p.946·1); bendrofluazide (p.827·3).
Hyperaldosteronism; hypertension; hypokalaemia; liver cirrhosis and ascites; oedema.

Salicairine Aerocid, Fr.
Salicaria.
Formerly contained salicaria and iron hydrate.
Diarrhoea.

Salicilato Attivato Ana Delalande, Ital.†.
Sodium salicylate (p.85·1); calcium chloride (p.1155·1); magnesium thiosulphate (p.996·3).
Musculoskeletal and joint disorders; pain.

Salicylin-P Key, Austral.†.
Salicylic acid (p.1090·2); podophyllum resin (p.1089·1).
Warts.

Sali-Decoderm
Merck, Aust.; Hermal, Ger.
Fluprednidene acetate (p.1042·2); salicylic acid (p.1090·2).
Scalp disorders (tincture); skin disorders.

Salidex Braun, Norw.
Anhydrous glucose (p.1343·3); sodium chloride (p.1162·2).
Carbohydrate source; fluid and electrolyte disorders.

Salidur Almirall, Spain.
Frusemide (p.871·1); triamterene (p.957·2).
Hypertension; oedema.

Salient Biomedica, Ital.†.
Ketoprofen (p.48·2).
Inflammation; musculoskeletal and joint disorders; pain.

Saliject Omega, Canad.†.
Sodium salicylate (p.85·1).
Sclerotherapy.

Salilax Orion, Swed.
Light magnesium oxide (p.1198·3).
Bowel evacuation.

Salimar-Bad L Li-il, Ger.
Sodium salicylate (p.85·1); salicylic acid (p.1090·2).
Bath additive; musculoskeletal and joint disorders.

Salinex
Charton, Canad.; Muro, USA.
Sodium chloride (p.1162·2).
Nasal hygiene.

Salinol Charton, Canad.
Macrogol (p.1597·3); propylene glycol (p.1622·1).
Nasal lubricant.

Salipran Evans, Fr.
Benorylate (p.21·2).
Fever; pain.

Sali-Prent Bayer, Ger.
Acebutolol hydrochloride (p.809·3); mefruside (p.902·2).
Hypertension.

Sali-Presinol Bayer, Ger.
Methyldopa (p.904·2); mefruside (p.902·2).
Hypertension.

Sali-Puren Isis Puren, Ger.
Triamterene (p.957·2); hydrochlorothiazide (p.885·2).
Heart failure; hypertension; oedema.

Sali-Raufuncton Minden, Ger.†.
Rauwolfia vomitoria; benzthiazide (p.828·1); squill; convallaria; oleander; adonis vernalis; potassium aspartate.
Hypertension.

Salirheuman Molimin, Ger.†.
Glycol salicylate (p.43·1); benzyl nicotinate (p.22·1); nonivamide (p.63·2).
Arthritis; frostbite; neuritis; neuromuscular pain.

Salisofar Clismi Sofar, Ital.†.
Mesalazine (p.1199·2).
Inflammatory bowel disease.

Sali-Spiroctan Boehringer Mannheim, Switz.
Spironolactone (p.946·1); buthiazide (p.835·2).
Hyperaldosteronism.

Salistoperm Ursapharm, Ger.
Salicylamide (p.82·3); benzocaine (p.1286·2).
Musculoskeletal, joint, peri-articular, and soft-tissue disorders; neuralgia.

Salisulf Gastroprotetto Giuliani, Ital.†.
Sulphasalazine (p.1215·2).
Crohn's disease; ulcerative colitis.

Salitanol Estreptomicina Quimpe, Spain.
Albumin tannate (p.1176·3); dihydrostreptomycin sulphate (p.202·2); sulphathiazole (p.257·1).
Gastro-intestinal infections.

Saliton Planta, Canad.
Salix (p.82·3).
Fever; pain.

Saliva Orthana
Note. This name is used for preparations of different composition.
Delta, Austral.†.
Mucins (p.1472·3); xylitol (p.1372·3); electrolytes (p.1147·1).
Saliva substitute.

Nycomed, UK.
Lozenges: Mucin (p.1472·3); xylitol (p.1372·3).
Oral spray: Mucin (p.1472·3); xylitol (p.1372·3); sodium fluoride (p.742·1).
Saliva substitute.

Salivace Penn, UK.
Carmellose sodium (p.1471·2); xylitol (p.1372·3); electrolytes (p.1147·1).
Dry mouth.

Salivart
Gebauer, Canad.; Gebauer, USA.
Carmellose sodium (p.1471·2); electrolytes (p.1147·1); sorbitol (p.1354·2).
Dry mouth.

Saliveze Wyvern, UK.
Electrolytes (p.1147·1).
Dry mouth.

Salivin Kabi, Swed.†.
Malic acid (p.1598·3); xylitol (p.1372·3).
Saliva stimulation.

Salivix Thames, UK.
Acacia (p.1470·2); malic acid (p.1598·3).
Salivary stimulant.

Salix Scandinavian Natural Health & Beauty, USA.
Artificial saliva.

Salmagne Fardi, Spain.
Magnesium citrate (p.1198·2); magnesium sulphate (p.1157·3); sodium bicarbonate (p.1153·2); tartaric acid (p.1634·3); mannitol (p.900·3).
Gastro-intestinal disorders.

Salmetedur Menarini, Ital.
Salmeterol xinafoate (p.761·2).
Bronchospastic disorders.

Salmocalcin Ripari-Gero, Ital.
Salcatonin (p.735·3).
Hypercalcaemia; osteoporosis; Paget's disease of bone; reflex sympathetic dystrophy.

Salmofar Lafare, Ital.
Salcatonin (p.735·3).
Hypercalcaemia; osteoporosis; Paget's disease of bone; reflex sympathetic dystrophy.

Salmundin Mundipharma, Ger.
Salbutamol (p.758·2) or salbutamol sulphate (p.758·2).
Obstructive airways disease.

Salocol Hauck, USA.
Aspirin (p.16·1); paracetamol (p.72·2); salicylamide (p.82·3); caffeine (p.749·3).
Pain.

Salodiur Gerot, Aust.
Triamterene (p.957·2); hydrochlorothiazide (p.885·2).
Hypertension; oedema.

Salofalk
Merck, Aust.; Axcan, Canad.; Falk, Ger.; Antigen, Irl.; Knoll, Ital.; Falk, Neth.; Falk, Switz.; Thames, UK.
Mesalazine (p.1199·2).
Inflammatory bowel disease.

Sal-Oil-T Syosset, USA.
Coal tar (p.1092·3); salicylic acid (p.1090·2).
Seborrhoea.

Salomol
Wolfs, Belg.†; Clonmel, Irl.
Salbutamol (p.758·2) or salbutamol sulphate (p.758·2).
Obstructive airways disease.

Salonair Salonpas, UK.
Methyl salicylate (p.55·2); *l*-menthol (p.1600·2); *d*-camphor (p.1557·2); benzyl nicotinate (p.22·1); glycol salicylate (p.43·1).
Muscle and joint pain.

Salongo Biosarto, Spain.
Oxiconazole nitrate (p.386·3).
Fungal skin infections.

Salonpas Farmila, Ital.
Liniment†: Menthol (p.1600·2); camphor (p.1557·2); thymol (p.1127·1); methyl salicylate (p.55·2).
Medicated bandage: Menthol (p.1600·2); methyl salicylate (p.55·2); camphor (p.1557·2); glycol salicylate (p.43·1); thymol (p.1127·1).
Topical spray: Methyl salicylate (p.55·2); menthol (p.1600·2); camphor (p.1557·2); benzyl nicotinate (p.22·1); glycol salicylate (p.43·1).
Bruises; musculoskeletal and joint pain.

Salphenyl Roberts, USA; Hauck, USA.
Phenylephrine hydrochloride (p.1066·2); paracetamol (p.72·2); chlorpheniramine maleate (p.405·1); salicylamide (p.82·3).
Upper respiratory-tract symptoms.

Sal-Plant Pedinol, USA.
Salicylic acid (p.1090·2).
Hyperkeratosis.

Salseb Draxis, Canad.
Salicylic acid (p.1090·2).

Salsitab Upsher-Smith, USA.
Salsalate (p.83·1).
Fever; inflammation; pain.

Salsyvase Ipex, Swed.
Salicylic acid (p.1090·2).
Formerly known as Salicylsyrevaselin.
Skin disorders.

Saltadol Lindopharm, Ger.
Potassium chloride; sodium chloride; sodium bicarbonate; glucose (p.1152·3).
Diarrhoea; oral rehydration therapy.

Saltermox Propan, S.Afr.
Amoxycillin (p.151·3).
Bacterial infections.

Salterpyn Propan, S.Afr.
Syrup: Paracetamol (p.72·2); codeine phosphate (p.26·1); promethazine hydrochloride (p.416·2).
Fever; pain.
Tablets: Paracetamol (p.72·2); codeine phosphate (p.26·1); caffeine (p.749·3); meprobamate (p.678·1).
Pain with tension.

Saltrates Uhlmann-Eyraud, Switz.
Cream: Triclosan (p.1127·2); methylchloroisothiazolinone (p.1118·3); menthol (p.1600·2); chamomile oil; hypericum oil (p.1590·1); melissa oil; lavender oil (p.1594·3).
Dry or painful feet.
Topical gel: Sodium hydroxide (p.1631·1); trometamol (p.1639·3).
Calluses; corns.

Saltrates Rodell Uhlmann-Eyraud, Switz.
Chamomile (p.1561·2); hypericum (p.1590·1); sodium bicarbonate (p.1153·2); anhydrous sodium carbonate (p.1630·2); sodium sesquicarbonate; sodium perborate (p.1125·2).
Foot disorders.

Sal-Tropine Hope, USA.
Atropine sulphate (p.455·1).

Saltucin
Boehringer Mannheim, Aust.; Boehringer Mannheim, Ger.
Buthiazide (p.835·2).
Diabetes insipidus; heart failure; hypertension; oedema; renal calculi.

Saltucin Co Boehringer Mannheim, S.Afr.†.
Buthiazide (p.835·2); reserpine (p.942·1); rescinnamine (p.942·1); raubasine (p.941·3); potassium chloride (p.1161·1).
Hypertension.

Salube Colgate Oral Care, Austral.
Artificial saliva.
Reduced salivary flow.

Saludopin SIT, Ital.
Methyldopa (p.904·2); buthiazide (p.835·2).
Hypertension.

Salures Pharmacia Upjohn, Swed.
Bendrofluazide (p.827·3).
Hypertension; oedema; renal calculi.

Salures-K Pharmacia Upjohn, Swed.
Bendrofluazide (p.827·3); potassium chloride (p.1161·1).
Hypertension; oedema; renal calculi.

Saluretin Zeneca, Switz.
Spironolactone (p.946·1); bendrofluazide (p.827·3).
Hyperaldosteronism; hypertension; oedema.

Saluric
Merck Sharp & Dohme, Irl.; Merck Sharp & Dohme, UK.
Chlorothiazide (p.839·1).
Hypertension; oedema.

Saluron Apothecon, USA.
Hydroflumethiazide (p.889·2).
Hypertension; oedema.

Salus Salushaus, Ger.
Rad. harpagophyti (p.27·2).
Tonic.

Salus Abfuhr-Tee Nr. 2 Salushaus, Ger.
Rose fruit (p.1365·2); chamomile (p.1561·2); calendula officinalis; buckthorn (p.1182·1); senna (p.1212·2); fennel (p.1579·1).
Constipation.

Salus Augenschutz-Kapseln Salushaus, Ger.
Myrtillus (p.1606·1); vitamin A palmitate (p.1359·2); riboflavine sodium phosphate (p.1362·1).
Hypersensitivity to light; nightblindness.

Salus Bronchial-Tee Nr.8 Salushaus, Ger.
Fennel (p.1579·1); calendula officinalis; lichen islandicus; verbascum; tilia (p.1637·3); primula flower; lamium album; thyme (p.1636·3); polygonum aviculare; raspberry leaf (p.1624·2).
Coughs and associated respiratory-tract disorders.

Salus Herz-Schutz-Kapseln Salushaus, Ger.
Crataegus (p.1568·2); alpha tocopheryl acetate (p.1369·2); magnesium complex with acid hydrolysate of maize starch.
Tonic.

Salus Kurbis-Tonikum Compositum Salushaus, Ger.†.
Cucurbita (p.1569·1); urtica (p.1642·3); dried bitter-orange peel (p.1610·3); poplar (p.1620·1); saw palmetto (p.1462·1); wheatgerm; buchu (p.1555·2); echinacea angustifolia (p.1574·2); vitamins.
Prostatic disorders.

Salus Leber-Galle-Tee Nr.18 Salushaus, Ger.
Cynara (p.1569·2); fennel (p.1579·1); chamomile (p.1561·2); taraxacum (p.1634·2); stoechados; calendula officinalis; achillea (p.1542·2); peppermint leaf (p.1208·1).
Liver and biliary disorders.

Salus Multi-Vitamin-Energetikum Salushaus, Ger.
Multivitamin preparation with plant extracts.

Salus Nerven-Schlaf-Tee Nr.22 Salushaus, Ger.
Chamomile (p.1561·2); bellis perrenis; paeonia officinalis; stoechados; fennel (p.1579·1); lupulus (p.1597·2); hypericum (p.1590·1); lavender (p.1594·3); melissa (p.1600·1); citrus sinensis.
Nervous disorders.

Salus Nieren-Blasen-Tee Nr.23 Salushaus, Ger.
Bearberry (p.1552·2); birch leaf (p.55·3); solidago virgaurea; calendula officinalis; centaurea cyanus; orthosiphon (p.1592·2); juniper (p.1592·2); equisetum (p.1575·1).
Diuretic.

Salus Rheuma-Tee Krautertee Nr. 12 Salushaus, Ger.
Birch leaf (p.55·3); urtica (p.1642·3); fennel (p.1579·1); taraxacum (p.1634·2); calendula officinalis; equisetum (p.1575·1); achillea (p.1542·2); juniper (p.1592·2).
Rheumatic disorders.

Salus Venen Krauter Dragees N Salushaus, Ger.
Aesculus (p.1543·3); melilotus.
Vascular disorders.

Salus Zinnkraut Salushaus, Ger.
Equisetum (p.1575·1).
Oedema.

Salusan Salushaus, Ger.
Crataegus (p.1568·2); mistletoe (p.1604·1); ammi visnaga fruit (p.1593·2); equisetum (p.1575·1); dried bitter-orange peel (p.1610·3); lemon peel; passion flower (p.1615·3); melissa (p.1600·1); valerian (p.1643·1); hypericum (p.1590·1); lupulus (p.1597·2); rosemary; cymbopogon citratus; bearberry (p.1552·2); wheat germ; tinct. germen. hordeoli.
Cardiovascular disorders.

Salus-Ol Salushaus, Ger.†.
Light liquid paraffin (p.1382·1).
Constipation; inflammatory bowel disease.

Salutensin Roberts, USA.
Hydroflumethiazide (p.889·2); reserpine (p.942·1).
Hypertension.

Salva Infantes Camps, Spain.
Magnesium carbonate (p.1198·1); magnesium sulphate (p.1157·3); betanaphthyl benzoate (p.98·3).
Gastro-intestinal disorders.

Salvacam Salvat, Spain.
Piroxicam (p.80·2).
Gout; musculoskeletal, joint, peri-articular, and soft-tissue disorders; pain.

Salvacolina Salvat, Spain.
Albumin tannate (p.1176·3); opium (p.70·3).
Formerly contained albumin tannate, dihydrostreptomycin sulphate, neomycin sulphate, opium, and papaverine hydrochloride.
Diarrhoea.

Salvacolina NN Salvat, Spain†.
Aluminium hydroxide (p.1177·3); atropine sulphate (p.455·1); hyoscyamine hydrobromide (p.464·2); neomycin sulphate (p.229·2); pectin (p.1474·1); aluminium glycinate (p.1177·2).
Gastro-intestinal infections.

Salvacolon Salvat, Spain.
Bacillus subtilis; vitamins and amino acids.
Cystitis; gastro-intestinal disorders; restoration of the gastro-intestinal flora.

Salvalion Normon, Spain.
Raubasine (p.941·3); almitrine (p.1477·2).
Cerebrovascular disorders; vestibular disorders.

Salvapen Salvat, Spain.
Amoxycillin trihydrate (p.151·3).
Bacterial infections.

Salvapen Mucolitico Salvat, Spain.
Amoxycillin trihydrate (p.151·3); bromhexine hydrochloride (p.1055·3).
Respiratory-tract infections.

Salvarina Salvat, Spain.
Caffeine (p.749·3); dimenhydrinate (p.408·2); ibuprofen (p.44·1).
Dysmenorrhoea.

Salvatrim Salvat, Spain.
Co-trimoxazole (p.196·3).
Bacterial infections.

Salvent Wolff, Ger.
Salbutamol (p.758·2).
Obstructive airways disease.

Salvesept Cederroth, Spain.
Alcohol (p.1099·1); chlorhexidine hydrochloride (p.1107·2).
Wound disinfection.

Salvi Cal E-G Baxter, Ger.
Glucose and electrolyte infusion.
Parenteral nutrition.

Salvi Cal GX Baxter, Ger.
Glucose monohydrate (p.1343·3); xylitol (p.1372·3).
Parenteral nutrition.

Salviamin Baxter, Ger.
A range of amino-acid, carbohydrate, and electrolyte infusions.
Parenteral nutrition.

Salviamin Hepar Baxter, Ger.
Amino-acid and electrolyte infusion.
Parenteral nutrition in liver disease.

Salviathymol N Galenika, Ger.
Sage oil; eucalyptus oil (p.1578·1); peppermint oil (p.1208·1); cinnamon oil (p.1564·2); clove oil (p.1565·2); fennel oil (p.1579·2); anise oil (p.1550·1); menthol (p.1600·2); thymol (p.1127·1).
Inflammatory disorders of the oropharynx.

Salviette H Whitehall, Ital.
Hamamelis water (p.1587·1); glycerol (p.1585·2).
Anal cleansing; haemorrhoids.

Salvilipid Baxter, Ger.
Soya oil (p.1355·1).
Contains egg lecithin.
Lipid infusion for parenteral nutrition.

Salvital Reckitt & Colman, Austral.
Magnesium sulphate (p.1157·3); sodium bicarbonate (p.1153·2); tartaric acid (p.1634·3).
Dyspepsia; nausea.

Salvituss FIRMA, Ital.
Levodropopizine (p.1059·2).
Coughs.

Salvizol med Hydrocortison A.L., Norw.†.
Dequalinium chloride (p.1112·1); hydrocortisone (p.1043·3).
Infected skin disorders.

Salvstrumpa Perstorp, Swed.
Zinc oxide (p.1096·2).
Skin ulcers; vascular disorders.

Salvyl Petrasch, Aust.
Undecenoic acid (p.389·2) sulphur (p.1091·2) complex; betanaphthol (p.98·3); salicylic acid (p.1090·2).
Acne; erythrasma; fungal skin infections.

Salvysat
Mayrhofer, Aust.; Ysatfabrik, Ger.
Sage leaf (p.1627·1).
Hyperhidrosis; mouth and throat inflammation.

Salycad Ducray, Fr.†.
Cade oil (p.1092·2); salicylic acid (p.1090·2); aluminium allantoinate.
Seborrhoea.

Salzone Wallace Mfg Chem., UK.
Paracetamol (p.72·2).
Fever; pain.

Samarin Sal de Frutas Cederroth, Spain†.
Sodium bicarbonate (p.1153·2); sodium carbonate (p.1630·2); disodium tartrate (p.1214·1); sodium potassium tartrate (p.1213·3).
Gastro-intestinal disorders.

Sambil Lacer, Spain.
Boldine (p.1554·1); hydroxymethylnicotinamide (p.1589·3).
Digestive-system disorders.

Sambuco (Specie Composta) Dynacren, Ital.; AFOM, Ital.
Tilia (p.1637·3); sambucus (p.1627·2); spiraea (p.1599·1); rose fruit (p.1365·2).
Respiratory-tract disorders.

Sambucus Complex Blackmores, Austral.
Sambucus (p.1627·2); euphrasia; echinacea angustifolia (p.1574·2); hydrastis (p.1588·2); euphorbia hirta; *d*-alpha tocopheryl acid succinate (p.1369·2); vitamin A acetate (p.1359·2).
Conjunctivitis; upper respiratory-tract disorders.

Samecin Savoma, Ital.†.
Doxycycline hydrochloride (p.202·3).
Bacterial infections.

Samedrin Savoma, Ital.†.
Cephradine (p.181·3).
Bacterial infections.

Same-Seb Savoma, Ital.
Colloidal sulphur (p.1091·2); salicylic acid (p.1090·2).
Acne; seborrhoea.

Samil-O_2 Samil, Ital.†.
Benzoyl peroxide (p.1079·2).
Skin disinfection.

Samilstin Novartis, Ital.
Octreotide (p.1255·2).
Acromegaly; diarrhoea associated with immunodeficiency; endocrinal tumours of the gastro-intestinal tract; pancreatic fistula; postoperative complications of pancreatic surgery.

Samyr Knoll, Ital.
Ademetionine sulphate tosylate (p.1543·1).
Depression.

Sanabex Farmatre, Ital.†.
Wild thyme; tolu balsam (p.1071·1); grindelia; cherry-laurel water.
Respiratory-tract disorders.

Sanabronchiol Falqui, Ital.
Dextromethorphan hydrobromide (p.1057·3).
Coughs.

Sanaden Reforzado Calmante Vitaminado, Spain.
Creosote (p.1057·3); benzocaine (p.1286·2); niaouli oil (p.1607·1).
Toothache.

Sanaderm Herbaline, Ital.
Echinacea (p.1574·2); calendula officinalis; viola tricolor; helichrysum italicum; bergamot oil (p.1553·1); lavender oil (p.1594·3); thyme oil (p.1637·1); geranium oil (p.1584·1).
Burns; skin irritation; wounds.

Sanadermil Vifor, Switz.
Hydrocortisone acetate (p.1043·3).
Skin disorders.

Sanadorn Jacoby, Aust.
Crataegus (p.1568·2).
Heart disorders.

Sanaform Esoform, Ital.
Benzalkonium chloride (p.1101·3).
Surface disinfection.

Sanalepsi N Roche, Switz.
Doxylamine succinate (p.410·1).
Hypersensitivity reactions; nervous disorders.

Sanalgin
Boehringer Ingelheim, Neth.; Gebro, Switz.
Paracetamol (p.72·2); propyphenazone (p.81·3); caffeine (p.749·3).
Fever; pain.

Sanalgit Gebro, Aust.†.
Paracetamol (p.72·2); propyphenazone (p.81·3); caffeine (p.749·3).
Fever; pain.

Sanalgutt-S Hormosan, Ger.†.
Phenazone (p.78·2); phosphoric acid.
Formerly contained phenazone, gelsemium, ignatia, belladonna, secale cornutum, caffeine, ascorbic acid, and phosphoric acid.
Fever; pain.

Sanamidol Inkeysa, Spain.
Omeprazole (p.1204·2).
Gastro-oesophageal reflux; peptic ulcer; Zollinger-Ellison syndrome.

Sanaprav Sankyo, Ital.
Pravastatin sodium (p.1277·1).
Arteriosclerosis; cardiovascular disorders; hypercholesterolaemia.

Sanasepton Yamanouchi, Ger.
Erythromycin (p.204·1), erythromycin estolate (p.204·1), or erythromycin ethyl succinate (p.204·2).
Bacterial infections.

Sanasma Serpero, Ital.†.
Reproterol hydrochloride (p.758·1).
Bronchopulmonary disorders.

Sanasthmax Glaxo Wellcome, Ger.
Beclomethasone dipropionate (p.1032·1).
Asthma; inflammatory respiratory-tract disorders.

Sanasthmyl Glaxo Wellcome, Ger.
Beclomethasone dipropionate (p.1032·1).
Asthma; inflammatory respiratory-tract disorders.

Sanatison Mono Parke, Davis, Ger.
Hydrocortisone (p.1043·3).
Burns; skin disorders.

Sanatogen
Key, Austral.; Roche Consumer, Irl.; Roche, S.Afr.; Roche Consumer, UK.
A range of vitamin, mineral, and nutritional preparations.

Sanato-Lax Hotz, Ger.†.
Liquid paraffin (p.1382·1).
Intestinal disorders.

Sanato-Lax-forte Hotz, Ger.†.
Liquid paraffin (p.1382·1); frangula (p.1193·2); cascara (p.1183·1); aloes (p.1177·1).
Bowel disorders.

Sanato-Rhev Hotz, Ger.
Camphor (p.1557·2); isopropyl alcohol (p.1118·2).
Muscle and joint pain; soft-tissue disorders; superficial circulatory disorders.

Sanatot SCAM, Ital.†.
Alkylaminoethylglycine hydrochloride (p.1112·3).
Surface disinfection.

Sanaven Luitpold, Ger.
A heparinoid (p.882·3); phenylephrine hydrochloride (p.1066·2).
Venous disorders.

Sanaven Venentabletten Luitpold, Ger.
Aesculus (p.1543·3).
Venous insufficiency.

Sanavitan S Bottger, Ger.
dl-Alpha tocopheryl acetate (p.1369·2).
Vitamin E deficiency.

Sanaxin Sanabo, Aust.
Cephalexin (p.178·2).
Bacterial infections.

Sanderson's Throat Specific Sandersons, UK.
Mixture: Acetic acid (p.1541·2); quassia (p.1624·1); squill (p.1070·1); capsicum (p.1559·2).
Pastilles: Honey (p.1345·3); squill vinegar (p.1070·1); capsicum (p.1559·2); tolu (p.1071·1); menthol (p.1600·2); cinnamic acid (p.1111·1); benzoic acid (p.1102·3); eucalyptus oil (p.1578·1).
Catarrh; sore throat.

Sandilax Lesvi, Spain†.
Plantago ovata (p.1194·2).
Constipation.

Sandimmun
Biochemie, Aust.; Sandoz, Aust.; Sanabo, Aust.; Novartis, Austral.; Sandoz, Belg.†; Sandoz, Fr.; Sandoz, Ger.; Sandoz, Irl.; Novartis, Ital.; Sandoz, Norw.; Novartis, S.Afr.; Sandoz, Spain; Novartis, Swed.; Sandoz, Switz.; Sandoz, UK.
Cyclosporin (p.519·1).
Atopic dermatitis; graft-versus-host disease; nephrotic syndrome; psoriasis; rheumatoid arthritis; transplant rejection; uveitis.

Sandimmune
Sandoz, Canad.; Novartis, Neth.; Sandoz, USA.
Cyclosporin (p.519·1).
Atopic dermatitis; graft-versus-host disease; nephrotic syndrome; psoriasis; rheumatoid arthritis; transplant rejection; uveitis.

Sandocal
Novartis, Austral.; Sandoz, Fr.; Sandoz, Irl.; Sandoz, UK.
Calcium lactate gluconate (p.1155·2); calcium carbonate (p.1182·1).
Hypocalcaemia; osteoporosis.

Sandoglobulin
Novartis, Austral.; Sandoz, Ger.; Sandoz, Irl.; Sandoz, Norw.; Sandoz, S.Afr.†; Novartis, Swed.; Novartis, UK; Sandoz, USA.
A normal immunoglobulin (p.1522·1).
Bone marrow transplantation; idiopathic thrombocytopenic purpura; immunodeficiency; Kawasaki disease; passive immunisation.

Sandoglobulina Sandoz, Ital.
A normal immunoglobulin (p.1522·1).
Idiopathic thrombocytopenic purpura; immunodeficiency; passive immunisation.

Sandoglobuline
Sandoz, Belg.; Sandoz, Fr.; Sandoz, Switz.
A normal immunoglobulin (p.1522·1).
Auto-immune disorders; hypogammaglobulinaemia; idiopathic thrombocytopenic purpura; Kawasaki disease; passive immunisation.

Sando-K
Sandoz, Irl.; Sandoz, UK.
Potassium bicarbonate (p.1153·1); potassium chloride (p.1161·1).
Hypokalaemia.

Sandolanid
Sandoz, Aust.; Sandoz, Ger.†.
Acetyldigoxin (p.812·3).
Arrhythmias.

Sandomigran
Sandoz, Aust.; Novartis, Austral.; Wander, Belg.; Sandoz, Canad.; Sandoz, Ger.; Sandoz, Ital.; Novartis, Neth.; Novartis, S.Afr.; Sandoz, Spain; Sandoz, Switz.†.
Pizotifen malate (p.449·1).
Migraine and other vascular headaches.

Sandomigrin
Sandoz, Norw.; Novartis, Swed.
Pizotifen malate (p.449·1).
Migraine and other vascular headaches.

Sandonorm
Sandoz, Aust.; Sandoz, Switz.
Bopindolol malonate (p.833·2).
Angina pectoris; hypertension.

Sandoparin Sandoz, Aust.
Certoparin sodium (p.839·1).
Thrombosis prophylaxis.

Sandoparine Sandoz, Switz.
Certoparin sodium (p.839·1).
Thrombosis prophylaxis.

Sandopart
Sandoz, Ital.; Sandoz, S.Afr.†; Sandoz, Switz.†.
Demoxytocin (p.1245·1).
Induction of labour; post-partum uterine involution; prevention of breast engorgement and mastitis; stimulation of lactation.

Sandopril Sandoz, Aust.
Spirapril hydrochloride (p.946·1).
Hypertension.

Sandoretic Sandoz, Switz.
Bopindolol malonate (p.833·2); chlorthalidone (p.839·3).
Hypertension.

Sandosource Wander, Ital.
Preparation for enteral nutrition.
Gastro-intestinal disorders.

Sandosource Peptide Sandoz Nutrition, Canad.
Preparation for enteral nutrition.

Sandostatin
Sandoz, Aust.; Novartis, Austral.; Sandoz, Canad.; Sandoz, Ger.; Sandoz, Irl.; Sandoz, Norw.; Novartis, S.Afr.; Sandoz, Spain; Novartis, Swed.; Novartis, UK; Sandoz, USA.
Octreotide (p.1255·2) or octreotide acetate (p.1255·1).
Acromegaly; AIDS-associated refractory diarrhoea; gastro-intestinal endocrine tumours; prevention of complications following pancreatic surgery.

Sandostatina Novartis, Ital.
Octreotide (p.1255·2).
Acromegaly; diarrhoea associated with immunodeficiency; endocrinal tumours of the gastro-intestinal tract; pancreatic fistulae; postoperative complications of pancreatic surgery.

Sandostatine
Sandoz, Belg.; Sandoz, Fr.; Novartis, Neth.; Sandoz, Switz.
Octreotide (p.1255·2) or octreotide acetate (p.1255·1).
Acromegaly; complications following pancreatic surgery; external fistulae of the pancreas and small intestine; gastro-intestinal neoplasms; refractory diarrhoea associated with HIV infection.

Sandothal Sandoz, S.Afr.†.
Thiopentone sodium (p.1233·1).
General anaesthesia.

Sandovac Sandoz, Aust.
An inactivated influenza vaccine (p.1515·2).
Active immunisation.

Sandoven
Sandoz, Aust.; Sandoz, Ital.†.
Dihydroergocristine mesylate (p.1571·3); esculoside (p.1543·3); rutin (p.1580·2).
Peripheral vascular disorders.

Sandovene Sandoz, S.Afr.†.
Dihydroergocristine (p.1571·3); esculoside (p.1543·3); rutin (p.1580·2).
Vascular disorders.

Sandovene f Sandoz, Switz.†.
Dihydroergocristine mesylate (p.1571·3); esculoside (p.1543·3); rutin (p.1580·2).
Vascular disorders.

Sandrena Organon, UK.
Oestradiol (p.1455·1).
Menopausal disorders.

Sandril Lilly, USA†.
Reserpine (p.942·1).

Sanein Prodes, Spain.
Aceclofenac (p.12·1).
Musculoskeletal, joint, and peri-articular disorders; pain.

Sanelor Chefaro, Belg.
Loratadine (p.413·1).
Allergic rhinitis; urticaria.

Sangen Casa Boots Healthcare, Ital.
Liquid: Benzethonium chloride (p.1102·3); benzalkonium chloride (p.1101·3).
Spray: Orthophenylphenol (p.1120·3); benzalkonium chloride (p.1101·3).
Surface disinfection.

Sangen Medical Boots, Ital.
Benzalkonium chloride (p.1101·3).
Personal hygiene.

Sangen Sapone Disinfettante Boots, Ital.
Triclocarban (p.1127·2).
Skin disinfection.

Sangenor Mundipharma, Aust.
Arginine aspartate (p.1334·2).
Tonic.

Sangerol Sandoz OTC, Switz.
Lignocaine hydrochloride (p.1293·2); muramidase hydrochloride (p.1604·3); tyrothricin (p.267·2).
Mouth and throat disorders.

Sanguisan N Coradol, Ger.
Homoeopathic preparation.

Sanguisorbis F Madaus, Ger.
Homoeopathic preparation.

Sangur-Test Boehringer Mannheim, Austral.
Test for blood in urine.

Sanhelios Capsules a la vitamine A Voigt, Switz.
Vitamin A palmitate (p.1359·2); wheat-germ oil.
Vitamin A deficiency.

Sanhelios Einschlaf Bregenzer, Aust.
Valerian root (p.1643·1); lupulus (p.1597·2).
Sleep disorders.

Sanhelios Leber-Galle Bregenzer, Aust.
Silybum marianum (p.993·3); turmeric (p.1001·3).
Digestive disorders; hepatobiliary disorders.

Sanhelios-Entwasserungsdragees Bregenzer, Aust.
Silver birch (p.1553·3).
Urinary-tract disorders.

Sanicel Squibb, Spain.
Amphotericin (p.372·2); tetracycline hydrochloride (p.259·1).
Vulvovaginal infections.

Sanicolax Sanico, Belg.
Phenolphthalein (p.1208·2); podophyllum (p.1089·1); aloin (p.1177·2); belladonna (p.457·1); hyoscyamus (p.464·3); nux vomica (p.1609·3).
Constipation.

Sanicopyrine Sanico, Belg.
Paracetamol (p.72·2).
Fever; pain.

Sanieb Puerto Galiano, Spain.
Glycine (p.1345·2); arginine (p.1334·1); brassica oleracea.
Gastro-intestinal disorders.

Sanifer Esseti, Ital.
Ferric sodium gluconate.
Anaemias; oligohaemia in infants.

Saniflor Dentifricio Esseti, Ital.
Benzydamine hydrochloride (p.21·3).
Gingivitis.

Saniflor Vena Esseti, Ital.
Benzydamine hydrochloride (p.21·3).
Peripheral vascular disorders.

Sanifolin Esseti, Ital.
Calcium folinate (p.1342·2).
Anaemias; antidote to folic acid antagonists; folate deficiency; reduction of aminopterin and methotrexate toxicity.

Sanifug Wolff, Ger.
Loperamide hydrochloride (p.1197·2).
Diarrhoea.

Sanipirina Bayropharm, Ital.†.
Paracetamol (p.72·2).
Fever; pain.

Sani-Supp G & W, USA.
Glycerol (p.1585·2).
Constipation.

Sanitube Sanitube, USA†.
Mercurous chloride (p.1601·3); hydroxyquinoline benzoate (p.1589·3).
Prevention of syphilis and gonorrhoea after sexual contact.

Sankombi Sanum-Kehlbeck, Ger.
Homoeopathic preparation.

Sanmigran Sandoz, Fr.
Pizotifen hydrochloride (p.449·2).
Migraine.

Sano Tuss Welti, Switz.
Emetine hydrochloride (p.582·2); ethylmorphine hydrochloride (p.36·1); ephedrine hydrochloride (p.1059·3); codeine phosphate (p.26·1); guaiphenesin (p.1061·3); cherry-laurel; tolu balsam (p.1071·1).
Catarrh; coughs.

Sano-Angin Amino, Switz.†.
Lignocaine hydrochloride (p.1293·2); chlorquinaldol (p.185·1).
Mouth and throat disorders.

Sanobamat Sanico, Belg.
Meprobamate (p.678·1).
Anxiety disorders; sleep disorders.

Sanocapt Sanol, Ger.†.
Aspirin (p.16·1).
Fever; pain.

Sanodin Byk Elmu, Spain.
Carbenoxolone sodium (p.1182·2).
Mouth ulcers.

Sanoformine Mayoly-Spindler, Fr.
Anhydrous copper sulphate (p.1338·1); sodium fluoride (p.742·1).
Disinfection of mucous membranes.

Sanogyl Pharmascience, Fr.
Pink toothpaste: Sodium monofluorophosphate (p.743·3); sodium fluoride (p.742·1).
White toothpaste: Sodium fluoride (p.742·1).
Formerly contained sodium fluoride and sodium monofluorophosphate.
Oral hygiene.

Sanogyl Bianco Berna, Ital.
Sodium monofluorophosphate (p.743·3); acetarsol sodium (p.578·2).
Gingivitis; oral hygiene.

Sanogyl Fluo Pharmascience, Fr.
Sodium monofluorophosphate (p.743·3); sodium fluoride (p.742·1).
Dental caries prophylaxis.

Sanogyl Junior Pharmascience, Fr.
Sodium monofluorophosphate (p.743·3); sodium fluoride (p.742·1).
Dental caries prophylaxis.

Sanoma Pierre Fabre, Ger.
Carisoprodol (p.1312·3).
Skeletal muscle spasm.

Sanomigran
Sandoz, Irl.; Sandoz, UK.
Pizotifen malate (p.449·1).
Migraine and other vascular headaches.

Sanopin N Wernigerode, Ger.†.
Conifer oil; camphor oil.
Respiratory-tract disorders.

Sanopinwern Wernigerode, Ger.
Eucalyptus oil (p.1578·1); oleum pini sylvestris.
Cold symptoms.

Sanoral
Note. This name is used for preparations of different composition.
Sanabo, Aust.
Tyrothricin (p.267·2); muramidase hydrochloride (p.1604·3); lignocaine hydrochloride (p.1293·2).
Mouth and throat inflammation.
Bioprogress, Ital.
Chlorhexidine gluconate (p.1107·2).
Mouth disinfection.

Sanorex
Sandoz, Austral.†; Sandoz, Canad.; Sandoz, Jpn; Sandoz, USA.
Mazindol (p.1482·1).
Obesity.

Sanostol Schmidgall, Aust.
Multivitamin preparation.

Sanovox Parisis, Spain†.
Aconite (p.1542·2); amylocaine hydrochloride (p.1286·1); sulphur (p.1091·2); borax (p.1554·2); sodium chlorate (p.1630·3).
Mouth and throat disorders.

Sanoxit Basotherm, Ger.
Benzoyl peroxide (p.1079·2).
Acne.

Sanox-N Chefaro, Neth.†.
Valerian (p.1643·1).
Nervous tension; nervousness.

Sans-Acne Galderma, Canad.
Erythromycin (p.204·1); alcohol (p.1099·1).
Acne.

Sansanal Rottapharm, Ger.
Captopril (p.836·3).
Heart failure; hypertension.

Sansert
Sandoz, Canad.; Sandoz, Swed.†; Sandoz, USA.
Methysergide maleate (p.448·1).
Vascular headache.

Sansion Colgate Oral Care, Austral.†.
A non-ionic phosphate-free equipment cleaning solution.

Sansudor Boehringer Ingelheim, Switz.
Aluminium chlorohydrex (p.1079·1).
Hyperhidrosis; intertrigo.

Santa Flora S Madaus, Ger.
Homoeopathic preparation.

Santaherba
Homeocan, Canad.; Lehning, Fr.
Homoeopathic preparation.

Santalyt Asche, Ger.
Sodium chloride; glucose; potassium chloride; sodium bicarbonate (p.1152·3).
Diarrhoea; oral rehydration therapy.

Santane A_4 Iphym, Fr.
Ulmaria flowers (p.1599·1); black currant leaf (p.1365·2); willow leaf (p.82·3); heather flowers; orange leaf; juniper berry (p.1592·2); chamomile flowers (p.1561·2); matricaria flowers (p.1561·2); vervain leaves.
Musculoskeletal disorders.

Santane C_6 Iphym, Fr.
Frangula bark (p.1193·2); senna leaf (p.1212·2); boldo leaf (p.1554·1); vervain leaf; peppermint leaf (p.1208·1); mallow flowers; cornflower flowers; pale rose flowers; caraway seed (p.1559·3).
Constipation.

Santane D_5 Iphym, Fr.
Melissa leaf (p.1600·1); origanum flowers; peppermint leaf (p.1208·1); fennel seed (p.1579·1); aniseed (p.1549·3); lupulus flowers (p.1597·2); matricaria flowers (p.1561·2); thyme flowers (p.1636·3); rosemary leaf; caraway seed (p.1559·3); cinnamon bark (p.1564·2).
Gastro-intestinal disorders.

Santane F_{10} Iphym, Fr.
Boldo leaf (p.1554·1); box leaf; peppermint leaf (p.1208·1); tetragonum leaf; marigold flowers; rosemary leaf; chamomile flowers (p.1561·2); caraway seed (p.1559·3); cinnamon bark (p.1564·2).
Hepato-biliary insufficiency.

Santane H_7 Iphym, Fr.
Mistletoe leaf (p.1604·1); olive leaf; crataegus flowers and leaf (p.1568·2); melilot flowers; marigold flowers; myrtillus berry (p.1606·1); peppermint leaf (p.1208·1); vervain leaves; broom flowers (p.1628·1); fennel seed (p.1579·1); sweet orange peel.
Hypertension.

Santane N_9 Iphym, Fr.
Tilia flowers (p.1637·3); crataegus flowers and leaves (p.1568·2); pale rose flowers; peppermint leaf (p.1208·1); melissa leaf (p.1600·1); bitter-orange leaves and buds; origanum flowers; lupulus flowers (p.1597·2); lavender flowers (p.1594·3).
Nervous disorders.

Santane O_1 Iphym, Fr.
Heather flowers; bearberry leaf (p.1552·2); peppermint leaf (p.1208·1); pulegium; ulmaria flowers (p.1599·1); rosemary leaf; mallow flowers; tilia flowers (p.1637·3); eucalyptus leaf (p.1578·1); laurel leaf; caraway seed (p.1559·3); bitter orange leaves.
Nutritional disorders.

Santane R_8 Iphym, Fr.
Bearberry leaf (p.1552·2); heather flowers; black currant leaf (p.1365·2); rosemary leaf; peppermint leaf (p.1208·1); broom flowers (p.1628·1); lavender flowers (p.1594·3); juniper berry (p.1592·2); thyme flowers

(p.1636·3); ulmaria flowers (p.1599·1); cinnamon bark (p.1564·2).
Kidney disorders.

Santane V_3 *Iphym, Fr.*
Artemisia leaf; peppermint leaf (p.1208·1); sage leaf (p.1627·1); crataegus flowers and leaf (p.1568·2); broom flowers (p.1628·1); green tea flowers (p.1645·1); cypress leaf; melilotus officinalis flower and leaf; sweet orange peel (p.1610·3); citrus aurantium leaf.
Vascular disorders.

Santasal N *Merckle, Ger.*
Aspirin (p.16·1).
Fever; pain.

Santasapina
Bioforce, Ger.; Bioforce, Switz.
Pine buds.
Upper-respiratory-tract disorders.

Santax S *Asche, Ger.*
Saccharomyces boulardii (p.1594·1).
Diarrhoea.

Santenol *Coop. Farm., Ital.*
Lefetamine hydrochloride (p.50·1).
Lignocaine hydrochloride (p.1293·2) is included in this preparation to alleviate the pain of injection.
Pain.

Santyl
Knoll, Canad.; Knoll, USA.
Collagenase (p.1566·3).
Debridement of dermal ulcers and severe burns.

Sanukehl D6 *Sanum-Kehlbeck, Ger.*
Homoeopathic preparation.

Sanuvis *Sanum-Kehlbeck, Ger.*
Homoeopathic preparation.

Sanvita Bronchial *Sanamed, Aust.*
Eucalyptus oil (p.1578·1); peppermint oil (p.1208·1); thyme oil (p.1637·1).
Catarrh; coughs.

Sanvita Enerlecit *Sanamed, Aust.*
Lecithin (p.1595·2); vitamins.
Tonic.

Sanvita Enerlecit-Tonikum mit Rosmarin *Sanamed, Aust.*
Lecithin (p.1595·2); rosemary.
Tonic.

Sanvita Herz *Sanamed, Aust.*
Crataegus (p.1568·2); rosemary.
Cardiovascular disorders.

Sanvita Leber-Galle *Sanamed, Aust.*
Cynara (p.1569·2); turmeric (p.1001·3).
Hepatobiliary disorders.

Sanvita Magen *Sanamed, Aust.*
Ginger (p.1193·2); caraway oil (p.1559·3); gentian root (p.1583·3).
Dyspepsia; motion sickness; nausea; vomiting.

Sanvita Verdauungstropfen *Strallhofer, Aust.*
Peppermint leaf (p.1208·1); gentian root (p.1583·3); caraway fruit (p.1559·3).
Gastro-intestinal disorders.

Sanvita-Entschlackungstonikum *Strallhofer, Aust.*
Parsley (p.1615·3); silver birch (p.1553·3); ononis (p.1610·2).
Diuresis.

Sanytol *Ideal, Fr.*
Bis(aminopropyl)laurylamine; permethrin (p.1409·2).
House dust mite acaricide.

Sanzur *Garec, S.Afr.*
Fluoxetine hydrochloride (p.284·1).
Anxiety disorders; bulimia nervosa; depression.

Sapec *Lichtwer, Ger.*
Garlic (p.1583·1).
Hyperlipidaemias.

Sapocitrosil *Citrosil, Ital.†.*
Benzalkonium chloride (p.1101·3).
Disinfection of skin, mucous membranes, and wounds.

Sapoderm
Note. This name is used for preparations of different composition.
Reckitt & Colman, Austral.
Triclosan (p.1127·2).
Skin cleansing.

Ingram & Bell, Canad.
Hexachlorophane (p.1115·2).
Antisepsis.

Saprol *Medecine Vegetale, Fr.†.*
Buchu (p.1555·2); boldo (p.1554·1); bearberry (p.1552·2); Bordeaux turpentine; salol (p.83·1); hexamine (p.216·1).
Adjunctive therapy of urogenital infections.

Sarapin *High Chemical, USA†.*
Sarracenia purpurea distillate (p.83·2).
Neuromuscular or neuralgic pain.

Saratoga *Blair, USA.*
Zinc oxide (p.1096·2); boric acid (p.1554·2); cineole (p.1564·1); peru balsam (p.1617·2).
Minor skin irritation.

Sarenin NT *Rohm, Ger.†.*
Saralasin acetate (p.943·1).
Preservation of renal function in kidneys for transplantation.

Sargenor
Sarget, Fr.; Asta Medica, Ital.; Asta Medica, Spain.
Arginine aspartate (p.1334·2).
Tonic.

Sargepirine *Sarget, Fr.*
Aspirin (p.16·1).
Glycine (p.1345·2) is included in some tablets in an attempt to limit adverse effects on the gastro-intestinal mucosa.
Fever; pain.

Saridon
Roche, Aust.; Roche, Belg.; Roche Nicholas, Ger.; Roche, Ital.; Roche Nicholas, Neth.; Roche Nicholas, Spain; Roche, Switz.
Paracetamol (p.72·2); propyphenazone (p.81·3); caffeine (p.749·3).
Formerly known as Saridon Neu in *Ger.*
Fever; pain.

Saridon senza Caffeina *Roche, Ital.†.*
Paracetamol (p.72·2); propyphenazone (p.81·3).
Fever; pain.

Sarilen *Normon, Spain.*
Roxatidine acetate (p.1212·2).
Gastro-oesophageal reflux; peptic ulcer.

Sarna *Stiefel, Austral.*
Camphor (p.1557·2); menthol (p.1600·2); phenol (p.1121·2).
Pruritus.

Sarna Anti-Itch *Stiefel, USA.*
Camphor (p.1557·2); menthol (p.1600·2).
Poison ivy; poison oak; pruritus; sunburn.

Sarna HC *Stiefel, Canad.*
Hydrocortisone (p.1043·3).
Skin disorders.

Sarna-P *Stiefel, Canad.*
Pramoxine hydrochloride (p.1298·2); camphor (p.1557·2); menthol (p.1600·2).
Skin irritation.

Sarnical *Perez Gimenez, Spain†.*
Sulphur (p.1091·2); peru balsam (p.1617·2).
Scabies.

Saroten
Lundbeck, Aust.; Bayer, Ger.; Lundbeck, S.Afr.; Lundbeck, Swed.; Lundbeck, Switz.
Amitriptyline hydrochloride (p.273·3).
Depression; nocturnal enuresis; pain; sleep disorders.

Sarotex
Lundbeck, Neth.; Lundbeck, Norw.
Amitriptyline hydrochloride (p.273·3).
Depression; nocturnal enuresis; pain.

Sarpan *Farge, Ital.†.*
Raubasine (p.941·3).
Vascular disorders.

Sarsaparol *Madaus, Ger.*
Homoeopathic preparation.

Sarsapsor *Ysatfabrik, Ger.*
Sarsaparilla (p.1627·2).
Psoriasis.

Sartol *Stiefel, Spain.*
Menthol (p.1600·2); camphor (p.1557·2).
Insect bites; skin disorders.

SAS *ICN, Canad.*
Sulphasalazine (p.1215·2).
Ulcerative colitis.

Saspryl *Inibsa, Spain.*
Aspirin (p.16·1).
Fever; musculoskeletal, joint and peri-articular disorders; pain; thrombo-embolism prophylaxis.

Sastid
Note. This name is used for preparations of different composition.
Stiefel, Canad.; Stiefel, S.Afr.; Stiefel, Spain.
Sulphur (p.1091·2); salicylic acid (p.1090·2).
Acne.

Stiefel, USA.
Precipitated sulphur (p.1091·2).
Formerly contained precipitated sulphur and salicylic acid.

Sastridex *Lindopharm, Ger.†.*
Flufenamic acid (p.41·3).
Dysmenorrhoea; inflammation; musculoskeletal and joint disorders.

Sasulen *Faes, Spain.*
Piroxicam (p.80·2).
Gout; musculoskeletal, joint, peri-articular, and soft-tissue disorders; pain.

Satina d *Bayer, Ger.†.*
Condensation products of albumin hydrolysate and fatty acids.
Skin disorders.

Satinique Anti-Dandruff *Amway, Canad.*
Pyrithione zinc (p.1089·3).

Sativol *Boiron, Canad.*
Homoeopathic preparation.

Sauerstoffbad Bastian *Bastian, Ger.†.*
Sodium percarbonate.
Bath additive; nervous disorders.

Saugella Antisettica *Guieu, Ital.†.*
Thyme (p.1636·3); sage (p.1627·1); whey.
Disinfection of the skin and genitals.

Saugella Salviettine *Guieu, Ital.*
Sage (p.1627·1); whey; lactic acid (p.1593·3).
Personal hygiene.

Saugella Uomo *Guieu, Ital.*
Helichrysum italicum; clove (p.1565·2).
Male personal hygiene.

Sauran *Abello, Spain.*
Citicoline (p.1564·3) or citicoline sodium (p.1564·3).
Cerebrovascular disorders.

Savacol Mouth and Throat Rinse *Colgate Oral Care, Austral.*
Chlorhexidine gluconate (p.1107·2).
Minor oral infections; mouth ulcers.

Savacol Throat Lozenges *Colgate Oral Care, Austral.†.*
Chlorhexidine hydrochloride (p.1107·2).
Throat infections.

Savarine *Zeneca, Fr.*
Proguanil hydrochloride (p.435·3); chloroquine phosphate (p.426·3).
Malaria.

Saventrine
Pharmax, Irl.; Restan, S.Afr.†; Pharmax, UK.
Isoprenaline hydrochloride (p.892·1).
Bradycardia; heart block; Stokes-Adams syndrome.

Savex *Sabex, Canad.*
Camphor (p.1557·2); menthol (p.1600·2).

Savex 15 *Sabex, Canad.*
SPF 15: Ethylhexyl *p*-methoxycinnamate (p.1487·1); oxybenzone (p.1487·3); camphor (p.1557·2).
Sunscreen.

Savex with PABA *Sabex, Canad.*
Padimate O (p.1488·1); camphor (p.1557·2); menthol (p.1600·2); salicylic acid (p.1090·2).
Sunscreen.

Savex Sunblock *Sabex, Canad.*
SPF 15: Padimate O (p.1488·1); oxybenzone (p.1487·3).
Sunscreen.

Savex with Sunscreen *Sabex, Canad.*
Camphor (p.1557·2); menthol (p.1600·2); salicylic acid (p.1090·2).

Saviosol *Green Cross, Jpn†.*
Dextran 40 (p.716·2) with electrolytes.
Circulatory disorders; plasma volume expansion; thrombosis.

Savloclens *Zeneca, S.Afr.†.*
Cetrimide (p.1105·2); chlorhexidine gluconate (p.1107·2).
Wound disinfection.

Savlodil
Zeneca, Canad.; Zeneca, Irl.†; Zeneca, Ital.†; Zeneca, S.Afr.†.
Cetrimide (p.1105·2); chlorhexidine gluconate (p.1107·2).
Wound disinfection.

Savlon
Note. This name is used for preparations of different composition.
Whitehall-Robins, Canad.
Cetrimide (p.1105·2).
Skin disorders.

Zeneca, Irl.†; Zeneca, Ital.†; Pharmedica, S.Afr.; Zeneca, Spain†.
Cetrimide (p.1105·2); chlorhexidine gluconate (p.1107·2) or chlorhexidine hydrochloride (p.1107·2).
Burns; disinfection; wounds.

Savlon Antiseptic *Boots, Austral.*
Cream; topical liquid: Cetrimide (p.1105·2); chlorhexidine (p.1107·2).
Topical disinfection.
Topical powder: Povidone-iodine (p.1123·3).
Fungal skin infections; skin abrasions; wounds.

Savlon Bath Oil *Zyma, UK†.*
Liquid paraffin (p.1382·1); wool alcohols (p.1385·2).
Dry skin.

Savlon Cream *Zyma, UK.*
Cetrimide (p.1105·2); chlorhexidine gluconate (p.1107·2).
Skin disinfection.

Savlon Dry *Zyma, UK.*
Povidone-iodine (p.1123·3).
Skin disinfection.

Savlon Hospital Concentrate
ICI, Austral.†; Zeneca, Canad.
Cetrimide (p.1105·2); chlorhexidine gluconate (p.1107·2).
Skin, surface, and instrument disinfection.

Savlon Liquid *Zyma, UK.*
Cetrimide (p.1105·2); chlorhexidine gluconate (p.1107·2).
Skin disinfection.

Savlon Medicated Powder *ICI, Austral.†.*
Hibitane chlorhexidine (p.1107·2).
Minor skin irritations.

Savlon Nappy Rash Cream *Zyma, UK†.*
Dimethicone (p.1384·2); cetrimide (p.1105·2).

Savlon Wound Wash *Zyma, UK.*
Chlorhexidine gluconate (p.1107·2).
Formerly known as Savlon Junior.
Skin disinfection.

Savoral *Sodietal, Fr.*
Preparation for enteral nutrition.

Sayomol *Cinfa, Spain.*
Promethazine hydrochloride (p.416·2).
Cutaneous hypersensitivity reactions.

Sazio *Zyma, Ital.†.*
Alginic acid (p.1470·3).
Appetite reduction.

SC-300 *Hamilton, Austral.*
Coconut oil derivatives (p.1383·3).
Barrier cream; skin cleansing.

Scabecid *Stiefel, Fr.*
Lindane (p.1407·2).
Pediculosis; scabies.

Scabene *Stiefel, Canad.*
Esdepallethrine (p.1406·1); piperonyl butoxide (p.1409·3).
Scabies.

Scadan *Miles, USA.*
Trimethyltetradecylammonium bromide (p.1105·3); stearyl dimethyl benzyl ammonium chloride.
Seborrhoea.

Scalpicin *Combe, USA.*
Hydrocortisone (p.1043·3); menthol (p.1600·2).

Scalpicin Anti-Dandruff Anti-Itch *Coombe, Canad.*
Menthol (p.1600·2); salicylic acid (p.1090·2).

Scalpicin Capilar *Combe, Spain.*
Hydrocortisone (p.1043·3).
Skin disorders.

Scalpvit *Kemiprogress, Ital.*
Vitamins, selenium, yeast, and amino acids.
Nutritional supplement.

Scandicain
Note. This name is used for preparations of different composition.
Astra, Aust.; Astra, Ger.; Astra, Switz.
Mepivacaine hydrochloride (p.1297·2).
Adrenaline acid tartrate (p.813·3) is included in some injections as a vasoconstrictor to diminish absorption and localise the effect of the local anaesthetic.
Local anaesthesia.

Astra, Ger.†.
Topical gel: Mepivacaine hydrochloride (p.1297·2); laureth 9 (p.1325·2).
Catheterisation; intubation; local anaesthesia.

Scandicain "N3" *Astra, Ger.†.*
Mepivacaine hydrochloride (p.1297·2).
Noradrenaline acid tartrate (p.924·1) is included in this preparation as a vasoconstrictor to diminish absorption and localise the effect of the local anaesthetic.
Local anaesthesia.

Scandicaine
Astra, Belg.; Astra, Neth.
Mepivacaine hydrochloride (p.1297·2).
Adrenaline acid tartrate (p.813·3) is included in some injections as a vasoconstrictor to diminish absorption and localise the effect of the local anaesthetic.
Local anaesthesia.

Scandine
Zambon, Belg.; Zambon, Ital.
Ibopamine hydrochloride (p.889·3).
Heart failure.

Scandinibsa *Inibsa, Spain.*
Mepivacaine hydrochloride (p.1297·2).
Adrenaline acid tartrate (p.813·3) is included in some injections as a vasoconstrictor to diminish absorption and localise the effect of the local anaesthetic.
Local anaesthesia.

Scandishake
Scientific Hospital Supplies, Irl.; Scientific Hospital Supplies, UK.
Food for special diets.
Cystic fibrosis; HIV infection; malignant neoplasms.

Scandonest
Austrodent, Aust.; Dental Warehouse, S.Afr.; Septodont, Switz.
Mepivacaine hydrochloride (p.1297·2).
Adrenaline (p.813·2) or noradrenaline acid tartrate (p.924·1) is included in some injections as a vasoconstrictor to diminish absorption and localise the effect of the local anaesthetic.
Local anaesthesia.

Scannotrast *Gerot, Aust.*
Barium sulphate (p.1003·1).
Radiographic contrast medium for CT scanning.

Scavenger *Aesculapius, Ital.*
Glutathione (p.983·1).
Alcohol or drug poisoning; ionising radiation trauma.

SCF *Searle, Austral.*
Sucralfate (p.1214·2).
Peptic ulcers.

Schamberg *Paddock, USA†; C & M, USA†.*
Zinc oxide (p.1096·2); menthol (p.1600·2); phenol (p.1121·2).
Pruritus.

Scheinpharm Artificial Tears *Schein, Canad.*
Polyvinyl alcohol (p.1474·2).

Scheinpharm Artificial Tears Plus *Schein, Canad.*
Polyvinyl alcohol (p.1474·2); povidone (p.1474·2).

Scheinpharm Testone-Cyp *Schein, Canad.*
Testosterone cypionate (p.1464·1).
Androgen.

Scheinpharm Triamcine-A *Schein, Canad.*
Triamcinolone acetonide (p.1050·2).
Corticosteroid.

Schericur
Schering, Aust.; Schering, Spain.
Hydrocortisone (p.1043·3).
Skin disorders.

Schering PC4 *Schering, UK.*
Norgestrel (p.1454·1); ethinyloestradiol (p.1445·1).
Postcoital oral contraceptive.

Scheriproct
Note. This name is used for preparations of different composition.
Schering, Aust.; Schering, Austral.; Schering, Belg.; Schering, Irl.; Schering, Norw.; Schering, S.Afr.
Prednisolone hexanoate (p.1048·1); cinchocaine hydrochloride (p.1289·2); clemizole undecanoate (p.406·3).
Anorectal disorders.

Schering, Ger.; Schering, Switz.; Schering, UK.
Prednisolone hexanoate (p.1048·1); cinchocaine hydrochloride (p.1289·2).
Formerly contained prednisolone hexanoate, clemizole undecanoate, and cinchocaine hydrochloride in *Switz.*
Anorectal disorders.

Schering, Spain.
Prednisolone (p.1048·1); cinchocaine hydrochloride (p.1289·2); menthol (p.1600·2).
Anorectal disorders.

Scheriproct N Schering, Swed.
Prednisolone hexanoate (p.1048·1); cinchocaine hydrochloride (p.1289·2).
Formerly contained prednisolone hexanoate, cinchocaine hydrochloride, and clemizole undecanoate.
Anorectal disorders.

Scherisolon Schering, Ger.†.
Prednisolone (p.1048·1) or prednisolone acetate (p.1048·1).
Corticosteroid.

Scherogel
Schering, Aust.; Schering, Belg.; Asche, Ger.; Schering, Ital.; Schering, Spain†.
Benzoyl peroxide (p.1079·2).
Acne.

Schias-Amaro Medicinale AFOM, Ital.
Rhubarb (p.1212·1); boldo (p.1554·1); cascara (p.1183·1).
Constipation; digestive disorders.

Schiwalys Hemofiltration Dicamed, Swed.
Electrolyte solution for haemofiltration (p.1151·1).
Some solutions also contain glucose.

Schlankheits-Unterstutzungstee Herbaknepp Kneipp, Ger.†.
Senna leaves; peppermint leaves; black tea; golden rod wort; lovage root; hibiscus flowers.
Herbal preparation.

Schlehepar N Hanosan, Ger.
Homoeopathic preparation.

Schleimhaut-Komplex Liebermann, Ger.
Homoeopathic preparation.

Schmerz-Dolgit Dolorgiet, Ger.
Ibuprofen (p.44·1).
Fever; pain; rheumatism.

Schmerzetten Salushaus, Ger.†.
Salix (p.82·3).
Fever; headache; rheumatism.

Schneckensaft N Hotz, Ger.
Thyme (p.1636·3); castanea vulgaris; limacin.
Bronchitis; coughs.

Schneckensirup Alsitan, Ger.
Alfalfa (p.1544·2); thyme (p.1636·3).
Cold symptoms.

schnupfen endrine Asche, Ger.
Xylometazoline hydrochloride (p.1071·2).
Nasal congestion.

Scholl Athlete's Foot Preparations Schering-Plough, Canad.
Tolnaftate (p.389·1).
Tinea pedis.

Scholl Corn, Callus Plaster Preparation Schering-Plough, Canad.
Salicylic acid (p.1090·2).
Calluses; corns.

Scholl Corn Salve Schering-Plough, Canad.
Salicylic acid (p.1090·2).
Calluses; corns.

Scholl 2-Drop Corn Remedy Schering-Plough, Canad.
Salicylic acid (p.1090·2).
Calluses; corns.

Scholl Dry Antiperspirant Foot Spray Schering-Plough, Canad.
Aluminium chlorohydrate (p.1078·3).
Foot odour; foot perspiration.

Scholl Wart Remover Schering-Plough, Canad.
Salicylic acid (p.1090·2).
Warts.

Scholl Zino Scholl, Canad.
Salicylic acid (p.1090·2).
Corns.

Schoolife Lifeplan, UK.
Multinutrient preparation.

Schoum Pharmygiene, Fr.
Fumitory (p.1581·3); ononis (p.1610·2); piscidia erythrina; sorbitol (p.1354·2); alverine citrate (p.1548·1).
Gastro-intestinal and kidney disorders.

Schrundensalbe - Dermi-cyl Liebermann, Ger.
Salicylic acid (p.1090·2).
Skin disorders.

Schupps Baldrian Sedativbad Schupp, Ger.
Valerian (p.1643·1); valerian oil; citronella oil (p.1565·1); lupulus (p.1597·2).
Bath additive; nervous disorders; sleep disorders.

Schupps Fichte-Menthol Olbad Schupp, Ger.
Norway spruce oil; eucalyptus oil (p.1578·1); menthol (p.1600·2).
Bath additive; catarrh.

Schupps Heilkrauter Erkaltungsbad Schupp, Ger.
Eucalyptus oil (p.1578·1); thyme oil (p.1637·1); peppermint oil (p.1208·1).
Bath additive; cold symptoms.

Schupps Heilkrauter Rheumabad Schupp, Ger.
Methyl salicylate (p.55·2); camphor (p.1557·2); rosemary oil (p.1626·2); Norway spruce oil; sage oil; juniper oil (p.1592·3).
Bath additive; musculoskeletal and joint disorders.

Schupps Kohlensaurebad Schupp, Ger.
Sodium bicarbonate (p.1153·2); aluminium sulphate (p.1548·1).
Bath additive; circulatory disorders; hypertension.

Schupps Latschenkiefer Olbad Schupp, Ger.
Pumilio pine oil (p.1623·3); pine-needle oil; Norway spruce oil; turpentine oil (p.1641·1); juniper oil (p.1592·3).
Bath additive; musculoskeletal and joint disorders; nervous disorders.

Schwarze-Salbe Lichtenstein, Ger.
Ichthammol (p.1083·3).
Skin disorders.

Schwedenjorg mild Mayrhofer, Aust.
Aloes (p.1177·1); angelica root; gentian root (p.1583·3); imperatoria root; galanga root; zedoary root; rosemary leaf; nutmeg (p.1609·2).
Gastro-intestinal disorders.

Schwedentrunk Infirmarius-Rovit, Ger.
Aloes (p.1177·1); senna (p.1212·2); manna (p.1199·1); myrrh (p.1606·1); angelica; carlina; gentian (p.1583·3); zedoary; camphor (p.1557·2); saffron (p.1001·1); theriacale; vitamin C (p.1365·2).
Gastro-intestinal disorders.

Schwedentrunk mit Ginseng Infirmarius-Rovit, Ger.
Aloes (p.1177·1); senna (p.1212·2); manna (p.1199·1); myrrh (p.1606·1); angelica; carlina; gentian (p.1583·3); zedoary; camphor (p.1557·2); saffron (p.1001·1); theriacale; vitamin C (p.1365·2); ginseng (p.1584·2).
Gastro-intestinal disorders.

Schwefelbad Dr Klopfer
Note. This name is used for preparations of different composition.
Nycomed, Aust.; Protina, Ger.
Sulphur (p.1091·2); sodium thiosulphate (p.996·2).
Bath additive; musculoskeletal and joint disorders; skin disorders.

Protina, Switz.
Zinc sulphide; sodium sulphite (p.1126·1); sodium bisulphite (p.1125·3); colloidal sulphur (p.1091·2); pine oil; turpentine oil (p.1641·1).
Formerly known as Bain Soufre du Dr Klopfer.
Circulatory disorders; hyperhidrosis; musculoskeletal and joint disorders; skin disorders.

Schwefelbad Saar CPF, Ger.
Sulphurated potash (p.1091·3).
Bath additive; rheumatic disorders; skin disorders.

Schwefel-Diasporal Protina, Ger.
Cream: Sulphur (p.1091·2).
Lotion†: Colloidal sulphur (p.1091·2); camphor (p.1557·2); alcohol.
Tincture†: Sulphur (p.1091·2); tannic acid (p.1634·2); formic acid (p.1581·3); salicylic acid (p.1090·2); cholesterol (p.1383·3).
Topical solution: Sulphur (p.1091·2); camphor (p.1557·2).
Skin disorders.

Schwohepan S Schwörer, Ger.
Silybum marianum (p.993·3); chelidonium majus.
Biliary and gastro-intestinal spasm; liver disorders.

Schwoneural Schwörer, Ger.
Homoeopathic preparation.

Schworheumal Schwörer, Ger.†.
Homoeopathic preparation.

Schworocard Schwörer, Ger.
Homoeopathic preparation.

Schworocor Schwörer, Ger.
Homoeopathic preparation.

Schworosin Schwörer, Ger.
Homoeopathic preparation.

Schworotox Schwörer, Ger.
Homoeopathic preparation.

Sciargo Potter's, UK.
Shepherds purse; wild carrot (p.1644·3); clivers (p.1565·2); bearberry (p.1552·2); juniper berry oil (p.1592·3).
Lumbago; sciatica.

Sciatalgen IRBI, Ital.†.
Vitamin B substances.
Nervous disorders; neuritis.

Scillacor Steigerwald, Ger.
Homoeopathic preparation.

Scillamiron Knoll, Ger.†.
Squill (p.1070·1).
Heart failure.

Scillase N Ziethen, Ger.
Squill (p.1070·1).
Cardiac disorders; oedema.

Scintadren Amersham International, UK.
Selenium-75 (p.1425·1) in the form of 6β-(methyl(^{75}Se)seleno)methyl-19-norcholest-5(10)-en-3β-ol.
Adrenal gland imaging.

Scintifor C Italfarmaco, Ital.†.
Indium (^{111}In) satumomab (p.1423·3).
Diagnosis of colorectal neoplasms.

Sciroppo Berta Berta, Ital.
Liquorice (p.1197·1); potassium guaiacolsulfonate (p.1068·3).
Catarrh; coughs.

Sciroppo Fenoglio AFOM, Ital.
Ferric ammonium citrate (p.1339·2).
Anaemias.

Sciroppo Merck all'Efetonina Bracco, Ital.
Racephedrine hydrochloride (Efetonina) (p.1060·1); thyme (p.1636·3).
Coughs; respiratory-tract disorders.

Sclane Llorente, Spain.
Betamethasone acetate (p.1033·2); betamethasone sodium phosphate (p.1033·3).
Corticosteroid.

Sclavo-Test P.P.D. Sclavo, Ital.†.
Tuberculin purified protein derivative (p.1640·2).
Detection of tuberculoprotein hypersensitivity.

Scleramin Ibirn, Ital.
Vinburnine phosphate (p.1644·1).
Cerebrovascular disorders.

Scleremo Therica, Fr.
Chrome alum (p.1562·2); glycerol (p.1585·2).
Varicose veins.

Scleril AGIPS, Ital.
Fenofibrate (p.1273·1).
Hyperlipidaemias.

Sclerocalcine Lehning, Fr.
Homoeopathic preparation.

Sclerodex Omega, Canad.†.
Glucose (p.1343·3); sodium chloride (p.1162·2); phenethyl alcohol (p.1121·1).
Sclerotherapy.

Sclerodine Omega, Canad.†.
Iodine (p.1493·1); sodium iodide (p.1493·2).
Sclerotherapy.

Scleromate Glenwood, USA.
Sodium morrhuate (p.1631·2).
Varicose veins.

S-Coaltar Ducray, Fr.
Coal tar (p.1092·3); salicylic acid (p.1090·2).
Dandruff.

Scoline
DBL, Austral.; Glaxo Wellcome, S.Afr.; Medeva, UK†.
Suxamethonium chloride (p.1319·1).
Depolarising neuromuscular blocker.

Scop Ciba-Geigy, Austral.†.
Hyoscine (p.462·3).
Motion sickness.

Scopace Hope, USA.
Hyoscine hydrobromide (p.462·3).
Parkinsonism.

Scope Procter & Gamble, USA.
Cetylpyridinium chloride (p.1106·2).
Minor mouth or throat irritation.

Scope with Oraseptate Procter & Gamble, Canad.
Cetylpyridinium chloride (p.1106·2); domiphen bromide (p.1112·3).
Oral hygiene.

Scopex Propan, S.Afr.; Mer-National, S.Afr.
Hyoscine butylbromide (p.462·3).
Dysmenorrhoea; smooth muscle spasm.

Scopex Co Propan, S.Afr.†.
Hyoscine butylbromide (p.462·3); dipyrone (p.35·1).
Gastro-intestinal spasm; urinary-tract spasm.

Scopoderm
Ciba-Geigy, Aust.; Ciba, Norw.; Novartis, Swed.
Hyoscine (p.462·3).
Motion sickness.

Scopoderm TTS
Ciba-Geigy, Fr.; Ciba, Ger.; Novartis, Neth.; Ciba-Geigy, S.Afr.†; Geigy, Switz.; Ciba, UK.
Hyoscine (p.462·3).
Motion sickness.

Scorbex Pharmacare Consumer, S.Afr.
Vitamin C (p.1365·2).
Vitamin C deficiency.

Scorbo-Betaine Fournier, Fr.†.
Betaine ascorbate (p.1553·2); betaine hydrate (p.1553·2).
Liver disorders.

Scordal Kattwiga, Ger.
Capsules: Herba teucrii.
Tonic.
Oral drops: Herba teucrii; magnesium chloride (p.1157·2).
Cardiovascular disorders; gastro-intestinal disorders.

Scorotox Kattwiga, Ger.
Homoeopathic preparation.

Scottopect Hafslund Nycomed, Aust.
Gel: Turpentine oil (p.1641·1); eucalyptus oil (p.1578·1); thyme oil (p.1637·1); menthol (p.1600·2); camphor (p.1557·2).
Oral drops: Thyme (p.1636·3).
Oral liquid: Thyme (p.1636·3); wild thyme; plantago lanceolata.
Bronchitis; catarrh.

Scott's Emulsion
Note. This name is used for preparations of different composition.
SmithKline Beecham Consumer, UK.
Cod-liver oil (p.1337·3); calcium hypophosphite; sodium hypophosphite.

SmithKline Beecham, USA.
Vitamins A and D.

Scot-Tussin Allergy Scot-Tussin, USA.
Diphenhydramine hydrochloride (p.409·1).

Scot-Tussin Cough & Cold Medicine Scot-Tussin, USA†.
Dextromethorphan hydrobromide (p.1057·3); chlorpheniramine maleate (p.405·1).
Coughs and cold symptoms.

Scot-Tussin Cough Formula Scot-Tussin, USA†.
Guaiphenesin (p.1061·3).
Coughs.

Scot-Tussin DM Scot-Tussin, USA.
Chlorpheniramine maleate (p.405·1); dextromethorphan hydrobromide (p.1057·3).
Coughs and cold symptoms.

Scot-Tussin DM Cough Chasers Scot-Tussin, USA.
Dextromethorphan hydrobromide (p.1057·3).
Coughs.

Scot-Tussin Expectorant Scot-Tussin, USA.
Guaiphenesin (p.1061·3).
Coughs.

Scot-Tussin Original 5-Action Scot-Tussin, USA.
Phenylephrine hydrochloride (p.1066·2); pheniramine maleate (p.415·3); sodium citrate (p.1153·2); sodium salicylate (p.85·1); caffeine citrate (p.749·3).
Upper respiratory-tract symptoms.

Scot-Tussin Senior Clear Scot-Tussin, USA.
Guaiphenesin (p.1061·3); dextromethorphan hydrobromide (p.1057·3).
Coughs.

SCR Pickles, UK.
Salicylic acid (p.1090·2).
Cradle cap.

Scriptogesic Propan-Vernleigh, S.Afr.†.
Paracetamol (p.72·2); codeine phosphate (p.26·1); caffeine (p.749·3); meprobamate (p.678·1).
Pain.

Scriptolyte Propan, S.Afr.
Potassium chloride; sodium chloride; sodium citrate; glucose (p.1152·3).
Diarrhoea; oral rehydration therapy.

Scripto-Metic Propan, S.Afr.
Prochlorperazine maleate (p.687·3).
Anxiety disorders; migraine; nausea and vomiting; vestibular disorders.

Scriptopam Propan-Vernleigh, S.Afr.†.
Diazepam (p.661·1).
Alcohol withdrawal syndrome; anxiety; premedication.

Scriptozone Pharmagen, S.Afr.†.
Phenylbutazone (p.79·2).
Ankylosing spondylitis.

SD-Hermal Hermal, Ger.
Clotrimazole (p.376·3).
Pityriasis versicolor; seborrhoeic dermatitis.

SDL SmithKline Beecham, Ger.
Allergen extracts (p.1545·1).
Hyposensitisation.

SDV Teomed, Switz.
Pollen allergen extracts (p.1545·1).
Hyposensitisation.

Sea Breeze Bristol-Myers Squibb, Canad.
Alcohol (p.1099·1); camphor (p.1557·2); benzoic acid (p.1102·3).
Skin cleansing.

Sea-Cal Bioceuticals, UK.
Calcium carbonate (p.1182·1).

Seacor SPA, Ital.
Omega-3 triglycerides (p.1276·1).
Hypertriglyceridaemia.

Seal & Heal Scholl, UK.
Salicylic acid (p.1090·2); camphor (p.1557·2).
Verrucas.

Sea-legs Seton, UK.
Meclozine hydrochloride (p.413·3).
Motion sickness.

Seale's Lotion C & M, USA.
Sulphur (p.1091·2); borax (p.1554·2); zinc oxide (p.1096·2).
Acne.

SeaMist Schein, USA.
Sodium chloride (p.1162·2).
Inflammation and dryness of nasal membranes.

Sea-Omega Rugby, USA.
Omega-3 marine triglycerides with vitamin E (p.1276·1).
Dietary supplement.

Search Stafford-Miller, UK.
Cetylpyridinium chloride (p.1106·2).
Oral hygiene.

Seatone Healthcrafts, UK.
Green-lipped mussel (p.1586·3).

Sebacide Paddock, USA†.
Skin cleanser.

Sebaklen Fumouze, Fr.
Xenysalate hydrochloride (p.1096·1).
Seborrhoeic dermatitis.

Seba-Nil Galderma, USA; Owen, USA.
Skin cleanser.
Acne.

Sebaquin Summers, USA†.
Di-iodohydroxyquinoline (p.581·1).
Scalp disorders.

Sebase Westbrook, UK.
A self-emulsifying base.

Sebasorb Summers, USA.
Sulphur (p.1091·2); salicylic acid (p.1090·2).
Acne.

Sebaveen Rydelle, Ital.
Avena (p.1551·3); salicylic acid (p.1090·2); carbocisteine (p.1056·3).
Seborrhoeic dermatitis.

Sebcur Dermtek, Canad.
Salicylic acid (p.1090·2).
Seborrhoea of the scalp.

Sebcur/T *Dermtek, Canad.*
Salicylic acid (p.1090·2); coal tar (p.1092·3).
Psoriasis of the scalp.

Sebercim *SmithKline Beecham, Ital.*
Norfloxacin (p.233·1).
Urinary-tract infections.

Sebex *Rugby, USA.*
Salicylic acid (p.1090·2); sulphur (p.1091·2).
Seborrhoea.

Sebex-T *Rugby, USA.*
Coal tar (p.1092·3); sulphur (p.1091·2); salicylic acid (p.1090·2).
Seborrhoea.

Sebirinse *Ego, Austral.*
Diacetyldimonium chloride; dexpanthenol (p.1570·3); phenethyl alcohol (p.1121·1).
Dandruff.

Sebitar *Ego, Austral.*
Tar (p.1092·3); coal tar (p.1092·3); salicylic acid (p.1090·2); undecylenamide (p.389·2).
Scalp disorders.

Sebizon *Schering, USA.*
Sulphacetamide sodium (p.252·2).
Bacterial skin infections; seborrhoeic dermatitis of the scalp.

Sebo Concept D/A *Marcel, Canad.*
Resorcinol (p.1090·1); salicylic acid (p.1090·2); sulphur (p.1091·2).

Sebo Creme *Widmer, Switz.*
Vitamins; urea (p.1095·2); triclosan (p.1127·2).
Acne; seborrhoea.

Sebo Lotion *Widmer, Switz.†.*
Cetrimonium bromide (p.1106·1); choline chloride (p.1337·1); sodium thiosulphate (p.996·2).
Scalp disorders.

Sebo Shampooing *Widmer, Switz.*
Pyrithione zinc (p.1089·3); sodium sulphosuccinated undecenoic acid monoethanolamide (p.389·2); triclosan (p.1127·2).
Scalp disorders.

Sebocalm *Gresval, Fr.†.*
Quillaia (p.1328·2).
Seborrhoea.

Seboderm *Sodip, Switz.†.*
Salicylic acid (p.1090·2); avena (p.1551·3); colloidal sulphur (p.1091·2); detergents.
Skin disorders.

Sebogel *Bergamon, Ital.†.*
Benzalkonium chloride (p.1101·3).
Skin cleansing.

Sebohermal
Note. This name is used for preparations of different composition.
Hermal, Ger.†.
Tincture: Oestradiol (p.1455·1); light ammonium bituminosulphonate (p.1083·3); resorcinol (p.1090·1).
Topical emulsion: Oestradiol (p.1455·1); light ammonium bituminosulphonate (p.1083·3).
Acne; seborrhoea.
Bruschettini, Ital.†.
Dienoestrol diacetate (p.1444·1); dimercaprol (p.979·2); ichthammol (p.1083·3); resorcinol (p.1090·1).
Skin disorders.

Sebo-Lenium *Winthrop, Switz.†.*
Selenium sulphide (p.1091·1).
Skin disorders.

Sebopona flussig *Hermal, Ger.†.*
Emollient.
Skin disorders.

Sebopona flussig mit Teer *Hermal, Ger.†.*
Coal tar distillate (p.1092·3).
Skin disorders.

Sebo-Psor *Widmer, Switz.*
Dexamethasone (p.1037·1); tretinoin (p.1093·3); urea (p.1095·2).
Scalp disorders.

Seborrol *Ego, Austral.*
Salicylic acid (p.1090·2); resorcinol (p.1090·1); undecylenamide (p.389·2).
Seborrhoea capitis; tinea capitis.

Seboval *Trans Canaderm, Canad.†.*
Propylene glycol (p.1622·1).
Pityriasis.

Sebucare *Westwood-Squibb, USA.*
Salicylic acid (p.1090·2).
Seborrhoea.

Sebulex
Westwood-Squibb, Canad.; Westwood-Squibb, USA.
Sulphur (p.1091·2); salicylic acid (p.1090·2).
Scalp disorders.

Sebulon
Westwood-Squibb, Canad.; Westwood-Squibb, USA†.
Pyrithione zinc (p.1089·3).
Scalp disorders.

Sebumselen *Llorente, Spain.*
Benzalkonium chloride (p.1101·3); selenium sulphide (p.1091·1).
Skin and scalp disorders.

Sebutone
Westwood-Squibb, Canad.; Westwood-Squibb, USA†.
Coal tar (p.1092·3); salicylic acid (p.1090·2); sulphur (p.1091·2).
Scalp disorders.

Secabiol *Normon, Spain.*
Carnitine (p.1336·2).
Cardiac disorders; carnitine deficiency.

Secaderm *Roche Consumer, UK†.*
Colophony (p.1567·1); melaleuca oil (p.1599·2); phenol (p.1121·2); terebene; turpentine oil (p.1641·1).
Chilblains.

Secadine *Xixia, S.Afr.*
Cimetidine (p.1183·2).
Gastro-intestinal disorders.

Secadrex
Rhone-Poulenc Rorer, Irl.; Rhone-Poulenc Rorer, Neth.; Rhone-Poulenc Rorer, S.Afr.; Italfarmaco, Spain; Akita, UK.
Acebutolol hydrochloride (p.809·3); hydrochlorothiazide (p.885·2).
Hypertension.

Secafobell *Dreluso, Ger.†.*
Belladonna (p.457·1); secale cornutum (p.1576·1); phenobarbitone (p.350·2).
Nervous disorders.

Secalan *Max Ritter, Switz.*
Chlorhexidine gluconate (p.1107·2); isopropyl alcohol (p.1118·2).
Minor skin lesions; skin disinfection.

Secale (Hevertoplex 147) *Hevert, Ger.*
Homoeopathic preparation.

Secale Med Complex *Dynamit, Aust.*
Homoeopathic preparation.

Secalip
Biotherapie, Fr.; Fournier SA, Spain.
Fenofibrate (p.1273·1).
Hyperlipidaemias.

Secalosan N *Hanosan, Ger.*
Homoeopathic preparation.

Secalysat EM *Ysatfabrik, Ger.*
Ergometrine maleate (p.1575·1).
Gynaecological bleeding.

Secaris *Pharmascience, Canad.*
Macrogol (p.1597·3); propylene glycol (p.1622·1).
Rhinitis.

Secerna *Fides, Ger.†.*
Urtica (p.1642·3); hamamelis (p.1587·1); arnica (p.1550·3); chamomile (p.1561·2); hypericum; graphites.
Tonic.

Seclin *Panthox & Burck, Ital.†.*
Dihexyverine hydrochloride (p.460·3).
Smooth muscle spasm.

Seclodin *Much, Ger.*
Ibuprofen (p.44·1).
Fever; pain.

Seconal
Lilly, Canad.; Lilly, Irl.; Lilly, S.Afr.; Lilly, UK; Lilly, USA.
Quinalbarbitone sodium (p.690·2).
Insomnia; sedative.

Secran *Scherer, USA†.*
Multivitamin preparation.

Secrebil *Isnardi, Ital.†.*
Piprozolin (p.1619·1).
Biliary-tract disorders.

Secrebil B *Wasserman, Spain†.*
Bile extract (p.1553·2); boldo (p.1554·1); rhubarb (p.1212·1).
Hepatobiliary disorders.

Secrepat *Knoll, Spain.*
Aluminium hydroxide (p.1177·3); calcium carbonate (p.1182·1); magnesium trisilicate (p.1199·1); aluminium glycinate (p.1177·2).
Gastro-intestinal hyperacidity.

Secrepina *Alonga, Spain.*
Omeprazole (p.1204·2) or omeprazole sodium (p.1204·2).
Gastro-oesophageal reflux; peptic ulcer; Zollinger-Ellison syndrome.

Secresol *Permamed, Switz.*
Acetylcysteine (p.1052·3).
Respiratory-tract disorders associated with increased or viscous mucus.

Secretil *Caber, Ital.*
Ambroxol hydrochloride (p.1054·3).
Respiratory-tract disorders.

Secron *De Witt, UK.*
Ephedrine hydrochloride (p.1059·3).
Nasal congestion.

Sectam *Locatelli, Ital.*
Latamoxef disodium (p.221·2).
Bacterial infections.

Sectral
Rhone-Poulenc Rorer, Aust.; Rhone-Poulenc Rorer, Belg.; Rhone-Poulenc Rorer, Canad.; Specia, Fr.; Rhone-Poulenc Rorer, Irl.; Rhone-Poulenc Rorer, Ital.; Rhone-Poulenc Rorer, Neth.; Rhone-Poulenc Rorer, S.Afr.; Italfarmaco, Spain; Rhone-Poulenc Rorer, Switz.; Akita, UK; Wyeth-Ayerst, USA.
Acebutolol hydrochloride (p.809·3).
Angina pectoris; arrhythmias; hypertension; myocardial infarction.

Sectrazide *Rhone-Poulenc Rorer, Belg.*
Acebutolol hydrochloride (p.809·3); hydrochlorothiazide (p.885·2).
Hypertension.

Secubar *Vita Elan, Spain.*
Lisinopril (p.898·2).
Heart failure; hypertension; myocardial infarction.

Secubar Diu *Vita Elan, Spain.*
Lisinopril (p.898·2); hydrochlorothiazide (p.885·2).
Hypertension.

Securgin *Menarini, Ital.*
Desogestrel (p.1443·3); ethinyloestradiol (p.1445·1).
Combined oral contraceptive.

Securon *Knoll, UK.*
Verapamil hydrochloride (p.960·3).
Angina pectoris; hypertension; myocardial infarction.

Securopen
Bayer, Aust.; Bayer, Austral.†; Bayer, Ger.; Bayer, Irl.; Bayer, Ital.; Bayer, Norw.; Bayer, UK.
Azlocillin sodium (p.156·1).
Pseudomonal infections.

Securpres *Poli, Ital.*
Indenolol hydrochloride (p.891·1).
Angina pectoris; arrhythmias; hypertension.

Seda Baxacor *Helopharm, Ger.†.*
Etafenone hydrochloride (p.866·3); meprobamate (p.678·1).
Cardiac disorders.

Seda Kneipp N *Kneipp, Ger.*
Valerian (p.1643·1); lupulus (p.1597·2).
Nervous disorders; sleep disorders.

Seda Nitro Mack *Mack, Illert., Ger.†.*
Glyceryl trinitrate (p.874·3); phenobarbitone (p.350·2).
Cardiac disorders.

Seda-baxacor *Sanus, Aust.†.*
Etafenone hydrochloride (p.866·3); meprobamate (p.678·1).
Angina pectoris; arrhythmias; heart failure.

Sedacalman *Schwarzwalder, Ger.*
Homoeopathic preparation.

Sedacollyre *Cooperation Pharmaceutique, Fr.*
Oxedrine tartrate (p.925·3); berberine hydrochloride (p.1553·1); benzododecinium bromide (p.1103·2).
Eye disorders.

Sedacoron *Ebewe, Aust.*
Amiodarone hydrochloride (p.820·1).
Arrhythmias.

Sedacur *Schaper & Brummer, Ger.*
Valerian (p.1643·1); lupulus (p.1597·2); melissa (p.1600·1).
Nervous disorders; sleep disorders.

Seda-Do *Grasler, Ger.*
Homoeopathic preparation.

Seda-Gel *Key, Austral.*
Lotion: Lignocaine (p.1293·2).
Oral gel: Choline salicylate (p.25·2); menthol (p.1600·2).
Painful mouth disorders.

Sedagin *Biocontrolfarm, Ital.*
Eschscholtzia californica.

Seda-Grandelat *Synpharma, Aust.*
Lupulus (p.1597·2); melissa leaf (p.1600·1).
Anxiety disorders.

Sedagul *Wild, Switz.*
Lignocaine hydrochloride (p.1293·2).
Local anaesthesia.

Sedahopf *Hennig, Ger.*
Valerian (p.1643·1); lupulus (p.1597·2).
Nervous disorders; sleep disorders.

Seda-ildamen *Asta Medica, Ger.†.*
Oxyfedrine hydrochloride (p.927·1); homofenazine hydrochloride (p.675·2).
Cardiac disorders.

Sedalande
Synthelabo, Belg.†; Delalande, Fr.†; Delalande, Ger.†; Synthelabo, Switz.†.
Fluanisone (p.670·1).
Psychiatric disorders.

Sedalint Baldrian *Sanofi Winthrop, Ger.*
Valerian root (p.1643·1).
Nervous disorders; sleep disorders.

Sedalint Kava *Sanofi Winthrop, Ger.*
Kava (p.1592·3).
Anxiety disorders.

Sedalipid *Steigerwald, Ger.*
Magnesium-pyridoxal-5′-phosphate-glutaminate.
Hyperlipidaemias.

Sedalium *Janssen, Spain†.*
Moperone (p.682·1); prozapine.
Extrapyramidal disorders; smooth muscle spasm.

Sedalmerck *Merck, Spain.*
Caffeine (p.749·3); ephedrine hydrochloride (p.1059·3); ethylmorphine hydrochloride (p.36·1); propyphenazone (p.81·3).
Pain.

Sedalozia *Plantes Tropicales, Fr.*
Crataegus (p.1568·2); eschscholtzia californica; valerian (p.1643·1).
Insomnia; nervous disorders.

Sedalpan *Teofarma, Ital.*
Methyl nicotinate (p.55·1); diethylamine salicylate (p.33·1).
Musculoskeletal, joint, and soft-tissue disorders.

Seda-Movicard *Ravensberg, Ger.†.*
Magnesium aspartate (p.1157·2); potassium aspartate (p.1161·3); adenosine triphosphate disodium salt (p.1543·2); troxerutin (p.1580·2); mistletoe (p.1604·1); crataegus (p.1568·2); phenobarbitone (p.350·2).
Cardiac disorders.

Sedanoct *Woelm, Ger.†.*
Tryptophan (p.310·2).
Sleep disorders.

Sedans *Ganassini, Ital.*
Amitriptyline hydrochloride (p.273·3); chlordiazepoxide hydrochloride (p.646·3).
Nervous disorders.

Sedanxol *Tropon, Ger.†.*
Zuclopenthixol hydrochloride (p.700·2).
Psychiatric disorders.

Sedapain
Note. This name is used for preparations of different composition.
Iyakuhin Kogyo, Jpn†.
Eptazocine hydrobromide (p.35·3).
Pain.
Garec, S.Afr.
Paracetamol (p.72·2); doxylamine succinate (p.410·1); caffeine (p.749·3); codeine phosphate (p.26·1).
Pain with tension.

Sedapap-10 *Mayrand, USA.*
Paracetamol (p.72·2); butalbital (p.644·3).
Pain.

Seda-Pasc N *Pascoe, Ger.†.*
Crataegus (p.1568·2); chamomile (p.1561·2); lupulus (p.1597·2); valerian (p.1643·1); melissa (p.1600·1); passion flower (p.1615·3); pyridoxine hydrochloride.
Nervous disorders; sleep disorders.

Seda-Plantina *Plantina, Ger.*
Valerian (p.1643·1); lupulus (p.1597·2); melissa (p.1600·1); passion flower (p.1615·3); rosemary.
Agitation; sleep disorders.

Sedaplus *Chephasaar, Ger.; Rosen, Ger.*
Doxylamine succinate (p.410·1).
Hypersensitivity reactions; nervous disorders; nocturnal enuresis; sleep disorders.

Sedapon D *Essex, Ger.†.*
Meprobamate (p.678·1); yohimbic acid (p.1645·3); belladonna alkaloids (p.457·1).
Psychiatric disorders; sleep disorders.

Seda-Quell *Key, Austral.†.*
Promethazine hydrochloride (p.416·2); paracetamol (p.72·2).
Formerly known as Seda-Gel Suspension.
Fever; pain.

Seda-Rash *Key, Austral.*
Zinc oxide (p.1096·2); castor oil (p.1560·2).
Eczema; heat rash; intertrigo; nappy rash.

Sedarene
Aerocid, Fr.
Capsules: Paracetamol (p.72·2); codeine phosphate (p.26·1).
Fever; pain.
Wintec, Fr.†.
Suppositories: Paracetamol (p.72·2); diethylsalicylamide (p.33·1); caffeine (p.749·3).
Fever; pain.

Sedariston *Steiner, Ger.*
Valerian root (p.1643·1); hypericum (p.1590·1); melissa leaf (p.1600·1).
Nervous disorders.

Sedariston Konzentrat *Steiner, Ger.*
Hypericum (p.1590·1); valerian root (p.1643·1).
Anxiety disorders; sleep disorders.

Sedartryl *Oberlin, Fr.*
Methyl nicotinate (p.55·1); amyl salicylate (p.15·3); salicylic acid (p.1090·2); menthol (p.1600·2); synthetic camphor (p.1557·2); turpentine oil (p.1641·1); volatile mustard oil (p.1605·3).
Musculoskeletal and joint pain.

Sedaselect *Dreluso, Ger.*
Homoeopathic preparation.

Sedaselect N *Dreluso, Ger.*
Lupulus (p.1597·2); valerian (p.1643·1); passion flower (p.1615·3); melissa (p.1600·1).
Nervous exhaustion and excitability; sleep disorders.

Sedasept
Note. This name is used for preparations of different composition.
Michaux, Belg.
Chlorhexidine gluconate (p.1107·2); lignocaine hydrochloride (p.1293·2).
Formerly contained acetarsol sodium, sulphanilamide, and thymol.
Mouth and throat disorders.
Sanico, Switz.
Cineole (p.1564·1); peppermint oil (p.1208·1); thyme oil (p.1637·1); menthol (p.1600·2); thymol (p.1127·1); methyl salicylate (p.55·2).
Dental inflammation; oral hygiene.

Sedaspir *Bride, Fr.*
Codeine phosphate (p.26·1); caffeine (p.749·3); aspirin (p.16·1).
Fever; pain.

Sedaspray *Cusi, Spain†.*
Ibuprofen aminoethanol (p.44·3).
Musculoskeletal disorders.

Seda-Stenocrat-N *Schwabe, Ger.†.*
Hyoscine hydrobromide (p.462·3); ammi visnaga (p.1593·2); crataegus leaves and fruit (p.1568·2).
Angina.

Sedasyx *Syxyl, Ger.*
Valerian (p.1643·1); lupulus (p.1597·2); melissa (p.1600·1).
Nervous disorders; sleep disorders.

Sedatermin *Hortel, Spain†.*
Paracetamol (p.72·2); propyphenazone (p.81·3).
Fever; pain.

Sedatif PC
Boiron, Canad.; Boiron, Fr.; Boiron, Switz.
Homoeopathic preparation.

Sedatif Tiber *Medecine Vegetale, Fr.*
Crataegus (p.1568·2); passion flower (p.1615·3); potassium bromide (p.1620·3); sodium bromide (p.1620·3).
Anxiety; insomnia.

Sedatol *Bonomelli, Ital.*
Capsules: Passion flower (p.1615·3); valerian (p.1643·1); crataegus (p.1568·2); chamomile (p.1561·2); piscidia.
Syrup: Passion flower (p.1615·3); chamomile (p.1561·2); crataegus (p.1568·2); piscidia; melissa (p.1600·1).
Insomnia.

Sedatonyl *Lipha Sante, Fr.*
Phenobarbitone (p.350·2); crataegus (p.1568·2).
Anxiety; insomnia.

Sedatruw S *Truw, Ger.*
Valerian (p.1643·1); lupulus (p.1597·2); melissa (p.1600·1).
Nervous disorders; sleep disorders.

Sedatuss *Trianon, Canad.*
Dextromethorphan hydrobromide (p.1057·3); chlorpheniramine maleate (p.405·1); guaiacol (p.1061·2); pseudoephedrine hydrochloride (p.1068·3).
Coughs.

Sedatuss DM *Trianon, Canad.*
Dextromethorphan hydrobromide (p.1057·3).

Sedazin *Lagap, Switz.†.*
Lorazepam (p.675·3).
Anxiety; premedication; sleep disorders.

Sedemol *Sopar, Belg.†.*
Althaea (p.1546·3); poppy capsule (p.1068·2); borax (p.1554·2); sodium fluoride (p.742·1); phenol (p.1121·2); chloral hydrate (p.645·3).
Mouth and throat disorders; whitlow.

Sedergine *Upsamedica, Belg.*
Aspirin (p.16·1); ascorbic acid (p.1365·2).
Fever; pain.

Sedergine C *Irmesan, Spain.*
Aspirin (p.16·1); ascorbic acid (p.1365·2).
Fever; pain.

Sediat *Pfleger, Ger.*
Diphenhydramine hydrochloride (p.409·1).
Sleep disorders.

Sedibaine *Marion Merrell, Fr.*
Strophanthus (p.951·1); phenobarbitone (p.350·2); hyoscyamus (p.464·3); crataegus (p.1568·2); ballota; valerian (p.1643·1); belladonna (p.457·1).
Nervous disorders.

Sedigrippal a la vitamine C *Boehringer Ingelheim, Fr.†.*
Paracetamol (p.72·2); potassium aspartate (p.1161·3); calcium ascorbate (p.1365·2); caffeine (p.749·3).
Cold symptoms; fever.

Sedilor *Dolisos, Canad.*
Homoeopathic preparation.

Sedinal *Rhone-Poulenc Rorer, Belg.*
Crataegus (p.1568·2); ballota; passion flower (p.1615·3).
Nervous disorders.

Sedinfant N *Biocur, Ger.*
Valerian (p.1643·1); lupulus (p.1597·2); passion flower (p.1615·3).
Agitation; excitability; sleep disorders.

Sedinol *Pharmacare Consumer, S.Afr.*
Doxylamine succinate (p.410·1); paracetamol (p.72·2); codeine phosphate (p.26·1); caffeine (p.749·3).
Pain and associated tension.

Sediomed S *Pfleger, Ger.†.*
Allobarbitone (p.640·3); phenobarbitone (p.350·2); valerian (p.1643·1); lupulus (p.1597·2); passion flower (p.1615·3).
Nervous disorders; sleep disorders.

Sedionbel *Alter, Spain†.*
Adenosine triphosphate (p.1543·2); cocarboxylase (p.1361·2); hydroxocobalamin (p.1363·3); ornithine hydrochloride (p.1352·3); pangamic acid (p.1614·1); pyridoxal phosphate (p.1363·1); dexamethasone phosphate (p.1037·2); uridine triphosphate (p.1641·3). Lignocaine hydrochloride (p.1293·2) is included in this preparation to alleviate the pain of injection.
Myopathies; neuralgias; neuritis; rheumatism.

Sedital *Vis, Ital.†.*
Phenytoin sodium (p.352·3); phenobarbitone (p.350·2).
Pain; sedative.

Sedizepan *Septa, Spain.*
Lorazepam (p.675·3).
Alcohol withdrawal syndrome; anxiety; epilepsy; insomnia; nausea; vomiting.

Sedlinct *Restan, S.Afr.†.*
Promethazine hydrochloride (p.416·2); ephedrine hydrochloride (p.1059·3); codeine phosphate (p.26·1).
Coughs.

Sedo *Rapide, Spain.*
Methadone (p.54·2).
Diamorphine detoxification; opioid withdrawal; pain.

Sedo Alufilm *Boots, Spain†.*
Metoclopramide hydrochloride (p.1200·3); almasilate (p.1177·1).
Gastro-intestinal disorders.

Sedobex *Ecobi, Ital.*
Sodium dibunate (p.1070·1); grindelia; cardamom (p.1560·1); lattuca sativa; sodium benzoate (p.1102·3).
Bronchial disorders; coughs.

Sedobrina *Vinas, Spain.*
Lormetazepam (p.677·1).
Insomnia.

Sedocalcio *Deca, Ital.*
Calcium lactate (p.1155·2); sodium benzoate (p.1102·3).
Mouth and throat disorders.

Sedocardin *Pfluger, Ger.*
Homoeopathic preparation.

Sedodermil *Vifor, Switz.*
Methyl anthranilate; pentyl valerate; bornyl salicylate (p.22·1); laurus nobilis oil; menthol (p.1600·2).
Musculoskeletal and joint pain.

Sedofarin *Pensa, Spain.*
Dequalinium chloride (p.1112·1); dexamethasone (p.1037·1); benzocaine (p.1286·2); tyrothricin (p.267·2).
Mouth and throat disorders.

Sedogelat *Metochem, Aust.*
Valerian root (p.1643·1); melissa leaf (p.1600·1); passion flower (p.1615·3).
Anxiety disorders; sleep disorders.

Sedol *OFF, Ital.*
Propyphenazone (p.81·3); caffeine (p.749·3).
Fever; influenza symptoms; neuralgia.

Sedonerva *Benvegna, Ital.†.*
Crataegus (p.1568·2); passion flower (p.1615·3); matricaria (p.1561·2); valerian (p.1643·1); boldo (p.1554·1); phenobarbitone (p.350·2); peptone.
Nervous disorders.

Sedonium *Lichtwer, Ger.*
Valerian (p.1643·1).
Agitation; insomnia.

Sedopal *Lehning, Fr.*
Crataegus (p.1568·2); eschscholtzia californica; melilotus officinalis.
Insomnia; nervous disorders.

Sedophon *Mayoly-Spindler, Fr.*
Ethylmorphine hydrochloride (p.36·1); aconite (p.1542·2); guaiphenesin (p.1061·3).
Coughs.

Sedopretten *Schoning-Berlin, Ger.*
Diphenhydramine hydrochloride (p.409·1).
Insomnia.

Sedopuer F *SIT, Ital.*
Passion flower (p.1615·3); valerian (p.1643·1); crataegus (p.1568·2); calcium glycerophosphate (p.1155·2).
Insomnia; nervous disorders.

Sedopulmina *Medosan, Ital.†.*
Pumilio pine oil (p.1623·3); cineole (p.1564·1); terpin monohydrate (p.1070·2).
Coughs.

Sedorrhoide *Lipha, Fr.*
Dodeclonium; benzocaine (p.1286·2); esculoside (p.1543·3); enoxolone (p.35·2).
Anorectal disorders.

Sedosan *Grossmann, Switz.*
Crataegus (p.1568·2); passion flower (p.1615·3).
Nervous disorders.

Sedosil *Vifor, Switz.*
Pimethixene (p.416·1).
Nervous disorders.

Sedotime *SmithKline Beecham, Spain.*
Ketazolam (p.675·2).
Anxiety; insomnia.

Sedotiren *Panthox & Burck, Ital.†.*
Isobutiacilic acid; phenobarbitone (p.350·2).
Hyperthyroidism.

Sedotosse *Panthox & Burck, Ital.†.*
Isoaminile citrate (p.1063·2).
Catarrh; coughs.

Sedotus *Valda, Ital.†.*
Dextromethorphan hydrobromide (p.1057·3).
Coughs.

Sedotussin
Note. This name is used for preparations of different composition.
UCB, Aust.; UCB, Ger.; Rodleben, Ger.; Vedim, Ger.
Pentoxyverine (p.1066·1), pentoxyverine citrate (p.1066·1), or pentoxyverine hydrochloride (p.1066·2).
Coughs.

UCB, Switz.
Oral drops: Pentoxyverine citrate (p.1066·1); terpin hydrate (p.1070·2); cineole (p.1564·1); menthol (p.1600·2); thymol (p.1127·1); guaiphenesin (p.1061·3).
Suppositories: Pentoxyverine (p.1066·1); terpin hydrate (p.1070·2); terpineol (p.1635·1); cineole (p.1564·1); guaiphenesin (p.1061·3).
Syrup: Pentoxyverine citrate (p.1066·1); terpin hydrate (p.1070·2); cineole (p.1564·1); menthol (p.1600·2); thyme (p.1636·3).
Coughs and associated respiratory-tract disorders.

Sedotussin Expectorans *UCB, Ger.*
Oral drops: Pentoxyverine citrate (p.1066·1); terpin (p.1070·2); cineole (p.1564·1); menthol (p.1600·2); thymol (p.1127·1); guaiphenesin (p.1061·3).
Suppositories†: Pentoxyverine (p.1066·1); cineole (p.1564·1); guaiphenesin (p.1061·3); methen-8-ol; terpin (p.1070·2).
Syrup: Pentoxyverine citrate (p.1066·1); terpin (p.1070·2); cineole (p.1564·1); menthol (p.1600·2); thyme (p.1636·3).
Coughs and associated respiratory-tract disorders.

Sedotussin Muco *UCB, Ger.; Rodleben, Ger.; Vedim, Ger.*
Carbocisteine (p.1056·3).
Respiratory-tract disorders with excess or viscous mucus.

Sedotussin plus *UCB, Ger.; Rodleben, Ger.; Vedim, Ger.*
Pentoxyverine citrate (p.1066·1); chlorpheniramine maleate (p.405·1).
Coughs.

Sedovalin *Streuli, Switz.†.*
Oral drops: Diphenhydramine hydrochloride (p.409·1); stramonium tincture (p.468·2); hyoscyamus tincture (p.464·3); valerian tincture (p.1643·1); cascara (p.1183·1).
Tablets: Diphenhydramine hydrochloride (p.409·1); belladonna (p.457·1); hyoscyamus (p.464·3); ballota; crataegus (p.1568·2); valerian (p.1643·1).
Nervous disorders.

Sedovegan *Wolff, Ger.*
Hypericum (p.1590·1).
Formerly contained phenobarbitone, quinine, quinidine, quinidine sulphate, cinchonine, cinchonine sulphate, and cinchonidine.
Depression; nervous disorders.

Sedovegan Novo *Wolff, Ger.*
Diphenhydramine hydrochloride (p.409·1).
Insomnia.

Sedovent *Schworer, Ger.*
Cinchona bark (p.1564·1); cinnamon (p.1564·2); dried bitter-orange peel (p.1610·3); achillea (p.1542·2); calamus (p.1556·1); gentian (p.1583·3).
Gastro-intestinal disorders.

Sedral *Banyu, Jpn.*
Cefadroxil (p.163·3).
Bacterial infections.

Seduan *Pharmed, Aust.†.*
Carbromal (p.645·2); bromisoval (p.643·1).
Anxiety disorders; depression; sleep disorders.

Sefralax *Corvi, Ital.†.*
Senna leaves (p.1212·2); frangula bark (p.1193·2); rhubarb root (p.1212·1).
Constipation.

Sefril
Bristol-Myers Squibb, Aust.; Bristol-Myers Squibb, Ger.†; Squibb, Switz.†.
Cephradine (p.181·3).
Bacterial infections.

Seftem *Shionogi, Jpn.*
Ceftibuten (p.175·1).
Bacterial infections.

Seglor
Sanofi Winthrop, Fr.; Synthelabo, Ital.
Dihydroergotamine mesylate (p.444·2).
Headache; migraine; orthostatic hypotension; peripheral vascular disorders; vertigo.

Segmentocut *Redel, Ger.†.*
Cajuput oil (p.1556·1); camphor (p.1557·2); menthol (p.1600·2); methyl salicylate (p.55·2); capsicum (p.1559·2).
Lumbago; myalgia; neuralgia; rheumatism; sciatica.

Segmentocut Thermo *Redel, Ger.*
Glycol salicylate (p.43·1); benzyl nicotinate (p.22·1).
Musculoskeletal, joint, and soft-tissue pain; superficial vascular disorders.

Seguril *Hoechst, Spain.*
Frusemide (p.871·1).
Hypertension; oedema.

Sejungin B *Bock, Ger.*
Homoeopathic preparation.

Seki *Zambon, Ital.*
Cloperastine fendizoate (p.1057·2) or cloperastine hydrochloride (p.1057·2).
Coughs.

Sekin *Sintesa, Belg.*
Cloperastine fendizoate (p.1057·2) or cloperastine hydrochloride (p.1057·2).
Coughs.

Sekisan *Daker Farmasimes, Spain.*
Cloperastine fendizoate (p.1057·2) or cloperastine hydrochloride (p.1057·2).
Coughs.

Sekretolin *Hoechst, Ger.*
Secretin hydrochloride (p.1628·1).
Diagnosis of pancreatic disorders and Zollinger-Ellison syndrome.

Sekretovit *Bender, Aust.*
Ambroxol hydrochloride (p.1054·3).
Respiratory-tract disorders.

Sekucid
Note. This name is used for preparations of different composition.
Paragerm, Fr.
Glutaraldehyde (p.1114·3).
Instrument disinfection.

Henkel, Ital.
Glutaraldehyde (p.1114·3); isopropyl alcohol (p.1118·2).
Instrument disinfection.

Sekudrill
Henkel, Ger.; Henkel, Ital.
Potassium hydroxide (p.1621·1); propylene glycol (p.1622·1).
Instrument disinfection.

Sekugerm *Henkel, Ital.*
Glutaraldehyde (p.1114·3); glyoxal (p.1115·1).
Disinfection of fibre-optic equipment; endoscope disinfection.

Sekumatic D *Henkel, Ital.*
Glutaraldehyde (p.1114·3); alcohol (p.1099·1); chloroform; acetone.
Instrument disinfection.

Sekumatic FD *Henkel, Ger.*
Glutaraldehyde (p.1114·3).
Instrument disinfection.

Sekumatic FDR *Henkel, Ger.*
Glucoprotamine; didecylmethylpoly(oxyethyl) ammonium propionate; tributyltetradecylphosphonium chloride.
Surface and instrument disinfection.

Sekundal *Rorer, Ger.†.*
Bromvaletone (p.643·1); carbromal (p.645·2).
Sleep disorders.

Sekundal-D *Rorer, Ger.†.*
Diphenhydramine hydrochloride (p.409·1).
Sleep disorders.

Sekusept *Henkel, Ger.*
Sodium perborate (p.1125·2); tetraacetyl ethylenediamine.
Instrument and surface disinfection.

Sekusept Extra N *Henkel, Ger.*
Benzalkonium chloride (p.1101·3); glutaraldehyde (p.1114·3).
Instrument disinfection.

Sekusept forte *Henkel, Ger.*
Formaldehyde (p.1113·2); glyoxal (p.1115·1); glutaraldehyde (p.1114·3); benzalkonium chloride (p.1101·3).
Instrument disinfection.

Sekusept N *Henkel, Ital.*
Sodium perborate (p.1125·2).
Instrument disinfection.

Sekusept Plus *Henkel, Ger.*
Glucoprotamine.
Instrument disinfection.

Sel D *SFPH, Fr.*
Sodium chloride; sodium phosphate; sodium sulphate.
Dietary salt substitute.

Sel d'Ems *Siemens, Switz.*
Natural sels d'Ems.
Upper-respiratory-tract disorders.

Selan *Iquinosa, Spain.*
Cefuroxime axetil (p.177·1).
Bacterial infections.

Selax *Odan, Canad.*
Docusate sodium (p.1189·3).
Constipation.

Selbex *Eisai, Jpn.*
Teprenone (p.1217·3).
Gastric ulcers; gastritis.

Sel'bis *Soekami, Fr.†.*
Potassium chloride; ammonium chloride; calcium formate; glutamic acid.
Dietary salt substitute.

Selcarbinol *Sella, Ital.†.*
Nicotinyl alcohol tartrate (p.915·3).
Hypertension.

Seldane
Hoechst Marion Roussel, Canad.; Hoechst Marion Roussel, UK; Merrell Dow, USA†.
Terfenadine (p.418·1).
Allergic rhinitis; hypersensitivity reactions.

Seldane-D *Marion Merrell Dow, USA†.*
Pseudoephedrine hydrochloride (p.1068·3); terfenadine (p.418·1).
Upper respiratory-tract symptoms.

Selecid *Alter, Spain†.*
Pivmecillinam hydrochloride (p.239·1).
Bacterial infections.

Selectafer N *Dreluso, Ger.*
Saccharated iron oxide (p.1353·2); cyanocobalamin (p.1363·3); folic acid (p.1340·3).
Primary and secondary anaemias; tonic.

Selectin *Bristol-Myers Squibb, Ital.*
Pravastatin sodium (p.1277·1).
Arteriosclerosis; cardiovascular disorders; hypercholesterolaemia.

Selectografin *Schering, Ital.*
Sodium diatrizoate (p.1003·2); meglumine diatrizoate (p.1003·2).
Contrast medium for urography and angiography.

Selectol
Gerot, Aust.; Pharmacia Upjohn, Belg.; Pharmacia Upjohn, Ger.; Rhone-Poulenc Rorer, Irl.; Rhone-Poulenc Rorer, Switz.
Celiprolol hydrochloride (p.838·3).
Angina pectoris; arrhythmias; hypertension.

Selectomycin *Grunenthal, Ger.*
Spiramycin (p.249·2).
Bacterial infections; toxoplasmosis.

Selecturon *Gerot, Aust.*
Celiprolol hydrochloride (p.838·3); chlorthalidone (p.839·3).
Hypertension.

Seledat *Master Pharma, Ital.*
Selegiline hydrochloride (p.1144·2).
Psychiatric disorders.

Selegam *Hexal, Ger.*
Selegiline hydrochloride (p.1144·2).
Parkinsonism.

Selegel *Ducray, Fr.*
Selenium sulphide (p.1091·1).
Seborrhoeic dermatitis.

Selektine *Bristol-Myers Squibb, Neth.*
Pravastatin sodium (p.1277·1).
Hypercholesterolaemia.

Selemax *Gazzoni, Ital.*
Selenium; betacarotene; vitamin E; vitamin C; zinc; copper.
Antioxidant nutritional supplement.

Selemite-B *Vitaplex, Austral.†.*
Selenomethionine.
Selenium deficiency.

Selen
Leopold, Aust.; Kabi, Swed.†.
Sodium selenite (p.1354·1).
Dietary supplement.

Selen + E *Kabi, Swed.†.*
Sodium selenite (p.1354·1); *dl*-alpha tocopheryl acetate (p.1369·2).
Dietary supplement.

Selenarell *Sanorell, Ger.*
Homoeopathic preparation.

selenase *GN, Ger.*
Sodium selenite (p.1354·1).
Selenium deficiency.

Selenica *Nikken, Jpn.*
Sodium valproate (p.361·2).
Epilepsy.

Selenion *Labcatal, Fr.*
Selenium (p.1353·3).
Muscular disorders; skin disorders.

Selenium Med Complex *Dynamit, Aust.*
Homoeopathic preparation.

Selenium-ACE
Richelet, Fr.; Pharmco, S.Afr.†; Wassen, UK.
Selenium yeast (p.1353·3); vitamins A, C, and E.

Seleno-6 *Solgar, UK.*
Selenomethionine.
Dietary supplement.

Selenokehl *Sanum-Kehlbeck, Ger.*
Homoeopathic preparation.

Selepain *Ducray, Fr.†.*
Selenium sulphide (p.1091·1).
Seborrhoeic dermatitis.

Sele-Pak *Smith & Nephew SoloPak, USA.*
Selenious acid (p.1353·3).
Parenteral nutrition.

Seleparina *Italfarmaco, Ital.*
Nadroparin calcium (p.914·1).
Thrombosis prophylaxis.

Selepark *Betapharm, Ger.*
Selegiline hydrochloride (p.1144·2).
Parkinsonism.

Selepen *Lyphomed, USA.*
Selenious acid (p.1353·3).
Parenteral nutrition.

Seles Beta *Schwarz, Ital.*
Atenolol (p.825·3).
Angina pectoris; hypertension.

Selestoject *Mayrand, USA†.*
Betamethasone sodium phosphate (p.1033·3).
Corticosteroid.

Selexid
Merck, Aust.; Leo, Belg.†; Leo, Canad.; Leo, Fr.; Leo, Irl.†; Leo, Norw.; Lovens, Swed.; Leo, Switz.†; Leo, UK†.
Mecillinam (p.223·3), pivmecillinam (p.238·3), or pivmecillinam hydrochloride (p.239·1).
Urinary-tract infections.

Selexidin *Leo, UK†.*
Mecillinam (p.223·3).
Bacterial infections.

Selezen *Teofarma, Ital.*
Imidazole salicylate (p.45·2).
Fever; inflammation; pain.

Selg *Promefarm, Ital.*
Macrogol 4000 (p.1598·2); electrolytes (p.1147·1).
Bowel evacuation; constipation.

Selgene *Alphapharm, Austral.*
Selegiline hydrochloride (p.1144·2).
Parkinsonism.

Selg-Esse *Promefarm, Ital.*
Macrogol 4000 (p.1598·2); simethicone (p.1213·1); electrolytes (p.1147·1).
Bowel evacuation.

Selgine *Zyma, Fr.*
Sodium chloride (p.1162·2); sel marin.
Mouth disorders.

Selide *Croce Bianca, Ital.†.*
Cefmolexin lysine.
Bacterial infections.

Selinol *Orion, Swed.*
Atenolol (p.825·3).
Angina pectoris; arrhythmias; hypertension.

Selipran
Bristol-Myers Squibb, Aust.; Bristol-Myers Squibb, Switz.
Pravastatin sodium (p.1277·1).
Hypercholesterolaemia.

Selit *GN, Ger.*
Sodium selenite (p.1354·1).
Selenium deficiency.

Selobloc *Lagap, Switz.†.*
Atenolol (p.825·3).
Angina pectoris; arrhythmias; hypertension.

Selokeen *Astra, Neth.*
Metoprolol succinate (p.908·2) or metoprolol tartrate (p.907·3).
Angina pectoris; arrhythmias; hypertension; hyperthyroidism; migraine; myocardial infarction.

Seloken
Astra, Aust.; Astra, Belg.; Astra, Fr.; Astra, Ital.; Astra, Norw.; Astra, Spain; Hassle, Swed.
Metoprolol succinate (p.908·2) or metoprolol tartrate (p.907·3).
Angina pectoris; arrhythmias; hypertension; hyperthyroidism; migraine; myocardial infarction.

Seloken retard Plus *Astra, Aust.*
Metoprolol succinate (p.908·2); hydrochlorothiazide (p.885·2).
Hypertension.

Seloken ZOC *Hassle, Swed.*
Metoprolol succinate (p.908·2).
Angina pectoris; arrhythmias; hypertension; migraine; myocardial infarction.

Selokomb *Astra, Neth.*
Metoprolol succinate (p.908·2) or metoprolol tartrate (p.907·3); hydrochlorothiazide (p.885·2).
Hypertension.

Selon *Serturner, Ger.*
Valerian (p.1643·1); lupulus (p.1597·2).
Agitation; sleep disorders.

Selopresin *Astra, Spain.*
Metoprolol tartrate (p.907·3); hydrochlorothiazide (p.885·2).
Hypertension.

Selozide
Astra, Belg.; Astra, Ital.
Metoprolol tartrate (p.907·3); hydrochlorothiazide (p.885·2).
Hypertension.

Selozok *Astra, Belg.*
Metoprolol succinate (p.908·2).
Angina pectoris; arrhythmias; hypertension; hyperthyroidism; migraine; myocardial infarction.

Selo-Zok *Astra, Norw.*
Metoprolol succinate (p.908·2).
Angina pectoris; arrhythmias; hypertension; migraine; myocardial infarction.

Selpar *Therabel, Ital.*
Selegiline hydrochloride (p.1144·2).
Parkinsonism.

Sels Calcaires Nutritifs *Weleda, Fr.*
Combination pack: Homoeopathic preparation.

Selsun
Abbott, Aust.; Abbott, Austral.; Abbott, Belg.; Abbott, Canad.; Abbott, Fr.; Abbott, Ger.; Abbott, Irl.; Abbott, Norw.; Abbott, S.Afr.†; Abbott, Swed.; Abbott, Switz.; Abbott, UK; Ross, USA.
Selenium sulphide (p.1091·1).
Dandruff; pityriasis versicolor; seborrhoeic dermatitis of the scalp.

Selsun Blu *Abbott, Ital.*
Selenium sulphide (p.1091·1).
Seborrhoeic dermatitis.

Selsun Trattamento *Abbott, Ital.†.*
Selenium sulphide (p.1091·1); menthol (p.1600·2).
Dandruff.

Selsun-R *Abbott, Neth.*
Selenium sulphide (p.1091·1).
Pityriasis versicolor.

Seltoc *Apomedica, Aust.*
Etenzamide (p.35·3); diphenhydramine hydrochloride (p.409·1); quinine hydrochloride (p.439·2); ascorbic acid (p.1365·2).
Cold symptoms.

Seltrans *Fresenius-Praxis, Ger.*
Sodium selenite (p.1354·1).
Selenium deficiency.

Selukos
Pharmacia Upjohn, Aust.; Pharmacia Upjohn, Ger.; ACO, Norw.; ACO, Swed.
Selenium sulphide (p.1091·1).
Scalp disorders.

Selvigon *Asta Medica, Aust.*
Pipazethate hydrochloride (p.1068·2).
Coughs.

Selvigon Hustensaft *Asta Medica, Ger.*
Pipazethate hydrochloride (p.1068·2).
Formerly known as Transpulmin N.
Coughs.

Selvjgon *Rhone-Poulenc Rorer, Ital.*
Pipazethate hydrochloride (p.1068·2).
Coughs.

Semap
Janssen-Cilag, Aust.; Janssen-Cilag, Belg.; Janssen-Cilag, Fr.; Janssen-Cilag, Neth.; Janssen-Cilag, Switz.
Penfluridol (p.684·3).
Psychoses.

Sembrina
Boehringer Mannheim, Ger.; Boehringer Mannheim, Neth.
Methyldopa (p.904·2).
Hypertension.

Sembrina-Saltucin *Boehringer Mannheim, Ger.†.*
Methyldopa (p.904·2); buthiazide (p.835·2).
Hypertension.

Semelciclina *Proter, Ital.†.*
Doxycycline hydrochloride (p.202·3).
Bacterial infections.

Semibiocin *Nycomed, Ger.†.*
Erythromycin (p.204·1) or erythromycin stearate (p.204·2).
Bacterial infections.

Semicid
Theraplix, Fr.; Whitehall, USA.
Nonoxinol 9 (p.1326·1).
Contraceptive.

Semi-Daonil
Hoechst Marion Roussel, Austral.; Hoechst Marion Roussel, Irl.; Hoechst Marion Roussel, S.Afr.†; Hoechst Marion Roussel, Switz.; Hoechst Marion Roussel, UK.
Glibenclamide (p.319·3).
Diabetes mellitus.

Semi-Euglucon
Boehringer Mannheim, Aust.; Hoechst, Aust.; Boehringer Mannheim, Neth.; Boehringer Mannheim, Switz.
Glibenclamide (p.319·3).
Diabetes mellitus.

Semi-Euglucon N *Boehringer Mannheim, Ger.; Hoechst, Ger.*
Glibenclamide (p.319·3).
Diabetes mellitus.

Semi-Gliben-Puren N *Isis Puren, Ger.*
Glibenclamide (p.319·3).
Diabetes mellitus.

Semilente
Novo Nordisk, Ger.; Squibb-Novo, USA†.
Insulin zinc suspension (bovine or porcine) (p.322·1).
Diabetes mellitus.

Semilente Iletin I *Lilly, USA†.*
Insulin zinc suspension (bovine and porcine) (p.322·1).
Diabetes mellitus.

Semilente Insulin *Novo Nordisk, Canad.†.*
Insulin zinc suspension (amorphous) (bovine and porcine) (p.322·1).
Diabetes mellitus.

Semilente MC
CSL-Novo, Austral.†; Novo Nordisk, Fr.; Novo Nordisk, Switz.
Insulin zinc suspension (amorphous) (porcine, monocomponent) (p.322·1).
Diabetes mellitus.

Semitard MC *Novo Nordisk, UK†.*
Insulin zinc suspension (amorphous) (porcine, monocomponent) (p.322·1).
Diabetes mellitus.

Sempera *Janssen-Cilag, Ger.; Glaxo Wellcome, Ger.*
Itraconazole (p.381·3).
Fungal infections.

Semprex
Glaxo Wellcome, Aust.; Glaxo Wellcome, Ital.; Glaxo Wellcome, Neth.; Glaxo Wellcome, S.Afr.; Glaxo Wellcome, Swed.; Wellcome, UK.
Acrivastine (p.401·3).
Allergic rhinitis; dermatological hypersensitivity reactions.

Semprex-D *Glaxo Wellcome, USA.*
Acrivastine (p.401·3); pseudoephedrine hydrochloride (p.1068·3).

Senacit *Chinosolfabrik, Ger.†.*
Sodium (3-(cyclohexenyl)-hydroxymethyl)phosphinate; multivitamins.

Senagar *Sigma, Austral.*
Senega and ammonia mixture, chloroform free.
Coughs.

Senamon *Rhone-Poulenc Rorer, Austral.†.*
Ammonium bicarbonate (p.1055·1); compound camphor spirit (p.1557·2); liquorice liquid extract (p.1197·1); concentrated senega infusion (p.1069·3); concentrated chloroform water.
Respiratory-tract disorders.

Sendoxan
Asta, Norw.; Asta Medica, Swed.
Cyclophosphamide (p.516·2).
Immune system disorders; malignant neoplasms.

Senecard *Metochem, Aust.*
Crataegus (p.1568·2).
Heart disorders.

Senecion *Klein, Ger.*
Senecio (p.1628·1); ascorbic acid (p.1365·2).
Haemorrhagic disorders.

Senefor *Pierre Fabre, Ital.*
Phosphatidylserine (p.1618·1).
Mental function impairment.

Senega *Kabi, Swed.†.*
Senega (p.1069·3); ammonium chloride (p.1055·2).
Coughs; sore throats.

Senega and Ammonia *McGloin, Austral.*
Ammonium bicarbonate (p.1055·1); camphor (p.1557·2); liquorice (p.1197·1); senega root (p.1069·3); ammonia solution (p.1548·3).
Cold symptoms.

Senetuss *Nelson, Austral.†.*
Ephedrine hydrochloride (p.1059·3); diphenhydramine hydrochloride (p.409·1); dihydrocodeine hydrochloride (p.34·2); senega and ammonia.
Coughs.

Seneuval *Qualiphar, Belg.*
Valerian (p.1643·1); melissa (p.1600·1).
Insomnia; nervousness.

Senexon *Rugby, USA.*
Senna (p.1212·2).
Constipation.

Senicor *Duopharm, Ger.*
Crataegus (p.1568·2).
Cardiac disorders.

Senilezol *Edwards, USA.*
Vitamin B substances with iron.

Senior *Strathmann, Ger.*
Pemoline (p.1484·1).
Mental function disorders.

Senioral *Semar, Spain.*
Clocinizine hydrochloride (p.406·3); phenylpropanolamine hydrochloride (p.1067·2).
Formerly contained buzepide metiodide, clocinizine hydrochloride, and pholcodine.
Nasal congestion.

Senioral Comp *Semar, Spain†.*
Clocinizine hydrochloride (p.406·3); phenylpropanolamine (p.1067·2); buzepide metiodide (p.459·2).
Nasal congestion.

Seniosan *Luitpold, Ger.†.*
Nicametate hydrogen tartrate; deanol hydrogen tartrate (p.1478·2); rutin (p.1580·2); fat-free, dried bovine spinal cord; vitamins.
Tonic.

Seniovita *Redel, Ger.*
Homoeopathic preparation.

Senlax *Intercare, UK.*
Senna (p.1212·2).
Constipation.

Senna-Gen *Goldline, USA.*
Senna (p.1212·2).
Constipation.

Sennatural *G & W, USA.*
Senna (p.1212·2).
Constipation.

Sennocol *Asta Medica, Neth.*
Senna (p.1212·2).
Constipation.

Senodin-AN *Bristol-Myers Squibb, Ital.*
Pheniramine maleate (p.415·3); codeine phosphate (p.26·1).
Coughs.

Senoger *Janssen-Cilag, Ital.†.*
Cinnarizine (p.406·1).
Vascular disorders.

Senokot
Reckitt & Colman, Austral.; Reckitts, Irl.; Reckitt & Colman, S.Afr.; Rovi, Spain†.
Sennosides A and B (p.1212·3).
Bowel evacuation; constipation.

Reckitt & Colman, Belg.; Purdue Frederick, Canad.; Sarget, Fr.; Nycomed, Norw.; Mundipharma, Switz.†; Reckitt & Colman, UK; Purdue Frederick, USA.
Senna (p.1212·2).
Bowel evacuation; constipation.

Senokot-S
Purdue Frederick, Canad.; Purdue Frederick, USA.
Senna (p.1212·2); docusate sodium (p.1189·3).
Constipation.

Senokotxtra *Purdue Frederick, USA.*
Senna (p.1212·2).
Constipation.

Senol *Bier, Ital.*
Cetrimonium bromide (p.1106·1).
Nipple disinfection.

Senolax
Neolab, Canad.
Sennosides A and B (p.1212·3).

Schein, USA†.
Senna (p.1212·2).
Constipation.

Senophile *Braun, Fr.*
Zinc oxide (p.1096·2); cholesteryl benzoate (p.1383·3).
Skin disorders.

Senro *Biosarto, Spain.*
Norfloxacin (p.233·1).
Gastro-enteritis; gonorrhoea; urinary-tract infections.

Sensaval *Lundbeck, Swed.*
Nortriptyline hydrochloride (p.300·2).
Depression.

Sensicutan *Harras-Curarina, Ger.*
Levomenol (p.1596·1); heparin sodium (p.879·3).
Skin disorders.

Sensifluid *Ducray, Fr.*
Avena (p.1551·3).
Soap substitute.

Sensifluor *Warner-Lambert, Ital.*
Sodium fluoride (p.742·1).
Dental caries prophylaxis; dental hypersensitivity.

Sensinerv *Redel, Ger.†.*
Wheat-germ; haemoglobin; malti; minerals; valerian; avena sativa; abrotanum.
Tonic.

Sensinerv forte *Redel, Ger.*
Valerian root (p.1643·1); lupulus (p.1597·2).
Nervous disorders; sleep disorders.

Sensiotin *Steigerwald, Ger.*
Homoeopathic preparation.

Sensit
Organon, Aust.; Thiemann, Ger.; Organon, Switz.
Fendiline hydrochloride (p.868·1).
Ischaemic heart disease.

Sensit-F *Organon, Ital.*
Fendiline hydrochloride (p.868·1).
Ischaemic heart disease; myocardial infarction.

Sensitive Eyes *Bausch & Lomb, USA.*
Range of solutions for contact lenses.

Sensitivity Protection Crest *Procter & Gamble, USA.*
Potassium nitrate (p.1123·1); sodium fluoride (p.742·1).
Sensitive teeth.

Sensivision au plantain *Chauvin, Fr.*
Plantain (p.1208·3).
Eye disorders.

Sensodent *Stafford-Miller, Switz.*
Strontium chloride (p.1633·1).
Hypersensitive teeth.

Sensodyne *Block, Canad.*
Strontium chloride (p.1633·1).
Hypersensitive teeth.

Sensodyne med *Salus, Aust.*
Strontium chloride (p.1633·1).
Dental hypersensitivity.

Sensodyne-F *Block, Canad.; Block, USA.*
Potassium nitrate (p.1123·1); sodium fluoride (p.742·1) or sodium monofluorophosphate (p.743·3).
Hypersensitive teeth.

Sensodyne-SC *Block, USA.*
Strontium chloride (p.1633·1).
Sensitive teeth.

SensoGARD *Block, USA.*
Benzocaine (p.1286·2).
Mouth and throat disorders.

Sensorcaine *Astra, Canad.; Astra, USA.*
Bupivacaine hydrochloride (p.1286·3).
Adrenaline (p.813·2) or adrenaline acid tartrate (p.813·3) is included in some injections as a vasoconstrictor to diminish absorption and localise the effect of the local anaesthetic.
Local anaesthesia.

Sential *Kabi Pharmacia, Canad.†.*
Hydrocortisone (p.1043·3); urea (p.1095·2).
Skin disorders.

Sential E *Pharmacia, UK†.*
Urea (p.1095·2); sodium chloride (p.1162·2).
Dry, pruritic skin.

Sential HC *Pharmacia, UK†.*
Urea (p.1095·2); hydrocortisone (p.1043·3); sodium chloride (p.1162·2).
Eczema.

Sential Hydrocortisone *Galderma, Belg.†.*
Hydrocortisone (p.1043·3).
Skin disorders.

Sepatren *Sumitomo, Jpn.*
Cefpiramide sodium (p.171·2).
Bacterial infections.

Sepazon *Sankyo, Jpn.*
Cloxazolam (p.657·3).
Anxiety states; premedication; sleep disorders.

Sepcen *Centrum, Spain.*
Ciprofloxacin hydrochloride (p.185·3).
Bacterial infections.

Sepdelen 7 *Hameln, Ger.†.*
Sodium tartrate (p.1214·1); dibasic sodium phosphate (p.1159·3); sodium sulphate (p.1213·3); tartaric acid (p.1634·3); sodium bicarbonate (p.1153·2); sodium citrate (p.1153·2); sodium dihydrogen citrate; sodium hydrogen tartrate.
Gout; liver and biliary-tract disorders; neuralgia; rheumatism; sciatica.

Sepik *Also, Ital.†.*
Aluminium clofibrate (p.1271·1).
Arteritis; cardiac disorders; disturbances of lipid metabolism.

Se-Power *Contassium Co., UK.*
Selenium yeast (p.1353·3); bilberry (p.1606·1); euphrasia; vitamin E (p.1369·1); zinc gluconate (p.1373·2); vitamin A (p.1358·1); riboflavine (p.1362·1).

Seprafilm *Genzyme, UK.*
Sodium hyaluronate (p.1630·3); carmellose (p.1471·2).
Prevention of surgical adhesions.

Sepso *Fink, Ger.†.*
Aluminium chloride (p.1078·3); ferric chloride (p.1579·3); bromosalicylic acid (p.1090·3); ammonium thiocyanate; salicylic acid (p.1090·2); isopropyl alcohol (p.1118·2).
Skin and mucous membrane disinfection.

Sepso J *Hofmann & Sommer, Ger.*
Povidone-iodine (p.1123·3).
Burns; skin, hand, and mucous membrane disinfection; wounds.

Septa *Circle, USA.*
Polymyxin B sulphate (p.239·1); neomycin sulphate (p.229·2); bacitracin (p.157·3).
Bacterial skin infections.

Septacef *Septa, Spain.*
Cephradine (p.181·3).
Bacterial infections.

Septacene *Prosana, Austral.†.*
Lignocaine (p.1293·2); calamine (p.1080·1); witch hazel (p.1587·1); vitamin A palmitate (p.1359·2); phenol liquid (p.1121·2); calcium pantothenate (p.1352·3); allantoin (p.1078·2); alpha tocopheryl acetate (p.1369·1); protein derivative; lanolin derivative.
Bites; minor burns; skin irritations.

Septacord *Muller Goppingen, Ger.*
Potassium aspartate (p.1161·3); magnesium aspartate (p.1157·2); crataegus (p.1568·2).
Cardiac disorders.

Septadine *Be-Tabs, S.Afr.*
Povidone-iodine (p.1123·3).
Minor throat infections; skin infections; wound and burn disinfection.

Septalibour *Ducray, Fr.*
Avena (p.1551·3); copper sulphate (p.1338·1); zinc sulphate (p.1373·2).
Cleansing of atopic skin.

Septanest *Ogna, Ital.; Septodont, Switz.*
Carticaine hydrochloride (p.1289·1).
Adrenaline acid tartrate (p.813·3) is included in this preparation as a vasoconstrictor to diminish absorption and localise the effect of the local anaesthetic.
Local anaesthesia.

Septasal *Septa, Spain†.*
Electrolyte preparation with glutamic acid.
Malnutrition; nutritional supplement in cardiac and renal disorders.

Septeal *Sinbio, Fr.*
Chlorhexidine gluconate (p.1107·2).
Skin and wound disinfection.

Septicol *Streuli, Switz.*
Chloramphenicol (p.182·1).
Bacterial eye infections.

Septicon *Ciba-Geigy, Aust.*
Combination pack: Lensept, hydrogen peroxide (p.1116·2); Lensrins NT, storage and rinsing solution.
Care of soft contact lenses.

Septicortin *Streuli, Switz.*
Cortisone acetate (p.1036·1); chloramphenicol (p.182·1).
Inflammatory eye infections.

Septidron *Hoechst Marion Roussel, S.Afr.*
Pipemidic acid (p.237·2).
Urinary-tract infections.

Septiline *Medecine Vegetale, Fr.†.*
Lithium carbonate; lithium benzoate; anhydrous sodium hydrogen phosphate; sodium bicarbonate; tartaric acid.
Aid to digestion.

Septimide *Nelson, Austral.†.*
Chlorhexidine (p.1107·2); cetrimide (p.1105·2).
Minor abrasions.

Septi-Soft *Calgon Vestal, USA.*
Triclosan (p.1127·2).
Skin cleanser.

Septisol
Note. This name is used for preparations of different composition.
Monot, Fr.
Salicylic acid (p.1090·2).
Chronic conjunctivitis.

Calgon Vestal, USA.
Foam: Hexachlorophane (p.1115·2).
Solution: Triclosan (p.1127·2).
Skin cleanser; skin disinfection.

Septivon *Scholl, Fr.*
Triclocarban (p.1127·2); detergents.
Skin and mucous membrane disinfection.

Septivon N *Scholl, Switz.*
Triclocarban (p.1127·2); cetrimonium chloride (p.1106·1).
Hand disinfection; minor skin lesions.

Septocipro *Lesvi, Spain.*
Ciprofloxacin hydrochloride (p.185·3) or ciprofloxacin lactate (p.185·3).
Bacterial infections.

Septolit *Henkel, Ger.*
Benzalkonium chloride (p.1101·3); oligo(di(iminoimidocarbonyl)iminohexamethylene).
Surface disinfection.

Septomandolo *IPA, Ital.*
Cephamandole nafate (p.180·1).
Lignocaine hydrochloride (p.1293·2) is included in the intramuscular injection to alleviate the pain of injection.
Bacterial infections.

Septomixine *Septodont, Switz.*
Dexamethasone (p.1037·1); polymyxin B sulphate (p.239·1); tyrothricin (p.267·2); neomycin sulphate (p.229·2).
Dental infections.

Septonsil *Pekana, Ger.*
Homoeopathic preparation.

Septopal *Merck, Aust.; Smith & Nephew, Austral.; Merck-Belgolabo, Belg.; Merck, Ger.; E. Merck, Irl.; Bracco, Ital.†; E. Merck, Neth.; E. Merck, Norw.; Merck, S.Afr.; Meda, Swed.; E. Merck, Switz.; E. Merck, UK.*
Gentamicin sulphate (p.212·1); polymethylmethacrylate-methylmethacrylate copolymer (p.1603·2).
Bacterial infections of bone and soft tissues.

Septosol *Xeragen, S.Afr.*
Phenol (p.1121·2).
Sore throat.

Septra *Glaxo Wellcome, Canad.; Glaxo Wellcome, USA.*
Co-trimoxazole (p.196·3).
Bacterial infections; Pneumocystis carinii pneumonia.

Septran *Glaxo Wellcome, S.Afr.*
Co-trimoxazole (p.196·3).
Bacterial infections.

Septrin *Glaxo Wellcome, Austral.; Wellcome, Irl.; Evans, Spain; Wellcome, UK.*
Co-trimoxazole (p.196·3).
Bacterial infections; Pneumocystis carinii pneumonia.

Sequennia *Wyeth Lederle, Aust.*
Red/brown tablets, conjugated oestrogens (p.1457·3); white tablets, medroxyprogesterone acetate (p.1448·3).
Menopausal disorders.

Sequilar *Schering, Aust.; Schering, Austral.; Schering, Ger.; Schering, Switz.*
Levonorgestrel (p.1454·1); ethinyloestradiol (p.1445·1).
28-Day packs also contain 7 inert tablets.
Biphasic oral contraceptive.

Sequilarum *Schering, Swed.†.*
Levonorgestrel (p.1454·1); ethinyloestradiol (p.1445·1).
Biphasic oral contraceptive.

Sequostat *Jenapharm, Ger.*
6 Tablets ethinyloestradiol (p.1445·1); 15 tablets ethinyloestradiol; norethisterone acetate (p.1453·1).
Sequential oral contraceptive.

Seracalm *Demopharm, Switz.*
Valerian (p.1643·1); melissa (p.1600·1); neroli oil (p.1606·3); lavender oil (p.1594·3).
Sleep disorders.

Seractil *Gebro, Aust.*
Dexibuprofen (p.44·3).
Fever; inflammation; musculoskeletal and joint disorders; pain.

Serad *Boehringer Mannheim, Ital.*
Sertraline hydrochloride (p.307·2).
Depression.

Seralbuman *ISI, Ital.*
Albumin (p.710·1).
Hypoalbuminaemia.

Seralgan *Lundbeck, Aust.*
Citalopram hydrobromide (p.281·1).
Pain.

Seranex sans codeine *Demopharm, Switz.*
Phenazone (p.78·2); propyphenazone (p.81·3); etenzamide (p.35·3); benzyl mandelate; caffeine (p.749·3).
Pain.

Ser-Ap-Es *Ciba, Canad.; Ciba, USA.*
Reserpine (p.942·1); hydralazine hydrochloride (p.883·2); hydrochlorothiazide (p.885·2).
Hypertension.

Seravit *Scientific Hospital Supplies, Irl.; Scientific Hospital Supplies, UK.*
Multivitamin, mineral, and carbohydrate preparation.
Nutritional supplement.

Serax *Wyeth-Ayerst, Canad.; Wyeth-Ayerst, USA.*
Oxazepam (p.683·2).
Alcohol withdrawal syndrome; anxiety.

Serc *Solvay, Austral.; Solvay, Canad.; Solvay, Fr.; Solvay, Irl.; Solvay, S.Afr.; Duphar, Spain; Solvay, UK.*
Betahistine hydrochloride (p.1553·1).
Ménière's disease; vestibular disorders.

Serdolect *Lundbeck, Irl.†; Lundbeck, Neth.†; Lundbeck, UK†.*
Sertindole (p.692·2).
Schizophrenia.

Serecor *Synthelabo, Fr.*
Hydroquinidine hydrochloride (p.889·3).
Arrhythmias.

Sereine *Optikem, USA.*
Range of solutions for hard contact lenses.

Sere-Mit *Mitim, Ital.*
Saw palmetto (p.1462·1).
Prostatic hyperplasia.

Seren *Vita, Ital.†.*
Chlordiazepoxide hydrochloride (p.646·3).
Alcohol withdrawal syndrome; anxiety.

Seren Vita *Synthelabo, Ital.†.*
Chlordiazepoxide hydrochloride (p.646·3).
Alcohol withdrawal syndrome; anxiety.

Serenace *Searle, Austral.; Baker Norton, Irl.; Searle, S.Afr.; Baker Norton, UK.*
Haloperidol (p.673·3).
Agitation; anxiety; childhood behaviour disorders; intractable hiccup; nausea and vomiting; neuroleptanalgesia; psychoses; Tourette syndrome.

Serenade *Alter, Spain.*
Nitrazepam (p.682·2).
Insomnia.

Serenal *Sankyo, Jpn.*
Oxazolam (p.684·1).
Anxiety states; premedication; sleep disorders.

Serenase
Note. This name is used for preparations of different composition.
Sintesa, Belg.
Lorazepam (p.675·3).
Anxiety; insomnia; premedication.

Lusofarmaco, Ital.
Haloperidol (p.673·3).
Alcohol withdrawal syndrome; hiccups; movement disorders; pain; psychoses; vomiting.

Serenity *Gerard House, UK.*
Lupulus (p.1597·2); passion flower (p.1615·3); valerian (p.1643·1); gentian (p.1583·3).
Agitation; nervousness.

Serenival *Chefaro Ardeval, Fr.*
Crataegus (p.1568·2); passion flower (p.1615·3); valerian (p.1643·1).
Insomnia; nervous disorders.

Serenoa Complex *Blackmores, Austral.*
Equisetum (p.1575·1); saw palmetto (p.1462·1) buchu (p.1555·2); *d*-alpha tocopheryl acid succinate (p.1369·2); zinc amino acid chelate (p.1373·3).
Prostate disorders; urinary-tract disorders.

Serenoa-C *Wassen, UK.*
Saw palmetto (p.1462·1); vitamins; minerals.

Serenol *Dolisos, Canad.*
Homoeopathic preparation.

Serentil *Sandoz, Canad.; Boehringer Ingelheim, USA.*
Mesoridazine besylate (p.678·2).
Alcohol withdrawal syndrome; psychoses.

Serepax *Wyeth, Austral.; Wyeth, Norw.; Akromed, S.Afr.; Wyeth Lederle, Swed.*
Oxazepam (p.683·2).
Alcohol withdrawal syndrome; anxiety disorders; insomnia.

Serepress *Formenti, Ital.*
Ketanserin tartrate (p.894·3).
Hypertension.

Sereprile *Synthelabo, Ital.*
Tiapride hydrochloride (p.696·1).
Gastro-intestinal dyskinesia; movement and behaviour disorders.

Sereprostat *Robapharm, Spain.*
Saw palmetto (p.1462·1).
Prostatic disorders.

Seresta *Wyeth Lederle, Belg.; Wyeth, Fr.; Wyeth, Neth.; Wyeth, Switz.*
Oxazepam (p.683·2).
Alcohol withdrawal syndrome; anxiety; sleep disorders.

Sereupin *Ravizza, Ital.*
Paroxetine hydrochloride (p.301·2).
Depression; obsessive-compulsive disorder; panic disorders.

Serevent *Glaxo Wellcome, Aust.; Glaxo Wellcome, Austral.; Glaxo Wellcome, Belg.; Glaxo Wellcome, Canad.; Glaxo Wellcome, Fr.; Glaxo Wellcome, Ger.; Allen & Hanburys, Irl.; Glaxo Wellcome, Ital.; Glaxo Wellcome, Neth.; Glaxo Wellcome, Norw.; Allen & Hanburys, S.Afr.; Glaxo Wellcome, Spain; Glaxo Wellcome, Swed.; Glaxo Wellcome, Switz.; Allen & Hanburys, UK; Glaxo Wellcome, USA.*
Salmeterol xinafoate (p.761·2).
Obstructive airways disease.

Serfabiotic *Serra Pamies, Spain.*
Metampicillin (p.224·3) or metampicillin sodium (p.224·3).
Bacterial infections.

Serfoxide *Morrith, Spain.*
Pyridoxine phosphoserinate (p.1363·1).
Chronic alcoholism; vitamin B_6 deficiency.

Sergast *Serturner, Ger.*
Turmeric (p.1001·3).
Digestive system disorders.

Seriel *Biogalenique, Fr.†.*
Tofisopam (p.696·3).
Alcohol withdrawal syndrome; anxiety.

Seriglutan B12 *Serpero, Ital.*
Amino-acid and vitamin B_{12} preparation.
Tonic.

Serlain *Roerig, Belg.*
Sertraline hydrochloride (p.307·2).
Depression; obsessive-compulsive disorder.

Sermaform *Lilly, Ger.†.*
Flurandrenolone (p.1042·2); clioquinol (p.193·2).
Infected skin disorders.

Sermaka *Lilly, Ger.*
Flurandrenolone (p.1042·2).
Skin disorders.

Sermaka N *Lilly, Ger.†.*
Flurandrenolone (p.1042·2); neomycin sulphate (p.229·2).
Infected skin disorders.

Sermidrina *Farmitalia Carlo Erba, Ital.†.*
Reserpine (p.942·1); hydrochlorothiazide (p.885·2); nicergoline (p.1607·1).
Hypertension.

Sermion *Pharmacia Upjohn, Aust.; Specia, Fr.; Pharmacia Upjohn, Ger.; Pharmacia Upjohn, Ital.; Kenfarma, Spain; Pharmacia Upjohn, Switz.*
Nicergoline (p.1607·1) or nicergoline tartrate (p.1607·1).
Cerebral and peripheral vascular disorders.

Serobif *Serono, Ital.*
Interferon beta (p.616·1).
Malignant neoplasms; viral infections.

Serocion *Sanwa, Jpn.*
Propagermanium (p.624·2).
Hepatitis B.

Seroclorina *Whitehall, Ital.†.*
Chloramine (p.1106·3).
Disinfection.

Serocryptin *Serono, Ital.†; Serono, Switz.*
Bromocriptine mesylate (p.1132·2).
Acromegaly; benign breast disorders; female infertility; galactorrhoea; lactation inhibition; male hypogonadism; menstrual disorders; parkinsonism; pituitary adenoma.

Serocytol *Serolab, Switz.*
A range of equine antisera raised against body tissues and organs.

Serofene *Serono, Ital.*
Clomiphene citrate (p.1439·2).
Amenorrhoea; anovulatory infertility; functional uterine haemorrhage; oligomenorrhoea; polycystic ovary syndrome.

Seromycin *Lilly, Canad.; Dura, USA.*
Cycloserine (p.198·3).
Bacterial infections of the urinary tract; tuberculosis.

Serophene *Serono, Aust.; Serono, Austral.; Serono, Canad.; Serono, Irl.; Serono, Neth.; Research Labs, S.Afr.; Serono, Switz.; Serono, UK; Serono, USA.*
Clomiphene citrate (p.1439·2).
Anovulatory infertility.

Serophy Monal, Fr.; Interdelta, Switz.
Sodium chloride (p.1162·2).
Rhinitis.

Seropram Lundbeck, Aust.; Lundbeck, Fr.; Lundbeck, Ital.; Lundbeck, Spain; Lundbeck, Switz.
Citalopram hydrobromide (p.281·1) or citalopram hydrochloride (p.281·1).
Depression; pain.

Seroquel Zeneca, UK; Zeneca, USA.
Quetiapine fumarate (p.690·1).
Psychoses.

Serosod Serono, Ital.†.
Orgotein (p.87·3).
Inflammation.

Serostim Serono, USA.
Somatropin (p.1249·3).
AIDS-related cachexia; growth hormone deficiency.

Serotone Yoshitomi, Jpn.
Azasetron hydrochloride (p.1179·1).
Nausea and vomiting associated with antineoplastic therapy.

Serotonyl ICT-Lodi, Ital.†.
Oxitriptan (p.301·2).
Serotonin-deficiency disorders.

Serotulle Seton, UK.
Chlorhexidine acetate (p.1107·2).
Wounds.

Serovit Zilliken, Ital.†.
Oxitriptan (p.301·2).
Depression; epilepsy (adjuvant); migraine; myoclonus; pain syndrome; parkinsonism (adjuvant); sleep disorders.

Seroxat SmithKline Beecham, Aust.; SK-RIT, Belg.; SmithKline Beecham, Ger.; SmithKline Beecham, Irl.; SmithKline Beecham, Ital.; SmithKline Beecham, Neth.; Novo Nordisk, Norw.; SmithKline Beecham, Spain; Novo Nordisk, Swed.; SmithKline Beecham, UK.
Paroxetine hydrochloride (p.301·2).
Depression; obsessive-compulsive disorder; panic disorders.

Serpalan Lannett, USA.
Reserpine (p.942·1).
Hypertension; psychoses.

Serpasil Ciba, Canad.; Ciba, Ital.†.
Reserpine (p.942·1).
Hypertension; psychoses.

Serpasil-Esidrix Ciba, Canad.†.
Reserpine (p.942·1); hydrochlorothiazide (p.885·2).
Hypertension.

Serpasil-Navidrex-K Ciba-Geigy, S.Afr.†.
Reserpine (p.942·1); cyclopenthiazide (p.845·2); potassium chloride (p.1161·1).
Hypertension.

Serpasol Ciba-Geigy, Spain†.
Reserpine (p.942·1).
Anxiety; hypertension; tension.

Serpax Wyeth, Ital.
Oxazepam (p.683·2).
Anxiety; depression; insomnia.

Serpens Lisapharma, Ital.
Saw palmetto (p.1462·1).
Prostatic hyperplasia.

Serrulatum Pfluger, Ger.†.
Saw palmetto (p.1462·1); echinacea angustifolia (p.1574·2).
Urinary-tract disorders.

Sertofren Geigy, Norw.†.
Desipramine hydrochloride (p.282·2).
Depression.

Serumar Armour, Ger.†.
A plasma protein fraction (p.726·3).
Hypoproteinaemia; hypovolaemia.

Serum-Cholinesterase Centeon, Ger.
Acetylcholinesterase (p.972·2).
Antidote to suxamethonium chloride; organophosphorus poisoning.

Serutan Menley & James, USA.
Psyllium (p.1194·2).
Constipation.

Servambutol Servipharm, Switz.†.
Ethambutol hydrochloride (p.207·2).
Tuberculosis.

Servamox Servipharm, Switz.
Amoxycillin trihydrate (p.151·3).
Bacterial infections.

Servanolol Servipharm, Switz.†.
Propranolol hydrochloride (p.937·1).
Angina pectoris; arrhythmias; hypertension; hyperthyroidism; migraine; myocardial infarction; obstructive hypertrophic cardiomyopathy; phaeochromocytoma; tremor.

Servatrin Lennon, S.Afr.
Timolol maleate (p.953·3); amiloride hydrochloride (p.819·2); hydrochlorothiazide (p.885·2).
Hypertension.

Servetinal Seid, Spain.
Aluminium hydroxide (p.1177·3); belladonna (p.457·1); calcium carbonate (p.1182·1); magnesium hydroxide (p.1198·2); sodium bicarbonate (p.1153·2).
Gastritis; gastro-intestinal hyperacidity.

Servicef Servipharm, Switz.
Cephazolin sodium (p.181·1).
Bacterial infections.

Servicillin Servipharm, Switz.†.
Ampicillin sodium (p.153·1) or ampicillin trihydrate (p.153·2).
Bacterial infections.

Serviclofen Servipharm, Switz.†.
Chloramphenicol (p.182·1).
Bacterial infections.

Servidipine Servipharm, Switz.†.
Nifedipine (p.916·2).
Angina pectoris; hypertension.

Servidoxyne Servipharm, Switz.†.
Doxycycline hydrochloride (p.202·3).
Bacterial infections.

Servidrat Servipharm, Switz.†.
Glucose; sodium chloride; potassium chloride; citric acid; sodium bicarbonate (p.1152·3).
Diarrhoea; oral rehydration therapy.

Servigenta Servipharm, Switz.
Gentamicin sulphate (p.212·1).
Bacterial infections.

Servimeta Servipharm, Switz.†.
Indomethacin (p.45·2).
Gout; inflammation; musculoskeletal, joint, and periarticular disorders; pain.

Servinaprox Servipharm, Switz.
Naproxen (p.61·2).
Inflammation; pain.

Serviprofen Servipharm, Switz.
Ibuprofen (p.44·1).
Inflammation; musculoskeletal and joint disorders; pain.

Servispor Servipharm, Switz.
Cephalexin (p.178·2).
Bacterial infections.

Servitamol Servipharm, Switz.
Salbutamol (p.758·2).
Asthma.

Servitenol Servipharm, Switz.
Atenolol (p.825·3).
Angina pectoris; hypertension; myocardial infarction.

Servitet Servipharm, Switz.†.
Tetracycline hydrochloride (p.259·1).
Bacterial infections.

Servitrocin Servipharm, Switz.
Erythromycin ethyl succinate (p.204·2) or erythromycin stearate (p.204·2).
Bacterial infections.

Servivit + M Servipharm, Switz.†.
Multivitamin and mineral preparation.

Servizol Servipharm, Switz.
Metronidazole (p.585·1) or metronidazole benzoate (p.585·1).
Anaerobic infections; protozoal infections.

Serzone Bristol-Myers Squibb, Austral.; Bristol-Myers Squibb, Canad.; Bristol-Myers Squibb, S.Afr.; Bristol-Myers Squibb, USA.
Nefazodone hydrochloride (p.299·3).
Depression.

Sesame Street McNeil Consumer, USA.
A range of vitamin preparations.

Sesden Tanabe, Jpn.
Timepidium bromide (p.469·1).
Premedication for examination of the gastro-intestinal tract or urinary system; smooth muscle spasm.

Sesquicillina ITA, Ital.†.
Ampicillin (p.153·1).
Bacterial infections.

Setamol Reckitt & Colman, Austral.; Reckitt & Colman, S.Afr.†.
Paracetamol (p.72·2).
Fever; pain.

Setamol Co Reckitt & Colman, S.Afr.†.
Paracetamol (p.72·2); codeine phosphate (p.26·1).
Pain.

Setin Schwulst, S.Afr.
Metoclopramide hydrochloride (p.1200·3).
Gastro-intestinal disorders.

Setlers Stafford-Miller, UK.
Calcium carbonate (p.1182·1).
Dyspepsia; flatulence.

Setlers Extra Strength Stafford-Miller, UK.
Aluminium hydroxide (p.1177·3); magnesium hydroxide (p.1198·2).
These ingredients can be described by the British Approved Name Co-magaldrox.

Setlers Tums SmithKline Beecham Consumer, Irl.
Calcium carbonate (p.1182·1).
Dyspepsia; flatulence; heartburn; nausea.

Setlers Wind-eze Stafford-Miller, UK.
Simethicone (p.1213·1).
Flatulence.

Setrilan Essex, Ital.
Spirapril hydrochloride (p.946·1).
Hypertension.

Seudotabs Parmed, USA.
Pseudoephedrine hydrochloride (p.1068·3).
Nasal congestion.

Seven Seas Seven Seas, UK.
A range of vitamin, mineral, and nutritional preparations.

Sevinol Schering-Plough, Belg.
Fluphenazine (p.672·1).
Anxiety; nausea; psychosis; vomiting.

Sevorane Abbott, Austral.; Abbott, Canad.; Abbott, Ger.; Abbott, Irl.; Abbott, Ital.; Abbott, Neth.; Abbott, Norw.; Abbott, Swed.; Abbott, Switz.
Sevoflurane (p.1231·3).
General anaesthesia.

Sevorex Tika, Swed.
Precipitated sulphur (p.1091·2); salicylic acid (p.1090·2).
Scalp disorders.

Sevredol Mundipharma, Ger.; Napp, Irl.; Asta Medica, Neth.; Asta Medica, Spain; Mundipharma, Switz.; Napp, UK.
Morphine sulphate (p.56·2).
Pain.

Sevrium Vinas, Spain.
Tetrabamate.
Alcohol withdrawal syndrome.

SFC Lotion Stiefel, USA.
Stearyl alcohol (p.1385·1).
Skin cleanser.

Sfigmoreg Lisapharma, Ital.†.
Hydrochlorothiazide (p.885·2); reserpine (p.942·1).
Hypertension; production of diuresis.

Sguardi Farmigea, Ital.
Benzalkonium chloride (p.1101·3).
Eye disinfection.

SH-206 Pharmascience, Canad.
Acetic acid (p.1541·2); camphor (p.1557·2).
Pediculosis.

SH 420 Schering, UK†.
Norethisterone acetate (p.1453·1).
Breast cancer.

Shade
Note. This name is used for preparations of different composition.
Schering-Plough, Canad.; Schering-Plough, USA.
SPF 15: Ethylhexyl *p*-methoxycinnamate (p.1487·1); oxybenzone (p.1487·3).
Sunscreen.

Schering-Plough, Canad.
SPF 25: Oxybenzone (p.1487·3); ethylhexyl *p*-methoxycinnamate (p.1487·1); octyl salicylate (p.1487·3).
Sunscreen.

Schering-Plough, Canad.; Schering-Plough, USA.
Lotion SPF 30; stick SPF 30: Ethylhexyl *p*-methoxycinnamate (p.1487·1); oxybenzone (p.1487·3); homosalate (p.1487·2); 2-ethylhexyl salicylate (p.1487·3).
Sunscreen.

Schering-Plough, USA.
Gel SPF 30: Ethylhexyl *p*-methoxycinnamate (p.1487·1); oxybenzone (p.1487·3); homosalate (p.1487·2).
Sunscreen.

Schering-Plough, Canad.; Schering-Plough, USA.
SPF 45: Ethylhexyl *p*-methoxycinnamate (p.1487·1); oxybenzone (p.1487·3); octocrylene (p.1487·3); 2-ethylhexyl salicylate (p.1487·3).
Sunscreen.

Shade UVAGuard Schering-Plough, USA.
Ethylhexyl *p*-methoxycinnamate (p.1487·1); avobenzone (p.1486·3); oxybenzone (p.1487·3).
Sunscreen.

Shak Iso Clintec, Fr.
Preparation for enteral nutrition.

Shaklee Dandruff Control Shaklee, Canad.
Pyrithione zinc (p.1089·3).

Shaklee Lip Protection Stick Shaklee, Canad.
SPF 15: Padimate O (p.1488·1); oxybenzone (p.1487·3).
Sunscreen.

Shaklee Sunscreen Shaklee, Canad.
SPF 30: Ethylhexyl *p*-methoxycinnamate (p.1487·1); octyl salicylate (p.1487·3); oxybenzone (p.1487·3).
Sunscreen.

Shamday Antiforfora Euroderm, Ital.
Piroctone olamine (p.1089·1); urtica (p.1642·3).
Seborrhoeic dermatitis.

Shampoo Antiparassitario al Piretro Cruz Verde Fastfarm, Ital.†.
Pyrethrum (p.1410·1); piperonyl butoxide (p.1409·3).
Pediculosis.

Shampoo Potenziato Cruz Verde Allo Zolfo Organico Fastfarm, Ital.†.
Mesulphen (p.1086·3).
Pediculosis.

Shampoo SDE Tar Schering-Plough, Ital.
Coal tar (p.1092·3).
Scalp disorders.

Shampoo SDE Zinc Schering-Plough, Ital.
Pyrithione zinc (p.1089·3).
Seborrhoeic dermatitis.

Shampooing Anti-Pelliculaire Atlas, Canad.
Pyrithione zinc (p.1089·3).

Shampooing extra-doux Widmer, Switz.
Triclosan (p.1127·2).
Scalp disorders.

Shampoux Qualiphar, Belg.
Permethrin (p.1409·2); piperonyl butoxide (p.1409·3).
Pediculosis.

Shampoux Repel Qualiphar, Belg.
(N-Butyl-N-acetyl)-3-ethylaminopropionate.
Pediculosis.

SHC Vitabiotics, UK†.
Multivitamin, mineral, and amino-acid preparation.

Sheik Schmid, Canad.
Nonoxinol 9 (p.1326·1).
Contraceptive.

Sheik Elite Schmid, USA.
Nonoxinol 9 (p.1326·1).
Contraceptive.

Shepard's Dermik, USA.
Emollient and moisturiser.

Shii-ta-ker Holistica, Fr.
Lentinus edodes.
Immunostimulant.

Shiomarin Shionogi, Jpn.
Latamoxef sodium (p.221·2).
Lignocaine (p.1293·2) is included in the intramuscular injection to alleviate the pain of injection.
Bacterial infections.

Shiseido Sun Protection Shiseido, Canad.
SPF 8: Ethylhexyl *p*-methoxycinnamate (p.1487·1).
Sunscreen.

Shiseido Sunblock Shiseido, Canad.
SPF 19: Ethylhexyl *p*-methoxycinnamate (p.1487·1); oxybenzone (p.1487·3).
Sunscreen.

Shiseido Sunblock Face Cream Shiseido, Canad.
Ethylhexyl *p*-methoxycinnamate (p.1487·1); oxybenzone (p.1487·3); 2-phenyl-1*H*=benzimidazole-5-sulphonic acid (p.1488·2); titanium dioxide (p.1093·3).
Sunscreen.

Shiseido Sunblock Lip Protection Shiseido, Canad.
Ethylhexyl *p*-methoxycinnamate (p.1487·1).
Sunscreen.

Shiseido Tanning Shiseido, Canad.
SPF 4: Ethylhexyl *p*-methoxycinnamate (p.1487·1).
Sunscreen.

Shiseido Translucent Sun Block Shiseido, Canad.
Ethylhexyl *p*-methoxycinnamate (p.1487·1); oxybenzone (p.1487·3); titanium dioxide (p.1093·3).
Sunscreen.

Shur-Seal Milex, USA.
Nonoxinol 9 (p.1326·1).
Contraceptive.

S-hydril Laves, Ger.†.
Sodium thiosulphate (p.996·2).
Poisoning with heavy metals, gases, cyanide, nitrides, nitrogen gases, carbon monoxide.

Sialin Sigmapharm, Aust.
Carmellose sodium (p.1471·2); electrolytes (p.1147·1).
Saliva substitute.

Sialor Solvay, Canad.
Anethole trithione (p.1549·3).
Dry mouth.

Siaten Italfarmaco, Spain.
Zopiclone (p.699·2).
Insomnia.

Sibelium Janssen-Cilag, Aust.; Janssen-Cilag, Belg.; Janssen-Ortho, Canad.; Janssen-Cilag, Fr.; Janssen-Cilag, Ger.; Janssen-Cilag, Irl.; Janssen-Cilag, Ital.; Janssen-Cilag, Neth.; Janssen-Cilag, S.Afr.; Esteve, Spain; Janssen-Cilag, Switz.
Flunarizine hydrochloride (p.411·1).
Migraine; nausea and vomiting; vestibular disorders.

Sibevit Delagrange, Spain†.
Pyridoxine (p.1363·1).
Acute alcoholism; convulsions in infants; drug-induced pyridoxine deficiency; Huntington's chorea.

Siblin Warner-Lambert, USA†.
Psyllium husk (p.1194·2).
Constipation.

Sical Rottapharm, Ital.; Rottapharm, Spain.
Salcatonin (p.735·3).
Hypercalcaemia; metastatic bone pain; Paget's disease of bone; postmenopausal osteoporosis.

Sicazine Smith & Nephew, Fr.
Silver sulphadiazine (p.247·3).
Burns; wounds.

Siccagent Bournonville, Belg.
Povidone (p.1474·2).
Dry eyes.

Siccalix Drossapharm, Switz.
Sea salt (p.1162·2); dexpanthenol (p.1570·3).
Nasal dryness.

Siccaprotect Croma, Aust.; Ursapharm, Ger.
Dexpanthenol (p.1570·3); polyvinyl alcohol (p.1474·2).
Dry eyes.

Sicca-Stulln Stulln, Ger.
Hypromellose (p.1473·1).
Dry eyes.

Siccatears Allergan, Neth.†.
White paraffin (p.1382·3); liquid paraffin (p.1382·1); Amerchol CAB.
Dry eyes.

Sicco Dresden, Ger.
Indapamide (p.890·2).
Hypertension.

Sicco-Gynaedron Artesan, Ger.†.
Aluminium magnesium silicate (p.1471·1).
Vaginitis.

Siccoral *Salus, Aust.*
Acetylcysteine (p.1052·3).
Respiratory-tract disorders associated with viscous mucus.

Sicef *Kemyos, Ital.*
Cephazolin sodium (p.181·1).
Lignocaine hydrochloride (p.1293·2) is included in this preparation to alleviate the pain of injection.
Bacterial infections.

Si-Cliss *SIFRA, Ital.*
Sorbitol (p.1354·2); sodium citrate (p.1153·2); sodium lauryl sulphoacetate (p.1468·3).
Constipation.

Sico Relax *Rottapharm, Spain.*
Diazepam (p.661·1).
Alcohol withdrawal syndrome; anxiety; epilepsy; general anaesthesia; insomnia; skeletal muscle spasm.

Sicombyl *Christiaens, Belg.*
Salicylic acid (p.1090·2).
Hygiene of the umbilicus in neonates.

Sic-Ophtal *Winzer, Ger.*
Hypromellose (p.1473·1).
Dry eyes.

Sicorten
Zyma, Aust.; Zyma, Belg.; Zyma, Ger.; Novartis, Neth.; Zyma, Spain; Max Ritter, Switz.
Halometasone monohydrate (p.1043·3).
Skin disorders.

Sicorten Plus
Zyma, Ger.; Ciba-Geigy, S.Afr.†; Zyma, Spain; Max Ritter, Switz.
Halometasone monohydrate (p.1043·3); triclosan (p.1127·2).
Infected skin disorders.

Sideck Shampoo Antiforfora *Sideck, Ital.†.*
Piroctone olamine (p.1089·1); matricaria (p.1561·2); copper usnate (p.1643·1); undecenoic acid (p.389·2).
Seborrhoeic dermatitis.

Sideritrina *Guieu, Ital.†.*
Cyanocobalamin (p.1363·3); ferrous gluconate (p.1340·1).
Iron-deficiency anaemia.

Siderofolin *Lifepharma, Ital.†.*
Iron succinyl-protein complex (p.1349·2); calcium folinate (p.1342·2).
Anaemias.

Sideroglobina *Pharmacia Upjohn, Ital.*
Ferritransferrin.
Iron-deficiency anaemia.

Sideros *Inverni della Beffa, Ital.†.*
Ferritin (p.1580·1).
Anaemias; oligohaemia of infancy.

Sidroga Brust-Husten-Tee *Jacoby, Aust.*
Althaea (p.1546·3); plantago lanceolata; thyme leaf (p.1636·3); aniseed (p.1549·3); orange flowers.
Catarrh; coughs.

Sidroga Erkaltungstee *Jacoby, Aust.*
Rose fruit (p.1365·2); wild thyme; chamomile flower (p.1561·2); sambucus (p.1627·2); tilia (p.1637·3).
Respiratory tract disorders.

Sidroga Herz-Kreislauf-Tee *Jacoby, Aust.*
Crataegus (p.1568·2); melissa leaf (p.1600·1); rosemary leaf; orange flowers; spearmint (p.1632·1).
Anxiety disorders; cardiac disorders.

Sidroga Kindertee *Jacoby, Aust.*
Fennel (p.1579·1); chamomile flower (p.1561·2); melissa leaf (p.1600·1); peppermint leaf (p.1208·1); tilia (p.1637·3).
Gastro-intestinal disorders; sleep disorders.

Sidroga Leber-Galle-Tee *Jacoby, Aust.*
Taraxacum (p.1634·2); silybum marianum fruit (p.993·3); achillea (p.1542·2); peppermint leaf (p.1208·1); caraway (p.1559·3).
Gastro-intestinal and biliary disorders.

Sidroga Magen-Darm-Tee *Jacoby, Aust.*
Calamus root (p.1556·1); centaury (p.1561·1); chamomile flower (p.1561·2); achillea (p.1542·2); melissa leaf (p.1600·1); spearmint (p.1632·1).
Gastro-intestinal disorders.

Sidroga Nerven- und Schlaftee *Jacoby, Aust.*
Lupulus (p.1597·2); melissa leaf (p.1600·1); valerian root (p.1643·1); spearmint (p.1632·1); orange flowers.
Anxiety disorders; sleep disorders.

Sidroga Nieren- und Blasentee *Jacoby, Aust.*
Bearberry leaf (p.1552·2); silver birch leaf (p.1553·3); solidago virgaurea; orthosiphon leaf (p.1592·2); couch-grass (p.1567·3); peppermint leaf (p.1208·1).
Urinary-tract disorders.

Sidroga Stoffwechseltee *Jacoby, Aust.*
Spearmint (p.1632·1); taraxacum (p.1634·2); urtica (p.1642·3); prunus spinosa.
Digestive disorders; renal disorders.

Siepex *Nattermann, Spain.*
Dextromethorphan hydrobromide (p.1057·3).
Cough.

Siero Antiofidico *Sclavo, Ital.*
European viper venom antiserum (p.1534·1).
European viper bite.

Sieropresol *Herdel, Ital.†.*
Methylprednisolone (p.1046·1).
Corticosteroid.

Siesta-I *Welti, Switz.*
Anhydrous citric acid (p.1564·3); tartaric acid (p.1634·3); magnesium sulphate (p.1157·3); sodium bicarbonate (p.1153·2).
Constipation.

Siete Mares Higado Bacal *Grifols, Spain.*
Cod-liver oil (p.1337·3); tocopherol.
Vitamin A and D deficiencies.

Sifamic *SIFI, Ital.*
Amikacin sulphate (p.150·2).
Eye infections.

Sificetina *SIFI, Ital.*
Chloramphenicol (p.182·1).
Eye infections.

Sificrom *SIFI, Ital.*
Sodium cromoglycate (p.762·1).
Conjunctivitis; keratoconjunctivitis.

Sifiviral *SIFI, Ital.*
Aciclovir (p.602·3).
Herpes simplex keratitis.

Siframin *SIFRA, Ital.*
Amino-acid infusion.
Parenteral nutrition.

Sigabloc *Kytta, Ger.*
Atenolol (p.825·3); chlorthalidone (p.839·3).
Hypertension.

Sigabroxol *Kytta, Ger.*
Ambroxol hydrochloride (p.1054·3).
Respiratory-tract disorders with increased or viscous mucus.

Sigacalm *Kytta, Ger.*
Oxazepam (p.683·2).
Anxiety; sleep disorders.

Sigacap Cor *Kytta, Ger.*
Captopril (p.836·3).
Heart failure; hypertension.

Sigacefal *Kytta, Ger.*
Cefaclor (p.163·2).
Bacterial infections.

Sigacimet *Kytta, Ger.*
Cimetidine (p.1183·2).
Aspiration syndrome; gastro-oesophageal reflux; peptic ulcer; Zollinger-Ellison syndrome.

Sigacora *Kytta, Ger.*
Isosorbide mononitrate (p.893·3).
Ischaemic heart disease; pulmonary hypertension.

Sigacyclat *Siegfried, Ger.†.*
Doxycycline fosfatex (p.202·3).
Bacterial infections.

Sigadoc *Kytta, Ger.*
Indomethacin (p.45·2).
Musculoskeletal and joint disorders; sports injuries.

Sigadoxin
Jacoby, Aust.; Kytta, Ger.; Siegfried, Switz.
Doxycycline hydrochloride (p.202·3).
Bacterial infections.

Sigafenac *Kytta, Ger.*
Diclofenac sodium (p.31·2).
Gout; inflammation; musculoskeletal and joint disorders; pain; sports injuries; superficial thrombophlebitis.

Sigamopen
Kytta, Ger.; Siegfried, Switz.†.
Amoxycillin (p.151·3) or amoxycillin trihydrate (p.151·3).
Bacterial infections.

Sigamuc *Kytta, Ger.*
Doxycycline hydrochloride (p.202·3); ambroxol hydrochloride (p.1054·3).
Bacterial infections of the respiratory tract.

Sigamucil *Kytta, Ger.*
Acetylcysteine (p.1052·3).
Respiratory-tract disorders associated with increased or viscous mucus.

Sigapaedil *Siegfried, Ger.†.*
Erythromycin (p.204·1).
Bacterial infections.

Sigaperidol
Kytta, Ger.; Siegfried, Switz.
Haloperidol (p.673·3).
Hyperactivity; pain; psychiatric disorders; vomiting.

Sigaprim
Kytta, Ger.; Siegfried, Switz.
Co-trimoxazole (p.196·3).
Bacterial infections; Pneumocystis carinii pneumonia.

Sigaprolol *Kytta, Ger.*
Metoprolol tartrate (p.907·3).
Arrhythmias; hypertension; migraine; myocardial infarction.

Sigapurol *Siegfried, Switz.*
Allopurinol (p.390·2).
Gout; hyperuricaemia; renal calculi.

Sigasalur *Kytta, Ger.*
Tablets: Frusemide (p.871·1).
Hypertension; oedema.

Sigma Relief *Sigma, Austral.*
Dextromethorphan hydrobromide (p.1057·3); pseudoephedrine hydrochloride (p.1068·3); guaiphenesin (p.1061·3); sodium citrate.
Cold symptoms; coughs.

Sigma Relief Chest Rub *Sigma, Austral.†.*
Menthol (p.1600·2); camphor (p.1557·2); eucalyptus oil (p.1578·1); thymol (p.1127·1); clove oil (p.1565·2); cedar wood oil; turpentine oil (p.1641·1).
Respiratory-tract congestion.

Sigma Relief Cold Tablets *Sigma, Austral.†.*
Codeine phosphate (p.26·1); paracetamol (p.72·2); pseudoephedrine hydrochloride (p.1068·3).
Cold symptoms; coughs.

Sigma Relief Junior *Sigma, Austral.*
Dextromethorphan (p.1057·3); pseudoephedrine hydrochloride (p.1068·3); sodium citrate.
Cold symptoms; coughs.

Sigmacort *Sigma, Austral.*
Hydrocortisone acetate (p.1043·3).
Inflammatory skin disorders.

Sigmafon *Lafare, Ital.*
Mebutamate (p.901·3).
Hypertension.

Sigmalin B_6 *Sigmapharm, Aust.*
Salicylamide (p.82·3); paracetamol (p.72·2); caffeine (p.749·3); pyridoxine hydrochloride (p.1362·3).
Fever; pain.

Sigmalin B_6 forte *Sigmapharm, Aust.*
Salicylamide (p.82·3); paracetamol (p.72·2); dextropropoxyphene hydrochloride (p.27·3); caffeine (p.749·3); pyridoxine hydrochloride (p.1362·3).
Fever; pain.

Sigmalin B_6 ohne Coffein *Sigmapharm, Aust.*
Salicylamide (p.82·3); paracetamol (p.72·2); pyridoxine hydrochloride (p.1362·3).
Fever; pain.

Sigman-Haustropfen *Sigmapharm, Aust.*
Peppermint oil (p.1208·1); caraway oil (p.1559·3); dexpanthenol (p.1570·3); chamomile flower (p.1561·2); condurango bark (p.1567·2); senna leaf (p.1212·2); frangula bark (p.1193·2); liquorice root (p.1197·1); absinthium (p.1541·1); gentian root (p.1583·3); bitter orange peel (p.1610·3).
Gastro-intestinal and biliary-tract disorders.

Sigmart *Chugai, Jpn.*
Nicorandil (p.915·3).
Angina pectoris.

Sigmetadine *Sigma, Austral.*
Cimetidine (p.1183·2).
Gastro-oesophageal reflux; peptic ulcer; Zollinger-Ellison syndrome.

Sigtab-M *Roberts, USA.*
Multivitamin and mineral preparation.

Siguent Hycor *Sigma, Austral.*
Hydrocortisone acetate (p.1043·3).
Inflammatory eye disorders.

Siguent Neomycin *Sigma, Austral.*
Neomycin sulphate (p.229·2).
Topical skin infections.

Siguran E plus *Mack, Illert., Ger.†.*
Paracetamol (p.72·2); caffeine (p.749·3).
Pain.

Siguran E retard *Mack, Illert., Ger.†.*
Aspirin (p.16·1); paracetamol (p.72·2); caffeine (p.749·3).
Cold symptoms; fever; pain.

Siguran N *Mack, Illert., Ger.†.*
Salicylamide (p.82·3); paracetamol (p.72·2); caffeine (p.749·3).
Cold symptoms; influenza; pain.

Silace
Tanta, Canad.; Silarx, USA.
Docusate sodium (p.1189·3).
Constipation.

Silace-C *Silarx, USA.*
Casanthranol (p.1182·3); docusate sodium (p.1189·3).
Constipation.

SilaClean 20/20 *Professional Supplies, USA.*
Cleansing solution for hard contact lenses.

Siladryl *Silarx, USA.*
Diphenhydramine hydrochloride (p.409·1).
Hypersensitivity reactions.

Silafed *Silarx, USA.*
Pseudoephedrine hydrochloride (p.1068·3); triprolidine hydrochloride (p.420·3).
Upper respiratory-tract symptoms.

Silaminic Cold *Silarx, USA.*
Phenylpropanolamine hydrochloride (p.1067·2); chlorpheniramine maleate (p.405·1).
Cold symptoms.

Silaminic Expectorant *Silarx, USA.*
Phenylpropanolamine hydrochloride (p.1067·2); guaiphenesin (p.1061·3).
Coughs.

Silapap *Silarx, USA.*
Paracetamol (p.72·2).
Fever; pain.

Silargetten *Bristol-Myers Squibb, Ger.†.*
Silver chloride (p.1629·2).
Infections of the oropharynx.

Silargin *Level, Spain†.*
Dimethicone (p.1213·1); magaldrate (p.1198·1).
Gastro-intestinal disorders.

Silarine *Vir, Spain.*
Silymarin (p.993·3).
Toxic hepatitis.

Silastic *Dow Corning, UK.*
Liquid silicone (p.1384·2); stannous octoate.
Open granulating wounds.

Silaxon *Restan, S.Afr.*
Sennosides A and B (p.1212·3).
Constipation.

Silbar *Sigma, Austral.†.*
Barrier cream.

Silberne *Brady, Aust.*
Cascara (p.1183·1); rhubarb (p.1212·1); ox bile (p.1553·2).
Constipation.

Silborina *Iema, Ital.†.*
Potassium guaiacolsulfonate (p.1068·3).
Coughs.

Silcocks Base *Ovelle, Irl.†.*
Ointment basis.

Silcon *Faulding, Austral.*
Barrier cream.

Sildec-DM *Silarx, USA.*
Carbinoxamine maleate (p.404·2); pseudoephedrine hydrochloride (p.1068·3); dextromethorphan hydrobromide (p.1057·3).
Coughs.

Sildicon-E *Silarx, USA.*
Phenylpropanolamine hydrochloride (p.1067·2); guaiphenesin (p.1061·3).
Coughs.

Silentan
Note. This name is used for preparations of different composition.
Krewel, Ger.
Nefopam hydrochloride (p.62·3).
Formerly contained diazepam and aspirin.
Pain.

Lubapharm, Switz.†.
Diazepam (p.661·1); dihydroergotamine tartrate (p.444·3); aspirin (p.16·1); caffeine (p.749·3).
Headache.

Silentan spezial *Krewel, Ger.†.*
Paracetamol (p.72·2); orphenadrine citrate (p.465·2).
Skeletal muscle spasm.

Silepar *Ibirn, Ital.*
Silymarin (p.993·3).
Liver disorders.

Silfedrine *Silarx, USA.*
Pseudoephedrine hydrochloride (p.1068·3).
Nasal congestion.

Silgastrin-T *Ethimed, S.Afr.†.*
Chlorprothixene (p.656·1); silgastrin gel.
Gastro-intestinal disorders.

Silibene *Merckle, Ger.*
Silybum marianum (p.993·3).
Liver disorders.

Silic 15 *Ego, Austral.*
Dimethicone 350 (p.1384·2).
Barrier preparation; dry skin.

Silic C *Ego, Austral.†.*
Clioquinol (p.193·2) in a barrier cream.
Infected dermatitis; topical candidal infections.

Silica L11 *Homeocan, Canad.*
Homoeopathic preparation.

Silicic Complex *Procare, Austral.*
Equisetum (p.1575·1); silica (p.1474·3); calcium (p.1155·1); potassium (p.1161·1).
Tissue repair.

Silicogamma *IBP, Ital.†.*
Dimethicone (p.1384·2); zinc stearate (p.1469·3).
Skin disorders.

Silicur *Biocur, Ger.*
Silybum marianum (p.993·3).
Liver disorders.

Silidermil *Fides, Spain.*
Ointment: Dimethicone (p.1384·2); zinc oxide (p.1096·2).
Topical powder: Cetylpyridinium chloride (p.1106·2); dimethicone (p.1384·2); zinc oxide (p.1096·2).
Skin disorders.

Siligaz
Bio-Sante, Canad.; Arkomedika, Fr.
Dimethicone (p.1213·1).
Abdominal distension; flatulence; gastro-oesophageal reflux.

Silimag *Faes, Spain.*
Magnesium trisilicate (p.1199·1).
Gastro-intestinal hyperacidity.

Silimarin *Benedetti, Ital.*
Silymarin (p.993·3).
Liver disorders.

Silimarit *Bionorica, Ger.*
Silybum marianum (p.993·3).
Liver disorders.

Silimazu *Farmasur, Spain.*
Silymarin (p.993·3).
Toxic hepatitis.

Sili-Met-San
Bio-Therabel, Belg.; UCB, Switz.
Dimethicone (p.1213·1); calcium pantothenate (p.1352·3).
Aid to radiologic examination; flatulence.

Silino *Robapharm, Ger.†.*
Diclofenac sodium (p.31·2).
Acute gout; inflammation; neuralgia; neuritis; rheumatism.

Siliprele *Herbaxt, Fr.*
Equisetum (p.1575·1).
Gastro-intestinal and renal disorders.

Silirex *Lampugnani, Ital.*
Silymarin (p.993·3).
Liver disorders.

Silisan *Lipha, Ital.*
Simethicone (p.1213·1); calcium pantothenate (p.1352·3).
Gastro-intestinal disorders associated with excess gas; preparation of the stomach for endoscopy and surgery.

Silkonol *Pharmacia Upjohn, Aust.*
Dimethicone (p.1213·1); zinc oxide (p.1096·2).
Barrier preparation.

Silliver *Abbott, Ital.*
Silymarin (p.993·3).
Liver disorders.

Sillix *Giuliani, Ital.*
Dried yeast (p.1373·1); vitamin B substances.

Sillix Donna *Giuliani, Ital.*
Minerals; dried yeast; vitamin E; vitamin B_6; folic acid.
Nutritional supplement.

Silmar
Hennig, Ger.
Silybum marianum (p.993·3).
Liver disorders.

Lebens, Ital.†.
Silymarin (p.993·3).
Liver disorders.

Silnet *Henkel, Ger.†.*
Alcohol (p.1099·1); isopropyl alcohol (p.1118·2).
Skin disinfection.

Silomat
Note. This name is used for preparations of different composition.
Bender, Aust.; Boehringer Ingelheim, Belg.; Boehringer Ingelheim, Fr.; Thomae, Ger.
Tablets; oral solution; injection: Clobutinol hydrochloride (p.1057·1).
Coughs.

Boehringer Ingelheim, Fr.
Syrup: Clobutinol hydrochloride (p.1057·1); ammonium chloride (p.1055·2); sodium benzoate (p.1102·3).
Coughs.

Silomat Compositum
Note. This name is used for preparations of different composition.
Boehringer Ingelheim, Ital.†.
Clobutinol hydrochloride (p.1057·1); orciprenaline sulphate (p.756·3); ammonium chloride (p.1055·2).
Coughs.

Boehringer Ingelheim, Swed.†.
Clobutinol hydrochloride (p.1057·1); orciprenaline sulphate (p.756·3).
Coughs.

Silomat DA *Boehringer Ingelheim, S.Afr.*
Clobutinol hydrochloride (p.1057·1); orciprenaline sulphate (p.756·3).
Formerly known as Silomat Composit.
Coughs.

Silomat-Fher *Boehringer Ingelheim, Ital.*
Clobutinol hydrochloride (p.1057·1).
Coughs.

Silon
Pharmacia, Canad.†; Perstorp, Swed.
Dimethicone (p.1384·2); zinc oxide (p.1096·2).
Barrier cream.

Siloxan *Nycomed, Norw.*
Dimethicone (p.1213·1).
Flatulence; postoperative intestinal gas retention.

Siloxyl *Martindale Pharmaceuticals, UK†.*
Oral suspension: Aluminium hydroxide (p.1177·3); simethicone (p.1213·1); light magnesium oxide (p.1198·3).
Tablets: Aluminium hydroxide (p.1177·3); simethicone (p.1213·1).
NOTE. There is no connection between Martindale, The Complete Drug Reference and Martindale Pharmaceuticals.
Dyspepsia; flatulence.

Silphen *Silarx, USA.*
Diphenhydramine hydrochloride (p.409·1).

Silphen DM *Silarx, USA.*
Dextromethorphan hydrobromide (p.1057·3).
Coughs.

Silphoscalin *Heilit, Ger.†.*
Ammi visnaga (p.1593·2); ephedra (p.1059·3); equisetum (p.1575·1); galeopsis; polygonum; primula root; senega (p.1069·3); sem. erucae; calcium gluconate (p.1155·2); calcium glycerophosphate (p.1155·2); calcium phosphate (p.1155·3); tilia (p.1637·3).
Respiratory-tract disorders.

Siltapp *Silarx, USA.*
Brompheniramine maleate (p.403·2); phenylpropanolamine hydrochloride (p.1067·2); dextromethorphan hydrobromide (p.1057·3).
Upper respiratory-tract symptoms.

Sil-Tex *Silarx, USA.*
Phenylephrine hydrochloride (p.1066·2); phenylpropanolamine hydrochloride (p.1067·2); guaiphenesin (p.1061·3).
Coughs.

Siltussin *Silarx, USA.*
Guaiphenesin (p.1061·3).
Coughs.

Siltussin DM *Silarx, USA.*
Guaiphenesin (p.1061·3); dextromethorphan hydrobromide (p.1057·3).
Coughs.

Siltussin-CF *Silarx, USA.*
Guaiphenesin (p.1061·3); phenylpropanolamine hydrochloride (p.1067·2); dextromethorphan hydrobromide (p.1057·3).
Coughs.

Silubin *Grunenthal, Switz.*
Buformin (p.319·1).
Diabetes mellitus.

Silubin Retard *Andromaco, Spain.*
Buformin (p.319·1).
Diabetes mellitus.

Silvadene
Hoechst Marion Roussel, Switz.; Hoechst Marion Roussel, USA.
Silver sulphadiazine (p.247·3).
Infected burns; skin ulcers.

Silvana *Molteni, Ital.*
Benzalkonium chloride (p.1101·3); glacial acetic acid (p.1541·2).
Skin disinfection.

Silvapin Aktiv-Tonic MMP *Pino, Ger.†.*
Isopropyl alcohol (p.1118·2); racemic menthol (p.1600·2); dementholised mint oil (p.1604·1); citronella oil (p.1565·1).
Circulatory disorders of the skin.

Silvapin Baldrianwurzel-Extrakt *Pino, Ger.†.*
Valerian (p.1643·1).
Bath additive; menopausal disorders; nervous symptoms.

Silvapin Brombaldrianbad *Pino, Ger.†.*
Potassium bromide (p.1620·3); valerian oil.
Bath additive; nervous disorders.

Silvapin Eichenrinden-Extrakt *Pino, Ger.†.*
Oak bark (p.1609·3).
Anorectal disorders; bath additive; skin disorders.

Silvapin Fichtennadel-Extrakt *Pino, Ger.†.*
Pine oil.
Bath additive; menopausal disorders; nervous symptoms; rheumatic disorders and arthritis.

Silvapin Franzbranntwein *Pino, Ger.†.*
Pine needle oil (p.1623·3); oleum templini; rosemary oil (p.1626·2); camphor (p.1557·2).
Muscle and joint pain; poor skin circulation.

Silvapin Heublumen/Krauter-Extrakt *Pino, Ger.†.*
Hay flower; sage oil; thyme oil (p.1637·1).
Bath additive; musculoskeletal, neuromuscular, and joint disorders.

Silvapin Kamillenbluten-Extrakt *Pino, Ger.†.*
Chamomile (p.1561·2).
Bath additive; skin disorders.

Silvapin Kohlensaurebad *Pino, Ger.†.*
Sodium bicarbonate (p.1153·2); aluminium sulphate (p.1548·1).
Bath additive; circulatory disorders.

Silvapin Kohlensaurebad F mit Fichtennadelol *Pino, Ger.†.*
Sodium bicarbonate (p.1153·2); pine oil; aluminium sulphate (p.1548·1).
Bath additive; circulatory disorders.

Silvapin Rosmarinblatter-Extrakt *Pino, Ger.†.*
Rosemary leaf.
Bath additive; muscular disorders; nervous disorders; peripheral circulatory disorders; skin disorders.

Silvapin Sauerstoffbad *Pino, Ger.†.*
Sodium percarbonate; copper sulphate (p.1338·1).
Bath additive; circulatory disorders; nervous disorders.

Silvapin Sauerstoffbad mit Fichtennadelol *Pino, Ger.†.*
Sodium percarbonate; pine oil; copper sulphate (p.1338·1).
Bath additive; circulatory disorders; nervous disorders.

Silvapin Weizenkleie-Extrakt *Pino, Ger.†.*
Wheat bran (p.1181·2).
Bath additive; skin disorders.

Silvazine *Smith & Nephew, Austral.*
Silver sulphadiazine (p.247·3); chlorhexidine gluconate (p.1107·2).
Prevention and treatment of infection in burns, leg ulcers, and pressure sores.

Silvederma *Aldo, Spain.*
Silver sulphadiazine (p.247·3).
Skin infections.

Silver-Nova T *Geymonat, Ital.†.*
Copper (p.1337·3); silver (p.1629·2).
Intra-uterine contraceptive device.

Silvertone *Resinag, Switz.*
Silver sulphadiazine (p.247·3).
Infected burns; infected wounds.

Silybum Complex *Blackmores, Austral.*
Silybum marianum (p.993·3); garlic (p.1583·1); taraxacum (p.1634·2); nicotinic acid (p.1351·2); sodium sulphate (p.1213·3).
Hypercholesterolaemia; liver and biliary-tract disorders.

Silyhexal *Hexal, Aust.*
Silybum marianum (p.993·3).
Liver disorders.

Simaal Gel 2 *Schein, USA.*
Aluminium hydroxide (p.1177·3); magnesium hydroxide (p.1198·2); simethicone (p.1213·1).
Hyperacidity.

Simactil *Rorer, Fr.†.*
Co-dergocrine mesylate (p.1566·1).
Cerebral and peripheral vascular disorders; mental function impairment in the elderly.

Simagel *Philopharm, Ger.*
Almasilate (p.1177·1).
Gastro-intestinal disorders.

Simaphil *Philopharm, Ger.*
Magaldrate (p.1198·1).
Gastro-intestinal disorders.

Simatin
Chemomedica, Aust.; Inibsa, Spain†.
Ethosuximide (p.344·3).
Absence seizures; myoclonic seizures.

Simatus *Radiumfarma, Ital.†.*
Oral drops: Dextromethorphan hydrobromide (p.1057·3); ammonium glycyrrhizinate (p.1055·2).
Syrup: Dextromethorphan hydrobromide (p.1057·3).
Coughs.

Simeco
Note. This name is used for preparations of different composition.
Whitehall, Austral.; Wyeth, UK.
Oral suspension: Aluminium hydroxide (p.1177·3); magnesium hydroxide (p.1198·2); simethicone (p.1213·1).
Dyspepsia; flatulence.

Whitehall, Austral.†.
Tablets: Aluminium hydroxide-magnesium carbonate co-dried gel (p.1178·2); simethicone (p.1213·1).
Gastro-intestinal disorders.

Wyeth, UK.
Tablets: Aluminium hydroxide-magnesium carbonate co-dried gel (p.1178·2); magnesium hydroxide (p.1198·2); simethicone (p.1213·1).
Dyspepsia; flatulence.

Simepar *Mepha, Switz.*
Silymarin (p.993·3); vitamin B substances.
Liver disorders.

Simic *Zyma, Switz.*
Urtica root (p.1642·3).
Benign prostatic hyperplasia.

Simil NF *Labima, Belg.*
Etenzamide (p.35·3).
Fever; pain.

Similac *Ross, USA.*
Low-mineral infant feed.
For infants predisposed to hypocalcaemia or requiring low mineral levels.

Similac LF *Abbott, Canad.*
Lactose-free infant feed.
Lactose intolerance.

Similasan I *Ocusoft, USA.*
Artificial tears.

Simoxil *Virginia, Ital.*
Amoxycillin trihydrate (p.151·3).
Bacterial infections.

Simp *Esoform, Ital.*
Chlorhexidine gluconate (p.1107·2); benzalkonium chloride (p.1101·3).
Skin and wound disinfection.

Simplamox *ISF, Ital.†.*
Amoxycillin trihydrate (p.151·3).
Bacterial infections.

Simple *Agepha, Aust.*
Disinfection and storage solution for contact lenses.

Simple Cleaner *Agepha, Aust.*
Cleaning solution for hard, gas permeable and soft contact lenses.

Simplene
Chauvin, Irl.; Smith & Nephew, S.Afr.; Chauvin, UK.
Adrenaline (p.813·2).
Open-angle glaucoma.

Simplet *Major, USA.*
Pseudoephedrine hydrochloride (p.1068·3); chlorpheniramine maleate (p.405·1); paracetamol (p.72·2).
Upper respiratory-tract symptoms.

Simplex *Nycomed, Norw.*
Liquid paraffin (p.1382·1); white soft paraffin (p.1382·3).
Sore and dry skin in the eyelid area.

Simplicity Plus *Rhone-Poulenc Rorer, Austral.†.*
Pregnancy test (p.1621·2).

Simplotan
G.P. Laboratories, Austral.; Pfizer, Ger.
Tinidazole (p.594·1).
Anaerobic bacterial infections; protozoal infections.

Simpottantacinque *Esoform, Ital.*
Benzalkonium chloride (p.1101·3); chlorhexidine gluconate (p.1107·2); alcohol (p.1099·1).
Disinfection of skin, hands, and wounds.

Simprox *Reig Jofre, Spain.*
Astemizole (p.402·1).
Hypersensitivity reactions.

Simpsons *Sestri, UK.*
Zinc stearate (p.1469·3); zinc oxide (p.1096·2); sublimed sulphur (p.1091·2); salicylic acid (p.1090·2).
Skin disorders.

Simron *SmithKline Beecham, USA†.*
Ferrous gluconate (p.1340·1).
Iron-deficiency anaemias.

Simron Plus *SmithKline Beecham, USA.*
Vitamin B substances with vitamin C, iron, and folic acid.

Simulcium G3 *Gandhour, Fr.*
Monomethyltrisilanol mannuronate.
Skin disorders.

Simulect
Novartis, UK; Novartis, USA.
Basiliximab (p.507·1).
Renal transplant rejection.

Sin Mareo x 4 *Calmante Vitaminado, Spain.*
Dimenhydrinate (p.408·2); belladonna (p.457·1).
Nausea; vertigo; vomiting.

Sinacarb *Amrad, Austral.*
Levodopa (p.1137·1); carbidopa (p.1136·1).
Parkinsonism.

Sinacet *UCM-Difme, Ital.†.*
Nutritional preparation.
Vomiting.

Si-Nade *SmithKline Beecham, S.Afr.*
Paracetamol (p.72·2); phenylpropanolamine hydrochloride (p.1067·2).
Cold and influenza symptoms; sinusitis.

Sinalfa *Abbott, Swed.*
Terazosin hydrochloride (p.952·1).
Benign prostatic hyperplasia; hypertension.

Sinapils *Pfeiffer, USA.*
Phenylpropanolamine hydrochloride (p.1067·2); chlorpheniramine maleate (p.405·1); paracetamol (p.72·2); caffeine (p.749·3).
Upper respiratory-tract symptoms.

Sinapisme Rigollot *Chefaro Ardeval, Fr.*
Defatted black mustard paper (p.1605·3).
Respiratory-tract congestion.

Sinapsan *Rodleben, Ger.; Vedim, Ger.*
Piracetam (p.1619·1).
Organic brain disorders.

Sinarest *Ciba, USA.*
Pseudoephedrine hydrochloride (p.1068·3); chlorpheniramine maleate (p.405·1); paracetamol (p.72·2).
Upper respiratory-tract symptoms.

Sinartrol *SPA, Ital.*
Piroxicam cinnamate (p.81·1).
Musculoskeletal and joint disorders.

Sinaryl *Homberger, Switz.*
Homoeopathic preparation.

Sinaspril-Paracetamol *Roche Nicholas, Neth.*
Paracetamol (p.72·2).
Fever; pain.

Sinassial *Fidia, Ital.†.*
Polysiagoside.
Polyneuropathy.

Sinaxamol *Roche, S.Afr.†.*
Styramate (p.1319·1); paracetamol (p.72·2).
Fever; pain; skeletal muscle spasm.

Sincomen
Schering, Belg.†; Farmades, Ital.†.
Spironolactone (p.946·1).
Hyperaldosteronism; hypertension; oedema.

Sincon *Tika, Swed.*
Polyvinyl alcohol (p.1474·2).
Dry eyes.

Sincosan *Omisan, Ital.*
Benzalkonium chloride (p.1101·3).
Surface disinfection.

Sincrivit *AGIPS, Ital.*
Multivitamin preparation.

Sine Fluor *Knoll, Spain†.*
Desonide (p.1036·3).
Skin disorders.

Sine-Aid *McNeil Consumer, USA†.*
Paracetamol (p.72·2); pseudoephedrine hydrochloride (p.1068·3).
Sinus headache.

Sine-Aid IB *McNeil Consumer, USA.*
Pseudoephedrine (p.1068·3); ibuprofen (p.44·1).

Sinecod
Therabel Pharma, Belg.; Zyma, Ger.†; Zyma, Spain†; Zyma, Switz.
Butamyrate citrate (p.1056·2).
Coughs.

Sinecod Bocca *Zyma, Ital.*
Benzoxonium chloride (p.1103·3).
Oral antiseptic.

Sinecod Tosse Fluidificante *Zyma, Ital.*
Carbocisteine (p.1056·3).
Catarrh; coughs.

Sinecod Tosse Sedativo *Novartis Consumer, Ital.*
Butamyrate citrate (p.1056·2).
Formerly known as Sinecod Tosse.
Coughs.

Sinedal *Synpharma, Switz.*
Propyphenazone (p.81·3); paracetamol (p.72·2); caffeine (p.749·3).
Fever; pain.

Sinedol *Corvi, Ital.†.*
Salicylamide (p.82·3).
Cold symptoms; fever; pain.

Sinedyston *Steiner, Ger.*
Co-dergocrine mesylate (p.1566·1); hypericum (p.1590·1).
Mental function disorders.

Sinefricol *Sanofi Winthrop, Spain.*
Caffeine (p.749·3); phenylephrine hydrochloride (p.1066·2); paracetamol (p.72·2); thenyldiamine hydrochloride (p.419·1).
Catarrh; influenza symptoms.

Sinegastrin *Ferrer, Spain.*
Almasilate (p.1177·1).
Formerly contained dimethicone, metoclopramide hydrochloride, oxethazaine, silodrate, and sorbitol.
Gastro-intestinal hyperacidity.

Sinemet
Merck Sharp & Dohme, Aust.; Merck Sharp & Dohme, Austral.; Merck Sharp & Dohme, Belg.; Du Pont, Canad.; Du Pont, Fr.; Du Pont, Irl.; Du Pont, Ital.; Merck Sharp & Dohme, Neth.; Merck Sharp & Dohme, Norw.; Merck Sharp & Dohme, S.Afr.; Du Pont, Spain; Merck Sharp & Dohme, Swed.; Merck Sharp & Dohme, Switz.; Du Pont Pharmaceuticals, UK; Du Pont, USA.
Carbidopa (p.1136·1); levodopa (p.1137·1).
These ingredients can be described by the British Approved Name Co-careldopa.
Parkinsonism.

Sine-Off
SmithKline Beecham, Switz.†; SmithKline Beecham Consumer, UK†.
Aspirin (p.16·1); chlorpheniramine maleate (p.405·1); phenylpropanolamine hydrochloride (p.1067·2).
Cold symptoms.

Sine-Off Allergy SmithKline Beecham Consumer, Canad.
Paracetamol (p.72·2); chlorpheniramine maleate (p.405·1); phenylpropanolamine hydrochloride (p.1067·2).

Sine-Off Maximum Strength Allergy/Sinus
SmithKline Beecham, USA.
Paracetamol (p.72·2); chlorpheniramine maleate (p.405·1); pseudoephedrine hydrochloride (p.1068·3).
Upper respiratory-tract symptoms.

Sine-Off Maximum Strength No Drowsiness Formula SmithKline Beecham Consumer, USA.
Paracetamol (p.72·2); pseudoephedrine hydrochloride (p.1068·3).
Upper respiratory-tract symptoms.

Sine-Off ND SmithKline Beecham Consumer, Canad.
Paracetamol (p.72·2); phenylpropanolamine hydrochloride (p.1067·2).

Sine-Off Sinus Medicine SmithKline Beecham Consumer, USA.
Aspirin (p.16·1); chlorpheniramine maleate (p.405·1); phenylpropanolamine hydrochloride (p.1067·2).
Upper respiratory-tract symptoms.

Sinepress Rolab, S.Afr.
Methyldopa (p.904·2).
Hypertension.

Sinequan
Pfizer, Aust.; Pfizer, Austral.; Pfizer, Belg.; Pfizer, Canad.; Pfizer, Fr.; Pfizer, Irl.; Pfizer, Neth.; Pfizer, Norw.; Pfizer, Spain; Pfizer, UK; Roerig, USA.
Doxepin hydrochloride (p.283·2).
Anxiety disorders; depression; peptic ulcer.

Sinergina Faes, Spain.
Phenytoin (p.352·3).
Formerly contained ascorbic acid, phenytoin, and phenobarbitone.
Epilepsy.

Sinergina S Faes, Spain†.
Phenytoin (p.352·3); phenobarbitone (p.350·2).
Epilepsy.

Sinesalin
Merck, Aust.†; ICI, Ger.†; Zeneca, Switz.
Bendrofluazide (p.827·3).
Hypertension; oedema.

Sinetus Sanico, Belg.†.
Noscapine hydrochloride (p.1065·2); potassium guaiacolsulfonate (p.1068·3); ipecacuanha (p.1062·2); red-poppy petal; tolu balsam (p.1071·1).
Coughs.

Sinevrile Serpero, Ital.
Hydroxocobalamin (p.1363·3); thiamine monophosphate chloride (p.1361·2).
Lignocaine hydrochloride (p.1293·2) is included in this preparation to alleviate the pain of injection.
Alcoholic neuritis; diabetic neuritis; neuritis; polyneuritis; sciatica; trigeminal neuralgia.

Sinex
Note. This name is used for preparations of different composition.
Richardson-Vicks, Austral.†.
Xylometazoline hydrochloride (p.1071·2); menthol; camphor; cineole.
Nasal congestion.

Lachartre, Fr.
Oxymetazoline hydrochloride (p.1065·3); menthol (p.1600·2); camphor (p.1557·2).
Congestion of the upper respiratory tract.

Richardson-Vicks, USA.
Phenylephrine hydrochloride (p.1066·2).
Nasal congestion.

Sinezan Esoform, Ital.†.
Diethyltoluamide (p.1405·1).
Insect repellent.

Sinfibrex Isnardi, Ital.†.
Simfibrate (p.1278·2).
Hyperlipidaemias.

Sinfrontal Muller Goppingen, Ger.
Homoeopathic preparation.

Singlet SmithKline Beecham Consumer, USA.
Pseudoephedrine hydrochloride (p.1068·3); chlorpheniramine maleate (p.405·1); paracetamol (p.72·2).
Upper respiratory-tract symptoms.

Singulair
Merck Sharp & Dohme, UK; Merck, USA.
Montelukast sodium (p.756·1).
Asthma.

Siniphen Singer, Switz.
Suppositories: Salicylamide (p.82·3); propyphenazone (p.81·3); caffeine (p.749·3); lignocaine hydrochloride (p.1293·2).
Tablets: Salicylamide (p.82·3); propyphenazone (p.81·3); caffeine (p.749·3).
Fever; pain.

Sinketol Locatelli, Ital.
Capsules; suppositories: Ketoprofen (p.48·2).
Injection†: Ketoprofen sodium (p.48·3).
Gout; musculoskeletal, joint, and peri-articular disorders.

Sinkron Ripari-Gero, Ital.
Citicoline sodium (p.1564·3).
Cerebrovascular disorders; mental function disorders.

Sinmol Maxfarma, Spain.
Paracetamol (p.72·2).
Fever; pain.

Sinogan Rhone-Poulenc Rorer, Spain.
Methotrimeprazine hydrochloride (p.679·1).
Anxiety; psychoses; schizophrenia.

Sinografin
Squibb Diagnostics, Canad.; Squibb Diagnostics, USA.
Meglumine diatrizoate (p.1003·2); meglumine iodipamide (p.1005·3).
Contrast medium for hysterosalpingography.

Sinolax-Milder Synpharma, Aust.
Fig (p.1193·2); fennel (p.1579·1); manna (p.1199·1).
Constipation; stool softener.

Sinophenin Rodleben, Ger.
Promazine hydrochloride (p.689·1).
Anxiety disorders; pain; pre- and postoperative sedative; pruritus; psychoses; sleep disorders; vomiting; withdrawal symptoms.

Sinosid SIFI, Ital.†.
Paromomycin sulphate (p.235·3).
Bacterial eye infections.

Sinotar Modern Health Products, UK.
Marshmallow root (p.1546·3); echinacea (p.1574·2); elderflower (p.1627·2).
Blocked sinuses; catarrh.

Sinovial IRBI, Ital.†.
Parsalmide (p.75·1).
Inflammation; pain.

Sinovula Asche, Ger.
Norethisterone (p.1453·1); ethinyloestradiol (p.1445·1).
Combined oral contraceptive.

Sinoxis Hosbon, Spain.
Buflomedil hydrochloride (p.834·2).
Vascular disorders.

Sinpro junior Bayer, Ger.†.
Paracetamol (p.72·2).
Fever; pain.

Sinpro-N Bayer, Ger.†.
Paracetamol (p.72·2).
Fever; pain.

Sinquan Pfizer, Ger.
Doxepin hydrochloride (p.283·2).
Depression; sleep disorders; withdrawal syndromes.

Sinquane Pfizer, Switz.
Doxepin hydrochloride (p.283·2).
Anxiety disorders; depression.

Sinrinal UCM-Difme, Ital.†.
Framycetin sulphate (p.210·3); hydrocortisone (p.1043·3); phenylpropanolamine hydrochloride (p.1067·2); phenylephrine hydrochloride (p.1066·2); lignocaine hydrochloride (p.1293·2).
Mouth and throat disorders.

Sinsurrene Parke, Davis, Ital.
Hydrocortisone sodium hemisuccinate (p.1044·1); deoxycortone sodium hemisuccinate (corticosterone) (p.1036·3); aldosterone sodium hemisuccinate (p.1031·3); prasterone sodium sulphate (p.1459·2).
Adrenal insufficiency.

Sintamin SIFRA, Ital.
Amino-acid infusion.
Parenteral nutrition.

Sintecilina Antibioticos, Spain†.
Ampicillin sodium (p.153·1).
Bacterial infections.

Sinteroid Crinos, Ital.†.
A heparinoid (p.882·3); clofibrate (p.1271·1).
Exudative diabetic retinopathy; hyperlipoproteinaemia; xanthomas.

Sinthrome
Ciba-Geigy, Irl.†; Alliance, UK.
Nicoumalone (p.916·1).
Thrombo-embolic disorders.

Sintisone Pharmacia, Swed.†.
Prednisolone steaglate (p.1048·2).
Corticosteroid.

Sintobil Molteni, Ital.
Fencibutirol (p.1578·3); boldo (p.1554·1); cascara (p.1183·1); frangula (p.1193·2).
Constipation.

Sintocalcin Biagini, Ital.
Elcatonin (p.735·3).
Hypercalcaemia; osteoporosis; Paget's disease of bone; reflex sympathetic dystrophy.

Sintocef Pulitzer, Ital.
Cefonicid sodium (p.167·2).
Lignocaine hydrochloride (p.1293·2) is included in the intramuscular injection to alleviate the pain of injection.
Bacterial infections.

Sintoclar Pulitzer, Ital.
Citicoline (p.1564·3).
Cerebrovascular disorders; mental function disorders.

Sintodian Pharmacia Upjohn, Ital.
Droperidol (p.668·2).
Anaesthesia; psychoses.

Sintolatt Lampugnani, Ital.
Lactulose (p.1195·3).
Constipation; disturbances in intestinal flora.

Sintolexyn ISF, Ital.†.
Cephalexin (p.178·2) or cephalexin lysine (p.178·3).
Bacterial infections.

Sintomodulina Italfarmaco, Ital.
Thymopentin (p.1637·2).
Immunodeficiency.

Sintonal Europharma, Spain.
Brotizolam (p.643·2).
Insomnia.

Sintopen Mitim, Ital.
Amoxycillin trihydrate (p.151·3).
Bacterial infections.

Sintotrat Bracco, Ital.
Hydrocortisone acetate (p.1043·3).
Skin disorders.

Sintrogel Roche Nicholas, Spain.
Aluminium hydroxide (p.1177·3); magnesium carbonate (p.1198·1); magnesium oxide (p.1198·3).
Formerly contained aluminium magnesium hydroxide, dimethicone, and magnesium oxide.
Gastro-intestinal hyperacidity.

Sintrom
Ciba-Geigy, Aust.; Ciba-Geigy, Belg.; Geigy, Canad.; Novartis, Fr.; Ciba, Ger.†; Ciba, Ital.; Ciba-Geigy, Spain; Geigy, Switz.
Nicoumalone (p.916·1).
Thrombo-embolic disorders.

Sintrom Mitis Novartis, Neth.
Nicoumalone (p.916·1).
Thrombo-embolic disorders.

Sinuc Biocur, Ger.
Hedera helix.
Catarrh.

Sinuclear
Note. A similar name is used for preparations of different composition.
Garec, S.Afr.
Paracetamol (p.72·2); phenylpropanolamine hydrochloride (p.1067·2).
Upper respiratory-tract congestion.

Sinu-Clear
Note. A similar name is used for preparations of different composition.
Warner Chilcott, USA†.
Triprolidine hydrochloride (p.420·3); pseudoephedrine hydrochloride (p.1068·3).

Sinufed Timecelles Roberts, USA.
Pseudoephedrine hydrochloride (p.1068·3); guaiphenesin (p.1061·3).
Coughs and cold symptoms; nasal congestion.

Sinuforton Sanofi Winthrop, Ger.
Capsules: Anise oil (p.1550·1); primula rhizome; thyme (p.1636·3).
Oral drops: Anise oil (p.1550·1); eucalyptus oil (p.1578·1); thyme (p.1636·3).
Sinusitis.

Sinugex Frega, Canad.
Diphenylpyraline hydrochloride (p.409·3); paracetamol (p.72·2); caffeine (p.749·3).

Sinuguard With Antihistamine Nelson, Austral.†.
Chlorpheniramine maleate (p.405·1); paracetamol (p.72·2); pseudoephedrine hydrochloride (p.1068·3); bioflavonoids complex (p.1580·1); ascorbic acid (p.1365·2); phenylephrine hydrochloride (p.1066·2).
Hay fever.

Sinuguard N/F Without Antihistamine Nelson, Austral.†.
Paracetamol (p.72·2); pseudoephedrine hydrochloride (p.1068·3); bioflavonoids complex (p.1580·1); ascorbic acid (p.1365·2); phenylephrine hydrochloride (p.1066·2).
Colds.

Sinulene Inverni della Beffa, Ital.†.
Acetoxolone aluminium (p.1176·2); aluminium hydroxide (p.1177·3); belladonna alkaloids (p.457·1); frangula bark (p.1193·2).
Gastro-duodenal inflammation; peptic ulcer.

Sinulin Carnrick, USA.
Paracetamol (p.72·2); chlorpheniramine maleate (p.405·1); phenylpropanolamine hydrochloride (p.1067·2).
Cold symptoms; nasal congestion.

Sinumax Janssen-Cilag, S.Afr.
Paracetamol (p.72·2); pseudoephedrine hydrochloride (p.1068·3).
Cold symptoms.

Sinumed Triomed, S.Afr.
Pseudoephedrine hydrochloride (p.1068·3).
Upper respiratory-tract congestion.

Sinumist-SR Hauck, USA.
Guaiphenesin (p.1061·3).
Coughs.

Sinupan Ion, USA.
Guaiphenesin (p.1061·3); phenylephrine hydrochloride (p.1066·2).
Coughs and cold symptoms; nasal congestion.

Sinupret
Austroplant, Aust.; Bionorica, Ger.
Gentian root (p.1583·3); primula flower; rumex acetosa; sambucus flower (p.1627·2); verbena officinalis.
Respiratory-tract inflammation.

Sinus
Note. This name is used for preparations of different composition.
Homeocan, Canad.
Homoeopathic preparation.

Boots, Spain†.
Injection: Ampicillin sodium (p.153·1); ampicillin benzathine (p.154·1); bromhexine hydrochloride (p.1055·3); chymotrypsin (p.1563·2).
Lignocaine hydrochloride (p.1293·2) is included in this preparation to alleviate the pain of injection.
Respiratory-tract infections.
Nasal spray: Oxymetazoline hydrochloride (p.1065·3).
Nasal or sinus congestion.
Tablets: Amoxycillin trihydrate (p.151·3); benzydamine hydrochloride (p.21·3); bromhexine hydrochloride (p.1055·3).
Respiratory-tract infections.

Sinus & Congestion Relief WestCan, Canad.
Pseudoephedrine hydrochloride (p.1068·3); paracetamol (p.72·2).

Sinus Excedrin Bristol-Myers Squibb, USA.
Paracetamol (p.72·2); pseudoephedrine hydrochloride (p.1068·3).
Nasal congestion.

Sinus and Hayfever Vita Glow, Austral.
Cochlearia armoracia; fenugreek (p.1579·3); ascorbic acid (p.1365·2); betacarotene (p.1335·2); zinc amino acid chelate (p.1373·3).
Hay fever; sinusitis; upper respiratory-tract congestion.

Sinus Inhalaciones Boots, Spain.
Camphor (p.1557·2); cineole (p.1564·1); peppermint oil (p.1208·1); oleum pini sylvestris; menthol (p.1600·2); eucalyptus oil (p.1578·1).
Upper-respiratory-tract congestion.

Sinus Medication Stanley, Canad.
Pseudoephedrine hydrochloride (p.1068·3); paracetamol (p.72·2).

Sinus Pain & Nasal Congestion Relief WestCan, Canad.
Pseudoephedrine hydrochloride (p.1068·3); paracetamol (p.72·2).

Sinus Symptoms Relief Brauer, Austral.
Homoeopathic preparation.

Sinusalia Boiron, Canad.
Homoeopathic preparation.

Sinuselect Dreluso, Ger.
Homoeopathic preparation.

Sinusitis Hevert N Hevert, Ger.
Homoeopathic preparation.

Sinusitis-Komplex Staufen, Ger.
Homoeopathic preparation.

Sinusol Richter, Aust.
Gentian root (p.1583·3); primula flower; verbena officinalis.
Catarrh.

Sinusol-B Kay, USA.
Brompheniramine maleate (p.403·2).
Hypersensitivity reactions.

Sinusol-Schleimlosender Tee Richter, Aust.
Primula flower; sambucus (p.1627·2); verbena.
Catarrh.

Sinuspax
Homeocan, Canad.; Lehning, Fr.
Homoeopathic preparation.

Sinus-Relief Major, USA.
Pseudoephedrine hydrochloride (p.1068·3); paracetamol (p.72·2).
Upper respiratory-tract symptoms.

Sinustat
Note. This name is used for preparations of different composition.
Xixia, S.Afr.
Paracetamol (p.72·2); phenylpropanolamine hydrochloride (p.1067·2).
Cold and influenza symptoms.

Murdock, USA†.
Pseudoephedrine hydrochloride (p.1068·3).

Sinustop Adcock Ingram Self Medication, S.Afr.†.
Nasal spray: Oxymetazoline hydrochloride (p.1065·3).
Nasal congestion.
Tablets: Paracetamol (p.72·2); phenylpropanolamine hydrochloride (p.1067·2); phenyltoloxamine citrate (p.416·1).
Cold and flu symptoms.

Sinustop with Codeine Adcock Ingram Self Medication, S.Afr.†.
Paracetamol (p.72·2); phenylpropanolamine hydrochloride (p.1067·2); phenyltoloxamine citrate (p.416·1); codeine phosphate (p.26·1).
Cold and flu symptoms.

Sinustop Pro Murdock, USA.
Pseudoephedrine hydrochloride (p.1068·3).
Nasal congestion.

Sinusyx Syxyl, Ger.
Homoeopathic preparation.

Sinutab
Note. This name is used for preparations of different composition.
Warner-Lambert Consumer, Belg.; Parke, Davis, S.Afr.
Paracetamol (p.72·2); phenyltoloxamine citrate (p.416·1); phenylpropanolamine hydrochloride (p.1067·2).
Cold and influenza symptoms; sinus headache.

Warner-Lambert, Irl.; Warner-Lambert, UK.
Paracetamol (p.72·2); phenylpropanolamine hydrochloride (p.1067·2).
Allergic rhinitis; cold and influenza symptoms; sinusitis.

Parke, Davis, S.Afr.
Nasal spray: Xylometazoline hydrochloride (p.1071·2).
Nasal congestion.

Warner-Lambert, Spain.
Chlorpheniramine maleate (p.405·1); paracetamol (p.72·2); pseudoephedrine hydrochloride (p.1068·3).
Fever; influenza and cold symptoms; pain.

Sinutab Antihistamine Warner-Lambert, Austral.†.
Paracetamol (p.72·2); pseudoephedrine hydrochloride (p.1068·3); chlorpheniramine maleate (p.405·1).
Upper respiratory-tract disorders.

Sinutab with Codeine
Note. This name is used for preparations of different composition.
Warner-Lambert, Austral.†; Parke, Davis, S.Afr.
Paracetamol (p.72·2); phenylpropanolamine hydrochloride (p.1067·2); phenyltoloxamine citrate (p.416·1); codeine phosphate (p.26·1).
Cold and influenza symptoms; sinus headache.

Warner-Lambert, Canad.
Paracetamol (p.72·2); pseudoephedrine hydrochloride (p.1068·3); chlorpheniramine maleate (p.405·1); codeine (p.26·1).
Cold symptoms; nasal congestion.

Sinutab Extra Strength *Warner-Lambert, Canad.*
Paracetamol (p.72·2); pseudoephedrine hydrochloride (p.1068·3); chlorpheniramine maleate (p.405·1).
Cold symptoms; nasal congestion.

Sinutab Maximum Strength Sinus Allergy *Parke, Davis, USA.*
Pseudoephedrine hydrochloride (p.1068·3); chlorpheniramine maleate (p.405·1); paracetamol (p.72·2).
Upper respiratory-tract symptoms.

Sinutab ND *Parke, Davis, S.Afr.*
Paracetamol (p.72·2); phenylpropanolamine hydrochloride (p.1067·2).
Cold and influenza symptoms.

Sinutab ND Daytime Formula *Warner-Lambert, Canad.†.*
Paracetamol (p.72·2); pseudoephedrine (p.1068·3).
Cold symptoms; nasal congestion.

Sinutab Nightime *Warner-Lambert, UK.*
Phenylpropanolamine (p.1067·2); paracetamol (p.72·2); phenyltoloxamine (p.416·1).
Congestion.

Sinutab Nighttime *Warner-Lambert, Canad.*
Paracetamol (p.72·2); diphenhydramine hydrochloride (p.409·1); pseudoephedrine hydrochloride (p.1068·3).
Formerly contained paracetamol, chlorpheniramine, and pseudoephedrine.
Cold symptoms; nasal congestion.

Sinutab No Drowsiness *Warner-Lambert, Canad.*
Paracetamol (p.72·2); pseudoephedrine hydrochloride (p.1068·3).
Cold symptoms; nasal congestion.

Sinutab Non-Drying *Glaxo Wellcome, USA.*
Pseudoephedrine hydrochloride (p.1068·3); guaiphenesin (p.1061·3).
Coughs.

Sinutab Regular *Warner-Lambert, Canad.*
Paracetamol (p.72·2); pseudoephedrine hydrochloride (p.1068·3); chlorpheniramine maleate (p.405·1).
Cold symptoms; nasal congestion.

Sinutab SA *Warner-Lambert, Canad.*
Paracetamol (p.72·2); phenylpropanolamine hydrochloride (p.1067·2); phenyltoloxamine citrate (p.416·1).
Cold symptoms; nasal congestion.

Sinutab Sinus Allergy and Pain Relief *Warner-Lambert, Austral.*
Paracetamol (p.72·2); pseudoephedrine hydrochloride (p.1068·3); chlorpheniramine maleate (p.405·1).
Formerly known as Sinutab with Antihistamine and Pseudoephedrine.
Upper respiratory-tract disorders.

Sinutab Sinus and Pain Relief *Warner-Lambert, Austral.*
Paracetamol (p.72·2); pseudoephedrine hydrochloride (p.1068·3).
Formerly known as Sinutab with Pseudoephedrine.
Upper respiratory-tract disorders.

Sinutab Sinus Relief *Warner-Lambert, Austral.†.*
Pseudoephedrine hydrochloride (p.1068·3).
Formerly known as Sinutab Decongestant.
Sinus disorders.

Sinutab Without Drowsiness *Warner-Lambert, USA.*
Pseudoephedrine hydrochloride (p.1068·3); paracetamol (p.72·2).
Upper respiratory-tract symptoms.

Sinutrex Extra Strength *Schein, USA.*
Pseudoephedrine hydrochloride (p.1068·3); chlorpheniramine maleate (p.405·1); paracetamol (p.72·2).
Upper respiratory-tract symptoms.

SINUvent *WE, USA.*
Phenylpropanolamine hydrochloride (p.1067·2); guaiphenesin (p.1061·3).
Coughs and cold symptoms; nasal congestion.

Sinuzets Cold and Flu Capsules *Boots, Austral.†.*
Pseudoephedrine hydrochloride (p.1068·3); phenylephrine hydrochloride (p.1066·2); paracetamol (p.72·2).
Colds.

Sinuzets Cold and Flu Capsules with Antihistamine *Boots, Austral.†.*
Pseudoephedrine hydrochloride (p.1068·3); phenylephrine hydrochloride (p.1066·2); diphenylpyraline hydrochloride (p.409·3); paracetamol (p.72·2).
Colds.

Sinuzets Forte Hayfever Capsules *Boots, Austral.†.*
Pseudoephedrine hydrochloride (p.1068·3); phenylephrine hydrochloride (p.1066·2).
Hay fever; rhinitis; sinusitis.

Sinvacor *Merck Sharp & Dohme, Ital.*
Simvastatin (p.1278·2).
Coronary arteriosclerosis; hyperlipidaemia; ischaemic heart disease.

Siofor *Berlin-Chemie, Ger.*
Metformin hydrochloride (p.330·1).
Diabetes mellitus.

Siopel
Zeneca, Irl.; Zeneca, S.Afr.; Zeneca, UK.
Cetrimide (p.1105·2); dimethicone 1000 (p.1384·2).
Barrier cream.

Siosol *Febena, Ger.*
Chelidonium majus.
Biliary and gastro-intestinal spasm.

Siozwo *Febena, Ger.†.*
Naphazoline hydrochloride (p.1064·2); laureth 9 (p.1325·2).
Catarrh; colds.

Siozwo N *Febena, Ger.*
Nasal ointment: Naphazoline hydrochloride (p.1064·2); peppermint oil (p.1208·1).
Catarrh; rhinitis.
Ointment: Bismuth subgallate (p.1180·2); hamamelis (p.1587·1); zinc oxide (p.1096·2).
Burns; skin disorders; wounds.

Siqualone
Bristol-Myers Squibb, Norw.; Bristol-Myers Squibb, Swed.
Fluphenazine decanoate (p.671·2) or fluphenazine hydrochloride (p.671·3).
Alcohol withdrawal syndrome; anxiety; nausea and vomiting; psychoses; senile agitation and confusion.

Siquil
Bristol-Myers Squibb, Belg.†; Bristol-Myers Squibb, Neth.
Fluopromazine hydrochloride (p.670·3).
Agitation; nausea and vomiting; premedication; psychoses; sedative.

Siran
Temmler, Ger.; Temmler, Switz.†.
Acetylcysteine (p.1052·3).
Respiratory-tract disorders with increased or viscous mucus.

Sirdalud
Sandoz, Aust.; Sandoz, Belg.; Sanofi Winthrop, Ger.; Novartis, Ital.; Novartis, Neth.; Sandoz, Spain; Sandoz, Switz.
Tizanidine hydrochloride (p.1322·1).
Skeletal muscle spasm; spasticity.

Sirenitas *Benvegna, Ital.†.*
Dibromotyrosine (p.1493·1); methimazole (p.1495·3); benactyzine (p.280·1); vitamins.
Anxiety; hyperthyroidism.

Sirigen *Adivar, Ital.*
Benzalkonium chloride (p.1101·3).
Disinfection of wounds and burns.

Sirinal *Woelm, Ger.†.*
Dequalinium chloride (p.1112·1); chlorquinaldol (p.185·1).
Inflammatory disorders and infections of the oropharynx; prophylaxis of influenza and colds.

Sirit *Stark, Ger.†.*
Dequalinium chloride (p.1112·1); tyrothricin (p.267·2); ascorbic acid (p.1365·2).
Infections of the oropharynx.

Sirmia Abfuhrkapseln *Niedermaier, Ger.*
Senna (p.1212·2); peppermint oil (p.1208·1); caraway oil (p.1559·3).
Constipation.

Sirmia Artischockenelixier N *Niedermaier, Ger.*
Cynara (p.1569·2); taraxacum (p.1634·2).
Hepatobiliary disorders.

Sirmia Knoblauchsaft N *Niedermaier, Ger.*
Garlic (p.1583·1).
Hyperlipidaemia.

Sirmiosta Nervenelixier N *Niedermaier, Ger.*
Melissa (p.1600·1); passion flower (p.1615·3); valerian (p.1643·1).
Agitation; insomnia.

Sirodex *Prospa, Switz.†.*
Dextromethorphan hydrobromide (p.1057·3); potassium guaiacolsulfonate (p.1068·3).
Coughs.

Sirodina *Clariana, Spain.*
Pyridoxine (p.1363·1); sulpiride (p.692·3).
Psychoses; vertigo.

Sirop Adrian a la pholcodine adulte *Doms-Adrian, Fr.†.*
Bromoform (p.1620·3); pholcodine (p.1068·1); cherry laurel; aconite (p.1542·2); tolu balsam (p.1071·1); Desessartz syrup.
Coughs.

Sirop Adrian a la pholcodine enfant *Doms-Adrian, Fr.†.*
Bromoform (p.1620·3); pholcodine (p.1068·1); tolu balsam (p.1071·1); Desessartz syrup.
Coughs.

Sirop antitussif Wyss a base de codeine *Wyss, Switz.*
Codeine phosphate (p.26·1); cherry-laurel; ipecacuanha (p.1062·2); senega root (p.1069·3); althaea (p.1546·3).
Coughs.

Sirop Boin *Picot, Fr.*
Codeine (p.26·1); menthol (p.1600·2); adrenaline (p.813·2); guaiacol (p.1061·2); aconite (p.1542·2); cherry laurel.
Respiratory disorders.

Sirop contre la toux nouvelle formule *Zeller, Switz.*
Hedera helix.
Bronchial disorders with viscous mucus.

Sirop Dentition *Sabex, Canad.*
Benzocaine (p.1286·2).

Sirop Des Vosges Caze *SmithKline Beecham, Fr.*
Pholcodine (p.1068·1).
Coughs.

Sirop DM *Marc-O, Canad.*
Dextromethorphan hydrobromide (p.1057·3).

Sirop Expectorant *Marc-O, Canad.*
Guaiphenesin (p.1061·3).

Sirop Famel *Etris, Fr.†.*
Lactocreosote (p.1057·3); calcium lactophosphate; codeine (p.26·1); aconite (p.1542·2).
Coughs.

Sirop Manceau *SmithKline Beecham, Fr.†.*
Senna (p.1212·2); pippin apple syrup.
Constipation.

Sirop Passi-Par *Parsenn, Switz.*
Passion flower (p.1615·3); crataegus (p.1568·2).
Anxiety; insomnia.

Sirop Pectoral adulte *Oberlin, Fr.*
Ethylmorphine hydrochloride (p.36·1); aconite (p.1542·2); bromoform (p.1620·3); sodium benzoate (p.1102·3); potassium guaiacolsulfonate (p.1068·3); cherry laurel; belladonna (p.457·1); drosera (p.1574·1); eucalyptus oil (p.1578·1); senega (p.1069·3); ipecacuanha (p.1062·2) tolu balsam (p.1071·1).
Coughs.

Sirop pectoral DP1 *DP-Medica, Switz.*
Guaiphenesin (p.1061·3); codeine phosphate (p.26·1); ephedrine hydrochloride (p.1059·3); sodium benzoate (p.1102·3); althaea (p.1546·3); tolu balsam (p.1071·1); plantain (p.1208·3); thyme (p.1636·3); pine buds; pectoral syrup.
Bronchitis; catarrh; coughs.

Sirop pectoral DP2, DP3 *DP-Medica, Switz.*
Guaiphenesin (p.1061·3); codeine phosphate (p.26·1); ephedrine hydrochloride (p.1059·3); sodium benzoate (p.1102·3); belladonna (p.457·1); althaea (p.1546·3); tolu balsam (p.1071·1); plantain (p.1208·3); thyme (p.1636·3); pine buds; pectoral syrup.
Bronchitis; catarrh; coughs.

Sirop Pectoral enfant *Oberlin, Fr.*
Sodium benzoate (p.1102·3); potassium guaiacolsulfonate (p.1068·3); sodium bromide (p.1620·3); drosera (p.1574·1); eucalyptus oil (p.1578·1); frangula (p.1193·2); ethylmorphine hydrochloride (p.36·1); tolu balsam (p.1071·1).
Coughs.

Sirop pour le sommeil *Zeller, Switz.*
Valerian (p.1643·1).
Sleep disorders.

Sirop S contre la toux et la bronchite *Synpharma, Switz.*
Codeine phosphate (p.26·1); drosera (p.1574·1); hyoscyamus (p.464·3); liquorice (p.1197·1) primula root.
Coughs.

Sirop Teyssedre *Bouteille, Fr.†.*
Calcium bromide (p.1620·3); chloral hydrate (p.645·3); calamint.
Irritability and sleep disorders in children.

Sirop Toux du Larynx *Qualiphar, Belg.*
Codeine phosphate (p.26·1); belladonna (p.457·1); aconite (p.1542·2); lobelia (p.1481·3); cherry-laurel water; drosera (p.1574·1); erysimin.
Coughs.

Sirop Wyss contre la toux *Wyss, Switz.*
Cherry-laurel; ipecacuanha (p.1062·2); senega root (p.1069·3); althaea (p.1546·3).
Coughs.

Siros *Janssen-Cilag, Ger.*
Itraconazole (p.381·3).
Vulvovaginal candidiasis.

Siroxyl
Rhone-Poulenc Rorer, Belg.; Sopar, Neth.†.
Carbocisteine (p.1056·3).
Respiratory-tract disorders.

Sirtal
Sanofi Winthrop, Aust.; Sanofi Winthrop, Ger.
Carbamazepine (p.339·2).
Alcohol withdrawal syndrome; bipolar disorder; diabetes insipidus; diabetic neuropathy; epilepsy; multiple sclerosis; neuralgia.

Sisare *Nourypharma, Ger.*
11 Tablets, oestradiol valerate (p.1455·2); 10 tablets, oestradiol valerate; medroxyprogesterone acetate (p.1448·3).
Menopausal disorders.

Sisobiotic *Von Boch, Ital.†.*
Sissomicin sulphate (p.248·1).
Bacterial infections.

Sisolline *Schering-Plough, Fr.†.*
Sissomicin sulphate (p.248·1).
Bacterial infections.

Sisomin *Max Farma, Ital.†.*
Sissomicin sulphate (p.248·1).
Bacterial infections.

Sisomina *Schering-Plough, Spain.*
Sissomicin sulphate (p.248·1).
Bacterial infections.

Sistalgin Compositum *Bracco, Ital.†.*
Pramiverine hydrochloride (p.1621·2); dipyrone (p.35·1).
Smooth muscle spasm.

Sisu-Dophilus Plus *Sisu, Canad.†.*
Lactobacillus acidophilus (p.1594·1); *Lactobacillus rhamnosus* (p.1594·1); *Lactobacillus bifidus* (p.1594·1); *Streptococcus faecium* (p.1594·1).
Establishment of healthy intestinal microflora.

Sita *Hoyer, Ger.*
Saw palmetto (p.1462·1).
Benign prostatic hyperplasia.

Sito-Lande *Synthelabo, Ger.*
Sitosterol (p.1279·3).
Hyperlipidaemias.

Sitosterol-B *Wassen, UK†.*
Sitosterols (p.1279·3); multivitamins; minerals.

Sitriol *Alphapharm, Austral.*
Calcitriol (p.1366·3).
Hypocalcaemia; osteoporosis.

Situalin *Formenti, Ital.*
Dexamethasone linoleate (p.1037·3).
Inflammatory skin disorders.

Situalin Antibiotico *Formenti, Ital.*
Dexamethasone linoleate (p.1037·3); bekanamycin sulphate (p.158·2).
Infected skin disorders.

Sitzmarks *Konsyl, USA.*
Polyvinyl chloride.
Contrast medium for gastro-intestinal radiography.

Sivastin *Sigma-Tau, Ital.*
Simvastatin (p.1278·2).
Coronary arteriosclerosis; hypercholesterolaemia; ischaemic heart disease.

SJ Liniment *International Dermatologicals, Canad.*
Methyl salicylate (p.55·2); menthol (p.1600·2); ammonia (p.1548·3); coal tar (p.1092·3).

Skeeter Stik *Triton, USA.*
Lignocaine (p.1293·2); phenol (p.1121·2).
Skin disorders.

Skelaxin *Carnrick, USA.*
Metaxalone (p.1316·1).
Painful musculoskeletal conditions.

Skelid
Sanofi Winthrop, Aust.; Sanofi Winthrop, Belg.; Sanofi Winthrop, Fr.; Sanofi Winthrop, Ger.; Sanofi Winthrop, Neth.; Sanofi, Swed.; Sanofi Winthrop, Switz.; Sanofi Winthrop, UK; Sanofi Winthrop, USA.
Disodium tiludronate (p.744·2).
Paget's disease of bone.

Skenan
UPSA, Fr.; Ethypharm, Ital.; Bristol-Myers Squibb, Neth.
Morphine sulphate (p.56·2).
Pain.

Skiacol *Alcon, Fr.*
Cyclopentolate hydrochloride (p.459·3).
Ophthalmic procedures.

Skiatropine *Novopharma, Switz.*
Atropine sulphate (p.455·1).
Eye disorders; production of cycloplegia and mydriasis.

Skid *Lichtenstein, Ger.*
Minocycline hydrochloride (p.226·2).

Skid E *Lichtenstein, Ger.*
Erythromycin (p.204·1).
Acne.

Skilar *Glaxo Allen, Ital.†.*
Econazole nitrate (p.377·2).
Bacterial and fungal infections of the skin.

Skilax *Prodes, Spain.*
Sodium picosulphate (p.1213·2).
Constipation.

Skin Bond Cement *Smith & Nephew, Austral.*
Appliance adhesive.

Skin Cleanser & Deodorizer *Arjo, Canad.*
Benzethonium chloride (p.1102·3).
Skin hygiene in incontinent patients.

Skin Cleansing *Cantassium Co., UK.*
Burdock (p.1594·2); senna (p.1212·2); fumitory (p.1581·3); clivers (p.1565·2).

Skin Clear *Potter's, UK.*
Ointment: Starch (p.1356·2); sublimed sulphur (p.1091·2); zinc oxide (p.1096·2).
Tablets: Echinacea root (p.1574·2).
Skin disorders.

Skin Conditioner & Bath Oil *Arjo, Canad.*
Light liquid paraffin (p.1382·1).
Dry skin; pruritus.

Skin Eruptions Mixture *Potter's, UK.*
Blue flag (p.1591·3); burdock root (p.1594·2); yellow dock; sarsaparilla (p.1627·2); buchu (p.1555·2); cascara (p.1183·1).
Skin disorders.

Skin Gel *Abbott, Austral.†.*
Appliance adhesive.

Skin Healing Cream *Brauer, Austral.*
Homoeopathic preparation.

Skin Prep *Smith & Nephew, Austral.*
Film dressing.

Skin Repair *Fisons Consumer, Austral.†.*
Emollient and barrier cream.

Skin Shield
Del, Canad.; Del, USA.
Dyclocaine hydrochloride (p.1292·3); benzethonium chloride (p.1102·3).
Liquid bandage.

Skin Tablets *Healthcrafts, UK.*
Burdock root (p.1594·2); wild pansy.
Eczema; skin blemishes.

Skin-Aid *Stiefel, Ger.†.*
Cream: Chloroxylenol (p.1111·1); resorcinol (p.1090·1); sulphur (p.1091·2).
Soap: Sulphonated plant oils.
Acne; seborrhoea.

Skinat *Zyma, Ital.*
Collagen (p.1566·3).
Prevention of scarring.

Skincalm *Noristan, S.Afr.†.*
Hydrocortisone (p.1043·3).
Skin disorders.

Skinicles *Skinicles, Canad.*
Hydroquinone (p.1083·1); padimate O (p.1488·1).

Skinman Intensiv *Henkel, Ger.*
Alcohol (p.1099·1); chlorhexidine gluconate (p.1107·2).
Skin disinfection.

Skinman Soft *Henkel, Ger.*
Isopropyl alcohol (p.1118·2); benzalkonium chloride (p.1101·3); undecenoic acid (p.389·2).
Skin disinfection.

Skinoren
Schering, Aust.; Schering, Austral.; Schering, Belg.; Schering, Fr.; Schering, Ger.; Schering, Ital.; Schering, Norw.; Schering, S.Afr.; Schering, Spain; Schering, Swed.; Schering, Switz.; Schering, UK.
Azelaic acid (p.1079·1).
Acne.

Skinsept F *Henkel, Ger.*
Isopropyl alcohol (p.1118·2); chlorhexidine gluconate (p.1107·2); hydrogen peroxide (p.1116·2).
Skin disinfection.

Skinsept G *Henkel, Ger.*
Alcohol (p.1099·1); isopropyl alcohol (p.1118·2).
Skin disinfection.

Skinsept Mucosa *Henkel, Ger.*
Alcohol (p.1099·1); hydrogen peroxide 30% (p.1116·2); chlorhexidine gluconate (p.1107·2).
Mucous membrane disinfection.

Skintex *Lloyd, Aimee, UK.*
Chloroxylenol (p.1111·1); camphor (p.1557·2).
Skin disorders.

Skin-vit *Pharmadass, UK.*
Multivitamin, mineral, and trace element preparation.

Skitz *Rorer, Austral.†.*
Benzoyl peroxide (p.1079·2).
Acne.

Sklerocedin N *Wolfer, Ger.†.*
Di-isopropylammonium dichloroacetate (p.854·1); orotic acid (p.1611·2).
Buzzing ears; forgetfulness; peripheral vascular disorders; poor concentration.

Sklerofibrat *Merckle, Ger.*
Bezafibrate (p.1268·2).
Hyperlipidaemias.

Skleromexe *Merckle, Ger.†.*
Clofibrate (p.1271·1).
Lipid disorders.

Sklerosol *Febena, Ger.*
Colloidal silicon dioxide (p.1475·1).
Arteriosclerosis; silicon deficiency.

Sklerovenol N *Febena, Ger.*
Aesculus (p.1543·3); rutoside sodium sulphate (p.1580·2).
Vascular disorders.

Sklerovitol *Lannacher, Aust.*
Vitamin B substances; rutin (p.1580·2).
Peripheral vascular disorders; reduced mental and physical capacity in the elderly; tonic.

Skopyl *Pharmacia Upjohn, Ger.†.*
Hyoscine methonitrate (p.463·1).
Smooth muscle spasms.

Sleep Aid
Tanta, Canad.; Numark, UK.
Diphenhydramine hydrochloride (p.409·1).
Insomnia.

Sleep Complex *Brauer, Austral.†.*
Homoeopathic preparation.

Sleep-eze 3 *Whitehall, USA.*
Diphenhydramine hydrochloride (p.409·1).
Insomnia.

Sleep-Eze D *Whitehall-Robins, Canad.*
Diphenhydramine hydrochloride (p.409·1).
Insomnia.

Sleepia *Pfizer Consumer, UK.*
Diphenhydramine hydrochloride (p.409·1).
Insomnia.

Sleeplessness & Insomnia Relief *Brauer, Austral.*
Homoeopathic preparation.

Sleepwell 2-nite *Rugby, USA.*
Diphenhydramine hydrochloride (p.409·1).
Insomnia.

Slendoll *Laser, S.Afr.†.*
Cathine hydrochloride (p.1478·1); betula; juniper oil (p.1592·3).
Obesity.

Slenz *SA Druggists, S.Afr.†.*
Cathine hydrochloride (p.1478·1).
Obesity.

Slepan *Staufen, Ger.*
Homoeopathic preparation.

Slim Mint
Note. This name is used for preparations of different composition.
Stella, Canad.
Benzocaine (p.1286·2); methylcellulose (p.1473·3).
Obesity.

Thompson, USA.
Benzocaine (p.1286·2).
Obesity.

Slim 'n Trim *Covan, S.Afr.*
Cathine (p.1478·1).
Obesity.

Slimase *Sessa, Ital.*
Enzymes and minerals.
Skin disorders.

Slim-Fast *Slim-Fast, Canad.†.*
Meal replacement.
Obesity.

Slimin *Zyma, Ger.†.*
Triamterene (p.957·2); hydrochlorothiazide (p.885·2).
Oedema.

SlimLinea *Bifarma, Ital.*
Bladderwrack (p.1554·1); betula (p.1553·3).

Slimmer *Baif, Ital.*
Piscidia erythrina; fucus vesiculosus; ananas sativa; equisetum arvense; betula alba; ononis spinosa; centalla asiatica; orthosiphon stamineus; ruscus aculeatus; lespedeza capitata.
Nutritional supplement.

Slim-Plan *Shaklee, Canad.†.*
Meal replacement.
Obesity.

Slimrite *Nelson, Austral.†.*
Phenylpropanolamine hydrochloride (p.1067·2); aloin (p.1177·2); ascorbic acid (p.1365·2); thiamine hydrochloride (p.1361·1); riboflavine (p.1362·1); calcium pantothenate (p.1352·3); nicotinamide (p.1351·2).
Obesity.

Slimswift Day Trim *Cantassium Co., UK†.*
Levoglutamide (p.1344·3); calcium ascorbate (p.1365·2); carnitine (p.1336·2); tyrosine (p.1357·3); phenylalanine (p.1353·1); vitamin B_6 (p.1362·3); chromium orotate.
Diet aid.

Slimswift Night Trim *Cantassium Co., UK†.*
Ornithine (p.1352·3); L-glycine (p.1345·2); vegetable protein hydrolysate; vitamin B substances.
Diet aid.

Slippery Elm Stomach Tablets *Potter's, UK.*
Slippery elm bark (p.1630·1); cinnamon oil (p.1564·2); clove oil (p.1565·2); peppermint oil (p.1208·1).
Dyspepsia.

Sloan *Warner-Lambert, Ital.*
Capsicum oleoresin; glycol monosalicylate (p.43·1); white camphor oil; pine oil; menthol (p.1600·2); eucalyptus oil (p.1578·1); benzyl nicotinate (p.22·1).
Musculoskeletal, joint, and soft-tissue pain.

Sloan Baume *Warner-Lambert Consumer, Switz.*
Ethyl nicotinate (p.36·1); menthol (p.1600·2); camphor (p.1557·2); methyl salicylate (p.55·2); capsicum oleoresin; eucalyptus oil (p.1578·1); pine oil; turpentine oil (p.1641·1).
Musculoskeletal and joint disorders.

Sloan Liniment *Warner-Lambert Consumer, Switz.*
Camphor (p.1557·2); methyl salicylate (p.55·2); capsicum oleoresin; pine oil; turpentine oil (p.1641·1).
Musculoskeletal and joint disorders.

Sloan's balsem *Warner-Lambert, Neth.*
Capsicum (p.1559·2); camphor (p.1557·2); benzyl nicotinate (p.22·1); glycol salicylate (p.43·1).
Muscle and joint pain.

Sloan's liniment
Note. This name is used for preparations of different composition.
Warner-Lambert, Neth.†.
Capsicum (p.1559·2); camphor (p.1557·2); methyl salicylate (p.55·2).
Muscle and joint pain.

Parke, Davis, Swed.†.
Capsicum oleoresin; methyl salicylate (p.55·2); camphor oil; pine oil; ammonia solution (p.1548·3); turpentine oil (p.1641·1).
Muscle pain.

Slo-Bid
Rhone-Poulenc Rorer, Austral.†; Rhone-Poulenc Rorer, Canad.; Rhone-Poulenc Rorer, USA.
Theophylline (p.765·1).
Obstructive airways disease.

Slofedipine *Sanofi Winthrop, UK.*
Nifedipine (p.916·2).
Angina pectoris; hypertension.

Slofenac *Sterwin, UK.*
Diclofenac sodium (p.31·2).

Slo-Indo *Generics, UK.*
Indomethacin (p.45·2).
Inflammation; pain.

Slo-Niacin *Upsher-Smith, USA.*
Nicotinic acid (p.1351·2).
Hyperlipidaemia (adjunct); nicotinic acid deficiency; pellagra.

Slo-Phyllin
Lipha, Irl.; Rorer, Ital.†; Lipha, UK; Rhone-Poulenc Rorer, USA.
Theophylline (p.765·1).
Obstructive airways disease.

Slo-Phyllin GG *Rorer, USA.*
Theophylline (p.765·1); guaiphenesin (p.1061·3).
Asthma; bronchospasm.

Sloprolol *CP Pharmaceuticals, UK†.*
Propranolol hydrochloride (p.937·1).
Anxiety; cardiac disorders; essential tremor; hypertension; migraine.

Slo-Salt-K *Mission Pharmacal, USA.*
Sodium chloride (p.1162·2); potassium chloride (p.1161·1).
Dehydration; heat prostration; sodium depletion; volume depletion.

Slow Release Mega C *Vita Glow, Austral.*
Calcium ascorbate (p.1365·2); ascorbic acid (p.1365·2).
Bruising; cold and influenza symptoms; maintenance of oral health; vitamin supplement; wounds.

Slow Release Mega Multi *Vita Glow, Austral.*
Multivitamin and mineral preparation.

Slow-Apresoline *Ciba, Switz.†.*
Hydralazine hydrochloride (p.883·2).
Heart failure; hypertension.

Slow-Fe
Novartis Consumer, Canad.; Ciba-Geigy, Irl.†; Ciba, UK; Ciba Consumer, USA.
Dried ferrous sulphate (p.1340·2).
Iron deficiency; iron-deficiency anaemia.

Slow-Fe Folic
Ciba Self Medication, Canad.; Ciba-Geigy, Irl.†; Ciba, UK.
Dried ferrous sulphate (p.1340·2); folic acid (p.1340·3).
Iron and folic acid deficiency in pregnancy.

Slow-K
Novartis, Austral.; Ciba, Canad.; Ciba-Geigy, Irl.; Novartis, Neth.; Novartis, S.Afr.; Alliance, UK; Summit, USA.
Potassium chloride (p.1161·1).
Hypokalaemia.

Slow-Mag
Merck, S.Afr.; Searle, USA.
Magnesium chloride (p.1157·2).
Magnesium deficiency.

Slow-Pren *Norton, UK†.*
Oxprenolol hydrochloride (p.926·2).
Angina pectoris; anxiety; hypertension.

Slow-Sodium
Novartis, Austral.; Ciba-Geigy, Irl.; Ciba, UK.
Sodium chloride (p.1162·2).
Hyponatraemia.

Slow-Trasicor
Ciba, Canad.; Ciba-Geigy, Irl.; Ciba-Geigy, S.Afr.†; Ciba, Switz.; Ciba, UK.
Oxprenolol hydrochloride (p.926·2).
Angina pectoris; anxiety; arrhythmias; hypertension; myocardial infarction.

Slow-Trasitensine *Ciba, Switz.*
Oxprenolol hydrochloride (p.926·2); chlorthalidone (p.839·3).
Hypertension.

Slozem *Lipha, UK.*
Diltiazem hydrochloride (p.854·2).
Angina pectoris; hypertension.

SLT *C & M, USA.*
Coal tar (p.1092·3); salicylic acid (p.1090·2); lactic acid (p.1593·3).
Seborrhoea.

SM-33 *Roche Consumer, Austral.*
Salicylic acid (p.1090·2); lignocaine (p.1293·2); tannic acid (p.1634·2); menthol (p.1600·2); thymol (p.1127·1); glycerol; alcohol.
Mouth ulcers; oral abrasions; teething and denture pain.

SM-33 Adult Formula *Roche Consumer, Austral.*
Lignocaine (p.1293·2); salicylic acid (p.1090·2); tannins; alcohol; rhubarb (p.1212·1).
Mouth ulcers; oral abrasions.

Smecta *IPSEN, Fr.*
Smectite beidellitique.
Gastro-intestinal disorders.

Smoke-Eze *Brauer, Austral.*
Homoeopathic preparation.

Smokeless *Inibsa, Spain.*
Lobeline sulphate (p.1481·3).
Aid to smoking withdrawal.

Smokerette *Medinex, Canad.*
Silver acetate (p.1629·2).
Aid to smoking withdrawal.

Smokescreen *Suisse, Austral.†.*
Vitamin, mineral, and amino acid supplement.

Smoking Withdrawal Support *Homeocan, Canad.*
Homoeopathic preparation.

Smok-Quit *Eagle, Austral.*
Homoeopathic preparation.

SMZ-TMP *Apothecon, USA.*
Co-trimoxazole (p.196·3).

Snake Bite *CSL, Austral.*
A range of monovalent and polyvalent snake antisera (brown snake, tiger snake, death adder, taipan, black snake) (p.1534·1).
Passive immunisation.

Snaplets-D *Baker Norton, USA.*
Phenylpropanolamine hydrochloride (p.1067·2); chlorpheniramine maleate (p.405·1).
Upper respiratory-tract symptoms.

Snaplets-DM *Baker Cummins, USA.*
Phenylpropanolamine hydrochloride (p.1067·2); dextromethorphan hydrobromide (p.1057·3).
Coughs and cold symptoms.

Snaplets-EX *Baker Cummins, USA.*
Phenylpropanolamine hydrochloride (p.1067·2); guaiphenesin (p.1061·3).
Coughs.

Snaplets-FR *Baker Cummins, USA.*
Paracetamol (p.72·2).
Pain.

Snaplets-Multi *Baker Cummins, USA.*
Phenylpropanolamine hydrochloride (p.1067·2); dextromethorphan hydrobromide (p.1057·3); chlorpheniramine maleate (p.405·1).
Coughs and cold symptoms.

Snelling Past *Farmades, Ital.†.*
Dietary fibre supplement.
Disorders of lipid and glucose metabolism.

Sno Phenicol
Chauvin, Irl.†; Chauvin, UK.
Chloramphenicol (p.182·1).
Bacterial eye infections.

Sno Pilo
Chauvin, Irl.†; Chauvin, UK.
Pilocarpine hydrochloride (p.1396·3).
Glaucoma; reduction of intra-ocular pressure before surgery; reversal of mydriasis.

Sno Pro *Scientific Hospital Supplies, Irl.*
Low-protein, low-phenylalanine food for special diets.
Disorders of amino-acid metabolism; milk substitute.

Sno Strips *Smith & Nephew, Irl.*
Test for tears before administration of ophthalmic medication.

Sno Tears
Chauvin, Irl.; Chauvin, UK.
Polyvinyl alcohol (p.1474·2).
Dry eyes.

Snooze Fast *BDI, USA.*
Diphenhydramine hydrochloride (p.409·1).
Insomnia.

Sno-Pro *Medifood-Trufood, Ital.*
Food for special diets.
Phenylketonuria; renal failure.

Snowfire *Pickles, UK.*
Benzoin (p.1634·1); citronella (p.1565·1); thyme oil (p.1637·1); lemon thyme (p.1636·3); clove oil (p.1565·2); cade oil (p.1092·2).
Chapped hands; chilblains.

SNP *Quatromed, S.Afr.*
Sodium nitroprusside hydrochloride.
Hypertension; production of controlled hypotension during surgery.

Snufflebabe *Pickles, UK.*
Menthol (p.1600·2); thyme oil (p.1637·1); eucalyptus oil (p.1578·1).
Congestion.

Snup *Karlspharma, Ger.†.*
Xylometazoline hydrochloride (p.1071·2).
Acute otitis media; catarrh; rhinitis.

Soaclens
Alcon, Austral.; Alcon, Canad.; Alcon, Fr.; Alcon, USA.
Soaking and wetting solution for hard and gas permeable contact lenses.

Sobelin *Pharmacia Upjohn, Ger.*
Clindamycin hydrochloride (p.191·1) or clindamycin palmitate hydrochloride (p.191·1) or clindamycin phosphate (p.191·1).
Bacterial infections.

Sobile *Alonga, Spain†.*
Oxazepam (p.683·2).
Anxiety; insomnia.

Sobrepin
Roche, Ital.; Tedec Meiji, Spain.
Sobrerol (p.1069·3).
Respiratory-tract disorders.

Sobrepin Amoxi *Zambeletti, Spain†.*
Amoxycillin trihydrate (p.151·3); sobrerol (p.1069·3).
Respiratory-tract infections.

Sobrepin Antibiotico *Corvi, Ital.†.*
Ampicillin (p.153·1); sobrerol (p.1069·3).
Bacterial infections of the respiratory tract; respiratory-tract congestion.

Sobrepin Respiro *Corvi, Ital.†.*
Sobrerol (p.1069·3); diprophylline (p.752·1).
Respiratory-tract disorders.

Sobril
Pharmacia Upjohn, Norw.; Pharmacia Upjohn, Swed.
Oxazepam (p.683·2).
Alcohol withdrawal syndrome; anxiety disorders; premedication; sleep disorders.

Sodex N *Woelm, Ger.*
Calcium carbonate (p.1182·1); magnesium hydroxide (p.1198·2).
Sodex formerly contained calcium carbonate, magnesium hydroxide, and bismuth subnitrate.
Gastro-intestinal disorders.

Sodibic *Rhone-Poulenc Rorer, Austral.*
Sodium bicarbonate (p.1153·2).
Bicarbonate replacement in renal failure.

Sodical Plus *Blackmores, Austral.†.*
Sodium phosphate (p.1159·3); iron phosphate; calcium phosphate (p.1155·3).

Sodiclo *Brissenco, S.Afr.*
Diclofenac sodium (p.31·2).
Inflammation; rheumatic disorders.

Sodinon *Boehringer Mannheim, Aust.*
Alginic acid (p.1470·3); aluminium hydroxide (p.1177·3); magnesium trisilicate (p.1199·1); sodium bicarbonate (p.1153·2).
Dyspepsia with reflux.

Sodiopen *CEPA, Spain.*
Benzylpenicillin sodium (p.159·3).
Bacterial infections.

Sodioral *CaDiGroup, Ital.*
Glucose; sodium chloride (p.1152·3).
Diarrhoea.

Sodip-phylline *Sodip, Switz.*
Theophylline (p.765·1).
Obstructive airways disease.

Sodipryl retard *Sodip, Switz.*
Naftidrofuryl oxalate (p.914·2).
Peripheral and cerebral vascular disorders.

Sodium Amytal
Lilly, Irl.; Lilly, UK.
Amylobarbitone sodium (p.641·3).
Insomnia; status epilepticus.

Sodium Edecrin *Merck Sharp & Dohme, USA.*
Sodium ethacrynate (p.866·3).
For rapid diuresis; oedema.

Sodium Sulamyd
Schering, Canad.; Schering, USA.
Sulphacetamide sodium (p.252·2).
Eye infections.

Sodium Uromiro *E. Merck, UK†.*
Sodium iodamide (p.1005·3).
Radiographic contrast medium.

Sodol Compound *Major, USA.*
Aspirin (p.16·1); carisoprodol (p.1312·3).
Musculoskeletal pain.

Sofargen *Sofar, Ital.*
Silver sulphadiazine (p.247·3).
Burns; ulcers.

Sofenol *C & M, USA.*
Emollient and moisturiser.

Soflax *Pharmascience, Canad.*
Docusate sodium (p.1189·3).
Constipation.

Soflax Fleet *Fleet, USA.*
Docusate sodium (p.1189·3).
Stool softener.

Soflax Overnight *Fleet, USA.*
Docusate sodium (p.1189·3); casanthranol (p.1182·3).
Constipation; stool softener.

Soflens *Bausch & Lomb, Fr.†.*
Disinfecting and soaking solution for soft contact lenses.

Sof/Pro-Clean *Sherman, USA.*
Cleansing solution for soft contact lenses.

Sofracort *Hoechst Marion Roussel, Canad.*
Framycetin sulphate (p.210·3); gramicidin (p.215·2); dexamethasone (p.1037·1).
Ear disorders; eye disorders.

Sofradex
Hoechst Marion Roussel, Austral.; Hoechst Marion Roussel, Irl.; Hoechst Marion Roussel, Neth.; Hoechst Marion Roussel, Norw.; Hoechst Marion Roussel, S.Afr.; Hoechst Marion Roussel, Swed.; Hoechst Marion Roussel, Switz.; Florizel, UK.
Dexamethasone (p.1037·1) or dexamethasone sodium *m*-sulphobenzoate (p.1037·2); framycetin sulphate (p.210·3); gramicidin (p.215·2).
Infected ear and eye disorders.

Sofraline *Hoechst Marion Roussel, Belg.*
Framycetin sulphate (p.210·3); naphazoline nitrate (p.1064·2).
Respiratory-tract disorders.

Soframycin
Note. This name is used for preparations of different composition.
Hoechst Marion Roussel, Austral.; Hoechst Marion Roussel, Canad.; Roussel, Irl.; Hoechst Marion Roussel, Neth.; Hoechst Marion Roussel, S.Afr.; Hoechst Marion Roussel, Switz.; Florizel, UK.
Eye/ear drops; eye/ear ointment: Framycetin sulphate (p.210·3).
Bacterial eye and ear infections.

Roussel, Austral.†; Hoechst Marion Roussel, Canad.
Nasal spray: Framycetin sulphate (p.210·3); gramicidin (p.215·2); phenylephrine hydrochloride (p.1066·2).
Bacterial nasal infections; nasal congestion.

Hoechst Marion Roussel, Austral.; Hoechst Marion Roussel, Canad.; Albert-Roussel, Ger.†; Hoechst Marion Roussel, Irl.; Roussel, S.Afr.†; Florizel, UK.
Ointment: Framycetin sulphate (p.210·3); gramicidin (p.215·2).
Bacterial skin infections.

Soframycine
Hoechst Marion Roussel, Belg.; Roussel, Fr.
Framycetin sulphate (p.210·3).
Bacterial infections.

Soframycine Hydrocortisone *Roussel, Fr.*
Framycetin sulphate (p.210·3); hydrocortisone (p.1043·3).
Bacterial infections with inflammation.

Soframycine Naphazoline *Roussel, Fr.*
Framycetin sulphate (p.210·3); naphazoline nitrate (p.1064·2).
Congestion and bacterial infection of the upper respiratory tract.

Sofrasolone *Hoechst Marion Roussel, Belg.*
Prednisolone acetate (p.1048·1); framycetin sulphate (p.210·3); naphazoline nitrate (p.1064·2).
Allergy or infections of the respiratory-tract.

Sofra-Tull
Albert-Roussel, Aust.; Albert-Roussel, Ger.; Hoechst, Ger.
Framycetin sulphate (p.210·3).
Infected skin disorders; wounds.

Sofra-Tulle
Hoechst Marion Roussel, Austral.; Hoechst Marion Roussel, Canad.; Hoechst Marion Roussel, Irl.; Roussel, Ital.†; Hoechst Marion Roussel, Neth.; Hoechst Marion Roussel, Norw.; Roussel, S.Afr.; Hoechst Marion Roussel, Swed.; Hoechst Marion Roussel, Switz.; Roussel, UK.
Framycetin sulphate (p.210·3).
Infected skin disorders; wounds.

Sofro *Alcon-Thilo, Ger.†.*
Sodium cromoglycate (p.762·1).
Allergic eye disorders.

SOF-T *Doetsch, Grether, Switz.*
Copper-wound plastic (p.1337·3).
Intra-uterine contraceptive device.

Soft Lips *Mentholatum, Canad.*
SPF 17: Ethylhexyl *p*-methoxycinnamate (p.1487·1); oxybenzone (p.1487·3); padimate O (p.1488·1); dimethicone (p.1384·2).
Sunscreen.

Soft Mate *Pilkington Barnes-Hind, USA.*
Range of solutions for soft contact lenses.

Soft Mate Comfort Drops *Allergan, Austral.*
Lubricating and cleansing solution.
Irritation and dryness occurring during contact lens wear.

Soft Mate Consept *Pilkington Barnes-Hind, USA.*
Hydrogen peroxide (p.1116·2).
Disinfecting solution for soft contact lenses.

Soft Mate Consept 1
Willvonseder, Aust.; Allergan, Austral.
Hydrogen peroxide (p.1116·2).
Cleansing and disinfecting solution for contact lenses.

Soft Mate Consept 2
Willvonseder, Aust.; Allergan, Austral.
Rinsing and neutralising solutions for contact lenses.

Soft Mate Daily Cleaning Solution *Allergan, Austral.*
Cleansing solution for soft contact lenses.

Soft Mate Enzyme Plus Cleaner *Pilkington Barnes-Hind, USA.*
Subtilisin-A.
Cleansing solution for soft contact lenses.

Soft Mate Hydrogen Peroxide *Barnes-Hind, Austral.†.*
Hydrogen peroxide (p.1116·2).
Disinfection of soft contact lenses.

Soft Mate Preservative Free Saline Solution
Barnes-Hind, Austral.†.
Rinsing and storage solution for soft contact lenses.

Soft Mate Saline Solution *Barnes-Hind, Austral.†.*
Rinsing and storage solution for soft contact lenses.

Soft Rinse 250 *SoftRinse, USA.*
Sodium chloride (p.1162·2).
Rinsing and storage solution for soft contact lenses.

Softa Man
Braun, Belg.†; Braun, Ger.; Braun, Ital.
Alcohol (p.1099·1); propyl alcohol (p.1124·2).
Hand disinfection.

Softab *Alcon, Austral.*
Sodium dichloroisocyanurate (p.1124·3).
Cleansing and sterilisation of soft contact lenses.

Softasept N *Braun, Ger.*
Alcohol (p.1099·1); isopropyl alcohol (p.1118·2).
Skin disinfection.

Softene *Rhone-Poulenc Rorer, Belg.*
Docusate sodium (p.1189·3); bisacodyl (p.1179·3).
Constipation.

Soft-Stress *Marlyn, USA†.*
Multivitamin and mineral preparation with iron and folic acid.

Softwash *Palmolive Skincare, Austral.*
Triclosan (p.1127·2).
Hand disinfection.

Softwear *Ciba Vision, Austral.*
Sodium chloride (p.1162·2).
Solution for contact lens care.

Sokaral *Allergan, Ger.†.*
Dexamethasone (p.1037·1).
Scalp disorders; skin disorders.

Soker *Medecine Vegetale, Fr.*
Aniseed (p.1549·3); star anise; condurango (p.1567·2); sodium hydrogen phosphate (p.1159·3); calcium carbonate (p.1182·1); magnesium oxide (p.1198·3).
Gastro-intestinal disorders.

Soklinal *Allergan, Ger.*
Phenylmercuric nitrate (p.1122·2).
Storage and rinsing solution for contact lenses.

Sol Dial Perit *Grifols, Spain†.*
Electrolytes; heparin (p.879·3); glucose or sorbitol (p.1151·1).
Peritoneal dialysis.

Sol Ringer And Farm *Andalucia, Spain†.*
Electrolyte infusion (p.1147·1).
Fluid and electrolyte depletion.

Sol Schoum *Expanscience, Spain.*
Boldo (p.1554·1); fumitory (p.1581·3); hamamelis (p.1587·1); melissa (p.1600·1); rhubarb (p.1212·1); piscidia; peppermint oil (p.1208·1); ethyl alcohol; glycerol; hydrastis canadensis (p.1588·2); electrolytes (p.1147·1).
Hepatobiliary disorders.

Sola Stick Broad Spectrum *Hamilton, Austral.*
SPF15+: Ethylhexyl *p*-methoxycinnamate (p.1487·1); avobenzone (p.1486·3).
Sunscreen.

Solacap *Lesvi, Spain.*
Fluconazole (p.378·1).
Vulvovaginal candidiasis.

Solacy
Serozym, Fr.; Wild, Switz.†.
Cystine (p.1339·1); sulphur (p.1091·2); vitamin A (p.1358·1); vitamin A acetate (p.1359·2); yeast (p.1373·1).
Upper respiratory-tract disorders.

Solamin
Note. This name is used for preparations of different composition.
Ardeypharm, Ger.†.
Oral drops: Ethaverine hydrochloride (p.1577·1); diphenhydramine hydrochloride (p.409·1); ephedrine hydrochloride (p.1059·3); hedera helix; guaiphenesin (p.1061·3); proxyphylline (p.757·3); anise oil (p.1550·1).
Bronchial asthma; bronchitis; cardiac asthma; dyspnoea; silicosis.

Pharmacia Upjohn, Ital.
Amino-acid infusion.
Parenteral nutrition.

Solan-M *Winzer, Ger.*
Vitamin A palmitate (p.1359·2).
Eye disorders.

Solantal *Fujisawa, Jpn.*
Tiaramide hydrochloride (p.89·2).
Inflammation; pain.

Solaquin
Note. This name is used for preparations of different composition.
ICN, Canad.
Hydroquinone (p.1083·1); roxadimate (p.1488·2); dioxybenzone (p.1487·1); oxybenzone (p.1487·3).
Skin hyperpigmentation.

ICN, USA.
Hydroquinone (p.1083·1).
Skin hyperpigmentation.

Solaquin Forte *ICN, USA.*
Cream: Hydroquinone (p.1083·1); roxadimate (p.1488·2); dioxybenzone (p.1487·1); oxybenzone (p.1487·3).
Topical gel: Hydroquinone (p.1083·1); roxadimate (p.1488·2); dioxybenzone (p.1487·1).
Skin hyperpigmentation.

Solar Block *Fisons Consumer, Austral.†.*
Padimate O (p.1488·1); oxybenzone (p.1487·3); avobenzone (p.1486·3).
Sunscreen.

Solarcaine
Note. This name is used for preparations of different composition.
Schering-Plough, Canad.; Schering-Plough, UK; Schering-Plough, USA.
Cream; lotion; topical spray: Benzocaine (p.1286·2); triclosan (p.1127·2).
Minor skin injuries; sunburn.

Schering-Plough, Spain.
Benzocaine (p.1286·2); hexachlorophane (p.1115·2).
Skin disorders.

Essex, Switz.
Lignocaine (p.1293·2).
Minor skin lesions and burns.

Schering-Plough, UK.
Topical gel: Aloe vera (p.1177·1); lignocaine (p.1293·2).
Cuts; insect bites; sunburn.

Solarcaine Aloe Extra Burn Relief *Schering-Plough, USA.*
Lignocaine (p.1293·2); aloe vera (p.1177·1).
Local anaesthesia.

Solarcaine Lidocaine *Schering-Plough, Canad.*
Lignocaine (p.1293·2) or lignocaine hydrochloride (p.1293·2).
Sunburn; wounds.

Solarcaine Stop Itch *Schering-Plough, Canad.*
Papain (p.1614·1).
Skin pain and irritation.

Solarex *Essex, Switz.†.*
Oxybenzone (p.1487·3); padimate O (p.1488·1).
Sunscreen.

Solart *Bioindustria, Ital.*
Acemetacin (p.12·2).
Musculoskeletal and joint disorders.

Solarub *Nelson, Austral.†.*
Methyl salicylate (p.55·2); menthol (p.1600·2); camphor (p.1557·2); capsicum oleoresin; eucalyptus oil (p.1578·1).
Topical analgesic and counter-irritant.

Solaskil *Specia, Fr.*
Levamisole hydrochloride (p.102·3).
Worm infections.

Solatene
Roche, Austral.†; Roche, USA†.
Betacarotene (p.1335·2).
Erythropoietic protoporphyria.

Solatran
Bencard, Belg.; SmithKline Beecham, S.Afr.; SmithKline Beecham, Switz.
Ketazolam (p.675·2).
Anxiety disorders; nervous disorders; skeletal muscle spasm.

Solaurit *Polcopharma, Austral.*
Homoeopathic preparation.

SolBar *Person & Covey, USA.*
SPF 15: Ethylhexyl *p*-methoxycinnamate (p.1487·1); oxybenzone (p.1487·3).
SPF 30: Octocrylene (p.1487·3); ethylhexyl *p*-methoxycinnamate (p.1487·1); oxybenzone (p.1487·3).
SPF 50: Oxybenzone (p.1487·3); ethylhexyl *p*-methoxycinnamate (p.1487·1); octocrylene (p.1487·3).
Sunscreen.

SolBar Plus
Note. This name is used for preparations of different composition.
Person & Covey, Canad.
SPF 15: Oxybenzone (p.1487·3); roxadimate (p.1488·2).
Sunscreen.

Person & Covey, USA†.
SPF 15: Oxybenzone (p.1487·3); dioxybenzone (p.1487·1); padimate O (p.1488·1).
Sunscreen.

Solclot *Sumitomo, Jpn.*
Duteplase (p.863·1).

Solcode *Reckitt & Colman, Austral.*
Aspirin (p.16·1); codeine phosphate (p.26·1).
Fever; pain.

Solcodein *Inibsa, Spain†.*
Codeine phosphate (p.26·1).
Coughs.

Solcoderm *Solco, Switz.*
Nitric acid (p.1609·1); glacial acetic acid (p.1541·2); oxalic acid dihydrate (p.1611·3); lactic acid (p.1593·3); copper nitrate trihydrate.
Benign skin growths.

Solco-Derman *Basotherm, Ger.*
Glacial acetic acid (p.1541·2); oxalic acid (p.1611·3); nitric acid (p.1609·1); lactic acid (p.1593·3); copper nitrate.
Skin disorders.

Solcogyn *Solco, Switz.*
Nitric acid (p.1609·1); glacial acetic acid (p.1541·2); oxalic acid dihydrate (p.1611·3); zinc nitrate hexahydrate.
Benign cervical lesions.

Solcort *Lebens, Ital.†.*
Suprarenal cortex (p.1050·1).
Endotoxic shock; postinfection convalescence; suprarenal insufficiency.

Solcoseryl
Chemieprodukte, Aust.; Sarget, Fr.†; Asta Medica, Ital.; Asta Medica, Neth.; Swisspharm, S.Afr.†; Berna, Spain; Solco, Switz.
Protein-free calf blood extract.
Burns; gastro-intestinal disorders; ulcers; vascular disorders; wounds.

Solcoseryl comp *Chemieprodukte, Aust.*
Protein-free calf blood extract; laureth 9 (p.1325·2).
Dental adhesive; mouth disorders.

Solcoseryl Dental
Oral-B, Ger.; Solco, Switz.
Protein-free calf blood concentrate; laureth 9 (p.1325·2).
Dental adhesive; mouth disorders.

Solcosplen *Strathmann, Ger.*
Calf spleen extract.
Menopausal disorders.

Solco-Trichovac
Note. This name is used for preparations of different composition.
Chemieprodukte, Aust.†.
A trichomonal vaccine (p.1536·3).
Active immunisation.

Solco, Switz.
Lactobacillus acidophilus (p.1594·1).
Vaginal infections.

SolcoUrovac
Stroschein, Ger.†; Solco, Switz.†.
Escherichia coli; *Proteus mirabilis*; *Proteus morganii*; *Klebsiella pneumoniae*; *Enterococcus faecalis* (p.1594·1).
Urinary-tract infections.

Soldactone
Searle, Belg.; Searle, Neth.; Searle, Norw.; Searle, S.Afr.†; Searle, Swed.; Searle, Switz.
Canrenoate potassium (p.836·2).
Hyperaldosteronism; hypokalaemia; oedema.

Soldesam *Farmacologico Milanese, Ital.*
Dexamethasone sodium phosphate (p.1037·2).
Corticosteroid.

Solecin *Echo, Ital.*
Soya lecithin (p.1595·2); wheat germ; gelatin (p.723·2); glycerol (p.1585·2); betacarotene (p.1335·2).
Nutritional supplement.

Soledexin *Cassella-med, Ger.†.*
Benzyl isothiocyanate (p.1552·3); cineole (p.1564·1).
Bacterial and candidal infections of the respiratory tract.

Soledum *Cassella-med, Ger.*
Cineole (p.1564·1).
Coughs and associated respiratory-tract disorders.

Soledum Balsam *Cassella-med, Ger.*
Cineole (p.1564·1).
Respiratory-tract disorders.

Soledum Hustensaft *Cassella-med, Ger.*
Thyme (p.1636·3).
Coughs.

Soledum Hustensaft N *Cassella-med, Ger.†.*
Liquorice (p.1197·1); thyme (p.1636·3); hedera helix; equisetum (p.1575·1); turion. pini; sodium benzoate (p.1102·3); ammonium chloride (p.1055·2); ammonia solution (p.1548·3).
Coughs and associated respiratory-tract disorders.

Soledum Hustentropfen *Cassella-med, Ger.*
Thyme (p.1636·3).
Coughs.

Soledum Hustentropfen N *Cassella-med, Ger.†.*
Ammonium chloride (p.1055·2); liquorice (p.1197·1); thyme (p.1636·3); equisetum (p.1575·1); hedera helix; turiones pini.
Coughs and associated respiratory-tract disorders.

Soledum med *Cassella-med, Ger.*
Chamomile oil.
Rhinitis.

Soledum Nasentropfen N *Cassella-med, Ger.†.*
Eucalyptus oil (p.1578·1); pine oil; chamomile oil.
Rhinitis.

Solex A15 *Dermol, USA.*
Padimate O (p.1488·1); oxybenzone (p.1487·3).
Sunscreen.

Soleze *Pickles, UK.*
Dibromopropamidine isethionate (p.1112·2); hydroviton.
Burns; sunburn.

Solfa *Takeda, Jpn.*
Amlexanox (p.749·1).
Allergic rhinitis; asthma.

Solfac EW *Bayer, Ital.*
Cyfluthrin (p.1404·1).
Insecticide.

Solfachinid *Bouty, Ital.†.*
Quinidine sulphate (p.939·1).
Arrhythmias.

Solfofil *Farmila, Ital.†.*
Sulphur (p.1091·2); hexachlorophane (p.1115·2).
Skin disinfection.

Solfomucil *Locatelli, Ital.*
Carbocisteine (p.1056·3).
Otorhinolaryngeal disorders; respiratory-tract congestion.

Solfoton *ECR, USA.*
Phenobarbitone (p.350·2).
Epilepsy; insomnia; sedative.

Solganal
Schering, Canad.; Schering, USA.
Aurothioglucose (p.20·2).
Rheumatoid arthritis.

Solgeretik
Bristol-Myers Squibb, Aust.; Bristol-Myers Squibb, Ger.†.
Nadolol (p.913·2); bendrofluazide (p.827·3).
Hypertension.

Solgol
Bristol-Myers Squibb, Aust.; Bristol-Myers Squibb, Ger.; Uriach, Spain.
Nadolol (p.913·2).
Angina pectoris; arrhythmias; hypertension; hyperthyroidism; migraine.

Solian
Synthelabo, Fr.; Lorex, UK.
Amisulpride (p.641·2).
Psychoses.

Solidago II/ 035 B *Phonix, Ger.†.*
Homoeopathic preparation.

Solidagoren N *Klein, Ger.*
Solidago virgaurea; potentilla anserina; equisetum (p.1575·1).
Renal disorders.

Solidagosan N *Hanosan, Ger.*
Homoeopathic preparation.

Solin S *Iromedica, Switz.†.*
Hypericum oil (p.1590·1); menthol (p.1600·2); camphor (p.1557·2); chamomile (p.1561·2); jecoris oil; peru balsam (p.1617·2); zinc oxide (p.1096·2).
Skin disorders; wounds.

Solinitrina *Berenguer Infale, Spain.*
Glyceryl trinitrate (p.874·3).
Angina pectoris; heart failure; induction of hypotension; myocardial infarction.

Solipid *Laevosan, Aust.*
Soya oil (p.1355·1).
Some preparations contain egg lecithin.
Lipid infusion for parenteral nutrition.

Solis *Galen, UK†.*
Diazepam (p.661·1).
Alcohol withdrawal syndrome; anxiety; epilepsy; insomnia; premedication; skeletal muscle spasm.

Solisan *Synpharma, Aust.*
Ononis root (p.1610·2); bearberry (p.1552·2); centaury (p.1561·1).
Urinary-tract disorders.

Solitab *Hermes, Ger.*
Magnesium trisilicate (p.1199·1).
Gastro-intestinal disorders associated with hyperacidity.

Solitacina *Lirca, Ital.†.*
Indomethacin (p.45·2); zolimidine.
Arthritis; gout.

Solium *Horner, Canad.†.*
Chlordiazepoxide hydrochloride (p.646·3).
Alcohol withdrawal syndrome; anxiety; tension.

Solivito N
Pharmacia Upjohn, Irl.; Pharmacia Upjohn, UK.
Water-soluble vitamin preparation.
Parenteral nutrition.

Soliwax *Martindale Pharmaceuticals, UK†.*
Docusate sodium (p.1189·3).
NOTE. There is no connection between Martindale, The Complete Drug Reference and Martindale Pharmaceuticals.
Ear wax removal.

Sol-Jod *Ecobi, Ital.*
Iodine (p.1493·1).
Oral antisepsis.

Solmucol
Genevrier, Fr.; Fidia, Ital.; Continental Ethicals, S.Afr.; IBSA, Switz.
Acetylcysteine (p.1052·3).
Eye disorders; paracetamol overdosage; respiratory-tract disorders.

Solo-care *Ciba Vision, Austral.*
Cleansing, rinsing, disinfecting and storing solution for soft contact lenses.

Solo-care Hard *Ciba Vision, Aust.*
Rinsing, storage and disinfecting solution for hard contact lenses.

Solo-care Soft *Ciba Vision, Aust.*
Rinsing. storage and disinfecting solution for soft contact lenses.

Solone
Note. This name is used for preparations of different composition.
Fawns & McAllan, Austral.
Prednisolone (p.1048·1).
Corticosteroid.

Boots, Spain†.
Dexamethasone sodium phosphate (p.1037·2).
Corticosteroid.

Solosin *Hoechst, Ger.*
Theophylline (p.765·1).
Obstructive airways disease.

SoloSite *Smith & Nephew, Austral.*
Carmellose sodium (p.1471·2); allantoin (p.1078·2).
Wounds.

Solotrim *Laevosan, Aust.*
Trimethoprim (p.265·1).
Bacterial infections.

Solovite *Solgar, UK.*
Multivitamin and mineral preparation.

Solozone *Palmolive Skincare, Austral.†.*
SPF15+: Ethylhexyl *p*-methoxycinnamate (p.1487·1); titanium dioxide (p.1093·3).
Sunscreen.

Solpadeine
SmithKline Beecham Consumer, Irl.; SmithKline Beecham Consumer, UK.
Paracetamol (p.72·2); codeine phosphate (p.26·1); caffeine (p.749·3).
Fever; pain.

Solpadeine Max *SmithKline Beecham Consumer, UK.*
Paracetamol (p.72·2); codeine phosphate (p.26·1).
These ingredients can be described by the British Approved Name Co-codamol.
Pain.

Solpadol
Sanofi Winthrop, Irl.; Sanofi Winthrop, UK.
Paracetamol (p.72·2); codeine phosphate (p.26·1).
These ingredients can be described by the British Approved Name Co-codamol 30/500.
Pain.

Solpaflex *SmithKline Beecham Consumer, UK.*
Tablets: Ibuprofen (p.44·1); codeine phosphate (p.26·1).
Fever; pain.
Topical gel: Ketoprofen (p.48·2).
Oedema; pain; peri-articular and soft-tissue disorders.

Solphyllex *Adcock Ingram, S.Afr.*
Theophylline (p.765·1); etofylline (p.753·1); diphenylpyraline hydrochloride (p.409·3); ammonium chloride (p.1055·2); sodium citrate (p.1153·2).
Coughs.

Solphyllin *Adcock Ingram, S.Afr.*
Theophylline (p.765·1); etofylline (p.753·1).
Obstructive airways disease.

Solplex 40 *SIFRA, Ital.*
Dextran 40 (p.716·2) in sodium chloride or glucose.
Plasma volume expansion.

Solplex 70 *SIFRA, Ital.*
Dextran 70 (p.717·1) in sodium chloride or glucose.
Plasma volume expansion; thrombosis prophylaxis.

Solprene *Farmigea, Ital.*
Prednisolone sodium phosphate (p.1048·1); neomycin sulphate (p.229·2).
Infected eye disorders.

Solprin *Reckitt & Colman, Austral.*
Aspirin (p.16·1).
Fever; inhibition of platelet aggregation; pain.

Solpurin *Salfa, Ital.†.*
Probenecid (p.394·3).
Gout; gouty arthritis; uricaemia.

Soltice *Chattem, USA.*
Methyl salicylate (p.55·2); camphor (p.1557·2); menthol (p.1600·2).
Muscle, joint, and soft-tissue pain; neuralgia.

Soltrim *Almirall, Spain.*
Sulphamethoxazole lysine (p.256·1); trimethoprim (p.265·1).
Bacterial infections.

Soltux *Corvi, Ital.†.*
Sobrerol (p.1069·3); chlophedianol (p.1057·1).
Coughs.

Solu Dacortin H *Merck, Spain.*
Prednisolone sodium succinate (p.1048·2).
Corticosteroid.

Solu Moderin *Upjohn, Spain.*
Methylprednisolone sodium succinate (p.1046·1).
Corticosteroid.

Solubacter
Pharmethic, Belg.†; Boots Healthcare, Fr.
Triclocarban (p.1127·2).
Disinfection of skin and mucous membranes.

Solubeol *Piette, Belg.*
Guaiphenesin (p.1061·3); phenoxyethanol (p.1122·2).
Solvent for painful intramuscular injections.

Solu-Biloptin
Schering, Ger.†; Schering, Spain†; Schering, UK.
Calcium iopodate (p.1007·3).
Contrast medium for biliary-tract radiography.

Solubiloptine *Schering, Fr.†.*
Calcium iopodate (p.1007·3).
Contrast medium for biliary-tract radiography.

Solubitrat
Note. This name is used for preparations of different composition.
Salus, Aust.
Silver birch leaf (p.1553·3); solidago virgaurea; orthosiphon leaf (p.1592·2); fennel oil (p.1578·1).
Urinary-tract disorders.

Heumann, Switz.†.
Orthosiphon (p.1592·2); solidago virgaurea; equisetum (p.1575·1); betula (p.1553·3); juniper oil (p.1592·3); fennel oil (p.1579·2).
Urinary-tract disorders.

Solucamphre
Note. This name is used for preparations of different composition.
Synthelabo, Belg.
Codeine (p.26·1); ethylmorphine (p.36·1); ephedrine (p.1059·3); piperazine hydrate (p.107·2); camsylic acid; aconite (p.1542·2); belladonna (p.457·1); ipecacuanha (p.1062·2); senna (p.1212·2).
Coughs.

Synthelabo, Fr.
Piperazine camsylate (p.108·1).
Hypotension.

Synthelabo, Switz.
Codeine camsylate (p.27·1); ethylmorphine camsylate (p.36·1); ephedrine camsylate (p.1060·1); belladonna (p.457·1); ipecacuanha (p.1062·2).
Coughs.

Solu-Celestan *Aesca, Aust.*
Betamethasone disodium phosphate (p.1033·3).
Corticosteroid.

Soluchrom *Cooperation Pharmaceutique, Fr.*
Mercurochrome sodium (p.1119·2).
Skin, burn and wound disinfection.

Solucion Fisio Nasal *PQS, Spain.*
Sodium chloride (p.1162·2).
Nasal congestion.

Solucionic *Diviser Aquilea, Spain.*
Povidone-iodine (p.1123·3).
Bacterial vaginosis.

Solucis *Aesculapius, Ital.*
Carbocisteine (p.1056·3).
Respiratory-tract disorders.

Solucort *Merck Sharp & Dohme-Chibret, Fr.*
Prednisolone sodium phosphate (p.1048·1).
Corticosteroid.

Solu-Cortef
Pharmacia Upjohn, Austral.; Pharmacia Upjohn, Belg.; Pharmacia Upjohn, Canad.; Pharmacia Upjohn, Irl.; Pharmacia Upjohn, Ital.; Pharmacia Upjohn, Neth.; Pharmacia Upjohn, Norw.; Pharmacia Upjohn, S.Afr.; Pharmacia Upjohn, Swed.; Pharmacia Upjohn, Switz.; Upjohn, UK; Upjohn, USA.
Hydrocortisone sodium succinate (p.1044·1).
Corticosteroid.

Solu-Dacortin *Merck, Aust.*
Prednisolone sodium succinate (p.1048·2).
Corticosteroid.

Soludacortin *Bracco, Ital.*
Prednisolone sodium succinate (p.1048·2).
Corticosteroid.

Solu-Dacortine
Merck-Belgolabo, Belg.; E. Merck, Switz.
Prednisolone sodium succinate (p.1048·2).
Corticosteroid.

Soludactone *Searle, Fr.*
Canrenoate potassium (p.836·2).
Hyperaldosteronism; hypokalaemia.

Soludecadron *Merck Sharp & Dohme-Chibret, Fr.*
Dexamethasone sodium phosphate (p.1037·2).
Corticosteroid.

Solu-Decortin-H *Merck, Ger.*
Prednisolone sodium succinate (p.1048·2).
Parenteral corticosteroid.

Soludial *Soludia, Fr.*
Sodium bicarbonate (p.1153·2).
Haemodialysis.

Soludor *Lehning, Fr.*
Homoeopathic preparation.

Solufen
Brovar, S.Afr.†; Whitehall-Robins, Switz.
Ibuprofen (p.44·1).
Fever; pain.

Solufena *UCB, Spain.*
Ibuprofen (p.44·1).
Fever; musculoskeletal, joint, and peri-articular disorders; pain.

Solufilina Sedante *BOI, Spain.*
Etamiphylline hydrochloride (p.753·1); phenobarbitone (p.350·2).
Obstructive airways disease; precordial pain.

Solufilina Simple *BOI, Spain.*
Etamiphylline hydrochloride (p.753·1).
Angina pectoris; heart failure; myocardial infarction; obstructive airways disease.

Solufina *BOI, Spain.*
Etamiphylline hydrochloride (p.753·1).
Cardiac disorders; obstructive airways disease.

Solu-Flur *Germiphene, Canad.*
Sodium fluoride (p.742·1).
Dental caries prophylaxis.

Solufos *Fermentaciones y Sintesis, Spain.*
Fosfomycin calcium (p.210·2) or fosfomycin sodium (p.210·2).
Lignocaine (p.1293·2) is included in the intramuscular injection to alleviate the pain of injection.
Bacterial infections.

Solugastril
Salus, Aust.; Heumann, Ger.; Heumann, Switz.†.
Aluminium hydroxide gel (p.1177·3); calcium carbonate (p.1182·1).
Gastro-intestinal disorders associated with hyperacidity.

Solugastryl *Oberlin, Fr.†.*
Anhydrous sodium sulphate (p.1213·3); anhydrous sodium hydrogen phosphate (p.1159·3); magnesium chloride (p.1157·2).
Gastro-intestinal disorders.

Solugel *Stiefel, Canad.*
Benzoyl peroxide (p.1079·2).
Acne.

Solu-Glyc *Erco pharm, Swed.†.*
Hydrocortisone sodium succinate (p.1044·1).
Corticosteroid.

Solu-Hepar N *Heumann, Ger.†.*
Boldo leaf (p.1554·1); chelidonium; silybum marianum (p.993·3); tolynol (p.1638·2); peppermint oil (p.1208·1).
Herbal tea.

Solumag
Kolassa, Aust.; Boehringer Ingelheim, Fr.; Geymonat, Ital.; Hexal, S.Afr.
Magnesium oxide (p.1198·3) or magnesium pidolate (p.1157·3).
Dysmenorrhoea; eclampsia and other obstetric disorders; nervous hyperexcitability associated with magnesium deficiency.

Solu-Medrol
Pharmacia Upjohn, Aust.; Pharmacia Upjohn, Austral.; Pharmacia Upjohn, Belg.; Pharmacia Upjohn, Canad.; Pharmacia Upjohn, Fr.; Pharmacia Upjohn, Ital.; Pharmacia Upjohn, Neth.; Pharmacia Upjohn, Norw.; Pharmacia Upjohn, S.Afr.; Pharmacia Upjohn, Swed.; Pharmacia Upjohn, Switz.; Upjohn, USA.
Methylprednisolone hemisuccinate (p.1046·1) or methylprednisolone sodium succinate (p.1046·1).
Corticosteroid.

Solu-Medrone
Pharmacia Upjohn, Irl.; Upjohn, Swed.†; Upjohn, UK.
Methylprednisolone sodium succinate (p.1046·1).
Corticosteroid.

Solumol *C & M, USA.*
Vehicle for topical preparations.

Solupemid *Recordati, Ital.†.*
Pipemidic acid (p.237·2).
Bacterial infections of the urinary tract; prostatitis.

Solupen
Note. This name is used for preparations of different composition.
Winzer, Ger.†.
Oxedrine tartrate (p.925·3); naphazoline hydrochloride (p.1064·2); antazoline hydrochloride (p.401·3).
Rhinitis.

Aristegui, Spain.
Doxycycline hydrochloride (p.202·3).
Bacterial infections.

Solupen Enzimatico *Aristegui, Spain.*
Doxycycline hydrochloride (p.202·3); chymotrypsin (p.1563·2); trypsin (p.1640·1).
Bacterial infections.

Solupen-D *Winzer, Ger.*
Oxedrine tartrate (p.925·3); naphazoline hydrochloride (p.1064·2); dexamethasone sodium phosphate (p.1037·2).
Rhinitis; sinusitis.

Solupred *Houde, Fr.*
Prednisolone sodium metasulphobenzoate (p.1048·1).
Corticosteroid.

Solupríck SQ *ALK, Swed.*
Allergen extracts (p.1545·1).
Diagnosis of hypersensitivity.

Solupsa *Upsamedica, Belg.*
Carbaspirin calcium (p.25·1).
Cardiovascular disorders; fever; inflammation; pain.

Solupsan *UPSA, Fr.*
Carbaspirin calcium (p.25·1).
Fever; myocardial infarction; pain; rheumatic disorders.

Solurex *Hyrex, USA.*
Dexamethasone acetate (p.1037·1) or dexamethasone sodium phosphate (p.1037·2).
Corticosteroid.

Solurrinol *Knoll, Spain.*
Potassium chlorate (p.1620·3); sodium bicarbonate (p.1153·2); sodium chloride (p.1162·2).
Upper-respiratory-tract disorders.

Solurutine Papaverine F. Retard *Synthelabo, Fr.*
Ethoxazorutoside (p.1580·1); ascorbic acid (p.1365·2); papaverine hydrochloride (p.1614·2).
Cerebral and peripheral vascular disorders.

Solus *Lifeplan, UK.*
Multivitamin, mineral, and nutritional preparation.

Solusprin *Knoll, Spain.*
Lysine aspirin (p.50·3).
Fever; musculoskeletal, joint and peri-articular disorders; pain; thrombo-embolism prophylaxis.

Solusteril *Urgo, Fr.*
Sodium dichloroisocyanurate (p.1124·3).
Infant feeding equipment disinfection.

Solustrep *Caps, S.Afr.*
Streptomycin sulphate (p.249·3).
Tuberculosis.

Solutio Cordes
Ichthyol, Aust.; Ichthyol, Ger.
Ictasol (p.1083·3).
Scalp disorders.

Solutio Cordes Dexa N *Ichthyol, Ger.*
Dexamethasone (p.1037·1).
Solutio Cordes Dexa contained ictasol and dexamethasone.
Scalp disorders.

Solution Buvable Hepatoum *Hepatoum, Fr.†.*
Anemone; turmeric (p.1001·3); chloroform (p.1220·3); peppermint oil (p.1208·1).
Gastro-intestinal disorders.

Solution ChKM du Prof Dr Walkhoff *Haupt, Switz.*
Parachlorophenol (p.1120·3); camphor (p.1557·2); menthol (p.1600·2).
Dental inflammation.

Solution de Rincage Trempage *Meram, Fr.†.*
Rinsing and soaking solution for contact lenses.

Solution Stago Diluee *Pharmadeveloppement, Fr.*
Boldo (p.1554·1); chamomile (p.1561·2); kinkeliba (p.1593·2); golden rod.
Digestive disorders.

Solutrast *Byk Gulden, Ger.*
Iopamidol (p.1007·1).
Radiographic contrast medium.

Solutricina *UCB, Ital.†.*
Tyrothricin (p.267·2).
Bacterial infections of the skin and mucous membranes.

Solutricine *Schieffer, Switz.*
Tyrothricin (p.267·2); ascorbic acid (p.1365·2).
Mouth and throat disorders.

Solutricine Tetracaine *Theraplix, Fr.*
Tyrothricin (p.267·2); amethocaine hydrochloride (p.1285·2).
Mouth and throat disorders.

Solutricine Vitamine C *Theraplix, Fr.*
Tyrothricin (p.267·2); ascorbic acid (p.1365·2).
Inflammation and infection of the mouth and throat.

Soluver *Dermtek, Canad.*
Salicylic acid (p.1090·2).
Verrucas.

Soluver Plus *Dermtek, Canad.*
Salicylic acid (p.1090·2); lactic acid (p.1593·3).
Warts.

Solu-Vetan NG cum Belladonna *Heumann, Ger.†.*
Belladonna (p.457·1); liquorice (p.1197·1); peppermint leaf (p.1208·1); peppermint oil (p.1208·1).
Gastro-intestinal spasm.

Soluvit
Pharmacia Upjohn, Belg.; Pharmacia Upjohn, Fr.; Pharmacia Upjohn, Ger.; Pharmacia Upjohn, Ital.; Pharmacia Upjohn, Norw.; Pharmacia Upjohn, S.Afr.; Pharmacia Upjohn, Swed.
Multivitamin preparation.
Parenteral nutrition.

Soluvit N
Hamilton, Austral.; Pharmacia Upjohn, Neth.; Pharmacia Upjohn, Switz.
Multivitamin preparation.
Parenteral nutrition.

Soluvit Neu *Pharmacia Upjohn, Aust.*
Multivitamin preparation.
Parenteral nutrition.

Soluvite *Pharmics, USA.*
Multivitamin preparation with fluoride (p.742·1).
Dental caries prophylaxis; dietary supplement.

Solu-Volon *Bristol-Myers Squibb, Aust.*
Triamcinolone acetonide dipotassium phosphate (p.1050·3).
Corticosteroid.

Soluzione Composta Alcoolica Saponosa di Coaltar *Bruni, Ital.*
Coal tar (p.1092·3); quillaia (p.1328·2); methyl salicylate (p.55·2); alcohol (p.1099·1).
Eczema.

Soluzione Darrow *Diaco, Ital.*
Electrolytes (p.1152·3).
Infantile diarrhoea.

Soluzione Schoum *Rhone-Poulenc Rorer, Ital.*
Fumitory (p.1581·3); ononis (p.1610·2); piscidia.
Painful spasm of the urinary and biliary tracts.

Solvazinc *Thames, UK.*
Zinc sulphate (p.1373·2).
Zinc deficiency.

Solvefort N *Stada, Ger.†.*
Bearberry leaf (p.1552·2); birch leaf; garden bean pod; solidago virgaurea; orthosiphon leaf (p.1592·2); equisetum (p.1575·1).
Urinary-tract disorders.

Solvelin *De Angeli, Ital.†.*
Bromhexine hydrochloride (p.1055·3); feprazone (p.41·2).
Respiratory-tract disorders.

Solvezink
Astra, Aust.; Stern, Ger.; Tika, Norw.; Tika, Swed.
Zinc sulphate (p.1373·2).
Acrodermatitis enteropathica; ulcers; wounds; zinc deficiency.

Solvipect *Nycomed, Norw.*
Guaiphenesin (p.1061·3); liquorice (p.1197·1).
Coughs.

Solvipect comp *Nycomed, Norw.*
Guaiphenesin (p.1061·3); liquorice (p.1197·1); ethylmorphine hydrochloride (p.36·1).
Coughs.

Solvobil *Recordati, Ital.*
Sodium cholate; nicotinamide (p.1351·2); boldo (p.1554·1); cascara (p.1183·1).
Constipation.

Solvolin *Genera, Switz.*
Bromhexine hydrochloride (p.1055·3).
Respiratory-tract disorders with viscous mucus.

Solvomed *Kwizda, Aust.*
Acetylcysteine (p.1052·3).
Bronchitis.

Solyptol *Faulding, Austral.*
Cream: Benzalkonium chloride (p.1101·3); allantoin (p.1078·2).
Soap: Triclosan (Irgasan) (p.1127·2).
Topical liquid: Pine oil; chloroxylenol (p.1111·1).
Abrasions; cuts; insect bites.

Som *Satori, Fr.*
A range of nutritional supplements.

Soma
Carter Horner, Canad.; Wallace, USA.
Carisoprodol (p.1312·3).
Musculoskeletal disorders.

Soma Complex *Teofarma, Ital.*
Carisoprodol (p.1312·3); dipyrone (p.35·1).
Musculoskeletal and joint disorders.

Soma Compound *Wallace, USA.*
Carisoprodol (p.1312·3); aspirin (p.16·1).
Musculoskeletal disorders.

Soma Compound with Codeine *Wallace, USA.*
Carisoprodol (p.1312·3); aspirin (p.16·1); codeine phosphate (p.26·1).
Musculoskeletal disorders.

Somac
Pharmacia Upjohn, Austral.; Byk Gulden, Norw.
Pantoprazole sodium (p.1207·3).
Gastro-oesophageal reflux; peptic ulcer; Zollinger-Ellison syndrome.

Somacur *Schering, Ital.†.*
Somatostatin (p.1261·1).
Gastro-intestinal haemorrhage.

Somadril
Dumex, Norw.; Dumex-Alpharma, Swed.
Carisoprodol (p.1312·3).
Pain; skeletal muscle spasm.

Somadril Comp
Dumex, Norw.†; Dumex-Alpharma, Swed.
Carisoprodol (p.1312·3); paracetamol (p.72·2); caffeine (p.749·3).
Musculoskeletal and joint disorders; pain.

Somagerol *Brenner-Efeka, Ger.*
Lorazepam (p.675·3).
Anxiety disorders; premedication; sleep disorders.

Somalgit *Inibsa, Spain.*
Carisoprodol (p.1312·3).
Skeletal muscle spasm.

Somanol *Braun, Swed.*
Sorbitol (p.1354·2); mannitol (p.900·3).
Urological irrigation.

Somarexin *Lalco, Canad.*
Vitamin B substances and iron.

Somarexin & C *Lalco, Canad.*
Vitamin B substances, vitamin C, calcium, and iron.

Somatarax *UCB, Spain.*
Brallobarbital calcium (p.643·1); hydroxyzine dihydrochloride (p.412·1); quinalbarbitone sodium (p.690·2).
Insomnia.

Somatin *Torrex, Aust.*
Somatostatin acetate (p.1261·1).
Gastro-intestinal haemorrhage; prevention of complications following pancreatic surgery.

Somatobiss
Bissendorf, Neth.†; Ferring, Switz.†.
Somatorelin acetate (p.1260·3).
Test of pituitary function.

Somatofalk *Falk, Neth.*
Somatostatin acetate (p.1261·1).
Gastro-intestinal haemorrhage.

Somatolan *Lannacher, Aust.*
Somatostatin acetate (p.1261·1).
Gastro-intestinal haemorrhage; prevention of complications following pancreatic surgery.

Somatoline *Manetti Roberts, Ital.*
Thyroxine (p.1498·3); aescin (p.1543·3).
Adipose states with cellulite.

Somatonorm
Pharmacia, Austral.†; Kabivitrum, Irl.†; Pierrel, Ital.†; Pharmacia, Spain†; Kabi, Swed.†.
Somatrem (p.1249·3).
Growth hormone deficiency; Turner's syndrome.

Somatron *Volchem, Ital.*
L-Arginine (p.1334·1); L-ornithine (p.1352·3).
Nutritional supplement.

Somatulina *Lasa, Spain.*
Lanreotide acetate (p.1252·3).
Acromegaly.

Somatuline
IPSEN Biotech, Fr.; Ipsen, UK.
Lanreotide acetate (p.1252·3).
Acromegaly; neuroendocrine tumours.

Somatyl *Teofarma, Ital.*
Betaine sodium aspartate (p.1553·2).
Digestive disorders.

Somazina
Ferrer, Spain; Ferrer, Switz.†.
Citicoline (p.1564·3) or citicoline sodium (p.1564·3).
Cerebrovascular disorders.

Sombril *Mallinckrodt, Spain†.*
Meglumine iothalamate (p.1008·1) or sodium iothalamate (p.1008·1).
Radiographic contrast medium.

Somelin *Sankyo, Jpn.*
Haloxazolam (p.675·1).
Insomnia.

Somiaton *Serono, Spain.*
Somatostatin acetate (p.1261·1).
Gastro-intestinal haemorrhage; pancreatic fistulae.

Sominex
Note. This name is used for preparations of different composition.
SmithKline Beecham Consumer, Canad.; SmithKline Beecham Consumer, USA.
Diphenhydramine hydrochloride (p.409·1).
Insomnia.

Seton, UK.
Promethazine hydrochloride (p.416·2).
Insomnia.

Sominex Pain Relief *SmithKline Beecham Consumer, USA.*
Diphenhydramine hydrochloride (p.409·1); paracetamol (p.72·2).
Insomnia.

Sommieres Au Pentavit B *Chauvin, Fr.†.*
Sodium iodide (p.1493·2); lithium iodide (p.295·1); calcium chloride (p.1155·1); vitamin B substances.
Cataracts.

Somnal *Wassermann, Ital.†.*
Flutemazepam.
Anxiety; insomnia.

Somnibel N *UCB, Ger.†.*
Nitrazepam (p.682·2).
Sleep disorders.

Somnil *Pharmacare Consumer, S.Afr.*
Doxylamine succinate (p.410·1).
Insomnia.

Somnipar *Rolab, S.Afr.*
Nitrazepam (p.682·2).
Insomnia.

Somnite
Norgine, Irl.; Norgine, UK.
Nitrazepam (p.682·2).
Insomnia.

Somnium
Note. This name is used for preparations of different composition.
Laevosan, Aust.; Medichemie, Switz.
Lorazepam (p.675·3); diphenhydramine hydrochloride (p.409·1).
Sleep disorders.

Reinecke, Ger.†.
Eschscholtzia californica; avena (p.1551·3); valerian (p.1643·1); lupulus (p.1597·2); passion flower (p.1615·3); dibasic potassium phosphate (p.1159·2); dibasic sodium phosphate (p.1159·3); dibasic magnesium phosphate.
Nervous disorders; sleep disorders.

Somnium forte *Reinecke, Ger.†.*
Eschscholtzia californica; valerian (p.1643·1); carbromal (p.645·2).
Sleep disorders.

Somnol *Carter Horner, Canad.*
Flurazepam monohydrochloride (p.672·2).
Insomnia.

Somnovit *Hosbon, Spain.*
Loprazolam (p.675·3).
Insomnia.

Somnubene *Merckle, Aust.*
Flunitrazepam (p.670·1).
Sleep disorders.

Somnupan C *Merckle, Ger.†.*
Cyclobarbitone calcium (p.660·2).
Sleep disorders.

Somnus *Gerard House, UK.*
Valerian (p.1643·1); lupulus (p.1597·2); wild lettuce (p.1645·1).
Insomnia.

Somnuvis S *Truw, Ger.*
Valerian (p.1643·1); lupulus (p.1597·2); passion flower (p.1615·3); kava (p.1592·3).
Nervous disorders; sleep disorders.

Somofillina *Fisons, Ital.†.*
Theophylline (p.765·1).
Bronchospastic disorders.

Somonal *Juste, Spain.*
Somatostatin acetate (p.1261·1).
Bleeding oesophageal varices; pancreatic fistulas.

Somophyllin
Fisons, Canad.†; Roche, S.Afr.†.
Theophylline (p.765·1).
Obstructive airways disease.

Somsanit *Kohler, Ger.*
Sodium oxybate (p.1232·2).
General anaesthesia.

Sonacide *Wyeth-Ayerst, Canad.*
Glutaraldehyde (p.1114·3).
Instrument disinfection.

Sonarex *Biotherax, Ger.†.*
Sodium chloride; glycerol; polysorbate 80.
Nasal lubricant for snoring.

Sondalis
Clintec-Sopharga, Fr.; Clintec, Ital.
A range of preparations for enteral nutrition.

Sone *Fawns & McAllan, Austral.*
Prednisone (p.1049·2).
Corticosteroid.

Soneryl
Rhone-Poulenc Rorer, Austral.†; Rhone-Poulenc Rorer, Irl.†; May & Baker, S.Afr.†; Hansam, UK.
Butobarbitone (p.645·1).
Insomnia.

Songar *Valeas, Ital.*
Triazolam (p.696·3).
Insomnia.

Sonicur *Kalifarma, Spain.*
Anethole trithione (p.1549·3).
Dry mouth.

Sonifilan *Kaken, Jpn.*
Sizofiran (p.561·3).
Radiotherapy enhancement for uterine cervical cancer.

Sonin *Lipha, Ger.*
Loprazolam (p.675·3).
Sleep disorders.

Soni-Slo
Helsinn Birex, Irl.; Lipha, Irl.; Lipha, UK.
Isosorbide dinitrate (p.893·1).
Angina pectoris.

Sonnenbraun *Twardy, Ger.*
Betacarotene (p.1335·2); biotin (p.1336·1); calcium pantothenate (p.1352·3).
Sunburn.

Sonodor *Vitafarma, Spain.*
Diphenhydramine hydrochloride (p.409·1); pyrithyldione (p.689·3).
Insomnia.

Sonotryl *Singer, Switz.*
Propyphenazone (p.81·3); paracetamol (p.72·2); caffeine (p.749·3); drofenine hydrochloride (p.460·3).
Painful smooth muscle spasm.

Sonsuur *Rolab, S.Afr.*
Cimetidine (p.1183·2).
Gastro-intestinal disorders.

Soor-Gel *Engelhard, Ger.*
Dequalinium salicylate (p.1112·1).
Fungal and bacterial mouth and throat infections.

Soorphenesin *Kade, Ger.*
Chlorphenesin (p.376·2).
Fungal and bacterial infections of the vagina.

Soothaderm *Pharmakon, USA.*
Mepyramine maleate (p.414·1); benzocaine (p.1286·2); zinc oxide (p.1096·2).
Pruritus.

Soothake Toothache Gel *Pickles, UK.*
Benzocaine (p.1286·2); clove oil (p.1565·2).
Gum or tooth pain.

Soothe *Alcon, USA.*
Tetrahydrozoline hydrochloride (p.1070·2).
Minor eye irritation.

Soothe Aid *Zee, Canad.*
Hexylresorcinol (p.1116·1).

Soothelip *Bayer, UK.*
Aciclovir (p.602·3).
Herpes labialis.

Soothe'n Heal *Mentholatum, Austral.*
Triethanolamine oleate; hydrous wool fat (p.1385·3); glycerol (p.1585·2).
Dry skin.

Soothers *Warner-Lambert, USA†.*
Menthol (p.1600·2).
Sore throat.

Soothex *Jamieson, Canad.*
Allantoin (p.1078·2).

Sootheye *Rhone-Poulenc Rorer, UK†.*
Zinc sulphate (p.1373·2).
Eye irritation.

Soov Bite *Ego, Austral.*
Lignocaine hydrochloride (p.1293·2); cetrimide (p.1105·2); menthol (p.1600·2).
Insect bites and stings.

Soov Burn *Ego, Austral.*
Lignocaine hydrochloride (p.1293·2); cetrimide (p.1105·2).
Minor burns; minor cuts; sunburn.

Soov Cream *Ego, Austral.*
Lignocaine hydrochloride (p.1293·2); cetrimide (p.1105·2); chlorhexidine gluconate (p.1107·2).
Haemorrhoids; minor cuts, abrasions, and burns; sunburn.

Soov Prickly Heat *Ego, Austral.*
Light liquid paraffin (p.1382·1); salicylic acid (p.1090·2); zinc oxide (p.1096·2).
Heat rash.

Sopalamin 3B *Rhone-Poulenc Rorer, Belg.*
Vitamin B substances.
Alcoholism; neurogenic pain; vitamin B deficiency.

Sopalamine 3B *Charton, Canad.*
Vitamin B substances.
Vitamin B deficiency.

Sopalamine 3B Plus *Charton, Canad.*
Multivitamin preparation.

Sopalamine 3B Plus C *Charton, Canad.*
Multivitamin preparation.

Sopamycetin *Charton, Canad.†.*
Chloramphenicol (p.182·1).
Bacterial infections of the ear and eye.

Sopamycetin/HC *Charton, Canad.†.*
Chloramphenicol (p.182·1); hydrocortisone acetate (p.1043·3).
Bacterial infections of the ear and eye.

Sopental *Continental Ethicals, S.Afr.†.*
Pentobarbitone sodium (p.685·1).
Insomnia; sedative.

Sophtal *Alcon, Fr.*
Eye drops: Salicylic acid (p.1090·2); chlorhexidine gluconate (p.1107·2).
Eye lotion: Salicylic acid (p.1090·2); borax (p.1554·2); rose water.
Eye disorders.

Sophtal-POS N *Ursapharm, Ger.*
Salicylic acid (p.1090·2).
Eye disorders.

Soporil *Duphar, Ger.†.*
Promethazine hydrochloride (p.416·2).
Antihistamine; sedative.

Soporin *Herbamed, Switz.*
Valerian (p.1643·1); passion flower (p.1615·3); lupulus (p.1597·2); melissa (p.1600·1).
Sleep disorders.

Soprol *Novalis, Fr.*
Bisoprolol fumarate (p.833·1).
Angina pectoris; hypertension.

Sopulmin *Farmochimica, Ital.*
Sobrerol (p.1069·3).
Respiratory-tract disorders.

Soraderm *Stafford-Miller, Norw.*
Coal tar (p.1092·3).
Psoriasis; seborrhoeic dermatitis.

Sorbacel
Note. This name is used for preparations of different composition.
Braun Fandre, Fr.†.
Oxidised cellulose (p.714·2).
Haemorrhage.
Hartmann, Ger.†.
Calcium cellulose polyuronate.
Capillary bleeding.

Sorbangil
Pharmacia Upjohn, Norw.; Pharmacia Upjohn, Swed.
Isosorbide dinitrate (p.893·1).
Angina pectoris; heart failure.

Sorbenor *Casen Fisons, Spain.*
Arginine aspartate (p.1334·2).
Tonic.

Sorbichew *Zeneca, UK.*
Isosorbide dinitrate (p.893·1).
Angina pectoris.

Sorbiclean *Allergan, Austral.†.*
Cleansing solution for contact lenses.

Sorbiclis *SIT, Ital.*
Sorbitol (p.1354·2); docusate sodium (p.1189·3).
Constipation.

Sorbid *Zeneca, UK.*
Isosorbide dinitrate (p.893·1).
Angina pectoris.

Sorbidilat
Astra, Aust.; Fresenius, Ger.†; Astra, Switz.
Isosorbide dinitrate (p.893·1).
Angina pectoris; heart failure; hypertension; myocardial infarction.

Sorbidin *Alphapharm, Austral.*
Isosorbide dinitrate (p.893·1).
Heart failure; ischaemic heart disease.

Sorbifen *Zyma, Aust.*
Chlorhexidine acetate (p.1107·2).
Prevention of wound infection.

Sorbifen Baby *Zyma, Aust.*
Lactose (p.1349·3).
Care of umbilicus.

Sorbilande *Delalande, Ital.†.*
Sorbitol (p.1354·2).
Constipation.

Sorbilax *Delta, Austral.*
Sorbitol (p.1354·2).
Constipation.

Sorbimon *Merckle, Aust.*
Isosorbide mononitrate (p.893·3).
Angina pectoris; heart failure; pulmonary hypertension.

Sorbisal *Allergan, Austral.*
Rinsing solution for soft contact lenses.

Sorbisterit
Leopold, Aust.; Fresenius, Ger.; Fresenius, Switz.
Calcium polystyrene sulphonate (p.974·3).
Hyperkalaemia.

Sorbitoxin *Novag, Spain†.*
Oral suspension: Aluminium hydroxide (p.1177·3); attapulgite (p.1178·3); dihydrostreptomycin sulphate (p.202·2); formosulphathiazole (p.210·1); neomycin sulphate (p.229·2); pectin (p.1474·1).
Tablets: Attapulgite (p.1178·3); dihydrostreptomycin sulphate (p.202·2); formosulphathiazole (p.210·1); neomycin sulphate (p.229·2); pectin (p.1474·1).
Infectious diarrhoea.

Sorbitrate
Zeneca, Belg.; Zeneca, Fr.†; Zeneca, UK; Zeneca, USA.
Isosorbide dinitrate (p.893·1).
Angina pectoris; heart failure.

Sorbitur *Baxter, Swed.*
Sorbitol (p.1354·2).
Bladder irrigation.

Sorbocetil *Ris, Ital.†.*
Cetylpyridinium chloride (p.1106·2).
Oral disinfection.

Sorbocitryl *Meram, Fr.†.*
Sorbitol (p.1354·2); monosodium citrate; trisodium citrate (p.1153·2).
Constipation; dyspepsia.

Sorbosan *Merck, Ger.†.*
Moxaverine hydrochloride (p.1604·3); sorbitol (p.1354·2).
Biliary disorders; gastro-intestinal disorders; liver disorders.

Sorbostyl *Synthelabo, Fr.†.*
Sorbitol (p.1354·2).
Postoperative ileus.

Sorbsan
Boots, Austral.; Braun Biotrol, Fr.; Braun, Ital.; Steriseal, UK.
Calcium alginate (p.714·1).
Burns; skin ulceration; wounds.

Sorciclina *Inexfa, Spain.*
Doxycycline hydrochloride (p.202·3); prolase.
Bacterial infections.

Sordinol *Lundbeck, Ital.*
Clopenthixol hydrochloride (p.700·2).
Anxiety; mental function disorders; psychoses.

Sore Throat Chewing Gum *Or-Dov, Austral.*
Dichlorobenzyl alcohol (p.1112·2); amylmetacresol (p.1101·3); vitamin C (p.1365·2).
Sore throat.

Sore Throat L39 *Homeocan, Canad.*
Homoeopathic preparation.

Sore Throat Lozenges *Sutton, Canad.*
Benzocaine (p.1286·2); menthol (p.1600·2).

Sore Throat Relief *Brauer, Austral.*
Homoeopathic preparation.

Sore Throats *Weleda, UK†.*
Homoeopathic preparation.

Sorgoa *Scheurich, Ger.*
Tolnaftate (p.389·1).
Fungal skin infections.

Sorgoran *Salus, Aust.*
Tolnaftate (p.389·1).
Fungal skin and nail infections.

Soriatane
Roche, Canad.; Roche, Fr.; Roche, USA.
Acitretin (p.1077·3).
Keratinisation disorders; psoriasis.

Soriflor *Nycomed, Swed.†.*
Diflorasone diacetate (p.1039·3).
Skin disorders.

Sormodren
Ebewe, Aust.; Knoll, Ger.; Knoll, Irl.†; Ravizza, Ital.; Knoll, Spain†.
Bornaprine hydrochloride (p.459·1).
Hyperhidrosis; parkinsonism.

Soropon *Purdue Frederick, Canad.*
Tyrothricin (p.267·2); triethanolamine polypeptide cocoate condensate (p.1639·2).
Scalp disorders.

Sorot
Petrasch, Aust.; Ravensberg, Ger.
Dequalinium chloride (p.1112·1).
Mouth and throat infections.

Sorot-comp *Ravensberg, Ger.†.*
Dequalinium chloride (p.1112·1); cetylpyridinium chloride (p.1106·2); menthol (p.1600·2); ascorbic acid (p.1365·2).
Mouth and throat infections.

Sorquetan *Basotherm, Ger.*
Tinidazole (p.594·1).
Bacterial or protozoal infections.

Sosegon *Sanofi Winthrop, Spain.*
Pentazocine (p.75·1), pentazocine hydrochloride (p.75·1), or pentazocine lactate (p.75·1).
Pain.

Sosenol *Adcock Ingram, S.Afr.*
Pentazocine (p.75·1).
Pain.

Sostril *Cascan, Ger.*
Ranitidine hydrochloride (p.1209·3).
Gastro-intestinal disorders.

Sotabeta *Betapharm, Ger.*
Sotalol hydrochloride (p.945·1).
Arrhythmias.

Sotacor
Bristol-Myers Squibb, Aust.; Bristol-Myers Squibb, Austral.; Bristol, Canad.; Bristol-Myers Squibb, Irl.; Bristol-Myers Squibb, Neth.; Bristol-Myers Squibb, Norw.; Bristol-Myers Squibb, S.Afr.; Bristol-Myers Squibb, Swed.; Bristol-Myers Squibb, UK.
Sotalol hydrochloride (p.945·1).
Angina pectoris; arrhythmias; hypertension; hyperthyroidism.

Sotacor/ASA *Bristol-Myers Squibb, Swed.†.*
Tablet I, sotalol hydrochloride (p.945·1); tablet II, aspirin (p.16·1).
Angina pectoris.

Sotahexal *Hexal, Ger.*
Sotalol hydrochloride (p.945·1).
Arrhythmias.

Sotalex
Bristol-Myers Squibb, Belg.; Allard, Fr.; Bristol-Myers Squibb, Ger.; Bristol-Myers Squibb, Ital.; Bristol-Myers Squibb, Switz.
Sotalol hydrochloride (p.945·1).
Angina pectoris; arrhythmias; hypertension; myocardial infarction.

Sotapor *Bristol-Myers, Spain.*
Sotalol hydrochloride (p.945·1).
Angina pectoris; arrhythmias; hypertension; myocardial infarction.

Sotaryt *Azupharma, Ger.*
Sotalol hydrochloride (p.945·1).
Arrhythmias.

Sota-saar *Rosen, Ger.*
Sotalol hydrochloride (p.945·1).
Arrhythmias.

Sotastad *Stada, Ger.*
Sotalol hydrochloride (p.945·1).
Arrhythmias.

Sotazide
Bristol-Myers Squibb, Irl.†; Bristol-Myers Squibb, S.Afr.†; Bristol-Myers Squibb, UK†.
Sotalol hydrochloride (p.945·1); hydrochlorothiazide (p.885·2).
Hypertension.

Sotaziden *Bristol, Ger.†.*
Sotalol hydrochloride (p.945·1); hydrochlorothiazide (p.885·2).
Hypertension.

Sotaziden N *Bristol-Myers Squibb, Ger.*
Nadolol (p.913·2); bendrofluazide (p.827·3).
Hypertension.

Sotorni *Ravensberg, Ger.†.*
Levopropoxyphene dibudinate (p.1063·3).
Coughs and associated respiratory-tract disorders.

Sotradecol *Elkins-Sinn, USA.*
Sodium tetradecyl sulphate (p.1469·2).
Varicose veins.

Soufrane *Sanofi Winthrop, Fr.*
Thenoate sodium (p.262·2).
Nasopharyngeal infections.

Soufrol *Max Ritter, Switz.*
Mesulphen (p.1086·3).
Musculoskeletal and joint disorders; skin disorders.

Soufrol TP *Max Ritter, Switz.*
Medicinal mud; sulphur (p.1091·2).
Musculoskeletal and joint disorders.

Soufrol ZNP *Max Ritter, Switz.*
Sulphur (p.1091·2); pyrithione zinc (p.1089·3).
Scalp disorders.

Sovarel *Normon, Spain.*
Almitrine (p.1477·2).
Respiratory depression.

Sovel *Geigy, Ger.*
Norethisterone acetate (p.1453·1).
Menstrual disorders.

Soventol
Ebewe, Aust.; Knoll, Ger.; Knoll, Neth.†.
Bamipine hydrochloride (p.403·2) or bamipine lactate (p.403·2).
Frostbite; hay fever; insect and jellyfish stings; pruritus; sunburn; urticaria.

Soventol C *Nordmark, Ger.†.*
Bamipine hydrochloride (p.403·2); levopropylhexedrine hydrochloride (p.1485·2).
Frostbite; hay fever; insect and jellyfish stings; pruritus; sunburn; urticaria.

Soventol Hydrocortison *Knoll, Ger.*
Hydrocortisone acetate (p.1043·3).
Insect stings; itchy eczema; sunburn; urticaria.

Soya Semp *Semper, Norw.†.*
Infant feed.
Intolerance to cow's milk, lactose, sucrose, and galactose.

Soyacal
Bieffe, Ital.†; Alpha Therapeutic, UK.
Soya oil (p.1355·1).
Contains egg phospholipids.
Lipid infusion for parenteral nutrition.

Soyalac *Nutricia-Luma Lindar, USA.*
Lactose-free soy protein infant feed.

Soypliment *Vitaplex, Austral.†.*
Soybean powder (p.1355·1).
Milk substitute in milk allergies.

SP *Sussex, UK.*
Paracetamol (p.72·2); caffeine (p.749·3); phenylephrine hydrochloride (p.1066·2).

SP Betaisodona *Mundipharma, Ger.*
Povidone-iodine (p.1123·3).
Hand disinfection; skin and mucous membrane disinfection.

Spabucol *Lagap, Ital.†.*
Trimebutine maleate (p.1639·3).
Gastro-intestinal disorders.

Spaciclina *SPA, Ital.*
Tetracycline hydrochloride (p.259·1).
Bacterial and protozoal infections.

Spagall *Donau, Aust.*
Tolynol nicotinate (p.1638·3); naphthylacetic acid (p.1606·2); caroverine (p.1560·1).
Hepatobiliary disorders.

Spagulax *Pharmafarm, Fr.*
Ispaghula husk (p.1194·2).
Constipation.

Spagulax au Citrate de Potassium *Pharmafarm, Fr.*
Ispaghula husk (p.1194·2); potassium citrate (p.1153·1).
Constipation.

Spagulax au Sorbitol *Pharmafarm, Fr.*
Ispaghula husk (p.1194·2); sorbitol (p.1354·2).
Constipation.

Spagulax K *SmithKline Beecham Consumer, Belg.†.*
Ispaghula husk (p.1194·2); potassium citrate (p.1153·1); potassium bicarbonate (p.1153·1).
Constipation.

Spagulax L *SmithKline Beecham Consumer, Belg.†.*
Ispaghula husk (p.1194·2); frangula bark (p.1193·2).
Constipation.

Spagulax M *SmithKline Beecham Consumer, Belg.†.*
Ispaghula husk (p.1194·2).
Constipation.

Spagulax S *SmithKline Beecham Consumer, Belg.†.*
Ispaghula husk (p.1194·2); sorbitol (p.1354·2).
Hepatobiliary disorders.

Spai *INTES, Ital.*
Sodium chloride; potassium chloride; calcium chloride; magnesium chloride; sodium acetate; sodium citrate (p.1147·1).
Adjunct in otorhinolaryngeal procedures; cleaning solution for contact lens; ocular irrigation.

Spalgin *SPA, Ital.*
Pipethanate ethobromide (p.467·1).
Premedication; smooth muscle spasticity.

Spalt
Note. This name is used for preparations of different composition.
Salus, Aust.
Phenazone salicylate (p.78·2); salicylamide (p.82·3); caffeine (p.749·3).
Pain.
Much, Ger.
Aspirin (p.16·1).
Cold symptoms; fever; pain.

Spalt A + P *Much, Ger.*
Aspirin (p.16·1); paracetamol (p.72·2).
Pain.

Spalt N
Note. This name is used for preparations of different composition.
Whitehall, Swed.
Phenazone (p.78·2).
Fever; pain.
Whitehall-Robins, Switz.
Paracetamol (p.72·2).
Fever; pain.

Spaltina *Merck, Spain†.*
Aspirin (p.16·1); caffeine (p.749·3); paracetamol (p.72·2).
Fever; pain.

Span C *Freeda, USA.*
Citrus bioflavonoids complex (p.1580·1); ascorbic acid (p.1365·2).
Capillary bleeding.

Spancap No. 1 *Vortech, USA.*
Dexamphetamine sulphate (p.1478·2).
Attention deficit disorder with hyperactivity; narcolepsy syndrome; obesity.

Span-FF *Lexis, USA†.*
Ferrous fumarate (p.1339·3).
Iron-deficiency anaemias.

Spanidin *Kayaku, Jpn.*
Gusperimus hydrochloride (p.538·2).
Renal transplant rejection.

Spanish Tummy Mixture *Potter's, UK.*
Blackberry root bark; catechu (p.1560·3).
Diarrhoea.

Span-K *Rhone-Poulenc Rorer, Austral.*
Potassium chloride (p.1161·1).
Potassium deficiency.

Spanor *Biotherapie, Fr.*
Doxycycline hydrochloride (p.202·3).
Bacterial infections.

Spara *Dainippon, Jpn.*
Sparfloxacin (p.248·2).
Bacterial infections.

Sparaplaie NA *Urgo, Fr.*
Benzalkonium chloride (p.1101·3).
Burns; wounds.

Sparheugin *Staufen, Ger.†.*
Homoeopathic preparation.

Sparheugol *Staufen, Ger.†.*
Homoeopathic preparation.

Sparine
Wyeth, Austral.; Wyeth, Irl.; Akromed, S.Afr.; Wyeth, UK; Wyeth-Ayerst, USA.
Promazine embonate (p.689·1) or promazine hydrochloride (p.689·1).
Drug withdrawal symptoms; hiccup; nausea; pain; premedication; psychoses; sedative; vomiting.

Spark *Medecine Vegetale, Fr.*
Frangula bark (p.1193·2); boldo leaf (p.1554·1); aloes (p.1177·1).
Constipation.

Sparkal GEA, Swed.
Hydrochlorothiazide (p.885·2); amiloride hydrochloride (p.819·2).
Hypertension; liver cirrhosis with ascites; oedema.

Sparkles Lafayette, USA.
Sodium bicarbonate (p.1153·2); citric acid (p.1564·3); simethicone (p.1213·1).
Adjunct in endoscopy; flatulence.

Spartiol Klein, Ger.
Sarothamnus scoparius (p.1628·1).
Arrhythmias.

Spartocina UCB, Ital.†.
Ferrous aspartate (p.1339·2).
Anaemias; muscle fatigue.

Spartocine Darci, Belg.
Ferrous aspartate (p.1339·2).
Iron-deficiency anaemias.

Spartocine N UCB, Ger.
Ferrous aspartate (p.1339·2).
Iron-deficiency anaemias.

Spasdilat N Rhenomed, Ger.†.
Oral liquid: Paracetamol (p.72·2); diprophylline (p.752·1); papaverine hydrochloride (p.1614·2).
Suppositories: Paracetamol (p.72·2); theobromine (p.765·1); papaverine (p.1614·2).
Tablets: Paracetamol (p.72·2); theobromine and sodium salicylate (p.765·1); papaverine hydrochloride (p.1614·2).
Peripheral and cerebral vascular disorders.

Spasen FIRMA, Ital.
Suppositories: Otilonium bromide (p.1611·2); lignocaine hydrochloride (p.1293·2).
Tablets: Otilonium bromide (p.1611·2).
The name Spasen was formerly used for a preparation containing fenalamide and aminopropylone.
Gastro-intestinal spasm.

Spasen Somatico FIRMA, Ital.
Otilonium bromide (p.1611·2); diazepam (p.661·1).
Painful gastro-intestinal spasm.

Spasfon
Bio-Therabel, Belg.; Lafon, Fr.
Phloroglucinol (p.1618·1); trimethylphloroglucinol (p.1618·1).
Smooth muscle spasm.

Spasfon-Lyoc Lafon, Fr.
Phloroglucinol (p.1618·1).
Smooth muscle spasm.

Spasgesic Legere, USA†.
Chlorzoxazone (p.1313·1); paracetamol (p.72·2).

Spasma Stella, Belg.
Morphine hydrochloride (p.56·1); hyoscine hydrobromide (p.462·3).
Biliary and renal colic; pain; premedication.

Spasmag Serozym, Fr.
Capsules; oral solution: Magnesium sulphate (p.1157·3); dried yeast (p.1373·1).
Injection: Magnesium sulphate (p.1157·3).
Eclampsia; magnesium deficiency.

Spasmalfher Fher, Spain†.
Suppositories: 1-(*p*-Ethoxyphenyl)-1-diethylamino-3-methyl-3-phenylpropane hydrochloride (p.1577·2); codeine phosphate (p.26·1); propyphenazone (p.81·3).
Tablets: 1-(*p*-Ethoxyphenyl)-1-diethylamino-3-methyl-3-phenylpropane hydrochloride (p.1577·2); caffeine (p.749·3); propyphenazone (p.81·3).
Pain.

Spasmalgan Apogepha, Ger.
Denaverine hydrochloride.
Smooth muscle spasm.

Spasmamide Composta Schering, Ital.†.
Fenalamide (p.1578·3); dipyrone (p.35·1).
Smooth muscle spasm.

Spasmamide Semplice Schering, Ital.†.
Fenalamide (p.1578·3).
Smooth muscle spasm.

Spasman Gastropharm, Ger.
Demelverine hydrochloride; benzhexol hydrochloride (p.457·3).
Smooth muscle spasm.

Spasmanodine Spirig, Switz.†.
Atropine methobromide (p.455·1); papaverine hydrochloride (p.1614·2); codeine phosphate (p.26·1); propyphenazone (p.81·3).
Pain due to smooth muscle spasm.

Spasmaverine Theraplix, Fr.
Suppositories: Alverine (p.1548·1); benzocaine (p.1286·2).
Tablets: Alverine citrate (p.1548·1).
Smooth muscle spasm.

Spasmend Restan, S.Afr.
Paracetamol (p.72·2); mephenesin (p.1315·3).
Pain; skeletal muscle spasm.

Spasmeridan UCB, Ital.
Diazepam (p.661·1); hyoscine methobromide (p.463·1).
Gastro-intestinal spasm.

Spasmex
Note. This name is used for preparations of different composition.
Pfleger, Ger.
Trospium chloride (p.1640·1).
Smooth muscle spasms; urinary incontinence.

Farmochimica, Ital.
Injection: Phloroglucinol (p.1618·1).
Tablets; suppositories: Phloroglucinol (p.1618·1); trimethylphloroglucinol (p.1618·1).
Painful spasm of the biliary and urinary tracts.

Spasmidenal Jolly-Jatel, Fr.
Crataegus (p.1568·2); valerian (p.1643·1); phenobarbitone (p.350·2).
Insomnia; nervous disorders.

Spasmine Jolly-Jatel, Fr.
Valerian (p.1643·1); crataegus (p.1568·2).
Insomnia; nervous disorders.

Spasmium Donau, Aust.
Caroverine (p.1560·1) or caroverine hydrochloride (p.1560·1).
Smooth muscle spasm.

Spasmium comp Donau, Aust.
Caroverine (p.1560·1); dipyrone (p.35·1); metamizole calcium (p.35·1).
Painful smooth muscle spasm.

Spasmo Claim Apomedica, Aust.
Turmeric (p.1001·3); benzyl mandelate; tolynol (p.1638·2); peppermint oil (p.1208·1); caraway oil (p.1559·3); fennel oil (p.1579·2); lemon oil (p.1595·3); camphor (p.1557·2); thymol (p.1127·1); guaiazulene (p.1586·3).
Gastro-intestinal disorders.

Spasmo Gallo Sanol Sanol, Ger.
Chelidonium majus; turmeric (p.1001·3).
Biliary and gastro-intestinal disorders.

Spasmo Gallo Sanol N Sanol, Ger.
Xenytropium bromide (p.469·3); ox bile (p.1553·2); aloes (p.1177·1).
Biliary disorders.

Spasmo Gallosanol Mayrhofer, Aust.
Xenytropium bromide (p.469·3); ox bile (p.1553·2); aloes (p.1177·1).
Biliary-tract disorders.

Spasmo Inalgon Neu Laevosan, Aust.
Dipyrone (p.35·1).
Painful smooth muscle spasm.

Spasmo Nierofu Hoyer, Ger.†.
Nitrofurantoin (p.231·3); phenazopyridine (p.79·1).
Urinary-tract infections.

Spasmo Nil Duchesnay, Canad.
Aluminium hydroxide (p.1177·3); magnesium trisilicate (p.1199·1); dicyclomine hydrochloride (p.460·1); simethicone (p.1213·1).

Spasmo-Aringal Harras-Curarina, Ger.†.
Aristolochia ringens.
Smooth muscle spasm.

Spasmo-Barbamin Streuli, Switz.
Propyphenazone (p.81·3); adiphenine hydrochloride; diphenhydramine hydrochloride (p.409·1).
Painful smooth muscle spasm.

Spasmo-Barbamine compositum Streuli, Switz.
Propyphenazone (p.81·3); adiphenine hydrochloride; diphenhydramine hydrochloride (p.409·1); codeine phosphate (p.26·1).
Painful smooth muscle spasm.

Spasmo-Bilicura Muller Goppingen, Ger.†.
Kava (p.1592·3); cynara (p.1569·2); silybum marianum (p.993·3); aloes (p.1177·1); frangula bark (p.1193·2); ox bile (p.1553·2); peppermint oil (p.1208·1); guaiazulene (p.1586·3); hyoscine methobromide (p.463·1); ethaverine hydrochloride (p.1577·1).
Biliary spasm; gastro-intestinal spasm.

Spasmo-Bomaleb Hevert, Ger.
Homoeopathic preparation.

Spasmo-Canulase
Novartis Consumer, S.Afr.; Wander OTC, Switz.
Cellulase (p.1561·1); pancreatin (p.1612·1); dimethicone (p.1213·1); sodium dehydrocholate (p.1570·3); methixene hydrochloride (p.465·1); pepsin (p.1616·3); glutamic acid hydrochloride (p.1344·3).
Gastro-intestinal disorders.

Spasmo-Canulase N Wander, Ger.†.
Methixene hydrochloride (p.465·1); dimethicone (p.1213·1); porcine pancreatin (p.1612·1).
Digestive system disorders.

Spasmo-CC Steiner, Ger.†.
Chelidonium majus; turmeric (p.1001·3).
Biliary-tract spasm.

Spasmo-Cibalgin Zyma, Switz.
Propyphenazone (p.81·3); drofenine hydrochloride (p.460·3).
Painful smooth muscle spasm.

Spasmo-Cibalgin comp Zyma, Switz.
Propyphenazone (p.81·3); drofenine hydrochloride (p.460·3); codeine phosphate (p.26·1).
Painful smooth muscle spasm.

Spasmo-Cibalgin compositum S Geigy, Ger.
Propyphenazone (p.81·3); drofenine hydrochloride (p.460·3); codeine phosphate (p.26·1).
Smooth muscle spasm.

Spasmo-Cibalgin S Geigy, Ger.
Propyphenazone (p.81·3); drofenine hydrochloride (p.460·3).
Smooth muscle spasm.

Spasmo-Cibalgina Ciba, Ital.
Propyphenazone (p.81·3); drofenine hydrochloride (p.460·3).
Painful smooth muscle spasm.

Spasmo-Cibalgine Ciba-Geigy, Belg.
Propyphenazone (p.81·3); drofenine hydrochloride (p.460·3).
Dysmenorrhoea; smooth muscle spasm.

Spasmocor Asta Medica, Aust.
Glyceryl trinitrate (p.874·3); pentaerythrityl tetranitrate (p.927·3); nicotinic acid (p.1351·2); benzyl mandelate.
Angina pectoris; heart failure; peripheral vascular spasm.

Spasmoctyl Menarini, Spain.
Otilonium bromide (p.1611·2).
Gastro-intestinal spasm; irritable bowel syndrome.

Spasmocyclon 3M, Ger.
Cyclandelate (p.845·2).
Cerebrovascular disorders; migraine; vestibular disorders.

Spasmodex Crinex, Fr.
Dihexyverine hydrochloride (p.460·3).
Gastro-intestinal disorders.

Spasmodil ABC, Ital.
Pipethanate ethobromide (p.467·1).
Gastro-intestinal spasm and hypermotility; premedication for endoscopy and radiography; urinary and biliary spasm and dyskinesia.

Spasmodil Complex ABC, Ital.†.
Procaine hydrochloride (p.1299·2); etamiphylline hydrochloride (p.753·1); methylbenactyzium bromide (p.465·2).
Biliary-tract disorders.

Spasmo-Entoxin N Klein & Steube, Ger.†.
Homoeopathic preparation.

Spasmofen Abigo, Swed.
Hyoscine methonitrate (p.463·1); papaverine hydrochloride (p.1614·2); morphine hydrochloride (p.56·1); noscapine hydrochloride (p.1065·2); codeine hydrochloride (p.26·1).
Pain; smooth muscle spasm.

Spasmofides S Fides, Ger.
Homoeopathic preparation.

Spasmoflex Rolab, S.Afr.
Paracetamol (p.72·2); chlormezanone (p.648·3).
Pain and associated tension.

Spasmo-Gentarol N UCB, Ger.†.
Ethaverine hydrochloride (p.1577·1); paracetamol (p.72·2); salicylamide (p.82·3); codeine phosphate (p.26·1); caffeine (p.749·3).
Migraine; smooth muscle spasms.

Spasmo-Granobil-Krampf- und Reizhusten
Synpharma, Aust.
Aniseed (p.1549·3); helianthus annuus; thyme (p.1636·3).
Coughs.

Spasmoject Mayrand, USA†.
Dicyclomine hydrochloride (p.460·1).
Functional bowel/irritable bowel syndrome.

Spasmolyt
Madaus, Aust.; Madaus, Ger.
Trospium chloride (p.1640·1).
Bladder function disorders; smooth muscle spasm.

Spasmomen
Menarini, Belg.; Menarini, Ital.
Otilonium bromide (p.1611·2).
Gastro-intestinal spasm; premedication for gastro-intestinal procedures.

Spasmomen Somatico Menarini, Ital.
Otilonium bromide (p.1611·2); diazepam (p.661·1).
Gastro-intestinal spasm.

Spasmo-Mucosolvan Thomae, Ger.
Clenbuterol hydrochloride (p.752·1); ambroxol hydrochloride (p.1054·3).
Respiratory tract disorders.

Spasmonal
Note. This name is used for preparations of different composition.
Trenker, Belg.
Mebeverine hydrochloride (p.1199·2).
Irritable bowel syndrome.

Norgine, Irl.; Norgine, UK.
Alverine citrate (p.1548·1).
Smooth muscle spasm.

Spasmo-Nervogastrol Heumann, Ger.
Butinoline phosphate (p.1555·3); calcium carbonate (p.1182·1); bismuth subnitrate (p.1180·2).
Gastro-intestinal disorders.

Spasmophen Lannett, USA†.
Atropine sulphate (p.455·1); hyoscine hydrobromide (p.462·3); hyoscyamine hydrobromide (p.464·2) or hyoscyamine sulphate (p.464·2); phenobarbitone (p.350·2).
Gastro-intestinal disorders.

Spasmoplus
Note. This name is used for preparations of different composition.
Ciba-Geigy, Aust.; Ciba-Geigy, Belg.
Propyphenazone (p.81·3); drofenine hydrochloride (p.460·3); codeine phosphate (p.26·1).
Painful smooth muscle spasm.

Ciba, Ital.
Propyphenazone (p.81·3); codeine phosphate (p.26·1).
Pain.

Spasmopriv
Note. This name is used for preparations of different composition.
Irex, Fr.
Mebeverine hydrochloride (p.1199·2).
Gastro-intestinal and biliary-tract spasm.

Synthelabo, Fr.†; Lusofarmaco, Ital.†.
Fenoverine (p.1579·2).
Smooth muscle spasm.

Spasmo-Rhoival Tosse, Ger.
Trospium chloride (p.1640·1).
Formerly contained dicyclomine hydrochloride.
Bladder function disorders.

Spasmosan TAD, Ger.†.
Phenazopyridine hydrochloride (p.78·3).
Urinary-tract pain.

Spasmosarto Biosarto, Spain.
Trospium chloride (p.1640·1).
Urinary incontinence.

Spasmosedine
Note. This name is used for preparations of different composition.
Pharmethic, Belg.
Phenobarbitone (p.350·2); quinine hydrobromide (p.439·2); crataegus (p.1568·2); meprobamate (p.678·1).
Arrhythmias; vascular spasm.

Theranol-Deglaude, Fr.
Crataegus (p.1568·2); phenobarbitone (p.350·2).
Formerly contained quinine hydrobromide, crataegus, and phenobarbitone.
Cardiac disorders; nervous disorders.

Spasmosol Streuli, Switz.
Injection: Mixed opium alkaloids (p.71·1); atropine sulphate (p.455·1); papaverine hydrochloride (p.1614·2).
Pain.
Oral drops†*:* Mixed opium alkaloids (p.71·1); atropine sulphate (p.455·1); papaverine hydrochloride (p.1614·2); phenazone (p.78·2).
Suppositories†*; tablets*†*:* Mixed opium alkaloids (p.71·1); atropine sulphate (p.455·1); papaverine hydrochloride (p.1614·2); propyphenazone (p.81·3).
Smooth muscle spasm.

Spasmo-Solugastril
Salus, Aust.; Heumann, Ger.
Aluminium hydroxide gel (p.1177·3); butinoline phosphate (p.1555·3); calcium carbonate (p.1182·1).
Gastro-intestinal disorders.

Spasmosyx N Syxyl, Ger.
Homoeopathic preparation.

Spasmo-Urgenin
Madaus, Aust.; Byk Madaus, S.Afr.; Madaus, Spain.
Trospium chloride (p.1640·1); echinacea angustifolia (p.1574·2); saw palmetto (p.1462·1).
Genito-urinary spasm; prostatic hyperplasia; prostatitis.

Spasmo-Urgenin Rectal Madaus, Spain†.
Trospium chloride (p.1640·1); buphenine hydrochloride (p.1555·3); echinacea angustifolia (p.1574·2); saw palmetto (p.1462·1).
Genito-urinary spasm; prostatic hyperplasia; prostatitis.

Spasmo-Urgenin TC Madaus, Ger.
Trospium chloride (p.1640·1).
Bladder function disorders.

Spasmo-Urgenine Neo Madaus, Switz.
Trospium chloride (p.1640·1).
Spasmo-Urgenine formerly contained sabal serrulata, echinacea angustifolia, and trospium chloride.
Urinary-tract disorders.

Spasmo-Uroclear Parke, Davis, Ger.†.
Nitrofurantoin (p.231·3); sulphadiazine (p.252·3); phenazopyridine hydrochloride (p.78·3).
Urinary-tract infections.

Spasmo-Urolong
Organon, Aust.; Thiemann, Ger.†; Sodip, Switz.†.
Nitrofurantoin (p.231·3); camylofin hydrochloride (p.1558·2).
Urinary-tract infections.

Spasquid Geneva, USA†.
Atropine sulphate (p.455·1); hyoscine hydrobromide (p.462·3); hyoscyamine hydrobromide (p.464·2) or hyoscyamine sulphate (p.464·2); phenobarbitone (p.350·2).
Gastro-intestinal disorders.

Spastrex Propan, S.Afr.
Oxyphenonium bromide (p.466·3).
Gastro-intestinal and urinary-tract spasm.

Spasuret Sanofi Winthrop, Ger.
Flavoxate hydrochloride (p.461·2).
Urinary-tract disorders.

Speciafoldine Specia, Fr.
Folic acid (p.1340·3).
Nutritional deficiency; prevention of neural tube disorders.

Special Defense Sun Block Clinique, Canad.
SPF 25: Titanium dioxide (p.1093·3).
Sunscreen.

Speci-Chol Pekana, Ger.
Homoeopathic preparation.

Species Carvi comp Weleda, Aust.
Aniseed (p.1549·3); urtica (p.1642·3); fennel (p.1579·1); caraway (p.1559·3).
Flatulence; gastro-intestinal cramp.

Species nervinae Kwizda, Aust.
Hypericum (p.1590·1); valerian (p.1643·1); melissa leaf (p.1600·1); peppermint leaf (p.1208·1).
Anxiety disorders; sleep disorders.

Spec-T
Note. This name is used for preparations of different composition.
Apothecon, USA.
Dextromethorphan hydrobromide (p.1057·3); benzocaine (p.1286·2).
Coughs.

Squibb, USA.
Benzocaine (p.1286·2).
Sore throat.

Spec-T Sore Throat/Decongestant *Apothecon, USA.*
Phenylpropanolamine hydrochloride (p.1067·2); phenylephrine hydrochloride (p.1066·2); benzocaine (p.1286·2).
Upper respiratory-tract symptoms.

Spectazole *Ortho Dermatological, USA.*
Econazole nitrate (p.377·2).
Cutaneous candidiasis; tinea versicolor.

Spectraban
Note. This name is used for preparations of different composition.
Stiefel, Ger.†; Stiefel, S.Afr.; Stiefel, UK†.
SPF 4: Padimate O (p.1488·1).
Sunscreen.

Stiefel, UK†.
SPF 10: Ethylhexyl *p*-methoxycinnamate (p.1487·1); oxybenzone (p.1487·3).
SPF 15: Padimate O (p.1488·1); aminobenzoic acid (p.1486·3).
SPF 25: Padimate O (p.1488·1); aminobenzoic acid (p.1486·3).
Sunscreen.

Spectraban Ultra
Note. This name is used for preparations of different composition.
Stiefel, Fr.†.
Padimate O (p.1488·1); oxybenzone (p.1487·3); avobenzone (p.1486·3).
Sunscreen.

Stiefel, UK.
SPF 17: Padimate O (p.1488·1); avobenzone (p.1486·3); oxybenzone (p.1487·3); titanium dioxide (p.1093·3).
Sunscreen.

Spectracil *Schwulst, S.Afr.*
Ampicillin trihydrate (p.153·2).
Bacterial infections.

Spectralgen 4 Grass Mix *Pharmacia, UK†.*
Allergen extracts of 4 grass pollens(p.1545·1).
Hyposensitisation.

Spectralgen Single Species *Pharmacia, UK†.*
Allergen extract of Timothy grass (p.1545·1).
Hyposensitisation.

Spectralgen 3 Tree Mix *Pharmacia, UK†.*
Allergen extracts of 3 tree pollens(p.1545·1).
Hyposensitisation.

Spectralys Hemofiltration 05, 23 *Schiwa, Swed.†.*
Electrolyte infusion (p.1151·1).
Haemofiltration.

Spectralys Hemofiltration 19, 20 *Schiwa, Swed.†.*
Electrolyte infusion with glucose (p.1151·1).
Haemofiltration.

Spectramedryn *Allergan, Ger.*
Medrysone (p.1045·3).
Allergic and inflammatory disorders of the eye.

Spectramox *Schwulst, S.Afr.*
Amoxycillin trihydrate (p.151·3).
Bacterial infections.

Spectrapain *Schwulst, S.Afr.*
Paracetamol (p.72·2); codeine phosphate (p.26·1).
Pain.

Spectrapain Forte *Schwulst, S.Afr.*
Paracetamol (p.72·2); codeine phosphate (p.26·1); caffeine (p.749·3); meprobamate (p.678·1).
Pain and associated tension.

Spectrasone *Schwulst, S.Afr.*
Erythromycin estolate (p.204·1).
Bacterial infections.

Spectratet *Schwulst, S.Afr.*
Oxytetracycline (p.235·1).
Bacterial infections.

Spectravit *Schwulst, S.Afr.†.*
Multivitamin and mineral preparation.

Spectrim *Schwulst, S.Afr.*
Co-trimoxazole (p.196·3).
Bacterial infections.

Spectro Derm *Spectropharm, Canad.*
Skin cleanser.
Cleansing of abraded and irritated skin.

Spectro Gluvs *Spectropharm, Canad.*
Barrier cream.

Spectro Gram *Spectropharm, Canad.*
Chlorhexidine gluconate (p.1107·2).
Disinfection of skin and hands.

Spectro Jel *Spectropharm, Canad.*
Skin cleanser.

Spectro Tar *Spectropharm, Canad.*
Shampoo: Chlorhexidine gluconate (p.1107·2); coal tar (p.1092·3).
Scalp disorders.
Skin wash: Coal tar (p.1092·3).
Eczema; psoriasis.

Spectrobid *Roerig, USA.*
Bacampicillin hydrochloride (p.157·2).
Bacterial infections.

Spectrocin *Iquinosa, Spain.*
Gramicidin (p.215·2); neomycin sulphate (p.229·2).
Skin infections.

Spectrocin Plus *Numark, USA.*
Neomycin sulphate (p.229·2); polymyxin B sulphate (p.239·1); bacitracin (p.157·3); lignocaine (p.1293·2).
Bacterial skin infections.

Spectro-Jel *Recsei, USA.*
Soap-free skin cleanser.

Spectroxyl *Ecosol, Switz.*
Amoxycillin (p.151·3).
Bacterial infections.

Spectrum
Note. This name is used for preparations of different composition.
KSL, Canad.
Multivitamin and mineral preparation.

Sigma-Tau, Ital.
Ceftazidime (p.173·3).
Bacterial infections.

Johnson & Johnson Medical, UK.
Alcohol (p.1099·1); quaternary ammonium compounds.
Formerly contained alcohol, chlorhexidine gluconate, and quaternary ammonium compounds.
Surface disinfection.

Specyton cartilage-parathyroide *Menarini, Fr.*
Cartilage and parathyroid antisera.
Arthritis.

Speda *Byk Gulden, Ger.†.*
Vinylbitone (p.698·2).
Sleep disorders.

Spedifen *Inpharzam, Switz.*
Ibuprofen (p.44·1).
Fever; inflammation; pain.

Spedralgin sans codeine *Demopharm, Switz.*
Paracetamol (p.72·2); phenazone (p.78·2); propyphenazone (p.81·3); caffeine (p.749·3).
Fever; pain.

Spedro *Demopharm, Switz.*
Codeine phosphate (p.26·1); ephedrine hydrochloride (p.1059·3); belladonna (p.457·1); ipecacuanha (p.1062·2); guaiphenesin (p.1061·3); sodium benzoate (p.1102·3); terpin hydrate (p.1070·2).
Coughs and associated respiratory-tract disorders.

Spektramox *Astra, Swed.*
Amoxycillin trihydrate (p.151·3); potassium clavulanate (p.190·2).
Bacterial infections.

Spencer's Bronchitis *McGloin, Austral.*
Ammonium chloride (p.1055·2); codeine phosphate (p.26·1); phenylpropanolamine hydrochloride (p.1067·2).
Cold symptoms; throat irritation.

Spenglersan *Apotheke Roten Krebs, Aust.*
An antisera.
Active and passive immunisation.

Spenglersan Kolloid *Meckel, Ger.*
Homoeopathic preparation.

Sperlisin *Inibsa, Spain†.*
Chlorosulphamoylbenzoate sodium (p.1120·1).
Vulvovaginal infections.

Spermargin *Isnardi, Ital.†.*
Arginine (p.1334·1).
Male infertility.

Spersacarbachol *Ciba Vision, Switz.*
Carbachol (p.1390·1).
Glaucoma; ocular hypertension.

Spersacarpin *Ciba Vision, Ger.*
Pilocarpine hydrochloride (p.1396·3).
Glaucoma; reversal of mydriasis.

Spersacarpine
Ciba Vision, Canad.†; Ciba Vision, Swed.†; Ciba Vision, Switz.
Pilocarpine hydrochloride (p.1396·3).
Glaucoma; ocular hypertension; production of miosis.

Spersacet *Ciba Vision, Switz.*
Sulphacetamide sodium (p.252·2).
Bacterial eye infections; dacryocystitis.

Spersacet C
Restan, S.Afr.; Ciba Vision, Switz.
Sulphacetamide sodium (p.252·2); chloramphenicol (p.182·1).
Eye infections; lachrymo-nasal irrigation.

Spersadex
Ciba Vision, Canad.†; Ciba Vision, Ger.; Ciba Vision, Norw.; Restan, S.Afr.; Ciba Vision, Switz.
Dexamethasone sodium phosphate (p.1037·2).
Inflammatory eye disorders.

Spersadex Comp
Ciba Vision, Ger.; Restan, S.Afr.; Ciba Vision, Switz.
Dexamethasone sodium phosphate (p.1037·2); chloramphenicol (p.182·1).
Inflammatory eye infections.

Spersadex med kloramfenikol *Ciba Vision, Norw.*
Dexamethasone sodium phosphate (p.1037·2); chloramphenicol (p.182·1).
Inflammatory eye infections.

Spersadexolin *Ciba Vision, Ger.*
Dexamethasone sodium phosphate (p.1037·2); chloramphenicol (p.182·1); tetrahydrozoline hydrochloride (p.1070·2).
Inflammatory eye infections.

Spersadexoline
Restan, S.Afr.; Ciba Vision, Switz.
Dexamethasone sodium phosphate (p.1037·2); chloramphenicol (p.182·1); tetrahydrozoline hydrochloride (p.1070·2).
Inflammatory eye infections.

Spersallerg
Ciba Vision, Ger.; Ciba Vision, Norw.; Restan, S.Afr.; Ciba Vision, Switz.
Antazoline hydrochloride (p.401·3); tetrahydrozoline hydrochloride (p.1070·2).
Conjunctivitis.

Spersamide *Restan, S.Afr.*
Sulphacetamide sodium (p.252·2).
Eye infections.

Spersanicol
Restan, S.Afr.; Ciba Vision, Switz.
Chloramphenicol (p.182·1).
Eye infections; lachrymo-nasal irrigation.

Spersanicol vitamine *Dispersa, Switz.†.*
Chloramphenicol (p.182·1); vitamin A acetate; calciferol.
Eye infections.

Spersantovit *Dispersa, Ger.†.*
Calcium pantothenate (p.1352·3); vitamin A acetate (p.1359·2).
Eye disorders.

Spersapolymyxin *Ciba Vision, Switz.*
Polymyxin B sulphate (p.239·1); neomycin sulphate (p.229·2).
Bacterial eye infections.

Spersatear *Restan, S.Afr.*
Hypromellose (p.1473·1).
Dry eyes.

Spersatropine *Restan, S.Afr.†.*
Atropine sulphate (p.455·1).
Ophthalmic diagnostic procedures.

Spersidu C *Dispersa, Ger.†.*
Idoxuridine (p.613·2); chloramphenicol (p.182·1).
Ophthalmic herpes simplex.

Spersin *Sigma, Austral.*
Ointment†: Neomycin sulphate (p.229·2); bacitracin (p.157·3); polymyxin B sulphate (p.239·1).
Topical powder: Polymyxin B sulphate (p.239·1); neomycin sulphate (p.229·2).
Skin infections.

Sperti Praparation H
Salus, Aust.; Much, Ger.
Yeast (p.1373·1); shark-liver oil.
Haemorrhoids.

Sperti Preparation H
Whitehall, Neth.; Whitehall-Robins, Switz.
Yeast (p.1373·1); shark-liver oil.
Haemorrhoids.

Speton *Trenker, Belg.†.*
Monalazone disodium (p.1120·1).
Spermicidal contraceptive.

Spevin *Arcis-Toledano, Fr.*
Cascara sagrada (p.1183·1); quassia amara (p.1624·1).
Constipation.

Spherex *Pharmacia Upjohn, Ger.*
Amilomer 25-45.
Adjuvant to antineoplastics in liver cancer.

Spherulin *ALK, USA.*
Coccidioidin (p.1566·1).
Skin test for coccidioidomycosis.

S.P.H.P. *Cantassium Co., UK.*
Prostate gland; spinal cord (p.1599·1); calcium hypophosphite; nicotinamide (p.1351·2); lecithin (p.1595·2); wheat germ; kola (p.1645·1); vitamin A (p.1358·1); vitamin D (p.1366·3).

Spidifen *Zambon, Spain†.*
Ibuprofen (p.44·1).
Fever; pain.

Spilan *Kanoldt, Ger.*
Hypericum (p.1590·1).
Anxiety disorders; depression.

Spir *Inava, Fr.*
Beclomethasone dipropionate (p.1032·1).
Asthma.

Spiractin
Alphapharm, Austral.; Lennon, S.Afr.
Spironolactone (p.946·1).
Hirsutism; hyperaldosteronism; hypertension; hypokalaemia; oedema.

Spiraphan *Kattwiga, Ger.*
Homoeopathic preparation.

Spirbon *Laevosan, Aust.*
Chlorphenoxamine hydrochloride (p.405·3); ephedrine hydrochloride (p.1059·3); emetine hydrochloride (p.582·2).
Respiratory-tract disorders.

Spireadosa *Chefaro Ardeval, Fr.†.*
Meadowsweet (p.1599·1).
Fever; pain.

Spiretic *DDSA Pharmaceuticals, UK.*
Spironolactone (p.946·1).

Spirial Antitraspirante *SVR, Ital.*
Aluminium chlorohydrate (p.1078·3).
Hyperhidrosis.

Spiricort *Spirig, Switz.*
Prednisolone (p.1048·1).
Corticosteroid.

Spiridazide *SIT, Ital.*
Spironolactone (p.946·1); hydrochlorothiazide (p.885·2).
Hyperaldosteronism.

Spirix
AFI, Norw.; Nycomed, Swed.
Spironolactone (p.946·1).
Hyperaldosteronism; hypertension; liver cirrhosis with ascites; oedema.

Spiro *CT, Ger.*
Spironolactone (p.946·1).
Heart failure; hyperaldosteronism; hypertension; liver cirrhosis; nephrotic syndrome; oedema.

Spiro comp *Ratiopharm, Ger.*
Spironolactone (p.946·1); frusemide (p.871·1).
Ascites; hyperaldosteronism; liver cirrhosis; oedema.

Spirobene *Merckle, Aust.*
Spironolactone (p.946·1).
Hyperaldosteronism; hypertension; oedema.

Spiro-Co *Norton, UK.*
Spironolactone (p.946·1); hydroflumethiazide (p.889·2).
These ingredients are present in such proportions that together they can be described by the British Approved Name Co-flumactone.
Heart failure.

Spiroctan
Boehringer Mannheim, Fr.; Boehringer Mannheim, Neth.†; Boehringer Mannheim, Switz.; Boehringer Mannheim, UK.
Canrenoate potassium (p.836·2) or spironolactone (p.946·1).
Adjuvant in myasthenia; ascites; heart failure; hyperaldosteronism; hypertension; oedema.

Spiroctan-M *Boehringer Mannheim, UK.*
Canrenoate potassium (p.836·2).
Ascites; hyperaldosteronism; oedema.

Spiroctazine *Boehringer Mannheim, Fr.*
Spironolactone (p.946·1); althiazide (p.819·1).
Hypertension; oedema.

Spiro-D *Sanorania, Ger.*
Spironolactone (p.946·1); frusemide (p.871·1).
Ascites; hyperaldosteronism; hypertension; oedema.

Spiroderm *Searle, Ital.*
Spironolactone (p.946·1).
Acne.

Spirodigal *Hormosan, Ger.†.*
β-Acetyldigoxin (p.812·3); spironolactone (p.946·1).
Heart failure.

Spiro-D-Tablinen *Sanorania, Ger.†.*
Spironolactone (p.946·1); frusemide (p.871·1).
Ascites; hyperaldosteronism; hypertension; oedema.

Spirofur *Bruno, Ital.*
Spironolactone (p.946·1); frusemide (p.871·1).
Hypertension; oedema.

Spirogel *Worndli, Switz.*
Camphor (p.1557·2); phenol (p.1121·2); cinnamic acid (p.1111·1); cinnamaldehyde; guaiacol (p.1061·2); phenazone (p.78·2); chlorbutol (p.1106·3); thymol iodide (p.1127·1); thymol (p.1127·1); anethole (p.1549·3); safrole; eugenol (p.1578·2).
Dental disorders.

Spirohexal *Hexal, Aust.*
Spironolactone (p.946·1).
Hyperaldosteronism; hypertension; oedema.

Spirolair *3M, Belg.*
Pirbuterol acetate (p.757·2).
Asthma; bronchitis; emphysema.

Spirolang *SIT, Ital.*
Spironolactone (p.946·1).
Hyperaldosteronism.

Spirolone *Berk, UK.*
Spironolactone (p.946·1).
Ascites; heart failure; nephrotic syndrome; oedema; primary hyperaldosteronism.

Spirometon *Belmac, Spain.*
Bendrofluazide (p.827·3); spironolactone (p.946·1).
Hypertension; oedema.

Spirono *Isis Puren, Ger.*
Spironolactone (p.946·1).
Ascites; hyperaldosteronism; oedema.

Spirono comp *Genericon, Aust.*
Spironolactone (p.946·1); frusemide (p.871·1).
Hyperaldosteronism; oedema.

Spironolacton Plus *Heumann, Ger.*
Spironolactone (p.946·1) frusemide (p.871·1).
Formerly known as Spironolacton Comp.
Ascites; oedema.

Spironone *Pharmafarm, Fr.*
Spironolactone (p.946·1).
Adjuvant in myasthenia; hyperaldosteronism; hypertension; oedema.

Spironothiazid
Henning, Ger.; Henning, Switz.
Spironolactone (p.946·1); hydrochlorothiazide (p.885·2).
Ascites; hyperaldosteronism; hypertension; oedema.

Spiropal *AFI, Norw.*
Spironolactone (p.946·1).
Hyperaldosteronism; hypertension; oedema.

Spiropent
Bender, Aust.; Thomae, Ger.; Boehringer Ingelheim, Ital.; Europharma, Spain.
Clenbuterol hydrochloride (p.752·1).
Obstructive airways disease.

Spirophar *Pharbiol, Fr.†.*
Spironolactone (p.946·1).
Hyperaldosteronism; hypertension; myasthenia; oedema.

Spiroprop *Searle, Irl.†.*
Propranolol hydrochloride (p.937·1); spironolactone (p.946·1).
Hypertension.

Spiroscand *Enapharm, Swed.*
Spironolactone (p.946·1).
Hyperaldosteronism; hypertension; liver cirrhosis with ascites; oedema.

Spirospare *Ashbourne, UK.*
Spironolactone (p.946·1).
Ascites; heart failure; nephrotic syndrome; oedema; primary hyperaldosteronism.

Spirostada comp *Stada, Ger.*
Spironolactone (p.946·1); bendrofluazide (p.827·3).
Ascites; hyperaldosteronism; hypertension; oedema.

Spiro-Tablinen *Sanorania, Ger.*
Spironolactone (p.946·1).
Ascites; hyperaldosteronism; oedema.

Spirotone *CP Protea, Austral.†.*
Spironolactone (p.946·1).

Spirsa *Alter, Spain.*
Chlorpheniramine maleate (p.405·1); phenylephrine hydrochloride (p.1066·2); paracetamol (p.72·2).
Cold and influenza symptoms.

Spitacid *Henkel, Ger.*
Alcohol (p.1099·1); isopropyl alcohol (p.1118·2); benzyl alcohol (p.1103·3).
Hand disinfection.

Spitaderm
Paragerm, Fr.; Henkel, Ger.†; Henkel, Ital.
Isopropyl alcohol (p.1118·2); chlorhexidine gluconate (p.1107·2); hydrogen peroxide (p.1116·2).
Skin disinfection.

Spitalen *Bencard, Belg.*
Virginiamycin (p.269·3); neomycin sulphate (p.229·2).
Bacterial infections.

Spizef
Grunenthal, Aust.; Takeda, Ger.
Cefotiam hydrochloride (p.170·2).
Lignocaine hydrochloride (p.1293·2) may be included in the intramuscular injection to alleviate the pain of injection.
Bacterial infections.

SPL *Delmont, USA.*
Two strains of lysed Staphylococcus aureus in solution (p.1535·1).
Staphylococcal infection.

Splenocarbine *Lesourd, Fr.*
Activated charcoal (p.972·2).
Gastro-intestinal disorders.

Splen-Uvocal *Stroschein, Ger.*
Spleen extract.
Immunotherapy.

Spolera
Note. This name is used for preparations of different composition.
OTW, Ger.
Acmellae ciliatae.
Insect stings; soft-tissue injuries.

Gebro, Switz.†.
Spilanthis oleraceae.
Skin trauma; soft-tissue trauma.

Spolera forte *OTW, Ger.†.*
Glycol salicylate (p.43·1).
Polyarthritis; rheumatic disorders; synovitis.

Spolera "plus" *Gebro, Switz.†.*
Spilanthis oleraceae; glycol salicylate (p.43·1).
Musculoskeletal and joint disorders; soft-tissue trauma.

Spolera therm *OTW, Ger.†.*
Diethylamine salicylate (p.33·1); benzyl nicotinate (p.22·1); oleum pini sylvestris (p.1623·3).
Myalgia; neuralgia; neuritis; pleuritis; rheumatic disorders.

Spondylon *Brenner-Efeka, Ger.*
Capsules: Ketoprofen (p.48·2).
Gout; inflammation; musculoskeletal and joint disorders; pain.
Embrocation: Methyl nicotinate (p.55·1); camphor (p.1557·2).
Formerly contained heparin sodium, methyl nicotinate and camphor.
Muscular and neuromuscular disorders.
Injection†: Dipyrone (p.35·1); lignocaine hydrochloride (p.1293·2).
Pain.

Spondylon N *Brenner-Efeka, Ger.†.*
Suppositories: Phenazone salicylate (p.78·2).
Formerly contained phenazone salicylate, methylpentynol, diphenhydramine hydrochloride, esculoside, and benzocaine.
Tablets: Phenazone salicylate (p.78·2); guaiphenesin (p.1061·3).
Musculoskeletal and joint disorders.

Spondylon S *Brenner-Efeka, Ger.†.*
Phenazone (p.78·2); salicylamide (p.82·3).
Musculoskeletal and joint disorders.

Spondylonal *Brenner-Efeka, Ger.*
Multivitamin preparation.

Spondyvit *Brenner-Efeka, Ger.; LAW, Ger.*
d-Alpha tocopheryl acetate (p.1369·2).
Vitamin E deficiency.

Spongostan
Johnson & Johnson, Aust.; Ethicon, Ital.; Novo Nordisk, S.Afr.†.
Gelatin (p.723·2).
Haemorrhage.

Sponsin *Farmasan, Ger.*
Co-dergocrine mesylate (p.1566·1).
Adjuvant for mental function disorders; cervical disc syndrome; hypertension.

Sponwiga *Kattwiga, Ger.*
Homoeopathic preparation.

Sporacid *IMS, Ital.*
Glutaraldehyde (p.1114·3).
Instrument disinfection.

Sporanox
Janssen-Cilag, Aust.; Janssen-Cilag, Austral.; Janssen-Cilag, Belg.; Janssen-Ortho, Canad.; Janssen-Cilag, Fr.; Janssen-Cilag, Irl.; Janssen-Cilag, Ital.; Janssen-Cilag, Norw.; Janssen-Cilag, S.Afr.; Janssen-Cilag, Spain; Janssen-Cilag, Swed.; Janssen-Cilag, Switz.; Janssen-Cilag, UK; Janssen, USA.
Itraconazole (p.381·3).
Fungal infections.

Sporcid *Fresenius, Ger.*
2-Alkoxi-3,4-dihydro-2-H-pyran aldehyde adduct; formaldehyde (p.1113·2); glyoxal (p.1115·1); ricinoleic acid propylamidotrimethylammonium methosulphate; oleylaminooxyethylate.
Instrument disinfection.

Sporex *IMS, Ital.*
Glutaraldehyde (p.1114·3).
Instrument disinfection.

Sporicidin *IMS, Ital.*
Glutaraldehyde-phenate complex (p.1114·3).
Instrument and surface disinfection.

Sporicidine *Peters, Fr.†.*
Phenate-glutaraldehyde complex (p.1114·3).
Instrument disinfection.

Sporidyn *Zoja, Ital.†.*
Cefotiam hydrochloride (p.170·2).
Bacterial infections.

Sporiline *Schering-Plough, Fr.*
Tolnaftate (p.389·1).
Fungal skin infections.

Sporol *Cantabria, Spain†.*
Cephalexin (p.178·2).
Bacterial infections.

Sport Sunblock *Avon, Canad.*
SPF 30: Ethylhexyl *p*-methoxycinnamate (p.1487·1); octyl salicylate (p.1487·3); oxybenzone (p.1487·3).
Sunscreen.

Sportenine *Boiron, Canad.*
Homoeopathic preparation.

Sportino *Harras-Curarina, Ger.*
Heparin sodium (p.879·3).
Soft-tissue injury; superficial vascular disorders.

Sportino Akut *Harras-Curarina, Ger.*
Glycol salicylate (p.43·1); arnica (p.1550·3).
Musculoskeletal, joint, and soft-tissue disorders.

Sportofit *Gry, Ger.†.*
Arnica (p.1550·3); heparin sodium (p.879·3).
Bruising; peripheral vascular disorders.

Sports Multi *Cenovis, Austral.*
Multivitamin and mineral preparation.

Sports Spray *Mentholatum, USA†.*
Methyl salicylate (p.55·2); menthol (p.1600·2); camphor (p.1557·2).
Muscle, joint, and soft-tissue pain; neuralgia.

Sportscreme
Stella, Canad.†; Thompson, USA.
Triethanolamine salicylate (p.1639·2).
Muscle, joint, and soft-tissue pain; neuralgia.

Sportscreme Ice *Thompson, USA.*
Menthol (p.1600·2).
Muscle, joint, and soft-tissue pain; neuralgia.

Sportsmega *Cantassium Co., UK.*
Multivitamin and mineral preparation.

Sportsvit *Schwulst, S.Afr.†.*
Multivitamin and mineral preparation.

Sportupac N *Terra-Bio, Ger.*
Aesculus (p.1543·3); aescin (p.1543·3); heparin sodium (p.879·3).
Myopathy; soft tissue injuries.

Sportusal *Permamed, Switz.*
Laureth 9 (p.1325·2); dimethyl sulphoxide (p.1377·2); heparin sodium (p.879·3); glycol salicylate (p.43·1); dexpanthenol (p.1570·3).
Soft-tissue trauma; superficial thrombophlebitis; varices.

Sportusal Spray sine heparino *Permamed, Switz.*
Laureth 9 (p.1325·2); dimethyl sulphoxide (p.1377·2); glycol salicylate (p.43·1); dexpanthenol (p.1570·3); menthol (p.1600·2); camphor (p.1557·2).
Soft-tissue disorders.

Sportz Sunscreen *Scott, Canad.*
SPF 15: Ethylhexyl *p*-methoxycinnamate (p.1487·1); octyl salicylate (p.1487·3); oxybenzone (p.1487·3).
Sunscreen.

Spotoway *Pure Plant Products, UK.*
Chlorhexidine (p.1107·2).
Skin irritation and spots.

Spraydil *SmithKline Beecham, Belg.†.*
Phenylephrine hydrochloride (p.1066·2).
Rhinitis.

Spray-n-Wake *Caprice Greystoke, USA.*
Caffeine (p.749·3).

Spray-on Bande *Eagle, Austral.*
Povidone and vinyl acetate copolymer.
Plastic skin preparation for colostomies and ileostomies.

Spray-Pax *SCAT, Fr.*
Pyrethrum (p.1410·1); piperonyl butoxide (p.1409·3).
Pediculosis.

Sprayrin *SIFI, Ital.†.*
Neomycin sulphate (p.229·2); gramicidin (p.215·2); triamcinolone (p.1050·2); phenylephrine hydrochloride (p.1066·2).
Inflammation of nasal mucous membranes.

Spray-Tish *Boehringer Ingelheim, Austral.*
Tramazoline hydrochloride (p.1071·1).
Nasal congestion.

Spray-ur-Cold *Caprice Greystoke, USA.*
Phenylpropanolamine hydrochloride (p.1067·2); dextromethorphan (p.1057·3); chlorpheniramine (p.405·2).

Spray-U-Thin *Caprice Greystoke, USA.*
Phenylpropanolamine hydrochloride (p.1067·2).

Spregal
Note. This name is used for preparations of different composition.
SCAT, Fr.
Esdepallethrine (p.1406·1); piperonyl butoxide (p.1409·3).
Scabies.

Wolff, Ger.
Bioallethrin (p.1402·3); piperonyl butoxide (p.1409·3).
Scabies.

Spren *Sigma, Austral.*
Aspirin (p.16·1).
Fever; inhibition of platelet aggregation; pain.

Spreor *Inava, Fr.*
Salbutamol (p.758·2).
Obstructive airways disease.

Sprilon
Perstorp, Irl.; Smith & Nephew Healthcare, UK.
Dimethicone (p.1384·2); zinc oxide (p.1096·2).
Barrier preparation; eczema; leg ulcers; pressure sores; skin fissures.

Sprucaine Spray *OTW, Ger.†.*
Amethocaine hydrochloride (p.1285·2); benzocaine (p.1286·2).
Local anaesthesia.

SPS *Carolina, USA.*
Sodium polystyrene sulphonate (p.995·3).
Hyperkalaemia.

S-P-T *Fleming, USA.*
Thyroid (porcine) (p.1496·3).
Hypothyroidism; thyroid cancer.

Spuman *Luitpold, Switz.†.*
Anhydrous calcium lactate (p.1155·2); lactose (p.1349·3).
Leucorrhoea.

Spuman a la camomille *Luitpold, Switz.†.*
Chamomile (p.1561·2); lactose (p.1349·3); saccharum amylaceum.
Leucorrhoea.

Spuman c. Acid. lactic. 5% *Luitpold, Ger.†.*
Calcium lactate (p.1155·2).
Regulation of vaginal pH.

Squad *Irex, Fr.*
Flavodate sodium (p.1580·1).
Menorrhagia; peripheral vascular disorders.

Squamasol
Ichthyol, Aust.; Ichthyol, Ger.
Salicylic acid (p.1090·2).
Scalp disorders.

Squa-med *Permamed, Switz.*
Pyrithione zinc (p.1089·3); sodium undecylamide MEA-sulphosuccinate; urea (p.1095·2).
Scalp disorders.

Squibb-HC *Bristol-Myers Squibb, Austral.*
Hydrocortisone acetate (p.1043·3).
Skin disorders.

Sqworm *Norgine, Austral.*
Mebendazole (p.104·1).
Enterobiasis.

SRA *Boots, Austral.†.*
Aspirin (p.16·1).
Osteoarthritis; rheumatoid arthritis.

SRC Expectorant *Edwards, USA.*
Pseudoephedrine hydrochloride (p.1068·3); guaiphenesin (p.1061·3); hydrocodone tartrate (p.43·1).
Coughs.

Srilane
Lipha, Belg.; Lipha Sante, Fr.
Idrocilamide (p.1315·3).
Skeletal muscle spasm; superficial phlebitis.

SRM-Rhotard
Research Labs, S.Afr.; Farmitalia Carlo Erba, UK†.
Morphine sulphate (p.56·2).
Pain.

SSD
Knoll, Canad.; Boots, USA.
Silver sulphadiazine (p.247·3).
Burns; wounds.

SSKI *Upsher-Smith, USA.*
Potassium iodide (p.1493·1).
Respiratory-tract disorders.

SS-Tab *Alra, USA.*
Sulphafurazole (p.253·3).

ST-52 *Asta Medica, Fr.*
Fosfestrol sodium (p.1447·1).
Prostatic cancer.

ST 37 *Menley & James, USA.*
Hexylresorcinol (p.1116·1).
Antiseptic.

St Bonifatius-Tee *Kolassa, Aust.*
Equisetum (p.1575·1); frangula bark (p.1193·2); senna leaf (p.1212·2); valerian root (p.1643·1); citrus aurantium; tilia flower (p.1637·3); boldo leaf (p.1554·1); juniper wood (p.1592·2); rhubarb (p.1212·1).
Diuretic; gastro-intestinal motility disorders.

S-T Cort *Scot-Tussin, USA.*
Hydrocortisone (p.1043·3).
Skin disorders.

S-T Forte *Scot-Tussin, USA.*
Hydrocodone tartrate (p.43·1); phenylephrine hydrochloride (p.1066·2); phenylpropanolamine hydrochloride (p.1067·2); pheniramine maleate (p.415·3); guaiphenesin (p.1061·3).
Coughs and cold symptoms; nasal congestion.

S-T Forte 2 *Scot-Tussin, USA.*
Chlorpheniramine maleate (p.405·1); hydrocodone tartrate (p.43·1).
Coughs and cold symptoms.

St. Jakobs-Balsam Mono *Palmicol, Ger.*
Zinc oxide (p.1096·2).
Skin disorders.

St James Balm *Medico-Biological Laboratories, UK.*
Zinc oxide (p.1096·2); ichthammol (p.1083·3); salicylic acid (p.1090·2); urea (p.1095·2).
Skin disorders.

St. Joseph Adult Chewable *Schering-Plough, USA.*
Aspirin (p.16·1).

St. Joseph Aspirin-Free for Children *Plough, USA.*
Paracetamol (p.72·2).
Fever; pain.

St. Joseph Cold Tablets For Children *Schering-Plough, USA.*
Phenylpropanolamine hydrochloride (p.1067·2); paracetamol (p.72·2).
Upper respiratory-tract symptoms.

St. Joseph Cough Suppressant *Schering-Plough, USA.*
Dextromethorphan hydrobromide (p.1057·3).
Coughs.

St Mary's Thistle Plus *Eagle, Austral.*
Silybum marianum (p.993·3); myrtillus (p.1606·1); taraxacum (p.1634·2).
Liver tonic; peripheral vascular disorders; psoriasis.

St Radegunder Abfuhrtee mild *Synpharma, Aust.*
Prunus spinosa; cichorium intybus; fennel (p.1579·1); mallow flower.
Constipation.

St Radegunder Beruhigungs- und Einschlaftee *Synpharma, Aust.*
Valerian root (p.1643·1); lupulus (p.1597·2); citrus aurantium; melissa leaf (p.1600·1).
Anxiety disorders; sleep disorders.

St Radegunder Blahungstreibender Tee *Synpharma, Aust.*
Fennel (p.1579·1); caraway (p.1559·3); peppermint leaf (p.1208·1); chamomile flower (p.1561·2).
Dyspepsia; flatulence.

St Radegunder Bronchialtee *Synpharma, Aust.*
Fennel (p.1579·1); thyme (p.1636·3); eucalyptus leaf (p.1578·1); veronica officinalis; verbascum flower.
Catarrh.

St Radegunder Entschlackungs-Elixier *Synpharma, Aust.*
Taraxacum (p.1634·2); pansy; manna (p.1199·1); bitter orange peel (p.1610·3); rose fruit (p.1365·2).
Diuretic.

St Radegunder Entwasserungs-Elixier *Synpharma, Aust.*
Silver birch (p.1553·3); equisetum (p.1575·1); urtica (p.1642·3).
Urinary-tract disorders.

St Radegunder Entwasserungstee *Synpharma, Aust.*
Ononis root (p.1610·2); silver birch (p.1553·3); equisetum (p.1575·1); urtica (p.1642·3).
Urinary-tract disorders.

St Radegunder Fiebertee *Synpharma, Aust.*
Tilia flower (p.1637·3); sambucus flower (p.1627·2); chamomile flower (p.1561·2); melissa leaf (p.1600·1).
Cold symptoms.

St Radegunder Herz-Kreislauf-Tonikum *Synpharma, Aust.*
Crataegus (p.1568·2); melissa leaf (p.1600·1); rosemary leaf.
Cardiac disorders.

St Radegunder Herz-Kreislauf-unterstutzender Tee *Synpharma, Aust.*
Crataegus (p.1568·2); rosemary leaf; melissa leaf (p.1600·1); lavender flower (p.1594·3).
Cardiac disorders.

St Radegunder Hustentee *Synpharma, Aust.*
Wild thyme; plantago lanceolata; althaea (p.1546·3); galeopsis ochroleuca; mallow flower.
Coughs.

St Radegunder Leber-Galle-Tee *Synpharma, Aust.*
Cichorium intybus root; taraxacum (p.1634·2); marrubium vulgare root (p.1063·3); peppermint leaf (p.1208·1).
Gastro-intestinal and biliary-tract disorders.

St Radegunder Magenberuhigungstee *Synpharma, Aust.*
Melissa leaf (p.1600·1); peppermint leaf (p.1208·1); fennel fruit (p.1579·1); mallow flower.
Gastro-intestinal disorders.

St Radegunder Nerventee *Synpharma, Aust.*
Melissa leaf (p.1600·1); valerian root (p.1643·1); lupulus (p.1597·2); delphinium consolida flower.
Nervous disorders; sleep disorders.

St Radegunder Nerven-Tonikum *Synpharma, Aust.*
Valerian root (p.1643·1); lupulus (p.1597·2); melissa leaf (p.1600·1).
Nervous disorders; sleep disorders.

St Radegunder Nierentee *Synpharma, Aust.*
Bearberry (p.1552·2); equisetum (p.1575·1); herniaria (p.1587·2) ononis (p.1610·2).
Urinary-tract disorders.

St Radegunder Reizmildernder Magentee *Synpharma, Aust.*
Chamomile flower (p.1561·2); mallow; fennel (p.1579·1); melissa leaf (p.1600·1).
Gastro-intestinal disorders.

St Radegunder Rosmarin-Wein *Synpharma, Aust.*
Rosemary leaf; melissa leaf (p.1600·1).
Circulatory disorders.

St Radegunder Tee gegen Durchfall *Synpharma, Aust.*
Hamamelis leaf (p.1587·1); strawberry; chamomile flower (p.1561·2); juglans regia fennel (p.1579·1).
Diarrhoea.

St Radegunder Thorasan-Krauterhustensaft *Synpharma, Aust.*
Primula root; thyme (p.1636·3); plantago lanceolata.
Catarrh; coughs.

St Radegunder Verdauungstee *Synpharma, Aust.*
Absinthium (p.1541·1); centaury (p.1561·1); bitter orange peel (p.1610·3); caraway (p.1559·3); gentian root (p.1583·3).
Gastro-intestinal disorders.

Stabicilline *Vifor, Switz.*
Syrup†: Benzathine penicillin (p.158·3).
Tablets: Phenoxymethylpenicillin potassium (p.236·2).
Bacterial infections.

Stabillin V-K *Boots, UK†.*
Phenoxymethylpenicillin potassium (p.236·2).
Bacterial infections.

Stablon *Ardix, Fr.*
Tianeptine sodium (p.308·2).
Depression.

Stacho N *Selz, Ger.†.*
Magnesium trisilicate (p.1199·1); aluminium hydroxide gel (p.1177·3); bismuth subnitrate (p.1180·2); sodium sulphate (p.1213·3); valerian (p.1643·1); frangula bark (p.1193·2); calamus (p.1556·1); chamomile (p.1561·2); fennel (p.1579·1); liquorice (p.1197·1); fennel oil (p.1579·2).
Gastro-intestinal disorders.

Stacho-Zym N *Kattwiga, Ger.*
Pancreatin (p.1612·1); enzymes from Aspergillus.
Digestive system disorders.

Stacillin *Schiapparelli Searle, Ital.†.*
Amoxycillin trihydrate (p.151·3); potassium clavulanate (p.190·2).
Bacterial infections.

Stada Reise-Dragees *Stada, Ger.†.*
Diphenhydramine hydrochloride (p.409·1); 8-chlorotheophylline.
Nausea; travel sickness; vertigo; vomiting.

Stadacain *Stada, Ger.†.*
Butoxycaine hydrochloride (p.1289·1).

Stadaglicin *Stada, Ger.†.*
Sodium cromoglycate (p.762·1).
Allergic eye disorders.

Stadalax *Stada, Ger.*
Bisacodyl (p.1179·3).
Constipation.

stadasan *Stada, Ger.†.*
Ibuprofen (p.44·1).
Pain.

stadasan Thermo *Stada, Ger.†.*
Liniment: Benzyl nicotinate (p.22·1); glycol salicylate (p.43·1); pine oil; rosemary oil (p.1626·2).
Ointment: Benzyl nicotinate (p.22·1); glycol salicylate (p.43·1).
Musculoskeletal and joint disorders.

Stadol
Bristol-Myers Squibb, Canad.; Apothecon, USA; Mead Johnson Laboratories, USA.
Butorphanol tartrate (p.24·1).
Pain.

Staficyn *FIRMA, Ital.*
Methicillin sodium (p.225·1).
Staphylococcal infections.

Stafilon *AGIPS, Ital.*
Methacycline hydrochloride (p.225·1).
Bacterial infections.

Stafoxil
Yamanouchi, Irl.; Yamanouchi, Neth.; Yamanouchi, UK.
Flucloxacillin sodium (p.209·2).
Bacterial infections.

Stafusid Antibiotico *Italfarmaco, Ital.†.*
Sodium fusidate (p.211·1).
Staphylococcal infections.

Stagesic *Huckaby, USA.*
Hydrocodone tartrate (p.43·1); paracetamol (p.72·2).
Pain.

Stagid *Merck-Clevenot, Fr.*
Metformin embonate (p.330·2).
Diabetes mellitus.

Stago
Note. This name is used for preparations of different composition.
Darci, Belg.†.
Ajuga reptans; anthemis nobilis (p.1561·2); boldo (p.1554·1); cinchona bark (p.1564·1); pini sylvestris; sarsaparilla (p.1627·2); euonymus (p.1192·1); barosma crenulata (p.1555·2); kinkeliba (p.1593·2).
Liver, kidney, and bladder pain.

Synthelabo, Switz.†.
Ajuga reptans; chamomile (p.1561·2); tilia alburnum (p.1637·3); barosma crenata (p.1555·2); combretum (p.1593·2); cinchona bark (p.1564·1); chelidonium majus; turmeric (p.1001·3); cynara (p.1569·2); boldo (p.1554·1); mint oil (p.1604·1).
Biliary-tract disorders; constipation; nausea.

Stagural *Stada, Ger.†.*
Norfenefrine hydrochloride (p.925·1).
Hypotension.

Stahist *Huckaby, USA.*
Phenylpropanolamine hydrochloride (p.1067·2); phenylephrine hydrochloride (p.1066·2); chlorpheniramine maleate (p.405·1); hyoscyamine sulphate (p.464·2); hyoscine hydrobromide (p.462·3); atropine sulphate (p.455·1).
Upper respiratory-tract symptoms.

Stalcin *Locatelli, Ital.*
Salcatonin (p.735·3).
Hypercalcaemia; osteoporosis; Paget's disease.

Stallergenes *Stallergenes, Switz.†.*
Allergen extracts (p.1545·1).
Hyposensitisation.

Stallergenes MRV *Stallergenes, Fr.*
Staphylococcus aureus; *Staphylococcus albus*; Streptococcus spp.; *Diplococcus pneumoniae*; *Haemophilus influenzae*; *Klebsiella pneumoniae*; *Moraxella (Branhamella) catarrhalis.*
Respiratory-tract infections.

Stallerpatch *Stallergenes, Switz.†.*
Allergen extracts (p.1545·1).
Hyposensitisation.

Staloral *Stallergenes, Switz.*
Pollen allergen extracts(p.1545·1).
Hyposensitisation.

Stamaril
Pasteur Merieux, Belg.; Pasteur Vaccins, Fr.; Pasteur Merieux, Ital.; Rhone-Poulenc Rorer, S.Afr.; Pasteur Merieux, Swed.; Pro Vaccine, Switz.
A yellow fever vaccine (17D strain) (p.1539·1).
Active immunisation.

Stamicina *Torre, Ital.†.*
Doxycycline hydrochloride (p.202·3).
Bacterial infections.

Stamoist E *Huckaby, USA.*
Pseudoephedrine hydrochloride (p.1068·3); guaiphenesin (p.1061·3).
Coughs.

Stamoist LA *Huckaby, USA.*
Phenylpropanolamine hydrochloride (p.1067·2); guaiphenesin (p.1061·3).
Coughs and cold symptoms; nasal congestion.

Stancare *Stanley, Canad.*
Wool fat (p.1385·3); liquid paraffin (p.1382·1).

Standacillin *Tyrol, Aust.*
Ampicillin sodium (p.153·1) or ampicillin trihydrate (p.153·2).
Bacterial infections.

Standard III *Aguettant, Fr.*
Electrolyte preparation (p.1147·1).
Parenteral nutrition.

Stangyl
Rhone-Poulenc Rorer, Aust.; Rhone-Poulenc Rorer, Ger.
Trimipramine maleate (p.310·1) or trimipramine mesylate (p.310·2).
Depression; pain.

Stanhexidine *Novopharm, Canad.*
Chlorhexidine (p.1107·2).

Stanilo *Pharmacia Upjohn, Ger.*
Spectinomycin hydrochloride (p.248·3).
Gonorrhoea.

Stanno-Bardane *Pharmacobel, Belg.*
Tin (p.1638·1); lappa (p.1594·2).
Staphylococcal infections.

Stapenor
Bayer, Aust.; Bayer, Ger.
Oxacillin sodium (p.234·2).
Staphylococcal infections.

Staphcillin *Apothecon, USA†.*
Methicillin sodium (p.225·1).
Bacterial infections.

Staphlipen *Lederle, UK†.*
Flucloxacillin sodium (p.209·2).
Formerly known as Staphcil.
Bacterial infections.

Staphycid *Beecham, Belg.*
Flucloxacillin magnesium (p.209·1) or flucloxacillin sodium (p.209·2).
Bacterial infections.

Staphylex
Alphapharm, Austral.; SmithKline Beecham, Ger.
Flucloxacillin magnesium (p.209·1) or flucloxacillin sodium (p.209·2).
Bacterial infections.

Staphylomycine *SmithKline Beecham, Fr.†.*
Virginiamycin (p.269·3).
Bacterial infections.

Staphypan
Berna, Ital.†; Berna, Switz.
Cell lysate of *Staphylococcus aureus.*
Staphylococcal infections.

Staporos
Cassenne, Fr.†; Hoechst Marion Roussel, Ital.†.
Calcitonin (pork) (p.735·3).
Bone metabolic disorders; hypercalcaemia.

Starasid *Kayaku, Jpn.*
Cytarabine ocfosfate (p.526·1).
Malignant neoplasms.

Starcef *FIRMA, Ital.*
Ceftazidime (p.173·3).
Bacterial infections.

Staril *Squibb, UK.*
Fosinopril sodium (p.870·3).
Heart failure; hypertension.

Starkungs- und Kraftigungstee *Bio-Reform, Aust.*
Achillea bitter orange peel; gentian; rosemary leaf; rose fruit.
Tonic.

Starlep *Farma Lepori, Spain.*
Metoclopramide glycyrrhizinate (p.1202·1); sodium bicarbonate (p.1153·2); tartaric acid (p.1634·3).
Gastritis, nausea; gastro-intestinal hyperacidity; hepatobiliary disorders; vomiting.

Star-Otic *Stellar, USA.*
Glacial acetic acid (p.1541·2); aluminium acetate (p.1547·3); boric acid (p.1554·2).
Ear infection.

Star-Pen *Sanabo, Aust.*
Benzathine phenoxymethylpenicillin (p.159·2) or phenoxymethylpenicillin potassium (p.236·2).
Bacterial infections.

Startonyl *Wyeth Lederle, Aust.*
Citicoline (p.1564·3).
Cerebrovascular disorders; head injury.

Stas Akut *Stada, Ger.*
Acetylcysteine (p.1052·3).
Respiratory-tract disorders with excess mucus.

Stas Erkaltungs-Salbe *Stada, Ger.*
Camphor (p.1557·2); eucalyptus oil (p.1578·1); pine needle oil.
Cold symptoms.

Stas Erkaltungs-Salbe Mild *Stada, Ger.*
Eucalyptus oil (p.1578·1); pine needle oil.
Cold symptoms.

Stas Gurgellosung *Stada, Ger.*
Hexetidine (p.1116·1).
Inflammatory disorders and infections of the oropharynx.

Stas Halsschmerz *Stada, Ger.*
Cetylpyridinium chloride(p.1106·2); dequalinium chloride (p.1112·1).
Bacterial infections of the mouth and throat.

Stas Halstabletten *Stada, Ger.†.*
Acriflavine (p.1098·3); butoxycaine hydrochloride (p.1289·1); tyrothricin (p.267·2); menthol (p.1600·2).
Mouth and throat disorders.

Stas Nasentropfen, Nasenspray *Stada, Ger.*
Xylometazoline hydrochloride (p.1071·2).
Rhinitis.

Stas-Hustenloser *Stada, Ger.*
Ambroxol hydrochloride (p.1054·3).
Respiratory-tract disorders associated with increased or viscous mucus.

Stas-Hustenstiller N *Stada, Ger.*
Clobutinol hydrochloride (p.1057·1).
Formerly contained oxeladin citrate.
Coughs.

Stasten C *UCM-Difme, Ital.†.*
Suprarenal cortex (p.1050·1); sodium ascorbate (p.1365·2); lignocaine hydrochloride (p.1293·2).
Adrenal insufficiency.

Statcillin *Pharmador, S.Afr.†.*
Ampicillin trihydrate (p.153·2).
Bacterial infections.

Stat-Crit *Wampole, USA.*
Test for haematocrit/haemoglobin measurement.

Statex *Pharmascience, Canad.*
Morphine sulphate (p.56·2).
Pain.

Staticin
Westwood-Squibb, Canad.; Westwood, USA.
Erythromycin (p.204·1).
Acne.

Staticine *Bristol-Myers Squibb, Switz.*
Erythromycin (p.204·1).
Acne.

Staticum *Uriach, Spain.*
Glisentide (p.321·1).
Diabetes mellitus.

Statobex *Lemmon, USA†.*
Phendimetrazine tartrate (p.1484·2).
Obesity.

Statrol
Note. This name is used for preparations of different composition.
Alcon, Belg.
Neomycin sulphate (p.229·2); polymyxin B sulphate (p.239·1).
Bacterial eye infections.

Alcon, Spain; Alcon, Switz.†.
Neomycin sulphate (p.229·2); polymyxin B sulphate (p.239·1); phenylephrine hydrochloride (p.1066·2).
Eye infections.

Statuss Expectorant *Huckaby, USA.*
Phenylpropanolamine hydrochloride (p.1067·2); codeine phosphate (p.26·1); guaiphenesin (p.1061·3).
Coughs.

Statuss Green *Huckaby, USA.*
Pheniramine maleate (p.415·3); mepyramine maleate (p.414·1); phenylephrine hydrochloride (p.1066·2); phenylpropanolamine hydrochloride (p.1067·2); hydrocodone tartrate (p.43·1).
Coughs and cold symptoms.

Staufen-Goldtropfen *Staufen, Ger.†.*
Homoeopathic preparation.

Staurodorm
Schoeller, Aust.†; Madaus, Belg.
Flurazepam (p.672·2).
Insomnia.

Staurodorm Neu *Dolorgiet, Ger.*
Flurazepam (p.672·2).
Sleep disorders.

Stay Moist Lip Conditioner *Stanback, USA.*
Padimate O (p.1488·1); oxybenzone (p.1487·3); aloe vera (p.1177·1); vitamin E (p.1369·1).

Stay Trim *Schering-Plough, USA.*
Phenylpropanolamine (p.1067·2).

Staycept Jelly *Roche Consumer, UK†.*
Octoxinol 9 (p.1326·2).
Contraceptive.

Staycept Pessaries *Roche Consumer, UK†.*
Nonoxinol 9 (p.1326·1).
Contraceptive.

Stay-Wet 3 *Sherman, USA.*
Cleansing, wetting, and soaking solution for gas permeable contact lenses.

Stay-Wet 4 *Sherman, USA.*
Wetting solutions for hard contact lenses.

STD
Faulding, Austral.; Intramed, S.Afr.
Sodium tetradecyl sulphate (p.1469·2).
Varicose veins.

Steclin
Bristol-Myers Squibb, Aust.; Bristol-Myers Squibb, Ger.†.
Tetracycline hydrochloride (p.259·1).
Amoebiasis; bacterial infections.

Steclin-V *Squibb, Austral.†.*
Tetracycline hydrochloride (p.259·1).
Bacterial infections.

Stediril
Wyeth Lederle, Belg.; Wyeth, Fr.; Wyeth, Ger.
Norgestrel (p.1454·1); ethinyloestradiol (p.1445·1).
Combined oral contraceptive; endometriosis; menstrual disorders.

Stediril 30
Wyeth Lederle, Belg.; Wyeth, Ger.; Wyeth, Neth.; Wyeth, Switz.
Levonorgestrel (p.1454·1); ethinyloestradiol (p.1445·1).
28-Day packs also contain 7 inert tablets.
Combined oral contraceptive.

Stediril D
Wyeth Lederle, Aust.; Wyeth Lederle, Belg.; Wyeth, Ger.; Wyeth, Switz.
Levonorgestrel (p.1454·1); ethinyloestradiol (p.1445·1).
Combined oral contraceptive; endometriosis; menstrual disorders.

Steicardin N *Steigerwald, Ger.*
Homoeopathic preparation.

Steicorton *Steigerwald, Ger.*
Crataegus (p.1568·2).
Heart failure.

Steigal *Steigerwald, Ger.*
Turmeric (p.1001·3); chelidonium majus.
Biliary colic.

Steinhoff's Fluid Esco Pin *Klever, Ger.†.*
Camphor (p.1557·2); rosemary oil; thyme oil; juniper oil; arnica; chamomile; rhus; ammonia solution.
Pain; rheumatism; sciatica.

Steiprostat *Steigerwald, Ger.*
Saw palmetto (p.1462·1).
Prostatic hyperplasia.

Steirocall *Steierl, Ger.*
Homoeopathic preparation.

Stelabid
Procter & Gamble, Aust.; SmithKline Beecham, Austral.†; SmithKline Beecham, Canad.; Rohm, Ger.†; SmithKline Beecham, Irl.; SmithKline Beecham, S.Afr.†.
Isopropamide iodide (p.464·3); trifluoperazine hydrochloride (p.697·3).
Gastro-intestinal disorders.

Stelazine
SmithKline Beecham, Austral.; SmithKline Beecham, Canad.; SmithKline Beecham, Irl.; SmithKline Beecham, S.Afr.; SmithKline Beecham, UK; SmithKline Beecham, USA.
Trifluoperazine hydrochloride (p.697·3).
Agitation; anxiety; nausea and vomiting; psychoses.

Stellachrome *Stella, Belg.†.*
Mercurochrome (p.1119·2).
Disinfection of skin and minor wounds or burns; skin disorders.

Stellacyl N *Sauter, Switz.†.*
Paracetamol (p.72·2); codeine hydrochloride (p.26·1) or codeine phosphate (p.26·1).
Fever; pain.

Stellacyl nouvelle formule *Roche, Switz.†.*
Paracetamol (p.72·2).
Fever; pain.

Stellamicina *Pierrel, Ital.*
Erythromycin estolate (p.204·1).
Bacterial infections.

Stellaphine *Stella, Belg.†.*
Morphine hydrochloride (p.56·1).
Pain.

Stellarid *SmithKline Beecham, Ital.†.*
Proscillaridin (p.938·1).
Heart failure.

Stellatropine *Stella, Belg.*
Atropine sulphate (p.455·1).
Arrhythmias; cholinesterase inhibitor intoxication; premedication.

Stellavit *Sauter, Switz.†.*
Multivitamin preparation.

Stellisept *Beiersdorf, Switz.*
Orthophenylphenol (p.1120·3); sodium lauryl sulphate (p.1468·3).
Skin and hand disinfection.

Stellorphine *Stella, Belg.*
Morphine hydrochloride (p.56·1).
Acute pulmonary oedema; pain; premedication; severe trauma.

Stemetic *Legere, USA†.*
Trimethobenzamide hydrochloride (p.420·1).

Stemetil
Rhone-Poulenc Rorer, Austral.; Rhone-Poulenc Rorer, Canad.; Rhone-Poulenc Rorer, Irl.; Rhone-Poulenc Rorer, Ital.; Rhone-Poulenc Rorer, Neth.; Rhone-Poulenc Rorer, Norw.; Rhone-Poulenc Rorer, S.Afr.; Rhone-Poulenc Rorer, Swed.; Castlemead, UK.
Prochlorperazine (p.687·3), prochlorperazine maleate (p.687·3), or prochlorperazine mesylate (p.687·3).
Alcohol and opioid withdrawal syndromes; anxiety; mania; migraine; nausea and vomiting; schizophrenia; vestibular disorders.

Stenabolin *AFI, Ital.†.*
Nandrolone phenylpropionate (p.1452·2).
Anabolic.

Stenobronchial *Giovanardi, Ital.*
Potassium guaiacolsulfonate (p.1068·3); wild thyme; tolu balsam (p.1071·1).
Coughs, catarrh.

Stenocor *Lagap, Ital.†.*
Dipyridamole (p.857·1).
Ischaemic heart disease.

Stenocrat *Schwabe, Ger.*
Ammi visnaga fruit (p.1593·2); crataegus leaves and fruit (p.1568·2).
Angina pectoris.

Stenodilate *Schwarz, Ital.†.*
Isosorbide dinitrate (p.893·1); pentaerythritol tetranitrate (p.927·3).
Ischaemic heart disease.

steno-loges N *Loges, Ger.*
Ammi visnaga (p.1593·2).
Cardiac disorders.

Stenoptin *Knoll, Ger.*
Verapamil hydrochloride (p.960·3); isosorbide dinitrate (p.893·1).
Cardiac disorders.

Steno-Valocordin *Promonta, Ger.†.*
Glyceryl trinitrate (p.874·3); bromisoval (p.643·1); phenobarbitone (p.350·2); lupulus (p.1597·2); peppermint oil (p.1208·1).
Angina pectoris.

Stensolo *Salfa, Ital.†.*
Meprobamate (p.678·1).
Anxiety.

Steocin *SoSe, Ital.*
Salcatonin (p.735·3).
Hypercalcaemia; osteoporosis; Paget's disease of bone.

Step 2 *GenDerm, USA.*
Benzyl alcohol (p.1103·3); formic acid (p.1581·3).
Aid to removal of lice eggs.

Sterac *Ivex, UK.*
Sodium chloride (p.1162·2).
Irrigation solution.
Sterile water.
Diluent for antiseptic solutions; wounds.

Steramin *Formenti, Ital.*
Benzalkonium chloride (p.1101·3).
Disinfection of wounds, burns, and mucous membranes.

Steramina G *Formenti, Ital.*
Benzalkonium chloride (p.1101·3).
Disinfection of wounds, burns, vagina, hands, instruments, surfaces, and skin.

Steranabol *Farmitalia Carlo Erba, Ger.†.*
Clostebol acetate (p.1440·2).
Anabolic; diabetic retinopathy; osteoporosis.

Steranabol Ritardo *Pharmacia Upjohn, Ital.*
Oxabolone cypionate (p.1458·2).
Osteoporosis.

Steranabol-Depot *Farmitalia Carlo Erba, Ger.†.*
Oxabolone cypionate (p.1458·2).
Anabolic; diabetic retinopathy; osteoporosis.

Steranios *Anios, Fr.*
Glutaraldehyde (p.1114·3).
Instrument disinfection.

Sterapred *Mayrand, USA.*
Prednisone (p.1049·2).
Corticosteroid.

Sterax
Galderma, Belg.; Galderma, Ger.; Galderma, Switz.
Desonide (p.1036·3).
Skin disorders.

Ster-Dex *Ciba Vision, Fr.*
Oxytetracycline (p.235·1); dexamethasone (p.1037·1).
Eye disorders.

Sterecyt
Kabi Pharmacia, Aust.†; Pharmacia Upjohn, Ger.†; Pharmacia, Swed.†; Pharmacia Upjohn, Switz.†.
Prednimustine (p.559·2).
Malignant neoplasms.

Stereocidin *Crinos, Ital.†.*
Bekanamycin sulphate (p.158·2).
Bacterial infections.

Stereocyt *Pharmacia Upjohn, Fr.†.*
Prednimustine (p.559·2).
Chronic lymphoid leukaemia; non-Hodgkin's lymphosarcoma.

Sterets *Seton, UK.*
Isopropyl alcohol (p.1118·2).
Skin disinfection.

Sterets H *Seton, UK.*
Isopropyl alcohol (p.1118·2); chlorhexidine acetate (p.1107·2).
Skin and instrument disinfection.

Sterexidine *Ivex, UK.*
Chlorhexidine gluconate (p.1107·2).
Antiseptic irrigation solution.

Steridol *Biocure, Ital.*
Chlorhexidine gluconate (p.1107·2); cetrimide (p.1105·2).
Disinfection.

Steridrolo *Molteni, Ital.*
Chloramine (p.1106·3).
Disinfection of wounds, burns, and external genitals.

Steridrolo a rapida idrolisi *Molteni, Ital.*
Halazone (p.1115·1).
Water purification.

Sterigel *Seton, UK.*
Hemicellulose (p.1472·1).
Ulcers; wounds.

Sterijet *Seton, UK.*
Sodium chloride (p.1162·2).
Wound irrigation.

Steril Zeta *Zeta, Ital.*
Cream: Triclosan (Irgasan) (p.1127·2); diacetyl-3,7,9-trihydroxy-8,9b-dimethyl-(9bh)-dibenzofuran-1-one; hamamelis virginiana (p.1587·1); cod-liver oil (p.1337·3).
Insect stings; wound disinfection.
Topical powder: Triclosan (Irgasan) (p.1127·2); 2,6-diacetyl-3,7,9-trihydroxy-8,9b-dimethyl-(9bh)-dibenzofuran-1-one; zinc oxide (p.1096·2); zinc stearate (p.1469·3).
Wound disinfection.

Sterilent *SIFI, Ital.*
Sterilising solution for hard contact lenses.

Sterilet T au Cuivre *Schering, Fr.†.*
Copper-wound plastic (p.1337·3).
Intra-uterine contraceptive device.

Steri-Lette *Gelflex, Austral.†.*
Eye lubricant and lens cleaner for extended-wear contact lenses.

Sterilite *Coventry, UK.*
Tar acids (p.1126·2).

Sterilix *Ircafarm, Ital.*
Benzalkonium chloride (p.1101·3).
Disinfection wounds and burns.

Sterillium
Beiersdorf, Fr.; Bode, Ger.
Mecetronium ethylsulphate (p.1119·1); isopropyl alcohol (p.1118·2); propyl alcohol (p.1124·2).
Skin disinfection.

Sterillium Virugard *Bode, Ger.*
Alcohol (p.1099·1).
Hand disinfection.

Sterilon
Bournonville, Belg.; Boots Healthcare, Neth.; Boots, Spain; Roter, Switz.†.
Chlorhexidine gluconate (p.1107·2) or chlorhexidine hydrochloride (p.1107·2).
Disinfection of skin, wounds, and objects.

Sterilys B 84 *Pharmalink, Swed.†.*
Electrolyte solution (p.1151·1).
Haemodialysis.

Sterimycine *Ciba Vision, Fr.*
Kanamycin sulphate (p.220·3); polymyxin B sulphate (p.239·1).
Eye infections.

SteriNail *Dr. Nordyke's, USA.*
Undecenoic acid (p.389·2); tolnaftate (p.389·1).
Fungal nail infections.

Steri-Neb Cromogen *Baker Norton, Irl.*
Sodium cromoglycate (p.762·1).
Asthma.

Steri-Neb Salamol *Norton Waterford, Irl.*
Salbutamol sulphate (p.758·2).
Obstructive airways disease.

Sterinet *Consol, Ital.*
Cetylpyridinium chloride (p.1106·2).
Skin and hand disinfection.

Sterinor
Heumann, Ger.; ABC, Ital.
Co-tetroxazine (p.196·3).
Bacterial infections.

Sterinova *Medentech, Irl.*
Sodium dichloroisocyanurate (p.1124·3).
Sterilisation of infant feeding equipment.

Steripaste *Seton, UK.*
Zinc oxide (p.1096·2).
Wounds.

Steripod Blue *Seton, UK.*
Sodium chloride (p.1162·2).
Irrigation solution.

Steripod Pink *Seton, UK.*
Chlorhexidine gluconate (p.1107·2).
Skin disinfection.

Steripod Yellow *Seton, UK.*
Chlorhexidine gluconate (p.1107·2); cetrimide (p.1105·2).
Skin disinfection.

Steri-Sal II *Gelflex, Austral.†.*
Chlorhexidine (p.1107·2); thiomersal (p.1126·3).
Soft contact lens sterilisation.

Steri-Soft *Gelflex, Austral.†.*
Methyl, ethyl, propyl, and butyl hydroxybenzoate (Nipastat).
Soft contact lens sterilisation.

Steri/Sol *Warner-Lambert, Canad.*
Hexetidine (p.1116·1).
Mouth and throat disorders.

Steri-Solv *Gelflex, Austral.†.*
Surfactant cleaner for soft contact lenses.

Sterispon *Allen & Hanburys, UK†.*
Gelatin (p.723·2).
Haemorrhage.

Steriwipe *Seton, UK†.*
Chlorhexidine acetate (p.1107·2); cetrimide (p.1105·2).
Skin disinfection.

Sterk hostesirup *Nycomed, Norw.*
Ethylmorphine hydrochloride (p.36·1); codeine phosphate (p.26·1).
Coughs.

Sterlane *Pharmascience, Fr.*
Tincture†: Lauryloxypropyl-β-aminobutyric acid; dodecylaminopropyl-β-aminobutyric acid; miristalkonium chloride (p.1119·3); alcohol (70%) (p.1099·1).
Topical solution; cream: Lauryloxypropyl-β-aminobutyric acid; dodecylaminopropyl-β-aminobutyric acid; miristalkonium chloride (p.1119·3).
Skin disinfection.

Stern Biene Fenchelhonig N *Roland, Ger.*
Fennel oil (p.1579·2).
Congestion; coughs; hoarseness.

Stern Biene Fenchelhonig N Sirup *Roland, Ger.*
Fennel oil (p.1579·2).
Congestion; coughs; hoarseness.

Stern Biene Fencheltee *Makara, Ger.†.*
Fennel (p.1579·1); anise (p.1549·3); coriander (p.1567·3); caraway (p.1559·3); fennel oil (p.1579·2); anise oil (p.1550·1); coriander oil (p.1567·3).
Flatulence; fluid loss; gastro-intestinal cramp.

Sternbiene-Fenchelhonig *Makara, Aust.*
Fennel oil (p.1579·2).
Coughs and cold symptoms.

Sterodelta *Metapharma, Ital.*
Diflorasone diacetate (p.1039·3).
Skin disorders.

Sterofrin *Alcon, Austral.*
Prednisolone acetate (p.1048·1).
Inflammatory and allergic eye disorders.

Sterofundin *Braun, Ger.*
Electrolyte infusion (p.1147·1).
Fluid and electrolyte disorders.

Sterofundin, Sterofundin K *Braun, Aust.*
Electrolyte infusion (p.1147·1).
Fluid and electrolyte disorders.

Sterofundin A
Braun, Aust.; Braun, Ger.†.
Potassium-free electrolyte infusion with glucose (p.1147·1).
Carbohydrate source; fluid and electrolyte disorders.

Sterofundin B, Sterofundin G, Sterofundin HG *Braun, Aust.*
Electrolyte infusion with glucose (p.1147·1).
Carbohydrate source; fluid and electrolyte disorders.

Sterofundin BG *Braun, Ger.*
Electrolyte infusion with glucose (p.1147·1).
Carbohydrate source; fluid and electrolyte disorders.

Sterofundin BX *Braun, Ger.*
Electrolyte infusion with xylitol (p.1147·1).
Carbohydrate source; fluid and electrolyte disorders.

Sterofundin Cal *Braun, Ger.†.*
Carbohydrate infusion with or without electrolytes.
Parenteral nutrition.

Sterofundin CD *Braun, Ger.†.*
Sodium chloride (p.1162·2); sodium bicarbonate (p.1153·2).
Diabetic coma.

Sterofundin CH *Braun, Ger.†.*
Arginine (p.1334·1); malic acid; sorbitol; sodium hydroxide; vitamins.
Liver disease.

Sterofundin CH compositum *Braun, Ger.†.*
Arginine (p.1334·1); malic acid; thioctic acid (p.1636·2); citiolone (p.1564·3); choline chloride (p.1337·1); sorbitol; sodium hydroxide; vitamins.
Liver disease.

Sterofundin F *Braun, Ger.†.*
Electrolyte infusion with fructose (p.1147·1).
Carbohydrate source; fluid and electrolyte disorders.

Sterofundin HEG *Braun, Ger.*
Electrolyte infusion with glucose (p.1147·1).
Carbohydrate source; fluid and electrolyte disorders.

Sterofundin HEX *Braun, Ger.†.*
Electrolyte infusion with malic acid and sorbitol (p.1147·1).
Fluid and electrolyte disorders.

Sterofundin HF *Braun, Ger.†.*
Electrolyte infusion with fructose (p.1147·1).
Carbohydrate source; fluid and electrolyte disorders.

Sterofundin HG *Braun, Ger.†.*
Electrolyte infusion with glucose (p.1147·1).
Carbohydrate source; fluid and electrolyte disorders.

Sterofundin K *Braun, Ger.†.*
Electrolyte infusion (p.1147·1).
Electrolyte disorders; metabolic disorders.

Sterofundin OH⁻ *Braun, Ger.†.*
Sodium lactate (p.1153·2); sorbitol (p.1354·2).
Metabolic acidosis.

Sterofundin R *Braun, Aust.*
Electrolyte infusion (p.1147·1) with rutin sodium sulphate (p.1580·2).
Fluid and electrolyte disorders.

Sterofundin VG *Braun, Ger.*
Electrolyte infusion with glucose (p.1147·1).
Carbohydrate source; fluid and electrolyte disorders.

Sterofundin VX *Braun, Ger.†.*
Electrolyte infusion with malic acid and sorbitol (p.1147·1).
Carbohydrate source; fluid and electrolyte disorders.

Sterogyl
Hoechst Marion Roussel, Belg.; Roussel, Fr.
Ergocalciferol (p.1367·1).
Vitamin D deficiency.

Sterolone *Francia, Ital.*
Fluocinolone acetonide (p.1041·1).
Skin disorders.

Steromien *Compu, S.Afr.*
Betamethasone (p.1033·2).
Corticosteroid.

Sterosan
Note. This name is used for preparations of different composition.
Lachifarma, Ital.
Benzalkonium chloride (p.1101·3); hydroxyiodophenol (p.1121·3).
Skin, wound, and burn disinfection.
Ciba-Geigy, Switz.†.
Chlorquinaldol (p.185·1).
Skin infections.

Steros-Anal
Bristol-Myers Squibb, Aust.; Bristol-Myers Squibb, Ger.; Squibb, Switz.†.
Triamcinolone acetonide (p.1050·2); lignocaine hydrochloride (p.1293·2).
Anorectal disorders.

Sterosan-Hydrocortisone *Ciba-Geigy, Swed.†.*
Chlorquinaldol (p.185·1); hydrocortisone (p.1043·3).
Infected eczema.

Sterox *Granelli, Ital.†.*
Dequalinium chloride (p.1112·1); enoxolone (p.35·2).
Mouth and throat disorders.

Steroxin *Geigy, Austral.†.*
Chlorquinaldol (p.185·1).
Bacterial and fungal skin infections.

Ster-Zac *Houghs Healthcare, UK.*
Bath additive: Triclosan (p.1127·2).
Topical powder; skin cleanser: Hexachlorophane (p.1115·2).
Skin disinfection.

Stesolid
Chemomedica, Aust.; Dumex, Ger.; Dumex, Irl.; Dumex, Neth.†; Dumex, Norw.; Lasa, Spain; Dumex-Alpharma, Swed.; Dumex, Switz.; Dumex, UK.
Diazepam (p.661·1).
Alcohol withdrawal syndrome; anxiety; convulsions; eclampsia; epilepsy; premedication; sedative; skeletal muscle spasm; sleep disorders; status epilepticus; tetanus.

Sthenorex
SCAT, Fr.; Sodip, Switz.†.
Allergen-free pollen extracts.
Tonic.

Stick Ecran Solaire *Clarins, Canad.*
SPF 19: Ethylhexyl *p*-methoxycinnamate (p.1487·1); oxybenzone (p.1487·3); titanium dioxide (p.1093·3).
Sunscreen.

Stick Ecran Total *Vichy, Canad.*
SPF 25: Ethylhexyl *p*-methoxycinnamate (p.1487·1); titanium dioxide (p.1093·3).
Sunscreen.

Stickoxydul *Hoechst, Ger.†.*
Nitrous oxide (p.1228·3).
Inhalational anaesthetic.

Stiedex *Stiefel, UK.*
Cream†: Desoxymethasone (p.1037·1).
Lotion: Desoxymethasone (p.1037·1); salicylic acid (p.1090·2).
Skin disorders.

Stiedex LP *Stiefel, UK.*
Desoxymethasone (p.1037·1).
Skin disorders.

StieLasan *Stiefel, Ger.†.*
Dithranol (p.1082·1); salicylic acid (p.1090·2).
Psoriasis.

Stiemazol
Stiefel, Ger.†; Stiefel, S.Afr.†.
Clotrimazole (p.376·3).
Fungal skin infections.

Stiemycin
Stiefel, Irl.; Stiefel, Neth.; Stiefel, S.Afr.; Stiefel, UK.
Erythromycin (p.204·1).
Acne.

Stiemycine
Salus, Aust.; Stiefel, Ger.; Stiefel, Switz.
Erythromycin (p.204·1).
Acne.

Stieva-A
Stiefel, Austral.; Stiefel, Canad.
Tretinoin (p.1093·3).
Acne.

Stievamycin Stiefel, Canad.
Tretinoin (p.1093·3); erythromycin (p.204·1).
Acne.

Stilamin
Serono, Aust.; Serono, Belg.†; Serono, Canad.; Serono, Ger.†; Serono, Ital.; Serono, Switz.
Somatostatin acetate (p.1261·1).
Biliary, pancreatic, and intestinal fistulae; diabetic ketoacidosis; gastro-intestinal haemorrhage; prevention of postoperative complications following pancreatic surgery; rheumatoid arthritis.

Stilaze Sandipro, Belg.
Lormetazepam (p.677·1).
Insomnia.

Stilene Warner-Lambert Consumer, Belg.
Dipropylene glycol salicylate; capsicum oleoresin.
Musculoskeletal, joint, nerve, and soft-tissue pain.

Stilex Vifor, Switz.
Cream: Mepyramine maleate (p.414·1); lignocaine hydrochloride (p.1293·2); calcium laevulinate (p.1155·2); menthol (p.1600·2).
Skin disorders.
Tablets†: Mepyramine maleate (p.414·1); caffeine (p.749·3).
Hypersensitivity reactions; pruritus.
Topical gel; fluigel; topical spray: Mepyramine maleate (p.414·1); lignocaine hydrochloride (p.1293·2); dexpanthenol (p.1570·3).
Skin disorders.

Stilla
Note. This name is used for preparations of different composition.
Phygiene, Fr.
Phenylephrine hydrochloride (p.1066·2); methylene blue (p.984·3).
Eye disorders.
Unipharma, Switz.†.
Tetrahydrozoline hydrochloride (p.1070·2).
Conjunctival irritation.

Stilla Decongestionante Angelini, Ital.
Tetrahydrozoline hydrochloride (p.1070·2).
Eye irritation.

Stilla Delicato Angelini, Ital.
Benzalkonium chloride (p.1101·3).
Eye disinfection; eye irritation.

Stillacor Wolff, Ger.
β-Acetyldigoxin (p.812·3).
Cardiac disorders.

Stillargol Mayoly-Spindler, Fr.
Silver protein (p.1629·3).
Infections of the eye and nose.

Stilline Berk, UK.
Selegiline hydrochloride (p.1144·2).
Parkinsonism.

Stilnoct
Synthelabo, Belg.; Lorex, Irl.; Lorex Synthelabo, Neth.; Synthelabo, Norw.; Astra, Swed.; Lorex, UK.
Zolpidem tartrate (p.698·3).
Insomnia.

Stilnox
Synthelabo, Aust.; Synthelabo, Fr.; Synthelabo, Ger.; Synthelabo, Ital.; Alonga, Spain; Synthelabo, Switz.
Zolpidem tartrate (p.698·3).
Insomnia.

Stilny
Boehringer Mannheim, Aust.; Will-Pharma, Belg.†.
Nordazepam (p.682·3).
Anxiety disorders; sleep disorders.

Stilpane Lennon, S.Afr.
Capsules: Paracetamol (p.72·2); codeine phosphate (p.26·1); meprobamate (p.678·1).
Pain and associated tension.
Syrup†: Paracetamol (p.72·2); codeine phosphate (p.26·1); promethazine (p.416·2).
Fever; pain.
Tablets: Paracetamol (p.72·2); codeine phosphate (p.26·1); caffeine (p.749·3); meprobamate (p.678·1).
Pain and associated tension.

Stilphostrol Miles, USA.
Fosfestrol (p.1447·1) or fosfestrol sodium (p.1447·1).
Prostatic cancer.

Stimate Armour, USA.
Desmopressin acetate (p.1245·2).
Diabetes insipidus; haemophilia A; von Willebrand's disease.

Stimlor Berk, UK.
Naftidrofuryl oxalate (p.914·2).
Cerebral and peripheral vascular disorders.

Stimol Roussel, Fr.
Citrulline malate (p.1337·2).
Asthenia.

Stimolcardio Panthox & Burck, Ital.†.
Dipyridamole (p.857·1).
Cardiac disorders.

Stimovul
Organon, Ger.†; Organon, Ital.†; Organon, Neth.†.
Epimestrol (p.1444·3).
Anovulatory infertility; amenorrhoea.

Stimtes Lilly, Ital.
Collagen (bovine) (p.1566·3).
Skin ulcers; wounds.

Stimufor Biocodex, Switz.†.
Citrulline malate (p.1337·2).
Tonic.

Stimul Medinova, Switz.
Pemoline (p.1484·1).
Fatigue; hyperactivity; narcoleptic syndrome.

Stimu-LH Roussel, Fr.
Gonadorelin (p.1247·2).
Diagnosis of hypothalamic-pituitary-gonadal dysfunction.

Stimu-TSH Roussel, Fr.
Protirelin (p.1259·1).
Diagnosis of hypothalamic-pituitary-thyroid dysfunction.

Stimuzim Biotekfarma, Ital.
Inosine pranobex (p.615·2).
Immunodeficiency; viral infections.

Stimycine Stiefel, Fr.
Erythromycin (p.204·1).
Acne.

Sting-Eze Wisconsin Pharmacal, USA.
Diphenhydramine hydrochloride (p.409·1); camphor (p.1557·2); phenol (p.1121·2); benzocaine (p.1286·2); cineole (p.1564·1).
Pruritus.

Sting-Kill Kiwi, USA.
Benzocaine (p.1286·2); menthol (p.1600·2).
Skin disorders.

Stingose
Warner-Lambert, Austral.; Boots, S.Afr.; Chancellor, UK.
Aluminium sulphate (p.1548·1).
Insect, plant, and jellyfish stings.

Stioxyl Sylak, Swed.
Benzoyl peroxide (p.1079·2).
Acne.

Stipo Repha, Ger.
Thuja; lycopodium; lemna min.; pulsatilla; mezereum; kal. bichrom.; hydrastis; benzocaine (p.1286·2); ephedrine hydrochloride (p.1059·3); naphazoline hydrochloride (p.1064·2).
Nasal disorders.

Stivane Beaufour, Fr.
Pirisudanol maleate (p.1619·2).
Tonic.

Stix Vifor, Switz.†.
Mepyramine maleate (p.414·1); amylocaine hydrochloride (p.1286·1); chloral hydrate (p.645·3); thymol (p.1127·1); menthol (p.1600·2).
Insect bites.

Stodal Boiron, Fr.
Homoeopathic preparation.

Stoffwechseldragees Molitor, Ger.†.
Papain (p.1614·1); caraway (p.1559·3); urtica (p.1642·3); fennel (p.1579·2); calamus (p.1556·1); antimonium crud.; sodium potassium tartrate (p.1213·3); sodium citrate (p.1153·2); sodium bicarbonate (p.1153·2).
Digestive system disorders.

Stofilan Christiaens, Belg.
Co-dergocrine mesylate (p.1566·1).
Mental function impairment.

STOI-X Apomedica, Aust.†.
Selenium disulphide (p.1091·1).
Dandruff.

Stoko Gard Stockhausen, USA.
Barrier cream.

Stolina Almirall, Spain.
Cyproheptadine cyclamate (p.407·3); amino acids and cyanocobalamin.
Anorexia; tonic; weight loss.

Stoma Anestesia Dental Bucca, Spain.
Potassium hydroxyquinoline sulphate (p.1621·1); lignocaine hydrochloride (p.1293·2).
Adrenaline (p.813·2) and noradrenaline acid tartrate (p.924·1) are included in this preparation as vasoconstrictors to diminish absorption and localise the effect of the local anaesthetic.
Local anaesthesia.

Stomaax Theralab, Canad.
Aluminium hydroxide (p.1177·3); magnesium hydroxide (p.1198·2).

Stomaax Plus Therapex, Canad.
Aluminium hydroxide (p.1177·3); magnesium hydroxide (p.1198·2); simethicone (p.1213·1).

Stomach Calm Brauer, Austral.
Homoeopathic preparation.

Stomach Mixture Potter's, UK.
Bismuth and ammonium citrate (p.1181·1); taraxacum (p.1634·2); gentian root (p.1583·3); rhubarb (p.1212·1).
Dyspepsia.

Stomachiagil Mindel, Ger.†.
Chelidonium majus; boldo (p.1554·1); curcuma zanthorrhiza; euonymus (p.1192·1); cynara (p.1569·2); ox bile (p.1553·2); scopolia carniolica root; aloes (p.1177·1); peppermint oil (p.1208·1).
Digestive system disorders.

Stomachicon N Syxyl, Ger.
Chamomile (p.1561·2); peppermint leaf (p.1208·1); caraway (p.1559·3); dried bitter-orange peel (p.1610·3).
Appetite loss; dyspepsia.

Stomachysat Burger Ysatfabrik, Ger.
Rhubarb (p.1212·1); absinthium (p.1541·1); achillea (p.1542·2); gnaphalium dioicum; peppermint leaves (p.1208·1).
Gastro-intestinal disorders.

Stomacine Plan, Switz.
Pepsin (p.1616·3); condurango (p.1567·2); cardamom (p.1560·1); quassia (p.1624·1).
Gastro-intestinal disorders.

Stomaform Michallik, Ger.†.
Aluminium glycinate (p.1177·2); bismuth subnitrate (p.1180·2); bismuth subgallate (p.1180·2); gentian root (p.1583·3); condurango bark (p.1567·2).
Gastro-intestinal disorders.

Stoma-Gastreu N R5 Reckeweg, Ger.
Homoeopathic preparation.

Stomagel N CPF, Ger.
Aluminium hydroxide gel (p.1177·3); magnesium oxide (p.1198·3).
Gastro-intestinal disorders.

Stomahesive
Note. This name is used for preparations of different composition.
Convatec, Austral.
Topical paste: Butyl monoester polymer with ethanol.
Colostomies and ileostomies.
Convatec, Austral.; ConvaTec, UK.
Wafer: Carmellose sodium (p.1471·2); gelatin (p.723·2); pectin (p.1474·1); polyisobutylene.
Colostomies and ileostomies.

Stom-Antiba Pharmastra, Fr.†.
Alum (p.1547·1); cherry laurel; chloral hydrate (p.645·3); procaine hydrochloride (p.1299·2); thymol (p.1127·1); salicylic acid (p.1090·2); chloroform (p.1220·3); arnica (p.1550·3); mint oil (p.1208·1).
Mouth disorders.

Stomaqualine GABA, Switz.†.
Allantoin (p.1078·2); aluminium chlorohydrate (p.1078·3); tannic acid (p.1634·2); dequalinium chloride (p.1112·1); amethocaine hydrochloride (p.1285·2).
Mouth and gum disorders.

Stomasal Mauermann, Ger.†.
Dried aluminium hydroxide (p.1177·3); dibasic sodium phosphate (p.1159·3); magnesium oxide (p.1198·3); lupulus (p.1597·2); peppermint leaf (p.1208·1); agrimony; calamus (p.1556·1); chlorophyllin (p.1000·1).
Gastro-intestinal disorders.

Stomasal Med Mauermann, Ger.
Aluminium hydroxide (p.1177·3); magnesium oxide (p.1198·3); lupulus (p.1597·2); peppermint leaf (p.1208·1); agrimony; calamus (p.1556·1); chlorophyllin (p.1000·1).
Gastro-intestinal disorders.

Stomax Hope, USA.
Bismuth subgallate (p.1180·2).
Control of ostomy odour.

Stomedine SmithKline Beecham Sante, Fr.
Cimetidine (p.1183·2).
Gastro-oesophageal reflux.

Stomet Sark, Ital.
Cimetidine (p.1183·2).
Gastric hyperacidity; gastro-intestinal haemorrhage; peptic ulcer; Zollinger-Ellison syndrome.

Stomidros Stomygen, Ital.
Calcium hydroxide (p.1556·3).
Dental capping; infection of the dental canal.

Stomigen forte Steiner, Ger.
Magnesium hydroxide (p.1198·2); calcium carbonate (p.1182·1).
Gastro-intestinal disorders.

Stomosan Vicente, Spain.
Bismuth subnitrate (p.1180·2); marrubium vulgare (p.1063·3); sodium bromide (p.1620·3); sodium citrate (p.1153·2).
Gastritis; gastro-intestinal hyperacidity; peptic ulcer.

Stomylex Stomygen, Ital.†.
Calcium oxide (p.1557·1).
Infection of the dental canal.

Stop Oral-B, USA.
Stannous fluoride (p.1632·2).
Dental caries prophylaxis.

Stop Espinilla Normaderm Capilares, Spain.
Benzoyl peroxide (p.1079·2).
Acne.

Stop Hemo
Brothier, Fr.; Brothier, Switz.; G-B-M, UK.
Calcium alginate (p.714·1).
Superficial haemorrhage.

Stopain Astra, Spain†.
Paracetamol (p.72·2).
Fever; pain.

Stopasthme Granions, Mon.†.
Ephedrine hydrochloride (p.1059·3).
Asthma.

Stopayne Adcock Ingram, S.Afr.
Syrup: Paracetamol (p.72·2); codeine phosphate (p.26·1); promethazine hydrochloride (p.416·2).
Tablets; capsules: Paracetamol (p.72·2); codeine phosphate (p.26·1); caffeine (p.749·3); meprobamate (p.678·1).
Fever; pain.

Stopitch Mer-National, S.Afr.
Hydrocortisone acetate (p.1043·3).
Skin disorders.

Stoppers Charwell Pharmaceuticals, UK.
Tobacco substitute.
Aid to smoking withdrawal.

Storzfen Lederle, USA.
Phenylephrine hydrochloride (p.1066·2).
Aid in eye examination; glaucoma; production of mydriasis.

Storzine Lederle, USA.
Pilocarpine hydrochloride (p.1396·3).
Glaucoma; production of miosis; raised intra-ocular pressure.

Storz-N-D Lederle, USA.
Neomycin (p.229·2); dexamethasone sodium phosphate (p.1037·2).
Infected eye disorders.

Storz-N-P-D Lederle, USA.
Neomycin (p.229·2); polymyxin B (p.239·3); dexamethasone (p.1037·1).
Infected eye disorders.

Storzolamide Storz, USA†.
Acetazolamide (p.810·3).

Storz-Sulf Lederle, USA.
Sulphacetamide sodium (p.252·2).
Eye infections.

Stovalid N Redel, Ger.
Peppermint leaves (p.1208·1); absinthium (p.1541·1); fennel (p.1579·1); chamomile (p.1561·2); anise (p.1549·3); caraway (p.1559·3); angelica root; calamus root (p.1556·1); gentian root (p.1583·3).
Gastro-intestinal disorders.

Stovaren Lifepharma, Ital.†.
Cefoxitin sodium (p.170·3).
Bacterial infections.

Stoxil
SmithKline Beecham Consumer, Austral.; SmithKline Beecham, S.Afr.†.
Idoxuridine (p.613·2).
Herpes simplex infections.

Stoxine SmithKline Beecham, Austral.†.
Povidone-iodine (p.1123·3).
Herpes simplex infections of the skin.

Straderm ITA, Ital.†.
Fluocinolone acetonide (p.1041·1).
Skin disorders.

Strains Ointment Nelson, UK.
Homoeopathic preparation.

Straminol Bracco, Ital.†.
Dodecarbonium chloride.
Mouth and throat infections.

Stranoval Teofarma, Ital.
Betamethasone valerate (p.1033·3); dextran sulphate (p.1571·1).
Peripheral vascular disorders; soft-tissue disorders.

Stratene
Gerda, Fr.; Sigma-Tau, Ital.†.
Cetiedil citrate (p.839·1).
Intermittent claudication.

S.trat.os Ghimas, Ital.†.
Clofibrate (p.1271·1); pyricarbate (p.1624·1).
Arteriosclerosis.

Strength Potter's, UK.
Damiana (p.1570·2); kola (p.1645·1); saw palmetto (p.1462·1).
Tonic.

Strepsils
Boots, Austral.; Boots Healthcare, Belg.; Boots Healthcare, Fr.; Boots Healthcare, Irl.; Boots Healthcare, Neth.; Boots, S.Afr.; Boots, Spain; Astra, Swed.; Crookes Healthcare, UK.
Dichlorobenzyl alcohol (p.1112·2); amylmetacresol (p.1101·3).
Sore throat.

Strepsils Anaesthetic Boots, Austral.†.
Lignocaine hydrochloride (p.1293·2); dichlorobenzyl alcohol (p.1112·2); amylmetacresol (p.1101·3).
Mouth ulcers; sore throat.

Strepsils con Vitamina C Boots, Spain.
Sodium ascorbate (p.1365·2); ascorbic acid (p.1365·2); dichlorobenzyl alcohol (p.1112·2); amylmetacresol (p.1101·3).
Sore throat.

Strepsils Direct Action Spray Crookes Healthcare, UK.
Lignocaine hydrochloride (p.1293·2).
Sore throat.

Strepsils Dual Action
Boots Healthcare, Irl.; Crookes Healthcare, UK.
Amylmetacresol (p.1101·3); dichlorobenzyl alcohol (p.1112·2); lignocaine (p.1293·2) or lignocaine hydrochloride (p.1293·2).
Sore throat.

Strepsils Eucalyptus Menthol Boots, S.Afr.
Dichlorobenzyl alcohol (p.1112·2); amylmetacresol (p.1101·3); menthol (p.1600·2).
Sore throat.

Strepsils Extra Crookes Healthcare, UK.
Hexylresorcinol (p.1116·1).
Sore throat.

Strepsils Menthol Boots Healthcare, Belg.
Dichlorobenzyl alcohol (p.1112·2); amylmetacresol (p.1101·3); menthol (p.1600·2).
Nasal congestion; sore throat.

Strepsils Menthol en Eucalyptus *Boots Healthcare, Neth.*
Amylmetacresol (p.1101·3); dichlorobenzyl alcohol (p.1112·2); menthol (p.1600·2); eucalyptus oil (p.1578·1).
Sore throat.

Strepsils Menthol Eucalyptus *Boots, Fr.†.*
Amylmetacresol (p.1101·3); dichlorobenzyl alcohol (p.1112·2); menthol (p.1600·2).
Sore throat.

Strepsils Miel-Citron *Boots Healthcare, Fr.*
Amylmetacresol (p.1101·3); dichlorobenzyl alcohol (p.1112·2).
Sore throat.

Strepsils Orange-C *Boots, S.Afr.*
Dichlorobenzyl alcohol (p.1112·2); amylmetacresol (p.1101·3); ascorbic acid (p.1365·2); menthol (p.1600·2).
Sore throat.

Strepsils Plus
Boots, Austral.; Boots, S.Afr.
Dichorobenzyl alcohol (p.1112·2); amylmetacresol (p.1101·3); lignocaine (p.1293·2) or lignocaine hydrochloride (p.1293·2).
Sore throat.

Strepsils Sinaasappel en Vitamine C *Boots Healthcare, Neth.*
Dichlorobenzyl alcohol (p.1112·2); amylmetacresol (p.1101·3); ascorbic acid (p.1365·2).
Sore throat.

Strepsils Soothing Honey & Lemon *Boots, S.Afr.*
Dichorobenzyl alcohol (p.1112·2); amylmetacresol (p.1101·3).
Sore throat.

Strepsils Vit C *Boots Healthcare, Belg.*
Dichlorobenzyl alcohol (p.1112·2); amylmetacresol (p.1101·3); ascorbic acid (p.1365·2); sodium ascorbate (p.1365·2).
Sore throat.

Strepsils Vitamin C *Boots Healthcare, Irl.*
Amylmetacresol (p.1101·3); dichlorobenzyl alcohol (p.1112·2); vitamin C (p.1365·2).
Sore throat.

Strepsils with Vitamin C *Crookes Healthcare, UK.*
Sodium ascorbate (p.1365·2); amylmetacresol (p.1101·3); dichlorobenzyl alcohol (p.1112·2).
Sore throat.

Strepsils Vitamine C *Boots Healthcare, Fr.*
Amylmetacresol (p.1101·3); dichlorobenzyl alcohol (p.1112·2); ascorbic acid (p.1365·2); sodium ascorbate (p.1365·2).
Sore throat.

Strepsilspray Lidocaine *Boots Healthcare, Fr.*
Amylmetacresol (p.1101·3); dichlorobenzyl alcohol (p.1112·2); lignocaine (p.1293·2).
Mouth and throat infections.

Streptan *Also, Ital.†.*
Streptomycin sulphate (p.249·3); menadiol sodium sulphate (p.1371·3); nicotinamide (p.1351·2).
Bacterial infections of the gastro-intestinal tract.

Streptase
Hoechst, Aust.; Hoechst Marion Roussel, Austral.; Hoechst Marion Roussel, Belg.; Hoechst Marion Roussel, Canad.; Hoechst, Fr.; Hoechst, Ger.; Hoechst Marion Roussel, Irl.; Hoechst Marion Roussel, Ital.; Behring, Neth.; Behring, Norw.; Hoechst Marion Roussel, S.Afr.; Hoechst, Spain; Hoechst Marion Roussel, Swed.; Centeon, Switz.; Hoechst Marion Roussel, UK; Astra, USA.
Streptokinase (p.948·2).
Thrombo-embolic disorders.

Streptocol *Molteni, Ital.*
Streptomycin sulphate (p.249·3).
Bacterial infections of the gastro-intestinal tract.

Strepto-Fatol *Fatol, Ger.*
Streptomycin sulphate (p.249·3).
Bacterial infections; tuberculosis.

Streptomagma *Wyeth, Ital.*
Oral suspension: Dried aluminium hydroxide (p.1177·3); heavy kaolin (p.1195·1); pectin (p.1474·1). *Tablets:* Activated attapulgite (p.1178·3); pectin (p.1474·1); dried aluminium hydroxide (p.1177·3).
Diarrhoea.

Strepto-Plus *Molteni, Ital.*
Co-trimoxazole (p.196·3).
Bacterial infections.

Streptosil con Neomicina-Fher *Boehringer Ingelheim, Ital.*
Neomycin sulphate (p.229·2); sulphathiazole (p.257·1).
Bacterial skin infections.

Streptosil L PMC *Fher, Ital.*
Benzalkonium chloride (p.1101·3).
Skin and hand disinfection.

Streptozyme
Carter-Wallace, Switz.; Wampole, USA.
Test for streptococcal extracellular antigens in blood, plasma, and serum.

Stresam *Biocodex, Fr.*
Etifoxin hydrochloride (p.669·3).
Anxiety.

Streso B *Eagle, Austral.†.*
Multivitamin, mineral, and nutritional preparation.

Stress *Homeocan, Canad.*
Homoeopathic preparation.

Stress 600 *Nion, USA.*
Multivitamin and mineral preparation.

Stress B Complex with Vitamins C & E *Pharmavite, Canad.*
Vitamin B substances, vitamin C, and vitamin E.

Stress B-Complex *Moore, USA.*
Multivitamin and mineral preparation.

Stress Formula
Wampole, Canad.; Nature's Bounty, USA.
A range of vitamin preparations.

Stress Formula B Compound plus Vitamin C *Quest, Canad.*
Vitamin B substances and vitamin C.

Stress Formula with Iron *Nature's Bounty, USA.*
Multivitamin preparation with iron and folic acid.

Stress Plex C *Jamieson, Canad.*
Vitamin B substances, vitamin C, and zinc.

Stress Relief *Brauer, Austral.*
Homoeopathic preparation.

Stress Tab *Shoppers Drug Mart, Canad.*
Vitamin B substances and vitamin C.

Stress Tablets *Drug Trading, Canad.*
Vitamin B substances and vitamin C.

Stresscaps
Lederle, Ger.†; Lederle, USA.
Vitamin B substances with vitamin C.

Stressease *Jamieson, Canad.*
Multivitamin and mineral preparation.

Stressen *Medosan, Ital.*
Amino-acid and vitamin preparation.
Tonic.

StressForm "605" with Iron *Nature's Bounty, USA.*
Multivitamin preparation with iron.

Stressgard *Miles, Canad.†.*
Multivitamin and mineral preparation.

Stresson
Bender, Aust.; Boehringer Ingelheim, Ger.†.
Bunitrolol hydrochloride (p.835·2).
Cardiac disorders; hypertension.

Stresstabs
Whitehall-Robins, Canad.; Lederle, USA.
A range of vitamin preparations with or without minerals.

Stresstein *Sandoz Nutrition, USA.*
Preparation for enteral nutrition.
Stress.

Striadyne *Wyeth, Fr.†.*
Adenosine triphosphate, disodium salt (p.1543·2).
Arrhythmias.

Striaton *Knoll, Ger.*
Levodopa (p.1137·1); carbidopa (p.1136·1).
Parkinsonism.

Striatridin *Opfermann, Ger.*
Alkylated fatty-acid esters of octadecyl alcohols; hydrolysed albumin; ethyl nicotinate (p.36·1).
Skin disorders.

Stri-Dex Antibacterial Cleansing *Sterling, USA.*
Triclosan (p.1127·2).

Stri-Dex Clear *Sterling, USA.*
Salicylic acid (p.1090·2).

Stridex Face Wash *Sterling Health, USA.*
Triclosan (p.1127·2).
Skin cleanser.

Stri-Dex Pads *Glenbrook, USA.*
Salicylic acid (p.1090·2); alcohol (p.1099·1).
Acne.

Stringan
Strallhofer, Aust.; Kabi, Switz.†.
Polyphloretin phosphate; phenylephrine (p.1066·2) or phenylephrine hydrochloride (p.1066·2).
Nasal congestion.

Strocain *Eisai, Jpn.*
Oxethazaine (p.1298·1).
Gastro-intestinal disorders.

Strodival
Merz & Schoeller, Aust.†; Herbert, Ger.
Ouabain (p.925·2).
Cardiac disorders.

Strofopan Vena *Simes, Ital.†.*
Strophanthin-K (p.951·1).
Heart failure.

Strogen *Strathmann, Ger.*
Saw palmetto (p.1462·1).
Prostatic hyperplasia.

Stromba
Sanofi Winthrop, Belg.; Sanofi Winthrop, Irl.; Sanofi Winthrop, Neth.; Sanofi Winthrop, UK.
Stanozolol (p.1462·2).
Anabolic; angioedema; cutaneous vasculitis; osteoporosis; Raynaud's syndrome; scleroderma; thrombo-embolic disorders.

Strombaject *Sanofi Winthrop, Belg.*
Stanozolol (p.1462·2).
Anabolic.

Stromectol
Merck Sharp & Dohme, Austral.; Merck, USA.
Ivermectin (p.101·1).
Onchocerciasis; strongyloidiasis.

Stromic *Strathmann, Ger.*
Solidago virgaurea.
Urinary-tract disorders.

217 Strong *Frosst, Canad.*
Aspirin (p.16·1); caffeine citrate (p.749·3).
Fever; inflammation; pain.

Stronglife *Pascoe, Ger.†.*
Homoeopathic preparation.

Strongus *Franconpharm, Ger.*
Garlic (p.1583·1).
Hyperlipidaemia.

Strophanon *Athenstaedt, Ger.†.*
Ouabain (p.925·2); convallaria (p.1567·2); crataegus (p.1568·2); camphor; saponin.
Cardiac disorders.

Strophanthus *Phytomed, Switz.*
Homoeopathic preparation.

Strophanthus-Strath *Strath-Labor, Ger.†.*
Convallaria (p.1567·2); crataegus (p.1568·2); digitalis purpura (p.848·3); strophanthus (p.951·1).
Cardiac disorders.

Stropheupas-forte *Pascoe, Ger.*
Homoeopathic preparation.

Strophocor N *Hennig, Ger.*
Ouabain (p.925·2).
Cardiac disorders.

Strotan *Strathmann, Ger.*
Agnus castus (p.1544·2).
Mastalgia; menstrual disorders.

Strovite *Everett, USA.*
A range of vitamin and mineral preparations.

Structolipid *Pharmacia Upjohn, Swed.*
Coconut oil (p.1383·3); soya oil (p.1355·1).
Contains egg phospholipid.
Lipid infusion for parenteral nutrition.

Structum
Robapharm, Fr.; Robapharm, Switz.
Sodium chondroitin sulphate (p.1562·2).
Arthroses.

Strumazol
Christiaens, Belg.; Nourypharma, Neth.
Methimazole (p.1495·3).
Hyperthyroidism.

Strumedical 400 *Henning, Ger.*
Diiodotyrosine (p.1493·1).
Iodine-deficiency disorders.

Strumetten *Roland, Ger.†.*
Homoeopathic preparation.

Strumex *Robugen, Ger.*
Sodium iodide (p.1493·2).
Iodine-deficiency disorders.

Stryphnasal *Serturner, Ger.*
Adrenalone hydrochloride (p.1543·3).
Formerly known as Stryphonasal.
Epistaxis.

Stuart Formula *J&J-Merck, USA.*
Multivitamin and mineral preparation with iron and folic acid.

Stuart Prenatal *Wyeth-Ayerst, USA.*
Multivitamin and mineral preparation with folic acid and iron.
Dietary supplement in pregnancy.

Stuartinic *J&J-Merck, USA.*
Ferrous fumarate (p.1339·3); vitamin B substances with vitamin C.
Iron-deficiency anaemias.

Stuartnatal 1+1 *Wyeth-Ayerst, USA.*
Multivitamin and mineral preparation with iron and folic acid.
Dietary supplement in pregnancy.

Stuartnatal Plus *Wyeth-Ayerst, USA.*
Multivitamin and mineral preparation.

Stubit *Pickles, UK.*
Nicotine (p.1607·2).
Aid to smoking withdrawal.

Stud 100 *Key, Austral.*
Lignocaine (p.1293·2).
Premature ejaculation.

Stugeron
Janssen-Cilag, Belg.; Janssen-Cilag, Irl.; Janssen-Cilag, Ital.; Janssen-Cilag, S.Afr.; Esteve, Spain; Janssen-Cilag, Switz.; Janssen-Cilag, UK; Johnson & Johnson MSD Consumer, UK.
Cinnarizine (p.406·1).
Cerebral and peripheral vascular disorders; migraine; motion sickness; nausea and vomiting; vestibular disorders.

Stullmaton *Stulln, Ger.*
Centaury (p.1561·1); arnica (p.1550·3); melissa (p.1600·1); chamomile (p.1561·2); absinthium (p.1541·1); spruce tips; trace elements.
Gastro-intestinal disorders.

Stutgeron
Janssen-Cilag, Aust.; Janssen-Cilag, Ger.
Cinnarizine (p.406·1).
Cerebral and peripheral vascular disorders; vestibular disorders.

Stutgeron-Digoxin *Janssen-Cilag, Ger.†.*
Cinnarizine (p.406·1); digoxin (p.849·3).
Cardiovascular disorders.

Stye *Del, USA†.*
Yellow mercuric oxide (p.1601·3).
Minor eye infections.

Stylo Sport *Lancome, Canad.*
SPF 15: Ethylhexyl *p*-methoxycinnamate (p.1487·1); titanium dioxide (p.1093·3).
Sunscreen.

Styptanon
Bender, Aust.; Organon, Switz.†.
Oestriol sodium succinate (p.1457·2).
Capillary haemorrhage.

Styptobion *Merck, Ger.†.*
Ascorbic acid (p.1365·2); menadiol dibutyrate (p.1371·3); rutin (p.1580·2).
Haemorrhagic disorders.

Stypto-Caine *Pedinol, USA.*
Aluminium chloride (p.1078·3); amethocaine (p.1285·2); hydroxyquinoline sulphate (p.1589·3).
Bleeding in minor wounds.

Styptysat *Ysatfabrik, Ger.*
Capsella bursa pastoris.
Haemorrhagic disorders.

Suadian *Schering, Ital.*
Naftifine hydrochloride (p.385·3).
Fungal skin and nail infections.

Sualyn *Vita, Spain.*
Bismuth subnitrate (p.1180·2); magnesium carbonate (p.1198·1); metoclopramide hydrochloride (p.1200·3); sorbitol (p.1354·2).
Gastric spasms; gastritis; nausea; peptic ulcer; vomiting.

Suamoxil *Cantabria, Spain.*
Amoxycillin trihydrate (p.151·3).
Bacterial infections.

Suaviter *Boehringer Mannheim, Ital.*
Aspartame (p.1335·1).
Sugar substitute.

Suavuret *Organon, Spain.*
Ethinyloestradiol (p.1445·1); desogestrel (p.1443·3).
Combined oral contraceptive; menstrual disorders.

Sub Tensin *Byk Elmu, Spain.*
Nitrendipine (p.923·1).
Hypertension.

Subcutin N *Ritsert, Ger.*
Benzocaine (p.1286·2).
Gastro-intestinal pain and inflammation.

Sublimaze
Janssen-Cilag, Austral.; Janssen-Ortho, Canad.; Janssen-Cilag, Irl.; Janssen-Cilag, S.Afr.; Janssen, UK; Janssen, USA.
Fentanyl citrate (p.38·1).
Adjunct to anaesthesia; neuroleptanalgesia; pain.

Sublivac B.E.S.T. *HAL, Neth.*
Allergen extracts (p.1545·1).
Hyposensitisation.

Subreum *Tosse, Ger.*
E. coli antigens.
Chronic polyarthritis.

Substi *Abbott, Fr.*
Preparation for enteral nutrition.

Substitol *Solvay, Aust.*
Oestradiol (p.1455·1).
Oestrogen deficiency.

Subutex *Schering-Plough, Fr.*
Buprenorphine hydrochloride (p.22·2).
Opioid withdrawal syndrome.

Sucaryl
Note. This name is used for preparations of different composition.
Abbott, Austral.; Abbott, Fr.
Calcium cyclamate (p.1338·3) or sodium cyclamate (p.1338·3); saccharin sodium (p.1353·3).
Sugar substitute.

Abbott, Canad.
Sodium cyclamate (p.1338·3) with or without glucose.
Sugar substitute.

Succicuran *Rodleben, Ger.*
Suxamethonium chloride (p.1319·1).
Depolarising neuromuscular blocker.

Succilate *Garec, S.Afr.*
Erythromycin estolate (p.204·1).
Bacterial infections.

Succin *Garec, S.Afr.*
Erythromycin ethyl succinate (p.204·2).
Bacterial infections.

Succinolin *Amino, Switz.*
Suxamethonium chloride (p.1319·1).
Depolarising neuromuscular blocker.

Succinyl
Asta Medica, Ger.†; Dagra, Neth.†; Asta Medica, Switz.†.
Suxamethonium chloride (p.1319·1).
Depolarising neuromuscular blocker.

Succosa *Tika, Swed.*
Sucralfate (p.1214·2).
Peptic ulcer.

Succus Cineraria Maritima *Walker Pharmacal, USA.*
Senecio (p.1628·1); hamamelis (p.1587·1); boric acid (p.1554·2).
Cataract opacity.

Sucontral *Harras-Curarina, Ger.*
Coutarea latiflora.
Diabetes mellitus (adjuvant).

Sucostrin *Apothecon, USA†.*
Suxamethonium chloride (p.1319·1).
Depolarising neuromuscular blocker.

Sucrabest *Hexal, Ger.*
Sucralfate (p.1214·2).
Peptic ulcer.

Sucrager *Ripari-Gero, Ital.*
Sucralfate (p.1214·2).
Gastritis; gastro-oesophageal reflux; peptic ulcer.

Sucraid *Orphan Medical, USA.*
Sacrosidase (p.1627·1).
Sucrase deficiency.

Sucral *Bioprogress, Ital.*
Sucralfate (p.1214·2).
Gastritis; gastro-oesophageal reflux; peptic ulcer.

Sucralan *Lannacher, Aust.*
Sucralfate (p.1214·2).
Gastro-oesophageal reflux; peptic ulcer.

Sucralbene *Merckle, Aust.*
Sucralfate (p.1214·2).
Gastro-oesophageal reflux; peptic ulcer; stress-related gastro-intestinal haemorrhage.

Sucralfin *Inverni della Beffa, Ital.*
Sucralfate (p.1214·2).
Gastritis; gastro-oesophageal reflux; peptic ulcer.

Sucramal *Sanofi Winthrop, Ital.*
Sucralfate (p.1214·2).
Gastritis; gastro-oesophageal reflux; peptic ulcer.

Sucraphil *Philopharm, Ger.*
Sucralfate (p.1214·2).
Gastro-oesophageal reflux; peptic ulcer.

Sucrate *Lisapharma, Ital.*
Sucralfate (p.1214·2).
Gastritis; gastro-oesophageal reflux; peptic ulcer.

Sucredulcor *Pierre Fabre, Fr.*
Saccharin (p.1353·2).
Sugar substitute.

Sucrets
Note. This name is used for preparations of different composition.
SmithKline Beecham Consumer, Canad.
Hexylresorcinol (p.1116·1).
Sore throat.

SmithKline Beecham Consumer, USA.
Dyclocaine hydrochloride (p.1292·3).
Sore throat.

Sucrets Cough Control
SmithKline Beecham Consumer, Canad.; SmithKline Beecham, USA.
Dextromethorphan (p.1057·3) or dextromethorphan hydrobromide (p.1057·3).
Coughs.

Sucrets 4-Hour Cough *SmithKline Beecham Consumer, USA.*
Dextromethorphan (p.1057·3).
Coughs.

Sucrets for Kids *SmithKline Beecham Consumer, Canad.*
Dyclocaine hydrochloride (p.1292·3).

Sucrets Sore Throat *SmithKline Beecham Consumer, USA.*
Hexylresorcinol (p.1116·1).
Sore throat.

Sucrinburck *Panthox & Burck, Ital.†.*
Fructose (p.1343·2); saccharin (p.1353·2).
Sugar substitute.

Suczulen *Minden, Ger.†.*
Liquorice (p.1197·1); guaiazulene (p.1586·3).
Gastro-intestinal disorders.

Suczulen compositum *Minden, Ger.†.*
Liquorice (p.1197·1); guaiazulene (p.1586·3); 2-pyrrolidinoethyl(2-phenylbicyclo(2.2.1)heptan-2-carboxylate) hydrochloride.
Gastro-intestinal disorders.

Suczulen mono *Knoll, Ger.*
Liquorice (p.1197·1).
Peptic ulcer.

Sudac *Errekappa, Ital.†.*
Sulindac (p.86·3).
Fever; inflammation; pain.

Sudafed
Warner-Lambert, Austral.; Wellcome, Belg.†; Warner-Lambert, Canad.; Glaxo Wellcome, Fr.; Calmic, Irl.; Warner-Lambert, Ital.; Glaxo Wellcome, S.Afr.; Wellcome, Spain†; Warner-Lambert, UK; Wellcome, USA.
Pseudoephedrine hydrochloride (p.1068·3).
Upper respiratory-tract congestion.

Sudafed Co *Warner-Lambert, UK.*
Pseudoephedrine hydrochloride (p.1068·3); paracetamol (p.72·2).
Fever; pain; upper respiratory-tract congestion.

Sudafed Cold & Cough
Note. This name is used for preparations of different composition.
Warner-Lambert, Canad.
Pseudoephedrine hydrochloride (p.1068·3); dextromethorphan hydrobromide (p.1057·3); paracetamol (p.72·2).
Coughs and cold symptoms.

Wellcome, USA.
Dextromethorphan hydrobromide (p.1057·3); pseudoephedrine hydrochloride (p.1068·3); paracetamol (p.72·2); guaiphenesin (p.1061·3).
Coughs and cold symptoms.

Sudafed Cold & Flu *Warner-Lambert, Canad.*
Paracetamol (p.72·2); dextromethorphan (p.1057·3); guaiphenesin (p.1061·3); pseudoephedrine hydrochloride (p.1068·3).
Coughs and cold symptoms.

Sudafed Cough *Wellcome, USA†.*
Pseudoephedrine hydrochloride (p.1068·3); dextromethorphan hydrobromide (p.1057·3); guaiphenesin (p.1061·3).
Coughs.

Sudafed DM *Warner-Lambert, Canad.*
Pseudoephedrine hydrochloride (p.1068·3); dextromethorphan hydrobromide (p.1057·3).
Cold symptoms; nasal congestion.

Sudafed Expectorant
Wellcome, Canad.†; Calmic, Irl.; Glaxo Wellcome, S.Afr.; Warner-Lambert, UK.
Pseudoephedrine hydrochloride (p.1068·3); guaiphenesin (p.1061·3).
Coughs; upper respiratory-tract congestion.

Sudafed Head Cold & Sinus *Warner-Lambert, Canad.*
Paracetamol (p.72·2); pseudoephedrine hydrochloride (p.1068·3).
Cold symptoms; sinus pain.

Sudafed Linctus *Warner-Lambert, UK.*
Dextromethorphan hydrobromide (p.1057·3); pseudoephedrine hydrochloride (p.1068·3).
Coughs; upper respiratory-tract congestion.

Sudafed Nasal Spray *Warner-Lambert, UK.*
Oxymetazoline hydrochloride (p.1065·3).
Nasal congestion.

Sudafed Plus
Note. This name is used for preparations of different composition.
Warner-Lambert, Austral.
Pseudoephedrine hydrochloride (p.1068·3); paracetamol (p.72·2); triprolidine hydrochloride (p.420·3).
Formerly known as Sudagesic.
Sinus disorders.

Warner-Lambert, UK.
Triprolidine hydrochloride (p.420·3); pseudoephedrine hydrochloride (p.1068·3).
Allergic rhinitis.

Wellcome, USA.
Pseudoephedrine hydrochloride (p.1068·3); chlorpheniramine maleate (p.405·1).
Upper respiratory-tract symptoms.

Sudafed Severe Cold *Wellcome, USA.*
Pseudoephedrine hydrochloride (p.1068·3); dextromethorphan hydrobromide (p.1057·3); paracetamol (p.72·2).
Coughs and cold symptoms.

Sudafed Sinus
Wellcome, Canad.†; Wellcome, USA.
Pseudoephedrine hydrochloride (p.1068·3); paracetamol (p.72·2).
Nasal congestion.

Sudagesic *Glaxo Wellcome, S.Afr.*
Pseudoephedrine hydrochloride (p.1068·3); paracetamol (p.72·2).
Cold and influenza symptoms.

Sudal *Atley, USA.*
Pseudoephedrine hydrochloride (p.1068·3); guaiphenesin (p.1061·3).
Coughs.

Sudermin *Interpharma, Spain†.*
Aluminium chlorohydrate (p.1078·3); nystatin (p.386·1); salicylic acid (p.1090·2).
Fungal skin infections; hyperhidrosis; intertrigo.

Sudex *Roberts, USA†.*
Pseudoephedrine hydrochloride (p.1068·3).
Formerly contained pseudoephedrine hydrochloride and guaiphenesin.
Nasal congestion.

Sudocrem
Tosara, Irl.; Tosara, UK.
Zinc oxide (p.1096·2); benzyl benzoate (p.1402·2); benzyl cinnamate; benzyl alcohol (p.1103·3).
Acne; bed sores; burns; chilblains; eczema; napkin rash; sunburn; wounds.

Sudodrin *ICN, Canad.*
Pseudoephedrine hydrochloride (p.1068·3).

Sudol *Coventry, UK.*
Tar acids (p.1126·2).

Sudosin *Medea, Spain.*
Formaldehyde (p.1113·2); lindane (p.1407·2); aminobenzoic acid (p.1486·3); salicylic acid (p.1090·2); talc; thymol (p.1127·1); lavender essence.
Skin disorders.

Suero Fisio Andal Farm *Andalucia, Spain†.*
Sodium chloride (p.1162·2).
Fluid and electrolyte depletion; hypovolaemia.

Suero Fisio Hayem Rapide *Bieffe, Spain†.*
Sodium chloride (p.1162·2).
Fluid and electrolyte depletion; hypovolaemia.

Suero Fisio Vitulia *Ern, Spain†.*
Sodium chloride (p.1162·2).
Fluid and electrolyte depletion; hypovolaemia.

Suero Fisiologico *IBYS, Spain†.*
Sodium chloride (p.1162·2).
Fluid and electrolyte depletion; hypovolaemia.

Suero Glucosalino *IBYS, Spain†.*
Sodium chloride infusion (p.1162·2) with glucose (p.1343·3).
Fluid and electrolyte depletion.

Suero Levoglusal Vitulia *Ern, Spain†.*
Electrolyte infusion with fructose (p.1147·1).
Carbohydrate source; fluid and electrolyte depletion.

Suero Potassico Bieffe ME *Bieffe, Spain.*
Potassium chloride (p.1161·1); sodium chloride (p.1162·2).
Diabetic ketoacidosis; hypokalaemia.

Suero Ringer And Farm *Andalucia, Spain†.*
Electrolyte infusion (p.1147·1).
Fluid and electrolyte depletion.

Suero Ringer Rapide *Bieffe, Spain†.*
Electrolyte infusion (p.1147·1).
Fluid and electrolyte depletion.

Sueroral *Casen Fleet, Spain.*
Glucose; potassium chloride; sodium bicarbonate; sodium chloride (p.1152·3).
Diarrhoea; oral rehydration therapy.

Sueroral Hiposodico *Casen Fleet, Spain.*
Glucose; potassium chloride; sucrose; sodium bicarbonate; sodium chloride (p.1152·3).
Diarrhoea; oral rehydration therapy.

Sufenta
Janssen-Cilag, Aust.; Janssen-Cilag, Belg.; Janssen-Ortho, Canad.; Janssen-Cilag, Fr.; Janssen-Cilag, Ger.; Janssen-Cilag, Neth.; Janssen-Cilag, Norw.; Janssen-Cilag, S.Afr.; Janssen-Cilag, Swed.; Janssen-Cilag, Switz.; Janssen, USA.
Sufentanil citrate (p.85·2).
General anaesthesia; pain.

Sufil *Elfar, Spain.*
Mebendazole (p.104·1).
Worm infections.

Sufortan *Farmades, Ital.†.*
Penicillamine (p.988·3).
Cystinuria; heavy-metal poisoning; hepatitis; rheumatoid arthritis; scleroderma; Wilson's disease.

Sufortanon *Asta Medica, Spain.*
Penicillamine (p.988·3).
Biliary cirrhosis; cystinuria; heavy-metal poisoning; rheumatoid arthritis; Wilson's disease.

Sufrexal
Janssen-Cilag, Belg.; Janssen-Cilag, Ital.; Janssen-Cilag, Switz.†.
Ketanserin tartrate (p.894·3).
Hypertension.

Sugar Bloc *Cantassium Co., UK.*
Gymnena sylvestre; chromium orotate (p.1611·2).
Diet aid.

Sugarbil *Novag, Spain.*
Cyclobutyrol sodium (p.1569·2); magnesium sulphate (p.1157·3); sorbitol (p.1354·2).
Constipation; hepatobiliary disorders.

Sugarceton *Novag, Spain.*
Calcium fructose diphosphate; hydroxocobalamin hydrochloride (p.1364·2); promethazine hydrochloride (p.416·2); thiamine phosphate (p.1361·2); trometamol acephyllinate (p.1640·1); trometamol thioctate (p.1640·1); sorbitol (p.1354·2); glucose (p.1343·3).
Acetonaemia; acidosis.

Sugarless C *Cenovis, Austral.; Vitelle, Austral.*
Ascorbic acid (p.1365·2); sodium ascorbate (p.1365·2).
Vitamin C supplement.

Sugast *Selvi, Ital.*
Sucralfate (p.1214·2).
Gastritis; gastro-oesophageal reflux; peptic ulcer.

Sugiran *Pensa, Spain.*
Alprostadil alfadex (p.1413·1).
Peripheral vascular disease.

Suguan *Hoechst Marion Roussel, Ital.*
Glibenclamide (p.319·3); phenformin hydrochloride (p.330·3).
Diabetes mellitus.

Suguan M *Hoechst Marion Roussel, Ital.*
Glibenclamide (p.319·3); metformin hydrochloride (p.330·1).
Diabetes mellitus.

Suismycetin *Lagap, Switz.†.*
Chloramphenicol (p.182·1) or chloramphenicol palmitate (p.182·2).
Bacterial infections.

Sulamid *Baldacci, Ital.*
Amisulpride (p.641·2).
Depression.

Sular
Zeneca, Neth.; Zeneca, USA.
Nisoldipine (p.922·3).
Angina pectoris; hypertension.

Sulartrene *NCSN, Ital.*
Sulindac (p.86·3).
Gout; musculoskeletal, joint, peri-articular, and soft-tissue disorders.

Sulazine
CP Protea, Austral.†; Chatfield Laboratories, UK.
Sulphasalazine (p.1215·2).
Inflammatory bowel disease; rheumatoid arthritis.

Sulcain *Shinyaku, Jpn.*
Ethyl *p*-piperidinoacetylaminobenzoate (p.1293·1).
Gastritis.

Sulcrate *Hoechst Marion Roussel, Canad.*
Sucralfate (p.1214·2).
Gastro-intestinal haemorrhage; peptic ulcer.

Suldex *Errekappa, Ital.†.*
Sulodexide (p.951·1).
Atherosclerosis; hyperlipidaemias.

Sulen *Farmacologico Milanese, Ital.*
Sulindac (p.86·3).
Gout; musculoskeletal, joint, and peri-articular disorders.

Suleo-C *Seton, UK.*
Carbaryl (p.1403·1).
Pediculosis.

Suleo-M *Seton, UK.*
Malathion (p.1407·3).
Pediculosis.

Sulf-10,-15 *Iolab, USA.*
Sulphacetamide sodium (p.252·2).
Eye infections.

Sulfa 10 *Asta Medica, Belg.*
Sulphacetamide sodium (p.252·2).
Bacterial eye infections.

Sulfableph N Liquifilm *Allergan, Ger.†.*
Sulphacetamide sodium (p.252·2).
Eye disorders.

Sulfac *Ocusoft, USA.*
Sulphacetamide sodium (p.252·2).
Bacterial eye infections.

Sulfacet
Note. This name is used for preparations of different composition.
Sanofi Winthrop, Ger.†.
Co-trimoxazole (p.196·3).
Bacterial infections.

Llorens, Spain.
Sulphacetamide sodium (p.252·2).
Bacterial eye infections.

Sulfacetam *Medical, Spain.*
Sulphacetamide sodium (p.252·2).
Eye infections.

Sulfacet-R
Dermik, Canad.; Dermik, USA.
Sulphacetamide sodium (p.252·2); sulphur (p.1091·2).
Acne; rosacea; seborrhoeic dermatitis.

Sulfactin Homburg *Asta Medica, Ger.†.*
Dimercaprol (p.979·2).
Arsenic and metal poisoning.

Sulfadeck *Sideck, Ital.†.*
Sulphur prolamine; collagen (p.1566·3); undecenoic acid (p.389·2).
Acne; seborrhoea.

Sulfadren *Biotrading, Ital.†.*
Sulphadimethoxine (p.253·2).
Bacterial infections.

Sulfadrina *Difa, Ital.†.*
Sulphadiazine sodium (p.252·3); ephedrine sulphate (p.1059·3).
Eye disorders.

Sulfalax Calcium *Major, USA.*
Docusate calcium (p.1189·3).
Constipation.

Sulfalex *De Angeli, Ital.†.*
Sulphamethoxypyridazine (p.256·2).
Bacterial infections.

Sulfamethoprim *Quad, USA.*
Co-trimoxazole (p.196·3).
Bacterial infections; Pneumocystis carinii pneumonia.

Sulfamylon *Bertek, USA.*
Mafenide acetate (p.223·2).
Burns.

Sulfarlem
Solvay, Belg.; Solvay, Canad.; Solvay, Fr.; UCM-Difme, Ital.†; Hoechst Marion Roussel, S.Afr.; Solvay, Switz.
Anethole trithione (p.1549·3).
Biliary-tract disorders; dry eye; dry mouth; hypersensitivity reactions; liver disorders.

Sulfarlem Choline *Solvay, Belg.*
Anethole trithione (p.1549·3); choline bitartrate (p.1337·1).
Liver disorders; steatosis.

Sulfarlem S 25 *Solvay, Belg.*
Anethole trithione (p.1549·3).
Dry mouth.

Sulfaryl *Zeneca, Belg.*
Acetarsol (p.578·2); sulphanilamide (p.256·3); sodium perborate (p.1125·2).
Mouth disorders.

Sulfa-Sedemol *Sopar, Belg.†.*
Sulphanilamide camsylate (p.256·3); phenol (p.1121·2); borax (p.1554·2); althaea (p.1546·3); poppy capsule (p.1068·2); sodium fluoride (p.742·1); chloral hydrate (p.645·3).
Mouth and throat disorders.

Sulfastop *Vis, Ital.†.*
Sulphadimethoxine (p.253·2).
Bacterial infections.

Sulfathalidin Estrepto *Andreu, Spain†.*
Streptomycin sulphate (p.249·3); phthalylsulphathiazole (p.237·1).
Gastro-intestinal infections.

Sulfathox *Pharmalab, S.Afr.†.*
Sulphadimethoxine (p.253·2).
Urinary-tract infections.

Sulfatiazol Dr. Andreu *Andreu, Spain†.*
Cholesterol; sulphathiazole (p.257·1); zinc oxide (p.1096·2).
Skin infections.

Sulfatrim DS *Schein, USA.*
Co-trimoxazole (p.196·3).
Bacterial infections; Pneumocystis carinii pneumonia.

Sulfa-Urolong *Thiemann, Ger.†.*
Nitrofurantoin (p.231·3); sulphadiazine (p.252·3).
Urinary-tract infections.

Sulfa-Uro-Tablinen *Sanorania, Ger.†.*
Nitrofurantoin (p.231·3); sulphadiazine (p.252·3).
Urinary-tract infections.

Sulfazine *Pinewood, Irl.†.*
Sulphasalazine (p.1215·2).
Crohn's disease; ulcerative colitis.

Sulfex *Charton, Canad.*
Sulphacetamide sodium (p.252·2).
Eye infections.

Sulfil *Cusi, Spain†.*
Mebendazole (p.104·1).
Nematode infections.

Sulfile *Poli, Ital.*
Arginine timonacicate (p.1334·2).
Liver disorders.

Sulfintestin Neom *Hosbon, Spain.*
Formosulphathiazole (p.210·1); neomycin sulphate (p.229·2).
Gastro-intestinal infections.

Sulfintestin Neomicina *Hosbon, Spain.*
Dihydrostreptomycin sulphate (p.202·2); formosulphathiazole (p.210·1); neomycin sulphate (p.229·2).
Gastro-intestinal infections.

Sulfiselen *Diviser Aquilea, Spain.*
Selenium sulphide (p.1091·1); thiram disulphide (p.1636·2).
Dandruff.

Sulfix *Allo Pro, Aust.*
Methylmethacrylate/polymethylmethacrylate (p.1603·2).
Bone cement.

Sulfoam *Kenwood, USA; Bradley, USA.*
Salicylic acid (p.1090·2).
Dandruff; seborrhoea.

Sulfo-Balmiral *Amino, Switz.†.*
Sodium thiosulphate (p.996·2); sodium sulphoricinoleate.
Musculoskeletal and joint disorders; skin disorders.

Sulfoform
Brady, Aust.†.
Triphenyl antimony sulphide (p.1095·2).

OTW, Ger.†.
Ointment: Triphenyl antimony sulphide (p.1095·2); salicylic acid (p.1090·2).
Topical application; topical oil; topical solution; topical powder: Triphenyl antimony sulphide (p.1095·2).
Skin disorders.

Sulfoil *C & M, USA.*
Soap-free skin cleanser.

Sulfolitruw *Truw, Ger.†.*
Serine (p.1354·2); methionine (p.984·2); cholic acid; vitamins; silybum marianum (p.993·3); viola tricolor; lycopodium; antimony sulphide; dried aluminium hydroxide (p.1177·3); sodium molybdate (p.1351·1); copper sulphate (p.1338·1); manganese hydrogen citrate (p.1351·1); zinc oxide (p.1096·2).
Liver disorders.

Sulfolitruw H *Truw, Ger.†.*
Silybum marianum (p.993·3).
Liver disorders.

Sulfona *Orsade, Spain.*
Dapsone (p.199·2).
Leprosy.

Sulfo-Olbad Cordes
Ichthyol, Ger.; Ichthyol, Switz.†.
Shale oil; soya oil (p.1355·1).
Bath additive; skin disorders.

Sulfopal *Bastian, Ger.†.*
Colloidal sulphur (p.1091·2); sodium humate.
Bath additive; musculoskeletal and joint disorders; skin disorders.

sulfopecticept *Sanol, Ger.†.*
Oral liquid: Sulphadiazine (p.252·3); dextromethorphan hydrobromide (p.1057·3); phenylephrine hydrochloride (p.1066·2); chlorpheniramine maleate (p.405·1); ammonium chloride (p.1055·2); menthol (p.1600·2).
Tablets: Sulphadiazine (p.252·3); dextromethorphan hydrobromide (p.1057·3); phenylephrine hydrochloride (p.1066·2); chlorpheniramine maleate (p.405·1).
Coughs associated with infections of the respiratory tract.

Sulfopino *Schoning-Berlin, Ger.*
Colloidal sulphur (p.1091·2).
Bath additive; joint disorders; neuralgia; skin disorders.

Sulfopiran *Panthox & Burck, Ital.†.*
Sulfaperin.
Bacterial infections.

Sulfopirimidina *Terapeutico, Ital.†.*
Sulfaperin.
Bacterial infections.

Sulforcin *Owen, USA.*
Sulphur (p.1091·2); resorcinol (p.1090·1).
Acne.

Sulforgan *Jolly-Jatel, Fr.†.*
Thiophenic oil.
Pulmonary disorders; rheumatic disorders.

Sulfo-Schwefelbad *Strallhofer, Aust.*
Sulphur (p.1091·2); sodium hydroxide (p.1631·1).
Musculoskeletal and joint disorders; skin disorders.

Sulfo-Selenium *Asta Medica, Belg.*
Hydrocortisone (p.1043·3); selenium disulphide (p.1091·1).
Squamous blepharitis.

Sulfosol *Waldheim, Aust.*
Sulphur (p.1091·2).
Inflammatory gynaecological disorders; musculoskeletal and joint disorders; skin disorders.

Sulfotar *Blucher-Schering, Ger.†.*
Birch tar (p.1092·2); colloidal sulphur (p.1091·2).
Eczema.

Sulfo-Thiorine Pantothenique *Plantier, Fr.†.*
Aerosol solution: Sodium thiosulphate (p.996·2); sodium pantothenate (p.1353·1).
Oral granules; tablets: Sulphur (p.1091·2); sodium thiosulphate (p.996·2); calcium pantothenate (p.1352·3).
Respiratory-tract infections.

Sulfotrim *Gea, Neth.†.*
Co-trimoxazole (p.196·3).
Bacterial infections.

Sulfotrimin *Combustin, Ger.†.*
Co-trimoxazole (p.196·3).
Bacterial infections.

Sulfoxyl
Note. This name is used for preparations of different composition.
Stiefel, Canad.; Stiefel, USA.
Benzoyl peroxide (p.1079·2); sulphur (p.1091·2).
Acne.

Sodip, Switz.†.
Aluminium sodium sulphosilicate; calcium sulphate (p.1557·1).
Respiratory-tract disorders.

Sulfredox *Jossa-Arznei, Ger.†.*
Oral granules: Aluminium sodium silicate (p.1178·3); sulphur (p.1091·2); calcium carbonate (p.1182·1); magnesium oxide (p.1198·3); sodium ascorbate; trace elements.
Tablets: Aluminium sodium silicate (p.1178·3); sulphur (p.1091·2); calcium carbonate (p.1182·1); sodium ascorbate; trace elements.
Digestive system disorders.

Sulfur Med Complex *Dynamit, Aust.*
Homoeopathic preparation.

Sulfuretten *Stulln, Ger.*
Sulphur (p.1091·2); sodium thiosulphate.
Dermatoses; lead, arsenic, or mercury poisoning; metabolic disorders.

Sulfuryl *Aerocid, Fr.*
Sulphurated aluminium sodium silicate (p.1178·3).
Respiratory-tract congestion.

Sulgan *Doetsch, Grether, Switz.*
Ointment; suppositories: Ethyl linoleate; ethyl linolenate; lignocaine hydrochloride (p.1293·2); dichlorobenzyl alcohol (p.1112·2); hamamelis (p.1587·1); camphor (p.1557·2); menthol (p.1600·2); triclosan (p.1127·2).
Wipes: Dichlorobenzyl alcohol (p.1112·2); lignocaine hydrochloride (p.1293·2); chamomile (p.1561·2); hamamelis (p.1587·1); camphor (p.1557·2); menthol (p.1600·2).
Anorectal disorders.

Sulgan 99 *Klosterfrau, Aust.*
Ointment; suppositories: Ethyl linoleate; ethyl linolenate; benzocaine (p.1286·2); dichlorobenzyl alcohol (p.1112·2); aluminium chlorohydrate (p.1078·3); hamamelis (p.1587·1); camphor (p.1557·2); menthol (p.1600·2); zinc oxide (p.1096·2).
Rectal wipes: Benzocaine (p.1286·2); dichlorobenzyl alcohol (p.1112·2); hamamelis (p.1587·1); chamomile water (p.1561·2); camphor (p.1557·2); menthol (p.1600·2).
Anorectal disorders.

Sulic *Crosara, Ital.*
Sulindac (p.86·3) or sulindac sodium (p.87·2).
Gout; musculoskeletal, joint, and peri-articular disorders; neuritis; sciatica.

Sulide *Virginia, Ital.*
Nimesulide (p.63·2).
Fever; inflammation; pain.

Sulindal *Merck Sharp & Dohme, Spain.*
Sulindac (p.86·3).
Gout; musculoskeletal, joint, and peri-articular disorders.

Sulinol *ICT, Ital.*
Sulindac (p.86·3).
Gout; musculoskeletal, joint, and peri-articular disorders; neuritis; sciatica.

Sulmasque *C & M, USA.*
Sulphur (p.1091·2).
Acne.

Sulmen *Menarini, Ital.†.*
Co-trimoxazole (p.196·3).
Bacterial infections.

Sulmetin *Semar, Spain.*
Injection: Magnesium sulphate (p.1157·3).
Procaine hydrochloride (p.1299·2) is included in the intramuscular injection to alleviate the pain of injection.
Convulsions; tachycardia; vertigo.
Oral solution†: Magnesium gluconate (p.1157·2); metoclopramide hydrochloride (p.1200·3); sorbitol (p.1354·2).
Formerly contained magnesium gluconate and metoclopramide hydrochloride.
Nausea and vomiting.

Sulmetin Papaver *Semar, Spain.*
Atropine methobromide (p.455·1); magnesium sulphate (p.1157·3); papaverine hydrochloride (p.1614·2); propyphenazone (p.81·3).
Pain due to smooth muscle spasm.

Sulmetin Papaverina *Semar, Spain.*
Injection: Magnesium sulphate (p.1157·3); papaverine hydrochloride (p.1614·2).
Procaine hydrochloride (p.1299·2) is included in the intramuscular injection to alleviate the pain of injection.
Convulsions; hypertension; smooth muscle spasm; tachycardia.
Tablets: Atropine methobromide (p.455·1); magnesium gluconate (p.1157·2); papaverine hydrochloride (p.1614·2); propyphenazone (p.81·3).
Pain due to smooth muscle spasm.

Sulmycin
Aesca, Aust.; Essex, Ger.
Gentamicin sulphate (p.212·1).
Bacterial infections.

Sulmycin mit Celestan-V *Essex, Ger.*
Gentamicin sulphate (p.212·1); betamethasone valerate (p.1033·3).
Infected skin disorders; otitis externa.

Suloves *Lampugnani, Ital.*
A heparinoid (p.882·3).
Thrombosis prophylaxis.

Sulp *Hexal, Ger.*
Sulpiride (p.692·3).
Depression; schizophrenia; vestibular disorders.

Sulparex *Bristol-Myers Squibb, UK.*
Sulpiride (p.692·3).
Schizophrenia.

Sulperazon *Pfizer, Aust.†.*
Sulbactam sodium (p.250·3); cefoperazone sodium (p.167·3).
Bacterial infections.

Sulphamezathine *Zeneca, Irl.†.*
Sulphadimidine (p.253·2).
Bacterial infections.

Sulpho-Lac *Doak, USA.*
Sulphur (p.1091·2); zinc sulphate (p.1373·2).
Acne.

Sulphonated Lauryls *Ronsheim & Moore, UK.*
A range of alkyl sulphates.

Sulphrin *Bausch & Lomb, USA†.*
Prednisolone acetate (p.1048·1); sulphacetamide sodium (p.252·2).
Eye inflammation with bacterial infection.

Sulpitil *Tillotts, UK.*
Sulpiride (p.692·3).
Schizophrenia.

Sulquipen *Bohm, Spain.*
Cephalexin (p.178·2).
Bacterial infections.

Sulreuma *Lebens, Ital.†.*
Sulindac (p.86·3).
Musculoskeletal and joint disorders; neuritis; sciatica.

Sulster *Akorn, USA.*
Sulphacetamide sodium (p.252·2); prednisolone sodium phosphate (p.1048·1).
Infected eye disorders.

Sultanol
Glaxo Wellcome, Aust.; Glaxo Wellcome, Ger.
Salbutamol (p.758·2) or salbutamol sulphate (p.758·2).
Obstructive airways disease.

Sulton *Geymonat, Ital.*
Calcium folinate (p.1342·2).
Anaemias; antidote to folic acid antagonists; reduction of aminopterin and methotrexate toxicity.

Sultrin
Janssen-Cilag, Austral.; Janssen-Cilag, Belg.; Janssen-Ortho, Canad.; Janssen-Cilag, Irl.; Janssen-Cilag, S.Afr.; Janssen-Cilag, Switz.†; Janssen-Cilag, UK; Ortho Pharmaceutical, USA.
Sulfabenzamide (p.251·1); sulphacetamide (p.252·2); sulphathiazole (p.257·1).
Cervicitis; vaginitis.

Sulvina *Inibsa, Spain†.*
Griseofulvin (p.380·2).
Fungal skin infections.

Sumacal
Wyeth-Ayerst, Canad.†.
Preparation for enteral nutrition.

Sherwood, USA.
Glucose polymers.
Carbohydrate source.

Sumadol *Italfarmaco, Ital.†.*
Sumatriptan succinate (p.450·1).
Migraine.

Sumial *Zeneca, Spain.*
Propranolol hydrochloride (p.937·1).
Angina pectoris; arrhythmias; hypertension; hyperthyroidism; migraine; myocardial infarction; obstructive cardiomyopathy; phaeochromocytoma; tremor.

Sumigrene *Sigma-Tau, Ital.*
Sumatriptan succinate (p.450·1).
Cluster headache; migraine.

Sumithrin *Sumitomo, Jpn†.*
Phenothrin (p.1409·2).
Pediculosis.

Summavit *Bioprogress, Ital.*
Multivitamin preparation.

Summer's Eve *Fleet, USA.*
A range of feminine hygiene preparations.

Summer's Eve Disposable
Note. This name is used for preparations of different composition.
Fleet, Austral.
Fresh Scent: Phenol (p.1121·2).
Herbal Scented; White Flowers; Hint of Musk: Octoxinol 9 (p.1326·2).
Vinegar and Water: Vinegar (p.1541·2).
Vaginal cleanser.

Fleet, USA.
Regular solution: Sodium citrate (p.1153·2); citric acid (p.1564·3); sodium benzoate (p.1102·3).
Scented solution: Sodium citrate (p.1153·2); citric acid (p.1564·3); sodium benzoate (p.1102·3); octoxinol 9 (p.1326·2).
Solution: Vinegar (p.1541·2).
Vaginal disorders.

Summer's Eve Feminine *Fleet, Austral.*
Topical liquid; topical spray: Soap substitute.
Vaginal hygiene.
Topical powder: Octoxinol 9 (p.1326·2); benzethonium chloride (p.1102·3).
Intertrigo; vaginal irritation.
Towelettes: Octoxinol 9 (p.1326·2).

Summer's Eve Medicated *Fleet, USA.*
Povidone-iodine (p.1123·3).
Vaginal disorders.

Summer's Eve Post-Menstrual *Fleet, USA.*
Sodium lauryl sulphate (p.1468·3); monobasic sodium phosphate (p.1159·3); dibasic sodium phosphate (p.1159·3); sodium chloride (p.1162·2); edetic acid (p.980·3).
Vaginal disorders.

Summicort *Benvegna, Ital.†.*
Methylprednisolone (p.1046·1).
Corticosteroid.

Sumycin *Apothecon, USA.*
Tetracycline hydrochloride (p.259·1).
Bacterial infections.

Sun Buffer *Clinique, Canad.*
SPF 15: Ethylhexyl *p*-methoxycinnamate (p.1487·1).
Sunscreen.

Sun Defense Lip Block *Norman, Canad.*
SPF 15: Ethylhexyl *p*-methoxycinnamate (p.1487·1); oxybenzone (p.1487·3).
Sunscreen.

Sun Defense Sunblock *Norman, Canad.*
SPF 25: Ethylhexyl *p*-methoxycinnamate (p.1487·1); homosalate (p.1487·2); octyl salicylate (p.1487·3); oxybenzone (p.1487·3).
Sunscreen.

Sun Defense Sunscreen *Norman, Canad.*
SPF 8: Ethylhexyl *p*-methoxycinnamate (p.1487·1); oxybenzone (p.1487·3).
Sunscreen.

Sun E45 *Crookes Healthcare, UK.*
Titanium dioxide (p.1093·3); zinc oxide (p.1096·2).
Sunscreen.

Sun Management Extensive Protection *Kay, Canad.*
Ethylhexyl *p*-methoxycinnamate (p.1487·1); octyl salicylate (p.1487·3); oxybenzone (p.1487·3).
Sunscreen.

Sun Management Intensive Protection *Kay, Canad.*
SPF 20: Ethylhexyl *p*-methoxycinnamate (p.1487·1); octyl salicylate (p.1487·3); oxybenzone (p.1487·3).
Sunscreen.

Sun Management Lip Protection *Kay, Canad.*
SPF 15: Ethylhexyl *p*-methoxycinnamate (p.1487·1); oxybenzone (p.1487·3).
Sunscreen.

Sun Management Sensible Protection *Kay, Canad.*
Ethylhexyl *p*-methoxycinnamate (p.1487·1); oxybenzone (p.1487·3).
Sunscreen.

Sun Pacer Protective *Amway, Canad.*
SPF 8: Oxybenzone (p.1487·3); padimate O (p.1488·1).
SPF 15: Ethylhexyl *p*-methoxycinnamate (p.1487·1); oxybenzone (p.1487·3); padimate O (p.1488·1).
SPF 30: Ethylhexyl *p*-methoxycinnamate (p.1487·1); oxybenzone (p.1487·3); padimate O (p.1488·1); titanium dioxide (p.1093·3).
Sunscreen.

Sun Pacer Sunless Tanning *Amway, Canad.*
SPF 15: Ethylhexyl *p*-methoxycinnamate (p.1487·1); octyl salicylate (p.1487·3); oxybenzone (p.1487·3).
Sunscreen.

Sun-Benz *Sun, Canad.*
Benzydamine hydrochloride (p.21·3).
Oropharyngeal mucositis; sore throat.

Sunblock *Estee Lauder, Canad.*
SPF 15; SPF 25: Titanium dioxide (p.1093·3).
Sunscreen.

Suncodin *Noristan, S.Afr.†.*
Syrup: Paracetamol (p.72·2); codeine phosphate (p.26·1).
Tablets: Paracetamol (p.72·2); codeine phosphate (p.26·1); phenyltoloxamine citrate (p.416·1); caffeine (p.749·3).
Fever; pain; sinus congestion.

Sundays Maximum Protection *Nutri-Metics, Canad.*
SPF 15: Avobenzone (p.1486·3); ethylhexyl *p*-methoxycinnamate (p.1487·1).
Sunscreen.

Sundown
Johnson & Johnson, Austral.; Johnson & Johnson, USA.
SPF 8; SPF 10; SPF 15; SPF 30: Ethylhexyl *p*-methoxycinnamate (p.1487·1); octyl salicylate (p.1487·3); oxybenzone (p.1487·3); titanium dioxide (p.1093·3).
Sunscreen.

Sundown Active *Johnson & Johnson, Austral.*
SPF15+: Titanium dioxide (p.1093·3); zinc oxide (p.1096·2).
Sunscreen.

Sundown with Insect Repellant *Johnson & Johnson, Austral.*
SPF15+: Ethylhexyl *p*-methoxycinnamate (p.1487·1); avobenzone (p.1486·3); titanium dioxide (p.1093·3); di-*N*-propyl isocinchomeronate; piperonyl butoxide (p.1409·3); octylbicycloheptene dicarboximide; pyrethrins.
Sunscreen and insect repellent.

Sundown Sport *Johnson & Johnson, USA.*
SPF 15: Zinc oxide (p.1096·2); titanium dioxide (p.1093·3).
Sunscreen.

Sundown Toddler *Johnson & Johnson, Austral.*
SPF15+: Ethylhexyl *p*-methoxycinnamate (p.1487·1); oxybenzone (p.1487·3); octyl salicylate (p.1487·3); avobenzone (p.1486·3).
Sunscreen.

SuNerven *Modern Health Products, UK.*
Motherwort (p.1604·2); vervain; valerian (p.1643·1); passion flower (p.1615·3).
Stresses and strains.

Sunfilter *Estee Lauder, Canad.*
SPF 15: Avobenzone (p.1486·3); ethylhexyl *p*-methoxycinnamate (p.1487·1); titanium dioxide (p.1093·3).
Sunscreen.

Suniderma *Farmacusi, Spain.*
Hydrocortisone aceponate (p.1044·2).
Skin disorders.

Sunkist *Ciba, USA.*
Ascorbic acid (p.1365·2).

SUNPRuF *C & M, USA.*
SPF 15: Ethylhexyl *p*-methoxycinnamate (p.1487·1); oxybenzone (p.1487·3).
SPF 17: Ethylhexyl *p*-methoxycinnamate (p.1487·1); octyl salicylate (p.1487·3).
Sunscreen.

Sunsan-Heillotion *Richter, Aust.*
Diphenhydramine hydrochloride (p.409·1); dexpanthenol (p.1570·3); allantoin (p.1078·2).
Inflammatory skin disorders; skin irritation.

Sunscreen *Hamilton, Austral.*
Cream SPF15+: Ethylhexyl *p*-methoxycinnamate (p.1487·1); avobenzone (p.1486·3); octyl salicylate (p.1487·3).
Formerly contained ethylhexyl*p*-methoxycinnamate and avobenzone.
Lotion-spray SPF15+: Ethylhexyl *p*-methoxycinnamate (p.1487·1); avobenzone (p.1486·3); oxybenzone (p.1487·3).
Milky lotion SPF 15+: 3-(4-Methylbenzylidene)bornan-2-one (p.1487·2); ethylhexyl *p*-methoxycinnamate (p.1487·1); avobenzone (p.1486·3).
Sunscreen.

Sunscreen Lotion
Note. This name is used for preparations of different composition.
Norwood, Canad.
SPF 8; SPF 15: Ethylhexyl *p*-methoxycinnamate (p.1487·1); oxybenzone (p.1487·3); titanium dioxide (p.1093·3).
SPF 45: Ethylhexyl *p*-methoxycinnamate (p.1487·1); octocrylene (p.1487·3); octyl salicylate (p.1487·3); oxybenzone (p.1487·3).
Sunscreen.
Therapex, Canad.
SPF 15: Avobenzone (p.1486·3); ethylhexyl *p*-methoxycinnamate (p.1487·1); oxybenzone (p.1487·3).
SPF 30: Avobenzone (p.1486·3); ethylhexyl *p*-methoxycinnamate (p.1487·1); oxybenzone (p.1487·3); titanium dioxide (p.1093·3).
Sunscreen.

Sunseekers *Avon, Canad.*
SPF 6; SPF30: Ethylhexyl *p*-methoxycinnamate (p.1487·1); octyl salicylate (p.1487·3); oxybenzone (p.1487·3).
SPF 8; SPF 15: Ethylhexyl *p*-methoxycinnamate (p.1487·1); oxybenzone (p.1487·3).
Sunscreen.

Sunsense *Ego, Austral.†.*
SPF15+: Titanium dioxide (p.1093·3); oxybenzone (p.1487·3); ethylhexyl *p*-methoxycinnamate (p.1487·1); avobenzone (p.1486·3).
Sunscreen.

Sunsense Aftersun *Ego, Austral.*
Emollient.
Dry skin.

Sunsense Daily Face *Ego, Austral.*
SPF 30+: Ethylhexyl *p*-methoxycinnamate (p.1487·1); titanium dioxide (p.1093·3); 3-(4-methylbenzylidene)bornan-2-one (p.1487·2).
Sunscreen.

Sunsense LIF *Ego, Austral.†.*
Ethylhexyl *p*-methoxycinnamate (p.1487·1); titanium dioxide (p.1093·3); avobenzone (p.1486·3).
Sunscreen.

Sunsense Lip Balm *Ego, Austral.*
SPF 30+: Ethylhexyl *p*-methoxycinnamate (p.1487·1); oxybenzone (p.1487·3); titanium dioxide (p.1093·3); avobenzone (p.1486·3).
Sunscreen.

Sunsense Low Irritant *Ego, Austral.*
SPF20: Titanium dioxide (p.1093·3).
Formerly known as Sunsensitive.
Sunscreen.

Sunsense Sport *Ego, Austral.*
SPF 30+: Ethylhexyl *p*-methoxycinnamate (p.1487·1); titanium dioxide (p.1093·3); oxybenzone (p.1487·3); 3-(4-methylbenzylidene)bornan-2-one (p.1487·2).
Sunscreen.

Sunsense and Sunsense Ultra *Ego, Austral.*
SPF 30+: Ethylhexyl *p*-methoxycinnamate (p.1487·1); oxybenzone (p.1487·3); titanium dioxide (p.1093·3).
Sunscreen.

Sunsense Toddler Milk *Ego, Austral.*
SPF30: Ethylhexyl *p*-methoxycinnamate (p.1487·1); oxybenzone (p.1487·3); isoamyl methoxycinnamate; titanium dioxide (p.1093·3).
Sunscreen.

Sunsmackers *Bonne Bell, Canad.*
SPF 6; SPF 30: Ethylhexyl *p*-methoxycinnamate (p.1487·1); oxybenzone (p.1487·3); padimate O (p.1488·1).
Sunscreen.

Sunspot
Note. This name is used for preparations of different composition.
Sunspot, Austral.
Salicylic acid (p.1090·2).
Hard skin; solar keratoses.
Surf Ski International, UK.
Camphor (p.1557·2); benzoin (p.1634·1); ethyl glycol.; benzalkonium chloride (p.1101·3); allantoin (p.1078·2); isopropyl alcohol (p.1118·2).
Herpes labialis.

Suotex *Pinewood, Irl.†.*
Paracetamol (p.72·2).
Fever; pain.

Supa C *Vitaplex, Austral.*
Calcium ascorbate (p.1365·2).
Vitamin C deficiency.

Supa-Boost *Vitaplex, Austral.*
Multivitamin and mineral preparation.

Supac *Mission Pharmacal, USA.*
Paracetamol (p.72·2); aspirin (p.16·1); caffeine (p.749·3).
Pain.

Supadol
Note. This name is used for preparations of different composition.
Whitehall, Fr.
Paracetamol (p.72·2); codeine phosphate (p.26·1).
Formerly contained paracetamol, papaverine hydrochloride, papaverine nicotinate, codeine hydrobromide, and homatropine methobromide.
Pain.
Sodip, Switz.†.
Paracetamol (p.72·2); papaverine hydrochloride (p.1614·2); papaverine nicotinate (p.1614·3); codeine hydrobromide (p.27·1); homatropine methobromide (p.462·2).
Pain; smooth muscle spasm.

Supadol Mono *Bios, Belg.†.*
Paracetamol (p.72·2).
Fever; pain.

Super Active Multi *Quest, Canad.*
Multivitamin and mineral preparation.

Super AO Formula *Seroyal, Canad.*
Betacarotene, selenium, vitamin C, vitamin D, and zinc.

Super B
Parke, Davis, Austral.†.
Vitamin B substances and nutritional preparation.
Vita Glow, Austral.
Vitamin B substances with ascorbic acid.
Formerly known as Super B Complex.
Dietary supplement.

Super B Complex *Sisu, Canad.*
Vitamin B substances.
Nutritional supplement.

Super B Extra *Roche Consumer, Austral.*
Vitamin B substances with ascorbic acid and minerals.
Dietary supplement.

Super B Plus *Vita Glow, Austral.*
Vitamin B substances, vitamin C, and mineral preparation.

Super B Plus Liver Tonic *Vita Glow, Austral.*
Silybum marianum (p.993·3); vitamins; minerals.
Dietary supplement; digestive system disorders.

Super Banish *Smith & Nephew, Austral.*
Silver nitrate (p.1629·2); ethylene thiourea.
Ostomy deodorant.

Super Cal-C Bio *Eagle, Austral.*
Calcium ascorbate (p.1365·2); bioflavonoids (p.1580·1).
Vitamin C deficiency.

Super Citro Cee *Marlyn, USA.*
Lemon bioflavonoids (p.1580·1); rutin (p.1580·2); ascorbic acid (p.1365·2); rose hips (p.1365·2).
Capillary bleeding.

Super Complex C *Approved Drug, USA.*
Hesperidin (p.1580·2); citrus bioflavonoids complex (p.1580·1); rutin (p.1580·2); ascorbic acid (p.1365·2); rose hips (p.1365·2); acerola (p.1001·1).
Capillary bleeding.

Super Cromer Orto *Normon, Spain.*
Mercurochrome (p.1119·2).
Wound disinfection.

Super D Perles *Roberts, USA.*
Vitamins A and D.

Super Daily *Lee-Adams, Canad.†.*
Multivitamin and mineral preparation.

Super Energex Plus *Sante Naturelle, Canad.*
Vitamin B substances, minerals, and kola.

Super Galanol *Lifeplan, UK.*
Borage oil (p.1582·1).
Nutritional supplement.

Super GammaOil Marine *Quest, UK.*
Evening primrose oil (p.1582·1); borage oil (p.1582·1); concentrated fish oil (p.1276·1).

Super GLA *Cantassium Co., UK.*
Gamma linolenic acid (from vegetable oils) (p.1582·1).

Super Hi Potency *Nion, USA.*
Multivitamin and mineral preparation.

Super Koki *Perez Gimenez, Spain†.*
Belladonna (p.457·1); sodium dibunate (p.1070·1); ethylmorphine (p.36·1); peppermint oil (p.1208·1); tyrothricin (p.267·2); menthol (p.1600·2).
Mouth and throat inflammation.

Super Malic *Optimox, USA.*
Malic acid (p.1598·3); magnesium (p.1157·2).

Super Mega B+C *Quest, UK.*
Vitamin B and C substances; valerian (p.1643·1); passion flower (p.1615·3); peppermint oil (p.1208·1); wood betony; black cohosh root (p.1563·3); scullcap; lupulus (p.1597·2); ginger root (p.1193·2).

Super Once A Day
Quest, Canad.; Quest, UK.
Multivitamin and mineral preparation.

Super Orti-Vite *Seroyal, Canad.*
Multivitamin and mineral preparation.

Super Plenamins
3M, Irl.; 3M, UK.
Multivitamin and mineral preparation.

Super Quints *Freeda, USA.*
Vitamin B substances.

Super Soluble Maxipro HBV *Scientific Hospital Supplies, Austral.*
Preparation for enteral nutrition.
Hypoproteinaemia.

Super Vita Vim *Jamieson, Canad.*
Multivitamin and mineral preparation.

Super Vitalex *Carmaran, Canad.*
Vitamin B substances and iron.

Super Wate-On *DDD, UK.*
Nutritional supplement with vitamins.

Super Weight Gain *Suisse, Austral.†.*
Nutritional supplement.

Super Weight Loss *Suisse, Austral.†.*
Nutritional supplement.

Superdophilus *Natren, USA.*
Lactobacillus acidophilus (p.1594·1).
Dietary supplement.

SuperEPA *Advanced Nutritional Technology, USA.*
Omega-3 marine triglycerides with vitamin E (p.1276·1).
Dietary supplement.

Superfade *Sunspot, Austral.*
Hydroquinone (p.1083·1); salicylic acid (p.1090·2); dexpanthenol (p.1570·3); padimate O (p.1488·1); vitamin E.
Skin hyperpigmentation.

Supergan *Waldheim, Aust.*
Dihydroergocristine mesylate (p.1571·3); reserpine (p.942·1); hydrochlorothiazide (p.885·2).
Hypertension.

Superlaxol *Labopharma, Ger.†.*
Senna leaves (p.1212·2).
Constipation.

Superlipid *Berenguer Infale, Spain.*
Probucol (p.1277·3).
Hyperlipidaemias.

Supermidone *Salfa, Ital.†.*
Nifenazone (p.63·1).
Musculoskeletal and joint disorders; neuralgia; neuritis.

Supermin *Vita Glow, Austral.*
Mineral and trace element preparation.

Supero *Italfarmaco, Ital.*
Cefuroxime sodium (p.177·1).
Lignocaine hydrochloride (p.1293·2) is included in the intramuscular injection to alleviate the pain of injection.
Bacterial infections.

Superol *Tendem, Neth.*
Hydroxyquinoline sulphate (p.1589·3).
Throat pain.

Superpeni *Roussel, Spain.*
Amoxycillin trihydrate (p.151·3).
Bacterial infections.

Superpeni Mucolitico *Roussel, Spain.*
Amoxycillin trihydrate (p.151·3); bromhexine hydrochloride (p.1055·3).
Respiratory-tract infections.

Superpep *Hermes, Ger.*
Dimenhydrinate (p.408·2).
Motion sickness; nausea; vomiting.

Superplex-T *Major, USA.*
Vitamin B substances with vitamin C.

Supertendin 3000 *SmithKline Beecham, Ger.†.*
Dexamethasone (p.1037·1); lignocaine hydrochloride (p.1293·2); diphenhydramine hydrochloride (p.409·1); cyanocobalamin (p.1363·3); pyridoxine hydrochloride (p.1362·3).
Painful inflammatory and degenerative disorders.

Supertendin 2000 N *Thiemann, Ger.*
Dexamethasone (p.1037·1); lignocaine hydrochloride (p.1293·2).
Painful inflammatory musculoskeletal and joint disorders.

Supertendin-Depot N *Thiemann, Ger.*
Dexamethasone acetate (p.1037·1); lignocaine hydrochloride (p.1293·2).
Musculoskeletal, joint, and peri-articular disorders; neuritis.

Superthiol *Francia, Ital.*
Carbocisteine (p.1056·3) or carbocisteine sodium (p.1056·3).
Respiratory-tract congestion.

Supertonic *Diafarm, Spain.*
Amino-acid preparation with cyanocobalamin.
Tonic.

Supervite C *Medinat, Austral.†.*
Calcium ascorbate (p.1365·2).
Vitamin C deficiency.

Supervite Multi-vitamins *Medinat, Austral.†.*
Multivitamin and mineral preparation.

Supervite Zinc Plus *Medinat, Austral.†.*
Vitamin and mineral preparation.

Supeudol *Sabex, Canad.*
Oxycodone hydrochloride (p.71·2).
Pain.

Suplasyn *Bioniche, Canad.*
Sodium hyaluronate (p.1630·3).
Synovial fluid replacement following arthrocentesis.

Suplena
Abbott, Canad.; Ross, USA.
Preparation for enteral nutrition.
Formerly known as Replena in the *USA.*

Suplevit *Riva, Canad.*
Multivitamin and mineral preparation.

Supo Gliz *Calmante Vitaminado, Spain.*
Glycerol (p.1585·2).
Constipation; laxative dependence.

Supo Kristal *CEPA, Spain.*
Glycerol (p.1585·2).
Constipation; laxative dependence.

Suppap *Raway, USA.*
Paracetamol (p.72·2).
Pain.

Suppla-Cal *NCI, USA.*
Supplemental nutrition bar.

Supplavit *3M, Belg.†.*
Multivitamin and mineral preparation.

Supplemaman *Yves Ponroy, Fr.*
Vitamin B substances, fatty acids, magnesium, and iron.
Nutritional supplement during pregnancy.

Supplevit Magnum *Woelm, Ger.*
Magnesium oxide (p.1198·3); alpha tocopheryl acetate (p.1369·1).
Vitamin E or magnesium deficiency.

Supplimen *Clintec, UK†.*
Preparation for enteral nutrition.

Suppolax *Wellcome, Belg.†.*
Docusate sodium (p.1189·3); sodium bicarbonate (p.1153·2); potassium acid tartrate (p.1209·1).
Constipation.

Suppomaline *Solvay, Fr.*
Belladonna (p.457·1); codeine phosphate (p.26·1); caffeine (p.749·3); paracetamol (p.72·2).
Fever; pain.

Suppoptanox *Byk, Fr.†.*
Vinylbitone (p.698·2).
Insomnia.

Suppositoires Midy *Clin Midy, Fr.†.*
Amylocaine hydrochloride (p.1286·1); benzocaine (p.1286·2); hamamelis (p.1587·1); aesculus (p.1543·3).
Anorectal disorders.

Supposte Midy *Midy, Ital.†.*
Benzocaine (p.1286·2); hamamelis (p.1587·1); aesculus (p.1543·3).
Anorectal disorders.

Supprelin *Roberts, USA.*
Histrelin acetate (p.1251·3).
Precocious puberty.

Suppress
Note. This name is used for preparations of different composition.
Stanley, Canad.
Diphenhydramine hydrochloride (p.409·1); codeine phosphate (p.26·1); ammonium chloride (p.1055·2).
Ferndale, USA.
Dextromethorphan hydrobromide (p.1057·3).
Coughs.

Supra Leodin *Byk Elmu, Spain†.*
Caffeine citrate (p.749·3); codeine phosphate (p.26·1); propyphenazone (p.81·3).
Fever; pain.

Supraalox *Rhone-Poulenc Rorer, Spain.*
Aluminium hydroxide (p.1177·3); magnesium hydroxide (p.1198·2).
Hyperacidity.

Supracaine *Hoechst Marion Roussel, Canad.*
Amethocaine (p.1285·2).
Oral soft-tissue pain; reduction of gag reflex.

Supracid *Asta Medica, Aust.*
Spironolactone (p.946·1); hydrochlorothiazide (p.885·2).
Hyperaldosteronism; hypertension; oedema.

Supracombin
Grunenthal, Aust.; Grunenthal, Ger.; Grunenthal, Switz.
Co-trimoxazole (p.196·3).
Bacterial infections; Pneumocystis carinii pneumonia.

Supracort *Amsa, Ital.†.*
Suprarenal cortex (p.1050·1).
Postoperative shock; tonic; toxicosis.

Supracyclin
Grunenthal, Aust.; Grunenthal, Ger.
Doxycycline (p.202·3) or doxycycline hydrochloride (p.202·3).
Bacterial infections.

Supracycline *Grunenthal, Switz.*
Doxycycline (p.202·3) or doxycycline hydrochloride (p.202·3).
Bacterial infections.

Supradyn
Roche, Aust.
Multivitamin preparation.

Roche Consumer, Austral.; Roche, Belg.; Roche Nicholas, Ger.; Roche, Ital.; Roche Nicholas, Neth.; Roche, S.Afr.†; Roche, Switz.; Roche Consumer, UK.
Multivitamin and mineral preparation.

Supradyn + Mineralien + Spurenelementen
Roche, Aust.
Multivitamin and mineral preparation.

Supradyne *Roche Nicholas, Fr.*
Multivitamin and mineral preparation.

Supragenta *Juste, Spain†.*
Gentamicin sulphate (p.212·1).
Bacterial infections.

Supragesic *Pharmaceutical Enterprises, S.Afr.*
Capsules: Paracetamol (p.72·2); codeine phosphate (p.26·1); caffeine (p.749·3); meprobamate (p.678·1).
Syrup: Paracetamol (p.72·2); codeine phosphate (p.26·1).
Fever; pain.

Supralef *Martin, Spain.*
Hydrocortisone acetate (p.1043·3).
Skin disorders.

Supralox
Theraplix, Fr.; Rhone-Poulenc Rorer, Ger.
Aluminium hydroxide gel (p.1177·3); magnesium hydroxide (p.1198·2).
Gastro-intestinal disorders.

Supramox
Grunenthal, Aust.; Grunenthal, Switz.
Amoxycillin (p.151·3) or amoxycillin trihydrate (p.151·3).
Bacterial infections.

Supramycin *Grunenthal, Ger.*
Tetracycline hydrochloride (p.259·1).
Bacterial infections.

Suprane
Pharmacia Upjohn, Aust.; Pharmacia Upjohn, Belg.; Pharmacia Upjohn, Ger.; Pharmacia Upjohn, Irl.; Pharmacia Upjohn, Ital.; Pharmacia Upjohn, Neth.; Pharmacia Upjohn, Norw.; Pharmacia Upjohn, Spain; Pharmacia Upjohn, Swed.; Pharmacia Upjohn, Switz.; Pharmacia Upjohn, UK; Ohmeda, USA.
Desflurane (p.1221·2).
General anaesthesia.

Suprapen *SmithKline Beecham, S.Afr.*
Amoxycillin (p.151·3); flucloxacillin (p.209·1).
Bacterial infections.

Suprarenin
Hoechst, Aust.; Hoechst, Ger.
Adrenaline hydrochloride (p.813·3).
Adjunct to local anaesthesia; circulatory collapse; hypersensitivity reactions; shock.

Suprastin *EGIS, Hung.*
Halopyramine hydrochloride (p.411·3).
Hypersensitivity reactions.

Supratonin *Grunenthal, Ger.*
Amezinium methylsulphate (p.819·1).
Hypotension.

Supraviran *Grunenthal, Ger.*
Aciclovir (p.602·3) or aciclovir sodium (p.602·3).
Herpesvirus infections.

Supravite
Nobel, Canad.; Pharmavite, Canad.
A range of vitamin preparations with or without minerals.

Supravite C *Nobel, Canad.*
Vitamin B substances, vitamin C, and iron.

Suprax
Rhone-Poulenc Rorer, Canad.; Klinge, Ger.; Rhone-Poulenc Rorer, Irl.; Cyanamid, Ital.; Lederle, UK; Lederle, USA.
Cefixime (p.165·3).
Bacterial infections.

Suprecur
Hoechst, Aust.; Hoechst, Ger.; Hoechst Marion Roussel, Irl.; Hoechst Marion Roussel, Neth.; Hoechst Marion Roussel, Norw.; Hoechst Marion Roussel, S.Afr.†; Hoechst, Spain; Hoechst Marion Roussel, Swed.; Shire, UK.
Buserelin acetate (p.1241·3).
Endometriosis; ovulation induction; prostatic cancer.

Suprefact
Behring, Aust.; Hoechst, Aust.; Hoechst Marion Roussel, Belg.; Hoechst Marion Roussel, Canad.; Hoechst, Fr.; Behringwerke, Ger.†; Hoechst Marion Roussel, Irl.; Hoechst Marion Roussel, Ital.; Hoechst Marion Roussel, Neth.; Hoechst Marion Roussel, Norw.; Hoechst Marion Roussel, S.Afr.; Hoechst, Spain; Hoechst Marion Roussel, Swed.; Hoechst Marion Roussel, Switz.; Shire, UK.
Buserelin acetate (p.1241·3).
Ovulation induction; prostatic cancer.

Suprenoat *Boehringer Mannheim, Aust.*
Spironolactone (p.946·1); buthiazide (p.835·2); reserpine (p.942·1).
Hypertension.

Supres *Frosst, Canad.*
Methyldopa (p.904·2); chlorothiazide (p.839·1).
Hypertension.

Supressin *Pfizer, Aust.*
Doxazosin mesylate (p.862·3).
Hypertension.

Suprexon
Ciba Vision, Ger.; Ciba Vision, Neth.; Ciba Vision, Switz.
Guanethidine monosulphate (p.878·1); adrenaline (p.813·2).
Glaucoma.

Sup-Rhinite *SmithKline Beecham Sante, Fr.*
Chlorpheniramine maleate (p.405·1); phenylephrine hydrochloride (p.1066·2).
Rhinopharyngeal congestion.

Suprimal *IPS, Neth.*
Meclozine hydrochloride (p.413·3).
Motion sickness.

Suprin
Note. This name is used for preparations of different composition.
Valeas, Ital.†.
Co-trimoxazole (p.196·3).
Bacterial infections.

Invamed, USA.
Aspirin (p.16·1); aluminium hydroxide (p.1177·3); magnesium oxide (p.1198·3).

Supristol
Gallier, Fr.†; Noristan, S.Afr.†; Iquinosa, Spain†.
Co-trifamole (p.196·3).
Bacterial infections; Pneumocystis carinii pneumonia.

Suprotide *Torre, Ital.*
Nutritional supplement.

Suralgan *Poli, Ital.*
Tiaprofenic acid (p.89·1).
Inflammation; pain.

Surazem *Pharmacia Upjohn, Neth.*
Diltiazem hydrochloride (p.854·2).
Hypertension.

Surbex
Abbott, Canad.; Abbott, USA.
A range of vitamin preparations.

Surbex plus Iron *Abbott, Canad.*
Vitamin B substances with ascorbic acid and ferrous sulphate.
Nutritional supplement.

Surbex plus Zinc *Abbott, Canad.*
Vitamin B substances with ascorbic acid and zinc sulphate.
Nutritional supplement.

Surbex T
Abbott, S.Afr.†; Abbott, UK†.
Vitamin B substances with vitamin C.

Surbronc
Boehringer Ingelheim, Belg.; Boehringer Ingelheim, Fr.
Ambroxol hydrochloride (p.1054·3).
Respiratory-tract congestion.

Surbu-Gen-T *Goldline, USA.*
Vitamin B substances with vitamin C.

SureLac *Caraco, USA.*
Tilactase (p.1637·3).
Lactose intolerance.

Sure-Lax *English Grains, UK.*
Yellow phenolphthalein (p.1208·2).
Constipation.

Surelen *Roche Nicholas, Fr.*
Nutritional supplement.
Tonic.

Surem
Note. This name is used for preparations of different composition.
Boehringer Mannheim, Spain.
Butalamine hydrochloride (p.835·2).
Vascular disorders.

Galen, UK†.
Nitrazepam (p.682·2).
Insomnia.

Sureptil
Synthelabo, Fr.; Delalande, Ital.†.
Cinnarizine (p.406·1); heptaminol acephyllinate (p.754·1).
Vascular disorders.

Sureskin *Euromedex, Fr.*
Carmellose sodium (p.1471·2); pectin (p.1474·1); gelatin (p.723·2).
Burns; ulcers; wounds.

Surfa-Base *Rougier, Canad.*
Emollient and vehicle.

Surfactal *Boehringer Ingelheim, Ital.*
Ambroxol hydrochloride (p.1054·3).
Neonatal surfactant deficiency; prevention of bronchopulmonary complications following surgery.

Surfacten *Tokyo Tanabe, Jpn.*
Bovine pulmonary extract (p.1622·3).
Respiratory distress syndrome.

Surfak
Hoechst Marion Roussel, Canad.; Upjohn, USA.
Docusate calcium (p.1189·3).
Constipation.

Surfalyse *Peters, Fr.†.*
Formaldehyde (p.1113·2); glutaraldehyde (p.1114·3); glyoxal (p.1115·1); quaternary ammonium compound.
Surface disinfection.

Surfexo Neonatal *Glaxo Wellcome, Fr.*
Colfosceril palmitate (p.1623·1).
Respiratory distress syndrome in premature infants.

Surfol *Stiefel, USA.*
Emollient.

Surfolase *Poli, Ital.*
Ambroxol acefyllinate (p.1054·3).
Obstructive airways disease.

Surfont *Ardeypharm, Ger.*
Mebendazole (p.104·1).
Worm infections.

Surfortan *Diepha, Fr.*
Amino acid, mineral, and vitamin preparation.
Tonic.

Surgam
Hoechst Marion Roussel, Austral.; Hoechst Marion Roussel, Belg.; Hoechst Marion Roussel, Canad.; Roussel, Fr.; Albert-Roussel, Ger.; Hoechst, Ger.; Hoechst Marion Roussel, Irl.; Hoechst Marion Roussel, Neth.; Hoechst Marion Roussel, S.Afr.; Hoechst Marion Roussel, Switz.; Florizel, UK.
Tiaprofenic acid (p.89·1) or tiaprofenic acid, trometamol salt (p.89·1).
Inflammation; musculoskeletal, joint, peri-articular, and soft-tissue disorders; pain.

Surgamic *Rorer, Spain.*
Tiaprofenic acid (p.89·1).
Inflammation; musculoskeletal, joint, and peri-articular disorders; pain.

Surgamyl *Corvi, Ital.*
Tiaprofenic acid (p.89·1).
Lignocaine (p.1293·2) is included in the intramuscular injection to alleviate the pain of injection.
Inflammation; pain.

Surgel *Ulmer, USA.*
Carmellose sodium (p.1471·2); propylene glycol (p.1622·1); glycerol (p.1585·2).
Vaginal lubricant.

Surgestone *Cassenne, Fr.*
Promegestone (p.1461·2).
Fibroids; mastalgia; menopausal disorders; menstrual disorders.

Surgicel
Johnson & Johnson Medical, Fr.; Johnson & Johnson Medical, UK; Johnson & Johnson Medical, USA.
Oxidised cellulose (p.714·2).
Haemorrhage.

Surgicoll *MBP, Ger.; Biodynamics, Ger.*
Collagen (p.1566·3).
Haemorrhage.

Surgident *Mini, Switz.*
Adrenaline hydrochloride (p.813·3).
Gingival haemorrhage.

Surheme *Lipha, Ital.†.*
Butalamine hydrochloride (p.835·2).
Vascular disorders.

Surifarm *Farmapros, Spain.*
Aluminium hydroxide (p.1177·3); dimethicone (p.1213·1); magnesium trisilicate (p.1199·1); metoclopramide (p.1202·1).
Gastro-intestinal disorders.

Suril *Ibirn, Ital.*
Sucralfate (p.1214·2).
Gastritis; gastro-oesophageal reflux; peptic ulcer.

Surlid *Hoechst Marion Roussel, Swed.*
Roxithromycin (p.247·1).
Bacterial infections.

Surmenalit *Foes, Spain.*
Sulbutiamine (p.1360·3).
Vitamin B1 deficiency.

Surmontil
Rhone-Poulenc Rorer, Austral.; Rhone-Poulenc Rorer, Belg.; Rhone-Poulenc Rorer, Canad.; Specia, Fr.; Rhone-Poulenc Rorer, Irl.; Rhone-Poulenc Rorer, Ital.; Rhone-Poulenc Rorer, Neth.; Rhone-Poulenc Rorer, Norw.; Rhone-Poulenc Rorer, S.Afr.; Rhone-Poulenc Rorer, Spain; Rhone-Poulenc Rorer, Swed.; Rhone-Poulenc Rorer, Switz.; Futuna, UK; Wyeth-Ayerst, USA.
Trimipramine (p.310·1), trimipramine maleate (p.310·1), or trimipramine mesylate (p.310·2).
Depression; pain; peptic ulcer.

Surmoruine *Bournonville, Belg.*
Cod-liver oil (p.1337·3).
Osteomalacia; osteoporosis; rickets; vitamin A and D deficiency.

Surnox *Roussel, Spain.*
Ofloxacin (p.233·3) or ofloxacin hydrochloride (p.234·1).
Bacterial infections.

Surplix *Vis, Ital.†.*
Imipramine hydrochloride (p.289·2).
Depression.

Surrenovis *Teofarma, Ital.†.*
Suprarenal cortex (p.1050·1); vitamins.
Acetonaemia; tonic; toxic states; vomiting.

Survanta
Abbott, Aust.; Abbott, Austral.; Abbott, Belg.; Abbott, Canad.; Abbott, Fr.; Abbott, Ger.; Abbott, Neth.; Abbott, S.Afr.; Abbott, Spain; Abbott, Switz.; Abbott, UK; Ross, USA.
Beractant (p.1623·1).
Neonatal respiratory distress syndrome.

Survanta-Vent
Abbott, Norw.; Abbott, Swed.
Beractant (p.1623·1).
Neonatal respiratory distress syndrome.

Survector
Eutherapie, Fr.; Stroder, Ital.; Danval, Spain.
Amineptine hydrochloride (p.273·2).
Depression.

Survimed *Fresenius, Switz.*
Range of preparations for enteral nutrition.

Survitine *Roche Nicholas, Fr.*
Multivitamin and mineral preparation.
Nutritional disorders.

Susano *Halsey, USA.*
Atropine sulphate (p.455·1); hyoscine hydrobromide (p.462·3); hyoscyamine hydrobromide (p.464·2) or hyoscyamine sulphate (p.464·2); phenobarbitone (p.350·2).
Gastro-intestinal disorders.

Suscard
Pharmax, Irl.; Pierrel, Ital.†; Astra, Norw.; Hassle, Swed.; Pharmax, UK.
Glyceryl trinitrate (p.874·3).
Angina pectoris; heart failure.

Suspendol *Merckle, Ger.†.*
Allopurinol (p.390·2).
Gout; hyperuricaemia.

Suspensie Tegen Overmatig Maagzuur *SAN, Neth.†.*
Aluminium oxide (p.1077·2); magnesium oxide (p.1198·3).
Eructation; heartburn.

Sus-Phrine *Forest Pharmaceuticals, USA.*
Adrenaline (p.813·2).
Asthma; bronchospasm.

Sustac
Pharmax, Irl.; Pharmax, UK.
Glyceryl trinitrate (p.874·3).
Angina pectoris.

Sustacal
Mead Johnson, Austral.; Mead Johnson, Canad.; Mead Johnson Nutritionals, USA.
A range of preparations for enteral nutrition.

Sustagen
Mead Johnson, Austral.; Mead Johnson, Canad.†; Mead Johnson Nutritionals, USA.
Range of preparations for enteral nutrition.

Sustaire *Pfizer, USA.*
Theophylline (p.765·1).
Asthma; bronchospastic disorders.

Sustamycin *Boehringer Mannheim, UK†.*
Tetracycline hydrochloride (p.259·1).
Bacterial infections.

Sustanon
Organon, Belg.; Organon, Ital.
Testosterone propionate (p.1464·2); testosterone phenylpropionate (p.1464·2); testosterone isocaproate (p.1464·2); testosterone decanoate (p.1464·1).
Androgen deficiency; male hypogonadism.

Sustanon 100
Organon, Austral.; Organon, Irl.; Organon, Neth.; Organon, UK.
Testosterone propionate (p.1464·2); testosterone phenylpropionate (p.1464·2); testosterone isocaproate (p.1464·2).
Androgen deficiency; female breast cancer; male osteoporosis.

Sustanon 250
Organon, Austral.; Organon, Irl.; Organon, Neth.; Donmed, S.Afr.; Organon, UK.
Testosterone propionate (p.1464·2); testosterone phenylpropionate (p.1464·2); testosterone isocaproate (p.1464·2); testosterone decanoate (p.1464·1).
Androgen deficiency; female breast cancer; male osteoporosis.

Sustein *Inibsa, Spain†.*
Papaverine monophosphoadenine (p.1614·3).
Cerebrovascular disorders.

Sustemial *Malesci, Ital.*
Ferrous gluconate (p.1340·1).
Anaemias; iron deficiency.

Sustenium *Malesci, Ital.*
Fosfocreatinine disodium (p.1581·3).
Muscle disorders.

Sustiva *Du Pont, USA.*
Efavirenz (p.609·3).
HIV Infection.

Sutilan *Cusi, Spain†.*
Tiopronin (p.997·2).
Liver disorders.

Sutril *Novag, Spain.*
Torasemide (p.956·3).
Hypertension; oedema.

Suvipen *Thera, Fr.*
Metampicillin sodium (p.224·3).
Bacterial infections.

Suxidina *Seid, Spain.*
Aspergillus oryzae; dimethicone (p.1213·1); metoclopramide hydrochloride (p.1200·3); oxazepam hemisuccinate (p.683·3).
Gastro-intestinal disorders.

Suxilep *Jenapharm, Ger.*
Ethosuximide (p.344·3).
Absence seizures.

Suxinutin
Parke, Davis, Aust.; Parke, Davis, Ger.; Parke, Davis, Swed.; Parke, Davis, Switz.
Ethosuximide (p.344·3).
Absence seizures.

SVC *May & Baker, S.Afr.†.*
Acetarsol (p.578·2).
Leucorrhoea; vaginal trichomoniasis.

Svedocain Sin Vasoconstr *Inibsa, Spain.*
Bupivacaine hydrochloride (p.1286·3).
Local anaesthesia.

Sveltosyl *Homberger, Switz.†.*
Homoeopathic preparation.

Swansol-Wundsalbe *Worwag, Ger.†.*
Zinc oxide (p.1096·2); cod-liver oil (p.1337·3).
Skin disorders.

Swarm *Pickles, UK.*
Hamamelis (p.1587·1); dibromopropamidine isethionate (p.1112·2); calamine (p.1080·1).
Insect bites.

Sweatosan N *Zyma, Ger.*
Sage (p.1627·1).
Hyperhidrosis.

Sween *Coloplast, UK.*
A deodorant for stoma care.

Sween Cream *Coloplast, USA.*
Barrier cream.

Sween Prep *Sween, USA†.*
Chloroxylenol (p.1111·1) in a protective film forming base.
Skin protectant.

Swim-Ear
Metapharma, Canad.; Fougera, USA.
Isopropyl alcohol (p.1118·2); glycerol (p.1585·2).
Ear disorders.

Swiss One *Swiss Herbal, Canad.*
Multivitamin and mineral preparation.

Swiss-Kal Eff *Byk Madaus, S.Afr.*
Potassium citrate (p.1153·1); potassium bicarbonate (p.1153·1).
Hypokalaemia in hyperchloraemic acidosis.

Swiss-Kal SR *Byk Madaus, S.Afr.*
Potassium chloride (p.1161·1).

Syaline-spray *Biosedra, Fr.†.*
Carmellose sodium (p.1471·2); sorbitol (p.1354·2); electrolytes (p.1147·1).
Artificial saliva.

Sygen *Fidia, Ital.†.*
Monosialoganglioside sodium (p.1582·3).
Cerebrovascular disorders.

Syllact *Wallace, USA.*
Psyllium husk (p.1194·2).
Constipation.

Syllamalt
Bouty, Ital.†; Wallace, USA.
Malt extract (p.1350·1); psyllium husk (p.1194·2).
Constipation.

Sylvemid *Weimer, Ger.†.*
Amitriptyline hydrochloride (p.273·3).
Depression.

Symadal *ankerpharm, Ger.*
Dimethicone 200 (p.1384·2).
Barrier preparation.

Symadine *Solvay, USA†.*
Amantadine hydrochloride (p.1129·2).
Drug-induced extrapyramidal disorders; influenza A; parkinsonism.

Symbial *Galderma, Neth.*
Urea (p.1095·2); sodium chloride (p.1162·2).
Skin disorders.

Symbioflor I *Symbiopharm, Ger.*
Cells and autolysate of *Enterococcus faecalis* (p.1594·1).
Immunotherapy.

Symbioflor 2 *Symbiopharm, Ger.*
Escherichia coli.
Gastro-intestinal disorders.

Symbioflor I *Peithner, Aust.*
Live cells and autolysate of *Enterococcus faecalis* (p.1594·1).
Gastro-intestinal disorders; infections.

Symbioflor II *Peithner, Aust.*
Live cells and autolysate of *Escherichia coli.*
Gastro-intestinal disorders; infections.

Symbioflor-Antigen *Symbiopharm, Ger.*
Escherichia coli.
Immunotherapy.

Symbol *Wassermann, Ital.†.*
Misoprostol (p.1419·3).
Peptic ulcer.

Symfona *Medichemie, Switz.†.*
Etofylline (p.753·1); buphenine hydrochloride (p.1555·3); vitamins.
Tonic.

Symfona N *Medichemie, Switz.*
Ginkgo biloba (p.1584·1).
Cerebrovascular disorders.

Symmetrel
Ciba-Geigy, Aust.†; Novartis, Austral.; Du Pont, Canad.; Geigy, Ger.†; Geigy, Irl.; Novartis, Neth.; Geigy, Norw.†; Novartis, S.Afr.; Ciba-Geigy, Swed.†; Geigy, Switz.; Alliance, UK; Du Pont, USA.
Amantadine hydrochloride (p.1129·2).
Drug-induced extrapyramidal disorders; herpes zoster; influenza A; parkinsonism.

Symoron *Yamanouchi, Neth.*
Methadone hydrochloride (p.53·2).
Opioid addiction; pain.

Sympalept *Streuli, Switz.*
Oxedrine tartrate (p.925·3).
Circulatory disorders; hypotension.

Sympaneurol *Lemoine, Fr.*
Phenobarbitone (p.350·2); crataegus (p.1568·2); passion flower (p.1615·3); valerian (p.1643·1).
Anxiety; sleep disorders.

Sympathyl *Innothera, Fr.*
Phenobarbitone (p.350·2); crataegus (p.1568·2).
Anxiety; sleep disorders.

Sympatocard *Boehringer Ingelheim, Ger.†.*
Oxedrine (p.925·2); pentetrazol (p.1484·2).
Hypotension.

Sympatol
Bender, Aust.; Boehringer Ingelheim, Ger.; Boehringer Ingelheim, Ital.; Boehringer Ingelheim, Switz.†.
Oxedrine tartrate (p.925·3).
Hypotension.

Sympatovit *Biotherax, Ger.†.*
Oxedrine tartrate (p.925·3); vitamin A; thiamine nitrate; riboflavine; cyanocobalamin; nicotinamide; sodium ascorbate; cholecalciferol.
Tonic.

Sympavagol *Monal, Fr.*
Passion flower (p.1615·3); crataegus (p.1568·2).
The tablets formerly contained phenobarbitone.
Nervous disorders.

Symphytum Ro-Plex (Rowo-776) *Pharmakon, Ger.*
Homoeopathic preparation.

Symphytum Ro-Plex (Rowo-777) *Pharmakon, Ger.†.*
Comfrey (p.1567·1); methyl nicotinate (p.55·1).
Inflammatory disorders.

Symphytum Ro-Plex T (Rowo-778) *Pharmakon, Ger.†.*
Homoeopathic preparation.

Symphytum-Komplex *Rodler, Ger.*
Homoeopathic preparation.

Symptofed *Propan, S.Afr.*
Pseudoephedrine hydrochloride (p.1068·3).
Upper respiratory-tract congestion.

Syn MD
Synthelabo, Belg.; Kramer, Switz.
Sorbitol (p.1354·2).
Bowel evacuation; constipation; dyspepsia.

Synacol CF *Roberts, USA.*
Dextromethorphan hydrobromide (p.1057·3); guaiphenesin (p.1061·3).
Coughs.

Synacort *Syntex, USA.*
Hydrocortisone (p.1043·3).
Skin disorders.

Synacthen
Ciba-Geigy, Aust.; Novartis, Austral.; Ciba-Geigy, Belg.; Ciba, Ger.; Ciba-Geigy, Irl.; Ciba, Ital.; Novartis, Neth.; Ciba, Norw.; Novartis, Swed.; Ciba, Switz.; Alliance, UK.
Tetracosactrin (p.1261·3), tetracosactrin acetate (p.1261·3), or tetracosactrin-zinc complex (p.1261·3).
Adrenocorticotrophic hormone; diagnosis of adrenocortical insufficiency; infantile spasms; multiple sclerosis.

Synacthen Depot
Ciba, Canad.; Ciba, Ger.; Ciba-Geigy, Irl.†; Novartis, S.Afr.; Alliance, UK.
Tetracosactrin acetate zinc phosphate complex (p.1261·3).
Adrenocorticotrophic hormone; diagnosis of adrenocortical insufficiency.

Synacthen Retard *Ciba, Switz.*
Tetracosactrin hexaacetate zinc complex (p.1261·3).
Adrenocorticotrophic hormone.

Synacthene *Ciba-Geigy, Fr.*
Tetracosactrin (p.1261·3).
Adrenocorticotrophic hormone; diagnosis of adrenocortical insufficiency.

Syn-A-Gen *Pharmacal, Switz.*
Nonoxinol 9 (p.1326·1).
Contraceptive.

Synagis *Medimmune, USA.*
Palivizumab (p.1532·1).
Respiratory syncytial virus infections.

Synalar
Grunenthal, Aust.; Yamanouchi, Belg.; Roche, Canad.; Cassenne, Fr.; Zeneca, Irl.; Yamanouchi, Neth.†; Zeneca, Norw.; Zeneca, S.Afr.; Yamanouchi, Spain; Zeneca, Swed.; Grunenthal, Switz.; Bioglan, UK; Syntex, USA.
Fluocinolone acetonide (p.1041·1).
Skin disorders.

Synalar Bi-Ophtalmic *Syntex, Belg.†.*
Fluocinolone acetonide (p.1041·1); neomycin sulphate (p.229·2); polymyxin B sulphate (p.239·1).
Eye disorders.

Synalar Bi-Otic
Yamanouchi, Belg.; Syntex, Canad.†; Syntex, Neth.
Fluocinolone acetonide (p.1041·1); neomycin sulphate (p.229·2); polymyxin B sulphate (p.239·1).
Inflammatory ear infections.

Synalar C
Zeneca, Irl.; Zeneca, S.Afr.; Bioglan, UK.
Fluocinolone acetonide (p.1041·1); clioquinol (p.193·2).
Infected skin disorders.

Synalar + DBO *Syntex, Neth.†.*
Fluocinolone acetonide (p.1041·1); broxyquinoline.
Skin disorders.

Synalar med Chinoform
Zeneca, Norw.; Zeneca, Swed.†.
Fluocinolone acetonide (p.1041·1); clioquinol (p.193·2).
Infected skin disorders; otitis externa.

Synalar N
Grunenthal, Aust.; Zeneca, Irl.; Zeneca, S.Afr.; Grunenthal, Switz.; Bioglan, UK.
Fluocinolone acetonide (p.1041·1); neomycin sulphate (p.229·2).
Infected skin disorders.

Synalar Nasal *Yamanouchi, Spain.*
Phenylephrine hydrochloride (p.1066·2); fluocinolone acetonide (p.1041·1); neomycin (p.229·2); polymyxin B sulphate (p.239·1).
Nasal congestion and infection.

Synalar Neomicina *Yamanouchi, Spain.*
Fluocinolone acetonide (p.1041·1); neomycin sulphate (p.229·2).
Infected skin disorders.

Synalar Neomycine *Cassenne, Fr.*
Fluocinolone acetonide (p.1041·1); neomycin sulphate (p.229·2).
Infected skin disorders.

Synalar Otico *Yamanouchi, Spain.*
Fluocinolone acetonide (p.1041·1); neomycin sulphate (p.229·2); polymyxin B sulphate (p.239·1).
Ear disorders.

Synalar Rectal *Yamanouchi, Spain.*
Bismuth subgallate (p.1180·2); fluocinolone acetonide (p.1041·1); lignocaine hydrochloride (p.1293·2); menthol (p.1600·2).
Anorectal disorders.

Synaleve *Mer-National, S.Afr.*
Capsules: Paracetamol (p.72·2); codeine phosphate (p.26·1); meprobamate (p.678·1).
Pain and associated tension.
Syrup: Paracetamol (p.72·2); codeine phosphate (p.26·1); promethazine hydrochloride (p.416·2).
Fever; pain.
Tablets: Paracetamol (p.72·2); codeine phosphate (p.26·1); caffeine (p.749·3); meprobamate (p.678·1).
Pain and associated tension.

Synalgo *Geymonat, Ital.*
Naproxen aminobutanol (p.62·1).
Musculoskeletal and joint disorders; neuralgia; sciatica.

Synalgos-DC *Wyeth-Ayerst, USA.*
Dihydrocodeine tartrate (p.34·1); aspirin (p.16·1); caffeine (p.749·3).
Pain.

Synamol *Syntex, Canad.†.*
Fluocinolone acetonide (p.1041·1).
Skin disorders.

Synap *Restan, S.Afr.*
Paracetamol (p.72·2); dextropropoxyphene napsylate (p.27·3); diphenhydramine hydrochloride (p.409·1); caffeine (p.749·3).
Pain.

Synapause
Organon, Fr.†; Nourypharma, Ger.†; Donmed, S.Afr.; Organon, Spain.
Oestriol succinate (p.1457·2).
Oestrogen deficiency.

Synapause E *Nourypharma, Ger.*
Oestriol (p.1457·2).
Menopausal disorders.

Synapause-E$_3$ *Organon, Neth.*
Oestriol (p.1457·2).
Female infertility; menopausal disorders; oestrogen deficiency.

Synarel
Searle, Austral.; Searle, Belg.; Searle, Canad.; Monsanto, Fr.; Searle, Irl.; Syntex, Neth.; Searle, S.Afr.; Searle, UK; Syntex, USA.
Nafarelin acetate (p.1254·2).
Endometriosis; ovarian stimulation; precocious puberty; uterine fibroids.

Synarela
Heumann, Ger.; Searle, Norw.; Searle, Swed.
Nafarelin acetate (p.1254·2).
Endometriosis; ovarian stimulation.

Synasteron *Syntex, Belg.†.*
Oxymetholone (p.1459·1).
Aplastic anaemias.

Syncarpin *Winzer, Ger.*
Pilocarpine borate (p.1396·3); neostigmine bromide (p.1393·3); naphazoline hydrochloride (p.1064·2).
Glaucoma.

Synchrodyn *Hoechst Marion Roussel, Ital.†.*
Alsactide.
Adrenocorticotrophic hormone deficiency; test for suprarenal cortex function.

Syncillin *Bayer, Ger.*
Azidocillin sodium (p.155·2).
Bacterial infections.

Syncortyl *Roussel, Fr.*
Deoxycortone acetate (p.1036·2).
Mineralocorticoid deficiency.

Syndette *Mer-National, S.Afr.*
Paracetamol (p.72·2); doxylamine succinate (p.410·1).
Fever; pain; sedative.

Syndol
Note. This name is used for preparations of different composition.
Seton, Irl.; Mer-National, S.Afr.; Hoechst Marion Roussel, UK.
Tablets: Paracetamol (p.72·2); codeine phosphate (p.26·1); doxylamine succinate (p.410·1); caffeine (p.749·3).
Fever; pain.
Mer-National, S.Afr.
Syrup: Paracetamol (p.72·2); doxylamine succinate (p.410·1); codeine phosphate (p.26·1).
Fever; pain with tension.

Synedil *Yamanouchi, Fr.*
Sulpiride (p.692·3).
Nervous disorders; psychoses.

Synemol *Syntex, USA.*
Fluocinolone acetonide (p.1041·1).
Skin disorders.

Synerbiol *Nutergia, Fr.*
Marine fish oil (p.1276·1).
Nutritional supplement.

Synerga *Laves, Ger.*
Peptide extract from *Escherichia coli.*
Allergies; neurodermatitis.

Synergistic Manganese *Quest, Canad.*
Manganese, vitamin A, and vitamin C.

Synergistic Selenium *Quest, Canad.*
Selenium, vitamin C, and vitamin E.

Synergomycin *Abbott, Ger.*
Erythromycin (p.204·1) or erythromycin ethyl succinate (p.204·2); bromhexine hydrochloride (p.1055·3).
Bacterial infections of the respiratory tract.

Synergon *Lipha Sante, Fr.*
Progesterone (p.1459·3); oestrone (p.1458·2).
Female infertility; menstrual disorders.

Synergyl *Monsanto, Fr.*
Multivitamin and mineral preparation.

Synerpril *Merck Sharp & Dohme, Swed.*
Enalapril maleate (p.863·2); hydrochlorothiazide (p.885·2).
Hypertension.

Syneudon *Krewel, Ger.*
Amitriptyline hydrochloride (p.273·3).
Depression; pain.

Synfase
Searle, Norw.; Searle, Swed.
Norethisterone (p.1453·1); ethinyloestradiol (p.1445·1).
Triphasic oral contraceptive.

Synflex
Syntex, Austral.†; Syncare, Canad.; Roche, Irl.; Recordati, Ital.; Roche, S.Afr.; Roche, UK.
Naproxen sodium (p.61·2).
Gout; musculoskeletal, joint, and peri-articular disorders; pain.

Syngel *Will-Pharma, Belg.*
Aluminium hydroxide-magnesium carbonate co-dried gel (p.1178·2); magnesium hydroxide (p.1198·2); magnesium trisilicate (p.1199·1); lignocaine hydrochloride (p.1293·2).
Gastritis; gastro-oesophageal reflux.

Syngynon *Jenapharm, Ger.*
Hydroxyprogesterone hexanoate (p.1448·1); oestradiol benzoate (p.1455·1).
Menstrual disorders.

Synkapton *Strallhofer, Aust.*
Ergotamine tartrate (p.445·3); dimenhydrinate (p.408·2); anhydrous caffeine (p.749·3).
Migraine and other vascular headaches.

Synkavit
Roche, Irl.†; Cambridge, UK.
Menadiol sodium phosphate (p.1370·3).
Factor VII deficiency; hypoprothrombinaemia.

Synmiol *Winzer, Ger.†.*
Idoxuridine (p.613·2).
Viral eye infections.

Synobel *Yamanouchi, Spain.*
Clioquinol (p.193·2); fluocinolone acetonide (p.1041·1).
Infected skin disorders.

Synophylate-GG *Schwarz, USA†.*
Theophylline sodium glycinate (p.772·2); guaiphenesin (p.1061·3).
Bronchospasm.

SynPharma Bronchial *Synpharma, Aust.*
Anise oil (p.1550·1); eucalyptus oil (p.1578·1); thyme oil (p.1637·1).
Catarrh; coughs.

Synpharma Instant-Blasen-und-Nierentee
Synpharma, Aust.
Silver birch (p.1553·3); equisetum (p.1575·1); urtica (p.1642·3).
Urinary-tract disorders.

Synpharma Instant-Nerventee *Synpharma, Aust.*
Valerian (p.1643·1); melissa leaf (p.1600·1); orange.
Nervous disorders; sleep disorders.

Synphase *Searle, UK.*
Ethinyloestradiol (p.1445·1); norethisterone (p.1453·1).
Triphasic oral contraceptive.

Synphasec *Grunenthal, Ger.*
Ethinyloestradiol (p.1445·1); norethisterone (p.1453·1).
Triphasic oral contraceptive.

Synphasic
Searle, Austral.; Searle, Canad.
Ethinyloestradiol (p.1445·1); norethisterone (p.1453·1).
28-Day packs also contain 7 inert tablets.
Triphasic oral contraceptive.

Synrelina *Searle, Switz.*
Nafarelin acetate (p.1254·2).
Endometriosis.

Syn-Rx *Adams, USA.*
Dark blue tablets, pseudoephedrine hydrochloride (p.1068·3); guaiphenesin (p.1061·3); light green tablets, guaiphenesin.
Cough and cold symptoms.

Syntaris
Roche, Aust.; Roche, Belg.; Syntex, Ger.; Roche, Ger.; Roche, Irl.; Recordati, Ital.; Syntex, Neth.; Roche, S.Afr.; Roche, Switz.; Roche Consumer, UK.
Flunisolide (p.1040·3).
Allergic rhinitis.

Syntaverin Merck, Spain†.
Dipyrone (p.35·1); pramiverine hydrochloride (p.1621·2).
Pain.

Syntestan Syntex, Ger.; Roche, Ger.
Cloprednol (p.1035·3).
Asthma; polyarthritis.

Synthamin
Baxter, Austral.; Baxter, Ger.†; Baxter, Irl.; Pharmacia Upjohn, S.Afr.; Clintec, Spain; Baxter, UK.
Amino-acid infusion with or without electrolytes.
Parenteral nutrition.

Synthamine Baxter, Switz.
Amino-acid infusion with or without electrolytes.
Parenteral nutrition.

Synthamix Clintec, UK†.
Amino-acid, glucose, and electrolyte infusion.
Parenteral nutrition.

Synthol
Note. This name is used for preparations of different composition.
Bournonville, Belg.; SmithKline Beecham, Fr.; Smith Kline & French, Switz.†.
Chloral hydrate (p.645·3); levomenthol (p.1600·2); resorcinol (p.1090·1); salicylic acid (p.1090·2); veratrol.
Mouth and throat disorders; musculoskeletal pain; neuralgias; soft-tissue trauma.

Synthol, Spain†.
Chloral hydrate (p.645·3); geranium oil (p.1584·1); lemon oil (p.1595·3); menthol (p.1600·2); resorcinol (p.1090·1); salicylic acid (p.1090·2); veratrol.
Mouth and throat and vaginal infections; musculoskeletal pain.

Synthroid
Knoll, Canad.; Knoll, USA.
Thyroxine sodium (p.1497·1).
Diagnosis of hyperthyroidism; hypothyroidism; thyroid-stimulating hormone suppression.

Syntocaine Sintetica, Switz.
Procaine hydrochloride (p.1299·2).
Local anaesthesia.

Syntocinon
Sandoz, Aust.; Novartis, Austral.; Sandoz, Belg.; Sandoz, Canad.†; Sandoz, Fr.; Sandoz, Ger.; Sandoz, Irl.; Sandoz, Ital.; Novartis, Neth.; Sandoz, Norw.; Novartis, S.Afr.; Sandoz, Spain; Novartis, Swed.; Sandoz, Switz.; Alliance, UK; Sandoz, USA†.
Oxytocin (p.1257·2).
Incomplete abortion; induction and maintenance of labour; lactation stimulation; mastitis; postpartum haemorrhage.

Syntometrin Sandoz, Ger.
Oxytocin (p.1257·2); methylergometrine maleate (p.1603·1).
Delivery of the placenta; postpartum haemorrhage.

Syntometrine
Novartis, Austral.; Sandoz, Irl.; Novartis, S.Afr.; Alliance, UK.
Ergometrine maleate (p.1575·1); oxytocin (p.1257·2).
Labour induction; postpartum haemorrhage.

Syntopressin
Sandoz, Irl.; Sandoz, UK.
Lypressin (p.1263·2).
Diabetes insipidus.

Syntrogel-4 Sauter, Switz.†.
Aluminium hydroxide-magnesium carbonate co-dried gel (p.1178·2); calcium carbonate (p.1182·1); magnesium hydroxide (p.1198·2); sodium bicarbonate (p.1153·2).
Heartburn; hyperchlorhydria.

Synuretic DDSA Pharmaceuticals, UK.
Hydrochlorothiazide (p.885·2); amiloride hydrochloride (p.819·2).
These ingredients can be described by the British Approved Name Co-amilozide.
Ascites; heart failure; hypertension.

Synureticum Medisa, Switz.
Spironolactone (p.946·1); hydrochlorothiazide (p.885·2).
Heart failure; hypertension; nephrotic syndrome; oedema.

Synvisc
Biomatrix, Canad.; Rhone-Poulenc Rorer, Canad.; Roche, Swed.; Wyeth-Ayerst, USA.
Hylan G-F 20 (p.1631·1).
Osteoarthritis of the knee.

Syprine Merck Sharp & Dohme, USA.
Trientine dihydrochloride (p.998·1).
Formerly known as Cuprid.
Wilson's disease.

Syracerin Beiersdorf, Ger.†.
Citric acid (p.1564·3); ammonium citrate (p.1055·2).
Skin disorders.

Syracol CF Roberts, USA.
Guaiphenesin (p.1061·3); dextromethorphan hydrobromide (p.1057·3).
Coughs.

Syracort Beiersdorf, Ger.†.
Fluocortolone (p.1041·3).
Scalp disorders; skin disorders.

Syralvit Calcio Clariana, Spain†.
Ascorbic acid (p.1365·2); calcium gluceptate (p.1155·1); calcium hypophosphite; ergocalciferol (p.1367·1); lysine.
Bone and dental disorders; calcium deficiency; osteomalacia; rickets.

Syraprim Wellcome, Spain†.
Trimethoprim (p.265·1).
Bacterial infections.

Syrea Medac, Ger.
Hydroxyurea (p.539·1).
Malignant neoplasms.

Syrup DM Therapex, Canad.
Dextromethorphan hydrobromide (p.1057·3).

Syrup DM-D Therapex, Canad.
Dextromethorphan hydrobromide (p.1057·3); pseudoephedrine hydrochloride (p.1068·3).

Syrup DM-D-E Therapex, Canad.
Dextromethorphan hydrobromide (p.1057·3); pseudoephedrine hydrochloride (p.1068·3); guaiphenesin (p.1061·3).

Syrup DM-E Therapex, Canad.
Dextromethorphan hydrobromide (p.1057·3); guaiphenesin (p.1061·3).

Syrvite Barre-National, USA; Major, USA; Moore, USA.
Multivitamin preparation.

Syscor
Bayer, Aust.; Bayer, Belg.; Bayer, Ital.; Bayer, Neth.; Zeneca, Spain; Bayer, Swed.; Zeneca, Switz.; Bayer, UK.
Nisoldipine (p.922·3).
Angina pectoris; hypertension.

Systen
Janssen-Cilag, Aust.; Janssen-Cilag, Belg.; Janssen-Cilag, Fr.; Janssen-Cilag, Ital.; Janssen-Cilag, Neth.; Janssen-Cilag, Switz.
Oestradiol (p.1455·1).
Menopausal disorders; osteoporosis.

Systepin Klinge, Irl.
Nifedipine (p.916·2).
Hypertension; ischaemic heart disease.

Systodin Nycomed, Norw.
Quinidine sulphate (p.939·1).
Arrhythmias.

Systral
Laevosan, Aust.; Lucien, Fr.†; Asta Medica, Ger.
Chlorphenoxamine hydrochloride (p.405·3).
Asthma; dysmenorrhoea; hypersensitivity reactions; migraine; motion sickness; nausea; rhinitis.

Systral C
Laevosan, Aust.; Asta Medica, Ger.†.
Chlorphenoxamine hydrochloride (p.405·3); caffeine (p.749·3).
Asthma; dysmenorrhoea; hypersensitivity reactions; migraine; motion sickness; nausea; rhinitis.

Systrason Laevosan, Aust.
Chlorphenoxamine (p.405·3); hydrocortisone acetate (p.1043·3).
Skin disorders.

Sytron Link, UK.
Sodium ironedetate (p.1354·2).
Iron-deficiency anaemia.

Syviman N Muller Goppingen, Ger.
Comfrey (p.1567·1); mistletoe (p.1604·1).
Joint disorders.

Syxyl-Vitamin-Comb Syxyl, Ger.
Vitamin B substances.
Vitamin B deficiency.

Szillosan Henk, Ger.†.
Squill (p.1070·1); convallaria (p.1567·2); crataegus (p.1568·2); adonis vernalis (p.1543·3).
Heart failure.

Szillosan forte Henk, Ger.
Squill (p.1070·1); crataegus (p.1568·2).
Heart failure.

T 21 MC, Ital.†.
Benzalkonium chloride (p.1101·3); benzethonium chloride (p.1102·3); didecyldimethylammonium chloride (p.1112·2).

T. Polio Merieux, Fr.
A tetanus and poliomyelitis (inactivated) vaccine (p.1536·3).
Active immunisation.

T 10 Sapone Chirurgico MC, Ital.†.
Ethyleneglycolphenylundecylenether benzoate; benzalkonium chloride (p.1101·3).
Hand disinfection.

T & T Antioxidant Procare, Austral.
Silybum marianum (p.993·3); camellia sinensis (p.1645·1).
Adjunct in detoxification regimens; exposure to chemical and environmental toxins and tobacco smoke; inflammation.

TA Baumpollen SmithKline Beecham, Ger.
Allergen extracts of tree pollen(p.1545·1).
Hyposensitisation.

TA Graserpollen SmithKline Beecham, Ger.
Allergen extracts of grass pollen(p.1545·1).
Hyposensitisation.

TA MIX SmithKline Beecham, Ger.
Allergen extracts of mixed pollens(p.1545·1).
Hyposensitisation.

Tab Vaccin Berna, Switz.†.
Salmonella typhi.
Formerly known as Vaccin Tab.
Active immunisation.

Tabalon Hoechst, Ger.
Ibuprofen (p.44·1).
Fever; inflammation; musculoskeletal and joint disorders; pain.

Tabanil Medinex, Canad.†.
Mouthwash; lozenges; dentifrice: Glycerolargentinate.
Throat spray: Silver glycerolate (p.1629·2).
Aid to smoking withdrawal.

Tabapax Arkopharma, Fr.†.
Tablets, nicotiana tabacum; capsules, valerian (p.1643·1).
Aid to smoking withdrawal.

Tab-A-Vite Major, USA.
A range of vitamin preparations.

Tabazur Theraplix, Fr.†.
Nicotine (p.1607·2).
Nicotine dependence.

Tabcin Bayer, Aust.
Ibuprofen (p.44·1).
Pain.

Tabiomyl Hoechst Marion Roussel, Belg.†.
Benfotiamine (p.1360·3).
Alcoholism; vitamin B_1 deficiency.

Tabletas Quimpe Quimpe, Spain.
Atropine methonitrate (p.455·1); codeine phosphate (p.26·1); diphenhydramine hydrochloride (p.409·1); ephedrine hydrochloride (p.1059·3); phenazone (p.78·2); propyphenazone (p.81·3).
Upper respiratory-tract disorders.

Tablettes pour la Gorge Medica Qualiphar, Belg.†.
Amylocaine hydrochloride (p.1286·1); benzocaine (p.1286·2); potassium chlorate (p.1620·3); borax (p.1554·2); menthol (p.1600·2).
Throat disorders.

Tabmint Roche Consumer, UK†.
Silver acetate (p.1629·2).
Aid to smoking withdrawal.

Taborcil Lacer, Spain.
Gemfibrozil (p.1273·3).
Hyperlipidaemias.

Tabotamp
Johnson & Johnson, Ger.; Ethicon, Ital.
Oxidised cellulose (p.714·2).
Surgical haemorrhage.

Tabritis Potter's, UK.
Elder flowers (p.1627·2); yarrow (p.1542·2); prickly ash bark (p.1645·3); burdock (p.1594·2); clivers (p.1565·2); poplar bark (p.1620·1); bearberry (p.1552·2).
Rheumatic pain and stiffness.

Tabron Parke, Davis, USA†.
Ferrous fumarate (p.1339·3); folic acid (p.1340·3); vitamins B, C, and E.
Docusate sodium (p.1189·3) is included in this preparation to reduce the constipating effects of iron.
Iron-deficiency anaemias.

Tab-Vita Nicholas, Austral.†.
Vitamin B substances with vitamin C.

Tac Allergan Herbert, USA.
Triamcinolone acetonide (p.1050·2).
Corticosteroid.

TAC Esofago Bracco, Ital.
Barium sulphate (p.1003·1).
Contrast medium for computerised tomography of the oesophagus.

Tacaryl Westwood-Squibb, USA†.
Methdilazine (p.414·2) or methdilazine hydrochloride (p.414·2).
Nasal allergies; pruritus.

Tace
Marion Merrell Dow, Belg.†; Marion Merrell, Spain; Marion Merrell Dow, Switz.†; Marion Merrell Dow, USA.
Chlorotrianisene (p.1439·2).
Female hypogonadism; menopausal disorders; postpartum breast engorgement; prostatic cancer; vulval and vaginal atrophy.

Tacef
Grunenthal, Aust.; Takeda, Ger.
Cefmenoxime hydrochloride (p.166·2).
Bacterial infections.

Tachipirina Angelini, Ital.
Paracetamol (p.72·2).
Fever; pain.

Tachmalcor Dresden, Ger.
Detajmium bitartrate.
Arrhythmias.

Tachmalin Dresden, Ger.
Ajmaline (p.817·1).
Arrhythmias.

TachoComb
Nycomed, Aust.; Nycomed, Ger.
Collagen (p.1566·3); fibrinogen (p.722·3); thrombin (p.728·1); aprotinin (p.711·3).
Haemorrhage.

Tacholiquin
Sigmapharm, Aust.; Bene, Ger.; Bene, Switz.†.
Tyloxapol (p.1329·2).
Respiratory-tract disorders.

Tachotop N Nycomed, Ger.
Collagen (p.1566·3).
Haemorrhagic disorders.

Tachydaron Dresden, Ger.
Amiodarone hydrochloride (p.820·1).
Arrhythmias.

Tachyfenon Dresden, Ger.
Propafenone hydrochloride (p.935·3).
Arrhythmias.

Tachynerg N Eberth, Ger.
Testosterone propionate (p.1464·2); benzyl nicotinate (p.22·1); camphor (p.1557·2); menthol (p.1600·2); lemon oil (p.1595·3).
Cardiac disorders.

Tachyrol Duphar, Irl.†.
Dihydrotachysterol (p.1366·3).
Vitamin D deficiencies.

Tachystin ankerpharm, Ger.
Dihydrotachysterol (p.1366·3).
Hypoparathyroidism.

Tachytalol Dresden, Ger.
Sotalol hydrochloride (p.945·1).
Arrhythmias.

Tacid-4 Roche, S.Afr.
Aluminium hydroxide-magnesium carbonate co-dried gel (p.1178·2); calcium carbonate (p.1182·1); magnesium hydroxide (p.1198·2); sodium bicarbonate (p.1153·2).
Hyperchlorhydria.

tactu-nerval Feldhoff, Ger.
Bovine testicular extract (p.1464·1); bovine placental extract.
Musculoskeletal disorders; peripheral circulatory disorders.

TAD Biomedica, Ital.
Glutathione sodium (p.983·1).
Alcohol or drug poisoning; ionising radiation damage.

TAD+ Seroyal, Canad.
Multivitamins with zinc.

Tadenan
Boehringer Mannheim, Aust.; Debat, Fr.; Fournier, Ital.; Debat, Switz.
Pygeum africanum (p.1461·3).
Benign prostatic hyperplasia.

Tafil Pharmacia Upjohn, Ger.
Alprazolam (p.640·3).
Anxiety disorders.

Tagagel SmithKline Beecham, Ger.
Cimetidine (p.1183·2).
Gastro-oesophageal reflux; peptic ulcer; Zollinger-Ellison syndrome.

Tagamet
SmithKline Beecham, Austral.; SK-RIT, Belg.; SmithKline Beecham, Canad.; SmithKline Beecham, Fr.; SmithKline Beecham, Ger.; SmithKline Beecham, Irl.; Smith Kline & French, Ital.; SmithKline Beecham, Neth.; SmithKline Beecham, Norw.; SmithKline Beecham, S.Afr.; Smith Kline & French, Spain; SmithKline Beecham, Swed.; SmithKline Beecham, Switz.; SmithKline Beecham, UK; SmithKline Beecham, USA.
Cimetidine (p.1183·2) or cimetidine hydrochloride (p.1185·3).
Acid aspiration; gastro-intestinal haemorrhage; gastro-oesophageal reflux; peptic ulcer; Zollinger-Ellison syndrome.

Tagamet Dual Action SmithKline Beecham Consumer, UK†.
Cimetidine (p.1183·2); sodium alginate (p.1470·3).
Heartburn.

TAGG Eagle, Austral.
Benzododecinium chloride (p.1103·2).
Deodorant detergent for ostomies.

Tagonis Janssen-Cilag, Ger.
Paroxetine hydrochloride (p.301·2).
Depression.

Taguinol Spyfarma, Spain.
Loperamide hydrochloride (p.1197·2).
Diarrhoea.

Tai Ginseng N Poehlmann, Switz.
Ginseng (p.1584·2); crataegus (p.1568·2); hypericum (p.1590·1); vitamins.
Tonic.

Taingel Ghimas, Ital.
Royal jelly; pollen; ginseng; eleutherococcus; dried yeast.
Nutritional supplement.

Tairal Rottapharm, Spain.
Famotidine (p.1192·1).
Gastro-oesophageal reflux; peptic ulcer; Zollinger-Ellison syndrome.

Takacillin Torii, Jpn†.
Lenampicillin hydrochloride (p.221·2).

Taka-Diastase Warner-Lambert, Ital.
Pepsin (p.1616·3); pancreatin (p.1612·1).
Formerly contained amylitic enzymes of *Aspergillus oryzae.*
Dyspepsia.

Takadispep Complex Cantabria, Spain.
Amylase (p.1549·1); dimethicone (p.1213·1); pancreatin (p.1612·1); papain (p.1614·1).
Aerophagia; digestive enzyme deficiency; dyspepsia; meteorism.

Takata Madariaga, Spain.
Aloin (p.1177·2); belladonna (p.457·1); phenolphthalein (p.1208·2).
Constipation.

Takepron Takeda, Jpn.
Lansoprazole (p.1196·2).
Gastro-oesophageal reflux; peptic ulcer; Zollinger-Ellison syndrome.

Takesulin Takeda, Jpn.
Cefsulodin sodium (p.173·2).
Mepivacaine hydrochloride (p.1297·2) is included in the intramuscular injection to alleviate the pain of injection.
Pseudomonal infections.

Taketiam
Takeda, Fr.
Cefotiam hydrochloride (p.170·2) or cefotiam hexetil hydrochloride (p.170·2).
Lignocaine hydrochloride (p.1293·2) is included in the intramuscular injection to alleviate the pain of injection.
Formerly known as Pansporine.

Bacterial infections.

Takus *Pharmacia Upjohn, Ger.*
Ceruletide tris(diethylamine) (p.1561·2).
Diagnostic agent; paralytic ileus; postoperative atony.

Talacen *Sanofi Winthrop, USA.*
Pentazocine hydrochloride (p.75·1); paracetamol (p.72·2).
Pain.

Talcid
Bayer, Aust.; Bayer, Ger.; Bayer, Spain; Bayer, Swed.†.
Hydrotalcite (p.1194·1).
Gastro-intestinal hyperacidity.

Talco Antihistam Calber *Pentafarm, Spain.*
Calamine (p.1080·1); zinc oxide (p.1096·2); bismuth subnitrate (p.1180·2); kaolin; diphenhydramine hydrochloride (p.409·1); menthol (p.1600·2); talc (p.1092·1).
Cutaneous hypersensitivity reactions.

Taleilcina *Rovi, Spain†.*
Erythromycin estolate (p.204·1).
Bacterial infections.

Talgo Odontalgico *Ern, Spain.*
Ethyl chloride (p.1292·3); trichlorethylene (p.1234·2).
Dental pain.

Talidat *Merck, Ger.*
Hydrotalcite (p.1194·1).
Gastro-intestinal disorders associated with hyperacidity; peptic ulcer.

Talis
Kali, Aust.†; Organon, Ger.
Metaclazepam hydrochloride (p.678·3).
Psychiatric disorders.

Talkosona *Vita, Spain.*
Benzalkonium chloride (p.1101·3); bismuth subnitrate (p.1180·2); dexamethasone (p.1037·1); talc; tannic acid (p.1634·2); zinc oxide (p.1096·2).
Skin infections with inflammation.

Talofen *Fournier, Ital.*
Promazine hydrochloride (p.689·1).
Anxiety; pain; psychoses; vomiting.

Taloxa
Aesca, Aust.; Schering-Plough, Fr.; Essex, Ger.; Schering-Plough, Ital.; Schering-Plough, Neth.; Schering-Plough, Spain; Schering-Plough, Swed.
Felbamate (p.345·3).
Epilepsy.

Taloxoral *Schering-Plough, Norw.*
Felbamate (p.345·3).
Epilepsy.

Talquissar *Vita, Spain.*
Bismuth subnitrate (p.1180·2); boric acid (p.1554·2); calamine (p.1080·1); talc (p.1092·1); tannic acid (p.1634·2).
Skin disorders.

Talquistina *Vita, Spain.*
Bismuth subnitrate (p.1180·2); boric acid (p.1554·2); calamine (p.1080·1); diphenhydramine hydrochloride (p.409·1); talc (p.1092·1); tannic acid (p.1634·2).
Cutaneous hypersensitivity reactions.

Talso
Sanofi Winthrop, Aust.; Sanofi Winthrop, Ger.
Saw palmetto (p.1462·1).
Benign prostatic hyperplasia.

Talsutin *Squibb, Ital.†.*
Tetracycline (p.259·1); amphotericin (p.372·2).
Bacterial and fungal infections of the vagina.

Talusin
Knoll, Austral.; Knoll, Ger.; Knoll, Irl.†; Knoll, Ital.†; Knoll, S.Afr.†; Meda, Swed.†; Knoll, Switz.
Proscillaridin (p.938·1).
Heart failure.

Taluvian
Ebewe, Aust.†; Knoll, Ger.†.
Proscillaridin (p.938·1); verapamil hydrochloride (p.960·3).
Cardiovascular disorders.

Talval *Lipha, Switz.*
Idrocilamide (p.1315·3).
Musculoskeletal and joint disorders.

Talvosilen
Sigmapharm, Aust.; Bene, Ger.
Codeine phosphate (p.26·1); paracetamol (p.72·2).
Pain.

Talvosilene *Milupa, Switz.*
Codeine phosphate (p.26·1); paracetamol (p.72·2).
Pain.

Talwin
Sanofi Winthrop, Canad.; Sanofi Winthrop, Ital.; Sanofi Winthrop, USA.
Pentazocine hydrochloride (p.75·1) or pentazocine lactate (p.75·1).
Adjunct to general anaesthesia; pain; premedication.

Talwin Compound *Sanofi Winthrop, USA.*
Pentazocine hydrochloride (p.75·1); aspirin (p.16·1).
Pain.

Talwin NX *Sanofi Winthrop, USA.*
Pentazocine hydrochloride (p.75·1).
Naloxone hydrochloride (p.986·2) is included in this preparation to discourage abuse.
Pain.

Talwin-Tab *Sanofi Winthrop, Ital.*
Pentazocine hydrochloride (p.75·1).
Pain.

Tam *Alacan, Spain.*
Ciprofloxacin hydrochloride (p.185·3).
Bacterial infections.

Tamanybonsan *Salushaus, Ger.*
Salix (p.82·3).
Fever; headache; rheumatic disorders.

Tamarine
Note. This name is used for preparations of different composition.
SmithKline Beecham Consumer, Belg.; Serono, Ital.; Whitehall-Robins, Switz.
Senna (p.1212·2); cassia (p.1183·1); tamarind (p.1217·3); coriander (p.1567·3); liquorice (p.1197·1).
Constipation.

SmithKline Beecham Sante, Fr.
Senna leaf (p.1212·2); tamarind (p.1217·3).
Constipation.

Tamarmanna *Benvegna, Ital.†.*
Senna (p.1212·2); manna (p.1199·1); sorbitol (p.1354·2).
Constipation.

Tamax *Laevosan, Aust.*
Tamoxifen citrate (p.563·3).
Breast cancer; endometrial cancer.

Tamaxin *Orion, Swed.*
Tamoxifen citrate (p.563·3).
Breast cancer.

Tambocor
3M, Austral.; 3M, Belg.; 3M, Canad.; 3M, Ger.; 3M, Irl.; 3M, Neth.; 3M, Norw.; 3M, S.Afr.; 3M, Swed.; 3M, Switz.; 3M, UK; 3M, USA.
Flecainide acetate (p.868·3).
Arrhythmias.

Tameran *Semar, Spain.*
Famotidine (p.1192·1).
Gastro-oesophageal reflux; peptic ulcer; Zollinger-Ellison syndrome.

Tametin *Caber, Ital.*
Cimetidine (p.1183·2).
Gastric hyperacidity; peptic ulcer; Zollinger-Ellison syndrome.

Tamik *Marcofina, Fr.*
Dihydroergotamine mesylate (p.444·2).
Migraine; orthostatic hypotension; peripheral venous insufficiency.

Tamin *Merck Sharp & Dohme, Spain.*
Famotidine (p.1192·1).
Gastro-oesophageal reflux; peptic ulcer; Zollinger-Ellison syndrome.

Tamine SR *Geneva, USA.*
Phenylpropanolamine hydrochloride (p.1067·2); phenylephrine hydrochloride (p.1066·2); brompheniramine maleate (p.403·2).
Upper respiratory-tract symptoms.

Tamizam *Zambon, Belg.*
Tamoxifen citrate (p.563·3).
Breast cancer; endometrial cancer.

Tamobeta *Betapharm, Ger.*
Tamoxifen citrate (p.563·3).
Breast cancer.

Tamofen
Gerot, Aust.; Rhone-Poulenc Rorer, Canad.; Rhone-Poulenc Rorer, Ger.; Pharmacia Upjohn, Irl.; Leiras, Norw.; Pharmacia Upjohn, UK.
Tamoxifen citrate (p.563·3).
Anovulatory infertility; breast cancer; endometrial cancer.

Tamofene *Bellon, Fr.*
Tamoxifen citrate (p.563·3).
Breast cancer.

Tamokadin *Kade, Ger.*
Tamoxifen citrate (p.563·3).
Breast cancer.

Tamone *Pharmacia Upjohn, Canad.*
Tamoxifen citrate (p.563·3).
Breast cancer.

Tamoplex
Lannacher, Aust.; Du Pont, Canad.†; Pharmachemie, S.Afr.
Tamoxifen citrate (p.563·3).
Breast cancer; endometrial cancer.

Tamosin *Sigma, Austral.*
Tamoxifen citrate (p.563·3).
Breast cancer.

Tamox
Gry, Ger.; Isis Puren, Ger.; Rowex, Irl.
Tamoxifen citrate (p.563·3).
Breast cancer; endometrial cancer.

Tamoxasta *Asta Medica, Ger.*
Tamoxifen citrate (p.563·3).
Breast cancer.

Tamoxen *Douglas, Austral.*
Tamoxifen citrate (p.563·3).
Breast cancer.

Tamoxigenat *Azupharma, Ger.*
Tamoxifen citrate (p.563·3).
Breast cancer.

Tamoximerck *Merck, Ger.*
Tamoxifen citrate (p.563·3).
Breast cancer.

Tamoxistad *Stada, Ger.*
Tamoxifen citrate (p.563·3).
Breast cancer.

Tampilen *Sabater, Spain†.*
Metampicillin sodium (p.224·3).
Bacterial infections.

Tamposit *Lappe, Ger.†.*
Aesculus (p.1543·3); hamamelis (p.1587·1); laureth 9 (p.1325·2); zinc oxide (p.1096·2); bismuth subnitrate (p.1180·2).
Anorectal disorders.

Tamposit N *Lappe, Ger.*
Laureth 9 (p.1325·2) zinc oxide (p.1096·2); bismuth subnitrate (p.1180·2).
Anorectal disorders.

Tampositoires B *Piraud, Switz.†.*
Belladonna (p.457·1); guaiazulene (p.1586·3); hamamelis (p.1587·1).
Anorectal disorders.

Tampositorien B *Lappe, Ger.†.*
Belladonna (p.457·1); guaiazulene (p.1586·3); hamamelis (p.1587·1).
Anorectal disorders.

Tampositorien H *Lappe, Ger.*
Hamamelis (p.1587·1).
Anorectal disorders.

Tampositorien mit Belladonna *Provita, Aust.*
Belladonna (p.457·1); guaiazulene (p.1586·3); hamamelis (p.1587·1).
Anorectal disorders.

Tampovagan *Co-Pharma, UK.*
Stilboestrol (p.1462·3); lactic acid (p.1593·3).
Postmenopausal vaginitis.

Tampovagan c. Acid. lact. *Sanofi Winthrop, Ger.*
Lactic acid (p.1593·3).
Vaginitis.

Tampovagan C-N N *Sanofi Winthrop, Ger.†.*
Hydrocortisone acetate (p.1043·3); neomycin sulphate (p.229·2); sulphathiazole (p.257·1).
Vaginal infections; vaginitis.

Tamuc *TAD, Ger.*
Acetylcysteine (p.1052·3).
Respiratory-tract disorders associated with increased or viscous mucus.

Tamyl *Formatrading, Ital.*
Propylene glycol cefatrizine (p.164·2).
Bacterial infections.

Tanac
Note. This name is used for preparations of different composition.
Del, Canad.
Topical gel: Allantoin (p.1078·2); dyclocaine hydrochloride (p.1292·3).
Topical liquid: Benzocaine (p.1286·2); benzalkonium chloride (p.1101·3); tannic acid (p.1634·2).

Del, USA.
Lipstick: Benzocaine (p.1286·2); tannic acid (p.1634·2); benzalkonium chloride (p.1101·3).
Sore lips.
Topical gel: Dyclocaine hydrochloride (p.1292·3); allantoin (p.1078·2).
Herpes labialis.
Topical liquid: Benzocaine (p.1286·2); benzalkonium chloride (p.1101·3).
Mouth ulcers; sore gums.

Tanac Dual Core *Del, USA.*
Benzocaine (p.1286·2); tannic acid (p.1634·2); allantoin (p.1078·2); benzalkonium chloride (p.1101·3); padimate O (p.1488·1).
Oral lesions.

Tanacet
McNeil Consumer, Canad.; Herbal Laboratories, UK.
Feverfew (p.447·3).
Migraine.

Tanadopa *Tanabe, Jpn.*
Docarpamine (p.861·1).
Circulatory insufficiency.

Tanafed *Horizon, USA.*
Chlorpheniramine tannate (p.405·2); pseudoephedrine tannate (p.1069·2).
Upper respiratory-tract symptoms.

Tanagel *Durban, Spain.*
Belladonna (p.457·1); gelatin tannate; opium (p.70·3).
Colitis; diarrhoea; gastroenteritis.

Tanagel Inf *Durban, Spain†.*
Gelatin tannate.
Diarrhoea.

Tanagel Papeles *Durban, Spain.*
Gelatin tannate.
Diarrhoea.

Tanakan *IPSEN, Fr.*
Ginkgo biloba (p.1584·1).
Mental function impairment in the elderly; peripheral vascular disorders.

Tanakene
Semar, Spain; Intersan, Switz.
Ginkgo biloba (p.1584·1).
Vascular disorders.

Tanalone *Labima, Belg.*
Albumin tannate (p.1176·3); pectin (p.1474·1).
Diarrhoea.

Tanasid *Rovifarma, Spain.*
Aluminium hydroxide (p.1177·3); sodium carbonate (p.1630·2).
Gastro-intestinal disorders.

Tanatril *Tanabe, Jpn.*
Imidapril hydrochloride (p.890·2).
Hypertension.

Tancolin *Roche Consumer, UK†.*
Dextromethorphan hydrobromide (p.1057·3); ascorbic acid (p.1365·2); citric acid (p.1564·3); sodium citrate (p.1153·2).
Formerly contained dextromethorphan hydrobromide, theophylline, and ascorbic acid.
Coughs.

Tandem Icon *Britpharm, UK.*
Pregnancy test (p.1621·2).

Tanderil
Ciba Vision, Aust.; Dispersa, Ger.†; Zyma, Irl.†; Ciba Vision, Switz.†; Zyma, UK†.
Oxyphenbutazone (p.72·1).
Eye disorders.

Tanderil Chloramphenicol *Zyma, Irl.†.*
Oxyphenbutazone (p.72·1); chloramphenicol (p.182·1).
Inflamed eye infections.

Tanganil
Pierre Fabre, Fr.; Rhone-Poulenc Rorer, Neth.†.
Acetylleucine (p.1542·1).
Vertigo.

Tangenol *Bucca, Spain.*
Eugenol (p.1578·2); procaine hydrochloride (p.1299·2); tannic acid (p.1634·2).
Dental disorders.

Tanidina *Robert, Spain.*
Ranitidine hydrochloride (p.1209·3).
Acid aspiration; gastro-intestinal haemorrhage; gastro-oesophageal reflux; peptic ulcer; Zollinger-Ellison syndrome.

Tannacomp *Knoll, Ger.*
Albumin tannate (p.1176·3); ethacridine lactate (p.1098·3).
Diarrhoea.

Tannalbin
Ebewe, Aust.; Knoll, Austral.†; Knoll, Ger.; Knoll, Neth.
Albumin tannate (p.1176·3).
Diarrhoea.

Tannamicina *Panthox & Burck, Ital.†.*
Kanamycin tannate (p.221·1).
Bacterial infections.

Tannidin Plus *GD, Ital.*
Betacarotene (p.1335·2); selenium (p.1353·3); vitamin E (p.1369·1).
Antioxidant.

Tannisol *GD, Ital.*
Betacarotene (p.1335·2).
Sunscreen.

Tannolact *Basotherm, Ger.*
Condensation product of urea-sodium cresolsulphonic acid.
Hyperhidrosis; skin disorders.

Tannolil *Li-il, Ger.*
Tannic acid (p.1634·2); aluminium sulphate (p.1548·1).
Haemorrhoids; hyperhidrosis; skin irritation.

Tannosynt
Note. This name is used for preparations of different composition.
Merck, Aust.
2,6-Bis-N' (2-hydroxy-3-sulpho-(ev. 5-methyl-)benzyl)-ureidomethyl-phenol(ev. p-cresol) disodium.
Skin disorders.

Hermal, Ger.
Tannic acid (p.1634·2).
Burns; hyperhidrosis; skin disorders.

Hermal, Switz.
Phenol cresol sulphonic acid-formaldehyde condensation product.
Formerly contained tannic acid or sodium tannate.
Skin disorders.

Tannovit *Difa, Ital.†.*
Benzalkonium chloride (p.1101·3); tannic acid (p.1634·2).
Disinfection of the nasal mucosa.

Tanoral *Parmed, USA.*
Phenylephrine tannate (p.1067·1); chlorpheniramine tannate (p.405·2); mepyramine tannate (p.414·1).
Upper respiratory-tract symptoms.

Tanrix
SmithKline Beecham, Aust.; SmithKline Beecham, Ital.
An adsorbed tetanus vaccine (p.1535·3).
Active immunisation.

Tantacol DM *Tanta, Canad.*
Phenylpropanolamine hydrochloride (p.1067·2); pheniramine maleate (p.415·3); mepyramine maleate (p.414·1); dextromethorphan hydrobromide (p.1057·3).
Cold symptoms; coughs.

Tantafed *Tanta, Canad.*
Pseudoephedrine hydrochloride (p.1068·3).

Tantaphen *Tanta, Canad.*
Paracetamol (p.72·2).
Fever; pain.

Tantapp *Tanta, Canad.*
Phenylephrine hydrochloride (p.1066·2); phenylpropanolamine hydrochloride (p.1067·2); brompheniramine maleate (p.403·2).

Tantol Skin Cleanser *Quatromed, S.Afr.*
Triclosan (p.1127·2); phenonip; phenoxyethanol (p.1122·2).
Skin disinfection.

Tantol Skin Lotion *Quatromed, S.Afr.*
Soap substitute.

Tantum
Note. This name is used for preparations of different composition.
Angelini, Aust.; 3M, Canad.; Angelini, Ital.; Organon, Neth.†; Donmed, S.Afr.†; Farma Lepori, Spain; Sauter, Switz.†.
Benzydamine hydrochloride (p.21·3).
Inflammation; pain; peripheral vascular disorders; soft-tissue disorders; thrombophlebitis; vaginitis.

Farma Lepori, Spain.
Throat spray: Benzydamine hydrochloride (p.21·3); hexamidine di-isethionate (p.1115·3).
Mouth and throat inflammation.

Tantum Ciclina *Farma Lepori, Spain.*
Benzydamine hydrochloride (p.21·3); tetracycline hydrochloride (p.259·1).
Acne; bacterial infections.

Tantum Verde
Solvay, Ger.; Farma Lepori, Spain.
Benzydamine hydrochloride (p.21·3).
Mouth and throat pain and inflammation.

Tanyl *Intramed, S.Afr.*
Fentanyl citrate (p.38·1).
Adjunct to general anaesthesia; pain.

Tanzal *Iquinosa, Spain.*
Oxatomide (p.415·1).
Hypersensitivity reactions.

TAO
Roerig, Belg.†; Roerig, USA.
Triacetyloleandomycin (p.264·3).
Bacterial infections.

Tapanol *Republic, USA.*
Paracetamol (p.72·2).
Fever; pain.

Tapazole
Lilly, Canad.; Lilly, Ital.; Lilly, S.Afr.†; Dista, Switz.; Lilly, USA.
Methimazole (p.1495·3).
Hyperthyroidism.

Taponoto *Parisis, Spain.*
Potassium carbonate.
Formerly contained potassium carbonate and thymol.
Removal of ear wax.

Tar Doak *Trans Canaderm, Canad.*
Coal tar (p.1092·3).
Skin disorders.

Tara Abfuhrsirup *Disperga, Aust.*
Senna (p.1212·2).
Bowel evacuation; stool softener.

Taractan
Roche, Ger.†; Roche, Ital.†; Roche, USA†.
Chlorprothixene (p.656·1), chlorprothixene hydrochloride (p.656·2), or chlorprothixene lactate (p.656·2) and chlorprothixene hydrochloride (p.656·2).
Psychoses.

Taradyl *Roche, Belg.*
Ketorolac trometamol (p.49·1).
Pain.

Taraleon *Zilly, Ger.*
Taraxacum (p.1634·2).
Biliary-tract disorders; diuretic; dyspepsia; loss of appetite.

Taraphilic *Medco, USA.*
Coal tar (p.1092·3).
Skin disorders.

Taraskon *Farmasan, Ger.†.*
Atenolol (p.825·3).
Cardiovascular disorders.

Taraxacum Med Complex *Dynamit, Aust.*
Homoeopathic preparation.

Tarband
Boots, Austral.; Seton, UK.
Coal tar (p.1092·3); zinc oxide (p.1096·2).
Medicated bandage.

Tarcil *SmithKline Beecham, Austral.*
Ticarcillin sodium (p.263·2).
Bacterial infections.

Tarcortin *Stafford-Miller, UK.*
Hydrocortisone (p.1043·3); coal tar (p.1092·3).
Skin disorders.

Tardan *Odan, Canad.*
Salicylic acid (p.1090·2); coal tar (p.1092·3).
Seborrhoea.

Tardigal *Beiersdorf-Lilly, Ger.†.*
Digitoxin (p.848·3).
Cardiac disorders.

Tardocillin *Bayer, Ger.*
Benzathine penicillin (p.158·3).
Tolycaine hydrochloride (p.1301·1) is included in this preparation to alleviate the pain of injection.
Long-term treatment of rheumatic fever.

Tardrox *Carlton Laboratories, UK†.*
Tar (p.1092·3); halquinol (p.215·3).

Tardurol *Procter & Gamble, Aust.*
Propranolol hydrochloride (p.937·1); triamterene (p.957·2); hydrochlorothiazide (p.885·2).
Hypertension.

Tardyferon
Germania, Aust.; Robapharm, Fr.; Pierre Fabre, Ger.; Pierre Fabre, Spain; Robapharm, Switz.
Ferrous sulphate (p.1340·2); mucoproteose.
Ascorbic acid (p.1365·2) is included in this preparation to increase the absorption and availability of iron.
Iron-deficiency; iron-deficiency anaemias.

Tardyferon B$_9$ *Robapharm, Fr.*
Ferrous sulphate (p.1340·2); folic acid (p.1340·3); mucoproteose.
Ascorbic acid (p.1365·2) is included in this preparation to increase the absorption and availability of iron.
Iron and folic acid deficiency.

Tardyferon-Fol
Germania, Aust.; Pierre Fabre, Ger.
Ferrous sulphate (p.1340·2); folic acid (p.1340·3).
Iron and folic acid deficiency; iron-deficiency anaemias.

Tareg *Novartis, Ital.*
Valsartan (p.960·2).
Hypertension.

Tarestin *Inibsa, Spain†.*
Dicyclomine hydrochloride (p.460·1).
Gastro-intestinal spasm.

Targel *Odan, Canad.*
Coal tar (p.1092·3).
Psoriasis.

Targel SA *Odan, Canad.*
Coal tar solution (p.1092·3); salicylic acid (p.1090·2).
Psoriasis.

Target
Note. This name is used for preparations of different composition.
Wyeth Lederle, Aust.; Much, Ger.; Lederle, Switz.
Felbinac (p.37·1) or felbinac iminobispropanol salt (p.37·1).
Musculoskeletal, joint, peri-articular, and soft-tissue disorders.

Lisapharma, Ital.
Atenolol (p.825·3); chlorthalidone (p.839·3).

Targocid
Wyeth Lederle, Aust.; Hoechst Marion Roussel, Austral.; Hoechst Marion Roussel, Belg.; Marion Merrell, Fr.; Hoechst, Ger.; Hoechst Marion Roussel, Irl.; Hoechst Marion Roussel, Neth.; Astra, Norw.; Hoechst Marion Roussel, S.Afr.; Marion Merrell, Spain; Astra, Swed.; Hoechst Marion Roussel, Switz.; Hoechst Marion Roussel, UK.
Teicoplanin (p.257·3).
Gram-positive bacterial infections.

Targophagin *Godecke, Ger.†.*
Silver protein acetyl tannate; benzocaine (p.1286·2); amethocaine hydrochloride (p.1285·2).
Mouth and throat disorders.

Targosid *Lepetit, Ital.*
Teicoplanin (p.257·3).
Gram-positive bacterial infections.

Tarisdin *Isdin, Spain.*
Coal tar (p.1092·3); salicylic acid (p.1090·2).
Skin disorders.

Tarisdin Cutaneo *Isdin, Spain†.*
Coal tar (p.1092·3).
Skin disorders.

Tarivid
Hoechst, Aust.; Hoechst Marion Roussel, Belg.; Hoechst, Ger.; Hoechst Marion Roussel, Irl.; Daiichi, Jpn; Hoechst Marion Roussel, Neth.; Hoechst Marion Roussel, Norw.; Hoechst Marion Roussel, S.Afr.; Hoechst, Spain; Hoechst Marion Roussel, Swed.; Hoechst Marion Roussel, Switz.; Hoechst Marion Roussel, UK.
Ofloxacin (p.233·3) or ofloxacin hydrochloride (p.234·1).
Bacterial infections.

Tarka
Knoll, Ger.; Knoll, Neth.; Knoll, UK; Knoll, USA.
Trandolapril (p.957·1); verapamil hydrochloride (p.960·3).
Hypertension.

Tarlene *Medco, USA.*
Coal tar (p.1092·3); salicylic acid (p.1090·2).
Seborrhoea.

Tarmed *Stiefel, Ital.*
Coal tar (p.1092·3).
Seborrhoeic dermatitis.

Taro Gel *Taro, Canad.*
Sterile lubricating jelly.

Ta-Ro-Cap *Soekami, Fr.†.*
Phenylmercuric nitrate (p.1122·2); benzethonium chloride (p.1102·3).
Contraceptive.

Taro-Sone *Taro, Canad.*
Betamethasone dipropionate (p.1033·3).
Skin disorders.

Tarphosyl *Stafford-Miller, Ital.†.*
Coal tar (p.1092·3).
Seborrhoeic dermatitis.

Tarseb *Draxis, Canad.*
Tar (p.1092·3).

Tarsum *Summers, USA.*
Coal tar (p.1092·3); salicylic acid (p.1090·2).
Seborrhoea.

Tasep *Septa, Spain.*
Cephazolin sodium (p.181·1).
Bacterial infections.

Tasmaderm *Roche, Switz.*
Motretinide (p.1088·3).
Acne.

Tasmar
Roche, Irl.†; Roche, Swed.†; Roche, UK†; Roche, USA.
Tolcapone (p.1146·1).
Parkinsonism.

Tasnon *Kolassa, Aust.*
Piperazine citrate (p.107·2).

Tasto *Roussel, Ital.†.*
Aloglutamol (p.1177·2).
Gastric hyperacidity.

Tasumicina *CEPA, Spain†.*
Calcium pantothenate (p.1352·3); kanamycin sulphate (p.220·3).
Bacterial infections.

Tathion *Yamanouchi, Jpn.*
Reduced glutathione (p.983·1).
Corneal disorders; hepatic disorders; leucopenia due to radiotherapy or chemotherapy; poisoning; radiation-induced inflammation of oral mucosa; skin disorders; vomiting.

Tatig *Bioindustria, Ital.*
Sertraline hydrochloride (p.307·2).
Depression.

Tationil *Boehringer Mannheim, Ital.*
Glutathione sodium (p.983·1).
Alcohol or drug poisoning; radiation trauma.

Tatum-T *Searle, USA†.*
Copper-wound polyethylene (p.1337·3).
Intra-uterine contraceptive device.

Taucor *Sigma-Tau, Spain.*
Lovastatin (p.1275·1).
Hyperlipidaemias.

Taucorten *Sigma-Tau, Ital.†.*
Triamcinolone aminobenzal benzamidoisobutyrate (p.1050·3).
Haemorrhoids; skin disorders.

Tauglicolo *SIT, Ital.*
Bromhexine hydrochloride (p.1055·3); potassium guaiacolsulfonate (p.1068·3).
Respiratory-tract congestion.

Tauliz *Hoechst Marion Roussel, Ital.*
Injection†: Piretanide sodium (p.931·3).
Tablets: Piretanide (p.931·3).
Hypertension; oedema.

Tauma *Vaillant, Ital.*
Salix (p.82·3); passion flower (p.1615·3); crataegus (p.1568·2).
Insomnia.

Tauredon
Byk, Aust.; Tosse, Ger.; Byk, Switz.
Sodium aurothiomalate (p.83·2).
Juvenile chronic arthritis; psoriatic arthritis; rheumatoid arthritis.

Tauro *Ravizza, Ital.*
Tauroursodeoxycholic acid (p.1642·1).
Gallstones.

Taurobetina *Zambon, Spain.*
Adenosine phosphate dipotassium (p.1543·2); cyanocobalamin (p.1363·3); pyridoxine hydrochloride (p.1362·3); uridine phosphate (p.1641·3); taurine (p.1635·1).
Lignocaine hydrochloride (p.1293·2) is included in the intramuscular injection to alleviate the pain of injection.
Neuromuscular metabolic disorders.

Taurolin
Chemomedica, Aust.; Hoechst, Ger.; Geistlich, Neth.†; Geistlich, Switz.
Taurolidine (p.257·2).
Bacterial infections.

Taursol *Wassermann, Ital.†.*
Tauroursodeoxycholic acid (p.1642·1).
Gallstones.

Tauval *Sigma-Tau, Spain.*
Valerian (p.1643·1).
Anxiety; insomnia.

Tauxolo *SIT, Ital.*
Ambroxol hydrochloride (p.1054·3).
Bronchial congestion.

Tavanic *Hoechst Marion Roussel, UK.*
Levofloxacin (p.221·2).
Bacterial infections.

Tavan-SP 54 *Hoechst Marion Roussel, S.Afr.*
Pentosan polysulphate sodium (p.928·1).
Hyperlipidaemias; thrombo-embolic disorders.

Tavegil
Sandoz, Ger.; Sandoz, Irl.; Novartis, Ital.; Novartis, Neth.; Sandoz, Spain; Sandoz, UK.
Clemastine fumarate (p.406·2).
Hypersensitivity reactions.

Tavegyl
Sandoz, Aust.; Sandoz, Austral.†; Sandoz, Norw.; Novartis Consumer, S.Afr.; Novartis, Swed.; Sandoz OTC, Switz.
Clemastine fumarate (p.406·2).
Hypersensitivity reactions.

Tavidan *Baldacci, Ital.*
Heparan sulphate (p.879·2).
Thrombosis prophylaxis.

Tavipec *Montavit, Aust.*
Spike lavender oil (p.1632·2).
Respiratory-tract disorders.

Tavist
Sandoz, Canad.; Sandoz, USA.
Clemastine fumarate (p.406·2).
Hypersensitivity reactions.

Tavist-1 *Sandoz, USA†.*
Clemastine fumarate (p.406·2).
Allergic rhinitis.

Tavist-D
Sandoz, Canad.; Sandoz, USA.
Clemastine fumarate (p.406·2); phenylpropanolamine hydrochloride (p.1067·2).
Allergic rhinitis; nasal congestion.

Tavolax *Singer, Switz.*
Aloes (p.1177·1); belladonna (p.457·1); matricaria (p.1561·2); cascara (p.1183·1); senna (p.1212·2); bisacodyl (p.1179·3); docusate sodium (p.1189·3).
Bowel evacuation; constipation.

Tavonin *VSM, Neth.*
Ginkgo biloba (p.1584·1).
Peripheral vascular disorders.

Tavor
Wyeth, Ger.; Wyeth, Ital.
Lorazepam (p.675·3).
Anxiety; depression; insomnia; premedication; status epilepticus.

Taxilan
Promonta, Ger.; Byk, Neth.
Perazine dimalonate (p.685·1).
Agitation; depression; mania; psychoses.

Taxol
Bristol-Myers Squibb, Aust.; Bristol-Myers Squibb, Austral.; Bristol-Myers Squibb, Belg.; Bristol-Myers Squibb, Canad.; Bristol-Myers Squibb, Fr.; Bristol-Myers Squibb, Ger.; Bristol-Myers Squibb, Irl.; Bristol-Myers Squibb, Ital.; Bristol-Myers Squibb, Neth.; Bristol-Myers Squibb, Norw.; Bristol-Myers Squibb, S.Afr.; Bristol-Myers, Spain; Bristol-Myers Squibb, Swed.; Bristol-Myers Squibb, Switz.; Bristol-Myers Squibb, UK; Bristol-Myers Squibb, USA.
Paclitaxel (p.556·3).
AIDS-related Kaposi's sarcoma; breast cancer; ovarian cancer.

Taxotere
Schoeller, Aust.; Rhone-Poulenc Rorer, Austral.; Rhone-Poulenc Rorer, Canad.; Bellon, Fr.; Rhone-Poulenc Rorer, Ger.; Rhone-Poulenc Rorer, Irl.; Rhone-Poulenc Rorer, Ital.; Rhone-Poulenc Rorer, Neth.; Rhone-Poulenc Rorer, Norw.; Rhone-Poulenc Rorer, S.Afr.; Rhone-Poulenc Rorer, Spain; Rhone-Poulenc Rorer, Swed.; Rhone-Poulenc Rorer, UK; Rhone-Poulenc Rorer, USA.
Docetaxel (p.529·1).
Breast cancer; lung cancer.

Tazac *Lilly, Austral.*
Nizatidine (p.1203·2).
Gastro-oesophageal reflux; peptic ulcer.

Tazicef *SmithKline Beecham, USA; Abbott, USA.*
Ceftazidime (p.173·3).
Bacterial infections.

Tazidime
Lilly, Canad.; Lilly, USA.
Ceftazidime (p.173·3).
Bacterial infections.

Tazobac
Lederle, Ger.; IRBI, Ital.; Lederle, Switz.
Piperacillin sodium (p.237·2); tazobactam sodium (p.257·3).
Bacterial infections.

Tazocel *Cyanamid, Spain.*
Piperacillin sodium (p.237·2); tazobactam sodium (p.257·3).
Bacterial infections.

Tazocilline *Lederle, Fr.*
Piperacillin sodium (p.237·2); tazobactam sodium (p.257·3).
Bacterial infections.

Tazocin
Lederle, Austral.; Wyeth Lederle, Belg.; Wyeth-Ayerst, Canad.; Wyeth, Irl.; Cyanamid, Ital.; Lederle, Neth.; Wyeth, S.Afr.; Wyeth Lederle, Swed.; Lederle, UK.
Piperacillin sodium (p.237·2); tazobactam sodium (p.257·3).
Lignocaine hydrochloride (p.1293·2) may be included in the intramuscular injection to alleviate the pain of injection.
Bacterial infections.

Tazonam *Wyeth Lederle, Aust.*
Piperacillin sodium (p.237·2); tazobactam sodium (p.257·3).
Bacterial infections.

Tazorac *Allergan, USA.*
Tazarotene (p.1093·2).
Acne; psoriasis.

T-BMP *Seroyal, Canad.*
Vitamin B$_1$ and choline tartrate.

Tb-Phlogin cum B$_6$ *Heyl, Ger.†.*
Isoniazid (p.218·1).
Pyridoxine hydrochloride (p.1362·3) is included in this preparation for the prophylaxis of peripheral neuropathy.
Tuberculosis.

TBV *Seroyal, Canad.*
Vitamin B$_1$, vitamin B$_3$, and magnesium.

3TC
Glaxo Wellcome, Austral.; Glaxo Wellcome, Switz.
Lamivudine (p.622·1).
HIV infection.

TCO *Seroyal, Canad.*
Vitamin and mineral preparation.

TCP *Pfizer Consumer, UK.*
Cream: Chloroxylenol (p.1111·1); triclosan (p.1127·2); chlorine (p.1109·3); iodine (p.1493·1); phenol (p.1121·2); sodium salicylate (p.85·1).
Minor skin disorders; skin disinfection.
Ointment: Chlorine (p.1109·3); iodine (p.1493·1); phenol (p.1121·2); sodium salicylate (p.85·1); methyl salicylate (p.55·2); precipitated sulphur (p.1091·2); tannic acid (p.1634·2); camphor (p.1557·2); salicylic acid (p.1090·2).
Haemorrhoids; minor skin disorders; pruritus.
Pastilles; liquid: Halogenated phenols; phenol (p.1121·2); sodium salicylate (p.85·1).
Minor skin disorders; mouth ulcers; sore throat.

T-Cypionate *Legere, USA†.*
Testosterone cypionate (p.1464·1).

TD Spray Iso Mack *Mack, Illert., Ger.*
Isosorbide dinitrate (p.893·1).
Cardiac disorders.

T-Diet *Jones, USA†.*
Phentermine hydrochloride (p.1484·3).

Td-Impfstoff *Chiron Behring, Ger.; Pasteur Merieux, Ger.*
An adsorbed diphtheria and tetanus vaccine (p.1508·1).
Active immunisation of older children and adults.

Td-Rix *SmithKline Beecham, Ger.*
An adsorbed diphtheria and tetanus vaccine (p.1508·1).
Active immunisation of older children and adults.

T-Dry *Jones, USA.*
Pseudoephedrine hydrochloride (p.1068·3); chlorpheniramine maleate (p.405·1).
Cold symptoms.

Td-Vaccinol *Procter & Gamble, Ger.*
An adsorbed diphtheria and tetanus vaccine (p.1508·1).
Active immunisation of older children and adults.

Te Anatoxal *Kwizda, Aust.*
A tetanus vaccine (p.1535·3).
Active immunisation.

T-E Cypionate *Legere, USA†.*
Testosterone cypionate (p.1464·1); oestradiol cypionate (p.1455·1).

Tealine *Arkopharma, Fr.*
Orthosiphon (p.1592·2); green tea (p.1645·1).
Slimming aid.

Tear Drop *Parmed, USA.*
Polyvinyl alcohol (p.1474·2).
Dry eyes.

Teardrops
Ciba Vision, Austral.; Ciba Vision, Canad.
Polyvinyl alcohol (p.1474·2); povidone (p.1474·2).
Dry eyes.

TearGard *Lee, USA.*
Hydroxyethylcellulose (p.1472·3).
Artificial tears.

Tear-Gel
Ciba Vision, Canad.; Restan, S.Afr.
Carbomer 940 (p.1471·2).
Dry eyes.

Teargen *Goldline, USA.*
Artificial tear solution.
Dry eyes.

Tearisol
Note. This name is used for preparations of different composition.
Inibsa, Spain†.
Benzalkonium chloride (p.1101·3).
Dry eyes.

Iolab, USA.
Hypromellose (p.1473·1).
Dry eyes.

Tears Again *Ocusoft, USA.*
Eye drops: Polyvinyl alcohol (p.1474·2).
Eye ointment: White soft paraffin (p.1382·3); liquid paraffin (p.1382·1).
Dry eyes.

Tears Again MC *Ocusoft, USA.*
Hypromellose (p.1473·1).
Dry eyes.

Tears Encore *Dioptic, Canad.*
Polysorbate 80 (p.1327·3).
Dry eyes.

Tears Humectante *Alcon, Spain.*
Dextran 70 (p.717·1); hypromellose (p.1473·1).
Dry eyes.

Tears Lubricante *Alcon, Spain.*
Wool fat (p.1385·3); white soft paraffin (p.1382·3).
Formerly known as Tears Gel.
Dry eyes.

Tears Naturale
Alcon, Austral.; Alcon, Belg.; Alcon, Canad.; Alcon, Irl.; Alcon, S.Afr.; Alcon, Switz.; Alcon, UK; Alcon, USA.
Dextran 70 (p.717·1); hypromellose (p.1473·1).
Dry eyes.

Tears Plus
Allergan, Austral.; Allergan, Canad.; Allergan, Neth.†; Allergan, S.Afr.; Allergan, Switz.; Allergan, USA.
Polyvinyl alcohol (p.1474·2); povidone (p.1474·2).
Dry eyes.

Tears Renewed *Akorn, USA.*
Eye drops: Dextran 70 (p.717·1); hypromellose (p.1473·1).
Eye ointment: White soft paraffin (p.1382·3); light liquid paraffin (p.1382·1).
Dry eyes.

Teatrois *Theranol-Deglaude, Fr.*
Tiratricol (p.1499·3).
Thyroid disorders.

Tebamide *G & W, USA.*
Trimethobenzamide hydrochloride (p.420·1).
Nausea and vomiting.

Tebege-Tannin *Laevosan, Aust.*
Tannic acid (p.1634·2); acriflavine (p.1098·3).
Anal fissures; burns; frostbite; infected skin disorders; sunburn; ulcers.

Tebertin *Berenguer Infale, Spain.*
Inosine (p.1591·1).
Digitalis intoxication; heart failure; hepatitis; radiation toxicity.

tebesium *Hefa, Ger.*
Isoniazid (p.218·1).
Pyridoxine hydrochloride (p.1362·3) is included in this preparation for the prophylaxis of peripheral neuropathy.
Tuberculosis.

tebesium-s *Hefa, Ger.*
Isoniazid (p.218·1).
Tuberculosis.

Tebetane Compuesto *Elfar, Spain.*
Alanine (p.1333·3); glycine (p.1345·2); glutamic acid (p.1344·3); prunus africana.
Prostatic disorders.

Tebloc *Lafare, Ital.*
Loperamide hydrochloride (p.1197·2).
Diarrhoea.

Tebofortan *Austroplant, Aust.*
Ginkgo biloba (p.1584·1).
Cerebral and peripheral vascular disorders.

Tebofortin *Schwabe, Switz.*
Ginkgo biloba (p.1584·1).
Tonic.

Tebonin
Austroplant, Aust.; Schwabe, Ger.
Ginkgo biloba (p.1584·1).
Cerebral and peripheral vascular disorders.

Tebraxin *Bracco, Ital.*
Rufloxacin hydrochloride (p.247·3).
Bacterial infections.

Tebrazid
Continental Pharma, Belg.; ICN, Canad.
Pyrazinamide (p.241·1).
Tuberculosis.

Tecfazolina *Bohm, Spain.*
Cephazolin sodium (p.181·1).
Lignocaine (p.1293·2) is included in this preparation to alleviate the pain of injection.
Bacterial infections.

Techneplex *Squibb Diagnostics, USA.*
Technetium-99m pentetate (p.1425·1).

TechneScan MAG3 *Byk Gulden, Ital.*
Technetium-99m betiatide (p.1425·1).
Evaluation of urinary-tract disorders.

Techniphylline *Techni-Pharma, Mon.†.*
Theophylline (p.765·1).
Asthma.

Tecipul *Mochida, Jpn†.*
Setiptiline maleate (p.308·1).
Depression.

Tecnal *Technilab, Canad.*
Butalbital (p.644·3); caffeine (p.749·3); aspirin (p.16·1).
Pain; tension.

Tecnal C *Technilab, Canad.*
Butalbital (p.644·3); caffeine (p.749·3); aspirin (p.16·1); codeine phosphate (p.26·1).
Pain; tension.

Tectivit *Rorer, Ger.†.*
Chlorophyllin copper complex (p.1000·1); acriflavine (p.1098·3); terra silicea (p.1474·3); colloidal silicon dioxide (p.1475·1).
Wounds.

Tecura *Polcopharma, Austral.†.*
Aesculus (p.1543·3).
Menopausal disorders; peripheral vascular disorders.

Teczem *Hoechst Marion Roussel, USA.*
Enalapril maleate (p.863·2); diltiazem maleate.
Hypertension.

Tedarol *Specia, Fr.†.*
Triamcinolone diacetate (p.1050·2).
Corticosteroid.

Tediprima *Estedi, Spain.*
Trimethoprim (p.265·1).
Genito-urinary infections.

Tedipulmo *Estedi, Spain.*
Terbutaline sulphate (p.764·1).
Obstructive airways disease.

Tedivax *SK-RIT, Belg.*
An adsorbed diphtheria and tetanus vaccine (p.1508·1).
Active immunisation.

Tedral
Parke, Davis, Canad.; Parke, Davis, S.Afr.†; Parke, Davis, Spain†; Parke, Davis, USA†.
Theophylline (p.765·1); ephedrine hydrochloride (p.1059·3); phenobarbitone (p.350·2).
Asthma; bronchospasm.

Tedralan *Labomed, Fr.*
Theophylline (p.765·1); racephedrine hydrochloride (p.1060·1); phenobarbitone (p.350·2).
Asthma; bronchospasm.

Tedrigen *Goldline, USA.*
Theophylline (p.765·1); ephedrine hydrochloride (p.1059·3); phenobarbitone (p.350·2).
Bronchospasm.

Tee gegen Durchfall nach Dr Bohmig *Bio-Reform, Aust.†.*
Tormentil root (p.1638·3); chamomile flower (p.1561·2); fragaria vesca; rubus fruticosus; raspberry leaf (p.1624·2).
Diarrhoea.

Teedex *Rice Steele, Irl.*
Paracetamol (p.72·2); diphenhydramine hydrochloride (p.409·1).
Fever; teething pain.

Teejel
Asta Medica, Belg.; Purdue Frederick, Canad.; Seton, Irl.
Choline salicylate (p.25·2).
Gum and mouth pain.

Teekanne Blasen- und Nierentee *Teekanne, Aust.*
Equisetum (p.1575·1); silver birch (p.1553·3); solidago virgaurea; ononis (p.1610·2); peppermint leaf (p.1208·1).
Urinary tract disorders.

Teekanne Erkaltungstee *Teekanne, Aust.*
Sambucus (p.1627·2); tilia (p.1637·3); thyme (p.1636·3).
Cold symptoms.

Teekanne Herz- und Kreislauftee *Teekanne, Aust.*
Crataegus (p.1568·2); rosemary; fennel (p.1579·1); spearmint (p.1632·1).
Cardiac disorders.

Teekanne Husten- und Brusttee *Teekanne, Aust.*
Fennel (p.1579·1); aniseed (p.1549·3); wild thyme; sage leaf (p.1627·1); thyme (p.1636·3).
Coughs.

Teekanne Leber- und Galletee *Teekanne, Aust.*
Fennel (p.1579·1); curcuma zanthorrhiza; chamomile (p.1561·2); taraxacum (p.1634·2).
Liver and biliary disorders.

Teekanne Magen- und Darmtee *Teekanne, Aust.*
Chamomile (p.1561·2); peppermint leaf (p.1208·1); cinnamon (p.1564·2); melissa leaf (p.1600·1).
Gastro-intestinal disorders.

Teekanne Schlaf- und Nerventee *Teekanne, Aust.*
Lavender (p.1594·3); peppermint leaf (p.1208·1); melissa (p.1600·1); valerian (p.1643·1).
Sleep disorders.

Teen Formula *Avon, Canad.*
Multivitamin and mineral preparation.

Teen Midol *Sterling, USA.*
Paracetamol (p.72·2); pamabrom (p.927·1).

Teen Vitamins *Adams, Canad.*
Multivitamin and mineral preparation.

Teer-Linola-Fett *Wolff, Ger.*
Coal tar (p.1092·3).
Skin disorders.

Teerol *Max Ritter, Switz.*
Coal tar (p.1092·3).
Skin disorders.

Teerol-H *Max Ritter, Switz.*
Coal tar (p.1092·3); allantoin (p.1078·2); triclosan (p.1127·2).
Scalp disorders.

Teerseife "Blucher-Schering" *Blucher-Schering, Ger.†.*
Birch tar.
Skin disorders.

Teerseife "Blucher-Schering" flussig *Blucher-Schering, Ger.†.*
Coal tar (p.1092·3).
Skin disorders.

Teetha *Nelson, UK.*
Homoeopathic preparation.
Formerly known as Teething Granules.

Teething Relief *Brauer, Austral.*
Homoeopathic preparation.

Teething Syrup *Sabex, Canad.†.*
Benzocaine (p.1286·2).
Teething pain.

Tefamin *Recordati, Ital.*
Aminophylline (p.748·1) or theophylline (p.765·1).
Asthma; bronchospasm.

Tefavinca *Bohm, Spain.*
Vincamine (p.1644·1).
Cerebral trauma; cerebrovascular disorders.

Tefilin *Hermal, Ger.*
Tetracycline hydrochloride (p.259·1).
Bacterial infections.

Tegasorb *3M, Fr.*
Carmellose (p.1471·2).
Burns; ulcers.

Tega-Vert *Ortega, USA.*
Dimenhydrinate (p.408·2).
Motion sickness.

Tegeline *Lab Francais du Fractionnement, Fr.*
A normal immunoglobulin (p.1522·1).
Hypogammaglobulinaemia; idiopathic thrombocytopenic purpura; Kawasaki disease; passive immunisation.

Tegens *Inverni della Beffa, Ital.*
Myrtillus (p.1606·1).
Capillary disorders.

Tegisec *Roussel, Spain.*
Fenproporex hydrochloride (p.1481·3).
Obesity.

Tegison
Roche, Canad.†; Roche, USA.
Etretinate (p.1082·2).
Keratinisation disorders; psoriasis.

Tego 2000 *Goldschmidt, UK.*
1-alkyl-1,5-diazapentane.
Surface disinfection.

Tego 103 G
Note. This name is used for preparations of different composition.
Goldschmidt, Ger.†.
Dodicin (p.1112·3); *N,N'*-didodecyl-3-carboxymethyl-3-azapentylen-(1,5)-diamine hydrochloride.
Fungal skin infections; surface disinfection.

Tego, Ital.†.
Alkylaminoethylglycine hydrochloride (p.1112·3).
Skin disinfection; surface disinfection.

Goldschmidt, UK†.
Dodicin (p.1112·3).
Surface disinfection.

Tego 103 S *Goldschmidt, Ger.†.*
Dodicin (p.1112·3).
Instrument disinfection; skin disinfection.

Tego Spray
Note. This name is used for preparations of different composition.
Goldschmidt, Ger.†.
Dodicin hydrochloride (p.1112·3); isopropyl alcohol (p.1118·2).
Hand disinfection.

Tego, Ital.†.
Dodicin (p.1112·3).
Surface disinfection.

Tegodor
Note. This name is used for preparations of different composition.
Goldschmidt, Ger.†; Goldschmidt, UK.
Benzalkonium chloride (p.1101·3); glutaraldehyde (p.1114·3); formaldehyde (p.1113·2).
Fungal skin infections; surface disinfection.

Tego, Ital.†.
Glutaraldehyde (p.1114·3); quaternary ammonium salts.
Instrument and surface disinfection.

Tegodor F *Goldschmidt, Ger.†.*
Benzalkonium chloride (p.1101·3); glutaraldehyde (p.1114·3); didecyldimethylammonium chloride (p.1112·2).
Surface disinfection.

Tegodor forte *Goldschmidt, Ger.†.*
Formaldehyde (p.1113·2); glutaraldehyde (p.1114·3); alkylbenzyldimethylammonium chloride (p.1101·3); glyoxal (p.1115·1).
Surface disinfection.

Tegofektol *Goldschmidt, Ger.†.*
Formaldehyde (p.1113·2); glutaraldehyde (p.1114·3); benzalkonium chloride (p.1101·3).
Surface disinfection.

Tegoment
Note. This name is used for preparations of different composition.
Goldschmidt, Ger.†.
Formaldehyde (p.1113·2); glutaraldehyde (p.1114·3); glyoxal (p.1115·1).
Surface disinfection.

Tego, Ital.†.
Glutaraldehyde (p.1114·3); glyoxal (p.1115·1).
Instrument disinfection.

Tegopen
Bristol, Canad.; Apothecon, USA†.
Cloxacillin sodium (p.195·2).
Bacterial infections.

Tegosinol *Goldschmidt, Ger.†.*
Formaldehyde (p.1113·2); glutaraldehyde (p.1114·3); glyoxal (p.1115·1).
Surface disinfection.

Tegra *Hermes, Ger.*
Garlic oil.
Hyperlipidaemias.

Tegretal *Geigy, Ger.*
Carbamazepine (p.339·2).
Alcohol withdrawal syndrome; bipolar disorder; epilepsy; neuralgias; neuropathies.

Tegretol
Ciba-Geigy, Aust.; Novartis, Austral.; Ciba-Geigy, Belg.; Geigy, Canad.; Ciba-Geigy, Fr.; Geigy, Irl.; Ciba, Ital.; Novartis, Neth.; Geigy, Norw.; Novartis, S.Afr.; Ciba-Geigy, Spain; Novartis, Swed.; Geigy, Switz.; Geigy, UK; Geigy, USA.
Carbamazepine (p.339·2).
Alcohol withdrawal syndrome; bipolar disorder; diabetes insipidus; diabetic neuropathy; epilepsy; mania; trigeminal neuralgia.

Tegrin
Block, Canad.; Reedco, USA.
Coal tar (p.1092·3).
Skin and scalp disorders.

Tegrin Medicated *Block, USA.*
Coal tar (p.1092·3).
Skin disorders.

Tegrin-HC *Block, USA.*
Hydrocortisone (p.1043·3).
Skin disorders.

Tegrin-LT *Block, USA.*
Pyrethrins; piperonyl butoxide (p.1409·3).

Tegunal *CEPA, Spain.*
Dimethicone (p.1384·2); benzethonium chloride (p.1102·3); talc (p.1092·1); zinc oxide (p.1096·2).
Skin disorders.

Teicomid *Hoechst Marion Roussel, Ital.*
Teicoplanin (p.257·3).
Gram-positive bacterial infections.

Teinture de Cocheux *Aguettant, Fr.†.*
Colchicum (p.394·2).
Gout.

Tejuntivo *Iquinosa, Spain.*
Oxaceprol (p.1611·3).
Musculoskeletal and joint disorders; soft tissue disorders; wounds.

Teknadone *Teknofarma, Ital.†.*
Carisoprodol (p.1312·3); nifenazone (p.63·1).
Musculoskeletal and joint disorders.

Telachlor *Major, USA†.*
Chlorpheniramine maleate (p.405·1).
Hypersensitivity reactions.

Teladar *Dermol, USA.*
Betamethasone dipropionate (p.1033·3).
Skin disorders.

Telament
Adcock Ingram Self Medication, S.Afr.†.
Chewable tablets: Simethicone (p.1213·1); atropine methobromide (p.455·1); magnesium carbonate (p.1198·1); dried aluminium hydroxide gel (p.1177·3).
Dyspepsia; flatulence.

Mer-National, S.Afr.
Oral drops: Simethicone (p.1213·1).
Colic; gripe.

Telbibur N *Fatol, Ger.*
Cyanocobalamin (p.1363·3); nicotinamide (p.1351·2); pyridoxine hydrochloride (p.1362·3).
Lignocaine hydrochloride (p.1293·2) is included in this preparation to alleviate the pain of injection.
Liver disorders.

Teldafed Albert-Roussel, Aust.
Terfenadine (p.418·1); pseudoephedrine hydrochloride (p.1068·3).
Allergic rhinitis.

Teldafen Hoechst Marion Roussel, Belg.
Terfenadine (p.418·1); pseudoephedrine hydrochloride (p.1068·3).
Allergic rhinitis.

Teldane
Hoechst Marion Roussel, Austral.; Marion Merrell, Fr.; Hoechst, Ger.; Lepetit, Ital.†; Hoechst Marion Roussel, Switz.
Terfenadine (p.418·1).
Hypersensitivity reactions.

Teldanex
Tika, Norw.; Tika, Swed.
Terfenadine (p.418·1).
Hypersensitivity reactions.

Teldrin SmithKline Beecham Consumer, USA.
Chlorpheniramine maleate (p.405·1).
Hypersensitivity reactions.

Telebar Guerbet, Fr.†.
Barium sulphate (p.1003·1).
Radiographic contrast medium.

Telebrix
Salus, Aust.; Codali, Belg.; Mallinckrodt, Canad.
Meglumine ioxitalamate (p.1009·1); sodium ioxitalamate (p.1009·1).
Contrast medium for CT scanning of the abdomen and pelvis.

Telebrix 12
Guerbet, Fr.; Guerbet, Ital.†; Guerbet, Neth.; Guerbet, Switz.†.
Sodium ioxitalamate (p.1009·1).
Radiographic contrast medium.

Telebrix 30
Guerbet, Fr.; Guerbet, Ital.; Guerbet, Neth.; Guerbet, Switz.†.
Meglumine ioxitalamate (p.1009·1).
Radiographic contrast medium.

Telebrix 35 Guerbet, Fr.
Meglumine ioxitalamate (p.1009·1); sodium ioxitalamate (p.1009·1).
Radiographic contrast medium.

Telebrix 38
Guerbet, Ital.; Guerbet, Neth.†; Guerbet, Switz.†.
Meglumine ioxitalamate (p.1009·1); sodium ioxitalamate (p.1009·1).
Radiographic contrast medium.

Telebrix 350 Guerbet, Neth.
Meglumine ioxitalamate (p.1009·1); sodium ioxitalamate (p.1009·1).
Radiographic contrast medium.

Telebrix Gastro
Codali, Belg.; Guerbet, Fr.; Byk Gulden, Ger.; Guerbet, Neth.; Guerbet, Switz.
Meglumine ioxitalamate (p.1009·1).
Contrast medium for gastro-intestinal radiography.

Telebrix Hystero
Codali, Belg.; Guerbet, Fr.
Meglumine ioxitalamate (p.1009·1); povidone.
Formerly known as Vasurix Polyvidone in *Belg.*
Contrast medium for hysterosalpingography and urinary-tract radiography.

Telebrix N 180 and 300 Byk Gulden, Ger.
Meglumine ioxitalamate (p.1009·1).
Contrast medium for urinary-tract radiography.

Telebrix N 350 and 380 Byk Gulden, Ger.†.
Meglumine ioxitalamate (p.1009·1); sodium ioxitalamate (p.1009·1).
Radiographic contrast medium.

Telebrix N 30 g and 45 g Byk Gulden, Ger.†.
Meglumine ioxitalamate (p.1009·1).
Radiographic contrast medium.

Telebrix Polyvidone Guerbet, Neth.
Meglumine ioxitalamate (p.1009·1); povidone.
Formerly known as Vasurix-Polyvidone.
Contrast medium for hysterosalpingography and urinary-tract radiography.

Telen Yamanouchi, Ger.
Tripotassium dicitratobismuthate (p.1180·2).
Duodenal ulcer.

Telepaque
Nycomed, Austral.; Sanofi Winthrop, Belg.†; Sanofi Winthrop, Canad.; Sanofi Winthrop, Irl.†; Sanofi Winthrop, UK; Nycomed, USA.
Iopanoic acid (p.1007·1).
Contrast medium for biliary-tract radiography.

Telergon II Codit, Ital.
Royal jelly (p.1626·3).
Nutritional supplement.

Telesol Lasa, Spain.
Oxitriptan (p.301·2).
Depression; myoclonus.

Tele-Stulln Stulln, Ger.
Actinoquinol sodium (p.1543·1); naphazoline nitrate (p.1064·2).
Eye disorders.

Telfast
Hoechst Marion Roussel, Austral.; Hoechst Marion Roussel, Swed.; Hoechst Marion Roussel, UK.
Fexofenadine hydrochloride (p.410·3).
Allergic rhinitis; urticaria.

Teline Hauck, USA†.
Tetracycline hydrochloride (p.259·1).
Bacterial infections.

Telo Cypro Relax, Ital.
Copper wire (p.1337·3).
Muscle spasm; musculoskeletal and joint disorders; pain; peripheral vascular disorders.

Telocort Rottapharm, Ital.†.
Ciclomethasone.
Asthma; bronchitis.

Temac Abbott, Swed.†.
Temafloxacin hydrochloride (p.258·2).
Bacterial infections.

Temador Sanico, Belg.
Temazepam (p.693·3).
Anxiety disorders; premedication; sleep disorders.

Temagin Beiersdorf, Ger.†.
Propyphenazone (p.81·3); etenzamide (p.35·3); caffeine (p.749·3).
Influenza; migraine; pain.

Temagin ASS Beiersdorf, Ger.†.
Aspirin (p.16·1).
Arthritis; cold symptoms; fever; inflammation; pain; rheumatism; thrombo-embolic disorders.

Temaril Allergan Herbert, USA†.
Trimeprazine tartrate (p.419·3).
Pruritus.

Temaz Quantum, USA†.
Temazepam (p.693·3).

Temaze Alphapharm, Austral.
Temazepam (p.693·3).
Insomnia.

Temazep CT, Ger.
Temazepam (p.693·3).
Sleep disorders.

Temazin Cold Trenier, USA.
Phenylpropanolamine hydrochloride (p.1067·2); chlorpheniramine maleate (p.405·1).
Upper respiratory-tract symptoms.

Temazine Pinewood, Irl.
Temazepam (p.693·3).
Insomnia.

Temesta
Wyeth Lederle, Aust.; Wyeth Lederle, Belg.; Wyeth, Fr.; Wyeth, Neth.; Wyeth Lederle, Swed.; Wyeth, Switz.
Lorazepam (p.675·3).
Alcohol withdrawal syndrome; anxiety; insomnia; nausea and vomiting; premedication; status epilepticus.

Temetex
Roche, Ger.†; Roche, Ital.; Roche, Spain†; Sauter, Switz.†.
Diflucortolone valerate (p.1039·3).
Skin disorders.

Temetex C Sauter, Switz.†.
Diflucortolone valerate (p.1039·3); chlorquinaldol (p.185·1).
Infected skin disorders.

Temetex Compositum Roche, Spain†.
Diflucortolone valerate (p.1039·3); chlorquinaldol (p.185·1).
Skin infections.

Temetex Excipiens Sauter, Switz.†.
Emollient.
Skin disorders.

Temgesic
Boehringer Mannheim, Aust.; Reckitt & Colman, Austral.; Schering-Plough, Belg.; Schering-Plough, Fr.; Boehringer Mannheim, Ger.; Reckitts, Irl.; Boehringer Mannheim, Ital.; Schering-Plough, Neth.; Reckitt & Colman, Norw.; Reckitt & Colman, S.Afr.; Meda, Swed.; Reckitt & Colman, Switz.; Reckitt & Colman, UK.
Buprenorphine hydrochloride (p.22·2).
Pain.

Temic Uno, Ital.
Cimetidine (p.1183·2).
Gastric hyperacidity; peptic ulcer; Zollinger-Ellison syndrome.

Temol Rolab, S.Afr.
Paracetamol (p.72·2).
Fever; pain.

Temopen
SmithKline Beecham, Ger.†; Bencard, UK†.
Temocillin sodium (p.258·3).
Bacterial infections.

Temovate Glaxo Wellcome, USA.
Clobetasol propionate (p.1035·2).
Skin disorders.

Temoxa Chinoin, Ital.†.
Oxolamine citrate (p.1065·3); amidopyrine (p.15·2).
Cold symptoms; respiratory-tract inflammation; rheumatism.

Temperal Prodes, Spain.
Paracetamol (p.72·2).
Fever; pain.

Tempil Temmler, Ger.
Ibuprofen (p.44·1).
Fever; pain.

Tempil N Temmler, Ger.
Diphenylpyraline hydrochloride (p.409·3); dimepropion hydrochloride (p.1572·1); aspirin (p.16·1).
Cold symptoms.

Templax Sanofi Winthrop, Spain†.
Chlordiazepoxide (p.646·3); homatropine methobromide (p.462·2).
Extrapyramidal disorders; gastro-intestinal disorders; smooth muscle spasm.

Tempo Thompson, USA.
Aluminium hydroxide (p.1177·3); magnesium hydroxide (p.1198·2); simethicone (p.1213·1); calcium carbonate (p.1182·1).
Hyperacidity.

Tempodia SmithKline Beecham Sante, Fr.
Ascorbic acid (p.1365·2).
Vitamin C deficiency.

Tempolax Hommel, Ger.
Bisacodyl (p.1179·3).
Bowel evacuation; constipation.

Temporinolo Hoechst Marion Roussel, Ital.
Phenylpropanolamine hydrochloride (p.1067·2); chlorpheniramine maleate (p.405·1).
Nasal congestion.

Temporol
Orion, Irl.; SMP, S.Afr.†.
Carbamazepine (p.339·2).
Alcohol withdrawal syndrome; deafferentation pain; epilepsy; trigeminal neuralgia.

Temposil Wyeth-Ayerst, Canad.
Calcium carbimide (p.1556·2).
Alcoholism.

Tempra
Mead Johnson, Austral.; Bristol-Myers Squibb, Belg.; Mead Johnson, Canad.; Mead Johnson Nutritionals, USA.
Paracetamol (p.72·2).
Fever; pain.

Tempra Cold Care Mead Johnson, Canad.†.
Paracetamol (p.72·2); pseudoephedrine hydrochloride (p.1068·3); dextromethorphan hydrobromide (p.1057·3).
Cold symptoms.

Temserin Frosst, Ger.†.
Timolol maleate (p.953·3).
Cardiac disorders; hypertension.

Temtabs Wyeth, Austral.
Temazepam (p.693·3).
Insomnia.

Tenacid Sigma-Tau, Ital.
Imipenem (p.216·3); cilastatin sodium (p.185·2).
Lignocaine hydrochloride (p.1293·2) is included in the intramuscular injection to alleviate the pain of injection.
Bacterial infections.

Tenat Helvepharm, Switz.
Atenolol (p.825·3).
Angina pectoris; arrhythmias; hypertension; myocardial infarction.

Tenben Galen, UK.
Atenolol (p.825·3); bendrofluazide (p.827·3).
Hypertension.

Ten-Bloka SA Druggists, S.Afr.
Atenolol (p.825·3).
Angina pectoris; hypertension.

Tencef Tedec Meiji, Spain.
Cefminox sodium (p.167·1).
Bacterial infections.

Tencet Hauck, USA.
Paracetamol (p.72·2); butalbital (p.644·3); caffeine (p.749·3).
Formerly known as G-1.
Pain.

Tenchlor
Berk, Irl.; SA Druggists, S.Afr.; Berk, UK.
Atenolol (p.825·3); chlorthalidone (p.839·3).
These ingredients can be described by the British Approved Name Co-tenidone.
Hypertension.

Tencon International Ethical, USA.
Paracetamol (p.72·2); butalbital (p.644·3).

Tendosimol Tendem, Neth.†.
Albumin tannate (p.1176·3).
Diarrhoea.

Tenelid Helsinn, Switz.†.
Guanabenz acetate (p.877·3).
Hypertension.

Teneretic Zeneca, Ger.
Atenolol (p.825·3); chlorthalidone (p.839·3).
Hypertension.

Tenex Robins, USA.
Guanfacine hydrochloride (p.879·1).
Hypertension.

Tenif
Zeneca, Belg.; Zeneca, UK.
Atenolol (p.825·3); nifedipine (p.916·2).
Angina pectoris; hypertension.

Tenitran Bioindustria, Ital.
Tenitramine (p.952·1).
Cardiac stenosis; ischaemic heart disease.

Ten-K Summit, USA.
Potassium chloride (p.1161·1).
Hypokalaemia; potassium depletion.

Tenkafruse CP Pharmaceuticals, UK.
Frusemide (p.871·1).
Hypercalcaemia; hypertension; oedema; oliguria.

Tenlol Amrad, Austral.
Atenolol (p.825·3).
Angina pectoris; arrhythmias; hypertension; myocardial infarction.

Teno BASF, Ger.
Atenolol (p.825·3).
Cardiac disorders; hypertension.

teno-basan Sagitta, Ger.†.
Atenolol (p.825·3).
Cardiovascular disorders.

Tenolin Technilab, Canad.
Atenolol (p.825·3).
Angina pectoris; hypertension.

Tenolone Lusofarmaco, Ital.
Atenolol (p.825·3); chlorthalidone (p.839·3).
Hypertension.

Tenol-Plus Vortech, USA.
Paracetamol (p.72·2); aspirin (p.16·1); caffeine (p.749·3).
Pain.

Tenopt Sigma, Austral.
Timolol maleate (p.953·3).
Glaucoma; ocular hypertension.

Tenordate Zeneca, Fr.
Nifedipine (p.916·2); atenolol (p.825·3).
Hypertension.

Tenoret
Zeneca, Irl.; Zeneca, S.Afr.†; Zeneca, UK.
Atenolol (p.825·3); chlorthalidone (p.839·3).
These ingredients can be described by the British Approved Name Co-tenidone.
Hypertension.

Tenoretic
Zeneca, Aust.; Zeneca, Belg.; Zeneca, Canad.; Zeneca, Irl.; Zeneca, Ital.; Zeneca, Neth.; Zeneca, S.Afr.; Zeneca, Spain; Zeneca, Switz.; Zeneca, UK; Zeneca, USA.
Atenolol (p.825·3); chlorthalidone (p.839·3).
These ingredients can be described by the British Approved Name Co-tenidone.
Hypertension.

Tenormin
Zeneca, Aust.; ICI, Austral.; Zeneca, Belg.; Zeneca, Canad.; Zeneca, Ger.; Zeneca, Irl.; Zeneca, Ital.; Zeneca, Neth.; Zeneca, Norw.; Zeneca, S.Afr.; Zeneca, Spain; Zeneca, Swed.; Zeneca, Switz.; Zeneca, UK; Zeneca, USA.
Atenolol (p.825·3).
Angina pectoris; arrhythmias; hypertension; hyperthyroidism; migraine; myocardial infarction.

Tenormine Zeneca, Fr.
Atenolol (p.825·3).
Angina pectoris; hypertension; myocardial infarction.

Ten-O-Six Bonne Bell, Canad.
Salicylic acid (p.1090·2).
Acne.

Tenox Orion, Irl.
Temazepam (p.693·3).
Insomnia; premedication.

Tenoxol Pulitzer, Ital.
Neltenexine (p.1065·1).
Respiratory-tract disorders.

Tensadiur Crinos, Ital.
Benazepril hydrochloride (p.827·1); hydrochlorothiazide (p.885·2).
Hypertension.

Tensan Klinge, Aust.
Nilvadipine (p.922·1).
Hypertension.

Tensanil Crinos, Ital.
Benazepril hydrochloride (p.827·1).
Hypertension.

Tensig Sigma, Austral.
Atenolol (p.825·3).
Angina pectoris; arrhythmias; hypertension; myocardial infarction.

Tensigradyl Lipha Sante, Fr.
Guabenxan sulphate (p.877·2); bemetizide (p.827·1).
Hypertension.

Tensilene Caber, Ital.†.
Oxprenolol hydrochloride (p.926·2); bencyclane fumarate (p.827·3).
Hypertension.

Tensilon
ICN, Canad.; Roche, Irl.†; Roche, S.Afr.; ICN, USA.
Edrophonium chloride (p.1392·2).
Diagnosis of myasthenia gravis; reversal of competitive neuromuscular blockade.

Tensin Rolab, S.Afr.
Spironolactone (p.946·1).
Ascites; oedema.

Tensiocomplet Medea, Spain.
Hydralazine hydrochloride (p.883·2); hydrochlorothiazide (p.885·2); reserpine (p.942·1).
Formerly contained chlorthalidone, dihydralazine hydrochloride, potassium gluconate, reserpine, rutin, xanthinol nicotinate, protoveratrine A, and protoveratrine B.
Hypertension.

Tensiomin-Cor Thiemann, Ger.
Captopril (p.836·3).
Heart failure; hypertension.

Tensionorme Leo, Fr.
Bendrofluazide (p.827·3); reserpine (p.942·1).
Hypertension.

Tensipine Ethical Generics, UK.
Nifedipine (p.916·2).
Angina pectoris; hypertension.

Tensiplex Francia, Ital.
Vinburnine phosphate (p.1644·1).
Cerebrovascular disorders; mental function impairment.

Tensitruw Truw, Ger.
Crataegus (p.1568·2).
Cardiac disorders.

Tensium DDSA Pharmaceuticals, UK.
Diazepam (p.661·1).
Alcohol withdrawal syndrome; anxiety; epilepsy; insomnia; premedication; skeletal muscle spasm.

Tenso Stop Esteve, Spain.
Fosinopril sodium (p.870·3).
Heart failure; hypertension.

Tensobon
Schwarz, Ger.; Schwarz, Switz.
Captopril (p.836·3).
Diabetic nephropathy; heart failure; hypertension.

Tensobon comp
Schwarz, Ger.; Schwarz, Switz.
Captopril (p.836·3); hydrochlorothiazide (p.885·2).
Heart failure; hypertension.

Tensocold *Smith & Nephew, Fr.†.*
Isoflurane (p.1225·1).
Formerly contained dichlorotetrafluoroethane.
Joint and muscle pain.

Tensodilen *Ciba Vision, Spain†.*
Dichlorphenamide (p.848·2).
Glaucoma; intra-ocular hypertension.

Tensoflux *Hennig, Ger.*
Bendrofluazide (p.827·3); amiloride hydrochloride (p.819·2).
Ascites; hypertension; oedema; renal calculi.

Tensogard *Mead Johnson, Ital.*
Fosinopril sodium (p.870·3).
Heart failure; hypertension.

Tensogradal *Berenguer Infale, Spain.*
Nitrendipine (p.923·1).
Hypertension.

Tensolve *Lennon, S.Afr.*
Paracetamol (p.72·2); diphenhydramine hydrochloride (p.409·1); codeine phosphate (p.26·1); caffeine (p.749·3).
Pain.

Tensophoril *Monot, Fr.†.*
Dopamine hydrochloride (p.861·1); boric acid; amylobarbitone (p.641·3); ascorbic acid (p.1365·2).
Asthenia; hypotension.

Tensoprel *Rubio, Spain.*
Captopril (p.836·3).
Diabetic nephropathy; heart failure; hypertension; myocardial infarction.

Tensopyn *Parke-Med, S.Afr.*
Paracetamol (p.72·2); codeine phosphate (p.26·1); doxylamine succinate (p.410·1); caffeine (p.749·3).
Pain and associated tension.

Tensostad *Stada, Ger.*
Captopril (p.836·3).
Heart failure; hypertension.

Tenso-Timelets *Temmler, Ger.†.*
Clonidine hydrochloride (p.841·2).
Hypertension.

Tensozide *Mead Johnson, Ital.*
Fosinopril sodium (p.870·3); hydrochlorothiazide (p.885·2).
Hypertension.

Tenstaten *IPSEN, Fr.*
Cicletanine hydrochloride (p.840·2).
Hypertension.

Tenston *Covan, S.Afr.*
Sustained-release capsules; sustained-release tablets: Paracetamol (p.72·2); caffeine (p.749·3); codeine phosphate (p.26·1); meprobamate (p.678·1).
Syrup: Promethazine hydrochloride (p.416·2); paracetamol (p.72·2); codeine phosphate (p.26·1).
Tablets: Aspirin (p.16·1); paracetamol (p.72·2); caffeine (p.749·3); codeine phosphate (p.26·1); meprobamate (p.678·1).
Fever; pain.

Tentroc *Boehringer Ingelheim, Spain†.*
Gemfibrozil (p.1273·3).
Hyperlipidaemias.

Tenuate
Hoechst Marion Roussel, Austral.; Hoechst Marion Roussel, Canad.; Lakeside, USA.
Diethylpropion hydrochloride (p.1479·3).
Obesity.

Tenuate Dospan
Hoechst Marion Roussel, Belg.; Marion Merrell, Fr.; Bruno, Ital.; Mer-National, S.Afr.; Hoechst Marion Roussel, UK†.
Diethylpropion hydrochloride (p.1479·3).
Obesity.

Tenuate Retard
Synomed, Ger.; Hoechst Marion Roussel, Switz.
Diethylpropion hydrochloride (p.1479·3).
Obesity.

Tenuatina *Rottapharm, Spain.*
Dihydroergotamine mesylate (p.444·2).
Circulatory disorders; migraine; orthostatic hypotension.

Tenutex *Recip, Swed.*
Disulfiram (p.1573·1); benzyl benzoate (p.1402·2).
Pediculosis; scabies.

Teobid *Vita, Ital.*
Theophylline (p.765·1).
Asthma; bronchospasm.

Teodelin *Leti, Spain.*
Theophylline (p.765·1).
Heart failure; obstructive airways disease; paroxysmal dyspnoea.

Teofilcolina *Salfa, Ital.†.*
Choline theophyllinate (p.751·3).
Asthma; cardiac disorders; production of diuresis.

Teofilcolina Sedativa *Salfa, Ital.†.*
Choline theophyllinate (p.751·3); phenobarbitone (p.350·2); papaverine hydrochloride (p.1614·2).
Asthma; cardiac disorders; production of diuresis.

Teogel *Cantabria, Spain†.*
Theophylline (p.765·1).
Obstructive airways disease.

Teolixir *Biogalenica, Spain.*
Theophylline (p.765·1).
Heart failure; obstructive airways disease; paroxysmal dyspnoea.

Teolixir Compositum *Biogalenica, Spain.*
Guaiphenesin (p.1061·3); prednisolone (p.1048·1); theophylline (p.765·1).
Obstructive airways disease.

Teonim *Teofarma, Ital.*
Nimesulide (p.63·2).
Fever; inflammation; pain.

Teonova *Corvi, Ital.*
Theophylline (p.765·1).
Obstructive airways disease.

Teoplus *Formenti, Ital.†.*
Theophylline (p.765·1).
Asthma; bronchospasm.

Teoptic
Ciba Vision, Irl.; Ciba Vision, Neth.; Ciba Vision, UK.
Carteolol hydrochloride (p.837·3).
Glaucoma; ocular hypertension.

Teoremac *Farmades, Ital.†.*
Glucametacin (p.42·3).
Musculoskeletal and joint disorders.

Teostellarid *SmithKline Beecham, Ital.†.*
Proscillaridin (p.938·1); etofylline (p.753·1).
Heart failure.

Teoval/R *Valeas, Ital.†.*
Theophylline (p.765·1).
Asthma; bronchospastic disorders.

Teovent
Pharmacia Upjohn, Norw.; Pharmacia Upjohn, Swed.
Choline theophyllinate (p.751·3).
Obstructive airways disease.

Teovit *Inexfa, Spain.*
Aceglutamide (p.1541·2); hydroxocobalamin acetate (p.1364·2); pyridoxine hydrochloride (p.1362·3); thiamine phosphate (p.1361·2).
Vitamin B deficiency.

Tepam *BASF, Ger.*
Tetrazepam (p.694·3).
Skeletal muscle tension and spasticity.

Tepanil *Riker, USA†.*
Diethylpropion hydrochloride (p.1479·3).
Obesity.

Tepavil *Prodes, Spain.*
Sulpiride (p.692·3).
Neuroses; psychoses; vertigo.

Tepazepan *Prodes, Spain.*
Diazepam (p.661·1); pyridoxine (p.1363·1); sulpiride (p.692·3).
Anxiety; neurosis; psychoses; psychosomatic disorders.

Tepilta
Wyeth Lederle, Aust.; Wyeth, Ger.; Wyeth, Spain.
Aluminium hydroxide gel (p.1177·3); light magnesium carbonate (p.1198·1) or magnesium hydroxide (p.1198·2); oxethazaine (p.1298·1).
Gastro-intestinal disorders.

Teproside *Malesci, Ital.†.*
Vincamine teprosilate (p.1644·1).
Cerebrovascular disorders; mental function disorders.

Teralithe *Specia, Fr.*
Lithium carbonate (p.290·3).
Bipolar disorder; schizophrenia.

Teramine *Legere, USA†.*
Phentermine hydrochloride (p.1484·3).

Teraprost *Malesci, Ital.*
Terazosin hydrochloride (p.952·1).
Benign prostatic hyperplasia.

Terazol
Janssen-Ortho, Canad.; Janssen-Cilag, Ital.†; Janssen-Cilag, S.Afr.; Janssen-Cilag, Swed.; Ortho Pharmaceutical, USA.
Terconazole (p.388·2).
Vulvovaginal candidiasis.

Terbasmin
Pharmacia Upjohn, Ital.†; Astra, Spain.
Terbutaline sulphate (p.764·1).
Obstructive airways disease; premature labour.

Terbasmin Expectorante *Astra, Spain.*
Guaiphenesin (p.1061·3); terbutaline sulphate (p.764·1).
Obstructive airways disease.

Terbintil *Spitzner, Ger.†.*
Bath additive: Methyl nicotinate (p.55·1); benzyl nicotinate (p.22·1); camphor (p.1557·2); Norway spruce oil.
Bath additive; frostbite; musculoskeletal and joint disorders; neuritis; peripheral circulatory disorders.
Topical application: Bornyl salicylate (p.22·1); ethyl salicylate (p.36·1); camphor (p.1557·2); methyl nicotinate (p.55·1); turpentine oil (p.1641·1).
Neuromuscular disorders; rheumatism; sports injuries.

Terbolan *Hoechst, Aust.*
Frusemide (p.871·1); reserpine (p.942·1).
Hypertension.

Terbuforton *Plantorgan, Ger.†.*
Terbutaline sulphate (p.764·1).
Obstructive airways disease.

Terbul *Hexal, Ger.*
Terbutaline sulphate (p.764·1).
Obstructive airways disease.

Terbuturmant *Desitin, Ger.*
Terbutaline sulphate (p.764·1).
Obstructive airways disease.

Tercian *Specia, Fr.*
Cyamemazine (p.660·2) or cyamemazine tartrate (p.660·2).
Aggression; anxiety; depression; psychoses.

Tercinol *Sopar, Belg.†.*
Phenol (p.1121·2); borax (p.1554·2); salicylic acid (p.1090·2); benzoic acid (p.1102·3).
Mouth and throat disorders; skin disorders.

Tercodine *Monot, Fr.†.*
Terpin (p.1070·2); codeine (p.26·1); cherry-laurel.
Respiratory-tract disorders.

Terconal *Italchimici, Ital.*
Terconazole (p.388·2).
Fungal balanitis; vulvovaginal candidiasis.

Terelit *Farmasan, Ger.*
Doxycycline hydrochloride (p.202·3); ambroxol hydrochloride (p.1054·3).
Respiratory-tract infections associated with increased or viscous mucus.

Terfedura *Durachemie, Ger.*
Terfenadine (p.418·1).
Hypersensitivity disorders.

Terfemundin *Mundipharma, Ger.*
Terfenadine (p.418·1).
Hypersensitivity disorders.

Terfen-Diolan *Engelhard, Ger.†.*
Terfenadine (p.418·1).
Hypersensitivity disorders.

Terfenor *Norton, S.Afr.*
Terfenadine (p.418·1).
Allergic rhinitis; allergic skin disorders.

Terfenor Antihistamine *Norton, UK.*
Terfenadine (p.418·1).
Allergic rhinitis; allergic skin disorders.

Terfex
Ciba Vision, Swed.†; Penn, UK.
Terfenadine (p.418·1).
Hypersensitivity reactions.

Terfium *Hexal, Ger.*
Terfenadine (p.418·1).
Hypersensitivity reactions.

Terfluzine
ICN, Canad.; Specia, Fr.; Rhone-Poulenc Rorer, Neth.
Trifluoperazine hydrochloride (p.697·3).
Agitation; bipolar disorder; psychoses.

Tergynan *Bouchara, Fr.*
Ternidazole (p.594·1); neomycin sulphate (p.229·2); nystatin (p.386·1); prednisolone sodium metasulphobenzoate (p.1048·1).
Vaginitis.

Teril
Alphapharm, Austral.; Taro, UK.
Carbamazepine (p.339·2).
Bipolar disorder; epilepsy; trigeminal neuralgia.

Terion *Lusofarmaco, Ital.†.*
Fominoben hydrochloride (p.1061·2).
Respiratory-tract disorders.

Terivalidin
Gerot, Aust.; Noristan, S.Afr.†.
Terizidone (p.259·1).
Bacterial infections.

Terizidon *Fatol, Ger.†.*
Terizidone (p.259·1).
Tuberculosis.

Terlane *Mundipharma, Aust.*
Terfenadine (p.418·1).
Hypersensitivity reactions.

Termalgin *Sandoz, Spain.*
Paracetamol (p.72·2).
Fever; pain.

Termalgin Codeina *Sandoz, Spain.*
Codeine phosphate (p.26·1); paracetamol (p.72·2).
Pain.

Termidon *Lepetit, Ital.†.*
Amidopyrine (p.15·2).
Cold symptoms; fever; inflammation of the ear, nose, and throat.

Termobalsamo *Procemsa, Ital.†.*
Capsicum oleoresin; camphor (p.1557·2); salicylic acid (p.1090·2).
Musculoskeletal and joint pain.

Termosan *Domenech Garcia, Spain.*
Camphor (p.1557·2); capsicum oleoresin; methyl salicylate (p.55·2); salicylic acid (p.1090·2); turpentine oil (p.1641·1); menthol (p.1600·2); lavender oil (p.1594·3); thyme oil (p.1637·1); eucalyptus oil (p.1578·1).
Muscle pain; soft-tissue disorders; upper respiratory-tract disorders.

Ternadin *Cantabria, Spain.*
Terfenadine (p.418·1).
Hypersensitivity reactions.

Ternelin *Sandoz, Jpn.*
Tizanidine hydrochloride (p.1322·1).
Myotonia; spastic paralysis.

Terneurine
Bristol-Myers Squibb, Belg.†; Allard, Fr.
Vitamin B substances.
Neuralgia; neuritis; vitamin B deficiency.

Teronac
Sandoz, Irl.†; Novartis, Neth.; Wander, S.Afr.†; Sandoz, Switz.; Sandoz, UK†.
Mazindol (p.1482·1).
Obesity.

Terpalate *Ferrer, Spain.*
Aluminium hydroxide (p.1177·3); attapulgite (p.1178·3); enoxolone aluminium (p.1191·3); magnesium oxide (p.1198·3); sodium citrate (p.1153·2).
Gastritis; gastro-intestinal hyperacidity; peptic ulcer.

Terpestrol H *Medopharm, Ger.*
Turpentine oil (p.1641·1).
Respiratory tract disorders.

Terpestrol-Inhalant *Pharmasal, Ger.†.*
Turpentine oil (p.1641·1); peppermint oil (p.1208·1); siberian fir oil; pumilio pine oil (p.1623·3).
Respiratory-tract disorders.

Terpine des Monts-Dore *Centropharm, Fr.*
Terpin (p.1070·2).
Coughs.

Terpine Gonnon
Gonnon, Fr.†.
Tablets: Terpin (p.1070·2); sodium benzoate (p.1102·3); codeine (p.26·1).
Respiratory-tract disorders.

Pharminter, Fr.
Oral liquid: Terpin (p.1070·2); tolu balsam (p.1071·1).
Respiratory-tract disorders.

Terpoin *Houghs Healthcare, UK.*
Codeine phosphate (p.26·1); menthol; cineole.
Coughs.

Terpone *Rosa-Phytopharma, Fr.*
Terpin (p.1070·2); Siberian fir oil; niaouli oil (p.1607·1); eucalyptus oil (p.1578·1).
Formerly contained semisynthetic oxide derivatives of terpene oils terpin, and quinine camsylate.
Respiratory-tract disorders.

Terponil *Vitafarma, Spain.*
Oxidised terpenes; terpin (p.1070·2).
Respiratory-tract disorders.

Terposen *Vir, Spain.*
Ranitidine hydrochloride (p.1209·3).
Acid aspiration; gastro-intestinal haemorrhage; gastro-oesophageal reflux; peptic ulcer; Zollinger-Ellison syndrome.

Terra-Cortril
Note. This name is used for preparations of different composition.
Pfizer, Aust.; Pfizer, Belg.; Pfizer, Irl.; Pfizer, Neth.†; Pfizer, Norw.; Pfizer, S.Afr.; Pfizer, Spain; Pfizer, Swed.; Pfizer, UK; Roerig, USA.
Oxytetracycline hydrochloride (p.235·1); hydrocortisone (p.1043·3) or hydrocortisone acetate (p.1043·3).
Infected skin disorders.

Pfizer, Belg.; Pfizer, Ger.; Pfizer, S.Afr.; Pfizer, Spain; Pfizer, Switz.; Pfizer, UK†.
Oxytetracycline hydrochloride (p.235·1); hydrocortisone (p.1043·3) or hydrocortisone acetate (p.1043·3); polymyxin B sulphate (p.239·1).
Infected eye, ear, and skin disorders.

Pfizer, Ger.†; Pfizer, Switz.†.
Oxytetracycline calcium (p.235·1); hydrocortisone (p.1043·3); polymyxin B sulphate (p.239·1).
Cervicitis; infected skin disorders; prophylaxis of urethral infections; sinusitis.

Terra-Cortril Gel Steraject met polymyxine-B *Pfizer, Neth.*
Oxytetracycline calcium (p.235·1); hydrocortisone (p.1043·3); polymyxin B sulphate (p.239·1).
Sinusitis.

Terracortril med polymyxin B *Pfizer, Swed.*
Oxytetracycline hydrochloride (p.235·1); hydrocortisone acetate (p.1043·3); polymyxin B sulphate (p.239·1).
Infected ear and eye disorders; otitis externa.

Terra-Cortril met polymyxine-B *Pfizer, Neth.*
Oxytetracycline hydrochloride (p.235·1); hydrocortisone acetate (p.1043·3); polymyxin B sulphate (p.239·1).
Blepharitis squamosa; inflammatory ear infections.

Terra-Cortril mit Gentamicin *Pfizer, Aust.*
Oxytetracycline calcium (p.235·1); gentamicin sulphate (p.212·1); hydrocortisone acetate (p.1043·3).
Bacterial infections and inflammation of the nose or genito-urinary tract.

Terra-Cortril mit Polymyxin B-Sulfat *Pfizer, Aust.*
Oxytetracycline calcium (p.235·1) or oxytetracycline hydrochloride (p.235·1); polymyxin B sulphate (p.239·1); hydrocortisone (p.1043·3).
Bacterial infections and inflammation of the nose and sinuses.

Terra-Cortril Nystatin
Pfizer, Irl.; Pfizer, UK.
Oxytetracycline calcium (p.235·1); hydrocortisone (p.1043·3); nystatin (p.386·1).
Infected skin disorders.

Terra-Cortril Polymyxin B *Pfizer, Norw.*
Oxytetracycline hydrochloride (p.235·1); hydrocortisone acetate (p.1043·3); polymyxin B sulphate (p.239·1).
Ear disorders.

Terralin *Schulke & Mayr, Ger.*
Benzalkonium chloride (p.1101·3); phenoxypropanol (p.1122·2).
Surface disinfection.

Terramicina *Pfizer, Spain.*
Ointment: Oxytetracycline hydrochloride (p.235·1); polymyxin B sulphate (p.239·1).
Tablets; injection; capsules; eye ointment: Oxytetracycline (p.235·1) or oxytetracycline hydrochloride (p.235·1).
Lignocaine (p.1293·2) is included in the injection to alleviate the pain of injection.
Bacterial infections.

Terramicina con Polimixina B Pomata Dermica *Pfizer, Ital.*†.
Oxytetracycline hydrochloride (p.235·1); polymyxin B sulphate (p.239·1).
Bacterial infections of the skin.

Terramycin
Note. This name is used for preparations of different composition.
Pfizer, Ger.; Pfizer, S.Afr.
Eye ointment; ointment; pessaries: Oxytetracycline hydrochloride (p.235·1); polymyxin B sulphate (p.239·1).
Bacterial infections.

Pfizer, S.Afr.†*; Pfizer, UK; Pfizer, USA; Roerig, USA.*
Capsules; injection; tablets: Oxytetracycline (p.235·1) or oxytetracycline hydrochloride (p.235·1).
Lignocaine (p.1293·2) is included in the injection to alleviate the pain of injection.
Bacterial infections.

Terramycin met polymyxine-B *Pfizer, Neth.*
Oxytetracycline hydrochloride (p.235·1); polymyxin B sulphate (p.239·1).
Bacterial infections.

Terramycin mit Polymyxin-B-Sulfat *Pfizer, Aust.*
Oxytetracycline hydrochloride (p.235·1); polymyxin B sulphate (p.239·1).
Bacterial infections of the eye or skin.

Terramycin Polymyxin B
Pfizer, Norw.; Pfizer, Swed.
Oxytetracycline hydrochloride (p.235·1); polymyxin B sulphate (p.239·1).
Bacterial skin and eye infections.

Terramycin with Polymyxin B *Roerig, USA*†.
Oxytetracycline hydrochloride (p.235·1); polymyxin B sulphate (p.239·1).
Bacterial vaginal infections; eye infections.

Terramycine
Note. This name is used for preparations of different composition.
Pfizer, Belg.†*; Pfizer, Switz.*†.
Capsules: Oxytetracycline hydrochloride (p.235·1).
Amoebic dysentery; bacterial infections.

Pfizer, Belg.; Pfizer, Switz.
Eye ointment; ointment; cream: Oxytetracycline hydrochloride (p.235·1); polymyxin B sulphate (p.239·1).
Eye infections; skin infections.

Pfizer, Fr.†.
Ointment; eye ointment: Oxytetracycline hydrochloride (p.235·1).
Bacterial infections.

Terramycine Solu-Retard *Pfizer, Fr.*
Oxytetracycline (p.235·1).
Lignocaine (p.1293·2) is included in this preparation to alleviate the pain of injection.
Bacterial infections.

Terranilo *Ifidesa Aristegui, Spain.*
Chymotrypsin (p.1563·2); tetracycline hydrochloride (p.259·1).
Bacterial infections.

Tersac *Trans Canaderm, Canad.*
Salicylic acid (p.1090·2); triclosan (p.1127·2).
Acne.

Tersaseptic
Note. This name is used for preparations of different composition.
Trans Canaderm, Canad.
Triclosan (p.1127·2).
Skin cleanser; skin disorders.

Doak, USA.
Soap substitute.

Tersa-Tar *Trans Canaderm, Canad.*
Coal tar (p.1092·3).
Psoriasis; seborrhoea.

Tersigat *3M, Fr.*
Oxitropium bromide (p.757·1).
Obstructive airways disease.

Tersulpha *Lennon, S.Afr.*†.
Sulphadiazine (p.252·3); sulfamerazine (p.251·3); sulphadimidine (p.253·2).
Bacterial infections.

Tertensif *Danval, Spain.*
Indapamide (p.890·2).
Hypertension; oedema.

Tertroxin
Boots, Austral.; Glaxo Wellcome, Irl.†*; Glaxo Wellcome, S.Afr.; Goldshield, UK.*
Liothyronine sodium (p.1495·1).
Hyperthyroidism; hypothyroidism; myxoedema coma.

Terzolin *Janssen-Cilag, Ger.*
Ketoconazole (p.383·1).
Pityriasis versicolor; seborrhoeic dermatitis.

Tesamone *Dunhall, USA.*
Testosterone (p.1464·1).
Androgen replacement therapy; delayed puberty.

Teslac
Bristol-Myers Squibb, Belg.†*; Bristol-Myers Oncology, USA.*
Testolactone (p.566·1).
Adjunct in breast cancer.

Teslascan
Nycomed, Swed.; Nycomed, USA.
Mangafodipir trisodium (p.1009·1).
Contrast medium for magnetic resonance imaging of the liver.

Tesoprel *Thiemann, Ger.*
Bromperidol (p.643·2) or bromperidol lactate (p.643·2).
Schizophrenia.

Tesos *Byk Elmu, Spain.*
Tetrydamine maleate (p.88·3).
Vaginitis.

Tespamin *Sumitomo, Jpn.*
Thiotepa (p.566·3).
Malignant neoplasms.

Tessalon *Forest Pharmaceuticals, USA.*
Benzonatate (p.1055·3).
Coughs.

Test Pack Plus *Abbott, UK.*
Pregnancy test (p.1621·2).

Testac *Medac, Ger.*
Flutamide (p.537·1).
Prostatic cancer.

Testandro *Redur, USA.*
Testosterone (p.1464·1).
Androgen replacement therapy; delayed puberty.

Tes-Tape
Aza, Austral.; Lilly, Canad.; Lilly, Irl.; Lilly, Ital.; Lilly, S.Afr.; Lilly, Switz.; Lilly, USA†.
Test for glucose in urine (p.1585·1).

testasa *Chefaro, Ger.*†.
Kola; muira-puama; yohimbe; alpha tocopheryl acetate.
Tonic.

testasa e *Chefaro, Ger.*
Yohimbe extract.
Male sexual exhaustion.

Testaval 90/4 *Legere, USA*†.
Testosterone enanthate (p.1464·1); oestradiol valerate (p.1455·2).

Test-Estro *Rugby, USA.*
Oestradiol cypionate (p.1455·1); testosterone cypionate (p.1464·1).
Menopausal vasomotor symptoms; prevention of postpartum breast engorgement.

Testes-Uvocal *Mulli, Ger.*†.
Testicular extract (p.1464·1).
Male menopausal disorders.

Testex *Byk Elmu, Spain.*
Testosterone cypionate (p.1464·1) or testosterone propionate (p.1464·2).
Aplastic anaemia; female breast cancer; lactation inhibition; male hypogonadism and androgen deficiency; osteoporosis.

Testiculi *Disperga, Aust.*
Testis extract (p.1464·1).
Androgen deficiency; hypogonadism.

Testiwop *Hor-Fer-Vit, Ger.*†.
Spleen extracts.
Tonic.

Testoderm *Alza, USA.*
Testosterone (p.1464·1).
Hypogonadism.

Testo-Enant *Geymonat, Ital.*
Testosterone enanthate (p.1464·1).
Androgenic; breast cancer; fibroids.

Testopel *Bartor Pharmacal, USA.*
Testosterone (p.1464·1).
Androgen deficiency; delayed puberty.

Testosterone Implants *Organon, UK.*
Testosterone (p.1464·1).
Male hypogonadism.

Testotard *Chephasaar, Ger.*
Flutamide (p.537·1).
Prostatic cancer.

Testotop
Stada, Aust.; Eastern Pharmaceuticals, UK†.
Testosterone (p.1464·1).
Testosterone deficiency.

Testoviron *Schering, Ital.*†.
Testosterone propionate (p.1464·2).
Androgenic; hyperfollicular states; hypogonadism.

Testoviron 100 *Schering, Aust.*
Testosterone propionate (p.1464·2); testosterone enanthate (p.1464·1).
Aplastic anaemia in men; female breast cancer; male hypogonadism; male impotence.

Testoviron 250 *Schering, Aust.*
Testosterone enanthate (p.1464·1).
Aplastic anaemia in men; female breast cancer; male hypogonadism; male impotence.

Testoviron Depot
Note. This name is used for preparations of different composition.
Schering, Belg.; Schering, Irl.; Schering, Neth.; Schering, Swed.; Schering, Switz.
Testosterone enanthate (p.1464·1).
Androgen deficiency in males; breast cancer.

Schering, Ital.
Testosterone enanthate (p.1464·1); testosterone propionate (p.1464·2).
Androgenic; breast cancer.

Testoviron Depot 50 *Schering, Ger.*
Testosterone enanthate (p.1464·1); testosterone propionate (p.1464·2).
Hypogonadism in men.

Testoviron Depot 100
Schering, Ger.; Schering, Neth.†*; Schering, Spain; Schering, Switz.*†.
Testosterone enanthate (p.1464·1); testosterone propionate (p.1464·2).
Female breast cancer; haemopoietic disorders; hepatic cirrhosis; male hypogonadism and androgen deficiency; osteoporosis.

Testoviron Depot 250
Schering, Ger.; Schering, Spain.
Testosterone enanthate (p.1464·1).
Female breast cancer; haemopoietic disorders; hepatic cirrhosis; male hypogonadism and androgen deficiency; osteoporosis.

Testovis *SIT, Ital.*
Methyltestosterone (p.1450·3) or testosterone propionate (p.1464·2).
Androgenic; breast disorders; fibroids; menstrual disorders.

Testpack hCG-Urine *Abbott, Irl.*
Pregnancy test (p.1621·2).

TestPack Plus hCG-Urine *Abbott, USA.*
Pregnancy test (p.1621·2).

Testred *ICN, USA.*
Capsules: Methyltestosterone (p.1450·3).
Injection†*:* Testosterone cypionate (p.1464·1).
Androgen replacement therapy; breast cancer; male hypogonadism; postpartum breast engorgement; prepubertal cryptorchidism.

Tesuloid *Squibb Diagnostics, USA.*
Technetium-99m sulphur colloid (p.1425·1).

Teta-Aktiv *Fresenius, Ger.*†.
Polyhexanide (p.1123·1); benzalkonium chloride (p.1101·3); cocosammoniumbetaine.
Surface disinfection.

Tetabulin
Immuno, Aust.; Immuno, Irl.; Immuno, Ital.; Immuno, UK.
A tetanus immunoglobulin (p.1535·2).
Formerly known as Humotet in the *UK*.
Passive immunisation.

Tetabuline
Immuno, Belg.; Immuno, Switz.
A tetanus immunoglobulin (p.1535·2).
Passive immunisation.

Tetagam
Centeon, Aust.; NBI, S.Afr.
A tetanus immunoglobulin (p.1535·2).
Passive immunisation.

Tetagam N *Centeon, Ger.; Chiron Behring, Ger.*
A tetanus immunoglobulin (p.1535·2).
Passive immunisation.

Tetagamma *Nuovo ISM, Ital.*
A tetanus immunoglobulin (p.1535·2).
Passive immunisation.

Tetaglobulin S *Merieux, Ger.*†.
A tetanus immunoglobulin (p.1535·2).
Passive immunisation.

Tetaglobuline *Merieux, Belg.*†.
A tetanus immunoglobulin (p.1535·2).
Passive immunisation.

Tetagloman *Octapharma, Aust.*†.
A tetanus immunoglobulin (p.1535·2).
Passive immunisation.

Tetagrip *Merieux, Fr.*
A tetanus and influenza vaccine (p.1536·3).
Active immunisation.

Tet-Aktiv *Tropon-Cutter, Ger.*†.
An adsorbed tetanus vaccine (p.1535·3).
Active immunisation.

Tetamer *Pasteur Merieux, Belg.*
An adsorbed tetanus vaccine (p.1535·3).
Active immunisation.

Tetamun SSW *SSW, Ger.; SmithKline Beecham, Ger.*
A tetanus vaccine (p.1535·3).
Active immunisation.

Tetanibys *Antibioticos, Spain*†.
A tetanus vaccine (p.1535·3).
Active immunisation.

Tetano Difter *Evans, Spain*†.
A diphtheria and tetanus vaccine (p.1508·1).
Active immunisation of infants and young children.

Tetanobulin S *Immuno, Ger.*
A tetanus immunoglobulin (p.1535·2).
Passive immunisation.

Tetanol
Hoechst, Aust.; Chiron Behring, Ger.; Behring, Ital.†.
An adsorbed tetanus vaccine (p.1535·3).
Active immunisation.

Tetanosimultan *Immuno, Aust.*
A tetanus immunoglobulin (p.1535·2).
Passive immunisation.

Tetanus-Gamma *Biagini, Ital.*
A tetanus immunoglobulin (p.1535·2).
Passive immunisation.

Teta-S *Fresenius, Ger.*
Didecylmethylalkoxiammonium propionate; cocospropylenediamineguanidinium diacetate; polyhexanide (p.1123·1).
Surface disinfection.

Tetasorbat SSW *SSW, Ger.; SmithKline Beecham, Ger.*
An adsorbed tetanus vaccine (p.1535·3).
Active immunisation.

Tetatox *Berna, Ital.*
An adsorbed tetanus vaccine (p.1535·3).
Active immunisation.

Tetavax
Merieux, Fr.; Pasteur Merieux, Ger.; Pasteur Merieux, Neth.; Rhone-Poulenc Rorer, S.Afr.; Pasteur Merieux, UK.
An adsorbed tetanus vaccine (p.1535·3).
Active immunisation.

Tetaven *Immuno, Ital.*
A tetanus immunoglobulin (p.1535·2).
Passive immunisation.

Tetavenin *Immuno, Aust.*
A tetanus immunoglobulin (p.1535·2).
Passive immunisation.

Tetavenine *Immuno, Switz.*†.
A tetanus immunoglobulin (p.1535·2).
Passive immunisation.

Tetefit Vitamin E *Medra, Aust.*
Alpha-tocopherol (p.1369·1).
Tonic.

Tetesept
Kolassa, Aust.
Balsam: Camphor (p.1557·2); menthol (p.1600·2); eucalyptus oil (p.1578·1); pumilio pine oil (p.1623·3); turpentine oil (p.1641·1); rosemary oil (p.1626·2); sage oil.
Coughs and cold symptoms.
Pastilles: Dequalinium chloride (p.1112·1); cetylpyridinium chloride (p.1106·2); hesperidin methyl chalcone (p.1580·2); ascorbic acid (p.1365·2).
Bacterial infections of the mouth and throat.

Medra, Aust.
Oral liquid: Plantago lanceolata.
Catarrh; coughs.

Tetesept Calcium *Medra, Aust.*
Calcium carbonate (p.1182·1).
Calcium supplement.

Tetesept Magnesium *Medra, Aust.*
Magnesium carbonate (p.1198·1).
Magnesium deficiency.

Tetesept Vitamin C *Medra, Aust.*
Ascorbic acid (p.1365·2).
Vitamin C deficiency.

Tethexal *Hexal, Ger.*
Tetrazepam (p.694·3).
Skeletal muscle tension and spasticity.

Tetmosol
Zeneca, Irl.†*; Zeneca, S.Afr.; ICI, UK*†.
Monosulfiram (p.1408·2).
Scabies.

Tetra Hubber *ICN, Spain.*
Tetracycline hydrochloride (p.259·1).
Bacterial infections.

Tetra Tripsin *Torlan, Spain.*
Novobiocin (p.233·3); protease; tetracycline phosphate (p.259·1).
Bacterial infections.

Tetrabakat *Dorsch, Ger.*†.
Tetracycline hydrochloride (p.259·1).
Bacterial infections.

Tetrabid-Organon *Organon, UK*†.
Tetracycline hydrochloride (p.259·1).
Bacterial infections.

Tetrabioptal *Farmila, Ital.*
Tetracycline (p.259·1) or tetracycline hydrochloride (p.259·1).
Bacterial infections of the eye.

Tetrablet *Makara, Ger.*†.
Tetracycline hydrochloride (p.259·1).
Bacterial infections.

Tetracap *Circle, USA.*
Tetracycline hydrochloride (p.259·1).
Bacterial infections.

Tetracem *Crown, S.Afr.*
Oxytetracycline (p.235·1).
Bacterial infections.

Tetrachel
Central, Irl.†*; Berk, UK.*
Tetracycline hydrochloride (p.259·1).
Amoebiasis; bacterial infections.

Tetracitro S *Chephasaar, Ger.*†.
Tetracycline hydrochloride (p.259·1).
Bacterial infections; infections with large viruses.

Tetracoq *Merieux, Fr.*
An adsorbed diphtheria, pertussis, tetanus, and poliomyelitis (inactivated) vaccine (p.1509·3).
Active immunisation.

Tetract-HIB
Pasteur Merieux, Belg.; Pasteur Merieux, Ital.
A diphtheria, tetanus, pertussis, and Haemophilus influenzae conjugate vaccine (p.1509·3).
Active immunisation.

Tetracycletten N *Voigt, Ger.*†.
Oxytetracycline hydrochloride (p.235·1).
Bacterial infections; infections with large viruses; toxoplasmosis.

Tetracyn *Pfizer, Canad.*
Tetracycline hydrochloride (p.259·1).
Bacterial infections.

Tetrafluor *Stomygen, Ital.*
Ammonium fluoride; potassium fluoride; sodium fluoride (p.742·1); sodium monofluorophosphate (p.743·3).
Oral hygiene.

Tetrafosammina *FIRMA, Ital.*
Tetracycline phosphate complex (p.259·1).
Bacterial infections.

Tetra-Gelomyrtol
Salus, Aust.; Pohl, Ger.
Oxytetracycline hydrochloride (p.235·1); myrtol.
Bronchitis; sinusitis.

Tetragynon
Schering, Ger.; Schering, Norw.; Schering, Swed.†*; Schering, Switz.*
Levonorgestrel (p.1454·1); ethinyloestradiol (p.1445·1).
Postcoital oral contraceptive.

Tetralan *Lannett, USA*†.
Tetracycline hydrochloride (p.259·1).
Bacterial infections.

Tetralen *CEPA, Spain†.*
Tetracycline hydrochloride (p.259·1).
Bacterial infections.

Tetralfa *Fournier SA, Spain†.*
Lymecycline (p.223·2); chymotrypsin (p.1563·2).
Bacterial infections.

Tetralution *Merckle, Ger.*
Tetracycline hydrochloride (p.259·1).
Bacterial infections.

Tetralysal
AB-Consult, Aust.; Galderma, Belg.; Galderma, Fr.; Pharmacia Upjohn, Norw.; Galderma, S.Afr.; Meda, Swed.; Galderma, UK.
Lymecycline (p.223·2).
Bacterial infections.

Tetram
Note. This name is used for preparations of different composition.
Nycomed, Norw.
Piroxicam (p.80·2).
Dysmenorrhoea; musculoskeletal and joint disorders.

Dunhall, USA†.
Tetracycline hydrochloride (p.259·1).
Bacterial infections.

Tetramdura *Durachemie, Ger.*
Tetrazepam (p.694·3).
Skeletal muscle spasm.

Tetramel *Lennon, S.Afr.*
Oxytetracycline hydrochloride (p.235·1).
Bacterial infections.

Tetramig *Biogalenique, Fr.†.*
Tetracycline hydrochloride (p.259·1).
Bacterial infections.

Tetramil *Farmigea, Ital.*
Tetrahydrozoline hydrochloride (p.1070·2); pheniramine maleate (p.415·3).
Conjunctivitis; eye irritation and congestion.

Tetramune
Wyeth-Ayerst, Canad.; Lederle, Switz.; Lederle, USA.
A diphtheria, tetanus, pertussis, and haemophilus influenzae vaccine (p.1509·3).
Active immunisation.

Tetramykoin *Boucher & Muir, Austral.†.*
Tetracycline hydrochloride (p.259·1).

Tetranase *Rottapharm, Fr.*
Oxytetracycline hydrochloride (p.235·1); bromelains (p.1555·1).
Bacterial infections.

Tetra-Ozothin *SmithKline Beecham, Ger.†.*
Tetracycline hydrochloride (p.259·1); oxidation product of turpentine oil "Landes" (p.1641·1); terpin hydrate (p.1070·2).
Bacterial infections of the respiratory tract.

Tetrapongyl *Gallier, Fr.†.*
Thyroid (p.1496·3).
Hypothyroidism.

Tetra-Proter *Proter, Ital.†.*
Tetracycline hydrochloride (p.259·1).
Bacterial infections.

Tetrarco
Richter, Aust.; ICN, Neth.†.
Tetracycline hydrochloride (p.259·1).
Bacterial infections.

Tetrarco Simple *Clarben, Spain†.*
Tetracycline phosphate complex (p.259·1).
Bacterial infections.

Tetra-saar *Chephasaar, Ger.*
Tetrazepam (p.694·3).
Skeletal muscle tension and spasticity.

Tetrasan *CEPA, Spain.*
Doxycycline hydrochloride (p.202·3).
Bacterial infections.

Tetraseptine *Andreabal, Switz.*
Tetracycline hydrochloride (p.259·1).
Bacterial infections.

Tetrasine *Optopics, USA.*
Tetrahydrozoline hydrochloride (p.1070·2).
Minor eye irritation.

Tetrasine Extra *Optopics, USA.*
Tetrahydrozoline hydrochloride (p.1070·2); macrogol 400 (p.1597·3).
Minor eye irritation.

Tetra-Tablinen
Wenig, Aust.; Sanorania, Ger.
Oxytetracycline hydrochloride (p.235·1).
Bacterial infections.

TetraTITER *Wyeth, S.Afr.*
A diphtheria, tetanus, pertussis, and haemophilus influenzae vaccine (p.1509·3).
Active immunisation.

Tetrazep *CT, Ger.*
Tetrazepam (p.694·3).
Skeletal muscle tension and spasticity.

Tetrazufre *Quimica Medica, Spain†.*
Sulphur (p.1091·2); tetrachloroethylene.
Seborrhoea.

Tetrex
Bristol-Myers Squibb, Austral.; Bristol-Myers Squibb, S.Afr.
Tetracycline hydrochloride (p.259·1).
Acne; adjunct in amoebiasis; bacterial infections.

Tetrex-F
Astra, Austral.†; Bristol-Myers Squibb, S.Afr.
Tetracycline hydrochloride (p.259·1); nystatin (p.386·1).
Bacterial infections; candidiasis.

Tet-Tox *CSL, Austral.*
An adsorbed tetanus vaccine (p.1535·3).
Active immunisation.

Tetuman
Kwizda, Aust.; Berna, Belg.; Berna, Ital.; Swisspharm, S.Afr.; Berna, Spain; Berna, Switz.
A tetanus immunoglobulin (p.1535·2).
Passive immunisation.

Tevax *SK-RIT, Belg.*
An adsorbed tetanus vaccine (p.1535·3).
Active immunisation.

Teveten
SmithKline Beecham, Irl.; SmithKline Beecham, Swed.
Eprosartan mesylate (p.865·3).
Hypertension.

Tevit *Benvegna, Ital.†.*
Testosterone hexahydrobenzoate (p.1465·3); *dl*-alpha tocopheryl acetate (p.1369·2).
Androgenic.

Texacort
GenDerm, Canad.; GenDerm, USA.
Hydrocortisone (p.1043·3).
Skin disorders.

Texodil *Cassenne, Fr.*
Cefotiam hexetil hydrochloride (p.170·2).
Bacterial infections of the respiratory-tract.

TFE *Seroyal, Canad.*
Vitamin A, vitamin E, and zinc.

TFT
Alcon-Thilo, Ger.; Bausch & Lomb, S.Afr.
Trifluridine (p.627·3).
Herpes simplex keratitis.

TFT Ophtiole
Tramedico, Belg.; Mann, Neth.
Trifluridine (p.627·3).
Herpes simplex keratitis.

T-GAM *Serotherapeutisches, Aust.†.*
A tetanus immunoglobulin (p.1535·2).
Passive immunisation.

T/Gel
Prof. Pharm. Corp., Canad.†; Neutrogena, UK.
Coal tar (p.1092·3).
Scalp disorders.

T-Gen *Goldline, USA.*
Trimethobenzamide hydrochloride (p.420·1).
Nausea and vomiting.

T-Gesic *Williams, USA.*
Paracetamol (p.72·2); hydrocodone tartrate (p.43·1).
Pain.

THA *Woods, Austral.*
Tacrine hydrochloride (p.1399·1).
Prolongation of depolarising neuromuscular blockade; respiratory stimulant; reversal of competitive neuromuscular blockade.

Thacapzol *Recip, Swed.*
Methimazole (p.1495·3).
Hyperthyroidism.

Thaden *Lennon, S.Afr.*
Dothiepin hydrochloride (p.283·1).
Depression.

Thalamonal
Janssen-Cilag, Aust.; Janssen-Cilag, Belg.; Janssen-Cilag, Ger.; Janssen-Cilag, Neth.; Janssen-Cilag, Switz.†; Janssen, UK†.
Droperidol (p.668·2); fentanyl citrate (p.38·1).
Anaesthesia; neuroleptanalgesia; premedication; vestibular disorders.

Thalaris *Charton, Canad.*
Sodium chloride (p.1162·2).
Oral hygiene.

Thalitone *Boehringer Ingelheim, USA.*
Chlorthalidone (p.839·3).
Hypertension; oedema.

Thalomid *Celgene, USA.*
Thalidomide (p.1635·2).
Erythema nodosum leprosum.

Tham *Abbott, Austral.*
Trometamol (p.1639·3).
Metabolic acidosis.

Thamacetat *Bellon, Fr.*
Trometamol (p.1639·3).
Metabolic acidosis.

Thamesol *Diaco, Ital.*
Trometamol (p.1639·3).
Metabolic acidosis.

t/h-basan *Schonenberger, Switz.*
Triamterene (p.957·2); hydrochlorothiazide (p.885·2).
Hypertension; oedema.

The Brioni *Husler, Switz.*
Sambucus (p.1627·2); melissa (p.1600·1); peppermint leaf (p.1208·1); senna (p.1212·2); fennel (p.1579·1); agrimony.
Constipation.

The Chambard-Tee *Brady, Aust.*
Senna leaf (p.1212·2); althaea leaf (p.1546·3); peppermint leaf (p.1208·1); melissa leaf (p.1600·1); hyssopus officinalis; anthyllidis flower; calendula officinalis; cyanae flower.
Bowel evacuation; constipation; stool softener.

The Franklin *Noveal, Switz.*
Senna (p.1212·2); couch-grass (p.1567·3); fennel (p.1579·1); melissa (p.1600·1); boldo (p.1554·1); hyssopus officinalis; cuminum cyminum; peppermint leaf (p.1208·1); aniseed (p.1549·3).
Constipation.

The Ginseng King *Codit, Ital.*
Fish milk; fish brain extract; cod-liver extract; myrtillus; acacia honey; fructose; ginseng.
Nutritional supplement.

The laxatif Solubilax *Heumann, Switz.*
Senna (p.1212·2); frangula bark (p.1193·2).
Bowel evacuation; constipation.

Thedox *Mer-National, S.Afr.*
Doxycycline polyphosphate sodium complex.
Bacterial infections.

Theelin *Parke, Davis, USA†.*
Oestrone (p.1458·2).
Abnormal uterine bleeding; breast cancer; female castration; female hypogonadism; menopausal vulval and vaginal atrophy; primary ovarian failure; prostatic cancer.

Theinol *Bailly, Fr.*
Sodium salicylate (p.85·1); phenazone (p.78·2); caffeine (p.749·3).
Fever; pain.

Theo *CT, Ger.*
Theophylline hydrate (p.765·1).
Obstructive airways disease.

Theo$_2$ *Galephar, Neth.†.*
Theophylline (p.765·1).
Bronchospasm.

Theo-24
Searle, Ital.; UCB, USA.
Theophylline (p.765·1).
Asthma; bronchospasm.

Theo Max *Desarrollo, Spain.*
Theophylline (p.765·1).
Heart failure; obstructive airways disease; paroxysmal dyspnoea.

Theobid Duracaps *Russ, USA.*
Theophylline (p.765·1).
Asthma; chronic bronchitis; emphysema.

Theo-Bronc *Rougier, Canad.*
Guaiphenesin (p.1061·3); potassium iodide (p.1493·1); theophylline (p.765·1); mepyramine maleate (p.414·1).
Obstructive airways disease.

Theocaradrin *Laevosan, Aust.*
Proscillaridin (p.938·1); theophylline hydrate (p.765·1).
Heart failure.

Theochron
Riva, Canad.; Inwood, USA; Lemmon, USA.
Theophylline (p.765·1).
Obstructive airways disease.

Theoclear *Schwarz, USA.*
Theophylline (p.765·1).
Asthma; bronchospasm.

Theodrine *Rugby, USA.*
Theophylline (p.765·1); ephedrine hydrochloride (p.1059·3); phenobarbitone (p.350·2).
Bronchospasm.

Theo-Dur
Astra, Austral.; Astra, Belg.; Astra, Canad.; Astra, Irl.; Recordati, Ital.; Astra, Norw.; Astra, S.Afr.; Pharmacia Upjohn, Spain; Draco, Swed.; Astra, UK; Key, USA.
Theophylline (p.765·1).
Heart failure; obstructive airways disease; paroxysmal dyspnoea.

Theogel *SAN, Ital.*
Royal jelly (p.1626·3).

Theo-Heptylon *Delalande, Ger.†.*
Heptaminol acephyllinate (p.754·1).
Cardiac and respiratory disorders.

Theohexal *Hexal, Aust.*
Theophylline (p.765·1).
Obstructive airways disease.

Theo-Hexanicit *Promed, Ger.†.*
Inositol nicotinate (p.891·3); heptaminol acephyllinate (p.754·1); bamethan sulphate (p.827·1).
Cerebral, coronary, and peripheral vascular disorders.

Theokal *Schaper & Brummer, Ger.†.*
Coumarin (p.1568·1); rutin sodium sulphate (p.1580·2) or troxerutin (p.1580·2); proxyphylline (p.757·3).
Cerebral and peripheral vascular disorders.

Theokombetin *Boehringer Mannheim, Ger.†.*
Strophanthin-K (p.951·1); diprophylline (p.752·1).
Cardiac disorders.

Theolair
3M, Belg.; 3M, Canad.; 3M, Fr.; 3M, Ger.; Synthelabo, Ital.; 3M, Neth.; 3M, Spain; 3M, Switz.; 3M, USA.
Theophylline (p.765·1).
Heart failure; obstructive airways disease; paroxysmal dyspnoea.

Theolan *Elan, Irl.*
Theophylline (p.765·1).
Bronchospasm.

Theo-Lanicor
Note. This name is used for preparations of different composition.
Boehringer Mannheim, Aust.; Boehringer Mannheim, Ger.†.
Tablets: Digoxin (p.849·3); theophylline hydrate (p.765·1); theobromine (p.765·1).
Cardiac disorders.

Boehringer Mannheim, Ger.†.
Oral liquid: Digoxin (p.849·3); proxyphylline (p.757·3); diprophylline (p.752·1).
Cardiac disorders.

Theo-Lanitop
Boehringer Mannheim, Aust.; Boehringer Mannheim, Ger.†.
Theophylline (p.765·1); medigoxin (p.902·1).
Heart failure.

Theolin *Astra, Neth.*
Theophylline (p.765·1).
Bronchospasm.

Theolong *Eisai, Jpn.*
Theophylline (p.765·1).
Obstructive airways disease.

Theomax DF *Barre-National, USA; Schein, USA.*
Theophylline (p.765·1); ephedrine sulphate (p.1059·3); hydroxyzine hydrochloride (p.412·1).
Bronchospasm.

Theon *Klinge, Switz.†.*
Theophylline (p.765·1).
Obstructive airways disease.

Theo-Organidin *Wallace, USA†.*
Theophylline (p.765·1); iodinated glycerol (p.1062·2).
Bronchial asthma and other bronchospastic disorders.

Theophen *Pharmacare Consumer, S.Afr.*
Theophylline (p.765·1); etofylline (p.753·1).
Obstructive airways disease.

Theophen Comp *Pharmacare Consumer, S.Afr.*
Theophylline (p.765·1); etofylline (p.753·1); diphenylpyraline hydrochloride (p.409·3); ammonium chloride (p.1055·2).
Coughs.

Theophyllard
Byk, Belg.; OPW, Ger.
Theophylline (p.765·1).
Obstructive airways disease.

Theophylline Sedative Bruneau *Synthelabo, Belg.†.*
Theophylline (p.765·1); butobarbitone (p.645·1).
Asthma; bronchospastic disorders.

Theoplus
Germania, Aust.; Byk Madaus, S.Afr.; Pierre Fabre, Spain.
Theophylline (p.765·1).
Heart failure; obstructive airways disease; paroxysmal dyspnoea.

Theo-Sav *Savage, USA†.*
Theophylline (p.765·1).
Asthma; bronchospasm.

Theospan-SR *Laser, USA.*
Theophylline (p.765·1).

Theospirex *Gebro, Aust.*
Theophylline (p.765·1) or theophylline sodium glycinate (p.772·2).
Obstructive airways disease.

Theo-SR *Rhone-Poulenc Rorer, Canad.*
Theophylline (p.765·1).
Obstructive airways disease.

Theostat
Note. This name is used for preparations of different composition.
Inava, Fr.; Laser, USA.
Theophylline (p.765·1).
Asthma; bronchospasm.

Lagamed, S.Afr.
Etofylline (p.753·1).
Obstructive airways disease.

Theo-Talusin
Knoll, Ger.†; Knoll, Switz.
Proscillaridin (p.938·1); etofylline (p.753·1).
Cardiac disorders.

Theotex *Terapeutico, Ital.*
Dodecarbonium chloride.
Personal hygiene; skin disinfection.

Theovent *Schering, USA.*
Theophylline (p.765·1).
Asthma; reversible bronchospasm.

Theo-X *Carnrick, USA.*
Theophylline (p.765·1).

Thephorin
Sinclair, Irl.; Sinclair, UK.
Phenindamine tartrate (p.415·2).
Hypersensitivity reactions.

Theprubicine *Bellon, Fr.*
Pirarubicin (p.558·1).
Breast cancer.

Thera Hematinic *Major, USA.*
Ferrous fumarate (p.1339·3); folic acid (p.1340·3); multivitamins and minerals.
Iron-deficiency anaemias.

Therabid *Mission Pharmacal, USA.*
Multivitamin preparation.

Therac *C & M, USA.*
Sulphur (p.1091·2); salicylic acid (p.1090·2).
Acne.

TheraCys *Connaught, USA.*
A BCG vaccine (p.1504·3).
Bladder cancer.

Theradol *Knoll, Neth.*
Tramadol hydrochloride (p.90·1).
Pain.

TheraFlu Flu and Cold *Sandoz, USA.*
Chlorpheniramine maleate (p.405·1); pseudoephedrine hydrochloride (p.1068·3); paracetamol (p.72·2).
Cold and flu symptoms.

TheraFlu Flu, Cold & Cough
Sandoz, Canad.; Sandoz, USA.
Chlorpheniramine maleate (p.405·1); pseudoephedrine hydrochloride (p.1068·3); paracetamol (p.72·2); dextromethorphan hydrobromide (p.1057·3).
Coughs and cold symptoms.

Thera-Flur *Colgate-Hoyt, USA.*
Sodium fluoride (p.742·1).
Dental caries prophylaxis.

Theragenerix *Goldline, USA.*
A range of vitamin preparations.

Theragenerix-H *Goldline, USA.*
Ferrous fumarate (p.1339·3); folic acid (p.1340·3); multivitamins and minerals.
Iron-deficiency anaemias.

Thera-gesic *Mission Pharmacal, USA.*
Methyl salicylate (p.55·2); menthol (p.1600·2).
Musculoskeletal soreness and discomfort; topical adjunct in arthritis, rheumatism, and bursitis.

Theragran *Mead Johnson Nutritionals, USA.*
A range of vitamin preparations.

Theragran AntiOxidant *Bristol-Myers Squibb, USA.*
Vitamins A, C, and E with minerals.

Theragran Hematinic *Apothecon, USA.*
Multivitamin and mineral preparation with iron and folic acid.
Iron-deficiency anaemias.

Theragran-M
Bristol-Myers Squibb, Belg.†; Bristol-Myers Squibb, S.Afr.
Multivitamin and mineral preparation.

Thera-Hist *Major, USA.*
Phenylpropanolamine hydrochloride (p.1067·2); chlorpheniramine maleate (p.405·1).
Upper respiratory-tract symptoms.

Theralen *Rhone-Poulenc Rorer, Swed.*
Trimeprazine tartrate (p.419·3).
Agitation; behaviour disorders; hypersensitivity reactions; premedication; sleep disorders; vomiting.

Theralene
Rhone-Poulenc Rorer, Belg.; Evans, Fr.; Rhone-Poulenc, Ger.†; Rhone-Poulenc Rorer, Switz.†.
Trimeprazine (p.419·3) or trimeprazine tartrate (p.419·3).
Agitation; cough; cramps; dystonias; hypersensitivity reactions; insomnia; premedication; pruritus; tics.

Theralene Pectoral
Rhone-Poulenc Rorer, Belg.; Theraplix, Fr.†.
Trimeprazine tartrate (p.419·3); ethylmorphine hydrochloride (p.36·1); ephedrine hydrochloride (p.1059·3); ammonium acetate (p.1055·1).
Coughs.

Theralene Pectoral Nourrisson *Evans, Fr.*
Trimeprazine tartrate (p.419·3); ammonium acetate (p.1055·1); sodium benzoate (p.1102·3); magnesium sulphate (p.1157·3); tolu balsam (p.1071·1).
Coughs.

Thera-M *Major, USA.*
Multivitamin preparation with minerals and folic acid.

Theramycin Z *Medicis, USA.*
Erythromycin (p.204·1).
Acne.

Theranyl *Abigo, Swed.*
Nicotinic acid (p.1351·2); salicylic acid (p.1090·2).
Musculoskeletal and joint disorders.

Therapeutic Bath *Goldline, USA.*
Emollient and moisturiser.

Therapeutic Bath Oil *Avant Garde, Canad.*
Liquid paraffin (p.1382·1).
Scott, Canad.
Liquid paraffin (p.1382·1); wool fat (p.1385·3).

Therapeutic Mineral Ice *Bristol-Myers Products, USA.*
Menthol (p.1600·2).
Muscle, joint, and soft-tissue pain; neuralgia.

Therapeutic Skin Lotion *Scott, Canad.*
Lanolin oil (p.1385·3); liquid paraffin (p.1382·1).

Therapeutic Soothing Ice *Jamieson, Canad.*
Methyl salicylate (p.55·2); camphor (p.1557·2); menthol (p.1600·2); eucalyptus oil (p.1578·1).

Therapin Halstabletten *Nattermann, Ger.†.*
Cetylpyridinium chloride (p.1106·2); ascorbic acid (p.1365·2).
Inflammatory disorders of the oropharynx.

Therapin Hustenloser *Nattermann, Ger.†.*
Ambroxol hydrochloride (p.1054·3).
Respiratory-tract disorders associated with increased or viscous mucus.

Therapin Schnupfentropfen/spray *Nattermann, Ger.†.*
Xylometazoline hydrochloride (p.1071·2).
Nasal congestion.

Theraplex T *Medicis, USA.*
Coal tar (p.1092·3).
Scalp disorders.

Theraplex Z *Medicis, USA.*
Pyrithione zinc (p.1089·3).
Dandruff; seborrhoeic dermatitis.

Therarubicin *Meiji, Jpn.*
Pirarubicin hydrochloride (p.558·1).
Malignant neoplasms.

Therasphere *Nordion, Canad.†.*
Yttrium-90 (p.1425·3) in glass microspheres.
Liver cancer.

Theravee *Vangard, USA.*
A range of vitamin preparations.

Theravee Hematinic *Vangard, USA.*
Iron (p.1346·1); folic acid (p.1340·3); multivitamins and minerals.
Iron-deficiency anaemias.

Theravim *Nature's Bounty, USA.*
A range of vitamin preparations.

Theravite *Barre-National, USA.*
Multivitamin preparation.

Therems *Rugby, USA.*
A range of vitamin preparations.

Therevac Plus *Jones, USA.*
Docusate sodium (p.1189·3); glycerol (p.1585·2); benzocaine (p.1286·2); soft soap (p.1468·1).
Constipation.

Therevac SB *Jones, USA.*
Docusate sodium (p.1189·3); glycerol (p.1585·2); soft soap (p.1468·1).
Constipation.

Thermal
Provita, Aust.; Alpharma, Norw.
Ethyl nicotinate (p.36·1); diethylamine salicylate (p.33·1).
Muscle and nerve pain.

Thermalife *Thermalife, Austral.*
Protein and trace metal complex (Peptophen).
Arthritic pain; bath additive; bed sores; emollient; muscular pain.

Thermalife C *Thermalife, Austral.*
Protein/trace metal complex (Peptophen); capsicum oleoresin.
Arthritic pain; muscular pain.

Thermazene *Sherwood, USA.*
Silver sulphadiazine (p.247·3).
Infected burns.

Thermazet *Zwintscher, Ger.†.*
Capsaicin (p.24·2); hamamelis (p.1587·1).
Angina; lumbago; neuralgia; rheumatism; sciatica.

Thermo Burger *Ysatfabrik, Ger.*
Capsicum extract (p.1559·2).
Musculoskeletal and joint disorders; soft-tissue injury.

Thermo Mobilisin *Luitpold, Ger.*
Flufenamic acid (p.41·3); a heparinoid (p.882·3); benzyl nicotinate (p.22·1).
Musculoskeletal and joint disorders; neuralgia.

Thermo Rub *Rolmex, Canad.*
Methyl salicylate (p.55·2); menthol (p.1600·2); cineole (p.1564·1).

Thermocutan *Streuli, Switz.*
Nonivamide (p.63·2); ethyl nicotinate (p.36·1); benzyl nicotinate (p.22·1); amidopyrine salicylate (p.15·2).
Chilblains; musculoskeletal, joint, peri-articular, and soft-tissue disorders.

Thermodent *Mentholatum, Austral.*
Potassium nitrate (p.1123·1); sodium monofluorophosphate (p.743·3).
Desensitising toothpaste.

Thermo-Gel *Prodemdis, Canad.*
Camphor (p.1557·2); menthol (p.1600·2); benzocaine (p.1286·2); thymol (p.1127·1).

Thermogene *Montefarmaco, Ital.*
Medicated dressing; ointment (water-soluble): Capsicum oleoresin.
Topical emulsion†; ointment (revulsive)†: Capsicum oleoresin; glycol salicylate (p.43·1).
Musculoskeletal and joint pain.

thermo-loges *Loges, Ger.*
Benzyl nicotinate (p.22·1); oleum pini sylvestris; rosemary oil (p.1626·2).
Circulatory disorders; musculoskeletal, joint, and soft-tissue disorders.

Thermo-Menthoneurin *Tosse, Ger.*
Glycol salicylate (p.43·1); benzyl nicotinate (p.22·1).
Musculoskeletal, joint, and peri-articular disorders; neuralgia.

Thermo-Menthoneurin Bad *Tosse, Ger.*
Glycol salicylate (p.43·1); benzyl nicotinate (p.22·1); methyl nicotinate (p.55·1).
Bath additive; musculoskeletal and joint disorders; peripheral circulatory disorders.

Thermo-Rheumon
Kolassa, Aust.; Bayer, Ger.
Etofenamate (p.36·3); benzyl nicotinate (p.22·1).
Musculoskeletal, joint, peri-articular, and soft-tissue disorders.

Thermo-Rub *Propan, S.Afr.*
Methyl salicylate (p.55·2).
Muscular pain; rheumatism.

Thermosan *Sanofi Winthrop, Ger.†.*
Ethanolamine salicylate; benzyl nicotinate (p.22·1); nonivamide (p.63·2).
Frostbite; muscular, neuromuscular, and joint disorders; peripheral vascular disorders.

Thermosenex *Brenner-Efeka, Ger.; LAW, Ger.*
Camphor (p.1557·2); glycol salicylate (p.43·1); benzyl nicotinate (p.22·1).
Musculoskeletal and joint disorders; neuralgia; sprains.

Theroxide *Medicis, USA†.*
Benzoyl peroxide (p.1079·2).

Thesit *Gepepharm, Ger.*
Laureth 9 (p.1325·2); mepivacaine hydrochloride (p.1297·2); benzalkonium chloride (p.1101·3).
Skin disorders.

Thesit P *Gepepharm, Ger.*
Laureth 9 (p.1325·2); promethazine hydrochloride (p.416·2); prednisolone acetate (p.1048·1).
Skin disorders.

Thevier *Glaxo Wellcome, Ger.*
Thyroxine sodium (p.1497·1).
Hypothyroidism.

Thex Forte *Lee, USA.*
Vitamin B and C preparation.

Thiacide *Beach, USA†.*
Hexamine mandelate (p.216·1); monobasic potassium phosphate (p.1159·3).

Thiamilate *Tyson, USA.*
Thiamine hydrochloride (p.1361·1).
Thiamine deficiency.

Thiaton *Hokuriku, Jpn.*
Tiquizium bromide (p.1638·2).
Smooth muscle spasm and hypermotility.

Thiazid-comp. *Wolff, Ger.*
Triamterene (p.957·2); hydrochlorothiazide (p.885·2).
Hypertension; oedema.

Thiazid-Wolff *Wolff, Ger.†.*
Hydrochlorothiazide (p.885·2).
Cardiovascular disorders; diabetes insipidus; renal calculi.

Thierry *Makara, Aust.*
Fennel oil (p.1579·2): purified honey (p.1345·3).
Catarrh; colds; coughs.

Thilo Tears *Bournonville, Belg.*
Carbomer (p.1471·2).
Dry eyes.

Thilo Wet *Agepha, Aust.*
A wetting solution for contact lenses.

Thiloadren *Agepha, Aust.*
Dipivefrine hydrochloride (p.1572·3); pilocarpine hydrochloride (p.1396·3).
Glaucoma.

Thiloadren N *Alcon-Thilo, Ger.*
Dipivefrine hydrochloride (p.1572·3); pilocarpine hydrochloride (p.1396·3).
Glaucoma.

Thilocanfol *Alcon-Thilo, Ger.*
Azidamfenicol (p.155·2).
Bacterial eye infections.

Thilocanfol C *Alcon-Thilo, Ger.*
Chloramphenicol (p.182·1).
Bacterial eye infections.

Thilocombin *Agepha, Aust.*
Theophylline (p.765·1); heptaminol (p.1587·2) or heptaminol hydrochloride (p.1587·2); nicotinyl alcohol (p.915·3) or nicotinyl alcohol tartrate (p.915·3).
Angina pectoris; migraine; peripheral, coronary, and cerebral vascular disorders; thrombo-embolic disorders.

Thilodigon
Agepha, Aust.; Alcon-Thilo, Ger.
Guanethidine monosulphate (p.878·1); dipivefrine hydrochloride (p.1572·3).
Glaucoma.

Thilorbin *Alcon-Thilo, Ger.*
Oxybuprocaine hydrochloride (p.1298·1); fluorescein sodium (p.1581·1).
Ophthalmic procedures.

Thilo-Tears
Alcon-Thilo, Ger.; Thilo, Neth.†; Alcon, Switz.
Carbomer (p.1471·2).
Dry eyes.

Thinz *Pharmacare Consumer, S.Afr.*
Cathine hydrochloride (p.1478·1).
Obesity.

Thiobitum *LAW, Ger.*
Ammonium bituminosulphonate (p.1083·3).
Skin disorders.

Thioctacid *Asta Medica, Ger.*
Thioctic acid (p.1636·2) or trometamol thioctate (p.1640·1).
Diabetic neuropathy.

Thiocyl *Alba, USA.*
Sodium thiosalicylate (p.85·2).

Thioderazine B I *Sanofi Winthrop, Spain†.*
Piperazine hydrate (p.107·2); thiamine (p.1361·2); thiourea; iodazine.
Fever; inflammation; pain.

Thioderon *Shionogi, Jpn.*
Mepitiostane (p.1450·1).
Breast cancer; renal anaemia.

Thiogamma *Worwag, Ger.*
Thioctic acid (p.1636·2).
Diabetic neuropathy.

Thiola
Coop. Farm., Ital.; Mission Pharmacal, USA.
Tiopronin (p.997·2).
Liver disorders; prevention of cystine renal calculi.

Thiophenicol *Sanofi Winthrop, Fr.*
Thiamphenicol (p.262·3) or thiamphenicol glycinate hydrochloride (p.262·3).
Bacterial infections.

Thiopheol *Biogalenique, Fr.†.*
Suppositories: Thiophene; colloidal sulphur (p.1091·2); cineole (p.1564·1); calcium pantothenate (p.1352·3).
Tablets: Thenoate lithium (p.262·2).
Respiratory-tract disorders.

Thioplex *Immunex, USA.*
Thiotepa (p.566·3).
Malignant neoplasms.

Thiopon *Amido, Fr.*
Thiophene oil.
Respiratory-tract inflammation.

Thiopon Balsamique *Amido, Fr.*
Thiophene oil; eucalyptus oil (p.1578·1); pine oil; niaouli oil (p.1607·1).
Upper respiratory-tract infections.

Thiopon Pantothenique *Amido, Fr.*
Thiophene oil; calcium pantothenate (p.1352·3).
Respiratory-tract inflammation.

Thioprine *Alphapharm, Austral.*
Azathioprine (p.505·3).
Autoimmune disorders; organ transplantation.

Thiopurinol *Bouchara, Fr.†.*
Tisopurine (p.396·3).
Gout; hyperuricaemia.

Thiorubrol *Adroka, Switz.*
Bath additive: Sodium thioricinol sulphonate; sodium thiosulphate (p.996·2); sodium sulphate (p.1213·3).
Bath oil: Triethanolamine thioricinol sulphate.
Muscle and joint pain; skin disorders.

Thiosedal *Zyma, Fr.*
Ethylmorphine hydrochloride (p.36·1); hyoscyamus (p.464·3); potassium guaiacolsulfonate (p.1068·3).
Coughs.

Thiosept *Terrapharm, Aust.*
Shale oil.
Hyperhidrosis; inflammation; musculoskeletal and joint disorders; peripheral vascular disorders; skin disorders.

Thiosol *Coop. Farm., Ital.*
Tiopronin (p.997·2).
Respiratory-tract congestion.

Thiosulfil Forte *Wyeth-Ayerst, USA.*
Sulphamethizole (p.254·2).
Urinary-tract infections.

Thiovalone *Eurorga, Fr.*
Tixocortol pivalate (p.1050·1); chlorhexidine acetate (p.1107·2).
Inflammation of the mouth and throat.

Thioxene *Esseti, Ital.*
Glutathione sodium (p.983·1).
Alcohol or drug poisoning; ionising radiation damage.

Thiozine *Pinewood, Irl.*
Thioridazine hydrochloride (p.695·1).
Anxiety; behaviour disorders; psychoses; senile confusion; tension.

Thirial *Plantes et Medecines, Fr.*
Garlic (p.1583·1).
Circulatory disorders.

Thiuretic *Warner Chilcott, USA.*
Hydrochlorothiazide (p.885·2).
Hypertension; oedema.

Thixo-Flur *Colgate Oral Care, Austral.*
Fluoride.

Thohelur I *Truw, Ger.*
Mineral preparation.

Thohelur II *Truw, Ger.*
Mineral preparation with cholecalciferol.

Thomaeamin GX E *Delta, Ger.*
Amino-acid, electrolyte, glucose, and xylitol infusion.
Parenteral nutrition.

Thomaeamin Hepar *Delta, Ger.*
Amino-acid infusion.
Parenteral nutrition in liver failure.

Thomaeamin n *Delta, Ger.*
Amino-acid and vitamin infusion with or without electrolytes.
Parenteral nutrition.

Thomaeamin n mit Kohlenhydraten und Elektrolyten *Thomae, Ger.†.*
Amino-acid, carbohydrate, electrolyte, and vitamin infusion.
Parenteral nutrition.

Thomaeamin nephro *Thomae, Ger.†.*
Amino-acid infusion.
Parenteral nutrition in renal disease.

Thomaeamin Pad *Delta, Ger.*
Amino-acid infusion.
Parenteral nutrition.

Thomaeamin X E *Delta, Ger.*
Amino-acid, electrolyte, and xylitol infusion.
Parenteral nutrition.

Thomaedex 40 *Delta, Ger.*
Dextran 40 (p.716·2) in sodium chloride.
Plasma volume expansion; thrombosis prophylaxis; vascular disorders.

Thomaedex 60 *Delta, Ger.*
Dextran 60 (p.716·3) in sodium chloride.
Plasma volume expansion; thrombosis prophylaxis.

Thomaegelin *Delta, Ger.*
Gelatin polysuccinate (p.723·2) in Ringer acetate.
Hypovolaemia.

Thomaejonin *Delta, Ger.*
A range of electrolyte infusions with or without carbohydrate (p.1147·1).
Fluid and electrolyte disorders.

Thomaemannit *Delta, Ger.*
Mannitol (p.900·3).
Fluid retention; renal failure.

Thomaetrisol *Thomae, Ger.†.*
Carbohydrate infusion.
Parenteral nutrition.

Thomaetrisol E *Thomae, Ger.†.*
Carbohydrate and electrolyte infusion.
Parenteral nutrition.

Thomapyrin
Bender, Aust.; Thomae, Ger.
Aspirin (p.16·1); paracetamol (p.72·2); caffeine (p.749·3).
Cold symptoms; fever; inflammation; pain.

Thomapyrin C *Thomae, Ger.*
Aspirin (p.16·1); paracetamol (p.72·2); ascorbic acid (p.1365·2).
Fever; inflammation; pain.

Thomapyrin mit Vitamin C Bender, Aust.
Aspirin (p.16·1); paracetamol (p.72·2); ascorbic acid (p.1365·2).
Cold symptoms.

Thomapyrine Boehringer Ingelheim, Switz.
Aspirin (p.16·1); paracetamol (p.72·2); caffeine (p.749·3).
Fever; pain.

Thomasin Apogepha, Ger.
Etilefrine hydrochloride (p.867·2).
Cardiovascular disorders; dumping syndrome.

Thombran Thomae, Ger.
Trazodone hydrochloride (p.308·3).
Depression.

Thorazine SmithKline Beecham, USA.
Chlorpromazine (p.649·1) or chlorpromazine hydrochloride (p.649·1).
Acute intermittent porphyria; adjunct in tetanus; bipolar disorder; hiccups; nausea and vomiting; premedication; psychoses; severe behavioural disorders in children.

Thoxaprim Pharmagen, S.Afr.†.
Co-trimoxazole (p.196·3).
Bacterial infections.

THR Seroyal, Canad.
Vitamin E, magnesium, and potassium.

Threamine DM Barre-National, USA.
Phenylpropanolamine hydrochloride (p.1067·2); chlorpheniramine maleate (p.405·1); dextromethorphan hydrobromide (p.1057·3).
Coughs and cold symptoms.

Throat Discs SmithKline Beecham, USA.
Capsicum (p.1559·2); peppermint oil (p.1208·1); liquid paraffin (p.1382·1).
Sore throat.

Throat Lozenges
Note. This name is used for preparations of different composition.
Novopharm, Canad.
Benzocaine (p.1286·2); cetylpyridinium chloride (p.1106·2).
Novopharm, Canad.
Cetylpyridinium chloride (p.1106·2).
Stanley, Canad.
Hexylresorcinol (p.1116·1).

Throaties Catarrh Pastilles Ernest Jackson, UK.
Menthol (p.1600·2); lemon oil (p.1595·3); eucalyptus (p.1578·1); honey (p.1345·3).

Throaties Family Cough Linctus Ernest Jackson, UK.
Ipecacuanha (p.1062·2); glycerol (p.1585·2); honey (p.1345·3); terpeneless lemon oil (p.1596·1); citric acid (p.1564·3).
Coughs.

Thrombace Drossapharm, Switz.
Aloxiprin (p.15·1).
Thrombo-embolic disorders.

Thrombareduct Azupharma, Ger.
Heparin sodium (p.879·3).
Soft-tissue injury.

Thrombate Bayer, Canad.
Antithrombin III (p.711·2).
Antithrombin III deficiency.

Thrombhibin Immuno, Aust.
Antithrombin III (p.711·2).
Antithrombin III deficiency.

Thrombimed Medice, Ger.†.
Heparin sodium (p.879·3); benzethonium chloride (p.1102·3); cetylpyridinium chloride (p.1106·2); urea (p.1095·2); laureth 9 (p.1325·2).
Skin trauma.

Thrombinar
Rhone-Poulenc Rorer, Austral.†; Jones, USA.
Thrombin (p.728·1).
Minor haemorrhage.

Thrombion Hofmann, Aust.
Heparin sodium (p.879·3); nicotinic acid (p.1351·2); diethylaminoethanol (p.1479·3).
Peripheral vascular disorders; soft-tissue injury.

Thrombo Holzinger, Aust.†.
Ammonium tri-β-oxyethylβ-oxypropan-α,β,γ-tricarbonate.

Thrombo ASS Lannacher, Aust.
Aspirin (p.16·1).
Thrombosis prophylaxis.

Thrombocid
Note. This name is used for preparations of different composition.
Sigmapharm, Aust.; Bene, Ger.; Bene, Switz.
Ointment: Pentosan polysulphate sodium (p.928·1); guaiazulene (p.1586·3); thymol (p.1127·1).
Soft-tissue disorders; superficial vascular disorders.
Bene, Ger.
Suppositories: Pentosan polysulphate sodium (p.928·1); aluminium monostearate; guaiazulene (p.1586·3).
Anorectal disorders.
Bene, Ger.; Bene, Switz.
Topical gel: Pentosan polysulphate sodium (p.928·1); rosemary oil (p.1626·2); pumilio pine oil (p.1623·3); melissa oil.
Soft-tissue disorders; superficial vascular disorders.
Lacer, Spain.
Pentosan polysulphate sodium (p.928·1); thymol (p.1127·1).
Burns; haemorrhoids; peripheral vascular disorders; soft-tissue disorders.

Thrombocoll Johnson & Johnson, Ger.
Thrombin (p.728·1).
Haemorrhage.

Thrombocutan Dorsch, Ger.†.
Heparin sodium (p.879·3); dexpanthenol (p.1570·3).
Skin trauma.

Thrombo-Enelbin N Cassella-med, Ger.†.
Ointment: Heparin sodium (p.879·3); salicylic acid (p.1090·2).
Topical gel: Heparin sodium (p.879·3); glycol salicylate (p.43·1).
Soft tissue injury; thrombotic disorders.

Thrombogen Johnson & Johnson Medical, USA.
Thrombin (p.728·1).
Bleeding from small blood vessels.

Thromboject Omega, Canad.†.
Sodium tetradecyl sulphate (p.1469·2).
Sclerotherapy.

Thrombophob
Note. This name is used for preparations of different composition.
Ebewe, Aust.; Knoll, Belg.†; Hoechst Marion Roussel, S.Afr.
Ointment: Heparin (p.879·3) or heparin sodium (p.879·3); benzyl nicotinate (p.22·1).
Soft-tissue injury; superficial vascular disorders.
Ebewe, Aust.; Knoll, Ger.; Immuno, Ger.; Hoechst Marion Roussel, S.Afr.; Knoll, Switz.†.
Injection; ointment; topical gel: Heparin (p.879·3) or heparin sodium (p.879·3).
Soft-tissue injuries; superficial vascular disorders; thrombo-embolic disorders.

Thrombophob-S Ebewe, Aust.
Heparin sodium (p.879·3).
Soft-tissue injury; superficial vascular disorders.

Thrombosantin Bender, Aust.
Dipyridamole (p.857·1); aspirin (p.16·1).
Thrombo-embolic disorders.

Thrombostat
Parke, Davis, Austral.; Parke, Davis, Canad.; Parke, Davis, USA.
Thrombin (p.728·1).
Minor haemorrhage.

Thrombo-Vetren Promonta, Ger.†.
Heparin sodium (p.879·3).
Thrombo-embolic disorders.

Thrombo-Wellcotest Wellcome, Austral.†.
Diagnostic test for fibrinogen degradation products in serum.

Thuja Med Complex Dynamit, Aust.
Homoeopathic preparation.

Thuja Oligoplex Madaus, Ger.
Homoeopathic preparation.

Thunas Bilettes Thuna, Canad.
Aloin (p.1177·2); cascara (p.1183·1); phenolphthalein (p.1208·2).

Thunas Hyperacidity Tablets Thuna, Canad.
Magnesium hydroxide (p.1198·2); aluminium hydroxide-magnesium carbonate co-dried gel (p.1178·2); simethicone (p.1213·1).

Thunas Laxative Thuna, Canad.
Cascara (p.1183·1); senna (p.1212·2); bryony; fennel (p.1579·1); liquorice (p.1197·1); juglans; leptandra.

Thunas Pile Thuna, Canad.
Benzocaine (p.1286·2); bismuth subcarbonate (p.1180·1); ephedrine sulphate (p.1059·3); zinc oxide (p.1096·2).
Haemorrhoids.

Thunas Salve for Rheumatic Pains Thuna, Canad.
Methyl salicylate (p.55·2); camphor (p.1557·2); menthol (p.1600·2).

Thunas Tab for Menstrual Pain Thuna, Canad.
Motherwort (p.1604·2); senecio (p.1628·1); sodium salicylate (p.85·1); teucrium scorodonia; viburnum.

Thybon Henning, Ger.
Liothyronine hydrochloride (p.1495·2).
Hypothyroidism.

Thylin Inibsa, Spain†.
Nifenazone (p.63·1).
Inflammation.

Thylline-GG Schein, USA†.
Diprophylline (p.752·1); guaiphenesin (p.1061·3).
Bronchospasm.

Thymi-Fips Lichtenstein, Ger.
Thyme (p.1636·3).
Respiratory-tract disorders.

Thymipin N Zyma, Ger.
Cream: Thyme (p.1636·3); camphor (p.1557·2); eucalyptus oil (p.1578·1).
Syrup; oral drops; suppositories: Thyme (p.1636·3).
Coughs and associated respiratory-tract disorders.

Thymitussin Medice, Ger.†.
Oral drops: Thyme (p.1636·3); chamomile (p.1561·2); chelidonium; drosera (p.1574·1); ethaverine (p.1577·1); thymol (p.1127·1); menthol (p.1600·2); camphor (p.1557·2); ephedrine sulphate (p.1059·3); potassium guaiacolsulfonate (p.1068·3).
Tablets: Althaea (p.1546·3); aniseed (p.1549·3); chelidonium; coltsfoot leaf (p.1057·2); lichen islandicus; thyme (p.1636·3); equisetum (p.1575·1); sage (p.1627·1); ethaverine hydrochloride (p.1577·1); calcium phosphate (p.1155·3); ephedrine sulphate (p.1059·3); liquorice root (p.1197·1); potassium guaiacolsulfonate (p.1068·3); dibasic magnesium phosphate trihydrate; sodium thiocyanate.
Coughs and associated respiratory-tract disorders.

Thymiverlan Verla, Ger.
Thyme (p.1636·3).
Respiratory-tract disorders.

Thymodrosin Gubler, Switz.
Guaiphenesin (p.1061·3); codeine phosphate (p.26·1); thyme (p.1636·3); drosera (p.1574·1); plantaginis; castanea vulgaris; ipecacuanha (p.1062·2); belladonna (p.457·1); liquorice (p.1197·1).
Coughs.

Thymo-Glanduretten Biosyn, Ger.
Bovine thymus extract.
Immunotherapy.

Thymoglobuline
Pasteur Merieux, Belg.; Imtix, Fr.; Rhone-Poulenc Rorer, S.Afr.; Rhone-Poulenc Rorer, Switz.
An antithymocyte immunoglobulin (rabbit) (p.504·2).
Immunosuppressive therapy; transplant rejection.

Thymoject Biosyn, Ger.
Bovine thymus extract.
Immunological disorders.

Thymophysin CytoChemia, Ger.
Thymus extract.
Immunotherapy.

Thymoval Smetana, Aust.
Primula; valerian (p.1643·1); thyme (p.1636·3).
Coughs.

Thymowied Wiedemann, Ger.
Thymus.
Immunotherapy.

Thymunes Eagle, Austral.
Thymus.

Thym-Uvocal Strathmann, Ger.
Calf thymus extract.
Immunotherapy.

Thypinone Abbott, USA.
Protirelin (p.1259·1).
Diagnostic assessment of thyroid function.

Thyranon Organon, Spain†.
Thyroid (p.1496·3).
Hypothyroidism.

Thyrar Rhone-Poulenc Rorer, USA.
Thyroid (bovine) (p.1496·3).
Hypothyroidism; thyroid cancer.

Thyrax
Organon, Belg.; Nourypharma, Neth.; Organon, Spain.
Thyroxine sodium (p.1497·1).
Euthyroid goitre; hypothyroidism; thyroid cancer.

Thyrefact Hoechst Marion Roussel, Swed.
Protirelin (p.1259·1).
Test of thyroid or pituitary-hypothalamic function; thyroid disorders.

Thyrel-TRH Ferring, USA.
Protirelin (p.1259·1).
Formerly called Relefact TRH.
Diagnostic assessment of thyroid function.

Thyreocomb N Berlin-Chemie, Ger.
Thyroxine (p.1498·3); potassium iodide (p.1493·1).
Thyreocomb formerly contained liothyronine, thyroxine, and potassium iodide.
Hypothyroidism.

Thyreogutt Austroplant, Aust.
Leonurus cardiaca (p.1604·2); lycopus europaeus.
Hyperthyroidism; mastalgia; tachycardia.

Thyreogutt mono Schwabe, Ger.
Leonurus cardiaca (p.1604·2).
Mastalgia; mild hyperthyroidism.

Thyreogutt-N Schwabe, Ger.†.
Leonurus cardiaca (p.1604·2); lycopus europaeus.
Hyperthyroidism; menopausal disorders; premenstrual mastalgia.

Thyreoid-Dispert Kali-Chemie, Ger.†.
Thyroid (p.1496·3).
Hypothyroidism; obesity.

Thyreoidinum Pfluger, Ger.†.
Homoeopathic preparation.

thyreo-loges Loges, Ger.
Homoeopathic preparation.

thyreo-loges N Loges, Ger.
Lycopus europaeus.
Hyperthyroidism.

Thyreo-Pasc N Pascoe, Ger.
Homoeopathic preparation.

Thyreostat Herbrand, Ger.†.
Methylthiouracil (p.1495·3).
Hyperthyroidism.

Thyreostat II Herbrand, Ger.; Berlin-Chemie, Ger.
Propylthiouracil (p.1496·2).
Hyperthyroidism.

Thyreotom Berlin-Chemie, Ger.
Liothyronine (p.1495·2); thyroxine (p.1498·3).
Hypothyroidism.

Thyrex Sanabo, Aust.
Thyroxine sodium (p.1497·1).
Hypothyroidism.

Thyro-Block
Carter Horner, Canad.; Wallace, USA.
Potassium iodide (p.1493·1).
Blockade of thyroid uptake of radioiodine.

Thyrojod depot Henning, Ger.†.
Potassium iodide (p.1493·1).
Iodine-deficiency disorders.

Thyrolar Forest Pharmaceuticals, USA.
Liothyronine sodium (p.1495·1); thyroxine sodium (p.1497·1).
Evaluation of thyroid function; hypothyroidism; TSH suppression.

Thyroliberin Merck, Ger.
Protirelin (p.1259·1).
Assessment of pituitary and thyroid function.

Thyroliberin TRH Merck, Aust.†.
Protirelin (p.1259·1).
Test for thyroid-pituitary function.

Thyronajod Henning, Ger.
Thyroxine sodium (p.1497·1); potassium iodide (p.1493·1).
Hypothyroidism.

Thyrophan (Rowo-222) Pharmakon, Ger.†.
Homoeopathic preparation.

Thyrotardin Henning, Ger.
Liothyronine hydrochloride (p.1495·2).
Hypothyroidism.

Thyrozol Merck, Ger.
Methimazole (p.1495·3).
Hyperthyroidism.

Thytropar
Rhone-Poulenc Rorer, Canad.†; Armour, USA.
Thyrotrophin (p.1262·1).
Diagnosis of hypothyroidism; thyroid cancer.

TI Baby Natural Fischer, USA.
SPF 16: Titanium dioxide (p.1093·3).
Sunscreen.

TI Lite Fischer, USA.
SPF 15: Ethylhexyl *p*-methoxycinnamate (p.1487·1); titanium dioxide (p.1093·3).
Sunscreen.

TI Screen
Fischer, USA†.
SPF 20+: Ethylhexyl *p*-methoxycinnamate (p.1487·1); oxybenzone (p.1487·3); 2-ethylhexyl salicylate (p.1487·3).
Sunscreen.
Pedinol, USA.
SPF 8; SPF 15: Ethylhexyl *p*-methoxycinnamate (p.1487·1); oxybenzone (p.1487·3).
SPF 30: Ethylhexyl *p*-methoxycinnamate (p.1487·1); oxybenzone (p.1487·3); octyl salicylate (p.1487·3); octocrylene (p.1487·3).
Sunscreen.

TI Screen Natural Pedinol, USA.
SPF 16: Titanium dioxide (p.1093·3).
Sunscreen.

Tia Doce Alba, USA.
Cyanocobalamin (p.1363·3); thiamine hydrochloride (p.1361·1).

Tiabrenolo NCSN, Ital.
Tiadenol (p.1279·3).
Hyperlipidaemias.

Tiacid Draxis, Canad.
Salicylic acid (p.1090·2); lactic acid (p.1593·3).

Tiaclar CT, Ital.†.
Tiadenol (p.1279·3).
Hyperlipidaemias.

Tiaden Malesci, Ital.
Tiadenol (p.1279·3).
Hyperlipidaemias.

Tiadilon Crinex, Fr.
Arginine tidiacicate (p.1334·2).
Liver disorders.

Tiadipona Knoll, Spain.
Bentazepam (p.642·3).
Anxiety; insomnia.

Tiakem Vita, Ital.
Diltiazem hydrochloride (p.854·2).
Hypertension; ischaemic heart disease.

Tiamate Hoechst Marion Roussel, USA.
Diltiazem maleate.
Angina pectoris; hypertension.

Tiamol Draxis, Canad.
Fluocinonide (p.1041·2).
Skin disorders.

Tiamon Mono Temmler, Ger.
Dihydrocodeine tartrate (p.34·1).
Coughs.

Tiapridal
Synthelabo, Belg.; Synthelabo, Fr.; Lorex Synthelabo, Neth.; Synthelabo, Switz.
Tiapride hydrochloride (p.696·1).
Aggression; agitation; choreic movements; drug-induced extrapyramidal disorders; pain.

Tiapridex Synthelabo, Ger.
Tiapride hydrochloride (p.696·1).
Parkinsonism and other hyperkinetic disorders.

Tiaprizal Delagrange, Spain.
Tiapride hydrochloride (p.696·1).
Anxiety; behaviour disorders; movement disorders; nausea and vomiting.

Tiaprorex Lampugnani, Ital.
Tiaprofenic acid (p.89·1).
Inflammation; pain.

Tiase Vedim, Ital.†.
Stepronin (p.1070·1).
Liver disorders.

Tiaterol Midy, Ital.†.
Tiadenol (p.1279·3).
Hyperlipidaemias.

Tiatral Sandoz, Switz.†.
Aloxiprin (p.15·1).
Thrombo-embolic disorders.

Tiatral 100 SR Sandoz, Switz.
Aspirin (p.16·1).
Thrombo-embolic disorders.

Tiazac Forest Pharmaceuticals, USA.
Diltiazem hydrochloride (p.854·2).
Angina pectoris; hypertension.

Tiazen Bioprogress, Ital.
Diltiazem hydrochloride (p.854·2).
Hypertension; ischaemic heart disease.

Tiazolidin Solvay, Ital.
Timonacic (p.1638·1).
Liver disorders.

Tiberal
Roche, Belg.; Roche, Fr.; Roche, Ital.; Roche, Switz.
Ornidazole (p.589·3).
Anaerobic bacterial infections; protozoal infections.

Ti-Bi Sisu, Canad.†.
Melaleuca oil (p.1599·2).
Disinfection of skin and wounds; vaginal hygiene.

Tibicorten
Stiefel, Fr.†; Sigma-Tau, Ital.†.
Triamcinolone benetonide (p.1050·3).
Haemorrhoids; skin disorders.

Tibicorten F Sigma-Tau, Ital.†.
Triamcinolone benetonide (p.1050·3); fusidic acid (p.211·1).
Skin disorders.

Tibinide Recip, Swed.
Isoniazid (p.218·1).
Tuberculosis.

Tibirox Roche, Ital.†.
Co-tetroxazine (p.196·3).
Bacterial infections.

Tiblex Fournier SA, Spain.
Sucralfate (p.1214·2).
Gastro-intestinal haemorrhage; peptic ulcer.

Tiburon Monot, Fr.
Ibuprofen (p.44·1).
Fever; musculoskeletal and joint disorders; pain; soft-tissue disorders.

Ticalma Kelemata, Ital.
Valerian root (p.1643·1).
Nervous disorders.

Ticar
SmithKline Beecham, Canad.; Link, UK†; SmithKline Beecham, USA.
Ticarcillin sodium (p.263·2).
Bacterial infections.

Ticarpen
SmithKline Beecham, Fr.; SmithKline Beecham, Neth.; SmithKline Beecham, Spain.
Ticarcillin sodium (p.263·2).
Bacterial infections.

Tice Organon, USA.
A BCG vaccine (p.1504·3).
Active immunisation; bladder cancer.

Ticillin CSL, Austral.†.
Ticarcillin sodium (p.263·2).
Bacterial infections.

Ticillina Lenza, Ital.†.
Talampicillin hydrochloride.
Bacterial infections.

Ticinil De Angeli, Ital.†.
Phenylbutazone (p.79·2).
Arthritis.

Ticinil Calcico Boehringer Ingelheim, Ital.†.
Phenylbutazone calcium (p.79·3).
Arthritis.

Ticlid
Syntex, Austral.; Sanofi Winthrop, Belg.; Roche, Canad.; Sanofi Winthrop, Fr.; Sanofi Winthrop, Norw.; Sanofi, Swed.; Sanofi Winthrop, Switz.; Sanofi Winthrop, UK; Syntex, USA.
Ticlopidine hydrochloride (p.953·1).
Stroke prophylaxis; thrombo-embolism prophylaxis.

Ticlodone
Sanofi Winthrop, Aust.; Sigma-Tau, Ital.; Berenguer Infale, Spain.
Ticlopidine hydrochloride (p.953·1).
Thrombo-embolism prophylaxis.

Ticloproge Proge, Ital.
Ticlopidine hydrochloride (p.953·1).
Thrombosis prophylaxis.

Ticlosan Von Boch, Ital.†.
Ticlopidine hydrochloride (p.953·1).
Thrombosis prophylaxis.

Ticoflex Uno, Ital.
Naproxen aminobutanol (p.62·1).
Gout; musculoskeletal, joint, peri-articular, and soft-tissue disorders; neuralgias.

Ticon Hauck, USA.
Trimethobenzamide hydrochloride (p.420·1).
Nausea and vomiting.

Tielle Johnson & Johnson Medical, UK.
Foamed hydrogel.
Wounds.

Tiempe DDSA Pharmaceuticals, UK.
Trimethoprim (p.265·1).

Tienam
Merck Sharp & Dohme, Belg.; Merck Sharp & Dohme-Chibret, Fr.; Merck Sharp & Dohme, Ital.; Merck Sharp & Dohme, Neth.; Merck Sharp & Dohme, Norw.; Merck Sharp & Dohme, S.Afr.; Merck Sharp & Dohme, Spain; Merck Sharp & Dohme, Swed.; Merck Sharp & Dohme, Switz.
Imipenem (p.216·3); cilastatin sodium (p.185·2).
Lignocaine hydrochloride (p.1293·2) may be included in the intramuscular injection to alleviate the pain of injection.
Bacterial infections.

Tienor Farmaka, Ital.
Clotiazepam (p.657·2).
Anxiety; insomnia; nervous disorders.

Tifell Bucca, Spain.
Cineole (p.1564·1); cresol (p.1111·2); eugenol (p.1578·2); formaldehyde (p.1113·2).
Mouth infections.

Tifenso Clinced, Aust.
Benzyl nicotinate (p.22·1); choline salicylate (p.25·2).

Tifomycine Roussel, Fr.†.
Chloramphenicol (p.182·1).
Bacterial infections.

Tifox Parekh, Ital.
Cefoxitin sodium (p.170·3).
Lignocaine hydrochloride (p.1293·2) is included in the intramuscular injection to alleviate the pain of injection.
Gram-negative bacterial infections.

TIG Horm Hormonchemie, Ger.†.
A tetanus immunoglobulin (p.1535·2).
Passive immunisation.

Tigan Roberts, USA.
Capsules; injection: Trimethobenzamide hydrochloride (p.420·1).
Suppositories: Trimethobenzamide hydrochloride (p.420·1); benzocaine (p.1286·2).
Nausea and vomiting.

Tigason
Roche, Austral.†; Roche, Fr.†; Roche, Ger.†; Roche, Irl.†; Roche, Ital.; Roche, S.Afr.†; Andreu, Spain†; Roche, Swed.†; Sauter, Switz.†; Roche, UK†.
Etretinate (p.1082·2).
Keratinisation disorders; psoriasis.

Tiger Balm Liquid LRC Products, UK.
Cajuput oil (p.1556·1); camphor (p.1557·2); cinnamon oil (p.1564·2); clove oil (p.1565·2); menthol (p.1600·2); peppermint oil (p.1208·1).
Muscle ache.

Tiger Balm Red
Note. This name is used for preparations of different composition.
Felton, Austral.
Cajuput oil (p.1556·1); camphor (p.1557·2); cassia oil (p.1560·2); clove oil (p.1565·2); menthol (p.1600·2).
Muscular aches and pains.

Haw Par, Canad.; LRC Products, UK.
Cajuput oil (p.1556·1); camphor (p.1557·2); cinnamon oil (p.1564·2); clove oil (p.1565·2); menthol (p.1600·2); peppermint oil (p.1208·1).
Muscle ache.

Tiger Balm White
Felton, Austral.; Haw Par, Canad.; LRC Products, UK.
Cajuput oil (p.1556·1); camphor (p.1557·2); clove oil (p.1565·2); menthol (p.1600·2); peppermint oil (p.1208·1).
Muscle ache.

Tiger Balsam Rot Klosterfrau, Aust.
Camphor (p.1557·2); menthol (p.1600·2); cajuput oil (p.1556·1); peppermint oil (p.1208·1); clove oil (p.1565·2); cinnamon oil (p.1564·2).
Muscle pain.

Tigidol Phytomedica, Fr.
Camphor (p.1557·2); menthol (p.1600·2); clove oil (p.1565·2); eucalyptus oil (p.1578·1); peppermint oil (p.1208·1); cinnamon oil (p.1564·2).
Pain.

Tigonal IBP, Ital.†.
Chlophedianol hydrochloride (p.1057·1).
Coughs.

Tijgerbalsem Dagra, Neth.†.
Ointment: Cajuput oil (p.1556·1); clove oil (p.1565·2); camphor (p.1557·2); menthol (p.1600·2); peppermint oil (p.1208·1).
Topical liquid: Cajuput oil (p.1556·1); camphor (p.1557·2); cinnamon oil (p.1564·2); clove oil (p.1565·2); menthol (p.1600·2); peppermint oil (p.1208·1); ammonia liquid.
Muscle and joint pain.

Tijgerolie Dagra, Neth.†.
Menthol (p.1600·2); methyl salicylate (p.55·2); camphor (p.1557·2); eucalyptus oil (p.1578·1); lavender oil (p.1594·3); chloroform.
Muscle and joint pain.

Tikacillin Tika, Swed.
Phenoxymethylpenicillin potassium (p.236·2).
Bacterial infections.

Tikalac Tika, Swed.†.
Lactulose (p.1195·3).
Constipation; hepatic encephalopathy.

Tiklid
Sanofi Winthrop, Aust.; Sanofi Winthrop, Ital.; Sanofi Winthrop, Spain.
Ticlopidine hydrochloride (p.953·1).
Thrombo-embolism prophylaxis.

Tiklyd Sanofi Winthrop, Ger.
Ticlopidine hydrochloride (p.953·1).
Thrombosis prophylaxis.

Tilad Casen Fisons, Spain.
Nedocromil sodium (p.756·2).
Asthma.

Tilade
Schoeller, Aust.; Rhone-Poulenc Rorer, Austral.; Rhone-Poulenc Rorer, Canad.; Specia, Fr.; Fisons, Ger.; Rhone-Poulenc Rorer, Ger.; Rhone-Poulenc Rorer, Irl.; Italchimici, Ital.; Fisons, Neth.; Rhone-Poulenc Rorer, S.Afr.; Fisons, Switz.; Pantheon, UK; Fisons, USA.
Nedocromil sodium (p.756·2).
Asthma.

Tilaren Midy Sanofi Winthrop, Spain†.
Tilia platyphyllos (p.1637·3).
Hepatobiliary disorders.

Tilarin
Schoeller, Aust.; Italchimici, Ital.; Fisons, Switz.; Fisons, UK.
Nedocromil sodium (p.756·2).
Allergic rhinitis.

Tilavist
Schoeller, Aust.; Specia, Fr.; Rhone-Poulenc Rorer, Irl.; Italchimici, Ital.; Fisons, Neth.; Casen Fisons, Spain; Rhone-Poulenc Rorer, Swed.; Fisons, Switz.
Nedocromil sodium (p.756·2).
Conjunctivitis.

Tilazem Parke, Davis, S.Afr.
Diltiazem hydrochloride (p.854·2).
Angina pectoris; hypertension.

Tilcotil
Roche, Aust.; Roche, Austral.; Roche, Belg.; Roche, Fr.; Roche, Ger.; Roche, Ital.; Roche, Neth.; Roche, S.Afr.; Andreu, Spain; Roche, Switz.
Tenoxicam (p.88·2).
Dysmenorrhoea; gout; musculoskeletal, joint and peri-articular disorders.

Tildiem
Synthelabo, Belg.; Synthelabo, Fr.; Lorex, Irl.; Synthelabo, Ital.; Lorex Synthelabo, Neth.; Lorex, UK.
Diltiazem hydrochloride (p.854·2).
Angina pectoris; arrhythmias; hypertension; myocardial ischaemia.

Tilene Francia, Ital.
Fenofibrate (p.1273·1).
Hyperlipidaemias.

Tilexim Select, Ital.
Cefuroxime axetil (p.177·1).
Bacterial infections.

Tilfilin Funk, Spain.
Carbocisteine (p.1056·3); chlorpheniramine maleate (p.405·1); phenylephrine hydrochloride (p.1066·2); choline theophyllinate (p.751·3).
Obstructive airways disease.

Tilidalor Hexal, Ger.
Tilidate hydrochloride (p.89·2).
Naloxone hydrochloride (p.986·2) is included in this preparation to discourage abuse.
Pain.

Tilitrate Parke, Davis, Spain.
Tilidate hydrochloride (p.89·2).
Pain.

Tilker Synthelabo Delagrange, Spain.
Diltiazem hydrochloride (p.854·2).
Angina pectoris; hypertension; myocardial infarction.

Till Tosi, Ital.
Triclosan (p.1127·2); alkylamidobetaine.
Personal hygiene.

Tiloryth Tillomed, UK.
Erythromycin (p.204·1).
Bacterial infections.

Ti-Lub Draxis, Canad.
Liquid paraffin (p.1382·1) or light liquid paraffin (p.1382·1).

Tilur Drossapharm, Switz.
Acemetacin (p.12·2).
Musculoskeletal and joint disorders; superficial thrombophlebitis.

Tilvis Roussel, Ital.†.
Oxolinic acid (p.235·1).
Bacterial infections of the genito-urinary tract.

TIM Seroyal, Canad.
Vitamins A, C, and E, and zinc.

Timacor Merck Sharp & Dohme-Chibret, Fr.
Timolol maleate (p.953·3).
Angina pectoris; hypertension; myocardial infarction.

Tim-Ak Dioptic, Canad.
Timolol maleate (p.953·3).
Raised intra-ocular pressure.

Timecef
Albert-Roussel, Aust.; Corvi, Ital.; Roussel, UK.
Cefodizime sodium (p.167·1).
Lignocaine hydrochloride (p.1293·2) is included in some intramuscular injections to alleviate the pain of injection.
Bacterial infections.

Timed Release C Jamieson, Canad.
Ascorbic acid (p.1365·2).

Timed Release Swiss One Swiss Herbal, Canad.
Multivitamin and mineral preparation.

Timedose B Plex Stanley, Canad.†.
Vitamin B substances.

Timedose B Plex C Stanley, Canad.†.
Vitamin B substances with vitamin C.

Timelit UCB, Ital.†.
Lofepramine hydrochloride (p.296·1).
Depression.

Timenten
SmithKline Beecham, Aust.; SmithKline Beecham, Switz.
Ticarcillin sodium (p.263·2); potassium clavulanate (p.190·2).
Bacterial infections.

Timentin
SmithKline Beecham, Austral.; Beecham, Belg.; SmithKline Beecham, Canad.; SmithKline Beecham, Irl.; SmithKline Beecham, Ital.; SmithKline Beecham, Neth.; Beecham Research, UK; SmithKline Beecham, USA.
Ticarcillin sodium (p.263·2); potassium clavulanate (p.190·2).
Lignocaine hydrochloride (p.1293·2) may be included in the intramuscular injection to alleviate the pain of injection.
Bacterial infections.

Timicon Merck Sharp & Dohme, Ital.
Timolol maleate (p.953·3); pilocarpine hydrochloride (p.1396·3).
Glaucoma; ocular hypertension.

T-Immun
Immuno, Aust.; Immuno, Ger.
A tetanus vaccine (p.1535·3).
Active immunisation.

Timo-Comod Ursapharm, Ger.
Timolol maleate (p.953·3).
Glaucoma; ocular hypertension.

Timodine
Reckitts, Irl.; Reckitt & Colman, UK.
Nystatin (p.386·1); hydrocortisone (p.1043·3).
Infected skin disorders.

Timoedo Mann, Ger.
Timolol maleate (p.953·3).
Glaucoma; ocular hypertension.

Timoftol Merck Sharp & Dohme, Spain.
Timolol maleate (p.953·3).
Glaucoma; ocular hypertension.

Timohexal Hexal, Ger.
Timolol maleate (p.953·3).
Cataracts; glaucoma; ocular hypertension.

Timolene Ellem, Ital.†.
Potassium guaiacolsulfonate (p.1068·3); sodium benzoate (p.1102·3); wild thyme; tolu balsam (p.1071·1).
Coughs; respiratory-tract disorders.

Timolide
Frosst, Canad.; Merck Sharp & Dohme, USA.
Timolol maleate (p.953·3); hydrochlorothiazide (p.885·2).
Hypertension.

Timomann Mann, Ger.
Timolol maleate (p.953·3).
Glaucoma; ocular hypertension.

Timonil
Desitin, Ger.; Desitin, Switz.; CP Pharmaceuticals, UK.
Carbamazepine (p.339·2).
Alcohol withdrawal syndrome; bipolar disorder; diabetic neuropathy; epilepsy; neuralgias.

Tim-Ophtal Winzer, Ger.
Timolol maleate (p.953·3).
Glaucoma; ocular hypertension.

Timopos COMOD Ursapharm, Ger.†.
Timolol maleate (p.953·3).
Glaucoma; ocular hypertension.

Timoptic
Merck Sharp & Dohme, Aust.; Merck Sharp & Dohme, Canad.; Merck Sharp & Dohme, Switz.; Merck Sharp & Dohme, USA.
Timolol maleate (p.953·3).
Glaucoma; ocular hypertension.

Timoptol
Frosst, Austral.; Merck Sharp & Dohme, Belg.; Merck Sharp & Dohme-Chibret, Fr.; Merck Sharp & Dohme, Irl.; Merck Sharp & Dohme, Ital.; Chibret, Neth.; Merck Sharp & Dohme, S.Afr.; Merck Sharp & Dohme, UK.
Timolol maleate (p.953·3).
Glaucoma; ocular hypertension.

Timoptol-XE Merck Sharp & Dohme, Austral.
Timolol maleate (p.953·3).
Glaucoma; ocular hypertension.

Timosin Sclavo, Ital.
Thymalfasin (p.1637·2).
Influenza in immunodeficient patients.

Timosine Chibret, Ger.
Timolol maleate (p.953·3).
Glaucoma; ocular hypertension.

Timpanalgesic Juventus, Spain†.
Benzocaine (p.1286·2); phenazone (p.78·2); tyrothricin (p.267·2).
External ear disorders.

Timpilo
Merck Sharp & Dohme, Aust.; Merck Sharp & Dohme, Austral.; Merck Sharp & Dohme, Belg.†; Merck Sharp & Dohme, Canad.; Merck Sharp & Dohme-Chibret, Fr.; Chibret, Ger.; Merck Sharp & Dohme, Norw.; Merck Sharp & Dohme, Swed.; Merck Sharp & Dohme, Switz.
Timolol maleate (p.953·3); pilocarpine hydrochloride (p.1396·3).
Glaucoma; ocular hypertension.

Timpilo-2 Chibret, Neth.
Timolol maleate (p.953·3); pilocarpine hydrochloride (p.1396·3).
Glaucoma; ocular hypertension.

Timpron Berk, UK.
Naproxen (p.61·2).
Gout; musculoskeletal and joint disorders.

Timulcer Nezel, Spain†.
Dimethicone (p.1213·1); gefarnate (p.1193·2); magnesium polygalacturonate; metoclopramide (p.1202·1).
Gastritis; gastro-oesophageal reflux; peptic ulcer; ulcerative colitis.

Timunox
Janssen-Cilag, Ger.†; Janssen-Cilag, Ital.
Thymopentin (p.1637·2) or thymopentin acetate.
Immunodeficiency disorders.

Tinacare Delta, Austral.†.
Tolnaftate (p.389·1).
Fungal skin infections.

Tinacidin Schering-Plough, Austral.†.
Tolnaftate (p.389·1).
Fungal skin infections.

Tinactin
Schering, Canad.; Schering-Plough, USA.
Tolnaftate (p.389·1).
Fungal skin infections.

Tinaderm
Schering-Plough, Austral.; Schering-Plough, Irl.; Schering-Plough, Ital.; Schering-Plough, S.Afr.; Schering-Plough, Spain; Schering-Plough, UK.
Tolnaftate (p.389·1).
Fungal skin infections.

Tinaderm Extra Schering-Plough, Austral.
Clotrimazole (p.376·3).
Fungal infections.

Tinaderm-M
Schering-Plough, Irl.; Schering-Plough, UK.
Tolnaftate (p.389·1); nystatin (p.386·1).
Fungal skin and nail infections.

Tinagel
Schering-Plough, Belg.; Schering-Plough, Neth.†.
Benzoyl peroxide (p.1079·2).
Acne.

Tinatox Brenner-Efeka, Ger.
Tolnaftate (p.389·1).
Fungal skin infections.

TinBen Ferndale, USA.
Barrier preparation.

TinCoBen Ferndale, USA.
Barrier preparation.

Tinctura Justi Pascoe, Ger.
Homoeopathic preparation.

Tindal Schering, USA†.
Acetophenazine maleate (p.640·2).
Psychoses.

Tine Test PPD Lederle-Praxis, USA.
Tuberculin purified protein derivative (p.1640·2).
Diagnosis of tuberculosis.

Tineafax
Note. This name is used for preparations of different composition.
Glaxo Wellcome, Aust.
Ointment: Zinc undecenoate (p.389·2); zinc naphthenate; mesulphen (p.1086·3); methyl salicylate (p.55·2); terpineol (p.1635·1).
Topical powder: Zinc undecenoate (p.389·2); methyl salicylate (p.55·2); eucalyptus oil (p.1578·1).
Douglas, Austral.; Wellcome, UK†.
Tolnaftate (p.389·1).
Tinea pedis.

Tinerol Roche, Spain.
Ornidazole (p.589·3).
Amoebiasis; anaerobic bacterial infections; giardiasis.

Ting Fisons, USA.
Tolnaftate (p.389·1).
Fungal skin infections.

Tinoran Diamant, Fr.†.
Demexiptiline hydrochloride (p.282·2).
Depression.

Tinset
Janssen-Cilag, Aust.; Janssen-Cilag, Belg.; Janssen-Cilag, Fr.; Janssen-Cilag, Ger.; Formenti, Ital.; Taxandria, Neth.; Janssen-Cilag, S.Afr.; Janssen-Cilag, Switz.†; Janssen, UK†.
Oxatomide (p.415·1).
Hypersensitivity reactions.

Tintorine Bipharma, Neth.
Salicylic acid (p.1090·2); lactic acid (p.1593·3).
Warts.

Tintu. Mertiolato Asens Asens, Spain.
Thiomersal (p.1126·3); ethanolamine.
Skin disinfection.

Tintura Stomatica Foletto, Ital.†.
Alpine herbs; rhubarb (p.1212·1).
Biliary-tract disorders.

Tinver Pilkington Barnes-Hind, USA.
Sodium thiosulphate (p.996·2); salicylic acid (p.1090·2); isopropyl alcohol (p.1118·2).
Pityriasis versicolor.

Tiobarbital Miro Palex, Spain.
Thiopentone sodium (p.1233·1).
Epilepsy; general anaesthesia.

Tiobec Pharmo-Natura, Ital.
Thioctic acid (p.1636·2); vitamins.
Neuropathies; nutritional supplement.

Tiocalmina Ottolenghi, Ital.
Potassium guaiacolsulfonate (p.1068·3); dropropizine (p.1059·2).
Coughs.

Tioclin Sterling Health, Spain†.
Oxymetazoline hydrochloride (p.1065·3).
Nasal congestion.

Tiocosol OFF, Ital.
Potassium guaiacolsulfonate (p.1068·3); sodium benzoate (p.1102·3); tolu balsam (p.1071·1); grindelia.
Bronchial congestion; coughs.

Tioctan
Aesca, Aust.; Fujisawa, Jpn.
Thioctic acid (p.1636·2).
Diabetic neuropathy; subacute necrotising encephalomyelopathy; thioctic acid deficiency; vestibular deafness.

Tioctidasi ISI, Ital.†.
Ethylenediamine thioctate (p.1636·2).
Liver disorders.

Tioderma Medici Domus, Ital.†.
Salicylic acid (p.1090·2); zinc oxide (p.1096·2); betanaphthol (p.98·3); benzyl benzoate (p.1402·2); colloidal sulphur (p.1091·2).
Dermatitis; scabies.

Tioglis Logifarm, Ital.†.
Tiopronin (p.997·2).
Liver disorders.

Tioguaialina Montefarmaco, Ital.
Potassium guaiacolsulfonate (p.1068·3).
Catarrh; coughs.

Tiomidone Edmond Pharma, Ital.†.
Amidopyrine γ-thiomethyl-α-hydroxybutyrate (p.15·2).
Musculoskeletal and joint disorders.

Tionamil Ogna, Ital.
Potassium guaiacolsulfonate (p.1068·3); sodium benzoate (p.1102·3); terpin hydrate (p.1070·2).
Coughs.

Tiopirin Farge, Ital.†.
Chlormezanone (p.648·3); amidopyrine (p.15·2).
Arthritis; fever; neuralgia; rheumatism.

Tiorfan Bioprojet, Fr.
Acetorphan (p.1176·2).
Diarrhoea.

Tioscina Inverni della Beffa, Ital.
Aescin (p.1543·3); thiocolchicoside (p.1322·1).
Inflammation; musculoskeletal and soft-tissue disorders.

Tiosulfan Inibsa, Spain†.
Sulphamethizole (p.254·2).
Urinary-tract infections.

Tioten Therabel, Ital.
Stepronin sodium (p.1070·1).
Respiratory-tract congestion.

Tiotil Abigo, Swed.
Propylthiouracil (p.1496·2).
Hyperthyroidism.

tiovalon Intersan, Ger.†.
Tixocortol pivalate (p.1050·1).
Allergic rhinitis.

Tiovalone Juste, Spain.
Tixocortol pivalate (p.1050·1).
Nasal polyps; rhinitis.

Tiparol Astra, Swed.
Tramadol hydrochloride (p.90·1).
Pain.

Tipeptid Pharmacia Upjohn, Fr.†.
Preparation for enteral nutrition.

Tiperal Clonmel, Irl.
Propranolol hydrochloride (p.937·1).
Angina pectoris; anxiety; arrhythmias; essential tremor; hypertension; migraine; phaeochromocytoma.

Tipodex Farmacusi, Spain.
Famotidine (p.1192·1).
Gastro-oesophageal reflux; peptic ulcer; Zollinger-Ellison syndrome.

Tiprocin Clonmel, Irl.
Erythromycin (p.204·1).
Bacterial infections.

Tipuric Clonmel, Irl.
Allopurinol (p.390·2).
Gout; prophylaxis of uric acid and calcium oxalate stones.

Tiracrin Geymonat, Ital.
Iodothyreoglobulin.
Hypothyroidism; obesity.

Tirend SmithKline Beecham, USA†.
Caffeine (p.749·3).
Fatigue.

Tirgon
Note. This name is used for preparations of different composition.
Woelm, Ger.†.
Suppositories: Bisacodyl (p.1179·3); docusate sodium (p.1189·3); sodium citrate (p.1153·2).
Topical gel: Docusate sodium (p.1189·3); sodium citrate (p.1153·2); sorbitol (p.1354·2).
Bowel evacuation; constipation.
Schieffer, Switz.†.
Bisacodyl (p.1179·3); frangula bark (p.1193·2); rhubarb root (p.1212·1); caraway fruit oil (p.1559·3); peppermint oil (p.1208·1).
Constipation.

Tirgon N Woelm, Ger.
Bisacodyl (p.1179·3).
Formerly contained frangula bark, rhubarb, caraway oil, peppermint oil, and bisacodyl.
Constipation.

Tirocetil Ale, Spain†.
Cetylpyridinium chloride (p.1106·2).
Mouth infections.

Tirocular Angelini, Ital.
Acetylcysteine (p.1052·3).
Corneal disorders; dry eyes.

Tirodex ISM, Ital.†.
Allergen extracts (p.1545·1).
Hyposensitisation.

Tirodril Estedi, Spain.
Methimazole (p.1495·3).
Hyperthyroidism.

Tirolaxo Alcala, Spain.
Docusate sodium (p.1189·3).
Constipation.

Tiroler Steinol Tiroler, Aust.
Yellow soft paraffin (p.1382·3); yellow beeswax (p.1383·1); hydrous wool fat (p.1385·3); white soft paraffin (p.1382·3).
Skin disorders.

Tirs Difa, Ital.
Benzalkonium chloride (p.1101·3); hypromellose (p.1473·1).
Dry eyes; eye disinfection.

Tisana Arnaldi Arnaldi-Uscio, Ital.
Senna (p.1212·2); frangula bark (p.1193·2); liquorice (p.1197·1); boldo leaves (p.1554·1); chinese rhubarb (p.1212·1); chelidonium; couch-grass root (p.1567·3); saponaria root; dulcamara (p.1574·2); melissa leaves (p.1600·1); angelica root; viola tricolor flowers.
Constipation.

Tisana Cisbey Geymonat, Ital.
Rhubarb (p.1212·1); liquorice (p.1197·1); couch-grass (p.1567·3); peppermint leaf (p.1208·1); parietaria; melissa (p.1600·1); fennel (p.1579·1); coriander (p.1567·3); mallow.
Digestive disorders; sleep disorders.

Tisana Kelemata Kelemata, Ital.
Tablets: Senna (p.1212·2).
Teabags; tea: Senna (p.1212·2); couch-grass (p.1567·3); guaiacum; hyssop; parietaria; peppermint (p.1208·1); sarsaparilla (p.1627·2); aniseed (p.1549·3); melissa (p.1600·1).
Constipation.

Tisane Antibiliaire et Stomachique Denolin, Belg.
Senna (p.1212·2); frangula bark (p.1193·2); althaea (p.1546·3); peppermint leaf (p.1208·1); cnicus benedictus (p.1565·3); rosemary; melilotus officinalis; liquorice (p.1197·1); calendula flower; mallow flower; fennel (p.1579·1); aniseed (p.1549·3); tilia (p.1637·3).
Biliary-tract congestion; digestive disorders.

Tisane antirhumatismale Sidroga, Switz.
Spearmint (p.1632·1); passion flower (p.1615·3); salix (p.82·3); stevia rebaudiana.
Rheumatism.

Tisane antirhumatismale "H" Hanseler, Switz.†.
Salix (p.82·3); spireaea ulmaria (p.1599·1); birch (p.1553·3); juniper (p.1592·2); liquorice (p.1197·1); couch-grass (p.1567·3); bearberry (p.1552·2); peppermint leaf (p.1208·1); centaurea cyanus; lavender flower (p.1594·3).
Musculoskeletal and joint disorders.

Tisane antiseptique diuretique Sidroga, Switz.†.
Angelica; birch (p.1553·3); boldo (p.1554·1); equisetum (p.1575·1); juglans regia; juniper (p.1592·2); levisticum officinale (p.1597·2); mallow flowers; peppermint leaf (p.1208·1); orthosiphon (p.1592·2); rose fruit (p.1365·2); tilia (p.1637·3); bearberry (p.1552·2).
Urinary-tract disorders.

Tisane antitussive et pectorale "H" Hanseler, Switz.†.
Calendula officinalis; centaurea cyanus; helichrysum arenarium; mallow flowers; red-poppy petal (p.1001·1); verbascum flowers; mallow leaves; althaea (p.1546·3); liquorice (p.1197·1); primula.
Respiratory-tract disorders.

Tisane Clairo Weleda, Fr.
Aniseed (p.1549·3); clove (p.1565·2); peppermint leaf (p.1208·1); senna leaflets (p.1212·2).
Constipation.

Tisane Contre la Tension Denolin, Belg.
Mistletoe (p.1604·1); frangula bark (p.1193·2); crataegus (p.1568·2); orthosiphonis stamineus (p.1592·2); bearberry (p.1552·2); curcuma zanthorrhiza; passion flower (p.1615·3); olive leaf; star anise; peppermint leaf (p.1208·1).
Hypertension.

Tisane contre les refroidissements Sidroga, Switz.
Rose fruit (p.1365·2); sambucus (p.1627·2); chamomile (p.1561·2); tilia (p.1637·3); wild thyme.
Cold symptoms.

Tisane d'allaitement "H" Hanseler, Switz.†.
Caraway (p.1559·3); fennel (p.1579·1); aniseed (p.1549·3); urtica (p.1642·3).
Low appetite.

Tisane Depurative "les 12 Plantes" Denolin, Belg.
Sarsaparilla (p.1627·2); lappa (p.1594·2); fumitory (p.1581·3); parietaria; saponaria; senna (p.1212·2); frangula bark (p.1193·2); liquorice (p.1197·1); peppermint leaf (p.1208·1); mallow flower; calendula flower; fennel (p.1579·1); angelica; star anise.
Digestive disorders; kidney disorders; skin eruptions.

Tisane des Familles Sterling Midy, Fr.†.
Equisetum (p.1575·1); tilia (p.1637·3); senna (p.1212·2); peppermint (p.1208·1); althaea (p.1546·3); liquorice (p.1197·1); parietaria; fennel (p.1579·1); melissa (p.1600·1); caraway (p.1559·3); sambucus (p.1627·2); ash; verbena; cynara (p.1569·2); boldo (p.1554·1); aniseed (p.1549·3); frangula (p.1193·2); meadowsweet (p.1599·1).
Constipation.

Tisane Digestive Weleda Weleda, Fr.
Achillaea (p.1542·2); aniseed (p.1549·3); caraway (p.1559·3); fennel (p.1579·1); chamomile (p.1561·2).
Gastro-intestinal disorders.

Tisane Diuretique Denolin, Belg.
Bearberry (p.1552·2); juniper (p.1592·2); spireae ulmaria (p.1599·1); fraxinus excelsior; cynodontis root; liquorice (p.1197·1); calendula flower; star anise; calluna; angelica; fennel (p.1579·1); tritici root.
Kidney and urinary disorders.

Tisane diuretique Sidroga, Switz.
Birch (p.1553·3); bean pods; urtica (p.1642·3); equisetum (p.1575·1).
Urinary-tract disorders.

Tisane diuretique "H" Hanseler, Switz.†.
Red-rose petal (p.1001·1); birch (p.1553·3); orthosiphon (p.1592·2); bearberry (p.1552·2); aniseed (p.1549·3); juniper (p.1592·2); equisetum (p.1575·1); levisticum officinale (p.1597·2).
Urinary-tract disorders.

Tisane gastrique "H" Hanseler, Switz.†.
Matricaria (p.1561·2); mallow flower; melissa (p.1600·1); senna (p.1212·2); aniseed (p.1549·3); caraway (p.1559·3); fennel (p.1579·1); absinthium (p.1541·1); sweet basil; peppermint leaf (p.1208·1); achillea (p.1542·2); gentian (p.1583·3); liquorice (p.1197·1); calamus (p.1556·1).
Carminative; digestive system disorders.

Tisane Grande Chartreuse Aerocid, Fr.
Marjoram; althaea (p.1546·3); liquorice (p.1197·1); senna (p.1212·2); frangula (p.1193·2); melissa (p.1600·1); peppermint (p.1208·1); ash; parietaria; coriander (p.1567·3).
Constipation; skin disorders of digestive origin.

Tisane hepatique et biliaire Sidroga, Switz.
Cynara (p.1569·2); boldo (p.1554·1); taraxacum (p.1634·2); silybum marianum (p.993·3); peppermint leaf (p.1208·1); achillea (p.1542·2).
Digestive system disorders.

Tisane hepatique et biliaire "H" Hanseler, Switz.†.
Matricaria (p.1561·2); boldo (p.1554·1); absinthium (p.1541·1); marrubium vulgare (p.1063·3); liquorice (p.1197·1); taraxacum (p.1634·2); turmeric (p.1001·3).
Digestive system disorders.

Tisane laxative Sidroga, Switz.
Frangula bark (p.1193·2); fennel (p.1579·1); senna (p.1212·2); star anise; liquorice (p.1197·1).
Constipation.

Tisane laxative H Hanseler, Switz.
Sambucus (p.1627·2); senna (p.1212·2); aniseed (p.1549·3); fennel (p.1579·1).
Constipation.

Tisane laxative Natterman no 13 Piraud, Switz.
Senna (p.1212·2); aniseed (p.1549·3); caraway (p.1559·3); coriander (p.1567·3); fennel (p.1579·1); juniper (p.1592·2); liquorice (p.1197·1).
Constipation.

Tisane laxative Natterman no 13 instant Piraud, Switz.
Senna (p.1212·2); liquorice (p.1197·1).
Constipation.

Tisane Mexicaine Medecine Vegetale, Fr.
Red vine leaf; boldo leaf (p.1554·1); frangula bark (p.1193·2); hyssop; rosemary; ash leaf; senna leaf (p.1212·2).
Venous-lymphatic insufficiency.

Tisane Natterman instantanee no 6 pour calmer les nerfs et lutter contre l'insomnie
Piraud, Switz.†.
Orange flower; lavender flower (p.1594·3); melissa (p.1600·1); liquorice (p.1197·1); lupulus (p.1597·2); valerian (p.1643·1).
Anxiety; sleep disorders; tension.

Tisane Obeflorine Lehning, Fr.
Bladderwrack (p.1554·1); senna leaflets (p.1212·2); liquorice root (p.1197·1); ash leaves.
Constipation.

Tisane Orientale Soker Medecine Vegetale, Fr.
Arenaria; parietaria; couch-grass root (p.1567·3); bearberry leaves (p.1552·2); maize stigmas.
Urinary infections; water retention.

Tisane Pectorale Denolin, Belg.
Poppy capsule (p.1068·2); star anise; liquorice (p.1197·1); carrageenan (p.1471·3); hedera terrestris; hyssop; angelica; althaea (p.1546·3); mallow flower; calendula flower; tilia (p.1637·3).
Coughs.

Tisane pectorale et antitussive Sidroga, Switz.
Sage (p.1627·1); althaea (p.1546·3); fennel (p.1579·1); iceland moss; red-poppy petal (p.1001·1); plantaginis; star anise; liquorice (p.1197·1); thyme (p.1636·3).
Coughs and congestion.

Tisane pectorale et bechique Natterman instantee no 9 Piraud, Switz.†.
Plantain (p.1208·3); primula rhizome; liquorice (p.1197·1); thyme oil (p.1637·1).
Respiratory-tract disorders.

Tisane Phlebosedol Lehning, Fr.
Aesculus bark (p.1543·3); clematis vitalba leaves; hamamelis leaves (p.1587·1); lesser celandine leaves; viburnum bark; piscidia bark; frangula bark (p.1193·2); senecio leaves (p.1628·1); alchemilla leaves.
Venous insufficiency disorders.

Tisane pour Dormir Denolin, Belg.
Poppy capsule (p.1068·2); citrus aurantium; chamomile romanae (p.1561·2); crataegus (p.1568·2); star anise; sage (p.1627·1); peppermint leaf (p.1208·1).
Insomnia; nervous disorders.

Tisane pour le coeur et la circulation Sidroga, Switz.
Birch (p.1553·3); motherwort (p.1604·2); spearmint (p.1632·1); melissa (p.1600·1); crataegus (p.1568·2).
Cardiac and circulatory disorders.

Tisane pour le coeur et la circulation "H" Hanseler, Switz.†.
Calendula officinalis; crataegus (p.1568·2); garlic (p.1583·1); cnicus benedictus (p.1565·3); leonurus cardiaca (p.1604·2); melissa (p.1600·1); peppermint leaf (p.1208·1); solidago virgaurea; viola tricolor; valerian (p.1643·1); lupulus (p.1597·2).
Cardiac disorders.

Tisane pour le Foie Denolin, Belg.
Curcuma zanthorrhiza; fabianae imbricatae; boldo (p.1554·1); cynara scolymus (p.1569·2); kinkeliba (p.1593·2); senna (p.1212·2); peppermint leaf

(p.1208·1); melissa (p.1600·1); aniseed (p.1549·3); verbena; liquorice (p.1197·1); tilia (p.1637·3); calendula flower.
Biliary-tract congestion; digestive disorders.

Tisane pour le sommeil et les nerfs *Sidroga, Switz.*
Valerian (p.1643·1); lupulus (p.1597·2); spearmint (p.1632·1); melissa (p.1600·1); orange flower.
Nervousness; sleep disorders.

Tisane pour les enfants *Sidroga, Switz.*
Fennel (p.1579·1); matricaria (p.1561·2); tilia (p.1637·3); melissa (p.1600·1); peppermint leaf (p.1208·1); verbena.
Agitation; muscular contractures; sleep disorders.

Tisane pour les reins et la vessie *Sidroga, Switz.*
Bearberry (p.1552·2); birch (p.1553·3); boldo (p.1554·1); angelica; rose fruit (p.1365·2); lovage; tilia (p.1637·3); mallow flowers; orthosiphon (p.1592·2); peppermint leaf (p.1208·1); equisetum (p.1575·1); juniper (p.1592·2); juglans regia.
Urinary-tract disorders.

Tisane pour les reins et la vessie "H" *Hanseler, Switz.†.*
Centaurea cyanus; birch (p.1553·3); black currant (p.1365·2); bearberry (p.1552·2); phaseolus vulgaris; equisetum (p.1575·1); solidago virgaurea; tilia (p.1637·3); rose fruit (p.1365·2); liquorice (p.1197·1); ononis (p.1610·2); parsley (p.1615·3).
Urinary-tract disorders.

Tisane pour l'estomac *Sidroga, Switz.*
Calamus (p.1556·1); matricaria (p.1561·2); spearmint (p.1632·1); melissa (p.1600·1); achillea (p.1542·2); centaury (p.1561·1).
Gastro-intestinal disorders.

Tisane Purgative *Denolin, Belg.*
Senna (p.1212·2); frangula bark (p.1193·2); peppermint leaf (p.1208·1); althaea (p.1546·3); fennel (p.1579·1); aniseed (p.1549·3); calendula flower; mallow flower; angelica; liquorice (p.1197·1); melissa (p.1600·1).
Constipation; digestive disorders.

Tisane relaxante *Sidroga, Switz.*
Valerian (p.1643·1); achillea (p.1542·2); lavender flower (p.1594·3); melissa (p.1600·1); passion flower (p.1615·3).
Nervous tension.

Tisane sedative et somnifere "H" *Hanseler, Switz.†.*
Matricaria (p.1561·2); lavender flower (p.1594·3); tilia (p.1637·3); aurantii folium; peppermint leaf (p.1208·1); melissa (p.1600·1); thyme (p.1636·3); clove (p.1565·2); majorana origanum; achillea (p.1542·2); valerian (p.1643·1).
Nervousness; sleep disorders.

Tisane Sedative Weleda *Weleda, Fr.*
Lavender (p.1594·3); valerian (p.1643·1); mallow flowers.
Insomnia; nervous disorders.

Tisane Touraine *Pharmacie Principale, Fr.*
Ash; verbena; asperule; parietaria; meadowsweet (p.1599·1); fragaria vesca; peppermint (p.1208·1); melissa (p.1600·1); frangula (p.1193·2); cornflower; senna (p.1212·2).
Constipation.

Tisanes de l'Abbe Hamon no 3 *Aerocid, Fr.*
Frangula (p.1193·2); viola; lily of the valley (p.1567·2); equisetum (p.1575·1); ash; meadowsweet (p.1599·1); maize; cornflower; hazel.
Arthritis; gout; pain; sciatica.

Tisanes de l'Abbe Hamon no 6 *Aerocid, Fr.*
Asperule; oranger; passion flower (p.1615·3); waterlily; sage (p.1627·1); marigold; mistletoe (p.1604·1); tilia (p.1637·3); lyciet.
Nervous disorders.

Tisanes de l'Abbe Hamon no 11 *Aerocid, Fr.*
Fucus (p.1554·1); rumex crispus; couch-grass (p.1567·3); liquorice (p.1197·1); hazel.
Obesity.

Tisanes de l'Abbe Hamon no 14 *Aerocid, Fr.*
Groundsel; achillea (p.1542·2); viburnum; shepherds purse; oak (p.1609·3); cypress; verveine; asperule; liquorice (p.1197·1); hazel; marigold; cornflower; snake weed.
Circulatory disorders.

Tisanes de l'Abbe Hamon no 15 *Aerocid, Fr.*
Inula helenium (p.1059·2); comfrey (p.1567·1); erysimum; marrube (p.1063·3); borage; bugloss; eucalyptus (p.1578·1); hazel; sticta pulmonaria.
Respiratory-tract disorders.

Tisanes de l'Abbe Hamon no 16 *Aerocid, Fr.*
Burdock (p.1594·2); carrot; centaury (p.1561·1); thistle-roland; scoparium (p.1628·1); gratiola; convallaria (p.1567·2); hazel; liquorice (p.1197·1).
Liver disorders.

Tisanes de l'Abbe Hamon no 17 *Aerocid, Fr.*
Globulaire; frangula (p.1193·2); mint (p.1632·1); mercurial; hazel; rhapontic rhubarb (p.1212·1).
Constipation.

Tisanes de l'Abbe Hamon no 18 *Aerocid, Fr.†.*
Inula helenium (p.1059·2); myrtle; geranium robertianum; mint (p.1632·1); hazel; violet.
Gastro-intestinal disorders.

TI-Screen Sunless *Pedinol, USA.*
SPF 17; SPF 23: Ethylhexyl *p*-methoxycinnamate (p.1487·1); oxybenzone (p.1487·3).
Sunscreen.

Tisept *Seton, UK.*
Cetrimide (p.1105·2); chlorhexidine gluconate (p.1107·2).
Skin disinfection.

Tisercin *Thiemann, Ger.*
Methotrimeprazine (p.679·1) or methotrimeprazine maleate (p.679·1).
Pain; psychoses.

Tisit *Pfeiffer, USA.*
Pyrethrins; piperonyl butoxide (p.1409·3).
Pediculosis.

TiSol *Parnell, USA.*
Benzyl alcohol (p.1103·3); menthol (p.1600·2).
Minor mouth or throat irritation.

Tispol S *Woelm, Ger.*
Propyphenazone (p.81·3); paracetamol (p.72·2).
Toothache.

Tisseel
Immuno, Canad.†; Immuno, Irl.; Omnimed, S.Afr.; Immuno, UK.
1 Vial, fibrinogen (p.722·3); fibronectin (p.1580·1); factor XIII (p.722·2); plasminogen (p.932·1); 1 vial, aprotinin (p.711·3); 1 vial, calcium chloride (p.1155·1); 2 vials, thrombin (p.728·1);
On mixing this forms a fibrin glue (p.722·2).
Available on a named-patient basis only in the *UK.*
Wounds.

Tisseel Duo Quick *Baxter, Swed.*
1 vial, fibrinogen (p.722·3); fibronectin (p.1580·1); factor XIII (p.722·2); plasminogen (p.932·1); aprotinin (p.711·3); 1 vial, calcium chloride (p.1155·1) 1 vial, thrombin (p.728·1); plasma protein (p.726·3); calcium chloride (p.1155·1)
On mixing this forms a fibrin glue (p.722·2).
Haemorrhage.

Tissucol
Immuno, Aust.; Immuno, Belg.; Immuno, Ital.; Immuno, Spain; Immuno, Switz.
1 Vial, fibrinogen (p.722·3); fibronectin (p.1580·1); factor XIII (p.722·2); plasminogen (p.932·1); 1 vial, aprotinin (p.711·3); 2 vials, thrombin (p.728·1); 1 vial, calcium chloride (p.1155·1);
On mixing this forms a fibrin glue (p.722·2).
Haemorrhage; wounds.

Tissucol Duo Quick *Immuno, Aust.*
1 vial, fibrinogen (p.722·3); fibronectin (p.1580·1); factor XIII (p.722·2); plasminogen (p.932·1); aprotinin (p.711·3); 1 vial, bovine thrombin (p.728·1); calcium chloride dihydrate (p.1155·1)
On mixing this forms a fibrin glue (p.722·2).
Wounds.

Tissucol Duo S *Immuno, Ger.*
Combination pack: 1 ampoule: plasma protein fraction (p.726·3); fibrinogen (p.722·3); fibronectin (p.1580·1); factor XIII (p.722·2); plasminogen (p.932·1); aprotinin (p.711·3); 1 ampoule: thrombin (p.728·1); calcium chloride (p.1155·1)
On mixing this forms a fibrin glue (p.722·2).
Wounds.

Tissucol Fibrinkleber tiefgefroren *Immuno, Ger.*
Combination pack: 1 ampoule: plasma protein fraction (p.726·3); fibrinogen (p.722·3); fibronectin (p.1580·1); factor XIII (p.722·2); plasminogen (p.932·1); 1 application set: aprotinin (p.711·3); calcium chloride (p.1155·1); lotion: calcium chloride; thrombin (p.728·1)
On mixing this forms a fibrin glue (p.722·2).
Wounds.

Tissucol-Kit *Immuno, Ger.*
Combination pack: 1 ampoule: plasma protein fraction (p.726·3); fibrinogen (p.722·3); fibronectin (p.1580·1); factor XIII (p.722·2); plasminogen (p.932·1); 1 ampoule: aprotinin (p.711·3); 2 ampoules: thrombin (p.728·1); 1 ampoule: calcium chloride (p.1155·1)
On mixing this forms a fibrin glue (p.722·2).
Wounds.

tissula-N *Hefa, Ger.†.*
Glucose monohydrate (p.1343·3); lecithin (p.1595·2).
Nasal irritation.

TissuVlies *Immuno, Ger.*
Collagen (p.1566·3).
Haemorrhage.

Tisuderma *Cinfa, Spain.*
Hydrocortisone acetate (p.1043·3); neomycin sulphate (p.229·2).
Skin infections with inflammation.

Tis-U-Sol *Baxter, USA.*
Electrolytes (p.1147·1).
Irrigation solution.

Titan
Note. This name is used for preparations of different composition.
Barnes-Hind, Austral.†; Pilkington Barnes-Hind, USA.
Cleansing solution for hard contact lenses.

Schmid, Canad.
Nonoxinol 9 (p.1326·1).
Contraceptive.

Titanoreine
Brunet, Fr.; Martin, Switz.
Ointment: Carrageenan (p.1471·3); titanium dioxide (p.1093·3); zinc oxide (p.1096·2); lignocaine (p.1293·2).
Anorectal disorders.

Brunet, Fr.; Martin, Switz.
Suppositories: Carrageenan (p.1471·3); titanium dioxide (p.1093·3); zinc oxide (p.1096·2).
Anorectal disorders.

Tition *Pharmazam, Spain.*
Reduced glutathione (p.983·1).
Hepatitis.

Titmus Losung 1 *Ciba Vision, Aust.*
Hydrogen peroxide (p.1116·2).
Disinfection and storage of contact lenses.

Titmus Losung 2 *Ciba Vision, Aust.*
Catalase (p.1560·3).
Neutralisation and rinsing of contact lenses.

Titralac
3M, Austral.; 3M, Canad.; Nycomed, Norw.; 3M, S.Afr.; 3M, UK.
Calcium carbonate (p.1182·1); glycine.
Calcium supplement; gastric hyperacidity; hyperphosphataemia.

Titralac Extra Strength *3M, USA.*
Calcium carbonate (p.1182·1).
Hyperacidity.

Titralac Plus *3M, USA.*
Calcium carbonate (p.1182·1); simethicone (p.1213·1).
Hyperacidity.

Titralgan *Berlin-Chemie, Ger.†.*
Phenazone (p.78·2); paracetamol (p.72·2); caffeine (p.749·3).
Pain.

Titrane *CEPA, Spain.*
Isosorbide mononitrate (p.893·3).
Angina pectoris; heart failure.

Ti-Tre *Teofarma, Ital.*
Liothyronine sodium (p.1495·1).
Hypothyroidism.

Titretta *Berlin-Chemie, Ger.*
Propyphenazone (p.81·3); codeine phosphate (p.26·1).
Pain.

Titretta analgica *Berlin-Chemie, Ger.†.*
Propyphenazone (p.81·3); codeine phosphate (p.26·1); caffeine (p.749·3).
Pain.

Titretta analgica B *Berlin-Chemie, Ger.†.*
Propyphenazone (p.81·3); codeine phosphate (p.26·1); atropine sulphate (p.455·1).
Pain; painful smooth muscle spasm.

Ti-U-Lac *Draxis, Canad.*
Urea (p.1095·2).

Ti-U-Lac HC *Draxis, Canad.*
Hydrocortisone (p.1043·3); urea (p.1095·2).
Skin disorders.

Tiurasin *Bouty, Ital.†.*
Oxolinic acid (p.235·1).
Gram-negative bacterial infections of the urinary tract.

Tiutol KF *Braun, Ital.†.*
Sodium hypochlorite (p.1124·3).
Disinfection of dialysis equipment.

Ti-UVA-B *Draxis, Canad.*
SPF 22: Ethylhexyl *p*-methoxycinnamate (p.1487·1); oxybenzone (p.1487·3).
Sunscreen.

Tivitis *Llorens, Spain.*
Gramicidin (p.215·2); methylene blue (p.984·3); neomycin sulphate (p.229·2); polymyxin B sulphate (p.239·1); tetrahydrozoline hydrochloride (p.1070·2).
Eye infections.

Tixair *Asta Medica, Fr.*
Acetylcysteine (p.1052·3).
Mucolytic in respiratory-tract disorders.

Tixobar *Astra, Austral.*
Barium sulphate (p.1003·1).
Radiography of gastro-intestinal tract.

Tixylix
Note. This name is used for preparations of different composition.
Rhone-Poulenc Rorer, Austral.; Rhone-Poulenc Rorer, S.Afr.
Promethazine hydrochloride (p.416·2); pholcodine (p.1068·1).
Formerly contained promethazine hydrochloride, pholcodine, and phenylpropanolamine hydrochloride.
Coughs.

Intercare, Irl.
Promethazine hydrochloride (p.416·2); pholcodine citrate (p.1068·1); phenylpropanolamine hydrochloride (p.1067·2).
Coughs.

Tixylix Catarrh *Intercare, UK.*
Diphenhydramine (p.409·1); menthol (p.1600·2).
Nasal congestion.

Tixylix Chest Rub *Rhone-Poulenc Rorer, Austral.*
Cineole (p.1564·1); terpineol (p.1635·1); pine oil; rosemary oil (p.1626·2); thyme oil (p.1637·1).
Nasal congestion.

Tixylix Chesty Cough *Intercare, UK.*
Guaiphenesin (p.1061·3).

Tixylix Cough & Cold *Intercare, UK.*
Pseudoephedrine hydrochloride (p.1068·3); chlorpheniramine maleate (p.405·1); pholcodine (p.1068·1).
Coughs.

Tixylix Daytime
Note. This name is used for preparations of different composition.
Rhone-Poulenc Rorer, Austral.
Pseudoephedrine hydrochloride (p.1068·3).
Upper respiratory-tract congestion.

Intercare, UK.
Pholcodine (p.1068·1).
Coughs.

Tixylix Inhalant *Intercare, UK.*
Camphor (p.1557·2); menthol (p.1600·2); turpentine oil (p.1641·1); eucalyptus oil (p.1578·1).
Nasal congestion.

Tixylix Night-Time *Intercare, UK.*
Promethazine hydrochloride (p.416·2); pholcodine (p.1068·1).
Formerly known as Tixylix Original.
Coughs.

Tixymol *Novartis Consumer, UK.*
Paracetamol (p.72·2).
Fever; pain.

T-KI *Seroyal, Canad.*
Vitamin A and vitamin C.

T-Koff *Williams, USA.*
Phenylpropanolamine hydrochloride (p.1067·2); phenylephrine hydrochloride (p.1066·2); chlorpheniramine maleate (p.405·1); codeine phosphate (p.26·1).
Coughs and cold symptoms.

T-LI *Seroyal, Canad.*
Vitamin B substances, vitamin C, copper, and iron.

TLM *Seroyal, Canad.*
Vitamin C and minerals.

T-LU *Seroyal, Canad.*
Vitamins A, C, and E.

T-MA *Seroyal, Canad.*
Vitamin A, vitamin E, and zinc.

T-Medevax *Ribosepharm, Ger.*
An adsorbed tetanus vaccine (p.1535·3).
Active immunisation.

TMP-ratiopharm *Ratiopharm, Ger.*
Trimethoprim (p.265·1).
Bacterial infections of the urinary tract.

TMS
TAD, Ger.; TAD, Switz.†.
Co-trimoxazole (p.196·3).
Bacterial infections.

Tobanum *Gedeon Richter, Hung.*
Cloranolol hydrochloride (p.844·3).
Cardiovascular disorders.

Tobi *Pathogenesis, USA.*
Tobramycin (p.264·1).
Pseudomonal infections in cystic fibrosis.

Tobispray *Boehringer Ingelheim, Austral.†.*
Tramazoline hydrochloride (p.1071·1); dexamethasone isonicotinate (p.1037·1).
Allergic rhinitis.

Tobra Gobens *Normon, Spain.*
Tobramycin sulphate (p.264·1).
Bacterial infections.

Tobra Laf *Palex, Spain†.*
Tobramycin sulphate (p.264·1).
Bacterial infections.

Tobra-cell *Cell Pharm, Ger.*
Tobramycin sulphate (p.264·1).
Bacterial infections.

Tobradex
Alcon, Belg.; Alcon, Canad.; Alcon, Ital.; Alcon, Neth.†; Alcon, S.Afr.; Alcon, Switz.; Alcon, USA.
Tobramycin (p.264·1); dexamethasone (p.1037·1).
Infected eye disorders.

Tobradistin *Dista, Spain.*
Tobramycin sulphate (p.264·1).
Bacterial infections.

Tobral *Alcon, Ital.*
Tobramycin (p.264·1).
Bacterial infections of the eye and external ear.

Tobralex
Alcon, Irl.; Alcon, UK†.
Tobramycin (p.264·1).
Bacterial eye infections.

Tobramaxin *Alcon-Thilo, Ger.*
Tobramycin (p.264·1).
Bacterial eye infections.

Tobrasix *Lilly, Aust.*
Tobramycin sulphate (p.264·1).
Bacterial infections.

Tobrasol *Ocusoft, USA.*
Tobramycin (p.264·1).
Bacterial eye infections.

Tobrex
Alcon, Aust.; Alcon, Austral.; Alcon, Belg.; Alcon, Canad.; Alcon, Fr.; FIRMA, Ital.; Alcon, Neth.†; Alcon, S.Afr.; Alcon, Spain; Alcon, Switz.; Alcon, USA.
Tobramycin (p.264·1) or tobramycin sulphate (p.264·1).
Bacterial infections.

Tocalfa
Note. This name is used for preparations of different composition.
Cipharm, Fr.
dl-Alpha tocopheryl acetate (p.1369·2).
Vitamin E deficiency.

Asta Medica, Ital.
dl-Alpha tocopheryl acetate (p.1369·2); retinol esters (p.1358·1).
Vitamin A and E deficiency.

Tocanol *Lyssia, Belg.†.*
Vitamin A (p.1358·1); vitamin E (p.1369·1).
Vitamin deficiencies.

Tocatherol *Triosol, Belg.†.*
Vitamin E (p.1369·1); vitamin A (p.1358·1).
Vitamin A and E deficiencies.

Toclase
UCB, Norw.; UCB, Swed.
Pentoxyverine citrate (p.1066·1) or pentoxyverine hydrochloride (p.1066·2).
Coughs.

Toco *Pharma 2000, Fr.*
Alpha tocopheryl acetate (p.1369·1).
Hyperlipidaemia.

Tocodrine *Medichemie, Switz.*
Buphenine hydrochloride (p.1555·3).
Inhibition of uterine contraction.

Tocoferina E *Lisapharma, Ital.†.*
d-Alpha tocopheryl acetate (p.1369·2).

Tocoferolo Bioglan Neopharmed, Ital.†.
d-Alpha tocopheryl acetate (p.1369·2).
Cardiac disorders; diabetes mellitus; muscular atrophy; peripheral vascular disorders; sterility.

Tocogen Gentili, Ital.†.
d-Alpha tocopheryl acetate (p.1369·2).
Cardiac stenosis; diabetes mellitus; disorders of the female reproductive system; muscular dystrophy; peripheral vascular disorders.

Tocogestan Theramex, Mon.
Hydroxyprogesterone enanthate (p.1448·1); progesterone (p.1459·3); *dl*-alpha tocopheryl palmitate (p.1370·1).
Premature labour; threatened abortion.

Tocolysan Byk Gulden, Ital.†.
Hexoprenaline sulphate (p.754·1).
Premature labour.

Tocomine Eurorga, Fr.
dl-Alpha tocopheryl acetate (p.1369·2).
Vitamin E deficiency.

Tocorell Sanorell, Ger.
d-Alpha tocopherol (p.1369·1).
Vitamin E deficiency.

Tocovenos Fresenius, Ger.
dl-Alpha tocopheryl acetate (p.1369·2).
Vitamin E deficiency.

Tocovital Steigerwald, Ger.
d-Alpha tocopheryl acetate (p.1369·2).
Vitamin E deficiency.

Todalgil Aldo, Spain.
Ibuprofen (p.44·1).
Fever; musculoskeletal, joint, and peri-articular disorders; pain.

Today
Wyeth-Ayerst, Canad.†; Wyeth, UK; Whitehall, USA.
Nonoxinol 9 (p.1326·1).
Contraceptive.

Tododermil Compuesto Organon, Spain.
Dexpanthenol (p.1570·3); erythromycin estolate (p.204·1); nystatin (p.386·1); triamcinolone acetonide (p.1050·2).
Infected skin disorders.

Tododermil Simple Organon, Spain†.
Dexpanthenol (p.1570·3); triamcinolone acetonide (p.1050·2).
Skin disorders.

Toepedo DDD, UK.
Benzoic acid (p.1102·3); salicylic acid (p.1090·2).
Fungal skin infections.

Toesen Ferring, Canad.†.
Oxytocin (p.1257·2).
Induction and stimulation of labour; postpartum haemorrhage.

Tofranil
Ciba-Geigy, Aust.; Novartis, Austral.; Ciba-Geigy, Belg.; Geigy, Canad.; Ciba-Geigy, Fr.; Geigy, Ger.; Geigy, Irl.; Ciba, Ital.; Novartis, Neth.; Geigy, Norw.; Novartis, S.Afr.; Ciba-Geigy, Spain; Novartis, Swed.; Geigy, Switz.; Novartis, UK; Geigy, USA.
Imipramine (p.289·2), imipramine embonate (p.289·2), or imipramine hydrochloride (p.289·2).
Depression; nocturnal enuresis; pain; panic attacks..

Tofranil-PM Geigy, USA.
Imipramine embonate (p.289·2).
Depression.

Togal
Note. This name is used for preparations of different composition.
Schoeller, Aust.; Togal, Ger.
Tablets: Aspirin (p.16·1); lithium citrate (p.290·3); quinine dihydrochloride (p.439·1).
Fever; inflammation; pain.

Togal, Ger.
Suppositories: Paracetamol (p.72·2).
Fever; pain.

Togal ASS
Togal, Ger.; Togal, Switz.
Aspirin (p.16·1).
Fever; inflammation; pain; thrombo-embolic disorders.

Togal ASS + C Togal, Switz.†.
Aspirin (p.16·1); ascorbic acid (p.1365·2); caffeine (p.749·3).
Fever; pain.

Togal Kopfschmerzbrause + Vit C Togal, Ger.
Aspirin (p.16·1); ascorbic acid (p.1365·2); caffeine (p.749·3).
Pain.

Togal N Togal, Ger.
Ibuprofen (p.44·1).
Fever; pain.

Togasan Togal, Ger.
dl-Alpha tocopheryl acetate (p.1369·2).
Vitamin E deficiency.

Togiren Lilly, Ger.†.
Erythromycin estolate (p.204·1).
Bacterial infections.

Togram Llorente, Spain†.
Ampicillin sodium (p.153·1).
Bacterial infections.

Toilax
Orion, Irl.; Ercopharm, Neth.†; Erco, Norw.; Orion, Swed.
Bisacodyl (p.1179·3).
Bowel evacuation; constipation.

Tokolysan Byk Gulden, Ger.†.
Hexoprenaline sulphate (p.754·1).
Prevention of labour.

Tolanase
Pharmacia Upjohn, Irl.; Upjohn, UK.
Tolazamide (p.333·2).
Diabetes mellitus.

Tolbet Corvi, Ital.†.
Bitolterol mesylate (p.749·2).
Asthma.

Tolectin
Janssen-Cilag, Aust.; Janssen-Cilag, Belg.; Janssen-Ortho, Canad.; Janssen-Cilag, Ger.†; Janssen-Cilag, Irl.; Janssen-Cilag, Ital.; Janssen-Cilag, Neth.; Janssen-Cilag, S.Afr.; Janssen-Cilag, Switz.; Janssen-Cilag, UK†; McNeil Pharmaceutical, USA.
Tolmetin (p.90·1) or tolmetin sodium (p.89·3).
Musculoskeletal, joint, peri-articular, and soft-tissue disorders.

Tolerabiotico Iquinosa, Spain†.
Erythromycin stearate (p.204·2).
Bacterial infections.

Tolerex
Sandoz Nutrition, Canad.; Procter & Gamble, USA.
Preparation for enteral nutrition.

Tolerzide Bristol-Myers Squibb, UK†.
Sotalol hydrochloride (p.945·1); hydrochlorothiazide (p.885·2).
Hypertension.

Tolexine Biorga, Fr.
Doxycycline (p.202·3).
Bacterial infections.

Tolfrinic Ascher, USA.
Ferrous fumarate (p.1339·3); cyanocobalamin (p.1363·3).
Vitamin C (p.1365·2) is included in this preparation to increase the absorption and availability of iron.
Iron-deficiency anaemias.

Tolid Dolorgiet, Ger.
Lorazepam (p.675·3).
Anxiety; sleep disorders.

Toliman Farmochimica, Ital.
Cinnarizine (p.406·1).
Cerebral and peripheral vascular disorders.

Tolinase
Upjohn, Belg.†; Upjohn, Neth.†; Pharmacia Upjohn, Swed.; Upjohn, USA.
Tolazamide (p.333·2).
Diabetes mellitus.

Tolindol Meuse, Belg.
Proglumetacin (p.81·2).
Musculoskeletal, joint, and peri-articular disorders.

Tollwutglobulin Pasteur Merieux, Ger.
A rabies immunoglobulin (p.1530·2).
Passive immunisation.

Tollwut-Impfstoff (HDC) Pasteur Merieux, Ger.
A rabies vaccine (human diploid cell) (p.1530·3).
Active immunisation.

Tolmicen Pharmacia Upjohn, Ital.
Tolciclate (p.388·3).
Fungal skin infections.

Tolodina Estedi, Spain.
Amoxycillin trihydrate (p.151·3).
Bacterial infections.

Tolopelon Daiichi, Jpn†.
Timiperone (p.696·2).

Tol-Tab Alra, USA.
Tolbutamide (p.333·2).

Toluidinblau Kohler, Ger.
Tolonium chloride (p.1638·2).
Methaemoglobinaemia.

Tolu-Sed DM Scherer, USA.
Dextromethorphan hydrobromide (p.1057·3); guaiphenesin (p.1061·3).
Coughs.

Tolvin Organon, Ger.
Mianserin hydrochloride (p.297·1).
Depression.

Tolvon
Organon, Aust.; Organon, Austral.; Organon, Irl.; Nourypharma, Neth.; Organon, Norw.; Organon, Swed.; Organon, Switz.
Mianserin hydrochloride (p.297·1).
Depression.

Tolyprin Du Pont, Ger.
Azapropazone (p.20·3).
Acute gout; inflammation; pain; rheumatism; soft-tissue disorders.

Tolzer, Jodquell-Dragees Jodquellen, Ger.†.
Sodium bromide; sodium iodide (p.1493·2); sodium chloride; magnesium carbonate; calcium carbonate; calcium; potassium bicarbonate; sodium; bicarbonate.
Iodine-deficiency disorders.

TOM Meyer, Fr.†.
Oestradiol benzoate (p.1455·1); tyrothricin (p.267·2).
Acne; oestrogen deficiency disorders with infection.

Tomabef Salus, Ital.
Cefoperazone sodium (p.167·3).
Lignocaine hydrochloride (p.1293·2) is included in this preparation to alleviate the pain of injection.
Bacterial infections.

Tomasl Croce Bianca, Ital.†.
Lysine aspirin (p.50·3).
Arthropathy; myalgia; pain; rheumatism.

Tomcor Croce Bianca, Ital.†.
Suprarenal cortex (p.1050·1).
Endotoxic shock; suprarenal cortex insufficiency; surgical stress; tonic.

Tomevit Spyfarma, Spain.
Adenosine triphosphate; arginine aspartate; glutathione; hydroxocobalamin; lysine hydrochloride; pyritinol hydrochloride.
Tonic.

Tomocat Lafayette, USA.
Barium sulphate (p.1003·1).
Contrast medium for gastro-intestinal radiography.

Tomudex
ICI, Austral.; Zeneca, Fr.; Zeneca, Irl.; Zeneca, Ital.; Zeneca, Neth.; Zeneca, UK.
Raltitrexed (p.560·1).
Colorectal cancer.

Ton Was Wasserman, Spain.
Vitamin B substances; ginseng (p.1584·2).
Tonic.

Tonactil Arkopharma, Fr.
Kola (p.1645·1); ginseng (p.1584·2).
Asthenia.

Tonactiv Herbaline, Ital.
Angelica; fennel (p.1579·1); laurus nobilis; aniseed (p.1549·3).
Depression; hypotension; tonic.

Tonamil Ecobi, Ital.
Thonzylamine (p.419·2).
Conjunctivitis; rhinitis; skin irritation.

Tonamyl Bolder, Ger.†.
Meprobamate (p.678·1); reserpine (p.942·1); kola (p.1645·1); faex med.
Psychiatric disorders; sleep disorders.

Tonaton N Luitpold, Ger.†.
Yohimbe; atropine methonitrate (p.455·1); ephedrine hydrochloride (p.1059·3).
Atonic bladder; impotence; prostatitis.

Tondinel H Pflüger, Ger.
Homoeopathic preparation.

Tonerg Angelini, Ital.
Pivagabine (p.306·3).
Depression.

Toness Angelini, Ital.
Proxazole citrate (p.1622·2).
Smooth muscle relaxant; vascular disorders.

Tonex Boehringer Ingelheim, Switz.
Amethocaine hydrochloride (p.1285·2); chamomile (p.1561·2); sage (p.1627·1); aluminium formate; mint oil (p.1604·1); menthol (p.1600·2).
Minor skin lesions; mouth disorders.

Tonexis
Clintec, Fr.; Clintec, Irl.; Clintec, Ital.; Nestle, UK.
A range of preparations for enteral nutrition.

Tonexis HP Clintec, Fr.
High-protein nutritional supplement.

Tonexol
Note. This name is used for preparations of different composition.
Krug, Aust.; Pharmaton, Switz.†.
Topical spray: Amethocaine hydrochloride (p.1285·2); ethacridine lactate (p.1098·3).
Mouth disorders.

Pharmaton, Switz.†.
Topical solution: Amethocaine hydrochloride (p.1285·2); ethacridine lactate (p.1098·3); phenol (p.1121·2).
Mouth disorders.

Tongill Sandoz, Aust.
Tyrothricin (p.267·2); muramidase hydrochloride (p.1604·3); lignocaine hydrochloride (p.1293·2).
Mouth and throat disorders.

Tonibral Adulte Bouchara, Fr.
Deanol hemisuccinate (p.1478·2).
Tonic.

Tonicalcium
Therabel Pharma, Belg.; Bouchara, Fr.
DL-Lysine ascorbate; calcium ascorbate (p.1365·2).
Vitamin C deficiency.

Tonico Juventus Juventus, Spain.
Cyproheptadine hydrochloride (p.407·2); cobamamide (p.1364·2).
Tonic.

Tonicol & ADC Multi-Pro, Canad.
Multivitamin and iron preparation.

Tonicum
Petrasch, Aust.
Vitamins; caffeine; lactic acid.
Tonic.

SIT, Ital.
Amino-acid and vitamin preparation.

Tonimol Herbes Universelles, Canad.
Multivitamin preparation.

Tonipan Alpharma, Norw.
Vitamin B substances with manganese.
Vitamin B deficiency.

Tonique D Demopharm, Switz.
Multivitamin and minerals with plant extracts.
Tonic.

Tonique Vegetal Lehning, Fr.
Homoeopathic preparation.

Tonique-B_{12} Roche, Switz.†.
Kola; cyanocobalamin; manganese; anhydrous disodium phosphate; liver extract.
Tonic.

Tonisan Dolisos, Fr.
Ginseng (p.1584·2); black tea (p.1645·1).
Tonic.

Tonitan Christiaens, Belg.†.
Lysine hydrochloride; nicotinamide; pyridoxine hydrochloride; sodium glycerophosphate; strychnine nitrate.
Tonic.

Tonizin Betapharm, Ger.
Hypericum (p.1590·1).
Anxiety; nervous disorders.

Ton-O_2 (Tonozwei) Voigt, Ger.†.
Heptaminol hydrochloride (p.1587·2); amphetaminil (p.1477·3); adenosine (p.812·3).
Hypotension.

Tonocalcin Searle, Ital.
Salcatonin (p.735·3).
Hypercalcaemia; osteoporosis; Paget's disease of bone; reflex sympathetic dystrophy.

Tonocaltin Zambon, Spain.
Salcatonin (p.735·3).
Hypercalcaemia; metastatic bone pain; Paget's disease of bone; postmenopausal osteoporosis.

Tonocard
Astra, Belg.†; Astra, Canad.; Astra, Irl.; Astra, Neth.; Hassle, Swed.; Astra, UK†; Astra Merck, USA.
Tocainide hydrochloride (p.955·1).
Ventricular arrhythmias.

Tonofolin Zyma, Ital.
Calcium folinate (p.1342·2).
Megaloblastic anaemias.

Tonoftal Essex, Ger.
Tolnaftate (p.389·1).
Fungal skin infections.

Tonogen ABC, Ital.
Haematoporphyrin hydrochloride (p.1587·1); cyanocobalamin (p.1363·3).
Tonic.

Tonoglutal Roche, Switz.
Glutamic acid; sodium hydroxybenzylphosphinate; ascorbic acid; magnesium glycerophosphate; thiamine nitrate.
Tonic.

Tonoliver 10000 ABC, Ital.†.
Nicotinamide (p.1351·2); riboflavine sodium phosphate (p.1362·1); thiamine hydrochloride (p.1361·1); cyanocobalamin (p.1363·3); calcium folinate (p.1342·2).
Anaemias; liver disorders; toxicosis; vitamin deficiency.

Tonoliver Ferro ABC, Ital.†.
Ferritin (p.1580·1); cyanocobalamin (p.1363·3); calcium folinate (p.1342·2).
Anaemias.

Tonopan
Sandoz, Aust.; Sandoz, Spain; Sandoz OTC, Switz.
Caffeine (p.749·3); dihydroergotamine mesylate (p.444·2); propyphenazone (p.81·3).
Migraine and other vascular headaches.

Tonopaque Lafayette, USA.
Barium sulphate (p.1003·1).
Contrast medium for gastro-intestinal radiography.

Tonoplantin Mono Palmicol, Ger.
Crataegus (p.1568·2).
Heart failure.

Tonoplus ABC, Ital.
Arginine oxoglurate (p.1334·2); aceglutamide (p.1541·2).
Tonic.

Tonopres Boehringer Ingelheim, Ger.
Dihydroergotamine mesylate (p.444·2).
Hypotension; migraine and other vascular headaches.

Tonoprotect Brenner-Efeka, Ger.
Atenolol (p.825·3).
Angina pectoris; arrhythmias; hypertension.

Tonovit Godecke, Ger.†.
Norfenefrine hydrochloride (p.925·1); vitamin A; thiamine nitrate; riboflavine; ascorbic acid; nicotinamide.
Hypotension.

Tonozime UTP Zyma, Spain†.
Capsules: Hydroxocobalamin acetate (p.1364·2); pyridoxine hydrochloride (p.1362·3); prosultiamine (p.1360·3); trisodium uridine triphosphate.
Oral powder: Cocarboxylase (p.1361·2); hydroxocobalamin acetate (p.1364·2); pyridoxine hydrochloride (p.1362·3); trisodium uridine triphosphate.
Muscular and neuromuscular disorders; polyneuritis.

Tonsilase Pejo, Ger.†.
Papain (p.1614·1); bacitracin (p.157·3); muramidase hydrochloride (p.1604·3); cetylpyridinium chloride (p.1106·2).
Upper respiratory tract infection and inflammation.

Tonsilase dolo Medice, Ger.
Benzocaine (p.1286·2); cetylpyridinium chloride (p.1106·2).
Mouth and throat disorders.

Tonsilgon-N Bionorica, Ger.
Althaea (p.1546·3); chamomile (p.1561·2); equisetum (p.1575·1); juglans regia; achillea (p.1542·2); oak bark (p.1609·3); taraxacum (p.1634·2).
Respiratory-tract infections.

Tonsillitis PMD Plantamed, Ger.
Homoeopathic preparation.

Tonsillol Merckle, Aust.
Dequalinium chloride (p.1112·1).
Mouth and throat infections.

Tonsillopas Pascoe, Ger.
Homoeopathic preparation.

Tonsillosan Spitzner, Ger.†.
Lactic acid (p.1593·3).
Oropharyngitis.

Tonsillosyx Syxyl, Ger.
Homoeopathic preparation.

Tonsiotren H DHU, Ger.
Homoeopathic preparation.

Tonum Funk, Spain.
Ketorolac trometamol (p.49·1).
Pain.

Tonus-forte-Tablinen Sanorania, Ger.
Etilefrine hydrochloride (p.867·2).
Hypotension.

Tonuvital Delalande, Fr.†.
Deanol bitartrate (p.1478·2); ribonucleic acid (p.1624·3).
Tonic.

Toose Juventus, Spain.
Co-trimoxazole (p.196·3).
Bacterial infections.

Toothache Gel Roberts, USA.
Benzocaine (p.1286·2); clove oil (p.1565·2).
Toothache.

3 in 1 Toothache Relief Dent, USA.
Benzocaine (p.1286·2).

Top Calcium Esseti, Ital.
Calcium carbonate (p.1182·1).
Calcium depletion; calcium supplement.

Top dent fluor Pharmalink, Swed.
Sodium fluoride (p.742·1).
Dental caries prophylaxis.

Top Fit-C Merck, Spain†.
Ascorbic acid (p.1365·2).
Adjunct in treatment of iron supplementation; vitamin C deficiency.

Top Mag Genevrier, Fr.
Magnesium pidolate (p.1157·3).
Magnesium deficiency.

Top Marks Lifeplan, UK.
Multinutrient preparation.

Topaal Sinbio, Fr.
Alginic acid (p.1470·3); colloidal aluminium hydroxide (p.1177·3); magnesium carbonate (p.1198·1); silicon dioxide (p.1474·3).
Gastro-oesophageal reflux.

Topal Novex Pharma, UK.
Aluminium hydroxide (p.1177·3); light magnesium carbonate (p.1198·1); alginic acid (p.1470·3).
Gastro-intestinal hyperacidity.

Topalgic Houde, Fr.
Tramadol hydrochloride (p.90·1).
Pain.

Topamax
Janssen-Cilag, Austral.; Janssen-Cilag, Irl.; Janssen-Cilag, S.Afr.; Janssen-Cilag, Switz.; Janssen-Cilag, UK; Ortho McNeil, USA.
Topiramate (p.360·2).
Epilepsy.

Topasel Europharma, Spain.
Algestone acetophenide (p.1439·1); oestradiol enanthate (p.1455·2).
Combined injectable contraceptive.

Topex Procter & Gamble, Austral.†.
Benzoyl peroxide (p.1079·2).
Acne.

Topfena GNR, Fr.
Ketoprofen (p.48·2).
Formerly known as Topfen.
Musculoskeletal, joint, peri-articular, and soft-tissue disorders.

"Topfer" Kinderbad mit Teer Topfer, Ger.†.
Wheat bran (p.1181·2); whey; coal tar sodium sulphonate; pine oil; rosemary oil (p.1626·2); sage oil; lavender oil (p.1594·3); matricaria oil.
Bath additive; skin disorders.

"Topfer" Teerkleiebad Topfer, Ger.†.
Wheat bran (p.1181·2); whey; coal tar sodium sulphonate; pine oil; rosemary oil (p.1626·2); sage oil; lavender oil (p.1594·3); matricaria oil.
Bath additive; skin disorders.

Topic Syntex, USA.
Benzyl alcohol (p.1103·3); camphor (p.1557·2); menthol (p.1600·2).
Pruritus.

Topicaina Organon, Spain.
Benzalkonium chloride (p.1101·3); butacaine sulphate (p.1288·3); butyl aminobenzoate (p.1289·1); cetrimide; (p.1106·1); benzocaine (p.1286·2) amethocaine hydrochloride (p.1285·2).
Local anaesthesia.

Topicaina Miro Andalucia, Spain†.
Benzalkonium chloride (p.1101·3); butacaine sulphate (p.1288·3); butyl aminobenzoate hydrochloride; cetalkonium bromide (p.1105·2); benzocaine (p.1286·2); amethocaine hydrochloride (p.1285·2).
Local anaesthesia.

Topicaine
Colgate Oral Care, Austral.; Hoechst Marion Roussel, Canad.
Benzocaine (p.1286·2).
Local anaesthesia.

Topicaldermo Derly, Spain†.
Thiomersal (p.1126·3).
Skin disinfection.

Topiclens Seton, UK†.
Sodium chloride (p.1162·2).
Irrigation solution.

Topico Denticion Vera Labitec, Spain.
Sodium bromide (p.1620·3); borax (p.1554·2); ethylene glycol (p.1577·3); musk; anemone pulsatilla; menthol.
Toothache.

Topicort
Hoechst Marion Roussel, Canad.; Roussel, Ital.†; Hoechst Marion Roussel, USA.
Desoxymethasone (p.1037·1).
Skin disorders.

Topicort Composto Roussel, Ital.†.
Desoxymethasone (p.1037·1); framycetin sulphate (p.210·3).
Skin disorders.

Topicorte
Hoechst Marion Roussel, Belg.; Roussel, Fr.; Hoechst Marion Roussel, Neth.
Desoxymethasone (p.1037·1).
Skin disorders.

Topicrem Rhone-Poulenc Rorer, Spain.
Triethanolamine salicylate (p.1639·2).
Peri-articular and soft-tissue disorders.

Topicycline
Pannoc, Belg.†; Monmouth, Irl.; Monmouth, UK; Procter & Gamble, USA.
Tetracycline hydrochloride (p.259·1); epitetracycline hydrochloride (p.261·1).
Acne.

Topifluor Eurofarmaco, Ital.†.
Fluocinolone acetonide (p.1041·1).
Skin disorders.

Topifram Roussel, Fr.
Desoxymethasone (p.1037·1); framycetin sulphate (p.210·3); gramicidin (p.215·2).
Infected skin disorders.

Topifug Wolff, Ger.†.
Desonide (p.1036·3).
Skin disorders.

Topilar
Syntex, Austral.†; Syntex, Fr.†; Bioglan, UK†.
Fluclorolone acetonide (p.1040·1).
Skin disorders.

Topilene Technilab, Canad.
Betamethasone dipropionate (p.1033·3).
Skin disorders.

Topimax
Janssen-Cilag, Norw.; Janssen-Cilag, Swed.
Topiramate (p.360·2).
Epilepsy.

Topinasal Stern, Ger.†.
Budesonide (p.1034·3).
Allergic rhinitis; nasal polyps.

Topionic Diviser Aquilea, Spain.
Povidone-iodine (p.1123·3).
Instrument disinfection; mouth and throat infections; skin, burn, and wound disinfection.

Topionic Gin Rius, Spain†.
Povidone-iodine (p.1123·3).
Leucorrhoea; vulvovaginitis.

Topisalen Hoechst Marion Roussel, Switz.†.
Desoxymethasone (p.1037·1); salicylic acid (p.1090·2).
Skin disorders.

Topisolon
Note. This name is used for preparations of different composition.
Albert-Roussel, Aust.; Hoechst, Ger.; Hoechst Marion Roussel, Irl.; Hoechst Marion Roussel, S.Afr.†; Knoll, Switz.
Desoxymethasone (p.1037·1).
Burns; skin disorders.

Hoechst, Ger.
Topical solution: Desoxymethasone (p.1037·1); salicylic acid (p.1090·2).
Scalp disorders; skin disorders.

Topisolon mit Salicylsaure Albert-Roussel, Aust.
Desoxymethasone (p.1037·1); salicylic acid (p.1090·2).
Skin disorders.

Topisone Technilab, Canad.
Betamethasone dipropionate (p.1033·3).
Skin disorders.

Topisporin Pharmafair, USA†.
Neomycin sulphate (p.229·2); polymyxin B sulphate (p.239·1); bacitracin zinc (p.157·3).

Topivate Xeragen, S.Afr.
Betamethasone valerate (p.1033·3).
Skin disorders.

Toplexil
Note. This name is used for preparations of different composition.
Rhone-Poulenc Rorer, Belg.; Theraplix, Fr.
Oxomemazine (p.415·2); guaiphenesin (p.1061·3); sodium benzoate (p.1102·3); paracetamol (p.72·2).
Coughs.

Rhone-Poulenc Rorer, Neth.
Oxomemazine (p.415·2); sodium benzoate (p.1102·3).
Formerly contained oxomemazine, guaiphenesin, and sodium benzoate.
Coughs.

Rhone-Poulenc Rorer, Switz.
Oxomemazine (p.415·2); guaiphenesin (p.1061·3); sodium benzoate (p.1102·3).
Coughs.

Top-Nitro Schering-Plough, Ital.
Glyceryl trinitrate (p.874·3).
Angina pectoris.

Topoderm N Gepepharm, Ger.
Diphenylpyraline hydrochloride (p.409·3); hydrocortisone (p.1043·3); neomycin sulphate (p.229·2).
Haemorrhoids; infected skin disorders; skin disorders.

Topol Warner-Lambert, Canad.†.
Calcium hydrogen phosphate (p.1155·3).
Stained teeth.

Topol with Fluoride Warner-Lambert, Canad.†.
Silicon dioxide (p.1474·3); aluminium oxide (p.1077·2); sodium monofluorophosphate (p.743·3).
Prevention of tooth decay.

Topol Gel with Fluoride Warner-Lambert, Canad.†.
Sodium monofluorophosphate (p.743·3); silicon dioxide (p.1474·3).
Prevention of tooth decay.

Toposar Pharmacia, USA.
Etoposide (p.532·3).
Small-cell lung cancer; testicular cancer.

Topostasin
Roche, Ger.†; Roche, Ital.†.
Thrombin (p.728·1).
Haemorrhagic disorders.

Toprec Theraplix, Fr.
Ketoprofen (p.48·2).
Fever; pain.

Toprek
Rhone-Poulenc Rorer, Aust.; Rhone-Poulenc Rorer, Belg.; Rhone-Poulenc Rorer, Ital.
Ketoprofen (p.48·2).
Musculoskeletal, joint, and peri-articular disorders; pain.

Toprol XL Astra, USA.
Metoprolol succinate (p.908·2).
Angina pectoris; hypertension.

Topromel Clonmel, Irl.
Metoprolol tartrate (p.907·3).
Angina pectoris; arrhythmias; hyperthyroidism; migraine; myocardial infarction.

Topsiton Triomed, S.Afr.
Vitamins; anhydrous caffeine; calcium gluconate; calcium citrate.
Tonic.

Topsym
Grunenthal, Aust.; Grunenthal, Ger.; Grunenthal, Switz.
Fluocinonide (p.1041·2).
Skin disorders.

Topsym polyvalent
Note. This name is used for preparations of different composition.
Grunenthal, Aust.; Grunenthal, Switz.
Fluocinonide (p.1041·2); gramicidin (p.215·2); neomycin sulphate (p.229·2); nystatin (p.386·1).
Infected skin disorders.

Grunenthal, Ger.
Fluocinonide (p.1041·2); neomycin sulphate (p.229·2); nystatin (p.386·1).
Infected skin disorders.

Topsymin Grunenthal, Switz.
Fluocinonide (p.1041·2).
Skin disorders.

Topsymin F Grunenthal, Aust.
Fluocinonide (p.1041·2).
Skin disorders.

Topsyn
Syntex, Canad.†; Recordati, Ital.
Fluocinonide (p.1041·2).
Skin disorders.

Topsyn Neomicina Recordati, Ital.†.
Fluocinonide (p.1041·2); neomycin sulphate (p.229·2).
Skin disorders.

Topsyne
Cassenne, Fr.; Yamanouchi, Neth.
Fluocinonide (p.1041·2).
Skin disorders.

Topsyne Neomycine Cassenne, Fr.
Fluocinonide (p.1041·2); neomycin sulphate (p.229·2).
Infected skin disorders.

Toptabs Sussex, UK.
Aspirin (p.16·1); caffeine (p.749·3).

Toquilone compositum Medichemie, Switz.
Methaqualone (p.678·3); diphenhydramine hydrochloride (p.409·1).
Sleep disorders.

Toradiur Boehringer Mannheim, Ital.
Torasemide sodium (p.956·3).
Ascites; heart failure; oedema; renal failure.

Toradol
Syntex, Austral.; Roche, Canad.; Syntex, Fr.†; Recordati, Ital.; Roche, Norw.; Roche, S.Afr.; Syntex, Spain; Syntex, Swed.; Syntex, Switz.; Roche, UK; Syntex, USA.
Ketorolac (p.49·3) or ketorolac trometamol (p.49·1).
Pain.

Toramin N Athenstaedt, Ger.†.
Oxeladin citrate (p.1065·3); etofylline (p.753·1); guaiphenesin (p.1061·3).
Airways infection; bronchitis; coughs; pertussis.

Toraseptol Lesvi, Spain.
Azithromycin (p.155·2).
Bacterial infections.

Torax Farmades, Ital.†.
Dextromethorphan hydrobromide (p.1057·3).
Coughs.

Torbetol
Note. This name is used for preparations of different composition.
Torbet, Irl.
Cetrimide (p.1105·2); benzalkonium chloride (p.1101·3); hexachlorophane (p.1115·2).
Acne.

Torbet Laboratories, UK.
Cetrimide (p.1105·2); chlorhexidine gluconate (p.1107·2).
Formerly contained hexachlorophane.
Acne.

Torecan
Sandoz, Aust.; Sandoz, Austral.†; Sandoz, Canad.†; Sandoz, Ger.; Sandoz, Irl.†; LPB, Ital.; Sandoz, Neth.†; Sandoz, Norw.†; Sandoz, Spain; Novartis, Swed.; Sandoz, Switz.; Sandoz, UK†; Roxane, USA.
Thiethylperazine (p.419·2), thiethylperazine malate (p.419·2), or thiethylperazine maleate (p.419·2).
Nausea; vestibular disorders; vomiting.

Torem
Berlin-Chemie, Ger.; Boehringer Mannheim, Neth.†; Boehringer Mannheim, Swed.; Boehringer Mannheim, Switz.; Boehringer Mannheim, UK.
Torasemide (p.956·3) or torasemide sodium (p.956·3).
Heart failure; hypertension; oedema; renal failure.

Torental
Hoechst Marion Roussel, Belg.; Hoechst, Fr.
Oxpentifylline (p.925·3).
Mental function impairment in the elderly; vascular disorders.

Torfan Abbott, Ital.
Dextromethorphan hydrobromide (p.1057·3); guaiphenesin (p.1061·3); carbinoxamine maleate (p.404·2).
Coughs.

Torfanolo Francia, Ital.†.
Dextromethorphan hydrobromide (p.1057·3); potassium guaiacolsulfonate (p.1068·3); oxedrine tartrate (p.925·3).
Coughs.

Toriac Rhone-Poulenc Rorer, Belg.
Loperamide hydrochloride (p.1197·2).
Diarrhoea.

Toriol Vita, Spain.
Ranitidine hydrochloride (p.1209·3).
Acid aspiration; gastro-intestinal haemorrhage; gastro-oesophageal reflux; peptic ulcer; Zollinger-Ellison syndrome.

Torlanbulina Antitenani Torlan, Spain.
A tetanus immunoglobulin (p.1535·2).
Passive immunisation.

Torlasporin Torlan, Spain.
Cephalexin (p.178·2).
Bacterial infections.

Tornacin Merck, Spain†.
Bile (p.1553·2); bromelains (p.1555·1); dimethicone (p.1213·1); pancreatin (p.1612·1).
Digestive enzyme deficiency; dyspepsia; hyperchlorhydria; meteorism.

Tornalate Dura, USA.
Bitolterol mesylate (p.749·2).
Asthma; bronchospasm.

Tornix Steierl, Ger.
Crataegus (p.1568·2); valerian (p.1643·1); passion flower (p.1615·3); rutin (p.1580·2).
Cardiac disorders.

Torrat
Boehringer Mannheim, Aust.; Boehringer Mannheim, Ger.; Boehringer Mannheim, Switz.†.
Metipranolol (p.906·2); buthiazide (p.835·2).
Hypertension.

Torrem Boehringer Mannheim, Belg.
Torasemide (p.956·3).
Hypertension; oedema.

Torvast Pfizer, Ital.
Atorvastatin calcium (p.1268·1).
Hyperlipidaemias.

Toryxil Baer, Ger.
Diclofenac sodium (p.31·2).
Inflammation; rheumatism.

T-OS Seroyal, Canad.
Calcium, molybdenum, and phosphorus.

Tos Mai Alcala, Spain.
Dextromethorphan hydrobromide (p.1057·3); benzocaine (p.1286·2); guaiacol (p.1061·2); sodium benzoate (p.1102·3).
Respiratory-tract disorders.

Toscal Abbott, Spain.
Syrup: Ammonium chloride (p.1055·2); tolu balsam (p.1071·1); dextromethorphan hydrobromide (p.1057·3); ephedrine hydrochloride (p.1059·3); ipecacuanha (p.1062·2).
Tablets: Carbinoxamine maleate (p.404·2); dextromethorphan hydrobromide (p.1057·3).
Respiratory-tract disorders.

Toscal Compuesto Abbott, Spain.
Ammonium chloride (p.1055·2); tolu balsam (p.1071·1); carbinoxamine maleate (p.404·2); dextromethorphan hydrobromide (p.1057·3); ephedrine hydrochloride (p.1059·3); ipecacuanha (p.1062·2).
Upper respiratory-tract disorders.

Tosdetan Martin, Spain.
Citiolone (p.1564·3); co-trimoxazole (p.196·3).
Respiratory-tract infections.

Tosdiazina Clariana, Spain.
Tolu balsam (p.1071·1); erythromycin stearate (p.204·2); guaiphenesin (p.1061·3).
Respiratory-tract infections.

Tosfriol *Derly, Spain.*
Dextromethorphan hydrobromide (p.1057·3).
Coughs.

Tosidrin *Fardi, Spain.*
Dihydrocodeine tartrate (p.34·1).
Formerly contained dihydrocodeine tartrate, drosera, guaiphenesin, nikethamide, and thyme.
Coughs; pain.

Tosifar *Ifidesa Aristegui, Spain.*
Fominoben hydrochloride (p.1061·2).
Respiratory-tract disorders.

Tosion Retard *Boots Healthcare, Neth.*
Dextromethorphan polistirex (p.1058·2).
Coughs.

Tosmilen *Sinclair, UK†.*
Demecarium bromide (p.1390·3).
Available on a named-patient basis only.
Raised intra-ocular pressure.

Tossamine *Sandoz OTC, Switz.*
Codeine phosphate (p.26·1); noscapine (p.1065·2).
Coughs.

Tossamine plus *Sandoz OTC, Switz.*
White capsules, codeine phosphate (p.26·1); noscapine (p.1065·2); methylephedrine hydrochloride (p.1064·1); blue capsules, codeine phosphate; noscapine; diphenhydramine hydrochloride (p.409·1).
Coughs.

Tossarel *Aerocid, Fr.*
Inula helenium (p.1059·2); marrubium (p.1063·3); terpin (p.1070·2); sodium benzoate (p.1102·3).
Coughs.

Tossemed *Iodosan, Ital.*
Dextromethorphan hydrobromide (p.1057·3); guaiphenesin (p.1061·3).
Coughs.

Tosuman
Berna, Ital.; Berna, Switz.
A pertussis immunoglobulin (p.1525·3).
Passive immunisation.

Totacef *Bristol-Myers Squibb, Ital.*
Cephazolin sodium (p.181·1).
Bacterial infections.

Totacillin *SmithKline Beecham, USA.*
Ampicillin trihydrate (p.153·2).
Bacterial infections.

Totacillin-N *SmithKline Beecham, USA†.*
Ampicillin sodium (p.153·1).
Bacterial infections.

Totaforte
Asta Medica, Belg.; Asta Medica, Neth.
Multivitamin and mineral preparation.

Total
Allergan, Austral.; Allergan, USA.
Cleansing, soaking and wetting solution for hard contact lenses.

Total Cover Sunblock *Clinique, Canad.*
SPF 30: Ethylhexyl *p*-methoxycinnamate (p.1487·1); homosalate (p.1487·2); octyl salicylate (p.1487·3); oxybenzone (p.1487·3).
Sunscreen.

Total Eclipse *Triangle, USA.*
SPF 15: Padimate O (p.1488·1); oxybenzone (p.1487·3); lisadimate (p.1487·2).
Sunscreen.

Total Eclipse Moisturizing *Triangle, USA.*
SPF 15: Padimate O (p.1488·1); oxybenzone (p.1487·3); octyl salicylate (p.1487·3).
Sunscreen.

Total Formula *Vitaline, USA.*
A range of vitamin preparations.

Total Woman *Vita Glow, Austral.*
A range of multivitamin and mineral preparations.
Dietary supplement.

Totalbloc *Australis, Austral.†.*
SPF15+: Padimate O (p.1487·3); oxybenzone (p.1487·3); avobenzone (p.1486·3).
Sunscreen.

Totalbloc Maximum Protection *Creative Brands, Austral.*
Escalol 507; oxybenzone (p.1487·3); avobenzone (p.1486·3).
Sunscreen.

TotalCare *Allergan, Ger.*
Disinfecting, storage, and moistening solution for contact lenses.

Totalciclina *Benvegna, Ital.†.*
Ampicillin trihydrate (p.153·2).
Bacterial infections.

Totalip *Guidotti, Ital.*
Atorvastatin calcium (p.1268·1).
Hyperlipidaemias.

Totamine *Clintec, Fr.*
Amino-acid, electrolyte, and vitamin infusion.
Parenteral nutrition.

Totamol *CP Pharmaceuticals, UK.*
Atenolol (p.825·3).
Angina pectoris; arrhythmias; hypertension.

Totapen *Bristol-Myers Squibb, Fr.*
Ampicillin sodium (p.153·1) or ampicillin trihydrate (p.153·2).
Bacterial infections.

Totaretic *CP Pharmaceuticals, UK.*
Atenolol (p.825·3); chlorthalidone (p.839·3).
These ingredients can be described by the British Approved Name Co-tenidone.
Hypertension.

Totavit *Seton, UK†.*
Multivitamin, mineral, and amino acid preparation.

Totephan *Paraphar, Fr.*
Gelatin (p.723·2); methionine (p.984·2); cystine (p.1339·1); vitamins and minerals.
Hair and nail tonic.

Tot'hema *Innothera, Fr.*
Ferrous gluconate (p.1340·1); manganese gluconate (p.1351·1); copper gluconate (p.1338·1).
Anaemia.

Totifen *Master Pharma, Ital.†.*
Ketotifen fumarate (p.755·2).
Asthma; bronchitis; rhinitis.

Totocillin
Bayer, Aust.†; Bayer, Ger.†.
Ampicillin sodium (p.153·1) or ampicillin trihydrate (p.153·2); dicloxacillin sodium (p.202·1) or oxacillin sodium (p.234·2).
Bacterial infections.

Totocortin *Winzer, Ger.*
Dexamethasone sodium phosphate (p.1037·2).
Eye disorders.

Totonik *Pharmaceutical Enterprises, S.Afr.*
Vitamins; potassium glycerophosphate; caffeine; ferrous sulphate.
Tonic.

Toulumad *Ceninter, Spain.*
Magnesium polygalacturonate.
Gastric hyperacidity; peptic ulcer.

Touristil *Janssen-Cilag, Belg.*
Cinnarizine (p.406·1); domperidone maleate (p.1191·1).
Dyspepsia; motion sickness; nausea; sleep disorders; vertigo; vomiting.

Touro A & H *Dartmouth, USA.*
Pseudoephedrine hydrochloride (p.1068·3); brompheniramine maleate (p.403·2).
Allergic rhinitis; nasal congestion.

Touro DM *Dartmouth, USA.*
Dextromethorphan hydrobromide (p.1057·3); guaiphenesin (p.1061·3).
Coughs.

Touro Ex *Dartmouth, USA.*
Guaiphenesin (p.1061·3).
Coughs.

Touro LA *Dartmouth, USA.*
Pseudoephedrine hydrochloride (p.1068·3); guaiphenesin (p.1061·3).
Coughs and cold symptoms.

Touxium *SMB, Belg.*
Dextromethorphan hydrobromide (p.1057·3).
Coughs.

Tovene *Solvay, Ger.*
Diosmin (p.1580·1).
Venous insufficiency.

Toxepasi *Boehringer Mannheim, Ital.*
Cogalactoisomerase sodium (p.1566·2).
Hyperbilirubinaemia.

Toxepasi Complex *Boehringer Mannheim, Ital.†.*
Cogalactoisomerase sodium (p.1566·2); glutathione (p.983·1); cyanocobalamin (p.1363·3).
Liver disorders.

Toxepasi Complex Forte *IBYS, Spain†.*
Reduced glutathione (p.983·1); meglumine (p.1599·2); cogalactoisomerase (p.1566·2).
Liver disorders.

Toxex *Pekana, Ger.*
Homoeopathic preparation.

Toxicol *Eagle, Austral.*
Vitamin B substances with mineral, herbal, and nutritional agents.

toxi-L 90 N *Loges, Ger.*
Homoeopathic preparation.

toxi-loges *Loges, Ger.*
Homoeopathic preparation.

toxi-loges C *Loges, Ger.†.*
Echinacea angustifolia; bryonia root; cinchona bark; eupatorium perfol.; baptisia; aconitum; ipecacuanha; ascorbic acid.
Tonic.

toxi-loges N *Loges, Ger.*
Homoeopathic preparation.

Toximer
Note. This name is used for preparations of different composition.
Merckle, Aust.
Suppositories: Paracetamol (p.72·2); codeine phosphate (p.26·1).
Tablets: Propyphenazone (p.81·3); paracetamol (p.72·2); codeine phosphate (p.26·1).
Fever; pain.

Merckle, Ger.†.
Etenzamide (p.35·3); paracetamol (p.72·2); caffeine (p.749·3); codeine phosphate (p.26·1).
Cold symptoms; neuralgia; pain; rheumatism; spasms.

Toximer C *Merckle, Ger.*
Paracetamol (p.72·2); caffeine (p.749·3).
Pain.

Toxiselect *Dreluso, Ger.*
Homoeopathic preparation.

Toxogonin
Merck, Aust.; Merck, Ger.; E. Merck, Neth.; Merck, S.Afr.; Meda, Swed.
Obidoxime chloride (p.988·3).
Organophosphorus pesticide poisoning.

Toxogonine *E. Merck, Switz.*
Obidoxime chloride (p.988·3).
Organophosphorus poisoning.

Toxorephan *Repha, Ger.†.*
Echinacea angustifolia (p.1574·2); stellaria media; marrubium vulgare (p.1063·3); belladonna; apis; lachesis.
Tonic.

TP-1
Serono, Ger.†; Serono, Ital.†; Serono, Spain.
Thymostimulin.
Immunotherapy.

T-PA *Seroyal, Canad.*
Vitamin D and minerals.

TPE 1800 GX *Pharmacia Upjohn, Ger.*
Amino-acid, carbohydrate, and electrolyte infusion.
Parenteral nutrition.

TPH *Clintec, Ital.*
Amino-acid infusion.
Parenteral nutrition for neonates and infants.

T-Phyl *Purdue Frederick, USA.*
Theophylline (p.765·1).
Asthma; bronchospasm.

TPN Additive *DBL, Austral.*
Electrolytes (p.1147·1).
Parenteral nutrition.

T-Quil *Legere, USA†.*
Diazepam (p.661·1).

Trac Tabs 2X *Hyrex, USA.*
Hexamine (p.216·1); salol (p.83·1); atropine sulphate (p.455·1); hyoscyamine sulphate (p.464·2); benzoic acid (p.1102·3); methylene blue (p.984·3).
Urinary-tract infections.

Tracel
Tracel, Austral.†.
Vitamin B_{12} with minerals.

Pharmacia Upjohn, Norw.; Pharmacia Upjohn, Swed.
Trace element infusion.
Parenteral nutrition.

Tracelyte *Lyphomed, USA.*
A range of trace element and electrolyte preparations (p.1147·1).
Parenteral nutrition.

Tracemate *Pharmy, Fr.*
Disodium edetate (p.980·1).
Hypocalcaemia provocation test.

Tracer bG *Boehringer Mannheim, USA.*
Test for glucose in blood (p.1585·1).

Tracer Glucose *Boehringer Mannheim, Fr.*
Test for glucose in blood (p.1585·1).

Tracheo Fresh *Rappai, Switz.*
Sea salt (p.1162·2); macrogol 300 (p.1598·2).
Tracheal lubricant; tracheostomy care.

Trachisan
Note. This name is used for preparations of different composition.
Engelhard, Ger.; Engelhard, Switz.
Lozenges: Chlorhexidine gluconate (p.1107·2); lignocaine hydrochloride (p.1293·2); tyrothricin (p.267·2).
Mouth and throat disorders.

Engelhard, Ger.
Mouthwash: Chlorhexidine gluconate (p.1107·2); lignocaine hydrochloride (p.1293·2).
Mouth and throat disorders.

Trachitol *Engelhard, Ger.*
Lignocaine hydrochloride (p.1293·2); propyl hydroxybenzoate (p.1117·2); alum (p.1547·1).
Infections of the upper-respiratory tract; inflammatory disorders of the oropharynx.

Trachyl *Monal, Fr.*
Ethylmorphine hydrochloride (p.36·1).
Coughs.

Tracitrans *Fresenius, Ger.*
Electrolyte and trace element preparation.
Parenteral nutrition.

Tracrium
Glaxo Wellcome, Aust.; Glaxo Wellcome, Austral.; Glaxo Wellcome, Belg.; Glaxo Wellcome, Canad.; Glaxo Wellcome, Fr.; Glaxo Wellcome, Ger.; Wellcome, Irl.; Glaxo Wellcome, Ital.; Glaxo Wellcome, Neth.; Glaxo Wellcome, Norw.; Glaxo Wellcome, S.Afr.; Wellcome, Spain; Glaxo Wellcome, Swed.; Wellcome, Switz.; Wellcome, UK; Glaxo Wellcome, USA.
Atracurium besylate (p.1304·3).
Competitive neuromuscular blocker.

Tractur *Damor, Ital.*
Pipemidic acid (p.237·2).
Bacterial infections of the urinary tract.

Tracutil
Braun, Ger.; Braun, Switz.
Mineral preparation.
Parenteral nutrition.

Tradella *Sanofi Winthrop, Ger.*
Oestradiol (p.1455·1).
Menopausal disorders.

Tradol *Isis Puren, Ger.*
Tramadol hydrochloride (p.90·1).
Pain.

Tradolan *Nordic, Swed.*
Tramadol hydrochloride (p.90·1).
Pain.

Tradon *Beiersdorf-Lilly, Ger.†.*
Pemoline (p.1484·1).
Stimulant.

Trafloxal
Tramedico, Belg.; Mann, Neth.
Ofloxacin (p.233·3).
Eye infections.

Trafuril
Note. This name is used for preparations of different composition.
Ciba-Geigy, Aust.†.
Thurfyl nicotinate; salen; methyl salicylate (p.55·2); camphor (p.1557·2); menthol (p.1600·2); salicylic acid (p.1090·2).
Musculoskeletal and joint disorders.

Ciba-Geigy, Swed.†.
Thurfyl nicotinate; methyl salicyloyl oxyacetate; ethyl salicyloyl oxyacetate; methyl salicylate (p.55·2); camphor (p.1557·2); menthol (p.1600·2).
Muscle pain.

Tralgiol *Boehringer Mannheim, Spain.*
Tramadol hydrochloride (p.90·1).
Pain.

Tralisin *FIRMA, Ital.†.*
Lymecycline (p.223·2).
Bacterial infections.

Trama *BASF, Ger.; Sanorania, Ger.*
Tramadol hydrochloride (p.90·1).
Pain.

Tramabeta *Betapharm, Ger.*
Tramadol hydrochloride (p.90·1).
Pain.

Tramadolor
Hexal, Ger.; Mepha, Switz.
Tramadol hydrochloride (p.90·1).
Pain.

Trama-Dorsch *Nycomed, Ger.*
Tramadol hydrochloride (p.90·1).
Pain.

Tramadura *Durachemie, Ger.*
Tramadol hydrochloride (p.90·1).
Pain.

Tramagetic
Azupharma, Ger.; Christiaens, Neth.
Tramadol hydrochloride (p.90·1).
Pain.

Tramagit *Krewel, Ger.*
Tramadol hydrochloride (p.90·1).
Pain.

Tramake
Galen, Irl.; Galen, UK.
Tramadol hydrochloride (p.90·1).
Pain.

Tramal
Grunenthal, Aust.; Grunenthal, Ger.; Grunenthal, Neth.; Boehringer Mannheim, S.Afr.; Grunenthal, Switz.
Tramadol hydrochloride (p.90·1).
Pain.

Tramamerck *Merck, Ger.*
Tramadol hydrochloride (p.90·1).
Pain.

Tramedphano *Medphano, Ger.*
Tramadol hydrochloride (p.90·1).
Pain.

Tramil
Note. This name is used for preparations of different composition.
Whitehall, Irl.
Paracetamol (p.72·2); caffeine (p.749·3).
Fever; pain.

Whitehall, UK.
Paracetamol (p.72·2).
Fever; pain.

Tramisal *Astier, Fr.*
Ginkgo biloba (p.1584·1).
Mental function impairment in the elderly; peripheral vascular disorders.

Tramundin *Mundipharma, Ger.*
Tramadol hydrochloride (p.90·1).
Pain.

Trancalgyl *Innothera, Fr.†.*
Etenzamide (p.35·3).
Fever; pain.

Trancocard *Benvegna, Ital.†.*
Dipyridamole (p.857·1).
Ischaemic heart disease.

Trancogesic *Sterling Winthrop, Fr.†.*
Aspirin (p.16·1); chlormezanone (p.648·3).
Pain; skeletal muscle spasm.

Trancopal
Sanofi Winthrop, Aust.†; Sanofi Winthrop, Belg.†; Sterling Winthrop, Fr.†; Sanofi Winthrop, Irl.†; Sanofi Winthrop, Neth.†; Sanofi Winthrop, Norw.†; Sanofi, Swed.†; Sanofi Winthrop, Switz.†; Sanofi Winthrop, UK†; Sanofi Winthrop, USA†.
Chlormezanone (p.648·3).
Anxiety; insomnia; skeletal muscle spasm.

Trancopal compositum
Sanofi Winthrop, Aust.†; Sanofi Winthrop, Switz.†.
Chlormezanone (p.648·3); paracetamol (p.72·2).
Musculoskeletal pain and spasm.

Trancopal Dolo *Sanofi Winthrop, Ger.*
Flupirtine maleate (p.42·1).
Pain.

Trandate
Glaxo Wellcome, Aust.; Glaxo Wellcome, Austral.; Glaxo Wellcome, Belg.; Roberts, Canad.; Glaxo Wellcome, Fr.; Cascan, Ger.†; Glaxo Wellcome, Ger.†; Allen & Hanburys, Irl.; Teofarma, Ital.; Glaxo Wellcome, Neth.; Glaxo Wellcome, Norw.; Glaxo Wellcome, S.Afr.; Dun-

can, Spain; Glaxo Wellcome, Swed.; Glaxo Wellcome, Switz.; Medeva, UK; Allen & Hanburys, USA.
Labetalol hydrochloride (p.896·1).
Angina pectoris; controlled hypotension during anaesthesia; hypertension.

Trandiur Teofarma, Ital.
Labetalol hydrochloride (p.896·1); chlorthalidone (p.839·3).
Hypertension.

Tranex Malesci, Ital.
Tranexamic acid (p.728·2).
Hyperfibrinolytic haemorrhage.

Trangorex Sanofi Winthrop, Spain.
Amiodarone hydrochloride (p.820·1).
Angina pectoris; arrhythmias.

Trankimazin Upjohn, Spain.
Alprazolam (p.640·3).
Anxiety.

Tran-Qil Rolab, S.Afr.
Lorazepam (p.675·3).
Anxiety.

Tranqipam Lennon, S.Afr.
Lorazepam (p.675·3).
Alcohol withdrawal syndrome; anxiety; premedication; sedative.

Tranquase Azupharma, Ger.
Diazepam (p.661·1).
Anxiety; muscular disorders; premedication.

Tranquax Berk, UK.
Clomipramine hydrochloride (p.281·2).
Depression; narcoleptic syndrome; obsessive-compulsive disorder.

Tranquil Pharmadass, UK.
Crataegus (p.1568·2); linden flower extract (p.1637·3); viburnum; hawthorn oil (p.1568·2).

Tranquiplex Vitaplex, Austral.†.
Vitamins and minerals; passion flower (p.1615·3); scutellaria; valerian (p.1643·1).

Tranquirax Rorer, Ital.†.
Bevonium methylsulphate; medazepam (p.677·3).
Gastro-intestinal disorders.

Tranquirit Rhone-Poulenc Rorer, Ital.
Diazepam (p.661·1).
Anxiety; epilepsy; insomnia; psychoses.

Tranquit Promonta, Ger.†.
Oxazolam (p.684·1).
Anxiety.

Tranquital Monal, Fr.
Valerian (p.1643·1); crataegus (p.1568·2).
Insomnia; nervous disorders.

Tranquo
Note. This name is used for preparations of different composition.
Boehringer Ingelheim, Belg.
Oxazepam (p.683·2).
Anxiety disorders.

Sanorania, Ger.†.
Diazepam (p.661·1).
Anxiety.

Tranquo-Buscopan
Boehringer Ingelheim, Belg.†; Boehringer Ingelheim, Ital.†.
Hyoscine butylbromide (p.462·3); oxazepam (p.683·2).
Gastro-intestinal disorders; hiccup.

Trans Act$_{LAT}$ Boots, S.Afr.
Flurbiprofen (p.42·1).
Musculoskeletal and joint disorders.

Trans Frac Cantassium Co., UK†.
Trans ferulic acid.

Transacalm Norgine, Fr.
Trimebutine maleate (p.1639·3).
Formerly called Transicalm.
Gastro-intestinal disorders.

Transact Lat Nordmark, Ital.
Flurbiprofen (p.42·1).
Musculoskeletal pain.

Transamin Daiichi, Jpn.
Tranexamic acid (p.728·2).
Haemorrhagic disorders; inflammation.

Transannon
Pharmacia Upjohn, Ger.; Pharmacia Upjohn, Switz.
21 Tablets, conjugated oestrogens (p.1457·3); 7 tablets, inactive.
Menopausal disorders.

Transbilix
Codali, Belg.; Guerbet, Fr.
Meglumine iodipamide (p.1005·3).
Contrast medium for biliary-tract radiography.

Transbronchin Asta Medica, Ger.
Carbocisteine (p.1056·3) or carbocisteine sodium (p.1056·3).
Respiratory-tract disorders associated with increased or viscous mucus.

Transcop Recordati, Ital.
Hyoscine (p.462·3).
Motion sickness.

Transderm Scop Ciba, USA.
Hyoscine (p.462·3).
Motion sickness.

Transdermal-NTG Warner Chilcott, USA.
Glyceryl trinitrate (p.874·3).
Angina pectoris.

Transderm-Nitro
Ciba, Canad.; Summit, USA.
Glyceryl trinitrate (p.874·3).
Angina pectoris.

Transderm-V Ciba, Canad.
Hyoscine (p.462·3).
Motion sickness.

Transene Sanofi Winthrop, Ital.
Potassium clorazepate (p.657·1).
Anxiety; insomnia; nervous disorders.

Transferal Ferrer, Spain.
Tocofibrate (p.1280·1).
Hyperlipidaemias.

Transfert Piam, Ital.
Carnitine (p.1336·2).
Carnitine deficiency; myocardial ischaemia.

Transfusine Adultos Semar, Spain†.
Embryo extract; gastric mucosa extract; muscle extract.
Tonic.

Transfusine Infantil Semar, Spain†.
Carnitine chloride; cyanocobalamin; embryo extract; gastric mucosa extract; muscle extract.
Tonic.

Transiderm-Nitro
Novartis, Austral.; Ciba-Geigy, Irl.; Novartis, Neth.; Ciba, Norw.; Novartis, Swed.; Ciba, UK.
Glyceryl trinitrate (p.874·3).
Angina pectoris; prophylaxis of phlebitis and extravasation.

Transil Malesci, Ital.†.
Tranexamic acid (p.728·2); ethamsylate (p.720·1).
Haemorrhage.

Transilane Innothera, Fr.
Purified hemicellulose from psyllium seeds (p.1194·2).
Constipation.

Transipeg
Roche, Belg.; Nicholas, Fr.
Macrogol 3350 (p.1598·2); electrolytes (p.1147·1).
Constipation.

Transitol Lincoln, Fr.
Refined soft paraffins (p.1382·3); liquid paraffin (p.1382·1).
Constipation.

Transix Christiaens, Belg.†.
Sennosides B (p.1212·3).
Constipation.

Translet Franklin Medical, UK.
Barrier cream.

Translet Plus One Rusch, UK.
A deodorant liquid for use with colostomies and ileostomies.

Translet Plus Two Rusch, UK.
A deodorant liquid for use with colostomies and ileostomies.

Translight Merck Sharp & Dohme-Chibret, Fr.
Tyloxapol (p.1329·2).
Hard contact lens cleaner.

Transmer Soekami, Fr.†.
Promethazine hydrochloride (p.416·2); ephedrine hydrochloride (p.1059·3).
Motion sickness.

Transmetil Knoll, Ital.
Ademetionine butanedisulphonate (p.1543·1).
Liver disorders.

Transoak Pabisch, Aust.
A rinsing and storage solution for hard and gas permeable contact lenses.

Transoddi Lipha Sante, Fr.
Cinametic acid (p.1563·3).
Gastro-intestinal disorders.

Transol Pabisch, Aust.
A wetting solution for hard and gas permeable contact lenses.

Trans-Plantar Westwood-Squibb, Canad.
Salicylic acid (p.1090·2).
Plantar warts.

Transpulmin Asta Medica, Ger.†.
Cineole (p.1564·1); camphor (p.1557·2); guaiacol (p.1061·2); laureth 9 (p.1325·2); sage oil; isothipendyl hydrochloride (p.412·2); matricaria flowers (p.1561·2).
Respiratory-tract disorders.

Transpulmin E Asta Medica, Ger.
Cineole (p.1564·1); menthol (p.1600·2); camphor (p.1557·2).
Respiratory-tract disorders.

Transpulmin Kinderbalsam S Asta Medica, Ger.
Eucalyptus oil (p.1578·1); oleum pini sylvestris.
Respiratory-tract disorders.

Transpulmina Gel Bayropharm, Ital.†.
Cineole (p.1564·1); menthol (p.1600·2); camphor (p.1557·2).
Catarrh; coughs.

Transpulmina Gola Bayer, Ital.
Dequalinium chloride (p.1112·1); menthol (p.1600·2); cineole (p.1564·1).
Mouth and throat infections.

Transpulmina Gola Nebulizzatore Bayropharm, Ital.†.
Dequalinium chloride (p.1112·1); cineole (p.1564·1); thyme oil (p.1637·1); mint oil (p.1604·1).
Respiratory-tract infections.

Transpulmina Rino Bayropharm, Ital.†.
Naphazoline hydrochloride (p.1064·2).
Nasal congestion.

Transpulmina Tosse Bayer, Ital.
Pastilles: Guaiphenesin (p.1061·3); menthol (p.1600·2); cineole (p.1564·1); camphor (p.1557·2).
Syrup: Guaiphenesin (p.1061·3); menthol (p.1600·2); cineole (p.1564·1).
Catarrh; coughs.

Transpulmine Asta Medica, Switz.†.
Cineole (p.1564·1); chamomile flowers (p.1561·2).
Respiratory-tract disorders.

Transulose Schwarz, Fr.
Lactulose (p.1195·3); liquid paraffin (p.1382·1); white soft paraffin (p.1382·3).
Constipation.

Transvane Reckitt & Colman, Belg.†.
Thurfyl salicylate (p.88·3); hexyl nicotinate (p.43·1); ethyl nicotinate (p.36·1); benzocaine (p.1286·2).
Musculoskeletal, joint, and soft-tissue disorders.

Transvasin
Seton, Irl.; Meda, Swed.; Seton, UK.
Ethyl nicotinate (p.36·1); hexyl nicotinate (p.43·1); thurfyl salicylate (p.88·3).
Formerly contained thurfyl salicylate, ethyl nicotinate, hexyl nicotinate, and benzocaine in *Irl.*
Rheumatic and muscular pain; sprains; strains.

Transvercid Pierre Fabre Sante, Fr.
Salicylic acid (p.1090·2).
Warts.

Trans-Ver-Sal
Westwood-Squibb, Canad.; Difa, Ital.
Salicylic acid (p.1090·2).
Calluses; verrucas.

Trans-Ver-Sal AdultPatch Doak, USA.
Salicylic acid (p.1090·2).
Verrucas.

Trans-Ver-Sal PediaPatch Doak, USA.
Salicylic acid (p.1090·2).
Formerly known as PediaPatch.
Warts.

Trans-Ver-Sal PlantarPatch Doak, USA.
Salicylic acid (p.1090·2).
Formerly known as Trans-Plantar.
Warts.

Trantalol Pinewood, Irl.
Atenolol (p.825·3).
Angina pectoris; arrhythmias; hypertension; myocardial infarction.

Tranxene
Glaxo Wellcome, Austral.; Sanofi Winthrop, Belg.; Abbott, Canad.; Sanofi Winthrop, Fr.; Boehringer Ingelheim, Irl.; Sanofi Winthrop, Neth.; Sanofi Omnimed, S.Afr.; Boehringer Ingelheim, UK; Abbott, USA.
Potassium clorazepate (p.657·1).
Agitation; alcohol withdrawal syndrome; anxiety disorders; premedication; tetany.

Tranxilen Kabi, Swed.†.
Potassium clorazepate (p.657·1).
Alcohol withdrawal syndrome; non-psychotic mental disorders.

Tranxilium
Sanofi Winthrop, Aust.; Sanofi Winthrop, Ger.; Sanofi Winthrop, Spain; Sanofi Winthrop, Switz.
Potassium clorazepate (p.657·1).
Agitation; anxiety; premedication; sleep disorders.

Tranxilium N Sanofi Winthrop, Ger.
Nordazepam (p.682·3).
Anxiety; sleep disorders.

Trapanal Byk Gulden, Ger.
Thiopentone sodium (p.1233·1).
General anaesthesia.

Traquivan Llorente, Spain.
Dihydrocodeine tartrate (p.34·1); co-trimoxazole (p.196·3).
Respiratory-tract infections.

Trasicor
Ciba-Geigy, Aust.; Ciba-Geigy, Austral.†; Ciba-Geigy, Belg.; Ciba, Canad.; Ciba-Geigy, Fr.; Ciba, Ger.; Ciba-Geigy, Irl.; Ciba, Ital.†; Novartis, Neth.; Ciba, Norw.; Novartis, S.Afr.; Ciba-Geigy, Spain; Ciba-Geigy, Swed.†; Ciba, Switz.; Ciba, UK.
Oxprenolol hydrochloride (p.926·2).
Angina pectoris; anxiety; arrhythmias; hypertension; hyperthyroidism; myocardial infarction; obstructive cardiomyopathy.

Trasicor Esidrix Ciba, Ger.†.
Combination pack: Trasicor: oxprenolol hydrochloride (p.926·2); Esidrix: hydrochlorothiazide (p.885·2).
Hypertension.

Trasidrex
Ciba-Geigy, Irl.; Novartis, S.Afr.; Ciba, UK.
Oxprenolol hydrochloride (p.926·2); cyclopenthiazide (p.845·2).
These ingredients can be described by the British Approved Name Co-prenozide.
Hypertension.

Trasipressol Ciba-Geigy, Fr.
Oxprenolol hydrochloride (p.926·2); dihydralazine sulphate (p.854·1).
Hypertension.

Trasitensin
Ciba-Geigy, Aust.; Ciba, Ger.; Ciba, Ital.; Ciba-Geigy, Spain.
Oxprenolol hydrochloride (p.926·2); chlorthalidone (p.839·3).
Hypertension.

Trasitensine
Ciba-Geigy, Fr.; Ciba, Switz.
Oxprenolol hydrochloride (p.926·2); chlorthalidone (p.839·3).
Hypertension.

Traspica Perez Gimenez, Spain†.
Ammonia solution (p.1548·3).
Bites and stings.

Trasylol
Bayer, Aust.; Bayer, Austral.; Bayer, Belg.; Bayer, Canad.; Bayer, Fr.; Bayer, Ger.; Bayer, Irl.†; Bayer, Ital.; Bayer, Neth.; Bayer, S.Afr.; Bayer, Swed.; Bayer, Switz.; Bayer, UK; Bayer, USA.
Aprotinin (p.711·3).
Hyperfibrinolytic haemorrhage; pulmonary embolism; reduction of blood loss in open heart surgery; shock.

Tratul Gerot, Aust.
Diclofenac (p.31·2) or diclofenac diethylamine (p.31·2) or diclofenac sodium (p.31·2).
Fever; gout; inflammation; musculoskeletal, joint, and peri-articular disorders; pain.

Trauma Relief Brauer, Austral.
Homoeopathic preparation.

TraumaCal
Mead Johnson, Austral.; Mead Johnson, Canad.†; Mead Johnson Nutritionals, USA.
Preparation for enteral nutrition.
Stress.

Traumacut Brenner-Efeka, Ger.†.
Methocarbamol (p.1316·1).
Muscle relaxant.

Trauma-cyl Liebermann, Ger.
Chamomile oil; sage oil; arnica (p.1550·3); aesculus (p.1543·3); hamamelis (p.1587·1).
Vascular disorders.

Trauma-cyl N Complex Liebermann, Ger.
Homoeopathic preparation.

Trauma-Dolgit Dolorgiet, Ger.
Ibuprofen (p.44·1).
Musculoskeletal and joint disorders; sports injuries.

Traumadyn Plantamed, Ger.
Homoeopathic preparation.

Traumafusin Pharmacia Upjohn, Aust.
Amino-acid and electrolyte infusion.
Parenteral nutrition.

Traumal Zyma, Ital.
Oxerutins (p.1580·2); a heparinoid (p.882·3).
Bruises; sprains.

Traumalgyl Pharmadeveloppement, Fr.
Phenylbutazone (p.79·2); mephenesin (p.1315·3); diethylamine salicylate (p.33·1); lignocaine (p.1293·2).
Musculoskeletal, joint, peri-articular, and soft-tissue disorders.

Traumalitan 3M, Ger.
Heparin sodium (p.879·3).
Skin trauma; thrombo-embolic disorders.

Traumalix Drossapharm, Switz.
Etofenamate (p.36·3).
Musculoskeletal, joint, peri-articular, and soft-tissue disorders.

Traumanase
Nattermann, Ger.; Rhone-Poulenc Rorer, Switz.
Bromelains (p.1555·1).
Inflammation with oedema.

Traumanase-cyclin Rorer, Ger.†.
Tetracycline hydrochloride (p.259·1); bromelains (p.1555·1).
Bacterial infections.

Traumaparil Madaus, Aust.
Aescin (p.1543·3).
Soft-tissue disorders.

Traumaplant Harras-Curarina, Ger.
Comfrey (p.1567·1).
Musculoskeletal and joint disorders; sports injuries; wounds.

Trauma-Puren Isis Puren, Ger.
Heparin sodium (p.879·3); menthol (p.1600·2); glycol salicylate (p.43·1).
Haematoma; inflammation; phlebitis.

Traumasalbe Provita, Aust.
Capsicum (p.1559·2); methyl salicylate (p.55·2); turpentine oil (p.1641·1).
Musculoskeletal, joint, peri-articular, and soft-tissue disorders.

Trauma-Salbe Rodler 301 N Woelm, Ger.
Camphor (p.1557·2); menthol (p.1600·2); methyl salicylate (p.55·2).
Cold symptoms; joint, muscular, and neuromuscular pain.

Trauma-Salbe Rodler 302 N Woelm, Ger.
Camphor (p.1557·2); turpentine oil (p.1641·1); eucalyptus oil (p.1578·1).
Formerly contained cayenne pepper, turpentine oil, and methyl salicylate.
Muscle and joint injuries.

Trauma-Salbe Rodler 303 N Woelm, Ger.
Camphor (p.1557·2).
Formerly contained cayenne pepper, camphor, menthol, and methyl salicylate.
Muscle and joint disorders.

Traumasenex Brenner-Efeka, Ger.
Glycol salicylate (p.43·1).
Rheumatism; soft-tissue disorders.

Traumasept Wolff, Ger.
Povidone-iodine (p.1123·3).
Burns; skin disinfection; ulcers; vaginal infections; wounds.

Traumasteril kohlenhydratfrei Fresenius, Ger.
Amino-acid and electrolyte infusion.
Parenteral nutrition.

Traumasteril mit Kohlenhydraten Fresenius, Ger.†.
Amino-acid, carbohydrate, and electrolyte infusion.
Parenteral nutrition.

Traumatociclina *Biomedica, Ital.*
Meclocycline sulfosalicylate (p.224·1).
Bacterial skin infections.

Traumeel S *Heel, Ger.*
Homoeopathic preparation.

Traumicid *Montefarmaco, Ital.*
Methylbenzethonium chloride (p.1119·3); chlorothymol (p.1111·1).
Wound disinfection.

Traumon
Kolassa, Aust.; Bayer, Ger.
Etofenamate (p.36·3).
Musculoskeletal, joint, peri-articular, and soft-tissue disorders.

Traumox *Medpro, S.Afr.*
Naproxen (p.61·2).
Dysmenorrhoea; gout; musculoskeletal and joint disorders.

Trausabun *Promonta, Ger.*†.
Melitracen hydrochloride (p.296·3) or melitracen mesylate (p.296·3).
Depression.

Trautil *CEPA, Spain.*
Cisapride (p.1187·1).
Gastro-oesophageal reflux; gastroparesis.

Travacalm *Hamilton, Austral.*
Dimenhydrinate (p.408·2); hyoscine hydrobromide (p.462·3); caffeine (p.749·3).
Motion sickness.

Travad *Baxter, Austral.*
Anhydrous monobasic sodium phosphate (p.1159·3); anhydrous dibasic sodium phosphate (p.1159·3).
Bowel evacuation; constipation.

Travamine *ICN, Canad.*
Dimenhydrinate (p.408·2).

Travase
Knoll, Canad.†; *Boots, USA*†.
Sutilains (p.1634·2).
Debridement of burns, ulcers, and wounds.

Travasept *Baxter, UK.*
Cetrimide (p.1105·2); chlorhexidine acetate (p.1107·2).
Skin disinfection.

Travasol *Clintec, USA.*
A range of amino-acid infusions.
Parenteral nutrition.

Travasol in Dextrose *Clintec, USA.*
Amino-acid and glucose infusion.
Parenteral nutrition.

Travasol with Electrolytes
Clintec, Canad.; Clintec, USA.
Amino-acid and electrolyte infusion.
Parenteral nutrition.

Travasol with Electrolytes and Dextrose *Clintec, Canad.*
Amino-acid, carbohydrate, and electrolyte infusion.
Parenteral nutrition.

Travasol without Electrolytes *Clintec, Canad.*
Amino-acid infusion.
Parenteral nutrition.

Travasorb *Clintec, USA.*
A range of preparations for enteral nutrition.

Travel Aid *WestCan, Canad.*
Dimenhydrinate (p.408·2).
Nausea; vomiting.

Travel Calm *Boots, UK; Unichem, UK.*
Hyoscine hydrobromide (p.462·3).
Motion sickness.

Travel Sickness *Cantassium Co., UK.*
Ginger (p.1193·2).

Travel Sickness Cocculus *Homeocan, Canad.*
Homoeopathic preparation.

Travel Tabs *WestCan, Canad.*
Dimenhydrinate (p.408·2).
Motion sickness.

Travel Well *Farmalider, Spain.*
Dimenhydrinate (p.408·2).
Motion sickness; vertigo.

Travelaide *Yauyip, Austral.*
Ginger (p.1193·2); cardamom (p.1560·1); slippery elm (p.1630·1).
Motion sickness.

Travel-Caps *English Grains, UK.*
Ginger (p.1193·2); calumba (p.1557·2); chamomile (p.1561·2).

Travel-Gum *Asta Medica, Aust.*
Dimenhydrinate (p.408·2).
Motion sickness.

Travelgum *Asta Medica, Ital.*
Dimenhydrinate (p.408·2).
Motion sickness.

Travella *Nelson, UK.*
Homoeopathic preparation.
Formerly known as Travel Sickness Tablets.

Travellers *Phillips Yeast, UK.*
Ginger (p.1193·2).
Motion sickness.

Travello
Pharmacia Upjohn, Norw.; Pharmacia Upjohn, Swed.
Loperamide hydrochloride (p.1197·2).
Diarrhoea.

Travelmate *Shoppers Drug Mart, Canad.*
Dimenhydrinate (p.408·2).

Traveltabs *Stanley, Canad.*
Dimenhydrinate (p.408·2).
Nausea; vomiting.

Travert
Pharmacia Upjohn, Norw.; Baxter, USA.
Invert sugar (p.1357·3); electrolytes (p.1147·1).
Carbohydrate source; fluid and electrolyte disorders.

Travisco *Master Pharma, Ital.*
Trapidil (p.957·2).
Ischaemic heart disease; prevention of restenosis following angioplasty.

Travocort
Schering, Aust.; Schering, Belg.; Schering, Ger.; Schering, Irl.; Schering, Ital.; Schering, S.Afr.; Schering, Switz.
Isoconazole nitrate (p.381·2); diflucortolone valerate (p.1039·3).
Inflamed fungal skin infections.

Travogen
Schering, Aust.; Schering, Austral.†; *Schering, Belg.; Schering, Ger.; Schering, Irl.*†; *Schering, Ital.; Schering, Neth.*†; *Schering, S.Afr.*†; *Schering, Switz.*
Isoconazole (p.381·2) or isoconazole nitrate (p.381·2).
Fungal skin infections.

Travogyn *Schering, UK.*
Isoconazole nitrate (p.381·2).
Fungal vaginal infections.

Trawell *Asta Medica, Switz.*
Dimenhydrinate (p.408·2).
Motion sickness.

Traxam
Whitehall, Irl.; Cyanamid, Ital.; Wyeth, UK; Whitehall, UK.
Felbinac (p.37·1).
Musculoskeletal, joint, and peri-articular disorders; soft tissue injuries; sprains.

Traxaton *Steigerwald, Ger.*
Oak bark (p.1609·3).
Diarrhoea.

Trazograf *Juste, Spain.*
Meglumine diatrizoate (p.1003·2); sodium diatrizoate (p.1003·2).
Radiographic contrast medium.

Trazolan
Continental Pharma, Belg.; Searle, Neth.
Trazodone hydrochloride (p.308·3).
Depression.

Trebi *Coop. Farm., Ital.*†.
Thiamine disulphide (p.1361·2); pyridoxine hydrochloride (p.1362·3); cyanocobalamin (p.1363·3).
Chronic alcoholism; neuralgias; neuritis.

Trecalmo *Bayer, Ger.*
Clotiazepam (p.657·2).
Anxiety; sleep disorders.

Trecator *Wyeth-Ayerst, USA.*
Ethionamide (p.208·2).
Tuberculosis.

Tredalat *Bayer, Ger.*
Nifedipine (p.916·2); acebutolol hydrochloride (p.809·3).
Angina pectoris; hypertension.

Tredemine *Bellon, Fr.*
Niclosamide (p.105·3).
Taeniasis.

Tredilat *Coop. Farm., Ital.*†.
Co-dergocrine mesylate (p.1566·1).
Cerebrovascular disorders; hypertension.

Trefocor *Malesci, Ital.*†.
Vitamin B substances.

Trefovital *Vaillant, Ital.*
Royal jelly (p.1626·3).
Nutritional supplement.

Tregor *Hormosan, Ger.*
Amantadine sulphate (p.1129·2).
Parkinsonism.

Treis-Ciclina *Ecobi, Ital.*†.
Methacycline hydrochloride (p.225·1).
Bacterial infections.

Treis-Micina *Ecobi, Ital.*†.
Triacetyloleandomycin (p.264·3).
Bacterial infections.

Treloc *Astra, Ger.*
Metoprolol tartrate (p.907·3); hydrochlorothiazide (p.885·2); hydralazine hydrochloride (p.883·2).
Hypertension.

Tremaril
LPB, Ital.; Sandoz, Spain†; *Wander, Switz.*†.
Methixene hydrochloride (p.465·1).
Drug-induced extrapyramidal disorders; parkinsonism; tremor.

Tremarit *Wander, Ger.*
Methixene hydrochloride (p.465·1).
Parkinsonism and other hyperkinetic disorders.

Tremblex
Janssen-Cilag, Belg.; Yamanouchi, Ital.†; *Janssen-Cilag, Neth.; Janssen-Cilag, Switz.*†.
Dexetimide hydrochloride (p.460·1).
Drug-induced extrapyramidal disorders; parkinsonism.

Tremetex *Laakefarmos, Swed.*†.
Methotrexate (p.547·1).
Malignant neoplasms.

Tremoforat *Klein, Ger.*
Belladonna (p.457·1).
Parkinsonism.

Tremonil
Sandoz, Irl.†; *Sandoz, UK*†.
Methixene hydrochloride (p.465·1).
Parkinsonism; senile tremor.

Tremoquil *Astra, Swed.*
Methixene hydrochloride (p.465·1).
Parkinsonism.

Trenantone *Takeda, Ger.*
Leuprorelin acetate (p.1253·1).
Prostatic cancer.

Trendar *Whitehall, USA*†.
Ibuprofen (p.44·1).
Fever; osteoarthritis; pain; rheumatoid arthritis.

Trendar PMS *Whitehall-Robins, Canad.*
Paracetamol (p.72·2); pamabrom (p.927·1); mepyramine maleate (p.414·1).
Premenstrual syndrome.

Trendinol *Vita Elan, Spain.*
Nitrendipine (p.923·1).
Hypertension.

Trentadil
Christiaens, Belg.; Evans, Fr.
Bamifylline hydrochloride (p.749·2).
Biliary dyskinesia; cardiovascular disorders; gastro-intestinal spasm; obstructive airways disease; respiratory insufficiency.

Trental
Albert-Roussel, Aust.; Hoechst Marion Roussel, Austral.; Hoechst Marion Roussel, Canad.; Albert-Roussel, Ger.; Hoechst, Ger.; Hoechst Marion Roussel, Irl.; Hoechst Marion Roussel, Ital.; Hoechst Marion Roussel, Neth.; Hoechst Marion Roussel, Norw.; Hoechst Marion Roussel, S.Afr.; Hoechst Marion Roussel, Switz.; Borg, UK; Hoechst, USA.
Oxpentifylline (p.925·3).
Angioneurotic disorders; cerebral and ocular vascular disorders; disorders of the inner ear; peripheral vascular disorders.

Trentovlane *Schering, Fr.*†.
Norethisterone acetate (p.1453·1); ethinyloestradiol (p.1445·1).
Combined oral contraceptive; dysmenorrhoea.

Treo
Note. This name is used for preparations of different composition.
Pharmacia Upjohn, Aust.; Pharmacia Upjohn, Swed.
Aspirin (p.16·1); caffeine (p.749·3).
Fever; pain.

Biopharm, USA.
SPF 8; SPF 15; SPF 30: Octocrylene (p.1487·3); ethylhexyl *p*-methoxycinnamate (p.1487·1); oxybenzone (p.1487·3); octyl salicylate (p.1487·3); citronella oil (p.1565·1).
Sunscreen.

Treo comp *Pharmacia Upjohn, Swed.*
Aspirin (p.16·1); codeine phosphate (p.26·1); caffeine (p.749·3).
Pain.

Treparin *NCSN, Ital.*
A heparinoid (p.882·3).
Thrombosis prophylaxis.

Trepidan *Max Farma, Ital.*
Prazepam (p.687·2).
Anxiety.

Trepiline *Lennon, S.Afr.*
Amitriptyline hydrochloride (p.273·3).
Depression.

Trepress
Ciba-Geigy, Aust.; Ciba, Ger.; Ciba, Switz.
Oxprenolol hydrochloride (p.926·2); hydralazine hydrochloride (p.883·2); chlorthalidone (p.839·3).
Hypertension.

Tres Orix Forte *Prodes, Spain.*
Cyproheptadine orotate (p.407·3); amino acids and vitamins.
Anorexia; tonic; weight loss.

Tresal *Tremedic, Swed.*
Sodium chloride (p.1162·2).
Irrigation solution.

Tresanil *ISF, Ital.*†.
Tritiozine (p.1217·3).
Gastric hypersecretion.

Tresium *Prodes, Spain.*
Bromhexine hydrochloride (p.1055·3); co-trimoxazole (p.196·3).
Respiratory-tract infections.

Tresleen *Pfizer, Aust.*
Sertraline hydrochloride (p.307·2).
Depression.

Tresos B *Eagle, Austral.*
Multivitamin, amino-acid, and mineral preparation.
Dietary supplement.

Tretinoine *Widmer, Switz.*
Tretinoin (p.1093·3); urea (p.1095·2); triclosan (p.1127·2).
Acne.

Tretinoine Kefrane *RoC, Fr.*
Tretinoin (p.1093·3).
Acne.

Treupel *Asta Medica, Switz.*†.
Codeine phosphate (p.26·1); aspirin (p.16·1); paracetamol (p.72·2).
Fever; pain.

Treupel comp *Asta Medica, Ger.*
Codeine phosphate (p.26·1); paracetamol (p.72·2).
Fever; pain.

Treupel mono *Asta Medica, Ger.*
Paracetamol (p.72·2).
Fever; pain.

Treupel N *Asta Medica, Switz.*
Paracetamol (p.72·2).
Fever; pain.

Treupel sans codeine *Asta Medica, Switz.*
Aspirin (p.16·1); paracetamol (p.72·2).
Fever; pain.

Treupel simplex *Asta Medica, Switz.*
Aspirin (p.16·1); paracetamol (p.72·2); ascorbic acid (p.1365·2).
Fever; pain.

Treupel-N *Asta Medica, Ger.*†.
Codeine phosphate (p.26·1); salicylamide (p.82·3); paracetamol (p.72·2).
Cold symptoms; fever; neuralgia; pain.

Treuphadol *Treupha, Switz.*
Paracetamol (p.72·2).
Fever; pain.

Treuphadol Plus *Treupha, Switz.*
Paracetamol (p.72·2); codeine phosphate (p.26·1).
Fever; pain.

Trevilor *Wyeth, Ger.*
Venlafaxine hydrochloride (p.311·2).
Depression.

Trevintix *CSL, Austral.*†.
Prothionamide (p.241·1).
Tuberculosis.

Trevis *Kabi, Swed.*†.
4 Strains of *Lactobacillus* (p.1594·1).
Diarrhoea.

Trewilor *Wyeth Lederle, Aust.*
Venlafaxine hydrochloride (p.311·2).
Depression.

Trexan *Du Pont, USA.*
Naltrexone hydrochloride (p.988·1).
Opioid dependence.

TRH Prem *Zyma, Spain*†.
Protirelin (p.1259·1).
Evaluation of thyroid function.

TRH UCB *UCB, Belg.*
Protirelin (p.1259·1).
Test of hypothalamic-pituitary-thyroid axis, prolactin secretion, growth hormone secretion.

TRH-Cambridge *Cambridge, UK.*
Protirelin (p.1259·1).
Now known as Protirelin.
Diagnosis of hypothalamic-pituitary-thyroid dysfunction.

Tri *Vita, Ital.*†.
Nitrazepam (p.682·2).
Insomnia.

Tri Hachemina *Medea, Spain.*
Inositol (p.1591·1); calcium pantothenate (p.1352·3); aminobenzoic acid (p.1486·3) or sodium aminobenzoate.
Infertility; skin disorders.

Tri Viaben *Schurholz, Ger.*†.
Bromopride (p.1181·3); dimethicone (p.1213·1); pepsin (p.1616·3); alpha amylase (p.1549·1); lipase.
Gastro-intestinal disorders.

Tri Vit with Fluoride *Barre-National, USA.*
Multivitamin preparation with fluoride (p.742·1).
Dental caries prophylaxis; dietary supplement.

Tri-Ac *Zyma, UK*†.
Ethyl lactate (p.1082·2); zinc sulphate (p.1373·2).
Acne.

Tri-Ac Medicated Cleanser *Zyma, UK*†.
Chlorhexidine gluconate (p.1107·2); alcohol (p.1099·1); cocamidopropyl betaine.

Triacana *Marcofina, Fr.*
Tiratricol (p.1499·3).
Thyroid disorders; treatment of cellulite.

Triacelluvax *Chiron, Ital.*
A diphtheria, tetanus, and acellular pertussis vaccine (p.1509·1).
Formerly known as Acelluvax DTP.
Active immunisation.

Triacet *Lemmon, USA.*
Triamcinolone acetonide (p.1050·2).
Skin disorders.

Triacilline *Beecham, Belg.*
Ticarcillin sodium (p.263·2).
Bacterial infections.

Triacomb *Technilab, Canad.*
Triamcinolone acetonide (p.1050·2); nystatin (p.386·1); neomycin sulphate (p.229·2); gramicidin (p.215·2).
Anal and vulvar pruritus; infected skin disorders.

Triad *UAD, USA.*
Butalbital (p.644·3); paracetamol (p.72·2); caffeine (p.749·3).

Triadapin *Novopharm, Canad.*
Doxepin hydrochloride (p.283·2).
Depression.

Tri-Adcortyl *Squibb, UK.*
Nystatin (p.386·1); triamcinolone acetonide (p.1050·2); neomycin sulphate (p.229·2); gramicidin (p.215·2).
Bacterial and fungal skin infections.

Triadene *Schering, UK.*
Ethinyloestradiol (p.1445·1); gestodene (p.1447·2).
Triphasic oral contraceptive.

Triaderm *Taro, Canad.*
Triamcinolone acetonide (p.1050·2).
Skin disorders.

Triafed *Schein, USA.*
Pseudoephedrine hydrochloride (p.1068·3); triprolidine hydrochloride (p.420·3).
Upper respiratory-tract symptoms.

Triafed with Codeine *Schein, USA.*
Pseudoephedrine hydrochloride (p.1068·3); triprolidine hydrochloride (p.420·3); codeine phosphate (p.26·1).
Coughs.

Triaformo *Cusi, Spain†.*
Clioquinol (p.193·2); triamcinolone acetonide (p.1050·2).
Infected skin disorders.

Triagynon *Schering, Spain.*
Levonorgestrel (p.1454·1); ethinyloestradiol (p.1445·1).
Triphasic oral contraceptive.

Trialix
Hoechst, Aust.; Hoechst Marion Roussel, Irl.; Hoechst Marion Roussel, Switz.
Ramipril (p.941·1); piretanide (p.931·3).
Hypertension.

Trialmin *Menarini, Spain.*
Gemfibrozil (p.1273·3).
Hyperlipidaemias.

Trialodine *Quantum, USA†.*
Trazodone hydrochloride (p.308·3).

Trialone *Janssen-Cilag, S.Afr.*
Miconazole nitrate (p.384·3); triamcinolone acetonide (p.1050·2); neomycin sulphate (p.229·2).
Infected skin disorders.

Trialyn DM *Trianon, Canad.*
Dextromethorphan hydrobromide (p.1057·3); diphenhydramine hydrochloride (p.409·1); ammonium chloride (p.1055·2).
Coughs.

Triam
Lichtenstein, Ger.; Hyrex, USA.
Triamcinolone acetonide (p.1050·2) or triamcinolone diacetate (p.1050·2).
Corticosteroid.

Triam-A *Hyrex, USA.*
Triamcinolone acetonide (p.1050·2).
Corticosteroid.

Triamaxco *Ashbourne, UK.*
Triamterene (p.957·2); hydrochlorothiazide (p.885·2).
These ingredients can be described by the British Approved Name Co-triamterzide.
Hypertension; oedema.

Triamcinair *Pharmafair, USA†.*
Triamcinolone acetonide (p.1050·2).

Triamco *Norton, UK.*
Hydrochlorothiazide (p.885·2); triamterene (p.957·2).
These ingredients can be described by the British Approved Name Co-triamterzide.
Hypertension; oedema.

Triamcort *Helvepharm, Switz.*
Triamcinolone acetonide (p.1050·2).
Corticosteroid.

TriamCreme *Lichtenstein, Ger.*
Triamcinolone acetonide (p.1050·2).
Skin disorders.

Triamer *Pasteur Merieux, Belg.*
An adsorbed diphtheria, tetanus, and pertussis vaccine (p.1509·1).
Active immunisation of infants and young children.

Triamgalen *Pharmagalen, Ger.*
Triamcinolone acetonide (p.1050·2).
Formerly known as Triamcort-Pharmagalen.
Allergic and inflammatory skin disorders.

Triamhexal *Hexal, Ger.*
Triamcinolone acetonide (p.1050·2).
Corticosteroid.

Triami *Sandoz, S.Afr.†.*
Phenylpropanolamine hydrochloride (p.1067·2); pheniramine maleate (p.415·3); mepyramine maleate (p.414·1); caffeine (p.749·3).
Nasal congestion; rhinitis; sinusitis.

Triaminic
Note. This name is used for preparations of different composition.
Wander, Belg.†; Novartis, Ital.; Wander, Switz.†.
Tablets: Phenylpropanolamine hydrochloride (p.1067·2); pheniramine maleate (p.415·3); mepyramine maleate (p.414·1); caffeine (p.749·3).
Cold symptoms; rhinitis.

Sandoz, Canad.
Paediatric oral drops: Pseudoephedrine hydrochloride (p.1068·3).

Sandoz, Canad.; Sandoz, Fr.; Novartis Consumer, S.Afr.; Wander, Switz.†.
Paediatric oral drops; syrup; tablets: Phenylpropanolamine hydrochloride (p.1067·2); pheniramine maleate (p.415·3); mepyramine maleate (p.414·1).
Nasal and sinus congestion.

Novartis, Ital.
Nasal spray: Chlorpheniramine maleate (p.405·1); oxymetazoline hydrochloride (p.1065·3).
Nasal congestion.

Sandoz Consumer, USA.
Phenylpropanolamine hydrochloride (p.1067·2); chlorpheniramine maleate (p.405·1).
Formerly contained mepyramine maleate, pheniramine maleate, and phenylpropanolamine hydrochloride.
Upper respiratory-tract symptoms.

Triaminic-12 *Sandoz Consumer, USA.*
Phenylpropanolamine hydrochloride (p.1067·2); chlorpheniramine maleate (p.405·1).
Cold symptoms.

Triaminic Allergy *Sandoz Consumer, USA.*
Phenylpropanolamine hydrochloride (p.1067·2); chlorpheniramine maleate (p.405·1).
Upper respiratory-tract symptoms.

Triaminic AM Cough & Decongestant Formula *Sandoz Consumer, USA.*
Pseudoephedrine hydrochloride (p.1068·3); dextromethorphan hydrobromide (p.1057·3).

Triaminic AM Decongestant Formula *Sandoz Consumer, USA.*
Pseudoephedrine hydrochloride (p.1068·3).

Triaminic Chewable *Sandoz Consumer, USA.*
Phenylpropanolamine hydrochloride (p.1067·2); chlorpheniramine maleate (p.405·1).
Upper respiratory-tract symptoms.

Triaminic Cold *Sandoz Consumer, USA.*
Phenylpropanolamine hydrochloride (p.1067·2); chlorpheniramine maleate (p.405·1).
Cold symptoms.

Triaminic Cold & Allergy *Sandoz, Canad.*
Phenylpropanolamine hydrochloride (p.1067·2); chlorpheniramine maleate (p.405·1).
Nasal and sinus congestion.

Triaminic Cold & Fever *Sandoz, Canad.*
Pseudoephedrine hydrochloride (p.1068·3); dextromethorphan hydrobromide (p.1057·3); paracetamol (p.72·2).

Triaminic Decongestant & Expectorant *Sandoz, Canad.*
Pseudoephedrine hydrochloride (p.1068·3); guaiphenesin (p.1061·3).

Triaminic DM
Note. This name is used for preparations of different composition.
Sandoz, Canad.
Dextromethorphan hydrobromide (p.1057·3).
Coughs.

Sandoz Consumer, USA.
Phenylpropanolamine hydrochloride (p.1067·2); dextromethorphan hydrobromide (p.1057·3).
Coughs and cold symptoms.

Triaminic DM Daytime *Sandoz, Canad.*
Dextromethorphan hydrobromide (p.1057·3); phenylpropanolamine hydrochloride (p.1067·2); guaiphenesin (p.1061·3).
Coughs and cold symptoms.

Triaminic DM Expectorant *Sandoz, Canad.*
Dextromethorphan hydrobromide (p.1057·3); pseudoephedrine hydrochloride (p.1068·3); chlorpheniramine maleate (p.405·1); guaiphenesin (p.1061·3).
Formerly contained dextromethorphan hydrobromide, phenylpropanolamine hydrochloride, pheniramine maleate, mepyramine maleate, and guaiphenesin.
Coughs; nasal congestion.

Triaminic DM Nighttime *Sandoz, Canad.*
Dextromethorphan hydrobromide (p.1057·3); chlorpheniramine maleate (p.405·1); pseudoephedrine hydrochloride (p.1068·3).
Coughs; nasal congestion.

Triaminic DM-D *Sandoz, Canad.*
Dextromethorphan hydrobromide (p.1057·3); pseudoephedrine hydrochloride (p.1068·3).
Coughs; nasal and sinus congestion.

Triaminic Expectorant
Note. This name is used for preparations of different composition.
Sandoz, Canad.
Pseudoephedrine hydrochloride (p.1068·3); chlorpheniramine maleate (p.405·1); guaiphenesin (p.1061·3).
Formerly contained phenylpropanolamine hydrochloride, pheniramine maleate, mepyramine maleate, and guaiphenesin.
Coughs; nasal congestion.

Sandoz Consumer, USA.
Phenylpropanolamine hydrochloride (p.1067·2); guaiphenesin (p.1061·3).
Coughs.

Triaminic Expectorant with Codeine *Sandoz Consumer, USA.*
Codeine phosphate (p.26·1); phenylpropanolamine hydrochloride (p.1067·2); guaiphenesin (p.1061·3).
Coughs.

Triaminic Expectorant DH
Sandoz, Canad.; Sandoz Consumer, USA.
Hydrocodone tartrate (p.43·1); phenylpropanolamine hydrochloride (p.1067·2); pheniramine maleate (p.415·3); mepyramine maleate (p.414·1); guaiphenesin (p.1061·3).
Coughs.

Triaminic Night Time Rub *Sandoz, Canad.*
Camphor (p.1557·2); eucalyptus oil (p.1578·1); menthol (p.1600·2).

Triaminic Nite Light *Sandoz Consumer, USA.*
Pseudoephedrine hydrochloride (p.1068·3); chlorpheniramine maleate (p.405·1); dextromethorphan hydrobromide (p.1057·3).
Coughs and cold symptoms.

Triaminic Oral Infant *Sandoz Consumer, USA.*
Phenylpropanolamine hydrochloride (p.1067·2); mepyramine maleate (p.414·1); pheniramine maleate (p.415·3).
Upper respiratory-tract symptoms.

Triaminic Pediatric Drops *Sandoz, Canad.*
Pseudoephedrine hydrochloride (p.1068·3).

Triaminic Sore Throat Formula *Sandoz Consumer, USA.*
Pseudoephedrine hydrochloride (p.1068·3); dextromethorphan hydrobromide (p.1057·3); paracetamol (p.72·2).
Coughs and cold symptoms.

Triaminicflu *Novartis, Ital.*
Paracetamol (p.72·2); pheniramine maleate (p.415·3); phenylephrine hydrochloride (p.1066·2).
Cold and influenza symptoms.

Triaminicin *Sandoz, Canad.*
Phenylpropanolamine hydrochloride (p.1067·2); mepyramine maleate (p.414·1); pheniramine maleate (p.415·3); paracetamol (p.72·2); caffeine (p.749·3).
Cold symptoms.

Triaminicin Cold, Allergy, Sinus *Sandoz Consumer, USA.*
Phenylpropanolamine hydrochloride (p.1067·2); chlorpheniramine maleate (p.405·1); paracetamol (p.72·2).
Upper respiratory-tract symptoms.

Triaminicol *Sandoz, Ital.†.*
Phenylpropanolamine hydrochloride (p.1067·2); pheniramine maleate (p.415·3); mepyramine maleate (p.414·1).
Cold symptoms; rhinitis.

Triaminicol DM *Sandoz, Canad.*
Pseudoephedrine hydrochloride (p.1068·3); chlorpheniramine maleate (p.405·1); dextromethorphan hydrobromide (p.1057·3).
Formerly contained phenylpropanolamine hydrochloride, mepyramine maleate, pheniramine maleate, and dextromethorphan hydrobromide.
Coughs; nasal congestion.

Triaminicol Multi-Symptom Cough and Cold *Sandoz Consumer, USA.*
Phenylpropanolamine hydrochloride (p.1067·2); chlorpheniramine maleate (p.405·1); dextromethorphan hydrobromide (p.1057·3).
Coughs and cold symptoms.

Triaminicol Multi-Symptom Relief *Sandoz Consumer, USA.*
Phenylpropanolamine hydrochloride (p.1067·2); chlorpheniramine maleate (p.405·1); dextromethorphan hydrobromide (p.1057·3).
Coughs and cold symptoms.

Triam-Injekt *Sanorania, Ger.*
Triamcinolone acetonide (p.1050·2).
Corticosteroid.

Triamolone *Forest Pharmaceuticals, USA.*
Triamcinolone diacetate (p.1050·2).
Corticosteroid.

Triamonide *Forest Pharmaceuticals, USA.*
Triamcinolone acetonide (p.1050·2).
Corticosteroid.

Triam-oral *Sanorania, Ger.*
Triamcinolone (p.1050·2).
Corticosteroid.

Triampur *Dresden, Ger.*
Triamterene (p.957·2); hydrochlorothiazide (p.885·2).
Heart failure; hypertension; oedema.

TriamSalbe *Lichtenstein, Ger.*
Triamcinolone acetonide (p.1050·2).
Skin disorders.

Triamteren comp
Genericon, Aust.; Ratiopharm, Ger.
Triamterene (p.957·2); hydrochlorothiazide (p.885·2).
Heart failure; hypertension; oedema.

Triamteren-H *3M, Ger.*
Triamterene (p.957·2); hydrochlorothiazide (p.885·2).
Heart failure; hypertension; oedema.

Triamteril Complex *Farmitalia Carlo Erba, Ital.†.*
Triamterene (p.957·2); hydrochlorothiazide (p.885·2).
Hypertension; oedema.

Trianal
Will-Pharma, Belg.; Will-Pharma, Neth.
Triamcinolone acetonide (p.1050·2); lignocaine hydrochloride (p.1293·2).
Haemorrhoids; pruritus ani.

Tri-Anemul *Medopharm, Ger.*
Triamcinolone acetonide (p.1050·2).
Skin disorders.

Triaprin *Dunhall, USA†.*
Paracetamol (p.72·2); butalbital (p.644·3).
Pain.

Triaprin-DC *Dunhall, USA†.*
Dihydrocodeine tartrate (p.34·1); paracetamol (p.72·2); salicylamide (p.82·3).

Triapten *LAW, Ger.; Wyeth, Ger.*
Foscarnet sodium (p.610·2).
Local herpes simplex virus infections.

Tri-Aqua *Pfeiffer, USA.*
Caffeine (p.749·3); buchu (p.1555·2); bearberry (p.1552·2); zea; triticum.
Oedema associated with premenstrual syndrome.

Triarese *Hexal, Ger.*
Triamterene (p.957·2); hydrochlorothiazide (p.885·2).
Heart failure; hypertension; oedema.

Triasox *Berna, Spain.*
Thiabendazole (p.110·1).
Worm infections.

Triasporin *Italfarmaco, Ital.*
Itraconazole (p.381·3).
Fungal infections.

Triastonal *Osterholz, Ger.*
Sitosterol (p.1279·3).
Benign prostatic hyperplasia.

Triatec
Hoechst, Fr.; Hoechst Marion Roussel, Ital.; Hoechst Marion Roussel, Norw.; Hoechst Marion Roussel, Swed.; Hoechst Marion Roussel, Switz.
Ramipril (p.941·1).
Heart failure; hypertension; myocardial infarction.

Triatec-8 *Trianon, Canad.*
Paracetamol (p.72·2); codeine phosphate (p.26·1); caffeine citrate (p.749·3).
Coughs; fever; pain.

Triatec-30 *Trianon, Canad.*
Paracetamol (p.72·2); codeine phosphate (p.26·1).
Coughs; fever; pain.

Triatec comp
Hoechst Marion Roussel, Swed.; Hoechst Marion Roussel, Switz.
Ramipril (p.941·1); hydrochlorothiazide (p.885·2).
Hypertension.

Triatec HCT *Hoechst Marion Roussel, Ital.*
Ramipril (p.941·1); hydrochlorothiazide (p.885·2).
Hypertension.

Triatop *Janssen-Cilag, Ital.*
Ketoconazole (p.383·1).
Scalp disorders.

Triaval *Orion, Switz.*
70 Tablets, oestradiol valerate (p.1455·2); 14 tablets, oestradiol valerate; medroxyprogesterone acetate (p.1448·3); 7 tablets, inert.
Menopausal disorders; osteoporosis.

Triavil
Merck Sharp & Dohme, Canad.; Merck Sharp & Dohme, USA.
Perphenazine (p.685·2); amitriptyline hydrochloride (p.273·3).
Mixed anxiety depressive states; schizophrenia.

Tri-A-Vite F *Major, USA.*
Multivitamin preparation with fluoride.

Triaz *Medicis, USA.*
Benzoyl peroxide (p.1079·2).
Acne.

Triazid *CT, Ger.*
Triamterene (p.957·2); hydrochlorothiazide (p.885·2).
Heart failure; hypertension; oedema.

Triazine *Lennon, S.Afr.†.*
Cyclizine hydrochloride (p.407·1).
Motion sickness; vertigo.

Tri-B3 *Rhone-Poulenc Rorer, Austral.†.*
Nicotinic acid (p.1351·2).
Hyperlipidaemias.

Triban *Great Southern, USA.*
Trimethobenzamide hydrochloride (p.420·1); benzocaine (p.1286·2).

Tribeton *Chemedica, Switz.*
Cyanocobalamin (p.1363·3) or hydroxocobalamin (p.1363·3); thiamine hydrochloride (p.1361·1); pyridoxine hydrochloride (p.1362·3).
Lignocaine hydrochloride (p.1293·2) is included in the injections to alleviate the pain of injection.
Alcoholism; nerve pain; neuritis; pain; vitamin B deficiency.

Tribilina *Farge, Ital.†.*
Cyclobutyrol sodium (p.1569·2); rhubarb (p.1212·1).
Gastro-intestinal disorders; liver disorders.

Tribiotic *3M, UK†.*
Neomycin sulphate (p.229·2); bacitracin zinc (p.157·3); polymyxin B sulphate (p.239·1).
Bacterial infections.

Tribiotic Plus *Thompson, USA.*
Polymyxin B sulphate (p.239·1); neomycin sulphate (p.229·2); bacitracin (p.157·3); lignocaine (p.1293·2).

Tribonat
Pharmacia Upjohn, Norw.; Pharmacia Upjohn, Swed.
Trometamol (p.1639·3); electrolytes (p.1147·1).
Buffer; metabolic and respiratory acidosis.

Tricandil
Prospa, Belg.; SPA, Ital.; Prospa, Switz.†.
Mepartricin (p.384·2).
Candidiasis; trichomoniasis.

Tricef
Note. This name is used for preparations of different composition.
Merck, Aust.; Astra, Swed.
Cefixime (p.165·3).
Bacterial infections.

Eurofarmaco, Ital.
Propylene glycol cefatrizine (p.164·2).
Bacterial infections.

Tricept *Cuprocept, S.Afr.*
Copper-wound plastic (p.1337·3).
Intra-uterine contraceptive device.

Trichazole *Intramed, S.Afr.; Lennon, S.Afr.*
Metronidazole (p.585·1).
Anaerobic bacterial infections; protozoal infections.

Trichex *Gerot, Aust.*
Metronidazole (p.585·1).
Gardnerella vaginalis infections; trichomoniasis.

Tri-Chlor *Gordon, USA.*
Trichloroacetic acid (p.1639·1).
Warts.

Trichlorol *Lysoform, Ger.*
Chloramine (p.1106·3).
Surface and hand disinfection.

Tricho Cordes *Ichthyol, Ger.†.*
Metronidazole (p.585·1).
Trichomoniasis.

Trichobiol *Therasophia, Fr.*
Amino-acid, mineral, vitamin, and herbal preparation.
Hair and nail disorders.

Tricho-Gynedron Noriston, S.Afr.†
Acetarsol sodium (p.578·2); sulphasomidine (p.257·1); borax (p.1554·2).
Vaginal trichomoniasis.

Trichotine Reed & Carnrick, USA.
Powder: Sodium lauryl sulphate (p.1468·3); sodium perborate (p.1125·2); sodium chloride (p.1162·2).
Solution: Sodium lauryl sulphate (p.1468·3); borax (p.1554·2); alcohol (p.1099·1).
Vaginal disorders.

Tri-Cicatrin Wellcome, UK†.
Neomycin sulphate (p.229·2); bacitracin zinc (p.157·3); nystatin (p.386·1); hydrocortisone (p.1043·3).
Skin disorders with bacterial or fungal infection.

Triciclor Wyeth, Spain.
Levonorgestrel (p.1454·1); ethinyloestradiol (p.1445·1).
Triphasic oral contraceptive.

Tricidine Warner-Lambert Consumer, Belg.
Tyrothricin (p.267·2); lignocaine hydrochloride (p.1293·2).
Mouth and throat disorders.

TriCilest Janssen-Cilag, Aust.
Norgestimate (p.1453·3); ethinyloestradiol (p.1445·1).
Formerly known as Ortrel.
Triphasic oral contraceptive.

Tricin Cusi, Spain†.
Bacitracin zinc (p.157·3); neomycin sulphate (p.229·2); triamcinolone acetonide (p.1050·2).
Infected skin disorders.

Tri-Clear Warner Chilcott, USA†.
Phenylpropanolamine hydrochloride (p.1067·2); chlorpheniramine maleate (p.405·1).

Tri-Clear Expectorant Warner Chilcott, USA†.
Phenylpropanolamine hydrochloride (p.1067·2); guaiphenesin (p.1061·3).

Tricloryl
Galen, Irl.; Glaxo Wellcome, S.Afr.†.
Triclofos (p.697·2) or triclofos sodium (p.697·2).
Hypnotic; sedative.

Triclose ICT, Ital.
Azanidazole (p.580·2).
Vaginal trichomoniasis.

Triclosept Houghs Healthcare, UK†.
Triclosan (p.1127·2).
Skin disinfection.

Tri-Co
Note. A similar name is used for preparations of different composition.
Garec, S.Afr.
Co-trimoxazole (p.196·3).
Bacterial infections.

Trico
Note. A similar name is used for preparations of different composition.
ICN, Spain†.
Minoxidil (p.910·3).
Alopecia androgenetica.

Tricodein
Chemieprodukte, Aust.; Solco, Ger.; Solco, Switz.
Codeine phosphate (p.26·1).
Coughs.

Tricodene Cough & Cold Pfeiffer, USA.
Mepyramine maleate (p.414·1); codeine phosphate (p.26·1).
Coughs and cold symptoms.

Tricodene Forte Pfeiffer, USA.
Phenylpropanolamine hydrochloride (p.1067·2); chlorpheniramine maleate (p.405·1); dextromethorphan hydrobromide (p.1057·3).
Coughs and cold symptoms.

Tricodene NN Pfeiffer, USA.
Phenylpropanolamine hydrochloride (p.1067·2); chlorpheniramine maleate (p.405·1); dextromethorphan hydrobromide (p.1057·3).
Coughs and cold symptoms.

Tricodene Pediatric Cough & Cold Pfeiffer, USA.
Phenylpropanolamine hydrochloride (p.1067·2); dextromethorphan hydrobromide (p.1057·3).
Coughs and cold symptoms.

Tricodene Sugar Free Pfeiffer, USA.
Chlorpheniramine maleate (p.405·1); dextromethorphan hydrobromide (p.1057·3).
Coughs and cold symptoms.

Tricofur Formenti, Ital.†.
Nifuroxime (p.386·1); furazolidone (p.583·1).
Bacterial, trichomonal, and candidal infections.

Tricol Softgels Ram, USA.
Omega-3 marine triglycerides (p.1276·1).

Tricolam Pfizer, Spain.
Tinidazole (p.594·1).
Anaerobic bacterial infections; protozoal infections.

Tri-Cold Labima, Belg.
Diphenylpyraline hydrochloride (p.409·3); phenylephrine hydrochloride (p.1066·2); terpin hydrate (p.1070·2).
Cold symptoms; hay fever; hypersensitivity reactions; nasal congestion; sinusitis.

Tricom Nutripharm, USA.
Pseudoephedrine hydrochloride (p.1068·3); chlorpheniramine maleate (p.405·1); paracetamol (p.72·2).
Upper respiratory-tract symptoms.

Tricomicin Inibsa, Spain†.
Hachimycin (p.381·2).
Fungal infections; trichomoniasis.

Tricomox Pinewood, Irl.
Co-trimoxazole (p.196·3).
Bacterial infections.

Tricor Abbott, USA.
Fenofibrate (p.1273·1).
Hyperlipidaemias.

Tricortale Bergamon, Ital.†.
Triamcinolone (p.1050·2).
Corticosteroid.

Tricortin Fidia, Ital.
Phosphatides (p.1595·2); cyanocobalamin (p.1363·3).
Lignocaine hydrochloride (p.1293·2) is included in this preparation to alleviate the pain of injection.
Mental function disorders.

Tricosal Invamed, USA.
Choline magnesium trisalicylate (p.25·2).

Tricowas B Wasserman, Spain.
Metronidazole (p.585·1).
Anaerobic bacterial infections; dracunculiasis; protozoal infections.

Tricoxidil Bioindustria, Ital.
Minoxidil (p.910·3).
Alopecia androgenetica.

Tri-Cyclen Janssen-Ortho, Canad.
Norgestimate (p.1453·3); ethinyloestradiol (p.1445·1).
Triphasic oral contraceptive.

Tridelta Ceccarelli, Ital.
Cholecalciferol (p.1366·3).
Vitamin deficiency.

Triderm
Note. This name is used for preparations of different composition.
Essex, Switz.
Betamethasone dipropionate (p.1033·3); clotrimazole (p.376·3); gentamicin sulphate (p.212·1).
Infected skin disorders.

Del-Ray, USA.
Triamcinolone acetonide (p.1050·2).
Skin disorders.

Triderm 5 Bio Nike ICIM, Ital.
Barrier preparation.

Tridesilon
Note. This name is used for preparations of different composition.
Bayer, Canad.; Klinge, Ger.†; Miles, USA.
Cream; ointment: Desonide (p.1036·3).
Skin disorders.

Miles, USA†.
Ear drops: Desonide (p.1036·3); acetic acid (p.1541·2).
Superficial ear infections with inflammation.

Tridesonit Dome-Hollister-Stier, Fr.
Desonide (p.1036·3).
Skin disorders.

Tridestra
Orion, Irl.; Orion, UK.
70 Tablets, oestradiol valerate (p.1455·2); 14 tablets, oestradiol valerate; medroxyprogesterone acetate (p.1448·3); 7 tablets, inert.
Menopausal disorders; osteoporosis.

Tridigestine Hepatoum Hepatoum, Fr.†.
Pepsin (p.1616·3); pancreatin (p.1612·1); amylase (p.1549·1).
Dyspepsia.

Tridil
Boots, Austral.†; Du Pont, Canad.; Du Pont, Irl.; Boots, S.Afr.; Du Pont Pharmaceuticals, UK†; Faulding, USA.
Glyceryl trinitrate (p.874·3).
Control of blood pressure during surgery; heart failure; ischaemic heart disease.

Tridin
Opfermann, Ger.; Rottapharm, Ital.
Levoglutamide monofluorophosphate or sodium monofluorophosphate (p.743·3); calcium gluconate (p.1155·2); calcium citrate (p.1155·1).
Osteoporosis.

Tridione
Abbott, Ger.†; Abbott, USA.
Troxidone (p.361·1).
Absence seizures; myoclonic seizures.

Tridodilan Roussel, Ital.†.
Injection: Hydroxocobalamin acetate (p.1364·2); thiamine monophosphate chloride (p.1361·2); pyridoxine hydrochloride (p.1362·3); lignocaine hydrochloride (p.1293·2).
Tablets: Hydroxocobalamin acetate (p.1364·2); benfotiamine (p.1360·3); pyridoxine hydrochloride (p.1362·3).
Neuralgias; neuritis.

Tridomose Hoechst Marion Roussel, S.Afr.
Gestrinone (p.1447·3).
Endometriosis.

Tridrate Bowel Evacuant Kit Lafayette, USA.
Combination pack: Magnesium citrate solution (p.1198·2); 3 bisacodyl tablets (p.1179·3); 1 bisacodyl suppository (p.1179·3).
Constipation.

Triella Janssen-Cilag, Fr.
Norethisterone (p.1453·1); ethinyloestradiol (p.1445·1).
Triphasic oral contraceptive.

Triene Schiapparelli, Ital.
Polyenacid.
Barrier preparation; burns; skin irritation; wounds.

Triette Brenner-Efeka, Ger.
Levonorgestrel (p.1454·1); ethinyloestradiol (p.1445·1).
Triphasic oral contraceptive.

Trifed Geneva, USA.
Pseudoephedrine hydrochloride (p.1068·3); triprolidine hydrochloride (p.420·3).
Upper respiratory-tract symptoms.

Trifed-C Cough Geneva, USA.
Pseudoephedrine hydrochloride (p.1068·3); codeine phosphate (p.26·1); triprolidine hydrochloride (p.420·3).
Coughs and cold symptoms.

Trifeme Wyeth, Austral.
21 Tablets, ethinyloestradiol (p.1445·1); levonorgestrel (p.1454·1); 7 tablets, inert.
Triphasic oral contraceptive.

Trifen Be-Tabs, S.Afr.
Triprolidine hydrochloride (p.420·3); pseudoephedrine hydrochloride (p.1068·3); codeine phosphate (p.26·1); guaiphenesin (p.1061·3).
Coughs.

Triferm-Sulfa Merckle, Swed.†.
Co-trimoxazole (p.196·3).
Bacterial infections; Pneumocystis carinii pneumonia.

Triferon Salus, Ital.
Thiamine hydrochloride (p.1361·1); pyridoxine hydrochloride (p.1362·3); hydroxocobalamin (p.1363·3).
Neuralgia; neuritis; post-infection paresis; vitamin B deficiency.

Tri-Filena Organon, Aust.
White tablets, oestradiol valerate (p.1455·2); blue tablets, oestradiol valerate; medroxyprogesterone acetate (p.1448·3); yellow tablets, inert.
Menopausal disorders.

Tri-Flor-Vite with Fluoride Everett, USA.
Multivitamin and fluoride preparation (p.742·1).

Triflucan Pfizer, Fr.
Fluconazole (p.378·1).
Candidiasis; cryptococcal meningitis.

Trifluid Otsuka, Jpn.
Carbohydrate and electrolyte infusion.
Parenteral nutrition.

Triflumann Mann, Ger.
Trifluridine (p.627·3).
Herpesvirus keratitis.

Trifolium Complex Blackmores, Austral.
Rumex crispus; taraxacum (p.1634·2); trifolium pratense (p.1624·2); lappa (p.1594·2); zinc amino acid chelate (p.1373·3); vitamin A acetate (p.1359·2).
Skin disorders.

Trifortal Merck, Spain†.
Pyridoxal phosphate (p.1363·1); pyridoxamine hydrochloride; pyridoxine hydrochloride (p.1362·3).
Vitamin B_6 deficiency.

Trifosfaneurina
Note. This name is used for preparations of different composition.
Bruschettini, Ital.†.
Cocarboxylase chloride (p.1361·2).
Cardiomyopathy; neuritis; vitamin B1 deficiency.

Farma Lepori, Spain.
Vitamin B substances.
Lignocaine (p.1293·2) is included in the injection to alleviate the pain of injection.

Trifyba
Sanofi Winthrop, Irl.; Sanofi Winthrop, UK.
Wheat grain extract (p.1181·2).
Bowel disorders; constipation; haemorrhoids; stoma management.

Triga Couvreur, Belg.†.
Felypressin (p.1246·3); chlorhexidine gluconate (p.1107·2).
Throat disorders.

Trigastril
Salus, Aust.; Heumann, Ger.
Aluminium hydroxide gel (p.1177·3); magnesium hydroxide (p.1198·2); calcium carbonate (p.1182·1).
Gastro-intestinal disorders.

Trigesic Squibb, USA.
Paracetamol (p.72·2); aspirin (p.16·1); caffeine (p.749·3).
Pain.

Trigger Polifarma, Ital.
Ranitidine hydrochloride (p.1209·3).
Gastric hyperacidity; gastro-oesophageal reflux; peptic ulcer; Zollinger-Ellison syndrome.

Triglobe
Astra, Aust.; Astra, Ger.; Astra, Spain.
Sulphadiazine (p.252·3); trimethoprim (p.265·1).
Bacterial infections.

Triglysal
Note. This name is used for preparations of different composition.
Gallier, Fr.†.
Basic aluminium glycinate (p.1177·2); magnesium trisilicate (p.1199·1); ammonium glycyrrhizinate (p.1055·2).
Gastric hyperacidity.

Inibsa, Spain†.
Aluminium glycinate (p.1177·2); magnesium trisilicate (p.1199·1).
Gastro-intestinal disorders.

Trigoa LAW, Ger.
Levonorgestrel (p.1454·1); ethinyloestradiol (p.1445·1).
Triphasic oral contraceptive.

Trigon Depot Squibb, Spain.
Triamcinolone acetonide (p.1050·2).
Corticosteroid.

Trigon Rectal Squibb, Spain.
Lignocaine (p.1293·2); triamcinolone acetonide (p.1050·2).
Anorectal disorders.

Trigon Topico Squibb, Spain.
Amphotericin (p.372·2); gramicidin (p.215·2); neomycin sulphate (p.229·2); triamcinolone acetonide (p.1050·2).
Infected skin disorders.

Trigonyl Hoyer, Ger.†.
Co-trimoxazole (p.196·3).
Bacterial infections.

Trigynon
Schering, Aust.; Schering, Belg.; Schering, Ital.; Schering, Neth.
Levonorgestrel (p.1454·1); ethinyloestradiol (p.1445·1).
Triphasic oral contraceptive.

Trigynovin Schering, Spain.
Gestodene (p.1447·2); ethinyloestradiol (p.1445·1).
Triphasic oral contraceptive.

TriHEMIC Lederle, USA.
Ferrous fumarate (p.1339·3); vitamin B_{12} substances (p.1363·3); intrinsic factor concentrate; folic acid (p.1340·3); vitamin E.
Vitamin C (p.1365·2) is included in this preparation to increase the absorption and availability of ferrous fumarate; docusate sodium (p.1189·3) is included to reduce the constipating effects of ferrous fumarate.
Anaemias.

Triherpine
Ciba Vision, Ital.; Ciba Vision, Switz.
Trifluridine (p.627·3).
Herpes simplex infections of the eye.

Trihexy Geneva, USA.
Benzhexol hydrochloride (p.457·3).
Parkinsonism.

TriHIBit Pasteur Merieux, USA.
A diphtheria, tetanus, acellular pertussis, and haemophilus influenzae vaccine (p.1509·3).
Active immunisation.

Trihistalex Wolfs, Belg.
Diphenhydramine hydrochloride (p.409·1); cinchocaine hydrochloride (p.1289·2); nicotinamide (p.1351·2).
Cutaneous hypersensitivity reactions; pain.

Trihistan Weifa, Norw.
Chlorcyclizine hydrochloride (p.404·3).
Hypersensitivity reactions; motion sickness; nausea; vertigo.

Tri-Hydroserpine Rugby, USA.
Hydrochlorothiazide (p.885·2); reserpine (p.942·1); hydralazine hydrochloride (p.883·2).
Hypertension.

Tri-Immunol
Wyeth-Ayerst, Canad.; Lederle-Praxis, USA.
An adsorbed diphtheria, tetanus, and pertussis vaccine (p.1509·1).
Active immunisation.

Triiodothyronine Injection Medeva, UK.
Liothyronine sodium (p.1495·1).
Myxoedema coma.

Tri-K Century, USA.
Potassium acetate (p.1161·1); potassium bicarbonate (p.1153·1); potassium citrate (p.1153·1).
Hypokalaemia; potassium depletion.

Trikacide Pharmascience, Canad.
Metronidazole (p.585·1).
Bacterial infections; protozoal infections.

Tri-Kort Keene, USA.
Triamcinolone acetonide (p.1050·2).
Corticosteroid.

Trilafon
Schering-Plough, Austral.†; Schering-Plough, Belg.; Schering, Canad.; Schering-Plough, Ital.; Schering-Plough, Neth.; Schering-Plough, Norw.; Scherag, S.Afr.; Schering-Plough, Swed.; Essex, Switz.; Schering, USA.
Perphenazine (p.685·2), perphenazine decanoate (p.685·3), or perphenazine enanthate (p.685·3).
Alcohol withdrawal syndrome; anxiety; behaviour disorders; depression; hiccup; nausea; pain; premedication; pruritus; psychoses; vomiting.

Trilagavit Lagap, Switz.†.
Thiamine hydrochloride (p.1361·1) or thiamine nitrate (p.1361·1); pyridoxine hydrochloride (p.1362·3); cyanocobalamin (p.1363·3).
Peripheral neuropathies.

Trilam Gerard, Irl.
Triazolam (p.696·3).
Insomnia.

Trileptal
Ciba-Geigy, Aust.; Ciba, Ital.; Novartis, Neth.; Novartis, S.Afr.; Geigy, Switz.
Oxcarbazepine (p.349·2).
Epilepsy.

Tri-Levlen Berlex, USA.
Levonorgestrel (p.1454·1); ethinyloestradiol (p.1445·1).
28-Day packs also contain 7 inert tablets.
Triphasic oral contraceptive.

Trilifan Schering-Plough, Fr.
Perphenazine enanthate (p.685·3).
Psychoses.

Trilisate
Purdue Frederick, Canad.; Napp, Irl.†; Napp, UK†; Purdue Frederick, USA.
Choline magnesium trisalicylate (p.25·2).
Fever; inflammation; musculoskeletal and joint disorders; pain.

Trillium Complex Blackmores, Austral.
Trillium erectum; geranium maculatum; hydrastis (p.1588·2); ginseng (p.1584·2); *d*-alpha tocopheryl acid succinate (p.1369·2).
Menorrhagia.

Triloc Astra, Aust.
Metoprolol tartrate (p.907·3); hydrochlorothiazide (p.885·2); hydralazine hydrochloride (p.883·2).
Hypertension.

Trilog Hauck, USA.
Triamcinolone acetonide (p.1050·2).
Corticosteroid.

Trilombrin Pfizer, Spain.
Pyrantel embonate (p.109·3).
Worm infections.

Trilone Hauck, USA.
Triamcinolone diacetate (p.1050·2).
Corticosteroid.

Triludan
Albert-Roussel, Aust.; Hoechst Marion Roussel, Belg.; Hoechst Marion Roussel, Irl.; Hoechst Marion Roussel, Ital.†; Hoechst Marion Roussel, Neth.; Hoechst Marion Roussel, S.Afr.; Marion Merrell, Spain; Hoechst Marion Roussel, Switz.; Hoechst Marion Roussel, UK.
Terfenadine (p.418·1).
Hypersensitivity reactions.

Trim Herdel, Ital.†.
Co-trimoxazole (p.196·3).
Bacterial infections.

Trimag Magis, Ital.†.
Oxitriptan (p.301·2).
Depression; Down's syndrome; epilepsy; insomnia; movement disorders; pain; parkinsonism; phenylketonuria; vascular headache.

Trimalcina Isnardi, Ital.†.
Amylase (p.1549·1); cellulase (p.1561·1); trypsin (p.1640·1); chymotrypsin (p.1563·2); lipase; dimethicone (p.1213·1); pepsin (p.1616·3).
Digestive disorders; dyspepsia; flatulence.

Trimanyl Tosse, Ger.†.
Trimethoprim (p.265·1).
Bacterial infections of the urinary tract.

Trimaran Benvegna, Ital.†.
Vitamin B substances.

Trimatrim Belphar, Belg.†.
Sulphadiazine (p.252·3); trimethoprim (p.265·1).
Bacterial infections.

Trimazide Major, USA.
Trimethobenzamide hydrochloride (p.420·1).
Nausea and vomiting.

Trimed Rorer, Ital.†.
Trimethoprim (p.265·1); sulfametopyrazine (p.251·3).
Bacterial infections.

Trimedat Italfarmaco, Ital.
Trimebutine maleate (p.1639·3).
Gastro-intestinal spasm; irritable bowel disease; oesophageal motility disorders.

Trimedil
Zyma, Aust.; Zyma, Belg.†; Zyma, Switz.†.
Paracetamol (p.72·2); phenylephrine hydrochloride (p.1066·2); dimethindene maleate (p.408·3); ascorbic acid (p.1365·2); oxerutins (p.1580·2).
Cold symptoms.

Trimedil N Zyma, Ger.†.
Dimethindene maleate (p.408·3); paracetamol (p.72·2).
Cold symptoms; influenza.

Trimetabol Uriach, Spain.
Cyproheptadine acephyllinate (p.407·3); amino acids and vitamins.
Anorexia; tonic; weight loss.

Trimetho comp Strallhofer, Aust.
Co-trimoxazole (p.196·3).
Bacterial infections.

Trimethox Caps, S.Afr.
Co-trimoxazole (p.196·3).
Bacterial infections.

Trimeton Schering-Plough, Ital.
Chlorpheniramine maleate (p.405·1).
Hypersensitivity reactions.

Trimetoprim-Sulfa Selena, Swed.†.
Co-trimoxazole (p.196·3).
Bacterial infections; Pneumocystis carinii pneumonia.

Trimin sulfa Astra, Swed.
Sulphadiazine (p.252·3); trimethoprim (p.265·1).
Urinary-tract infections.

Triminol Cough Rugby, USA.
Phenylpropanolamine hydrochloride (p.1067·2); chlorpheniramine maleate (p.405·1); dextromethorphan hydrobromide (p.1057·3).
Coughs and cold symptoms.

Tri-Minulet
Wyeth Lederle, Aust.; Wyeth, Austral.; Wyeth Lederle, Belg.; Wyeth, Fr.; Wyeth, Irl.; Wyeth, Ital.; Wyeth, Neth.; Akromed, S.Afr.; Wyeth, Spain; Wyeth, Switz.†; Wyeth, UK.
Gestodene (p.1447·2); ethinyloestradiol (p.1445·1).
28-Day packs also contain 7 inert tablets.
Triphasic oral contraceptive.

TriMix E Pharmacia Upjohn, Aust.
Amino-acid, carbohydrate, lipid (from soya oil (p.1355·1)), and electrolyte infusion.
Contains egg lecithin.
Parenteral nutrition.

Trimogal Lagap, UK.
Trimethoprim (p.265·1).
Bronchitis; urinary-tract infections.

Trimoks Docmed, S.Afr.
Co-trimoxazole (p.196·3).
Bacterial infections.

Trimolex Zurich, S.Afr.†.
Amiloride hydrochloride (p.819·2); hydrochlorothiazide (p.885·2).
Hypertension; oedema.

Trimonase Tosi, Ital.
Tinidazole (p.594·1).
Amoebiasis; giardiasis; trichomoniasis.

Trimonil
Desitin, Norw.; Desitin, Swed.
Carbamazepine (p.339·2).
Alcohol withdrawal syndrome; bipolar disorder; diabetes insipidus; diabetic neuropathy; epilepsy; mania; trigeminal neuralgia.

Trimono Procter & Gamble, Ger.
Trimethoprim (p.265·1).
Bacterial infections of the urinary tract.

Trimopan Berk, UK.
Trimethoprim (p.265·1).
Urinary- and respiratory-tract infections.

Trimo-San Milex, USA.
Hydroxyquinoline sulphate (p.1589·3); boric acid (p.1554·2); borax (p.1554·2); sodium lauryl sulphate (p.1468·3); glycerol (p.1585·2).
Vaginal deodoriser.

Trimovate Glaxo, UK.
Clobetasone butyrate (p.1035·3); oxytetracycline calcium (p.235·1); nystatin (p.386·1).
Skin disorders with bacterial or fungal infection.

Trimovax
Pasteur, Fr.†; Pasteur Merieux, Ital.; Rhone-Poulenc Rorer, S.Afr.; Merieux, Switz.†.
A measles, mumps, and rubella vaccine (Schwarz, Urabe Am-9, and Wistar RA 27/3M strains respectively) (p.1519·3).
Active immunisation.

Trimox Apothecon, USA.
Amoxycillin trihydrate (p.151·3).
Bacterial infections.

Trimoxol Yamanouchi, Neth.
Co-trimoxazole (p.196·3).
Bacterial infections; Pneumocystis carinii pneumonia.

Trimpex Roche, USA.
Trimethoprim (p.265·1).
Urinary-tract infections.

Trimstat Laser, USA.
Phendimetrazine tartrate (p.1484·2).
Obesity.

Trimysten Bellon, Fr.†.
Clotrimazole (p.376·3).
Erythrasma; fungal infections.

Trimzol Schwulst, S.Afr.
Co-trimoxazole (p.196·3).
Bacterial infections.

Trinagesic Propan, S.Afr.
Meprobamate (p.678·1); paracetamol (p.72·2); codeine phosphate (p.26·1).
Pain and associated tension.

Trinalin
Schering, Canad.; Schering, USA.
Azatadine maleate (p.402·3); pseudoephedrine sulphate (p.1068·3).
Allergic rhinitis; Eustachian tube congestion; nasal congestion.

Trind Mead Johnson Nutritionals, USA.
Phenylpropanolamine hydrochloride (p.1067·2); chlorpheniramine maleate (p.405·1).
Upper respiratory-tract symptoms.

Tri-Nefrin Extra Strength Pfeiffer, USA.
Phenylpropanolamine hydrochloride (p.1067·2); chlorpheniramine maleate (p.405·1).
Upper respiratory-tract symptoms.

Trinevrina B6 Guidotti, Ital.
Thiamine hydrochloride (p.1361·1); pyridoxine hydrochloride (p.1362·3); cyanocobalamin (p.1363·3).
Lignocaine hydrochloride (p.1293·2) is included in the intramuscular injection to alleviate the pain of injection.
Neuralgias; neuritis; radiation sickness; toxicosis.

Triniagar Daker Farmasimes, Spain.
Mebutizide (p.901·3); triamterene (p.957·2).
Hypertension; oedema.

Trinidex Diaco, Ital.
Glucose and vitamin infusion.
Parenteral nutrition.

Triniol Syntex, Spain.
Injection: Paramethasone acetate (p.1047·3); paramethasone disodium phosphate (p.1047·3).
Tablets†: Paramethasone acetate (p.1047·3).
Corticosteroid.

Trinipatch
Synthelabo, Fr.; Lorex Synthelabo, Neth.
Glyceryl trinitrate (p.874·3).
Angina pectoris.

Triniplas Novartis, Ital.
Glyceryl trinitrate (p.874·3).
Angina pectoris.

Triniton Apogepha, Ger.
Dihydralazine sulphate (p.854·1); hydrochlorothiazide (p.885·2); reserpine (p.942·1).
Hypertension.

Trinitran Theraplix, Fr.†.
Glyceryl trinitrate (p.874·3).
Angina pectoris; heart failure.

Trinitrina Pharmacia Upjohn, Ital.
Glyceryl trinitrate (p.874·3).
Angina pectoris; cardiac stenosis.

Trinitrine Sodip, Switz.
Glyceryl trinitrate (p.874·3).
Angina pectoris; heart failure; pulmonary oedema.

Trinitrosan Merck, Ger.
Glyceryl trinitrate (p.874·3).
Heart failure; hypertensive crisis; myocardial infarction.

Trinordiol
Wyeth Lederle, Aust.; Wyeth Lederle, Belg.; Wyeth, Fr.; Wyeth, Ger.; Wyeth, Irl.; Wyeth, Ital.; Wyeth, Neth.; Wyeth, Norw.; Wyeth Lederle, Swed.; Wyeth, Switz.; Wyeth, UK.
Levonorgestrel (p.1454·1); ethinyloestradiol (p.1445·1).
28-Day packs also contain 7 inert tablets.
Triphasic oral contraceptive.

Tri-Norinyl Syntex, USA.
Norethisterone (p.1453·1); ethinyloestradiol (p.1445·1).
28-Day packs also contain 7 inert tablets.
Triphasic oral contraceptive.

TRI-Normin Zeneca, Ger.
Atenolol (p.825·3); chlorthalidone (p.839·3); hydralazine hydrochloride (p.883·2).
Hypertension.

Trinovum
Janssen-Cilag, Aust.; Janssen-Cilag, Belg.; Janssen-Cilag, Ger.; Janssen-Cilag, Irl.; Janssen-Cilag, Ital.; Janssen-Cilag, Neth.; Janssen-Cilag, S.Afr.; Janssen-Cilag, Swed.; Janssen-Cilag, Switz.; Cilag, UK.
Norethisterone (p.1453·1); ethinyloestradiol (p.1445·1).
28-Day packs also contain 7 inert tablets.
Triphasic oral contraceptive.

Trinsicon
Lilly, Aust.; Lilly, Canad.†; Lilly, S.Afr.; UCB, USA.
Vitamin B $_{12}$ (p.1363·3); ferrous fumarate (p.1339·3); folic acid (p.1340·3); intrinsic factor.
Vitamin C (p.1365·2) is included in this preparation to increase the absorption and availability of iron.
Anaemias.

Trinsicon M Russ, USA†.
Liver-stomach concentrate; vitamin B_{12}; ferrous fumarate (p.1339·3).
Ascorbic acid (p.1365·2) is included in this preparation to increase the absorption and availability of iron.
Anaemias.

Trinuride Wolfs, Belg.†.
Pheneturide (p.350·1); phenytoin sodium (p.352·3); phenobarbitone (p.350·2).
Epilepsy.

Triocaps Vifor, Switz.
Chlorpheniramine maleate (p.405·1); phenylephrine hydrochloride (p.1066·2).
Upper-respiratory-tract disorders.

Triocetin OFF, Ital.
Triacetyloleandomycin (p.264·3).
Bacterial infections.

Triodeen Schering, Neth.
Gestodene (p.1447·2); ethinyloestradiol (p.1445·1).
Triphasic oral contraceptive.

Trioden ED Schering, Austral.
21 Tablets, gestodene (p.1447·2); ethinyloestradiol (p.1445·1); 7 tablets, inert.
Triphasic oral contraceptive.

Triodena Schering, Aust.
Gestodene (p.1447·2); ethinyloestradiol (p.1445·1).
Triphasic oral contraceptive.

Triodene
Schering, Belg.; Schering, Irl.; Schering, S.Afr.
Gestodene (p.1447·2); ethinyloestradiol (p.1445·1).
28-Day packs also contain 7 inert tablets.
Triphasic oral contraceptive.

Triodurin
Pharmacia Upjohn, Aust.; Kabi, Swed.†.
Polyoestriol phosphate (p.1459·2).
Mepivacaine hydrochloride (p.1297·2) is included in this preparation to alleviate the pain of injection.
Menopausal disorders; oestrogen deficiency.

Triofan Vifor, Switz.
Xylometazoline hydrochloride (p.1071·2); carbocisteine (p.1056·3).
Upper-respiratory-tract disorders.

Triofed Barre-National, USA.
Pseudoephedrine hydrochloride (p.1068·3); triprolidine hydrochloride (p.420·3).
Upper respiratory-tract symptoms.

Triofusin Kabi Pharmacia, Ger.†.
Carbohydrate infusion.
Parenteral nutrition.

Triofusin E Kabi Pharmacia, Ger.†.
Carbohydrate and electrolyte infusion.
Parenteral nutrition.

Triogene Medecine Vegetale, Fr.
Kola (p.1645·1); gentian (p.1583·3); magnesium chloride (p.1157·2); ferrous gluconate (p.1340·1).
Tonic.

Triogesic
Intercare, Irl.; Intercare, UK.
Phenylpropanolamine hydrochloride (p.1067·2); paracetamol (p.72·2).
Nasal congestion.

Triogestena Schering, Aust.
Gestodene (p.1447·2); ethinyloestradiol (p.1445·1).
Triphasic oral contraceptive.

Triogestin Wyeth Lederle, Aust.
Gestodene (p.1447·2); ethinyloestradiol (p.1445·1).
Triphasic oral contraceptive.

Triolandren
Ciba-Geigy, Swed.†; Ciba, Switz.†.
Testosterone propionate (p.1464·2); testosterone valerianate; testosterone undecenoate (p.1465·3).
Anaemias; androgen deficiency in males; breast cancer in females; excessive growth in boys.

Triolax Herbes Universelles, Canad.
Aloin (p.1177·2); cascara (p.1183·1); phenolphthalein (p.1208·2); bile salts (p.1553·2).

Triolinctus Intercare, UK†.
Pholcodine (p.1068·1); pseudoephedrine hydrochloride (p.1068·3); chlorpheniramine maleate (p.405·1).
Coughs.

Triolix Day-time Drug Houses Austral., Austral.†.
Dextromethorphan hydrobromide (p.1057·3); pseudoephedrine hydrochloride (p.1068·3); paracetamol (p.72·2).
Cold symptoms.

Triolix Night-time Drug Houses Austral., Austral.†.
Dextromethorphan hydrobromide (p.1057·3); pseudoephedrine hydrochloride (p.1068·3); paracetamol (p.72·2); chlorpheniramine maleate (p.405·1).
Cold symptoms.

TRI-OM OM, Switz.
Magnesium aluminium silicate (p.1471·1); calcium aluminium silicate (p.1178·3).
Gastro-intestinal disorders.

Triomar Prism, UK.
Omega-3 triglycerides (p.1276·1).

Triomer Vifor, Switz.
Sterile sea water (p.1162·2).
Nasal disorders.

Triomin Triomed, S.Afr.
Minocycline hydrochloride (p.226·2).
Bacterial infections.

Triominic
Note. This name is used for preparations of different composition.
Intercare, Irl.; Intercare, UK.
Phenylpropanolamine hydrochloride (p.1067·2); pheniramine maleate (p.415·3).
Allergic rhinitis; nasal congestion.

Sandoz, Spain.
Phenylpropanolamine hydrochloride (p.1067·2); pheniramine maleate (p.415·3); mepyramine maleate (p.414·1).
Nasal congestion.

Trionetta
Schering, Norw.; Schering, Swed.
Levonorgestrel (p.1454·1); ethinyloestradiol (p.1445·1).
28-Day packs also contain 7 inert tablets.
Triphasic oral contraceptive.

Trioplex Triomed, S.Afr.†.
Multivitamin and mineral preparation.

Triosorbon E. Merck, UK†.
Gluten-free preparation for enteral nutrition.

Triospan Extractum, Hung.
Isopropamide iodide (p.464·3); drotaverine hydrochloride (p.1574·2); phenobarbitone (p.350·2).
Smooth muscle spasm.

Triostat SmithKline Beecham, USA.
Liothyronine sodium (p.1495·1).
Evaluation of thyroid function; hypothyroidism.

Triotann Invamed, USA; Duramed, USA.
Phenylephrine tannate (p.1067·1); mepyramine tannate (p.414·1); chlorpheniramine tannate (p.405·2).
Allergic rhinitis; nasal congestion.

Tri-Otic Pharmics, USA.
Chloroxylenol (p.1111·1); pramoxine hydrochloride (p.1298·2); hydrocortisone (p.1043·3).
Inflammatory ear infections.

Triovex Kabi, Swed.†.
Oestriol (p.1457·2).
Menopausal disorders.

Triovit Lane, UK.
A vitamin A, C, and D preparation.

Tripac-Cyano Covan, S.Afr.
4 Vials, sodium thiosulphate (p.996·2); 2 vials, sodium nitrite (p.995·2); 6 vials, amyl nitrite (p.974·2).
Cyanide poisoning.

Tripacel Connaught, Canad.
An adsorbed diphtheria, tetanus, and pertussis vaccine (p.1509·1).
Active immunisation.

Tri-Pain Ferndale, USA.
Paracetamol (p.72·2); aspirin (p.16·1); salicylamide (p.82·3); caffeine (p.749·3).
Pain.

Tripalgen Cold Barre-National, USA.
Phenylpropanolamine hydrochloride (p.1067·2); chlorpheniramine maleate (p.405·1).
Upper respiratory-tract symptoms.

Triparen Otsuka, Jpn.
Carbohydrate and electrolyte infusion.
Parenteral nutrition.

Triparsean Tecnobio, Spain.
Piketoprofen (p.80·1) or piketoprofen hydrochloride (p.80·1).
Peri-articular and soft-tissue disorders.

Tripedia Connaught, USA.
A diphtheria, tetanus, and acellular pertussis vaccine (p.1509·1).
Active immunisation of infants and young children.

Triperidol
Janssen, Belg.†; Janssen-Cilag, Fr.; Janssen-Cilag, Ger.; Lagap, UK.
Trifluperidol hydrochloride (p.698·1).
Psychoses.

Tripervan Bellon, Fr.†.
Vincamine (p.1644·1).
Cerebrovascular disorders; mental function impairment in the elderly.

Triphacycline Tripharma, Switz.
Tetracycline chloride (p.259·1).
Bacterial infections.

Triphasil
Wyeth, Austral.; Wyeth-Ayerst, Canad.; Akromed, S.Afr.; Wyeth-Ayerst, USA.
Levonorgestrel (p.1454·1); ethinyloestradiol (p.1445·1).
28-Day packs also contain 7 inert tablets.
Triphasic oral contraceptive.

Tri-Phen-Chlor TR Rugby, USA.
Phenylpropanolamine hydrochloride (p.1067·2); phenylephrine hydrochloride (p.1066·2); chlorpheniramine maleate (p.405·1); phenyltoloxamine citrate (p.416·1).
Upper respiratory-tract symptoms.

Triphenyl Rugby, USA.
Phenylpropanolamine hydrochloride (p.1067·2); chlorpheniramine maleate (p.405·1).
Upper respiratory-tract symptoms.

Triphenyl Expectorant Rugby, USA.
Phenylpropanolamine hydrochloride (p.1067·2); guaiphenesin (p.1061·3).
Coughs.

Triphosmag Boehringer Ingelheim, Fr.
Adenosine triphosphate (p.1543·2); phosphoric acid (p.1618·1); dibasic sodium phosphate (p.1159·3); magnesium chloride (p.1157·2); magnesium glycerophosphate (p.1157·2).
Tonic.

Triple Antibiotic Dixon-Shane, USA; Geneva, USA; Marsam, USA; Goldline, USA; Lannett, USA; Moore, USA; NMC, USA; Parmed, USA; Rugby, USA; Schein, USA.
Polymyxin B sulphate (p.239·1); neomycin sulphate (p.229·2); bacitracin (p.157·3).
Bacterial skin infections.

Triple Antigen CSL, Austral.
An adsorbed diphtheria, tetanus, and pertussis vaccine (p.1509·1).
Active immunisation.

Triple Care Smith & Nephew, Austral.
Emollient and skin cleanser.
Skin disorders associated with incontinence.

Triple Care Cleanser Smith & Nephew, USA.
Benzethonium chloride (p.1102·3); glycerol (p.1585·2); aloe vera (p.1177·1).
Removal of urine and faeces.

Triple Care Extra Protective Cream Smith & Nephew, USA.
Zinc oxide (p.1096·2); soft paraffin (p.1382·3); chloroxylenol (p.1111·1).
Protection of skin from incontinence.

Triple Care Protective Cream Smith & Nephew, USA.
Zinc oxide (p.1096·2); aloe vera (p.1177·1); allantoin (p.1078·2).
Protection of skin from incontinence.

Triple Sulfa Fougera, USA; Goldline, USA; Major, USA; NMC, USA; Rugby, USA; Schein, USA.
Sulphathiazole (p.257·1); sulphacetamide (p.252·2); sulfabenzamide (p.251·1).
Vaginitis due to Gardnerella vaginalis.

Triple Sulfa No 2 Rugby, USA†.
Sulphadiazine (p.252·3); sulfamerazine (p.251·3); sulphadimidine (p.253·2).
Bacterial infections.

Triple X Carter, USA.
Pyrethrins; piperonyl butoxide (p.1409·3).
Pediculosis.

Triplex Streuli, Switz.†.
Codeine phosphate (p.26·1); aspirin (p.16·1); paracetamol (p.72·2).
Fever; pain.

Triplex sans codeine Streuli, Switz.†.
Aspirin (p.16·1); paracetamol (p.72·2).
Fever; pain.

Triplice Midy, Ital.†.
Aspirin (p.16·1); paracetamol (p.72·2); caffeine (p.749·3).
Fever; pain.

Triposed Halsey, USA.
Pseudoephedrine hydrochloride (p.1068·3); triprolidine hydrochloride (p.420·3).
Upper respiratory-tract symptoms.

Triprim
Merckle, Aust.; Glaxo Wellcome, Austral.; Roche, S.Afr.
Trimethoprim (p.265·1).
Urinary-tract infections.

Triprimix Ashbourne, UK.
Trimethoprim (p.265·1).
Bacterial infections.

Triprofed ICN, Canad.
Pseudoephedrine hydrochloride (p.1068·3); triprolidine hydrochloride (p.420·3).

Tri-Profen 3M, Austral.
Ibuprofen (p.44·1).
Inflammation; musculoskeletal and joint disorders; pain.

Triptafen
Goldshield, Irl.; Forley, UK.
Amitriptyline hydrochloride (p.273·3); perphenazine (p.685·2).
Mixed anxiety depressive states.

Triptene IRBI, Ital.†.
Oxitriptan (p.301·2).
Depression; Down's syndrome; epilepsy; headache; insomnia; movement disorders; pain; parkinsonism; phenylketonuria.

Triptil Merck Sharp & Dohme, Canad.
Protriptyline hydrochloride (p.306·3).
Depression.

Triptizol Merck Sharp & Dohme, Ital.
Amitriptyline hydrochloride (p.273·3).
Depression.

Tript-OH
Sigma-Tau, Ital.; Sigma-Tau, Switz.
Oxitriptan (p.301·2).
Depression; Down's syndrome; epilepsy; headache; insomnia; migraine; movement disorders; pain; parkinsonism; phenylketonuria.

Triptone Del, USA.
Dimenhydrinate (p.408·2).
Motion sickness.

Triptum Inpharzam, Switz.†.
Oxitriptan (p.301·2).
Depression; migraine; myoclonus; sleep disorders.

Triquilar
Schering, Austral.; Berlex, Canad.; Schering, Ger.; Schering, Switz.
Levonorgestrel (p.1454·1); ethinyloestradiol (p.1445·1).
28-Day packs also contain 7 inert tablets.
Triphasic oral contraceptive.

Tririnol Biomedica, Ital.
Xylometazoline hydrochloride (p.1071·2); dequalinium chloride (p.1112·1).
Cold symptoms; sinusitis.

Trirutin Strathmann, Ger.
Heparin sodium (p.879·3).
Skin trauma; vascular disorders.

Trirutin N Strathmann, Ger.
Troxerutin (p.1580·2).
Formerly contained troxerutin and etofylline.
Vascular disorders.

Tris
Leopold, Aust.; Braun, Ger.
Trometamol (p.1639·3).
Citrate intoxication following blood transfusion; metabolic acidosis; respiratory acidosis.

Trisalgina Molteni, Ital.
Dipyrone (p.35·1).
Fever; pain.

Trisdine Delta, Austral.†.
Chlorhexidine gluconate (p.1107·2).
Urinary catheter care.

Trisekvens
Novo Nordisk, Norw.; Novo Nordisk, Swed.
18 Tablets, oestradiol (p.1455·1); 10 tablets, oestradiol; norethisterone acetate (p.1453·1).
Menopausal disorders; osteoporosis.

Triseptil Gedis, Ital.
Chlorhexidine gluconate (p.1107·2).
Hand disinfection.

Trisequens
Note. This name is used for preparations of different composition.
Novo Nordisk, Aust.; Novo Nordisk, Austral.; Novo Nordisk, Belg.; Novo Nordisk, Fr.; Novo Nordisk, Ger.; Novo Nordisk, Irl.; Novo Nordisk, Ital.; Novo Nordisk, Neth.; Novo Nordisk, S.Afr.; Novo Nordisk, UK.
18 Tablets, oestradiol (p.1455·1); 10 tablets, oestradiol; norethisterone acetate (p.1453·1).
Formerly contained oestradiol and oestriol, and oestradiol, oestriol, and norethisterone acetate.
Menopausal disorders.

Novo Nordisk, Switz.
18 Tablets, oestradiol (p.1455·1); oestriol (p.1457·2); 10 tablets, oestradiol; oestriol; norethisterone acetate (p.1453·1).
Menopausal disorders; osteoporosis.

Trisibam Sanofi Winthrop, Belg.†.
Gel complex of: silicon dioxide hydrate (p.1474·3); bismuth oxide hydrate (p.1180·1); aluminium hydroxide (p.1177·3); magnesium oxide hydrate (p.1198·3); sodium hydroxide (p.1631·1).
Gastro-intestinal disorders associated with hyperacidity.

Trisiston Jenapharm, Ger.
Ethinyloestradiol (p.1445·1); levonorgestrel (p.1454·1).
Triphasic oral contraceptive.

Trisolvit Chauvin, Fr.
Tocophersolan (p.1370·1); sodium ascorbate (p.1365·2); ethoxazorutoside (p.1580·1).
Vascular eye disorders.

Trisoralen
Dermatech, Austral.; ICN, Canad.; Lifepharma, Ital.; Restan, S.Afr.†; ICN, USA.
Trioxsalen (p.1095·1).
Intolerance to sunlight; vitiligo.

Trisorcin Merckle, Ger.
Penicillamine (p.988·3).
Cystinuria; heavy-metal poisoning; polyarthritis; scleroderma; Wilson's disease.

Trisorcin B_6 N Merckle, Ger.†.
Penicillamine (p.988·3); pyridoxine hydrochloride.
Cystinuria; heavy-metal poisoning; hepatitis; inflammatory disorders; Wilson's disease.

Trisporal Janssen, Neth.
Itraconazole (p.381·3).
Fungal infections.

Trissil Piam, Ital.
Silymarin (p.993·3).
Liver disorders.

Tri-Statin II Rugby, USA.
Triamcinolone acetonide (p.1050·2); nystatin (p.386·1).
Skin disorders.

TriStep Asche, Ger.
Levonorgestrel (p.1454·1); ethinyloestradiol (p.1445·1).
Triphasic oral contraceptive.

Tristoject Mayrand, USA.
Triamcinolone diacetate (p.1050·2).
Corticosteroid.

Trisulfamid Weifa, Norw.
Sulphadiazine (p.252·3); sulphadimidine(p.253·2); sulphaurea (p.257·2).
Bacterial infections of the urinary tract.

Trisulfaminic Shepherd, Canad.
Phenylpropanolamine hydrochloride (p.1067·2); pheniramine maleate (p.415·3); mepyramine maleate (p.414·1); sulphadiazine (p.252·3); sulfamerazine (p.251·3); sulphadimidine (p.253·2).
Congestion and infections of the upper respiratory-tract.

Trisulpha Pharmalab, S.Afr.†.
Sulphadiazine (p.252·3); sulfamerazine (p.251·3); sulphathiazole (p.257·1).
Bacterial infections.

Trisyn Baker Cummins, Canad.
Fluocinonide (p.1041·2); procinonide (p.1049·3); ciprocinonide (p.1035·2).
Skin disorders.

Tritace
Hoechst, Aust.; Hoechst Marion Roussel, Austral.; Hoechst Marion Roussel, Belg.; Hoechst Marion Roussel, Irl.; Hoechst Marion Roussel, Neth.; Hoechst Marion Roussel, S.Afr.; Hoechst, UK.
Ramipril (p.941·1).
Heart failure; hypertension; myocardial infarction.

Tritamyl Procea, Irl.†.
Gluten- and lactose-free food for special diets.
Gluten sensitivity.

Tritamyl PK Procea, Irl.†.
Gluten-, lactose-, and protein-free food for special diets.
Amino acid metabolic disorders; gluten sensitivity; liver disorders; renal failure.

Tritan Eon, USA.
Chlorpheniramine tannate (p.405·2); mepyramine tannate (p.414·1); phenylephrine tannate (p.1067·1).
Allergic rhinitis; nasal congestion.

Tri-Tannate Rugby, USA.
Phenylephrine tannate (p.1067·1); chlorpheniramine tannate (p.405·2); mepyramine tannate (p.414·1).
Upper respiratory-tract symptoms.

Tri-Tannate Plus Pediatric Rugby, USA.
Phenylephrine tannate (p.1067·1); ephedrine tannate (p.1060·1); chlorpheniramine tannate (p.405·2); pentoxyverine tannate (p.1066·2).
Coughs and cold symptoms.

Tritanrix SmithKline Beecham, Ital.
A diphtheria, tetanus, and pertussis vaccine (p.1509·1).
Active immunisation.

Tritanrix-DTPw SmithKline Beecham, Aust.
A diphtheria, tetanus and pertussis vaccine (p.1509·1).
Active immunisation.

Tritar Triomed, S.Afr.†.
Tar (p.1092·3); coal tar (p.1092·3); cade oil (p.1092·2).
Seborrhoeic dermatitis.

Tritazide
Hoechst, Aust.; Hoechst Marion Roussel, Neth.
Ramipril (p.941·1); hydrochlorothiazide (p.885·2).
Hypertension.

Tritec Glaxo Wellcome, USA.
Ranitidine bismutrex (p.1211·2).
Peptic ulcer.

Tritet Akromed, S.Afr.
Tetracycline hydrochloride (p.259·1); chlortetracycline hydrochloride (p.185·1); demeclocycline hydrochloride (p.201·2).
Bacterial infections.

Tri-Thiazid Stada, Ger.
Triamterene (p.957·2); hydrochlorothiazide (p.885·2).
Hypertension; oedema.

Tri-Thiazid Reserpin Stada, Ger.
Triamterene (p.957·2); hydrochlorothiazide (p.885·2); reserpine (p.942·1).
Hypertension.

Tritin Schering-Plough, Canad.†.
Tolnaftate (p.389·1).
Tinea pedis.

Tri-Torrat Boehringer Mannheim, Ger.
Metipranolol (p.906·2); buthiazide (p.835·2); dihydralazine sulphate (p.854·1).
Hypertension.

Trittico
Angelini, Aust.; Angelini, Ital.; ACRAF, Switz.
Trazodone hydrochloride (p.308·3).
Depression; neuroleptanalgesia; pain; premedication.

Triv Boyle, USA.
Hydroxyquinoline sulphate (p.1589·3); alkyl aryl sulphonate; edetic acid (p.980·3); sodium sulphate (p.1213·3).
Vaginal disorders.

Trivacuna Leti, Spain.
A diphtheria, tetanus, and pertussis vaccine (p.1509·1).
Active immunisation of infants and young children.

Trivastal
Eutherapie, Fr.; Servier, Ger.
Piribedil (p.1143·2) or piribedil mesylate (p.1143·2).
Extrapyramidal disorders; mental function impairment in the elderly; peripheral vascular disorders; vascular eye disorders.

Trivastan Stroder, Ital.
Piribedil (p.1143·2).
Vascular disorders.

Trivax
Wellcome, Irl.; Medeva, UK†.
A diphtheria, tetanus, and pertussis vaccine (p.1509·1).
Active immunisation.

Trivax-AD
Wellcome, Irl.; Medeva, UK.
An adsorbed diphtheria, tetanus, and pertussis vaccine (p.1509·1).
Active immunisation.

Trivax-Hib SmithKline Beecham, UK.
A diphtheria, tetanus, pertussis, and haemophilus influenzae vaccine (p.1509·3).
Active immunisation.

Trive
Clintec, Fr.; Clintec, Spain.
Amino-acid, carbohydrate and lipid (from soya oil (p.1355·1)) infusion.
Parenteral nutrition.

Trivemil Clintec, Ital.
An amino-acid, lipid, and carbohydrate preparation.
Parenteral nutrition.

Tri-Vi-Flor
Mead Johnson, Canad.; Mead Johnson Nutritionals, USA.
A range of vitamin preparations with fluoride (p.742·1).
Dental caries prophylaxis; dietary supplement.

Trivina
Continental Ethicals, S.Afr.; Orion, Swed.
White tablets, oestradiol valerate (p.1455·2); blue tablets oestradiol valerate; medroxyprogesterone acetate (p.1448·3); yellow tablets, inert.
Menopausal disorders; osteoporosis.

Triviraten
Berna, Ital.; Swisspharm, S.Afr.; Berna, Spain; Berna, Switz.
A measles, mumps, and rubella vaccine (Edmonston-Zagreb, Rubini, and RA 27/3 strains respectively) (p.1519·3).
Active immunisation.

Tri-Vi-Sol
Mead Johnson, Canad.; Mead Johnson Nutritionals, USA.
Multivitamin preparation.

Tri-Vi-Sol with Fluoride Mead Johnson, Canad.
Multivitamin preparation with fluoride (p.742·1).
Dental caries prophylaxis; vitamin supplement.

Tri-Vi-Sol with Iron Mead Johnson Nutritionals, USA.
Multivitamin preparation with iron.

Tri-Vitamin Schein, USA.
Vitamins A, C, and D.

Trivitamin Fluoride Drops Schein, USA.
Multivitamin preparation with fluoride (p.742·1).

Trivitan Merck, Spain.
Pyridoxine (p.1363·1); vitamin A (p.1358·1); tocopherol (p.1369·2).
Hyperkeratosis; keratoconjunctivitis; rhinitis; tonic; xerophthalmia.

Trivitepar B12 Damor, Ital.†.
Cyanocobalamin (p.1363·3); folic acid (p.1340·3); nicotinamide (p.1351·2); ascorbic acid (p.1365·2).
Liver disorders; neuralgia.

Trivitol Wenig, Aust.
Vitamins; caffeine; kola.
Tonic.

Tri-Wycillina Pharmacia Upjohn, Ital.
Benzathine penicillin (p.158·3); benzylpenicillin potassium (p.159·2); procaine penicillin (p.240·2).
Bacterial infections; rheumatism; syphilis.

T-Rix SmithKline Beecham, Ger.†.
Adsorbed tetanus vaccine (p.1535·3).
Active immunisation.

Trixidine Asta Medica, Ital.
Propylene glycol cefatrizine (p.164·2).
Bacterial infections.

Trixilan Pulitzer, Ital.
Propylene glycol cefatrizine (p.164·2).
Bacterial infections.

Trizima Madaus, Spain†.
Bromelains (p.1555·1); cellulase (p.1561·1); amylase (p.1549·1); dimethicone (p.1213·1); pancreatin (p.1612·1); papain (p.1614·1); valethamate bromide (p.469·3); dehydrocholic acid (p.1570·2).
Digestive enzyme deficiency; dyspepsia; hepatobiliary dyskinesia; meteorism.

Trizina Francia, Ital.
Propylene glycol cefatrizine (p.164·2).
Bacterial infections.

Trizymal Pharmethic, Belg.†.
Pancreatin (p.1612·1); *Schizomycetii fermentum*; ox bile extract (p.1553·2).
Pancreatic insufficiency.

Trobicin
Pharmacia Upjohn, Aust.; Pharmacia Upjohn, Austral.; Pharmacia Upjohn, Belg.; Pharmacia Upjohn, Canad.; Pharmacia Upjohn, Irl.; Pharmacia Upjohn, Ital.; Pharmacia Upjohn, Norw.†; Pharmacia Up-

john, S.Afr.; Pharmacia Upjohn, Swed.; Pharmacia Upjohn, Switz.; Upjohn, UK; Upjohn, USA.
Spectinomycin hydrochloride (p.248·3).
Gonorrhoea.

Trobicine *Pharmacia Upjohn, Fr.*
Spectinomycin hydrochloride (p.248·3).
Gonorrhoea.

Troc *Melisana, Belg.†.*
Aspirin (p.16·1); diphenhydramine salicylate (p.409·2); caffeine hydrate (p.750·1); codeine phosphate (p.26·1).
Cold symptoms; fever; headache.

Troca Cationi *Pharma-Natura, Ital.*
Magnesium; potassium; zinc (p.1147·1).
Mineral deficiencies; stress; viral infections.

Trocaine *Roberts, USA.*
Benzocaine (p.1286·2).
Sore throat.

Trocal *Roberts, USA.*
Dextromethorphan hydrobromide (p.1057·3).
Coughs.

Trochain *Propan, S.Afr.*
Cetrimide (p.1105·2); benzocaine (p.1286·2).
Sore throat.

Trocurine *Labatec, Switz.†.*
Sustained-release capsules: Nitrofurantoin (p.231·3).
Tablets; syrup: Nitrofurantoin (p.231·3); pyridoxine hydrochloride (p.1362·3).
Urinary-tract infections.

Trofalgon *Madariaga, Spain.*
Cyanocobalamin (p.1363·3); muramidase hydrochloride (p.1604·3).
Formerly contained cobamamide and muramidase hydrochloride.
Tonic.

Trofi Milina *Europharma, Spain.*
Capsules: Phospholipids; pyridoxine hydrochloride (p.1362·3).
Injection: Cyanocobalamin (p.1363·3); phospholipids. Lignocaine hydrochloride (p.1293·2) is included in this preparation to alleviate the pain of injection.
Dystonia; tonic.

Trofinerv *Fidia, Ital.*
Omega-3 marine triglycerides (p.1276·1); vitamins.
Nutritional supplement.

Trofo 5 *Uniderm, Ital.*
Zinc oxide (p.1096·2); cod-liver oil (p.1337·3); hyaluronic acid; chamomile oil.
Skin disorders.

Trofocalcium *Fournier, Ital.*
Vitamin and calcium preparation.
Calcium depletion; metabolic bone disorders.

Trofodermin *Carlo Erba OTC, Ital.*
Clostebol (p.1440·2); neomycin sulphate (p.229·2).
Skin trauma.

Trofomed *Trofomed, Ital.*
Royal jelly (p.1626·3).

Troforex Pepsico *Reig Jofre, Spain.*
Cyproheptadine hydrochloride (p.407·2); amino acids and hydroxocobalamin; pepsin (p.1616·3).
Tonic.

Trofoseptine *Boehringer Ingelheim, Fr.†.*
Clostebol acetate (p.1440·2); neomycin sulphate (p.229·2).
Ulcers; wounds.

Trojan *Carter Horner, Canad.*
Nonoxinol 9 (p.1326·1).
Contraceptive.

Trolic *Garec, S.Afr.*
Prednisone (p.1049·2).
Corticosteroid.

Trolovol
Bayer, Fr.; Asta Medica, Ger.
Penicillamine (p.988·3).
Chronic polyarthritis; cystinuria; heavy-metal poisoning; rheumatoid arthritis; scleroderma; Wilson's disease.

Tromacaps *Madaus, Ger.†.*
Benzyl isothiocyanate (p.1552·3).
Bacterial infections.

Tromalyt *Madaus, Spain.*
Aspirin (p.16·1).
Thrombosis prophylaxis.

Tromasin SA *Parke, Davis, S.Afr.†.*
Papain (p.1614·1).
Inflammation; oedema.

Trombenox *Menarini, Ital.*
Enoxaparin sodium (p.864·2).
Thrombo-embolic disorders.

Tromboliquine *Organon Teknika, Neth.†.*
Heparin sodium (p.879·3).
Thrombo-embolic disorders.

Trombovar
Therapex, Canad.; Promedica, Fr.; Bouty, Ital.; Promedica, Neth.†.
Sodium tetradecyl sulphate (p.1469·2).
Cysts; oesophageal varices; tuberous angioma; varicose veins.

Trombufen *Trommsdorff, Ger.†.*
Ibuprofen (p.44·1).
Musculoskeletal and joint disorders.

Trombyl *Pharmacia Upjohn, Swed.*
Aspirin (p.16·1).
Angina pectoris; myocardial infarction; prevention of cerebrovascular ischaemia.

Tromcardin *Trommsdorff, Ger.*
Potassium aspartate (p.1161·3); magnesium aspartate (p.1157·2).
Cardiac disorders; potassium and magnesium deficiency.

Tromexane *Geigy, Fr.†.*
Ethyl biscoumacetate (p.867·1).
Thrombo-embolic disorders.

Tromgallol *Jacoby, Aust.*
Cyclobutyrol sodium (p.1569·2); cynarine (p.1569·3); sorbitol (p.1354·2); magnesium sulphate dihydrate (p.1157·3).
Hepatobiliary disorders.

Tromir *Ibirn, Ital.*
Heparan sulphate (p.879·2).
Thrombosis prophylaxis.

Tromlipon *Trommsdorff, Ger.*
Thioctic acid (p.1636·2) or trometamol thioctate (p.1640·1).
Diabetic neuropathy.

Trommcardin *Jacoby, Aust.*
Potassium aspartate hemihydrate (p.1161·3); magnesium aspartate tetrahydrate (p.1157·2).
Arrhythmias; digitalis intoxication; heart failure; potassium and magnesium deficiency.

Tromscillan *Trommsdorff, Ger.†.*
Proscillaridin (p.938·1); potassium aspartate (p.1161·3); magnesium aspartate (p.1157·2).
Heart failure.

Tronan *Boehringer Mannheim, Ital.*
Heparan sulphate (p.879·2).
Thrombosis prophylaxis.

Tronolane *Ross, USA.*
Cream: Pramoxine hydrochloride (p.1298·2); zinc oxide (p.1096·2).
Suppositories: Pramoxine hydrochloride (p.1298·2); pramoxine (p.1298·2); zinc oxide (p.1096·2).
Haemorrhoids.

Tronotene *Abbott, Ital.*
Pramoxine hydrochloride (p.1298·2).
Burns; haemorrhoids; pruritus.

Tronothane
Abbott, Canad.†; Abbott, Fr.; Abbott, USA.
Pramoxine hydrochloride (p.1298·2).
Local anaesthesia.

Tronoxal *Funk, Spain.*
Ifosfamide (p.540·2).
Malignant neoplasms.

Tropamine *Matrix, USA†.*
Multivitamin, amino acid, and mineral preparation.

Tropargal *Alonga, Spain.*
Diazepam (p.661·1); nortriptyline hydrochloride (p.300·2).
Depression with anxiety or agitation.

Troparin *Biochemie, Aust.*
Certoparin sodium (p.839·1).
Thrombo-embolism prophylaxis.

Troparin compositum *Biochemie, Aust.*
Certoparin sodium (p.839·1); dihydroergotamine mesylate (p.444·2).
Lignocaine hydrochloride (p.1293·2) is included in this preparation to alleviate the pain of injection.
Thrombo-embolism prophylaxis.

Tropax *Noristan, S.Afr.†.*
Phenobarbitone (p.350·2); hyoscyamine sulphate (p.464·2); atropine sulphate (p.455·1); hyoscine hydrobromide (p.462·3).
Gastro-intestinal disorders; urinary-tract spasm.

Tropergen *Norgine, UK.*
Diphenoxylate hydrochloride (p.1189·1).
Atropine sulphate (p.455·1) is included in this preparation to discourage abuse.
These ingredients can be described by the British Approved Name Co-phenotrope.
Diarrhoea.

Tropex *Rowa, Irl.*
Phenazone (p.78·2).
Ear wax removal; otitis media.

Trophamine
Pharmacia Upjohn, Spain; McGaw, USA.
Amino-acid infusion.
Parenteral nutrition.

Trophicard *Kohler-Pharma, Ger.*
Potassium aspartate (p.1161·3); magnesium aspartate (p.1157·2).
Cardiac disorders; magnesium or potassium deficiency.

Trophicreme *Sanofi Winthrop, Fr.*
Oestriol (p.1457·2).
Postmenopausal vulvovaginal disorders.

Trophiderm *Brothier, Fr.*
Calcium alginate (p.714·1).
Ulcers.

Trophigil *Sanofi Winthrop, Fr.*
Lactobacillus acidophilus (p.1594·1); oestriol (p.1457·2); progesterone (p.1459·3).
Atrophic vaginitis; pre- and postoperative gynaecological care.

Trophires
Note. This name is used for preparations of different composition.
Sanofi Winthrop, Fr.
Suppositories: Eucalyptus oil (p.1578·1); thenoate sodium (p.262·2).
Formerly contained camphor, myrtle oil, eucalyptus oil, and thenoate sodium.
Respiratory-tract disorders.
Syrup: Pholcodine (p.1068·1); thenoate sodium (p.262·2); eucalyptus oil (p.1578·1).
Coughs.
Semar, Spain.
Capsules: Thenoate sodium (p.262·2).
Bronchitis.
Nasal drops: Cineole (p.1564·1); Cupressus sempervirens oil; myrtle oil; thenoate sodium (p.262·2).
Nasal cleansing.
Suppositories; syrup: Pholcodine (p.1068·1).
Trophires suppositories formerly contained camphor, cineole, pholcodine, myrtle oil, paracetamol, and thenoate sodium. Trophires syrup formerly contained cineole, pholcodine, and thenoate sodium.
Cough.

Trophires Compose *Sanofi Winthrop, Fr.*
Paracetamol (p.72·2); eucalyptus oil (p.1578·1); thenoate sodium (p.262·2).
Formerly contained camphor, myrtle oil, eucalyptus oil, thenoate sodium, paracetamol, and pholcodine.
Fever; respiratory-tract disorders.

Trophires Rectal Lact *Semar, Spain†.*
Cineole (p.1564·1); myrtle oil; paracetamol (p.72·2); thenoate sodium (p.262·2).
Respiratory-tract disorders.

Troph-Iron *Menley & James, USA†.*
Ferric pyrophosphate (p.1339·2); vitamin B substances.
Iron-deficiency anaemias.

Trophite *Menley & James, USA†.*
Vitamin B substances.

Trophobolene *Theramex, Mon.*
Estrapronicate (p.1444·3); nandrolone undecanoate (p.1452·2); hydroxyprogesterone enanthate (p.1448·1).
Anabolic; osteoporosis.

Trophysan *Clintec, Fr.*
Amino-acid, carbohydrate, mineral, and vitamin infusion.
Enteral and parenteral nutrition.

Tropicacyl *Akorn, USA.*
Tropicamide (p.469·2).
Induction of mydriasis and cycloplegia.

Tropical Blend *Schering-Plough, Canad.*
Oxybenzone (p.1487·3).
Sunscreen.

Tropical Blend Dark Tanning *Schering-Plough, USA.*
SPF 2: Homosalate (p.1487·2).
Lotion SPF 4: Ethylhexyl *p*-methoxycinnamate (p.1487·1); oxybenzone (p.1487·3).
Oil SPF 4: Padimate O (p.1488·1); oxybenzone (p.1487·3).
Sunscreen.

Tropical Blend Dry Oil *Schering-Plough, USA.*
SPF 2: Homosalate (p.1487·2).
SPF 4: Homosalate (p.1487·2); oxybenzone (p.1487·3).
Sunscreen.

Tropical Blend Tan Magnifier *Schering-Plough, USA.*
SPF 2; SPF 4: Triethanolamine salicylate (p.1639·2).
Sunscreen.

Tropical Gold Dark Tanning *Goldline, USA.*
SPF 2: Ethylhexyl *p*-methoxycinnamate (p.1487·1); padimate O (p.1488·1).
SPF 4: Ethylhexyl *p*-methoxycinnamate (p.1487·1); oxybenzone (p.1487·3).
Sunscreen.

Tropical Gold Sunblock *Goldline, USA.*
SPF 15: Ethylhexyl *p*-methoxycinnamate (p.1487·1); oxybenzone (p.1487·3).
SPF 30: Ethylhexyl *p*-methoxycinnamate (p.1487·1); octyl salicylate (p.1487·3); homosalate (p.1487·2); oxybenzone (p.1487·3).
Sunscreen.

Tropical Gold Sunscreen *Goldline, USA.*
SPF 8: Ethylhexyl *p*-methoxycinnamate (p.1487·1); oxybenzone (p.1487·3).
Sunscreen.

Tropicol *Bournonville, Belg.*
Tropicamide (p.469·2).
Production of mydriasis.

Tropimil *Farmigea, Ital.*
Tropicamide (p.469·2).
Production of mydriasis and cycloplegia.

Tropiovent *Ashbourne, UK.*
Ipratropium bromide (p.754·2).
Obstructive airways disease.

Tropi-Storz *Lederle, USA.*
Tropicamide (p.469·2).
Production of mydriasis and cycloplegia.

Tropium *DDSA Pharmaceuticals, UK.*
Chlordiazepoxide hydrochloride (p.646·3).
Alcohol withdrawal syndrome; anxiety.

Tropoderm *Kolassa, Aust.*
Neomycin sulphate (p.229·2); diphenylpyraline hydrochloride (p.409·3); buphenine hydrochloride (p.1555·3); hydrocortisone (p.1043·3).

Trosid *Pfizer, Spain.*
Tioconazole (p.388·3).
Trosid pessaries formerly contained fluconazole.
Fungal skin and nail infections; vulvovaginal candidiasis.

Trospi *Medac, Ger.*
Trospium chloride (p.1640·1).
Urinary-tract disorders.

Trosyd
Note. This name is used for preparations of different composition.
Pfizer, Aust.; Pfizer, Canad.; Pfizer, Fr.; Roerig, Ital.; Pfizer, S.Afr.; Pfizer, Switz.
Tioconazole (p.388·3).
Fungal and bacterial infections of the skin, nails, and vagina.
Pfizer, Switz.†.
Topical solution: Tioconazole (p.388·3); undecenoic acid (p.389·2).
Fungal and bacterial infections of the skin and nails.

Trosyl
Pfizer, Irl.; Pfizer, UK.
Tioconazole (p.388·3).
Fungal and bacterial infections of the nails.

Trovan *Pfizer, USA.*
Injection: Alatrofloxacin mesylate (p.150·1).
Tablets: Trovafloxacin mesylate (p.267·1).
Bacterial infections.

Troxazole *Propan, S.Afr.*
Co-trimoxazole (p.196·3).
Bacterial infections.

Troxeven *Kreussler, Ger.*
Troxerutin (p.1580·2).
Venous disorders.

Troymycetin *Noristan, S.Afr.†.*
Chloramphenicol (p.182·1).
Bacterial infections.

Trozocina *Sigma-Tau, Ital.*
Azithromycin (p.155·2).
Bacterial infections.

True Test
Abello, Ger.; Glaxo Wellcome, USA.
Adhesive patches impregnated with a range of potential allergens (p.1545·1).
Sensitivity test for contact allergies.

Trufree
Cantassium Co., UK.
Tablets: Multivitamin and mineral preparation.
Cantassium Co., UK.
Gluten-free, wheat-free flours for special diets.
Gluten sensitivity.

Truphylline *G & W, USA.*
Aminophylline (p.748·1).
Asthma; bronchospasm.

Trusopt
Merck Sharp & Dohme, Aust.; Merck Sharp & Dohme, Austral.; Merck Sharp & Dohme, Belg.; Merck Frosst, Canad.; Merck Sharp & Dohme-Chibret, Fr.; Chibret, Ger.; Merck Sharp & Dohme, Irl.; Merck Sharp & Dohme, Ital.; Merck Sharp & Dohme, Neth.; Merck Sharp & Dohme, Norw.; Merck Sharp & Dohme, S.Afr.; Merck Sharp & Dohme, Spain; Merck Sharp & Dohme, Swed.; Merck Sharp & Dohme, Switz.; Merck Sharp & Dohme, UK; Merck, USA.
Dorzolamide hydrochloride (p.862·3).
Glaucoma; ocular hypertension.

Trust *Edmond Pharma, Ital.†.*
Benzocaine (p.1286·2); chlorhexidine gluconate (p.1107·2).
Burns; erythema.

Truw-Gold *Truw, Ger.†.*
Homoeopathic preparation.

Truxal
Lundbeck, Aust.; Lundbeck, Belg.†; Promonta, Ger.; Lundbeck, Neth.; Lundbeck, Norw.; Lundbeck, Swed.; Lundbeck, Switz.
Chlorprothixene (p.656·1), chlorprothixene acetate (p.656·2), chlorprothixene citrate (p.656·2), or chlorprothixene hydrochloride (p.656·2).
Alcohol and drug withdrawal syndromes; anxiety disorders; behaviour disorders in children; bipolar disorder; neuroses; pain; psychoses; skin irritation; sleep disorders; vomiting.

Truxaletten
Lundbeck, Aust.; Promonta, Ger.†; Lundbeck, Switz.
Chlorprothixene (p.656·1) or chlorprothixene hydrochloride (p.656·2).
Alcohol and drug withdrawal syndromes; anxiety disorders; behaviour disorders in children; neuroses; nocturnal enuresis; pain; psychiatric disorders; sleep disorders; vomiting.

Truxalettes *Lundbeck, Belg.†.*
Chlorprothixene hydrochloride (p.656·2).
Agitation; pain; psychosis.

Tryasol *Wernigerode, Ger.*
Codeine phosphate (p.26·1).
Coughs.

Trymex *Savage, USA†.*
Triamcinolone acetonide (p.1050·2).

Tryptan *ICN, Canad.*
Tryptophan (p.310·2).
Adjunct in treatment of depression.

Tryptanol
Frosst, Austral.; Merck Sharp & Dohme, S.Afr.
Amitriptyline embonate (p.273·3) or amitriptyline hydrochloride (p.273·3).
Depression; nocturnal enuresis.

Tryptine *Amrad, Austral.*
Amitriptyline hydrochloride (p.273·3).
Depression; nocturnal enuresis.

Tryptizol
Merck Sharp & Dohme, Aust.; Merck Sharp & Dohme, Belg.; Morson, Irl.; Merck Sharp & Dohme, Neth.; Merck Sharp & Dohme, Norw.; Merck Sharp & Dohme, Spain; Merck Sharp & Dohme, Swed.; Merck Sharp & Dohme, Switz.; Morson, UK.
Amitriptyline embonate (p.273·3) or amitriptyline hydrochloride (p.273·3).
Bulimia; depression; nocturnal enuresis; postherpetic neuralgia.

Tryptoferm *Gaschler, Ger.*
Pancreatin (p.1612·1).
Inflammatory disorders.

Trypto-Sleep *Vitaplex, Austral.†.*
Tryptophan (p.310·2), vitamin B substances; minerals.
Insomnia.

Trysul *Savage, USA.*
Sulphathiazole (p.257·1); sulphacetamide (p.252·2); sulfabenzamide (p.251·1).
Vaginitis due to Gardnerella vaginalis.

T-Stat
Westwood-Squibb, Canad.; Westwood-Squibb, USA.
Erythromycin (p.204·1).
Acne.

TTD-B$_3$-B$_4$ *AJC, Fr.*
Disulfiram (p.1573·1); nicotinamide (p.1351·2); adenine (p.1543·2).
Alcoholism.

Tubarine
Wellcome, Canad.†; Wellcome, Ital.†; Calmic, UK†.
Tubocurarine chloride (p.1322·3).
Competitive neuromuscular blocker.

Tubergen-Test
Chiron Behring, Ger.; Berna, Switz.†.
Tuberculin (p.1640·2).
Sensitivity test.

Tuberol
Note. This name is used for preparations of different composition.
Bouteille, Fr.†.
Paediatric syrup: Sodium benzoate (p.1102·3); potassium guaiacolsulfonate (p.1068·3); sodium bromide (p.1620·3); chloral hydrate (p.645·3); senega (p.1069·3); belladonna (p.457·1); codeine (p.26·1); Desessartz syrup.
Syrup: Melaleuca oil (p.1599·2); codeine (p.26·1); aconite (p.1542·2); belladonna (p.457·1); sodium benzoate (p.1102·3); benzoic acid (p.1102·3); turpentine; cherry-laurel; opium (p.70·3).
Coughs.
Topical liquid; ointment: Thymol (p.1127·1); cajuput oil (p.1556·1); marjoram oil; niaouli oil (p.1607·1); cineole (p.1564·1); turpentine oil (p.1641·1).
Minor respiratory disorders.
Rolab, S.Afr.
Ethambutol hydrochloride (p.207·2); isoniazid (p.218·1).
Tuberculosis.

Tubersol
Parisis, Spain; Connaught, USA.
Tuberculin purified protein derivative (p.1640·2).
Diagnosis of tuberculosis.

Tucks
Note. This name is used for preparations of different composition.
Warner-Lambert, Canad.; Glaxo Wellcome, USA.
Pads; gel: Hamamelis (p.1587·1); glycerol (p.1585·2).
Perianal cleansing.
Warner-Wellcome, USA†.
Cream: Hamamelis (p.1587·1).
Anorectal disorders; vaginal irritation.

Tuclase
Bios, Belg.; UCB, Ital.; UCB, Neth.
Pentoxyverine citrate (p.1066·1) or pentoxyverine hydrochloride (p.1066·2).
Coughs.

Tudcabil *Pharmacia Upjohn, Ital.*
Tauroursodeoxycholic acid (p.1642·1).
Biliary disorders.

Tufemin *Ravensberg, Ger.*
Multivitamin preparation with iron.
Anaemias; iron and vitamin deficiency.

Tuinal
Lilly, Canad.; Lilly, Irl.; Lilly, S.Afr.†; Lilly, UK; Lilly, USA.
Quinalbarbitone sodium (p.690·2); amylobarbitone sodium (p.641·3).
Insomnia; sedative.

Tulgrasum Antibiotico *Knoll, Spain.*
Bacitracin zinc (p.157·3) neomycin sulphate (p.229·2); polymyxin B sulphate (p.239·1).
Skin disorders.

Tulgrasum Cicatrizante *Knoll, Spain.*
Glycine; benzyl benzoate (p.1402·2); benzalkonium chloride (p.1101·3); amino acids.
Skin disorders.

Tulip *Upjohn, Spain.*
Flurbiprofen (p.42·1).
Musculoskeletal, joint, and peri-articular disorders; pain.

Tulle Gras Lumiere
Solvay, Belg.; Solvay, Fr.; Hefa, Ger.
Peru balsam (p.1617·2).
Burns; wounds.

Tulotract *Ardeypharm, Ger.*
Lactulose (p.1195·3).
Constipation; hepatic encephalopathy; salmonella enteritis.

Tumarol *Renapharm, Switz.*
Camphor (p.1557·2); menthol (p.1600·2); cedar atlant. oil; eucalyptus oil (p.1578·1); turpentine oil (p.1641·1); thymol (p.1127·1).
Cold symptoms.

Tumarol Kinderbalsam *Robugen, Ger.*
Eucalyptus oil (p.1578·1); oleum pini sylvestris.
Cold symptoms.

Tumarol-N *Robugen, Ger.*
Camphor (p.1557·2); menthol (p.1600·2); eucalyptus oil (p.1578·1).
Cold symptoms.

Tumasan *Robugen, Ger.†.*
Bismuth salicylate (p.1180·1); calcium carbonate (p.1182·1).
Formerly contained bismuth subgallate, bismuth salicylate, calcium carbonate, magnesium oxide, white clay, and magnesium peroxide.
Gastro-intestinal disorders.

Tumoglin *Pfluger, Ger.†.*
Homoeopathic preparation.

Tums
SmithKline Beecham Consumer, Canad.; SmithKline Beecham Consumer, UK; SmithKline Beecham Consumer, USA.
Calcium carbonate (p.1182·1).
Hyperacidity.

Tums Plus *SmithKline Beecham, USA.*
Calcium carbonate (p.1182·1); simethicone (p.1213·1).

Tundrax *Tecnobio, Spain.*
Pseudoephedrine hydrochloride (p.1068·3); ebastine (p.410·2).
Allergic rhinitis.

Tuplix *Iquinosa, Spain†.*
Cortobenzolone (p.1034·1).
Skin disorders.

Turbatherm *Torfwerk Einfeld, Ger.*
Peat.
Gastro-intestinal disorders; musculoskeletal and joint disorders.

Turbinal *Valeas, Ital.*
Beclomethasone dipropionate (p.1032·1).
Rhinitis.

Turbocalcin *SmithKline Beecham, Ital.*
Elcatonin (p.735·3).
Hypercalcaemia; osteoporosis; Paget's disease of bone; reflex sympathetic dystrophy.

Turexan Capilla *Turimed, Switz.*
Cetrimonium bromide (p.1106·1); urea (p.1095·2); dexpanthenol (p.1570·3).
Scalp disorders.

Turexan Creme *Turimed, Switz.*
Undecenoic acid (p.389·2); zinc undecenoate (p.389·2).
Barrier cream; skin disorders.

Turexan Douche *Turimed, Switz.*
Undecenoic acid (p.389·2).
Skin disorders; soap substitute.

Turexan Emulsion *Turimed, Switz.*
Undecenoic acid (p.389·2); zinc undecenoate (p.389·2); triclosan (p.1127·2).
Skin disorders; soap substitute.

Turexan Lotion *Turimed, Switz.*
Urea (p.1095·2); dexpanthenol (p.1570·3).
Skin disorders.

Turfa *BASF, Ger.*
Triamterene (p.957·2); hydrochlorothiazide (p.885·2).
Hypertension; oedema.

Turgostad *Stada, Ger.†.*
Heparin (p.879·3); benzyl nicotinate (p.22·1); arnica flower (p.1550·3).
Skin trauma.

Turicard *Jenapharm, Ger.*
Glyceryl trinitrate (p.874·3).
Cardiac disorders.

Turigeran *Jenapharm, Ger.†.*
Multivitamin preparation.
Geriatric disorders.

Turimonit *Jenapharm, Ger.*
Isosorbide mononitrate (p.893·3).
Cardiac disorders.

Turimycin *Jenapharm, Ger.*
Clindamycin hydrochloride (p.191·1).
Bacterial infections.

Turineurin *Jenapharm, Ger.*
Hypericum (p.1590·1).
Psychiatric disorders.

Turiplex *Jenapharm, Ger.*
Cucurbita (p.1569·1).
Urinary-tract disorders.

Turisan *Turimed, Switz.*
Cetrimonium bromide (p.1106·1).
Skin disinfection; skin infections.

Turisteron *Jenapharm, Ger.*
Ethinyloestradiol propanesulphonate (p.1445·1).
Prostatic cancer.

Turixin *SmithKline Beecham, Ger.*
Calcium mupirocin (p.227·3).
Nasal carriage of staphylococci.

Turkadon *Bioiberica, Spain.*
Chondroitin sulphate (p.1562·2).
Arteriosclerosis; thrombo-embolic disorders.

Turoptin
Ciba Vision, Ital.; Ciba Vision, Switz.
Metipranolol (p.906·2).
Glaucoma; ocular hypertension.

Turpentine White Liniment *McGloin, Austral.*
Turpentine oil (p.1641·1); camphor (p.1557·2).
Muscle pain.

Tusben *Benedetti, Ital.*
Dimemorfan phosphate (p.1058·3).
Coughs.

Tuscalman
Note. This name is used for preparations of different composition.
Kwizda, Aust.; Berna, Ital.; Berna, Switz.
Oral drops; suppositories: Noscapine hydrochloride (p.1065·2); guaiphenesin (p.1061·3).
Respiratory-tract disorders.
Berna, Spain.
Suppositories†: Guaiphenesin (p.1061·3); noscapine hydrochloride (p.1065·2); salicylamide (p.82·3).
Syrup; infant suppositories: Noscapine hydrochloride (p.1065·2).
Formerly contained guaiphenesin and noscapine hydrochloride.
Respiratory-tract disorders.
Berna, Switz.
Syrup: Noscapine hydrochloride (p.1065·2); guaiphenesin (p.1061·3); althaea (p.1546·3).
Respiratory-tract disorders.

Tuscodin *Knoll, Austral.†.*
Dihydrocodeine tartrate (p.34·1); chlorhexidine hydrochloride (p.1107·2); lignocaine hydrochloride (p.1293·2).
Sore throat.

Tuselin Expectorante *Knoll, Spain.*
Alloclamide hydrochloride (p.1054·3); ammonium chloride (p.1055·2); carbocisteine (p.1056·3); phenylephrine hydrochloride (p.1066·2); ipecacuanha (p.1062·2).
Respiratory-tract disorders.

Tusibron *Kenwood, USA.*
Guaiphenesin (p.1061·3).
Coughs.

Tusibron-DM *Kenwood, USA.*
Guaiphenesin (p.1061·3); dextromethorphan hydrobromide (p.1057·3).
Coughs.

Tusitinas *Pensa, Spain.*
Dextromethorphan hydrobromide (p.1057·3).
Cough.

Tusofren *Prodes, Spain.*
Dropropizine (p.1059·2).
Coughs.

Tusorama *Boehringer Mannheim, Spain.*
Dextromethorphan hydrobromide (p.1057·3).
Coughs.

Tusquelin *Circle, USA.*
Phenylpropanolamine hydrochloride (p.1067·2); dextromethorphan hydrobromide (p.1057·3); phenylephrine hydrochloride (p.1066·2); chlorpheniramine maleate (p.405·1); ipecacuanha (p.1062·2); potassium guaiacolsulfonate (p.1068·3).
Coughs and cold symptoms.

Tusquit *Xixia, S.Afr.*
Diphenhydramine hydrochloride (p.409·1); ammonium chloride (p.1055·2).
Coughs.

Tuss *Disperga, Aust.*
Wild thyme; castanea vulgaris.
Coughs and viscous mucus.

Tuss Hustenstiller *Rentschler, Ger.*
Dextromethorphan hydrobromide (p.1057·3).
Coughs.

Tussafed *Everett, USA.*
Carbinoxamine maleate (p.404·2); pseudoephedrine hydrochloride (p.1068·3); dextromethorphan hydrobromide (p.1057·3).
Coughs and cold symptoms.

Tussafed HC *Everett, USA.*
Hydrocodone tartrate (p.43·1); phenylephrine hydrochloride (p.1066·2); guaiphenesin (p.1061·3).
Coughs.

Tussafin Expectorant *Rugby, USA.*
Pseudoephedrine hydrochloride (p.1068·3); guaiphenesin (p.1061·3); hydrocodone tartrate (p.43·1).
Coughs.

Tussafug
Robugen, Ger.; Medipharm, Switz.
Benproperine embonate (p.1055·2) or benproperine phosphate (p.1055·2).
Coughs.

Tuss-Allergine Modified TD *Rugby, USA.*
Phenylpropanolamine hydrochloride (p.1067·2); caramiphen edisylate (p.1056·2).
Coughs.

Tussamag
Note. This name is used for preparations of different composition.
Montavit, Aust.
Ointment: Spike lavender oil (p.1632·2); eucalyptus oil (p.1578·1); turpentine oil (p.1641·1); camphor (p.1557·2).
Oral liquid: Thyme (p.1636·3); castanea vulgaris.
Bronchitis; catarrh; coughs.
Teofarma, Ital.
Wild thyme; castaneae leaves.
Respiratory-tract congestion.

Tussamag Codeintropfen *CT, Ger.*
Codeine phosphate (p.26·1).
Coughs.

Tussamag Complex *Teofarma, Ital.*
Wild thyme; dropropizine (p.1059·2).
Coughs.

Tussamag Erkaltungsbalsam N *CT, Ger.*
Eucalyptus oil (p.1578·1); oleum pini sylvestris.
Catarrh.

Tussamag Halstabletten *CT, Ger.*
Benzocaine (p.1286·2); menthol (p.1600·2); peppermint oil (p.1208·1); eucalyptus oil (p.1578·1).
Pain, inflammation, and infection of the mouth and throat.

Tussamag Hustensaft N *CT, Ger.*
Thyme (p.1636·3).
Bronchitis; catarrh; coughs.

Tussamag Hustentropfen N *CT, Ger.*
Thyme (p.1636·3).
Bronchitis; catarrh; coughs.

Tussamag mit Codein und Ephedrin *Montavit, Aust.*
Codeine phosphate (p.26·1); ephedrine hydrochloride (p.1059·3).
Bronchitis; catarrh; coughs.

Tussamed *Hexal, Ger.*
Clobutinol hydrochloride (p.1057·1).
Coughs.

Tussaminic C *Sandoz, Canad.*
Codeine phosphate (p.26·1); phenylpropanolamine hydrochloride (p.1067·2); mepyramine maleate (p.414·1); pheniramine maleate (p.415·3).
Coughs.

Tussaminic DH *Sandoz, Canad.*
Hydrocodone tartrate (p.43·1); phenylpropanolamine hydrochloride (p.1067·2); mepyramine maleate (p.414·1); pheniramine maleate (p.415·3).
Coughs.

Tussanil Compositum *Vifor, Switz.*
Noscapine (p.1065·2); drosera (p.1574·1); liquorice (p.1197·1); eucalyptus oil (p.1578·1); peppermint oil (p.1208·1).
Coughs.

Tussanil DH *Misemer, USA.*
Syrup: Phenylephrine hydrochloride (p.1066·2); chlorpheniramine maleate (p.405·1); hydrocodone tartrate (p.43·1).
Tablets: Phenylpropanolamine hydrochloride (p.1067·2); hydrocodone tartrate (p.43·1); guaiphenesin (p.1061·3).
Coughs and cold symptoms.

Tussanil N *Vifor, Switz.*
Noscapine hydrochloride (p.1065·2).
Coughs.

Tussanil Plain *Misemer, USA.*
Phenylephrine hydrochloride (p.1066·2); chlorpheniramine maleate (p.405·1).
Upper respiratory-tract symptoms.

Tussantiol *Medisa, Switz.*
Carbocisteine (p.1056·3).
Respiratory-tract disorders with increased mucus.

Tussanyl *Giovanardi, Ital.*
Potassium guaiacolsulfonate (p.1068·3); grindelia.
Catarrh; coughs.

Tussar-2 *Rhone-Poulenc Rorer, USA.*
Codeine phosphate (p.26·1); guaiphenesin (p.1061·3); pseudoephedrine hydrochloride (p.1068·3).
Coughs.

Tussar DM *Rorer, USA.*
Dextromethorphan hydrobromide (p.1057·3); chlorpheniramine maleate (p.405·1); pseudoephedrine hydrochloride (p.1068·3).
Coughs and cold symptoms.

Tussar SF *Rhone-Poulenc Rorer, USA.*
Codeine phosphate (p.26·1); guaiphenesin (p.1061·3); pseudoephedrine hydrochloride (p.1068·3).
Coughs.

Tussa-Tablinen *Sanorania, Ger.*
Pentoxyverine citrate (p.1066·1).
Coughs.

Tusscodin *Lannacher, Aust.*
Nicocodine hydrochloride (p.1065·1).
Coughs.

Tuss-DM *Hyrex, USA.*
Dextromethorphan hydrobromide (p.1057·3); guaiphenesin (p.1061·3).
Coughs.

Tusselix *Propan-Vernleigh, S.Afr.†.*
Terpin hydrate (p.1070·2); tolu syrup (p.1071·1); squill (p.1070·1).
Coughs.

Tusselix Cough Silencers *Key, Austral.†.*
Dextromethorphan hydrobromide (p.1057·3); lignocaine hydrochloride (p.1293·2).
Coughs; sore throat.

Tussend *Monarch, USA.*
Hydrocodone tartrate (p.43·1); pseudoephedrine hydrochloride (p.1068·3); chlorpheniramine maleate (p.405·1).
Coughs.

Tusseval *Marco Viti, Ital.†.*
Piperidione (p.1068·2).
Coughs.

Tussgen *Goldline, USA.*
Hydrocodone tartrate (p.43·1); pseudoephedrine hydrochloride (p.1068·3).
Coughs and cold symptoms.

Tuss-Genade Modified *Goldline, USA.*
Phenylpropanolamine hydrochloride (p.1067·2); caramiphen edisylate (p.1056·2).
Coughs.

Tussibron *Sella, Ital.*
Oxolamine citrate (p.1065·3).
Coughs.

Tussidermil N *Li-il, Ger.*
Eucalyptus oil (p.1578·1).
Catarrh; musculoskeletal and joint disorders.

Tussidyl *Tika, Swed.*
Dextromethorphan hydrobromide (p.1057·3).
Coughs.

Tussifama *FAMA, Ital.†.*
Dextromethorphan hydrobromide (p.1057·3); guaiphenesin (p.1061·3).
Coughs.

Tussifed Warner-Lambert, Fr.
Triprolidine hydrochloride (p.420·3); dextromethorphan hydrobromide (p.1057·3).
Formerly contained triprolidine hydrochloride, pseudoephedrine hydrochloride, and dextromethorphan hydrobromide.
Coughs.

Tussiflex Kemyos, Ital.
Oxeladin citrate (p.1065·3); terpin hydrate (p.1070·2).
Coughs.

Tussiflorin forte Pascoe, Ger.
Hedera helix; primula root; thyme (p.1636·3).
Respiratory-tract disorders.

Tussiflorin N Pascoe, Ger.
Polygonum aviculare; sanicula europaea; galeopsis ochroleuca; equisetum (p.1575·1); primula rhizome.
Coughs and associated respiratory-tract disorders.

Tussigon Daniels, USA.
Hydrocodone tartrate (p.43·1); homatropine methobromide (p.462·2).
Coughs and cold symptoms.

Tussilinct Restan, S.Afr.
Diphenhydramine hydrochloride (p.409·1); codeine phosphate (p.26·1); ammonium chloride (p.1055·2); sodium citrate (p.1153·2).
Coughs.

Tussimed Propan, S.Afr.
Diphenhydramine hydrochloride (p.409·1); codeine phosphate (p.26·1); ammonium chloride (p.1055·2); sodium citrate (p.1153·2); menthol (p.1600·2).
Coughs.

Tussimed Expectorant Propan-Vernleigh, S.Afr.†.
Diphenhydramine hydrochloride (p.409·1); ammonium chloride (p.1055·2); sodium citrate (p.1153·2); menthol (p.1600·2).
Coughs.

Tussimont Pharmonta, Aust.
Ointment: Camphor (p.1557·2); menthol (p.1600·2); eucalyptus oil (p.1578·1).
Oral drops: Ammonium chloride (p.1055·2); thyme (p.1636·3); plantago lanceolata.
Oral liquid: Senega (p.1069·3); thyme (p.1636·3).
Coughs and cold symptoms.

Tussinfant N Biocur, Ger.
Primula root; thyme (p.1636·3).
Cold symptoms.

Tussinfantum Jossa-Arznei, Ger.†.
Thyme (p.1636·3); primula rhizome; sodium phytate (p.995·3); oxeladin citrate (p.1065·3); guaiphenesin (p.1061·3); glycerol (p.1585·2).
Coughs.

Tussinol G.P. Laboratories, Austral.
Pholcodine (p.1068·1).
Coughs.

Tussionex Rhone-Poulenc Rorer, Canad.
Hydrocodone resin complex; phenyltoloxamine resin complex (p.416·1).
Coughs.

Tussionex Pennkinetic Fisons, USA.
Hydrocodone polistirex (p.43·2); chlorpheniramine polistirex (p.405·2).
Coughs and cold symptoms.

Tussi-Organidin Horner, Canad.†.
Iodinated glycerol (p.1062·2); codeine phosphate (p.26·1); chlorpheniramine maleate (p.405·1).
Coughs.

Tussi-Organidin DM NR Wallace, USA.
Guaiphenesin (p.1061·3); dextromethorphan hydrobromide (p.1057·3).
Tussi-Organidin DM formerly contained iodinated glycerol and dextromethorphan hydrobromide.
Coughs.

Tussi-Organidin NR Wallace, USA.
Codeine phosphate (p.26·1); guaiphenesin (p.1061·3).
Tussi-Organidin formerly contained codeine phosphate and iodinated glycerol.
Coughs.

Tussipax Therica, Fr.
Oral solution: Ethylmorphine hydrochloride (p.36·1); codeine (p.26·1).
Formerly contained ethylmorphine hydrochloride, codeine, bromoform, and maidenhair fern.
Syrup: Ethylmorphine hydrochloride (p.36·1); codeine (p.26·1); tolu balsam (p.1071·1); pectoral concentrate.
Formerly contained ethylmorphine hydrochloride, codeine, bromoform, tolu balsam, and pectoral concentrate.
Tablets: Ethylmorphine hydrochloride (p.36·1); codeine (p.26·1).
Formerly contained ethylmorphine hydrochloride, codeine, bromoform, drosera, and maidenhair fern.
Coughs.

Tussipax a l'Euquinine Therica, Fr.
Ethylmorphine hydrochloride (p.36·1); codeine (p.26·1); pine oil; eucalyptus oil (p.1578·1); quinine ethyl carbonate (p.439·1).
Coughs.

Tussipect
Note. This name is used for preparations of different composition.
Qualiphar, Belg.
Dextromethorphan hydrobromide (p.1057·3).
Coughs.

Beiersdorf-Lilly, Ger.
Thyme (p.1636·3); liquorice (p.1197·1); saponin; cetylpyridinium chloride (p.1106·2); peppermint oil (p.1208·1); menthol (p.1600·2); anethole (p.1549·3); eucalyptus oil (p.1578·1); camphor (p.1557·2).
Coughs and associated respiratory-tract disorders.

Tussipect A Beiersdorf-Lilly, Ger.†.
Ambroxol hydrochloride (p.1054·3).
Bronchopulmonary secretory disorders.

Tussipect Codein Beiersdorf-Lilly, Ger.†.
Codeine phosphate (p.26·1).
Formerly contained codeine phosphate, ephedrine hydrochloride, and thyme.
Coughs and associated respiratory-tract disorders.

Tussipect mit Codein Beiersdorf-Lilly, Ger.†.
Codeine (p.26·1); saponin; ephedrine hydrochloride (p.1059·3); thyme (p.1636·3).
Coughs and associated respiratory-tract disorders.

Tussipect mono Beiersdorf-Lilly, Ger.†.
Codeine phosphate (p.26·1).
Coughs.

Tussipect N Beiersdorf-Lilly, Ger.†.
Ephedrine hydrochloride (p.1059·3); thyme (p.1636·3).
Coughs and associated respiratory-tract disorders.

Tussiplex Vifor, Switz.
Chlorpheniramine maleate (p.405·1); phenylephrine hydrochloride (p.1066·2); pholcodine (p.1068·1); guaiphenesin (p.1061·3).
Coughs.

Tussiprene Zambeletti, Ital.†.
Orciprenaline (p.756·3); calcium iodide (p.1056·2).
Bronchitis.

Tussirex Scot-Tussin, USA.
Codeine phosphate (p.26·1); pheniramine maleate (p.415·3); phenylephrine hydrochloride (p.1066·2); sodium citrate (p.1153·2); sodium salicylate (p.85·1); caffeine citrate (p.749·3); menthol (p.1600·2).
Coughs.

Tussisana N Muller Goppingen, Ger.
Homoeopathic preparation.

Tussisedal Elerte, Fr.
Noscapine (p.1065·2); promethazine (p.416·2); polysorbate 85 (Tween 85).
Coughs.

Tussistin DHU, Ger.
Homoeopathic preparation.

Tussistin N DHU, Ger.
Homoeopathic preparation.

Tussitot Restan, S.Afr.
Diphenhydramine hydrochloride (p.409·1); codeine phosphate (p.26·1); ammonium chloride (p.1055·2); sodium citrate (p.1153·2).
Coughs.

Tussiverlan Verla, Ger.
Acetylcysteine (p.1052·3).
Formerly contained butethamate citrate, diphenylpyraline hydrochloride, guaiphenesin, plantago lanceolata, and thyme.
Respiratory-tract disorders with viscous mucus.

Tuss-LA Hyrex, USA.
Pseudoephedrine hydrochloride (p.1068·3); guaiphenesin (p.1061·3).
Coughs.

Tusso BASF, Ger.
Ambroxol hydrochloride (p.1054·3).
Respiratory-tract disorders with increased or viscous mucus.

tusso-basan Sagitta, Ger.†.
Ambroxol hydrochloride (p.1054·3).
Respiratory-tract disorders associated with increased or viscous mucus.

Tussodan DM Odan, Canad.
Dextromethorphan hydrobromide (p.1057·3); pseudoephedrine hydrochloride (p.1068·3).

Tusso-DM Everett, USA†.
Dextromethorphan hydrobromide (p.1057·3); iodinated glycerol (p.1062·2).
Coughs.

Tussogest Extended-Release Major, USA.
Phenylpropanolamine hydrochloride (p.1067·2); caramiphen edisylate (p.1056·2).
Coughs.

Tussoglobin
Behringwerke, Ger.†; Behring, Ital.†.
A pertussis immunoglobulin (p.1525·3).
Passive immunisation.

Tussol Nycomed, Norw.
Guaiphenesin (p.1061·3); ammonium chloride (p.1055·2); liquorice (p.1197·1); ammonium glycyrrhizinate (p.1055·2).
Coughs.

Tussolvina Bioindustria, Ital.
Nepinalone hydrochloride (p.1065·1).
Coughs.

Tussoretard Klinge, Ger.†.
Capsules: Daytime capsules, codeine phosphate (p.26·1); DL-*N*-methylephedrine hydrochloride (p.1064·1); noscapine (p.1065·2); night-time capsules, codeine phosphate (p.26·1); diphenhydramine hydrochloride (p.409·1); noscapine (p.1065·2).
Oral liquid: Codeine phosphate (p.26·1); noscapine (p.1065·2).
Coughs and associated respiratory-tract disorders.

Tussoretard SN Klinge, Ger.
Codeine phosphate (p.26·1).
Coughs.

Tussoretardin Klinge, Aust.
White tablets, pentoxyverine citrate (p.1066·1); methylephedrine hydrochloride (p.1064·1); blue tablets, pentoxyverine citrate; diphenhydramine hydrochloride (p.409·1).
Coughs.

Tuss-Ornade SmithKline Beecham, USA†.
Caramiphen edisylate (p.1056·2); phenylpropanolamine hydrochloride (p.1067·2).
Coughs and cold symptoms.

Tusstat Century, USA.
Diphenhydramine hydrochloride (p.409·1).
Coughs.

Tussycalm Rhone-Poulenc Rorer, Ital.
Dextromethorphan hydrobromide (p.1057·3).
Coughs.

Tutofusin
Pharmacia Upjohn, Aust.
Electrolyte infusion with glucose (p.1147·1).
Carbohydrate source; fluid and electrolyte disorders.

Pharmacia Upjohn, Ger.
Electrolyte infusion (p.1147·1).
Fluid and electrolyte disorders; peritoneal irrigation.

Tutofusin BG Pharmacia Upjohn, Ger.
Electrolyte solution with glucose (p.1147·1).
Carbohydrate source; fluid and electrolyte disorders.

Tutofusin BX Pharmacia Upjohn, Ger.
Electrolyte infusion with xylitol (p.1147·1).
Carbohydrate source; fluid and electrolyte disorders.

Tutofusin CH Kabi Pharmacia, Ger.†.
Electrolytes; xylitol; amino acids; thioctic acid (p.1636·2); vitamins.
Liver disease.

Tutofusin HL Kabi Pharmacia, Ger.†.
Electrolyte infusion with fructose (p.1147·1).
Carbohydrate source; fluid and electrolyte disorders.

Tutofusin K 10 Kabi Pharmacia, Ger.†.
Electrolyte infusion (p.1147·1).
Fluid and electrolyte disorders.

Tutofusin K 80 Kabi Pharmacia, Ger.†.
Electrolyte infusion with xylitol and glucose (p.1147·1).
Potassium deficiency in cardiac disorders.

Tutofusin L 5 Kabi Pharmacia, Ger.†.
Electrolyte infusion with fructose (p.1147·1).
Carbohydrate source; fluid and electrolyte disorders.

Tutofusin LC Kabi Pharmacia, Ger.†.
Electrolytes; sorbitol; choline chloride (p.1337·1); amino acids; citiolone (p.1564·3); thioctic acid (p.1636·2); anhydrous orotic acid; vitamins.
Liver disease.

Tutofusin Malat Kabi Pharmacia, Ger.†.
Electrolyte infusion with xylitol (p.1147·1).
Carbohydrate source; fluid and electrolyte disorders.

Tutofusin OP Pharmacia Upjohn, Ger.
Electrolyte infusion (p.1147·1).
Fluid and electrolyte disorders.

Tutofusin OP G Pharmacia Upjohn, Ger.
Electrolyte infusion with glucose (p.1147·1).
Carbohydrate source; fluid and electrolyte disorders.

Tutofusin OP S Kabi Pharmacia, Ger.†.
Electrolyte infusion with sorbitol (p.1147·1).
Carbohydrate source; fluid and electrolyte disorders.

Tutofusin OP X Pharmacia Upjohn, Ger.
Electrolyte infusion with xylitol (p.1147·1).
Carbohydrate source; fluid and electrolyte disorders.

Tutofusin Pad Pharmacia Upjohn, Ger.†.
Electrolyte solution with glucose (p.1147·1).

Tutofusin S Pharmacia Upjohn, Ger.
Sodium chloride (p.1162·2); sodium acetate (p.1153·1); sorbitol (p.1354·2).
Fluid retention; renal failure.

Tutoplast Dura E. Merck, UK†.
Absorbable collagen from dehydrated human dura mater (p.1566·3).
Repair or closure of body tissue.

Tutoseral Streuli, Switz.
Electrolyte infusion (p.1147·1).
Fluid and electrolyte disorders.

Tuttomycin Mago, Ger.†.
Framycetin sulphate (p.210·3).
Pyococcal skin infections.

Tuttozem N Strathmann, Ger.
Dexamethasone (p.1037·1).
Burns; skin disorders.

Tux Warner-Lambert Consumer, Belg.
Ethylmorphine hydrochloride (p.36·1); codeine phosphate (p.26·1); ephedrine hydrochloride (p.1059·3); guaiphenesin (p.1061·3); sodium benzoate (p.1102·3); sodium camsylate; polygala (p.1069·3); senna (p.1212·2); tolu balsam (p.1071·1).
Colds; coughs; respiratory disorders.

Tuxi Weifa, Norw.
Pholcodine (p.1068·1).
Coughs.

Tuxidrin Weifa, Norw.
Pholcodine (p.1068·1); ephedrine (p.1059·3).
Coughs.

Tuxium Galephar, Fr.
Dextromethorphan hydrobromide (p.1057·3).
Coughs.

Tuzanil Bohm, Spain.
Prunus africana.
Prostatic adenoma.

T-Vaccinol Rohm, Ger.†.
An adsorbed tetanus vaccine (p.1535·3).
Active immunisation.

TVC-2 Dandruff Shampoo Dermol, USA.
Pyrithione zinc (p.1089·3).

T-Vites Freeda, USA.
Multivitamin preparation with minerals.

T-Wellcovax Wellcopharm, Ger.†.
An adsorbed tetanus vaccine (p.1535·3).
Active immunisation.

Twice-A-Day Major, USA.
Oxymetazoline hydrochloride (p.1065·3).
Nasal congestion.

Twilite Pfeiffer, USA.
Diphenhydramine hydrochloride (p.409·1).
Insomnia.

Twin-K Boots, USA.
Potassium gluconate (p.1161·1); potassium citrate (p.1153·1).
Hypokalaemia; potassium depletion.

Twinrix
SmithKline Beecham, Austral.; SmithKline Beecham, Fr.; SmithKline Beecham, Ger.; SmithKline Beecham, Irl.; SmithKline Beecham, Ital.; SmithKline Beecham, Neth.; SmithKline Beecham, Swed.; SmithKline Beecham, UK.
An inactivated hepatitis A vaccine and recombinant hepatitis B vaccine (p.1515·1).
Separate preparations are available for infants and children and for adults.
Active immunisation.

Twocal Abbott, Ital.
Preparation for enteral nutrition.

Twocal HN
Abbott, Austral.; Ross, USA.
High calorie, high nitrogen lactose-free preparation for enteral nutrition.

Two-Dyne Hyrex, USA†.
Paracetamol (p.72·2); caffeine (p.749·3); butalbital (p.644·3).
Pain.

Two's Company Family Planning Sales, UK†.
Nonoxinol 9 (p.1326·1).
Contraceptive.

Tyco Beta, Ital.†.
Hamamelis water; rose water; matricaria water; sodium sulphate; benzalkonium chloride.
Eye irritation.

Ty-Cold Major, USA.
Chlorpheniramine maleate (p.405·1); dextromethorphan hydrobromide (p.1057·3); paracetamol (p.72·2); pseudoephedrine hydrochloride (p.1068·3).
Coughs and cold symptoms.

Tycopan Lilly, USA†.
Multivitamin preparation.

Tydamine Lennon, S.Afr.
Trimipramine (p.310·1).
Anxiety disorders; depression; nocturnal enuresis.

Tylenol
Johnson & Johnson, Aust.; Johnson & Johnson, Austral.; McNeil Consumer, Canad.; Johnson & Johnson, Irl.; Janssen-Cilag, S.Afr.; Abello, Spain; Janssen-Cilag, Switz.; McNeil Consumer, USA.
Paracetamol (p.72·2).
Fever; pain.

Tylenol Aches & Strains McNeil Consumer, Canad.
Chlorzoxazone (p.1313·1); paracetamol (p.72·2).
Muscular aches and strains.

Tylenol Allergy Sinus
Johnson & Johnson, Austral.; McNeil Consumer, Canad.
Paracetamol (p.72·2); chlorpheniramine maleate (p.405·1); pseudoephedrine hydrochloride (p.1068·3).
Allergy symptoms; sinus pain and congestion.

Tylenol with Codeine
McNeil Consumer, Canad.; McNeil Pharmaceutical, USA.
Paracetamol (p.72·2); codeine phosphate (p.26·1).
Fever; pain.

Tylenol with Codeine No 4 McNeil, Canad.
Paracetamol (p.72·2); codeine phosphate (p.26·1).
Fever; pain.

Tylenol with Codeine No 1, No 2, or No 3
McNeil, Canad.
Paracetamol (p.72·2); caffeine (p.749·3); codeine phosphate (p.26·1).
Fever; pain.

Tylenol Cold Effervescent McNeil Consumer, USA†.
Paracetamol (p.72·2); phenylpropanolamine hydrochloride (p.1067·2); chlorpheniramine maleate (p.405·1).
Upper respiratory-tract symptoms.

Tylenol Cold & Flu
Note. This name is used for preparations of different composition.
Johnson & Johnson, Austral.
Paracetamol (p.72·2); pseudoephedrine hydrochloride (p.1068·3); dextromethorphan hydrobromide (p.1057·3); chlorpheniramine maleate (p.405·1).
Cold and influenza symptoms.

Janssen-Cilag, S.Afr.
Paracetamol (p.72·2); chlorpheniramine maleate (p.405·1); pseudoephedrine hydrochloride (p.1068·3).
Allergic rhinitis; cold symptoms.

Tylenol Cold & Flu Non-Drowsy Johnson & Johnson, Austral.
Paracetamol (p.72·2); pseudoephedrine hydrochloride (p.1068·3); dextromethorphan hydrobromide (p.1057·3).
Cold and influenza symptoms.

Tylenol Cold and Flu Powder McNeil Consumer, Canad.
Paracetamol (p.72·2); chlorpheniramine maleate (p.405·1); pseudoephedrine hydrochloride (p.1068·3); dextromethorphan hydrobromide (p.1057·3).
Cold symptoms.

Tylenol Cold Medication McNeil Consumer, Canad.
Paracetamol (p.72·2); chlorpheniramine maleate (p.405·1); pseudoephedrine hydrochloride (p.1068·3).
Cold symptoms.

Tylenol Cold Medication (Daytime) *McNeil Consumer, Canad.*
Paracetamol (p.72·2); pseudoephedrine hydrochloride (p.1068·3); dextromethorphan hydrobromide (p.1057·3).
Cold symptoms.

Tylenol Cold Medication DM *McNeil Consumer, Canad.*
Paracetamol (p.72·2); chlorpheniramine maleate (p.405·1); pseudoephedrine hydrochloride (p.1068·3); dextromethorphan hydrobromide (p.1057·3).
Cold symptoms.

Tylenol Cold Medication (Nighttime) *McNeil Consumer, Canad.*
Paracetamol (p.72·2); chlorpheniramine maleate (p.405·1); pseudoephedrine hydrochloride (p.1068·3); dextromethorphan hydrobromide (p.1057·3).
Cold symptoms.

Tylenol Cold No Drowsiness *McNeil Consumer, USA.*
Paracetamol (p.72·2); pseudoephedrine hydrochloride (p.1068·3); dextromethorphan hydrobromide (p.1057·3).
Coughs and cold symptoms.

Tylenol Cold Severe Congestion *McNeil Consumer, USA.*
Paracetamol (p.72·2); pseudoephedrine hydrochloride (p.1068·3); dextromethorphan hydrobromide (p.1057·3); guaiphenesin (p.1061·3).
Coughs and cold symptoms.

Tylenol Cough *McNeil Consumer, Canad.*
Paracetamol (p.72·2); dextromethorphan hydrobromide (p.1057·3).
Coughs; fever; pain; sore throat.

Tylenol Cough with Decongestant *McNeil Consumer, Canad.*
Paracetamol (p.72·2); dextromethorphan hydrobromide (p.1057·3); pseudoephedrine hydrochloride (p.1068·3).
Coughs; fever; nasal congestion; pain; sore throat.

Tylenol Flu Night Time *McNeil Consumer, USA.*
Paracetamol (p.72·2); diphenhydramine hydrochloride (p.409·1); pseudoephedrine hydrochloride (p.1068·3).

Tylenol Flu No Drowsiness *McNeil Consumer, USA.*
Paracetamol (p.72·2); dextromethorphan hydrobromide (p.1057·3); pseudoephedrine hydrochloride (p.1068·3).

Tylenol Night Pain *Janssen-Cilag, S.Afr.*
Paracetamol (p.72·2); diphenhydramine hydrochloride (p.409·1).
Insomnia with pain.

Tylenol Severe Allergy *McNeil Consumer, USA.*
Paracetamol (p.72·2); diphenhydramine hydrochloride (p.409·1).
Cold symptoms.

Tylenol Sinus *Johnson & Johnson, Austral.*
Paracetamol (p.72·2); pseudoephedrine hydrochloride (p.1068·3).
Sinus and nasal congestion; sinus pain.

Tylenol Sinus Medication *McNeil Consumer, Canad.*
Paracetamol (p.72·2); pseudoephedrine hydrochloride (p.1068·3).
Cold symptoms; sinus.

Tylex
Note. This name is used for preparations of different composition.
Janssen-Cilag, Ger.†.
Carbinoxamine maleate (p.404·2); paracetamol (p.72·2); phenylephrine hydrochloride (p.1066·2).
Cold symptoms.
Schwarz, Irl.; Schwarz, UK.
Paracetamol (p.72·2); codeine phosphate (p.26·1).
These ingredients can be described by the British Approved Name Co-codamol 30/500.
Pain.

Tyliculine *Amino, Switz.†.*
Oestradiol benzoate (p.1455·1); tyrothricin (p.267·2).
Atrophic vaginitis; prophylaxis of cracked nipples.

Tylosterone *Lilly, USA†.*
Stilboestrol (p.1462·3); methyltestosterone (p.1450·3).

Tylox *McNeil Pharmaceutical, USA.*
Oxycodone hydrochloride (p.71·2); paracetamol (p.72·2).
Pain.

Tymasil *Brocades, UK†.*
Natamycin (p.385·3).
Allergy to house-dust mite.

Tymelyt
Lundbeck, Aust.; Lundbeck, Belg.; Lundbeck, Swed.
Lofepramine hydrochloride (p.296·1).
Depression.

Tymium *Sauter, Switz.†.*
Febarbamate (p.670·1).
Agitation; depression; dysphoria; emotional disorders; mental function disorders in the elderly.

Tympagesic *Savage, USA.*
Phenylephrine hydrochloride (p.1066·2); phenazone (p.78·2); benzocaine (p.1286·2).
Earache.

Tympalgine *Therabel Pharma, Belg.*
Phenazone (p.78·2); procaine hydrochloride (p.1299·2).
Otitis.

Typherix *SmithKline Beecham, UK.*
A typhoid vaccine (VI capsular polysaccharide) (p.1536·3).
Active immunisation.

Typhidrall *Biocine, Ital.†.*
An adsorbed typhoid-paratyphoid A and B vaccine.
Active immunisation.

Typhim Vi
Serotherapeutisches, Aust.; CSL, Austral.; Merieux, Belg.; Connaught, Canad.; Pasteur Vaccins, Fr.; Pasteur Merieux, Ger.; Pasteur Merieux, Irl.; Pasteur Merieux, Ital.; Pasteur Merieux, Neth.; Pasteur Merieux, Norw.; Rhone-Poulenc Rorer, S.Afr.; Pasteur Merieux, Swed.; Pasteur Merieux, UK; Connaught, USA.
A typhoid vaccine (Vi capsular polysaccharide) (p.1536·3).
Active immunisation.

Typhoral L *Chiron Behring, Ger.*
A live oral typhoid vaccine (p.1536·3).
Active immunisation.

Typh-Vax *CSL, Austral.*
A typhoid vaccine (attenuated Ty21a Berna strain) (p.1536·3).
Active immunisation.

Tyrcine *Oberlin, Fr.*
Tyrothricin (p.267·2); amethocaine hydrochloride (p.1285·2).
Mouth and throat disorders.

Tyrex *Ross, USA.*
Phenylalanine- and tyrosine-free preparation for enteral nutrition.
Tyrosinaemia type II.

Tyrocane *Seton, UK†.*
Tyrothricin (p.267·2); benzocaine (p.1286·2); cetylpyridinium chloride (p.1106·2).
Sore throat.

Tyrocane Junior *Seton, UK†.*
Cetylpyridinium chloride (p.1106·2).
Sore throat.

Tyrocombine *Synpharma, Switz.*
Ointment: Tyrothricin (p.267·2); neomycin sulphate (p.229·2); benzethonium chloride (p.1102·3).
Topical powder†: Tyrothricin (p.267·2); neomycin sulphate (p.229·2); benzethonium chloride (p.1102·3); sulphathiazole (p.257·1).
Infected skin disorders; infected wounds.

Tyrodone *Major, USA.*
Hydrocodone tartrate (p.43·1); pseudoephedrine hydrochloride (p.1068·3).

Tyro-Drops *Centrapharm, Belg.*
Tyrothricin (p.267·2); lignocaine hydrochloride (p.1293·2).
Mouth and throat disorders.

Tyrogel *Mer-National, S.Afr.†.*
Tyrothricin (p.267·2); hydroxypolyethoxy dodecan (p.1325·2).
Burns; wounds.

Tyromex *Ross, USA.*
Methionine-, phenylalanine-, and tyrosine-free infant feed.
Tyrosinaemia type I.

Tyroneomicin *Alcala, Spain.*
Bacitracin zinc (p.157·3); benzocaine (p.1286·2); hydrocortisone acetate (p.1043·3); neomycin sulphate (p.229·2); potassium chlorate (p.1620·3).
Mouth and throat disorders.

Tyropenicilin R *Ale, Spain†.*
Bacitracin (p.157·3); benzylpenicillin sodium (p.159·3); benzocaine (p.1286·2); potassium chlorate (p.1620·3); menthol (p.1600·2).
Mouth and throat disorders.

Tyroqualine *Spirig, Switz.*
Tyrothricin (p.267·2); dequalinium chloride (p.1112·1); lignocaine hydrochloride (p.1293·2).
Mouth and throat disorders.

Tyroseng *Eagle, Austral.*
Tyrosine (p.1357·3); eleutherococcus senticosis (p.1584·2); calcium glycerophosphate (p.1155·2); phosphatidyl choline (p.1618·1); vitamin B substances.
Dietary supplement.

Tyrosin S *SmithKline Beecham, Ger.*
Mixed allergen extracts (p.1545·1).
Hyposensitisation.

Tyrosirinal *Woelm, Ger.†.*
Tyrothricin (p.267·2); dequalinium chloride (p.1112·1); chlorquinaldol (p.185·1).
Inflammatory disorders and infections of the oropharynx.

Tyrosolvetten *Tosse, Ger.*
Cetylpyridinium chloride (p.1106·2); benzocaine (p.1286·2).
Mouth and throat disorders.

Tyrosolvetten-C *Tosse, Ger.*
Cetylpyridinium chloride (p.1106·2); ascorbic acid (p.1365·2).
Inflammatory disorders and infection of the oropharynx.

Tyrosolvin
Lundbeck, Aust.; Lundbeck, Switz.†.
Tyrothricin (p.267·2); cetylpyridinium chloride (p.1106·2).
Bacterial infections.

Tyrosum *Summers, USA.*
Skin cleanser.

Tyrosur *Engelhard, Ger.*
Topical gel: Tyrothricin (p.267·2); cetylpyridinium chloride (p.1106·2).
Topical powder: Tyrothricin (p.267·2).
Infected skin disorders; infected wounds and burns.

Tyrothricin *Streuli, Switz.*
Tyrothricin (p.267·2); ethacridine lactate (p.1098·3); lignocaine hydrochloride (p.1293·2); menthol (p.1600·2); mint oil (p.1604·1).
Mouth and throat disorders.

Tyrothricin comp *Provita, Aust.*
Tyrothricin (p.267·2); neomycin sulphate (p.229·2); benzalkonium chloride (p.1101·3); benzocaine (p.1286·2).
Mouth and throat disorders.

Tyrothricine + Gramicidine *Pharmacal, Switz.*
Tyrothricin (p.267·2); gramicidin (p.215·2); amethocaine hydrochloride (p.1285·2); benzethonium chloride (p.1102·3).
Mouth and throat disorders.

Tyrothricine Lafran *Lafran, Fr.*
Tyrothricin (p.267·2); butyl aminobenzoate (p.1289·1).
Mouth and throat disorders.

Tyrozets
Merck Sharp & Dohme, Irl.; Johnson & Johnson MSD Consumer, UK.
Tyrothricin (p.267·2); benzocaine (p.1286·2).
Mouth and throat disorders.

Tyzine
Pfizer, Ger.; Pfizer, Switz.; Kenwood, USA.
Tetrahydrozoline hydrochloride (p.1070·2).
Nasal congestion.

Tyzine compositum *Pfizer, Ger.†.*
Tetrahydrozoline hydrochloride (p.1070·2); prednisolone (p.1048·1); neomycin sulphate (p.229·2).
Rhinitis; sinusitis.

UAA *Econo Med, USA.*
Hexamine (p.216·1); salol (p.83·1); atropine sulphate (p.455·1); hyoscyamine sulphate (p.464·2); benzoic acid (p.1102·3); methylene blue (p.984·3).
Urinary-tract infections.

UAD Cream or Lotion *UAD, USA†.*
Clioquinol (p.193·2); hydrocortisone (p.1043·3).

UAD-Otic *UAD, USA.*
Hydrocortisone (p.1043·3); neomycin sulphate (p.229·2); polymyxin B sulphate (p.239·1).
Bacterial ear infections.

Ubicarden *Locatelli, Ital.*
Ubidecarenone (p.1641·2).
Cardiac disorders; coenzyme Q10 deficiency.

Ubicardio *Tosi, Ital.*
Ubidecarenone (p.1641·2).
Cardiac disorders; coenzyme Q10 deficiency.

Ubicor
Note. This name is used for preparations of different composition.
Magis, Ital.
Ubidecarenone (p.1641·2).
Cardiac disorders; coenzyme Q10 deficiency.
Siegfried, Switz.†.
Diltiazem hydrochloride (p.854·2).
Angina pectoris; hypertension; myocardial infarction.

Ubidenone *Esseti, Ital.*
Ubidecarenone (p.1641·2).
Cardiac disorders; coenzyme Q10 deficiency.

Ubidex *OFF, Ital.*
Ubidecarenone (p.1641·2).
Cardiac disorders; coenzyme Q10 deficiency.

Ubifactor *San Carlo, Ital.*
Ubidecarenone (p.1641·2).
Cardiac disorders; coenzyme Q10 deficiency.

Ubilab *Del Saz & Filippini, Ital.*
Ubidecarenone (p.1641·2).
Cardiac disorders.

Ubimaior *Master Pharma, Ital.*
Ubidecarenone (p.1641·2).
Cardiac disorders; coenzyme Q10 deficiency.

Ubisan *Lebens, Ital.†.*
Ubidecarenone (p.1641·2).
Cardiac disorders; coenzyme Q10 deficiency.

Ubisint *Francia, Ital.*
Ubidecarenone (p.1641·2).
Coenzyme Q10 deficiency: cardiac disorders.

Ubistesin
Espe, Aust.; Espe, Ger.; Espe, Switz.
Carticaine hydrochloride (p.1289·1).
Adrenaline hydrochloride (p.813·3) is included in this preparation as a vasoconstrictor to diminish absorption and localise the effect of the local anaesthetic.
Local anaesthesia.

Ubiten *Zilliken, Ital.*
Ubidecarenone (p.1641·2).
Cardiac disorders; coenzyme Q10 deficiency.

Ubivis *AGIPS, Ital.*
Ubidecarenone (p.1641·2).
Cardiac disorders; coenzyme Q10 deficiency.

Ubixal *Foletto, Ital.†.*
Ubidecarenone (p.1641·2).
Cardiac disorders; coenzyme Q10 deficiency.

Ubretid
Hafslund Nycomed, Aust.; Rhone-Poulenc Rorer, Austral.†; Nycomed, Ger.; Rhone-Poulenc Rorer, Irl.; Christiaens, Neth.; Roche, S.Afr.; Nycomed, Switz.; Rorer, UK.
Distigmine bromide (p.1391·1).
Constipation; intestinal motility disorders; myasthenia gravis; urinary retention.

Ucecal
UCB, Aust.; UCB, Spain.
Salcatonin (p.735·3).
Hypercalcaemia; hyperparathyroidism; immobilisation; metastatic bone pain; osteoporosis; Paget's disease of bone; pancreatic disorders; reflex sympathetic dystrophy; vitamin D intoxication.

Ucee *Brenner-Efeka, Ger.†.*
Calendula officinalis; hypericum (p.1590·1); wheatgerm oil; calendula oil; zinc oxide (p.1096·2).
Ulcers; wounds.

Ucee D *Kytta, Ger.*
Dexpanthenol (p.1570·3).
Skin lesions.

Ucemine PP *Darci, Belg.*
Nicotinamide (p.1351·2).
Vitamin PP deficiency.

Ucephan *McGaw, USA.*
Sodium benzoate (p.1102·3); sodium phenylacetate (p.1631·3).
Hyperammonaemia.

Ucerax *UCB, UK.*
Hydroxyzine hydrochloride (p.412·1).
Anxiety; pruritus.

UCG-Beta
Carter-Wallace, Austral.†; Horner, Canad.†.
Pregnancy test (p.1621·2).

UCG-Slide
Carter-Wallace, Austral.†; Wampole, USA.
Pregnancy test (p.1621·2).

Ucine *Ashbourne, UK.*
Sulphasalazine (p.1215·2).
Inflammatory bowel disease.

U-Cort *Thames, USA.*
Hydrocortisone acetate (p.1043·3).
Skin disorders.

Udepasi-50 *Aandersen, Ital.†.*
Cogalactoisomerase sodium trihydrate (p.1566·2).
Hepatic insufficiency; impaired glucuronidation.

Udetox *San Carlo, Ital.†.*
Cogalactoisomerase sodium trihydrate (p.1566·2).
Hepatitis.

Udicil *Pharmacia Upjohn, Ger.*
Cytarabine (p.525·2).
Malignant neoplasms.

Udicit *CT, Ital.†.*
Cogalactoisomerase sodium trihydrate (p.1566·2).
Liver disorders.

Udima *Dermapharm, Ger.*
Minocycline hydrochloride (p.226·2).
Bacterial infections.

Udima Ery *Dermapharm, Ger.*
Erythromycin (p.204·1).
Acne.

Udrik *Albert-Roussel, Ger.; Hoechst, Ger.*
Trandolapril (p.957·1).
Hypertension.

UFT
Taiho, Jpn.; Miquel Otsuka, Spain.
Tegafur (p.565·2); uracil.
Malignant neoplasms.

Ugurol
Bayer, Ger.; Bayer, Ital.
Tranexamic acid (p.728·2).
Hyperfibrinolytic haemorrhage.

Ujostabil *Felgentrager, Ger.*
Ammonium polystyrene sulphonate; potassium polystyrene sulphonate (p.992·2); magnesium polystyrene sulphonate; sodium polystyrene sulphonate (p.995·3).
Renal calculi.

Ukidan
Serono, Aust.; Serono, Austral.; Serono, Ger.†; Serono, Ital.; Research Labs, S.Afr.; Serono, Swed.; Serono, Switz.; Serono, UK.
Urokinase (p.959·3).
Intra-ocular haemorrhage; thrombo-embolic disorders.

Ulcaid *Seton, UK†.*
Oral gel: Lignocaine (p.1293·2); cetylpyridinium chloride (p.1106·2); alcohol (p.1099·1).
Tablets: Tyrothricin (p.267·2); benzocaine (p.1286·2); cetylpyridinium chloride (p.1106·2).
Mouth disorders.

Ulcar *Houde, Fr.*
Sucralfate (p.1214·2).
Peptic ulcer.

Ulcedin *AGIPS, Ital.*
Cimetidine (p.1183·2).
Gastric hyperacidity; gastro-oesophageal reflux; peptic ulcer; Zollinger-Ellison syndrome.

Ulcefate *Abbott, S.Afr.*
Sucralfate (p.1214·2).
Gastritis; peptic ulcer.

Ulceral *Tedec Meiji, Spain.*
Omeprazole (p.1204·2).
Gastro-oesophageal reflux; peptic ulcer; Zollinger-Ellison syndrome.

Ulcerease *Med-Derm, USA.*
Liquefied phenol (p.1121·2).
Mouth and throat pain.

Ulcerlmin *Chugai, Jpn.*
Sucralfate (p.1214·2).
Gastritis; peptic ulcer.

Ulcerone *Pharmaplan, S.Afr.*
Tripotassium dicitratobismuthate (p.1180·2).
Peptic ulcer.

Ulcesep *Centrum, Spain.*
Omeprazole (p.1204·2).
Gastro-oesophageal reflux; peptic ulcer; Zollinger-Ellison syndrome.

Ulcesium *Zambon, Ital.†.*
Fentonium bromide (p.461·2).
Preparation for urography/duodenography; visceral spasms; vomiting.

Ulcestop *Metapharma, Ital.*
Cimetidine hydrochloride (p.1185·3).
Gastro-oesophageal reflux; peptic ulcer; Zollinger-Ellison syndrome.

Ulcetab *Noristan, S.Afr.†.*
Sucralfate (p.1214·2).
Gastritis; gastro-oesophageal reflux; peptic ulcer.

Ulcetic *Noristan, S.Afr.†.*
Sucralfate (p.1214·2).
Gastritis; gastro-oesophageal reflux; peptic ulcer.

Ulcetrax *Salvat, Spain.*
Famotidine (p.1192·1).
Gastro-oesophageal reflux; peptic ulcer; Zollinger-Ellison syndrome.

Ulcex *Guidotti, Ital.*
Ranitidine hydrochloride (p.1209·3).
Gastritis or duodenitis associated with acid hypersecretion; gastro-oesophageal reflux; peptic ulcer; Zollinger-Ellison syndrome.

Ulcim *Noristan, S.Afr.†.*
Cimetidine (p.1183·2).
Gastro-intestinal disorders.

Ulcin *Ibirn, Ital.*
Pirenzepine hydrochloride (p.467·1).
Gastroduodenitis; peptic ulcer.

Ulco -cyl Ho-Len-Complex *Liebermann, Ger.*
Homoeopathic preparation.

Ulcodina *SoSe, Ital.*
Cimetidine (p.1183·2).
Gastritis and duodenitis associated with acid hypersecretion; gastro-oesophageal reflux; peptic ulcer; Zollinger-Ellison syndrome.

Ulcofalk *Pirri, Ital.†.*
Cimetidine (p.1183·2).
Gastritis and duodenitis associated with acid hypersecretion; gastro-oesophageal reflux; peptic ulcer; Zollinger-Ellison syndrome.

Ulcogant
Merck, Aust.; Merck-Belgolabo, Belg.; Merck, Ger.; Lipha, Ger.; E. Merck, Neth.; E. Merck, Switz.
Sucralfate (p.1214·2).
Gastro-oesophageal reflux; peptic ulcer; stress-related gastro-intestinal haemorrhage.

Ulcol *Alphapharm, Austral.†.*
Sulphasalazine (p.1215·2).
Crohn's disease; ulcerative colitis.

Ulcolind Amoxi *Lindopharm, Ger.*
Amoxycillin trihydrate (p.151·3).
Bacterial infections.

Ulcolind H_2 *Lindopharm, Ger.*
Cimetidine (p.1183·2).
Acid aspiration syndrome; gastro-oesophageal reflux; peptic ulcer; Zollinger-Ellison syndrome.

Ulcolind Metro *Lindopharm, Ger.*
Metronidazole (p.585·1).
Anaerobic bacterial infections; protozoal infections.

Ulcolind N *Lindopharm, Ger.†.*
Bismuth aluminate (p.1180·1); magnesium trisilicate (p.1199·1); liquorice (p.1197·1).
Gastro-intestinal disorders.

Ulcolind Rani *Lindopharm, Ger.*
Ranitidine hydrochloride (p.1209·3).
Aspiration syndrome; gastro-intestinal haemorrhage; gastro-oesophageal reflux; peptic ulcer; Zollinger-Ellison syndrome.

Ulcolind Wismut *Lindopharm, Ger.*
Bismuth salicylate (p.1180·1).
Gastritis; peptic ulcer.

Ulcomedina *Pharmaland, Ital.*
Cimetidine (p.1183·2).
Gastritis and duodenitis associated with acid hypersecretion; gastro-oesophageal reflux; peptic ulcer; Zollinger-Ellison syndrome.

Ulcomet *Italfarmaco, Ital.†.*
Cimetidine hydrochloride (p.1185·3).
Gastritis and duodenitis associated with acid hypersecretion; gastro-oesophageal reflux; peptic ulcer; Zollinger-Ellison syndrome.

Ulcometin *Merckle, Aust.*
Cimetidine (p.1183·2) or cimetidine hydrochloride (p.1185·3).
Acid aspiration syndrome; gastro-intestinal haemorrhage; gastro-oesophageal reflux disease; hypersensitivity reactions; peptic ulcer; Zollinger-Ellison syndrome.

Ulcometion *Juventus, Spain.*
Omeprazole (p.1204·2).
Gastro-oesophageal reflux; peptic ulcer; Zollinger-Ellison syndrome.

ulcominerase *GN, Ger.†.*
Bismuth aluminate (p.1180·1); magnesium hydroxide (p.1198·2); magnesium trisilicate (p.1199·1); calcium carbonate (p.1182·1).
Gastritis; peptic ulcer.

Ulcopir *Aesculapius, Ital.*
Pirenzepine hydrochloride (p.467·1).
Gastro-intestinal disorders.

Ulcoprotect *Azupharma, Ger.*
Pirenzepine hydrochloride (p.467·1).
Gastro-intestinal disorders.

Ulcosafe *BASF, Ger.*
Pirenzepine hydrochloride (p.467·1).
Gastro-intestinal disorders.

Ulcosal *Lilly, Spain.*
Nizatidine (p.1203·2).
Gastro-oesophageal reflux; peptic ulcer.

Ulcostad *Stada, Aust.*
Cimetidine (p.1183·2) or cimetidine hydrochloride (p.1185·3).
Acid aspiration syndrome; gastro-intestinal haemorrhage; gastro-oesophageal reflux disease; hypersensitivity reactions; peptic ulcer; Zollinger-Ellison syndrome.

Ulcosyntex *Francia, Ital.†.*
Pirenzepine hydrochloride (p.467·1).
Peptic ulcer.

Ulcotenal *Recordati Elmu, Spain.*
Pantoprazole sodium (p.1207·3).
Gastro-oesophageal reflex; peptic ulcer.

Ulcotest *Makara, Ger.†.*
Silver colloid; aluminium hydroxide (p.1177·3); bismuth subnitrate (p.1180·2); heavy magnesium carbonate (p.1198·1); dibasic magnesium phosphate; hamamelis (p.1587·1); valerian (p.1643·1); trace elements.
Gastro-intestinal disorders.

Ulcotris *ISF, Ital.†.*
Trometamol (p.1639·3); alginic acid (p.1470·3).
Gastritis; gastro-oesophageal reflux; hyperacidity; peptic ulcer.

Ulcotruw N *Truw, Ger.*
Peppermint leaf (p.1208·1); liquorice (p.1197·1); chamomile (p.1561·2).
Gastro-intestinal disorders.

Ulcubloc *Wolff, Ger.*
Cimetidine (p.1183·2).
Acid aspiration syndrome; gastro-oesophageal reflux; peptic ulcer; Zollinger-Ellison syndrome.

Ulcufato *Berenguer Infale, Spain.*
Sucralfate (p.1214·2).
Gastro-intestinal haemorrhage; peptic ulcer.

Ulcuforton *Plantorgan, Ger.†.*
Pirenzepine hydrochloride (p.467·1).
Gastro-intestinal disorders.

Ulcumel *Mack, Illert., Ger.†.*
Injection: Procaine-*N*-glucoside hydrochloride (p.1299·2); phenobarbitone (p.350·2); atropine sulphate (p.455·1).
Tablets: Bismuth aluminate (p.1180·1).
Gastro-intestinal disorders.

Ulcu-Pasc *Pascoe, Ger.*
Liquorice (p.1197·1); chamomile (p.1561·2).
Gastro-intestinal disorders.

Ulcurilen *Austroplant, Aust.*
Allantoin (p.1078·2); neomycin sulphate (p.229·2); chlorocresol (p.1110·3); alpha tocopherol acetate (p.1369·2).
Ulcers; wounds.

Ulcurilen N *Spitzner, Ger.*
Ointment: Allantoin (p.1078·2); chlorocresol (p.1110·3); neomycin sulphate (p.229·2).
Topical powder: Allantoin (p.1078·2); neomycin sulphate (p.229·2); alpha-tocopheryl acetate (p.1369·2).
Infected skin disorders; wounds.

Ulcusan *Kwizda, Aust.*
Famotidine (p.1192·1).
Acid aspiration syndrome; gastro-intestinal haemorrhage; gastro-oesophageal reflux; peptic ulcer; stress-related ulcer; Zollinger-Ellison syndrome.

Ulcus-Tablinen *Sanorania, Ger.†.*
Carbenoxolone sodium (p.1182·2).
Peptic ulcer.

Ulcyte *Alphapharm, Austral.*
Sucralfate (p.1214·2).
Peptic ulcer.

Ulfon *Lafon, Fr.*
Aldioxa (p.1078·2); alcloxa (p.1078·2); calcium carbonate (p.1182·1).
Formerly contained aldioxa, alcloxa, and homatropine methobromide.
Gastro-intestinal disorders.

Ulgarine *Byk Elmu, Spain.*
Famotidine (p.1192·1).
Gastro-oesophageal reflux; peptic ulcer; Zollinger-Ellison syndrome.

Ulgastrin *Dolorgiet, Ger.†.*
Liquorice (p.1197·1); bismuth subnitrate (p.1180·2); aluminium sodium silicate (p.1178·3); anhydrous sodium sulphate (p.1213·3).
Gastro-intestinal disorders.

Ulgastrin Bis *Dolorgiet, Ger.*
Bismuth subnitrate (p.1180·2).
Formerly contained liquorice, bismuth subnitrate, aluminium sodium silicate, anhydrous sodium sulphate, and belladonna.
Gastritis; peptic ulcer.

Ulgastrin Neu *Dolorgiet, Ger.*
Liquorice (p.1197·1).
Peptic ulcer.

Ulgastrin Rollkur Neu *Dolorgiet, Ger.†.*
Liquorice (p.1197·1); bismuth subnitrate (p.1180·2).
Formerly contained liquorice, bismuth subnitrate, aluminium sodium silicate, anhydrous sodium sulphate, and colloidal silicon dioxide.
Gastro-intestinal disorders.

Ulgastrin-Lac *Dolorgiet, Ger.†.*
Calcium carbonate (p.1182·1); magnesium hydroxide (p.1198·2); bismuth subnitrate (p.1180·2); fat-free milk powder.
Gastro-intestinal disorders.

Ulgescum *Dolorgiet, Ger.*
Pirenzepine hydrochloride (p.467·1).
Gastro-intestinal disorders.

Ulis *Lafare, Ital.*
Cimetidine (p.1183·2).
Gastritis and duodenitis associated with acid hypersecretion; gastro-oesophageal reflux; peptic ulcer; Zollinger-Ellison syndrome.

Ulkobrin *Salus, Ital.†.*
Ranitidine hydrochloride (p.1209·3).
Gastro-oesophageal reflux; peptic ulcer; Zollinger-Ellison syndrome.

Ulkowis *Temmler, Ger.*
Bismuth subnitrate (p.1180·2).
Dyspepsia; peptic ulcer.

Ulkusal *TAD, Ger.*
Cimetidine (p.1183·2).
Aspiration syndrome; gastro-oesophageal reflux; peptic ulcer; Zollinger-Ellison syndrome.

Ullus Blasen-Nieren-Tee N *Polypharm, Ger.*
Birch leaf (p.1553·3); solidago virgaurea; ononis (p.1610·2).
Urinary-tract disorders.

Ullus Galle-Tee N *Polypharm, Ger.*
Taraxacum (p.1634·2); peppermint leaf (p.1208·1); cynara (p.1569·2).
Gastro-intestinal spasm.

Ullus Kapseln N *Polypharm, Ger.*
Liquorice (p.1197·1); chamomile (p.1561·2).
Gastro-intestinal disorders.

Ullus Magen-Tee N *Polypharm, Ger.*
Fennel (p.1579·1); peppermint leaf (p.1208·1).
Dyspepsia.

Ulmet *Ace, S.Afr.†.*
Cimetidine (p.1183·2).
Gastro-intestinal disorders.

Ulone *3M, Canad.*
Chlophedianol hydrochloride (p.1057·1).
Coughs.

Ulpir *IBP, Ital.†.*
Pirenzepine hydrochloride (p.467·1).
Peptic ulcer.

ULR-LA *Geneva, USA.*
Phenylpropanolamine hydrochloride (p.1067·2); guaiphenesin (p.1061·3).
Coughs and cold symptoms; nasal congestion.

Ulsal *Gebro, Aust.*
Ranitidine hydrochloride (p.1209·3).
Acid aspiration syndrome; gastro-intestinal haemorrhage; gastro-oesophageal reflux; peptic ulcer; stress-related ulcer; Zollinger-Ellison syndrome.

Ulsanic *Continental Ethicals, S.Afr.*
Sucralfate (p.1214·2).
Gastritis; gastro-oesophageal reflux; peptic ulcer.

Ulso *ULSO, Irl.†.*
Bismuth ammonium citrate (p.1181·1).
Peptic ulcer.

Ultacit *Hoechst Marion Roussel, Neth.*
Hydrotalcite (p.1194·1).
Gastro-intestinal disorders associated with hyperacidity.

Ultacite *Roche Nicholas, Fr.*
Hydrotalcite (p.1194·1).
Gastro-intestinal disorders.

Ultane
Abbott, S.Afr.; Abbott, USA.
Sevoflurane (p.1231·3).
General anaesthesia.

Ultec *Berk, UK.*
Cimetidine (p.1183·2).
Dyspepsia; heartburn.

Ultexiv *Alcon-Thilo, Ger.*
Triamcinolone acetonide (p.1050·2); neomycin sulphate (p.229·2); gramicidin (p.215·2).
Eye disorders.

Ultilac N *Gastropharm, Ger.*
Almasilate (p.1177·1); calcium carbonate (p.1182·1); skimmed milk powder.
Gastro-intestinal disorders.

Ultimag *Mirren, S.Afr.*
Magnesium chloride (p.1157·2); zinc oxide (p.1096·2).
Magnesium and zinc supplement.

Ultimate Multi Vitamin and Mineral Formula *Suisse, Austral.†.*
Multivitamin, mineral, and nutritional agent preparation.

Ultimex *Ciba, Ital.†.*
Poloxalene iodide (p.1326·3); sodium iodide (p.1493·2).
Skin and wound disinfection.

Ultin *Rentschler, Ger.†.*
Bismuth aluminate (p.1180·1).
Gastritis; peptic ulcer.

Ultiva
Glaxo Wellcome, Fr.; Glaxo Wellcome, Ger.; Zeneca, Ger.; Glaxo Wellcome, Ital.; Glaxo Wellcome, Neth.; Glaxo Wellcome, UK; Glaxo Wellcome, USA.
Remifentanil hydrochloride (p.82·1).
Analgesia in anaesthesia.

Ultra *Medgenix, Belg.*
Sulphacetamide sodium (p.252·2).
Infected skin lesions.

Ultra Adsorb *Lainco, Spain.*
Adsorbent carbon (p.972·2).
Diarrhoea.

Ultra Augenschutz *Provita, Aust.*
Actinoquinol sodium (p.1543·1).
Protection of the eyes from ultraviolet radiation.

Ultra Clearasil *Procter & Gamble (H&B Care), UK†.*
Benzoyl peroxide (p.1079·2).
Acne.

Ultra Derm *Baker Cummins, USA.*
Emollient and moisturiser.

Ultra Levura *Upsamedica, Spain.*
Saccharomyces boulardii (p.1594·1).
Restoration of the gastro-intestinal flora.

Ultra Mide
Baker Cummins, Canad.; Baker Cummins, USA.
Urea (p.1095·2).
Dry skin; hyperkeratosis.

Ultra Tears *Alcon, USA.*
Hypromellose (p.1473·1).
Dry eyes.

Ultra Vita Time *Nature's Bounty, USA.*
Multivitamin and mineral preparation with iron and folic acid.

Ultrabas *Schering, Ger.*
Emollient.
Diluent for Ultralan ointment.

Ultrabase
Schering, S.Afr.; Schering, UK.
Emollient.
Dry skin; pharmaceutical diluent.

Ultrabion *Sabater, Spain.*
Capsules†: Ampicillin trihydrate (p.153·2).
Injection: Ampicillin sodium (p.153·1); ampicillin benzathine (p.154·1).
Bacterial infections.

Ultrabion Balsamico *Sabater, Spain.*
Ampicillin sodium (p.153·1); ampicillin benzathine (p.154·1); niaouli oil (p.1607·1); guaiphenesin (p.1061·3).
Respiratory-tract infections.

ULTRAbrom PD *WE, USA.*
Pseudoephedrine hydrochloride (p.1068·3); brompheniramine maleate (p.403·2).
Upper respiratory-tract symptoms.

Ultracain
Hoechst, Ger.; Normon, Spain.
Carticaine or carticaine hydrochloride (p.1289·1).
Adrenaline (p.813·2) is included in some injections as a vasoconstrictor to diminish absorption and localise the effect of the local anaesthetic.
Local anaesthesia.

Ultracain Dental *Hoechst, Aust.*
Carticaine hydrochloride (p.1289·1).
Adrenaline hydrochloride (p.813·3) is included in this preparation as a vasoconstrictor to diminish absorption and localise the effect of the local anaesthetic.
Local anaesthesia.

Ultracain D-S
Hoechst, Ger.; Novaxa, Ital.; Hoechst Marion Roussel, Neth.
Carticaine hydrochloride (p.1289·1).
Adrenaline hydrochloride (p.813·3) is included in this preparation as a vasoconstrictor to diminish absorption and localise the effect of the local anaesthetic.
Local anaesthesia.

Ultracain Hyperbaar *Hoechst Marion Roussel, Neth.*
Carticaine hydrochloride (p.1289·1).
Local anaesthesia.

Ultracain Hyperbar *Hoechst, Ger.*
Carticaine hydrochloride (p.1289·1).
Local anaesthesia.

Ultracaine D-S
Hoechst Marion Roussel, Canad.; Hoechst Marion Roussel, Switz.
Carticaine hydrochloride (p.1289·1).
Adrenaline (p.813·2) or adrenaline hydrochloride (p.813·3) is included in this preparation as a vasoconstrictor to diminish absorption and localise the effect of the local anaesthetic.
Local anaesthesia.

Ultracain-Suprarenin *Hoechst, Ger.*
Carticaine hydrochloride (p.1289·1).
Adrenaline hydrochloride (p.813·3) is included in this preparation as a vasoconstrictor to diminish absorption and localise the effect of the local anaesthetic.
Local anaesthesia.

Ultracal
Mead Johnson, Austral.; Mead Johnson Nutritionals, USA.
Preparation for enteral nutrition.

UltraCare
Allergan, Canad.; Allergan, USA.
Disinfecting solution, hydrogen peroxide solution 3% (p.1116·2); neutralising tablets, catalase (p.1560·3).
Contact lens care.

UltraCare Daily Cleaner *Allergan, Canad.*
Cleaning solution for soft contact lenses.

Ultracef
Bristol-Myers Squibb, Irl.; Bristol, USA†.
Cefadroxil (p.163·3).
Bacterial infections.

Ultracholine *Tyson, USA†.*
Phosphatidyl choline and phospholipid (p.1618·1).

Ultracillin *Caps, S.Afr.*
Benzathine penicillin (p.158·3); benzylpenicillin sodium (p.159·3); procaine penicillin (p.240·2).
Bacterial infections.

Ultra-Clear-A-Med *Procter & Gamble, Aust.*
Benzoyl peroxide (p.1079·2).
Acne.

Ultracort *Ripari-Gero, Ital.†.*
Suprarenal cortex (p.1050·1).
Adrenocortical insufficiency; endotoxic shock.

The symbol † denotes a preparation no longer actively marketed

Ultracorten *Ciba, Ger.†.*
Prednisone (p.1049·2).
Oral corticosteroid.

Ultracortene-H *Ciba, Switz.*
Prednisolone sodium tetrahydrophthalate (p.1049·1).
Corticosteroid.

Ultracorten-H *Ciba, Ger.†.*
Prednisolone sodium tetrahydrophthalate (p.1049·1).
Parenteral corticosteroid.

Ultracortenol
Ciba Vision, Aust.; Ciba Vision, Ger.; Ciba Vision, Neth.; Ciba Vision, Norw.; Ciba Vision, Swed.; Ciba Vision, Switz.
Prednisolone acetate (p.1048·1) or prednisolone pivalate (p.1048·1).
Inflammatory eye disorders.

Ultra-Demoplas *Godecke, Ger.*
Dexamethasone (p.1037·1); prednisolone (p.1048·1); lignocaine hydrochloride (p.1293·2).
Musculoskeletal and joint disorders.

Ultraderm *Ecobi, Ital.*
Fluocinolone acetonide (p.1041·1).
Skin disorders.

Ultraderme *Biocodex, Fr.*
Saccharomyces boulardii (p.1594·1).
Seborrhoea.

Ultradil
Schering, Irl.†; Schering, Ital.†.
Fluocortolone hexanoate (p.1041·3); fluocortolone pivalate (p.1041·3).
Skin disorders.

Ultradil Plain *Schering, UK†.*
Fluocortolone hexanoate (p.1041·3); fluocortolone pivalate (p.1041·3).
Skin disorders.

Ultradol *Procter & Gamble, Canad.*
Etodolac (p.36·2).
Osteoarthritis; rheumatoid arthritis.

Ultra-Freeda *Freeda, USA.*
Multivitamin and mineral preparation.

Ultra-K *Rhone-Poulenc Rorer, Belg.*
Potassium gluconate (p.1161·1).
Potassium depletion.

Ultralan
Note. This name is used for preparations of different composition.
Schering, Aust.; Schering, Ger.; Schering, Ital.; Schering, Spain†.
Tablets: Fluocortolone (p.1041·3).
Corticosteroid.

Schering, Aust.; Schering, Austral.†; Schering, Belg.†; Schering, Fr.; Schering, Ger.; Schering, Irl.†; Schering, Ital.; Schering, Neth.; Schering, Switz.
Topical preparations: Fluocortolone (p.1041·3) or fluocortolone pivalate (p.1041·3); fluocortolone hexanoate (p.1041·3).
Skin disorders.

Schering, Irl.†.
Ointment: Fluocortolone pivalate (p.1041·3); fluocortolone hexanoate (p.1041·3); clemizole hexachlorophane (p.406·3).
Skin disorders.

Schering, Spain†.
Eye drops: Chloramphenicol (p.182·1); fluocortolone pivalate (p.1041·3).
Eye disorders.

Elan, USA.
Lactose-free, gluten-free preparation for enteral nutrition.

Ultralan M *Schering, Spain.*
Fluocortolone (p.1041·3).
Skin disorders.

Ultralan-crinale *Schering, Ger.*
Fluocortolone pivalate (p.1041·3); salicylic acid (p.1090·2).
Scalp disorders; skin disorders.

Ultralanum *Schering, Swed.†.*
Fluocortolone (p.1041·3) or fluocortolone pivalate (p.1041·3); fluocortolone hexanoate (p.1041·3).
Skin disorders.

Ultralanum Plain *Schering, UK.*
Fluocortolone (p.1041·3) or fluocortolone pivalate (p.1041·3); fluocortolone hexanoate (p.1041·3).
Skin disorders.

Ultralente
Novo Nordisk, Ger.; Novo Nordisk, USA.
Insulin zinc suspension (crystalline) (bovine, monocomponent) (p.322·1).
Diabetes mellitus.

Ultralente Iletin I *Lilly, USA†.*
Insulin zinc suspension (bovine and porcine) (p.322·1).
Diabetes mellitus.

Ultralente Insulin *Novo Nordisk, Canad.†.*
Insulin zinc suspension (crystalline) (bovine and porcine) (p.322·1).
Diabetes mellitus.

Ultralente MC
Novo Nordisk, Austral.; Novo Nordisk, Belg.; Novo Nordisk, Fr.; Novo Nordisk, Switz.
Insulin zinc suspension (crystalline) (bovine, monocomponent) (p.322·1).
Diabetes mellitus.

Ultralente U *Novo Nordisk, USA†.*
Insulin zinc suspension, extended (bovine) (p.322·1).
Diabetes mellitus.

Ultra-Levure
Biocodex, Fr.; Biocodex, Switz.
Saccharomyces boulardii (p.1594·1).
Diarrhoea.

Ultralexin *Almirall, Spain†.*
Cephalexin (p.178·2) or cephalexin lysine (p.178·3).
Bacterial infections.

Ultram *Ortho McNeil, USA.*
Tramadol hydrochloride (p.90·1).
Pain.

Ultra-Mag *Germania, Aust.*
Magnesium gluconate (p.1157·2).
Magnesium deficiency.

Ultra-Mg *Rhone-Poulenc Rorer, Belg.*
Magnesium gluconate (p.1157·2).
Magnesium deficiency; neuromuscular hyperexcitability.

Ultramicina *Lisapharma, Ital.*
Fosfomycin calcium (p.210·2) or fosfomycin disodium (p.210·2).
Lignocaine hydrochloride (p.1293·2) is included in the intramuscular injection to alleviate the pain of injection.
Bacterial infections.

Ultramop *Canderm, Canad.*
Methoxsalen (p.1086·3).
Psoriasis; vitiligo.

Ultramox *Restan, S.Afr.*
Amoxycillin trihydrate (p.151·3).
Bacterial infections.

Ultramoxil *Hosbon, Spain†.*
Amoxycillin trihydrate (p.151·3); potassium clavulanate (p.190·2).
Bacterial infections.

Ultrapenil *Vir, Spain.*
Ampicillin sodium (p.153·1); ampicillin benzathine (p.154·1).
Bacterial infections.

Ultraplex 31 *Presselin, Ger.*
Homoeopathic preparation.

Ultraproct
Note. This name is used for preparations of different composition.
Schering, Aust.; Schering, Austral.; Schering, Belg.; Schering, Irl.; Schering, Spain†.
Fluocortolone pivalate (p.1041·3); fluocortolone hexanoate (p.1041·3); cinchocaine hydrochloride (p.1289·2); clemizole undecanoate (p.406·3).
Anorectal disorders.

Schering, Fr.; Schering, Ger.; Schering, Ital.; Schering, Neth.†; Schering, Switz.; Schering, UK.
Fluocortolone pivalate (p.1041·3); fluocortolone hexanoate (p.1041·3); cinchocaine hydrochloride (p.1289·2).
Formerly contained fluocortolone pivalate, fluocortolone hexanoate, cinchocaine hydrochloride, and clemizole undecanoate in *Ital.*
Anorectal disorders.

Ultrapyrin
Nycomed, Aust.†; Rorer, Ger.†.
Dextropropoxyphene hydrochloride (p.27·3); paracetamol (p.72·2); etenzamide (p.35·3).
Cold symptoms; pain.

Ultraquin *Canderm, Canad.*
Hydroquinone (p.1083·1); padimate O (p.1488·1); oxybenzone (p.1487·3).
Skin hyperpigmentation; sunscreen.

Ultraquin Plain *Canderm, Canad.*
Hydroquinone (p.1083·1).
Skin hyperpigmentation.

Ultraquinol *Schering, Aust.*
Fluocortolone pivalate (p.1041·3); fluocortolone hexanoate (p.1041·3); chlorquinaldol (p.185·1).
Infected skin disorders.

Ultra-R *Therapex, Canad.*
Barium sulphate (p.1003·1).
Contrast medium for radiography of the small bowel.

Ultra-scope *Fresenius, Ger.†.*
Glutaraldehyde (p.1114·3); glyoxal (p.1115·1).
Instrument disinfection.

Ultrase
Jouveinal, Canad.; Scandipharm, USA.
Pancrelipase (p.1613·3).
Pancreatic enzyme deficiency.

Ultrasep *Rivadis, Fr.*
Glutaraldehyde (p.1114·3); didecyldimethylammonium chloride (p.1112·2).
Surface disinfection.

Ultrasept *Genpharm, S.Afr.†.*
Co-trimoxazole (p.196·3).
Bacterial infections.

Ultrasine *Schering, Ger.*
Emollient base.
Skin disorders.

Ultrasol-F *Fresenius, Ger.*
Formaldehyde (p.1113·2); glyoxal (p.1115·1); glutaraldehyde (p.1114·3); benzalkonium chloride (p.1101·3).
Surface disinfection.

Ultrasol-K *Fresenius, Ger.†.*
Didecyldimethylammonium chloride (p.1112·2); benzalkonium chloride (p.1101·3).
Surface disinfection.

Ultrasol-S *Fresenius, Ger.*
Formaldehyde (p.1113·2); glyoxal (p.1115·1); glutaraldehyde (p.1114·3); benzalkonium chloride (p.1101·3).
Surface disinfection.

Ultrasol-spezial *Fresenius, Ger.†.*
Glutaraldehyde (p.1114·3); glyoxal (p.1115·1); quaternary ammonium compounds.
Surface disinfection.

Ultratard
Novo Nordisk, Irl.; Novo Nordisk, Neth.; Novo Nordisk, Norw.; Novo Nordisk, Spain; Novo Nordisk, Swed.
Insulin zinc suspension (human, monocomponent, pyr) (p.322·1).
Formerly known as Human Ultratard in *Irl.*
Diabetes mellitus.

Ultratard HM
Novo Nordisk, Aust.; Novo Nordisk, Austral.; Novo Nordisk, Belg.; Novo Nordisk, Fr.; Novo Nordisk, Ger.; Novo Nordisk, Ital.; Novo Nordisk, S.Afr.; Novo Nordisk, Switz.
Insulin zinc suspension (crystalline) (human, monocomponent, pyr) (p.322·1).
Diabetes mellitus.

Ultra-Tears *Alcon, Switz.*
Hypromellose (p.1473·1).
Dry eyes.

Ultrathon *3M, UK.*
Diethyltoluamide (p.1405·1).
Insect repellent.

Ultravate
Westwood-Squibb, Canad.; Westwood-Squibb, USA.
Halobetasol propionate (p.1043·2).
Skin disorders.

Ultraviro C *Covan, S.Afr.*
Aspirin (p.16·1); caffeine (p.749·3); ascorbic acid (p.1365·2); chlorpheniramine maleate (p.405·1).
Cold symptoms; fever; pain.

Ultravisin *Farmigea, Ital.*
Myrtillus (p.1606·1); *dl*-alpha tocopheryl acetate (p.1369·2).
Vascular retinopathy; vision disorders.

Ultravist
Schering, Aust.; Schering, Austral.; Schering, Belg.; Berlex, Canad.; Schering, Fr.; Schering, Ger.; Schering, Ital.; Schering, Neth.; Schering, Norw.; Schering, S.Afr.; Schering, Spain; Schering, Swed.; Schering, Switz.; Schering, UK; Berlex, USA.
Iopromide (p.1007·3).
Radiographic contrast medium.

Ultravite with Minerals *Stanley, Canad.*
Multivitamin and mineral preparation.

Ultrazole *Rolab, S.Afr.*
Co-trimoxazole (p.196·3).
Bacterial infections.

Ultrazyme
Allergan, Austral.; Allergan, Canad.; Allergan, USA.
Subtilisin-A.
Cleanser for soft contact lenses.

Ultren *Salus, Aust.*
Vitamin A acetate (p.1359·2); ascorbic acid (p.1365·2).
Cold and influenza symptoms; vitamin deficiency.

Ultrex *Parke, Davis, Fr.†.*
Pyrithione zinc (p.1089·3).
Seborrhoea.

Ultrex a l'Huile de Cade *Pharmeurop, Fr.†.*
Cade oil (p.1092·2).
Scalp disorders.

Ultrex Shampooing Antipelliculaire d'Entretien *Pharmeurop, Fr.†.*
Piroctone olamine (p.1089·1).
Seborrhoeic dermatitis.

Ultroxim *Duncan, Ital.†.*
Cefuroxime sodium (p.177·1).
Bacterial infections.

Ulxit *Tyrol, Aust.*
Nizatidine (p.1203·2).
Gastro-oesophageal reflux; peptic ulcer.

Umadren *Montavit, Aust.*
Skin wash: Undecenoic acid polydiethanolamide (p.389·2).
Topical gel: Undecenoic acid monoethanolamide (p.389·2); diphenhydramine hydrochloride (p.409·1).
Topical powder: Undecenoic acid polydiethanolamide (p.389·2); diphenhydramine hydrochloride (p.409·1); paraformaldehyde (p.1121·1).
Fungal skin infections.

Uman-Big *Biagini, Ital.*
A hepatitis B immunoglobulin (p.1512·3).
Passive immunisation.

Uman-Cig *Biagini, Ital.*
A cytomegalovirus immunoglobulin (p.1507·1).
Passive immunisation.

Uman-Complex-IX-VI *Biagini, Ital.†.*
Factor IX (p.721·3).
Deficiency of factors II, VII, IX or X.

Uman-Cry DI *Biagini, Ital.†.*
Factor VIII (p.720·3).
Factor VIII deficiency.

Uman-Fibrin *Biagini, Ital.*
Fibrinogen (p.722·3).
Hypofibrinogenaemia.

Uman-Gal E *Biagini, Ital.*
Antilymphocyte immunoglobulin (horse) (p.504·2).
Immunosuppressant therapy.

Uman-Gamma *Biagini, Ital.*
A normal immunoglobulin (p.1522·1).
Hypogammaglobulinaemia; passive immunisation.

Uman-Serum *Biagini, Ital.*
Plasma protein fraction (p.726·3).
Hypoproteinaemia; shock.

Uman-Vzig *Biagini, Ital.*
A varicella-zoster immunoglobulin (p.1538·1).
Passive immunisation.

Umatrope *Lilly, Fr.*
Somatropin (p.1249·3).
Growth hormone deficiency; Turner's syndrome.

Umbradol *Salvat, Spain.*
Salsalate (p.83·1).
Fever; musculoskeletal, joint and peri-articular disorders; pain.

Umbrium *Kwizda, Aust.*
Diazepam (p.661·1).
Anxiety disorders; skeletal muscle spasm; sleep disorders.

Umckaloabo *Iso, Ger.*
Pelargonium reniforme/sidoides.
Upper respiratory-tract infections.

Umoril *Synthelabo, Ital.*
Toloxatone (p.308·2).
Depression.

Umprel *Sandoz, Aust.*
Bromocriptine mesylate (p.1132·2).
Parkinsonism.

Umuline Profil 10, 20, 30, 40, and 50 *Lilly, Fr.*
Mixtures of neutral insulin injection (human, prb) 10%, 20%, 30%, 40%, and 50% and isophane insulin injection (human, prb) 90%, 80%, 70%, 60%, and 50% respectively (p.322·1).
Diabetes mellitus.

Umuline Protamine Isophane (NPH) *Lilly, Fr.*
Isophane insulin injection (human, prb) (p.322·1).
Diabetes mellitus.

Umuline Rapide *Lilly, Fr.*
Neutral insulin injection (human, prb) (p.322·1).
Diabetes mellitus.

Umuline Zinc *Lilly, Fr.*
Insulin zinc suspension (human, prb) (crystalline) (p.322·1).
Diabetes mellitus.

Umuline Zinc Compose *Lilly, Fr.*
Insulin zinc suspension (human, prb) (amorphous 30%, crystalline 70%) (p.322·1).
Diabetes mellitus.

Unacid *Pfizer, Ger.*
Sulbactam sodium (p.250·3); ampicillin sodium (p.153·1).
Bacterial infections.

Unacid PD *Pfizer, Ger.*
Sultamicillin (p.257·2) or sultamicillin tosylate (p.257·2).
Bacterial infections.

Unacide *Pfizer, Switz.†.*
Sultamicillin tosylate (p.257·2).
Bacterial infections.

Unacil *FIRMA, Ital.*
Doxycycline hydrochloride (p.202·3).
Bacterial infections.

Unacim *Jouveinal, Fr.*
Injection: Sulbactam sodium (p.250·3); ampicillin sodium (p.153·1).
Lignocaine hydrochloride (p.1293·2) is included in the intramuscular injection to alleviate the pain of injection.
Tablets: Sultamicillin tosylate (p.257·2).
Bacterial infections.

Unakalm
Pharmacia Upjohn, Belg.; Pharmacia Upjohn, Neth.
Ketazolam (p.675·2).
Anxiety.

Un-Alfa *Leo, Fr.*
Alfacalcidol (p.1366·3).
Hypocalcaemia; hypoparathyroidism; renal osteodystrophy; rickets.

Unasyn
Note. This name is used for preparations of different composition.
Pfizer, Aust.; Pfizer, Ital.; Pfizer, Spain; Roerig, USA.
Injection: Ampicillin sodium (p.153·1); sulbactam sodium (p.250·3).
Lignocaine hydrochloride (p.1293·2) may be included in the intramuscular injection to alleviate the pain of injection.
Bacterial infections.

Pfizer, Aust.; Pfizer, Ital.; Pfizer, Spain; Pfizer, UK†.
Tablets; oral suspension: Sultamicillin (p.257·2) or sultamicillin tosylate (p.257·2).
Bacterial infections.

Unat
Boehringer Mannheim, Ger.; Boehringer Mannheim, S.Afr.
Torasemide (p.956·3) or torasemide sodium (p.956·3).
Hypertension; oedema; renal insufficiency.

Unatol *Streuli, Switz.*
Vitamin A palmitate (p.1359·2); dexpanthenol (p.1570·3); allantoin (p.1078·2).
Nasal disorders.

Undecilendermina *Granata, Ital.†.*
Undecenoic acid (p.389·2); zinc undecenoate (p.389·2).
Fungal skin infections.

Undehache *Genove, Spain†.*
Propionic acid (p.387·1); sodium aminobenzoate undecylenic acid.
Fungal skin infections.

Undestor
Organon, Belg.; Organon, Swed.
Testosterone undecanoate (p.1464·2).
Male hypogonadism.

Undetin *Recordati, Ital.†.*
Undecenoic acid (p.389·2); zinc caprylate (p.1610·1); calcium propionate (p.387·1); salicylic acid (p.1090·2).
Fungal skin infections.

Undex Schieffer, Switz.†.
Cream: Tolnaftate (p.389·1); undecenoic acid (p.389·2); zinc undecenoate (p.389·2); calcium lactate (p.1155·2); urea (p.1095·2).
Topical liquid: Triclosan (p.1127·2); undecenoic acid (p.389·2); triacetine; benzethonium chloride (p.1102·3); dexpanthenol (p.1570·3).
Topical powder: Tolnaftate (p.389·1); undecenoic acid (p.389·2); zinc undecenoate (p.389·2); calcium lactate (p.1155·2).
Topical spray: Tolnaftate (p.389·1); polyethylene glycol undecenoate; triclocarban (p.1127·2).
Tinea pedis.

Unergol Poli, Ital.
Dihydroergocristine mesylate (p.1571·3).
Hyperprolactinaemia; inhibition of lactation.

Unex Amarum Repha, Ger.
Gentian (p.1583·3); absinthium (p.1541·1); ginger (p.1193·2).
Gastro-intestinal disorders.

Unexym MD Repha, Ger.
Pancreatin (p.1612·1); papain (p.1614·1); betaine hydrochloride (p.1553·2).
Digestive disorders.

Unexym N Repha, Ger.†.
Pancreatin (p.1612·1); papain (p.1614·1); pepsin (p.1616·3); betaine hydrochloride (p.1553·2).
Digestive system disorders.

Ung Vernleigh Propan, S.Afr.
Sulphanilamide (p.256·3); mercurochrome (p.1119·2); peru balsam (p.1617·2); cod-liver oil (p.1337·3).
Burns; wounds.

Unguentacid-Salbe Mucos, Ger.
Linoleic acid triglyceride; vitamin A palmitate (p.1359·2); *dl*-alpha tocopheryl acetate (p.1369·2).
Skin disorders; ulcers; wounds.

Unguentine Mentholatum, USA.
Aerosol†: Benzocaine (p.1286·2).
Local anaesthesia.
Ointment: Phenol (p.1121·2); zinc oxide (p.1096·2); eucalyptus oil (p.1578·1); thyme oil (p.1637·1).
Pain in minor burns.

Unguentine Plus Mentholatum, USA.
Lignocaine hydrochloride (p.1293·2); chloroxylenol (p.1111·1); phenol (p.1121·2).
Skin disorders.

Unguento Callicida Naion Puerto Galiano, Spain.
Lactic acid (p.1593·3); salicylic acid (p.1090·2).
Callosities.

Unguento Morryth SmithKline Beecham, Spain.
Salicylic acid (p.1090·2).
Formerly known as Callicida Unguento Morri.
Calluses.

Unguentolan Heyl, Ger.
Cod-liver oil (p.1337·3).
Anorectal disorders; burns; ulcers; wounds.

Unguentum Bossi Doak, USA.
Ammoniated mercury (p.1086·3); hexamine sulfosalicylate; coal tar (p.1092·3).
Skin disorders.

Unguentum Lactisol Galactopharm, Ger.
Lactic acid (p.1593·3).
Skin disorders; wounds.

Unguentum Lymphaticum PGM, Ger.
Hemlock; colchicum (p.394·2); digitalis (p.848·3); podophyllum (p.1089·1); hyoscyamus (p.464·3); calendula officinalis.
Lymphatic disorders.

Unguentum M Crookes Healthcare, UK.
Emollient.
Formerly known as Unguentum Merck.
Pharmaceutical diluent.

Unguentum Merck Whitehall, Irl.; E. Merck, Irl.
Emollient.
Barrier cream; dry skin; pharmaceutical vehicle.

Unguentum Truw Truw, Ger.
Homoeopathic preparation.

Ungvita Roche Consumer, Austral.
Cream: Vitamin A palmitate (p.1359·2); calamine (p.1080·1); a dimethicone (p.1384·2).
Ointment: Fish-liver oil; vitamin A palmitate (p.1359·2).
Skin disorders.

Uni Derm United, USA†.
Wool fat (p.1385·3).
Dry, sensitive, and irritated skin.

Uni Masdil Esteve, Spain.
Diltiazem hydrochloride (p.854·2).
Angina pectoris; hypertension; myocardial infarction.

Uni Salve
Smith & Nephew, Austral.; United, USA†.
Soft paraffin (p.1382·3).
Barrier cream; minor skin irritations.

Uni-Ace URL, USA.
Paracetamol (p.72·2).

Unibac Lilly, Belg.
Dirithromycin (p.202·2).
Bacterial infections.

Unibar Therapex, Canad.
Barium sulphate (p.1003·1).
Radiographic contrast medium.

Unibaryt
Note. This name is used for preparations of different composition.
Goldham, Ger.
Effervescent tablets: Sodium bicarbonate (p.1153·2); anhydrous citric acid (p.1564·3); simethicone (p.1213·1).
Adjuvant to double contrast radiography; diagnostic agent.
Procter & Gamble, Aust.; Goldham, Ger.
Oral liquid: Barium sulphate (p.1003·1).
Contrast medium for gastro-intestinal radiography.

Unibase Warner Chilcott, USA.
Vehicle for topical preparations.

Uni-Bent Cough URL, USA.
Diphenhydramine hydrochloride (p.409·1).

Unibloc
Kohler, Ger.†; Roche, Neth.
Atenolol (p.825·3).
Angina pectoris; arrhythmias; hypertension; myocardial infarction.

Unicaine Bournonville, Belg.
Oxybuprocaine hydrochloride (p.1298·1).
Local anaesthesia.

Unicam Master Pharma, Ital.†.
Piroxicam pivalate (p.81·1).
Musculoskeletal and joint disorders.

Unicap
Upjohn, UK; Upjohn, USA.
A range of vitamin preparations.

Unicap M Upjohn, UK†.
Multivitamin and mineral preparation.

Unicap T
Upjohn, Austral.†; Upjohn, UK†.
Multivitamin and mineral preparation.

Unicare United, USA†.
Allantoin (p.1078·2); dimethicone (p.1384·2).
Dry, chapped, and irritated skin.

Unicef Ripari-Gero, Ital.
Cefonicid sodium (p.167·2).
Lignocaine hydrochloride (p.1293·2) is included in this preparation to alleviate the pain of injection.
Bacterial infections.

Unichol Merck, Aust.
Hymecromone (p.1589·3).
Biliary-tract disorders.

Unicid Prospa, Ital.
Cefonicid sodium (p.167·2).
Lignocaine hydrochloride (p.1293·2) is included in the intramuscular injection to alleviate the pain of injection.
Bacterial infections.

Unicilina Pharmacia Upjohn, Spain.
Benzylpenicillin sodium (p.159·3).
Bacterial infections.

Unicomplex-T & M Rugby, USA.
Multivitamin and mineral preparation with iron and folic acid.

Uni-Decon URL, USA.
Phenylpropanolamine hydrochloride (p.1067·2); phenylephrine hydrochloride (p.1066·2); chlorpheniramine maleate (p.405·1); phenyltoloxamine citrate (p.416·1).
Upper respiratory-tract symptoms.

Uniderm
Note. This name is used for preparations of different composition.
Smith & Nephew, Austral.
Moisturiser.
Schering-Plough, Swed.
Hydrocortisone (p.1043·3).
Anogenital pruritus; eczema.

Unidermo Uniderm, Ital.
Lactic acid (p.1593·3); collagen (p.1566·3).
Skin cleansing.

Unidie Morrith, Spain.
Cefonicid sodium (p.167·2).
Bacterial infections.

Unidipin Pharmacia Upjohn, Aust.
Nifedipine (p.916·2).
Angina pectoris; hypertension.

Unidipine Pharmacia Upjohn, Switz.†.
Nifedipine (p.916·2).
Hypertension.

Unidor Synthelabo Delagrange, Spain.
Aspirin (p.16·1); caffeine (p.749·3).
Fever; pain.

Unidox
Yamanouchi, Belg.; Yamanouchi, Neth.
Doxycycline (p.202·3).
Bacterial infections.

Uni-Dur
Schering-Plough, S.Afr.; Key, USA.
Theophylline (p.765·1).
Obstructive airways disease.

Unifer Tosi, Ital.
Saccharated iron oxide (p.1353·2).
Iron deficiency anaemias.

Unifiber Hickam, USA.
Powdered cellulose (p.1472·2).
Constipation.

Uniflox Bayer, Fr.
Ciprofloxacin hydrochloride (p.185·3).
Cystitis; gonococcal urethritis.

Uniflu with Gregovite C Unigreg, UK.
Uniflu tablets, phenylephrine hydrochloride (p.1066·2); caffeine (p.749·3); codeine phosphate (p.26·1); diphenhydramine hydrochloride (p.409·1); paracetamol (p.72·2); Gregovite C tablets, ascorbic acid (p.1365·2).
Cold symptoms.

Uniflu & Gregovite C Unigreg, Irl.
Uniflu tablets, paracetamol (p.72·2); codeine phosphate (p.26·1); caffeine (p.749·3); diphenhydramine hydrochloride (p.409·1); phenylephrine hydrochloride (p.1066·2); Gregovite C tablets, ascorbic acid (p.1365·2).
Colds and influenza symptoms.

Unifyl
Mundipharma, Aust.; Mundipharma, Switz.
Theophylline (p.765·1).
Obstructive airways disease.

Unigal Solido Uniderm, Ital.†.
Sulphur (p.1091·2); lactic acid (p.1593·3).
Acne; skin cleansing.

Unigam Norgine, UK.
Evening primrose oil (p.1582·1).
Atopic eczema; mastalgia.

Unigamol Norgine, Ger.
Evening primrose oil (p.1582·1).
Atopic eczema.

Unigest Unigreg, UK.
Aluminium hydroxide (p.1177·3); dimethicone (p.1213·1).
Gastro-intestinal disorders.

Uniget Chibret, Ger.†.
Timolol maleate (p.953·3).
Glaucoma; ocular hypertension.

Unigyn Uniderm, Ital.
Lactic acid (p.1593·3).
Personal hygiene; vaginal douche.

Unihep
Leo, Irl.; Leo, UK.
Heparin sodium (p.879·3).
Thrombo-embolic disorders.

Uniket Lacer, Spain.
Isosorbide mononitrate (p.893·3).
Angina pectoris; heart failure.

Unik-Zoru Therapex, Canad.
Tartaric acid (p.1634·3); sodium bicarbonate (p.1153·2).
Diagnostic agent.

Unilair
3M, Ger.; 3M, Neth.
Theophylline (p.765·1) or theophylline sodium glycinate (p.772·2).
Obstructive airways disease.

Unilarm Ciba Vision, Fr.
Sodium chloride (p.1162·2).
Dry eye.

Unilax Ascher, USA.
Docusate sodium (p.1189·3); phenolphthalein (p.1208·2).
Constipation.

Uniloc
AFI, Norw.; Nycomed, Swed.
Atenolol (p.825·3).
Angina pectoris; arrhythmias; hypertension; hyperthyroidism; migraine; myocardial infarction.

Unilong Byk Elmu, Spain.
Theophylline (p.765·1).
Heart failure; obstructive airways disease; paroxysmal dyspnoea.

Unimaalox Rhone-Poulenc Rorer, Spain.
Aluminium hydroxide (p.1177·3); magnesium hydroxide (p.1198·2).
Gastro-intestinal hyperacidity.

Unimox Propan, S.Afr.
Amoxycillin (p.151·3).
Bacterial infections.

Uniparin
Rhone-Poulenc Rorer, Austral.; CP Pharmaceuticals, Irl.; CP Pharmaceuticals, UK.
Heparin calcium (p.879·3) or heparin sodium (p.879·3).
Thrombo-embolic disorders.

Unipen
Wyeth-Ayerst, Canad.†; Wyeth-Ayerst, USA.
Nafcillin sodium (p.228·1).
Bacterial infections.

Uniphyl
Purdue Frederick, Canad.; Adcock Ingram, S.Afr.; Purdue Frederick, USA.
Theophylline (p.765·1).
Obstructive airways disease.

Uniphyllin Mundipharma, Ger.
Theophylline (p.765·1) or theophylline sodium glycinate (p.772·2).
Obstructive airways disease.

Uniphyllin Continus
Napp, Irl.; Napp, UK.
Theophylline (p.765·1).
Bronchospasm; cardiac asthma; heart failure.

Unipine XL Ethical Generics, UK.
Nifedipine (p.916·2).
Hypertension.

Uniplus Angelini, Ital.
Suppositories: Oxolamine citrate (p.1065·3); propyphenazone (p.81·3).
Tablets†: Oxolamine phosphate (p.1065·3); propyphenazone (p.81·3).
Influenza symptoms; oral inflammation; otorhinolaryngeal inflammation; tracheobronchitis.

Unipres Solvay, USA†.
Hydrochlorothiazide (p.885·2); reserpine (p.942·1); hydralazine hydrochloride (p.883·2).
Hypertension.

Unipril Astra, Ital.
Ramipril (p.941·1).
Heart failure; hypertension.

Uniquin
Biochemie, Aust.; Wassermann, Ital.; Searle, S.Afr.
Lomefloxacin hydrochloride (p.222·2).
Bacterial infections.

Uniretic Schwarz, USA.
Moexipril hydrochloride (p.912·1); hydrochlorothiazide (p.885·2).
Hypertension.

Uniroid Unigreg, UK.
Hydrocortisone (p.1043·3); neomycin sulphate (p.229·2); polymyxin B sulphate (p.239·1); cinchocaine hydrochloride (p.1289·2).
Anorectal disorders.

Uniroid-HC Unigreg, UK.
Cinchocaine hydrochloride (p.1289·2); hydrocortisone (p.1043·3).
Anorectal disorders.

Unisal Merck Sharp & Dohme, Switz.
Diflunisal (p.33·2).
Inflammation; pain.

Uniscrub Seton, UK.
Chlorhexidine gluconate (p.1107·2).
Skin disinfection.

Unisept Seton, UK.
Chlorhexidine gluconate (p.1107·2).
Skin disinfection.

Unisoil Therapex, Canad.
Castor oil (p.1560·2).
Constipation.

Unisol
Agepha, Aust.
Disinfecting and storage solution for contact lenses.
Alcon, USA.
Rinsing and storage solutions for soft contact lenses.

Unisolve Smith & Nephew, Austral.
Dipropylene glycol methylether; isopropyl alcohol (p.1118·2); isoparaffin.
Formerly contained VM & P naphtha and trichloroethane.
Medical adhesive remover.

Unisom
Note. This name is used for preparations of different composition.
Pfizer, Austral.; Pfizer, Canad.
Diphenhydramine hydrochloride (p.409·1).
Insomnia.
Rovifarma, Spain.
Doxylamine succinate (p.410·1).
Insomnia.

Unisom-2 Pfizer, Canad.
Doxylamine succinate (p.410·1).
Insomnia.

Unisom Nighttime Sleep-Aid Pfizer, USA.
Doxylamine succinate (p.410·1).
Insomnia.

Unisom with Pain Relief Pfizer, USA.
Paracetamol (p.72·2); diphenhydramine hydrochloride (p.409·1).
Insomnia; pain.

Unisom-C Pfizer, Canad.
Diphenhydramine hydrochloride (p.409·1).
Insomnia.

Unisomnia Unigreg, UK.
Nitrazepam (p.682·2).
Insomnia.

Unistep hCG Orion, USA.
Pregnancy test (p.1621·2).

United Soft Guard Smith & Nephew, Austral.†.
Carmellose (p.1471·2); polyisobutylene; pectin (p.1474·1).
Skin protection; wounds.

Uni-Tranxene Sanofi Winthrop, Belg.
Dipotassium clorazepate (p.657·1).
Anxiety; mixed depression and anxiety.

Unitrim Master Pharma, Ital.
Brodimoprim (p.162·1).
Otorhinolaryngeal infections; respiratory-tract infections.

Unitrol Republic, USA.
Phenylpropanolamine hydrochloride (p.1067·2).
Obesity.

Unitul Complex Bama, Spain.
Sodium acexamate (p.1542·1); silver sulphadiazine (p.247·3).
Burns; ulcers; wounds.

Unitulle
Hoechst Marion Roussel, Austral.; Cassenne, Fr.
White soft paraffin (p.1382·3).
Wounds.

Unituss HC URL, USA.
Hydrocodone tartrate (p.43·1); phenylephrine hydrochloride (p.1066·2); chlorpheniramine maleate (p.405·1).
Upper respiratory-tract symptoms.

Uni-tussin URL, USA.
Guaiphenesin (p.1061·3).
Coughs.

Uni-tussin DM *URL, USA.*
Dextromethorphan hydrobromide (p.1057·3); guaiphenesin (p.1061·3).
Coughs.

Univasc *Schwarz, USA.*
Moexipril hydrochloride (p.912·1).
Hypertension.

Univer
Rorer, Spain†; Elan, UK.
Verapamil hydrochloride (p.960·3).
Angina pectoris; hypertension.

Universal Concentration Tablets *Universal, S.Afr.*
Caffeine (p.749·3).
Fatigue.

Universal Earache Drops *Universal, S.Afr.*
Phenazone (p.78·2); procaine hydrochloride (p.1299·2); potassium hydroxyquinoline sulphate (p.1621·1).
Ear disorders.

Universal Eye Drops *Universal, S.Afr.*
Phenylephrine hydrochloride (p.1066·2); boric acid (p.1554·2).
Eye inflammation; eye irritation.

Universal Nasal Drops *Universal, S.Afr.*
Phenylephrine hydrochloride (p.1066·2); naphazoline nitrate (p.1064·2).
Allergic rhinitis; sinusitis.

Universal Throat Lollies *Universal, S.Afr.*
Cetylpyridinium chloride (p.1106·2).
Mouth and throat infections.

Univol *Carter Horner, Canad.*
Aluminium hydroxide (p.1177·3); magnesium hydroxide (p.1198·2).
Gastro-intestinal disorders associated with hyperacidity.

Uniwash *Smith & Nephew, Austral.*
Skin cleanser.

Unixime *FIRMA, Ital.*
Cefixime (p.165·3).
Bacterial infections.

Unizink *Kohler-Pharma, Ger.*
Zinc aspartate.
Zinc deficiency.

Uno-Enantone *Takeda, Ger.*
Leuprorelin acetate (p.1253·1).
Prostatic cancer.

Unotex N feminin *Bilgast, Ger.*
Homoeopathic preparation.

Unotex N masculin *Bilgast, Ger.*
Homoeopathic preparation.

Upelva *Pekana, Ger.*
Homoeopathic preparation.

Uplex *Madaus, Ger.†.*
Bismuth subgallate (p.1180·2); magnesium oxide (p.1198·3).
Hyperchlorhydria.

Upsa C
Upsamedica, Belg.; Upsamedica, Spain.
Ascorbic acid (p.1365·2).
Adjunct in treatment of iron supplementation; methaemoglobinaemia; vitamin C deficiency.

Upsa Plus *Upsamedica, Ital.*
Oxolamine citrate (p.1065·3); propyphenazone (p.81·3).
Influenza symptoms; respiratory-tract inflammation.

Upsadex *Irmesan, Spain.*
Doxylamine succinate (p.410·1); sodium bromide; dibasic sodium phosphate; sodium sulphate (p.1147·1).
Anxiety disorders; insomnia.

Upsalgin C *Upsamedica, Switz.*
Aspirin (p.16·1); ascorbic acid (p.1365·2).
Fever; pain.

Upsalgina *Upsamedica, Spain.*
Aspirin (p.16·1).
Fever; inflammation; pain; thrombosis prophylaxis.

Upset Stomach *Homeocan, Canad.*
Homoeopathic preparation.

Uracid
Note. This name is used for preparations of different composition.
Hassle, Swed.
Aluminium hydroxide (p.1177·3); calcium carbonate (p.1182·1).
Heartburn; hyperphosphataemia; peptic ulcer.

Wesley, USA.
Methionine (p.984·2).
Odour, dermatitis, and ulceration in incontinent adults.

Uractazide *Prospa, Belg.*
Hydrochlorothiazide (p.885·2); spironolactone (p.946·1).
Hypertension; oedema.

Uractone
Prospa, Belg.; SPA, Ital.
Spironolactone (p.946·1).
Hyperaldosteronism; hypertension; oedema.

Ural *Abbott, Austral.*
Sodium bicarbonate (p.1153·2); anhydrous sodium citrate (p.1153·2); anhydrous citric acid (p.1564·3); tartaric acid (p.1634·3).
Gastric hyperacidity; urinary alkalinisation.

Uralgin *Ceccarelli, Ital.*
Nalidixic acid (p.228·2).
Gram-negative bacterial infections of the urinary tract.

Uralyt *Madaus, Spain.*
Arnica (p.1550·3); convallaria (p.1567·2); equisetum arvense (p.1575·1); rubia tinctorum; solidago virgaurea; echinacea angustifolia (p.1574·2); magnesium phosphate (p.1157·3).
Renal calculi.

Uralyt Urato *Madaus, Spain.*
Citric acid (p.1564·3); aescin (p.1543·3); potassium citrate (p.1153·1); ruberitric acid; sodium citrate (p.1153·2).
Hypocitraturia; renal calculi; renal tubular acidosis.

Uralyt-Kalium *Madaus, Ger.†.*
Potassium bicarbonate (p.1153·1); citric acid (p.1564·3).
Renal calculi.

Uralyt-U
Madaus, Aust.; Madaus, Belg.; Madaus, Ger.; Ibi, Ital.; Byk Madaus, S.Afr.; Madaus, Switz.
Potassium sodium hydrogen citrate.
Cystinuria; porphyria cutanea tarda; renal calculi; urinary alkalinisation.

Urantin *Xixia, S.Afr.*
Nitrofurantoin (p.231·3).
Urinary-tract infections.

Urantoin *DDSA Pharmaceuticals, UK.*
Nitrofurantoin (p.231·3).

Uraplex *Madaus, Spain.*
Trospium chloride (p.1640·1).
Urinary incontinence.

Uraprene *Ibi, Ital.†.*
Urapidil fumarate (p.959·2) or urapidil hydrochloride (p.959·2).
Hypertension; hypertensive emergencies.

Urarthone *Lehning, Fr.*
Homoeopathic preparation.

Urasal *Carter Horner, Canad.*
Hexamine (p.216·1).
Urinary-tract infections.

Uraseptine Rogier *Gallier, Fr.†.*
Hexamine (p.216·1); hexamine anhydromethylenecitrate (p.216·2); piperazine hydrate (p.107·2); sodium benzoate (p.1102·3); lithium benzoate (p.1596·3).
Urinary-tract infections.

Urathone *Homeocan, Canad.*
Homoeopathic preparation.

Urbadan *Roussel, Neth.†.*
Clobazam (p.656·3).
Anxiety.

Urbal *Merck, Spain.*
Sucralfate (p.1214·2).
Gastro-intestinal haemorrhage; peptic ulcer.

Urbanol *Roussel, S.Afr.*
Clobazam (p.656·3).
Alcohol withdrawal syndrome; anxiety; premedication.

Urbanyl
Synthelabo, Fr.; Hoechst Marion Roussel, Switz.
Clobazam (p.656·3).
Alcohol withdrawal syndrome; anxiety; epilepsy.

Urbason
Hoechst, Aust.; Hoechst, Ger.; Hoechst Marion Roussel, Ital.†; Hoechst, Spain; Hoechst Marion Roussel, Switz.
Methylprednisolone (p.1046·1), methylprednisolone acetate (p.1046·1), or methylprednisolone sodium succinate (p.1046·1).
Corticosteroid.

Urbi Medi-Test *Macherey Nagel Duren, S.Afr.*
Test for bilirubin and urobilinogen in urine.

Urbilat *Hor-Fer-Vit, Ger.†.*
Meprobamate (p.678·1).
Depression; sleep disorders.

Urdes *Errekappa, Ital.*
Ursodeoxycholic acid (p.1642·1).
Biliary disorders.

Urdox *CP Pharmaceuticals, UK.*
Ursodeoxycholic acid (p.1642·1).
Cholesterol gallstones.

Urdrim *Urbion, Spain.*
Astemizole (p.402·1).
Hypersensitivity reactions.

Ureacin *Pedinol, USA.*
Urea (p.1095·2).
Dry skin; hyperkeratosis; nail dissolution and destruction.

Ureaphil *Abbott, USA.*
Urea (p.1095·2).
Cerebral oedema; raised intra-ocular pressure.

Ureata S *Fides, Ger.*
Urea (p.1095·2); alpha tocopheryl acetate (p.1369·1).
Skin disorders; ulcers.

Urecare *Delta, Austral.*
Urea (p.1095·2).
Dry skin disorders.

Urecholine
Merck Sharp & Dohme, Austral.; Frosst, Canad.; Merck Sharp & Dohme, Ital.; Merck Sharp & Dohme, S.Afr.; Merck Sharp & Dohme, USA.
Bethanechol chloride (p.1389·3).
Gastro-oesophageal reflux; neurogenic bladder; urinary retention.

Urecortyn *Roussel, Ital.†.*
Hydrocortisone acetate (p.1043·3).
Skin disorders.

Urederm *Hamilton, Austral.*
Urea (p.1095·2).
Dry skin conditions.

Uredimin *Andreabal, Switz.*
Allopurinol (p.390·2).
Gout; hyperuricaemia; renal calculi.

Uree *Riva, Canad.*
Urea (p.1095·2).

Uregyt *Medphano, Ger.*
Ethacrynic acid (p.866·3).
Refractory oedema.

Urelium Neu *Europharm, Aust.*
Ammi visnaga fruit (p.1593·2); solidago virgaurea; taraxacum (p.1634·2); aescin (p.1543·3).
Renal calculi.

Urem
Mayrhofer, Aust.†; Kade, Ger.
Ibuprofen (p.44·1) or ibuprofen sodium (p.44·3).
Fever; inflammation; musculoskeletal and joint disorders; pain.

Uremiase *Nogues, Fr.*
Kinkéliba (p.1593·2); calcium carbonate (p.1182·1).
Formerly contained silica, cholesterol, tricalcium phosphate, dibasic sodium phosphate, sodium chloride, kidney extract, combretum micranthum, heavy chalk.
Gastro-intestinal disorders.

Uremide
Alphapharm, Austral.; Propan, S.Afr.
Frusemide (p.871·1).
Hypertension; oedema.

Uremol *Trans Canaderm, Canad.*
Urea (p.1095·2).
Skin disorders.

Uremol-HC *Trans Canaderm, Canad.*
Hydrocortisone acetate (p.1043·3); urea (p.1095·2).
Skin disorders.

Ureotop *Dermapharm, Ger.*
Urea (p.1095·2).
Skin disorders.

Ureotop + VAS *Dermapharm, Ger.*
Urea (p.1095·2); tretinoin (p.1093·3).
Skin keratinisation disorders.

Urepasina *Radiumfarma, Ital.†.*
Cogalactoisomerase sodium (p.1566·2).
Liver disorders.

Urethra-Steril *Wild, Switz.†.*
Neomycin sulphate (p.229·2); sulphathiazole (p.257·1); diethylaminoethyl parabutylaminobenzoate hydrochloride.
Skin infections; urethritis; vulvovaginal infections.

Uretral *Scharper, Ital.†.*
Dexamethasone sodium phosphate (p.1037·2); amethocaine hydrochloride (p.1285·2); neomycin sulphate (p.229·2).
Inflammation and infection of the urinary tract; uroscopy.

Uretrim *TAD, Ger.*
Trimethoprim (p.265·1).
Urinary-tract infections.

Urex
Note. This name is used for preparations of different composition.
Fawns & McAllan, Austral.
Frusemide (p.871·1).
Hypertension; oedema; renal failure.

3M, USA.
Hexamine hippurate (p.216·1).
Urinary-tract infections.

Urfadyn
Note. This name is used for preparations of different composition.
Zambon, Fr.†.
Nifurtoinol (p.231·3); dried aluminium hydroxide gel (p.1177·3).
Urinary-tract infections.

Zambon, Ital.†.
Nifurtoinol (p.231·3).
Urinary-tract infections.

Urfadyn PL *Zambon, Belg.*
Nifurtoinol (p.231·3).
Urinary-tract infections.

Urfadyne *Inpharzam, Switz.*
Nifurtoinol (p.231·3).
Urinary-tract infections.

Urfamycin *Zambon, Spain.*
Thiamphenicol (p.262·3) or thiamphenicol glycinate hydrochloride (p.262·3).
Bacterial infections.

Urfamycine
Zambon, Belg.; Zambon, Ger.†; Inpharzam, Switz.
Thiamphenicol (p.262·3) or thiamphenicol glycinate hydrochloride (p.262·3).
Bacterial infections.

Urgenin
Note. This name is used for preparations of different composition.
Madaus, Aust.; Polcopharma, Austral.; Madaus, Belg.; Madaus, Ger.†.
Echinacea angustifolia or echinacea purpurea (p.1574·2); saw palmetto (p.1462·1).
Prostatic and urinary-tract disorders.

Madaus, Spain.
Echinacea angustifolia (p.1574·2); esculoside (p.1543·3); saw palmetto (p.1462·1).
Prostatic and urinary-tract disorders.

Urgenin Cucurbitae oleum *Madaus, Ger.*
Cucurbita seed oil.
Benign prostatic hyperplasia; urinary-tract disorders.

Urgenine *Madaus, Switz.*
Echinacea purpurea (p.1574·2); saw palmetto (p.1462·1).
Bladder irritability; prostatitis.

Urgo Pangen *Madaus, Aust.*
Collagen (p.1566·3).
Haemorrhage.

Urgocall *Fournier SA, Spain.*
Salicylic acid (p.1090·2).
Calluses; corns.

Urgomed *Urgo, Fr.*
Carmellose (p.1471·2).
Burns; wounds.

Urgo-N Huhneraugenpflaster *Fournier, Ger.*
Salicylic acid (p.1090·2).
Calluses; corns; warts.

Urgospray
Urgo, Fr.†; Fournier SA, Spain†.
Chlorhexidine gluconate (p.1107·2).
Skin disinfection; wounds.

Uriben *Rosemont, UK.*
Nalidixic acid (p.228·2).
Urinary-tract infections.

Uribenz *RAN, Ger.*
Allopurinol (p.390·2).
Gout; hyperuricaemia.

Uricedin *Stroschein, Ger.†.*
Citric acid (p.1564·3); anhydrous sodium sulphate (p.1213·3); sodium bicarbonate (p.1153·2).
Digestive disorders.

Uricemil *Molteni, Ital.*
Allopurinol (p.390·2).
Hyperuricaemia.

Uricodue *IFI, Ital.*
Allopurinol (p.390·2); benziodarone (p.393·1).
Hyperuricaemia.

Uriconorme *Streuli, Switz.*
Allopurinol (p.390·2).
Gout; hyperuricaemia; renal calculi.

Uricovac *Sanofi Winthrop, Aust.*
Benzbromarone (p.392·3).
Gout; hyperuricaemia; psoriasis; psoriatic arthritis.

Uricovac comp *Sanofi Winthrop, Ger.†.*
Benzbromarone (p.392·3); allopurinol (p.390·2).
Gout; hyperuricaemia.

Uricozyme
Sanofi Winthrop, Fr.; Sanofi Winthrop, Ital.
Urate oxidase (p.396·3).
Hyperuricaemia.

Uridasi *Coli, Ital.†.*
Cogalactoisomerase sodium (p.1566·2).
Liver disorders.

Urideal *Plantes et Medecines, Fr.*
Pilosella.
Gastro-intestinal disorders; renal disorders.

Uridinvit Forte *Gibipharma, Ital.†.*
Cocarboxylase (p.1361·2); cyanocobalamin (p.1363·3); pyridoxine hydrochloride (p.1362·3).
Neuralgias; neuritis; polyneuritis.

Uridion *Gentili, Ital.*
Isobromindione (p.394·3).
Gout; hyperuricaemia.

Uridon Modified *Rugby, USA.*
Hexamine (p.216·1); salol (p.83·1); atropine sulphate (p.455·1); hyoscyamine sulphate (p.464·2); benzoic acid (p.1102·3); methylene blue (p.984·3).
Urinary-tract infections.

Uridoz *Therabel, Fr.*
Fosfomycin trometamol (p.210·2).
Cystitis.

Uridurine *Zambon, Neth.†.*
Nifurtoinol (p.231·3).
Urinary-tract infections.

Uriflex *Galen, UK†.*
Citric acid (p.1564·3).
Bladder wash.

Uriflex C *Seton, UK.*
Chlorhexidine gluconate (p.1107·2).
Urinary catheter care.

Uriflex G *Seton, UK.*
Citric acid (p.1564·3); sodium bicarbonate (p.1153·2); light magnesium oxide (p.1198·3); disodium edetate (p.980·1).
Urinary catheter care.

Uriflex R *Seton, UK.*
Citric acid (p.1564·3); light magnesium carbonate (p.1198·1); gluconolactone; disodium edetate (p.980·1).
Urinary catheter care.

Uriflex S *Seton, UK.*
Sodium chloride (p.1162·2).
Urinary catheter care.

Uriflex W *Seton, UK.*
Sterile pyrogen free water.
Urinary catheter care.

Uri-Flor *AGIPS, Ital.*
Nalidixic acid (p.228·2).
Gram-negative bacterial infections of the urinary tract.

Urifugan *IRBI, Ital.†.*
Allopurinol (p.390·2); benzbromarone (p.392·3).
Hyperuricaemia.

Uriginex *Repha, Ger.†.*
Birch leaf; salix; fig; cowberry; herb. apii; meadowsweet; senna; orthosiphon; juniper; juglans regia; sodium salicylate (p.85·1); colchic. autum.
Blood disorders; hyperuricaemia; musculoskeletal and joint disorders.

Uriginex Urtica *Repha, Ger.*
Urtica (p.1642·3).
Rheumatic disorders.

Urihesive *Convatec, Austral.*
Medical adhesive.

Urimar-T *Marnel, USA.*
Hexamine (p.216·1); monobasic sodium phosphate (p.1159·3); salol (p.83·1); methylene blue (p.984·3); hyoscyamine sulphate (p.464·2).
Urinary-tract infections.

Urimiodin *Francia, Ital.†.*
Trisodium uridine triphosphate anhydrous; cyanocobalamin (p.1363·3).
Muscular disorders.

Urinase *Eagle, Austral.*
Saw palmetto (p.1462·1); echinacea (p.1574·2); maize; buchu (p.1555·2); hydrastis (p.1588·2); sassafras; bearberry (p.1552·2); minerals.
Prostatitis; urinary bladder disorders.

Urinex (nouvelle formule) *Kern, Switz.*
Birch (p.1553·3); buchu (p.1555·2); barbiflore; bearberry (p.1552·2); haricot bean; equisetum (p.1575·1); solidago virgaurea; meadowsweet (p.1599·1); calamus (p.1556·1); calendula officinalis.
Urinary-tract disorders.

Urinol *Lennon, S.Afr.†.*
Allopurinol (p.390·2).
Gout; hyperuricaemia.

Urinorm *Sanofi Winthrop, Spain.*
Benzbromarone (p.392·3).
Hyperuricaemia.

Urion
Zambon, Fr.; Byk Gulden, Ger.
Alfuzosin hydrochloride (p.817·2).
Benign prostatic hyperplasia.

Uri-Plus Rubia *Homeocan, Canad.*
Homoeopathic preparation.

Uripurinol *Azupharma, Ger.*
Allopurinol (p.390·2).
Gout; hyperuricaemia.

Urirex-K *Pharmador, S.Afr.†.*
Hydrochlorothiazide (p.885·2); potassium chloride (p.1161·1).
Hypertension; oedema.

Urisal *Sterling Winthrop, UK†.*
Sodium citrate dihydrate (p.1153·2).
Cystitis.

Urisan *Tedec Meiji, Spain.*
Pipemidic acid (p.237·2).
Urinary-tract infections.

Urisec *Odan, Canad.*
Urea (p.1095·2).
Dry skin conditions.

Urised *PolyMedica, USA.*
Hexamine (p.216·1); salol (p.83·1); methylene blue (p.984·3); benzoic acid (p.1102·3); atropine sulphate (p.455·1); hyoscyamine sulphate (p.464·2).
Lower urinary-tract infection or spasm.

Urisedamine *PolyMedica, USA.*
Hexamine mandelate (p.216·1); hyoscyamine (p.464·2).
Urinary-tract infections.

Urispas
Byk, Aust.; Byk, Belg.; Pharmascience, Canad.; Negma, Fr.; Roche, Irl.; Byk, Neth.; Searle, S.Afr.; Galenica, Switz.; Roche, UK; SmithKline Beecham, USA.
Flavoxate hydrochloride (p.461·2).
Urinary-tract disorders.

Uristix
Bayer Diagnostics, Austral.; Bayer, Canad.; Ames, Irl.; Ames, S.Afr.; Bayer Diagnostics, UK; Bayer, USA.
Test for glucose and protein in urine.

Uristix 2 *Bayer Diagnostici, Ital.*
Test for leucocytes and nitrites in urine.

Uristix 4
Bayer Diagnostics, Austral.†; Bayer, Canad.; Ames, S.Afr.; Bayer, USA.
Test for glucose, protein, nitrite, and leucocytes in urine.

Uritest *Bayer Diagnostics, Fr.*
Test for leucocytes, nitrites, glucose, and protein in urine.

Uritest 2 *Bayer Diagnostics, Fr.*
Test for leucocytes and nitrites in urine.

Uri-Tet *American Urologicals, USA†.*
Oxytetracycline hydrochloride (p.235·1).
Bacterial infections.

Uritol *Horner, Canad.†.*
Frusemide (p.871·1).
Hypertension; oedema.

Uritrate
Parke, Davis, Belg.; Parke, Davis, Ital.†.
Oxolinic acid (p.235·1).
Genito-urinary-tract infections.

Urizide *Rolab, S.Afr.*
Triamterene (p.957·2); hydrochlorothiazide (p.885·2).
Hypertension; oedema.

Urizone *Adcock Ingram, S.Afr.*
Fosfomycin trometamol (p.210·2).
Urinary-tract Escherichia coli infections.

Uro 3000 *Aguettant, Fr.*
Sodium chloride (p.1162·2), water, or glycine (p.1345·2) for irrigation.

Uro Angiografin *Schering, Spain.*
Meglumine diatrizoate (p.1003·2).
Radiographic contrast medium.

Uro Fink *Fink, Ger.*
Silver birch leaf (p.1553·3); solidago virgaurea; orthosiphon leaf (p.1592·2); black currant leaf (p.1365·2); bearberry (p.1552·2).
Urinary-tract disorders.

Uroalpha *Debat, Fr.†.*
Thymoxamine hydrochloride (p.952·2).
Benign prostatic hyperplasia.

Urobacid *Tyrol, Aust.*
Norfloxacin (p.233·1).
Bacterial infections.

Urobactam *Esteve, Spain.*
Aztreonam (p.156·3).
Bacterial infections.

Urobak *Shionogi, USA.*
Sulphamethoxazole (p.254·3).
Bacterial infections.

Uro-Beniktol N *Byk, Switz.*
Neomycin sulphate (p.229·2).
Uro-Beniktol formerly contained neomycin sulphate and sulphamethizole.
Urinary-tract infections.

Urobilistix
Bayer Diagnostics, Austral.†; Ames, S.Afr.; Ames, UK†.
Test for urobilinogen in urine.

Urobiotic-250 *Pfizer, USA†.*
Oxytetracycline hydrochloride (p.235·1); sulphamethizole (p.254·2); phenazopyridine hydrochloride (p.78·3).
Urinary-tract infections.

Uroc *Lampugnani, Ital.*
Cinoxacin (p.185·2).
Urinary-tract infections.

Urocarb *Hamilton, Austral.*
Bethanechol chloride (p.1389·3).
Neurogenic bladder; urinary retention.

Urocarf *SPA, Ital.*
Carfecillin sodium (p.163·1).
Urinary-tract infections.

Urocaudal *Pan Quimica, Spain.*
Triamterene (p.957·2).
Hypertension; hypokalaemia; oedema.

Urocaudal Tiazida *Pan Quimica, Spain.*
Hydrochlorothiazide (p.885·2); triamterene (p.957·2).
Hypertension; oedema.

Urocedulamin *Cedona, Neth.†.*
Hexamine mandelate (p.216·1).
Urinary-tract infections.

Uro-Cephoral *Merck, Ger.*
Cefixime (p.165·3).
Bacterial infections.

Urocid *Ist. Chim. Inter., Ital.†.*
Probenecid (p.394·3).
Gout; hyperuricaemia.

Urocit-K *Mission Pharmacal, USA.*
Potassium citrate (p.1153·1).
Urinary alkalinising agent.

Uroclear *Parke, Davis, Ger.†.*
Nitrofurantoin (p.231·3); sulphadiazine (p.252·3).
Urinary-tract infections.

Uro-Coli *Roussel, Ital.†.*
Nitroxoline (p.233·1).
Urinary-tract infections.

Urocridin *Fresenius, Ger.*
Ethacridine lactate (p.1098·3).
Bladder irrigation for urinary-tract infections.

Uroctal *Funk, Spain.*
Norfloxacin (p.233·1).
Gastro-enteritis; gonorrhoea; urinary-tract infections.

Urodene *OFF, Ital.*
Pipemidic acid (p.237·2).
Urinary-tract infections.

Urodie *Abbott, Ital.*
Terazosin hydrochloride (p.952·1).
Benign prostatic hyperplasia.

Urodil *Selz, Ger.†.*
Nitrofurantoin (p.231·3).
Urinary-tract infections.

Urodil Blasen-Nieren Arzneitee *Selz, Ger.*
Orthosiphon (p.1592·2); ononis (p.1610·2); birch leaf (p.1553·3); solidago virgaurea; fennel (p.1579·1); rose fruit (p.1365·2); peppermint leaf (p.1208·1); calendula officinalis; liquorice (p.1197·1).
Urinary-tract disorders.

Urodil N *Selz, Ger.†.*
Calcium-(RS)-mandelate (p.223·3); ammonium chloride (p.1055·2); salol (p.83·1); squill (p.1070·1); santalum album; stoechados flowers; ononis (p.1610·2); silver birch leaf (p.1553·3); herniaria (p.1587·2); jaborandi; buchu (p.1555·2); phaseolis vulgaris; bearberry (p.1552·2).
Urinary-tract disorders.

Urodil phyto *Selz, Ger.*
Birch leaves (p.1553·3); solidago virgaurea; orthosiphon (p.1592·2).
Urinary-tract disorders.

Urodil S *Selz, Ger.†.*
Squill (p.1070·1); santalum album; stoechados flowers; ononis (p.1610·2); birch leaves (p.1553·3); herniaria (p.1587·2); jaborandi; buchu (p.1555·2); phaseolis vulgaris; bearberry (p.1552·2).
Urinary-tract infections.

Urodin *Streuli, Switz.*
Nitrofurantoin (p.231·3).
Urinary-tract infections.

Urodine *Interstate Drug Exchange, USA†; Schein, USA†.*
Phenazopyridine hydrochloride (p.78·3).
Irritation of the lower urinary tract.

Urodyn *Bionorica, Ger.*
Solidago virgaurea.
Urinary-tract disorders.

Uroflex *Vifor Medical, Switz.*
Range of solutions for catheter care.

Uroflo *Abbott, Aust.*
Terazosin hydrochloride (p.952·1).
Benign prostatic hyperplasia.

Urogesic *Edwards, USA.*
Phenazopyridine hydrochloride (p.78·3).
Irritation of the lower urinary tract.

Urogesic Blue *Edwards, USA.*
Hexamine (p.216·1); monobasic sodium phosphate (p.1159·3); salol (p.83·1); methylene blue (p.984·3); hyoscyamine sulphate (p.464·2).
Urinary-tract infections.

Urogliss *Hoechst Marion Roussel, Neth.*
Chlorhexidine hydrochloride (p.1107·2); lignocaine hydrochloride (p.1293·2).
Catheterisation.

Urogliss-S *Hoechst Marion Roussel, Neth.*
Chlorhexidine hydrochloride (p.1107·2).
Catheterisation.

Urogobens Antiespasmo *Normon, Spain.*
Phenazopyridine hydrochloride (p.78·3); nitrofurantoin (p.231·3); hyoscine butylbromide (p.462·3).
Urinary-tract infections; urinary-tract spasm.

Urografin
Schering, Aust.; Schering, Ger.; Schering, Ital.†; Schering, Neth.; Schering, S.Afr.; Schering, Spain; Schering, Swed.; Schering, Switz.; Schering, UK.
Meglumine diatrizoate (p.1003·2); sodium diatrizoate (p.1003·2).
Radiographic contrast medium.

Urografin 310M *Schering, UK†.*
Meglumine diatrizoate (p.1003·2).
Radiographic contrast medium.

Urogram *FIRMA, Ital.*
Nalidixic acid (p.228·2).
Gram-negative bacterial infections of the genito-urinary tract.

Uro-KP-Neutral *Star, USA.*
Mineral preparation.
Phosphorus supplement.

Urol *Hoyer, Ger.†.*
Rubia tinctorum; ammi visnaga (p.1593·2); solidago virgaurea; taraxacum (p.1634·2); aescin (p.1543·3).
Urinary-tract disorders.

uro-L 90 *Loges, Ger.*
Homoeopathic preparation.

Urol mono *Hoyer, Ger.*
Solidago virgaurea.
Urinary-tract disorders.

Urolene Blue *Star, USA.*
Methylene blue (p.984·3).
Cyanide poisoning; cystitis; urethritis; drug-induced methaemoglobinaemia.

Urolin *Salus, Ital.†.*
Chlorthalidone (p.839·3).
Hypertension; oedema.

Urolisa *Lisapharma, Ital.†.*
Nitrofurantoin (p.231·3).
Urinary-tract infections.

Urologicum *Plantamed, Ger.*
Homoeopathic preparation.

Urolong
Organon, Aust.; Thiemann, Ger.†; Sodip, Switz.†.
Nitrofurantoin (p.231·3).
Bacterial infections of the urinary tract.

Urolucosil
Lundbeck, Aust.; Parke, Davis, Austral.†; Lundbeck, Belg.†; Lundbeck, Switz.†.
Sulphamethizole (p.254·2).
Bacterial infections of the urinary tract.

Uro-Mag *Blaine, USA.*
Magnesium oxide (p.1198·3).
Hyperacidity; magnesium deficiency.

Urombrine *Dagra, Neth.†.*
Meglumine iodamide (p.1005·3).
Radiographic contrast medium.

Urombrine 420 *Dagra, Neth.†.*
Meglumine iodamide (p.1005·3); sodium iodamide (p.1005·3).
Pyelography.

Urometron *Pharmagen, S.Afr.†.*
Metronidazole (p.585·1).
Anaerobic bacterial infections; protozoal infections.

Uromil *IPRAD, Fr.*
Piperazine (p.107·2); hexamine (p.216·1); anhydrous dibasic sodium phosphate (p.1159·3); morpholine mandelate; theophylline (p.765·1).
Urinary alkaliniser.

Uromiro
Gerot, Aust.; Bristol-Myers Squibb, Ger.†; Bracco, Switz.
Meglumine iodamide (p.1005·3).
Radiographic contrast medium.

Uromiro 300 *E. Merck, UK†.*
Meglumine iodamide (p.1005·3).
Radiographic contrast medium.

Uromiro 340 and 420 *Bracco, Ital.*
Meglumine iodamide (p.1005·3); sodium iodamide (p.1005·3).
Radiographic contrast medium.

Uromiro 24%, 36%, and 300 *Bracco, Ital.*
Meglumine iodamide (p.1005·3).
Radiographic contrast medium.

Uromiro 340, 380, and 420 *E. Merck, UK†.*
Meglumine iodamide (p.1005·3); sodium iodamide (p.1005·3).
Radiographic contrast medium.

Uromiro 300 Sodico *Bracco, Ital.*
Sodium iodamide (p.1005·3).
Radiographic contrast medium.

Uromitexan
Asta Medica, Aust.; Asta Medica, Austral.; Asta Medica, Belg.; Bristol, Canad.; Asta Medica, Fr.; Asta Medica, Ger.; Asta Medica, Irl.; Asta Medica, Ital.; Asta Medica, Neth.; Asta, Norw.; Hoechst Marion Roussel, S.Afr.; Pras, Spain; Asta Medica, Swed.; Asta Medica, Switz.; Asta Medica, UK.
Mesna (p.983·3).
Prevention of urotoxicity due to oxazaphosphorine antineoplastics.

Uromont *Montavit, Aust.*
Dexamethasone (p.1037·1); chlorhexidine hydrochloride (p.1107·2); lignocaine hydrochloride (p.1293·2).
Stricture prevention following transurethral procedures.

Uro-Munal *OM, Ger.*
Escherichia coli.
Urinary-tract disorders.

Uromycin *Farco, Ger.†.*
Neomycin sulphate (p.229·2); lignocaine hydrochloride (p.1293·2).
Urinary-tract infections.

Uromykol *Hoyer, Ger.*
Clotrimazole (p.376·3).
Fungal infections of skin and genito-urinary tract.

Uronase *Mochida, Jpn†.*
Urokinase (p.959·3).
Myocardial infarction.

Uro-Nebacetin N *Byk Gulden, Ger.*
Neomycin sulphate (p.229·2).
Formerly contained neomycin sulphate and sulphamethizole.
Urinary-tract infections.

Uronefrex
Therabel Pharma, Belg.; Cassenne, Fr.; Robert, Spain.
Acetohydroxamic acid (p.1541·3).
Adjunct in urinary-tract infections with urea-splitting organisms; renal calculi due to bacterial urease.

Uronid *Recordati Elmu, Spain.*
Flavoxate hydrochloride (p.461·2).
Urinary-tract disorders.

Uronorm *Wassermann, Ital.*
Cinoxacin (p.185·2).
Urinary-tract infections.

Uropan *Eurofarmaco, Ital.†.*
Nalidixic acid (p.228·2).
Genito-urinary-tract infections.

Uro-Pasc *Pascoe, Ger.*
Solidago virgaurea; taraxacum (p.1634·2).
Urinary-tract disorders.

Uro-pH Control *Apothecary, USA.*
Cranberry (p.1568·2); vitamin C (p.1365·2).

Uro-Phosphate *ECR, USA.*
Hexamine (p.216·1); monobasic sodium phosphate (p.1159·3).
Urinary-tract infections.

Uropimid *CT, Ital.*
Pipemidic acid (p.237·2).
Urinary-tract infections.

Uropipedil *Fournier SA, Spain.*
Pipemidic acid (p.237·2).
Urinary-tract infections.

Uropir *Salus, Ital.†.*
Piromidic acid (p.238·2).
Bacterial infections.

Uroplant Forte *Biomo, Ger.*
Solidago virgaurea.
Urinary-tract disorders.

Uroplus
Note. This name is used for preparations of different composition.
Kwizda, Aust.
Allopurinol (p.390·2); benzbromarone (p.392·3).
Gout; hyperuricaemia.

Shionogi, USA.
Co-trimoxazole (p.196·3).
Bacterial infections; Pneumocystis carinii pneumonia.

Uro-Pos *Ursapharm, Ger.*
Urtica (p.1642·3).
Prostatic hyperplasia.

Uro-Pract *Ebewe, Aust.*
Sodium chloride (p.1162·2).
Bladder irrigation; maintenance of bladder catheters.

Uro-Pract N *Fresenius, Ger.*
Sodium chloride (p.1162·2).
Maintenance of bladder catheters.

Uropurat *Kwizda, Aust.*
Bearberry (p.1552·2); herniaria (p.1587·2); equisetum (p.1575·1); ononis (p.1610·2).
Urinary-tract disorders.

Uropyrine *Pharmacobel, Belg.*
Phenazopyridine hydrochloride (p.78·3).
Urinary-tract disorders.

Uroqid-Acid *Beach, USA.*
Hexamine mandelate (p.216·1); monobasic sodium phosphate monohydrate (p.1159·3).
Urinary-tract infections.

Uroquidan *Serono, Spain.*
Urokinase (p.959·3).
Intra-ocular haemorrhage; thrombo-embolic disorders.

Uro-Ripirin *Pharmacia Upjohn, Ger.*
Emepronium carrageenate (p.461·1).
Urinary-tract disorders.

Urosan *AGIPS, Ital.*
Pipemidic acid (p.237·2).
Urinary-tract infections.

Uro-Selz *Selz, Ger.†.*
Nitrofurantoin (p.231·3).
Urinary-tract infections.

Urosetic *Finmedical, Ital.*
Pipemidic acid (p.237·2).
Urinary-tract infections.

Urosin
Boehringer Mannheim, Aust.; Boehringer Mannheim, Ger.
Allopurinol (p.390·2).
Gout; hyperuricaemia; renal calculi.

Urosiphon *Pierre Fabre, Fr.*
Orthosiphon stamineus (p.1592·2).
Diuretic; slimming aid.

Urospasmon
Note. This name is used for preparations of different composition.
Heumann, Switz.†.
Capsules: Nitrofurantoin (p.231·3); sulphadiazine (p.252·3).
Urinary-tract infections.
Heumann, Ger.; Heumann, Switz.†.
Tablets: Nitrofurantoin (p.231·3); sulphadiazine (p.252·3); phenazopyridine hydrochloride (p.78·3).
Urinary-tract infections.

Urospasmon sine *Heumann, Ger.*
Nitrofurantoin (p.231·3); sulphadiazine (p.252·3).
Urinary-tract infections.

Urospasmon sine phenazopyridino *Salus, Aust.*
Nitrofurantoin (p.231·3); sulphadiazine (p.252·3).

Urostei *Steigerwald, Ger.*
Birch leaf (p.1553·3); solidago virgaurea; orthosiphon (p.1592·2).
Urinary-tract disorders.

Urosten *Glaxo Allen, Ital.†.*
Pipemidic acid (p.237·2).
Urinary-tract infections.

Uro-Stilloson *Farco, Ger.*
Dexamethasone (p.1037·1); lignocaine hydrochloride (p.1293·2); chlorhexidine gluconate (p.1107·2).
Urinary-tract disorders.

Uro-Tablinen *Sanorania, Ger.*
Nitrofurantoin (p.231·3).
Urinary-tract infections.

Uro-Tainer *Braun, Belg.*
Chlorhexidine acetate (p.1107·2) or sodium chloride (p.1162·2).
Urinary catheter care; urinary-bladder lavage.

Uro-Tainer M *CliniMed, UK.*
Sodium chloride (p.1162·2).
Vehicle for intravesical administration of drugs.

Uro-Tainer Solutio R
Braun, Belg.†; Vifor Medical, Switz.
Citric acid monohydrate (p.1564·3); gluconolactone; light magnesium carbonate (p.1198·1).
Urinary catheter care.

Uro-Tainer Solution R *CliniMed, UK.*
Citric acid (p.1564·3); light magnesium carbonate (p.1198·1); gluconolactone.
Urinary catheter care.

Uro-Tainer Suby G
Braun, Belg.†; Vifor Medical, Switz.; CliniMed, UK.
Citric acid (p.1564·3); light magnesium oxide (p.1198·3); sodium bicarbonate (p.1153·2).
Urinary catheter care.

Uro-Tarivid *Hoechst, Ger.*
Ofloxacin (p.233·3).
Urinary-tract infections.

Uro-Trac *Apothecary, USA.*
Phenazopyridine hydrochloride (p.78·3).

Urotractan *Klinge, Ger.*
Hexamine hippurate (p.216·1).
Hyperhidrosis; urinary-tract infections.

Urotractin *SmithKline Beecham, Ital.*
Pipemidic acid (p.237·2).
Urinary-tract infections.

Urotrate *Parke, Davis, Fr.*
Oxolinic acid (p.235·1).
Urinary-tract infections.

Urotruw S *Truw, Ger.*
Homoeopathic preparation.

Uroval *FIRMA, Ital.*
Pipemidic acid (p.237·2).
Genito-urinary-tract infections.

Urovalidin *Bracco, Ital.†.*
Terizidone (p.259·1).
Urinary-tract infections.

Uro-Vaxom
Sanofi Winthrop, Ger.; OM, Switz.
Lysed immuno-active fraction of *Escherichia coli.*
Urinary-tract infections.

Urovison
Schering, Aust.; Schering, Ger.; Schering, Ital.†; Schering, Neth.
Meglumine diatrizoate (p.1003·2); sodium diatrizoate (p.1003·2).
Radiographic contrast medium.

Urovist
Schering, Ger.†; Berlex, USA.
Meglumine diatrizoate (p.1003·2) or sodium diatrizoate (p.1003·2).
Radiographic contrast medium.

Uroxacin *Malesci, Ital.*
Cinoxacin (p.185·2).
Urinary-tract infections.

UroXatral *Synthelabo, Ger.*
Alfuzosin hydrochloride (p.817·2).
Benign prostatic hyperplasia.

Urozyl-SR *Restan, S.Afr.*
Allopurinol (p.390·2).
Gout; hyperuricaemia.

Urprosan *Biohorm, Spain.*
Finasteride (p.1446·1).
Benign prostatic hyperplasia.

Ursacol *Zambon, Ital.*
Ursodeoxycholic acid (p.1642·1).
Biliary-tract disorders.

Ursilon *Ibi, Ital.*
Ursodeoxycholic acid (p.1642·1).
Biliary-tract disorders.

Ursinus Inlay-Tabs *Sandoz, USA.*
Pseudoephedrine hydrochloride (p.1068·3); aspirin (p.16·1).
Upper respiratory-tract symptoms.

Urso
Heumann, Ger.; Tokyo Tanabe, Jpn.
Ursodeoxycholic acid (p.1642·1).
Biliary-tract disorders; cholesterol gallstones; gastro-intestinal disorders; hepatic disorders; hyperlipidaemia.

Urso Mix *Fresenius, Ger.*
Chenodeoxycholic acid (p.1562·1); ursodeoxycholic acid (p.1642·1).
Cholesterol gallstones.

Ursobil *ABC, Ital.; Unibios, Ital.*
Ursodeoxycholic acid (p.1642·1).
Biliary-tract disorders.

Ursobilane *Estedi, Spain.*
Ursodeoxycholic acid (p.1642·1).
Gallstones.

Ursochol
Zambon, Belg.; Zambon, Ger.; Zambon, Neth.; Zambon, Spain; Inpharzam, Switz.
Ursodeoxycholic acid (p.1642·1).
Cholesterol gallstones; primary biliary cirrhosis.

Ursodamor *Damor, Ital.*
Sodium succinate ursodeoxycholate (p.1642·1).
Biliary-tract disorders.

Ursodiol *Bioprogress, Ital.*
Ursodeoxycholic acid (p.1642·1).
Biliary-tract disorders.

Ursofalk
Merck, Aust.; Codali, Belg.; Jouveinal, Canad.; Falk, Ger.; Antigen, Irl.; Knoll, Ital.; Falk, Neth.; Meda, Swed.; Falk, Switz.; Thames, UK.
Ursodeoxycholic acid (p.1642·1).
Cholesterol gallstones; primary biliary cirrhosis.

Ursofalk + Chenofalk *Falk, Ger.*
White capsules, ursodeoxycholic acid (Ursofalk) (p.1642·1); yellow-orange capsules, chenodeoxycholic acid (Chenofalk) (p.1562·1).
Cholesterol gallstones.

Ursoflor *SoSe, Ital.*
Ursodeoxycholic acid (p.1642·1).
Biliary-tract disorders.

Ursogal *Galen, UK.*
Ursodeoxycholic acid (p.1642·1).
Cholesterol gallstones.

Ursolac *Salus, Ital.*
Ursodeoxycholic acid (p.1642·1).
Biliary-tract disorders.

Ursolisin *Magis, Ital.*
Ursodeoxycholic acid (p.1642·1).
Biliary-tract disorders.

Ursolite *Vita, Spain.*
Ursodeoxycholic acid (p.1642·1).
Gallstones.

Ursolvan *Synthelabo, Fr.*
Ursodeoxycholic acid (p.1642·1).
Cholestasis; cholesterol gallstones.

Urson *Ripari-Gero, Ital.*
Sodium succinate ursodeoxycholate (p.1642·1).
Biliary-tract disorders.

Ursoproge *Proge, Ital.*
Ursodeoxycholic acid (p.1642·1).
Biliary-tract disorders.

Ursotan *Hoechst Marion Roussel, S.Afr.*
Ursodeoxycholic acid (p.1642·1).
Cholesterol gallstones.

Urtias *BASF, Ger.*
Allopurinol (p.390·2).
Gout; hyperuricaemia.

Urtica Plus *Europharm, Aust.*
Urtica (p.1642·3).
Urinary-tract disorders.

Urtica Plus N *Hoyer, Ger.*
Urtica (p.1642·3).
Benign prostatic hyperplasia.

Urticalcin
Bioforce, Canad.; Bioforce, Ger.; Bioforce, Switz.
Homoeopathic preparation.

Urticaprostat Uno *Azupharma, Ger.*
Urtica (p.1642·3).
Benign prostatic hyperplasia.

Urticur *Biocur, Ger.*
Urtica (p.1642·3).
Benign prostatic hyperplasia.

Urtipret *Bionorica, Ger.*
Urtica (p.1642·3).
Stage I/II prostatic adenoma.

Urtosal *Lifepharma, Ital.†.*
Salicylamide (p.82·3).
Fever; pain.

Urupan *Merckle, Ger.*
Dexpanthenol (p.1570·3).
Wounds.

Uskan
Desitin, Ger.; Cimex, Switz.
Oxazepam (p.683·2).
Anxiety; sleep disorders.

Usneabasan *Sanum-Kehlbeck, Ger.*
Homoeopathic preparation.

Ustilakehl *Sanum-Kehlbeck, Ger.*
Homoeopathic preparation.

Ustimon
Sigmapharm, Aust.; Lacer, Spain.
Hexobendine hydrochloride (p.883·1).
Cardiac disorders.

Ustionil *ICT, Ital.†.*
Silver sulphadiazine (p.247·3).
Burns; skin ulcers.

Utabon *Uriach, Spain.*
Oxymetazoline hydrochloride (p.1065·3).
Nasal congestion.

Utefos *Almirall, Spain.*
Tegafur (p.565·2).
Gastric and pancreatic cancer.

Uteplex *Wyeth, Fr.*
Trisodium uridine triphosphate.
Musculoskeletal disorders.

Uticort *Parke, Davis, USA†.*
Betamethasone benzoate (p.1033·3).
Skin disorders.

Uticox *Squibb, Spain.*
Meloxicam (p.52·1).
Osteoarthritis; rheumatoid arthritis.

Utilin *Sanum-Kehlbeck, Ger.*
Bacillus subtilis.
Immunotherapy.

Utilin N *Sanum-Kehlbeck, Ger.*
Bacillus subtilis.
Gout; musculoskeletal and joint disorders; skin disorders.

Utilin "S" *Sanum-Kehlbeck, Ger.*
Mycobacterium phlei.
Immunotherapy.

Utinor
Neopharmed, Ital.; Merck Sharp & Dohme, UK.
Norfloxacin (p.233·1).
Bacterial infections of the urinary tract.

Utk Uno *TAD, Ger.*
Urtica (p.1642·3).
Benign prostatic hyperplasia.

Utopar *Solvay, Norw.†.*
Ritodrine hydrochloride (p.1625·3).
Premature labour; uterine hypermotility in labour.

Utovlan *Searle, UK.*
Norethisterone (p.1453·1).
Breast cancer; endometriosis; menstrual disorders.

Utrogestan
Piette, Belg.; Besins-Iscovesco, Fr.; Hoechst Marion Roussel, Irl.; Seid, Spain; Besins-Iscovesco, Switz.
Progesterone (p.1459·3).
Benign breast disorders; female infertility; menopausal disorders; menstrual disorders; premature labour; threatened or recurring abortion.

UV Face Block Broad Spectrum Cream *ICI, Austral.†.*
SPF15+: Ethylhexyl *p*-methoxycinnamate (p.1487·1); oxybenzone (p.1487·3); avobenzone (p.1486·3).
Sunscreen.

UV Face Broad Spectrum *Boots, Austral.†.*
SPF15+: Ethylhexyl *p*-methoxycinnamate (p.1487·1); phenylbenzimidazole sulphonic acid (p.1488·2); titanium dioxide (p.1093·3).
Sunscreen.

UV Lip Block Broad Spectrum Stick - Water Resistant *Palmolive Skincare, Austral.†.*
SPF15+: Ethylhexyl *p*-methoxycinnamate (p.1487·1); oxybenzone (p.1487·3); avobenzone (p.1486·3).
Sunscreen.

UV Protectant *Norwood, Canad.*
SPF 15: Avobenzone (p.1486·3); ethylhexyl *p*-methoxycinnamate (p.1487·1); oxybenzone (p.1487·3).
Sunscreen.

UV Triplegard Broad Spectrum - Water Resistant
Boots, Austral.
Lotion SPF15+: Ethylhexyl *p*-methoxycinnamate (p.1487·1); oxybenzone (p.1487·3); titanium dioxide (p.1093·3).
Sunscreen.
Palmolive Skincare, Austral.†.
Stick SPF15+: Ethylhexyl *p*-methoxycinnamate (p.1487·1); oxybenzone (p.1487·3); avobenzone (p.1486·3).
Sunscreen.

UV Triplegard Clear *Boots, Austral.†.*
Ethylhexyl *p*-methoxycinnamate (p.1487·1); octyl salicylate (p.1487·3); oxybenzone (p.1487·3).
Sunscreen.

UV Triplegard Low Allergenic *Boots, Austral.*
SPF15+: Titanium dioxide (p.1093·3).
Sunscreen.

UV Triplegard Sunscreen Cream - Water Resistant *Boots, Austral.*
SPF15+: Ethylhexyl *p*-methoxycinnamate (p.1487·1); oxybenzone (p.1487·3); titanium dioxide (p.1093·3).
Sunscreen.

UV Triplegard Sunstick *Boots, Austral.*
SPF 15+: Ethylhexyl *p*-methoxycinnamate (p.1487·1); octocrylene (p.1487·3); zinc oxide (p.1096·2).
Sunscreen.

UV Tripleguard Toddler Block Broad Spectrum Lotion - Water Resistant *Boots, Austral.*
SPF15+: Ethylhexyl *p*-methoxycinnamate (p.1487·1); oxybenzone (p.1487·3); titanium dioxide (p.1093·3).
Sunscreen.

UV Water Sport *Boots, Austral.*
SPF15+: Ethylhexyl *p*-methoxycinnamate (p.1487·1); titanium dioxide (p.1093·3).
Sunscreen.

Uvacin *Lichtwer, UK.*
Taraxacum (p.1634·2); bearberry (p.1552·2).
Female bladder discomfort.

Uvacnyl *Galderma, Fr.†.*
Benzoyl peroxide (p.1079·2); 2-phenyl-1*H*-benzimidazole-5-sulphonic acid (p.1488·2).
Acne.

Uvalysat *Ysatfabrik, Ger.*
Bearberry leaf (p.1552·2).
Urinary-tract infections.

Uvamine retard *Mepha, Switz.*
Nitrofurantoin (p.231·3).
Urinary-tract infections.

Uva-Ursi Complex *Blackmores, Austral.*
Taraxacum (p.1634·2); galium aparine (p.1565·2); bearberry (p.1552·2); buchu (p.1555·2).
Bloating; dysuria; fluid retention; prostatitis; renal calculi; urethritis.

Uva-Ursi Plus *Eagle, Austral.*
Bearberry (p.1552·2); parsley (p.1615·3); taraxacum (p.1634·2); zanthoxylum (p.1645·3).
Cystitis; fluid retention.

Uvavit *Kolassa, Aust.*
Multivitamin and mineral preparation.
Nutritional supplement in pregnancy.

Uvedose *Crinex, Fr.*
Cholecalciferol (p.1366·3).
Vitamin D deficiency.

Uveline *Martin, Fr.*
Methylhydroxyquinoline methylsulphate (p.1603·2).
Eye disorders.

Uvestat *Bournonville, Belg.*
Methylhydroxyquinoline methylsulphate (p.1603·2).
Light-induced eye irritation.

Uvesterol *Crinex, Fr.*
Multivitamin preparation.

Uvesterol D *Crinex, Fr.*
Ergocalciferol (p.1367·1).
Vitamin D deficiency.

UVGuard *Schering-Plough, Canad.*
Ethylhexyl *p*-methoxycinnamate (p.1487·1); avobenzone (p.1486·3); oxybenzone (p.1487·3).
Sunscreen.

Uvicin *Steigerwald, Ger.*
Homoeopathic preparation.

Uvicol *Alcon, Fr.*
Actinoquinol (p.1543·1); oxedrine hydrochloride (p.925·3); borax (p.1554·2).
Eye disorders.

Uvilon *Bayer, Ital.†.*
Piperazine hydrate (p.107·2).
Ascariasis; enterobiasis.

Uvimag B$_6$ *Laphal, Fr.*
Magnesium glycerophosphate (p.1157·2); pyridoxine hydrochloride (p.1362·3).
Vitamin and mineral supplementation.

Uvirgan Mono *Kanoldt, Ger.*
Cucurbita (p.1569·1).
Urinary-tract disorders.

Uvirgan N *Kanoldt, Ger.*
Urtica (p.1642·3); cucurbita (p.1569·1); ononis (p.1610·2).
Formerly contained urtica, cucurbita, ononis, and bearberry.
Urinary-tract disorders.

Uvistat *Windsor, UK.*
SPF 6; SPF 8: Mexenone (p.1487·2); ethylhexyl *p*-methoxycinnamate (p.1487·1).
SPF 10: Mexenone (p.1487·2); ethylhexyl *p*-methoxycinnamate (p.1487·1); avobenzone (p.1486·3); titanium dioxide (p.1093·3).
SPF 15: Ethylhexyl *p*-methoxycinnamate (p.1487·1); avobenzone (p.1486·3).
Sunscreen.

Uvistat Babysun Cream *Windsor, UK.*
SPF 12: Mexenone (p.1487·2); ethylhexyl *p*-methoxycinnamate (p.1487·1).
Sunscreen.

Uvistat Lipscreen *Windsor, Irl.*
SPF 15: Mexenone (p.1487·2); avobenzone (p.1486·3); titanium dioxide (p.1093·3).
Sunscreen.

Uvistat Sun Cream *Windsor, Irl.*
SPF 8; SPF 10; SPF 15; SPF 20; SPF 30: Mexenone (p.1487·2); ethylhexyl *p*-methoxycinnamate

(p.1487·1); avobenzone (p.1486·3); titanium dioxide (p.1093·3).
Sunscreen.

Uvistat UV Protectant Windsor, Irl.
SPF 6; SPF 8; SPF 15: Mexenone (p.1487·2); ethylhexyl *p*-methoxycinnamate (p.1487·1); avobenzone (p.1486·3); titanium dioxide (p.1093·3).
Sunscreen.

Uvistik Air Link, Austral.†.
Ethylhexyl *p*-methoxycinnamate (p.1487·1); avobenzone (p.1486·3).
Sunscreen.

Uwobletten Hevert, Ger.†.
Homoeopathic preparation.

V Infusionslosung Baxter, Ger.
Electrolyte infusion (p.1147·1).
Fluid and electrolyte disorders.

Vac Anticatar Hermes Iny Organon, Spain†.
Haemophilus influenzae; *Streptococcus pneumoniae*; *Klebsiella pneumoniae*; *Moraxella (Branhamella) catarrhalis*; *Staphylococcus aureus*; *Streptococcus pyogenes*; *Streptococcus viridans*.
Respiratory-tract infections.

Vac Anticatarral Hermes Organon, Spain†.
Haemophilus influenzae; *Klebsiella pneumoniae*; *Streptococcus pneumoniae*; *Streptococcus sp.*; *Moraxella (Branhamella) catarrhalis*.
Respiratory-tract infections.

Vac Anticatarral Leti Leti, Spain†.
Pneumococcus; *Staphylococcus*; *Streptococcus*; *Klebsiella pneumoniae*; *Moraxella (Branhamella) catarrhalis*.
Respiratory-tract infections.

Vac Anticatarral Llte Evans, Spain†.
Moraxella (Branhamella) catarrhalis; *Staphylococcus*; *Streptococcus*; *Pneumococcus*; *Klebsiella pneumoniae*; *Haemophilus influenzae*.
Respiratory-tract infections.

Vac Anticatarral P Davis Parke, Davis, Spain†.
Injection: Moraxella (Branhamella) catarrhalis; *Klebsiella pneumoniae*; *Diplococcus pneumoniae*; *Haemophilus influenzae*; *Streptococcus*; phenol.
Tablets (prophylaxis): Diplococcus pneumoniae; *Streptococcus*; *Staphylococcus*; *Moraxella (Branhamella) catarrhalis*; *Haemophilus influenzae*.
Tablets (treatment): Diplococcus pneumoniae; *Streptococcus*; *Staphylococcus aureus*; *Moraxella (Branhamella) catarrhalis*; *Haemophilus influenzae*; *Klebsiella pneumoniae*; *Corynebacterium diphtheriae*.
Respiratory-tract infections.

Vac Anticolerica Llorente, Spain†.
A cholera vaccine (p.1506·2).
Active immunisation.

Vac Antidift Tet Llte Ev Evans, Spain†.
A diphtheria and tetanus vaccine (p.1508·1).
Active immunisation of infants and young children.

Vac Antigripal Sanofi, Spain; Leti, Spain.
An influenza vaccine (p.1515·2).
Active immunisation.

Vac Antimenin AC Llorente, Spain†.
A meningococcal vaccine (groups A and C) (p.1520·3).
Active immunisation.

Vac Antiparotiditis Pasteur Merieux, Spain.
A mumps vaccine (p.1521·2).
Active immunisation.

Vac Antipolio Or Evans, Spain; Alcala, Spain.
An oral poliomyelitis vaccine (p.1528·2).
Active immunisation.

Vac Antipolio Oral Glaxo Wellcome, Spain.
An oral poliomyelitis vaccine (p.1528·2).
Active immunisation.

Vac Antirrabica Rhone-Poulenc Rorer, Spain.
A rabies vaccine (p.1530·3).
Active immunisation.

Vac Antirrub Llorente, Spain†.
A rubella vaccine (RA 27/3) (p.1532·3).
Active immunisation.

Vac Antirrubeola Evans, Spain; Rhone-Poulenc Rorer, Spain; Smith Kline & French, Spain.
A rubella vaccine (RA 27/3) (p.1532·3).
Active immunisation.

Vac Antirubeola Leti, Spain†.
A rubella vaccine (p.1532·3).
Active immunisation.

Vac Antisaramp Llorente, Spain†.
A measles vaccine (Schwarz strain) (p.1517·3).
Active immunisation.

Vac Antitet Llorente, Spain†.
An adsorbed tetanus vaccine (p.1535·3).
Active immunisation.

Vac Antitetanica Evans, Spain.
A tetanus vaccine (p.1535·3).
Active immunisation.

Vac Antitifica Llorente, Spain†.
A typhoid vaccine (p.1536·3).
Active immunisation.

Vac Polio Sabin Smith Kline & French, Spain.
An oral poliomyelitis vaccine (p.1528·2).
Active immunisation.

Vac Poliomielitica Berna, Spain.
An oral poliomyelitis vaccine (p.1528·2).
Active immunisation.

Vac Tab Berna Berna, Spain†.
A typhoid vaccine (p.1536·3).
Active immunisation.

Vac Triple MSD Merck Sharp & Dohme, Spain.
A measles, mumps, and rubella vaccine (attenuated Enders, Jeryl Lynn, and Wistar RA 27/3 strains respectively) (p.1519·3).
Formerly known as Vac Anti Sar Rub Par.
Active immunisation.

Vaccin Catarrhal
Berna, Belg.; Berna, Switz.†.
An inactivated vaccine containing: pneumococci; *Staphylococcus aureus*; *Staphylococcus albus*; streptococci; *Klebsiella pneumoniae*; *Branhamella catarrhalis*; *Haemophilus influenzae*.
Upper respiratory-tract infections.

Vaccin DTCP Pasteur Vaccins, Fr.
An adsorbed diphtheria, tetanus, pertussis, and poliomyelitis (inactivated) vaccine (p.1509·3).
Active immunisation.

Vaccin DTP Pasteur Vaccins, Fr.
A diphtheria, tetanus, and poliomyelitis (inactivated) vaccine (p.1510·1).
Active immunisation.

Vaccin Tab Berna, Switz.
A typhoid vaccine (p.1536·3).
Active immunisation.

Vaccin TP Pasteur Vaccins, Fr.
A tetanus and poliomyelitis (inactivated) vaccine (p.1536·3).
Active immunisation.

Vaccino Antipiogeno Bruschettini, Ital.
A vaccine prepared from *Staphylococcus aureus*, *Pseudomonas aeruginosa*, *Escherichia coli*, *Streptococcus pyogenes*, and *Streptococcus pneumoniae*.
Active immunisation against pyogenic bacterial infections.

Vaccino Antipneumocatarrale Bruschettini, Ital.
A vaccine prepared from *Streptococcus pneumoniae*, *Streptococcus pyogenes*, *Haemophilus influenzae*, and *Branhamella catarrhalis*.
Bacterial infections of the respiratory tract.

Vaccino Difto Tetano ISI, Ital.
An adsorbed diphtheria and tetanus vaccine (p.1508·1).
Active immunisation.

Vaccino DPT ISI, Ital.
An adsorbed diphtheria, tetanus, and pertussis vaccine (p.1509·1).
Active immunisation.

Vaccino Tab Te Nuovo ISM, Ital.
A typhoid, paratyphoid A and B, and tetanus vaccine (p.1537·3).
Active immunisation.

Vacubucal Evans, Spain†.
Haemophilus influenzae; *Klebsiella pneumoniae*; *Staphylococcus aureus*; *Streptococcus pneumoniae*; *Moraxella (Branhamella) catarrhalis*.
Respiratory-tract infections.

Vacudol Xixia, S.Afr.
Paracetamol (p.72·2); codeine phosphate (p.26·1); promethazine hydrochloride (p.416·2).
Fever; pain.

Vacudol Forte Xixia, S.Afr.
Paracetamol (p.72·2); codeine phosphate (p.26·1); caffeine (p.749·3); meprobamate (p.678·1).
Pain and associated tension.

Vacuosa Ultra Adsorb Lainco, Spain†.
Activated charcoal (p.972·2); lactose (p.1349·3).
Diarrhoea; enteritis.

Vademin-Z Roberts, USA; Hauck, USA.
Multivitamin and mineral preparation.

Vadicate Inkeysa, Spain.
Vincamine hydrochloride (p.1644·1).
Cerebral trauma; cerebrovascular disorders.

Vadilex Synthelabo, Fr.
Ifenprodil tartrate (p.890·1).
Arteriopathy.

Vadol Phyteia, Switz.
Aspirin (p.16·1); caffeine (p.749·3).
Fever; pain.

Vadolax Ogna, Ital.
Cascara (p.1183·1); cynara (p.1569·2).
Constipation.

Vagantin Palmicol, Ger.
Methantheline bromide (p.465·1).
Gastro-intestinal disorders.

Vagantyl Pierre Fabre, Fr.†.
Homatropine methobromide (p.462·2); hyoscine oxide hydrobromide (p.463·2); pyridoxine hydrochloride (p.1362·3).
Motion sickness.

Vagarsol Lennon, S.Afr.
Di-iodohydroxyquinoline (p.581·1); cetylpyridinium chloride (p.1106·2); aminacrine hydrochloride (p.1098·3); boric acid (p.1554·2).
Vaginal infections.

Vagicillin Schur, Ger.
Neomycin sulphate (p.229·2).
Vaginal infections.

Vagifem
Novo Nordisk, Aust.; Novo Nordisk, Austral.; Novo Nordisk, Belg.; Novo Nordisk, Ger.; Novo Nordisk, Irl.; Novo Nordisk, Ital.; Novo Nordisk, Neth.; Novo Nordisk, S.Afr.; Novo Nordisk, Swed.; Novo Nordisk, Switz.; Novo Nordisk, UK.
Oestradiol (p.1455·1).
Atrophic vaginitis.

Vagiflor Asche, Ger.
Lactobacillus acidophilus (p.1594·1).
Disorders of the vaginal flora; vaginitis.

Vagi-Hex Drossapharm, Switz.
Hexetidine (p.1116·1).
Vaginitis.

Vagilen Farmigea, Ital.
Metronidazole (p.585·1).
Trichomoniasis.

Vagimid Apogepha, Ger.
Metronidazole (p.585·1).
Anaerobic bacterial infections; protozoal infections.

Vaginex
Schmid, Canad.; QHP, USA.
Tripelennamine hydrochloride (p.420·2).
External vaginal irritation.

Vaginyl DDSA Pharmaceuticals, UK.
Metronidazole (p.585·1).

Vagisec Schmid, USA†.
Polyoxyethylene nonyl phenol; sodium edetate (p.980·1); docusate sodium (p.1189·3).
Vaginal disorders.

Vagisec Plus Schmid, USA†.
Polyoxyethylene nonyl phenol; edetic acid (p.980·3); docusate sodium (p.1189·3); aminacrine hydrochloride (p.1098·3).
Vaginal disorders.

Vagisil
Note. This name is used for preparations of different composition.
Combe, Canad.; Combe, USA.
Cream: Benzocaine (p.1286·2); resorcinol (p.1090·1).
Skin disorders.

Combe, USA.
Topical powder: Aloes (p.1177·1); liquid paraffin (p.1382·1); benzethonium chloride (p.1102·3).
Vaginal disorders.

CCM, Ital.
Lignocaine (p.1293·2); chlorothymol (p.1111·1).
Anal and vulvar pruritus.

Combe, UK.
Lignocaine (p.1293·2).
Pruritus vulvae.

Vagistat Bristol-Myers Squibb, USA.
Tioconazole (p.388·3).
Vulvovaginal candidiasis.

Vagmycin Bristol-Myers Squibb, S.Afr.
Tetracycline (p.259·1); amphotericin (p.372·2).
Vaginal infections.

Vagoclyss Grossmann, Switz.
Lactic acid (p.1593·3).
Vaginal infections and irritation.

Vagogastrin Benvegna, Ital.†.
Oxyphencyclimine hydrochloride (p.466·3).
Gastro-intestinal disorders.

Vagogernil Benvegna, Ital.†.
Gefarnate (p.1193·2).
Duodenitis; gastritis; peptic ulcer.

Vagolisal Biotekfarma, Ital.
Cimetidine (p.1183·2).
Gastritis and duodenitis associated with acid hypersecretion; peptic ulcer.

Vago-med Stroschein, Ger.†.
Oestriol (p.1457·2).
Oestrogen deficiency disorders.

Vagomine Qualiphar, Belg.
Dimenhydrinate (p.408·2).
Motion sickness; nausea; vertigo; vomiting.

Vagostabyl Leurquin, Fr.
Crataegus (p.1568·2); calcium lactate (p.1155·2); melissa (p.1600·1); magnesium thiosulphate (p.996·3).
Nervous disorders.

Vagostal Cantabria, Spain.
Famotidine (p.1192·1).
Gastro-oesophageal reflux; peptic ulcer; Zollinger-Ellison syndrome.

Valase Herdel, Ital.†.
Stepronin sodium (p.1070·1).
Liver disorders.

Valatux Farmacologico Milanese, Ital.
Dextromethorphan hydrobromide (p.1057·3).
Coughs.

Valaxona Schaper & Brummer, Ger.†.
Diazepam (p.661·1).
Anxiety; insomnia; muscular disorders.

Valbil
Rohm, Aust.†; Procter & Gamble, Ger.
Febuprol (p.1578·3).
Biliary-tract disorders.

Valclair Sinclair, UK.
Diazepam (p.661·1).
Alcohol withdrawal syndrome; anxiety; epilepsy; premedication; skeletal muscle spasm.

Valda
Note. This name is used for preparations of different composition.
Bayer, Canad.
Menthol (p.1600·2); cineole (p.1564·1); thymol (p.1127·1); terpin hydrate (p.1070·2); guaiacol (p.1061·2).
Coughs.

SmithKline Beecham Sante, Fr.; SmithKline Beecham, Irl.†; Sterling Health, UK.
Menthol (p.1600·2); cineole (p.1564·1); thymol (p.1127·1); terpineol (p.1635·1); guaiacol (p.1061·2).
Upper respiratory-tract disorders.

Valda F3 Sterling Midy, Ital.
Potassium fluoride; sodium fluoride (p.742·1); ciclimenol; enoxolone (p.35·2).
Dental disorders.

Valda Mal de Gorge Sterling Midy, Fr.†.
Lignocaine hydrochloride (p.1293·2); cicliomenol; enoxolone (p.35·2).
Upper respiratory-tract disorders.

Valda Rhinite Sterling Midy, Fr.†.
Phenylpropanolamine hydrochloride (p.1067·2); phenylephrine hydrochloride (p.1066·2); paracetamol (p.72·2).
Upper respiratory-tract disorders.

Valda Septol SmithKline Beecham Sante, Fr.
Menthol (p.1557·2); cineole (p.1564·1); enoxolone (p.35·2); cicliomenol.
Mouth and throat infections.

Valdatos Sterling Health, Spain.
Dextromethorphan hydrobromide (p.1057·3).
Cough.

Valderma Roche Consumer, Irl.
Cream: Potassium hydroxyquinoline sulphate (p.1621·1); chlorocresol (p.1110·3).
Skin disorders.
Soap: Triclocarban (p.1127·2).
Acne.

Valderma Active Roche Consumer, UK†.
Benzoyl peroxide (p.1079·2).
Acne.

Valderma Cream Roche Consumer, UK.
Potassium hydroxyquinoline sulphate (p.1621·1); chlorocresol (p.1110·3).
Acne.

Valderma Soap Roche Consumer, UK.
Triclocarban (p.1127·2).
Acne.

Valdig-N Burger Ysatfabrik, Ger.
Convallaria (p.1567·2).
Heart failure.

Valdispert
Kali, Aust.†; Solvay, Belg.; Solvay, Ger.; Solvay, Neth.; Solvay, Spain; Solvay, Switz.
Valerian (p.1643·1).
Anxiety; insomnia; nervous disorders.

Valdispert comp Solvay, Ger.
Valerian (p.1643·1); lupulus (p.1597·2).
Anxiety; sleep disorders.

Valdorm Valeas, Ital.
Flurazepam monohydrochloride (p.672·2).
Insomnia.

Valeans Valeas, Ital.
Alprazolam (p.640·3).
Anxiety.

Valena N Spreewald, Ger.
Hypericum (p.1590·1); passion flower (p.1615·3); valerian (p.1643·1).
Anxiety; depression.

Valenac Shire, UK†.
Diclofenac sodium (p.31·2).
Gout; inflammation; musculoskeletal disorders; pain.

Valerbe Saunier-Daguin, Fr.
Valerian (p.1643·1); vitamins.
Aid to smoking withdrawal.

Valerecen Abigo, Swed.
Valerian (p.1643·1).
Sedative.

Valergen Hyrex, USA†.
Oestradiol valerate (p.1455·2).
Female castration; female hypogonadism; menopausal vasomotor symptoms; prevention of breast engorgement; primary ovarian failure; prostatic cancer; vulval and vaginal atrophy.

Valeria-Fordine Darci, Belg.†.
Valerian (p.1643·1); passion flower (p.1615·3); hyoscyamus (p.464·3); quassia (p.1624·1); condurango (p.1567·2); crataegus (p.1568·2); citrus aurantium.
Anxiety; circulatory disorders; dyspnoea; neurovegetative disorders; tonic.

Valerial Zambon, Belg.
Valerian (p.1643·1).
Sleep disorders.

Valerian Vitaplex, Austral.
Leonurus cardiaca (p.1604·2); valerian (p.1643·1); scutellaria; populus (p.1620·1); capsicum (p.1559·2).
Herbal sedative.

Valerian Compound Gerard House, UK.
Lupulus (p.1597·2); passion flower (p.1615·3); valerian (p.1643·1); wild lettuce (p.1645·1); jamaican dogwood.
Restlessness.

Valerian Plus Herbal Plus Formula 12 Vitelle, Austral.
Valerian (p.1643·1); scutellaria; passion flower (p.1615·3); dibasic potassium phosphate (p.1159·2); magnesium oxide (p.1198·3).
Insomnia; smooth muscle spasm.

Valeriana comp Hevert, Ger.
Diphenhydramine hydrochloride (p.409·1); pericarpium aurantii (p.1610·3); chamomile (p.1561·2); lupulus (p.1597·2); kava (p.1592·3); valerian (p.1643·1); peppermint oil (p.1208·1).
Nervous disorders; sleep disorders.

Valeriana forte Hevert, Ger.
Diphenhydramine hydrochloride (p.409·1); valerian (p.1643·1); lupulus (p.1597·2).
Sedative.

Valeriana mild Hevert, Ger.
Valerian (p.1643·1); passion flower (p.1615·3); lupulus (p.1597·2).
Nervous disorders; sleep disorders.

Valeriana Orto *Normon, Spain.*
Valerian (p.1643·1).
Anxiety; insomnia.

Valeriana-Digitalysat (Valdig) *Ysatfabrik, Ger.†.*
Valerian root (p.1643·1); peppermint leaf; digitalis purpurea leaf (p.848·3).
Cardiac disorders.

Valeriana-Strath *Strath-Labor, Ger.†.*
Crataegus (p.1568·2); lavender flower (p.1594·3); lupulus (p.1597·2); melissa (p.1600·1); valerian (p.1643·1).
Nervous system disorders.

Valerina Day Time *Lichtwer, UK.*
Valerian (p.1643·1); melissa (p.1600·1).
Stress.

Valerina Night-Time *Lichtwer, UK.*
Valerian (p.1643·1); lupulus (p.1597·2); melissa (p.1600·1).
Insomnia.

Valerocalma *Piam, Ital.*
Centranthus ruber.
Insomnia; sedative.

Valeromill *Pierrel, Ital.†.*
Valerian (p.1643·1); matricaria (p.1561·2).
Nervousness.

Valertest *Hyrex, USA.*
Oestradiol valerate (p.1455·2); testosterone enanthate (p.1464·1).
Menopausal vasomotor symptoms; prevention of postpartum breast engorgement.

Valesporin *Valles Mestre, Spain†.*
Cephalexin (p.178·2).
Bacterial infections.

Valette *Jenapharm, Ger.*
Ethinyloestradiol (p.1445·1); dienogest (p.1444·1).
Combined oral contraceptive.

Valin Baldrian *Salus, Aust.*
Valerian (p.1643·1); citronella oil (p.1565·1).
Nervous disorders; sleep disorders.

Valinor *Clintec, Fr.*
Amino-acid infusion.
Parenteral nutrition.

Valiquid *Roche, Ger.*
Diazepam (p.661·1).
Muscular disorders; psychiatric disorders; sleep disorders.

Valisone
Schering, Canad.; Schering, USA.
Betamethasone valerate (p.1033·3).
Scalp and skin disorders.

Valisone-G *Schering, Canad.*
Betamethasone valerate (p.1033·3); gentamicin sulphate (p.212·1).
Infected skin disorders.

Valitran *FIRMA, Ital.†.*
Diazepam (p.661·1).
Anxiety; epilepsy.

Valium
Roche, Aust.; Roche, Austral.; Roche, Belg.; Roche, Canad.; Roche, Fr.; Roche, Ger.; Roche, Irl.; Roche, Ital.; Roche, Neth.; Roche, Norw.; Roche, S.Afr.; Andreu, Spain; Roche, Swed.; Roche, Switz.; Roche, UK; Roche Products, USA.
Diazepam (p.661·1).
Alcohol withdrawal syndrome; anxiety disorders; convulsions; eclampsia; epilepsy; general anaesthesia; panic attacks; premedication; sedative; skeletal muscle spasm; sleep disorders; spasticity; status epilepticus; tetanus.

Vallene *Simes, Ital.†.*
Mebutamate (p.901·3).
Hypertension.

Vallene Complex *Daker Farmasimes, Spain†.*
Mebutamate (p.901·3); mebutizide (p.901·3); picodralazine (p.930·2).
Hypertension.

Vallergan
Rhone-Poulenc Rorer, Austral.; Rhone-Poulenc Rorer, Irl.; Rhone-Poulenc Rorer, Norw.; Rhone-Poulenc Rorer, S.Afr.; Castlemead, UK.
Trimeprazine tartrate (p.419·3).
Premedication; pruritus; sleep disorders; urticaria.

Vallizina *Simes, Ital.†.*
Mebutamate (p.901·3); dihydralazine tartrate (p.854·1); hydrochlorothiazide (p.885·2).
Hypertension.

Valmagen *UCM-Difme, Ital.†.*
Cimetidine (p.1183·2).
Gastro-oesophageal reflux; peptic ulcer; Zollinger-Ellison syndrome.

Valmane
Solvay, Aust.; Solvay, Ger.; Vemedia, Neth.†; Ethimed, S.Afr.†.
Valerian (p.1643·1) or valepotriates (p.1643·1).
Anxiety disorders.

Valmarin Bad N *Hoernecke, Ger.*
Citronella oil (p.1565·1).
Bath additive; insomnia; nervous disorders.

Valobonin
Note. This name is used for preparations of different composition.
Hanseler, Ger.†.
Valerian (p.1643·1); crataegus (p.1568·2); passion flower (p.1615·3); lupulus (p.1597·2).
Sleeplessness.
Hanseler, Switz.†.
Valerian (p.1643·1); lupulus (p.1597·2); passion flower (p.1615·3); melissa (p.1600·1).
Sedative.

Valocordin *Meuselbach, Ger.†.*
Phenobarbitone (p.350·2).
Formerly contained phenobarbitone, bromisoval, lupulus, and peppermint oil.
Nervous disorders.

Valocordin-Diazepam *Krewel, Ger.*
Diazepam (p.661·1).
Anxiety disorders; sleep disorders.

Valoid
Wellcome, Irl.; Glaxo Wellcome, S.Afr.; Wellcome, UK.
Cyclizine hydrochloride (p.407·1) or cyclizine lactate (p.407·1).
Nausea; vestibular disorders; vomiting.

Valomenth *Tosse, Ger.†.*
Valerian (p.1643·1); peppermint leaf (p.1208·1).
Nervous disorders.

Valometten *Hormosan, Ger.†.*
Valerian (p.1643·1); calcium isovalerate; menthol (p.1600·2).
Nervous disorders; sleeplessness.

Valontan
Recordati, Ital.; Zambon, Spain†.
Dimenhydrinate (p.408·2).
Motion sickness; vertigo.

Valopride
Celafar, Ital.; Delagrange, Spain†.
Bromopride (p.1181·3).
Gastro-intestinal disorders.

Valoron
Parke, Davis, Belg.; Parke, Davis, S.Afr.; Parke, Davis, Switz.
Tilidate hydrochloride (p.89·2).
Pain.

Valoron N *Godecke, Ger.*
Tilidate hydrochloride (p.89·2).
Naloxone hydrochloride (p.986·2) is included in this preparation to discourage abuse.
Pain.

Valpeda *Roche Consumer, UK.*
Halquinol (p.215·3).
Skin disorders.

Valpiform *General Dietary, UK.*
A range of gluten-free foods.

Valpinax *Crinos, Ital.*
Octatropine methylbromide (p.465·2); diazepam (p.661·1).
Gastro-intestinal spasm.

Val-Plus *Edmond Pharma, Ital.*
Valerian (p.1643·1); passion flower (p.1615·3).
Insomnia; sedative.

Valpro *Alphapharm, Austral.*
Sodium valproate (p.361·2).
Epilepsy.

Valrelease *Roche, USA†.*
Diazepam (p.661·1).
Alcohol withdrawal syndrome; anxiety; premedication; skeletal muscle spasm; status epilepticus.

Valrox *Shire, UK†.*
Naproxen (p.61·2).
Dysmenorrhoea; gout; musculoskeletal disorders.

Valsera *Polifarma, Ital.*
Flunitrazepam (p.670·1).
Insomnia.

Valstar *Anthra, USA.*
Valrubicin.
Bladder cancer.

Valtran *Parke, Davis, Belg.*
Tilidate hydrochloride (p.89·2).
Naloxone hydrochloride (p.986·2) is included in this preparation to discourage abuse.
Pain.

Valtrax *Valeas, Ital.*
Diazepam (p.661·1); isopropamide iodide (p.464·3).
Gastro-intestinal spasm.

Valtrex
Glaxo Wellcome, Aust.; Glaxo Wellcome, Austral.; Glaxo Wellcome, Canad.; Glaxo Wellcome, Ger.; Hoechst, Ger.; Wellcome, Irl.; Glaxo Wellcome, Norw.; Wellcome, Spain; Glaxo Wellcome, Swed.; Wellcome, Switz.; Wellcome, UK; Wellcome, USA.
Valaciclovir hydrochloride (p.628·1).
Herpesvirus infections.

Val-Uno *Edmond Pharma, Ital.*
Valerian (p.1643·1).
Insomnia; sedative.

Valverde contre les douleurs *Ciba-Geigy, Switz.†.*
Salix (p.82·3); cinchona bark (p.1564·1); petasites root; kola (p.1645·1).
Pain.

Valverde Dragees laxatives *Zyma, Switz.*
Fig (p.1193·2); senna (p.1212·2); petasites root.
Constipation.

Valverde Dragees pour la detente nerveuse *Zyma, Switz.*
Petasites root; passion flower (p.1615·3); valerian (p.1643·1); melissa (p.1600·1).
Nervous disorders.

Valverde Dragees pour le coeur *Zyma, Switz.*
Crataegus leaves and fruit (p.1568·2); passion flower (p.1615·3); lupulus (p.1597·2); valerian root (p.1643·1).
Cardiac disorders.

Valverde Dragees pour le sommeil N *Zyma, Switz.*
Lupulus (p.1597·2); valerian root (p.1643·1).
Sleep disorders.

Valverde Ginkgo Vital *Zyma, Switz.*
Ginkgo biloba (p.1584·1).
Tonic.

Valverde Gouttes pour le coeur *Zyma, Switz.*
Crataegus leaves and fruit (p.1568·2); passion flower (p.1615·3).
Cardiac disorders.

Valverde Hyperval *Zyma, Switz.*
Hypericum (p.1590·1).
Anxiety; tension.

Valverde Sirop contre la toux *Zyma, Switz.*
Hedera helix.
Respiratory-tract disorders associated with excess mucus.

Valverde Sirop laxatif *Zyma, Switz.*
Fig (p.1193·2); senna (p.1212·2).
Constipation.

Valverde Sirop pour le sommeil *Zyma, Switz.*
Valerian (p.1643·1).
Sleep disorders.

Valverde Tablettes contre la toux *Zyma, Switz.*
Hedera helix.
Respiratory-tract disorders associated with excess mucus.

Vamin
Pharmacia Upjohn, Aust.; Pharmacia Upjohn, Austral.; Pharmacia Upjohn, Belg.; Pharmacia Upjohn, Canad.; Pharmacia Upjohn, Irl.; Pharmacia Upjohn, Neth.; Pharmacia Upjohn, Norw.; Pharmacia Upjohn, Swed.; Pharmacia Upjohn, UK.
Amino-acid infusion with or without electrolytes.
Parenteral nutrition.

Vamin con Glucosa *Pharmacia, Spain.*
Amino-acid infusion with glucose and electrolytes.
Parenteral nutrition.

Vamin Electrolyte Free *Pharmacia Upjohn, S.Afr.*
Amino-acid infusion.
Parenteral nutrition.

Vamin Glucose
Pharmacia Upjohn, Austral.; Pharmacia Upjohn, Belg.; Pharmacia Upjohn, Irl.; Pharmacia Upjohn, Neth.; Pharmacia Upjohn, S.Afr.; Pharmacia Upjohn, UK.
Amino-acid, carbohydrate, and electrolyte infusion.
Parenteral nutrition.

Vamin Infant *Kabivitrum, Irl.†.*
Amino-acid infusion.
Parenteral nutrition.

Vamin mit Glukose *Pharmacia Upjohn, Aust.*
Amino-acid, electrolyte, and glucose infusion.
Parenteral nutrition.

Vamin N
Pharmacia Upjohn, Austral.; Kabi Pharmacia, Belg.†.
Amino-acid and electrolyte infusion.
Parenteral nutrition.

Vamina *Pharmacia Upjohn, Switz.*
Amino-acid infusion.
Parenteral nutrition.

Vamina Glucose *Pharmacia Upjohn, Switz.*
Amino-acid, carbohydrate, and electrolyte infusion.
Parenteral nutrition.

Vamine *Pharmacia Upjohn, Fr.*
Amino-acid and electrolyte infusion with or without glucose.
Parenteral nutrition.

Vamin-Glukos
Pharmacia Upjohn, Norw.; Pharmacia Upjohn, Swed.
Amino-acid, carbohydrate, and electrolyte infusion.
Parenteral nutrition.

Vaminolac
Pharmacia Upjohn, Norw.; Pharmacia Upjohn, Swed.
Amino-acid infusion.
Parenteral nutrition.

Vaminolact
Pharmacia Upjohn, Aust.; Pharmacia Upjohn, Belg.; Pharmacia Upjohn, Fr.; Pharmacia Upjohn, Irl.; Pharmacia Upjohn, Neth.; Pharmacia Upjohn, Switz.; Pharmacia Upjohn, UK.
Amino-acid infusion.
Parenteral nutrition.

Vancenase
Schering, Canad.; Schering, USA.
Beclomethasone dipropionate (p.1032·1).
Nasal polyps; rhinitis.

Vanceril
Schering, Canad.; Schering, USA.
Beclomethasone dipropionate (p.1032·1).
Asthma.

VANCO *Cell Pharm, Ger.; Reusch, Ger.*
Vancomycin hydrochloride (p.267·2).
Bacterial infections.

Vancocin
Lilly, Austral.; Lilly, Belg.; Lilly, Canad.; Lilly, Irl.; Lilly, Neth.; Lilly, Norw.; Lilly, S.Afr.; Lilly, Swed.; Lilly, Switz.; Lilly, UK; Lilly, USA.
Vancomycin hydrochloride (p.267·2).
Antibiotic-associated colitis; bacterial infections.

Vancocina *Lilly, Ital.*
Vancomycin hydrochloride (p.267·2).
Bacterial infections.

Vancocine *Lilly, Fr.*
Vancomycin hydrochloride (p.267·2).
Bacterial infections.

Vancoled
Lederle, Austral.; Wyeth Lederle, Swed.†; Lederle, USA.
Vancomycin hydrochloride (p.267·2).
Bacterial infections.

Vancor *Adria, USA†.*
Vancomycin hydrochloride (p.267·2).
Staphylococcal infections.

Vancoscand *Scand Pharm, Swed.*
Vancomycin hydrochloride (p.267·2).
Gram-positive bacterial infections.

Vandol *Schering-Plough, S.Afr.*
Vitamin A (p.1358·1); vitamin D (p.1366·3).
Skin disorders.

Vandral *Wyeth, Spain.*
Venlafaxine hydrochloride (p.311·2).
Depression.

Vanex Expectorant *Abana, USA.*
Pseudoephedrine hydrochloride (p.1068·3); guaiphenesin (p.1061·3); hydrocodone tartrate (p.43·1).
Coughs.

Vanex Forte *Abana, USA.*
Phenylpropanolamine hydrochloride (p.1067·2); phenylephrine hydrochloride (p.1066·2); chlorpheniramine maleate (p.405·1); mepyramine maleate (p.414·1).
Upper respiratory-tract symptoms.

Vanex Forte-R *Schwarz, USA.*
Phenylpropanolamine hydrochloride (p.1067·2); chlorpheniramine maleate (p.405·1).
Upper respiratory-tract disorders.

Vanex Grape *Abana, USA.*
Dihydrocodeine tartrate (p.34·1); phenylephrine hydrochloride (p.1066·2); phenylpropanolamine hydrochloride (p.1067·2); chlorpheniramine maleate (p.405·1).
Coughs and congestion.

Vanex-HD *Abana, USA.*
Phenylephrine hydrochloride (p.1066·2); chlorpheniramine maleate (p.405·1); hydrocodone tartrate (p.43·1).
Coughs and cold symptoms.

Vanex-LA *Abana, USA†.*
Phenylpropanolamine hydrochloride (p.1067·2); guaiphenesin (p.1061·3).
Coughs.

Vanicream *Pharmaceutical Specialties, USA.*
Vehicle for topical preparations.

Vanidene *Asta Medica, Belg.*
Cyclovalone (p.1569·2).
Liver disorders; skin disorders; vomiting with ketonuria.

Vanilone *Ienapharm, Fr.*
Cyclovalone (p.1569·2).
Dyspepsia.

Vanoxide *Dermik, USA.*
Benzoyl peroxide (p.1079·2).
Acne.

Vanoxide-HC
Rhone-Poulenc Rorer Consumer, Canad.†; Dermik, USA.
Benzoyl peroxide (p.1079·2); hydrocortisone (p.1043·3).
Skin disorders.

Vanquin
Warner-Lambert, Belg.†; Warner-Lambert, Canad.; Warner-Lambert, Ital.; Warner-Lambert, Norw.; Parke, Davis, Swed.
Viprynium embonate (p.111·2).
Enterobiasis.

Vanquish *Glenbrook, USA.*
Aspirin (p.16·1); paracetamol (p.72·2); caffeine (p.749·3).
Aluminium hydroxide (p.1177·3) and magnesium hydroxide (p.1198·2) are included in this preparation in an attempt to limit adverse effects on the gastro-intestinal mucosa.
Pain.

Vansil
Pfizer, Fr.†; Pfizer, UK†; Pfizer, USA.
Oxamniquine (p.106·2).
Schistosomiasis.

Vantaggio *Gazzoni, Ital.*
Aspartame (p.1335·1).
Sugar substitute.

Vantin *Upjohn, USA.*
Cefpodoxime proxetil (p.172·1).
Bacterial infections.

Vap Air *Drug Trading, Canad.*
Camphor (p.1557·2); eucalyptus oil (p.1578·1); menthol (p.1600·2); pumilio pine oil (p.1623·3); thymol (p.1127·1).

Vapex *Roche Consumer, UK†.*
Menthol (p.1600·2).
Nasal congestion.

Vapin *Lacer, Spain.*
Octatropine methylbromide (p.465·2).
Adjunct in peptic ulcer; gastro-intestinal spasm; irritable bowel syndrome.

Vapin Complex *Lacer, Spain.*
Dipyrone (p.35·1); octatropine methylbromide (p.465·2).
Gastro-intestinal spasm; pain.

Vapo-Myrtol *Marion Merrell, Fr.*
Borneol; menthol (p.1600·2); myrtle oil; niaouli oil (p.1607·1); thyme oil (p.1637·1); cineole (p.1564·1).
Respiratory-tract congestion.

Vaponefrin
Rhone-Poulenc Rorer, Canad.; Fisons, USA.
Racepinephrine (p.815·2) or racepinephrine hydrochloride (p.815·2).
Bronchospasm.

Vapor Flay *Herbaline, Ital.*
Cymbopogon nardus oil; geranium oil (p.1584·1); pinus pinaster oil; verbena citriodora oil; peppermint oil (p.1208·1).
Insect repellent.

Vapor Sol *Difa, Ital.†.*
Naphazoline nitrate (p.1064·2); colloidal sulphur (p.1091·2); cineole (p.1564·1); terpin hydrate (p.1070·2).
Inhalant for nose and throat.

Vapores Pyt *Fardi, Spain.*
Peru balsam (p.1617·2); cupressus sempervirens; eucalyptus (p.1578·1); niaouli oil (p.1607·1); diplotaxis tenuifolia; abies pectinata; pinus sylvestris; beech.
Upper respiratory-tract congestion.

Vaporisateur Medicamente
Note. This name is used for preparations of different composition.
Alsi, Canad.
Camphor (p.1557·2); cineole (p.1564·1); menthol (p.1600·2); thymol (p.1127·1).
Multi-Pro, Canad.
Camphor (p.1557·2); eucalyptus oil (p.1578·1); menthol (p.1600·2); thymol (p.1127·1).

Vaporisateur Nasal Decongestionnant *Prodemdis, Canad.*
Xylometazoline hydrochloride (p.1071·2).

Vaporizing Colds Rub *Scott, Canad.*
Camphor (p.1557·2); eucalyptus oil (p.1578·1); menthol (p.1600·2).

Vaporizing Ointment *Prodemdis, Canad.*
Camphor (p.1557·2); cedar; eucalyptus oil (p.1578·1); menthol (p.1600·2); nutmeg oil (p.1609·3); thymol (p.1127·1); turpentine.

Vapour Rub
Note. This name is used for preparations of different composition.
Mentholatum, UK.
Menthol (p.1600·2); camphor (p.1557·2); methyl salicylate (p.55·2).
Nasal congestion; rheumatic and muscular pain; skin irritation.
Numark, UK.
Eucalyptus oil (p.1578·1); camphor (p.1557·2); menthol (p.1600·2).

VAQTA
CSL, Austral.; Pasteur Merieux, Ger.; Chiron Behring, Ger.; Pasteur Merieux, UK; Merck, USA.
A hepatitis A vaccine (p.1512·2).
Active immunisation.

Varacillin *Kanebo, Jpn†.*
Lenampicillin hydrochloride (p.221·2).

Varecort *Zyma, Switz.†.*
Prednisolone pivalate (p.1048·1); oxerutins (p.1580·2); hexachlorophane (p.1115·2).
Anorectal disorders.

Varemoid
Novartis, Austral.; Novartis Consumer, S.Afr.; Zyma, Switz.
Oxerutins (p.1580·2).
Anorectal disorders.

Variargil *Italfarmaco, Spain.*
Trimeprazine tartrate (p.419·3).
Hypersensitivity skin disorders.

Varibiotic
Cyanamid, Ital.†; Cyanamid, Spain.
Demeclocycline hydrochloride (p.201·2); streptodornase (p.1632·3); streptokinase (p.948·2).
Bacterial infections.

Varicella
SmithKline Beecham, Aust.; SmithKline Beecham, Switz.†.
A varicella zoster vaccine (OKA strain) (p.1538·2).
Active immunisation.

Varicellon *Centeon, Ger.; Chiron Behring, Ger.*
A varicella-zoster immunoglobulin (p.1538·1).
Passive immunisation.

Varicex
Note. This name is used for preparations of different composition.
Stella, Belg.†.
Zinc oxide (p.1096·2); calcium chloride (p.1155·1).
Medicated dressing.
Lohmann, Ital.
Zinc oxide (p.1096·2).
Medicated dressing.

Variclene *Dermal Laboratories, UK†.*
Brilliant green (p.1104·2); lactic acid (p.1593·3).
Skin ulcers.

varico sanol Beincreme *Sanol, Ger.†.*
8-Bis-(6-diethylaminomethylrutin)-methane-aescin (p.1543·3); heparin (p.879·3); hamamelis (p.1587·1).
Skin trauma.

varico sanol forte *Sanol, Ger.†.*
8-Bis-(6-diethylaminomethylrutin)-methane-aescin (p.1543·3); hesperidin complex (p.1580·2); hamamelis (p.1587·1); thiamine nitrate (p.1361·1).
Vascular disorders.

Varicocid *Kreussler, Ger.†.*
Sodium morrhuate (p.1631·2); benzyl alcohol (p.1103·3).
Haemorrhoids; varicose veins.

Varicogel *Schiapparelli, Ital.*
Aesculus (p.1543·3); hamamelis (p.1587·1).
Peripheral vascular disorders.

Varicose Ointment *Potter's, UK.*
Cade oil (p.1092·2); hamamelis (p.1587·1); zinc oxide (p.1096·2).
Skin irritation due to varicosity.

Varicylum *Chemosan, Aust.*
Hamamelis (p.1587·1); chamomile oil; arnica (p.1550·3).
Skin disorders; soft-tissue disorders.

Varicylum N *Liebermann, Ger.*
Homoeopathic preparation.

Varicylum S *Liebermann, Ger.*
Chamomile oil; sage oil; arnica (p.1550·3); aesculus (p.1543·3); hamamelis (p.1587·1).
Haemorrhoids; soft-tissue injury; vascular disorders.

Varidasa *Cyanamid, Spain.*
Streptodornase (p.1632·3); streptokinase (p.948·2).
Inflammation; tissue damage.

Varidase
Cyanamid, Aust.; Lederle, Austral.; Wyeth Lederle, Belg.; Lederle, Ger.; Wyeth, Irl.; Cyanamid, Ital.; Lederle, Neth.; Wyeth, Norw.; Wyeth, S.Afr.; Wyeth Lederle, Swed.; Wyeth, UK.
Streptokinase (p.948·2); streptodornase (p.1632·3).
Bruising; haematoma; inflammation; local removal of blood clots and purulent matter; oedema.

Varigloban *Kreussler, Ger.*
Sodium iodide (p.1493·2); iodine (p.1493·1).
Haemorrhoids; varicose veins.

Variglobin *Globopharm, Switz.*
Sodium iodide (p.1493·2); iodine (p.1493·1).
Varicose veins.

Varihes
Laevosan, Aust.; Laevosan, Switz.
Hetastarch (p.724·1).
Hypovolaemia.

Varihesive *ConvaTec, UK.*
Carmellose sodium (p.1471·2); gelatin (p.723·2); pectin (p.1474·1); polyisobutylene.
Leg ulcers.

Varihesive Hydroactive *Convatec, Switz.*
Carmellose sodium (p.1471·2); gelatin (p.723·2); pectin (p.1474·1).
Burns; skin ulcers; wounds.

Varilisin *Knoll, Belg.*
Collagenase (p.1566·3).
Debridement of necrotic ulcers.

Varilrix
SK-RIT, Belg.; SmithKline Beecham, Ger.; Dresden, Ger.; SmithKline Beecham, Swed.; SmithKline Beecham, Switz.
A live attenuated varicella-zoster vaccine (OKA strain) (p.1538·2).
Formerly known as Varicella-RIT in *Ger.*
Active immunisation.

Varismil *Veris, Spain†.*
Hidrosmin.
Peripheral vascular disorders.

Varitan N *Godecke, Ger.*
Bismuth subgallate (p.1180·2); zinc oxide (p.1096·2); laureth 9 (p.1325·2).
Anorectal disorders.

Varitect
Biotest, Aust.; Biotest, Ger.; Intra Pharma, Irl.; Biotest, Ital.; Biotest, Switz.
A varicella-zoster immunoglobulin (p.1538·1).
Passive immunisation.

Varivax *Merck, USA.*
A live varicella vaccine (Oka/Merck) (p.1538·2).
Active immunisation.

Varlane *Schering, Belg.*
Fluocortin butyl (p.1041·3).
Burns; skin disorders; stings.

Varnoline
Organon, Fr.; Intervet, Switz.†.
Desogestrel (p.1443·3); ethinyloestradiol (p.1445·1).
28-Day packs also contain 7 inert tablets.
Combined oral contraceptive.

Varonina *Perez Gimenez, Spain†.*
Multivitamin, mineral, and amino-acid preparation.
Tonic.

Varson *Almirall, Spain.*
Nicergoline (p.1607·1).
Vascular disorders.

Vartmedel *Kabi, Swed.†.*
Salicylic acid (p.1090·2); lactic acid (p.1593·3).
Warts.

Var-Zeta *Alfa Biotech, Ital.*
A varicella-zoster immunoglobulin (p.1538·1).
Passive immunisation.

Vas
Note. This name is used for preparations of different composition.
Elexsam, Austral.†.
Methyl nicotinate (p.55·1).
Peripheral vascular disorders.
Geymonat, Ital.
Heparan sulphate (p.879·2).
Thrombosis prophylaxis.
Sclavo, Ital.†.
A catarrh vaccine.
Catarrh; complications of influenza.

Vasad *Shire, UK†.*
Nifedipine (p.916·2).
Angina pectoris; hypertension; Raynaud's syndrome.

Vasa-Gastreu N R63 *Reckeweg, Ger.*
Homoeopathic preparation.

Vasagin *Salus, Ital.†.*
Pyricarbate (p.1624·1).
Angiopathies.

Vasan *Also, Ital.†.*
Ginkgo biloba (p.1584·1).
Peripheral vascular insufficiency.

Vasaten *Shire, UK†.*
Atenolol (p.825·3).
Angina pectoris; arrhythmias; hypertension; migraine; myocardial infarction.

Vascace
Roche, Irl.; Roche, UK.
Cilazapril (p.840·3).
Heart failure; hypertension.

Vascal *Schwarz, Ger.*
Isradipine (p.894·2).
Hypertension.

Vascardin
Nicholas, Irl.†; Nicholas, UK†.
Isosorbide dinitrate (p.893·1).
Angina pectoris; heart failure.

Vascase *Roche, Neth.*
Cilazapril (p.840·3).
Hypertension.

Vascase Plus *Roche, Neth.*
Cilazapril (p.840·3); hydrochlorothiazide (p.885·2).
Hypertension.

Vascocitrol *Jumer, Fr.*
Citroflavonoids (p.1580·1); ascorbic acid (p.1365·2); light magnesium carbonate (p.1198·1).
Venous insufficiency.

Vascoman *Takeda, Ital.*
Manidipine dihydrochloride (p.900·2).
Hypertension.

Vascor *McNeil Pharmaceutical, USA.*
Bepridil hydrochloride (p.828·2).
Angina pectoris.

Vascoray
Rovi, Spain†; Mallinckrodt, USA.
Meglumine iothalamate (p.1008·1); sodium iothalamate (p.1008·1).
Radiographic contrast medium.

Vascoril *Delalande, Ital.†.*
Cinepazet maleate (p.841·1).
Coronary circulatory disorders.

Vascular Cream *Brauer, Austral.†.*
Homoeopathic preparation.

Vasculat
Bender, Aust.; Boehringer Ingelheim, Ger.†; Boehringer Ingelheim, Ital.†; Boehringer Ingelheim, Spain; Boehringer Ingelheim, Switz.†.
Bamethan sulphate (p.827·1).
Cerebral and peripheral vascular disorders.

Vasculene *Lebens, Ital.†.*
Flunarizine hydrochloride (p.411·1).
Migraine; vascular disorders; vertigo.

Vasculine *Desbergers, Canad.*
Multivitamin and mineral preparation.

Vascumine *Bottu, Fr.†.*
Tocopheryl acetate (p.1369·1); troxerutin (p.1580·2).
Peripheral vascular disorders.

Vascunormyl *Alcon, Fr.*
Cyclandelate (p.845·2).
Vascular disorders.

Vasdilat *MDM, Ital.*
Isosorbide mononitrate (p.893·3).
Ischaemic heart disease.

Vaselastica *Inibsa, Spain†.*
Amine oxidase; lipase; tyrosinase.
Arteriosclerosis.

Vaselina Boricada *Brum, Spain; Calmante Vitaminado, Spain; Orravan, Spain; Puerto Galiano, Spain.*
Boric acid (p.1554·2); white soft paraffin (p.1382·3).
Skin disorders.

Vaselina Mentolada *Brum, Spain; Puerto Galiano, Spain.*
White soft paraffin (p.1382·3); menthol (p.1600·2).
Skin disorders.

Vaseline
Lever Pond's, Canad.; Chesebrough-Pond's, UK.
White soft paraffin (p.1382·3).
Minor skin disorders.

Vaseline Gomenolee *Gomenol, Fr.*
Niaouli oil (p.1607·1); white soft paraffin.
Irritation of skin and mucous membranes.

Vaseline Intensive Care *Chesebrough-Pond's, USA.*
SPF4; SPF 8; SPF 15: Ethylhexyl *p*-methoxycinnamate (p.1487·1); oxybenzone (p.1487·3).
SPF 25: Ethylhexyl *p*-methoxycinnamate (p.1487·1); oxybenzone (p.1487·3); 2-ethylhexyl salicylate (p.1487·3).
SPF 30: Ethylhexyl *p*-methoxycinnamate (p.1487·1); oxybenzone (p.1487·3); 2-ethylhexyl salicylate (p.1487·3); titanium dioxide (p.1093·3).
Sunscreen.

Vaseline Intensive Care Active Sport *Chesebrough-Pond's, USA.*
SPF 8; SPF 15: Ethylhexyl *p*-methoxycinnamate (p.1487·1); oxybenzone (p.1487·3).
Sunscreen.

Vaseline Intensive Care Baby *Chesebrough-Pond's, USA.*
SPF 15: Titanium dioxide (p.1093·3); zinc oxide (p.1096·2).
SPF 30+: Ethylhexyl *p*-methoxycinnamate (p.1487·1); oxybenzone (p.1487·3); 2-ethylhexyl salicylate (p.1487·3); titanium dioxide (p.1093·3).
Sunscreen.

Vaseline Intensive Care Blockout *Chesebrough-Pond's, USA.*
SPF 40: Padimate (p.1487·3); ethylhexyl *p*-methoxycinnamate (p.1487·1); oxybenzone (p.1487·3); 2-ethylhexyl salicylate (p.1487·3); titanium dioxide (p.1093·3).
Sunscreen.

Vaseline Intensive Care No Burn No Bite *Chesebrough-Pond's, USA.*
SPF 8; SPF 15: Ethylhexyl *p*-methoxycinnamate (p.1487·1); oxybenzone (p.1487·3).
Sunscreen.

Vaseline Lip Therapy *Lever Pond's, Canad.*
SPF 15: Ethylhexyl *p*-methoxycinnamate (p.1487·1); oxybenzone (p.1487·3); white soft paraffin.
Sunscreen.

Vaseretic
Frosst, Canad.; Merck Sharp & Dohme, USA.
Enalapril maleate (p.863·2); hydrochlorothiazide (p.885·2).
Hypertension.

Vasesana-Vasoregulans *Hotz, Ger.*
Aesculus (p.1543·3); mistletoe (p.1604·1); crataegus (p.1568·2); hamamelis (p.1587·1); arnica (p.1550·3); silybum marianum (p.993·3).
Haemorrhoids; vascular disorders.

Vasetic *Shire, UK†.*
Amiloride hydrochloride (p.819·2); hydrochlorothiazide (p.885·2).
These ingredients can be described by the British Approved Name Co-amilozide.
Heart failure; hepatic cirrhosis; hypertension.

Vaslan *Faes, Spain.*
Isradipine (p.894·2).
Hypertension.

Vasmol *Sabater, Spain†.*
Pyricarbate (p.1624·1).
Arteriosclerosis; peripheral vascular disorders.

vasoatherolip *Schwarz, Ger.†.*
Aluminium clofibrate (p.1271·1); nicotinic acid (p.1351·2).
Hyperlipidaemias.

Vasobral
Logeais, Fr.; Geymonat, Ital.
Dihydroergocryptine mesylate (p.1571·3); caffeine (p.749·3).
Cerebral and peripheral vascular disorders; headache.

Vasobrix *Guerbet, Fr.†.*
Ethanolamine ioxitalamate (p.1009·1); meglumine ioxitalamate (p.1009·1).
Contrast medium for radiography.

Vasoc *Lindopharm, Ger.†.*
Benzarone (p.1552·3).
Vascular disorders.

Vasocalm *Fournier, Fr.†.*
Black currant (p.1365·2); papaverine hydrochloride (p.1614·2); meprobamate (p.678·1).
Vascular disorders.

Vasocardol *Marion Merrell Dow, Austral.†.*
Diltiazem hydrochloride (p.854·2).
Angina pectoris; hypertension.

Vasocedine *Qualiphar, Belg.*
Naphazoline nitrate (p.1064·2).
Nasal congestion.

Vasocet *Cipharm, Fr.*
Cetiedil citrate (p.839·1).
Vascular disorders.

Vasocidin
Ciba Vision, Canad.; Iolab, USA.
Prednisolone acetate (p.1048·1) or prednisolone sodium phosphate (p.1048·1); sulphacetamide sodium (p.252·2).
Formerly contained prednisolone sodium phosphate, phenylephrine hydrochloride, and sulphacetamide sodium in *Canad.*
Eye inflammation with bacterial infection.

Vasocil *Aesculapius, Ital.†.*
Pyricarbate (p.1624·1).
Retinopathies; vasculitis obliterans; venous ulcers.

VasoClear *Iolab, USA.*
Naphazoline hydrochloride (p.1064·2); polyvinyl alcohol (p.1474·2).
Minor eye irritation.

VasoClear A *Iolab, USA.*
Naphazoline hydrochloride (p.1064·2); zinc sulphate (p.1373·2).
Eye irritation.

Vasocon
Ciba Vision, Canad.; Iolab, USA.
Naphazoline hydrochloride (p.1064·2).
Eye irritation.

Vasocon Ant *Ciba Vision, Spain.*
Naphazoline nitrate (p.1064·2); neomycin sulphate (p.229·2); zinc sulphate (p.1373·2).
Eye congestion; eye infections.

Vasocon-A
Ciba Vision, Canad.; Ciba Vision, UK†; Iolab, USA.
Naphazoline hydrochloride (p.1064·2); antazoline phosphate (p.401·3).
Eye irritation.

Vasoconstr *Ciba Vision, Spain.*
Naphazoline (p.1064·2); zinc sulphate (p.1373·2).
Eye irritation.

Vasoconstrictor Pensa *Pensa, Spain.*
Naphazoline hydrochloride (p.1064·2).
Nasal congestion.

Vasocor *Bio-Therabel, Belg.†.*
Indenolol hydrochloride (p.891·1).
Angina pectoris; arrhythmias; hypertension.

Vasoderm *Taro, USA.*
Fluocinonide (p.1041·2).
Skin disorders.

Vasodexa *Llorens, Spain.*
Dexamethasone sodium succinate (p.1037·3); tetrahydrozoline hydrochloride (p.1070·2).
Inflammatory eye disorders.

Vasodilan *Apothecon, USA.*
Isoxsuprine hydrochloride (p.1592·1).
Cerebrovascular disorders; peripheral vascular disorders.

Vaso-Dilatan *Agepha, Aust.*
Tolazoline hydrochloride (p.956·1).
Vascular disorders.

Vasodin *Teofarma, Ital.*
Nicardipine hydrochloride (p.915·1).
Angina pectoris; heart failure; hypertension.

Vasodistal *Delalande, Ital.†.*
Cinepazide maleate (p.841·1).
Arteriopathies.

Vaso-E-Bion *Strathmann, Ger.*
Troxerutin (p.1580·2); *dl*-alpha tocopheryl acetate (p.1369·2).
Vascular disorders.

Vasofed
Antigen, Irl.; Garec, S.Afr.
Nifedipine (p.916·2).
Angina pectoris; hypertension.

Vasofen *Allergan, Ital.*
Chloramphenicol sodium hemisuccinate (p.182·2); phenylephrine (p.1066·2); mepyramine maleate (p.414·1).
Eye disorders.

Vasofilo *Benvegna, Ital.†.*
Gallbladder wall extract; xenbucin; dehydrocholic acid (p.1570·2); pyridoxine (p.1363·1).
Hypercholesterolaemia.

Vasoforte N *Krugmann, Ger.*
Aesculus (p.1543·3).
Vascular disorders.

Vasofrinic *Trianon, Canad.*
Chlorpheniramine maleate (p.405·1); pseudoephedrine hydrochloride (p.1068·3).
Respiratory congestion.

Vasofrinic Plus *Trianon, Canad.*
Dextromethorphan hydrobromide (p.1057·3); guaiphenesin (p.1061·3); chlorpheniramine maleate (p.405·1); pseudoephedrine hydrochloride (p.1068·3).
Coughs; respiratory congestion.

Vasogen
Pharmax, Irl.; Pharmax, UK.
Dimethicone (p.1384·2); zinc oxide (p.1096·2); calamine (p.1080·1).
Barrier cream.

Vasolan *Eisai, Jpn.*
Verapamil hydrochloride (p.960·3).
Angina pectoris; arrhythmias; ischaemic heart disease; myocardial infarction.

Vasolastine *Enzypharm, Neth.†.*
Triacylglycerol lipase; acyl-CoA-dehydrogenase; amino oxidase; monophenol monoxygenase.
Myocardial infarction; vascular disease.

Vasolate *Napp, Irl.†.*
Naftidrofuryl oxalate (p.914·2).
Peripheral and cerebral vascular disorders.

Vasolator *Sanwa, Jpn.*
Glyceryl trinitrate (p.874·3).
Angina pectoris.

Vasolipid
Braun, Norw.; Braun, Swed.
Soya oil (p.1355·1); medium-chain triglycerides.
Contains egg lecithin.
Lipid infusion for parenteral nutrition.

Vasomil *Lennon, S.Afr.*
Verapamil hydrochloride (p.960·3).
Angina pectoris; arrhythmias.

Vasomotal *Solvay, Ger.*
Betahistine hydrochloride (p.1553·1).
Ménière's disease; vertigo; vestibular disorders.

Vasonase *Syntex, Spain.*
Nicardipine hydrochloride (p.915·1).
Angina pectoris; cerebrovascular disorders; hypertension.

Vasonett *INTES, Ital.*
Vincamine (p.1644·1).
Cerebrovascular insufficiency.

Vasonicit *IBIS, Ital.†.*
Inositol nicotinate (p.891·3); pyridoxine hydrochloride (p.1362·3).
Hemicrania; hypercholesterolaemia; hyperlipidaemias; myocardial ischaemia; peripheral and cerebral vascular disorders; restless leg syndrome; varicose ulcers.

Vasonicit Composto *IBIS, Ital.†.*
Inositol nicotinate (p.891·3); pyridoxine hydrochloride (p.1362·3); buphenine.
Peripheral vascular disorders.

Vasonit *Lannacher, Aust.*
Oxpentifylline (p.925·3).
Peripheral vascular disorders.

Vasopos N *Ursapharm, Ger.*
Tetrahydrozoline hydrochloride (p.1070·2).
Eye disorders.

Vasopresina *Sandoz, Spain.*
Lypressin (p.1263·2).
Diabetes insipidus.

Vasopressin
Sandoz, Ger.; Sandoz, S.Afr.†; Sandoz, Swed.†.
Lypressin (p.1263·2).
Diabetes insipidus.

Vasopressine
Sandoz, Neth.†; Sandoz, Switz.†.
Lypressin (p.1263·2).
Diabetes insipidus; variceal haemorrhage.

Vasorbate *Arcana, Aust.*
Isosorbide dinitrate (p.893·1).
Angina pectoris; heart failure; myocardial infarction; pulmonary hypertension.

Vasorema *Inverni della Beffa, Ital.*
Heparan sulphate (p.879·2).
Thrombosis prophylaxis.

Vasoretic *Merck Sharp & Dohme, Ital.*
Enalapril maleate (p.863·2); hydrochlorothiazide (p.885·2).
Hypertension.

Vasorinil *Farmila, Ital.*
Tetrahydrozoline hydrochloride (p.1070·2).
Nasal congestion.

Vasosan *Felgentrager, Ger.*
Cholestyramine (p.1269·3).
Hyperlipidaemias.

Vasosterone *Angelini, Ital.*
Hydrocortisone (p.1043·3); tetrahydrozoline hydrochloride (p.1070·2).
Nasal congestion.

Vasosterone Antibiotico *Angelini, Ital.*
Hydrocortisone acetate (p.1043·3); tetrahydrozoline hydrochloride (p.1070·2); neomycin sulphate (p.229·2); gramicidin (p.215·2).
Rhinitis.

Vasosterone Collirio *Angelini, Ital.*
Hydrocortisone acetate (p.1043·3); tetrahydrozoline hydrochloride (p.1070·2); neomycin sulphate (p.229·2).
Eye disorders.

Vasosterone Oto *Angelini, Ital.*
Flumethasone pivalate (p.1040·3); gentamicin sulphate (p.212·1).
Formerly contained hydrocortisone, tetrahydrozoline hydrochloride, neomycin sulphate, and gramicidin.
Otitis externa.

Vasosulf
Ciba Vision, Canad.; Iolab, USA.
Sulphacetamide sodium (p.252·2); phenylephrine hydrochloride (p.1066·2).
Bacterial eye infections.

Vasosuprina Ilfi *Lusofarmaco, Ital.*
Isoxsuprine hydrochloride (p.1592·1).
Premature labour; threatened abortion.

Vasotec
Frosst, Canad.; Merck Sharp & Dohme, USA.
Enalapril maleate (p.863·2) or enalaprilat (p.863·2).
Heart failure; hypertension.

Vasoton *NCSN, Ital.*
Dihydroergocristine mesylate (p.1571·3).
Cerebral and peripheral vascular disorders; dopamine deficiency; headache; hypertension; migraine.

Vasotonin *Merz, Ger.*
Capsules: Aesculus (p.1543·3).
Haemorrhoids; vascular disorders.
Topical gel: Arnica (p.1550·3).
Musculoskeletal, joint, and soft-tissue disorders; superficial thrombophlebitis.

Vasotonin forte *Merz, Ger.*
Aesculus (p.1543·3); mofebutazone (p.56·1).
Superficial thrombophlebitis.

Vasotonin S *Merz, Ger.†.*
Aesculus (p.1543·3); thiamine hydrochloride.
Vascular disorders.

Vasotonin Serol *Merz, Ger.†.*
Aesculus (p.1543·3); arnica (p.1550·3).
Vascular disorders.

Vasovitol *Lannacher, Aust.*
Vitamin A palmitate (p.1359·2); alpha tocopherol acetate (p.1369·2).
Vitamin A and E deficiency.

Vasoxine
Glaxo Wellcome, Aust.; Wellcome, Irl.; Wellcome, UK.
Methoxamine hydrochloride (p.903·3).
Hypotension.

Vasoxyl
Glaxo Wellcome, Canad.; Wellcome, USA.
Methoxamine hydrochloride (p.903·3).
Control of blood pressure during surgery; postoperative collapse; supraventricular tachycardia.

Vasperdil *Lacer, Spain.*
Ethamivan (p.1480·3); etofylline (p.753·1); hexobendine hydrochloride (p.883·1).
Cerebrovascular disorders; circulatory disorders.

Vaspit
Asche, Ger.; Schering, Ital.; Schering, Spain.
Fluocortin butyl (p.1041·3).
Skin disorders.

Vastarel
Biopharma, Fr.; Servier, Irl.; Stroder, Ital.
Trimetazidine hydrochloride (p.959·2).
Angina pectoris; neurosensorial ischaemia.

Vasten *Specia, Fr.*
Pravastatin sodium (p.1277·1).
Hyperlipidaemias.

Vastensium *Salvat, Spain.*
Nitrendipine (p.923·1).
Hypertension.

Vastin *Astra, Austral.*
Fluvastatin sodium (p.1273·2).
Hypercholesterolaemia.

Vastocin *Coli, Ital.†.*
Fosfomycin calcium (p.210·2).
Bacterial infections.

Vastribil *Farmasan, Ger.*
Troxerutin (p.1580·2).
Vascular disorders.

Vasylox *Douglas, Austral.*
Oxymetazoline hydrochloride (p.1065·3); cineole (p.1564·1); menthol (p.1600·2).
Allergic rhinitis; nasal congestion; sinusitis.

Vasylox Junior *Douglas, Austral.†.*
Methoxamine hydrochloride (p.903·3).
Nasal congestion; rhinitis.

Vasyrol *Shire, UK†.*
Dipyridamole (p.857·1).
Thrombo-embolic disorders.

Vatran *Valeas, Ital.*
Diazepam (p.661·1).
Nervous tension; psychosomatic disorders; skeletal muscle spasm.

Vatrasin *Sanofi, Spain.*
Nicardipine hydrochloride (p.915·1).
Angina pectoris; cerebrovascular disorders; hypertension.

Vaxem Hib *Chiron, Ital.†.*
A Haemophilus influenzae conjugate vaccine (p.1511·1).
Active immunisation.

Vaxicoq *Merieux, Fr.*
An adsorbed pertussis vaccine (p.1526·1).
Active immunisation.

Vaxicum N *Worwag, Ger.*
Camphor oil (p.1557·2); rosemary oil (p.1626·2); laureth 9 (p.1325·2).
Musculoskeletal, joint, peri-articular, and soft-tissue disorders; neuralgia.

Vaxidina *VAAS, Ital.*
Chlorhexidine gluconate (p.1107·2).
Skin disinfection; wound disinfection.

Vaxigrip
Serotherapeutisches, Aust.; Rhone-Poulenc Rorer, Austral.†; Pasteur Merieux, Belg.; Merieux, Fr.; Pasteur Merieux, Ital.; Pasteur Merieux, Neth.; Pasteur Merieux, Norw.; Rhone-Poulenc Rorer, S.Afr.; Meda, Swed.
An inactivated influenza vaccine (split virion) (p.1515·2).
Active immunisation.

Vaxipar *Biocine, Ital.*
A mumps vaccine (Urabe strain) (p.1521·2).
Active immunisation.

Vaxitiol *Bouty, Ital.*
A suspension of intestinal bacteria (E. coli, enterococci, staphylococci, Proteus vulgaris) in a sulphur-containing medium.
Gastro-intestinal infections; genito-urinary infections.

Vazigam *NBI, S.Afr.*
A varicella-zoster immunoglobulin (p.1538·1).
Passive immunisation.

VCF *Apothecus, USA.*
Nonoxinol 9 (p.1326·1).
Contraceptive.

V-Cil-K
Lilly, Irl.†; Lilly, S.Afr.
Phenoxymethylpenicillin potassium (p.236·2).
Bacterial infections.

V-Cillin K
Lilly, Canad.; Lilly, USA†.
Phenoxymethylpenicillin potassium (p.236·2).
Bacterial infections.

V-Dec-M *Seatrace, USA.*
Pseudoephedrine hydrochloride (p.1068·3); guaiphenesin (p.1061·3).
Coughs.

Veclam *Malesci, Ital.*
Clarithromycin (p.189·1).
Bacterial infections.

Vectarion
Servier, Belg.; Eutherapie, Fr.; Servier, Ger.; Servier, Irl.; Servier, Spain.
Almitrine dimesylate (p.1477·2).
Respiratory insufficiency.

Vectavir
SmithKline Beecham, Austral.; Beecham, Belg.; SmithKline Beecham, Ger.; SmithKline Beecham, Swed.; SmithKline Beecham, UK.
Penciclovir (p.624·1).
Herpes labialis.

Vectrin *Warner Chilcott, USA.*
Minocycline hydrochloride (p.226·2).
Bacterial infections.

Vectrine *Pharma 2000, Fr.*
Erdosteine (p.1060·3).
Respiratory-tract congestion.

Vedrin *Polifarma, Ital.*
Xanthinol nicotinate (p.971·1).
Peripheral vascular disorders.

Veekay *Pharmador, S.Afr.†.*
Phenoxymethylpenicillin potassium (p.236·2).
Bacterial infections.

Veetids *Apothecon, USA.*
Phenoxymethylpenicillin potassium (p.236·2).
Bacterial infections.

Vega *Ono, Jpn.*
Ozagrel hydrochloride (p.1612·1).
Asthma.

Vegadeine *Warner-Lambert, Fr.*
Aspirin (p.16·1); paracetamol (p.72·2); codeine phosphate (p.26·1).
Fever; pain.

Veganin
Note. This name is used for preparations of different composition.
Parke, Davis, Aust.; Warner-Lambert, Irl.; Warner-Lambert, Spain; Warner-Lambert, UK.
Aspirin (p.16·1); paracetamol (p.72·2); codeine phosphate (p.26·1).
Fever; pain.

Warner-Lambert, Austral.
Aspirin (p.16·1); codeine phosphate (p.26·1).
Fever; pain.

Veganin 3 *Parke, Davis, S.Afr.*
Aspirin (p.16·1); paracetamol (p.72·2); codeine phosphate (p.26·1).
Fever; pain.

Veganine
Note. This name is used for preparations of different composition.
Warner-Lambert Consumer, Belg.
Aspirin (p.16·1); paracetamol (p.72·2); codeine phosphate (p.26·1).
Fever; pain.

Warner-Lambert, Fr.
Paracetamol (p.72·2); caffeine (p.749·3).
Formerly contained aspirin, paracetamol and codeine phosphate.
Fever; pain.

Vegebaby *Clintec, Fr.*
Infant feed.
Milk intolerance.

Vegebom
Note. This name is used for preparations of different composition.
Bournonville, Belg.†.
Cineole (p.1564·1); cajuput oil (p.1556·1); sassafras oil (p.1627·3); cedar wood oil; camphor (p.1557·2); menthol (p.1600·2); nutmeg oil (p.1609·3).
Muscle injury; skin irritation and pain; wounds.

Jessel, Fr.
Cineole (p.1564·1); cajuput oil (p.1556·1); cedar oil; nutmeg oil (p.1609·3); sassafras oil (p.1627·3); camphor (p.1557·2); menthol (p.1600·2); bay-laurel oil.
Haemorrhoids; skin disorders.

Vegebyl *Roche, Ital.*
Boldo (p.1554·1); cynara (p.1569·2); rhubarb (p.1212·1); cascara (p.1183·1); chamomile (p.1561·2).
Constipation; digestive disorders.

Vegelact
Diepal, Fr.; Bonomelli, Ital.†.
Infant feed.
Milk intolerance.

Vegelax *Biologiques de l'Ile-de-France, Fr.*
Senna (p.1212·2); boldo (p.1554·1); cynara (p.1569·2).
Formerly contained frangula, cascara, senna, boldo, cynara, belladonna, aloes, scammony, and rhubarb.
Constipation.

Vegelose *Clintec, Fr.*
Gluten-free, milk-free nutritional supplement.

Vegesan *Mack, Switz.*
Nordazepam (p.682·3).
Anxiety disorders.

Vegetable Cough Remover *Potter's, UK.*
Black cohosh (p.1563·3); ipecacuanha (p.1062·2); lobelia (p.1481·3); pleurisy root; scullcap; elecampane (p.1059·2); horehound (p.1063·3); hyssop.
Coughs.

Vegetal Tonic *Homeocan, Canad.*
Homoeopathic preparation.

Vegetalin *Genove, Spain.*
Bearberry (p.1552·2); senna (p.1212·2); coriander (p.1567·3); hyssop; sage (p.1627·1).
Constipation.

Vegetallumina *Recordati, Ital.*
Camphor (p.1557·2); aluminium subacetate (p.1547·3); methyl salicylate (p.55·2); thyme oil (p.1637·1).
Soft-tissue and peri-articular disorders.

Vegetarian Protein Supplement *Neo-Life, Austral.*
Nutritional supplement.

Vegetex *Modern Health Products, UK.*
Celery (p.1561·1); buckbean (p.1601·2); black cohosh (p.1563·3).
Muscular pain.

Vegetoserum
Jumer, Fr.
Adult syrup: Ethylmorphine hydrochloride (p.36·1); grindelia.
Formerly contained ethylmorphine hydrochloride, aconite, belladonna, grindelia, and cherry-laurel.

Medgenix, Fr.†.
Paediatric syrup: Ethylmorphine hydrochloride (p.36·1); liquorice (p.1197·1); orange flowers.
Coughs.

Vegicap Vegetarian *Solgar, UK.*
Multivitamin and mineral preparation.

Vegomed *Athenstaedt, Ger.†.*
Phenobarbitone (p.350·2); benzyl mandelate; belladonna (p.457·1); silybum marianum (p.993·3).
Agitation; motion sickness; sleep disorders; stress.

Vehem *Sandoz, Fr.*
Teniposide (p.565·3).
Malignant neoplasms.

Vehiculan NF *Krugmann, Ger.†.*
Glycol salicylate (p.43·1); benzyl nicotinate (p.22·1); laureth 9 (p.1325·2).
Musculoskeletal and joint disorders; sports injuries; superficial thrombophlebitis.

Veil *Blake, UK.*
A covering cream.
Concealment of birth marks, scars, and disfiguring skin disease.

Veinamitol
Negma, Belg.; Negma, Fr.
Troxerutin (p.1580·2).
Haemorrhoids; venous insufficiency.

Veinobiase
Note. This name is used for preparations of different composition.
Fournier, Fr.†.
Black currant (p.1365·2); ruscus; ascorbic acid (p.1365·2).
Peripheral vascular disorders.
Fournier SA, Spain.
Ascorbic acid (p.1365·2); ruscus aculeatus; gooseberry.
Anorectal disorders; peripheral vascular disorders; premenstrual syndrome.

Veinoconfort *Yves Ponroy, Fr.*
Vitamin C substances (p.1365·2).
Circulatory disorders.

Veinoglobuline
Merieux, Belg.†; Merieux, Fr.†; Pasteur Merieux, Neth.†.
A normal immunoglobulin (p.1522·1).
Hypogammaglobulinaemia; idiopathic thrombocytopenic purpura; passive immunisation.

Veinosane *Dolisos, Fr.*
Melilotus officinalis; red vine leaf.
Haemorrhoids; venous insufficiency.

Veinosclerol *Kreussler, Fr.*
Laureth 9 (p.1325·2).
Varicose veins.

Veinostase *Richelet, Fr.*
Aesculus (p.1543·3); hamamelis (p.1587·1); cupressus sempervirens; ascorbic acid (p.1365·2).
Haemorrhoids; vascular disorders.

Veinotonyl *Lipha Sante, Fr.*
Aesculus (p.1543·3); metesculetol sodium (p.1602·3).
Peripheral vascular disorders.

Velamox *SmithKline Beecham, Ital.*
Amoxycillin sodium (p.151·3) or amoxycillin trihydrate (p.151·3).
Bacterial infections.

Velamox D *SmithKline Beecham, Ital.†.*
Amoxycillin (p.151·3); dicloxacillin (p.201·3).
Bacterial infections.

Velasulin *Novo Nordisk, Ger.*
Neutral insulin injection (crystalline) (porcine, highly-purified) (p.322·1).
Diabetes mellitus.

Velasulin Human *Novo Nordisk, Ger.*
Insulin injection (human) (p.322·1).
Diabetes mellitus.

Velaten *Corvi, Ital.*
Sulphamethoxypyridazine (p.256·2); trimethoprim (p.265·1).
Bacterial infections; Pneumocystis carinii pneumonia.

Velbacil *Pfizer, Spain.*
Bacampicillin hydrochloride (p.157·2).
Bacterial infections.

Velban *Lilly, USA.*
Vinblastine sulphate (p.569·1).
Malignant neoplasms.

Velbe
Lilly, Aust.; Lilly, Austral.; Lilly, Belg.; Lilly, Canad.; Lilly, Fr.; Lilly, Ger.; Lilly, Ital.; Lilly, Neth.; Lilly, Norw.; Lilly, Swed.; Lilly, Switz.; Lilly, UK.
Vinblastine sulphate (p.569·1).
Malignant neoplasms.

Velicin *Henkel, Ger.†.*
Orthophenylphenol (p.1120·3); chlorocresol (p.1110·3).
Instrument and surface disinfection.

Veliten *Wyeth, Fr.*
Vitamins; rutin (p.1580·2).
Vascular disorders.

Velmonit *Esteve, Spain.*
Ciprofloxacin hydrochloride (p.185·3) or ciprofloxacin lactate (p.185·3).
Bacterial infections.

Velocef
Squibb, Ital.†; Squibb, Spain.
Cephradine (p.181·3).
Bacterial infections.

Velodan *Vita, Spain.*
Loratadine (p.413·1).
Hypersensitivity reactions.

Velonarcon *Dresden, Ger.*
Ketamine hydrochloride (p.1226·2).
General anaesthesia; pain; status asthmaticus.

Velopural *Optimed, Ger.*
Hydrocortisone acetate (p.1043·3).
Skin disorders.

Velosef
Bristol-Myers Squibb, Belg.; Squibb, Canad.†; Bristol-Myers Squibb, Irl.; Bristol-Myers Squibb, Neth.; Squibb, UK; Apothecon, USA.
Cephradine (p.181·3).
Bacterial infections.

Velosulin
Novo Nordisk, Aust.†; Novo Nordisk, Irl.†; Wellcome, Irl.†; Novo Nordisk, UK; Glaxo Wellcome, UK; Nordisk, USA†.
Insulin injection (porcine, highly purified) (p.322·1).
Diabetes mellitus.
Novo Nordisk, Neth.; Novo Nordisk, Norw.; Novo Nordisk, Swed.
Insulin injection (human, emp) (p.322·1).
Diabetes mellitus.

Velosulin HM
Novo Nordisk, Aust.; Novo Nordisk, Switz.
Insulin injection (human, monocomponent) (p.322·1).
Diabetes mellitus.

Velosulin Human *Novo Nordisk, Canad.†.*
Insulin injection (human, emp) (p.322·1).
Diabetes mellitus.

Velosulin Human BR *Novo Nordisk, USA.*
Insulin injection (human, emp) (p.322·1).
Diabetes mellitus.

Velosulin Humana *Nordisk, Spain†.*
Insulin injection (human) (p.322·1).
Diabetes mellitus.

Velosulin MC *Novo Nordisk, Switz.*
Insulin injection (porcine, monocomponent) (p.322·1).
Diabetes mellitus.

Velosulin (Regular) *Novo Nordisk, Canad.†.*
Insulin injection (porcine, highly purified) (p.322·1).
Diabetes mellitus.

Velosuline *Novo Nordisk, Fr.†.*
Insulin injection (porcine, highly purified) (p.322·1).
Diabetes mellitus.

Velosuline Humaine *Novo Nordisk, Fr.†.*
Insulin injection (human, emp, highly purified) (p.322·1).
Diabetes mellitus.

Velosuline Humanum *Novo Nordisk, Belg.*
Insulin injection (human, emp) (p.322·1).
Diabetes mellitus.

Veltane *Lannett, USA.*
Brompheniramine maleate (p.403·2).
Hypersensitivity reactions.

Veltex *Vesta, S.Afr.*
Diclofenac sodium (p.31·2).
Gout; inflammation; musculoskeletal and joint disorders; pain.

Velvachol *Owen-Galderma, USA.*
Vehicle for topical preparations.

Velvelan *Merck Sharp & Dohme, Canad.; Frosst, Canad.*
Urea (p.1095·2).
Dry skin disorders.

Venachlor *Lennon, S.Afr.†.*
Atenolol (p.825·3); chlorthalidone (p.839·3).
Hypertension.

Venacol *Llorens, Spain.*
Aescin (p.1543·3); esculoside (p.1543·3); heparin sodium (p.879·3); ruscogenin (p.1627·1).
Oedema; peripheral vascular disorders.

Venacton *Klein, Ger.*
Aesculus (p.1543·3); scoparium (p.1628·1); hypericum (p.1590·1); silybum marianum (p.993·3); hamamelis (p.1587·1).
Haemorrhoids; paraesthesias; vascular disorders.

Venactone *Lepetit, Ital.*
Canrenoate potassium (p.836·2).
Hyperaldosteronism; hypertension.

Venagil *Logifarm, Ital.†.*
Benzarone (p.1552·3).
Capillary bleeding; capillary fragility.

Venalisin *AGIPS, Ital.*
Tribenoside (p.1638·3).
Haemorrhoids; thrombophlebitis; varicose veins.

Venalitan *3M, Ger.*
Topical gel: Heparin sodium (p.879·3).
Skin trauma.

Venalitan N *3M, Ger.*
Heparin sodium (p.879·3).
Venalitan formerly contained heparin sodium and benzyl nicotinate.
Skin trauma.

Venalot
Note. This name is used for preparations of different composition.
Boots, Belg.†.
Coumarin (p.1568·1); troxerutin (p.1580·2).
Lymphoedema.
Schaper & Brummer, Ger.
Injection: Coumarin (p.1568·1); rutoside sodium sulphate (p.1580·2).
Formerly contained melilotus and rutoside sodium sulphate.
Vascular disorders.
Liniment†: Melilotus; heparin sodium (p.879·3).
Skin trauma.
Sustained-release tablets: Coumarin (p.1568·1); troxerutin (p.1580·2).
Haemorrhoids; vascular disorders.
Tablets: Melilotus.
Formerly contained melilotus and rutoside.
Haemorrhoids; venous insufficiency.
S & B, Neth.†.
Melilotus; rutin (p.1580·2).
Peripheral vascular disorders.
Asta Medica, Switz.
Liniment: Melilotus; heparin (p.879·3).
Peripheral vascular disorders.
Sustained-release tablets: Coumarin (p.1568·1).
Formerly contained coumarin and troxerutin.
Lymphoedema.
Schaper & Brummer, Switz.†.
Capsules; injection: Melilotus; rutin (p.1580·2) or rutin sodium sulphate (p.1580·2).
Peripheral vascular disorders.

Venalot mono *Schaper & Brummer, Ger.*
Coumarin (p.1568·1).
Soft-tissue injury.

Venapulse *Lennon, S.Afr.†.*
Atenolol (p.825·3).
Angina pectoris; hypertension.

Venbig *Biagini, Ital.*
A hepatitis B immunoglobulin (p.1512·3).
Passive immunisation.

Vencipon *Artesan, Ger.*
Ephedrine hydrochloride (p.1059·3); phenolphthalein (p.1208·2).
Obesity.

Vendal *Lannacher, Aust.*
Morphine hydrochloride (p.56·1).
Pain.

Ven-Detrex
Therabel Pharma, Belg.; Zyma, Switz.†.
Diosmin (p.1580·1).
Peripheral vascular disorders.

Venelbin *Hoechst, Ger.*
Dihydroergotamine mesylate (p.444·2); troxerutin (p.1580·2).
Vascular disorders.

Venelbin N *Hoechst, Ger.*
Heparin sodium (p.879·3).
Venelbin formerly contained heparin sodium and troxerutin.
Superficial vascular disorders.

Venen-Dragees *CT, Ger.*
Aesculus (p.1543·3).
Venous insufficiency.

Venen-Fluid *CT, Ger.*
Aesculus (p.1543·3).
Phlebitis; soft-tissue injury; varices.

Venen-Salbe *Eu Rho, Ger.*
Aesculus (p.1543·3); arnica (p.1550·3).
Haemorrhoids; soft-tissue injury; venous insufficiency.

Venen-Salbe N *CT, Ger.*
Aesculus (p.1543·3); esculoside (p.1543·3).
Bruising; oedema; varices.

Venen-Tabletten *Stada, Ger.*
Aesculus (p.1543·3).
Venous insufficiency.

Venentabs *Ratiopharm, Ger.*
Aesculus (p.1543·3).
Venous insufficiency.

Venen-Tropfen *Eu Rho, Ger.*
Aesculus (p.1543·3).
Haemorrhoids; thrombosis prophylaxis; venous insufficiency.

Venex *Recordati, Ital.†.*
Tribenoside (p.1638·3).
Haemorrhoids; thrombophlebitis; varicose veins.

Venimmun
Centeon, Aust.; Centeon, Ger.; Centeon, Ital.
A normal immunoglobulin (p.1522·1).
Hypogammaglobulinaemia; idiopathic thrombocytopenic purpura; passive immunisation.

Veniten *Whitehall-Robins, Switz.*
Troxerutin (p.1580·2).
Peripheral vascular disorders.

Venitrin *Astra, Ital.*
Glyceryl trinitrate (p.874·3).
Angina pectoris; hypertensive crises; left-ventricular failure; myocardial infarction.

Venium *Lubapharm Phlebologie, Switz.*
Coumarin (p.1568·1).
Lymphoedema.

Veno *Waldheim, Aust.*
Troxerutin (p.1580·2); dihydroergotamine tartrate (p.444·3).
Chronic venous insufficiency.

Veno SL *Ursapharm, Ger.*
Troxerutin (p.1580·2).
Vascular disorders.

Venobene *Merckle, Aust.*
Heparin sodium (p.879·3); dexpanthenol (p.1570·3).
Anorectal disorders; soft-tissue injury; superficial vascular disorders.

Venobiase *Fournier, Ger.*
Ruscus aculeatus rhizome; black currant (p.1365·2).
Vascular disorders.

Venobiase mono *Fournier, Ger.*
Ruscus aculeatus rhizome.
Haemorrhoids; venous insufficiency.

Veno-biomo *Biomo, Ger.*
Aesculus (p.1543·3).
Thrombo-embolic disorders; venous insufficiency.

Venocaina *Braun, Spain.*
Procaine hydrochloride (p.1299·2).
Local anaesthesia.

Venodin *Tosi, Ital.*
Tribenoside (p.1638·3).
Haemorrhoids; thrombophlebitis; varicose veins.

Venofer *Vifor International, Switz.*
Saccharated iron oxide (p.1353·2).
Iron deficiency.

Venoflavan *Zyma, Spain†.*
Beclomethasone dipropionate (p.1032·1); tyrothricin (p.267·2); sulodexide (p.951·1).
Anorectal disorders.

Venoflexil *Nycomed, Ger.†.*
Heparin sodium (p.879·3).
Formerly contained aescin, dexpanthenol, and glycol salicylate.
Skin trauma.

Venofusin Glucosalina *Pharmacia, Spain†.*
Sodium chloride infusion (p.1162·2) with glucose.
Fluid and electrolyte depletion.

Venofusin Ringer Rest *Pharmacia, Spain†.*
Electrolyte infusion (p.1147·1) with glucose.
Fluid and electrolyte depletion.

Venogal S *Chinosolfabrik, Ger.*
Aesculus (p.1543·3).
Inflammation; vascular disorders.

Venogamma Anti-Rho (D) *Alfa Biotech, Ital.*
An anti-D immunoglobulin (p.1503·2).
Prevention of rhesus sensitisation.

Venogamma Polivalente *Alfa Biotech, Ital.*
A normal immunoglobulin (p.1522·1).
Hypogammaglobulinaemia; passive immunisation.

Venoglobulin
Alpha Therapeutic, UK†; Alpha Therapeutic, USA.
A normal immunoglobulin (p.1522·1).
Idiopathic thrombocytopenic purpura; immunodeficiency; Kawasaki disease.

Venoglobulina *Merieux, Ital.†.*
A normal immunoglobulin (p.1522·1).
Idiopathic thrombocytopenia; passive immunisation.

Veno-Hexanicit *Promed, Ger.*
Inositol nicotinate (p.891·3); heptaminol hydrochloride (p.1587·2); troxerutin (p.1580·2).
Inflammation; oedema; vascular disorders; vascular headache.

Veno-Kattwiga N *Kattwiga, Ger.*
Aescin (p.1543·3); procaine hydrochloride (p.1299·2).
Vascular disorders.

veno-L 90 N *Loges, Ger.*
Homoeopathic preparation.

Venolen *Farmacologico Milanese, Ital.*
Troxerutin (p.1580·2).
Haemorrhoids; varicose veins.

Venomil
SmithKline Beecham, Ger.; Miles, USA.
Venoms of bee, wasp, hornet, yellow jacket, and mixed vespids (p.1545·1).
Hyposensitisation.

Venopirin *Green Cross, Jpn†.*
Lysine aspirin (p.50·3).
Fever; neuralgia; pain.

Venoplant
Note. This name is used for preparations of different composition.
Austroplant, Aust.; Schwabe, Ger.†; Also, Ital.†.
Injection: Aesculus (p.1543·3).
Inflammation; menstrual disorders; thrombo-embolic disorders.
Also, Ital.†; Schwabe, Neth.†; Semar, Spain.
Tablets; oral drops: Silybum marianum (p.993·3); aesculus (p.1543·3); hamamelis (p.1587·1).
Vascular disorders.
Schwabe, Ger.
Cream: Hamamelis (p.1587·1).
Skin inflammation; varices.
Schwabe, Ger.
Delayed-release tablets: Aesculus (p.1543·3).
Venous insufficiency.
Schwabe, Ger.†.
Ointment: Heparin (p.879·3); aesculus (p.1543·3).
Skin trauma.
Schwabe, Ger.
Topical gel: Aescin (p.1543·3); heparin sodium (p.879·3); glycol salicylate (p.43·1).
Soft-tissue injury; venous insufficiency.
Semar, Spain.
Ointment: Aesculus (p.1543·3); hamamelis (p.1587·1); heparin (p.879·3).
Peripheral vascular disorders.

Venoplant N *Schwabe, Switz.*
Aesculus (p.1543·3); heparin (p.879·3).
Vascular disorders.

Venoplant plus *Schwabe, Ger.†.*
Aesculus (p.1543·3).
Vascular disorders.

Venoplus *Also, Ital.*
Aesculus (p.1543·3); hamamelis (p.1587·1); silybum marianum (p.993·3).
Alterations in capillary permeability; varicose veins; venous dilatation.

Venopyronum *Knoll, Ger.*
Aesculus (p.1543·3).
Venous insufficiency.

Venopyronum N *Knoll, Ger.*
Aesculus (p.1543·3).
Venous insufficiency.

Venopyronum N triplex *Minden, Ger.*
Aesculus (p.1543·3); squill (p.1070·1); convallaria (p.1567·2); oleander (p.1610·1); adonis vernalis (p.1543·3).
Venopyronum triplex formerly contained aesculus, squill, convallaria, oleander, adonis vernalis, and rutoside.
Vascular disorders.

Venoruton
Zyma, Aust.; Zyma, Belg.; Zyma, Ger.; Zyma, Ital.; Novartis Consumer, Neth.; Zyma, Spain; Zyma, Switz.
Oxerutins (p.1580·2).
Chronic venous insufficiency; diabetic retinopathy; haemorrhoids; peripheral vascular disorders.

Venoruton Heparin Zyma, Ger.
Heparin sodium (p.879·3).
Superficial vascular disorders.

Venos Dry Cough SmithKline Beecham Consumer, UK.
Liquid glucose (p.1343·3); treacle; anise oil (p.1550·1); capsicum tincture (p.1559·2); camphor (p.1557·2).
Coughs.

Venos Expectorant SmithKline Beecham Consumer, UK.
Guaiphenesin (p.1061·3); glucose liquid (p.1343·3); treacle; anise oil (p.1550·1); capsicum tincture (p.1559·2); camphor (p.1557·2).
Coughs.

Venos Honey & Lemon SmithKline Beecham Consumer, UK.
Glucose (p.1343·3); honey (p.1345·3); lemon juice.
Formerly contained ammonium chloride and ipecacuanha.
Coughs.

Venosan
Mack, Illert., Ger.†; Binesa, Spain; Mack, Switz.
Inositol nicotinate (p.891·3); pholedrine sulphate (p.930·2); troxerutin (p.1580·2).
Vascular disorders.

Venoselect Dreluso, Ger.
Homoeopathic preparation.

Venosin Klinge, Aust.
Capsules; ointment; oral drops: Aesculus (p.1543·3).
Topical gel: Aescin (p.1543·3); heparin sodium (p.879·3); glycol salicylate (p.43·1).
Chronic venous insufficiency; haemorrhoids; oedema; superficial vascular disorders; thrombosis prophylaxis.

Venosmil Faes, Spain.
Hidrosmin.
Peripheral vascular disorders.

Venosmine Geymonat, Ital.
Diosmin (p.1580·1).
Peripheral vascular disorders.

Venostasin
Klinge, Aust.†.
Capsules; ointment; oral drops: Aesculus (p.1543·3).
Chronic venous insufficiency; haemorrhoids; menorrhagia; soft-tissue injury; thrombosis prophylaxis.
Topical gel: Aescin (p.1543·3); heparin sodium (p.879·3); glycol salicylate (p.43·1).
Chronic venous insufficiency; soft-tissue injury.
Klinge, Ger.
Controlled-release capsules; oral drops; tablets; ointment: Aesculus (p.1543·3).
Inflammation; venous insufficiency.
Topical gel: Aescin (p.1543·3); heparin sodium (p.879·3); glycol salicylate (p.43·1).
Soft-tissue injury; vascular disorders.

Venostasin comp Klinge, Switz.†.
Aescin (p.1543·3); heparin sodium (p.879·3); glycol salicylate (p.43·1).
Peripheral vascular disorders.

Venostasin special Klinge, Switz.†.
Aesculus (p.1543·3).
Peripheral vascular disorders.

Veno-Tablinen Sanorania, Ger.†.
Bamethan sulphate (p.827·1); ruscus aculeatus.
Vascular disorders.

Veno-Tebonin N Schwabe, Ger.
Ginkgo biloba (p.1584·1); heptaminol hydrochloride (p.1587·2); troxerutin (p.1580·2).
Haemorrhoids; vascular disorders.

Venothromb Alcon-Thilo, Ger.†.
Ointment: Heparin (p.879·3); aesculus (p.1543·3); thiamine hydrochloride; essential fatty acids; benzyl nicotinate (p.22·1).
Skin trauma.
Tablets: Hesperidin methyl chalcone (p.1580·2); aesculus (p.1543·3); thiamine hydrochloride.
Vascular disorders.

Venotop Sandoz, Aust.
Dihydroergotamine tartrate (p.444·3); troxerutin (p.1580·2).
Chronic venous insufficiency.

Venotrauma Also, Ital.
Aesculus (p.1543·3); hamamelis (p.1587·1); heparin sodium (p.879·3).
Soft-tissue disorders.

Venotrulan comp Truw, Ger.†.
Garlic (p.1583·1).
Vascular disorders.

Venotrulan Compositum Truw, Ger.†.
Aesculus (p.1543·3); nicotinic acid (p.1351·2); rutin (p.1580·2); etofylline (p.753·1).
Peripheral, coronary, and central circulatory disorders.

Venotrulan N Truw, Ger.
Aesculus (p.1543·3).
Venotrulan formerly contained aesculus, hamamelis, collinsonia, and paeonia officinalis.
Venous insufficiency.

Venovit Bifarma, Ital.
Ruscus; hamamelis (p.1587·1); aesculus (p.1543·3).
Venous insufficiency.

Vent Retard BOI, Spain.
Theophylline (p.765·1).
Heart failure; obstructive airways disease; paroxysmal dyspnoea.

Ventadur Evans, Spain.
Salbutamol sulphate (p.758·2).
Obstructive airways disease; premature labour.

Ventamol Pinewood, Irl.
Salbutamol (p.758·2).
Obstructive airways disease.

Venteze SA Druggists, S.Afr.
Salbutamol (p.758·2) or salbutamol sulphate (p.758·2).
Obstructive airways disease.

Ventide
Glaxo Wellcome, Aust.; Glaxo, Fr.†; Allen & Hanburys, UK.
Salbutamol (p.758·2) or salbutamol sulphate (p.758·2); beclomethasone dipropionate (p.1032·1).
Obstructive airways disease.

Ventilat Thomae, Ger.
Oxitropium bromide (p.757·1).
Obstructive airways disease.

Ventimax Norton, S.Afr.
Salbutamol (p.758·2).
Obstructive airways disease.

Ventnaze SA Druggists, S.Afr.
Beclomethasone dipropionate (p.1032·1).
Hayfever; rhinitis.

Ventodisk
Glaxo Wellcome, Canad.; Allen & Hanburys, S.Afr.; Glaxo Wellcome, Switz.
Salbutamol sulphate (p.758·2).
Obstructive airways disease.

Ventodisks
Glaxo Wellcome, Fr.; Allen & Hanburys, Irl.; Allen & Hanburys, UK.
Salbutamol sulphate (p.758·2).
Obstructive airways disease.

Ventolase Juste, Spain.
Clenbuterol hydrochloride (p.752·1).
Obstructive airways disease.

Ventolin
Allen & Hanburys, Austral.; Glaxo Wellcome, Austral.; Glaxo Wellcome, Belg.; Glaxo Wellcome, Canad.; Allen & Hanburys, Irl.; Glaxo Wellcome, Ital.; Glaxo Wellcome, Neth.; Allen & Hanburys, S.Afr.; Glaxo Wellcome, Spain; Glaxo Wellcome, Switz.; Allen & Hanburys, UK; Glaxo Wellcome, USA.
Salbutamol (p.758·2) or salbutamol sulphate (p.758·2).
Obstructive airways disease; premature labour; status asthmaticus.

Ventolin Espettorante Glaxo Wellcome, Ital.
Salbutamol sulphate (p.758·2); guaiphenesin (p.1061·3).
Bronchial congestion; bronchospasm.

Ventolin Flogo Glaxo Wellcome, Ital.
Beclomethasone dipropionate (p.1032·1); salbutamol (p.758·2).
Obstructive airways disease.

Ventolin plus Glaxo Wellcome, Switz.†.
Salbutamol (p.758·2); beclomethasone dipropionate (p.1032·1).
Asthma.

Ventoline
Glaxo Wellcome, Fr.; Glaxo Wellcome, Norw.; Glaxo Wellcome, Swed.
Salbutamol (p.758·2) or salbutamol sulphate (p.758·2).
Obstructive airways disease.

Ventracid N Repha, Ger.
Sodium bicarbonate (p.1153·2); pancreatin (p.1612·1); curcuma (p.1001·3).
Gastro-intestinal disorders.

Ventricon N Syxyl, Ger.
Bismuth subnitrate (p.1180·2); calcium carbonate (p.1182·1); magnesium oxide (p.1198·3).
Gastro-intestinal disorders.

ventri-loges Loges, Ger.
Lycopodium; taraxacum (p.1634·2); silybum marianum (p.993·3); aesculus (p.1543·3); abrotanum; absinthium (p.1541·1); calamamus (p.1556·1); gentian (p.1583·3).
Gastro-intestinal disorders.

Ventrimarin Novo Steigerwald, Ger.
Absinthium (p.1541·1); gentian (p.1583·3); angelica.
Gastro-intestinal disorders.

Ventrodigest Hormosan, Ger.†.
Valerian (p.1643·1); cnicus benedictus (p.1565·3); gentian (p.1583·3); menyanthes (p.1601·2); centaury (p.1561·1); caraway (p.1559·3); aniseed (p.1549·3); arnica (p.1550·3); chamomile (p.1561·2); fennel (p.1579·1); peppermint leaf (p.1208·1).
Gastro-intestinal disorders.

Ventrodynat Rhenomed, Ger.†.
Ethaverine (p.1577·1); magnesium trisilicate (p.1199·1); aluminium hydroxide gel (p.1177·3); liquorice (p.1197·1).
Gastro-intestinal disorders.

Ventrovis Truw, Ger.†.
Chlorophyllin; carbo veget.; peppermint oil (p.1208·1); lactose; aluminium hydroxide gel (p.1177·3); angelica; zedoary; clove (p.1565·2); lavender (p.1594·3); herba majorana; wild thyme sage (p.1627·1); peppermint leaf (p.1208·1); terra san.
Gastro-intestinal disorders.

Ventrux Bigmar, Switz.
Enterococcus faecium (p.1594·1).
Gastro-intestinal disorders; restoration of intestinal flora.

Ventzone SA Druggists, S.Afr.
Beclomethasone dipropionate (p.1032·1).
Asthma.

Venustas Lozione Antiforfora BPR, Ital.
Cinchona succirubra (p.1564·1).
Seborrhoeic dermatitis.

Venustas Lozione Caduta BPR, Ital.
Arnica (p.1550·3).
Alopecia.

Venustas Shampoo per Capelli con Forfora e/o Grassi BPR, Ital.
Urtica (p.1642·3).
Seborrhoeic dermatitis.

Venyl Plantes et Medecines, Fr.
Ruscus aculeatus; hesperidin methyl chalcone (p.1580·2); ascorbic acid (p.1365·2).
Haemorrhoids; peripheral vascular disorders.

Vepar Savio, Ital.
Heparan sulphate (p.879·2).
Peripheral vascular disorders.

Vepenicillin Scand Pharm, Swed.†.
Phenoxymethylpenicillin potassium (p.236·2).
Bacterial infections.

Vepesid
Bristol-Myers Squibb, Aust.; Bristol-Myers Squibb, Austral.; Bristol-Myers Squibb, Belg.; Bristol, Canad.; Bristol-Myers Squibb, Ger.; Bristol-Myers Squibb, Irl.; Bristol-Myers Squibb, Ital.; Bristol-Myers Squibb, Neth.; Bristol-Myers Squibb, Norw.; Bristol-Myers Squibb, S.Afr.; Bristol-Myers, Spain; Bristol-Myers Squibb, Swed.; Bristol-Myers Squibb, Switz.; Bristol-Myers Squibb, UK; Bristol-Myers Oncology, USA.
Etoposide (p.532·3).
Malignant neoplasms.

Vepeside Sandoz, Fr.
Etoposide (p.532·3).
Malignant neoplasms.

Vera CT, Ger.; Heumann, Ger.; BASF, Ger.
Verapamil hydrochloride (p.960·3).
Angina pectoris; arrhythmias; hypertension.

Verabeta Betapharm, Ger.
Verapamil hydrochloride (p.960·3).
Angina pectoris; arrhythmias; hypertension.

Veracaps Sigma, Austral.
Verapamil hydrochloride (p.960·3).
Angina pectoris; hypertension.

Veracapt Ebewe, Aust.
Verapamil hydrochloride (p.960·3); captopril (p.836·3).
Hypertension.

Veracim Cimex, Switz.
Verapamil hydrochloride (p.960·3).
Arrhythmias; ischaemic heart disease.

Veracolate
Note. This name is used for preparations of different composition.
Warner-Lambert, Austral.†.
Sodium tauroglycocholate; cascara (p.1183·1); phenolphthalein (p.1208·2); capsicum oleoresin.
Biliary-tract disorders; constipation.
Parke, Davis, S.Afr.
Cascara sagrada (p.1183·1); phenolphthalein (p.1208·2).
Formerly contained bile salts, cascara sagrada, phenolphthalein, and capsicum oleoresin.
Constipation.
Numark, USA.
Cascara (p.1183·1); phenolphthalein (p.1208·2); capsicum oleoresin.

Veractil Rhone-Poulenc Rorer, Norw.†.
Methotrimeprazine embonate (p.679·2) or methotrimeprazine maleate (p.679·1).
Alcohol withdrawal syndrome; insomnia; pain; pruritus; psychoses.

Veracur
Typharm, Irl.; Typharm, UK.
Formaldehyde (p.1113·2).
Warts.

Veradurat Pohl, Ger.†.
Verapamil hydrochloride (p.960·3).
Angina pectoris; arrhythmias; hypertension.

Verahexal
Hexal, Ger.; Hexal, S.Afr.
Verapamil hydrochloride (p.960·3).
Angina pectoris; arrhythmias; hypertension.

Verakard AFI, Norw.
Verapamil hydrochloride (p.960·3).
Angina pectoris; arrhythmias; hypertension.

Veralgit Krewel, Ger.†.
Aspirin (p.16·1); codeine phosphate (p.26·1); caffeine (p.749·3).
Pain.

Veralipril Sanofi Winthrop, Ital.
Veralipride (p.698·1).
Menopausal disorders.

Veraloc Orion, Swed.
Verapamil hydrochloride (p.960·3).
Angina pectoris; arrhythmias; hypertension; myocardial infarction.

Veramex Sanofi Winthrop, Ger.
Verapamil hydrochloride (p.960·3).
Cardiac disorders; hypertension.

Veramil Orion, Irl.
Verapamil hydrochloride (p.960·3).
Angina pectoris; arrhythmias; hypertension.

Veramon Sofar, Ital.
Propyphenazone (p.81·3); paracetamol (p.72·2).
Fever; pain.

Veranorm Isis Puren, Ger.
Verapamil hydrochloride (p.960·3).
Angina pectoris; arrhythmias; hypertension.

Verapabene Merckle, Aust.
Verapamil hydrochloride (p.960·3).
Angina pectoris; arrhythmias; heart failure; hypertension; hypertrophic obstructive cardiomyopathy.

Verapress Dexcel, UK.
Verapamil hydrochloride (p.960·3).
Angina pectoris; hypertension.

Veraptin Lagap, Switz.†.
Verapamil hydrochloride (p.960·3).
Angina; arrhythmias; hypertension; myocardial infarction.

Verasifar Siphar, Switz.
Verapamil hydrochloride (p.960·3).
Hypertension.

Veratensin Farma Lepori, Spain.
Verapamil hydrochloride (p.960·3).
Angina pectoris; arrhythmias; hypertension.

Veratide Procter & Gamble, Ger.
Verapamil hydrochloride (p.960·3); triamterene (p.957·2); hydrochlorothiazide (p.885·2).
Hypertension.

Veratran Murat, Fr.
Clotiazepam (p.657·2).
Alcohol withdrawal syndrome; anxiety.

Veratrum Med Complex Dynamit, Aust.
Homoeopathic preparation.

Verax Tosi, Ital.
Benzydamine hydrochloride (p.21·3).
Fever; inflammation; pain; peripheral vascular disorders; vulvovaginal disorders.

Verazinc Forest Pharmaceuticals, USA.
Zinc sulphate (p.1373·2).
Dietary supplement.

Verbascum Complex Blackmores, Austral.
Verbascum thapsus; marrubium vulgare (p.1063·3); asclepias tuberosa; liquorice (p.1197·1); ascorbic acid (p.1365·2); vitamin A acetate (p.1359·2).
Respiratory system disorders.

Verbesol ICT, Ital.
L-Verbenone.
Respiratory-tract disorders.

Verbex Istoria, Ital.
L-verbenone.
Respiratory-tract disorders.

Verboril Select, Ital.†.
L-Verbenone.
Respiratory-tract disorders.

Vercef Ranbaxy, S.Afr.
Cefaclor (p.163·2).
Bacterial infections.

Vercite Abbott, Ital.
Pipobroman (p.558·1).
Chronic myeloid leukaemia; polycythaemia vera.

Vercyte
Abbott, Fr.; Abbott, USA†.
Pipobroman (p.558·1).
Chronic myeloid leukaemia; polycythaemia vera.

Verdal Falqui, Ital.
Aspirin (p.16·1); paracetamol (p.72·2); caffeine (p.749·3).
Fever; influenza symptoms; pain.

Verecolene Maggioni, Ital.†.
Oral drops: Cascara (p.1183·1); frangula bark (p.1193·2); senna (p.1212·2); docusate sodium (p.1189·3).
Syrup: Fencibutirol (p.1578·3); frangula (p.1193·2); rhubarb (p.1212·1); cascara (p.1183·1).
Constipation.

Verecolene Complesso Maggioni, Ital.†.
Fencibutirol (p.1578·3); frangula (p.1193·2); rhubarb (p.1212·1); cascara (p.1183·1); phenolphthalein (p.1208·2).
Constipation.

Verel Yamanouchi, Ital.
Salicylic acid (p.1090·2); lactic acid (p.1593·3).
Hard skin; verrucas; warts.

Verelait Valda, Ital.
Lactulose (p.1195·3).
Constipation.

Verelan
Wyeth-Ayerst, Canad.; Elan, Irl.; Lederle, USA.
Verapamil hydrochloride (p.960·3).
Angina pectoris; arrhythmias; hypertension.

Verexamil Laevosan, Aust.
Verapamil hydrochloride (p.960·3).
Angina pectoris; arrhythmias; hypertension.

Vergentan Synthelabo, Ger.
Alizapride hydrochloride (p.1176·3).
Nausea and vomiting; radiation sickness.

Vergeturine Vigan, Fr.
Vitamins.
Skin disorders.

Vergon Marnel, USA.
Meclozine hydrochloride (p.413·3).

Vericap Cuxson, Gerrard, UK†.
Podophyllum resin (p.1089·1); linseed oil (p.1596·2).
Warts.

Vericaps Ovelle, Irl.
Salicylic acid (p.1090·2).
Warts.

Vericardine Laleuf, Fr.
Phenobarbitone (p.350·2); crataegus (p.1568·2).
Formerly contained papaverine hydrochloride, quinine hydrobromide, phenobarbitone, and crataegus.
Anxiety; insomnia; nervous disorders.

Veriderm *Lachifarma, Ital.*
Sulphur (p.1091·2).
Seborrhoea.

Veriga *Frega, Canad.*
Piperazine citrate (p.107·2).

Verimex *Vachon, Canad.*
Piperazine citrate (p.107·2).

Verintex *Pekana, Ger.*
Homoeopathic preparation.

Verintex N *Pekana, Ger.*
Homoeopathic preparation.

Veripaque
Sanofi Winthrop, Irl.†; Sanofi Winthrop, UK.
Oxyphenisatin (p.1207·2).
Barium enema adjunct; bowel evacuation.

Verisop *Gerard, Irl.*
Verapamil hydrochloride (p.960·3).
Angina pectoris; hypertension; supraventricular tachycardia.

Verla-3 *Verla, Ger.†.*
Propyphenazone (p.81·3); caffeine (p.749·3).
Fever; pain.

Verladyn *Verla, Ger.*
Dihydroergotamine mesylate (p.444·2).
Hypotension; migraine and related vascular headaches.

Verla-Lipon *Verla, Ger.*
Thioctic acid (p.1636·2) or ethylenediamine thioctate (p.1636·2).
Diabetic polyneuropathy.

Verlapyrin N *Verla, Ger.†.*
Paracetamol (p.72·2).
Formerly contained paracetamol, salicylamide, and diphenhydramine hydrochloride.
Fever; pain.

Vermi *Quimpe, Spain.*
Piperazine adipate (p.107·2).
Worm infections.

Vermicet *Sanofi Winthrop, Ger.†.*
Isosorbide dinitrate (p.893·1).
Cardiac disorders.

Vermicidin *Rivopharm, Switz.†.*
Mebendazole (p.104·1).
Worm infections.

Vermifuge *Sorin-Maxim, Fr.*
Piperazine hydrate (p.107·2); sodium bromide (p.1620·3).
Intestinal nematode infections.

Vermox
Janssen-Cilag, Austral.; Janssen-Cilag, Belg.; Janssen-Ortho, Canad.; Janssen-Cilag, Ger.; Janssen-Cilag, Irl.; Janssen-Cilag, Ital.; Janssen-Cilag, Neth.; Janssen-Cilag, Norw.; Janssen-Cilag, S.Afr.; Janssen-Cilag, Swed.; Janssen-Cilag, Switz.; Janssen, UK.; Janssen, USA.
Mebendazole (p.104·1).
Worm infections.

Vernacycline-V *Propan-Vernleigh, S.Afr.†.*
Oxytetracycline hydrochloride (p.235·1); vitamin B substances.
Bacterial infections.

Vernelan *Verla, Ger.*
Magnesium aspartate hydrobromide (p.677·3).
Psychiatric disorders; sleep disorders.

Vernies *Parke, Davis, Spain.*
Glyceryl trinitrate (p.874·3).
Angina pectoris; heart failure; myocardial infarction.

Vernleigh Baby Cream *Propan, S.Afr.; Mer-National, S.Afr.*
Zinc oxide (p.1096·2); starch; boric acid.
Skin disorders.

Vernthol *Propan-Vernleigh, S.Afr.†.*
Theophylline (p.765·1).
Obstructive airways disease.

Verolax *Angelini, Ital.*
Glycerol (p.1585·2).
Constipation.

Veroptinstada *Stada, Ger.*
Verapamil hydrochloride (p.960·3).
Cardiac disorders; hypertension.

Verorab *Rhone-Poulenc Rorer, S.Afr.*
Rabies vaccine (p.1530·3).
Formerly known as Imovax Rabies Vero.
Active immunisation.

Verospiron *Hormosan, Ger.*
Spironolactone (p.946·1).
Oedema.

Veroxil *Baldacci, Ital.*
Indapamide (p.890·2).
Hypertension.

Verpamil *Rolab, S.Afr.†.*
Verapamil hydrochloride (p.960·3).
Angina; arrhythmias.

Verra-med *Permamed, Switz.*
Tretinoin (p.1093·3); salicylic acid (p.1090·2); dimethyl sulphoxide (p.1377·2).
Warts.

Verr-Canth *C & M, USA†; Palisades, USA†.*
Cantharidin (p.1559·2).
Removal of benign epithelial growths.

Verrex *C & M, USA†; Palisades, USA†.*
Salicylic acid (p.1090·2); podophyllum resin (p.1089·1).
Removal of benign epithelial growths.

Verruca Treatment *Numark, UK.*
Salicylic acid (p.1090·2).

Verrucid *Pharmagalen, Ger.*
Salicylic acid (p.1090·2).
Hyperkeratotic skin disorders.

Verrucosal *Monal, Fr.*
Salicylic acid (p.1090·2).
Warts.

Verrufilm *Isopharm, Fr.*
Lactic acid (p.1593·3); salicylic acid (p.1090·2).
Warts.

Verrugon *Pickles, UK.*
Salicylic acid (p.1090·2).
Hard skin; warts.

Verrulyse-Methionine
Bournonville, Belg.
Calcium glycerophosphate (p.1155·2); ferric glycerophosphate (p.1586·2); manganese glycerophosphate (p.1586·2); magnesium glycerophosphate (p.1157·2); magnesium oxide (p.1198·3); methionine (p.984·2).
Warts.

Saunier-Daguin, Fr.
Magnesium oxide (p.1198·3); methionine (p.984·2); calcium glycerophosphate (p.1155·2); ferric glycerophosphate (p.1586·2); manganese glycerophosphate (p.1586·2).
Warts.

Verrumal
Hermal, Ger.; Hermal, Switz.
Fluorouracil (p.534·3); salicylic acid (p.1090·2); dimethyl sulphoxide (p.1377·2).
Warts.

Verrupor *Sella, Ital.*
Trichloroacetic acid (p.1639·1).
Hard skin; verrucas; warts.

Verrusol *C & M, USA†; Palisades, USA†.*
Salicylic acid (p.1090·2); podophyllum resin (p.1089·1); cantharidin (p.1559·2).
Removal of benign epithelial growths.

Versacaps *Seatrace, USA.*
Pseudoephedrine hydrochloride (p.1068·3); guaiphenesin (p.1061·3).
Coughs.

Versacort *Angelini, Ital.†.*
Bendacort (p.1033·2).
Skin disorders.

Versal
Nycomed, Norw.; Pro Medica, Swed.
Loratadine (p.413·1).
Allergic conjunctivitis; allergic rhinitis; hypersensitivity reactions.

Versed
Roche, Canad.; Roche, USA.
Midazolam hydrochloride (p.679·3).
General anaesthesia; premedication.

Versel *Trans Canaderm, Canad.*
Selenium sulphide (p.1091·1).
Fungal skin infections.

Versiclear *Hope, USA.*
Sodium thiosulphate (p.996·2); salicylic acid (p.1090·2).
Fungal infections.

Versol
Note. This name is used for preparations of different composition.
Gerbex, Canad.
Piperazine (p.107·2).

Aguettant, Fr.
Sodium chloride (p.1162·2) or water for irrigation.

Verstadol *Bristol-Myers, Spain.*
Butorphanol tartrate (p.24·1).
Pain; premedication.

Versus
Angelini, Aust.; Angelini, Ital.
Bendazac (p.21·1).
Skin disorders.

Vertab *UAD, USA.*
Dimenhydrinate (p.408·2).

Vertebralon N *Rentschler, Ger.†.*
Glycol salicylate (p.43·1); nonivamide (p.63·2); salicylic acid (p.1090·2).
Formerly contained glycol salicylate, nonivamide, salicylic acid, heparin, and suprarenal cortex extract.
Muscle and joint disorders.

Vertigex *Farmades, Ital.†.*
Vitamin A; *dl*-alpha tocopherol; cinnarizine (p.406·1).
Atherosclerosis; menopausal disorders; vertigo.

Vertigoheel *Heel, Ger.*
Homoeopathic preparation.

Vertigo-Hevert *Hevert, Ger.*
Homoeopathic preparation.

Vertigon
Smith Kline & French, Irl.†; SmithKline Beecham, UK†.
Prochlorperazine maleate (p.687·3).
Anxiety; nausea; vestibular disorders; vomiting.

Vertigopas *Pascoe, Ger.*
Homoeopathic preparation.

Vertigo-Vomex *Yamanouchi, Ger.*
Dimenhydrinate (p.408·2).
Vertigo; vestibular disorders.

Vertigum *Liade, Spain.*
Dixyrazine (p.668·2); inositol nicotinate (p.891·3); pyridoxine hydrochloride (p.1362·3).
Vertigo.

Vertin *Alba, USA.*
Meclozine hydrochloride (p.413·3).

Vertirosan *Sigmapharm, Aust.*
Dimenhydrinate (p.408·2).
Migraine; motion sickness; nausea and vomiting; vestibular disorders.

Vertirosan Vitamin B_6 *Sigmapharm, Aust.*
Dimenhydrinate (p.408·2); pyridoxine hydrochloride (p.1362·3).
Migraine; motion sickness; nausea and vomiting; vestibular disorders.

Vertiserc *Solvay, Ital.*
Betahistine hydrochloride (p.1553·1).
Vestibular disorders.

Verucasep
Galen, Irl.; Galen, UK†.
Glutaraldehyde (p.1114·3).
Warts.

Verucca Removal System *Scholl, UK.*
Salicylic acid (p.1090·2).
Verrucas.

Verucca Treatment *Seton, UK†.*
Salicylic acid (p.1090·2).

Verucid
Yamanouchi, Ital.; Nycomed, Norw.
Salicylic acid (p.1090·2); lactic acid (p.1593·3).
Hard skin; verrucas; warts.

Verufil *Stiefel, Spain.*
Lactic acid (p.1593·3); salicylic acid (p.1090·2).
Warts.

Verunec 3 *Savoma, Ital.*
Salicylic acid (p.1090·2); lactic acid (p.1593·3); urea (p.1095·2).
Hard skin; verrucas; warts.

Verus *OTW, Ger.†.*
Mistletoe (p.1604·1); crataegus (p.1568·2); convallaria (p.1567·2); adonis vernalis (p.1543·3); sage (p.1627·1); juniper (p.1592·2); arnica (p.1550·3).
Hypertension.

Verutal *Stiefel, Fr.*
Glutaraldehyde (p.1114·3).
Warts.

Vesadol *Janssen-Cilag, Fr.*
Haloperidol (p.673·3); buzepide metiodide (p.459·2).
Gastro-intestinal spasms associated with anxiety.

Vesagex
Rybar, Irl.; Shire, UK.
Cetrimide (p.1105·2).
Skin injuries, irritation, and inflammation.

Vesalium
Janssen-Cilag, Aust.; Janssen-Cilag, Belg.; Lusofarmaco, Ital.†; Janssen-Cilag, Switz.†.
Haloperidol (p.673·3); isopropamide bromide (p.464·3) or isopropamide iodide (p.464·3).
Anxiety; gastro-intestinal and biliary spasm; psychosomatic disorders; sleep disturbances; urogenital spasm; vertigo.

Vesanoid
Roche, Austral.; Roche, Canad.; Roche, Fr.; Roche, Ger.; Roche, Ital.; Roche, Neth.; Roche, Norw.; Roche, S.Afr.; Roche, Swed.; Roche, Switz.; Roche, UK; Roche, USA.
Tretinoin (p.1093·3).
Acute promyelocytic leukaemia.

Vesdil
Astra, Ger.; Promed, Ger.; Astra, Switz.
Ramipril (p.941·1).
Heart failure; hypertension; myocardial infarction.

Vesdil plus *Astra, Ger.; Promed, Ger.*
Ramipril (p.941·1); hydrochlorothiazide (p.885·2).
Hypertension.

Vesiform S *Dispersa, Ger.†.*
Oxybuprocaine hydrochloride (p.1298·1).
Ophthalmic procedures.

Vesilax *Frega, Canad.*
Cascara (p.1183·1); phenolphthalein (p.1208·2); bile salts (p.1553·2); pancreatin (p.1612·1); papain (p.1614·1).

Vesirig *Aguettant, Fr.*
Sodium chloride (p.1162·2).
Lavage and irrigation.

Vesistol *Inverni della Beffa, Ital.†.*
Amrinone (p.823·2).
Heart failure.

Vesix *Nycomed, Neth.†.*
Frusemide (p.871·1).
Hypertension; oedema.

Vesparax
Note. This name is used for preparations of different composition.
UCB, Belg.; UCB, Ital.†; UCB, Neth.; UCB, S.Afr.
Hydroxyzine (p.412·2); brallobarbital (p.643·1); quinalbarbitone (p.690·2).
Insomnia.

UCB, Ger.†.
Etodroxizine maleate (p.670·1); brallobarbital calcium (p.643·1); quinalbarbitone sodium (p.690·2).
Sleep disorders.

Vesprin *Apothecon, USA; Princeton, USA.*
Fluopromazine hydrochloride (p.670·3).
Nausea; psychoses; vomiting.

Vessel Due F *Wassermann, Ital.*
Sulodexide (p.951·1).
Thrombosis prophylaxis.

Vessiflex *Schiapparelli, Ital.*
Sulodexide (p.951·1); aminopropylone (p.15·2).
Inflammation; injuries associated with pain and swelling.

Vetedol *Robert, Spain.*
Benorylate (p.21·2).
Fever; musculoskeletal, joint, and peri-articular disorders; pain.

Vethoine *Wolfs, Belg.*
Phenytoin (p.352·3); phenobarbitone (p.350·2); cascara (p.1183·1).
Epilepsy.

Vetren
Note. This name is used for preparations of different composition.
Byk, Aust.; Byk Gulden, Ger.; Roland, Ger.
Injection; ointment; topical gel: Heparin sodium (p.879·3).
Soft tissue injury; superficial vascular disorders.

Promonta, Ger.†.
Ointment: Heparin sodium (p.879·3); dexpanthenol (p.1570·3).
Skin trauma.

Vetuss HC *Cypress, USA.*
Hydrocodone tartrate (p.43·1); phenylephrine hydrochloride (p.1066·2); phenylpropanolamine hydrochloride (p.1067·2); mepyramine maleate (p.414·1); pheniramine maleate (p.415·3).
Coughs and related respiratory-tract disorders.

Vexol
Alcon, Canad.; Alcon, USA.
Rimexolone (p.1050·1).
Inflammatory eye disorders.

Veybirol-Tyrothyricine *Veyron-Froment, Fr.*
Solution A: formaldehyde (p.1113·2); solution B: tyrothricin (p.267·2).
Mouth infections.

VG Capsules *Med. Prod. Panam., USA†.*
Multivitamin and mineral preparation.
Vitamin and mineral deficiencies.

V-Gan *Hauck, USA†.*
Promethazine hydrochloride (p.416·2).
Hypersensitivity reactions; motion sickness; nausea; postoperative pain (adjunct); sedative; vomiting.

Via Mal *Byk Gulden, Ital.*
Aspirin (p.16·1); caffeine (p.749·3).
Aluminium hydroxide (p.1177·3) is included in this preparation in an attempt to limit the adverse effects of aspirin on the gastro-intestinal mucosa.
Fever; pain.

Via Mal Trauma Gel *Byk Gulden, Ital.*
Diethylamine salicylate (p.33·1); heparin sodium (p.879·3); menthol (p.1600·2).
Soft-tissue disorders.

Viaben *Synthelabo, Ger.†.*
Bromopride (p.1181·3) or bromopride hydrochloride (p.1181·3).
Gastro-intestinal disorders.

Viacin *Garec, S.Afr.*
Doxycycline hydrochloride (p.202·3).
Bacterial infections.

Viadent *Carter Horner, Canad.*
Mouthwash: Sanguinaria (p.1627·2).
Toothpaste: Sanguinaria (p.1627·2); sodium monofluorophosphate (p.743·3).
Dental plaque; gingivitis.

Viaderm-KC *Taro, Canad.*
Triamcinolone acetonide (p.1050·2); neomycin sulphate (p.229·2); nystatin (p.386·1); gramicidin (p.215·2).
Infected skin disorders.

Viadetres *Alacan, Spain.*
Hydroxocobalamin (p.1363·3); pyridoxine dihydrochloride (p.1362·3); prosultiamine (p.1360·3).
Vitamin B deficiency.

Viafen *Zyma, Ital.*
Bufexamac (p.22·2).
Dermatitis; pruritus.

Viaggio *Vifor, Switz.*
Dimenhydrinate (p.408·2); atropine sulphate (p.455·1); hyoscyamine sulphate (p.464·2); hyoscine hydrobromide (p.462·3); caffeine (p.749·3).
Motion sickness; nausea; vomiting.

Viagra
Pfizer, UK; Pfizer, USA.
Sildenafil citrate (p.1629·1).
Impotence.

Vial's tonischer Wein *Eberth, Ger.*
Calcium phospholactate; beef extract; cinchonine; wine.
Tonic.

Viamicina *Benvegna, Ital.†.*
Triacetyloleandomycin (p.264·3).
Bacterial infections.

Viamon *Nadeau, Canad.*
Multivitamin and mineral preparation.

Viapres *Zambon, Ital.*
Lacidipine (p.897·1).
Hypertension.

Viarin *Byk, Neth.†.*
Beclomethasone dipropionate (p.1032·1).
Rhinitis.

Viarox
Byk Gulden, Ger.; Schering-Plough, Norw.†; Schering-Plough, S.Afr.
Beclomethasone dipropionate (p.1032·1).
Allergic rhinitis; nasal polyps; obstructive airways disease.

Viartril *Rottapharm, Ital.†.*
Glucosamine sulphate (p.1585·1); glucosamine hydriodide (p.1585·1).
Arthritis.

Viaspan *Du Pont, Canad.*
Solution for flushing and cold storage of donor organs.

Viatine *Essex, Spain.*
Loratadine (p.413·1).
Hypersensitivity reactions.

Viavent *Byk Madaus, S.Afr.*
Salbutamol sulphate (p.758·2).
Obstructive airways disease.

Viazem XL *Du Pont Pharmaceuticals, UK.*
Diltiazem hydrochloride (p.854·2).
Hypertension.

Vibalgan *Doms-Adrian, Fr.*
Hydroxocobalamin acetate (p.1364·2); cobamamide (p.1364·2).
Neuralgias and neuropathies.

Vibalt *Roerig, Belg.†.*
Multivitamin preparation.

Vibeline *Promesa, Spain†.*
Visnadine (p.964·2).
Vascular disorders.

Viberol Tirotricina *Organon, Spain.*
Formaldehyde (p.1113·2); tyrothricin (p.267·2).
Mouth and throat inflammation.

Vibolex *Chephasaar, Ger.†.*
Vitamin B substances.
Vitamin B deficiency.

Vibrabron *Pfizer, Aust.*
Doxycycline hydrochloride (p.202·3); ambroxol hydrochloride (p.1054·3).
Bacterial infections of the respiratory tract.

Vibracare *Pfizer, Belg.*
Doxycycline carrageenate (p.203·2).
Bacterial infections.

Vibracina *Pfizer, Spain.*
Doxycycline hydrochloride (p.202·3).
Bacterial infections.

Vibramycin
Pfizer, Aust.; Pfizer, Austral.; Pfizer, Canad.; Pfizer, Ger.; Invicta, Irl.; Pfizer, Neth.; Pfizer, Norw.; Pfizer, S.Afr.; Pfizer, Swed.; Invicta, UK; Pfizer, USA; Roerig, USA.
Doxycycline (p.202·3), doxycycline calcium (p.202·3), doxycycline carrageenate (p.203·2), or doxycycline hydrochloride (p.202·3).
Bacterial infections.

Vibramycin D *Invicta, UK.*
Doxycycline (p.202·3).
Bacterial infections.

Vibramycine
Note. This name is used for preparations of different composition.
Pfizer, Belg.; Pfizer, Switz.
Doxycycline (p.202·3) or doxycycline hydrochloride (p.202·3).
Bacterial infections; malaria.

Vibramycine N *Pfizer, Fr.*
Doxycycline (p.202·3).
Bacterial infections.

Vibra-S *Pfizer, Neth.*
Doxycycline (p.202·3).
Bacterial infections.

Vibratab *Pfizer, Belg.*
Doxycycline (p.202·3).
Bacterial infections.

Vibra-Tabs
Pfizer, Austral.; Pfizer, Canad.; Pfizer, USA.
Doxycycline hydrochloride (p.202·3).
Acne; bacterial infections; intestinal amoebiasis.

Vibratussal *Pfizer, Ger.†.*
Doxycycline hydrochloride (p.202·3); codeine polistirex (p.27·1).
Coughs associated with infections of the respiratory-tract.

Vibraveineuse
Pfizer, Fr.; Pfizer, Switz.
Doxycycline hydrochloride (p.202·3).
Bacterial infections.

Vibravenos
Pfizer, Aust.; Pfizer, Ger.
Doxycycline hydrochloride (p.202·3).
Bacterial infections.

Vibravenosa *Pfizer, Spain.*
Doxycycline hydrochloride (p.202·3).
Bacterial infections.

Vibrocil
Note. This name is used for preparations of different composition.
Zyma, Aust.; Zyma, Belg.; Zyma, Ger.; Zyma, Ital.; Zyma, Switz.
Nasal gel; nasal spray; nasal drops: Dimethindene maleate (p.408·3); phenylephrine (p.1066·2).
Rhinitis; sinusitis.

Zyma, Irl.†; Novartis Consumer, S.Afr.; Zyma, UK†.
Nasal gel; nasal spray; nasal drops: Dimethindene maleate (p.408·3); phenylephrine (p.1066·2); neomycin sulphate (p.229·2).
Rhinitis; sinusitis.

Zyma, Belg.
Capsules: Pseudoephedrine hydrochloride (p.1068·3); dimethindene maleate (p.408·3).
Allergic rhinitis; sinusitis; vasomotor rhinitis.

Vibrocil cN *Zyma, Ger.†.*
Dimethindene maleate (p.408·3); phenylephrine (p.1066·2); neomycin sulphate (p.229·2).
Rhinitis.

Vibrocil-S *Novartis Consumer, S.Afr.*
Dimethindene maleate (p.408·3); phenylephrine (p.1066·2).
Nasal and sinus congestion.

Vibtil
Bio-Therabel, Belg.; Lafon, Fr.
Tilia (p.1637·3).
Digestive disorders.

Viburcol *Heel, Ger.*
Homoeopathic preparation.

Viburnum Complex *Blackmores, Austral.*
Viburnum opulus; cimicifuga (p.1563·3); angelica sinensis pulsatilla (p.1623·3); *d*-alpha tocopheryl acid succinate (p.1369·2).
Gynaecological disorders; muscle cramp.

Vicam *Keene, USA.*
Vitamin B substances.
Parenteral nutrition.

Vicapan N *Merckle, Ger.*
Cyanocobalamin (p.1363·3).
Vitamin B deficiency.

Vi-Caps *Grossmann, Switz.*
Multivitamin and mineral preparation.

Vicard
Nycomed, Aust.†; Abbott, Switz.†.
Terazosin hydrochloride (p.952·1).
Hypertension.

Vicedent *Terramin, Aust.*
Ascorbic acid (p.1365·2).
Gum disorders.

Vicemex *Cimex, Switz.*
Ascorbic acid (p.1365·2).
Vitamin C deficiency; vitamin C supplement.

Vici *Monico, Ital.*
Ascorbic acid (p.1365·2).
Vitamin C deficiency.

Vicilan *Zeneca, Ital.*
Viloxazine hydrochloride (p.312·1).
Depression.

Vicitina *CT, Ital.*
Ascorbic acid (p.1365·2).
Gingivitis; stomatitis; vitamin C deficiency.

Vicks Action *Procter & Gamble, UK.*
Ibuprofen (p.44·1); pseudoephedrine (p.1068·3).
Cold symptoms.

Vicks Blue Drops *Procter & Gamble, Austral.*
Menthol (p.1600·2); peppermint oil (p.1208·1).
Throat irritation.

Vicks Cetamium Vit/C *Procter & Gamble, Ital.†.*
Menthol (p.1600·2); cetylpyridinium chloride (p.1106·2); ascorbic acid (p.1365·2).
Coughs; sore throat.

Vicks Children's Chloraseptic *Procter & Gamble, USA.*
Lozenges: Benzocaine (p.1286·2).
Throat spray: Phenol (p.1121·2).
Sore throat.

Vicks Children's NyQuil Allergy/Head Cold *Richardson-Vicks, USA.*
Pseudoephedrine hydrochloride (p.1068·3); chlorpheniramine maleate (p.405·1).
Upper respiratory-tract symptoms.

Vicks Children's NyQuil Night-time Cold/Cough Liquid *Richardson-Vicks, USA.*
Chlorpheniramine maleate (p.405·1); pseudoephedrine hydrochloride (p.1068·3); dextromethorphan hydrobromide (p.1057·3).
Coughs and cold symptoms.

Vicks Childrens Vaposyrup *Procter & Gamble, UK†.*
Dextromethorphan hydrobromide (p.1057·3).
Coughs.

Vicks Chloraseptic
Procter & Gamble, Irl.; Procter & Gamble (H&B Care), UK; Procter & Gamble, USA.
Phenol (p.1121·2).
Oral hygiene; sore throat.

Vicks Chloraseptic Sore Throat *Procter & Gamble, USA.*
Benzocaine (p.1286·2); menthol (p.1600·2).
Sore throat.

Vicks Cold Care *Procter & Gamble (H&B Care), UK.*
Paracetamol (p.72·2); dextromethorphan (p.1057·3); phenylpropanolamine (p.1067·2).
Cold symptoms.

Vicks Cough Drops *Procter & Gamble, USA.*
Menthol (p.1600·2).
Sore throat.

Vicks Cough Silencers *Richardson-Vicks, USA.*
Dextromethorphan hydrobromide (p.1057·3); benzocaine (p.1286·2).
Coughs.

Vicks Cough Syrup
Note. This name is used for preparations of different composition.
Procter & Gamble, Austral.
Pentoxyverine citrate (p.1066·1); sodium citrate (p.1153·2); menthol (p.1600·2).
Coughs.

Procter & Gamble, Canad.
Ephedrine (p.1059·3); guaiphenesin (p.1061·3); pentoxyverine citrate (p.1066·1).

Vicks 44D Cough & Head Congestion *Procter & Gamble, USA.*
Dextromethorphan hydrobromide (p.1057·3); pseudoephedrine hydrochloride (p.1068·3).
Coughs and cold symptoms.

Vicks DayQuil *Richardson-Vicks, USA.*
Pseudoephedrine hydrochloride (p.1068·3); dextromethorphan hydrobromide (p.1057·3); guaiphenesin (p.1061·3); paracetamol (p.72·2).
Coughs.

Vicks DayQuil Allergy Relief *Procter & Gamble, USA.*
Phenylpropanolamine hydrochloride (p.1067·2); brompheniramine maleate (p.403·2).

Vicks DayQuil Sinus Pressure & Congestion Relief *Procter & Gamble, USA†.*
Phenylpropanolamine hydrochloride (p.1067·2); guaiphenesin (p.1061·3).

Vicks DayQuil Sinus Pressure & Pain Relief *Procter & Gamble, USA.*
Pseudoephedrine hydrochloride (p.1068·3); paracetamol (p.72·2).

Vicks Decongestive Cough Syrup *Richardson-Vicks, Austral.†.*
Pentoxyverine citrate (p.1066·1); ephedrine sulphate (p.1059·3); sodium citrate (p.1153·2); menthol (p.1600·2).
Pentoxyverine citrate is omitted in Victoria state.
Coughs; nasal congestion.

Vicks Dry Hacking Cough *Procter & Gamble, USA.*
Dextromethorphan hydrobromide (p.1057·3).
Formerly known as Vicks Formula 44.
Coughs.

Vicks 44E *Procter & Gamble, USA.*
Dextromethorphan hydrobromide (p.1057·3); guaiphenesin (p.1061·3).
Coughs.

Vicks Expectorant *Procter & Gamble (H&B Care), UK.*
Guaiphenesin (p.1061·3); cetylpyridinium chloride (p.1106·2); sodium citrate (p.1153·2).
Coughs.

Vicks Formel 44 *Procter & Gamble, Switz.*
Dextromethorphan (p.1057·3); benzocaine (p.1286·2); cetylpyridinium chloride (p.1106·2); menthol (p.1600·2); peppermint oil (p.1208·1).
Coughs; sore throat.

Vicks Formula 44 *Procter & Gamble, Spain.*
Anethole (p.1549·3); cetylpyridinium chloride (p.1106·2); dextromethorphan (p.1057·3); benzocaine (p.1286·2); peppermint oil (p.1208·1); menthol (p.1600·2).
Respiratory-tract disorders.

Vicks Formula 44 Cough Control Discs *Richardson-Vicks, USA.*
Dextromethorphan hydrobromide (p.1057·3); benzocaine (p.1286·2).
Coughs.

Vicks Formule 44 *Procter & Gamble, Belg.†.*
Dextromethorphan hydrobromide (p.1057·3); doxylamine succinate (p.410·1).
Coughs.

Vicks Gola *Procter & Gamble, Ital.†.*
Menthol (p.1600·2); ascorbic acid (p.1365·2); cetylpyridinium chloride (p.1106·2); eucalyptus oil (p.1578·1); camphor (p.1557·2).
Mouth and throat disorders.

Vicks Headclear *Procter & Gamble, Austral.†.*
Pseudoephedrine hydrochloride (p.1068·3); paracetamol (p.72·2); chlorpheniramine maleate (p.405·1).
Cold, influenza, and sinus symptoms.

Vicks Headclear Nondrowsy *Procter & Gamble, Austral.†.*
Pseudoephedrine hydrochloride (p.1068·3); paracetamol (p.72·2).
Cold, influenza, and sinus symptoms.

Vicks Inalante *Procter & Gamble, Ital.*
Menthol (p.1600·2); camphor (p.1557·2); methyl salicylate (p.55·2); pine oil.
Nasal congestion.

Vicks Inhalador *Procter & Gamble, Spain.*
Camphor (p.1557·2); methyl salicylate (p.55·2); sassafras oil (p.1627·3); menthol (p.1600·2); bornyl acetate (p.1555·1).
Nasal obstruction.

Vicks Inhaler
Note. This name is used for preparations of different composition.
Procter & Gamble, Austral.; Procter & Gamble (H&B Care), UK.
Menthol (p.1600·2); camphor (p.1557·2); methyl salicylate (p.55·2); pumilio pine oil (p.1623·3).
Nasal congestion.

Procter & Gamble, Canad.
Menthol (p.1600·2); camphor (p.1557·2).
Nasal congestion.

Procter & Gamble, Irl.
Menthol (p.1600·2); camphor (p.1557·2); pine needle oil.
Nasal congestion.

Vicks Inhaler N *Procter & Gamble, Switz.*
Menthol (p.1600·2); camphor (p.1557·2); methyl salicylate (p.55·2); pine needle oil.
Nasal congestion.

Vicks 44M Cold, Flu & Cough LiquiCaps *Procter & Gamble, USA.*
Dextromethorphan hydrobromide (p.1057·3); pseudoephedrine hydrochloride (p.1068·3); chlorpheniramine maleate (p.405·1); paracetamol (p.72·2).

Vicks Medinait
Procter & Gamble, Ital.; Alter, Spain†; Procter & Gamble, Switz.
Dextromethorphan hydrobromide (p.1057·3); doxylamine succinate (p.410·1); ephedrine sulphate (p.1059·3); paracetamol (p.72·2).
Cold and influenza symptoms.

Vicks Medinite *Procter & Gamble (H&B Care), UK.*
Dextromethorphan (p.1057·3); doxylamine (p.410·1); ephedrine (p.1059·3); paracetamol (p.72·2).
Cold symptoms.

Vicks Menthol Cough Drops *Procter & Gamble, USA.*
Menthol (p.1600·2); thymol (p.1127·1); eucalyptus oil (p.1578·1); camphor (p.1557·2); tolu balsam (p.1071·1).
Sore throat.

Vicks 44 Non-Drowsy Cold & Cough LiquiCaps *Procter & Gamble, USA.*
Dextromethorphan hydrobromide (p.1057·3); pseudoephedrine hydrochloride (p.1068·3).

Vicks NyQuil LiquiCaps *Richardson-Vicks, USA.*
Dextromethorphan hydrobromide (p.1057·3); paracetamol (p.72·2); pseudoephedrine hydrochloride (p.1068·3); doxylamine succinate (p.410·1).
Coughs and cold symptoms.

Vicks NyQuil Multi-Symptom Cold Flu Relief *Procter & Gamble, USA.*
Pseudoephedrine hydrochloride (p.1068·3); doxylamine succinate (p.410·1); dextromethorphan hydrobromide (p.1057·3); paracetamol (p.72·2).
Cold symptoms.

Vicks Original Cough Syrup for Chesty Coughs *Procter & Gamble, Irl.*
Guaiphenesin (p.1061·3); cetylpyridinium chloride (p.1106·2); sodium citrate (p.1153·2).
Coughs.

Vicks Pastilles *Lachartre, Fr.†.*
Camphor (p.1557·2); menthol (p.1600·2); eucalyptus oil (p.1578·1); thymol (p.1127·1); tolu balsam (p.1071·1); benzyl alcohol (p.1103·3).
Sore throats.

Vicks Pectoral *Procter & Gamble, Ital.†.*
Pentoxyverine citrate (p.1066·1); guaiphenesin (p.1061·3).
Coughs.

Vicks Pediatric Formula 44d Dry Hacking Cough & Head Congestion *Procter & Gamble, USA.*
Pseudoephedrine hydrochloride (p.1068·3); dextromethorphan hydrobromide (p.1057·3).
Formerly known as Vicks Formula 44d Pediatric.
Coughs and cold symptoms.

Vicks Pediatric Formula 44E *Richardson-Vicks, USA.*
Dextromethorphan hydrobromide (p.1057·3); guaiphenesin (p.1061·3).
Coughs.

Vicks Pediatric Formula 44m Multi-Symptom Cough & Cold *Richardson-Vicks, USA.*
Pseudoephedrine hydrochloride (p.1068·3); dextromethorphan hydrobromide (p.1057·3); chlorpheniramine maleate (p.405·1).
Coughs and cold symptoms.

Vicks Rhume *Lachartre, Fr.*
Ibuprofen (p.44·1); pseudoephedrine hydrochloride (p.1068·3).
Rhinitis.

Vicks Sinex
Note. This name is used for preparations of different composition.
Procter & Gamble, Austral.; Procter & Gamble, Ital.; Procter & Gamble, Switz.; Procter & Gamble (H&B Care), UK.
Oxymetazoline hydrochloride (p.1065·3); menthol (p.1600·2); camphor (p.1557·2); cineole (p.1564·1).
Nasal congestion.

Procter & Gamble, Belg.; Procter & Gamble, Canad.; Procter & Gamble, Irl.
Oxymetazoline hydrochloride (p.1065·3).
Nasal congestion.

Richardson-Vicks, Neth.
Oxymetazoline hydrochloride (p.1065·3); menthol (p.1600·2); camphor (p.1557·2); eucalyptus oil (p.1578·1).
Cold symptoms.

Vicks Sinex 12-Hour *Procter & Gamble, USA.*
Oxymetazoline hydrochloride (p.1065·3).
Formerly known as Sinex Long Acting.
Nasal congestion.

Vicks Sirop *Lachartre, Fr.†.*
Pentoxyverine citrate (p.1066·1); guaiphenesin (p.1061·3); sodium citrate (p.1153·2).
Coughs.

Vicks Soulagil *Lachartre, Fr.†.*
Oral spray: Lignocaine hydrochloride (p.1293·2); cetylpyridinium chloride (p.1106·2); dequalinium chloride (p.1112·1).
Pastilles: Cetylpyridinium chloride (p.1106·2); ascorbic acid (p.1365·2); sodium ascorbate (p.1365·2); menthol (p.1600·2); peppermint oil (p.1208·1); benzyl alcohol (p.1103·3).
Sore throats.

Vicks Spray *Procter & Gamble, Spain.*
Camphor (p.1557·2); cineole (p.1564·1); oxymetazoline hydrochloride (p.1065·3); menthol (p.1600·2).
Nasal congestion.

Vicks Throat Drops
Procter & Gamble, Austral.; Procter & Gamble, Canad.
Menthol (p.1600·2).
Coughs; throat irritation.

Vicks Tosse Fluidificante *Procter & Gamble, Ital.*
Guaiphenesin (p.1061·3).
Respiratory-tract congestion.

Vicks Tosse Pastiglie *Procter & Gamble, Ital.*
Dextromethorphan (p.1057·3).
Coughs.

Vicks Tosse Sedativo *Procter & Gamble, Ital.*
Dextromethorphan hydrobromide (p.1057·3).
Coughs.

Vicks Toux Seche *Lachartre, Fr.*
Dextromethorphan hydrobromide (p.1057·3).
Coughs.

Vicks Ultra Chloraseptic *Procter & Gamble (H&B Care), UK.*
Benzocaine (p.1286·2).
Sore throat.

Vicks Vapodrops *Procter & Gamble, Austral.*
Menthol (p.1600·2); eucalyptus oil (p.1578·1).
Nasal congestion; sore throat.

Vicks Vapodrops with Butter and Menthol *Procter & Gamble, Austral.*
Menthol (p.1600·2).
Nasal congestion; sore throat.

Vicks Vapor Inhaler *Richardson-Vicks, USA.*
Levmetamfetamine (p.1063·3).
Nasal congestion.

Vicks Vaporub
Note. This name is used for preparations of different composition.
Procter & Gamble, Austral.
Menthol (p.1600·2); camphor (p.1557·2); eucalyptus oil (p.1578·1); turpentine oil (p.1641·1); nutmeg oil (p.1609·3); cedar leaf oil.
Cold symptoms.

Procter & Gamble, Belg.; Lachartre, Fr.; Procter & Gamble, Spain; Procter & Gamble, Swed.; Procter & Gamble, Switz.
Camphor (p.1557·2); menthol (p.1600·2); thymol (p.1127·1); cedar leaf oil; eucalyptus oil (p.1578·1); nutmeg oil (p.1609·3); turpentine oil (p.1641·1).
Upper respiratory-tract congestion.

Procter & Gamble, Canad.
Camphor (p.1557·2); menthol (p.1600·2); eucalyptus oil (p.1578·1).
Cold symptoms.

Procter & Gamble, Irl.; Procter & Gamble, Ital.; Euromed, Ital.; Procter & Gamble (H&B Care), UK.
Menthol (p.1557·2); camphor (p.1600·2); eucalyptus oil (p.1578·1); turpentine oil (p.1641·1).
Upper respiratory-tract congestion.

Richardson-Vicks, Neth.
Menthol (p.1600·2); camphor (p.1557·2); eucalyptus oil (p.1578·1); cedar wood oil; turpentine oil; thymol (p.1127·1).
Cold and influenza symptoms.

Procter & Gamble, USA.
Camphor (p.1557·2); menthol (p.1600·2); eucalyptus oil (p.1578·1); cedar leaf oil.

Vicks Vapsiroop *Richardson-Vicks, Neth.*
Dextromethorphan hydrobromide (p.1057·3).
Coughs.

Vicks Vaposyrup *Procter & Gamble, Canad.*
Menthol (p.1600·2).

Vicks Vaposyrup Antitussif *Procter & Gamble, Belg.*
Dextromethorphan (p.1057·3) or dextromethorphan hydrobromide (p.1057·3).
Coughs.

Vicks Vaposyrup for chesty coughs *Procter & Gamble (H&B Care), UK.*
Guaiphenesin (p.1061·3).
Coughs.

Vicks Vaposyrup for chesty coughs and nasal congestion *Procter & Gamble (H&B Care), UK†.*
Phenylpropanolamine (p.1067·2); guaiphenesin (p.1061·3).
Coughs.

Vicks Vaposyrup for dry coughs *Procter & Gamble (H&B Care), UK.*
Dextromethorphan hydrobromide (p.1057·3).
Coughs.

Vicks Vaposyrup for dry coughs and nasal congestion *Procter & Gamble (H&B Care), UK†.*
Phenylpropanolamine (p.1067·2); dextromethorphan (p.1057·3).
Coughs.

Vicks Vaposyrup Expectorant
Procter & Gamble, Belg.; Lachartre, Fr.
Guaiphenesin (p.1061·3).
Coughs; respiratory-tract congestion.

Vicks Vaposyrup toux seche *Lachartre, Fr.*
Dextromethorphan hydrobromide (p.1057·3).
Coughs.

Vicks Vatronol *Richardson-Vicks, USA†.*
Ephedrine sulphate (p.1059·3).
Nasal congestion.

Vicks Victors Dual Action Cough Drops *Richardson-Vicks, USA.*
Menthol (p.1600·2); eucalyptus oil (p.1578·1).

Vicks vitamine C pastilles *Lachartre, Fr.†.*
Menthol (p.1600·2); eucalyptus oil (p.1578·1); camphor (p.1557·2); thymol (p.1127·1); tolu balsam (p.1071·1); ascorbic acid (p.1365·2); sodium ascorbate (p.1365·2); benzyl alcohol (p.1103·3).
Sore throats.

Vicnas *Semar, Spain.*
Norfloxacin (p.233·1).
Gastroenteritis; gonorrhoea; urinary-tract infections.

Vicodin *Knoll, USA.*
Hydrocodone tartrate (p.43·1); paracetamol (p.72·2).
Pain.

Vicodin Tuss *Knoll, USA.*
Hydrocodone tartrate (p.43·1); guaiphenesin (p.1061·3).
Coughs.

Vicomin A C *Warner-Lambert, Spain.*
Ascorbic acid (p.1365·2); vitamin A (p.1358·1).
Deficiency of vitamins A and C.

Vicon *UCB, USA.*
A range of vitamin preparations.

Vicoprofen *Knoll, USA.*
Hydrocodone tartrate (p.43·1); ibuprofen (p.44·1).
Pain.

Victan
Sanofi Winthrop, Belg.; Sanofi Winthrop, Fr.; Midy, Ital.†.
Ethyl loflazepate (p.669·3).
Alcohol withdrawal syndrome; anxiety disorders.

Victogon *Normon, Spain.*
Amino acids and vitamins; isoniazid (p.218·1).
Anorexia; tonic; weight loss.

Vi-Daylin
Ross, Canad.†; Abbott, S.Afr.†; Abbott, UK; Ross, USA.
A range of vitamin preparations.

Vi-Daylin with Minerals *Abbott, S.Afr.*
Multivitamin and mineral preparation.

Vi-Daylin/F *Ross, USA.*
A range of vitamin and fluoride (p.742·1) preparations.

Vi-De₃
Salus, Aust.; Sandoz, Switz.
Cholecalciferol (p.1366·3).
Hypoparathyroidism; osteomalacia; rickets; tetany.

Videne *Adams, UK.*
Povidone-iodine (p.1123·3).
Burns; skin disinfection; wounds.

Video
Note. This name is used for preparations of different composition.
Monot, Fr.
Phenylephrine hydrochloride (p.1066·2); rutin sodium sulphate (p.1580·2).
Conjunctivitis.

Farmila, Ital.
Benzalkonium chloride (p.1101·3).
Eye disinfection.

Video Capsule con Mirtillo *Farmila, Ital.*
Vitamin E; magnesium; betacarotene; selenium; myrtillus.
Antioxidant nutritional supplement.

Video-Net *Interdelta, Switz.*
Phenylephrine hydrochloride (p.1066·2); rutin sodium sulphate (p.1580·2).
Eye irritation.

Videorelax *SIFI, Ital.*
Chlorhexidine gluconate (p.1107·2); tilia (p.1637·3); chamomile (p.1561·2).
Eye disinfection; eye irritation.

Viderm *Ganassini, Ital.*
Hydroxyquinoline sulphate (p.1589·3); enoxolone (p.35·2).
Wound disinfection.

Vidermina *Ganassini, Ital.*
Copper usnate (p.1643·1).
Vaginal disinfection.

Videx
Bristol-Myers Squibb, Aust.; Bristol-Myers Squibb, Austral.; Bristol-Myers Squibb, Belg.; Bristol, Canad.; Bristol-Myers Squibb, Fr.; Bristol-Myers Squibb, Ger.; Bristol-Myers Squibb, Irl.; Bristol-Myers Squibb, Ital.; Bristol-Myers Squibb, Neth.; Bristol-Myers Squibb, Norw.; Bristol-Myers Squibb, S.Afr.; Bristol-Myers, Spain; Bristol-Myers Squibb, Swed.; Bristol-Myers Squibb, Switz.; Bristol-Myers Squibb, UK; Bristol-Myers Squibb, USA.
Didanosine (p.607·3).
HIV infection.

Vi-Dieci *Teknofarma, Ital.†.*
Multivitamin preparation.

Vidirakt N *Mann, Ger.†.*
Sodium iodide (p.1493·2); thiamine hydrochloride (p.1361·1); sodium pantothenate (p.1353·1).
Eye disorders.

Vidirakt S *Mann, Ger.*
Povidone (p.1474·2).
Dry eyes.

Vidisept N *Mann, Ger.*
Povidone (p.1474·2).
Dry eyes.

Vidiseptal EDO Sine *Mann, Ger.*
Tetrahydrozoline hydrochloride (p.1070·2).
Eye irritation and inflammation.

Vidisic
Riel, Aust.; Tramedico, Belg.; Mann, Ger.; Mann, Irl.; Mann, Neth.
Carbomer (p.1471·2).
Dry eyes.

Vidopen
Berk, Irl.; Berk, UK.
Ampicillin (p.153·1) or ampicillin trihydrate (p.153·2).
Bacterial infections.

Vidora
Wyeth, Fr.; Wyeth, Ital.†.
Indoramin hydrochloride (p.891·1).
Hypertension; migraine.

Vie Ca Rad *Multi-Pro, Canad.*
Betacarotene, selenium, vitamin C, and vitamin E.

Vier-Winde-Tee *Fresenius, Ger.†.*
Caraway (p.1559·3); aniseed (p.1549·3); peppermint leaf (p.1208·1); matricaria flowers (p.1561·2); chamomile flowers (p.1561·2).
Gastro-intestinal disorders.

Vifenac *Vifor, Switz.*
Diclofenac epolamine (p.32·3).
Musculoskeletal and joint disorders.

Vig *Key, Austral.*
Guarana (p.1645·1); ginseng (p.1584·2); ginkgo biloba (p.1584·1).
Tonic.

Vigam S *BPL, UK.*
A normal immunoglobulin (p.1522·1).
Hypogammaglobulinaemia; idiopathic thrombocytopenic purpura.

Vigantol *Merck, Ger.*
Cholecalciferol (p.1366·3).
Vitamin D deficiency.

Vigantoletten
Note. This name is used for preparations of different composition.
Merck, Aust.†.
Cholecalciferol-cholesterin.
Rickets prophylaxis.

Merck, Ger.
Cholecalciferol (p.1366·3).
Vitamin D deficiency.

Vigar N *Agpharm, Switz.†.*
Yeast.
Digestive disorders; skin disorders.

Vigem *Pharmavite, Canad.*
Vitamin B substances.

Vigencial *Estedi, Spain.*
Alcohol (p.1099·1); benzalkonium chloride (p.1101·3); dexpanthenol (p.1570·3); crystal violet (p.1111·2).
Aphthous ulcers; impetigo; infected wounds; mouth inflammation; skin ulcers.

Vigigan *Rhone-Poulenc Rorer, Switz.†.*
Mequitazine (p.414·2).
Hypersensitivity reactions.

Vigilia *Grands Espaces, Fr.*
Tilia (p.1637·3); verbena.
Sedative.

Vigilon *Seton, UK.*
Polyethylene oxide (p.1474·1).
Hydrogel dressing; wounds.

Vigiten *Wyeth Lederle, Belg.*
Lorazepam (p.675·3).
Anxiety disorders; depression; mixed anxiety-depression; obsessive-compulsive disorder.

Vigodana *Madaus, S.Afr.†.*
Vitamin E; orotic acid; procaine hydrochloride; haematoporphyrin; magnesium l-aspartate; magnesium oxide; dried magnesium sulphate.
Tonic.

Vigodana N *Loges, Ger.*
Alpha tocopheryl acetate; orotic acid; haematoporphyrin; magnesium aspartate; magnesium oxide; dried magnesium sulphate.
Tonic.

Vigogel *Farmetrusca, Ital.*
Royal jelly (p.1626·3); liver extract; dried yeast (p.1373·1).

Vigomar Forte *Marlop, USA.*
Multivitamin and mineral preparation with iron.

Vigoplus *Gazzoni, Ital.*
Maltodextrin; fructose; vitamins; minerals.
Nutritional supplement.

Vigoran *Golaz, Switz.*
Ginseng (p.1584·2); deanol hydrogen tartrate (p.1478·2); magnesium orotate (p.1611·2).
Tonic.

Vigorsan *Albert-Roussel, Ger.; Hoechst, Ger.*
Cholecalciferol (p.1366·3).
Vitamin D deficiency.

Vigortol *Rugby, USA.*
Multivitamin and mineral preparation.

Vigoton A *Milanfarma, Ital.†.*
Multivitamin preparation.

Vigour S *Restan, S.Afr.*
Haematoporphyrin; cyanocobalamin; caffeine; yeast extract.
Tonic.

Vigovit C *Janssen-Cilag, Ital.†.*
Ascorbic acid (p.1365·2).

Vigranon B *Wallace Mfg Chem., UK.*
Vitamin B preparation.

Vikaman *Disperga, Aust.*
Menadione sodium bisulphite (p.1370·3).
Haemorrhage.

Vilan
Lannacher, Aust.; Nourypharma, Neth.; Synmedic, Switz.
Nicomorphine hydrochloride (p.63·1).
Pain; premedication; smooth muscle spasm.

Villescon *Boehringer Ingelheim, UK†.*
Prolintane hydrochloride (p.1485·1); thiamine hydrochloride (p.1361·1); riboflavine sodium phosphate (p.1362·1); pyridoxine hydrochloride (p.1362·3); nicotinamide (p.1351·2).
Tonic.

Vi-Medin *Sabex, Canad.†.*
Benzethonium chloride (p.1102·3).
Formerly contained methylbenzethonium chloride.
Deodorant; hyperhidrosis.

Vimeral *ICN, Canad.*
Multivitamin and mineral preparation.

Viminate *Barre-National, USA.*
Multivitamin and mineral preparation.

Vi-Mono-Tab *Nuovo ISM, Ital.†.*
A typhoid-paratyphoid A & B vaccine.
Active immunisation.

Vin Tonique de Vial *Eberth, Switz.*
Cinchona alkaloids (p.1564·1); calcium phosphate (p.1155·3); lactic acid (p.1593·3); beef extract; sweet wine.
Tonic.

Vinatal *Triomed, S.Afr.*
Multivitamin and mineral preparation.

Vinca *Genodex, Fr.*
Vincamine (p.1644·1).
Mental function impairment in the elderly.

Vinca minor *Hausmann, Switz.†.*
Vincamine (p.1644·1).
Cerebrovascular disorders.

Vincacen *Centrum, Spain.*
Vincamine (p.1644·1).
Cerebral trauma; cerebrovascular disorders.

Vincadar *Hoechst Marion Roussel, Ital.*
Vincamine (p.1644·1).
Cerebrovascular disorders.

Vinca-Dil *Lepetit, Ital.†.*
Vincamine (p.1644·1).
Cerebrovascular disorders.

Vincafarm *Radiumfarma, Ital.†.*
Vincamine (p.1644·1).
Cerebrovascular disorders.

Vincafolina *Lampugnani, Ital.*
Vincamine (p.1644·1).
Cerebrovascular disorders.

Vincafor *Pharmafarm, Fr.*
Vincamine (p.1644·1).
Mental function impairment in the elderly.

Vincalen *FIRMA, Ital.†.*
Vincamine (p.1644·1).
Cerebrovascular disorders.

Vincamas *Pan Quimica, Spain†.*
Vincamine (p.1644·1).
Cerebrovascular disorders.

Vincamidol *Magis, Ital.†.*
Vincamine (p.1644·1).
Cerebrovascular disorders.

Vincaminol *Alacan, Spain.*
Vincamine (p.1644·1).
Cerebral trauma; cerebrovascular disorders.

Vincapront *Mack, Illert., Ger.*
Vincamine (p.1644·1).
Ménière's disease; metabolic and circulatory disorders of the brain, retina, and inner ear.

Vinca-Ri *INTES, Ital.*
Vincamine hydrochloride (p.1644·1).
Disorders of cerebral, ocular, and vestibular perfusion.

Vincarutine *Pharbiol, Fr.*
Vincamine (p.1644·1); rutin (p.1580·2).
Mental function impairment in the elderly.

Vincasar PFS *Adria, USA.*
Vincristine sulphate (p.570·1).
Malignant neoplasms.

Vinca-Tablinen *Sanorania, Ger.*
Vincamine (p.1644·1).
Circulatory disorders of the brain, retina, and inner ear; Ménière's disease.

Vinca-Treis *Ecobi, Ital.*
Vincamine (p.1644·1).
Cerebrovascular disorders.

Vincavix *Llorens, Spain†.*
Vincamine (p.1644·1).
Cerebral trauma; cerebrovascular disorders.

Vincent's Powders *Roche Consumer, Austral.*
Aspirin (p.16·1).
Fever; pain.

Vinci *Bayropharm, Ital.†.*
Ascorbic acid (p.1365·2).

Vincigrip *Salvat, Spain.*
Chlorpheniramine maleate (p.405·1); phenylpropanolamine hydrochloride (p.1067·2); paracetamol (p.72·2).
Cold and influenza symptoms; fever; pain.

Vincigrip Balsamico *Salvat, Spain.*
Guaiphenesin (p.1061·3); paracetamol (p.72·2).
Influenza and cold symptoms; sinusitis.

Vincimax *Synthelabo, Fr.*
Vincamine (p.1644·1).
Cerebrovascular disorders; mental function impairment in the elderly.

Vinciseptil Otico *Salvat, Spain.*
Benzydamine hydrochloride (p.21·3); fluocinolone acetonide (p.1041·1); neomycin sulphate (p.229·2); polymyxin B sulphate (p.239·1); amethocaine hydrochloride (p.1285·2).
Ear disorders.

Vinco *OTW, Ger.†.*
Senna (p.1212·2).
Bowel evacuation; constipation.

Vinco Forte *OTW, Ger.*
Bisacodyl (p.1179·3).
Constipation.

Vinco V *OTW, Ger.†.*
Bisacodyl (p.1179·3); aloes (p.1177·1); frangula bark (p.1193·2).
Constipation.

Vinco-Abfuhrperlen *OTW, Ger.*
Bisacodyl (p.1179·3).
Constipation.

Vincosedan *Reig Jofre, Spain.*
Diazepam (p.661·1).
Contains pyridoxine.
Alcohol withdrawal syndrome; anxiety; febrile convulsions; insomnia; skeletal muscle spasm.

Vincosona *Reig Jofre, Spain.*
Diflorasone diacetate (p.1039·3).
Skin disorders.

Vincrisul *Lilly, Spain.*
Vincristine sulphate (p.570·1).
Malignant neoplasms.

Vinopepsin *Terrapharm, Aust.*
Pepsin (p.1616·3); absinthium (p.1541·1).
Gastro-intestinal disorders.

Vinsal *Salus, Ital.*
Vincamine (p.1644·1).
Cerebrovascular disorders.

Vintene *Clintec, Fr.*
Amino-acid infusion.
Parenteral nutrition.

Vi-Nutro Drops VCA *Bergamon, Ital.†.*
Multivitamin preparation.

Vinzam *Funk, Spain.*
Azithromycin (p.155·2).
Bacterial infections.

Viobeta *IDI, Ital.*
Betamethasone valero-acetate (p.1034·1); clioquinol (p.193·2).
Infected skin disorders.

Viocidina *IDI, Ital.*
Clioquinol (p.193·2); cod-liver oil (p.1337·3).
Infected skin disorders.

Viocort *Lennon, S.Afr.*
Hydrocortisone acetate (p.1043·3); di-iodohydroxyquinoline (p.581·1).
Skin disorders.

Viodenum *Iquinosa, Spain.*
Hidrosmin.
Peripheral vascular disorders.

Viodine *Pharmacia Upjohn, Austral.*
Povidone-iodine (p.1123·3).
Skin infections; sore throat; viral lesions.

Viodor *Lennon, S.Afr.*
Di-iodohydroxyquinoline (p.581·1); benzocaine (p.1286·2).
Skin infections with pruritus.

Vioform
Sigma, Austral.†; Ciba, Canad.; FLAWA, Switz.; Ciba, USA.
Clioquinol (p.193·2).
Infected skin disorders.

Vioform-Hydrocortisone
Sigma, Austral.†; Ciba, Canad.; Zyma, Irl.; Zyma, UK; Ciba, USA†.
Clioquinol (p.193·2); hydrocortisone (p.1043·3).
Skin disorders.

Viogen-C *Goldline, USA.*
Vitamin B substances with vitamin C and minerals.

Viogencianol *Aprofa, Spain†.*
Crystal violet (p.1111·2).
Skin disorders.

Viokase
Note. This name is used for preparations of different composition.
Wyeth, Austral.; Continental Ethicals, S.Afr.; Robins, USA.
Pancreatin (porcine) (p.1612·1).
Cystic fibrosis; pancreatic insufficiency.

Wolfs, Belg.; Axcan, Canad.
Pancrelipase (p.1613·3).
Pancreatic insufficiency.

Viola Pommade a l'huile d'amandes *Priorin, Switz.†.*
Viola tricolor; coltsfoot flower (p.1057·2); achillea (p.1542·2); veronica officinalis; couch-grass (p.1567·3); zinc oxide (p.1096·2); almond oil (p.1546·2).
Skin disorders.

Violgen *INTES, Ital.*
Crystal violet (p.1111·2); lactic acid (p.1593·3).
Vulvovaginitis.

Vioneurin *Continental Pharma, Belg.*
Vitamin B substances.
Neuralgia; polyneuritis in chronic alcoholism; vitamin B deficiency.

Viplex *Riva, Canad.*
Vitamin B substances, iron, and liver extract.

Vipracutan *Chinosolfabrik, Ger.†.*
Vipera ammodytes toxin; methyl salicylate (p.55·2); camphor (p.1557·2); menthol (p.1600·2).
Bruising; rheumatic and nerve disorders.

Vipral *Sanofi Winthrop, Spain†.*
Aciclovir (p.602·3).
Herpesvirus infections.

Vipratox *Serum-Werk Bernburg, Ger.*
Vipera ammodytes toxin; methyl salicylate (p.55·2); camphor (p.1557·2).
Musculoskeletal, joint, and soft-tissue disorders; neuralgias.

Vipro *Scientific Hospital Supplies, UK.*
Preparation for enteral nutrition.

Viprotene *Fermenti, Ital.†.*
Nutritional preparation.

Vipsogal *Harley Street Supplies, UK.*
Betamethasone dipropionate (p.1033·3); fluocinonide (p.1041·2); gentamicin sulphate (p.212·1); salicylic acid (p.1090·2); panthenol (p.1571·1).
Available on a named-patient basis only.
Skin disorders.

Viquin Forte *ICN, USA.*
Hydroquinone (p.1083·1); padimate O (p.1488·1); dioxybenzone (p.1487·1); oxybenzone (p.1487·3).
Hyperpigmentation; sunscreen.

Vira-A
Parke, Davis, Austral.; Parke, Davis, Canad.†; Parke, Davis, Fr.†; Parke, Davis, Irl.†; Parke, Davis, Spain†; Parke, Davis, USA.
Vidarabine (p.628·2).
Herpesvirus infections.

Viraban *Faulding, Austral.*
Povidone-iodine (p.1123·3).
Viral sore throat.

Virac *Crosara, Ital.*
Inosine pranobex (p.615·2).
Immunodeficiency; viral infections.

Viracept
Roche, UK; Agouron, USA.
Nelfinavir mesylate (p.623·1).
HIV infection.

Viractin *JB Williams, USA.*
Amethocaine (p.1285·2) or amethocaine hydrochloride (p.1285·2).
Topical anaesthesia.

Virafer *Rhone-Poulenc Rorer, Ital.*
Multivitamin and mineral preparation.

Viraferon
Schering-Plough, Fr.; Schering-Plough, Spain; Schering-Plough, UK.
Interferon alfa-2b (p.615·3).
Anogenital warts; hepatitis B; hepatitis C; malignant neoplasms.

Viralin *Magis, Ital.*
Inosine pranobex (p.615·2).
Viral infections.

Viramid *Wassermann, Ital.*
Tribavirin (p.626·2).
Viral bronchiolitis.

Vira-MP *Sinbio, Fr.; Pierre Fabre, Fr.*
Vidarabine sodium phosphate (p.629·1).
Chronic active viral hepatitis B; recurrent genital herpes infection.

Viramune
Boehringer Ingelheim, Austral.; Boehringer Ingelheim, UK; Roxane, USA.
Nevirapine (p.623·2).
HIV infection.

Viranol *American Dermal, USA†.*
Topical gel: Salicylic acid (p.1090·2).
Topical solution: Salicylic acid (p.1090·2); lactic acid (p.1593·3).
Warts.

Virasolve *Warner-Lambert, Austral.*
Idoxuridine (p.613·2); lignocaine hydrochloride (p.1293·2); benzalkonium chloride (p.1101·3).
Herpes simplex infections of the mouth and skin.

Virasorb *Seton, UK.*
Aciclovir (p.602·3).
Herpes labialis.

Virax *Isis Puren, Ger.*
Aciclovir (p.602·3).
Herpesvirus infections.

Virazid
ICN, Spain; ICN, UK.
Tribavirin (p.626·2).
Respiratory syncytial virus bronchiolitis.

Virazide
Dermatech, Austral.; Ciba, Ital.†.
Tribavirin (p.626·2).
Respiratory syncytial virus bronchiolitis.

Virazole
Sanico, Belg.; ICN, Canad.; Thomae, Ger.†; Antigen, Irl.†; ICN, Neth.†; Swedish Orphan, Swed.; Sanofi Winthrop, Switz.†; ICN, USA.
Tribavirin (p.626·2).
Respiratory syncytial virus infections.

Virdex *Fulton, Ital.*
Ergotamine tartrate (p.445·3); caffeine (p.749·3); amidopyrine (p.15·2).
Migraine.

Viregyt *Thiemann, Ger.*
Amantadine hydrochloride (p.1129·2).
Parkinsonism.

Virelon C *Chiron Behring, Ger.*
An inactivated poliomyelitis vaccine (p.1528·2).
Active immunisation.

Virexen
Will-Pharma, Belg.; Vinas, Spain; Vinas, Switz.
Idoxuridine (p.613·2) in dimethyl sulphoxide.
Herpesvirus infections of the skin and mucous membranes.

Virgamelis *Pascoe, Ger.*
Hamamelis (p.1587·1).
Skin irritation; wounds.

Virgan *Thea, Fr.*
Ganciclovir (p.612·3).
Herpes eye infections.

Virgilocard *Salus, Aust.*
Crataegus (p.1568·2); absinthium (p.1541·1).
Cardiac disorders in the elderly.

Virginiana Gocce Verdi *Kelemata, Ital.*
Naphazoline nitrate (p.1064·2).
Eye congestion.

Virherpes *Pensa, Spain.*
Aciclovir (p.602·3) or aciclovir sodium (p.602·3).
Herpesvirus infections.

Viridal
Schwarz, Irl.; Schwarz, UK.
Alprostadil alfadex (p.1413·1).
Impotence.

Viridex *Transpharma, Fr.†.*
Arginine (p.1334·1); L-aspartic acid (p.1335·1); L-glutamic acid (p.1344·3).
Asthenia.

Virilon *Star, USA.*
Capsules: Methyltestosterone (p.1450·3).
Injection†: Testosterone cypionate (p.1464·1).
Androgen replacement therapy; breast cancer; male hypogonadism; postpartum breast engorgement; prepubertal cryptorchidism.

Virivac *SBL, Swed.*
A measles, mumps, and rubella vaccine (Enders Edmonston B, Jeryl Lynn B, and RA 27/3 strains respectively) (p.1519·3).
Active immunisation.

Virlix
Synthelabo, Fr.; Mediolanum, Ital.; Lacer, Spain.
Cetirizine hydrochloride (p.404·2).
Hypersensitivity reactions.

Virmen *Menarini, Spain.*
Aciclovir (p.602·3) or aciclovir sodium (p.602·3).
Herpesvirus infections.

Virobin *Bock, Ger.*
Homoeopathic preparation.

Virobis *Ethimed, S.Afr.†.*
Cream: Moroxydine hydrochloride (p.623·1); cetrimide (p.1105·2); diphenhydramine hydrochloride (p.409·1).
Tablets: Moroxydine hydrochloride (p.623·1); atropine methonitrate (p.455·1); hyoscine methonitrate (p.463·1).
Viral infections.

Virofral *Ferrosan, Swed.*
Amantadine hydrochloride (p.1129·2).
Influenza A; parkinsonism.

Viro-Med *Whitehall, USA.*
Chlorpheniramine maleate (p.405·1); dextromethorphan hydrobromide (p.1057·3); paracetamol (p.72·2); pseudoephedrine hydrochloride (p.1068·3).
Coughs and cold symptoms.

Viromidin *Cusi, Spain.*
Trifluridine (p.627·3).
Herpes simplex infections of the eye.

Viron Wart Lotion *Odan, Canad.*
Glacial acetic acid (p.1541·2); lactic acid (p.1593·3); salicylic acid (p.1090·2).
Verrucae.

Vironox *Iketon, Ital.*
Nonoxinol 9 (p.1326·1); chloroxylenol (p.1111·1).
Disinfection.

Viropect *DHU, Ger.*
Homoeopathic preparation.

Virophta *Allergan, Fr.*
Trifluridine (p.627·3).
Viral infections of the eye.

Viroptic
Glaxo Wellcome, Canad.; Glaxo Wellcome, USA; Monarch, USA.
Trifluridine (p.627·3).
Herpesvirus infections.

Virormone *Ferring, UK.*
Testosterone propionate (p.1464·2).
Breast cancer; male hypogonadism.

Virostat *Janssen-Ortho, Canad.*
Edoxudine (p.609·2).
Genital herpes simplex infections.

Virovir *Opus, UK.*
Aciclovir (p.602·3).
Herpesvirus infections.

Virpex *Ayerst, Belg.†.*
Idoxuridine (p.613·2) in dimethyl sulphoxide.
Herpesvirus infections of the skin and genitals.

Virubact *Medisculab, Ger.*
Homoeopathic preparation.

Virucid *Hofmann, Aust.*
Amantadine hydrochloride (p.1129·2).
Influenza A; parkinsonism.

Virucida Idu *Cusi, Spain†.*
Idoxuridine (p.613·2).
Herpes keratitis; herpes keratoconjunctivitis.

Virudermin
Schmidgall, Aust.†; Robugen, Ger.; Renapharm, Switz.
Zinc sulphate (p.1373·2).
Herpes labialis.

Virudin *Bracco, Ital.*
Foscarnet sodium (p.610·2).
Cytomegalovirus retinitis.

Virudox *Bioglan, UK†.*
Idoxuridine (p.613·2) in dimethyl sulphoxide.
Herpes simplex and zoster infections of the skin.

Virulex *Drossapharm, Switz.*
Chelidonium.
Herpes labialis.

Viru-Merz
Kolassa, Aust.; Bio-Therabel, Belg.; Merz, Ger.; Merz, Neth.
Tromantadine hydrochloride (p.628·1).
Herpesvirus infections.

Viru-Merz Serol *Merz, Switz.*
Tromantadine hydrochloride (p.628·1).
Herpesvirus infections of the skin and mucous membranes.

Virunguent
Hermal, Ger.; Hermal, Switz.
Idoxuridine (p.613·2).
Herpes simplex infections of the skin and mucous membranes.

Virunguent-P
Hermal, Ger.; Hermal, Switz.†.
Idoxuridine (p.613·2); prednisolone (p.1048·1).
Herpes simplex infections of the skin and mucous membranes.

Virupos *Ursapharm, Ger.*
Aciclovir (p.602·3).
Herpes simplex eye infections.

Viru-Salvysat *Ysatfabrik, Ger.*
Sage (p.1627·1).
Mouth and throat infections.

Viruseen *Hommel, Ger.*
Aciclovir (p.602·3).
Herpesvirus infections.

Viruserol
Zyma, Ital.; Lacer, Spain.
Tromantadine hydrochloride (p.628·1).
Herpesvirus infections of the skin and mucous membranes.

Virustat
Delagrange, Belg.†; Goupil, Fr.†.
Moroxydine hydrochloride (p.623·1).
Herpesvirus infections.

Virustop *Pulitzer, Ital.*
Inosine pranobex (p.615·2).
Immunodeficiency; viral infections.

Viruxan *Sigma-Tau, Ital.*
Inosine pranobex (p.615·2).
Immunodeficiency; viral infections.

Visadron
Bender, Aust.; Boehringer Ingelheim, Belg.; Basotherm, Ger.; Boehringer Ingelheim, Ital.; Boehringer Ingelheim, Neth.†; Fher, Spain.
Phenylephrine hydrochloride (p.1066·2).
Conjunctival irritation.

Visaline *Novopharma, Switz.*
Buphenine hydrochloride (p.1555·3); betacarotene (p.1335·2); alpha tocopherol (p.1369·1); ascorbic acid (p.1365·2).
Eye disorders.

Visano N *Kade, Ger.*
Meprobamate (p.678·1).
Anxiety disorders; gastro-intestinal disorders; insomnia.

VisanoCor N *Kade, Ger.*
Pentaerythritol tetranitrate (p.927·3); diphenhydramine hydrochloride (p.409·1).
VisanoCor formerly contained pentaerythritol tetranitrate, meprobamate, diphenhydramine hydrochloride, and nicotinic acid.
Cardiac disorders.

Visatear *Pfizer, Canad.*
Macrogol 400 (p.1598·2).
Dry eye.

Viscal *Zoja, Ital.*
Metoclopramide hydrochloride (p.1200·3).
Digestive disorders.

Viscalox *Pharmatec, S.Afr.†.*
Dried aluminium hydroxide gel (p.1177·3); magnesium hydroxide (p.1198·2); simethicone (p.1213·1).
Gastro-intestinal disorders.

Viscasan *Bioforce, Ger.*
Homoeopathic preparation.

Visceralgina *SIT, Ital.†.*
Tiemonium iodide (p.468·3).
Visceral spasms; vomiting.

Visceralgine
Exel, Belg.; Riom, Fr.
Tiemonium iodide (p.468·3) or tiemonium methylsulphate (p.468·3).
Smooth muscle spasms.

Visceralgine Compositum *Exel, Belg.*
Tiemonium iodide (p.468·3); dipyrone (p.35·1); codeine phosphate (p.26·1).
Smooth muscle spasm 1411 2.

Visceralgine Forte *Riom, Fr.*
Injection: Tiemonium methylsulphate (p.468·3); dipyrone (p.35·1).
Suppositories; tablets: Tiemonium methylsulphate (p.468·3); dipyrone (p.35·1); codeine phosphate (p.26·1).
Pain; smooth muscle spasms.

Visclair
Sinclair, Irl.; Sinclair, UK.
Methyl cysteine hydrochloride (p.1064·1).
Bronchitis; respiratory-tract disorders with excessive or viscous mucus.

Viscoat
Alcon, Aust.; Alcon, Austral.; Alcon, Belg.; Alcon, Fr.; Alcon-Thilo, Ger.; Alcon, Ital.; Alcon, S.Afr.; Alcon, Swed.†; Alcon, Switz.; Alcon, UK; Alcon, USA.
Sodium chondroitin (p.1562·2); sodium hyaluronate (p.1630·3).
Adjunct in ocular surgery.

Viscobande *Smith & Nephew, Fr.†.*
Gelatin; glycerol; zinc oxide (p.1096·2).
Skin disorders.

Viscocort *Bournonville, Belg.*
Prednisolone acetate (p.1048·1); chloramphenicol (p.182·1).
Infected inflammatory ear disorders.

Viscolex *Pinewood, Irl.*
Carbocisteine (p.1056·3).
Respiratory-tract disorders with excessive or viscous mucus.

Viscomucil *ABC, Ital.*
Ambroxol hydrochloride (p.1054·3).
Respiratory-tract congestion.

Visconisan N *Hanosan, Ger.*
Homoeopathic preparation.

Viscopaste PB7
Smith & Nephew, Irl.; Smith & Nephew, Ital.; Smith & Nephew, S.Afr.; Smith & Nephew, UK.
Zinc oxide (p.1096·2).
Medicated bandage.

Visc-Ophtal sine *Winzer, Ger.†.*
Hypromellose (p.1473·1).
Dry eyes.

Viscophyll *Meuselbach, Ger.*
Mistletoe (p.1604·1); bladderwrack (p.1554·1).
Circulatory disorders.

Viscor *Ital Suisse, Ital.†.*
Dipyridamole (p.857·1).
Disorders of platelet aggregation.

Viscorapas Duo *Pascoe, Ger.*
Convallaria (p.1567·2); crataegus (p.1568·2).
Heart failure.

Viscotears
Ciba Vision, Austral.; Ciba Vision, Norw.; Ciba Vision, Spain; Ciba Vision, Swed.; Ciba Vision, Switz.; Ciba Vision, UK.
Carbomer 940 (p.1471·2).
Dry eyes.

Viscoteina *Iquinosa, Spain.*
Carbocisteine (p.1056·3).
Respiratory-tract congestion.

Viscotiol
Evans, Fr.; Searle, Ital.
Letosteine (p.1063·2).
Respiratory-tract congestion.

Viscotirs *Ciba Vision, Ital.*
Carbomer (p.1471·2).
Dry eyes.

Viscotraan *Covan, S.Afr.*
Hypromellose (p.1473·1).
Contact lens lubricant; dry eyes.

Viscratyl *DHU, Ger.†.*
Homoeopathic preparation.

Viscum album H *Pfluger, Ger.*
Homoeopathic preparation.

Viscysat *Ysatfabrik, Ger.*
Mistletoe (p.1604·1).
Hypertension.

Visergil
LPB, Ital.; Sandoz, Spain.
Co-dergocrine mesylate (p.1566·1); thioridazine (p.695·1) or thioridazine hydrochloride (p.695·1).
Anxiety with depression; cerebrovascular disorders.

Vi-Siblin
Warner-Lambert, Norw.; Parke, Davis, Swed.
Ispaghula husk (p.1194·2).
Constipation; irritable bowel syndrome.

Vi-Siblin S *Parke, Davis, Swed.*
Ispaghula husk (p.1194·2); sorbitol (p.1354·2).
Constipation; irritable bowel syndrome.

Visidex II *Ames, UK†.*
Test for glucose in blood (p.1585·1).

Visinal *Stada, Ger.*
Valerian (p.1643·1); lupulus (p.1597·2); passion flower (p.1615·3).
Nervous disorders; sleep disorders.

Visine
Pfizer, Austral.; Mack, Belg.; Pfizer, Canad.; Restiva, Ital.; Pfizer, Neth.†; Pfizer, Switz.; Pfizer, USA†.
Tetrahydrozoline hydrochloride (p.1070·2).
Eye irritation.

Visine Allergy
Pfizer, Austral.; Pfizer, Canad.
Tetrahydrozoline hydrochloride (p.1070·2); zinc sulphate (p.1373·2).
Formerly known as Visine Plus in *Austral.* and Visine AC in *Canad.*
Eye irritation.

Visine Allergy Relief *Pfizer, USA.*
Tetrahydrozoline hydrochloride (p.1070·2); zinc sulphate (p.1373·2).
Formerly called Visine AC.
Eye irritation.

Visine LR *Pfizer, USA.*
Oxymetazoline hydrochloride (p.1065·3).
Eye irritation.

Visine Moisturizing
Pfizer, Canad.; Pfizer, USA.
Tetrahydrozoline hydrochloride (p.1070·2); macrogol 400 (p.1598·2).
Formerly called Visine Extra.
Eye irritation.

Visine Revive *Pfizer, Austral.*
Tetrahydrozoline hydrochloride (p.1070·2); macrogol 400 (p.1598·2).
Dry eyes; eye irritation.

Visine True Tears *Pfizer, Canad.*
Macrogol 400 (p.1598·2).

Visine Workplace *Pfizer, Canad.*
Oxymetazoline hydrochloride (p.1065·3).
Formerly known as Visine LR.
Eye irritation.

Visiodose *Cooperation Pharmaceutique, Fr.*
Chlorhexidine gluconate (p.1107·2); phenylephrine hydrochloride (p.1066·2).
Conjunctivitis.

Visioglobina *Morrith, Spain†.*
Ocular antiserum (equine).
Eye disorders.

Visiolyre *Urgo, Fr.*
Cadmium sulphate (p.1555·3); zinc sulphate (p.1373·2); phenylephrine hydrochloride (p.1066·2).
Eye disorders.

Vision Care Enzymatic Cleaner *Alcon, USA.*
Pancreatin (p.1612·1).
Cleansing solution for soft contact lenses.

Visionace *Vitabiotics, UK.*
Vitamin, mineral, and nutrient preparation.
Eye disorders.

Visipaque
Nycomed, Aust.; Sanofi Winthrop, Canad.; Nycomed, Fr.; Nycomed, Ger.; Nycomed, Ital.; Nycomed, Neth.; Nycomed Imaging, Norw.; Nycomed, Spain; Nycomed, Swed.; Nycomed, Switz.; Nycomed, UK; Nycomed, USA.
Iodixanol (p.1006·2).
Radiographic contrast medium.

Viskaldix
Sandoz, Aust.; Sandoz, Belg.; Sandoz, Fr.; Sandoz, Ger.; Sandoz, Irl.; Novartis, Neth.; Wander, S.Afr.†; Sandoz, Switz.; Sandoz, UK.
Pindolol (p.931·1); clopamide (p.844·2).
Hypertension.

Viskazide *Sandoz, Canad.*
Pindolol (p.931·1); hydrochlorothiazide (p.885·2).
Hypertension.

Viskeen *Novartis, Neth.*
Pindolol (p.931·1).
Cardiovascular disorders.

Visken
Sandoz, Aust.; Novartis, Austral.; Sandoz, Belg.; Sandoz, Canad.; Sandoz, Fr.; Wander, Ger.; Sandoz, Irl.; Sandoz, Ital.; Sandoz, Norw.; Novartis, S.Afr.; Novartis, Swed.; Sandoz, UK; Sandoz, USA.
Pindolol (p.931·1).
Angina pectoris; anxiety; arrhythmias; hypertension.

Viskene *Sandoz, Switz.*
Pindolol (p.931·1).
Cardiac disorders; hypertension.

Viskenit
Sandoz, Aust.; Sandoz, Switz.†.
Pindolol (p.931·1); isosorbide dinitrate (p.893·1).
Angina pectoris.

Viskoferm *Nordic, Swed.*
Acetylcysteine (p.1052·3).
Bronchitis.

Visopt *Sigma, Austral.*
Phenylephrine (p.1066·2).
Eye irritation and congestion.

Vispring *Rovifarma, Spain.*
Tetrahydrozoline hydrochloride (p.1070·2).
Conjunctival congestion; eye irritation.

Vistacarpin *Allergan, Ger.*
Pilocarpine hydrochloride (p.1396·3).
Glaucoma; production of miosis.

Vistacon *Hauck, USA†.*
Hydroxyzine hydrochloride (p.412·1).
Anxiety; hypersensitivity reactions.

Vistacrom
Allergan, Austral.†; Allergan, Canad.; Allergan, S.Afr.
Sodium cromoglycate (p.762·1).
Allergic conjunctivitis; vernal keratoconjunctivitis.

Vistafrin *Allergan, Spain.*
Phenylephrine hydrochloride (p.1066·2).
Conjunctival congestion; eye irritation.

Vistagan
Allergan, Aust.; Allergan, Ger.; Allergan, Ital.; Allergan, Switz.
Levobunolol hydrochloride (p.897·3).
Glaucoma; ocular hypertension.

Vistaject *Mayrand, USA†.*
Hydroxyzine hydrochloride (p.412·1).
Anxiety; hypersensitivity reactions.

Vistajunctin *Allergan, Switz.†.*
Neomycin sulphate (p.229·2); polymyxin B sulphate (p.239·1).
Eye infections.

Vistalbalon *Allergan, Ger.*
Naphazoline hydrochloride (p.1064·2).
Eye disorders.

Vista-Methasone *Martindale Pharmaceuticals, UK.*
Betamethasone sodium phosphate (p.1033·3).
NOTE. There is no connection between Martindale, The Complete Drug Reference and Martindale Pharmaceuticals.
Inflammatory disorders of the ear, eye, or nose.

Vista-Methasone N
Daniels, Irl.; Martindale Pharmaceuticals, UK.
Betamethasone sodium phosphate (p.1033·3); neomycin sulphate (p.229·2).
NOTE. There is no connection between Martindale, The Complete Drug Reference and Martindale Pharmaceuticals.
Inflammatory disorders of the ear, eye, or nose with bacterial infection.

Vistamycin *Meiji, Jpn.*
Ribostamycin sulphate (p.242·2).
Bacterial infections.

Vistaquel *Pasadena, USA†.*
Hydroxyzine hydrochloride (p.412·1).
Anxiety; hypersensitivity reactions.

Vistaran *Merck Sharp & Dohme, Spain†.*
Clobetasone butyrate (p.1035·3).
Eye disorders.

Vistaril
Roerig, Swed.†; Roerig, USA.
Hydroxyzine embonate (p.411·3) or hydroxyzine hydrochloride (p.412·1).
Anxiety; premedication; pruritus; sedative.

Vistazine *Keene, USA.*
Hydroxyzine hydrochloride (p.412·1).
Anxiety; hypersensitivity reactions.

Vistide
Pharmacia Upjohn, UK; Gilead, USA.
Cidofovir (p.606·3).
Cytomegalovirus retinitis.

Vistimon *Jenapharm, Ger.*
Mesterolone (p.1450·1).
Androgen deficiency.

Vistofilm *Allergan, Ger.*
Polyvinyl alcohol (p.1474·2).
Wetting solution for contact lenses.

Vistosan *Allergan, Ger.*
Phenylephrine hydrochloride (p.1066·2).
Eye disorders.

Vistoxyn
Allergan, Ger.; Allergan, Switz.
Oxymetazoline hydrochloride (p.1065·3).
Conjunctivitis; eye irritation.

Visual-Eyes *Optopics, USA.*
Electrolyte solution (p.1147·1).
Eye irrigation.

Visublefarite
Pharmec, Ital.; Merck Sharp & Dohme, Spain.
Betamethasone (p.1033·2); sulphacetamide sodium (p.252·2); tetrahydrozoline phosphate (p.1070·3).
Eye disorders.

Visucloben *Pharmec, Ital.*
Clobetasone butyrate (p.1035·3).
Eye disorders.

Visucloben Antibiotico *Merck Sharp & Dohme, Ital.*
Clobetasone butyrate (p.1035·3); bekanamycin sulphate (p.158·2).
Eye inflammation.

Visucloben Decongestionante *Merck Sharp & Dohme, Ital.*
Clobetasone butyrate (p.1035·3); tetrahydrozoline hydrochloride (p.1070·2).
Conjunctivitis.

Visuglican *Merck Sharp & Dohme, Ital.*
Sodium cromoglycate (p.762·1); chlorpheniramine maleate (p.405·1).
Conjunctivitis.

Visumetazone *Merck Sharp & Dohme, Ital.*
Dexamethasone (p.1037·1).
Inflammatory eye disorders.

Visumetazone Antibiotico *Merck Sharp & Dohme, Ital.*
Bekanamycin sulphate (p.158·2); tetrahydrozoline hydrochloride (p.1070·2); betamethasone (p.1033·2).
Eye infections associated with inflammation and congestion.

Visumetazone Antistaminico *Merck Sharp & Dohme, Ital.*
Dexamethasone (p.1037·1); chlorpheniramine maleate (p.405·1).
Conjunctivitis.

Visumetazone Decongestionante *Merck Sharp & Dohme, Ital.*
Dexamethasone (p.1037·1); tetrahydrozoline hydrochloride (p.1070·2).
Conjunctivitis; eye congestion; scleritis.

Visumicina *Pharmec, Ital.*
Bekanamycin sulphate (p.158·2); tetrahydrozoline hydrochloride (p.1070·2).
Bacterial eye infections.

Visumidriatic *Merck Sharp & Dohme, Ital.*
Tropicamide (p.469·2).
Production of mydriasis.

Visumidriatic Antiflogistico *Merck Sharp & Dohme, Ital.*
Betamethasone (p.1033·2); tropicamide (p.469·2).
Inflammatory eye disorders.

Visumidriatic Fenilefrina *Merck Sharp & Dohme, Ital.*
Tropicamide (p.469·2); phenylephrine hydrochloride (p.1066·2).
Production of mydriasis.

Visuphrine N in der Ophtiole *Mann, Ger.†.*
Antazoline hydrochloride (p.401·3).
Eye disorders.

Visustrin *Merck Sharp & Dohme, Ital.*
Tetrahydrozoline hydrochloride (p.1070·2); methylene blue (p.984·3).
Conjunctival oedema; eye irritation; hyperaemia.

Visutensil *Pharmec, Ital.*
Guanethidine monosulphate (p.878·1).
Glaucoma.

Vit Eparin *Teofarma, Ital.*
Heparin sodium (p.879·3); tocopheryl acetate (p.1369·1).
Ocular haemorrhage and its sequelae.

Vita 3
Ciba Vision, Fr.; Ciba Vision, Switz.
Phenylephrine hydrochloride (p.1066·2); rutin sodium sulphate (p.1580·2).
Conjunctivitis; eye irritation.

Vita 21 *Cambridge Laboratories, Austral.†.*
Multivitamin and mineral preparation.

Vita B *Faure, Fr.†.*
Thiamine hydrochloride (p.1361·1); riboflavine (p.1362·1); nicotinamide (p.1351·2).
Eye disorders.

Vita 3B *Riva, Canad.*
Vitamin B substances.

Vita 3B + C *Riva, Canad.*
Vitamin B substances with vitamin C.

Vita B Complex *Nutri-Metics, Canad.*
Vitamin B substances.

Vita B plus C *Romilo, Canad.*
Vitamin B substances and vitamin C.

Vita Bar *Shaklee, Canad.†.*
Dietary supplement.

Vita Bee *Rugby, USA.*
Multivitamin preparation.

Vita Buer-G-plus *Byk Roland, Switz.†.*
Capsules: Multivitamin and mineral preparation with kola and ginseng.
Oral liquid: Multivitamin and mineral preparation with ginseng.
Tonic.

Vita Buerlecithin *Roland, Ger.*
Lecithin (p.1595·2); vitamins.
Tonic.

Vita Buerlecithine *Byk Roland, Switz.†.*
Vitamin B preparation with lecithin (p.1595·2).
Tonic.

Vita Cris *Cris Flower, Ital.*
Multivitamin preparation.
Nutritional supplement.

Vita Day *Jamieson, Canad.*
Multivitamin and mineral preparation.

Vita Disc *Vita Glow, Austral.†.*
Vitamins and minerals; bromelains (p.1555·1); papain (p.1614·1).
Musculoskeletal disorders.

Vita Ferin C *Geistlich, Switz.*
Multivitamin and mineral preparation.

Vita Gerine *Geistlich, Switz.*
Deanol orotate; vitamins; minerals; rutin; choline bitartrate.
Tonic.

Vita Glow Calcium *Vita Glow, Austral.†.*
Pure oyster shell powder; cholecalciferol (p.1366·3).
Calcium deficiency.

Vita Glow Sports Supplement *Vita Glow, Austral.†.*
Combination pack: Multivitamin preparation; mineral preparation.

Vita Menal *Alacan, Spain.*
Cyproheptadine hydrochloride (p.407·2); amino acids; cyanocobalamin; fosforylethanolamine.
Tonic.

Vita Plex *Sante Naturelle, Canad.*
Multivitamin and mineral preparation.

Vita Stress *Vita Pharm, Canad.*
Multivitamin preparation.

Vita Truw *Truw, Ger.*
Multivitamin and mineral preparation.

Vita Vim *Jamieson, Canad.*
Multivitamin and mineral preparation.

Vitabact
Ciba Vision, Fr.; Ciba Vision, Switz.
Picloxydine dihydrochloride (p.1123·1).
Bacterial eye infections.

Vitaber A E *Llorens, Spain.*
Di-isopropylammonium dichloroacetate (p.854·1); vitamin A acetate (p.1359·2); tocopheryl acetate (p.1369·1).
Deficiency of vitamins A and E; eye disorders; habitual abortion; infertility; skin disorders.

Vitaber PP + E *Llorens, Spain.*
Tocopheryl nicotinate (p.1280·1).
Hyperlipidaemias.

Vitabese *Legere, USA†.*
Multivitamin preparation.

Vitabil Composto *IBP, Ital.†.*
Nicotinamide (p.1351·2); inositol (p.1591·1); boldo (p.1554·1); cynara (p.1569·2); frangula (p.1193·2); chelidonium.
Constipation.

Vitableu *Ciba Vision, Fr.*
Methylene blue (p.984·3).
Ocular antiseptic.

Vita-Bob *Scot-Tussin, USA.*
Multivitamin preparation.

Vita-Brachont *Azupharma, Ger.*
Cyanocobalamin (p.1363·3).
Lignocaine hydrochloride (p.1293·2) is included in this preparation to alleviate the pain of injection.
Arthritis; neuralgia; neuritis; vitamin B_{12} deficiency.

Vita-C
Shaklee, Canad.; Freeda, USA.
Ascorbic acid (p.1365·2).
Scurvy; vitamin C deficiency.

Vita-C R15 *Reckeweg, Ger.*
Homoeopathic preparation.

Vita-Cal Plus *Shaklee, Canad.*
Multivitamin and mineral preparation.

VitaCarn *Kendall McGaw, USA.*
Carnitine (p.1336·2).
Carnitine deficiency.

Vitacarpine *Faure, Fr.†.*
Pilocarpine nitrate (p.1396·3).
Glaucoma.

Vitace *Pascoe, Ger.*
Multivitamin preparation.

Vita-Ce *Pharmacal, Switz.*
Ascorbic acid (p.1365·2).
Vitamin C deficiency; vitamin C supplement.

Vitacemil *Soekami, Fr.†.*
Ascorbic acid (p.1365·2).
Vitamin C deficiency.

Vitacic *Ciba Vision, Fr.*
Adenosine (p.812·3); thymidine (p.1637·2); cytidine; uridine (p.1641·3); disodium guanylate (p.1573·1).
Corneal damage.

Vitacim *Cimex, Switz.†.*
d-Alpha tocopherol (p.1369·1).
Vitamin E deficiency.

Vitaclair *Faure, Fr.†.*
Sodium lauryl sulphate (p.1468·3); sodium edetate (p.980·1).
Contact lens cleanser.

Vitacontact *Faure, Fr.†.*
Chlorhexidine gluconate (p.1107·2).
Disinfection of corneal lenses and ocular prostheses.

Vitacrecil *Vinas, Spain.*
Cystine (p.1339·1).
Alopecia; nail disorders; skin disorders.

Vitacuivre *Ipropharm, Fr.†.*
Ascorbic acid (p.1365·2); copper (p.1337·3).

Vitaday Forte *Pharmadex, Canad.†.*
Multivitamin and mineral preparation.

Vitaday Junior *Pharmadex, Canad.†.*
Multivitamin preparation.

Vita-Dermacide *CS, Fr.*
Nicotinamide (p.1351·2); glutamic acid (p.1344·3); tryptophan (p.310·2).
Irritative dermatitis.

Vita-Diem *Seven Seas, UK.*
Multivitamin preparation.

Vitadral *Wernigerode, Ger.*
Vitamin A palmitate (p.1359·2).
Vitamin A deficiency.

Vita-Drops *Pharma Plus, Switz.†.*
Multivitamin preparation.

Vit-A-Drops *Vision, USA.*
Vitamin A (p.1358·1).
Dry eyes.

Vitadye
Dermatech, Austral.; ICN, Canad.†.
Dihydroxyacetone (p.1081·2).
Vitiligo.

Vita-E
Shaklee, Canad.; Bioglan, UK.
Vitamin E (p.1369·1).
Dietary supplement.

Vita-E Plus Selenium *Shaklee, Canad.*
Vitamin E (p.1369·1); selenium (p.1353·3).
Dietary supplement.

Vitaendil C K P *Wasserman, Spain.*
Ascorbic acid (p.1365·2); menadione (p.1370·3); rutin (p.1580·2).
Haemorrhage.

Vitafardi C B12 *Fardi, Spain.*
Ascorbic acid (p.1365·2); hydroxocobalamin (p.1363·3).
Deficiency of vitamins B_{12} and C.

Vitafem *Vita Pharm, Canad.*
Multivitamin and mineral preparation.

Vitafer *Frega, Canad.*
Vitamin B substances and iron.

Vita-Feron *Vitaline, USA.*
Iron (p.1346·1); folic acid (p.1340·3); vitamin B_{12} (p.1363·3).

Vitaferro *LAW, Ger.*
Ferrous sulphate (p.1340·2).
Iron deficiency.

Vitafissan *Uhlmann-Eyraud, Switz.*
Caseine hydrolysate (Labiline); vitamins A, D, and E; linoleic acid (p.1582·1); linolenic acid.
Skin disorders.

Vitafol *Everett, USA.*
Syrup: Ferric pyrophosphate (p.1339·2); folic acid (p.1340·3); vitamin B substances.
Tablets: Ferrous fumarate (p.1339·3); folic acid (p.1340·3); multivitamins and minerals.
Iron-deficiency anaemias.

Vitaforce *Pharma-Natura, S.Afr.†.*
Multivitamin and mineral preparation.

Vitaforce Carotene A *Pharma-Natura, S.Afr.†.*
Betacarotene (p.1335·2).
Vitamin A deficiencies.

Vitaforce Forti-Plus *Pharma-Natura, S.Afr.†.*
Multivitamins; minerals; amino acids; kelp (p.1593·1).

Vitaforce 21-Plus *Pharma-Natura, S.Afr.†.*
Multivitamins; minerals; kelp (p.1593·1); lecithin (p.1595·2); rose fruit (p.1365·2); rutin (p.1580·2); wheatgerm oil; yeast (p.1373·1).

Vitaforce Sylvacal *Pharma-Natura, S.Afr.†.*
Cuttle-fish bone.
Calcium supplement.

Vitagama Fluor *Almirall, Spain.*
Sodium fluoride (p.742·1); multivitamins and minerals.
Vitamin and fluoride deficiencies.

Vitagama Fluor Complex *Almirall, Spain.*
Multivitamin preparation with ferrous sulphate (p.1340·2).
Vitamin and iron deficiency.

Vita-Gard *Neo-Life, Austral.*
Multivitamin and mineral preparation.

Vita-Gerin
Chemomedica, Aust.; Cassella-med, Ger.
Deanol orotate; magnesium orotate; vitamins; minerals; rutin; adenosine; choline bitartrate.
Tonic.

Vitaglow Executive Anti Stress *Vita Glow, Austral.†.*
Scutellaria; passion flower (p.1615·3); lupulus (p.1597·2); vitamin B substances and ascorbic acid.
Anxiety; pain; stress; tension.

Vitaglow Herbal Laxative *Vita Glow, Austral.†.*
Aloes (p.1177·1); cascara (p.1183·1); senna (p.1212·2); ginger (p.1193·2); cardamom (p.1560·1); peppermint oil (p.1208·1).
Constipation.

Vitaglow Herbal Stress *Vita Glow, Austral.†.*
Valerian (p.1643·1); scutellaria; mistletoe (p.1604·1); passion flower (p.1615·3); lupulus (p.1597·2); avena (p.1551·3).
Anxiety; stress; tension.

Vitaglow Primetime *Vita Glow, Austral.†.*
Multivitamin and mineral preparation.
Dietary supplement.

Vitaglow Selemite B Tablets *Vita Glow, Austral.*
Selenium (p.1353·3); dried yeast (p.1373·1).
Selenium deficiency.

Vitaglow Smoke Stop *Vita Glow, Austral.†.*
Homoeopathic preparation.

Vitagutt Knoblauch *Schwarzhaupt, Ger.*
Garlic oil.
Circulatory disorders.

Vitagutt Vitamin E *Schwarzhaupt, Ger.*
dl-Alpha tocopheryl acetate (p.1369·2).
Vitamin E deficiency.

Vita-Hefe S *Fides, Ger.†.*
Echinacea ang.; fagopyrum; hepar sulf.; silicea; sulfur; dried yeast.

Vita-Hexin *Streuli, Switz.*
Chlorhexidine gluconate (p.1107·2); vitamin A palmitate (p.1359·2); cod-liver oil (p.1337·3); zinc oxide (p.1096·2).
Skin lesions.

Vita-Iodurol *Ciba Vision, Fr.*
Potassium iodide (p.1493·1); calcium chloride (p.1155·1); magnesium chloride (p.1157·2); cysteine hydrochloride (p.1338·3); glutathione (p.983·1); thiamine hydrochloride (p.1361·1); nicotinic acid (p.1351·2).
Cataract.

Vita-Iodurol ATP *Ciba Vision, Fr.*
Potassium iodide (p.1493·1); calcium chloride (p.1155·1); magnesium chloride (p.1157·2); cysteine hydrochloride (p.1338·3); glutathione (p.983·1); thiamine hydrochloride (p.1361·1); nicotinic acid (p.1351·2); adenosine triphosphate sodium (p.1543·2).
Cataract.

Vitaject *Syxyl, Ger.*
Thiamine hydrochloride (p.1361·1); pyridoxine hydrochloride (p.1362·3); cyanocobalamin (p.1363·3).
Vitamin B deficiency.

Vita-Kid
Solgar, UK; Solgar, USA.
Multivitamin preparation.

Vital *Lalco, Canad.*
Multivitamin and mineral preparation.

Vital Eyes
Note. This name is used for preparations of different composition.
Ciba Vision, UK.
Lavender (p.1594·3); orange flower; hamamelis (p.1587·1); euphrasia.
Eye irritation.

Allergan, USA.
A multivitamin and mineral preparation.

Vital Floramin *Bennett, UK.*
Mineral preparation.
Immune stimulant.

Vital High Nitrogen *Ross, USA.*
Lactose-free preparation for enteral nutrition.

Vital HN
Abbott, Austral.; Abbott, Canad.
Preparation for enteral nutrition.

Vitalag *Lagap, Switz.†.*
Multivitamin preparation.

Vit-Alboform *Merckle, Ger.†.*
Cyanocobalamin (p.1363·3).
Vitamin B deficiency.

Vital-Dragees (Rowo-540) *Pharmakon, Ger.†.*
Colae; muira puama; ferr. pomat.; nuphar luteum; agnus cast.; eryngium; caladium; calc. glycerinophosph.; ferr. glycerinophosph.; ferr. peptonat.; chinin ferrocitric.; magnes. hypophosphoric.; natr. hypophosphoric.; lecithinium ex ovo; testes; cerebellum; medulla ossium rubra; hypophysis cerebri; acid. picronitric.; cantharis; natr. formicic.
Tonic.

Vita-Lea *Shaklee, Canad.*
Multivitamin and mineral preparation.
Dietary supplement.

Vitaleph *Aleph, Ital.*
Nutritional supplement.

Vitalerina *Polifarma, Ital.†.*
Multivitamin preparation.

Vitalets *Freeda, USA.*
Multivitamin and mineral preparation with iron.

Vitalgine *Medecine Vegetale, Fr.*
Hamamelis (p.1587·1); viburnum.
Haemorrhoids; peripheral vascular disorders.

Vitaline *Bioglan, Austral.*
Lysine (p.1350·1); zinc oxide (p.1096·2).
Herpes simplex lesions.

Vitalion *Biagini, Ital.†.*
Inosine (p.1591·1); cyanocobalamin (p.1363·3); ascorbic acid (p.1365·2); suprarenal cortex (p.1050·1).
Lignocaine (p.1293·2) is included in this preparation to alleviate the pain of injection.
Liver disorders; tonic.

Vitalipid
Pharmacia Upjohn, Belg.; Pharmacia Upjohn, Ger.; Pharmacia Upjohn, Ital.; Pharmacia, Neth.†; Pharmacia Upjohn, Norw.; Pharmacia Upjohn, S.Afr.; Pharmacia Upjohn, Swed.
Vitamins A, D_2, E, and K_1 for infusion.
Parenteral nutrition.

Vitalipid N
Baxter, Austral.; Pharmacia Upjohn, Switz.
Vitamins A, D_2, E, and K_1 for infusion.
Parenteral nutrition.

Vitalipid Neu *Pharmacia Upjohn, Aust.*
Vitamins A, D, E, and K for infusion.
Contains egg lipid.
Parenteral nutrition.

Vitalipide *Pharmacia Upjohn, Fr.*
Vitamins A, D_2, E, and K_1 for infusion.
Parenteral nutrition.

Vitalize *Scot-Tussin, USA.*
Ferric pyrophosphate (p.1339·2); vitamin B substances with L-lysine.
Iron-deficiency anaemias.

Vital-Kapseln *Ratiopharm, Ger.*
Eleutherococcus senticosis (p.1584·2).
Tonic.

Vitalmix *Montefarmaco, Ital.*
Myrtillus (p.1606·1); eleutherococcus (p.1584·2); soya; royal jelly (p.1626·3); wheat germ; extract of citrus fruits; honey (p.1345·3); fructose (p.1343·2).
Nutritional supplement.

Vitalux
Ciba Vision, Fr.; Ciba Vision, Ital.
A multivitamin and mineral preparation.
Eye disorders.

Vitalyt *Polcopharma, Austral.†.*
Garlic (p.1583·1); wheat germ.

Vitamag *Columbia, S.Afr.*
Vitamin B substances; magnesium; zinc.
Vitamin and mineral supplement.

Vitamax *Medosan, Ital.†.*
Multivitamin preparation.

Vita-Mefren *Zyma, Belg.*
Chlorhexidine gluconate (p.1107·2); vitamin A palmitate (p.1359·2).
Burns; infected skin disorders; wounds.

Vitamen *Beta, Ital.*
Protein and multivitamin preparation.

Vita-Merfen *Zyma, Switz.†.*
Phenylmercuric borate (p.1122·2); cod-liver oil (p.1337·3).
Skin disorders.

Vita-Merfen N *Zyma, Ger.†.*
Phenylmercuric acetate (p.1122·2); halibut-liver oil (p.1345·3).
Skin disorders.

Vita-Merfen (nouveau) *Max Ritter, Switz.*
Chlorhexidine gluconate (p.1107·2); benzoxonium chloride (p.1103·3); vitamin A (p.1358·1).
Minor wounds and burns.

Vitamfenicolo *Allergan, Ital.*
Chloramphenicol (p.182·1) or chloramphenicol sodium succinate (p.182·2).
Bacterial eye infections.

Vitamin B 15 *Kattwiga, Ger.†.*
Thiamine hydrochloride (p.1361·1); sodium pangamate (p.1614·1).
Vitamin B deficiency.

Vitamin B12 forte *Hevert, Ger.*
Cyanocobalamin (p.1363·3).
Vitamin B deficiency.

Vitamin C *Lane, UK.*
Rose fruit (p.1365·2); acerola cherry (p.1001·1); ascorbic acid (p.1365·2).
Formerly known as Top C.
Vitamin C deficiency.

Vitamin C-Calcium *Herbrand, Ger.*
Calcium carbonate (p.1182·1); ascorbic acid (p.1365·2).
Calcium deficiency; cold symptoms.

Vitamin F *Klosterfrau, Aust.*
Ethyl linoleate.
Skin disorders; wounds.

Vitamina F99 Topica *Vitafarma, Spain.*
Peru balsam (p.1617·2); vitamin F.
Skin disorders.

Vitaminas Lorenzini *Maxfarma, Spain.*
Multivitamin and mineral preparation with ginseng.

Vitamine 15 *Solco, Switz.*
Multivitamin and mineral preparation.

Vitamine F99 *Doetsch, Grether, Switz.*
Ethyl linoleate; ethyl linolenate.
Burns; skin disorders; wounds.

Vitamineral *ACO, Swed.*
Multivitamin and mineral preparation.

Vitaminex *Ferrer, Spain.*
Nucleosides; vitamins.
Tonic.

Vitaminic A-D *Asta Medica, Belg.*
Vitamin A (p.1358·1); ergocalciferol (p.1367·1).
Conjunctivitis; corneal burns and wounds; dry eyes.

Vitaminol *Bio-Sante, Canad.*
Multivitamin and mineral preparation.

Vitaminorum *Sigma, Austral.*
Multivitamin preparation.

Vitamins Only *Solgar, UK.*
Multivitamin preparation.

Vitamorrhuine *Medgenix, Belg.*
Cod-liver oil (p.1337·3); vitamin A acetate (p.1359·2); cholecalciferol (p.1366·3).
Burns; skin disorders; wounds.

Vitamucin B Complesso *Salfa, Ital.†.*
Intrinsic factor; vitamin B complex.
Anaemias.

Vitamucin con Ferro *Salfa, Ital.†.*
Intrinsic factor; cyanocobalamin (p.1363·3); crystalline ferrous sulphate (p.1340·2); ascorbic acid (p.1365·2); folic acid (p.1340·3).
Anaemias.

Vitamucin Semplice *Salfa, Ital.†.*
Intrinsic factor; cyanocobalamin (p.1363·3).
Anaemias.

Vitan *Antigen, Irl.*
Multivitamin or multivitamin and mineral preparation.

Vit-A-N *Farmigea, Ital.*
Vitamin A acetate (p.1359·2).
Corneal ulcer; keratitis; keratoconjunctivitis.

Vitanal *Klever, Ger.†.*
Liquorice; saponaria; senna; parietaria; melissa; frangula bark; fennel; coriander; viola; sassafras; consolida maj.; rad. gei urbani; ginseng; cinchona bark; vitamins.
Tonic.

Vitaneed
Wyeth-Ayerst, Canad.†; Sherwood, USA.
Preparation for enteral nutrition.

Vitanevril Fort *Clin Midy, Fr.†.*
Benfotiamine (p.1360·3).
Vitamin B_1 deficiency.

Vitantial *Delagrange, Spain†.*
Thiamine hydrochloride (p.1361·1).
Vitamin B_1 deficiency.

Vitanumonyl *Teral, USA.*
Injection: Vitamin A palmitate (p.1359·2); ergocalciferol (p.1367·1); cineole (p.1564·1).
Oral liquid: Potassium guaiacolsulfonate (p.1068·3); dextromethorphan hydrobromide (p.1057·3); mepyramine maleate (p.414·1); phenylephrine hydrochloride (p.1066·2).
Coughs.

Vitanumonyl Pediatric *Teral, USA.*
Dextromethorphan hydrobromide (p.1057·3); phenylephrine hydrochloride (p.1066·2).
Coughs.

Vitapan *Provita, Aust.*
Cod-liver oil (p.1337·3); cholecalciferol (p.1366·3).
Vitamin A and D deficiency.

Vitapantol *Davigo, Belg.*
Calcium pantothenate (p.1352·3); vitamin A acetate (p.1359·2); nicotinamide (p.1351·2).
Nasal disorders.

Vitaphakol
Ciba Vision, Fr.; Cusi, Spain; Ciba Vision, Switz.
Cytochrome C (p.1570·1); sodium succinate (p.1632·1); adenosine (p.812·3); nicotinamide (p.1351·2); sorbitol (p.1354·2).
Cataracts.

Vitaphakol N *Ciba Vision, Ger.†.*
Adenosine (p.812·3); cytochrome C (p.1570·1); nicotinamide (p.1351·2).
Cataracts.

Vitaplex
Provita, Aust.; Kabi, Swed.†.
Multivitamin preparation.

Vitaplex comp *Pharmacia Upjohn, Swed.*
Multivitamin preparation with iron.

Vitaplex Digestive Enzyme Formula *Vitaplex, Austral.†.*
Bromelains (p.1555·1); papain (p.1614·1); pancreatin (p.1612·1); betaine hydrochloride (p.1553·2); liquorice (p.1197·1).

Vitaplex mineral *Pharmacia Upjohn, Swed.*
Multivitamin and mineral preparation.

Vitaplex PMT *Vitaplex, Austral.†.*
Vitamin B substances; minerals; leonurus cardiaca (p.1604·2); buchu (p.1555·2).
Premenstrual syndrome.

Vita-Plus *Scot-Tussin, USA.*
A range of vitamin and mineral preparations.

Vitaplus B Plus *Mer-National, S.Afr.*
Vitamin B substances; vitamin C; calcium.
Vitamin and calcium supplement.

Vitaplus C Plus *Mer-National, S.Afr.*
Ascorbic acid (p.1365·2); calcium (p.1155·1).
Vitamin C and calcium deficiencies.

Vita-Plus E *Scot-Tussin, USA.*
Vitamin E (p.1369·1).
Vitamin E deficiency.

Vita-PMS *Bajamar, USA.*
Multivitamin and mineral preparation.

Vitarex *Pasadena, USA.*
Multivitamin and mineral preparation with iron.

Vitargenol *Ciba Vision, Fr.*
Silver protein (p.1629·3).
Eye disorders.

Vitarnin *Grossmann, Switz.*
Multivitamin and mineral preparation.

Vitarubin *Streuli, Switz.*
Cyanocobalamin (p.1363·3) or hydroxocobalamin acetate (p.1364·2).
Anaemias; neurological disorders; vitamin B_{12} deficiency.

Vitarutine *Ciba Vision, Fr.*
Rutin sodium sulphate (p.1580·2); nicotinamide (p.1351·2).
Eye disorders.

Vitasana-Lebenstropfen *Hotz, Ger.*
Gentian; calamus; menyanthes; melissa; achillea; peppermint leaf; crataegus; rosemary; rue; lupulus; valerian; juniper; aniseed; fennel; caraway; herba marjoranae.
Tonic.

Vita-Schlanktropfen *Schuck, Ger.*
Cathine hydrochloride (p.1478·1).
Formerly contained cathine hydrochloride, caffeine sodium benzoate, nikethamide, and vitamin B substances.
Obesity.

Vitascorbol *Theraplix, Fr.*
Ascorbic acid (p.1365·2) with or without sodium ascorbate (p.1365·2).
Vitamin C deficiency.

Vitasedine *Ciba Vision, Fr.*
Phenylephrine hydrochloride (p.1066·2); zinc sulphate (p.1373·2).
Eye disorders.

Vitaseptine *Ciba Vision, Fr.*
Sulphacetamide sodium (p.252·2).
Formerly contained sulphacetamide sodium, zinc sulphate, sodium iodide, and nicotinamide.
Eye infections.

Vitaseptol *Ciba Vision, Fr.*
Thiomersal (p.1126·3).
Ocular antiseptic.

Vitasic
Germania, Aust.; Wider, Ger.†.
Adenosine (p.812·3); thymidine (p.1637·2); cytidine; uridine (p.1641·3); disodium guanylate (p.1573·1).
Eye disorders.

VitaSohn *Antonetto, Ital.*
Multivitamin and mineral preparation.

Vitasol *Faure, Fr.†.*
Sodium chloride (p.1162·2).
Contact lens care.

Vitasprint *Poli, Ital.*
DL-Phosphoserine; cyanocobalamin (p.1363·3); levoglutamide (p.1344·3).
Tonic.

Vitasprint B_{12} *Brenner-Efeka, Ger.; LAW, Ger.*
Levoglutamide (p.1344·3); DL-phosphoserine; cyanocobalamin (p.1363·3).
Vitamin B deficiency.

Vitasprint Complex
Poli, Ital.; Poli, Switz.
L-Phosphoserine; arginine hydrochloride (p.1334·1); L-phosphothreonine; levoglutamide (p.1344·3); hydroxocobalamin (p.1363·3).
Tonic.

Vita-Squares *Neo-Life, Austral.*
Multivitamin and mineral preparation.

Vitatabs *Lederle, Switz.†.*
Multivitamin preparation.

Vitathion
Note. This name is used for preparations of different composition.
Eutherapie, Belg.
Ascorbic acid (p.1365·2); glutathione (p.983·1); adenosine triphosphate (p.1543·2); thiamine (p.1361·2); inositocalcium; haemoglobin (p.723·3).
Asthenia; vitamin deficiency.

Servier, Fr.
Ascorbic acid (p.1365·2); thiamine hydrochloride (p.1361·1); inositocalcium.
Asthenia.

Vita-Thion *Servier, S.Afr.*
Vitamins; glutathione; haemoglobin; sodium adenosine triphosphate; calcium inositol hexaphosphate.
Tonic.

Vitathion-ATP *Servier, Canad.*
Ascorbic acid (p.1365·2); adenosine triphosphate (p.1543·2); calcium inositohexaphosphate; glutathione (p.983·1); haemoglobin (p.723·3); magnesium inositohexaphosphate; thiamine (p.1361·2).
Stress conditions.

Vitathone *Seton, UK†.*
Methyl nicotinate (p.55·1).
Chilblains.

Vitatona *Brauer, Austral.*
Angelica; ascorbic acid (p.1365·2); cola nitida (p.1645·1); vitamin B substances; hypericum (p.1590·1); ginseng (p.1584·2); urtica urens (p.1642·3); aurum muriaticum; calcarea phosphorica; ferrum metallicum; ferrum phosphoricum; kali phosphoricum; magnesia phosphorica; phosphoric acid.
Tonic.

Vitatonin *Pharmacia Upjohn, Swed.*
Multivitamins; caffeine (p.749·3); vin. vermuth.; alcohol.
Tonic.

Vitatropine *Faure, Fr.†.*
Atropine sulphate (p.455·1).
Ocular inflammatory disorders; production of cycloplegia.

Vitavox Pastillas *Escaned, Spain.*
Camphor (p.1557·2); cineole (p.1564·1); chlorophyll (p.1000·1); ephedrine hydrochloride (p.1059·3); niaouli oil (p.1607·1); menthol (p.1600·2); sulphanilamide sodium mesylate (p.256·3); peppermint (p.1208·1).
Mouth and throat inflammation.

Vitawund *Zyma, Aust.*
Chlorhexidine gluconate (p.1107·2); halibut-liver oil (p.1345·3).
Burns; wounds.

Vitaxicam *Robert, Spain.*
Piroxicam (p.80·2).
Gout; musculoskeletal, joint, peri-articular, and soft-tissue disorders; pain.

Vitazell *Tosse, Ger.†.*
Multivitamin preparation.

Vita-Zinc *Vitaplex, Austral.†.*
Zinc gluconate (p.1373·2); vitamins and minerals.
Zinc deficiency.

Vitazinc *Ciba Vision, Fr.*
Zinc sulphate (p.1373·2).
Formerly contained zinc sulphate and thiamine hydrochloride.
Ocular antiseptic.

Viteax *Medinova, Switz.†.*
Vitamin A acetate (p.1359·2); tocopheryl acetate (p.1369·1).
Dietary supplement; vitamin A deficiency.

Vitec *Pharmaceutical Specialties, USA.*
dl-Alpha tocopheryl acetate (p.1369·2).
Skin disorders.

Vitecaf *SIFI, Ital.*
Eye drops: Rolitetracycline (p.247·1); chloramphenicol (p.182·1).
Eye ointment: Tetracycline hydrochloride (p.259·1); chloramphenicol (p.182·1); calcium pantothenate (p.1352·3).
Infected eye disorders.

Vitef *Teofarma, Ital.*
Polyenacid.
Skin disorders.

Vitenur *Nycomed, Ger.†.*
Acetylcysteine (p.1052·3).
Formerly contained theophylline, ephedrine hydrochloride, and guaiphenesin.
Respiratory-tract disorders with viscous mucus.

Viteril *Panthox & Burck, Ital.†.*
Vitamin E (p.1369·1).
Hypertension; lactation insufficiency; male infertility; muscular disorders; threatened and habitual abortion.

Viternum *Juste, Spain.*
Cyproheptadine pyridoxal phosphate (p.407·3).
Allergic rhinitis; anorexia; urticaria.

Viterra
Restiva, Ital.; Pfizer, Spain.
Multivitamin and mineral preparation.

Vitestable *Alcor, Spain.*
Royal jelly; ginseng; tocopherol.
Tonic.

Vithera *Roerig, Belg.†.*
Multivitamin and mineral preparation.

Vitialgin *Boots Healthcare, Ital.*
Propyphenazone (p.81·3); paracetamol (p.72·2).
Fever; pain.

Vitinoin *Pharmascience, Canad.*
Tretinoin (p.1093·3).
Acne.

Vitintra
Kabi Pharmacia, Ger.†; Pharmacia Upjohn, Neth.
Multivitamin infusion.
Parenteral nutrition.

Vitiron *Mepha, Switz.*
Multivitamin, mineral, and amino-acid preparation.

Vitiveine *Arkopharma, Fr.*
Red vine.
Haemorrhoids; peripheral vascular disorders.

Vitlan *Marco Viti, Ital.†.*
Wool fat (p.1385·3).
Barrier cream; moisturiser.

Vitlipid N
Pharmacia Upjohn, Irl.; Pharmacia Upjohn, UK.
Vitamins A, D_2, E, and K_1 for infusion.
Parenteral nutrition.

Vito Bronches *Duchesnay, Canad.*
Diphenylpyraline hydrochloride (p.409·3); dextromethorphan hydrobromide (p.1057·3); potassium iodide (p.1493·1); sodium citrate (p.1153·2).

Vit-O_2 (Vitozwei) *Voigt, Ger.†.*
Amphetaminil (p.1477·3); inositol nicotinate (p.891·3).
Tonic.

Vitobasan N *BASF, Ger.*
Thiamine hydrochloride (p.1361·1); pyridoxine hydrochloride (p.1362·3).
Nervous system disorders.

Vitobronchial *Biotrading, Ital.†.*
Potassium guaiacolsulfonate (p.1068·3); ephedrine hydrochloride (p.1059·3).
Catarrh; coughs.

Vitogen *Stanley, Canad.*
A range of vitamin preparations with or without minerals.

Vitogen Spectrum *Shoppers Drug Mart, Canad.*
Multivitamin and mineral preparation.

Vit-o-Mar *Asta Medica, Ger.*
Silybum marianum (p.993·3).
Liver disorders.

Viton *Menadier, Ger.†.*
Halibut-liver oil (p.1345·3).
Vitamin A and D deficiency.

Vitosal *Ziethen, Ger.*
Vitamins; rutoside sulphuric acid ester sodium salt (p.1580·2); arnica (p.1550·3); sage (p.1627·1); peppermint oil (p.1208·1).
Gum disorders.

Vit-Porphyrin *Teofarma, Ital.*
Haematoporphyrin dihydrochloride (p.1587·1); nicotinamide (p.1351·2).
Tonic.

Vitrace *Columbia, S.Afr.*
Multivitamin and mineral preparation.
Tonic.

Vitraday *Lifeplan, UK.*
Multinutrient preparation.

Vitrafem *Lifeplan, UK.*
Multinutrient preparation.

Vitrasert
Chiron, UK; Chiron, USA.
Ganciclovir (p.612·3).
Cytomegalovirus retinitis.

Vitravene *Isis, USA.*
Fomivirsen sodium.
Cytomegalovirus retinitis.

Vitrax *Allergan, Fr.*
Sodium hyaluronate (p.1630·3).
Adjunct in eye surgery.

Vitreolent *Ciba Vision, Switz.*
Potassium iodide (p.1493·1); sodium iodide (p.1493·2).
Eye disorders.

Vitreolent N *Ciba Vision, Ger.†.*
Potassium iodide (p.1493·1); sodium iodide (p.1493·2).
Cataracts.

Vitreolent Plus *Ciba Vision, Ger.*
Cytochrome C (p.1570·1); adenosine (p.812·3); nicotinamide (p.1351·2).
Cataracts.

Vitreosan *DMG, Ital.*
Potassium bicarbonate; magnesium chloride; vitamin C.
Nutritional supplement.

Vitrimix
Pharmacia Upjohn, Norw.; Pharmacia Upjohn, Swed.; Pharmacia Upjohn, Switz.
Amino-acid, glucose, and lipid (from soya oil (p.1355·1)) infusion.
Contains fractionated egg lecithin.
Parenteral nutrition.

Vitrimix KV
Pharmacia Upjohn, Fr.; Pharmacia Upjohn, Irl.; Pharmacia Upjohn, Neth.; Pharmacia Upjohn, UK.
Amino acid, carbohydrate, and lipid (from soya oil (p.1355·1)) infusion.
Contains fractionated egg phospholipids.
Parenteral nutrition.

Vitrite *Seven Seas, UK.*
Multivitamin preparation.

Vitron-C *Ciba, USA†.*
Ferrous fumarate (p.1339·3).
Ascorbic acid (p.1365·2) is included in this preparation to increase the absorption and availability of iron.
Iron-deficiency anaemias.

Vitrosups *Llorens, Spain.*
Glycerol (p.1585·2).
Constipation; laxative dependence.

Vit-u-pept *Plantina, Ger.*
Weisskohl; bismuth subcarbonate (p.1180·1); heavy magnesium carbonate (p.1198·1); sodium bicarbonate (p.1153·2).
Gastro-intestinal disorders.

Vivactil *Merck Sharp & Dohme, USA.*
Protriptyline hydrochloride (p.306·3).
Depression.

Viva-Drops *Ocusoft, USA.*
Polysorbate 80 (p.1327·3); vitamin A palmitate (p.1359·2).
Dry eyes.

Vival *Alpharma, Norw.*
Diazepam (p.661·1).
Alcohol withdrawal syndrome; anxiety; convulsions; premedication; sedative; skeletal muscle spasm; sleep disorders.

Vivalan
Zeneca, Belg.; Menarini, Belg.; Zeneca, Fr.; Zeneca, Ger.; Zeneca, UK.
Viloxazine hydrochloride (p.312·1).
Depression.

Vivalen *Sanofi Winthrop, Spain†.*
Adenosine phosphate; vitamins; calcium gluceptate; lysine hydrochloride; potassium aspartate; hypophosphorous acid.
Hypocalcaemia; tonic.

Vivamyne *Whitehall, Fr.*
Multivitamin and mineral preparation.

Vivapryl *Asta Medica, UK.*
Selegiline hydrochloride (p.1144·2).
Parkinsonism.

Vivarin *SmithKline Beecham Consumer, USA.*
Caffeine (p.749·3).
Fatigue.

Vivarint
Zeneca, Aust.; Zeneca, Spain.
Viloxazine hydrochloride (p.312·1).
Depression.

Vivatec
Merck Sharp & Dohme, Norw.; Merck Sharp & Dohme, Swed.
Lisinopril (p.898·2).
Heart failure; hypertension; myocardial infarction.

Vivatec Comp *Merck Sharp & Dohme, Norw.*
Lisinopril (p.898·2); hydrochlorothiazide (p.885·2).
Hypertension.

Vivelle
Ciba, Canad.; Ciba, USA.
Oestradiol (p.1455·1).
Menopausal disorders; oestrogen deficiency; osteoporosis.

Vivena HA *Dieterba, Ital.*
Infant feed.
Cow's milk intolerance.

Vivene *Aerocid, Fr.*
Aesculus (p.1543·3); troxerutin (p.1580·2).
Formerly contained buphenine hydrochloride, aesculus, troxerutin.
Haemorrhoids; peripheral vascular disorders.

Vivicil *Andreu, Spain†.*
Netilmicin (p.231·2).
Bacterial infections.

Vividrin
Riel, Aust.; Tramedico, Belg.; Mann, Ger.; Mann, Irl.; Mann, Neth.; Bausch & Lomb, S.Afr.; Novex Pharma, UK.
Sodium cromoglycate (p.762·1).
Allergic conjunctivitis; allergic rhinitis; asthma.

Vividrin comp *Mann, Ger.*
Sodium cromoglycate (p.762·1); xylometazoline hydrochloride (p.1071·2).
Allergic rhinitis.

Vividrin mit Terfenadin *Mann, Ger.*
Terfenadine (p.418·1).
Hypersensitivity reactions.

Vividyl *Lilly, Ital.*
Nortriptyline hydrochloride (p.300·2).
Depression.

Vivimed
Note. This name is used for preparations of different composition.
Riel, Aust.
Propyphenazone (p.81·3); paracetamol (p.72·2); caffeine (p.749·3).
Fever; pain.

Mann, Ger.
Paracetamol (p.72·2).
Fever; pain.

Mann, Irl.
Paracetamol (p.72·2); caffeine (p.749·3).
Pain.

Vivin C
Menarini, Ital.; Alter, Spain.
Aspirin (p.16·1); ascorbic acid (p.1365·2).
Cold and influenza symptoms; fever; pain.

Vivinox
Note. This name is used for preparations of different composition.
Riel, Aust.
Valerian (p.1643·1); lupulus (p.1597·2); mistletoe (p.1604·1).
Anxiety disorders.

Mann, Ger.
Valerian (p.1643·1); lupulus (p.1597·2); passion flower (p.1615·3).
Nervous disorders.

Vivinox Stark *Mann, Ger.*
Diphenhydramine hydrochloride (p.409·1).
Sleep disorders.

Vivinox-Schlafdragees *Mann, Ger.*
Diphenhydramine hydrochloride (p.409·1); valerian (p.1643·1); lupulus (p.1597·2).
Sleep disorders.

Vivioptal
Mann, Irl.; Pharma-Global, UK.
Multivitamin and mineral preparation.

Viviplus *Mann, Ger.*
Hypericum (p.1590·1).
Anxiety; depression.

ViviRhin S *Mann, Ger.*
Xylometazoline hydrochloride (p.1071·2).
Nasal congestion.

Vivisun *Mann, Ger.*
Diphenhydramine hydrochloride (p.409·1); laureth 9 (p.1325·2).
Hypersensitivity reactions of the skin.

Vivol *Carter Horner, Canad.*
Diazepam (p.661·1).
Anxiety; sedative.

Vivonex
Sandoz Nutrition, Canad.; Procter & Gamble, USA.
Preparation for enteral nutrition.

Vivotif
Kwizda, Aust.; Berna, Belg.; Berna, Canad.; Hormosan, Ger.; Evans Medical, Irl.; Berna, Ital.; Berna, Norw.; Swisspharm, S.Afr.; Berna, Spain; Cortec, Swed.; Berna, Switz.; Medeva, UK; Berna, USA.
A live oral typhoid vaccine (p.1536·3).
Active immunisation.

Vivox *Nativelle, Ital.†.*
Pyridoxal phosphate (p.1363·1).
Pyridoxine deficiency.

Vivural *Procter & Gamble, Ger.*
Calcium carbonate (p.1182·1).
Calcium deficiency.

Vi-Zac *UCB, USA.*
Multivitamin and mineral preparation.

Vizam *Amrad, Austral.*
Doxycycline hydrochloride (p.202·3).
Bacterial infections; malaria.

Vizax *Essex, Ital.*
Isepamicin (p.218·1).
Bacterial infections.

Viz-On *Opus, UK.*
Sodium cromoglycate (p.762·1).
Allergic conjunctivitis.

V-Lax *Century, USA.*
Psyllium hydrophilic mucilloid (p.1194·2).
Constipation.

Vlemasque *Rhone-Poulenc Rorer, Canad.†.*
Sulphurated lime (p.1091·3).
Acne.

VM-2000 *Solgar, UK.*
Multivitamin and mineral preparation.

Voalla *Maruho, Jpn.*
Dexamethasone valerate (p.1037·3).
Skin disorders.

Vobaderm *Hermal, Ger.†.*
Fluprednidene acetate (p.1042·2).
Skin disorders.

Vobaderm Basiscreme *Hermal, Ger.†.*
Colloidal silicon dioxide (p.1475·1); medium-chain triglycerides; glycerol monostearate; liquid paraffin; propylene glycol; polysorbate 40; cetostearyl alcohol; sorbic acid; white soft paraffin.
Skin disorders.

Vobaderm Plus *Hermal, Ger.†.*
Cream; topical paste: Fluprednidene acetate (p.1042·2); chlorquinaldol (p.185·1).
Tincture: Fluprednidene acetate (p.1042·2); coal tar (p.1092·3).
Skin disorders.

Vocadys *Chemineau, Fr.*
Codeine (p.26·1); lignocaine hydrochloride (p.1293·2); erysimum.
Formerly contained codeine, amethocaine hydrochloride, and aconite.
Sore throat.

Vocalzone *Kestrel, UK.*
Menthol (p.1600·2); peppermint oil (p.1208·1); myrrh (p.1606·1); liquorice (p.1197·1).
Throat irritation.

Vogalen *Italfarmaco, Spain†.*
Metopimazine (p.1202·3).
Nausea and vomiting; vestibular disorders.

Vogalene
Rhone-Poulenc Rorer, Belg.; Schwarz, Fr.
Metopimazine (p.1202·3).
Nausea and vomiting.

Volamin *Volchem, Ital.*
Amino-acid preparation.
Fatigue; liver disorders.

Volcolon *Parke, Davis, Neth.*
Plantago ovata (p.1194·2).
Constipation.

Voldal *Genevar, Fr.*
Diclofenac sodium (p.31·2).
Dysmenorrhoea; musculoskeletal, joint, and peri-articular disorders; renal colic.

Volital *Laboratories for Applied Biology, UK†.*
Pemoline (p.1484·1).
Hyperactivity in children.

Vollmers praparierter gruner *Salushaus, Ger.*
Avena sativa (p.1551·3); urtica (p.1642·3); hypericum (p.1590·1); alchemilla.
Digestive disorders; nervous disorders; oedema; urinary-tract disorders.

Volmac *Glaxo Wellcome, Ger.*
Salbutamol sulphate (p.758·2).
Obstructive airways disease.

Volmax
Glaxo Wellcome, Canad.†; Glaxo Allen, Ital.; Allen & Hanburys, S.Afr.; Glaxo Wellcome, Switz.; Allen & Hanburys, UK; Muro, USA.
Salbutamol sulphate (p.758·2).
Obstructive airways disease.

Vologen *Antigen, Irl.*
Diclofenac sodium (p.31·2).
Gout; inflammation; musculoskeletal, joint, and peri-articular disorders; pain.

Volon
Bristol-Myers Squibb, Aust.; Bristol-Myers Squibb, Ger.
Triamcinolone (p.1050·2).
Corticosteroid.

Volon A
Bristol-Myers Squibb, Aust.; Bristol-Myers Squibb, Ger.
Triamcinolone acetonide (p.1050·2) or triamcinolone acetonide dipotassium phosphate (p.1050·3).
Corticosteroid.

Volon A antibiotikahaltig *Bristol-Myers Squibb, Aust.*
Triamcinolone acetonide (p.1050·2); neomycin sulphate (p.229·2); gramicidin (p.215·2).
Eye disorders.

Volon A antibiotikahaltig N *Bristol-Myers Squibb, Ger.*
Triamcinolone acetonide (p.1050·2); neomycin sulphate (p.229·2).
Skin disorders.

Volon A Tinktur N *Bristol-Myers Squibb, Ger.*
Triamcinolone acetonide (p.1050·2); salicylic acid (p.1090·2).
Otitis externa; skin disorders.

Volon A-Rhin neu *Bristol-Myers Squibb, Ger.*
Triamcinolone acetonide (p.1050·2); phenylephrine hydrochloride (p.1066·2).
Rhinitis; sinusitis.

Volon A-Schuttelmix *Bristol-Myers Squibb, Ger.*
Triamcinolone acetonide (p.1050·2); zinc oxide (p.1096·2).
Skin disorders.

Volon A-Zinklotion *Bristol-Myers Squibb, Aust.*
Triamcinolone acetonide (p.1050·2); zinc oxide (p.1096·2).
Skin disorders.

Volonimat *Bristol-Myers Squibb, Ger.*
Triamcinolone acetonide (p.1050·2).
Skin disorders.

Volonimat N *Bristol-Myers Squibb, Ger.*
Triamcinolone acetonide (p.1050·2).
Skin disorders.

Volonimat Plus N *Bristol-Myers Squibb, Ger.*
Triamcinolone acetonide (p.1050·2); nystatin (p.386·1).
Eczema with secondary yeast infection.

Volraman *Eastern Pharmaceuticals, UK.*
Diclofenac sodium (p.31·2).
Gout; inflammation; musculoskeletal disorders; pain.

Volsaid *Trinity, UK.*
Diclofenac sodium (p.31·2).
Inflammation; musculoskeletal, joint, and peri-articular disorders; pain.

Voltamicin
Ciba Vision, Ital.; Ciba Vision, Switz.
Diclofenac sodium (p.31·2); gentamicin (p.214·1) or gentamicin sulphate (p.212·1).
Bacterial eye infections and inflammation.

Voltaren
Ciba-Geigy, Aust.; Novartis, Austral.; Ciba-Geigy, Belg.; Geigy, Canad.; Geigy, Ger.; Ciba, Ital.; Novartis, Ital.; Novartis, Neth.; Geigy, Norw.; Novartis, S.Afr.; Ciba Vision, Spain; Ciba-Geigy, Spain; Novartis, Swed.; Ciba Vision, USA; Geigy, USA.
Diclofenac (p.31·2), diclofenac cholestyramine (p.32·3), diclofenac diethylamine (p.31·2), diclofenac potassium (p.31·2), or diclofenac sodium (p.31·2).
Adjunct in cataract surgery; gout; inflammation; inflammatory eye disorders; musculoskeletal, joint, periarticular, and soft-tissue disorders; oedema; pain; renal and biliary colic.

Voltaren Emulgel *Ciba-Geigy, Spain.*
Diclofenac diethylamine (p.31·2).
Peri-articular and soft-tissue disorders.

Voltaren Ophtha
Ciba Vision, Austral.; Ciba Vision, Canad.; Ciba Vision, Ger.
Diclofenac sodium (p.31·2).
Postoperative eye inflammation; prevention of miosis during cataract surgery.

Voltaren T *Novartis, Swed.*
Diclofenac potassium (p.31·2).
Pain.

Voltarene
Ciba Vision, Fr.; Ciba-Geigy, Fr.; Geigy, Switz.
Diclofenac diethylamine (p.31·2), diclofenac resinate (p.31·2), or diclofenac sodium (p.31·2).
Dysmenorrhoea; eye pain; inflammation following eye surgery; inhibition of intraoperative miosis; musculoskeletal, joint, and peri-articular disorders; oedema; renal colic.

Voltarene Emulgel *Geigy, Switz.*
Diclofenac diethylamine (p.31·2).
Musculoskeletal, joint, peri-articular and soft-tissue disorders.

Voltarene Ophtha *Ciba Vision, Switz.*
Diclofenac sodium (p.31·2).
Eye disorders.

Voltarene Rapide *Geigy, Switz.*
Diclofenac potassium (p.31·2).
Inflammation; pain.

Voltarol
Geigy, Irl.; Geigy, UK.
Diclofenac (p.31·2), diclofenac diethylamine (p.31·2), or diclofenac sodium (p.31·2).
Gout; inflammation; musculoskeletal, joint, peri-articular, and soft-tissue disorders; pain.

Voltarol Ophtha *Ciba Vision, UK.*
Diclofenac sodium (p.31·2).
Inflammation and pain following eye surgery; inhibition of peroperative miosis.

Voltax *Poehlmann, Ger.*
Phospholipids; muira-puama; adenosine; vitamins.
Tonic.

Voltil *Ardeypharm, Ger.*
Protein-free extract of bovine spleen.
Gastro-intestinal disorders; peripheral and cerebral vascular disorders; skin disorders.

Voltric *UCB, Spain.*
Cetirizine hydrochloride (p.404·2).
Hypersensitivity reactions of the eye.

Volutine *Geymonat, Ital.*
Fenofibrate (p.1273·1).
Hyperlipidaemias.

Vomacur *Hexal, Ger.*
Dimenhydrinate (p.408·2).
Motion sickness; nausea; vertigo; vomiting.

Vomex A *Yamanouchi, Ger.*
Injection; suppositories; syrup; sustained-release capsules; sustained-release tablets; tablets: Dimenhydrinate (p.408·2).
Tablets†: Dimenhydrinate (p.408·2); caffeine (p.749·3).
Nausea; premedication; vestibular disorders; vomiting.

Vomifene *Vesta, S.Afr.*
Buclizine hydrochloride (p.404·1); pyridoxine (p.1363·1).
Motion sickness; nausea; vertigo; vomiting.

Vomistop *Weimer, Ger.†.*
Diphenylpyraline hydrochloride (p.409·3); pyridoxine hydrochloride (p.1362·3).
Motion sickness; vomiting.

Vontrol *SmithKline Beecham, USA†.*
Diphenidol hydrochloride (p.1189·1).
Nausea and vomiting; vertigo.

Vonum
Note. This name is used for preparations of different composition.
Gerot, Aust.
Indomethacin (p.45·2); laureth 9 (p.1325·2).
Musculoskeletal, joint, and soft-tissue disorders.
Lichtenstein, Ger.†.
Indomethacin (p.45·2) or meglumine indomethacin (p.46·3).
Inflammation; musculoskeletal and joint disorders; pain.

Vonum cutan *Lichtenstein, Ger.†.*
Indomethacin (p.45·2); laureth 9 (p.1325·2).
Musculoskeletal and joint disorders.

Vorigeno *Inibsa, Spain.*
Hyoscine hydrobromide (p.462·3).
Motion sickness.

VoSoL
Note. This name is used for preparations of different composition.
Carter-Wallace, Austral.
Propylene glycol diacetate (p.1328·2).
Otitis externa.
Carter Horner, Canad.; Wallace, USA.
Propylene glycol diacetate (p.1328·2); acetic acid (p.1541·2); benzethonium chloride (p.1102·3).
Otitis externa.

VoSoL HC
Carter Horner, Canad.; Wallace, USA.
Propylene glycol diacetate (p.1328·2); acetic acid (p.1541·2); benzethonium chloride (p.1102·3); hydrocortisone (p.1043·3).
Otitis externa.

Voxaletas *Clariana, Spain†.*
Aluminium hydroxide (p.1177·3); magnesium trisilicate (p.1199·1); liquorice (p.1197·1); aluminium glycinate (p.1177·2).
Gastro-intestinal disorders.

Voxpax
Homeocan, Canad.; Lehning, Fr.
Homoeopathic preparation.

Voxsuprine *Major, USA.*
Isoxsuprine hydrochloride (p.1592·1).
Cerebrovascular and peripheral vascular disorders.

Vraap *Inverni della Beffa, Ital.*
Vincamine (p.1644·1).
Disorders of cerebral, ocular, and vestibular circulation.

V-Tablopen *Dresden, Ger.*
Phenoxymethylpenicillin potassium (p.236·2).
Bacterial infections.

Vueffe *Baldacci, Ital.*
Peptides derived from the hydrolysis of bovine factor VIII (p.720·3).
Haemorrhage.

Vulcase *Pharmascience, Fr.*
Aloes (p.1177·1).
Formerly contained sulphur, bile, belladonna, aloes, and liquorice.
Constipation.

Vulna *Wiedenmann, Switz.†.*
Ichthammol (p.1083·3); zinc oxide (p.1096·2); titanium dioxide (p.1093·3); linseed oil (p.1596·2).
Skin disorders.

Vulneral *Sanofi Winthrop, Ger.†.*
Lignocaine hydrochloride (p.1293·2); allantoin (p.1078·2); dexpanthenol (p.1570·3).
Burns; skin disorders; wounds.

Vulnoagil *Agil, Ger.†.*
Hamamelis (p.1587·1); ol. jecoris; panthenol (p.1571·1).
Skin disorders.

Vulnostad *Stada, Ger.†.*
Benzethonium chloride (p.1102·3); lignocaine hydrochloride (p.1293·2); allantoin (p.1078·2); dexpanthenol (p.1570·3).
Skin disorders.

Vulnostimulin *Dermapharm, Ger.*
Wheat germ.
Burns; wounds.

Vulnotox *Serturner, Ger.†.*
Chlorophyll (p.1000·1); chlorophyllin copper complex (p.1000·1).
Burns; skin disorders; wounds.

Vulpuran *Rosch & Handel, Aust.*
Lead plaster-mass (p.1595·2); chamomile oil; hypericum oil (p.1590·1); cod-liver oil (p.1337·3); elemi; colophony (p.1567·1); emplastrum minii; turpentine oil (p.1641·1); peru balsam (p.1617·2); oxycholesterin.
Furuncles; ulcers; wounds.

Vumon
Bristol-Myers Squibb, Aust.; Bristol-Myers Squibb, Austral.; Bristol-Myers Squibb, Belg.; Bristol, Canad.; Bristol-Myers Squibb, Ital.; Bristol-Myers Squibb, Neth.; Bristol-Myers Squibb, S.Afr.; Bristol-Myers, Spain; Bristol-Myers Squibb, Swed.; Bristol-Myers Squibb, Switz.†; Bristol-Myers Oncology, USA.
Teniposide (p.565·3).
Malignant neoplasms.

Vuxolin *Farmitalia, Spain†.*
Clebopride malate (p.1188·2).
Gastro-oesophageal reflux; gastroparesis; nausea and vomiting.

VVS *Econo Med, USA.*
Sulphathiazole (p.257·1); sulphacetamide (p.252·2); sulfabenzamide (p.251·1).
Vaginitis due to Gardnerella vaginalis.

Vysorel *Novipharm, Ger.*
Mistletoe (p.1604·1).
Malignant neoplasms.

Vytone *Dermik, USA.*
Hydrocortisone (p.1043·3); di-iodohydroxyquinoline (p.581·1).

W5 *Aquamaid, UK.*
Multivitamin and mineral preparation.

Wake-Up Tablets *Adrem, Canad.*
Caffeine (p.749·3).
Stimulant.

Wampole Bronchial Cough Syrup *Wampole, Canad.*
Ammonium chloride (p.1055·2); aralia racemosa; poplar buds (p.1620·1); sanguinaria (p.1627·2); senega (p.1069·3); white pine; wild cherry (p.1644·3).

Wandonorm *Wander, Ger.*
Bopindolol malonate (p.833·2).
Hypertension.

Waran *Nycomed, Swed.*
Warfarin sodium (p.964·2).
Thrombo-embolic disorders.

Warfilone *Frosst, Canad.*
Warfarin sodium (p.964·2).
Thrombo-embolic disorders.

WariActiv *Ritter, Ger.*
Ethyl chloride (p.1292·3).
Topical anaesthesia.

Warix *Drossapharm, Switz.*
Podophyllotoxin (p.1089·1).
Anogenital warts.

Warme-Gel *Ratiopharm, Ger.*
Glycol salicylate (p.43·1); benzyl nicotinate (p.22·1).
Musculoskeletal, joint, and soft-tissue disorders; neuralgia; peripheral vascular disorders.

Warm-Up *Pharmco, S.Afr.*
Methyl salicylate (p.55·2); menthol (p.1600·2); eucalyptus oil (p.1578·1); turpentine oil (p.1641·1).
Muscular pain and stiffness.

Warondo Ekzemsalbe *Warondo, Ger.†.*
Salicylic acid (p.1090·2); zinc oxide (p.1096·2).
Skin disorders.

Warondo Psoriasissalbe *Warondo, Ger.†.*
Dithranol (p.1082·1); salicylic acid (p.1090·2).
Psoriasis.

Warondo-Abfuhrtee *Warondo, Ger.†.*
Rad. liquir.; flor. malv. silv.; flor. sambuci.; fol. menth. pip.; fol. farfarae; fol. sennae.
Herbal preparation.

Warondo-Flechtensalbe *Warondo, Ger.†.*
Salicylic acid (p.1090·2); ammoniumsulfobitol (p.1083·3); glycerol (p.1585·2); zinc oxide (p.1096·2).
Fungal infections.

Warondo-Wundsalbe *Warondo, Ger.†.*
Salicylic acid (p.1090·2); ichthammol (p.1083·3); zinc oxide (p.1096·2); arnica (p.1550·3); calendula officinalis; hypericum (p.1590·1).
Ulcers; wounds.

Wart Remover
Cress, Canad.; Stiefel, USA; Glades, USA; Rugby, USA.
Salicylic acid (p.1090·2).

Wart Solvent
Numark, UK†; Seton, UK†.
Glacial acetic acid (p.1541·2).

Wartec
Wellcome, Austral.†; Carter Horner, Canad.; Strathmann, Ger.; Perstorp, Norw.; Pharmafrica, S.Afr.; Fides, Spain; Perstorp, Swed.
Podophyllotoxin (p.1089·1).
Anogenital warts.

Wartex *Pickles, UK.*
Salicylic acid (p.1090·2).
Warts.

Warticon
Schwarz, Irl.; Perstorp, UK.
Podophyllotoxin (p.1089·1).
Genital warts.

Wartkil *Parke, Davis, Austral.†.*
Salicylic acid (p.1090·2); lactic acid (p.1593·3); podophyllum resin (p.1089·1).
Warts.

Wart-Off
Note. This name is used for preparations of different composition.
Nelson, Austral.†.
Salicylic acid (p.1090·2); lactic acid (p.1593·3); podophyllum resin (p.1089·1).
Warts.

Pfizer, USA.
Salicylic acid (p.1090·2).
Warts.

Warz-ab Extor Ohropax, Switz.
Salicylic acid (p.1090·2); lactic acid (p.1593·3); castor oil (p.1560·2).
Calluses; corns; warts.

Warzen-Alldahin Roha, Ger.
Salicylic acid (p.1090·2); lactic acid (p.1593·3).
Skin disorders.

Warzenmittel Salus, Aust.
Monochloroacetic acid.
Warts.

Warzin Rosch & Handel, Aust.
Lactic acid (p.1593·3).
Warts.

Wasacne IFI, Ital.†.
Thioxolone (p.1093·3).
Acne.

Wash E45 Crookes Healthcare, UK.
Soap substitute.
Dry skin.

Wasp-Eze Seton, UK.
Ointment: Antazoline hydrochloride (p.401·3).
Topical spray: Mepyramine maleate (p.414·1); benzocaine (p.1286·2).
Insect bites; stings.

Wasserdermina Wasserman, Spain†.
Benzoxiquine salicylate; dexamethasone (p.1037·1); neomycin sulphate (p.229·2); retinol; tyrothricin (p.267·2); tolnaftate (p.389·1); pyridoxine; ergocalciferol; tocopherol; vitamin F.
Infected skin disorders.

Wassermicina IFI, Ital.†.
Methacycline hydrochloride (p.225·1).
Bacterial infections.

Water Babies
Schering-Plough, Canad.; Schering-Plough, USA.
SPF 15: Ethylhexyl *p*-methoxycinnamate (p.1487·1); oxybenzone (p.1487·3).
Sunscreen.

Schering-Plough, Canad.†.
SPF 25: Oxybenzone (p.1487·3); ethylhexyl *p*-methoxycinnamate (p.1487·1); octyl salicylate (p.1487·3).
Sunscreen.

Schering-Plough, Canad.; Schering-Plough, USA.
SPF 30; SPF 45: Homosalate (p.1487·2); oxybenzone (p.1487·3); ethylhexyl *p*-methoxycinnamate (p.1487·1); octyl salicylate (p.1487·3).
Sunscreen.

Schering-Plough, USA.
SPF 45: Ethylhexyl *p*-methoxycinnamate (p.1487·1); oxybenzone (p.1487·3); octocrylene (p.1487·3); 2-ethylhexyl salicylate (p.1487·3).
Sunscreen.

Water Babies Little Licks Schering-Plough, USA.
SPF 30: Ethylhexyl *p*-methoxycinnamate (p.1487·1); oxybenzone (p.1487·3); 2-ethylhexyl salicylate (p.1487·3).
Sunscreen.

Water Naturtabs Larkhall Laboratories, UK.
Bladderwrack (p.1554·1); burdock (p.1594·2); ground ivy; clivers (p.1565·2).

Water Relief Tablets Healthcrafts, UK.
Bladderwrack (p.1554·1); clivers (p.1565·2); ground ivy; burdock (p.1594·2).
Water retention.

Waterbabies UVGuard Schering-Plough, Canad.
SPF 15: Avobenzone (p.1486·3); ethylhexyl *p*-methoxycinnamate (p.1487·1); oxybenzone (p.1487·3).
SPF 30: Avobenzone (p.1486·3); ethylhexyl *p*-methoxycinnamate (p.1487·1); octyl salicylate (p.1487·3); oxybenzone (p.1487·3).
Sunscreen.

Waterbury's Compound Parke, Davis, Austral.†.
Creosote (p.1057·3); guaiacol (p.1061·2); malt extract (p.1350·1); glucose; sodium hypophosphite; ferric manganese peptonate; wild cherry (p.1644·3); gentian root (p.1583·3).
Coughs; tonic.

Waterlex Gerard House, UK.
Taraxacum (p.1634·2); equisetum (p.1575·1); bearberry (p.1552·2).
Water retention.

Wax Aid Seton, UK†.
Paradichlorobenzene (p.1615·2); chlorbutol (p.1106·3); turpentine oil (p.1641·1).
Ear wax removal.

Waxsol
Norgine, Austral.; Norgine, Irl.; Norgine, UK.
Docusate sodium (p.1189·3).
Ear wax removal.

Waxsol NF Norgine, S.Afr.
Docusate sodium (p.1189·3).
Ear wax removal.

Waxwane Thornton & Ross, UK.
Turpentine oil (p.1641·1); terpineol (p.1635·1); chloroxylenol (p.1111·1).
Ear wax removal.

4-Way Cold Tablets Bristol-Myers Products, USA.
Paracetamol (p.72·2); phenylpropanolamine hydrochloride (p.1067·2); chlorpheniramine maleate (p.405·1).
Upper respiratory-tract symptoms.

4-Way Fast Acting Bristol-Myers Products, USA.
Phenylephrine hydrochloride (p.1066·2); naphazoline hydrochloride (p.1064·2); mepyramine maleate (p.414·1).
Nasal congestion.

4-Way Long Lasting Bristol-Myers Products, USA.
Oxymetazoline hydrochloride (p.1065·3).
Nasal congestion.

WCS Dusting Powder Weleda, UK.
Arnica montana (p.1550·3); calendula officinalis; echinacea angustifolia (p.1574·2); silica (p.1474·3); stibium met. praep.
Wounds.

Webber Antibiotic Cold Sore Ointment Novartis Consumer, Canad.
Polymyxin B sulphate (p.239·1); tyrothricin (p.267·2); camphor (p.1557·2); menthol (p.1600·2); benzocaine (p.1286·2).
Herpes labialis.

Webber E plus 3 Novartis Consumer, Canad.
Betacarotene, selenium, vitamin C, and vitamin E.

Wechseltee Smetana, Aust.
Passion flower (p.1615·3); valerian (p.1643·1); lupulus (p.1597·2); hypericum (p.1590·1); melissa (p.1600·1); crataegus (p.1568·2); mistletoe (p.1604·1).
Anxiety disorders; menopausal disorders; nervousness; sleep disorders.

Wehdryl Hauck, USA†.
Diphenhydramine hydrochloride (p.409·1).
Motion sickness; parkinsonism.

Wehgen Hauck, USA†.
Oestrone (p.1458·2).
Abnormal uterine bleeding; breast cancer; female castration; female hypogonadism; menopausal vulval and vaginal atrophy; primary ovarian failure; prostatic cancer.

Weh-less Hauck, USA.
Phendimetrazine tartrate (p.1484·2).
Obesity.

Weiche Zinkpaste Lichtenstein, Ger.
Zinc oxide (p.1096·2).
Skin disorders; wounds.

Weifapenin Weifa, Norw.
Phenoxymethylpenicillin potassium (p.236·2).
Bacterial infections.

Weight Control Homeocan, Canad.
Homoeopathic preparation.

Weight Watchers Punto Dieterba, Ital.
Oral granules: Fructose (p.1343·2); sorbitol (p.1354·2); aspartame (p.1335·1).
Tablets: Aspartame (p.1335·1).
Sugar substitute.

Weightrol Vortech, USA.
Phendimetrazine tartrate (p.1484·2).
Obesity.

Weimerquin Weimer, Ger.
Chloroquine phosphate (p.426·3).
Malaria.

Wellbutrin Glaxo Wellcome, USA.
Bupropion hydrochloride (p.280·1).
Depression.

Wellconal Glaxo Wellcome, S.Afr.
Dipipanone hydrochloride (p.34·3); cyclizine hydrochloride (p.407·1).
Pain.

Wellcoprim
Glaxo Wellcome, Aust.; Glaxo Wellcome, Belg.; Glaxo Wellcome, Fr.; Glaxo Wellcome, Neth.; Wellcome, Norw.†; Glaxo Wellcome, Swed.†.
Trimethoprim (p.265·1) or trimethoprim lactate (p.266·2).
Bacterial infections.

WellcoTIG Wellcopharm, Ger.†.
A tetanus immunoglobulin (p.1535·2).
Passive immunisation.

Wellcovorin Glaxo Wellcome, USA.
Calcium folinate (p.1342·2).
Megaloblastic anaemias; overdosage of folic acid antagonists.

Welldorm
Smith & Nephew, Irl.†; Smith & Nephew Pharmaceuticals, UK.
Chloral betaine (p.645·2) or chloral hydrate (p.645·3).
Formerly contained dichloralphenazone.
Insomnia.

Wellferon
Glaxo Wellcome, Aust.; Glaxo Wellcome, Canad.; Glaxo Wellcome, Ital.; Wellcome, Spain; Glaxo Wellcome, Swed.; Wellcome, Switz.; Glaxo Wellcome, UK.
Interferon alfa-n1 (lns) (p.615·3).
Anogenital warts; chronic active hepatitis; chronic myeloid leukaemia; hairy-cell leukaemia; juvenile laryngeal papillomatosis.

Wellman Vitabiotics, UK.
Multivitamin and mineral preparation.

Welltrivax Evans, Spain†.
A diphtheria, tetanus, and pertussis vaccine (p.1509·1).
Active immunisation of infants and young children.

Wellvone
Glaxo Wellcome, Aust.; Glaxo Wellcome, Austral.; Glaxo Wellcome, Belg.; Glaxo Wellcome, Fr.; Glaxo Wellcome, Ger.; Glaxo Wellcome, Ital.; Glaxo Wellcome, Neth.; Glaxo Wellcome, S.Afr.; Glaxo Wellcome, Swed.; Wellcome, Switz.; Wellcome, UK.
Atovaquone (p.579·3).
Pneumocystis carinii pneumonia.

Wellwoman Potter's, UK.
Herbal tea: Tilia (p.1637·3); scullcap; yarrow (p.1542·2); bearberry (p.1552·2).
Tablets: Yarrow (p.1542·2); motherwort (p.1604·2); tilia (p.1637·3); scullcap; valerian (p.1643·1).
Tonic.

Werdo Worwag, Ger.†.
Riboflavine (p.1362·1) or riboflavine sodium phosphate (p.1362·1).
Riboflavine deficiency.

Wescodyne Ciba, Ital.†.
Nonylphenoxypolyglycolether-iodate complex.
Surface disinfection.

Westcort
Westwood-Squibb, Canad.; Westwood-Squibb, USA.
Hydrocortisone valerate (p.1044·1).
Skin disorders.

White Cloverine Medtech, USA.
Barrier preparation.

White Lady Funk, Spain†.
Moisturiser.
Dry hands and skin.

Wibi
Galderma, Canad.; Galderma, USA.
Moisturiser.

Wibophorin Pfluger, Ger.
Homoeopathic preparation.

Wibotin H Pfluger, Ger.
Homoeopathic preparation.

Wick Daymed Erkaltungs Wick, Ger.
Capsules: Dextromethorphan hydrobromide (p.1057·3); paracetamol (p.72·2); phenylpropanolamine hydrochloride (p.1067·2).
Oral liquid: Paracetamol (p.72·2); guaiphenesin (p.1061·3); phenylephrine hydrochloride (p.1066·2); ascorbic acid (p.1365·2).
Cold symptoms.

Wick Erkaltungs-Saft fur die Nacht Procter & Gamble, Aust.
Doxylamine succinate (p.410·1); ephedrine sulphate (p.1059·3); dextromethorphan hydrobromide (p.1057·3); paracetamol (p.72·2).
Cold symptoms.

Wick Formel 44 Procter & Gamble, Aust.
Dextromethorphan (p.1057·3).
Coughs.

Wick Formel 44 Plus Hustenloser
Procter & Gamble, Aust.; Wick, Ger.
Guaiphenesin (p.1061·3).
Bronchitis; catarrh; coughs.

Wick Formel 44 plus Husten-Pastillen S Wick, Ger.
Dextromethorphan (p.1057·3).
Catarrh; coughs.

Wick Formel 44 Plus Hustenstiller
Procter & Gamble, Aust.; Wick, Ger.
Dextromethorphan hydrobromide (p.1057·3).
Coughs.

Wick Hustensaft Procter & Gamble, Aust.
Dextromethorphan hydrobromide (p.1057·3); doxylamine succinate (p.410·1); sodium citrate (p.1153·2).
Coughs.

Wick Inhalierstift N Wick, Ger.
Menthol (p.1600·2); camphor (p.1557·2).
Nasal congestion.

Wick Kinder Formel 44 Husten-Loser Wick, Ger.
Guaiphenesin (p.1061·3).
Catarrh; coughs.

Wick Kinder Formel 44 Husten-Stiller Wick, Ger.
Dextromethorphan hydrobromide (p.1057·3).
Coughs.

Wick Medinait Wick, Ger.
Doxylamine succinate (p.410·1); ephedrine sulphate (p.1059·3); dextromethorphan hydrobromide (p.1057·3); paracetamol (p.72·2).
Cold symptoms.

Wick Sinex
Note. This name is used for preparations of different composition.
Procter & Gamble, Aust.
Oxymetazoline hydrochloride (p.1065·3); menthol (p.1600·2); camphor (p.1557·2).
Cold symptoms.

Wick, Ger.
Oxymetazoline hydrochloride (p.1065·3).
Catarrh; rhinitis.

Wick Sulagil Wick, Ger.
Lignocaine (p.1293·2); dequalinium chloride (p.1112·1); cetylpyridinium chloride (p.1106·2).
Mouth and throat inflammation and infection.

Wick Vapo Sirup Procter & Gamble, Aust.
Menthol (p.1600·2).
Catarrh; coughs.

Wick Vaporub
Procter & Gamble, Aust.
Menthol (p.1600·2); camphor (p.1557·2); eucalyptus oil (p.1578·1); nutmeg oil (p.1609·3); cedar wood oil; turpentine oil (p.1641·1); thymol (p.1127·1).
Catarrh; coughs and cold symptoms.

Wick, Ger.
Cream: Menthol (p.1600·2); camphor (p.1557·2); cineole (p.1564·1); turpentine oil (p.1641·1).
Ointment: Menthol (p.1600·2); camphor (p.1557·2); eucalyptus oil (p.1578·1); turpentine oil (p.1641·1).
Catarrh; cold symptoms; coughs.

Wick Vaposyrup Wick, Ger.
Menthol (p.1600·2).
Bronchitis; coughs.

Wiedimmun Wiedemann, Ger.
Injection: Homoeopathic preparation.
Oral drops: Echinacea purpurea (p.1574·2).
Respiratory-tract infections.

Wigraine
Note. This name is used for preparations of different composition.
Organon, Canad.
Ergotamine tartrate (p.445·3); belladonna alkaloids (p.457·1); caffeine (p.749·3).
Migraine and other vascular headaches.

Organon, USA.
Ergotamine tartrate (p.445·3); caffeine (p.749·3).
Vascular headache.

Willlong Will-Pharma, Belg.
Glyceryl trinitrate (p.874·3).
Angina pectoris; heart failure.

Willospon
Will-Pharma, Belg.; Will-Pharma, Neth.
Gelatin foam (p.723·2).
Haemostatic dressing.

Willospon Forte Will-Pharma, Neth.
Collagen (p.1566·3).
Haemostatic dressing.

Willowbark Plus Herbal Formula 11 Vitelle, Austral.
Scutallaria; harpagophytum procumbens (p.27·2); salix (p.82·3).
Headache.

Wilprafen Yamanouchi, Ger.
Josamycin (p.220·2) or josamycin propionate (p.220·2).
Bacterial infections.

Winar Artesan, Ger.†.
Liver extract; vitamin B substances.
Appetite disorders.

Winasma Sanofi Winthrop, Spain†.
Ephedrine sulphate (p.1059·3); phenobarbitone (p.350·2); theophylline (p.765·1).
Obstructive airways disease.

Wincoram
Note. This name is used for preparations of different composition.
Sanofi Winthrop, Ger.; Sanofi Winthrop, Spain.
Amrinone (p.823·2) or amrinone lactate (p.823·1).
Heart failure.

Windol Dermapharm, Ger.
Bufexamac (p.22·2).
Inflammatory skin disorders.

Windol Basisbad Dermapharm, Ger.
Liquid paraffin (p.1382·1); soya oil (p.1355·1).
Skin disorders.

Windtreibender Tee Bio-Reform, Aust.
Fennel (p.1579·1); chamomile flower (p.1561·2); caraway (p.1559·3); achillea (p.1542·2); peppermint leaf (p.1208·1).
Flatulence.

WinGel Winthrop Consumer, USA†.
Hexitol-stabilised aluminium-magnesium hydroxide (p.1198·1).
Dyspepsia.

Wink Pharmco, S.Afr.
Naphazoline nitrate (p.1064·2); phenylephrine hydrochloride (p.1066·2).
Eye irritation.

40 Winks Roberts, USA.
Diphenhydramine hydrochloride (p.409·1).
Insomnia.

Winlomylon Adcock Ingram, S.Afr.
Nalidixic acid (p.228·2).
Urinary-tract infections.

Winobanin Sanofi Winthrop, Ger.
Danazol (p.1441·3).
Angioedema; benign breast disorders; endometriosis.

Winpain Brunel, S.Afr.
Paracetamol (p.72·2).
Fever; pain.

Winpred ICN, Canad.
Prednisone (p.1049·2).
Corticosteroid.

WinRho Cangene, Canad.
An anti-D immunoglobulin (p.1503·2).
Prevention of rhesus sensitisation.

Winseptic Winthrop, Austral.†.
Orthophenylphenol (p.1120·3); *N*-soya-*N*-ethyl morpholinium ethosulphate.
Surface disinfectant.

Winsprin SmithKline Beecham Consumer, Austral.†.
Aspirin (p.16·1).
Fever; pain.

Winstrol
Zambon, Ital.†; Zambon, Spain; Sanofi Winthrop, USA.
Stanozolol (p.1462·2).
Anabolic; anaemia associated with renal insufficiency; female breast cancer; hereditary angioedema; osteoporosis.

Wintomylon Sanofi Winthrop, Spain†.
Nalidixic acid (p.228·2).
Urinary-tract infections.

Winton Sanofi Winthrop, Spain.
Aluminium hydroxide (p.1177·3); magnesium hydroxide (p.1198·2).
Gastro-intestinal hyperacidity.

Wintonin Sanofi Winthrop, Ger.
Gepefrine tartrate (p.874·3).
Orthostatic hypotension.

Winuron *Sanofi Winthrop, Ger.*†.
Acrosoxacin (p.150·1).
Gonorrhoea.

Wisamt *Procter & Gamble, Aust.*
Resorcinol (p.1090·1); sulphur (p.1091·2).
Acne.

Wisamt N
Rohm, Ger.†.
Cream: Alcohol (p.1099·1); sulphur (p.1091·2); resorcinol (p.1090·1).
Topical powder: Sulphur (p.1091·2); resorcinol (p.1090·1).
Acne.

Wismut comp *Ratiopharm, Ger.*
Bismuth subcarbonate (p.1180·1); anhydrous aluminium hydroxide (p.1177·3); dimethicone (p.1213·1); magnesium trisilicate gel (p.1199·1).
Gastro-intestinal disorders.

Witch Doctor
Fleet, Austral.; De Witt, UK.
Hamamelis (p.1587·1).
Insect bites; skin irritation.

Witch Stik *Fleet, Austral.*
Hamamelis (p.1587·1).
Insect bites; skin irritation.

Witch Sunsore *De Witt, UK.*
Hamamelis (p.1587·1).
Sunburn.

Witte Kruis *Asta Medica, Neth.*
Paracetamol (p.72·2); caffeine (p.749·3).
Fever; pain.

Wobe-Mugos *Mucos, Aust.*
Proteolytic enzymes from bovine pancreas; calf thymus; pisum sativum; lens esculenta; papain (p.1614·1).
Adjunct to treatment of malignant neoplasms.

Wobe-Mugos E *Mucos, Ger.*
Trypsin (p.1640·1); chymotrypsin (p.1563·2); papain (p.1614·1).
Lignocaine hydrochloride (p.1293·2) is included in the injection to alleviate the pain of injection.
Malignant neoplasms; skin disorders; viral infections; wounds.

Wobe-Mugos Th *Mucos, Ger.*
Trypsin (p.1640·1); papain (p.1614·1); bovine thymus extract.
Malignant neoplasms; viral infections.

Wobenzimal *Vitafarma, Spain.*
Ointment: Papaya enzymes; lens sculenta enzymes; pisum sativum enzymes; pancreatin (p.1612·1); retinol (p.1358·1); thyme (p.1636·3); tocopherol (p.1369·1); vitamin F.
Tablets: Papaya; lens sculenta; pisum sativum; pancreatin (p.1612·1); thyme (p.1636·3).
Inflammation; oedema; peripheral vascular disorders.

Wobenzym *Mucos, Aust.*
Pancreatin (p.1612·1); papain (p.1614·1); bromelains (p.1555·1); trypsin (p.1640·1); lipase; amylase (p.1549·1); chymotrypsin (p.1563·2); rutin (p.1580·2).
Inflammation; oedema.

Wobenzym N *Mucos, Ger.*
Ointment: Bromelains (p.1555·1); trypsin (p.1640·1).
Tablets: Pancreatin (p.1612·1); bromelains (p.1555·1); papain (p.1614·1); protease; trypsin (p.1640·1); chymotrypsin (p.1563·2); rutin (p.1580·2).
Inflammation; oedema; thrombotic disorders.

Woloderma
Adroka, Switz.†.
Bath additive: Almond oil (p.1546·2); liquid paraffin (p.1382·1).
Adroka, Switz.†.
Soap substitute.
Wolo, Switz.†.
Topical lotion: Sodium lactate (p.1153·2); almond oil (p.1546·2).
Skin disorders.

Wolotherm *Wolo, Switz.*†.
Medicinal mud.
Musculoskeletal disorders.

Woman Adds *Cantassium Co., UK*†.
Multivitamin and mineral preparation.

Woman Formula *Avon, Canad.*
Multivitamin and mineral preparation.

Woman Kind *Windsor, UK.*
Pyridoxine (p.1363·1).
Premenstrual syndrome.

Women's Daily Formula *Kavon, USA.*
Multivitamin and mineral preparation with iron and folic acid.

Women's Formula Herbal Formula 3 *Vitelle, Austral.*
Angelica; cimicifuga (p.1563·3); caulophyllum thalictroides; pulsatilla (p.1623·3); agnus castus (p.1544·2).
Menstrual disorders.

Wonder Ice *Pedinol, USA.*
Menthol (p.1600·2).
Muscle, joint, and soft-tissue pain; neuralgia.

Wondra *Richardson-Vicks, USA.*
Emollient and moisturiser.

Woodwards Baby Chest Rub *Seton, UK.*
Menthol (p.1600·2); eucalyptus (p.1578·1).
Nasal congestion and catarrh.

Woodwards Gripe Water
Woodwards, Canad.; Seton, UK.
Terpeneless dill seed oil (p.1572·1); sodium bicarbonate (p.1153·2).
Wind in infants.

Woodwards Nappy Rash Ointment *Seton, UK.*
Zinc oxide (p.1096·2); cod-liver oil (p.1337·3).
Nappy rash.

Woodwards Teething Gel *Seton, UK.*
Lignocaine hydrochloride (p.1293·2).
Teething.

Worisetten *Kneipp, Ger.*†.
Cape aloe (p.1177·1); fennel (p.1579·1).
Constipation.

Worisetten S *Kneipp, Ger.*†.
Senna (p.1212·2).
Constipation.

Worishofener Dronalax *Dronania, Ger.*†.
Cape aloe (p.1177·1); fennel (p.1579·1); caraway (p.1559·3).
Constipation.

Worishofener Leber- und Gallensteinmittel Dr. Kleinschrod *Dronania, Ger.*†.
Chelidonium majus; turmeric (p.1001·3); agrimony; taraxacum (p.1634·2); berberis; silybum marinum (p.993·3); cichorium intybus; frangula bark (p.1193·2); raphany root; caraway (p.1559·3); achillea (p.1542·2); sage (p.1627·1).
Biliary-tract disorders.

Worishofener Nervenpflege Dr. Kleinschrod
Dronania, Ger.†.
Potentilla anserina; dried bitter-orange peel (p.1610·3); crataegus (p.1568·2); scoparium (p.1628·1); lupulus (p.1597·2); hypericum (p.1590·1); melissa (p.1600·1); achillea (p.1542·2); valerian (p.1643·1); mistletoe (p.1604·1); dried yeast (p.1373·1).
Nervous agitation.

Worishofener Nieren- und Blasenmittel Dr. Kleinschrod *Dronania, Ger.*†.
Bearberry (p.1552·2); phaseolus vulgaris; calluna vulgaris; rose fruit (p.1365·2); gentian (p.1583·3); equisetum (p.1575·1); orthosiphon (p.1592·2); solidago virgaurea; rad. carlinae; sage (p.1627·1); herb. basilici; birch leaves (p.1553·3); juniper (p.1592·2); rosemary; raphany root.
Urinary-tract disorders.

Worm *De Witt, UK.*
Piperazine citrate (p.107·2).
Worm infections.

Wormelix *Noristan, S.Afr.*†.
Piperazine citrate (p.107·2).
Ascariasis; enterobiasis.

Wormex *Sussex, UK.*
Piperazine citrate (p.107·2).

Wormgo *Pharmacare Consumer, S.Afr.*
Mebendazole (p.104·1).
Worm infections.

Wright's Vaporizing Fluid *LRC Products, UK.*
Chlorocresol (p.1110·3).
Congestion.

Wrinkle Defence *Sunspot, Austral.*
Oxybenzone (p.1487·3); ethylhexyl *p*-methoxycinnamate (p.1487·1) in a moisturising base.
Emollient; sunscreen.

Wulnasin *ECR, Switz.*†.
Cetylpyridinium chloride (p.1106·2); allantoin (p.1078·2); dexpanthenol (p.1570·3); lignocaine hydrochloride (p.1293·2).
Skin lesions.

Wund- und Brand-Gel Eu Rho *Eu Rho, Ger.*
Lignocaine hydrochloride (p.1293·2); allantoin (p.1078·2); cetylpyridinium chloride (p.1106·2); dexpanthenol (p.1570·3).
Burns; wounds.

Wund- und Heilsalbe *LAW, Ger.*
Dexpanthenol (p.1570·3).
Formerly contained bismuth subnitrate, allantoin, and hamamelis.
Skin disorders.

Wundesin *Zyma, Aust.*
Povidone-iodine (p.1123·3).
Wounds.

Wyamine *Wyeth-Ayerst, USA.*
Mephentermine sulphate (p.902·2).
Hypotension; shock.

Wyamycin *Wyeth-Ayerst, USA*†.
Erythromycin stearate (p.204·2).

Wyanoids *Wyeth-Ayerst, USA.*
Ephedrine sulphate (p.1059·3); belladonna extract (p.457·1); boric acid (p.1554·2); zinc oxide (p.1096·2); bismuth oxyiodide (p.1181·1); bismuth subcarbonate (p.1180·1); peru balsam (p.1617·2).
Anorectal disorders.

Wyanoids Relief Factor *Wyeth-Ayerst, USA.*
Live yeast cell derivative (p.1373·1); shark-liver oil.
Haemorrhoids.

Wycillin
Wyeth-Ayerst, Canad.†*; Wyeth-Ayerst, USA.*
Procaine penicillin (p.240·2).
Bacterial infections.

Wycillina *Pharmacia Upjohn, Ital.*
Benzathine penicillin (p.158·3).
Bacterial infections.

Wydase
Wyeth-Ayerst, Canad.; Wyeth-Ayerst, USA.
Hyaluronidase (p.1588·1).
Adjunct in subcutaneous urography; adjuvant to increase the absorption and dispersion of drugs; hypodermoclysis.

Wydora *Brenner-Efeka, Ger.*
Indoramin hydrochloride (p.891·1).
Hypertension.

Wygesic *Wyeth-Ayerst, USA.*
Dextropropoxyphene hydrochloride (p.27·3); paracetamol (p.72·2).
Fever; pain.

Wylaxine *Whitehall, Belg.*
Bisoxatin acetate (p.1181·2).
Bowel evacuation; constipation.

Wymox *Wyeth-Ayerst, USA.*
Amoxycillin trihydrate (p.151·3).
Bacterial infections.

Wypicil *Wyeth, Belg.*†.
Ciclacillin (p.185·2).
Bacterial infections.

Wypresin *Wyeth Lederle, Aust.*
Indoramin hydrochloride (p.891·1).
Hypertension.

Wysoy
Wyeth, Irl.; Wyeth, UK.
Lactose-free food for special diets.
Cows' milk or lactose intolerance; galactokinase deficiency; galactosaemia.

Wytensin
Wyeth Lederle, Aust.; Wyeth, Ger.†*; Wyeth-Ayerst, USA.*
Guanabenz acetate (p.877·3).
Hypertension.

X-Adene *GNR, Fr.*
Procaine hydrochloride (p.1299·2); vitamin B substances; polymerised sodium deoxyribonucleate.
Tonic.

Xal
Wolfs, Belg.; Soekami, Fr.†*; Adima, Switz.*†.
Potassium chloride; ammonium chloride; calcium formate; glutamic acid (p.1147·1).
Dietary salt substitute.

Xalatan
Pharmacia Upjohn, Austral.; Pharmacia Upjohn, Ital.; Pharmacia Upjohn, Neth.; Pharmacia Upjohn, Swed.; Pharmacia Upjohn, UK; Pharmacia, USA.
Latanoprost (p.1419·2).
Glaucoma; ocular hypertension.

xam *Woelm, Ger.*†.
Multivitamin preparation.

Xamamina *Bracco, Ital.*
Dimenhydrinate (p.408·2).
Motion sickness.

Xanax
Upjohn, Austral.; Pharmacia Upjohn, Belg.; Pharmacia Upjohn, Canad.; Pharmacia Upjohn, Fr.; Pharmacia Upjohn, Ger.; Pharmacia Upjohn, Irl.; Pharmacia Upjohn, Ital.; Pharmacia Upjohn, Neth.; Pharmacia Upjohn, Switz.; Pharmacia Upjohn, UK; Upjohn, USA.
Alprazolam (p.640·3).
Alcohol withdrawal syndrome; anxiety disorders; mixed anxiety-depression; panic attacks.

Xanbon *Kissei, Jpn.*
Ozagrel sodium (p.1612·1).
Cerebral thrombosis; cerebral vasospasm.

Xanef *Merck Sharp & Dohme, Ger.*
Enalapril maleate (p.863·2) or enalaprilat (p.863·2).
Heart failure; hypertension.

Xanomel *Clonmel, Irl.*
Ranitidine hydrochloride (p.1209·3).
Gastric hyperacidity; gastro-oesophageal reflux; peptic ulcer; Zollinger-Ellison syndrome.

Xanor
Pharmacia Upjohn, Aust.; Pharmacia Upjohn, Norw.; Pharmacia Upjohn, S.Afr.; Pharmacia Upjohn, Swed.
Alprazolam (p.640·3).
Anxiety disorders.

Xanpervit *Passauer, Ger.*†.
Potassium orotate (p.1611·2); vitamins.
Diabetes mellitus; liver disorders; vitamin-B deficiency.

Xantervit *SIFI, Ital.*
Xanthopterin; multivitamins.
Ocular trauma and lesions.

Xantervit Antibiotico *SIFI, Ital.*
Xanthopterin; chloramphenicol (p.182·1); multivitamins.
Ocular trauma and lesions.

Xantervit Eparina *SIFI, Ital.*
Xanthopterin; heparin sodium (p.879·3); multivitamins.
Ocular burns.

Xanthium
SMB, Belg.; Galephar, Fr.
Theophylline (p.765·1).
Obstructive airways disease.

Xanthomax *Ashbourne, UK.*
Allopurinol (p.390·2).

Xantium *Cyanamid, Ital.*
Protirelin tartrate (p.1259·3).
Neurological deficit.

Xantivent *Essex, Switz.*
Theophylline (p.765·1).
Bronchospasm.

Xanturenasi *Teofarma, Ital.*
Pyridoxine hydrochloride (p.1362·3).

Xanturic *Pharmafarm, Fr.*†.
Allopurinol (p.390·2).
Gout; hyperuricaemia; renal calculi.

Xapro *Jenapharm, Ger.*
Oestriol (p.1457·2).
Vulvovaginal disorders.

Xarator *Parke, Davis, Ital.*
Atorvastatin calcium (p.1268·1).
Hyperlipidaemias.

Xatral
Synthelabo, Fr.; Lorex, Irl.; Synthelabo, Ital.; Lorex Synthelabo, Neth.; Astra, Swed.; Synthelabo, Switz.; Lorex, UK.
Alfuzosin hydrochloride (p.817·2).
Benign prostatic hyperplasia.

Xefo *Nycomed, Swed.*
Lornoxicam (p.50·3).
Inflammation; musculoskeletal and joint disorders; pain.

Xeloda *Roche, USA.*
Capecitabine (p.510·3).
Breast cancer.

Xenalon *Mepha, Switz.*
Spironolactone (p.946·1).
Hyperaldosteronism.

Xenar *Wassermann, Ital.*
Naproxen (p.61·2).
Musculoskeletal, joint, peri-articular, and soft-tissue disorders; neuralgia.

Xenetix
Guerbet, Fr.; Guerbet, Ger.; Guerbet, Ital.; Guerbet, Neth.; Gothia, Swed.; Guerbet, Switz.
Iobitridol (p.1005·2).
Radiographic contrast medium.

Xenical *Roche, UK.*
Orlistat (p.1611·1).
Obesity.

Xenid *Biogalenique, Fr.*
Diclofenac epolamine (p.32·3) or diclofenac sodium (p.31·2).
Dysmenorrhoea; musculoskeletal, joint, and peri-articular disorders; renal colic.

Xenopan *Mundipharma, Aust.*
Naproxen (p.61·2).
Gout; inflammation; musculoskeletal, joint, and peri-articular disorders; pain.

Xepin *Bioglan, UK.*
Doxepin hydrochloride (p.283·2).
Pruritus.

Xerac *Person & Covey, USA*†.
Sulphur (p.1091·2).
Acne; oily skin.

Xerac AC *Person & Covey, USA.*
Aluminium chloride (p.1078·3); alcohol (p.1099·1).
Acne; antiperspirant; skin cleanser.

Xerac BP *Person & Covey, USA*†.
Benzoyl peroxide (p.1079·2).
Acne.

Xeracil *Xeragen, S.Afr.*
Amoxycillin (p.151·3).
Bacterial infections.

Xeramax *Xeragen, S.Afr.*
Syrup: Paracetamol (p.72·2); codeine phosphate (p.26·1); promethazine hydrochloride (p.416·2).
Fever; pain.
Tablets: Paracetamol (p.72·2); codeine phosphate (p.26·1); caffeine (p.749·3); meprobamate (p.678·1).
Pain with tension.

Xeramel *Xeragen, S.Afr.*
Erythromycin estolate (p.204·1).
Bacterial infections.

Xeraspor *Xeragen, S.Afr.*
Clotrimazole (p.376·3).
Fungal skin infections; vulvovaginal candidiasis.

Xerazole *Xeragen, S.Afr.*
Co-trimoxazole (p.196·3).
Bacterial infections.

Xerenal *Kwizda, Aust.*
Dothiepin hydrochloride (p.283·1).
Depression.

Xerial *SVR, Ital.*
Urea (p.1095·2); allantoin (p.1078·2); emollients.
Dry skin.

Xeroderm *Dermol, USA.*
Emollient.

Xerogesic *Crown, S.Afr.*
Paracetamol (p.72·2); codeine phosphate (p.26·1); caffeine (p.749·3); meprobamate (p.678·1).
Pain and associated tension.

Xeroprim *Crown, S.Afr.*
Co-trimoxazole (p.196·3).
Bacterial infections.

Xerotens *Covan, S.Afr.*
Doxylamine succinate (p.410·1); paracetamol (p.72·2); codeine phosphate (p.26·1); caffeine (p.749·3).
Pain and associated tension.

Xerumenex
Asta Medica, Belg.; Asta Medica, Neth.
Triethanolamine polypeptide oleate-condensate (p.1639·2).
Cleansing of external ear before otoscopy; removal of impacted ear wax.

Xflu
SmithKline Beecham, Austral.; SmithKline Beecham, S.Afr.
An inactivated influenza vaccine (split virion) (p.1515·2).
Active immunisation.

Xibornol Prodes *Prodes, Spain.*
Oral suspension: Bromhexine hydrochloride (p.1055·3); chlophedianol hydrochloride (p.1057·1); xibornol (p.270·3).

Suppositories: Camphor (p.1557·2); niaouli oil (p.1607·1); xibornol (p.270·3).
Respiratory-tract disorders.

Xicil *Rottapharm, Spain.*
Glucosamine sulphate (p.1585·1).
Rheumatic disorders.

Xillin *Laser, S.Afr.†.*
Amoxycillin trihydrate (p.151·3).
Bacterial infections.

Xilo-Mynol *Molteni, Ital.*
Lignocaine hydrochloride (p.1293·2).
Adrenaline acid tartrate (p.813·3) is included in this preparation as a vasoconstrictor to diminish absorption and localise the effect of the local anaesthetic.
Local anaesthesia.

Xilonibsa *Inibsa, Spain.*
Lignocaine hydrochloride (p.1293·2).
Adrenaline acid tartrate (p.813·3) is included in this preparation as a vasoconstrictor to diminish absorption and localise the effect of the local anaesthetic.
Local anaesthesia.

Xilorroidal *Rovi, Spain†.*
Peru balsam (p.1617·2); bismuth subgallate (p.1180·2); hydrocortisone (p.1043·3); lignocaine hydrochloride (p.1293·2); neomycin sulphate (p.229·2); salicylic acid (p.1090·2); adrenaline (p.813·2).
Anorectal disorders.

Ximicina *Rottapharm, Ital.†.*
Doxycycline hydrochloride (p.202·3).
Bacterial infections.

Ximovan *Rhone-Poulenc Rorer, Ger.; Nattermann, Ger.*
Zopiclone (p.699·2).
Insomnia.

Xitadil *Irex, Fr.†.*
Viquidil hydrochloride (p.1644·2).
Cerebrovascular disorders.

xitix *Woelm, Ger.†.*
Ascorbic acid (p.1365·2); sodium ascorbate (p.1365·2).
Vitamin C deficiency.

Xival *Bayropharm, Ital.†.*
Propyphenazone (p.81·3); caffeine (p.749·3); sodium benzoate (p.1102·3).
Headache; pain.

Xmet, Thre, Val, Isoleu Analog *Scientific Hospital Supplies, Austral.*
Infant feed.
Methylmalonic acidaemia; propionic acidaemia.

XP Analog *Scientific Hospital Supplies, Austral.*
Food for special diets.
Phenylketonuria.

XP Maxamaid *Scientific Hospital Supplies, Austral.*
Food for special diets.
Phenylketonuria.

XP Maxamum *Scientific Hospital Supplies, Austral.*
Food for special diets.
Phenylketonuria.

X-Praep *Asta Medica, Neth.*
Sennosides (p.1212·3).
Bowel evacuation; constipation.

X-Prep
Mundipharma, Aust.; Mundipharma, Ger.; Asta Medica, Ital.; Nycomed, Norw.; Mundipharma, Switz.; Gray, USA.
Senna (p.1212·2).
Bowel evacuation.

Purdue Frederick, Canad.; Asta Medica, Fr.; Adcock Ingram, S.Afr.; Asta Medica, Spain.
Sennosides A and B (p.1212·3).
Bowel evacuation.

X-Prep Bowel Evacuant Kit-1 *Gray, USA.*
Combination pack: 2 tablets, standardised senna concentrate (p.1212·2); docusate sodium (p.1189·3) (Senokot-S); 1 bottle, senna fruit (X-Prep); 1 suppository, bisacodyl (Rectolax) (p.1179·3).
Bowel evacuation.

X-Prep Bowel Evacuant Kit-2 *Gray, USA.*
Combination pack: 1 dose oral granules, effervescent citrate/magnesium sulphate (Citralax) (p.1153·2) (p.1157·3); 1 bottle, senna fruit (X-Prep) (p.1212·2); 1 suppository, bisacodyl (Rectolax) (p.1179·3).
Bowel evacuation.

X-Seb
Baker Cummins, Canad.; Baker Cummins, USA.
Salicylic acid (p.1090·2).
Skin and scalp disorders.

X-Seb Plus
Baker Cummins, Canad.; Baker Cummins, USA.
Pyrithione zinc (p.1089·3); salicylic acid (p.1090·2).
Scalp disorders.

X-Seb T
Baker Cummins, Canad.; Baker Cummins, USA.
Salicylic acid (p.1090·2); coal tar (p.1092·3).
Seborrhoea.

X-Seb T Plus
Baker Cummins, Canad.; Baker Cummins, USA.
Salicylic acid (p.1090·2); coal tar (p.1092·3); menthol (p.1600·2).
Scalp disorders.

X-Tar *Dormer, Canad.*
Salicylic acid (p.1090·2); coal tar solution (p.1092·3); menthol (p.1600·2).
Scalp disorders.

X-trozine *Rexar, USA.*
Phendimetrazine tartrate (p.1484·2).

Xuprin *Solvay, Aust.*
Isoxsuprine resinate (p.1592·1).
Peripheral vascular disorders.

Xuret *Galen, UK†.*
Metolazone (p.907·2).
Hypertension.

Xycam *Lennon, S.Afr.*
Piroxicam (p.80·2).
Gout; musculoskeletal and joint disorders.

Xylanaest *Gebro, Aust.*
Lignocaine hydrochloride (p.1293·2).
Adrenaline (p.813·2) is included in some injections as a vasoconstrictor to diminish absorption and localise the effect of the local anaesthetic.
Local anaesthesia.

Xylesine *Amino, Switz.*
Lignocaine hydrochloride (p.1293·2).
Local anaesthesia.

Xylestesin
Espe, Aust.; Espe, Switz.
Lignocaine (p.1293·2); cetrimonium bromide (p.1106·1).
Local anaesthesia.

Xylestesin Pumpspray *Espe, Ger.*
Lignocaine (p.1293·2); cetrimonium bromide.
Local anaesthesia.

Xylestesin, Xylestesin-F *Espe, Ger.*
Lignocaine hydrochloride (p.1293·2).
Noradrenaline hydrochloride (p.924·2) is included in this preparation as a vasoconstrictor to diminish absorption and localise the effect of the local anaesthetic.
Local anaesthesia.

Xylestesina *Davidall Florence, Ital.†.*
Injection: Lignocaine hydrochloride (p.1293·2).
Noradrenaline (p.924·1) is included in this preparation as a vasoconstrictor to diminish absorption and localise the effect of the local anaesthetic.
Spray: Lignocaine (p.1293·2); cetrimonium bromide (p.1106·1).
Local anaesthesia.

Xylestesina S *Davidall Florence, Ital.†.*
Lignocaine hydrochloride (p.1293·2).
Adrenaline (p.813·2) and noradrenaline (p.924·1) are included in this preparation as vasoconstrictors to diminish absorption and localise the effect of the local anaesthetic.
Local anaesthesia.

Xylestesin-A, Xylestesin centro *Espe, Ger.*
Lignocaine hydrochloride (p.1293·2).
Adrenaline hydrochloride (p.813·3) is included in this preparation as a vasoconstrictor to diminish absorption and localise the effect of the local anaesthetic.
Local anaesthesia.

Xylestesin-F *Espe, Switz.*
Lignocaine hydrochloride (p.1293·2).
Noradrenaline hydrochloride (p.924·2) is included in this preparation as a vasoconstrictor to diminish absorption and localise the effect of the local anaesthetic.
Local anaesthesia.

Xylestesin-S *Espe, Ger.*
Lignocaine hydrochloride (p.1293·2).
Noradrenaline hydrochloride (p.924·2) and adrenaline hydrochloride (p.813·3) are included in this preparation as vasoconstrictors to diminish absorption and localise the effect of the local anaesthetic.
Local anaesthesia.

Xylestesin-S "special" *Espe, Switz.*
Lignocaine hydrochloride (p.1293·2).
Adrenaline hydrochloride (p.813·3) and noradrenaline hydrochloride (p.924·2) are included in this preparation as vasoconstrictors to diminish absorption and localise the effect of the local anaesthetic.
Local anaesthesia.

Xylo *CT, Ger.*
Xylometazoline hydrochloride (p.1071·2).
Nasal congestion.

Xylocain
Note. This name is used for preparations of different composition.
Astra, Aust.; Astra, Ger.; Astra, Norw.; Astra, Swed.; Astra, Switz.
Lignocaine (p.1293·2) or lignocaine hydrochloride (p.1293·2).
Adrenaline (p.813·2) or adrenaline acid tartrate (p.813·3) is included in some injections as a vasoconstrictor to diminish absorption and localise the effect of the local anaesthetic.
Local anaesthesia.

Astra, Ger.†.
Ointment; suppositories: Lignocaine (p.1293·2); hydrocortisone acetate (p.1043·3); aluminium diacetate hydroxide; zinc oxide (p.1096·2).
Anorectal disorders.

Xylocain CO_2 *Astra, Switz.*
Lignocaine (p.1293·2); carbon dioxide.
Local anaesthesia.

Xylocain f.d. Kardiologie *Astra, Ger.*
Lignocaine hydrochloride (p.1293·2).
Arrhythmias; status epilepticus.

Xylocain tung *Astra, Swed.*
Lignocaine hydrochloride (p.1293·2).
Local anaesthesia.

Xylocaina
Note. This name is used for preparations of different composition.
Astra, Ital.; Inibsa, Spain.
Lignocaine (p.1293·2) or lignocaine hydrochloride (p.1293·2).
Adrenaline acid tartrate (p.813·3) is included in some injections as a vasoconstrictor to diminish absorption and localise the effect of the local anaesthetic.
Local anaesthesia; pain.

Xylocaine
Note. This name is used for preparations of different composition.
Astra, Austral.; Astra, Belg.; Astra, Canad.; Astra, Fr.; Astra, Irl.; Astra, Neth.; Astra, S.Afr.; Astra, UK; Astra, USA.
Lignocaine (p.1293·2) or lignocaine hydrochloride (p.1293·2).
Adrenaline (p.813·2) or adrenaline tartrate (p.813·3) is included in some injections as a vasoconstrictor to diminish absorption and localise the effect of the local anaesthetic.
Local anaesthesia; ventricular arrhythmias.

Xylocaine Accordion *Astra, UK.*
Lignocaine hydrochloride (p.1293·2).
Local anaesthesia.

Xylocaine Heavy
Astra, Austral.; Adcock Ingram, S.Afr.
Lignocaine hydrochloride (p.1293·2).
Local anaesthesia.

Xylocaine Jelly with Hibitane *Astra, Austral.*
Lignocaine hydrochloride (p.1293·2); chlorhexidine gluconate (p.1107·2).
Catheterisation; endoscopy; local anaesthesia.

Xylocaine 2% Plain *Astra, UK.*
Lignocaine hydrochloride (p.1293·2).
Formerly known as Lignostab.
Local anaesthesia.

Xylocaine Special Adhesive *Astra, Austral.*
Lignocaine hydrochloride (p.1293·2).
Topical anaesthesia in dentistry.

Xylocaine Visqueuse *Astra, Belg.*
Lignocaine hydrochloride (p.1293·2).
Adjunct in radiology and endoscopy; painful oral and oesophageal conditions.

Xylocard
Astra, Aust.; Astra, Austral.; Astra, Belg.; Astra, Canad.; Astra, Fr.; Astra, Irl.; Astra, Neth.; Astra, Norw.; Hassle, Swed.; Astra, Switz.; Astra, UK.
Lignocaine hydrochloride (p.1293·2).
Status epilepticus; ventricular arrhythmias.

Xylocitin *Jenapharm, Ger.*
Lignocaine hydrochloride (p.1293·2).
Adrenaline acid tartrate (p.813·3) is included in some injections as a vasoconstrictor to diminish absorption and localise the effect of the local anaesthetic.
Local anaesthesia.

Xylo-Comod *Ursapharm, Ger.*
Xylometazoline hydrochloride (p.1071·2).
Nasal congestion.

Xylonest
Astra, Ger.; Astra, Switz.
Prilocaine hydrochloride (p.1298·3).
Adrenaline acid tartrate (p.813·3) or felypressin (p.1246·3) is included in some injections as a vasoconstrictor to diminish absorption and localise the effect of the local anaesthetic.
Local anaesthesia.

Xylonest-Octapressin *Astra, Switz.*
Prilocaine hydrochloride (p.1298·3).
Felypressin (p.1246·3) is included in this preparation as a vasoconstrictor to diminish absorption and localise the effect of the local anaesthetic.
Local anaesthesia.

Xyloneural
Gebro, Aust.; Strathmann, Ger.; Gebro, Switz.
Lignocaine hydrochloride (p.1293·2).
Headache; local anaesthesia; migraine; tinnitus; vertigo.

Xylonibsa *Inibsa, Spain.*
Cetylpyridinium chloride (p.1106·2); lignocaine hydrochloride (p.1293·2).
Formerly known as Xylocaina.
Local anaesthesia.

Xylonor
Note. This name is used for preparations of different composition.
Ogna, Ital.; Septodont, Switz.
Injection: Lignocaine hydrochloride (p.1293·2).
Noradrenaline acid tartrate (p.924·1), adrenaline acid tartrate (p.813·3), or noradrenaline acid tartrate and adrenaline (p.813·2) are included in some injections as vasoconstrictors to diminish absorption and localise the effect of the local anaesthetic.
Local anaesthesia.

Austrodent, Aust.
Topical spray: Lignocaine (p.1293·2); cetrimide (p.1105·2).
Local anaesthesia.

Ogna, Ital.; Prats, Spain; Septodont, Switz.
Topical solution; pellets; topical spray: Lignocaine (p.1293·2) or lignocaine hydrochloride (p.1293·2); cetrimonium bromide (p.1106·1).
Local anaesthesia.

Xylonor Especial *Prats, Spain.*
Lignocaine hydrochloride (p.1293·2).
Adrenaline (p.813·2) and noradrenaline acid tartrate (p.924·1) are included in this preparation as vasoconstrictors to diminish absorption and localise the effect of the local anaesthetic.
Local anaesthesia.

Xylonor 2% Sin Vasoconst *Prats, Spain.*
Lignocaine hydrochloride (p.1293·2).
Local anaesthesia.

Xylo-Pfan
Pharmacia Upjohn, Canad.; Adria, USA.
Xylose (p.1645·2).
Diagnosis of malabsorption.

Xyloproct
Note. This name is used for preparations of different composition.
Astra, Austral.; Astra, Belg.; Astra, Irl.; Astra, Ital.; Astra, Neth.; Astra, Norw.; Tika, Swed.; Astra, UK.
Lignocaine (p.1293·2); hydrocortisone acetate (p.1043·3); aluminium acetate (p.1547·3); zinc oxide (p.1096·2).
Anorectal disorders; pruritus vulvae.

Astra, Irl.
Suppositories: Lignocaine (p.1293·2); hydrocortisone acetate (p.1043·3).
Anorectal disorders.

Xylose-BMS *Bio-Medical, UK.*
Xylose (p.1645·2).
Formerly known as Xylomed.
Diagnosis of malabsorption.

Xylotocan *Astra, Ger.*
Tocainide hydrochloride (p.955·1).
Ventricular arrhythmias.

Xylotox
Adcock Ingram, S.Afr.; Astra, UK.
Lignocaine hydrochloride(p.1293·2).
Adrenaline (p.813·2), adrenaline acid tartrate (p.813·3), or noradrenaline (p.924·1) is included in some preparations as a vasoconstrictor to diminish absorption and localise the effect of the local anaesthetic.
Local anaesthesia.

Yacutin *Merck, Spain.*
Benzyl benzoate (p.1402·2); lindane (p.1407·2).
Pediculosis; scabies.

Yadalan *Llorente, Spain.*
A nonoxinol (p.1326·1).
Contraceptive.

Yakona N *Rentsch, Switz.*
Hypericum (p.1590·1); kava (p.1592·3).
Anxiety; nervous tension.

Yal
Jacoby, Aust.; Trommsdorff, Ger.; Gebro, Switz.
Docusate sodium (p.1189·3); sorbitol (p.1354·2).
Bowel evacuation; constipation.

Yamalen *Marion Merrell Dow, Belg.†.*
Aspirin (p.16·1); paracetamol (p.72·2); dextropropoxyphene (p.27·3); caffeine (p.749·3); chlorpheniramine (p.405·2).
Fever; pain.

Yamalen New *Hoechst Marion Roussel, Belg.*
Dextropropoxyphene hydrochloride (p.27·3); paracetamol (p.72·2).
Pain.

Yamatetan *Yamanouchi, Jpn.*
Cefotetan disodium (p.170·1).
Lignocaine (p.1293·2) is included in the intramuscular injection to alleviate the pain of injection.
Bacterial infections.

Yatrox *Vita, Spain.*
Ondansetron hydrochloride (p.1206·2).
Nausea and vomiting.

Yeast Clear *Dolisos, Canad.*
Homoeopathic preparation.

Yeast Vite *Seton, UK.*
Caffeine (p.749·3); vitamin B substances; dried yeast (p.1373·1).
Tonic.

Yeast-Gard Advanced Sensitive Formula
Lake, USA†.
Benzocaine (p.1286·2); benzalkonium chloride (p.1101·3); aloe vera (p.1177·1); vitamin E (p.1369·1).
Vaginal irritation.

Yeast-Gard Maximum Strength Formula
Lake, USA†.
Benzocaine (p.1286·2); resorcinol (p.1090·1).
Vaginal irritation.

Yeast-Gard Medicated *Lake, USA.*
Povidone-iodine (p.1123·3).
Vaginal irritation.

Yeast-X *Fleet, USA.*
Powder: Corn starch (p.1356·2); zinc oxide (p.1096·2).
Suppositories: Pulsatilla (p.1623·3).

Yectofer *Astra, Spain.*
Iron sorbitol (p.1349·1).
Anaemias.

Yectofer Compuesto *Knoll, Spain†.*
Iron sorbitol (p.1349·1); hydroxocobalamin acetate (p.1364·2); folic acid (p.1340·3).
Anaemias.

Yedoc *Ciba Vision, Switz.*
Gentamicin sulphate (p.212·1).
Bacterial eye infections.

Yelets *Freeda, USA.*
Ferrous fumarate (p.1339·3); folic acid (p.1340·3); multivitamins and minerals.
Iron-deficiency anaemias.

Yendol *Faes, Spain.*
Caffeine (p.749·3); chlorpheniramine maleate (p.405·1); paracetamol (p.72·2); salicylamide (p.82·3).
Upper-respiratory-tract disorders.

Yermonil
Ciba-Geigy, Aust.; Geigy, Ger.; Ciba, Switz.
Ethinyloestradiol (p.1445·1); lynoestrenol (p.1448·2).
Combined oral contraceptive.

Yestamin *English Grains, UK.*
Vitamin B substances.

Yewtaxan *Pharmachemie, S.Afr.*
Paclitaxel (p.556·3).
Breast cancer; ovarian cancer.

YF-Vax *Connaught, USA.*
A yellow fever vaccine (p.1539·1).
Active immunisation.

Yocon Glenwood, Canad.; Glenwood, Ger.; Glenwood, USA.
Yohimbine hydrochloride (p.1645·3).
Impotence.

Yodo Tio Calci Cusi, Spain.
Calcium chloride (p.1155·1); potassium iodide (p.1493·1); sodium thiosulphate (p.996·2); sodium iodide (p.1493·2).
Eye disorders.

Yodocortison Boots, Spain†.
Povidone-iodine (p.1123·3); prednisolone (p.1048·1).
Mouth and throat inflammation; mouth ulcers; skin infection.

Yodos Wasserman, Spain†.
Iodine peptonisate.
Arteriosclerosis; hypertension; obstructive airways disease; thrombophlebitis.

Yodoxin Glenwood, USA.
Di-iodohydroxyquinoline (p.581·1).
Intestinal amoebiasis.

Yoguis C Ale, Spain†.
Ascorbic acid (p.1365·2).
Adjunct in treatment of iron supplementation; vitamin C deficiency.

Yoguito Ale, Spain†.
Cineole (p.1564·1); oleum pinus sylvestris; menthol (p.1600·2).
Throat irritation.

Yohimex Kramer, USA.
Yohimbine hydrochloride (p.1645·3).
Male impotence.

Yomesan Bayer, Austral.†; Bayer, Belg.; Bayer, Ger.; Bayer, Ital.; Bayer, Neth.; Bayer, S.Afr.; Bayer, Swed.; Bayer, UK.
Niclosamide (p.105·3).
Diphyllobothriasis; taeniasis.

Yomesane Bayer, Switz.†.
Niclosamide (p.105·3).
Taeniasis.

Yomogi Stroschein, Ger.†.
Lactobacillus acidophilus (p.1594·1).
Gastro-intestinal disorders.

Your Choice Amcon, USA.
Saline rinsing and storage solutions for soft contact lenses (p.1162·2).

Yovis Formenti, Ital.
Streptococcus salivarius subsp. *thermophilus; Bifidobacterium breve; B. infantis; B. longum; Lactobacillus acidophilus; L. plantarum; L. casei; L. delbrueckii* subsp. *bulgaricus; Streptococcus faecium* (p.1594·1).
Disturbance of gastro-intestinal flora.

Ypsiloheel Heel, Ger.
Homoeopathic preparation.

YSE Chatelut, Fr.
Zinc phosphate (p.1373·3); nux vomica (p.1609·3); kola (p.1645·1).
Tonic.

YSE Glutamique Chatelut, Fr.
Zinc phosphate (p.1373·3); glutamic acid (p.1344·3); nux vomica (p.1609·3); kola (p.1645·1).
Tonic.

Ysol Bournonville, Belg.†.
Acetic acid (p.1541·2); camphor (p.1557·2).
Pediculosis.

Ysol 206 Rabi & Solabo, Fr.
Acetic acid (p.1541·2); camphor (p.1557·2); Java citronella oil (p.1565·1); sodium lauryl sulphate (p.1468·3).
Pediculosis.

Yugu Prats, Spain†.
Venous plexus.
Vascular disorders.

Yurelax ICN, Spain.
Cyclobenzaprine hydrochloride (p.1313·2).
Skeletal muscle spasm.

Yutopar Solvay, Austral.; Bristol, Canad.; Solvay, Irl.; Schering, S.Afr.†; Solvay, UK; Astra, USA.
Ritodrine hydrochloride (p.1625·3).
Fetal distress; premature labour.

Yxin Pfizer, Ger.
Tetrahydrozoline hydrochloride (p.1070·2).
Eye disorders.

Z Span Goldshield, UK.
Zinc sulphate (p.1373·2).
Zinc deficiency.

Zacam Fournier, Ital.
Piroxicam (p.80·2).
Musculoskeletal, joint, and peri-articular disorders.

Zacin Bioglan, UK.
Capsaicin (p.24·2).
Osteoarthritis.

Z-Acne Vita Glow, Austral.
Cream†: Zinc oxide (p.1096·2); panthenol (p.1571·1); triclosan (p.1127·2); biosulphur (p.1091·2); alcloxa (p.1078·2).
Tablets: Zinc amino acid chelate (p.1373·3); vitamins and minerals.
Acne.

Zactin Alphapharm, Austral.
Fluoxetine hydrochloride (p.284·1).
Depression.

Zadine Schering-Plough, Austral.
Azatadine maleate (p.402·3).
Hypersensitivity reactions.

Zadipina SmithKline Beecham, Ital.
Nisoldipine (p.922·3).
Angina pectoris; hypertension.

Zaditen Sanabo, Aust.; Wander, Belg.; Sandoz, Canad.; Sandoz, Fr.; Wander, Ger.; Sandoz, Irl.; Novartis, Ital.; Sandoz, Jpn.; Novartis, Neth.; Novartis, S.Afr.; Sandoz, Switz.; Sandoz, UK.
Ketotifen fumarate (p.755·2).
Asthma; bronchitis; hypersensitivity reactions.

Zadorine Mepha, Switz.
Doxycycline hydrochloride (p.202·3).
Bacterial infections.

Zadstat Lederle, UK.
Metronidazole (p.585·1).
Anaerobic bacterial infections; protozoal infections.

Zadyl Thera, Fr.
Cephradine (p.181·3).
Bacterial infections.

Zaedoc Ashbourne, UK.
Ranitidine hydrochloride (p.1209·3).
Acid aspiration; dyspepsia; gastro-intestinal haemorrhage; gastro-oesophageal reflux; peptic ulcer; Zollinger-Ellison syndrome.

Zafen Zambon, Neth.
Ibuprofen (p.44·1).
Fever; inflammation; musculoskeletal, joint, and peri-articular disorders; pain.

Zafor Mepha, Switz.
Chlorzoxazone (p.1313·1); paracetamol (p.72·2).
Painful skeletal muscle spasm.

Zagam Specia, Fr.; Rhone-Poulenc Rorer, S.Afr.; Rhone-Poulenc Rorer, Switz.; Rhone-Poulenc Rorer, USA.
Sparfloxacin (p.248·2).
Bacterial infections.

Zagyl Xixia, S.Afr.
Metronidazole (p.585·1).
Anaerobic bacterial infections; protozoal infections.

Zahnerol N Dr Janssen, Ger.
Benzocaine (p.1286·2).
Zahnerol formerly contained benzocaine, guaiazulene, laureth 9, and sodium fluoride.
Dental disorders.

Zahnungstropfen Escatitona Madaus, Ger.
Homoeopathic preparation.

Zalain Trommsdorff, Ger.; Robert, Spain.
Sertaconazole nitrate (p.387·2).
Fungal skin infections.

Zalig Fournier, Ital.
Propionyl erythromycin mercaptosuccinate (p.206·2).
Bacterial infections.

Zalvor Glaxo Wellcome, Belg.
Permethrin (p.1409·2).
Scabies.

Zamadol Asta Medica, UK.
Tramadol hydrochloride (p.90·1).
Pain.

Zambesil Gentili, Ital.
Chlorthalidone (p.839·3).
Hypertension; oedema.

Zam-Buk
Note. This name is used for preparations of different composition.
Key, Austral.
Eucalyptus oil (p.1578·1); camphor (p.1557·2); sassafras oil (p.1627·3); thyme oil (p.1637·1); colophony (p.1567·1).
Minor skin disorders.

Roche, S.Afr.
Eucalyptus oil (p.1578·1); camphor (p.1557·2); thyme oil (p.1637·1); sassafras oil (p.1627·3).
Burns; chapped hands; insect bites; muscular pain; pruritus; wounds.

Roche Consumer, UK†.
Eucalyptus oil (p.1578·1); thyme oil (p.1637·1); camphor (p.1557·2); colophony (p.1567·1).
Skin abrasions; wounds.

Zamene Menarini, Spain.
Deflazacort (p.1036·2).
Corticosteroid.

Zamocillin Simes, Ital.†.
Amoxycillin trihydrate (p.151·3).
Bacterial infections.

Zamocilline Zambon, Fr.
Amoxycillin (p.151·3).
Bacterial infections.

Zanaflex Athena Neurosciences, UK; Athena Neurosciences, USA.
Tizanidine hydrochloride (p.1322·1).
Skeletal muscle spasticity.

Zandine Duncan, Flockhart, Irl.
Ranitidine hydrochloride (p.1209·3).
Gastric hyperacidity; gastro-oesophageal reflux; peptic ulcer; Zollinger-Ellison syndrome.

Zanidip Napp, UK.
Lercanidipine hydrochloride (p.897·3).
Hypertension.

Zanitrin Bristol-Myers Squibb, Ital.†.
Propylene glycol cefatrizine (p.164·2).
Bacterial infections.

Zanizal Italfarmaco, Ital.
Nizatidine (p.1203·2).
Gastro-oesophageal reflux; peptic ulcer.

Zanosar Pharmacia Upjohn, Canad.; Pharmacia Upjohn, Fr.; Upjohn, Neth.†; Upjohn, USA.
Streptozocin (p.562·1).
Pancreatic cancer.

Zantac Glaxo Wellcome, Aust.; Glaxo Wellcome, Austral.; Glaxo Wellcome, Belg.; Glaxo Wellcome, Canad.; Glaxo Wellcome, Irl.; Glaxo Wellcome, Ital.; Glaxo Wellcome, Neth.; Glaxo Wellcome, Norw.; Glaxo Wellcome, S.Afr.; Glaxo Wellcome, Spain; Glaxo Wellcome, Swed.; Glaxo, UK; Glaxo Wellcome, USA.
Ranitidine hydrochloride (p.1209·3).
Aspiration syndromes; gastric hyperacidity; gastro-intestinal haemorrhage; gastro-oesophageal reflux; peptic ulcer; Zollinger-Ellison syndrome.

Zantic Glaxo Wellcome, Ger.; Glaxo Wellcome, Switz.
Ranitidine hydrochloride (p.1209·3).
Gastro-intestinal disorders associated with hyperacidity; premedication.

Zantrene Lederle, Fr.†.
Bisantrene hydrochloride (p.507·3).
Malignant neoplasms.

Zantryl Ion, USA.
Phentermine hydrochloride (p.1484·3).

Zanzevia Milanfarma, Ital.†.
Plate: Bioallethrin (p.1402·3); piperonyl butoxide (p.1409·3).
Spiral: Bioallethrin (p.1402·3).
Insecticide.

Zanzipik Tipomark, Ital.
Diethyltoluamide (p.1405·1).
Insect repellent.

ZAP Germiphene, Canad.†.
Benzocaine (p.1286·2); amethocaine (p.1285·2).
Local anaesthesia.

Zaperin Sanabo, Aust.
Salbutamol (p.758·2).
Asthma; bronchoconstriction.

Zappelin Iso, Ger.
Homoeopathic preparation.

Zarent Italchimici, Ital.
Nedocromil sodium (p.756·2); salbutamol sulphate (p.758·2).
Obstructive airways disease.

Zariviz Hoechst Marion Roussel, Ital.
Cefotaxime sodium (p.168·2).
Lignocaine hydrochloride (p.1293·2) is included in the intramuscular injection to alleviate the pain of injection.
Bacterial infections.

Zarondan Warner-Lambert, Norw.
Ethosuximide (p.344·3).
Absence seizures.

Zarontin Parke, Davis, Austral.; Parke, Davis, Belg.; Parke, Davis, Canad.; Parke, Davis, Fr.; Parke, Davis, Irl.; Parke, Davis, Ital.; Parke, Davis, Neth.; Parke, Davis, S.Afr.; Parke, Davis, Spain; Parke, Davis, UK; Parke, Davis, USA.
Ethosuximide (p.344·3).
Absence seizures.

Zaroxolyn Rhone-Poulenc Rorer, Canad.; Heumann, Ger.; Rhone-Poulenc Rorer, Irl.; Teofarma, Ital.; Novartis, S.Afr.; Sanofi, Swed.; Fisons, USA.
Metolazone (p.907·2).
Hypertension; oedema; renal impairment.

Zaroxolyne Sandoz, Switz.
Metolazone (p.907·2).
Hypertension; oedema.

Zartan Dartmouth, USA†.
Cephalexin (p.178·2).

Zascal Albert, S.Afr.†.
Lacidipine (p.897·1).
Hypertension.

Zasten Sandoz, Spain.
Ketotifen (p.755·3).
Allergic rhinitis; asthma.

Zatinol Efarmes, Spain.
Paracetamol (p.72·2).
Fever; pain.

Zatofug Wolff, Ger.
Ketotifen fumarate (p.755·2).
Asthma; hypersensitivity reactions.

Zavedos Pharmacia Upjohn, Aust.; Pharmacia Upjohn, Austral.; Pharmacia Upjohn, Belg.; Pharmacia Upjohn, Fr.; Pharmacia Upjohn, Ger.; Pharmacia Upjohn, Irl.; Pharmacia Upjohn, Ital.; Pharmacia Upjohn, Neth.; Pharmacia Upjohn, Norw.; Pharmacia Upjohn, S.Afr.; Kenfarma, Spain; Pharmacia Upjohn, Swed.; Pharmacia Upjohn, Switz.; Farmitalia Carlo Erba, UK.
Idarubicin hydrochloride (p.540·1).
Malignant neoplasms.

Zaxopam Quantum, USA†.
Oxazepam (p.683·2).

Z-Bec
Note. This name is used for preparations of different composition.
Whitehall-Robins, Canad.
Multivitamin preparation with zinc sulphate (p.1373·2).

Robins, USA.
Multivitamin and mineral preparation.

ZBM Blackmores, Austral.
Zinc amino acid chelate (p.1373·3); vitamins and minerals.
Zinc deficiency.

ZBT Glenwood, USA.
Talc (p.1092·1); liquid paraffin (p.1382·1).
Nappy rash.

Ze Caps Everett, USA.
Zinc gluconate (p.1373·2); vitamin E (p.1369·1).
Dietary supplement.

ZeaSorb
Note. This name is used for preparations of different composition.
Stiefel, Austral.; Stiefel, Canad.; Stiefel, Ger.; Stiefel, Irl.
Chloroxylenol (p.1111·1); aldioxa (p.1078·2); cellulose (p.1472·1).
Bromhidrosis; hyperhidrosis; intertrigo.

Stiefel, Fr.
Cellulose (p.1472·1); aldioxa (p.1078·2); magnesium silicate (p.1473·3).
Hyperhidrosis.

Stiefel, S.Afr.†; Stiefel, UK.
Chloroxylenol (p.1111·1); aldioxa (p.1078·2).
Bromhidrosis; hyperhidrosis; intertrigo; prophylaxis of fungal skin infections.

ZeaSorb AF
Note. This name is used for preparations of different composition.
Stiefel, Canad.
Tolnaftate (p.389·1).
Fungal skin infections.

Stiefel, USA.
Miconazole nitrate (p.384·3).
Fungal skin infections.

Zebeta Lederle, USA.
Bisoprolol fumarate (p.833·1).
Hypertension.

Zeclar Abbott, Fr.
Clarithromycin (p.189·1).
Bacterial infections.

Zecnil Ferring, Ital.
Somatostatin acetate (p.1261·1).
Diabetic ketoacidosis; gastro-intestinal haemorrhage; pancreatic surgery.

Zeddan Mediolanum, Ital.
Trandolapril (p.957·1).
Hypertension.

Zedene C Whitehall, Fr.
Multivitamin and mineral preparation.

Zedolac Maggioni, Ital.†.
Etodolac (p.36·2).
Rheumatic joint disorders.

Zeefra Doms-Adrian, Fr.
Cephradine (p.181·3).
Bacterial infections.

Zeel Heel, Ger.
Homoeopathic preparation.

Zefazone Upjohn, USA.
Cefmetazole sodium (p.166·2).
Bacterial infections.

Zefirol Bayer, Ital.
Benzalkonium chloride (p.1101·3).
Disinfection of skin, mucous membranes, and wounds; surface disinfection.

Zeisin 3M, Ger.
Pirbuterol acetate (p.757·2).
Obstructive airways disease.

Zelapar Athena Neurosciences, UK.
Selegiline hydrochloride (p.1144·2).
Parkinsonism.

Zeliderm Vinas, Spain.
Azelaic acid (p.1079·1).
Acne.

Zelis Prospa, Ital.
Piroxicam cinnamate (p.81·1).
Musculoskeletal and joint disorders.

Zelitrex Glaxo Wellcome, Fr.; Glaxo Wellcome, Neth.; Glaxo Wellcome, S.Afr.
Valaciclovir hydrochloride (p.628·1).
Herpesvirus infections.

Zellaforte Zellaforte, Switz.
Multivitamin and mineral preparation.

Zellaforte N Plus Eurim, Ger.
Nikethamide calcium thiocyanate (p.1483·3); inositol nicotinate (p.891·3); pholedrine sulphate (p.930·2).
Tonic.

Zellaforte plus Chemieprodukte, Aust.
Procaine hydrochloride; haematoporphyrin; ferrous sulphate; vitamins.
Tonic.

Zeller-Augenwasser Herchemie, Aust.†.
Saffron (p.1001·1); fennel oil (p.1579·2); zinc sulphate (p.1373·2).
Eye inflammation and irritation.

Zemide Wyeth, Ger.
Tamoxifen citrate (p.563·3).
Breast cancer.

Zemplar Abbott, USA.
Paricalcitol (p.1368·1).
Hyperparathyroidism.

Zemtard Bartholomew Rhodes, UK.
Diltiazem hydrochloride (p.854·2).
Angina pectoris; hypertension.

Zemuron Organon, Canad.; Organon, USA.
Rocuronium bromide (p.1318·2).
Competitive neuromuscular blocker.

Zen Select, Ital.
Piroxicam cinnamate (p.81·1).
Musculoskeletal and joint disorders.

Zenalb BPL, UK.
Albumin (p.710·1).
Burns; hypoalbuminaemia; hypovolaemic shock.

Zenapax Roche, USA.
Daclizimab (p.527·1).
Renal transplant rejection.

Zenavan Wyeth, Spain.
Etofenamate (p.36·3).
Pain; peri-articular disorders.

Zenit Pulitzer, Ital.†.
Pivagabine (p.306·3).
Depression.

Zenoxone Biorex, UK.
Hydrocortisone (p.1043·3).

Zensyls Ernest Jackson, UK.
Benzalkonium chloride (p.1101·3).
Sore throat.

Zentavion Vita, Spain.
Azithromycin (p.155·2).
Bacterial infections.

Zentel
SmithKline Beecham, Austral.; SmithKline Beecham, Fr.; SmithKline Beecham, Ital.; SmithKline Beecham, S.Afr.; SmithKline Beecham, Switz.
Albendazole (p.96·2).
Worm infections.

Zentinic Lilly, USA†.
Multivitamin preparation with iron.

Zentramin Bastian N Bastian, Ger.
Electrolyte preparation (p.1147·1).

Zentron Lilly, USA†.
Multivitamin preparation with iron.

Zentropil Knoll, Ger.
Phenytoin (p.352·3) or phenytoin sodium (p.352·3).
Epilepsy.

Zepelin
Bender, Aust.; Boehringer Ingelheim, Ital.
Feprazone (p.41·2).
Inflammation; musculoskeletal and joint disorders; pain.

Zepelindue Boehringer Ingelheim, Ital.
Ketoprofen lysine (p.48·3).
Inflammation; musculoskeletal, joint, peri-articular, and soft-tissue disorders; pain.

Zephiran
Sanofi Winthrop, Canad.; Sanofi Winthrop, USA.
Benzalkonium chloride (p.1101·3).
Eye, bladder, urethra, and body cavity irrigation; skin, mucous membrane, wound, instrument, and surface disinfection; vaginal douching.

Zephirol Bayer, Ger.†.
Benzalkonium chloride (p.1101·3).
Instrument disinfection; skin disinfection.

Zepholin Klinge, Irl.
Theophylline (p.765·1).
Bronchospasm.

Zephrex Sanofi Winthrop, USA.
Pseudoephedrine hydrochloride (p.1068·3); guaiphenesin (p.1061·3).
Coughs.

Zerinetta-Fher Boehringer Ingelheim, Ital.
Paracetamol (p.72·2); phenylpropanolamine hydrochloride (p.1067·2); chlorpheniramine maleate (p.405·1).
Cold and influenza symptoms.

Zerinol-Fher Boehringer Ingelheim, Ital.
Paracetamol (p.72·2); phenylpropanolamine hydrochloride (p.1067·2); chlorpheniramine maleate (p.405·1).
Formerly contained feprazone, paracetamol, phenylpropanolamine hydrochloride, and chlorpheniramine maleate.
Cold and influenza symptoms.

Zerit
Bristol-Myers Squibb, Austral.; Bristol-Myers Squibb, Canad.; Bristol-Myers Squibb, Fr.; Bristol-Myers Squibb, Ger.; Bristol-Myers Squibb, Irl.; Bristol-Myers Squibb, Ital.; Bristol-Myers Squibb, Neth.; Bristol-Myers, Spain; Bristol-Myers Squibb, Swed.; Bristol-Myers Squibb, Switz.; Bristol-Myers Squibb, UK; Bristol-Myers Squibb, USA.
Stavudine (p.625·3).
HIV infection.

Zeropyn Pharmco, S.Afr.
Paracetamol (p.72·2); codeine phosphate (p.26·1).
Fever; pain.

Zestabs Suisse, Austral.†.
Royal jelly (p.1626·3); pollen; ginseng (p.1584·2); fo-ti-tieng; gotu cola (p.1080·3); sarsaparilla (p.1627·2).
Nutritional supplement.

Zesties Pharmatec, S.Afr.†.
Multivitamin preparation.

Zestoretic
Zeneca, Aust.; Zeneca, Belg.; Zeneca, Canad.; Zeneca, Fr.; Zeneca, Irl.; Zeneca, Ital.; Zeneca, Neth.; Zeneca, Norw.; Zeneca, S.Afr.; Zeneca, Spain; Zeneca, Swed.; Zeneca, Switz.; Zeneca, UK; Zeneca, USA.
Lisinopril (p.898·2); hydrochlorothiazide (p.885·2).
Hypertension.

Zestril
ICI, Austral.; Zeneca, Belg.; Zeneca, Canad.; Zeneca, Fr.; Zeneca, Irl.; Zeneca, Ital.; Zeneca, Neth.; Zeneca, Norw.; Zeneca, S.Afr.; Zeneca, Spain; Zeneca, Swed.; Zeneca, Switz.; Zeneca, UK; Zeneca, USA.
Lisinopril (p.898·2).
Diabetic nephropathy; heart failure; hypertension; myocardial infarction.

Zet 26 V Zwintscher, Ger.†.
Aloes (p.1177·1); senna (p.1212·2); frangula bark (p.1193·2).
Constipation.

Zeta N Bergamon, Ital.
Usnic acid (p.1643·1).
Vaginal disinfection.

Zeta-Bat Zeta, Ital.†.
Cetylpyridinium chloride (p.1106·2); aesculus (p.1543·3); magnesium thiosulphate (p.996·3).
Skin cleansing; skin irritation.

Zetacef Menarini, Ital.†.
Cephalexin (p.178·2).
Bacterial infections.

Zetacef-lis Menarini, Ital.†.
Cephalexin lysine (p.178·3).
Bacterial infections.

Zeta-Foot Zeta, Ital.†.
Cream: Usnic acid (p.1643·1); salicylic acid (p.1090·2); undecenoic acid (p.389·2); aluminium acetate (p.1547·3).
Topical powder: Usnic acid (p.1643·1); undecenoic acid (p.389·2); aluminium oxide (p.1077·2); zinc stearate (p.1469·3); zinc oxide (p.1096·2); kaolin (p.1195·1).
Hyperhidrosis and odour of the feet.

Zetamicin Menarini, Ital.
Netilmicin sulphate (p.231·1).
Bacterial infections.

Zetar
Dermik, Canad.; Dermik, USA.
Coal tar (p.1092·3).
Skin disorders.

Zetavit Zeta, Ital.
Multivitamin and mineral preparation.

Zetran Hauck, USA†.
Diazepam (p.661·1).
Anxiety; epilepsy; skeletal muscle spasm.

Zettagall V Zwintscher, Ger.†.
Chelidonium majus; turmeric (p.1001·3); centaury (p.1561·1); taraxacum (p.1634·2).
Biliary disorders; gastro-intestinal disorders.

Zettaviran Zwintscher, Ger.†.
Procaine hydrochloride (p.1299·2); sodium pangamate (p.1614·1).
Circulatory disorders; muscle and joint disorders.

Z-gen Goldline, USA.
Multivitamin and mineral preparation.

Ziac Lederle, USA.
Bisoprolol fumarate (p.833·1); hydrochlorothiazide (p.885·2).
Hypertension.

Zibren Purophama, Ital.
Acetylcarnitine or acetylcarnitine hydrochloride (p.1542·1).
Cerebrovascular disorders; peripheral neuropathy.

Ziclin Knoll, S.Afr.
Gliclazide (p.320·1).
Diabetes mellitus.

Zida-Co Opus, UK.
Amiloride hydrochloride (p.819·2); hydrochlorothiazide (p.885·2).
These ingredients can be described by the British Approved Name Co-amilozide.
Heart failure; hepatic cirrhosis; hypertension.

Zidoval 3M, UK.
Metronidazole (p.585·1).
Bacterial vaginosis.

Zidovit IBP, Ital.†.
Cobamamide (p.1364·2).
Tonic.

Zienam
Merck Sharp & Dohme, Aust.; Merck Sharp & Dohme, Ger.
Imipenem monohydrate (p.216·3); cilastatin sodium (p.185·2).
Lignocaine hydrochloride (p.1293·2) may be included in the intramuscular injection to alleviate the pain of injection.
Bacterial infections.

Zig C Falqui, Ital.
Ascorbic acid (p.1365·2).

Ziks Nnodum, USA.
Methyl salicylate (p.55·2); menthol (p.1600·2); capsaicin (p.24·2).
Musculoskeletal, joint, and soft-tissue disorders; neuralgia.

Zilabrace Zila, USA†.
Benzocaine (p.1286·2).

Zilactin
Note. This name is used for preparations of different composition.
Bausch & Lomb, Canad.
Benzyl alcohol (p.1103·3).
Formerly contained tannic acid.
Lip lesions; mouth ulcers.

Zila, USA.
Tannic acid (p.1634·2).
Canker sores; herpes labialis.

Zilactin-B Medicated Zila, USA.
Benzocaine (p.1286·2).
Sore throats.

Zilactin-L Zila, USA.
Lignocaine (p.1293·2).

ZilaDent Zila, USA†.
Benzocaine (p.1286·2).
Local anaesthesia.

Zildem Parke-Med, S.Afr.
Diltiazem hydrochloride (p.854·2).
Angina pectoris; hypertension.

Zilden Searle, Ital.
Diltiazem hydrochloride (p.854·2).
Angina pectoris; heart failure; myocardial infarction.

Zileze Opus, UK.
Zopiclone (p.699·2).
Insomnia.

Zimadoce Rubio, Spain.
Cobamamide (p.1364·2).
Tonic.

Zimetin Lagap, Switz.†.
Cimetidine (p.1183·2).
Gastro-oesophageal reflux; peptic ulcer; Zollinger-Ellison syndrome.

Zimeton Ital Suisse, Ital.†.
Cogalactoisomerase sodium (p.1566·2).
Liver disorders.

Zimocel Ilex, Ital.
Dried yeast (p.1373·1).

Zimor Rubio, Spain.
Omeprazole (p.1204·2).
Gastro-oesophageal reflux; peptic ulcer; Zollinger-Ellison syndrome.

Zimospuma Baldacci, Ital.
Bovine fibrin (p.722·2).
Haemorrhage.

Zimotrombina Baldacci, Ital.
Thrombin (porcine) (p.728·1).
Haemorrhage.

Zimovane
Rhone-Poulenc Rorer, Irl.; Rhone-Poulenc Rorer, UK.
Zopiclone (p.699·2).
Insomnia.

Zimox Pharmacia Upjohn, Ital.
Amoxycillin trihydrate (p.151·3).
Bacterial infections.

Zinacef
Glaxo Wellcome, Belg.; Glaxo Wellcome, Canad.; Hoechst, Ger.; Glaxo Wellcome, Ger.; Glaxo Wellcome, Irl.; Glaxo Wellcome, Neth.; Glaxo Wellcome, Norw.; Glaxo Wellcome, S.Afr.; Glaxo Wellcome, Swed.; Glaxo Wellcome, Switz.; Glaxo, UK; Glaxo Wellcome, USA.
Cefuroxime sodium (p.177·1).
Bacterial infections.

Zinaderm Technilab, Canad.
Zinc oxide (p.1096·2).
Skin disorders.

Zinadiur SmithKline Beecham, Ital.
Benazepril hydrochloride (p.827·1); hydrochlorothiazide (p.885·2).
Hypertension.

Zinadril SmithKline Beecham, Ital.
Benazepril hydrochloride (p.827·1).
Heart failure; hypertension.

Zinaf SoSe, Ital.
Propylene glycol cefatrizine (p.164·2).
Bacterial infections.

Zinamide
Merck Sharp & Dohme, Austral.; Merck Sharp & Dohme, Irl.; Merck Sharp & Dohme, UK.
Pyrazinamide (p.241·1).
Tuberculosis.

Zinat Glaxo Wellcome, Switz.
Cefuroxime axetil (p.177·1).
Bacterial infections.

Zinc + C250 Vitaplex, Austral.
Zinc amino acid chelate (p.1373·3); ascorbic acid (p.1365·2).
Zinc deficiency.

Zinc C Plus Vita Glow, Austral.
Zinc amino acid chelate (p.1373·3); ascorbic acid (p.1365·2); vitamin B substances.
Inflammation; skin disorders; wounds.

Zinc Cream White McGloin, Austral.
SPF15+: Zinc oxide (p.1096·2).
Burns; nappy rash; skin abrasions; skin irritation; sunscreen.

Zinc in der Ophtiole Mann, Ger.†.
Zinc lactate; ephedrine (p.1059·3).
Eye disorders.

Zinc Plus
Cenovis, Austral.; Vitelle, Austral.
Zinc amino acid chelate (p.1373·3); vitamins and minerals.
Zinc deficiency.

Bio-Health, UK.
Zinc gluconate; vitamin B_6; magnesium.

Zinc Supplement Vitaplex, Austral.
Zinc gluconate (p.1373·2); vitamins and minerals.
Zinc deficiency.

Zinc Zenith Eagle, Austral.
Zinc gluconate (p.1373·2); zinc amino acid chelate (p.1373·3); alfalfa (p.1544·2); ascorbic acid (p.1365·2); maltase (p.1546·2); pyridoxine hydrochloride (p.1362·3); minerals.
Zinc, vitamin C and vitamin B_6 supplement.

Zincaband
Boots, Austral.; Smith & Nephew, Swed.; Seton, UK.
Zinc oxide (p.1096·2).
Medicated bandage.

Zinca-Pak Smith & Nephew SoloPak, USA.
Zinc sulphate (p.1373·2).
Additive for intravenous total parenteral nutrition solutions.

Zincaps Rhone-Poulenc Rorer, Austral.
Zinc sulphate (p.1373·2).
Zinc deficiency.

Zincate Paddock, USA.
Zinc sulphate (p.1373·2).
Dietary supplement.

Zincfrin
Alcon, Austral.; Alcon, Belg.; Alcon, Canad.; Alcon-Thilo, Ger.; Alcon, Neth.†; Alcon, S.Afr.†; Alcon, Spain; Alcon, Swed.; Alcon, Switz.; Alcon, USA.
Phenylephrine hydrochloride (p.1066·2); zinc sulphate (p.1373·2).
Eye irritation.

Zincfrin Antihistaminicum Alcon, Belg.
Antazoline phosphate (p.401·3); naphazoline hydrochloride (p.1064·2); zinc sulphate (p.1373·2).
Formerly known as Zincfrin-A.
Conjunctival congestion; eye irritation.

Zincfrin-A
Alcon, Canad.; Alcon, S.Afr.†; Alcon, Switz.†.
Antazoline phosphate (p.401·3); naphazoline hydrochloride (p.1064·2); zinc sulphate (p.1373·2).
Allergic conjunctivitis.

Zinc-Ichtyol Asta Medica, Belg.
Zinc oxide (p.1096·2); ichthammol (p.1083·3).
Blepharitis; eczema and pruritus of the eye.

Zinc-Imizol Farmigea, Ital.
Zinc sulphate (p.1373·2); naphazoline nitrate (p.1064·2).
Conjunctivitis, alone or associated with blepharitis.

Zinco All' Acqua Lachifarma, Ital.; Sella, Ital.
Zinc oxide (p.1096·2).
Skin disorders.

Zincoderm Taro, Canad.
Zinc oxide (p.1096·2).

Zincofax Warner-Lambert, Canad.
Zinc oxide (p.1096·2).
Nappy rash.

Zincoimidazyl Allergan, Ital.†.
Antazoline sulphate (p.402·1); naphazoline nitrate (p.1064·2); zinc sulphate (p.1373·2); procaine hydrochloride (p.1299·2).
Allergic conjunctivitis.

Zincold 23 Vitalia, UK.
Zinc gluconate (p.1373·2); ascorbic acid (p.1365·2).
Colds.

Zincomed Medo, UK†.
Zinc sulphate (p.1373·2).
Zinc deficiency.

Zincometil Farmila, Ital.
Benzalkonium chloride (p.1101·3); zinc sulphate (p.1373·2).
Eye disinfection.

Zincon Lederle, USA.
Pyrithione zinc (p.1089·3).
Scalp disorders.

Zincoral Mavi, Ital.
Zinc and copper supplement.

Zincosin Vis, Ital.†.
Resorcinol (p.1090·1); zinc phenolsulphonate (p.1096·3); lignocaine hydrochloride (p.1293·2).
Eye infections.

Zincosol Bioceuticals, UK.
Zinc sulphate (p.1373·2).

Zincotape Lohmann, Ital.
Zinc oxide (p.1096·2).
Medicated dressing.

Zincotex Lohmann, Ital.
Zinc oxide (p.1096·2).
Medicated dressing.

Zincstic Vitalia, UK.
Zinc oxide (p.1096·2); titanium dioxide (p.1093·3).
Sunscreen.

Zinctrace Rorer, Austral.†.
Zinc chloride (p.1373·1).
Zinc deficiency.

Zincum val plus Hevert, Ger.†.
Diphenhydramine hydrochloride (p.409·1); aconit. nap.; ambra; castoreum; cimicifuga; cocculus; coffea; conium; convallaria; cypripedium; hypericum; ignatia; kava-kava; mitchella; moschus; nux vomica; ol. anisi; passiflora; platinum; valeriana; zincum val.
Nervous disorders; sleep disorders.

Zincum valerianicum-Hevert Hevert, Ger.
Homoeopathic preparation.

Zincvit Kenwood, USA.
Multivitamin and mineral preparation.

Zinecard
Pharmacia Upjohn, Canad.; Pharmacia, USA.
Dexrazoxane (p.978·3) or dexrazoxane hydrochloride (p.978·3).
Prevention of doxorubicin cardiotoxicity.

Zineryt
Yamanouchi, Belg.; Hermal, Ger.; Yamanouchi, Irl.; Yamanouchi, Ital.; Yamanouchi, Neth.; Yamanouchi, UK.
Erythromycin (p.204·1); zinc acetate (p.1646·2).
Acne.

Zinga Ashbourne, UK.
Nizatidine (p.1203·2).
Gastro-oesophageal reflux; peptic ulcer.

Zinkamin Falk, Ger.
Bis(L-histadinato) zinc (p.1373·3).
Zinc deficiency.

Zink-D *Artesan, Ger.; Cassella-med, Ger.*
Zinc gluconate (p.1373·2).
Zinc deficiency.

Zinkit *Worwag, Ger.*
Zinc sulphate (p.1373·2).
Zinc deficiency.

Zink'N'Swim *Or-Dov, Austral.*
SPF 15+: Zinc oxide (p.1096·2).
Sunscreen.

Zink'N'Swim Fluorescent *Or-Dov, Austral.*
SPF 15+: Zinc oxide (p.1096·2).
Sunscreen.

Zinkokehl *Sanum-Kehlbeck, Ger.*
Homoeopathic preparation.

Zinkolie *Boots Healthcare, Neth.*
Zinc oxide (p.1096·2).
Skin disorders.

Zinkorell *Sanorell, Ger.*
Homoeopathic preparation.

Zinkorot *Worwag, Ger.*
Zinc orotate (p.1373·3).
Zinc deficiency.

Zinkosalb *Hilarys, Canad.*
Salicylic acid (p.1090·2); zinc oxide (p.1096·2).

zinkotase *GN, Ger.*
Zinc aspartate.
Zinc deficiency.

Zinkzalf *Boots Healthcare, Neth.*
Zinc oxide (p.1096·2).
Skin disorders.

Zinnat
Glaxo Wellcome, Aust.; Glaxo Wellcome, Belg.; Glaxo Wellcome, Fr.; Glaxo Wellcome, Ger.; Glaxo Wellcome, Irl.; Glaxo Wellcome, Ital.; Glaxo Wellcome, Neth.; Glaxo Wellcome, S.Afr.; Glaxo Wellcome, Spain; Glaxo Wellcome, Swed.; Glaxo, UK.
Cefuroxime axetil (p.177·1) or cefuroxime sodium (p.177·1).
Lignocaine hydrochloride (p.1293·2) is included in some intramuscular injections to alleviate the pain of injection.
Formerly known as Curoxime in *Fr.*
Bacterial infections.

Zintona
Bender, Aust.; Pharmaton, Ger.; GPL, Switz.
Ginger (p.1193·2).
Digestive system disorders; gastric pain; motion sickness; vomiting.

Zinvit *Vita Glow, Austral.*
Zinc sulphate (p.1373·2); magnesium sulphate (p.1157·3); vitamin B substances.
Herpes labialis; mouth ulcers; skin disorders; wounds; zinc deficiency.

Zinvit C *Vita Glow, Austral.*
Zinc sulphate (p.1373·2); magnesium sulphate (p.1157·3); ascorbic acid (p.1365·2).
Herpes labialis; mouth ulcers; skin disorders; wounds.

Zinvit G *Vita Glow, Austral.*
Zinc sulphate (p.1373·2); magnesium sulphate (p.1157·3); vitamin B substances.
Skin disorders; zinc deficiency.

Zipzoc *Smith & Nephew Healthcare, UK.*
Zinc oxide (p.1096·2) impregnated stocking.
Leg ulcers.

Ziradryl *Parke, Davis, USA.*
Diphenhydramine hydrochloride (p.409·1); zinc oxide (p.1096·2); camphor (p.1557·2).
Pruritus.

Zirkulin Beruhigungs-Tee *Schulke & Mayr, Aust.*
Lupulus (p.1597·2).
Restlessness; sleep disorders.

Zirtec *UCB, Ital.*
Cetirizine hydrochloride (p.404·2).
Conjunctivitis; rhinitis; urticaria.

Zirtek
UCB, Irl.; UCB, UK.
Cetirizine hydrochloride (p.404·2).
Allergic rhinitis; pruritus; urticaria.

Zispin
Organon, Irl.; Organon, UK.
Mirtazapine (p.298·2).
Depression.

Zita *Eastern Pharmaceuticals, UK.*
Cimetidine (p.1183·2).
Gastro-intestinal disorders associated with hyperacidity.

Zitazonium *Thiemann, Ger.*
Tamoxifen citrate (p.563·3).
Breast cancer.

Zithromax
Pfizer, Aust.; Pfizer, Austral.; Pfizer, Canad.; Pfizer, Fr.; Mack, Illert., Ger.; Bayer, Ger.; Pfizer, Irl.; Pfizer, Neth.; Pfizer, S.Afr.; Pfizer, Switz.; Pfizer, UK; Pfizer, USA.
Azithromycin (p.155·2).
Bacterial infections.

Zitoxil *Italfarmaco, Ital.*
Zipeprol hydrochloride (p.1071·3).
Coughs.

Zitrix *Metapharma, Ital.*
Propylene glycol cefatrizine (p.164·2).
Bacterial infections.

Zitromax
Pfizer, Belg.; Pfizer, Ital.; Pfizer, Spain.
Azithromycin (p.155·2).
Bacterial infections.

ZN 220 *Covan, S.Afr.*
Zinc sulphate (p.1373·2).
Wounds.

ZNP
Stiefel, Canad.; Stiefel, Fr.; Stiefel, Ital.; Stiefel, USA.
Pyrithione zinc (p.1089·3).
Scalp disorders; seborrhoeic dermatitis.

Zobacide *Garec, S.Afr.*
Metronidazole (p.585·1).
Anaerobic bacterial infections; protozoal infections.

Zocor
Merck Sharp & Dohme, Austral.; Merck Sharp & Dohme, Belg.; Frosst, Canad.; Merck Sharp & Dohme-Chibret, Fr.; Dieckmann, Ger.; Merck Sharp & Dohme, Irl.; Neopharmed, Ital.; Merck Sharp & Dohme, Neth.; Merck Sharp & Dohme, Norw.; Merck Sharp & Dohme, S.Afr.; Merck Sharp & Dohme, Spain; Merck Sharp & Dohme, Switz.; Merck Sharp & Dohme, UK; Merck Sharp & Dohme, USA.
Simvastatin (p.1278·2).
Hypercholesterolaemia; ischaemic heart disease.

Zocord
Merck Sharp & Dohme, Aust.; Merck Sharp & Dohme, Swed.
Simvastatin (p.1278·2).
Hypercholesterolaemia.

Zodeac *Econo Med, USA.*
Ferrous fumarate (p.1339·3); folic acid (p.1340·3); multivitamins and minerals.
Iron-deficiency anaemias.

Zoff
Note. This name is used for preparations of different composition.
Smith & Nephew, Austral.
Adhesive plaster remover.

Smith & Nephew Pharmaceuticals, UK.
Trichloroethane (p.1381·2).
Adhesive plaster removal.

Zofran
Glaxo Wellcome, Aust.; Glaxo Wellcome, Austral.; Glaxo Wellcome, Belg.; Glaxo Wellcome, Canad.; Glaxo Wellcome, Ger.; Glaxo Wellcome, Irl.; Glaxo Wellcome, Ital.; Glaxo Wellcome, Neth.; Glaxo Wellcome, Norw.; Glaxo Wellcome, S.Afr.; Glaxo Wellcome, Spain; Glaxo Wellcome, Swed.; Glaxo Wellcome, Switz.; Glaxo Wellcome, UK; Glaxo Wellcome, USA.
Ondansetron or ondansetron hydrochloride (p.1206·2).
Nausea and vomiting induced by cytotoxics or radiotherapy; postoperative nausea and vomiting.

Zok-Zid *Astra, Belg.*
Metoprolol succinate (p.908·2); hydrochlorothiazide (p.885·2).
Hypertension.

Zoladex
Zeneca, Aust.; ICI, Austral.; Zeneca, Belg.; Zeneca, Canad.; Zeneca, Fr.; Zeneca, Ger.; Zeneca, Irl.; Zeneca, Ital.; Zeneca, Neth.; Zeneca, Norw.; Zeneca, S.Afr.; Zeneca, Spain; Zeneca, Swed.; Zeneca, Switz.; Zeneca, UK; Zeneca, USA.
Goserelin acetate (p.1249·1).
Breast cancer; endometriosis; female infertility; presurgical endometrial thinning; prostatic cancer; uterine fibroids.

Zolben
Ciba-Geigy, Spain.
Paracetamol (p.72·2).
Fever; pain.

Zyma, Switz.
Paracetamol (p.72·2).
Fever; pain.

Zolben C *Zyma, Switz.*
Paracetamol (p.72·2); ascorbic acid (p.1365·2).
Fever; pain.

Zoleptil *Knoll, UK.*
Zotepine (p.700·1).
Schizophrenia.

Zolerol *Rolab, S.Afr.*
Metronidazole (p.585·1).
Anaerobic bacterial infections; protozoal infections.

Zolicef
Laevosan, Aust.; Apothecon, USA.
Cephazolin sodium (p.181·1).
Lignocaine hydrochloride (p.1293·2) may be included in the intramuscular injection to alleviate the pain of injection.
Bacterial infections.

Zolin
Note. This name is used for preparations of different composition.
San Carlo, Ital.
Cephazolin sodium (p.181·1).
Lignocaine hydrochloride (p.1293·2) is included in the intramuscular injection to alleviate the pain of injection.
Bacterial infections.

ACO, Swed.
Oxymetazoline hydrochloride (p.1065·3).
Rhinitis; sinusitis.

Zolina *Llorens, Spain.*
Boric acid (p.1554·2); naphazoline hydrochloride (p.1064·2).
Eye irritation.

Zoliparin *Mann, Ger.*
Aciclovir (p.602·3).
Herpes simplex eye infections.

Zolisint *Benedetti, Ital.*
Cephazolin sodium (p.181·1).
Lignocaine hydrochloride (p.1293·2) is included in this preparation to alleviate the pain of injection.
Bacterial infections.

Zolival *Septa, Spain.*
Cephazolin sodium (p.181·1).
Bacterial infections.

Zoloft
Pfizer, Aust.; Pfizer, Austral.; Pfizer, Canad.; Pfizer, Fr.; Roerig, Ital.; Pfizer, Neth.; Pfizer, Norw.; Pfizer, S.Afr.; Pfizer, Swed.; Pfizer, Switz.; Roerig, USA.
Sertraline hydrochloride (p.307·2).
Depression; obsessive-compulsive disorder.

Zoltum *Bellon, Fr.*
Omeprazole (p.1204·2).
Gastro-oesophageal reflux; peptic ulcer; Zollinger-Ellison syndrome.

Zolyse *Alcon, Switz.†.*
Chymotrypsin (p.1563·2).
Cataract surgery.

Zomacton
Ferring, Belg.; Ferring, Ger.; Ferring, Irl.; Ferring, Ital.; Ferring, Neth.; Ferring, Spain; Ferring, Swed.; Ferring, UK.
Somatropin (p.1249·3).
Growth hormone deficiency; Turner's syndrome.

Zomig
Zeneca, Swed.; Zeneca, UK; Zeneca, USA.
Zolmitriptan (p.452·1).
Migraine.

Zomorph *Link, UK.*
Morphine sulphate (p.56·2).
Pain.

Zonalon
GenDerm, Canad.; GenDerm, USA.
Doxepin hydrochloride (p.283·2).
Pruritus.

Zoncef *AGIPS, Ital.*
Cefoperazone sodium (p.167·3).
Lignocaine hydrochloride (p.1293·2) is included in the intramuscular injection to alleviate the pain of injection.
Bacterial infections.

Zone-A *UAD, USA†.*
Hydrocortisone acetate (p.1043·3); pramoxine (p.1298·2).

Zoniden *IRBI, Ital.†.*
Tioconazole (p.388·3).
Fungal infections.

Zonite *Menley & James, USA.*
Benzalkonium chloride (p.1101·3); edetic acid (p.980·3); sodium acetate (p.1153·1); propylene glycol (p.1622·1); menthol (p.1600·2); thymol (p.1127·1).
Vaginal disorders.

Zonivent *Ashbourne, UK.*
Beclomethasone dipropionate (p.1032·1).
Rhinitis.

Zonk *Wander Health Care, Switz.†.*
Food for special diets.
Appetite reduction; fibre supplement.

Zonulasi *Merck Sharp & Dohme, Ital.†.*
Chymotrypsin (p.1563·2).
Eye surgery.

Zonulysin
Covan, S.Afr.†; Henleys, UK†.
Chymotrypsin (p.1563·2).
Adjunct in cataract extraction.

Zoo Chews *Hall, Canad.*
Multivitamin preparation.

Zoo Chews with Iron *Hall, Canad.*
Multivitamin preparation with iron.

Zopax *Cipla-Medpro, S.Afr.*
Alprazolam (p.640·3).
Anxiety disorders.

Zophren *Glaxo Wellcome, Fr.*
Ondansetron hydrochloride (p.1206·2).
Nausea and vomiting.

Zorac
Allergan, Swed.; Allergan, UK.
Tazarotene (p.1093·2).
Psoriasis.

Zoref *Duncan, Ital.*
Cefuroxime axetil (p.177·1).
Bacterial infections.

Zoroxin
Merck Sharp & Dohme, Aust.; Merck Sharp & Dohme, Belg.
Norfloxacin (p.233·1).
Bacterial infections.

ZORprin *Boots, USA.*
Aspirin (p.16·1).
Fever; osteoarthritis; pain; rheumatoid arthritis.

Zoru
Codali, Belg.†; Maruishi, Neth.†.
Tartaric acid (p.1634·3); sodium bicarbonate (p.1153·2); simethicone (p.1213·1).
Gastro-intestinal radiography.

Zostrix
Knoll, Austral.; GenDerm, Canad.; GenDerm, USA.
Capsaicin (p.24·2).
Diabetic neuropathy; osteoarthritis; postherpetic neuralgia; rheumatoid arthritis.

Zostrum
Basotherm, Ger.; Boehringer Ingelheim, Irl.
Idoxuridine (p.613·2) in dimethyl sulphoxide.
Herpesvirus infections.

Zosyn *Lederle, USA.*
Piperacillin sodium (p.237·2); tazobactam sodium (p.257·3).
Bacterial infections.

Zoto-HC *Horizon, USA.*
Chloroxylenol (p.1111·1); pramoxine hydrochloride (p.1298·2); hydrocortisone (p.1043·3).
Formerly known as Xotic.
Ear disorders.

Zoton
Lederle, Austral.; Wyeth, Irl.; Cyanamid, Ital.; Wyeth, UK.
Lansoprazole (p.1196·2).
Gastro-oesophageal reflux; peptic ulcer; Zollinger-Ellison syndrome.

Zovia *Watson, USA.*
Ethinyloestradiol (p.1445·1); ethynodiol diacetate (p.1445·3).
28-Day packs also contain 7 inert tablets.
Combined oral contraceptive.

Zovir *Glaxo Wellcome, Swed.†.*
Aciclovir (p.602·3).
Herpes simplex and zoster infections.

Zovirax
Glaxo Wellcome, Aust.; Warner-Lambert, Austral.; Glaxo Wellcome, Austral.; Glaxo Wellcome, Belg.; Warner-Lambert Consumer, Belg.; Glaxo Wellcome, Canad.; Glaxo Wellcome, Fr.; Warner-Lambert, Ger.; Glaxo Wellcome, Ger.; Wellcome, Irl.; Warner-Lambert, Irl.; Glaxo Wellcome, Ital.; Glaxo Wellcome, Neth.; Glaxo Wellcome, Norw.; Glaxo Wellcome, S.Afr.; Wellcome, Spain; Glaxo Wellcome, Swed.; Wellcome, Switz.; Glaxo Wellcome, UK; Glaxo Wellcome, USA.
Aciclovir (p.602·3) or aciclovir sodium (p.602·3).
Cytomegalovirus infections; herpesvirus infections.

Zoxil *Xixia, S.Afr.*
Amoxycillin trihydrate (p.151·3).
Bacterial infections.

Zoxin *Opus, UK.*
Flucloxacillin sodium (p.209·2).
Gram-positive bacterial infections.

ZP 11 *Revlon, Canad.*
Pyrithione zinc (p.1089·3).

Z-Pam *Rolab, S.Afr.*
Temazepam (p.693·3).
Hypnotic.

Z-Plus *Dormer, Canad.*
Pyrithione zinc (p.1089·3); menthol (p.1600·2).
Seborrhoeic dermatitis.

ZSC *Sigma, Austral.*
Zinc oxide (p.1096·2); starch (p.1356·2); chlorphenesin (p.376·2).
Hyperhidrosis; nappy rash; skin irritation.

Z.Stop *Chancellor, UK†.*
Ethohexadiol (p.1406·1).
Insect repellent.

Zuk Hepagel, Zuk Hepasalbe *Tosse, Ger.†.*
Heparin sodium (p.879·3).
Vascular skin disorders.

Zuk Rheuma *Tosse, Ger.; Roland, Ger.*
Glycol salicylate (p.43·1).
Musculoskeletal, joint, peri-articular, and soft-tissue disorders.

Zuk Thermo *Tosse, Ger.; Roland, Ger.*
Glycol salicylate (p.43·1); benzyl nicotinate (p.22·1).
Musculoskeletal and joint disorders.

Zumenon
Kali, Aust.; Solvay, Belg.; Solvay, Neth.; Solvay, UK.
Oestradiol (p.1455·1).
Menopausal disorders; osteoporosis.

Zumeston *Duphar, Neth.†.*
28 Zumenon tablets, oestradiol (p.1455·1); 14 Duphaston tablets, dydrogesterone (p.1444·2).
Menopausal disorders.

Zunden *Luitpold, Ital.*
Piroxicam (p.80·2).
Rheumatic disorders.

Zurcal *Nycomed, Aust.*
Pantoprazole sodium (p.1207·3).
Gastro-oesophageal reflux; peptic ulcer.

Zurcale *Exel, Belg.*
Pantoprazole sodium (p.1207·3).
Gastro-oesophageal reflux; peptic ulcer.

Zwitsalax/N *Roche Nicholas, Neth.*
Bisacodyl (p.1179·3).
Constipation.

Zwitsanal *Roche Nicholas, Neth.*
Bismuth subnitrate (p.1180·2); zinc oxide (p.1096·2); lignocaine (p.1293·2).
Haemorrhoids.

Zwitsavit-D *Roche Nicholas, Neth.*
Calcium carbonate (p.1182·1); cholecalciferol (p.1366·3).
Calcium or vitamin D deficiency.

Zyban *Glaxo Wellcome, USA.*
Bupropion hydrochloride (p.280·1).
Aid to smoking withdrawal.

Zyclir *Amrad, Austral.*
Aciclovir (p.602·3) or aciclovir sodium (p.602·3).
Herpesvirus infections; HIV infection.

Zyderm
Collagen, Aust.; Collagen, Austral.; Collagen, Fr.; Collagen, Ger.
Collagen (p.1566·3).
Lignocaine (p.1293·2) is included in this preparation to alleviate the pain of injection.
Skin contour defects.

Zydol
Searle, Irl.; Searle, UK.
Tramadol hydrochloride (p.90·1).
Pain.

Zydone *Du Pont, USA.*
Hydrocodone tartrate (p.43·1); paracetamol (p.72·2).
Pain.

Zygout *Amrad, Austral.*
Allopurinol (p.390·2).
Gout; hyperuricaemia; renal calculi.

Zykolat-EDO *Mann, Ger.*
Cyclopentolate hydrochloride (p.459·3).
Production of cycloplegia and mydriasis.

Zyloprim
Glaxo Wellcome, Austral.; Glaxo Wellcome, Canad.; Glaxo Wellcome, S.Afr.; Wellcome, USA.
Allopurinol (p.390·2).
Calcium oxalate calculi; gout; hyperuricaemia.

Zyloric
Glaxo Wellcome, Aust.; Glaxo Wellcome, Belg.; Glaxo Wellcome, Fr.; Glaxo Wellcome, Ger.; Wellcome, Irl.; Glaxo Wellcome, Ital.; Glaxo Wellcome, Neth.; Glaxo Wellcome, Norw.; Wellcome, Spain; Glaxo Wellcome, Swed.; Wellcome, Switz.; Wellcome, UK.
Allopurinol (p.390·2).
Gout; hyperuricaemia; uric acid or calcium oxalate stones.

Zymacap *Roberts, USA.*
Multivitamin preparation.

Zyma-D2 *Zyma, Fr.*
Ergocalciferol (p.1367·1).
Vitamin D deficiency.

Zymafluor
Gebro, Aust.; Zyma, Belg.†; Novartis, Fr.; Zyma, Ger.; Zyma, Ital.; Novartis Consumer, Neth.; Novartis Consumer, S.Afr.; Zyma, Switz.; Zyma, UK†.
Sodium fluoride (p.742·1).
Dental caries prophylaxis.

Zymafluor D *Zyma, Ger.*
Sodium fluoride (p.742·1); cholecalciferol (p.1366·3).
Dental caries prophylaxis; rickets.

Zymafluor-Calcium *Zyma, Ger.†.*
Sodium fluoride (p.742·1); calcium citrate (p.1155·1); calcium phosphate (p.1155·3).
Dental caries prophylaxis.

Zymase *Organon, USA.*
Pancrelipase (p.1613·3).
Pancreatic enzyme deficiency.

Zymelin *AFI, Norw.*
Xylometazoline hydrochloride (p.1071·2).
Otitis; rhinitis; sinusitis.

Zymizinc *Aguettant, Fr.*
Zinc gluconate (p.1373·2).
Zinc deficiency.

Zymoplex
SCAT, Fr.; Sodip, Switz.
Pancreatic protease and amylase; enzymes of *Aspergillus oryzae*; amylase (p.1549·1); protease; cellulase (p.1561·1); lipase; dimethicone (p.1213·1).
Dyspepsia; flatulence.

Zynedo-B *Weimer, Ger.†.*
Guaiacol (p.1061·2); cineole (p.1564·1); camphor (p.1557·2); thymol (p.1127·1); quinine (p.439·1).
Respiratory-tract disorders.

Zynedo-K *Weimer, Ger.†.*
Guaiacol (p.1061·2); cineole (p.1564·1); menthol (p.1600·2); camphor (p.1557·2); thymol (p.1127·1); quinine (p.439·1).
Respiratory-tract disorders.

Zynox *Intramed, S.Afr.*
Naloxone hydrochloride (p.986·2).
Opioid toxicity.

Zyplast
Collagen, Aust.; Collagen, Austral.; Collagen, Fr.; Collagen, Ger.
Collagen (p.1566·3).
Lignocaine (p.1293·2) is included in this preparation to alleviate the pain of injection.
Skin contour defects.

Zyprexa
Lilly, Austral.; Lilly, Ger.; Lilly, Irl.; Lilly, Neth.; Lilly, Norw.; Lilly, S.Afr.; Lilly, Spain; Lilly, Swed.; Lilly, UK; Lilly, USA.
Olanzapine (p.683·1).
Psychoses.

Zyrlex *UCB, Swed.*
Cetirizine hydrochloride (p.404·2).
Allergic conjunctivitis; allergic rhinitis; urticaria.

Zyrtec
UCB, Aust.; Faulding, Austral.; UCB, Belg.; UCB, Fr.; UCB, Ger.; Rodleben, Ger.; Vedim, Ger.; UCB, Neth.; UCB, Norw.; UCB, S.Afr.; UCB, Spain; UCB, Switz.
Cetirizine hydrochloride (p.404·2).
Hypersensitivity reactions.

Zytrim
Isis Puren, Ger.
Azathioprine (p.505·3).
Auto-immune disorders; organ transplantation.

Directory of Manufacturers

The names and addresses of the manufacturers or distributors of the products and proprietary medicines mentioned in Martindale are listed below in alphabetical order of the abbreviated names used in Part 3.

3M, Austral. 3M Pharmaceuticals Pty Ltd, 9-15 Chilvers Rd, Thornleigh, NSW 2120, Australia.

3M, Belg. 3M Pharma N.V./S.A., Hermeslaan 7, 1831 Diegem, Belgium.

3M, Canad. 3M Pharmaceuticals, P.O. Box 5757, London, Ontario, N6A 4T1, Canada.

3M, Fr. Laboratoires 3M Santé, 3 rue Danton, 92245 Malakoff Cedex, France.

3M, Ger. 3M Medica, Gelsenkirchener Strasse 11, Postfach: 1462, 46322 Borken, Germany.

3M, Irl. See *United Drug, Irl.*

3M, Ital. 3M Italia s.p.a., S. Felice, Segrate (MI), 20100 Milan, Italy.

3M, Neth. 3M Pharma Nederland B.V., Postbus 193, 2300 AD Leiden, Netherlands.

3M, Norw. 3M Pharma, Hvamv.6, Postboks 100, 2013 Skjetten, Norway.

3M, S.Afr. 3M, P.O. Box 10465, Johannesburg 2000, S. Africa.

3M, Spain. 3M España, Juan Ignacio Luca de Tena 19-25, 28027 Madrid, Spain.

3M, Swed. 3M Pharma, 191 89 Sollentuna, Sweden.

3M, Switz. See *Synthelabo, Switz.*

3M, UK. 3M Health Care, Morley St, Loughborough, Leics, LE11 1EP, UK.

3M, USA. 3M Riker, 3M Health Care Group, 225-IN-07 3M Center, St Paul, MN 55144, USA.

Aaciphar, Belg. Aaciphar S.A., AKZO Building, Ave Marnix 13, 1000 Brussels, Belgium.

Aandersen, Ital. Aandersen Farmaceutisk Institut s.p.a., Italy.

Abana, USA. Abana Pharmaceuticals Inc., P.O. Box 360388, Birmingham, AL 35236, USA.

Abatron, UK. Abatron Ltd, Chapel St, Potton, Sandy, Beds, SG1 G2PT, UK.

Abbe Chaupitre, Fr. Laboratoires d'Homéopathie Complexe Abbé Chaupitre LHC, 91 av. J.-B. Clement, 92100 Boulogne, France.

Abbott, Aust. Abbott GmbH, Diefenbachgasse 35, 1150 Vienna, Austria.

Abbott, Austral. Abbott Australasia Pty Ltd, P.O. Box 101, Cronulla, NSW 2230, Australia.

Abbott, Belg. Abbott S.A., Parc Scientifique, Rue du Bosquet 2, 1348 Ottignies-Louvain-la-Neuve, Belgium.

Abbott, Canad. Abbott Laboratories Ltd, P.O. Box 6150, Station A, Montreal, Quebec, H3C 3K6, Canada.

Abbott, Fr. Abbott-France, 12 rue de la Couture, Silic 233, 94528 Rungis Cedex, France.

Abbott, Ger. Abbott GmbH, Max-Planck-Ring 2, Postfach: 2103, 65011 Wiesbaden, Germany.

Abbott, Irl. Abbott Laboratories, Ireland Ltd, 1 Broomhill Business Park, Tallaght, Dublin 24, Ireland.

Abbott, Ital. Abbott s.p.a., 04010 Campoverde (Latina), Italy.

Abbott, Neth. Abbott B.V., Postbus 727, 2132 WT Hoofddorp, Netherlands.

Abbott, Norw. Abbott Norge, Nesoyv.4, Postboks 123, 1361 Billingstad, Norway.

Abbott, S.Afr. Abbott Laboratories South Africa (Pty) Ltd, P.O. Box 1616, Johannesburg 2000, S. Africa.

Abbott, Spain. Abbott, Josefa Valcarcel 48, 28027 Madrid, Spain.

Abbott, Swed. Abbott Scandinavia AB, Box 1074, 164 21 Kista-Stockholm, Sweden.

Abbott, Switz. Abbott SA, Gewerbestrasse 5, 6330 Cham, Switzerland.

Abbott, UK. Abbott Laboratories Ltd, Abbott House, Norden Rd, Maidenhead, Berkshire, SL6 4XE, UK.

Abbott, USA. Abbott Laboratories, North Chicago, IL 60064, USA.

ABC, Ital. Istituto Biologico Chemioterapico ABC s.p.a., Via Crescentino 25, 10154 Turin, Italy.

AB-Consult, Aust. AB-Consult GmbH, Eichenstrasse 32, 1120 Vienna, Austria.

Abello, Ger. Abello Deutschland Pharma GmbH, Postfach: 1320, 53310 Bornheim, Germany.

Abello, Spain. Abello, Josefa Valcarcel 38, 28027 Madrid, Spain.

Abic, Neth. See *Multipharma, Neth.*

Abigo, Swed. Abigo Medical AB, 436 32 Askim, Sweden.

Abiogen, Ital. Abiogen Pharma srl, Via G Fabbrioni 6, 00191 Rome, Italy.

Abnoba, Ger. Abnoba Heilmittel GmbH, Hohenzollernstr. 16, 75177 Pforzheim, Germany.

Ace, S.Afr. Ace, S. Africa.

Acme, USA. Acme United Corp., 75 Kings Highway Cutoff, Fairfield, CT 06430, USA.

ACO, Norw. See *Pharmacia Upjohn, Norw.*

ACO, Swed. ACO AB, Box 30064, 112 87 Stockholm, Sweden.

ACP, Belg. See *Therabel Pharma, Belg.*

ACRAF, Switz. ACRAF AG, Case postale 1067, 1701 Fribourg-Moncor, Switzerland.

Acro, Ital. Acro srl, Via Boccaccio 45, 20123 Milan, Italy.

ACT, Fr. Laboratoire ACT, 6 rue Paul-Baudry, 75008 Paris, France.

Actipharm, Switz. Actipharm S.àr.l., 42-4 rue Prevost-Martin, 1211 Geneva 9, Switzerland.

Acupharm, S.Afr. Acupharm, S. Africa.

Acusan, Ger. Acusan GmbH, Rheinstr. 219, 76532 Baden-Baden, Germany.

Adam, Mon. Laboratoires Adam, Les Flots Bleu, 16 rue du Gabian, B.P. 662, MC 98013 Monaco, Monaco.

Adams, Canad. See *Warner-Lambert, Canad.*

Adams, UK. Adams Healthcare Ltd, Lotherton Way, Garforth, Leeds, W Yorkshire, LS25 2JY, UK.

Adams, USA. Adams Laboratories, 14801 Sovereign Road, Ft Worth, TX 76155, USA.

Adcock Ingram, S.Afr. Adcock Ingram Laboratories Ltd, Private Bag 1, Industria 2042, S. Africa.

Adcock Ingram, UK. Adcock Ingram (UK), Premier House, 29 Rutland St, Leicester, LE1 1RE, UK.

Adcock Ingram Generics, S.Afr. See *Adcock Ingram, S.Afr.*

Adcock Ingram Self Medication, S.Afr. See *Adcock Ingram, S.Afr.*

Adenylchemie, Ger. Adenylchemie GmbH, 79090 Freiburg, Germany.

Adima, Switz. Adima SA, Case postale 1065, 1701 Fribourg, Switzerland.

Adivar, Ital. Angelini Distribuzioni Varie spa, Viale Amelia 70, 00181 Rome, Italy.

Adler, Aust. Adler-Apotheke, Wahringer Strasse 149, 1180 Vienna, Austria.

Adler, Switz. Adler Apotheke, Untertor 39, Postfach 1241, 8401 Winterthur, Switzerland.

Adolphs, USA. Adolphs, 75 Merritt Blvd, Trumbull, CT 06611, USA.

Adrem, Canad. Adrem Ltd, 140 Renfrew Dr, Ste 205, Markham, Ontario, L3R 6B3, Canada.

Adria, USA. Adria Laboratories, Division of Erbamont Inc., P.O. Box 16529, Columbus, OH 43216, USA.

Adroka, Switz. Adroka SA, Case postale, 4123 Allschwil 1, Switzerland.

Advanced Care, USA. Advanced Care Products, Route 202, P.O. Box 610, Raritan, NJ 08869, USA.

Advanced Nutritional Technology, USA. Advanced Nutritional Technology Inc., 6988 Sierra Court, Dublin, CA 94568-2641, USA.

Advil, Austral. Advil Pty Ltd, P.O. Box 4082, Doncaster Heights, Vic 3109, Australia.

Aeroceuticals, USA. See *Graham-Field, USA.*

Aerocid, Fr. Laboratoires de l'Aérocid, 248 bis, rue Gabriel-Peri, 94230 Cachan, France.

Aesca, Aust. Aesca, chemisch-pharmazeutische Fabrik GmbH, Badener Strasse 23, 2514 Traiskirchen, Austria.

Aesculapius, Ital. Aesculapius Farmaceutici s.r.l., Via Cozzaglio 24, 25125 Brescia, Italy.

AFI, Ital. Azienda Farmaceutica Italiana s.r.l., Via A. de Gasperi 47, 21040 Sumirago (VA), Italy.

AFI, Norw. See *Nycomed, Norw.*

AFOM, Ital. AFOM Laboratorio Farmacogeno s.r.l., Via Torino 448, 10032 Brandizzo, Italy.

Agamadon, Ger. Agamadon Biol.-Pharm.-Praparate W. Hild Nachf., Postfach: 1565, 61215 Bad Nauheim, Germany.

Agepha, Aust. Agepha GmbH, Guntherstrasse 11, 1150 Vienna, Austria.

Agil, Ger. Agil-Pharma, Dr R. Lang, Marienplatz, 8948 Mindelheim, Germany.

AGIPS, Ital. AGIPS Farmaceutici s.r.l., Via Amendola 4, 16035 Rapallo (GE), Italy.

Agouron, USA. Agouron Pharmaceuticals Inc., 10350 North Torrey Pines Rd, La Jolla, CA 92037-1020, USA.

Agpharm, Switz. Agpharm AG, Postfach, 4123 Allschwil 1, Switzerland.

Agropharm, UK. Agropharm Ltd, Buckingham House, Church Rd, Penn, High Wycombe, Bucks, HP10 8LN, UK.

Agua del Carmen, Spain. Agua del Carmen, Avda Estanislao Figueras 4, 43003 Tarragona, Spain.

Aguettant, Fr. Laboratoires Aguettant, Parc scientifique Tony-Garnier, 1 rue Alexander-Fleming, 69007 Lyon, France.

AHP, Neth. AHP Pharma B.V., Postbus 255, 2130 AG Hoofddorp, Netherlands.

AHP, Switz. AHP (Schweiz) AG, Grafenauweg 10, 6301 Zug, Switzerland.

Aima, Ital. See *ISI, Ital.*

Air Link, Austral. Air Link Sales & Marketing Pty Ltd, P.O. Box 538, Sunnybank, Qld 4109, Australia.

AJC, Fr. Laboratoires AJC, Usine de Fontaury, 16120 Chateauneuf, France.

Akita, UK. See *McGregor Cory, UK.*

Akko, Ital. Akko Italiana s.r.l., Via A. Friggeri 174/176, 00136 Rome, Italy.

Akorn, Canad. See *Dioptic, Canad.*

Akorn, USA. Akorn, Inc., 100 Akorn Drive, Abita Springs, LA 70420, USA.

AkPharma, USA. AkPharma Inc., 6840 Old Egg Harbor Road, P.O. Box 111, Pleasantville, NJ 08232, USA.

Akripan, Aust. Akripan GmbH, Johann-Wiesmayer-Gasse 17, 2332 Hennersdorf, Austria.

Akromed, S.Afr. Akromed Products (Pty) Ltd, P.O. Box 42, Isando 1600, S. Africa.

A.L., Norw. Apothekernes Laboratorium A.S., Harbitzalleen 3, Postboks 158 Skoyen, 0212 Oslo, Norway.

Alacan, Spain. Alacan, Capricornio 5, 03006 Alicante, Spain.

Alba, USA. See *Bart, USA.*

Albert, Canad. Albert Pharma Inc., 4300 rue Garand, Ville St-Laurent, Quebec, H4R 2A3, Canada.

Albert, S.Afr. See *Hoechst Marion Roussel, S.Afr.*

Albert-Roussel, Aust. Albert-Roussel Pharma GmbH, Altmannsdorfer Strasse 104, 1121 Vienna, Austria.

Albert-Roussel, Ger. Albert-Roussel Pharma GmbH, Abraham-Lincoln-Strasse 38-42, Postfach: 1160, 65001 Wiesbaden, Germany.

Albright & Wilson, UK. Albright & Wilson Ltd, Detergents Group, P.O. Box 3, 210-222 Hagley Rd West, Oldbury, Warley, West Midlands, B68 0NN, UK.

Alcala, Spain. Laboratorios Alcala Farma SL, Carretera M-300 Km 29.920, Alcala de Henares, 28802 Madrid, Spain.

Alckamed, Ital. Alckamed s.r.l., Via Benedetto Marcello 24, 20124 Milano, Italy.

Alclin, S.Afr. Alclin, S. Africa.

Alcon, Aust. Alcon Ophthalmika GmbH, Mariahilfer Strasse 121b, 1060 Vienna, Austria.

Alcon, Austral. Alcon Laboratories (Australia) Pty Ltd, Allambie Grove Park, 25 Frenchs Forest Rd, Frenchs Forest, NSW 2086, Australia.

Alcon, Belg. Alcon-Couvreur S.A., Rijksweg 14, 2870 Puurs, Belgium.

Alcon, Canad. Alcon Canada Inc., 2145 Meadowpine Blvd, Mississauga, Ontario, L5N 6R8, Canada.

Alcon, Fr. Laboratoires Alcon, 4 rue Henri-Ste-Claire-Deville, 92563 Rueil-Malmaison, France.

Alcon, Ger. See *Alcon-Thilo, Ger.*

Alcon, Irl. See *Allphar, Irl.*

Alcon, Ital. Alcon Italia s.p.a., Palazzo CD/1 Via Roma 108, 20060 Cassina de Pecchi (MI), Italy.

Alcon, Neth. See *Bipharma, Neth.*

Alcon, Norw. Alcon Norge AS, Billingstadsletta 13, Slependen, Postboks 22, 1301 Sandvika, Norway.

Alcon, S.Afr. Alcon Laboratories (South Africa) (Pty) Ltd, P.O. Box 3198, Randburg 2125, S. Africa.

Alcon, Spain. Alcon Iberhis, Cta Fuencarral Alcobendas K.15.4, Alcobendas, 28100 Madrid, Spain.

Alcon, Swed. Alcon Lakemedel Nordiska AB, Box 12233, 102 26 Stockholm, Sweden.

Alcon, Switz. Alcon Pharmaceuticals Ltd, Case postale 104, 6330 Cham, Switzerland.

Alcon, UK. Alcon Laboratories (UK) Ltd, Imperial Way, Watford, Herts, WD2 4YR, UK.

Alcon, USA. Alcon Laboratories Inc., 6201 South Freeway, P.O. Box 6600, Fort Worth, TX 76134, USA.

Alcon-Thilo, Ger. Alcon Pharma GmbH, Blankreutestr. 1, Postfach: 560, 79005 Freiburg, Germany.

Alcor, Spain. Alcor, Cervantes 24, 28014 Madrid, Spain.

Alcusal, Austral. Alcusal Inc. Pty Ltd, 12 Mahogany Drive, New Lambton, NSW 2302, Australia.

Aldo, Spain. Aldo Union, Angel Guimera 123-5, Esplugas de Llobregat, 08950 Barcelona, Spain.

Ale, Spain. Ale Pedemonte, Pasaje Jaime Roig 26-8, 08028 Barcelona, Spain.

Alembic Products, UK. Alembic Products Ltd, Unit A, Brymau 2 Estate, River Lane, Saltney, Chester, Cheshire, CH4 8RQ, UK.

Aleph, Ital. Aleph, s.p.a., Via Gregorio VII 466, 00165 Rome, Italy.

Alfa Biotech, Ital. Alfa Biotech s.p.a., Via Castagnetta 7, 00040 Pomezia (Roma), Italy.

Alfa Farmaceutici, Ital. See *Wassermann, Ital.*

Alfarma, Spain. Alfarma, Acanto 22, Planta 12, 28045 Madrid, Spain.

Alifarma, Ital. Alifarma s.r.l., Via Piane 64, 47040 Coriano (RN), Italy.

Aliud, Ger. Aliud Pharma GmbH & Co. KG, Postfach: 1380, 89146 Laichingen, Germany.

ALK, Norw. See *Nycomed, Norw.*

ALK, Swed. ALK Sverige AB, Smorhalevagen 3, 434 42 Kungsbacka, Sweden.

ALK, UK. ALK (UK), 8 Bennett Rd, Reading, Berks, RG2 0QX, UK.

ALK, USA. ALK Laboratories Inc., 27 Village Lane, Wallingford, CT 06492, USA.

Allard, Fr. See *Bristol-Myers Squibb, Fr.*

Allcock, Norw. See *Nycomed, Norw.*

Allen, Aust. See *Glaxo Wellcome, Aust.*

Allen, Spain. Allen Farmaceutica, Dr Severo Ochoa S/N, Tres Cantos, 28760 Madrid, Spain.

Allen & Hanburys, Austral. See *Glaxo Wellcome, Austral.*

Allen & Hanburys, Irl. See *Glaxo Wellcome, Irl.*

Allen & Hanburys, S.Afr. See *Glaxo, S.Afr.*

Allen & Hanburys, UK. Allen & Hanburys Ltd, Horsenden House, Oldfield Lane North, Greenford, Middx, UB6 0HE, UK.

Allen & Hanburys, USA. Allen & Hanburys, Division of Glaxo Inc., Five Moore Drive, Research Triangle Park, North Carolina, NC 27709, USA.

Allerbio, Fr. Laboratoires Allerbio, 55270 Varennes-en-Argonne, France.

Allerex, Canad. Allerex Laboratory Ltd, 580 Terry Fox Drive, Suite 408, Kanata, Ontario, K2L 4B9, Canada.

Allergan, Aust. Pharm Allergan GmbH, Landstrasser Hauptstrasse 60, 1030 Vienna, Austria.

Allergan, Austral. Allergan Australia Pty Ltd, Locked Bag 514, Frenchs Forest, NSW 2086, Australia.

Allergan, Belg. Allergan S.A., Meir 44a, 2000 Antwerp, Belgium.

Allergan, Canad. Allergan Inc., 625 Cochrane Dr., Suite 1000, Markham, Ontario, L3R 9R9, Canada.

Allergan, Fr. Allergan France, Font de l'Orme, av Dr Maurice-Donat, B.P. 42, 06251 Mougins Cdx, France.

Allergan, Ger. Pharm-Allergan GmbH, Rudolf-Plank-Strasse 31, Postfach: 100661, 76260 Ettlingen, Germany.

Allergan, Irl. Allergan Ltd, Pharmapark, California Heights, Dublin 20, Ireland.

Allergan, Ital. Allergan s.p.a., Via Costarica 20/22, 00040 Pomezia (Rome), Italy.

Allergan, Neth. See *Bournonville, Neth.*

Allergan, Norw. Allergan A/S, Industriv. 33, Postboks 276, 1300 Sandvika, Norway.

Allergan, S.Afr. Allergan Pharmaceuticals, P.O. Box 1517, Johannesburg 2000, S. Africa.

Allergan, Spain. Allergan, Avda Industria 24, Tres Cantos, 28760 Madrid, Spain.

Allergan, Swed. Allergan Norden AB, Business Campus, 194 81 Upplands Vasby, Sweden.

Allergan, Switz. Allergan AG, Feldmoosstrasse 6, 8853 Lachen, Switzerland.

Allergan, UK. Allergan Ltd, Crown Centre, Coronation Rd, Cressex Industrial Estate, High Wycombe, Bucks, UK.

Allergan, USA. Allergan Pharmaceuticals Inc., 2525 Dupont Dr., P.O. Box 19534, Irvine, CA 92713-9534, USA.

Allergan Herbert, USA. See *Allergan, USA.*

Allergomed, Switz. Allergomed AG, Ringstrasse 29, Postfach 117, 4106 Therwil, Switzerland.

Allergopharma, Ger. Allergopharma Joachim Ganzer KG, Hermann-Korner-Strasse 52, Postfach: 1109, 21462 Reinbek, Germany.

Allergopharma, Switz. See *Allergomed, Switz.*

Allga, Aust. Allga-Pharma GmbH, Am Barentobel 215, 6942 Krumbach, Austria.

Alliance, UK. Alliance Pharmaceuticals Ltd, Avonbridge House, Bath Rd, Chippenham, Wilts, SN15 2BB, UK.

Alliance, USA. Alliance Pharmaceuticals, 3040 Science Park Rd, San Diego, CA 92121, USA.

Allo Pro, Aust. Allo Pro GmbH, Enzersdorfer Strasse 12A, 2340 Modling, Austria.

Allphar, Irl. Allphar Services Ltd, Belgard Rd, Tallaght, Dublin 24, Ireland.

Allud, Ger. Allud Pharma GmbH & Co KG, Postfach: 1380, 89146 Laichingen, Germany.

Almed, Switz. Divapharma Chur AG, Abteilung Almed, Ankerstrasse 53, 8026 Zurich, Switzerland.

Almirall, Spain. Almirall, Rda Gral Mitre 151, 08022 Barcelona, Spain.

Alonga, Spain. Alonga, Alcala 434-6, 28027 Madrid, Spain.

Alpha Laboratories, UK. Alpha Laboratories Ltd, 40 Parham Drive, Eastleigh, Hants, SO5 4NU, UK.

Alpha Therapeutic, Ger. Alpha Therapeutic GmbH, Siemensstr. 18, Postfach: 1107, 63201 Langen, Germany.

Alpha Therapeutic, Ital. Alpha Therapeutic Italia s.p.a., Via Carducci 62d, 56010 Ghezzano (PI), Italy.

Alpha Therapeutic, Swed. Alpha Therapeutic Scandinavia, Box 124, 619 00 Trosa, Sweden.

Alpha Therapeutic, UK. Alpha Therapeutic UK Ltd, Howlett Way, Fison Way Industrial Estate, Thetford, Norfolk, IP24 1HZ, UK.

Alpha Therapeutic, USA. Alpha Therapeutic Corp., 5555 Valley Blvd, Los Angeles, CA 90032, USA.

Alphapharm, Austral. Alphapharm Pty Ltd, P.O. Box 36, Camperdown, NSW 2050, Australia.

Alpharma, Norw. Alpharma AS, Harbitzalleen 3, Postboks 158 Skoyen, 0212 Oslo, Norway.

Alpharma, USA. Alpharma USPD, 7205 Windsor Blvd, Baltimore, MD 21244-2654, USA.

Alpinamed, Switz. Alpinamed AG, Pharmazeutische Produkte, 9306 Freidorf, Switzerland.

Alra, USA. Alra Laboratories Inc., 3850 Clearview Court, Gurnee, IL 60031, USA.

Alsi, Canad. Alsi Cie Ltee, 150 rue Seigneuriale, Beauport, QC, G1E 3B3, Canada.

Alsitan, Ger. Alsitan WE Ronneburg GmbH, Buhl 16-18, 86926 Greifenberg, Germany.

Also, Ital. Also s.p.a., Viale Monte Rosa 96, 20149 Milan, Italy.

Alte Kreis, Aust. Alte Kreis-Apotheke, Untere Hauptstrasse 1, 7100 Neusiedl am See, Austria.

Alter, Spain. Alter, Mateo Inurria 30, 28036 Madrid, Spain.

Althin, Swed. Althin Medical Norden AB, Box 508, S-183 25 Taby, Sweden.

Altimed, Canad. Altimed Phamaceutical Co., 2100 Syntex Court, Mississauga, Ontario, L5N 3X4, Canada.

Alva, USA. Alva Laboratories, 6625 Avondale Ave, Chicago, IL 60631, USA.

Alza, Switz. See *Biomed, Switz.*

Alza, USA. Alza Corporation, 950 Page Mill Rd, P.O. Box 10950, Palo Alto, CA 94304-0802, USA.

Ambix, USA. Ambix Laboratories Inc., 210 Orchard St, East Rutherford, NJ 07073, USA.

Amcon, USA. Amcon Laboratories, 40 N Rock Hill Rd, St Louis, MO 63119, USA.

American Dermal, USA. American Dermal Corp., 51 Apple Tree Lane, P.O. Box 900, Plumsteadville, PA 18949-0900, USA.

American Lecithin, USA. American Lecithin Co, 115 Hurley Rd, Unit 2B, Oxford, CT 06478, USA.

American Medical, USA. American Medical, USA.

American Red Cross, USA. American Red Cross, National Headquarters, Washington, District of Columbia, DC 20006, USA.

American Regent, USA. American Regent, subsidiary Luitpold Pharm. Inc., 1 Luitpold Drive, Shirley, NY 11967, USA.

American Urologicals, USA. American Urologicals Inc., 10031 Pines Blvd, Suite 216, Pembroke Pines, FL 33024, USA.

Amersham, Canad. Amersham Canada Ltd, 1166 South Service Rd West, Oakville, Ontario, L6L 5T7, Canada.

Amersham, Fr. Laboratoires Amersham France, 12 av des Tropiques, B.P. 144, 91944 Les Ulis Cdx, France.

Amersham, Ital. Amersham Italia s.r.l., Via M.F. Quintiliano 30, 20138 Milan, Italy.

Amersham, Spain. Amersham Iberica, Bambu 38, 28036 Madrid, Spain.

Amersham, USA. See *Medi-Physics, USA.*

Amersham International, UK. Amersham International PLC, Amersham Place, Little Chalfont, Bucks, HP7 9NA, UK.

Ames, Irl. Ames, Division Bayer Diagnostics, Pharmapark, Chapelizod, Dublin 20, Ireland.

Ames, S.Afr. See *Bayer, S.Afr.*

Ames, UK. See *Bayer, UK.*

Ames, USA. Ames Division, Miles Laboratories Inc., 1127 Myrtle St, P.O. Box 70, Elkhart, IN 46515, USA.

Amgen, Austral. Amgen Australia Pty Ltd, P.O. Box 410, North Ryde, NSW 2113, Australia.

Amgen, Canad. Amgen Canada Inc., 6733 Mississauga Rd, Ste 303, Mississauga, Ontario, L5N 6J5, Canada.

Amgen, Ger. Amgen GmbH, Riesstrasse 25, 80992 Munich, Germany.

Amgen, Swed. Amgen AB, Box 34107, 100 26 Stockholm, Sweden.

Amgen, USA. Amgen Inc., 1900 Oak Terrace Lane, Thousand Oaks, CA 91320, USA.

Amide, USA. Amide Pharmaceuticals Inc., 101 E. Main Street, Little Falls, NJ 07424, USA.

Amido, Fr. Laboratoires Amido, 37 av Gabriel-Peri, 92500 Rueil-Malmaison, France.

Amino, Switz. Amino SA, Althofstrasse 12, 5432 Neuenhof, Switzerland.

Ampharco, USA. Ampharco, USA.

Amrad, Austral. Amrad Pharmaceuticals Pty Ltd, 17-27 Cotham Rd, Kew, Vic. 3101, Australia.

Amsa, Ital. Amsa s.r.l., Passeggiata Ripetta 22, 00186 Rome, Italy.

Amsco, USA. Amsco Scientific, Division of American Sterilizer Co., 1002 Lufkin Rd, PO Box 747, Apex, North Carolina, NC 27502, USA.

Amway, Canad. Amway of Canada Ltd, 375 Exeter Rd, P.O. Box 5706, London, Ontario, N6A 4S5, Canada.

Anaquest, USA. Anaquest, 110 Allen Rd, Liberty Corner, NJ 07938, USA.

Anatomia, UK. Anatomia, 21 Hampstead Road, Euston Centre, London, NW1 3JA, UK.

Andalucia, Spain. Andalucia Farmaceutica, C/Huelma, 5 Polg. los Olivares, 23009 Jaen, Spain.

Andersen, Norw. Jan F. Andersen AS, Postboks 1132 Flattum, 3501 Hønefoss, Norway.

Andreabal, Switz. Andreabal AG, Rudolfstrasse 2, 4054 Basel, Switzerland.

Andreu, Spain. Andreu, Travesera de Corts 39-43, 08028 Barcelona, Spain.

Andromaco, Spain. Andromaco, Dr Zamenhof 36, 28027 Madrid, Spain.

Angelini, Aust. Angelini Arzneimittelvertrieb GmbH, Taborstrasse 13, 1020 Vienna, Austria.

Angelini, Ital. Aziende Chimiche Riunite Angelini Francesco s.p.a., Viale Amelia 70, 00181 Rome, Italy.

Anglo-French Laboratories, Canad. Anglo-French Laboratories, Canada.

Anifer, Aust. Anifer Hausmittel GmbH, 5081 Salzburg-Anif, Austria.

Anios, Fr. Laboratoires Anios, Pave du Moulin, 59260 Lille-Hellemmes, France.

ankerpharm, Ger. ankerpharm GmbH, Theodor-Neubauer-Strasse 33/36, Postfach: 83, 07392 Rudolstadt, Germany.

Anpharm, UK. Anpharm UK, 82 Waterloo Rd, Hillside, Southport, Merseyside, PR8 4QW, UK.

Anphar-Rolland, Fr. See *Lipha Sante, Fr.*

Ansell, Canad. Ansell Canada Inc., 105 Lauder St, Cowansville, QC, J2K 2K8, Canada.

Antibioticos, Spain. See *Pharmacia Upjohn, Spain.*

Antigen, Irl. Antigen Pharmaceuticals Ltd, 54 Northumberland Rd, Dublin 4, Ireland.

Antigen, UK. Antigen Pharmaceuticals Ltd, Trafalgar House, Union St, Southport, Merseyside, PR9 0QS, UK.

Antipiol, Ital. Laboratorio di Chimica Medica dell' Antipiol s.n.c., Via S. Benigno 26, 10154 Turin, Italy.

Antistress, Switz. Antistress, Aktiengesellschaft für Gesundheitsschutz, Postfach 44, 8640 Rapperswil, Switzerland.

Antonetto, Ital. Marco Antonetto s.p.a., Via Arsenale 29, 10121 Turin, Italy.

Apogepha, Ger. Apogepha Arzneimittel GmbH, Kyffhauserstrasse 27, Postfach: 190155, 01281 Dresden, Germany.

Apomedica, Aust. Apomedica GmbH, Roseggerkai 3, 8011 Graz, Austria.

Apotex, Canad. Apotex Inc., 150 Signet Dr., Weston, Ontario, M9L 1T9, Canada.

Apotex, S.Afr. Apotex, S. Africa.

Apothecary, USA. Apothecary Products Inc., 11531 Rupp Drive, Burnsville, MN 55337, USA.

Apothecon, USA. See *Bristol-Myers Squibb, USA.*

Apothecus, USA. Apothecus Inc., 20 Audrye Ave, Oyster Bay, NY 11771, USA.

Apotheke Erzengel Michael, Aust. Apotheke zum Erzengel Michael, Sechshauser Strasse 9, 1150 Vienna, Austria.

Apotheke Gnadenmutter, Aust. Apotheke zur Gnadenmutter, Hauptplatz 4, 8630 Mariazell, Austria.

Apotheke Heiligen Brigitta, Aust. Apotheke zur Heiligen Brigitta, Wallensteinplatz 2, 1200 Vienna, Austria.

Apotheke Heiligen Dreifaltigkeit, Aust. Apotheke zur Heiligen Dreifaltigkeit, Kirchengasse 5, 2460 Bruck a. d. Leitha, Austria.

Apotheke Heiligen Josef, Aust. Apotheke zum Heiligen Josef, Doblinger Hauptstrasse 64, 1190 Vienna, Austria.

Apotheke Heiligen Rupertus, Aust. Apotheke zum Heiligen Rupertus, Maxglaner Hauptstrasse 13, 5020 Salzburg, Austria.

Apotheke Roten Krebs, Aust. Apotheke zum Roten Krebs, Lichtensteg 4, 1011 Vienna, Austria.

Approved Drug, USA. See *Health for Life, USA.*

Approved Prescription Services, UK. Approved Prescription Services Ltd, 18 Bruntcliffe Way, Morley, Leeds, LS27 0JG, UK.

Aprofa, Spain. Aprofa, Plg. Glorias Catalanas 15, Tarrasa, 08223 Barcelona, Spain.

APS, Ger. APS-Apotheker H. Starke Pharma GmbH, Bahnhofstr. 7, Postfach: 11 38, 82301 Starnberg, Germany.

Aqualab, Fr. Lab. Aqualab, ZAP du Lattay, 53240 Andouille, France.

Aquamaid, UK. Aquamaid Co. Ltd, 225 Putney Bridge Rd, London, SW15 2PY, UK.

Arcana, Aust. Arcana GmbH, Zimbagasse 5, 1147 Vienna, Austria.

Arcana, S.Afr. Arcana (Pty) Ltd, P.O. Box 1998, Halfway House 1685, S. Africa.

Arcis-Toledano, Fr. Laboratoires Arcis-Tolédano, 6 bd Suchet, 75016 Paris, France.

Arco, USA. Arco Pharmaceuticals Inc., 105 Orville Dr., Bohemia, NY 11716, USA.

Arcola, USA. Arcola Laboratories, 500 Arcola Rd, Collegeville, Pennsylvania, PA 19426-0107, USA.

Arcolab, Switz. Arcolab Ltd, 28 chemin du Grand-Puits, 1217 Meyrin 2/Geneva, Switzerland.

Ardern, UK. Ardern Healthcare Ltd, Pipers Brook Farm, Eastham, Tenbury Wells, Worcs, WR15 8NP, UK.

Ardeypharm, Ger. Ardeypharm GmbH Pharmazeutische Fabrik, Loerfeldstr. 20, Postfach: 1153, 58303 Herdekke, Germany.

Ardeypharm, Switz. See *Medipharm, Switz.*

Ardix, Fr. Ardix Medical, 27 rue du Pont, 92200 Neuilly-sur-Seine, France.

Areu, Spain. Areu, Ctra Madrid Valencia, Km 23.5, Arganda del Rey, 28500 Madrid, Spain.

Arik, Fr. Laboratoires Arik, 35 av. Saint-Jean, 06400 Cannes, France.

Aristegui, Spain. See *Ifidesa Aristegui, Spain.*

Arjo, Canad. Arjo Canada Inc., 277 Cree Cres., Winnipeg, Manitoba, R3J 3X4, Canada.

Arkochim, Spain. Arkochim España, Meneses 2, 28045 Madrid, Spain.

Arkofarm, Ital. Arkofarm srl, L.go Olgiata 15 Is 28/A, 00123 Rome, Italy.

Arkomedika, Fr. Laboratoires Arkomédika, B.P. 28, 06511 Carros Cdx, France.

Arkopharma, Fr. Laboratoires Arkopharma, B.P. 28, 06511 Carros Cedex, France.

Arkopharma, Switz. See *Naturpharma, Switz.*

Arkopharma, UK. Arkopharma UK Ltd, 6 Redlands Centre, Redlands, Coulsden, Surrey, CR5 2HT, UK.

Armour, Ger. See *Centeon, Ger.*

Armour, USA. Armour Pharmaceutical Co., Division of Rhone-Poulenc Rorer, 500 Arcola Rd, P.O. Box 1200, Collegeville, PA 19426-0107, USA.

Arnaldi-Uscio, Ital. Colonia della Salute Carlo Arnaldi s.p.a., Via Carlo Arnaldi 6, 16030 Uscio (GE), Italy.

Arrow, USA. Arrow, USA.

Artesan, Ger. Artesan Pharma GmbH, Wendlandstrasse 1, Postfach: 1142, 29431 Luchow, Germany.

Artesan, Switz. See *Lubapharm, Switz.*

Arteva, Ger. Arteva Pharma GmbH, Postfach: 1126, 82116 Gauting, Germany.

Artsana, Ital. Artsana spa, SS dei Giovi Km 7, 22070 Casnate con Bernate (CO), Italy.

Artu, Neth. Artu Biologicals Europe B.V., Postbus 612, 8200 AP Lelystad, Netherlands.

Arun, UK. Arun Pharmaceuticals Ltd, Delta House, Southwood Cres, Southwood Business Park, Farnborough, Hants, GU14 0NL, UK.

Arza, Spain. Arza, Spain.

A.S., Ger. A.S. Biologische und pharmazeutische Produkte GmbH, Kandelstrasse 10, Postfach: 1206, 79196 Kirchzarten, Germany.
Asahi, Jpn. Asahi Chemical Industry Co. Ltd, 5-13 Shibaura 4-chome, Minato-ku, Tokyo 108, Japan.
Asche, Ger. Asche AG, Fischers Allee 49-59, Postfach: 50 01 32, 22701 Hamburg, Germany.
Ascher, USA. B.F. Ascher & Co. Inc., 15501 W 109th St, Lenexa, KS 66219, USA.
Ascot, Austral. Ascot Pharmaceuticals Pty Ltd, P.O. Box 79, Croydon, NSW 2132, Australia.
Asens, Spain. Asens, Alava 61, 08005 Barcelona, Spain.
Ashbourne, UK. Ashbourne Pharmaceuticals Ltd, Scaldwell Rd, Industrial Estate (North), Brixworth, Northampton, NN6 9EN, UK.
Asid Bonz, Ger. Asid Bonz GmbH, Postfach: 1140, 71001 Boblingen, Germany.
Askit, UK. Askit Laboratories Ltd, 93 Saracen St, Glasgow, G22 5HX, UK.
Aspro-Nicholas, Aust. See *Roche, Aust.*
Associated Dental, UK. Associated Dental Products Ltd, Purton, Swindon, Wilts, SN5 9HT, UK.
Associated Hospital Supply, UK. Associated Hospital Supply, Sherwood Rd, Aston Fields, Bromsgrove, Worcs, B60 3DR, UK.
Association Nationale, Fr. Association Nationale pour la distribution des fractions plasmatiques humaines, 37 rue Violet, 75015 Paris, France.
Asta, Norw. See *Sunde, Norw.*
Asta Medica, Aust. Asta Medica Arzneimittel GmbH, Neustiftgasse 119, 1070 Vienna, Austria.
Asta Medica, Austral. Asta Medica Australasia Pty Ltd, P.O. Box 1305, Parramatta, NSW 2124, Australia.
Asta Medica, Belg. Asta Medica S.A., Rue de l'Etuve 77-81, 1000 Brussels, Belgium.
Asta Medica, Fr. Laboratoire Asta Medica, Av J-F-Kennedy, 33701 Merignac Cdx, France.
Asta Medica, Ger. Asta Medica AG/Asta Pharma AG, Weismullerstr. 45, Postfach: 100105, 60001 Frankfurt a.M., Germany.
Asta Medica, Irl. See *Asta Medica, UK.*
Asta Medica, Ital. Asta Medica s.p.a., Via Zanella 3/5, 20133 Milan, Italy.
Asta Medica, Neth. Asta Medica B.V., Postbus 171, 1110 BC Diemen, Netherlands.
Asta Medica, Spain. Asta Medica, Avda de Fuentemar 27 (Plg Indus), Coslada, 28820 Madrid, Spain.
Asta Medica, Swed. Asta Medica AB, Kemistvagen 17, 183 79 Taby, Sweden.
Asta Medica, Switz. ASTA Medica AG, Hegnaustrasse 60, 8602 Wangen/ZH, Switzerland.
Asta Medica, UK. ASTA Medica Ltd, ASTA House, 168 Cowley Rd, Cambridge, Cambs, CB4 4DL, UK.
Astier, Fr. See *URPAC, Fr.*
Astra, Aust. Astra GmbH, Sudtiroler Strasse 6, 4020 Linz, Austria.
Astra, Austral. Astra Pharmaceuticals Pty Ltd, P.O. Box 131, North Ryde, NSW 2113, Australia.
Astra, Belg. Astra Pharmaceuticals S.A., Rue Egide Van Ophem 110, 1180 Brussels, Belgium.
Astra, Canad. Astra Pharma Inc., 1004 Middlegate Rd, Mississauga, Ontario, L4Y 1M4, Canada.
Astra, Fr. Laboratoires Astra France, Groupe Pharmaceutique Astra Suède, 1 place Renault, 92844 Rueil-Malmaison cdx, France.
Astra, Ger. Astra GmbH, 22876 Wedel, Germany.
Astra, Irl. Astra Pharmaceuticals (Ireland) Ltd, 32 Fitzwilliam Square, Dublin 2, Ireland.
Astra, Ital. Astra Farmaceutici s.p.a., Via Messina 38 Torre A, 20157 Milan, Italy.
Astra, Neth. Astra Pharmaceutica B.V., Postbus 599, 2700 AN Zoetermeer, Netherlands.
Astra, Norw. Astra Norge AS, Skarersletta 50, Postboks 1, 1471 Skårer, Norway.
Astra, S.Afr. See *Keatings, S.Afr.*
Astra, Spain. Astra España, Mestre Joan Corrales 95-105, Esplugues de Llobregat, 08950 Barcelona, Spain.
Astra, Swed. Astra Läkemedel AB, 151 85 Sodertalje, Sweden.
Astra, Switz. Astra Pharmaceutica SA, Kanalstrasse 6, 8953 Dietikon, Switzerland.
Astra, UK. Astra Pharmaceuticals Ltd, Home Park Estate, Kings Langley, Herts, WD4 8DH, UK.
Astra, USA. Astra Pharmaceutical Products Inc., 50 Otis St, Westboro, MA 01581-4428, USA.
Astra Merck, USA. Astra Merck, 725 Chesterbrook Blvd, Wayne, PA 19087-5677, USA.
Astra Tech, Norw. See *Astra, Norw.*
Astra Tech, Swed. Astra Tech AB, Box 14, 431 21 Molndal, Sweden.
Astra Tech, UK. Astra Tech Ltd, PO Box 13, Stroud, Gloucestershire, GL5 3DL, UK.
Athena Neurosciences, UK. Athena Neurosciences (Europe) Ltd, 1 Meadway Court, Rutherford Close, Stevenage, Herts, SG1 2EF, UK.
Athena Neurosciences, USA. Athena Neurosciences Inc., 800 F Gateway Blvd, South San Francisco, California, CA 94080, USA.
Athenstaedt, Ger. Athenstaedt GmbH & Co. KG, Panrepel 11, Postfach: 450255, 28296 Bremen, Germany.
Athenstaedt, Switz. See *Drossapharm, Switz.*
Atlantic, Thai. Atlantic Pharmaceutical Co. Ltd., 2038 Sukumvit Rd., Bangkok 10250, Thailand.
Atlas, Canad. Laboratoire Atlas, 5750 Metropolitan E, Bur 200, St-Leonard, QC, H1S 1A7, Canada.
Atley, USA. Atley Pharmaceuticals, 340 South Richardson Rd, Ste. 1, Ashland, Virginia, VA 23005, USA.
Atzinger, Ger. Dr. Atzinger Pharmazeutische Fabrik, Dr. Atzinger Str. 5, Postfach: 1129, 94001 Passau, Germany.
Augot, Fr. Laboratoires Augot, 26 rue de Beauregard, 03400 Yzeure, France.
Australis, Austral. Australis Marketing Corporation Pty. Ltd, P.O. Box 752, Cheltenham, Vic. 3192, Australia.
Austrodent, Aust. Austrodent HandelsGmbH, Seidengasse 42, 1070 Vienna, Austria.
Austroflex, Aust. Austroflex Pharma, Schikanedergasse 12, 1040 Vienna, Austria.
Austroplant, Aust. Austroplant-Arzneimittel GmbH, Richard-Strauss-Strasse 13, 1232 Vienna, Austria.
Avant Garde, Canad. Avant-Garde Cosmetics Ltd, 3503 Griffith, St-Laurent, Quebec, H4T 1W5, Canada.
Avantgarde, Ital. Avantgarde s.p.a., Gruppo Sigma Tau, Via Treviso 4, 00040 Pomezia (Rome), Italy.
Avon, Canad. Avon Canada Inc., 5500 Trans Canada Hwy, Pointe-Claire, Quebec, H9R 1B6, Canada.
AVP, USA. AVP, USA.
Axcan, Canad. Axcan Pharma Inc., 597 Laurier Blvd, Mont St-Hilaire, Quebec, J3H 4X8, Canada.
Ayerst, Belg. See *Wyeth, Belg.*
Ayerst, USA. Ayerst Laboratories, Division of American Home Products Corp., 685 Third Ave, New York, NY 10017-4071, USA.
Aza, Austral. Aza Research Pty Ltd, 112 Wharf Rd, West Ryde, NSW 2114, Australia.
Azuchemie, Ger. Azuchemie, Dr med. R. Muller GmbH, Dieselstrasse 5, Postfach: 100126, 7016 Gerlingen, Germany.
Azupharma, Ger. Azupharma GmbH, Dieselstrasse 5, Postfach: 100126, 70826 Gerlingen, Germany.
Bach, UK. Bach Flower Remedies Ltd, 6 Suffolk Way, Abingdon, Oxon, OX14 5JX, UK.
Bad Heilbrunner, Ger. Bad Heilbrunner Reform-Diat-Arznei GmbH & Co., Postfach: 40, 83667 Bad Heilbrunn, Germany.
Baer, Ger. Chemisch-pharmazeutische Fabrik Dr Baer KG GmbH & Co., Ehrwalder Strasse 21, Postfach: 701669, 81316 Munich, Germany.
Baif, Ital. Baif International Products, New York s.n.c., Corso Europa 183, 16132 Genoa, Italy.
Bailey, UK. Robert Bailey & Sons, Dysart St, Great Moor, Stockport, Cheshire, UK.
Bailleul, Fr. Laboratoires Bailleul, 7 rue Michelet, 93364 Neuilly-Plaisance Cdx, France.
Bailly, Fr. Laboratoires Bailly S.P.E.A.B., 350 rue Lecourbe, 75015 Paris, France.
Bajamar, USA. Bajamar Chemical Co. Inc., 9609 Dielman Rock Island, St Louis, MO 63132, USA.
Baker Cummins, Canad. Baker Cummins Inc., 16751 Hymus Blvd, Kirkland, Quebec, H9H 3L4, Canada.
Baker Cummins, USA. Baker/Cummins, Division of Ivax, 8800 NW 36th Street, Miami, FL 33178-2404, USA.
Baker Norton, Irl. See *Norton Waterford, Irl.*
Baker Norton, UK. See *Norton, UK.*
Baker Norton, USA. Baker Norton Pharm. Inc., subsidiary of Ivax, 8800 NW 36th St, Miami, FL 33178-2404, USA.
Baldacci, Ital. Laboratori Baldacci s.p.a., Via S. Michele Scalzi 73, 56100 Pisa, Italy.
Balneopharm, Ger. Balneopharm Cohrdes & Co. OHG, Hanosanstr. 1, Postfach: 120164, 30808 Garbsen, Germany.
Bama, Spain. Bama Geve, Avda Diagonal 456, 08006 Barcelona, Spain.
Banana Boat, Canad. See *Playtex, Canad.*
Bano, Aust. Mag. J. Bano chem.-pharmazeutische Präparate, 6580 St Anton/Arlberg 485, Austria.
Banyu, Jpn. Banyu Pharmaceutical Co. Ltd, 9-3 Shimo-Meguro 2-chome, Meguro-ku, Tokyo 153, Japan.
Bard, UK. Bard Ltd, Forest House, Brighton Rd, Crawley, West Sussex, RH11 1BP, UK.
Barnes-Hind, Austral. See *Pilkington Barnes-Hind, Austral.*
Barnes-Hind, Switz. See *Dispersa, Switz.*
Barr, USA. Barr Laboratories Inc., 2 Quaker Rd, Pomona, NY 01970, USA.
Barre-National, USA. Barre-National Inc., 7502 Windsor Blvd, Baltimore, MD 21207, USA.
Barrere, Austral. Barrere Surgical Co., P.O. Box A84, Sydney South, NSW 2000, Australia.
Barry, Ital. Barry Italia s.r.l., Via Sardegna 40, Fizzonasco Pieve Emanuele (MI), Italy.
Bart, USA. A.J. Bart Inc., Gurabo Industrial Park, P.O. Box 813, Gurabo, PR 00658, Puerto Rico.
Bartholomew Rhodes, UK. Bartholomew Rhodes Ltd, Victor Barns, Hill Farm, Brixworth, Northants, NN6 9DQ, UK.
Bartor Pharmacal, USA. Bartor Pharmacal Co., 70 High St, Rye, NY 10580, USA.
Basel, USA. See *Ciba-Geigy, USA.*
BASF, Ger. BASF Generics GmbH, Gottlieb-Daimler-Str. 10, 68165 Mannheim, Germany.
Basotherm, Ger. Basotherm GmbH, Eichendorffweg 5, Postfach: 1254, 88396 Biberach an der Riss, Germany.
Basotherm, Switz. See *Boehringer Ingelheim, Switz.*
Bastian, Ger. Bastian-Werk GmbH, August-Exter-Strasse 4, Postfach: 600161, 81201 Munich, Germany.
Bastian, Switz. See *Globopharm, Switz.*
Bausch & Lomb, Austral. Bausch & Lomb (Australia) Pty Ltd, Level 4, 113 Wicks Rd, North Ryde, NSW 2113, Australia.
Bausch & Lomb, Canad. Bausch & Lomb Canada Inc., 85 Leek Cres., Richmond Hill, Ontario, L4B 3B3, Canada.
Bausch & Lomb, Fr. Laboratoires Bausch & Lomb, route de Levis-Saint-Nom, B.P. 51, 78320 Le Mesnil-Saint-Denis, France.
Bausch & Lomb, S.Afr. Bausch & Lomb, S. Africa.
Bausch & Lomb, UK. Bausch & Lomb UK Ltd, 106 London Rd, Kingston-upon-Thames, Surrey, KT2 6TN, UK.
Bausch & Lomb, USA. Bausch & Lomb Inc., Professional Products Division, 1400 N. Goodman St, Rochester, NY14692, USA.
Bauxili, Spain. Bauxili, Nueva 52, Igualada, 08700 Barcelona, Spain.
Baxenden, UK. Baxenden Chemicals Ltd, Union Lane, Droitwich, Worcs, WR9 9BB, UK.
Baxter, Aust. Baxter Vertrieb f. medizinische und pharmazeutische Produkte, Richard-Strauss-Strasse 33, 1232 Vienna, Austria.
Baxter, Austral. Baxter Healthcare Pty Ltd, P.O. Box 88, Toongabbie, NSW 2146, Australia.
Baxter, Belg. Baxter S.A., Rue Colonel Bourg 105 B, 1140 Evere, Belgium.
Baxter, Canad. Baxter Corporation, 2390 Argentia Rd, Mississauga, Ontario, L5N 3P1, Canada.
Baxter, Fr. Baxter SA, 6 av Louis-Pasteur, B.P. 56, 78311 Maurepas, France.
Baxter, Ger. Baxter Deutschland GmbH, Edisonstr. 3-4, Postfach: 1165, 85701 Unterschleissheim, Germany.
Baxter, Irl. Baxter Healthcare Ltd, 7 Deansgrange Industrial Estate, Blackrock, Co. Dublin, Ireland.
Baxter, Ital. Baxter s.p.a., Viale Tiziano 25, 00196 Rome, Italy.
Baxter, Spain. Baxter, Dels Gremis 7, Polig. Inds. Vara de Cuart, 46014 Valencia, Spain.
Baxter, Swed. Baxter Medical AB, Box 63, 164 94 Kista, Sweden.
Baxter, Switz. Baxter AG, Postfach 2412, Industriestrasse 31, 8305 Dietlikon, Switzerland.
Baxter, UK. Baxter Healthcare Ltd, Caxton Way, Thetford, Norfolk, IP24 3SE, UK.
Baxter, USA. Baxter Healthcare Corp., Route 120 and Wilson Rd, Round Lake, IL 60073, USA.
Bayer, Aust. Bayer Austria GmbH, Am Heumarkt 10, Postfach 10, 1037 Vienna, Austria.
Bayer, Austral. Bayer Australia Ltd (Health Care Business Group), 875 Pacific Highway, P.O. Box 903, Pymble, NSW 2073, Australia.
Bayer, Belg. Bayer S.A., Division Pharma, Ave Louise 143, 1050 Brussels, Belgium.
Bayer, Canad. Bayer Inc., 77 Belfield Rd, Etobicoke, Ontario, M9W 1G6, Canada.
Bayer, Fr. Bayer-Pharma, 13 rue Jean-Jaures, 92807 Puteaux cdx, France.
Bayer, Ger. Bayer AG, Pharma Deutschland, 51368 Leverkusen, Germany.
Bayer, Irl. Bayer (Ireland) Ltd, Kill O' the Grange, Dun Laoghaire, Co. Dublin, Ireland.
Bayer, Ital. Bayer s.p.a., Viale Certosa 126, 20156 Milan, Italy.
Bayer, Neth. Bayer B.V., Postbus 80, 3640 AB Mijdrecht, Netherlands.
Bayer, Norw. Bayer AS, Brennav 18, Skyttafeltet, Nittedal, Postboks 114, 1483 Skytta, Norway.
Bayer, S.Afr. Bayer-Miles (Pty) Ltd, P.O. Box 198, Isando 1600, S. Africa.
Bayer, Spain. Bayer, Calabria 268, 08029 Barcelona, Spain.
Bayer, Swed. Bayer Sverige AB, Box 5237, 402 24 Goteborg, Sweden.
Bayer, Switz. Bayer (Schweiz) AG, Pharma, Case postale, 8045 Zurich, Switzerland.
Bayer, UK. Bayer plc, Pharmaceutical Business Group, Ethical Products, Bayer House, Strawberry Hill, Newbury, Berks, RG13 1JA, UK.
Bayer, USA. Bayer Corp., 400 Morgan Lane, West Haven, CT 06516, USA.
Bayer Consumer, UK. See *Bayer, UK.*
Bayer Diagnostici, Ital. Bayer Diagnostici s.p.a., Via Grosio 10, 20151 Milan, Italy.
Bayer Diagnostics, Austral. See *Bayer, Austral.*
Bayer Diagnostics, Fr. Bayer Diagnostics, Tour Bayer, 13 rue Jean-Jaures, 92807 Puteaux Cdx, France.
Bayer Diagnostics, Switz. See *Bayer, Switz.*
Bayer Diagnostics, UK. See *Bayer, UK.*
Baypharm, Austral. See *Bayer, Austral.*
Bayrol, Ger. Bayrol Chemische Fabrik GmbH, Lochhamer Str. 29, Postfach: 700260 in 8000 Munich 70, 8033 Martinsreid b. Munich, Germany.
Bayropharm, Ger. See *Bayer, Ger.*
Bayropharm, Ital. Bayropharm Italiana s.r.l., Gruppo Bayer, Viale Certosa 210, 20156 Milan, Italy.
BC Lutz, Switz. BCLutz Company, Pharmaceutical Products Switzerland, Rebwiesstrasse 58, P.O. Box, 8702 Zollikon, Switzerland.
BCL, Switz. See *BC Lutz, Switz.*
BCS, Fr. See *CSP, Fr.*
BDH, USA. BDH Inc., 9410 St Catherine Ave, Cleveland, OH 44104, USA.
BDI, USA. BDI Pharmaceuticals, Inc., P.O. Box 78610, Indianapolis, IN 46278-0610, USA.
Beach, USA. Beach Pharmaceuticals, Division of Beach Products Inc., 5220 S Manhattan Ave, Tampa, FL 33611, USA.
Beaufour, Fr. Laboratoires Beaufour, 24 rue Erlanger, 75016 Paris, France.
Beaufour, Switz. See *Uhlmann-Eyraud, Switz.*
Becker, Aust. Becker, Vienna, Austria.

Beckerath, Ger. M. v. Beckerath GmbH Pharmavertrieb, Postfach: 305, 47703 Krefeld, Germany.

Becton, Dickinson, Canad. Becton, Dickinson Microbiology Systems, 2464 South Sheridan Way, Mississauga, Ontario, L5J 2M8, Canada.

Becton Dickinson, USA. Becton Dickinson & Co., 1 Becton Drive, Franklin Lanes, NJ 07417-1881, USA.

Beecham, Belg. See *SmithKline Beecham, Belg.*

Beecham, Irl. See *SmithKline Beecham, Irl.*

Beecham, S.Afr. See *SmithKline Beecham, S.Afr.*

Beecham, Spain. See *SmithKline Beecham, Spain.*

Beecham Research, UK. See *SmithKline Beecham, UK.*

Befelka, Ger. Befelka-Arzneimittel, Parkstr. 6 b, Postfach: 1351, 49003 Osnabruck, Germany.

Behring, Aust. See *Centeon, Aust.*

Behring, Ital. Istituto Behring s.p.a., S.S. 17, Km.22, 67019 Scoppito (AQ), Italy.

Behring, Neth. See *Hoechst Marion Roussel, Neth.*

Behring, Norw. See *Hoechst Marion Roussel, Norw.*

Behringwerke, Ger. See *Centeon, Ger.*

Beiersdorf, Aust. Beiersdorf GmbH, Laxenburger Strasse 151, 1101 Vienna, Austria.

Beiersdorf, Austral. Beiersdorf Australia Ltd, P.O. Box 139, North Ryde, NSW 2113, Australia.

Beiersdorf, Canad. See *Smith & Nephew, Canad.*

Beiersdorf, Fr. Laboratoires Pharmaceutiques Beiersdorf Medical, 1 rue des Sources, 77545 Savigny-le-Temple Cdx, France.

Beiersdorf, Ger. Beiersdorf AG, Unnastrasse 48, 20245 Hamburg, Germany.

Beiersdorf, Irl. See *Mayrs, Irl.*

Beiersdorf, Ital. Beiersdorf s.p.a., Via Eraclito 30, 20128 Milan, Italy.

Beiersdorf, Switz. Beiersdorf AG Medical, Aliothstrasse 40, 4142 Munchenstein 2, Switzerland.

Beiersdorf, UK. Beiersdorf UK Ltd, Yeomans Drive, Blakelands, Milton Keynes, Bucks, MK14 5LS, UK.

Beiersdorf, USA. Beiersdorf Inc., P.O. Box 5529, Norwalk, CT 06856-5529, USA.

Beiersdorf-Lilly, Ger. Beiersdorf-Lilly GmbH, Wiesingerweg 25, Postfach: 201852, 20243 Hamburg, Germany.

Beige, S.Afr. See *Brunel, S.Afr.*

Beldenta, Switz. Beldenta-Anstalt, Birkenweg 6, FL-9490 Vaduz, Switzerland.

Bellon, Belg. See *Wellcome, Belg.*

Bellon, Fr. Laboratoires Bellon Rhône-Poulenc Rorer,, 15 rue de la Vanne, 92120 Montrouge, France.

Belmac, Fr. Laboratoires Belmac S.A., France.

Belmac, Spain. Belmac, Montearagon 9, 28033 Madrid, Spain.

Belphar, Belg. See *Continental Pharma, Belg.*

Benarth, Canad. Produits Pharmaceutiques Benarth, 118 rue St-Odilon, Beauce Nord, Quebec, G0S 3A0, Canada.

Bencard, Belg. S.A. Bencard, Rue du Tilleul 13, 1332 Genval, Belgium.

Bencard, Canad. Bencard Allergy Laboratories, A SmithKline Beecham Company, 1345 Fewster Dr., Mississauga, Ontario, L4W 2A5, Canada.

Bencard, Irl. See *SmithKline Beecham, Irl.*

Bencard, Neth. See *SmithKline Beecham, Neth.*

Bencard, S.Afr. See *Beecham, S.Afr.*

Bencard, UK. See *SmithKline Beecham, UK.*

Bender, Aust. Bender & Co. GmbH, Dr Boehringer-Gasse 5-11, 1121 Vienna, Austria.

Bene, Ger. bene-Arzneimittel GmbH, Herterichstrasse 1, Postfach: 710269, 81452 Munich, Germany.

Bene, Switz. See *Max Ritter, Switz.*

Benedetti, Ital. Benedetti s.p.a., Vicolo de'Bacchettoni 3, 51100 Pistoia (PT), Italy.

Bengue, Irl. See *Syntex, Irl.*

Beni-med, Ger. beni-med Naturliche Heilmittel GmbH & Co. Vertriebs KG, Griegstr. 14A, 14193 Berlin, Germany.

Bennett, UK. Bennett Natural Products, Wheelton, Chorley, Lancs, PR6 8EP, UK.

Benvegna, Ital. Neoterapici Benvegna s.r.l., Via M. Amari 15, 90139 Palermo, Italy.

Benzon, Swed. See *Nycomed, Swed.*

Berenguer Infale, Spain. Berenguer Infale, Trabajo S/N, Sant Just Desvern, 08960 Barcelona, Spain.

Bergaderm, Fr. Laboratoires Bergaderm, France.

Bergamon, Ital. Bergamon s.r.l., Via di Cancelliera 60, 00040 Ariccia (Rome), Italy.

Berk, Irl. See *Rhone-Poulenc Rorer, Irl.*

Berk, UK. Berk Pharmaceuticals Ltd, 18 Bruntcliffe Way, Morley, Leeds, LS27 0JG, UK.

Berlex, Canad. Berlex Canada Inc., 2260 32nd Ave, Lachine, Quebec, H8T 3H4, Canada.

Berlex, USA. Berlex Laboratories Inc., 110 East Hanover Ave, Cedar Knolls, NJ 07927, USA.

Berlin-Chemie, Ger. Berlin-Chemie AG, Glienicker Weg 125, Postfach: 1108, 12474 Berlin, Germany.

Berna, Belg. See *Zyma, Belg.*

Berna, Canad. See *Berna, USA.*

Berna, Ital. Istituto Sieroterapico Berna s.r.l., Via Bellinzona 39, 22100 Como, Italy.

Berna, Norw. See *Bostad, Norw.*

Berna, Spain. Berna, P Castellana 163, 28046 Madrid, Spain.

Berna, Switz. Schweiz. Serum- & Impfinstitut, Postfach, 3001 Bern, Switzerland.

Berna, USA. Berna Products Corp., 4216 Ponce de Leon Blvd, Coral Gables, FL 33146, USA.

Bernhauer, Aust. Mr W Bernhauer OHG, Stadtplatz 7, 4400 Steyr, Austria.

Berta, Ital. Berta s.r.l., Via Andrea Doria 7, 20124 Milan, Italy.

Bertek, USA. Bertek Pharmaceuticals Inc, Sugar Land, TX 77478, USA.

Bescansa, Spain. Bescansa, Pl. Inds. Tambre-via Pasteur 8, Santiago de Compostela, 15890 La Coruna, Spain.

Besins-Iscovesco, Fr. Laboratoires Besins-Iscovesco, 5 rue du Bourg-l'Abbé, 75003 Paris, France.

Besins-Iscovesco, Switz. See *Golaz, Switz.*

Beta, Ital. Laboratorio Biologico Chemioterapico Beta s.r.l., Via IV Novembre 171/3, 25080 Prevalle, Italy.

Be-Tabs, S.Afr. Be-Tabs Pharmaceuticals (Pty) Ltd, P.O. Box 43486, Industria 2042, S. Africa.

Betafar, Spain. Betafar, Camino de Gozquez S/N, Valdemoro, 28340 Madrid, Spain.

Betapharm, Ger. Betapharm Arzneimittel GmbH, Steinerne Furt 78, 86167 Augsburg, Germany.

Beutlich, USA. Beutlich L.P., 7149 North Austin Ave, Niles, IL 60714, USA.

BHR, UK. BHR Pharmaceuticals Ltd, 41 Centenary Business Centre, Hammond Close, Attleborough Fields Industrial Estate, Nuneaton, Warks, CV11 6RY, UK.

Biagini, Ital. Farma Biagini s.p.a., 55020 Castelvecchio Pascoli (LU), Italy.

Bichsel, Switz. Laboratorium Dr G Bichsel AG, Bahnhofstrasse 5a, 3800 Interlaken, Switzerland.

Bicther, Spain. See *Inkeysa, Spain.*

Bieffe, Ital. Bieffe Medital s.p.a., Via Nuova Provinciale, 23034 Grosotto (SO), Italy.

Bieffe, Spain. Bieffe Medital, Ctra Biescas S/NC, Sabinanigo, 22666 Huesca, Spain.

Bieffe, Switz. Bieffe Medital SpA, Via S Balestra 27, 6900 Lugano, Switzerland.

Bier, Ital. Bier Farmaceutici s.n.c. di Pepe G. e Frattolino R., Via Cupa Capodichino 19, 80144 Naples, Italy.

Bifarma, Ital. Bifarma Fitoterapici di Bignardi Sergio, Via Pallia 5, 20139 Milan, Italy.

Bigmar, Switz. Bigmar Pharmaceuticals SA, Via Pian Scairolo 6, 6917 Barbengo, Switzerland.

Bilgast, Ger. Bilgast Arzneimittel Vertriebs GmbH, Postfach: 1205, 67502 Worms, Germany.

Bilosa, Aust. Bilosa GmbH & Co. KG, Burgerstrasse 15, 6020 Innsbruck, Austria.

Binesa, Spain. Binesa, Principe de Vergara 109, 28002 Madrid, Spain.

Bio2, Fr. Laboratoires Bio2, 99 bvd des Belges, 69006 Lyon, France.

Biobasal, Switz. Biobasal AG, Eulerstrasse 55, 4003 Basel, Switzerland.

Bioceuticals, UK. Bioceuticals Ltd, 26 Zennor Rd, London, SW12 0PS, UK.

Bio-Chemical, Canad. Bio-Chemical Laboratory Inc., Division of Technilab Inc., Canada.

Biochemie, Aust. Biochemie GmbH, 6250 Kundl, Austria.

Biochimici, Ital. Biochimici PSN, Via Viadagola 30, 40050 Quarto Inferiore (BO), Italy.

Biocine, Ital. See *Chiron Vaccines, Ital.*

Biocodex, Fr. Laboratoires Biocodex, 19 rue Barbès, 92126 Montrouge Cedex, France.

Biocodex, Switz. See *Biomed, Switz.*

Biocontrolfarm, Ital. Biocontrolfarm s.n.c., Via dell'Epomeo 72, 80126 Naples, Italy.

Biocur, Ger. See *Hexal, Ger.*

Biocure, Ital. Biocure s.r.l., Via Ricordi 21, 20131 Milan, Italy.

BioDevelopment, USA. BioDevelopment, USA.

Biodynamics, Ger. Biodynamics International (Deutschland) GmbH, Wetterkreuz 19a, 91058 Erlangen, Germany.

Bio-Familia, Switz. bio-familia AG, Hochwertige Nahrungsmittel, 6072 Sachseln, Switzerland.

Biofilm, USA. Biofilm Inc., 3121 Scott St 1707 Vista, CA 92083-8323, USA.

Bioflora, Aust. Bioflora GmbH, Teichweg 2, 5400 Hallein, Austria.

Bioforce, Canad. Bioforce Canada Inc., 4001 blvd Cote Vertu, St-Laurent, Quebec, H4R 1R5, Canada.

Bioforce, Ger. Bioforce GmbH, Postfach: 40, 78441 Constance, Germany.

Bioforce, Switz. Bioforce AG, Postfach 76, 9325 Roggwil/TG, Switzerland.

Biogalenica, Spain. Biogalenica, Ramon Trias Fargas 7-11, Marina Village, 08005 Barcelona, Spain.

Biogalenique, Fr. Laboratoires Biogalénique, Groupe Rhône-Poulenc Rorer, 82 rue Curial, 75019 Paris, France.

Biogam, Switz. See *Serolab, Switz.*

Bio-Garten, Aust. Bio-Garten, Flatschacher Strasse 57, 9020 Klagenfurt, Austria.

Biogen, Neth. Biogen, Strawinskylaan 305, 1077 XX Amsterdam, Netherlands.

Biogen, UK. Biogen Ltd, Ocean House, The Ring, Bracknell, Berks, RG12 1AX, UK.

Biogen, USA. Biogen, 14 Cambridge Center, Cambridge, MA 02142, USA.

Biogena, Ital. Valetudo s.r.l., Divisione Biogena, Via Ghiaie 6, 24030 Presezzo (BG), Italy.

BioGenex, USA. BioGenex Laboratories, 4600 Norris Canyon Rd, Ste. 400, San Ramon, California, CA 94583, USA.

Bioglan, Austral. Bioglan Ltd, 8/10 Yalgar Rd, Yalgar Business Park, Sydney-Kirrawee, NSW 2232, Australia.

Bioglan, Irl. Bioglan Ireland Ltd, 151 Baldoyle Industrial Estate, Dublin 13, Ireland.

Bioglan, Norw. Bioglan AS, Postboks 1865 Gulset, 3705 Skien, Norway.

Bioglan, Swed. Bioglan AB, Box 50310, 202 13 Malmo, Sweden.

Bioglan, UK. Bioglan Laboratories Ltd, 1 The Cam Centre, Wilbury Way, Hitchin, Herts, SG4 0TW, UK.

Bioglan, USA. Bioglan Pharma, 4902 Eisenhower Blvd, Suite 150, Tampa, FL 33634, USA.

Bio-Health, UK. Bio-Health Ltd, Culpeper Close, Medway City Estate, Rochester, Kent, ME2 4HU, UK.

Biohorm, Spain. Biohorm, Dega Bahi 67, 08026 Barcelona, Spain.

Biohorma, Ital. Biohorma Italia srl, Via del Mare 32 N/1, 00040 Pomezia (RM), Italy.

Bioiberica, Spain. Bioiberica, Ctra N-II Km 680.6, Palafolls, 08389 Barcelona, Spain.

Bioindustria, Ital. Bioindustria Farmaceutici s.p.a., Via Valbondione 113, 00188 Rome, Italy.

Biokanol, Ger. Biokanol Arzneimittel GmbH, Postfach: 2454, 76414 Rastatt, Germany.

Biolac, Swed. Biolac AB, Box 22057, 250 22 Helsingborg, Sweden.

Bioline, USA. See *Goldline, USA.*

BioImmun, Ger. BioImmunPharma Loh GmbH, Alte Weinstr. 1, Postfach: 1243, 61282 Bad Homburg, Germany.

Biologici Italia, Ital. Biologici Italia Laboratories s.r.l., Via Cavour 41/3, 20026 Novate Milanese (MI), Italy.

Biologiques de l'Ile-de-France, Fr. Laboratoires Biologiques de l'Ile-de-France S.A., 45 rue de Clichy, 75009 Paris, France.

Biomatrix, Canad. Biomatrix Medical Canada Inc., 275 av Labrosse, Pointe-Claire, Quebec, H9R 1A3, Canada.

Biomed, Switz. Biomed AG, Uberlandstrasse 199, Postfach, 8600 Dubendorf, Switzerland.

Biomedica, Ital. Biomedica Foscama Industria Chimico Farmaceutica s.p.a., Via Tiburtina Km. 14.5, 00131 Rome, Italy.

Biomedical, Ital. Biomedical di L. Imbriani, Via Novara 31, 20013 Magenta (MI), Italy.

Bio-Medical, UK. Bio-Medical Services Ltd, 6 Riverview Rd, Beverley, North Humberside, HU17 0LD, UK.

Biomerica, USA. Biomerica Inc., 1533 Monrovia Ave, Newport Beach, California, CA 92663, USA.

Biomo, Ger. Biomo Natur-Medizin GmbH, Lendersbergstr. 86, 53721 Siegburg, Germany.

Bioniche, Canad. Bioniche Inc., 383 Sovereign Rd, London, Ontario, N6M 1A3, Canada.

Bionorica, Ger. Bionorica GmbH, Kerschensteinerstr. 11-15, Postfach: 1851, 92308 Neumarkt/Opf, Germany.

Bio-Oil Research, Irl. See *Allphar, Irl.*

Bio-Oil Research, UK. Bio-Oil Research Ltd, The Hawthorns, 64 Welsh Row, Nantwich, Cheshire, CW5 5EU, UK.

Biopha, Fr. Laboratoires Dermopharmaceutiques Biopha, 15 rue Ampere, 91748 Massy cdx, France.

Biopharm, USA. Bio-Pharm Inc, 10 H Runway Rd, Levittown, PA 19057, USA.

Biopharma, Fr. Biopharma, 29 rue du Pont, 92200 Neuilly-sur-Seine, France.

Biopharma, Ital. Biopharma s.r.l., Via delle Gerbere, 00040 Santa Palomba (RM), Italy.

Biophytarom, Fr. Laboratoires Biophytarom, Cap 18, 43 rue de l'Evangile, 75886 Paris Cdx 18, France.

Bioprogress, Ital. Bioprogress s.p.a., Via Aurelia 58, 00165 Rome, Italy.

Bioprojet, Fr. Bioprojet Pharma, 9 rue Rameau, 75002 Paris, France.

Bio-Reform, Aust. Bio-Reform-Gesellsch., Apotheker Pichler & Co., Flatschacher Str. 57, 9020 Klagenfurt, Austria.

Bioresearch, Spain. Bioresearch, Avda de Burgos 91, Edi. 4, 28050 Madrid, Spain.

Biorex, Switz. Biorex AG, Neuzitliche Ernährung, 9642 Ebnat-Kappel, Switzerland.

Biorex, UK. Biorex Laboratories Ltd, 2 Crossfield Chambers, Gladbeck Way, Enfield, Middx, EN2 7HT, UK.

Biorga, Fr. Laboratoires Biorga, 1 rue Blaise-Pascal, Bat C, Parc de Pissaloup, 78190 Trappes, France.

Bios, Belg. Bios Coutelier S.A., Chaussee de Waterloo 935-7, 1180 Brussels, Belgium.

Bio-Sante, Canad. Les Laboratoires Bio-Sante, 3564 rue Griffith, St-Laurent, QC, H4C 1A7, Canada.

Biosarto, Spain. Biosarto, FOC 68-82, 08030 Barcelona, Spain.

Biosedra, Fr. Laboratoires Biosédra, 6 rue du Rempart, B.P. 611, 27406 Louviers Cdx, France.

Biosyn, Ger. biosyn Arzneimittel GmbH, Schorndorfer Strasse 32, Postfach: 1246, 70702 Fellbach, Germany.

Bio-Tech, USA. Bio-Tech, P.O. Box 1992, Fayetteville, AR 72702, USA.

Biotekfarma, Ital. Biotekfarma bkf s.r.l., Via di Tre Cannelle 12, 00040 Pomezia (Rome), Italy.

Biotel, USA. Biotel Corporation, 366 Madison Ave 1506, New York, NY 10017, USA.

Biotene, Austral. See *Advil, Austral.*

Biotest, Aust. Biotest Pharmazeutika GmbH, Einsiedlergasse 58, Postfach 8, 1053 Vienna, Austria.

Biotest, Ger. Biotest Pharma GmbH, Landsteinerstr. 3-5, Postfach: 401108, 63276 Dreieich, Germany.

Biotest, Ital. Biotest s.r.l., Via L. da Vinci 43, 20090 Trezzano sul Naviglio (MI), Italy.

Biotest, Switz. Biotest (Schweiz) AG, Bahnhofstrasse 18, Postfach, 5504 Othmarsingen, Switzerland.

Bio-Therabel, Belg. Bio-Therabel S.A., Rue Egide Van Ophem 110, 1180 Brussels, Belgium.

Biotherapie, Fr. Laboratoires Biotherapie, 88 rue Danton, 92400 Courbevoie, France.

Biotherax, Ger. See *Boehringer Ingelheim, Ger.*

Biotherm, Canad. See *Cosmair, Canad.*

Biotrading, Ital. Biotrading Co. s.r.l., Italy.

Bio-Transfusion, Fr. Bio-Transfusion, ZAC Paris Nord II, 117 av des Nations, B.P. 60079, 95973 Roissy-Charles-de-Gaulle Cdx, France.
Biotrol, Fr. See *Braun Biotrol, Fr.*
Biovac, S.Afr. Biovac, S. Africa.
Biovital, Austral. Biovital Pty. Ltd, 24-10 Yalgar Road, Kirrawee, NSW 2232, Australia.
Bipharma, Neth. Bipharma B.V., Postbus 151, 1380 AD Weesp, Netherlands.
Bira, USA. BIRA Corp., 2525 Quicksilver, McDonald, PA 15057, USA.
Birchwood, USA. Birchwood Laboratories Inc., 7900 Fuller Rd, Eden Prairie, MN 53344, USA.
Bird, USA. Bird Corp., 1100 Bird Center Drive, Palm Springs, CA 92262, USA.
Biscova, Ger. Biscova Fabrik Pharmaz. Praparate, Guntherstrasse 31, Postfach: 810150, 30501 Hannover, Germany.
Bissendorf, Neth. See *Byk, Neth.*
Blackmores, Austral. Blackmores Ltd, P.O. Box 258, Balgowlah, NSW 2093, Australia.
Blackmores, UK. Blackmores UK, 37 Rotasckild Rd, Chiswick, London, W4 5HT, UK.
Blaine, USA. Blaine Co. Inc., 2700 Dixie Highway, Fort Mitchell, KY 41017, USA.
Blair, USA. Blair Laboratories Inc., 100 Connecticut Ave, Norwalk, CT 06856, USA.
Blairex, USA. Blairex Labs Inc., P.O. Box 2127, Columbus, IN 47202-2127, USA.
Blake, UK. Thomas Blake & Co., The Byre House, Fearby, Nr Masham, N. Yorks, HG4 4NF, UK.
Blend-a-med, Ger. Blend-a-med Forschung, Zweigniederlassung der Procter & Gamble GmbH, Sulzbacher Str. 40, Postfach: 2503, 65818 Schwalbach, Germany.
Blend-a-pharm, Fr. Laboratoires Blend-a-pharm, 104 av Charles-de-Gaulle, B.P. 210, 92200 Neuilly-sur-Seine, France.
Blistex, Canad. Blistex Ltd, 2395 Drew Rd, Mississauga, Ontario, L5S 1A1, Canada.
Blistex, USA. Blistex Inc., 1800 Swift Drive, Oak Brook, IL 60521, USA.
Block, Canad. Block Drug Co. (Canada) Ltd, 7600 Danbro Cres., Mississauga, Ontario, L5N 6L6, Canada.
Block, Ger. Block Drug Company Inc., Postfach: 101146, 40831 Ratingen, Germany.
Block, USA. Block Drug Company, Inc., 257 Cornelison Avenue, Jersey City, NJ 07302, USA.
Blucher-Schering, Ger. Blücher-Schering GmbH & Co., Rademacherstrasse 2, Postfach: 1630, 23505 Lubeck, Germany.
Blue Cross, Ital. Blue Cross s.r.l., SS 156 Km 50, 04010 Borgo S Michele (LT), Italy.
BML, Austral. BML Pharmaceuticals Pty Ltd, P.O. Box 31, Arncliffe, NSW 2205, Australia.
BOC, UK. The BOC Group PLC, Chertsey Rd, Windlesham, Surrey, GU20 6HJ, UK.
Bock, Ger. W Bock GmbH & Co. KG, Postfach: 1163, 64679 Einhausen, Germany.
Bock, USA. See *Sanofi Winthrop, USA.*
Bode, Ger. Bode Chemie Hamburg, Melanchthonstrasse 27, Postfach: 540709, 22507 Hamburg, Germany.
Body Spring, Ital. Body Spring s.r.l., Via E. Fermi 3, Loc. Sotto Moscal, 37010 Affi (VR), Italy.
Boehringer Ingelheim, Aust. Boehringer Ingelheim International GmbH, D-55216 Ingelheim am Rhein, Austria.
Boehringer Ingelheim, Austral. Boehringer Ingelheim Pty Ltd, 50 Broughton Road, P.O. Box 1100, Artarmon, NSW 2064, Australia.
Boehringer Ingelheim, Belg. Boehringer Ingelheim S.A., Vesalius Science Park, Avenue Ariane 16, 1200 Brussels, Belgium.
Boehringer Ingelheim, Canad. Boehringer Ingelheim (Canada) Ltd, 5180 South Service Rd, Burlington, Ontario, L7L 5H4, Canada.
Boehringer Ingelheim, Fr. Boehringer Ingelheim France, 37-9 rue Boissiere, 75116 Paris, France.
Boehringer Ingelheim, Ger. Boehringer Ingelheim KG, Binger Strasse, Postfach: 200, 55216 Ingelheim, Germany.
Boehringer Ingelheim, Irl. Boehringer Ingelheim Ltd, 31 Sandyford Industrial Estate, Dublin 18, Ireland.
Boehringer Ingelheim, Ital. Boehringer Ingelheim Italia s.p.a., Via Pellicceria 10, 50123 Florence, Italy.
Boehringer Ingelheim, Jpn. Nippon Boehringer Ingelheim Co. Ltd, 3-10-1 Yato, Kawanishi, Hyogo Prefecture 666-01, Japan.
Boehringer Ingelheim, Neth. Boehringer Ingelheim B.V., Postbus 8037, 1802 KA Alkmaar, Netherlands.
Boehringer Ingelheim, Norw. Boehringer Ingelheim International GmbH, Informasjonskontor Norge, Drengsrudbekken 25, Postboks 405, 1371 Asker, Norway.
Boehringer Ingelheim, S.Afr. Boehringer Ingelheim (Pty) Ltd, Private Bag X3032, Randburg 2125, S. Africa.
Boehringer Ingelheim, Spain. Boehringer Ingelheim, Pablo Alcover 31-3, 08017 Barcelona, Spain.
Boehringer Ingelheim, Swed. Boehringer Ingelheim AB, Box 44, 127 21 Skarholmen, Sweden.
Boehringer Ingelheim, Switz. Boehringer Ingelheim (Schweiz) GmbH, Dufourstrasse 54, 4002 Basel, Switzerland.
Boehringer Ingelheim, UK. Boehringer Ingelheim Ltd, Ellesfield Ave, Bracknell, Berks, RG12 4YS, UK.
Boehringer Ingelheim, USA. Boehringer Ingelheim Pharmaceuticals Inc., 90 East Ridge, P.O. Box 368, Ridgefield, CT 06877, USA.
Boehringer Mannheim, Aust. Boehringer Mannheim Gmbh Wien, Engelhorngasse 3, 1210 Vienna, Austria.
Boehringer Mannheim, Austral. Boehringer Mannheim Australia Pty Ltd, 31 Victoria Avenue, Castle Hill, NSW 2154, Australia.
Boehringer Mannheim, Belg. Boehringer Mannheim Belgium S.A., Avenue des Croix de Guerre 90, 1120 Brussels, Belgium.
Boehringer Mannheim, Canad. Boehringer Mannheim (Canada) Ltd, 201 Armand-Frappier Blvd, Laval, Quebec, H7V 4A2, Canada.
Boehringer Mannheim, Fr. Laboratoires Boehringer Mannheim France Pharma SA, 2 av. du Vercors, B.P. 59, 38242 Meylan Cedex, France.
Boehringer Mannheim, Ger. Boehringer Mannheim GmbH, Sandhofer Strasse 116, 68305 Mannheim, Germany.
Boehringer Mannheim, Irl. Boehringer Mannheim Ireland, Valentine House, Temple Road, Blackrock, Co. Dublin, Ireland.
Boehringer Mannheim, Ital. Boehringer Mannheim Italia s.p.a., Viale GB Stucchi 110, 20052 Monza (MI), Italy.
Boehringer Mannheim, Jpn. Boehringer Mannheim KK, 10-11 Toranomon 3-chome, Minato-ku, Tokyo 105, Japan.
Boehringer Mannheim, Neth. Boehringer Mannheim B.V., Postbus 1007, 1300 BA Almere, Netherlands.
Boehringer Mannheim, Norw. See *Organon, Norw.*
Boehringer Mannheim, S.Afr. Boehringer Mannheim (SA) (Pty) Ltd, P.O. Box 51927, Randburg 2125, S. Africa.
Boehringer Mannheim, Spain. Boehringer Mannheim, Venus, 72 Polg. Indus. Colon II, Terrassa, 08228 Barcelona, Spain.
Boehringer Mannheim, Swed. Boehringer Mannheim Scandinavia AB, Box 147, 161 26 Bromma 1, Sweden.
Boehringer Mannheim, Switz. Boehringer Mannheim (Schweiz) SA, Industriestrasse, 6343 Rotkreuz, Switzerland.
Boehringer Mannheim, UK. Boehringer Mannheim (Pharmaceuticals), Simpson Parkway, Kirkton Campus, Livingston, West Lothian, UK.
Boehringer Mannheim, USA. Boehringer Mannheim, 9115 Hague Rd, P.O. Box 50100, Indianapolis, IN 46250-0100, USA.
Boehringer Mannheim Diagnostics, Irl. See *Boehringer Mannheim Diagnostics, UK.*
Boehringer Mannheim Diagnostics, UK. Boehringer Mannheim (Diagnostics & Biochemicals), Bell Lane, Lewes, East Sussex, BN7 1LG, UK.
Boehringer Mannheim Diagnostics, USA. See *Boehringer Mannheim, USA.*
Boffi, Ital. Eredi di Antonio Boffi s.n.c., Via Lorenzo Magalotti 6, 00197 Rome, Italy.
Bohm, Spain. Bohm, Molina Seca 23 Plg. Cobo Calleja, Fuenlabrada, 28940 Madrid, Spain.
BOI, Spain. Biologicos Organicos Industriales, Polig Ind Sur, Papiol, 08754 Barcelona, Spain.
Boileau & Boyd, Irl. Boileau & Boyd Ltd, 11a Parkmore Estate, Walkinstown, Dublin 12, Ireland.
Boiron, Canad. Boiron Homeopathie Inc., 816 rue Guimond, Longueil, Quebec, J4G 1T5, Canada.
Boiron, Fr. Boiron, 20 rue de la Liberation, 69110 Sainte-Foy-les-Lyon, France.
Boiron, Switz. See *Serolab, Switz.*
Boizot, Spain. Boizot, San Antonio Maria Claret 173, 08041 Barcelona, Spain.
Bolder, Ger. Bolder Arzneimittel GmbH, Koblenzer Strasse 65, Postfach: 510505, 50941 Cologne, Germany.
Boniscontro & Gazzone, Ital. Lab. Prod. Farm. Boniscontro & Gazzone s.r.l., Via Tiburtina 1004, 00156 Rome, Italy.
Bonne Bell, Canad. Bonne Bell of Canada, 6711 Mississauga Rd, Ste 602, Mississauga, Ontario, L5N 2W3, Canada.
Bonnington, Austral. See *SmithKline Beecham Consumer, Austral.*
Bonomelli, Ital. Bonomelli s.r.l., Via Montecuccoli 1, 22042 Dolzago (LC), Italy.
Boots, Austral. The Boots Co. (Australia) Pty Ltd, P.O. Box 120, Carlingford, NSW 2118, Australia.
Boots, Belg. See *Knoll, Belg.*
Boots, Fr. See *Knoll, Fr.*
Boots, Ger. See *Kanoldt, Ger.*
Boots, Ital. Boots Italia s.p.a., Via Lorenteggio 270/A, 20152 Milan, Italy.
Boots, Neth. Boots Pharmaceuticals B.V., Postbus 502, 1200 AM Hilversum, Netherlands.
Boots, S.Afr. Boots Healthcare (SA) (Pty) Ltd, 33 Kelly Rd, Meerlust Building, Meerzicht Business Park, Jet Park 1469, S. Africa.
Boots, Spain. Boots Pharmaceuticals, Avda de Burgos 91, 28050 Madrid, Spain.
Boots, Switz. See *Doetsch, Grether, Switz.*
Boots, UK. The Boots Co. PLC, 1 Thane Rd West, Nottingham, NG2 3AA, UK.
Boots, USA. Boots Pharmaceuticals Inc., 8800 Ellerbe Rd, P.O. Box 6750, Shreveport, LA 71106, USA.
Boots Healthcare, Belg. Boots Healthcare S.A., 't Hofveld 6d, 1702 Groot-Bijgaarden, Belgium.
Boots Healthcare, Fr. Laboratoires Boots Healthcare, 49 rue de Bitche, B.P. 66, 92404 Courbevoie Cedex, France.
Boots Healthcare, Irl. Boots Healthcare Ltd, Parkview House, Beech Hill Office Campus, Clonskeagh, Dublin 4, Ireland.
Boots Healthcare, Ital. Boots Healthcare Marco Viti Farmaceutici s.p.a., Via Tarantelli 15, 22076 Mozzate (CO), Italy.
Boots Healthcare, Neth. Boots Healthcare B.V., Postbus 5236, 1410 AE Naarden, Netherlands.
Boots Healthcare, Spain. Boots Healthcare, Avda de Europa 24, Edificio Torona, Alcobendas, 28109 Madrid, Spain.
Boots-Flint, USA. Boots-Flint Inc., 300 Tri-State International Center, Suite 200, Lincolnshire, IL 60015, USA.
Borg, UK. Borg Medicare Ltd, P.O. Box 99, Hitchin, Herts, SG5 2GF, UK.
Bostad, Norw. Sindre-Jacob Bostad, Kongensg 15, Postboks 449 sentrum, 0104 Oslo, Norway.
Bottger, Ger. Böttger GmbH Pharmazeutische und Kosmetische Praparate, Paulsborner Strasse 2, Postfach: 310320, 10633 Berlin, Germany.
Bottu, Fr. See *Pharmuka, Fr., RP-LABO, Fr., Specia, Fr.,* and *Theraplix, Fr.*
Bouchara, Fr. Laboratoires du Dr E. Bouchara, 68 rue Marjolin, 92302 Levallois-Perret, France.
Bouchara, Switz. See *Golaz, Switz.*
Bouchara Sante, Fr. Laboratoires Bouchara Santé Active, 68 rue Marjolin, B.P. 67, 92302 Levallois-Perret Cdx, France.
Bouchard, Fr. Laboratoires Bouchard, 11-13 rue de la Loge, B.P. 100, 94265 Fresnes Cedex, France.
Boucher & Muir, Austral. Boucher & Muir Pty Ltd, P.O. Box 333, North Sydney, NSW 2059, Australia.
Bouhon, Ger. Apotheker Walter Bouhon GmbH & Co. KG, Fuldaer Strasse 10, Postfach: 920131, 90266 Nurnberg, Germany.
Bournonville, Belg. Bournonville Pharma S.A., Parc Industriel de la Vallee du Hain, Ave de l'Industrie 11, 1420 Braine-l'Alleud, Belgium.
Bournonville, Neth. Bournonville-Pharma B.V., De Steiger 196, 1351 AV Almere, Netherlands.
Bouteille, Fr. Laboratoires Bouteille, 7 rue des Belges, 87000 Limoges, France.
Bouty, Ital. s.p.a. Italiana Laboratori Bouty, Via Vanvitelli 4, 20129 Milan, Italy.
Bowman, USA. Bowman Pharmaceuticals Inc., 119 Schroyer Ave SW, Canton, OH 44702, USA.
Boxo, Ger. Boxo-Pharm Arzneimittel GmbH, Postfach: 103951, 40030 Dusseldorf, Germany.
Boyle, USA. Boyle & Co. Pharmaceuticals, 1613 Chelsea Rd, San Marino, CA 91108, USA.
BPL, UK. Bio Products Laboratory, Dagger Lane, Elstree, Borehamwood, Herts, WD6 3BX, UK.
BPR, Ital. BPR International srl, Via della Fornace 1, 20010 Pogliano Milanese (MI), Italy.
BR Pharmaceuticals, UK. BR Pharmaceuticals Ltd, 21 Chapeltown, Pudsey, Leeds, West Yorks, LS28 7RZ, UK.
Bracco, Ital. Bracco s.p.a., Via E. Folli 50, 20134 Milan, Italy.
Bracco, Switz. See *Sintetica, Switz.,* and *Uhlmann-Eyraud, Switz.*
Bracco, UK. Bracco Diagnostics, UK.
Bracco, USA. Bracco Diagnostics, P.O. Box 5225, Princeton, NJ 08543, USA.
Bracey, UK. J Bracey, 209 Menlove Ave, Liverpool, Merseyside, UK.
Bradford Chemists Alliance, UK. Bradford Chemists Alliance Ltd, UK.
Bradley, Canad. See *Galen, Canad.*
Bradley, USA. Bradley Pharmaceutical Inc., 383 Rt. 46W, Fairfield, New Jersey, NJ 07006-2402, USA.
Brady, Aust. Brady C. KG, Horlgasse 5, 1092 Vienna, Austria.
Bragg, UK. J.L. Bragg (Ipswich) Ltd, 30 Greyfriars Rd, Ipswich, Suffolk, IP1 1UP, UK.
Braintree, USA. Braintree Laboratories Inc., P.O. Box 361, Braintree, MA 02184, USA.
Brandt, Switz. See *Uhlmann-Eyraud, Switz.*
Brauer, Austral. Brauer Biotherapies Pty Ltd, P.O. Box 234, Tanunda, SA 5352, Australia.
Braun, Aust. Braun Austria GmbH, In den Langackern 5, 2344 Maria Enzersdorf, Austria.
Braun, Belg. B. Braun Pharma S.A., Woluwelaan 140 b, 1831 Diegem, Belgium.
Braun, Fr. B Braun Medical SA, 204 av du Mal-Juin, B.P. 331, 92107 Boulogne Cdx, France.
Braun, Ger. B. Braun Melsungen AG, Carl-Braun-Strasse 1, Postfach: 1110 + 1120, 34209 Melsungen, Germany.
Braun, Irl. B. Braun Medical Ltd, 3 Naas Rd Industrial Park, Dublin 12, Ireland.
Braun, Ital. B. Braun Milano s.p.a., Via V. da Seregno 14, 20161 Milan, Italy.
Braun, Norw. B. Braun Medical A/S, Bjellandv. 12, 3173 Vear, Norway.
Braun, Spain. Braun Medical, Ctra Tarrasa S/N Km 21.6, Rubi, 08191 Barcelona, Spain.
Braun, Swed. B. Braun Medical AB, Box 4045, 17104 Solna, Sweden.
Braun, Switz. B. Braun Medical AG, Sparte Pharma, Rechenstrasse 27, Postfach, 9001 St Gallen, Switzerland.
Braun, UK. B. Braun Medical Ltd, 13/14 Farmbrough Close, Aylesbury Vale Industrial Park, Aylesbury, Bucks, HP20 1DQ, UK.
Braun Biotrol, Fr. B Braun Biotrol SA, 69 rue de la Grange-aux-Belles, 75010 Paris, France.
Braun Fandre, Fr. B Braun Fandre SA, ZI, rue Lavoisier, B.P. 41, 54713 Ludres Cdx, France.
Braun Surgical, Switz. B. Braun Surgical AG, Postfach 427, 8212 Neuhausen, Switzerland.
Breckenridge, USA. Breckenridge Pharmaceutical Inc, P.O. Box 206, Boca Raton, FL 33429, USA.
Bregenzer, Aust. Bregenzer Herbert, Am Damm 20, 6820 Frastanz, Austria.
Brenner-Efeka, Ger. Brenner-Efeka Pharma GmbH, Schleebruggenkamp 15, Postfach: 8807, 48136 Munster, Germany.
Bride, Fr. See *Cooperation Pharmaceutique, Fr.*
Bridoux, Fr. Laboratoires Bridoux, 6 rue Salengro, 62160 Bully-les-Mines, France.

Brioschi, Canad. Brioschi Inc., 465 Fenmar Drive, Weston, ON, M9L 2R6, Canada.
Bripharm, Irl. See *Yamanouchi, Irl.*
Brissenco, S.Afr. Brissenco, S. Africa.
Bristol, Canad. See *Bristol-Myers Squibb, Canad.*
Bristol, Ger. See *Bristol-Myers Squibb, Ger.*
Bristol, Ital. See *Bristol-Myers Squibb, Ital.*
Bristol, USA. See *Bristol-Myers Squibb, USA.*
Bristol-Myers, Austral. See *Bristol-Myers Squibb, Austral.*
Bristol-Myers, Spain. Bristol Myers, Campus Empresarial Jose Ma Churruca, Almansa 101, 28040 Madrid, Spain.
Bristol-Myers Oncology, USA. Bristol-Myers Oncology Division, Bristol-Myers Co., 2404 Pennsylvania St, Evansville, IN 47721, USA.
Bristol-Myers Products, USA. See *Bristol-Myers Squibb, USA.*
Bristol-Myers Squibb, Aust. Bristol-Myers Squibb GmbH, Columbusgasse 4, 1100 Vienna, Austria.
Bristol-Myers Squibb, Austral. Bristol-Myers Squibb Pharmaceuticals Pty Ltd, P.O. Box 39, Noble Park, Vic. 3174, Australia.
Bristol-Myers Squibb, Belg. Bristol-Myers Squibb Belgium S.A., Waterloo Office Park, Building I, Dreve Richelle 161, 1410 Waterloo, Belgium.
Bristol-Myers Squibb, Canad. Bristol-Myers Squibb Canada Inc., 2365 Cote de Liesse Rd, Montreal, Quebec, H4N 2M7, Canada.
Bristol-Myers Squibb, Fr. Bristol-Myers Squibb, La Grande Arche Nord, 92044 Paris-La-Defense cdx, France.
Bristol-Myers Squibb, Ger. Bristol-Myers Squibb GmbH, Volkartstrasse 83, 80636 Munich, Germany.
Bristol-Myers Squibb, Irl. Bristol-Myers Squibb Pharmaceuticals, Watery Lane, Swords, Co. Dublin, Ireland.
Bristol-Myers Squibb, Ital. Bristol-Myers Squibb s.p.a., Via Paolo di Dono 73, 00143 Rome, Italy.
Bristol-Myers Squibb, Neth. Bristol-Myers Squibb, Postbus 514, 3440 AM Woerden, Netherlands.
Bristol-Myers Squibb, Norw. Bristol-Myers Squibb Norway Ltd, Sandviksv. 26, Postboks 464, 1322 Hovik, Norway.
Bristol-Myers Squibb, S.Afr. Bristol-Myers Squibb (Pty) Ltd, S. Africa.
Bristol-Myers Squibb, Swed. Bristol-Myers Squibb AB, Box 15200, 161 15 Bromma, Sweden.
Bristol-Myers Squibb, Switz. Bristol-Myers Squibb AG, Neuhofstrasse 6, 6340 Baar, Switzerland.
Bristol-Myers Squibb, UK. Bristol-Myers Squibb Pharmaceuticals Ltd, Bristol-Myers Squibb House, 141-149 Staines Road, Hounslow, Middlesex, TW3 3JA, UK.
Bristol-Myers Squibb, USA. Bristol-Myers Squibb, 2400 w Lloyd Expressway, Evansville, IN 47721-0001, USA.
Britannia Pharmaceuticals, Irl. See *Clonmel, Irl.*
Britannia Pharmaceuticals, UK. Britannia Pharmaceuticals Ltd, Forum House, 41-75 Brighton Rd, Redhill, Surrey, RH1 6YS, UK.
BritCair, UK. See *Bristol-Myers Squibb, UK.*
BritHealth, UK. BritHealth Limited, Weltech Centre, Ridgeway, Welwyn Garden City, Herts, AL7 2AA, UK.
Britisfarma, Spain. Britisfarma, Pza Carlos Trias Bertran 4, 28020 Madrid, Spain.
British Pharmaceuticals, Austral. See *Organon, Austral.*
Britpharm, UK. Britpharm Laboratories Ltd, Kramer Mews, London, SW5 9JL, UK.
Broad, UK. Broad Laboratories plc, UK.
Brocades, Ital. See *Yamanouchi, Ital.*
Brocades, Neth. Brocades Pharma B.V., Elisabethhof 17, 2353 EW Leiderdorp, Netherlands.
Brocades, UK. See *Yamanouchi, UK.*
Brocchieri, Ital. Stabilimento Chimico Farmaceutico dr. L. Brocchieri s.r.l., Via Tiburtina Km. 14.4, 00131 Rome, Italy.
Bronchosirum, Canad. Bronchosirum Inc. 15 JF Kennedy, Bur 10, St-Jerome, QC, J7Y 4B4, Canada.
Brothier, Fr. Laboratoires Brothier, 41 rue de Neuilly, 92000 Nanterre, France.
Brothier, Switz. See *Uhlmann-Eyraud, Switz.*
Brovar, S.Afr. Brovar S & P (Pty) Ltd, P.O. Box 11434, Johannesburg 2000, S. Africa.
Bruco, Ital. Nuova Farmaceutici Bruco s.r.l., Via XXV Aprile 69, 18100 Imperia, Italy.
Brum, Spain. Brum, Quevedo 4, Oviedo, 33012 Asturias, Spain.
Brunel, S.Afr. Brunel Laboratories (Pty) Ltd, P.O. Box 23103, Innesdale 0031, S. Africa.
Brunet, Fr. See *Martin, Fr.*
Bruni, Ital. Bruni Dr. Domenico (Farmacia), Via Anfossi 9, 20135 Milan, Italy.
Brunnengraber, Ger. Dr Christian Brunnengräber GmbH, Germany.
Bruno, Ital. Bruno Farmaceutici srl, V.le Castello della Magnana 38, 00148 Rome, Italy.
Bruschettini, Ital. Bruschettini s.r.l., Via Isonzo 6, 16147 Genova, Italy.
Bruschettini, Switz. See *Galenica, Switz.*
BTG, USA. BTG Pharmaceuticals, 70 Wood Ave South, Iselin, NJ 08830, USA.
Bucaneve, Ital. Bucaneve Medicinali s.r.l., Via Sercognani 15, 20156 Milan, Italy.
Bucca, Spain. Bucca, Juan Alvarez Mendizabal 43, 28008 Madrid, Spain.
Buckley, Canad. W.K. Buckley Ltd, 84 Wingold Ave, Toronto, ON, M6B 1P5, Canada.
Buffington, USA. Buffington, USA.
Byk, Aust. Byk Österreich Pharma GmbH, Ketzergasse 200, 1235 Vienna, Austria.
Byk, Belg. Byk Belga S.A., Rue Anatole France 115-121/Bte 5, 1030 Brussels, Belgium.
Byk, Fr. Laboratoires Byk France S.A., 593 rte de Boissise, 77350 le Mee-sur-Seine, France.
Byk, Neth. Byk Nederland B.V., Postbus 61, 1160 AB Zwanenburg, Netherlands.
Byk, Switz. Byk AG, Bachstrasse 10, 8280 Kreuzlingen, Switzerland.
Byk Elmu, Spain. Byk Elmu, Ctra Nacional III, Km 23, Arganda del Rey, 28500 Madrid, Spain.
Byk Gulden, Ger. Byk Gulden Lomberg Chemische Fabrik GmbH, Byk-Gulden-Strasse 2, Postfach: 100310, 78403 Constance, Germany.
Byk Gulden, Ital. Byk Gulden Italia s.p.a., Via Giotto 1, 20032 Cormano (MI), Italy.
Byk Gulden, Norw. See *Orphan, Norw.*
Byk Gulden, S.Afr. Byk Gulden Pharmaceuticals, P.O. Box 1476, Randburg 2125, S. Africa.
Byk Leo, Spain. Byk Leo Lab. Farm., Ctra N-III Km 23, Arganda del Rey, 28500 Madrid, Spain.
Byk Madaus, S.Afr. Byk Madaus, S. Africa.
Byk Roland, Switz. Byk Roland GmbH, Bachstrasse 10, 8280 Kreuzlingen, Switzerland.
Byly, Spain. Byly, Avda Guipuzcoa 159, 08020 Barcelona, Spain.
C & M, USA. C & M Pharmacal Inc., 1721 Maple Lane, Hazel Park, MI 48030-1215, USA.
Caber, Ital. Farmaceutici Caber s.p.a., Via Cavour 11, 44022 Comacchio (FE), Italy.
Cabon, Ital. Cabon s.p.a., Via Melchiorre Gioia 168, 20125 Milan, Italy.
CaDiGroup, Ital. Ca.Di.Group srl, Via Pieve Tesino 75, 00124 Rome, Italy.
Cahill May Roberts, Irl. Cahill May Roberts Ltd, P.O. Box 1090, Chapelizod, Dublin 20, Ireland.
Calgon Vestal, USA. Calgon Vestal Laboratories, P.O. Box 147, St. Louis, MO 63166-0147, USA.
Callegari, Ital. Callegari s.p.a., Via Adamello 2/A, 43100 Parma, Italy.
Calmante Vitaminado, Spain. See *Perez Gimenez, Spain.*
Calmic, Irl. See *Glaxo Wellcome, Irl.*
Calmic, UK. See *Wellcome, UK.*
Calmic, USA. See *Wellcome, USA.*
Cal-White, USA. Cal-White Mineral Co., 7700 SE Beaverton Hillside Hwy, Portland, OR 97225, USA.
Camall, USA. Camall Inc., P.O. Box 307, Romeo, MI 48065-0307, USA.
Cambridge, UK. Cambridge Laboratories, division of Selfcare Diagnostics Ltd, Richmond House, Old Brewery Court, Sandyford Lane, Newcastle-upon -Tyne, NE2 1XG, UK.
Cambridge Laboratories, Austral. Cambridge Laboratories Pty Ltd, 397 Little Lonsdale St, Melbourne, Vic. 3000, Australia.
Camcos, Canad. Camcos Distributing Inc., 5334 Yonge St, Ste 1416, Toronto, Ontario, M2N 6M2, Canada.
Camps, Spain. Camps, Planeta 39, 08012 Barcelona, Spain.
Can-Am Care, USA. Can Am Care Corp, Cimetra Industrial Park, Chazy, NY 12921, USA.
Canderm, Canad. Canderm Pharmacal Ltd, 5353 boul. Thimens, St-Laurent, Quebec, H4R 2H4, Canada.
Candioli, Ital. Istituto Candioli Profilattico & Farmaceutico s.p.a., Via Manzoni 2, 10092 Torino Beinasco, Italy.
Cangene, Canad. Cangene Corp., 104 Chancellor Matheson Rd, Winnipeg, Manitoba, R3T 5Y3, Canada.
Cantabria, Spain. Cantabria, Ctra de Cazona Adarzo S/N, Santander, 39011 Cantabria, Spain.
Cantassium Co., UK. The Cantassium Company, 225 Putney Bridge Rd, London, SW15 2PY, UK.
Capilares, Spain. Productos Capilares, Lopez Bravo 78, Plg. Ind. Villalonquejar, 09080 Burgos, Spain.
Caprice Greystoke, USA. Caprice Greystoke, 1259 Activity Drive, Vista, CA 92083, USA.
Caps, S.Afr. Caps Pharmaceuticals (SA) (Pty) Ltd, P.O. Box 2801, Johannesburg 2000, S. Africa.
Caraco, USA. Caraco Pharmaceutical Labs, 1150 Elijah McCoy Drive, Detroit, MI 48202, USA.
Cardel, Fr. Laboratoires Cardel, 16-32 rue Henri-Regnault, 92400 Courbevoie, France.
Cardinaux, Canad. Cardinaux Enrg, 5420 Pasquier, Laval, QC, H7K 3K3, Canada.
Care, USA. Care Technologies Inc., 55 Holly Hill Lane, Greenwich, CT 06830, USA.
Carlo Erba, Ital. Farmitalia Carlo Erba s.r.l., Gruppo Ferruzzi-Erbamont, Via C. Imbonati 24, 20159 Milan, Italy.
Carlo Erba OTC, Ital. Carlo Erba OTC s.p.a., Via Robert Koch 1.2, 20152 Milan, Italy.
Carlton Laboratories, UK. Carlton Laboratories (UK) Ltd, UK.
Carmaran, Canad. Carmaran, 1467 Cunard, Chomedey-Laval, QC, H7S 2H8, Canada.
Carme, USA. Carme Inc., 84 Galli, Novato, CA 94949, USA.
Carnation, USA. Carnation, 800 North Brand Blvd, Glendale, CA 91203, USA.
Carnrick, USA. Carnrick Laboratories Inc., 65 Horse Hill Rd, Cedar Knolls, NJ 07927, USA.
Carolina, USA. Carolina Medical Products Co., P.O. Box 147, Farmville, NC 27828, USA.
Carter, USA. Carter Products, Half Acre Rd, P.O. Box 1001, Cranbury, NJ 08512-0181, USA.
Carter Horner, Canad. Carter Horner Inc., 6600 Kitimat Rd, Mississauga, Ontario, L5N 1L9, Canada.
Carter-Wallace, Austral. Carter Wallace (Australia) Pty Ltd, P.O. Box 216, Brookvale, NSW 2100, Australia.
Carter-Wallace, Switz. See *Doetsch, Grether, Switz.*
Carter-Wallace, UK. Carter-Wallace Ltd, Wear Bay Rd, Folkestone, Kent, UK.
Cascan, Ger. Cascan GmbH & Co. KG, Hohenstaufenstr. 7, Postfach: 1907, 65009 Wiesbaden, Germany.
Cascapharm, Ger. Cascapharm GmbH & Co., Hohenstaufenstr. 7, Postfach 1968, 65009 Wiesbaden, Germany.
Casen Fisons, Spain. Casen Fisons, Autovia de Logrono, Km 13300, Utebo, 50180 Zaragoza, Spain.
Casen Fleet, Spain. Casen Fleet, Autovia de Logrono Km 13.3, Utebo, 50180 Zaragoza, Spain.
Cassella-med, Ger. Cassella-med GmbH, Gereonsmuhlengasse 1, Postfach: 100624, 50446 Cologne, Germany.
Cassella-med, Ital. Cassella-med Italiana s.p.a., Via G. Frua 26, 20146 Milan, Italy.
Cassella-med, Switz. Cassella-med AG, Steinentorstrasse 19, 4051 Basel, Switzerland.
Cassella-Riedel, Ger. See *Hoechst, Ger.*
Cassenne, Austral. Cassenne Pty. Ltd, Locked Bag No. 30, Pennant Hills, NSW 2120, Australia.
Cassenne, Fr. Laboratoires Cassenne, 1 terrasse Bellini, 92800 Puteaux, France.
Castlemead, UK. See *Distriphar, UK.*
CCD, Fr. Laboratoires CCD, 60 rue Pierre-Charron, 75008 Paris, France.
CCM, Ger. CCM Pharma Ltd, Rheinstr. 219, 76532 Baden-Baden, Germany.
CCM, Ital. CCM Pharma s.r.l., Via F. Ferruccio 6, 20145 Milan, Italy.
CCP, Irl. CCP, Ireland, Ireland.
CCS, Swed. CCS Clean Chemical Sweden AB, Tunavagen 277 B, 781 73 Borlange, Sweden.
Ceccarelli, Ital. Ceccarelli A. & C. dei F.lli dr. Tanganelli, Via G. Caponsacchi 31, 50126 Florence, Italy.
Cedar Health, UK. Cedar Health Ltd, Pepper Rd, Hazel Grove, Stockport, Cheshire, SK7 5BW, UK.
Cederroth, Norw. Cederroth A/S, Postboks 23, 3174 Revetal, Norway.
Cederroth, Spain. Cederroth, Leon 57 (Pol. Ind. Cobo Calleja), Fuenlabrada, 28947 Madrid, Spain.
Cedona, Neth. Cedona Pharmaceuticals B.V., Netherlands.
Cefak, Ger. Cefak Arzneimittel, Chem.-pharm. Fabrik Dr. Brand & Co. KG Nachf., Postfach: 1360, 87403 Kempten, Germany.
Celafar, Ital. CE.LA.FAR s.r.l., C.so Peschiera 337, 10141 Turin, Italy.
Celgene, USA. Celgene Corp., 7 Powder Horn Drive, Warren, NJ 07059, USA.
Cell Pharm, Ger. cell pharm Gesellschaft für pharmazeutische und diagnostische Präparate mbH, Feodor-Lynen-Str. 23, 30625 Hannover, Germany.
Celsius, Ital. Celsius s.p.a., Via Grandi snc, 20090 Caleppio di Settala (MI), Italy.
Cenci, USA. HR Cenci Labs Inc., P.O. Box 12524, Fresno, CA 93778-2524, USA.
Ceninter, Spain. Ceninter, Roma 19, 28028 Madrid, Spain.
Cenovis, Austral. Cenovis Pty Ltd, P.O. Box 31, Arncliffe, NSW 2205, Australia.
Centeon, Aust. Centeon Pharma GmbH, Altmannsdorfer Strasse 104, 1121 Vienna, Austria.
Centeon, Ger. Centeon Pharma GmbH, Postfach: 1230, 35002 Marburg (Lahn), Germany.
Centeon, Irl. See *Centeon, UK.*
Centeon, Ital. Centeon s.p.a., V.le Gran Sasso 18/A, 20131 Milan, Italy.
Centeon, Neth. Centeon GmbH, Postbus 192, 1380 AD Weesp, Netherlands.
Centeon, Norw. See *Centeon, Swed.*
Centeon, Spain. Centeon, Ronda General Mitre 72-4, 08017 Barcelona, Spain.
Centeon, Swed. Centeon AB, Hjortgatan 3 B, 223 50 Lund, Sweden.
Centeon, Switz. See *Hoechst Marion Roussel, Switz.*
Centeon, UK. Centeon Ltd, Centeon House, Market Place, Haywards Heath, West Sussex, RH16 1DB, UK.
Centeon, USA. Centeon, 1020 First Ave, King of Prussia, PA 19406-1310, USA.
Center Laboratories, USA. Center Laboratories, Division of EM Pharmaceuticals Inc., 35 Channel Dr., Port Washington, NY 11050, USA.
Centocor, Fr. Laboratoires Centocor France, France.
Centocor, Neth. Centocor Europe B.V., Einsteinweg 101, 2333 CB Leiden, Netherlands.
Centocor, Norw. See *Lilly, Norw.*
Centocor, UK. See *Centocor, Neth.*
Centocor, USA. Centocor, Inc., 200 Great Valley Pkwy, Malvern, PA 19355, USA.
Central, Irl. Central Laboratories Ltd, 31 Ravensrock Rd, Sandyford Industrial Estate, Foxrock, Dublin 18, Ireland.
Central Pharmaceuticals, USA. See *Schwarz, USA.*
Centrapharm, Belg. Centrapharm S.A.-N.V., Chaussee de Gand 615, 1080 Brussels, Belgium.
Centrapharm, Fr. Laboratoires Centrapharm, 35 rue de la Chapelle, 63450 Saint-Amant-Tallende, France.
Centrum, Spain. Centrum, Sagitario 12, 03006 Alicante, Spain.

Century, USA. Century Pharmaceuticals Inc., 10377 Hague Rd, Indianapolis, IN 46256, USA.

CEPA, Spain. Compañia Española de la Penicilina y Antibioticos, Po. de la Castellana 141-15, Edif. Cuzco IV, 28046 Madrid, Spain.

Cephalon, UK. Cephalon UK Ltd, 11-13 Frederick Sanger Rd, Surrey Research Park, Guildford, Surrey, GU2 5YD, UK.

Cermak, Aust. Dr Cermak, Austria.

Cernitin, Switz. Cernitin SA, Via Pian Scairolo 6, 6917 Barbengo, Switzerland.

Cetylite, USA. Cetylite Industries Inc., P.O. Box CN6, 9051 River Rd, Pennsauken, NJ 08110, USA.

Ceuta, UK. Ceuta Healthcare Ltd, Hill House, 41 Richmond Hill, Bournemouth, Dorset, BH2 6HS, UK.

Chancellor, UK. Chancellor Group Ltd, Abbey House, Wrexham Industrial Estate, Wrexham, Clwyd, LL13 9PW, UK.

Charton, Canad. Charton Laboratories, Division of Herdt & Charton Inc., 7400 boul. des Galeries d'Anjou, Bureau 600, Anjou, Quebec, H1M 3S9, Canada.

Charwell Pharmaceuticals, Irl. See *Allphar, Irl.*

Charwell Pharmaceuticals, UK. Charwell Pharmaceuticals Ltd, Charwell House, Wilsom Rd, Alton, Hants, GU34 2TJ, UK.

Chatelut, Fr. Laboratoires Chatelut, 36170 St-Benoit-du-Sault, France.

Chatfield Laboratories, UK. Chatfield Laboratories, Kramer Mews, London, SW5 9JL, UK.

Chattem, Canad. Chattem (Canada) Inc., 2220 Argentia Rd, Mississauga, Ontario, L5N 2K7, Canada.

Chattem, USA. Chattem Consumer Products, 1715 W 38th St, Chattanooga, TN 37409, USA.

Chauvin, Fr. Laboratoires Chauvin, 416 rue Samuel-Morse, B.P. 1174, 34009 Montpellier Cedex, France.

Chauvin, Irl. See *Cahill May Roberts, Irl.*

Chauvin, UK. Chauvin Pharmaceuticals Ltd, Bampton Rd, Harold Hill, Romford, Essex, RM3 8SL, UK.

Chefaro, Belg. Chefaro S.A., AKZO Building, Ave Marnix 13, 1000 Brussels, Belgium.

Chefaro, Fr. See *Roche Nicholas, Fr.*

Chefaro, Ger. Deutsche Chefaro Pharma GmbH, Wirrigen 25, Postfach: 449, 45725 Waltrop, Germany.

Chefaro, Neth. Chefaro Nederland B.V., Keileweg 8, 3029 BS Rotterdam, Netherlands.

Chefaro, UK. Chefaro Proprietaries Ltd, Science Park, Milton Rd, Cambridge, CB4 4FL, UK.

Chefaro Ardeval, Fr. Chefaro-Ardeval, 164 rue Ambroise Croizat, B.P. 143, 93204 St Denis Cdx 01, France.

Chelsea, USA. Chelsea Laboratories, USA.

Chemdorf, Spain. Chemdorf, Gran Via de Carlos III 94, 08028 Barcelona, Spain.

Chemedica, Switz. Chemedica SA, Postfach 240, 1896 Vouvry, Switzerland.

Chemieprodukte, Aust. Chemieprodukte, Dipl.-Ing. Beindl, Mullner Hauptstrasse 1, 5020 Salzburg, Austria.

Chemil, Ital. Chemil Farmaceutici s.r.l., Via Praglia 15, 10044 Pianezza (TO), Italy.

Chemineau, Fr. Laboratoires Chemineau, 93 rte de Monnaie, 37210 Vouvray, France.

Cheminova, Spain. See *Euroexim, Spain.*

Chemomedica, Aust. Chemomedica-Creutzberg & Co., Wipplingerstrasse 19, 1013 Vienna, Austria.

Chemosan, Aust. Chemosan, Villach, Austria.

Chepharin, Aust. Hauser Paul-Chepharin, Flatschacher Strasse 57, 9020 Klagenfurt, Austria.

Chephasaar, Ger. Chephasaar, Chem.-pharm. Fabrik GmbH, Muhlstrasse 50, Postfach: 4120, 66376 St Ingbert, Germany.

Chesebrough-Pond's, UK. Chesebrough-Pond's Ltd, P.O. Box IDY, Hesket House, Portman Square, London, W1A 1DY, UK.

Chesebrough-Pond's, USA. Chesebrough-Pond's Inc., 33 Benedict Place, Greenwich, Connecticut, CT 06830, USA.

Cheshire, UK. Cheshire Cosmetics Ltd, Cromet House, 1 Gunco Lane, Macclesfield, Cheshire, SK11 7JX, UK.

Chibret, Ger. Chibret Pharmazeutische GmbH (MSD-Gruppe), Lindenplatz 1, Postfach: 1202, 85530 Haar, Germany.

Chibret, Neth. See *Merck Sharp & Dohme, Neth.*

Chiesi, Ital. Chiesi Farmaceutici s.p.a., Via Palermo 26/A, 43100 Parma, Italy.

Chiesi, Neth. See *Multipharma, Neth.*

Chiesi, Switz. See *Lucchini, Switz.*

Chinoin, Hung. Chinoin Pharmaceutical and Chemical Works Ltd, P.O. Box 110, 1325 Budapest, Hungary.

Chinoin, Ital. Chinoin s.p.a., Via Zanella 3/5, 20133 Milan, Italy.

Chinosolfabrik, Ger. Chinosolfabrik (Zweigniederlassung der Riedel-de Haen AG), Wunstorfer Strasse 40, Postfach: 100262, 30918 Seelze, Germany.

Chiron, Fr. Chiron France, 10 rue Chevreul, 92150 Suresnes, France.

Chiron, Irl. See *Cahill May Roberts, Irl.*

Chiron, Ital. Chiron Italia s.r.l., Via Cimarosa 4, 20144 Milan, Italy.

Chiron, Neth. Chiron B.V., Postbus 23023, 1100 DM Amsterdam, Netherlands.

Chiron, Spain. Chiron Iberia, Edificio Dublin, Parque Emp. San Fernando, San Fernando de Henares, 28831 Madrid, Spain.

Chiron, UK. Chiron UK Ltd, Salamander Quay West, Park Lane, Harefield, Middlesex, UB9 6NY, UK.

Chiron, USA. Chiron Therapeutics, 4560 Horton St, Emeryville, CA 94608, USA.

Chiron Behring, Ger. Chiron Behring GmbH & Co, Schimmersfeld 5, 40880 Rattingen, Germany.

Chiron Vaccines, Ital. Chiron Vaccines, Divisione Chiron s.p.a., Via Fiorentina 1, 53100 Siena, Italy.

Chlorella, UK. Chlorella Products Ltd, UK.

Choay, Fr. See *Sanofi Winthrop, Fr.*

Chong Kun Dang, Ital. Chong Kun Dang Italia spa, Fraz. Domodossolina, 20070 Borgo S Giovanni (MI), Italy.

Christiaens, Belg. Christiaens Pharma S.A., Chaussee de Gand 615, 1080 Brussels, Belgium.

Christiaens, Neth. Christiaens B.V., Postbus 3458, 4800 DL Breda, Netherlands.

Chugai, Jpn. Chugai Pharmaceutical Co. Ltd, 1-9 Kyobashi 2-chome, Chuo-ku, Tokyo 104, Japan.

Chugai, UK. Chugai Pharma UK, Mulliner House, Flanders Rd, Turnham Green, London, W4 1NN, UK.

Ciba, Canad. Ciba Pharmaceuticals, Division of Ciba-Geigy Canada Ltd, 6860 Century Ave, Mississauga, Ontario, L5N 2W5, Canada.

Ciba, Ger. Ciba-Geigy GmbH, Ciba Pharma, Oflinger Strasse 44, Postfach: 1160/1180, 79662 Wehr, Germany.

Ciba, Ital. Ciba Geigy s.p.a., 21040 Origgio (VA), Italy.

Ciba, Neth. Ciba-Geigy B.V., Postbus 241, 6800 LZ Arnhem, Netherlands.

Ciba, Norw. See *Novartis, Norw.*

Ciba, Switz. See *Ciba-Geigy, Switz.*

Ciba, UK. Ciba-Geigy Pharmaceuticals, Wimblehurst Rd, Horsham, West Sussex, RH12 4AB, UK.

Ciba, USA. See *Ciba-Geigy, USA.*

Ciba Cancer Care, Ger. See *Ciba, Ger.*

Ciba Consumer, USA. Ciba Consumer Pharmaceuticals, Division of Ciba-Geigy Corp., Mack Woodbridge II, 581 Main Street, Woodbridge, NJ 07095, USA.

Ciba Self Medication, Canad. Ciba Self Medication, Division of Ciba-Geigy Canada Ltd, P.O. Box 2000, Mississauga, Ontario, L5M 5N3, Canada.

Ciba Vision, Aust. Ciba Vision GmbH, Modecenterstrasse 14, 1030 Vienna, Austria.

Ciba Vision, Austral. Ciba Vision Australia Pty Ltd, Private Bag 100, Baulkham Hills Business Centre, Baulkham Hills, NSW 2153, Australia.

Ciba Vision, Belg. Ciba Vision, Belgium.

Ciba Vision, Canad. Ciba Vision Ophthalmics, 2150 Torquay Mews, Mississauga, Ontario, L5N 2M6, Canada.

Ciba Vision, Fr. Laboratoires Ciba Vision, 8 rue Colomies, B.P. 1129, 31036 Toulouse Cdx, France.

Ciba Vision, Ger. Ciba Vision Ophthalmics GmbH, Argelsrieder Feld 5, Postfach: 1262, 82231 Wessling, Germany.

Ciba Vision, Irl. See *United Drug, Irl.*

Ciba Vision, Ital. Ciba Vision s.r.l., gruppo Ciba Geigy, Via E Filiberto 130, 00185 Rome, Italy.

Ciba Vision, Neth. Ciba Vision Ophtha Nederland, Postbus 3126, 4800 DC Breda, Netherlands.

Ciba Vision, Norw. Ciba Vision Norge AS, Postboks 24, 3601 Kongsberg, Norway.

Ciba Vision, Spain. Ciba Vision, Valnecia 307, 08009 Barcelona, Spain.

Ciba Vision, Swed. Ciba Vision AB, Datavagen 24, 436 32 Askim, Sweden.

Ciba Vision, Switz. Ciba Vision AG, Freiburgstrasse 572, 3172 Niederwangen/BE, Switzerland.

Ciba Vision, UK. Ciba Vision Ophthalmics, Flanders Road, Hedge End, Southampton, Hampshire, SO3 3LG, UK.

Ciba Vision, USA. Ciba Vision Corporation, 2910 Amwiler Court, Atlanta, GA 30360, USA.

Ciba-Geigy, Aust. Ciba-Geigy GmbH, Breitenfurter Strasse 251, 1231 Vienna, Austria.

Ciba-Geigy, Austral. Ciba-Geigy Australia Ltd, P.O. Box 4, Wentworthville, NSW 2145, Australia.

Ciba-Geigy, Belg. See *Novartis, Belg.*

Ciba-Geigy, Fr. Laboratoires Ciba-Geigy, 2 et 4 rue Lionel-Terray, 92506 Rueil-Malmaison, France.

Ciba-Geigy, Ger. See *Ciba, Ger.*

Ciba-Geigy, Irl. See *Novartis, Irl.*

Ciba-Geigy, S.Afr. Ciba-Geigy (Pty) Ltd, P.O. Box 92, Isando 1600, S. Africa.

Ciba-Geigy, Spain. See *Novartis, Spain.*

Ciba-Geigy, Swed. Ciba-Geigy AB, Division Läkemedel, Box 605, 421 26 V Frolunda, Sweden.

Ciba-Geigy, Switz. Ciba-Geigy SA, Pharma Schweiz, Reinacherstrasse 115, Case postale, 4002 Basel, Switzerland.

Ciba-Geigy, USA. Ciba-Geigy Corporation, 556 Morris Ave, Summit, NJ 07901, USA.

Ciccarelli, Ital. Farmaceutici dott. Ciccarelli s.p.a., Via Clemente Prudenzio 13, 20138 Milan, Italy.

Cidan, Spain. Cidan, Ulldecona 69, Benicarlo, 12580 Castellon, Spain.

Cielle, Ital. Farma Cielle srl, Via Michele Amari 15, 90139 Palermo, Italy.

Cilag, Belg. Cilag S.A., Belgium.

Cilag, Ger. Cilag GmbH, Otto-Volger-Strasse 17, Postfach: 1229, 65838 Sulzbach/Taunus, Germany.

Cilag, Ital. Cilag Farmaceutici s.r.l., V. M. Buonarroti 23, 20093 Cologno Monzese (MI), Italy.

Cilag, Neth. Cilag S.A., Postbus 90240, 5000 LT Tilburg, Netherlands.

Cilag, Swed. See *Janssen-Cilag, Swed.*

Cilag, UK. Cilag Ltd, P.O. Box 79, Saunderton, High Wycombe, Bucks, HP14 4HJ, UK.

Cimex, Switz. Cimex AG, Chem. und pharmaz. Produkte, Birsweg 2, 4253 Liesberg 1, Switzerland.

Cinfa, Spain. Cinfa, Olaz-Chipi 10, Poligono Areta, Huarte-Pamplona, 31620 Navarra, Spain.

Cipharm, Fr. Laboratoires Cipharm, 69 rue Ampere, 75017 Paris, France.

Cipla-Medpro, S.Afr. Cipla-Medpro, S. Africa.

Circle, USA. Circle Pharmaceuticals Inc., 10377 Hague Rd, Indianapolis, IN 46256, USA.

CIS, Ital. CIS Diagnostici spa, Via E Mattei 1, 13049 Tronzano Vercellese (VC), Italy.

Citrosil, Ital. Citrosil Sanitas s.p.a., Via Antonio da Noli 4, 50127 Florence, Italy.

Clarben, Spain. Clarben, Vallermoso 28, 28015 Madrid, Spain.

Clariana, Spain. Clariana Pico, Ctra Cruz Negra 78, Carlet, 46240 Valencia, Spain.

Clarins, Canad. See *Lippens, Canad.*

Clement, Fr. Laboratoires Clément, La Boursidiere, B.P. 150, 92357 Le Plessis-Robinson cdx, France.

Clement Thionville, Fr. Laboratoires Clément-Thionville, 6 rue Joffre, B.P. 30028, 57101 Thionville Cedex, France.

Clements Stansen, Austral. Clements Stansen Medical, P.O. Box 110, North Ryde, NSW 2113, Australia.

Clin Midy, Fr. See *Sanofi Winthrop, Fr.*

Clinced, Aust. Clinced HandelsGmbH, Sandweg 8, 8071 Gossendorf, Austria.

CliniMed, UK. CliniMed Ltd, Cavell House, Knaves Beech Way, Loudwater, High Wycombe, Bucks, HP10 9QY, UK.

Clinique, Canad. See *Estee Lauder, Canad.*

Clintec, Canad. Clintec Nutrition Company, affiliated with Baxter Healthcare Corporation and Nestlé S.A., 6733 Mississauga Rd, Suite 502, Mississauga, Ontario, L5N 6J5, Canada.

Clintec, Fr. Clintec Nutrition Clinique (affiliation a Baxter Healthcare Corp. & Nestlé S.A.), 2 rue Troyon, 92316 Sevres cdx, France.

Clintec, Irl. See *Baxter, Irl.*

Clintec, Ital. Clintec s.r.l., Viale Tiziano 25, 00196 Rome, Italy.

Clintec, Spain. Clintec Nutricion, Parque Empresarial San Fernando, Edif. Londres, San Fernando de Henares, 28830 Madrid, Spain.

Clintec, UK. See *Baxter, UK,* and *Nestle, UK.*

Clintec, USA. Clintec Nutrition Company, affiliate of Baxter Healthcare Corp., 1425 Lake Cook Rd, LC11-03, Deerfield, IL 60015, USA.

Clintec-Sopharga, Fr. Clintec-Sopharga, Laboratoires Sopharga, 2 rue Troyon, 92316 Sevres Cdx, France.

Clonmel, Irl. Clonmel Healthcare Ltd, Waterford Rd, Clonmel, Co. Tipperary, Ireland.

COB, Belg. COB & Cie S.A., Ave Albert Giraud 115, 1030 Brussels, Belgium.

Cochon, Fr. Laboratoires Cochon-Tradiphar, ZI, ruche des 2 Lys, 59280 Armentieres, France.

Codali, Belg. Codali S.A., Avenue Henri Dunant 31, 1140 Brussels, Belgium.

Codit, Ital. Codit s.n.c. di Piccinini & C., Via Dronero 2, 10144 Turin, Italy.

Colgate Oral Care, Austral. Colgate Oral Care, 345 George St, Sydney, NSW 2000, Australia.

Colgate-Hoyt, USA. See *Colgate-Palmolive, USA.*

Colgate-Oral, USA. See *Colgate-Palmolive, USA.*

Colgate-Palmolive, Canad. Colgate Palmolive Canada, 99 Vanderhoof Ave, Toronto, Ontario, M4G 2H6, Canada.

Colgate-Palmolive, Ital. Colgate Palmolive spa, Via Giorgione 59/63, 00147 Rome, Italy.

Colgate-Palmolive, UK. Colgate-Palmolive Ltd, Guilford Business Park, Middleton Rd, Guildford, Surrey, GU2 5LZ, UK.

Colgate-Palmolive, USA. Colgate-Palmolive Co., 1 Colgate Way, Canton, MA 02021, USA.

Coli, Ital. Farmaceutici Coli s.r.l., Via Campobello 15, 00040 Pomezia (Rome), Italy.

Coll, Spain. Coll Farma, Napoles 166, 08013 Barcelona, Spain.

Collado, Spain. Collado, Varsovia 47-51, 08026 Barcelona, Spain.

Collagen, Aust. Collagen Vertrieb Biomedizinischer Produkte GmbH, Esslinger Hauptstrasse 81-7, 1228 Vienna, Austria.

Collagen, Austral. Collagen Biomedical Pty. Ltd, P.O. Box 1175, Auburn, NSW 2144, Australia.

Collagen, Fr. Collagen France, 113 rue Victor Hugo, 92300 Levallois-Perret, France.

Collagen, Ger. Collagen GmbH, Carl-Zeiss-Ring 7a, 85737 Ismaning, Germany.

Collagen, Ital. Collagen Research Center srl, Via Innocenzo XI 41, 00165 Rome, Italy.

Collins Elixir, UK. Collins Elixir Co., 2 Sprowston Rd, Norwich, Norfolk, NR3 4QN, UK.

Coloplast, Fr. Laboratoires Coloplast, 58 rue Roger-Salengro, Peripole 126, 94126 Fontenay-s-Bois Cedex, France.

Coloplast, Switz. Coloplast AG, Eurobusiness Center, Euro 1, Blegistrasse 1, 6343 Rotkreuz, Switzerland.

Coloplast, UK. Coloplast Ltd, Peterborough Business Park, Peterborough, PE2 0FX, UK.

Coloplast, USA. Coloplast, Plaza VII, Suite 3400, 45 South Seventh St, Minneapolis, Minnesota 55402, USA.

Columbia, S.Afr. Columbia Pharmaceuticals (Pty) Ltd, P.O. Box 7026, Bonaero Park 1622, S. Africa.

Columbia, USA. Columbia Laboratories Inc., 2665 South Bayshore Drive, Miami, FL 33133, USA.

Combe, Canad. See *Stuart House, Canad.*

Combe, Spain. Combe Europa, Orense 58, 28020 Madrid, Spain.

Combe, UK. Combe International Ltd, 17 Lansdowne Rd, Croydon, Surrey, CR9 2AU, UK.

Combe, USA. Combe Inc., 1101 Westchester Ave, White Plains, NY 10604, USA.

Combustin, Ger. Combustin Vertrieb Pharm. Präparate GmbH, Kolpingstr. 19, Postfach: 1242, 88382 Biberach an der Riss, Germany.

Commerce, USA. See *Del, USA.*

Compu, S.Afr. Compu, S. Africa.

Concord, UK. Concord Pharmaceuticals Ltd, 16 Leaden Close, Leaden Roding, Dunmow, Essex, CM6 1SD, UK.

Connaught, Canad. Connaught Laboratories Ltd, 1755 Steeles Ave West, North York, Ontario, M2R 3T4, Canada.

Connaught, Norw. See *Pasteur Merieux, Norw.*

Connaught, USA. Connaught Laboratories Inc., Swiftwater, PA 18370, USA.

Consol, Ital. Consol srl, Via Alessandro Brisse 27, 00149 Rome, Italy.

Consolidated Chemicals, Irl. See *Whelehan, Irl.*

Consolidated Chemicals, UK. Consolidated Chemicals Ltd, The Industrial Estate, Wrexham, Clwyd, LL13 9PS, UK.

Continental, Spain. Continental Farmaceutica, La Granja 30, Pol. Ind. Alcobendas, 28100 Madrid, Spain.

Continental, USA. Continental Consumer Products, Division of Continental Fragrances, 770 Forest Suite B, Birmingham, Michigan, MI 48009, USA.

Continental Ethicals, S.Afr. Continental Ethicals (Division of S.A. Druggists Ltd), P.O. Box 4493, Randburg 2125, S. Africa.

Continental Pharma, Belg. Continental Pharma Inc., Ave de Tervuren 270-2, Bte 24, 1150 Brussels, Belgium.

Continental Pharma, Switz. See *Vifor, Switz.*

Convatec, Austral. Convatec Australia, a Division of Bristol-Myers Squibb, 606 Hawthorn Road, East Brighton, Vic. 3187, Australia.

Convatec, Fr. Laboratoires Convatec, La Grande Arche Nord, 92044 Paris-La Defense, France.

Convatec, Irl. ConvaTec, Ireland.

Convatec, Ital. Convatec, Divisione della Bristol-Myers Squibb spa, Via Paolo di Dono 73, 00142 Rome, Italy.

Convatec, Switz. See *Bristol-Myers Squibb, Switz.*

ConvaTec, UK. See *Bristol-Myers Squibb, UK.*

Cook-Waite, USA. Cook-Waite Laboratories Inc., USA.

Coombe, Canad.

Coop. Farm., Ital. Cooperativa Farmaceutica Società Cooperativa a.r.l., Via Passione 8, 20122 Milan, Italy.

Cooperation Pharmaceutique, Fr. Cooperation Pharmaceutique Francaise, 77020 Melun cdx, France.

Coopervision, Canad. Coopervision Inc., 100 McPherson St, Markham, Ontario, L3R 3V6, Canada.

CooperVision, Irl. Cooper Vision (Ireland), Ireland.

Co-Pharma, UK. Co-Pharma Limited, Talbot House, 17 Church Street, Rickmansworth, Hertfordshire, WD3 1DE, UK.

Copley, USA. Copley Pharmaceutical Inc., 25 John Road, Canton, MA 02021, USA.

Cor Therapeutics, USA. Cor Therapeutics, USA.

Coradol, Ger. Coradol-Pharma GmbH, Eupener Strasse 159, 50933 Cologne, Germany.

corax, Ger. corax pharma GmbH, Lendersbergstr. 86, 53721 Siegburg, Germany.

Cortec, Swed. Cortec Medical AB, Torggatan 4, 211 40 Malmo, Sweden.

Cortecs, Irl. See *Cortecs, UK.*

Cortecs, UK. Cortecs International Ltd., The Old Blue School, Lower Square, Isleworth, Middlesex, TW7 6RL, UK.

Cortissone, Ital. Cortissone srl, Via Melzi d'Eril 29, 20154 Milan, Italy.

Cortunon, Canad. Cortunon Inc., Canada.

Corvi, Ital. Camillo Corvi s.p.a., Via R Lepetit 8, 20020 Lainate (MI), Italy.

Coryne de Bruynes, Mon. Laboratoires Coryne de Bruynes, 9 av Prince-Hereditaire-Albert, MC 98000 Monaco, Monaco.

Cos Farma, Ital. Cos Farma, Via di Portonaccio 23/B, 00159 Rome, Italy.

Cosmair, Canad. Cosmair Canada Inc., 4895 Hickmore, St-Laurent, Quebec, H4T 1K5, Canada.

Cosmetique Active, Switz. Cosmétique Active (Suisse) SA, Rietstrasse 14, 8108 Dallikon, Switzerland.

Couvreur, Belg. Couvreur Pharma S.A., Avenue de Schiphol 2, 1140 Brussels, Belgium.

Covan, S.Afr. Covan Pharmaceutical Products (Pty) Ltd, P.O. Box 155, Rosslyn 0200, S. Africa.

Coventry, UK. Coventry Chemicals Ltd, Woodhams Rd, Siskin Drive, Coventry, CV3 4FX, UK.

Cow & Gate, Irl. Cow & Gate Nutricia Ireland Ltd, 1B Sandyford Business Centre, Burton Hall Road, Dublin 18, Ireland.

Cow & Gate, UK. Cow & Gate Nutricia Ltd, White Horse Business Park, Trowbridge, Wilts, BA14 0XQ, UK.

Cox, Irl. See *Cox, UK.*

Cox, UK. A.H. Cox & Co. Ltd, Whiddon Valley, Barnstaple, Devon, EX32 8NS, UK.

CP Pharmaceuticals, Irl. See *Cahill May Roberts, Irl.*

CP Pharmaceuticals, UK. CP Pharmaceuticals Ltd, Red Willow Rd, Wrexham Industrial Estate, Wrexham, Clwyd, LL13 9PX, UK.

CP Protea, Austral. See *Protea, Austral.*

CPB, Belg. See *Rhone-Poulenc Rorer, Belg.*

CPF, Ger. C.P.F, Chemisch-pharmazeutische Fabrik GmbH, Heinrich-Bocking-Strasse 6-8, 66121 Saarbrucken, Germany.

Crawford, UK. Crawford Pharmaceuticals, 71a High St, Stony Stratford, Milton Keynes, MK11 1BA, UK.

Creapharm, Fr. Laboratoires Creapharm, France.

Creative Brands, Austral. Creative Brands Pty Ltd, P.O. Box 1435, Clayton South, Vic 3169, Australia.

Creighton, USA. Creighton Products Corp., 59 Route 10, East Hanover, NJ 07936-1080, USA.

Creme d'Orient, Fr. Laboratoires Crème d'Orient, 81 rue de l'Amiral-Roussin, 75015 Paris, France.

Cress, Canad. Cress Laboratories, P.O. Box 222, Kitchener, ON, N2G 3X9, Canada.

Crinex, Fr. Laboratoires Crinex, B.P. 337, 92541 Montrouge Cedex, France.

Crinos, Ital. Crinos Industria Farmacobiologica s.p.a., Piazza XX Settembre 2, 22079 Villaguardia (CO), Italy.

Cris Flower, Ital. Cris Flower International snc, Via Livorno 61, 00162 Rome, Italy.

Croce Bianca, Ital. Laboratorio Biochimico Croce Bianca s.r.l., Via Milano 141, 20021 Baranzate di Bollate (MI), Italy.

Croda, UK. Croda International PLC, Cowick Hall, Snaith, Goole, North Humberside, DN14 9AA, UK.

Croma, Aust. Croma-Pharma GmbH, Industriezeile 6, 2100 Leobendorf, Austria.

Crookes, Irl. See *Boots Healthcare, Irl.*

Crookes Healthcare, UK. Crookes Healthcare Ltd, P.O. Box 94, 1 Thane Rd West, Nottingham, NG2 3AA, UK.

Crookes Laboratories, UK. Crookes Laboratories Ltd, Thane Rd, Nottingham, NG2 3AA, UK.

Crosara, Ital. Laboratorio Farmaco Biologico Crosara s.p.a., Via Campobello 15, 00040 Pomezia (Rome), Italy.

Crown, S.Afr. Crown Laboratories Ltd, 767 Waterkloof Rd, Waterkloof, Pretoria 0181, Transvaal, S. Africa.

Cruz, Spain. Fernandez de la Cruz, Crta Sevilla Malaga Km 5.6, Alcala de Guadaira, 41500 Seville, Spain.

CS, Fr. Laboratoires CS Dermatologie, 35 rue d'Artois, 75008 Paris, France.

CSL, Austral. CSL Ltd, 45 Poplar Road, Parkville, Vic. 3052, Australia.

CSL-Novo, Austral. See *Novo Nordisk, Austral.*

CSP, Fr. CSP, ZI de la Barogne, B.P. 44, 77230 Moussy-le-Neuf, France.

CT, Ger. ct-Arzneimittel Chemische Tempelhof GmbH, Postfach: 420331, 12063 Berlin, Germany.

CT, Ital. C.T., Laboratorio Farmaceutico s.r.l., Via D. Alighieri 69-71, 18038 Sanremo (IM), Italy.

CTS Dental, UK. C.T.S. Dental Supplies, UK.

Cullen & Davison, UK. Cullen & Davison Ltd, 52 Lurgan Rd, Portadown, Craigavon, Co Armagh, BT63 5QG, UK.

Culver, Austral. Alberto Culver (Australia) Pty Ltd, P.O. Box 253, Parramatta, NSW 2150, Australia.

Cumberland, USA. Cumberland Packing Corp., 35 Old Ridgefield Rd, P.O. Box 7688, Willton, CT 06897, USA.

Cumino, Switz. Cumino GmbH, Switzerland.

Cupal, UK. See *Seton, UK.*

Cupharma, UK. Cupharma Ltd, Winkton House, Wynnswick Rd, Seer Green, Beaconsfield, Bucks, HP9 2XW, UK.

Cuprocept, S.Afr. Cuprocept SA, P.O. Box 400, New Germany 3620, S. Africa.

Curasan, Ger. curasan Pharma GmbH, Lindigstr. 4, 63801 Kleinostheim, Germany.

Cusi, Spain. Cusi, Ctra Nacional II, Km 632, El Masnou, 08320 Barcelona, Spain.

Cusi, UK. See *Dominion, UK.*

Cussons, UK. Cussons (UK) Ltd, Kersal Vale, Manchester, M7 0GL, UK.

Cutter, UK. Cutter Laboratories, Division of Miles Ltd, Stoke Court, Stoke Poges, Slough, SL2 4LY, UK.

Cutter, USA. Cutter Biological, Division of Miles Inc., 400 Morgan Lane, West Haven, CT 06516, USA.

Cuxson, Gerrard, UK. Cuxson, Gerrard & Co. (IMS) Ltd, Oldbury, Warley, West Midlands, B69 3BB, UK.

Cyanamid, Aust. Cyanamid GmbH, Tendlergasse 13, 1090 Vienna, Austria.

Cyanamid, Belg. Cyanamid Benelux S.A., Parc Scientifique, Rue du Bosquet 15, 1348 Louvain-la-Neuve, Belgium.

Cyanamid, Ital. Cyanamid Italia s.p.a., Zona Ind. Via F Gorgone, 95030 Catania, Italy.

Cyanamid, Spain. Cyanamid Iberica, Cristobal Bordiu 35, 28003 Madrid, Spain.

Cyanamid, Swed. Cyanamid Nordiska AB, Rissneleden 136, 172 48 Sundbyberg, Sweden.

Cyanamid, UK. Cyanamid of Great Britain Ltd, Fareham Rd, Gosport, Hants, PO13 0AS, UK.

Cyanamid, USA. American Cyanamid Co., P.O. Box 400, Princeton, NJ 08540, USA.

Cyclin, USA. Cyclin Pharmaceuticals Inc., 429 Gammon Place, Madison, WI 53715, USA.

Cypress, USA. Cypress Pharmaceutical, 135 Industrial Blvd, Madison, MS 39110, USA.

CytoChemia, Ger. CytoChemia Biologisch-Pharmazeutische Präparate GmbH, Burgerstock 7, 79241 Ihringen, Germany.

Cytogen, USA. Cytogen, 600 College Rd East, Princeton, NJ 08540, USA.

Cytosol Ophthalmics, USA. Cytosol Ophthalmics, 55 Messina Drive, Braintree, MA 02184, USA.

Czarniak, Austral. Czarniak Pharmaceuticals Pty Ltd, Australia.

DAB, Swed. DAB Dental AB, Box 423, 194 04 Upplands Vasby, Sweden.

Dagra, Neth. Dagra-Pharma B.V., Postbus 171, 1110 BC Diemen, Netherlands.

Daiichi, Jpn. Daiichi Pharmaceutical Co. Ltd, 16-13 Kita-Kasai 1-chome, Edogawa ku, Tokyo 134, Japan.

Daiichi, USA. Daiichi, USA.

Dainippon, Jpn. Dainippon Pharmaceutical Co. Ltd, 6-8 Doshomachi 2-chome, Chuo-ku, Osaka 541, Japan.

Daker Farmasimes, Spain. Daker Farmasimes, C/Trabajo S/N, Sant Just Desvern, 08960 Barcelona, Spain.

Dakota, Fr. Laboratoires Dakota Pharm, Europarc, 33 rue Auguste-Perret, 94042 Creteil Cdx, France.

Dakryon, USA. Dakryon Pharmaceuticals, 2579 S Loop, Suite 8, Lubbock, TX 79423-1400, USA.

Dallmann, Ger. Dallmann & Co., Fabrik chem.-pharm. Präparate, Zehntenhofstrasse 14-16, Postfach: 130307, 65091 Wiesbaden, Germany.

Dal-Med, USA. Dal-Med Pharmaceuticals Inc., USA.

Dal-Vita, Austral. Dal-Vita Products Pty Ltd, P.O. Box 477, Manly, NSW 2095, Australia.

Damor, Ital. Farmaceutici Damor s.p.a., Strada S.M. a Cubito 27, 80145 Naples, Italy.

Danbury, USA. Danbury Pharmacal Inc., 131 West St, P.O. Box 296, Danbury, CT 06810, USA.

Daniels, Canad. David D Daniels Ltd, P.O. Box 9, 62 Boychuk Rd, Elliot Lake, Ontario, P5A 2S9, Canada.

Daniels, Irl. See *Boileau & Boyd, Irl.*

Daniels, USA. Daniels Pharmaceuticals Inc., 2527 25th Avenue North, St Petersburg, FL 33713-3999, USA.

Dannorth, Canad. Dannorth Laboratories Inc., 225 Duncan Mill Rd, Ste 400, Toronto, On, M3B 3K9, Canada.

Danval, Spain. Danval, Avda de los Madronos 33, 28043 Madrid, Spain.

Darci, Belg. Darci Pharma S.A., Chaussee de Waterloo 935-7, 1180 Brussels, Belgium.

Darcy, Fr. Laboratoires Darcy, 3-5 rue Diderot, 92003 Nanterre, France.

Dartmouth, USA. Dartmouth Pharmaceuticals Inc., 37 Pine Hill Lane, Marion, MA 02738, USA.

Davidall Florence, Ital. Davidall Florence s.r.l., Italy.

Davigo, Belg. Davigo s.p.r.l., Rue de l'Ourchet 17, 1367 Bomal, Belgium.

Davis & Geck, UK. Davis & Geck, A division of Cyanamid of Great Britain Ltd, Fareham Rd, Gosport, Hants, PO13 0AS, UK.

Davis & Geck, USA. Davis & Geck, 1 Cyanamid Plaza, Wayne, NJ 07470, USA.

Day, Ital. Day Farma sas di Franco Tovecci & C, Via Alessandro Manzoni 227, 80123 Naples, Italy.

Dayton, USA. Dayton Laboratories Inc., 3307 NW 74 Ave, Miami, FL 33122, USA.

DB, Fr. Laboratoires DB Pharma, 1 bis, rue du cdt-Riviere, 94210 La Varenne-St-Hilaire, France.

DB, Switz. See *Uhlmann-Eyraud, Switz.*

DBL, Austral. David Bull Laboratories Pty Ltd, P.O. Box 394, Mulgrave North, Vic. 3170, Australia.

DCG, Swed. DCG Farmaceutiska AB, Box 2123, 421 02 Vastra Frolunda, Sweden.

DDC, UK. DDC (London) Ltd, 6 Clifton Gdns, London, W9 1DT, UK.

DDD, UK. DDD Ltd, 94 Rickmansworth Rd, Watford, Herts, WD1 7JJ, UK.

DDSA Pharmaceuticals, UK. DDSA Pharmaceuticals Ltd, 310 Old Brompton Rd, London, SW5 9JQ, UK.

De Angeli, Ital. Istituto De Angeli Ph s.p.a., Via Lorenzini 8, 20139 Milan, Italy.

De Witt, Irl. See *Mayrs, Irl.*

De Witt, UK. E.C. De Witt & Co. Ltd, Tudor Rd, Manor Park, Runcorn, Cheshire, WA7 1SZ, UK.

Debat, Fr. Laboratoires Debat, 153 rue de Buzenval, 92380 Garches, France.

Debat, Norw. See *Meda, Norw.*

Debat, Switz. See *Schwarz, Switz.*

Deca, Ital. Laboratorio Chimico Deca s.r.l., Via Balzaretti 17, 20133 Milan, Italy.

Declimed, Ger. Declimed Zweigniederlassung der Desitin Arzneimittel GmbH, Weg beim Jager 214, Postfach: 630109, 2000 Hamburg 63, Germany.

Deklerht, USA. Deklerht, USA.

Del, Canad. Del Pharmaceutics (Canada) Inc., 25 Morrow Rd, Barrie, ON, L4N 3V7, Canada.

Del, Switz. See *Para-Pharma, Switz.*

Del, USA. Del Pharmaceuticals Inc., 163 E Bethpage Rd, Plainview, NY 11803, USA.

Del Saz & Filippini, Ital. Farmaceutici Del Saz & Filippini s.r.l., Via Dei Pestagalli 7, 20138 Milan, Italy.

Delagrange, Belg. See *Synthelabo, Belg.*

Delagrange, Fr. Laboratoires Delagrange, Groupe Synthélabo (Lignage), 1 av Pierre-Brossolette, 91380 Chilly-Mazarin, France.

Delagrange, Neth. See *Pharmexport, Neth.*

Delagrange, Port. See *Infar, Port.*

Delagrange, Spain. See *Synthelabo Delagrange, Spain.*

Delagrange, Switz. Laboratories Delagrange (Schweiz) AG, Switzerland.

Delalande, Fr. Laboratoires Delalande, groupe Synthélabo (Carrion, Vaillant Defresne), France.

Delalande, Ger. See *Synthelabo, Ger.*

Delalande, Ital. Laboratori Delalande Isnardi s.p.a., Via XXV Aprile 69, 18100 Imperia, Italy.

Delalande, Switz. Lab. Delalande S.A., Switzerland.

Delamac, Austral. Delamac Pharmaceuticals Pty Ltd, P.O. Box 125, Spring Hill, Qld 4004, Australia.

Delandale, Irl. See *Lorex, Irl.*

Delandale, UK. Delandale Laboratories Ltd, Lunar House, Globe Park, Marlow, Bucks, SL7 1LW, UK.

Delmont, USA. Delmont Laboratories Inc., P.O. Box 269, Swarthmore, PA 19081, USA.

Del-Ray, USA. Del-Ray Laboratory Inc,, 22 20th Ave NW, Birmingham, AL 35215, USA.

Delta, Aust. Delta Arzneimittel, Gastebgasse 5-13, 1231 Vienna, Austria.

Delta, Austral. Delta West Pty Ltd, Technology Park, 15 Brodie Hall Drive, Bentley, WA 6102, Australia.

Delta, Ger. Delta-Pharma GmbH, Postfach: 7064, 72783 Pfullingen, Germany.

Delta BKB, Ital. Delta BKB s.n.c. di Benassati Emilio & C., V.le Emilio Po 224, 41100 Modena, Italy.

Delta Laboratories, Irl. Delta Laboratories Ltd, Ireland.

delta pronatura, Ger. delta pronatura Dr. Krauss & Dr. Beckmann GmbH & Co., Hans-Bockler-Str. 5, Postfach: 1255, 63232 Neu-Isenburg, Germany.

Demopharm, Switz. Demopharm AG, Werkstrasse 27, Postfach 363, 3250 Lyss, Switzerland.

Dendron, UK. See *DDD, UK.*

Dendy, Austral. Dendy Pharmaceuticals, 44 Cromer St, East Brighton, Vic. 3187, Australia.

Denolin, Belg. Denolin S.A., Rue des Goujons 152, 1070 Brussels, Belgium.

Dent, USA. C.S. Dent & Co. Division, The Grandpa Brands Co., 317 E. Eighth St, Cincinnati, Ohio, OH 45202, USA.

Dentaid, Spain. Dentaid, Parque Tecno del Valle, Ronda Can Fatjo 10, Cerdanyola, 08290 Barcelona, Spain.

Dental Health Products, UK. Dental Health Products Ltd, Pearl Assurance House, Mill St, Maidstone, Kent, ME15 6XH, UK.

Dental Warehouse, S.Afr. Dental Warehouse, S. Africa.

Dentalica, Ital. Dentalica s.p.a., Via Rimini 22, 20142 Milan, Italy.

Dentinox, Ger. Dentinox Gesellschaft für Pharmazeutische Präparate Lenk & Schuppan, Nunsdorfer Ring 19, Postfach: 480 369, 12253 Berlin, Germany.

Dentinox, Switz. See *Renapharm, Switz.*

Dentoria, Fr. Laboratoires Dentoria, 22 av Galilee, 92350 Le Plessis-Robinson, France.

Dentox, UK. Dentox Ltd, Hillmeadow, Lighthorne, Warwick, CV35 0AB, UK.

DEP, USA. DEP Corp., 2101 East Via Arado, Rancho Dominguez, CA 90220, USA.

DePuy, UK. DePuy Healthcare, Millshaw House, Manor Hill Lane, Leeds, LS11 8LQ, UK.

Derly, Spain. Derly, Avenida de la Industria 30, Alcobendas, 28100 Madrid, Spain.

Dermacare, Austral. Dermacare Pty Ltd, G.P.O. Box 2264, Sydney, NSW 2001, Australia.

Dermaide, USA. Dermaide Research Corp., P.O. Box 562, Palos Heights, IL 60463, USA.

Dermal Laboratories, Irl. See *Cahill May Roberts, Irl.*

Dermal Laboratories, UK. Dermal Laboratories Ltd, Tatmore Place, Gosmore, Hitchin, Herts, SG4 7QR, UK.

Dermalife, Ital. Dermalife s.p.a., Viale Tre Venezie 44-46, 35043 Monselice (PD), Italy.

Dermamend, UK. Dermamend, UK.

Dermapharm, Ger. Dermapharm GmbH Arzneimittel, Postfach: 1131, 82153 Grafelfing, Germany.

Dermatech, Austral. Dermatech Laboratories, Unit 12/6, Gladstone Rd, Castle Hill, NSW 2154, Australia.

Dermik, Canad. Dermik Laboratories Canada Inc., 6205 Airport Rd, Building B, Suite 100, Mississauga, Ontario, L4V 1E1, Canada.

Dermik, USA. Dermik Laboratories Inc., 500 Arcola Rd, P.O. Box 1200, Collegeville, PA 19426-0107, USA.

Dermofarma, Ital. Dermofarma Italia s.r.l., Via Beata Francesca 10, 83100 Avellino, Italy.

Dermol, USA. Dermol Pharmaceuticals Inc., 3807 Roswell Rd, Marietta, GA 30062, USA.

Dermon, Ital. Dermon s.p.a., Via Roma 165, 00040 Pomezia (Rome), Italy.

Dermophil Indien, Fr. Laboratoires du Dermophil Indien, B.P. 9, 61600 La Ferte-Mace, France.

Dermophil Indien, Switz. See *Uhlmann-Eyraud, Switz.*

Dermtek, Canad. Dermtek Pharmaceuticals Ltd, 1600 Trans Canada Highway, Dorval, Quebec, H9P 1H7, Canada.

Desarrollo, Spain. Desarrollo Farma y Cosmeticos, Pa de la Castellana 143, 28046 Madrid, Spain.

Desbergers, Canad. Desbergers Ltd, 8480 boul. Saint-Laurent, Montreal, Quebec, H2P 2M6, Canada.

Desitin, Ger. Desitin Arzneimittel GmbH, Weg beim Jager 214, Postfach: 63 01 64, 22311 Hamburg, Germany.

Desitin, Norw. Desitin Pharma AS, Niels Leuchsv. 99, 1343 Eiksmarka, Norway.

Desitin, Swed. Desitin Pharma AB, Box 2064, 431 02 Molndal, Sweden.

Desitin, Switz. See *Schwarz, Switz.*

Desopharmex, Switz. Desopharmex AG, Muttenzerstrasse 107, 4133 Pratteln 1, Switzerland.

Dessau, Ger. Pharma Dessau GmbH, Luxemburgstr. 8, 06846 Dessau, Germany.

Deverge, Ital. Devergè Medicina e Medicalizzazione s.r.l., C.so Casale 206, 10132 Turin, Italy.

Dexcel, UK. Dexcel Pharma Ltd, Bishop Crewe House, North St, Daventry, Northants, NN11 5PN, UK.

Dexo, Fr. Laboratoires Dexo, 31 rue d'Arras, 92000 Nanterre, France.

Dexo, Switz. See *Interlabo, Switz.*

Dexter, Spain. Dexter Farmaceutica, Avda Virgen de Montserrat 215, 08026 Barcelona, Spain.

Dey, USA. Dey Laboratories Inc., 10246 Miller Rd, Dallas, TX 75238, USA.

DHN, Fr. Lab. DHN, Division Nutrition Clinique, La Boisiniere, BP 16, 35530 Survon-sur-Vilaine, France.

DHU, Ger. Deutsche Homöopathie-Union, Ottostr. 24, Postfach: 410280, 76202 Karlsruhe, Germany.

Diabetylin, Ger. Diabetylingesellschaft Nachf. Apotheker Hans Meixner GmbH & Co., Ludwig-Merckle-Strasse 3, 89143 Blaubeuren, Germany.

Diaco, Ital. Laboratori Diaco Biomedicali spa, Via Flavia 124, 34147 Trieste, Italy.

Diadin, Ger. Diadin-Gesellschaft Chemisches Laboratorium GmbH, Ludwig Merckle-Str. 3, 89143 Blaubeuren, Germany.

Diafarm, Spain. Diafarm, Bernat de Rocaberti 17, Sabadell, 08205 Barcelona, Spain.

Dial, USA. The Dial Corp., 15101 North Scottsdale Rd, Scottsdale, AZ 85254-2199, USA.

Diamant, Fr. Laboratoires Diamant, 1 terrasse Bellini, 92800 Puteaux, France.

Dibropharm, Ger. Dibropharm, Postfach: 110, 76481 Baden-Baden, Germany.

Dicamed, Swed. Dicamed AB, Djupdalsvagen 24, 192 51 Sollentuna, Sweden.

Dickinson, USA. E.E. Dickinson Co., 2 Enterprise Drive, Shelton, Connecticut, CT 06484, USA.

Dicofarm, Ital. Dicofarm s.p.a., Via F. Saverio Nitti 11/15, 00191 Rome, Italy.

Dieckmann, Ger. Dieckmann Arzneimittel GmbH (MSD-Gruppe), Lindenplatz 1, Postfach: 1202, 85530 Haar, Germany.

Diedenhofen, Ger. Diedenhofen GmbH, Otto-von-Guericke-Strasse 1, Postfach: 1252, 53730 St Augustin/Bonn, Germany.

Diele, Fr. Diele Distripharma, 18 av Albert-Einstein, 93152 Le Blanc-Mesnil Cdx, France.

Diepal, Fr. Diépal-NSA, B.P. 432, 69654 Villefranche-sur-Saone Cedex, France.

Diepha, Fr. Laboratoires Diepha, 26 rue de l'Industrie, 92400 Corbevoie, France.

Dietavigor, Ital. Dietavigor s.r.l., Viale Certosa 40, 20155 Milan, Italy.

Dieterba, Ital. Dieterba, Via Migliara 45, 04100 Latina, Italy.

Dietetique et Sante, Fr. Laboratoires Diététique et Santé, groupe Sandoz, B.P. 106, 31250 Revel, France.

Diethelm, Switz. Diethelm & Co. SA, Case postale, 8052 Zurich, Switzerland.

Difa, Ital. Difa-Cooper s.p.a., Via Milano 160, 21042 Caronno Pertusella (VA), Italy.

Difer, Ital. Difer Industrie Farmaceutiche Triestine s.r.l., Via della Zonta 2, 34122 Trieste, Italy.

Diftersa, Spain. Diftersa, San Juan 20, Manlleu, 08560 Barcelona, Spain.

Dignos, Ger. Dignos-Chemie GmbH, Zielstattstrasse 21, Postfach: 70 04 60, 81304 Munich, Germany.

Dimportex, Spain. Dimportex, Deba Bahi 67, 08026 Barcelona, Spain.

Diophar, Fr. Diophar, ZAC des Cerisiers, 69380 Lozanne, France.

Dioptic, Canad. Dioptic Laboratories, Division of Akorn Pharmaceuticals Canada Ltd, 144 Steelcase Rd W, Markham, Ontario, L3R 3J9, Canada.

Disperga, Aust. Dr C Szalagyl Disperga GmbH, Josefstadter Strasse 43, 1080 Vienna, Austria.

Dispersa, Ger. See *Ciba Vision, Ger.*

Dispersa, Switz. Dispersa SA, Case postale, 8442 Hettlingen, Switzerland.

Dissolvurol, Mon. Laboratoires Dissolvurol, Le Minerve, av. Crovetto, B.P. 332 Monte-Carlo, 98006 Monaco Cdx, Monaco.

Dista, Austral. See *Lilly, Austral.*

Dista, Belg. See *Lilly, Belg.*

Dista, Irl. See *Lilly, Irl.*

Dista, Neth. See *Lilly, Neth.*

Dista, S.Afr. See *Lilly, S.Afr.*

Dista, Spain. Dista, Avenida de la Industria 30, Alcobendas, 28100 Madrid, Spain.

Dista, Switz. See *Schweiz. Serum & Impfinstitut, Switz.*

Dista, UK. Dista Products Ltd, Kingsclere Rd, Basingstoke, Hants, RG21 2XA, UK.

Dista, USA. Dista Products Company, Division of Eli Lilly & Co., Lilly Corporate Center, Indianapolis, IN 46285, USA.

Distri B3, Fr. Laboratoires Distri B3, 3 rue Bugeaud, 13003 Marseille, France.

Distriborg, Fr. Distriborg, 217 chem. du Grand-Revoyet, 69561 St-Genis-Laval, France.

Distriphar, UK. Distriphar, Broadwater Park, Denham, Uxbridge, Middx, UB9 5HP, UK.

Divapharma, Ger. Divapharma-Knufinke Arzneimittel-werk GmbH, 12274 Berlin, Germany.

Divinal, Ger. Divinal Arzneimittel GmbH, Rathausplatz 5, Postfach: 2108, 83423 Bad Reichenhall, Germany.

Diviser Aquilea, Spain. Diviser Aquilea, Pedro IV 84, 08005 Barcelona, Spain.

Divpharm, S.Afr. Divpharm, S. Africa.

Dixon-Shane, USA. Dixon-Shane Inc., 256 Geiger Rd, Philadelphia, PA 19115, USA.

DMG, Ger. DMG Chemisch-Pharmazeutische Fabrik GmbH, Postfach: 530104, 22531 Hamburg, Germany.

DMG, Ital. DMG Italia srl, Via Portoferraio 18, 00182 Rome, Italy.

Doak, USA. Doak Dermatologics, 383 Route 46 West, Fairfield, NJ 07004-2402, USA.

Docmed, S.Afr. Docmed, S. Africa.

Doerenkamp, Ger. Doerenkamp GmbH, Gereonsmuhlengasse 3, 50670 Cologne, Germany.

Doerr, Ger. Dr. Doerr-Pharma GmbH & Co. KG, Wurzburger Str 9, Postfach: 270102, 01171 Dresden, Germany.

Doetsch, Grether, Switz. Doetsch, Grether AG, 4002 Basel, Switzerland.

Dojin Iyaku, Jpn. Dojin Iyaku, 5-2-2 Yayoicho, Nakano-ku, Tokyo, Japan.

Dolisos, Canad. Dolisos, 1400 Hocquart, St-Bruno, QC, J3V 6E1, Canada.

Dolisos, Fr. Laboratoires Dolisos, 71 rue Beaubourg, 75003 Paris, France.

Dolisos, Ital. Dolisos Italia s.r.l., Laboratoires de Pharmacologie Homeopathique, Via Carlo Poma s.n.c., 00040 Pomezia (Rome), Italy.

Dolorgiet, Ger. Dolorgiet GmbH & Co. KG, Otto-von-Guericke-Str. 1, Postfach: 1252, 53730 St. Augustin/Bonn, Germany.

Dolorgiet, Switz. See *Mundipharma, Switz.*

Dome, Switz. See *Diethelm, Switz.*

Dome-Hollister-Stier, Fr. See *Bayer, Fr.*

Domenech Garcia, Spain. Domenech Garcia, San Martin 88, Cerdanyola del Valles, 08290 Barcelona, Spain.

Dominion, Irl. See *Dominion, UK.*

Dominion, UK. Dominion Pharma Ltd, Dominion House, Lion Lane, Haslemere, Surrey, GU27 1JL, UK.

Dompe, Ital. Dompè Farmaceutici s.p.a., Via San Martino 12, 20122 Milan, Italy.

Dompe Biotec, Ital. Dompè Biotec s.p.a., Via Santa Lucia 4, 20122 Milan, Italy.

Doms, Switz. See *Actipharm, Switz.*

Doms-Adrian, Fr. Laboratoires Doms-Adrian, 4 rue Ficatier, 92400 Courbevoie, France.

Don Baxter, Ital. Laboratori Don Baxter s.p.a., Via Flavia 124, 34147 Trieste, Italy.

Donau, Aust. Donau-Pharmazie-Cehasol GmbH, Industriegasse 7, 1230 Vienna, Austria.

Donell DerMedex, USA. Donell DerMedex, 342 Madison Ave, Suite 1422, New York, NY 10173, USA.

Donini, Ital. Donini s.r.l., Via Ecce Homo 18, 37054 Nogara (VR), Italy.

Donmed, S.Afr. Donmed Pharmaceuticals, S. Africa.

Dormer, Canad. Dormer Laboratories Inc., 91 Kelfield St, Unit 5, Rexdale, Ontario, M9W 5A3, Canada.

Dorom, Ital. Dorom s.r.l., Piazza Agrippa 1, 20141 Milan, Italy.

Dorsch, Ger. Dorsch GmbH, Lochhamer Schlag 10, Postfach: 1131, 82153 Grafelfing, Germany.

Doskar, Aust. Doskar Mag. Martin Pharm. Produkte, Schottenring 14, 1010 Vienna, Austria.

Douglas, Austral. Douglas Pharmaceuticals Aust. Ltd, 4 Packard Avenue, Castle Hill, NSW 2154, Australia.

Dow, Canad. See *Marion Merrell Dow, Canad.*

Dow, USA. See *Marion Merrell Dow, USA.*

Dow Corning, UK. Dow Corning Ltd, Kings Court, 185 Kings Rd, Reading, Berks, RG1 4EX, UK.

Dox-Al, Ital. Dox-Al s.p.a., Via E Fermi 2, 20050 Correzzana (MI), Italy.

DP-Medica, Switz. DP-Medica SA Pharmazeutische Produkte, Case postale 238, Fribourg, Switzerland.

DPT, USA. DPT, USA.

Dr Janssen, Ger. Dr. Werner Janssen Nachf. Chem.-pharm. Produkte GmbH, Grenzstrasse 2, Postfach: 1160, 53333 Meckenheim, Germany.

Dr. Nordyke's, USA. Dr. Nordyke's Laboratory, 1650 Palma Drive, Suite 102, Ventura, California, CA 93003, USA.

Draco, Swed. Draco Läkemedel AB, Box 2, 221 00 Lund, Sweden.

Draxis, Canad. Draxis Health Inc., 6870 Goreway Dr, Mississauga, Ontario, L4V 1P1, Canada.

Dreluso, Ger. Dreluso Pharmazeutika, Dr Elten & Sohn GmbH, Marktplatz 5, Postfach: 140, 31833 Hessisch Oldendorf, Germany.

drepharm, Ger. drepharm GmbH Laage, Bahnhofstrasse 13, Postfach: 39, 18293 Laage, Germany.

Dresden, Ger. Arzneimittelwerk Dresden GmbH, Meissner Strasse 35, Postfach: 010131/010132, 01435 Radebeul, Germany.

Dreveny, Aust. Dr. Dreveny, Mag. pharm. & Co. OHG, Herrandgasse 7, 8010 Graz, Austria.

Drogenhansa, Aust. Drogenhansa, Drogerie und Reformwaren GmbH, Michelbeuerngasse 9 A, 1090 Vienna, Asutria.

Dronania, Ger. Dronania Naturheilmittel GmbH, Karl-Benz-Strasse 3, Postfach: 1244, 8939 Bad Worishofen, Germany.

Drossapharm, Switz. Drossapharm SA, Drosselstrasse 47, 4059 Basel, Switzerland.

Drug Houses Austral., Austral. Drug Houses of Australia Pty Ltd, Australia.

Drug Research, Ital. D.R. Drug Research s.r.l., Via Podgora 9, 20122 Milan, Italy.

Drug Trading, Canad. Drug Trading Co. Ltd, 795 Pharmacy Ave, Scarborough, Ontario, M1L 3K2, Canada.

Du Pont, Aust. See *Du Pont, Belg.*

Du Pont, Belg. See *Therabel Pharma, Belg.*

Du Pont, Canad. Du Pont Pharma, Suite 180, 2655 North Sheridan Way, Mississauga, Ontario, L5K 2P8, Canada.

Du Pont, Fr. Du Pont Pharma S.A., 137 rue de l'Universite, 75007 Paris, France.

Du Pont, Ger. Du Pont Pharma GmbH, 61352 Bad Homburg v.d.H., Germany.

Du Pont, Irl. See *United Drug, Irl.*

Du Pont, Ital. Du Pont Pharma Italia s.r.l., Via de Conti 2A, 50123 Florence, Italy.

Du Pont, Norw. See *Meda, Norw.*

Du Pont, Spain. Du Pont Pharma, Albacete 5, 1 Planta, 28027 Madrid, Spain.

Du Pont, Swed. See *Meda, Swed.*

Du Pont, Switz. See *Opopharma, Switz.*

Du Pont, USA. du Pont Pharmaceuticals, E.I. du Pont de Nemours & Co. Inc., Wilmington, DE 19898, USA.

Du Pont Pharmaceuticals, UK. Du Pont Pharmaceuticals Ltd, Wedgwood Way, Stevenage, Herts, SG1 4QN, UK.

Duchesnay, Canad. Duchesnay Inc., 2925 boul. Industriel, Chomedey-Laval, Quebec, H7L 3W9, Canada.
Ducray, Fr. Laboratoires Ducray, Pierre Fabre Cosmétique, 45 place Abel-Gance, 92654 Boulogne, France.
Dukron, Ital. Dukron Italiana s.r.l., 04010 Campoverde (LT), Italy.
Dumex, Ger. Dumex GmbH, Larchenstrasse 12, 61118 Bad Vilbel, Germany.
Dumex, Irl. See *Allphar, Irl.*
Dumex, Neth. Dumex B.V., Bothalaan 2, 1217 JP Hilversum, Netherlands.
Dumex, Norw. See *Alpharma, Norw.*
Dumex, Switz. Dumex AG, Baarerstrasse 10, 6300 Zug, Switzerland.
Dumex, UK. Dumex Ltd, Longwick Rd, Princes Risborough, Aylesbury, Bucks, HP17 9UZ, UK.
Dumex-Alpharma, Swed. Dumex Alpharma AB, Nordenflychtsvagen 74, 112 89 Stockholm, Sweden.
Duncan, Ital. Duncan Farmaceutici s.p.a., Via A. Fleming 2, 37100 Verona, Italy.
Duncan, Spain. See *Glaxo Wellcome, Spain.*
Duncan, Flockhart, Austral. See *Glaxo Wellcome, Austral.*
Duncan, Flockhart, Irl. See *Glaxo Wellcome, Irl.*
Dunhall, USA. Dunhall Pharmaceuticals Inc., Highway 59N, P.O. Box 100, Gravette, AR 72736, USA.
Duopharm, Ger. Duopharm GmbH, Grassingerstr. 9, 83043 Bad Aibling, Germany.
Duphar, Ger. See *Solvay, Ger.*
Duphar, Irl. See *Solvay, Irl.*
Duphar, Neth. See *Solvay, Neth.*
Duphar, Spain. Duphar, Avda Diagonal 507-9, 08029 Barcelona, Spain.
Duphar, UK. See *Solvay, UK.*
Dura, USA. Dura Pharmaceuticals, 5880 Pacific Center Blvd, San Diego, CA 92121, USA.
Durachemie, Ger. durachemie GmbH & Co. KG, Schleebruggenkamp 15, Postfach: 8808, 48136 Munster, Germany.
Duramed, USA. Duramed Pharmaceuticals, 5040 Lester Rd, Cincinnati, OH 45213, USA.
Durban, Spain. Durban, Santos Zarate 20, 04004 Almeria, Spain.
Durbin, UK. Durbin B.S. Ltd, 240 Northolt Rd, South Harrow, Middx, HA2 8DU, UK.
Dyckerhoff, Ger. Laboratorium Prof. Dr. H. Dyckerhoff GmbH & Co., Robert-Perthel-Strasse 49, 50739 Cologne (Longerich), Germany.
Dynacren, Ital. Dynacren Laboratorio Farmaceutico del Dott. A. Francioni e di M. Gerosa s.r.l., Via P Nenni 12, 28053 Castelletto Ticino (NO), Italy.
Dynamed, S.Afr. Dynamed, S. Africa.
Dynamit, Aust. Dynamit Nobel Wien GmbH, 8813 St Lamprecht, Austria.
Dynapharm, USA. Dynapharm Inc., P.O. Box 2141, Del Mar, CA 92014, USA.
Dynathera, Fr. See *Labodynathera, Fr.*
E. Merck, Irl. See *Lipha, Irl.*
E. Merck, Neth. E. Merck Nederland B.V., Postbus 8198, 1005 AD Amsterdam, Netherlands.
E. Merck, Norw. See *Meda, Norw.*
E. Merck, Swed. See *Meda, Swed.*
E. Merck, Switz. E. Merck (Schweiz) AG, Ruchligstrasse 20, 8953 Dietikon, Switzerland.
E. Merck, UK. E. Merck Pharmaceuticals, division of Merck Ltd, Winchester Road, Four Marks, Alton, Hants, GU34 5HG, UK.
Eagle, Austral. Eagle Pharmaceuticals Pty Ltd, 6/15 Carrington Rd, Castle Hill, NSW 2154, Australia.
Eastern Pharmaceuticals, UK. Eastern Pharmaceuticals Ltd, Coomb House, St. John's Rd, Isleworth, Middlesex, TW7 6NA, UK.
Eberth, Ger. Dr. Friedrich Eberth Nachf., Kick-Rasel-Strasse 23/25, Postfach: 8, 92250 Schnaittenbach, Germany.
Eberth, Switz. See *Uhlmann-Eyraud, Switz.*
Ebewe, Aust. Ebewe Arzneimittel GmbH, 4866 Unterach am Attersee, Austria.
Ebi, Switz. Ebi-Pharm AG, Lindachstrasse 8c, 3038 Kirchlindach, Switzerland.
Echo, Ital. Echo s.r.l., Via della Mattonaia 15, 50121 Florence, Italy.
Ecobi, Ital. Farmaceutici Ecobi s.a.s., Via E. Bazzano 26, 16019 Ronco Scrivia (GE), Italy.
Econo Med, USA. Econo Med Pharmaceuticals Inc., P.O. Box 3303, Burlington, NC 27215, USA.
Ecosol, Switz. Ecosol AG, Postfach 7332, 8032 Zurich, Switzerland.
ECR, Switz. ECR Pharma AG, Bosch 104, 6331 Hunenberg/ZG, Switzerland.
ECR, USA. ECR Pharmaceuticals, Division of Claiborne Robins Co., Inc., P.O. Box 71600, Richmond, VA 23255, USA.
Ecupharma, Ital. Ecupharma s.r.l., Via Mazzini 20, 20123 Milan, Italy.
Edmond Pharma, Ital. Edmond Pharma s.r.l., Via dei Giovi 131, 20037 Paderno Dugnano (MI), Italy.
Edwards, USA. Edwards Pharmacal Inc., P.O. Drawer 129, Osceola, AR 72370-9990, USA.
Efamed, S.Afr. Efamed (Pty) Ltd, S. Africa.
Efamol, Canad. Efamol Research Inc., Annapolis Valley Industrial Park, P.O. Box 818, Unit 2, Chipman Drive, Kentville, Nova Scotia, B4N 4H8, Canada.
Efamol, UK. Efamol Ltd, Units 26-9, Surrey Technology Centre, The Research Park, Guildford, Surrey, GU2 5YH, UK.
Efarmes, Spain. Efarmes, Pasaje de las Torres 11, 08025 Barcelona, Spain.
EF-EM-ES, Aust. Ef-EM-ES - Dr Smetana & Co., Scheidlstrasse 28, 1180 Vienna, Austria.
Effcon, USA. Effcon Laboratories Inc., 1800 Sandy Plains Pkwy, Marietta, Georgia, GA 30066, USA.
Effik, Fr. Laboratoires Effik, Burospace 7, rte de Gisy, 91571 Bievres cdx, France.
Effik, Spain. Effik, Avda de Burgos 91, 28050 Madrid, Spain.
EGIS, Hung. EGIS Pharmaceuticals, P.O. Box 100, 1475 Budapest, Hungary.
Ego, Austral. Ego Pharmaceuticals Pty Ltd, 21-31 Malcolm Rd, Braeside, Vic. 3195, Australia.
EGS, Ger. EGS Pharma Vertrieb, Schulstr. 38, 19125 Chemnitz, Germany.
Ehrenhofer, Aust. Dr. F. Ehrenhöfer GmbH, Triester Strasse 36, 2620 Neunkirchen, Austria.
Ehrmann, Aust. Ehrmann Apotheker Mag. pharm. Liselotte GmbH, Obertrumer Landstr. 7, 5201 Seekirchen, Austria.
Eifelfango, Ger. Eifelfango GmbH & Co. KG chem.-pharm. Werke, Ringener Strasse 45, Postfach: 100365, 53441 Bad Neuenahr-Ahrweiler, Germany.
Eifelfango, Switz. See *Agpharm, Switz.*
Eisai, Jpn. Eisai Co. Ltd, 5-5-5 Koishikawa, Bunkyo-ku, Tokyo 112-88, Japan.
Eisai, UK. Eisai Ltd, Hammersmith International Ctr, 3 Shortlands, 2nd Floor, London, W6 8EE, UK.
Eladon, UK. Eladon Ltd, 63 High St, Bangor, Gwynedd, LL57 1NT, UK.
Elan, Irl. See *Knoll, Irl.*
Elan, UK. Elan Pharma, Lambert Court, Chestnut Ave, Eastleigh, Hants, SO5 3ZQ, UK.
Elan, USA. Elan Corp., 1300 Gould Dr, Gainesville, GA 30504, USA.
Elder, Neth. See *ICN, Neth.*
Elder, UK. Don Elder Products Ltd, Unit 15, Chiltonian Industrial Estate, 203 Manor Lane, London, SE12 0TX, UK.
Electramed, Irl. Electramed Ireland Ltd, 2 Kinsealy Business Park, Malahide Rd, Co. Dublin, Ireland.
Electrolactil, Spain. Electrolactil, Ciscar 26, 46005 Valencia, Spain.
Elerte, Fr. Laboratoires des Réalisations Thérapeutiques Elerté, 181-3 rue Andre-Karman, B.P. 101, 93303 Aubervilliers Cedex, France.
Elexsam, Austral. Elexsam International, 5 Berowra Waters Road, Berowra, NSW 2081, Australia.
Elfar, Spain. Elfar Drag, Guzman el Bueno, 133 Edif Britannia, 28942 Madrid, Spain.
Eliovit, Ital. Laboratori Eliovit s.a.s., Via Marsala 31/C, 25100 Brescia, Italy.
Elkins-Sinn, USA. Elkins-Sinn Inc., A subsidiary of A.H. Robins Co., 2 Esterbrook Lane, Cherry Hill, NJ 08003-4099, USA.
Ellem, Ital. See *Pierre Fabre, Ital.*
Elmu, Spain. See *Byk Leo, Spain.*
Emonta, Aust. Emonta Arznei- u. Körperpflegemittel GmbH, 6522 Prutz 36, Austria.
Enapharm, Swed. Enapharm AB, Box 30, 745 21 Enkoping, Sweden.
Endo, Canad. See *Du Pont, Canad.*
Engelhard, Ger. Karl Engelhard, Fabrik pharm. Präparate GmbH & Co. KG, Sandweg 94, Postfach: 100824, 60008 Frankfurt, Germany.
Engelhard, Switz. See *Pharmakos, Switz.*
Engelshof, Aust. Engelshof-Apotheke, Leystrasse 19-21, 1200 Vienna, Austria.
English Grains, UK. English Grains Ltd, Swains Park Industrial Estate, Park Rd, Overseal, Burton-on-Trent, Staffs, UK.
Enviroderm, USA. Enviroderm, USA.
Enzon, USA. Enzon, Inc., 40 Kingsbridge Rd, Piscataway, NJ 08854, USA.
Enzypharm, Aust. Enzypharm GmbH, Piaristengasse 29, 1080 Vienna, Austria.
Enzypharm, Neth. Enzypharm B.V., Amersfoortsestraat 65, 3769 AE Soesterberg, Netherlands.
Eon, USA. Eon Labs Manufacturing Inc., 227-15 North Conduit Ave, Laurelton, NY 11413, USA.
Epifarma, Ital. Epifarma s.a.s., Via San Rocco 6, 85033 Episcopia (Pz), Italy.
Epipharm, Aust. Epipharm GmbH, Herrenstrasse 2, 4020 Linz, Austria.
Erco, Norw. See *Orion, Norw.*
Erco pharm, Swed. See *Orion, Swed.*
Ercopharm, Aust. See *Ercopharm, Denm.*
Ercopharm, Denm. Ercopharm A/S, Boegeskovvej 9, 3490 Kvistgaard, Denmark.
Ercopharm, Neth. See *Multipharma, Neth.*
Ercopharm, Switz. See *Orion, Switz.*
Ern, Spain. Ern, Pedro IV 499, 08020 Barcelona, Spain.
Ernest Jackson, UK. Ernest Jackson & Co. Ltd, Crediton, Devon, EX17 3AP, UK.
Erredici, Ital. Erredici, Italy.
Errekappa, Ital. Errekappa Euroterapici s.p.a., Via C. Menotti 1/A, 20129 Milan, Italy.
Escaned, Spain. Escaned, Tomas Breton 46, 28045 Madrid, Spain.
ESI, USA. ESI Pharma, PO Box 41502, Philadelphia, PA 19101, USA.
Esoform, Ital. Esoform s.r.l., Viale del Lavoro 10, 45100 Rovigo, Italy.
Esparma, Ger. esparma pharmazeutische Fabrik GmbH, Lutherstr. 1-2, Postfach 1461, 39045 Magdeburg, Germany.
Espe, Aust. Espe HandelsGmbH, Marokkanergasse 9/8, 1030 Vienna, Austria.
Espe, Ger. ESPE Dental-Medezin GmbH & Co. KG, Griesberg 2, 82229 Seefeld, Germany.
Espe, Switz. Espe AG, Baumackerstrasse 46, Postfach 8360, 8050 Zurich, Switzerland.
Esplanade, Aust. Esplanade-Apotheke, Esplanade 18, 4820 Bad Ischl, Austria.
Esplanade, Fr. Pharmaceutique de l'Esplanade, 34 route d'Ecully, BP 94, 69573 Dardilly Cdx, France.
Esseti, Ital. Esseti Farmaceutici s.p.a., Via Cavalli di Bronzo 41, 80046 S. Giorgio a Cremano (NA), Italy.
Essex, Ger. Essex Pharma GmbH, Thomas-Dehler-Strasse 27, Postfach: 830347, 81703 Munich, Germany.
Essex, Ital. Essex Italia SpA, Via Serio 1, 20141 Milan, Italy.
Essex, Spain. See *Schering-Plough, Spain.*
Essex, Switz. Essex Chemie AG, Case postale 2769, 6002 Luzern, Switzerland.
Essilor, Aust. Essilor-Swarovski GmbH, Hasengasse 56, 1100 Vienna, Austria.
Estedi, Spain. Estedi, Montseny 41, 08012 Barcelona, Spain.
Estee Lauder, Canad. Estee Lauder Cosmetics Ltd, 161 Commander Blvd, Agincourt, Ontario, M1S 3K9, Canada.
Esteve, Spain. Esteve, Avda Virgen Montserrat 221, 08041 Barcelona, Spain.
Etajesa, Fr. Etajesa, 14 av. Edouard-Vaillant, 93698 Pantin Cedex, France.
Etapharm, Aust. Etapharm GmbH, Vormosergasse 3, 1190 Vienna, Austria.
Ethex, USA. Ethex Corporation, 10888 Metro Court, St Louis, Missouri, MO 63043-2413, USA.
Ethical Generics, UK. Ethical Generics Ltd, West Point, 46-8 West St, Newbury, Berks, RG14 1BD, UK.
Ethical Research, Irl. See *Ethical Research, UK.*
Ethical Research, UK. Ethical Research Marketing, 3A Landgate, Rye, East Sussex, TN31 7LH, UK.
Ethicare, Austral. Ethicare Pharmaceuticals Pty Ltd, 259 Walcott St, Mount Lawley, WA 6050, Australia.
Ethicon, Ger. Ethicon GmbH & Co. KG, Robert-Koch-Strasse 1, 22851 Norderstedt, Germany.
Ethicon, Ital. Ethicon s.p.a., 00040 Pratica di Mare Pomezia (Rome), Italy.
Ethimed, S.Afr. See *Noristan, S.Afr.*
Ethipharm, Canad. Ethipharm International, 2 boul. Crepeau, St-Laurent, Quebec, H4N 1M7, Canada.
Ethitek, USA. Ethitek Pharmaceuticals Co., 7701 North Austin, Skokie, IL 60077, USA.
Ethypharm, Ital. Ethypharm srl, Viale Monza 196, 20128 Milan, Italy.
Etris, Fr. Etris, 14 rue de la Comète, 75007 Paris, France.
Eu Rho, Ger. Eu.Rho. Pharma, Sudfeld 1a, 59174 Kamen, Germany.
Eugal, Ital. Laboratorio Chimico Farmaceutico Eugal s.r.l., Via Fabbriche 18, 15069 Serravalle Scrivia (AL), Italy.
Eulactol, S.Afr. Eulactol (Pty) Ltd, P.O. Box 3265, Randburg 2125, S. Africa.
Eumedica, Belg. Eumedica, Belgium.
Eumedica, Switz. Eumedica, Switzerland.
Eumedis, Belg. See *Bio-Therabel, Belg.*
Eumedis, Fr. Laboratoires Eumédis, 22 rue Rennequin, 75017 Paris, France.
Eurim, Ger. Eurim-Pharm GmbH, Ganselehen 4-5, 83451 Piding, Germany.
Eurocetus, UK. See *Chiron, UK.*
Eurochimica, Ital. Eurochimica, Via F.P. Volpe 37, 84100 Salerno, Italy.
Euroderm, Ital. Euroderm, Via Laurentina Km 28 800, 00040 Ardea (RM), Italy.
Euroderma, UK. Euroderma Ltd, The Old Coach House, 34 Elm Rd, Chessington, Surrey, KT9 1AW, UK.
Eurodrug, Aust. Eurodrug GmbH, Hoesselgasse 20, Postfach 43, 9802 Spittal/Drau, Austria.
Euroexim, Spain. Euroexim, C/Emilio Munoz 15, 28037 Madrid, Spain.
Eurofarmaco, Ital. Eurofarmaco s.r.l., Via Aurelia 58, 00166 Rome, Italy.
Euromed, Ital. Euromed s.r.l., Via Napoli 101, Pianura, 80126 Naples, Italy.
Euromedex, Fr. Lab. Euromedex, 24 rue des Tuileries, ZI, BP 80, 67460 Souffel-weyersheim, France.
Europharm, Aust. Europharm, Jochen-Rindt-Strasse 23, 1230 Vienna, Austria.
Europharm, S.Afr. See *Luitpold, S.Afr.*
Europharma, Spain. Europharma, Pablo Alcover 31-3, 08017 Barcelona, Spain.
Europhta, Mon. Laboratoires Europhta, 6 av Prince-Hereditaire-Albert, 98000 Monaco, Monaco.
Eurorga, Fr. Eurorga, 11-13 rue de la Loge, B.P. 100, 94265 Fresnes Cedex, France.
Eurospital, Ital. Eurospital s.p.a., Via Flavia 122, 34147 Trieste, Italy.
Eutherapie, Belg. Eutherapie Benelux S.A., Blvd International 57, 1070 Brussels, Belgium.
Eutherapie, Fr. Euthérapie, 27 rue du Pont, 92200 Neuilly-sur-Seine Cdx, France.
Evans, Fr. Laboratoires Evans Medical, 6 pl Boulnois, 75017 Paris, France.
Evans, Neth. See *Glaxo Wellcome, Neth.*
Evans, Spain. Evans Medical España, Caleruega 81, 28033 Madrid, Spain.
Evans Medical, Irl. See *Wellcome, Irl.*
Evans Medical, Norw. See *Mericon, Norw.*
Evapharm, Ital. Evapharm s.r.l., Via Bolognola 47, 00138 Rome, Italy.
Evening Primrose Oil Co., UK. Evening Primrose Oil Co. Ltd, Chaplin House, Widewater Place, Moorhall Rd, Harefield, Uxbridge, Middx, UB9 6NS, UK.
Everest, Canad. Everest Pharmaceuticals Ltd, Canada.
Everett, USA. Everett Laboratories Inc., 76 Franklin St, East Orange, NJ 07017, USA.
Evers, Ger. Pharmazeutische Fabrik Evers & Co. GmbH, Siemensstrasse 4, Postfach: 1334, 25403 Pinneberg, Germany.
Exel, Belg. Exel Pharma S.A.-N.V., Chaussee de Gand 615, 1080 Brussels, Belgium.
Exflora, Fr. Laboratoires Exflora, 26 rue du Mont-Roti, 78550 Houdan, France.
Exflora, Switz. See *Uhlmann-Eyraud, Switz.*
Expancience, Spain. Expancience, Alava 6, Pol. Ind. San Roque, Arganda del Rey, 28500 Madrid, Spain.

Expanpharm, Fr. Laboratoires Expanpharm, 18 rue du Dr Ragnaud, 16000 Angouleme, France.

Expharma, Ital. ExPharma srl, Riviera Francia 3/A, 35127 Padua, Italy.

Extractum, Hung. Extractum Pharma Rt, Gyogyszer Business Center, 1047 Budapest, Hungary.

E-Z-EM, Neth. See *Rooster, Neth.*

E-Z-EM, UK. E-Z-EM Ltd, 1230 High Rd, London, N20 0LH, UK.

F5 Profas, Spain. F5 Profas, Pastora Imperio 3, 28036 Madrid, Spain.

FAB, Ital. Fidia Advanced Biopolymers srl, Via Ponte della Fabbrica 3/A, 35031 Abano Terme (PD), Italy.

Fabrigen, Canad. See *Technilab, Canad.*

Face, Ital. Face Laboratori Farmaceutici s.r.l., Via Albisola 49, 16163 Genova-Bolzaneto, Italy.

Fader, Spain. Fader, Castaner 15, 08006 Barcelona, Spain.

Faes, Spain. Faes, Maximo Aguirre 14, Lejona, 48940 Vizcaya, Spain.

Falafi, Spain. Falafi, Ramon Llull 6, Consell (Mallorca), 07330 Baleares, Spain.

Falk, Ger. Dr. Falk Pharma GmbH, Leinenweberstr. 5, Postfach: 6529, 79041 Freiburg, Germany.

Falk, Neth. See *Tramedico, Neth.*

Falk, Switz. See *Phardi, Switz.*

Falqui, Ital. Falqui Prodotti Farmaceutici s.p.a., Via Sabotino 19/2, 20135 Milan, Italy.

FAMA, Ital. F.A.M.A. s.r.l., Istituto Chimico Biologico, Via A. Sauli 21, 20127 Milan, Italy.

Family Planning Sales, UK. Family Planning Sales Ltd, 28 Kelburne Rd, Cowley, Oxford, OX4 3SZ, UK.

Farbo, Ital. Farbo s.n.c. del dott. Donato Mele & C., Via Stelvio 12/18, 20021 Ospiate di Bollate (MI), Italy.

Farco, Ger. Farco-Pharma GmbH Pharmazeutische Präparate, Mathias-Bruggen-Str. 82, Postfach: 300433, 50774 Cologne, Germany.

Farco, Irl. See *Boileau & Boyd, Irl.*

Fardi, Spain. Fardi, Grassot 16, 08025 Barcelona, Spain.

Farex, Canad. Laboratoire Farex Enrg, 5750 boul. Metropolitan E, Bur 200, St-Leonard, QC, H1S 1A7, Canada.

Farge, Ital. Farge, Via Tortona 12, 16139 Genoa, Italy.

Farley, UK. Farley Health Products Ltd, P.O. Box 94, 1 Thane Rd West, Nottingham, Notts, NG2 3AA, UK.

Farma Lepori, Spain. Farma Lepori, Osio 7-9, 08034 Barcelona, Spain.

Farmabel, Belg. Farmabel C.V., Kortrijksesteenweg 323/2, 8530 Harelbeke, Belgium.

Farmacologico Milanese, Ital. Laboratorio Farmacologico Milanese s.r.l., Via Monterosso 273, 21042 Caronno Pertusella (VA), Italy.

Farmacusi, Spain. Farmacusi, Marina 16-18, Torre Mapfre, 08005 Barcelona, Spain.

Farmades, Ital. Farmades s.p.a., Via di Tor Cervara 282, 00155 Rome, Italy.

Farmagan, Ital. Farmagan s.a., Via Vitalis di Giovanni 34, 47031 Galazzano (Rep. S. Marino), Italy.

Farmaka, Ital. Farmaka s.r.l. Laboratori Farmaceutici, Via Vetreria 1, 22070 Grandate (CO), Italy.

Farmalider, Spain. Farmalider, C/ Aragoneses 9, Alcobendas, 28100 Madrid, Spain.

Farmalyoc, Fr. Laboratoires Farmalyoc, 5 rue Charles-Martigny, 94700 Maisons-Alfort, France.

Farmanova, Ital. Farmanova AFM s.r.l., Via Flaminia 287 Sc. A. int.10, 00196 Rome, Italy.

Farmapros, Spain. Farmapros, Aribau 180, 08036 Barcelona, Spain.

Farmarekord, Ital. Farmarekord srl, Via Bracciano 7, 20098 San Giuliano Milanese (MI), Italy.

Farmasan, Ger. Farmasan Arzneimittel GmbH & Co., Pforzheimer Str. 5, Postfach: 410440, 76204 Karlsruhe, Germany.

Farmasur, Spain. Farmasur, Pol. Store, C/H 28-A, 41008 Seville, Spain.

Farmatrading, Ital. Farmatrading s.r.l., Via Pisacane 26, 20016 Pero (MI), Italy.

Farmatre, Ital. Farma 3 s.r.l., Via Solferino 42, 20036 Meda (MI), Italy.

Farmec, Ital. Farmec s.n.c., Via E Fermi, Settimo, 37026 Pescantina (VR), Italy.

Farmetrusca, Ital. Farmetrusca s.a.s. di C. Pini e C., Via G. di Vittorio, 50029 Tavarnuzze (FI), Italy.

Farmigea, Ital. Farmigea s.p.a., Industria Chimico Farmaceutica, Via Carmignani 2, 56127 Pisa, Italy.

Farmila, Ital. Farmila-Farmaceutici Milano s.r.l., Via E. Fermi 50, 20019 Settimo Milanese (MI), Italy.

Farmitalia, Spain. Pharmacia Farmitalia, Antonio Lopez, 28026 Madrid, Spain.

Farmitalia Carlo Erba, Aust. Farmitalia Carlo Erba GmbH, Karlsplatz 1, 1010 Vienna, Austria.

Farmitalia Carlo Erba, Fr. See *Pharmacia Upjohn, Fr.*

Farmitalia Carlo Erba, Ger. See *Pharmacia Upjohn, Ger.*

Farmitalia Carlo Erba, Ital. Farmitalia Carlo Erba s.r.l., Gruppo Ferruzzi-Erbamont, Via C. Imbonati 24, 20159 Milan, Italy.

Farmitalia Carlo Erba, UK. Farmitalia Carlo Erba Ltd, Italia House, 23 Grosvenor Rd, St. Albans, Herts, AL1 3AW, UK.

Farmochimica, Ital. La Farmochimica Italiana s.r.l., Via Milanese 20, 20099 Sesto San Giovanni (MI), Italy.

Farmoderm, Ital. Farmoderm Divisione Farmaceutica di Bioderm s.r.l., Via Magellano 3, 20158 Milan, Italy.

Fastfarm, Ital. Fastfarm Italia s.p.a., Via Del Rione Sirignano 6, 80121 Naples, Italy.

Fater, Ital. Fater s.p.a., Via Italica 101, 65127 Pescara, Italy.

Fatol, Aust. Fatol Arzneimittel GmbH, Robert-Koch-Strasse, D-66578 Schiffweiler, Austria.

Fatol, Ger. Fatol Arzneimittel GmbH, Robert-Koch-Strasse, Postfach: 1260, 66573 Schiffweiler, Germany.

Faulding, Austral. Faulding Pharmaceuticals, P.O. Box 746, Salisbury, SA 5108, Australia.

Faulding, Canad. Faulding (Canada) Inc., 334 Aime-Vincent, Vaudreuil, Quebec, J7V 5V5, Canada.

Faulding, UK. Faulding Pharmaceuticals Plc, Spartan Close, Tachbrook Park, Warwick, Warcks, CV34 6RS, UK.

Faulding, USA. Faulding, 200 Elmora Ave, Elizabeth, NJ 07207, USA.

Faure, Fr. Laboratoires H. Faure. See *Ciba Vision, Fr.*

Fawns & McAllan, Austral. Fawns & McAllan, 96 Merrindale Drive, Croydon, Vic. 3136, Australia.

Febena, Ger. Febena GmbH Fabrik pharm. Präparate, Oskar-Jager-Str. 115, Postfach: 300127, 50771 Cologne, Germany.

Feldhoff, Ger. W. Feldhoff & Comp. Arzneimittel GmbH, Nutzleber Feld 2, Postfach: 100137, 99855 Gotha, Germany.

Felgentrager, Ger. Dr. Felgenträger & Co. Öko-chem. und Pharma GmbH, Zerbster Str. 7a, Postfach: 238, 06855 Rosslau, Germany.

Felton, Austral. Felton, Grimwade & Bickford Pty Ltd, P.O. Box 74, Oakleigh South, Vic. 3167, Australia.

Fennings, UK. Fennings Pharmaceuticals, 46 London Rd, Horsham, West Sussex, RH12 2DT, UK.

Fenton, UK. Fenton Pharmaceuticals Ltd, 4J Portman Mansions, Chiltern St, London, W1M 1LF, UK.

Fermenta, Swed. See *Ferring, Swed.*

Fermentaciones y Sintesis, Spain. Fermentaciones y Sintesis, Castellon 23, 28001 Madrid, Spain.

Fermenti, Ital. Istituto Italiano Fermenti s.p.a., Via Beldiletto 1, 20142 Milan, Italy.

Ferndale, USA. Ferndale Laboratories Inc., 780 West Eight Mile Rd, Ferndale, MI 48220, USA.

Ferrer, Spain. Ferrer Farma, Gran Via Carlos III 94, 08028 Barcelona, Spain.

Ferrer, Switz. See *Lucchini, Switz.*

Ferring, Belg. Ferring S.A., Vlamingstraat 4, 8560 Wevelgem, Belgium.

Ferring, Canad. Ferring Inc., 515 Consumers Rd, Suite 304, North York, Ontario, M2J 4Z2, Canada.

Ferring, Fr. Laboratoires Ferring, 7 rue Jean-Baptiste-Clement, 94250 Gentilly, France.

Ferring, Ger. Ferring Arzneimittel GmbH, Wittland 11, Postfach: 2145, 24020 Kiel, Germany.

Ferring, Irl. See *Allphar, Irl.*

Ferring, Ital. Ferring s.r.l., Via Corti 11, 20133 Milano, Italy.

Ferring, Neth. Ferring B.V., Postbus 184, 2130 AD Hoofddorp, Netherlands.

Ferring, Norw. Ferring Legemidler AS, Postboks 4445 Torshov, 0403 Oslo, Norway.

Ferring, Spain. Ferring, Paseo de la Habana 15, 28036 Madrid, Spain.

Ferring, Swed. Ferring AB, Box 30047, 200 61 Malmo, Sweden.

Ferring, Switz. Ferring SA, Hochbordstrasse 9, 8600 Dubendorf, Switzerland.

Ferring, UK. Ferring Pharmaceuticals Ltd, Greville House, Hatton Rd, Feltham, Middx, TW14 9PX, UK.

Ferring, USA. Ferring Laboratories Inc., 75 Montebello Rd, Suffern, NY 10901, USA.

Ferrosan, Swed. Ferrosan AB, Grynbodgatan 14, 211 33 Malmo, Sweden.

Fertin, Norw. See *Meda, Norw.*

FertiPro, Irl. See *Electramed, Irl.*

Fher, Ital. Fher, Divisione della Boehringer Ingelheim, Casella Postale, 50100 Florence, Italy.

Fher, Spain. Fher, Pablo Alcover 31-7, 08017 Barcelona, Spain.

Fibertone, USA. Fibertone Co., 14851 N Scottsdale Rd, Scottsdale, AZ 85254, USA.

Fides, Ger. Fides Vertrieb pharm. Präparate GmbH, Bahnackerstrasse 16 a, Postfach: 309, 76482 Baden-Baden, Germany.

Fides, Spain. See *Rottapharm, Spain.*

Fidia, Ital. Fidia, Farmaceutici Italiani Derivati Industriali e Affini s.p.a., Via Ponte d/Fabbrica 3/A, 35031 Abano Terme (Padua), Italy.

Fielding, USA. The Fielding Co., P.O. Box 2186, 94 Weldon Parkway, Maryland Heights, MO 63043, USA.

Fink, Ger. Fink GmbH, Hermannstr. 7, Postfach: 1464, 77804 Buhl, Germany.

Finmedical, Ital. Finmedical srl, Vicolo De Bacchettoni 1a, 51100 Pistoia, Italy.

Fiori, Ital. Dr F & C Fiori snc, Corso San Maurizio 35, 10124 Turin, Italy.

FIRMA, Ital. Fabbr. Ital. Ritrov. Medic. Aff. s.p.a., Via di Scandicci 37, 50143 Florence, Italy.

Fischer, USA. Fischer Pharmaceuticals Inc., 165 Gibraltar Court, Sunnyvale, CA 94089, USA.

Fiske, USA. Fiske Industries, 527 Route 303, Orangeburg, NY 10962, USA.

Fisons, Aust. Fisons Austria GmbH, An den langen Lussen 1/6/1, 1190 Vienna, Austria.

Fisons, Austral. Fisons Pharmaceuticals, P.O. Box 191, Castle Hill, NSW 2154, Australia.

Fisons, Belg. See *Rhone-Poulenc Rorer, Belg.*

Fisons, Canad. See *Rhone-Poulenc Rorer, Canad.*

Fisons, Fr. See *Specia, Fr.*

Fisons, Ger. Fisons Arzneimittel GmbH, Nattermannallee 1, Postfach: 350120, 50792 Cologne, Germany.

Fisons, Irl. See *Rhone-Poulenc Rorer, Irl.*

Fisons, Ital. Fisons Italchimici s.p.a., V.le Castello d/Magliana 38, 00148 Rome, Italy.

Fisons, Neth. Fisons B.V., Postbus 982, 1180 AZ Amstelveen, Netherlands.

Fisons, Switz. See *Rhone-Poulenc Rorer, Switz.*

Fisons, UK. Fisons PLC, Pharmaceutical Division, 12 Derby Rd, Loughborough, Leics, LE11 0BB, UK.

Fisons, USA. Fisons Corporation, Two Preston Court, Bedford, MA 01730, USA.

Fisons Consumer, Austral. Fisons Consumer Health Division of Fisons Pty Ltd, 6 Chilvers Road, Thornleigh, NSW 2120, Australia.

Fisons Consumer, USA. See *Ciba Consumer, USA.*

Fitobucaneve, Ital. Fitobucaneve srl, Via Galvani 25/27, 20018 Sedriano (MI), Italy.

Fitodorfarma, Ital. Fitodorfarma s.a.s., Sezione Erboristeria, Via Genova 28, 21052 Busto Arsizio (VA), Italy.

Fitolife, Ital. Laboratorio Fitolife srl, Via Domiziana km 55, 80072 Arco Felice (NA), Italy.

Flanders, USA. Flanders Inc., P.O. Box 39143, Northbridge Station, Charleston, SC 29407, USA.

FLAWA, Switz. FLAWA Schweizer Verbandstoff- und Wattefabriken AG, Badstrasse 43, 9230 Flawil, Switzerland.

Fleet, Austral. C.B. Fleet Co. (Aust) Pty Ltd, P.O. Box 64, Mentone, Vic 3194, Australia.

Fleet, Neth. See *Tramedico, Neth.*

Fleet, USA. C.B. Fleet Co. Inc., 4615 Murray Pl., Lynchburg, VA 24502-2235, USA.

Fleming, USA. Fleming & Co., 1600 Fenpark Dr., Fenton, MO 63026, USA.

Flora, Canad. Flora Mfg & Dist. Ltd, 7400 Fraser Park Drive, Burnaby, BC, V5J 5B9, Canada.

Florafaun, Austral. Florafaun Pty Ltd, 12/231 Balcatta Road, Balcatta, WA 6021, Australia.

Florizel, UK. Florizel Ltd, P.O. Box 138, Stevenage, Herts, SG2 8YN, UK.

Fluoritab, USA. Fluoritab Corp., P.O. Box 507, Temperance, MI 48182-0507, USA.

Foletto, Ital. A Foletto di Foletto Alberto & C s.n.c., Via Cassoni 3, 38060 Pieve di Ledro (Trento), Italy.

Forest Laboratories, USA. Forest Laboratories, 150 East 58th St, New York, NY 10155, USA.

Forest Pharmaceuticals, USA. Forest Pharmaceuticals Inc., 13622 Lakefront Drive, St Louis, MO 63045, USA.

Forley, UK. Forley Ltd, 54 Hillbury Ave, Harrow, Middlesex, HA3 8EW, UK.

Formenti, Ital. Prodotti Formenti s.r.l., Via Correggio 43, 20149 Milan, Italy.

Fornet, Fr. Laboratoires Fornet, 68 rue Jean-Jacques-Rousseau, 75001 Paris, France.

Fougera, USA. E. Fougera & Co., Division of Altana Inc., 60 Baylis Rd, Melville, NY 11747, USA.

Four Macs, Austral. Four Macs Pty Ltd, 78 Burns Rd, Wahroonga, NSW 2076, Australia.

Fournier, Belg. Fournier Pharma S.A., Rue des Trois Arbres 16b, 1180 Brussels, Belgium.

Fournier, Canad. Fournier Pharma Inc., 1010 Sherbrooke St W, P.O. Box 16, 19th Floor, Montreal, Quebec, H3A 2R7, Canada.

Fournier, Fr. Laboratoires Fournier, 9 rue Petitot, 21000 Dijon, France.

Fournier, Ger. Fournier Pharma GmbH, Justus-von-Liebig Str. 16, Postfach: 1145, 66272 Sulzbach, Germany.

Fournier, Ital. Fournier Pierrel Farma s.p.a., Palazzo Caravaggio, Via Cassanese 224, 20090 Segrate (MI), Italy.

Fournier, Spain. Fournier Iberica, Ctra de Navarra S/N, Hernani, 20120 Guipuzcoa, Spain.

Fournier, Switz. See *Schwarz, Switz.*

Fournier, UK. Fournier Pharmaceuticals Ltd, 19-20 Progress Business Centre, Whittle Parkway, Slough, SL1 6DQ, UK.

Fournier SA, Spain. Fournier SA, Euronova 3, Rda Poniente 16, Tres Cantos, 28760 Madrid, Spain.

Fox, UK. Charles H. Fox Ltd, 22 Tavistock St, London, WC2E 7PY, UK.

Francia, Ital. Francia Farmaceutici Industria Farmaco Biologica s.r.l., Via dei Pestagalli 7, 20138 Milan, Italy.

Franconpharm, Ger. franconpharm Arzneimittel GmbH, Alexandrinenstr. 1, 96450 Coburg, Germany.

Franklin Medical, UK. Franklin Medical Ltd, P.O. Box 138, Turnpike Rd, High Wycombe, Bucks, HP12 3NB, UK.

Freeda, USA. Freeda Vitamins Inc., 36 E 41st St, New York, NY 10017-6203, USA.

Frega, Canad. See *Pharmalab, Canad.*

Frere, Belg. Frere & Cie S.A., Ave des Noisetiers 7, 1170 Brussels, Belgium.

Fresenius, Belg. Fresenius S.A., Molenberglei 7, 2627 Schelle, Belgium.

Fresenius, Fr. Fresenius France, 6 rue du Rempart, BP 611, 27406 Louviers cdx, France.

Fresenius, Ger. Fresenius AG, 61343 Bad Homburg v. d. H., Germany.

Fresenius, Norw. See *Meda, Norw.*

Fresenius, Spain. Fresenius Medical Care, Pol. Ind. Pinares Llanos, Cerrajeros 6 Nave-30, 28670 Madrid, Spain.

Fresenius, Switz. Fresenius SA, Case postale, 6370 Stans, Switzerland.

Fresenius, UK. Fresenius Ltd, 6/7 Christleton Court, Stuart Rd, Manor Park, Runcorn, Cheshire, WA7 1ST, UK.

Fresenius-Klinik, Ger. See *Fresenius, Ger.*

Fresenius-Praxis, Ger. See *Fresenius, Ger.*

Frika, Aust. Frika GmbH, Erdbergstrasse 8, 1031 Vienna, Austria.

Frosst, Austral. See *Merck Sharp & Dohme, Austral.*

Frosst, Canad. Frosst, Division of Merck Frosst Canada Inc., P.O. Box 1005, Pointe-Claire-Dorval, Quebec, H9R 4P8, Canada.

Frosst, Ger. See *MSD Chibropharm, Ger.*
Frosst, Neth. Frosst, divisie van Merck Sharp & Dohme B.V., Waarderweg 39, 2031 BN Haarlem, Netherlands.
Fruit of the Earth, Canad. Fruit of the Earth, Canada.
Fuca, Fr. Laboratoires Fuca, 1 bis, rue de Plaisance, 94732 Nogent-sur-Marne Cedex, France.
Fuji, Jpn. Fuji Chemical Industry Co Ltd, 3-3 Uchikanda, 1-Chome, Chiyoda-ku, Tokyo 101, Japan.
Fuji, Swed. Fuji Film Sverige AB, Box 23086, 104 35 Stockholm, Sweden.
Fujisawa, Canad. Fujisawa Canada Inc., 625 Cochrane Dr., Suite 800, Markham, Ontario, L3R 9R9, Canada.
Fujisawa, Fr. Fujisawa, Le Clemenceau II, 215 av Georges-Clemenceau, 92024 Nanterre cdx, France.
Fujisawa, Ger. Fujisawa GmbH, Postfach: 800628, 81606 Munich, Germany.
Fujisawa, Irl. See *Fujisawa, UK.*
Fujisawa, Jpn. Fujisawa Pharmaceutical Co. Ltd, 4-7 Doshomachi 3-chome, Chuo-ku, Osaka 541, Japan.
Fujisawa, Spain. Fujisawa, Sor Angela de la Cruz 2 No 3, Planta 13, 28020 Madrid, Spain.
Fujisawa, Swed. Fujisawa Scandinavia, Skeppsbron 5-6, 411 21 Goteborg, Sweden.
Fujisawa, UK. Fujisawa Ltd, 8th Floor, CP House, 97-107 Uxbridge Rd, London, W5 5TL, UK.
Fujisawa, USA. Fujisawa Pharmaceutical Co., Fujisawa USA Inc., 3 Parkway North Center, Deerfield, IL 600 15-2548, USA.
Fulton, Ital. Fulton Medicinali s.r.l., Via Edison 68/70, 20019 Settimo Milanese (MI), Italy.
Fulton, USA. Fulton, USA.
Fumedica, Ger. Fumedica Arzneimittel GmbH, Postfach: 101649, 44606 Herne, Germany.
Fumouze, Fr. Laboratoires Fumouze, 7 place des Martyrs, 92110 Clichy, France.
Funk, Spain. Funk, San Juan 9, Manlleu, 08037 Barcelona, Spain.
Futuna, UK. Futuna Ltd, 57 Masonfield, Bamberbridge, Preston, Lancs, PR5 8HP, UK.
G & W, USA. G & W Laboratories Inc., 111 Coolidge St, South Plainfield, NJ 07080, USA.
GABA, Switz. GABA AG, Pharmazeutische und kosmetische Präparate, Grabetsmattweg, 4106 Therwil, Switzerland.
Galactina, Switz. Galactina AG, Birkenweg 1-8, 3123 Belp, Switzerland.
Galactopharm, Ger. Galactopharm Hans Sanders, Sudstr. 10, Postfach: 1429, 49746 Sogel, Germany.
Galderma, Austral. Galderma Australia Pty. Ltd, P.O. Box 502, Frenchs Forest, NSW 2086, Australia.
Galderma, Belg. Galderma Belgilux S.A., Lodderstraat 8, Bus 2, 2880 Bornem, Belgium.
Galderma, Canad. Galderma Canada Inc., 5025 Orbitor Dr, Bldg 6, Suite 400, Mississauga, Ontario, L4W 4Y5, Canada.
Galderma, Fr. Laboratoires Galderma, 20 av. Andre-Malraux, 92309 Levallois-Perret Cdx, France.
Galderma, Ger. Galderma Laboratorium GmbH, Sasbacher Strasse 10, 79111 Freiburg i. Br., Germany.
Galderma, Irl. See *Galderma, UK.*
Galderma, Ital. Galderma Italia s.p.a., Palazzo Sirio, Ingresso 3, 20041 Agrate Brianza (MI), Italy.
Galderma, Neth. Galderma S.A., Avelingen-West 5, 4202 MS Gorinchem, Netherlands.
Galderma, S.Afr. Galderma, S. Africa.
Galderma, Spain. Galderma, Ctra Fuencarral-Alcobendas Km 15.4, Alcobendas, 28100 Madrid, Spain.
Galderma, Switz. Galderma SA, Sinserstrasse 47, Postfach 492, 6330 Cham, Switzerland.
Galderma, UK. Galderma Ltd, Imperial Way, Watford, Herts, WD2 4YR, UK.
Galderma, USA. Galderma Laboratories Inc., Suite 300, 3000 Alta Mesa Blvd, P.O. Box 331329, Fort Worth, TX 76163, USA.
Galen, Canad. Galen Group, 7305 Woodbine Ave, Unit 5, Markham, Ontario, L3R 3V7, Canada.
Galen, Irl. See *Allphar, Irl.*
Galen, UK. Galen Ltd, 19 Lower Seagoe Industrial Estate, Portadown, Craigavon, Armagh, BT63 5QD, UK.
Galenica, Switz. Galenica Vertretungen AG, Untermattweg 8, 3001 Bern, Switzerland.
Galenika, Ger. Galenika Dr. Hetterich GmbH, Gebhardtstrasse 5, Postfach: 1753, 90707 Furth/Bayern, Germany.
Galephar, Fr. Laboratoires Galephar, ZI de Krafft, bat B, 67150 Erstein, France.
Galephar, Neth. See *Zambon, Neth.*
Galepharma, Spain. Galepharma Iberica, Balmes 127, San Adrian de Besos, 08930 Barcelona, Spain.
Gallia, Fr. See *Diepal, Fr.*
Gallier, Fr. Laboratoires Gallier, 40 rue Lecuyer, 93300 Aubervilliers, France.
Galmeda, Ger. Galmeda GmbH, Ostmerheimer Strasse 198, Postfach: 910353, 51073 Cologne, Germany.
Galpharm, UK. Gal Pharm International, Hugh House, Foundry Street, Birds Royd Lane, Brighouse, West Yorkshire, HD6 1LW, UK.
Galway, Irl. Galway Laboratories, Oughterard, Co. Galway, Ireland.
Gambar, Ital. Laboratori Gambar s.r.l., Via Bolognola 45, 00138 Rome, Italy.
Gambro, Swed. Gambro Lundia AB, Box 10101, 220 10 Lund, Sweden.
Gambro, USA. Gambro Inc., 1185 Oak St, Lakewood, CO 80215, USA.
Ganassini, Ital. Istituto Ganassini s.p.a. di Ricerche Biochimiche, Via Gaggia 16, 20139 Milan, Italy.
Gandhour, Fr. Laboratoires Gandhour, 1 bis rue de Plaisance, 94732 Nogent-sur-Marne Cedex, France.
Garant, Ital. Laboratorio Chimico Garant s.r.l., Via Melzi d'Eril 29, 20154 Milan, Italy.
Garcia Suarez, Spain. Garcia Suarez, CID 3, 28001 Madrid, Spain.
Garec, S.Afr. Garec Pharmaceuticals, P.O. Box 1123, Halfway House 1685, S. Africa.
Garnier, UK. Garnier, 30 Kensington Church St, London, W8 4HA, UK.
Gaschler, Ger. Pharma Laboratorium S.M. Gaschler GmbH, Postfach: 4012, 88119 Lindau, Germany.
Gastropharm, Ger. Gastropharm GmbH Arzneimittel, Postfach: 2051, 37010 Gottingen, Germany.
Gate, USA. Gate Pharmaceuticals, 650 Cathill Rd, Sellersville, PA 18960, USA.
Gazzoni, Ital. Gazzoni s.r.l., Via Ilio Barontini 16/20, 40138 Bologna, Italy.
G-B-M, UK. G-B-M Ltd, P.O. Box 69, Godalming, Surrey, GU7 2PB, UK.
GD, Ital. GD Tecnologie Interdisciplinari Farmaceutiche s.r.l., Via Augusto Gaudenzi 29, 00163 Rome, Italy.
Gea, Neth. See *Multipharma, Neth.*
Gea, Norw. See *Pharmacia Upjohn, Norw.*
GEA, Swed. GEA Farmaceutisk Fabrik AB, Berga Alle 1 E, 254 52 Helsingborg, Sweden.
Gea, Switz. See *Globopharm, Switz.,* and *Luitpold, Switz.*
Gebauer, Canad. See *BDH, USA.*
Gebauer, USA. Gebauer Chemical Co., 9410 St Catherine Ave, Cleveland, OH 44104, USA.
Gebro, Aust. Gebro Broschek GmbH, Tirol, 6391 Fieberbrunn, Austria.
Gebro, Switz. Gebro Pharma SA, Oristalstrasse 87a, 4410 Liestal, Switzerland.
Gedeon Richter, Hung. Chemical Works of Gedeon Richter Ltd, P.O. Box 27, 1475 Budapest, Hungary.
Gedis, Ital. Gedis s.r.l., Via Vezzolano 15, 10153 Turin, Italy.
Geigy, Austral. See *Ciba-Geigy, Austral.*
Geigy, Canad. See *Ciba, Canad.*
Geigy, Fr. See *Ciba-Geigy, Fr.*
Geigy, Ger. See *Ciba, Ger.*
Geigy, Irl. See *Novartis, Irl.*
Geigy, Norw. See *Novartis, Norw.*
Geigy, Switz. See *Ciba-Geigy, Switz.*
Geigy, UK. See *Ciba, UK.*
Geigy, USA. Geigy Pharmaceuticals, Division of Ciba-Geigy Corporation, Ardsley, NY 10502, USA.
Geistlich, Irl. Geistlich Pharma, 36 Lower Stephen Street, Dublin 2, Ireland.
Geistlich, Neth. See *Multipharma, Neth.*
Geistlich, Switz. Geistlich-Pharma, 6110 Wolhusen, Switzerland.
Geistlich, UK. Geistlich Sons Ltd, Newton Bank, Long Lane, Chester, CH2 3QZ, UK.
Gelflex, Austral. Gelflex Australia, P.O. Box 716, West Perth, WA 6005, Australia.
Gelos, Spain. Gelos, Joan XXIII 10, Esplugues de Llobregat, 08950 Barcelona, Spain.
Geminis, Spain. Geminis, Gran Via de las Corts, Catalanes 764, 08013 Barcelona, Spain.
Gencon, USA. Gencon, 6116 N Central Expy 200, Dallas, TX 75206, USA.
GenDerm, Canad. GenDerm Canada Inc., 355 rue McCaffrey, St-Laurent, Quebec, H4T 1Z7, Canada.
GenDerm, USA. GenDerm Corp., 600 Knightsbridge Parkway, Lincolnshire, IL 60069, USA.
Genentech, USA. Genentech Inc., 460 Point San Bruno Blvd, South San Francisco, CA 94080, USA.
Genera, Switz. Genera Pharma AG, Hilariweg 9, Postfach, 4501 Solothurn, Switzerland.
General Dietary, UK. General Dietary Ltd, P.O. Box 38, Kingston upon Thames, Surrey, KT2 7YP, UK.
Genericon, Aust. Genericon Pharma GmbH, Schlossplatz 1, 8502 Lannach, Austria.
Generics, UK. Generics (UK) Ltd, 12 Station Close, Potters Bar, Herts, EN6 1TL, UK.
Genetics Institute, USA. Genetics Institute, USA.
Geneva, USA. Geneva Pharmaceuticals, 2599 W Midway Blvd, P.O. Box 469, Broomfield, CO 80038-0469, USA.
Genevar, Fr. Genevar, 95 av de la Chataigneraie, 92503 Rueil-Malmaison, France.
Genevrier, Fr. Laboratoires Génévrier, B.P. 47, 06901 Sophia Antipolis Cdx, France.
Gen-King, USA. See *Kinray, USA.*
Genodex, Fr. Lab. Genodex, 15 av de Breteuil, 75007 Paris, France.
Genove, Spain. Genove, Prat de la Manta 54, Hospitalet de Llobregat, 08902 Barcelona, Spain.
Genpharm, Canad. Genpharm Inc., 37 Advance Rd, Etobicoke, Ontario, M8Z 2S6, Canada.
Genpharm, S.Afr. Genpharm Pharmaceuticals CC, P.O. Box 607, Rivonia 2128, S. Africa.
Gensia, Irl. See *Sanofi Winthrop, Irl.*
Gensia, Swed. See *Gensia, UK.*
Gensia, Switz. See *Opopharma, Switz.*
Gensia, UK. Gensia Automedics Ltd, Unit 31, Wellington Business Park, Dukes Ride, Crowthorne, Berks, RG45 6LS, UK.
Gensia, USA. Gensia Laboratories Ltd, 19 Hughes, Irvine, CA 92718-1902, USA.
Gentili, Ital. Istituto Gentili s.p.a., Via Mazzini 112, 56125 Pisa, Italy.
Genzyme, Ger. Genzyme GmbH, Rontgenstr. 4, 63755 Alzenau, Germany.
Genzyme, Ital. Genzyme Therapeutics srl, Via Scaglia Est 144, 41100 Modena, Italy.
Genzyme, Spain. Genzyme BV, Camino de las Vinas 7, San Sebastian de los Reyes, 28708 Madrid, Spain.
Genzyme, UK. Genzyme Therapeutics, 37 Hollands Rd, Haverhill, Suffolk, CB9 8PU, UK.
Genzyme, USA. Genzyme Corp., 1 Kendall Square, Cambridge, MA 02139, USA.
Gepepharm, Ger. gepepharm GmbH, Lendersbergstr. 86, 53721 Siegburg, Germany.
Gerard, Irl. Gerard Laboratories, 36 Baldoyle Industrial Estate, Dublin 13, Ireland.
Gerard House, UK. Gerard House Ltd, Mulberry Court, Stour Rd, Christchurch, Dorset, BH23 1PS, UK.
Gerbex, Canad. Gerbex Inc. Produits, 331 rue Principale, St-Thomas d'Aquin, QC, J0H 2A0, Canada.
Gerbiol, Fr. Laboratoires Gerbiol, Tour PFA, La Defense 10, Cdx 43, 92076 Paris-La-Defense, France.
Gerda, Fr. Laboratoires Gerda, 6 rue Childebert, 69002 Lyon, France.
Geriatric Pharm. Corp., USA. Geriatric Pharmaceutical Corp., 6 Industrial Way W, Eatontown, NJ 07724, USA.
Gerlach, Ger. Eduard Gerlach GmbH, Backerstrasse 4-8, Postfach: 12 49, 32292 Lubbecke, Germany.
Germania, Aust. Germania Pharmazeutika GmbH, Schuselkagasse 8, 1150 Vienna, Austria.
Germiphene, Canad. Germiphene Corporation, P.O. Box 1748, Brantford, Ontario, N3T 5V7, Canada.
Gerot, Aust. Gerot Pharmazeutika GmbH, Arnethgasse 3, 1160 Vienna, Austria.
Gerot, Switz. See *Byk, Switz.*
Gersthofer, Aust. Gersthofer-Apotheke, Gersthofer Strasse 61, 1180 Vienna, Austria.
Gewo, Ger. Gewo Chemie GmbH, Schneidweg 5, Postfach: 110164, 76487 Baden-Baden, Germany.
Geymonat, Ital. Geymonat s.p.a., Via S. Anna 2, 03012 Anagni (FR), Italy.
Geymonat, Switz. See *Lucchini, Switz.*
Ghimas, Ital. Ghimas s.p.a., Via R. Fucini 2, 40033 Casalecchio di Reno (BO), Italy.
Gibipharma, Ital. Gibipharma s.p.a., Via Carlo Pisacane 7, 20016 Pero (Milan), Italy.
GiEnne, Ital. GiEnne, Italy.
Gifrer Barbezat, Fr. Laboratoires Gifrer Barbezat, B.P. 165, 69151 Decines Cedex, France.
Gilbert, Fr. Laboratoires Gilbert, av. du General-de-Gaulle, B.P.115, 14204 Herouville-Saint-Clair, France.
Gilead, USA. Gilead Sciences Inc., 333 Lakeside Drive, Foster City, CA 94404, USA.
Gingi-Pak, Switz. See *Beldenta, Switz.*
Giovanardi, Ital. Giovanardi Farmaceutico s.n.c. del Dr Benito Giovanardi e Figli, Via Sapeto 28, 16132 Genoa, Italy.
Gisand, Switz. Gisand AG, Schlaflistrasse 14, 3013 Bern, Switzerland.
Giuliani, Ital. Giuliani s.p.a., Via Palagi 2, 20129 Milan, Italy.
Giuliani, Switz. Giuliani SA, via Riviera 21, 6976 Castagnola-Lugano, Switzerland.
Giulini, Ger. See *Solvay, Ger.*
Glades, USA. Glades Pharmaceuticals, 255 Alhambra Circle, Suite 1000, Coral Gables, FL 33134, USA.
Glaxo, Belg. See *Glaxo Wellcome, Belg.*
Glaxo, Fr. See *Glaxo Wellcome, Fr.*
Glaxo, S.Afr. Glaxo South Africa (Pty) Ltd, P.O. Box 3388, Halfway House 1685, S. Africa.
Glaxo, UK. Glaxo Laboratories Ltd, Greenford Rd, Greenford, Middx, UB6 0HE, UK.
Glaxo, USA. See *Glaxo Wellcome, USA.*
Glaxo Allen, Ital. See *Glaxo Wellcome, Ital.*
Glaxo Wellcome, Aust. Glaxo Wellcome Pharma GmbH, Albert-Schweitzer-Gasse 6, A-1140 Vienna, Austria.
Glaxo Wellcome, Austral. Glaxo-Wellcome, P.O. Box 168, Boronia, Vic 3155, Australia.
Glaxo Wellcome, Belg. Glaxo Wellcome Belgium S.A., Blvd du Triomphe 172, 1160 Brussels, Belgium.
Glaxo Wellcome, Canad. Glaxo Wellcome Inc., 7333 Mississauga Rd North, Mississauga, Ontario, L5N 6L4, Canada.
Glaxo Wellcome, Fr. Laboratoires Glaxo Wellcome, 43 rue Vineuse, 75764 Paris cdx 16, France.
Glaxo Wellcome, Ger. Glaxo Wellcome GmbH & Co, Industriestrasse 32-36, Postfach: 1460/1465, 23834 Bad Oldesloe, Germany.
Glaxo Wellcome, Irl. Glaxo WellcomeLtd, P.O. Box 700, Grange Rd, Rathfarnham, Dublin 16, Ireland.
Glaxo Wellcome, Ital. Glaxo Wellcome s.p.a., Via A. Fleming 2, 37135 Verona, Italy.
Glaxo Wellcome, Neth. Glaxo Wellcome B.V., Postbus 780, 3700 AT Zeist, Netherlands.
Glaxo Wellcome, Norw. Glaxo Wellcome A/S, Sandakerv.114A, Postboks 4312 Torshov, 0402 Oslo, Norway.
Glaxo Wellcome, S.Afr. Glaxo Wellcome South Africa (Pty) Ltd, 44 Old Pretoria Rd, Halfway House, Midrand, Gauteng, South Africa.
Glaxo Wellcome, Spain. Glaxo Wellcome, Severo Ochoa 2, Tres Cantos, 28760 Madrid, Spain.
Glaxo Wellcome, Swed. Glaxo Wellcome AB, Box 528, S-183 25 Taby, Sweden.
Glaxo Wellcome, Switz. Glaxo Wellcome AG, Bahnhofstrasse 5, Postfach, 3322 Schonbuhl/Bern, Switzerland.
Glaxo Wellcome, UK. Glaxo Wellcome, Stockley Park, Uxbridge, Middx, UB11 1BT, UK.
Glaxo Wellcome, USA. Glaxo Wellcome Inc., Five Moore Drive, Research Triangle Park, NC 27709, USA.
Glenbrook, USA. Glenbrook Laboratories, Division of Sterling Drug Inc., 90 Park Ave, New York, NY 10016, USA.
Glenwood, Canad. Glenwood Laboratories Canada Ltd, 2406 Speers Rd, Oakville, Ontario, L6L 5M2, Canada.

Glenwood, Ger. Glenwood GmbH Pharmazeutische Erzeugnisse, Riedener Weg 23, Postfach: 1261, 82302 Starnberg, Germany.

Glenwood, Switz. See *Galenica, Switz.*

Glenwood, UK. Glenwood Laboratories Ltd, Unit D, Jenkins Dale, Chatham, Kent, ME4 5RD, UK.

Glenwood, USA. Glenwood Inc., 83 North Summit St, Tenafly, NJ 07670, USA.

Globopharm, Aust. Globopharm, Vienna, Austria.

Globopharm, Switz. Globopharm SA, Gewerbestrasse 12, 8132 Egg, Switzerland.

GN, Ger. G.N. Pharm Arzneimittel GmbH, Schorndorfer Strasse 32, Postfach: 1440, 70704 Fellbach, Germany.

GNR, Fr. Lab. GNR-pharma, 37 rue de la Plaine, 75020 Paris, France.

Go Travel, UK. Go Travel Products, UK.

Godecke, Ger. Gödecke AG, Postfach: 100250, 10562 Berlin, Germany.

Golaz, Switz. Laboratoire Golaz SA, Ch. du Devent, 1024 Ecublens/VD, Switzerland.

Gold Cross, UK. See *Searle, UK.*

Goldcrest, UK. Goldcrest Pharmaceuticals Ltd, UK.

Golden Neo-Life Diamite, Austral. Golden Neo-Life Diamite International Pty Ltd, 21 Webster Drive, Caboolture, Qld 4510, Australia.

Golden Pride, Canad. Golden Pride, 60 Colonnade Rd, Nepean, ON, K2E 7J6, Canada.

Goldham, Ger. Goldham Arzneimittel GmbH, Wasserberg 11, 86441 Zusmarshausen, Germany.

Goldline, USA. Goldline Laboratories Inc., 1900 W Commercial Blvd, Ft Lauderdale, FL 33309, USA.

Goldschmidt, Ger. Th. Goldschmidt AG, Goldschmidtstrasse 100, Postfach: 101461, 45116 Essen, Germany.

Goldschmidt, Switz. See *Desopharmex, Switz.*

Goldschmidt, UK. Th. Goldschmidt Ltd, UK.

Goldshield, Irl. See *Allphar, Irl.*

Goldshield, UK. Goldshield Pharmaceuticals Ltd, Bensham House, 324 Bensham Lane, Thornton Heath, Surrey, CR7 7EQ, UK.

Gomenol, Fr. Laboratoires du Gomenol, 48 rue des Petites-Écuries, 75010 Paris, France.

Gonnon, Fr. Laboratoires Gonnon, France.

Goodys, USA. Goody's Manufacturing Corp., 436 Salt St, Winston Salem, NC 27108, USA.

Gordon, USA. Gordon Laboratories, 6801 Ludlow St, Upper Darby, PA 19082-1694, USA.

Gothia, Swed. Gothia Läkemedel AB, Bolshedens Industrivag 20, 427 50 Billdal, Sweden.

Goupil, Fr. See *Synthelabo, Fr.*

Goupil, Ital. Goupil Italia s.p.a., Via S. Paolo 13, 20121 Milan, Italy.

Goupil, Spain. Goupil Iberica, Avda Industria 31, Alcobendas, 28100 Madrid, Spain.

G.P. Laboratories, Austral. See *Pfizer, Austral.*

GPL, Switz. GPL Ginsana Products Lugano SA, Case postale, 6903 Lugano, Switzerland.

Grafton, UK. Grafton International, 5-12 Birchbrook Park, Shenstone, Staffs, WS14 0DJ, UK.

Graham-Field, USA. Graham-Field Inc., 400 Rabro Drive East, Hauppauge, NY 11788, USA.

Granata, Ital. Granata Medicinali Affini, Via Valtellina 2, 20159 Milan, Italy.

Grandel-Synpharma, Ger. Dr Grandel GmbH - Vertrieb Syn-Pharma GmbH, Pfladergasse 7-13, Postfach: 111649, 86041 Augsburg, Germany.

Grands Espaces, Fr. Les Grands Espaces Therapeutiques, BP 6054, 34030 Montpelier cdx, France.

Granelli, Ital. Laboratori E. Granelli s.p.a. Divisione OTC Synthelabo, Via Rivoltana 13, 20090 Limito (MI), Italy.

Granions, Mon. Laboratoires des Granions, 7 rue de l'Industrie, 98000 Monaco, Monaco.

Grasler, Ger. grasler pharma GmbH, Postfach: 17, 82284 Grafrath, Germany.

Gray, USA. Gray Pharmaceutical Co., Affiliate of The Purdue Frederick Co., 100 Connecticut Ave, Norwalk, CT 06856, USA.

Great Southern, USA. Great Southern Laboratories, 10863 Rockley Rd, Houston, TX 77099, USA.

Green Cross, Jpn. The Green Cross Corporation, 3-3 Imabashi 1-chome, Chuo-ku, Osaka 541, Japan.

Green Turtle Bay Vitamin Co., USA. The Green Turtle Bay Vitamin Co., P.O. Box 642, Summit, NJ 07902, USA.

Gresval, Fr. Laboratoires Gresval, 2 rue Thimonnier, 75009 Paris, France.

Gricar, Ital. Industria Chimico Farmaceutica Gricar Chemical srl, Via S Giuseppe 18/20, 20047 Brugherio (MI), Italy.

Grifols, Spain. Grifols, Can Guasch 2 Pol. Levante, Parets del Valles, 08150 Barcelona, Spain.

Gripp, Ger. Hermann Gripp Chem. pharm. Laboratorium, Oberaltenallee 16, Postfach: 760428, 2000 Hamburg 76, Germany.

Grossmann, Switz. Dr Grossmann AG, Pharmaca, Hardstrasse 25, Postfach 914, 4127 Birsfelden/Basel, Switzerland.

Grunenthal, Aust. Grünenthal GmbH, Wolfganggasse 45-7, 1120 Vienna, Austria.

Grunenthal, Ger. Grünenthal GmbH Aachen, Steinfeldstrasse 2, 52222 Stolberg, Germany.

Grunenthal, Neth. See *Byk, Neth.*

Grunenthal, Switz. Grünenthal Pharma AG, 8756 Mitlodi/Glarus, Switzerland.

Gry, Ger. Gry-Pharma GmbH, Kandelstr. 10, Postfach: 1206, 79196 Kirchzarten, Germany.

Gry, Switz. See *Galenica, Switz.*

GS, S.Afr. GS Pharmaceuticals, P.O. Box 1123, Halfway House 1685, S. Africa.

Guardian, Canad. See *Pharmascience, Canad.*

Guardian, USA. Guardian Laboratories, A division of United-Guardian Inc., 230 Marcus Blvd, P.O. Box 2500, Smithtown, NY 11787, USA.

Gubler, Switz. Dr AW Gubler, Petersgraben 5, 4051 Basel, Switzerland.

Guerbet, Fr. Laboratoires Guerbet, 15 rue des Vanesses, B.P. 50400, 95943 Roissy-Charles-de-Gaulle Cdx, France.

Guerbet, Ger. Guerbet GmbH, Otto-Volger Strasse 11, Postfach: 1240, 65838 Sulzbach/Ts, Germany.

Guerbet, Ital. See *Farmades, Ital.*

Guerbet, Neth. Guerbet Nederland B.V., Avelingen West 28c, 4202 MS Gorinchem, Netherlands.

Guerbet, Norw. See *Partner, Norw.*

Guerbet, Switz. Guerbet AG, Winterthurerstrasse 92, 8006 Zurich, Switzerland.

Guidotti, Ital. Laboratori Guidotti s.p.a., Via Trieste 40, 56126 Pisa, Italy.

Guieu, Fr. Laboratoires Guieu France, ZI de la Barogne, 77230 Moussy-le-Neuf, France.

Guieu, Ital. Laboratori Guieu s.p.a., Via Lomellina 10, 20133 Milan, Italy.

Guigoz, Ital. Guigoz, Via le Richard 5, 20143 Milan, Italy.

Gynetics, USA. Gynetics, USA.

Gynopharma, USA. Gynopharma Inc., 50 Division St, Somerville, NJ 08876, USA.

Haemacure, Canad. Haemacure Corp., 16771 ch. Ste-Marie, Kirkland, Quebec, H9H 5H3, Canada.

Hafslund Nycomed, Aust. Hafslund Nycomed Pharma AG, St Peter-Strasse 25, 4010 Linz, Austria.

Hafslund Nycomed, Switz. Hafslund Nycomed Pharma AG, Moosacherstrasse 14, Au, 8820 Wadenswil, Switzerland.

Hal, Ger. Hal Allergie GmbH, Kolner Landstr. 34 a, Postfach: 130450, 40554 Dusseldorf, Germany.

HAL, Neth. HAL Allergenen Laboratorium B.V., Postbus 1007, 2001 BA Haarlem, Netherlands.

Halal, UK. Halal Pharmaceuticals Ltd, 7 Oxford St, Manchester, M1 4WX, UK.

Hall, Canad. Hall Laboratories Ltd, 207-13060 80th Ave, Surrey, British Columbia, V3W 3B2, Canada.

Halsey, USA. Halsey Drug Co, 1827 Pacific St, Brooklyn, NY 11233, USA.

Hameln, Ger. Pharma Hameln Infusionen GmbH, Langes Feld 13, 31789 Hameln, Germany.

Hamilton, Austral. Hamilton Pharmaceuticals Pty Ltd, G.P.O. Box 7, Adelaide, SA 5001, Australia.

Hanosan, Ger. Hanosan GmbH Pharmazeutische Fabrik, Hanosanstr. 1, Postfach: 120164, 30808 Garbsen, Germany.

Hansam, UK. Hansam Healthcare Ltd, 60 Ondine Rd, London, SE15 4EB, UK.

Hanseler, Ger. Hänseler GmbH, Gottlieb-Daimler-Strasse 1, Postfach: 5628, 78435 Constance a. B., Germany.

Hanseler, Switz. Hänseler AG, Industriestrasse 35, 9100 Herisau, Switzerland.

Hargell, Canad. Hargell Ltd, 5050 Dufferin St, Ste 108, Downsview, Ontario, M3H 5T5, Canada.

Harley Street Supplies, UK. Harley Street Supplies, 26 Paddington St, London, W1M 3RF, UK.

Harras-Curarina, Ger. Harras-Pharma-Curarina Arzneimittel GmbH (Vertrieb), Harras 15, 81373 Munich, Germany.

Hartmann, Ger. Paul Hartmann AG Verbandstoff-Fabriken, Paul-Hartmann-Strasse 12, Postfach: 14 20, 89504 Heidenheim (Brenz), Germany.

Harvey-Scruton, UK. Harvey-Scruton Ltd, 4 Barker Lane, York, UK.

Hasenclever, Ger. Waldemar Hasenclever GmbH, Germany.

Hassle, Norw. See *Astra, Norw.*

Hassle, Swed. Hässle Läkemedel AB, 431 83 Molndal, Sweden.

Hauck, USA. See *Roberts, USA.*

Haupt, Switz. Medidenta AG, Schachenstrasse 2, 9016 St Gallen, Switzerland.

Hausmann, Irl. See *Clonmel, Irl.*

Hausmann, Switz. Laboratoires Hausmann SA, Case postale, 9001 St Gallen, Switzerland.

Haw Par, Canad. Haw Par Brothers International Ltd, P.O. Box 4129, Vancouver, BC, V6B 3Z6, Canada.

Health & Medical, USA. See *Graham-Field, USA.*

Health Care Products, USA. Health Care Products, 369 Bayview Ave, Amityville, New York, NY 11701, USA.

Health for Life, USA. Health for Life Brands Inc., 1643 E Genesee St, Syracuse, NY 13210, USA.

Health Perception, UK. Health Perception Ltd (UK), Woodbine Stores Cottage, Chavey Down Rd, Winkfield Row, Bracknell, Berks, RG42 7NY, UK.

Healthcrafts, UK. Healthcrafts Ltd, Beaver House, York Close, Byfleet, Surrey, KT14 7HN, UK.

Healtheze, UK. Healtheze Ltd, Burleigh Manor, Peel Rd, Douglas, Isle of Man, UK.

Healthfirst, USA. Healthfirst Corp., 22316 70th Ave W, Mountlake Terrace, WA 98043, USA.

Healthline, USA. Healthline Laboratories Inc., 1601 Brookfield Ave, Ste A1, Green Bay, WI 54313-8855, USA.

Heel, Ger. Biologische Heilmittel Heel GmbH, Dr-Reckeweg-Str. 2-4, Postfach: 729, 76484 Baden-Baden, Germany.

Hefa, Ger. Hefa Pharma Vertriebs GmbH & Co. KG, Bahnhof 1-3, Postfach: 1252, 59355 Werne, Germany.

Heilit, Ger. Heilit Arzneimittel GmbH, Danziger Strasse 5, Postfach: 1248, 21452 Reinbek, Germany.

Hek, Ger. Hek Pharma GmbH, Sellhopsweg 1, Postfach: 610425, 2000 Hamburg 61, Germany.

Helago, Ger. Helago-Pharma GmbH, Koblenzer Strasse 93, Postfach: 200652, 53136 Bonn, Germany.

Helena, USA. Helena Laboratories, 1530 Lindbergh Dr, P.O. Box 752, Beaumont, TX 77704, USA.

Helixor, Ger. Helixor Heilmittel GmbH & Co., Hofgut Fischermuhle, Postfach: 8, 72344 Rosenfeld, Germany.

Helopharm, Ger. Helopharm W. Petrik GmbH & Co. KG, Waldstrasse 23-24, 13403 Berlin, Germany.

Helsinn, Switz. Helsinn Pharma AG, Switzerland.

Helsinn Birex, Irl. Helsinn Birex Pharmaceuticals Ltd, Unit 4, Heather Industrial Park, Heather Rd, Sandyford Industrial Estate, Dublin 18, Ireland.

Helvepharm, Switz. Helvepharm AG, Route Andre-Piller 2, Postfach 76, 1762 Givisiez, Switzerland.

HemispheRx, USA. HemispheRx, 1617 John F Kennedy Blvd, Philadelphia, PA 19103, USA.

Henk, Ger. See *Dolorgiet, Ger.*

Henkel, Ger. Henkel Hygiene GmbH, Reisholzer Werftstr. 36-42, Postfach: 130406, 40554 Dusseldorf, Germany.

Henkel, Ital. Henkel Ecolab s.p.a., Via Paracelso 6, 20041 Agrate Brianza (MI), Italy.

Henleys, UK. Henleys Medical Supplies Ltd, Brownfields, Welwyn Garden City, Herts, AL7 1AN, UK.

Hennig, Ger. Hennig Arzneimittel GmbH & Co. KG, Liebigstrasse 1-2, Postfach: 1240, 65433 Florsheim am Main, Germany.

Henning, Ger. Henning Berlin GmbH, Komturstrasse 58-62, Postfach: 420732, 12067 Berlin, Germany.

Henning, Switz. See *Marion Merrell Dow, Switz.*

Henning Walldorf, Ger. Dr. Georg Friedrich Henning, Chemische Fabrik Walldorf GmbH, Robert-Bosch-Strasse 62, Postfach: 1232, 69183 Walldorf, Germany.

Hepatoum, Fr. Laboratoires Hepatoum, B.P. 5, 03270 Saint-Yorre, France.

Herbal Laboratories, UK. Herbal Laboratories Ltd, Pierpoint House, 1 Beach Rd, St Annes-on-Sea, Lancs, FY8 2NR, UK.

Herbaline, Ital. Herbaline snc di Ugo Venara & C, Via dell'Artigianato 13, 13040 Rovasenda (VC), Italy.

Herbamed, Switz. Herbamed AG, Untere Au, 9055 Buhler, Switzerland.

Herbapharm, Ger. Herbapharm GmbH, Postfach: 1211, 79326 Teningen, Germany.

Herbaxt, Fr. Laboratoires Herbaxt, Z.I. Nord, bat 5, 77200 Torcy, France.

Herbert, Canad. L Herbert Dist., 5157 boul Pierre Bernard, Montreal, QC, H1K 2R8, Canada.

Herbert, Ger. Herbert Arzneimittel GmbH, Kreuzberger Ring 13, 65205 Wiesbaden, Germany.

Herbes Universelles, Canad. Herbes Universelles, 7 70e Ave O, Blainville, QC, J7C 1R7, Canada.

Herbrand, Ger. Dr Herbrand KG, chem.-pharm. Werk, Brambachstrasse 31, Postfach: 1107, 77717 Gengenbach, Germany.

Herchemie, Aust. Herchemie, Hasnerstrasse 7, 9020 Klagenfurt, Austria.

Hercon, USA. Hercon Laboratories Corp., York, PA 17405, USA.

Herdel, Ital. Herdel s.r.l., Italy.

Hermal, Ger. Hermal Kurt Herrmann (Merck-Gruppe), Scholtzstr. 3, 21465 Reinbek, Germany.

Hermal, Neth. See *E. Merck, Neth.*

Hermal, Norw. See *Meda, Norw.*

Hermal, Switz. See *E. Merck, Switz.*

Hermal, USA. Hermal Pharmaceutical Laboratories Inc., Route 145, Oak Hill, NY 12460, USA.

Hermes, Ger. Hermes Arzneimittel GmbH, Georg-Kalb-Strasse 5-8, 82049 Grosshesselohe/Munich, Germany.

Herzpunkt, Ger. Herzpunkt-Pharma GmbH, Binger Strasse 80, Postfach: 1220, 56136 Boppard/Bad Salzig, Germany.

Hestag, Aust. Hestag GmbH, Kreitnergasse 1-3, 1171 Vienna, Austria.

Heumann, Ger. Heumann Pharma GmbH, Heideloffstrasse 18-28, Postfach: 2260, 90009 Nurnberg, Germany.

Heumann, Switz. See *Searle, Switz.*

Hevert, Ger. Hevert-Arzneimittel GmbH & Co. KG, Eckweilerstrasse 10-12, Postfach: 61, 55560 Nussbaum bei Bad Sobernheim, Germany.

Hexal, Aust. Hexal Pharma GmbH, Wolfganggasse 45-7, 1120 Vienna, Austria.

Hexal, Austral. Hexal, Australia.

Hexal, Ger. Hexal AG, Industriestr. 25, Postfach: 1263, 83602 Holzkirchen, Germany.

Hexal, S.Afr. Hexal, S. Africa.

Heyl, Ger. Heyl Chemisch-pharmazeutische Fabrik GmbH & Co. KG, Goerzallee 253, 14167 Berlin, Germany.

Hickam, USA. Dow B. Hickam Inc., P.O. Box 2006, Sugar Land, TX 77487-2006, USA.

High Chemical, USA. High Chemical Co., Division of Day & Frick Inc., 1760 N Howard St, Philadelphia, PA 19122, USA.

Hilarys, Canad. Hilarys Salemaster Ltd, 330 Esna Park Drive, Unit 38, Markham, ON, L3R 1H3, Canada.

Hill, USA. Hill Dermaceuticals Inc., P.O. Box 149283, Orlando, FL 32814, USA.

Hillcross, UK. Hillcross Pharmaceuticals, Talbot St, Briercliffe, Burnley, Lancs, BB10 2JY, UK.

Himmel, USA. Himmel Pharmaceuticals Inc., P.O. Box 5479, Lake Worth, FL 33466-5479, USA.

Hirsch, USA. Hirsch Industries Inc., 4912 West Broad St, Richmond, VA 23230-0974, USA.
Hobein, Ger. Dr. Hobein & Co. Nachf. GmbH Arzneimittel, Grenzstrasse 2, Postfach: 1160, 53333 Meckenheim, Germany.
Hochstetter, Aust. Hochstetter & Co. GmbH, Brahmsplatz 4, 1040 Vienna, Austria.
Hoechst, Aust. Hoechst Austria AG, Altmannsdorfer Strasse 104, 1121 Vienna, Austria.
Hoechst, Austral. See *Hoechst Marion Roussel, Austral.*
Hoechst, Belg. See *Hoechst Marion Roussel, Belg.*
Hoechst, Canad. See *Hoechst Marion Roussel, Canad.*
Hoechst, Fr. Laboratoires Hoechst, Tour Roussel-Hoechst, 1 terrasse Bellini, 92910 Paris-La-Defense cdx, France.
Hoechst, Ger. Hoechst AG, Hoechst Marion Roussel Deutschland, Konigsteiner Str. 10, Postfach: 1109, 65796 Bad Soden am Ts, Germany.
Hoechst, Neth. See *Hoechst Marion Roussel, Neth.*
Hoechst, Spain. See *Hoechst Marion Roussel, Spain.*
Hoechst, Swed. See *Hoechst Marion Roussel, Swed.*
Hoechst, UK. See *Hoechst Roussel, UK.*
Hoechst, USA. See *Hoechst Roussel, USA.*
Hoechst Marion Roussel, Austral. Hoechst Marion Roussel (Australia) Pty Ltd, 27 Sirus Rd, Lane Cove, NSW 2066, Australia.
Hoechst Marion Roussel, Belg. Hoechst Marion Roussel SA, Extensa Square, Rue Colonel Bourg 155, 1140 Brussels, Belgium.
Hoechst Marion Roussel, Canad. Hoechst Marion Roussel Canada Inc., 2150 St-Elzear Blvd W, Laval, Quebec, H7L 4A8, Canada.
Hoechst Marion Roussel, Irl. Hoechst Marion Roussel Ireland Ltd, Cookstown Industrial Estate, Tallaght, Dublin 24, Ireland.
Hoechst Marion Roussel, Ital. Hoechst Marion Roussel Italia s.p.a., Via Marco Ulio Traiano 18, 20149 Milan, Italy.
Hoechst Marion Roussel, Neth. Hoechst Marion Roussel B.V., Postbus 100, 3870 CC Hoevelaken, Netherlands.
Hoechst Marion Roussel, Norw. Hoechst Marion Roussel AS, Okernveien 145, Postboks 232 Okern, N-0510 Oslo, Norway.
Hoechst Marion Roussel, S.Afr. Hoechst Marion Roussel Pharmaceuticals (Pty) Ltd, S. Africa.
Hoechst Marion Roussel, Spain. Hoechst Marion Roussel, Ronda General Mitre 72-4, 08017 Barcelona, Spain.
Hoechst Marion Roussel, Swed. Hoechst Marion Roussel AB, Bryggvagen 16-18, 117 68 Stockholm, Sweden.
Hoechst Marion Roussel, Switz. Hoechst Marion Roussel, a divivsion of Hoechst-Pharma SA, Herostrasse 7, 8048 Zurich, Switzerland.
Hoechst Marion Roussel, UK. Hoechst Marion Roussel, Broadwater Park, Denham, Uxbridge, Middx, UB9 5HP, UK.
Hoechst Marion Roussel, USA. Hoechst Marion Roussel, P.O. Box 9627, Kansas City, MO 64134, USA.
Hoechst Roussel, UK. See *Hoechst Marion Roussel, UK.*
Hoechst Roussel, USA. Hoechst-Roussel Pharm. Inc., Route 202-6, P.O. Box 2500, Somerville, NJ 08876-1258, USA.
Hoernecke, Ger. Carl Hoernecke GmbH Magdeburg Fabrik chem. pharm. Praparate, Halberstadter Chaussee 22, 39116 Magdeburg, Germany.
Hofmann, Aust. Hofmann Pharma GmbH & Co. KG, Postfach 7, 5081 Anif 36 (Salzburg), Austria.
Hofmann & Sommer, Ger. Hofmann & Sommer GmbH & Co. KG Chemisch-phamazeutische Fabrik, Lindenstr. 11, 07426 Konigsee, Germany.
Hogapharm, Switz. Hogapharm AG, Unterdorf 8, 6403 Kussnacht am Rigi, Switzerland.
Hogil, USA. Hogil Pharmaceutical Corporation, 1 Byram Brook Place, Armonk, New York, NY 10504, USA.
Hokuriku, Jpn. Hokuriku Seiyaku Co. Ltd, 25-5 Sendagaya 5-chome, Shibuya-ku, Tokyo 151, Japan.
Holistica, Fr. Laboratoires Holistica International, 6 parc des Jalassieres, 13510 Eguilles, France.
Hollborn, Ger. Dr K Hollborn & Sohne GmbH & Co. KG, Brahestr. 13, 04347 Leipzig, Germany.
Hollister-Stier, USA. See *MGI, USA.*
Holloway, USA. Holloway Pharmaceuticals Inc., USA.
Holsten, Ger. Holsten Pharma GmbH, Burgerstock, 79241 Ihringen, Germany.
Holzinger, Aust. Dr. et Mr. L. Holzinger pharm. Erzeugungs- und Vertrieb GmbH, Matznergasse 17, 1140 Vienna, Austria.
Homberger, Switz. Laboratoire du Dr E Homberger SA, 10 place du Bourg-de-Four, 1204 Geneva, Switzerland.
Home, Ital. Home Products Italiana s.p.a., Via Puccini 3, 20121 Milan, Italy.
Home Diagnostics, USA. Home Diagnostics Inc., USA.
Homeocan, Canad. Homeocan, 1900 rue Ste-Catherine E, Montreal, QC, H2K 2H5, Canada.
Homeopathie Boribel, Fr. See *Plantes et Medecines, Fr.*
Homeopathie Complexe, Fr. See *Abbe Chaupitre, Fr.*
Homme de Fer, Fr. Laboratoires de l'Homme de Fer, 2 pl. de l'Homme de Fer, 67000 Strasbourg, France.
Hommel, Ger. Chemische Werke Hommel GmbH, Carl-Sonnenschein-Str. 32a, Postfach: 1662, 59336 Ludinghausen, Germany.
Hope, USA. Hope Pharmaceuticals, 2961 W. MacArthur Blvd, Suite 130, Santa Ana, California, CA 92704, USA.
Hor-Fer-Vit, Ger. HorFerVit Pharma GmbH, H.-Brockmann Str. 81, Postfach: 2329, 26013 Oldenburg, Germany.
Horizon, USA. Horizon Pharmaceutical Corp, 1125 Northmeadow Parkway, Suite 130, Roswell, Georgia, GA 30076, USA.
Hormonchemie, Ger. Hormon-Chemie München GmbH, Freisinger Landstrasse 74, Postfach: 450361, 8000 Munich 45, Germany.
Hormosan, Ger. Hormosan-Kwizda GmbH, Wilhelmshoher Strasse 106, Postfach: 600340, 60333 Frankfurt/Main, Germany.
Horner, Canad. See *Carter Horner, Canad.*
Hortel, Spain. Hortel, +34a de Cieza 58, Abaran, 30550 Murcia, Spain.
Hosbon, Spain. Hosbon, Ronda General Mitre 72-4, 08017 Barcelona, Spain.
Hospamed, Swed. Hospamed AB, Box 721, 503 16 Boras, Sweden.
Hotz, Ger. Dr. W. Hotz & Co. KG Nachf., Gartenstrasse 33, Postfach: 2104, D-61250 Usingen, Germany.
Houde, Fr. Laboratoires Houdé, 1 Terrasse Bellini, 92910 Paris-La Defense cdx, France.
Houghs Healthcare, UK. Houghs Healthcare Ltd, 22 Chapel St, Levenshulme, Manchester, M19 3PT, UK.
Hoveler, Aust. Höveler Mag. & Co. GmbH, Mosham 40, 4943 Geinberg, Austria.
Howmedica, Switz. Howmedica Jaquet Orthopedie SA, Case postale 725, 1212 Grand-Lancy 1/GE, Switzerland.
Hoyer, Ger. Hoyer GmbH & Co. Pharmazeutische Präparate, Alfred-Nobel-Str. 10, 40789 Monheim, Germany.
Huckaby, USA. Huckaby Pharmacal Inc., 104 E Main St, LaGrange, KY 40031, USA.
Hudson, USA. Hudson Corp., 90 Orville Drive, Bohemia, NY 11716, USA.
Hughes & Hughes, UK. Hughes & Hughes Ltd, Unit 1F, Lowmoor Industrial Estate, Tonedale, Wellington, Somerset, TA21 0AZ, UK.
Huls, Ger. See *Athenstaedt, Ger.*
Humana, Ital. Humana Italia s.p.a., Via Boscovich 55, 20124 Milan, Italy.
Husler, Switz. Franz Hüsler AG, Pharmazeutische Präparate, Chriesbaumstrasse 2, 8604 Volketswil, Switzerland.
Hyde, Canad. Hyde Pharmaceuticals, Canada.
Hydro, Swed. Hydro Pharma AB, Box 50310, 202 13 Malmo, Sweden.
Hyland, USA. Baxter Hyland, Division of Baxter Healthcare, 550 North Brand Blvd, Glendale, CA 91203, USA.
Hylands, Canad. Hylands, 2360 Argentia Rd, Mississauga, Ontario, L5N 3P1, Canada.
Hypoguard, UK. Hypoguard (UK) Ltd, Dock Lane, Melton, Woodbridge, Suffolk, IP12 1PE, UK.
Hyrex, USA. Hyrex Pharmaceuticals, 3494 Democrat Rd, P.O. Box 18385, Memphis, TN 38118, USA.
I Farmacologia, Spain. I Farmacologia Española, Po de la Castellana 141, Edif. Cuzco IV, 28046 Madrid, Spain.
IAF Biovac, Canad. IAF Biovac Inc., P.O. Box 70, Laval, Quebec, H7N 4Z2, Canada.
Iatric, USA. Iatric Corp, 2330 S Industrial Park Drive, Tempe, AZ 85282-1893, USA.
Ibi, Ital. Istituto Biochimico Italiano Giovanni Lorenzini s.p.a., Via Ripamonti 332/4, 20141 Milan, Italy.
Ibirn, Ital. Istituto Bioterapico Nazionale s.r.l., Via V. Grassi 9/11/13/15, 00155 Rome, Italy.
IBIS, Ital. Istituto Biochimico Sperimentale s.p.a., Italy.
IBP, Ital. Istituto Biochimico Pavese s.p.a., Viale Certosa 10, 27100 Pavia, Italy.
IBSA, Ital. Ibsa Farmaceutici Italia srl, Viale Bianca Maria 31, 20122 Milan, Italy.
IBSA, Switz. Institut Biochimique SA, Via al Ponte 13, 6903 Lugano, Switzerland.
IBYS, Spain. Instituto de Biologia y Sueroterapia, Antonio Lopez 111, 28026 Madrid, Spain.
Ichthyol, Aust. Österreichische Ichthyol GmbH nunmehr KG, 6100 Seefeld/Tirol, Austria.
Ichthyol, Ger. Ichthyol-Gesellschaft Cordes, Hermanni & Co., Sportallee 85, Postfach: 630361, 22313 Hamburg, Germany.
Ichthyol, Switz. See *Diethelm, Switz.*
ICI, Austral. ICI Australia Operations Pty Ltd, P.O. Box 4311, Melbourne, Vic. 3001, Australia.
ICI, Ger. See *Zeneca, Ger.*
ICI, Ital. See *Zeneca, Ital.*
ICI, Neth. See *Zeneca, Neth.*
ICI, UK. See *Zeneca, UK.*
ICIM, Ital. Istituto Chimico Italiano Milano s.a.s., Via Peloritana 28, SS Varesina, 20024 Garbagnate M.se (MI), Italy.
ICN, Canad. ICN Canada Ltd, 1956 rue Bourdon, Montreal, Quebec, H4M 1V1, Canada.
ICN, Neth. ICN Pharmaceuticals Holland B.V., Stephensonstraat 45, 2723 RM Zoetermeer, Netherlands.
ICN, Spain. ICN Iberica, Casanova 27-31, Corbera de Llobregat, 08757 Barcelona, Spain.
ICN, UK. ICN Pharmaceuticals Inc., Eagle House, Peregrine Business Park, Gomm Rd, High Wycombe, Bucks, HP13 7DL, UK.
ICN, USA. ICN Pharmaceuticals Inc., ICN Plaza, 3300 Hyland Ave, Costa Mesa, CA 92626, USA.
ICT, Ital. Istituto Chemioterapico s.p.a., Strada Bobbiese 108, 29100 Piacenza, Italy.
ICT-Lodi, Ital. See *ICT, Ital.*
Ideal, Fr. Ideal, 65 rue Alexandre-Dumas, BP 53, 69513 Vaulx-en-Velin cdx, France.
IDEC, USA. IDEC Pharmaceuticals, 11011 Torreyana Rd, San Diego, CA 92121, USA.
Iderne, Fr. Laboratoires Michel Iderne, Dpt Unipharma, Parc d'activites Rosenmeer, 67560 Rosheim, France.
IDI, Ital. IDI Farmaceutici s.p.a., Via dei Castelli Romani 83/85, 00040 Pomezia (Rome), Italy.
IDIS, UK. IDIS Ltd World Medicines, The Common, Potten End, Berkhamstead, Herts, HP4 2QF, UK.
Ido, Fr. Laboratoires Ido, 8-10 passage Beslay, 75011 Paris, France.
Iema, Ital. Iema s.r.l., Via Adelasio 33, 24020 Ranica (BG), Italy.
Ienapharm, Fr. Iénapharm, 41 rue d'Iena, 16000 Angouleme, France.
IFCI, Ital. Industria Clonesystems s.p.a., Via Dei Fornaciai 24, 40129 Bologna, Italy.
Ifesa, Spain. See *Astra, Spain.*
IFI, Ital. Istituto Farmacoterapico Italiano s.p.a., Via Paolo Frisi 23, 00197 Rome, Italy.
Ifidesa Aristegui, Spain. Ifidesa Aristegui, Alameda de Urquijo 27 1, Bilbao, 48008 Vizcaya, Spain.
Iketon, Ital. Iketon Farmaceutici s.r.l., Via Cassanese 224, 20090 Segrate (MI), Italy.
Ilex, Ital. Ilex Italiana s.r.l., Via Milano 160, 21042 Caronno Pertusella (VA), Italy.
Illa, Ger. ILLA Healthcare GmbH, Bahnhofstr. 15, 82515 Wolfratshausen, Germany.
Imba, Spain. Imba, Paseo Padre Feijoo 14, Ceuto, 11702 Cadiz, Spain.
Imeco, Swed. IMECO AB, 151 85 Sodertalje, Sweden.
I-Med, Canad. I-Med Pharma Inc., 3869 Sources Blvd, Suite 200, Dollard des Ormeaux, Quebec, H9B 2A2, Canada.
Immunex, USA. Immunex, 51 University St, Seattle, WA 98101, USA.
Immuno, Aust. Immuno AG, Industriestrasse 67, 1220 Vienna, Austria.
Immuno, Belg. S.A. Immuno, Rue Emile Feron 153, 1060 Brussels, Belgium.
Immuno, Canad. Immuno Canada Ltd, 6635 Kitimat Rd, Suite 30, Mississauga, Ontario, L5N 6J2, Canada.
Immuno, Fr. Immuno France SA, Parc d'Innovation, bd Gonthier-d'Andernach, 67400 Ilkirch-Graffenstaden, France.
Immuno, Ger. Immuno GmbH, Breitspiel 13, Postfach: 103080, 69020 Heidelberg, Germany.
Immuno, Irl. See *Allphar, Irl.*
Immuno, Ital. Immuno s.p.a., Via Cocchi 7-9, 56121 Pisa, Italy.
Immuno, Spain. Immuno, San Sebastian S/N, Sant Just Desvern, 08960 Barcelona, Spain.
Immuno, Swed. See *Baxter, Swed.*
Immuno, Switz. Immuno SA, Chriesbaumstrasse 2, 8604 Volketswil/ZH, Switzerland.
Immuno, UK. See *Baxter, UK.*
Immuno, USA. Immuno-U.S. Inc., 1200 Parkdale Road, Rochester, MI 48307, USA.
Immunomedics, USA. Immunomedics, 300 American Rd, Morris Plains, NJ 07950, USA.
Impharm, UK. Impharm Nationwide Ltd, Valley House, Britannia Business Park, Union Rd, Bolton, Lancs, BL2 2HP, UK.
IMS, Canad. International Medication Systems of Canada Ltd, 406 Watline Ave, Mississauga, Ontario, L4Z 1X2, Canada.
IMS, Ital. International Medical Service s.r.l., Via Lauretina Km 26500, 00040 Pomezia (RM), Italy.
IMS, UK. International Medication Systems (UK) Ltd, 11 Royal Oak Way South, Daventry, Northants, NN11 5PJ, UK.
IMS, USA. I.M.S. Ltd, 1886 Santa Anita Ave, South El Monte, CA 91733, USA.
Imtix, Fr. Imtix, Pasteur Merieux, 58 av Leclerc, 69007 Lyon, France.
Imtix, Ital. Imtix srl, Via Winckelmann 2, 20146 Milan, Italy.
Imtix, Neth. Imtix B.V., Postbus 2207, 1180 EE Amstelveen, Netherlands.
InAgra, USA. InAgra, USA.
Inava, Fr. Laboratoires Inava, département médical de Pierre-Fabre Médicament, 45 place Abel-Gance, 92100 Boulogne, France.
Inergie, Fr. Laboratoires Inergie, 42 rue de Longvic, 21300 Chenove, France.
Inexfa, Spain. Inexfa, Ctra Nacional 340, Km 28, Orihuela, 03300 Alicante, Spain.
Infar, Port. Infar - Indústria Farmacêutica, Lda, Estrada de circunvalacao, Rameiras, Alges, 1495 Lisbon, Portugal.
Infectopharm, Ger. Infectopharm Arzneimittel und Consilium GmbH, Von-Humboldt-Str. 1, 64646 Heppenheim, Germany.
Infirmarius-Rovit, Ger. Pharmazeutische Fabrik Infirmarius-Rovit GmbH, Eislinger Str. 66, Postfach: 1155, 73080 Salach, Germany.
Ingram & Bell, Canad. Ingram & Bell Inc., 20 Bond Ave, Don Mills, Ontario, M3B 1L9, Canada.
Inibsa, Spain. Inibsa, Ctra Sabadell Granollers Km 14.5, Llissa de Vall, 08185 Barcelona, Spain.
Inkeysa, Spain. Inkeysa, Juan XXIII 15, Esplugas de Llobregat, 08950 Barcelona, Spain.
Innotech, Fr. Sté du groupe Innothéra Industries, Innotech International, 7-9 av Francois-Vincent-Raspail, B.P. 32, 94111 Arcueil cdx, France.
Innothera, Fr. Sté du groupe Innothéra Industries, 10 ave P.-Vaillant-Couturier, B.P. 35, 94111 Arcueil Cdx, France.
Innothera, Switz. See *Interlabo, Switz.*
Innovex, UK. See *Novex Pharma, UK.*
InnoVisions, USA. Innovisions Inc., 6065 Frantz Rd, Suite 202, Dublin, OH 43017, USA.
Innovite, USA. Innovite, USA.
Innoxa, UK. Innoxa (England) Ltd, UK.
Inorgan, Switz. Inorgan SA, Case postale 162, 1215 Geneva 15, Switzerland.
Inpharma, Norw. Inpharma a.s., Industrig 15, Postboks 663, 3412 Lierstranda, Norway.
Inpharma, Swed. See *Inpharma, Norw.*

Inpharzam, Switz. Inpharzam SA, PO Box 200, 6814 Cadempino, Switzerland.
Instituto Farmacologico, Spain. Instituto Farmacologico, Ramallosa-Teo, Santiago de Compostela, 15883 La Coruna, Spain.
Intercare, Irl. See *Mayrs, Irl.*
Intercare, UK. Intercare Products Ltd, 7 The Business Centre, Molly Millars Lane, Wokingham, Berks, RG11 2QZ, UK.
Interdelta, Switz. Interdelta SA, Case postale 460, 1701 Fribourg, Switzerland.
Interfarma, Ital. Interfarma Farmaceutici s.r.l., Via Vivaldi 16, 35030 Selvazzano Dentro (PD), Italy.
Interlabo, Switz. Interlabo SA, Case postale 8, 42/44 rue Prevost-Martin, 1211 Geneva 9, Switzerland.
Intermedica, Switz. Intermedica SA Pharmazeutische Produkte, 91 rue de Lausanne, Case postale 238, 1701 Fribourg, Switzerland.
Intermuti, Ger. intermuti pharma GmbH, Postfach: 100662, 40770 Monheim, Germany.
International Dermatologicals, Canad. International Dermatologicals Inc., 1940 Lonsdale Ave, Ste 217A, Vancouver, BC, V7M 2K2, Canada.
International Ethical, USA. International Ethical Labs, Reparto Metropolitano, Rio Piedras, PR 00921, USA.
International Pharmaceutical, USA. See *Marion Laboratories, USA.*
International Research, Austral. International Research Pharmaceuticals, 1/32 Leighton Place, Hornsby, NSW 2077, Australia.
Interpharm, Aust. Interpharm GmbH, Effingergasse 21, 1160 Vienna, Austria.
Interpharma, Spain. Interpharma, Santa Rosa 6, Santa Coloma de Gramanet, 08921 Barcelona, Spain.
Intersan, Ger. Intersan, Institut fur pharmazeutische und klinische Forschung GmbH, Einsteinstrasse 30, Postfach: 413, 76258 Ettlingen, Germany.
Intersan, Switz. See *Uhlmann-Eyraud, Switz.*
Interstate Drug Exchange, USA. Interstate Drug Exchange, 1500 New Horizons Blvd, Amityville, NY 11701-1130, USA.
Intervet, Switz. Intervet AG, Postfach 129, Churerstrasse 160b, 8808 Pfaffikon SZ, Switzerland.
INTES, Ital. Industria Terapeutica Splendore, Oftalmoterapica ALFA, Via F.lli Bandiera 26, 80026 Casoria (NA), Italy.
Intra Pharma, Irl. Intra Pharma Ltd, 86 Broomhill Road, Tallaght, Dublin 24, Ireland.
Intramed, S.Afr. Intramed, S. Africa.
Intraveno, Irl. IntraVeno Healthcare Ltd, 86 Broomhill Rd, Tallaght, Dublin 24, Ireland.
Invamed, USA. Invamed Inc., 2400 Rt 130 North, Dayton, NJ 08810, USA.
Inverdia, Swed. Inverdia AB, Vretenvagen 8, 171 54 Solna, Sweden.
Inverni della Beffa, Ital. Inverni della Beffa s.p.a. (Gruppo Synthelabo), Via Rivoltana 13, 20090 Segrate (MI), Italy.
Invicta, Irl. See *Pfizer, Irl.*
Invicta, UK. See *Pfizer, UK.*
Invitech, UK. Invitech Ltd, 15 Witney Way, Boldon Business Park, Tyne & Wear, NE35 9PE, UK.
Inwood, USA. Inwood Laboratories, Subsidiary of Forest Laboratories, 300 Prospect St, Inwood, NY 11696, USA.
Iodosan, Ital. Iodosan S.p.A., Via Zambeletti, 20021 Baranzate di Bollate (MI), Italy.
Iolab, Canad. Iolab Pharmaceuticals, 1421 Lansdowne St W., Peterborough, Ontario, K9J 7B9, Canada.
Iolab, Norw. See *Johnson & Johnson, Norw.*
Iolab, USA. Iolab Pharmaceuticals, 500 Iolab Drive, Claremont, CA 91711, USA.
Iomed, USA. Iomed Laboratories, Inc., 7425 Pebble Drive, Fort Worth, TX 76118, USA.
Ion, USA. Ion Laboratories Inc., 7431 Pebble Drive, Fort Worth, TX 76118, USA.
Ioquin, Austral. See *Alcon, Austral.*
IPA, Ital. International Pharmaceuticals Associated s.r.l., Via del Casale Cavallari 53, 00156 Rome, Italy.
Ipex, Swed. Ipex Medical AB, Box 1266, 172 25 Sundbyberg, Sweden.
IPFI, Ital. I.P.F.I., Industria Farmaceutica s.r.l., Via Egadi 7, 20144 Milan, Italy.
Iphym, Fr. Laboratoires Iphym, chemin de la Sereine, B.P. 243, 01704 Beynost Cedex, France.
IPIT, Ital. Ist. Profil. Ital. s.r.l., Via Valletta 58, 10040 Leini (TO), Italy.
IPRAD, Fr. Laboratoires I.P.R.A.D., 42-52 rue de l'Aqueduc, 75010 Paris, France.
Ipropharm, Fr. Laboratoires Ipropharm, 192 av de Lodeve, 34000 Montpellier, France.
IPS, Neth. IPS, Beeldschermweg 6b, 3821 AH Amersfoort, Netherlands.
Ipsen, Belg. N.V. Ipsen S.A., Maaltecenter, Blok A, Derbystraat 201, 9051 Gent, Belgium.
IPSEN, Fr. Institut de Produits de Synthèse et d'Extraction Naturelle, 24 rue Erlanger, 75781 Paris Cdx 16, France.
Ipsen, Irl. Ipsen Pharmaceuticals Ltd, 7 Upper Leeson St, Dublin 4, Ireland.
Ipsen, Ital. Ipsen s.p.a., Via Ripamonti 332/4, 20141 Milano, Italy.
Ipsen, UK. Ipsen Ltd, 1 Bath Rd, Maidenhead, Berks, SL6 4UH, UK.
IPSEN Biotech, Fr. IPSEN/Biotech, 24 rue Erlanger, 75781 Paris Cdx, France.
Ipso, Ital. Ipso-Pharma, Via San Rocco 6, 85033 Episcopia (PZ), Italy.
Iquinosa, Spain. Iquinosa, Alpedrete 24, 28045 Madrid, Spain.
IRBI, Ital. IRBI s.p.a., Via Pontina 28, 00040 Pomezia (Rome), Italy.
Ircafarm, Ital. Ircafarm s.r.l., Societa del Gruppo Restiva, SS 156 Km 50, 04010 Borgo S Michele (LT), Italy.
Irex, Fr. Laboratoires Irex, B.P. 28, 13713 La Penne-sur-Huveaune cdx, France.
Irmed, Ital. Istituto Ricerche Mediche s.r.l., Via della Consortia 17, 37100 Verona, Italy.
Irmesan, Spain. Irmesan, Ronda de Poniente 2, Edificio Euronova 2A, Tres Cantos, 28760 Madrid, Spain.
Iromedica, Switz. Iromedica SA, Haggenstrasse 45, 9014 St Gallen, Switzerland.
Isdin, Spain. Isdin, Av. Diagonal 520, 08006 Barcelona, Spain.
ISF, Ital. ISF s.p.a., Italy.
ISI, Ital. Istituto Sierovaccinogeno Italiano s.p.a., 55020 Castelvecchio Pascoli (LU), Italy.
Isis, Ger. Isis Pharma GmbH, Postfach: 200557, 08005 Zwickau, Germany.
Isis, UK. Isis Products Ltd, Gough Lane, Bamber Bridge, Preston, Lancs, PR5 6AQ, UK.
Isis, USA. Isis Pharm, USA.
Isis Puren, Ger. See *Isis, Ger.*
ISM, Ital. Ist. Sieroterapico Milanese S. Belfanti, Via Darwin 22, 20143 Milan, Italy.
Ismunit, Ital. Istituto Immunologico Italiano s.r.l., Via Castagnetta 7, 00040 Pomezia (Rome), Italy.
Isnardi, Ital. Pietro Isnardi & C. s.p.a., Via XXV Aprile 69, 18100 Imperia Oneglia, Italy.
Iso, Ger. Iso-Arzneimittel GmbH & Co. KG, Bunsenstrasse 6-10, Postfach: 447, 76258 Ettlingen, Germany.
Isopharm, Fr. Laboratoires Isopharm, 1 rue Blaise-Pascal, Parc de Pissaloup, 78190 Trappes, France.
Isotec, Fr. Isotec, BP 220, 78051 Saint-Quentin-en-Yvelines Cdx, France.
Ist. Chim. Inter., Ital. Istituto Chimico Internazionale Dr. Giuseppe Rende s.r.l., Via Salaria 1240, 00138 Rome, Italy.
Istoria, Ital. Istoria Farmaceutici s.p.a., Riviera Francia 3/A, 35127 Padova, Italy.
ITA, Ital. Istituto Terapeutico Ambrosiano s.r.l., Italy.
Ital Suisse, Ital. Ital Suisse Co. s.a.s. di Giancarlo Ceroni & C., Italy.
Italchimici, Ital. Italchimici s.p.a., Via Pontina Km 29000, No 5, 00040 Pomezia (RM), Italy.
Italfarmaco, Ital. Italfarmaco s.p.a., Viale Fulvio Testi 330, 20126 Milan, Italy.
Italfarmaco, Spain. Italfarmaco, San Rafael 3, Alcobendas, 28100 Madrid, Spain.
Italzama, Ital. Italzama, Via Leonardo da Vinci 75, 00016 Monterotondo Scalo (RM), Italy.
Ivamed, Ger. IVAmed Arzneimittel GmbH, Janderstr. 9, 68199 Mannheim, Germany.
Ivex, UK. Ivex Pharmaceuticals, Division of the Galen Group, Old Belfast Rd, Millbrook, Larne, Co. Antrim, BT40 2SH, UK.
IVP, Ital. Istituto Vaccinogeno Pozzi s.p.a., Via Petriccio 27, 53100 Siena, Italy.
Iyakuhin Kogyo, Jpn. Nihon Iyakuhin Kogyo Co. Ltd, 1-6-21 Sogata, Toyama-shi, Toyama 930, Japan.
Jaapharm, Canad. Jaapharm, 200 Trowers Rd, Unit 1, Woodbridge, ON, L4L 5Z7, Canada.
Jacobs, UK. Jacobs Bakery Ltd, Suttons Business Park, Earley, Reading, Berks, RG6 1AZ, UK.
Jacobus, USA. Jacobus Pharmaceutical Co. Inc., 37 Cleveland Lane, P.O. Box 5290, Princeton, NJ 08540, USA.
Jacoby, Aust. Jacoby Pharmazeutika GmbH, Teichweg 2, 5400 Hallein-Kaltenhausen, Austria.
Jacomedic, Norw. Jacomedic AS, Sjog 11, 1516 Moss, Norway.
Jaldes, Fr. Laboratoires Jaldes, La Chaze, B.P. 84, 07600 Vals-Les-Bains, France.
Jamieson, Canad. C.E. Jamieson & Co. (Dom.) Ltd, 4025 Rhodes Drive, Windsor, Ontario, N8W 5B5, Canada.
Jamol, USA. Jamol Laboratories Inc., 13 Ackerman Ave, Emerson, NJ 07630, USA.
Jan, Canad. Jan Distributing, 100 West Beaver Creek Rd, Unit 2, Richmond Hill, Ontario, L4B 1H4, Canada.
Janpharm, S.Afr. See *Janssen-Cilag, S.Afr.*
Janssen, Belg. See *Janssen-Cilag, Belg.*
Janssen, Canad. See *Janssen-Ortho, Canad.*
Janssen, Ger. See *Janssen-Cilag, Ger.*
Janssen, Neth. See *Janssen-Cilag, Neth.*
Janssen, Spain. See *Janssen-Cilag, Spain.*
Janssen, Swed. See *Janssen-Cilag, Swed.*
Janssen, UK. See *Janssen-Cilag, UK.*
Janssen, USA. Janssen Pharmaceutical Inc., 1125 Trenton-Harbourton Road, P.O. Box 200, Titusville, NJ 08560, USA.
Janssen-Cilag, Aust. Janssen-Cilag Pharma Vertrieb GmbH, Pfarrgasse 75, 1232 Vienna, Austria.
Janssen-Cilag, Austral. Janssen-Cilag Pty Ltd, Locked Bag 30, P.O. Lane Cove, NSW 2066, Australia.
Janssen-Cilag, Belg. Janssen-Cilag S.A., Uitbreidingstraat 2, 2600 Berchem, Belgium.
Janssen-Cilag, Fr. Janssen-Cilag SA, 17 rue de l'Ancienne-Mairie, 92513 Boulogne-Billancourt cdx, France.
Janssen-Cilag, Ger. Janssen-Cilag GmbH, Postfach, 41457 Neuss, Germany.
Janssen-Cilag, Irl. Janssen-Cilag Ltd, Pharmapark, Chapelizod, Dublin 20, Ireland.
Janssen-Cilag, Ital. Janssen-Cilag s.p.a., Via M Buonarroti 23, 20093 Cologno Monzese (MI), Italy.
Janssen-Cilag, Neth. Janssen-Cilag B.V., Postbus 90240, 5000 LT Tilburg, Netherlands.
Janssen-Cilag, Norw. Janssen-Cilag AS, Postboks 143 Holmlia, 1203 Oslo, Norway.
Janssen-Cilag, S.Afr. Janssen-Cilag Pharmaceutica (Pty) Ltd, P.O. Box 785939, Sandton 2146, S. Africa.
Janssen-Cilag, Spain. Janssen-Cilag, P. de las Doce Estrellas 5-7, Campo de Naciones, 28042 Madrid, Spain.
Janssen-Cilag, Swed. Janssen-Cilag AB, Box 7073, 192 07 Sollentuna, Sweden.
Janssen-Cilag, Switz. Janssen-Cilag AG, Sihlbruggstrasse 111, CH-6341 Baar, Switzerland.
Janssen-Cilag, UK. Janssen-Cilag Ltd, P.O. Box 79, Saunderton, High Wycombe, Bucks, HP14 4HJ, UK.
Janssen-Ortho, Canad. Janssen-Ortho Inc., 19 Green Belt Drive, North York, Ontario, M3C 1L9, Canada.
Jauntal, Aust. Jauntal-Apotheke, Bleiburger Strasse 16, 9141 Eberndorf, Austria.
JB Williams, USA. J. B. Williams Co. Inc., 65 Harriston Road, Glen Rock, New Jersey, NJ 07452, USA.
JCP, Canad. JCP Laboratories Inc., P.O. Box 403, St-Martin Branch, Laval, QC, H7S 2A4, Canada.
Jenapharm, Ger. Jenapharm GmbH, Otto-Schott-Strasse 15, 07745 Jena, Germany.
Jergens, USA. Jergens, USA.
Jessel, Fr. Laboratoires Jessel-Végébom S.A., 59 av. d'Iena, 75116 Paris, France.
JHC Healthcare, UK. See *Distriphar, UK.*
J&J, S.Afr. See *Janssen-Cilag, S.Afr.*
J&J-Merck, USA. See *Johnson & Johnson Medical, USA,* and *Merck Sharp & Dohme, USA.*
JMI, USA. JMI-Canton Pharmaceuticals, 119 Schroyer Ave SW, Canton, OH 44702, USA.
Jodquellen, Ger. Jodquellen AG, Ludwigstrasse 14, Postfach: 2148, 83640 Bad Tolz, Germany.
John Wyeth, Irl. John Wyeth & Brother Ltd, 765 South Circular Rd, Islandbridge, Dublin 8, Ireland.
Johnson, Canad. S.C. Johnson and Son Ltd, 1 Webster St, Brantford, Ontario, N3T 5R1, Canada.
Johnson & Johnson, Aust. Johnson & Johnson GmbH, Weisslhofweg 9, 5400 Hallein, Austria.
Johnson & Johnson, Austral. Johnson & Johnson Medical Pty Ltd, P.O. Box 134, North Ryde, NSW 2113, Australia.
Johnson & Johnson, Canad. Johnson & Johnson Inc., 7101 Notre Dame St, Montreal, Quebec, H1N 2G4, Canada.
Johnson & Johnson, Ger. Johnson & Johnson Medical GmbH, Oststrasse 1, Postfach: 1680, 22806 Norderstedt, Germany.
Johnson & Johnson, Irl. Johnson & Johnson (Ireland) Ltd, Belgard Rd, Tallaght, Dublin 24, Ireland.
Johnson & Johnson, Ital. Johnson & Johnson Divisione Farmacia s.p.a., 00040 S. Palomba, Pomezia (Rome), Italy.
Johnson & Johnson, Norw. Johnson & Johnson AB, Ravnsborgv 52, 1364 Hvalstad, Norway.
Johnson & Johnson, Spain. Johnson Johnson, Ctra Madrid-Valencia Km 24.7, Arganda del Rey, 28500 Madrid, Spain.
Johnson & Johnson, Swed. Johnson & Johnson AB, 191 84 Sollentuna, Sweden.
Johnson & Johnson, Switz. Johnson & Johnson SA, Rotzenbuhlstrasse 55, 8957 Spreitenbach 1, Switzerland.
Johnson & Johnson, UK. Johnson & Johnson Ltd, Foundation Park, Rocksborough Way, Maidenhead, Berks, SL6 3UG, UK.
Johnson & Johnson, USA. Johnson & Johnson, Grandview Rd, Skillman, NJ 08558-9418, USA.
Johnson & Johnson Medical, Fr. Laboratoires Johnson & Johnson Médical, 1 Centrale Parc, av Sully-Prudhomme, 92298 Chatenay-Malabry cdx, France.
Johnson & Johnson Medical, UK. Johnson & Johnson Medical, Coronation Rd, Ascot, Berks, SL5 9EY, UK.
Johnson & Johnson Medical, USA. Johnson & Johnson Medical Inc., 2500 Arbrook Blvd, Arlington, TX 76014, USA.
Johnson & Johnson MSD Consumer, UK. Johnson & Johnson MSD Consumer Pharmaceuticals, Enterprise House, Station Rd, Loudwater, High Wycombe, Bucks, HP10 9UF, UK.
Jolly-Jatel, Fr. Laboratoires Jolly-Jatel, 28 av. Carnot, 78100 Saint-Germain-en-Laye, France.
Jones, USA. Jones Medical Industries Inc., P.O. Box 46903, St Louis, MO 63146-6903, USA.
Jorba, Spain. Jorba, Josefa Valcarcel 30, 28027 Madrid, Spain.
Jossa-Arznei, Ger. See *Hexal, Ger.*
Jouveinal, Canad. Jouveinal Inc., 3339 Griffith St, St Laurent, Quebec, H4T 1W5, Canada.
Jouveinal, Fr. Laboratoires Jouveinal, 1 rue des Moissons, B.P. 100, 94265 Fresnes Cdx, France.
Jouveinal, Switz. See *Actipharm, Switz.*
Juanola, Spain. Juanola, Marti 131, 08024 Barcelona, Spain.
Jukunda, Ger. Jukunda Naturarzneimittel Dr Ludwig Schmitt GmbH & Co. KG, Postfach: 1330, 82142 Planegg, Germany.
Jumer, Fr. Laboratoires Jumer, 40 rue Lecuyer, 93300 Aubervilliers, France.
Juste, Spain. Juste, Julio Camba 7, 28028 Madrid, Spain.
Juventus, Spain. Juventus, Valentin Beato 44, 28037 Madrid, Spain.
Juvex, Fr. Laboratoires Juvex, B.P. 11, 36110 Levroux, France.
Kabi, Irl. See *Pharmacia Upjohn, Irl.*
Kabi, S.Afr. See *Keatings, S.Afr.*
Kabi, Swed. See *Pharmacia, Swed.*
Kabi, Switz. See *Pharmacia Upjohn, Switz.*
Kabi, UK. Kabi Pharmacia Ltd, Davy Ave, Knowlhill, Milton Keynes, MK5 8PH, UK.
Kabi Pharmacia, Aust. See *Pharmacia Upjohn, Aust.*
Kabi Pharmacia, Austral. See *Pharmacia Upjohn, Austral.*
Kabi Pharmacia, Belg. See *Pharmacia Upjohn, Belg.*
Kabi Pharmacia, Canad. See *Pharmacia, Canad.*
Kabi Pharmacia, Ger. See *Pharmacia Upjohn, Ger.*

Kabi Pharmacia, Neth. See *Hoechst Marion Roussel, Neth.*

Kabi Pharmacia, USA. Kabi Pharmacia, 800 Centennial Avenue, P.O. Box 1327, Piscataway, NJ 08855, USA.

Kabivitrum, Irl. See *Pharmacia Upjohn, Irl.*

KabiVitrum, UK. See *Kabi, UK.*

Kabivitrum, USA. KabiVitrum Inc., 160 Industrial Drive, Franklin, OH 45005, USA.

Kade, Ger. Dr Kade Pharmazeutische Fabrik GmbH, Rigistrasse 2, Postfach: 480209, 12252 Berlin, Germany.

Kade, S.Afr. See *Rhone-Poulenc Rorer, S.Afr.*

Kade, Switz. See *Doetsch, Grether, Switz.*

Kaken, Jpn. Kaken Pharmaceutical Co. Ltd, 4-8-14 Nihonbashi Honcho, Chuo-ku, Tokyo 103, Japan.

Kali, Aust. Kali Pharma GmbH, Donaustrasse 106, 3400 Klosterneuburg, Austria.

Kali-Chemie, Ger. See *Solvay, Ger.*

Kali-Chemie, Swed. See *Meda, Swed.*

Kalifarma, Spain. Kalifarma, Avda Diagonal 507-9, 08029 Barcelona, Spain.

Kallergen, Ital. Kallergen s.r.l., Via IV Novembre 76, 20019 Settimo Milanese (MI), Italy.

Kalopharma, Ital. Kalopharma s.p.a., Italy.

Kamfarma, Switz. Kamfarma SA, 6928 Manno, Switzerland.

Kanebo, Jpn. Kanebo, 1-3-12 Motoakasaka, Minato-ku, Tokyo, Japan.

Kanoldt, Ger. Kanoldt Arzneimittel GmbH, Kohlplatte 21-3, 89420 Hochstadt (Donau), Germany.

Kario, Fr. Laboratoires Kario-Derlka S.A., 224 av. Hoff, B.P. 59, 01302 Belley Cdx, France.

Karlspharma, Ger. Karlspharma Pharmazeutische Produkte GmbH, Germany.

Karrer, Ger. Hans Karrer GmbH, Postfach: 1296, 86330 Konigsbrunn, Germany.

Katadyn, Fr. Katadyn France, B.P. 39, 77680 Roissy-en-Brie, France.

Kattwiga, Ger. Pharm. Fabrik Kattwiga GmbH, Grenze 30, Postfach: 2567, 48514 Nordhorn-Brandlecht, Germany.

Kavon, USA. Kavon, USA.

Kay, Canad. Mary Kay Cosmetics Ltd, 2020 Meadowvale Blvd, Mississauga, Ontario, L5N 6Y2, Canada.

Kay, USA. Kay, USA.

Kayaku, Jpn. Nippon Kayaku Co. Ltd, 11-2 Fujimi 1-chome, Chiyoda-ku, Tokyo 102, Japan.

KBR, Ital. Kroton Biologic Researches s.r.l., Corso Vittorio Emanuele 73, 88074 Crotone (CZ), Italy.

Keatings, S.Afr. See *Adcock Ingram, S.Afr.*

Keene, USA. Keene Pharmaceuticals Inc., 333 S. Mockingbird, P.O. Box 7, Keene, TX 76059, USA.

Keimdiat, Ger. Keimdiät GmbH - Vertrieb Synpharma GmbH, Pfladergasse 7-13, Postfach: 111649, 8900 Augsburg, Germany.

Kelco International, UK. Kelco International Ltd, Waterfield, Tadworth, Surrey, KT20 5HQ, UK.

Kelemata, Ital. Kelemata s.p.a., Via S Quintino 28, 10121 Turin, Italy.

Kemiflor, Swed. Kemiflor AB, Box 7245, 103 89 Stockholm, Sweden.

Kemiprogress, Ital. Kemiprogress s.r.l., Via Aurelia 58, 00165 Rome, Italy.

Kemyos, Ital. Kemyos Biomedical Research s.r.l., Via Tre Cannelle 12, 00040 Pomezia (RM), Italy.

Kendall, Spain. Kendall Institute, Narciso Monturiol 2, Sant Just Desvern, 08960 Barcelona, Spain.

Kendall, UK. Kendall Healthcare Products-Europe, 2 Elmwood, Chineham Business Park, Crockford Lane, Basingstoke, Hants, RG24 0WG, UK.

Kendall McGaw, Canad. Kendall McGaw Canada, P.O. Box 570, 1100 Curity Ave, Peterborough, Ontario, K9J 6Z6, Canada.

Kendall McGaw, USA. Kendall McGaw Pharmaceutical Inc., 2525 McGaw Ave, Irvine, CA 92714-5895, USA.

Kendon, UK. Kendon International Ltd, 8-14 Orsman Rd, London, N1 5QJ, UK.

Kenfarma, Spain. Kenfarma, Antonio Lopez 109, 28026 Madrid, Spain.

Kenral, Austral. See *Pharmacia Upjohn, Austral.*

Kenral, Canad. See *Altimed, Canad.*

Kent, UK. Kent Pharmaceuticals Ltd, Letraset Site, Wotton Rd, Ashford, Kent, TN23 2LL, UK.

Kenwood, USA. Kenwood Laboratories, Division of Bradley Pharmaceuticals Inc., 383 Route 46 West, Fairfield, NJ 07006-2402, USA.

Kerifarm, Spain. Kerifarm, Spain.

Kern, Switz. E Kern AG Pharmazeutische Krauterspezialitaten, Hauptstrasse 23, 8867 Niederumen, Switzerland.

Kestrel, UK. Kestrel Healthcare Ltd, 21a Hyde St, Winchester, Hants, SO23 7DR, UK.

Kettelhack Riker, Ger. See *3M, Ger.*

Key, Austral. Key Pharmaceuticals Pty Ltd, P.O. Box 121, Concord West, NSW 2138, Australia.

Key, Canad. Key, Division of Schering Canada Inc., 3535 Transcanada Hwy, Pointe-Claire, Quebec, H9R 1B4, Canada.

Key, USA. Key Pharmaceuticals Inc., Galloping Hill Rd, Kenilworth, NJ 07033, USA.

Kin, Spain. Kin, Granada 123, 08018 Barcelona, Spain.

Kingswood, USA. Kingswood Labs Inc., 10375 Hague Rd, Indianapolis, IN 46256, USA.

Kinray, USA. Kinray, 152-35 10th Ave, Whitestone, NY 11357, USA.

Kinsmor, Canad. Kinsmor Pharmaceuticals Canada Inc., 210 Binnington Court, Kingston, Ontario, K7M 8N1, Canada.

Kirin, Jpn. Kirin Brewery Co. Ltd, Nikko Motoyoyogi Building, 30-13 Motoyoyogi-cho, Shibuya-ku, Tokyo 151, Japan.

Kirkman, USA. Kirkman Sales Co., PO Box 1009, Wilsonville, Oregon, OR 97070, USA.

Kissei, Jpn. Kissei Pharmaceutical Co. Ltd, 19-48 Yoshino, Matsumoto-City, Nagano-Pref. 399, Japan.

Kiwi, USA. Kiwi Brands, Inc., Division of Sara Lee Corporation, 447 Old Swede Rd, Douglassville, Pennsylvania, PA 19518-1239, USA.

Klein, Ger. Dr Gustav Klein, Steinenfeld 3, Postfach: 1165, 77732 Zell-Harmersbach, Germany.

Klein & Steube, Ger. Klein & Steube Entoxin GmbH, Steinfeldweg 13, Postfach: 1418, 77804 Buhl, Germany.

Klemenz, Ger. Klemenz GmbH, Hermann-Burkhardt-Strasse 3, Postfach: 7269, 72785 Pfullingen, Germany.

Klever, Ger. F. W. Klever GmbH, Hauptstrasse 20, 84168 Aham/Ndb., Germany.

KLI, USA. KLI Corp., 1119 Third Ave SW, Carmel, IN 46032, USA.

Klinge, Aust. Klinge Pharma GmbH, Hietzinger Hauptstrasse 64, 1132 Vienna, Austria.

Klinge, Ger. Klinge Pharma GmbH, Berg-am-Laim-Str. 129, Postfach: 801063, 81610 Munich, Germany.

Klinge, Irl. Klinge Pharmaceuticals & Co., 52 James Place East, Dublin 2, Ireland.

Klinge, Switz. Klinge Pharma AG, Bachstrasse 10, 8280 Kreuzlingen, Switzerland.

Klinge Munich, Switz. See *Ridupharm, Switz.*

Klinge-Nattermann, Ger. See *Isis, Ger.*

Klosterfrau, Aust. Maria Clementine Martin Klosterfrau GmbH, Doerenkampgasse 11, 1105 Vienna, Austria.

Klosterfrau, Ger. Maria Clementine Martin Klosterfrau Vertriebsgesellschaft mbH, 50606 Cologne, Germany.

Klus, Switz. Klus-Apotheke, F & Dr J Fröhlich-Decurtins, Hegibachstrasse 102, 8032 Zurich, Switzerland.

Kneipp, Ger. Kneipp-Werke, 97064 Wurzburg, Germany.

Knoll, Austral. Knoll Australia Pty Ltd, 15 Orion Rd, Lane Cove, NSW 2066, Australia.

Knoll, Belg. Knoll Belgium S.A., Avenue Hamoir 14, 1180 Brussels, Belgium.

Knoll, Canad. Knoll Pharma Inc., 100 Allstate Parkway, Suite 600, Markham, Ontario, L3R 6H3, Canada.

Knoll, Fr. Laboratoires Knoll France, 49 av Georges-Pompidou, 92300 Levallois-Perret, France.

Knoll, Ger. Knoll Deutschland GmbH, Rathausplatz 10-12, Postfach: 210660, 67006 Ludwigshafen, Germany.

Knoll, Irl. Knoll Ltd, United Drug House, Belgard Rd, Tallaght, Dublin 24, Ireland.

Knoll, Ital. Knoll Farmaceutici s.p.a., Via Europa 35, 20053 Muggio, Italy.

Knoll, Neth. Knoll B.V., Postbus 22622, 1100 DC Amsterdam, Netherlands.

Knoll, Norw. See *Meda, Norw.*, and *Astra, Norw.*

Knoll, S.Afr. Knoll Pharmaceuticals (South Africa) (Ptg) Ltd, P.O. Box 3030, Halfway House 1685, S. Africa.

Knoll, Spain. Knoll Made, Avda de Burgos 91, 28050 Madrid, Spain.

Knoll, Switz. Knoll SA, Case postale 631, 4410 Liestal, Switzerland.

Knoll, UK. Knoll Ltd, 9 Castle Quay, Castle Boulevard, Nottingham, Notts, NG7 1FW, UK.

Knoll, USA. Knoll Pharmaceuticals, Unit of BASF K&F Corp., 30 North Jefferson Rd, Whippany, NJ 07981, USA.

Koch, Aust. Edmund Koch, Biol. Heilmittel, Herrenstrasse 2, 4010 Linz, Austria.

Kohler, Aust. Dr Köhler Pharma GmbH, Steckhovengasse 17, 1130 Vienna, Austria.

Kohler, Ger. Dr Franz Köhler Chemie GmbH, Neue Bergstrasse 3-7, Postfach: 1117, 64659 Alsbach-Hahnlein, Germany.

Kohler, Neth. See *Tramedico, Neth.*

Kohler-Pharma, Ger. Köhler Vertrieb Pharma GmbH, Neue Bergstr. 3, Postfach: 1222, 64660 Alsbach, Germany.

Kolassa, Aust. Dr. Kolassa & Merz GmbH, Gastgebgasse 5-13, 1230 Vienna, Austria.

Kollerics, Aust. Kollerics Helmut, Hauptstrasse 25, 8061 St Radegund, Austria.

Kondon, USA. Kondon Manufacturing, Croswell, MI 48422, USA.

Konsyl, USA. Konsyl Pharmaceuticals, 4200 South Hulen, Suite 513, Ft Worth, TX 76109, USA.

KOS, USA. Kos Pharmaceuticals Inc, Miami, FL 33131, USA.

Kottas-Heldenberg, Aust. Kottas-Heldenberg Mag. R.U. Sohn, Bauernmarkt 24, 1014 Vienna, Austria.

Kowa, Jpn. Kowa, 3-6-29 Nishiki, Naka-ku, Nagoya-shi, Japan.

Kramer, Switz. Kramer-Pharma AG, 46 ave des Boveresses, 1000 Lausanne 21, Switzerland.

Kramer, USA. Kramer Laboratories Inc., 8778 SW 8th St, Miami, FL 33174, USA.

Kreussler, Fr. Laboratoire Kreussler Pharma, 2 rue de la Haye, Le Dome, BP 10901, 95731 Roissy-Charles-de-Gaulle cdx, France.

Kreussler, Ger. Chemische Fabrik Kreussler & Co. GmbH, Rheingaustrasse 87-93, Postfach: 120454, 65082 Wiesbaden, Germany.

Kreussler, Switz. See *Globopharm, Switz.*

Krewel, Ger. Krewel Meuselbach GmbH, Krewelstrasse 2, Postfach: 1263, 53775 Eitorf, Germany.

Krewel, Switz. See *Lubapharm, Switz.*

Kronans, Swed. Kronans Farm. & Kem. Laboratorium, Box 1266, 172 25 Sundbyberg, Sweden.

Kropf, Switz. Dr A & M Kropf-Schenk, Apotheke und Laboratorium Gstaad, Hauptstrasse, 3780 Gstaad, Switzerland.

Krug, Aust. Dr et Mag. Gilbert Krug GmbH, Bernardgasse 26, 1070 Vienna, Austria.

Krugmann, Ger. Krugmann GmbH, Mundipharma-Strasse 4, Postfach: 1350, 65533 Limburg (Lahn), Germany.

KSL, Canad. KSL Laboratories, 117-260 West Esplanade, North Vancouver, British Columbia, V7M 3G7, Canada.

Kunzle, Switz. Kräuterpfarrer Künzle AG, 6648 Minusio, Switzerland.

Kur und Stadtapotheke, Aust. Kur- und Stadtapotheke, Oberer Stadtplatz 5, 6060 Hall in Tirol, Austria.

Kureha, Jpn. Kureha Chemical Industry Co. Ltd, 3-25-1 Hyakunin-cho, Shinjuku-ku, Tokyo 169, Japan.

Kwizda, Aust. F. Joh. Kwizda Chemische Fabrik, Dr.-Karl-Lueger-Ring 6, 1011 Vienna, Austria.

Kwizda, Switz. See *Schwarz, Switz.*

Kyorin, Jpn. Kyorin Pharmaceutical Co. Ltd, 5 Kanda Surugadai 2-chome, Chiyoda-ku, Tokyo 101, Japan.

Kyowa, Jpn. Kyowa Hakko Kogyo Co. Ltd, 1-6-1 Ohtemachi, Chiyoda-ku, Tokyo 100, Japan.

Kyowa, UK. Kyowa Hakko (UK) Ltd, County Mark House, 50 Regent Street, London, W1R 6LP, UK.

Kytta, Ger. Kytta-Siegfried Pharma GmbH, Robert-Koch-Strasse 2, Postfach: 1260, 72272 Alpirsbach, Germany.

Laakefarmos, Swed. See *Orion, Swed.*

LAB, Switz. See *Schonenberger, Switz.*

Lab Francais du Fractionnement, Fr. Lab Francais du Fractionnement et des Biotechnologies, 3 av des Tropiques, BP 305, 91958 Les Ulis cdx, France.

Lab Line, Ital. Lab-Line s.p.a., Via Donizetti 5, 20090 Assago (MI), Italy.

Labatec, Switz. Labatec-Pharma SA, Case postale 62, 27 rue du Cardinal-Journet, 1217 Meyrin 2, Switzerland.

Labaz, Fr. See *Sanofi Winthrop, Fr.*

Labaz, Spain. See *Sanofi Winthrop, Spain.*

Labcatal, Fr. Laboratoires Labcatal, 7 rue Roger Salengro, B.P. 305, 92541 Montrouge Cdx, France.

Labcatal, Switz. See *Oligosol, Switz.*

Labima, Belg. Labima S.A., Ave Van Volxem 328, 1190 Brussels, Belgium.

Labitec, Spain. Labitec, Lope de Rueda 46, 28009 Madrid, Spain.

Labodynathera, Fr. Laboratoires Labodynathéra Groupe Doms-Adrian, 26 rue de l'Industrie, 92400 Courbevoie, France.

Labomed, Fr. Labomed, ZAC des Cerisiers, 69380 Lozanne, France.

Labopharma, Ger. Labopharma, Chemisch- pharmazeutische Fabrik GmbH, Nordhauser Strasse 30, 1000 Berlin 10, Germany.

Labor, Aust. Labor Buchrucker, Aschacher Strasse 1, 4100 Ottensheim, Austria.

Laboratories for Applied Biology, Irl. See *Boileau & Boyd, Irl.*

Laboratories for Applied Biology, UK. Laboratories for Applied Biology Ltd, 91 Amhurst Park, London, N16 5DR, UK.

Lacer, Spain. Lacer, Cerdena 346-50, 08025 Barcelona, Spain.

Lachartre, Fr. Laboratoires Lachartre, 104 av. Charles-de-Gaulle, 92200 Neuilly-sur-Seine, France.

Lachifarma, Ital. Lachifarma s.r.l., Laboratorio Chimico Farmaceutico Salentino, S.S. 16, Zona Industriale, 73010 Zollino (LE), Italy.

Lacteol, Switz. See *Uhlmann-Eyraud, Switz.*

Lacteol du Dr Boucard, Fr. Laboratoires du Lactéol du Dr Boucard, Route de Bu, B.P. 41, 78550 Houdan, France.

Laevosan, Aust. Laevosan GmbH, Estermannstrasse 17, 4020 Linz, Austria.

Laevosan, Switz. Laevosan International AG, Dufourstrasse 32, 8008 Zurich, Switzerland.

Lafar, Ital. Lafar, Via Noto 7, 20141 Milan, Italy.

Lafare, Ital. Laboratorio Farmaceutico Reggiano s.r.l., Via S.B. Cozzolino 77, 80056 Ercolano Resina (NA), Italy.

Lafayette, USA. Lafayette Pharmacal Inc., 4200 South Hulen St, Fort Worth, TX 76109, USA.

Lafon, Fr. Laboratoires Lafon, 19 ave du Professeur Cadiot, B.P. 22, 94701 Maisons-Alfort Cdx, France.

Lafon-Ratiopharm, Fr. Laboratoires Lafon-Ratiopharm, 5 rue Charles-Martigny, B.P. 42, 94702 Maisons-Alfort Cdx, France.

Lafran, Fr. Laboratoires Lafran, 1 rte des Stains, 94387 Bonneuil/Marne Cdx, France.

Lagamed, S.Afr. Lagamed (Pty) Ltd, P.O. Box 553, Isando 1600, S. Africa.

Lagap, Ital. Lagap Italiana s.r.l., Via Doberdo 16, 20126 Milan, Italy.

Lagap, Switz. Lagap Pharmaceuticals SA, Postfach 7, 6943 Vezia, Switzerland.

Lagap, UK. Lagap Pharmaceuticals Ltd, Woolmer Way, Bordon, Hants, GU35 9QE, UK.

Lainco, Spain. Lainco, Avda Bizet 8-12, Rubi, 08191 Barcelona, Spain.

Lake, USA. Lake Consumer Products Inc., 625 Forest Edge Dr, Vernon Hills, Illinois, IL 60061, USA.

Lakeside, USA. See *Marion Merrell Dow, USA.*

Lalco, Canad. See *Nobel, Canad.*

Laleuf, Fr. Societe d'exploitation des Laboratoires Laleuf, 45 rue de Clichy, 75009 Paris, France.

Lambda, USA. See *Bart, USA.*

Lampugnani, Ital. Lampugnani Farmaceutici s.p.a., Via Gramsci 4, 20014 Nerviano (Milan), Italy.

Lancome, Canad. See *Cosmair, Canad.*

Lander, Canad. Lander Co. Canada Ltd, 275 Finchdene Square, Scarborough, ON, M1X 1C7, Canada.

Landerlan, Spain. Landerlan, Spain.

Landmark, Canad. Landmark Medical Systems Ltd, 7 Main St, Unionville, Ontario, L3R 2E5, Canada.

Lane, UK. G.R. Lane Health Products Ltd, Sisson Rd, Gloucester, GL1 3QB, UK.

Lannacher, Aust. Lannacher Heilmittel GmbH, Schlossplatz 1, 8502 Lannach, Austria.

Lannett, USA. Lannett Inc., 9000 State Rd, Philadelphia, PA 19136, USA.

Lanzas, Spain. Lanzas, Laurea Miro 395, Sant Feliu de Llobregat, 08980 Barcelona, Spain.

Laphal, Fr. Laboratoires Laphal, B.P. 7, 13718 Allauch cdx, France.

Lappe, Ger. Produpharm Lappe GmbH, Senefelderstrasse 44, Postfach: 200529, 51435 Bergisch Gladbach, Germany.

Laproquifar, Spain. Laproquifar, Las Carolinas 13, 08012 Barcelona, Spain.

L'Arguenon, Fr. L'Arguenon International - S.E.R.B. Laboratoires, 53 rue Villiers de l'Isle Adam, 75020 Paris, France.

Larkhall Laboratories, UK. Larkhall Laboratories, 225 Putney Bridge Rd, London, SW15 2PY, UK.

Laroche Navarron, Belg. See *Roche, Belg.*

Laroche Navarron, Neth. See *Bournonville, Neth.*

Lasa, Spain. Lasa, Ctra Laurea Miro 385, Sant Feliu de Llobregat, 08980 Barcelona, Spain.

Laser, S.Afr. Laser (Pty) Ltd, S. Africa.

Laser, USA. Laser Inc., 2000 N. Main St, P.O. Box 905, Crown Point, IN 46307, USA.

Latema, Fr. See *Solvay, Fr.*

Laves, Ger. Laves-Arzneimittel GmbH, Barbarastrasse 14, 30952 Ronnenberg, Germany.

Lavomat, Swed. Lavomat AB, Sweden.

Lavoris-Dep, Canad. Lavoris-Dep, Canada.

LAW, Ger. Leipziger Arzneimittelwerk GmbH (LAW), Elisabeth-Schumacher-Strasse 54-6, Postfach: 041, 04301 Leipzig, Germany.

LCA, Fr. Laboratoire LCA, 8 rue Jean-Antoine-de-Baif, 75013 Paris, France.

LDM, Fr. LDM Santé, 2 pl Edmond-Puyo, B.P. 129, 29600 Morlaix, France.

Le Marchand, Fr. Laboratoires Le Marchand, 2 bis rue Moussard, 28600 Luisant, France.

Lebeh, USA. Lebeh, USA.

Lebens, Ital. Leben's s.r.l., Via Rovigo 1, 00161 Rome, Italy.

LED, Fr. Laboratoires d'Evolution Dermatologique, rue Albert-Caquot, Residence Petra C-Bat Arithmos, 06560 Sophia Antipolis, France.

Lederle, Austral. See *Wyeth, Austral.*

Lederle, Fr. Laboratoires Lederle, Le Wilson 2, 80 av du Pdt-Wilson, 92031 Paris-La Defense cdx, France.

Lederle, Ger. Lederle Arzneimittel GmbH & Co., Schleebruggenkamp 15, Postfach: 8808, 48136 Munster, Germany.

Lederle, Jpn. Lederle (Japan), Ltd, Central Post Office Box 957, Tokyo 104, Japan.

Lederle, Neth. See *AHP, Neth.*

Lederle, Norw. Lederle Informasjonskontor, Dronningensg. 40, Postboks 138 Sentrum, 0102 Oslo, Norway.

Lederle, S.Afr. Lederle Laboratories (Division of S.A. Cyanamid (Pty) Ltd), P.O. Box 58, Isando 1600, S. Africa.

Lederle, Switz. See *AHP, Switz.*

Lederle, UK. Lederle Laboratories, Fareham Rd, Gosport, Hants, PO13 0AS, UK.

Lederle, USA. Lederle Laboratories, Division of American Cyanamid Co., Pearl River, NY 10965, USA.

Lederle Consumer, Canad. See *Whitehall-Robins, Canad.*

Lederle-Praxis, USA. See *Cyanamid, USA.*

Ledi, Ital. Laboratori Eudermici Italiani s.r.l., Via Augusto Gaudenzi 29, 00163 Rome, Italy.

Lee, USA. Lee Pharmaceuticals, 1444 Santa Anita Blvd, South Elmonte, California, CA 91733, USA.

Lee-Adams, Canad. Lee-Adams Laboratories, Division of Pharmascience Inc., 8400 Darnley Rd, Montreal, Quebec, H4T 1M4, Canada.

Leeming, USA. Leeming Division, Pfizer Inc., 100 Jefferson Rd, Parsippany, NJ 07054, USA.

Lefevre, Fr. Laboratoires du Dr J. Lefèvre-Albrenor S.A., 82 rue National, 57350 Stiring-Wendel, France.

Legere, USA. Legere Pharmaceuticals, 7326 E. Evans Rd, Scottsdale, AZ 85260, USA.

Legon, Ital. Legon Farmaceutici s.r.l., Via Antonio Nibby 18, 00161 Rome, Italy.

Lehn & Fink, USA. See *Personal Care, USA.*

Lehning, Fr. Laboratoires Lehning, 1 place Arsene-Vigeant, B.P. 30326, 57007 Metz Cedex 1, France.

Leiras, Norw. Leiras Norge AS, Bogstadv. 6, 0355 Oslo, Norway.

Leiras, Swed. Leiras AB, Box 23138, 104 35 Stockholm, Sweden.

Lemmon, USA. Lemmon Co., P.O. Box 630, Sellersville, PA 18960, USA.

Lemoine, Fr. Laboratoires Lemoine, 13 rue Faraday, BP 13, 41260 La-Chaussee-Saint-Victor, France.

Lemstam, Austral. Lemstam Pharmaceutical, 57 Gladesville Drive, Kilsyth, Vic. 3137, Australia.

Lennod, USA. Lennod, USA.

Lennon, S.Afr. See *SA Druggists, S.Afr.*

Lennon, UK. Lennon Pharmaceuticals, Tuition House, 27/37 St George's Rd, Wimbledon, London, SW19 4EU, UK.

Lensa, Spain. Lensa, Potosi 2-4, 08030 Barcelona, Spain.

Lentheric Morny, UK. Lentheric Morny Ltd, UK.

Lenza, Ital. Farmaceutici Lenza s.r.l., Italy.

Leo, Belg. Leo Pharma S.A., Excelsiorlaan 40-2, 1930 Zaventem, Belgium.

Leo, Canad. Leo Laboratories Canada Ltd, 555 Kingston Rd W., Ajax, Ontario, L1S 6M1, Canada.

Leo, Fr. Laboratoires Leo, B.P. 311, 78054 St-Quentin-Yvelines Cdx, France.

Leo, Ger. Leo GmbH, Pharmazeutische Produkte, Einsteinstr. 18, 63303 Dreieich, Germany.

Leo, Irl. Leo Laboratories Ltd, 285 Cashel Rd, Dublin 12, Ireland.

Leo, Neth. Leo Pharmaceutical Products B.V., Postbus 51, 1380 AB Weesp, Netherlands.

Leo, Norw. Løvens kemiske Fabrik, Ramstadsletta 15, Postboks 103, 1322 Hovik, Norway.

Leo, S.Afr. See *Adcock Ingram, S.Afr.*

Leo, Switz. Leo Pharmaceutical Products Sarath Ltd, Eggbuhlstrasse 28, 8052 Zurich, Switzerland.

Leo, UK. Leo Pharmaceuticals, Longwick Rd, Princes Risborough, Bucks, HP27 9RR, UK.

Leopold, Aust. Leopold Pharma GmbH, Hafnerstrasse 36, 8055 Graz, Austria.

Lepetit, Ital. Gruppo Lepetit s.p.a., Via R Lepetit 8, 20020 Lainate (MI), Italy.

Leppin, S.Afr. Leppin, S. Africa.

Lersa, Spain. Lersa, Spain.

Lesourd, Fr. Laboratoires Gabriel Lesourd, 6 rue Sainte-Isaure, 75018 Paris, France.

Lesvi, Spain. Lesvi, Plg. Ind. Can Pelegri S/N, Castellbisbal, 08755 Barcelona, Spain.

Leti, Spain. Leti, Gran Via de las Corts Catalanes 184, 08004 Barcelona, Spain.

Leurquin, Fr. Laboratoires Leurquin Mediolanum, 68-84 rue Ampere, 93330 Neuilly-sur-Marne, France.

Level, Spain. Level, Pedro-IV 499, 08020 Barcelona, Spain.

Lever Pond's, Canad. Lever Pond's Canada, 1 Sunlight Park, Toronto, ON, M4M 1B6, Canada.

Lexis, USA. Lexis Laboratories, P.O. Box 202887, Austin, TX 78720, USA.

Leyh, Ger. Leyh Pharma GmbH, Gewerbegebeit Baierstal, 98596 Trusetal, Germany.

Liade, Spain. See *Boots, Spain.*

Liberman, Spain. Liberman, Spain.

Lichtenheldt, Ger. Lichtenheldt GmbH, Pharmazeutische Fabrik, Justus-Liebig-Weg 1, 23812 Wahlstedt, Germany.

Lichtenstein, Ger. Lichtenstein Pharmazeutica GmbH, Bergpflege 45, Postfach: 2191, 56107 Lahnstein/Rhein, Germany.

Lichtwer, Fr. Laboratoires Lichtwer, France.

Lichtwer, Ger. Lichtwer Pharma GmbH, Wallenroder Strasse 8-10, Postfach: 260326, 13413 Berlin, Germany.

Lichtwer, Switz. See *Adroka, Switz.*

Lichtwer, UK. Lichtwer Pharma UK, Regency House, Dedmere Rd, Marlow, Bucks, SL7 1FJ, UK.

Liebermann, Ger. Pharma Liebermann GmbH, Hauptstrasse 27, Postfach: 49, 89421 Gundelfingen/Do., Germany.

Lierac, Fr. Laboratoires Liérac, 99 rue du Faubourg Saint-Honore, 75008 Paris, France.

Life, Ger. Life Pharma Vertriebs mbH, Mainstr. 3, 67141 Neuhofen, Germany.

Life Essence, UK. See *Elder, UK.*

Lifepharma, Ital. Lifepharma s.p.a., Via Carducci 27, 20099 Sesto San Giovanni (MI), Italy.

Lifeplan, UK. Lifeplan Products, Elizabethan Way, Lutterworth, Leics, LE17 4ND, UK.

Lifesavers, Canad. Lifesavers Canada, Division of Hershey Can Inc., 100 Cumberland Ave, Hamilton, ON, L8M 1Z1, Canada.

Lifescan, Fr. Lab. Lifescan, ZAC Paris-Nord II, BP 50042, 69 rue de la Belle-Etoile, 95946 Roissy cdx, France.

LifeScan, USA. Lifescan, 1000 Gibraltar, Milpitas, CA 95035-6312, USA.

Ligand, Canad. See *Ligand, USA.*

Ligand, USA. Ligand Pharmaceuticals Inc., 9393 Towne Centre Drive, San Diego, CA 92121, USA.

Li-il, Ger. Li-iL GmbH Arzneimittel, Postfach: 300115, 01131 Dresden, Germany.

Lilly, Aust. Eli Lilly GmbH (Austria), Barichgasse 40-2, 1030 Vienna, Austria.

Lilly, Austral. Eli Lilly Australia Pty Ltd, 112 Wharf Rd, West Ryde, NSW 2114, Australia.

Lilly, Belg. Eli Lilly Benelux S.A., Rue de l'Etuve 52/bte 1, 1000 Brussels, Belgium.

Lilly, Canad. Eli Lilly Canada Inc., 3650 Danforth Ave, Scarborough, Ontario, M1N 2E8, Canada.

Lilly, Fr. Lilly France, 203 bureaux de la Colline, 92213 Saint-Cloud, France.

Lilly, Ger. Lilly Deutschland GmbH, Saalburgstr. 153, 61350 Bad Homburg, Germany.

Lilly, Irl. Eli Lilly & Co. (Ireland) Ltd, 44 Fitzwilliam Place, Dublin 2, Ireland.

Lilly, Ital. Eli Lilly Italia s.p.a., Via Gramsci 731/733, 50019 Sesto Fiorentino (FI), Italy.

Lilly, Neth. Eli Lilly Nederland, Krijtwal 17-23, 3432 ZT Nieuwegein, Netherlands.

Lilly, Norw. Eli Lilly Norway A.S, PB 6090 Etterstad, 0601 Oslo, Norway.

Lilly, S.Afr. Eli Lilly (SA) (Pty) Ltd, P.O. Box 98, Isando 1600, S. Africa.

Lilly, Spain. Lilly, Avda de la Industria 30, Alcobendas, 28100 Madrid, Spain.

Lilly, Swed. Eli Lilly Sweden AB, Box 30037, 104 25 Stockholm, Sweden.

Lilly, Switz. Eli Lilly (Suisse) SA, 16 Ch. des Coquelicots, Case postale 580, 1214 Vernier/GE, Switzerland.

Lilly, UK. Eli Lilly & Co. Ltd, Kingsclere Rd, Basingstoke, Hants, RG21 2XA, UK.

Lilly, USA. Eli Lilly & Co., Lilly Corporate Center, Indianapolis, IN 46285, USA.

Lina, UK. Lina Trading Ltd, P.O. Box 2341, London, W1A 2NZ, UK.

Lincoln, Fr. Laboratoires Lincoln, 16 rue de la Cure, 75016 Paris, France.

Lindopharm, Ger. Lindopharm GmbH, Neustrasse 82, Postfach: 560, 40705 Hilden, Germany.

Lineafarm, Spain. Lineafarm, Spain.

Lineamedica, Ital. Lineamedica spa, Via Gian Galeazzo 16, 20136 Milan, Italy.

Link, Irl. See *United Drug, Irl.,* and *Intra Pharma, Irl.*

Link, UK. Link Pharmaceuticals Ltd, 51 Bishopric, Horsham, West Sussex, RH12 1QJ, UK.

Linobion, Aust. Linobion Chem.-pharm. Laboratorium, Kardinal-Nagl-Platz 1, 1030 Vienna, Austria.

Linotar, Austral. Linotar Pty Ltd, P.O. Box 17, Terrey Hills, NSW 2084, Australia.

Linton, S.Afr. M Linton, S. Africa.

Lioh, Canad. Lioh Inc., Canada.

Lion, Jpn. Lion, 1-3-7 Honjyo, Sumida-ku, Tokyo, Japan.

Lipha, Belg. Lipha s.a., Brusselsesteenweg 288, 3090 Overijse, Belgium.

Lipha, Fr. See *Lipha Sante, Fr.,* and *Monot, Fr.*

Lipha, Ger. Lipha Arzneimittel GmbH, Zeche Katharina 6, Postfach: 130326, 45293 Essen, Germany.

Lipha, Irl. See *Helsinn Birex, Irl.*

Lipha, Ital. Lipha s.p.a., Via G. Garibaldi 80/82, 50041 Calenzano (FI), Italy.

Lipha, Norw. See *Meda, Norw.*

Lipha, Switz. Lipha Pharma AG, Ruchligstrasse 20, Postfach 496, 8953 Dietikon, Switzerland.

Lipha, UK. Lipha Pharmaceuticals Ltd, Harrier House, High St, Yiewsley, West Drayton, Middx, UB7 7QG, UK.

Lipha Sante, Fr. Lipha Santé, 34 rue St-Romain, 69008 Lyon, France.

Lipomed, UK. Lipomed Ltd, UK.

Liposome Company, Irl. See *Central, Irl.*

Liposome Company, Swed. See *Liposome Company, UK.*

Liposome Company, UK. The Liposome Company Ltd, Bechtel House, 245 Hammersmith Rd, London, W6 8DP, UK.

Lippens, Canad. Lippens Inc., 4757 Blvd Poirier, St-Laurent, Quebec, H4R 2A4, Canada.

Liquipharm, USA. Liquipharm, 10716 McCune Avenue, Los Angeles, CA 90034, USA.

Lirca, Ital. See *Synthelabo, Ital.*

Lisapharma, Ital. Lisapharma s.p.a., Via Licinio 11, 22036 Erba (Como), Italy.

Lizofarm, Ital. Lizofarm s.r.l., Via D. Millelire 13, 20147 Milan, Italy.

Llano, Spain. Llano, Spain.

Llorens, Spain. Llorens, Ciudad de Balaguer 7-11, 08022 Barcelona, Spain.

Llorente, Spain. Llorente, Ctra el Pardo Km 1, 28035 Madrid, Spain.

Lloyd, Aimee, UK. Lloyd, Aimee & Co. Ltd, Kingsend House, 44 Kingsend, Ruislip, Middx, HA4 7DA, UK.

Locatelli, Ital. Farmaceutici Locatelli s.r.l., Via Campobello 15, 00040 Pomezia (Rome), Italy.

Lodim, Switz. Lodim distribution Sagl, Via al Bosco 8, Casella postale 60, 6942 Savosa, Switzerland.

Lofarma, Ital. Laboratorio Farmaceutico Lofarma s.r.l., Viale Cassala 40, 20143 Milan, Italy.

Lofthouse of Fleetwood, Canad. See *TFB, Canad.*

Lofthouse of Fleetwood, UK. Lofthouse of Fleetwood Ltd, Maritime St, Fleetwood, Lancs, FY7 7LP, UK.

Logeais, Fr. Laboratoires Jacques Logeais, 71 ave du Général-de-Gaulle, 92130 Issy-les-Moulineaux, France.

Loges, Ger. Dr. Loges & Co. GmbH Arzneimittel, Schutzenstrasse 5, Postfach: 1262, 21412 Winsen (Luhe), Germany.

Logifarm, Ital. Logifarm s.r.l., Italy.

Logomed, Ger. Logomed Pharma GmbH, Eckenheimer Landstr. 100-4, Postfach 11 13 53, 60048 Frankfurt/Main, Germany.

Logos, S.Afr. Logos Pharmaceuticals, Private Bag 3, Halfway House 1685, S. Africa.

Lohmann, Ger. Lohmann GmbH & Co. KG, Postfach: 2343, 56515 Neuwied, Germany.

Lohmann, Ital. Lohmann Medical Italia s.r.l., Via E. Fermi 4, 35030 Sarmeola di Rubano, Italy.

Lomapharm, Ger. Lomapharm, Rudolf Lohmann GmbH KG Pharmazeutische Fabrik, Langes Feld 5, Postfach: 1210, 31857 Emmerthal, Germany.

London Drugs, Canad. London Drugs Ltd, 12831 Horseshoe Place, Richmond, British Colombia, V7A 4X5, Canada.

L'Oreal, Canad. See *Cosmair, Canad.*

Lorenz, Ger. Lorenz Arzneimittel GmbH, Laupendahler Landstrasse 5, Postfach: 164305, 4300 Essen-Werden 16, Germany.

Lorex, Irl. See *Allphar, Irl.*

Lorex, UK. Lorex Synthelabo Ltd, Lunar House, Globe Park, Marlow, Bucks, Sl7 1LW, UK.

Lorex Synthelabo, Irl. See *Allphar, Irl.*

Lorex Synthelabo, Neth. Lorex Synthélabo B.V., Postbus 1401, 3600 BK Maarssen, Netherlands.

Lorvic, Canad. Lorvic, Canada.

Lorvic, USA. Lorvic Corp., 8810 Frost Ave, St Louis, MO 63134-1095, USA.

Lotus, USA. Lotus Biochemical, PO Box 3586, 7335 Lee Highway, Radford, Virginia, VA 24143, USA.

Lovens, Swed. Lövens Läkemedel AB, Box 404, 201 24 Malmo, Sweden.

Loveridge, UK. J.M. Loveridge PLC, Southbrook Rd, Southampton, SO9 3LT, UK.

LPB, Ital. LPB Istituto Farmaceutico s.p.a., Via C Arconati 1, 20135 Milan, Italy.

LRC Products, UK. LRC Products Ltd, North Circular Rd, London, E4 8QA, UK.

Lu Chem, USA. Lu Chem Pharmaceuticals Inc., 8910 Linwood Ave, P.O. Box 6038, Shreveport, LA 71106, USA.

Lubapharm, Switz. Lubapharm SA, Ringstrasse 29, Postfach 434, 4106 Therwil, Switzerland.

Lubapharm Phlebologie, Switz. Lubapharm AG, Postfach 348, 4144 Arlesheim, Switzerland.

Lucchini, Ital. Lucchini Italiana s.r.l., Via S. Anna 2, 03012 Anagni (FR), Italy.

Lucchini, Switz. Lab Lucchini SA, 8 rue de la Coulouvreniere, 1204 Geneva, Switzerland.

Luchon, Fr. Laboratoires de Luchon, 22 bd Dardenne, 31110 Luchon, France.

Lucien, Fr. See *Therabel, Fr.*

Luhr-Lehrs, Ger. A Lühr-Lehrs Arzneimittel & Praventivprodukte, Postfach: 300884, 50778 Cologne, Germany.

Luitpold, Aust. Luitpold Pharmazeutika GmbH, Effingergasse 21, 1160 Vienna, Austria.

Luitpold, Austral. See *Organon, Austral.*

Luitpold, Belg. See *Will-Pharma, Belg.*

Luitpold, Ger. Luitpold Pharma GmbH, Zielstattstrasse 9, 81379 Munich, Germany.

Luitpold, Ital. Luitpold s.p.a., Via Montecassiano 157, 00156 Rome, Italy.

Luitpold, Neth. See *Will-Pharma, Neth.*

Luitpold, Norw. See *Weiders, Norw.*

Luitpold, S.Afr. Luitpold, S. Africa.

Luitpold, Switz. Luitpold AG, Industriestrasse 7, 8117 Fallanden, Switzerland.

Lundbeck, Aust. Lundbeck-Arzneimittel GmbH, Brigittagasse 22-6, Postfach 201, 1201 Vienna, Austria.

Lundbeck, Austral. Lundbeck Australia Pty Ltd, P.O. Box 6300, Baulkham Hills Business Centre, NSW 2153, Australia.

Lundbeck, Belg. Lundbeck S.A., Luchthavenlaan 20, 1800 Vilvoorde, Belgium.

Lundbeck, Canad. Lundbeck Canada Inc., 413 St-Jacques St W, Suite FB-230, Montreal, Quebec, H2Y 1N9, Canada.

Lundbeck, Fr. Laboratoires Lundbeck, 37 av Pierre-1er-de-Serbie, 75008 Paris, France.

Lundbeck, Irl. Lundbeck (Ireland) Ltd, Leopardstown Office Park, Sandyford Industrial Estate, Foxrock, Dublin 18, Ireland.

Lundbeck, Ital. Lundbeck Italia s.p.a., Via Fara 35, 20124 Milan, Italy.

Lundbeck, Neth. Lundbeck B.V., Postbus 12021, 1100 AA Amsterdam Z.O., Netherlands.

Lundbeck, Norw. H. Lundbeck A/S, Lysaker torg 10, 1324 Lysaker, Norway.

Lundbeck, S.Afr. Lundbeck South Africa, P.O. Box 2357, Randburg 2125, S. Africa.

Lundbeck, Spain. Lundbeck España, Avda Diagonal 605, 08028 Barcelona, Spain.

Lundbeck, Swed. H. Lundbeck AB, Box 23, 250 53 Helsingborg, Sweden.

Lundbeck, Switz. Lundbeck (Schweiz) AG, Cherstrasse 4, Postfach, 8152 Opfikon-Glattbrugg, Switzerland.

Lundbeck, UK. Lundbeck Ltd, Sunningdale House, Caldecotte Lake Business Park, Caldecotte, Milton Keynes, MK7 8LF, UK.

Lunsco, USA. Lunsco Inc., Route 2, P.O. Box 62, Pulaski, VA 24301, USA.

Luond, Switz. Pharma Lüönd, Bahnhofstrasse 17-19, 8280 Kreuzlingen, Switzerland.

Lusofarmaco, Ital. Istituto Lusofarmaco d'Italia s.p.a., Via Carnia 26, 20132 Milan, Italy.

Lusty, UK. Lusty's Natural Products Ltd, Sisson Rd, Gloucester, GL1 3OB, UK.

Lutsia, Fr. Laboratoires Lutsia, Tour Roussel-Hoechst, 1 terrasse Bellini, 92910 Paris-La Defense Cdx 3, France.

Lutsia, Ital. See *Boots Healthcare, Ital.*

Luvabec, Canad. Luvabec Laboratories Inc., 11177 rue Hamon, Montreal, Quebec, H3M 3E4, Canada.

Luvos, Ger. Heilerde-Gesellschaft Luvos Just GmbH & Co., Otto-Hahn-Strasse 23, Postfach: 47, 6382 Friedrichsdorf 2, Germany.

Lyocentre, Fr. Laboratoires Lyocentre, 15004 Aurillac Cdx, France.

Lyphomed, USA. See *Fujisawa, USA.*

Lysoform, Ger. Lysoform Dr. Hans Rosemann GmbH, Kaiser-Wilhelm-Strasse 133, Postfach: 460120, 12211 Berlin, Germany.

Lyssia, Belg. Lyssia S.A., Blvd Emile Bockstael 122, 1020 Brussels, Belgium.

Lyssia, Ger. See *Solvay, Ger.*

Mabo, Spain. Mabo, Caminode Carriles SN, Coslada, 28820 Madrid, Spain.

Macarthur, Austral. Macarthur Research, a division of Syntex Australia, P.O. Box 255, Dee Why, NSW 2099, Australia.

Macarthys, UK. Macarthys Medical Ltd, UK.

Macherey Nagel Duren, S.Afr. See *Pharmaceutical Enterprises, S.Afr.*

Mack, Belg. See *Vitalpharma, Belg.*

Mack, Neth. See *Astra, Neth.*

Mack, Switz. Mack Pharma, Fluelastrasse 7, Case postale, 8048 Zurich, Switzerland.

Mack, Illert., Ger. Heinrich Mack Nachf., ein Unternehmen der Pfizer-Gruppe, Heinrich-Mack-Strasse 35, Postfach: 2064, 89252 Illertissen, Germany.

Macsil, USA. Macsil Inc., P.O. Box 29276, Philadelphia, PA 19125-0976, USA.

Madariaga, Spain. Madariaga, Bocangel 21, 28028 Madrid, Spain.

Madaus, Aust. Madaus GmbH, Lienfeldergasse 91-3, 1171 Vienna, Austria.

Madaus, Belg. Madaus Pharma S.A., Rue des Trois-Arbres 16, 1180 Brussels, Belgium.

Madaus, Fr. Laboratoires Madaus, 60 bis, rue de Bellevue, 92100 Boulogne, France.

Madaus, Ger. Madaus AG, Ostmerheimer Strasse 198, 51109 Cologne, Germany.

Madaus, Neth. See *Byk, Neth.*

Madaus, S.Afr. Madaus Pharmaceuticals (Pty) Ltd, S. Africa.

Madaus, Spain. Madaus Cerafarm, Foc 68-82, 08038 Barcelona, Spain.

Madaus, Switz. See *Biomed, Switz.*

Maggioni, Ital. Maggioni S.p.A., Via Zambeletti, 20021 Baranzate di Bollate (MI), Italy.

Magis, Ital. Magis Farmaceutici s.p.a., Via Cacciamali 34-36-38, Zona Ind. (Loc. Noce), 25125 Brescia, Italy.

Magistra, Switz. Laboratoires Magistra SA, 28 Chemin du Grand-Puits, Case postale 122, 1217 Meyrin 2/Geneva, Switzerland.

Mago, Ger. Mago Dr Bischoff Magdalinski & Co. Herstellung u. Vertrieb pharm. Spezialitäten GmbH & Co. KG, Manteuffelstrasse 7, 44623 Herne, Germany.

Mahdeen, Canad. Mahdeen Memahdeen Mediceuticals, Division of Canmax Labs, 4255 Sherwoodtowne Blvd, Ste 322, Mississauga, Ontario, L4Z 1Y5, Canada.

Maizena, Ger. Maizena Diat GmbH, Knorrstrasse 1, Postffach: 2650, 7100 Heilbronn, Germany.

Major, USA. Major Pharmaceutical Corp., 1640 W Fulton St, Chicago, IL 60612, USA.

Makara, Aust. Makara Pharm GmbH, 6234 Brandenberg 19C, Austria.

Makara, Ger. Makara GmbH, Pharmazeutische Fabrik, Industriestrasse 6, Postfach: 1161, 5173 Aldenhoven, Germany.

Malam, UK. Malam Laboratories Ltd, 37 Oakwood Rise, Heaton, Bolton, BL1 5EE, UK.

Malesci, Ital. Malesci Istituto Farmacobiologico s.p.a., Via Lungo l'Ema 7, 50015 Bagno a Ripoli (FI), Italy.

Mallard, USA. Mallard Medical Products, 81 Corbett Way, Eatontown, NJ 07724-2264, USA.

Mallinckrodt, Aust. Mallinckrodt Medical GmbH, Strasse 7, Obj. 58/B/5, 2355 Wiener Neudorf, Austria.

Mallinckrodt, Austral. Mallinckrodt Medical Pty Ltd, P.O. Box 944, Mt Waverley, Vic. 3149, Australia.

Mallinckrodt, Canad. Mallinckrodt Medical Inc., 7500 Transcanada Highway, Pointe-Claire, Quebec, H9R 5H8, Canada.

Mallinckrodt, Ger. Mallinckrodt Medical GmbH, Josef-Dietzgen-Strasse 1-3, Postfach: 1462, 53761 Hennef, Germany.

Mallinckrodt, Spain. Mallinckrodt Iberica, Avda San Pablo 28, Coslada, 28820 Madrid, Spain.

Mallinckrodt, USA. Mallinckrodt Inc., 675 McDonnell Blvd, P.O. Box 5840, St Louis, MO 63147, USA.

Mandri, Spain. Mandri, Pau Claris 182, 08037 Barcelona, Spain.

Manetti Roberts, Ital. L. Manetti H. Roberts & C. per Azioni, Via Pellicceria 8, 50123 Florence, Italy.

Mann, Ger. Dr Gerhard Mann, Chem.-pharm. Fabrik GmbH, Brunsbutteler Damm 165-73, 13581 Berlin, Germany.

Mann, Irl. See *Pharma-Global, Irl.*

Mann, Neth. See *Tramedico, Neth.*

Mann, S.Afr. See *Restan, S.Afr.*

Manne, USA. Manne, P.O. Box 825, Johns Island, SC 29457, USA.

Manx, UK. Manx Pharma Ltd, Manx House, Spectrum Business Estate, Maidstone, Kent, ME15 9YP, UK.

Manzoni, Ital. Lab. G Manzoni & C. s.r.l., Via S Anna 2, 03012 Anagni (FR), Italy.

Marano, Ital. Marano Benito, Via E Vittorini, Villa Scalea, 90147 Palermo, Italy.

Marbot, Switz. Dr C Marbot AG, Amselweg 3, 3422 Kirchberg, Switzerland.

Marcel, Canad. Les Cosmetiques Marcel de Sevres, 1777 Lavoisier, Ste-Julie, Quebec, J3E 1Y6, Canada.

Marc-O, Canad. Marc-O Inc. Produits, 3175 rue Girard, Trois-Rivieres, QC, G8Z 2M5, Canada.

Marco Viti, Ital. Marco Viti Farmaceutici s.p.a., Via Tarantelli 15, 22076 Mozzate (CO), Italy.

Marcofina, Fr. Laboratoires Marcofina, 48 bis, rue des Belles-Feuilles, 75116 Paris, France.

Marion Laboratories, USA. See *Marion Merrell Dow, USA.*

Marion Merrell, Fr. Marion Merrell SA, 1 terrasse Bellini, 92800 Puteaux, France.

Marion Merrell, Spain. See *Hoechst Marion Roussel, Spain.*

Marion Merrell Dow, Austral. See *Hoechst Marion Roussel, Austral.*

Marion Merrell Dow, Belg. See *Hoechst Marion Roussel, Belg.*

Marion Merrell Dow, Canad. See *Hoechst Marion Roussel, Canad.*

Marion Merrell Dow, Ger. See *Hoechst, Ger.*

Marion Merrell Dow, Switz. See *Hoechst Marion Roussel, Switz.*

Marion Merrell Dow, UK. See *Hoechst Marion Roussel, UK.*

Marion Merrell Dow, USA. Marion Merrell Dow Inc., Marion Park Drive, P.O. Box 9627, Kansas City, MO 64134-0627, USA.

Marlin, USA. Marlin Industries, P.O. Box 560, Grover City, CA 93483-0560, USA.

Marlop, USA. Marlop Pharm Inc., 5704 Mosholu Ave, Bronx, NY 10471, USA.

Marlyn, USA. Marlyn Company Inc., 14851 North Scottsdale Road, Scottsdale, AZ 85254, USA.

Marnel, USA. Marnel Pharmaceuticals Inc., 206 Luke Drive, Lafayette, LA 70506, USA.

Marpa, Austral. Marpa, Australia.

Marrero, Spain. Marrero Perez, General Bravo 39, Pol. Industrial, Telde, 35200 Las Palmas, Spain.

Marsam, USA. Marsam Pharmaceuticals Inc., P.O. Box 1022, Cherry Hill, NJ 08034, USA.

Martec, USA. Martec Pharmaceutical Inc., 1800 N Topping Ave, Kansas City, MO 64120-1228, USA.

Martin, Fr. Laboratoires Jean-Paul Martin, Le Comte, 03340 Bessay-sur-Allier, France.

Martin, Spain. B Martin Pharma, Centro Empresarial el Planto, Ochandiano 6, 28023 Madrid, Spain.

Martin, Switz. See *Schonenberger, Switz.*

Martindale Pharmaceuticals, UK. Martindale Pharmaceuticals Ltd, Bampton Rd, Harold Hill, Romford, Essex, RM3 8UG, UK. NOTE. There is no connection between Martindale, The Complete Drug Reference and Martindale Pharmaceuticals.

Martinez Llenas, Spain. Martinez Llenas, Afueras del Barrio de Santa Ines, La Roca del Valles, 08430 Barcelona, Spain.

Martini, Ital. Martini Tommaso, Viale C. Felice 101, 00185 Rome, Italy.

Maruho, Jpn. Maruho Co. Ltd, 6-24 Nakatsu 1-chome, Kita-ku, Osaka 531, Japan.

Maruishi, Neth. See *Rooster, Neth.*

Mason, USA. Mason Pharmaceuticals Inc., 4425 Jamboree, Suite 250, Newport Beach, CA 92660, USA.

Mastelli, Ital. Mastelli s.r.l., Via Bussana Vecchia 32, 18032 Sanremo (IM), Italy.

Master Pharma, Ital. Master Pharma s.r.l., Via Firenze 8/A, 43100 Parma, Italy.

Mathieu, Canad. JL Mathieu Cie Ltee, 1225 Volta, Bur 100, Boucherville, QC, J4B 7M7, Canada.

Matrix, UK. Matrix Pharmaceutical Ltd, Selbourne House, Mill Lane, Alton, Hants, GU34 2QJ, UK.

Matrix, USA. Matrix Laboratories, 1430 O'Brian Drive, Suite G, Menlo Park, CA 94025, USA.

Mauermann, Ger. Mauermann-Arzneimittel, Franz Mauermann oHG, Heinrich-Knote-Strasse 2, Postfach: 20, 82341 Pocking, Germany.

Maurer, Ger. Maurer-Pharma GmbH, Ursulinenstrasse 55, 66111 Saarbrucken, Germany.

Mavi, Ital. Mavi Sud s.r.l., V.le dell'Industria 1, 04011 Aprilia (LT), Italy.

Max Farma, Ital. Max Farma, Via Pisacane 7, 20016 Pero (MI), Italy.

Max Ritter, Switz. Max Ritter Pharma SA, Prangins, Case postale 340, Avenue du Mont-Blanc, 1196 Gland, Switzerland.

Maxfarma, Spain. Maxfarma, Salamanca 13, 28020 Madrid, Spain.

Maxwell, S.Afr. Maxwell Pharm-Jhb, S. Africa.

May & Baker, Austral. See *Rhone-Poulenc Rorer, Austral.*

May & Baker, Canad. See *Rhone-Poulenc Rorer, Canad.*

May & Baker, S.Afr. See *Rhone-Poulenc Rorer, S.Afr.*

May & Baker, UK. May & Baker Pharmaceuticals, Rhone Poulenc Ltd, Rainham Rd South, Dagenham, Essex, RM10 7XS, UK.

Mayoly-Spindler, Fr. Laboratoires Mayoly-Spindler, 6 av de l'Europe, 78400 Chatou, France.

Mayoly-Spindler, Switz. See *Uhlmann-Eyraud, Switz.*

Mayrand, USA. Mayrand Inc., 4 Dundas Circle, P.O. Box 8869, Greensboro, NC 27419, USA.

Mayrhofer, Aust. Mayrhofer Pharmazeutika, Herrenstrasse 2, 4010 Linz, Austria.

Mayrs, Irl. David Mayrs Ltd, Broombridge Industrial Estate, Dublin 11, Ireland.

MBP, Ger. Medical Biomaterial Products GmbH, Postfach: 144, 19304 Neustadt-Glewe, Germany.

MC, Ital. Off. Prod. Presidi Medico Chirurgici s.r.l., S.S. 106, 89040 Portigliola (RC), Italy.

McGaw, USA. American McGaw Laboratories, American Hospital Supply Corp., 2525 McGaw Ave, Irvine, CA 92714, USA.

McGloin, Austral. J. McGloin Pty Ltd, P.O. Box 294, Kings Grove, NSW 2208, Australia.

McGregor, USA. McGregor Pharmaceuticals Inc., 8420 Ulmenton Rd, Suite 305, Largo, FL 34641, USA.

McGregor Cory, UK. McGregor Cory, Middleton Rd, Banbury, Oxon, OX16 8RS, UK.

McHenry, USA. McHenry Labs Inc., 118 N Wells, Lee Building, Edna, TX 77957, USA.

MCM, S.Afr. MCM, S. Africa.

McNeil, Canad. See *Janssen-Ortho, Canad.*

McNeil Consumer, Canad. McNeil Consumer Products Co., 890 Woodlawn Rd W., Guelph, Ontario, N1K 1A5, Canada.

McNeil Consumer, USA. McNeil Consumer Products Co., Camp Hill Rd, Fort Washington, PA 19034, USA.

McNeil Pharmaceutical, USA. McNeil Pharmaceutical, McNeilab Inc., Spring House, PA 19477, USA.

MCR, USA. MCR American Pharmaceuticals, 120 Summit Parkway, Suite 101, Birmingham, AL 35209, USA.

MDM, Ital. MDM s.r.l., Via Milanese 20, 20099 Sesto San Giovanni (MI), Italy.

MDR, USA. MDR Fitness Corp., 5207 NW 163rd St, Miami, FL 33014, USA.

ME Pharmaceuticals, USA. ME Pharmaceuticals Inc., 2800 Southeast Parkway, Richmond, IN 47375, USA.

Mead Johnson, Austral. See *Bristol-Myers Squibb, Austral.*

Mead Johnson, Canad. Mead Johnson Canada, Division of Bristol-Myers Squibb Canada Inc., 333 Preston Ave, Ottawa, Ontario, K1S 5N4, Canada.

Mead Johnson, Fr. Mead Johnson France, Division de Bristol-Myers Squibb, 33 av du Mal-de-Lattre-de-Tassigny, 94120 Fontenay-sous-Bois, France.

Mead Johnson, Ger. Mead Johnson Arzneimittel, Niederlassung der Bristol-Myers GmbH, Germany.

Mead Johnson, Ital. Mead Johnson s.p.a., Via Paolo di Dono 73, 000142 Rome, Italy.

Mead Johnson Laboratories, USA. See *Bristol-Myers Squibb, USA.*

Mead Johnson Nutritionals, UK. See *Bristol-Myers Squibb, UK.*

Mead Johnson Nutritionals, USA. See *Bristol-Myers Squibb, USA.*

Mead Johnson Oncology, USA. See *Bristol-Myers Squibb, USA.*

Mead Johnson Pharmaceutical, USA. See *Bristol-Myers Squibb, USA.*

Meckel, Ger. Meckel-Spenglersan GmbH, Postfach: 1418, 77804 Buhl, Germany.

Med Fabrik, Ger. Med Fabrik chemisch-pharmazeutischer Praparate J. Carl Pflüger GmbH & Co., Neukollnische Allee 146/148, Postfach: 440358, 1000 Berlin 44, Germany.

Med. Prod. Panam., USA. Medical Products Panamericana Inc., P.O. Box 771, Coral Gables, FL 33134, USA.

Meda, Norw. Meda A/S, Bjerkas Industriomrade, 3470 Slemmestad, Norway.

Meda, Swed. Meda AB, Box 138, 401 22 Goteborg, Sweden.

Medac, Ger. medac Gesellschaft fur klinische Spezialpraparate mbH, Fehlandstrasse 3, Postfach: 303629, 20312 Hamburg, Germany.

Medchem, S.Afr. Medchem, S. Africa.

Medco, USA. Medco Laboratories Inc., P.O. Box 864, Sioux City, IA 51102, USA.

Med-Derm, USA. Med-Derm Pharmaceuticals, P.O. Box 5193, Kingsport, TN 37663, USA.

Medea, Spain. Medea, Santa Carolina 53-9, 08025 Barcelona, Spain.

Medecine Vegetale, Fr. Laboratoires Médecine Végétale, 89 rue Salvador-Allende, 95870 Bezons, France.

Medefield, Austral. Medefield Pty Ltd, 19 Dickson Ave, Artarmon, NSW 2064, Australia.

Medentech, Irl. Medentech Ltd, Whitemill Industrial Estate, Whitemill Rd, Wexford, Ireland.

Medeva, UK. Medeva Pharma, 318 High St North, Dunstable, Beds, LU6 1BE, UK.

Medeva, USA. Medeva Pharmaceuticals, 755 Jefferson Rd, Rochester, NY 14623-0000, USA.

Medgenix, Belg. Medgenix Benelux N.V., Vliegveld 21, 8560 Wevelgem, Belgium.

Medgenix, Fr. Medgenix Pharma, La Boursidiere, B.P. 150, 92357 Le Plessis-Robinson, France.

Medial, Neth. See *Will-Pharma, Neth.*

Medibel, Switz. Laboratoire Medibel SA, Case postale 2631, 1211 Geneva 2 Cornavin, Switzerland.

Medica, Neth. Medica B.V., Lederstraat 1, 5223 AW's-Hertogenbosch, Netherlands.

Medical, Spain. Medical, Virgen de las Angustias 2, 14006 Cordoba, Spain.

Medical Research, Austral. Medical Research (Australia) Pty Ltd, P.O. Box 6025, Parramatta BC, NSW 2150, Australia.

Medice, Ger. Medice, Chem.-pharm. Fabrik Pütter GmbH & Co. KG, Kuhloweg 37-9, Postfach: 2063, 58634 Iserlohn, Germany.

Medice, Switz. See *Ridupharm, Switz.*

Medichemie, Neth. See *Vemedia, Neth.*

Medichemie, Switz. Medichemie AG, Postfach 3650, 4002 Basel, Switzerland.

Medici, Ital. Lab. Farm. Dr Medici s.r.l., Localita Tor Maggiore-Santa Palomba, 00040 Pomezia (Rome), Italy.

Medici Domus, Ital. Medici Domus s.r.l., Via Egeo 8, 10134 Turin, Italy.

Medicis, USA. Medicis Dermatologics Inc., Medicis Pharmaceutical Corp., 4343 E Camelback Rd, Phoenix, AZ 85018-2700, USA.

Medico-Biological Laboratories, UK. Medico-Biological Laboratories Ltd, Kingsend House, 44 Kingsend, Ruislip, Middx, HA4 7DA, UK.

Medicone, USA. Medicone Co., USA.

Medicopharm, Aust. Medicopharm Dr H Sorgo GmbH, Thimiggasse 25, 1180 Vienna, Austria.

Medidom, Switz. Laboratoire Medidom SA, Ave de Champel 24, Case postale 13, 1211 Geneva 12, Switzerland.

Medifood-Trufood, Ital. Medifood-Trufood Italia s.r.l., Via Balbi 31/1, 16126 Genoa, Italy.

Medika, Ger. Medika Lizenz Pharmaz. Praparate, Am Alten Weg 20, 82041 Oberhaching, Germany.

MediMar, UK. MediMar Laboratories, Sarum House, 17 The Queensway, Chalfont St Peter, Bucks, SL9 8NB, UK.

Medimmune, USA. Medimmune Inc., 35 West Watkins Mill Rd, Gaithersburg, MD 20878, USA.

Medimpex, UK. Medimpex UK Ltd, 127 Shirland Rd, London, W9 2EP, UK.

Medinat, Austral. See *Drug Houses Austral., Austral.*

Medinat, Fr. Medinat sarl, 48 av de la Republique, 78500 Sartrouville, France.

Medinaturals, UK. Medinaturals, 37 Limpsfield Rd, Sanderstead, Surrey, CR2 9LA, UK.

Medinex, Canad. Medinex Ltd, 2 boul. Crepeau, Saint-Laurent, Quebec, H4N 1M7, Canada.

Medinova, Switz. Medinova SA, Eggbuhlstrasse 14, 8052 Zurich, Switzerland.

Medinsa, Spain. Medinsa, Doctor Zamenhof 36, 28027 Madrid, Spain.

Mediolanum, Ital. Mediolanum Farmaceutici s.p.a., Via S.G. Cottolengo 15-31, 20143 Milan, Italy.

Medipharm, Switz. Medipharm SA, Rue du Chateau 3, 1636 Broc, Switzerland.

Medipharma, Ger. Medipharma Homburg GmbH, Michelinstr. 10, Postfach: 1455, 66405 Homburg, Germany.

Medi-Physics, USA. Medi-Physics Inc., Amersham Healthcare, 2636 S Clearbrook Drive, Arlington Heights, Il 60005, USA.

Medi-Plex, USA. Medi-Plex Pharmaceuticals Inc., P.O. Box 71600, Richmond, VA 23255-1600, USA.

Medirel, Switz. Medirel SA, Redondello, 6982 Agno, Switzerland.

Medisa, Switz. Medisa AG, Postfach 446, 6343 Rotkreuz, Switzerland.

Medisan, Canad. See *Pharmacia Upjohn, Canad.*

Medisan, Swed. Medisan Pharmaceuticals AB, AR 4, 741 74 Uppsala, Sweden.

Medisculab, Ger. medisculab Arzneimittel GmbH, Postfach: 1628, 70706 Fellbach, Germany.

MediSense, Canad. MediSense, 6535 Millcreek Dr, Unit 41, Mississauga, Ontario, L5N 2M2, Canada.

Medisense, UK. Medisense Britain Ltd, 17 The Courtyard, Gorsey Lane, Coleshill, Birmingham, West Midlands, B46 1JAR, UK.

Medivis, Ital. Medivis srl, Corso Italia 171, 95127 Catania, Italy.

Medix, Fr. Laboratoires Médix, 18 rue Saint-Mathieu, 78550 Houdan, France.

Medix, Spain. Medix, Alcala 431, 28027 Madrid, Spain.

Mednostica, S.Afr. Mednostica, S. Africa.

Medo, UK. Medo Pharmaceuticals Ltd, East St, Chesham, Bucks, HP5 1DG, UK.

Medopharm, Ger. Medopharm Arzneimittelwerk, Dr. Zillich GmbH & Co., Drosselgasse 5, Postfach: 1380, 82155 Grafelfing, Germany.

Medosan, Ital. Medosan s.r.l., Industrie Biochimiche Riunite, Via di Cancelliera 12, 00040 Cecchina (RM), Italy.

Medphano, Ger. medphano Arzneimittel GmbH, Maienbergstr. 10, 15562 Rudersdorf, Germany.

Medpro, S.Afr. Medpro, S. Africa.

Medra, Aust. Medra Handels-GmbH, Gastgebgasse 5-13, 1230 Vienna, Austria.

Medtech, Canad. Medtech Lab, 330 Esna Park Drive, Markham, ON, L3R 1H3, Canada.

Medtech, USA. Medtech Laboratories Inc., 3510 N Lake Creek, POB 1108, Jackson, WY 83011-1108, USA.

Mega Vitamin, Austral. Mega Vitamin Laboratories Pty Ltd, 5 Tahlee St, Burwood, NSW 2134, Australia.

Meiji, Jpn. Meiji Seika Kaisha Ltd, 4-16 Kyobashi 2-chome, Chuo-ku, Tokyo 104, Japan.

Mein, Spain. Mein, Dr. Ferran 4, Vilassar de Dalt, 08339 Barcelona, Spain.

Melisana, Belg. Melisana S.A., ave du Four a Briques 1, 1140 Brussels, Belgium.

Melisana, Switz. Melisana AG, Ankerstrasse 53, 8026 Zurich, Switzerland.

Mellin, Ital. Mellin, Div. Dietetica Star, Via Matteotti 142, 20041 Agrate Brianza (MI), Italy.

Men, Spain. Men, Perello 21, 08005 Barcelona, Spain.

Menadier, Ger. Menadier Heilmittel GmbH, Fischers Allee 49-59, Postfach: 501004, 22710 Hamburg, Germany.

Menarini, Belg. Menarini Benelux S.A., Belgicastraat 4, 1930 Zaventem, Belgium.

Menarini, Fr. Menarini France, 21 rue du Pont-des-Halles, Delta 109, 94536 Rungis Cdx, France.

Menarini, Ital. A. Menarini Industrie Farmaceutiche Riunite s.r.l., Via Sette Santi 3, 50131 Florence, Italy.

Menarini, Neth. Menarini Benelux, Postbus 189, 3440 AD Woerden, Netherlands.

Menarini, Spain. Menarini, Alfonso XII 587, Badalona, 08912 Barcelona, Spain.

Mendelejeff, Ital. Stabilimento Chimico Farmaceutico Mendelejeff s.r.l., Via Aurelia 58, 00165 Rome, Italy.

Menley & James, USA. Menley & James Laboratories Inc., 100 Tournament Drive, Horsham, PA 19044, USA.

Mennen, USA. Mennen Co., Hanover Ave, Morristown, NJ 07962-1928, USA.

Mentholatum, Austral. Mentholatum Pty Ltd, P.O. Box 398, Mulgrave North, Vic. 3170, Australia.

Mentholatum, Canad. Mentholatum Co. of Canada Ltd, 20 Lewis St, Fort Erie, ON, L2A 5M6, Canada.

Mentholatum, UK. The Mentholatum Co. Ltd, 1 Redwood Ave, Peel Park Campus, East Kilbride, Glasgow, G74 5PF, UK.

Mentholatum, USA. Mentholatum Inc., 1360 Niagara St, Buffalo, NY 14213, USA.

Mepha, Switz. Mepha Pharma AG, Pharmazeutische Forschung, Entwicklung und Produktion, Postfach 445, 4147 Aesch/BL, Switzerland.

Mepra-Pharm, UK. Mepra-pharm, P.O. Box 4, Rickmansworth, Herts, WD3 4AU, UK.

Meram, Fr. Laboratoires Meram, 4 bd Malesherbes, 75008 Paris, France.

Merck, Aust. Merck GmbH, Zimbagasse 5, 1147 Vienna, Austria.

Merck, Ger. Merck KGaA, Frankfurter Strasse 250, 64271 Darmstadt, Germany.

Merck, S.Afr. Merck Pharmaceuticals (South Africa) (Pty) Ltd, P.O. Box 1998, Midrand City 1685, S. Africa.

Merck, Spain. Merck Farma Quimica, Poligono Merck, Mollet del Valles, 08100 Barcelona, Spain.

Merck, USA. Merck & Co., P.O. Box 4, West Point, PA 19486, USA.

Merck Frosst, Canad. Merck Frosst Canada Inc., P.O. Box 1005, Pointe-Claire, Dorval, Quebec, H9R 4P8, Canada.

Merck Sharp & Dohme, Aust. Merck Sharp & Dohme GmbH, Gunoldstrasse 14, 1190 Vienna, Austria.

Merck Sharp & Dohme, Austral. Merck Sharp & Dohme (Australia) Pty Ltd, P.O. Box 79, Granville, NSW 2142, Australia.

Merck Sharp & Dohme, Belg. Merck Sharp & Dohme B.V., Chaussee de Waterloo 1135, 1180 Brussels, Belgium.

Merck Sharp & Dohme, Canad. Merck Sharp & Dohme Canada, Division of Merck Frosst Canada Inc., P.O. Box 1005, Pointe-Claire-Dorval, Quebec, H9R 4P8, Canada.

Merck Sharp & Dohme, Ger. MSD Sharp & Dohme GmbH, Lindenplatz 1, Postfach: 1202, 85530 Haar, Germany.

Merck Sharp & Dohme, Irl. See *Cahill May Roberts, Irl.*

Merck Sharp & Dohme, Ital. Merck Sharp & Dohme (Italia) s.p.a., Via G. Fabbroni 6, 00191 Rome, Italy.

Merck Sharp & Dohme, Neth. Merck Sharp & Dohme B.V., Postbus 581, 2003 PC Haarlem, Netherlands.

Merck Sharp & Dohme, Norw. MSD (Norge) A/S, Solbakken 1, Postboks 458 Brakeroya, 3002 Drammen, Norway.

Merck Sharp & Dohme, S.Afr. Merck Sharp & Dohme, S. Africa.

Merck Sharp & Dohme, Spain. Merck Sharp & Dohme, Josefa Valcarcel 38, 28027 Madrid, Spain.

Merck Sharp & Dohme, Swed. Merck Sharp & Dohme (Sweden) AB, Box 7125, 191 07 Sollentuna, Sweden.

Merck Sharp & Dohme, Switz. Merck Sharp & Dohme-Chibret SA, Niederlassung von Merck & Co., Inc., USA, Schaffhauserstrasse 136, Postfach, 8152 Glattbrugg, Switzerland.

Merck Sharp & Dohme, UK. Merck Sharp & Dohme Ltd, Hertford Rd, Hoddesdon, Herts, EN11 9BU, UK.

Merck Sharp & Dohme, USA. Merck Sharp & Dohme, Division of Merck & Co. Inc., West Point, PA 19486, USA.

Merck Sharp & Dohme-Chibret, Fr. Laboratoires Merck Sharp & Dohme-Chibret, 3 ave Hoche, 75114 Paris, France.

Merck-Belgolabo, Belg. Merck-Belgolabo N.V./S.A., Brusselsesteenweg 288, 3090 Overijse, Belgium.

Merck-Clevenot, Fr. Laboratoires Merck-Clévenot, 5-9 rue Anquetil, 94736 Nogent-sur-Marne Cdx, France.

Merck-Clevenot, Switz. See *Interlabo, Switz.*

Merckle, Aust. Merckle Ludwig GmbH, Albert-Schweitzer-Gasse 3, 1140 Vienna, Austria.

Merckle, Ger. Merckle GmbH, Ludwig-Merckle-Strasse 3, Postfach: 1161, 89135 Blaubeuren, Germany.

Merckle, Swed. See *Ferring, Swed.*

Merckle-Diadin, Ger. See *Merckle, Ger.*

Mericon, Norw. Mericon AS, Postboks 1865 Gulset, 3705 Skien, Norway.

Mericon, USA. Mericon Industries Inc., 8819 N Pioneer Rd, Peoria, IL 61615, USA.

Merieux, Belg. See *Pasteur Merieux, Belg.*

Merieux, Fr. Mérieux MSD, PM-MSD, SNC, Halle Borie, 8 rue Jonas-Salk, 69367 Lyon cdx 7, France.

Merieux, Ger. See *Pasteur Merieux, Ger.*

Merieux, Ital. See *Pasteur Merieux, Ital.*

Merieux, Switz. See *Pasteur Merieux, Switz.*

Merieux, UK. See *Pasteur Merieux, UK.*

Merlin, UK. Merlin Pharmaceuticals Ltd, 11 Picardy Street, Belvedere, Kent, DA17 5QQ, UK.

Mer-National, S.Afr. Mer-National (Pty) Ltd, P.O. Box 2432, Randburg 2125, S. Africa.

Merrell Dow, Canad. See *Hoechst Marion Roussel, Canad.*

Merrell Dow, Spain. See *Hoechst Marion Roussel, Spain.*

Merrell Dow, USA. See *Marion Merrell Dow, USA.*

Merz, Ger. Merz & Co., GmbH & Co., Eckenheimer Landstrasse 100-4, Postfach: 111353, 60048 Frankfurt (Main), Germany.

Merz, Neth. See *Hoechst Marion Roussel, Neth.*

Merz, Switz. See *Adroka, Switz.*

Merz & Schoeller, Aust. Merz & Schoeller GmbH, Industriegasse 7, 1230 Vienna, Austria.

Meta Fackler, Ger. meta Biologische Heilmittel Fackler KG, Bogenstr. 3, Postfach: 210226, 30402 Hannover, Germany.

Metapharma, Canad. Metapharma, 10 Corinne Court, Vaughan, Ontario, L4K 4T7, Canada.

Metapharma, Ital. Metapharma s.p.a., Via Pontina 100, 04011 Aprilia (LT), Italy.

Metochem, Aust. Metochem - Dr Partisch & Co., Jochen-Rindt-Strasse 23, 1230 Vienna, Austria.

Met-Rx, USA. Met-Rx Substrate Technology, USA.

Meuse, Belg. Laboratoires de la Meuse S.A., Rue Egide Van Ophem 110, 1180 Brussels, Belgium.

Meuselbach, Ger. See *Krewel, Ger.*

Meyer, Fr. Laboratoires Meyer, 54510 Tomblaine-Nancy, France.

MGI, USA. MGI Pharma Inc., 9900 Bren Road East, Ste. 300E, Minneapolis, Minnesota, MN 55343-9667, USA.

Miba, Ital. Miba Prodotti Chimici e Farmaceutici s.p.a., Via Falzarego 8, 20021 Ospiate di Bollate (MI), Italy.

Michallik, Ger. Fritz Osk. Michallik GmbH & Co., Kisslingweg 60, Postfach: 1362, 75403 Muhlacker, Germany.

Michaux, Belg. See *Sanico, Belg.*

Mickan, Ger. Mickan Arzneimittel GmbH, Industriestrasse 5, Postfach: 210940, 76159 Karlsruhe, Germany.

Midro, Ger. Midro Lörrach GmbH, Postfach: 2006, 79510 Lorrach, Germany.

Midy, Ital. See *Sanofi Winthrop, Ital.*

Milana, Ital. Milana s.r.l., Via A de Gasperi 239, 90146 Palermo, Italy.

Milance, USA. Milance, USA.

Milanfarma, Ital. Milanfarma s.p.a., Piazzale S Turr 5, 20149 Milan, Italy.

Miles, Canad. See *Bayer, Canad.*

Miles, Ital. See *Bayer Diagnostici, Ital.*

Miles, USA. Miles Inc., Pharmaceutical Division, 400 Morgan Lane, West Haven, Connecticut, CT 06516, USA.

Miles Consumer Healthcare, USA. See *MGI, USA.*

Miles Laboratories, USA. See *MGI, USA.*

Milex, Canad. See *Milex, USA.*

Milex, USA. Milex Products Inc., 5915 Northwest Highway, Chicago, IL 60631, USA.

Miller, USA. Miller Pharmacal Group Inc., 350 Randy Rd, Unit 2, Carol Stream, IL 60188, USA.

Millot-Solac, Fr. See *Sanofi Winthrop, Fr.*

Milo, Spain. Milo, Av. Constitucion 18, Nave 6, Cuarte de Huerva, 50080 Zaragoza, Spain.

Milupa, Aust. Milupa GmbH, Postfach 2, 5412 Puch, Austria.

Milupa, Fr. Milupa, 40 rue Jean-Jaures, 93176 Bagnolet Cdx, France.

Milupa, Irl. Milupa Ltd, 1B Sandyford Business Centre, Burton Hall Rd, Dublin 18, Ireland.

Milupa, Ital. Milupa s.p.a., Via Marsala 40, 21013 Gallarate (VA), Italy.

Milupa, Switz. Milupa SA, 1564 Domdidier, Switzerland.

Milupa, UK. Milupa Ltd, Milupa House, Uxbridge Rd, Hillingdon, Middx, UB10 0NE, UK.

Mindel, Ger. Mindel-Pharma Apoth. Dr. Rudolf Lang, Marienplatz, 8948 Mindelheim, Germany.

Minden, Ger. See *Knoll, Ger.*

Mini, Switz. Bernardo Mini & Co, Loretostrasse 5, 6300 Zug, Switzerland.

Minophagen, Jpn. Minophagen Pharmaceutical Co., 10-22 Akasaka 8-chome, Minato-ku, Tokyo 107, Japan.

Miquel Garriga, Spain. Miquel Garriga, Joaquin Costa 18, Montgat, 08390 Barcelona, Spain.

Miquel Otsuka, Spain. Miquel Otsuka, Santany 16, 08016 Barcelona, Spain.

Mirren, S.Afr. Mirren (Pty) Ltd, P.O. Box 87607, Houghton 2041, S. Africa.

Misemer, USA. Misemer Pharmaceuticals Inc., 4553 S Campbell, Springfield, MO 65810-5918, USA.

Mission Pharmacal, USA. Mission Pharmacal Co., 1325 East Durango, P.O. Box 1676, San Antonio, TX 78210, USA.

Mitchell, UK. Mitchell International Pharmaceuticals Ltd, Unit 7, Kingston House Estate, Portsmouth Road, Thames Ditton, Surrey, KT6 5QG, UK.

Mitim, Ital. Mitim s.r.l., Via Rodi 27, 25126 Brescia, Italy.

Mitsubishi, Jpn. Mitsubishi Chemical Corp., 2-24 Higashishinagawa 2-chome, Shinagawa, Tokyo 140, Japan.

Mitsui, Jpn. Mitsui Seiyaku, Asahi Building, 3-12-2 Nihonbashi, Chuo-ku, Tokyo, Japan.

Mletzko, Ger. "Mletzko" Fabrik pharmazeutischer Praparate, Haferstrasse 42, Postfach: 72, 4520 Melle 1, Germany.

Mochida, Jpn. Mochida Pharmaceutical Co. Ltd, 7 Yotsuya 1-chome, Shinjuku-ku, Tokyo 160, Japan.

Modern Health Products, UK. Modern Health Products Ltd, Sisson Rd, Gloucester, GL1 3QB, UK.

Molimin, Ger. Molimin Arzneimittel GmbH, 96101 Hallstadt/Ofr., Germany.

Molitor, Ger. Molitor Pharma GmbH, Bielefelder Strasse 17, Postfach: 2208, 33350 Rheda-Wiedenbruck, Germany.

Molnlycke, Swed. Mölnlycke Clinical Products AB, 405 03 Goteborg, Sweden.

Molteni, Ital. Molteni L. & C. dei F.lli Alitti Società Esercizio s.p.a., Via Pisana 458, 50018 Scandicci (FI), Italy.

Monal, Fr. Laboratoires Monal, Groupe Sandoz, 5 et 7 rue Salvador-Allende, 91127 Palaiseau Cdx, France.

Monal, Neth. See *Bournonville, Neth.*

Monarch, USA. Monarch Pharmaceuticals, 355 Beecham St, Bristol, TN 37620, USA.

Monico, Ital. Jacopo Monico Laboratorio Chimico Biologico s.r.l., Casa Fondata nel 1883, Via Orlanda 10, Ponte Pietra, 30173 Venezia-Mestre (VE), Italy.

Monik, Spain. Monik, Avda de la Playa 1, Conil de la Frontera, 11140 Cadiz, Spain.

Monin, Fr. Laboratoires Monin-Chanteaud, Parc Euromedecine II, rue de la Valsiere, 34099 Montpellier Cdx 5, France.

Monmouth, Irl. See *Allphar, Irl.*

Monmouth, UK. Monmouth Pharmaceuticals, 4 Chancellor Court, 20 Priestley Rd, The Surrey Research Park, Guildford, Surrey, GU2 5YP, UK.

Mono, S.Afr. Mono, S. Africa.

Monoclonal Antibodies, USA. See *Quidel, USA.*

Monot, Fr. Monot, 34 rue St-Romain, 69008 Lyon, France.

Monsanto, Austral. Monsanto Australia Ltd, P.O. Box 1380, Crows Nest, NSW 2065, Australia.

Monsanto, Fr. Monsanto France SA, division Searle, 52 rue Marcel-Dassault, 92514 Boulogne-Billancourt cdx, France.

Monsanto, Ital. Monsanto Italiana s.p.a., Divisione Searle Farmaceutici, Via Walter Tobagi 8, 20068 Peschiera Borromeo (MI), Italy.

Montavit, Aust. Montavit GmbH, Salzbergstrasse 96, 6060 Absam, Austria.

Montefarmaco, Ital. Montefarmaco s.p.a., Via G. Galilei 7, 20016 Pero (MI), Italy.

Moore, USA. H.L. Moore Drug Exchange Inc., 389 John Downey Dr., New Britain, CT 06050, USA.

Morado, Ital. Morado s.p.a., Via Cacciamali 36, 25125 Brescia, Italy.

Moraz, UK. See *Impharm, UK.*

Moreau, Fr. Catherine Moreau SARL, 105 chemin de Suzon, 33400 Talence, France.

Morigi, Ital. Dr. Morigi s.r.l., Via Adelasio 33, 24020 Ranica (BG), Italy.

Morrith, Spain. Morrith, Valle de la Fuenfria 3, 28034 Madrid, Spain.

Morson, Irl. See *Cahill May Roberts, Irl.*

Morson, UK. Thomas Morson Pharmaceuticals, Hertford Rd, Hoddesdon, Herts, EN11 9BU, UK.

Morton Grove, USA. Morton Grove Pharmaceuticals Inc., 6451 West Main St, Morton Grove, IL 60053, USA.

Morton Salt, USA. Morton Salt, 100 N Riverside Plaza, Chicago, IL 60606-1597, USA.

MPS, Austral. MPS Laboratories (Australia) Pty. Ltd, 8 Kinane Street, Brighton, Vic. 3186, Australia.

MSD Chibropharm, Ger. See *Merck Sharp & Dohme, Ger.*

Much, Ger. Much Pharma GmbH, Memeler Str. 30, Postfach: 1462, 42758 Haan, Germany.

Mucos, Aust. Mucos EmulsionsGmbH, Leberstrasse 96, 1110 Vienna, Austria.

Mucos, Ger. Mucos Pharma GmbH & Co., Malvenweg 2, Postfach: 1380, 82524 Geretsried, Germany.

Muller Goppingen, Ger. Chemisch-Pharmazeutische Fabrik Göppingen Carl Müller, Apotheker, GmbH & Co. KG, Bahnhofstrasse 33-35 & 40, Postfach: 869, 73008 Goppingen, Germany.

Mulli, Ger. Dr Mulli Pharma GmbH & Co. KG, Otto-Hahn-Str. 2, Postfach: 1252, 79390 Neuenberg, Germany.

Multipharma, Neth. Multipharma B.V., Gemeenschapspolderweg 28, 1382 GR Weesp, Netherlands.

Multi-Pro, Canad. Multi-Pro Inc, Division of Les Distributions, 2113-E Blvd St-Regis, Dollard des Ormeaux, QC, H9B 2M9, Canada.

Mundipharma, Aust. Mundipharma GmbH, Apollogasse 16-18, 1072 Vienna, Austria.

Mundipharma, Ger. Mundipharma GmbH, Mundipharma-Strasse 2, Postfach: 1350, 65533 Limburg (Lahn), Germany.

Mundipharma, Switz. Mundipharma Pharmaceutical Co, St Alban Rheinweg 74, 4006 Basel, Switzerland.

Mundipharma Proter, Ital. Mundipharma Proter s.r.l., Via Lambro 36, 20090 Opera (MI), Italy.

Murat, Fr. Laboratoires Murat, 160 rue de Paris, 92771 Boulogne-Billancourt, France.

Murdock, USA. Murdock Pharmaceuticals Inc., 1400 Mountain Springs Park, Springville, UT 84663, USA.

Muro, USA. Muro Pharmaceutical Inc., 890 East St, Tewksbury, MA 01876-9987, USA.

MVM, Fr. Lab MVM, 14 rue Guynemer, 92380 Garches, France.

Mykal, UK. Mykal Industries Ltd, Farnsworth House, Morris Close, Park Farm Industrial Estate, Wellingborough, Northants, NN8 6XF, UK.

Myplan, UK. Myplan Ltd, Manor House, 12a Castle St, Berkhamsted, Herts, HP4 2BQ, UK.

MZ, S.Afr. MZ, S. Africa.

Nadeau, Canad. Nadeau Laboratory Ltd, 8480 boul. Saint-Laurent, Montreal, Quebec, H2P 2M6, Canada.

Nadinola, Canad. See *Hargell, Canad.*

NAM, Ger. NAM Neukönigsförder Arzneimittel GmbH, Moorbeker Strasse 35, 26197 Grossenkneten, Germany.

Napp, Irl. Napp Laboratories Ltd, 54 Fitzwilliam Square, Dublin 2, Ireland.

Napp, UK. Napp Laboratories Ltd, Cambridge Science Park, Milton Rd, Cambridge, CB4 4GW, UK.

Nasmark, Canad. Nasmark Inc., 5650 Tomken Rd, Unit 12, Mississauga, ON, L4W 4P1, Canada.

Nastech, USA. Nastech Pharmaceutical Co. Inc., 1 Shields Drive, Route 2, Box 30, Bennington, Vermont, VT 05201, USA.

Nat Druggists, S.Afr. Nat Druggists, S. Africa.

National Care, Canad. National Care, Canada.

Nativelle, Ital. See *Procter & Gamble, Ital.*

Nativelle, Switz. See *Interdelta, Switz.*

Natren, USA. Natren Inc., 3105 Willow Lane, Westlake Village, CA 91361, USA.

Nattermann, Ger. A. Nattermann & Cie. GmbH (Rhône-Poulenc-Rorer), Nattermannallee 1, Postfach: 350120, 50792 Cologne, Germany.

Nattermann, Neth. See *Rhone-Poulenc Rorer, Neth.*

Nattermann, S.Afr. See *Rhone-Poulenc Rorer, S.Afr.*

Nattermann, Spain. Nattermann, Avda de Leganes 62, Alcorcon, 28925 Madrid, Spain.

Nattermann Tee-Arznei, Ger. See *Nattermann, Ger.*

Natura Line, Switz. Natura Line, Via dei Somazzi 12, 6932 Breganzona, Switzerland.

Natural Touch, UK. Natural Touch Ltd, 7 Dragoon House, Hussar Court, Brambles Farm, Waterlooville, Hants, PO7 7SE, UK.

Naturarzneimittel, Ger. Naturarzneimittel Regneri GmbH & Co. KG, Postfach: 100225, 76256 Ettlingen, Germany.

Nature's Bounty, USA. Nature's Bounty Inc., 90 Orville Drive, Bohemia, NY 11716, USA.

Naturpharma, Switz. Naturpharma SA, 5d route des Jeunes, Case postale 8, 1211 Geneva 26, Switzerland.

Naturwaren, Ital. Naturwaren Madaus s.r.l., Via Giotto 23, 39100 Bolzano, Italy.

Navarro, Spain. Navarro Ruiz, Azcona 31, 28028 Madrid, Spain.

NBF-Lanes, Ital. NBF-Lanes srl, Corso di Porta Vittoria 14, 20122 Milan, Italy.

NBI, S.Afr. NBI, S. Africa.

NCI, USA. NCI Medical Foods, USA.

NCSN, Ital. NCSN Farmaceutici s.r.l., Via Tiburtina Km 14.400, 00131 Rome, Italy.

Nefro, Aust. Nefro Pharma GrosshandelsGmbH, Jochingergasse 33, 2100 Korneuburg, Austria.

Negma, Belg. See *Vitalpharma, Belg.*

Negma, Fr. Laboratoires Negma, Immeuble Strasbourg, av de l'Europe, Toussus-le-Noble 78771, France.

Nella, UK. Nella Pharmaceutical Products Ltd, 63 Jenkin Rd, Sheffield, S9 1DS, UK.

Nelson, Austral. Nelson Laboratories (Sales) Pty Ltd, P.O. Box 210, Ermington, NSW 2115, Australia.

Nelson, UK. A Nelson & Co. Ltd, 5 Endeavour Way, Wimbledon, London, SW19 9UH, UK.

Neo Abello, Ital. Neo Abello spa, Via Falzarego 8, 20021 Bollate (MI), Italy.

Neo Laboratories, UK. Neo Laboratories Ltd, Standard House, 16-22 Epworth Street, London, EC2A 4DL, UK.

Neolab, Canad. Néolab Inc., 5476 Upper Lachine Rd, Montreal, Quebec, H4A 2A4, Canada.

Neo-Life, Austral. See *Golden Neo-Life Diamite, Austral.*

Neomed, Switz. Neomed AG, Route Andre-Piller 2, Case postale 76, 1762 Givisiez, Switzerland.

Neopharmed, Ital. Neopharmed s.p.a., Via Giovanni Fabbroni 6, 00191 Rome, Italy.

Neos-Donner, Ger. See *Optimed, Ger.*

NeoStrata, USA. NeoStrata Co. Inc., 4 Research Way, Princeton, NJ 08540, USA.

Nephron, USA. Nephron Pharmaceuticals Corp., 4121 SW 34th St, Orlando, FL 32811-6458, USA.

Nephro-Tech, USA. Nephro-Tech, Inc., P.O. Box 14703, Lenexa, KS 66285, USA.

Nestle, Austral. Nestle Australia Ltd, 60 Bathurst St, Sydney, NSW 2000, Australia.

Nestle, Canad. Nestle Canada Inc., 25 Sheppard Ave W, North York, Ontario, M2N 6S8, Canada.

Nestle, Fr. Nestlé, 7 bd Pierre-Carle, B.P. 900, Noisiel, 77446 Marne-la-Vallee cdx 2.

Nestle, Ital. Nestlè Italiana s.p.a., Via Richard 5, 20143 Milan, Italy.

Nestle, Norw. A/S Nestlé Norge, Barnematavd., Postboks 595, 1301 Sandvika, Norway.

Nestle, S.Afr. Nestlé Infant and Dietetic Services, P.O. Box 50616, Randburg 2125, S. Africa.

Nestle, Switz. Nestlé Produkte AG, Postfach 352, 1800 Vevey, Switzerland.

Nestle, UK. The Nestlé Co. Ltd, St George's House, Croydon, CR9 1NR, UK.

Neuners, Aust. Neuner's Kräuterprodukte GmbH, Oberndorf 60, 6322 Kirchbichl, Austria.

Neurex, USA. Neurex, USA.

NeuroGenesis, USA. NeuroGenesis/Matrix Tech. Inc., USA.

Neusc, Spain. Neusc, Apartado de Correos 11, 08500 Barcelona, Spain.

Neutrogena, UK. Neutrogena (UK) Ltd, 2 Mansfield Rd, South Croydon, Surrey, CR2 6HN, UK.

Neutrogena, USA. Neutrogena Corp., 5760 W 96th St, Los Angeles, CA 90045-5595, USA.

Neutrogena Dermatologics, USA. Neutrogena Dermatologics, Division of Neutrogena Corp., 5755 West 96th St, P.O. Box 45036, Los Angeles, CA 90045, USA.

Neutron Technology, USA. Neutron Technology Corp, 877 Main St, Boise, ID 83702, USA.

New Farma, Ital. New Farma Soc. Coop. a.r.l., Via Umberto 20, 95030 Sant'Agata li Battiati (CT), Italy.

New World Trading Corporation, USA. New World Trading Corporation, PO Box 952, DeBary, Florida, FL 32713, USA.

Newport, Irl. Newport Synthesis Ltd, Baldoyle Industrial Estate, Dublin 13, Ireland.

Newton, UK. Newton Chemical Ltd, 2 Mansfield Rd, South Croydon, Surrey, CR2 6HN, UK.

Nexstar, Belg. Nexstar Pharmaceuticals Inc., Laarstraat 16, 2610 Wilrijk, Belgium.

Nexstar, Ital. Nexstar Pharmaceuticals Italia s.r.l., Via G Frua 16, 20146 Milan, Italy.

Nexstar, UK. Nexstar Pharmaceuticals Ltd, The Quorum, Barnwell Rd, Cambridge, CB5 8RE, UK.

Nexstar, USA. Nexstar, 2860 Wilderness Place, Boulder, CO 80301, USA.

Nextar, Neth. Nextar Pharmaceuticals B.V., Postbus 6313, 6074 ZG Melick, Netherlands.

Nextar, Spain. Nextar Farmaceutica, Paseo de la Castellana 139, 28046 Madrid, Spain.

Nezel, Spain. Nezel, Av. Diagonal 507, 08029 Barcelona, Spain.

Niche, USA. Niche Pharmaceuticals Inc, 200 N Oak St, P.O. Box 449, Roanoake, TX 76262, USA.

Nicholas, Austral. See *Roche, Austral.*

Nicholas, Fr. See *Roche Nicholas, Fr.*

Nicholas, Ger. See *Guerbet, Ger.*

Nicholas, Irl. See *Roche, Irl.*

Nicholas, Neth. See *Roche Nicholas, Neth.*, and *Guerbet, Neth.*

Nicholas, Swed. See *Meda, Swed.*

Nicholas, Switz. See *Searle, Switz.*

Nicholas, UK. See *Roche, UK.*

Nicodent, Austral. See *Advil, Austral.*

Niedermaier, Ger. Dr Niedermaier GmbH, Taufkirchner Strasse 59, 85662 Hohenbrunn bei Munich, Germany.

Nigy, Fr. Laboratoires Nigy, 116 av. des Champs-Elysees, 75008 Paris, France.

Nihon, Jpn. Nihon Pharmaceutical Co. Ltd, 9-8 Higashikanda 1-chome, Chiyoda-ku, Tokyo 101, Japan.

Nikken, Jpn. Nikken Chemicals Co., Ltd, 4-14 Tsukiji 5-chome, Chuo-ku, Tokyo 104, Japan.

Nion, USA. Nion Corp., 15501 First St, Irwindale, CA 91706, USA.

Niverpharm, Fr. Laboratoires Niverpharm, ZI des Taupieres, rue Francis-Garnier, 58000 Nevers, France.

NM, Swed. NM Pharma AB, 112 87 Stockholm, Sweden.

NMC, USA. NMC Labs, 70-36 83rd St, Glendale, NY 11385, USA.

Nnodum, USA. Nnodum, USA.

Nobel, Canad. Nobel Pharm Enrg, 2615 pl. Chasse, Montreal, QC, H1Y 2C3, Canada.

Nogues, Fr. Laboratoires Noguès, 43 rue de Neuilly, 92000 Nanterre, France.

Nogues, Switz. See *Uhlmann-Eyraud, Switz.*

Nomax, USA. Nomax Inc., 40 North Rock Hill Rd, St Louis, MO 63119, USA.

Norcliff Thayer, USA. See *SmithKline Beecham, USA.*

Nordic, Canad. See *Marion Merrell Dow, Canad.*

Nordic, Swed. See *Ferring, Swed.*

Nordic, UK. See *Ferring, UK.*

Nordion, Canad. Nordion International Inc., 447 March Rd, Kanata, Ontario, K2K 1X8, Canada.

Nordisk, Fr. See *Novo Nordisk, Fr.*

Nordisk, Spain. See *Novo Nordisk, Spain.*

Nordisk, USA. See *Novo Nordisk, USA.*

Nordmark, Ger. See *Knoll, Ger.*

Nordmark, Ital. Nordmark Farmaceutici s.p.a., Via Lorenteggio 270/A, 20152 Milan, Italy.

Nordmark, Neth. See *Knoll, Neth.*

Norgine, Austral. Norgine Pty Ltd, 25 Small St, Hampton, Vic. 3188, Australia.

Norgine, Belg. Norgine S.A., Belview Building, Berkenlaan 7, Bus 2, 1831 Diegem, Belgium.

Norgine, Fr. Laboratoires Norgine Pharma, 23 avenue de Neuilly, 75116 Paris, France.

Norgine, Ger. Norgine GmbH, Schwarzenborn 4, Postfach: 1840, 35007 Marburg, Germany.

Norgine, Irl. See *United Drug, Irl.*

Norgine, Ital. Norgine Italia srl, Via Panzini 13, 20145 Milan, Italy.

Norgine, Neth. Norgine B.V., Postbox 10552, 1001 EN Amsterdam, Netherlands.

Norgine, S.Afr. Norgine (Pty) Ltd, P.O. Box 781247, Sandton 2146, S. Africa.

Norgine, Switz. Norgine AG, Bosch 37, 6331 Hunenberg, Switzerland.

Norgine, UK. Norgine Ltd, Widewater Place, Moorhall Rd, Harefield, Uxbridge, Middx, UB9 6NS, UK.

Noristan, S.Afr. Noristan Laboratories (Pty) Ltd, Private Bag X516, Silverton 0127, S. Africa.

Noristan Generica, S.Afr. See *Noristan, S.Afr.*

Norit, Neth. See *Vemedia, Neth.*

Norma, UK. Norma Chemicals Ltd, Standard House, 16-22 Epworth St, London, EC2A 4DL, UK.

Norman, Canad. Merle Norman, Canada.

Normon, Spain. Normon, Nierenberg 10, 28002 Madrid, Spain.

Norpharma, Norw. See *Andersen, Norw.*

Norstar, USA. Norstar Consumer, 206 Pegasus Ave, Northvale, NJ 07647, USA.

Northampton Medical, USA. See *UCB, USA.*

Norton, S.Afr. Norton, S. Africa.

Norton, UK. H.N. Norton & Co. Ltd, Gemini House, Flex Meadow, Harlow, Essex, CM19 5TJ, UK.

Norton Waterford, Irl. Norton Waterford Ltd, Waterford Industrial Estate, Waterford, Ireland.

Norwood, Canad. Norwood, Canada.

Nourypharma, Ger. Nourypharma GmbH, Mittenheimer Strasse 62, 85764 Oberschleissheim, Germany.

Nourypharma, Neth. Nourypharma Nederland B.V., Postbus 20, 5340 BH Oss, Netherlands.

Nourypharma, Switz. See *Orion, Switz.*

Nova Argentia, Ital. Nova Argentia Industria Farmaceutica s.r.l., Via G. Pascoli 1, 20064 Gorgonzola (MI), Italy.

Novag, Spain. Novag, Gran Via de Carlos III 94, 08028 Barcelona, Spain.

Novalac, Fr. Novalac, 209 rue de l'Universite, 75007 Paris, France.

Novalis, Fr. See *Lederle, Fr.*

Novartis, Austral. Novartis Pharmaceuticals Pty Ltd, P.O. Box 101, North Ryde, NSW 2113, Australia.

Novartis, Belg. Novartis Pharma N.V./S.A., Chaussee de Haecht 226, 1030 Brussels, Belgium.

Novartis, Fr. Novartis Pharma SA, 2-4 rue Lionel-Terray, 92500 Rueil-Malmaison, France.

Novartis, Irl. Novartis Ireland Ltd, Beech House, Beech Hill Office Campus, Clonskeagh, Dublin 4, Ireland.

Novartis, Ital. Novartis Farma spa, SS 233 (Varesina) km 20.5, 21040 Origgio (VA), Italy.

Novartis, Neth. Novartis Pharma B.V., Postbus 241, 6800 LZ Arnhem, Netherlands.

Novartis, Norw. Novartis Norge AS, Brynsalleen 4, Postboks 237 Okern, 0510 Oslo, Norway.

Novartis, S.Afr. Novartis, S. Africa.

Novartis, Spain. Novartis Farmaceutica, Gran Via Corts Catalanes 764, 08013 Barcelona, Spain.

Novartis, Swed. Novartis Sverige AB, Box 1150, 183 11 Taby, Sweden.

Novartis, UK. Novartis Pharmaceuticals UK Ltd, Frimley Business Park, Frimley, Camberley, Surrey, GU16 5SG, UK.

Novartis, USA. Novartis, 556 Morris Ave, Summit, NJ 07901, USA.

Novartis Consumer, Belg. Novartis Consumer Health Benelux N.V./S.A., Rue de Wand 211-13, 1020 Brussels, Belgium.

Novartis Consumer, Canad. Novartis Consumer Health Canada Inc., 2233 Argentia Rd, Ste 205, Mississauga, ON, L5N 2X7, Canada.

Novartis Consumer, Ital. Novartis Consumer Health spa, Strada Statale 233 km 20.5, 21040 Orrigio (VA), Italy.

Novartis Consumer, Neth. Novartis Consumer Health Benelux, Postbus 1070, 4801 BB Breda, Netherlands.

Novartis Consumer, S.Afr. Novartis Consumer, S. Africa.

Novartis Consumer, UK. Novartis Consumer Health, Wimblehurst Rd, Horsham, West Sussex, RH12 4AB, UK.

Novartis Nutrition, Spain. See *Novartis, Spain.*

Novartis Nutrition, Swed. Novartis Nutrition, Box 4, 171 18 Solna, Sweden.

Novaxa, Ital. Novaxa s.p.a., Via Aquileja 49, 20092 Cinisello Balsamo (MI), Italy.

Noveal, Switz. See *Uhlmann-Eyraud, Switz.*

Noven, USA. Noven Pharmaceuticals, 13300 SW 128th St, Miami, FL 33186, USA.

Novex Pharma, UK. Novex Pharma Ltd, Innovex House, Marlow Park, Marlow, Bucks, SL7 1TB, UK.

Novipharm, Aust. Novipharm GmbH, Klagenfurter Strasse 164, 9210 Portschach, Austria.

Novipharm, Ger. Novipharm GmbH, Haidachstrasse 29/7/43, 75181 Pforzheim, Germany.

Novo Nordisk, Aust. Novo-Nordisk Pharma GmbH, Universitatsstrasse 11, 1010 Vienna, Austria.

Novo Nordisk, Austral. Novo Nordisk Pharmaceuticals Pty. Ltd, P.O. Box 6086, Parramatta Business Centre, NSW 2150, Australia.

Novo Nordisk, Belg. Novo Nordisk Pharma S.A., Riverside Business Park, Blvd International 55, 1070 Brussels, Belgium.

Novo Nordisk, Canad. Novo Nordisk Canada Inc., 2700 Matheson Blvd E, 3rd Floor, West Tower, Mississauga, Ontario, L4W 4V9, Canada.

Novo Nordisk, Fr. Novo Nordisk Pharmaceutique, 32 rue de Bellevue, 92773 Boulogne-Billancourt, France.

Novo Nordisk, Ger. Novo Nordisk Pharma GmbH, Brucknerstrasse 1, Postfach: 2840, 55018 Mainz, Germany.

Novo Nordisk, Irl. Novo-Nordisk Pharmaceuticals Ltd, 3/4 Upper Pembroke St, Dublin 2, Ireland.

Novo Nordisk, Ital. Novo Nordisk Farmaceutici s.p.a., Via Elio Vitorini 129, 00144 Rome (RM), Italy.

Novo Nordisk, Neth. Novo Nordisk Farma, Postbus 443, 2400 AK Alphen ald Rijn, Netherlands.

Novo Nordisk, Norw. Novo Nordisk Pharma AS, Hauger Skolev. 16, Postboks 24, 1351 Rud, Norway.

Novo Nordisk, S.Afr. Novo-Nordisk (Pty) Ltd, P.O. Box 783155, Sandton 2146, S. Africa.

Novo Nordisk, Spain. Novo Nordisk, Calereuga 102, 28033 Madrid, Spain.

Novo Nordisk, Swed. Novo Nordisk Pharma AB, Box 50587, 202 15 Malmo, Sweden.

Novo Nordisk, Switz. Novo Nordisk Pharma AG, Untere Heslibachstrasse 46, Postfach, 8700 Kusnacht/ZH, Switzerland.

Novo Nordisk, UK. Novo Nordisk Pharmaceuticals Ltd, Novo Nordisk House, Broadfield Park, Brighton Rd, Pease Pottage, Crawley, West Sussex, RH11 9RT, UK.

Novo Nordisk, USA. Novo/Nordisk Pharm. Inc., 100 Overlook Center, Suite 200, Princeton, NJ 08540, USA.

Novocol, USA. Novocol Chemical Mfr Co., P.O. Box 11926, Wilmington, DE 19850, USA.

Novogaleno, Ital. Novogaleno srl, Via Michelangelo Schipa 91, 80122 Naples, Italy.

Novopharm, Canad. Novopharm Ltd, 30 Nably Court, Scarborough, Ontario, M1B 2K9, Canada.

Novopharma, Switz. Novopharma AG, Sumpfstrasse 3, CH-6312 Steinhausen/ZG, Switzerland.

Nucare, UK. Nucare Plc, Raebarn House, 86 Northolt Rd, Harrow, Middx, HA2 0EL, UK.

Numark, UK. Numark Management Ltd, 5/6 Fairway Court, Amber Close, Tamworth Business Park, Tamworth, Staffs, B77 4RP, UK.

Numark, USA. NUmark Laboratories Inc., P.O. Box 6321, Edison, NJ 08818, USA.

Nuovo, Ital. Nuovo Consorzio Sanitario Nazionale s.r.l., Via Svetonio 6, 00136 Rome, Italy.

Nuovo ISM, Ital. Nuovo Istituto Sieroterapico Milanese s.r.l., Viale Tunisia 39, 20124 Milan, Italy.

Nu-Pharm, Canad. Nu-Pharm Inc., 380 Elgin Mills Rd East, Richmond Hill, Ontario, L4C 5H2, Canada.

Nutergia, Fr. Laboratoires Nutergia, B.P. 52, 12700 Capdenac, France.

Nutraceuticals, UK. Nutraceuticals Ltd, 4 Castle House, Kirtley Drive, Nottingham, NG7 1LD, UK.

Nutraloric, USA. Nutraloric, 350 N Lantana, Unit G1, Camarillo, CA 93010, USA.

Nutricia, Austral. Nutricia Australia Pty Ltd, P.O. Box 666, Castle Hill, NSW 2154, Australia.

Nutricia, Fr. Laboratoires Nutricia, L'Europeen, 4 rue Joseph-Monier, 92859 Rueil-Malmaison Cdx, France.

Nutricia, Irl. Nutricia Ireland Ltd, 18 Sandyford Business Centre, Burton Hall Rd, Dublin 18, Ireland.

Nutricia, Ital. Nutricia s.p.a., Via Fosse Adreatine 4, 20092 Cinisello Balsamo (MI), Italy.

Nutricia, UK. See *Cow & Gate, UK.*

Nutricia-Luma Lindar, USA. Nutricia-Luma Lindar, USA.

Nutrimed, Fr. Nutrimed Medic System, 6/10 rue Mirabeau, 75016 Paris, France.

Nutri-Metics, Canad. Nutri-Metics International (Can) Ltd, 3915-16 Ave SE, Calgary, AB, T2C 1V5, Canada.

Nutripharm, USA. Nutripharm Laboratories Inc., Salem Industrial Park, Building 5, Lebanon, NJ 08833, USA.

Nutripharm Elgi, Fr. Laboratoires Nutripharm Elgi, B.P. 432, 365 rue Philippe-Heron, 69654 Villefranche-sur-Saone Cdx, France.

Nyal, Austral. See *SmithKline Beecham Consumer, Austral.*

Nycomed, Aust. Nycomed-Heilmittelwerke Wien GmbH, Triester Strasse 50, 1102 Vienna, Austria.

Nycomed, Austral. Nycomed Australia, Level 6, 1 Railway St, Chatswood, NSW 2067, Australia.

Nycomed, Belg. Nycomed S.A., Chaussee de Gand 615, 1080 Brussels, Belgium.

Nycomed, Fr. Laboratoires Nycomed SA, Centre d'affaires et d'activites Tolbiac-Massena, 25 quai Panhard-et-Levassor, CE no. 19, 75644 Paris Cdx 13, France.

Nycomed, Ger. Nycomed Arzneimittel GmbH, Fraunhoferstr. 7, Postfach: 1209, 85730 Ismaning b. Munich, Germany.

Nycomed, Ital. Nycomed s.p.a., Piazza S Eustorgio 2, 20122 Milan, Italy.

Nycomed, Neth. Nycomed B.V., Postbus 3458, 4800 DL Breda, Netherlands.

Nycomed, Norw. Nycomed Pharma AS, Slemdalsv. 37, Postboks 5012 Majorstua, 0301 Oslo, Norway.

Nycomed, Spain. Nycomed, Avda Pio XII 99, 28036 Madrid, Spain.

Nycomed, Swed. Nycomed AB, Box 1215, 181 24 Lidingo, Sweden.

Nycomed, Switz. Nycomed AG, Moosacherstrassestrasse 14, Au, 8820 Wadenswil, Switzerland.

Nycomed, UK. Nycomed (UK) Ltd, Nycomed House, 2111 Coventry Rd, Sheldon, Birmingham, B26 3EA, UK.

Nycomed, USA. Nycomed, 101 Carnegie Center, Prinston, NJ 08540-6231, USA.

Nycomed Imaging, Norw. Nycomed Imaging AS, Nycov. 2, Postboks 4220 Torshov, 0401 Oslo, Norway.

Oakhurst, USA. Oakhurst Co., 3000 Hempstead Turnpike, Levittown, NY 11756, USA.

Oberlin, Fr. Laboratoires Oberlin, 304 av du Docteur Jean-Bru, 47000 Agen, France.

Oclassen, USA. Oclassen Pharmaceuticals Inc., 100 Pelican Way, San Rafael, CA 94901, USA.

O'Connor, USA. See *Columbia, USA.*

Octapharma, Aust. Octapharma Pharmazeutika, Oberlaaer Strasse 235, 1100 Vienna, Austria.

Octapharma, Ger. Octapharma Vertrieb von Plasmaderivaten GmbH, Bahnhofstrasse 43, Postfach: 1464, 40739 Langenfeld, Germany.

Octapharma, Norw. Octapharma A.S., Rustad, 2090 Hurdal, Norway.

Octapharma, Swed. Octapharma Scandinavia, Box 69, 182 07 Stocksund, Sweden.

Octapharma, Switz. Octapharma AG, Haus im Park, 8866 Ziegelbrucke, Switzerland.

Octapharma, UK. Octapharma Ltd, Olton Bridge, 245 Warwick Rd, Solihull, West Midlands, B92 7AH, UK.

Ocumed, USA. Ocumed Inc., 119 Harrison Ave, Roseland, NJ 07068, USA.

Ocusoft, USA. Ocusoft, P.O. Box 429, Richmond, TX 77406-0429, USA.

Odan, Canad. Odan Laboratories Ltd, 847 McCaffrey St, St Laurent, Quebec, H4T 1N3, Canada.

Odontopharm, Switz. Odontopharm AG, Engestrasse 23, 3000 Bern 26, Switzerland.

Oenobiol, Fr. Lab. Oenobiol, 59 bd Exelmans, 75781 Paris cdx 16, France.

OFF, Ital. Officina Farmaceutica Fiorentina s.r.l. Istituto Biochimico, Quart. Varignano 12-14, 55049 Viareggio (Lucca), Italy.

Oftalmiso, Spain. Oftalmiso, Spain.

Ogna, Ital. Giovanni Ogna & Figli s.p.a., Via Figini 41, 20053 Muggio (MI), Italy.

Ohm, USA. Ohm Laboratories Inc., P.O. Box 279, Franklin Park, NJ 08823, USA.

Ohmeda, USA. Ohmeda, subsidiary of BOC Health Care, Inc., P.O. Box 804, Liberty Corner, NJ 07938-0804, USA.

Ohropax, Switz. See *Uhlmann-Eyraud, Switz.*

Oligosol, Switz. Oligosol AG, Untermattweg 8, 3001 Bern, Switzerland.

OM, Ger. Deutsche OM Arzneimittel GmbH, Houiller Platz 17, 61381 Friedrichsdorf/Ts, Germany.

OM, Switz. Laboratoire OM SA, 22 rue du Bois-du-Lan, 1217 Meyrin 2/Geneva, Switzerland.

Omega, Canad. Omega Laboratories Ltd, 11177 rue Hamon, Montreal, Quebec, H3M 3A2, Canada.

Omega, Spain. Omega Farmaceutica, Ronda General Mitre 151, 08022 Barcelona, Spain.

Omegin, Ger. Omegin Dr Schmidgall GmbH & Co. KG, Postfach: 1164, 73253 Kongen, Germany.

Omida, Switz. Omida AG, Homoopathische Heilmittel, Erlistrasse 2, 6403 Kussnacht aR, Switzerland.

Omisan, Ital. Omisan Farmaceutici di Antonio Vona & C sas, Via Scarperia 33, 00146 Rome, Italy.

Omnimed, S.Afr. OmniMed (Pty) Ltd, P.O. Box 42128, Fordsburg 2033, S. Africa.

Ono, Jpn. Ono Pharmaceutical Co. Ltd, 1-5 Doshomachi 2-chome, Chuo-ku, Osaka 541, Japan.

Opfermann, Ger. Opfermann Arzneimittel GmbH, Robert-Koch-Strasse 2, Postfach: 1420, 51658 Wiehl, Germany.

Ophtapharma, Canad. Ophtapharma Canada Inc., 1100 Cremazie E, Suite 708, Montreal, Quebec, H2P 2X2, Canada.

Opocalcium, Fr. Laboratoires de l'Opocalcium, 423 rue Audemars, ZI, 78530 Buc, France.

Opocalcium, Switz. See *Uhlmann-Eyraud, Switz.*

Opopharma, Switz. Opopharma SA, Kirchgasse 42, 8001 Zurich, Switzerland.

Opsia, Fr. Laboratoires Opsia Pharma, ZAC de la Bourgade, BP 711, rue Max-Planck, 31683 Toulouse Labege Cdx, France.

Optikem, USA. Optikem International Inc., 2172 S Jason St, Denver, CO 80223, USA.

Optimed, Ger. Optimed Pharma GmbH, Alfred-Nobel-Str. 5, Postfach: 1345, 50203 Frechen, Germany.

Optimox, USA. Optimox Inc., 2720 Monterey St, Suite 406, Torrance, CA 90503, USA.

Optopics, USA. Optopics Laboratories Corp., 32 Main St, P.O. Box 210, Fairton, NJ 08320-0210, USA.

Opus, S.Afr. Opus Pharmaceuticals (Pty) Ltd, P.O.Box 78618, Sandton 2146, S. Africa.

Opus, UK. Opus Pharmaceuticals Ltd, Tuition House, 27/37 St George's Rd, Wimbledon, London, SW19 4DS, UK.

OPW, Ger. Oranienburger Pharmawerk GmbH (OPW), Lehnitzstrasse 70-98, Postfach: 100244, 16502 Oranienburg, Germany.

Oral-B, Austral. Oral-B Laboratories Pty Ltd, P.O. Box 957, North Sydney, NSW 2060, Australia.

Oral-B, Canad. Oral-B Laboratories Inc., 974 Lakeshore Rd E., Mississauga, Ontario, L5E 1E4, Canada.

Oral-B, Ger. Oral-B Laboratories GmbH, Russelsheimer Str. 22, Postfach: 190340, 60090 Frankfurt/M., Germany.

Oral-B, Irl. Oral-B, Ireland.

Oral-B, Ital. Oral-B Laboratories Italy, Via Beato Angelico 1, 21047 Saronno (VA), Italy.

Oral-B, UK. Oral-B Laboratories Ltd, Gatehouse Rd, Aylesbury, Bucks, HP19 3ED, UK.

Oral-B, USA. Oral-B Labs Inc., 1 Lagoon Drive, Redwood City, CA 94065, USA.

Oramon, Ger. Oramon Arzneimittel GmbH, Mittelstrasse 18, Postfach: 1461, 88464 Laupheim, Germany.

Ordesa, Spain. Ordesa, Ctra Enlace con Prat S/N, Sant Boi de Llobregat, 08830 Barcelona, Spain.

Or-Dov, Austral. Or-Dov Pharmaceuticals Pty Ltd, P.O. Box 172, Doncaster, Vic. 3108, Australia.

Organon, Aust. Organon GmbH, Siebenbrunnengasse 21/D/IV, 1050 Vienna, Austria.

Organon, Austral. Organon (Australia) Pty Ltd, Private Bag 25, Lane Cove, NSW 2066, Australia.

Organon, Belg. Organon Belge S.A., AKZO Building, Ave Marnix 13, 1050 Brussels, Belgium.

Organon, Canad. Organon Canada Ltd, 200 Consilium Place, Ste 700, Scarborough, Ontario, M1H 3E4, Canada.

Organon, Fr. Organon, B.P. 144, 93204 Saint-Denis Cdx 01, France.

Organon, Ger. Organon GmbH, Mittenheimer Strasse 62, 85764 Oberschleissheim, Germany.

Organon, Irl. See *United Drug, Irl.*

Organon, Ital. Organon Italia s.p.a., Via Ostilia 15, 00184 Rome, Italy.

Organon, Neth. Organon Nederland B.V., Postbus 20, 5340 BH Oss, Netherlands.

Organon, Norw. Organon A/S, Roykenv.70, Postboks 324, 1371 Asker, Norway.

Organon, Spain. Organon Hermes, Castello 1, Pol. Ind. las Salinas, Sant Boi de Llobregat, 08830 Barcelona, Spain.

Organon, Swed. Organon AB, Box 5076, 426 05 V Frolunda, Sweden.

Organon, Switz. Organon SA, Churerstrasse 160b, 8808 Pfaffikon/SZ, Switzerland.

Organon, UK. Organon Laboratories Ltd, Cambridge Science Park, Milton Rd, Cambridge, CB4 4FL, UK.

Organon, USA. Organon Inc., 375 Mount Pleasant Ave, West Orange, NJ 07052, USA.

Organon Teknika, Austral. Organon Teknika Pty Ltd, Unit 13, 5 Hudson Ave, Castle Hill, NSW 2154, Australia.

Organon Teknika, Belg. Organon Teknika N.V., Veedijk 58, 2300 Turnhout, Belgium.

Organon Teknika, Canad. Organon Teknika Inc., 30 North Wind Place, Scarborough, Ontario, M1S 3R5, Canada.

Organon Teknika, Fr. Organon Teknika, 5 av. des Pres, B.P. 26, 94267 Fresnes Cedex, France.

Organon Teknika, Ger. Organon Teknika Medizinische Produkte GmbH, Wernher-von-Braun-Strasse 18, Postfach: 1280, 69209 Eppelheim, Germany.

Organon Teknika, Irl. See *Organon Teknika, UK.*

Organon Teknika, Ital. Organon Teknika s.p.a., Via Ostilia 15, 00184 Rome, Italy.

Organon Teknika, Neth. Organon Teknika Nederland B.V., Postbus 23, 5280 AA Boxtel, Netherlands.

Organon Teknika, Norw. See *Organon, Norw.*

Organon Teknika, Spain. Organon Teknika, Castello 1, Sant Boi de Llobregat, 08830 Barcelona, Spain.

Organon Teknika, Swed. Organon Teknika AB, Hantverksvagen 15, 436 33 Askim, Sweden.

Organon Teknika, Switz. Organon Teknika AG, Postfach 129, 8808 Pfaffikon/SZ, Switzerland.

Organon Teknika, UK. Organon-Teknika Ltd, Cambridge Science Park, Milton Rd, Cambridge, CB4 4FL, UK.

Organon Teknika, USA. Organon Teknika Corporation, 100 Akzo Ave, Durham, North Carolina, NC 27704, USA.

Original Additions, UK. Original Additions (Beauty Products) Ltd, 1 Elystan Business Centre, Springfield Rd, Hayes, Middx, UB4 0UJ, UK.

Orion, Ger. Orion Pharma GmbH, Albert-Einstein-Ring 1, 22761 Hamburg, Germany.

Orion, Irl. See *Allphar, Irl.*

Orion, Norw. Orion Pharma AS, Ulvenv 84, Postboks 52 Okern, 0508 Oslo, Norway.

Orion, Swed. Orion Pharma AB, Box 334, 192 30 Sollentuna, Sweden.

Orion, Switz. Orion Pharma AG, Untermuli 11, 6300 Zug, Switzerland.

Orion, UK. Orion Pharma UK Ltd, 1st Floor Leat House, Overbridge Square, Hambridge Lane, Newbury, Berks, RG14 5UX, UK.

Orion, USA. Orion Diagnostica, 71 Veronica Ave., P.O. Box 218, Somerset, NJ 08875-0218, USA.

OroClean, Switz. OroClean-Chemie AG, Buelstrasse 17, 8330 Pfaffikon/ZH, Switzerland.

Orphan, Austral. Orphan, Australia.

Orphan, Fr. Orphan Europe, Imm Le Guillaumet, 92046 Paris-La Defense, France.

Orphan, Norw. Orphan Norge, Tverkjeglav 11, 1440 Drobak, Norway.

Orphan Europe, UK. Orphan Europe (UK) Ltd, 32 Bell St, Henley-on-Thames, Oxfordshire, RG9 2BH, UK.

Orphan Medical, USA. Orphan Medical, 13911 Ridgedale Drive, Minnetonka, MN 55305, USA.

Orravan, Spain. Orravan, Marco Aurelio 18-20, 08006 Barcelona, Spain.

Orsade, Spain. Orsade, Avda Virgen de Montserrat 221, 08026 Barcelona, Spain.

Ortega, USA. Ortega, USA.

Ortho, Canad. See *Janssen-Ortho, Canad.*

Ortho, Ital. Ortho Clinical Diagnostics spa, Via Volta 16, 20093 Cologno Monzese (MI), Italy.

Ortho, UK. See *Cilag, UK.*

Ortho Biotech, USA. See *Ortho Pharmaceutical, USA.*

Ortho Dermatological, USA. Ortho Pharmaceutical Corp., Dermatological Division, Route 202, P.O. Box 300, Raritan, NJ 08869-0602, USA.

Ortho Diagnostic, UK. Ortho Diagnostic Systems Ltd, Enterprise House, Station Rd, Loudwater, High Wycombe, Bucks, HP10 9UF, UK.

Ortho McNeil, USA. See *Ortho Pharmaceutical, USA.*

Ortho Pharmaceutical, USA. Ortho Pharmaceutical Corp., Raritan, NJ 08869, USA.

Ortho-Cilag, UK. See *Cilag, UK.*

Ortis, Ital. Ortis Italia s.r.l., Via Maroncelli 62/64, Padua, Italy.

Osterholz, Ger. Pharma Osterholz GmbH, Postfach: 100662, 40770 Monheim, Germany.

Osterreichisches Institut, Aust. Österreichisches Institut fur Hämoderivate, Vienna, Austria.

OTC, Spain. OTC-Iberica, President Lluis Companys 16, Santa Coloma de Gramanet, 08921 Barcelona, Spain.

Otifarma, Ital. Otifarma s.p.a., Via Martiri d/la Liberta 34, 43058 Sorbolo (PR), Italy.

Otosan, Ital. Otosan, Via Balzella 75, 47100 Forli, Italy.

Otsuka, Jpn. Otsuka Pharmaceutical Co. Ltd, Kanda Building 2, 2-2 Tsukasa-cho, Kanda, Chiyoda-ku, Tokyo 101, Japan.

Otsuka, USA. Otsuka America Pharmaceutical, 1201 Third Avenue, Ste. 5300, Seattle, WA 98101, USA.

Ottolenghi, Ital. Dr. Ottolenghi & C. s.r.l., Via Cuneo 5, 10028 Trofarello (TO), Italy.

OTW, Ger. Organotherapeutische Werke GmbH (OTW), Carl-Zeiss-Strasse 4, Postfach: 100225, 76256 Ettlingen, Germany.

Outdoor Recreations, USA. Outdoor Recreations, USA.

Ovelle, Irl. Ovelle Ltd, Industrial Estate, Coe's Rd, Dundalk, Co. Louth, Ireland.

Overta, Aust. Overta, Austria.

Owen, USA. See *Galderma, USA.*

Owen-Galderma, USA. See *Galderma, USA.*

Oxford Nutrition, UK. Oxford Nutrition Ltd, P.O. Box 31, Oxford, OX4 3UH, UK.

Oxford Pharmaceuticals, UK. Oxford Pharmaceuticals Ltd, Masters House, 5 Sandridge Close, Harrow, Middx, HA1 1XD, UK.

Oxo, Switz. See *Doetsch, Grether, Switz.*

Oykol, Spain. Oykol, Valentin Beato 44, 28037 Madrid, Spain.

Pabisch, Aust. Pabisch GmbH, Baldassgasse 5, 1217 Vienna, Austria.

Paddock, USA. Paddock Laboratories Inc., 3940 Quebec Ave North, Minneapolis, MN 55427, USA.

Padma, Switz. Padma AG, für tibetische Heilmittel, Dammstrasse 29, 8702 Zollikon, Switzerland.

Padma, UK. Padma 28 UK Ltd, Pepper Rd, Bramhall Moor Lane, Hazel Grove, Stockport, Cheshire, SK7 5BW, UK.

Padro, Spain. Padro, C de la Marina 208, 08013 Barcelona, Spain.

Paedpharm, Austral. Paedpharm Pty Ltd, P.O. Box 6533, East Perth, WA 6892, Australia.

Paesel, Ger. Paesel & Lorei GmbH & Co., Moselstr. 2B, 63452 Hanau, Germany.

Pagni, Ital. See *Parke, Davis, Ital.*

Paines & Byrne, Irl. See *United Drug, Irl.*

Paines & Byrne, UK. Paines & Byrne Ltd, Brocades House, Pyrford Rd, West Byfleet, Surrey, KT14 6RA, UK.

Palex, Spain. Palex, C/ Huelma 5, Pol. Ind. Olivares, 23009 Jaen, Spain.

Palisades, USA. See *Glenwood, USA.*

Palmicol, Ger. Palmicol Arzneimittel GmbH, Gartenstr. 33, 61250 Usingen, Germany.

Palmolive Skincare, Austral. Palmolive Skincare Laboratories, G.P.O. Box 3964, Sydney, NSW 2001, Australia.

Pal-Pak, USA. Pal-Pak Inc., 1201 LIberty St, P.O. Box 299, Allentown, PA 18105, USA.

Pan America, USA. Pan America Labs, P.O. Box 8950, Mandeville, LA 70470-8950, USA.

Pan Quimica, Spain. Pan Quimica Farmaceutica, Rufino Gonzalez 50, 28037 Madrid, Spain.

Panax, Switz. Panax Import, F Ruckstuhl & Co., Bergtalweg 2a, 9500 Wil, Switzerland.

Panderma, Aust. Panderma Arzneimittel GmbH, Hernalser Hauptstrasse 114/41, 1170 Vienna, Austria.

Pannoc, Belg. Pannoc Chemie S.A., Lammerdries 23, B.P. 70, 2250 Olen, Belgium.

Panpharma, Fr. Laboratoires Panpharma, Z.I. du Clairay Luitre, 35133 Fougeres, France.

Panpharma, UK. Panpharma Ltd, Panpharma House, White Lion Rd, Little Chalfont, Amersham, Bucks, HP7 9LP, UK.

Pantene, Austral. See *Richardson-Vicks, Austral.*

Pantheon, UK. Pantheon Healthcare Ltd, Studio 8, 48 Tierney Rd, London, SW2 4QS, UK.

Panthox & Burck, Ital. Panthox & Burck s.p.a., Istituto Biochimico Italo Svizzero, Italy.

Panto, Spain. Panto Farma, Pedro IV 84, 08005 Barcelona, Spain.

Panzera, Ital. Farmaceutici G.B. Panzera s.r.l., Via De Sanctis 71, 20141 Milan, Italy.

Par, USA. Par Pharmaceutical Inc., One Ram Ridge Rd, Spring Valley, NY 10977, USA.

Paragerm, Fr. Laboratoires Paragerm, Z.I., 3e rue, B.P. 68, 06511 Carros, France.

Paraphar, Fr. Laboratoires Paraphar, 10 rue Varet, 75015 Paris, France.

Para-Pharma, Switz. Para-Pharma AG, c/o Investarit AG, Freigutstrasse 16, Postfach, 8027 Zurich, Switzerland.

Parekh, Ital. Parekh Chemicals Italia S.p.A., Fraz. Domodossolina, 20070 Borgo S Giovanni (MI), Italy.

Parisis, Spain. Parisis, Juan de Juanes 8, 28007 Madrid, Spain.

Parke, Davis, Aust. Parke-Davis GmbH, Ketzergasse 118, Postfach 35, 1234 Vienna, Austria.

Parke, Davis, Austral. Parke Davis Pty Ltd, P.O. Box 42, Taren Point, NSW 2229, Australia.

Parke, Davis, Belg. Parke-Davis, Division of Warner-Lambert (Belgium) S.A., Excelsiorlaan 75-7, 1930 Zaventem, Belgium.

Parke, Davis, Canad. Parke-Davis, P.O. Box 2200, Station A, Scarborough, Ontario, M1K 5C9, Canada.

Parke, Davis, Fr. Parke, Davis, 11 av. Dubonnet, 92407 Courbevoie Cdx, France.

Parke, Davis, Ger. Parke-Davis GmbH, 79090 Freiburg, Germany.

Parke, Davis, Irl. Parke Davis, Pottery Rd, Dun Laoghaire, Co. Dublin, Ireland.

Parke, Davis, Ital. Parke Davis s.p.a., Via C. Colombo 1, 20020 Lainate (Milan), Italy.

Parke, Davis, Neth. Parke-Davis, Postbus 3008, 2130 KA Hoofddorp, Netherlands.

Parke, Davis, S.Afr. See *Warner, S.Afr.*

Parke, Davis, Spain. Parke Davis, Plg. Ind. Manso Mateu S-N, Prat de Llobregat, 08820 Barcelona, Spain.

Parke, Davis, Swed. Parke-Davis, Division of Warner Lambert Nordic AB, Box 4130, 171 04 Solna, Sweden.

Parke, Davis, Switz. See *Warner-Lambert, Switz.*, and *Uhlmann-Eyraud, Switz.*

Parke, Davis, UK. Parke-Davis Medical, Mitchell House, Southampton Rd, Eastleigh, Hants, SO5 5RY, UK.

Parke, Davis, USA. Parke-Davis, Division of Warner-Lambert Co., 201 Tabor Rd, Morris Plains, NJ 07950, USA.

Parke Davis-Wellcome, Austral. See *Wellcome, Austral.*

Parke-Med, S.Afr. Parke-Med, S. Africa.

Parkfields, UK. Parkfields Sterile Supply Unit, Pond Lane, Parkfields, Wolverhampton, West Midlands, WV2 1HL, UK.

Parmed, USA. Parmed Pharmaceuticals Inc., 4220 Hyde Park Blvd, Niagara Falls, NY 14305, USA.

Parnell, USA. Parnell Pharmaceuticals, Inc., Larkspur Landing Circle, Larkspur, CA 94939, USA.

Parsenn, Switz. Parsenn-Produkte AG, Hauptstrasse 1, 7240 Kublis, Switzerland.

Parthenon, USA. Parthenon Company Inc., 3311 W. 2400 South, Salt Lake City, Utah, UT 84119, USA.

Partner, Norw. Partner Farma AS, Postboks 77 Leirdal, 1008 Oslo, Norway.

Pasadena, USA. Pasadena Research Labs Inc., P.O. Box 5136, San Clemente, CA 92674-5136, USA.

Pascoe, Ger. Pascoe Pharmazeutische Präparate GmbH, Schiffenberger Weg 55, Postfach: 100755, 35337 Giessen, Germany.

Passauer, Ger. Herbert J Passauer GmbH, Chem.-Pharm. Fabrik, Kirchhainer Damm 62, Postfach: 490248, 12282 Berlin, Germany.

Pastaba, Fr. See *Monal, Fr.*

Pasteur, Fr. See *Merieux, Fr.*, and *Pasteur Vaccins, Fr.*

Pasteur Merieux, Austral. Pasteur Merieux Australia, a division of Merieux UK Ltd, 35 Cotham Road, Kew, Vic. 3101, Australia.

Pasteur Merieux, Belg. Pasteur Merieux MSD, Ave Jules Bordet 13, 1140 Brussels, Belgium.

Pasteur Merieux, Ger. Pasteur Merieux MSD GmbH, Paul-Ehrlich-Str. 1, Postfach: 1468, 69172 Leimen, Germany.

Pasteur Merieux, Irl. Pasteur Merieux MSD Ltd, Burton Hall Park, Sandyford Industrial Estate, Dublin 18, Ireland.

Pasteur Merieux, Ital. Pasteur Merieux MSD s.p.a., Via di Villa Troili 56, 00163 Rome, Italy.

Pasteur Merieux, Neth. Pasteur Merieux MSD, Postbus 512, 1180 AM Amstelveen, Netherlands.

Pasteur Merieux, Norw. See *Meda, Norw.*

Pasteur Merieux, Spain. Pasteur Merieux MSD, Josefa Valcarcel 40, 28027 Madrid, Spain.

Pasteur Merieux, Swed. See *Meda, Swed.*

Pasteur Merieux, Switz. See *Rhone-Poulenc Rorer, Switz.*

Pasteur Merieux, UK. Pasteur Merieux MSD Ltd, Clivemont House, Clivemont Rd, Maidenhead, Berks, SL6 7BU, UK.

Pasteur Merieux, USA. See *Connaught, USA.*

Pasteur Vaccins, Fr. Pasteur Vaccins, 3 av. Pasteur, B.P. 10, 92430 Marnes-la-Coquette, France.

Pastor Farina, Ital. Pastor Farina s.r.l., Via Garibaldi 69, 22100 Como, Italy.

Patentex, Ger. Patentex GmbH, Marschnerstr. 8-10, Postfach: 111353, 60048 Frankfurt/Main, Germany.

Patentex, Switz. See *Adroka, Switz.*

Pathogenesis, USA. PathoGenesis Corp., USA.

Pautrat, Fr. Laboratoires Pautrat, P.P.D.H. S.A., 247 bis rue des Pyrenees, 75020 Paris, France.

PCR, Ger. PCR Arzneimittel GmbH, Wielandstr. 7, 53173 Bonn, Germany.

PD Pharm, S.Afr. PD Pharm, S. Africa.

Pearson, Ital. Guglielmo Pearson s.r.l., Via delle Fabbriche 40, 16158 Genova-Voltri (GE), Italy.

Pedinol, USA. Pedinol Pharmacal Inc., 30 Banfi Plaza North, Farmingdale, NY 11735, USA.

Pedi-Pak, Canad. Pedi-Pak Products Canada Inc., 700 Lawrence Ave W, Ste 125, Toronto, ON, M6A 3B4, Canada.

Peithner, Aust. Dr Peithner KG, Richard Strauss-Strasse 13, 1232 Vienna, Austria.

Pejo, Ger. Pejo Heilmittel- u. Diat GmbH & Co. KG, Kuhloweg 37-39, Postfach: 2162, 5860 Iserlohn, Germany.

Pekana, Ger. Pekana Naturheilmittel GmbH, Postfach: 1262, 88350 Kisslegg/Allgau, Germany.

Pelayo, Spain. Pelayo, Tallers 16, 08001 Barcelona, Spain.

Penederm, Canad. See *Pharmascience, Canad.*

Penederm, USA. Penederm Inc., 320 Lakeside Drive, Suite A, Foster City, CA 94404, USA.

Penn, Irl. See *Central, Irl.*

Penn, UK. Penn Pharmaceuticals Ltd, Buckingham House, Church Rd, Penn, High Wycombe, Bucks, HP10 8LN, UK.

Pensa, Spain. Pensa, Av. Virgen de Montserrat 215, 08026 Barcelona, Spain.

Pentaderm, Ital. Pentaderm Industria Chimica e Farmaceutica s.r.l., Via Nazionale Pentimele 157, 89121 Reggio Calabria, Italy.

Pentafarm, Spain. Pentafarm, Galileo 250, 08028 Barcelona, Spain.

Pentapharm, Switz. Pentapharm SA, Engelgasse 109, 4002 Basle, Switzerland.

Perez Gimenez, Spain. Calmante Vitaminado, S.A., Laboratorios Perez Gimenez, Glorieta Perez Gimenez 1, 14007 Cordoba, Spain.

Perfecta, Switz. Perfecta AG, Gewerbestrasse 16, 3065 Bolligen-Station, Switzerland.

Pergam, Ital. Pergam s.r.l., Via Gradisca 8, 20151 Milan, Italy.

Permamed, Switz. Permamed AG, Ringstrasse 29, Postfach 360, 4106 Therwil, Switzerland.

Person & Covey, Canad. Person & Covey, Canada.

Person & Covey, USA. Person & Covey Inc., 616 Allen Ave, Glendale, CA 91201, USA.

Personal Care, USA. Personal Care Group Inc., 1 Paragon Drive, Montvale, NJ 07645, USA.

Perstorp, Irl. See *Cahill May Roberts, Irl.*

Perstorp, Norw. See *Solveig Ekeberg, Norw.*

Perstorp, Swed. Perstorp Pharma, Forskningsbyn Ideon, Beta 4, 223 70 Lund, Sweden.

Perstorp, Switz. See *Adroka, Switz.*

Perstorp, UK. Perstorp Pharma Ltd, Wound Care Division, Studio 1, Intec 2, Wade Road, Basingstoke, Hampshire, RG24 8NE, UK.

Pertussin, USA. Pertussin Laboratories, USA.

Peters, Fr. Laboratoires Peters, ZI Les Vignes, 42 rue Benoit-Frachon, 93000 Bobigny Cedex, France.

Petrasch, Aust. Mr Petrasch GmbH & Co. KG und Petrasch-Pharma GmbH, Schlachthausstrasse 3, 6850 Dornbirn, Austria.

Petrus, Austral. Petrus Pharmaceuticals, P.O. Box 41, Midland, Perth, WA 6936, Australia.

Pfeiffer, USA. Pfeiffer Company, PO Box 100, Wilkes-Barre, PA 18773, USA.

Pfizer, Aust. Pfizer Corporation Austria GmbH, Mondscheingasse 16, 1070 Vienna, Austria.

Pfizer, Austral. Pfizer Pty Ltd, P.O. Box 57, West Ryde, NSW 2114, Australia.

Pfizer, Belg. Pfizer S.A., Rue Leon Theodor 102, 1090 Brussels, Belgium.

Pfizer, Canad. Pfizer Canada Inc., P.O. Box 800, Pointe-Claire-Dorval, Quebec, H9R 4V2, Canada.

Pfizer, Fr. Laboratoires Pfizer, 86 rue de Paris, 91407 Orsay Cdx, France.

Pfizer, Ger. Pfizer GmbH, Pfizerstrasse 1, Postfach: 4949, 76032 Karlsruhe, Germany.

Pfizer, Irl. Pfizer Pharmaceuticals, Pharmapark, Chapelizod, Dublin 20, Ireland.

Pfizer, Ital. Pfizer Italiana s.p.a., Via Valbondione 113, 00188 Rome, Italy.

Pfizer, Neth. Pfizer B.V., Postbus 37, 2900 AA Capelle a/d Ijssel, Netherlands.

Pfizer, Norw. Pfizer A/S, Strandv. 55, 1324 Lysaker, Norway.

Pfizer, S.Afr. Pfizer Laboratories (Pty) Ltd, P.O. Box 783720, Sandton 2146, S. Africa.

Pfizer, Spain. Pfizer, Principe de Vergara 109, 28002 Madrid, Spain.

Pfizer, Swed. Pfizer AB, Box 501, 183 25 Taby, Sweden.

Pfizer, Switz. Pfizer SA, Case postale, 8048 Zurich, Switzerland.

Pfizer, UK. Pfizer Ltd, Sandwich, Kent, CT13 9NJ, UK.

Pfizer, USA. Pfizer Laboratories Division, Pfizer Inc., 235 East 42nd St, New York, NY 10017, USA.

Pfizer Consumer, UK. Pfizer Consumer Healthcare, Wilsom Rd, Alton, Hants, GU34 2TJ, UK.

Pfleger, Ger. Dr R. Pfleger Chemische Fabrik GmbH, 96045 Bamberg, Germany.

Pfluger, Ger. Homöopathisches Laboratorium A. Pflüger GmbH, Bielefelder Strasse 17, Postfach: 2129, 33374 Rheda-Wiedenbruck, Germany.

Pfrimmer, Ger. See *Kabi Pharmacia, Ger.*

Pfrimmer Nutricia, Switz. See *Uhlmann-Eyraud, Switz.*

PGM, Ger. PGM Pharmazeutische Gesellschaft mbH & Co. Munchen, Furstenstr 6, 80333 Munchen, Germany.

Pharbiol, Fr. Laboratoires Pharbiol, ZAC des Cerisiers, 69380 Lozanne, France.

Phardi, Switz. Phardi AG, Postfach 3650, 4002 Basel, Switzerland.

Pharkos, Ital. Pharkos s.r.l., Via Appia Km.54,700, 04012 Cisterna di Latina (LT), Italy.

Pharma 2000, Fr. Laboratoires Pharma 2000, Immeuble Strasbourg, av de l'Europe, Toussus-le-Noble, 78771 Magny-les-Hameaux cdx, France.

Pharma Health, UK. Pharma Health Care Ltd, 186 South Ealing Road, London, W5 4RJ, UK.

Pharma Nord, Irl. See *Electramed, Irl.*

Pharma Plus, Switz. Pharma Plus SA, 6814 Lamone, Switzerland.

Pharma Tek, USA. Pharma Tek Inc., P.O. Box 1920, Huntington, NY 11743-0568, USA.

Pharmacal, Switz. Pharmacal SA, Case postale 1065, 1701 Fribourg, Switzerland.

Pharmacare Consumer, S.Afr. Pharmacare Consumer, S. Africa.

Pharmacel, USA. Pharmacel Laboratory Inc., 203 South Coolidge Ave, Tampa, Florida, FL 33609, USA.

Pharmaceutical Basics, USA. See *Rosemont, USA.*

Pharmaceutical Enterprises, S.Afr. Pharmaceutical Enterprises (Pty) Ltd, P.O. Box 201, Howard Place 7450, S. Africa.

Pharmaceutical Specialties, USA. Pharmaceutical Specialties Inc., P.O. Box 6298, Rochester, MN 55903, USA.

Pharmachemie, S.Afr. Pharmachemie, S. Africa.

Pharmacia, Austral. See *Pharmacia Upjohn, Austral.*

Pharmacia, Canad. See *Pharmacia Upjohn, Canad.*

Pharmacia, Neth. See *Pharmacia Upjohn, Neth.*

Pharmacia, S.Afr. See *Keatings, S.Afr.*

Pharmacia, Spain. See *Pharmacia Upjohn, Spain.*

Pharmacia, Swed. See *Pharmacia Upjohn, Swed.*

Pharmacia, UK. See *Pharmacia Upjohn, UK.*

Pharmacia, USA. See *Kabi Pharmacia, USA.*

Pharmacia Upjohn, Aust. Pharmacia & Upjohn Handels GmbH, Oberlaaer Strasse 251, 1100 Vienna, Austria.

Pharmacia Upjohn, Austral. Pharmacia & Upjohn Pty Ltd, P.O. Box 46, Rydalmere, NSW 2116, Australia.

Pharmacia Upjohn, Belg. Pharmacia & Upjohn N.V./S.A., Rue de la Fusee 66, 1130 Brussels, Belgium.

Pharmacia Upjohn, Canad. Pharmacia & Upjohn Inc., 865 York Mills Rd, Don Mills, Ontario, M3B 1Y6, Canada.

Pharmacia Upjohn, Fr. Pharmacia & Upjohn SA, B.P. 210, 78051 St-Quentin-Yvelines Cdx, France.

Pharmacia Upjohn, Ger. Pharmacia & Upjohn GmbH, Hofmannstr. 26, 91051 Erlangen, Germany.

Pharmacia Upjohn, Irl. Pharmacia & Upjohn, P.O. Box 1752, Airways Industrial Estate, Dublin 17, Ireland.

Pharmacia Upjohn, Ital. Pharmacia & Upjohn s.p.a., Via Robert Koch 1.2, 20152 Milan, Italy.

Pharmacia Upjohn, Neth. Pharmacia & Upjohn B.V., Postbus 17, 3440 AA Woerden, Netherlands.

Pharmacia Upjohn, Norw. Pharmacia & Upjohn AS, Gjerdrumsvei 10B, N-0486 Oslo, Norway.

Pharmacia Upjohn, S.Afr. Pharmacia Upjohn (Pty) Ltd, P.O. Box 246, Isando 1600, S. Africa.

Pharmacia Upjohn, Spain. Pharmacia Upjohn, Ctra de Gracia a Manresa Km 15, Sant Cugat del Valles, 08190 Barcelona, Spain.

Pharmacia Upjohn, Swed. Pharmacia & Upjohn Sverige AB, 112 87 Stockholm, Sweden.

Pharmacia Upjohn, Switz. Pharmacia & Upjohn AG, Lagerstrasse 14, 8600 Dubendorf, Switzerland.

Pharmacia Upjohn, UK. Pharmacia & Upjohn, Davy Ave, Knowlhill, Milton Keynes, Bucks, MK5 8PH, UK.

Pharmacia Upjohn, USA. Pharmacia & Upjohn, P.O. Box 16529, Columbus, OH 43216-6529, USA.

Pharmacie Centrale des Hopitaux, Fr. Pharmacie Centrale des Hopitaux.

Pharmacie de France, Switz. See *Doetsch, Grether, Switz.*

Pharmacie Principale, Fr. Pharmacie Principale, 53 rue Nationale, 37011 Tours Cdx, France.

Pharmacobel, Belg. S.A. Laboratoires Belges Pharmacobel, Ave de Scheut 46-50, 1070 Brussels, Belgium.

Pharmadass, UK. Pharmadass Ltd, 16 Aintree Rd, Greenford, Middx, UB6 7LA, UK.

Pharmadeveloppement, Fr. Pharmadéveloppement, 7 rue Valentin-Hauy, 75015 Paris, France.

Pharmadex, Canad. Pharmadex Laboratories Inc., 745 Place Fortier, Suite 307, Ville St-Laurent, Quebec, H4L 5A6, Canada.

Pharmador, S.Afr. See *Protea, S.Afr.*

Pharmafair, USA. See *Bausch & Lomb, USA.*

Pharmafarm, Fr. Laboratoires Pharmafarm, 46 rue Boissiere, 75116 Paris, France.

Pharmafrica, S.Afr. Pharmafrica, S. Africa.

Pharmagalen, Ger. Pharmagalen GmbH, Wittland 13, Postfach: 3764, 24036 Kiel, Germany.

Pharmagen, S.Afr. Pharmagen, S. Africa.

Pharma-Global, Irl. Pharma-Global Ltd, Hudson Rd, Sandycove, Co. Dublin, Ireland.

Pharma-Global, UK. Pharma-Global (UK) Ltd, 39 Earls Court Rd, Kensington, London, W8 6ED, UK.

Pharmagyne, Fr. Pharmagyne S.A., 28 rue de la Chapelle, 75018 Paris, France.

Pharmakon, Ger. Pharmakon Arzneimittel GmbH, Albert-Schweitzer-Str. 52-4, Postfach: 60, 67592 Florsheim-Dalsheim, Germany.

Pharmakon, Switz. Pharmakon SA, Burglistrasse 39, 8304 Wallisellen, Switzerland.

Pharmakon, USA. Pharmakon Laboratories Inc., 6050 Jet Port Industrial Blvd, Tampa, FL 33634, USA.

Pharmakos, Switz. Pharmakos AG, Lowenstrasse 59, 8001 Zurich, Switzerland.

Pharmalab, Canad. Pharmalab (1982) Inc., 8750 boul. de-la-Rive-Sud, Levis, QC, G6V 6N6, Canada.

Pharmalab, S.Afr. See *Noristan, S.Afr.*

Pharmalab, Spain. Pharmalab, Valls y Taberner 2, 08006 Barcelona, Spain.

Pharmaland, Ital. Pharmaland, Via Ronco Mauro 16/B, 47031 Dogana Repubblica San Marino, Italy.

Pharmalink, Swed. Pharmalink Basläkemedel AB, 171 83 Solna, Sweden.

Pharma-Natura, Ital. Pharma Natura srl, Via Vicinale di Parabiago, 20014 Nerviano (MI), Italy.

Pharma-Natura, S.Afr. Pharma-Natura (Pty) Ltd, P.O. Box 5502, Johannesburg 2000, S. Africa.

Pharmaplan, S.Afr. Pharmaplan, S. Africa.

Pharmarecord, Ital. Pharmarecord s.r.l., Via Laurentina Km 24.730, 00040 Pomezia (Roma), Italy.

Pharmark, UK. Pharmark Ltd, 7 Windermere Rd, High Street, West Wickham, Kent, BR4 9AN, UK.

Pharmasal, Ger. Pharmasal Chem.-Pharm. Fabrik H. Franzke KG, Drosselgasse 5, Postfach: 1380, 82155 Grafelfing, Germany.

Pharmascience, Canad. Pharmascience Inc., 8400 Darnley Rd, Montreal, Quebec, H4T 1M4, Canada.

Pharmascience, Fr. Laboratoires Pharmascience, 73 bd de la Mission-Marchand, 92400 Courbevoie, France.

Pharmasette, Ital. Pharmasette di Paolo Donati e C. s.a.s., Via Anna Faustina 15, 00153 Rome, Italy.

Pharmastra, Fr. Pharmastra, Usines Chimiques et Pharmaceutiques deStrasbourg, 40 rue du Canal, 67460 Souffelweyersheim, France.

Pharmatec, Neth. See *Multipharma, Neth.*

Pharmatec, S.Afr. Pharmatec Ltd, P.O. Box 23222, Claremont 7735, S. Africa.

Pharmaton, Ger. Pharmaton GmbH, Postfach: 1660, 88386 Biberach, Germany.

Pharmaton, S.Afr. See *Swisspharm, S.Afr.*

Pharmaton, Switz. Pharmaton SA, 6934 Bioggio, Switzerland.

Pharmavite, Canad. Pharmavite Corp., 1151 Gorham St, Newmarket, ON, L3Y 7V1, Canada.

Pharmax, Irl. See *Allphar, Irl.*

Pharmax, UK. Pharmax Ltd, Bourne Rd, Bexley, Kent, DA5 1NX, UK.

Pharmazam, Spain. Pharmazam, Pol. Ind. Urvasa, Sta Perpetua de Mogoda, 08130 Barcelona, Spain.

Pharmco, S.Afr. Pharmco Holdings Ltd., 16a Drake Ave, Eastleigh Ridge, Edenvale 1609, S. Africa.

Pharmec, Ital. Pharmec s.r.l., Via Canino 21, 00191 Rome, Italy.

Pharmed, Aust. Pharmed, Sackstrasse 4, 8011 Graz, Austria.

Pharmedica, S.Afr. Pharmedica Laboratories (Pty) Ltd, P.O. Box 87, East London 5200, Cape Province, S. Africa.

Pharmel, Canad. Pharmel Inc., 8699 8e Ave, Montreal, QC, H1Z 2X4, Canada.

Pharmethic, Belg. Pharmethic S.A., Rue de Vivier 89-93, 1050 Brussels, Belgium.

Pharmeurop, Fr. See *Parke, Davis, Fr.*

Pharmexco, UK. Pharmexco Ltd, 5-6 Zennor Rd, London, SW12 0PS, UK.

Pharmexport, Neth. Pharmexport B.V., Netherlands.

Pharmics, USA. Pharmics Inc., P.O. Box 27554, Salt Lake City, UT 84127, USA.

Pharminfant, Ger. Pharminfant Gesellschaft fur die Therapie im Kindes- und Jugendalter mbH, Mittelstrasse 18, Postfach: 320, 7958 Laupheim, Germany.

Pharminter, Fr. Laboratoires Pharminter, 34 rue St-Romain, 69008 Lyon, France.

Pharmochem, Austral. Pharmochem (Australia) Pty. Ltd, P.O. Box 146, Ashburton, Vic. 3147, Australia.

Pharmonta, Aust. Pharmonta Mag. pharm. Dr Fischer, Montanastrasse 7, Steiermark, 8112 Gratwein, Austria.

Pharmotech, Austral. Pharmotech (Australia) Pty Ltd, P.O. Box 580, Elsternwick, Vic 3185, Australia.

Pharmuka, Fr. See *Bellon, Fr.*

Pharmy, Fr. Laboratoires Pharmy II, 20-22 pl Charles-de-Gaulle, 78100 St-Germain-en-Laye, France.

Pharmygiene, Fr. Laboratoires Pharmygiène, La Boursidiere, B.P. 150, 92357 Le Plessis-Robinson, France.

Phillips Yeast, UK. Phillips Yeast Products Ltd, Park Royal Rd, London, NW10 7JX, UK.

Philopharm, Ger. Philopharm GmbH, Groperntor 20, Postfach: 15, 06484 Quedlinburg, Germany.

Phoenix Health, UK. Phoenix Health Ltd, UK.

Phonix, Ger. Phönix Laboratorium GmbH, Benzstrasse 10, Postfach: 20, 71145 Bondorf, Germany.

Phygiene, Fr. Laboratoires Phygiène, 11-13 rue de la Loge, B.P. 100, 94265 Fresnes cdx, France.

Phyteia, Switz. Phyteia AG, Drosselstrasse 47, 4059 Basel, Switzerland.

Phytomed, Switz. Phytomed Armand Kilchherr, 3415 Hasle bei Burgdorf, Switzerland.

Phytomedica, Fr. Laboratoires Phytomedica, Parc d'activites de Pichaury, 535 rue Pierre-Simon Laplace, ZI Les Milles, 13791 Aix-en-Provence Cdx 3, France.

Phytopharma, Ger. Phytopharma Apotheker Paul Regneri GmbH & Co. KG, Roonstr. 23 a, Postfach: 2940, 7500 Karlsruhe 1, Germany.

Phytosolba, Fr. Laboratoires Phytosolba, 89 rue Salvador-Allende, 95871 Bezons, France.

Piam, Ital. Vecchi & C. Piam di G. Assereto, E. Maragliano e C. s.a.p.a., Via Padre G. Semeria 5, 16131 Genoa, Italy.

Pickles, UK. J. Pickles & Sons, Beech House, 62 High St, Knaresborough, North Yorkshire, HG5 0EA, UK.

Picot, Fr. Laboratoires des Produits Picot, 189 quai Lucien-Lheureux, B.P. 83, 62102 Calais Cdx, France.

Picot, Switz. See *Ridupharm, Switz.*

Pierre Fabre, Fr. Laboratoires Pierre Fabre, Départmentmédical de Pierre Fabre Médicament, 45 place Abel-Gance, 92100 Boulogne, France.

Pierre Fabre, Ger. Pierre Fabre Pharma GmbH, Jechtinger Str. 13, Postfach: 6769, 79043 Freiburg, Germany.

Pierre Fabre, Ital. Pierre Fabre Italia s.p.a., Via G.G. Winckelmann 1, 20146 Milan, Italy.

Pierre Fabre, Spain. Pierre Fabre, Ramon Trias Fargas 7-11, 08005 Barcelona, Spain.

Pierre Fabre, Swed. Pierre Fabre Pharma Norden AB, Box 349, 192 30 Sollentuna, Sweden.

Pierre Fabre, Switz. Pierre Fabre (Suisse) SA, Route Sous-Riette 21, 1023 Crissier, Switzerland.

Pierre Fabre, UK. Pierre Fabre Ltd, UK.

Pierre Fabre Medikosma, Ger. See *Pierre Fabre, Ger.*

Pierre Fabre Sante, Fr. See *Pierre Fabre, Fr.*

Pierrel, Ital. Pierrel s.p.a., Via G di Vittorio 10, 20094 Corsico (MI), Italy.

Pietrasanta, Ital. Pietrasanta Pharma s.r.l., Via S. Francesco 67, 55049 Viareggio, Italy.

Piette, Belg. Lab. Piette International S.A., Groot-Bijgaardenstraat 128, 1620 Drogenbos, Belgium.

Pilkington Barnes-Hind, Austral. Pilkington Barnes-Hind Pty. Ltd, P.O. Box 422, Brookvale, NSW 2100, Australia.

Pilkington Barnes-Hind, USA. Pilkington Barnes-Hind, 810 Kifer Rd, Sunnyvale, CA 94086-5200, USA.

Pinewood, Irl. Pinewood Laboratories Ltd, Ballymacarby, Clonmel, Co. Tipperary, Ireland.

Pinewood, UK. See *Pinewood, Irl.*

Piniol, Switz. Piniol AG, Pharmazeutische Spezialitäten, Erlistrasse 2, 6403 Kussnacht aR, Switzerland.

Pino, Ger. Pino Pharmazeutische Praparate GmbH, Hohenzollernring 127-9, Postfach: 501406, 22714 Hamburg, Germany.

Pionneau, Fr. Laboratoires Pionneau, 33870 Vayres, France.

Piraud, Switz. Piraud AG, Zurcherstrasse 68, 8800 Thalwil, Switzerland.

Pirri, Ital. Istituto Pirri s.r.l., Via Puccini 3, 20121 Milan, Italy.

Plan, Switz. Laboratoires Plan SA, Chemin des Sellieres, 1219 Aire-Geneva, Switzerland.

Planta, Canad. Planta Dei Pharma, P.O. Box 415, Route 105, Nackawic, NB, E0H 1P0, Canada.

Plantamed, Ger. Plantamed Arzneimittel GmbH, Postfach: 1861, 92308 Neumarkt/Opf., Germany.

Plantes et Medecines, Fr. Laboratoires Plantes et Médecines, Le Payrat, 46000 Cahors, France.

Plantes Tropicales, Fr. Laboratoires de Plantes Tropicales, 24 rue Jouffroy d'Abbans, 75017 Paris, France.

Plantier, Fr. Laboratoires du Dr Plantier, Groupe Asta Medica, av. J.-F. Kennedy, 33700 Merignac Cdx, France.

Plantina, Ger. Plantina GmbH Biologische Arzneimittel, Czernyring 22/10, Postfach: 104129, 69031 Heidelberg, Germany.

Plantorgan, Ger. Plantorgan GmbH & Co OHG, Hornbusch 1, Postfach: 1463, 26151 Bad Zwischenahn, Germany.

Plantorgan, Neth. See *Bipharma, Neth.*

Plants, Ital. Plants, Laboratorio della Dott.ssa Luisa Coletta, Via V d'Amore 4, 98100 Messina, Italy.

Plasmon, Ital. Plasmon Dietetici Alimentari s.p.a., Corso Garibaldi 97/99, 20121 Milan, Italy.

Playtex, Canad. Playtex Ltd, 124 Fourth Ave, Arnprior, Ontario, K7S 1Z4, Canada.

Plevifarma, Spain. Plevifarma, Fernando Puig 58,60, 08023 Barcelona, Spain.

Plough, USA. Plough Inc., 3030 Jackson Ave, Memphis, TN 38151, USA.

PMC, Austral. PMC Pharma, Australia.

Poehlmann, Ger. Dr Poehlmann & Co. GmbH, Postfach: 1365, 58303 Herdecke, Germany.

Poehlmann, Switz. See *Renapharm, Switz.*

Pohl, Ger. G. Pohl-Boskamp GmbH & Co., Kieler Strasse 11, Postfach: 1253, 25550 Hohenlockstedt, Germany.

Pohl, Neth. See *Tramedico, Neth.*

Pohl, Norw. See *Meda, Norw.*

Pohl, Switz. See *Lubapharm, Switz.*

Poirier, Fr. Laboratoires Patrick Poirier, ZI Saint-Malo, B.P. 37, 37320 Esvres, France.

Polcopharma, Austral. Polcopharma Polley F & Co. Pty Ltd, P.O. Box 100, Epping, NSW 2121, Australia.

Poli, Ital. Poli Industria Chimica s.p.a., Via Volturno 48, 20089 Quinto de Stampi-Rozzano (MI), Italy.

Poli, Switz. See *Adroka, Switz.*

Polidis, Fr. Ste Polidis, 7 rue Gallieni, 93500 Rueil-Malmaison, France.

Polifarma, Ital. Polifarma s.p.a., Via Tor Sapienza 138, 00155 Rome, Italy.

Polive, Fr. Laboratoires Polivé SNC, 19-23 bd Georges-Clemenceau, 92400 Courbevoie, France.

Poly, USA. Poly Pharm, USA.

PolyMedica, USA. PolyMedica Pharmaceuticals, 2 Constitution Way, Woburn, MA 01801, USA.

Polymer Technology, USA. Polymer Technology Corp., 100 Research Drive, Wilmington, MA 01887, USA.

Polypharm, Ger. Polypharm GmbH, Rosslerstr. 88, Postfach: 101144, 64211 Darmstadt, Germany.

Pons, Spain. Pons, Mayor 27, 25007 Lerida, Spain.

Potter's, UK. Potter's (Herbal Supplies) Ltd, Leyland Mill Lane, Wigan, Lancs, WN1 2SB, UK.

Poythress, USA. See *ECR, USA.*

PQS, Spain. PQS Farma, Ctra Madrid-Cadiz Km 554.4, Dos Hermanas, 41700 Seville, Spain.

Pras, Spain. Pras Farma, C/Del Pont Reixat 5, Sant Just Desvern, 08960 Barcelona, Spain.

Prats, Spain. Prats, Traversa del Dalt 44, 08024 Barcelona, Spain.

Pred, Fr. Laboratoires Pred, Chemin de Nuisement, ZI des 150 Arpents, 28500 Vernouillet, France.

Premier, USA. Premier Inc., Greenwich, CT 06831, USA.

Presselin, Ger. Presselin Arzneimittel GmbH & Co. KG, Bahnhofstrasse 12, Postfach: 1346, 32270 Kirchlengern, Germany.

Prevention et Biologie, Fr. Prévention et Biologie SA, 29-33 rue de Metz, 94170 Le Perreux, France.

Princeton, USA. Princeton Pharmaceutical Products (A Squibb Co.), P.O. Box 4500, Princeton, NJ 08543-4500, USA.

Priorin, Switz. Priorin SA, Switzerland.

Priory, Irl. Priory Pharmaceuticals Ltd, 4 Priory Hall, Stillorgan Road, Co. Dublin, Ireland.

Prism, UK. Prism Healthcare, Medihealth House, Wycombe 3, Boundary Rd, Loudwater, High Wycombe, Buckinghamshire, HP10 9PN, UK.

Pro Doc, Canad. Pro Doc (Laboratories) Ltd, 2925 Industrial Blvd, Laval, Quebec, H7L 3W9, Canada.

Pro Medica, Swed. Pro Medica AB, Box 27190, 102 52 Stockholm, Sweden.

Pro Vaccine, Switz. Pro Vaccine AG, Grabenstrasse 42, 6301 Zug, Switzerland.

Procare, Austral. See *Biovital, Austral.*

Procea, Irl. Procea, Alexandra Rd, Dublin 1, Ireland.

Procemsa, Ital. Farmaceutici Procemsa s.r.l., Via Mentana 10, 10042 Nichelino (TO), Italy.

Procter & Gamble, Aust. Procter & Gamble Austria GmbH, Mariahilfer Strasse 77-9, 1061 Vienna, Austria.

Procter & Gamble, Austral. Procter & Gamble Australia Pty Ltd, Locked Bag No. 75, Parramatta, NSW 2124, Australia.

Procter & Gamble, Belg. Procter & Gamble Pharmaceuticals S.A., Temselaan 100, 1853 Strombeek Bever, Belgium.

Procter & Gamble, Canad. Procter & Gamble Inc., P.O. Box 355, Station A, Toronto, Ontario, M5W 1C5, Canada.

Procter & Gamble, Fr. Procter & Gamble Pharmaceuticals France, 96 av Charles-de-Gaulle, 92201 Neuilly-sur-Seine cdx, France.

Procter & Gamble, Ger. Procter & Gamble Pharmaceuticals Germany GmbH, Dr. Otto-Rohm-Str. 2-4, Postfach: 100161, 64201 Darmstadt, Germany.

Procter & Gamble, Irl. See *United Drug, Irl.*

Procter & Gamble, Ital. Procter & Gamble Italia s.p.a., Viale C Pavese 385, 00144 Rome, Italy.

Procter & Gamble, Neth. Procter & Gamble Pharmaceuticals, Postbus 2507, 3000 CM Rotterdam, Netherlands.

Procter & Gamble, Norw. See *Roche, Norw.*

Procter & Gamble, Spain. Procter & Gamble, Av. Partenon 16-18, Campo Naciones, 28042 Madrid, Spain.

Procter & Gamble, Swed. Procter & Gamble Scandinavia Inc., Box 15, 164 93 Kista, Sweden.

Procter & Gamble, Switz. Procter & Gamble AG, 1 rue du Pre-de-la-Bichette, 1211 Geneva 2, Switzerland.

Procter & Gamble, UK. Procter & Gamble Pharmaceuticals UK Ltd, Lovett House, Lovett Rd, Staines, Middx, TW18 3AZ, UK.

Procter & Gamble, USA. Procter & Gamble, P.O. Box 171, Cincinnati, OH 45201, USA.

Procter & Gamble (H&B Care), UK. Procter & Gamble (Health & Beauty Care) Ltd, Rusham Park, Whitehall Lane, Egham, Surrey, TW20 9NW, UK.

Prodemdis, Canad. Prodemdis Enrg, 4355 boul. Sir Wilfred Laurier, St-Hubert, QC, J3Y 3X3, Canada.

Prodes, Spain. Prodes, Trabajo S/N, San Justo de Desvern, 08960 Barcelona, Spain.

Produits Dentaires, Switz. Produits Dentaires SA, 18 rue des Bosquets, 1800 Vevey, Switzerland.

Prof. Pharm. Corp., Canad. Professional Pharmaceutical Corporation, 9200 Cote-de-Liesse Rd, Lachine, Quebec, H8T 1A1, Canada.

Professional Health, Canad. Professional Health Products, 4307-49 St, Innisfail, AB, T4G 1P3, Canada.

Professional Supplies, USA. See *SoftRinse, USA.*

Proge, Ital. Proge Farm srl, Via Croce 4, 28065 Cerano (NO), Italy.

Progest, Ital. Progest Industria Chimica s.r.l., Corso Trieste 109, 00198 Rome, Italy.

Promed, Ger. Promed Arzneimittel GmbH, 22876 Wedel, Germany.

Promedica, Fr. Laboratoires Promedica, 13 rue Faraday, 41260 La Chaussee-St-Victor, France.

Promedica, Neth. See *Multipharma, Neth.*

Promedical, Ital. Promedical srl, Via G Greco 8, 90017 Santa Flavia (PA), Italy.

Promefarm, Ital. Promefarm s.r.l., Corso Indipendenza 6, 20129 Milan, Italy.

Promesa, Spain. Promesa, Loas Cedros, S/N Polg. Industrial, Paracuellos del Jarma, 28860 Madrid, Spain.

Promonta, Ger. See *Promonta Lundbeck, Ger.*

Promonta Lundbeck, Ger. Promonta Lundbeck Arzneimittel GmbH & Co, Amsinckstr. 57-61, Postfach: 105126, 20035 Hamburg, Germany.

Pro-Nat, Fr. Pro-Nat SA, 26 rue Castagnary, 75015 Paris, France.

Propan, S.Afr. Propan Zurich, P.O. Box 200, Isando 1600, Transvaal, S. Africa.

Propan-Vernleigh, S.Afr. See *Propan, S.Afr.*

Propharm, S.Afr. Propharm, S. Africa.

Prophin, Ital. Laboratorio Prophin s.r.l., Via Lambro 36, 20090 Opera (MI), Italy.

Prosana, Austral. Prosana Laboratories Pty Ltd, Australia.

Prosintex, Ital. Prosintex Industrie Chimiche Italiane s.r.l., Via E Fermi 20/26, 20019 Settimo Milanese (MI), Italy.

Prospa, Belg. Prospa S.A., Blvd Brand Whitlock 156, 1200 Brussels, Belgium.

Prospa, Ital. Prospa Italia s.r.l., Milanofiori Palazzo E 2, 20090 Assago (MI), Italy.

Prospa, Switz. Prospa SA, Case postale 284, 1401 Yverdon-les-Bains, Switzerland.

Protea, Austral. Protea Pharmaceuticals, A Division of Fisons Pty Ltd, Australia.

Protea, S.Afr. Protea Pharm (Pty) Ltd, P.O. Box 422, East London 5200, S. Africa.

Protec, UK. Protec Health Ltd, 5 Priory Court, Poulton, Cirencester, Gloucs, GL7 5JB, UK.

Proter, Ital. See *Mundipharma Proter, Ital.*

Protina, Ger. Protina Pharmazeutische GmbH, Adalperostr. 30, Postfach: 1253, 85730 Ismaning, Germany.

Protina, Switz. See *Doetsch, Grether, Switz.*

Provita, Aust. Provita HandelsGmbH, Albrechtsbergergasse 13, 1120 Vienna, Austria.

Puerto Galiano, Spain. Puerto Galiano, Cea Bermudez 18, 28003 Madrid, Spain.

Pulitzer, Ital. Pulitzer Italiana s.r.l., Via Tiburtina 1004, 00156 Rome, Italy.

Pulsion, Ger. Pulsion Verwaltungs GmbH & Co. Medizintechnik KG, Kirchenstr. 88, 81675 Munich, Germany.

Purdue Frederick, Canad. Purdue Frederick Inc., 575 Granite Court, Pickering, Ontario, L1W 3W8, Canada.

Purdue Frederick, USA. The Purdue Frederick Co., 100 Connecticut Ave, Norwalk, CT 06856, USA.

Pure Plant Products, UK. Pure Plant Products, UK.

Puropharma, Ital. Puropharma s.r.l., Via Correggio 43, 20149 Milan, Italy.

QHP, USA. Quality Health Products Inc., P.O. Box 31, Yaphank, NY 11980, USA.

Quad, USA. Quad Pharmaceuticals Inc., USA.

Qualimed, Austral. See *Hoechst Marion Roussel, Austral.*

Qualiphar, Belg. Lab. Qualiphar S.A., Rijksweg 9, 2880 Bornem, Belgium.

Qualitest, USA. Qualitest Products Inc., 1236 Jordan Rd, Huntsville, AL 35811, USA.

Quality Formulations, USA. Quality Formulations Inc., P.O. Box 827, Zachary, LA 70791-0827, USA.

Quantum, USA. Quantum Pharmics Ltd, USA.

Quatromed, S.Afr. Quatromed, S. Africa.

Queisser, Ger. Queisser Pharma GmbH & Co., Postfach: 2456, 24914 Flensburg, Germany.

Quest, Canad. Quest Vitamin Supplies, 1781 West 75th Ave., Vancouver, British Columbia, V6P 6P2, Canada.

Quest, UK. Quest Vitamins Ltd, 8 Venture Way, Aston Science Park, Birmingham, B7 4AP, UK.

Quick-Med, S.Afr. Quick-Med, S. Africa.

Quidel, Fr. Lab. Quidel, 1 rue de Rome, 93561 Rosny-sous-Bois cdx, France.

Quidel, USA. Quidel Corp., 10165 McKellar Court, San Diego, CA 92121, USA.

Quimica Medica, Spain. La Quimica Medica, San Juan Bosco 55, 08017 Barcelona, Spain.

Quimifar, Spain. Quimifar, Cadaques 30, La Llagosta, 08120 Barcelona, Spain.

Quimpe, Spain. Quimpe, Cruz 47-9, Alhaurin el Grande, 29120 Malaga, Spain.

Quinoderm, Switz. See *Golaz, Switz.*

Quinoderm, UK. Quinoderm Ltd, Manchester Rd, Oldham, Lancs, OL8 4PB, UK.

Rabi & Solabo, Fr. Laboratoires Rabi & Solabo, BP 19, 56 av Laplace, 94111 Arcueil Cdx, France.

Rachelle, USA. Rachelle, USA.

Radiumfarma, Ital. Radiumfarma s.r.l., Laboratori Farmaco Biologici, Via Carnevali 111, 20158 Milan, Italy.

Ragionieri, Ital. Dr R.R. Ragionieri s.p.a, Via Corsi Salviati 27, 50019 Sesto Fiorentino (FI), Italy.

Rahslog, USA. Rahslog, USA.

Raith, Aust. Dr Ch Raith GmbH, Friedlgasse 21, 1190 Vienna, Austria.

Ram, USA. Ram Laboratories, Division of Bradley Pharmaceuticals Inc., 3300 University Drive, Coral Springs, FL 33065, USA.

Ramelco, Canad. Ramelco Ltd, Subsidiary of Maltby Ltd, 306 Dawlish Ave, Toronto, Ontario, M4N 1J5, Canada.

Ramini, Ital. Ramini s.r.l., Via Sacco e Vanzetti 10, 60131 Ancona, Italy.

Ramon Sala, Spain. Ramon Sala, Paris 174, 08036 Barcelona, Spain.

RAN, Ger. RAN Novesia AG Arzneimittel, Hurtgener Strasse 6, Postfach: 101 243, 41412 Neuss/Rhein, Germany.

Ranbaxy, S.Afr. Ranbaxy, S. Africa.

Randob, USA. Randob Laboratories Ltd, P.O. Box 440, Cornwall, NY 12518, USA.

Rapide, Spain. See *Bieffe, Spain.*

Rappai, Switz. Dr F. Rappai Pharmazeutika, Case postale, 8952 Schlieren-Zurich, Switzerland.

Ratiopharm, Ger. ratiopharm GmbH, Graf-Arco-Str. 3, Postfach: 3380, 89023 Ulm-Donautal, Germany.

Ratiopharm, Spain. Ratiopharm, Sor Angela de la Cruz 6, 28020 Madrid, Spain.

Ravasini, Ital. Stabilimenti Chimico-Farmaceutici Dott. R. Ravasini & C.ia s.p.a., Via Ostilia 15, 00184 Rome, Italy.

Ravensberg, Ger. Ravensberg GmbH Chemische Fabrik, Schneckenburgstrasse 46, Postfach: 101743, 78417 Constance, Germany.

Ravizza, Ital. Ravizza Farmaceutici s.p.a., Via Europa 35, 20053 Muggio (MI), Italy.

Ravizza, Neth. See *Will-Pharma, Neth.*

Raway, USA. Raway Pharmacal Inc., 15 Granit Rd, Accord, NY 12404-0047, USA.

Rawleigh, Canad. Rawleigh, 60 Colonnade Rd, Nepean, ON, K2E 7J6, Canada.

R&D, USA. R & D Laboratories Inc., 4204 Glencoe Ave, Marina Del Rey, CA 90292-5612, USA.

RDC, Ital. Laboratori Ricerche Dermo Cosmetiche s.r.l., Via G. Armellini 37, 00143 Rome, Italy.

Realdyme, Fr. Sté Réaldyme, 28700 Garancieres-en-Beauce, France.

Reall, Switz. Medical Concepts Reall-YS Sárl, Ave Villardin 22, 1009 Pully, Switzerland.

Realpharma, Ger. realpharma Geschaftsbereich der Dolorgiet Arzneimittel, Postfach: 1252, 53730 St Augustin/Bonn, Germany.

Recip, Norw. See *Pharmacia Upjohn, Norw.*

Recip, Swed. Recip AB, Branningevagen 12, 120 54 Arsta, Sweden.

Recipe, Aust. Recipe GmbH, Sudtiroler Strasse 6, 4020 Linz, Austria.

Reckeweg, Ger. Pharmazeutische Fabrik Dr. Reckeweg & Co. GmbH, Berliner Ring 32, Postfach: 1661, 64606 Bensheim, Germany.

Reckitt & Colman, Austral. Reckitt & Colman Pharmaceuticals, P.O. Box 138, West Ryde, NSW 2114, Australia.

Reckitt & Colman, Belg. Reckitt & Colman S.A., Allee de la Recherche 20, 1070 Brussels, Belgium.

Reckitt & Colman, Norw. See *Meda, Norw.*, and *Nycomed, Norw.*

Reckitt & Colman, S.Afr. R & C Pharmaceuticals (Pty) Ltd, P.O. Box 31069, Merebank 4059, S. Africa.

Reckitt & Colman, Spain. Reckitt & Colman, Plaza Cuidad Salta 4, 28016 Madrid, Spain.

Reckitt & Colman, Switz. See *Desopharmex, Switz.*

Reckitt & Colman, UK. Reckitt & Colman Products Ltd, Dansom Lane, Hull, HU8 7DS, UK.

Reckitt & Colman, USA. Reckitt & Colman, 1901 Huguenot Rd, Suite 110, Richmond, VA 23235, USA.

Reckitts, Irl. Reckitt's (Ireland) Ltd, P.O. Box 730, Cloverhill Industrial Estate, Clondalkin, Dublin 22, Ireland.

Recofarma, Ital. Recofarma s.r.l., Via Mediana Cisterna 4, 04010 Campoverde di Aprilia (LT), Italy.

Recordati, Ital. Recordati Industria Chimica e Farmaceutica S.p.a., Via Civitali 1, 20148 Milan, Italy.

Recordati Elmu, Spain. Recordati Elmu SL, Ctra N-III Km 23, Arganda del Rey, 28500 Madrid, Spain.

Recsei, USA. Recsei Laboratories, 330 S Kellogg, Building M, Goleta, CA 93117-3875, USA.

Redel, Ger. Julius Redel Cesra-Arzneimittelfabrik GmbH & Co., Braunmattstr. 20, Postfach: 20 20, 76490 Baden-Baden, Germany.

Redi-Products, USA. Redi-Products Labs Inc., P.O. Box 237, Prichard, WV 25555, USA.

Redur, USA. Redur, USA.

Reed & Carnrick, Canad. Reed & Carnrick, Division of Block Drug Co. (Canada) Ltd, 7600 Danbro Cres., Mississauga, Ontario, L5N 6L6, Canada.

Reed & Carnrick, Neth. See *Byk, Neth.*

Reed & Carnrick, USA. Reed & Carnrick, 257 Cornelison Ave, Jersey City, NJ 07302, USA.

Reedco, USA. Reedco, USA.

Reese, USA. The Reese Chemical Co., 10617 Frank Ave, Cleveland, OH 44106, USA.

Regal, Canad. Regal Pharmaceuticals, Division of Bradcan Corp., 900 Harrington Court, Burlington, Ontario, L7N 3N4, Canada.

Regenaplex, Ger. Regenaplex-Arzneispezialitäten GmbH, Robert-Bosch-Str. 3, Postfach: 5609, 78435 Constance, Germany.

Regina, UK. Regina Royal Jelly Ltd, 2a Alexandra Grove, Finchley, London, N12 8NU, UK.

Reid-Rowell, USA. Reid-Rowell, 901 Sawyer Rd, Marietta, GA 30062, USA.

Reig Jofre, Spain. Reig Jofre, Pl. I. Margall 41, 08024 Barcelona, Spain.

Reinecke, Ger. Georg A. Reinecke GmbH & Co. KG, Weidendamm 15, Postfach: 4945, 30049 Hannover, Germany.

Reith & Petrasch, Ger. Reith & Petrasch GmbH, Postfach: 25, 77836 Rheinmunster, Germany.

Relax, Ital. Relax Health Care srl, Corso Sempione 36, 20154 Milan, Italy.

Renal Systems, USA. Renal Systems, USA.

Renapharm, Switz. Renapharm S.A., Rue du Chateau 3, 1636 Broc, Switzerland.

Rentsch, Switz. Hans Rentsch AG Pharmazeutische Produkte, Trogenerstrasse 5, 9042 Speicher, Switzerland.

Rentschler, Ger. Dr. Rentschler Arzneimittel GmbH & Co., Mittelstrasse 18, Postfach: 1461, 88464 Laupheim, Germany.

Repha, Ger. Repha GmbH Biologische Arzneimittel, Alt-Godshorn 87, Postfach: 1180, 30832 Langenhagen, Germany.

Republic, USA. Republic Drug Co., P.O. Box 807, Buffalo, NY 14207, USA.

Requa, USA. Requa Inc., 1 Seneca Place, P.O. Box 4008, Greenwich, CT 06830, USA.

Research Industries Corp., USA. Research Industries Corporation, Pharmaceutical Division, 6864 South 300 West, Midvale, UT 84047, USA.

Research Labs, S.Afr. Research Labs, S. Africa.

Resinag, Switz. Resinag AG, Oberer Steisteg 18, 6430 Schwyz, Switzerland.

Respa, USA. Respa Pharmaceuticals Inc., PO Box 88222, Carol Stream, Illinois, IL 60188, USA.

Restan, S.Afr. Restan Laboratories (Pty) Ltd, P.O. Box 41286, Craighall 2024, S. Africa.

Restiva, Ital. Restiva s.r.l., Via Valbondione 113, 00188 Rome, Italy.

Retrain, Spain. Retrain, Alfonso XII 587, Badalona, 08912 Barcelona, Spain.

Retsews, USA. Retsews, USA.

Retterspitz, Ger. Retterspitz GmbH, Laufer Strasse 17-19, Postfach: 47, 90567 Schwaig, Germany.

Reuabuen, USA. Reuabuen, USA.

Reusch, Ger. Pharma Reusch GmbH, Celsiusstr. 43, 53125 Bonn, Germany.

Revlon, Canad. Revlon Canada Inc., 2501 Stanfield Rd, Mississauga, Ontario, L4Y 1R9, Canada.

Revlon, UK. Revlon International Corp., 86 Brook St, London W1Y 2BA, UK.

Rexar, USA. Rexar Pharmacal Corp., 396 Rockaway Ave, Valley Stream, NY 11581, USA.

Rhein-Pharma, Ger. Rhein-Pharma GmbH, Brauereistrasse, Postfach: 2080, 68721 Schwetzingen, Germany.

Rhenomed, Ger. Rhenomed Arzneimittel GmbH, Luth.-Kirch.-Str. 69/71, Postfach: 130662, 47758 Krefeld, Germany.

Rhodiapharm, Canad. See *Rhone-Poulenc Rorer, Canad.*

Rhone Poulenc Chemicals, UK. Rhone-Poulenc Chemicals, Poleacre Lane, Woodley, Stockport, Cheshire, SK6 1PQ, UK.

Rhone-Poulenc, Ger. See *Rhone-Poulenc Rorer, Ger.*

Rhone-Poulenc, Ital. See *Rhone-Poulenc Rorer, Ital.*

Rhone-Poulenc Rorer, Aust. Rhone-Poulenc Rorer, Grinzinger Allee 18-20, 1190 Vienna, Austria.

Rhone-Poulenc Rorer, Austral. Rhone-Poulenc Rorer Australia Pty Ltd, Private Bag 6263, Baulkham Hills Business Centre, Baulkham Hills, NSW 2153, Australia.

Rhone-Poulenc Rorer, Belg. Rhone-Poulenc Rorer S.A., Blvd Sylvain Dupuis 243, B 3, 1070 Brussels, Belgium.

Rhone-Poulenc Rorer, Canad. Rhône-Poulenc Rorer Canada Inc., 4707 rue Levy, Ville Saint-Laurent, Quebec, H4R 2P9, Canada.

Rhone-Poulenc Rorer, Fr. Rhone-Poulenc Rorer, 20 ave Raymond Aron, Tri 350, 92165 Antony Cedex, France.

Rhone-Poulenc Rorer, Ger. Rhone-Poulenc Rorer GmbH, Postfach: 350120, 50792 Cologne, Germany.

Rhone-Poulenc Rorer, Irl. Rhone Poulenc Rorer (Ireland) Ltd, 14 Deansgrange Industrial Estate, Blackrock, Co. Dublin, Ireland.

Rhone-Poulenc Rorer, Ital. Rhone-Poulenc Rorer s.p.a., Viale Europa 11, 21040 Origgio (VA), Italy.

Rhone-Poulenc Rorer, Neth. Rhône-Poulenc Rorer B.V., Postbus 982, 1180 AZ Amstelveen, Netherlands.

Rhone-Poulenc Rorer, Norw. Rhône-Poulenc Rorer, Eiksv 110, Postboks 24, 1345 Osteras, Norway.

Rhone-Poulenc Rorer, S.Afr. Rhône-Poulenc Rorer SA (Pty) Ltd, P.O. Box 1130, Port Elizabeth 6000, S. Africa.

Rhone-Poulenc Rorer, Spain. Rhone Poulenc Rorer, Avda Leganes 62, Alcorcon-Leganes, 28925 Madrid, Spain.

Rhone-Poulenc Rorer, Swed. Rhone-Poulenc Rorer AB, Box 33, 250 53 Helsingborg, Sweden.

Rhone-Poulenc Rorer, Switz. Rhône-Poulenc Rorer AG, Zurcherstrasse 68, 8800 Thalwil, Switzerland.

Rhone-Poulenc Rorer, UK. Rhone-Poulenc Rorer Ltd, RPR House, 50 Kings Hill Ave, Kings Hill, West Malling, Kent, ME19 4AH, UK.

Rhone-Poulenc Rorer, USA. Rhone-Poulenc Rorer Pharmaceuticals Inc., 500 Arcola Rd, P.O. Box 1200, Collegeville, PA 19426-0107, USA.

Rhone-Poulenc Rorer Consumer, Canad. See *Rhone-Poulenc Rorer, Canad.*

Rho-Pharm, Canad. See *Rhone-Poulenc Rorer, Canad.*

Ribosepharm, Ger. See *Klinge, Ger.*

Rice Steele, Irl. Rice Steele Sales Ltd, Cookstown Industrial Estate, Tallaght, Dublin 24, Ireland.

Richard, Fr. Laboratoires Richard, 26740 Sauzet, France.

Richardson-Vicks, Austral. Richardson-Vicks Pty Ltd, P.O. Box 95, Villawood, NSW 2163, Australia.

Richardson-Vicks, Neth. Richardson-Vicks B.V., Postbus 1345, 3000 BH Rotterdam, Netherlands.

Richardson-Vicks, USA. Richardson-Vicks Inc., Health Care Products Division, P.O. Box 599, Cincinnati, OH 45202, USA.

Richardson-Vicks Personal Care, USA. See *Richardson-Vicks, USA.*

Richelet, Fr. Laboratoires Richelet, 15 rue La Perouse, 75116 Paris, France.

Richelin, S.Afr. Richelin Pharmaceuticals (Pty) Ltd, P.O. Box 4857, Johannesburg 2000, S. Africa.

Richmond, Canad. See *Rivex, Canad.*

Richmond Ophthalmics, Canad. See *Rivex, Canad.*

Richter, Aust. Richter Pharma, Feldgasse 19, 4600 Wels, Austria.

Richwood, USA. Richwood Pharmaceutical Inc., P.O. Box 6497, Florence, KY 41022, USA.

Rico, USA. See *Bart, USA.*

R.I.D., USA. R.I.D. Inc., 525 Mednik Ave, Los Angeles, California, CA 90022, USA.

Ridupharm, Switz. Ridupharm, Emil Frey-Strasse 99, 4142 Munchenstein, Switzerland.

Riel, Aust. Riel GmbH & Co. KG, Gasselberg 53-4, 8564 Krottendorf-Gaisfeld, Austria.

Riker, Austral. See *3M, Austral.*

Riker, S.Afr. See *3M, S.Afr.*

Riker, UK. See *3M, UK.*

Riker, USA. See *3M, USA.*

Rima, UK. Rima Pharmaceuticals Ltd, 214-16 St James's Rd, Croydon, Surrey, CR0 2BW, UK.

Rinnerthaler, Aust. Rinnerthaler Zahnwaren HandelsGmbH, Drogengrosshandel, Lenaustrasse 10, 4021 Linz, Austria.

Riom, Fr. Riom Laboratoires-C.E.R.M., 63203 Riom Cedex, France.

Ripari-Gero, Ital. Istituto Farmaco Biologico Ripari-Gero s.p.a., Via Montarioso 11, 53035 Monteriggioni (SI), Italy.

Ris, Ital. Ris-Farma s.r.l., Italy.

Ritsert, Ger. Dr. E. Ritsert GmbH & Co. KG, Klausenweg 12, Postfach: 1254, 69402 Eberbach, Germany.

Ritter, Ger. Walter Ritter GmbH & Co., Spaldingstrasse 110 B, Postfach: 105464, 20037 Hamburg, Germany.

Rius, Spain. Rius Garriga, Pujadas 95, 08005 Barcelona, Spain.

Riva, Canad. Laboratoire Riva Inc., 660 Industrial Blvd, Blainville, Quebec, J7C 3V4, Canada.

Rivadis, Fr. Laboratoires Rivadis, B.P. 111, Impasse du Petit-Rose, ZI de Louzy, 79103 Thouars Cdx, France.

Rivex, Canad. Rivex Pharma Inc., 3-305 Industrial Parkway S, Aurora, Ontario, L4G 6X7, Canada.

Rivopharm, Switz. Rivopharm SA, 6928 Manno, Switzerland.

RKG, Ital. RKG srl, Via Ciro Menotti 1/A, 20129 Milan, Italy.

RMC, Canad. RMC Group, 5080 Timberlea Blvd, Ste 42, Mississauga, ON, L4W 4M2, Canada.

Robapharm, Fr. Laboratoires Robapharm, dpt médical de PierreFabre Médicament, 45 place Abel-Gance, 92100 Boulogne, France.

Robapharm, Ger. See *Pierre Fabre, Ger.*

Robapharm, Spain. Robapharm España, Ramon Trias Fargas 7-11, Edif Marina Village, 08005 Barcelona, Spain.

Robapharm, Switz. Robapharm SA, Sempacherstrasse 43, Postfach, 4008 Basel, Switzerland.

Robert, Spain. Robert, Gran via de Carlos III 98, 08028 Barcelona, Spain.

Robert & Carriere, Canad. See *Anglo-French Laboratories, Canad.*

Roberts, Canad. Roberts Pharmaceutical Canada Inc., 2430 Medowpines Blvd, Unit 105, Mississauga, Ontario, L5N 6S2, Canada.

Roberts, USA. Roberts Pharmaceutical Corp., Meridian Center III, 6-G Industrial Way West, Eatontown, NJ 07724, USA.

Roberts & Sheppey, UK. Roberts & Sheppey (Melrose) Ltd, Manor Farm House, Ickford, Aylesbury, Bucks, HP18 9JB, UK.

Robins, Austral. See *Whitehall, Austral.*

Robins, Irl. See *Whitehall, Irl.*

Robins, Swed. See *Wyeth Lederle, Swed.*

Robins, Switz. See *Whitehall-Robins, Switz.*

Robins, USA. See *Whitehall-Robins, USA.*

Robinson, UK. Robinson Healthcare, Hipper House, Chesterfield, Derbyshire, S40 1YF, UK.

Robugen, Ger. Robugen GmbH Pharmazeutische Fabrik, Alleenstrasse 22-6, Postfach: 266, 73703 Esslingen, Germany.

RoC, Fr. RoC S.A., 50 rue de Seine, 92703 Colombes Cdx, France.

Roc, UK. Laboratoires RoC UK Ltd, Foundation Park, Roxborough Way, Maidenhead, Berks, SL6 3UG, UK.

Roche, Arg. Roche S.A.Q. e I., Fray Justo Sarmiento 2350, 1636 Olivos, Buenos Aires, Argentina.

Roche, Aust. Hoffmann-La Roche Wein GmbH, Jacquingasse 16-18, 1030 Vienna, Austria.
Roche, Austral. Roche Products Pty Ltd, P.O. Box 255, Dee Why, NSW 2099, Australia.
Roche, Belg. Roche S.A., Rue Dante 75, 1070 Brussels, Belgium.
Roche, Braz. Produtos Roche Quimicos e Farmaceuticos S.A., Brazil.
Roche, Canad. Hoffmann-La Roche Ltd, 2455 Meadowpine Blvd, Mississauga, Ontario, L5N 6L7, Canada.
Roche, Ecuad. Roche, Ave 10 de Agosto No 5133, Edif. Urania 5to. piso, Quito, Ecuador.
Roche, Fr. Produits Roche, 52 bd du Parc, 92521 Neuilly-sur-Seine Cdx, France.
Roche, Ger. Hoffmann-La Roche AG, Emil-Barell-Strasse 1, Postfach: 1270, 79630 Grenzach-Wyhlen, Germany.
Roche, Irl. Roche Pharmaceuticals (Ireland) Ltd, 3 Richview, Clonskeagh, Dublin 14, Ireland.
Roche, Ital. Roche s.p.a., Piazza Durante 11, 20131 Milan, Italy.
Roche, Jpn. Nihon Roche, 6-1 Shiba 2-chome, Minato-ku, Tokyo 105, Japan.
Roche, Neth. Roche Nederland B.V., Postbus 42, 3640 AA Mijdrecht, Netherlands.
Roche, Norw. Roche Norge A/S, Kristoffer Robinsv. 13, Postboks 41 Haugenstua, 0915 Oslo, Norway.
Roche, S.Afr. Roche Products (Pty) Ltd, P.O. Box 4589, Johannesburg 2000, S. Africa.
Roche, Spain. Roche, Ctra Carabanchel Andalucia S/N, 28025 Madrid, Spain.
Roche, Swed. Roche AB, Box 47327, 100 74 Stockholm, Sweden.
Roche, Switz. Roche Pharma (Schweiz) AG, Schonmattstrasse 2, 4153 Reinach, Switzerland.
Roche, UK. Roche Products Ltd, P.O. Box 8, Welwyn Garden City, Herts, AL7 3AY, UK.
Roche, USA. Roche Laboratories, Division of Hoffmann-La Roche Inc., Nutley, NJ 07110, USA.
Roche Consumer, Austral. See *Roche, Austral.*
Roche Consumer, Belg. See *Roche, Belg.*
Roche Consumer, Irl. See *Roche, Irl.*
Roche Consumer, UK. See *Roche, UK.*
Roche Dermatologics, USA. Roche Dermatologics, Division of Hoffmann-La Roche Inc., Overlook at Great Notch, 150 Clove Rd, Little Falls, NJ 07424, USA.
Roche Nicholas, Fr. Laboratoires Roche Nicholas, 74240 Gaillard, France.
Roche Nicholas, Ger. Roche Nicholas Deutschland GmbH, Postfach: 72, 65813 Eppstein-Bremthal, Germany.
Roche Nicholas, Neth. Roche Nicholas B.V., Postbus 23, 5530 AA Bladel, Netherlands.
Roche Nicholas, Spain. Roche Nicholas, Trav. de les Corts 39-43, 08028 Barcelona, Spain.
Roche Posay, Switz. See *Cosmetique Active, Switz.*
Roche Products, USA. Roche Products Inc., Manati, 00701, Puerto Rico.
Roche-Posay, Fr. Laboratoires Pharmaceutiques Roche-Posay, B.P. 23, 86270 La Roche-Posay, France.
Rodleben, Ger. Rodleben Pharma GmbH, Waldchen 19, Postfach: 205, 06855 Rosslau, Germany.
Rodler, Ger. See *Woelm, Ger.*
Roerig, Belg. See *Pfizer, Belg.*
Roerig, Ital. Roerig Farmaceutici Italiana s.r.l., Società del Gruppo Pfizer, Via Valbondione 113, 00188 Rome, Italy.
Roerig, Swed. Roerig AB, Box 501, 183 25 Taby, Sweden.
Roerig, USA. Roerig, Division of Pfizer Inc., 235 East 42nd St, New York, NY 10017, USA.
Roger, Spain. Roger, Santiago Ramon y Cajal 6, Molins de Rei, 08750 Barcelona, Spain.
Rogers, Canad. Rogers Pharmaceuticals Ltd, 330 Marwood Drive, Oshawa, ON, L1H 8B4, Canada.
Roha, Ger. roha Arzneimittel GmbH, Rockwinkeler Heerstrasse 100, Postfach: 330340, 28333 Bremen, Germany.
Roha, Irl. See *Pharma-Global, Irl.*
Roha, Switz. See *Adroka, Switz.*
Rohm, Aust. Röhm Pharma GmbH, Tendlergasse 13, 1090 Vienna, Austria.
Rohm, Ger. Röhm Pharma GmbH, Dr-Otto-Röhm-Strasse 2-4, Postfach: 100161, 64201 Darmstadt, Germany.
Rohm, S.Afr. See *Noristan, S.Afr.*
Rolab, S.Afr. Rolab (Pty) Ltd, P.O. Box 154, Isando 1600, S. Africa.
Roland, Ger. Roland Arzneimittel GmbH, Bargkoppelweg 66, Postfach: 730820, 22128 Hamburg, Germany.
Rolland, Switz. See *Lipha, Switz.*
Rolmex, Canad. Rolmex International Inc., 1155 rue Samuel Morse, C.P. 1005, Boucherville, QC, J4B 7L1, Canada.
Romigal, Ger. Romigal-Werk, Galileiplatz 2, 81679 Munich, Germany.
Romilo, Canad. Romilo Labs, 2807 LeCorbusier, Laval, Quebec, H7L 4J5, Canada.
Ronsheim & Moore, UK. Ronsheim & Moore, Division of Hickson & Welch Ltd, Ings Lane, Castleford, West Yorkshire, WF10 2JT, UK.
Rooster, Neth. J.H. Rooster & Zn. B.V., Netherlands.
Roques, Fr. Laboratoires Roques, 31 rue Jules-Guesde, 92130 Issy-les-Moulineaux, France.
Rorer, Austral. See *Rhone-Poulenc Rorer, Austral.*
Rorer, Canad. See *Rhone-Poulenc Rorer, Canad.*
Rorer, Fr. See *Bellon, Fr.*, and *Specia, Fr.*
Rorer, Ger. See *Rhone-Poulenc Rorer, Ger.*
Rorer, Irl. See *Rhone-Poulenc Rorer, Irl.*
Rorer, Ital. See *Rhone-Poulenc Rorer, Ital.*
Rorer, Norw. See *Inpharma, Norw.*
Rorer, Spain. See *Rhone-Poulenc Rorer, Spain.*
Rorer, UK. See *Rhone-Poulenc Rorer, UK.*
Rorer, USA. See *Rhone-Poulenc Rorer, USA.*
Rosa-Phytopharma, Fr. Laboratoires Rosa-Phytopharma, 68 rue Jean-Jaques-Rousseau, 75001 Paris, France.
Rosa-Phytopharma, Switz. See *Golaz, Switz.*
Rosch & Handel, Aust. Rösch & Handel, Gudrunstrasse 150, 1100 Vienna, Austria.
Rosco, Norw. See *Andersen, Norw.*
Rosemont, UK. Rosemont Pharmaceuticals Ltd, Rosemont House, Yorkdale Industrial Park, Braithwaite St, Leeds, West Yorks, LS11 9XE, UK.
Rosemont, USA. Rosemont Pharmaceutical Corp., 301 South Cherokee St, Denver, CO 80223, USA.
Rosen, Ger. Rosen Pharma GmbH, Muhlstr. 50, 66386 St Ingbert, Germany.
Ross, Canad. See *Abbott, Canad.*
Ross, UK. Ross Products, Abbott House, Norden House, Maidenhead, Berks, SL6 4XE, UK.
Ross, USA. Ross Laboratories, Division of Abbott Laboratories, Columbus, OH 43216, USA.
Roter, Switz. See *Galenica, Switz.*
Roterpharma, Irl. Roterpharma, Ireland.
Roterpharma, UK. Roterpharma Ltd, UK.
Rotexmedica, Ger. Rotexmedica GmbH Arzneimittelwerk, Bunsenstrasse 4, Postfach: 1266, 22943 Trittau, Germany.
Rotta, Ital. Rotta Research Laboratorium s.p.a., Via Valosa di Sopra 7/9, 20052 Monza (MI), Italy.
Rottapharm, Fr. Laboratoires Rottapharm, 6 rue Casimir-Delavigne, 75006 Paris, France.
Rottapharm, Ger. Rottapharm GmbH Arzneimittel, Postfach: 1420, 51658 Wiehl, Germany.
Rottapharm, Ital. Rottapharm s.r.l., Via Valosa di Sopra 9, 20052 Monza (MI), Italy.
Rottapharm, Spain. Rottapharm, Ctra Barcelona 2, Almacera, 46132 Valencia, Spain.
Rougier, Canad. Rougier Inc., 8480 boul. Saint-Laurent, Montreal, Quebec, H2P 2M6, Canada.
Roussel, Austral. See *Hoechst Marion Roussel, Austral.*
Roussel, Fr. See *Hoechst, Fr.*
Roussel, Irl. See *Hoechst Marion Roussel, Irl.*
Roussel, Ital. See *Hoechst Marion Roussel, Ital.*
Roussel, Neth. See *Hoechst Marion Roussel, Neth.*
Roussel, S.Afr. See *Hoechst Marion Roussel, S.Afr.*
Roussel, Spain. See *Hoechst Marion Roussel, Spain.*
Roussel, Switz. See *Hoechst Marion Roussel, Switz.*
Roussel, UK. See *Hoechst Marion Roussel, UK.*
Rovi, Spain. Rovi, Julian Camarillo 35, 28037 Madrid, Spain.
Rovifarma, Spain. Rovifarma, Principe de Vergara 109, 28007 Madrid, Spain.
Rowa, Ger. Rowa-Wagner GmbH & Co. KG Arzneimittelfabrik, Frankenforster Strasse 77, Postfach: 100556, 51405 Bergisch-Gladbach, Germany.
Rowa, Irl. Rowa Pharmaceuticals Ltd, Bantry, Co. Cork, Ireland.
Rowa, UK. See *Rowa, Irl.*
Rowex, Irl. See *Rowa, Irl.*
Roxane, USA. Roxane Laboratories Inc., P.O. Box 16532, Columbus, OH 43216, USA.
Royal Childrens Hospital, Austral. Royal Children's Hospital, Flemington Rd, Parkeville, Vic 3052, Australia.
RP-LABO, Fr. RP-LABO, France.
RTA, Switz. Laboratoire RTA, La Bruyere A, 1817 Fontanivent, Switzerland.
Rubio, Spain. Rubio, Berlines 39, 08022 Barcelona, Spain.
Rugby, USA. Rugby Laboratories Inc., 20 Nassau Ave, Rockville Center, New York, NY 11570, USA.
Rupertus, Aust. St Rupertus-Apotheke, Markt 107, 5090 Lofer, Austria.
Rusch, UK. Rüsch UK Ltd, PO Box 138, Cressex Industrial Estate, High Wycombe, Bucks, HP12 3NB, UK.
Russ, USA. See *UCB, USA.*
Rybar, Irl. See *Cahill May Roberts, Irl.*
Rybar, UK. See *Shire, UK.*
Rydelle, Fr. Lab. Rydelle Johnson, ZA du Vert-Galant, 10 rue St-Hilaire, 95310 Saint-Ouen-l'Aumone, France.
Rydelle, Ital. Rydelle Laboratories Business, Johnson Wax s.p.a., P.le M. Burke 3, 20020 Arese (MI), Italy.
Rydelle, USA. Rydelle Laboratories Inc., Subsidiary of S.C. Johnson & Son Inc., 1525 Howe St, Racine, WI 53403, USA.
Rystan, USA. Rystan Co. Inc., 47 Center Ave, P.O. Box 214, Little Falls, NJ 07424-0214, USA.
S & B, Neth. See *Multipharma, Neth.*
S & K, Ger. S & K Pharma, Schumann & Kohl GmbH, Bahnhofstr. 4-6, 66706 Perl, Germany.
SA Druggists, S.Afr. South African Druggists Pharma, P.O. Box 2251, Randberg 2125, S. Africa.
SA Druggists Self Med, S.Afr. See *SA Druggists, S.Afr.*
Saba, Ital. Saba, Via Salbertrand 21, 10146 Turin, Italy.
Sabater, Spain. Sabater J., Los Centelles 7, 46006 Valencia, Spain.
Sabax, S.Afr. See *Adcock Ingram, S.Afr.*
Sabex, Canad. Sabex Inc., 145 rue Jules-Leger, Boucherville, Quebec, J4B 7K8, Canada.
Sagitta, Ger. Sagitta Arzneimittel GmbH, Frühlingstrasse 7, Postfach: 1262, 83618 Feldkirchen-Westerham, Germany.
Salf, Ital. Salf Laboratorio Farmacologico s.p.a., Via G. d'Alzano 12, 24122 Bergamo, Italy.
Salfa, Ital. Salfa, Biochimici dr. Ferranti s.a.s., Via del Castellano 47, 60129 Ancona, Italy.
Salmon, Switz. Salmon Pharma GmbH, St Jakobs-Strasse 96, Postfach, 4002 Basel, Switzerland.
Salonpas, UK. Salonpas (UK) Ltd, Unit B, 32a Eveline Rd, Mitchum, Surrey, CR4 3LE, UK.
Salt, UK. Salt & Son Ltd, Saltair House, Lord St, Heartlands, Birmingham, B7 4DS, UK.
Salters, S.Afr. Salters, S. Africa.
Salud, Spain. Salud, Joaquin Costa 26, 28002 Madrid, Spain.
Salus, Aust. Salus-Braumapharm GmbH, Industriegasse 7, Postfach 8, 1231 Vienna, Austria.
Salus, Ital. Salus Researches s.p.a., Via Aurelia 58, 00165 Rome, Italy.
Salusa, S.Afr. Salusa (Pty) Ltd, Private Bag X516, Silverton 0127, S. Africa.
Salushaus, Ger. Salus-Haus Dr. med. Otto Greither Nachf. GmbH & Co KG, Bahnhofstrasse 24, Postfach: 1180, 83044 Bruckmuhl/Mangfall (Obb.), Germany.
Salutas, Ger. Salutas Fahlberg-List Pharma GmbH, Alt Salbke 60-3, Postfach: 11, 39049 Magdeburg, Germany.
Salvat, Spain. Salvat, Gall 30, Esplugas de Llobregat, 08950 Barcelona, Spain.
Salvator, Aust. Salvator-Apotheke, Zimmermannplatz 1, 1090 Vienna, Austria.
Salver, Fr. See *Cooperation Pharmaceutique, Fr.*
Samil, Ital. Samil s.p.a., Via Piemonte 32, 00187 Rome, Italy.
SAN, Ital. S.A.N. s.a.s., Viale Corsica 92, 50127 Florence 710 Italy.
SAN, Neth. Samenwerkende Apothekers Nederland B.V., Europalaan 2, 3526 KS Utrecht, Netherlands.
San Carlo, Ital. S. Carlo Farmaceutici s.p.a., Tor Maggiore, 00040 S. Palomba Pomezia (Rome), Italy.
Sanabo, Aust. Sanabo Wien GmbH, Brunner Strasse 59, 1235 Vienna, Austria.
Sanamed, Aust. Sanamed Import- und HandelsGmbH, Steckhovengasse 9, 1130 Vienna, Austria.
Sandersons, UK. Sandersons (Chemists) Ltd, 37 Oakwood Rise, Heaton, Bolton, BL1 5EE, UK.
Sandipro, Belg. Sandipro S.A.-N.V., Chaussee de Gand 615, 1080 Brussels, Belgium.
Sandoz, Aust. Sandoz GmbH, Brunnerstrasse 59, 1235 Vienna, Austria.
Sandoz, Austral. See *Novartis, Austral.*
Sandoz, Belg. See *Novartis, Belg.*
Sandoz, Canad. Sandoz Canada Inc., Pharmaceutical Division, 385 boul. Bouchard, Dorval, Quebec, H9R 4P5, Canada.
Sandoz, Fr. Laboratoires Sandoz, 14 bd Richelieu, 92500 Rueil-Malmaison, France.
Sandoz, Ger. Sandoz AG, Deutschherrnstrasse 15, 90327 Nurnberg, Germany.
Sandoz, Irl. See *Novartis, Irl.*
Sandoz, Ital. Sandoz Prodotti Farmaceutici s.p.a., Via C. Arconati 1, 20135 Milan, Italy.
Sandoz, Jpn. Sandoz Yakuhin KK, 17-30 Nishi-Azabu 4-chome, Minato-ku, Tokyo 106, Japan.
Sandoz, Neth. Sandoz B.V., Postbus 91, 5400 AB Uden, Netherlands.
Sandoz, Norw. See *Novartis, Norw.*
Sandoz, S.Afr. Sandoz Products (Pty) Ltd, P.O. Box 371, Randburg 2125, S. Africa.
Sandoz, Spain. See *Novartis, Spain.*
Sandoz, Swed. See *Novartis, Swed.*
Sandoz, Switz. Sandoz-Wander Pharma AG, Sudbahnhofstrasse 14 D, Postfach, 3001 Bern, Switzerland.
Sandoz, UK. See *Novartis, UK.*
Sandoz, USA. Sandoz Pharmaceuticals Corp., Dorsey Division, Sandoz Division, Route 10, East Hanover, NJ 07936, USA.
Sandoz Consumer, USA. See *Sandoz, USA.*
Sandoz Nutrition, Canad. Sandoz Nutrition Corporation, 1621 McEwen Dr., Unit 50, Whitby, Ontario, L1N 9A5, Canada.
Sandoz Nutrition, Spain. See *Novartis Nutrition, Spain.*
Sandoz Nutrition, USA. Clinical Nutrition Division, Sandoz Nutrition Corp., 5320 West 23rd St, P.O. Box 370, Minneapolis, MN 55440, USA.
Sandoz OTC, Switz. See *Sandoz, Switz.*
Sanico, Belg. Sanico N.V., Industrieterrein IV, Veedijk 59, 2300 Turnhout, Belgium.
Sanico, Switz. See *Uhlmann-Eyraud, Switz.*
Sanitalia, Ital. Sanitalia s.n.c. di Lavarra G. & C., Strada dei Tadini 5, 10131 Turin, Italy.
Sanitas, Ital. Sanitas Italia s.r.l., Via G Argento 37, 80141 Naples, Italy.
Sanitube, USA. Sanitube Co., 19 Concord St, S Norwalk, CT 06854, USA.
Sankyo, Austral. See *Searle, Austral.*
Sankyo, Ital. Sankyo Pharma Italia spa, Via Montecassiano 157, 00156 Rome, Italy.
Sankyo, Jpn. Sankyo Co. Ltd, 5-1 Nihonbashi-Honcho 3-chome, Chuo-ku, Tokyo 103, Japan.
Sanofi, Spain. See *Sanofi Winthrop, Spain.*
Sanofi, Swed. Sanofi Winthrop AB, Box 1403, 171 27 Solna, Sweden.
Sanofi, UK. See *Sanofi Winthrop, UK.*
Sanofi Animal Health, UK. Sanofi Animal Health Ltd, 7 Awberry Court, Hatters Lane, Watford, Herts, WD1 8YJ, UK.
Sanofi Labaz, Neth. See *Sanofi Winthrop, Neth.*
Sanofi Midy, Neth. See *Sterling Health, Neth.*

Sanofi Omnimed, S.Afr. Sanofi Omnimed, S. Africa.
Sanofi Winthrop, Aust. Sanofi Winthrop GmbH, Koppstrasse 116/4, 1160 Vienna, Austria.
Sanofi Winthrop, Austral. Sanofi Winthrop, Riverview Park Estate, 166 Epping Rd, Lane Cove, NSW 2066, Australia.
Sanofi Winthrop, Belg. Sanofi-Winthrop S.A., Ave de la Metrologie 5, 1130 Brussels, Belgium.
Sanofi Winthrop, Canad. Sanofi Winthrop, 90 Allstate Parkway, Markham, Ontario, L3R 6H3, Canada.
Sanofi Winthrop, Fr. Sanofi Winthrop, 9 rue de Pdt-Allende, 94258 Gentilly Cdx, France.
Sanofi Winthrop, Ger. Sanofi Winthrop GmbH, Augustenstrasse 10, Postfach: 200134, 80001 Munich, Germany.
Sanofi Winthrop, Irl. Sanofi Winthrop Ireland Ltd, United Drug House, Belgard Rd, Tallaght, Dublin 24, Ireland.
Sanofi Winthrop, Ital. Sanofi Winthrop s.p.a., Via G.B. Piranesi 38, 20137 Milan, Italy.
Sanofi Winthrop, Neth. Sanofi Winthrop, Postbus 97, 3140 AB Maassluis, Netherlands.
Sanofi Winthrop, Norw. Sanofi Winthrop AS, Baerumsv 473, 1351 Rud, Norway.
Sanofi Winthrop, Spain. Sanofi Winthrop, Ctra Batlloria A, Hostalric Km 1.4, Rielu I Viabrea, 17404 Girona, Spain.
Sanofi Winthrop, Switz. Sanofi Winthrop AG, Jurastrasse 2, 4142 Munchenstein, Switzerland.
Sanofi Winthrop, UK. Sanofi Winthrop Ltd, 1 Onslow St, Guildford, Surrey, GU1 4YS, UK.
Sanofi Winthrop, USA. Sanofi Winthrop Pharm., 90 Park Ave, New York, NY 10016, USA.
Sanol, Ger. Sanol GmbH, Alfred-Nobel-Strasse 10, Postfach: 100662, 40770 Monheim, Germany.
Sanopharm, Switz. Sanopharm AG, Postplatz 44, 7000 Chur, Switzerland.
Sanorania, Ger. Sanorania Pharma GmbH, Berliner Ring 89, 64625 Bensheim, Germany.
Sanorania, Switz. See *Medipharm, Switz.*
Sanoreform, Ger. Sanoreform GmbH, Postfach: 1365, 58303 Herdecke, Germany.
Sanorell, Ger. Sanorell Pharma GmbH & Co., Rechtmurgstr. 27, 72270 Baiersbronn-Obertal, Germany.
Sante Naturelle, Canad. Sante Naturelle AG Ltee, 369 Charles Peguy, La Prairie, QC, J5R 3E8, Canada.
Santen, Jpn. Santen Seiyaku, 3-9-19 Shimoshinjyo, Higashiyodogawa-ku, Osaka, Japan.
Santen, Swed. Santen Pharma AB, 171 45 Solna, Sweden.
Santiveri, Spain. Santiveri, Encuny 8, 08038 Barcelona, Spain.
Sanum-Kehlbeck, Ger. Sanum-Kehlbeck GmbH & Co. KG, Hasseler Steinweg 9-12, Postfach: 1355, 27316 Hoya, Germany.
Sanus, Aust. Sanus, Lehmanngasse 21, 1235 Vienna, Austria.
Sanwa, Jpn. Sanwa Kagaku Kenkyusho Co Ltd, 35 Higashisotobori-cho, Higashi-ku, Nagoya 461, Japan.
Saphar, S.Afr. See *Adcock Ingram Self Medication, S.Afr.*
Saprochi, Switz. Saprochi SA, Chemin de la Cretaux, Case postale 327, 1196 Gland/VD, Switzerland.
Sarget, Fr. Laboratoires Sarget Pharma, ave J.-F. Kennedy, 33701 Mérignac Cdx, France.
Sark, Ital. Sark spa, Via Zambeletti, 20021 Baranzate di Bollate (MI), Italy.
Sarm, Ital. Soc. An. Ritrovati Medicinali s.r.l., Via Tiburtina Km 18,300, 00012 Guidonia (Rome), Italy.
Satori, Fr. Lab. Satori International, Parc d'activite de Limonest, 540 allee des Hetres, 69760 Limonest, France.
Saunier-Daguin, Fr. Laboratoires Saunier-Daguin, 2 rue Marechal-Foch, 45370 Clery-St-Andre, France.
Sauter, Austral. See *Roche, Austral.*
Sauter, Switz. Lab. Sauter S.A., Case postale 224, 1211 Geneva 28, Switzerland.
Savage, USA. Savage Laboratories, Division of Atlanta Inc., 60 Baylis Road, P.O. Box 2006, Melville, NY 11747, USA.
Savio, Ital. Istituto Biochimico Nazionale Savio s.r.l., Via E. Bazzano 14, 16019 Ronco Scrivia (GE), Italy.
Savoma, Ital. Savoma Medicinali s.p.a., Via Baganza 2/A, 43100 Parma, Italy.
SBL, Swed. SBL Vaccin AB, 105 21 Stockholm, Sweden.
SCAM, Ital. Società Costruttrice Albatros Modena s.r.l., Via Bellaria 164, 41050 S. Maria di Mugnano (MO), Italy.
Scand Pharm, Swed. Scandinavian Pharmaceuticals-Generics AB, Box 6198, 102 30 Stockholm, Sweden.
Scandinavian Natural Health & Beauty, USA. Scandinavian Natural Health & Beauty Products Inc., 13 North Seventh St, Perkasie, Pennsylvania, PA 18944, USA.
Scandipharm, USA. Scandipharm Inc., 22 Inverness Center Pkwy, Suite 310, Birmingham, AL 35242, USA.
Scania, Swed. Scania Dental AB, Box 5, 741 21 Knivsta, Sweden.
SCAT, Fr. Societé de Conception et d'Applications-Thérapeutiques, La Boursidiere, B.P. 150, 92357 Le Plessis-Robinson, France.
SCAT, Neth. See *Byk, Neth.*
SCAT, Switz. See *Doetsch, Grether, Switz.*
Schaffer, USA. Schaffer Laboratories, 1058 North Allen Ave, Pasadena, California, CA 91104, USA.
Schaper & Brummer, Ger. Schaper & Brümmer GmbH & Co. KG, Bahnhofstrasse 35, Postfach: 611160, 38251 Salzgitter (Ringelheim), Germany.
Schaper & Brummer, Switz. See *Cumino, Switz.*
Scharper, Ital. Scharper s.p.a., Italy.
Schein, Canad. Schein Pharmaceutical Canada Inc., 77 Belfield Rd, Etobicoke, Ontario, M9W 1G9, Canada.
Schein, UK. Schein Rexodent, 25-7 Merrick Rd, Southall, Middx, UB2 4AU, UK.
Schein, USA. Schein Pharmaceutical Inc., 5 Harbor Park Dr., Port Washington, NY 11050, USA.
Scherag, S.Afr. Scherag (Pty) Ltd, P.O. Box 46, Isando 1600, S. Africa.
Scherax, Ger. Scherax Arzneimittel GmbH, Sulldorfer Landstrasse 128, Postfach: 550940, 22569 Hamburg, Germany.
Scherer, Ital. R.P. Scherer s.p.a., Via Nettunese Km. 20,100, 04011 Aprilia (Latina), Italy.
Scherer, USA. Scherer Laboratories Inc., 16200 N Dallas Parkway, Suite 165, Dallas, TX 75248, USA.
Schering, Aust. Schering-Wien GmbH, Scheringgasse 2, 1141 Vienna, Austria.
Schering, Austral. Schering Pty Ltd, 27-31 Doody Street, Alexandria, NSW 2015, Australia.
Schering, Belg. Schering S.A., J.E. Mommaertslaan 14, P.B.8, 1831 Diegem, Belgium.
Schering, Canad. Schering Canada Inc., 3535 Transcanada Hwy, Pointe-Claire, Quebec, H9R 1B4, Canada.
Schering, Fr. Schering, rue de Toufflers, B.P. 69, 59452 Lys-lez-Lannoy Cdx, France.
Schering, Ger. Schering Aktiengesellschaft, Mullerstrasse 178, 13353 Berlin, Germany.
Schering, Irl. Schering A.G., 44 Dartmouth Square, Dublin 6, Ireland.
Schering, Ital. Schering s.p.a., Via E. Schering 19-21, 20090 Segrate (MI), Italy.
Schering, Jpn. Schering, Japan.
Schering, Neth. Schering Nederland B.V., Postbus 116, 1380 AC Weesp, Netherlands.
Schering, Norw. Schering Norge A/S, Ringsv 3, Postboks 180, 1321 Stabekk, Norway.
Schering, S.Afr. Schering (Pty) Ltd, P.O. Box 5278, Halfway House 1685, S. Africa.
Schering, Spain. Schering, Mendez Alvaro 55, 28045 Madrid, Spain.
Schering, Swed. Schering Nordiska AB, Box 23117, 104 35 Stockholm, Sweden.
Schering, Switz. Schering (Schweiz) AG, Postfach 766, 8010 Zurich, Switzerland.
Schering, UK. Schering Health Care Ltd, The Brow, Burgess Hill, West Sussex, RH15 9NE, UK.
Schering, USA. Schering Corporation, Galloping Hill Rd, Kenilworth, NJ 07033, USA.
Schering-Plough, Austral. Schering-Plough Pty Ltd, P.O. Box 231, Baulkham Hills, NSW 2153, Australia.
Schering-Plough, Belg. Schering-Plough S.A., Rue de Stalle 67, 1180 Brussels, Belgium.
Schering-Plough, Canad. Schering-Plough Healthcare Products Canada Inc., 6400 Northam Dr., Mississauga, ON, L4V 1J1, Canada.
Schering-Plough, Fr. Schering-Plough, 92 rue Baudin, 92307 Levallois-Perret Cdx, France.
Schering-Plough, Irl. See *Pharmacia Upjohn, Irl.*
Schering-Plough, Ital. Schering Plough s.p.a., Via Ripamonti 89, 20141 Milan, Italy.
Schering-Plough, Neth. Schering-Plough B.V., Postbus 70, 1180 AB Amstelveen, Netherlands.
Schering-Plough, Norw. Schering-Plough A/S, Ankerv. 209, 1343 Eiksmarka, Norway.
Schering-Plough, S.Afr. Schering-Plough, S. Africa.
Schering-Plough, Spain. Schering Plough, Ctra Burgos Km 36, San Agustin de Guadalix, 28750 Madrid, Spain.
Schering-Plough, Swed. Schering-Plough AB, Box 27190, 102 52 Stockholm, Sweden.
Schering-Plough, UK. Schering-Plough Ltd, Schering-Plough House, Shire Park, Welwyn Garden City, Herts, AL7 1TW, UK.
Schering-Plough, USA. Schering-Plough Corp., 110 Allen Rd, Liberty Corner, NJ 07938, USA.
Scheurich, Ger. E. Scheurich Pharma GmbH, Strassburger Strasse 77, Postfach: 1361, 77763 Appenweier, Germany.
Schiapparelli, Ital. Schiapparelli Farmaceutici s.p.a., Viale Sarca 223, 20126 Milan, Italy.
Schiapparelli Searle, Ital. See *Searle, Ital.*
Schiapparelli Searle, USA. See *Searle, USA.*
Schieffer, Aust. Dr Schieffer Arzneimittel GmbH, Gansterergasse 12, 1160 Vienna, Austria.
Schieffer, Ger. Dr Schieffer Arzneimittel GmbH, Postfach: 350120, 50792 Koln, Germany.
Schieffer, Switz. Dr Schieffer AG, Zurcherstrasse 68, 8800 Thalwil, Switzerland.
Schiwa, Ger. Schiwa GmbH, Kattenvenner Str. 32, Postfach: 1180, 4519 Glandorf, Germany.
Schiwa, Swed. See *Dicamed, Swed.*
Schmid, Canad. Julius Schmid Canada Ltd, 100 Courtland Ave, Concord, ON, L4K 3T6, Canada.
Schmid, USA. Schmid Products Co., P.O. Box 4703, Sarasota, FL 34230, USA.
Schmidgall, Aust. Dr A & L Schmidgall chem.-pharm. Fabrik, Wolfganggasse 45-7, 1121 Vienna, Austria.
Schoeller, Aust. Schoeller-Pharma GmbH, Industriegasse 7, 1230 Vienna, Austria.
Scholl, Fr. Laboratoires Scholl, 13 bis av. de l'Escouvrier, B.P. 585, 95205 Sarcelles Cdx, France.
Scholl, Switz. Scholl AG, Sternenhofstrasse 15A, 4153 Reinach 1, Switzerland.
Scholl, UK. Scholl Consumer Products Ltd, 475 Capability Green, Luton, Beds, LU1 3LU, UK.
Scholl, USA. Scholl Inc., 3030 Jackson Ave, Memphis, TN 38151, USA.
Schonenberger, Switz. Schönenberger Pharma AG, Schachenstrasse 24, 5012 Schonenwerd, Switzerland.
Schoning-Berlin, Ger. Richard Schöning oHG, Pharmazeutische Präparate, Porschestrasse 22-24, Postfach: 420463, 12064 Berlin, Germany.
Schuck, Ger. Schuck GmbH, Industriestrasse 11, Postfach: 100265, 90564 Schwaig b. Nurnberg, Germany.
Schulke & Mayr, Aust. Schülke & Mayr GmbH, Zieglergasse 8/3, 1070 Vienna, Austria.
Schulke & Mayr, Ger. Schülke & Mayr GmbH, Heidbergstr. 100, 22846 Norderstedt, Germany.
Schulke & Mayr, Switz. See *Diethelm, Switz.*
Schupp, Ger. Schupp GmbH & Co., Postfach: 840, 72238 Freudenstadt, Germany.
Schur, Ger. Schur Pharmazeutika GmbH & Co. KG, Schorlemerstr. 68, 40547 Dusseldorf, Germany.
Schurholz, Ger. See *Synthelabo, Ger.*
Schutz, Aust. Maria Schutz Apotheke, Reinprechtsdorfer Strasse 2, 1050 Vienna, Austria.
Schwab, Ger. Dr Schwab GmbH, Berg-am-Laim-Strasse 129, Postfach: 801507, 81615 Munich, Germany.
Schwabe, Ger. Dr Willmar Schwabe GmbH & Co., Willmar-Schwabe-Strasse 4, Postfach: 410925, 76209 Karlsruhe, Germany.
Schwabe, Neth. See *VSM, Neth.*
Schwabe, Switz. Schwabe Pharma AG, Spezialist für Phytopharmaka, Erlistrasse 2, 6403 Kussnacht aR, Switzerland.
Schwabe-Curamed, Ger. Dr Willmar Schwabe GmbH & Co. Abt. Curamed Pharma GmbH, Pforzheimer Strasse 5, Postfach: 410229, 76202 Karlsruhe, Germany.
Schwarz, Fr. Laboratoires Schwarz Pharma, 235 av Le Jour-se-Leve, 92100 Boulogne-Billancourt, France.
Schwarz, Ger. Schwarz Pharma Deutschland GmbH, Alfred-Nobel-Strasse 10, Postfach: 100662, 40770 Monheim, Germany.
Schwarz, Irl. See *Allphar, Irl.*
Schwarz, Ital. Schwarz Pharma s.p.a., Via Felice Casati 16, 20124 Milan, Italy.
Schwarz, Switz. Schwarz Pharma AG, Hammerstrasse 23, 4410 Liestal, Switzerland.
Schwarz, UK. Schwarz Pharma Ltd, Schwarz House, East St, Chesham, Bucks, HP5 1DG, UK.
Schwarz, USA. Schwarz Pharma Inc., P.O. Box 2038, Milwaukee, WI 53201, USA.
Schwarzhaupt, Aust. Schwarzhaupt GmbH, Nordwestbahnstrasse 101, 1200 Vienna, Austria.
Schwarzhaupt, Ger. Kommanditgesellschaft Schwarzhaupt GmbH & Co., Sachsenring 37-47, 50677 Cologne, Germany.
Schwarzwalder, Ger. Schwarzwalder Natur-Heilmittel, Marktplatz 4, 93183 Kallmunz, Germany.
Schweiz. Serum & Impfinstitut, Switz. See *Berna, Switz.*
Schworer, Ger. Pharma Schwörer GmbH, Goethestrasse 29, Postfach: 1111, 69257 Wiesenbach, Germany.
Schwulst, S.Afr. Geo Schwulst Laboratories (Pty) Ltd, P.O. Box 38481, Booysens 2016, S. Africa.
Sciencex, Fr. Laboratoires Sciencex, 1 rue Edmond-Guillout, 75015 Paris, France.
Scientific, S.Afr. Scientific Pharmaceuticals (Pty) Ltd, P.O. Box 4261, Randburg 2125, S. Africa.
Scientific Hospital Supplies, Austral. Scientific Hospital Supplies, 12 Hope St, Ermington, NSW 2115, Australia.
Scientific Hospital Supplies, Irl. Scientific Hospital Supplies (Ireland) Ltd, 23b Moyle Road, Dublin Industrial Estate, Finglas, Dublin 11, Ireland.
Scientific Hospital Supplies, UK. Scientific Hopsital Supplies Ltd, 38 Queensland St, Liverpool, L7 3JG, UK.
Scimat, UK. See *Bailey, UK.*
Sclavo, Ital. Sclavo s.p.a., Via Fiorentina 1, 53100 Siena, Italy.
Scotia, S.Afr. See *Searle, S.Afr.*
Scott, Canad. Scott Chemical Canada, Division of Lander Co. Canada Ltd, 275 Finchdene Square, Scarborough, ON, M1X 1C7.
Scot-Tussin, USA. Scot-Tussin Pharmacal Co. Inc., 50 Clemence St, Cranston, RI 02920-0217, USA.
SCS, USA. SCS Pharmaceuticals, P.O. Box 5110, Chicago, IL 60680, USA.
SCT, Ital. S.C.T. s.n.c. di G. Boccheni & C., Via Liberta 21, 10095 Grugliasco (TO), Italy.
Searle, Austral. See *Monsanto, Austral.*
Searle, Belg. See *Continental Pharma, Belg.*
Searle, Canad. Searle Canada, a unit of Monsanto Canada Inc., 400 Iroquois Shore Rd, Oakville, Ontario, L6H 1M5, Canada.
Searle, Fr. See *Monsanto, Fr.*
Searle, Ger. G.D. Searle Vertrieb: Heumann Pharma GmbH & Co, Heideloffstrasse 18-28, Postfach: 2260, 8500 Nurenburg, Germany.
Searle, Irl. Searle, Bray Industrial Estate, Pinewood Close, Bray, Co. Wicklow, Ireland.
Searle, Ital. See *Monsanto, Ital.*
Searle, Neth. Searle Nederland B.V., Postbus 1402, 3600 BK Maarssen, Netherlands.
Searle, Norw. Searle, Division of Monsanto Norge A/S, Fornebuv. 37, 1324 Lysaker, Norway.
Searle, S.Afr. G.D. Searle (SA) (Pty) Ltd, P.O. Box 11128, Johannesburg 2000, S. Africa.
Searle, Spain. Searle Iberica, La Granja 30 (Polg. Ind.), Alcobendas, 28100 Madrid, Spain.
Searle, Swed. Searle Scandinavia, Division of Monsanto Sverige AB, Hastvagen 4A, 212 35 Malmo, Sweden.

Searle, Switz. Searle SA, 1170 Aubonne, Switzerland.

Searle, UK. Searle Pharmaceuticals, P.O. Box 53, Lane End Rd, High Wycombe, Bucks, HP12 4HL, UK.

Searle, USA. G.D. Searle & Co., 4901 Searle Pkwy, Skokie, IL 60077, USA.

Seatrace, USA. The Seatrace Co., P.O. Box 363, Gadsden, AL 35902, USA.

Sedifa, Mon. Laboratoires Sédifa, 4 av. Prince-Hereditaire-Albert, Fontvieille, MC 98000 Monaco, Monaco.

Segix, Ital. Segix Italia spa, Via del Mare 36, 00040 Pomezia (RM), Italy.

Seid, Spain. Seid, Ctra Sabadell Granollers Km 15, Llissa de Vall, 08185 Barcelona, Spain.

Select, Ital. Select Pharma s.p.a., Via Pontina 100, 04011 Aprilia (LT), Italy.

Selena, Swed. Selena Läkemedel AB, Box 1266, 172 25 Sundbyberg, Sweden.

Sella, Ital. Sella A. Lab. Chim. Farm. s.r.l., Via Vicenza 2, 36015 Schio (Vicenza), Italy.

Selmag, Switz. Selmag-Weibel, Bergackerweg 4, 3054 Schupfen/BE, Switzerland.

Selvi, Ital. Selvi Laboratorio Bioterapico s.p.a., Via Lisbona 23, 00198 Rome, Italy.

Selz, Ger. Pharma Selz GmbH, Albert-Schweitzer Str. 52-4, Postfach: 60, 67592 Florsheim-Dalsheim, Germany.

Semar, Spain. Semar, Avda Litoral Mar 12-14, 08005 Barcelona, Spain.

Semper, Norw. See *Nycomed, Norw.*

Sempio, Ital. Farmaceutici Sempio, Via Nino Bixio 1, 21040 Carnago (VA), Italy.

Senju, Jpn. Senju Pharmaceutical Co., Ltd, 5-8 Hiranomachi 2-chome, Chuo-ku, Osaka 541, Japan.

Sepharma, Ital. Sepharma srl, Via Walter Tobagi 8, 20068 Peschiera Borromeo (MI), Italy.

Septa, Spain. Septa Chemifarma, Sierra Guadarrama 11, Pol. Ind. 2, San Fernando de Henares, 28850 Madrid, Spain.

Septfons, Fr. Moulin de Regime de Septfons, 03290 Dompierre-sur-Besbre, France.

Septodont, Switz. See *Odontopharm, Switz.*

Sequus, Aust. See *Sequus, UK.*

Sequus, UK. Sequus Pharmaceuticals Inc., 10 Barley Mow Passage, London, W4 4PH, UK.

Sequus, USA. Sequus Pharmaceuticals Inc., 960 Hamilton Court, Menlo Park, CA 94025, USA.

Serag-Wiessner, Ger. Serag-Wiessner GmbH & Co. KG, Kugelfang 8-12, Postfach: 1140, 95112 Naila, Germany.

SERB, Fr. See *L'Arguenon, Fr.*

Seres, USA. Seres Laboratories Inc., 3331 Industrial Dr., P.O. Box 470, Santa Rosa, CA 95402, USA.

Serolab, Switz. Serolab SA, En Marin, CP36, Ch. de la Vulliette 4, 1000 Lausanne 25, Switzerland.

Serolam, Fr. Laboratoires Sérolam, 30 rue Armand Silvestre, 92400 Courbevoie, France.

Serono, Aust. Serono Pharm. Präparate GmbH, Wienerbergstrasse 7, 1100 Vienna, Austria.

Serono, Austral. Serono Australia Pty. Ltd, Allambie Grove Business Park, Warrington Rd, Frenchs Forest, NSW 2086, Australia.

Serono, Belg. Laboratoires Serono Benelux S.A., Belgium.

Serono, Canad. Serono Canada Inc., 1075 North Service Rd, Suite 100, Oakville, Ontario, L6M 2G2, Canada.

Serono, Fr. Laboratoires Serono, L'Arche du Parc, 738 rue Yves-Kermen, 92658 Boulogne Cdx, France.

Serono, Ger. Serono Pharma GmbH, Gutenbergstrasse 5, Postfach: 1507, 85705 Unterschleissheim, Germany.

Serono, Irl. See *Allphar, Irl.*

Serono, Ital. Industria Farmaceutica Serono s.p.a., Via Casilina 125, 00176 Rome, Italy.

Serono, Neth. Serono Benelux, Koninginnegracht 28, 2514 AB Den Haag, Netherlands.

Serono, Norw. Serono Nordic AB, Solheimsv. 32, 1473 Skarer, Norway.

Serono, Spain. Serono, Maria de Molina 40, 28006 Madrid, Spain.

Serono, Swed. Serono Nordic AB, Box 1803, 171 21 Solna, Sweden.

Serono, Switz. Laboratoires Serono SA, 1170 Aubonne, Switzerland.

Serono, UK. Serono Laboratories (UK) Ltd, 99 Bridge Road East, Welwyn Garden City, Herts, AL7 1BG, UK.

Serono, USA. Serono Laboratories Inc., 280 Pond St, Randolph, MA 02368, USA.

Serono OTC, Ital. See *Serono, Ital.*

Serotherapeutisches, Aust. Serotherapeutisches Institut, Richard-Strauss-Strasse 33, 1232 Vienna, Austria.

Seroyal, Canad. Seroyal, Canada.

Serozym, Fr. Laboratoires Serozym, 30 rue Armand-Silvestre, 92400 Courbevoie, France.

SERP, Mon. S.E.R.P., 3 rue Princesse-Florestine, MC 98000 Monaco, Monaco.

Serpero, Ital. Serpero Industria Galenica Milanese s.p.a., Viale L. Maino 40, 20129 Milan, Italy.

Serra Pamies, Spain. Serra Pamies, Ctra de Castellvell 24, Reus, 43206 Tarragona, Spain.

Serturner, Ger. Sertürner Arzneimittel GmbH, Stadtring Nordhorn 113, Postfach: 2761, 33257 Gutersloh, Germany.

Serum-Werk Bernburg, Ger. Serum-Werk Bernburg AG, Hallesche Landstrasse 105 b, Postfach: 1263, 06392 Bernburg, Germany.

Servier, Aust. Servier Pharma, Vienna, Austria.

Servier, Austral. Servier Laboratories (Aust.) Pty Ltd, P.O. Box 196, Hawthorn, Vic. 3122, Australia.

Servier, Belg. Servier Benelux S.A., Blvd International 57, 1070 Brussels, Belgium.

Servier, Canad. Servier Canada Inc., 235 blvd Armand-Frappier, Laval, Quebec, H7V 4A7, Canada.

Servier, Fr. Laboratoires Servier, 22 rue Garnier, 92200 Neuilly-sur-Seine, France.

Servier, Ger. Servier Deutschland GmbH, Westendstrasse 170, 80686 Munich, Germany.

Servier, Irl. Servier Laboratories (Ireland) Ltd, AMEV House, Temple Rd, Blackrock, Co. Dublin, Ireland.

Servier, Ital. Servier Italia s.p.a., Via degli Aldobrandeschi 107, 00163 Rome, Italy.

Servier, Neth. Servier Nederland B.V., Postbus 672, 2300 AR Leiden, Netherlands.

Servier, S.Afr. Servier Laboratories (SA) (Pty) Ltd, P.O. Box 930, Rivonia 2128, S. Africa.

Servier, Spain. Servier, Avda de Madronos 33, 28043 Madrid, Spain.

Servier, Switz. Servier (Suisse) SA, 21, rue de Veyrot, 1217 Meyrin 1, Switzerland.

Servier, UK. Servier Laboratories Ltd, Fulmer Hall, Windmill Rd, Fulmer, Slough, Bucks, SL3 6HH, UK.

Servipharm, Switz. Servipharm AG, Postfach, 4002 Basel, Switzerland.

Sessa, Ital. Sessa Carlo s.p.a., Viale Gramsci 212, 20099 Sesto S. Giovanni (MI), Italy.

Sestri, UK. Sestri (Sales) Ltd, Kingsend House, 44 Kingsend, Ruislip, Middx, HA4 7DA, UK.

Seton, Irl. See *Intraveno, Irl.*

Seton, UK. Seton Healthcare Group plc, Tubiton House, Medlock St, Oldham, Lancs, OL1 3HS, UK.

Seven Seas, UK. Seven Seas Health Care Ltd, Marfleet, Kingston-Upon-Hull, HU9 5NJ, UK.

SFPH, Fr. S.F.P.H., 13 rue de l'Epinette, 77165 St-Soupplets, France.

Shaklee, Canad. Shaklee Canada Inc., 952 Century Dr, Burlington, Ontario, L7L 5P2, Canada.

Sharpe, Austral. Sharpe Laboratories Pty Ltd, 12 Hope Street, Ermington, NSW 2115, Australia.

Shepherd, Canad. Shepherd Pharmaceuticals Inc., 3332 Yonge St, P.O. Box 94018, Toronto, Ontario, M4N 3R1, Canada.

Sherman, USA. Sherman Pharmaceuticals Inc., P.O. Box 1377, Mandeville, LA 70470-1377, USA.

Sherwood, USA. Sherwood Laboratories Inc., 1601 E 31st St, Willoughby, OH 44094, USA.

Shin Poong, Kor. Shin Poong Pharm. Co., Korea.

Shinyaku, Jpn. Nippon Shinyaku Co. Ltd, 14 Nishinosho-Monguchi-cho, Kisshoin, Minami-ku, Kyoto 601, Japan.

Shionogi, Ger. Shionogi & Co. GmbH, Germany.

Shionogi, Jpn. Shionogi & Co. Ltd, 1-8 Dosho-machi 3-chome, Chuo-ku, Osaka 541, Japan.

Shionogi, USA. Shionogi USA Inc., 3848 Carson St, Suite 206, Torrance, CA 90503, USA.

Shire, Irl. See *Cahill May Roberts, Irl.*

Shire, UK. Shire Pharmaceuticals Ltd, Fosse House, East Anton Court, Icknield Way, Andover, Hants, SP10 5RG, UK.

Shiseido, Canad. Shiseido Cosmetics Ltd Canada, 486 Queen St E, Ste 212, Toronto, Ontario, M5A 1T7, Canada.

Shoppers Drug Mart, Canad. Shoppers Drug Mart, 225 Yorkland Blvd, Willowdale, ON, M2J 4Y7, Canada.

SHS, USA. SHS/Scientific Hospital Supplies, 9600 Medical Center Drive, Suite 102, Rockville, MD 20850, USA.

Sicor, Ital. Sicor, Via Terrazzano 77, 20017 Rho (MI), Italy.

Sideck, Ital. Sideck Farmaceutici s.r.l., Via Tremestieri II Trav. 16, 95030 Mascalucia (CT), Italy.

Sidroga, Switz. Sidroga AG, Postfach 524, 4800 Zofingen, Switzerland.

Siegfried, Ger. Siegfried Pharma GmbH, Mumpferfährstr. 68, Postfach: 1141, 79702 Bad Sackingen, Germany.

Siegfried, Swed. See *Thore Solum, Swed.*

Siegfried, Switz. Siegfried Pharma AG, 4800 Zofingen, Switzerland.

Siemens, Ger. Siemens & Co., Heilwasser und Quellenprodukte des Staatsbades Bad Ems GmbH & Co. KG, Arzbacher Strasse 78, 56130 Bad Ems, Germany.

Siemens, Switz. See *Adroka, Switz.*

Sifarma, Ital. Sifarma s.p.a., Via Brunelleschi 12, 20146 Milan, Italy.

SIFI, Ital. Società Industria Farmaceutica Italiana s.p.a., Via N. Coviello 15/B, 95128 Catania, Italy.

SIFRA, Ital. SIFRA Farmaceutici Verona s.p.a., Via Camagre 41/43, 37063 Isola della Scala (VR), Italy.

Sigma, Austral. Sigma Pharmaceuticals Pty Ltd, 96 Merrindale Drive, Croydon, Vic. 3136, Australia.

Sigmapharm, Aust. Sigmapharm, Dr H Punzengruber und Dr H Pichler, Leystrasse 129, 1204 Vienna, Austria.

Sigmapharm, Switz. See *Ridupharm, Switz.*

Sigma-Tau, Canad. See *Sigma-Tau, USA.*

Sigma-Tau, Fr. Sigma-Tau France, 5 av de Verdun, 94202 Ivry sur Seine, France.

Sigma-Tau, Ger. Sigma Tau GmbH, Peinz-Georg Str. 126, 40479 Dusseldorf, Germany.

Sigma-Tau, Ital. Sigma Tau s.p.a., Via Pontina Km. 30,400, 00040 Pomezia (Rome), Italy.

Sigma-Tau, Spain. Sigma Tau, Pl. Ind. Azque, Parcelas 13-14, Alcala de Henares, 28806 Madrid, Spain.

Sigma-Tau, Switz. Sigma-Tau Pharma AG, Luzernerstrasse 2, 4800 Zofingen, Switzerland.

Sigma-Tau, USA. Sigma-Tau Pharmaceuticals Inc., 800 S Frederick Ave, Gaithersburg, MD 20877-4150, USA.

Silarx, USA. Silarx Pharmaceuticals Inc., 15 West St, Spring Valley, NY 10977, USA.

Silhouette, Aust. Silhouette International GmbH, Ellbognerstrasse 24, 4020 Linz, Austria.

Simcare, UK. Simcare, Peter Rd, Lancing, West Sussex, BN15 8TJ, UK.

Simes, Ital. Simes s.p.a., Italy.

Simons, Ger. Georg Simons GmbH & Co., Bunsenstrasse 5, Postfach: 1465, 82143 Planegg/Martinsried, Germany.

Sinax, Ital. Sinax s.p.a., Via Ponte della Fabbrica 3/B, 35031 Abano Terme (PD), Italy.

Sinbio, Fr. Laboratoires Sinbio, Dept médical dePierre Fabre Médicament, 45 place Abel-Gance, 92100 Boulogne, France.

Sinclair, Irl. See *Allphar, Irl.*

Sinclair, UK. Sinclair Pharmaceuticals Ltd, Borough Rd, Godalming, Surrey, GU7 2AB, UK.

Singer, Switz. Pharma-Singer AG, Windeggstrasse 2, 8867 Niederurnen, Switzerland.

Sintesa, Belg. Sintesa S.A.-N.V., Blvd de la Woluwe 34, Bte 11, 1200 Brussels, Belgium.

Sintetica, Switz. Sintetica SA, San Martino, casella postale 223, 6850 Mendrisio, Switzerland.

Siphar, Switz. Siphar SA, Casella postale 32, 6814 Cadempino, Switzerland.

Sirmeta, Austral. Sirmeta, Australia.

Sisu, Canad. Sisu Enterprises Ltd, 312-8495 Ontario St, Vancouver, British Columbia, V5X 3E8, Canada.

SIT, Ital. Specialità Igienico Terapeutiche s.r.l., C.so Cavour 70, 27035 Mede (Pavia), Italy.

Skinicles, Canad. Skinicles Ltd, 150 Priscilla Ave, P.O. Box 1655, Toronto, Ontario, M6S 3W3, Canada.

SK-RIT, Belg. See *SmithKline Beecham, Belg.*

Slim-Fast, Canad. Slim-Fast Nutritional Foods International, 407-220 Duncan Mill Rd, Don Mills, Ontario, M3B 3J5, Canada.

Smaller, Spain. Smaller, Sagitario 12, 03006 Alicante, Spain.

SMB, Belg. Lab. S.M.B. S.A., rue de la Pastorale 26-28, 1080 Brussels, Belgium.

Smetana, Aust. See *EF-EM-ES, Aust.*

Smith & Nephew, Austral. Smith & Nephew Pty Ltd, P.O. Box 150, Clayton, Vic. 3168, Australia.

Smith & Nephew, Canad. Smith & Nephew Inc., 2100, 52e Ave, Lachine, Quebec, H8T 2Y5, Canada.

Smith & Nephew, Fr. Smith & Nephew, 25 bd Alexandre-Oyon, 72019 Le Mans cdx, France.

Smith & Nephew, Irl. Smith & Nephew Medical, Pottery Rd, Kill O' the Grange, Dun Laoghaire, Co. Dublin, Ireland.

Smith & Nephew, Ital. Smith & Nephew s.r.l., Viale Colleoni 13, 20041 Agrate Brianza (MI), Italy.

Smith & Nephew, Norw. Smith & Nephew AS, Postboks 224, 1360 Nesbru.

Smith & Nephew, S.Afr. Smith & Nephew Pharmaceuticals (Pty) Ltd, P.O. Box 92, Pinetown 3600, S. Africa.

Smith & Nephew, Swed. Smith & Nephew Scandinavia AB, Box 143, 431 22 Molndal, Sweden.

Smith & Nephew, UK. Smith & Nephew Medical Ltd, P.O. Box 81, 101 Hessle Rd, Hull, HU3 2BN, UK.

Smith & Nephew, USA. Smith & Nephew United, 11775 Starkey Rd, Largo, FL 34643, USA.

Smith & Nephew Healthcare, UK. Smith & Nephew Healthcare Ltd, Healthcare House, Goulton St, Hull, HU3 4DJ, UK.

Smith & Nephew Pharmaceuticals, UK. See *Smith & Nephew Healthcare, UK.*

Smith & Nephew SoloPak, USA. See *SoloPak, USA.*

Smith Kline & French, Irl. See *SmithKline Beecham, Irl.*

Smith Kline & French, Ital. See *SmithKline Beecham, Ital.*

Smith Kline & French, Spain. See *SmithKline Beecham, Spain.*

Smith Kline & French, Switz. See *SmithKline Beecham, Switz.*

SmithKline Beecham, Aust. SmithKline Beecham Pharma GmbH, Hietzinger Hauptstrasse 55 A, 1130 Vienna, Austria.

SmithKline Beecham, Austral. SmithKline Beecham International Pharmaceuticals, Private Mail Bag 34, Dandenong, Vic. 3175, Australia.

SmithKline Beecham, Belg. SmithKline Beecham Pharma S.A., Rue du Tilleul 13, 1332 Genval, Belgium.

SmithKline Beecham, Canad. SmithKline Beecham Pharma Inc., 2030 Bristol Circle, Oakville, Ontario, L6H 5V2, Canada.

SmithKline Beecham, Fr. SmithKline Beecham Laboratoires Pharmaceutiques, 6 esplanade Charles-de-Gaulle, 92731 Nanterre Cdx, France.

SmithKline Beecham, Ger. SmithKline Beecham Pharma GmbH, Leopoldstrasse 175, Postfach: 401642, 80716 Munich, Germany.

SmithKline Beecham, Irl. SmithKline Beecham Pharmaceuticals, Corig Ave, Dun Laoghaire, Co. Dublin, Ireland.

SmithKline Beecham, Ital. SmithKline Beecham s.p.a., Via Zambeletti, 20021 Baranzate di Bollate (MI), Italy.

SmithKline Beecham, Neth. SmithKline Beecham Farma, Postbus 3120, 2280 GC Rijswijk, Netherlands.

SmithKline Beecham, Norw. SmithKline Beecham Pharmaceuticals, Solheimv. 112, Postboks 134, 1471 Skarer, Norway.

SmithKline Beecham, S.Afr. SmithKline Beecham Pharmaceuticals, P.O. Box 347, Bergvlei 2012, S. Africa.

SmithKline Beecham, Spain. SmithKline Beecham, Valle de la Fuenfria 3, 28034 Madrid, Spain.
SmithKline Beecham, Swed. SmithKline Beecham Pharmaceuticals AB, Box 4092, 171 04 Solna, Sweden.
SmithKline Beecham, Switz. SmithKline Beecham AG, 3174 Thorishaus, Switzerland.
SmithKline Beecham, UK. SmithKline Beecham Pharmaceuticals, Mundells, Welwyn Garden City, Herts, AL7 1EY, UK.
SmithKline Beecham, USA. SmithKline Beecham Pharmaceuticals, P.O. Box 7929, Philadelphia, PA 19103, USA.
SmithKline Beecham Consumer, Austral. SmithKline Beecham International (Consumer Healthcare), P.O. Box 3, Ermington, NSW 2115, Australia.
SmithKline Beecham Consumer, Belg. See *SmithKline Beecham, Belg.*
SmithKline Beecham Consumer, Canad. See *SmithKline Beecham, Canad.*
SmithKline Beecham Consumer, Irl. See *SmithKline Beecham, Irl.*
SmithKline Beecham Consumer, Neth. SmithKline Beecham Consumer Healthcare, Postbus 394, 1180 AJ Amstelveen, Netherlands.
SmithKline Beecham Consumer, Switz. See *SmithKline Beecham, Switz.*
SmithKline Beecham Consumer, UK. SmithKline Beecham Consumer Healthcare UK, SB House, Great West Rd, Brentford, Middx, TW8 9BD, UK.
SmithKline Beecham Consumer, USA. SmithKline Beecham Consumer Brands, Unit of SmithKline Beecham Inc., 100 Beecham Dr., Pittsburgh, PA 15205, USA.
SmithKline Beecham Drinks, UK. See *SmithKline Beecham, UK.*
SmithKline Beecham Sante, Fr. Laboratoires SmithKline Beecham Pharmacie Santé, 5 esplanade Charles-de-Gaulle, B.P. 306, 92003 Nanterre cdx, France.
SmithKline Diagnostics, USA. SmithKline Diagnostics, 225 Baypoint Parkway, San Jose, CA 95134-1622, USA.
SMP, S.Afr. SMP, S. Africa.
Socopharm, Fr. Socopharm, Chemin de Marcy, 58800 Corbigny, France.
Sodia, Fr. Laboratoires Sodia, 12 rue Lafage, 51200 Epernay, France.
Sodietal, Fr. Laboratoires Sodiétal, BP 100, 29260 Ploudaniel, France.
Sodilac, Fr. Sodilac, Le Wilson 2, 80 av du President-Wilson, Puteaux 92031 Paris-La Defense, France.
Sodip, Switz. Sodip SA, 11 rue Alphonse-Large, 1217 Meyrin 1, Switzerland.
Soekami, Fr. See *Roche Nicholas, Fr.*
Sofar, Ital. Sofar Farmaceutici s.p.a., Via Ramazzini 5, 20129 Milan, Italy.
SoftRinse, USA. SoftRinse Corp., 2411 Third St South, Wisconsin Rapids, WI 54494, USA.
Sohan, Canad. Sohan Chemicals Ltd, 70 Gibson Drive, Unit 14, Markham, ON, L3R 2Z3, Canada.
Sokosi, Switz. Sokosi Pharma SA, Via General Guisan 6, 6830 Chiasso, Switzerland.
Solar, Canad. Solar Cosmetics, Canada.
Solco, Ger. Solco GmbH, Salzwerkstrasse 7, Postfach: 110, 79633 Grenzach-Wyhlen, Germany.
Solco, Switz. Solco Basel SA, Ruhrbergstrasse 21, 4127 Birsfelden, Switzerland.
Solea, Ital. Solea s.a.s., Via Cassoli 22, 42100 Reggio Emilia, Italy.
Solent, UK. Solent Diagnostics, 27 Silver Birch Ave, Fareham, Hants, PO14 1SZ, UK.
Solgar, UK. Solgar Vitamins Ltd, Solgar House, Chiltern Commerce Centre, Asheridge Rd, Chesham, Bucks, UK.
Solgar, USA. Solgar Vitamin Co. Inc., P.O. Box 330, Lynbrook, NY 11563, USA.
Solmer, Switz. Solmer SA, Postfach 100, 6976 Lugano-Castagnola, Switzerland.
SoloPak, USA. SoloPak Pharmaceuticals Inc., 1845 Tonne Rd, Elk Grove Village, IL 60007-5125, USA.
Soludia, Fr. Laboratoires Soludia, Route de Revel, 31450 Fourquevaux, France.
Solvay, Aust. Solvay Pharma GmbH, Donaustrasse 106, 3400 Klosterneuburg, Austria.
Solvay, Austral. Solvay Pharmaceuticals, Locked Bag 1070, Pymble, NSW 2073, Australia.
Solvay, Belg. Solvay Pharma & Cie S.N.C., Boulevard Emile Bockstael 122, 1020 Brussels, Belgium.
Solvay, Canad. Solvay Pharma Inc., 50 Venture Drive, Unit 1, Scarborough, Ontario, M1B 3L6, Canada.
Solvay, Fr. Solvay Pharma, 42 rue Rouget-de-Lisle, B.P. 22, 92151 Suresnes cdx, France.
Solvay, Ger. Solvay Arzneimittel GmbH, Postfach: 220, 30002 Hannover, Germany.
Solvay, Irl. Solvay Healthcare Ltd, Belgard Rd, Tallaght, Dublin 24, Ireland.
Solvay, Ital. Solvay Pharma s.p.a., Via Marco Polo 38, 10095 Grugliasco (TO), Italy.
Solvay, Neth. Solvay Pharma B.V., Postbus 501, 1380 AM Weesp, Netherlands.
Solvay, Norw. See *Meda, Norw.*
Solvay, S.Afr. Solvay, S. Africa.
Solvay, Spain. Solvay Farma, Avda Diagonal 507-9, 08029 Barcelona, Spain.
Solvay, Switz. Solvay Pharma AG, Untermattweg 8, CH-3027 Bern, Switzerland.
Solvay, UK. Solvay Healthcare, Hamilton House, Gaters Hill, West End, Southampton, Hants, SO18 3JD, UK.
Solvay, USA. Solvay, 901 Sawyer Road, Marietta, GA 30062-2224, USA.
Solvay Duphar, Swed. See *Meda, Swed.*
Solveig Ekeberg, Norw. Advokat Solveig Ekeberg, Radmann Halmrastv 2, Postboks 296, 1301 Sandvika, Norway.
Solymes, Fr. Laboratoires Solymès, 1 terrasse Bellini, 92910 Paris-La Defense Cdx, France.
Somerset, USA. Somerset Pharmaceuticals, 777 S Harbour Island Blvd 880, Tampa, FL 33602, USA.
Sopar, Belg. Sopar Pharma S.A., Blvd Sylvain Dupuis 243, 1070 Brussels, Belgium.
Sopar, Neth. See *Will-Pharma, Neth.*
Sorin, Ital. Sorin Radiofarmaci, Italy.
Sorin-Maxim, Fr. Laboratoires Sorin-Maxim, rue Claude-Bernard, 12700 Capdenac, France.
SoSe, Ital. So.Se. Pharm s.r.l., Via dei castelli Romani 22, 00040 Pomezia (Rome), Italy.
SPA, Ital. Società Prodotti Antibiotici s.p.a., Via Biella 8, 20143 Milan, Italy.
SPAD, Fr. Laboratoires Spécialités Pour l'Art Dentaire, B.P. 7, 21801 Quetigny Cdx, France.
Specia, Fr. Specia, Groupe Rhône-Poulenc-Rorer, 15 rue de la Vanne, 92120 Montrouge, France.
Spectra Nova, Swed. Spectra Nova AB, Box 937, S-75109 Uppsala, Sweden.
Spectropharm, Canad. Spectropharm Inc., 6700 Cote de Liesse, Suite 207, Ville St Laurent, Quebec, H4T 1E3, Canada.
Speywood, Swed. See *Speywood, UK.*
Speywood, Switz. See *Opopharma, Switz.*
Speywood, UK. Speywood Laboratories Ltd, Ash Rd, Wrexham Industrial Estate, Wrexham, Clwyd, UK.
Speywood, USA. Speywood Pharmaceuticals Inc, 27 Maple St, Milford, Massachusetts 01757-3650, USA.
Spiphar, Belg. Ets Spiphar S.P.R.L., Ave de la Couronne 114A, 1050 Brussels, Belgium.
Spirig, Switz. Spirig AG, Pharmazeutische Präparate, 4622 Egerkingen, Switzerland.
Spitzner, Ger. W. Spitzner, Arzneimittelfabrik GmbH, Bunsenstrasse 6-10, Postfach: 763, 76261 Ettlingen, Germany.
Splenodex, Fr. Laboratoires Recherche Thérapeutique-Splénodex, 4 av. Maurice-Leroy, 77310 Ponthierry, France.
Spodefell, UK. Spodefell Ltd, 5 Inverness Mews, London, W2 3QJ, UK.
Spreewald, Ger. Spreewald Pharma GmbH, Kuschkower Str. 9, 15910 Groditsch, Germany.
Spyfarma, Spain. Spyfarma, Ctra Sevilla Malaga Km 9.5 Km, Alcala de Guadaira, 41500 Seville, Spain.
Squibb, Austral. See *Bristol-Myers Squibb, Austral.*
Squibb, Canad. See *Bristol-Myers Squibb, Canad.*
Squibb, Ital. See *Bristol-Myers Squibb, Ital.*
Squibb, Neth. See *Bristol-Myers Squibb, Neth.*
Squibb, Spain. Squibb, Josep Anselm Clave 95, Esplugas De Llobregat, 08950 Barcelona, Spain.
Squibb, Switz. See *Bristol-Myers Squibb, Switz.*
Squibb, UK. See *Bristol-Myers Squibb, UK.*
Squibb, USA. See *Bristol-Myers Squibb, USA.*
Squibb Diagnostics, Canad. See *Bristol-Myers Squibb, Canad.*
Squibb Diagnostics, USA. Squibb Diagnostics, P.O. Box 4500, Princeton, NJ 08543-4500, USA.
Squibb-Heyden, Ger. See *Bristol-Myers Squibb, Ger.*
Squibb-Novo, USA. See *Bristol-Myers Squibb, USA.*
SRK, Switz. See *ZLB, Switz.*
SS, Jpn. SS Pharmaceutical, Japan.
SSW, Ger. Sächsisches Serumwerk GmbH, Zirkusstrasse 40, Postfach: 120227, 01003 Dresden, Germany.
St Laurent, Canad. See *Romilo, Canad.*
Stada, Aust. Stada Arzneimittel GmbH, 5081 Salzburg-Anif, Austria.
Stada, Ger. Stada Arzneimittel AG, Stadastrasse 2-18, Postfach: 1260, 61102 Bad Vilbel, Germany.
Stada, Switz. Stada Arzneimittel (Schweiz) AG, Route Andre-Piller 2, Case postale 76, 1762 Givisiez, Switzerland.
Stadapharm, Ger. See *Stada, Ger.*
Stafford-Miller, Austral. Stafford Miller Ltd, Locked Bag 185, Milperra, NSW 2214, Australia.
Stafford-Miller, Fr. Laboratoires Stafford-Miller, 1 bd Victor, 75015 Paris, France.
Stafford-Miller, Irl. See *Intra Pharma, Irl.*
Stafford-Miller, Ital. Stafford-Miller s.r.l., Via Correggio 19, 20149 Milan, Italy.
Stafford-Miller, Norw. See *Searle, Norw.*
Stafford-Miller, Spain. Stafford Miller, Pol. Ind. Malpica C/C 102-7, 50016 Zaragoza, Spain.
Stafford-Miller, Switz. See *Doetsch, Grether, Switz.*
Stafford-Miller, UK. Stafford-Miller Ltd, Stafford-Miller House, Broadwater Rd, Welwyn Garden City, Herts, AL7 3SP, UK.
Stafford-Miller Continental, Belg. Stafford-Miller Continental N.V.-S.A., Nijverhaidsstraat 9, 2260 Oevel, Belgium.
Stallergenes, Belg. Stallergenes Belgium S.A., Rue de Tilleul 13, 1332 Genval, Belgium.
Stallergenes, Fr. Stallergènes SA, 7 allee des Platanes, 94264 Fresnes Cdx, France.
Stallergenes, Switz. Lab. des Stallergènes Sàrl, 17C rue Vautier, case postale 1331, 1227 Carouge, Switzerland.
Stanback, USA. Stanback Co., PO Box 1669, Salisbury, North Carolina, NC 28145-1669, USA.
Standard Drug, USA. Standard Drug Company, P.O. Box 710, Riverton, IL 62561, USA.
Stanley, Canad. Stanley Pharmaceuticals Ltd, 1353 Main St, N. Vancouver, British Columbia, V7J 1C5, Canada.
Star, USA. Star Pharmaceuticals Inc., 1990 NW 44th St, Pompano Beach, FL 33064-1278, USA.
Stark, Ger. H. C. Stark GmbH Chemische Fabrik, Schneckenburgstrasse 46, Postfach: 101743, 78417 Constance, Germany.
Staufen, Ger. Staufen-Pharma GmbH & Co., Bahnhofstrasse 35, Postfach: 1143, 73011 Goppingen, Germany.
STD, Irl. See *STD Pharmaceutical Products, UK.*
STD Pharmaceutical Products, UK. STD Pharmaceutical Products Ltd, Fields Yard, Plough Lane, Hereford, HR4 0EL, UK.
Steierl, Ger. Steierl-Pharma GmbH, Muhlfelder Str. 48, Postfach: 1268, 82207 Herrsching, Germany.
Steigerwald, Ger. Steigerwald Arzneimittelwerk GmbH, Havelstrasse 5, Postfach: 101345, 64213 Darmstadt, Germany.
Steigerwald, Switz. See *Hanseler, Switz.*
Steiner, Ger. Steiner & Co. Deutsche Arzneimittel Gesellschaft, Ostpreussendamm 72/74, Postfach: 520, 12175 Berlin, Germany.
Steiner, Switz. See *Drossapharm, Switz.*
Stella, Belg. Lab. Stella S.A., Rue des Pontons 25, 4032 Chenee (Liege), Belgium.
Stella, Canad. Stella Pharmaceutical Co. Ltd, 407-220 Duncan Mill Rd, Don Mills, Ontario, M3B 3J5, Canada.
Stellar, USA. Stellar Pharmacal Corp., 1990 NW 44th St, Pompano Beach, FL 33064-1278, USA.
Steris, USA. Steris Laboratories Inc., 620 N 51st Ave, Phoenix, AZ 85043, USA.
Steriseal, UK. Steriseal Ltd, 26-7 Thornhill Rd, North Moons Moat, Redditch, Worcs, B98 9NL, UK.
Sterling, Canad. Sterling Products Ltd, Division of Sterling Drug, Canada.
Sterling, Neth. See *Sterling Health, Neth.*
Sterling, USA. See *Sterling Health, USA.*
Sterling Health, Austral. See *SmithKline Beecham Consumer, Austral.*
Sterling Health, Belg. See *SmithKline Beecham, Belg.*
Sterling Health, Neth. Sterling Health VOF, Netherlands.
Sterling Health, Spain. Sterling health, Avda Diagonal 618, 6, 08021 Barcelona, Spain.
Sterling Health, Swed. Sterling Health AB, Box 1403, 171 27 Solna, Sweden.
Sterling Health, Switz. Sterling Health AG, Postfach, 4002 Basel, Switzerland.
Sterling Health, UK. See *SmithKline Beecham, UK.*
Sterling Health, USA. Sterling Health, 99 Cherry Hill Rd, Parsippany, NJ 07054-1102, USA.
Sterling Midy, Fr. See *SmithKline Beecham Sante, Fr.*
Sterling Midy, Ital. Sterling Midy s.p.a., Viale Ortles 12, 20139 Milan, Italy.
Sterling Research, UK. See *Sanofi Winthrop, UK.*
Sterling Winthrop, Fr. See *Sanofi Winthrop, Fr.*
Sterling Winthrop, Spain. See *Sanofi Winthrop, Spain.*
Sterling Winthrop, Swed. See *Sterling Health, Swed.*
Sterling Winthrop, UK. See *Sanofi Winthrop, UK.*
Stern, Ger. Pharma-stern GmbH, 22876 Wedel, Germany.
Sterwin, UK. Sterwin Medicines, 1 Onslow St, Guildford, Surrey, GU1 4YS, UK.
Stickley, Canad. E.L. Stickley & Co. Ltd, P.O. Box 1748, Brantford, Ontario, N3T 5V7, Canada.
Stiefel, Austral. Stiefel Laboratories Pty Ltd, Unit 14, 5 Salisbury Road, Castle Hill, NSW 2154, Australia.
Stiefel, Canad. Stiefel Canada Inc., 6635 boul. Henri-Bourassa Ouest, Montreal, Quebec, H4R 1E1, Canada.
Stiefel, Fr. Laboratoires Stiefel, Z.I. du Petit Nanterre, 15 rue des Grands Pres, 92000 Nanterre, France.
Stiefel, Ger. Stiefel Laboratorium GmbH, Muhlheimer Strasse 231, 63075 Offenbach am Main, Germany.
Stiefel, Irl. See *Allphar, Irl.*
Stiefel, Ital. Stiefel Laboratories s.r.l., Via Calabria 15, 20090 Redecesio di Segrate (MI), Italy.
Stiefel, Neth. See *Bipharma, Neth.*
Stiefel, Norw. See *Jacomedic, Norw.*
Stiefel, S.Afr. Stiefel Laboratories SA (Pty) Ltd, P.O. Box 27114, Benrose 2011, S. Africa.
Stiefel, Spain. Stiefel, Soledad 37, San Martin de la Vega, 28330 Madrid, Spain.
Stiefel, Switz. Stiefel Laboratorium AG, c/o Micucci Treuhand AG, Romertorstrasse 1, 8404 Winterthur, Switzerland.
Stiefel, UK. Stiefel Laboratories (UK) Ltd, Holtspur Lane, Wooburn Green, High Wycombe, Bucks, HP10 0AU, UK.
Stiefel, USA. Stiefel Laboratories Inc., Route 145, Oak Hill, NY 12422, USA.
Stockhausen, USA. Stockhausen Inc., 2408 Doyle St, Greensboro, NC 27406, USA.
Stomygen, Ital. Gruppo Stomygen s.r.l., Via F. Jorini 69, 00149 Rome, Italy.
Storz, Austral. Storz Ophthalmics, 5 Gibbon Rd, Baulkham Hills, NSW 2153, Australia.
Storz, Belg. Storz Ophthalmics, a division of AHP Pharma, Rue du Bosquet 15, 1348 Louvain-la-Neuve, Belgium.
Storz, Canad. Storz, division of Wyeth-Ayerst Canada Inc., 1200 Aerowood Dr., Suite 24, Mississauga, Ontario, L4W 2S7, Canada.
Storz, Fr. See *Lederle, Fr.*
Storz, Irl. See *Whelehan, Irl.*
Storz, Norw. See *Lederle, Norw.*
Storz, Swed. See *Cyanamid, Swed.*
Storz, UK. See *Cyanamid, UK.*
Storz, USA. Storz Ophthalmic Pharmaceuticals, 3365 Tree Court Industrial Blvd, St Louis, MO 63122-6694, USA.

Stotzer, Switz. Stotzer AG, Jura-Apotheke Bern, Breitenrainplatz 40, 3000 Bern 22, Switzerland.
Strallhofer, Aust. Dr. Till Strallhofer Mag., St-Veit-Gasse 56, 1030 Vienna, Austria.
Strath-Labor, Ger. Strath-Labor GmbH, Strath-Strasse 5-7, Postfach: 20, 93093 Donaustauf, Germany.
Strathmann, Ger. Strathmann AG & Co., Sellhopsweg 1, 22459 Hamburg, Germany.
Stratus, USA. Stratus Pharmaceuticals Inc., P.O. Box 4632, Miami, FL 33265, USA.
Streuli, Switz. G. Streuli & Co. SA, 8730 Uznach, Switzerland.
Strickland, Canad. See *Hargell, Canad.*
Stroder, Ital. Ist. Farmaco Biologico Stroder s.r.l., Via di Ripoli 207/V, 50126 Florence, Italy.
Stroschein, Ger. Pharma Stroschein GmbH, Sellhopsweg 1, Postfach: 610425, 22421 Hamburg, Germany.
Strunz & Korber, Aust. Strunz & Körber OHG, Austria.
Stuart, USA. Stuart Pharmaceuticals, Division of ICI Americas Inc., Wilmington, DE 19897, USA.
Stuart House, Canad. Stuart House, 77 Rivalda Rd, Weston, ON, M9M 2M6, Canada.
Stulln, Ger. Pharma Stulln GmbH, Werksweg 2, Postfach: 1127, 92501 Nabburg, Germany.
Stulln, Switz. See *Galenica, Switz.*
Substantia, Fr. See *Parke, Davis, Fr.*
Sudmedica, Ger. Südmedica GmbH, Chemisch-pharmazeutische Fabrik, Ehrwalder Strasse 21, Postfach: 701669, 81316 Munich, Germany.
Suisse, Austral. Suisse Naturopathics Pty Ltd, Australia.
Sumitomo, Jpn. Sumitomo Pharmaceuticals Co. Ltd, 27 Kandasurugadai 3-chome, Chiyoda-ku, Tokyo 101, Japan.
Summers, USA. Summers Laboratories Inc., Morris Rd, Ft Washington, PA 19034, USA.
Summit, USA. Summit Pharmaceuticals, Division of Ciba-Geigy Corporation, 556 Morris Avenue, Summit, NJ 07901, USA.
Sun, Canad. Sun Pharmaceutical Industries Inc., 1111 Flint Rd, Unit 23, Downsview, Ontario, M3J 3C7, Canada.
Sun Life, Fr. Lab. Sun Life, 33 rue Fortuny, 75017 Paris, France.
Sunde, Norw. Advokat Jens A. Sunde, Tidemandsg. 40, 0260 Oslo, Norway.
Sunfresh, Canad. Sunfresh Ltd, 22 St Clair Ave E, Toronto, ON, M4T 2S8, Canada.
Sunspot, Austral. Sunspot Products Pty Ltd, 303/20 Bungan Street, Mona Vale, NSW 2103, Australia.
Superfos Biosector, Norw. Superfos Kjemi Norge AS, Tvetenv 6, Postboks 6335 Etterstad, 0604 Oslo, Norway.
Supergen, USA. Supergen Inc., 2 Annabel Lane, Suite 220, San Ramon, CA 94583, USA.
Surf Ski International, UK. Surf Ski International Ltd, Atlantique, Grande Route Des Mielles, St Ouen, Jersey, Channel Islands, UK.
Survival Technology, USA. Survival Technology Inc., 2275 Research Blvd, Rockville, MD 20850, USA.
Sussex, UK. Sussex Pharmaceutical Ltd, Charlwoods Rd, East Grinstead, Sussex, RH19 2HL, UK.
Sutton, Canad. HJ Sutton Industries Ltd, 433 rue Ste-Helene, Montreal, QC, H2Y 2L1, Canada.
Svenska Dental, Swed. Svenska Dental Instrument AB, Box 723, 194 27 Upplands Vasby, Sweden.
SVR, Ital. SVR Italia, Via Ca Rossa 10, 35010 Limena (PD), Italy.
Swedish Orphan, Swed. Swedish Orphan AB, Drottninggatan 98, 111 60 Stockholm, Sweden.
Sween, USA. Sween Corp., Sween Building, P.O. Box 980, Lake Crystal, MN 56055, USA.
Swiss Herbal, Canad. Swiss Herbal Remedies Ltd, 35 Leek Cres, Richmond Hill, Ontario, L4B 4C2, Canada.
SwissHealth, UK. SwissHealth, UK.
Swissphar, Neth. See *Will-Pharma, Neth.*
Swisspharm, S.Afr. Swisspharm (Pty) Ltd, S. Africa.
Sylak, Swed. Sylak AB, Box 1228, 600 42 Norrkoping, Sweden.
Symbiopharm, Ger. SymbioPharm GmbH, Postfach: 1765, 35727 Herborn, Germany.
Syncare, Canad. See *Altimed, Canad.*
Synlab, Fr. Laboratoires Synlab, 15 rue de l'Hotel-de-Ville, 92200 Neuilly-sur-Seine, France.
Synmedic, Switz. Synmedic AG, Seebahnstrasse 85, Postfach, 8036 Zurich, Switzerland.
Synomed, Ger. Synomed GmbH, Postfach: 880, 25308 Elmshorn, Germany.
Synpharma, Aust. Synpharma GmbH, pharmaz. u. diätet. Erzeugnisse, Mayrwies 56, Postfach 4, 5023 Salzburg, Austria.
Synpharma, Switz. Synpharma SA, Case postale, 9240 Uzwil, Switzerland.
Syntex, Austral. Syntex Australia Ltd, P.O. Box 255, Dee Why, NSW 2099, Australia.
Syntex, Belg. Syntex S.A., Belgium.
Syntex, Canad. See *Roche, Canad.*
Syntex, Fr. Laboratoires Syntex, 20 rue Jean-Jaures, 92800 Puteaux, France.
Syntex, Ger. Syntex Arzneimittel GmbH, Emil-Barell-Strasse 1, Postfach: 1270, 79630 Grenzach-Wyhlen, Germany.
Syntex, Irl. See *Roche, Irl.*
Syntex, Neth. Syntex B.V., Postbus 3171, 2280 GD Rijswijk, Netherlands.
Syntex, S.Afr. Syntex Pharmaceuticals (Pty) Ltd, P.O. Box 89566, Lyndhurst, S. Africa.
Syntex, Spain. Syntex Latino, Severo Ochoa 13 (Pol. Ind.), Leganes, 28914 Madrid, Spain.
Syntex, Swed. Syntex Nordica AB, Box 19003, 152 25 Sodertalje, Sweden.
Syntex, Switz. See *Uhlmann-Eyraud, Switz.*
Syntex, UK. See *Roche, UK.*
Syntex, USA. See *Roche, USA.*
Synthelabo, Aust. Synthelabo-Byk Pharma Vertrieb GmbH, Ketzergassse 200, 1235 Vienna, Austria.
Synthelabo, Belg. Synthelabo Belgium S.A., Ave de Schiphol 2, 1140 Brussels, Belgium.
Synthelabo, Fr. Laboratoires Synthélabo France, 22 av. Galilee, 92350 Le Plessis-Robinson, France.
Synthelabo, Ger. Synthelabo Arzneimittel GmbH, Lindberghstrasse 1, Postfach: 1554, 82171 Puchheim, Germany.
Synthelabo, Ital. Synthelabo s.p.a., Via Rivoltana 35, 20090 Limito (MI), Italy.
Synthelabo, Norw. See *Astra, Norw.*
Synthelabo, Switz. Synthélabo-Pharma SA, Case postale 45, 1000 Lausanne 21, Switzerland.
Synthelabo Delagrange, Spain. Synthelabo Delagrange, Avda de la Industria 31, Alcobendas, 28100 Madrid, Spain.
Synthes, Aust. Synthes GmbH, Karolingerstrasse 16, 5035 Salzburg, Austria.
Synthol, Spain. Synthol Cientifical, Roca Umbert 17, Hospitalet de Llobregat, 08907 Barcelona, Spain.
Syosset, USA. Syosset Laboratories Inc., 150 Eileen Way, Syosset, NY 11791, USA.
Syxyl, Ger. Syxyl Petereit GmbH & Co. KG, Flamweg 132/134, Postfach: 880, 25308 Elmshorn, Germany.
Taco, Ger. Taco-GmbH, Chem.-Pharm. Fabrik, Alte Heerstrasse 76, Postfach: 2146, 53744 St. Augustin, Germany.
TAD, Ger. TAD Pharmazeutisches Werk GmbH, Heinz-Lohmann-Strasse 5, Postfach: 720, 27457 Cuxhaven, Germany.
TAD, Switz. See *Grossmann, Switz.*
Tafir, Spain. Tafir, Trifon Pedrero 4-6, 28019 Madrid, Spain.
Taiho, Jpn. Taiho Pharmaceutical Co. Ltd, 27 Kandanishiki-cho 1-chome, Chiyoda-ku, Tokyo 101, Japan.
Takeda, Aust. Takeda Pharma GmbH, Siedengasse 33-5, 1070 Vienna, Austria.
Takeda, Fr. Laboratoires Takeda, 15 quai de Dion-Bouton, 92816 Puteaux Cdx, France.
Takeda, Ger. Takeda Pharma GmbH, Victoriaallee 3-5, Postfach: 1607, 52017 Aachen, Germany.
Takeda, Ital. Takeda Italia Farmaceutici s.p.a., Via Giovannino 7, 95126 Catania, Italy.
Takeda, Jpn. Takeda Chemical Industries Ltd, 1-1 Doshomachi 4-chome, Chuo-ku, Osaka 541, Japan.
Tanabe, Jpn. Tanabe Seiyaku Co. Ltd, 2-10 Doshomachi 3-chome, Chuo-ku, Osaka 541, Japan.
Tanning Research, Canad. See *Tropic Suncare, Canad.*
Tanning Research, USA. Tanning Research Labs Inc., 1190 US 1 North, Ormond Beach, FL 32174, USA.
Tanta, Canad. Tanta Pharmaceuticals Inc., 1009 Burns St East, Whitby, Ontario, L1N 6A6, Canada.
TAP, USA. TAP Pharmaceuticals, 1400 Sheridan Rd, North Chicago, IL 60064, USA.
Taphlan, Switz. See *Serolab, Switz.*
Taranis, Fr. Taranis, 6 rue de Trésor, 75004 Paris, France.
Taro, Canad. Taro Pharmaceuticals Inc., 130 East Drive, Bramalea, Ontario, L6T 1C3, Canada.
Taro, UK. Taro Pharmaceuticals (UK) Ltd, 10 Lincolns Inn Fields, London, WC2A 3BP, UK.
Taro, USA. Taro Pharmaceuticals USA Inc., 6 Skyline Drive, Hawthorne, NY 10532-9998, USA.
Taxandria, Neth. Taxandria Pharmaceutica B.V., Postbus 90241, 5000 LV Tilburg, Netherlands.
Tebib, Spain. Tebib, Castello 57, 28001 Madrid, Spain.
Tec, USA. Tec Laboratories Inc., 615 Water Ave. S.E., PO Box 1958, Albany, OR 97321, USA.
Tecefarma, Spain. Tecefarma, Guifre 724, Badalona, 08912 Barcelona, Spain.
Technicon, S.Afr. Technicon Laboratories, P.O. Box 150, Maraisburg 1700, S. Africa.
Technilab, Canad. Technilab Inc., 17800 Lapointe St, Mirabel, Quebec, J7J 1P3, Canada.
Techni-Pharma, Mon. Techni-Pharma, 7 rue de l'Industrie, B.P. 717, MC 98000 Monaco Cdx, Monaco.
Tecnobio, Spain. Tecnobio, Rda Gral Mitre 151, 08022 Barcelona, Spain.
Tecnodif, Fr. Laboratoires Tecnodif, 44 rue du Moulin, 57480 Sierck-Les-Bains, France.
Tedec Meiji, Spain. Tedec Meiji Farma S.A., Poligono Industrial de Coslada, Camino de Carriles S/N, 28820 Madrid, Spain.
Teekanne, Aust. Teekanne GmbH, Munchner Bundesstrasse 120, 5021 Salzburg, Austria.
Tego, Ital. Tego Italiana s.r.l. Prodotti Chimici, Viale Campania 33, 20133 Milan, Italy.
Teikoku, Jpn. Teikoku Hormone Mfg Co. Ltd, 5-1 Akasaka 2-chome, Minato-ku, Tokyo 107, Japan.
Teknofarma, Ital. Teknofarma s.p.a., S. Bertolla Abb. Stura 14, 10156 Turin, Italy.
Telluride, USA. Telluride Pharm. Corp, 146 Flanders Drive, Hillsborough, NJ 08876-4656, USA.
Temmler, Ger. Temmler Pharma GmbH, Temmlerstrasse 2, Postfach: 2269, 35010 Marburg/Lahn, Germany.
Temmler, Switz. See *Doetsch, Grether, Switz.*
Tendem, Neth. Tendem B.V., Postbus 190, 8000 AD Zwolle, Netherlands.
Tendem-Haco, Neth. See *Tendem, Neth.*
Tender, Canad. Tender Corp. Canada, 18 Alliance Blvd, Unit 10, Barrie, Ontario, L4M 5A5, Canada.
Tentan, Switz. Tentan AG, Fuchsweidweg 11, 4852 Rothrist, Switzerland.
Teofarma, Ital. Teofarma, Via F.lli Cervi 5, 27100 Valle Salimbene (PV), Italy.
Teomed, Switz. Teomed AG, Tumigerstrasse 71, Postfach 20, CH-8606 Greifensee, Switzerland.
Teral, USA. See *Bart, USA.*
Terapeutico, Ital. Labor. Terapeutico M.R. s.r.l., Via Domenico Veneziano 13, 50143 Florence, Italy.
Terme di Chianciano, Ital. Terme di Chianciano s.p.a., Via delle Rose 12, 53042 Chianciano Terme (Siena), Italy.
Terme di Montecatini, Ital. Terme di Montecatini s.p.a., Viale Marconi 7, 51016 Montecatini Terme (PT), Italy.
Terme di Salsomaggiore, Ital. Terme di Salsomaggiore s.p.a., Via Roma 9, 43039 Salsomaggiore Terme (Parma), Italy.
Terme Sirmione, Ital. Terme Sirmione spa, Piazza Castello 12, 25019 Sirmione (BS), Italy.
Terra-Bio, Ger. Terra-Bio-Chemie GmbH, Ekkebertstrasse 28, 79117 Freiburg i. Br., Germany.
Terramin, Aust. Terramin Pharma GmbH & Co. KEG, 5571 Maria Pfarr 135, Austria.
Terrapharm, Aust. Terrapharm Pharm. Produktions- und HandelsGmbH, Braunlichgasse 40-2, 2700 Wiener Neustadt, Austria.
Teva, USA. See *Hoechst Marion Roussel, USA.*
TFB, Canad. TFB & Associates Ltd, Canada.
Thackray, UK. See *DePuy, UK.*
Thames, UK. Thames Laboratories Ltd, Abbey House, Wrexham Industrial Estate, Wrexham, Clwyd, LL13 9PW, UK.
Thames, USA. Thames Pharmacal Co. Inc., 2100 Fifth Ave, Ronkonkoma, NY 11779, USA.
Thea, Fr. Laboratoires Théa, 12 rue Louis-Bleriot, ZI du Brezet, B.P. 72 Saint Jean, 63016 Clermont-Ferrand cdx 1, France.
Thea, Spain. Thea, Balmes 49, 08007 Barcelona, Spain.
Thepenier, Fr. Laboratoires Thépénier, 10 rue Clapeyron, 75008 Paris, France.
Thepenier, Switz. See *Uhlmann-Eyraud, Switz.*
Thera, Fr. Laboratoires Thera France, 61 rue Lecuyer, B.P. 63, 93302 Aubervilliers cdx, France.
Therabel, Fr. Laboratoires Théabel Lucien Pharma, 15 rue de l'Hotel-de-Ville, 92522 Neuilly-sur-Seine cdx, France.
Therabel, Ital. Therabel Pharma s.p.a., Via Passione 8, 20122 Milan, Italy.
Therabel Pharma, Belg. Therabel Pharma S.A., Rue Egide Van Ophen 110, 1180 Brussels, Belgium.
Theralab, Canad. See *Therapex, Canad.*
Theramex, Mon. Laboratoires Théramex, 6 av. Prince-Hereditaire-Albert, B.P. 59, MC 98007 Monaco Cdx, Monaco.
Theranol-Deglaude, Fr. Laboratoires Theranol-Deglaude, 58 ave Aristide Briand, B.P. 140, 92223 Bagneux, France.
Therapex, Canad. Therapex, Division of E-Z-EM Canada Inc., 11 100 rue Colbert, Ville d'Anjou, Quebec, H1J 2M9, Canada.
Theraplix, Fr. Théraplix - Rhône-Poulenc Rorer, 46-52 rue Albert, 75640 Paris Cdx 13, France.
Therasophia, Fr. Lab. Therasophia, BP 122, 06334 Grasse cdx, France.
Therica, Fr. Laboratoires Thérica, 15 av. Henry Dunant, 27400 Louviers, France.
Thermalife, Austral. Thermalife International Pharmaceuticals Ltd, 391 Oxford Street, Mt Hawthorn, WA 6016, Australia.
Therval, Fr. Therval Medical, 29 rue du Pont, 92200 Neuilly-sur-Seine, France.
Thiemann, Ger. Thiemann Arzneimittel GmbH, Wirrigen 25, Postfach: 440, 45725 Waltrop, Germany.
Thilo, Neth. See *Bournonville, Neth.*
Thomae, Ger. Dr Karl Thomae GmbH, Birkendorfer Strasse 65, 88397 Biberach/Riss, Germany.
Thompson, UK. Thompson Medical Co. Ltd, Riding Court, Riding Court Rd, Datchet, Slough, Berks, SL3 9JT, UK.
Thompson, USA. Thompson Medical Co. Inc., 919 Third Ave, New York, NY 10022, USA.
Thore Solum, Swed. Thore Solum, Nonnens vag 6, 451 50 Uddevalla, Sweden.
Thornton & Ross, UK. Thornton & Ross Ltd, Linthwaite Laboratories, Huddersfield, HD7 5QH, UK.
Thuasne, Fr. Thuasne SA, 6 rue des Marronniers, B.P. 243, 92307 Levallois-Perret Cdx, France.
Thuna, Canad. Thuna Herbal Remedies Ltd, 298 Danforth Ave, Toronto, ON, M4K 1N6, Canada.
Thylmer, Belg. Thylmer S.A., Belgium.
Tican, Canad. Tican Pharmaceuticals Ltd, 100 Blvd St-Joseph O, Montreal, Quebec, H2T 2P6, Canada.
Tika, Norw. See *Astra, Norw.*
Tika, Swed. Tika Läkemedel AB, Box 2, 221 00 Lund, Sweden.
Tillomed, UK. Tillomed Laboratories Ltd, Unit 2, Campus 5, Letchworth Business Park, Letchworth, Herts, SG6 2JF, UK.
Tillotts, Switz. Tillotts Pharma AG, Hauptstrasse 27, 4417 Ziefen, Switzerland.
Tillotts, UK. Tillotts Laboratories, Unit 24, Henlow Trading Estate, Henlow, Beds, SG16 6DS, UK.
Time-Cap, USA. Time-Cap Labs Inc., 7 Michael Ave, Farmingdale, NY 11735, USA.
Tipomark, Ital. Tipomark s.r.l., Via Ippolito Nievi 28/1, 20145 Milan, Italy.
Tiroler, Aust. Tiroler Steinölwerke OHG, 6213 Pertisau am Achensee, Tirol, Austria.
Tissot, Fr. Laboratoires du Dr Tissot, 34 bd de Clichy, 75018 Paris, France.

Tissot, Switz. See *Uhlmann-Eyraud, Switz.*
Togal, Ger. Togal-Werk AG, Postfach: 860760, 81634 Munich, Germany.
Togal, Switz. Togal-Werk SA, Via Val Gersa 4, 6900 Lugano-Massagno, Switzerland.
Tokyo Tanabe, Jpn. Tokyo Tanabe Co. Ltd, 2-6 Nihonbashi-Honcho 2-chome, Chuo-ku, Tokyo 103, Japan.
Topfer, Ger. Töpfer GmbH, Heisingerstrasse 6, Postfach: 1180, 87460 Dietmannsried, Germany.
Toray, Jpn. Toray Industries Inc., 2-1 Nihonbashi-Muromachi 2-chome, Chuo-ku, Tokyo 103, Japan.
Torbet, Irl. See *Allphar, Irl.*
Torbet Laboratories, UK. Torbet Laboratories, Pearl Assurance House, Mill St, Maidstone, Kent, ME15 6XH, UK.
Torch, USA. Torch Laboratories Inc., USA.
Torfwerk Einfeld, Ger. Torfwerk Einfeld Carl Hornung, Seekamp 2, Postfach: 2667, 24516 Neumunster, Germany.
Torii, Jpn. Torii Yakuhin, 3-3-14 Hon-cho, Nihonbashi, Chuo-ku, Tokyo, Japan.
Torlan, Spain. Torlan, Ctra Barcelona 135-B, Cerdenola del Valles, 08290 Barcelona, Spain.
Torre, Ital. Dr. A. Torre Farmaceutici s.r.l., Viale E. Forlanini 15, 20134 Milan, Italy.
Torrens, Spain. Torrens, Camino del Hospital S/N, Olesa de Bonevalls, 08739 Barcelona, Spain.
Torrex, Aust. Torrex Pharma GmbH, Lange Gasse 76/16, 1080 Vienna, Austria.
Tosara, Irl. Tosara Products Ltd, Unit 146, Baldoyle Industrial Estate, Dublin 13, Ireland.
Tosara, UK. Tosara Products (UK) Ltd, P.O. Box 5, 70 Picton Rd, Liverpool, L15 4NS, UK.
Tosi, Ital. Tosi Dr A Farmaceutici s.r.l., C.so della Vittoria 12/B, 28100 Novara, Italy.
Tosse, Ger. E. Tosse & Co. mbH, Friedrich-Ebert-Damm 101, Postfach: 701648, 22016 Hamburg, Germany.
Toulade, Fr. Laboratoires Toulade, av. du Dr-Aubry, 76280 Criquetot-L'Esneval, France.
Tracel, Austral. Tracel Australia Pty Ltd, P.O. Box 152, Mt Hawthorn, WA 6016, Australia.
Tramedico, Belg. Tramedico S.A., Europark-Oost 34, PB 50, 9100 Sint-Niklaas, Belgium.
Tramedico, Neth. Tramedico B.V., Postbus 192, 1380 AD Weesp, Netherlands.
Trans Canaderm, Canad. See *Stiefel, Canad.*
Transpharma, Fr. Transpharma, France.
Travenol, UK. Travenol Laboratories Ltd, Caxton Way, Thetford, Norfolk, IP24 3SE, UK.
Travenol, USA. Travenol Laboratories Inc., One Baxter Parkway, Deerfield, IL 60015, USA.
Treiner, USA. Treiner Co, USA.
Tremedic, Swed. Tremedic AB, Faktorvagen 13, 434 37 Kungsbacka, Sweden.
Trenier, USA. Trenier, USA.
Trenka, Switz. See *Uhlmann-Eyraud, Switz.*
Trenker, Belg. Lab. Pharm. Trenker S.A., Ave Dolez 480-2, 1180 Brussels, Belgium.
Treupha, Switz. Treupha SA, Zurcherstrasse 59, 5401 Baden, Switzerland.
Triangle, USA. Triangle Labs Inc., 1000 Robins Rd, Lynchburg, VA 24504-3558, USA.
Trianon, Canad. Trianon Laboratories Inc., 660 Blvd Industriel, Blainville, Quebec, J7C 3V4, Canada.
Trimedal, Switz. Trimedal AG, Postfach, 8306 Bruttisellen, Switzerland.
Trimen, USA. Trimen Laboratories Inc., USA.
Trinity, UK. Trinity Pharmaceuticals Ltd, Tuition House, 27/37 St George's Rd, Wimbledon, London, SW19 4DS, UK.
Triomed, S.Afr. Triomed, P.O. Box 309, Bellville 7530, S. Africa.
Triosol, Belg. Triosol S.A., Blvd Emile Bockstael 122, 1020 Brussels, Belgium.
Tripharma, Switz. Tripharma AG, 8730 Uznach, Switzerland.
Triton, USA. Triton Consumer Products, Inc., Division of M. George Research, Inc., 561 West Golf, Arlington Heights, Illinois, IL 60005, USA.
Trofomed, Ital. Trofomed s.r.l., Via IV Novembre 7, 70020 Cassano delle Murge (BA), Italy.
Trommsdorff, Ger. Trommsdorff GmbH & Co. Arzneimittel, Trommsdorffstrasse 2-6, 52475 Alsdorf, Germany.
Tropic Suncare, Canad. Tropic Suncare Canada Ltd, 344 Sovereign Rd, London, Ontario, N6M 1A3, Canada.
Tropon, Ger. See *Bayer, Ger.*
Tropon-Cutter, Ger. See *Bayer, Ger.*
Truw, Ger. Truw-Arzneimittel GmbH, Alfred-Nobel-Str. 5, Postfach: 1345, 50203 Frechen, Germany.
Truxton, USA. C.O. Truxton Inc., P.O. Box 1594, Camden, NJ 08101, USA.
Tsumura, Jpn. Tsumura, Japan.
Turimed, Switz. Turimed SA, Hertistrasse 8, 8304 Wallisellen, Switzerland.
Twardy, Aust. Twardy GmbH, Handelskai 388, 1020 Vienna, Austria.
Twardy, Ger. Astrid Twardy GmbH, Liebigstrasse 18, 65439 Florsheim/Main, Germany.
Tweezerman, USA. Tweezerman, 55 Sea Cliff Ave, Glen Cove, New York, NY 11542, USA.
Typharm, Irl. See *Boileau & Boyd, Irl.*
Typharm, UK. Typharm Ltd, 14 Parkstone Rd, Poole, Dorset, UK.
Tyrol, Aust. Tyrol Pharma GmbH, Brunner Strasse 59, 1235 Vienna, Austria.
Tyson, USA. Tyson & Associates Inc., 12832 Chadron Avenue, Hawthorne, CA 90250, USA.
UAD, USA. UAD Laboratories Inc., P.O. Box 10587, 8339 Highway 18, Jackson, MS 39289-0587, USA.
UB Interpharm, Switz. UB Interpharm SA, 36 av Cardinal-Mermillod, 1227 Carouge/GE, Switzerland.
UBI, USA. UBI Corp., 2920 NW Boca Raton Blvd, Boca Raton, FL 33431, USA.
UCB, Aust. UCB Pharma GmbH, Hauffgasse 3-5, 1110 Vienna, Austria.
UCB, Belg. UCB Pharma S.A., Chaussee de Waterloo 935-7, 1180 Brussels, Belgium.
UCB, Fr. UCB Pharma S.A., 21 rue de Neuilly, 92003 Nanterre, France.
UCB, Ger. UCB GmbH, Huttenstrasse 205, Postfach: 1340, 50142 Kerpen, Germany.
UCB, Irl. See *United Drug, Irl.*
UCB, Ital. Laboratori UCB s.p.a., Via Praglia 15, 10044 Pianezza (TO), Italy.
UCB, Neth. UCB Pharma B.V., Postbus 6851, 4802 HW Breda, Netherlands.
UCB, Norw. See *Searle, Norw.*
UCB, S.Afr. UCB SA (Pty) Ltd, P.O. Box 31036, Braamfontein 2017, S. Africa.
UCB, Spain. UCB, Santiago Ramon y Cajal 6, Molins de Rei, 08750 Barcelona, Spain.
UCB, Swed. UCB Pharma AB (Sweden), 212 25 Malmo, Sweden.
UCB, Switz. UCB-Pharma AG, Pharmazeutische Produkte, Klosbachstrasse 2, 8032 Zurich, Switzerland.
UCB, UK. UCB Pharma Ltd, Star House, 60 Clarendon Rd, Watford, Herts, WD1 1DJ, UK.
UCB, USA. UCB Pharmaceuticals. Inc., P.O.Box 4410, Hampton VA 23664-0410, USA.
UCM-Difme, Ital. See *Solvay, Ital.*
Ucyclyd, USA. Ucyclyd Pharma Inc., 10819 Gilroy Rd, Suite 100, Hunt Valley, MD 21031, USA.
Ueno, Jpn. Ueno Fine Chemicals Industry Ltd, 5-5 Nihonbashi-Honcho 3-chome, Chuoku, Tokyo 103, Japan.
Uhlmann-Eyraud, Switz. F. Uhlmann-Eyraud SA, 28 ch. du Grand-Puits, 1217 Meyrin 2/Geneva, Switzerland.
Ulmer, USA. Ulmer Pharmacal Co., 2440 Fernbrook Lane, Minneapolis, MN 55441, USA.
Ulrich, Ital. D Ulrich spa, Str. del Pascolo 3, 10126 Turin, Italy.
ULSO, Irl. ULSO Laboratories Ltd, 283 South Richmond St, Dublin 2, Ireland.
Ultrapharm, UK. Ultrapharm Ltd, Kenton House, 21 New St, Henley-on-Thames, Oxon, RG9 2PB, UK.
Ungar, Aust. Ungar-Apotheke zur Göttlichen Vorsehung, Ungargasse 14, 1030 Vienna, Austria.
Unibios, Ital. Istituto Biologico Chemioterapico s.p.a., Via S Pellico 3, 28069 Trecate (NO), Italy.
Unibios, Spain. Unibios, Spain.
Unichem, UK. Unichem Ltd, Unichem House, Cox Lane, Chessington, Surrey, UK.
Uniderm, Ital. Uniderm Farmaceutici s.r.l., Via G. Armandi 64, 00126 Rome Acilia, Italy.
Unifarma, Spain. Unifarma, Mino 8, 08022 Barcelona, Spain.
Unigreg, Irl. See *United Drug, Irl.*
Unigreg, UK. Unigreg Ltd, Enterprise House, 181-9 Garth Rd, Morden, Surrey, SM4 4LL, UK.
Unimed, USA. Unimed Inc., 2150 E. Blake Cook Road, Buffalo Grove, IL 60089, USA.
Unipack, Aust. Unipack GmbH, Braunlichgasse 40-2, 2700 Wiener Neustadt, Austria.
Unipath, UK. Unipath Ltd, Norse Rd, Bedford, MK41 0QG, UK.
Unipharma, Switz. Unipharma SA, 6917 Barbengo, Switzerland.
Unitech, Irl. See *United Drug, Irl.*
United, USA. United Medical, Division of Pfizer Hospital Products Group Inc., 11775 Starkey Rd, Largo, FL 34643-4799, USA.
United Drug, Irl. United Drug, United Drug House, Belgard Rd, Tallaght, Dublin 24, Ireland.
Universal, S.Afr. Universal Pharmaceuticals (Pty) Ltd, P.O. Box 33068, Jeppestown 2043, S. Africa.
Uno, Ital. Farma Uno s.r.l., Via Conforti 42, 84083 Castel San Giorgio (SA), Italy.
Upjohn, Austral. See *Pharmacia Upjohn, Austral.*
Upjohn, Belg. See *Pharmacia Upjohn, Belg.*
Upjohn, Ger. See *Pharmacia Upjohn, Ger.*
Upjohn, Irl. See *Pharmacia Upjohn, Irl.*
Upjohn, Jpn. Upjohn, Japan.
Upjohn, Neth. See *Pharmacia Upjohn, Neth.*
Upjohn, Spain. See *Pharmacia Upjohn, Spain.*
Upjohn, Swed. See *Pharmacia Upjohn, Swed.*
Upjohn, Switz. See *Pharmacia Upjohn, Switz.*
Upjohn, UK. See *Pharmacia Upjohn, UK.*
Upjohn, USA. See *Pharmacia Upjohn, USA.*
UPSA, Fr. Laboratoires UPSA, 128 rue Danton, 92500 Rueil-Malmaison, France.
Upsamedica, Belg. Upsamedica S.A., Rue Colonel Bourg 127-9, 1140 Brussels, Belgium.
Upsamedica, Ital. Upsamedica s.p.a., Via Agnello 18, 20121 Milan, Italy.
Upsamedica, Spain. Upsamedica, Carretera General de Ulia 31, San Sebastian, 20013 Guipuzcoa, Spain.
Upsamedica, Switz. Upsamedica SA, Neuhofstrasse 6, 6341 Baar, Switzerland.
Upsher-Smith, USA. Upsher-Smith Laboratories Inc., 14905 23rd Ave North, Minneapolis, MN 55447, USA.
Urbion, Spain. Urbion Farma, Avda Portugal, Parcela 85, Aranada de Duero, 09400 Burgos, Spain.
Urgentum, Swed. Urgentum AB, Ideon Industriparken, St Lars vag 41, 222 70 Lund, Sweden.
Urgo, Fr. Laboratoires Urgo, B.P. 157, 42 rue de Longvic, 21300 Chenove, France.
Uriach, Spain. Uriach, Dega Bahi 59, 08026 Barcelona, Spain.
URL, USA. United Research Laboratories, 4629 Adams Ave, Philadelphia, PA 19124, USA.
URPAC, Fr. URPAC-Astier, 24 rue Erlanger, 75781 Paris Cdx 16, France.
Ursapharm, Ger. Ursapharm Arzneimittel GmbH, Industriestrasse, Postfach: 400151, 66057 Saarbrucken, Germany.
US Bioscience, Norw. See *Orphan, Norw.*
US Bioscience, USA. US Bioscience, One Tower Bridge, 100 Front St, Suite 400, West Conshohocken, PA 19428, USA.
US Pharmaceutical, USA. US Pharmaceutical Corp., 2500 Park Central Blvd, Decatur, GA 30035, USA.
VAAS, Ital. V.A.A.S. s.r.l., Via Siena 268, 47030 Capocolle di Bertinoro (FO), Italy.
Vaccina, S.Afr. Vaccina, S. Africa.
Vachon, Canad. Vachon, Canada.
Vaillant, Ital. Laboratori Italiani Vaillant s.r.l., Via Mascagni 55, 21040 Cislago (VA), Italy.
Valda, Canad. See *Bayer, Canad.*
Valda, Ital. Valda Laboratori Farmaceutici s.p.a., Via Zambeletti, 20021 Baranzate di Bollate (MI), Italy.
Vale, USA. The Vale Chemical Co. Inc., USA.
Valeas, Ital. Valeas s.p.a., Via Vallisneri 10, 20133 Milan, Italy.
Valles Mestre, Spain. Valles Mestre, Av. Generalitat 181, Viladecans, 08840 Barcelona, Spain.
ValMed, USA. ValMed Inc., 203 Southwest Cutoff, Northboro, MA 01532, USA.
Valmo, Canad. Lab. Valmo Enrg, 1000 boul. Industriel, Chambly, QC, J3L 3H9, Canada.
Valtec, Canad. See *Omega, Canad.*
Vangard, USA. Vangard Labs Inc., P.O. Box 1268, Glasgow, KY 42142-1268, USA.
Vectem, Spain. Vectem, Wagner 22 (Pol. Can Jardi), Rubi, 08191 Barcelona, Spain.
Vedim, Fr. Laboratoires Vedim, 7 rue Diderot, 92003 Nanterre, France.
Vedim, Ger. Vedim Pharma GmbH, Postfach: 1340, 50142 Kerpen, Germany.
Vedim, Ital. Vedim Pharma srl, Via Praglia 15, 10044 Pianezza (TO), Italy.
Vegetal, Ital. Vegetal Progress s.r.l., Localita Novaro 8, 10070 Devesi di Cierie (TO), Italy.
Vemedia, Neth. Vemedia B.V., Postbus 502, 1380 AN Weesp, Netherlands.
Veris, Spain. Veris, C/Juan Bravo 47, 28006 Madrid, Spain.
Verkos, Spain. Verkos, Ctra Zaragoza Logrono Km 20.2, Pinseque, 50298 Zaragoza, Spain.
Verla, Ger. Verla-Pharm, Arzneimittelfabrik, Apotheker H.J. v. Ehrlich GmbH & Co. KG, Hauptstrasse 98, Postfach: 1261, 82324 Tutzing, Germany.
Verla, Switz. See *Biomed, Switz.*
Vernleigh, S.Afr. See *Propan, S.Afr.*
Vesta, S.Afr. Vesta Medicines (Pty) Ltd, S. Africa.
Veyron-Froment, Fr. Laboratoires Veyron et Froment, 30 rue Benedit, 13248 Marseille Cdx 04, France.
VFZ, Switz. Verbandstoff-Fabrik Zurich AG, Tamperlistrasse 3, 8117 Fallanden, Zurich, Switzerland.
Via, Switz. Via Marketing & Promotion SA, Via Ponte Tresa 7-7A, 6924 Sorengo, Switzerland.
Vicente, Spain. Vicente Dr., Cartagena 113, 28002 Madrid, Spain.
Vichy, Canad. See *Cosmair, Canad.*
Vick International, Ital. Vick International s.p.a., V.le Cesare Pavese 385, 00144 Rome, Italy.
Vifor, Switz. Vifor SA, Case Postale 1067, 1701 Fribourg-Moncor, Switzerland.
Vifor International, Switz. Vifor (International) AG, Pharmazeutische Spezialitäten, Rechenstrasse 37, Postfach, 9001 St Gallen, Switzerland.
Vifor Medical, Switz. Vifor Medical SA, 9 route de Sorge, Case postale 161, 1023 Crissier, Switzerland.
Vigan, Fr. Laboratoires Vigan et Cie, 6 rue Salneuve, 75017 Paris, France.
Vilardell, Spain. Vilardell, Constitucion 66-8, Les Grases, San Feliu de Llobregat, 08980 Barcelona, Spain.
Vinas, Spain. Viñas, Provenza 386, 08025 Barcelona, Spain.
Vinas, Switz. See *Golaz, Switz.*
Vingmed, Norw. Vingmed AS, Fornebuv 3, Postboks 8, 1324 Lysaker, Norway.
Vir, Spain. Vir, Cardenal Mendoza 42, 28011 Madrid, Spain.
Virginia, Ital. Virginia Farmaceutici s.r.l., P.zza Amendola 3, 20149 Milan, Italy.
Virgo Healthcare, Austral. Virgo Healthcare, Unit 2, 85-7 Moore St, Leichhardt, NSW 2040, Australia.
Vis, Ital. Vis Farmaceutici, Istituto Scientifico delle Venezie s.p.a., Viale dell'industria 54, 35129 Padua, Italy.
Vision, USA. Vision Pharmaceuticals Inc., P.O. Box 400, Mitchell, SD 57301-0400, USA.
Vita, Ital. Laboratori Farmaceutici Vita s.r.l., Via Rivoltana 32, 20090 Limito (MI), Italy.
Vita, Spain. Vita, Avda de Barcelona 69, San Juan Despi, 08970 Barcelona, Spain.
Vita Elan, Spain. See *Vita, Spain.*
Vita Glow, Austral. Vita Glow Pty Ltd, P.O. Box 172, Balgowah, NSW 2093, Australia.
Vita Health, Canad. Vita Health Co. (1985) Ltd, 150 Beghin Ave, Winnipeg, Manitoba, R2J 3W2, Canada.
Vita Pharm, Canad. Vita Pharm Canada Ltd, 2835 Kew Dr., Windsor, Ontario, N8T 3B7, Canada.
Vitabiotics, Irl. See *Allphar, Irl.*
Vitabiotics, UK. Vitabiotics Ltd, Vitabiotics House, 3 Bashley Rd, London, NW10 6SU, UK.

Vitafarma, Spain. Vitafarma, Alto de los Robles 12, San Sebastian, 20080 Guipuzcoa, Spain.
Vital Health, UK. Vital Health Innovations Ltd, The Coach House, St Michael's Wildhill Rd, Woodside, Herefordshire, AL9 6DL, UK.
Vitalia, UK. Vitalia Ltd, Paradise, Hemel Hempstead, Herts, HP2 4TF, UK.
Vitaline, Norw. See *Vingmed, Norw.*
Vitaline, UK. Vitaline Pharmaceuticals UK Ltd, Tower House, 6 Tower Court, Horns Lane, Princes Risborough, Bucks, HP27 0AJ, UK.
Vitaline, USA. Vitaline Formulas, 722 Jefferson Ave, Ashland, OR 97520, USA.
Vitalpharma, Belg. S.A. Vitalpharma Astra N.V., Rue Egide Van Ophem 110, 1180 Brussels, Belgium.
Vitaplex, Austral. Vitaplex Products, P.O. Box 270, Gymea, NSW 2227, Australia.
Vitelle, Austral. Vitelle Health Company Pty. Ltd, P.O. Box 31, Arncliffe, NSW 2205, Australia.
Vitorgan, Ger. vitOrgan Arzneimittel GmbH, Brunnweisenstrasse 21, Postfach: 4240, 73745 Ostfildern, Germany.
Viviar, Spain. Viviar, Pista de Ademuz Km 9.4, Paterna, 46980 Valencia, Spain.
Vivus, USA. Vivus Inc, 545 Middlefield Rd, Menlo Park, CA 94025, USA.
Voigt, Ger. Dr med. Hans Voigt GmbH, Mundipharma Strasse 4, Postfach: 1350, 65533 Limburg/Lahn, Germany.
Voigt, Switz. Voigt & Co AG, Hofstrasse 50, 8590 Romanshorn, Switzerland.
Volchem, Ital. Volchem, Via E Dandolo 14, 35010 Grossa di Gazzo (PD), Italy.
Von Boch, Ital. Von Boch Arzneimittel s.r.l. Istituto Farmacobiologico, Via Rovigo 1, 00161 Rome, Italy.
Vortech, USA. Vortech Pharmaceuticals, 6851 Chase Rd, Dearborn, MI 48126, USA.
VSM, Neth. VSM Geneesmiddelen B.V., Postbus 9321, 1800 GH Alkmaar, Netherlands.
Wakefield, USA. Wakefield Pharmaceuticals, Inc., 1050 Cambridge Square, Suite C, Alpharetta, GA 30201, USA.
Wala, Ger. Wala-Heilmittel GmbH, Bosslerweg 2, Postfach: 1191, 73085 Eckwalden/Bad Boll, Germany.
Waldheim, Aust. Waldheim Pharmazeutika GmbH, Boltzmanngasse 11, 1090 Vienna, Austria.
Waldheim, Ger. Waldheim Pharmatec GmbH, Liebrechstr. 58, 30519 Hannover, Germany.
Walker Pharmacal, USA. Walker Pharmacal Co., 4200 Laclede Ave, St Louis, MO 63108, USA.
Wallace, USA. Wallace Laboratories, Division of Carter-Wallace Inc., P.O. Box 1, Cranbury, NJ 08512, USA.
Wallace Mfg Chem., UK. Wallace Manufacturing Chemists Ltd, Standard House, 16-22 Epworth St, London, EC2A 4DL, UK.
Wallis, UK. Wallis Laboratory, Laposte Way, Luton, Beds, LU4 8EF, UK.
Wampole, Canad. Wampole Inc., 6299 Airport Rd, Suite 200, Mississauga, Ontario, L4V 1N3, Canada.
Wampole, USA. Wampole Laboratories, Division of Carter-Wallace Inc., Half Acre Rd, PO Box 1001, Cranbury, New Jersey, NJ 08515-0181, USA.
Wander, Aust. Wander, Vienna, Austria.
Wander, Belg. See *Novartis, Belg.*
Wander, Ger. Wander Pharma GmbH, Deutschherrnstrasse 15, 90327 Nurnberg, Germany.
Wander, Ital. Wander s.p.a., Via Meucci 39, 20128 Milan, Italy.
Wander, Neth. See *Sandoz, Neth.*
Wander, S.Afr. See *Sandoz, S.Afr.*
Wander, Switz. See *Sandoz, Switz.*
Wander Health Care, Switz. Wander AG Health Care, Postfach, 3001 Bern, Switzerland.
Wander OTC, Switz. See *Sandoz, Switz.*
Wanskerne, UK. Wanskerne Ltd, 31 High Cross Street, St Austell, Cornwall, PL25 4AN, UK.
Warner, S.Afr. Warner-Lambert South Africa (Pty) Ltd, Private Bag X6, Tokai 7966, S. Africa.
Warner Chilcott, USA. Warner Chilcott Laboratories, Division of Warner-Lambert Co., 201 Tabor Rd, Morris Plains, NJ 07950, USA.
Warner-Lambert, Austral. See *Parke, Davis, Austral.*
Warner-Lambert, Belg. Warner-Lambert Consumer Healthcare s.c.a., Exelsiorlaan 75-7, 1930 Zaventem, Belgium.
Warner-Lambert, Canad. See *Warner-Wellcome, Canad.*
Warner-Lambert, Fr. Warner-Lambert Santé Grand Public, 11 av Dubonnet, 92407 Courbevoie cdx, France.
Warner-Lambert, Ger. Warner-Lambert Consumer Healthcare GmbH, Wohlerstr. 9, 79108 Freiburg, Germany.
Warner-Lambert, Irl. Warner-Lambert Consumer Healthcare, Pottery Rd, Dun Laoghaire, Co. Dublin, Ireland.
Warner-Lambert, Ital. Warner Lambert Consumer Healthcare S.Comp.p.A., Via de Gasperi 17-19, 20020 Lainate (MI), Italy.
Warner-Lambert, Neth. Warner-Lambert Consumer Healthcare B.V., Saturnusstraat 1, 2132 HB Hoofddorp, Netherlands.
Warner-Lambert, Norw. See *Yamanouchi, Norw.*
Warner-Lambert, Spain. Warner Lambert Consumer Health, Pol. Ind. Manso Mateu SN, Prat de Llobregat, 08820 Barcelona, Spain.
Warner-Lambert, Swed. Warner-Lambert Consumer Healthcare, Division of Warner Lambert Nordic AB, Box 4130, 171 04 Solna, Sweden.
Warner-Lambert, Switz. Warner-Lambert (Schweiz) AG, Blegistrasse 11a, 6341 Baar, Switzerland.
Warner-Lambert, UK. Warner-Lambert Consumer HealthCare, Lambert Court, Chestnut Ave, Eastleigh, Hants, SO53 3ZQ, UK.
Warner-Lambert, USA. Warner-Lambert Co., Consumer Health Products Group, 201 Tabor Rd, Morris Plains, NJ 07950, USA.
Warner-Lambert Confectionery, UK. See *Warner-Wellcome, UK.*
Warner-Lambert Consumer, Belg. See *Parke, Davis, Belg.*
Warner-Lambert Consumer, Switz. See *Warner-Lambert, Switz.*
Warner-Wellcome, Canad. Warner Wellcome Consumer Health Products, P.O. Box 2200, Station A, Scarborough, Ontario, M1K 5C9, Canada.
Warner-Wellcome, Ger. See *Warner-Lambert, Ger.*
Warner-Wellcome, Spain. Warner Wellcome Consumer Health, Pol. Ind. Manso Mateu S/N, Prat de Llobregat, 08820 Barcelona, Spain.
Warner-Wellcome, UK. See *Warner-Lambert, UK.*
Warner-Wellcome, USA. See *Warner-Lambert, USA.*
Warondo, Ger. Pharmazeutische Fabrik Lengerich Walther Ronsdorf Nachf. (Warondo), Poststrasse 24, Postfach: 1468, 49514 Lengerich, Germany.
Wassen, Ital. Wassen Italia srl, Via Melzi d'Eril 38, 20154 Milan, Italy.
Wassen, UK. Wassen International Ltd, 14 The Mole, Business Park, Leatherhead, Surrey, KT22 7BA, UK.
Wasserman, Spain. Wasserman, Avda San Antonio M. Claret 173, 08041 Barcelona, Spain.
Wassermann, Ital. Alfa Wassermann s.p.a., Contrada Sant'Emidio, 65020 Alanno (PE), Italy.
Waterhouse, UK. J. Waterhouse & Co. Ltd, Standard House, 5th Floor, 16-22 Epworth St, London, EC2A 4DL, UK.
Watson, USA. Watson Laboratories, 132-A Business Center Drive, Corona, CA 91720, USA.
Watsons, Canad. Watsons Pharmaceuticals, 3 Ontario St, Port Hope, Ontario, L1A 3T5, Canada.
Waymar, Canad. Waymar Pharmaceuticals Inc., 330 Marwood Dr., Unit 4, Oshawa, Ontario, L1H 8B4, Canada.
WE, USA. WE Pharmaceuticals Inc, P.O. Box 1142, Ramona, CA 92065, USA.
Weber & Weber, Ger. Weber & Weber GmbH, Herrschinger Strasse 33, Postfach: 20, 82263 Inning/Ammersee, Germany.
Weider, UK. Weider Nutrition Ltd, Howard Way, Newport Pagnell, Bucks, MK16 9PY, UK.
Weiders, Norw. Weiders Farmasøytiske A/S, Hausmannsgt 6, Postboks 9113 Gronland, 0133 Oslo, Norway.
Weifa, Norw. See *Weiders, Norw.*
Weimer, Ger. Weimer Pharma GmbH, Steingerust 30, Postfach: 2454, 76414 Rastatt, Germany.
Weimer, Switz. Weimer Pharma AG, Diepold-Schillingstrasse 14a, 6004 Luzern, Switzerland.
Weinco, Spain. Weinco, Cobo Calleja-Torre del Bierzo 29, Fuenlabrada, 28947 Madrid, Spain.
Welcker-Lyster, Canad. Welcker-Lyster Ltd, 8480 boul. Saint-Laurent, Montreal, Quebec, H2P 2M6, Canada.
Weleda, Aust. Weleda GmbH & Co. KG, Gauermanngasse 2-4, 1010 Vienna, Austria.
Weleda, Fr. Laboratoires Weleda, 9 rue Eugene-Jung, 68330 Huningue, France.
Weleda, Ger. Weleda AG-Heilmittelbetriebe, Mohlerstrasse 3-5, Postfach: 1309/1320, 73503 Schwabisch Gmund, Germany.
Weleda, UK. Weleda (UK) Ltd, Heanor Rd, Ilkeston, Derbyshire, DE7 8DR, UK.
Wellcome, Austral. See *Glaxo Wellcome, Austral.*
Wellcome, Belg. See *Glaxo Wellcome, Belg.*
Wellcome, Canad. See *Glaxo Wellcome, Canad.*
Wellcome, Fr. See *Glaxo Wellcome, Fr.*
Wellcome, Irl. See *Glaxo Wellcome, Irl.*
Wellcome, Ital. See *Glaxo Wellcome, Ital.*
Wellcome, Norw. See *Glaxo Wellcome, Norw.*
Wellcome, Spain. See *Glaxo Wellcome, Spain.*
Wellcome, Switz. See *Glaxo Wellcome, Switz.*
Wellcome, UK. See *Glaxo Wellcome, UK.*
Wellcome, USA. See *Glaxo Wellcome, USA.*
Wellcome Diagnostics, UK. Wellcome Diagnostics, A Division of The Wellcome Foundation Ltd, Temple Hill, Dartford, DA1 5AH, UK.
Wellcopharm, Ger. See *Glaxo Wellcome, Ger.*
Welti, Switz. Dr Heinz Welti AG, Fabrik chemisch-pharmazeutischer Produkte, Althofstrasse 12, 5432 Neuenhof, Switzerland.
Wenig, Aust. Mr JW Wenig GmbH, Lange Gasse 35 a, 1080 Vienna, Austria.
Wernigerode, Ger. Pharma Wernigerode GmbH, Muhlental 42, Postfach: 35, 38841 Wernigerode/Harz, Germany.
Wesley, USA. The Wesley Pharmacal Co. Inc., 114 Railroad Drive, Ivyland, PA 18974, USA.
Westbrook, UK. Westbrook Lanolin Co., Argonaut Works, Laisterdyke, Bradford, BD4 8AU, UK.
WestCan, Canad. See *Vita Health, Canad.*
Westermans, S.Afr. Westermans, S. Africa.
Western Medical, USA. Western Medical, USA.
Westward, Canad. Westward Dist., Canada.
Westwood, USA. Westwood Pharmaceuticals Inc., 100 Forest Ave, Buffalo, NY 14213, USA.
Westwood-Squibb, Canad. See *Bristol-Myers Squibb, Canad.*
Westwood-Squibb, USA. See *Bristol-Myers Squibb, USA.*
Wharton, Ital. Wharton s.r.l., Via Ragazzi del 99 n.5, 40133 Bologna, Italy.
Whelehan, Irl. Whelehan T.P. Son & Co. Ltd, North Rd, Finglas, Dublin 11, Ireland.
Whitby, USA. See *UCB, USA.*
Whitehall, Austral. Whitehall Laboratories (Aust) Pty. Ltd, Private Bag 1, Punchbowl, NSW 2196, Australia.
Whitehall, Belg. Whitehall Benelux s.a., Rue du Bosquet 15, 1348 Louvain-la-Neuve, Belgium.
Whitehall, Canad. See *Whitehall-Robins, Canad.*
Whitehall, Fr. Whitehall, 80 av du pdt-Wilson, 92031 Paris-La Defense cdx, France.
Whitehall, Irl. Whitehall Laboratories Ltd, 765 South Circular Rd, Islandbridge, Dublin 8, Ireland.
Whitehall, Ital. Whitehall Italia s.p.a., Via Puccini 3, 20121 Milan, Italy.
Whitehall, Neth. Whitehall Laboratoria, Sophialaan 25, 1075 BL Amsterdam, Netherlands.
Whitehall, Norw. See *Wyeth, Norw.*
Whitehall, S.Afr. Whitehall, S. Africa.
Whitehall, Swed. Whitehall Nordiska, Box 344, 191 30 Sollentuna, Sweden.
Whitehall, UK. Whitehall Laboratories Ltd, Huntercombe Lane South, Taplow, Maidenhead, Berks, SL6 0PH, UK.
Whitehall, USA. See *Whitehall-Robins, USA.*
Whitehall-Robins, Canad. Whitehall-Robins Inc., 5975 Whittle Ave, Mississauga, Ontario, L4Z 3M6, Canada.
Whitehall-Robins, Switz. Whitehall-Robins AG, Grafenauweg 10, 6301 Zug 7, Switzerland.
Whitehall-Robins, USA. Whitehall Robins, Five Giralda Farms, Madison, NJ 07940-0871, USA.
Wick, Ger. Wick Pharma Zweigniederlassung der Procter & Gamble GmbH, Postfach, 65823 Schwalbach, Germany.
Wider, Ger. Dr. Wider GmbH & Co., Brennerstrasse 48, Postfach: 1862, 71208 Leonberg, Germany.
Widmer, Aust. Louis Widmer GmbH, Itzlinger Hauptstrasse 34, 5020 Salzburg, Austria.
Widmer, Ger. Louis Widmer GmbH, Grossmattstr. 11, Postfach: 1266, 79602 Rheinfelden, Germany.
Widmer, Switz. Dermatologica Widmer, Laboratoires Louis Widmer AG, 8048 Zurich, Switzerland.
Wiedemann, Ger. Wiedemann Pharma GmbH, Pilotyweg 14, 82541 Munsing, Germany.
Wiedenmann, Switz. Wiedenmann SA, Switzerland.
Wigglesworth, UK. Wigglesworth (1982) Ltd, Cunard Rd, North Acton, London, NW10 6PN, UK.
Wild, Switz. Dr Wild & Co. SA, Lange Gasse 4, 4002 Basel, Switzerland.
Willen, USA. See *Baker Norton, USA.*
Williams, USA. Williams T.E. Pharm. Inc., USA.
Will-Pharma, Belg. Will-Pharma S.A., Rue du Manil 80, 1301 Wavre, Belgium.
Will-Pharma, Neth. Will-Pharma B.V., Postbus 30, 1160 AA Zwanenburg, Netherlands.
Willvonseder, Aust. Willvonseder & Marchesani, Heinrich-v-Buol-Gasse, Postfach 45, 1211 Vienna, Austria.
Windsor, Irl. See *Allphar, Irl.*
Windsor, UK. Windsor Healthcare Ltd, Ellesfield Ave, Bracknell, Berks, RG12 4YS, UK.
Wintec, Fr. Wintec Pharma, France.
Winthrop, Austral. See *SmithKline Beecham Consumer, Austral.*
Winthrop, Belg. Winthrop S.A., Ave du Martin-Pecheur 19-31, 1170 Brussels, Belgium.
Winthrop, Neth. See *Sterling Health, Neth.*, and *Sanofi Winthrop, Neth.*
Winthrop, Switz. Winthrop AG, Niederlassung Schülke & Mayr-Produkte, Obere Zaune 12, 8001 Zurich, Switzerland.
Winthrop, USA. Winthrop Pharmaceuticals, 90 Park Ave, New York, NY 10016, USA.
Winthrop Consumer, USA. Winthrop Consumer Products, Division of Sterling Drug Inc., 90 Park Ave, New York, NY 10016, USA.
Winzer, Ger. Dr Winzer Pharma GmbH, Ilzweg 7, Postfach: 1234, 82134 Olching, Germany.
Wisconsin Pharmacal, USA. Wisconsin Pharmacal Co., USA.
Woelm, Ger. Woelm Pharma GmbH & Co., Rhondorfer Str 80, 53604 Bad Honnef, Germany.
Wolfer, Ger. Otto A.H. Wölfer GmbH, Herrenhaus Kluvensiek, 24796 Bovenau, Germany.
Wolff, Ger. Dr. August Wolff Arzneimittel GmbH & Co., Sudbrackstrasse 56, Postfach: 103251 + 53, 33532 Bielefeld, Germany.
Wolfs, Belg. Wolfs N.V., Industriepark West 68, 9100 Sint-Niklaas, Belgium.
Wolo, Switz. Wolo SA, Eggbühlstrasse 20, 8052 Zurich, Switzerland.
Woods, Austral. H.W. Woods Pty Ltd, P.O. Box 5, Huntingdale, Vic. 3166, Australia.
Woodward, USA. Woodward Laboratories, Inc., 10357 Los Alamitos Blvd, Los Alamitos, CA 90720, USA.
Woodwards, Canad. See *Schmid, Canad.*
Worndli, Switz. Labor Worndli, Postfach 53, 5300 Turgi, Switzerland.

Worwag, Ger. Wörwag Pharma GmbH, Calwer Str. 7, 71034 Boblingen, Germany.

Wybert, Ger. Wybert GmbH, Postfach: 2520, 79515 Lorrach, Germany.

Wyeth, Austral. Wyeth Pharmaceuticals, Division of Wyeth Australia Pty Ltd, P.O Box 9, Baulkham Hills, NSW 2153, Australia.

Wyeth, Belg. See *Wyeth Lederle, Belg.*

Wyeth, Fr. Laboratoires Wyeth France, Le Wilson II, 80 av du Pdt-Wilson, Puteaux, 92031 Paris-La Defense cdx, France.

Wyeth, Ger. Wyeth-Pharma GmbH, Schleebruggenkamp 15, Postfach: 8808, 48136 Munster, Germany.

Wyeth, Irl. Wyeth Laboratories, 765 South Circular Road, Dublin 8, Ireland.

Wyeth, Ital. Wyeth s.p.a., Via Nettunense 90, 04011 Aprilia (LT), Italy.

Wyeth, Neth. See *AHP, Neth.*

Wyeth, Norw. Wyeth Lederle Norge, Drammensv 145A, Postboks 313 Skoyen, 02125 Oslo, Norway.

Wyeth, S.Afr. Wyeth, S. Africa.

Wyeth, Spain. Wyeth Orfi, Baronesa de Malda 73, Esplugas de Llobregat, 08950 Barcelona, Spain.

Wyeth, Switz. See *AHP, Switz.*

Wyeth, UK. Wyeth Laboratories, Huntercombe Lane South, Taplow, Maidenhead, Berks, SL6 0PH, UK.

Wyeth Health, Austral. See *Wyeth, Austral.*

Wyeth Lederle, Aust. Wyeth-Lederle Pharma GmbH, Storchengasse 1, 1150 Vienna, Austria.

Wyeth Lederle, Belg. Wyeth Lederle, a division of AHP Pharma, Rue du Bosquet 15, 1348 Louvain-la-Neuve, Belgium.

Wyeth Lederle, Swed. Wyeth Lederle Nordiska AB, Box 1822, 171 24 Solna, Sweden.

Wyeth-Ayerst, Canad. Wyeth-Ayerst Canada Inc., 1025 Marcel Laurin Blvd, Saint-Laurent, Quebec, H4R 1J6, Canada.

Wyeth-Ayerst, USA. Wyeth-Ayerst Laboratories, P.O. Box 8299, Philadelphia, PA 19101, USA.

Wyss, Switz. Wyss Pharma AG, Riedstrasse 1, 6330 Cham, Switzerland.

Wyvern, UK. Wyvern Medical Ltd, P.O. Box 17, Ledbury, Herefordshire, HR8 2ES, UK.

Xeragen, S.Afr. Xeragen, S. Africa.

Xixia, S.Afr. Xixia, S. Africa.

Yamanouchi, Belg. Yamanouchi Pharma B.V., Riverside Business Park, Blvd International 55, Bte 7, B-1070 Brussels, Belgium.

Yamanouchi, Fr. Yamanouchi Pharma, 10 pl de la Coupole, 94220 Charenton-le-Pont, France.

Yamanouchi, Ger. Yamanouchi Pharma GmbH, Hertzstr. 2-4, 69126 Heidelberg, Germany.

Yamanouchi, Irl. See *United Drug, Irl.*

Yamanouchi, Ital. Yamanouchi Pharma s.p.a., Via delle Industrie 2, 20061 Carugate (MI), Italy.

Yamanouchi, Jpn. Yamanouchi Pharmaceutical Co. Ltd, 3-11 Nihonbashi-Honcho 2-chome, Chuo-ku, Tokyo 103, Japan.

Yamanouchi, Neth. Yamanouchi Pharma, Postbus 108, 2350 AC Leiderdorp, Netherlands.

Yamanouchi, Norw. Yamanouchi Pharma, Solbrav 47, 1370 Asker, Norway.

Yamanouchi, S.Afr. Yamanouchi, S. Africa.

Yamanouchi, Spain. Yamanouchi Pharma, Ochandiano 6 C, Empresarial El Plantio, 28023 Madrid, Spain.

Yamanouchi, Swed. Yamanouchi Pharma AB, Hans Michelsensgatan 1B, 211 20 Malmo, Sweden.

Yamanouchi, Switz. See *Doetsch, Grether, Switz.*

Yamanouchi, UK. Yamanouchi Pharma Ltd, Yamanouchi House, Pyrford Rd, West Byfleet, Weybridge, Surrey, KT14 6RA, UK.

Yauyip, Austral. Yauyip Pty. Ltd, Suite 503 Cliveden, 4 Bridge Street, NSW 2000, Australia.

Yer, Spain. Yer, Av. de les Flors S/N, Sant Joan Despi, 08970 Barcelona, Spain.

Yorkshire Pharmaceuticals, UK. Yorkshire Pharmaceuticals Ltd, KAM House, 87 Horton Grange Rd, Bradford, West Yorkshire, BD7 3AH, UK.

Yoshitomi, Jpn. Yoshitomi Pharmaceutical Industries Ltd, 6-9 Hiranomachi 2-chome, Chuo-ku, Osaka 541, Japan.

Young, Canad. WF Young Inc, 1225 rue Volta, Boucherville, QC, J4B 7M7, Canada.

Young, USA. Young Pharmaceuticals Inc., 1840 Berlin Turnpike, Wethersfield, CT 06109, USA.

Young Again Products, USA. Young Again Products, 43 Randolph Rd, 125 Silver Spring, MD 20904, USA.

Ysatfabrik, Ger. Johannes Bürger Ysatfabrik GmbH, Herzog-Julius-Strasse 81/83, Postfach: 1544, 38657 Bad Harzburg, Germany.

Yves Ponroy, Fr. Institut de recherche biologique Yves Ponroy, 78340 Les Clayessous-Bois, France.

Zambeletti, Ital. Dr. L. Zambeletti s.p.a., Via Zambeletti, 20021 Baranzate (MI), Italy.

Zambeletti, Spain. See *Tedec Meiji, Spain.*

Zambon, Belg. Zambon S.A., Ave R Vandendriessche 18, B 1, 1150 Brussels, Belgium.

Zambon, Fr. Laboratoires Zambon France, 46 av du General Leclerc, 92517 Boulogne cdx, France.

Zambon, Ger. Zambon GmbH, Lochhamer Schlag 17, Postfach: 1602, 82158 Grafelfing, Germany.

Zambon, Ital. Zambon Italia s.r.l., Via della Chimica 9, 36100 Vicenza, Italy.

Zambon, Neth. Zambon Nederland BV, Postbus 1312, 3800 BH Amersfoort, Netherlands.

Zambon, Spain. Zambon, Maresme S/N (Pol. Ind. Urvasa), Santa Perpetua de Mogoda, 08130 Barcelona, Spain.

Zee, Canad. Zee Medical Canada, P.O. Box 1266, Stn T, Calgary, AB, T2H 2H6, Canada.

Zellaforte, Switz. Zellaforte Vertriebsanstalt, Auststrasse 52, FL-9490 Vaduz, Switzerland.

Zeller, Switz. Max Zeller Söhne AG, Pflanzliche Heilmittel, Seeblickstrasse 4, Postfach 29, 8590 Romanshorn, Switzerland.

Zeneca, Aust. Zeneca Österreich GmbH, Schwarzenbergplatz 7, 1037 Vienna, Austria.

Zeneca, Belg. Zeneca N.V., Schaessestraat 15, 9070 Destelbergen, Belgium.

Zeneca, Canad. Zeneca Pharma Inc., 2505 Meadowvale Blvd, Mississauga, Ontario, L5N 5R7, Canada.

Zeneca, Fr. Zeneca-Pharma, 1 rue des Chauffours, B.P. 127, 95022 Cergy Cdx, France.

Zeneca, Ger. Zeneca GmbH, Otto-Hahn-Strasse, Postfach: 2080, 68721 Schwetzingen, Germany.

Zeneca, Irl. Zeneca Pharma, P.O. Box 245A, College Park House, 20 Nassau St, Dublin 2, Ireland.

Zeneca, Ital. Zeneca s.p.a., Via F Sforza, Palazzo Volta, 20080 Basiglio (MI), Italy.

Zeneca, Neth. Zeneca Farma, Postbus 4136, 2980 GC Ridderkerk, Netherlands.

Zeneca, Norw. Zeneca AS, Skysstasjon 14, Postboks 275 Skoyen, 1371 Asker, Norway.

Zeneca, S.Afr. Zeneca Pharmaceuticals, Private Bag X7, Gallo Manor 2052, S. Africa.

Zeneca, Spain. Zeneca Farma, Josefa Valcarcel 3-5, 28027 Madrid, Spain.

Zeneca, Swed. Zeneca AB, Box 453, 401 27 Goteborg, Sweden.

Zeneca, Switz. Zeneca AG, Landenbergstrasse 34, 6002 Luzern, Switzerland.

Zeneca, UK. Zeneca Pharma, King's Court, Water Lane, Wilmslow, Cheshire, SK9 5AZ, UK.

Zeneca, USA. Zeneca Inc., Concord Pike and Murphy Rd, Wilmington, Delaware, DE 19897, USA.

Zenith, USA. Zenith Laboratories Inc., 140 LeGrand Ave, Northvale, NJ 07647, USA.

Zenyaku, Jpn. Zenyaku Kogyo Co. Ltd, 6-15 Otsuka 5-chome, Bunkyo-ku, Tokyo 112, Japan.

Zeppenfeldt, Ger. H Zeppenfeldt KG, Postfach: 2540, 79515 Lorrach, Germany.

Zeta, Ital. Zeta Farmaceutici s.p.a., Via Galvani 10, 36066 Sandrigo (VI), Italy.

Ziethen, Ger. Ziethen, Tengstrasse 26, Postfach: 249, 80751 Munich, Germany.

Zila, USA. Zila Pharmaceuticals Inc., 5227 N. 7th Street, Phoenix, AZ 85014, USA.

Zilliken, Ital. Zilliken s.p.a., Viale Fulvio Testi 326, 20126 Milan, Italy.

Zilly, Ger. Fritz Zilly GmbH, Eckbergstrasse 18, Postfach: 1318, 76502 Baden-Baden, Germany.

ZLB, Switz. ZLB Zentrallaboratorium, Blutspendedienst SRK, Wankdorfstrasse 10, 3000 Bern 22, Switzerland.

Zoja, Ital. See *Formenti, Ital.*

Zollweiden, Switz. Zollweiden Apotheke, Baselstrasse 71, 4142 Munchenstein, Switzerland.

Zurich, S.Afr. Zurich, S. Africa.

Zwintscher, Ger. Zwintscher Pharma GmbH, Roonstrasse 23a, Postfach: 2940, 7500 Karlsruhe 1, Germany.

Zyma, Aust. Zyma-Gebro Arzneimittel GmbH, Bahnhofbichl 13, 6391 Fieberbrunn, Austria.

Zyma, Belg. See *Novartis Consumer, Belg.*

Zyma, Fr. Laboratoires Zyma, Tour Albert 1er, 65 av. de Colmar, 92507 Rueil-Malmaison Cdx, France.

Zyma, Ger. Zyma GmbH, Zielstattstrasse 40, Postfach: 701980, 81366 Munich, Germany.

Zyma, Irl. See *Ciba-Geigy, Irl.*

Zyma, Ital. Zyma s.p.a., Corso Italia 13, 21047 Saronno (VA), Italy.

Zyma, Norw. See *Novartis, Norw.*

Zyma, Spain. Zyma Farmaceutica, Suiza 9-11, 08023 Barcelona, Spain.

Zyma, Swed. See *Ciba-Geigy, Swed.*

Zyma, Switz. Zyma SA, Nyon, Case postale 340, Avenue du Mont-Blanc, 1196 Gland, Switzerland.

Zyma, UK. Zyma Healthcare, Mill Road, Holmwood, Nr Dorking, Surrey, RH5 4NU, UK.

General Index

Entries cover drugs (by monograph title, other approved names, synonyms, and chemical names), diseases (by disease treatment review title and associated terms), and proprietary preparations (by proprietary or brand name). They are arranged alphabetically in word-by-word order. Page references give both the page and column number as in 476·1, where 476 represents the page number and the figure 1 indicates that the entry will be found in column 1 of that page. There is no column number when the entry is in a table.

B

D

E

F

G

I

K

L

M

N

P

Q

S

U

V

X

Y

Z